EXPERT

ICD-10-CM Expert for Home Health & Hospice

The complete official code set

Codes valid from October 1, 2019
through September 30, 2020

2020

Publisher's Notice

The *ICD-10-CM Expert for Home Health and Hospice: The Complete Official Code Set* is designed to be an accurate and authoritative source regarding coding. Every reasonable effort has been made to ensure accuracy and completeness of the content. However, Optum360 makes no guarantee, warranty, or representation that this publication is accurate, complete or without errors. It is understood that Optum360 is not rendering any legal or other professional services or advice in this publication and that Optum360 bears no liability for any results or consequences that may arise from the use of this book.

Please address all correspondence to:
Optum360
2525 Lake Park Blvd.
West Valley City, UT 84120

Acknowledgments

Marianne Randall, CPC, *Product Manager*
Karen Schmidt, BSN, *Technical Director*
Anita Schmidt, BS, RHIA, AHIMA-approved ICD-10-CM/PCS Trainer, *Clinical Technical Editor*
Karen Krawzik, RHIT, CCS, AHIMA-approved ICD-10-CM/PCS Trainer, *Clinical Technical Editor*
Peggy Willard, CCS, AHIMA-approved ICD-10-CM/PCS Trainer, *Clinical Technical Editor*
Leanne Patterson, CPC, *Clinical Technical Editor*
LaJuana Green, RHIA, CCS, *Clinical Technical Editor*
Stacy Perry, *Manager, Desktop Publishing*
Lisa Singley, *Project Manager*
Tracy Betzler, *Senior Desktop Publishing Specialist*
Hope M. Dunn, *Senior Desktop Publishing Specialist*
Katie Russell, *Desktop Publishing Specialist*
Kate Holden, *Editor*

Our Commitment to Accuracy

Optum360 is committed to producing accurate and reliable materials.

To report corrections, please visit www.optum360coding.com/accuracy or email accuracy@optum.com. You can also reach customer service by calling 1.800.464.3649, option 1.

Anita Schmidt, BS, RHIA, AHIMA-approved ICD-10-CM/PCS Trainer

Ms. Schmidt has expertise in ICD-10-CM/PCS, DRG, and CPT with more than 15 years' experience in coding in multiple settings, including inpatient, observation, and same-day surgery. Her experience includes analysis of medical record documentation, assignment of ICD-10-CM and PCS codes, and DRG validation. She has conducted training for ICD-10-CM/PCS and electronic health record. She has also collaborated with clinical documentation specialists to identify documentation needs and potential areas for physician education. Most recently she has been developing content for resource and educational products related to ICD-10-CM, ICD-10-PCS, DRG, and CPT. Ms. Schmidt is an AHIMA-approved ICD-10-CM/PCS trainer and is an active member of the American Health Information Management Association (AHIMA) and the Minnesota Health Information Management Association (MHIMA).

Karen Krawzik, RHIT, CCS, AHIMA-approved ICD-10-CM/PCS Trainer

Ms. Krawzik has expertise in ICD-10-CM, ICD-9-CM, CPT/HCPCS, DRG, and data quality and analytics, with more than 30 years' experience coding in multiple settings, including inpatient, observation, ambulatory surgery, ancillary, and emergency room. She has served as a DRG analyst and auditor of commercial and government payer claims, as a contract administrator, and worked on a team providing enterprise-wide conversion of the ICD-9-CM code set to ICD-10. More recently, she has been developing print and electronic content related to ICD-10-CM and ICD-10-PCS coding systems, MS-DRGs, and HCCs. Ms. Krawzik is credentialed by the American Health Information Management Association (AHIMA) as a Registered Health Information Technician (RHIT) and a Certified Coding Specialist (CCS) and is an AHIMA-approved ICD-10-CM/PCS trainer. She is an active member of AHIMA and the Missouri Health Information Management Association.

2020 ICD-10-CM Official Guidelines for Coding and Reporting

Optum360 is pleased to provide you with this 2020 ICD-10-CM code book that INCLUDES the 2020 Official Guidelines for Coding and Reporting.

Contents

Contents

Preface

ICD-10-CM Official Preface

This FY 2020 update of the International Statistical Classification of Diseases and Related Health Problems, 10th revision, Clinical Modification (ICD-10-CM) is being published by the United States government in recognition of its responsibility to promulgate this classification throughout the United States for morbidity coding. The International Statistical Classification of Diseases and Related Health Problems, 10th Revision (ICD-10), published by the World Health Organization (WHO), is the foundation of ICD-10-CM. ICD-10 continues to be the classification used in cause-of-death coding in the United States. The ICD-10-CM is comparable with the ICD-10. The WHO Collaborating Center for the Family of International Classifications in North America, housed at the Centers for Disease Control and Prevention's National Center for Health Statistics (NCHS), has responsibility for the implementation of ICD and other WHO-FIC classifications and serves as a liaison with the WHO, fulfilling international obligations for comparable classifications and the national health data needs of the United States. The historical background of ICD and ICD-10 can be found in the Introduction to the International Classification of Diseases and Related Health Problems (ICD-10), 2010, World Health Organization, Geneva, Switzerland.

ICD-10-CM is the United States' clinical modification of the World Health Organization's ICD-10. The term "clinical" is used to emphasize the modification's intent: to serve as a useful tool in the area of classification of morbidity data for indexing of health records, medical care review, and ambulatory and other health care programs, as well as for basic health statistics. To describe the clinical picture of the patient the codes must be more precise than those needed only for statistical groupings and trend analysis.

Characteristics of ICD-10-CM

ICD-10-CM far exceeds its predecessors in the number of concepts and codes provided. The disease classification has been expanded to include health-related conditions and to provide greater specificity at the sixth and seventh character level. The sixth and seventh characters are not optional and are intended for use in recording the information documented in the clinical record.

ICD-10-CM extensions, interpretations, modifications, addenda, or errata other than those approved by the Centers for Disease Control and Prevention are not to be considered official and should not be utilized. Continuous maintenance of the ICD-10-CM is the responsibility of the aforementioned agencies. However, because the ICD-10-CM represents the best in contemporary thinking of clinicians, nosologists, epidemiologists, and statisticians from both public and private sectors, when future modifications are considered, advice will be sought from all stakeholders.

All official authorized addenda since the last complete update (October 1, 2019) have been included in this revision. For more detailed information please see the complete official authorized addenda to ICD-10-CM, including the "ICD-10-CM Official Guidelines for Coding and Reporting," and a description of the ICD-10-CM updating and maintenance process.

How to Use ICD-10-CM Expert for Home Health and Hospice 2020

Introduction

ICD-10-CM Expert for Home Health and Hospice: The Complete Official Code Set is your definitive coding resource, combining the work of the National Center for Health Statistics (NCHS), Centers for Medicare and Medicaid Services (CMS), American Hospital Association (AHA), and Optum360 experts to provide the information you need for coding accuracy.

The International Classification of Diseases, 10th Revision, Clinical Modification (ICD-10-CM), is an adaptation of ICD-10, copyrighted by the World Health Organization (WHO). The development and maintenance of this clinical modification (CM) is the responsibility of the NCHS as authorized by WHO. Any new concepts added to ICD-10-CM are based on an established update process through the collaboration of WHO's Update and Revision Committee and the ICD-10-CM Coordination and Maintenance Committee.

In addition to the ICD-10-CM classification, other official government source information has been included in this manual. Depending on the source, updates to information may be annual or quarterly. This manual provides the most current information that was available at the time of publication. For updates to the source documents that may have occurred after this manual was published, please refer to the following:

- **National Center for Health Statistics (NCHS), International Classification of Diseases, Tenth Revision, Clinical Modification (ICD-10-CM)**

  https://www.cdc.gov/nchs/icd/icd10cm.htm

  https://www.cms.gov/Medicare/Coding/ICD10/2020-ICD-10-CM.html

- **Centers for Medicare and Medicaid Services (CMS) Integrated Outpatient Code Editor (IOCE), version 20.2**

  https://www.cms.gov/Medicare/Coding/OutpatientCodeEdit/OCEQtrReleaseSpecs.html

- **Centers for Medicare & Medicaid Services (CMS) Home Health Patient-Driven Groupings Model (PDGM)**

  https://www.cms.gov/Medicare/Medicare-Fee-for-Service-Payment/HomeHealthPPS/HH-PDGM.html

- **Centers for Medicare & Medicaid Services (CMS) Hospice Quality Reporting Requirements**

  https://www.cms.gov/Medicare/Medicare-Fee-for-Service-Payment/Hospice/Hospice-Regulations-and-Notices.html?DLSort=3&DLEntries=10&DLPage=1&DLSortDir=descending

- **American Hospital Association (AHA) Coding Clinics**

  https://www.codingclinicadvisor.com/

The official NCHS ICD-10-CM classification includes three main sections: the guidelines, the indexes, and the tabular list, all of which make up the bulk of this coding manual. To complement the classification, Optum360's coding experts have incorporated Medicare-related coding edits and proprietary features, such as supplementary notations, coding tools, and appendixes, into a comprehensive and easy-to-use reference. This publication is organized as follows:

What's New for 2020

This section provides a high-level overview of the changes made to the ICD-10-CM official code set for fiscal 2020, identifying codes that have been added and deleted from the classification, codes that had validity changes as a result of these additions and deletions, as well as codes that had revisions to their descriptions. All changes are based on the 2020 official addendum, posted June 20, 2019, by the National Center for Health Statistics (NCHS), the agency charged with maintaining and updating ICD-10-CM. NCHS is part of the Centers for Disease Control and Prevention (CDC).

Conversion Table

The conversion table was developed by National Center for Healthcare Statistics (NCHS) to help facilitate data retrieval as new codes are added to the ICD-10-CM classification. This table provides a crosswalk from each FY 2020 new code to the equivalent code(s) assigned prior to October 1, 2019, for that particular diagnosis or condition. For the full conversion table, including code crosswalks before October 1, 2019, refer to the 2020 Conversion Table zip file at https://www.cms.gov/Medicare/Coding/ICD10/2020-ICD-10-CM.html.

10 Steps to Correct Coding

This step-by-step tutorial walks the coder through the process of finding the correct code — from locating the code in the official indexes to verifying the code in the tabular section — while following applicable conventions, guidelines, and instructional notes. Specific examples are provided with detailed explanations of each coding step along with advice for proper sequencing.

Official ICD-10-CM Guidelines for Coding and Reporting

This section provides the full official conventions and guidelines regulating the appropriate assignment and reporting of ICD-10-CM codes. These conventions and guidelines are published by the U.S. Department of Health and Human Services (DHHS) and approved by the cooperating parties (American Health Information Management Association [AHIMA], National Center for Health Statistics [NCHS], Centers for Disease Control and Prevention [CDC], and the American Hospital Association [AHA]).

Indexes

Index to Diseases and Injuries

The Index to Diseases and Injuries is arranged in alphabetic order by terms specific to a disease, condition, illness, injury, eponym, or abbreviation as well as terms that describe circumstances other than a disease or injury that may require attention from a health care professional.

Neoplasm Table

The Neoplasm Table is arranged in alphabetic order by anatomical site. Codes are then listed in individual columns based upon the histological behavior (malignant, in situ, benign, uncertain, or unspecified) of the neoplasm.

Table of Drugs and Chemicals
The Table of Drugs and Chemicals is arranged in alphabetic order by the specific drug or chemical name. Codes are listed in individual columns based upon the associated intent (poisoning, adverse effect, or underdosing).

External Causes Index
The External Causes Index is arranged in alphabetic order by main terms that describe the cause, the intent, the place of occurrence, the activity, and the status of the patient at the time the injury occurred or health condition arose.

Index Notations

With
The word "with" or "in" should be interpreted to mean "associated with" or "due to." The classification presumes a causal relationship between the two conditions linked by these terms in the index. These conditions should be coded as related even in the absence of provider documentation explicitly linking them unless the documentation clearly states the conditions are unrelated or when another guideline specifically requires a documented linkage between two conditions (e.g., the sepsis guideline for "acute organ dysfunction that is not clearly associated with the sepsis"). For conditions not specifically linked by these relational terms in the classification or when a guideline requires explicit documentation of a linkage between two conditions, provider documentation must link the conditions to code them as related.

The word "with" in the index is sequenced immediately following the main term, not in alphabetical order.

> **Dermatopolymyositis** M33.9Ø
>   with
>   myopathy M33.92
>   respiratory involvement M33.91
>   specified organ involvement NEC M33.99
>   in neoplastic disease — *see also* Neoplasm D49.9 *[M36.Ø]*

See
When the instruction "see" follows a term in the index, it indicates that another term must be referenced to locate the correct code.

> **Hematoperitoneum** — *see* Hemoperitoneum

See Also
The instructional note "see also" simply provides alternative terms the coder may reference that may be useful in determining the correct code but are not necessary to follow if the main term supplies the appropriate code.

> **Hematinuria** — *see also* Hemaglobinuria
>   malarial B5Ø.8

Default Codes
In the index, the default code is the code listed next to the main term and represents the condition most commonly associated with that main term. This code may be assigned when documentation does not support reporting a more specific code. Alternatively, it may provide an unspecified code for the condition.

> **Headache** R51
>   allergic NEC G44.89
>   associated with sexual activity G44.82
>   chronic daily R51

Parentheses
Parentheses in the indexes enclose nonessential modifiers, supplementary words that may be present or absent in the statement of a disease without affecting the code.

> **Pseudomeningocele** (cerebral) (infective) (post-traumatic) G96.19
>   postprocedural (spinal) G97.82

Brackets
ICD-10-CM has a coding convention addressing code assignment for manifestations that occur as a result of an underlying condition. This convention requires the underlying condition to be sequenced first, followed by the code or codes for the associated manifestation. In the index, italicized codes in brackets identify manifestation codes.

> **Polyneuropathy** (peripheral) G62.9
>   alcoholic G62.1
>   amyloid (Portuguese) E85.1 *[G63]*
>   transthyretin-related (ATTR) familial E85.1 *[G63]*

Shaded Guides
Exclusive vertical shaded guides in the Index to Diseases and Injuries and External Causes Index help the user easily follow the indent levels for the subentries under a main term. Sequencing rules may apply depending on the level of indent for separate subentries.

> **Hemicrania**
>   congenital malformation Q00.0
>   continua G44.51
>   meaning migraine — *see also* Migraine G43.909
>   paroxysmal G44.039
>   chronic G44.049
>   intractable G44.041
>   not intractable G44.049
>   episodic G44.039
>   intractable G44.031
>   not intractable G44.039
>   intractable G44.031
>   not intractable G44.039

Following References
The Index to Diseases and Injuries includes following references to assist in locating out-of-sequence codes in the tabular list. Out-of-sequence codes contain an alphabetic character (letter) in the third- or 4th-character position. These codes are placed according to the classification rules — according to condition — not according to alphabetic or numeric sequencing rules.

> **Carcinoma** (malignant) — *see also* Neoplasm, by site, malignant
>   neuroendocrine — *see also* Tumor, neuroendocrine
>   high grade, any site C7A.1 *(following* C75)
>   poorly differentiated, any site C7A.1 *(following* C75)

Additional Character Required
The Index to Diseases and Injuries, Neoplasm Table, and External Causes Index provide an icon after certain codes to signify to the user that additional characters are required to make the code valid. The tabular list should be consulted for appropriate character selection.

> **Fall, falling** (accidental) W19 ☑
>   building W2Ø.1 ☑

Tabular List of Diseases

ICD-10-CM codes and descriptions are arranged numerically within the tabular list of diseases with 19 separate chapters providing codes associated with a particular body system or nature of injury or disease. There is also a chapter providing codes for external causes of an injury or health conditions and finally a chapter for codes that address encounters with healthcare facilities for circumstances other than a disease or injury.

Code and Code Descriptions

ICD-10-CM is an alphanumeric classification system that contains categories, subcategories, and valid codes. The first character is always a letter with any additional characters represented by either a letter or number. A three-character category without further subclassification is equivalent to a valid three-character code. Valid codes may be three, four, five, six, or seven characters in length, with each level of subdivision after a three-character category representing a subcategory. The final level of subdivision is a valid code.

Boldface

Boldface type is used for all codes and descriptions in the tabular list.

Italics

Italicized type is used to identify manifestation codes, those codes that should not be reported as first-listed diagnoses.

Deleted Text

~~Strikethrough~~ on a code and code description indicates a deletion from the classification for the current year.

Key Word

Green font is used throughout the Tabular List of Diseases to differentiate the key words that appear in similar code descriptions in a given category or subcategory. The key word convention is used only in those categories in which there are multiple codes with very similar descriptions with only a few words that differentiate them.

For example, refer to the list of codes below from category H55:

> ☑4ᵗʰ **H55 Nystagmus and other** irregular eye movements
> ☑5ᵗʰ **H55.Ø Nystagmus**
> **H55.ØØ Unspecified nystagmus**
> **H55.Ø1** Congenital **nystagmus**
> **H55.Ø2** Latent **nystagmus**
> **H55.Ø3** Visual deprivation **nystagmus**
> **H55.Ø4** Dissociated **nystagmus**
> **H55.Ø9 Other forms of nystagmus**

The portion of the code description that appears in green font in the tabular list helps the coder quickly identify the key terms and the correct code. This convention is especially useful when the codes describe laterality, such as the following codes from subcategory H40.22:

> ☑6ᵗʰ **H4Ø.22** Chronic **angle-closure glaucoma**
> Chronic primary angle-closure glaucoma
> ☑7ᵗʰ **H4Ø.221 Chronic angle-closure glaucoma,** right **eye**
> ☑7ᵗʰ **H4Ø.222 Chronic angle-closure glaucoma,** left **eye**
> ☑7ᵗʰ **H4Ø.223 Chronic angle-closure glaucoma,** bilateral
> ☑7ᵗʰ **H4Ø.229 Chronic angle-closure glaucoma, unspecified eye**

Tabular Notations

Official parenthetical notes as well as Optum360's supplementary notations are provided at the chapter, code block, category, subcategory, and individual code level to help the user assign proper codes. The information in the notation can apply to one or more codes depending on where the citation is placed.

Official Notations

Includes Notes

The word `INCLUDES` appears immediately under certain categories to further define, clarify, or give examples of the content of a code category.

Inclusion Terms

Lists of inclusion terms are included under certain codes. These terms indicate some of the conditions for which that code number may be used. Inclusion terms may be synonyms with the code title, or, in the case of "other specified" codes, the terms may also provide a list of various conditions included within a classification code. The inclusion terms are not exhaustive. The index may provide additional terms that may also be assigned to a given code.

Excludes Notes

ICD-10-CM has two types of excludes notes. Each note has a different definition for use. However, they are similar in that they both indicate that codes excluded from each other are independent of each other.

Excludes 1

An `EXCLUDES 1` note is a "pure" excludes. It means "NOT CODED HERE!" An Excludes 1 note indicates mutually exclusive codes: two conditions that cannot be reported together. An Excludes1 note indicates that the code excluded should never be used at the same time as the code above the Excludes1 note. An Excludes1 is used when two conditions cannot occur together, such as a congenital form versus an acquired form of the same condition.

An exception to the Excludes 1 definition is when the two conditions are unrelated to each other. If it is not clear whether the two conditions involving an Excludes 1 note are related or not, query the provider. For example, code F45.8 Other somatoform disorders, has an Excludes 1 note for "sleep related teeth grinding (G47.63)" because "teeth grinding" is an inclusion term under F45.8. Only one of these two codes should be assigned for teeth grinding. However, psychogenic dysmenorrhea is also an inclusion term under F45.8, and a patient could have both this condition and sleep-related teeth grinding. In this case, the two conditions are clearly unrelated to each other, so it would be appropriate to report F45.8 and G47.63 together.

Excludes 2

An `EXCLUDES 2` note means "NOT INCLUDED HERE." An Excludes 2 note indicates that although the excluded condition is not part of the condition it is excluded from, a patient may have both conditions at the same time. Therefore, when an Excludes 2 note appears under a code, it may be acceptable to use both the code and the excluded code together if supported by the medical documentation.

Note

The term "NOTE" appears as an icon and precedes the instructional information. These notes function as alerts to highlight coding instructions within the text.

Code First/Use additional code

These instructional notes provide sequencing instruction. They may appear independently of each other or to designate certain etiology/manifestation paired codes. These instructions signal the coder that an additional code should be reported to provide a more complete picture of that diagnosis.

In etiology/manifestation coding, ICD-10-CM requires the underlying condition to be sequenced first, followed by the manifestation. In these situations, codes with "In diseases classified elsewhere" in the code description are never permitted as a first-listed or principal diagnosis code and must be sequenced following the underlying condition code.

Code Also

A "code also" note alerts the coder that more than one code may be required to fully describe the condition. The sequencing depends on the circumstances of the encounter. Factors that may determine sequencing include severity and reason for the encounter.

Revised Text

The revised text ▶◀ "bow ties" alert the user to changes in official notations for the current year. Revised text may include the following:

- A change in a current parenthetical description
- A change in the code(s) associated with a current parenthetical note
- A change in how a current parenthetical note is classified (e.g., an Excludes 1 note that changed to an Excludes 2 note)
- Addition of a new parenthetical note(s) to a code

Deleted Text

~~Strikethrough~~ on official notations indicate a deletion from the classification for the current year.

Optum360 Notations

AHA Coding Clinic Citations

Coding Clinics are official American Hospital Associated (AHA) publications that provide coding advice specific to ICD-10-CM and ICD-10-PCS.

These citations identify the year, quarter, and page number of one or more *Coding Clinic* publications that may have coding advice relevant to a particular code or group of codes. With the most current citation listed first, these notations are preceded by the symbol **AHA:** and appear in purple type.

I15.1	Hypertension secondary to other renal disorders
	AHA: 2016, 3Q, 22

Definitions

Definitions explain a specific term, condition, or disease process in layman's terms. These notations are preceded by the symbol **DEF:** and appear in purple type.

✓5ᵗ	M51.4 Schmorl's nodes
	DEF: Irregular bone defect in the margin of the vertebral body that causes herniation into the end plate of the vertebral body.

Coding Tips

The tips in the tabular list offer coding advice that is not readily available within the ICD-10-CM classification. It may relate official coding guidelines, indexing nuances, or advice from *AHA's Coding Clinic for ICD-10-CM/PCS*. These notations are preceded by the symbol **TIP:** and appear in brown type.

P15.8	Other specified birth injuries
	TIP: Use for any injury of newborn from scalpel.

Icons

Note: The following icons are placed to the left of the code.

● **New Code**
Codes that have been added to the classification system for the current year.

▲ **Revised Code Title**
Codes that have had a change to their description or validity change for the current year. For additional information on codes with validity changes, see the "What's New" section.

☑ **Additional Characters Required**

☑4ᵗ This symbol indicates that the code requires a 4th character.

☑5ᵗ This symbol indicates that the code requires a 5th character.

☑6ᵗ This symbol indicates that the code requires a 6th character.

☑7ᵗ This symbol indicates that the code requires a 7th character.

✓5ᵗ	H60.3 Other infective otitis externa
✓6ᵗ	H60.31 Diffuse otitis externa
	H60.311 Diffuse otitis externa, right ear
	H60.312 Diffuse otitis externa, left ear
	H60.313 Diffuse otitis externa, bilateral
	H60.319 Diffuse otitis externa, unspecified ear

✓x7ᵗ **Placeholder Alert**
This symbol indicates that the code requires a 7th character following the placeholder "X". Codes with fewer than six characters that require a 7th character must contain placeholder "X" to fill in the empty character(s).

✓x7ᵗ	T16.1 Foreign body in right ear

Note: The following icons are placed to the right of the code description.

Age Edits

Codes intended for a specific age group based on CMS IOCE designations, v20.2.

Ⓝ **Newborn Age: 0**
These diagnoses are intended for newborns and neonates and the patient's age must be 0 years.

N47.0	Adherent prepuce, newborn	Ⓝ♂

Ⓟ **Pediatric Age: 0-17**
These diagnoses are intended for children and the patient's age must be between 0 and 17 years.

L21.1	Seborrheic infantile dermatitis	Ⓟ

Ⓜ **Maternity Age: 12-55**
These diagnoses are intended for childbearing patients between the age of 12 and 55 years.

O02.9	Abnormal product of conception, unspecified	Ⓜ♀

Ⓐ **Adult Age: 15-124**
These diagnoses are intended for patients between the age of 15 and 124 years.

R54	Age-related physical debility	Ⓐ
	Frailty	
	Old age	
	Senescence	
	Senile asthenia	
	Senile debility	
	EXCLUDES 1 age-related cognitive decline (R41.81)	
	sarcopenia (M62.84)	
	senile psychosis (F03)	
	senility NOS (R41.81)	

Sex Edits

Codes intended for a specific sex based on CMS IOCE designations, v20.2.

♂ **Male diagnosis only**

Q98.0	Klinefelter syndrome karyotype 47, XXY	♂

♀ **Female diagnosis only**

N35.12	Postinfective urethral stricture, not elsewhere classified, female	♀

CL Comorbidity Low

This symbol identifies secondary diagnosis codes that are considered a low comorbidity relative to the primary diagnosis. When at least one comorbidity-low diagnosis is reported on a home health claim, the period of care receives a low comorbidity payment adjustment. For a comprehensive list of all comorbidity-low diagnosis codes, refer to appendix H, "Patient-Driven Groupings Model (PDGM) Comorbid Conditions," at the back of this book.

| G62.1 | Alcoholic polyneuropathy | CL |

CH Comorbidity High

This symbol identifies secondary diagnosis codes that are considered a high comorbidity relative to the primary diagnosis. When at least two comorbidity-high diagnoses are reported on a home health claim, the period of care receives a high comorbidity payment adjustment. For a comprehensive list of all comorbidity-high diagnosis codes, refer to appendix H, "Patient-Driven Groupings Model (PDGM) Comorbid Conditions," at the back of this book.

| F33.Ø | Major depressive disorder, recurrent, mild | CH |

NC Dx Noncancer Diagnosis

This symbol indicates a noncancer diagnosis that may satisfy the medical necessity criteria for Medicare coverage of hospice care. The diagnosis alone does not support medical necessity but represents one of the many factors that establish medical necessity. For more detailed explanation of the noncancer diagnosis policies for hospice care, please refer to appendix J, "Hospice Criteria for Medicare Coverage on Noncancer Hospice Care," at the back of this book.

I51.5	Myocardial degeneration	NC Dx
	Fatty degeneration of heart or myocardium	
	Myocardial disease	
	Senile degeneration of heart or myocardium	

PDx PDx Symbol

This symbol identifies a Z code that generally is for use as a first-listed (or principal) diagnosis only but may be used as an additional diagnosis if the patient has more than one encounter on the same day or there is more than one reason for the encounter.

The instructions for Z code use contained in the ICD-10-CM official coding guidelines identify those Z codes that can be used only as a PDx. All other Z codes may either be SDx or PDx, depending upon circumstances of the encounter, by meeting the definition of first-listed or principal diagnosis, and by following any specific Z code guidelines in section I.C.21 a-c. The responsibility of those assigning the Z codes as PDx is to make sure the circumstances of the encounter meet the definition of first-listed or principal diagnosis, follow all coding instructions, and follow the Z code specific guidelines. Optum360 does not include any SDx edit since there is no official source for it and the Z code use is determined by circumstances of the encounter.

Note: Please note that the Z code "principal or first-listed only" designation and the Z codes that may be principal or first-listed diagnoses included in the official coding guidelines (section 1.C.21.c.16) are consistent with reporting guidelines for health care encounters *excluding acute care inpatient admissions*. In addition, hospice claims billed for both inpatient and outpatient hospice services may not assign any Z code as a primary or first-listed diagnosis under any condition. To report hospice services, both inpatient and outpatient, the claim must list as primary or first listed the condition resulting in a terminal diagnosis with life

expectancy of six months or less. Hospices may assign Z codes to the claim as secondary codes at their discretion to provide additional information regarding a patient's overall condition.

| Z51.12 | Encounter for antineoplastic immunotherapy | PDx |

Color Bars

Manifestation Code

Codes defined as manifestation codes based on CMS IOCE designations v20.2, appear in italic type, with a blue color bar over the code description. A manifestation cannot be reported as a first-listed code; it is sequenced as a secondary diagnosis with the underlying disease code listed first.

| G32.89 | *Other specified degenerative disorders of nervous system in diseases classified elsewhere* |
| | Degenerative encephalopathy in diseases classified elsewhere |

Unspecified Diagnosis

Codes that appear with a gray color bar over the alphanumeric code identify unspecified diagnoses. These codes should be used in limited circumstances, when neither the diagnostic statement nor the documentation provides enough information to assign a more specific diagnosis code. The abbreviation NOS, "not otherwise specified," in the tabular list may be interpreted as "unspecified."

| GØ3.9 | Meningitis, unspecified |
| | Arachnoiditis (spinal) NOS |

Chapter-Level Notations

Chapter-specific Guidelines with Coding Examples
Each chapter begins with the Official Guidelines for Coding and Reporting specific to that chapter, where provided. Coding examples specific to outpatient care settings have been provided to illustrate the coding and/or sequencing guidance in these guidelines.

Muscle and Tendon Table
ICD-10-CM categorizes certain muscles and tendons in the upper and lower extremities by their action (e.g., extension or flexion) as well as their anatomical location. The Muscle/Tendon table is provided at the beginning of chapter 13 and chapter 19 to help users when code selection depends on the action of the muscle and/or tendon.

Note: This table is not all-inclusive, and proper code assignment should be based on the provider's documentation.

Appendixes
The additional resources described below have been included as appendixes for this book. These resources further instruct the professional coder on the appropriate application of the ICD-10-CM code set.

Appendix A: Valid 3-character ICD-10-CM Codes
The user may consult this table to confirm that no further specificity, such as the use of 4th, 5th, 6th or 7th characters or placeholders (X), is necessary. All ICD-10-CM codes that are valid at the three-character level are listed.

Appendix B: Pharmacology List 2020
This reference is a comprehensive but not all-inclusive list of pharmacological agents used to treat acute and/or chronic conditions. Drugs are listed in alphabetical order by their brand and/or generic names along with their drug action and indications for which they may commonly be prescribed. Some drugs have also been mapped to their appropriate Z code for long-term drug use.

Appendix C: Z Codes for Long-Term Drug Use with Associated Drugs

This resource correlates Z codes that are used to identify current long-term drug use with a list of drugs that are typically categorized to that class of drug.

Note: These tables are not all-inclusive but list some of the more commonly used drugs.

Appendix D: Z Codes Only as Principal/First-Listed Diagnosis

Chapter 21, Factors Influencing Health Status and Contact with Health Services, provides codes to deal with encounters for circumstances other than a disease or injury. Many of these codes may be reported *only* as the principal/first listed diagnosis. This resource lists all of these codes in one table for quick and easy reference to ensure accurate reporting.

Appendix E: Qualifications for Medicare Coverage of Home Health Services

Medicare coverage for home health services is subject to specific criteria the patient must meet to qualify for coverage. This resource summarizes the coverage requirements provided in the Medicare Benefit Policy Manual (Pub. 100-02), chapter 7, "Home Health Services."

Appendix F: Overview of the Patient-Driven Groupings Model (PDGM)

The Patient-Driven Groupings Model (PDGM) is a case-mix classification model used to calculate payments for home health services. The model comprises broad payment categories that are further refined and adjusted depending primarily on the patient's clinical characteristics. This resource looks at the overall structure of the PDGM and defines the elements used to categorize a patient into a case-mix group for appropriate payment.

Appendix G: OASIS Diagnosis Guidance

This resource addresses the reporting and coding of diagnoses on the Outcome and Assessment Information Set (OASIS-D), specifically items M1021, M1023, and M1028. The official source for this information can be found in the OASIS-D Guidance Manual, chapter 3.

Appendix H: Patient-Driven Groupings Model (PDGM) Comorbid Conditions

This resource provides a comprehensive list of the ICD-10-CM codes that are considered comorbidities that interact with the primary diagnosis for the PDGM. If one of the reported secondary diagnosis codes is identified in the comorbidity low list, the period of care would receive a low comorbidity payment adjustment. If at least two of the reported secondary diagnosis codes are identified in the comorbidity high list, the period of care would receive a high comorbidity adjustment.

Appendix I: Patient-Driven Groupings Model (PDGM) Return-to-Provider Code List

This resource provides a comprehensive list of the ICD-10-CM codes that do not map to one of the 12 clinical grouping categories and therefore are not acceptable as the primary reason for home health care. These codes lack either the certainty or specificity required to properly categorize a resident under PDGM or describe underlying conditions that cannot be the main reason for home health care. When one of these codes is listed as the primary reason diagnosis code on the OASIS-D or as the principal diagnosis on the claim, the form should be returned to the provider to select an appropriate ICD-10-CM diagnosis code using the clinical grouping list provided by CMS.

Appendix J: Hospice Criteria for Medicare Coverage on Noncancer Hospice Care

This resource provides the requirements that must be met for an individual to be recommended and covered for hospice care; in particular, when a patient does not have a cancer diagnosis.

Appendix K: Hospice Diagnosis and Quality Reporting Guidance

This resource provides an overview of the FY 2019 hospice rule, including a summary of the major provisions regarding diagnosis reporting as well as quality measures and data submission requirements for the Hospice Quality Reporting Program.

Appendix L: Coding Issues for Long-Term Care (LTC)

This resource identifies coding and reporting issues that may be encountered in the long-term (post-acute) care setting. Specific case scenarios along with the applicable ICD-10-CM code or codes and rationales are provided.

Illustrations

This section includes illustrations of normal anatomy with ICD-10-CM-specific terminology.

What's New for 2020

Official Updates

The official ICD-10-CM addendum was posted to the Centers for Medicare and Medicaid Services (CMS) website on June 20, 2019, identifying the changes to the ICD-10-CM code set for fiscal 2020, effective October 1, 2019, to September 30, 2020. These changes were made by the agency charged with maintaining and updating the ICD-10-CM code set, the National Center for Health Statistics (NCHS), a section of the Centers for Disease Control and Prevention (CDC). A summary of the changes is provided below:

15 Codes with a Change in Validity

Note: Validity changes are the result of codes being added to or deleted from the classification. Codes that change from valid to invalid allow the creation of a new subcategory to which new codes can be assigned that provide greater detail about the condition. Codes that change from invalid to valid are the result of subcategory codes being deleted from the classification, when the detail provided in those codes is no longer required.

Valid to Invalid

D81.3	I48.1	I48.2	Q66.0	Q66.1
Q66.21	Q66.22	Q66.3	Q66.4	Q66.7
Q66.9	Q79.6	Q87.1	R82.8	

Invalid to Valid
H81.4

7 Codes Deleted from the Classification

H81.41	Vertigo of central origin, right ear
H81.42	Vertigo of central origin, left ear
H81.43	Vertigo of central origin, bilateral
H81.49	Vertigo of central origin, unspecified ear
T67.0XXA	Heatstroke and sunstroke, initial encounter
T67.0XXD	Heatstroke and sunstroke, subsequent encounter
T67.0XXS	Heatstroke and sunstroke, sequela

273 New Codes Added to the Classification

D75.A	Glucose-6-phosphate dehydrogenase (G6PD) deficiency without anemia
D81.30	Adenosine deaminase deficiency, unspecified
D81.31	Severe combined immunodeficiency due to adenosine deaminase deficiency
D81.32	Adenosine deaminase 2 deficiency
D81.39	Other adenosine deaminase deficiency
I26.93	Single subsegmental pulmonary embolism without acute cor pulmonale
I26.94	Multiple subsegmental pulmonary emboli without acute cor pulmonale
I48.11	Longstanding persistent atrial fibrillation
I48.19	Other persistent atrial fibrillation
I48.20	Chronic atrial fibrillation, unspecified
I48.21	Permanent atrial fibrillation
I80.241	Phlebitis and thrombophlebitis of right peroneal vein
I80.242	Phlebitis and thrombophlebitis of left peroneal vein
I80.243	Phlebitis and thrombophlebitis of peroneal vein, bilateral
I80.249	Phlebitis and thrombophlebitis of unspecified peroneal vein
I80.251	Phlebitis and thrombophlebitis of right calf muscular vein
I80.252	Phlebitis and thrombophlebitis of left calf muscular vein
I80.253	Phlebitis and thrombophlebitis of calf muscular vein, bilateral
I80.259	Phlebitis and thrombophlebitis of unspecified calf muscular vein
I82.451	Acute embolism and thrombosis of right peroneal vein
I82.452	Acute embolism and thrombosis of left peroneal vein
I82.453	Acute embolism and thrombosis of peroneal vein, bilateral
I82.459	Acute embolism and thrombosis of unspecified peroneal vein
I82.461	Acute embolism and thrombosis of right calf muscular vein
I82.462	Acute embolism and thrombosis of left calf muscular vein
I82.463	Acute embolism and thrombosis of calf muscular vein, bilateral
I82.469	Acute embolism and thrombosis of unspecified calf muscular vein
I82.551	Chronic embolism and thrombosis of right peroneal vein
I82.552	Chronic embolism and thrombosis of left peroneal vein
I82.553	Chronic embolism and thrombosis of peroneal vein, bilateral
I82.559	Chronic embolism and thrombosis of unspecified peroneal vein
I82.561	Chronic embolism and thrombosis of right calf muscular vein
I82.562	Chronic embolism and thrombosis of left calf muscular vein
I82.563	Chronic embolism and thrombosis of calf muscular vein, bilateral
I82.569	Chronic embolism and thrombosis of unspecified calf muscular vein
L89.006	Pressure-induced deep tissue damage of unspecified elbow
L89.016	Pressure-induced deep tissue damage of right elbow
L89.026	Pressure-induced deep tissue damage of left elbow
L89.106	Pressure-induced deep tissue damage of unspecified part of back
L89.116	Pressure-induced deep tissue damage of right upper back
L89.126	Pressure-induced deep tissue damage of left upper back
L89.136	Pressure-induced deep tissue damage of right lower back
L89.146	Pressure-induced deep tissue damage of left lower back
L89.156	Pressure-induced deep tissue damage of sacral region
L89.206	Pressure-induced deep tissue damage of unspecified hip
L89.216	Pressure-induced deep tissue damage of right hip
L89.226	Pressure-induced deep tissue damage of left hip
L89.306	Pressure-induced deep tissue damage of unspecified buttock
L89.316	Pressure-induced deep tissue damage of right buttock
L89.326	Pressure-induced deep tissue damage of left buttock
L89.46	Pressure-induced deep tissue damage of contiguous site of back, buttock and hip
L89.506	Pressure-induced deep tissue damage of unspecified ankle
L89.516	Pressure-induced deep tissue damage of right ankle
L89.526	Pressure-induced deep tissue damage of left ankle
L89.606	Pressure-induced deep tissue damage of unspecified heel

L89.616	Pressure-induced deep tissue damage of right heel
L89.626	Pressure-induced deep tissue damage of left heel
L89.816	Pressure-induced deep tissue damage of head
L89.896	Pressure-induced deep tissue damage of other site
L89.96	Pressure-induced deep tissue damage of unspecified site
N63.15	Unspecified lump in the right breast, overlapping quadrants
N63.25	Unspecified lump in the left breast, overlapping quadrants
N99.85	Post endometrial ablation syndrome
Q66.00	Congenital talipes equinovarus, unspecified foot
Q66.01	Congenital talipes equinovarus, right foot
Q66.02	Congenital talipes equinovarus, left foot
Q66.10	Congenital talipes calcaneovarus, unspecified foot
Q66.11	Congenital talipes calcaneovarus, right foot
Q66.12	Congenital talipes calcaneovarus, left foot
Q66.211	Congenital metatarsus primus varus, right foot
Q66.212	Congenital metatarsus primus varus, left foot
Q66.219	Congenital metatarsus primus varus, unspecified foot
Q66.221	Congenital metatarsus adductus, right foot
Q66.222	Congenital metatarsus adductus, left foot
Q66.229	Congenital metatarsus adductus, unspecified foot
Q66.30	Other congenital varus deformities of feet, unspecified foot
Q66.31	Other congenital varus deformities of feet, right foot
Q66.32	Other congenital varus deformities of feet, left foot
Q66.40	Congenital talipes calcaneovalgus, unspecified foot
Q66.41	Congenital talipes calcaneovalgus, right foot
Q66.42	Congenital talipes calcaneovalgus, left foot
Q66.70	Congenital pes cavus, unspecified foot
Q66.71	Congenital pes cavus, right foot
Q66.72	Congenital pes cavus, left foot
Q66.90	Congenital deformity of feet, unspecified, unspecified foot
Q66.91	Congenital deformity of feet, unspecified, right foot
Q66.92	Congenital deformity of feet, unspecified, left foot
Q79.60	Ehlers-Danlos syndrome, unspecified
Q79.61	Classical Ehlers-Danlos syndrome
Q79.62	Hypermobile Ehlers-Danlos syndrome
Q79.63	Vascular Ehlers-Danlos syndrome
Q79.69	Other Ehlers-Danlos syndromes
Q87.11	Prader-Willi syndrome
Q87.19	Other congenital malformation syndromes predominantly associated with short stature
R11.15	Cyclical vomiting syndrome unrelated to migraine
R82.81	Pyuria
R82.89	Other abnormal findings on cytological and histological examination of urine
S02.121A	Fracture of orbital roof, right side, initial encounter for closed fracture
S02.121B	Fracture of orbital roof, right side, initial encounter for open fracture
S02.121D	Fracture of orbital roof, right side, subsequent encounter for fracture with routine healing
S02.121G	Fracture of orbital roof, right side, subsequent encounter for fracture with delayed healing
S02.121K	Fracture of orbital roof, right side, subsequent encounter for fracture with nonunion
S02.121S	Fracture of orbital roof, right side, sequela
S02.122A	Fracture of orbital roof, left side, initial encounter for closed fracture
S02.122B	Fracture of orbital roof, left side, initial encounter for open fracture
S02.122D	Fracture of orbital roof, left side, subsequent encounter for fracture with routine healing
S02.122G	Fracture of orbital roof, left side, subsequent encounter for fracture with delayed healing
S02.122K	Fracture of orbital roof, left side, subsequent encounter for fracture with nonunion
S02.122S	Fracture of orbital roof, left side, sequela
S02.129A	Fracture of orbital roof, unspecified side, initial encounter for closed fracture
S02.129B	Fracture of orbital roof, unspecified side, initial encounter for open fracture
S02.129D	Fracture of orbital roof, unspecified side, subsequent encounter for fracture with routine healing
S02.129G	Fracture of orbital roof, unspecified side, subsequent encounter for fracture with delayed healing
S02.129K	Fracture of orbital roof, unspecified side, subsequent encounter for fracture with nonunion
S02.129S	Fracture of orbital roof, unspecified side, sequela
S02.831A	Fracture of medial orbital wall, right side, initial encounter for closed fracture
S02.831B	Fracture of medial orbital wall, right side, initial encounter for open fracture
S02.831D	Fracture of medial orbital wall, right side, subsequent encounter for fracture with routine healing
S02.831G	Fracture of medial orbital wall, right side, subsequent encounter for fracture with delayed healing
S02.831K	Fracture of medial orbital wall, right side, subsequent encounter for fracture with nonunion
S02.831S	Fracture of medial orbital wall, right side, sequela
S02.832A	Fracture of medial orbital wall, left side, initial encounter for closed fracture
S02.832B	Fracture of medial orbital wall, left side, initial encounter for open fracture
S02.832D	Fracture of medial orbital wall, left side, subsequent encounter for fracture with routine healing
S02.832G	Fracture of medial orbital wall, left side, subsequent encounter for fracture with delayed healing
S02.832K	Fracture of medial orbital wall, left side, subsequent encounter for fracture with nonunion
S02.832S	Fracture of medial orbital wall, left side, sequela
S02.839A	Fracture of medial orbital wall, unspecified side, initial encounter for closed fracture
S02.839B	Fracture of medial orbital wall, unspecified side, initial encounter for open fracture
S02.839D	Fracture of medial orbital wall, unspecified side, subsequent encounter for fracture with routine healing
S02.839G	Fracture of medial orbital wall, unspecified side, subsequent encounter for fracture with delayed healing
S02.839K	Fracture of medial orbital wall, unspecified side, subsequent encounter for fracture with nonunion
S02.839S	Fracture of medial orbital wall, unspecified side, sequela

S02.841A	Fracture of lateral orbital wall, right side, initial encounter for closed fracture
S02.841B	Fracture of lateral orbital wall, right side, initial encounter for open fracture
S02.841D	Fracture of lateral orbital wall, right side, subsequent encounter for fracture with routine healing
S02.841G	Fracture of lateral orbital wall, right side, subsequent encounter for fracture with delayed healing
S02.841K	Fracture of lateral orbital wall, right side, subsequent encounter for fracture with nonunion
S02.841S	Fracture of lateral orbital wall, right side, sequela
S02.842A	Fracture of lateral orbital wall, left side, initial encounter for closed fracture
S02.842B	Fracture of lateral orbital wall, left side, initial encounter for open fracture
S02.842D	Fracture of lateral orbital wall, left side, subsequent encounter for fracture with routine healing
S02.842G	Fracture of lateral orbital wall, left side, subsequent encounter for fracture with delayed healing
S02.842K	Fracture of lateral orbital wall, left side, subsequent encounter for fracture with nonunion
S02.842S	Fracture of lateral orbital wall, left side, sequela
S02.849A	Fracture of lateral orbital wall, unspecified side, initial encounter for closed fracture
S02.849B	Fracture of lateral orbital wall, unspecified side, initial encounter for open fracture
S02.849D	Fracture of lateral orbital wall, unspecified side, subsequent encounter for fracture with routine healing
S02.849G	Fracture of lateral orbital wall, unspecified side, subsequent encounter for fracture with delayed healing
S02.849K	Fracture of lateral orbital wall, unspecified side, subsequent encounter for fracture with nonunion
S02.849S	Fracture of lateral orbital wall, unspecified side, sequela
S02.85XA	Fracture of orbit, unspecified, initial encounter for closed fracture
S02.85XB	Fracture of orbit, unspecified, initial encounter for open fracture
S02.85XD	Fracture of orbit, unspecified, subsequent encounter for fracture with routine healing
S02.85XG	Fracture of orbit, unspecified, subsequent encounter for fracture with delayed healing
S02.85XK	Fracture of orbit, unspecified, subsequent encounter for fracture with nonunion
S02.85XS	Fracture of orbit, unspecified, sequela
T50.911A	Poisoning by multiple unspecified drugs, medicaments and biological substances, accidental (unintentional), initial encounter
T50.911D	Poisoning by multiple unspecified drugs, medicaments and biological substances, accidental (unintentional), subsequent encounter
T50.911S	Poisoning by multiple unspecified drugs, medicaments and biological substances, accidental (unintentional), sequela
T50.912A	Poisoning by multiple unspecified drugs, medicaments and biological substances, intentional self-harm, initial encounter
T50.912D	Poisoning by multiple unspecified drugs, medicaments and biological substances, intentional self-harm, subsequent encounter
T50.912S	Poisoning by multiple unspecified drugs, medicaments and biological substances, intentional self-harm, sequela
T50.913A	Poisoning by multiple unspecified drugs, medicaments and biological substances, assault, initial encounter
T50.913D	Poisoning by multiple unspecified drugs, medicaments and biological substances, assault, subsequent encounter
T50.913S	Poisoning by multiple unspecified drugs, medicaments and biological substances, assault, sequela
T50.914A	Poisoning by multiple unspecified drugs, medicaments and biological substances, undetermined, initial encounter
T50.914D	Poisoning by multiple unspecified drugs, medicaments and biological substances, undetermined, subsequent encounter
T50.914S	Poisoning by multiple unspecified drugs, medicaments and biological substances, undetermined, sequela
T50.915A	Adverse effect of multiple unspecified drugs, medicaments and biological substances, initial encounter
T50.915D	Adverse effect of multiple unspecified drugs, medicaments and biological substances, subsequent encounter
T50.915S	Adverse effect of multiple unspecified drugs, medicaments and biological substances, sequela
T50.916A	Underdosing of multiple unspecified drugs, medicaments and biological substances, initial encounter
T50.916D	Underdosing of multiple unspecified drugs, medicaments and biological substances, subsequent encounter
T50.916S	Underdosing of multiple unspecified drugs, medicaments and biological substances, sequela
T67.01XA	Heatstroke and sunstroke, initial encounter
T67.01XD	Heatstroke and sunstroke, subsequent encounter
T67.01XS	Heatstroke and sunstroke, sequela
T67.02XA	Exertional heatstroke, initial encounter
T67.02XD	Exertional heatstroke, subsequent encounter
T67.02XS	Exertional heatstroke, sequela
T67.09XA	Other heatstroke and sunstroke, initial encounter
T67.09XD	Other heatstroke and sunstroke, subsequent encounter
T67.09XS	Other heatstroke and sunstroke, sequela
Y35.009A	Legal intervention involving unspecified firearm discharge, unspecified person injured, initial encounter
Y35.009D	Legal intervention involving unspecified firearm discharge, unspecified person injured, subsequent encounter
Y35.009S	Legal intervention involving unspecified firearm discharge, unspecified person injured, sequela
Y35.019A	Legal intervention involving injury by machine gun, unspecified person injured, initial encounter
Y35.019D	Legal intervention involving injury by machine gun, unspecified person injured, subsequent encounter
Y35.019S	Legal intervention involving injury by machine gun, unspecified person injured, sequela
Y35.029A	Legal intervention involving injury by handgun, unspecified person injured, initial encounter
Y35.029D	Legal intervention involving injury by handgun, unspecified person injured, subsequent encounter
Y35.029S	Legal intervention involving injury by handgun, unspecified person injured, sequela
Y35.039A	Legal intervention involving injury by rifle pellet, unspecified person injured, initial encounter
Y35.039D	Legal intervention involving injury by rifle pellet, unspecified person injured, subsequent encounter

Y35.039S	Legal intervention involving injury by rifle pellet, unspecified person injured, sequela
Y35.049A	Legal intervention involving injury by rubber bullet, unspecified person injured, initial encounter
Y35.049D	Legal intervention involving injury by rubber bullet, unspecified person injured, subsequent encounter
Y35.049S	Legal intervention involving injury by rubber bullet, unspecified person injured, sequela
Y35.099A	Legal intervention involving other firearm discharge, unspecified person injured, initial encounter
Y35.099D	Legal intervention involving other firearm discharge, unspecified person injured, subsequent encounter
Y35.099S	Legal intervention involving other firearm discharge, unspecified person injured, sequela
Y35.109A	Legal intervention involving unspecified explosives, unspecified person injured, initial encounter
Y35.109D	Legal intervention involving unspecified explosives, unspecified person injured, subsequent encounter
Y35.109S	Legal intervention involving unspecified explosives, unspecified person injured, sequela
Y35.119A	Legal intervention involving injury by dynamite, unspecified person injured, initial encounter
Y35.119D	Legal intervention involving injury by dynamite, unspecified person injured, subsequent encounter
Y35.119S	Legal intervention involving injury by dynamite, unspecified person injured, sequela
Y35.129A	Legal intervention involving injury by explosive shell, unspecified person injured, initial encounter
Y35.129D	Legal intervention involving injury by explosive shell, unspecified person injured, subsequent encounter
Y35.129S	Legal intervention involving injury by explosive shell, unspecified person injured, sequela
Y35.199A	Legal intervention involving other explosives, unspecified person injured, initial encounter
Y35.199D	Legal intervention involving other explosives, unspecified person injured, subsequent encounter
Y35.199S	Legal intervention involving other explosives, unspecified person injured, sequela
Y35.209A	Legal intervention involving unspecified gas, unspecified person injured, initial encounter
Y35.209D	Legal intervention involving unspecified gas, unspecified person injured, subsequent encounter
Y35.209S	Legal intervention involving unspecified gas, unspecified person injured, sequela
Y35.219A	Legal intervention involving injury by tear gas, unspecified person injured, initial encounter
Y35.219D	Legal intervention involving injury by tear gas, unspecified person injured, subsequent encounter
Y35.219S	Legal intervention involving injury by tear gas, unspecified person injured, sequela
Y35.299A	Legal intervention involving other gas, unspecified person injured, initial encounter
Y35.299D	Legal intervention involving other gas, unspecified person injured, subsequent encounter
Y35.299S	Legal intervention involving other gas, unspecified person injured, sequela
Y35.309A	Legal intervention involving unspecified blunt objects, unspecified person injured, initial encounter
Y35.309D	Legal intervention involving unspecified blunt objects, unspecified person injured, subsequent encounter
Y35.309S	Legal intervention involving unspecified blunt objects, unspecified person injured, sequela
Y35.319A	Legal intervention involving baton, unspecified person injured, initial encounter
Y35.319D	Legal intervention involving baton, unspecified person injured, subsequent encounter
Y35.319S	Legal intervention involving baton, unspecified person injured, sequela
Y35.399A	Legal intervention involving other blunt objects, unspecified person injured, initial encounter
Y35.399D	Legal intervention involving other blunt objects, unspecified person injured, subsequent encounter
Y35.399S	Legal intervention involving other blunt objects, unspecified person injured, sequela
Y35.409A	Legal intervention involving unspecified sharp objects, unspecified person injured, initial encounter
Y35.409D	Legal intervention involving unspecified sharp objects, unspecified person injured, subsequent encounter
Y35.409S	Legal intervention involving unspecified sharp objects, unspecified person injured, sequela
Y35.419A	Legal intervention involving bayonet, unspecified person injured, initial encounter
Y35.419D	Legal intervention involving bayonet, unspecified person injured, subsequent encounter
Y35.419S	Legal intervention involving bayonet, unspecified person injured, sequela
Y35.499A	Legal intervention involving other sharp objects, unspecified person injured, initial encounter
Y35.499D	Legal intervention involving other sharp objects, unspecified person injured, subsequent encounter
Y35.499S	Legal intervention involving other sharp objects, unspecified person injured, sequela
Y35.819A	Legal intervention involving manhandling, unspecified person injured, initial encounter
Y35.819D	Legal intervention involving manhandling, unspecified person injured, subsequent encounter
Y35.819S	Legal intervention involving manhandling, unspecified person injured, sequela
Y35.831A	Legal intervention involving a conducted energy device, law enforcement official injured, initial encounter
Y35.831D	Legal intervention involving a conducted energy device, law enforcement official injured, subsequent encounter
Y35.831S	Legal intervention involving a conducted energy device, law enforcement official injured, sequela
Y35.832A	Legal intervention involving a conducted energy device, bystander injured, initial encounter
Y35.832D	Legal intervention involving a conducted energy device, bystander injured, subsequent encounter
Y35.832S	Legal intervention involving a conducted energy device, bystander injured, sequela
Y35.833A	Legal intervention involving a conducted energy device, suspect injured, initial encounter
Y35.833D	Legal intervention involving a conducted energy device, suspect injured, subsequent encounter
Y35.833S	Legal intervention involving a conducted energy device, suspect injured, sequela

What's New for 2020 *(vertical side tab)*

Y35.839A	Legal intervention involving a conducted energy device, unspecified person injured, initial encounter
Y35.839D	Legal intervention involving a conducted energy device, unspecified person injured, subsequent encounter
Y35.839S	Legal intervention involving a conducted energy device, unspecified person injured, sequela
Y35.99XA	Legal intervention, means unspecified, unspecified person injured, initial encounter
Y35.99XD	Legal intervention, means unspecified, unspecified person injured, subsequent encounter
Y35.99XS	Legal intervention, means unspecified, unspecified person injured, sequela
Z01.020	Encounter for examination of eyes and vision following failed vision screening without abnormal findings
Z01.021	Encounter for examination of eyes and vision following failed vision screening with abnormal findings
Z11.7	Encounter for testing for latent tuberculosis infection
Z22.7	Latent tuberculosis
Z71.84	Encounter for health counseling related to travel
Z86.002	Personal history of in-situ neoplasm of other and unspecified genital organs
Z86.003	Personal history of in-situ neoplasm of oral cavity, esophagus and stomach
Z86.004	Personal history of in-situ neoplasm of other and unspecified digestive organs
Z86.005	Personal history of in-situ neoplasm of middle ear and respiratory system
Z86.006	Personal history of melanoma in-situ
Z86.007	Personal history of in-situ neoplasm of skin
Z86.15	Personal history of latent tuberculosis infection
Z96.82	Presence of neurostimulator

30 Code Descriptions Revised

Note: Each code is listed with its revised description only. Please refer to the full FY 2020 official addenda code files at https://www.cms.gov/Medicare/Coding/ICD10/2020-ICD-10-CM.html for the specific changes made to the codes listed.

B96.21	Shiga toxin-producing Escherichia coli [E. coli] [STEC] O157 as the cause of diseases classified elsewhere
B96.22	Other specified Shiga toxin-producing Escherichia coli [E. coli] [STEC] as the cause of diseases classified elsewhere
B96.23	Unspecified Shiga toxin-producing Escherichia coli [E. coli] [STEC] as the cause of diseases classified elsewhere
G43.A0	Cyclical vomiting, in migraine, not intractable
G43.A1	Cyclical vomiting, in migraine, intractable
I70.238	Atherosclerosis of native arteries of right leg with ulceration of other part of lower leg
I70.248	Atherosclerosis of native arteries of left leg with ulceration of other part of lower leg
J44.0	Chronic obstructive pulmonary disease with (acute) lower respiratory infection
M50.120	Mid-cervical disc disorder, unspecified level
M66.88	Spontaneous rupture of other tendons, other sites

M67.839	Other specified disorders of synovium and tendon, unspecified wrist
M77.50	Other enthesopathy of unspecified foot and ankle
M77.51	Other enthesopathy of right foot and ankle
M77.52	Other enthesopathy of left foot and ankle
N35.814	Other anterior urethral stricture, male
R82.993	Hyperuricosuria
T40.906A	Underdosing of unspecified psychodysleptics [hallucinogens], initial encounter
T40.906D	Underdosing of unspecified psychodysleptics [hallucinogens], subsequent encounter
T40.906S	Underdosing of unspecified psychodysleptics [hallucinogens], sequela
T40.996A	Underdosing of other psychodysleptics [hallucinogens], initial encounter
T40.996D	Underdosing of other psychodysleptics [hallucinogens], subsequent encounter
T40.996S	Underdosing of other psychodysleptics [hallucinogens], sequela
T44.1X6A	Underdosing of other parasympathomimetics [cholinergics], initial encounter
T44.1X6D	Underdosing of other parasympathomimetics [cholinergics], subsequent encounter
T44.1X6S	Underdosing of other parasympathomimetics [cholinergics], sequela
V43.13XA	Car passenger injured in collision with pick-up truck in nontraffic accident, initial encounter
V43.13XD	Car passenger injured in collision with pick-up truck in nontraffic accident, subsequent encounter
V43.13XS	Car passenger injured in collision with pick-up truck in nontraffic accident, sequela
Z45.42	Encounter for adjustment and management of neurostimulator
Z68.43	Body mass index (BMI) 50.0-59.9, adult

Proprietary Updates

The following proprietary features have also been added:

- 40+ new definitions that describe, in lay terms, a specific condition or disease process

- 40+ new coding tips that provide coding advice beyond the code classification

- Updated *AHA Coding Clinic* references through second quarter 2019

- New edits related to home health Patient-Driven Groupings Model (PDGM)

- Several new appendixes outlining various aspects of the home health PDGM

Conversion Table of ICD-10-CM Codes

Code Assignment Beginning 10/1/2019	Previous Code(s) Assignment	Code Assignment Beginning 10/1/2019	Previous Code(s) Assignment	Code Assignment Beginning 10/1/2019	Previous Code(s) Assignment
D75.A	D55.0	L89.316	L89.310	S02.121A	S02.19A*
D81.30	D81.3	L89.326	L89.320	S02.121B	S02.19B*
D81.31	D81.3	L89.46	L89.45	S02.121D	S02.19D*
D81.32	D81.3	L89.506	L89.500	S02.121G	S02.19G*
D81.39	D81.3	L89.516	L89.510	S02.121K	S02.19K*
H81.4	H81.41–H81.43; H81.49	L89.526	L89.520	S02.121S	S02.19S*
		L89.606	L89.600	S02.122A	S02.19A*
I26.93	I26.99	L89.616	L89.610	S02.122B	S02.19B*
I26.94	I26.99	L89.626	L89.620	S02.122D	S02.19D*
I48.11	I48.1	L89.816	L89.810	S02.122G	S02.19G*
I48.19	I48.1	L89.896	L89.890	S02.122K	S02.19K*
I48.20	I48.2	L89.96	L89.95	S02.122S	S02.19S*
I48.21	I48.2	N63.15	N63.11–N63.14	S02.129A	S02.19A*
I80.241	I80.291	N63.25	N63.21–N63.24	S02.129B	S02.19B*
I80.242	I80.292	N99.85	N99.89	S02.129D	S02.19D*
I80.243	I80.293	Q66.00	Q66.0	S02.129G	S02.19G*
I80.249	I80.299	Q66.01	Q66.0	S02.129K	S02.19K*
I80.251	I80.291	Q66.02	Q66.0	S02.129S	S02.19S*
I80.252	I80.292	Q66.10	Q66.1	S02.831A	S02.81XA
I80.253	I80.293	Q66.11	Q66.1	S02.831B	S02.81XB
I80.259	I80.299	Q66.12	Q66.1	S02.831D	S02.81XD
I82.451	I80.491	Q66.211	Q66.21	S02.831G	S02.81XG
I82.452	I80.492	Q66.212	Q66.21	S02.831K	S02.81XK
I82.453	I80.493	Q66.219	Q66.21	S02.831S	S02.81XS
I82.459	I80.499	Q66.221	Q66.22	S02.832A	S02.82XA
I82.461	I80.491	Q66.222	Q66.22	S02.832B	S02.82XB
I82.462	I80.492	Q66.229	Q66.22	S02.832D	S02.82XD
I82.463	I80.493	Q66.30	Q66.3	S02.832G	S02.82XG
I82.469	I80.499	Q66.31	Q66.3	S02.832K	S02.82XK
I82.551	I80.591	Q66.32	Q66.3	S02.832S	S02.82XS
I82.552	I80.592	Q66.40	Q66.4	S02.839A	S02.80XA
I82.553	I80.593	Q66.41	Q66.4	S02.839B	S02.80XB
I82.559	I80.599	Q66.42	Q66.4	S02.839D	S02.80XD
I82.561	I80.591	Q66.70	Q66.7	S02.839G	S02.80XG
I82.562	I80.592	Q66.71	Q66.7	S02.839K	S02.80XK
I82.563	I80.593	Q66.72	Q66.7	S02.839S	S02.80XS
I82.569	I80.599	Q66.90	Q66.9	S02.841A	S02.81XA
L89.006	L89.000	Q66.91	Q66.9	S02.841B	S02.81XB
L89.016	L89.010	Q66.92	Q66.9	S02.841D	S02.81XD
L89.026	L89.020	Q79.60	Q79.6	S02.841G	S02.81XG
L89.106	L89.100	Q79.61	Q79.6	S02.841K	S02.81XK
L89.116	L89.110	Q79.62	Q79.6	S02.841S	S02.81XS
L89.126	L89.120	Q79.63	Q79.6	S02.842A	S02.82XA
L89.136	L89.130	Q79.69	Q79.6	S02.842B	S02.82XB
L89.146	L89.140	Q87.11	Q87.1	S02.842D	S02.82XD
L89.156	L89.150	Q87.19	Q87.1	S02.842G	S02.82XG
L89.206	L89.200	R11.15	K31.89 and a code from R11-	S02.842K	S02.82XK
L89.216	L89.210			S02.842S	S02.82XS
L89.226	L89.220	R82.81	R82.8	S02.849A	S02.80XA
L89.306	L89.300	R82.89	R82.8	S02.849B	S02.80XB

Conversion Table of ICD-10-CM Codes

Code Assignment Beginning 10/1/2019	Previous Code(s) Assignment	Code Assignment Beginning 10/1/2019	Previous Code(s) Assignment	Code Assignment Beginning 10/1/2019	Previous Code(s) Assignment
S02.849D	S02.80XD	Y35.029A	None	Y35.409D	None
S02.849G	S02.80XG	Y35.029D	None	Y35.409S	None
S02.849K	S02.80XK	Y35.029S	None	Y35.419A	None
S02.849S	S02.80XS	Y35.039A	None	Y35.419D	None
S02.85XA	S02.80XA	Y35.039D	None	Y35.419S	None
S02.85XB	S02.80XB	Y35.039S	None	Y35.499A	None
S02.85XD	S02.80XD	Y35.049A	None	Y35.499D	None
S02.85XG	S02.80XG	Y35.049D	None	Y35.499S	None
S02.85XK	S02.80XK	Y35.049S	None	Y35.819A	None
S02.85XS	S02.80XS	Y35.099A	None	Y35.819D	None
T50.911A	T50.991A	Y35.099D	None	Y35.819S	None
T50.911D	T50.991D	Y35.099S	None	Y35.831A	Y35.891A
T50.911S	T50.991S	Y35.109A	None	Y35.831D	Y35.891D
T50.912A	T50.992A	Y35.109D	None	Y35.831S	Y35.891S
T50.912D	T50.992D	Y35.109S	None	Y35.832A	Y35.892A
T50.912S	T50.992S	Y35.119A	None	Y35.832D	Y35.892D
T50.913A	T50.993A	Y35.119D	None	Y35.832S	Y35.892S
T50.913D	T50.993D	Y35.119S	None	Y35.833A	Y35.893A
T50.913S	T50.993S	Y35.129A	None	Y35.833D	Y35.893D
T50.914A	T50.994A	Y35.129D	None	Y35.833S	Y35.893S
T50.914D	T50.994D	Y35.129S	None	Y35.839A	None
T50.914S	T50.994S	Y35.199A	None	Y35.839D	None
T50.915A	T50.995A	Y35.199D	None	Y35.839S	None
T50.915D	T50.995D	Y35.199S	None	Y35.99XA	None
T50.915S	T50.995S	Y35.209A	None	Y35.99XD	None
T50.916A	T50.996A	Y35.209D	None	Y35.99XS	None
T50.916D	T50.996D	Y35.209S	None	Z01.020	Z01.00
T50.916S	T50.996S	Y35.219A	None	Z01.021	Z01.01
T67.01XA	T67.0XXA	Y35.219D	None	Z11.7	Z11.1
T67.01XD	T67.0XXD	Y35.219S	None	Z22.7	R76.11
T67.01XS	T67.0XXS	Y35.299A	None	Z71.84	Z71.89
T67.02XA	T67.0XXA	Y35.299D	None	Z86.002	Z86.008
T67.02XD	T67.0XXD	Y35.299S	None	Z86.003	Z86.008
T67.02XS	T67.0XXS	Y35.309A	None	Z86.004	Z86.008
T67.09XA	T67.0XXA	Y35.309D	None	Z86.005	Z86.008
T67.09XD	T67.0XXD	Y35.309S	None	Z86.006	Z86.008
T67.09XS	T67.0XXS	Y35.319A	None	Z86.007	Z86.008
Y35.009A	None	Y35.319D	None	Z86.15	R76.11
Y35.009D	None	Y35.319S	None	Z96.82	Z96.89
Y35.009S	None	Y35.399A	None		
Y35.019A	None	Y35.399D	None		
Y35.019D	None	Y35.399S	None		
Y35.019S	None	Y35.409A	None		

* These codes are listed exactly as found in the official conversion table from the CDC.

10 Steps to Correct Coding

Follow the 10 steps below to correctly code encounters for health care services.

Step 1: Identify the reason for the visit or encounter (i.e., a sign, symptom, diagnosis and/or condition).
The medical record documentation should accurately reflect the patient's condition, using terminology that includes specific diagnoses and symptoms or clearly states the reasons for the encounter.

Choosing the main term that best describes the reason chiefly responsible for the service provided is the most important step in coding. If symptoms are present and documented but a definitive diagnosis has not yet been determined, code the symptoms. *For outpatient cases, do not code conditions that are referred to as "rule out," "suspected," "probable," or "questionable."* Diagnoses often are not established at the time of the initial encounter/visit and may require two or more visits to be established. Code only what is documented in the available outpatient records and only to the highest degree of certainty known at the time of the patient's visit. For inpatient medical records, uncertain diagnoses may be reported if documented at the time of discharge.

Step 2: After selecting the reason for the encounter, consult the alphabetic index.
The most critical rule is to begin code selection in the alphabetic index. Never turn first to the tabular list. The index provides cross-references, essential and nonessential modifiers, and other instructional notations that may not be found in the tabular list.

Step 3: Locate the main term entry.
The alphabetic index lists conditions, which may be expressed as nouns or eponyms, with critical use of adjectives. Some conditions known by several names have multiple main entries. Reasons for encounters may be located under general terms such as admission, encounter, and examination. Other general terms such as history, status (post), or presence (of) can be used to locate other factors influencing health.

Step 4: Scan subterm entries.
Scan the subterm entries, as appropriate, being sure to review continued lines and additional subterms that may appear in the next column or on the next page. Shaded vertical guidelines in the index indicate the indentation level for each subterm in relation to the main terms.

Step 5: Pay close attention to index instructions.
- Parentheses ( ) enclose nonessential modifiers, terms that are supplementary words or explanatory information that may or may not appear in the diagnostic statement and do not affect code selection.

- Brackets [ ] enclose manifestation codes that can be used only as secondary codes to the underlying condition code immediately preceding it. If used, manifestation codes must be reported with the appropriate etiology codes.

- Default codes are listed next to the main term and represent the condition most commonly associated with the main term or the unspecified code for the main term.

- "*See*" cross-references, identified by italicized type and "code by" cross-references indicate that another term *must be referenced* to locate the correct code.

- "*See also*" cross-references, identified by italicized type, provide alternative terms that may be useful to look up but *are not mandatory*.

- "Omit code" cross-references identify instances when a code is not applicable depending on the condition being coded.

- "With" subterms are listed out of alphabetic order and identify a presumed causal relationship between the two conditions they link.

- "Due to" subterms identify a relationship between the two conditions they link.

- "NEC," abbreviation for "not elsewhere classified," follows some main terms or subterms and indicates that there is no specific code for the condition even though the medical documentation may be very specific.

- "NOS," abbreviation for "not otherwise specified," follows some main terms or subterms and is the equivalent of unspecified; NOS signifies that the information in the medical record is insufficient for assigning a more specific code.

- *Following* references help coders locate alphanumeric codes that are out of sequence in the tabular section.

- Check-additional-character symbols flag codes that require additional characters to make the code valid; the characters available to complete the code should be verified in the tabular section.

Step 6: Choose a potential code and locate it in the tabular list.
To prevent coding errors, always use both the alphabetic index (to identify a code) and the tabular list (to verify a code), as the index does not include the important instructional notes found in the tabular list. An added benefit of using the tabular list, which groups like things together, is that while looking at one code in the list, a coder might see a more specific one that would have been missed had the coder relied solely on the alphabetic index. Additionally, many of the codes require a fourth, fifth, sixth, or seventh character to be valid, and many of these characters can be found only in the tabular list.

Step 7: Read all instructional material in the tabular section.
The coder must follow any Includes, Excludes 1 and Excludes 2 notes, and other instructional notes, such as "Code first" and "Use additional code," listed in the tabular list for the chapter, category, subcategory, and subclassification levels of code selection that direct the coder to use a different or additional code. Any codes in the tabular range A00.0-through T88.9- may be used to identify the diagnostic reason for the encounter. The tabular list encompasses many codes describing disease and injury classifications (e.g., infectious and parasitic diseases, neoplasms, symptoms, nervous and circulatory system etc.).

Codes that describe symptoms and signs, as opposed to definitive diagnoses, should be reported when an established diagnosis has not been made (confirmed) by the physician. Chapter 18 of the ICD-10-CM code book, "Symptoms, Signs, and Abnormal Clinical and Laboratory Findings, Not Elsewhere Classified" (codes R00.--R99), contains many, but not all, codes for symptoms.

ICD-10-CM classifies encounters with health care providers for circumstances other than a disease or injury in chapter 21, "Factors Influencing Health Status and Contact with Health Services" (codes Z00–Z99). Circumstances other than a disease or injury often are recorded as chiefly responsible for the encounter.

A code is invalid if it does not include the full number of characters (greatest level of specificity) required. Codes in ICD-10-CM can contain from three to seven alphanumeric characters. A three-character code is to be used only if the category is not further subdivided into four-, five-, six-, or seven-character codes. Placeholder character X is used as part of an alphanumeric code to allow for future expansion and as a placeholder for empty characters in a code that requires a seventh character but has no fourth, fifth, or sixth character. Note that certain categories require seventh characters that apply to all codes in that category. Always check the category level for applicable seventh characters for that category.

Step 8: Consult the official ICD-10-CM conventions and guidelines.
The *ICD-10-CM Official Guidelines for Coding and Reporting* govern the use of certain codes. These guidelines provide both general and chapter-specific coding guidance.

Step 9: Confirm and assign the code.
Having reviewed all relevant information concerning the possible code choices, assign the code that most completely describes the condition.

Repeat steps 1 through 9 for all additional documented conditions that meet the following criteria:

- They exist at the time of the visit *AND*
- They require or affect patient care, treatment, or management

Step 10: Sequence codes correctly.
Sequencing is the order in which the codes are listed on the claim. List first the ICD-10-CM code for the diagnosis, condition, problem, or other reason for the encounter/visit that is shown in the medical record to be chiefly responsible for the services provided. List additional codes that describe any coexisting conditions. Follow the official coding guidelines (see the guidelines, section II, "Selection of Principal Diagnosis"; section III, "Reporting Additional Diagnoses"; and section IV, "Diagnostic Coding and Reporting Guidelines for Outpatient Services") on proper sequencing of codes.

Coding Examples

Diagnosis: Anorexia
Step 1: The reason for the encounter was the condition, anorexia.

Step 2: Consult the alphabetic index.

Step 3: Locate the main term "Anorexia."

Step 4: Two possible subterms are available, "hysterical" and "nervosa." Neither is documented in this instance, however, so they cannot be used in code selection.

Step 5: The code listed next to the main term is called the default code selection. Because the two subentries (essential modifiers) do not apply in this instance, the default code (R63.0) should be used.

Step 6: Turn to code R63.0 in the tabular list and read all instructional notes.

Step 7: The Excludes 1 note at code R63.0 indicates that anorexia nervosa and loss of appetite determined to be of nonorganic origin should be reported with a code from chapter 5. The diagnostic statement does not describe the condition as anorexia nervosa, however, and does not indicate that the anorexia is of a nonorganic origin. There is no further division of the category past the fourth-character subcategory. Therefore, code R63.0 is at the highest level of specificity.

Step 8: Review of official guideline I.C.18 indicates that a symptom code is appropriate when a more definitive diagnosis is not documented.

Step 9: The default code, R63.0 Anorexia, is the correct code selection.

Repeat steps 1 through 9 for any concomitant diagnoses.

Step 10: Since anorexia is listed as the chief reason for the health care encounter, the first-listed, or principal, diagnosis is R63.0. Note that this is a chapter 18 symptom code but can be assigned for both inpatient and outpatient records since the provider did not establish a more definitive diagnosis, according to sections II.A and IV.D.

Diagnosis: Acute bronchitis
Step 1: The reason for the encounter was the condition, acute bronchitis.

Step 2: Consult the alphabetic index.

Step 3: Locate the main term "Bronchitis."

Step 4: There is a subterm for "acute or subacute." Additional subterms are not included in the diagnostic statement.

Step 5: Review the instructional notes. Nonessential modifiers (with bronchospasm or obstruction) are terms that do not affect code assignment. Since no other subterms indented under "acute" apply here, the code listed next to this subentry—in this case J20.9—should be chosen.

Step 6: Turn to code J20.9 in the tabular list and read all instructional notes.

Step 7: The Includes note under category J20 lists alternative terms for acute bronchitis. Note that the list is not exhaustive but is only a representative selection of diagnoses that are included in the subcategory. The Excludes 1 note refers to category J40 for bronchitis and tracheobronchitis NOS. There are several conditions in the Excludes 2 notes that, if applicable, can be coded in addition to this code.

Note that the codes included in J20 represent acute bronchitis due to various infectious organisms that could be selected if identified in the documentation. In this case, the organism was not identified and there is no further division of the category past the fourth character subcategory. Therefore, code J20.9 is at the highest level of specificity.

Step 8: Review of official guideline I.C.10 provides no additional information affecting the code selected.

Step 9: Assign code J20.9 Acute bronchitis, unspecified.

Repeat steps 1 through 9 for any concomitant diagnoses.

Step 10: In the absence of additional diagnoses that may affect sequencing, code J20.9 should be sequenced as the first-listed, or principal, diagnosis.

Diagnosis: Cerebellar ataxia in myxedema
Step 1: The reason for the encounter was the condition, cerebellar ataxia.

Step 2: Consult the alphabetic index.

Step 3: Locate the main term "Ataxia."

Step 4: Available subterms include "cerebellar (hereditary)," with additional indented subterms for "in" and "myxedema," all essential modifiers that are included in the diagnostic statement. Two codes are provided, E03.9 and G13.2, the latter of which is in brackets.

Step 5: Note the nonessential modifier (in parentheses) after the subterm cerebellar includes the term "hereditary." Because it is in parentheses, this term is not required in the diagnostic statement for this subentry to apply. The brackets around G13.2 identify this code as a manifestation of the condition described by code E03.9 and indicate that the two must be reported together and sequencing rules apply.

Step 6: Locate codes E03.9 and G13.2 in the tabular list, and read all instructional notes.

Step 7: For code E03.9, there are no instructional notes in the tabular list at the category E03 or code level that indicate that this condition should be coded elsewhere in the classification or that additional codes are required. Without further information from the diagnostic statement, myxedema, not otherwise specified (NOS), is appropriately reported with code E03.9 Hypothyroidism, unspecified, according to the inclusion term at this code.

Code G13.2 in the tabular list has an instructional note to "Code first underlying disease," which includes conditions found in category E03.-. Based on this note, codes E03.9 and G13.2 are to be coded together, with G13.2 listed only as a secondary diagnosis. This correlates with what the alphabetic index indicated. As there is no further division of codes in category G13 beyond the fourth character, G13.2 is at the highest level of specificity.

Step 8: Although there are some general conventions, such as how to interpret brackets in the alphabetic index, no chapter-specific guidelines apply to this coding scenario.

Step 9: Assign codes E03.9 Hypothyroidism, unspecified, and G13.2 Systemic atrophy primarily affecting the central nervous system in myxedema.

Repeat steps 1 through 9 for any concomitant diagnoses.

Step 10: Based on the alphabetic index and tabular instructional notations, code E03.9 should be sequenced as the first-listed, or principal, diagnosis followed by G13.2 as a secondary diagnosis.

Diagnosis: Decubitus ulcer of right elbow with skin loss and necrosis of subcutaneous tissue

Step 1: The reason for the encounter was the condition, decubitus ulcer.

Step 2: Consult the alphabetic index.

Step 3: Locate the main term "Ulcer."

Step 4: For the subterm "decubitus," there is no code provided or additional subterms indented, but a cross-reference is listed.

Step 5: The italicized cross-reference instructs the coder to "*see* Ulcer, pressure, by site."

Repeat steps 3 through 5 for the cross-reference.

Step 3: Locate the main term "Ulcer."

Step 4: Review the subentries for the subterm "pressure." The next level of indent lists either the site of the ulcer or the specific stage of the ulcer (stage 1–4, unstageable, and unspecified stages). The diagnostic statement provides the site, right elbow, and the extent of tissue damage (skin loss and necrosis of subcutaneous tissue) but does not specifically state that the ulcer is stage 1, stage 2, etc. Nonessential modifiers (in parentheses) at each stage include a description of the typical extent of damage at each stage. For example, stage 1 describes "pre-ulcer skin changes limited to persistent focal edema." Based on the documentation in the record, the coder can correlate the documentation to the nonessential modifiers and choose the specific stage from the index. The coder can also go directly to the body site, choosing the stage of the ulcer after reviewing the code options and instructional notations in the tabular list.

The diagnostic statement indicates that the extent of the damage to the elbow includes skin loss and necrosis of subcutaneous tissue, coinciding with the nonessential modifier next to the subentry "stage 3." The body site of elbow (L89.0-) is listed as another level of indent with other body sites.

Step 5: Note that code L89.0 is followed by a dash and an additional-character-required icon, which indicate that more characters are needed to complete the code. From here, the tabular listing for L89.0- can be consulted.

Step 6: Locate code L89.0- in the tabular list and read all instructional notes.

Step 7: The tabular listing at category L89 has an Includes note for "decubitus ulcer," which confirms that category L89 is the appropriate category to represent what is documented in the diagnostic statement.

Several Excludes 2 notes are also listed at the category level. Excludes 2 notes represent conditions that can occur concomitantly with the decubitus ulcer and can be coded in addition to code L89, if supported by the documentation.

The subcategory codes under L89.0 indicate that the fifth character describes laterality. Locate the right elbow at subcategory L89.01. See that an additional sixth character to specify the stage of the ulcer is now needed to complete the code. The stage can be determined either by the specific documentation of the stage (e.g., stage 1, stage 2) or, in this case, a description that matches one of the inclusion terms that follow

each stage code. For example, the diagnostic description in this case of "skin loss and necrosis of the subcutaneous tissue" matches the inclusion term under L89.013 Pressure ulcer of right elbow, stage 3. No additional characters are required because code L89.013 is at its highest level of specificity.

Step 8: The official guidelines contain quite a bit of information relating to pressure ulcers in chapter-specific guideline I.C.12 as well as information in general guideline I.B.14. These and any other pertinent guidelines should be reviewed to ensure appropriate code assignment.

Step 9: Assign code L89.013 Pressure ulcer of right elbow, stage 3.

Repeat steps 1 through 9 for any concomitant diagnoses.

Step 10: Since the decubitus ulcer is listed as the chief reason for the health care encounter, the first-listed, or principal, diagnosis is L89.013. However, according to the code first instructional note at the L89 category level, gangrene (I96) would be sequenced before the pressure ulcer if it were documented.

Diagnosis: Emergency department visit for bimalleolar fracture of the right ankle due to trauma

Step 1: The reason for the encounter was the condition, bimalleolar fracture.

Step 2: Consult the alphabetic index.

Step 3: Locate the main term "Fracture." Note that many main terms represent fractures: "Fracture, burst," "Fracture, chronic," "Fracture, insufficiency," "Fracture, nontraumatic NEC," "Fracture, pathological," and "Fracture, traumatic." Since the diagnostic statement specifically states that this fracture was the result of trauma, the main term "Fracture, traumatic" should be used.

Step 4: Subterms that should be referenced are "ankle" and "bimalleolar (displaced)," which lists code S82.84-.

Step 5: A nonessential modifier (in parentheses) next to the term bimalleolar for "displaced" indicates that S82.84- is the default category unless the fracture is specifically identified as "nondisplaced."

Note that code S82.84- is followed by a dash and an additional-character icon, both of which indicate that more characters are required. From here, the tabular list can be consulted.

Step 6: Locate code S82.84- in the tabular list and read all instructional notes.

Step: 7 The instructional notes at category S82 indicate that fractures not specified as displaced or nondisplaced default to displaced and that fractures not designated as open or closed default to closed. Additional instructional notes can be found at the category level but none pertain to the current scenario.

Read through the subcategory codes under S82.84, and note that the sixth character specifies displaced or nondisplaced and laterality. Based on the index nonessential modifier (displaced) and the code note at category S82, code selection should identify a displaced fracture of the right side. A displaced bimalleolar fracture of the right lower leg is coded to S82.841.

To complete the code, a seventh character must be assigned to identify the type of encounter (initial, subsequent, or sequela) and whether the fracture is open or closed. Most of the codes in category S82 require a seventh character represented in the list at the category level. However, it is important to note that some subcategories have their own specific set of seventh characters. In this instance, subcategory S82.84- does not have a unique set of seventh characters and the list provided at the category level should be used. Without documentation of the fracture being open, the tabular notation indicates that the default is closed. Character A, representing "initial encounter for closed fracture," listed in the box at the category level is the most appropriate option.

Step 8: Assign code S82.841A Displaced bimalleolar fracture of right lower leg, initial encounter for closed fracture.

Repeat steps 1 through 9 for any concomitant diagnoses.

Step 9: Review chapter-specific guideline I.C.19. and any other official conventions or guidelines to ensure appropriate code assignment.

Step 10: Additional codes can be applied to relate the specific cause of the injury, the place of occurrence, the activity of the patient at the time of the injury, and the patient's status, when this information is available in the record. However, coding this information is voluntary and reporting requirements depend on state mandates and/or facility-specific reporting requirements. If assigned, the external cause codes should be reported as secondary diagnoses only with the injury (fracture) sequenced first. Most codes in chapter 20, "External Causes of Morbidity," require a seventh character to identify the type of encounter. The seventh character assigned to an external cause code should match the seventh character of the code assigned for the associated injury or condition for the encounter.

2020 ICD-10-CM Official Guidelines for Coding and Reporting

Narrative changes appear in **bold** text

Items underlined have been moved within the guidelines since the FY 2019 version

Italics are used to indicate revisions to heading changes

The Centers for Medicare and Medicaid Services (CMS) and the National Center for Health Statistics (NCHS), two departments within the U.S. Federal Government's Department of Health and Human Services (DHHS) provide the following guidelines for coding and reporting using the International Classification of Diseases, 10th Revision, Clinical Modification (ICD-10-CM). These guidelines should be used as a companion document to the official version of the ICD-10-CM as published on the NCHS website. The ICD-10-CM is a morbidity classification published by the United States for classifying diagnoses and reason for visits in all health care settings. The ICD-10-CM is based on the ICD-10, the statistical classification of disease published by the World Health Organization (WHO).

These guidelines have been approved by the four organizations that make up the Cooperating Parties for the ICD-10-CM: the American Hospital Association (AHA), the American Health Information Management Association (AHIMA), CMS, and NCHS.

These guidelines are a set of rules that have been developed to accompany and complement the official conventions and instructions provided within the ICD-10-CM itself. The instructions and conventions of the classification take precedence over guidelines. These guidelines are based on the coding and sequencing instructions in the Tabular List and Alphabetic Index of ICD-10-CM, but provide additional instruction. Adherence to these guidelines when assigning ICD-10-CM diagnosis codes is required under the Health Insurance Portability and Accountability Act (HIPAA). The diagnosis codes (Tabular List and Alphabetic Index) have been adopted under HIPAA for all healthcare settings. A joint effort between the healthcare provider and the coder is essential to achieve complete and accurate documentation, code assignment, and reporting of diagnoses and procedures. These guidelines have been developed to assist both the healthcare provider and the coder in identifying those diagnoses that are to be reported. The importance of consistent, complete documentation in the medical record cannot be overemphasized. Without such documentation accurate coding cannot be achieved. The entire record should be reviewed to determine the specific reason for the encounter and the conditions treated.

The term encounter is used for all settings, including hospital admissions. In the context of these guidelines, the term provider is used throughout the guidelines to mean physician or any qualified health care practitioner who is legally accountable for establishing the patient's diagnosis. Only this set of guidelines, approved by the Cooperating Parties, is official.

The guidelines are organized into sections. Section I includes the structure and conventions of the classification and general guidelines that apply to the entire classification, and chapter-specific guidelines that correspond to the chapters as they are arranged in the classification. Section II includes guidelines for selection of principal diagnosis for non-outpatient settings. Section III includes guidelines for reporting additional diagnoses in non-outpatient settings. Section IV is for outpatient coding and reporting. It is necessary to review all sections of the guidelines to fully understand all of the rules and instructions needed to code properly.

Section I. Conventions, general coding guidelines and chapter specific guidelines

The conventions, general guidelines and chapter-specific guidelines are applicable to all health care settings unless otherwise indicated. The conventions and instructions of the classification take precedence over guidelines.

A. Conventions for the ICD-10-CM

The conventions for the ICD-10-CM are the general rules for use of the classification independent of the guidelines. These conventions are incorporated within the Alphabetic Index and Tabular List of the ICD-10-CM as instructional notes.

1. **The Alphabetic Index and Tabular List**

   The ICD-10-CM is divided into the Alphabetic Index, an alphabetical list of terms and their corresponding code, and the Tabular List, a structured list of codes divided into chapters based on body system or condition. The Alphabetic Index consists of the following parts: the Index of Diseases and Injury, the Index of External Causes of Injury, the Table of Neoplasms and the Table of Drugs and Chemicals.

   See Section I.C2. General guidelines

   See Section I.C.19. Adverse effects, poisoning, underdosing and toxic effects

2. **Format and Structure:**

   The ICD-10-CM Tabular List contains categories, subcategories and codes. Characters for categories, subcategories and codes may be either a letter or a number. All categories are 3 characters. A three-character category that has no further subdivision is equivalent to a code. Subcategories are either 4 or 5 characters. Codes may be 3, 4, 5, 6 or 7 characters. That is, each level of subdivision after a category is a subcategory. The final level of subdivision is a code. Codes that have applicable 7th characters are still referred to as codes, not subcategories. A code that has an applicable 7th character is considered invalid without the 7th character.

   The ICD-10-CM uses an indented format for ease in reference.

3. **Use of codes for reporting purposes**

   For reporting purposes only codes are permissible, not categories or subcategories, and any applicable 7th character is required.

4. **Placeholder character**

   The ICD-10-CM utilizes a placeholder character "X". The "X" is used as a placeholder at certain codes to allow for future expansion. An example of this is at the poisoning, adverse effect and underdosing codes, categories T36-T50.

   Where a placeholder exists, the X must be used in order for the code to be considered a valid code.

5. **7th Characters**

   Certain ICD-10-CM categories have applicable 7th characters. The applicable 7th character is required for all codes within the category, or as the notes in the Tabular List instruct. The 7th character must always be the 7th character in the data field. If a code that requires a 7th character is not 6 characters, a placeholder X must be used to fill in the empty characters.

6. **Abbreviations**
   a. **Alphabetic Index abbreviations**
      NEC "Not elsewhere classifiable"

      This abbreviation in the Alphabetic Index represents "other specified." When a specific code is not available for a condition, the Alphabetic Index directs the coder to the "other specified" code in the Tabular List.

      NOS "Not otherwise specified"

      This abbreviation is the equivalent of unspecified.

   b. **Tabular List abbreviations**
      NEC "Not elsewhere classifiable"

      This abbreviation in the Tabular List represents "other specified". When a specific code is not available for a condition, the Tabular List includes an NEC entry under a code to identify the code as the "other specified" code.

      NOS "Not otherwise specified"

      This abbreviation is the equivalent of unspecified.

7. **Punctuation**
   [ ] Brackets are used in the Tabular List to enclose synonyms, alternative wording or explanatory phrases. Brackets are used in the Alphabetic Index to identify manifestation codes.

   ( ) Parentheses are used in both the Alphabetic Index and Tabular List to enclose supplementary words that may be present or absent in the statement of a disease or procedure without affecting the code number to which it is assigned. The terms within the parentheses are referred to as nonessential modifiers. The nonessential modifiers in the Alphabetic Index to Diseases apply to subterms following a main term except when a nonessential modifier and a subentry are mutually exclusive, the subentry takes precedence. For example, in the ICD-10-CM Alphabetic Index under the main term Enteritis, "acute" is a nonessential modifier and "chronic" is a subentry. In this case, the nonessential modifier "acute" does not apply to the subentry "chronic".

   : Colons are used in the Tabular List after an incomplete term which needs one or more of the modifiers following the colon to make it assignable to a given category.

8. **Use of "and"**

   See Section I.A.14. Use of the term "And"

9. **Other and Unspecified codes**
   a. **"Other" codes**

      Codes titled "other" or "other specified" are for use when the information in the medical record provides detail for which a specific code does not exist. Alphabetic Index entries with NEC in the line designate "other" codes in the Tabular List. These Alphabetic Index entries represent specific disease entities for which no specific code exists so the term is included within an "other" code.

   b. **"Unspecified" codes**

      Codes titled "unspecified" are for use when the information in the medical record is insufficient to assign a more specific code. For those categories for which an unspecified code is not provided, the "other specified" code may represent both other and unspecified.

      See Section I.B.18 Use of Signs/Symptom/Unspecified Codes

10. **Includes Notes**

    This note appears immediately under a three character code title to further define, or give examples of, the content of the category.

11. **Inclusion terms**

    List of terms is included under some codes. These terms are the conditions for which that code is to be used. The terms may be synonyms of the code title, or, in the case of "other specified" codes, the terms are a list of the various conditions assigned to that code. The inclusion terms are not necessarily exhaustive. Additional terms found only in the Alphabetic Index may also be assigned to a code.

12. **Excludes Notes**

    The ICD-10-CM has two types of excludes notes. Each type of note has a different definition for use but they are all similar in that they indicate that codes excluded from each other are independent of each other.

    a. **Excludes1**

       A type 1 Excludes note is a pure excludes note. It means "NOT CODED HERE!" An Excludes1 note indicates that the code excluded should never be used at the same time as the code above the Excludes1 note. An Excludes1 is used when two conditions cannot occur together, such as a congenital form versus an acquired form of the same condition.

       An exception to the Excludes1 definition is the circumstance when the two conditions are unrelated to each other. If it is not clear whether the two conditions involving an Excludes1 note are related or not, query the provider. For example, code F45.8, Other somatoform disorders, has an Excludes1 note for "sleep related teeth grinding (G47.63)," because "teeth grinding" is an inclusion term under F45.8. Only one of these two codes should be assigned for teeth grinding. However psychogenic dysmenorrhea is also an inclusion term under F45.8, and a patient could have both this condition and sleep related teeth grinding. In this case, the two conditions are clearly unrelated to each other, and so it would be appropriate to report F45.8 and G47.63 together.

b. Excludes2

A type 2 Excludes note represents "Not included here." An excludes2 note indicates that the condition excluded is not part of the condition represented by the code, but a patient may have both conditions at the same time. When an Excludes2 note appears under a code, it is acceptable to use both the code and the excluded code together, when appropriate.

13. Etiology/manifestation convention ("code first", "use additional code" and "in diseases classified elsewhere" notes)

Certain conditions have both an underlying etiology and multiple body system manifestations due to the underlying etiology. For such conditions, the ICD-10-CM has a coding convention that requires the underlying condition be sequenced first, if applicable, followed by the manifestation. Wherever such a combination exists, there is a "use additional code" note at the etiology code, and a "code first" note at the manifestation code. These instructional notes indicate the proper sequencing order of the codes, etiology followed by manifestation.

In most cases the manifestation codes will have in the code title, "in diseases classified elsewhere." Codes with this title are a component of the etiology/ manifestation convention. The code title indicates that it is a manifestation code. "In diseases classified elsewhere" codes are never permitted to be used as first-listed or principal diagnosis codes. They must be used in conjunction with an underlying condition code and they must be listed following the underlying condition. See category F02, Dementia in other diseases classified elsewhere, for an example of this convention.

There are manifestation codes that do not have "in diseases classified elsewhere" in the title. For such codes, there is a "use additional code" note at the etiology code and a "code first" note at the manifestation code, and the rules for sequencing apply.

In addition to the notes in the Tabular List, these conditions also have a specific Alphabetic Index entry structure. In the Alphabetic Index both conditions are listed together with the etiology code first followed by the manifestation codes in brackets. The code in brackets is always to be sequenced second.

An example of the etiology/manifestation convention is dementia in Parkinson's disease. In the Alphabetic Index, code G20 is listed first, followed by code F02.80 or F02.81 in brackets. Code G20 represents the underlying etiology, Parkinson's disease, and must be sequenced first, whereas code F02.80 and F02.81 represent the manifestation of dementia in diseases classified elsewhere, with or without behavioral disturbance.

"Code first" and "Use additional code" notes are also used as sequencing rules in the classification for certain codes that are not part of an etiology/ manifestation combination.

See Section I.B.7. Multiple coding for a single condition.

14. "And"

The word "and" should be interpreted to mean either "and" or "or" when it appears in a title.

For example, cases of "tuberculosis of bones", "tuberculosis of joints" and "tuberculosis of bones and joints" are classified to subcategory A18.0, Tuberculosis of bones and joints.

15. "With"

The word "with" or "in" should be interpreted to mean "associated with" or "due to" when it appears in a code title, the Alphabetic Index (either under a main term or subterm), or an instructional note in the Tabular List. The classification presumes a causal relationship between the two conditions linked by these terms in the Alphabetic Index or Tabular List. These conditions should be coded as related even in the absence of provider documentation explicitly linking them, unless the documentation clearly states the conditions are unrelated or when another guideline exists that specifically requires a documented linkage between two conditions (e.g., sepsis guideline for "acute organ dysfunction that is not clearly associated with the sepsis").

For conditions not specifically linked by these relational terms in the classification or when a guideline requires that a linkage between two conditions be explicitly documented, provider documentation must link the conditions in order to code them as related.

The word "with" in the Alphabetic Index is sequenced immediately following the main term **or subterm**, not in alphabetical order.

16. "See" and "See Also"

The "see" instruction following a main term in the Alphabetic Index indicates that another term should be referenced. It is necessary to go to the main term referenced with the "see" note to locate the correct code.

A "see also" instruction following a main term in the Alphabetic Index instructs that there is another main term that may also be referenced that may provide additional Alphabetic Index entries that may be useful. It is not necessary to follow the "see also" note when the original main term provides the necessary code.

17. "Code also" note

A "code also" note instructs that two codes may be required to fully describe a condition, but this note does not provide sequencing direction. The sequencing depends on the circumstances of the encounter.

18. Default codes

A code listed next to a main term in the ICD-10-CM Alphabetic Index is referred to as a default code. The default code represents that condition that is most commonly associated with the main term, or is the unspecified code for the condition. If a condition is documented in a medical record (for example, appendicitis) without any additional information, such as acute or chronic, the default code should be assigned.

19. Code assignment and Clinical Criteria

The assignment of a diagnosis code is based on the provider's diagnostic statement that the condition exists. The provider's statement that the patient has a particular condition is sufficient. Code assignment is not based on clinical criteria used by the provider to establish the diagnosis.

B. General Coding Guidelines

1. Locating a code in the ICD-10-CM

To select a code in the classification that corresponds to a diagnosis or reason for visit documented in a medical record, first locate the term in the Alphabetic Index, and then verify the code in the Tabular List. Read and be guided by instructional notations that appear in both the Alphabetic Index and the Tabular List.

It is essential to use both the Alphabetic Index and Tabular List when locating and assigning a code. The Alphabetic Index does not always provide the full code, including laterality and any applicable 7th character can only be done in the Tabular List. A dash (-) at the end of an Alphabetic Index entry indicates that additional characters are required. Even if a dash is not included at the Alphabetic Index entry, it is necessary to refer to the Tabular List to verify that no 7th character is required.

2. Level of Detail in Coding

Diagnosis codes are to be used and reported at their highest number of characters available.

ICD-10-CM diagnosis codes are composed of codes with 3, 4, 5, 6 or 7 characters. Codes with three characters are included in ICD-10-CM as the heading of a category of codes that may be further subdivided by the use of fourth and/or fifth characters and/or sixth characters, which provide greater detail.

A three-character code is to be used only if it is not further subdivided. A code is invalid if it has not been coded to the full number of characters required for that code, including the 7th character, if applicable.

3. Code or codes from A00.0 through T88.9, Z00-Z99.8

The appropriate code or codes from A00.0 through T88.9, Z00-Z99.8 must be used to identify diagnoses, symptoms, conditions, problems, complaints or other reason(s) for the encounter/visit.

4. Signs and symptoms

Codes that describe symptoms and signs, as opposed to diagnoses, are acceptable for reporting purposes when a related definitive diagnosis has not been established (confirmed) by the provider. Chapter 18 of ICD-10-CM, Symptoms, Signs, and Abnormal Clinical and Laboratory Findings, Not Elsewhere Classified (codes R00.0 - R99) contains many, but not all, codes for symptoms.

See Section I.B.18 Use of Signs/Symptom/Unspecified Codes

5. Conditions that are an integral part of a disease process

Signs and symptoms that are associated routinely with a disease process should not be assigned as additional codes, unless otherwise instructed by the classification.

6. Conditions that are not an integral part of a disease process

Additional signs and symptoms that may not be associated routinely with a disease process should be coded when present.

7. Multiple coding for a single condition

In addition to the etiology/manifestation convention that requires two codes to fully describe a single condition that affects multiple body systems, there are other single conditions that also require more than one code. "Use additional code" notes are found in the Tabular List at codes that are not part of an etiology/manifestation pair where a secondary code is useful to fully describe a condition. The sequencing rule is the same as the etiology/manifestation pair, "use additional code" indicates that a secondary code should be added, if known.

For example, for bacterial infections that are not included in chapter 1, a secondary code from category B95, Streptococcus, Staphylococcus, and Enterococcus, as the cause of diseases classified elsewhere, or B96, Other bacterial agents as the cause of diseases classified elsewhere, may be required to identify the bacterial organism causing the infection. A "use additional code" note will normally be found at the infectious disease code, indicating a need for the organism code to be added as a secondary code.

"Code first" notes are also under certain codes that are not specifically manifestation codes but may be due to an underlying cause. When there is a "code first" note and an underlying condition is present, the underlying condition should be sequenced first, if known.

"Code, if applicable, any causal condition first" notes indicate that this code may be assigned as a principal diagnosis when the causal condition is unknown or not applicable. If a causal condition is known, then the code for that condition should be sequenced as the principal or first-listed diagnosis.

Multiple codes may be needed for sequela, complication codes and obstetric codes to more fully describe a condition. See the specific guidelines for these conditions for further instruction.

8. Acute and Chronic Conditions

If the same condition is described as both acute (subacute) and chronic, and separate subentries exist in the Alphabetic Index at the same indentation level, code both and sequence the acute (subacute) code first.

9. Combination Code

A combination code is a single code used to classify:

> Two diagnoses, or

> A diagnosis with an associated secondary process (manifestation)

> A diagnosis with an associated complication

Combination codes are identified by referring to subterm entries in the Alphabetic Index and by reading the inclusion and exclusion notes in the Tabular List.

Assign only the combination code when that code fully identifies the diagnostic conditions involved or when the Alphabetic Index so directs. Multiple coding should not be used when the classification provides a combination code that clearly identifies all of the elements documented in the diagnosis. When the combination code lacks necessary specificity in describing the manifestation or complication, an additional code should be used as a secondary code.

10. Sequela (Late Effects)

A sequela is the residual effect (condition produced) after the acute phase of an illness or injury has terminated. There is no time limit on when a sequela code can be used. The residual may be apparent early, such as in cerebral infarction, or it may occur months or years later, such as that due to a previous injury. Examples of sequela include: scar formation resulting from a burn, deviated septum due to a nasal fracture, and infertility due to tubal occlusion from old tuberculosis. Coding of sequela generally requires two codes sequenced in the following order: the condition or nature of the sequela is sequenced first. The sequela code is sequenced second.

An exception to the above guidelines are those instances where the code for the sequela is followed by a manifestation code identified in the Tabular List and title, or the sequela code has been expanded (at the fourth, fifth or sixth character levels) to include the manifestation(s). The code for the acute phase of an illness or injury that led to the sequela is never used with a code for the late effect.

See Section I.C.9. Sequelae of cerebrovascular disease

See Section I.C.15. Sequelae of complication of pregnancy, childbirth and the puerperium

See Section I.C.19. Application of 7th characters for Chapter 19

11. Impending or Threatened Condition

Code any condition described at the time of discharge as "impending" or "threatened" as follows:

> If it did occur, code as confirmed diagnosis.

> If it did not occur, reference the Alphabetic Index to determine if the condition has a subentry term for "impending" or "threatened" and also reference main term entries for "Impending" and for "Threatened."

> If the subterms are listed, assign the given code.

> If the subterms are not listed, code the existing underlying condition(s) and not the condition described as impending or threatened.

12. Reporting Same Diagnosis Code More than Once

Each unique ICD-10-CM diagnosis code may be reported only once for an encounter. This applies to bilateral conditions when there are no distinct codes identifying laterality or two different conditions classified to the same ICD-10-CM diagnosis code.

13. Laterality

Some ICD-10-CM codes indicate laterality, specifying whether the condition occurs on the left, right or is bilateral. If no bilateral code is provided and the condition is bilateral, assign separate codes for both the left and right side. If the side is not identified in the medical record, assign the code for the unspecified side.

When a patient has a bilateral condition and each side is treated during separate encounters, assign the "bilateral" code (as the condition still exists on both sides), including for the encounter to treat the first side. For the second encounter for treatment after one side has previously been treated and the condition no longer exists on that side, assign the appropriate unilateral code for the side where the condition still exists (e.g., cataract surgery performed on each eye in separate encounters). The bilateral code would not be assigned for the subsequent encounter, as the patient no longer has the condition in the previously-treated site. If the treatment on the first side did not completely resolve the condition, then the bilateral code would still be appropriate.

14. Documentation *by Clinicians Other than the Patient's Provider*

Code assignment is based on the documentation by patient's provider (i.e., physician or other qualified healthcare practitioner legally accountable for establishing the patient's diagnosis). There are a few exceptions, such as codes for the Body Mass Index (BMI), depth of non-pressure chronic ulcers, pressure ulcer stage, coma scale, and NIH stroke scale (NIHSS) codes, code assignment may be based on medical record documentation from clinicians who are not the patient's provider (i.e., physician or other qualified healthcare practitioner legally accountable for establishing the patient's diagnosis), since this information is typically documented by other clinicians involved in the care of the patient (e.g., a dietitian often documents the BMI, a nurse often documents the pressure ulcer stages, and an emergency medical technician often documents the coma scale). However, the associated diagnosis (such as overweight, obesity, acute stroke, or pressure ulcer) must be documented by the patient's provider. If there is conflicting medical record documentation, either from the same clinician or different clinicians, the patient's attending provider should be queried for clarification.

For social determinants of health, such as information found in categories Z55-Z65, Persons with potential health hazards related to socioeconomic and psychosocial circumstances, code assignment may be based on medical record documentation from clinicians involved in the care of the patient who are not the patient's provider since this information represents social information, rather than medical diagnoses.

The BMI, coma scale, NIHSS codes and categories Z55-Z65 should only be reported as secondary diagnoses.

15. Syndromes

Follow the Alphabetic Index guidance when coding syndromes. In the absence of Alphabetic Index guidance, assign codes for the documented manifestations of the syndrome. Additional codes for manifestations that are not an integral part of the disease process may also be assigned when the condition does not have a unique code.

16. Documentation of Complications of Care

Code assignment is based on the provider's documentation of the relationship between the condition and the care or procedure, unless otherwise instructed by the classification. The guideline extends to any complications of care, regardless of the chapter the code is located in. It is important to note that not all conditions that occur during or following medical care or surgery are classified as complications. There must be a cause-and-effect relationship between the care provided and the condition, and an indication in the documentation that it is a complication. Query the provider for clarification, if the complication is not clearly documented.

17. Borderline Diagnosis

If the provider documents a "borderline" diagnosis at the time of discharge, the diagnosis is coded as confirmed, unless the classification provides a specific entry (e.g., borderline diabetes). If a borderline condition has a specific index entry in ICD-10-CM, it should be coded as such. Since borderline conditions are not uncertain diagnoses, no distinction is made between the care setting (inpatient versus outpatient). Whenever the documentation is unclear regarding a borderline condition, coders are encouraged to query for clarification.

18. Use of Sign/Symptom/Unspecified Codes

Sign/symptom and "unspecified" codes have acceptable, even necessary, uses. While specific diagnosis codes should be reported when they are supported by the available medical record documentation and clinical knowledge of the patient's health condition, there are instances when signs/symptoms or unspecified codes are the best choices for accurately reflecting the healthcare encounter. Each healthcare encounter should be coded to the level of certainty known for that encounter.

If a definitive diagnosis has not been established by the end of the encounter, it is appropriate to report codes for sign(s) and/or symptom(s) in lieu of a definitive diagnosis. When sufficient clinical information isn't known or available about a particular health condition to assign a more specific code, it is acceptable to report the appropriate "unspecified" code (e.g., a diagnosis of pneumonia has been determined, but not the specific type). Unspecified codes should be reported when they are the codes that most accurately reflect what is known about the patient's condition at the time of that particular encounter. It would be inappropriate to select a specific code that is not supported by the medical record documentation or conduct medically unnecessary diagnostic testing in order to determine a more specific code.

19. Coding for Healthcare Encounters in Hurricane Aftermath

a. Use of External Cause of Morbidity Codes

An external cause of morbidity code should be assigned to identify the cause of the injury(ies) incurred as a result of the hurricane. The use of external cause of morbidity codes is supplemental to the application of ICD-10-CM codes. External cause of morbidity codes are never to be recorded as a principal diagnosis (first-listed in non-inpatient settings). The appropriate injury code should be sequenced before any external cause codes. The external cause of morbidity codes capture how the injury or health condition happened (cause), the intent (unintentional or accidental; or intentional, such as suicide or assault), the place where the event occurred, the activity of the patient at the time of the event, and the person's status (e.g., civilian, military). They should not be assigned for encounters to treat hurricane victims' medical conditions when no injury, adverse effect or poisoning is involved. External cause of morbidity codes should be assigned for each encounter for care and treatment of the injury. External cause of morbidity codes may be assigned in all health care settings. For the purpose of capturing complete and accurate ICD-10-CM data in the aftermath of the hurricane, a healthcare setting should be considered as any location where medical care is provided by licensed healthcare professionals.

b. Sequencing of External Causes of Morbidity Codes

Codes for cataclysmic events, such as a hurricane, take priority over all other external cause codes except child and adult abuse and terrorism and should be sequenced before other external cause of injury codes. Assign as many external cause of morbidity codes as necessary to fully explain each cause. For example, if an injury occurs as a result of a building collapse during the hurricane, external cause codes for both the hurricane and the building collapse should be assigned, with the external causes code for hurricane being sequenced as the first external cause code. For injuries incurred as a direct result of the hurricane, assign the appropriate code(s) for the injuries, followed by the code X37.0-, Hurricane (with the appropriate 7th character), and any other applicable external cause of injury codes. Code X37.0- also should be assigned when an injury is incurred as a result of flooding caused by a levee breaking related to the hurricane. Code X38.-, Flood (with the appropriate 7th character), should be assigned when an injury is from flooding resulting directly from the storm. Code X36.0.-, Collapse of dam or man-made structure, should not be assigned when the cause of the collapse is due to the hurricane. Use of code X36.0- is limited to collapses of man-made structures due to earth surface movements, not due to storm surges directly from a hurricane.

c. Other External Causes of Morbidity Code Issues

For injuries that are not a direct result of the hurricane, such as an evacuee that has incurred an injury as a result of a motor vehicle accident, assign the appropriate external cause of morbidity code(s) to

describe the cause of the injury, but do not assign code X37.0-, Hurricane. If it is not clear whether the injury was a direct result of the hurricane, assume the injury is due to the hurricane and assign code X37.0-, Hurricane, as well as any other applicable external cause of morbidity codes. In addition to code X37.0-, Hurricane, other possible applicable external cause of morbidity codes include:

W54.0-, Bitten by dog

X30-, Exposure to excessive natural heat

X31-, Exposure to excessive natural cold

X38-, Flood

d. Use of Z codes

Z codes (other reasons for healthcare encounters) may be assigned as appropriate to further explain the reasons for presenting for healthcare services, including transfers between healthcare facilities. The ICD-10-CM Official Guidelines for Coding and Reporting identify which codes maybe assigned as principal or first-listed diagnosis only, secondary diagnosis only, or principal/first-listed or secondary (depending on the circumstances). Possible applicable Z codes include:

Z59.0, Homelessness

Z59.1, Inadequate housing

Z59.5, Extreme poverty

Z75.1, Person awaiting admission to adequate facility elsewhere

Z75.3, Unavailability and inaccessibility of health-care facilities

Z75.4, Unavailability and inaccessibility of other helping agencies

Z76.2, Encounter for health supervision and care of other healthy infant and child

Z99.12, Encounter for respirator [ventilator] dependence during power failure

The external cause of morbidity codes and the Z codes listed above are not an all-inclusive list. Other codes may be applicable to the encounter based upon the documentation. Assign as many codes as necessary to fully explain each healthcare encounter. Since patient history information may be very limited, use any available documentation to assign the appropriate external cause of morbidity and Z codes.

C. Chapter-Specific Coding Guidelines

In addition to general coding guidelines, there are guidelines for specific diagnoses and/or conditions in the classification. Unless otherwise indicated, these guidelines apply to all health care settings. Please refer to Section II for guidelines on the selection of principal diagnosis.

1. Chapter 1: Certain Infectious and Parasitic Diseases (A00-B99)

a. Human Immunodeficiency Virus (HIV) Infections

1) Code only confirmed cases

Code only confirmed cases of HIV infection/illness. This is an exception to the hospital inpatient guideline Section II, H.

In this context, "confirmation" does not require documentation of positive serology or culture for HIV; the provider's diagnostic statement that the patient is HIV positive, or has an HIV-related illness is sufficient.

2) Selection and sequencing of HIV codes

(a) Patient admitted for HIV-related condition

If a patient is admitted for an HIV-related condition, the principal diagnosis should be B20, Human immunodeficiency virus [HIV] disease followed by additional diagnosis codes for all reported HIV-related conditions.

(b) Patient with HIV disease admitted for unrelated condition

If a patient with HIV disease is admitted for an unrelated condition (such as a traumatic injury), the code for the unrelated condition (e.g., the nature of injury code) should be the principal diagnosis. Other diagnoses would be B20 followed by additional diagnosis codes for all reported HIV-related conditions.

(c) Whether the patient is newly diagnosed

Whether the patient is newly diagnosed or has had previous admissions/encounters for HIV conditions is irrelevant to the sequencing decision.

(d) Asymptomatic human immunodeficiency virus

Z21, Asymptomatic human immunodeficiency virus [HIV] infection status, is to be applied when the patient without any documentation of symptoms is listed as being "HIV positive," "known HIV," "HIV test positive," or similar terminology. Do not use this code if the term "AIDS" is used or if the patient is treated for any HIV-related illness or is described as having any condition(s) resulting from his/her HIV positive status; use B20 in these cases.

(e) Patients with inconclusive HIV serology

Patients with inconclusive HIV serology, but no definitive diagnosis or manifestations of the illness, may be assigned code R75, Inconclusive laboratory evidence of human immunodeficiency virus [HIV].

(f) Previously diagnosed HIV-related illness

Patients with any known prior diagnosis of an HIV-related illness should be coded to B20. Once a patient has developed an HIV-related illness, the patient should always be assigned code B20 on every subsequent admission/encounter. Patients previously diagnosed with any HIV illness (B20) should never be assigned to R75 or Z21, Asymptomatic human immunodeficiency virus [HIV] infection status.

(g) HIV Infection in Pregnancy, Childbirth and the Puerperium

During pregnancy, childbirth or the puerperium, a patient admitted (or presenting for a health care encounter) because of an HIV-related illness should receive a principal diagnosis code of O98.7-, Human immunodeficiency [HIV] disease complicating pregnancy, childbirth and the puerperium, followed by B20 and the code(s) for the HIV-related illness(es). Codes from Chapter 15 always take sequencing priority.

Patients with asymptomatic HIV infection status admitted (or presenting for a health care encounter) during pregnancy, childbirth, or the puerperium should receive codes of O98.7- and Z21.

(h) Encounters for testing for HIV

If a patient is being seen to determine his/her HIV status, use code Z11.4, Encounter for screening for human immunodeficiency virus [HIV]. Use additional codes for any associated high risk behavior.

If a patient with signs or symptoms is being seen for HIV testing, code the signs and symptoms. An additional counseling code Z71.7, Human immunodeficiency virus [HIV] counseling, may be used if counseling is provided during the encounter for the test.

When a patient returns to be informed of his/her HIV test results and the test result is negative, use code Z71.7, Human immunodeficiency virus [HIV] counseling.

If the results are positive, see previous guidelines and assign codes as appropriate.

b. Infectious agents as the cause of diseases classified to other chapters

Certain infections are classified in chapters other than Chapter 1 and no organism is identified as part of the infection code. In these instances, it is necessary to use an additional code from Chapter 1 to identify the organism. A code from category B95, Streptococcus, Staphylococcus, and Enterococcus as the cause of diseases classified to other chapters, B96, Other bacterial agents as the cause of diseases classified to other chapters, or B97, Viral agents as the cause of diseases classified to other chapters, is to be used as an additional code to identify the organism. An instructional note will be found at the infection code advising that an additional organism code is required.

c. Infections resistant to antibiotics

Many bacterial infections are resistant to current antibiotics. It is necessary to identify all infections documented as antibiotic resistant. Assign a code from category Z16, Resistance to antimicrobial drugs, following the infection code only if the infection code does not identify drug resistance.

d. Sepsis, Severe Sepsis, and Septic Shock

1) Coding of Sepsis and Severe Sepsis

(a) Sepsis

For a diagnosis of sepsis, assign the appropriate code for the underlying systemic infection. If the type of infection or causal organism is not further specified, assign code A41.9, Sepsis, unspecified organism.

A code from subcategory R65.2, Severe sepsis, should not be assigned unless severe sepsis or an associated acute organ dysfunction is documented.

(i) Negative or inconclusive blood cultures and sepsis

Negative or inconclusive blood cultures do not preclude a diagnosis of sepsis in patients with clinical evidence of the condition; however, the provider should be queried.

(ii) Urosepsis

The term urosepsis is a nonspecific term. It is not to be considered synonymous with sepsis. It has no default code in the Alphabetic Index. Should a provider use this term, he/she must be queried for clarification.

(iii) Sepsis with organ dysfunction

If a patient has sepsis and associated acute organ dysfunction or multiple organ dysfunction (MOD), follow the instructions for coding severe sepsis.

(iv) Acute organ dysfunction that is not clearly associated with the sepsis

If a patient has sepsis and an acute organ dysfunction, but the medical record documentation indicates that the acute organ dysfunction is related to a medical condition other than the sepsis, do not assign a code from subcategory R65.2, Severe sepsis. An acute organ dysfunction must be associated with the sepsis in order to assign the severe sepsis code. If the documentation is not clear as to whether an acute organ dysfunction is related to the sepsis or another medical condition, query the provider.

(b) Severe sepsis

The coding of severe sepsis requires a minimum of 2 codes: first a code for the underlying systemic infection, followed by a code from subcategory R65.2, Severe sepsis. If the causal organism is not documented, assign code A41.9, Sepsis, unspecified organism, for the infection. Additional code(s) for the associated acute organ dysfunction are also required.

Due to the complex nature of severe sepsis, some cases may require querying the provider prior to assignment of the codes.

2) Septic shock

(a) Septic shock generally refers to circulatory failure associated with severe sepsis, and therefore, it represents a type of acute organ dysfunction.

For cases of septic shock, the code for the systemic infection should be sequenced first, followed by code R65.21, Severe sepsis with septic shock or code T81.12, Postprocedural septic shock. Any additional codes for the other acute organ dysfunctions should also be assigned. As noted in the sequencing instructions in the Tabular List, the code for septic shock cannot be assigned as a principal diagnosis.

3) Sequencing of severe sepsis

If severe sepsis is present on admission, and meets the definition of principal diagnosis, the underlying systemic infection should be assigned as principal diagnosis followed by the appropriate code from subcategory R65.2 as required by the sequencing rules in the Tabular List. A code from subcategory R65.2 can never be assigned as a principal diagnosis.

When severe sepsis develops during an encounter (it was not present on admission), the underlying systemic infection and the appropriate code from subcategory R65.2 should be assigned as secondary diagnoses.

Severe sepsis may be present on admission, but the diagnosis may not be confirmed until sometime after admission. If the documentation is not clear whether severe sepsis was present on admission, the provider should be queried.

4) Sepsis *or* severe sepsis with a localized infection

If the reason for admission is sepsis or severe sepsis and a localized infection, such as pneumonia or cellulitis, a code(s) for the underlying systemic infection should be assigned first and the code for the localized infection should be assigned as a secondary diagnosis. If the patient has severe sepsis, a code from subcategory R65.2 should also be assigned as a secondary diagnosis. If the patient is admitted with a localized infection, such as pneumonia, and sepsis/severe sepsis doesn't develop until after admission, the localized infection should be assigned first, followed by the appropriate sepsis/severe sepsis codes.

5) **Sepsis due to a postprocedural infection**

(a) **Documentation of causal relationship**

As with all postprocedural complications, code assignment is based on the provider's documentation of the relationship between the infection and the procedure.

(b) **Sepsis due to a postprocedural infection**

For infections following a procedure, a code from T81.40, to T81.43 Infection following a procedure, or a code from O86.00 to O86.03, Infection of obstetric surgical wound, that identifies the site of the infection should be coded first, if known. Assign an additional code for sepsis following a procedure (T81.44) or sepsis following an obstetrical procedure (O86.04). Use an additional code to identify the infectious agent. If the patient has severe sepsis, the appropriate code from subcategory R65.2 should also be assigned with the additional code(s) for any acute organ dysfunction.

For infections following infusion, transfusion, therapeutic injection, or immunization, a code from subcategory T80.2, Infections following infusion, transfusion, and therapeutic injection, or code T88.0-, Infection following immunization, should be coded first, followed by the code for the specific infection. If the patient has severe sepsis, the appropriate code from subcategory R65.2 should also be assigned, with the additional codes(s) for any acute organ dysfunction.

(c) **Postprocedural infection and postprocedural septic shock**

If a postprocedural infection has resulted in postprocedural septic shock, assign the codes indicated above for sepsis due to a postprocedural infection, followed by code T81.12-, Postprocedural septic shock. Do not assign code R65.21, Severe sepsis with septic shock. Additional code(s) should be assigned for any acute organ dysfunction.

6) **Sepsis and severe sepsis associated with a noninfectious process (condition)**

In some cases a noninfectious process (condition), such as trauma, may lead to an infection which can result in sepsis or severe sepsis. If sepsis or severe sepsis is documented as associated with a noninfectious condition, such as a burn or serious injury, and this condition meets the definition for principal diagnosis, the code for the noninfectious condition should be sequenced first, followed by the code for the resulting infection. If severe sepsis is present, a code from subcategory R65.2 should also be assigned with any associated organ dysfunction(s) codes. It is not necessary to assign a code from subcategory R65.1, Systemic inflammatory response syndrome (SIRS) of non-infectious origin, for these cases.

If the infection meets the definition of principal diagnosis, it should be sequenced before the non-infectious condition. When both the associated non-infectious condition and the infection meet the definition of principal diagnosis, either may be assigned as principal diagnosis.

Only one code from category R65, Symptoms and signs specifically associated with systemic inflammation and infection, should be assigned. Therefore, when a non-infectious condition leads to an infection resulting in severe sepsis, assign the appropriate code from subcategory R65.2, Severe sepsis. Do not additionally assign a code from subcategory R65.1, Systemic inflammatory response syndrome (SIRS) of non-infectious origin.

See Section I.C.18. SIRS due to non-infectious process

7) **Sepsis and septic shock complicating abortion, pregnancy, childbirth, and the puerperium**

See Section I.C.15. Sepsis and septic shock complicating abortion, pregnancy, childbirth and the puerperium

8) **Newborn sepsis**

See Section I.C.16. f. Bacterial sepsis of Newborn

e. **Methicillin Resistant Staphylococcus aureus (MRSA) Conditions**

1) **Selection and sequencing of MRSA codes**

(a) **Combination codes for MRSA infection**

When a patient is diagnosed with an infection that is due to methicillin resistant *Staphylococcus aureus* (MRSA), and that infection has a combination code that includes the causal organism (e.g., sepsis, pneumonia) assign the appropriate combination code for the condition (e.g., code A41.02, Sepsis due to Methicillin resistant Staphylococcus aureus or code J15.212, Pneumonia due to Methicillin resistant Staphylococcus aureus). Do not assign code B95.62, Methicillin resistant Staphylococcus aureus infection as the cause of diseases classified elsewhere, as an additional code, because the combination code includes the type of infection and the MRSA organism. Do not assign a code from subcategory Z16.11, Resistance to penicillins, as an additional diagnosis.

See Section C.1. for instructions on coding and sequencing of sepsis and severe sepsis.

(b) **Other codes for MRSA infection**

When there is documentation of a current infection (e.g., wound infection, stitch abscess, urinary tract infection) due to MRSA, and that infection does not have a combination code that includes the causal organism, assign the appropriate code to identify the condition along with code B95.62, Methicillin resistant Staphylococcus aureus infection as the cause of diseases classified elsewhere for the MRSA infection. Do not assign a code from subcategory Z16.11, Resistance to penicillins.

(c) **Methicillin susceptible Staphylococcus aureus (MSSA) and MRSA colonization**

The condition or state of being colonized or carrying MSSA or MRSA is called colonization or carriage, while an individual person is described as being colonized or being a carrier. Colonization means that MSSA or MSRA is present on or in the body without necessarily causing illness. A positive MRSA colonization test might be documented by the provider as "MRSA screen positive" or "MRSA nasal swab positive".

Assign code Z22.322, Carrier or suspected carrier of Methicillin resistant Staphylococcus aureus, for patients documented as having MRSA colonization. Assign code Z22.321, Carrier or suspected carrier of Methicillin susceptible Staphylococcus aureus, for patients documented as having MSSA colonization. Colonization is not necessarily indicative of a disease process or as the cause of a specific condition the patient may have unless documented as such by the provider.

(d) **MRSA colonization and infection**

If a patient is documented as having both MRSA colonization and infection during a hospital admission, code Z22.322, Carrier or suspected carrier of Methicillin resistant Staphylococcus aureus, and a code for the MRSA infection may both be assigned.

f. **Zika virus infections**

1) **Code only confirmed cases**

Code only a confirmed diagnosis of Zika virus (A92.5, Zika virus disease) as documented by the provider. This is an exception to the hospital inpatient guideline Section II, H. In this context, "confirmation" does not require documentation of the type of test performed; the **provider's** diagnostic statement that the condition is confirmed is sufficient. This code should be assigned regardless of the stated mode of transmission.

If the provider documents "suspected", "possible" or "probable" Zika, do not assign code A92.5. Assign a code(s) explaining the reason for encounter (such as fever, rash, or joint pain) or Z20.821, Contact with and (suspected) exposure to Zika virus.

2. **Chapter 2: Neoplasms (C00-D49)**
General guidelines

Chapter 2 of the ICD-10-CM contains the codes for most benign and all malignant neoplasms. Certain benign neoplasms, such as prostatic adenomas, may be found in the specific body system chapters. To properly code a neoplasm it is necessary to determine from the record if the neoplasm is benign, in-situ, malignant, or of uncertain histologic behavior. If malignant, any secondary (metastatic) sites should also be determined.

Primary malignant neoplasms overlapping site boundaries

A primary malignant neoplasm that overlaps two or more contiguous (next to each other) sites should be classified to the subcategory/code .8 ('overlapping lesion'), unless the combination is specifically indexed elsewhere. For multiple neoplasms of the same site that are not contiguous such as tumors in different quadrants of the same breast, codes for each site should be assigned.

Malignant neoplasm of ectopic tissue

Malignant neoplasms of ectopic tissue are to be coded to the site of origin mentioned, e.g., ectopic pancreatic malignant neoplasms involving the stomach are coded to malignant neoplasm of pancreas, unspecified (C25.9).

The neoplasm table in the Alphabetic Index should be referenced first. However, if the histological term is documented, that term should be referenced first, rather than going immediately to the Neoplasm Table, in order to determine which column in the Neoplasm Table is appropriate. For example, if the documentation indicates "adenoma," refer to the term in the Alphabetic Index to review the entries under this term and the instructional note to "see also neoplasm, by site, benign." The table provides the proper code based on the type of neoplasm and the site. It is important to select the proper column in the table that corresponds to the type of neoplasm. The Tabular List should then be referenced to verify that the correct code has been selected from the table and that a more specific site code does not exist.

See Section I.C.21. Factors influencing health status and contact with health services, Status, for information regarding Z15.0, codes for genetic susceptibility to cancer.

a. Treatment directed at the malignancy

If the treatment is directed at the malignancy, designate the malignancy as the principal diagnosis.

The only exception to this guideline is if a patient admission/encounter is solely for the administration of chemotherapy, immunotherapy or external beam radiation therapy, assign the appropriate Z51.-- code as the first-listed or principal diagnosis, and the diagnosis or problem for which the service is being performed as a secondary diagnosis.

b. Treatment of secondary site

When a patient is admitted because of a primary neoplasm with metastasis and treatment is directed toward the secondary site only, the secondary neoplasm is designated as the principal diagnosis even though the primary malignancy is still present.

c. Coding and sequencing of complications

Coding and sequencing of complications associated with the malignancies or with the therapy thereof are subject to the following guidelines:

1) Anemia associated with malignancy

When admission/encounter is for management of an anemia associated with the malignancy, and the treatment is only for anemia, the appropriate code for the malignancy is sequenced as the principal or first-listed diagnosis followed by the appropriate code for the anemia (such as code D63.0, Anemia in neoplastic disease).

2) Anemia associated with chemotherapy, immunotherapy and radiation therapy

When the admission/encounter is for management of an anemia associated with an adverse effect of the administration of chemotherapy or immunotherapy and the only treatment is for the anemia, the anemia code is sequenced first followed by the appropriate codes for the neoplasm and the adverse effect (T45.1X5-, Adverse effect of antineoplastic and immunosuppressive drugs).

When the admission/encounter is for management of an anemia associated with an adverse effect of radiotherapy, the anemia code should be sequenced first, followed by the appropriate neoplasm code and code Y84.2, Radiological procedure and radiotherapy as the cause of abnormal reaction of the patient, or of later complication, without mention of misadventure at the time of the procedure.

3) Management of dehydration due to the malignancy

When the admission/encounter is for management of dehydration due to the malignancy and only the dehydration is being treated (intravenous rehydration), the dehydration is sequenced first, followed by the code(s) for the malignancy.

4) Treatment of a complication resulting from a surgical procedure

When the admission/encounter is for treatment of a complication resulting from a surgical procedure, designate the complication as the principal or first-listed diagnosis if treatment is directed at resolving the complication.

d. Primary malignancy previously excised

When a primary malignancy has been previously excised or eradicated from its site and there is no further treatment directed to that site and there is no evidence of any existing primary malignancy at that site, a code from category Z85, Personal history of malignant neoplasm, should be used to indicate the former site of the malignancy. Any mention of extension, invasion, or metastasis to another site is coded as a secondary malignant neoplasm to that site. The secondary site may be the principal or first-listed **diagnosis** with the Z85 code used as a secondary code.

e. Admissions/Encounters involving chemotherapy, immunotherapy and radiation therapy

1) Episode of care involves surgical removal of neoplasm

When an episode of care involves the surgical removal of a neoplasm, primary or secondary site, followed by adjunct chemotherapy or radiation treatment during the same episode of care, the code for the neoplasm should be assigned as principal or first-listed diagnosis.

2) Patient admission/encounter solely for administration of chemotherapy, immunotherapy and radiation therapy

If a patient admission/encounter is solely for the administration of chemotherapy, immunotherapy or external beam radiation therapy assign code Z51.0, Encounter for antineoplastic radiation therapy, or Z51.11, Encounter for antineoplastic chemotherapy, or Z51.12, Encounter for antineoplastic immunotherapy as the first-listed or principal diagnosis. If a patient receives more than one of these therapies during the same admission more than one of these codes may be assigned, in any sequence.

The malignancy for which the therapy is being administered should be assigned as a secondary diagnosis.

If a patient admission/encounter is for the insertion or implantation of radioactive elements (e.g., brachytherapy) the appropriate code for the malignancy is sequenced as the principal or first-listed diagnosis. Code Z51.0 should not be assigned.

3) Patient admitted for radiation therapy, chemotherapy or immunotherapy and develops complications

When a patient is admitted for the purpose of external beam radiotherapy, immunotherapy or chemotherapy and develops complications such as uncontrolled nausea and vomiting or dehydration, the principal or first-listed diagnosis is Z51.0, Encounter for antineoplastic radiation therapy, or Z51.11, Encounter for antineoplastic chemotherapy, or Z51.12, Encounter for antineoplastic immunotherapy followed by any codes for the complications.

When a patient is admitted for the purpose of insertion or implantation of radioactive elements (e.g., brachytherapy)and develops complications such as uncontrolled nausea and vomiting or dehydration, the principal or first-listed diagnosis is the appropriate code for the malignancy followed by any codes for the complications.

f. Admission/encounter to determine extent of malignancy

When the reason for admission/encounter is to determine the extent of the malignancy, or for a procedure such as paracentesis or thoracentesis, the primary malignancy or appropriate metastatic site is designated as the principal or first-listed diagnosis, even though chemotherapy or radiotherapy is administered.

g. Symptoms, signs, and abnormal findings listed in Chapter 18 associated with neoplasms

Symptoms, signs, and ill-defined conditions listed in Chapter 18 characteristic of, or associated with, an existing primary or secondary site malignancy cannot be used to replace the malignancy as principal or first-listed diagnosis, regardless of the number of admissions or encounters for treatment and care of the neoplasm.

See section I.C.21. Factors influencing health status and contact with health services, Encounter for prophylactic organ removal.

h. Admission/encounter for pain control/management

See Section I.C.6. for information on coding admission/encounter for pain control/management.

i. **Malignancy in two or more noncontiguous sites**
A patient may have more than one malignant tumor in the same organ. These tumors may represent different primaries or metastatic disease, depending on the site. Should the documentation be unclear, the provider should be queried as to the status of each tumor so that the correct codes can be assigned.

j. **Disseminated malignant neoplasm, unspecified**
Code C80.0, Disseminated malignant neoplasm, unspecified, is for use only in those cases where the patient has advanced metastatic disease and no known primary or secondary sites are specified. It should not be used in place of assigning codes for the primary site and all known secondary sites.

k. **Malignant neoplasm without specification of site**
Code C80.1, Malignant (primary) neoplasm, unspecified, equates to Cancer, unspecified. This code should only be used when no determination can be made as to the primary site of a malignancy. This code should rarely be used in the inpatient setting.

l. **Sequencing of neoplasm codes**
1) **Encounter for treatment of primary malignancy**
If the reason for the encounter is for treatment of a primary malignancy, assign the malignancy as the principal/first-listed diagnosis. The primary site is to be sequenced first, followed by any metastatic sites.

2) **Encounter for treatment of secondary malignancy**
When an encounter is for a primary malignancy with metastasis and treatment is directed toward the metastatic (secondary) site(s) only, the metastatic site(s) is designated as the principal/first-listed diagnosis. The primary malignancy is coded as an additional code.

3) **Malignant neoplasm in a pregnant patient**
When a pregnant woman has a malignant neoplasm, a code from subcategory O9A.1-, Malignant neoplasm complicating pregnancy, childbirth, and the puerperium, should be sequenced first, followed by the appropriate code from Chapter 2 to indicate the type of neoplasm.

4) **Encounter for complication associated with a neoplasm**
When an encounter is for management of a complication associated with a neoplasm, such as dehydration, and the treatment is only for the complication, the complication is coded first, followed by the appropriate code(s) for the neoplasm.

The exception to this guideline is anemia. When the admission/encounter is for management of an anemia associated with the malignancy, and the treatment is only for anemia, the appropriate code for the malignancy is sequenced as the principal or first-listed diagnosis followed by code D63.0, Anemia in neoplastic disease.

5) **Complication from surgical procedure for treatment of a neoplasm**
When an encounter is for treatment of a complication resulting from a surgical procedure performed for the treatment of the neoplasm, designate the complication as the principal/first-listed diagnosis. See **the** guideline regarding the coding of a current malignancy versus personal history to determine if the code for the neoplasm should also be assigned.

6) **Pathologic fracture due to a neoplasm**
When an encounter is for a pathological fracture due to a neoplasm, and the focus of treatment is the fracture, a code from subcategory M84.5, Pathological fracture in neoplastic disease, should be sequenced first, followed by the code for the neoplasm.

If the focus of treatment is the neoplasm with an associated pathological fracture, the neoplasm code should be sequenced first, followed by a code from M84.5 for the pathological fracture.

m. **Current malignancy versus personal history of malignancy**
When a primary malignancy has been excised but further treatment, such as an additional surgery for the malignancy, radiation therapy or chemotherapy is directed to that site, the primary malignancy code should be used until treatment is completed.

When a primary malignancy has been previously excised or eradicated from its site, there is no further treatment (of the malignancy) directed to that site, and there is no evidence of any existing primary malignancy at that site, a code from category Z85, Personal history of malignant neoplasm, should be used to indicate the former site of the malignancy.

Subcategories Z85.0 – Z85.7 should only be assigned for the former site of a primary malignancy, not the site of a secondary malignancy. Codes from subcategory Z85.8-, may be assigned for the former site(s) of either a primary or secondary malignancy included in this subcategory.
See Section I.C.21. Factors influencing health status and contact with health services, History (of)

n. **Leukemia, Multiple Myeloma, and Malignant Plasma Cell Neoplasms in remission versus personal history**
The categories for leukemia, and category C90, Multiple myeloma and malignant plasma cell neoplasms, have codes indicating whether or not the leukemia has achieved remission. There are also codes Z85.6, Personal history of leukemia, and Z85.79, Personal history of other malignant neoplasms of lymphoid, hematopoietic and related tissues. If the documentation is unclear as to whether the leukemia has achieved remission, the provider should be queried.
See Section I.C.21. Factors influencing health status and contact with health services, History (of)

o. **Aftercare following surgery for neoplasm**
See Section I.C.21. Factors influencing health status and contact with health services, Aftercare

p. **Follow-up care for completed treatment of a malignancy**
See Section I.C.21. Factors influencing health status and contact with health services, Follow-up

q. **Prophylactic organ removal for prevention of malignancy**
See Section I.C. 21, Factors influencing health status and contact with health services, Prophylactic organ removal

r. **Malignant neoplasm associated with transplanted organ**
A malignant neoplasm of a transplanted organ should be coded as a transplant complication. Assign first the appropriate code from category T86.-, Complications of transplanted organs and tissue, followed by code C80.2, Malignant neoplasm associated with transplanted organ. Use an additional code for the specific malignancy.

3. **Chapter 3: Disease of the blood and blood-forming organs and certain disorders involving the immune mechanism (D50-D89)**
Reserved for future guideline expansion

4. **Chapter 4: Endocrine, Nutritional, and Metabolic Diseases (E00-E89)**
a. **Diabetes mellitus**
The diabetes mellitus codes are combination codes that include the type of diabetes mellitus, the body system affected, and the complications affecting that body system. As many codes within a particular category as are necessary to describe all of the complications of the disease may be used. They should be sequenced based on the reason for a particular encounter. Assign as many codes from categories E08 – E13 as needed to identify all of the associated conditions that the patient has.

1) **Type of diabetes**
The age of a patient is not the sole determining factor, though most type 1 diabetics develop the condition before reaching puberty. For this reason type 1 diabetes mellitus is also referred to as juvenile diabetes.

2) **Type of diabetes mellitus not documented**
If the type of diabetes mellitus is not documented in the medical record the default is E11.-, Type 2 diabetes mellitus.

3) **Diabetes mellitus and the use of insulin and oral hypoglycemics**
If the documentation in a medical record does not indicate the type of diabetes but does indicate that the patient uses insulin, code E11-, Type 2 diabetes mellitus, should be assigned. An additional code should be assigned from category Z79 to identify the long-term (current) use of insulin or oral hypoglycemic drugs. If the patient is treated with both oral medications and insulin, only the code for long-term (current) use of insulin should be assigned. Code Z79.4 should not be assigned if insulin is given temporarily to bring a type 2 patient's blood sugar under control during an encounter.

4) **Diabetes mellitus in pregnancy and gestational diabetes**
See Section I.C.15. Diabetes mellitus in pregnancy.
See Section I.C.15. Gestational (pregnancy induced) diabetes

5) Complications due to insulin pump malfunction

(a) Underdose of insulin due to insulin pump failure

An underdose of insulin due to an insulin pump failure should be assigned to a code from subcategory T85.6, Mechanical complication of other specified internal and external prosthetic devices, implants and grafts, that specifies the type of pump malfunction, as the principal or first-listed code, followed by code T38.3X6-, Underdosing of insulin and oral hypoglycemic [antidiabetic] drugs. Additional codes for the type of diabetes mellitus and any associated complications due to the underdosing should also be assigned.

(b) Overdose of insulin due to insulin pump failure

The principal or first-listed code for an encounter due to an insulin pump malfunction resulting in an overdose of insulin, should also be T85.6-, Mechanical complication of other specified internal and external prosthetic devices, implants and grafts, followed by code T38.3X1-, Poisoning by insulin and oral hypoglycemic [antidiabetic] drugs, accidental (unintentional).

6) Secondary diabetes mellitus

Codes under categories E08, Diabetes mellitus due to underlying condition, E09, Drug or chemical induced diabetes mellitus, and E13, Other specified diabetes mellitus, identify complications/manifestations associated with secondary diabetes mellitus. Secondary diabetes is always caused by another condition or event (e.g., cystic fibrosis, malignant neoplasm of pancreas, pancreatectomy, adverse effect of drug, or poisoning).

(a) Secondary diabetes mellitus and the use of insulin or oral hypoglycemic drugs

For patients with secondary diabetes mellitus who routinely use insulin or oral hypoglycemic drugs, an additional code from category Z79 should be assigned to identify the long-term (current) use of insulin or oral hypoglycemic drugs. If the patient is treated with both oral medications and insulin, only the code for long-term (current) use of insulin should be assigned. Code Z79.4 should not be assigned if insulin is given temporarily to bring a secondary diabetic patient's blood sugar under control during an encounter.

(b) Assigning and sequencing secondary diabetes codes and its causes

The sequencing of the secondary diabetes codes in relationship to codes for the cause of the diabetes is based on the Tabular List instructions for categories E08, E09 and E13.

(i) Secondary diabetes mellitus due to pancreatectomy

For postpancreatectomy diabetes mellitus (lack of insulin due to the surgical removal of all or part of the pancreas), assign code E89.1, Postprocedural hypoinsulinemia. Assign a code from category E13 and a code from subcategory Z90.41, Acquired absence of pancreas, as additional codes.

(ii) Secondary diabetes due to drugs

Secondary diabetes may be caused by an adverse effect of correctly administered medications, poisoning or sequela of poisoning.

See section I.C.19.e for coding of adverse effects and poisoning, and section I.C.20 for external cause code reporting.

5. Chapter 5: Mental, Behavioral and Neurodevelopmental disorders (F01–F99)

a. Pain disorders related to psychological factors

Assign code F45.41, for pain that is exclusively related to psychological disorders. As indicated by the Excludes 1 note under category G89, a code from category G89 should not be assigned with code F45.41.

Code F45.42, Pain disorders with related psychological factors, should be used with a code from category G89, Pain, not elsewhere classified, if there is documentation of a psychological component for a patient with acute or chronic pain.

See Section I.C.6. Pain

b. Mental and behavioral disorders due to psychoactive substance use

1) In Remission

Selection of codes for "in remission" for categories F10-F19, Mental and behavioral disorders due to psychoactive substance use (categories F10-F19 with -.11, -.21) requires the provider's clinical judgment. The appropriate codes for "in remission" are assigned only on the basis of provider documentation (as defined in the Official Guidelines for Coding and Reporting), unless otherwise instructed by the classification.

Mild substance use disorders in early or sustained remission are classified to the appropriate codes for substance abuse in remission, and moderate or severe substance use disorders in early or sustained remission are classified to the appropriate codes for substance dependence in remission.

2) Psychoactive Substance Use, Abuse and Dependence

When the provider documentation refers to use, abuse and dependence of the same substance (e.g. alcohol, opioid, cannabis, etc.), only one code should be assigned to identify the pattern of use based on the following hierarchy:

- If both use and abuse are documented, assign only the code for abuse
- If both abuse and dependence are documented, assign only the code for dependence
- If use, abuse and dependence are all documented, assign only the code for dependence
- If both use and dependence are documented, assign only the code for dependence.

3) Psychoactive Substance Use, Unspecified

As with all other unspecified diagnoses, the codes for unspecified psychoactive substance use (F10.9-, F11.9-, F12.9-, F13.9-, F14.9-, F15.9-, F16.9-, F18.9-, F19.9-) should only be assigned based on provider documentation and when they meet the definition of a reportable diagnosis (see Section III, Reporting Additional Diagnoses). These codes are to be used only when the psychoactive substance use is associated with a physical, mental or behavioral disorder, and such a relationship is documented by the provider.

c. Factitious Disorder

Factitious disorder imposed on self or Munchausen's syndrome is a disorder in which a person falsely reports or causes his or her own physical or psychological signs or symptoms. For patients with documented factitious disorder on self or Munchausen's syndrome, assign the appropriate code from subcategory F68.1-, Factitious disorder imposed on self.

Munchausen's syndrome by proxy (MSBP) is a disorder in which a caregiver (perpetrator) falsely reports or causes an illness or injury in another person (victim) under his or her care, such as a child, an elderly adult, or a person who has a disability. The condition is also referred to as "factitious disorder imposed on another" or "factitious disorder by proxy." The perpetrator, not the victim, receives this diagnosis. Assign code F68.A, Factitious disorder imposed on another, to the perpetrator's record. For the victim of a patient suffering from MSBP, assign the appropriate code from categories T74, Adult and child abuse, neglect and other maltreatment, confirmed, or T76, Adult and child abuse, neglect and other maltreatment, suspected.

See Section I.C.19.f. Adult and child abuse, neglect and other maltreatment

6. Chapter 6: Diseases of the Nervous System (G00-G99)

a. Dominant/nondominant side

Codes from category G81, Hemiplegia and hemiparesis, and subcategories G83.1, Monoplegia of lower limb, G83.2, Monoplegia of upper limb, and G83.3, Monoplegia, unspecified, identify whether the dominant or nondominant side is affected. Should the affected side be documented, but not specified as dominant or nondominant, and the classification system does not indicate a default, code selection is as follows:

- For ambidextrous patients, the default should be dominant.
- If the left side is affected, the default is non-dominant.
- If the right side is affected, the default is dominant.

b. Pain - Category G89

1) General coding information

Codes in category G89, Pain, not elsewhere classified, may be used in conjunction with codes from other categories and chapters to provide more detail about acute or chronic pain and neoplasm-related pain, unless otherwise indicated below.

If the pain is not specified as acute or chronic, post-thoracotomy, postprocedural, or neoplasm-related, do not assign codes from category G89.

A code from category G89 should not be assigned if the underlying (definitive) diagnosis is known, unless the reason for the encounter is pain control/ management and not management of the underlying condition.

When an admission or encounter is for a procedure aimed at treating the underlying condition (e.g., spinal fusion, kyphoplasty), a code for the underlying condition (e.g., vertebral fracture, spinal stenosis) should be assigned as the principal diagnosis. No code from category G89 should be assigned.

(a) Category G89 Codes as Principal or First-Listed Diagnosis

Category G89 codes are acceptable as principal diagnosis or the first-listed code:

- When pain control or pain management is the reason for the admission/encounter (e.g., a patient with displaced intervertebral disc, nerve impingement and severe back pain presents for injection of steroid into the spinal canal). The underlying cause of the pain should be reported as an additional diagnosis, if known.
- When a patient is admitted for the insertion of a neurostimulator for pain control, assign the appropriate pain code as the principal or first-listed diagnosis. When an admission or encounter is for a procedure aimed at treating the underlying condition and a neurostimulator is inserted for pain control during the same admission/encounter, a code for the underlying condition should be assigned as the principal diagnosis and the appropriate pain code should be assigned as a secondary diagnosis.

(b) Use of Category G89 Codes in Conjunction with Site Specific Pain Codes

(i) Assigning Category G89 and Site-Specific Pain Codes

Codes from category G89 may be used in conjunction with codes that identify the site of pain (including codes from chapter 18) if the category G89 code provides additional information. For example, if the code describes the site of the pain, but does not fully describe whether the pain is acute or chronic, then both codes should be assigned.

(ii) Sequencing of Category G89 Codes with Site-Specific Pain Codes

The sequencing of category G89 codes with site-specific pain codes (including chapter 18 codes), is dependent on the circumstances of the encounter/admission as follows:

- If the encounter is for pain control or pain management, assign the code from category G89 followed by the code identifying the specific site of pain (e.g., encounter for pain management for acute neck pain from trauma is assigned code G89.11, Acute pain due to trauma, followed by code M54.2, Cervicalgia, to identify the site of pain).
- If the encounter is for any other reason except pain control or pain management, and a related definitive diagnosis has not been established (confirmed) by the provider, assign the code for the specific site of pain first, followed by the appropriate code from category G89.

2) Pain due to devices, implants and grafts
See Section I.C.19. Pain due to medical devices

3) Postoperative Pain

The provider's documentation should be used to guide the coding of postoperative pain, as well as Section III. Reporting Additional Diagnoses and Section IV. Diagnostic Coding and Reporting in the Outpatient Setting.

The default for post-thoracotomy and other postoperative pain not specified as acute or chronic is the code for the acute form.

Routine or expected postoperative pain immediately after surgery should not be coded.

(a) Postoperative pain not associated with specific postoperative complication

Postoperative pain not associated with a specific postoperative complication is assigned to the appropriate postoperative pain code in category G89.

(b) Postoperative pain associated with specific postoperative complication

Postoperative pain associated with a specific postoperative complication (such as painful wire sutures) is assigned to the appropriate code(s) found in Chapter 19, Injury, poisoning, and certain other consequences of external causes. If appropriate, use additional code(s) from category G89 to identify acute or chronic pain (G89.18 or G89.28).

4) Chronic pain

Chronic pain is classified to subcategory G89.2. There is no time frame defining when pain becomes chronic pain. The provider's documentation should be used to guide use of these codes.

5) Neoplasm Related Pain

Code G89.3 is assigned to pain documented as being related, associated or due to cancer, primary or secondary malignancy, or tumor. This code is assigned regardless of whether the pain is acute or chronic.

This code may be assigned as the principal or first-listed code when the stated reason for the admission/encounter is documented as pain control/pain management. The underlying neoplasm should be reported as an additional diagnosis.

When the reason for the admission/encounter is management of the neoplasm and the pain associated with the neoplasm is also documented, code G89.3 may be assigned as an additional diagnosis. It is not necessary to assign an additional code for the site of the pain.

See Section I.C.2 for instructions on the sequencing of neoplasms for all other stated reasons for the admission/encounter (except for pain control/pain management).

6) Chronic pain syndrome

Central pain syndrome (G89.0) and chronic pain syndrome (G89.4) are different than the term "chronic pain," and therefore codes should only be used when the provider has specifically documented this condition.

See Section I.C.5. Pain disorders related to psychological factors

7. Chapter 7: Diseases of the Eye and Adnexa (H00-H59)
a. Glaucoma

1) Assigning Glaucoma Codes

Assign as many codes from category H40, Glaucoma, as needed to identify the type of glaucoma, the affected eye, and the glaucoma stage.

2) Bilateral glaucoma with same type and stage

When a patient has bilateral glaucoma and both eyes are documented as being the same type and stage, and there is a code for bilateral glaucoma, report only the code for the type of glaucoma, bilateral, with the seventh character for the stage.

When a patient has bilateral glaucoma and both eyes are documented as being the same type and stage, and the classification does not provide a code for bilateral glaucoma (i.e. subcategories H40.10 and H40.20) report only one code for the type of glaucoma with the appropriate seventh character for the stage.

3) Bilateral glaucoma stage with different types or stages

When a patient has bilateral glaucoma and each eye is documented as having a different type or stage, and the classification distinguishes laterality, assign the appropriate code for each eye rather than the code for bilateral glaucoma.

When a patient has bilateral glaucoma and each eye is documented as having a different type, and the classification does not distinguish laterality (i.e. subcategories H40.10 and H40.20), assign one code for each type of glaucoma with the appropriate seventh character for the stage.

When a patient has bilateral glaucoma and each eye is documented as having the same type, but different stage, and the classification does not distinguish laterality (i.e. subcategories H40.10 and H40.20), assign a code for the type of glaucoma for each eye with the seventh character for the specific glaucoma stage documented for each eye.

4) Patient admitted with glaucoma and stage evolves during the admission
If a patient is admitted with glaucoma and the stage progresses during the admission, assign the code for highest stage documented.

5) Indeterminate stage glaucoma
Assignment of the seventh character "4" for "indeterminate stage" should be based on the clinical documentation. The seventh character "4" is used for glaucomas whose stage cannot be clinically determined. This seventh character should not be confused with the seventh character "Ø", unspecified, which should be assigned when there is no documentation regarding the stage of the glaucoma.

b. Blindness
If "blindness" or "low vision" of both eyes is documented but the visual impairment category is not documented, assign code H54.3, Unqualified visual loss, both eyes. If "blindness" or "low vision" in one eye is documented but the visual impairment category is not documented, assign a code from H54.6-, Unqualified visual loss, one eye. If "blindness" or "visual loss" is documented without any information about whether one or both eyes are affected, assign code H54.7, Unspecified visual loss.

8. Chapter 8: Diseases of the Ear and Mastoid Process (H60-H95)
Reserved for future guideline expansion

9. Chapter 9: Diseases of the Circulatory System (I00-I99)

a. Hypertension
The classification presumes a causal relationship between hypertension and heart involvement and between hypertension and kidney involvement, as the two conditions are linked by the term "with" in the Alphabetic Index. These conditions should be coded as related even in the absence of provider documentation explicitly linking them, unless the documentation clearly states the conditions are unrelated.

For hypertension and conditions not specifically linked by relational terms such as "with," "associated with" or "due to" in the classification, provider documentation must link the conditions in order to code them as related.

1) Hypertension with Heart Disease
Hypertension with heart conditions classified to I50.- or I51.4-I51.7, I51.89, I51.9, are assigned to a code from category I11, Hypertensive heart disease. Use additional code(s) from category I50, Heart failure, to identify the type(s) of heart failure in those patients with heart failure.

The same heart conditions (I50.-, I51.4-I51.7, I51.89, I51.9) with hypertension are coded separately if the provider has documented they are unrelated to the hypertension. Sequence according to the circumstances of the admission/encounter.

2) Hypertensive Chronic Kidney Disease
Assign codes from category I12, Hypertensive chronic kidney disease, when both hypertension and a condition classifiable to category N18, Chronic kidney disease (CKD), are present. CKD should not be coded as hypertensive if the provider indicates the CKD is not related to the hypertension.

The appropriate code from category N18 should be used as a secondary code with a code from category I12 to identify the stage of chronic kidney disease.

See Section I.C.14. Chronic kidney disease.

If a patient has hypertensive chronic kidney disease and acute renal failure, an additional code for the acute renal failure is required.

3) Hypertensive Heart and Chronic Kidney Disease
Assign codes from combination category I13, Hypertensive heart and chronic kidney disease, when there is hypertension with both heart and kidney involvement. If heart failure is present, assign an additional code from category I50 to identify the type of heart failure.

The appropriate code from category N18, Chronic kidney disease, should be used as a secondary code with a code from category I13 to identify the stage of chronic kidney disease.

See Section I.C.14. Chronic kidney disease.

The codes in category I13, Hypertensive heart and chronic kidney disease, are combination codes that include hypertension, heart

disease and chronic kidney disease. The Includes note at I13 specifies that the conditions included at I11 and I12 are included together in I13. If a patient has hypertension, heart disease and chronic kidney disease, then a code from I13 should be used, not individual codes for hypertension, heart disease and chronic kidney disease, or codes from I11 or I12.

For patients with both acute renal failure and chronic kidney disease, an additional code for acute renal failure is required.

4) Hypertensive Cerebrovascular Disease
For hypertensive cerebrovascular disease, first assign the appropriate code from categories I60-I69, followed by the appropriate hypertension code.

5) Hypertensive Retinopathy
Subcategory H35.Ø, Background retinopathy and retinal vascular changes, should be used with a code from category I10- I15, Hypertensive disease to include the systemic hypertension. The sequencing is based on the reason for the encounter.

6) Hypertension, Secondary
Secondary hypertension is due to an underlying condition. Two codes are required: one to identify the underlying etiology and one from category I15 to identify the hypertension. Sequencing of codes is determined by the reason for admission/encounter.

7) Hypertension, Transient
Assign code RØ3.Ø, Elevated blood pressure reading without diagnosis of hypertension, unless patient has an established diagnosis of hypertension. Assign code O13.-, Gestational [pregnancy-induced] hypertension without significant proteinuria, or O14.-, Pre-eclampsia, for transient hypertension of pregnancy.

8) Hypertension, Controlled
This diagnostic statement usually refers to an existing state of hypertension under control by therapy. Assign the appropriate code from categories I10-I15, Hypertensive diseases.

9) Hypertension, Uncontrolled
Uncontrolled hypertension may refer to untreated hypertension or hypertension not responding to current therapeutic regimen. In either case, assign the appropriate code from categories I10-I15, Hypertensive diseases.

10) Hypertensive Crisis
Assign a code from category I16, Hypertensive crisis, for documented hypertensive urgency, hypertensive emergency or unspecified hypertensive crisis. Code also any identified hypertensive disease (I10-I15). The sequencing is based on the reason for the encounter.

11) Pulmonary Hypertension
Pulmonary hypertension is classified to category I27, Other pulmonary heart diseases. For secondary pulmonary hypertension (I27.1, I27.2-), code also any associated conditions or adverse effects of drugs or toxins. The sequencing is based on the reason for the encounter, except for adverse effects of drugs (See Section I.C.19.e.).

b. Atherosclerotic Coronary Artery Disease and Angina
ICD-10-CM has combination codes for atherosclerotic heart disease with angina pectoris. The subcategories for these codes are I25.11, Atherosclerotic heart disease of native coronary artery with angina pectoris and I25.7, Atherosclerosis of coronary artery bypass graft(s) and coronary artery of transplanted heart with angina pectoris.

When using one of these combination codes it is not necessary to use an additional code for angina pectoris. A causal relationship can be assumed in a patient with both atherosclerosis and angina pectoris, unless the documentation indicates the angina is due to something other than the atherosclerosis.

If a patient with coronary artery disease is admitted due to an acute myocardial infarction (AMI), the AMI should be sequenced before the coronary artery disease.

See Section I.C.9. Acute myocardial infarction (AMI)

c. Intraoperative and Postprocedural Cerebrovascular Accident
Medical record documentation should clearly specify the cause-and-effect relationship between the medical intervention and the cerebrovascular accident in order to assign a code for intraoperative or postprocedural cerebrovascular accident.

Proper code assignment depends on whether it was an infarction or hemorrhage and whether it occurred intraoperatively or postoperatively. If it was a cerebral hemorrhage, code assignment depends on the type of procedure performed.

d. Sequelae of Cerebrovascular Disease

1) Category I69, Sequelae of Cerebrovascular disease

Category I69 is used to indicate conditions classifiable to categories I60-I67 as the causes of sequela (neurologic deficits), themselves classified elsewhere. These "late effects" include neurologic deficits that persist after initial onset of conditions classifiable to categories I60-I67. The neurologic deficits caused by cerebrovascular disease may be present from the onset or may arise at any time after the onset of the condition classifiable to categories I60-I67.

Codes from category I69, Sequelae of cerebrovascular disease, that specify hemiplegia, hemiparesis and monoplegia identify whether the dominant or nondominant side is affected. Should the affected side be documented, but not specified as dominant or nondominant, and the classification system does not indicate a default, code selection is as follows:

- For ambidextrous patients, the default should be dominant.
- If the left side is affected, the default is non-dominant.
- If the right side is affected, the default is dominant.

2) Codes from category I69 with codes from I60-I67

Codes from category I69 may be assigned on a health care record with codes from I60-I67, if the patient has a current cerebrovascular disease and deficits from an old cerebrovascular disease.

3) Codes from category I69 and Personal history of transient ischemic attack (TIA) and cerebral infarction (Z86.73)

Codes from category I69 should not be assigned if the patient does not have neurologic deficits.

See Section I.C.21. 4. History (of) for use of personal history codes

e. Acute myocardial infarction (AMI)

1) Type 1 ST elevation myocardial infarction (STEMI) and non-ST elevation myocardial infarction (NSTEMI)

The ICD-10-CM codes for type 1 acute myocardial infarction (AMI) identify the site, such as anterolateral wall or true posterior wall. Subcategories I21.0-I21.2 and code I21.3 are used for type 1 ST elevation myocardial infarction (STEMI). Code I21.4, Non-ST elevation (NSTEMI) myocardial infarction, is used for type 1 non ST elevation myocardial infarction (NSTEMI) and nontransmural MIs.

If a type 1 NSTEMI evolves to STEMI, assign the STEMI code. If a type 1 STEMI converts to NSTEMI due to thrombolytic therapy, it is still coded as STEMI.

For encounters occurring while the myocardial infarction is equal to, or less than, four weeks old, including transfers to another acute setting or a postacute setting, and the myocardial infarction meets the definition for "other diagnoses" (see Section III, Reporting Additional Diagnoses), codes from category I21 may continue to be reported. For encounters after the 4 week time frame and the patient is still receiving care related to the myocardial infarction, the appropriate aftercare code should be assigned, rather than a code from category I21. For old or healed myocardial infarctions not requiring further care, code I25.2, Old myocardial infarction, may be assigned.

2) Acute myocardial infarction, unspecified

Code I21.9, Acute myocardial infarction, unspecified, is the default for unspecified acute myocardial infarction or unspecified type. If only type 1 STEMI or transmural MI without the site is documented, assign code I21.3, ST elevation (STEMI) myocardial infarction of unspecified site.

3) AMI documented as nontransmural or subendocardial but site provided

If an AMI is documented as nontransmural or subendocardial, but the site is provided, it is still coded as a subendocardial AMI.

See Section I.C.21.3 for information on coding status post administration of tPA in a different facility within the last 24 hours.

4) Subsequent acute myocardial infarction

A code from category I22, Subsequent ST elevation (STEMI) and non-ST elevation (NSTEMI) myocardial infarction, is to be used when a patient who has suffered a type 1 or unspecified AMI has a new AMI within the 4 week time frame of the initial AMI. A code from category I22 must be used in conjunction with a code from

category I21. The sequencing of the I22 and I21 codes depends on the circumstances of the encounter.

Do not assign code I22 for subsequent myocardial infarctions other than type 1 or unspecified. For subsequent type 2 AMI assign only code I21.A1. For subsequent type 4 or type 5 AMI, assign only code I21.A9.

If a subsequent myocardial infarction of one type occurs within 4 weeks of a myocardial infarction of a different type, assign the appropriate codes from category I21 to identify each type. Do not assign a code from I22. Codes from category I22 should only be assigned if both the initial and subsequent myocardial infarctions are type 1 or unspecified.

5) Other Types of Myocardial Infarction

The ICD-10-CM provides codes for different types of myocardial infarction. Type 1 myocardial infarctions are assigned to codes I21.0-I21.4.

Type 2 myocardial infarction (myocardial infarction due to demand ischemia or secondary to ischemic **im**balance), is assigned to code I21.A1, Myocardial infarction type 2 with the underlying cause **coded first**. Do not assign code I24.8, Other forms of acute ischemic heart disease, for the demand ischemia. **If** a type 2 AMI is described as NSTEMI or STEMI, only assign code I21.A1. Codes I21.01-I21.4 should only be assigned for type 1 AMIs.

Acute myocardial infarctions type 3, 4a, 4b, 4c and 5 are assigned to code I21.A9, Other myocardial infarction type.

The "Code also" and "Code first" notes should be followed related to complications, and for coding of postprocedural myocardial infarctions during or following cardiac surgery.

10. Chapter 10: Diseases of the Respiratory System (J00-J99)

a. Chronic Obstructive Pulmonary Disease [COPD] and Asthma

1) Acute exacerbation of chronic obstructive bronchitis and asthma

The codes in categories J44 and J45 distinguish between uncomplicated cases and those in acute exacerbation. An acute exacerbation is a worsening or a decompensation of a chronic condition. An acute exacerbation is not equivalent to an infection superimposed on a chronic condition, though an exacerbation may be triggered by an infection.

b. Acute Respiratory Failure

1) Acute respiratory failure as principal diagnosis

A code from subcategory J96.0, Acute respiratory failure, or subcategory J96.2, Acute and chronic respiratory failure, may be assigned as a principal diagnosis when it is the condition established after study to be chiefly responsible for occasioning the admission to the hospital, and the selection is supported by the Alphabetic Index and Tabular List. However, chapter-specific coding guidelines (such as obstetrics, poisoning, HIV, newborn) that provide sequencing direction take precedence.

2) Acute respiratory failure as secondary diagnosis

Respiratory failure may be listed as a secondary diagnosis if it occurs after admission, or if it is present on admission, but does not meet the definition of principal diagnosis.

3) Sequencing of acute respiratory failure and another acute condition

When a patient is admitted with respiratory failure and another acute condition, (e.g., myocardial infarction, cerebrovascular accident, aspiration pneumonia), the principal diagnosis will not be the same in every situation. This applies whether the other acute condition is a respiratory or nonrespiratory condition. Selection of the principal diagnosis will be dependent on the circumstances of admission. If both the respiratory failure and the other acute condition are equally responsible for occasioning the admission to the hospital, and there are no chapter-specific sequencing rules, the guideline regarding two or more diagnoses that equally meet the definition for principal diagnosis *(Section II, C.)* may be applied in these situations.

If the documentation is not clear as to whether acute respiratory failure and another condition are equally responsible for occasioning the admission, query the provider for clarification.

c. Influenza due to certain identified influenza viruses

Code only confirmed cases of influenza due to certain identified influenza viruses (category J09), and due to other identified influenza virus (category J10). This is an exception to the hospital inpatient guideline Section II, H. (Uncertain Diagnosis).

In this context, "confirmation" does not require documentation of positive laboratory testing specific for avian or other novel influenza A or other identified influenza virus. However, coding should be based on the provider's diagnostic statement that the patient has avian influenza, or other novel influenza A, for category J09, or has another particular identified strain of influenza, such as H1N1 or H3N2, but not identified as novel or variant, for category J10.

If the provider records "suspected" or "possible" or "probable" avian influenza, or novel influenza, or other identified influenza, then the appropriate influenza code from category J11, Influenza due to unidentified influenza virus, should be assigned. A code from category J09, Influenza due to certain identified influenza viruses, should not be assigned nor should a code from category J10, Influenza due to other identified influenza virus.

d. Ventilator associated Pneumonia

1) Documentation of Ventilator associated Pneumonia
As with all procedural or postprocedural complications, code assignment is based on the provider's documentation of the relationship between the condition and the procedure.

Code J95.851, Ventilator associated pneumonia, should be assigned only when the provider has documented ventilator associated pneumonia (VAP). An additional code to identify the organism (e.g., Pseudomonas aeruginosa, code B96.5) should also be assigned. Do not assign an additional code from categories J12-J18 to identify the type of pneumonia.

Code J95.851 should not be assigned for cases where the patient has pneumonia and is on a mechanical ventilator and the provider has not specifically stated that the pneumonia is ventilator-associated pneumonia. If the documentation is unclear as to whether the patient has a pneumonia that is a complication attributable to the mechanical ventilator, query the provider.

2) Ventilator associated Pneumonia Develops after Admission
A patient may be admitted with one type of pneumonia (e.g., code J13, Pneumonia due to Streptococcus pneumonia) and subsequently develop VAP. In this instance, the principal diagnosis would be the appropriate code from categories J12-J18 for the pneumonia diagnosed at the time of admission. Code J95.851, Ventilator associated pneumonia, would be assigned as an additional diagnosis when the provider has also documented the presence of ventilator associated pneumonia.

11. Chapter 11: Diseases of the Digestive System (K00-K95)
Reserved for future guideline expansion

12. Chapter 12: Diseases of the Skin and Subcutaneous Tissue (L00-L99)
a. Pressure ulcer stage codes
1) Pressure ulcer stages
Codes in category L89, Pressure ulcer, identify the site and stage of the pressure ulcer.

The ICD-10-CM classifies pressure ulcer stages based on severity, which is designated by stages 1-4, deep tissue pressure injury, unspecified stage and unstageable.

Assign as many codes from category L89 as needed to identify all the pressure ulcers the patient has, if applicable.

See Section I.B.14 for pressure ulcer stage documentation by clinicians other than patient's provider

2) Unstageable pressure ulcers
Assignment of the code for unstageable pressure ulcer (L89.--0) should be based on the clinical documentation. These codes are used for pressure ulcers whose stage cannot be clinically determined (e.g., the ulcer is covered by eschar or has been treated with a skin or muscle graft). This code should not be confused with the codes for unspecified stage (L89.--9). When there is no documentation regarding the stage of the pressure ulcer, assign the appropriate code for unspecified stage (L89.--9).

3) Documented pressure ulcer stage
Assignment of the pressure ulcer stage code should be guided by clinical documentation of the stage or documentation of the terms found in the Alphabetic Index. For clinical terms describing the stage that are not found in the Alphabetic Index, and there is no documentation of the stage, the provider should be queried.

4) Patients admitted with pressure ulcers documented as healed
No code is assigned if the documentation states that the pressure ulcer is completely healed at the time of admission.

5) Pressure ulcers documented as healing
Pressure ulcers described as healing should be assigned the appropriate pressure ulcer stage code based on the documentation in the medical record. If the documentation does not provide information about the stage of the healing pressure ulcer, assign the appropriate code for unspecified stage.

If the documentation is unclear as to whether the patient has a current (new) pressure ulcer or if the patient is being treated for a healing pressure ulcer, query the provider.

For ulcers that were present on admission but healed at the time of discharge, assign the code for the site and stage of the pressure ulcer at the time of admission.

6) Patient admitted with pressure ulcer evolving into another stage during the admission
If a patient is admitted to an inpatient hospital with a pressure ulcer at one stage and it progresses to a higher stage, two separate codes should be assigned: one code for the site and stage of the ulcer on admission and a second code for the same ulcer site and the highest stage reported during the stay.

7) Pressure-induced deep tissue damage
For pressure-induced deep tissue damage or deep tissue pressure injury, assign only the appropriate code for pressure-induced deep tissue damage (L89.--6).

b. Non-Pressure Chronic Ulcers
1) Patients admitted with non-pressure ulcers documented as healed
No code is assigned if the documentation states that the non-pressure ulcer is completely healed at the time of admission.

2) Non-pressure ulcers documented as healing
Non-pressure ulcers described as healing should be assigned the appropriate non-pressure ulcer code based on the documentation in the medical record. If the documentation does not provide information about the severity of the healing non-pressure ulcer, assign the appropriate code for unspecified severity.

If the documentation is unclear as to whether the patient has a current (new) non-pressure ulcer or if the patient is being treated for a healing non-pressure ulcer, query the provider.

For ulcers that were present on admission but healed at the time of discharge, assign the code for the site and severity of the non-pressure ulcer at the time of admission.

3) Patient admitted with non-pressure ulcer that progresses to another severity level during the admission
If a patient is admitted to an inpatient hospital with a non-pressure ulcer at one severity level and it progresses to a higher severity level, two separate codes should be assigned: one code for the site and severity level of the ulcer on admission and a second code for the same ulcer site and the highest severity level reported during the stay.

See Section I.B.14 for pressure ulcer stage documentation by clinicians other than patient's provider

13. Chapter 13: Diseases of the Musculoskeletal System and Connective Tissue (M00-M99)
a. Site and laterality
Most of the codes within Chapter 13 have site and laterality designations. The site represents the bone, joint or the muscle involved. For some conditions where more than one bone, joint or muscle is usually involved, such as osteoarthritis, there is a "multiple sites" code available. For categories where no multiple site code is provided and more than one bone, joint or muscle is involved, multiple codes should be used to indicate the different sites involved.

1) Bone versus joint
For certain conditions, the bone may be affected at the upper or lower end, (e.g., avascular necrosis of bone, M87, Osteoporosis, M80, M81). Though the portion of the bone affected may be at the joint, the site designation will be the bone, not the joint.

b. Acute traumatic versus chronic or recurrent musculoskeletal conditions
Many musculoskeletal conditions are a result of previous injury or trauma to a site, or are recurrent conditions. Bone, joint or muscle conditions that are the result of a healed injury are usually found in chapter 13. Recurrent bone, joint or muscle conditions are also usually found in chapter 13. Any current, acute injury should be coded to the

appropriate injury code from chapter 19. Chronic or recurrent conditions should generally be coded with a code from chapter 13. If it is difficult to determine from the documentation in the record which code is best to describe a condition, query the provider.

c. Coding of Pathologic Fractures

7th character A is for use as long as the patient is receiving active treatment for the fracture. While the patient may be seen by a new or different provider over the course of treatment for a pathological fracture, assignment of the 7th character is based on whether the patient is undergoing active treatment and not whether the provider is seeing the patient for the first time.

7th character D is to be used for encounters after the patient has completed active treatment for the fracture and is receiving routine care for the fracture during the healing or recovery phase. The other 7th characters, listed under each subcategory in the Tabular List, are to be used for subsequent encounters for treatment of problems associated with the healing, such as malunions, nonunions, and sequelae.

Care for complications of surgical treatment for fracture repairs during the healing or recovery phase should be coded with the appropriate complication codes.

See Section I.C.19. Coding of traumatic fractures.

d. Osteoporosis

Osteoporosis is a systemic condition, meaning that all bones of the musculoskeletal system are affected. Therefore, site is not a component of the codes under category M81, Osteoporosis without current pathological fracture. The site codes under category M80, Osteoporosis with current pathological fracture, identify the site of the fracture, not the osteoporosis.

1) Osteoporosis without pathological fracture

Category M81, Osteoporosis without current pathological fracture, is for use for patients with osteoporosis who do not currently have a pathologic fracture due to the osteoporosis, even if they have had a fracture in the past. For patients with a history of osteoporosis fractures, status code Z87.310, Personal history of (healed) osteoporosis fracture, should follow the code from M81.

2) Osteoporosis with current pathological fracture

Category M80, Osteoporosis with current pathological fracture, is for patients who have a current pathologic fracture at the time of an encounter. The codes under M80 identify the site of the fracture. A code from category M80, not a traumatic fracture code, should be used for any patient with known osteoporosis who suffers a fracture, even if the patient had a minor fall or trauma, if that fall or trauma would not usually break a normal, healthy bone.

14. Chapter 14: Diseases of Genitourinary System (N00-N99)
a. Chronic kidney disease
1) Stages of chronic kidney disease (CKD)

The ICD-10-CM classifies CKD based on severity. The severity of CKD is designated by stages 1-5. Stage 2, code N18.2, equates to mild CKD; stage 3, code N18.3, equates to moderate CKD; and stage 4, code N18.4, equates to severe CKD. Code N18.6, End stage renal disease (ESRD), is assigned when the provider has documented end-stage-renal disease (ESRD).

If both a stage of CKD and ESRD are documented, assign code N18.6 only.

2) Chronic kidney disease and kidney transplant status

Patients who have undergone kidney transplant may still have some form of chronic kidney disease (CKD) because the kidney transplant may not fully restore kidney function. Therefore, the presence of CKD alone does not constitute a transplant complication. Assign the appropriate N18 code for the patient's stage of CKD and code Z94.0, Kidney transplant status. If a transplant complication such as failure or rejection or other transplant complication is documented, see section I.C.19.g for information on coding complications of a kidney transplant. If the documentation is unclear as to whether the patient has a complication of the transplant, query the provider.

3) Chronic kidney disease with other conditions

Patients with CKD may also suffer from other serious conditions, most commonly diabetes mellitus and hypertension. The sequencing of the CKD code in relationship to codes for other contributing conditions is based on the conventions in the Tabular List.

See I.C.9. Hypertensive chronic kidney disease.

See I.C.19. Chronic kidney disease and kidney transplant complications.

15. Chapter 15: Pregnancy, Childbirth, and the Puerperium (O00-O9A)
a. General Rules for Obstetric Cases
1) Codes from chapter 15 and sequencing priority

Obstetric cases require codes from chapter 15, codes in the range O00-O9A, Pregnancy, Childbirth, and the Puerperium. Chapter 15 codes have sequencing priority over codes from other chapters. Additional codes from other chapters may be used in conjunction with chapter 15 codes to further specify conditions. Should the provider document that the pregnancy is incidental to the encounter, then code Z33.1, Pregnant state, incidental, should be used in place of any chapter 15 codes. It is the provider's responsibility to state that the condition being treated is not affecting the pregnancy.

2) Chapter 15 codes used only on the maternal record

Chapter 15 codes are to be used only on the maternal record, never on the record of the newborn.

3) Final character for trimester

The majority of codes in Chapter 15 have a final character indicating the trimester of pregnancy. The timeframes for the trimesters are indicated at the beginning of the chapter. If trimester is not a component of a code, it is because the condition always occurs in a specific trimester, or the concept of trimester of pregnancy is not applicable. Certain codes have characters for only certain trimesters because the condition does not occur in all trimesters, but it may occur in more than just one.

Assignment of the final character for trimester should be based on the provider's documentation of the trimester (or number of weeks) for the current admission/encounter. This applies to the assignment of trimester for pre-existing conditions as well as those that develop during or are due to the pregnancy. The provider's documentation of the number of weeks may be used to assign the appropriate code identifying the trimester.

Whenever delivery occurs during the current admission, and there is an "in childbirth" option for the obstetric complication being coded, the "in childbirth" code should be assigned.

4) Selection of trimester for inpatient admissions that encompass more than one trimester

In instances when a patient is admitted to a hospital for complications of pregnancy during one trimester and remains in the hospital into a subsequent trimester, the trimester character for the antepartum complication code should be assigned on the basis of the trimester when the complication developed, not the trimester of the discharge. If the condition developed prior to the current admission/encounter or represents a pre-existing condition, the trimester character for the trimester at the time of the admission/encounter should be assigned.

5) Unspecified trimester

Each category that includes codes for trimester has a code for "unspecified trimester." The "unspecified trimester" code should rarely be used, such as when the documentation in the record is insufficient to determine the trimester and it is not possible to obtain clarification.

6) 7th character for Fetus Identification

Where applicable, a 7th character is to be assigned for certain categories (O31, O32, O33.3 - O33.6, O35, O36, O40, O41, O60.1, O60.2, O64, and O69) to identify the fetus for which the complication code applies.

Assign 7th character "0":

- For single gestations
- When the documentation in the record is insufficient to determine the fetus affected and it is not possible to obtain clarification.
- When it is not possible to clinically determine which fetus is affected.

b. Selection of OB Principal or First-listed Diagnosis
1) Routine outpatient prenatal visits

For routine outpatient prenatal visits when no complications are present, a code from category Z34, Encounter for supervision of normal pregnancy, should be used as the first-listed diagnosis. These codes should not be used in conjunction with chapter 15 codes.

2) **Supervision of High-Risk Pregnancy**
Codes from category O09, Supervision of high-risk pregnancy, are intended for use only during the prenatal period. For complications during the labor or delivery episode as a result of a high-risk pregnancy, assign the applicable complication codes from Chapter 15. If there are no complications during the labor or delivery episode, assign code O80, Encounter for full-term uncomplicated delivery.

For routine prenatal outpatient visits for patients with high-risk pregnancies, a code from category O09, Supervision of high-risk pregnancy, should be used as the first-listed diagnosis. Secondary chapter 15 codes may be used in conjunction with these codes if appropriate.

3) **Episodes when no delivery occurs**
In episodes when no delivery occurs, the principal diagnosis should correspond to the principal complication of the pregnancy which necessitated the encounter. Should more than one complication exist, all of which are treated or monitored, any of the complication codes may be sequenced first.

4) **When a delivery occurs**
When an obstetric patient is admitted and delivers during that admission, the condition that prompted the admission should be sequenced as the principal diagnosis. If multiple conditions prompted the admission, sequence the one most related to the delivery as the principal diagnosis. A code for any complication of the delivery should be assigned as an additional diagnosis. In cases of cesarean delivery, if the patient was admitted with a condition that resulted in the performance of a cesarean procedure, that condition should be selected as the principal diagnosis. If the reason for the admission was unrelated to the condition resulting in the cesarean delivery, the condition related to the reason for the admission should be selected as the principal diagnosis.

5) **Outcome of delivery**
A code from category Z37, Outcome of delivery, should be included on every maternal record when a delivery has occurred. These codes are not to be used on subsequent records or on the newborn record.

c. **Pre-existing conditions versus conditions due to the pregnancy**
Certain categories in Chapter 15 distinguish between conditions of the mother that existed prior to pregnancy (pre-existing) and those that are a direct result of pregnancy. When assigning codes from Chapter 15, it is important to assess if a condition was pre-existing prior to pregnancy or developed during or due to the pregnancy in order to assign the correct code.

Categories that do not distinguish between pre-existing and pregnancy-related conditions may be used for either. It is acceptable to use codes specifically for the puerperium with codes complicating pregnancy and childbirth if a condition arises postpartum during the delivery encounter.

d. **Pre-existing hypertension in pregnancy**
Category O10, Pre-existing hypertension complicating pregnancy, childbirth and the puerperium, includes codes for hypertensive heart and hypertensive chronic kidney disease. When assigning one of the O10 codes that includes hypertensive heart disease or hypertensive chronic kidney disease, it is necessary to add a secondary code from the appropriate hypertension category to specify the type of heart failure or chronic kidney disease.

See Section I.C.9. Hypertension.

e. **Fetal Conditions Affecting the Management of the Mother**
1) **Codes from categories O35 and O36**
Codes from categories O35, Maternal care for known or suspected fetal abnormality and damage, and O36, Maternal care for other fetal problems, are assigned only when the fetal condition is actually responsible for modifying the management of the mother, i.e., by requiring diagnostic studies, additional observation, special care, or termination of pregnancy. The fact that the fetal condition exists does not justify assigning a code from this series to the mother's record.

2) **In utero surgery**
In cases when surgery is performed on the fetus, a diagnosis code from category O35, Maternal care for known or suspected fetal abnormality and damage, should be assigned identifying the fetal condition. Assign the appropriate procedure code for the procedure performed.

No code from Chapter 16, the perinatal codes, should be used on the mother's record to identify fetal conditions. Surgery performed in utero on a fetus is still to be coded as an obstetric encounter.

f. **HIV Infection in Pregnancy, Childbirth and the Puerperium**
During pregnancy, childbirth or the puerperium, a patient admitted because of an HIV-related illness should receive a principal diagnosis from subcategory O98.7-, Human immunodeficiency [HIV] disease complicating pregnancy, childbirth and the puerperium, followed by the code(s) for the HIV-related illness(es).

Patients with asymptomatic HIV infection status admitted during pregnancy, childbirth, or the puerperium should receive codes of O98.7- and Z21, Asymptomatic human immunodeficiency virus [HIV] infection status.

g. **Diabetes mellitus in pregnancy**
Diabetes mellitus is a significant complicating factor in pregnancy. Pregnant women who are diabetic should be assigned a code from category O24, Diabetes mellitus in pregnancy, childbirth, and the puerperium, first, followed by the appropriate diabetes code(s) (E08-E13) from Chapter 4.

h. **Long term use of insulin and oral hypoglycemics**
See section I.C.4.a.3 for information on the long term use of insulin and oral hypoglycemic.

i. **Gestational (pregnancy induced) diabetes**
Gestational (pregnancy induced) diabetes can occur during the second and third trimester of pregnancy in women who were not diabetic prior to pregnancy. Gestational diabetes can cause complications in the pregnancy similar to those of pre-existing diabetes mellitus. It also puts the woman at greater risk of developing diabetes after the pregnancy. Codes for gestational diabetes are in subcategory O24.4, Gestational diabetes mellitus. No other code from category O24, Diabetes mellitus in pregnancy, childbirth, and the puerperium, should be used with a code from O24.4.

The codes under subcategory O24.4 include diet controlled, insulin controlled, and controlled by oral hypoglycemic drugs. If a patient with gestational diabetes is treated with both diet and insulin, only the code for insulin-controlled is required. If a patient with gestational diabetes is treated with both diet and oral hypoglycemic medications, only the code for "controlled by oral hypoglycemic drugs" is required. Code Z79.4, Long-term (current) use of insulin or code Z79.84, Long-term (current) use of oral hypoglycemic drugs, should not be assigned with codes from subcategory O24.4.

An abnormal glucose tolerance in pregnancy is assigned a code from subcategory O99.81, Abnormal glucose complicating pregnancy, childbirth, and the puerperium.

j. **Sepsis and septic shock complicating abortion, pregnancy, childbirth and the puerperium**
When assigning a chapter 15 code for sepsis complicating abortion, pregnancy, childbirth, and the puerperium, a code for the specific type of infection should be assigned as an additional diagnosis. If severe sepsis is present, a code from subcategory R65.2, Severe sepsis, and code(s) for associated organ dysfunction(s) should also be assigned as additional diagnoses.

k. **Puerperal sepsis**
Code O85, Puerperal sepsis, should be assigned with a secondary code to identify the causal organism (e.g., for a bacterial infection, assign a code from category B95-B96, Bacterial infections in conditions classified elsewhere). A code from category A40, Streptococcal sepsis, or A41, Other sepsis, should not be used for puerperal sepsis. If applicable, use additional codes to identify severe sepsis (R65.2-) and any associated acute organ dysfunction.

l. **Alcohol, tobacco and drug use during pregnancy, childbirth and the puerperium**
1) **Alcohol use during pregnancy, childbirth and the puerperium**
Codes under subcategory O99.31, Alcohol use complicating pregnancy, childbirth, and the puerperium, should be assigned for any pregnancy case when a mother uses alcohol during the pregnancy or postpartum. A secondary code from category F10, Alcohol related disorders, should also be assigned to identify manifestations of the alcohol use.

2) **Tobacco use during pregnancy, childbirth and the puerperium**
Codes under subcategory O99.33, Smoking (tobacco) complicating pregnancy, childbirth, and the puerperium, should

be assigned for any pregnancy case when a mother uses any type of tobacco product during the pregnancy or postpartum. A secondary code from category F17, Nicotine dependence, should also be assigned to identify the type of nicotine dependence.

3) Drug use during pregnancy, childbirth and the puerperium
Codes under subcategory O99.32, Drug use complicating pregnancy, childbirth, and the puerperium, should be assigned for any pregnancy case when a mother uses drugs during the pregnancy or postpartum. This can involve illegal drugs, or inappropriate use or abuse of prescription drugs. Secondary code(s) from categories F11-F16 and F18-F19 should also be assigned to identify manifestations of the drug use.

m. Poisoning, toxic effects, adverse effects and underdosing in a pregnant patient
A code from subcategory O9A.2, Injury, poisoning and certain other consequences of external causes complicating pregnancy, childbirth, and the puerperium, should be sequenced first, followed by the appropriate injury, poisoning, toxic effect, adverse effect or underdosing code, and then the additional code(s) that specifies the condition caused by the poisoning, toxic effect, adverse effect or underdosing.
See Section I.C.19. Adverse effects, poisoning, underdosing and toxic effects.

n. Normal Delivery, Code O80
1) Encounter for full term uncomplicated delivery
Code O80 should be assigned when a woman is admitted for a full-term normal delivery and delivers a single, healthy infant without any complications antepartum, during the delivery, or postpartum during the delivery episode. Code O80 is always a principal diagnosis. It is not to be used if any other code from chapter 15 is needed to describe a current complication of the antenatal, delivery, or **postnatal** period. Additional codes from other chapters may be used with code O80 if they are not related to or are in any way complicating the pregnancy.

2) Uncomplicated delivery with resolved antepartum complication
Code O80 may be used if the patient had a complication at some point during the pregnancy, but the complication is not present at the time of the admission for delivery.

3) Outcome of delivery for O80
Z37.0, Single live birth, is the only outcome of delivery code appropriate for use with O80.

o. The Peripartum and Postpartum Periods
1) Peripartum and Postpartum periods
The postpartum period begins immediately after delivery and continues for six weeks following delivery. The peripartum period is defined as the last month of pregnancy to five months postpartum.

2) Peripartum and postpartum complication
A postpartum complication is any complication occurring within the six-week period.

3) Pregnancy-related complications after 6 week period
Chapter 15 codes may also be used to describe pregnancy-related complications after the peripartum or postpartum period if the provider documents that a condition is pregnancy related.

4) Admission for routine postpartum care following delivery outside hospital
When the mother delivers outside the hospital prior to admission and is admitted for routine postpartum care and no complications are noted, code Z39.0, Encounter for care and examination of mother immediately after delivery, should be assigned as the principal diagnosis.

5) Pregnancy associated cardiomyopathy
Pregnancy associated cardiomyopathy, code O90.3, is unique in that it may be diagnosed in the third trimester of pregnancy but may continue to progress months after delivery. For this reason, it is referred to as peripartum cardiomyopathy. Code O90.3 is only for use when the cardiomyopathy develops as a result of pregnancy in a woman who did not have pre-existing heart disease.

p. Code O94, Sequelae of complication of pregnancy, childbirth, and the puerperium
1) Code O94
Code O94, Sequelae of complication of pregnancy, childbirth, and the puerperium, is for use in those cases when an initial

complication of a pregnancy develops a sequelae requiring care or treatment at a future date.

2) After the initial postpartum period
This code may be used at any time after the initial postpartum period.

3) Sequencing of Code O94
This code, like all sequela codes, is to be sequenced following the code describing the sequelae of the complication.

q. Termination of Pregnancy and Spontaneous abortions
1) Abortion with Liveborn Fetus
When an attempted termination of pregnancy results in a liveborn fetus, assign code Z33.2, Encounter for elective termination of pregnancy and a code from category Z37, Outcome of Delivery.

2) Retained Products of Conception following an abortion
Subsequent encounters for retained products of conception following a spontaneous abortion or elective termination of pregnancy, without complications are assigned O03.4, Incomplete spontaneous abortion without complication, or code O07.4, Failed attempted termination of pregnancy without complication. This advice is appropriate even when the patient was discharged previously with a discharge diagnosis of complete abortion. If the patient has a specific complication associated with the spontaneous abortion or elective termination of pregnancy in addition to retained products of conception, assign the appropriate complication **code (e.g., O03.-, O04.-, O07.-)** instead of code O03.4 or O07.4

3) Complications leading to abortion
Codes from Chapter 15 may be used as additional codes to identify any documented complications of the pregnancy in conjunction with codes in categories in O04, O07 and O08.

r. Abuse in a pregnant patient
For suspected or confirmed cases of abuse of a pregnant patient, a code(s) from subcategories O9A.3, Physical abuse complicating pregnancy, childbirth, and the puerperium, O9A.4, Sexual abuse complicating pregnancy, childbirth, and the puerperium, and O9A.5, Psychological abuse complicating pregnancy, childbirth, and the puerperium, should be sequenced first, followed by the appropriate codes (if applicable) to identify any associated current injury due to physical abuse, sexual abuse, and the perpetrator of abuse.
See Section I.C.19. Adult and child abuse, neglect and other maltreatment.

16. Chapter 16: Certain Conditions Originating in the Perinatal Period (P00-P96)
For coding and reporting purposes the perinatal period is defined as before birth through the 28th day following birth. The following guidelines are provided for reporting purposes.

a. General Perinatal Rules
1) Use of Chapter 16 Codes
Codes in this chapter are <u>never</u> for use on the maternal record. Codes from Chapter 15, the obstetric chapter, are never permitted on the newborn record. Chapter 16 codes may be used throughout the life of the patient if the condition is still present.

2) Principal Diagnosis for Birth Record
When coding the birth episode in a newborn record, assign a code from category Z38, Liveborn infants according to place of birth and type of delivery, as the principal diagnosis. A code from category Z38 is assigned only once, to a newborn at the time of birth. If a newborn is transferred to another institution, a code from category Z38 should not be used at the receiving hospital.
A code from category Z38 is used only on the newborn record, not on the mother's record.

3) Use of Codes from other Chapters with Codes from Chapter 16
Codes from other chapters may be used with codes from chapter 16 if the codes from the other chapters provide more specific detail. Codes for signs and symptoms may be assigned when a definitive diagnosis has not been established. If the reason for the encounter is a perinatal condition, the code from chapter 16 should be sequenced first.

4) Use of Chapter 16 Codes after the Perinatal Period
Should a condition originate in the perinatal period, and continue throughout the life of the patient, the perinatal code should continue to be used regardless of the patient's age.

5) Birth process or community acquired conditions

If a newborn has a condition that may be either due to the birth process or community acquired and the documentation does not indicate which it is, the default is due to the birth process and the code from Chapter 16 should be used. If the condition is community-acquired, a code from Chapter 16 should not be assigned.

6) Code all clinically significant conditions

All clinically significant conditions noted on routine newborn examination should be coded. A condition is clinically significant if it requires:

- clinical evaluation; or
- therapeutic treatment; or
- diagnostic procedures; or
- extended length of hospital stay; or
- increased nursing care and/or monitoring; or
- has implications for future health care needs

Note: The perinatal guidelines listed above are the same as the general coding guidelines for "additional diagnoses," except for the final point regarding implications for future health care needs. Codes should be assigned for conditions that have been specified by the provider as having implications for future health care needs.

b. Observation and Evaluation of Newborns for Suspected Conditions not Found

1) Use of Z05 codes

Assign a code from category Z05, Observation and evaluation of newborns and infants for suspected conditions ruled out, to identify those instances when a healthy newborn is evaluated for a suspected condition that is determined after study not to be present. Do not use a code from category Z05 when the patient has identified signs or symptoms of a suspected problem; in such cases code the sign or symptom.

2) Z05 on other than the birth record

A code from category Z05 may also be assigned as a principal or first-listed code for readmissions or encounters when the code from category Z38 code no longer applies. Codes from category Z05 are for use only for healthy newborns and infants for which no condition after study is found to be present.

3) Z05 on a birth record

A code from category Z05 is to be used as a secondary code after the code from category Z38, Liveborn infants according to place of birth and type of delivery.

c. Coding Additional Perinatal Diagnoses

1) Assigning codes for conditions that require treatment

Assign codes for conditions that require treatment or further investigation, prolong the length of stay, or require resource utilization.

2) Codes for conditions specified as having implications for future health care needs

Assign codes for conditions that have been specified by the provider as having implications for future health care needs.

Note: This guideline should not be used for adult patients.

d. Prematurity and Fetal Growth Retardation

Providers utilize different criteria in determining prematurity. A code for prematurity should not be assigned unless it is documented. Assignment of codes in categories P05, Disorders of newborn related to slow fetal growth and fetal malnutrition, and P07, Disorders of newborn related to short gestation and low birth weight, not elsewhere classified, should be based on the recorded birth weight and estimated gestational age.

When both birth weight and gestational age are available, two codes from category P07 should be assigned, with the code for birth weight sequenced before the code for gestational age.

e. Low birth weight and immaturity status

Codes from category P07, Disorders of newborn related to short gestation and low birth weight, not elsewhere classified, are for use for a child or adult who was premature or had a low birth weight as a newborn and this is affecting the patient's current health status.

See Section I.C.21. Factors influencing health status and contact with health services, Status.

f. Bacterial Sepsis of Newborn

Category P36, Bacterial sepsis of newborn, includes congenital sepsis. If a perinate is documented as having sepsis without documentation

of congenital or community acquired, the default is congenital and a code from category P36 should be assigned. If the P36 code includes the causal organism, an additional code from category B95, Streptococcus, Staphylococcus, and Enterococcus as the cause of diseases classified elsewhere, or B96, Other bacterial agents as the cause of diseases classified elsewhere, should not be assigned. If the P36 code does not include the causal organism, assign an additional code from category B96. If applicable, use additional codes to identify severe sepsis (R65.2-) and any associated acute organ dysfunction.

g. Stillbirth

Code P95, Stillbirth, is only for use in institutions that maintain separate records for stillbirths. No other code should be used with P95. Code P95 should not be used on the mother's record.

17. Chapter 17: Congenital malformations, deformations, and chromosomal abnormalities (Q00-Q99)

Assign an appropriate code(s) from categories Q00-Q99, Congenital malformations, deformations, and chromosomal abnormalities when a malformation/deformation or chromosomal abnormality is documented. A malformation/deformation/or chromosomal abnormality may be the principal/first-listed diagnosis on a record or a secondary diagnosis.

When a malformation/deformation or chromosomal abnormality does not have a unique code assignment, assign additional code(s) for any manifestations that may be present.

When the code assignment specifically identifies the malformation/deformation or chromosomal abnormality, manifestations that are an inherent component of the anomaly should not be coded separately. Additional codes should be assigned for manifestations that are not an inherent component.

Codes from Chapter 17 may be used throughout the life of the patient. If a congenital malformation or deformity has been corrected, a personal history code should be used to identify the history of the malformation or deformity. Although present at birth, **a** malformation/deformation/or chromosomal abnormality may not be identified until later in life. Whenever the condition is diagnosed by the **provider**, it is appropriate to assign a code from codes Q00-Q99. For the birth admission, the appropriate code from category Z38, Liveborn infants, according to place of birth and type of delivery, should be sequenced as the principal diagnosis, followed by any congenital anomaly codes, Q00- Q99.

18. Chapter 18: Symptoms, signs, and abnormal clinical and laboratory findings, not elsewhere classified (R00-R99)

Chapter 18 includes symptoms, signs, abnormal results of clinical or other investigative procedures, and ill-defined conditions regarding which no diagnosis classifiable elsewhere is recorded. Signs and symptoms that point to a specific diagnosis have been assigned to a category in other chapters of the classification.

a. Use of symptom codes

Codes that describe symptoms and signs are acceptable for reporting purposes when a related definitive diagnosis has not been established (confirmed) by the provider.

b. Use of a symptom code with a definitive diagnosis code

Codes for signs and symptoms may be reported in addition to a related definitive diagnosis when the sign or symptom is not routinely associated with that diagnosis, such as the various signs and symptoms associated with complex syndromes. The definitive diagnosis code should be sequenced before the symptom code.

Signs or symptoms that are associated routinely with a disease process should not be assigned as additional codes, unless otherwise instructed by the classification.

c. Combination codes that include symptoms

ICD-10-CM contains a number of combination codes that identify both the definitive diagnosis and common symptoms of that diagnosis.

When using one of these combination codes, an additional code should not be assigned for the symptom.

d. Repeated falls

Code R29.6, Repeated falls, is for use for encounters when a patient has recently fallen and the reason for the fall is being investigated.

Code Z91.81, History of falling, is for use when a patient has fallen in the past and is at risk for future falls. When appropriate, both codes R29.6 and Z91.81 may be assigned together.

e. Coma scale

The coma scale codes (R40.2-) can be used in conjunction with traumatic brain injury codes, acute cerebrovascular disease or sequelae of cerebrovascular disease codes. These codes are primarily for use by trauma registries, but they may be used in any setting where this information is collected. The coma scale may also be used to assess the status of the central nervous system for other non-trauma conditions, such as monitoring patients in the intensive care unit regardless of medical condition. The coma scale codes should be sequenced after the diagnosis code(s).

These codes, one from each subcategory, are needed to complete the scale. The 7th character indicates when the scale was recorded. The 7th character should match for all three codes.

At a minimum, report the initial score documented on presentation at your facility. This may be a score from the emergency medicine technician (EMT) or in the emergency department. If desired, a facility may choose to capture multiple coma scale scores.

Assign code R40.24, Glasgow coma scale, total score, when only the total score is documented in the medical record and not the individual score(s).

Do not report codes for individual or total Glasgow coma scale scores for a patient with a medically induced coma or a sedated patient.

See Section I.B.14 for coma scale documentation by clinicians other than patient's provider

f. Functional quadriplegia
GUIDELINE HAS BEEN DELETED EFFECTIVE OCTOBER 1, 2017

g. SIRS due to Non-Infectious Process
The systemic inflammatory response syndrome (SIRS) can develop as a result of certain non-infectious disease processes, such as trauma, malignant neoplasm, or pancreatitis. When SIRS is documented with a noninfectious condition, and no subsequent infection is documented, the code for the underlying condition, such as an injury, should be assigned, followed by code R65.10, Systemic inflammatory response syndrome (SIRS) of non-infectious origin without acute organ dysfunction, or code R65.11, Systemic inflammatory response syndrome (SIRS) of non-infectious origin with acute organ dysfunction. If an associated acute organ dysfunction is documented, the appropriate code(s) for the specific type of organ dysfunction(s) should be assigned in addition to code R65.11. If acute organ dysfunction is documented, but it cannot be determined if the acute organ dysfunction is associated with SIRS or due to another condition (e.g., directly due to the trauma), the provider should be queried.

h. Death NOS
Code R99, Ill-defined and unknown cause of mortality, is only for use in the very limited circumstance when a patient who has already died is brought into an emergency department or other healthcare facility and is pronounced dead upon arrival. It does not represent the discharge disposition of death.

i. NIHSS Stroke Scale
The NIH stroke scale (NIHSS) codes (R29.7- -) can be used in conjunction with acute stroke codes (I63) to identify the patient's neurological status and the severity of the stroke. The stroke scale codes should be sequenced after the acute stroke diagnosis code(s).

At a minimum, report the initial score documented. If desired, a facility may choose to capture multiple stroke scale scores.

See Section I.B.14 for NIHSS stroke scale documentation by clinicians other than patient's provider

19. Chapter 19: Injury, poisoning, and certain other consequences of external causes (S00-T88)

a. Application of 7th Characters in Chapter 19
Most categories in chapter 19 have a 7th character requirement for each applicable code. Most categories in this chapter have three 7th character values (with the exception of fractures): A, initial encounter, D, subsequent encounter and S, sequela. Categories for traumatic fractures have additional 7th character values. While the patient may be seen by a new or different provider over the course of treatment for an injury, assignment of the 7th character is based on whether the patient is undergoing active treatment and not whether the provider is seeing the patient for the first time.

For complication codes, active treatment refers to treatment for the condition described by the code, even though it may be related to an earlier precipitating problem. For example, code T84.50XA, Infection and inflammatory reaction due to unspecified internal joint prosthesis, initial encounter, is used when active treatment is provided for the infection, even though the condition relates to the prosthetic device, implant or graft that was placed at a previous encounter.

7th character "A", initial encounter is used for each encounter where the patient is receiving active treatment for the condition.

7th character "D" subsequent encounter is used for encounters after the patient has completed active treatment of the condition and is receiving routine care for the condition during the healing or recovery phase.

The aftercare Z codes should not be used for aftercare for conditions such as injuries or poisonings, where 7th characters are provided to identify subsequent care. For example, for aftercare of an injury, assign the acute injury code with the 7th character "D" (subsequent encounter).

7th character "S", sequela, is for use for complications or conditions that arise as a direct result of a condition, such as scar formation after a burn. The scars are sequelae of the burn. When using 7th character "S", it is necessary to use both the injury code that precipitated the sequela and the code for the sequela itself. The "S" is added only to the injury code, not the sequela code. The 7th character "S" identifies the injury responsible for the sequela. The specific type of sequela (e.g. scar) is sequenced first, followed by the injury code.

See Section I.B.10 Sequelae, (Late Effects)

b. Coding of Injuries
When coding injuries, assign separate codes for each injury unless a combination code is provided, in which case the combination code is assigned. Codes from category T07, Unspecified multiple injuries should not be assigned in the inpatient setting unless information for a more specific code is not available. Traumatic injury codes (S00-T14.9) are not to be used for normal, healing surgical wounds or to identify complications of surgical wounds.

The code for the most serious injury, as determined by the provider and the focus of treatment, is sequenced first.

1) Superficial injuries
Superficial injuries such as abrasions or contusions are not coded when associated with more severe injuries of the same site.

2) Primary injury with damage to nerves/blood vessels
When a primary injury results in minor damage to peripheral nerves or blood vessels, the primary injury is sequenced first with additional code(s) for injuries to nerves and spinal cord (such as category S04), and/or injury to blood vessels (such as category S15). When the primary injury is to the blood vessels or nerves, that injury should be sequenced first.

3) Iatrogenic injuries
Injury codes from Chapter 19 should not be assigned for injuries that occur during, or as a result of, a medical intervention. Assign the appropriate complication code(s).

c. Coding of Traumatic Fractures
The principles of multiple coding of injuries should be followed in coding fractures. Fractures of specified sites are coded individually by site in accordance with both the provisions within categories S02, S12, S22, S32, S42, S49, S52, S59, S62, S72, S79, S82, S89, S92 and the level of detail furnished by medical record content.

A fracture not indicated as open or closed should be coded to closed. A fracture not indicated whether displaced or not displaced should be coded to displaced.

More specific guidelines are as follows:

1) Initial vs. subsequent encounter for fractures
Traumatic fractures are coded using the appropriate 7th character for initial encounter (A, B, C) for each encounter where the patient is receiving active treatment for the fracture. The appropriate 7th character for initial encounter should also be assigned for a patient who delayed seeking treatment for the fracture or nonunion.

Fractures are coded using the appropriate 7th character for subsequent care for encounters after the patient has completed active treatment of the fracture and is receiving routine care for the fracture during the healing or recovery phase.

Care for complications of surgical treatment for fracture repairs during the healing or recovery phase should be coded with the appropriate complication codes.

Care of complications of fractures, such as malunion and nonunion, should be reported with the appropriate 7th character for subsequent care with nonunion (K, M, N,) or subsequent care with malunion (P, Q, R).

Malunion/nonunion: The appropriate 7th character for initial encounter should also be assigned for a patient who delayed seeking treatment for the fracture or nonunion.

The open fracture designations in the assignment of the 7th character for fractures of the forearm, femur and lower leg, including ankle are based on the Gustilo open fracture classification. When the Gustilo classification type is not specified for an open fracture, the 7th character for open fracture type I or II should be assigned (B, E, H, M, Q).

A code from category M80, not a traumatic fracture code, should be used for any patient with known osteoporosis who suffers a fracture, even if the patient had a minor fall or trauma, if that fall or trauma would not usually break a normal, healthy bone.

See Section I.C.13. Osteoporosis.

The aftercare Z codes should not be used for aftercare for traumatic fractures. For aftercare of a traumatic fracture, assign the acute fracture code with the appropriate 7th character.

2) Multiple fractures sequencing
Multiple fractures are sequenced in accordance with the severity of the fracture.

3) Physeal fractures
For physeal fractures, assign only the code identifying the type of physeal fracture. Do not assign a separate code to identify the specific bone that is fractured.

d. Coding of Burns and Corrosions
The ICD-10-CM makes a distinction between burns and corrosions. The burn codes are for thermal burns, except sunburns, that come from a heat source, such as a fire or hot appliance. The burn codes are also for burns resulting from electricity and radiation. Corrosions are burns due to chemicals. The guidelines are the same for burns and corrosions.

Current burns (T20-T25) are classified by depth, extent and by agent (X code). Burns are classified by depth as first degree (erythema), second degree (blistering), and third degree (full-thickness involvement). Burns of the eye and internal organs (T26-T28) are classified by site, but not by degree.

1) Sequencing of burn and related condition codes
Sequence first the code that reflects the highest degree of burn when more than one burn is present.

   a. When the reason for the admission or encounter is for treatment of external multiple burns, sequence first the code that reflects the burn of the highest degree.

   b. When a patient has both internal and external burns, the circumstances of admission govern the selection of the principal diagnosis or first-listed diagnosis.

   c. When a patient is admitted for burn injuries and other related conditions such as smoke inhalation and/or respiratory failure, the circumstances of admission govern the selection of the principal or first-listed diagnosis.

2) Burns of the same anatomic site
Classify burns of the same anatomic site and on the same side but of different degrees to the subcategory identifying the highest degree recorded in the diagnosis (e.g., for second and third degree burns of right thigh, assign only code T24.311-).

3) Non-healing burns
Non-healing burns are coded as acute burns.
Necrosis of burned skin should be coded as a non-healed burn.

4) Infected *burn*
For any documented infected burn site, use an additional code for the infection.

5) Assign separate codes for each burn site
When coding burns, assign separate codes for each burn site. Category T30, Burn and corrosion, body region unspecified is extremely vague and should rarely be used.

Codes for burns of "multiple sites" should only be assigned when the medical record documentation does not specify the individual sites.

6) Burns and corrosions classified according to extent of body surface involved
Assign codes from category T31, Burns classified according to extent of body surface involved, or T32, Corrosions classified according to extent of body surface involved, when the site of the burn is not specified or when there is a need for additional data. It is advisable to use category T31 as additional coding when needed to provide data for evaluating burn mortality, such as that needed by burn units. It is also advisable to use category T31 as an additional code for reporting purposes when there is mention

of a third-degree burn involving 20 percent or more of the body surface.

Categories T31 and T32 are based on the classic "rule of nines" in estimating body surface involved: head and neck are assigned nine percent, each arm nine percent, each leg 18 percent, the anterior trunk 18 percent, posterior trunk 18 percent, and genitalia one percent. Providers may change these percentage assignments where necessary to accommodate infants and children who have proportionately larger heads than adults, and patients who have large buttocks, thighs, or abdomen that involve burns.

7) Encounters for treatment of sequela of burns
Encounters for the treatment of the late effects of burns or corrosions (i.e., scars or joint contractures) should be coded with a burn or corrosion code with the 7th character "S" for sequela.

8) Sequelae with a late effect code and current burn
When appropriate, both a code for a current burn or corrosion with 7th character "A" or "D" and a burn or corrosion code with 7th character "S" may be assigned on the same record (when both a current burn and sequelae of an old burn exist). Burns and corrosions do not heal at the same rate and a current healing wound may still exist with sequela of a healed burn or corrosion.

See Section I.B.10 Sequela (Late Effects)

9) Use of an external cause code with burns and corrosions
An external cause code should be used with burns and corrosions to identify the source and intent of the burn, as well as the place where it occurred.

e. Adverse Effects, Poisoning, Underdosing and Toxic Effects
Codes in categories T36-T65 are combination codes that include the substance that was taken as well as the intent. No additional external cause code is required for poisonings, toxic effects, adverse effects and underdosing codes.

1) Do not code directly from the Table of Drugs
Do not code directly funderdosinrom the Table of Drugs and Chemicals. Always refer back to the Tabular List.

2) Use as many codes as necessary to describe
Use as many codes as necessary to describe completely all drugs, medicinal or biological substances.

3) If the same code would describe the causative agent
If the same code would describe the causative agent for more than one adverse reaction, poisoning, toxic effect or underdosing, assign the code only once.

4) If two or more drugs, medicinal or biological substances
If two or more drugs, medicinal or biological substances are **taken**, code each individually unless a combination code is listed in the Table of Drugs and Chemicals.

If multiple unspecified drugs, medicinal or biological substances were taken, assign the appropriate code from subcategory T50.91, Poisoning by, adverse effect of and underdosing of multiple unspecified drugs, medicaments and biological substances.

5) The occurrence of drug toxicity is classified in ICD-10-CM as follows:

   (a) Adverse Effect
When coding an adverse effect of a drug that has been correctly prescribed and properly administered, assign the appropriate code for the nature of the adverse effect followed by the appropriate code for the adverse effect of the drug (T36-T50). The code for the drug should have a 5th or 6th character "5" (for example T36.0X5-) Examples of the nature of an adverse effect are tachycardia, delirium, gastrointestinal hemorrhaging, vomiting, hypokalemia, hepatitis, renal failure, or respiratory failure.

   (b) Poisoning
When coding a poisoning or reaction to the improper use of a medication (e.g., overdose, wrong substance given or taken in error, wrong route of administration), first assign the appropriate code from categories T36-T50. The poisoning codes have an associated intent as their 5th or 6th character (accidental, intentional self-harm, assault and undetermined. If the intent of the poisoning is unknown or unspecified, code the intent as accidental intent. The undetermined

intent is only for use if the documentation in the record specifies that the intent cannot be determined. Use additional code(s) for all manifestations of poisonings.

If there is also a diagnosis of abuse or dependence of the substance, the abuse or dependence is assigned as an additional code.

Examples of poisoning include:

(i) Error was made in drug prescription
Errors made in drug prescription or in the administration of the drug by provider, nurse, patient, or other person.

(ii) Overdose of a drug intentionally taken
If an overdose of a drug was intentionally taken or administered and resulted in drug toxicity, it would be coded as a poisoning.

(iii) Nonprescribed drug taken with correctly prescribed and properly administered drug
If a nonprescribed drug or medicinal agent was taken in combination with a correctly prescribed and properly administered drug, any drug toxicity or other reaction resulting from the interaction of the two drugs would be classified as a poisoning.

(iv) Interaction of drug(s) and alcohol
When a reaction results from the interaction of a drug(s) and alcohol, this would be classified as poisoning.

See Section I.C.4. if poisoning is the result of insulin pump malfunctions.

(c) Underdosing

Underdosing refers to taking less of a medication than is prescribed by a provider or a manufacturer's instruction. Discontinuing the use of a prescribed medication on the patient's own initiative (not directed by the patient's provider) is also classified as an underdosing. For underdosing, assign the code from categories T36-T50 (fifth or sixth character "6").

Codes for underdosing should never be assigned as principal or first-listed codes. If a patient has a relapse or exacerbation of the medical condition for which the drug is prescribed because of the reduction in dose, then the medical condition itself should be coded.

Noncompliance (Z91.12-, Z91.13- and Z91.14-) or complication of care (Y63.6-Y63.9) codes are to be used with an underdosing code to indicate intent, if known.

(d) Toxic Effects

When a harmful substance is ingested or comes in contact with a person, this is classified as a toxic effect. The toxic effect codes are in categories T51-T65.

Toxic effect codes have an associated intent: accidental, intentional self-harm, assault and undetermined.

f. Adult and child abuse, neglect and other maltreatment

Sequence first the appropriate code from categories T74, Adult and child abuse, neglect and other maltreatment, confirmed) or T76, Adult and child abuse, neglect and other maltreatment, suspected) for abuse, neglect and other maltreatment, followed by any accompanying mental health or injury code(s).

If the documentation in the medical record states abuse or neglect it is coded as confirmed (T74.-). It is coded as suspected if it is documented as suspected (T76.-).

For cases of confirmed abuse or neglect an external cause code from the assault section (X92-Y09) should be added to identify the cause of any physical injuries. A perpetrator code (Y07) should be added when the perpetrator of the abuse is known. For suspected cases of abuse or neglect, do not report external cause or perpetrator code.

If a suspected case of abuse, neglect or mistreatment is ruled out during an encounter code Z04.71, Encounter for examination and observation following alleged physical adult abuse, ruled out, or code Z04.72, Encounter for examination and observation following alleged child physical abuse, ruled out, should be used, not a code from T76.

If a suspected case of alleged rape or sexual abuse is ruled out during an encounter code Z04.41, Encounter for examination and observation following alleged adult rape or code Z04.42, Encounter for examination and observation following alleged child rape, should be used, not a code from T76.

If a suspected case of forced sexual exploitation or forced labor exploitation is ruled out during an encounter, code Z04.81, Encounter

for examination and observation of victim following forced sexual exploitation, or code Z04.82, Encounter for examination and observation of victim following forced labor exploitation, should be used, not a code from T76.

See Section I.C.15. Abuse in a pregnant patient.

g. Complications of care

1) General guidelines for complications of care

(a) Documentation of complications of care

See Section I.B.16. for information on documentation of complications of care.

2) Pain due to medical devices

Pain associated with devices, implants or grafts left in a surgical site (for example painful hip prosthesis) is assigned to the appropriate code(s) found in Chapter 19, Injury, poisoning, and certain other consequences of external causes. Specific codes for pain due to medical devices are found in the T code section of the ICD-10-CM. Use additional code(s) from category G89 to identify acute or chronic pain due to presence of the device, implant or graft (G89.18 or G89.28).

3) Transplant complications

(a) Transplant complications other than kidney

Codes under category T86, Complications of transplanted organs and tissues, are for use for both complications and rejection of transplanted organs. A transplant complication code is only assigned if the complication affects the function of the transplanted organ. Two codes are required to fully describe a transplant complication: the appropriate code from category T86 and a secondary code that identifies the complication.

Pre-existing conditions or conditions that develop after the transplant are not coded as complications unless they affect the function of the transplanted organs.

See I.C.21. for transplant organ removal status

See I.C.2. for malignant neoplasm associated with transplanted organ.

(b) Kidney transplant complications

Patients who have undergone kidney transplant may still have some form of chronic kidney disease (CKD) because the kidney transplant may not fully restore kidney function. Code T86.1- should be assigned for documented complications of a kidney transplant, such as transplant failure or rejection or other transplant complication. Code T86.1- should not be assigned for post kidney transplant patients who have chronic kidney (CKD) unless a transplant complication such as transplant failure or rejection is documented. If the documentation is unclear as to whether the patient has a complication of the transplant, query the provider.

Conditions that affect the function of the transplanted kidney, other than CKD, should be assigned a code from subcategory T86.1, Complications of transplanted organ, Kidney, and a secondary code that identifies the complication.

For patients with CKD following a kidney transplant, but who do not have a complication such as failure or rejection, *see section I.C.14. Chronic kidney disease and kidney transplant status.*

4) Complication codes that include the external cause

As with certain other T codes, some of the complications of care codes have the external cause included in the code. The code includes the nature of the complication as well as the type of procedure that caused the complication. No external cause code indicating the type of procedure is necessary for these codes.

5) Complications of care codes within the body system chapters

Intraoperative and postprocedural complication codes are found within the body system chapters with codes specific to the organs and structures of that body system. These codes should be sequenced first, followed by a code(s) for the specific complication, if applicable.

Complication codes from the body system chapters should be assigned for intraoperative and postprocedural complications (e.g., the appropriate complication code from chapter 9 would be assigned for a vascular intraoperative or postprocedural complication) unless the complication is specifically indexed to a T code in chapter 19.

20. Chapter 20: External Causes of Morbidity (V00-Y99)

The external causes of morbidity codes should never be sequenced as the first-listed or principal diagnosis.

External cause codes are intended to provide data for injury research and evaluation of injury prevention strategies. These codes capture how the injury or health condition happened (cause), the intent (unintentional or accidental; or intentional, such as suicide or assault), the place where the event occurred the activity of the patient at the time of the event, and the person's status (e.g., civilian, military).

There is no national requirement for mandatory ICD-10-CM external cause code reporting. Unless a provider is subject to a state-based external cause code reporting mandate or these codes are required by a particular payer, reporting of ICD-10-CM codes in Chapter 20, External Causes of Morbidity, is not required. In the absence of a mandatory reporting requirement, providers are encouraged to voluntarily report external cause codes, as they provide valuable data for injury research and evaluation of injury prevention strategies.

a. General External Cause Coding Guidelines

1) **Used with any code in the range of A00.0-T88.9 Z00-Z99**
   An external cause code may be used with any code in the range of A00.0-T88.9, Z00-Z99, classification that represents a health condition due to an external cause. Though they are most applicable to injuries, they are also valid for use with such things as infections or diseases due to an external source, and other health conditions, such as a heart attack that occurs during strenuous physical activity.

2) **External cause code used for length of treatment**
   Assign the external cause code, with the appropriate 7th character (initial encounter, subsequent encounter or sequela) for each encounter for which the injury or condition is being treated.
   Most categories in chapter 20 have a 7th character requirement for each applicable code. Most categories in this chapter have three 7th character values: A, initial encounter, D, subsequent encounter and S, sequela. While the patient may be seen by a new or different provider over the course of treatment for an injury or condition, assignment of the 7th character for external cause should match the 7th character of the code assigned for the associated injury or condition for the encounter.

3) **Use the full range of external cause codes**
   Use the full range of external cause codes to completely describe the cause, the intent, the place of occurrence, and if applicable, the activity of the patient at the time of the event, and the patient's status, for all injuries, and other health conditions due to an external cause.

4) **Assign as many external cause codes as necessary**
   Assign as many external cause codes as necessary to fully explain each cause. If only one external code can be recorded, assign the code most related to the principal diagnosis.

5) **The selection of the appropriate external cause code**
   The selection of the appropriate external cause code is guided by the Alphabetic Index of External Causes and by Inclusion and Exclusion notes in the Tabular List.

6) **External cause code can never be a principal diagnosis**
   An external cause code can never be a principal (first-listed) diagnosis.

7) **Combination external cause codes**
   Certain of the external cause codes are combination codes that identify sequential events that result in an injury, such as a fall which results in striking against an object. The injury may be due to either event or both. The combination external cause code used should correspond to the sequence of events regardless of which caused the most serious injury.

8) **No external cause code needed in certain circumstances**
   No external cause code from Chapter 20 is needed if the external cause and intent are included in a code from another chapter (e.g. T36.0X1- Poisoning by penicillins, accidental (unintentional)).

b. Place of Occurrence Guideline

Codes from category Y92, Place of occurrence of the external cause, are secondary codes for use after other external cause codes to identify the location of the patient at the time of injury or other condition.

Generally, a place of occurrence code is assigned only once, at the initial encounter for treatment. However, in the rare instance that a new injury occurs during hospitalization, an additional place of occurrence code may be assigned. No 7th characters are used for Y92.

Do not use place of occurrence code Y92.9 if the place is not stated or is not applicable.

c. Activity Code

Assign a code from category Y93, Activity code, to describe the activity of the patient at the time the injury or other health condition occurred.

An activity code is used only once, at the initial encounter for treatment. Only one code from Y93 should be recorded on a medical record.

The activity codes are not applicable to poisonings, adverse effects, misadventures or sequela.

Do not assign Y93.9, Unspecified activity, if the activity is not stated.

A code from category Y93 is appropriate for use with external cause and intent codes if identifying the activity provides additional information about the event.

d. Place of Occurrence, Activity, and Status Codes Used with other External Cause Code

When applicable, place of occurrence, activity, and external cause status codes are sequenced after the main external cause code(s). Regardless of the number of external cause codes assigned, generally there should be only one place of occurrence code, one activity code, and one external cause status code assigned to an encounter. However, in the rare instance that a new injury occurs during hospitalization, an additional place of occurrence code may be assigned.

e. If the Reporting Format Limits the Number of External Cause Codes

If the reporting format limits the number of external cause codes that can be used in reporting clinical data, report the code for the cause/intent most related to the principal diagnosis. If the format permits capture of additional external cause codes, the cause/intent, including medical misadventures, of the additional events should be reported rather than the codes for place, activity, or external status.

f. Multiple External Cause Coding Guidelines

More than one external cause code is required to fully describe the external cause of an illness or injury. The assignment of external cause codes should be sequenced in the following priority:

If two or more events cause separate injuries, an external cause code should be assigned for each cause. The first-listed external cause code will be selected in the following order:

External codes for child and adult abuse take priority over all other external cause codes.

See Section I.C.19., Child and Adult abuse guidelines.

External cause codes for terrorism events take priority over all other external cause codes except child and adult abuse.

External cause codes for cataclysmic events take priority over all other external cause codes except child and adult abuse and terrorism.

External cause codes for transport accidents take priority over all other external cause codes except cataclysmic events, child and adult abuse and terrorism.

Activity and external cause status codes are assigned following all causal (intent) external cause codes.

The first-listed external cause code should correspond to the cause of the most serious diagnosis due to an assault, accident, or self-harm, following the order of hierarchy listed above.

g. Child and Adult Abuse Guideline

Adult and child abuse, neglect and maltreatment are classified as assault. Any of the assault codes may be used to indicate the external cause of any injury resulting from the confirmed abuse.

For confirmed cases of abuse, neglect and maltreatment, when the perpetrator is known, a code from Y07, Perpetrator of maltreatment and neglect, should accompany any other assault codes.

See Section I.C.19. Adult and child abuse, neglect and other maltreatment

h. Unknown or Undetermined Intent Guideline

If the intent (accident, self-harm, assault) of the cause of an injury or other condition is unknown or unspecified, code the intent as accidental intent. All transport accident categories assume accidental intent.

2020 ICD-10-CM Official Guidelines for Coding and Reporting

1) **Use of undetermined intent**
External cause codes for events of undetermined intent are only for use if the documentation in the record specifies that the intent cannot be determined.

i. **Sequelae (Late Effects) of External Cause Guidelines**
1) **Sequelae external cause codes**
Sequela are reported using the external cause code with the 7th character "S" for sequela. These codes should be used with any report of a late effect or sequela resulting from a previous injury.
See Section I.B.10 Sequela (Late Effects)

2) **Sequela external cause code with a related current injury**
A sequela external cause code should never be used with a related current nature of injury code.

3) **Use of sequela external cause codes for subsequent visits**
Use a late effect external cause code for subsequent visits when a late effect of the initial injury is being treated. Do not use a late effect external cause code for subsequent visits for follow-up care (e.g., to assess healing, to receive rehabilitative therapy) of the injury when no late effect of the injury has been documented.

j. **Terrorism Guidelines**
1) **Cause of injury identified by the Federal Government (FBI) as terrorism**
When the cause of an injury is identified by the Federal Government (FBI) as terrorism, the first-listed external cause code should be a code from category Y38, Terrorism. The definition of terrorism employed by the FBI is found at the inclusion note at the beginning of category Y38. Use additional code for place of occurrence (Y92.-). More than one Y38 code may be assigned if the injury is the result of more than one mechanism of terrorism.

2) **Cause of an injury is suspected to be the result of terrorism**
When the cause of an injury is suspected to be the result of terrorism a code from category Y38 should not be assigned. Suspected cases should be classified as assault.

3) **Code Y38.9, Terrorism, secondary effects**
Assign code Y38.9, Terrorism, secondary effects, for conditions occurring subsequent to the terrorist event. This code should not be assigned for conditions that are due to the initial terrorist act.

It is acceptable to assign code Y38.9 with another code from Y38 if there is an injury due to the initial terrorist event and an injury that is a subsequent result of the terrorist event.

k. **External Cause Status**
A code from category Y99, External cause status, should be assigned whenever any other external cause code is assigned for an encounter, including an Activity code, except for the events noted below. Assign a code from category Y99, External cause status, to indicate the work status of the person at the time the event occurred. The status code indicates whether the event occurred during military activity, whether a non-military person was at work, whether an individual including a student or volunteer was involved in a non-work activity at the time of the causal event.

A code from Y99, External cause status, should be assigned, when applicable, with other external cause codes, such as transport accidents and falls. The external cause status codes are not applicable to poisonings, adverse effects, misadventures or late effects.

Do not assign a code from category Y99 if no other external cause codes (cause, activity) are applicable for the encounter.

An external cause status code is used only once, at the initial encounter for treatment. Only one code from Y99 should be recorded on a medical record.

Do not assign code Y99.9, Unspecified external cause status, if the status is not stated.

21. **Chapter 21: Factors influencing health status and contact with health services (Z00-Z99)**
Note: The chapter specific guidelines provide additional information about the use of Z codes for specified encounters.

a. **Use of Z Codes in Any Healthcare Setting**
Z codes are for use in any healthcare setting. Z codes may be used as either a first-listed (principal diagnosis code in the inpatient setting) or secondary code, depending on the circumstances of the encounter. Certain Z codes may only be used as first-listed or principal diagnosis.

b. **Z Codes Indicate a Reason for an Encounter**
Z codes are not procedure codes. A corresponding procedure code must accompany a Z code to describe any procedure performed.

c. **Categories of Z Codes**
1) **Contact/Exposure**
Category Z20 indicates contact with, and suspected exposure to, communicable diseases. These codes are for patients who do not show any sign or symptom of a disease but are suspected to have been exposed to it by close personal contact with an infected individual or are in an area where a disease is epidemic.

Category Z77, Other contact with and (suspected) exposures hazardous to health, indicates contact with and suspected exposures hazardous to health.

Contact/exposure codes may be used as a first-listed code to explain an encounter for testing, or, more commonly, as a secondary code to identify a potential risk.

2) **Inoculations and vaccinations**
Code Z23 is for encounters for inoculations and vaccinations. It indicates that a patient is being seen to receive a prophylactic inoculation against a disease. Procedure codes are required to identify the actual administration of the injection and the type(s) of immunizations given. Code Z23 may be used as a secondary code if the inoculation is given as a routine part of preventive health care, such as a well-baby visit.

3) **Status**
Status codes indicate that a patient is either a carrier of a disease or has the sequelae or residual of a past disease or condition. This includes such things as the presence of prosthetic or mechanical devices resulting from past treatment. A status code is informative, because the status may affect the course of treatment and its outcome. A status code is distinct from a history code. The history code indicates that the patient no longer has the condition.

A status code should not be used with a diagnosis code from one of the body system chapters, if the diagnosis code includes the information provided by the status code. For example, code Z94.1, Heart transplant status, should not be used with a code from subcategory T86.2, Complications of heart transplant. The status code does not provide additional information. The complication code indicates that the patient is a heart transplant patient.

For encounters for weaning from a mechanical ventilator, assign a code from subcategory J96.1, Chronic respiratory failure, followed by code Z99.11, Dependence on respirator [ventilator] status.

The status Z codes/categories are:

Z14   Genetic carrier

Genetic carrier status indicates that a person carries a gene, associated with a particular disease, which may be passed to offspring who may develop that disease. The person does not have the disease and is not at risk of developing the disease.

Z15   Genetic susceptibility to disease

Genetic susceptibility indicates that a person has a gene that increases the risk of that person developing the disease.

Codes from category Z15 should not be used as principal or first-listed codes. If the patient has the condition to which he/she is susceptible, and that condition is the reason for the encounter, the code for the current condition should be sequenced first. If the patient is being seen for follow-up after completed treatment for this condition, and the condition no longer exists, a follow-up code should be sequenced first, followed by the appropriate personal history and genetic susceptibility codes. If the purpose of the encounter is genetic counseling associated with procreative management, code Z31.5, Encounter for genetic counseling, should be assigned as the first-listed code, followed by a code from category Z15. Additional codes should be assigned for any applicable family or personal history.

Z16   Resistance to antimicrobial drugs

This code indicates that a patient has a condition that is resistant to antimicrobial drug treatment. Sequence the infection code first.

Z17   Estrogen receptor status

Z18   Retained foreign body fragments

Z19   Hormone sensitivity malignancy status

Z21   Asymptomatic HIV infection status

This code indicates that a patient has tested positive for HIV but has manifested no signs or symptoms of the disease.

Z22   Carrier of infectious disease

Carrier status indicates that a person harbors the specific organisms of a disease without manifest symptoms and is capable of transmitting the infection.

Z28.3   Underimmunization status

Z33.1   Pregnant state, incidental

This code is a secondary code only for use when the pregnancy is in no way complicating the reason for visit. Otherwise, a code from the obstetric chapter is required.

Z66   Do not resuscitate

This code may be used when it is documented by the provider that a patient is on do not resuscitate status at any time during the stay.

Z67   Blood type

Z68   Body mass index (BMI)

BMI codes should only be assigned when **there is an associated, reportable diagnosis (such as obesity).** Do not assign BMI codes during pregnancy.

See Section I.B.14 for BMI documentation by clinicians other than the patient's provider.

Z74.Ø1   Bed confinement status

Z76.82   Awaiting organ transplant status

Z78   Other specified health status

Code Z78.1, Physical restraint status, may be used when it is documented by the provider that a patient has been put in restraints during the current encounter. Please note that this code should not be reported when it is documented by the provider that a patient is temporarily restrained during a procedure.

Z79   Long-term (current) drug therapy

Codes from this category indicate a patient's continuous use of a prescribed drug (including such things as aspirin therapy) for the long-term treatment of a condition or for prophylactic use. It is not for use for patients who have addictions to drugs. This subcategory is not for use of medications for detoxification or maintenance programs to prevent withdrawal symptoms in patients with drug dependence (e.g., methadone maintenance for opiate dependence). Assign the appropriate code for the drug dependence instead.

Assign a code from Z79 if the patient is receiving a medication for an extended period as a prophylactic measure (such as for the prevention of deep vein thrombosis) or as treatment of a chronic condition (such as arthritis) or a disease requiring a lengthy course of treatment (such as cancer). Do not assign a code from category Z79 for medication being administered for a brief period of time to treat an acute illness or injury (such as a course of antibiotics to treat acute bronchitis).

Z88   Allergy status to drugs, medicaments and biological substances

Except: Z88.9, Allergy status to unspecified drugs, medicaments and biological substances status

Z89   Acquired absence of limb

Z9Ø   Acquired absence of organs, not elsewhere classified

Z91.Ø-   Allergy status, other than to drugs and biological substances

Z92.82   Status post administration of tPA (rtPA) in a different facility within the last 24 hours prior to admission to a current facility

Assign code Z92.82, Status post administration of tPA (rtPA) in a different facility within the last 24 hours prior to admission to current facility, as a secondary diagnosis when a patient is received by transfer into a facility and documentation indicates they were administered tissue plasminogen activator (tPA) within the last 24 hours prior to admission to the current facility.

This guideline applies even if the patient is still receiving the tPA at the time they are received into the current facility.

The appropriate code for the condition for which the tPA was administered (such as cerebrovascular disease or myocardial infarction) should be assigned first.

Code Z92.82 is only applicable to the receiving facility record and not to the transferring facility record.

Z93   Artificial opening status

Z94   Transplanted organ and tissue status

Z95   Presence of cardiac and vascular implants and grafts

Z96   Presence of other functional implants

Z97   Presence of other devices

Z98   Other postprocedural states

Assign code Z98.85, Transplanted organ removal status, to indicate that a transplanted organ has been previously removed. This code should not be assigned for the encounter in which the transplanted organ is removed. The complication necessitating removal of the transplant organ should be assigned for that encounter.

See section I.C19. for information on the coding of organ transplant complications.

Z99   Dependence on enabling machines and devices, not elsewhere classified

Note: Categories Z89-Z9Ø and Z93-Z99 are for use only if there are no complications or malfunctions of the organ or tissue replaced, the amputation site or the equipment on which the patient is dependent.

4)   History (of)

There are two types of history Z codes, personal and family. Personal history codes explain a patient's past medical condition that no longer exists and is not receiving any treatment, but that has the potential for recurrence, and therefore may require continued monitoring.

Family history codes are for use when a patient has a family member(s) who has had a particular disease that causes the patient to be at higher risk of also contracting the disease.

Personal history codes may be used in conjunction with follow-up codes and family history codes may be used in conjunction with screening codes to explain the need for a test or procedure. History codes are also acceptable on any medical record regardless of the reason for visit. A history of an illness, even if no longer present, is important information that may alter the type of treatment ordered.

The history Z code categories are:

Z8Ø   Family history of primary malignant neoplasm

Z81   Family history of mental and behavioral disorders

Z82   Family history of certain disabilities and chronic diseases (leading to disablement)

Z83   Family history of other specific disorders

Z84   Family history of other conditions

Z85   Personal history of malignant neoplasm

Z86   Personal history of certain other diseases

Z87   Personal history of other diseases and conditions

Z91.4-   Personal history of psychological trauma, not elsewhere classified

Z91.5   Personal history of self-harm

Z91.81 History of falling

Z91.82 Personal history of military deployment

Z92   Personal history of medical treatment

Except: Z92.Ø, Personal history of contraception

Except: Z92.82, Status post administration of tPA (rtPA) in a different facility within the last 24 hours prior to admission to a current facility

5)   Screening

Screening is the testing for disease or disease precursors in seemingly well individuals so that early detection and treatment can be provided for those who test positive for the disease (e.g., screening mammogram).

The testing of a person to rule out or confirm a suspected diagnosis because the patient has some sign or symptom is a diagnostic examination, not a screening. In these cases, the sign or symptom is used to explain the reason for the test.

A screening code may be a first-listed code if the reason for the visit is specifically the screening exam. It may also be used as an additional code if the screening is done during an office visit for other health problems. A screening code is not necessary if the screening is inherent to a routine examination, such as a pap smear done during a routine pelvic examination.

Should a condition be discovered during the screening then the code for the condition may be assigned as an additional diagnosis.

The Z code indicates that a screening exam is planned. A procedure code is required to confirm that the screening was performed.

The screening Z codes/categories:

Z11 Encounter for screening for infectious and parasitic diseases

Z12 Encounter for screening for malignant neoplasms

Z13 Encounter for screening for other diseases and disorders
     Except: Z13.9, Encounter for screening, unspecified

Z36 Encounter for antenatal screening for mother

6) Observation

There are three observation Z code categories. They are for use in very limited circumstances when a person is being observed for a suspected condition that is ruled out. The observation codes are not for use if an injury or illness or any signs or symptoms related to the suspected condition are present. In such cases the diagnosis/symptom code is used with the corresponding external cause code.

The observation codes are to be used as principal diagnosis only. The only exception to this is when the principal diagnosis is required to be a code from category Z38, Liveborn infants according to place of birth and type of delivery. Then a code from category Z05, Encounter for observation and evaluation of newborn for suspected diseases and conditions ruled out, is sequenced after the Z38 code. Additional codes may be used in addition to the observation code, but only if they are unrelated to the suspected condition being observed.

Codes from subcategory Z03.7, Encounter for suspected maternal and fetal conditions ruled out, may either be used as a first-listed or as an additional code assignment depending on the case. They are for use in very limited circumstances on a maternal record when an encounter is for a suspected maternal or fetal condition that is ruled out during that encounter (for example, a maternal or fetal condition may be suspected due to an abnormal test result). These codes should not be used when the condition is confirmed. In those cases, the confirmed condition should be coded. In addition, these codes are not for use if an illness or any signs or symptoms related to the suspected condition or problem are present. In such cases the diagnosis/symptom code is used.

Additional codes may be used in addition to the code from subcategory Z03.7, but only if they are unrelated to the suspected condition being evaluated.

Codes from subcategory Z03.7 may not be used for encounters for antenatal screening of mother. *See Section I.C.21. Screening.*

For encounters for suspected fetal condition that are inconclusive following testing and evaluation, assign the appropriate code from category O35, O36, O40 or O41.

The observation Z code categories:

Z03 Encounter for medical observation for suspected diseases and conditions ruled out

Z04 Encounter for examination and observation for other reasons
     Except: Z04.9, Encounter for examination and observation for unspecified reason

Z05 Encounter for observation and evaluation of newborn for suspected diseases and conditions ruled out

7) Aftercare

Aftercare visit codes cover situations when the initial treatment of a disease has been performed and the patient requires continued care during the healing or recovery phase, or for the long-term consequences of the disease. The aftercare Z code should not be used if treatment is directed at a current, acute disease. The diagnosis code is to be used in these cases. Exceptions to this rule are codes Z51.0, Encounter for antineoplastic radiation therapy, and codes from subcategory Z51.1, Encounter for antineoplastic chemotherapy and immunotherapy. These codes are to be first-listed, followed by the diagnosis code when a patient's encounter is solely to receive radiation therapy, chemotherapy, or immunotherapy for the treatment of a neoplasm. If the reason for the encounter is more than one type of antineoplastic therapy, code Z51.0 and a code from subcategory Z51.1 may be assigned together, in which case one of these codes would be reported as a secondary diagnosis.

The aftercare Z codes should also not be used for aftercare for injuries. For aftercare of an injury, assign the acute injury code with the appropriate 7th character (for subsequent encounter).

The aftercare codes are generally first-listed to explain the specific reason for the encounter. An aftercare code may be used as an additional code when some type of aftercare is provided in addition to the reason for admission and no diagnosis code is applicable. An example of this would be the closure of a colostomy during an encounter for treatment of another condition.

Aftercare codes should be used in conjunction with other aftercare codes or diagnosis codes to provide better detail on the specifics of an aftercare encounter visit, unless otherwise directed by the classification. The sequencing of multiple aftercare codes depends on the circumstances of the encounter.

Certain aftercare Z code categories need a secondary diagnosis code to describe the resolving condition or sequelae. For others, the condition is included in the code title.

Additional Z code aftercare category terms include fitting and adjustment, and attention to artificial openings.

Status Z codes may be used with aftercare Z codes to indicate the nature of the aftercare. For example, code Z95.1, Presence of aortocoronary bypass graft, may be used with code Z48.812, Encounter for surgical aftercare following surgery on the circulatory system, to indicate the surgery for which the aftercare is being performed. A status code should not be used when the aftercare code indicates the type of status, such as using Z43.0, Encounter for attention to tracheostomy, with Z93.0, Tracheostomy status.

The aftercare Z category/codes:

Z42 Encounter for plastic and reconstructive surgery following medical procedure or healed injury

Z43 Encounter for attention to artificial openings

Z44 Encounter for fitting and adjustment of external prosthetic device

Z45 Encounter for adjustment and management of implanted device

Z46 Encounter for fitting and adjustment of other devices

Z47 Orthopedic aftercare

Z48 Encounter for other postprocedural aftercare

Z49 Encounter for care involving renal dialysis

Z51 Encounter for other aftercare and medical care

8) Follow-up

The follow-up codes are used to explain continuing surveillance following completed treatment of a disease, condition, or injury. They imply that the condition has been fully treated and no longer exists. They should not be confused with aftercare codes, or injury codes with a 7th character for subsequent encounter, that explain ongoing care of a healing condition or its sequelae. Follow-up codes may be used in conjunction with history codes to provide the full picture of the healed condition and its treatment. The follow-up code is sequenced first, followed by the history code.

A follow-up code may be used to explain multiple visits. Should a condition be found to have recurred on the follow-up visit, then the diagnosis code for the condition should be assigned in place of the follow-up code.

The follow-up Z code categories:

Z08   Encounter for follow-up examination after completed treatment for malignant neoplasm

Z09   Encounter for follow-up examination after completed treatment for conditions other than malignant neoplasm

Z39   Encounter for maternal postpartum care and examination

9) **Donor**

Codes in category Z52, Donors of organs and tissues, are used for living individuals who are donating blood or other body tissue. These codes are only for individuals donating for others, not for self-donations. They are not used to identify cadaveric donations.

10) **Counseling**

Counseling Z codes are used when a patient or family member receives assistance in the aftermath of an illness or injury, or when support is required in coping with family or social problems.

The counseling Z codes/categories:

Z30.0-   Encounter for general counseling and advice on contraception

Z31.5   Encounter for procreative genetic counseling

Z31.6-   Encounter for general counseling and advice on procreation

Z32.2   Encounter for childbirth instruction

Z32.3   Encounter for childcare instruction

Z69   Encounter for mental health services for victim and perpetrator of abuse

Z70   Counseling related to sexual attitude, behavior and orientation

Z71   Persons encountering health services for other counseling and medical advice, not elsewhere classified

Note: Code Z71.84, Encounter for health counseling related to travel, is to be used for health risk and safety counseling for future travel purposes.

Z76.81   Expectant mother prebirth pediatrician visit

11) **Encounters for Obstetrical and Reproductive Services**
See Section I.C.15. Pregnancy, Childbirth, and the Puerperium, for further instruction on the use of these codes.

Z codes for pregnancy are for use in those circumstances when none of the problems or complications included in the codes from the Obstetrics chapter exist (a routine prenatal visit or postpartum care). Codes in category Z34, Encounter for supervision of normal pregnancy, are always first-listed and are not to be used with any other code from the OB chapter.

Codes in category Z3A, Weeks of gestation, may be assigned to provide additional information about the pregnancy. Category Z3A codes should not be assigned for pregnancies with abortive outcomes (categories O00-O08), elective termination of pregnancy (code Z33.2), nor for postpartum conditions, as category Z3A is not applicable to these conditions. The date of the admission should be used to determine weeks of gestation for inpatient admissions that encompass more than one gestational week.

The outcome of delivery, category Z37, should be included on all maternal delivery records. It is always a secondary code. Codes in category Z37 should not be used on the newborn record.

Z codes for family planning (contraceptive) or procreative management and counseling should be included on an obstetric record either during the pregnancy or the postpartum stage, if applicable.

Z codes/categories for obstetrical and reproductive services:

Z30   Encounter for contraceptive management

Z31   Encounter for procreative management

Z32.2   Encounter for childbirth instruction

Z32.3   Encounter for childcare instruction

Z33   Pregnant state

Z34   Encounter for supervision of normal pregnancy

Z36   Encounter for antenatal screening of mother

Z3A   Weeks of gestation

Z37   Outcome of delivery

Z39   Encounter for maternal postpartum care and examination

Z76.81   Expectant mother prebirth pediatrician visit

12) **Newborns and Infants**
See Section I.C.16. Newborn (Perinatal) Guidelines, for further instruction on the use of these codes.

Newborn Z codes/categories:

Z76.1   Encounter for health supervision and care of foundling

Z00.1-   Encounter for routine child health examination

Z38   Liveborn infants according to place of birth and type of delivery

13) **Routine and Administrative Examinations**

The Z codes allow for the description of encounters for routine examinations, such as, a general check-up, or, examinations for administrative purposes, such as, a pre-employment physical. The codes are not to be used if the examination is for diagnosis of a suspected condition or for treatment purposes. In such cases the diagnosis code is used. During a routine exam, should a diagnosis or condition be discovered, it should be coded as an additional code. Pre-existing and chronic conditions and history codes may also be included as additional codes as long as the examination is for administrative purposes and not focused on any particular condition.

Some of the codes for routine health examinations distinguish between "with" and "without" abnormal findings. Code assignment depends on the information that is known at the time the encounter is being coded. For example, if no abnormal findings were found during the examination, but the encounter is being coded before test results are back, it is acceptable to assign the code for "without abnormal findings." When assigning a code for "with abnormal findings," additional code(s) should be assigned to identify the specific abnormal finding(s).

Pre-operative examination and pre-procedural laboratory examination Z codes are for use only in those situations when a patient is being cleared for a procedure or surgery and no treatment is given.

The Z codes/categories for routine and administrative examinations:

Z00   Encounter for general examination without complaint, suspected or reported diagnosis

Z01   Encounter for other special examination without complaint, suspected or reported diagnosis

Z02   Encounter for administrative examination
Except: Z02.9, Encounter for administrative examinations, unspecified

Z32.0-   Encounter for pregnancy test

14) **Miscellaneous Z *Codes***

The miscellaneous Z codes capture a number of other health care encounters that do not fall into one of the other categories. Certain of these codes identify the reason for the encounter; others are for use as additional codes that provide useful information on circumstances that may affect a patient's care and treatment.

Prophylactic Organ Removal

For encounters specifically for prophylactic removal of an organ (such as prophylactic removal of breasts due to a genetic susceptibility to cancer or a family history of cancer), the principal or first-listed code should be a code from category Z40, Encounter for prophylactic surgery, followed by the appropriate codes to identify the associated risk factor (such as genetic susceptibility or family history).

If the patient has a malignancy of one site and is having prophylactic removal at another site to prevent either a new primary malignancy or metastatic disease, a code for the malignancy should also be assigned in addition to a code from subcategory Z40.0, Encounter for prophylactic surgery for risk factors related to malignant neoplasms. A Z40.0 code should not be assigned if the patient is having organ removal for treatment of a malignancy, such as the removal of the testes for the treatment of prostate cancer.

Miscellaneous Z codes/categories:

Z28	Immunization not carried out
	Except: Z28.3, Underimmunization status
Z29	Encounter for other prophylactic measures
Z40	Encounter for prophylactic surgery
Z41	Encounter for procedures for purposes other than remedying health state
	Except: Z41.9, Encounter for procedure for purposes other than remedying health state, unspecified
Z53	Persons encountering health services for specific procedures and treatment, not carried out
Z55	Problems related to education and literacy
Z56	Problems related to employment and unemployment
Z57	Occupational exposure to risk factors
Z58	Problems related to physical environment
Z59	Problems related to housing and economic circumstances
Z60	Problems related to social environment
Z62	Problems related to upbringing
Z63	Other problems related to primary support group, including family circumstances
Z64	Problems related to certain psychosocial circumstances
Z65	Problems related to other psychosocial circumstances
Z72	Problems related to lifestyle
	Note: These codes should be assigned only when the documentation specifies that the patient has an associated problem
Z73	Problems related to life management difficulty
Z74	Problems related to care provider dependency
	Except: Z74.01, Bed confinement status
Z75	Problems related to medical facilities and other health care
Z76.0	Encounter for issue of repeat prescription
Z76.3	Healthy person accompanying sick person
Z76.4	Other boarder to healthcare facility
Z76.5	Malingerer [conscious simulation]
Z91.1-	Patient's noncompliance with medical treatment and regimen
Z91.83	Wandering in diseases classified elsewhere
Z91.84-	Oral health risk factors
Z91.89	Other specified personal risk factors, not elsewhere classified

See Section I.B.14 for Z55-Z65 Persons with potential health hazards related to socioeconomic and psychosocial circumstances, documentation by clinicians other than the patient's provider.

15) Nonspecific Z *Codes*

Certain Z codes are so non-specific, or potentially redundant with other codes in the classification, that there can be little justification for their use in the inpatient setting. Their use in the outpatient setting should be limited to those instances when there is no further documentation to permit more precise coding. Otherwise, any sign or symptom or any other reason for visit that is captured in another code should be used.

Nonspecific Z codes/categories:

Z02.9	Encounter for administrative examinations, unspecified
Z04.9	Encounter for examination and observation for unspecified reason
Z13.9	Encounter for screening, unspecified
Z41.9	Encounter for procedure for purposes other than remedying health state, unspecified
Z52.9	Donor of unspecified organ or tissue
Z86.59	Personal history of other mental and behavioral disorders
Z88.9	Allergy status to unspecified drugs, medicaments and biological substances status
Z92.0	Personal history of contraception

16) Z Codes That May Only be Principal/First-Listed Diagnosis

The following Z codes/categories may only be reported as the principal/first-listed diagnosis, except when there are multiple encounters on the same day and the medical records for the encounters are combined:

Z00	Encounter for general examination without complaint, suspected or reported diagnosis
	Except: Z00.6
Z01	Encounter for other special examination without complaint, suspected or reported diagnosis
Z02	Encounter for administrative examination
Z03	Encounter for medical observation for suspected diseases and conditions ruled out
Z04	Encounter for examination and observation for other reasons
Z33.2	Encounter for elective termination of pregnancy
Z31.81	Encounter for male factor infertility in female patient
Z31.83	Encounter for assisted reproductive fertility procedure cycle
Z31.84	Encounter for fertility preservation procedure
Z34	Encounter for supervision of normal pregnancy
Z39	Encounter for maternal postpartum care and examination
Z38	Liveborn infants according to place of birth and type of delivery
Z40	Encounter for prophylactic surgery
Z42	Encounter for plastic and reconstructive surgery following medical procedure or healed injury
Z51.0	Encounter for antineoplastic radiation therapy
Z51.1-	Encounter for antineoplastic chemotherapy and immunotherapy
Z52	Donors of organs and tissues
	Except: Z52.9, Donor of unspecified organ or tissue
Z76.1	Encounter for health supervision and care of foundling
Z76.2	Encounter for health supervision and care of other healthy infant and child
Z99.12	Encounter for respirator [ventilator] dependence during power failure

Section II. Selection of Principal Diagnosis

The circumstances of inpatient admission always govern the selection of principal diagnosis. The principal diagnosis is defined in the Uniform Hospital Discharge Data Set (UHDDS) as "that condition established after study to be chiefly responsible for occasioning the admission of the patient to the hospital for care."

The UHDDS definitions are used by hospitals to report inpatient data elements in a standardized manner. These data elements and their definitions can be found in the July 31, 1985, Federal Register (Vol. 50, No, 147), pp. 31038-40.

Since that time the application of the UHDDS definitions has been expanded to include all non-outpatient settings (acute care, short term, long term care and psychiatric hospitals; home health agencies; rehab facilities; nursing homes, etc). The UHDDS definitions also apply to hospice services (all levels of care).

In determining principal diagnosis, coding conventions in the ICD-10-CM, the Tabular List and Alphabetic Index take precedence over these official coding guidelines.

(See Section I.A., Conventions for the ICD-10-CM)

The importance of consistent, complete documentation in the medical record cannot be overemphasized. Without such documentation the application of all coding guidelines is a difficult, if not impossible, task.

A. Codes for symptoms, signs, and ill-defined conditions

Codes for symptoms, signs, and ill-defined conditions from Chapter 18 are not to be used as principal diagnosis when a related definitive diagnosis has been established.

B. Two or more interrelated conditions, each potentially meeting the definition for principal diagnosis.

When there are two or more interrelated conditions (such as diseases in the same ICD-10-CM chapter or manifestations characteristically associated with a certain disease) potentially meeting the definition of principal diagnosis, either condition may be sequenced first, unless the circumstances of the admission, the therapy provided, the Tabular List, or the Alphabetic Index indicate otherwise.

C. Two or more diagnoses that equally meet the definition for principal diagnosis

In the unusual instance when two or more diagnoses equally meet the criteria for principal diagnosis as determined by the circumstances of admission, diagnostic workup and/or therapy provided, and the Alphabetic Index, Tabular List, or another coding guidelines does not provide sequencing direction, any one of the diagnoses may be sequenced first.

D. Two or more comparative or contrasting conditions

In those rare instances when two or more contrasting or comparative diagnoses are documented as "either/or" (or similar terminology), they are coded as if the diagnoses were confirmed and the diagnoses are sequenced according to the circumstances of the admission. If no further determination can be made as to which diagnosis should be principal, either diagnosis may be sequenced first.

E. A symptom(s) followed by contrasting/comparative diagnoses

GUIDELINE HAS BEEN DELETED EFFECTIVE OCTOBER 1, 2014

F. Original treatment plan not carried out

Sequence as the principal diagnosis the condition, which after study occasioned the admission to the hospital, even though treatment may not have been carried out due to unforeseen circumstances.

G. Complications of surgery and other medical care

When the admission is for treatment of a complication resulting from surgery or other medical care, the complication code is sequenced as the principal diagnosis. If the complication is classified to the T80-T88 series and the code lacks the necessary specificity in describing the complication, an additional code for the specific complication should be assigned.

H. Uncertain Diagnosis

If the diagnosis documented at the time of discharge is qualified as "probable," "suspected," "likely," "questionable," "possible," or "still to be ruled out," **"compatible with," "consistent with,"** or other similar terms indicating uncertainty, code the condition as if it existed or was established. The bases for these guidelines are the diagnostic workup, arrangements for further workup or observation, and initial therapeutic approach that correspond most closely with the established diagnosis.

Note: This guideline is applicable only to inpatient admissions to short-term, acute, long-term care and psychiatric hospitals.

I. Admission from Observation Unit

1. Admission Following Medical Observation

When a patient is admitted to an observation unit for a medical condition, which either worsens or does not improve, and is subsequently admitted as an inpatient of the same hospital for this same medical condition, the principal diagnosis would be the medical condition which led to the hospital admission.

2. Admission Following Post-Operative Observation

When a patient is admitted to an observation unit to monitor a condition (or complication) that develops following outpatient surgery, and then is subsequently admitted as an inpatient of the same hospital, hospitals should apply the Uniform Hospital Discharge Data Set (UHDDS) definition of principal diagnosis as "that condition established after study to be chiefly responsible for occasioning the admission of the patient to the hospital for care."

J. Admission from Outpatient Surgery

When a patient receives surgery in the hospital's outpatient surgery department and is subsequently admitted for continuing inpatient care at the same hospital, the following guidelines should be followed in selecting the principal diagnosis for the inpatient admission:

- If the reason for the inpatient admission is a complication, assign the complication as the principal diagnosis.
- If no complication, or other condition, is documented as the reason for the inpatient admission, assign the reason for the outpatient surgery as the principal diagnosis.
- If the reason for the inpatient admission is another condition unrelated to the surgery, assign the unrelated condition as the principal diagnosis.

K. Admissions/Encounters for Rehabilitation

When the purpose for the admission/encounter is rehabilitation, sequence first the code for the condition for which the service is being performed. For example, for an admission/encounter for rehabilitation for right-sided dominant hemiplegia following a cerebrovascular infarction, report code I69.351, Hemiplegia and hemiparesis following cerebral infarction affecting right dominant side, as the first-listed or principal diagnosis.

If the condition for which the rehabilitation service is being provided is no longer present, report the appropriate aftercare code as the first-listed or principal diagnosis, unless the rehabilitation service is being provided following an injury. For rehabilitation services following active treatment of an injury, assign the injury code with the appropriate seventh character for subsequent encounter as the first-listed or principal diagnosis. For example, if a patient with severe degenerative osteoarthritis of the hip, underwent hip replacement and the current encounter/admission is for rehabilitation, report code Z47.1, Aftercare following joint replacement surgery, as the first-listed or principal diagnosis. If the patient requires rehabilitation post hip replacement for right intertrochanteric femur fracture, report code S72.141D, Displaced intertrochanteric fracture of right femur, subsequent encounter for closed fracture with routine healing, as the first-listed or principal diagnosis.

See Section I.C.21.c.7, Factors influencing health states and contact with health services, Aftercare.

See Section I.C.19.a for additional information about the use of 7th characters for injury codes.

Section III. Reporting Additional Diagnoses

GENERAL RULES FOR OTHER (ADDITIONAL) DIAGNOSES

For reporting purposes the definition for "other diagnoses" is interpreted as additional conditions that affect patient care in terms of requiring:

> clinical evaluation; or
> therapeutic treatment; or
> diagnostic procedures; or
> extended length of hospital stay; or
> increased nursing care and/or monitoring.

The UHDDS item #11-b defines Other Diagnoses as "all conditions that coexist at the time of admission, that develop subsequently, or that affect the treatment received and/or the length of stay. Diagnoses that relate to an earlier episode which have no bearing on the current hospital stay are to be excluded." UHDDS definitions apply to inpatients in acute care, short-term, long term care and psychiatric hospital setting. The UHDDS definitions are used by acute care short-term hospitals to report inpatient data elements in a standardized manner. These data elements and their definitions can be found in the July 31, 1985, Federal Register (Vol. 50, No, 147), pp. 31038-40.

Since that time the application of the UHDDS definitions has been expanded to include all non-outpatient settings (acute care, short term, long term care and psychiatric hospitals; home health agencies; rehab facilities; nursing homes, etc). The UHDDS definitions also apply to hospice services (all levels of care).

The following guidelines are to be applied in designating "other diagnoses" when neither the Alphabetic Index nor the Tabular List in ICD-10-CM provide direction. The listing of the diagnoses in the patient record is the responsibility of the attending provider.

A. Previous conditions

If the provider has included a diagnosis in the final diagnostic statement, such as the discharge summary or the face sheet, it should ordinarily be coded. Some providers include in the diagnostic statement resolved conditions or diagnoses and status-post procedures from previous admission that have no bearing on the current stay. Such conditions are not to be reported and are coded only if required by hospital policy.

However, history codes (categories Z80-Z87) may be used as secondary codes if the historical condition or family history has an impact on current care or influences treatment.

B. Abnormal findings

Abnormal findings (laboratory, x-ray, pathologic, and other diagnostic results) are not coded and reported unless the provider indicates their clinical significance. If the findings are outside the normal range and the attending provider has ordered other tests to evaluate the condition or prescribed treatment, it is appropriate to ask the provider whether the abnormal finding should be added.

Please note: This differs from the coding practices in the outpatient setting for coding encounters for diagnostic tests that have been interpreted by a provider.

C. Uncertain Diagnosis

If the diagnosis documented at the time of discharge is qualified as "probable," "suspected," "likely," "questionable," "possible," or "still to be ruled out," **"compatible with," "consistent with,"** or other similar terms indicating uncertainty, code the condition as if it existed or was established. The bases for these guidelines are the diagnostic workup, arrangements for further workup or observation, and initial therapeutic approach that correspond most closely with the established diagnosis.

Note: This guideline is applicable only to inpatient admissions to short-term, acute, long-term care and psychiatric hospitals.

Section IV.Diagnostic Coding and Reporting Guidelines for Outpatient Services

These coding guidelines for outpatient diagnoses have been approved for use by hospitals/ providers in coding and reporting hospital-based outpatient services and provider-based office visits. Guidelines in Section I, Conventions, general coding guidelines and chapter-specific guidelines, should also be applied for outpatient services and office visits.

Information about the use of certain abbreviations, punctuation, symbols, and other conventions used in the ICD-10-CM Tabular List (code numbers and titles), can be found in Section IA of these guidelines, under "Conventions Used in the Tabular List." Section I.B. contains general guidelines that apply to the entire classification. Section I.C. contains chapter-specific guidelines that correspond to the chapters as they are arranged in the classification. Information about the correct sequence to use in finding a code is also described in Section I.

The terms encounter and visit are often used interchangeably in describing outpatient service contacts and, therefore, appear together in these guidelines without distinguishing one from the other.

Though the conventions and general guidelines apply to all settings, coding guidelines for outpatient and provider reporting of diagnoses will vary in a number of instances from those for inpatient diagnoses, recognizing that:

The Uniform Hospital Discharge Data Set (UHDDS) definition of principal diagnosis does not apply to hospital-based outpatient services and provider-based office visits.

Coding guidelines for inconclusive diagnoses (probable, suspected, rule out, etc.) were developed for inpatient reporting and do not apply to outpatients.

A. Selection of first-listed condition

In the outpatient setting, the term first-listed diagnosis is used in lieu of principal diagnosis.

In determining the first-listed diagnosis the coding conventions of ICD-10-CM, as well as the general and disease specific guidelines take precedence over the outpatient guidelines.

Diagnoses often are not established at the time of the initial encounter/visit. It may take two or more visits before the diagnosis is confirmed.

The most critical rule involves beginning the search for the correct code assignment through the Alphabetic Index. Never begin searching initially in the Tabular List as this will lead to coding errors.

1. Outpatient Surgery

When a patient presents for outpatient surgery (same day surgery), code the reason for the surgery as the first-listed diagnosis (reason for the encounter), even if the surgery is not performed due to a contraindication.

2. Observation Stay

When a patient is admitted for observation for a medical condition, assign a code for the medical condition as the first-listed diagnosis.

When a patient presents for outpatient surgery and develops complications requiring admission to observation, code the reason for the surgery as the first reported diagnosis (reason for the encounter), followed by codes for the complications as secondary diagnoses.

B. Codes from A00.0 through T88.9, Z00-Z99

The appropriate code(s) from A00.0 through T88.9, Z00-Z99 must be used to identify diagnoses, symptoms, conditions, problems, complaints, or other reason(s) for the encounter/visit.

C. Accurate reporting of ICD-10-CM diagnosis codes

For accurate reporting of ICD-10-CM diagnosis codes, the documentation should describe the patient's condition, using terminology which includes specific diagnoses as well as symptoms, problems, or reasons for the encounter. There are ICD-10-CM codes to describe all of these.

D. Codes that describe symptoms and signs

Codes that describe symptoms and signs, as opposed to diagnoses, are acceptable for reporting purposes when a diagnosis has not been established (confirmed) by the provider. Chapter 18 of ICD-10-CM, Symptoms, Signs, and Abnormal Clinical and Laboratory Findings Not Elsewhere Classified (codes R00-R99) contain many, but not all codes for symptoms.

E. Encounters for circumstances other than a disease or injury

ICD-10-CM provides codes to deal with encounters for circumstances other than a disease or injury. The Factors Influencing Health Status and Contact with Health Services codes (Z00-Z99) are provided to deal with occasions when circumstances other than a disease or injury are recorded as diagnosis or problems.

See Section I.C.21. Factors influencing health status and contact with health services.

F. Level of Detail in Coding

1. ICD-10-CM codes with 3, 4, 5, 6 or 7 characters

ICD-10-CM is composed of codes with 3, 4, 5, 6 or 7 characters. Codes with three characters are included in ICD-10-CM as the heading of a category of codes that may be further subdivided by the use of fourth, fifth, sixth or seventh characters to provide greater specificity.

2. Use of full number of characters required for a code

A three-character code is to be used only if it is not further subdivided. A code is invalid if it has not been coded to the full number of characters required for that code, including the 7th character, if applicable.

G. ICD-10-CM code for the diagnosis, condition, problem, or other reason for encounter/visit

List first the ICD-10-CM code for the diagnosis, condition, problem, or other reason for encounter/visit shown in the medical record to be chiefly responsible for the services provided. List additional codes that describe any coexisting conditions. In some cases the first-listed diagnosis may be a symptom when a diagnosis has not been established (confirmed) by the **provider**.

H. Uncertain diagnosis

Do not code diagnoses documented as "probable", "suspected," "questionable," "rule out," **"compatible with," "consistent with,"** or "working diagnosis" or other similar terms indicating uncertainty. Rather, code the condition(s) to the highest degree of certainty for that encounter/visit, such as symptoms, signs, abnormal test results, or other reason for the visit.

Please note: This differs from the coding practices used by short-term, acute care, long-term care and psychiatric hospitals.

I. Chronic diseases

Chronic diseases treated on an ongoing basis may be coded and reported as many times as the patient receives treatment and care for the condition(s)

J. Code all documented conditions that coexist

Code all documented conditions that coexist at the time of the encounter/visit, and require or affect patient care treatment or management. Do not code conditions that were previously treated and no longer exist. However, history codes (categories Z80-Z87) may be used as secondary codes if the historical condition or family history has an impact on current care or influences treatment.

K. Patients receiving diagnostic services only

For patients receiving diagnostic services only during an encounter/visit, sequence first the diagnosis, condition, problem, or other reason for encounter/visit shown in the medical record to be chiefly responsible for the outpatient services provided during the encounter/visit. Codes for other diagnoses (e.g., chronic conditions) may be sequenced as additional diagnoses.

For encounters for routine laboratory/radiology testing in the absence of any signs, symptoms, or associated diagnosis, assign Z01.89, Encounter for other specified special examinations. If routine testing is performed during the same encounter as a test to evaluate a sign, symptom, or diagnosis, it is appropriate to assign both the Z code and the code describing the reason for the non-routine test.

For outpatient encounters for diagnostic tests that have been interpreted by a physician, and the final report is available at the time of coding, code any confirmed or definitive diagnosis(es) documented in the interpretation. Do not code related signs and symptoms as additional diagnoses.

Please note: This differs from the coding practice in the hospital inpatient setting regarding abnormal findings on test results.

L. Patients receiving therapeutic services only

For patients receiving therapeutic services only during an encounter/visit, sequence first the diagnosis, condition, problem, or other reason for encounter/visit shown in the medical record to be chiefly responsible for the outpatient services provided during the encounter/visit. Codes for other diagnoses (e.g., chronic conditions) may be sequenced as additional diagnoses.

The only exception to this rule is that when the primary reason for the admission/encounter is chemotherapy or radiation therapy, the appropriate Z code for the service is listed first, and the diagnosis or problem for which the service is being performed listed second.

M. Patients receiving preoperative evaluations only
For patients receiving preoperative evaluations only, sequence first a code from subcategory Z01.81, Encounter for pre-procedural examinations, to describe the pre-op consultations. Assign a code for the condition to describe the reason for the surgery as an additional diagnosis. Code also any findings related to the pre-op evaluation.

N. Ambulatory surgery
For ambulatory surgery, code the diagnosis for which the surgery was performed. If the postoperative diagnosis is known to be different from the preoperative diagnosis at the time the diagnosis is confirmed, select the postoperative diagnosis for coding, since it is the most definitive.

O. Routine outpatient prenatal visits
See Section I.C.15. Routine outpatient prenatal visits.

P. Encounters for general medical examinations with abnormal findings
The subcategories for encounters for general medical examinations, Z00.0- and encounter for routine child health examination, Z00.12-, provide codes for with and without abnormal findings. Should a general medical examination result in an abnormal finding, the code for general medical examination with abnormal finding should be assigned as the first-listed diagnosis. An examination with abnormal findings refers to a condition/diagnosis that is newly identified or a change in severity of a chronic condition (such as uncontrolled hypertension, or an acute exacerbation of chronic obstructive pulmonary disease) during a routine physical examination. A secondary code for the abnormal finding should also be coded.

Q. Encounters for routine health screenings
See Section I.C.21. Factors influencing health status and contact with health services, Screening

Appendix I. Present on Admission Reporting Guidelines

Introduction
These guidelines are to be used as a supplement to the *ICD-10-CM Official Guidelines for Coding and Reporting* to facilitate the assignment of the Present on Admission (POA) indicator for each diagnosis and external cause of injury code reported on claim forms (UB-04 and 837 Institutional).

These guidelines are not intended to replace any guidelines in the main body of the *ICD-10-CM Official Guidelines for Coding and Reporting*. The POA guidelines are not intended to provide guidance on when a condition should be coded, but rather, how to apply the POA indicator to the final set of diagnosis codes that have been assigned in accordance with Sections I, II, and III of the official coding guidelines. Subsequent to the assignment of the ICD-10-CM codes, the POA indicator should then be assigned to those conditions that have been coded.

As stated in the Introduction to the *ICD-10-CM Official Guidelines for Coding and Reporting,* a joint effort between the healthcare provider and the coder is essential to achieve complete and accurate documentation, code assignment, and reporting of diagnoses and procedures. The importance of consistent, complete documentation in the medical record cannot be overemphasized. Medical record documentation from any provider involved in the care and treatment of the patient may be used to support the determination of whether a condition was present on admission or not. In the context of the official coding guidelines, the term "provider" means a physician or any qualified healthcare practitioner who is legally accountable for establishing the patient's diagnosis.

These guidelines are not a substitute for the provider's clinical judgment as to the determination of whether a condition was/was not present on admission. The provider should be queried regarding issues related to the linking of signs/symptoms, timing of test results, and the timing of findings.

Please see the CDC website for the detailed list of ICD-10-CM codes that do not require the use of a POA indicator (https://www.cdc.gov/nchs/icd/icd10cm.htm). The codes and categories on this exempt list are for circumstances regarding the healthcare encounter or factors influencing health status that do not represent a current disease or injury or that describe conditions that are always present on admission.

General Reporting Requirements
All claims involving inpatient admissions to general acute care hospitals or other facilities that are subject to a law or regulation mandating collection of present on admission information

Present on admission is defined as present at the time the order for inpatient admission occurs -- conditions that develop during an outpatient encounter, including emergency department, observation, or outpatient surgery, are considered as present on admission.

POA indicator is assigned to principal and secondary diagnoses (as defined in Section II of the Official Guidelines for Coding and Reporting) and the external cause of injury codes.

Issues related to inconsistent, missing, conflicting or unclear documentation must still be resolved by the provider.

If a condition would not be coded and reported based on UHDDS definitions and current official coding guidelines, then the POA indicator would not be reported.

Reporting Options
    Y - Yes
    N - No
    U - Unknown
    W – Clinically undetermined
    Unreported/Not used – (Exempt from POA reporting)

Reporting Definitions
    Y = present at the time of inpatient admission
    N = not present at the time of inpatient admission
    U = documentation is insufficient to determine if condition is present on admission
    W = provider is unable to clinically determine whether condition was present on admission or not

Timeframe for POA Identification and Documentation
There is no required timeframe as to when a provider (per the definition of "provider" used in these guidelines) must identify or document a condition to be present on admission. In some clinical situations, it may not be possible for a provider to make a definitive diagnosis (or a condition may not be recognized or reported by the patient) for a period of time after admission. In some cases it may be several days before the provider arrives at a definitive diagnosis. This does not mean that the condition was not present on admission. Determination of whether the condition was present on admission or not will be based on the applicable POA guideline as identified in this document, or on the provider's best clinical judgment.

If at the time of code assignment the documentation is unclear as to whether a condition was present on admission or not, it is appropriate to query the provider for clarification.

Assigning the POA Indicator
Condition is on the "Exempt from Reporting" list
    Leave the "present on admission" field blank if the condition is on the list of ICD-10-CM codes for which this field is not applicable. This is the only circumstance in which the field may be left blank.

POA Explicitly Documented
    Assign Y for any condition the provider explicitly documents as being present on admission.
    Assign N for any condition the provider explicitly documents as not present at the time of admission.

Conditions diagnosed prior to inpatient admission
    Assign "Y" for conditions that were diagnosed prior to admission (example: hypertension, diabetes mellitus, asthma)

Conditions diagnosed during the admission but clearly present before admission
    Assign "Y" for conditions diagnosed during the admission that were clearly present but not diagnosed until after admission occurred.
    Diagnoses subsequently confirmed after admission are considered present on admission if at the time of admission they are documented as suspected, possible, rule out, differential diagnosis, or constitute an underlying cause of a symptom that is present at the time of admission.

Condition develops during outpatient encounter prior to inpatient admission
    Assign Y for any condition that develops during an outpatient encounter prior to a written order for inpatient admission.

Documentation does not indicate whether condition was present on admission
    Assign "U" when the medical record documentation is unclear as to whether the condition was present on admission. "U" should not be routinely assigned and used only in very limited circumstances. Coders are encouraged to query the providers when the documentation is unclear.

Documentation states that it cannot be determined whether the condition was or was not present on admission

Assign "W" when the medical record documentation indicates that it cannot be clinically determined whether or not the condition was present on admission.

Chronic condition with acute exacerbation during the admission

If a single code identifies both the chronic condition and the acute exacerbation, see POA guidelines pertaining to codes that contain multiple clinical concepts.

If a single code only identifies the chronic condition and not the acute exacerbation (e.g., acute exacerbation of chronic leukemia), assign "Y."

Conditions documented as possible, probable, suspected, or rule out at the time of discharge

If the final diagnosis contains a possible, probable, suspected, or rule out diagnosis, and this diagnosis was based on signs, symptoms or clinical findings suspected at the time of inpatient admission, assign "Y."

If the final diagnosis contains a possible, probable, suspected, or rule out diagnosis, and this diagnosis was based on signs, symptoms or clinical findings that were not present on admission, assign "N".

Conditions documented as impending or threatened at the time of discharge

If the final diagnosis contains an impending or threatened diagnosis, and this diagnosis is based on symptoms or clinical findings that were present on admission, assign "Y".

If the final diagnosis contains an impending or threatened diagnosis, and this diagnosis is based on symptoms or clinical findings that were not present on admission, assign "N".

Acute and Chronic Conditions

Assign "Y" for acute conditions that are present at time of admission and N for acute conditions that are not present at time of admission.

Assign "Y" for chronic conditions, even though the condition may not be diagnosed until after admission.

If a single code identifies both an acute and chronic condition, see the POA guidelines for codes that contain multiple clinical concepts.

Codes That Contain Multiple Clinical Concepts

Assign "N" if at least one of the clinical concepts included in the code was not present on admission (e.g., COPD with acute exacerbation and the exacerbation was not present on admission; gastric ulcer that does not start bleeding until after admission; asthma patient develops status asthmaticus after admission).

Assign "Y" if all of the clinical concepts included in the code were present on admission (e.g., duodenal ulcer that perforates prior to admission).

For infection codes that include the causal organism, assign "Y" if the infection (or signs of the infection) were present on admission, even though the culture results may not be known until after admission (e.g., patient is admitted with pneumonia and the provider documents Pseudomonas as the causal organism a few days later).

Same Diagnosis Code for Two or More Conditions

When the same ICD-10-CM diagnosis code applies to two or more conditions during the same encounter (e.g. two separate conditions classified to the same ICD-10-CM diagnosis code):

Assign "Y" if all conditions represented by the single ICD-10-CM code were present on admission (e.g. bilateral unspecified age-related cataracts).

Assign "N" if any of the conditions represented by the single ICD-10-CM code was not present on admission (e.g. traumatic secondary and recurrent hemorrhage and seroma is assigned to a single code T79.2, but only one of the conditions was present on admission).

Obstetrical conditions

Whether or not the patient delivers during the current hospitalization does not affect assignment of the POA indicator. The determining factor for POA assignment is whether the pregnancy complication or obstetrical condition described by the code was present at the time of admission or not.

If the pregnancy complication or obstetrical condition was present on admission (e.g., patient admitted in preterm labor), assign "Y".

If the pregnancy complication or obstetrical condition was not present on admission (e.g., 2nd degree laceration during delivery, postpartum hemorrhage that occurred during current hospitalization, fetal distress develops after admission), assign "N".

If the obstetrical code includes more than one diagnosis and any of the diagnoses identified by the code were not present on admission assign "N". (e.g., Category O11, Pre-existing hypertension with pre-eclampsia)

Perinatal conditions

Newborns are not considered to be admitted until after birth. Therefore, any condition present at birth or that developed in utero is considered present at admission and should be assigned "Y". This includes conditions that occur during delivery (e.g., injury during delivery, meconium aspiration, exposure to streptococcus B in the vaginal canal).

Congenital conditions and anomalies

Assign "Y" for congenital conditions and anomalies except for categories Q00-Q99, Congenital anomalies, which are on the exempt list. Congenital conditions are always considered present on admission.

External cause of injury codes

Assign "Y" for any external cause code representing an external cause of morbidity that occurred prior to inpatient admission (e.g., patient fell out of bed at home, patient fell out of bed in emergency room prior to admission)

Assign "N" for any external cause code representing an external cause of morbidity that occurred during inpatient hospitalization (e.g., patient fell out of hospital bed during hospital stay, patient experienced an adverse reaction to a medication administered after inpatient admission).

ICD-10-CM Index to Diseases and Injuries

A

Aarskog's syndrome Q87.19
Abandonment — *see* Maltreatment
Abasia (-astasia) (hysterical) F44.4
Abderhalden-Kaufmann-Lignac syndrome (cystinosis) E72.04
Abdomen, abdominal — *see also* condition
  muscle deficiency syndrome Q79.4
  angina K55.1
  acute R10.0
Abdominalgia — *see* Pain, abdominal
Abduction contracture, hip or other joint — *see*
  Contraction, joint
Aberrant (congenital) — *see also* Malposition, congenital
  hepatic duct Q44.5
  endocrine gland NEC Q89.2
  breast Q83.8
  artery (peripheral) Q27.8
    basilar NEC Q28.1
    cerebral Q28.3
    coronary Q24.5
    digestive system Q27.8
    eye Q15.8
    lower limb Q27.8
    precerebral Q28.1
    pulmonary Q25.79
    renal Q27.2
    retina Q14.1
    specified site NEC Q27.8
    subclavian Q27.8
    upper limb Q27.8
    vertebral Q28.1
  adrenal gland Q89.1
  pancreas Q45.3
  parathyroid gland Q89.2
  pituitary gland Q89.2
  sebaceous glands, mucous membrane, mouth, congenital Q38.6
  spleen Q89.09
  subclavian artery Q27.8
  thymus (gland) Q89.2
  thyroid gland Q89.2
  vein (peripheral) NEC Q27.8
    cerebral Q28.3
    digestive system Q27.8
    lower limb Q27.8
    precerebral Q28.1
    specified site NEC Q27.8
    upper limb Q27.8
Aberration
  distantial — *see* Disturbance, visual
  mental F99
Abetalipoproteinemia E78.6
Abiotrophy R68.89
Ablatio, ablation
  retinae — *see* Detachment, retina
Ablepharia, ablepharon Q10.3
Abnormal, abnormality, abnormalities — *see also*
  Anomaly
  acid-base balance (mixed) E87.4
  albumin R77.0
  alphafetoprotein R77.2
  alveolar ridge K08.9
  anatomical relationship Q89.9
  apertures, congenital, diaphragm Q79.1
  auditory perception H93.29- ☑
    diplacusis — *see* Diplacusis
    hyperacusis — *see* Hyperacusis
    recruitment — *see* Recruitment, auditory
    threshold shift — *see* Shift, auditory threshold
  autosomes Q99.9
    fragile site Q95.5
  basal metabolic rate R94.8
  biosynthesis, testicular androgen E29.1
  bleeding time R79.1
  blood level (of)
    cobalt R79.0
    copper R79.0
    iron R79.0
    lithium R78.89
    magnesium R79.0

Abnormal, abnormality, abnormalities — *continued*
  blood level — *continued*
    mineral NEC R79.0
    zinc R79.0
  blood pressure
    elevated R03.0
    low reading (nonspecific) R03.1
  blood sugar R73.09
  blood-gas level R79.81
  bowel sounds R19.15
    absent R19.11
    hyperactive R19.12
  brain scan R94.02
  breathing R06.9
  caloric test R94.138
  cerebrospinal fluid R83.9
    cytology R83.6
    drug level R83.2
    enzyme level R83.0
    hormones R83.1
    immunology R83.4
    microbiology R83.5
    nonmedicinal level R83.3
    specified type NEC R83.8
  chemistry, blood R79.9
    C-reactive protein R79.82
    drugs — *see* Findings, abnormal, in blood
    gas level R79.81
    minerals R79.0
    pancytopenia D61.818
    PTT R79.1
    specified NEC R79.89
    toxins — *see* Findings, abnormal, in blood
  chest sounds (friction) (rales) R09.89
  chromosome, chromosomal Q99.9
    with more than three X chromosomes, female Q97.1
    analysis result R89.8
      bronchial washings R84.8
      cerebrospinal fluid R83.8
      cervix uteri NEC R87.89
      nasal secretions R84.8
      nipple discharge R89.8
      peritoneal fluid R85.89
      pleural fluid R84.8
      prostatic secretions R86.8
      saliva R85.89
      seminal fluid R86.8
      sputum R84.8
      synovial fluid R89.8
      throat scrapings R84.8
      vagina R87.89
      vulva R87.89
      wound secretions R89.8
    dicentric replacement Q93.2
    ring replacement Q93.2
    sex Q99.8
      female phenotype Q97.9
        specified NEC Q97.8
      male phenotype Q98.9
        specified NEC Q98.8
      structural male Q98.6
    specified NEC Q99.8
  clinical findings NEC R68.89
  coagulation D68.9
    newborn, transient P61.6
    profile R79.1
    time R79.1
  communication — *see* Fistula
  conjunctiva, vascular H11.41- ☑
  coronary artery Q24.5
  cortisol-binding globulin E27.8
  course, eustachian tube Q17.8
  creatinine clearance R94.4
  cytology
    anus R85.619
      atypical squamous cells cannot exclude high grade squamous intraepithelial lesion (ASC-H) R85.611
      atypical squamous cells of undetermined significance (ASC-US) R85.610
      cytologic evidence of malignancy R85.614

Abnormal, abnormality, abnormalities — *continued*
  cytology — *continued*
    anus — *continued*
      high grade squamous intraepithelial lesion (HGSIL) R85.613
      human papillomavirus (HPV) DNA test
        high risk positive R85.81
        low risk postive R85.82
      inadequate smear R85.615
      low grade squamous intraepithelial lesion (LGSIL) R85.612
      satisfactory anal smear but lacking transformation zone R85.616
      specified NEC R85.618
      unsatisfactory smear R85.615
    female genital organs — *see* Abnormal, Papanicolaou (smear)
  dark adaptation curve H53.61
  dentofacial NEC — *see* Anomaly, dentofacial
  development, developmental Q89.9
    central nervous system Q07.9
  diagnostic imaging
    abdomen, abdominal region NEC R93.5
    biliary tract R93.2
    bladder R93.41
    breast R92.8
    central nervous system NEC R90.89
    cerebrovascular NEC R90.89
    coronary circulation R93.1
    digestive tract NEC R93.3
    gastrointestinal (tract) R93.3
    genitourinary organs R93.89
    head R93.0
    heart R93.1
    intrathoracic organ NEC R93.89
    kidney R93.42- ☑
    limbs R93.6
    liver R93.2
    lung (field) R91.8
    musculoskeletal system NEC R93.7
    renal pelvis R93.41
    retroperitoneum R93.5
    site specified NEC R93.89
    skin and subcutaneous tissue R93.89
    skull R93.0
    testis R93.81- ☑
    ureter R93.41
    urinary organs specified NEC R93.49
  direction, teeth, fully erupted M26.30
  ear ossicles, acquired NEC H74.39- ☑
    ankylosis — *see* Ankylosis, ear ossicles
    discontinuity — *see* Discontinuity, ossicles, ear
    partial loss — *see* Loss, ossicles, ear (partial)
  Ebstein Q22.5
  echocardiogram R93.1
  echoencephalogram R90.81
  echogram — *see* Abnormal, diagnostic imaging
  electrocardiogram [ECG] [EKG] R94.31
  electroencephalogram [EEG] R94.01
  electrolyte — *see* Imbalance, electrolyte
  electromyogram [EMG] R94.131
  electro-oculogram [EOG] R94.110
  electrophysiological intracardiac studies R94.39
  electroretinogram [ERG] R94.111
  erythrocytes
    congenital, with perinatal jaundice D58.9
  feces (color) (contents) (mucus) R19.5
  finding — *see* Findings, abnormal, without diagnosis
  fluid
    amniotic — *see* Abnormal, specimen, specified
    cerebrospinal — *see* Abnormal, cerebrospinal fluid
    peritoneal — *see* Abnormal, specimen, digestive organs
    pleural — *see* Abnormal, specimen, respiratory organs
    synovial — *see* Abnormal, specimen, specified
    thorax (bronchial washings) (pleural fluid) — *see* Abnormal, specimen, respiratory organs
    vaginal — *see* Abnormal, specimen, female genital organs
  form
    teeth K00.2

Abnormal, abnormality, abnormalities —
    continued
  form — *continued*
    uterus — *see* Anomaly, uterus
  function studies
    auditory R94.120
    bladder R94.8
    brain R94.09
    cardiovascular R94.30
    ear R94.128
    endocrine NEC R94.7
    eye NEC R94.118
    kidney R94.4
    liver R94.5
    nervous system
      central NEC R94.09
      peripheral NEC R94.138
    pancreas R94.8
    placenta R94.8
    pulmonary R94.2
    special senses NEC R94.128
    spleen R94.8
    thyroid R94.6
    vestibular R94.121
  gait — *see* Gait
    hysterical F44.4
  gastrin secretion E16.4
  globulin R77.1
    cortisol-binding E27.8
    thyroid-binding E07.89
  glomerular, minor — *see also* N00-N07 with fourth
    character .0 N05.0
  glucagon secretion E16.3
  glucose tolerance (test) (non-fasting) R73.09
  gravitational (G) forces or states (effect of) T75.81 ☑
  hair (color) (shaft) L67.9
    specified NEC L67.8
  hard tissue formation in pulp (dental) K04.3
  head movement R25.0
  heart
    rate R00.9
      ·specified NEC R00.8
    shadow R93.1
    sounds NEC R01.2
  hemoglobin (disease) — *see also* Disease, hemoglobin
    D58.2
    trait — *see* Trait, hemoglobin, abnormal
  histology NEC R89.7
  immunological findings R89.4
    in serum R76.9
      specified NEC R76.8
  increase in appetite R63.2
  involuntary movement — *see* Abnormal, movement,
    involuntary
  jaw closure M26.51
  karyotype R89.8
  kidney function test R94.4
  knee jerk R29.2
  leukocyte (cell) (differential) NEC D72.9
  liver function test R94.5
  loss of
    height R29.890
    weight R63.4
  mammogram NEC R92.8
    calcification (calculus) R92.1
    microcalcification R92.0
  Mantoux test R76.11
  movement (disorder) — *see also* Disorder, movement
    head R25.0
    involuntary R25.9
      fasciculation R25.3
      of head R25.0
      spasm R25.2
      specified type NEC R25.8
      tremor R25.1
  myoglobin (Aberdeen) (Annapolis) R89.7
  neonatal screening P09
  oculomotor study R94.113
  palmar creases Q82.8
  Papanicolaou (smear)
    anus R85.619
      atypical squamous cells cannot exclude high
        grade squamous intraepithelial lesion
        (ASC-H) R85.611
      atypical squamous cells of undetermined signif-
        icance (ASC-US) R85.610
      cytologic evidence of malignancy R85.614

Abnormal, abnormality, abnormalities —
    continued
  Papanicolaou — *continued*
    anus — *continued*
      high grade squamous intraepithelial lesion
        (HGSIL) R85.613
      human papillomavirus (HPV) DNA test
        high risk positive R85.81
        low risk postive R85.82
      inadequate smear R85.615
      low grade squamous intraepithelial lesion (LGSIL)
        R85.612
      satisfactory anal smear but lacking transforma-
        tion zone R85.616
      specified NEC R85.618
      unsatisfactory smear R85.615
    bronchial washings R84.6
    cerebrospinal fluid R83.6
    cervix R87.619
      atypical squamous cells cannot exclude high
        grade squamous intraepithelial lesion
        (ASC-H) R87.611
      atypical squamous cells of undetermined signif-
        icance (ASC-US) R87.610
      cytologic evidence of malignancy R87.614
      high grade squamous intraepithelial lesion
        (HGSIL) R87.613
      inadequate smear R87.615
      low grade squamous intraepithelial lesion (LGSIL)
        R87.612
      non-atypical endometrial cells R87.618
      satisfactory cervical smear but lacking transfor-
        mation zone R87.616
      specified NEC R87.618
      thin preparaton R87.619
      unsatisfactory smear R87.615
    nasal secretions R84.6
    nipple discharge R89.6
    peritoneal fluid R85.69
    pleural fluid R84.6
    prostatic secretions R86.6
    saliva R85.69
    seminal fluid R86.6
    sites NEC R89.6
    sputum R84.6
    synovial fluid R89.6
    throat scrapings R84.6
    vagina R87.629
      atypical squamous cells cannot exclude high
        grade squamous intraepithelial lesion
        (ASC-H) R87.621
      atypical squamous cells of undetermined signif-
        icance (ASC-US) R87.620
      cytologic evidence of malignancy R87.624
      high grade squamous intraepithelial lesion
        (HGSIL) R87.623
      inadequate smear R87.625
      low grade squamous intraepithelial lesion (LGSIL)
        R87.622
      specified NEC R87.628
      thin preparation R87.629
      unsatisfactory smear R87.625
    vulva R87.69
    wound secretions R89.6
  partial thromboplastin time (PTT) R79.1
  pelvis (bony) — *see* Deformity, pelvis
  percussion, chest (tympany) R09.89
  periods (grossly) — *see* Menstruation
  phonocardiogram R94.39
  plantar reflex R29.2
  plasma
    protein R77.9
      specified NEC R77.8
    viscosity R70.1
  pleural (folds) Q34.0
  posture R29.3
  product of conception O02.9
    specified type NEC O02.89
  prothrombin time (PT) R79.1
  pulmonary
    artery, congenital Q25.79
    function, newborn P28.89
    test results R94.2
  pulsations in neck R00.2
  pupillary H21.56- ☑
    function (reaction) (reflex) — *see* Anomaly, pupil,
      function
  radiological examination — *see* Abnormal, diagnostic
    imaging

Abnormal, abnormality, abnormalities —
    continued
  red blood cell(s) (morphology) (volume) R71.8
  reflex — *see* Reflex
  renal function test R94.4
  response to nerve stimulation R94.130
  retinal correspondence H53.31
  retinal function study R94.111
  rhythm, heart — *see also* Arrhythmia
  saliva — *see* Abnormal, specimen, digestive organs
  scan
    kidney R94.4
    liver R93.2
    thyroid R94.6
  secretion
    gastrin E16.4
    glucagon E16.3
  semen, seminal fluid — *see* Abnormal, specimen, male
    genital organs
  serum level (of)
    acid phosphatase R74.8
    alkaline phosphatase R74.8
    amylase R74.8
    enzymes R74.9
      specified NEC R74.8
    lipase R74.8
    triacylglycerol lipase R74.8
  shape
    gravid uterus — *see* Anomaly, uterus
  sinus venosus Q21.1
  size, tooth, teeth K00.2
  spacing, tooth, teeth, fully erupted M26.30
  specimen
    digestive organs (peritoneal fluid) (saliva) R85.9
      cytology R85.69
      drug level R85.2
      enzyme level R85.0
      histology R85.7
      hormones R85.1
      immunology R85.4
      microbiology R85.5
      nonmedicinal level R85.3
      specified type NEC R85.89
    female genital organs (secretions) (smears) R87.9
      cytology R87.69
        cervix R87.619
          human papillomavirus (HPV) DNA test
            high risk positive R87.810
            low risk positive R87.820
          inadequate (unsatisfactory) smear
            R87.615
          non-atypical endometrial cells R87.618
          specified NEC R87.618
        vagina R87.629
          human papillomavirus (HPV) DNA test
            high risk positive R87.811
            low risk positive R87.821
          inadequate (unsatisfactory) smear
            R87.625
        vulva R87.69
      drug level R87.2
      enzyme level R87.0
      histological R87.7
      hormones R87.1
      immunology R87.4
      microbiology R87.5
      nonmedicinal level R87.3
      specified type NEC R87.89
    male genital organs (prostatic secretions) (semen)
      R86.9
      cytology R86.6
      drug level R86.2
      enzyme level R86.0
      histological R86.7
      hormones R86.1
      immunology R86.4
      microbiology R86.5
      nonmedicinal level R86.3
      specified type NEC R86.8
    nipple discharge — *see* Abnormal, specimen, spec-
      ified
    respiratory organs (bronchial washings) (nasal secre-
      tions) (pleural fluid) (sputum) R84.9
      cytology R84.6
      drug level R84.2
      enzyme level R84.0
      histology R84.7
      hormones R84.1
      immunology R84.4

Abnormal, abnormality, abnormalities —
  continued
  specimen — *continued*
    respiratory organs — *continued*
      microbiology R84.5
      nonmedicinal level R84.3
      specified type NEC R84.8
    specified organ, system and tissue NOS R89.9
      cytology R89.6
      drug level R89.2
      enzyme level R89.0
      histology R89.7
      hormones R89.1
      immunology R89.4
      microbiology R89.5
      nonmedicinal level R89.3
      specified type NEC R89.8
    synovial fluid — *see* Abnormal, specimen, specified
    thorax (bronchial washings) (pleural fluids) — *see*
      Abnormal, specimen, respiratory organs
    vagina (secretion) (smear) R87.629
    vulva (secretion) (smear) R87.69
    wound secretion — *see* Abnormal, specimen,
      specified
  spermatozoa — *see* Abnormal, specimen, male genital
    organs
  sputum (amount) (color) (odor) R09.3
  stool (color) (contents) (mucus) R19.5
    bloody K92.1
    guaiac positive R19.5
  synchondrosis Q78.8
  thermography — *see also* Abnormal, diagnostic
    imaging R93.89
  thyroid-binding globulin E07.89
  tooth, teeth (form) (size) K00.2
  toxicology (findings) R78.9
  transport protein E88.09
  tumor marker NEC R97.8
  ultrasound results — *see* Abnormal, diagnostic imaging
  umbilical cord complicating delivery O69.9 ☑
  urination NEC R39.198
  urine (constituents) R82.90
    bile R82.2
    cytological examination R82.89
    drugs R82.5
    fat R82.0
    glucose R81
    heavy metals R82.6
    hemoglobin R82.3
    histological examination R82.89
    ketones R82.4
    microbiological examination (culture) R82.79
    myoglobin R82.1
    positive culture R82.79
    protein — *see* Proteinuria
    specified substance NEC R82.998
      chromoabnormality NEC R82.91
    substances nonmedical R82.6
  uterine hemorrhage — *see* Hemorrhage, uterus
  vectorcardiogram R94.39
  visually evoked potential (VEP) R94.112
  white blood cells D72.9
    specified NEC D72.89
  X-ray examination — *see* Abnormal, diagnostic imaging
Abnormity (any organ or part) — *see* Anomaly
Abocclusion M26.29
  hemolytic disease (newborn) P55.1
  incompatibility reaction ABO — *see* Complication(s),
    transfusion, incompatibility reaction, ABO
Abolition, language R48.8
Aborter, habitual or recurrent — *see* Loss (of), pregnancy, recurrent
Abortion (complete) (spontaneous) O03.9
  with
    retained products of conception — *see* Abortion,
      incomplete
  attempted (elective) (failed) O07.4
    complicated by O07.30
      afibrinogenemia O07.1
      cardiac arrest O07.36
      chemical damage of pelvic organ(s) O07.34
      circulatory collapse O07.31
      cystitis O07.38
      defibrination syndrome O07.1
      electrolyte imbalance O07.33
      embolism (air) (amniotic fluid) (blood clot) (fat)
        (pulmonary) (septic) (soap) O07.2
      endometritis O07.0

Abortion — *continued*
  attempted — *continued*
    complicated by — *continued*
      genital tract and pelvic infection O07.0
      hemolysis O07.1
      hemorrhage (delayed) (excessive) O07.1
      infection
        genital tract or pelvic O07.0
        urinary tract tract O07.38
      intravascular coagulation O07.1
      laceration of pelvic organ(s) O07.34
      metabolic disorder O07.33
      oliguria O07.32
      oophoritis O07.0
      parametritis O07.0
      pelvic peritonitis O07.0
      perforation of pelvic organ(s) O07.34
      renal failure or shutdown O07.32
      salpingitis or salpingo-oophoritis O07.0
      sepsis O07.37
      shock O07.31
      specified condition NEC O07.39
      tubular necrosis (renal) O07.32
      uremia O07.32
      urinary tract infection O07.38
      venous complication NEC O07.35
        embolism (air) (amniotic fluid) (blood clot)
          (fat) (pulmonary) (septic) (soap) O07.2
  complicated (by) (following) O03.80
    afibrinogenemia O03.6
    cardiac arrest O03.86
    chemical damage of pelvic organ(s) O03.84
    circulatory collapse O03.81
    cystitis O03.88
    defibrination syndrome O03.6
    electrolyte imbalance O03.83
    embolism (air) (amniotic fluid) (blood clot) (fat)
      (pulmonary) (septic) (soap) O03.7
    endometritis O03.5
    genital tract and pelvic infection O03.5
    hemolysis O03.6
    hemorrhage (delayed) (excessive) O03.6
    infection
      genital tract or pelvic O03.5
      urinary tract O03.88
    intravascular coagulation O03.6
    laceration of pelvic organ(s) O03.84
    metabolic disorder O03.83
    oliguria O03.82
    oophoritis O03.5
    parametritis O03.5
    pelvic peritonitis O03.5
    perforation of pelvic organ(s) O03.84
    renal failure or shutdown O03.82
    salpingitis or salpingo-oophoritis O03.5
    sepsis O03.87
    shock O03.81
    specified condition NEC O03.89
    tubular necrosis (renal) O03.82
    uremia O03.82
    urinary tract infection O03.88
    venous complication NEC O03.85
      embolism (air) (amniotic fluid) (blood clot) (fat)
        (pulmonary) (septic) (soap) O03.7
  failed — *see* Abortion, attempted
  habitual or recurrent N96
    with current abortion — *see* categories O03-O04
    without current pregnancy N96
    care in current pregnancy O26.2- ☑
  incomplete (spontaneous) O03.4
    complicated (by) (following) O03.30
      afibrinogenemia O03.1
      cardiac arrest O03.36
      chemical damage of pelvic organ(s) O03.34
      circulatory collapse O03.31
      cystitis O03.38
      defibrination syndrome O03.1
      electrolyte imbalance O03.33
      embolism (air) (amniotic fluid) (blood clot) (fat)
        (pulmonary) (septic) (soap) O03.2
      endometritis O03.0
      genital tract and pelvic infection O03.0
      hemolysis O03.1
      hemorrhage (delayed) (excessive) O03.1
      infection
        genital tract or pelvic O03.0
        urinary tract O03.38
      intravascular coagulation O03.1
      laceration of pelvic organ(s) O03.34

Abortion — *continued*
  incomplete — *continued*
    complicated — *continued*
      metabolic disorder O03.33
      oliguria O03.32
      oophoritis O03.0
      parametritis O03.0
      pelvic peritonitis O03.0
      perforation of pelvic organ(s) O03.34
      renal failure or shutdown O03.32
      salpingitis or salpingo-oophoritis O03.0
      sepsis O03.37
      shock O03.31
      specified condition NEC O03.39
      tubular necrosis (renal) O03.32
      uremia O03.32
      urinary infection O03.38
      venous complication NEC O03.35
        embolism (air) (amniotic fluid) (blood clot)
          (fat) (pulmonary) (septic) (soap) O03.2
  induced (encounter for) Z33.2
    complicated by O04.80
      afibrinogenemia O04.6
      cardiac arrest O04.86
      chemical damage of pelvic organ(s) O04.84
      circulatory collapse O04.81
      cystitis O04.88
      defibrination syndrome O04.6
      electrolyte imbalance O04.83
      embolism (air) (amniotic fluid) (blood clot) (fat)
        (pulmonary) (septic) (soap) O04.7
      endometritis O04.5
      genital tract and pelvic infection O04.5
      hemolysis O04.6
      hemorrhage (delayed) (excessive) O04.6
      infection
        genital tract or pelvic O04.5
        urinary tract O04.88
      intravascular coagulation O04.6
      laceration of pelvic organ(s) O04.84
      metabolic disorder O04.83
      oliguria O04.82
      oophoritis O04.5
      parametritis O04.5
      pelvic peritonitis O04.5
      perforation of pelvic organ(s) O04.84
      renal failure or shutdown O04.82
      salpingitis or salpingo-oophoritis O04.5
      sepsis O04.87
      shock O04.81
      specified condition NEC O04.89
      tubular necrosis (renal) O04.82
      uremia O04.82
      urinary tract infection O04.88
      venous complication NEC O04.85
        embolism (air) (amniotic fluid) (blood clot)
          (fat) (pulmonary) (septic) (soap) O04.7
  missed O02.1
  spontaneous — *see* Abortion (complete) (spontaneous)
    threatened O20.0
  threatened (spontaneous) O20.0
  tubal O00.10- ☑
    with intrauterine pregnancy O00.11- ☑
Abortus fever A23.1
Aboulomania F60.7
Abrami's disease D59.8
Abramov-Fiedler myocarditis (acute isolated myocarditis) I40.1
Abrasion T14.8 ☑
  abdomen, abdominal (wall) S30.811 ☑
  alveolar process S00.512 ☑
  ankle S90.51- ☑
  antecubital space — *see* Abrasion, elbow
  anus S30.817 ☑
  arm (upper) S40.81- ☑
  auditory canal — *see* Abrasion, ear
  auricle — *see* Abrasion, ear
  axilla — *see* Abrasion, arm
  back, lower S30.810 ☑
  breast S20.11- ☑
  brow S00.81 ☑
  buttock S30.810 ☑
  calf — *see* Abrasion, leg
  canthus — *see* Abrasion, eyelid
  cheek S00.81 ☑
    internal S00.512 ☑
  chest wall — *see* Abrasion, thorax
  chin S00.81 ☑

Abrasion — *continued*
- clitoris S30.814 ☑
- cornea S05.0- ☑
- costal region — *see* Abrasion, thorax
- dental K03.1
- digit(s)
  - foot — *see* Abrasion, toe
  - hand — *see* Abrasion, finger
- ear S00.41- ☑
- elbow S50.31- ☑
- epididymis S30.813 ☑
- epigastric region S30.811 ☑
- epiglottis S10.11 ☑
- esophagus (thoracic) S27.818 ☑
  - cervical S10.11 ☑
- eyebrow — *see* Abrasion, eyelid
- eyelid S00.21- ☑
- face S00.81 ☑
- finger(s) S60.41- ☑
  - index S60.41- ☑
  - little S60.41- ☑
  - middle S60.41- ☑
  - ring S60.41- ☑
- flank S30.811 ☑
- foot (except toe(s) alone) S90.81- ☑
  - toe — *see* Abrasion, toe
- forearm S50.81- ☑
  - elbow only — *see* Abrasion, elbow
- forehead S00.81 ☑
- genital organs, external
  - female S30.816 ☑
  - male S30.815 ☑
- groin S30.811 ☑
- gum S00.512 ☑
- hand S60.51- ☑
- head S00.91 ☑
  - ear — *see* Abrasion, ear
  - eyelid — *see* Abrasion, eyelid
  - lip S00.511 ☑
  - nose S00.31 ☑
  - oral cavity S00.512 ☑
  - scalp S00.01 ☑
  - specified site NEC S00.81 ☑
- heel — *see* Abrasion, foot
- hip S70.21- ☑
- inguinal region S30.811 ☑
- interscapular region S20.419 ☑
- jaw S00.81 ☑
- knee S80.21- ☑
- labium (majus) (minus) S30.814 ☑
- larynx S10.11 ☑
- leg (lower) S80.81- ☑
  - knee — *see* Abrasion, knee
  - upper — *see* Abrasion, thigh
- lip S00.511 ☑
- lower back S30.810 ☑
- lumbar region S30.810 ☑
- malar region S00.81 ☑
- mammary — *see* Abrasion, breast
- mastoid region S00.81 ☑
- mouth S00.512 ☑
- nail
  - finger — *see* Abrasion, finger
  - toe — *see* Abrasion, toe
- nape S10.81 ☑
- nasal S00.31 ☑
- neck S10.91 ☑
  - specified site NEC S10.81 ☑
  - throat S10.11 ☑
- nose S00.31 ☑
- occipital region S00.01 ☑
- oral cavity S00.512 ☑
- orbital region — *see* Abrasion, eyelid
- palate S00.512 ☑
- palm — *see* Abrasion, hand
- parietal region S00.01 ☑
- pelvis S30.810 ☑
- penis S30.812 ☑
- perineum
  - female S30.814 ☑
  - male S30.815 ☑
- periocular area — *see* Abrasion, eyelid
- phalanges
  - finger — *see* Abrasion, finger
  - toe — *see* Abrasion, toe
- pharynx S10.11 ☑

Abrasion — *continued*
- pinna — *see* Abrasion, ear
- popliteal space — *see* Abrasion, knee
- prepuce S30.812 ☑
- pubic region S30.810 ☑
- pudendum
  - female S30.816 ☑
  - male S30.815 ☑
- sacral region S30.810 ☑
- scalp S00.01 ☑
- scapular region — *see* Abrasion, shoulder
- scrotum S30.813 ☑
- shin — *see* Abrasion, leg
- shoulder S40.21- ☑
- skin NEC T14.8 ☑
- sternal region S20.319 ☑
- submaxillary region S00.81 ☑
- submental region S00.81 ☑
- subungual
  - finger(s) — *see* Abrasion, finger
  - toe(s) — *see* Abrasion, toe
- supraclavicular fossa S10.81 ☑
- supraorbital S00.81 ☑
- temple S00.81 ☑
- temporal region S00.81 ☑
- testis S30.813 ☑
- thigh S70.31- ☑
- thorax, thoracic (wall) S20.91 ☑
  - back S20.41- ☑
  - front S20.31- ☑
- throat S10.11 ☑
- thumb S60.31- ☑
- toe(s) (lesser) S90.416 ☑
  - great S90.41- ☑
- tongue S00.512 ☑
- tooth, teeth (dentifrice) (habitual) (hard tissues) (occupational) (ritual) (traditional) K03.1
- trachea S10.11 ☑
- tunica vaginalis S30.813 ☑
- tympanum, tympanic membrane — *see* Abrasion, ear
- uvula S00.512 ☑
- vagina S30.814 ☑
- vocal cords S10.11 ☑
- vulva S30.814 ☑
- wrist S60.81- ☑

Abrism — *see* Poisoning, food, noxious, plant
Abruptio placentae O45.9- ☑
- with
  - afibrinogenemia O45.01- ☑
  - coagulation defect O45.00- ☑
    - specified NEC O45.09- ☑
  - disseminated intravascular coagulation O45.02- ☑
  - hypofibrinogenemia O45.01- ☑
- specified NEC O45.8- ☑
Abruption, placenta — *see* Abruptio placentae
Abscess (connective tissue) (embolic) (fistulous) (infective) (metastatic) (multiple) (pernicious) (pyogenic) (septic) L02.91
- with
  - diverticular disease (intestine) K57.80
    - with bleeding K57.81
    - large intestine K57.20
      - with
        - bleeding K57.21
        - small intestine K57.40
          - with bleeding K57.41
    - small intestine K57.00
      - with
        - bleeding K57.01
        - large intestine K57.40
          - with bleeding K57.41
  - lymphangitis — *code by* site under Abscess
- abdomen, abdominal
  - cavity K65.1
  - wall L02.211
- abdominopelvic K65.1
- accessory sinus — *see* Sinusitis
- adrenal (capsule) (gland) E27.8
- alveolar K04.7
  - with sinus K04.6
- amebic A06.4
  - brain (and liver or lung abscess) A06.6
  - genitourinary tract A06.82
  - liver (without mention of brain or lung abscess) A06.4
  - lung (and liver) (without mention of brain abscess) A06.5

Abscess — *continued*
- amebic — *continued*
  - specified site NEC A06.89
  - spleen A06.89
- anaerobic A48.0
- ankle — *see* Abscess, lower limb
- anorectal K61.2
- antecubital space — *see* Abscess, upper limb
- antrum (chronic) (Highmore) — *see* Sinusitis, maxillary
- anus K61.0
- apical (tooth) K04.7
  - with sinus (alveolar) K04.6
- appendix K35.33
- areola (acute) (chronic) (nonpuerperal) N61.1
  - puerperal, postpartum or gestational — *see* Infection, nipple
- arm (any part) — *see* Abscess, upper limb
- artery (wall) I77.89
- atheromatous I77.2
- auricle, ear — *see* Abscess, ear, external
- axilla (region) L02.41- ☑
  - lymph gland or node L04.2
- back (any part, except buttock) L02.212
- Bartholin's gland N75.1
  - with
    - abortion — *see* Abortion, by type complicated by, sepsis
    - ectopic or molar pregnancy O08.0
  - following ectopic or molar pregnancy O08.0
- Bezold's — *see* Mastoiditis, acute
- bilharziasis B65.1
- bladder (wall) — *see* Cystitis, specified type NEC
- bone (subperiosteal) — *see also* Osteomyelitis, specified type NEC
  - accessory sinus (chronic) — *see* Sinusitis
  - chronic or old — *see* Osteomyelitis, chronic
  - jaw (lower) (upper) M27.2
  - mastoid — *see* Mastoiditis, acute, subperiosteal
  - petrous — *see* Petrositis
  - spinal (tuberculous) A18.01
    - nontuberculous — *see* Osteomyelitis, vertebra
- bowel K63.0
- brain (any part) (cystic) (otogenic) G06.0
  - amebic (with abscess of any other site) A06.6
  - gonococcal A54.82
  - pheomycotic (chromomycotic) B43.1
  - tuberculous A17.81
- breast (acute) (chronic) (nonpuerperal) N61.1
  - newborn P39.0
  - puerperal, postpartum, gestational — *see* Mastitis, obstetric, purulent
- broad ligament N73.2
  - acute N73.0
  - chronic N73.1
- Brodie's (localized) (chronic) M86.8X- ☑
- bronchi J98.09
- buccal cavity K12.2
- bulbourethral gland N34.0
- bursa M71.00
  - ankle M71.07- ☑
  - elbow M71.02- ☑
  - foot M71.07- ☑
  - hand M71.04- ☑
  - hip M71.05- ☑
  - knee M71.06- ☑
  - multiple sites M71.09
  - pharyngeal J39.1
  - shoulder M71.01- ☑
  - specified site NEC M71.08
  - wrist M71.03- ☑
- buttock L02.31
- canthus — *see* Blepharoconjunctivitis
- cartilage — *see* Disorder, cartilage, specified type NEC
- cecum K35.33
- cerebellum, cerebellar G06.0
  - sequelae G09
- cerebral (embolic) G06.0
  - sequelae G09
- cervical (meaning neck) L02.11
  - lymph gland or node L04.0
- cervix (stump) (uteri) — *see* Cervicitis
- cheek (external) L02.01
  - inner K12.2
- chest J86.9
  - with fistula J86.0
  - wall L02.213
- chin L02.01
- choroid — *see* Inflammation, chorioretinal

Abscess — *continued*
circumtonsillar J36
cold (lung) (tuberculous) — *see also* Tuberculosis, abscess, lung
   articular — *see* Tuberculosis, joint
colon (wall) K63.0
colostomy K94.02
conjunctiva — *see* Conjunctivitis, acute
cornea H16.31- ☑
corpus
   cavernosum N48.21
   luteum — *see* Oophoritis
Cowper's gland N34.0
cranium G06.0
cul-de-sac (Douglas') (posterior) — *see* Peritonitis, pelvic, female
cutaneous — *see* Abscess, by site
dental K04.7
   with sinus (alveolar) K04.6
dentoalveolar K04.7
   with sinus K04.6
diaphragm, diaphragmatic K65.1
Douglas' cul-de-sac or pouch — *see* Peritonitis, pelvic, female
Dubois A50.59
ear (middle) — *see also* Otitis, media, suppurative
   acute — *see* Otitis, media, suppurative, acute
   external H60.0- ☑
entamebic — *see* Abscess, amebic
enterostomy K94.12
epididymis N45.4
epidural G06.2
   brain G06.0
   spinal cord G06.1
epiglottis J38.7
epiploon, epiploic K65.1
erysipelatous — *see* Erysipelas
esophagus K20.8
ethmoid (bone) (chronic) (sinus) J32.2
external auditory canal — *see* Abscess, ear, external
extradural G06.2
   brain G06.0
     sequelae G09
   spinal cord G06.1
extraperitoneal K68.19
eye — *see* Endophthalmitis, purulent
eyelid H00.03- ☑
face (any part, except ear, eye and nose) L02.01
fallopian tube — *see* Salpingitis
fascia M72.8
fauces J39.1
fecal K63.0
femoral (region) — *see* Abscess, lower limb
filaria, filarial — *see* Infestation, filarial
finger (any) — *see also* Abscess, hand
   nail — *see* Cellulitis, finger
foot L02.61- ☑
forehead L02.01
frontal sinus (chronic) J32.1
gallbladder K81.0
genital organ or tract
   female (external) N76.4
   male N49.9
     multiple sites N49.8
     specified NEC N49.8
gestational mammary O91.11- ☑
gestational subareolar O91.11- ☑
gingival — *see* Periodontitis, localized
gland, glandular (lymph) (acute) — *see* Lymphadenitis, acute
gluteal (region) L02.31
gonorrheal — *see* Gonococcus
groin L02.214
gum — *see* Periodontitis, localized
hand L02.51- ☑
head NEC L02.811
   face (any part, except ear, eye and nose) L02.01
heart — *see* Carditis
heel — *see* Abscess, foot
helminthic — *see* Infestation, helminth
hepatic (cholangitic) (hematogenic) (lymphogenic) (pylephlebitic) K75.0
   amebic A06.4
hip (region) — *see* Abscess, lower limb
horseshoe K61.31
ileocecal K35.33
ileostomy (bud) K94.12
iliac (region) L02.214

Abscess — *continued*
iliac — *continued*
   fossa K35.33
infraclavicular (fossa) — *see* Abscess, upper limb
inguinal (region) L02.214
   lymph gland or node L04.1
intersphincteric K61.4
intestine, intestinal NEC K63.0
   rectal K61.1
intra-abdominal — *see also* Abscess, peritoneum K65.1
   following procedure T81.43 ☑
     obstetrical O86.03
   postprocedural T81.49 ☑
     retroperitoneal K68.11
intracranial G06.0
intramammary — *see* Abscess, breast
intramuscular, following procedure T81.42 ☑
   obstetrical O86.02
intraorbital — *see* Abscess, orbit
intraperitoneal K65.1
intrasphincteric (anus) K61.4
intraspinal G06.1
intratonsillar J36
ischiorectal (fossa) (specified NEC) K61.39
jaw (bone) (lower) (upper) M27.2
joint — *see* Arthritis, pyogenic or pyemic
   spine (tuberculous) A18.01
     nontuberculous — *see* Spondylopathy, infective
kidney N15.1
   with calculus N20.0
     with hydronephrosis N13.6
   puerperal (postpartum) O86.21
knee — *see also* Abscess, lower limb
   joint M00.9
labium (majus) (minus) N76.4
lacrimal
   caruncle — *see* Inflammation, lacrimal, passages, acute
   gland — *see* Dacryoadenitis
   passages (duct) (sac) — *see* Inflammation, lacrimal, passages, acute
lacunar N34.0
larynx J38.7
lateral (alveolar) K04.7
   with sinus K04.6
leg (any part) — *see* Abscess, lower limb
lens H27.8
lingual K14.0
   tonsil J36
lip K13.0
Littre's gland N34.0
liver (cholangitic) (hematogenic) (lymphogenic) (pylephlebitic) (pyogenic) K75.0
   amebic (due to Entamoeba histolytica) (dysenteric) (tropical) A06.4
     with
       brain abscess (and liver or lung abscess) A06.6
       lung abscess A06.5
loin (region) L02.211
lower limb L02.41- ☑
lumbar (tuberculous) A18.01
   nontuberculous L02.212
lung (miliary) (putrid) J85.2
   with pneumonia J85.1
     due to specified organism (see Pneumonia, in (due to))
   amebic (with liver abscess) A06.5
     with
       brain abscess A06.6
       pneumonia A06.5
lymph, lymphatic, gland or node (acute) — *see also* Lymphadenitis, acute
   mesentery I88.0
malar M27.2
mammary gland — *see* Abscess, breast
marginal, anus K61.0
mastoid — *see* Mastoiditis, acute
maxilla, maxillary M27.2
   molar (tooth) K04.7
     with sinus K04.6
   premolar K04.7
   sinus (chronic) J32.0
mediastinum J85.3
meibomian gland — *see* Hordeolum
meninges G06.2
mesentery, mesenteric K65.1
mesosalpinx — *see* Salpingitis
mons pubis L02.215

Abscess — *continued*
mouth (floor) K12.2
muscle — *see* Myositis, infective
myocardium I40.0
nabothian (follicle) — *see* Cervicitis
nasal J32.9
nasopharyngeal J39.1
navel L02.216
   newborn P38.9
     with mild hemorrhage P38.1
     without hemorrhage P38.9
neck (region) L02.11
   lymph gland or node L04.0
nephritic — *see* Abscess, kidney
nipple N61.1
   associated with
     lactation — *see* Pregnancy, complicated by
     pregnancy — *see* Pregnancy, complicated by
nose (external) (fossa) (septum) J34.0
   sinus (chronic) — *see* Sinusitis
omentum K65.1
operative wound T81.49 ☑
orbit, orbital — *see* Cellulitis, orbit
otogenic G06.0
ovary, ovarian (corpus luteum) — *see* Oophoritis
oviduct — *see* Oophoritis
palate (soft) K12.2
   hard M27.2
palmar (space) — *see* Abscess, hand
pancreas (duct) — *see* Pancreatitis, acute
parafrenal N48.21
parametric, parametrium N73.2
   acute N73.0
   chronic N73.1
paranephric N15.1
parapancreatic — *see* Pancreatitis, acute
parapharyngeal J39.0
pararectal K61.1
parasinus — *see* Sinusitis
parauterine — *see also* Disease, pelvis, inflammatory N73.2
paravaginal — *see* Vaginitis
parietal region (scalp) L02.811
parodontal — *see* Periodontitis, aggressive, localized
parotid (duct) (gland) K11.3
   region K12.2
pectoral (region) L02.213
pelvis, pelvic
   female — *see* Disease, pelvis, inflammatory
   male, peritoneal K65.1
penis N48.21
   gonococcal (accessory gland) (periurethral) A54.1
perianal K61.0
periapical K04.7
   with sinus (alveolar) K04.6
periappendicular K35.33
pericardial I30.1
pericecal K35.33
pericemental — *see* Periodontitis, aggressive, localized
pericholecystic — *see* Cholecystitis, acute
pericoronal — *see* Periodontitis, aggressive, localized
peridental — *see* Periodontitis, aggressive, localized
perimetric — *see also* Disease, pelvis, inflammatory N73.2
perinephric, perinephritic — *see* Abscess, kidney
perineum, perineal (superficial) L02.215
   urethra N34.0
periodontal (parietal) — *see* Periodontitis, aggressive, localized
   apical K04.7
periosteum, periosteal — *see also* Osteomyelitis, specified type NEC
   with osteomyelitis — *see also* Osteomyelitis, specified type NEC
     acute — *see* Osteomyelitis, acute
     chronic — *see* Osteomyelitis, chronic
peripharyngeal J39.0
peripleuritic J86.9
   with fistula J86.0
periprostatic N41.2
perirectal K61.1
perirenal (tissue) — *see* Abscess, kidney
perisinuous (nose) — *see* Sinusitis
peritoneum, peritoneal (perforated) (ruptured) K65.1
   with appendicitis — *see also* Appendicitis K35.33
   pelvic
     female — *see* Peritonitis, pelvic, female
     male K65.1

Abscess — continued
  peritoneum, peritoneal — continued
    postoperative T81.49 ☑
    puerperal, postpartum, childbirth O85
    tuberculous A18.31
  peritonsillar J36
  perityphlic K35.33
  periureteral N28.89
  periurethral N34.0
    gonococcal (accessory gland) (periurethral) A54.1
  periuterine — see also Disease, pelvis, inflammatory N73.2
  perivesical — see Cystitis, specified type NEC
  petrous bone — see Petrositis
  phagedenic NOS L02.91
    chancroid A57
  pharynx, pharyngeal (lateral) J39.1
  pilonidal L05.01
  pituitary (gland) E23.6
  pleura J86.9
    with fistula J86.0
  popliteal — see Abscess, lower limb
  postcecal K35.33
  postlaryngeal J38.7
  postnasal J34.0
  postoperative (any site) — see also Infection, postoperative wound T81.49 ☑
    retroperitoneal K68.11
  postpharyngeal J39.0
  posttonsillar J36
  post-typhoid A01.09
  pouch of Douglas — see Peritonitis, pelvic, female
  premammary — see Abscess, breast
  prepatellar — see Abscess, lower limb
  prostate N41.2
    gonococcal (acute) (chronic) A54.22
  psoas muscle K68.12
  puerperal — code by site under Puerperal, abscess
  pulmonary — see Abscess, lung
  pulp, pulpal (dental) K04.01
    irreversible K04.02
    reversible K04.01
  rectovaginal septum K63.0
  rectovesical — see Cystitis, specified type NEC
  rectum K61.1
  renal — see Abscess, kidney
  retina — see Inflammation, chorioretinal
  retrobulbar — see Abscess, orbit
  retrocecal K65.1
  retrolaryngeal J38.7
  retromammary — see Abscess, breast
  retroperitoneal NEC K68.19
    postprocedural K68.11
  retropharyngeal J39.0
  retrouterine — see Peritonitis, pelvic, female
  retrovesical — see Cystitis, specified type NEC
  root, tooth K04.7
    with sinus (alveolar) K04.6
  round ligament — see also Disease, pelvis, inflammatory N73.2
  rupture (spontaneous) NOS L02.91
  sacrum (tuberculous) A18.01
    nontuberculous M46.28
  salivary (duct) (gland) K11.3
  scalp (any part) L02.811
  scapular — see Osteomyelitis, specified type NEC
  sclera — see Scleritis
  scrofulous (tuberculous) A18.2
  scrotum N49.2
  seminal vesicle N49.0
  septal, dental K04.7
    with sinus (alveolar) K04.6
  serous — see Periostitis
  shoulder (region) — see Abscess, upper limb
  sigmoid K63.0
  sinus (accessory) (chronic) (nasal) — see also Sinusitis
    intracranial venous (any) G06.0
  Skene's duct or gland N34.0
  skin — see Abscess, by site
  specified site NEC L02.818
  spermatic cord N49.1
  sphenoidal (sinus) (chronic) J32.3
  spinal cord (any part) (staphylococcal) G06.1
    tuberculous A17.81
  spine (column) (tuberculous) A18.01
    epidural G06.1
    nontuberculous — see Osteomyelitis, vertebra
  spleen D73.3

Abscess — continued
  spleen — continued
    amebic A06.89
  stitch T81.41 ☑
    following an obstetric procedure O86.01
  subarachnoid G06.2
    brain G06.0
    spinal cord G06.1
  subareolar — see Abscess, breast
  subcecal K35.33
  subcutaneous — see also Abscess, by site
    following procedure T81.41 ☑
      obstetrical O86.01
    pheomycotic (chromomycotic) B43.2
  subdiaphragmatic K65.1
  subdural G06.2
    brain G06.0
      sequelae G09
    spinal cord G06.1
  sub-fascial, following an obstetrical procedure O86.02
  subgaleal L02.811
  subhepatic K65.1
  sublingual K12.2
    gland K11.3
  submammary — see Abscess, breast
  submandibular (region) (space) (triangle) K12.2
    gland K11.3
  submaxillary (region) L02.01
    gland K11.3
  submental L02.01
    gland K11.3
  subperiosteal — see Osteomyelitis, specified type NEC
  subphrenic K65.1
    following an obstetrical procedure O86.03
    postoperative T81.43 ☑
  suburethral N34.0
  sudoriparous L75.8
  supraclavicular (fossa) — see Abscess, upper limb
  supralevator K61.5
  suprapelvic, acute N73.0
  suprarenal (capsule) (gland) E27.8
  sweat gland L74.8
  tear duct — see Inflammation, lacrimal, passages, acute
  temple L02.01
  temporal region L02.01
  temporosphenoidal G06.0
  tendon (sheath) M65.00
    ankle M65.07- ☑
    foot M65.07- ☑
    forearm M65.03- ☑
    hand M65.04- ☑
    lower leg M65.06- ☑
    pelvic region M65.05- ☑
    shoulder region M65.01- ☑
    specified site NEC M65.08
    thigh M65.05- ☑
    upper arm M65.02- ☑
  testis N45.4
  thigh — see Abscess, lower limb
  thorax J86.9
    with fistula J86.0
  throat J39.1
  thumb — see also Abscess, hand
    nail — see Cellulitis, finger
  thymus (gland) E32.1
  thyroid (gland) E06.0
  toe (any) — see also Abscess, foot
    nail — see Cellulitis, toe
  tongue (staphylococcal) K14.0
  tonsil(s) (lingual) J36
  tonsillopharyngeal J36
  tooth, teeth (root) K04.7
    with sinus (alveolar) K04.6
    supporting structures NEC — see Periodontitis, aggressive, localized
  trachea J39.8
  trunk L02.219
    abdominal wall L02.211
    back L02.212
    chest wall L02.213
    groin L02.214
    perineum L02.215
    umbilicus L02.216
  tubal — see Salpingitis
  tuberculous — see Tuberculosis, abscess
  tubo-ovarian — see Salpingo-oophoritis
  tunica vaginalis N49.1
  umbilicus L02.216

Abscess — continued
  upper
    limb L02.41- ☑
    respiratory J39.8
  urethral (gland) N34.0
  urinary N34.0
  uterus, uterine (wall) — see also Endometritis
    ligament — see also Disease, pelvis, inflammatory N73.2
    neck — see Cervicitis
  uvula K12.2
  vagina (wall) — see Vaginitis
  vaginorectal — see Vaginitis
  vas deferens N49.1
  vermiform appendix K35.33
  vertebra (column) (tuberculous) A18.01
    nontuberculous — see Osteomyelitis, vertebra
  vesical — see Cystitis, specified type NEC
  vesico-uterine pouch — see Peritonitis, pelvic, female
  vitreous (humor) — see Endophthalmitis, purulent
  vocal cord J38.3
  von Bezold's — see Mastoiditis, acute
  vulva N76.4
  vulvovaginal gland N75.1
  web space — see Abscess, hand
  wound T81.49 ☑
  wrist — see Abscess, upper limb
Absence (of) (organ or part) (complete or partial)
  adrenal (gland) (congenital) Q89.1
    acquired E89.6
  albumin in blood E88.09
  alimentary tract (congenital) Q45.8
    upper Q40.8
  alveolar process (acquired) — see Anomaly, alveolar
  ankle (acquired) Z89.44- ☑
  anus (congenital) Q42.3
    with fistula Q42.2
  aorta (congenital) Q25.41
  appendix, congenital Q42.8
  arm (acquired) Z89.20- ☑
    above elbow Z89.22- ☑
      congenital (with hand present) — see Agenesis, arm, with hand present
        and hand — see Agenesis, forearm, and hand
    below elbow Z89.21- ☑
      congenital (with hand present) — see Agenesis, arm, with hand present
        and hand — see Agenesis, forearm, and hand
    congenital — see Defect, reduction, upper limb
    shoulder (following explantation of shoulder joint prosthesis) (joint) (with or without presence of antibiotic-impregnated cement spacer) Z89.23- ☑
      congenital (with hand present) — see Agenesis, arm, with hand present
  artery (congenital) (peripheral) Q27.8
    brain Q28.3
    coronary Q24.5
    pulmonary Q25.79
    specified NEC Q27.8
    umbilical Q27.0
  atrial septum (congenital) Q21.1
  auditory canal (congenital) (external) Q16.1
  auricle (ear), congenital Q16.0
  bile, biliary duct, congenital Q44.5
  bladder (acquired) Z90.6
    congenital Q64.5
  bowel sounds R19.11
  brain Q00.0
    part of Q04.3
  breast(s) (and nipple(s)) (acquired) Z90.1- ☑
    congenital Q83.8
  broad ligament Q50.6
  bronchus (congenital) Q32.4
  canaliculus lacrimalis, congenital Q10.4
  cerebellum (vermis) Q04.3
  cervix (acquired) (with uterus) Z90.710
    with remaining uterus Z90.712
    congenital Q51.5
  chin, congenital Q18.8
  cilia (congenital) Q10.3
    acquired — see Madarosis
  clitoris (congenital) Q52.6
  coccyx, congenital Q76.49
  cold sense R20.8
  congenital
    lumen — see Atresia
    organ or site NEC — see Agenesis

☑ Additional Character Required — Refer to the Tabular List for Character Selection
▽ Subterms under main terms may continue to next column or page

Absence — *continued*
  congenital — *continued*
    septum — *see* Imperfect, closure
  corpus callosum Q04.0
  cricoid cartilage, congenital Q31.8
  diaphragm (with hernia), congenital Q79.1
  digestive organ(s) or tract, congenital Q45.8
    acquired NEC Z90.49
    upper Q40.8
  ductus arteriosus Q28.8
  duodenum (acquired) Z90.49
    congenital Q41.0
  ear, congenital Q16.9
    acquired H93.8- ☑
    auricle Q16.0
    external Q16.0
    inner Q16.5
    lobe, lobule Q17.8
    middle, except ossicles Q16.4
      ossicles Q16.3
    ossicles Q16.3
  ejaculatory duct (congenital) Q55.4
  endocrine gland (congenital) NEC Q89.2
    acquired E89.89
  epididymis (congenital) Q55.4
    acquired Z90.79
  epiglottis, congenital Q31.8
  esophagus (congenital) Q39.8
    acquired (partial) Z90.49
  eustachian tube (congenital) Q16.2
  extremity (acquired) Z89.9
    congenital Q73.0
    knee (following explantation of knee joint prosthesis) (joint) (with or without presence of antibiotic-impregnated cement spacer) Z89.52- ☑
    lower (above knee) Z89.619
      below knee Z89.51- ☑
    upper — *see* Absence, arm
  eye (acquired) Z90.01
    congenital Q11.1
    muscle (congenital) Q10.3
  eyeball (acquired) Z90.01
  eyelid (fold) (congenital) Q10.3
    acquired Z90.01
  face, specified part NEC Q18.8
  fallopian tube(s) (acquired) Z90.79
    congenital Q50.6
  family member (causing problem in home) NEC — *see also* Disruption, family Z63.32
  femur, congenital — *see* Defect, reduction, lower limb, longitudinal, femur
  fibrinogen (congenital) D68.2
    acquired D65
  finger(s) (acquired) Z89.02- ☑
    congenital — *see* Agenesis, hand
  foot (acquired) Z89.43- ☑
    congenital — *see* Agenesis, foot
  forearm (acquired) — *see* Absence, arm, below elbow
  gallbladder (acquired) Z90.49
    congenital Q44.0
  gamma globulin in blood D80.1
    hereditary D80.0
  genital organs
    acquired (female) (male) Z90.79
    female, congenital Q52.8
      external Q52.71
      internal NEC Q52.8
    male, congenital Q55.8
  genitourinary organs, congenital NEC
    female Q52.8
    male Q55.8
  globe (acquired) Z90.01
    congenital Q11.1
  glottis, congenital Q31.8
  hand and wrist (acquired) Z89.11- ☑
    congenital — *see* Agenesis, hand
  head, part (acquired) NEC Z90.09
  heat sense R20.8
  hip (following explantation of hip joint prosthesis) (joint) (with or without presence of antibiotic-impregnated cement spacer) Z89.62- ☑
  hymen (congenital) Q52.4
  ileum (acquired) Z90.49
    congenital Q41.2
  immunoglobulin, isolated NEC D80.3
    IgA D80.2
    IgG D80.3
    IgM D80.4

Absence — *continued*
  incus (acquired) — *see* Loss, ossicles, ear
    congenital Q16.3
  inner ear, congenital Q16.5
  intestine (acquired) (small) Z90.49
    congenital Q41.9
      specified NEC Q41.8
    large Z90.49
      congenital Q42.9
        specified NEC Q42.8
  iris, congenital Q13.1
  jejunum (acquired) Z90.49
    congenital Q41.1
  joint
    acquired
      hip (following explantation of hip joint prosthesis) (with or without presence of antibiotic-impregnated cement spacer) Z89.62- ☑
      knee (following explantation of knee joint prosthesis) (with or without presence of antibiotic-impregnated cement spacer) Z89.52- ☑
      shoulder (following explantation of shoulder joint prosthesis) (with or without presence of antibiotic-impregnated cement spacer) Z89.23- ☑
    congenital NEC Q74.8
  kidney(s) (acquired) Z90.5
    congenital Q60.2
      bilateral Q60.1
      unilateral Q60.0
  knee (following explantation of knee joint prosthesis) (joint) (with or without presence of antibiotic-impregnated cement spacer) Z89.52- ☑
  labyrinth, membranous Q16.5
  larynx (congenital) Q31.8
    acquired Z90.02
  leg (acquired) (above knee) Z89.61- ☑
    below knee (acquired) Z89.51- ☑
    congenital — *see* Defect, reduction, lower limb
  lens (acquired) — *see also* Aphakia
    congenital Q12.3
    post cataract extraction Z98.4- ☑
  limb (acquired) — *see* Absence, extremity
  lip Q38.6
  liver (congenital) Q44.7
  lung (fissure) (lobe) (bilateral) (unilateral) (congenital) Q33.3
    acquired (any part) Z90.2
  menstruation — *see* Amenorrhea
  muscle (congenital) (pectoral) Q79.8
    ocular Q10.3
  neck, part Q18.8
  neutrophil — *see* Agranulocytosis
  nipple(s) (with breast(s)) (acquired) Z90.1- ☑
    congenital Q83.2
  nose (congenital) Q30.1
    acquired Z90.09
  organ
    of Corti, congenital Q16.5
    or site, congenital NEC Q89.8
      acquired NEC Z90.89
  osseous meatus (ear) Q16.4
  ovary (acquired)
    bilateral Z90.722
    congenital
      bilateral Q50.02
      unilateral Q50.01
    unilateral Z90.721
  oviduct (acquired)
    bilateral Z90.722
    congenital Q50.6
    unilateral Z90.721
  pancreas (congenital) Q45.0
    acquired Z90.410
      complete Z90.410
      partial Z90.411
      total Z90.410
  parathyroid gland (acquired) E89.2
    congenital Q89.2
  patella, congenital Q74.1
  penis (congenital) Q55.5
    acquired Z90.79
  pericardium (congenital) Q24.8
  pituitary gland (congenital) Q89.2
    acquired E89.3
  prostate (acquired) Z90.79
    congenital Q55.4

Absence — *continued*
  pulmonary valve Q22.0
  punctum lacrimale (congenital) Q10.4
  radius, congenital — *see* Defect, reduction, upper limb, longitudinal, radius
  rectum (congenital) Q42.1
    with fistula Q42.0
    acquired Z90.49
  respiratory organ NOS Q34.9
  rib (acquired) Z90.89
    congenital Q76.6
  sacrum, congenital Q76.49
  salivary gland(s), congenital Q38.4
  scrotum, congenital Q55.29
  seminal vesicles (congenital) Q55.4
    acquired Z90.79
  septum
    atrial (congenital) Q21.1
    between aorta and pulmonary artery Q21.4
    ventricular (congenital) Q20.4
  sex chromosome
    female phenotype Q97.8
    male phenotype Q98.8
  skull bone (congenital) Q75.8
    with
      anencephaly Q00.0
      encephalocele — *see* Encephalocele
      hydrocephalus Q03.9
        with spina bifida — *see* Spina bifida, by site, with hydrocephalus
      microcephaly Q02
  spermatic cord, congenital Q55.4
  spine, congenital Q76.49
  spleen (congenital) Q89.01
    acquired Z90.81
  sternum, congenital Q76.7
  stomach (acquired) (partial) Z90.3
    congenital Q40.2
  superior vena cava, congenital Q26.8
  teeth, tooth (congenital) K00.0
    acquired (complete) K08.109
      class I K08.101
      class II K08.102
      class III K08.103
      class IV K08.104
      due to
        caries K08.139
          class I K08.131
          class II K08.132
          class III K08.133
          class IV K08.134
        periodontal disease K08.129
          class I K08.121
          class II K08.122
          class III K08.123
          class IV K08.124
        specified NEC K08.199
          class I K08.191
          class II K08.192
          class III K08.193
          class IV K08.194
        trauma K08.119
          class I K08.111
          class II K08.112
          class III K08.113
          class IV K08.114
      partial K08.409
        class I K08.401
        class II K08.402
        class III K08.403
        class IV K08.404
        due to
          caries K08.439
            class I K08.431
            class II K08.432
            class III K08.433
            class IV K08.434
          periodontal disease K08.429
            class I K08.421
            class II K08.422
            class III K08.423
            class IV K08.424
          specified NEC K08.499
            class I K08.491
            class II K08.492
            class III K08.493
            class IV K08.494
          trauma K08.419
            class I K08.411

Absence — *continued*
- teeth, tooth — *continued*
  - acquired — *continued*
    - partial — *continued*
      - due to — *continued*
        - trauma — *continued*
          - class II K08.412
          - class III K08.413
          - class IV K08.414
  - tendon (congenital) Q79.8
  - testis (congenital) Q55.0
    - acquired Z90.79
  - thumb (acquired) Z89.01- ☑
    - congenital — *see* Agenesis, hand
  - thymus gland Q89.2
  - thyroid (gland) (acquired) E89.0
    - cartilage, congenital Q31.8
    - congenital E03.1
  - toe(s) (acquired) Z89.42- ☑
    - with foot — *see* Absence, foot and ankle
    - congenital — *see* Agenesis, foot
    - great Z89.41- ☑
  - tongue, congenital Q38.3
  - trachea (cartilage), congenital Q32.1
  - transverse aortic arch, congenital Q25.49
  - tricuspid valve Q22.4
  - umbilical artery, congenital Q27.0
  - upper arm and forearm with hand present, congenital — *see* Agenesis, arm, with hand present
  - ureter (congenital) Q62.4
    - acquired Z90.6
  - urethra, congenital Q64.5
  - uterus (acquired) Z90.710
    - with cervix Z90.710
    - with remaining cervical stump Z90.711
    - congenital Q51.0
  - uvula, congenital Q38.5
  - vagina, congenital Q52.0
  - vas deferens (congenital) Q55.4
    - acquired Z90.79
  - vein (peripheral) congenital NEC Q27.8
    - cerebral Q28.3
    - digestive system Q27.8
    - great Q26.8
    - lower limb Q27.8
    - portal Q26.5
    - precerebral Q28.1
    - specified site NEC Q27.8
    - upper limb Q27.8
  - vena cava (inferior) (superior), congenital Q26.8
  - ventricular septum Q20.4
  - vertebra, congenital Q76.49
  - vulva, congenital Q52.71
  - wrist (acquired) Z89.12- ☑

Absorbent system disease I87.8

Absorption
- carbohydrate, disturbance K90.49
- chemical — *see* Table of Drugs and Chemicals
  - through placenta (newborn) P04.9
    - environmental substance P04.6
    - nutritional substance P04.5
    - obstetric anesthetic or analgesic drug P04.0
- drug NEC — *see* Table of Drugs and Chemicals
  - addictive
    - through placenta (newborn) — *see also* Newborn, affected by, maternal, use of P04.40
      - cocaine P04.41
      - hallucinogens P04.42
      - specified drug NEC P04.49
  - medicinal
    - through placenta (newborn) P04.19
  - through placenta (newborn) P04.19
    - obstetric anesthetic or analgesic drug P04.0
- fat, disturbance K90.49
  - pancreatic K90.3
- noxious substance — *see* Table of Drugs and Chemicals
- protein, disturbance K90.49
- starch, disturbance K90.49
- toxic substance — *see* Table of Drugs and Chemicals
- uremic — *see* Uremia

Abstinence symptoms, syndrome
- alcohol F10.239
  - with delirium F10.231
- cocaine F14.23
- neonatal P96.1
- nicotine — *see* Dependence, drug, nicotine, with, withdrawal
- opioid F11.93

Abstinence symptoms, syndrome — *continued*
- opioid — *continued*
  - with dependence F11.23
- psychoactive NEC F19.939
  - with
    - delirium F19.931
    - dependence F19.239
      - with
        - delirium F19.231
        - perceptual disturbance F19.232
      - uncomplicated F19.230
    - perceptual disturbance F19.932
  - uncomplicated F19.930
- sedative F13.939
  - with
    - delirium F13.931
    - dependence F13.239
      - with
        - delirium F13.231
        - perceptual disturbance F13.232
      - uncomplicated F13.230
    - perceptual disturbance F13.932
  - uncomplicated F13.930
- stimulant NEC F15.93
  - with dependence F15.23

Abulia R68.89

Abulomania F60.7

Abuse
- adult — *see* Maltreatment, adult
  - as reason for
    - couple seeking advice (including offender) Z63.0
- alcohol (non-dependent) F10.10
  - with
    - anxiety disorder F10.180
    - intoxication F10.129
      - with delirium F10.121
      - uncomplicated F10.120
    - mood disorder F10.14
    - other specified disorder F10.188
    - psychosis F10.159
      - delusions F10.150
      - hallucinations F10.151
    - sexual dysfunction F10.181
    - sleep disorder F10.182
    - unspecified disorder F10.19
  - counseling and surveillance Z71.41
  - in remission (early) (sustained) F10.11
- amphetamine (or related substance) — *see also* Abuse, drug, stimulant NEC
  - stimulant NEC F15.10
    - with
      - anxiety disorder F15.180
      - intoxication F15.129
        - with
          - delirium F15.121
          - perceptual disturbance F15.122
- analgesics (non-prescribed) (over the counter) F55.8
- antacids F55.0
- antidepressants — *see* Abuse, drug, psychoactive NEC
- anxiolytic — *see* Abuse, drug, sedative
- barbiturates — *see* Abuse, drug, sedative
- caffeine — *see* Abuse, drug, stimulant NEC
- cannabis, cannabinoids — *see* Abuse, drug, cannabis
- child — *see* Maltreatment, child
- cocaine — *see* Abuse, drug, cocaine
- drug NEC (non-dependent) F19.10
  - with sleep disorder F19.182
  - amphetamine type — *see* Abuse, drug, stimulant NEC
  - analgesics (non-prescribed) (over the counter) F55.8
  - antacids F55.0
  - antidepressants — *see* Abuse, drug, psychoactive NEC
  - anxiolytics — *see* Abuse, drug, sedative
  - barbiturates — *see* Abuse, drug, sedative
  - caffeine — *see* Abuse, drug, stimulant NEC
  - cannabis F12.10
    - with
      - anxiety disorder F12.180
      - intoxication F12.129
        - with
          - delirium F12.121
          - perceptual disturbance F12.122
        - uncomplicated F12.120
      - other specified disorder F12.188
      - psychosis F12.159
        - delusions F12.150
        - hallucinations F12.151

Abuse — *continued*
- drug — *continued*
  - cannabis — *continued*
    - with — *continued*
      - unspecified disorder F12.19
    - in remission (early) (sustained) F12.11
  - cocaine F14.10
    - with
      - anxiety disorder F14.180
      - intoxication F14.129
        - with
          - delirium F14.121
          - perceptual disturbance F14.122
        - uncomplicated F14.120
      - mood disorder F14.14
      - other specified disorder F14.188
      - psychosis F14.159
        - delusions F14.150
        - hallucinations F14.151
      - sexual dysfunction F14.181
      - sleep disorder F14.182
      - unspecified disorder F14.19
    - in remission (early) (sustained) F14.11
  - counseling and surveillance Z71.51
  - hallucinogen F16.10
    - with
      - anxiety disorder F16.180
      - flashbacks F16.183
      - intoxication F16.129
        - with
          - delirium F16.121
          - perceptual disturbance F16.122
        - uncomplicated F16.120
      - mood disorder F16.14
      - other specified disorder F16.188
      - perception disorder, persisting F16.183
      - psychosis F16.159
        - delusions F16.150
        - hallucinations F16.151
      - unspecified disorder F16.19
    - in remission (early) (sustained) F16.11
  - hashish — *see* Abuse, drug, cannabis
  - herbal or folk remedies F55.1
  - hormones F55.3
  - hypnotics — *see* Abuse, drug, sedative
  - in remission (early) (sustained) F19.11
  - inhalant F18.10
    - with
      - anxiety disorder F18.180
      - dementia, persisting F18.17
      - intoxication F18.129
        - with delirium F18.121
        - uncomplicated F18.120
      - mood disorder F18.14
      - other specified disorder F18.188
      - psychosis F18.159
        - delusions F18.150
        - hallucinations F18.151
      - unspecified disorder F18.19
    - in remission (early) (sustained) F18.11
  - laxatives F55.2
  - LSD — *see* Abuse, drug, hallucinogen
  - marihuana — *see* Abuse, drug, cannabis
  - morphine type (opioids) — *see* Abuse, drug, opioid
  - opioid F11.10
    - with
      - intoxication F11.129
        - with
          - delirium F11.121
          - perceptual disturbance F11.122
        - uncomplicated F11.120
      - mood disorder F11.14
      - other specified disorder F11.188
      - psychosis F11.159
        - delusions F11.150
        - hallucinations F11.151
      - sexual dysfunction F11.181
      - sleep disorder F11.182
      - unspecified disorder F11.19
    - in remission (early) (sustained) F11.11
  - PCP (phencyclidine) (or related substance) — *see* Abuse, drug, hallucinogen
  - psychoactive NEC F19.10
    - with
      - amnestic disorder F19.16
      - anxiety disorder F19.180
      - dementia F19.17
      - intoxication F19.129

Abuse — *continued*
  drug — *continued*
    psychoactive — *continued*
      with — *continued*
        intoxication — *continued*
          with
            delirium F19.121
            perceptual disturbance F19.122
          uncomplicated F19.120
        mood disorder F19.14
        other specified disorder F19.188
        psychosis F19.159
          delusions F19.150
          hallucinations F19.151
        sexual dysfunction F19.181
        sleep disorder F19.182
        unspecified disorder F19.19
    sedative, hypnotic or anxiolytic F13.10
      with
        anxiety disorder F13.180
        intoxication F13.129
          with delirium F13.121
          uncomplicated F13.120
        mood disorder F13.14
        other specified disorder F13.188
        psychosis F13.159
          delusions F13.150
          hallucinations F13.151
        sexual dysfunction F13.181
        sleep disorder F13.182
        unspecified disorder F13.19
      in remission (early) (sustained) F13.11
    solvent — *see* Abuse, drug, inhalant
    steroids F55.3
    stimulant NEC F15.10
      with
        anxiety disorder F15.180
        intoxication F15.129
          with
            delirium F15.121
            perceptual disturbance F15.122
          uncomplicated F15.120
        mood disorder F15.14
        other specified disorder F15.188
        psychosis F15.159
          delusions F15.150
          hallucinations F15.151
        sexual dysfunction F15.181
        sleep disorder F15.182
        unspecified disorder F15.19
      in remission (early) (sustained) F15.11
    tranquilizers — *see* Abuse, drug, sedative
    vitamins F55.4
  hallucinogens — *see* Abuse, drug, hallucinogen
  hashish — *see* Abuse, drug, cannabis
  herbal or folk remedies F55.1
  hormones F55.3
  hypnotic — *see* Abuse, drug, sedative
  inhalant — *see* Abuse, drug, inhalant
  laxatives F55.2
  LSD — *see* Abuse, drug, hallucinogen
  marihuana — *see* Abuse, drug, cannabis
  morphine type (opioids) — *see* Abuse, drug, opioid
  non-psychoactive substance NEC F55.8
    antacids F55.0
    folk remedies F55.1
    herbal remedies F55.1
    hormones F55.3
    laxatives F55.2
    steroids F55.3
    vitamins F55.4
  opioids — *see* Abuse, drug, opioid
  PCP (phencyclidine) (or related substance) — *see* Abuse, drug, hallucinogen
  physical (adult) (child) — *see* Maltreatment
  psychoactive substance — *see* Abuse, drug, psychoactive NEC
  psychological (adult) (child) — *see* Maltreatment
  sedative — *see* Abuse, drug, sedative
  sexual — *see* Maltreatment
  solvent — *see* Abuse, drug, inhalant
  steroids F55.3
  vitamins F55.4
Acalculia R48.8
  developmental F81.2
Acanthamebiasis (with) B60.10
  conjunctiva B60.12
  keratoconjunctivitis B60.13

Acanthamebiasis — *continued*
  meningoencephalitis B60.11
  other specified B60.19
Acanthocephaliasis B83.8
Acanthocheilonemiasis B74.4
Acanthocytosis E78.6
Acantholysis L11.9
Acanthosis (acquired) (nigricans) L83
  benign Q82.8
  congenital Q82.8
  seborrheic L82.1
    inflamed L82.0
  tongue K14.3
Acapnia E87.3
Acarbia E87.2
Acardia, acardius Q89.8
Acardiacus amorphus Q89.8
Acardiotrophia I51.4
Acariasis B88.0
  scabies B86
Acarodermatitis (urticarioides) B88.0
Acarophobia F40.218
Acatalasemia, acatalasia E80.3
Acathisia (drug induced) G25.71
Accelerated atrioventricular conduction I45.6
Accentuation of personality traits (type A) Z73.1
Accessory (congenital)
  adrenal gland Q89.1
  anus Q43.4
  appendix Q43.4
  atrioventricular conduction I45.6
  auditory ossicles Q16.3
  auricle (ear) Q17.0
  biliary duct or passage Q44.5
  bladder Q64.79
  blood vessels NEC Q27.9
    coronary Q24.5
  bone NEC Q79.8
  breast tissue, axilla Q83.1
  carpal bones Q74.0
  cecum Q43.4
  chromosome(s) NEC (nonsex) Q92.9
    with complex rearrangements NEC Q92.5
      seen only at prometaphase Q92.8
    13 — *see* Trisomy, 13
    18 — *see* Trisomy, 18
    21 — *see* Trisomy, 21
    partial Q92.9
    sex
      female phenotype Q97.8
  coronary artery Q24.5
  cusp(s), heart valve NEC Q24.8
    pulmonary Q22.3
  cystic duct Q44.5
  digit(s) Q69.9
  ear (auricle) (lobe) Q17.0
  endocrine gland NEC Q89.2
  eye muscle Q10.3
  eyelid Q10.3
  face bone(s) Q75.8
  fallopian tube (fimbria) (ostium) Q50.6
  finger(s) Q69.0
  foreskin N47.8
  frontonasal process Q75.8
  gallbladder Q44.1
  genital organ(s)
    female Q52.8
      external Q52.79
      internal NEC Q52.8
    male Q55.8
  genitourinary organs NEC Q89.8
    female Q52.8
    male Q55.8
  hallux Q69.2
  heart Q24.8
    valve NEC Q24.8
      pulmonary Q22.3
  hepatic ducts Q44.5
  hymen Q52.4
  intestine (large) (small) Q43.4
  kidney Q63.0
  lacrimal canal Q10.6
  leaflet, heart valve NEC Q24.8
  ligament, broad Q50.6
  liver Q44.7
    duct Q44.5
  lobule (ear) Q17.0
  lung (lobe) Q33.1

Accessory — *continued*
  muscle Q79.8
  navicular of carpus Q74.0
  nervous system, part NEC Q07.8
  nipple Q83.3
  nose Q30.8
  organ or site not listed — *see* Anomaly, by site
  ovary Q50.31
  oviduct Q50.6
  pancreas Q45.3
  parathyroid gland Q89.2
  parotid gland (and duct) Q38.4
  pituitary gland Q89.2
  preauricular appendage Q17.0
  prepuce N47.8
  renal arteries (multiple) Q27.2
  rib Q76.6
    cervical Q76.5
  roots (teeth) K00.2
  salivary gland Q38.4
  sesamoid bones Q74.8
    foot Q74.2
    hand Q74.0
  skin tags Q82.8
  spleen Q89.09
  sternum Q76.7
  submaxillary gland Q38.4
  tarsal bones Q74.2
  teeth, tooth K00.1
  tendon Q79.8
  thumb Q69.1
  thymus gland Q89.2
  thyroid gland Q89.2
  toes Q69.2
  tongue Q38.3
  tooth, teeth K00.1
  tragus Q17.0
  ureter Q62.5
  urethra Q64.79
  urinary organ or tract NEC Q64.8
  uterus Q51.28
  vagina Q52.10
  valve, heart NEC Q24.8
    pulmonary Q22.3
  vertebra Q76.49
  vocal cords Q31.8
  vulva Q52.79
Accident
  birth — *see* Birth, injury
  cardiac — *see* Infarct, myocardium
  cerebral I63.9
  cerebrovascular (embolic) (ischemic) (thrombotic) I63.9
    aborted I63.9
    hemorrhagic — *see* Hemorrhage, intracranial, intracerebral
    old (without sequelae) Z86.73
      with sequelae (of) — *see* Sequelae, infarction, cerebral
  coronary — *see* Infarct, myocardium
  craniovascular I63.9
  vascular, brain I63.9
Accidental — *see* condition
Accommodation (disorder) — *see also* condition
  hysterical paralysis of F44.89
  insufficiency of H52.4
  paresis — *see* Paresis, of accommodation
  spasm — *see* Spasm, of accommodation
Accouchement — *see* Delivery
Accreta placenta O43.21- ☑
Accretio cordis (nonrheumatic) I31.0
Accretions, tooth, teeth K03.6
Acculturation difficulty Z60.3
Accumulation secretion, prostate N42.89
Acephalia, acephalism, acephalus, acephaly Q00.0
Acephalobrachia monster Q89.8
Acephalochirus monster Q89.8
Acephalogaster Q89.8
Acephalostomus monster Q89.8
Acephalothorax Q89.8
Acerophobia F40.298
Acetonemia R79.89
  in Type 1 diabetes E10.10
    with coma E10.11
Acetonuria R82.4
Achalasia (cardia) (esophagus) K22.0
  congenital Q39.5
  pylorus Q40.0
  sphincteral NEC K59.8

Ache(s) — see Pain
Acheilia Q38.6
Achil' obursitis — see Tendinitis, Achilles
Achillodynia — see Tendinitis, Achilles
Achlorhydria, achlorhydric (neurogenic) K31.83
  anemia D50.8
  diarrhea K31.83
  psychogenic F45.8
  secondary to vagotomy K91.1
Achluophobia F40.228
Acholia K82.8
Acholuric jaundice (familial) (splenomegalic) — see also
  Spherocytosis
  acquired D59.8
Achondrogenesis Q77.0
Achondroplasia (osteosclerosis congenita) Q77.4
Achroma, cutis L80
Achromat (ism), achromatopsia (acquired) (congenital)
  H53.51
Achromia, congenital — see Albinism
Achromia parasitica B36.0
Achylia gastrica K31.89
  psychogenic F45.8
Acid
  burn — see Corrosion
  deficiency
    amide nicotinic E52
    ascorbic E54
    folic E53.8
    nicotinic E52
    pantothenic E53.8
  intoxication E87.2
  peptic disease K30
  phosphatase deficiency E83.39
  stomach K30
    psychogenic F45.8
Acidemia E87.2
  argininosuccinic E72.22
  isovaleric E71.110
  metabolic (newborn) P19.9
    first noted before onset of labor P19.0
    first noted during labor P19.1
    noted at birth P19.2
  methylmalonic E71.120
  pipecolic E72.3
  propionic E71.121
Acidity, gastric (high) K30
  psychogenic F45.8
Acidocytopenia — see Agranulocytosis
Acidocytosis D72.1
Acidopenia — see Agranulocytosis
Acidosis (lactic) (respiratory) E87.2
  in Type 1 diabetes E10.10
    with coma E10.11
  kidney, tubular N25.89
  lactic E87.2
  metabolic NEC E87.2
    with respiratory acidosis E87.4
    hyperchloremic, of newborn P74.421
    late, of newborn P74.0
  mixed metabolic and respiratory, newborn P84
  newborn P84
  renal (hyperchloremic) (tubular) N25.89
  respiratory E87.2
    complicated by
      metabolic
        acidosis E87.4
        alkalosis E87.4
Aciduria
  4-hydroxybutyric E72.81
  argininosuccinic E72.22
  gamma-hydroxybutyric E72.81
  glutaric (type I) E72.3
    type II E71.313
    type III E71.5- ☑
  orotic (congenital) (hereditary) (pyrimidine deficiency)
    E79.8
    anemia D53.0
Acladiosis (skin) B36.0
Aclasis, diaphyseal Q78.6
Acleistocardia Q21.1
Aclusion — see Anomaly, dentofacial, malocclusion
Acne L70.9
  artificialis L70.8
  atrophica L70.2
  cachecticorum (Hebra) L70.8
  conglobata L70.1
  cystic L70.0

Acne — continued
  decalvans L66.2
  excoriée (des jeunes filles) L70.5
  frontalis L70.0
  indurata L70.0
  infantile L70.4
  keloid L73.0
  lupoid L70.2
  necrotic, necrotica (miliaris) L70.2
  neonatal L70.4
  nodular L70.0
  occupational L70.8
  picker's L70.5
  pustular L70.0
  rodens L70.2
  rosacea L71.9
  specified NEC L70.8
  tropica L70.3
  varioliformis L70.2
  vulgaris L70.0
Acnitis (primary) A18.4
Acosta's disease T70.29 ☑
Acoustic — see condition
Acousticophobia F40.298
Acquired — see also condition
  immunodeficiency syndrome (AIDS) B20
Acrania Q00.0
Acroangiodermatitis I78.9
Acroasphyxia, chronic I73.89
Acrobystitis N47.7
Acrocephalopolysyndactyly Q87.0
Acrocephalosyndactyly Q87.0
Acrocephaly Q75.0
Acrochondrohyperplasia — see Syndrome, Marfan's
Acrocyanosis I73.89
  newborn P28.2
    meaning transient blue hands and feet — omit code
Acrodermatitis L30.8
  atrophicans (chronica) L90.4
  continua (Hallopeau) L40.2
  enteropathica (hereditary) E83.2
  Hallopeau's L40.2
  infantile papular L44.4
  perstans L40.2
  pustulosa continua L40.2
  recalcitrant pustular L40.2
Acrodynia — see Poisoning, mercury
Acromegaly, acromegalia E22.0
Acromelalgia I73.81
Acromicria, acromikria Q79.8
Acronyx L60.0
Acropachy, thyroid — see Thyrotoxicosis
Acroparesthesia (simple) (vasomotor) I73.89
Acropathy, thyroid — see Thyrotoxicosis
Acrophobia F40.241
Acroposthitis N47.7
Acroscleriasis, acroscleroderma, acrosclerosis — see
  Sclerosis, systemic
Acrosphacelus I96
Acrospiroma, eccrine — see Neoplasm, skin, benign
Acrostealgia — see Osteochondropathy
Acrotrophodynia — see Immersion
ACTH ectopic syndrome E24.3
Actinic — see condition
Actinobacillosis, actinobacillus A28.8
  mallei A24.0
  muris A25.1
Actinomyces israelii (infection) — see Actinomycosis
Actinomycetoma (foot) B47.1
Actinomycosis, actinomycotic A42.9
  with pneumonia A42.0
  abdominal A42.1
  cervicofacial A42.2
  cutaneous A42.89
  gastrointestinal A42.1
  pulmonary A42.0
  sepsis A42.7
  specified site NEC A42.89
Actinoneuritis G62.82
Action, heart
  disorder I49.9
  irregular I49.9
    psychogenic F45.8
Activated protein C resistance D68.51
Activation
  mast cell (disorder) (syndrome) D89.40
    idiopathic D89.42

Activation — continued
  mast cell — continued
    monoclonal D89.41
    secondary D89.43
    specified type NEC D89.49
Active — see condition
Acute — see also condition
  abdomen R10.0
  gallbladder — see Cholecystitis, acute
Acyanotic heart disease (congenital) Q24.9
Acystia Q64.5
Adair-Dighton syndrome (brittle bones and blue sclera,
  deafness) Q78.0
Adamantinoblastoma — see Ameloblastoma
Adamantinoma — see also Cyst, calcifying odontogenic
  long bones C40.90
    lower limb C40.2- ☑
    upper limb C40.0- ☑
  malignant C41.1
    jaw (bone) (lower) C41.1
      upper C41.0
  tibial C40.2- ☑
Adamantoblastoma — see Ameloblastoma
Adams-Stokes (-Morgagni) disease or syndrome I45.9
Adaption reaction — see Disorder, adjustment
Addiction — see also Dependence F19.20
  alcohol, alcoholic (ethyl) (methyl) (wood) (without re-
    mission) F10.20
    with remission F10.21
  drug — see Dependence, drug
  ethyl alcohol (without remission) F10.20
    with remission F10.21
  heroin — see Dependence, drug, opioid
  methyl alcohol (without remission) F10.20
    with remission F10.21
  methylated spirit (without remission) F10.20
    with remission F10.21
  morphine (-like substances) — see Dependence, drug,
    opioid
  nicotine — see Dependence, drug, nicotine
  opium and opioids — see Dependence, drug, opioid
  tobacco — see Dependence, drug, nicotine
Addison-Biermer anemia (pernicious) D51.0
Addisonian crisis E27.2
Addison's
  anemia (pernicious) D51.0
  disease (bronze) or syndrome E27.1
    tuberculous A18.7
  keloid L94.0
Addison-Schilder complex E71.528
Additional — see also Accessory
  chromosome(s) Q99.8
    21 — see Trisomy, 21
    sex — see Abnormal, chromosome, sex
Adduction contracture, hip or other joint — see
  Contraction, joint
Adenitis — see also Lymphadenitis
  acute, unspecified site L04.9
  axillary I88.9
    acute L04.2
    chronic or subacute I88.1
  Bartholin's gland N75.8
  bulbourethral gland — see Urethritis
  cervical I88.9
    acute L04.0
    chronic or subacute I88.1
  chancroid (Hemophilus ducreyi) A57
  chronic, unspecified site I88.1
  Cowper's gland — see Urethritis
  due to Pasteurella multocida (P. septica) A28.0
  epidemic, acute B27.09
  gangrenous L04.9
  gonorrheal NEC A54.89
  groin I88.9
    acute L04.1
    chronic or subacute I88.1
  infectious (acute) (epidemic) B27.09
  inguinal I88.9
    acute L04.1
    chronic or subacute I88.1
  lymph gland or node, except mesenteric I88.9
    acute — see Lymphadenitis, acute
    chronic or subacute I88.1
  mesenteric (acute) (chronic) (nonspecific) (subacute)
    I88.0
  parotid gland (suppurative) — see Sialoadenitis
  salivary gland (any) (suppurative) — see Sialoadeniti
  scrofulous (tuberculous) A18.2

Adenitis — *continued*
 Skene's duct or gland — *see* Urethritis
 strumous, tuberculous A18.2
 subacute, unspecified site I88.1
 sublingual gland (suppurative) — *see* Sialoadenitis
 submandibular gland (suppurative) — *see* Sialoadenitis
 submaxillary gland (suppurative) — *see* Sialoadenitis
 tuberculous — *see* Tuberculosis, lymph gland
 urethral gland — *see* Urethritis
 Wharton's duct (suppurative) — *see* Sialoadenitis
Adenoacanthoma — *see* Neoplasm, malignant, by site
Adenoameloblastoma — *see* Cyst, calcifying odontogenic
Adenocarcinoid (tumor) — *see* Neoplasm, malignant,
 by site
Adenocarcinoma — *see also* Neoplasm, malignant, by
 site
 acidophil
 specified site — *see* Neoplasm, malignant, by site
 unspecified site C75.1
 adrenal cortical C74.0- ☑
 alveolar — *see* Neoplasm, lung, malignant
 apocrine
 breast — *see* Neoplasm, breast, malignant
 in situ
 breast D05.8- ☑
 specified site NEC — *see* Neoplasm, skin, in situ
 unspecified site D04.9
 specified site NEC — *see* Neoplasm, skin, malignant
 unspecified site C44.99
 basal cell
 specified site — *see* Neoplasm, skin, malignant
 unspecified site C08.9
 basophil
 specified site — *see* Neoplasm, malignant, by site
 unspecified site C75.1
 bile duct type C22.1
 liver C22.1
 specified site NEC — *see* Neoplasm, malignant, by
 site
 unspecified site C22.1
 bronchiolar — *see* Neoplasm, lung, malignant
 bronchioloalveolar — *see* Neoplasm, lung, malignant
 ceruminous C44.29- ☑
 cervix, in situ — *see also* Carcinoma, cervix uteri, in situ
 D06.9
 chromophobe
 specified site — *see* Neoplasm, malignant, by site
 unspecified site C75.1
 diffuse type
 specified site — *see* Neoplasm, malignant, by site
 unspecified site C16.9
 duct
 infiltrating
 with Paget's disease — *see* Neoplasm, breast,
 malignant
 specified site — *see* Neoplasm, malignant, by
 site
 unspecified site (female) C50.91- ☑
 male C50.92- ☑
 specified site — *see* Neoplasm, malignant, by site
 unspecified site
 female C56.9
 male C61
 eosinophil
 specified site — *see* Neoplasm, malignant, by site
 unspecified site C75.1
 follicular
 with papillary C73
 moderately differentiated C73
 specified site — *see* Neoplasm, malignant, by site
 trabecular C73
 unspecified site C73
 well differentiated C73
 Hurthle cell C73
 in
 adenomatous
 polyposis coli C18.9
 infiltrating duct
 with Paget's disease — *see* Neoplasm, breast, malignant
 specified site — *see* Neoplasm, by site, malignant
 unspecified site (female) C50.91- ☑
 male C50.92- ☑
 inflammatory
 specified site — *see* Neoplasm, by site, malignant
 unspecified site (female) C50.91- ☑

Adenocarcinoma — *continued*
 inflammatory — *continued*
 unspecified site — *continued*
 male C50.92- ☑
 intestinal type
 specified site — *see* Neoplasm, by site, malignant
 unspecified site C16.9
 intracystic papillary
 intraductal
 breast D05.1- ☑
 noninfiltrating
 breast D05.1- ☑
 papillary
 with invasion
 specified site — *see* Neoplasm, by site,
 malignant
 unspecified site (female) C50.91- ☑
 male C50.92- ☑
 breast D05.1- ☑
 specified site NEC — *see* Neoplasm, in situ,
 by site
 unspecified site D05.1- ☑
 specified site NEC — *see* Neoplasm, in situ, by
 site
 unspecified site D05.1- ☑
 papillary
 with invasion
 specified site — *see* Neoplasm, malignant, by
 site
 unspecified site (female) C50.91- ☑
 male C50.92- ☑
 breast D05.1- ☑
 specified site — *see* Neoplasm, in situ, by site
 unspecified site D05.1- ☑
 specified site NEC — *see* Neoplasm, in situ, by site
 unspecified site D05.1- ☑
 islet cell
 with exocrine, mixed
 specified site — *see* Neoplasm, malignant, by
 site
 unspecified site C25.9
 pancreas C25.4
 specified site NEC — *see* Neoplasm, malignant, by
 site
 unspecified site C25.4
 lobular
 in situ
 breast D05.0- ☑
 specified site NEC — *see* Neoplasm, in situ, by
 site
 unspecified site D05.0- ☑
 specified site — *see* Neoplasm, malignant, by site
 unspecified site (female) C50.91- ☑
 male C50.92- ☑
 mucoid — *see also* Neoplasm, malignant, by site
 cell
 specified site — *see* Neoplasm, malignant, by
 site
 unspecified site C75.1
 nonencapsulated sclerosing C73
 papillary
 with follicular C73
 follicular variant C73
 intraductal (noninfiltrating)
 with invasion
 specified site — *see* Neoplasm, malignant, by
 site
 unspecified site (female) C50.91- ☑
 male C50.92- ☑
 breast D05.1- ☑
 specified site NEC — *see* Neoplasm, in situ, by
 site
 unspecified site D05.1- ☑
 serous
 specified site — *see* Neoplasm, malignant, by
 site
 unspecified site C56.9
 papillocystic
 specified site — *see* Neoplasm, malignant, by site
 unspecified site C56.9
 pseudomucinous
 specified site — *see* Neoplasm, malignant, by site
 unspecified site C56.9
 renal cell C64- ☑
 sebaceous — *see* Neoplasm, skin, malignant
 serous — *see also* Neoplasm, malignant, by site

Adenocarcinoma — *continued*
 serous — *see also* Neoplasm, malignant, by site —
 continued
 papillary
 specified site — *see* Neoplasm, malignant, by
 site
 unspecified site C56.9
 sweat gland — *see* Neoplasm, skin, malignant
 water-clear cell C75.0
Adenocarcinoma-in-situ — *see also* Neoplasm, in situ,
 by site
 breast D05.9- ☑
Adenofibroma
 clear cell — *see* Neoplasm, benign, by site
 endometrioid D27.9
 borderline malignancy D39.10
 malignant C56- ☑
 mucinous
 specified site — *see* Neoplasm, benign, by site
 unspecified site D27.9
 papillary
 specified site — *see* Neoplasm, benign, by site
 unspecified site D27.9
 prostate — *see* Enlargement, enlarged, prostate
 serous
 specified site — *see* Neoplasm, benign, by site
 unspecified site D27.9
 specified site — *see* Neoplasm, benign, by site
 unspecified site D27.9
Adenofibrosis
 breast — *see* Fibroadenosis, breast
 endometrioid N80.0
Adenoiditis (chronic) J35.02
 with tonsillitis J35.03
 acute J03.90
 recurrent J03.91
 specified organism NEC J03.80
 recurrent J03.81
 staphylococcal J03.80
 recurrent J03.81
 streptococcal J03.00
 recurrent J03.01
Adenoids — *see* condition
Adenolipoma — *see* Neoplasm, benign, by site
Adenolipomatosis, Launois-Bensaude E88.89
Adenolymphoma
 specified site — *see* Neoplasm, benign, by site
 unspecified site D11.9
Adenoma — *see also* Neoplasm, benign, by site
 acidophil
 specified site — *see* Neoplasm, benign, by site
 unspecified site D35.2
 acidophil-basophil, mixed
 specified site — *see* Neoplasm, benign, by site
 unspecified site D35.2
 adrenal (cortical) D35.00
 clear cell D35.00
 compact cell D35.00
 glomerulosa cell D35.00
 heavily pigmented variant D35.00
 mixed cell D35.00
 alpha-cell
 pancreas D13.7
 specified site NEC — *see* Neoplasm, benign, by site
 unspecified site D13.7
 alveolar D14.30
 apocrine
 breast D24- ☑
 specified site NEC — *see* Neoplasm, skin, benign,
 by site
 unspecified site D23.9
 basal cell D11.9
 basophil
 specified site — *see* Neoplasm, benign, by site
 unspecified site D35.2
 basophil-acidophil, mixed
 specified site — *see* Neoplasm, benign, by site
 unspecified site D35.2
 beta-cell
 pancreas D13.7
 specified site NEC — *see* Neoplasm, benign, by site
 unspecified site D13.7
 bile duct D13.4
 common D13.5
 extrahepatic D13.5
 intrahepatic D13.4
 specified site NEC — *see* Neoplasm, benign, by site
 unspecified site D13.4

Adenoma — *continued*
  black D35.00
  bronchial D38.1
    cylindroid type — *see* Neoplasm, lung, malignant
  ceruminous D23.2- ☑
  chief cell D35.1
  chromophobe
    specified site — *see* Neoplasm, benign, by site
    unspecified site D35.2
  colloid
    specified site — *see* Neoplasm, benign, by site
    unspecified site D34
  duct
  eccrine, papillary — *see* Neoplasm, skin, benign
  endocrine, multiple
    single specified site — *see* Neoplasm, uncertain
        behavior, by site
    two or more specified sites D44- ☑
    unspecified site D44.9
  endometrioid — *see also* Neoplasm, benign
    borderline malignancy — *see* Neoplasm, uncertain
        behavior, by site
  eosinophil
    specified site — *see* Neoplasm, benign, by site
    unspecified site D35.2
  fetal
    specified site — *see* Neoplasm, benign, by site
    unspecified site D34
  follicular
    specified site — *see* Neoplasm, benign, by site
    unspecified site D34
  hepatocellular D13.4
  Hurthle cell D34
  islet cell
    pancreas D13.7
    specified site NEC — *see* Neoplasm, benign, by site
    unspecified site D13.7
  liver cell D13.4
  macrofollicular
    specified site — *see* Neoplasm, benign, by site
    unspecified site D34
  malignant, malignum — *see* Neoplasm, malignant, by
      site
  microcystic
    pancreas D13.6
    specified site NEC — *see* Neoplasm, benign, by site
    unspecified site D13.6
  microfollicular
    specified site — *see* Neoplasm, benign, by site
    unspecified site D34
  mucoid cell
    specified site — *see* Neoplasm, benign, by site
    unspecified site D35.2
  multiple endocrine
    single specified site — *see* Neoplasm, uncertain
        behavior, by site
    two or more specified sites D44- ☑
    unspecified site D44.9
  nipple D24- ☑
  papillary — *see also* Neoplasm, benign, by site
    eccrine — *see* Neoplasm, skin, benign, by site
  Pick's tubular
    specified site — *see* Neoplasm, benign, by site
    unspecified site
      female D27.9
      male D29.20
  pleomorphic
    carcinoma in — *see* Neoplasm, salivary gland, ma-
        lignant
      specified site — *see* Neoplasm, malignant, by
          site
      unspecified site C08.9
  polypoid — *see also* Neoplasm, benign
    adenocarcinoma in — *see* Neoplasm, malignant, by
        site
    adenocarcinoma in situ — *see* Neoplasm, in situ, by
        site
  prostate — *see* Neoplasm, benign, prostate
  rete cell D29.20
  sebaceous — *see* Neoplasm, skin, benign
  Sertoli cell
    specified site — *see* Neoplasm, benign, by site
    unspecified site
      female D27.9
      male D29.20
  skin appendage — *see* Neoplasm, skin, benign
  sudoriferous gland — *see* Neoplasm, skin, benign
  sweat gland — *see* Neoplasm, skin, benign

Adenoma — *continued*
  testicular
    specified site — *see* Neoplasm, benign, by site
    unspecified site
      female D27.9
      male D29.20
  tubular — *see also* Neoplasm, benign, by site
    adenocarcinoma in — *see* Neoplasm, malignant, by
        site
    adenocarcinoma in situ — *see* Neoplasm, in situ, by
        site
    Pick's
      specified site — *see* Neoplasm, benign, by site
      unspecified site
        female D27.9
        male D29.20
  tubulovillous — *see also* Neoplasm, benign, by site
    adenocarcinoma in — *see* Neoplasm, malignant, by
        site
    adenocarcinoma in situ — *see* Neoplasm, in situ, by
        site
  villous — *see* Neoplasm, uncertain behavior, by site
    adenocarcinoma in — *see* Neoplasm, malignant, by
        site
    adenocarcinoma in situ — *see* Neoplasm, in situ, by
        site
  water-clear cell D35.1
Adenomatosis
  endocrine (multiple) E31.20
    single specified site — *see* Neoplasm, uncertain
        behavior, by site
  erosive of nipple D24- ☑
  pluriendocrine — *see* Adenomatosis, endocrine
  pulmonary D38.1
    malignant — *see* Neoplasm, lung, malignant
  specified site — *see* Neoplasm, benign, by site
  unspecified site D12.6
Adenomatous
  goiter (nontoxic) E04.9
    with hyperthyroidism — *see* Hyperthyroidism, with,
        goiter, nodular
    toxic — *see* Hyperthyroidism, with, goiter, nodular
Adenomyoma — *see also* Neoplasm, benign, by site
  prostate — *see* Enlarged, prostate
Adenomyometritis N80.0
Adenomyosis N80.0
Adenopathy (lymph gland) R59.9
  generalized R59.1
  inguinal R59.0
  localized R59.0
  mediastinal R59.0
  mesentery R59.0
  syphilitic (secondary) A51.49
  tracheobronchial R59.0
    tuberculous A15.4
      primary (progressive) A15.7
  tuberculous — *see also* Tuberculosis, lymph gland
    tracheobronchial A15.4
      primary (progressive) A15.7
Adenosalpingitis — *see* Salpingitis
Adenosarcoma — *see* Neoplasm, malignant, by site
Adenosclerosis I88.8
Adenosis (sclerosing) breast — *see* Fibroadenosis, breast
Adenovirus, as cause of disease classified elsewhere
  B97.0
Adentia (complete) (partial) — *see* Absence, teeth
Adherent — *see also* Adhesions
  labia (minora) N90.89
  pericardium (nonrheumatic) I31.0
    rheumatic I09.2
  placenta (with hemorrhage) O72.0
    without hemorrhage O73.0
  prepuce, newborn N47.0
  scar (skin) L90.5
  tendon in scar L90.5
Adhesions, adhesive (postinfective) K66.0
  with intestinal obstruction K56.50
    complete K56.52
    incomplete K56.51
    partial K56.51
  abdominal (wall) — *see* Adhesions, peritoneum
  appendix K38.8
  bile duct (common) (hepatic) K83.8
  bladder (sphincter) N32.89
  bowel — *see* Adhesions, peritoneum
  cardiac I31.0
    rheumatic I09.2
  cecum — *see* Adhesions, peritoneum

Adhesions, adhesive — *continued*
  cervicovaginal N88.1
    congenital Q52.8
    postpartal O90.89
    old N88.1
  cervix N88.1
  ciliary body NEC — *see* Adhesions, iris
  clitoris N90.89
  colon — *see* Adhesions, peritoneum
  common duct K83.8
  congenital — *see also* Anomaly, by site
    fingers — *see* Syndactylism, complex, fingers
    omental, anomalous Q43.3
    peritoneal Q43.3
    tongue (to gum or roof of mouth) Q38.3
  conjunctiva (acquired) H11.21- ☑
    congenital Q15.8
  cystic duct K82.8
  diaphragm — *see* Adhesions, peritoneum
  due to foreign body — *see* Foreign body
  duodenum — *see* Adhesions, peritoneum
  ear
    middle H74.1- ☑
  epididymis N50.89
  epidural — *see* Adhesions, meninges
  epiglottis J38.7
  eyelid H02.59
  female pelvis N73.6
  gallbladder K82.8
  globe H44.89
  heart I31.0
    rheumatic I09.2
  ileocecal (coil) — *see* Adhesions, peritoneum
  ileum — *see* Adhesions, peritoneum
  intestine — *see also* Adhesions, peritoneum
    with obstruction K56.50
      complete K56.52
      incomplete K56.51
      partial K56.51
  intra-abdominal — *see* Adhesions, peritoneum
  iris H21.50- ☑
    anterior H21.51- ☑
    goniosynechiae H21.52- ☑
    posterior H21.54- ☑
    to corneal graft T85.898 ☑
  joint — *see* Ankylosis
    knee M23.8X ☑
    temporomandibular M26.61- ☑
  labium (majus) (minus), congenital Q52.5
  liver — *see* Adhesions, peritoneum
  lung J98.4
  mediastinum J98.59
  meninges (cerebral) (spinal) G96.12
    congenital Q07.8
    tuberculous (cerebral) (spinal) A17.0
  mesenteric — *see* Adhesions, peritoneum
  nasal (septum) (to turbinates) J34.89
  ocular muscle — *see* Strabismus, mechanical
  omentum — *see* Adhesions, peritoneum
  ovary N73.6
    congenital (to cecum, kidney or omentum) Q50.39
  paraovarian N73.6
  pelvic (peritoneal)
    female N73.6
      postprocedural N99.4
    male — *see* Adhesions, peritoneum
    postpartal (old) N73.6
    tuberculous A18.17
  penis to scrotum (congenital) Q55.8
  periappendiceal — *see also* Adhesions, peritoneum
  pericardium (nonrheumatic) I31.0
    focal I31.8
    rheumatic I09.2
    tuberculous A18.84
  pericholecystic K82.8
  perigastric — *see* Adhesions, peritoneum
  periovarian N73.6
  periprostatic N42.89
  perirectal — *see* Adhesions, peritoneum
  perirenal N28.89
  peritoneum, peritoneal (postinfective) K66.0
    with obstruction (intestinal) K56.50
      complete K56.52
      incomplete K56.51
      partial K56.51
    congenital Q43.3
    pelvic, female N73.6
      postprocedural N99.4

☑ **Additional Character Required** — Refer to the Tabular List for Character Selection   ▽ **Subterms under main terms may continue to next column or page**

Adhesions, adhesive — *continued*
  peritoneum, peritoneal — *continued*
    postpartal, pelvic N73.6
    postprocedural K66.0
    to uterus N73.6
  peritubal N73.6
  periureteral N28.89
  periuterine N73.6
  perivesical N32.89
  perivesicular (seminal vesicle) N50.89
  pleura, pleuritic J94.8
    tuberculous NEC A15.6
  pleuropericardial J94.8
  postoperative (gastrointestinal tract) K66.0
    with obstruction — *see also* Obstruction, intestine,
      postoperative K91.30
    due to foreign body accidentally left in wound —
      see Foreign body, accidentally left during a
      procedure
    pelvic peritoneal N99.4
    urethra — *see* Stricture, urethra, postprocedural
    vagina N99.2
  postpartal, old (vulva or perineum) N90.89
  preputial, prepuce N47.5
  pulmonary J98.4
  pylorus — *see* Adhesions, peritoneum
  sciatic nerve — *see* Lesion, nerve, sciatic
  seminal vesicle N50.89
  shoulder (joint) — *see* Capsulitis, adhesive
  sigmoid flexure — *see* Adhesions, peritoneum
  spermatic cord (acquired) N50.89
    congenital Q55.4
  spinal canal G96.12
  stomach — *see* Adhesions, peritoneum
  subscapular — *see* Capsulitis, adhesive
  temporomandibular M26.61- ☑
  tendinitis (*see also* Tenosynovitis, specified type NEC)
    shoulder — *see* Capsulitis, adhesive
  testis N44.8
  tongue, congenital (to gum or roof of mouth) Q38.3
    acquired K14.8
  trachea J39.8
  tubo-ovarian N73.6
  tunica vaginalis N44.8
  uterus N73.6
    internal N85.6
    to abdominal wall N73.6
  vagina (chronic) N89.5
    postoperative N99.2
  vitreomacular H43.82- ☑
  vitreous H43.89
  vulva N90.89
Adiaspiromycosis B48.8
Adie (-Holmes) **pupil or syndrome** — *see* Anomaly,
  pupil, function, tonic pupil
Adiponecrosis neonatorum P83.88
Adiposis — *see also* Obesity
  cerebralis E23.6
  dolorosa E88.2
Adiposity — *see also* Obesity
  heart — *see* Degeneration, myocardial
  localized E65
Adiposogenital dystrophy E23.6
Adjustment
  disorder — *see* Disorder, adjustment
  implanted device — *see* Encounter (for), adjustment
    (of)
  prosthesis, external — *see* Fitting
  reaction — *see* Disorder, adjustment
Administration of tPA (rtPA) in a different facility within
  the last 24 hours prior to admission to current facility Z92.82
Admission (for) — *see also* Encounter (for)
  adjustment (of)
    artificial
      arm Z44.00- ☑
        complete Z44.01- ☑
        partial Z44.02- ☑
      eye Z44.2 ☑
      leg Z44.10- ☑
        complete Z44.11- ☑
        partial Z44.12- ☑
    brain neuropacemaker Z46.2
      implanted Z45.42
    breast
      implant Z45.81 ☑
      prosthesis (external) Z44.3 ☑

Admission — *continued*
  adjustment — *continued*
    colostomy belt Z46.89
    contact lenses Z46.0
    cystostomy device Z46.6
    dental prosthesis Z46.3
    device NEC
      abdominal Z46.89
      implanted Z45.89
        cardiac Z45.09
          defibrillator (with synchronous cardiac
            pacemaker) Z45.02
          pacemaker (cardiac resynchronization
            therapy (CRT-P)) Z45.018
            pulse generator Z45.010
          resynchronization therapy defibrillator
            (CRT-D) Z45.02
        hearing device Z45.328
          bone conduction Z45.320
          cochlear Z45.321
        infusion pump Z45.1
        nervous system Z45.49
          CSF drainage Z45.41
          hearing device — *see* Admission, adjust-
            ment, device, implanted, hearing
            device
          neuropacemaker Z45.42
          visual substitution Z45.31
        specified NEC Z45.89
        vascular access Z45.2
        visual substitution Z45.31
      nervous system Z46.2
        implanted — *see* Admission, adjustment,
          device, implanted, nervous system
    orthodontic Z46.4
    prosthetic Z44.9
      arm — *see* Admission, adjustment, artificial,
        arm
      breast Z44.3 ☑
      dental Z46.3
      eye Z44.2 ☑
      leg — *see* Admission, adjustment, artificial,
        leg
      specified type NEC Z44.8
    substitution
      auditory Z46.2
        implanted — *see* Admission, adjustment,
          device, implanted, hearing device
      nervous system Z46.2
        implanted — *see* Admission, adjustment,
          device, implanted, nervous system
      visual Z46.2
        implanted Z45.31
    urinary Z46.6
  hearing aid Z46.1
    implanted — *see* Admission, adjustment, device,
      implanted, hearing device
  ileostomy device Z46.89
  intestinal appliance or device NEC Z46.89
  neuropacemaker (brain) (peripheral nerve) (spinal
    cord) Z46.2
    implanted Z45.42
  orthodontic device Z46.4
  orthopedic (brace) (cast) (device) (shoes) Z46.89
  pacemaker (cardiac resynchronization therapy (CRT-
    P))
    cardiac Z45.018
      pulse generator Z45.010
    nervous system Z46.2
      implanted Z45.42
  portacath (port-a-cath) Z45.2
  prosthesis Z44.9
    arm — *see* Admission, adjustment, artificial, arm
    breast Z44.3 ☑
    dental Z46.3
    eye Z44.2 ☑
    leg — *see* Admission, adjustment, artificial, leg
    specified NEC Z44.8
  spectacles Z46.0
  aftercare — *see also* Aftercare Z51.89
    postpartum
      immediately after delivery Z39.0
      routine follow-up Z39.2
    radiation therapy (antineoplastic) Z51.0
  attention to artificial opening (of) Z43.9
    artificial vagina Z43.7
    colostomy Z43.3
    cystostomy Z43.5

Admission — *continued*
  attention to artificial opening — *continued*
    enterostomy Z43.4
    gastrostomy Z43.1
    ileostomy Z43.2
    jejunostomy Z43.4
    nephrostomy Z43.6
    specified site NEC Z43.8
      intestinal tract Z43.4
      urinary tract Z43.6
    tracheostomy Z43.0
    ureterostomy Z43.6
    urethrostomy Z43.6
  breast augmentation or reduction Z41.1
  breast reconstruction following mastectomy Z42.1
  change of
    dressing (nonsurgical) Z48.00
    neuropacemaker device (brain) (peripheral nerve)
      (spinal cord) Z46.2
      implanted Z45.42
    surgical dressing Z48.01
  circumcision, ritual or routine (in absence of diagnosis)
    Z41.2
  clinical research investigation (control) (normal com-
    parison) (participant) Z00.6
  contraceptive management Z30.9
  cosmetic surgery NEC Z41.1
  counseling — *see also* Counseling
    dietary Z71.3
    gestational carrier Z31.7
    HIV Z71.7
    human immunodeficiency virus Z71.7
    nonattending third party Z71.0
    procreative management NEC Z31.69
  delivery, full-term, uncomplicated O80
    cesarean, without indication O82
  desensitization to allergens Z51.6
  dietary surveillance and counseling Z71.3
  ear piercing Z41.3
  examination at health care facility (adult) — *see also*
    Examination Z00.00
    with abnormal findings Z00.01
    clinical research investigation (control) (normal
      comparison) (participant) Z00.6
    dental Z01.20
      with abnormal findings Z01.21
    donor (potential) Z00.5
    ear Z01.10
      with abnormal findings NEC Z01.118
    eye Z01.00
      with abnormal findings Z01.01
      following failed vision screening Z01.020
        with abnormal findings Z01.021
    general, specified reason NEC Z00.8
    hearing Z01.10
      with abnormal findings NEC Z01.118
      infant or child (over 28 days old) Z00.129
        with abnormal findings Z00.121
    postpartum checkup Z39.2
    psychiatric (general) Z00.8
      requested by authority Z04.6
    vision Z01.00
      with abnormal findings Z01.01
      following failed vision screening Z01.020
        with abnormal findings Z01.021
      infant or child (over 28 days old) Z00.129
        with abnormal findings Z00.121
  fitting (of)
    artificial
      arm — *see* Admission, adjustment, artificial, arm
      eye Z44.2 ☑
      leg — *see* Admission, adjustment, artificial, leg
    brain neuropacemaker Z46.2
      implanted Z45.42
    breast prosthesis (external) Z44.3 ☑
    colostomy belt Z46.89
    contact lenses Z46.0
    cystostomy device Z46.6
    dental prosthesis Z46.3
    dentures Z46.3
    device NEC
      abdominal Z46.89
      nervous system Z46.2
        implanted — *see* Admission, adjustment,
          device, implanted, nervous system
    orthodontic Z46.4
    prosthetic Z44.9
      breast Z44.3 ☑

Admission — *continued*
- fitting — *continued*
  - device — *continued*
    - prosthetic — *continued*
      - dental Z46.3
      - eye Z44.2 ☑
    - substitution
      - auditory Z46.2
        - implanted — *see* Admission, adjustment, device, implanted, hearing device
      - nervous system Z46.2
        - implanted — *see* Admission, adjustment, device, implanted, nervous system
      - visual Z46.2
        - implanted Z45.31
  - hearing aid Z46.1
  - ileostomy device Z46.89
  - intestinal appliance or device NEC Z46.89
  - neuropacemaker (brain) (peripheral nerve) (spinal cord) Z46.2
    - implanted Z45.42
  - orthodontic device Z46.4
  - orthopedic device (brace) (cast) (shoes) Z46.89
  - prosthesis Z44.9
    - arm — *see* Admission, adjustment, artificial, arm
    - breast Z44.3 ☑
    - dental Z46.3
    - eye Z44.2 ☑
    - leg — *see* Admission, adjustment, artificial, leg
    - specified type NEC Z44.8
  - spectacles Z46.0
- follow-up examination Z09
- intrauterine device management Z30.431
  - initial prescription Z30.014
- mental health evaluation Z00.8
  - requested by authority Z04.6
- observation — *see* Observation
- Papanicolaou smear, cervix Z12.4
  - for suspected malignant neoplasm Z12.4
- plastic and reconstructive surgery following medical procedure or healed injury NEC Z42.8
- plastic surgery, cosmetic NEC Z41.1
- postpartum observation
  - immediately after delivery Z39.0
  - routine follow-up Z39.2
- poststerilization (for restoration) Z31.0
  - aftercare Z31.42
- procreative management Z31.9
- prophylactic (measure) — *see also* Encounter, prophylactic measures
  - organ removal Z40.00
    - breast Z40.01
    - fallopian tube(s) Z40.03
      - with ovary(s) Z40.02
    - ovary(s) Z40.02
    - specified organ NEC Z40.09
    - testes Z40.09
  - vaccination Z23
- psychiatric examination (general) Z00.8
  - requested by authority Z04.6
- radiation therapy (antineoplastic) Z51.0
- reconstructive surgery following medical procedure or healed injury NEC Z42.8
- removal of
  - cystostomy catheter Z43.5
  - drains Z48.03
  - dressing (nonsurgical) Z48.00
  - implantable subdermal contraceptive Z30.46
  - intrauterine contraceptive device Z30.432
  - neuropacemaker (brain) (peripheral nerve) (spinal cord) Z46.2
    - implanted Z45.42
  - staples Z48.02
  - surgical dressing Z48.01
  - sutures Z48.02
  - ureteral stent Z46.6
- respirator [ventilator] use during power failure Z99.12
- restoration of organ continuity (poststerilization) Z31.0
  - aftercare Z31.42
- sensitivity test — *see also* Test, skin
  - allergy NEC Z01.82
  - Mantoux Z11.1
- tuboplasty following previous sterilization Z31.0
  - aftercare Z31.42
- vasoplasty following previous sterilization Z31.0
  - aftercare Z31.42
- vision examination Z01.00
  - with abnormal findings Z01.01

Admission — *continued*
- vision examination — *continued*
  - following failed vision screening Z01.020
    - with abnormal findings Z01.021
  - infant or child (over 28 days old) Z00.129
    - with abnormal findings Z00.121
- waiting period for admission to other facility Z75.1

Adnexitis (suppurative) — *see* Salpingo-oophoritis
Adolescent X-linked adrenoleukodystrophy E71.521
Adrenal (gland) — *see* condition
Adrenalism, tuberculous A18.7
Adrenalitis, adrenitis E27.8
- autoimmune E27.1
- meningococcal, hemorrhagic A39.1
Adrenarche, premature E27.0
Adrenocortical syndrome — *see* Cushing's, syndrome
Adrenogenital syndrome E25.9
- acquired E25.8
- congenital E25.0
- salt loss E25.0
Adrenogenitalism, congenital E25.0
Adrenoleukodystrophy E71.529
- neonatal E71.511
- X-linked E71.529
  - Addison only phenotype E71.528
  - Addison-Schilder E71.528
  - adolescent E71.521
  - adrenomyeloneuropathy E71.522
  - childhood cerebral E71.520
  - other specified E71.528
Adrenomyeloneuropathy E71.522
Adventitious bursa — *see* Bursopathy, specified type NEC
Adverse effect — *see* Table of Drugs and Chemicals, categories T36-T50, with 6th character 5
Advice — *see* Counseling
Adynamia (episodica) (hereditary) (periodic) G72.3
Aeration lung imperfect, newborn — *see* Atelectasis
Aerobullosis T70.3 ☑
Aerocele — *see* Embolism, air
Aerodermectasia
- subcutaneous (traumatic) T79.7 ☑
Aerodontalgia T70.29 ☑
Aeroembolism T70.3 ☑
Aerogenes capsulatus infection A48.0
Aero-otitis media T70.0 ☑
Aerophagy, aerophagia (psychogenic) F45.8
Aerophobia F40.228
Aerosinusitis T70.1 ☑
Aerotitis T70.0 ☑
Affection — *see* Disease
Afibrinogenemia — *see also* Defect, coagulation D68.8
- acquired D65
- congenital D68.2
- following ectopic or molar pregnancy O08.1
- in abortion — *see* Abortion, by type, complicated by, afibrinogenemia
- puerperal O72.3
African
- sleeping sickness B56.9
- tick fever A68.1
- trypanosomiasis B56.9
  - gambian B56.0
  - rhodesian B56.1
Aftercare — *see also* Care Z51.89
- following surgery (for) (on)
  - amputation Z47.81
  - attention to
    - drains Z48.03
    - dressings (nonsurgical) Z48.00
      - surgical Z48.01
    - sutures Z48.02
  - circulatory system Z48.812
  - delayed (planned) wound closure Z48.1
  - digestive system Z48.815
  - explantation of joint prosthesis (staged procedure)
    - hip Z47.32
    - knee Z47.33
    - shoulder Z47.31
  - genitourinary system Z48.816
  - joint replacement Z47.1
  - neoplasm Z48.3
  - nervous system Z48.811
  - oral cavity Z48.814
  - organ transplant
    - bone marrow Z48.290
    - heart Z48.21
    - heart-lung Z48.280

Aftercare — *continued*
- following surgery — *continued*
  - organ transplant — *continued*
    - kidney Z48.22
    - liver Z48.23
    - lung Z48.24
    - multiple organs NEC Z48.288
    - specified NEC Z48.298
  - orthopedic NEC Z47.89
  - planned wound closure Z48.1
  - removal of internal fixation device Z47.2
  - respiratory system Z48.813
  - scoliosis Z47.82
  - sense organs Z48.810
  - skin and subcutaneous tissue Z48.817
  - specified body system
    - circulatory Z48.812
    - digestive Z48.815
    - genitourinary Z48.816
    - nervous Z48.811
    - oral cavity Z48.814
    - respiratory Z48.813
    - sense organs Z48.810
    - skin and subcutaneous tissue Z48.817
    - teeth Z48.814
  - specified NEC Z48.89
  - spinal Z47.89
  - teeth Z48.814
- fracture — *code to* fracture with seventh character D
- involving
  - removal of
    - drains Z48.03
    - dressings (nonsurgical) Z48.00
    - staples Z48.02
    - surgical dressings Z48.01
    - sutures Z48.02
  - neuropacemaker (brain) (peripheral nerve) (spinal cord) Z46.2
    - implanted Z45.42
  - orthopedic NEC Z47.89
- postprocedural — *see* Aftercare, following surgery
After-cataract — *see* Cataract, secondary
Agalactia (primary) O92.3
- elective, secondary or therapeutic O92.5
Agammaglobulinemia (acquired (secondary)) (nonfamilial) D80.1
- with
  - immunoglobulin-bearing B-lymphocytes D80.1
  - lymphopenia D81.9
- autosomal recessive (Swiss type) D80.0
- Bruton's X-linked D80.0
- common variable (CVAgamma) D80.1
- congenital sex-linked D80.0
- hereditary D80.0
- lymphopenic D81.9
- Swiss type (autosomal recessive) D80.0
- X-linked (with growth hormone deficiency) (Bruton) D80.0
Aganglionosis (bowel) (colon) Q43.1
Age (old) — *see* Senility
Agenesis
- adrenal (gland) Q89.1
- alimentary tract (complete) (partial) NEC Q45.8
  - upper Q40.8
- anus, anal (canal) Q42.3
  - with fistula Q42.2
- aorta Q25.41
- appendix Q42.8
- arm (complete) Q71.0- ☑
  - with hand present Q71.1- ☑
- artery (peripheral) Q27.9
  - brain Q28.3
  - coronary Q24.5
  - pulmonary Q25.79
  - specified NEC Q27.8
  - umbilical Q27.0
- auditory (canal) (external) Q16.1
- auricle (ear) Q16.0
- bile duct or passage Q44.5
- bladder Q64.5
- bone Q79.9
- brain Q00.0
  - part of Q04.3
- breast (with nipple present) Q83.8
  - with absent nipple Q83.0
- bronchus Q32.4
- canaliculus lacrimalis Q10.4
- carpus — *see* Agenesis, hand

☑ **Additional Character Required** — Refer to the Tabular List for Character Selection
☷ **Subterms under main terms may continue to next column or page**

Agenesis — *continued*
  cartilage Q79.9
  cecum Q42.8
  cerebellum Q04.3
  cervix Q51.5
  chin Q18.8
  cilia Q10.3
  circulatory system, part NOS Q28.9
  clavicle Q74.0
  clitoris Q52.6
  coccyx Q76.49
  colon Q42.9
    specified NEC Q42.8
  corpus callosum Q04.0
  cricoid cartilage Q31.8
  diaphragm (with hernia) Q79.1
  digestive organ(s) or tract (complete) (partial) NEC
      Q45.8
    upper Q40.8
  ductus arteriosus Q28.8
  duodenum Q41.0
  ear Q16.9
    auricle Q16.0
    lobe Q17.8
  ejaculatory duct Q55.4
  endocrine (gland) NEC Q89.2
  epiglottis Q31.8
  esophagus Q39.8
  eustachian tube Q16.2
  eye Q11.1
    adnexa Q15.8
    eyelid (fold) Q10.3
  face
    bones NEC Q75.8
    specified part NEC Q18.8
  fallopian tube Q50.6
  femur — *see* Defect, reduction, lower limb, longitudi-
      nal, femur
  fibula — *see* Defect, reduction, lower limb, longitudinal,
      fibula
  finger (complete) (partial) — *see* Agenesis, hand
  foot (and toes) (complete) (partial) Q72.3- ☑
  forearm (with hand present) — *see* Agenesis, arm, with
      hand present
    and hand Q71.2- ☑
  gallbladder Q44.0
  gastric Q40.2
  genitalia, genital (organ(s))
    female Q52.8
      external Q52.71
      internal NEC Q52.8
    male Q55.8
  glottis Q31.8
  hair Q84.0
  hand (and fingers) (complete) (partial) Q71.3- ☑
  heart Q24.8
    valve NEC Q24.8
      pulmonary Q22.0
  hepatic Q44.7
  humerus — *see* Defect, reduction, upper limb
  hymen Q52.4
  ileum Q41.2
  incus Q16.3
  intestine (small) Q41.9
    large Q42.9
      specified NEC Q42.8
  iris (dilator fibers) Q13.1
  jaw M26.09
  jejunum Q41.1
  kidney(s) (partial) Q60.2
    bilateral Q60.1
    unilateral Q60.0
  labium (majus) (minus) Q52.71
  labyrinth, membranous Q16.5
  lacrimal apparatus Q10.4
  larynx Q31.8
  leg (complete) Q72.0- ☑
    with foot present Q72.1- ☑
    lower leg (with foot present) — *see* Agenesis, leg,
        with foot present
      and foot Q72.2- ☑
  lens Q12.3
  limb (complete) Q73.0
    lower — *see* Agenesis, leg
    upper — *see* Agenesis, arm
  lip Q38.0
  liver Q44.7
  lung (fissure) (lobe) (bilateral) (unilateral) Q33.3

Agenesis — *continued*
  mandible, maxilla M26.09
  metacarpus — *see* Agenesis, hand
  metatarsus — *see* Agenesis, foot
  muscle Q79.8
    eyelid Q10.3
    ocular Q15.8
  musculoskeletal system NEC Q79.8
  nail(s) Q84.3
  neck, part Q18.8
  nerve Q07.8
  nervous system, part NEC Q07.8
  nipple Q83.2
  nose Q30.1
  nuclear Q07.8
  organ
    of Corti Q16.5
    or site not listed — *see* Anomaly, by site
  osseous meatus (ear) Q16.1
  ovary
    bilateral Q50.02
    unilateral Q50.01
  oviduct Q50.6
  pancreas Q45.0
  parathyroid (gland) Q89.2
  parotid gland(s) Q38.4
  patella Q74.1
  pelvic girdle (complete) (partial) Q74.2
  penis Q55.5
  pericardium Q24.8
  pituitary (gland) Q89.2
  prostate Q55.4
  punctum lacrimale Q10.4
  radioulnar — *see* Defect, reduction, upper limb
  radius — *see* Defect, reduction, upper limb, longitudi-
      nal, radius
  rectum Q42.1
    with fistula Q42.0
  renal Q60.2
    bilateral Q60.1
    unilateral Q60.0
  respiratory organ NEC Q34.8
  rib Q76.6
  roof of orbit Q75.8
  round ligament Q52.8
  sacrum Q76.49
  salivary gland Q38.4
  scapula Q74.0
  scrotum Q55.29
  seminal vesicles Q55.4
  septum
    atrial Q21.1
    between aorta and pulmonary artery Q21.4
    ventricular Q20.4
  shoulder girdle (complete) (partial) Q74.0
  skull (bone) Q75.8
    with
      anencephaly Q00.0
      encephalocele — *see* Encephalocele
      hydrocephalus Q03.9
        with spina bifida — *see* Spina bifida, by site,
            with hydrocephalus
      microcephaly Q02
  spermatic cord Q55.4
  spinal cord Q06.0
  spine Q76.49
  spleen Q89.01
  sternum Q76.7
  stomach Q40.2
  submaxillary gland(s) (congenital) Q38.4
  tarsus — *see* Agenesis, foot
  tendon Q79.8
  testicle Q55.0
  thymus (gland) Q89.2
  thyroid (gland) E03.1
    cartilage Q31.8
  tibia — *see* Defect, reduction, lower limb, longitudinal,
      tibia
  tibiofibular — *see* Defect, reduction, lower limb, speci-
      fied type NEC
  toe (and foot) (complete) (partial) — *see* Agenesis, foot
  tongue Q38.3
  trachea (cartilage) Q32.1
  ulna — *see* Defect, reduction, upper limb, longitudinal,
      ulna
  upper limb — *see* Agenesis, arm
  ureter Q62.4
  urethra Q64.5

Agenesis — *continued*
  urinary tract NEC Q64.8
  uterus Q51.0
  uvula Q38.5
  vagina Q52.0
  vas deferens Q55.4
  vein(s) (peripheral) Q27.9
    brain Q28.3
    great NEC Q26.8
    portal Q26.5
  vena cava (inferior) (superior) Q26.8
  vermis of cerebellum Q04.3
  vertebra Q76.49
  vulva Q52.71
Ageusia R43.2
Agitated — *see* condition
Agitation R45.1
Aglossia (congenital) Q38.3
Aglossia-adactylia syndrome Q87.0
Aglycogenosis E74.00
Agnosia (body image) (other senses) (tactile) R48.1
  developmental F88
  verbal R48.1
    auditory R48.1
      developmental F80.2
    developmental F80.2
  visual (object) R48.3
Agoraphobia F40.00
  with panic disorder F40.01
  without panic disorder F40.02
Agrammatism R48.8
Agranulocytopenia — *see* Agranulocytosis
Agranulocytosis (chronic) (cyclical) (genetic) (infantile)
      (periodic) (pernicious) — *see also* Neutropenia
      D70.9
  congenital D70.0
  cytoreductive cancer chemotherapy sequela D70.1
  drug-induced D70.2
    due to cytoreductive cancer chemotherapy D70.1
  due to infection D70.3
  secondary D70.4
    drug-induced D70.2
      due to cytoreductive cancer chemotherapy D70.1
Agraphia (absolute) R48.8
  with alexia R48.0
  developmental F81.81
Ague (dumb) — *see* Malaria
Agyria Q04.3
Ahumada-del Castillo syndrome E23.0
Aichomophobia F40.298
AIDS (related complex) B20
Ailment heart — *see* Disease, heart
Ailurophobia F40.218
AIN — *see* Neoplasia, intraepithelial, anal
Ainhum (disease) L94.6
AIPHI (acute idiopathic pulmonary hemorrhage in infants
      (over 28 days old)) R04.81
Air
  anterior mediastinum J98.2
  compressed, disease T70.3 ☑
  conditioner lung or pneumonitis J67.7
  embolism (artery) (cerebral) (any site) T79.0 ☑
    with ectopic or molar pregnancy O08.2
    due to implanted device NEC — *see* Complications,
        by site and type, specified NEC
    following
      abortion — *see* Abortion by type, complicated
          by, embolism
      ectopic or molar pregnancy O08.2
    infusion, therapeutic injection or transfusion
        T80.0 ☑
    in pregnancy, childbirth or puerperium — *see* Em-
        bolism, obstetric
    traumatic T79.0 ☑
  hunger, psychogenic F45.8
  rarefied, effects of — *see* Effect, adverse, high altitude
  sickness T75.3 ☑
Airplane sickness T75.3 ☑
Akathisia (drug-induced) (treatment-induced) G25.71
  neuroleptic induced (acute) G25.71
  tardive G25.71
Akinesia R29.898
Akinetic mutism R41.89
Akureyri's disease G93.3
Alactasia, congenital E73.0
Alagille's syndrome Q44.7
Alastrim B03

Albers-Schönberg syndrome Q78.2
Albert's syndrome — see Tendinitis, Achilles
Albinism, albino E70.30
    with hematologic abnormality E70.339
        Chédiak-Higashi syndrome E70.330
        Hermansky-Pudlak syndrome E70.331
        other specified E70.338
    I E70.320
    II E70.321
    ocular E70.319
        autosomal recessive E70.311
        other specified E70.318
        X-linked E70.310
    oculocutaneous E70.329
        other specified E70.328
        tyrosinase (ty) negative E70.320
        tyrosinase (ty) positive E70.321
    other specified E70.39
Albinismus E70.30
Albright (-McCune)(-Sternberg) syndrome Q78.1
Albuminous — see condition
Albuminuria, albuminuric (acute) (chronic) (subacute)
        — see also Proteinuria R80.9
    complicating pregnancy — see Proteinuria, gestational
    with
        gestational hypertension — see Pre-eclampsia
        pre-existing hypertension — see Hypertension,
            complicating pregnancy, pre-existing,
            with, pre-eclampsia
    gestational — see Proteinuria, gestational
    with
        gestational hypertension — see Pre-eclampsia
        pre-existing hypertension — see Hypertension,
            complicating pregnancy, pre-existing,
            with, pre-eclampsia
    orthostatic R80.2
    postural R80.2
    pre-eclamptic — see Pre-eclampsia
    scarlatinal A38.8
Albuminurophobia F40.298
Alcaptonuria E70.29
Alcohol, alcoholic, alcohol-induced
    addiction (without remission) F10.20
        with remission F10.21
    amnestic disorder, persisting F10.96
        with dependence F10.26
    anxiety disorder F10.980
    bipolar and related disorder F10.94
    brain syndrome, chronic F10.97
        with dependence F10.27
    cardiopathy I42.6
    counseling and surveillance Z71.41
        family member Z71.42
    delirium (acute) (tremens) (withdrawal) F10.231
        with intoxication F10.921
            in
                abuse F10.121
                dependence F10.221
    dementia F10.97
        with dependence F10.27
    depressive disorder F10.94
    deterioration F10.97
        with dependence F10.27
    hallucinosis (acute) F10.951
        in
            abuse F10.151
            dependence F10.251
    insanity F10.959
    intoxication (acute) (without dependence) F10.129
        with
            delirium F10.121
            dependence F10.229
                with delirium F10.221
                uncomplicated F10.220
            uncomplicated F10.120
    jealousy F10.988
    Korsakoff's, Korsakov's, Korsakow's F10.26
    liver K70.9
        acute — see Disease, liver, alcoholic, hepatitis
    major neurocognitive disorder, amnestic-confabulatory
        type F10.96
    major neurocognitive disorder, nonamnestic-confabu-
        latory type F10.97
    mania (acute) (chronic) F10.959
    mild neurocognitive disorder F10.988
    paranoia, paranoid (type) psychosis F10.950
    pellagra E52

Alcohol, alcoholic, alcohol-induced — continued
    poisoning, accidental (acute) NEC — see Table of Drugs
        and Chemicals, alcohol, poisoning
    psychosis — see Psychosis, alcoholic
    psychotic disorder F10.959
    sexual dysfunction F10.981
    sleep disorder F10.982
    withdrawal (without convulsions) F10.239
        with delirium F10.231
Alcoholism (chronic) (without remission) F10.20
    with
        psychosis — see Psychosis, alcoholic
        remission F10.21
    Korsakov's F10.96
        with dependence F10.26
Alder (-Reilly) **anomaly or syndrome** (leukocyte granu-
    lation) D72.0
Aldosteronism E26.9
    familial (type I) E26.02
    glucocorticoid-remediable E26.02
    primary (due to (bilateral) adrenal hyperplasia) E26.09
    primary NEC E26.09
    secondary E26.1
    specified NEC E26.89
Aldosteronoma D44.10
Aldrich (-Wiskott) **syndrome** (eczema-thrombocytope-
    nia) D82.0
Alektorophobia F40.218
Aleppo boil B55.1
Aleukemic — see condition
Aleukia
    congenital D70.0
    hemorrhagica D61.9
        congenital D61.09
    splenica D73.1
Alexia R48.0
    developmental F81.0
    secondary to organic lesion R48.0
Algoneurodystrophy M89.00
    ankle M89.07- ☑
    foot M89.07- ☑
    forearm M89.03- ☑
    hand M89.04- ☑
    lower leg M89.06- ☑
    multiple sites M89.0- ☑
    shoulder M89.01- ☑
    specified site NEC M89.08
    thigh M89.05- ☑
    upper arm M89.02- ☑
Algophobia F40.298
Alienation, mental — see Psychosis
Alkalemia E87.3
Alkalosis E87.3
    metabolic E87.3
        with respiratory acidosis E87.4
        of newborn P74.41
    respiratory E87.3
Alkaptonuria E70.29
Allen-Masters syndrome N83.8
Allergy, allergic (reaction) (to) T78.40 ☑
    air-borne substance NEC (rhinitis) J30.89
    alveolitis (extrinsic) J67.9
        due to
            Aspergillus clavatus J67.4
            Cryptostroma corticale J67.6
            organisms (fungal, thermophilic actinomycete)
                growing in ventilation (air conditioning)
                systems J67.7
        specified type NEC J67.8
    anaphylactic reaction or shock T78.2 ☑
    angioneurotic edema T78.3 ☑
    animal (dander) (epidermal) (hair) (rhinitis) J30.81
    bee sting (anaphylactic shock) — see Toxicity, venom,
        arthropod, bee
    biological — see Allergy, drug
    colitis — see also Colitis, allergic K52.29
    dander (animal) (rhinitis) J30.81
    dandruff (rhinitis) J30.81
    dental restorative material (existing) K08.55
    dermatitis — see Dermatitis, contact, allergic
    diathesis — see History, allergy
    drug, medicament & biological (any) (external) (inter-
        nal) T78.40 ☑
        correct substance properly administered — see Ta-
            ble of Drugs and Chemicals, by drug, adverse
            effect

Allergy, allergic — continued
    drug, medicament & biological — continued
        wrong substance given or taken NEC (by accident)
            — see Table of Drugs and Chemicals, by drug,
            poisoning
    due to pollen J30.1
    dust (house) (stock) (rhinitis) J30.89
        with asthma — see Asthma, allergic extrinsic
    eczema — see Dermatitis, contact, allergic
    epidermal (animal) (rhinitis) J30.81
    feathers (rhinitis) J30.89
    food (any) (ingested) NEC T78.1 ☑
        anaphylactic shock — see Shock, anaphylactic, due
            to food
        dermatitis — see Dermatitis, due to, food
        dietary counseling and surveillance Z71.3
        in contact with skin L23.6
        rhinitis J30.5
        status (without reaction) Z91.018
            eggs Z91.012
            milk products Z91.011
            peanuts Z91.010
            seafood Z91.013
            specified NEC Z91.018
    gastrointestinal — see also specific type of allergic re-
        action
        meaning colitis — see also Colitis, allergic K52.29
        meaning gastroenteritis — see also Gastroenteritis,
            allergic K52.29
        meaning other adverse food reaction not elsewhere
            classified T78.1 ☑
    grain J30.1
    grass (hay fever) (pollen) J30.1
        asthma — see Asthma, allergic extrinsic
    hair (animal) (rhinitis) J30.81
    history (of) — see History, allergy
    horse serum — see Allergy, serum
    inhalant (rhinitis) J30.89
        pollen J30.1
    kapok (rhinitis) J30.89
    medicine — see Allergy, drug
    milk protein — see also Allergy, food Z91.011
        anaphylactic reaction T78.07 ☑
        dermatitis L27.2
        enterocolitis syndrome K52.21
        enteropathy K52.22
        gastroenteritis K52.29
        gastroesophageal reflux — see also Reaction, ad-
            verse, food K21.9
            with esophagitis K21.0
        proctocolitis K52.82
    nasal, seasonal due to pollen J30.1
    pneumonia J82
    pollen (any) (hay fever) J30.1
        asthma — see Asthma, allergic extrinsic
    primrose J30.1
    primula J30.1
    proctocolitis K52.82
    purpura D69.0
    ragweed (hay fever) (pollen) J30.1
        asthma — see Asthma, allergic extrinsic
    rose (pollen) J30.1
    seasonal NEC J30.2
    Senecio jacobae (pollen) J30.1
    serum — see also Reaction, serum T80.69 ☑
        anaphylactic shock T80.59 ☑
    shock (anaphylactic) T78.2 ☑
        due to
            administration of blood and blood products
                T80.51 ☑
            adverse effect of correct medicinal substance
                properly administered T88.6 ☑
            immunization T80.52 ☑
            serum NEC T80.59 ☑
            vaccination T80.52 ☑
    specific NEC T78.49 ☑
    tree (any) (hay fever) (pollen) J30.1
        asthma — see Asthma, allergic extrinsic
    upper respiratory J30.9
    urticaria L50.0
    vaccine — see Allergy, serum
    wheat — see Allergy, food
Allescheriasis B48.2
Alligator skin disease Q80.9
Allocheiria, allochiria R20.8
Almeida's disease — see Paracoccidioidomycosis
Alopecia (hereditaria) (seborrheica) L65.9

☑ Additional Character Required — Refer to the Tabular List for Character Selection   Subterms under main terms may continue to next column or page

Alopecia — *continued*
androgenic L64.9
drug-induced L64.0
specified NEC L64.8
areata L63.9
ophiasis L63.2
specified NEC L63.8
totalis L63.0
universalis L63.1
cicatricial L66.9
specified NEC L66.8
circumscripta L63.9
congenital, congenitalis Q84.0
due to cytotoxic drugs NEC L65.8
mucinosa L65.2
postinfective NEC L65.8
postpartum L65.0
premature L64.8
specific (syphilitic) A51.32
specified NEC L65.8
syphilitic (secondary) A51.32
totalis (capitis) L63.0
universalis (entire body) L63.1
X-ray L58.1
Alpers' disease G31.81
Alpine sickness T70.29 ☑
Alport syndrome Q87.81
ALTE (apparent life threatening event) **in newborn and infant** R68.13
Alteration (of), **Altered**
awareness
transient R40.4
unintended under general anesthesia, during procedure T88.53 ☑
mental status R41.82
pattern of family relationships affecting child Z62.898
sensation
following
cerebrovascular disease I69.998
cerebral infarction I69.398
intracerebral hemorrhage I69.198
nontraumatic intracranial hemorrhage NEC I69.298
specified disease NEC I69.898
subarachnoid hemorrhage I69.098
Alternating — *see* condition
Altitude, high (effects) — *see* Effect, adverse, high altitude
Aluminosis (of lung) J63.0
Alveolitis
allergic (extrinsic) — *see* Pneumonitis, hypersensitivity
due to
Aspergillus clavatus J67.4
Cryptostroma corticale J67.6
fibrosing (cryptogenic) (idiopathic) J84.112
jaw M27.3
sicca dolorosa M27.3
Alveolus, alveolar — *see* condition
Alymphocytosis D72.810
thymic (with immunodeficiency) D82.1
Alymphoplasia, thymic D82.1
Alzheimer's disease or sclerosis — *see* Disease, Alzheimer's
Amastia (with nipple present) Q83.8
with absent nipple Q83.0
Amathophobia F40.228
Amaurosis (acquired) (congenital) — *see also* Blindness
fugax G45.3
hysterical F44.6
Leber's congenital H35.50
uremic — *see* Uremia
Amaurotic idiocy (infantile) (juvenile) (late) E75.4
Amaxophobia F40.248
Ambiguous genitalia Q56.4
Amblyopia (congenital) (ex anopsia) (partial) (suppression) H53.00- ☑
anisometropic — *see* Amblyopia, refractive
deprivation H53.01- ☑
hysterical F44.6
nocturnal — *see also* Blindness, night
vitamin A deficiency E50.5
refractive H53.02- ☑
strabismic H53.03- ☑
suspect H53.04- ☑
tobacco H53.8
toxic NEC H53.8
uremic — *see* Uremia
Ameba, amebic (histolytica) — *see also* Amebiasis

Ameba, amebic — *continued*
abscess (liver) A06.4
Amebiasis A06.9
with abscess — *see* Abscess, amebic
acute A06.0
chronic (intestine) A06.1
with abscess — *see* Abscess, amebic
cutaneous A06.7
cutis A06.7
cystitis A06.81
genitourinary tract NEC A06.82
hepatic — *see* Abscess, liver, amebic
intestine A06.0
nondysenteric colitis A06.2
skin A06.7
specified site NEC A06.89
Ameboma (of intestine) A06.3
Amelia Q73.0
lower limb — *see* Agenesis, leg
upper limb — *see* Agenesis, arm
Ameloblastoma — *see also* Cyst, calcifying odontogenic
long bones C40.9- ☑
lower limb C40.2- ☑
upper limb C40.0- ☑
malignant C41.1
jaw (bone) (lower) C41.1
upper C41.0
tibial C40.2- ☑
Amelogenesis imperfecta K00.5
nonhereditaria (segmentalis) K00.4
Amenorrhea N91.2
hyperhormonal E28.8
primary N91.0
secondary N91.1
Amentia — *see* Disability, intellectual
Meynert's (nonalcoholic) F04
American
leishmaniasis B55.2
mountain tick fever A93.2
Ametropia — *see* Disorder, refraction
AMH (asymptomatic microscopic hematuria) R31.21
Amianthosis J61
Amimia R48.8
Amino-acid disorder E72.9
anemia D53.0
Aminoacidopathy E72.9
Aminoaciduria E72.9
Amnesia R41.3
anterograde R41.1
auditory R48.8
dissociative F44.0
with dissociative fugue F44.1
hysterical F44.0
postictal in epilepsy — *see* Epilepsy
psychogenic F44.0
retrograde R41.2
transient global G45.4
Amnes(t)ic syndrome (post-traumatic) F04
induced by
alcohol F10.96
with dependence F10.26
psychoactive NEC F19.96
with
abuse F19.16
dependence F19.26
sedative F13.96
with dependence F13.26
Amnion, amniotic — *see* condition
Amnionitis — *see* Pregnancy, complicated by
Amok F68.8
Amoral traits F60.89
Amphetamine (or other stimulant) **-induced**
anxiety disorder F15.980
bipolar and related disorder F15.94
delirium F15.921
depressive disorder F15.94
obsessive-compulsive and related disorder F15.988
psychotic disorder F15.959
sexual dysfunction F15.981
sleep disorder F15.982
stimulant withdrawal F15.23
Ampulla
lower esophagus K22.8
phrenic K22.8
Amputation — *see also* Absence, by site, acquired
neuroma (postoperative) (traumatic) — *see* Complications, amputation stump, neuroma

Amputation — *continued*
stump (surgical)
abnormal, painful, or with complication (late) — *see* Complications, amputation stump
healed or old NOS Z89.9
traumatic (complete) (partial)
arm (upper) (complete) S48.91- ☑
at
elbow S58.01- ☑
partial S58.02- ☑
shoulder joint (complete) S48.01- ☑
partial S48.02- ☑
between
elbow and wrist (complete) S58.11- ☑
partial S58.12- ☑
shoulder and elbow (complete) S48.11- ☑
partial S48.12- ☑
partial S48.92- ☑
breast (complete) S28.21- ☑
partial S28.22- ☑
clitoris (complete) S38.211 ☑
partial S38.212 ☑
ear (complete) S08.11- ☑
partial S08.12- ☑
finger (complete) (metacarpophalangeal) S68.11- ☑
index S68.11- ☑
little S68.11- ☑
middle S68.11- ☑
partial S68.12- ☑
index S68.12- ☑
little S68.12- ☑
middle S68.12- ☑
ring S68.12- ☑
ring S68.11- ☑
thumb — *see* Amputation, traumatic, thumb
transphalangeal (complete) S68.61- ☑
index S68.61- ☑
little S68.61- ☑
middle S68.61- ☑
partial S68.62- ☑
index S68.62- ☑
little S68.62- ☑
middle S68.62- ☑
ring S68.62- ☑
ring S68.61- ☑
foot (complete) S98.91- ☑
at ankle level S98.01- ☑
partial S98.02- ☑
midfoot S98.31- ☑
partial S98.32- ☑
partial S98.92- ☑
forearm (complete) S58.91- ☑
at elbow level (complete) S58.01- ☑
partial S58.02- ☑
between elbow and wrist (complete) S58.11- ☑
partial S58.12- ☑
partial S58.92- ☑
genital organ(s) (external)
female (complete) S38.211 ☑
partial S38.212 ☑
male
penis (complete) S38.221 ☑
partial S38.222 ☑
scrotum (complete) S38.231 ☑
partial S38.232 ☑
testes (complete) S38.231 ☑
partial S38.232 ☑
hand (complete) (wrist level) S68.41- ☑
finger(s) alone — *see* Amputation, traumatic, finger
partial S68.42- ☑
thumb alone — *see* Amputation, traumatic, thumb
transmetacarpal (complete) S68.71- ☑
partial S68.72- ☑
head
ear — *see* Amputation, traumatic, ear
nose (partial) S08.812 ☑
complete S08.811 ☑
part S08.89 ☑
scalp S08.0 ☑
hip (and thigh) (complete) S78.91- ☑
at hip joint (complete) S78.01- ☑
partial S78.02- ☑
between hip and knee (complete) S78.11- ☑
partial S78.12- ☑

Amputation — *continued*
  traumatic — *continued*
    hip — *continued*
      partial S78.92- ☑
    labium (majus) (minus) (complete) S38.21- ☑
      partial S38.21- ☑
    leg (lower) S88.91- ☑
      at knee level S88.01- ☑
        partial S88.02- ☑
      between knee and ankle S88.11- ☑
        partial S88.12- ☑
      partial S88.92- ☑
    nose (partial) S08.812 ☑
      complete S08.811 ☑
    penis (complete) S38.221 ☑
      partial S38.222 ☑
    scrotum (complete) S38.231 ☑
      partial S38.232 ☑
    shoulder — *see* Amputation, traumatic, arm
      at shoulder joint — *see* Amputation, traumatic, arm, at shoulder joint
    testes (complete) S38.231 ☑
      partial S38.232 ☑
    thigh — *see* Amputation, traumatic, hip
    thorax, part of S28.1 ☑
      breast — *see* Amputation, traumatic, breast
    thumb (complete) (metacarpophalangeal) S68.01- ☑
      partial S68.02- ☑
      transphalangeal (complete) S68.51- ☑
        partial S68.52- ☑
    toe (lesser) S98.13- ☑
      great S98.11- ☑
        partial S98.12- ☑
      more than one S98.21- ☑
        partial S98.22- ☑
      partial S98.14- ☑
    vulva (complete) S38.211 ☑
      partial S38.212 ☑
Amputee (bilateral) (old) Z89.9
Amsterdam dwarfism Q87.19
Amusia R48.8
  developmental F80.89
Amyelencephalus, amyelencephaly Q00.0
Amyelia Q06.0
Amygdalitis — *see* Tonsillitis
Amygdalolith J35.8
Amyloid heart (disease) E85.4 *[I43]*
Amyloidosis (generalized) (primary) E85.9
  with lung involvement E85.4 *[J99]*
  familial E85.2
  genetic E85.2
  heart E85.4 *[I43]*
  hemodialysis-associated E85.3
  light chain (AL) E85.81
  liver E85.4 *[K77]*
  localized E85.4
  neuropathic heredofamilial E85.1
  non-neuropathic heredofamilial E85.0
  organ limited E85.4
  Portuguese E85.1
  pulmonary E85.4 *[J99]*
  secondary systemic E85.3
  senile systemic (SSA) E85.82
  skin (lichen) (macular) E85.4 *[L99]*
  specified NEC E85.89
  subglottic E85.4 *[J99]*
  wild-type transthyretin-related (ATTR) E85.82
Amylopectinosis (brancher enzyme deficiency) E74.03
Amylophagia — *see* Pica
Amyoplasia congenita Q79.8
Amyotonia M62.89
  congenita G70.2
Amyotrophia, amyotrophy, amyotrophic G71.8
  congenita Q79.8
  diabetic — *see* Diabetes, amyotrophy
  lateral sclerosis G12.21
  neuralgic G54.5
  spinal progressive G12.25
Anacidity, gastric K31.83
  psychogenic F45.8
Anaerosis of newborn P28.89
Analbuminemia E88.09
Analgesia — *see* Anesthesia
Analphalipoproteinemia E78.6
Anaphylactic
  purpura D69.0

Anaphylactic — *continued*
  shock or reaction — *see* Shock, anaphylactic
Anaphylactoid shock or reaction — *see* Shock, anaphylactic
Anaphylactoid syndrome of pregnancy O88.01- ☑
Anaphylaxis — *see* Shock, anaphylactic
Anaplasia cervix — *see also* Dysplasia, cervix N87.9
Anaplasmosis, human A77.49
Anarthria R47.1
Anasarca R60.1
  cardiac — *see* Failure, heart, congestive
  lung J18.2
  newborn P83.2
  nutritional E43
  pulmonary J18.2
  renal N04.9
Anastomosis
  aneurysmal — *see* Aneurysm
  arteriovenous ruptured brain I60.8
    intracerebral I61.8
    intraparenchymal I61.8
    intraventricular I61.5
    subarachnoid I60.8
  intestinal K63.89
    complicated NEC K91.89
      involving urinary tract N99.89
  retinal and choroidal vessels (congenital) Q14.8
Anatomical narrow angle H40.03- ☑
Ancylostoma, ancylostomiasis (braziliense) (caninum) (ceylanicum) (duodenale) B76.0
  Necator americanus B76.1
Andersen's disease (glycogen storage) E74.09
Anderson-Fabry disease E75.21
Andrews' disease (bacterid) L08.89
Androblastoma
  benign
    specified site — *see* Neoplasm, benign, by site
    unspecified site
      female D27.9
      male D29.20
  malignant
    specified site — *see* Neoplasm, malignant, by site
    unspecified site
      female C56.9
      male C62.90
  specified site — *see* Neoplasm, uncertain behavior, by site
  tubular
    with lipid storage
      specified site — *see* Neoplasm, benign, by site
      unspecified site
        female D27.9
        male D29.20
    specified site — *see* Neoplasm, benign, by site
    unspecified site
      female D27.9
      male D29.20
  unspecified site
    female D39.10
    male D40.10
Androgen insensitivity syndrome — *see also* Syndrome, androgen insensitivity E34.50
Androgen resistance syndrome — *see also* Syndrome, androgen insensitivity E34.50
Android pelvis Q74.2
  with disproportion (fetopelvic) O33.3 ☑
    causing obstructed labor O65.3
Androphobia F40.290
Anectasis, pulmonary (newborn) — *see* Atelectasis
Anemia (essential) (general) (hemoglobin deficiency) (infantile) (primary) (profound) D64.9
  with (due to) (in)
    disorder of
      anaerobic glycolysis D55.2
      pentose phosphate pathway D55.1
    koilonychia D50.9
  achlorhydric D50.8
  achrestic D53.1
  Addison (-Biermer) (pernicious) D51.0
  agranulocytic — *see* Agranulocytosis
  amino-acid-deficiency D53.0
  aplastic D61.9
    congenital D61.09
    drug-induced D61.1
    due to
      drugs D61.1
      external agents NEC D61.2

Anemia — *continued*
  aplastic — *continued*
    due to — *continued*
      infection D61.2
      radiation D61.2
    idiopathic D61.3
    red cell (pure) D60.9
      chronic D60.0
      congenital D61.01
      specified type NEC D60.8
      transient D60.1
    specified type NEC D61.89
    toxic D61.2
  aregenerative
    congenital D61.09
  asiderotic D50.9
  atypical (primary) D64.9
  Baghdad spring D55.0
  Balantidium coli A07.0
  Biermer's (pernicious) D51.0
  blood loss (chronic) D50.0
    acute D62
  bothriocephalus B70.0 *[D63.8]*
  brickmaker's B76.9 *[D63.8]*
  cerebral I67.89
  childhood D58.9
  chlorotic D50.8
  chronic
    blood loss D50.0
    hemolytic D58.9
      idiopathic D59.9
    simple D53.9
  chronica congenita aregenerativa D61.09
  combined system disease NEC D51.0 *[G32.0]*
    due to dietary vitamin B12 deficiency D51.3 *[G32.0]*
  complicating pregnancy, childbirth or puerperium — *see* Pregnancy, complicated by (management affected by), anemia
  congenital P61.4
    aplastic D61.09
    due to isoimmunization NOS P55.9
    dyserythropoietic, dyshematopoietic D64.4
    following fetal blood loss P61.3
    Heinz body D58.2
    hereditary hemolytic NOS D58.9
    pernicious D51.0
    spherocytic D58.0
  Cooley's (erythroblastic) D56.1
  cytogenic D51.0
  deficiency D53.9
    2, 3 diphosphoglycurate mutase D55.2
    2, 3 PG D55.2
    6 phosphogluconate dehydrogenase D55.1
    6-PGD D55.1
    amino-acid D53.0
    combined B12 and folate D53.1
    enzyme D55.9
      drug-induced (hemolytic) D59.2
      glucose-6-phosphate dehydrogenase (G6PD) D55.0
      glycolytic D55.2
      nucleotide metabolism D55.3
      related to hexose monophosphate (HMP) shunt pathway NEC D55.1
      specified type NEC D55.8
    erythrocytic glutathione D55.1
    folate D52.9
      dietary D52.0
      drug-induced D52.1
    folic acid D52.9
      dietary D52.0
      drug-induced D52.1
    G SH D55.1
    G6PD D55.0
    GGS-R D55.1
    glucose-6-phosphate dehydrogenase D55.0
    glutathione reductase D55.1
    glyceraldehyde phosphate dehydrogenase D55.2
    hexokinase D55.2
    iron D50.9
      secondary to blood loss (chronic) D50.0
    nutritional D53.9
      with
        poor iron absorption D50.8
        specified deficiency NEC D53.8
    phosphofructo-aldolase D55.2
    phosphoglycerate kinase D55.2
    PK D55.2
    protein D53.0

Anemia — *continued*
deficiency — *continued*
pyruvate kinase D55.2
transcobalamin II D51.2
triose-phosphate isomerase D55.2
vitamin B12 NOS D51.9
dietary D51.3
due to
intrinsic factor deficiency D51.0
selective vitamin B12 malabsorption with proteinuria D51.1
pernicious D51.0
specified type NEC D51.8
Diamond-Blackfan (congenital hypoplastic) D61.01
dibothriocephalus B70.0 *[D63.8]*
dimorphic D53.1
diphasic D53.1
Diphyllobothrium (Dibothriocephalus) B70.0 *[D63.8]*
due to (in) (with)
antineoplastic chemotherapy D64.81
blood loss (chronic) D50.0
acute D62
chemotherapy, antineoplastic D64.81
chronic disease classified elsewhere NEC D63.8
chronic kidney disease D63.1
deficiency
amino-acid D53.0
copper D53.8
folate (folic acid) D52.9
dietary D52.0
drug-induced D52.1
molybdenum D53.8
protein D53.0
zinc D53.8
dietary vitamin B12 deficiency D51.3
disorder of
glutathione metabolism D55.1
nucleotide metabolism D55.3
drug — *see Anemia, by type — see also* Table of Drugs and Chemicals
end stage renal disease D63.1
enzyme disorder D55.9
fetal blood loss P61.3
fish tapeworm (D.latum) infestation B70.0 *[D63.8]*
hemorrhage (chronic) D50.0
acute D62
impaired absorption D50.9
loss of blood (chronic) D50.0
acute D62
myxedema E03.9 *[D63.8]*
Necator americanus B76.1 *[D63.8]*
prematurity P61.2
selective vitamin B12 malabsorption with protein-uria D51.1
transcobalamin II deficiency D51.2
Dyke-Young type (secondary) (symptomatic) D59.1
dyserythropoietic (congenital) D64.4
dyshematopoietic (congenital) D64.4
Egyptian B76.9 *[D63.8]*
elliptocytosis — *see* Elliptocytosis
enzyme-deficiency, drug-induced D59.2
epidemic — *see also* Ancylostomiasis B76.9 *[D63.8]*
erythroblastic
familial D56.1
newborn — *see also* Disease, hemolytic P55.9
of childhood D56.1
erythrocytic glutathione deficiency D55.1
erythropoietin-resistant anemia (EPO resistant anemia) D63.1
Faber's (achlorhydric anemia) D50.9
factitious (self-induced blood letting) D50.0
familial erythroblastic D56.1
Fanconi's (congenital pancytopenia) D61.09
favism D55.0
fish tapeworm (D. latum) infestation B70.0 *[D63.8]*
folate (folic acid) deficiency D52.9
glucose-6-phosphate dehydrogenase (G6PD) deficiency D55.0
glutathione-reductase deficiency D55.1
goat's milk D52.0
granulocytic — *see* Agranulocytosis
Heinz body, congenital D58.2
hemolytic D58.9
acquired D59.9
with hemoglobinuria NEC D59.6
autoimmune NEC D59.1
infectious D59.4
specified type NEC D59.8

Anemia — *continued*
hemolytic — *continued*
acquired — *continued*
toxic D59.4
acute D59.9
due to enzyme deficiency specified type NEC D55.8
Lederer's D59.1
autoimmune D59.1
drug-induced D59.0
chronic D58.9
idiopathic D59.9
cold type (secondary) (symptomatic) D59.1
congenital (spherocytic) — *see* Spherocytosis
due to
cardiac conditions D59.4
drugs (nonautoimmune) D59.2
autoimmune D59.0
enzyme disorder D55.9
drug-induced D59.2
presence of shunt or other internal prosthetic device D59.4
familial D58.9
hereditary D58.9
due to enzyme disorder D55.9
specified type NEC D55.8
specified type NEC D58.8
idiopathic (chronic) D59.9
mechanical D59.4
microangiopathic D59.4
nonautoimmune D59.4
drug-induced D59.2
nonspherocytic
congenital or hereditary NEC D55.8
glucose-6-phosphate dehydrogenase deficiency D55.0
pyruvate kinase deficiency D55.2
type
I D55.1
II D55.2
type
I D55.1
II D55.2
secondary D59.4
autoimmune D59.1
specified (hereditary) type NEC D58.8
Stransky-Regala type — *see also* Hemoglobinopathy D58.8
symptomatic D59.4
autoimmune D59.1
toxic D59.4
warm type (secondary) (symptomatic) D59.1
hemorrhagic (chronic) D50.0
acute D62
Herrick's D57.1
hexokinase deficiency D55.2
hookworm B76.9 *[D63.8]*
hypochromic (idiopathic) (microcytic) (normoblastic) D50.9
due to blood loss (chronic) D50.0
acute D62
familial sex-linked D64.0
pyridoxine-responsive D64.3
sideroblastic, sex-linked D64.0
hypoplasia, red blood cells D61.9
congenital or familial D61.01
hypoplastic (idiopathic) D61.9
congenital or familial (of childhood) D61.01
hypoproliferative (refractory) D61.9
idiopathic D64.9
aplastic D61.3
hemolytic, chronic D59.9
in (due to) (with)
chronic kidney disease D63.1
end stage renal disease D63.1
failure, kidney (renal) D63.1
neoplastic disease — *see also* Neoplasm D63.0
intertropical — *see also* Ancylostomiasis D63.8
iron deficiency D50.9
secondary to blood loss (chronic) D50.0
acute D62
specified type NEC D50.8
Joseph-Diamond-Blackfan (congenital hypoplastic) D61.01
Lederer's (hemolytic) D59.1
leukoerythroblastic D61.82
macrocytic D53.9
nutritional D52.0
tropical D52.8

Anemia — *continued*
malarial — *see also* Malaria B54 *[D63.8]*
malignant (progressive) D51.0
malnutrition D53.9
marsh — *see also* Malaria B54 *[D63.8]*
Mediterranean (with other hemoglobinopathy) D56.9
megaloblastic D53.1
combined B12 and folate deficiency D53.1
hereditary D53.1
nutritional D52.0
orotic aciduria D53.0
refractory D53.1
specified type NEC D53.1
megalocytic D53.1
microcytic (hypochromic) D50.9
due to blood loss (chronic) D50.0
acute D62
familial D56.8
microdrepanocytosis D57.40
microelliptopoikilocytic (Rietti-Greppi- Micheli) D56.9
miner's B76.9 *[D63.8]*
myelodysplastic D46.9
myelofibrosis D75.81
myelogenous D64.89
myelopathic D64.89
myelophthisic D61.82
myeloproliferative D47.Z9 (*following* D47.4)
newborn P61.4
due to
ABO (antibodies, isoimmunization, maternal/fetal incompatibility) P55.1
Rh (antibodies, isoimmunization, maternal/fetal incompatibility) P55.0
following fetal blood loss P61.3
posthemorrhagic (fetal) P61.3
nonspherocytic hemolytic — *see* Anemia, hemolytic, nonspherocytic
normocytic (infectional) D64.9
due to blood loss (chronic) D50.0
acute D62
myelophthisic D61.82
nutritional (deficiency) D53.9
with
poor iron absorption D50.8
specified deficiency NEC D53.8
megaloblastic D52.0
of prematurity P61.2
orotaciduric (congenital) (hereditary) D53.0
osteosclerotic D64.89
ovalocytosis (hereditary) — *see* Elliptocytosis
paludal — *see also* Malaria B54 *[D63.8]*
pernicious (congenital) (malignant) (progressive) D51.0
pleochromic D64.89
of sprue D52.8
posthemorrhagic (chronic) D50.0
acute D62
newborn P61.3
postoperative (postprocedural)
due to (acute) blood loss D62
chronic blood loss D50.0
specified NEC D64.9
postpartum O90.81
pressure D64.89
progressive D64.9
malignant D51.0
pernicious D51.0
protein-deficiency D53.0
pseudoleukemica infantum D64.89
pure red cell D60.9
congenital D61.01
pyridoxine-responsive D64.3
pyruvate kinase deficiency D55.2
refractory D46.4
with
excess of blasts D46.20
1 (RAEB 1) D46.21
2 (RAEB 2) D46.22
in transformation (RAEB T) — *see* Leukemia, acute myeloblastic
hemochromatosis D46.1
sideroblasts (ring) (RARS) D46.1
megaloblastic D53.1
sideroblastic D46.1
sideropenic D50.9
without ring sideroblasts, so stated D46.0
without sideroblasts without excess of blasts D46.0
Rietti-Greppi-Micheli D56.9
scorbutic D53.2

Anemia — continued

secondary to
  blood loss (chronic) D50.0
    acute D62
  hemorrhage (chronic) D50.0
    acute D62
semiplastic D61.89
sickle-cell — see Disease, sickle-cell
sideroblastic D64.3
  hereditary D64.0
  hypochromic, sex-linked D64.0
  pyridoxine-responsive NEC D64.3
  refractory D46.1
  secondary (due to)
    disease D64.1
    drugs and toxins D64.2
  specified type NEC D64.3
sideropenic (refractory) D50.9
  due to blood loss (chronic) D50.0
    acute D62
simple chronic D53.9
specified type NEC D64.89
spherocytic (hereditary) — see Spherocytosis
splenic D64.89
splenomegalic D64.89
stomatocytosis D58.8
syphilitic (acquired) (late) A52.79 [D63.8]
target cell D64.89
thalassemia D56.9
thrombocytopenic — see Thrombocytopenia
toxic D61.2
tropical B76.9 [D63.8]
  macrocytic D52.8
tuberculous A18.89 [D63.8]
vegan D51.3
vitamin
  B12 deficiency (dietary) pernicious D51.0
  B6-responsive D64.3
von Jaksch's D64.89
Witts' (achlorhydric anemia) D50.8

Anemophobia F40.228
Anencephalus, anencephaly Q00.0
Anergasia — see Psychosis, organic
Anesthesia, anesthetic R20.0
  complication or reaction NEC — see also Complications,
    anesthesia T88.59 ☑
    due to
      correct substance properly administered — see
        Table of Drugs and Chemicals, by drug,
        adverse effect
      overdose or wrong substance given — see Table
        of Drugs and Chemicals, by drug, poison-
        ing
      unintended awareness under general anesthesia
        during procedure T88.53 ☑
      personal history of Z92.84
  cornea H18.81- ☑
  dissociative F44.6
  functional (hysterical) F44.6
  hyperesthetic, thalamic G89.0
  hysterical F44.6
  local skin lesion R20.0
  sexual (psychogenic) F52.1
  shock (due to) T88.2 ☑
  skin R20.0
  testicular N50.9
Anetoderma (maculosum) (of) L90.8
  Jadassohn-Pellizzari L90.2
  Schweniger-Buzzi L90.1
Aneurin deficiency E51.9
Aneurysm (anastomotic) (artery) (cirsoid) (diffuse) (false)
    (fusiform) (multiple) (saccular) I72.9
  abdominal (aorta) I71.4
    ruptured I71.3
    syphilitic A52.01
  aorta, aortic (nonsyphilitic) I71.9
    abdominal I71.4
      ruptured I71.3
    arch I71.2
      ruptured I71.1
    arteriosclerotic I71.9
      ruptured I71.8
    ascending I71.2
      ruptured I71.1
    congenital Q25.43
    descending I71.9
      abdominal I71.4
        ruptured I71.3

Aneurysm — continued

aorta, aortic — continued
  descending — continued
    ruptured I71.8
    thoracic I71.2
      ruptured I71.1
  root Q25.43
    ruptured I71.8
  sinus, congenital Q25.43
  syphilitic A52.01
  thoracic I71.2
    ruptured I71.1
  thoracoabdominal I71.6
    ruptured I71.5
  thorax, thoracic (arch) I71.2
    ruptured I71.1
  transverse I71.2
    ruptured I71.1
  valve (heart) — see also Endocarditis, aortic I35.8
arteriosclerotic I72.9
  cerebral I67.1
    ruptured — see Hemorrhage, intracranial, sub-
      arachnoid
arteriovenous (congenital) — see also Malformation,
    arteriovenous
  acquired I77.0
    brain I67.1
      ruptured — see Aneurysm, arteriovenous,
        brain, ruptured
    coronary I25.41
    pulmonary I28.0
  brain Q28.2
    ruptured I60.8
      intracerebral I61.8
      intraparenchymal I61.8
      intraventricular I61.5
      subarachnoid I60.8
  peripheral — see Malformation, arteriovenous, pe-
    ripheral
  precerebral vessels Q28.0
  specified site NEC — see also Malformation, arteri-
    ovenous
    acquired I77.0
basal — see Aneurysm, brain
basilar (trunk) I72.5
berry (congenital) (nonruptured) I67.1
  ruptured I60.7
brain I67.1
  arteriosclerotic I67.1
    ruptured — see Hemorrhage, intracranial, sub-
      arachnoid
  arteriovenous (congenital) (nonruptured) Q28.2
    acquired I67.1
      ruptured — see Aneurysm, arteriovenous,
        brain, ruptured I60.8
      ruptured — see Aneurysm, arteriovenous, brain,
        ruptured I60.8
  berry (congenital) (nonruptured) I67.1
    ruptured — see also Hemorrhage, intracranial,
      subarachnoid I60.7
  congenital Q28.3
    ruptured I60.7
  meninges I67.1
    ruptured I60.8
  miliary (congenital) (nonruptured) I67.1
    ruptured — see also Hemorrhage, intracranial,
      subarachnoid I60.7
  mycotic I33.0
  ruptured — see Aneurysm, arteriovenous, brain,
    ruptured I60.8
  syphilitic (hemorrhage) A52.05
cardiac (false) — see also Aneurysm, heart I25.3
carotid artery (common) (external) I72.0
  internal (intracranial) I67.1
    extracranial portion I72.0
  ruptured into brain I60.0- ☑
  syphilitic A52.09
    intracranial A52.05
cavernous sinus I67.1
  arteriovenous (congenital) (nonruptured) Q28.3
    ruptured I60.8
celiac I72.8
central nervous system, syphilitic A52.05
cerebral — see Aneurysm, brain
chest — see Aneurysm, thorax
circle of Willis I67.1
  congenital Q28.3
    ruptured I60.6

Aneurysm — continued

circle of Willis — continued
  ruptured I60.6
common iliac artery I72.3
congenital (peripheral) Q27.8
  aorta (root) (sinus) Q25.43
  brain Q28.3
    ruptured I60.7
  coronary Q24.5
  digestive system Q27.8
  lower limb Q27.8
  pulmonary Q25.79
  retina Q14.1
  specified site NEC Q27.8
  upper limb Q27.8
conjunctiva — see Abnormality, conjunctiva, vascular
conus arteriosus — see Aneurysm, heart
coronary (arteriosclerotic) (artery) I25.41
  arteriovenous, congenital Q24.5
  congenital Q24.5
  ruptured — see Infarct, myocardium
  syphilitic A52.06
  vein I25.89
cylindroid (aorta) I71.9
  ruptured I71.8
  syphilitic A52.01
ductus arteriosus Q25.0
endocardial, infective (any valve) I33.0
femoral (artery) (ruptured) I72.4
gastroduodenal I72.8
gastroepiploic I72.8
heart (wall) (chronic or with a stated duration of over
    4 weeks) I25.3
  valve — see Endocarditis
hepatic I72.8
iliac (common) (artery) (ruptured) I72.3
infective I72.9
  endocardial (any valve) I33.0
innominate (nonsyphilitic) I72.8
  syphilitic A52.09
interauricular septum — see Aneurysm, heart
interventricular septum — see Aneurysm, heart
intrathoracic (nonsyphilitic) I71.2
  ruptured I71.1
  syphilitic A52.01
lower limb I72.4
lung (pulmonary artery) I28.1
mediastinal (nonsyphilitic) I72.8
  syphilitic A52.09
miliary (congenital) I67.1
  ruptured — see Hemorrhage, intracerebral, sub-
    arachnoid, intracranial
mitral (heart) (valve) I34.8
mural — see Aneurysm, heart
mycotic I72.9
  endocardial (any valve) I33.0
  ruptured, brain — see Hemorrhage, intracerebral,
    subarachnoid
myocardium — see Aneurysm, heart
neck I72.0
pancreaticoduodenal I72.8
patent ductus arteriosus Q25.0
peripheral NEC I72.8
  congenital Q27.8
    digestive system Q27.8
    lower limb Q27.8
    specified site NEC Q27.8
    upper limb Q27.8
popliteal (artery) (ruptured) I72.4
precerebral
  congenital (nonruptured) Q28.1
  specified site, NEC I72.5
pulmonary I28.1
  arteriovenous Q25.72
    acquired I28.0
  syphilitic A52.09
  valve (heart) — see Endocarditis, pulmonary
racemose (peripheral) I72.9
  congenital — see Aneurysm, congenital
radial I72.1
Rasmussen NEC A15.0
renal (artery) I72.2
retina — see also Disorder, retina, microaneurysms
  congenital Q14.1
  diabetic — see E08-E13 with .3-
sinus of Valsalva Q25.49
specified NEC I72.8
spinal (cord) I72.8

— continued
　continued
ic (hemorrhage) A52.09
8
n (artery) (ruptured) I72.8
tic A52.09
esenteric I72.8
aorta) A52.01
nervous system A52.05
nital (late) A50.54 *[I79.0]*
spinal A52.09
dominal (aorta) I71.6
ed I71.5
tic A52.01
oracic (aorta) (arch) (nonsyphilitic) I71.2
ed I71.1
tic A52.01
(complication) (early), specified site — *see*
　ry, blood vessel
heart) (valve) I07.8
1
b (ruptured) I72.1
vular — *see* Endocarditis
— *see also* Varix I86.8
nital Q27.8
estive system Q27.8
er limb Q27.8
cified site NEC Q27.8
er limb Q27.8
— *see* Aneurysm, heart
artery I72.6
EC I72.8
syndrome Q93.51

s, angiectopia I99.8
.6
ranulomatous M30.1
sitivity M31.0
ng M31.9
ied NEC M31.8
system, granulomatous I67.7
ack) (cardiac) (chest) (heart) (pectoris) (syn-
e) (vasomotor) I20.9

sclerotic heart disease — *see* Arteriosclerosis,
　coronary (artery),
mented spasm I20.1
al K55.1
ed — *see* Angina, unstable
cytic — *see* Agranulocytosis
stic — *see* Angina, with documented spasm
s B08.5
o — *see* Angina, unstable
s J05.0
.9
effort — *see* Angina, unstable
tic, membranous A36.0
nt I20.8
e, chronic J37.0
g acute myocardial infarction I23.7
ous diphtheritic A36.0
al K55.1
K12.2
s K12.2
nt diphtheritic A36.0
anous J05.0
theritic A36.0
nt's A69.1
ric K55.1
tic — *see* Mononucleosis, infectious
— *see* Angina, specified NEC
onous J36
theritic A36.0
arctional I23.7
rctional — *see* Angina, unstable
tal — *see* Angina, with documented spasm
sive — *see* Angina, unstable
membranous A69.1
ous, diphtheritic A36.0
nduced — *see* Angina, with documented spasm
d NEC I20.8
20.8
rdia — *see* Angina, specified NEC
us, diphtheritic A36.2
36
is J05.0
e I20.0
— *see* Angina, with documented spasm

Angina — *continued*
　Vincent's A69.1
　worsening effort — *see* Angina, unstable
Angioblastoma — *see* Neoplasm, connective tissue,
　uncertain behavior
Angiocholecystitis — *see* Cholecystitis, acute
Angiocholitis — *see also* Cholecystitis, acute K83.09
Angiodysgenesis spinalis G95.19
Angiodysplasia (cecum) (colon) K55.20
　with bleeding K55.21
　duodenum (and stomach) K31.819
　　with bleeding K31.811
　stomach (and duodenum) K31.819
　　with bleeding K31.811
Angioedema (allergic) (any site) (with urticaria) T78.3 ☑
　hereditary D84.1
Angioendothelioma — *see* Neoplasm, uncertain behav-
　ior, by site
　benign D18.00
　　intra-abdominal D18.03
　　intracranial D18.02
　　skin D18.01
　　specified site NEC D18.09
　bone — *see* Neoplasm, bone, malignant
　Ewing's — *see* Neoplasm, bone, malignant
Angioendotheliomatosis C85.8- ☑
Angiofibroma — *see also* Neoplasm, benign, by site
　juvenile
　　specified site — *see* Neoplasm, benign, by site
　　unspecified site D10.6
Angiohemophilia (A) (B) D68.0
Angioid streaks (choroid) (macula) (retina) H35.33
Angiokeratoma — *see* Neoplasm, skin, benign
　corporis diffusum E75.21
Angioleiomyoma — *see* Neoplasm, connective tissue,
　benign
Angiolipoma — *see also* Lipoma
　infiltrating — *see* Lipoma
Angioma — *see also* Hemangioma, by site
　capillary I78.1
　hemorrhagicum hereditaria I78.0
　intra-abdominal D18.03
　intracranial D18.02
　malignant — *see* Neoplasm, connective tissue, malig-
　　nant
　plexiform D18.00
　　intra-abdominal D18.03
　　intracranial D18.02
　　skin D18.01
　　specified site NEC D18.09
　senile I78.1
　serpiginosum L81.7
　skin D18.01
　specified site NEC D18.09
　spider I78.1
　stellate I78.1
　venous Q28.3
Angiomatosis Q82.8
　bacillary A79.89
　encephalotrigeminal Q85.8
　hemorrhagic familial I78.0
　hereditary familial I78.0
　liver K76.4
Angiomyolipoma — *see* Lipoma
Angiomyoliposarcoma — *see* Neoplasm, connective
　tissue, malignant
Angiomyoma — *see* Neoplasm, connective tissue, benign
Angiomyosarcoma — *see* Neoplasm, connective tissue,
　malignant
Angiomyxoma — *see* Neoplasm, connective tissue, un-
　certain behavior
Angioneurosis F45.8
Angioneurotic edema (allergic) (any site) (with urticaria)
　T78.3 ☑
　hereditary D84.1
Angiopathia, angiopathy I99.9
　cerebral I67.9
　　amyloid E85.4 *[I68.0]*
　diabetic (peripheral) — *see* Diabetes, angiopathy
　peripheral I73.9
　　diabetic — *see* Diabetes, angiopathy
　　specified type NEC I73.89
　retinae syphilitica A52.05
　retinalis (juvenilis)
　　diabetic — *see* Diabetes, retinopathy
　　proliferative — *see* Retinopathy, proliferative
Angiosarcoma — *see also* Neoplasm, connective tissue,
　malignant

Angiosarcoma — *continued*
　liver C22.3
Angiosclerosis — *see* Arteriosclerosis
Angiospasm (peripheral) (traumatic) (vessel) I73.9
　brachial plexus G54.0
　cerebral G45.9
　cervical plexus G54.2
　nerve
　　arm — *see* Mononeuropathy, upper limb
　　　axillary G54.0
　　　median — *see* Lesion, nerve, median
　　　ulnar — *see* Lesion, nerve, ulnar
　　axillary G54.0
　　leg — *see* Mononeuropathy, lower limb
　　median — *see* Lesion, nerve, median
　　plantar — *see* Lesion, nerve, plantar
　　ulnar — *see* Lesion, nerve, ulnar
Angiospastic disease or edema I73.9
Angiostrongyliasis
　due to
　　Parastrongylus
　　　cantonensis B83.2
　　　costaricensis B81.3
　intestinal B81.3
Anguillulosis — *see* Strongyloidiasis
Angulation
　cecum — *see* Obstruction, intestine
　coccyx (acquired) — *see also* subcategory M43.8 ☑
　　congenital NEC Q76.49
　femur (acquired) — *see also* Deformity, limb, specified
　　type NEC, thigh
　　congenital Q74.2
　intestine (large) (small) — *see* Obstruction, intestine
　sacrum (acquired) — *see also* subcategory M43.8 ☑
　　congenital NEC Q76.49
　sigmoid (flexure) — *see* Obstruction, intestine
　spine — *see* Dorsopathy, deforming, specified NEC
　tibia (acquired) — *see also* Deformity, limb, specified
　　type NEC, lower leg
　　congenital Q74.2
　ureter N13.5
　　with infection N13.6
　wrist (acquired) — *see also* Deformity, limb, specified
　　type NEC, forearm
　　congenital Q74.0
Angulus infectiosus (lips) K13.0
Anhedonia R45.84
　sexual F52.0
Anhidrosis L74.4
Anhydration E86.0
Anhydremia E86.0
Anidrosis L74.4
Aniridia (congenital) Q13.1
Anisakiasis (infection) (infestation) B81.0
Anisakis larvae infestation B81.0
Aniseikonia H52.32
Anisocoria (pupil) H57.02
　congenital Q13.2
Anisocytosis R71.8
Anisometropia (congenital) H52.31
Ankle — *see* condition
Ankyloblepharon (eyelid) (acquired) — *see also* Ble-
　pharophimosis
　filiforme (adnatum) (congenital) Q10.3
　total Q10.3
Ankyloglossia Q38.1
Ankylosis (fibrous) (osseous) (joint) M24.60
　ankle M24.67- ☑
　arthrodesis status Z98.1
　cricoarytenoid (cartilage) (joint) (larynx) J38.7
　dental K03.5
　ear ossicles H74.31- ☑
　elbow M24.62- ☑
　foot M24.67- ☑
　hand M24.64- ☑
　hip M24.65- ☑
　incostapedial joint (infectional) — *see* Ankylosis, ear
　　ossicles
　jaw (temporomandibular) M26.61- ☑
　knee M24.66- ☑
　lumbosacral (joint) M43.27
　postoperative (status) Z98.1
　produced by surgical fusion, status Z98.1
　sacro-iliac (joint) M43.28
　shoulder M24.61- ☑
　spine (joint) — *see also* Fusion, spine
　　spondylitic — *see* Spondylitis, ankylosing

Ankylosis — *continued*
  surgical Z98.1
  temporomandibular M26.61- ☑
  tooth, teeth (hard tissues) K03.5
  wrist M24.63- ☑
Ankylostoma — *see* Ancylostoma
Ankylostomiasis — *see* Ancylostomiasis
Ankylurethria — *see* Stricture, urethra
Annular — *see also* condition
  detachment, cervix N88.8
  organ or site, congenital NEC — *see* Distortion
  pancreas (congenital) Q45.1
Anodontia (complete) (partial) (vera) K00.0
  acquired K08.10 ☑
Anomaly, anomalous (congenital) (unspecified type)
      Q89.9
  abdominal wall NEC Q79.59
  acoustic nerve Q07.8
  adrenal (gland) Q89.1
  Alder (-Reilly) (leukocyte granulation) D72.0
  alimentary tract Q45.9
    upper Q40.9
  alveolar M26.70
    hyperplasia M26.79
        mandibular M26.72
        maxillary M26.71
    hypoplasia M26.79
        mandibular M26.74
        maxillary M26.73
    ridge (process) M26.79
    specified NEC M26.79
  ankle (joint) Q74.2
  anus Q43.9
  aorta (arch) NEC Q25.40
    coarctation (preductal) (postductal) Q25.1
  aortic cusp or valve Q23.9
  appendix Q43.8
  apple peel syndrome Q41.1
  aqueduct of Sylvius Q03.0
    with spina bifida — *see* Spina bifida, with hydro-
          cephalus
  arm Q74.0
  arteriovenous NEC
    coronary Q24.5
    gastrointestinal Q27.33
      acquired — *see* Angiodysplasia
  artery (peripheral) Q27.9
    basilar NEC Q28.1
    cerebral Q28.3
    coronary Q24.5
    digestive system Q27.8
    eye Q15.8
    great Q25.9
        specified NEC Q25.8
    lower limb Q27.8
    peripheral Q27.9
        specified NEC Q27.8
    pulmonary NEC Q25.79
    renal Q27.2
    retina Q14.1
    specified site NEC Q27.8
    subclavian Q27.8
        origin Q25.48
    umbilical Q27.0
    upper limb Q27.8
    vertebral NEC Q28.1
  aryteno-epiglottic folds Q31.8
  atrial
    bands or folds Q20.8
    septa Q21.1
  atrioventricular
    excitation I45.6
    septum Q21.0
  auditory canal Q17.8
  auricle
    ear Q17.8
        causing impairment of hearing Q16.9
    heart Q20.8
  Axenfeld's Q15.0
  back Q89.9
  band
    atrial Q20.8
    heart Q24.8
    ventricular Q24.8
  Bartholin's duct Q38.4
  biliary duct or passage Q44.5
  bladder Q64.70
    absence Q64.5

Anomaly, anomalous — *continued*
  bladder — *continued*
    diverticulum Q64.6
    exstrophy Q64.10
        cloacal Q64.12
        extroversion Q64.19
        specified type NEC Q64.19
        supravesical fissure Q64.11
    neck obstruction Q64.31
    specified type NEC Q64.79
  bone Q79.9
    arm Q74.0
    face Q75.9
    leg Q74.2
    pelvic girdle Q74.2
    shoulder girdle Q74.0
    skull Q75.9
      with
          anencephaly Q00.0
          encephalocele — *see* Encephalocele
          hydrocephalus Q03.9
            with spina bifida — *see* Spina bifida, by
                  site, with hydrocephalus
          microcephaly Q02
  brain (multiple) Q04.9
    vessel Q28.3
  breast Q83.9
  broad ligament Q50.6
  bronchus Q32.4
  bulbus cordis Q21.9
  bursa Q79.9
  canal of Nuck Q52.4
  canthus Q10.3
  capillary Q27.9
  cardiac Q24.9
    chambers Q20.9
        specified NEC Q20.8
    septal closure Q21.9
        specified NEC Q21.8
    valve NEC Q24.8
        pulmonary Q22.3
  cardiovascular system Q28.8
  carpus Q74.0
  caruncle, lacrimal Q10.6
  cascade stomach Q40.2
  cauda equina Q06.3
  cecum Q43.9
  cerebral Q04.9
    vessels Q28.3
  cervix Q51.9
  Chédiak-Higashi (-Steinbrinck) (congenital gigantism
        of peroxidase granules) E70.330
  cheek Q18.9
  chest wall Q67.8
    bones Q76.9
  chin Q18.9
  chordae tendineae Q24.8
  choroid Q14.3
    plexus Q07.8
  chromosomes, chromosomal Q99.9
    D (1) — *see* condition, chromosome 13
    E (3) — *see* condition, chromosome 18
    G — *see* condition, chromosome 21
    sex
        female phenotype Q97.8
        gonadal dysgenesis (pure) Q99.1
        Klinefelter's Q98.4
        male phenotype Q98.9
        Turner's Q96.9
    specified NEC Q99.8
  cilia Q10.3
  circulatory system Q28.9
  clavicle Q74.0
  clitoris Q52.6
  coccyx Q76.49
  colon Q43.9
  common duct Q44.5
  communication
    coronary artery Q24.5
    left ventricle with right atrium Q21.0
  concha (ear) Q17.3
  connection
    portal vein Q26.5
    pulmonary venous Q26.4
        partial Q26.3
        total Q26.2
    renal artery with kidney Q27.2
  cornea (shape) Q13.4
  coronary artery or vein Q24.5

Anomaly, anomalous — *continued*
  cranium — *see* Anomaly, skull
  cricoid cartilage Q31.8
  cystic duct Q44.5
  dental
    alveolar — *see* Anomaly, alveolar
    arch relationship M26.20
        specified NEC M26.29
  dentofacial M26.9
    alveolar — *see* Anomaly, alveolar
    dental arch relationship M26.20
        specified NEC M26.29
    functional M26.50
        specified NEC M26.59
    jaw size M26.00
        macrogenia M26.05
        mandibular
          hyperplasia M26.03
          hypoplasia M26.04
        maxillary
          hyperplasia M26.01
          hypoplasia M26.02
        microgenia M26.06
        specified type NEC M26.09
    jaw-cranial base relationship M26.10
        asymmetry M26.12
          maxillary M26.11
        specified type NEC M26.19
    malocclusion M26.4
        dental arch relationship NEC M26..
        jaw size — *see* Anomaly, dentofac'
        jaw-cranial base relationship — *se*
              dentofacial, jaw-cranial base
    specified type NEC M26.89
    temporomandibular joint M26.60- ☑
        adhesions M26.61- ☑
        ankylosis M26.61- ☑
        arthralgia M26.62- ☑
        articular disc M26.63- ☑
        specified type NEC M26.69
    tooth position, fully erupted M26.30
        specified NEC M26.39
  dermatoglyphic Q82.8
  diaphragm (apertures) NEC Q79.1
  digestive organ(s) or tract Q45.9
    lower Q43.9
    upper Q40.9
  distance, interarch (excessive) (inadequa◼
  distribution, coronary artery Q24.5
  ductus
    arteriosus Q25.0
    botalli Q25.0
  duodenum Q43.9
  dura (brain) Q04.9
    spinal cord Q06.9
  ear (external) Q17.9
    causing impairment of hearing Q16.9
    inner Q16.5
    middle (causing impairment of hearin◼
        ossicles Q16.3
  Ebstein's (heart) (tricuspid valve) Q22.5
  ectodermal Q82.9
  Eisenmenger's (ventricular septal defect) ◼
  ejaculatory duct Q55.4
  elbow Q74.0
  endocrine gland NEC Q89.2
  epididymis Q55.4
  epiglottis Q31.8
  esophagus Q39.9
  eustachian tube Q17.8
  eye Q15.9
    anterior segment Q13.9
        specified NEC Q13.89
    posterior segment Q14.9
        specified NEC Q14.8
    ptosis (eyelid) Q10.0
    specified NEC Q15.8
  eyebrow Q18.8
  eyelid Q10.3
    ptosis Q10.0
  face Q18.9
    bone(s) Q75.9
  fallopian tube Q50.6
  fascia Q79.9
  femur NEC Q74.2
  fibula NEC Q74.2
  finger Q74.0
  fixation, intestine Q43.3

☑ **Additional Character Required** — Refer to the Tabular List for Character Selection   ᵂ **Subterms under main terms may continue to next colu◼**

Anomaly, anomalous — *continued*
- flexion (joint) NOS Q74.9
  - hip or thigh Q65.89
- foot NEC Q74.2
  - varus (congenital) Q66.3- ☑
- foramen
  - Botalli Q21.1
  - ovale Q21.1
- forearm Q74.0
- forehead Q75.8
- form, teeth K00.2
- fovea centralis Q14.1
- frontal bone — *see* Anomaly, skull
- gallbladder (position) (shape) (size) Q44.1
- Gartner's duct Q52.4
- gastrointestinal tract Q45.9
- genitalia, genital organ(s) or system
  - female Q52.9
    - external Q52.70
    - internal NOS Q52.9
  - male Q55.9
    - hydrocele P83.5
    - specified NEC Q55.8
- genitourinary NEC
  - female Q52.9
  - male Q55.9
- Gerbode Q21.0
- glottis Q31.8
- granulation or granulocyte, genetic (constitutional) (leukocyte) D72.0
- gum Q38.6
- gyri Q07.9
- hair Q84.2
- hand Q74.0
- hard tissue formation in pulp K04.3
- head — *see* Anomaly, skull
- heart Q24.9
  - auricle Q20.8
  - bands or folds Q24.8
  - fibroelastosis cordis I42.4
  - obstructive NEC Q22.6
  - patent ductus arteriosus (Botalli) Q25.0
  - septum Q21.9
    - auricular Q21.1
    - interatrial Q21.1
    - interventricular Q21.0
      - with pulmonary stenosis or atresia, dextraposition of aorta and hypertrophy of right ventricle Q21.3
    - specified NEC Q21.8
    - ventricular Q21.0
      - with pulmonary stenosis or atresia, dextraposition of aorta and hypertrophy of right ventricle Q21.3
  - tetralogy of Fallot Q21.3
  - valve NEC Q24.8
    - aortic
      - bicuspid valve Q23.1
      - insufficiency Q23.1
      - stenosis Q23.0
        - subaortic Q24.4
    - mitral
      - insufficiency Q23.3
      - stenosis Q23.2
    - pulmonary Q22.3
      - atresia Q22.0
      - insufficiency Q22.2
      - stenosis Q22.1
        - infundibular Q24.3
        - subvalvular Q24.3
    - tricuspid
      - atresia Q22.4
      - stenosis Q22.4
  - ventricle Q20.8
- heel NEC Q74.2
- Hegglin's D72.0
- hemianencephaly Q00.0
- hemicephaly Q00.0
- hemicrania Q00.0
- hepatic duct Q44.5
- hip NEC Q74.2
- hourglass stomach Q40.2
- humerus Q74.0
- hydatid of Morgagni
  - female Q50.5
  - male (epididymal) Q55.4
    - testicular Q55.29
- hymen Q52.4
- hypersegmentation of neutrophils, hereditary D72.0

Anomaly, anomalous — *continued*
- hypophyseal Q89.2
- ileocecal (coil) (valve) Q43.9
- ileum Q43.9
- ilium NEC Q74.2
- integument Q84.9
  - specified NEC Q84.8
- interarch distance (excessive) (inadequate) M26.25
- intervertebral cartilage or disc Q76.49
- intestine (large) (small) Q43.9
  - with anomalous adhesions, fixation or malrotation Q43.3
- iris Q13.2
- ischium NEC Q74.2
- jaw — *see* Anomaly, dentofacial
  - alveolar — *see* Anomaly, alveolar
- jaw-cranial base relationship — *see* Anomaly, dentofacial, jaw-cranial base relationship
- jejunum Q43.8
- joint Q74.9
  - specified NEC Q74.8
- Jordan's D72.0
- kidney(s) (calyx) (pelvis) Q63.9
  - artery Q27.2
  - specified NEC Q63.8
- Klippel-Feil (brevicollis) Q76.1
- knee Q74.1
- labium (majus) (minus) Q52.70
- labyrinth, membranous Q16.5
- lacrimal apparatus or duct Q10.6
- larynx, laryngeal (muscle) Q31.9
  - web (bed) Q31.0
- lens Q12.9
- leukocytes, genetic D72.0
  - granulation (constitutional) D72.0
- lid (fold) Q10.3
- ligament Q79.9
  - broad Q50.6
  - round Q52.8
- limb Q74.9
  - lower NEC Q74.2
    - reduction deformity — *see* Defect, reduction, lower limb
  - upper Q74.0
- lip Q38.0
- liver Q44.7
  - duct Q44.5
- lower limb NEC Q74.2
- lumbosacral (joint) (region) Q76.49
  - kyphosis — *see* Kyphosis, congenital
  - lordosis — *see* Lordosis, congenital
- lung (fissure) (lobe) Q33.9
- mandible — *see* Anomaly, dentofacial
- maxilla — *see* Anomaly, dentofacial
- May (-Hegglin) D72.0
- meatus urinarius NEC Q64.79
- meningeal bands or folds Q07.9
  - constriction of Q07.8
  - spinal Q06.9
- meninges Q07.9
  - cerebral Q04.8
  - spinal Q06.9
- meningocele Q05.9
- mesentery Q45.9
- metacarpus Q74.0
- metatarsus NEC Q74.2
- middle ear Q16.4
  - ossicles Q16.3
- mitral (leaflets) (valve) Q23.9
  - insufficiency Q23.3
  - specified NEC Q23.8
  - stenosis Q23.2
- mouth Q38.6
- Müllerian — *see also* Anomaly, by site
  - uterus NEC Q51.818
- multiple NEC Q89.7
- muscle Q79.9
  - eyelid Q10.3
- musculoskeletal system, except limbs Q79.9
- myocardium Q24.8
- nail Q84.6
- narrowness, eyelid Q10.3
- nasal sinus (wall) Q30.8
- neck (any part) Q18.9
- nerve Q07.9
  - acoustic Q07.8
  - optic Q07.8
- nervous system (central) Q07.9

Anomaly, anomalous — *continued*
- nipple Q83.9
- nose, nasal (bones) (cartilage) (septum) (sinus) Q30.9
  - specified NEC Q30.8
- ocular muscle Q15.8
- omphalomesenteric duct Q43.0
- opening, pulmonary veins Q26.4
- optic
  - disc Q14.2
  - nerve Q07.8
- opticociliary vessels Q13.2
- orbit (eye) Q10.7
- organ Q89.9
  - of Corti Q16.5
- origin
  - artery
    - innominate Q25.8
    - pulmonary Q25.79
    - renal Q27.2
    - subclavian Q25.48
- osseous meatus (ear) Q16.1
- ovary Q50.39
- oviduct Q50.6
- palate (hard) (soft) NEC Q38.5
- pancreas or pancreatic duct Q45.3
- papillary muscles Q24.8
- parathyroid gland Q89.2
- paraurethral ducts Q64.79
- parotid (gland) Q38.4
- patella Q74.1
- Pelger-Huët (hereditary hyposegmentation) D72.0
- pelvic girdle NEC Q74.2
- pelvis (bony) NEC Q74.2
  - rachitic E64.3
- penis (glans) Q55.69
- pericardium Q24.8
- peripheral vascular system Q27.9
- Peter's Q13.4
- pharynx Q38.8
- pigmentation L81.9
  - congenital Q82.8
- pituitary (gland) Q89.2
- pleural (folds) Q34.0
- portal vein Q26.5
  - connection Q26.5
- position, tooth, teeth, fully erupted M26.30
  - specified NEC M26.39
- precerebral vessel Q28.1
- prepuce Q55.69
- prostate Q55.4
- pulmonary Q33.9
  - artery NEC Q25.79
  - valve Q22.3
    - atresia Q22.0
    - insufficiency Q22.2
    - specified type NEC Q22.3
    - stenosis Q22.1
      - infundibular Q24.3
      - subvalvular Q24.3
  - venous connection Q26.4
    - partial Q26.3
    - total Q26.2
- pupil Q13.2
  - function H57.00
    - anisocoria H57.02
    - Argyll Robertson pupil H57.01
    - miosis H57.03
    - mydriasis H57.04
    - specified type NEC H57.09
    - tonic pupil H57.05- ☑
- pylorus Q40.3
- radius Q74.0
- rectum Q43.9
- reduction (extremity) (limb)
  - femur (longitudinal) — *see* Defect, reduction, lower limb, longitudinal, femur
  - fibula (longitudinal) — *see* Defect, reduction, lower limb, longitudinal, fibula
  - lower limb — *see* Defect, reduction, lower limb
  - radius (longitudinal) — *see* Defect, reduction, upper limb, longitudinal, radius
  - tibia (longitudinal) — *see* Defect, reduction, lower limb, longitudinal, tibia
  - ulna (longitudinal) — *see* Defect, reduction, upper limb, longitudinal, ulna
  - upper limb — *see* Defect, reduction, upper limb
- refraction — *see* Disorder, refraction
- renal Q63.9

Anomaly, anomalous — continued
renal — continued
  artery Q27.2
  pelvis Q63.9
    specified NEC Q63.8
respiratory system Q34.9
  specified NEC Q34.8
retina Q14.1
rib Q76.6
  cervical Q76.5
Rieger's Q13.81
rotation — see Malrotation
  hip or thigh Q65.89
round ligament Q52.8
sacroiliac (joint) NEC Q74.2
sacrum NEC Q76.49
  kyphosis — see Kyphosis, congenital
  lordosis — see Lordosis, congenital
saddle nose, syphilitic A50.57
salivary duct or gland Q38.4
scapula Q74.0
scrotum — see Malformation, testis and scrotum
sebaceous gland Q82.9
seminal vesicles Q55.4
sense organs NEC Q07.8
sex chromosomes NEC — see also Anomaly, chromo-
    somes
  female phenotype Q97.8
  male phenotype Q98.9
shoulder (girdle) (joint) Q74.0
sigmoid (flexure) Q43.9
simian crease Q82.8
sinus of Valsalva Q25.49
skeleton generalized Q78.9
skin (appendage) Q82.9
skull Q75.9
  with
    anencephaly Q00.0
    encephalocele — see Encephalocele
    hydrocephalus Q03.9
      with spina bifida — see Spina bifida, by site,
        with hydrocephalus
    microcephaly Q02
specified organ or site NEC Q89.8
spermatic cord Q55.4
spine, spinal NEC Q76.49
  column NEC Q76.49
    kyphosis — see Kyphosis, congenital
    lordosis — see Lordosis, congenital
  cord Q06.9
  nerve root Q07.8
spleen Q89.09
  agenesis Q89.01
stenonian duct Q38.4
sternum NEC Q76.7
stomach Q40.3
submaxillary gland Q38.4
tarsus NEC Q74.2
tendon Q79.9
testis — see Malformation, testis and scrotum
thigh NEC Q74.2
thorax (wall) Q67.8
  bony Q76.9
throat Q38.8
thumb Q74.0
thymus gland Q89.2
thyroid (gland) Q89.2
  cartilage Q31.8
tibia NEC Q74.2
  saber A50.56
toe Q74.2
tongue Q38.3
tooth, teeth K00.9
  eruption K00.6
  position, fully erupted M26.30
  spacing, fully erupted M26.30
trachea (cartilage) Q32.1
tragus Q17.9
tricuspid (leaflet) (valve) Q22.9
  atresia or stenosis Q22.4
  Ebstein's Q22.5
Uhl's (hypoplasia of myocardium, right ventricle) Q24.8
ulna Q74.0
umbilical artery Q27.0
union
  cricoid cartilage and thyroid cartilage Q31.8
  thyroid cartilage and hyoid bone Q31.8
  trachea with larynx Q31.8

Anomaly, anomalous — continued
upper limb Q74.0
urachus Q64.4
ureter Q62.8
  obstructive NEC Q62.39
    cecoureterocele Q62.32
    orthotopic ureterocele Q62.31
urethra Q64.70
  absence Q64.5
  double Q64.74
  fistula to rectum Q64.73
  obstructive Q64.39
    stricture Q64.32
  prolapse Q64.71
  specified type NEC Q64.79
urinary tract Q64.9
uterus Q51.9
  with only one functioning horn Q51.4
uvula Q38.5
vagina Q52.4
valleculae Q31.8
valve (heart) NEC Q24.8
  coronary sinus Q24.5
  inferior vena cava Q24.8
  pulmonary Q22.3
  sinus coronario Q24.5
  venae cavae inferioris Q24.8
vas deferens Q55.4
vascular Q27.9
  brain Q28.3
  ring Q25.45
vein(s) (peripheral) Q27.9
  brain Q28.3
  cerebral Q28.3
  coronary Q24.5
  developmental Q28.3
  great Q26.9
    specified NEC Q26.8
vena cava (inferior) (superior) Q26.9
venous — see Anomaly, vein(s)
venous return Q26.8
ventricular
  bands or folds Q24.8
  septa Q21.0
vertebra Q76.49
  kyphosis — see Kyphosis, congenital
  lordosis — see Lordosis, congenital
vesicourethral orifice Q64.79
vessel(s) Q27.9
  optic papilla Q14.2
  precerebral Q28.1
vitelline duct Q43.0
vitreous body or humor Q14.0
vulva Q52.70
wrist (joint) Q74.0
Anomia R48.8
Anonychia (congenital) Q84.3
  acquired L60.8
Anophthalmos, anophthalmus (congenital) (globe)
  Q11.1
  acquired Z90.01
Anopia, anopsia H53.46- ☑
  quadrant H53.46- ☑
Anorchia, anorchism, anorchidism Q55.0
Anorexia R63.0
  hysterical F44.89
  nervosa F50.00
    atypical F50.9
    binge-eating type F50.2
      with purging F50.02
    restricting type F50.01
Anorgasmy, psychogenic (female) F52.31
  male F52.32
Anosmia R43.0
  hysterical F44.6
  postinfectional J39.8
Anosognosia R41.89
Anosteoplasia Q78.9
Anovulatory cycle N97.0
Anoxemia R09.02
  newborn P84
Anoxia (pathological) R09.02
  altitude T70.29 ☑
  cerebral G93.1
    complicating
      anesthesia (general) (local) or other sedation
        T88.59 ☑
        in labor and delivery O74.3

Anoxia — continued
cerebral — continued
  complicating — continued
    anesthesia or other sedation — continued
      in pregnancy O29.21- ☑
      postpartum, puerperal O89.2
    delivery (cesarean) (instrumental) O75.4
    during a procedure G97.81
    newborn P84
    resulting from a procedure G97.82
  due to
    drowning T75.1 ☑
    high altitude T70.29 ☑
  heart — see Insufficiency, coronary
  intrauterine P84
  myocardial — see Insufficiency, coronary
  newborn P84
  spinal cord G95.11
  systemic (by suffocation) (low content in atmosphere)
    — see Asphyxia, traumatic
Anteflexion — see Anteversion
Antenatal
  care (normal pregnancy) Z34.90
  screening (encounter for) of mother — see also En-
    counter, antenatal screening Z36.9
Antepartum — see condition
Anterior — see condition
Antero-occlusion M26.220
Anteversion
  cervix — see Anteversion, uterus
  femur (neck), congenital Q65.89
  uterus, uterine (cervix) (postinfectional) (postpartal,
    old) N85.4
    congenital Q51.818
    in pregnancy or childbirth — see Pregnancy, com-
      plicated by
Anthophobia F40.228
Anthracosilicosis J60
Anthracosis (lung) (occupational) J60
  lingua K14.3
Anthrax A22.9
  with pneumonia A22.1
  cerebral A22.8
  colitis A22.2
  cutaneous A22.0
  gastrointestinal A22.2
  inhalation A22.1
  intestinal A22.2
  meningitis A22.8
  pulmonary A22.1
  respiratory A22.1
  sepsis A22.7
  specified manifestation NEC A22.8
Anthropoid pelvis Q74.2
  with disproportion (fetopelvic) O33.0
Anthropophobia F40.10
  generalized F40.11
Antibodies, maternal (blood group) — see Isoimmuniza-
    tion, affecting management of pregnancy
  anti-D — see Isoimmunization, affecting management
    of pregnancy, Rh
  newborn P55.0
Antibody
  anticardiolipin R76.0
    with
      hemorrhagic disorder D68.312
      hypercoagulable state D68.61
  antiphosphatidylglycerol R76.0
    with
      hemorrhagic disorder D68.312
      hypercoagulable state D68.61
  antiphosphatidylinositol R76.0
    with
      hemorrhagic disorder D68.312
      hypercoagulable state D68.61
  antiphosphatidylserine R76.0
    with
      hemorrhagic disorder D68.312
      hypercoagulable state D68.61
  antiphospholipid R76.0
    with
      hemorrhagic disorder D68.312
      hypercoagulable state D68.61
Anticardiolipin syndrome D68.61
Anticoagulant, circulating (intrinsic) — see also Disor-
    der, hemorrhagic D68.318
  drug-induced (extrinsic) — see also Disorder, hemor-
    rhagic D68.32

Anticoagulant, circulating — *continued*
  iatrogenic D68.32
Antidiuretic hormone syndrome E22.2
Antimonial cholera — *see* Poisoning, antimony
Antiphospholipid
  antibody
    with hemorrhagic disorder D68.312
    syndrome D68.61
Antisocial personality F60.2
Antithrombinemia — *see* Circulating anticoagulants
Antithromboplastinemia D68.318
Antithromboplastinogenemia D68.318
Antitoxin complication or reaction — *see* Complications, vaccination
Antlophobia F40.228
Antritis J32.0
  maxilla J32.0
    acute J01.00
      recurrent J01.01
  stomach K29.60
    with bleeding K29.61
Antrum, antral — *see* condition
Anuria R34
  calculous (impacted) (recurrent) — *see also* Calculus, urinary N20.9
  following
    abortion — *see* Abortion by type complicated by, renal failure
    ectopic or molar pregnancy O08.4
  newborn P96.0
  postprocedural N99.0
  postrenal N13.8
  traumatic (following crushing) T79.5 ☑
Anus, anal — *see* condition
Anusitis K62.89
Anxiety F41.9
  depression F41.8
  episodic paroxysmal F41.0
  generalized F41.1
  hysteria F41.8
  neurosis F41.1
  panic type F41.0
  reaction F41.1
  separation, abnormal (of childhood) F93.0
  specified NEC F41.8
  state F41.1
Aorta, aortic — *see* condition
Aortectasia — *see* Ectasia, aorta
  with aneurysm — *see* Aneurysm, aorta
Aortitis (nonsyphilitic) (calcific) I77.6
  arteriosclerotic I70.0
  Doehle-Heller A52.02
  luetic A52.02
  rheumatic — *see* Endocarditis, acute, rheumatic
  specific (syphilitic) A52.02
  syphilitic A52.02
    congenital A50.54 *[I79.1]*
Apathetic thyroid storm — *see* Thyrotoxicosis
Apathy R45.3
Apeirophobia F40.228
Apepsia K30
  psychogenic F45.8
Aperistalsis, esophagus K22.0
Apertognathia M26.29
Apert's syndrome Q87.0
Aphagia R13.0
  psychogenic F50.9
Aphakia (acquired) (postoperative) H27.0- ☑
  congenital Q12.3
Aphasia (amnestic) (global) (nominal) (semantic) (syntactic) R47.01
  acquired, with epilepsy (Landau-Kleffner syndrome) — *see* Epilepsy, specified NEC
  auditory (developmental) F80.2
  developmental (receptive type) F80.2
    expressive type F80.1
    Wernicke's F80.2
  following
    cerebrovascular disease I69.920
      cerebral infarction I69.320
      intracerebral hemorrhage I69.120
      nontraumatic intracranial hemorrhage NEC I69.220
      specified disease NEC I69.820
      subarachnoid hemorrhage I69.020
  primary progressive G31.01 *[F02.80]*
    with behavioral disturbance G31.01 *[F02.81]*
  progressive isolated G31.01 *[F02.80]*

Aphasia — *continued*
  progressive isolated — *continued*
    with behavioral disturbance G31.01 *[F02.81]*
  sensory F80.2
  syphilis, tertiary A52.19
  Wernicke's (developmental) F80.2
Aphonia (organic) R49.1
  hysterical F44.4
  psychogenic F44.4
Aphthae, aphthous — *see also* condition
  Bednar's K12.0
  cachectic K14.0
  epizootic B08.8
  fever B08.8
  oral (recurrent) K12.0
  stomatitis (major) (minor) K12.0
  thrush B37.0
  ulcer (oral) (recurrent) K12.0
    genital organ(s) NEC
      female N76.6
      male N50.89
    larynx J38.7
Apical — *see* condition
Apiphobia F40.218
Aplasia — *see also* Agenesis
  abdominal muscle syndrome Q79.4
  alveolar process (acquired) — *see* Anomaly, alveolar
    congenital Q38.6
  aorta (congenital) Q25.41
  axialis extracorticalis (congenita) E75.29
  bone marrow (myeloid) D61.9
    congenital D61.01
  brain Q00.0
    part of Q04.3
  bronchus Q32.4
  cementum K00.4
  cerebellum Q04.3
  cervix (congenital) Q51.5
  congenital pure red cell D61.01
  corpus callosum Q04.0
  cutis congenita Q84.8
  erythrocyte congenital D61.01
  extracortical axial E75.29
  eye Q11.1
  fovea centralis (congenital) Q14.1
  gallbladder, congenital Q44.0
  iris Q13.1
  labyrinth, membranous Q16.5
  limb (congenital) Q73.8
    lower — *see* Defect, reduction, lower limb
    upper — *see* Agenesis, arm
  lung, congenital (bilateral) (unilateral) Q33.3
  pancreas Q45.0
  parathyroid-thymic D82.1
  Pelizaeus-Merzbacher E75.29
  penis Q55.5
  prostate Q55.4
  red cell (with thymoma) D60.9
    acquired D60.9
      due to drugs D60.9
    adult D60.9
    chronic D60.0
    congenital D61.01
    constitutional D61.01
    due to drugs D60.9
    hereditary D61.01
    of infants D61.01
    primary D61.01
    pure D61.01
      due to drugs D60.9
    specified type NEC D60.8
    transient D60.1
  round ligament Q52.8
  skin Q84.8
  spermatic cord Q55.4
  spleen Q89.01
  testicle Q55.0
  thymic, with immunodeficiency D82.1
  thyroid (congenital) (with myxedema) E03.1
  uterus Q51.0
  ventral horn cell Q06.1
Apnea, apneic (of) (spells) R06.81
  newborn NEC P28.4
    obstructive P28.4
    sleep (central) (obstructive) (primary) P28.3
    prematurity P28.4
  sleep G47.30
    central (primary) G47.31

Apnea, apneic — *continued*
  sleep — *continued*
    central — *continued*
      idiopathic G47.31
      in conditions classified elsewhere G47.37
    obstructive (adult) (pediatric) G47.33
      hypopnea G47.33
    primary central G47.31
    specified NEC G47.39
Apneumatosis, newborn P28.0
Apocrine metaplasia (breast) — *see* Dysplasia, mammary, specified type NEC
Apophysitis (bone) — *see also* Osteochondropathy
  calcaneus M92.8
  juvenile M92.9
Apoplectiform convulsions (cerebral ischemia) I67.82
Apoplexia, apoplexy, apoplectic
  adrenal A39.1
  heart (auricle) (ventricle) — *see* Infarct, myocardium
  heat T67.01 ☑
  hemorrhagic (stroke) — *see* Hemorrhage, intracranial
  meninges, hemorrhagic — *see* Hemorrhage, intracranial, subarachnoid
  uremic N18.9 *[I68.8]*
Appearance
  bizarre R46.1
  specified NEC R46.89
  very low level of personal hygiene R46.0
Appendage
  epididymal (organ of Morgagni) Q55.4
  intestine (epiploic) Q43.8
  preauricular Q17.0
  testicular (organ of Morgagni) Q55.29
Appendicitis (pneumococcal) (retrocecal) K37
  with
    gangrene K35.891
    perforation NOS K35.32
    peritoneal abscess K35.33
    peritonitis NEC K35.33
      generalized (with perforation or rupture) K35.20
        with abscess K35.21
      localized K35.30
        with
          gangrene K35.31
          perforation K35.32
            and abscess K35.33
    rupture (with localized peritonitis) K35.32
  acute (catarrhal) (fulminating) (gangrenous) (obstructive) (retrocecal) (suppurative) K35.80
    with
      gangrene K35.891
      peritoneal abscess K35.33
      peritonitis NEC K35.33
        generalized (with perforation or rupture) K35.20
          with abscess K35.21
        localized K35.30
          with
            gangrene K35.31
            perforation K35.32
              and abscess K35.33
    specified NEC K35.890
      with gangrene K35.891
  amebic A06.89
  chronic (recurrent) K36
  exacerbation — *see* Appendicitis, acute
  gangrenous — *see* Appendicitis, acute
  healed (obliterative) K36
  interval K36
  neurogenic K36
  obstructive K36
  recurrent K36
  relapsing K36
  ruptured NOS (with localized peritonitis) K35.32
  subacute (adhesive) K36
  subsiding K36
  suppurative — *see* Appendicitis, acute
  tuberculous A18.32
Appendicopathia oxyurica B80
Appendix, appendicular — *see also* condition
  epididymis Q55.4
  Morgagni
    female Q50.5
    male (epididymal) Q55.4
      testicular Q55.29
  testis Q55.29
Appetite
  depraved — *see* Pica

Appetite — *continued*
excessive R63.2
lack or loss — *see also* Anorexia R63.0
nonorganic origin F50.89
psychogenic F50.89
perverted (hysterical) — *see* Pica
Apple peel syndrome Q41.1
Apprehension state F41.1
Apprehensiveness, abnormal F41.9
Approximal wear K03.0
Apraxia (classic) (ideational) (ideokinetic) (ideomotor) (motor) (verbal) R48.2
following
cerebrovascular disease I69.990
cerebral infarction I69.390
intracerebral hemorrhage I69.190
nontraumatic intracranial hemorrhage NEC I69.290
specified disease NEC I69.890
subarachnoid hemorrhage I69.090
oculomotor, congenital H51.8
Aptyalism K11.7
Apudoma — *see* Neoplasm, uncertain behavior, by site
Aqueous misdirection H40.83- ☑
Arabicum elephantiasis — *see* Infestation, filarial
Arachnitis — *see* Meningitis
Arachnodactyly — *see* Syndrome, Marfan's
Arachnoiditis (acute) (adhesive) (basal) (brain) (cerebrospinal) — *see* Meningitis
Arachnophobia F40.210
Arboencephalitis, Australian A83.4
Arborization block (heart) I45.5
ARC (AIDS-related complex) B20
Arch
aortic Q25.49
bovine Q25.49
Arches — *see* condition
Arcuate uterus Q51.810
Arcuatus uterus Q51.810
Arcus (cornea) senilis — *see* Degeneration, cornea, senile
Arc-welder's lung J63.4
Areflexia R29.2
Areola — *see* condition
Argentaffinoma — *see also* Neoplasm, uncertain behavior, by site
malignant — *see* Neoplasm, malignant, by site
syndrome E34.0
Argininemia E72.21
Arginosuccinic aciduria E72.22
Argyll Robertson phenomenon, pupil or syndrome (syphilitic) A52.19
atypical H57.09
nonsyphilitic H57.09
Argyria, argyriasis
conjunctival H11.13- ☑
from drug or medicament — *see* Table of Drugs and Chemicals, by substance
Argyrosis, conjunctival H11.13- ☑
Arhinencephaly Q04.1
Ariboflavinosis E53.0
Arm — *see* condition
Arnold-Chiari disease, obstruction or syndrome (type II) Q07.00
with
hydrocephalus Q07.02
with spina bifida Q07.03
spina bifida Q07.01
with hydrocephalus Q07.03
type III — *see* Encephalocele
type IV Q04.8
Aromatic amino-acid metabolism disorder E70.9
specified NEC E70.8
Arousals, confusional G47.51
Arrest, arrested
cardiac I46.9
complicating
abortion — *see* Abortion, by type, complicated by, cardiac arrest
anesthesia (general) (local) or other sedation — *see* Table of Drugs and Chemicals, by drug
in labor and delivery O74.2
in pregnancy O29.11- ☑
postpartum, puerperal O89.1
delivery (cesarean) (instrumental) O75.4
due to
cardiac condition I46.2
specified condition NEC I46.8

Arrest, arrested — *continued*
cardiac — *continued*
intraoperative I97.71- ☑
newborn P29.81
personal history, successfully resuscitated Z86.74
postprocedural I97.12- ☑
obstetric procedure O75.4
cardiorespiratory — *see* Arrest, cardiac
circulatory — *see* Arrest, cardiac
deep transverse O64.0 ☑
development or growth
bone — *see* Disorder, bone, development or growth
child R62.50
tracheal rings Q32.1
epiphyseal
complete
femur M89.15- ☑
humerus M89.12- ☑
tibia M89.16- ☑
ulna M89.13- ☑
forearm M89.13- ☑
specified NEC M89.13- ☑
ulna — *see* Arrest, epiphyseal, by type, ulna
lower leg M89.16- ☑
specified NEC M89.168
tibia — *see* Arrest, epiphyseal, by type, tibia
partial
femur M89.15- ☑
humerus M89.12- ☑
tibia M89.16- ☑
ulna M89.13- ☑
specified NEC M89.18
granulopoiesis — *see* Agranulocytosis
growth plate — *see* Arrest, epiphyseal
heart — *see* Arrest, cardiac
legal, anxiety concerning Z65.3
physeal — *see* Arrest, epiphyseal
respiratory R09.2
newborn P28.81
sinus I45.5
spermatogenesis (complete) — *see* Azoospermia
incomplete — *see* Oligospermia
transverse (deep) O64.0 ☑
Arrhenoblastoma
benign
specified site — *see* Neoplasm, benign, by site
unspecified site
female D27.9
male D29.20
malignant
specified site — *see* Neoplasm, malignant, by site
unspecified site
female C56.9
male C62.90
specified site — *see* Neoplasm, uncertain behavior, by site
unspecified site
female D39.10
male D40.10
Arrhythmia (auricle) (cardiac) (juvenile) (nodal) (reflex) (sinus) (supraventricular) (transitory) (ventricle) I49.9
block I45.9
extrasystolic I49.49
newborn
bradycardia P29.12
occurring before birth P03.819
before onset of labor P03.810
during labor P03.811
tachycardia P29.11
psychogenic F45.8
specified NEC I49.8
vagal R55
ventricular re-entry I47.0
Arrillaga-Ayerza syndrome (pulmonary sclerosis with pulmonary hypertension) I27.0
Arsenical pigmentation L81.8
from drug or medicament — *see* Table of Drugs and Chemicals
Arsenism — *see* Poisoning, arsenic
Arterial — *see* condition
Arteriofibrosis — *see* Arteriosclerosis
Arteriolar sclerosis — *see* Arteriosclerosis
Arteriolith — *see* Arteriosclerosis
Arteriolitis I77.6
necrotizing, kidney I77.5
renal — *see* Hypertension, kidney
Arteriolosclerosis — *see* Arteriosclerosis

Arterionephrosclerosis — *see* Hypertension, kidney
Arteriopathy I77.9
cerebral autosomal dominant, with subcortical infarcts and leukoencephalopathy (CADASIL) I67.850
Arteriosclerosis, arteriosclerotic (diffuse) (obliterans) (of) (senile) (with calcification) I70.90
aorta I70.0
arteries of extremities — *see* Arteriosclerosis, extremities
brain I67.2
bypass graft
coronary — *see* Arteriosclerosis, coronary, bypass graft
extremities — *see* Arteriosclerosis, extremities, bypass graft
cardiac — *see* Disease, heart, ischemic, atherosclerotic
cardiopathy — *see* Disease, heart, ischemic, atherosclerotic
cardiorenal — *see* Hypertension, cardiorenal
cardiovascular — *see* Disease, heart, ischemic, atherosclerotic
carotid — *see also* Occlusion, artery, carotid I65.2- ☑
central nervous system I67.2
cerebral I67.2
cerebrovascular I67.2
coronary (artery)
due to
calcified coronary lesion (severely) I25.84
lipid rich plaque I25.83
bypass graft I25.810
with
angina pectoris I25.709
with documented spasm I25.701
specified type NEC I25.708
unstable I25.700
ischemic chest pain I25.709
autologous artery I25.810
with
angina pectoris I25.729
with documented spasm I25.721
specified type I25.728
unstable I25.720
ischemic chest pain I25.729
autologous vein I25.810
with
angina pectoris I25.719
with documented spasm I25.711
specified type I25.718
unstable I25.710
ischemic chest pain I25.719
nonautologous biological I25.810
with
angina pectoris I25.739
with documented spasm I25.731
specified type I25.738
unstable I25.730
ischemic chest pain I25.739
specified type NEC I25.810
with
angina pectoris I25.799
with documented spasm I25.791
specified type I25.798
unstable I25.790
ischemic chest pain I25.799
native vessel
with
angina pectoris I25.119
with documented spasm I25.111
specified type NEC I25.118
unstable I25.110
ischemic chest pain I25.119
transplanted heart I25.811
bypass graft I25.812
with
angina pectoris I25.769
with documented spasm I25.761
specified type I25.768
unstable I25.760
ischemic chest pain I25.769
native coronary artery I25.811
with
angina pectoris I25.759
with documented spasm I25.751
specified type I25.758
unstable I25.750
ischemic chest pain I25.759
extremities (native arteries) I70.209
bypass graft I70.309

Arteriosclerosis, arteriosclerotic — *continued*
  extremities — *continued*
    bypass graft — *continued*
      autologous vein graft I70.409
        leg I70.409
          with
            gangrene (and intermittent claudication, rest pain and ulcer) I70.469
            intermittent claudication I70.419
            rest pain (and intermittent claudication) I70.429
          bilateral I70.403
            with
              gangrene (and intermittent claudication, rest pain and ulcer) I70.463
              intermittent claudication I70.463
              rest pain (and intermittent claudication) I70.423
            specified type NEC I70.493
          left I70.402
            with
              gangrene (and intermittent claudication, rest pain and ulcer) I70.462
              intermittent claudication I70.412
              rest pain (and intermittent claudication) I70.422
              ulceration (and intermittent claudication and rest pain) I70.449
                ankle I70.443
                calf I70.442
                foot site NEC I70.445
                heel I70.444
                lower leg NEC I70.448
                midfoot I70.444
                thigh I70.441
            specified type NEC I70.492
          right I70.401
            with
              gangrene (and intermittent claudication, rest pain and ulcer) I70.461
              intermittent claudication I70.411
              rest pain (and intermittent claudication) I70.421
              ulceration (and intermittent claudication and rest pain) I70.439
                ankle I70.433
                calf I70.432
                foot site NEC I70.435
                heel I70.434
                lower leg NEC I70.438
                midfoot I70.434
                thigh I70.431
            specified type NEC I70.491
        specified type NEC I70.499
      specified NEC I70.408
        with
          gangrene (and intermittent claudication, rest pain and ulcer) I70.468
          intermittent claudication I70.418
          rest pain (and intermittent claudication) I70.428
          ulceration (and intermittent claudication and rest pain) I70.45
        specified type NEC I70.498
    leg I70.309
      with
        gangrene (and intermittent claudication, rest pain and ulcer) I70.369
        intermittent claudication I70.319
        rest pain (and intermittent claudication) I70.329
      bilateral I70.303
        with
          gangrene (and intermittent claudication, rest pain and ulcer) I70.363
          intermittent claudication I70.313
          rest pain (and intermittent claudication) I70.323
        specified type NEC I70.393
      left I70.302
        with
          gangrene (and intermittent claudication, rest pain and ulcer) I70.362
          intermittent claudication I70.312
          rest pain (and intermittent claudication) I70.322

Arteriosclerosis, arteriosclerotic — *continued*
  extremities — *continued*
    bypass graft — *continued*
      leg — *continued*
        left — *continued*
          with — *continued*
            ulceration (and intermittent claudication and rest pain) I70.349
              ankle I70.343
              calf I70.342
              foot site NEC I70.345
              heel I70.344
              lower leg NEC I70.348
              midfoot I70.344
              thigh I70.341
          specified type NEC I70.392
        right I70.301
          with
            gangrene (and intermittent claudication, rest pain and ulcer) I70.361
            intermittent claudication I70.311
            rest pain (and intermittent claudication) I70.321
            ulceration (and intermittent claudication and rest pain) I70.339
              ankle I70.333
              calf I70.332
              foot site NEC I70.335
              heel I70.334
              lower leg NEC I70.338
              midfoot I70.334
              thigh I70.331
          specified type NEC I70.391
      specified type NEC I70.399
    nonautologous biological graft I70.509
      leg I70.509
        with
          gangrene (and intermittent claudication, rest pain and ulcer) I70.569
          intermittent claudication I70.519
          rest pain (and intermittent claudication) I70.529
      bilateral I70.503
        with
          gangrene (and intermittent claudication, rest pain and ulcer) I70.563
          intermittent claudication I70.513
          rest pain (and intermittent claudication) I70.523
        specified type NEC I70.593
      left I70.502
        with
          gangrene (and intermittent claudication, rest pain and ulcer) I70.562
          intermittent claudication I70.512
          rest pain (and intermittent claudication) I70.522
          ulceration (and intermittent claudication and rest pain) I70.549
            ankle I70.543
            calf I70.542
            foot site NEC I70.545
            heel I70.544
            lower leg NEC I70.548
            midfoot I70.544
            thigh I70.541
        specified type NEC I70.592
      right I70.501
        with
          gangrene (and intermittent claudication, rest pain and ulcer) I70.561
          intermittent claudication I70.511
          rest pain (and intermittent claudication) I70.521
          ulceration (and intermittent claudication and rest pain) I70.539
            ankle I70.533
            calf I70.532
            foot site NEC I70.535
            heel I70.534
            lower leg NEC I70.538
            midfoot I70.534
            thigh I70.531
        specified type NEC I70.591
      specified type NEC I70.599
    specified NEC I70.508

Arteriosclerosis, arteriosclerotic — *continued*
  extremities — *continued*
    bypass graft — *continued*
      nonautologous biological graft — *continued*
        specified — *continued*
          with
            gangrene (and intermittent claudication, rest pain and ulcer) I70.568
            intermittent claudication I70.518
            rest pain (and intermittent claudication) I70.528
            ulceration (and intermittent claudication and rest pain) I70.55
          specified type NEC I70.598
      nonbiological graft I70.609
        leg I70.609
          with
            gangrene (and intermittent claudication, rest pain and ulcer) I70.669
            intermittent claudication I70.619
            rest pain (and intermittent claudication) I70.629
        bilateral I70.603
          with
            gangrene (and intermittent claudication, rest pain and ulcer) I70.663
            intermittent claudication I70.613
            rest pain (and intermittent claudication) I70.623
          specified type NEC I70.693
        left I70.602
          with
            gangrene (and intermittent claudication, rest pain and ulcer) I70.662
            intermittent claudication I70.612
            rest pain (and intermittent claudication) I70.622
            ulceration (and intermittent claudication and rest pain) I70.649
              ankle I70.643
              calf I70.642
              foot site NEC I70.645
              heel I70.644
              lower leg NEC I70.648
              midfoot I70.644
              thigh I70.641
          specified type NEC I70.692
        right I70.601
          with
            gangrene (and intermittent claudication, rest pain and ulcer) I70.661
            intermittent claudication I70.611
            rest pain (and intermittent claudication) I70.621
            ulceration (and intermittent claudication and rest pain) I70.639
              ankle I70.633
              calf I70.632
              foot site NEC I70.635
              heel I70.634
              lower leg NEC I70.638
              midfoot I70.634
              thigh I70.631
          specified type NEC I70.691
        specified type NEC I70.699
      specified NEC I70.608
        with
          gangrene (and intermittent claudication, rest pain and ulcer) I70.668
          intermittent claudication I70.618
          rest pain (and intermittent claudication) I70.628
          ulceration (and intermittent claudication and rest pain) I70.65
        specified type NEC I70.698
    specified graft NEC I70.709
      leg I70.709
        with
          gangrene (and intermittent claudication, rest pain and ulcer) I70.769
          intermittent claudication I70.719
          rest pain (and intermittent claudication) I70.729
      bilateral I70.703

⏷ Subterms under main terms may continue to next column or page   ☑ **Additional Character Required — Refer to the Tabular List for Character Selection**   **27**

Arteriosclerosis, arteriosclerotic — *continued*
extremities — *continued*
bypass graft — *continued*
specified graft — *continued*
leg — *continued*
bilateral — *continued*
with
gangrene (and intermittent claudication, rest pain and ulcer) I70.763
intermittent claudication I70.713
rest pain (and intermittent claudication) I70.723
specified type NEC I70.793
left I70.702
with
gangrene (and intermittent claudication, rest pain and ulcer) I70.762
intermittent claudication I70.712
rest pain (and intermittent claudication) I70.722
ulceration (and intermittent claudication and rest pain) I70.749
ankle I70.743
calf I70.742
foot site NEC I70.745
heel I70.744
lower leg NEC I70.748
midfoot I70.744
thigh I70.741
specified type NEC I70.792
right I70.701
with
gangrene (and intermittent claudication, rest pain and ulcer) I70.761
intermittent claudication I70.711
rest pain (and intermittent claudication) I70.721
ulceration (and intermittent claudication and rest pain) I70.739
ankle I70.733
calf I70.732
foot site NEC I70.735
heel I70.734
lower leg NEC I70.738
midfoot I70.734
thigh I70.731
specified type NEC I70.791
specified type NEC I70.799
specified NEC I70.708
with
gangrene (and intermittent claudication, rest pain and ulcer) I70.768
intermittent claudication I70.718
rest pain (and intermittent claudication) I70.728
ulceration (and intermittent claudication and rest pain) I70.75
specified type NEC I70.798
specified NEC I70.308
with
gangrene (and intermittent claudication, rest pain and ulcer) I70.368
intermittent claudication I70.318
rest pain (and intermittent claudication) I70.35
ulceration (and intermittent claudication and rest pain) I70.35
specified type NEC I70.398
leg I70.209
with
gangrene (and intermittent claudication, rest pain and ulcer) I70.269
intermittent claudication I70.219
rest pain (and intermittent claudication) I70.229
bilateral I70.203
with
gangrene (and intermittent claudication, rest pain and ulcer) I70.263
intermittent claudication I70.213
rest pain (and intermittent claudication) I70.223
specified type NEC I70.293
left I70.202

Arteriosclerosis, arteriosclerotic — *continued*
extremities — *continued*
leg — *continued*
left — *continued*
with
gangrene (and intermittent claudication, rest pain and ulcer) I70.262
intermittent claudication I70.212
rest pain (and intermittent claudication) I70.222
ulceration (and intermittent claudication and rest pain) I70.249
ankle I70.243
calf I70.242
foot site NEC I70.245
heel I70.244
lower leg NEC I70.248
midfoot I70.244
thigh I70.241
specified type NEC I70.292
right I70.201
with
gangrene (and intermittent claudication, rest pain and ulcer) I70.261
intermittent claudication I70.211
rest pain (and intermittent claudication) I70.221
ulceration (and intermittent claudication and rest pain) I70.239
ankle I70.233
calf I70.232
foot site NEC I70.235
heel I70.234
lower leg NEC I70.238
midfoot I70.234
thigh I70.231
specified type NEC I70.291
specified type NEC I70.299
specified site NEC I70.208
with
gangrene (and intermittent claudication, rest pain and ulcer) I70.268
intermittent claudication I70.218
rest pain (and intermittent claudication) I70.228
ulceration (and intermittent claudication and rest pain) I70.25
specified type NEC I70.298
generalized I70.91
heart (disease) — *see* Arteriosclerosis, coronary (artery),
kidney — *see* Hypertension, kidney
medial — *see* Arteriosclerosis, extremities
mesenteric (artery) K55.1
Mönckeberg's — *see* Arteriosclerosis, extremities
myocarditis I51.4
peripheral (of extremities) — *see* Arteriosclerosis, extremities
pulmonary (idiopathic) I27.0
renal (arterioles) — *see also* Hypertension, kidney
artery I70.1
retina (vascular) I70.8 *[H35.0-]* ✓
specified artery NEC I70.8
spinal (cord) G95.19
vertebral (artery) I67.2
Arteriospasm I73.9
Arteriovenous — *see* condition
Arteritis I77.6
allergic M31.0
aorta (nonsyphilitic) I77.6
syphilitic A52.02
aortic arch M31.4
brachiocephalic M31.4
brain I67.7
syphilitic A52.04
cerebral I67.7
in systemic lupus erythematosus M32.19
listerial A32.89
syphilitic A52.04
tuberculous A18.89
coronary (artery) I25.89
rheumatic I01.8
chronic I09.89
syphilitic A52.06
cranial (left) (right), giant cell M31.6
deformans — *see* Arteriosclerosis
giant cell NEC M31.6
with polymyalgia rheumatica M31.5
necrosing or necrotizing M31.9

Arteritis — *continued*
necrosing or necrotizing — *continued*
specified NEC M31.8
nodosa M30.0
obliterans — *see* Arteriosclerosis
pulmonary I28.8
rheumatic — *see* Fever, rheumatic
senile — *see* Arteriosclerosis
suppurative I77.2
syphilitic (general) A52.09
brain A52.04
coronary A52.06
spinal A52.09
temporal, giant cell M31.6
young female aortic arch syndrome M31.4
Artery, arterial — *see also* condition
abscess I77.89
single umbilical Q27.0
Arthralgia (allergic) — *see also* Pain, joint
in caisson disease T70.3 ✓
temporomandibular M26.62- ✓
Arthritis, arthritic (acute) (chronic) (nonpyogenic) (subacute) M19.90
allergic — *see* Arthritis, specified form NEC
ankylosing (crippling) (spine) — *see also* Spondylitis, ankylosing
sites other than spine — *see* Arthritis, specified NEC
atrophic — *see* Osteoarthritis
spine — *see* Spondylitis, ankylosing
back — *see* Spondylopathy, inflammatory
blennorrhagic (gonococcal) A54.42
Charcot's — *see* Arthropathy, neuropathic
diabetic — *see* Diabetes, arthropathy, neuropathic
syringomyelic G95.0
chylous (filarial) — *see also* category M01 B74.9
climacteric (any site) NEC — *see* Arthritis, specified form NEC
crystal (-induced) — *see* Arthritis, in, crystals
deformans — *see* Osteoarthritis
degenerative — *see* Osteoarthritis
due to or associated with
acromegaly E22.0
brucellosis — *see* Brucellosis
caisson disease T70.3 ✓
diabetes — *see* Diabetes, arthropathy
dracontiasis — *see also* category M01 B72
enteritis NEC
regional — *see* Enteritis, regional
erysipelas — *see also* category M01 A46
erythema
epidemic A25.1
nodosum L52
filariasis NOS B74.9
glanders A24.0
helminthiasis — *see also* category M01 B83.9
hemophilia D66 *[M36.2]*
Henoch- (Schönlein) purpura D69.0 *[M36.4]*
human parvovirus — *see also* category M01 B97
infectious disease NEC M01 ✓
leprosy (see also category M01) — *see also* Leprosy A30.9
Lyme disease A69.23
mycobacteria — *see also* category M01 A31.8
parasitic disease NEC — *see also* category M01 B89
paratyphoid fever (see also category M01) — *see also* Fever, paratyphoid A01.4
rat bite fever — *see also* category M01 A25.1
regional enteritis — *see* Enteritis, regional
respiratory disorder NOS J98.9
serum sickness — *see also* Reaction, serum T80.69 ✓
syringomyelia G95.0
typhoid fever A01.04
epidemic erythema A25.1
febrile — *see* Fever, rheumatic
gonococcal A54.42
gouty (acute) — *see* Gout
in (due to)
acromegaly — *see also* subcategory M14.8- E22.0
amyloidosis — *see also* subcategory M14.8- E85.4
bacterial disease — *see also* subcategory M01 A49.9
Behçet's syndrome M35.2
caisson disease — *see also* subcategory M14.8- T70.3 ✓
coliform bacilli (Escherichia coli) — *see* Arthritis, in, pyogenic organism NEC

✓ Additional Character Required — Refer to the Tabular List for Character Selection ▽ Subterms under main terms may continue to next column or page

Arthritis, arthritic — *continued*
in — *continued*
  crystals M11.9
    dicalcium phosphate — *see* Arthritis, in, crystals, specified type NEC
    hydroxyapatite M11.0- ☑
    pyrophosphate — *see* Arthritis, in, crystals, specified type NEC
    specified type NEC M11.80
      ankle M11.87- ☑
      elbow M11.82- ☑
      foot joint M11.87- ☑
      hand joint M11.84- ☑
      hip M11.85- ☑
      knee M11.86- ☑
      multiple sites M11.8- ☑
      shoulder M11.81- ☑
      vertebrae M11.88
      wrist M11.83- ☑
  dermatoarthritis, lipoid E78.81
  dracontiasis (dracunculiasis) — *see also* category M01 B72
  endocrine disorder NEC — *see also* subcategory M14.8- E34.9
  enteritis, infectious NEC — *see also* category M01 A09
    specified organism NEC — *see also* category M01 A08.8
  erythema
    multiforme — *see also* subcategory M14.8- L51.9
    nodosum — *see also* subcategory M14.8- L52
  gout — *see* Gout
  helminthiasis NEC — *see also* category M01 B83.9
  hemochromatosis — *see also* subcategory M14.8- E83.118
  hemoglobinopathy NEC D58.2 *[M36.3]*
  hemophilia NEC D66 *[M36.2]*
  Hemophilus influenzae M00.8- ☑ *[B96.3]*
  Henoch (-Schönlein) purpura D69.0 *[M36.4]*
  hyperparathyroidism NEC — *see also* subcategory M14.8- E21.3
  hypersensitivity reaction NEC T78.49 ☑ *[M36.4]*
  hypogammaglobulinemia — *see also* subcategory M14.8- D80.1
  hypothyroidism NEC — *see also* subcategory M14.8- E03.9
  infection — *see* Arthritis, pyogenic or pyemic
    spine — *see* Spondylopathy, infective
  infectious disease NEC M01 ☑
  leprosy — *see also* category M01 A30.9
  leukemia NEC C95.9- ☑ *[M36.1]*
  lipoid dermatoarthritis E78.81
  Lyme disease A69.23
  Mediterranean fever, familial — *see also* subcategory M14.8- M04.1
  Meningococcus A39.83
  metabolic disorder NEC — *see also* subcategory M14.8- E88.9
  multiple myelomatosis C90.0- ☑ *[M36.1]*
  mumps B26.85
  mycosis NEC — *see also* category M01 B49
  myelomatosis (multiple) C90.0- ☑ *[M36.1]*
  neurological disorder NEC G98.0
  ochronosis — *see also* subcategory M14.8- E70.29
  O'nyong-nyong — *see also* category M01 A92.1
  parasitic disease NEC — *see also* category M01 B89
  paratyphoid fever — *see also* category M01 A01.4
  Pseudomonas — *see* Arthritis, pyogenic, bacterial NEC
  psoriasis L40.50
  pyogenic organism NEC — *see* Arthritis, pyogenic, bacterial NEC
  Reiter's disease — *see* Reiter's disease
  respiratory disorder NEC — *see also* subcategory M14.8- J98.9
  reticulosis, malignant — *see also* subcategory M14.8- C86.0
  rubella B06.82
  Salmonella (arizonae) (cholerae-suis) (enteritidis) (typhimurium) A02.23
  sarcoidosis D86.86
  specified bacteria NEC — *see* Arthritis, pyogenic, bacterial NEC
  sporotrichosis B42.82
  syringomyelia G95.0
  thalassemia NEC D56.9 *[M36.3]*
  tuberculosis — *see* Tuberculosis, arthritis

Arthritis, arthritic — *continued*
in — *continued*
  typhoid fever A01.04
  urethritis, Reiter's — *see* Reiter's disease
  viral disease NEC — *see also* category M01 B34.9
infectious or infective — *see also* Arthritis, pyogenic or pyemic
  spine — *see* Spondylopathy, infective
juvenile M08.90
  with systemic onset — *see* Still's disease
  ankle M08.97- ☑
  elbow M08.92- ☑
  foot joint M08.97- ☑
  hand joint M08.94- ☑
  hip M08.95- ☑
  knee M08.96- ☑
  multiple site M08.99
  pauciarticular M08.40
    ankle M08.47- ☑
    elbow M08.42- ☑
    foot joint M08.47- ☑
    hand joint M08.44- ☑
    hip M08.45- ☑
    knee M08.46- ☑
    shoulder M08.41- ☑
    vertebrae M08.48
    wrist M08.43- ☑
  psoriatic L40.54
  rheumatoid — *see* Arthritis, rheumatoid, juvenile
  shoulder M08.91- ☑
  specified type NEC M08.80
    ankle M08.87- ☑
    elbow M08.82- ☑
    foot joint M08.87- ☑
    hand joint M08.84- ☑
    hip M08.85- ☑
    knee M08.86- ☑
    multiple site M08.89
    shoulder M08.81- ☑
    specified joint NEC M08.88
    vertebrae M08.88
    wrist M08.83- ☑
  wrist M08.93- ☑
meaning osteoarthritis — *see* Osteoarthritis
meningococcal A39.83
menopausal (any site) NEC — *see* Arthritis, specified form NEC
mutilans (psoriatic) L40.52
mycotic NEC — *see also* category M01 B49
neuropathic (Charcot) — *see* Arthropathy, neuropathic
  diabetic — *see* Diabetes, arthropathy, neuropathic
  nonsyphilitic NEC G98.0
  syringomyelic G95.0
ochronotic — *see also* subcategory M14.8- E70.29
palindromic (any site) — *see* Rheumatism, palindromic
pneumococcal M00.10
  ankle M00.17- ☑
  elbow M00.12- ☑
  foot joint — *see* Arthritis, pneumococcal, ankle
  hand joint M00.14- ☑
  hip M00.15- ☑
  knee M00.16- ☑
  multiple site M00.19
  shoulder M00.11- ☑
  vertebra M00.18
  wrist M00.13- ☑
postdysenteric — *see* Arthropathy, postdysenteric
postmeningococcal A39.84
postrheumatic, chronic — *see* Arthropathy, postrheumatic, chronic
primary progressive — *see also* Arthritis, specified form NEC
  spine — *see* Spondylitis, ankylosing
psoriatic L40.50
purulent (any site except spine) — *see* Arthritis, pyogenic or pyemic
  spine — *see* Spondylopathy, infective
pyogenic or pyemic (any site except spine) M00.9
  bacterial NEC M00.80
    ankle M00.87- ☑
    elbow M00.82- ☑
    foot joint — *see* Arthritis, pyogenic, bacterial NEC, ankle
    hand joint M00.84- ☑
    hip M00.85- ☑
    knee M00.86- ☑
    multiple site M00.89

Arthritis, arthritic — *continued*
pyogenic or pyemic — *continued*
  bacterial — *continued*
    shoulder M00.81- ☑
    vertebra M00.88
    wrist M00.83- ☑
  pneumococcal — *see* Arthritis, pneumococcal
  spine — *see* Spondylopathy, infective
  staphylococcal — *see* Arthritis, staphylococcal
  streptococcal — *see* Arthritis, streptococcal NEC
    pneumococcal — *see* Arthritis, pneumococcal
reactive — *see* Reiter's disease
rheumatic — *see also* Arthritis, rheumatoid
  acute or subacute — *see* Fever, rheumatic
rheumatoid M06.9
  with
    carditis — *see* Rheumatoid, carditis
    endocarditis — *see* Rheumatoid, carditis
    heart involvement NEC — *see* Rheumatoid, carditis
    lung involvement — *see* Rheumatoid, lung
    myocarditis — *see* Rheumatoid, carditis
    myopathy — *see* Rheumatoid, myopathy
    pericarditis — *see* Rheumatoid, carditis
    polyneuropathy — *see* Rheumatoid, polyneuropathy
    rheumatoid factor — *see* Arthritis, rheumatoid, seropositive
    splenoadenomegaly and leukopenia — *see* Felty's syndrome
    vasculitis — *see* Rheumatoid, vasculitis
    visceral involvement NEC — *see* Rheumatoid, arthritis, with involvement of organs NEC
  juvenile (with or without rheumatoid factor) M08.00
    ankle M08.07- ☑
    elbow M08.02- ☑
    foot joint M08.07- ☑
    hand joint M08.04- ☑
    hip M08.05- ☑
    knee M08.06- ☑
    multiple site M08.09
    shoulder M08.01- ☑
    vertebra M08.08
    wrist M08.03- ☑
  seronegative M06.00
    ankle M06.07- ☑
    elbow M06.02- ☑
    foot joint M06.07- ☑
    hand joint M06.04- ☑
    hip M06.05- ☑
    knee M06.06- ☑
    multiple site M06.09
    shoulder M06.01- ☑
    vertebra M06.08
    wrist M06.03- ☑
  seropositive M05.9
    specified NEC M05.80
      ankle M05.87- ☑
      elbow M05.82- ☑
      foot joint M05.87- ☑
      hand joint M05.84- ☑
      hip M05.85- ☑
      knee M05.86- ☑
      multiple sites M05.89
      shoulder M05.81- ☑
      vertebra — *see* Spondylitis, ankylosing
      wrist M05.83- ☑
    without organ involvement M05.70
      ankle M05.77- ☑
      elbow M05.72- ☑
      foot joint M05.77- ☑
      hand joint M05.74- ☑
      hip M05.75- ☑
      knee M05.76- ☑
      multiple sites M05.79
      shoulder M05.71- ☑
      vertebra — *see* Spondylitis, ankylosing
      wrist M05.73- ☑
  specified type NEC M06.80
    ankle M06.87- ☑
    elbow M06.82- ☑
    foot joint M06.87- ☑
    hand joint M06.84- ☑
    hip M06.85- ☑
    knee M06.86- ☑
    multiple site M06.89

Arthritis, arthritic — *continued*
  rheumatoid — *continued*
    specified type — *continued*
      shoulder M06.81- ☑
      vertebra M06.88
      wrist M06.83- ☑
    spine — *see* Spondylitis, ankylosing
  rubella B06.82
  scorbutic — *see also* subcategory M14.8- E54
  senile or senescent — *see* Osteoarthritis
  septic (any site except spine) — *see* Arthritis, pyogenic or pyemic
    spine — *see* Spondylopathy, infective
  serum (nontherapeutic) (therapeutic) — *see* Arthropathy, postimmunization
  specified form NEC M13.80
    ankle M13.87- ☑
    elbow M13.82- ☑
    foot joint M13.87- ☑
    hand joint M13.84- ☑
    hip M13.85- ☑
    knee M13.86- ☑
    multiple site M13.89
    shoulder M13.81- ☑
    specified joint NEC M13.88
    wrist M13.83- ☑
  spine — *see also* Spondylopathy, inflammatory
    infectious or infective NEC — *see* Spondylopathy, infective
    Marie-Strümpell — *see* Spondylitis, ankylosing
    pyogenic — *see* Spondylopathy, infective
    rheumatoid — *see* Spondylitis, ankylosing
    traumatic (old) — *see* Spondylopathy, traumatic
    tuberculous A18.01
  staphylococcal M00.00
    ankle M00.07- ☑
    elbow M00.02- ☑
    foot joint — *see* Arthritis, staphylococcal, ankle
    hand joint M00.04- ☑
    hip M00.05- ☑
    knee M00.06- ☑
    multiple site M00.09
    shoulder M00.01- ☑
    vertebra M00.08
    wrist M00.03- ☑
  streptococcal NEC M00.20
    ankle M00.27- ☑
    elbow M00.22- ☑
    foot joint — *see* Arthritis, streptococcal, ankle
    hand joint M00.24- ☑
    hip M00.25- ☑
    knee M00.26- ☑
    multiple site M00.29
    shoulder M00.21- ☑
    vertebra M00.28
    wrist M00.23- ☑
  suppurative — *see* Arthritis, pyogenic or pyemic
  syphilitic (late) A52.16
    congenital A50.55 [M12.80]
  syphilitica deformans (Charcot) A52.16
  temporomandibular M26.69
  toxic of menopause (any site) — *see* Arthritis, specified form NEC
  transient — *see* Arthropathy, specified form NEC
  traumatic (chronic) — *see* Arthropathy, traumatic
  tuberculous A18.02
    spine A18.01
  uratic — *see* Gout
  urethritica (Reiter's) — *see* Reiter's disease
  vertebral — *see* Spondylopathy, inflammatory
  villous (any site) — *see* Arthropathy, specified form NEC
Arthrocele — *see* Effusion, joint
Arthrodesis status Z98.1
Arthrodynia — *see also* Pain, joint
Arthrodysplasia Q74.9
Arthrofibrosis, joint — *see* Ankylosis
Arthrogryposis (congenital) Q68.8
  multiplex congenita Q74.3
Arthrokatadysis M24.7
Arthropathy — *see also* Arthritis M12.9
  Charcot's — *see* Arthropathy, neuropathic
    diabetic — *see* Diabetes, arthropathy, neuropathic
    syringomyelic G95.0
  cricoarytenoid J38.7
  crystal (-induced) — *see* Arthritis, in, crystals
  diabetic NEC — *see* Diabetes, arthropathy

Arthropathy — *continued*
  distal interphalangeal, psoriatic L40.51
  enteropathic M07.60
    ankle M07.67- ☑
    elbow M07.62- ☑
    foot joint M07.67- ☑
    hand joint M07.64- ☑
    hip M07.65- ☑
    knee M07.66- ☑
    multiple site M07.69
    shoulder M07.61- ☑
    vertebra M07.68
    wrist M07.63- ☑
  following intestinal bypass M02.00
    ankle M02.07- ☑
    elbow M02.02- ☑
    foot joint M02.07- ☑
    hand joint M02.04- ☑
    hip M02.05- ☑
    knee M02.06- ☑
    multiple site M02.09
    shoulder M02.01- ☑
    vertebra M02.08
    wrist M02.03- ☑
  gouty — *see also* Gout
    in (due to)
      Lesch-Nyhan syndrome E79.1 [M14.8-] ☑
      sickle-cell disorders D57- ☑ [M14.8-] ☑
  hemophilic NEC D66 [M36.2]
    in (due to)
      hyperparathyroidism NEC E21.3 [M14.8-] ☑
      metabolic disease NOS E88.9 [M14.8-] ☑
  in (due to)
    acromegaly E22.0 [M14.8-] ☑
    amyloidosis E85.4 [M14.8-] ☑
    blood disorder NOS D75.9 [M36.3]
    diabetes — *see* Diabetes, arthropathy
    endocrine disease NOS E34.9 [M14.8-] ☑
    erythema
      multiforme L51.9 [M14.8-] ☑
      nodosum L52 [M14.8-] ☑
    hemochromatosis E83.118 [M14.8-] ☑
    hemoglobinopathy NEC D58.2 [M36.3]
    hemophilia NEC D66 [M36.2]
    Henoch-Schönlein purpura D69.0 [M36.4]
    hyperthyroidism E05.90 [M14.8-] ☑
    hypothyroidism E03.9 [M14.8-] ☑
    infective endocarditis I33.0 [M12.80]
    leukemia NEC C95.9- ☑ [M36.1]
    malignant histiocytosis C96.A [M36.1]
    metabolic disease NOS E88.9 [M14.8-] ☑
    multiple myeloma C90.0- ☑ [M36.1]
    neoplastic disease NOS (*see also* Neoplasm) D49.9 [M36.1]
    nutritional deficiency — *see also* subcategory M14.8- E63.9
    psoriasis NOS L40.50
    sarcoidosis D86.86
    syphilis (late) A52.77
      congenital A50.55 [M12.80]
    thyrotoxicosis — *see also* subcategory M14.8-E05.90
    ulcerative colitis K51.90 [M07.60]
    viral hepatitis (postinfectious) NEC B19.9 [M12.80]
    Whipple's disease — *see also* subcategory M14.8-K90.81
  Jaccoud — *see* Arthropathy, postrheumatic, chronic
  juvenile — *see* Arthritis, juvenile
    psoriatic L40.54
  mutilans (psoriatic) L40.52
  neuropathic (Charcot) M14.60
    ankle M14.67- ☑
    diabetic — *see* Diabetes, arthropathy, neuropathic
    elbow M14.62- ☑
    foot joint M14.67- ☑
    hand joint M14.64- ☑
    hip M14.65- ☑
    knee M14.66- ☑
    multiple site M14.69
    nonsyphilitic NEC G98.0
    shoulder M14.61- ☑
    syringomyelic G95.0
    vertebra M14.68
    wrist M14.63- ☑
  osteopulmonary — *see* Osteoarthropathy, hypertrophic, specified NEC

Arthropathy — *continued*
  postdysenteric M02.10
    ankle M02.17- ☑
    elbow M02.12- ☑
    foot joint M02.17- ☑
    hand joint M02.14- ☑
    hip M02.15- ☑
    knee M02.16- ☑
    multiple site M02.19
    shoulder M02.11- ☑
    vertebra M02.18
    wrist M02.13- ☑
  postimmunization M02.20
    ankle M02.27- ☑
    elbow M02.22- ☑
    foot joint M02.27- ☑
    hand joint M02.24- ☑
    hip M02.25- ☑
    knee M02.26- ☑
    multiple site M02.29
    shoulder M02.21- ☑
    vertebra M02.28
    wrist M02.23- ☑
  postinfectious NEC B99 ☑ [M12.80]
    in (due to)
      enteritis due to Yersinia enterocolitica A04.6 [M12.80]
      syphilis A52.77
      viral hepatitis NEC B19.9 [M12.80]
  postrheumatic, chronic (Jaccoud) M12.00
    ankle M12.07- ☑
    elbow M12.02- ☑
    foot joint M12.07- ☑
    hand joint M12.04- ☑
    hip M12.05- ☑
    knee M12.06- ☑
    multiple site M12.09
    shoulder M12.01- ☑
    specified joint NEC M12.08
    vertebrae M12.08
    wrist M12.03- ☑
  psoriatic NEC L40.59
    interphalangeal, distal L40.51
  reactive M02.9
    in (due to)
      infective endocarditis I33.0 [M02.9]
    specified type NEC M02.80
      ankle M02.87- ☑
      elbow M02.82- ☑
      foot joint M02.87- ☑
      hand joint M02.84- ☑
      hip M02.85- ☑
      knee M02.86- ☑
      multiple site M02.89
      shoulder M02.81- ☑
      vertebra M02.88
      wrist M02.83- ☑
  specified form NEC M12.80
    ankle M12.87- ☑
    elbow M12.82- ☑
    foot joint M12.87- ☑
    hand joint M12.84- ☑
    hip M12.85- ☑
    knee M12.86- ☑
    multiple site M12.89
    shoulder M12.81- ☑
    specified joint NEC M12.88
    vertebrae M12.88
    wrist M12.83- ☑
  syringomyelic G95.0
  tabes dorsalis A52.16
  tabetic A52.16
  transient — *see* Arthropathy, specified form NEC
  traumatic M12.50
    ankle M12.57- ☑
    elbow M12.52- ☑
    foot joint M12.57- ☑
    hand joint M12.54- ☑
    hip M12.55- ☑
    knee M12.56- ☑
    multiple site M12.59
    shoulder M12.51- ☑
    specified joint NEC M12.58
    vertebrae M12.58
    wrist M12.53- ☑
Arthropyosis — *see* Arthritis, pyogenic or pyemic

☑ **Additional Character Required** — Refer to the Tabular List for Character Selection   ▽ **Subterms under main terms may continue to next column or page**

Arthrosis (deformans) (degenerative) (localized) — see also Osteoarthritis M19.90
 spine — see Spondylosis
Arthus' phenomenon or reaction T78.41 ✓
 due to
 drug — see Table of Drugs and Chemicals, by drug
Articular — see condition
Articulation, reverse (teeth) M26.24
Artificial
 insemination complication — see Complications, artificial, fertilization
 opening status (functioning) (without complication) Z93.9
 anus (colostomy) Z93.3
 colostomy Z93.3
 cystostomy Z93.50
 appendico-vesicostomy Z93.52
 cutaneous Z93.51
 specified NEC Z93.59
 enterostomy Z93.4
 gastrostomy Z93.1
 ileostomy Z93.2
 intestinal tract NEC Z93.4
 jejunostomy Z93.4
 nephrostomy Z93.6
 specified site NEC Z93.8
 tracheostomy Z93.0
 ureterostomy Z93.6
 urethrostomy Z93.6
 urinary tract NEC Z93.6
 vagina Z93.8
 vagina status Z93.8
Arytenoid — see condition
Asbestosis (occupational) J61
Ascariasis B77.9
 with
 complications NEC B77.89
 intestinal complications B77.0
 pneumonia, pneumonitis B77.81
Ascaridosis, ascaridiasis — see Ascariasis
Ascaris (infection) (infestation) (lumbricoides) — see Ascariasis
Ascending — see condition
ASC-H (atypical squamous cells cannot exclude high grade squamous intraepithelial lesion on cytologic smear)
 anus R85.611
 cervix R87.611
 vagina R87.621
Aschoff's bodies — see Myocarditis, rheumatic
Ascites (abdominal) R18.8
 cardiac — see also Failure, heart, right I50.810
 chylous (nonfilarial) I89.8
 filarial — see Infestation, filarial
 due to
 cirrhosis, alcoholic K70.31
 hepatitis
 alcoholic K70.11
 chronic active K71.51
 S. japonicum B65.2
 heart — see also Failure, heart, right I50.810
 malignant R18.0
 pseudochylous R18.8
 syphilitic A52.74
 tuberculous A18.31
ASC-US (atypical squamous cells of undetermined significance on cytologic smear)
 anus R85.610
 cervix R87.610
 vagina R87.620
Aseptic — see condition
Asherman's syndrome N85.6
Asialia K11.7
Asiatic cholera — see Cholera
Asimultagnosia (simultanagnosia) R48.3
Askin's tumor — see Neoplasm, connective tissue, malignant
Asocial personality F60.2
Asomatognosia R41.4
Aspartylglucosaminuria E77.1
Asperger's disease or syndrome F84.5
Aspergilloma — see Aspergillosis
Aspergillosis (with pneumonia) B44.9
 bronchopulmonary, allergic B44.81
 disseminated B44.7
 generalized B44.7
 pulmonary NEC B44.1
 allergic B44.81
 invasive B44.0

Aspergillosis — continued
 specified NEC B44.89
 tonsillar B44.2
Aspergillus (flavus) (fumigatus) (infection) (terreus) — see Aspergillosis
Aspermatogenesis — see Azoospermia
Aspermia (testis) — see Azoospermia
Asphyxia, asphyxiation (by) R09.01
 antenatal P84
 birth P84
 bunny bag — see Asphyxia, due to, mechanical threat to breathing, trapped in bed clothes
 crushing S28.0 ✓
 drowning T75.1 ✓
 gas, fumes, or vapor — see Table of Drugs and Chemicals
 inhalation — see Inhalation
 intrauterine P84
 local I73.00
 with gangrene I73.01
 mucus — see also Foreign body, respiratory tract, causing asphyxia
 newborn P84
 pathological R09.01
 postnatal P84
 mechanical — see Asphyxia, due to, mechanical threat to breathing
 prenatal P84
 reticularis R23.1
 strangulation — see Asphyxia, due to, mechanical threat to breathing
 submersion T75.1 ✓
 traumatic T71.9 ✓
 due to
 crushed chest S28.0 ✓
 foreign body (in) — see Foreign body, respiratory tract, causing asphyxia
 low oxygen content of ambient air T71.20 ✓
 due to
 being trapped in
 low oxygen environment T71.29 ✓
 in car trunk T71.221 ✓
 circumstances undetermined T71.224 ✓
 done with intent to harm by
 another person T71.223 ✓
 self T71.222 ✓
 in refrigerator T71.231 ✓
 circumstances undetermined T71.234 ✓
 done with intent to harm by
 another person T71.233 ✓
 self T71.232 ✓
 cave-in T71.21 ✓
 mechanical threat to breathing (accidental) T71.191 ✓
 circumstances undetermined T71.194 ✓
 done with intent to harm by
 another person T71.193 ✓
 self T71.192 ✓
 hanging T71.161 ✓
 circumstances undetermined T71.164 ✓
 done with intent to harm by
 another person T71.163 ✓
 self T71.162 ✓
 plastic bag T71.121 ✓
 circumstances undetermined T71.124 ✓
 done with intent to harm by
 another person T71.123 ✓
 self T71.122 ✓
 smothering
 in furniture T71.151 ✓
 circumstances undetermined T71.154 ✓
 done with intent to harm by
 another person T71.153 ✓
 self T71.152 ✓
 under
 another person's body T71.141 ✓
 circumstances undetermined T71.144 ✓
 done with intent to harm T71.143 ✓
 pillow T71.111 ✓
 circumstances undetermined T71.114 ✓
 done with intent to harm by
 another person T71.113 ✓

Asphyxia, asphyxiation — continued
 traumatic — continued
 due to — continued
 mechanical threat to breathing — continued
 smothering — continued
 under — continued
 pillow — continued
 done with intent to harm by — continued
 self T71.112 ✓
 trapped in bed clothes T71.131 ✓
 circumstances undetermined T71.134 ✓
 done with intent to harm by
 another person T71.133 ✓
 self T71.132 ✓
 vomiting, vomitus — see Foreign body, respiratory tract, causing asphyxia
Aspiration
 amniotic (clear) fluid (newborn) P24.10
 with
 pneumonia (pneumonitis) P24.11
 respiratory symptoms P24.11
 blood
 newborn (without respiratory symptoms) P24.20
 with
 pneumonia (pneumonitis) P24.21
 respiratory symptoms P24.21
 specified age NEC — see Foreign body, respiratory tract
 bronchitis J69.0
 food or foreign body (with asphyxiation) — see Asphyxia, food
 liquor (amnii) (newborn) P24.10
 with
 pneumonia (pneumonitis) P24.11
 respiratory symptoms P24.11
 meconium (newborn) (without respiratory symptoms) P24.00
 with
 pneumonitis (pneumonitis) P24.01
 respiratory symptoms P24.01
 milk (newborn) (without respiratory symptoms) P24.30
 with
 pneumonia (pneumonitis) P24.31
 respiratory symptoms P24.31
 specified age NEC — see Foreign body, respiratory tract
 mucus — see also Foreign body, by site, causing asphyxia
 newborn P24.10
 with
 pneumonia (pneumonitis) P24.11
 respiratory symptoms P24.11
 neonatal P24.9
 specific NEC (without respiratory symptoms) P24.80
 with
 pneumonia (pneumonitis) P24.81
 respiratory symptoms P24.81
 newborn P24.9
 specific NEC (without respiratory symptoms) P24.80
 with
 pneumonia (pneumonitis) P24.81
 respiratory symptoms P24.81
 pneumonia J69.0
 pneumonitis J69.0
 syndrome of newborn — see Aspiration, by substance, with pneumonia
 vernix caseosa (newborn) P24.80
 with
 pneumonia (pneumonitis) P24.81
 respiratory symptoms P24.81
 vomitus — see also Foreign body, respiratory tract
 newborn (without respiratory symptoms) P24.30
 with
 pneumonia (pneumonitis) P24.31
 respiratory symptoms P24.31
Asplenia (congenital) Q89.01
 postsurgical Z90.81
Assam fever B55.0
Assault, sexual — see Maltreatment
Assmann's focus NEC A15.0
Astasia (-abasia) (hysterical) F44.4
Asteatosis cutis L85.3
Astereognosia, astereognosis R48.1
Asterixis R27.8
 in liver disease K71.3
Asteroid hyalitis — see Deposit, crystalline
Asthenia, asthenic R53.1

◄ Subterms under main terms may continue to next column or page   ✓ Additional Character Required — Refer to the Tabular List for Character Selection   31

Arthrosis — Asthenia, asthenic

Asthenia, asthenic — *continued*
  cardiac — *see also* Failure, heart I50.9
    psychogenic F45.8
  cardiovascular — *see also* Failure, heart I50.9
    psychogenic F45.8
  heart — *see also* Failure, heart I50.9
    psychogenic F45.8
  hysterical F44.4
  myocardial — *see also* Failure, heart I50.9
    psychogenic F45.8
  nervous F48.8
  neurocirculatory F45.8
  neurotic F48.8
  psychogenic F48.8
  psychoneurotic F48.8
  psychophysiologic F48.8
  reaction (psychophysiologic) F48.8
  senile R54
Asthenopia — *see also* Discomfort, visual
  hysterical F44.6
  psychogenic F44.6
Asthenospermia — *see* Abnormal, specimen, male
  genital organs
Asthma, asthmatic (bronchial) (catarrh) (spasmodic)
  J45.909
  with
    chronic obstructive bronchitis J44.9
      with
        acute lower respiratory infection J44.0
        exacerbation (acute) J44.1
    chronic obstructive pulmonary disease J44.9
      with
        acute lower respiratory infection J44.0
        exacerbation (acute) J44.1
    exacerbation (acute) J45.901
    hay fever — *see* Asthma, allergic extrinsic
    rhinitis, allergic — *see* Asthma, allergic extrinsic
    status asthmaticus J45.902
  allergic extrinsic J45.909
    with
      exacerbation (acute) J45.901
      status asthmaticus J45.902
  atopic — *see* Asthma, allergic extrinsic
  cardiac — *see* Failure, ventricular, left
  cardiobronchial I50.1
  childhood J45.909
    with
      exacerbation (acute) J45.901
      status asthmaticus J45.902
  chronic obstructive J44.9
    with
      acute lower respiratory infection J44.0
      exacerbation (acute) J44.1
  collier's J60
  cough variant J45.991
  detergent J69.8
  due to
    detergent J69.8
    inhalation of fumes J68.3
  eosinophilic J82
  extrinsic, allergic — *see* Asthma, allergic extrinsic
  grinder's J62.8
  hay — *see* Asthma, allergic extrinsic
  heart I50.1
  idiosyncratic — *see* Asthma, nonallergic
  intermittent (mild) J45.20
    with
      exacerbation (acute) J45.21
      status asthmaticus J45.22
  intrinsic, nonallergic — *see* Asthma, nonallergic
  Kopp's E32.8
  late-onset J45.909
    with
      exacerbation (acute) J45.901
      status asthmaticus J45.902
  mild intermittent J45.20
    with
      exacerbation (acute) J45.21
      status asthmaticus J45.22
  mild persistent J45.30
    with
      exacerbation (acute) J45.31
      status asthmaticus J45.32
  Millar's (laryngismus stridulus) J38.5
  miner's J60
  mixed J45.909
    with
      exacerbation (acute) J45.901

Asthma, asthmatic — *continued*
  mixed — *continued*
    with — *continued*
      status asthmaticus J45.902
  moderate persistent J45.40
    with
      exacerbation (acute) J45.41
      status asthmaticus J45.42
  nervous — *see* Asthma, nonallergic
  nonallergic (intrinsic) J45.909
    with
      exacerbation (acute) J45.901
      status asthmaticus J45.902
  persistent
    mild J45.30
      with
        exacerbation (acute) J45.31
        status asthmaticus J45.32
    moderate J45.40
      with
        exacerbation (acute) J45.41
        status asthmaticus J45.42
    severe J45.50
      with
        exacerbation (acute) J45.51
        status asthmaticus J45.52
  platinum J45.998
  pneumoconiotic NEC J64
  potter's J62.8
  predominantly allergic J45.909
  psychogenic F54
  pulmonary eosinophilic J82
  red cedar J67.8
  Rostan's I50.1
  sandblaster's J62.8
  sequoiosis J67.8
  severe persistent J45.50
    with
      exacerbation (acute) J45.51
      status asthmaticus J45.52
  specified NEC J45.998
  stonemason's J62.8
  thymic E32.8
  tuberculous — *see* Tuberculosis, pulmonary
  Wichmann's (laryngismus stridulus) J38.5
  wood J67.8
Astigmatism (compound) (congenital) H52.20- ☑
  irregular H52.21- ☑
  regular H52.22- ☑
Astraphobia F40.220
Astroblastoma
  specified site — *see* Neoplasm, malignant, by site
  unspecified site C71.9
Astrocytoma (cystic)
  anaplastic
    specified site — *see* Neoplasm, malignant, by site
    unspecified site C71.9
  fibrillary
    specified site — *see* Neoplasm, malignant, by site
    unspecified site C71.9
  fibrous
    specified site — *see* Neoplasm, malignant, by site
    unspecified site C71.9
  gemistocytic
    specified site — *see* Neoplasm, malignant, by site
    unspecified site C71.9
  juvenile
    specified site — *see* Neoplasm, malignant, by site
    unspecified site C71.9
  pilocytic
    specified site — *see* Neoplasm, malignant, by site
    unspecified site C71.9
  piloid
    specified site — *see* Neoplasm, malignant, by site
    unspecified site C71.9
  protoplasmic
    specified site — *see* Neoplasm, malignant, by site
    unspecified site C71.9
  specified site NEC — *see* Neoplasm, malignant, by site
  subependymal D43.2
    giant cell
      specified site — *see* Neoplasm, uncertain behavior, by site
      unspecified site D43.2
    specified site — *see* Neoplasm, uncertain behavior, by site
    unspecified site D43.2
  unspecified site C71.9

Astroglioma
  specified site — *see* Neoplasm, malignant, by site
  unspecified site C71.9
Asymbolia R48.8
Asymmetry — *see also* Distortion
  between native and reconstructed breast N65.1
  face Q67.0
  jaw (lower) — *see* Anomaly, dentofacial, jaw-cranial
    base relationship, asymmetry
Asynergia, asynergy R27.8
  ventricular I51.89
Asystole (heart) — *see* Arrest, cardiac
At risk
  for
    dental caries Z91.849
      high Z91.843
      low Z91.841
      moderate Z91.842
    falling Z91.81
Ataxia, ataxy, ataxic R27.0
  acute R27.8
  brain (hereditary) G11.9
  cerebellar (hereditary) G11.9
    with defective DNA repair G11.3
    alcoholic G31.2
    early-onset G11.1
    in
      alcoholism G31.2
      myxedema E03.9 *[G13.2]*
      neoplastic disease — *see also* Neoplasm
        D49.9 *[G32.81]*
      specified disease NEC G32.81
    late-onset (Marie's) G11.2
  cerebral (hereditary) G11.9
  congenital nonprogressive G11.0
  family, familial — *see* Ataxia, hereditary
  following
    cerebrovascular disease I69.993
      cerebral infarction I69.393
      intracerebral hemorrhage I69.193
      nontraumatic intracranial hemorrhage NEC
        I69.293
      specified disease NEC I69.893
      subarachnoid hemorrhage I69.093
  Friedreich's (heredofamilial) (cerebellar) (spinal) G11.1
  gait R26.0
    hysterical F44.4
  general R27.8
  gluten M35.9 *[G32.81]*
    with celiac disease K90.0 *[G32.81]*
  hereditary G11.9
    with neuropathy G60.2
    cerebellar — *see* Ataxia, cerebellar
    spastic G11.4
    specified NEC G11.8
    spinal (Friedreich's) G11.1
  heredofamilial — *see* Ataxia, hereditary
  Hunt's G11.1
  hysterical F44.4
  locomotor (progressive) (syphilitic) (partial) (spastic)
    A52.11
  diabetic — *see* Diabetes, ataxia
  Marie's (cerebellar) (heredofamilial) (late-onset) G11.2
  nonorganic origin F44.4
  nonprogressive, congenital G11.0
  psychogenic F44.4
  Roussy-Lévy G60.0
  Sanger-Brown's (hereditary) G11.2
  spastic hereditary G11.4
  spinal
    hereditary (Friedreich's) G11.1
    progressive (syphilitic) A52.11
  spinocerebellar, X-linked recessive G11.1
  telangiectasia (Louis-Bar) G11.3
Ataxia-telangiectasia (Louis-Bar) G11.3
Atelectasis (massive) (partial) (pressure) (pulmonary)
  J98.11
  newborn P28.10
    due to resorption P28.11
    partial P28.19
    primary P28.0
    secondary P28.19
  primary (newborn) P28.0
  tuberculous — *see* Tuberculosis, pulmonary
Atelocardia Q24.9
Atelomyelia Q06.1

☑ **Additional Character Required** — **Refer to the Tabular List for Character Selection**   ▽ Subterms under main terms may continue to next column or pa[ge]

Atheroembolism

of
    extremities
        lower I75.02- ☑
        upper I75.01- ☑
    kidney I75.81
    specified NEC I75.89

Atheroma, atheromatous — *see also* Arteriosclerosis I70.90
    aorta, aortic I70.0
        valve — *see also* Endocarditis, aortic I35.8
    aorto-iliac I70.0
    artery — *see* Arteriosclerosis
    basilar (artery) I67.2
    carotid (artery) (common) (internal) I67.2
    cerebral (arteries) I67.2
    coronary (artery) I25.10
        with angina pectoris — *see* Arteriosclerosis, coronary (artery),
    degeneration — *see* Arteriosclerosis
    heart, cardiac — *see* Disease, heart, ischemic, atherosclerotic
    mitral (valve) I34.8
    myocardium, myocardial — *see* Disease, heart, ischemic, atherosclerotic
    pulmonary valve (heart) — *see also* Endocarditis, pulmonary I37.8
    tricuspid (heart) (valve) I36.8
    valve, valvular — *see* Endocarditis
    vertebral (artery) I67.2

Atheromatosis — *see* Arteriosclerosis

Atherosclerosis — *see also* Arteriosclerosis
    coronary
        artery I25.10
            with angina pectoris — *see* Arteriosclerosis, coronary (artery),
            due to
                calcified coronary lesion (severely) I25.84
                lipid rich plaque I25.83
        transplanted heart I25.811
            bypass graft I25.812
                with angina pectoris — *see* Arteriosclerosis, coronary (artery),
            native coronary artery I25.811
                with angina pectoris — *see* Arteriosclerosis, coronary (artery),

Athetosis (acquired) R25.8
    bilateral (congenital) G80.3
    congenital (bilateral) (double) G80.3
    double (congenital) G80.3
    unilateral R25.8

Athlete's
    foot B35.3
    heart I51.7

Athrepsia E41

Athyrea (acquired) — *see also* Hypothyroidism
    congenital E03.1

Atonia, atony, atonic
    bladder (sphincter) (neurogenic) N31.2
    capillary I78.8
    cecum K59.8
        psychogenic F45.8
    colon — *see* Atony, intestine
    congenital P94.2
    esophagus K22.8
    intestine K59.8
        psychogenic F45.8
    stomach K31.89
        neurotic or psychogenic F45.8
    uterus (during labor) O62.2
        with hemorrhage (postpartum) O72.1
        postpartum (with hemorrhage) O72.1
            without hemorrhage O75.89

Atopy — *see* History, allergy

Atransferrinemia, congenital E88.09

Atresia, atretic
    alimentary organ or tract NEC Q45.8
        upper Q40.8
    ani, anus, anal (canal) Q42.3
        with fistula Q42.2
    aorta (ring) Q25.29
    aortic (orifice) (valve) Q23.0
        arch Q25.21
        congenital with hypoplasia of ascending aorta and defective development of left ventricle (with mitral stenosis) Q23.4
        in hypoplastic left heart syndrome Q23.4
    aqueduct of Sylvius Q03.0

Atresia, atretic — *continued*
    aqueduct of Sylvius — *continued*
        with spina bifida — *see* Spina bifida, with hydrocephalus
    artery NEC Q27.8
        cerebral Q28.3
        coronary Q24.5
        digestive system Q27.8
        eye Q15.8
        lower limb Q27.8
        pulmonary Q25.5
        specified site NEC Q27.8
        umbilical Q27.0
        upper limb Q27.8
    auditory canal (external) Q16.1
    bile duct (common) (congenital) (hepatic) Q44.2
        acquired — *see* Obstruction, bile duct
    bladder (neck) Q64.39
        obstruction Q64.31
    bronchus Q32.4
    cecum Q42.8
    cervix (acquired) N88.2
        congenital Q51.828
        in pregnancy or childbirth — *see* Anomaly, cervix, in pregnancy or childbirth
            causing obstructed labor O65.5
    choana Q30.0
    colon Q42.9
        specified NEC Q42.8
    common duct Q44.2
    cricoid cartilage Q31.8
    cystic duct Q44.2
        acquired K82.8
            with obstruction K82.0
    digestive organs NEC Q45.8
    duodenum Q41.0
    ear canal Q16.1
    ejaculatory duct Q55.4
    epiglottis Q31.8
    esophagus Q39.0
        with tracheoesophageal fistula Q39.1
    eustachian tube Q17.8
    fallopian tube (congenital) Q50.6
        acquired N97.1
    follicular cyst N83.0- ☑
    foramen of
        Luschka Q03.1
            with spina bifida — *see* Spina bifida, with hydrocephalus
        Magendie Q03.1
            with spina bifida — *see* Spina bifida, with hydrocephalus
    gallbladder Q44.1
    genital organ
        external
            female Q52.79
            male Q55.8
        internal
            female Q52.8
            male Q55.8
    glottis Q31.8
    gullet Q39.0
        with tracheoesophageal fistula Q39.1
    heart valve NEC Q24.8
        pulmonary Q22.0
        tricuspid Q22.4
    hymen Q52.3
        acquired (postinfective) N89.6
    ileum Q41.2
    intestine (small) Q41.9
        large Q42.9
            specified NEC Q42.8
    iris, filtration angle Q15.0
    jejunum Q41.1
    lacrimal apparatus Q10.4
    larynx Q31.8
    meatus urinarius Q64.33
    mitral valve Q23.2
        in hypoplastic left heart syndrome Q23.4
    nares (anterior) (posterior) Q30.0
    nasopharynx Q34.8
    nose, nostril Q30.0
        acquired J34.89
    organ or site NEC Q89.8
    osseous meatus (ear) Q16.1
    oviduct (congenital) Q50.6
        acquired N97.1
    parotid duct Q38.4
        acquired K11.8

Atresia, atretic — *continued*
    pulmonary (artery) Q25.5
        valve Q22.0
    pulmonic Q22.0
    pupil Q13.2
    rectum Q42.1
        with fistula Q42.0
    salivary duct Q38.4
        acquired K11.8
    sublingual duct Q38.4
        acquired K11.8
    submandibular duct Q38.4
        acquired K11.8
    submaxillary duct Q38.4
        acquired K11.8
    thyroid cartilage Q31.8
    trachea Q32.1
    tricuspid valve Q22.4
    ureter Q62.10
        pelvic junction Q62.11
        vesical orifice Q62.12
    ureteropelvic junction Q62.11
    ureterovesical orifice Q62.12
    urethra (valvular) Q64.39
        stricture Q64.32
    urinary tract NEC Q64.8
    uterus Q51.818
        acquired N85.8
    vagina (congenital) Q52.4
        acquired (postinfectional) (senile) N89.5
    vas deferens Q55.3
    vascular NEC Q27.8
        cerebral Q28.3
        digestive system Q27.8
        lower limb Q27.8
        specified site NEC Q27.8
        upper limb Q27.8
    vein NEC Q27.8
        digestive system Q27.8
        great Q26.8
        lower limb Q27.8
        portal Q26.5
        pulmonary Q26.4
            partial Q26.3
            total Q26.2
        specified site NEC Q27.8
        upper limb Q27.8
    vena cava (inferior) (superior) Q26.8
    vesicourethral orifice Q64.31
    vulva Q52.79
        acquired N90.5

Atrichia, atrichosis — *see* Alopecia

Atrophia — *see also* Atrophy
    cutis senilis L90.8
        due to radiation L57.8
    gyrata of choroid and retina H31.23
    senilis R54
        dermatological L90.8
            due to radiation (nonionizing) (solar) L57.8
    unguium L60.3
        congenita Q84.6

Atrophie blanche (en plaque) (de Milian) L95.0

Atrophoderma, atrophodermia (of) L90.9
    diffusum (idiopathic) L90.4
    maculatum L90.8
        et striatum L90.8
            due to syphilis A52.79
        syphilitic A51.39
    neuriticum L90.8
    Pasini and Pierini L90.3
    pigmentosum Q82.1
    reticulatum symmetricum faciei L66.4
    senile L90.8
        due to radiation (nonionizing) (solar) L57.8
    vermiculata (cheeks) L66.4

Atrophy, atrophic (of)
    adrenal (capsule) (gland) E27.49
        primary (autoimmune) E27.1
    alveolar process or ridge (edentulous) K08.20
    anal sphincter (disuse) N81.84
    appendix K38.8
    arteriosclerotic — *see* Arteriosclerosis
    bile duct (common) (hepatic) K83.8
    bladder N32.89
        neurogenic N31.8
    blanche (en plaque) (of Milian) L95.0
    bone (senile) NEC — *see also* Disorder, bone, specified type NEC

⬑ Subterms under main terms may continue to next column or page   ☑ Additional Character Required — Refer to the Tabular List for Character Selection   33

Atheroembolism — Atrophy, atrophic

Atrophy, atrophic — *continued*
- bone — *see also* Disorder, bone, specified type — *continued*
  - due to
    - tabes dorsalis (neurogenic) A52.11
- brain (cortex) (progressive) G31.9
  - frontotemporal circumscribed G31.01 *[F02.80]*
    - with behavioral disturbance G31.01 *[F02.81]*
  - senile NEC G31.1
- breast N64.2
  - obstetric — *see* Disorder, breast, specified type NEC
- buccal cavity K13.79
- cardiac — *see* Degeneration, myocardial
- cartilage (infectional) (joint) — *see* Disorder, cartilage, specified NEC
- cerebellar — *see* Atrophy, brain
- cerebral — *see* Atrophy, brain
- cervix (mucosa) (senile) (uteri) N88.8
  - menopausal N95.8
- Charcot-Marie-Tooth G60.0
- choroid (central) (macular) (myopic) (retina) H31.10- ☑
  - diffuse secondary H31.12- ☑
  - gyrate H31.23
  - senile H31.11- ☑
- ciliary body — *see* Atrophy, iris
- conjunctiva (senile) H11.89
- corpus cavernosum N48.89
- cortical — *see* Atrophy, brain
- cystic duct K82.8
- Déjérine-Thomas G23.8
- disuse NEC — *see* Atrophy, muscle
- Duchenne-Aran G12.21
- ear H93.8- ☑
- edentulous alveolar ridge K08.20
- endometrium (senile) N85.8
  - cervix N88.8
- enteric K63.89
- epididymis N50.89
- eyeball — *see* Disorder, globe, degenerated condition, atrophy
- eyelid (senile) — *see* Disorder, eyelid, degenerative
- facial (skin) L90.9
- fallopian tube (senile) N83.32- ☑
  - with ovary N83.33- ☑
- fascioscapulohumeral (Landouzy- Déjérine) G71.02
- fatty, thymus (gland) E32.8
- gallbladder K82.8
- gastric K29.40
  - with bleeding K29.41
- gastrointestinal K63.89
- glandular I89.8
- globe H44.52- ☑
- gum — *see* Recession, gingival
- hair L67.8
- heart (brown) — *see* Degeneration, myocardial
- hemifacial Q67.4
  - Romberg G51.8
- infantile E41
  - paralysis, acute — *see* Poliomyelitis, paralytic
- intestine K63.89
- iris (essential) (progressive) H21.26- ☑
  - specified NEC H21.29
- kidney (senile) (terminal) — *see also* Sclerosis, renal N26.1
  - congenital or infantile Q60.5
    - bilateral Q60.4
    - unilateral Q60.3
  - hydronephrotic — *see* Hydronephrosis
- lacrimal gland (primary) H04.14- ☑
  - secondary H04.15- ☑
- Landouzy-Déjérine G71.02
- laryngitis, infective J37.0
- larynx J38.7
- Leber's optic (hereditary) H47.22
- lip K13.0
- liver (yellow) K72.90
  - with coma K72.91
  - acute, subacute K72.00
    - with coma K72.01
  - chronic K72.10
    - with coma K72.11
- lung (senile) J98.4
- macular (dermatological) L90.8
  - syphilitic, skin A51.39
    - striated A52.79
- mandible (edentulous) K08.20
  - minimal K08.21
  - moderate K08.22

Atrophy, atrophic — *continued*
- mandible — *continued*
  - severe K08.23
- maxilla K08.20
  - minimal K08.24
  - moderate K08.25
  - severe K08.26
- muscle, muscular (diffuse) (general) (idiopathic) (primary) M62.50
  - ankle M62.57- ☑
  - Duchenne-Aran G12.21
  - foot M62.57- ☑
  - forearm M62.53- ☑
  - hand M62.54- ☑
  - infantile spinal G12.0
  - lower leg M62.56- ☑
  - multiple sites M62.59
  - myelopathic — *see* Atrophy, muscle, spinal
  - myotonic G71.11
  - neuritic G58.9
  - neuropathic (peroneal) (progressive) G60.0
  - pelvic (disuse) N81.84
  - peroneal G60.0
  - progressive (bulbar) G12.21
    - adult G12.1
    - infantile (spinal) G12.0
    - spinal G12.25
      - adult G12.1
      - infantile G12.0
  - pseudohypertrophic G71.02
  - shoulder region M62.51- ☑
  - specified site NEC M62.58
  - spinal G12.9
    - adult form G12.1
    - Aran-Duchenne G12.21
    - childhood form, type II G12.1
    - distal G12.1
    - hereditary NEC G12.1
    - infantile, type I (Werdnig-Hoffmann) G12.0
    - juvenile form, type III (Kugelberg- Welander) G12.1
    - progressive G12.25
    - scapuloperoneal form G12.1
    - specified NEC G12.8
  - syphilitic A52.78
  - thigh M62.55- ☑
  - upper arm M62.52- ☑
- myocardium — *see* Degeneration, myocardial
- myometrium (senile) N85.8
  - cervix N88.8
- myopathic NEC — *see* Atrophy, muscle
- myotonia G71.11
- nail L60.3
- nasopharynx J31.1
- nerve — *see also* Disorder, nerve
  - abducens — *see* Strabismus, paralytic, sixth nerve
  - accessory G52.8
  - acoustic or auditory H93.3 ☑
  - cranial G52.9
    - eighth (auditory) H93.3 ☑
    - eleventh (accessory) G52.8
    - fifth (trigeminal) G50.8
    - first (olfactory) G52.0
    - fourth (trochlear) — *see* Strabismus, paralytic, fourth nerve
    - second (optic) H47.20
    - sixth (abducens) — *see* Strabismus, paralytic, sixth nerve
    - tenth (pneumogastric) (vagus) G52.2
    - third (oculomotor) — *see* Strabismus, paralytic, third nerve
    - twelfth (hypoglossal) G52.3
  - hypoglossal G52.3
  - oculomotor — *see* Strabismus, paralytic, third nerve
  - olfactory G52.0
  - optic (papillomacular bundle)
    - syphilitic (late) A52.15
      - congenital A50.44
  - pneumogastric G52.2
  - trigeminal G50.8
  - trochlear — *see* Strabismus, paralytic, fourth nerve
  - vagus (pneumogastric) G52.2
- neurogenic, bone, tabetic A52.11
- nutritional E41
- old age R54
- olivopontocerebellar G23.8
- optic (nerve) H47.20
  - glaucomatous H47.23- ☑

Atrophy, atrophic — *continued*
- optic — *continued*
  - hereditary H47.22
  - primary H47.21- ☑
  - specified type NEC H47.29- ☑
  - syphilitic (late) A52.15
    - congenital A50.44
- orbit H05.31- ☑
- ovary (senile) N83.31- ☑
  - with fallopian tube N83.33- ☑
- oviduct (senile) — *see* Atrophy, fallopian tube
- palsy, diffuse (progressive) G12.22
- pancreas (duct) (senile) K86.89
- parotid gland K11.0
- pelvic muscle N81.84
- penis N48.89
- pharynx J39.2
- pluriglandular E31.8
  - autoimmune E31.0
- polyarthritis M15.9
- prostate N42.89
- pseudohypertrophic (muscle) G71.02
- renal — *see also* Sclerosis, renal N26.1
- retina, retinal (postinfectional) H35.89
- rhinitis J31.0
- salivary gland K11.0
- scar L90.5
- sclerosis, lobar (of brain) G31.09 *[F02.80]*
  - with behavioral disturbance G31.09 *[F02.81]*
- scrotum N50.89
- seminal vesicle N50.89
- senile R54
  - due to radiation (nonionizing) (solar) L57.8
- skin (patches) (spots) L90.9
  - degenerative (senile) L90.8
  - due to radiation (nonionizing) (solar) L57.8
  - senile L90.8
- spermatic cord N50.89
- spinal (acute) (cord) G95.89
  - muscular — *see* Atrophy, muscle, spinal
  - paralysis G12.20
    - acute — *see* Poliomyelitis, paralytic
    - meaning progressive muscular atrophy G12.25
- spine (column) — *see* Spondylopathy, specified NEC
- spleen (senile) D73.0
- stomach K29.40
  - with bleeding K29.41
- striate (skin) L90.6
  - syphilitic A52.79
- subcutaneous L90.9
- sublingual gland K11.0
- submandibular gland K11.0
- submaxillary gland K11.0
- Sudeck's — *see* Algoneurodystrophy
- suprarenal (capsule) (gland) E27.49
  - primary E27.1
- systemic affecting central nervous system in
  - myxedema E03.9 *[G13.2]*
  - neoplastic disease — *see also* Neoplasm D49.9 *[G13.1]*
  - specified disease NEC G13.8
- tarso-orbital fascia, congenital Q10.3
- testis N50.0
- thenar, partial — *see* Syndrome, carpal tunnel
- thymus (fatty) E32.8
- thyroid (gland) (acquired) E03.4
  - with cretinism E03.1
  - congenital (with myxedema) E03.1
- tongue (senile) K14.8
  - papillae K14.4
- trachea J39.8
- tunica vaginalis N50.89
- turbinate J34.89
- tympanic membrane (nonflaccid) H73.82- ☑
  - flaccid H73.81- ☑
- upper respiratory tract J39.8
- uterus, uterine (senile) N85.8
  - cervix N88.8
  - due to radiation (intended effect) N85.8
    - adverse effect or misadventure N99.89
- vagina (senile) N95.2
- vas deferens N50.89
- vascular I99.8
- vertebra (senile) — *see* Spondylopathy, specified N
- vulva (senile) N90.5
- Werdnig-Hoffmann G12.0
- yellow — *see* Failure, hepatic

Attack, attacks
    with alteration of consciousness (with automatisms) — see Epilepsy, localization-related, symptomatic, with complex partial seizures
    Adams-Stokes I45.9
    akinetic — see Epilepsy, generalized, specified NEC
    angina — see Angina
    atonic — see Epilepsy, generalized, specified NEC
    benign shuddering G25.83
    cataleptic — see Catalepsy
    coronary — see Infarct, myocardium
    cyanotic, newborn P28.2
    drop NEC R55
    epileptic — see Epilepsy
    heart — see infarct, myocardium
    hysterical F44.9
    jacksonian — see Epilepsy, localization-related, symptomatic, with simple partial seizures
    myocardium, myocardial — see Infarct, myocardium
    myoclonic — see Epilepsy, generalized, specified NEC
    panic F41.0
    psychomotor — see Epilepsy, localization-related, symptomatic, with complex partial seizures
    salaam — see Epilepsy, spasms
    schizophreniform, brief F23
    shuddering, benign G25.83
    Stokes-Adams I45.9
    syncope R55
    transient ischemic (TIA) G45.9
        specified NEC G45.8
    unconsciousness R55
        hysterical F44.89
    vasomotor R55
    vasovagal (paroxysmal) (idiopathic) R55
    without alteration of consciousness — see Epilepsy, localization-related, symptomatic, with simple partial seizures
Attention (to)
    artificial
        opening (of) Z43.9
            digestive tract NEC Z43.4
                colon Z43.3
                ilium Z43.2
                stomach Z43.1
            specified NEC Z43.8
            trachea Z43.0
            urinary tract NEC Z43.6
                cystostomy Z43.5
                nephrostomy Z43.6
                ureterostomy Z43.6
                urethrostomy Z43.6
            vagina Z43.7
    colostomy Z43.3
    cystostomy Z43.5
    deficit disorder or syndrome F98.8
        with hyperactivity — see Disorder, attention-deficit hyperactivity
    gastrostomy Z43.1
    ileostomy Z43.2
    jejunostomy Z43.4
    nephrostomy Z43.6
    surgical dressings Z48.01
    sutures Z48.02
    tracheostomy Z43.0
    ureterostomy Z43.6
    urethrostomy Z43.6
Attrition
    gum — see Recession, gingival
    tooth, teeth (excessive) (hard tissues) K03.0
Atypical, atypism — see also condition
    cells (on cytolgocial smear) (endocervical) (endometrial) (glandular)
        cervix R87.619
        vagina R87.629
    cervical N87.9
    endometrium N85.9
        hyperplasia N85.00
    parenting situation Z62.9
Auditory — see condition
Aujeszky's disease B33.8
Aurantiasis, cutis E67.1
Auricle, auricular — see also condition
    cervical Q18.2
Auriculotemporal syndrome G50.8
Austin Flint murmur (aortic insufficiency) I35.1
Australian
    Q fever A78
    X disease A83.4

Autism, autistic (childhood) (infantile) F84.0
    atypical F84.9
    spectrum disorder F84.0
Autodigestion R68.89
Autoerythrocyte sensitization (syndrome) D69.2
Autographism L50.3
Autoimmune
    disease (systemic) M35.9
    inhibitors to clotting factors D68.311
    lymphoproliferative syndrome [ALPS] D89.82
    thyroiditis E06.3
Autointoxication R68.89
Automatism G93.89
    with temporal sclerosis G93.81
    epileptic — see Epilepsy, localization-related, symptomatic, with complex partial seizures
    paroxysmal, idiopathic — see Epilepsy, localization-related, symptomatic, with complex partial seizures
Autonomic, autonomous
    bladder (neurogenic) N31.2
    hysteria seizure F44.5
Autosensitivity, erythrocyte D69.2
Autosensitization, cutaneous L30.2
Autosome — see condition by chromosome involved
Autotopagnosia R48.1
Autotoxemia R68.89
Autumn — see condition
Avellis' syndrome G46.8
Aversion
    oral R63.3
        newborn P92.- ☑
        nonorganic origin F98.2 ☑
    sexual F52.1
Aviator's
    disease or sickness — see Effect, adverse, high altitude
    ear T70.0 ☑
Avitaminosis (multiple) — see also Deficiency, vitamin
    E56.9
    B E53.9
        with
            beriberi E51.11
            pellagra E52
    B2 E53.0
    B6 E53.1
    B12 E53.8
    D E55.9
        with rickets E55.0
    G E53.0
    K E56.1
    nicotinic acid E52
AVNRT (atrioventricular nodal re-entrant tachycardia) I47.1
AVRT (atrioventricular nodal re-entrant tachycardia) I47.1
Avulsion (traumatic)
    blood vessel — see Injury, blood vessel
    bone — see Fracture, by site
    cartilage — see also Dislocation, by site
        symphyseal (inner), complicating delivery O71.6
    external site other than limb — see Wound, open, by site
    eye S05.7- ☑
    head (intracranial)
        external site NEC S08.89 ☑
        scalp S08.0 ☑
    internal organ or site — see Injury, by site
    joint — see also Dislocation, by site
        capsule — see Sprain, by site
    kidney S37.06- ☑
    ligament — see Sprain, by site
    limb — see also Amputation, traumatic, by site
        skin and subcutaneous tissue — see Wound, open, by site
    muscle — see Injury, muscle
    nerve (root) — see Injury, nerve
    scalp S08.0 ☑
    skin and subcutaneous tissue — see Wound, open, by site
    spleen S36.032 ☑
    symphyseal cartilage (inner), complicating delivery O71.6
    tendon — see Injury, muscle
    tooth S03.2 ☑
Awareness of heart beat R00.2
Axenfeld's
    anomaly or syndrome Q15.0
    degeneration (calcareous) Q13.4

Axilla, axillary — see also condition
    breast Q83.1
Axonotmesis — see Injury, nerve
Ayerza's disease or syndrome (pulmonary artery sclerosis with pulmonary hypertension) I27.0
Azoospermia (organic) N46.01
    due to
        drug therapy N46.021
        efferent duct obstruction N46.023
        infection N46.022
        radiation N46.024
        specified cause NEC N46.029
        systemic disease N46.025
Azotemia R79.89
    meaning uremia N19
Aztec ear Q17.3
Azygos
    continuation inferior vena cava Q26.8
    lobe (lung) Q33.1

B

Baastrup's disease — see Kissing spine
Babesiosis B60.0
Babington's disease (familial hemorrhagic telangiectasia) I78.0
Babinski's syndrome A52.79
Baby
    crying constantly R68.11
    floppy (syndrome) P94.2
Bacillary — see condition
Bacilluria R82.71
Bacillus — see also Infection, bacillus
    abortus infection A23.1
    anthracis infection A22.9
    coli infection — see also Escherichia coli B96.20
    Flexner's A03.1
    mallei infection A24.0
    Shiga's A03.0
    suipestifer infection — see Infection, salmonella
Back — see condition
Backache (postural) M54.9
    sacroiliac M53.3
    specified NEC M54.89
Backflow — see Reflux
Backward reading (dyslexia) F81.0
Bacteremia R78.81
    with sepsis — see Sepsis
Bactericholia — see Cholecystitis, acute
Bacterid, bacteride (pustular) L40.3
Bacterium, bacteria, bacterial
    agent NEC, as cause of disease classified elsewhere B96.89
    in blood — see Bacteremia
    in urine — see Bacteriuria
Bacteriuria, bacteruria R82.71
    asymptomatic R82.71
Bacteroides
    fragilis, as cause of disease classified elsewhere B96.6
Bad
    heart — see Disease, heart
    trip
        due to drug abuse — see Abuse, drug, hallucinogen
        due to drug dependence — see Dependence, drug, hallucinogen
Baelz's disease (cheilitis glandularis apostematosa) K13.0
Baerensprung's disease (eczema marginatum) B35.6
Bagasse disease or pneumonitis J67.1
Bagassosis J67.1
Baker's cyst — see Cyst, Baker's
Bakwin-Krida syndrome (metaphyseal dysplasia) Q78.5
Balancing side interference M26.56
Balanitis (circinata) (erosiva) (gangrenosa) (phagedenic) (vulgaris) N48.1
    amebic A06.82
    candidal B37.42
    due to Haemophilus ducreyi A57
    gonococcal (acute) (chronic) A54.23
    xerotica obliterans N48.0
Balanoposthitis N47.6
    gonococcal (acute) (chronic) A54.23
    ulcerative (specific) A63.8
Balanorrhagia — see Balanitis
Balantidiasis, balantidiosis A07.0
Bald tongue K14.4
Baldness — see also Alopecia
    male-pattern — see Alopecia, androgenic

Balkan grippe A78
Balloon disease — *see* Effect, adverse, high altitude
Balo's disease (concentric sclerosis) G37.5
Bamberger-Marie disease — *see* Osteoarthropathy, hypertrophic, specified type NEC
Bancroft's filariasis B74.0
Band(s)
  adhesive — *see* Adhesions, peritoneum
  anomalous or congenital — *see also* Anomaly, by site
    heart (atrial) (ventricular) Q24.8
    intestine Q43.3
    omentum Q43.3
  cervix N88.1
  constricting, congenital Q79.8
  gallbladder (congenital) Q44.1
  intestinal (adhesive) — *see* Adhesions, peritoneum
  obstructive
    intestine K56.50
      complete K56.52
      incomplete K56.51
      partial K56.51
    peritoneum K56.50
      complete K56.52
      incomplete K56.51
      partial K56.51
  periappendiceal, congenital Q43.3
  peritoneal (adhesive) — *see* Adhesions, peritoneum
  uterus N73.6
    internal N85.6
  vagina N89.5
Bandemia D72.825
Bandl's ring (contraction), complicating delivery O62.4
Bangkok hemorrhagic fever A91
Bang's disease (brucella abortus) A23.1
Bankruptcy, anxiety concerning Z59.8
Bannister's disease T78.3 ☑
  hereditary D84.1
Banti's disease or syndrome (with cirrhosis) (with portal hypertension) K76.6
Bar, median, prostate — *see* Enlargement, enlarged, prostate
Barcoo disease or rot — *see* Ulcer, skin
Barlow's disease E54
Barodontalgia T70.29 ☑
Baron Münchausen syndrome — *see* Disorder, factitious
Barosinusitis T70.1 ☑
Barotitis T70.0 ☑
Barotrauma T70.29 ☑
  odontalgia T70.29 ☑
  otitic T70.0 ☑
  sinus T70.1 ☑
Barraquer (-Simons) **disease or syndrome** (progressive lipodystrophy) E88.1
Barré-Guillain disease or syndrome G61.0
Barrel chest M95.4
Barré-Liéou syndrome (posterior cervical sympathetic) M53.0
Barrett's
  disease — *see* Barrett's, esophagus
  esophagus K22.70
    with dysplasia K22.719
      high grade K22.711
      low grade K22.710
    without dysplasia K22.70
  syndrome — *see* Barrett's, esophagus
  ulcer K22.10
    with bleeding K22.11
    without bleeding K22.10
Bársony (-Polgár) (-Teschendorf) **syndrome** (corkscrew esophagus) K22.4
Barth syndrome E78.71
Bartholinitis (suppurating) N75.8
  gonococcal (acute) (chronic) (with abscess) A54.1
Bartonellosis A44.9
  cutaneous A44.1
  mucocutaneous A44.1
  specified NEC A44.8
  systemic A44.0
Barton's fracture S52.56- ☑
Bartter's syndrome E26.81
Basal — *see* condition
Basan's (hidrotic) ectodermal dysplasia Q82.4
Baseball finger — *see* Dislocation, finger
Basedow's disease (exophthalmic goiter) — *see* Hyperthyroidism, with, goiter
Basic — *see* condition

Basilar — *see* condition
Bason's (hidrotic) ectodermal dysplasia Q82.4
Basopenia — *see* Agranulocytosis
Basophilia D72.824
Basophilism (cortico-adrenal) (Cushing's) (pituitary) E24.0
Bassen-Kornzweig disease or syndrome E78.6
Bat ear Q17.5
Bateman's
  disease B08.1
  purpura (senile) D69.2
Bathing cramp T75.1 ☑
Bathophobia F40.248
Batten (-Mayou) **disease** E75.4
  retina E75.4 *[H36]*
Batten-Steinert syndrome G71.11
Battered — *see* Maltreatment
Battey Mycobacterium infection A31.0
Battle exhaustion F43.0
Battledore placenta O43.19- ☑
Baumgarten-Cruveilhier cirrhosis, disease or syndrome K74.69
Bauxite fibrosis (of lung) J63.1
Bayle's disease (general paresis) A52.17
Bazin's disease (primary) (tuberculous) A18.4
Beach ear — *see* Swimmer's, ear
Beaded hair (congenital) Q84.1
Béal conjunctivitis or syndrome B30.2
Beard's disease (neurasthenia) F48.8
Beat(s)
  atrial, premature I49.1
  ectopic I49.49
  elbow — *see* Bursitis, elbow
  escaped, heart I49.49
  hand — *see* Bursitis, hand
  knee — *see* Bursitis, knee
  premature I49.40
    atrial I49.1
    auricular I49.1
    supraventricular I49.1
Beau's
  disease or syndrome — *see* Degeneration, myocardial
  lines (transverse furrows on fingernails) L60.4
Bechterev's syndrome — *see* Spondylitis, ankylosing
Becker's
  cardiomyopathy I42.8
  disease
    idiopathic mural endomyocardial disease I42.3
    myotonia congenita, recessive form G71.12
  dystrophy G71.01
  pigmented hairy nevus D22.5
Beck's syndrome (anterior spinal artery occlusion) I65.8
Beckwith-Wiedemann syndrome Q87.3
Bed confinement status Z74.01
Bed sore — *see* Ulcer, pressure, by site
Bedbug bite(s) — *see* Bite(s), by site, superficial, insect
Bedclothes, asphyxiation or suffocation by — *see* Asphyxia, traumatic, due to, mechanical, trapped
Bednar's
  aphthae K12.0
  tumor — *see* Neoplasm, malignant, by site
Bedridden Z74.01
Bedsore — *see* Ulcer, pressure, by site
Bedwetting — *see* Enuresis
Bee sting (with allergic or anaphylactic shock) — *see* Toxicity, venom, arthropod, bee
Beer drinker's heart (disease) I42.6
Begbie's disease (exophthalmic goiter) — *see* Hyperthyroidism, with, goiter
Behavior
  antisocial
    adult Z72.811
    child or adolescent Z72.810
  disorder, disturbance — *see* Disorder, conduct
  disruptive — *see* Disorder, conduct
  drug seeking Z76.5
  inexplicable R46.2
  marked evasiveness R46.5
  obsessive-compulsive R46.81
  overactivity R46.3
  poor responsiveness R46.4
  self-damaging (life-style) Z72.89
  sleep-incompatible Z72.821
  slowness R46.4
  specified NEC R46.89
  strange (and inexplicable) R46.2
  suspiciousness R46.5
  type A pattern Z73.1

Behavior — *continued*
  undue concern or preoccupation with stressful event R46.6
  verbosity and circumstantial detail obscuring reason for contact R46.7
Behçet's disease or syndrome M35.2
Behr's disease — *see* Degeneration, macula
Beigel's disease or morbus (white piedra) B36.2
Bejel A65
Bekhterev's syndrome — *see* Spondylitis, ankylosing
Belching — *see* Eructation
Bell's
  mania F30.8
  palsy, paralysis G51.0
    infant or newborn P11.3
  spasm G51.3- ☑
Bence Jones albuminuria or proteinuria NEC R80.3
Bends T70.3 ☑
Benedikt's paralysis or syndrome G46.3
Benign — *see also* condition
  prostatic hyperplasia — *see* Hyperplasia, prostate
Bennett's fracture (displaced) S62.21- ☑
Benson's disease — *see* Deposit, crystalline
Bent
  back (hysterical) F44.4
  nose M95.0
    congenital Q67.4
Bereavement (uncomplicated) Z63.4
Bergeron's disease (hysterical chorea) F44.4
Berger's disease — *see* Nephropathy, IgA
Beriberi (dry) E51.11
  heart (disease) E51.12
  polyneuropathy E51.11
  wet E51.12
    involving circulatory system E51.11
Berlin's disease or edema (traumatic) S05.8X- ☑
Berlock (berloque) **dermatitis** L56.2
Bernard-Horner syndrome G90.2
Bernard-Soulier disease or thrombopathia D69.1
Bernhardt (-Roth) **disease** — *see* Mononeuropathy, lower limb, meralgia paresthetica
Bernheim's syndrome — *see* Failure, heart, right
Bertielliasis B71.8
Berylliosis (lung) J63.2
Besnier-Boeck (-Schaumann) **disease** — *see* Sarcoidosis
Besnier's
  lupus pernio D86.3
  prurigo L20.0
Bestiality F65.89
Best's disease H35.50
Betalipoproteinemia, broad or floating E78.2
Beta-mercaptolactate-cysteine disulfiduria E72.09
Betting and gambling Z72.6
  pathological (compulsive) F63.0
Bezoar T18.9 ☑
  intestine T18.3 ☑
  stomach T18.2 ☑
Bezold's abscess — *see* Mastoiditis, acute
Bianchi's syndrome R48.8
Bicornate or bicornis uterus Q51.3
  in pregnancy or childbirth O34.00
    causing obstructed labor O65.5
Bicuspid aortic valve Q23.1
Biedl-Bardet syndrome Q87.89
Bielschowsky (-Jansky) **disease** E75.4
Biermer's (pernicious) **anemia or disease** D51.0
Biett's disease L93.0
Bifid (congenital)
  apex, heart Q24.8
  clitoris Q52.6
  kidney Q63.8
  nose Q30.2
  patella Q74.1
  scrotum Q55.29
  toe NEC Q74.2
  tongue Q38.3
  ureter Q62.8
  uterus Q51.3
  uvula Q35.7
Biforis uterus (suprasimplex) Q51.3
Bifurcation (congenital)
  gallbladder Q44.1
  kidney pelvis Q63.8
  renal pelvis Q63.8
  rib Q76.6
  tongue, congenital Q38.3
  trachea Q32.1

☑ **Additional Character Required** — **Refer to the Tabular List for Character Selection**   ▽ **Subterms under main terms may continue to next column or page**

Bifurcation — *continued*
  ureter Q62.8
  urethra Q64.74
  vertebra Q76.49
Big spleen syndrome D73.1
Bigeminal pulse R00.8
Bilateral — *see* condition
Bile
  duct — *see* condition
  pigments in urine R82.2
Bilharziasis — *see also* Schistosomiasis
  chyluria B65.0
  cutaneous B65.3
  galacturia B65.0
  hematochyluria B65.0
  intestinal B65.1
  lipemia B65.9
  lipuria B65.0
  oriental B65.2
  piarhemia B65.9
  pulmonary NOS B65.9 [J99]
    pneumonia B65.9 [J17]
  tropical hematuria B65.0
  vesical B65.0
Biliary — *see* condition
Bilirubin metabolism disorder E80.7
  specified NEC E80.6
Bilirubinemia, familial nonhemolytic E80.4
Bilirubinuria R82.2
Biliuria R82.2
Bilocular stomach K31.2
Binswanger's disease I67.3
Bird
  face Q75.8
  fancier's disease or lung J67.2
Birth
  complications in mother — *see* Delivery, complicated
  compression during NOS P15.9
  defect — *see* Anomaly
  immature (less than 37 completed weeks) — *see*
    Preterm, newborn
    extremely (less than 28 completed weeks) — *see*
      Immaturity, extreme
  inattention, at or after — *see* Maltreatment, child, ne-
    glect
  injury NOS P15.9
    basal ganglia P11.1
    brachial plexus NEC P14.3
    brain (compression) (pressure) P11.2
    central nervous system NOS P11.9
    cerebellum P11.1
    cerebral hemorrhage P10.1
    external genitalia P15.5
    eye P15.3
    face P15.4
    fracture
      bone P13.9
        specified NEC P13.8
      clavicle P13.4
      femur P13.2
      humerus P13.3
      long bone, except femur P13.3
      radius and ulna P13.3
      skull P13.0
      spine P11.5
      tibia and fibula P13.3
    intracranial P11.2
      laceration or hemorrhage P10.9
        specified NEC P10.8
    intraventricular hemorrhage P10.2
    laceration
      brain P10.1
      by scalpel P15.8
      peripheral nerve P14.9
    liver P15.0
    meninges
      brain P11.1
      spinal cord P11.5
    nerve
      brachial plexus P14.3
      cranial NEC (except facial) P11.4
      facial P11.3
      peripheral P14.9
      phrenic (paralysis) P14.2

Birth — *continued*
  injury — *continued*
    paralysis
      facial nerve P11.3
      spinal P11.5
    penis P15.5
    rupture
      spinal cord P11.5
    scalp P12.9
    scalpel wound P15.8
    scrotum P15.5
    skull NEC P13.1
      fracture P13.0
    specified type NEC P15.8
    spinal cord P11.5
    spine P11.5
    spleen P15.1
    sternomastoid (hematoma) P15.2
    subarachnoid hemorrhage P10.3
    subcutaneous fat necrosis P15.6
    subdural hemorrhage P10.0
    tentorial tear P10.4
    testes P15.5
    vulva P15.5
  lack of care, at or after — *see* Maltreatment, child, ne-
    glect
  neglect, at or after — *see* Maltreatment, child, neglect
  palsy or paralysis, newborn, NOS (birth injury) P14.9
  premature (infant) — *see* Preterm, newborn
  shock, newborn P96.89
  trauma — *see* Birth, injury
  weight
    low (2499 grams or less) — *see* Low, birthweight
      extremely (999 grams or less) — *see* Low, birth-
        weight, extreme
    4000 grams to 4499 grams P08.1
    4500 grams or more P08.0
Birthmark Q82.5
Birt-Hogg-Dube syndrome Q87.89
Bisalbuminemia E88.09
Biskra's button B55.1
Bite(s) (animal) (human)
  abdomen, abdominal
    wall S31.159 ☑
      with penetration into peritoneal cavity
        S31.659 ☑
      epigastric region S31.152 ☑
        with penetration into peritoneal cavity
          S31.652 ☑
      left
        lower quadrant S31.154 ☑
          with penetration into peritoneal cavity
            S31.654 ☑
        upper quadrant S31.151 ☑
          with penetration into peritoneal cavity
            S31.651 ☑
      periumbilic region S31.155 ☑
        with penetration into peritoneal cavity
          S31.655 ☑
      right
        lower quadrant S31.153 ☑
          with penetration into peritoneal cavity
            S31.653 ☑
        upper quadrant S31.150 ☑
          with penetration into peritoneal cavity
            S31.650 ☑
      superficial NEC S30.871 ☑
        insect S30.861 ☑
  alveolar (process) — *see* Bite, oral cavity
  amphibian (venomous) — *see* Venom, bite, amphibian
  animal — *see also* Bite, by site
    venomous — *see* Venom
  ankle S91.05- ☑
    superficial NEC S90.57- ☑
      insect S90.56- ☑
  antecubital space — *see* Bite, elbow
  anus S31.835 ☑
    superficial NEC S30.877 ☑
      insect S30.867 ☑
  arm (upper) S41.15- ☑
    lower — *see* Bite, forearm
    superficial NEC S40.87- ☑
      insect S40.86- ☑
  arthropod NEC — *see* Venom, bite, arthropod
  auditory canal (external) (meatus) — *see* Bite, ear
  auricle, ear — *see* Bite, ear
  axilla — *see* Bite, arm

Bite(s) — *continued*
  back — *see also* Bite, thorax, back
    lower S31.050 ☑
      with penetration into retroperitoneal space
        S31.051 ☑
      superficial NEC S30.870 ☑
        insect S30.860 ☑
  bedbug — *see* Bite(s), by site, superficial, insect
  breast S21.05- ☑
    superficial NEC S20.17- ☑
      insect S20.16- ☑
  brow — *see* Bite, head, specified site NEC
  buttock S31.805 ☑
    left S31.825 ☑
    right S31.815 ☑
    superficial NEC S30.870 ☑
      insect S30.860 ☑
  calf — *see* Bite, leg
  canaliculus lacrimalis — *see* Bite, eyelid
  canthus, eye — *see* Bite, eyelid
  centipede — *see* Toxicity, venom, arthropod, centipede
  cheek (external) S01.45- ☑
    internal — *see* Bite, oral cavity
    superficial NEC S00.87 ☑
      insect S00.86 ☑
  chest wall — *see* Bite, thorax
  chigger B88.0
  chin — *see* Bite, head, specified site NEC
  clitoris — *see* Bite, vulva
  costal region — *see* Bite, thorax
  digit(s)
    hand — *see* Bite, finger
    toe — *see* Bite, toe
  ear (canal) (external) S01.35- ☑
    superficial NEC S00.47- ☑
      insect S00.46- ☑
  elbow S51.05- ☑
    superficial NEC S50.37- ☑
      insect S50.36- ☑
  epididymis — *see* Bite, testis
  epigastric region — *see* Bite, abdomen
  epiglottis — *see* Bite, neck, specified site NEC
  esophagus, cervical S11.25 ☑
    superficial NEC S10.17 ☑
      insect S10.16 ☑
  eyebrow — *see* Bite, eyelid
  eyelid S01.15- ☑
    superficial NEC S00.27- ☑
      insect S00.26- ☑
  face NEC — *see* Bite, head, specified site NEC
  finger(s) S61.259 ☑
    with
      damage to nail S61.359 ☑
    index S61.258 ☑
      with
        damage to nail S61.358 ☑
      left S61.251 ☑
        with
          damage to nail S61.351 ☑
      right S61.250 ☑
        with
          damage to nail S61.350 ☑
      superficial NEC S60.478 ☑
        insect S60.46- ☑
    little S61.25- ☑
      with
        damage to nail S61.35- ☑
      superficial NEC S60.47- ☑
        insect S60.46- ☑
    middle S61.25- ☑
      with
        damage to nail S61.35- ☑
      superficial NEC S60.47- ☑
        insect S60.46- ☑
    ring S61.25- ☑
      with
        damage to nail S61.35- ☑
      superficial NEC S60.47- ☑
        insect S60.46- ☑
    superficial NEC S60.479 ☑
      insect S60.469 ☑
    thumb — *see* Bite, thumb
  flank — *see* Bite, abdomen, wall
  flea — *see* Bite, by site, superficial, insect
  foot (except toe(s) alone) S91.35- ☑
    superficial NEC S90.87- ☑

Bite(s) — *continued*
  foot(s alone) — *continued*
    superficial — *continued*
      insect S90.86- ☑
    toe — *see* Bite, toe
  forearm S51.85- ☑
    elbow only — *see* Bite, elbow
    superficial NEC S50.87- ☑
      insect S50.86- ☑
  forehead — *see* Bite, head, specified site NEC
  genital organs, external
    female S31.552
      superficial NEC S30.876 ☑
        insect S30.866 ☑
      vagina and vulva — *see* Bite, vulva
    male S31.551
      penis — *see* Bite, penis
      scrotum — *see* Bite, scrotum
      superficial NEC S30.875 ☑
        insect S30.865 ☑
      testes — *see* Bite, testis
  groin — *see* Bite, abdomen, wall
  gum — *see* Bite, oral cavity
  hand S61.45- ☑
    finger — *see* Bite, finger
    superficial NEC S60.57- ☑
      insect S60.56- ☑
    thumb — *see* Bite, thumb
  head S01.95 ☑
    cheek — *see* Bite, cheek
    ear — *see* Bite, ear
    eyelid — *see* Bite, eyelid
    lip — *see* Bite, lip
    nose — *see* Bite, nose
    oral cavity — *see* Bite, oral cavity
    scalp — *see* Bite, scalp
    specified site NEC S01.85 ☑
      superficial NEC S00.87 ☑
        insect S00.86 ☑
    superficial NEC S00.97 ☑
      insect S00.96 ☑
    temporomandibular area — *see* Bite, cheek
  heel — *see* Bite, foot
  hip S71.05- ☑
    superficial NEC S70.27- ☑
      insect S70.26- ☑
  hymen S31.45 ☑
  hypochondrium — *see* Bite, abdomen, wall
  hypogastric region — *see* Bite, abdomen, wall
  inguinal region — *see* Bite, abdomen, wall
  insect — *see* Bite, by site, superficial, insect
  instep — *see* Bite, foot
  interscapular region — *see* Bite, thorax, back
  jaw — *see* Bite, head, specified site NEC
  knee S81.05- ☑
    superficial NEC S80.27- ☑
      insect S80.26- ☑
  labium (majus) (minus) — *see* Bite, vulva
  lacrimal duct — *see* Bite, eyelid
  larynx S11.015 ☑
    superficial NEC S10.17 ☑
      insect S10.16 ☑
  leg (lower) S81.85- ☑
    ankle — *see* Bite, ankle
    foot — *see* Bite, foot
    knee — *see* Bite, knee
    superficial NEC S80.87- ☑
      insect S80.86- ☑
    toe — *see* Bite, toe
    upper — *see* Bite, thigh
  lip S01.551 ☑
    superficial NEC S00.571 ☑
      insect S00.561 ☑
  lizard (venomous) — *see* Venom, bite, reptile
  loin — *see* Bite, abdomen, wall
  lower back — *see* Bite, back, lower
  lumbar region — *see* Bite, back, lower
  malar region — *see* Bite, head, specified site NEC
  mammary — *see* Bite, breast
  marine animals (venomous) — *see* Toxicity, venom, marine animal
  mastoid region — *see* Bite, head, specified site NEC
  mouth — *see* Bite, oral cavity
  nail
    finger — *see* Bite, finger
    toe — *see* Bite, toe

Bite(s) — *continued*
  nape — *see* Bite, neck, specified site NEC
  nasal (septum) (sinus) — *see* Bite, nose
  nasopharynx — *see* Bite, head, specified site NEC
  neck S11.95 ☑
    involving
      cervical esophagus — *see* Bite, esophagus, cervical
      larynx — *see* Bite, larynx
      pharynx — *see* Bite, pharynx
      thyroid gland S11.15 ☑
      trachea — *see* Bite, trachea
    specified site NEC S11.85 ☑
      superficial NEC S10.87 ☑
        insect S10.86 ☑
    superficial NEC S10.97 ☑
      insect S10.96 ☑
    throat S11.85 ☑
      superficial NEC S10.17 ☑
        insect S10.16 ☑
  nose (septum) (sinus) S01.25 ☑
    superficial NEC S00.37 ☑
      insect S00.36 ☑
  occipital region — *see* Bite, scalp
  oral cavity S01.552 ☑
    superficial NEC S00.572 ☑
      insect S00.562 ☑
  orbital region — *see* Bite, eyelid
  palate — *see* Bite, oral cavity
  palm — *see* Bite, hand
  parietal region — *see* Bite, scalp
  pelvis S31.050 ☑
    with penetration into retroperitoneal space S31.051
    superficial NEC S30.870 ☑
      insect S30.860 ☑
  penis S31.25 ☑
    superficial NEC S30.872 ☑
      insect S30.862 ☑
  perineum
    female — *see* Bite, vulva
    male — *see* Bite, pelvis
  periocular area (with or without lacrimal passages) — *see* Bite, eyelid
  phalanges
    finger — *see* Bite, finger
    toe — *see* Bite, toe
  pharynx S11.25 ☑
    superficial NEC S10.17 ☑
      insect S10.16 ☑
  pinna — *see* Bite, ear
  poisonous — *see* Venom
  popliteal space — *see* Bite, knee
  prepuce — *see* Bite, penis
  pubic region — *see* Bite, abdomen, wall
  rectovaginal septum — *see* Bite, vulva
  red bug B88.0
  reptile NEC — *see also* Venom, bite, reptile
    nonvenomous — *see* Bite, by site
    snake — *see* Venom, bite, snake
  sacral region — *see* Bite, back, lower
  sacroiliac region — *see* Bite, back, lower
  salivary gland — *see* Bite, oral cavity
  scalp S01.05 ☑
    superficial NEC S00.07 ☑
      insect S00.06 ☑
  scapular region — *see* Bite, shoulder
  scrotum S31.35 ☑
    superficial NEC S30.873 ☑
      insect S30.863 ☑
  sea-snake (venomous) — *see* Toxicity, venom, snake, sea snake
  shin — *see* Bite, leg
  shoulder S41.05- ☑
    superficial NEC S40.27- ☑
      insect S40.26- ☑
  snake — *see also* Venom, bite, snake
    nonvenomous — *see* Bite, by site
  spermatic cord — *see* Bite, testis
  spider (venomous) — *see* Toxicity, venom, spider
    nonvenomous — *see* Bite, by site, superficial, insect
  sternal region — *see* Bite, thorax, front
  submaxillary region — *see* Bite, head, specified site NEC
  submental region — *see* Bite, head, specified site NEC

Bite(s) — *continued*
  subungual
    finger(s) — *see* Bite, finger
    toe — *see* Bite, toe
  superficial — *see* Bite, by site, superficial
  supraclavicular fossa S11.85 ☑
  supraorbital — *see* Bite, head, specified site NEC
  temple, temporal region — *see* Bite, head, specified site NEC
  temporomandibular area — *see* Bite, cheek
  testis S31.35 ☑
    superficial NEC S30.873 ☑
      insect S30.863 ☑
  thigh S71.15- ☑
    superficial NEC S70.37- ☑
      insect S70.36- ☑
  thorax, thoracic (wall) S21.95 ☑
    back S21.25- ☑
      with penetration into thoracic cavity S21.45- ☑
    breast — *see* Bite, breast
    front S21.15- ☑
      with penetration into thoracic cavity S21.35- ☑
    superficial NEC S20.97 ☑
      back S20.47- ☑
      front S20.37- ☑
      insect S20.96 ☑
        back S20.46- ☑
        front S20.36- ☑
  throat — *see* Bite, neck, throat
  thumb S61.05- ☑
    with
      damage to nail S61.15- ☑
    superficial NEC S60.37- ☑
      insect S60.36- ☑
  thyroid S11.15 ☑
    superficial NEC S10.87 ☑
      insect S10.86 ☑
  toe(s) S91.15- ☑
    with
      damage to nail S91.25- ☑
    great S91.15- ☑
      with
        damage to nail S91.25- ☑
    lesser S91.15- ☑
      with
        damage to nail S91.25- ☑
    superficial NEC S90.47- ☑
      great S90.47- ☑
      insect S90.46- ☑
        great S90.46- ☑
  tongue S01.552 ☑
  trachea S11.025 ☑
    superficial NEC S10.17 ☑
      insect S10.16 ☑
  tunica vaginalis — *see* Bite, testis
  tympanum, tympanic membrane — *see* Bite, ear
  umbilical region S31.155 ☑
  uvula — *see* Bite, oral cavity
  vagina — *see* Bite, vulva
  venomous — *see* Venom
  vocal cords S11.035 ☑
    superficial NEC S10.17 ☑
      insect S10.16 ☑
  vulva S31.45 ☑
    superficial NEC S30.874 ☑
      insect S30.864 ☑
  wrist S61.55- ☑
    superficial NEC S60.87- ☑
      insect S60.86- ☑
Biting, cheek or lip K13.1
Biventricular failure (heart) I50.82
Björck (-Thorson) **syndrome** (malignant carcinoid) E34.
Black
  death A20.9
  eye S00.1- ☑
  hairy tongue K14.3
  heel (foot) S90.3- ☑
  lung (disease) J60
  palm (hand) S60.22- ☑
Blackfan-Diamond anemia or syndrome (congeni
  hypoplastic anemia) D61.01
Blackhead L70.0
Blackout R55
Bladder — *see* condition
Blast (air) (hydraulic) (immersion) (underwater)
  blindness S05.8X- ☑

☑ Additional Character Required — Refer to the Tabular List for Character Selection   ▽ Subterms under main terms may continue to next column or pa

Blast — *continued*
  injury
    abdomen or thorax — *see* Injury, by site
    ear (acoustic nerve trauma) — *see* Injury, nerve,
      acoustic, specified type NEC
  syndrome NEC T70.8 ☑
Blastoma — *see* Neoplasm, malignant, by site
  pulmonary — *see* Neoplasm, lung, malignant
Blastomycosis, blastomycotic B40.9
  Brazilian — *see* Paracoccidioidomycosis
  cutaneous B40.3
  disseminated B40.7
  European — *see* Cryptococcosis
  generalized B40.7
  keloidal B48.0
  North American B40.9
  primary pulmonary B40.0
  pulmonary B40.2
    acute B40.0
    chronic B40.1
  skin B40.3
  South American — *see* Paracoccidioidomycosis
  specified NEC B40.89
Bleb(s) R23.8
  emphysematous (lung) (solitary) J43.9
  endophthalmitis H59.43
  filtering (vitreous), after glaucoma surgery Z98.83
  inflamed (infected), postprocedural H59.40
    stage 1 H59.41
    stage 2 H59.42
    stage 3 H59.43
  lung (ruptured) J43.9
    congenital — *see* Atelectasis
    newborn P25.8
  subpleural (emphysematous) J43.9
Blebitis, postprocedural H59.40
  stage 1 H59.41
  stage 2 H59.42
  stage 3 H59.43
Bleeder (familial) (hereditary) — *see* Hemophilia
Bleeding — *see also* Hemorrhage
  anal K62.5
  anovulatory N97.0
  atonic, following delivery O72.1
  capillary I78.8
    puerperal O72.2
  contact (postcoital) N93.0
  due to uterine subinvolution N85.3
  ear — *see* Otorrhagia
  excessive, associated with menopausal onset N92.4
  familial — *see* Defect, coagulation
  following intercourse N93.0
  gastrointestinal K92.2
  hemorrhoids — *see* Hemorrhoids
  intermenstrual (regular) N92.3
    irregular N92.1
  intraoperative — *see* Complication, intraoperative,
      hemorrhage
  irregular N92.6
  menopausal N92.4
  newborn, intraventricular — *see* Newborn, affected
      by, hemorrhage, intraventricular
  nipple N64.59
  nose R04.0
  ovulation N92.3
  perimenopausal N92.4
  postclimacteric N95.0
  postcoital N93.0
  postmenopausal N95.0
  postoperative — *see* Complication, postprocedural,
      hemorrhage
  preclimacteric N92.4
  pre-pubertal vaginal N93.1
  puberty (excessive, with onset of menstrual periods)
      N92.2
  rectum, rectal K62.5
    newborn P54.2
  tendencies — *see* Defect, coagulation
  throat R04.1
  tooth socket (post-extraction) K91.840
  umbilical stump P51.9
  uterus, uterine NEC N93.9
    climacteric N92.4
    dysfunctional or functional N93.8
    menopausal N92.4
    preclimacteric or premenopausal N92.4
    unrelated to menstrual cycle N93.9
  vagina, vaginal (abnormal) N93.9

Bleeding — *continued*
  vagina, vaginal — *continued*
    dysfunctional or functional N93.8
    newborn P54.6
    pre-pubertal N93.1
  vicarious N94.89
Blennorrhagia, blennorrhagic — *see* Gonorrhea
Blennorrhea (acute) (chronic) — *see also* Gonorrhea
  inclusion (neonatal) (newborn) P39.1
  lower genitourinary tract (gonococcal) A54.00
  neonatorum (gonococcal ophthalmia) A54.31
Blepharelosis — *see* Entropion
Blepharitis (angularis) (ciliaris) (eyelid) (marginal)
      (nonulcerative) H01.009
  herpes zoster B02.39
  left H01.006
    lower H01.005
    upper H01.004
    upper and lower H01.00B
  right H01.003
    lower H01.002
    upper H01.001
    upper and lower H01.00A
  squamous H01.029
    left H01.026
      lower H01.025
      upper H01.024
      upper and lower H01.02B
    right H01.023
      lower H01.022
      upper H01.021
      upper and lower H01.02A
  ulcerative H01.019
    left H01.016
      lower H01.015
      upper H01.014
      upper and lower H01.01B
    right H01.013
      lower H01.012
      upper H01.011
      upper and lower H01.01A
Blepharochalasis H02.30
  congenital Q10.0
  left H02.36
    lower H02.35
    upper H02.34
  right H02.33
    lower H02.32
    upper H02.31
Blepharoclonus H02.59
Blepharoconjunctivitis H10.50- ☑
  angular H10.52- ☑
  contact H10.53- ☑
  ligneous H10.51- ☑
Blepharophimosis (eyelid) H02.529
  congenital Q10.3
  left H02.526
    lower H02.525
    upper H02.524
  right H02.523
    lower H02.522
    upper H02.521
Blepharoptosis H02.40- ☑
  congenital Q10.0
  mechanical H02.41- ☑
  myogenic H02.42- ☑
  neurogenic H02.43- ☑
  paralytic H02.43- ☑
Blepharopyorrhea, gonococcal A54.39
Blepharospasm G24.5
  drug induced G24.01
Blighted ovum O02.0
Blind — *see also* Blindness
  bronchus (congenital) Q32.4
  loop syndrome K90.2
    congenital Q43.8
  sac, fallopian tube (congenital) Q50.6
  spot, enlarged — *see* Defect, visual field, localized,
      scotoma, blind spot area
  tract or tube, congenital NEC — *see* Atresia, by site
Blindness (acquired) (congenital) (both eyes) H54.0X- ☑
  blast S05.8X- ☑
  color — *see* Deficiency, color vision
  concussion S05.8X- ☑
  cortical H47.619
    left brain H47.612
    right brain H47.611
  day H53.11

Blindness — *continued*
  due to injury (current episode) S05.9- ☑
    sequelae — *code to* injury with seventh character
      S
  eclipse (total) — *see* Retinopathy, solar
  emotional (hysterical) F44.6
  face H53.16
  hysterical F44.6
  legal (both eyes) (USA definition) H54.8
  mind R48.8
  night H53.60
    abnormal dark adaptation curve H53.61
    acquired H53.62
    congenital H53.63
    specified type NEC H53.69
    vitamin A deficiency E50.5
  one eye (other eye normal) H54.40
    left (normal vision on right) H54.42- ☑
      low vision on right H54.12- ☑
      low vision, other eye H54.10
    right (normal vision on left) H54.41- ☑
      low vision on left H54.11- ☑
  psychic R48.8
  river B73.01
  snow — *see* Photokeratitis
  sun, solar — *see* Retinopathy, solar
  transient — *see* Disturbance, vision, subjective, loss,
      transient
  traumatic (current episode) S05.9- ☑
  word (developmental) F81.0
    acquired R48.0
    secondary to organic lesion R48.0
Blister (nonthermal)
  abdominal wall S30.821 ☑
  alveolar process S00.522 ☑
  ankle S90.52- ☑
  antecubital space — *see* Blister, elbow
  anus S30.827 ☑
  arm (upper) S40.82- ☑
  auditory canal — *see* Blister, ear
  auricle — *see* Blister, ear
  axilla — *see* Blister, arm
  back, lower S30.820 ☑
  beetle dermatitis L24.89
  breast S20.12- ☑
  brow S00.82 ☑
  calf — *see* Blister, leg
  canthus — *see* Blister, eyelid
  cheek S00.82 ☑
    internal S00.522 ☑
  chest wall — *see* Blister, thorax
  chin S00.82 ☑
  costal region — *see* Blister, thorax
  digit(s)
    foot — *see* Blister, toe
    hand — *see* Blister, finger
  due to burn — *see* Burn, by site, second degree
  ear S00.42- ☑
  elbow S50.32- ☑
  epiglottis S10.12 ☑
  esophagus, cervical S10.12 ☑
  eyebrow — *see* Blister, eyelid
  eyelid S00.22- ☑
  face S00.82 ☑
  fever B00.1
  finger(s) S60.429 ☑
    index S60.42- ☑
    little S60.42- ☑
    middle S60.42- ☑
    ring S60.42- ☑
  foot (except toe(s) alone) S90.82- ☑
    toe — *see* Blister, toe
  forearm S50.82- ☑
    elbow only — *see* Blister, elbow
  forehead S00.82 ☑
  fracture — *omit code*
  genital organ
    female S30.826 ☑
    male S30.825 ☑
  gum S00.522 ☑
  hand S60.52- ☑
  head S00.92 ☑
    ear — *see* Blister, ear
    eyelid — *see* Blister, eyelid
    lip S00.521 ☑
    nose S00.32 ☑

Blister — *continued*
 head — *continued*
  oral cavity S00.522 ☑
  scalp S00.02 ☑
  specified site NEC S00.82 ☑
 heel — *see* Blister, foot
 hip S70.22- ☑
 interscapular region S20.429 ☑
 jaw S00.82 ☑
 knee S80.22- ☑
 larynx S10.12 ☑
 leg (lower) S80.82- ☑
  knee — *see* Blister, knee
  upper — *see* Blister, thigh
 lip S00.521 ☑
 malar region S00.82 ☑
 mammary — *see* Blister, breast
 mastoid region S00.82 ☑
 mouth S00.522 ☑
 multiple, skin, nontraumatic R23.8
 nail
  finger — *see* Blister, finger
  toe — *see* Blister, toe
 nasal S00.32 ☑
 neck S10.92 ☑
  specified site NEC S10.82 ☑
  throat S10.12 ☑
 nose S00.32 ☑
 occipital region S00.02 ☑
 oral cavity S00.522 ☑
 orbital region — *see* Blister, eyelid
 palate S00.522 ☑
 palm — *see* Blister, hand
 parietal region S00.02 ☑
 pelvis S30.820 ☑
 penis S30.822 ☑
 periocular area — *see* Blister, eyelid
 phalanges
  finger — *see* Blister, finger
  toe — *see* Blister, toe
 pharynx S10.12 ☑
 pinna — *see* Blister, ear
 popliteal space — *see* Blister, knee
 scalp S00.02 ☑
 scapular region — *see* Blister, shoulder
 scrotum S30.823 ☑
 shin — *see* Blister, leg
 shoulder S40.22- ☑
 sternal region S20.329 ☑
 submaxillary region S00.82 ☑
 submental region S00.82 ☑
 subungual
  finger(s) — *see* Blister, finger
  toe(s) — *see* Blister, toe
 supraclavicular fossa S10.82 ☑
 supraorbital S00.82 ☑
 temple S00.82 ☑
 temporal region S00.82 ☑
 testis S30.823 ☑
 thermal — *see* Burn, second degree, by site
 thigh S70.32- ☑
 thorax, thoracic (wall) S20.92 ☑
  back S20.42- ☑
  front S20.32- ☑
 throat S10.12 ☑
 thumb S60.32- ☑
 toe(s) S90.42- ☑
  great S90.42- ☑
 tongue S00.522 ☑
 trachea S10.12 ☑
 tympanum, tympanic membrane — *see* Blister, ear
 upper arm — *see* Blister, arm (upper)
 uvula S00.522 ☑
 vagina S30.824 ☑
 vocal cords S10.12 ☑
 vulva S30.824 ☑
 wrist S60.82- ☑
Bloating R14.0
Bloch-Sulzberger disease or syndrome Q82.3
Block, blocked
 alveolocapillary J84.10
 arborization (heart) I45.5
 arrhythmic I45.9
 atrioventricular (incomplete) (partial) I44.30
  with atrioventricular dissociation I44.2
   complete I44.2

Block, blocked — *continued*
 atrioventricular — *continued*
  complete — *continued*
   congenital Q24.6
  congenital Q24.6
  first degree I44.0
  second degree (types I and II) I44.1
  specified NEC I44.39
  third degree I44.2
  types I and II I44.1
 auriculoventricular — *see* Block, atrioventricular
 bifascicular (cardiac) I45.2
 bundle-branch (complete) (false) (incomplete) I45.4
  bilateral I45.2
  left I44.7
   with right bundle branch block I45.2
   hemiblock I44.60
    anterior I44.4
    posterior I44.5
   incomplete I44.7
    with right bundle branch block I45.2
  right I45.10
   with
    left bundle branch block I45.2
    left fascicular block I45.2
   specified NEC I45.19
  Wilson's type I45.19
 cardiac I45.9
 conduction I45.9
  complete I44.2
 fascicular (left) I44.60
  anterior I44.4
  posterior I44.5
  right I45.0
  specified NEC I44.69
 foramen Magendie (acquired) G91.1
  congenital Q03.1
   with spina bifida — *see* Spina bifida, by site, with hydrocephalus
 heart I45.9
  bundle branch I45.4
   bilateral I45.2
  complete (atrioventricular) I44.2
  congenital Q24.6
  first degree (atrioventricular) I44.0
  second degree (atrioventricular) I44.1
  specified type NEC I45.5
  third degree (atrioventricular) I44.2
 hepatic vein I82.0
 intraventricular (nonspecific) I45.4
  bundle branch
   bilateral I45.2
 kidney N28.9
  postcystoscopic or postprocedural N99.0
 Mobitz (types I and II) I44.1
 myocardial — *see* Block, heart
 nodal I45.5
 organ or site, congenital NEC — *see* Atresia, by site
 portal (vein) I81
 second degree (types I and II) I44.1
 sinoatrial I45.5
 sinoauricular I45.5
 third degree I44.2
 trifascicular I45.3
 tubal N97.1
 vein NOS I82.90
 Wenckebach (types I and II) I44.1
Blockage — *see* Obstruction
Blocq's disease F44.4
Blood
 constituents, abnormal R78.9
 disease D75.9
 donor — *see* Donor, blood
 dyscrasia D75.9
  with
    abortion — *see* Abortion, by type, complicated by, hemorrhage
    ectopic pregnancy O08.1
    molar pregnancy O08.1
   following ectopic or molar pregnancy O08.1
   newborn P61.9
   puerperal, postpartum O72.3
 flukes NEC — *see* Schistosomiasis
 in
   feces K92.1
    occult R19.5
   urine — *see* Hematuria
 mole O02.0

Blood — *continued*
 occult in feces R19.5
 pressure
  decreased, due to shock following injury T79.4 ☑
  examination only Z01.30
  fluctuating I99.8
  high — *see* Hypertension
   borderline R03.0
   incidental reading, without diagnosis of hypertension R03.0
  low — *see also* Hypotension
   incidental reading, without diagnosis of hypotension R03.1
 spitting — *see* Hemoptysis
 staining cornea — *see* Pigmentation, cornea, stromal
 transfusion
  reaction or complication — *see* Complications, transfusion
 type
  A (Rh positive) Z67.10
   Rh negative Z67.11
  AB (Rh positive) Z67.30
   Rh negative Z67.31
  B (Rh positive) Z67.20
   Rh negative Z67.21
  O (Rh positive) Z67.40
   Rh negative Z67.41
  Rh (positive) Z67.90
   negative Z67.91
 vessel rupture — *see* Hemorrhage
 vomiting — *see* Hematemesis
Blood-forming organs, disease D75.9
Bloodgood's disease — *see* Mastopathy, cystic
Bloom (-Machacek)(-Torre) **syndrome** Q82.8
Blount's disease or osteochondrosis — *see* Osteochondrosis, juvenile, tibia
Blue
 baby Q24.9
 diaper syndrome E72.09
 dome cyst (breast) — *see* Cyst, breast
 dot cataract Q12.0
 nevus D22.9
 sclera Q13.5
  with fragility of bone and deafness Q78.0
 toe syndrome I75.02- ☑
Blueness — *see* Cyanosis
Blues, postpartal O90.6
 baby O90.6
Blurring, visual H53.8
Blushing (abnormal) (excessive) R23.2
BMI — *see* Body, mass index
Boarder, hospital NEC Z76.4
 accompanying sick person Z76.3
 healthy infant or child Z76.2
  foundling Z76.1
Bockhart's impetigo L01.02
Bodechtel-Guttman disease (subacute sclerosing panencephalitis) A81.1
Boder-Sedgwick syndrome (ataxia-telangiectasia) G11
Body, bodies
 Aschoff's — *see* Myocarditis, rheumatic
 asteroid, vitreous — *see* Deposit, crystalline
 cytoid (retina) — *see* Occlusion, artery, retina
 drusen (degenerative) (macula) (retinal) — *see also* Degeneration, macula, drusen
  optic disc — *see* Drusen, optic disc
 foreign — *see* Foreign body
 loose
  joint, except knee — *see* Loose, body, joint
   knee M23.4- ☑
  sheath, tendon — *see* Disorder, tendon, specified type NEC
 mass index (BMI)
  adult
   19.9 or less Z68.1
   20.0-20.9 Z68.20
   21.0-21.9 Z68.21
   22.0-22.9 Z68.22
   23.0-23.9 Z68.23
   24.0-24.9 Z68.24
   25.0-25.9 Z68.25
   26.0-26.9 Z68.26
   27.0-27.9 Z68.27
   28.0-28.9 Z68.28
   29.0-29.9 Z68.29
   30.0-30.9 Z68.30
   31.0-31.9 Z68.31
   32.0-32.9 Z68.32

ody, bodies — *continued*
  mass index — *continued*
    adult — *continued*
        33.0-33.9 Z68.33
        34.0-34.9 Z68.34
        35.0-35.9 Z68.35
        36.0-36.9 Z68.36
        37.0-37.9 Z68.37
        38.0-38.9 Z68.38
        39.0-39.9 Z68.39
        40.0-44.9 Z68.41
        45.0-49.9 Z68.42
        50.0-59.9 Z68.43
        60.0-69.9 Z68.44
        70 and over Z68.45
    pediatric
      5th percentile to less than 85th percentile for age Z68.52
      85th percentile to less than 95th percentile for age Z68.53
      greater than or equal to ninety-fifth percentile for age Z68.54
      less than fifth percentile for age Z68.51
  Mooser's A75.2
  rice — *see also* Loose, body, joint
    knee M23.4- ☑
  rocking F98.4
oeck's
  disease or sarcoid — *see* Sarcoidosis
  lupoid (miliary) D86.3
oerhaave's syndrome (spontaneous esophageal rupture) K22.3
oggy
  cervix N88.8
  uterus N85.8
oil — *see also* Furuncle, by site
  Aleppo B55.1
  Baghdad B55.1
  Delhi B55.1
  lacrimal
    gland — *see* Dacryoadenitis
    passages (duct) (sac) — *see* Inflammation, lacrimal, passages, acute
  Natal B55.1
  orbit, orbital — *see* Abscess, orbit
  tropical B55.1
old hives — *see* Urticaria
ombé, iris — *see* Membrane, pupillary
one — *see* condition
onnevie-Ullrich syndrome — *see also* Turner's syndrome Q87.19
onnier's syndrome H81.8 ☑
onvale dam fever T73.3
ony block of joint — *see* Ankylosis
OOP (bronchiolitis obliterans organized pneumonia) J84.89
orderline
  diabetes mellitus R73.03
  hypertension R03.0
  osteopenia M85.8- ☑
  pelvis, with obstruction during labor O65.1
  personality F60.3
orna disease A83.9
ornholm disease B33.0
oston exanthem A88.0
otalli, ductus (patent) (persistent) Q25.0
othriocephalus latus infestation B70.0
otulism (foodborne intoxication) A05.1
  infant A48.51
  non-foodborne A48.52
  wound A48.52
ouba — *see* Yaws
ouchard's nodes (with arthropathy) M15.2
ouffée délirante F23
ouillaud's disease or syndrome (rheumatic heart disease) I01.9
ourneville's disease Q85.1
outonniere deformity (finger) — *see* Deformity, finger, boutonniere
ouveret (-Hoffmann) **syndrome** (paroxysmal tachycardia) I47.9
ovine heart — *see* Hypertrophy, cardiac
owel — *see* condition
owen's
  dermatosis (precancerous) — *see* Neoplasm, skin, in situ
  disease — *see* Neoplasm, skin, in situ

Bowen's — *continued*
  epithelioma — *see* Neoplasm, skin, in situ
  type
    epidermoid carcinoma-in-situ — *see* Neoplasm, skin, in situ
    intraepidermal squamous cell carcinoma — *see* Neoplasm, skin, in situ
Bowing
  femur — *see also* Deformity, limb, specified type NEC, thigh
    congenital Q68.3
  fibula — *see also* Deformity, limb, specified type NEC, lower leg
    congenital Q68.4
  forearm — *see* Deformity, limb, specified type NEC, forearm
  leg(s), long bones, congenital Q68.5
  radius — *see* Deformity, limb, specified type NEC, forearm
  tibia — *see also* Deformity, limb, specified type NEC, lower leg
    congenital Q68.4
Bowleg(s) (acquired) M21.16- ☑
  congenital Q68.5
  rachitic E64.3
Boyd's dysentery A03.2
Brachial — *see* condition
Brachycardia R00.1
Brachycephaly Q75.0
Bradley's disease A08.19
Bradyarrhythmia, cardiac I49.8
Bradycardia (sinoatrial) (sinus) (vagal) R00.1
  neonatal P29.12
  reflex G90.09
  tachycardia syndrome I49.5
Bradykinesia R25.8
Bradypnea R06.89
Bradytachycardia I49.5
Brailsford's disease or osteochondrosis — *see* Osteochondrosis, juvenile, radius
Brain — *see also* condition
  death G93.82
  syndrome — *see* Syndrome, brain
Branched-chain amino-acid disorder E71.2
Branchial — *see* condition
  cartilage, congenital Q18.2
Branchiogenic remnant (in neck) Q18.0
Brandt's syndrome (acrodermatitis enteropathica) E83.2
Brash (water) R12
Bravais-jacksonian epilepsy — *see* Epilepsy, localization-related, symptomatic, with simple partial seizures
Braxton Hicks contractions — *see* False, labor
Brazilian leishmaniasis B55.2
BRBPR K62.5
Break, retina (without detachment) H33.30- ☑
  with retinal detachment — *see* Detachment, retina
  horseshoe tear H33.31- ☑
  multiple H33.33- ☑
  round hole H33.32- ☑
Breakdown
  device, graft or implant — *see also* Complications, by site and type, mechanical T85.618 ☑
    arterial graft NEC — *see* Complication, cardiovascular device, mechanical, vascular
    breast (implant) T85.41 ☑
    catheter NEC T85.618 ☑
      cystostomy T83.010 ☑
      dialysis (renal) T82.41 ☑
        intraperitoneal T85.611 ☑
      Hopkins T83.018 ☑
      ileostomy T83.018 ☑
      infusion NEC T82.514 ☑
        cranial T85.610- ☑
        epidural T85.610 ☑
        intrathecal T85.610 ☑
        spinal T85.610 ☑
        subarachnoid T85.610 ☑
        subdural T85.610 ☑
      nephrostomy T83.012 ☑
      urethral indwelling T83.011 ☑
      urinary NEC T83.018 ☑
      urostomy T83.018 ☑
    electronic (electrode) (pulse generator) (stimulator)
      bone T84.310 ☑
      cardiac T82.119 ☑
        electrode T82.110 ☑

Breakdown — *continued*
  device, graft or implant — *see also* Complications, by site and type, mechanical — *continued*
    electronic — *continued*
      cardiac — *continued*
        pulse generator T82.111 ☑
        specified type NEC T82.118 ☑
      nervous system — *see* Complication, prosthetic device, mechanical, electronic nervous system stimulator
      urinary — *see* Complication, genitourinary, device, urinary, mechanical
    fixation, internal (orthopedic) NEC — *see* Complication, fixation device, mechanical
    gastrointestinal — *see* Complications, prosthetic device, mechanical, gastrointestinal device
    genital NEC T83.418 ☑
      intrauterine contraceptive device T83.31 ☑
      penile prosthesis (cylinder) (implanted) (pump) (resevoir) T83.410 ☑
      testicular prosthesis T83.411 ☑
    heart NEC — *see* Complication, cardiovascular device, mechanical
    intrathecal infusion pump T85.615 ☑
    joint prosthesis — *see* Complications..., joint prosthesis,internal, mechanical, by site
    nervous system, specified device NEC T85.615 ☑
    ocular NEC — *see* Complications, prosthetic device, mechanical, ocular device
    orthopedic NEC — *see* Complication, orthopedic, device, mechanical
    specified NEC T85.618 ☑
    subcutaneous device pocket
      nervous system prosthetic device, implant, or graft T85.890 ☑
      other internal prosthetic device, implant, or graft T85.898 ☑
    sutures, permanent T85.612 ☑
      used in bone repair — *see* Complications, fixation device, internal (orthopedic), mechanical
    urinary NEC T83.118 ☑
      graft T83.21 ☑
      sphincter, implanted T83.111 ☑
      stent (ileal conduit) (nephroureteral) T83.113 ☑
      ureteral indwelling T83.112 ☑
    vascular NEC — *see* Complication, cardiovascular device, mechanical
    ventricular intracranial shunt T85.01 ☑
  nervous F48.8
  perineum O90.1
  respirator J95.850
    specified NEC J95.859
  ventilator J95.850
    specified NEC J95.859
Breast — *see also* condition
  buds E30.1
    in newborn P96.89
  dense R92.2
  nodule — *see also* Lump, breast N63.0
Breath
  foul R19.6
  holder, child R06.89
  holding spell R06.89
  shortness R06.02
Breathing
  labored — *see* Hyperventilation
  mouth R06.5
    causing malocclusion M26.5 ☑
  periodic R06.3
    high altitude G47.32
Breathlessness R06.81
Breda's disease — *see* Yaws
Breech presentation (mother) O32.1 ☑
  causing obstructed labor O64.1 ☑
  footling O32.8 ☑
    causing obstructed labor O64.8 ☑
  incomplete O32.8 ☑
    causing obstructed labor O64.8 ☑
Breisky's disease N90.4
Brennemann's syndrome I88.0
Brenner
  tumor (benign) D27.9
    borderline malignancy D39.1- ☑
    malignant C56 ☑
    proliferating D39.1- ☑
Bretonneau's disease or angina A36.0
Breus' mole O02.0

Brevicollis Q76.49
Brickmakers' anemia B76.9 *[D63.8]*
Bridge, myocardial Q24.5
Bright red blood per rectum (BRBPR) K62.5
Bright's disease — *see also* Nephritis
  arteriosclerotic — *see* Hypertension, kidney
Brill (-Zinsser) **disease** (recrudescent typhus) A75.1
Brill-Symmers' disease C82.90
Brion-Kayser disease — *see* Fever, parathyroid
Briquet's disorder or syndrome F45.0
Brissaud's
  infantilism or dwarfism E23.0
  motor-verbal tic F95.2
Brittle
  bones disease Q78.0
  nails L60.3
    congenital Q84.6
Broad — *see also* condition
  beta disease E78.2
  ligament laceration syndrome N83.8
Broad- or floating-betalipoproteinemia E78.2
Brock's syndrome (atelectasis due to enlarged lymph
  nodes) J98.19
Brocq-Duhring disease (dermatitis herpetiformis) L13.0
Brodie's abscess or disease M86.8X- ☑
Broken
  arches — *see also* Deformity, limb, flat foot
  arm (meaning upper limb) — *see* Fracture, arm
  back — *see* Fracture, vertebra
  bone — *see* Fracture
  implant or internal device — *see* Complications, by site
    and type, mechanical
  leg (meaning lower limb) — *see* Fracture, leg
  nose S02.2 ☑
  tooth, teeth — *see* Fracture, tooth
Bromhidrosis, bromidrosis L75.0
Bromidism, bromism G92
  due to
    correct substance properly administered — *see* Table of Drugs and Chemicals, by drug, adverse effect
    overdose or wrong substance given or taken — *see* Table of Drugs and Chemicals, by drug, poisoning
  chronic (dependence) F13.20
Bromidrosiphobia F40.298
Bronchi, bronchial — *see* condition
Bronchiectasis (cylindrical) (diffuse) (fusiform) (localized)
  (saccular) J47.9
  with
    acute
      bronchitis J47.0
      lower respiratory infection J47.0
    exacerbation (acute) J47.1
  congenital Q33.4
  tuberculous NEC — *see* Tuberculosis, pulmonary
Bronchiolectasis — *see* Bronchiectasis
Bronchiolitis (acute) (infective) (subacute) J21.9
  with
    bronchospasm or obstruction J21.9
    influenza, flu or grippe — *see* Influenza, with, respiratory manifestations NEC
  chemical (chronic) J68.4
    acute J68.0
  chronic (fibrosing) (obliterative) J44.9
  due to
    external agent — *see* Bronchitis, acute, due to
    human metapneumovirus J21.1
    respiratory syncytial virus (RSV) J21.0
    specified organism NEC J21.8
  fibrosa obliterans J44.9
  influenzal — *see* Influenza, with, respiratory manifestations NEC
  obliterans J42
    with organizing pneumonia (BOOP) J84.89
  obliterative (chronic) (subacute) J44.9
    due to fumes or vapors J68.4
    due to chemicals, gases, fumes or vapors (inhalation) J68.4
  respiratory, interstitial lung disease J84.115
Bronchitis (diffuse) (fibrinous) (hypostatic) (infective) (membranous) J40
  with
    influenza, flu or grippe — *see* Influenza, with, respiratory manifestations NEC
    obstruction (airway) (lung) J44.9
    tracheitis (l5 years of age and above) J40

Bronchitis — *continued*
  with — *continued*
    tracheitis — *continued*
      acute or subacute J20.9
      chronic J42
      under l5 years of age J20.9
  acute or subacute (with bronchospasm or obstruction) J20.9
    with
      bronchiectasis J47.0
      chronic obstructive pulmonary disease J44.0
    chemical (due to gases, fumes or vapors) J68.0
    due to
      fumes or vapors J68.0
      Haemophilus influenzae J20.1
      Mycoplasma pneumoniae J20.0
      radiation J70.0
      specified organism NEC J20.8
      Streptococcus J20.2
      virus
        coxsackie J20.3
        echovirus J20.7
        parainfluenzae J20.4
        respiratory syncytial (RSV) J20.5
        rhinovirus J20.6
    viral NEC J20.8
  allergic (acute) J45.909
    with
      exacerbation (acute) J45.901
      status asthmaticus J45.902
  arachidic T17.528 ☑
  aspiration (due to fumes or vapors) J68.0
  asthmatic J45.9 ☑
    chronic J44.9
      with
        acute lower respiratory infection J44.0
        exacerbation (acute) J44.1
  capillary — *see* Pneumonia, broncho
  caseous (tuberculous) A15.5
  Castellani's A69.8
  catarrhal (l5 years of age and above) J40
    acute — *see* Bronchitis, acute
    chronic J41.0
    under l5 years of age J20.9
  chemical (acute) (subacute) J68.0
    chronic J68.4
    due to fumes or vapors J68.0
      chronic J68.4
  chronic J42
    with
      airways obstruction J44.9
      tracheitis (chronic) J42
    asthmatic (obstructive) J44.9
    catarrhal J41.0
    chemical (due to fumes or vapors) J68.4
    due to
      chemicals, gases, fumes or vapors (inhalation) J68.4
      radiation J70.1
      tobacco smoking J41.0
    emphysematous J44.9
    mucopurulent J41.1
    non-obstructive J41.0
    obliterans J44.9
    obstructive J44.9
    purulent J41.1
    simple J41.0
  croupous — *see* Bronchitis, acute
  due to gases, fumes or vapors (chemical) J68.0
  emphysematous (obstructive) J44.9
  exudative — *see* Bronchitis, acute
  fetid J41.1
  grippal — *see* Influenza, with, respiratory manifestations NEC
  in those under l5 years age — *see* Bronchitis, acute
    chronic — *see* Bronchitis, chronic
  influenzal — *see* Influenza, with, respiratory manifestations NEC
  mixed simple and mucopurulent J41.8
  moulder's J62.8
  mucopurulent (chronic) (recurrent) J41.1
    acute or subacute J20.9
    simple (mixed) J41.8
  obliterans (chronic) J44.9
  obstructive (chronic) (diffuse) J44.9
  pituitous J41.1
  pneumococcal, acute or subacute J20.2

Bronchitis — *continued*
  pseudomembranous, acute or subacute — *see* Bronchitis, acute
  purulent (chronic) (recurrent) J41.1
    acute or subacute — *see* Bronchitis, acute
  putrid J41.1
  senile (chronic) J42
  simple and mucopurulent (mixed) J41.8
  smokers' J41.0
  spirochetal NEC A69.8
  subacute — *see* Bronchitis, acute
  suppurative (chronic) J41.1
    acute or subacute — *see* Bronchitis, acute
  tuberculous A15.5
  under l5 years of age — *see* Bronchitis, acute
    chronic — *see* Bronchitis, chronic
  viral NEC, acute or subacute — *see also* Bronchitis, acute J20.8
Bronchoalveolitis J18.0
Bronchoaspergillosis B44.1
Bronchocele meaning goiter E04.0
Broncholithiasis J98.09
  tuberculous NEC A15.5
Bronchomalacia J98.09
  congenital Q32.2
Bronchomycosis NOS B49 *[J99]*
  candidal B37.1
Bronchopleuropneumonia — *see* Pneumonia, broncho
Bronchopneumonia — *see* Pneumonia, broncho
Bronchopneumonitis — *see* Pneumonia, broncho
Bronchopulmonary — *see* condition
Bronchopulmonitis — *see* Pneumonia, broncho
Bronchorrhagia (see Hemoptysis)
Bronchorrhea J98.09
  acute J20.9
  chronic (infective) (purulent) J42
Bronchospasm (acute) J98.01
  with
    bronchiolitis, acute J21.9
    bronchitis, acute (conditions in J20) — *see* Bronchitis, acute
  due to external agent — *see* condition, respiratory, acute, due to
  exercise induced J45.990
Bronchospirochetosis A69.8
  Castellani A69.8
Bronchostenosis J98.09
Bronchus — *see* condition
Brontophobia F40.220
Bronze baby syndrome P83.88
Brooke's tumor — *see* Neoplasm, skin, benign
Brown enamel of teeth (hereditary) K00.5
Brown's sheath syndrome H50.61- ☑
Brown-Séquard disease, paralysis or syndrome G83.81
Bruce sepsis A23.0
Brucellosis (infection) A23.9
  abortus A23.1
  canis A23.3
  dermatitis A23.9
  melitensis A23.0
  mixed A23.8
  sepsis A23.9
    melitensis A23.0
    specified NEC A23.8
  suis A23.2
Bruck-de Lange disease Q87.19
Bruck's disease — *see* Deformity, limb
BRUE (brief resolved unexplained event) R68.13
Brugsch's syndrome Q82.8
Bruise (skin surface intact) — *see also* Contusion
  with
    open wound — *see* Wound, open
  internal organ — *see* Injury, by site
  newborn P54.5
  scalp, due to birth injury, newborn P12.3
  umbilical cord O69.5 ☑
Bruit (arterial) R09.89
  cardiac R01.1
Brush burn — *see* Abrasion, by site
Bruton's X-linked agammaglobulinemia D80.0
Bruxism
  psychogenic F45.8
  sleep related G47.63
Bubbly lung syndrome P27.0
Bubo I88.8
  blennorrhagic (gonococcal) A54.89

☑ **Additional Character Required** — Refer to the Tabular List for Character Selection   ▽ **Subterms under main terms may continue to next column or pa**

Bubo — *continued*
  chancroidal A57
  climatic A55
  due to Haemophilus ducreyi A57
  gonococcal A54.89
  indolent (nonspecific) I88.8
  inguinal (nonspecific) I88.8
    chancroidal A57
    climatic A55
    due to H. ducreyi A57
    infective I88.8
  scrofulous (tuberculous) A18.2
  soft chancre A57
  suppurating — *see* Lymphadenitis, acute
  syphilitic (primary) A51.0
    congenital A50.07
  tropical A55
  virulent (chancroidal) A57
Bubonic plague A20.0
Bubonocele — *see* Hernia, inguinal
Buccal — *see* condition
Buchanan's disease or osteochondrosis M91.0
Buchem's syndrome (hyperostosis corticalis) M85.2
Bucket-handle fracture or tear (semilunar cartilage)
   — *see* Tear, meniscus
Budd-Chiari syndrome (hepatic vein thrombosis) I82.0
Budgerigar fancier's disease or lung J67.2
Buds
  breast E30.1
    in newborn P96.89
Buerger's disease (thromboangiitis obliterans) I73.1
Bulbar — *see* condition
Bulbus cordis (left ventricle) (persistent) Q21.8
Bulimia (nervosa) F50.2
  atypical F50.9
  normal weight F50.9
Bulky
  stools R19.5
  uterus N85.2
Bulla (e) R23.8
  lung (emphysematous) (solitary) J43.9
    newborn P25.8
Bullet wound — *see also* Wound, open
  fracture — *code as* Fracture, by site
  internal organ — *see* Injury, by site
Bundle
  branch block (complete) (false) (incomplete) — *see*
    Block, bundle-branch
  of His — *see* condition
Bunion M21.61- ☑
  tailor's M21.62- ☑
Bunionette M21.62- ☑
Buphthalmia, buphthalmos (congenital) Q15.0
Burdwan fever B55.0
Buried
  penis (congenital) Q55.64
    acquired N48.83
  roots K08.3
Burke's syndrome K86.89
Burkitt
  cell leukemia C91.0- ☑
  lymphoma (malignant) C83.7- ☑
    small noncleaved, diffuse C83.7- ☑
    spleen C83.77
    undifferentiated C83.7- ☑
  tumor C83.7- ☑
  type
    acute lymphoblastic leukemia C91.0- ☑
    undifferentiated C83.7- ☑
Burn (electricity) (flame) (hot gas, liquid or hot object)
  (radiation) (steam) (thermal) T30.0
  abdomen, abdominal (muscle) (wall) T21.02 ☑
    first degree T21.12 ☑
    second degree T21.22 ☑
    third degree T21.32 ☑
  above elbow T22.039 ☑
    first degree T22.139 ☑
    left T22.032 ☑
      first degree T22.132 ☑
      second degree T22.232 ☑
      third degree T22.332 ☑
    right T22.031 ☑
      first degree T22.131 ☑
      second degree T22.231 ☑
      third degree T22.331 ☑
    second degree T22.239 ☑

Burn — *continued*
  above elbow — *continued*
    third degree T22.339 ☑
  acid (caustic) (external) (internal) — *see* Corrosion, by
    site
  alimentary tract NEC T28.2 ☑
    esophagus T28.1 ☑
    mouth T28.0 ☑
    pharynx T28.0 ☑
  alkaline (caustic) (external) (internal) — *see* Corrosion,
    by site
  ankle T25.019 ☑
    first degree T25.119 ☑
    left T25.012 ☑
      first degree T25.112 ☑
      second degree T25.212 ☑
      third degree T25.312 ☑
    multiple with foot — *see* Burn, lower, limb, multiple,
      ankle and foot
    right T25.011 ☑
      first degree T25.111 ☑
      second degree T25.211 ☑
      third degree T25.311 ☑
    second degree T25.219 ☑
    third degree T25.319 ☑
  anus — *see* Burn, buttock
  arm (lower) (upper) — *see* Burn, upper, limb
  axilla T22.049 ☑
    first degree T22.149 ☑
    left T22.042 ☑
      first degree T22.142 ☑
      second degree T22.242 ☑
      third degree T22.342 ☑
    right T22.041 ☑
      first degree T22.141 ☑
      second degree T22.241 ☑
      third degree T22.341 ☑
    second degree T22.249 ☑
    third degree T22.349 ☑
  back (lower) T21.04 ☑
    first degree T21.14 ☑
    second degree T21.24 ☑
    third degree T21.34 ☑
    upper T21.03 ☑
      first degree T21.13 ☑
      second degree T21.23 ☑
      third degree T21.33 ☑
  blisters — *code as* Burn, second degree, by site
  breast(s) — *see* Burn, chest wall
  buttock(s) T21.05 ☑
    first degree T21.15 ☑
    second degree T21.25 ☑
    third degree T21.35 ☑
  calf T24.039 ☑
    first degree T24.139 ☑
    left T24.032 ☑
      first degree T24.132 ☑
      second degree T24.232 ☑
      third degree T24.332 ☑
    right T24.031 ☑
      first degree T24.131 ☑
      second degree T24.231 ☑
      third degree T24.331 ☑
    second degree T24.239 ☑
    third degree T24.339 ☑
  canthus (eye) — *see* Burn, eyelid
  caustic acid or alkaline — *see* Corrosion, by site
  cervix T28.3 ☑
  cheek T20.06 ☑
    first degree T20.16 ☑
    second degree T20.26 ☑
    third degree T20.36 ☑
  chemical (acids) (alkalines) (caustics) (external) (internal) — *see* Corrosion, by site
  chest wall T21.01 ☑
    first degree T21.11 ☑
    second degree T21.21 ☑
    third degree T21.31 ☑
  chin T20.03 ☑
    first degree T20.13 ☑
    second degree T20.23 ☑
    third degree T20.33 ☑
  colon T28.2 ☑
  conjunctiva (and cornea) — *see* Burn, cornea
  cornea (and conjunctiva) T26.1- ☑
    chemical — *see* Corrosion, cornea

Burn — *continued*
  corrosion (external) (internal) — *see* Corrosion, by site
  deep necrosis of underlying tissue — *code as* Burn,
    third degree, by site
  dorsum of hand T23.069 ☑
    first degree T23.169 ☑
    left T23.062 ☑
      first degree T23.162 ☑
      second degree T23.262 ☑
      third degree T23.362 ☑
    right T23.061 ☑
      first degree T23.161 ☑
      second degree T23.261 ☑
      third degree T23.361 ☑
    second degree T23.269 ☑
    third degree T23.369 ☑
  due to ingested chemical agent — *see* Corrosion, by
    site
  ear (auricle) (external) (canal) T20.01 ☑
    first degree T20.11 ☑
    second degree T20.21 ☑
    third degree T20.31 ☑
  elbow T22.029 ☑
    first degree T22.129 ☑
    left T22.022 ☑
      first degree T22.122 ☑
      second degree T22.222 ☑
      third degree T22.322 ☑
    right T22.021 ☑
      first degree T22.121 ☑
      second degree T22.221 ☑
      third degree T22.321 ☑
    second degree T22.229 ☑
    third degree T22.329 ☑
  epidermal loss — *code as* Burn, second degree, by site
  erythema, erythematous — *code as* Burn, first degree,
    by site
  esophagus T28.1 ☑
  extent (percentage of body surface)
    less than 10 percent T31.0
    10-19 percent T31.10
      with 0-9 percent third degree burns T31.10
      with 10-19 percent third degree burns T31.11
    20-29 percent T31.20
      with 0-9 percent third degree burns T31.20
      with 10-19 percent third degree burns T31.21
      with 20-29 percent third degree burns T31.22
    30-39 percent T31.30
      with 0-9 percent third degree burns T31.30
      with 10-19 percent third degree burns T31.31
      with 20-29 percent third degree burns T31.32
      with 30-39 percent third degree burns T31.33
    40-49 percent T31.40
      with 0-9 percent third degree burns T31.40
      with 10-19 percent third degree burns T31.41
      with 20-29 percent third degree burns T31.42
      with 30-39 percent third degree burns T31.43
      with 40-49 percent third degree burns T31.44
    50-59 percent T31.50
      with 0-9 percent third degree burns T31.50
      with 10-19 percent third degree burns T31.51
      with 20-29 percent third degree burns T31.52
      with 30-39 percent third degree burns T31.53
      with 40-49 percent third degree burns T31.54
      with 50-59 percent third degree burns T31.55
    60-69 percent T31.60
      with 0-9 percent third degree burns T31.60
      with 10-19 percent third degree burns T31.61
      with 20-29 percent third degree burns T31.62
      with 30-39 percent third degree burns T31.63
      with 40-49 percent third degree burns T31.64
      with 50-59 percent third degree burns T31.65
      with 60-69 percent third degree burns T31.66
    70-79 percent T31.70
      with 0-9 percent third degree burns T31.70
      with 10-19 percent third degree burns T31.71
      with 20-29 percent third degree burns T31.72
      with 30-39 percent third degree burns T31.73
      with 40-49 percent third degree burns T31.74
      with 50-59 percent third degree burns T31.75
      with 60-69 percent third degree burns T31.76
      with 70-79 percent third degree burns T31.77
    80-89 percent T31.80
      with 0-9 percent third degree burns T31.80
      with 10-19 percent third degree burns T31.81
      with 20-29 percent third degree burns T31.82
      with 30-39 percent third degree burns T31.83

Subterms under main terms may continue to next column or page   ☑ Additional Character Required — Refer to the Tabular List for Character Selection   43

Bubo — Burn

☑ **Additional Character Required — Refer to the Tabular List for Character Selection**   ▽ **Subterms under main terms may continue to next column or page**

Burn — continued
  lower — continued
    limb — continued
      right — continued
        second degree T24.201 ☑
          third degree T24.301 ☑
      second degree T24.209 ☑
      thigh — see Burn, thigh
      third degree T24.309 ☑
      toe — see Burn, toe
  lung (with larynx and trachea) T27.1 ☑
  mouth T28.0 ☑
  neck T20.07 ☑
    first degree T20.17 ☑
    second degree T20.27 ☑
    third degree T20.37 ☑
  nose (septum) T20.04 ☑
    first degree T20.14 ☑
    second degree T20.24 ☑
    third degree T20.34 ☑
  ocular adnexa — see Burn, eye
  orbit region — see Burn, eyelid
  palm T23.059 ☑
    first degree T23.159 ☑
    left T23.052 ☑
      first degree T23.152 ☑
      second degree T23.252 ☑
      third degree T23.352 ☑
    right T23.051 ☑
      first degree T23.151 ☑
      second degree T23.251 ☑
      third degree T23.351 ☑
    second degree T23.259 ☑
    third degree T23.359 ☑
  partial thickness — code as Burn, degree, by site
  pelvis — see Burn, trunk
  penis — see Burn, genital organs, external, male
  perineum
    female — see Burn, genital organs, external, female
    male — see Burn, genital organs, external, male
  periocular area — see Burn, eyelid
  pharynx T28.0 ☑
  rectum T28.2 ☑
  respiratory tract T27.3 ☑
    larynx — see Burn, larynx
    specified part NEC T27.2 ☑
    trachea — see Burn, trachea
  sac, lacrimal — see Burn, eye, specified site NEC
  scalp T20.05 ☑
    first degree T20.15 ☑
    second degree T20.25 ☑
    third degree T20.35 ☑
  scapular region T22.069 ☑
    first degree T22.169 ☑
    left T22.062 ☑
      first degree T22.162 ☑
      second degree T22.262 ☑
      third degree T22.362 ☑
    right T22.061 ☑
      first degree T22.161 ☑
      second degree T22.261 ☑
      third degree T22.361 ☑
    second degree T22.269 ☑
    third degree T22.369 ☑
  sclera — see Burn, eye, specified site NEC
  scrotum — see Burn, genital organs, external, male
  shoulder T22.059 ☑
    first degree T22.159 ☑
    left T22.052 ☑
      first degree T22.152 ☑
      second degree T22.252 ☑
      third degree T22.352 ☑
    right T22.051 ☑
      first degree T22.151 ☑
      second degree T22.251 ☑
      third degree T22.351 ☑
    second degree T22.259 ☑
    third degree T22.359 ☑
  stomach T28.2 ☑
  temple — see Burn, head
  testis — see Burn, genital organs, external, male
  thigh T24.019 ☑
    first degree T24.119 ☑
    left T24.012 ☑
      first degree T24.112 ☑
      second degree T24.212 ☑

Burn — continued
  thigh — continued
    left — continued
      third degree T24.312 ☑
    right T24.011 ☑
      first degree T24.111 ☑
      second degree T24.211 ☑
      third degree T24.311 ☑
    second degree T24.219 ☑
    third degree T24.319 ☑
  thorax (external) — see Burn, trunk
  throat (meaning pharynx) T28.0 ☑
  thumb(s) T23.019 ☑
    first degree T23.119 ☑
    left T23.012 ☑
      first degree T23.112 ☑
      second degree T23.212 ☑
      third degree T23.312 ☑
    multiple sites with fingers T23.049 ☑
      first degree T23.149 ☑
      left T23.042 ☑
        first degree T23.142 ☑
        second degree T23.242 ☑
        third degree T23.342 ☑
      right T23.041 ☑
        first degree T23.141 ☑
        second degree T23.241 ☑
        third degree T23.341 ☑
      second degree T23.249 ☑
      third degree T23.349 ☑
    right T23.011 ☑
      first degree T23.111 ☑
      second degree T23.211 ☑
      third degree T23.311 ☑
    second degree T23.219 ☑
    third degree T23.319 ☑
  toe T25.039 ☑
    first degree T25.139 ☑
    left T25.032 ☑
      first degree T25.132 ☑
      second degree T25.232 ☑
      third degree T25.332 ☑
    right T25.031 ☑
      first degree T25.131 ☑
      second degree T25.231 ☑
      third degree T25.331 ☑
    second degree T25.239 ☑
    third degree T25.339 ☑
  tongue T28.0 ☑
  tonsil(s) T28.0 ☑
  trachea T27.0 ☑
    with lung T27.1 ☑
  trunk T21.00 ☑
    abdominal wall — see Burn, abdominal wall
    anus — see Burn, buttock
    axilla — see Burn, upper limb
    back — see Burn, back
    breast — see Burn, chest wall
    buttock — see Burn, buttock
    chest wall — see Burn, chest wall
    first degree T21.10 ☑
    flank — see Burn, abdominal wall
    genital
      female — see Burn, genital organs, external, female
      male — see Burn, genital organs, external, male
    groin — see Burn, abdominal wall
    interscapular region — see Burn, back, upper
    labia — see Burn, genital organs, external, female
    lower back — see Burn, back
    penis — see Burn, genital organs, external, male
    perineum
      female — see Burn, genital organs, external, female
      male — see Burn, genital organs, external, male
    scapula region — see Burn, scapular region
    scrotum — see Burn, genital organs, external, male
    second degree T21.20 ☑
    specified site NEC T21.09 ☑
      first degree T21.19 ☑
      second degree T21.29 ☑
      third degree T21.39 ☑
    testes — see Burn, genital organs, external, male
    third degree T21.30 ☑
    upper back — see Burn, back, upper
    vulva — see Burn, genital organs, external, female

Burn — continued
  unspecified site with extent of body surface involved
    specified
    less than 10 percent T31.0
    10-19 percent (0-9 percent third degree) T31.10
      with 10-19 percent third degree T31.11
    20-29 percent (0-9 percent third degree) T31.20
      with
        10-19 percent third degree T31.21
        20-29 percent third degree T31.22
    30-39 percent (0-9 percent third degree) T31.30
      with
        10-19 percent third degree T31.31
        20-29 percent third degree T31.32
        30-39 percent third degree T31.33
    40-49 percent (0-9 percent third degree) T31.40
      with
        10-19 percent third degree T31.41
        20-29 percent third degree T31.42
        30-39 percent third degree T31.43
        40-49 percent third degree T31.44
    50-59 percent (0-9 percent third degree) T31.50
      with
        10-19 percent third degree T31.51
        20-29 percent third degree T31.52
        30-39 percent third degree T31.53
        40-49 percent third degree T31.54
        50-59 percent third degree T31.55
    60-69 percent (0-9 percent third degree) T31.60
      with
        10-19 percent third degree T31.61
        20-29 percent third degree T31.62
        30-39 percent third degree T31.63
        40-49 percent third degree T31.64
        50-59 percent third degree T31.65
        60-69 percent third degree T31.66
    70-79 percent (0-9 percent third degree) T31.70
      with
        10-19 percent third degree T31.71
        20-29 percent third degree T31.72
        30-39 percent third degree T31.73
        40-49 percent third degree T31.74
        50-59 percent third degree T31.75
        60-69 percent third degree T31.76
        70-79 percent third degree T31.77
    80-89 percent (0-9 percent third degree) T31.80
      with
        10-19 percent third degree T31.81
        20-29 percent third degree T31.82
        30-39 percent third degree T31.83
        40-49 percent third degree T31.84
        ·50-59 percent third degree T31.85
        60-69 percent third degree T31.86
        70-79 percent third degree T31.87
        80-89 percent third degree T31.88
    90 percent or more (0-9 percent third degree) T31.90
      with
        10-19 percent third degree T31.91
        20-29 percent third degree T31.92
        30-39 percent third degree T31.93
        40-49 percent third degree T31.94
        50-59 percent third degree T31.95
        60-69 percent third degree T31.96
        70-79 percent third degree T31.97
        80-89 percent third degree T31.98
        90-99 percent third degree T31.99
  upper limb T22.00 ☑
    above elbow — see Burn, above elbow
    axilla — see Burn, axilla
    elbow — see Burn, elbow
    first degree T22.10 ☑
    forearm — see Burn, forearm
    hand — see Burn, hand
    interscapular region — see Burn, back, upper
    multiple sites T22.099 ☑
      first degree T22.199 ☑
      left T22.092 ☑
        first degree T22.192 ☑
        second degree T22.292 ☑
        third degree T22.392 ☑
      right T22.091 ☑
        first degree T22.191 ☑
        second degree T22.291 ☑
        third degree T22.391 ☑
      second degree T22.299 ☑
      third degree T22.399 ☑
    scapular region — see Burn, scapular region
    second degree T22.20 ☑

Burn — *continued*
  upper limb — *continued*
    shoulder — *see* Burn, shoulder
    third degree T22.30 ☑
    wrist — *see* Burn, wrist
  uterus T28.3 ☑
  vagina T28.3 ☑
  vulva — *see* Burn, genital organs, external, female
  wrist T23.079 ☑
    first degree T23.179 ☑
    left T23.072 ☑
      first degree T23.172 ☑
      second degree T23.272 ☑
      third degree T23.372 ☑
    multiple sites with hand T23.099 ☑
      first degree T23.199 ☑
      left T23.092 ☑
        first degree T23.192 ☑
        second degree T23.292 ☑
        third degree T23.392 ☑
      right T23.091 ☑
        first degree T23.191 ☑
        second degree T23.291 ☑
        third degree T23.391 ☑
      second degree T23.299 ☑
      third degree T23.399 ☑
    right T23.071 ☑
      first degree T23.171 ☑
      second degree T23.271 ☑
      third degree T23.371 ☑
    second degree T23.279 ☑
    third degree T23.379 ☑
Burnett's syndrome E83.52
Burning
  feet syndrome E53.9
  sensation R20.8
  tongue K14.6
Burn-out (state) Z73.0
Burns' disease or osteochondrosis — *see* Osteochon-
    drosis, juvenile, ulna
Bursa — *see* condition
Bursitis M71.9
  Achilles — *see* Tendinitis, Achilles
  adhesive — *see* Bursitis, specified NEC
  ankle — *see* Enthesopathy, lower limb, ankle, specified
    type NEC
  calcaneal — *see* Enthesopathy, foot, specified type NEC
  collateral ligament, tibial — *see* Bursitis, tibial collateral
  due to use, overuse, pressure — *see also* Disorder, soft
    tissue, due to use, specified type NEC
    specified NEC — *see* Disorder, soft tissue, due to
      use, specified NEC
  Duplay's M75.0
  elbow NEC M70.3- ☑
    olecranon M70.2- ☑
  finger — *see* Disorder, soft tissue, due to use, specified
    type NEC, hand
  foot — *see* Enthesopathy, foot, specified type NEC
  gonococcal A54.49
  gouty — *see* Gout
  hand M70.1- ☑
  hip NEC M70.7- ☑
    trochanteric M70.6- ☑
  infective NEC M71.10
    abscess — *see* Abscess, bursa
    ankle M71.17- ☑
    elbow M71.12- ☑
    foot M71.17- ☑
    hand M71.14- ☑
    hip M71.15- ☑
    knee M71.16- ☑
    multiple sites M71.19
    shoulder M71.11- ☑
    specified site NEC M71.18
    wrist M71.13- ☑
  ischial — *see* Bursitis, hip
  knee NEC M70.5- ☑
    prepatellar M70.4- ☑
  occupational NEC — *see also* Disorder, soft tissue, due
    to, use
  olecranon — *see* Bursitis, elbow, olecranon
  pharyngeal J39.1
  popliteal — *see* Bursitis, knee
  prepatellar M70.4- ☑
  radiohumeral M77.8
  rheumatoid M06.20

Bursitis — *continued*
  rheumatoid — *continued*
    ankle M06.27- ☑
    elbow M06.22- ☑
    foot joint M06.27- ☑
    hand joint M06.24- ☑
    hip M06.25- ☑
    knee M06.26- ☑
    multiple site M06.29
    shoulder M06.21- ☑
    vertebra M06.28
    wrist M06.23- ☑
  scapulohumeral — *see* Bursitis, shoulder
  semimembranous muscle (knee) — *see* Bursitis, knee
  shoulder M75.5-
    adhesive — *see* Capsulitis, adhesive
  specified NEC M71.50
    ankle M71.57- ☑
    due to use, overuse or pressure — *see* Disorder, soft
      tissue, due to, use
    elbow M71.52- ☑
    foot M71.57- ☑
    hand M71.54- ☑
    hip M71.55- ☑
    knee M71.56- ☑
    shoulder — *see* Bursitis, shoulder
    specified site NEC M71.58
    tibial collateral M76.4- ☑
    wrist M71.53- ☑
  subacromial — *see* Bursitis, shoulder
  subcoracoid — *see* Bursitis, shoulder
  subdeltoid — *see* Bursitis, shoulder
  syphilitic A52.78
  Thornwaldt, Tornwaldt J39.2
  tibial collateral M76.4- ☑
  toe — *see* Enthesopathy, foot, specified type NEC
  trochanteric (area) — *see* Bursitis, hip, trochanteric
  wrist — *see* Bursitis, hand
Bursopathy M71.9
  specified type NEC M71.80
    ankle M71.87- ☑
    elbow M71.82- ☑
    foot M71.87- ☑
    hand M71.84- ☑
    hip M71.85- ☑
    knee M71.86- ☑
    multiple sites M71.89
    shoulder M71.81- ☑
    specified site NEC M71.88
    wrist M71.83- ☑
Burst stitches or sutures (complication of surgery)
    T81.31 ☑
  external operation wound T81.31 ☑
  internal operation wound T81.32 ☑
Buruli ulcer A31.1
Bury's disease L95.1
Buschke's
  disease B45.3
  scleredema — *see* Sclerosis, systemic
Busse-Buschke disease B45.3
Buttock — *see* condition
Button
  Biskra B55.1
  Delhi B55.1
  oriental B55.1
Buttonhole deformity (finger) — *see* Deformity, finger,
    boutonniere
Bwamba fever A92.8
Byssinosis J66.0
Bywaters' syndrome T79.5 ☑

C

Cachexia R64
  cancerous R64
  cardiac — *see* Disease, heart
  dehydration E86.0
  due to malnutrition R64
  exophthalmic — *see* Hyperthyroidism
  heart — *see* Disease, heart
  hypophyseal E23.0
  hypopituitary E23.0
  lead — *see* Poisoning, lead
  malignant R64
  marsh — *see* Malaria
  nervous F48.8

Cachexia — *continued*
  old age R54
  paludal — *see* Malaria
  pituitary E23.0
  renal N28.9
  saturnine — *see* Poisoning, lead
  senile R54
  Simmonds' E23.0
  splenica D73.0
  strumipriva E03.4
  tuberculous NEC — *see* Tuberculosis
CADASIL (cerebral autosomal dominant arteriopathy with
    subcortical infarcts and leukoencephalopathy)
    I67.850
Café, au lait spots L81.3
Caffeine-induced
  anxiety disorder F15.980
  sleep disorder F15.982
Caffey's syndrome Q78.8
Caisson disease T70.3 ☑
Cake kidney Q63.1
Caked breast (puerperal, postpartum) O92.79
Calabar swelling B74.3
Calcaneal spur — *see* Spur, bone, calcaneal
Calcaneo-apophysitis M92.8
Calcareous — *see* condition
Calcicosis J62.8
Calciferol (vitamin D) deficiency E55.9
  with rickets E55.0
Calcification
  adrenal (capsule) (gland) E27.49
    tuberculous E35 *[B90.8]*
  aorta I70.0
  artery (annular) — *see* Arteriosclerosis
  auricle (ear) — *see* Disorder, pinna, specified type NE
  basal ganglia G23.8
  bladder N32.89
    due to Schistosoma hematobium B65.0
  brain (cortex) — *see* Calcification, cerebral
  bronchus J98.09
  bursa M71.40
    ankle M71.47- ☑
    elbow M71.42- ☑
    foot M71.47- ☑
    hand M71.44- ☑
    hip M71.45- ☑
    knee M71.46- ☑
    multiple sites M71.49
    shoulder M75.3- ☑
    specified site NEC M71.48
    wrist M71.43- ☑
  cardiac — *see* Degeneration, myocardial
  cerebral (cortex) G93.89
    artery I67.2
  cervix (uteri) N88.8
  choroid plexus G93.89
  conjunctiva — *see* Concretion, conjunctiva
  corpora cavernosa (penis) N48.89
  cortex (brain) — *see* Calcification, cerebral
  dental pulp (nodular) K04.2
  dentinal papilla K00.4
  fallopian tube N83.8
  falx cerebri G96.19
  gallbladder K82.8
  general E83.59
  heart — *see also* Degeneration, myocardial
    valve — *see* Endocarditis
  idiopathic infantile arterial (IIAC) Q28.8
  intervertebral cartilage or disc (postinfective) — *see*
    Disorder, disc, specified NEC
  intracranial — *see* Calcification, cerebral
  joint — *see* Disorder, joint, specified type NEC
  kidney N28.89
    tuberculous N29 *[B90.1]*
  larynx (senile) J38.7
  lens — *see* Cataract, specified NEC
  lung (active) (postinfectional) J98.4
    tuberculous B90.9
  lymph gland or node (postinfectional) I89.8
    tuberculous — *see also* Tuberculosis, lymph glan
      B90.8
  mammographic R92.1
  massive (paraplegic) — *see* Myositis, ossificans, in,
    quadriplegia
  medial — *see* Arteriosclerosis, extremities
  meninges (cerebral) (spinal) G96.19
  metastatic E83.59

alcification — *continued*
  Mönckeberg's — *see* Arteriosclerosis, extremities
  muscle M61.9
    due to burns — *see* Myositis, ossificans, in, burns
    paralytic — *see* Myositis, ossificans, in, quadriplegia
    specified type NEC M61.40
      ankle M61.47- ☑
      foot M61.47- ☑
      forearm M61.43- ☑
      hand M61.44- ☑
      lower leg M61.46- ☑
      multiple sites M61.49
      pelvic region M61.45- ☑
      shoulder region M61.41- ☑
      specified site NEC M61.48
      thigh M61.45- ☑
      upper arm M61.42- ☑
  myocardium, myocardial — *see* Degeneration, myocardial
  ovary N83.8
  pancreas K86.89
  penis N48.89
  periarticular — *see* Disorder, joint, specified type NEC
  pericardium — *see also* Pericarditis I31.1
  pineal gland E34.8
  pleura J94.8
    postinfectional J94.8
    tuberculous NEC B90.9
  pulpal (dental) (nodular) K04.2
  sclera H15.89
  spleen D73.89
  subcutaneous L94.2
  suprarenal (capsule) (gland) E27.49
  tendon (sheath) — *see also* Tenosynovitis, specified type NEC
    with bursitis, synovitis or tenosynovitis — *see* Tendinitis, calcific
  trachea J39.8
  ureter N28.89
  uterus N85.8
  vitreous — *see* Deposit, crystalline
alcified — *see* Calcification
alcinosis (interstitial) (tumoral) (universalis) E83.59
  with Raynaud's phenomenon, esophageal dysfunction, sclerodactyly, telangiectasia (CREST syndrome) M34.1
  circumscripta (skin) L94.2
  cutis L94.2
alciphylaxis — *see also* Calcification, by site E83.59
alcium
  deposits — *see* Calcification, by site
  metabolism disorder E83.50
  salts or soaps in vitreous — *see* Deposit, crystalline
alciuria R82.994
alculi — *see* Calculus
alculosis, intrahepatic — *see* Calculus, bile duct
alculus, calculi, calculous
  ampulla of Vater — *see* Calculus, bile duct
  anuria (impacted) (recurrent) — *see also* Calculus, urinary N20.9
  appendix K38.1
  bile duct (common) (hepatic) K80.50
    with
      calculus of gallbladder — *see* Calculus, gallbladder and bile duct
      cholangitis K80.30
        with
          cholecystitis — *see* Calculus, bile duct, with cholecystitis
          obstruction K80.31
        acute K80.32
          with
            chronic cholangitis K80.36
              with obstruction K80.37
            obstruction K80.33
        chronic K80.34
          with
            acute cholangitis K80.36
              with obstruction K80.37
            obstruction K80.35
      cholecystitis (with cholangitis) K80.40
        with obstruction K80.41
        acute K80.42
          with
            chronic cholecystitis K80.46
              with obstruction K80.47
            obstruction K80.43
        chronic K80.44

Calculus, calculi, calculous — *continued*
  bile duct — *continued*
    with — *continued*
      cholecystitis — *continued*
        chronic — *continued*
          with
            acute cholecystitis K80.46
              with obstruction K80.47
            obstruction K80.45
  biliary — *see also* Calculus, gallbladder
    specified NEC K80.80
    with obstruction K80.81
  bilirubin, multiple — *see* Calculus, gallbladder
  bladder (encysted) (impacted) (urinary) (diverticulum) N21.0
  bronchus J98.09
  calyx (kidney) (renal) — *see* Calculus, kidney
  cholesterol (pure) (solitary) — *see* Calculus, gallbladder
  common duct (bile) — *see* Calculus, bile duct
  conjunctiva — *see* Concretion, conjunctiva
  cystic N21.0
    duct — *see* Calculus, gallbladder
  dental (subgingival) (supragingival) K03.6
  diverticulum
    bladder N21.0
    kidney N20.0
  epididymis N50.89
  gallbladder K80.20
    with
      bile duct calculus — *see* Calculus, gallbladder and bile duct
      cholecystitis K80.10
        with obstruction K80.11
        acute K80.00
          with
            chronic cholecystitis K80.12
              with obstruction K80.13
            obstruction K80.01
        chronic K80.10
          with
            acute cholecystitis K80.12
              with obstruction K80.13
            obstruction K80.11
        specified NEC K80.18
          with obstruction K80.19
      obstruction K80.21
  gallbladder and bile duct K80.70
    with
      cholecystitis K80.60
        with obstruction K80.61
        acute K80.62
          with
            chronic cholecystitis K80.66
              with obstruction K80.67
            obstruction K80.63
        chronic K80.64
          with
            acute cholecystitis K80.66
              with obstruction K80.67
            obstruction K80.65
      obstruction K80.71
  hepatic (duct) — *see* Calculus, bile duct
  ileal conduit N21.8
  intestinal (impaction) (obstruction) K56.49
  kidney (impacted) (multiple) (pelvis) (recurrent) (staghorn) N20.0
    with calculus, ureter N20.2
    congenital Q63.8
  lacrimal passages — *see* Dacryolith
  liver (impacted) — *see* Calculus, bile duct
  lung J98.4
  mammographic R92.1
  nephritic (impacted) (recurrent) — *see* Calculus, kidney
  nose J34.89
  pancreas (duct) K86.89
  parotid duct or gland K11.5
  pelvis, encysted — *see* Calculus, kidney
  prostate N42.0
  pulmonary J98.4
  pyelitis (impacted) (recurrent) N20.0
    with hydronephrosis N13.6
  pyelonephritis (impacted) (recurrent) — *see* category N20 ☑
    with hydronephrosis N13.6
  renal (impacted) (recurrent) — *see* Calculus, kidney
  salivary (duct) (gland) K11.5
  seminal vesicle N50.89
  staghorn — *see* Calculus, kidney

Calculus, calculi, calculous — *continued*
  Stensen's duct K11.5
  stomach K31.89
  sublingual duct or gland K11.5
    congenital Q38.4
  submandibular duct, gland or region K11.5
  submaxillary duct, gland or region K11.5
  suburethral N21.8
  tonsil J35.8
  tooth, teeth (subgingival) (supragingival) K03.6
  tunica vaginalis N50.89
  ureter (impacted) (recurrent) N20.1
    with calculus, kidney N20.2
      with hydronephrosis N13.2
        with infection N13.6
  urethra (impacted) N21.1
  urinary (duct) (impacted) (passage) (tract) N20.9
    with hydronephrosis N13.2
      with infection N13.6
    in (due to)
      lower N21.9
        specified NEC N21.8
  vagina N89.8
  vesical (impacted) N21.0
  Wharton's duct K11.5
  xanthine E79.8 *[N22]*
Calicectasis N28.89
Caliectasis N28.89
California
  disease B38.9
  encephalitis A83.5
Caligo cornea — *see* Opacity, cornea, central
Callositas, callosity (infected) L84
Callus (infected) L84
  bone — *see* Osteophyte
    excessive, following fracture — *code as* Sequelae of fracture
CALME (childhood asymmetric labium majus enlargement) N90.61
Calorie deficiency or malnutrition — *see also* Malnutrition E46
Calvé-Perthes disease — *see* Legg-Calvé-Perthes disease
Calvé's disease — *see* Osteochondrosis, juvenile, spine
Calvities — *see* Alopecia, androgenic
Cameroon fever — *see* Malaria
Camptocormia (hysterical) F44.4
Camurati-Engelmann syndrome Q78.3
Canal — *see also* condition
  atrioventricular common Q21.2
Canaliculitis (lacrimal) (acute) (subacute) H04.33- ☑
  Actinomyces A42.89
  chronic H04.42- ☑
Canavan's disease E75.29
Canceled procedure (surgical) Z53.9
  because of
    contraindication Z53.09
      smoking Z53.01
    left against medical advice (AMA) Z53.29
    patient's decision Z53.20
      for reasons of belief or group pressure Z53.1
      specified reason NEC Z53.29
    specified reason NEC Z53.8
Cancer — *see also* Neoplasm, by site, malignant
  bile duct type liver C22.1
  blood — *see* Leukemia
  breast — *see also* Neoplasm, breast, malignant C50.91- ☑
  hepatocellular C22.0
  lung — *see also* Neoplasm, lung, malignant C34.90
  ovarian — *see also* Neoplasm ovary, malignant C56.9
  unspecified site (primary) C80.1
Cancer (o)phobia F45.29
Cancerous — *see* Neoplasm, malignant, by site
Cancrum oris A69.0
Candidiasis, candidal B37.9
  balanitis B37.42
  bronchitis B37.1
  cheilitis B37.83
  congenital P37.5
  cystitis B37.41
  disseminated B37.7
  endocarditis B37.6
  enteritis B37.82
  esophagitis B37.81
  intertrigo B37.2
  lung B37.1
  meningitis B37.5

Candidiasis, candidal — *continued*
  mouth B37.Ø
  nails B37.2
  neonatal P37.5
  onychia B37.2
  oral B37.Ø
  osteomyelitis B37.89
  otitis externa B37.84
  paronychia B37.2
  perionyxis B37.2
  pneumonia B37.1
  proctitis B37.82
  pulmonary B37.1
  pyelonephritis B37.49
  sepsis B37.7
  skin B37.2
  specified site NEC B37.89
  stomatitis B37.Ø
  systemic B37.7
  urethritis B37.41
  urogenital site NEC B37.49
  vagina B37.3
  vulva B37.3
  vulvovaginitis B37.3
Candidid L3Ø.2
Candidosis — *see* Candidiasis
Candiru infection or infestation B88.8
Canities (premature) L67.1
  congenital Q84.2
Canker (mouth) (sore) K12.Ø
  rash A38.9
Cannabinosis J66.2
Cannabis induced
  anxiety disorder F12.98Ø
  psychotic disorder F12.959
  sleep disorder F12.988
Canton fever A75.9
Cantrell's syndrome Q87.89
Capillariasis (intestinal) B81.1
  hepatic B83.8
Capillary — *see* condition
Caplan's syndrome — *see* Rheumatoid, lung
Capsule — *see* condition
Capsulitis (joint) — *see also* Enthesopathy
  adhesive (shoulder) M75.Ø- ☑
  hepatic K65.8
  labyrinthine — *see* Otosclerosis, specified NEC
  thyroid EØ6.9
Caput
  crepitus Q75.8
  medusae I86.8
  succedaneum P12.81
Car sickness T75.3 ☑
Carapata (disease) A68.Ø
Carate — *see* Pinta
Carbon lung J6Ø
Carbuncle LØ2.93
  abdominal wall LØ2.231
  anus K61.Ø
  auditory canal, external — *see* Abscess, ear, external
  auricle ear — *see* Abscess, ear, external
  axilla LØ2.43- ☑
  back (any part) LØ2.232
  breast N61.1
  buttock LØ2.33
  cheek (external) LØ2.Ø3
  chest wall LØ2.233
  chin LØ2.Ø3
  corpus cavernosum N48.21
  ear (any part) (external) (middle) — *see* Abscess, ear, external
  external auditory canal — *see* Abscess, ear, external
  eyelid — *see* Abscess, eyelid
  face NEC LØ2.Ø3
  femoral (region) — *see* Carbuncle, lower limb
  finger — *see* Carbuncle, hand
  flank LØ2.231
  foot LØ2.63- ☑
  forehead LØ2.Ø3
  genital — *see* Abscess, genital
  gluteal (region) LØ2.33
  groin LØ2.234
  hand LØ2.53- ☑
  head NEC LØ2.831
  heel — *see* Carbuncle, foot
  hip — *see* Carbuncle, lower limb
  kidney — *see* Abscess, kidney

Carbuncle — *continued*
  knee — *see* Carbuncle, lower limb
  labium (majus) (minus) N76.4
  lacrimal
    gland — *see* Dacryoadenitis
    passages (duct) (sac) — *see* Inflammation, lacrimal, passages, acute
  leg — *see* Carbuncle, lower limb
  lower limb LØ2.43- ☑
  malignant A22.Ø
  navel LØ2.236
  neck LØ2.13
  nose (external) (septum) J34.Ø
  orbit, orbital — *see* Abscess, orbit
  palmar (space) — *see* Carbuncle, hand
  partes posteriores LØ2.33
  pectoral region LØ2.233
  penis N48.21
  perineum LØ2.235
  pinna — *see* Abscess, ear, external
  popliteal — *see* Carbuncle, lower limb
  scalp LØ2.831
  seminal vesicle N49.Ø
  shoulder — *see* Carbuncle, upper limb
  specified site NEC LØ2.838
  temple (region) LØ2.Ø3
  thumb — *see* Carbuncle, hand
  toe — *see* Carbuncle, foot
  trunk LØ2.239
    abdominal wall LØ2.231
    back LØ2.232
    chest wall LØ2.233
    groin LØ2.234
    perineum LØ2.235
    umbilicus LØ2.236
  umbilicus LØ2.236
  upper limb LØ2.43- ☑
  urethra N34.Ø
  vulva N76.4
Carbunculus — *see* Carbuncle
Carcinoid (tumor) — *see* Tumor, carcinoid
Carcinoidosis E34.Ø
Carcinoma (malignant) — *see also* Neoplasm, by site, malignant
  acidophil
    specified site — *see* Neoplasm, malignant, by site
    unspecified site C75.1
  acidophil-basophil, mixed
    specified site — *see* Neoplasm, malignant, by site
    unspecified site C75.1
  adnexal (skin) — *see* Neoplasm, skin, malignant
  adrenal cortical C74.Ø- ☑
  alveolar — *see* Neoplasm, lung, malignant
    cell — *see* Neoplasm, lung, malignant
  ameloblastic C41.1
    upper jaw (bone) C41.Ø
  apocrine
    breast — *see* Neoplasm, breast, malignant
    specified site NEC — *see* Neoplasm, skin, malignant
    unspecified site C44.99
  basal cell (pigmented) (*see also* Neoplasm, skin, malignant) C44.91
    fibro-epithelial — *see* Neoplasm, skin, malignant
    morphea — *see* Neoplasm, skin, malignant
    multicentric — *see* Neoplasm, skin, malignant
  basaloid
  basal-squamous cell, mixed — *see* Neoplasm, skin, malignant
  basophil
    specified site — *see* Neoplasm, malignant, by site
    unspecified site C75.1
  basophil-acidophil, mixed
    specified site — *see* Neoplasm, malignant, by site
    unspecified site C75.1
  basosquamous — *see* Neoplasm, skin, malignant
  bile duct
    with hepatocellular, mixed C22.Ø
    liver C22.1
    specified site NEC — *see* Neoplasm, malignant, by site
    unspecified site C22.1
  branchial or branchiogenic C1Ø.4
  bronchial or bronchogenic — *see* Neoplasm, lung, malignant
  bronchiolar — *see* Neoplasm, lung, malignant
  bronchioloalveolar — *see* Neoplasm, lung, malignant

Carcinoma — *continued*
  C cell
    specified site — *see* Neoplasm, malignant, by site
    unspecified site C73
  ceruminous C44.29- ☑
  cervix uteri
    in situ DØ6.9
      endocervix DØ6.Ø
      exocervix DØ6.1
      specified site NEC DØ6.7
  chorionic
    specified site — *see* Neoplasm, malignant, by site
    unspecified site
      female C58
      male C62.9Ø
  chromophobe
    specified site — *see* Neoplasm, malignant, by site
    unspecified site C75.1
  cloacogenic
    specified site — *see* Neoplasm, malignant, by site
    unspecified site C21.2
  diffuse type
    specified site — *see* Neoplasm, malignant, by site
    unspecified site C16.9
  duct (cell)
    with Paget's disease — *see* Neoplasm, breast, malignant
    infiltrating
      with lobular carcinoma (in situ)
        specified site — *see* Neoplasm, malignant, by site
        unspecified site (female) C5Ø.91- ☑
          male C5Ø.92- ☑
      specified site — *see* Neoplasm, malignant, by site
      unspecified site (female) C5Ø.91- ☑
        male C5Ø.92- ☑
  ductal
    with lobular
      specified site — *see* Neoplasm, malignant, by site
      unspecified site (female) C5Ø.91- ☑
        male C5Ø.92- ☑
  ductular, infiltrating
    specified site — *see* Neoplasm, malignant, by site
    unspecified site (female) C5Ø.91- ☑
      male C5Ø.92- ☑
  embryonal
    liver C22.7
  endometrioid
    specified site — *see* Neoplasm, malignant, by site
    unspecified site
      female C56.9
      male C61
  eosinophil
    specified site — *see* Neoplasm, malignant, by site
    unspecified site C75.1
  epidermoid — *see also* Neoplasm, skin, malignant
    in situ, Bowen's type — *see* Neoplasm, skin, in situ
  fibroepithelial, basal cell — *see* Neoplasm, skin, malignant
  follicular
    with papillary (mixed) C73
    moderately differentiated C73
    pure follicle C73
    specified site — *see* Neoplasm, malignant, by site
    trabecular C73
    unspecified site C73
    well differentiated C73
  generalized, with unspecified primary site C8Ø.Ø
  glycogen-rich — *see* Neoplasm, breast, malignant
  granulosa cell C56- ☑
  hepatic cell C22.Ø
  hepatocellular C22.Ø
    with bile duct, mixed C22.Ø
    fibrolamellar C22.Ø
  hepatocholangiolitic C22.Ø
  Hurthle cell C73
  in
    adenomatous
      polyposis coli C18.9
    pleomorphic adenoma — *see* Neoplasm, salivary glands, malignant
    situ — *see* Carcinoma-in-situ

☑ **Additional Character Required** — Refer to the Tabular List for Character Selection   ▼ Subterms under main terms may continue to next column or pa●

Carcinoma — *continued*
- infiltrating
  - duct
    - with lobular
      - specified site — *see* Neoplasm, malignant, by site
      - unspecified site (female) C50.91- ☑
        - male C50.92- ☑
    - with Paget's disease — *see* Neoplasm, breast, malignant
    - specified site — *see* Neoplasm, malignant
    - unspecified site (female) C50.91- ☑
      - male C50.92- ☑
  - ductular
    - specified site — *see* Neoplasm, malignant
    - unspecified site (female) C50.91- ☑
      - male C50.92- ☑
  - lobular
    - specified site — *see* Neoplasm, malignant
    - unspecified site (female) C50.91- ☑
      - male C50.92- ☑
- inflammatory
  - specified site — *see* Neoplasm, malignant
  - unspecified site (female) C50.91- ☑
    - male C50.92- ☑
- intestinal type
  - specified site — *see* Neoplasm, malignant, by site
  - unspecified site C16.9
- intracystic
  - noninfiltrating — *see* Neoplasm, in situ, by site
- intraductal (noninfiltrating)
  - with Paget's disease — *see* Neoplasm, breast, malignant
    - breast D05.1- ☑
  - papillary
    - with invasion
      - specified site — *see* Neoplasm, malignant, by site
      - unspecified site (female) C50.91- ☑
        - male C50.92- ☑
    - breast D05.1- ☑
    - specified site NEC — *see* Neoplasm, in situ, by site
    - unspecified site (female) D05.1- ☑
  - specified site NEC — *see* Neoplasm, in situ, by site
  - unspecified site (female) D05.1- ☑
- intraepidermal — *see* Neoplasm, in situ
  - squamous cell, Bowen's type — *see* Neoplasm, skin, in situ
- intraepithelial — *see* Neoplasm, in situ, by site
  - squamous cell — *see* Neoplasm, in situ, by site
- intraosseous C41.1
  - upper jaw (bone) C41.0
- islet cell
  - with exocrine, mixed
    - specified site — *see* Neoplasm, malignant, by site
    - unspecified site C25.9
  - pancreas C25.4
  - specified site NEC — *see* Neoplasm, malignant, by site
  - unspecified site C25.4
- juvenile, breast — *see* Neoplasm, breast, malignant
- large cell
  - small cell
    - specified site — *see* Neoplasm, malignant, by site
    - unspecified site C34.90
- Leydig cell (testis)
  - specified site — *see* Neoplasm, malignant, by site
  - unspecified site
    - female C56.9
    - male C62.90
- lipid-rich (female) C50.91- ☑
  - male C50.92- ☑
- liver cell C22.0
- liver NEC C22.7
- lobular (infiltrating)
  - with intraductal
    - specified site — *see* Neoplasm, malignant, by site
    - unspecified site (female) C50.91- ☑
      - male C50.92- ☑
  - noninfiltrating
    - breast D05.0- ☑
    - specified site NEC — *see* Neoplasm, in situ, by site

Carcinoma — *continued*
- lobular — *continued*
  - noninfiltrating — *continued*
    - unspecified site D05.0- ☑
  - specified site — *see* Neoplasm, malignant, by site
  - unspecified site (female) C50.91- ☑
    - male C50.92- ☑
- medullary
  - with
    - amyloid stroma
      - specified site — *see* Neoplasm, malignant, by site
      - unspecified site C73
    - lymphoid stroma
      - specified site — *see* Neoplasm, malignant, by site
      - unspecified site (female) C50.91- ☑
        - male C50.92- ☑
- Merkel cell C4A.9 (*following* C43)
  - anal margin C4A.51 (*following* C43)
  - anal skin C4A.51 (*following* C43)
  - canthus C4A.1- ☑ (*following* C43)
  - ear and external auricular canal C4A.2- ☑ (*following* C43)
  - external auricular canal C4A.2- ☑ (*following* C43)
  - eyelid, including canthus C4A.1- ☑ (*following* C43)
  - face C4A.30 (*following* C43)
    - specified NEC C4A.39 (*following* C43)
  - hip C4A.7- ☑ (*following* C43)
  - lip C4A.0 (*following* C43)
  - lower limb, including hip C4A.7- ☑ (*following* C43)
  - neck C4A.4 (*following* C43)
  - nodal presentation C7B.1 (*following* C75)
  - nose C4A.31 (*following* C43)
  - overlapping sites C4A.8 (*following* C43)
  - perianal skin C4A.51 (*following* C43)
  - scalp C4A.4 (*following* C43)
  - secondary C7B.1 (*following* C75)
  - shoulder C4A.6- ☑ (*following* C43)
  - skin of breast C4A.52 (*following* C43)
  - trunk NEC C4A.59 (*following* C43)
  - upper limb, including shoulder C4A.6- ☑ (*following* C43)
  - visceral metastatic C7B.1 (*following* C75)
- metastatic — *see* Neoplasm, secondary, by site
- metatypical — *see* Neoplasm, skin, malignant
- morphea, basal cell — *see* Neoplasm, skin, malignant
- mucoid
  - cell
    - specified site — *see* Neoplasm, malignant, by site
    - unspecified site C75.1
- neuroendocrine — *see also* Tumor, neuroendocrine
  - high grade, any site C7A.1 (*following* C75)
  - poorly differentiated, any site C7A.1 (*following* C75)
- nonencapsulated sclerosing C73
- noninfiltrating
  - intracystic — *see* Neoplasm, in situ, by site
  - intraductal
    - breast D05.1- ☑
    - papillary
      - breast D05.1- ☑
      - specified site NEC — *see* Neoplasm, in situ, by site
      - unspecified site D05.1- ☑
    - specified site — *see* Neoplasm, in situ, by site
    - unspecified site D05.1- ☑
  - lobular
    - breast D05.0- ☑
    - specified site NEC — *see* Neoplasm, in situ, by site
    - unspecified site (female) D05.0- ☑
- oat cell
  - specified site — *see* Neoplasm, malignant, by site
  - unspecified site C34.90
- odontogenic C41.1
  - upper jaw (bone) C41.0
- papillary
  - with follicular (mixed) C73
  - follicular variant C73
  - intraductal (noninfiltrating)
    - with invasion
      - specified site — *see* Neoplasm, malignant, by site
      - unspecified site (female) C50.91- ☑
        - male C50.92- ☑
    - breast D05.1- ☑

Carcinoma — *continued*
- papillary — *continued*
  - intraductal — *continued*
    - specified site NEC — *see* Neoplasm, in situ, by site
    - unspecified site D05.1- ☑
  - serous
    - specified site — *see* Neoplasm, malignant, by site
    - surface
      - specified site — *see* Neoplasm, malignant, by site
      - unspecified site C56.9
    - unspecified site C56.9
- papillocystic
  - specified site — *see* Neoplasm, malignant, by site
  - unspecified site C56.9
- parafollicular cell
  - specified site — *see* Neoplasm, malignant, by site
  - unspecified site C73
- pilomatrix — *see* Neoplasm, skin, malignant
- pseudomucinous
  - specified site — *see* Neoplasm, malignant, by site
  - unspecified site C56.9
- renal cell C64- ☑
- Schmincke — *see* Neoplasm, nasopharynx, malignant
- Schneiderian
  - specified site — *see* Neoplasm, malignant, by site
  - unspecified site C30.0
- sebaceous — *see* Neoplasm, skin, malignant
- secondary — *see also* Neoplasm, secondary, by site
  - Merkel cell C7B.1 (*following* C75)
- secretory, breast — *see* Neoplasm, breast, malignant
- serous
  - papillary
    - specified site — *see* Neoplasm, malignant, by site
    - unspecified site C56.9
  - surface, papillary
    - specified site — *see* Neoplasm, malignant, by site
    - unspecified site C56.9
- Sertoli cell
  - specified site — *see* Neoplasm, malignant, by site
  - unspecified site C62.90
    - female C56.9
    - male C62.90
- skin appendage — *see* Neoplasm, skin, malignant
- small cell
  - fusiform cell
    - specified site — *see* Neoplasm, malignant, by site
    - unspecified site C34.90
  - intermediate cell
    - specified site — *see* Neoplasm, malignant, by site
    - unspecified site C34.90
  - large cell
    - specified site — *see* Neoplasm, malignant, by site
    - unspecified site C34.90
- solid
  - with amyloid stroma
    - specified site — *see* Neoplasm, malignant, by site
    - unspecified site C73
  - microinvasive
    - specified site — *see* Neoplasm, malignant, by site
    - unspecified site C53.9
- sweat gland — *see* Neoplasm, skin, malignant
- theca cell C56.- ☑
- thymic C37
- unspecified site (primary) C80.1
- water-clear cell C75.0

Carcinoma-in-situ — *see also* Neoplasm, in situ, by site
- breast NOS D05.9- ☑
  - specified type NEC D05.8- ☑
- epidermoid — *see also* Neoplasm, in situ, by site
  - with questionable stromal invasion
    - cervix D06.9
    - specified site NEC — *see* Neoplasm, in situ, by site
    - unspecified site D06.9
  - Bowen's type — *see* Neoplasm, skin, in situ
- intraductal
  - breast D05.1- ☑
  - specified site NEC — *see* Neoplasm, in situ, by site

Carcinoma-in-situ — *continued*
  intraductal — *continued*
    unspecified site D05.1- ☑
  lobular
    with
      infiltrating duct
        breast (female) C50.91- ☑
          male C50.92- ☑
        specified site NEC — *see* Neoplasm, malignant
        unspecified site (female) C50.91- ☑
          male C50.92- ☑
      intraductal
        breast D05.8- ☑
        specified site NEC — *see* Neoplasm, in situ,
          by site
        unspecified site (female) D05.8- ☑
    breast D05.0- ☑
    specified site NEC — *see* Neoplasm, in situ, by site
    unspecified site D05.0- ☑
  squamous cell — *see also* Neoplasm, in situ, by site
    with questionable stromal invasion
      cervix D06.9
      specified site NEC — *see* Neoplasm, in situ, by
        site
      unspecified site D06.9
Carcinomaphobia F45.29
Carcinomatosis C80.0
  peritonei C78.6
  unspecified site (primary) (secondary) C80.0
Carcinosarcoma — *see* Neoplasm, malignant, by site
  embryonal — *see* Neoplasm, malignant, by site
Cardia, cardial — *see* condition
Cardiac — *see also* condition
  death, sudden — *see* Arrest, cardiac
  pacemaker
    in situ Z95.0
    management or adjustment Z45.018
  tamponade I31.4
Cardialgia — *see* Pain, precordial
Cardiectasis — *see* Hypertrophy, cardiac
Cardiochalasia K21.9
Cardiomalacia I51.5
Cardiomegalia glycogenica diffusa E74.02 *[I43]*
Cardiomegaly — *see also* Hypertrophy, cardiac
  congenital Q24.8
  glycogen E74.02 *[I43]*
  idiopathic I51.7
Cardiomyoliposis I51.5
Cardiomyopathy (familial) (idiopathic) I42.9
  alcoholic I42.6
  amyloid E85.4 *[I43]*
    transthyretin-related (ATTR) familial E85.4 *[I43]*
  arteriosclerotic — *see* Disease, heart, ischemic,
    atherosclerotic
  beriberi E51.12
  cobalt-beer I42.6
  congenital I42.4
  congestive I42.0
  constrictive NOS I42.5
  dilated I42.0
  due to
    alcohol I42.6
    beriberi E51.12
    cardiac glycogenosis E74.02 *[I43]*
    drugs I42.7
    external agents NEC I42.7
    Friedreich's ataxia G11.1
    myotonia atrophica G71.11 *[I43]*
    progressive muscular dystrophy G71.09 *[I43]*
  glycogen storage E74.02 *[I43]*
  hypertensive — *see* Hypertension, heart
  hypertrophic (nonobstructive) I42.2
    obstructive I42.1
      congenital Q24.8
  in
    Chagas' disease (chronic) B57.2
      acute B57.0
    sarcoidosis D86.85
  ischemic I25.5
  metabolic E88.9 *[I43]*
    thyrotoxic E05.90 *[I43]*
      with thyroid storm E05.91 *[I43]*
  newborn I42.8
    congenital I42.4
  non-ischemic — *see also* by cause I42.8
  nutritional E63.9 *[I43]*
    beriberi E51.12

Cardiomyopathy — *continued*
  obscure of Africa I42.8
  peripartum O90.3
  postpartum O90.3
  restrictive NEC I42.5
  rheumatic I09.0
  secondary I42.9
  specified NEC I42.8
  stress induced I51.81
  takotsubo I51.81
  thyrotoxic E05.90 *[I43]*
    with thyroid storm E05.91 *[I43]*
  toxic NEC I42.7
  transthyretin-related (ATTR) familial amyloid E85.4
  tuberculous A18.84
  viral B33.24
Cardionephritis — *see* Hypertension, cardiorenal
Cardionephropathy — *see* Hypertension, cardiorenal
Cardionephrosis — *see* Hypertension, cardiorenal
Cardiopathia nigra I27.0
Cardiopathy — *see also* Disease, heart I51.9
  idiopathic I42.9
  mucopolysaccharidosis E76.3 *[I52]*
Cardiopericarditis — *see* Pericarditis
Cardiophobia F45.29
Cardiorenal — *see* condition
Cardiorrhexis — *see* Infarct, myocardium
Cardiosclerosis — *see* Disease, heart, ischemic,
  atherosclerotic
Cardiosis — *see* Disease, heart
Cardiospasm (esophagus) (reflex) (stomach) K22.0
  congenital Q39.5
    with megaesophagus Q39.5
Cardiostenosis — *see* Disease, heart
Cardiosymphysis I31.0
Cardiovascular — *see* condition
Carditis (acute) (bacterial) (chronic) (subacute) I51.89
  meningococcal A39.50
  rheumatic — *see* Disease, heart, rheumatic
  rheumatoid — *see* Rheumatoid, carditis
  viral B33.20
Care (of) (for) (following)
  child (routine) Z76.2
  family member (handicapped) (sick)
    creating problem for family Z63.6
    provided away from home for holiday relief Z75.5
    unavailable, due to
      absence (person rendering care) (sufferer) Z74.2
      inability (any reason) of person rendering care
        Z74.2
  foundling Z76.1
  holiday relief Z75.5
  improper — *see* Maltreatment
  lack of (at or after birth) (infant) — *see* Maltreatment,
    child, neglect
  lactating mother Z39.1
  palliative Z51.5
  postpartum
    immediately after delivery Z39.0
    routine follow-up Z39.2
  respite Z75.5
  unavailable, due to
    absence of person rendering care Z74.2
    inability (any reason) of person rendering care Z74.2
  well-baby Z76.2
Caries
  bone NEC A18.03
  dental (dentino enamel junction) (early childhood) (of
    dentine) (pre-eruptive) (recurrent) (to the pulp)
    K02.9
    arrested (coronal) (root) K02.3
    chewing surface
      limited to enamel K02.51
      penetrating into dentin K02.52
      penetrating into pulp K02.53
    coronal surface
      chewing surface
        limited to enamel K02.51
        penetrating into dentin K02.52
        penetrating into pulp K02.53
      pit and fissure surface
        limited to enamel K02.51
        penetrating into dentin K02.52
        penetrating into pulp K02.53
      smooth surface
        limited to enamel K02.61
        penetrating into dentin K02.62
        penetrating into pulp K02.63

Caries — *continued*
  dental — *continued*
    pit and fissure surface
      limited to enamel K02.51
      penetrating into dentin K02.52
      penetrating into pulp K02.53
    primary, cervical origin K02.52
    root K02.7
    smooth surface
      limited to enamel K02.61
      penetrating into dentin K02.62
      penetrating into pulp K02.63
  external meatus — *see* Disorder, ear, external, specified
    type NEC
  hip (tuberculous) A18.02
  initial (tooth)
    chewing surface K02.51
    pit and fissure surface K02.51
    smooth surface K02.61
  knee (tuberculous) A18.02
  labyrinth H83.8 ☑
  limb NEC (tuberculous) A18.03
  mastoid process (chronic) — *see* Mastoiditis, chronic
    tuberculous A18.03
  middle ear H74.8 ☑
  nose (tuberculous) A18.03
  orbit (tuberculous) A18.03
  ossicles, ear — *see* Abnormal, ear ossicles
  petrous bone — *see* Petrositis
  root (dental) (tooth) K02.7
  sacrum (tuberculous) A18.01
  spine, spinal (column) (tuberculous) A18.01
  syphilitic A52.77
    congenital (early) A50.02 *[M90.80]*
  tooth, teeth — *see* Caries, dental
  tuberculous A18.03
  vertebra (column) (tuberculous) A18.01
Carious teeth — *see* Caries, dental
Carneous mole O02.0
Carnitine insufficiency E71.40
Carotenemia (dietary) E67.1
Carotenosis (cutis) (skin) E67.1
Carotid body or sinus syndrome G90.01
Carotidynia G90.01
Carpal tunnel syndrome — *see* Syndrome, carpal tunnel
Carpenter's syndrome Q87.0
Carpopedal spasm — *see* Tetany
Carr-Barr-Plunkett syndrome Q97.1
Carrier (suspected) of
  amebiasis Z22.1
  bacterial disease NEC Z22.39
    diphtheria Z22.2
    intestinal infectious NEC Z22.1
      typhoid Z22.0
    meningococcal Z22.31
    sexually transmitted Z22.4
    specified NEC Z22.39
    staphylococcal (Methicillin susceptible) Z22.321
      Methicillin resistant Z22.322
    streptococcal Z22.338
      group B Z22.330
        complicating pregnancy or delivery
          O99.82- ☑
    typhoid Z22.0
  cholera Z22.1
  diphtheria Z22.2
  gastrointestinal pathogens NEC Z22.1
  genetic Z14.8
    cystic fibrosis Z14.1
    hemophilia A (asymptomatic) Z14.01
      symptomatic Z14.02
  gestational, pregnant Z33.1
  gonorrhea Z22.4
  HAA (hepatitis Australian-antigen) B18.8
  HB (c)(s)-AG B18.1
  hepatitis (viral) B18.9
    Australia-antigen (HAA) B18.8
    B surface antigen (HBsAg) B18.1
      with acute delta- (super)infection B17.0
    C B18.2
    specified NEC B18.8
  human T-cell lymphotropic virus type-1 (HTLV-1) infec-
    tion Z22.6
  infectious organism Z22.9
    specified NEC Z22.8
  meningococci Z22.31
  Salmonella typhosa Z22.0
  serum hepatitis — *see* Carrier, hepatitis

Carrier of — *continued*
  staphylococci (Methicillin susceptible) Z22.321
    Methicillin resistant Z22.322
  streptococci Z22.338
    group B Z22.330
      complicating pregnancy or delivery O99.82- ☑
  syphilis Z22.4
  typhoid Z22.0
  venereal disease NEC Z22.4
Carrion's disease A44.0
Carter's relapsing fever (Asiatic) A68.1
Cartilage — *see* condition
Caruncle (inflamed)
  conjunctiva (acute) — *see* Conjunctivitis, acute
  labium (majus) (minus) N90.89
  lacrimal — *see* Inflammation, lacrimal, passages
  myrtiform N89.8
  urethral (benign) N36.2
Cascade stomach K31.2
Caseation lymphatic gland (tuberculous) A18.2
Cassidy (-Scholte) syndrome (malignant carcinoid) E34.0
Castellani's disease A69.8
Castration, traumatic, male S38.231 ☑
Casts in urine R82.998
Cat
  cry syndrome Q93.4
  ear Q17.3
  eye syndrome Q92.8
Catabolism, senile R54
Catalepsy (hysterical) F44.2
  schizophrenic F20.2
Cataplexy (idiopathic) — *see* Narcolepsy
Cataract (cortical) (immature) (incipient) H26.9
  with
    neovascularization — *see* Cataract, complicated
  age-related — *see* Cataract, senile
  anterior
    and posterior axial embryonal Q12.0
    pyramidal Q12.0
  associated with
    galactosemia E74.21 *[H28]*
    myotonic disorders G71.19 *[H28]*
  blue Q12.0
  central Q12.0
  cerulean Q12.0
  complicated H26.20
    with
      neovascularization H26.21- ☑
      ocular disorder H26.22- ☑
      glaucomatous flecks H26.23- ☑
  congenital Q12.0
  coraliform Q12.0
  coronary Q12.0
  crystalline Q12.0
  diabetic — *see* Diabetes, cataract
  drug-induced H26.3- ☑
  due to
    ocular disorder — *see* Cataract, complicated
    radiation H26.8
  electric H26.8
  extraction status Z98.4- ☑
  glass-blower's H26.8
  heat ray H26.8
  heterochromic — *see* Cataract, complicated
  hypermature — *see* Cataract, senile, morgagnian type
  in (due to)
    chronic iridocyclitis — *see* Cataract, complicated
    diabetes — *see* Diabetes, cataract
    endocrine disease E34.9 *[H28]*
    eye disease — *see* Cataract, complicated
    hypoparathyroidism E20.9 *[H28]*
    malnutrition-dehydration E46 *[H28]*
    metabolic disease E88.9 *[H28]*
    myotonic disorders G71.19 *[H28]*
    nutritional disease E63.9 *[H28]*
  infantile — *see* Cataract, presenile
  irradiational — *see* Cataract, specified NEC
  juvenile — *see* Cataract, presenile
  malnutrition-dehydration E46 *[H28]*
  morgagnian — *see* Cataract, senile, morgagnian type
  myotonic G71.19 *[H28]*
  myxedema E03.9 *[H28]*
  nuclear
    embryonal Q12.0
    sclerosis — *see* Cataract, senile, nuclear
  presenile H26.00- ☑
    combined forms H26.06- ☑

Cataract — *continued*
  presenile — *continued*
    cortical H26.01- ☑
    lamellar — *see* Cataract, presenile, cortical
    nuclear H26.03- ☑
    specified NEC H26.09
    subcapsular polar (anterior) H26.04- ☑
      posterior H26.05- ☑
    zonular — *see* Cataract, presenile, cortical
  secondary H26.40
    Soemmering's ring H26.41- ☑
    specified NEC H26.49- ☑
    to eye disease — *see* Cataract, complicated
  senile H25.9
    brunescens — *see* Cataract, senile, nuclear
    combined forms H25.81- ☑
    coronary — *see* Cataract, senile, incipient
    cortical H25.01- ☑
    hypermature — *see* Cataract, senile, morgagnian type
    incipient (mature) (total) H25.09- ☑
      cortical — *see* Cataract, senile, cortical
      subcapsular — *see* Cataract, senile, subcapsular
    morgagnian type (hypermature) H25.2- ☑
    nuclear (sclerosis) H25.1- ☑
    polar subcapsular (anterior) (posterior) — *see* Cataract, senile, incipient
    punctate — *see* Cataract, senile, incipient
    specified NEC H25.89
    subcapsular polar (anterior) H25.03- ☑
      posterior H25.04- ☑
  snowflake — *see* Diabetes, cataract
  specified NEC H26.8
  toxic — *see* Cataract, drug-induced
  traumatic H26.10- ☑
    localized H26.11- ☑
    partially resolved H26.12- ☑
    total H26.13- ☑
  zonular (perinuclear) Q12.0
Cataracta — *see also* Cataract
  brunescens — *see* Cataract, senile, nuclear
  centralis pulverulenta Q12.0
  complicata — *see* Cataract, complicated
  congenita Q12.0
  coralliformis Q12.0
  coronaria Q12.0
  diabetic — *see* Diabetes, cataract
  membranacea
    accreta — *see* Cataract, secondary
    congenita Q12.0
  nigra — *see* Cataract, senile, nuclear
  sunflower — *see* Cataract, complicated
Catarrh, catarrhal (acute) (febrile) (infectious) (inflammation) — *see also* condition J00
  bronchial — *see* Bronchitis
  chest — *see* Bronchitis
  chronic J31.0
  due to congenital syphilis A50.03
  enteric — *see* Enteritis
  eustachian H68.009
  fauces — *see* Pharyngitis
  gastrointestinal — *see* Enteritis
  gingivitis K05.00
    nonplaque induced K05.01
    plaque induced K05.00
  hay — *see* Fever, hay
  intestinal — *see* Enteritis
  larynx, chronic J37.0
  liver B15.9
    with hepatic coma B15.0
  lung — *see* Bronchitis
  middle ear, chronic — *see* Otitis, media, nonsuppurative, chronic, serous
  mouth K12.1
  nasal (chronic) — *see* Rhinitis
  nasobronchial J31.1
  nasopharyngeal (chronic) J31.1
    acute J00
  pulmonary — *see* Bronchitis
  spring (eye) (vernal) — *see* Conjunctivitis, acute, atopic
  summer (hay) — *see* Fever, hay
  throat J31.2
  tubotympanal — *see also* Otitis, media, nonsuppurative
    chronic — *see* Otitis, media, nonsuppurative, chronic, serous
Catatonia (schizophrenic) F20.2

Catatonic
  disorder due to known physiologic condition F06.1
  schizophrenia F20.2
  stupor R40.1
Cat-scratch — *see also* Abrasion
  disease or fever A28.1
Cauda equina — *see* condition
Cauliflower ear M95.1- ☑
Causalgia (upper limb) G56.4- ☑
  lower limb G57.7- ☑
Cause
  external, general effects T75.89 ☑
Caustic burn — *see* Corrosion, by site
Cavare's disease (familial periodic paralysis) G72.3
Cave-in, injury
  crushing (severe) — *see* Crush
  suffocation — *see* Asphyxia, traumatic, due to low oxygen, due to cave-in
Cavernitis (penis) N48.29
Cavernositis N48.29
Cavernous — *see* condition
Cavitation of lung — *see also* Tuberculosis, pulmonary
  nontuberculous J98.4
Cavities, dental — *see* Caries, dental
Cavity
  lung — *see* Cavitation of lung
  optic papilla Q14.2
  pulmonary — *see* Cavitation of lung
Cavovarus foot, congenital Q66.1- ☑
Cavus foot (congenital) Q66.7- ☑
  acquired — *see* Deformity, limb, foot, specified NEC
Cazenave's disease L10.2
Cecitis K52.9
  with perforation, peritonitis, or rupture K65.8
Cecoureterocele Q62.32
Cecum — *see* condition
Celiac
  artery compression syndrome I77.4
  disease (with steatorrhea) K90.0
  infantilism K90.0
Cell(s), cellular — *see also* condition
  in urine R82.998
Cellulitis (diffuse) (phlegmonous) (septic) (suppurative) L03.90
  abdominal wall L03.311
  anaerobic A48.0
  ankle — *see* Cellulitis, lower limb
  anus K61.0
  arm — *see* Cellulitis, upper limb
  auricle (ear) — *see* Cellulitis, ear
  axilla L03.11- ☑
  back (any part) L03.312
  breast (acute) (nonpuerperal) (subacute) N61.0
    nipple N61.0
  broad ligament
    acute N73.0
  buttock L03.317
  cervical (meaning neck) L03.221
  cervix (uteri) — *see* Cervicitis
  cheek (external) L03.211
    internal K12.2
  chest wall L03.313
  chronic L03.90
  clostridial A48.0
  corpus cavernosum N48.22
  digit
    finger — *see* Cellulitis, finger
    toe — *see* Cellulitis, toe
  Douglas' cul-de-sac or pouch
    acute N73.0
  drainage site (following operation) T81.49 ☑
  ear (external) H60.1- ☑
  eosinophilic (granulomatous) L98.3
  erysipelatous — *see* Erysipelas
  external auditory canal — *see* Cellulitis, ear
  eyelid — *see* Abscess, eyelid
  face NEC L03.211
  finger (intrathecal) (periosteal) (subcutaneous) (subcuticular) L03.01- ☑
  foot — *see* Cellulitis, lower limb
  gangrenous — *see* Gangrene
  genital organ NEC
    female (external) N76.4
    male N49.9
      multiple sites N49.8
      specified NEC N49.8
  gluteal (region) L03.317

Cellulitis — *continued*
- gonococcal A54.89
- groin L03.314
- hand — *see* Cellulitis, upper limb
- head NEC L03.811
  - face (any part, except ear, eye and nose) L03.211
- heel — *see* Cellulitis, lower limb
- hip — *see* Cellulitis, lower limb
- jaw (region) L03.211
- knee — *see* Cellulitis, lower limb
- labium (majus) (minus) — *see* Vulvitis
- lacrimal passages — *see* Inflammation, lacrimal, passages
- larynx J38.7
- leg — *see* Cellulitis, lower limb
- lip K13.0
- lower limb L03.11- ☑
  - toe — *see* Cellulitis, toe
- mouth (floor) K12.2
- multiple sites, so stated L03.90
- nasopharynx J39.1
- navel L03.316
  - newborn P38.9
    - with mild hemorrhage P38.1
    - without hemorrhage P38.9
- neck (region) L03.221
- nipple (acute) (nonpuerperal) (subacute) N61.0
- nose (septum) (external) J34.0
- orbit, orbital H05.01- ☑
- palate (soft) K12.2
- pectoral (region) L03.313
- pelvis, pelvic (chronic)
  - female — *see also* Disease, pelvis, inflammatory N73.2
    - acute N73.0
  - following ectopic or molar pregnancy O08.0
  - male K65.0
- penis N48.22
- perineal, perineum L03.315
- periorbital L03.213
- perirectal K61.1
- peritonsillar J36
- periurethral N34.0
- periuterine — *see also* Disease, pelvis, inflammatory N73.2
  - acute N73.0
- pharynx J39.1
- preseptal L03.213
- rectum K61.1
- retroperitoneal K68.9
- round ligament
  - acute N73.0
- scalp (any part) L03.811
- scrotum N49.2
- seminal vesicle N49.0
- shoulder — *see* Cellulitis, upper limb
- specified site NEC L03.818
- submandibular (region) (space) (triangle) K12.2
  - gland K11.3
- submaxillary (region) K12.2
  - gland K11.3
- thigh — *see* Cellulitis, lower limb
- thumb (intrathecal) (periosteal) (subcutaneous) (subcuticular) — *see* Cellulitis, finger
- toe (intrathecal) (periosteal) (subcutaneous) (subcuticular) L03.03- ☑
- tonsil J36
- trunk L03.319
  - abdominal wall L03.311
  - back (any part) L03.312
  - buttock L03.317
  - chest wall L03.313
  - groin L03.314
  - perineal, perineum L03.315
  - umbilicus L03.316
- tuberculous (primary) A18.4
- umbilicus L03.316
- upper limb L03.11- ☑
  - axilla — *see* Cellulitis, axilla
  - finger — *see* Cellulitis, finger
  - thumb — *see* Cellulitis, finger
- vaccinal T88.0 ☑
- vocal cord J38.3
- vulva — *see* Vulvitis
- wrist — *see* Cellulitis, upper limb

Cementoblastoma, benign — *see* Cyst, calcifying odontogenic
Cementoma — *see* Cyst, calcifying odontogenic

Cementoperiostitis — *see* Periodontitis
Cementosis K03.4
Central auditory processing disorder H93.25
Central pain syndrome G89.0
Cephalematocele, cephal (o)hematocele
- newborn P52.8
  - birth injury P10.8
- traumatic — *see* Hematoma, brain
Cephalematoma, cephalhematoma (calcified)
- newborn (birth injury) P12.0
- traumatic — *see* Hematoma, brain
Cephalgia, cephalalgia — *see also* Headache
- histamine G44.009
  - intractable G44.001
  - not intractable G44.009
- trigeminal autonomic (TAC) NEC G44.099
  - intractable G44.091
  - not intractable G44.099
Cephalic — *see* condition
Cephalitis — *see* Encephalitis
Cephalocele — *see* Encephalocele
Cephalomenia N94.89
Cephalopelvic — *see* condition
Cerclage (with cervical incompetence) in pregnancy — *see* Incompetence, cervix, in pregnancy
Cerebellitis — *see* Encephalitis
Cerebellum, cerebellar — *see* condition
Cerebral — *see* condition
Cerebritis — *see* Encephalitis
Cerebro-hepato-renal syndrome Q87.89
Cerebromalacia — *see* Softening, brain
- sequelae of cerebrovascular disease I69.398
Cerebroside lipidosis E75.22
Cerebrospasticity (congenital) G80.1
Cerebrospinal — *see* condition
Cerebrum — *see* condition
Ceroid-lipofuscinosis, neuronal E75.4
Cerumen (accumulation) (impacted) H61.2- ☑
Cervical — *see also* condition
- auricle Q18.2
- dysplasia in pregnancy — *see* Abnormal, cervix, in pregnancy or childbirth
- erosion in pregnancy — *see* Abnormal, cervix, in pregnancy or childbirth
- fibrosis in pregnancy — *see* Abnormal, cervix, in pregnancy or childbirth
- fusion syndrome Q76.1
- rib Q76.5
- shortening (complicating pregnancy) O26.87- ☑
Cervicalgia M54.2
Cervicitis (acute) (chronic) (nonvenereal) (senile (atrophic)) (subacute) (with ulceration) N72
- with
  - abortion — *see* Abortion, by type complicated by genital tract and pelvic infection
  - ectopic pregnancy O08.0
  - molar pregnancy O08.0
- chlamydial A56.09
- gonococcal A54.03
- herpesviral A60.03
- puerperal (postpartum) O86.11
- syphilitic A52.76
- trichomonal A59.09
- tuberculous A18.16
Cervicocolpitis (emphysematosa) — *see also* Cervicitis N72
Cervix — *see* condition
Cesarean delivery, previous, affecting management of pregnancy O34.219
- classical (vertical) scar O34.212
- low transverse scar O34.211
Céstan (-Chenais) paralysis or syndrome G46.3
Céstan-Raymond syndrome I65.8
Cestode infestation B71.9
- specified type NEC B71.8
Cestodiasis B71.9
Chabert's disease A22.9
Chacaleh E53.8
Chafing L30.4
Chagas' (-Mazza) disease (chronic) B57.2
- with
  - cardiovascular involvement NEC B57.2
  - digestive system involvement B57.30
    - megacolon B57.32
    - megaesophagus B57.31
    - other specified B57.39
  - megacolon B57.32

Chagas'disease — *continued*
- with — *continued*
  - megaesophagus B57.31
  - myocarditis B57.2
  - nervous system involvement B57.40
    - meningitis B57.41
    - meningoencephalitis B57.42
    - other specified B57.49
  - specified organ involvement NEC B57.5
- acute (with) B57.1
  - cardiovascular NEC B57.0
  - myocarditis B57.0
Chagres fever B50.9
Chairridden Z74.09
Chalasia (cardiac sphincter) K21.9
Chalazion H00.19
- left H00.16
  - lower H00.15
  - upper H00.14
- right H00.13
  - lower H00.12
  - upper H00.11
Chalcosis — *see also* Disorder, globe, degenerative, chalcosis
- cornea — *see* Deposit, cornea
- crystalline lens — *see* Cataract, complicated
- retina H35.89
Chalicosis (pulmonum) J62.8
Chancre (any genital site) (hard) (hunterian) (mixed) (primary) (seronegative) (seropositive) (syphilitic) A51.0
- congenital A50.07
- conjunctiva NEC A51.2
- Ducrey's A57
- extragenital A51.2
- eyelid A51.2
- lip A51.2
- nipple A51.2
- Nisbet's A57
- of
  - carate A67.0
  - pinta A67.0
  - yaws A66.0
- palate, soft A51.2
- phagedenic A57
- simple A57
- soft A57
  - bubo A57
  - palate A51.2
- urethra A51.0
- yaws A66.0
Chancroid (anus) (genital) (penis) (perineum) (rectum) (urethra) (vulva) A57
Chandler's disease (osteochondritis dissecans, hip) — *see* Osteochondritis, dissecans, hip
Change(s) (in) (of) — *see also* Removal
- arteriosclerotic — *see* Arteriosclerosis
- bone — *see also* Disorder, bone
  - diabetic — *see* Diabetes, bone change
- bowel habit R19.4
- cardiorenal (vascular) — *see* Hypertension, cardiorenal
- cardiovascular — *see* Disease, cardiovascular
- circulatory I99.9
- cognitive (mild) (organic) R41.89
- color, tooth, teeth
  - during formation K00.8
  - posteruptive K03.7
- contraceptive device Z30.433
- corneal membrane H18.30
  - Bowman's membrane fold or rupture H18.31- ☑
  - Descemet's membrane
    - fold H18.32- ☑
    - rupture H18.33- ☑
- coronary — *see* Disease, heart, ischemic
- degenerative, spine or vertebra — *see* Spondylosis
- dental pulp, regressive K04.2
- dressing (nonsurgical) Z48.00
  - surgical Z48.01
- heart — *see* Disease, heart
- hip joint — *see* Derangement, joint, hip
- hyperplastic larynx J38.7
- hypertrophic
  - nasal sinus J34.89
  - turbinate, nasal J34.3
  - upper respiratory tract J39.8
- indwelling catheter Z46.6
- inflammatory — *see also* Inflammation
  - sacroiliac M46.1

Change(s) — *continued*
job, anxiety concerning Z56.1
joint — *see* Derangement, joint
life — *see* Menopause
mental status R41.82
minimal (glomerular) — *see also* N00-N07 with fourth
    character .0 N05.0
myocardium, myocardial — *see* Degeneration, myocar-
    dial
of life — *see* Menopause
pacemaker Z45.018
    pulse generator Z45.010
personality (enduring) F68.8
    due to (secondary to)
        general medical condition F07.0
    secondary (nonspecific) F60.89
regressive, dental pulp K04.2
renal — *see* Disease, renal
retina H35.9
    myopic — *see also* Myopia, degenerative H44.2- ☑
sacroiliac joint M53.3
senile — *see also* condition R54
sensory R20.8
skin R23.9
    acute, due to ultraviolet radiation L56.9
        specified NEC L56.8
    chronic, due to nonionizing radiation L57.9
        specified NEC L57.8
    cyanosis R23.0
    flushing R23.2
    pallor R23.1
    petechiae R23.3
    specified change NEC R23.8
    swelling — *see* Mass, localized
    texture R23.4
trophic
    arm — *see* Mononeuropathy, upper limb
    leg — *see* Mononeuropathy, lower limb
vascular I99.9
vasomotor I73.9
voice R49.9
    psychogenic F44.4
    specified NEC R49.8
Changing sleep-work schedule, affecting sleep
    G47.26
Changuinola fever A93.1
Chapping skin T69.8 ☑
Charcot-Marie-Tooth disease, paralysis or syndrome
    G60.0
Charcot's
arthropathy — *see* Arthropathy, neuropathic
cirrhosis K74.3
disease (tabetic arthropathy) A52.16
joint (disease) (tabetic) A52.16
    diabetic — *see* Diabetes, with, arthropathy
    syringomyelic G95.0
syndrome (intermittent claudication) I73.9
CHARGE association Q89.8
Charley-horse (quadriceps) M62.831
    traumatic (quadriceps) S76.11- ☑
Charlouis' disease — *see* Yaws
Cheadle's disease E54
Checking (of)
cardiac pacemaker (battery) (electrode(s)) Z45.018
    pulse generator Z45.010
implantable subdermal contraceptive Z30.46
intrauterine contraceptive device Z30.431
wound Z48.0- ☑
    due to injury — code to Injury, by site, using appro-
        priate seventh character for subsequent en-
        counter
Check-up — *see* Examination
Chédiak-Higashi (-Steinbrinck) **syndrome** (congenital
    gigantism of peroxidase granules) E70.330
Cheek — *see* condition
Cheese itch B88.0
Cheese-washer's lung J67.8
Cheese-worker's lung J67.8
Cheilitis (acute) (angular) (catarrhal) (chronic) (exfoliative)
    (gangrenous) (glandular) (infectional) (suppurative)
    (ulcerative) (vesicular) K13.0
actinic (due to sun) L56.8
    other than from sun L59.8
candidal B37.83
Cheilodynia K13.0
Cheiloschisis — *see* Cleft, lip
Cheilosis (angular) K13.0
with pellagra E52

Cheilosis — *continued*
due to
    vitamin B2 (riboflavin) deficiency E53.0
Cheiromegaly M79.89
Cheiropompholyx L30.1
Cheloid — *see* Keloid
Chemical burn — *see* Corrosion, by site
Chemodectoma — *see* Paraganglioma, nonchromaffin
Chemosis, conjunctiva — *see* Edema, conjunctiva
Chemotherapy (session) (for)
cancer Z51.11
neoplasm Z51.11
Cherubism M27.8
Chest — *see* condition
Cheyne-Stokes breathing (respiration) R06.3
Chiari's
disease or syndrome (hepatic vein thrombosis) I82.0
malformation
    type I G93.5
    type II — *see* Spina bifida
    net Q24.8
Chicago disease B40.9
Chickenpox — *see* Varicella
Chiclero ulcer or sore B55.1
Chigger (infestation) B88.0
Chignon (disease) B36.8
newborn (from vacuum extraction) (birth injury) P12.1
Chilaiditi's syndrome (subphrenic displacement, colon)
    Q43.3
Chilblain(s) (lupus) T69.1 ☑
Child
custody dispute Z65.3
Childbirth — *see* Delivery
Childhood
cerebral X-linked adrenoleukodystrophy E71.520
period of rapid growth Z00.2
Chill(s) R68.83
with fever R50.9
congestive in malarial regions B54
without fever R68.83
Chilomastigiasis A07.8
Chimera 46,XX/46,XY Q99.0
Chin — *see* condition
Chinese dysentery A03.9
Chionophobia F40.228
Chitral fever A93.1
Chlamydia, chlamydial A74.9
cervicitis A56.09
conjunctivitis A74.0
cystitis A56.01
endometritis A56.11
epididymitis A56.19
female
    pelvic inflammatory disease A56.11
    pelviperitonitis A56.11
orchitis A56.19
peritonitis A74.81
pharyngitis A56.4
proctitis A56.3
psittaci (infection) A70
salpingitis A56.11
sexually-transmitted infection NEC A56.8
specified NEC A74.89
urethritis A56.01
vulvovaginitis A56.02
Chlamydiosis — *see* Chlamydia
Chloasma (skin) (idiopathic) (symptomatic) L81.1
eyelid H02.719
    hyperthyroid E05.90 *[H02.719]*
        with thyroid storm E05.91 *[H02.719]*
    left H02.716
        lower H02.715
        upper H02.714
    right H02.713
        lower H02.712
        upper H02.711
Chloroma C92.3- ☑
Chlorosis D50.9
Egyptian B76.9 *[D63.8]*
miner's B76.9 *[D63.8]*
Chlorotic anemia D50.8
Chocolate cyst (ovary) N80.1
Choked
disc or disk — *see* Papilledema
on food, phlegm, or vomitus NOS — *see* Foreign body,
    by site
while vomiting NOS — *see* Foreign body, by site

Chokes (resulting from bends) T70.3 ☑
Choking sensation R09.89
Cholangiectasis K83.8
Cholangiocarcinoma
with hepatocellular carcinoma, combined C22.0
    liver C22.1
specified site NEC — *see* Neoplasm, malignant, by site
unspecified site C22.1
Cholangiohepatitis K83.8
due to fluke infestation B66.1
Cholangiohepatoma C22.0
Cholangiolitis (acute) (chronic) (extrahepatic) (gan-
    grenous) (intrahepatic) K83.09
paratyphoidal — *see* Fever, paratyphoid
typhoidal A01.09
Cholangioma D13.4
malignant — *see* Cholangiocarcinoma
Cholangitis (ascending) (recurrent) (secondary) (stenos-
    ing) (suppurative) K83.09
with calculus, bile duct — *see* Calculus, bile duct, with
    cholangitis
chronic nonsuppurative destructive K74.3
primary K83.09
    sclerosing K83.01
sclerosing K83.09
Cholecystectasia K82.8
Cholecystitis K81.9
with
    calculus, stones in
        bile duct (common) (hepatic) — *see* Calculus,
            bile duct, with cholecystitis
        cystic duct — *see* Calculus, gallbladder, with
            cholecystitis
        gallbladder — *see* Calculus, gallbladder, with
            cholecystitis
        choledocholithiasis — *see* Calculus, bile duct, with
            cholecystitis
        cholelithiasis — *see* Calculus, gallbladder, with
            cholecystitis
    gangrene of gallbladder K82.A1
    perforation of gallbladder K82.A2
acute (emphysematous) (gangrenous) (suppurative)
    K81.0
    with
        calculus, stones in
            cystic duct — *see* Calculus, gallbladder, with
                cholecystitis, acute
            gallbladder — *see* Calculus, gallbladder, with
                cholecystitis, acute
        choledocholithiasis — *see* Calculus, bile duct,
            with cholecystitis, acute
        cholelithiasis — *see* Calculus, gallbladder, with
            cholecystitis, acute
    chronic cholecystitis K81.2
        with gallbladder calculus K80.12
            with obstruction K80.13
chronic K81.1
    with acute cholecystitis K81.2
        with gallbladder calculus K80.12
            with obstruction K80.13
emphysematous (acute) — *see* Cholecystitis, acute
gangrenous — *see* Cholecystitis, acute
paratyphoidal, current A01.4
suppurative — *see* Cholecystitis, acute
typhoidal A01.09
Cholecystolithiasis — *see* Calculus, gallbladder
Choledochitis (suppurative) K83.09
Choledocholith — *see* Calculus, bile duct
Choledocholithiasis (common duct) (hepatic duct) —
    see Calculus, bile duct
cystic — *see* Calculus, gallbladder
typhoidal A01.09
Cholelithiasis (cystic duct) (gallbladder) (impacted)
    (multiple) — *see* Calculus, gallbladder
bile duct (common) (hepatic) — *see* Calculus, bile duct
hepatic duct — *see* Calculus, bile duct
specified NEC K80.80
    with obstruction K80.81
Cholemia — *see also* Jaundice
familial (simple) (congenital) E80.4
Gilbert's E80.4
Choleperitoneum, choleperitonitis K65.3
Cholera (Asiatic) (epidemic) (malignant) A00.9
antimonial — *see* Poisoning, antimony
classical A00.0
due to Vibrio cholerae 01 A00.9
    biovar cholerae A00.0

Cholera — *continued*
due to Vibrio cholerae Ø1 — *continued*
  biovar eltor AØØ.1
  el tor AØØ.1
el tor AØØ.1
Cholerine — *see* Cholera
Cholestasis NEC K83.1
with hepatocyte injury K71.Ø
due to total parenteral nutrition (TPN) K76.89
pure K71.Ø
Cholesteatoma (ear) (middle) (with reaction) H71.9- ☑
attic H71.Ø- ☑
external ear (canal) H6Ø.4- ☑
mastoid H71.2- ☑
postmastoidectomy cavity (recurrent) — *see* Complications, postmastoidectomy, recurrent cholesteatoma
recurrent (postmastoidectomy) — *see* Complications, postmastoidectomy, recurrent cholesteatoma
tympanum H71.1- ☑
Cholesteatosis, diffuse H71.3- ☑
Cholesteremia E78.ØØ
Cholesterin in vitreous — *see* Deposit, crystalline
Cholesterol
deposit
  retina H35.89
  vitreous — *see* Deposit, crystalline
elevated (high) E78.ØØ
  with elevated (high) triglycerides E78.2
    screening for Z13.22Ø
imbibition of gallbladder K82.4
Cholesterolemia (essential) (pure) E78.ØØ
familial E78.Ø1
hereditary E78.Ø1
Cholesterolosis, cholesterosis (gallbladder) K82.4
cerebrotendinous E75.5
Cholocolic fistula K82.3
Choluria R82.2
Chondritis M94.8X9
aurical H61.Ø3- ☑
costal (Tietze's) M94.Ø
external ear H61.Ø3- ☑
patella, posttraumatic — *see* Chondromalacia, patella
pinna H61.Ø3- ☑
purulent M94.8X- ☑
tuberculous NEC A18.Ø2
  intervertebral A18.Ø1
Chondroblastoma — *see also* Neoplasm, bone, benign
malignant — *see* Neoplasm, bone, malignant
Chondrocalcinosis M11.2Ø
ankle M11.27- ☑
elbow M11.22- ☑
familial M11.1Ø
  ankle M11.17- ☑
  elbow M11.12- ☑
  foot joint M11.17- ☑
  hand joint M11.14- ☑
  hip M11.15- ☑
  knee M11.16- ☑
  multiple site M11.19
  shoulder M11.11- ☑
  vertebrae M11.18
  wrist M11.13- ☑
foot joint M11.27- ☑
hand joint M11.24- ☑
hip M11.25- ☑
knee M11.26- ☑
multiple site M11.29
shoulder M11.21- ☑
specified type NEC M11.2Ø
  ankle M11.27- ☑
  elbow M11.22- ☑
  foot joint M11.27- ☑
  hand joint M11.24- ☑
  hip M11.25- ☑
  knee M11.26- ☑
  multiple site M11.29
  shoulder M11.21- ☑
  vertebrae M11.28
  wrist M11.23- ☑
vertebrae M11.28
wrist M11.23- ☑
Chondrodermatitis nodularis helicis or anthelicis — *see* Perichondritis, ear
Chondrodysplasia Q78.9
with hemangioma Q78.4
calcificans congenita Q77.3

Chondrodysplasia — *continued*
fetalis Q77.4
metaphyseal (Jansen's) (McKusick's) (Schmid's) Q78.8
punctata Q77.3
Chondrodystrophy, chondrodystrophia (familial) (fetalis) (hypoplastic) Q78.9
calcificans congenita Q77.3
myotonic (congenital) G71.13
punctata Q77.3
Chondroectodermal dysplasia Q77.6
Chondrogenesis imperfecta Q77.4
Chondrolysis M94.35- ☑
Chondroma — *see also* Neoplasm, cartilage, benign
juxtacortical — *see* Neoplasm, bone, benign
periosteal — *see* Neoplasm, bone, benign
Chondromalacia (systemic) M94.2Ø
acromioclavicular joint M94.21- ☑
ankle M94.27- ☑
elbow M94.22- ☑
foot joint M94.27- ☑
glenohumeral joint M94.21- ☑
hand joint M94.24- ☑
hip M94.25- ☑
knee M94.26- ☑
  patella M22.4- ☑
multiple sites M94.29
patella M22.4- ☑
rib M94.28
sacroiliac joint M94.259
shoulder M94.21- ☑
sternoclavicular joint M94.21- ☑
vertebral joint M94.28
wrist M94.23- ☑
Chondromatosis — *see also* Neoplasm, cartilage, uncertain behavior
internal Q78.4
Chondromyxosarcoma — *see* Neoplasm, cartilage, malignant
Chondro-osteodysplasia (Morquio-Brailsford type) E76.219
Chondro-osteodystrophy E76.29
Chondro-osteoma — *see* Neoplasm, bone, benign
Chondropathia tuberosa M94.Ø
Chondrosarcoma — *see* Neoplasm, cartilage, malignant
juxtacortical — *see* Neoplasm, bone, malignant
mesenchymal — *see* Neoplasm, connective tissue, malignant
myxoid — *see* Neoplasm, cartilage, malignant
Chordee (nonvenereal) N48.89
congenital Q54.4
gonococcal A54.Ø9
Chorditis (fibrinous) (nodosa) (tuberosa) J38.2
Chordoma — *see* Neoplasm, vertebral (column), malignant
Chorea (chronic) (gravis) (posthemiplegic) (senile) (spasmodic) G25.5
with
  heart involvement IØ2.Ø
    active or acute (conditions in IØ1-) IØ2.Ø
    rheumatic IØ2.9
      with valvular disorder IØ2.Ø
    rheumatic heart disease (chronic) (inactive)(quiescent) — *code to* rheumatic heart condition involved
drug-induced G25.4
habit F95.8
hereditary G1Ø
Huntington's G1Ø
hysterical F44.4
minor IØ2.9
  with heart involvement IØ2.Ø
progressive G25.5
  hereditary G1Ø
rheumatic (chronic) IØ2.9
  with heart involvement IØ2.Ø
Sydenham's IØ2.9
  with heart involvement — *see* Chorea, with rheumatic heart disease
  nonrheumatic G25.5
Choreoathetosis (paroxysmal) G25.5
Chorioadenoma (destruens) D39.2
Chorioamnionitis O41.12- ☑
Chorioangioma D26.7
Choriocarcinoma — *see* Neoplasm, malignant, by site
combined with
  embryonal carcinoma — *see* Neoplasm, malignant, by site

Choriocarcinoma — *continued*
combined with — *continued*
  other germ cell elements — *see* Neoplasm, malignant, by site
  teratoma — *see* Neoplasm, malignant, by site
specified site — *see* Neoplasm, malignant, by site
unspecified site
  female C58
  male C62.9Ø
Chorioencephalitis (acute) (lymphocytic) (serous) A87.2
Chorioepithelioma — *see* Choriocarcinoma
Choriomeningitis (acute) (lymphocytic) (serous) A87.2
Chorionepithelioma — *see* Choriocarcinoma
Chorioretinitis — *see also* Inflammation, chorioretinal
disseminated — *see also* Inflammation, chorioretinal, disseminated
  in neurosyphilis A52.19
Egyptian B76.9 *[D63.8]*
focal — *see also* Inflammation, chorioretinal, focal
histoplasmic B39.9 *[H32]*
in (due to)
  histoplasmosis B39.9 *[H32]*
  syphilis (secondary) A51.43
    late A52.71
  toxoplasmosis (acquired) B58.Ø1
    congenital (active) P37.1 *[H32]*
  tuberculosis A18.53
juxtapapillary, juxtapapillaris — *see* Inflammation, chorioretinal, focal, juxtapapillary
leprous A3Ø.9 *[H32]*
miner's B76.9 *[D63.8]*
progressive myopia (degeneration) — *see also* Myopia, degenerative H44.2- ☑
syphilitic (secondary) A51.43
  congenital (early) A5Ø.Ø1 *[H32]*
    late A5Ø.32
  late A52.71
tuberculous A18.53
Chorioretinopathy, central serous H35.71- ☑
Choroid — *see* condition
Choroideremia H31.21
Choroiditis — *see* Chorioretinitis
Choroidopathy — *see* Disorder, choroid
Choroidoretinitis — *see* Chorioretinitis
Choroidoretinopathy, central serous — *see* Chorioretinopathy, central serous
Christian-Weber disease M35.6
Christmas disease D67
Chromaffinoma — *see also* Neoplasm, benign, by site
malignant — *see* Neoplasm, malignant, by site
Chromatopsia — *see* Deficiency, color vision
Chromhidrosis, chromidrosis L75.1
Chromoblastomycosis — *see* Chromomycosis
Chromoconversion R82.91
Chromomycosis B43.9
brain abscess B43.1
cerebral B43.1
cutaneous B43.Ø
skin B43.Ø
specified NEC B43.8
subcutaneous abscess or cyst B43.2
Chromophytosis B36.Ø
Chromosome — *see* Anomaly, by chromosome involved
D (1) — *see* Anomaly, chromosome 13
E (3) — *see* Anomaly, chromosome 18
G — *see* Anomaly, chromosome 21
Chromotrichomycosis B36.8
Chronic — *see* condition
fracture — *see* Fracture, pathological
Churg-Strauss syndrome M3Ø.1
Chyle cyst, mesentery I89.8
Chylocele (nonfilarial) I89.8
filarial — *see also* Infestation, filarial B74.9 *[N51]*
tunica vaginalis N5Ø.89
  filarial — *see also* Infestation, filarial B74.9 *[N51]*
Chylomicronemia (fasting) (with hyperprebetalipoproteinemia) E78.3
Chylopericardium I31.3
acute I3Ø.9
Chylothorax (nonfilarial) I89.8
filarial — *see also* Infestation, filarial B74.9 *[J91.8]*
Chylous — *see* condition
Chyluria (nonfilarial) R82.Ø
due to
  bilharziasis B65.Ø
  Brugia (malayi) B74.1
    timori B74.2

Chyluria — *continued*
  due to — *continued*
    schistosomiasis (bilharziasis) B65.0
    Wuchereria (bancrofti) B74.0
    filarial — *see* Infestation, filarial
Cicatricial (deformity) — *see* Cicatrix
Cicatrix (adherent) (contracted) (painful) (vicious) — *see also* Scar L90.5
  adenoid (and tonsil) J35.8
  alveolar process M26.79
  anus K62.89
  auricle — *see* Disorder, pinna, specified type NEC
  bile duct (common) (hepatic) K83.8
  bladder N32.89
  bone — *see* Disorder, bone, specified type NEC
  brain G93.89
  cervix (postoperative) (postpartal) N88.1
  common duct K83.8
  cornea H17.9
    tuberculous A18.59
  duodenum (bulb), obstructive K31.5
  esophagus K22.2
  eyelid — *see* Disorder, eyelid function
  hypopharynx J39.2
  lacrimal passages — *see* Obstruction, lacrimal
  larynx J38.7
  lung J98.4
  middle ear H74.8 ☑
  mouth K13.79
  muscle M62.89
    with contracture — *see* Contraction, muscle NEC
  nasopharynx J39.2
  palate (soft) K13.79
  penis N48.89
  pharynx J39.2
  prostate N42.89
  rectum K62.89
  retina — *see* Scar, chorioretinal
  semilunar cartilage — *see* Derangement, meniscus
  seminal vesicle N50.89
  skin L90.5
    infected L08.89
    postinfective L90.5
    tuberculous B90.8
  specified site NEC L90.5
  throat J39.2
  tongue K14.8
  tonsil (and adenoid) J35.8
  trachea J39.8
  tuberculous NEC B90.9
  urethra N36.8
  uterus N85.8
  vagina N89.8
    postoperative N99.2
  vocal cord J38.3
  wrist, constricting (annular) L90.5
CIDP (chronic inflammatory demyelinating polyneuropathy) G61.81
CIN — *see* Neoplasia, intraepithelial, cervix
CINCA (chronic infantile neurological, cutaneous and articular syndrome) M04.2
Cinchonism — *see* Deafness, ototoxic
  correct substance properly administered — *see* Table of Drugs and Chemicals, by drug, adverse effect
  overdose or wrong substance given or taken — *see* Table of Drugs and Chemicals, by drug, poisoning
Circle of Willis — *see* condition
Circular — *see* condition
Circulating anticoagulants — *see also* Disorder, hemorrhagic D68.318
  due to drugs — *see also* Disorder, hemorrhagic D68.32
  following childbirth O72.3
Circulation
  collateral, any site I99.8
  defective (lower extremity) I99.9
    congenital Q28.9
  embryonic Q28.9
  failure (peripheral) R57.9
    newborn P29.89
  fetal, persistent P29.38
  heart, incomplete Q28.9
Circulatory system — *see* condition
Circulus senilis (cornea) — *see* Degeneration, cornea, senile
Circumcision (in absence of medical indication) (ritual) (routine) Z41.2
Circumscribed — *see* condition
Circumvallate placenta O43.11- ☑

Cirrhosis, cirrhotic (hepatic) (liver) K74.60
  alcoholic K70.30
    with ascites K70.31
  atrophic — *see* Cirrhosis, liver
  Baumgarten-Cruveilhier K74.69
  biliary (cholangiolitic) (cholangitic) (hypertrophic) (obstructive) (pericholangiolitic) K74.5
    due to
      Clonorchiasis B66.1
      flukes B66.3
    primary K74.3
    secondary K74.4
  cardiac (of liver) K76.1
  Charcot's K74.3
  cholangiolitic, cholangitic, cholestatic (primary) K74.3
  congestive K76.1
  Cruveilhier-Baumgarten K74.69
  cryptogenic (liver) K74.69
  due to
    hepatolenticular degeneration E83.01
    Wilson's disease E83.01
    xanthomatosis E78.2
  fatty K76.0
    alcoholic K70.0
  Hanot's (hypertrophic) K74.3
  hepatic — *see* Cirrhosis, liver
  hypertrophic K74.3
  Indian childhood K74.69
  kidney — *see* Sclerosis, renal
  Laennec's K70.30
    with ascites K70.31
    alcoholic K70.30
      with ascites K70.31
    nonalcoholic K74.69
  liver K74.60
    alcoholic K70.30
      with ascites K70.31
      fatty K70.0
    congenital P78.81
    syphilitic A52.74
  lung (chronic) J84.10
  macronodular K74.69
    alcoholic K70.30
      with ascites K70.31
  micronodular K74.69
    alcoholic K70.30
      with ascites K70.31
  mixed type K74.69
  monolobular K74.3
  nephritis — *see* Sclerosis, renal
  nutritional K74.69
    alcoholic K70.30
      with ascites K70.31
  obstructive — *see* Cirrhosis, biliary
  ovarian N83.8
  pancreas (duct) K86.89
  pigmentary E83.110
  portal K74.69
    alcoholic K70.30
      with ascites K70.31
  postnecrotic K74.69
    alcoholic K70.30
      with ascites K70.31
  pulmonary J84.10
  renal — *see* Sclerosis, renal
  spleen D73.2
  stasis K76.1
  Todd's K74.3
  unilobar K74.3
  xanthomatous (biliary) K74.5
    due to xanthomatosis (familial) (metabolic) (primary) E78.2
Cistern, subarachnoid R93.0
Citrullinemia E72.23
Citrullinuria E72.23
Civatte's disease or poikiloderma L57.3
Clam digger's itch B65.3
Clammy skin R23.1
Clap — *see* Gonorrhea
Clarke-Hadfield syndrome (pancreatic infantilism) K86.89
Clark's paralysis G80.9
Clastothrix L67.8
Claude Bernard-Horner syndrome G90.2
  traumatic — *see* Injury, nerve, cervical sympathetic
Claude's disease or syndrome G46.3
Claudicatio venosa intermittens I87.8
Claudication (intermittent) I73.9

Claudication — *continued*
  cerebral (artery) G45.9
  spinal cord (arteriosclerotic) G95.19
    syphilitic A52.09
  venous (axillary) I87.8
Claustrophobia F40.240
Clavus (infected) L84
Clawfoot (congenital) Q66.89
  acquired — *see* Deformity, limb, clawfoot
Clawhand (acquired) — *see also* Deformity, limb, clawhand
  congenital Q68.1
Clawtoe (congenital) Q66.89
  acquired — *see* Deformity, toe, specified NEC
Clay eating — *see* Pica
Cleansing of artificial opening — *see* Attention to, artificial, opening
Cleft (congenital) — *see also* Imperfect, closure
  alveolar process M26.79
  branchial (persistent) Q18.2
    cyst Q18.0
      fistula Q18.0
      sinus Q18.0
  cricoid cartilage, posterior Q31.8
  cyst Q18.0
    fistula Q18.0
    sinus Q18.0
  foot Q72.7 ☑
  hand Q71.6 ☑
  lip (unilateral) Q36.9
    with cleft palate Q37.9
      hard Q37.1
        with soft Q37.5
      soft Q37.3
        with hard Q37.5
    bilateral Q36.0
      with cleft palate Q37.8
        hard Q37.0
          with soft Q37.4
        soft Q37.2
          with hard Q37.4
    median Q36.1
  nose Q30.2
  palate Q35.9
    with cleft lip (unilateral) Q37.9
      bilateral Q37.8
    hard Q35.1
      with
        cleft lip (unilateral) Q37.1
          bilateral Q37.0
        soft Q35.5
          with cleft lip (unilateral) Q37.5
            bilateral Q37.4
    medial Q35.5
    soft Q35.3
      with
        cleft lip (unilateral) Q37.3
          bilateral Q37.2
        hard Q35.5
          with cleft lip (unilateral) Q37.5
            bilateral Q37.4
  penis Q55.69
  scrotum Q55.29
  thyroid cartilage Q31.8
  uvula Q35.7
Cleidocranial dysostosis Q74.0
Cleptomania F63.2
Clicking hip (newborn) R29.4
Climacteric (female) — *see also* Menopause
  arthritis (any site) NEC — *see* Arthritis, specified form NEC
  depression (single episode) F32.89
    recurrent episode F33.8
  male (symptoms) (syndrome) NEC N50.89
  melancholia (single episode) F32.89
    recurrent episode F33.8
  paranoid state F22
  polyarthritis NEC — *see* Arthritis, specified form NEC
  symptoms (female) N95.1
Clinical research investigation (clinical trial) (control subject) (normal comparison) (participant) Z00.6
Clitoris — *see* condition
Cloaca (persistent) Q43.7
Clonorchiasis, clonorchis infection (liver) B66.1
Clonus R25.8
Closed bite M26.29
Clostridium (C.) **perfringens, as cause of disease classified elsewhere** B96.7

▽ Subterms under main terms may continue to next column or page   ☑ Additional Character Required — Refer to the Tabular List for Character Selection   55

Chyluria — Clostridium

Closure
- congenital, nose Q30.0
- cranial sutures, premature Q75.0
- defective or imperfect NEC — *see* Imperfect, closure
- fistula, delayed — *see* Fistula
- foramen ovale, imperfect Q21.1
- hymen N89.6
- interauricular septum, defective Q21.1
- interventricular septum, defective Q21.0
- lacrimal duct — *see also* Stenosis, lacrimal, duct
  - congenital Q10.5
- nose (congenital) Q30.0
  - acquired M95.0
- of artificial opening — *see* Attention to, artificial, opening
- vagina N89.5
- valve — *see* Endocarditis
- vulva N90.5

Clot (blood) — *see also* Embolism
- artery (obstruction) (occlusion) — *see* Embolism
- bladder N32.89
- brain (intradural or extradural) — *see* Occlusion, artery, cerebral
- circulation I74.9
- heart — *see also* Infarct, myocardium
  - not resulting in infarction I51.3
- vein — *see* Thrombosis

Clouded state R40.1
- epileptic — *see* Epilepsy, specified NEC
- paroxysmal — *see* Epilepsy, specified NEC

Cloudy antrum, antra J32.0
Clouston's (hidrotic) **ectodermal dysplasia** Q82.4
Clubbed nail pachydermoperiostosis M89.40 *[L62]*
Clubbing of finger(s) (nails) R68.3
Clubfinger R68.3
- congenital Q68.1
Clubfoot (congenital) Q66.89
- acquired — *see* Deformity, limb, clubfoot
- equinovarus Q66.0- ☑
- paralytic — *see* Deformity, limb, clubfoot
Clubhand (congenital) (radial) Q71.4- ☑
- acquired — *see* Deformity, limb, clubhand
Clubnail R68.3
- congenital Q84.6
Clump, kidney Q63.1
Clumsiness, clumsy child syndrome F82
Cluttering F80.81
Clutton's joints A50.51 *[M12.80]*
Coagulation, intravascular (diffuse) (disseminated) — *see also* Defibrination syndrome
- complicating abortion — *see* Abortion, by type, complicated by, intravascular coagulation
- following ectopic or molar pregnancy O08.1
Coagulopathy — *see also* Defect, coagulation
- consumption D65
- intravascular D65
  - newborn P60
Coalition
- calcaneo-scaphoid Q66.89
- tarsal Q66.89
Coalminer's
- elbow — *see* Bursitis, elbow, olecranon
- lung or pneumoconiosis J60
Coalworker's lung or pneumoconiosis J60
Coarctation
- aorta (preductal) (postductal) Q25.1
- pulmonary artery Q25.71
Coated tongue K14.3
Coats' disease (exudative retinopathy) — *see* Retinopathy, exudative
Cocaine-induced
- anxiety disorder F14.980
- bipolar and related disorder F14.94
- depressive disorder F14.94
- obsessive-compulsive and related disorder F14.988
- psychotic disorder F14.959
- sexual dysfunction F14.981
- sleep disorder F14.982
Cocainism — *see* Disorder, cocaine use
Coccidioidomycosis B38.9
- cutaneous B38.3
- disseminated B38.7
- generalized B38.7
- meninges B38.4
- prostate B38.81
- pulmonary B38.2
  - acute B38.0

Coccidioidomycosis — *continued*
- pulmonary — *continued*
  - chronic B38.1
- skin B38.3
- specified NEC B38.89
Coccidioidosis — *see* Coccidioidomycosis
Coccidiosis (intestinal) A07.3
Coccydynia, coccygodynia M53.3
Coccyx — *see* condition
Cochin-China diarrhea K90.1
Cockayne's syndrome Q87.19
Cocked up toe — *see* Deformity, toe, specified NEC
Cock's peculiar tumor L72.3
Codman's tumor — *see* Neoplasm, bone, benign
Coenurosis B71.8
Coffee-worker's lung J67.8 ☑
Cogan's syndrome H16.32- ☑
- oculomotor apraxia H51.8
Coitus, painful (female) N94.10
- male N53.12
- psychogenic F52.6
Cold J00
- with influenza, flu, or grippe — *see* Influenza, with, respiratory manifestations NEC
- agglutinin disease or hemoglobinuria (chronic) D59.1
- bronchial — *see* Bronchitis
- chest — *see* Bronchitis
- common (head) J00
- effects of T69.9 ☑
  - specified effect NEC T69.8 ☑
- excessive, effects of T69.9 ☑
  - specified effect NEC T69.8 ☑
- exhaustion from T69.8 ☑
- exposure to T69.9 ☑
  - specified effect NEC T69.8 ☑
- head J00
- injury syndrome (newborn) P80.0
- on lung — *see* Bronchitis
- rose J30.1
- sensitivity, auto-immune D59.1
- symptoms J00
- virus J00
Coldsore B00.1
Colibacillosis A49.8
- as the cause of other disease — *see also* Escherichia coli B96.20
- generalized A41.50
Colic (bilious) (infantile) (intestinal) (recurrent) (spasmodic) R10.83
- abdomen R10.83
  - psychogenic F45.8
- appendix, appendicular K38.8
- bile duct — *see* Calculus, bile duct
- biliary — *see* Calculus, bile duct
- common duct — *see* Calculus, bile duct
- cystic duct — *see* Calculus, gallbladder
- Devonshire NEC — *see* Poisoning, lead
- gallbladder — *see* Calculus, gallbladder
- gallstone — *see* Calculus, gallbladder
  - gallbladder or cystic duct — *see* Calculus, gallbladder
- hepatic (duct) — *see* Calculus, bile duct
- hysterical F45.8
- kidney N23
- lead NEC — *see* Poisoning, lead
- mucous K58.9
  - with diarrhea K58.0
  - psychogenic F54
- nephritic N23
- painter's NEC — *see* Poisoning, lead
- pancreas K86.89
- psychogenic F45.8
- renal N23
- saturnine NEC — *see* Poisoning, lead
- ureter N23
- urethral N36.8
  - due to calculus N21.1
- uterus NEC N94.89
  - menstrual — *see* Dysmenorrhea
- worm NOS B83.9
Colicystitis — *see* Cystitis
Colitis (acute) (catarrhal) (chronic) (noninfective) (hemorrhagic) — *see also* Enteritis K52.9
- allergic K52.29
  - with
    - food protein-induced enterocolitis syndrome K52.21

Colitis — *continued*
- allergic — *continued*
  - with — *continued*
    - proctocolitis K52.82
- amebic (acute) — *see also* Amebiasis A06.0
  - nondysenteric A06.2
- anthrax A22.2
- bacillary — *see* Infection, Shigella
- balantidial A07.0
- Clostridium difficile
  - not specified as recurrent A04.72
  - recurrent A04.71
- coccidial A07.3
- collagenous K52.831
- cystica superficialis K52.89
- dietary counseling and surveillance (for) Z71.3
- dietetic — *see also* Colitis, allergic K52.29
- drug-induced K52.1
- due to radiation K52.0
- eosinophilic K52.82
- food hypersensitivity — *see also* Colitis, allergic K52.29
- giardial A07.1
- granulomatous — *see* Enteritis, regional, large intestine
- indeterminate, so stated K52.3
- infectious — *see* Enteritis, infectious
- ischemic K55.9
  - acute (subacute) — *see also* Ischemia, intestine, acute K55.039
  - chronic K55.1
  - due to mesenteric artery insufficiency K55.1
  - fulminant (acute) — *see also* Ischemia, intestine, acute K55.039
- left sided K51.50
  - with
    - abscess K51.514
    - complication K51.519
      - specified NEC K51.518
    - fistula K51.513
    - obstruction K51.512
    - rectal bleeding K51.511
- lymphocytic K52.832
- membranous
  - psychogenic F54
- microscopic K52.839
  - specified NEC K52.838
- mucous — *see* Syndrome, irritable, bowel
  - psychogenic F54
- noninfective K52.9
  - specified NEC K52.89
- polyposa — *see* Polyp, colon, inflammatory
- protozoal A07.9
- pseudomembranous
  - not specified as recurrent A04.72
  - recurrent A04.71
- pseudomucinous — *see* Syndrome, irritable, bowel
- regional — *see* Enteritis, regional, large intestine
  - infectious A09
- segmental — *see* Enteritis, regional, large intestine
- septic — *see* Enteritis, infectious
- spastic K58.9
  - with diarrhea K58.0
  - psychogenic F54
- staphylococcal A04.8
  - foodborne A05.0
- subacute ischemic — *see also* Ischemia, intestine, acute K55.039
- thromboulcerative — *see also* Ischemia, intestine, acute K55.039
- toxic NEC K52.1
  - due to Clostridium difficile
    - not specified as recurrent A04.72
    - recurrent A04.71
- transmural — *see* Enteritis, regional, large intestine
- trichomonal A07.8
- tuberculous (ulcerative) A18.32
- ulcerative (chronic) K51.90
  - with
    - complication K51.919
      - abscess K51.914
      - fistula K51.913
      - obstruction K51.912
      - rectal bleeding K51.911
      - specified complication NEC K51.918
  - enterocolitis — *see* Enterocolitis, ulcerative
  - ileocolitis — *see* Ileocolitis, ulcerative
  - mucosal proctocolitis — *see* Proctocolitis, mucosal
  - proctitis — *see* Proctitis, ulcerative
  - pseudopolyposis — *see* Polyp, colon, inflammatory

Colitis — continued
- ulcerative — continued
  - psychogenic F54
  - rectosigmoiditis — see Rectosigmoiditis, ulcerative
  - specified type NEC K51.80
    - with
      - complication K51.819
        - abscess K51.814
        - fistula K51.813
        - obstruction K51.812
        - rectal bleeding K51.811
        - specified complication NEC K51.818

Collagenosis, collagen disease (nonvascular) (vascular) M35.9
- cardiovascular I42.8
- reactive perforating L87.1
- specified NEC M35.8

Collapse R55
- adrenal E27.2
- cardiorespiratory R57.0
- cardiovascular R57.0
  - newborn P29.89
- circulatory (peripheral) R57.9
  - during or after labor and delivery O75.1
  - following ectopic or molar pregnancy O08.3
  - newborn P29.89
- during or
  - after labor and delivery O75.1
  - resulting from a procedure, not elsewhere classified T81.10 ☑
- external ear canal — see Stenosis, external ear canal
- general R55
- heart — see Disease, heart
- heat T67.1 ☑
- hysterical F44.89
- labyrinth, membranous (congenital) Q16.5
- lung (massive) — see also Atelectasis J98.19
  - pressure due to anesthesia (general) (local) or other sedation T88.2
    - during labor and delivery O74.1
    - in pregnancy O29.02- ☑
    - postpartum, puerperal O89.09
- myocardial — see Disease, heart
- nervous F48.8
- neurocirculatory F45.8
- nose M95.0
- postoperative T81.10 ☑
- pulmonary — see also Atelectasis J98.19
  - newborn — see Atelectasis
- trachea J39.8
- tracheobronchial J98.09
- valvular — see Endocarditis
- vascular (peripheral) R57.9
  - during or after labor and delivery O75.1
  - following ectopic or molar pregnancy O08.3
  - newborn P29.89
- vertebra M48.50- ☑
  - cervical region M48.52- ☑
  - cervicothoracic region M48.53- ☑
  - in (due to)
    - metastasis — see Collapse, vertebra, in, specified disease NEC
    - osteoporosis — see also Osteoporosis M80.88 ☑
      - cervical region M80.88 ☑
      - cervicothoracic region M80.88 ☑
      - lumbar region M80.88 ☑
      - lumbosacral region M80.88 ☑
      - multiple sites M80.88 ☑
      - occipito-atlanto-axial region M80.88 ☑
      - sacrococcygeal region M80.88 ☑
      - thoracic region M80.88 ☑
      - thoracolumbar region M80.88 ☑
    - specified disease NEC M48.50- ☑
      - cervical region M48.52- ☑
      - cervicothoracic region M48.53- ☑
      - lumbar region M48.56- ☑
      - lumbosacral region M48.57- ☑
      - occipito-atlanto-axial region M48.51- ☑
      - sacrococcygeal region M48.58- ☑
      - thoracic region M48.54- ☑
      - thoracolumbar region M48.55- ☑
  - lumbar region M48.56- ☑
  - lumbosacral region M48.57- ☑
  - occipito-atlanto-axial region M48.51- ☑
  - sacrococcygeal region M48.58- ☑
  - thoracic region M48.54- ☑
  - thoracolumbar region M48.55- ☑

Collateral — see also condition
- circulation (venous) I87.8
- dilation, veins I87.8

Colles' fracture S52.53- ☑

Collet (-Sicard) syndrome G52.7

Collier's asthma or lung J60

Collodion baby Q80.2

Colloid nodule (of thyroid) (cystic) E04.1

Coloboma (iris) Q13.0
- eyelid Q10.3
- fundus Q14.8
- lens Q12.2
- optic disc (congenital) Q14.2
  - acquired H47.31- ☑

Coloenteritis — see Enteritis

Colon — see condition

Colonization
- MRSA (Methicillin resistant Staphylococcus aureus) Z22.322
- MSSA (Methicillin susceptible Staphylococcus aureus) Z22.321
- status — see Carrier (suspected) of

Coloptosis K63.4

Color blindness — see Deficiency, color vision

Colostomy
- attention to Z43.3
- fitting or adjustment Z46.89
- malfunctioning K94.03
- status Z93.3

Colpitis (acute) — see Vaginitis

Colpocele N81.5

Colpocystitis — see Vaginitis

Colpospasm N94.2

Column, spinal, vertebral — see condition

Coma R40.20
- with
  - motor response (none) R40.231 ☑
    - abnormal extensor posturing to pain or noxious stimuli (< 2 years of age) R40.232 ☑
    - abnormal flexure posturing to pain or noxious stimuli (0-5 years of age) R40.233 ☑
    - extensor posturing to pain or noxious stimuli (2-5 years of age) R40.232 ☑
    - flexion/decorticate posturing (< 2 years of age) R40.233 ☑
    - localizes pain (2-5 years of age) R40.235 ☑
    - normal or spontaneous movement (< 2 years of age) R40.236 ☑
    - obeys commands (2-5 years of age) R40.236 ☑
    - score of
      - 1 R40.231 ☑
      - 2 R40.232 ☑
      - 3 R40.233 ☑
      - 4 R40.234 ☑
      - 5 R40.235 ☑
      - 6 R40.236 ☑
    - withdraws from pain or noxious stimuli (0-5 years of age) R40.234 ☑
    - withdraws to touch (< 2 years of age) R40.235 ☑
  - opening of eyes (never) R40.211 ☑
    - in response to
      - pain R40.212 ☑
      - sound R40.213 ☑
    - score of
      - 1 R40.211 ☑
      - 2 R40.212 ☑
      - 3 R40.213 ☑
      - 4 R40.214 ☑
    - spontaneous R40.214 ☑
  - verbal response (none) R40.221 ☑
    - confused conversation R40.224 ☑
    - cooing or babbling or crying appropriately (<2 years of age) R40.225 ☑
    - inappropriate crying or screaming (< 2 years of age) R40.223 ☑
    - inappropriate words (2-5 years of age) R40.224 ☑
    - incomprehensible sounds (2-5 years of age) R40.222 ☑
    - incomprehensible words R40.222 ☑
    - irritable cries (< 2 years of age) R40.224 ☑
    - moans/grunts to pain; restless (< 2 years old) R40.222 ☑
    - oriented R40.225 ☑
    - score of
      - 1 R40.221 ☑
      - 2 R40.222 ☑

Coma — continued
- with — continued
  - verbal response — continued
    - score of — continued
      - 3 R40.223 ☑
      - 4 R40.224 ☑
      - 5 R40.225 ☑
    - screaming (2-5 years of age) R40.223 ☑
    - uses appropriate words (2-5 years of age) R40.225 ☑
- eclamptic — see Eclampsia
- epileptic — see Epilepsy
- Glasgow, scale score — see Glasgow coma scale
- hepatic — see Failure, hepatic, by type, with coma
- hyperglycemic (diabetic) — see Diabetes, by type, with hyperosmolarity, with coma
- hyperosmolar (diabetic) — see Diabetes, by type, with hyperosmolarity, with coma
- hypoglycemic (diabetic) — see Diabetes, by type, with hypoglycemia, with coma
  - nondiabetic E15
- in diabetes — see Diabetes, coma
- insulin-induced — see Coma, hypoglycemic
- ketoacidotic (diabetic) — see Diabetes, by type, with ketoacidosis, with coma
- myxedematous E03.5
- newborn P91.5
- persistent vegetative state R40.3
- specified NEC, without documented Glasgow coma scale score, or with partial Glasgow coma scale score reported R40.244 ☑

Comatose — see Coma

Combat fatigue F43.0

Combined — see condition

Comedo, comedones (giant) L70.0

Comedocarcinoma — see also Neoplasm, breast, malignant
- noninfiltrating
  - breast D05.8- ☑
  - specified site — see Neoplasm, in situ, by site
  - unspecified site D05.8- ☑

Comedomastitis — see Ectasia, mammary duct

Comminuted fracture — code as Fracture, closed

Common
- arterial trunk Q20.0
- atrioventricular canal Q21.2
- atrium Q21.1
- cold (head) J00
- truncus (arteriosus) Q20.0
- variable immunodeficiency — see Immunodeficiency, common variable
- ventricle Q20.4

Commotio, commotion (current)
- brain — see Injury, intracranial, concussion
- cerebri — see Injury, intracranial, concussion
- retinae S05.8X- ☑
- spinal cord — see Injury, spinal cord, by region
- spinalis — see Injury, spinal cord, by region

Communication
- between
  - base of aorta and pulmonary artery Q21.4
  - left ventricle and right atrium Q20.5
  - pericardial sac and pleural sac Q34.8
  - pulmonary artery and pulmonary vein, congenital Q25.72
- congenital between uterus and digestive or urinary tract Q51.7

Compartment syndrome (deep) (posterior) (traumatic) T79.A0 ☑ (following T79.7)
- abdomen T79.A3 ☑ (following T79.7)
- lower extremity (hip, buttock, thigh, leg, foot, toes) T79.A2 ☑ (following T79.7)
- nontraumatic
  - abdomen M79.A3 (following M79.7)
  - lower extremity (hip, buttock, thigh, leg, foot, toes) M79.A2- ☑ (following M79.7)
  - specified site NEC M79.A9 (following M79.7)
  - upper extremity (shoulder, arm, forearm, wrist, hand, fingers) M79.A1- ☑ (following M79.7)
- specified site NEC T79.A9 ☑ (following T79.7)
- upper extremity (shoulder, arm, forearm, wrist, hand, fingers) T79.A1- ☑ (following T79.7)

Compensation
- failure — see Disease, heart
- neurosis, psychoneurosis — see Disorder, factitious

Complaint — see also Disease
- bowel, functional K59.9

↻ Subterms under main terms may continue to next column or page   ☑ Additional Character Required — Refer to the Tabular List for Character Selection   57

Colitis — Complaint

Complaint — *continued*
  bowel, functional — *continued*
    psychogenic F45.8
  intestine, functional K59.9
    psychogenic F45.8
  kidney — *see* Disease, renal
  miners' J60
Complete — *see* condition
Complex
  Addison-Schilder E71.528
  cardiorenal — *see* Hypertension, cardiorenal
  Costen's M26.69
  disseminated mycobacterium avium- intracellulare
    (DMAC) A31.2
  Eisenmenger's (ventricular septal defect) I27.83
  hypersexual F52.8
  jumped process, spine — *see* Dislocation, vertebra
  primary, tuberculous A15.7
  Schilder-Addison E71.528
  subluxation (vertebral) M99.19
    abdomen M99.19
    acromioclavicular M99.17
    cervical region M99.11
    cervicothoracic M99.11
    costochondral M99.18
    costovertebral M99.18
    head region M99.10
    hip M99.15
    lower extremity M99.16
    lumbar region M99.13
    lumbosacral M99.13
    occipitocervical M99.10
    pelvic region M99.15
    pubic M99.15
    rib cage M99.18
    sacral region M99.14
    sacrococcygeal M99.14
    sacroiliac M99.14
    specified NEC M99.19
    sternochondral M99.18
    sternoclavicular M99.17
    thoracic region M99.12
    thoracolumbar M99.12
    upper extremity M99.17
  Taussig-Bing (transposition, aorta and overriding pulmonary artery) Q20.1
Complication(s) (from) (of)
  accidental puncture or laceration during a procedure (of) — *see* Complications, intraoperative (intraprocedural), puncture or laceration
  amputation stump (surgical) (late) NEC T87.9
    dehiscence T87.81
    infection or inflammation T87.40
      lower limb T87.4- ☑
      upper limb T87.4- ☑
    necrosis T87.50
      lower limb T87.5- ☑
      upper limb T87.5- ☑
    neuroma T87.30
      lower limb T87.3- ☑
      upper limb T87.3- ☑
    specified type NEC T87.89
  anastomosis (and bypass) — *see also* Complications, prosthetic device or implant
    intestinal (internal) NEC K91.89
      involving urinary tract N99.89
    urinary tract (involving intestinal tract) N99.89
    vascular — *see* Complications, cardiovascular device or implant
  anesthesia, anesthetic — *see also* Anesthesia, complication T88.59
    brain, postpartum, puerperal O89.2
    cardiac
      in
        labor and delivery O74.2
        pregnancy O29.19- ☑
      postpartum, puerperal O89.1
    central nervous system
      in
        labor and delivery O74.3
        pregnancy O29.29- ☑
      postpartum, puerperal O89.2
    difficult or failed intubation T88.4 ☑
      in pregnancy O29.6- ☑
    failed sedation (conscious) (moderate) during procedure T88.52 ☑
    general, unintended awareness during procedure T88.53 ☑

Complication(s) — *continued*
  anesthesia, anesthetic — *see also* Anesthesia, complication — *continued*
    hyperthermia, malignant T88.3 ☑
    hypothermia T88.51 ☑
    intubation failure T88.4 ☑
    malignant hyperthermia T88.3 ☑
    pulmonary
      in
        labor and delivery O74.1
        pregnancy NEC O29.09- ☑
      postpartum, puerperal O89.09
    shock T88.2 ☑
    spinal and epidural
      in
        labor and delivery NEC O74.6
          headache O74.5
        pregnancy NEC O29.5X- ☑
      postpartum, puerperal NEC O89.5
        headache O89.4
    unintended awareness under general anesthesia during procedure T88.53 ☑
  anti-reflux device — *see* Complications, esophageal anti-reflux device
  aortic (bifurcation) graft — *see* Complications, graft, vascular
  aortocoronary (bypass) graft — *see* Complications, coronary artery (bypass) graft
  aortofemoral (bypass) graft — *see* Complications, extremity artery (bypass) graft
  arteriovenous
    fistula, surgically created T82.9 ☑
      embolism T82.818 ☑
      fibrosis T82.828 ☑
      hemorrhage T82.838 ☑
      infection or inflammation T82.7 ☑
      mechanical
        breakdown T82.510 ☑
        displacement T82.520 ☑
        leakage T82.530 ☑
        malposition T82.520 ☑
        obstruction T82.590 ☑
        perforation T82.590 ☑
        protrusion T82.590 ☑
      pain T82.848 ☑
      specified type NEC T82.898 ☑
      stenosis T82.858 ☑
      thrombosis T82.868 ☑
    shunt, surgically created T82.9 ☑
      embolism T82.818 ☑
      fibrosis T82.828 ☑
      hemorrhage T82.838 ☑
      infection or inflammation T82.7 ☑
      mechanical
        breakdown T82.511 ☑
        displacement T82.521 ☑
        leakage T82.531 ☑
        malposition T82.521 ☑
        obstruction T82.591 ☑
        perforation T82.591 ☑
        protrusion T82.591 ☑
      pain T82.848 ☑
      specified type NEC T82.898 ☑
      stenosis T82.858 ☑
      thrombosis T82.868 ☑
  arthroplasty — *see* Complications, joint prosthesis
  artificial
    fertilization or insemination N98.9
      attempted introduction (of)
        embryo in embryo transfer N98.3
        ovum following in vitro fertilization N98.2
      hyperstimulation of ovaries N98.1
      infection N98.0
      specified NEC N98.8
    heart T82.9 ☑
      embolism T82.817 ☑
      fibrosis T82.827 ☑
      hemorrhage T82.837 ☑
      infection or inflammation T82.7 ☑
      mechanical
        breakdown T82.512 ☑
        displacement T82.522 ☑
        leakage T82.532 ☑
        malposition T82.522 ☑
        obstruction T82.592 ☑
        perforation T82.592 ☑

Complication(s) — *continued*
  artificial — *continued*
    heart — *continued*
      mechanical — *continued*
        protrusion T82.592 ☑
      pain T82.847 ☑
      specified type NEC T82.897 ☑
      stenosis T82.857 ☑
      thrombosis T82.867 ☑
    opening
      cecostomy — *see* Complications, colostomy
      colostomy — *see* Complications, colostomy
      cystostomy — *see* Complications, cystostomy
      enterostomy — *see* Complications, enterostomy
      gastrostomy — *see* Complications, gastrostomy
      ileostomy — *see* Complications, enterostomy
      jejunostomy — *see* Complications, enterostomy
      nephrostomy — *see* Complications, stoma, urinary tract
      tracheostomy — *see* Complications, tracheostomy
      ureterostomy — *see* Complications, stoma, urinary tract
      urethrostomy — *see* Complications, stoma, urinary tract
  balloon implant or device
    gastrointestinal T85.9 ☑
      embolism T85.818 ☑
      fibrosis T85.828 ☑
      hemorrhage T85.838 ☑
      infection and inflammation T85.79 ☑
      pain T85.848 ☑
      specified type NEC T85.898 ☑
      stenosis T85.858 ☑
      thrombosis T85.868 ☑
    vascular (counterpulsation) T82.9 ☑
      embolism T82.818 ☑
      fibrosis T82.828 ☑
      hemorrhage T82.838 ☑
      infection or inflammation T82.7 ☑
      mechanical
        breakdown T82.513 ☑
        displacement T82.523 ☑
        leakage T82.533 ☑
        malposition T82.523 ☑
        obstruction T82.593 ☑
        perforation T82.593 ☑
        protrusion T82.593 ☑
      pain T82.848 ☑
      specified type NEC T82.898 ☑
      stenosis T82.858 ☑
      thrombosis T82.868 ☑
  bariatric procedure
    gastric band procedure K95.09
      infection K95.01
    specified procedure NEC K95.89
      infection K95.81
  bile duct implant (prosthetic) T85.9 ☑
    embolism T85.818 ☑
    fibrosis T85.828 ☑
    hemorrhage T85.838 ☑
    infection and inflammation T85.79 ☑
    mechanical
      breakdown T85.510 ☑
      displacement T85.520 ☑
      malfunction T85.510 ☑
      malposition T85.520 ☑
      obstruction T85.590 ☑
      perforation T85.590 ☑
      protrusion T85.590 ☑
      specified NEC T85.590 ☑
    pain T85.848 ☑
    specified type NEC T85.898 ☑
    stenosis T85.858 ☑
    thrombosis T85.868 ☑
  bladder device (auxiliary) — *see* Complications, genitourinary, device or implant, urinary system
  bleeding (postoperative) — *see* Complication, postoperative, hemorrhage
    intraoperative — *see* Complication, intraoperative, hemorrhage
  blood vessel graft — *see* Complications, graft, vascular
  bone
    device NEC T84.9 ☑
      embolism T84.81 ☑
      fibrosis T84.82 ☑

Complication(s) — *continued*
  bone — *continued*
    device — *continued*
      hemorrhage T84.83 ☑
      infection or inflammation T84.7 ☑
      mechanical
        breakdown T84.318 ☑
        displacement T84.328 ☑
        malposition T84.328 ☑
        obstruction T84.398 ☑
        perforation T84.398 ☑
        protrusion T84.398 ☑
      pain T84.84 ☑
      specified type NEC T84.89 ☑
      stenosis T84.85 ☑
      thrombosis T84.86 ☑
    graft — *see* Complications, graft, bone
    growth stimulator (electrode) — *see* Complications, electronic stimulator device, bone
    marrow transplant — *see* Complications, transplant, bone, marrow
  brain neurostimulator (electrode) — *see* Complications, electronic stimulator device, brain
  breast implant (prosthetic) T85.9 ☑
    capsular contracture T85.44 ☑
    embolism T85.818 ☑
    fibrosis T85.828 ☑
    hemorrhage T85.838 ☑
    infection and inflammation T85.79 ☑
    mechanical
      breakdown T85.41 ☑
      displacement T85.42 ☑
      leakage T85.43 ☑
      malposition T85.42 ☑
      obstruction T85.49 ☑
      perforation T85.49 ☑
      protrusion T85.49 ☑
      specified NEC T85.49 ☑
    pain T85.848 ☑
    specified type NEC T85.898 ☑
    stenosis T85.858 ☑
    thrombosis T85.868 ☑
  bypass — *see also* Complications, prosthetic device or implant
    aortocoronary — *see* Complications, coronary artery (bypass) graft
    arterial — *see also* Complications, graft, vascular
      extremity — *see* Complications, extremity artery (bypass) graft
  cardiac — *see also* Disease, heart
    device, implant or graft T82.9 ☑
      embolism T82.817 ☑
      fibrosis T82.827 ☑
      hemorrhage T82.837 ☑
      infection or inflammation T82.7 ☑
        valve prosthesis T82.6 ☑
      mechanical
        breakdown T82.519 ☑
          specified device NEC T82.518 ☑
        displacement T82.529 ☑
          specified device NEC T82.528 ☑
        leakage T82.539 ☑
          specified device NEC T82.538 ☑
        malposition T82.529 ☑
          specified device NEC T82.528 ☑
        obstruction T82.599 ☑
          specified device NEC T82.598 ☑
        perforation T82.599 ☑
          specified device NEC T82.598 ☑
        protrusion T82.599 ☑
          specified device NEC T82.598 ☑
      pain T82.847 ☑
      specified type NEC T82.897 ☑
      stenosis T82.857 ☑
      thrombosis T82.867 ☑
  cardiovascular device, graft or implant T82.9 ☑
    aortic graft — *see* Complications, graft, vascular
    arteriovenous
      fistula, artificial — *see* Complication, arteriovenous, fistula, surgically created
      shunt — *see* Complication, arteriovenous, shunt, surgically created
    artificial heart — *see* Complication, artificial, heart
    balloon (counterpulsation) device — *see* Complication, balloon implant, vascular

Complication(s) — *continued*
  cardiovascular device, graft or implant — *continued*
    carotid artery graft — *see* Complications, graft, vascular
    coronary bypass graft — *see* Complication, coronary artery (bypass) graft
    dialysis catheter (vascular) — *see* Complication, catheter, dialysis
    electronic T82.9 ☑
      electrode T82.9 ☑
        embolism T82.817 ☑
        fibrosis T82.827 ☑
        hemorrhage T82.837 ☑
        infection T82.7 ☑
        mechanical
          breakdown T82.110 ☑
          displacement T82.120 ☑
          leakage T82.190 ☑
          obstruction T82.190 ☑
          perforation T82.190 ☑
          protrusion T82.190 ☑
          specified type NEC T82.190 ☑
        pain T82.847 ☑
        specified NEC T82.897 ☑
        stenosis T82.857 ☑
        thrombosis T82.867 ☑
      embolism T82.817 ☑
      fibrosis T82.827 ☑
      hemorrhage T82.837 ☑
      infection T82.7 ☑
      mechanical
        breakdown T82.119 ☑
        displacement T82.129 ☑
        leakage T82.199 ☑
        obstruction T82.199 ☑
        perforation T82.199 ☑
        protrusion T82.199 ☑
        specified type NEC T82.199 ☑
      pain T82.847 ☑
      pulse generator T82.9 ☑
        embolism T82.817 ☑
        fibrosis T82.827 ☑
        hemorrhage T82.837 ☑
        infection T82.7 ☑
        mechanical
          breakdown T82.111 ☑
          displacement T82.121 ☑
          leakage T82.191 ☑
          obstruction T82.191 ☑
          perforation T82.191 ☑
          protrusion T82.191 ☑
          specified type NEC T82.191 ☑
        pain T82.847 ☑
        specified NEC T82.897 ☑
        stenosis T82.857 ☑
        thrombosis T82.867 ☑
      specified condition NEC T82.897 ☑
      specified device NEC T82.9 ☑
        embolism T82.817 ☑
        fibrosis T82.827 ☑
        hemorrhage T82.837 ☑
        infection T82.7 ☑
        mechanical
          breakdown T82.118 ☑
          displacement T82.128 ☑
          leakage T82.198 ☑
          obstruction T82.198 ☑
          perforation T82.198 ☑
          protrusion T82.198 ☑
          specified type NEC T82.198 ☑
        pain T82.847 ☑
        specified NEC T82.897 ☑
        stenosis T82.857 ☑
        thrombosis T82.867 ☑
      stenosis T82.857 ☑
      thrombosis T82.867 ☑
    extremity artery graft — *see* Complication, extremity artery (bypass) graft
    femoral artery graft — *see* Complication, extremity artery (bypass) graft
    heart
      transplant — *see* Complication, transplant, heart
      valve — *see* Complication, prosthetic device, heart valve
        graft — *see* Complication, heart, valve, graft

Complication(s) — *continued*
  cardiovascular device, graft or implant — *continued*
    heart-lung transplant — *see* Complication, transplant, heart, with lung
    infection or inflammation T82.7 ☑
    umbrella device — *see* Complication, umbrella device, vascular
    vascular graft (or anastomosis) — *see* Complication, graft, vascular
  carotid artery (bypass) graft — *see* Complications, graft, vascular
  catheter (device) NEC — *see also* Complications, prosthetic device or implant
    cranial infusion
      infection and inflammation T85.735 ☑
      mechanical
        breakdown T85.610 ☑
        displacement T85.620 ☑
        leakage T85.630 ☑
        malfunction T85.690 ☑
        malposition T85.620 ☑
        obstruction T85.690 ☑
        perforation T85.690 ☑
        protrusion T85.690 ☑
        specified NEC T85.690 ☑
    cystostomy T83.9 ☑
      embolism T83.81 ☑
      fibrosis T83.82 ☑
      hemorrhage T83.83 ☑
      infection and inflammation T83.510 ☑
      mechanical
        breakdown T83.010 ☑
        displacement T83.020 ☑
        leakage T83.030 ☑
        malposition T83.020 ☑
        obstruction T83.090 ☑
        perforation T83.090 ☑
        protrusion T83.090 ☑
        specified NEC T83.090 ☑
      pain T83.84 ☑
      specified type NEC T83.89 ☑
      stenosis T83.85 ☑
      thrombosis T83.86 ☑
    dialysis (vascular) T82.9 ☑
      embolism T82.818 ☑
      fibrosis T82.828 ☑
      hemorrhage T82.838 ☑
      infection and inflammation T82.7 ☑
      intraperitoneal — *see* Complications, catheter, intraperitoneal
      mechanical
        breakdown T82.41 ☑
        displacement T82.42 ☑
        leakage T82.43 ☑
        malposition T82.42 ☑
        obstruction T82.49 ☑
        perforation T82.49 ☑
        protrusion T82.49 ☑
      pain T82.848 ☑
      specified type NEC T82.898 ☑
      stenosis T82.858 ☑
      thrombosis T82.868 ☑
    epidural infusion T85.9 ☑
      embolism T85.810 ☑
      fibrosis T85.820 ☑
      hemorrhage T85.830 ☑
      infection and inflammation T85.735 ☑
      mechanical
        breakdown T85.610 ☑
        displacement T85.620 ☑
        leakage T85.630 ☑
        malfunction T85.610 ☑
        malposition T85.620 ☑
        obstruction T85.690 ☑
        perforation T85.690 ☑
        protrusion T85.690 ☑
        specified NEC T85.690 ☑
      pain T85.840 ☑
      specified type NEC T85.890 ☑
      stenosis T85.850 ☑
      thrombosis T85.860 ☑
    intraperitoneal dialysis T85.9 ☑
      embolism T85.818 ☑
      fibrosis T85.828 ☑
      hemorrhage T85.838 ☑
      infection and inflammation T85.71 ☑

Index

Complication — Complication

Complication(s) — *continued*
  catheter — *see also* Complications, prosthetic device or implant — *continued*
    intraperitoneal dialysis — *continued*
      mechanical
        breakdown T85.611 ☑
        displacement T85.621 ☑
        leakage T85.631 ☑
        malfunction T85.611 ☑
        malposition T85.621 ☑
        obstruction T85.691 ☑
        perforation T85.691 ☑
        protrusion T85.691 ☑
        specified NEC T85.691 ☑
      pain T85.848 ☑
      specified type NEC T85.898 ☑
      stenosis T85.858 ☑
      thrombosis T85.868 ☑
    intrathecal infusion
      infection and inflammation T85.735 ☑
      mechanical
        breakdown T85.610 ☑
        displacement T85.620 ☑
        leakage T85.630 ☑
        malfunction T85.690 ☑
        malposition T85.620 ☑
        obstruction T85.690 ☑
        perforation T85.690 ☑
        protrusion T85.690 ☑
        specified NEC T85.690 ☑
    intravenous infusion T82.9 ☑
      embolism T82.818 ☑
      fibrosis T82.828 ☑
      hemorrhage T82.838 ☑
      infection or inflammation T82.7 ☑
      mechanical
        breakdown T82.514 ☑
        displacement T82.524 ☑
        leakage T82.534 ☑
        malposition T82.524 ☑
        obstruction T82.594 ☑
        perforation T82.594 ☑
        protrusion T82.594 ☑
      pain T82.848 ☑
      specified type NEC T82.898 ☑
      stenosis T82.858 ☑
      thrombosis T82.868 ☑
    spinal infusion
      infection and inflammation T85.735 ☑
      mechanical
        breakdown T85.610 ☑
        displacement T85.620 ☑
        leakage T85.630 ☑
        malfunction T85.690 ☑
        malposition T85.620 ☑
        obstruction T85.690 ☑
        perforation T85.690 ☑
        protrusion T85.690 ☑
        specified NEC T85.690 ☑
    subarachnoid infusion
      infection and inflammation T85.735 ☑
      mechanical
        breakdown T85.610 ☑
        displacement T85.620 ☑
        leakage T85.630 ☑
        malfunction T85.690 ☑
        malposition T85.620 ☑
        obstruction T85.690 ☑
        perforation T85.690 ☑
        protrusion T85.690 ☑
        specified NEC T85.690 ☑
    subdural infusion T85.9 ☑
      embolism T85.810 ☑
      fibrosis T85.820 ☑
      hemorrhage T85.830 ☑
      infection and inflammation T85.735 ☑
      mechanical
        breakdown T85.610 ☑
        displacement T85.620 ☑
        leakage T85.630 ☑
        malfunction T85.610 ☑
        malposition T85.620 ☑
        obstruction T85.690 ☑
        perforation T85.690 ☑
        protrusion T85.690 ☑
        specified NEC T85.690 ☑

Complication(s) — *continued*
  catheter — *see also* Complications, prosthetic device or implant — *continued*
    subdural infusion — *continued*
      pain T85.840 ☑
      specified type NEC T85.890 ☑
      stenosis T85.850 ☑
      thrombosis T85.860 ☑
    urethral T83.9 ☑
      displacement T83.028 ☑
      embolism T83.81 ☑
      fibrosis T83.82 ☑
      hemorrhage T83.83 ☑
      indwelling
        breakdown T83.011 ☑
        displacement T83.021 ☑
        infection and inflammation T83.511 ☑
        leakage T83.031 ☑
        specified complication NEC T83.091 ☑
      infection and inflammation T83.511 ☑
      leakage T83.038 ☑
      malposition T83.028 ☑
      mechanical
        breakdown T83.011 ☑
        obstruction (mechanical) T83.091 ☑
      pain T83.84 ☑
      perforation T83.091 ☑
      protrusion T83.091 ☑
      specified type NEC T83.091 ☑
      stenosis T83.85 ☑
      thrombosis T83.86 ☑
    urinary NEC
      breakdown T83.018 ☑
      displacement T83.028 ☑
      infection and inflammation T83.518 ☑
      leakage T83.038 ☑
      specified complication NEC T83.098 ☑
  cecostomy (stoma) — *see* Complications, colostomy
  cesarean delivery wound NEC O90.89
    disruption O90.0
    hematoma O90.2
    infection (following delivery) O86.00
  chemotherapy (antineoplastic) NEC T88.7 ☑
  chin implant (prosthetic) — *see* Complication, prosthetic device or implant, specified NEC
  circulatory system I99.8
    intraoperative I97.88
    postprocedural I97.89
      following cardiac surgery — *see also* Infarct, myocardium, associated with revascularization procedure I97.19-
        postcardiotomy syndrome I97.0
      hypertension I97.3
      lymphedema after mastectomy I97.2
      postcardiotomy syndrome I97.0
      specified NEC I97.89
  colostomy (stoma) K94.00
    hemorrhage K94.01
    infection K94.02
    malfunction K94.03
    mechanical K94.03
    specified complication NEC K94.09
  contraceptive device, intrauterine — *see* Complications, intrauterine, contraceptive device
  cord (umbilical) — *see* Complications, umbilical cord
  corneal graft — *see* Complications, graft, cornea
  coronary artery (bypass) graft T82.9 ☑
    atherosclerosis — *see* Arteriosclerosis, coronary (artery),
    embolism T82.818 ☑
    fibrosis T82.828 ☑
    hemorrhage T82.838 ☑
    infection and inflammation T82.7 ☑
    mechanical
      breakdown T82.211 ☑
      displacement T82.212 ☑
      leakage T82.213 ☑
      malposition T82.212 ☑
      obstruction T82.218 ☑
      perforation T82.218 ☑
      protrusion T82.218 ☑
      specified NEC T82.218 ☑
    pain T82.848 ☑
    specified type NEC T82.898 ☑
    stenosis T82.858 ☑
    thrombosis T82.868 ☑

Complication(s) — *continued*
  counterpulsation device (balloon), intra-aortic — *see* Complications, balloon implant, vascular
  cystostomy (stoma) N99.518
    catheter — *see* Complications, catheter, cystostomy
    hemorrhage N99.510
    infection N99.511
    malfunction N99.512
    specified type NEC N99.518
  delivery — *see also* Complications, obstetric O75.9
    procedure (instrumental) (manual) (surgical) O75.4
    specified NEC O75.89
  dialysis (peritoneal) (renal) — *see also* Complications, infusion
    catheter (vascular) — *see* Complication, catheter, dialysis
    peritoneal, intraperitoneal — *see* Complications, catheter, intraperitoneal
  dorsal column (spinal) neurostimulator — *see* Complications, electronic stimulator device, spinal cord
  drug NEC T88.7 ☑
  ear procedure — *see also* Disorder, ear
    intraoperative H95.88
      hematoma — *see* Complications, intraoperative, hemorrhage (hematoma) (of), ear
      hemorrhage — *see* Complications, intraoperative, hemorrhage (hematoma) (of), ear
      laceration — *see* Complications, intraoperative, puncture or laceration..., ear
      specified NEC H95.88
    postoperative H95.89
      external ear canal stenosis H95.81- ☑
      hematoma — *see* Complications, postprocedural, hematoma (of), ear
      hemorrhage — *see* Complications, postprocedural, hemorrhage (of), ear
      postmastoidectomy — *see* Complications, postmastoidectomy
      seroma — *see* Complications, postprocedural, seroma (of), mastoid process
      specified NEC H95.89
  ectopic pregnancy O08.9
    damage to pelvic organs O08.6
    embolism O08.2
    genital infection O08.0
    hemorrhage (delayed) (excessive) O08.1
    metabolic disorder O08.5
    renal failure O08.4
    shock O08.3
    specified type NEC O08.0
    venous complication NEC O08.7
  electronic stimulator device
    bladder (urinary) — *see* Complications, electronic stimulator device, urinary
    bone T84.9 ☑
      breakdown T84.310 ☑
      displacement T84.320 ☑
      embolism T84.81 ☑
      fibrosis T84.82 ☑
      hemorrhage T84.83 ☑
      infection or inflammation T84.7 ☑
      malfunction T84.310 ☑
      malposition T84.320 ☑
      mechanical NEC T84.390 ☑
      obstruction T84.390 ☑
      pain T84.84 ☑
      perforation T84.390 ☑
      protrusion T84.390 ☑
      specified type NEC T84.89 ☑
      stenosis T84.85 ☑
      thrombosis T84.86 ☑
    brain T85.9 ☑
      embolism T85.810 ☑
      fibrosis T85.820 ☑
      hemorrhage T85.830 ☑
      infection and inflammation T85.731 ☑
      mechanical
        breakdown T85.110 ☑
        displacement T85.120 ☑
        leakage T85.190 ☑
        malposition T85.120 ☑
        obstruction T85.190 ☑
        perforation T85.190 ☑
        protrusion T85.190 ☑
        specified NEC T85.190 ☑
      pain T85.840 ☑
      specified type NEC T85.890 ☑

Complication(s) — *continued*
  electronic stimulator device — *continued*
    brain — *continued*
      stenosis T85.850 ☑
      thrombosis T85.860 ☑
    cardiac (defibrillator) (pacemaker) — *see* Complications, cardiovascular device or implant, electronic
    generator (brain) (gastric) (peripheral) (sacral) (spinal)
      breakdown T85.113 ☑
      displacement T85.123 ☑
      leakage T85.193 ☑
      malposition T85.123 ☑
      obstruction T85.193 ☑
      perforation T85.193 ☑
      protrusion T85.193 ☑
      specified type NEC T85.193 ☑
    muscle T84.9
      breakdown T84.418 ☑
      displacement T84.428 ☑
      embolism T84.81 ☑
      fibrosis T84.82 ☑
      hemorrhage T84.83 ☑
      infection or inflammation T84.7 ☑
      mechanical NEC T84.498 ☑
      pain T84.84 ☑
      specified type NEC T84.89 ☑
      stenosis T84.85 ☑
      thrombosis T84.86 ☑
    nervous system T85.9 ☑
      brain — *see* Complications, electronic stimulator device, brain
      cranial nerve — *see* Complications, electronic stimulator device, peripheral nerve
      embolism T85.810 ☑
      fibrosis T85.820 ☑
      gastric nerve — *see* Complications, electronic stimulator device, peripheral nerve
      hemorrhage T85.830 ☑
      infection and inflammation T85.738 ☑
      mechanical
        breakdown T85.118 ☑
        displacement T85.128 ☑
        leakage T85.199 ☑
        malposition T85.128 ☑
        obstruction T85.199 ☑
        perforation T85.199 ☑
        protrusion T85.199 ☑
        specified NEC T85.199 ☑
      pain T85.840 ☑
      peripheral nerve — *see* Complications, electronic stimulator device, peripheral nerve
      sacral nerve — *see* Complications, electronic stimulator device, peripheral nerve
      specified type NEC T85.890 ☑
      spinal cord — *see* Complications, electronic stimulator device, spinal cord
      stenosis T85.850 ☑
      thrombosis T85.860 ☑
      vagal nerve — *see* Complications, electronic stimulator device, peripheral nerve
    peripheral nerve T85.9 ☑
      embolism T85.810 ☑
      fibrosis T85.820 ☑
      hemorrhage T85.830 ☑
      infection and inflammation T85.732 ☑
      mechanical
        breakdown T85.111 ☑
        displacement T85.121 ☑
        leakage T85.191 ☑
        malposition T85.121 ☑
        obstruction T85.191 ☑
        perforation T85.191 ☑
        protrusion T85.191 ☑
        specified NEC T85.191 ☑
      pain T85.840 ☑
      specified type NEC T85.890 ☑
      stenosis T85.850 ☑
      thrombosis T85.860 ☑
    spinal cord T85.9 ☑
      embolism T85.810 ☑
      fibrosis T85.820 ☑
      hemorrhage T85.830 ☑
      infection and inflammation T85.733 ☑

Complication(s) — *continued*
  electronic stimulator device — *continued*
    spinal cord — *continued*
      mechanical
        breakdown T85.112 ☑
        displacement T85.122 ☑
        leakage T85.192 ☑
        malposition T85.122 ☑
        obstruction T85.192 ☑
        perforation T85.192 ☑
        protrusion T85.192 ☑
        specified NEC T85.192 ☑
      pain T85.840 ☑
      specified type NEC T85.890 ☑
      stenosis T85.850 ☑
      thrombosis T85.860 ☑
    urinary T83.9 ☑
      embolism T83.81 ☑
      fibrosis T83.82 ☑
      hemorrhage T83.83 ☑
      infection and inflammation T83.598 ☑
      mechanical
        breakdown T83.110 ☑
        displacement T83.120 ☑
        malposition T83.120 ☑
        perforation T83.190 ☑
        protrusion T83.190 ☑
        specified NEC T83.190 ☑
      pain T83.84 ☑
      specified type NEC T83.89 ☑
      stenosis T83.85 ☑
      thrombosis T83.86 ☑
  electroshock therapy T88.9 ☑
    specified NEC T88.8 ☑
  endocrine E34.9
    postprocedural
      adrenal hypofunction E89.6
      hypoinsulinemia E89.1
      hypoparathyroidism E89.2
      hypopituitarism E89.3
      hypothyroidism E89.0
      ovarian failure E89.40
        asymptomatic E89.40
        symptomatic E89.41
      specified NEC E89.89
      testicular hypofunction E89.5
  endodontic treatment NEC M27.59
  enterostomy (stoma) K94.10
    hemorrhage K94.11
    infection K94.12
    malfunction K94.13
    mechanical K94.13
    specified complication NEC K94.19
  episiotomy, disruption O90.1
  esophageal anti-reflux device T85.9 ☑
    embolism T85.818 ☑
    fibrosis T85.828 ☑
    hemorrhage T85.838 ☑
    infection and inflammation T85.79 ☑
    mechanical
      breakdown T85.511 ☑
      displacement T85.521 ☑
      malfunction T85.511 ☑
      malposition T85.521 ☑
      obstruction T85.591 ☑
      perforation T85.591 ☑
      protrusion T85.591 ☑
      specified NEC T85.591 ☑
    pain T85.848 ☑
    specified type NEC T85.898 ☑
    stenosis T85.858 ☑
    thrombosis T85.868 ☑
  esophagostomy K94.30
    hemorrhage K94.31
    infection K94.32
    malfunction K94.33
    mechanical K94.33
    specified complication NEC K94.39
  extracorporeal circulation T80.90 ☑
  extremity artery (bypass) graft T82.9 ☑
    arteriosclerosis — *see* Arteriosclerosis, extremities, bypass graft
    embolism T82.818 ☑
    fibrosis T82.828 ☑
    hemorrhage T82.838 ☑
    infection and inflammation T82.7 ☑

Complication(s) — *continued*
  extremity artery graft — *continued*
    mechanical
      breakdown T82.318 ☑
        femoral artery T82.312 ☑
      displacement T82.328 ☑
        femoral artery T82.322 ☑
      leakage T82.338 ☑
        femoral artery T82.332 ☑
      malposition T82.328 ☑
        femoral artery T82.322 ☑
      obstruction T82.398 ☑
        femoral artery T82.392 ☑
      perforation T82.398 ☑
        femoral artery T82.392 ☑
      protrusion T82.398 ☑
        femoral artery T82.392 ☑
    pain T82.848 ☑
    specified type NEC T82.898 ☑
    stenosis T82.858 ☑
    thrombosis T82.868 ☑
  eye H57.9
    corneal graft — *see* Complications, graft, cornea
    implant (prosthetic) T85.9 ☑
      embolism T85.818 ☑
      fibrosis T85.828 ☑
      hemorrhage T85.838 ☑
      infection and inflammation T85.79 ☑
      mechanical
        breakdown T85.318 ☑
        displacement T85.328 ☑
        leakage T85.398 ☑
        malposition T85.328 ☑
        obstruction T85.398 ☑
        perforation T85.398 ☑
        protrusion T85.398 ☑
        specified NEC T85.398 ☑
      pain T85.848 ☑
      specified type NEC T85.898 ☑
      stenosis T85.858 ☑
      thrombosis T85.868 ☑
    intraocular lens — *see* Complications, intraocular lens
    orbital prosthesis — *see* Complications, orbital prosthesis
  female genital N94.9
    device, implant or graft NEC — *see* Complications, genitourinary, device or implant, genital tract
  femoral artery (bypass) graft — *see* Complication, extremity artery (bypass) graft
  fixation device, internal (orthopedic) T84.9 ☑
    infection and inflammation T84.60 ☑
      arm T84.61- ☑
        humerus T84.61- ☑
        radius T84.61- ☑
        ulna T84.61- ☑
      leg T84.629 ☑
        femur T84.62- ☑
        fibula T84.62- ☑
        tibia T84.62- ☑
      specified site NEC T84.89 ☑
      spine T84.63 ☑
    mechanical
      breakdown
        limb T84.119 ☑
          carpal T84.210 ☑
          femur T84.11- ☑
          fibula T84.11- ☑
          humerus T84.11- ☑
          metacarpal T84.210 ☑
          metatarsal T84.213 ☑
          phalanx
            foot T84.213 ☑
            hand T84.210 ☑
          radius T84.11- ☑
          tarsal T84.213 ☑
          tibia T84.11- ☑
          ulna T84.11- ☑
        specified bone NEC T84.218 ☑
        spine T84.216 ☑
      displacement
        limb T84.129 ☑
          carpal T84.220 ☑
          femur T84.12- ☑
          fibula T84.12- ☑
          humerus T84.12- ☑

▽ Subterms under main terms may continue to next column or page   ☑ Additional Character Required — Refer to the Tabular List for Character Selection   61

Complication — Complication

Complication(s) — *continued*
fixation device, internal — *continued*
  mechanical — *continued*
    displacement — *continued*
      limb — *continued*
        metacarpal T84.220 ☑
        metatarsal T84.223 ☑
        phalanx
          foot T84.223 ☑
          hand T84.220 ☑
        radius T84.12-
        tarsal T84.223 ☑
        tibia T84.12- ☑
        ulna T84.12-
        specified bone NEC T84.228 ☑
      spine T84.226 ☑
    malposition — *see* Complications, fixation device, internal, mechanical, displacement
    obstruction — *see* Complications, fixation device, internal, mechanical, specified type NEC
    perforation — *see* Complications, fixation device, internal, mechanical, specified type NEC
    protrusion — *see* Complications, fixation device, internal, mechanical, specified type NEC
    specified type NEC
      limb T84.199 ☑
        carpal T84.290 ☑
        femur T84.19- ☑
        fibula T84.19- ☑
        humerus T84.19- ☑
        metacarpal T84.290 ☑
        metatarsal T84.293 ☑
        phalanx
          foot T84.293 ☑
          hand T84.290 ☑
        radius T84.19- ☑
        tarsal T84.293 ☑
        tibia T84.19- ☑
        ulna T84.19- ☑
        specified bone NEC T84.298 ☑
      vertebra T84.296 ☑
  specified type NEC T84.89 ☑
    embolism T84.81 ☑
    fibrosis T84.82 ☑
    hemorrhage T84.83 ☑
    pain T84.84 ☑
    specified complication NEC T84.89 ☑
    stenosis T84.85 ☑
    thrombosis T84.86 ☑
following
  acute myocardial infarction NEC I23.8
    aneurysm (false) (of cardiac wall) (of heart wall) (ruptured) I23.3
    angina I23.7
    atrial
      septal defect I23.1
      thrombosis I23.6
    cardiac wall rupture I23.3
    chordae tendinae rupture I23.4
    defect
      septal
        atrial (heart) I23.1
        ventricular (heart) I23.2
    hemopericardium I23.0
    papillary muscle rupture I23.5
    rupture
      cardiac wall I23.3
        with hemopericardium I23.0
      chordae tendineae I23.4
      papillary muscle I23.5
    specified NEC I23.8
    thrombosis
      atrium I23.6
      auricular appendage I23.6
      ventricle (heart) I23.6
    ventricular
      septal defect I23.2
      thrombosis I23.6
  ectopic or molar pregnancy O08.9
    cardiac arrest O08.81
    sepsis O08.82
    specified type NEC O08.89
    urinary tract infection O08.83
  termination of pregnancy — *see* Abortion
gastrointestinal K92.9
  bile duct prosthesis — *see* Complications, bile duct implant

Complication(s) — *continued*
gastrointestinal — *continued*
  esophageal anti-reflux device — *see* Complications, esophageal anti-reflux device
  postoperative
    colostomy — *see* Complications, colostomy
    dumping syndrome K91.1
    enterostomy — *see* Complications, enterostomy
    gastrostomy — *see* Complications, gastrostomy
    malabsorption NEC K91.2
    obstruction — *see also* Obstruction, intestine, postoperative K91.30
    postcholecystectomy syndrome K91.5
    specified NEC K91.89
    vomiting after GI surgery K91.0
  prosthetic device or implant
    bile duct prosthesis — *see* Complications, bile duct implant
    esophageal anti-reflux device — *see* Complications, esophageal anti-reflux device
    specified type NEC
      embolism T85.818 ☑
      fibrosis T85.828 ☑
      hemorrhage T85.838 ☑
      mechanical
        breakdown T85.518 ☑
        displacement T85.528 ☑
        malfunction T85.518 ☑
        malposition T85.528 ☑
        obstruction T85.598 ☑
        perforation T85.598 ☑
        protrusion T85.598 ☑
        specified NEC T85.598 ☑
      pain T85.848 ☑
      specified complication NEC T85.898 ☑
      stenosis T85.858 ☑
      thrombosis T85.868 ☑
gastrostomy (stoma) K94.20
  hemorrhage K94.21
  infection K94.22
  malfunction K94.23
  mechanical K94.23
  specified complication NEC K94.29
genitourinary
  device or implant T83.9 ☑
    genital tract T83.9 ☑
      infection or inflammation T83.69 ☑
      intrauterine contraceptive device — *see* Complications, intrauterine, contraceptive device
      mechanical — *see* Complications, by device, mechanical
      mesh — *see* Complications, prosthetic device or implant, mesh
      penile prosthesis — *see* Complications, prosthetic device, penile
      specified type NEC T83.89 ☑
        embolism T83.81 ☑
        fibrosis T83.82 ☑
        hemorrhage T83.83 ☑
        pain T83.84 ☑
        specified complication NEC T83.89 ☑
        stenosis T83.85 ☑
        thrombosis T83.86 ☑
      vaginal mesh — *see* Complications, prosthetic device or implant, mesh
    urinary system T83.9 ☑
      cystostomy catheter — *see* Complication, catheter, cystostomy
      electronic stimulator — *see* Complications, electronic stimulator device, urinary
      indwelling urethral catheter — *see* Complications, catheter, urethral, indwelling
      infection or inflammation T83.598 ☑
        indwelling urethral catheter T83.511 ☑
      kidney transplant — *see* Complication, transplant, kidney
      organ graft — *see* Complication, graft, urinary organ
      specified type NEC T83.89 ☑
        embolism T83.81 ☑
        fibrosis T83.82 ☑
        hemorrhage T83.83 ☑
        mechanical T83.198 ☑
          breakdown T83.118 ☑
          displacement T83.128 ☑
          malfunction T83.118 ☑

Complication(s) — *continued*
genitourinary — *continued*
  device or implant — *continued*
    urinary system — *continued*
      specified type — *continued*
        mechanical — *continued*
          malposition T83.128 ☑
          obstruction T83.198 ☑
          perforation T83.198 ☑
          protrusion T83.198 ☑
          specified NEC T83.198 ☑
        sphincter implant — *see* Complications, implant, urinary sphincter
        sphincter, implanted T83.191 ☑
        stent (ileal conduit) (nephroureteral) T83.193 ☑
          pain T83.84 ☑
          specified complication NEC T83.89 ☑
          stenosis T83.85 ☑
          thrombosis T83.86 ☑
          ureteral indwelling T83.192 ☑
  postprocedural
    pelvic peritoneal adhesions N99.4
    renal failure N99.0
    specified NEC N99.89
    stoma — *see* Complications, stoma, urinary tract
    urethral stricture — *see* Stricture, urethra, postprocedural
    vaginal
      adhesions N99.2
      vault prolapse N99.3
graft (bypass) (patch) — *see also* Complications, prosthetic device or implant
  aorta — *see* Complications, graft, vascular
  arterial — *see* Complication, graft, vascular
  bone T86.839
    failure T86.831
    infection T86.832
    mechanical T84.318 ☑
      breakdown T84.318 ☑
      displacement T84.328 ☑
      protrusion T84.398 ☑
      specified type NEC T84.398 ☑
    rejection T86.830
    specified type NEC T86.838
  carotid artery — *see* Complications, graft, vascular
  cornea T86.849
    failure T86.841
    infection T86.842
    mechanical T85.398 ☑
      breakdown T85.318 ☑
      displacement T85.328 ☑
      protrusion T85.398 ☑
      specified type NEC T85.398 ☑
    rejection T86.840
    retroprosthetic membrane T85.398 ☑
    specified type NEC T86.848
  femoral artery (bypass) — *see* Complication, extremity artery (bypass) graft
  genital organ or tract — *see* Complications, genitourinary, device or implant, genital tract
  muscle T84.9 ☑
    breakdown T84.410 ☑
    displacement T84.420 ☑
    embolism T84.81 ☑
    fibrosis T84.82 ☑
    hemorrhage T84.83 ☑
    infection and inflammation T84.7 ☑
    mechanical NEC T84.490 ☑
    pain T84.84 ☑
    specified type NEC T84.89 ☑
    stenosis T84.85 ☑
    thrombosis T84.86 ☑
  nerve — *see* Complication, prosthetic device or implant, specified NEC
  skin — *see* Complications, prosthetic device or implant, skin graft
  tendon T84.9 ☑
    breakdown T84.410 ☑
    displacement T84.420 ☑
    embolism T84.81 ☑
    fibrosis T84.82 ☑
    hemorrhage T84.83 ☑
    infection and inflammation T84.7 ☑
    mechanical NEC T84.490 ☑
    pain T84.84 ☑
    specified type NEC T84.89 ☑

☑ Additional Character Required — Refer to the Tabular List for Character Selection   ▽ Subterms under main terms may continue to next column or page

Complication(s) — *continued*
  graft — *see also* Complications, prosthetic device or
      implant — *continued*
    tendon — *continued*
      stenosis T84.85 ☑
      thrombosis T84.86 ☑
    urinary organ T83.9 ☑
      embolism T83.81 ☑
      fibrosis T83.82 ☑
      hemorrhage T83.83 ☑
      infection and inflammation T83.598 ☑
        indwelling urethral catheter T83.511 ☑
      mechanical
        breakdown T83.21 ☑
        displacement T83.22 ☑
        erosion T83.24 ☑
        exposure T83.25 ☑
        leakage T83.23 ☑
        malposition T83.22 ☑
        obstruction T83.29 ☑
        perforation T83.29 ☑
        protrusion T83.29 ☑
        specified NEC T83.29 ☑
      pain T83.84 ☑
      specified type NEC T83.89 ☑
      stenosis T83.85 ☑
      thrombosis T83.86 ☑
    vascular T82.9 ☑
      embolism T82.818 ☑
      femoral artery — *see* Complication, extremity
          artery (bypass) graft
      fibrosis T82.828 ☑
      hemorrhage T82.838 ☑
      mechanical
        breakdown T82.319 ☑
          aorta (bifurcation) T82.310 ☑
          carotid artery T82.311 ☑
          specified vessel NEC T82.318 ☑
        displacement T82.329 ☑
          aorta (bifurcation) T82.320 ☑
          carotid artery T82.321 ☑
          specified vessel NEC T82.328 ☑
        leakage T82.339 ☑
          aorta (bifurcation) T82.330 ☑
          carotid artery T82.331 ☑
          specified vessel NEC T82.338 ☑
        malposition T82.329 ☑
          aorta (bifurcation) T82.320 ☑
          carotid artery T82.321 ☑
          specified vessel NEC T82.328 ☑
        obstruction T82.399 ☑
          aorta (bifurcation) T82.390 ☑
          carotid artery T82.391 ☑
          specified vessel NEC T82.398 ☑
        perforation T82.399 ☑
          aorta (bifurcation) T82.390 ☑
          carotid artery T82.391 ☑
          specified vessel NEC T82.398 ☑
        protrusion T82.399 ☑
          aorta (bifurcation) T82.390 ☑
          carotid artery T82.391 ☑
          specified vessel NEC T82.398 ☑
      pain T82.848 ☑
      specified complication NEC T82.898 ☑
      stenosis T82.858 ☑
      thrombosis T82.868 ☑
  heart I51.9
    assist device
      infection and inflammation T82.7 ☑
    following acute myocardial infarction — *see* Com-
        plications, following, acute myocardial infarc-
        tion
    postoperative — *see* Complications, circulatory
        system
    transplant — *see* Complication, transplant, heart
        and lung(s) — *see* Complications, transplant,
        heart, with lung
    valve
      graft (biological) T82.9 ☑
        embolism T82.817 ☑
        fibrosis T82.827 ☑
        hemorrhage T82.837 ☑
        infection and inflammation T82.7 ☑
        mechanical T82.228 ☑
          breakdown T82.221 ☑
          displacement T82.222 ☑

Complication(s) — *continued*
  heart — *continued*
    valve — *continued*
      graft — *continued*
        mechanical — *continued*
          leakage T82.223 ☑
          malposition T82.222 ☑
          obstruction T82.228 ☑
          perforation T82.228 ☑
          protrusion T82.228 ☑
        pain T82.847 ☑
        specified type NEC T82.897 ☑
        stenosis T82.857 ☑
        thrombosis T82.867 ☑
      prosthesis T82.9 ☑
        embolism T82.817 ☑
        fibrosis T82.827 ☑
        hemorrhage T82.837 ☑
        infection or inflammation T82.6 ☑
        mechanical T82.09 ☑
          breakdown T82.01 ☑
          displacement T82.02 ☑
          leakage T82.03 ☑
          malposition T82.02 ☑
          obstruction T82.09 ☑
          perforation T82.09 ☑
          protrusion T82.09 ☑
        pain T82.847 ☑
        specified type NEC T82.897 ☑
          mechanical T82.09 ☑
        stenosis T82.857 ☑
        thrombosis T82.867 ☑
  hematoma
    intraoperative — *see* Complication, intraoperative,
        hemorrhage
    postprocedural — *see* Complication, postprocedu-
        ral, hematoma
  hemodialysis — *see* Complications, dialysis
  hemorrhage
    intraoperative — *see* Complication, intraoperative,
        hemorrhage
    postprocedural — *see* Complication, postprocedu-
        ral, hemorrhage
  ileostomy (stoma) — *see* Complications, enterostomy
  immunization (procedure) — *see* Complications, vacci-
      nation
  implant — *see also* Complications, by site and type
    urinary sphincter T83.9 ☑
      embolism T83.81 ☑
      fibrosis T83.82 ☑
      hemorrhage T83.83 ☑
      infection and inflammation T83.591 ☑
      mechanical
        breakdown T83.111 ☑
        displacement T83.121 ☑
        leakage T83.191 ☑
        malposition T83.121 ☑
        obstruction T83.191 ☑
        perforation T83.191 ☑
        protrusion T83.191 ☑
        specified NEC T83.191 ☑
      pain T83.84 ☑
      specified type NEC T83.89 ☑
      stenosis T83.85 ☑
      thrombosis T83.86 ☑
  infusion (procedure) T80.90 ☑
    air embolism T80.0 ☑
    blood — *see* Complications, transfusion
    catheter — *see* Complications, catheter
    infection T80.29 ☑
    pump — *see* Complications, cardiovascular, device
        or implant
    sepsis T80.29 ☑
    serum reaction — *see also* Reaction, serum
        T80.69 ☑
      anaphylactic shock — *see also* Shock, anaphylac-
          tic T80.59 ☑
    specified type NEC T80.89 ☑
  inhalation therapy NEC T81.81 ☑
  injection (procedure) T80.90 ☑
    drug reaction — *see* Reaction, drug
    infection T80.29 ☑
    sepsis T80.29 ☑
    serum (prophylactic) (therapeutic) — *see* Complica-
        tions, vaccination
    specified type NEC T80.89 ☑

Complication(s) — *continued*
  injection — *continued*
    vaccine (any) — *see* Complications, vaccination
    inoculation (any) — *see* Complications, vaccination
  insulin pump
    infection and inflammation T85.72 ☑
    mechanical
      breakdown T85.614 ☑
      displacement T85.624 ☑
      leakage T85.633 ☑
      malposition T85.624 ☑
      obstruction T85.694 ☑
      perforation T85.694 ☑
      protrusion T85.694 ☑
      specified NEC T85.694 ☑
  intestinal pouch NEC K91.858
  intraocular lens (prosthetic) T85.9 ☑
    embolism T85.818 ☑
    fibrosis T85.828 ☑
    hemorrhage T85.838 ☑
    infection and inflammation T85.79 ☑
    mechanical
      breakdown T85.21 ☑
      displacement T85.22 ☑
      malposition T85.22 ☑
      obstruction T85.29 ☑
      perforation T85.29 ☑
      protrusion T85.29 ☑
      specified NEC T85.29 ☑
    pain T85.848 ☑
    specified type NEC T85.898 ☑
    stenosis T85.858 ☑
    thrombosis T85.868 ☑
  intraoperative (intraprocedural)
    cardiac arrest — *see also* Infarct, myocardium, asso-
        ciated with revascularization procedure
      during cardiac surgery I97.710
      during other surgery I97.711
    cardiac functional disturbance NEC — *see also* In-
        farct, myocardium, associated with revascular-
        ization procedure
      during cardiac surgery I97.790
      during other surgery I97.791
    hemorrhage (hematoma) (of)
      circulatory system organ or structure
        during cardiac bypass I97.411
        during cardiac catheterization I97.410
        during other circulatory system procedure
            I97.418
        during other procedure I97.42
      digestive system organ
        during procedure on digestive system K91.61
        during procedure on other organ K91.62
      ear
        during procedure on ear and mastoid process
            H95.21
        during procedure on other organ H95.22
      endocrine system organ or structure
        during procedure on endocrine system organ
            or structure E36.01
        during procedure on other organ E36.02
      eye and adnexa
        during ophthalmic procedure H59.11- ☑
        during other procedure H59.12- ☑
      genitourinary organ or structure
        during procedure on genitourinary organ or
            structure N99.61
        during procedure on other organ N99.62
      mastoid process
        during procedure on ear and mastoid process
            H95.21
        during procedure on other organ H95.22
      musculoskeletal structure
        during musculoskeletal surgery M96.810
        during non-orthopedic surgery M96.811
        during orthopedic surgery M96.810
      nervous system
        during a nervous system procedure G97.31
        during other procedure G97.32
      respiratory system
        during other procedure J95.62
        during procedure on respiratory system organ
            or structure J95.61
      skin and subcutaneous tissue
        during a dermatologic procedure L76.01
        during a procedure on other organ L76.02
      spleen
        during a procedure on other organ D78.02

Complication(s) — *continued*
  intraoperative — *continued*
    hemorrhage — *continued*
      spleen — *continued*
        during a procedure on the spleen D78.01
      puncture or laceration (accidental) (unintentional) (of)
        brain
          during a nervous system procedure G97.48
          during other procedure G97.49
        circulatory system organ or structure
          during circulatory system procedure I97.51
          during other procedure I97.52
        digestive system
          during procedure on digestive system K91.71
          during procedure on other organ K91.72
        ear
          during procedure on ear and mastoid process H95.31
          during procedure on other organ H95.32
        endocrine system organ or structure
          during procedure on endocrine system organ or structure E36.11
          during procedure on other organ E36.12
        eye and adnexa
          during ophthalmic procedure H59.21- ☑
          during other procedure H59.22- ☑
        genitourinary organ or structure
          during procedure on genitourinary organ or structure N99.71
          during procedure on other organ N99.72
        mastoid process
          during procedure on ear and mastoid process H95.31
          during procedure on other organ H95.32
        musculoskeletal structure
          during musculoskeletal surgery M96.820
          during non-orthopedic surgery M96.821
          during orthopedic surgery M96.820
        nervous system
          during a nervous system procedure G97.48
          during other procedure G97.49
        respiratory system
          during other procedure J95.72
          during procedure on respiratory system organ or structure J95.71
        skin and subcutaneous tissue
          during a dermatologic procedure L76.11
          during a procedure on other organ L76.12
        spleen
          during a procedure on other organ D78.12
          during a procedure on the spleen D78.11
    specified NEC
      circulatory system I97.88
      digestive system K91.81
      ear H95.88
      endocrine system E36.8
      eye and adnexa H59.88
      genitourinary system N99.81
      mastoid process H95.88
      musculoskeletal structure M96.89
      nervous system G97.81
      respiratory system J95.88
      skin and subcutaneous tissue L76.81
      spleen D78.81
  intraperitoneal catheter (dialysis) (infusion) — *see* Complications, catheter, intraperitoneal
  intrathecal infusion pump
    infection and inflammation T85.738 ☑
    mechanical
      breakdown T85.615 ☑
      displacement T85.625 ☑
      leakage T85.635 ☑
      malfunction T85.695 ☑
      malposition T85.625 ☑
      obstruction T85.695 ☑
      perforation T85.695 ☑
      protrusion T85.695 ☑
      specified NEC T85.695 ☑
  intrauterine
    contraceptive device
      embolism T83.81 ☑
      fibrosis T83.82 ☑
      hemorrhage T83.83 ☑
      infection and inflammation T83.69 ☑
      mechanical
        breakdown T83.31 ☑
        displacement T83.32 ☑

Complication(s) — *continued*
  intrauterine — *continued*
    contraceptive device — *continued*
      mechanical — *continued*
        malposition T83.32 ☑
        obstruction T83.39 ☑
        perforation T83.39 ☑
        protrusion T83.39 ☑
        specified NEC T83.39 ☑
      pain T83.84 ☑
      specified type NEC T83.89 ☑
      stenosis T83.85 ☑
      thrombosis T83.86 ☑
    procedure (fetal), to newborn P96.5
  jejunostomy (stoma) — *see* Complications, enterostomy
  joint prosthesis, internal T84.9 ☑
    breakage (fracture) T84.01- ☑
    dislocation T84.02- ☑
    fracture T84.01- ☑
    infection or inflammation T84.50 ☑
      hip T84.5- ☑
      knee T84.5- ☑
      specified joint NEC T84.59 ☑
    instability T84.02- ☑
    malposition — *see* Complications, joint prosthesis, mechanical, displacement
    mechanical
      breakage, broken T84.01- ☑
      dislocation T84.02- ☑
      fracture T84.01- ☑
      instability T84.02- ☑
      leakage — *see* Complications, joint prosthesis, mechanical, specified NEC
      loosening T84.039 ☑
        hip T84.03- ☑
        knee T84.03- ☑
        specified joint NEC T84.038 ☑
      obstruction — *see* Complications, joint prosthesis, mechanical, specified NEC
      perforation — *see* Complications, joint prosthesis, mechanical, specified NEC
      osteolysis T84.059 ☑
        hip T84.05- ☑
        knee T84.05- ☑
        other specified joint T84.058 ☑
      periprosthetic T84.059 ☑
      protrusion — *see* Complications, joint prosthesis, mechanical, specified NEC
      specified complication NEC T84.099 ☑
        hip T84.09- ☑
        knee T84.09- ☑
        other specified joint T84.098 ☑
      subluxation T84.02- ☑
      wear of articular bearing surface T84.069 ☑
        hip T84.06- ☑
        knee T84.06- ☑
        other specified joint T84.068 ☑
    specified joint NEC T84.89 ☑
      embolism T84.81 ☑
      fibrosis T84.82 ☑
      hemorrhage T84.83 ☑
      pain T84.84 ☑
      specified complication NEC T84.89 ☑
      stenosis T84.85 ☑
      thrombosis T84.86 ☑
    subluxation T84.02- ☑
  kidney transplant — *see* Complications, transplant, kidney
  labor O75.9
    specified NEC O75.89
  liver transplant (immune or nonimmune) — *see* Complications, transplant, liver
  lumbar puncture G97.1
    cerebrospinal fluid leak G97.0
    headache or reaction G97.1
  lung transplant — *see* Complications, transplant, lung and heart — *see* Complications, transplant, lung, with heart
  male genital N50.9
    device, implant or graft — *see* Complications, genitourinary, device or implant, genital tract
    postprocedural or postoperative — *see* Complications, genitourinary, postprocedural
    specified NEC N99.89

Complication(s) — *continued*
  mastoid (process) procedure
    intraoperative H95.88
      hematoma — *see* Complications, intraoperative, hemorrhage (hematoma) (of), mastoid process
      hemorrhage — *see* Complications, intraoperative, hemorrhage (hematoma) (of), mastoid process
      laceration — *see* Complications, intraoperative, puncture or laceration, mastoid process
      specified NEC H95.88
    postmastoidectomy — *see* Complications, postmastoidectomy
    postoperative H95.89
      external ear canal stenosis H95.81 ☑
      hematoma — *see* Complications, postprocedural, hematoma (of), mastoid process
      hemorrhage — *see* Complications, postprocedural, hemorrhage (of), mastoid process
      postmastoidectomy — *see* Complications, postmastoidectomy
      seroma — *see* Complications, postprocedural, seroma (of), mastoid process
      specified NEC H95.89
  mastoidectomy cavity — *see* Complications, postmastoidectomy
  mechanical — *see* Complications, by site and type, mechanical
  medical procedures — *see also* Complication(s), intraoperative T88.9 ☑
  metabolic E88.9
    postoperative E89.89
    specified NEC E89.89
  molar pregnancy NOS O08.9
    damage to pelvic organs O08.6
    embolism O08.2
    genital infection O08.0
    hemorrhage (delayed) (excessive) O08.1
    metabolic disorder O08.5
    renal failure O08.4
    shock O08.3
    specified type NEC O08.0
    venous complication NEC O08.7
  musculoskeletal system — *see also* Complication, intraoperative (intraprocedural), by site
    device, implant or graft NEC — *see* Complications, orthopedic, device or implant
    internal fixation (nail) (plate) (rod) — *see* Complications, fixation device, internal
    joint prosthesis — *see* Complications, joint prosthesis
    post radiation M96.89
      kyphosis M96.2
      scoliosis M96.5
      specified complication NEC M96.89
    postoperative (postprocedural) M96.89
      with osteoporosis — *see* Osteoporosis
      fracture following insertion of device — *see* Fracture, following insertion of orthopedic implant, joint prosthesis or bone plate
      joint instability after prosthesis removal M96.89
      lordosis M96.4
      postlaminectomy syndrome NEC M96.1
        kyphosis M96.3
      pseudarthrosis M96.0
      specified complication NEC M96.89
  nephrostomy (stoma) — *see* Complications, stoma, urinary tract, external NEC
  nervous system G98.8
    central G96.9
    device, implant or graft — *see also* Complication, prosthetic device or implant, specified NEC
      electronic stimulator (electrode(s)) — *see* Complications, electronic stimulator device
      specified NEC
        infection and inflammation T85.738 ☑
        mechanical T85.695 ☑
          breakdown T85.615 ☑
          displacement T85.625 ☑
          leakage T85.635 ☑
          malfunction T85.695 ☑
          malposition T85.625 ☑
          obstruction T85.695 ☑
          perforation T85.695 ☑
          protrusion T85.695 ☑
          specified NEC T85.695 ☑

☑ Additional Character Required — Refer to the Tabular List for Character Selection   ▽ Subterms under main terms may continue to next column or page

Complication(s) — *continued*
- nervous system — *continued*
  - device, implant or graft — *see also* Complication, prosthetic device or implant, specified — *continued*
    - ventricular shunt — *see* Complications, ventricular shunt
    - electronic stimulator (electrode(s)) — *see* Complications, electronic stimulator device
  - postprocedural G97.82
    - intracranial hypotension G97.2
    - specified NEC G97.82
    - spinal fluid leak G97.0
- newborn, due to intrauterine (fetal) procedure P96.5
- nonabsorbable (permanent) sutures — *see* Complication, sutures, permanent
- obstetric O75.9
  - procedure (instrumental) (manual) (surgical) specified NEC O75.4
  - specified NEC O75.89
  - surgical wound NEC O90.89
    - hematoma O90.2
    - infection O86.00
- ocular lens implant — *see* Complications, intraocular lens
- ophthalmologic
  - postprocedural bleb — *see* Blebitis
- orbital prosthesis T85.9 ☑
  - embolism T85.818 ☑
  - fibrosis T85.828 ☑
  - hemorrhage T85.838 ☑
  - infection and inflammation T85.79 ☑
  - mechanical
    - breakdown T85.31- ☑
    - displacement T85.32- ☑
    - malposition T85.32- ☑
    - obstruction T85.39- ☑
    - perforation T85.39- ☑
    - protrusion T85.39- ☑
    - specified NEC T85.39- ☑
  - pain T85.848 ☑
  - specified type NEC T85.898 ☑
  - stenosis T85.858 ☑
  - thrombosis T85.868 ☑
- organ or tissue transplant (partial) (total) — *see* Complications, transplant
- orthopedic — *see also* Disorder, soft tissue
  - device or implant T84.9 ☑
    - bone
      - device or implant — *see* Complication, bone, device NEC
      - graft — *see* Complication, graft, bone
    - breakdown T84.418 ☑
    - displacement T84.428 ☑
    - electronic bone stimulator — *see* Complications, electronic stimulator device, bone
    - embolism T84.81 ☑
    - fibrosis T84.82 ☑
    - fixation device — *see* Complication, fixation device, internal
    - hemorrhage T84.83 ☑
    - infection or inflammation T84.7 ☑
    - joint prosthesis — *see* Complication, joint prosthesis, internal
    - malfunction T84.418 ☑
    - malposition T84.428 ☑
    - mechanical NEC T84.498 ☑
    - muscle graft — *see* Complications, graft, muscle
    - obstruction T84.498 ☑
    - pain T84.84 ☑
    - perforation T84.498 ☑
    - protrusion T84.498 ☑
    - specified complication NEC T84.89 ☑
    - stenosis T84.85 ☑
    - tendon graft — *see* Complications, graft, tendon
    - thrombosis T84.86 ☑
  - fracture (following insertion of device) — *see* Fracture, following insertion of orthopedic implant, joint prosthesis or bone plate
  - postprocedural M96.89
    - fracture — *see* Fracture, following insertion of orthopedic implant, joint prosthesis or bone plate
    - postlaminectomy syndrome NEC M96.1
      - kyphosis M96.3
      - lordosis M96.4

Complication(s) — *continued*
- orthopedic — *see also* Disorder, soft tissue — *continued*
  - postprocedural — *continued*
    - postradiation
      - kyphosis M96.2
      - scoliosis M96.5
    - pseudarthrosis post-fusion M96.0
    - specified type NEC M96.89
- pacemaker (cardiac) — *see* Complications, cardiovascular device or implant, electronic
- pancreas transplant — *see* Complications, transplant, pancreas
- penile prosthesis (implant) — *see* Complications, prosthetic device, penile
- perfusion NEC T80.90 ☑
- perineal repair (obstetrical) NEC O90.89
  - disruption O90.1
  - hematoma O90.2
  - infection (following delivery) O86.09
- phototherapy T88.9 ☑
  - specified NEC T88.8 ☑
- postmastoidectomy NEC H95.19- ☑
  - cyst, mucosal H95.13- ☑
  - granulation H95.12- ☑
  - inflammation, chronic H95.11- ☑
  - recurrent cholesteatoma H95.0- ☑
- postoperative — *see* Complications, postprocedural
  - circulatory — *see* Complications, circulatory system
  - ear — *see* Complications, ear
  - endocrine — *see* Complications, endocrine
  - eye — *see* Complications, eye
  - lumbar puncture G97.1
    - cerebrospinal fluid leak G97.0
  - nervous system (central) (peripheral) — *see* Complications, nervous system
  - respiratory system — *see* Complications, respiratory system
- postprocedural — *see also* Complications, surgical procedure
  - cardiac arrest — *see also* Infarct, myocardium, associated with revascularization procedure
    - following cardiac surgery I97.120
    - following other surgery I97.121
  - cardiac functional disturbance NEC — *see also* Infarct, myocardium, associated with revascularization procedure
    - following cardiac surgery I97.190
    - following other surgery I97.191
  - cardiac insufficiency
    - following cardiac surgery I97.110
    - following other surgery I97.111
  - chorioretinal scars following retinal surgery H59.81- ☑
  - following cataract surgery
    - cataract (lens) fragments H59.02- ☑
    - cystoid macular edema H59.03- ☑
    - specified NEC H59.09- ☑
    - vitreous (touch) syndrome H59.01- ☑
  - heart failure
    - following cardiac surgery I97.130
    - following other surgery I97.131
  - hematoma (of)
    - circulatory system organ or structure
      - following cardiac bypass I97.631
      - following cardiac catheterization I97.630
      - following other circulatory system procedure I97.638
      - following other procedure I97.621
    - digestive system
      - following procedure on digestive system K91.870
      - following procedure on other organ K91.871
    - ear
      - following other procedure H95.52
      - following procedure on ear and mastoid process H95.51
    - endocrine system
      - following endocrine system procedure E89.820
      - following other procedure E89.821
    - eye and adnexa
      - following ophthalmic procedure H59.33- ☑
      - following other procedure H59.34- ☑
    - genitourinary organ or structure
      - following procedure on genitourinary organ or structure N99.840
      - following procedure on other organ N99.841

Complication(s) — *continued*
- postprocedural — *see also* Complications, surgical procedure — *continued*
  - hematoma — *continued*
    - mastoid process
      - following other procedure H95.52
      - following procedure on ear and mastoid process H95.51
    - musculoskeletal structure
      - following musculoskeletal surgery M96.840
      - following non-orthopedic surgery M96.841
      - following orthopedic surgery M96.840
    - nervous system
      - following nervous system procedure G97.61
      - following other procedure G97.62
    - respiratory system
      - following other procedure J95.861
      - following procedure on respiratory system organ or structure J95.860
    - skin and subcutaneous tissue
      - following dermatologic procedure L76.31
      - following procedure on other organ L76.32
    - spleen
      - following procedure on other organ D78.32
      - following procedure on the spleen D78.31
  - hemorrhage (of)
    - circulatory system organ or structure
      - following cardiac bypass I97.611
      - following cardiac catheterization I97.610
      - following other circulatory system procedure I97.618
      - following other procedure I97.620
    - digestive system
      - following procedure on digestive system K91.840
      - following procedure on other organ K91.841
    - ear
      - following other procedure H95.42
      - following procedure on ear and mastoid process H95.41
    - endocrine system
      - following endocrine system procedure E89.810
      - following other procedure E89.811
    - eye and adnexa
      - following ophthalmic procedure H59.31- ☑
      - following other procedure H59.32- ☑
    - genitourinary organ or structure
      - following procedure on genitourinary organ or structure N99.820
      - following procedure on other organ N99.821
    - mastoid process
      - following other procedure H95.42
      - following procedure on ear and mastoid process H95.41
    - musculoskeletal structure
      - following musculoskeletal surgery M96.830
      - following non-orthopedic surgery M96.831
      - following orthopedic surgery M96.830
    - nervous system
      - following nervous system procedure G97.51
      - following other procedure G97.52
    - respiratory system
      - following a respiratory system procedure J95.830
      - following other procedure J95.831
    - skin and subcutaneous tissue
      - following a procedure on other organ L76.22
      - following dermatologic procedure L76.21
    - spleen
      - following procedure on other organ D78.22
      - following procedure on the spleen D78.21
  - seroma (of)
    - circulatory system organ or structure
      - following cardiac bypass I97.641
      - following cardiac catheterization I97.640
      - following other circulatory system procedure I97.648
      - following other procedure I97.622
    - digestive system
      - following procedure on digestive system K91.872
      - following procedure on other organ K91.873
    - ear
      - following other procedure H95.54
      - following procedure on ear and mastoid process H95.53

Complication(s) — *continued*
- postprocedural — *see also* Complications, surgical procedure — *continued*
  - seroma — *continued*
    - endocrine system
      - following endocrine system procedure E89.822
      - following other procedure E89.823
    - eye and adnexa
      - following ophthalmic procedure H59.35- ☑
      - following other procedure H59.36- ☑
    - genitourinary organ or structure
      - following procedure on genitourinary organ or structure N99.842
      - following procedure on other organ N99.843
    - mastoid process
      - following other procedure H95.54
      - following procedure on ear and mastoid process H95.53
    - musculoskeletal structure
      - following musculoskeletal surgery M96.842
      - following non-orthopedic surgery M96.843
      - following orthopedic surgery M96.842
    - nervous system
      - following nervous system procedure G97.63
      - following other procedure G97.64
    - respiratory system
      - following other procedure J95.863
      - following procedure on respiratory system organ or structure J95.862
    - skin and subcutaneous tissue
      - following dermatologic procedure L76.33
      - following procedure on other organ L76.34
    - spleen
      - following procedure on other organ D78.34
      - following procedure on the spleen D78.33
  - specified NEC
    - circulatory system I97.89
    - digestive K91.89
    - ear H95.89
    - endocrine E89.89
    - eye and adnexa H59.89
    - genitourinary N99.89
    - mastoid process H95.89
    - metabolic E89.89
    - musculoskeletal structure M96.89
    - nervous system G97.82
    - respiratory system J95.89
    - skin and subcutaneous tissue L76.82
    - spleen D78.89
- pregnancy NEC — *see* Pregnancy, complicated by
- prosthetic device or implant T85.9 ☑
  - bile duct — *see* Complications, bile duct implant
  - breast — *see* Complications, breast implant
  - bulking agent
    - ureteral
      - erosion T83.714 ☑
      - exposure T83.724 ☑
    - urethral
      - erosion T83.713 ☑
      - exposure T83.723 ☑
  - cardiac and vascular NEC — *see* Complications, cardiovascular device or implant
  - corneal transplant — *see* Complications, graft, cornea
  - electronic nervous system stimulator — *see* Complications, electronic stimulator device
  - epidural infusion catheter — *see* Complications, catheter, epidural
  - esophageal anti-reflux device — *see* Complications, esophageal anti-reflux device
  - genital organ or tract — *see* Complications, genitourinary, device or implant, genital tract
    - specified NEC T83.79- ☑
  - heart valve — *see* Complications, heart, valve, prosthesis
  - infection or inflammation T85.79 ☑
    - intestine transplant T86.892
    - liver transplant T86.43
    - lung transplant T86.812
    - pancreas transplant T86.892
    - skin graft T86.822
  - intraocular lens — *see* Complications, intraocular lens
  - intraperitoneal (dialysis) catheter — *see* Complications, catheter, intraperitoneal
  - joint — *see* Complications, joint prosthesis, internal
  - mechanical NEC T85.698 ☑

Complication(s) — *continued*
- prosthetic device or implant — *continued*
  - mechanical — *continued*
    - dialysis catheter (vascular) — *see also* Complication, catheter, dialysis, mechanical
      - peritoneal — *see* Complication, catheter, intraperitoneal, mechanical
    - gastrointestinal device T85.598 ☑
    - ocular device T85.398 ☑
    - subdural (infusion) catheter T85.690 ☑
    - suture, permanent T85.692 ☑
      - that for bone repair — *see* Complications, fixation device, internal (orthopedic), mechanical
    - ventricular shunt
      - breakdown T85.01 ☑
      - displacement T85.02 ☑
      - leakage T85.03 ☑
      - malposition T85.02 ☑
      - obstruction T85.09 ☑
      - perforation T85.09 ☑
      - protrusion T85.09 ☑
      - specified NEC T85.09 ☑
  - mesh
    - erosion (to surrounding organ or tissue) T83.718 ☑
      - urethral (into pelvic floor muscles) T83.712 ☑
      - vaginal (into pelvic floor muscles) T83.711 ☑
    - exposure (into surrounding organ or tissue) T83.728 ☑
      - urethral (through urethral wall) T83.722 ☑
      - vaginal (into vagina) (through vaginal wall) T83.721 ☑
  - orbital — *see* Complications, orbital prosthesis
  - penile T83.9 ☑
    - embolism T83.81 ☑
    - fibrosis T83.82 ☑
    - hemorrhage T83.83 ☑
    - infection and inflammation T83.61 ☑
    - mechanical
      - breakdown T83.410 ☑
      - displacement T83.420 ☑
      - leakage T83.490 ☑
      - malposition T83.420 ☑
      - obstruction T83.490 ☑
      - perforation T83.490 ☑
      - protrusion T83.490 ☑
      - specified NEC T83.490 ☑
    - pain T83.84 ☑
    - specified type NEC T83.89 ☑
    - stenosis T83.85 ☑
    - thrombosis T83.86 ☑
  - prosthetic materials NEC
    - erosion (to surrounding organ or tissue) T83.718 ☑
    - exposure (into surrounding organ or tissue) T83.728 ☑
  - skin graft T86.829
    - artificial skin or decellularized allodermis
      - embolism T85.818 ☑
      - fibrosis T85.828 ☑
      - hemorrhage T85.838 ☑
      - infection and inflammation T85.79 ☑
      - mechanical
        - breakdown T85.613 ☑
        - displacement T85.623 ☑
        - malfunction T85.613 ☑
        - malposition T85.623 ☑
        - obstruction T85.693 ☑
        - perforation T85.693 ☑
        - protrusion T85.693 ☑
        - specified NEC T85.693 ☑
      - pain T85.848 ☑
      - specified type NEC T85.898 ☑
      - stenosis T85.858 ☑
      - thrombosis T85.868 ☑
    - failure T86.821
    - infection T86.822
    - rejection T86.820
    - specified NEC T86.828
  - sling
    - urethral (female) (male)
      - erosion T83.712 ☑
      - exposure T83.722 ☑
  - specified NEC T85.9 ☑
    - embolism T85.818 ☑

Complication(s) — *continued*
- prosthetic device or implant — *continued*
  - specified — *continued*
    - fibrosis T85.828 ☑
    - hemorrhage T85.838 ☑
    - infection and inflammation T85.79 ☑
    - mechanical
      - breakdown T85.618 ☑
      - displacement T85.628 ☑
      - leakage T85.638 ☑
      - malfunction T85.618 ☑
      - malposition T85.628 ☑
      - obstruction T85.698 ☑
      - perforation T85.698 ☑
      - protrusion T85.698 ☑
      - specified NEC T85.698 ☑
    - pain T85.848 ☑
    - specified type NEC T85.898 ☑
    - stenosis T85.858 ☑
    - thrombosis T85.868 ☑
  - subdural infusion catheter — *see* Complications, catheter, subdural
  - sutures — *see* Complications, sutures
  - urinary organ or tract NEC — *see* Complications, genitourinary, device or implant, urinary system
  - vascular — *see* Complications, cardiovascular device or implant
  - ventricular shunt — *see* Complications, ventricular shunt (device)
- puerperium — *see* Puerperal
- puncture, spinal G97.1
  - cerebrospinal fluid leak G97.0
  - headache or reaction G97.1
- pyelogram N99.89
- radiation
  - kyphosis M96.2
  - scoliosis M96.5
- reattached
  - extremity (infection) (rejection)
    - lower T87.1X- ☑
    - upper T87.0X- ☑
  - specified body part NEC T87.2
- reconstructed breast
  - asymmetry between native and reconstructed breast N65.1
  - deformity N65.0
  - disproportion between native and reconstructed breast N65.1
  - excess tissue N65.0
  - misshappen N65.0
- reimplant NEC — *see also* Complications, prosthetic device or implant
  - limb (infection) (rejection) — *see* Complications, reattached, extremity
  - organ (partial) (total) — *see* Complications, transplant
  - prosthetic device NEC — *see* Complications, prosthetic device
- renal N28.9
  - allograft — *see* Complications, transplant, kidney
  - dialysis — *see* Complications, dialysis
- respirator
  - mechanical J95.850
    - specified NEC J95.859
- respiratory system J98.9
  - device, implant or graft — *see* Complication, prosthetic device or implant, specified NEC
  - lung transplant — *see* Complications, prosthetic device or implant, lung transplant
  - postoperative J95.89
    - air leak J95.812
    - Mendelson's syndrome (chemical pneumonitis) J95.4
    - pneumothorax J95.811
    - pulmonary insufficiency (acute) (after nonthoracic surgery) J95.2
      - chronic J95.3
      - following thoracic surgery J95.1
    - respiratory failure (acute) J95.821
      - acute and chronic J95.822
    - specified NEC J95.89
    - subglottic stenosis J95.5
    - tracheostomy complication — *see* Complications, tracheostomy
  - therapy T81.89 ☑
- sedation during labor and delivery O74.9

Complication(s) — *continued*
  sedation during labor and delivery — *continued*
    cardiac O74.2
    central nervous system O74.3
    pulmonary NEC O74.1
  shunt — *see also* Complications, prosthetic device or implant
    arteriovenous — *see* Complications, arteriovenous, shunt
    ventricular (communicating) — *see* Complications, ventricular shunt
  skin
    graft T86.829
      failure T86.821
      infection T86.822
      rejection T86.820
      specified type NEC T86.828
  spinal
    anesthesia — *see* Complications, anesthesia, spinal
    catheter (epidural) (subdural) — *see* Complications, catheter
    puncture or tap G97.1
      cerebrospinal fluid leak G97.0
      headache or reaction G97.1
  stent
    bile duct — *see* Complications, bile duct prosthesis
    ureteral indwelling
      breakdown T83.112 ☑
      displacement T83.122 ☑
      leakage T83.192 ☑
      malposition T83.122 ☑
      obstruction T83.192 ☑
      perforation T83.192 ☑
      protrusion T83.192 ☑
      specified NEC T83.192 ☑
    urinary NEC (ileal conduit) (nephroureteral) T83.193 ☑
      embolism T83.81 ☑
      fibrosis T83.82 ☑
      hemorrhage T83.83 ☑
      infection and inflammation T83.593 ☑
      mechanical
        breakdown T83.113 ☑
        displacement T83.123 ☑
        leakage T83.193 ☑
        malposition T83.123 ☑
        obstruction T83.193 ☑
        perforation T83.193 ☑
        protrusion T83.193 ☑
        specified NEC T83.193 ☑
      pain T83.84 ☑
      specified type NEC T83.89 ☑
      stenosis T83.85 ☑
      thrombosis T83.86 ☑
    vascular
      end stent stenosis — *see* Restenosis, stent
      in stent stenosis — *see* Restenosis, stent
  stoma
    digestive tract
      colostomy — *see* Complications, colostomy
      enterostomy — *see* Complications, enterostomy
      esophagostomy — *see* Complications, esophagostomy
      gastrostomy — *see* Complications, gastrostomy
    urinary tract N99.528
      continent N99.538
        hemorrhage N99.530
        herniation N99.533
        infection N99.531
        malfunction N99.532
        specified type NEC N99.538
        stenosis N99.534
      cystostomy — *see* Complications, cystostomy
      external NOS N99.528
      hemorrhage N99.520
      herniation N99.523
      incontinent N99.528
        hemorrhage N99.520
        herniation N99.523
        infection N99.521
        malfunction N99.522
        specified type NEC N99.528
        stenosis N99.524
      infection N99.521
      malfunction N99.522
      specified type NEC N99.528
      stenosis N99.524

Complication(s) — *continued*
  stomach banding — *see* Complication(s), bariatric procedure
  stomach stapling — *see* Complication(s), bariatric procedure
  surgical material, nonabsorbable — *see* Complication, suture, permanent
  surgical procedure (on) T81.9 ☑
    amputation stump (late) — *see* Complications, amputation stump
    cardiac — *see* Complications, circulatory system
    cholesteatoma, recurrent — *see* Complications, postmastoidectomy, recurrent cholesteatoma
    circulatory (early) — *see* Complications, circulatory system
    digestive system — *see* Complications, gastrointestinal
    dumping syndrome (postgastrectomy) K91.1
    ear — *see* Complications, ear
    elephantiasis or lymphedema I97.89
      postmastectomy I97.2
    emphysema (surgical) T81.82 ☑
    endocrine — *see* Complications, endocrine
    eye — *see* Complications, eye
    fistula (persistent postoperative) T81.83 ☑
    foreign body inadvertently left in wound (sponge) (suture) (swab) — *see* Foreign body, accidentally left during a procedure
    gastrointestinal — *see* Complications, gastrointestinal
    genitourinary NEC N99.89
    hematoma
      intraoperative — *see* Complication, intraoperative, hemorrhage
      postprocedural — *see* Complication, postprocedural, hematoma
    hemorrhage
      intraoperative — *see* Complication, intraoperative, hemorrhage
      postprocedural — *see* Complication, postprocedural, hemorrhage
    hepatic failure K91.82
    hyperglycemia (postpancreatectomy) E89.1
    hypoinsulinemia (postpancreatectomy) E89.1
    hypoparathyroidism (postparathyroidectomy) E89.2
    hypopituitarism (posthypophysectomy) E89.3
    hypothyroidism (post-thyroidectomy) E89.0
    intestinal obstruction — *see also* Obstruction, intestine, postoperative K91.30
    intracranial hypotension following ventricular shunting (ventriculostomy) G97.2
    lymphedema I97.89
      postmastectomy I97.2
    malabsorption (postsurgical) NEC K91.2
      osteoporosis — *see* Osteoporosis, postsurgical malabsorption
    mastoidectomy cavity NEC — *see* Complications, postmastoidectomy
    metabolic E89.89
      specified NEC E89.89
    musculoskeletal — *see* Complications, musculoskeletal system
    nervous system (central) (peripheral) — *see* Complications, nervous system
    ovarian failure E89.40
      asymptomatic E89.40
      symptomatic E89.41
    peripheral vascular — *see* Complications, surgical procedure, vascular
    postcardiotomy syndrome I97.0
    postcholecystectomy syndrome K91.5
    postcommissurotomy syndrome I97.0
    postgastrectomy dumping syndrome K91.1
    postlaminectomy syndrome NEC M96.1
      kyphosis M96.3
    postmastectomy lymphedema syndrome I97.2
    postmastoidectomy cholesteatoma — *see* Complications, postmastoidectomy, recurrent cholesteatoma
    postvagotomy syndrome K91.1
    postvalvulotomy syndrome I97.0
    pulmonary insufficiency (acute) J95.2
      chronic J95.3
      following thoracic surgery J95.1
    reattached body part — *see* Complications, reattached
    respiratory — *see* Complications, respiratory system
    shock (hypovolemic) T81.19 ☑

Complication(s) — *continued*
  surgical procedure — *continued*
    spleen (postoperative) D78.89
      intraoperative D78.81
    stitch abscess T81.41
    subglottic stenosis (postsurgical) J95.5
    testicular hypofunction E89.5
    transplant — *see* Complications, organ or tissue transplant
    urinary NEC N99.89
    vaginal vault prolapse (posthysterectomy) N99.3
    vascular (peripheral)
      artery T81.719 ☑
        mesenteric T81.710 ☑
        renal T81.711 ☑
        specified NEC T81.718 ☑
      vein T81.72 ☑
    wound infection T81.49 ☑
  suture, permanent (wire) NEC T85.9 ☑
    with repair of bone — *see* Complications, fixation device, internal
    embolism T85.818 ☑
    fibrosis T85.828 ☑
    hemorrhage T85.838 ☑
    infection and inflammation T85.79 ☑
    mechanical
      breakdown T85.612 ☑
      displacement T85.622 ☑
      malfunction T85.612 ☑
      malposition T85.622 ☑
      obstruction T85.692 ☑
      perforation T85.692 ☑
      protrusion T85.692 ☑
      specified NEC T85.692 ☑
    pain T85.848 ☑
    specified type NEC T85.898 ☑
    stenosis T85.858 ☑
    thrombosis T85.868 ☑
  tracheostomy J95.00
    granuloma J95.09
    hemorrhage J95.01
    infection J95.02
    malfunction J95.03
    mechanical J95.03
    obstruction J95.03
    specified type NEC J95.09
    tracheo-esophageal fistula J95.04
  transfusion (blood) (lymphocytes) (plasma) T80.92 ☑
    air emblism T80.0 ☑
    circulatory overload E87.71
    febrile nonhemolytic transfusion reaction R50.84
    hemochromatosis E83.111
    hemolysis T80.89 ☑
    hemolytic reaction (antigen unspecified) T80.919 ☑
    incompatibility reaction (antigen unspecified) T80.919 ☑
      ABO T80.30 ☑
        delayed serologic (DSTR) T80.39 ☑
        hemolytic transfusion reaction (HTR) (unspecified time after transfusion) T80.319 ☑
          acute (AHTR) (less than 24 hours after transfusion) T80.310 ☑
          delayed (DHTR) (24 hours or more after transfusion) T80.311 ☑
        specified NEC T80.39 ☑
      acute (antigen unspecified) T80.910 ☑
      delayed (antigen unspecified) T80.911 ☑
      delayed serologic (DSTR) T80.89 ☑
      non-ABO (minor antigens) (Duffy) (K) (Kell) (Kidd) (Lewis) (M) (N) (P) (S) T80.A0 ☑ (*following T80.4*)
        delayed serologic (DSTR) T80.A9 ☑ (*following T80.4*)
        hemolytic transfusion reaction (HTR) (unspecified time after transfusion) T80.A19 ☑ (*following T80.4*)
          acute (AHTR) (less than 24 hours after transfusion) T80.A10 ☑ (*following T80.4*)
          delayed (DHTR) (24 hours or more after transfusion) T80.A11 ☑ (*following T80.4*)
        specified NEC T80.A9 ☑ (*following T80.4*)
      Rh (antigens) (C) (c) (D) (E) (e)) (factor) T80.40 ☑
        delayed serologic (DSTR) T80.49 ☑
        hemolytic transfusion reaction (HTR) (unspecified time after transfusion) T80.419 ☑

Complication(s) — *continued*
  transfusion — *continued*
    incompatibility reaction — *continued*
      Rh — *continued*
        hemolytic transfusion reaction — *continued*
          acute (AHTR) (less than 24 hours after transfusion) T80.410 ☑
          delayed (DHTR) (24 hours or more after transfusion) T80.411 ☑
          specified NEC T80.49 ☑
    infection T80.29 ☑
      acute T80.22- ☑
    reaction NEC T80.89 ☑
    sepsis T80.29 ☑
    shock T80.89 ☑
  transplant T86.90
    bone T86.839
      failure T86.831
      infection T86.832
      rejection T86.830
      specified type NEC T86.838
    bone marrow T86.00
      failure T86.02
      infection T86.03
      rejection T86.01
      specified type NEC T86.09
    cornea T86.849
      failure T86.841
      infection T86.842
      rejection T86.840
      specified type NEC T86.848
    failure T86.92
    heart T86.20
      with lung T86.30
      cardiac allograft vasculopathy T86.290
        failure T86.32
        infection T86.33
        rejection T86.31
        specified type NEC T86.39
      failure T86.22
      infection T86.23
      rejection T86.21
      specified type NEC T86.298
    infection T86.93
    intestine T86.859
      failure T86.851
      infection T86.852
      rejection T86.850
      specified type NEC T86.858
    kidney T86.10
      failure T86.12
      infection T86.13
      rejection T86.11
      specified type NEC T86.19
    liver T86.40
      failure T86.42
      infection T86.43
      rejection T86.41
      specified type NEC T86.49
    lung T86.819
      with heart T86.30
        failure T86.32
        infection T86.33
        rejection T86.31
        specified type NEC T86.39
      failure T86.811
      infection T86.812
      rejection T86.810
      specified type NEC T86.818
    malignant neoplasm C80.2
    pancreas T86.899
      failure T86.891
      infection T86.892
      rejection T86.890
      specified type NEC T86.898
    peripheral blood stem cells T86.5
    post-transplant lymphoproliferative disorder (PTLD) D47.Z1 (*following* D47.4)
    rejection T86.91
    skin T86.829
      failure T86.821
      infection T86.822
      rejection T86.820
      specified type NEC T86.828
    specified
      tissue T86.899
        failure T86.891

Complication(s) — *continued*
  transplant — *continued*
    specified — *continued*
      tissue — *continued*
        infection T86.892
        rejection T86.890
        specified type NEC T86.898
      type NEC T86.99
    stem cell (from peripheral blood) (from umbilical cord) T86.5
    umbilical cord stem cells T86.5
  trauma (early) T79.9
    specified NEC T79.8
  ultrasound therapy NEC T88.9 ☑
  umbilical cord NEC
    complicating delivery O69.9 ☑
      specified NEC O69.89 ☑
  umbrella device, vascular T82.9 ☑
    embolism T82.818 ☑
    fibrosis T82.828 ☑
    hemorrhage T82.838 ☑
    infection or inflammation T82.7 ☑
    mechanical
      breakdown T82.515 ☑
      displacement T82.525 ☑
      leakage T82.535 ☑
      malposition T82.525 ☑
      obstruction T82.595 ☑
      perforation T82.595 ☑
      protrusion T82.595 ☑
    pain T82.848 ☑
    specified type NEC T82.898 ☑
    stenosis T82.858 ☑
    thrombosis T82.868 ☑
  urethral catheter — *see* Complications, catheter, urethral, indwelling
  vaccination T88.1 ☑
    anaphylaxis NEC T80.52 ☑
    arthropathy — *see* Arthropathy, postimmunization
    cellulitis T88.0 ☑
    encephalitis or encephalomyelitis G04.02
    infection (general) (local) NEC T88.0 ☑
    meningitis G03.8
    myelitis G04.02
    protein sickness T80.62 ☑
    rash T88.1 ☑
    reaction (allergic) T88.1 ☑
      serum T80.62 ☑
    sepsis T88.0 ☑
    serum intoxication, sickness, rash, or other serum reaction NEC T80.62 ☑
      anaphylactic shock T80.52 ☑
    shock (allergic) (anaphylactic) T80.52 ☑
    vaccinia (generalized) (localized) T88.1 ☑
  vas deferens device or implant — *see* Complications, genitourinary, device or implant, genital tract
  vascular I99.9
    device or implant T82.9 ☑
      embolism T82.818 ☑
      fibrosis T82.828 ☑
      hemorrhage T82.838 ☑
      infection or inflammation T82.7 ☑
      mechanical
        breakdown T82.519 ☑
          specified device NEC T82.518 ☑
        displacement T82.529 ☑
          specified device NEC T82.528 ☑
        leakage T82.539 ☑
          specified device NEC T82.538 ☑
        malposition T82.529 ☑
          specified device NEC T82.528 ☑
        obstruction T82.599 ☑
          specified device NEC T82.598 ☑
        perforation T82.599 ☑
          specified device NEC T82.598 ☑
        protrusion T82.599 ☑
          specified device NEC T82.598 ☑
      pain T82.848 ☑
      specified type NEC T82.898 ☑
      stenosis T82.858 ☑
      thrombosis T82.868 ☑
    dialysis catheter — *see* Complication, catheter, dialysis
    following infusion, therapeutic injection or transfusion T80.1 ☑
    graft T82.9 ☑

Complication(s) — *continued*
  vascular — *continued*
    graft — *continued*
      embolism T82.818 ☑
      fibrosis T82.828 ☑
      hemorrhage T82.838 ☑
      mechanical
        breakdown T82.319 ☑
          aorta (bifurcation) T82.310 ☑
          carotid artery T82.311 ☑
          specified vessel NEC T82.318 ☑
        displacement T82.329 ☑
          aorta (bifurcation) T82.320 ☑
          carotid artery T82.321 ☑
          specified vessel NEC T82.328 ☑
        leakage T82.339 ☑
          aorta (bifurcation) T82.330 ☑
          carotid artery T82.331 ☑
          specified vessel NEC T82.338 ☑
        malposition T82.329 ☑
          aorta (bifurcation) T82.320 ☑
          carotid artery T82.321 ☑
          specified vessel NEC T82.328 ☑
        obstruction T82.399 ☑
          aorta (bifurcation) T82.390 ☑
          carotid artery T82.391 ☑
          specified vessel NEC T82.398 ☑
        perforation T82.399 ☑
          aorta (bifurcation) T82.390 ☑
          carotid artery T82.391 ☑
          specified vessel NEC T82.398 ☑
        protrusion T82.399 ☑
          aorta (bifurcation) T82.390 ☑
          carotid artery T82.391 ☑
          specified vessel NEC T82.398 ☑
      pain T82.848 ☑
      specified complication NEC T82.898 ☑
      stenosis T82.858 ☑
      thrombosis T82.868 ☑
    postoperative — *see* Complications, postoperative, circulatory
  vena cava device (filter) (sieve) (umbrella) — *see* Complications, umbrella device, vascular
  ventilation therapy NEC T81.81 ☑
  ventilator
    mechanical J95.850
      specified NEC J95.859
  ventricular (communicating) shunt (device) T85.9 ☑
    embolism T85.810 ☑
    fibrosis T85.820 ☑
    hemorrhage T85.830 ☑
    infection and inflammation T85.730 ☑
    mechanical
      breakdown T85.01 ☑
      displacement T85.02 ☑
      leakage T85.03 ☑
      malposition T85.02 ☑
      obstruction T85.09 ☑
      perforation T85.09 ☑
      protrusion T85.09 ☑
      specified NEC T85.09 ☑
    pain T85.840 ☑
    specified type NEC T85.890 ☑
    stenosis T85.850 ☑
    thrombosis T85.860 ☑
  wire suture, permanent (implanted) — *see* Complications, suture, permanent

Compressed air disease T70.3 ☑
Compression
  with injury — *code by* Nature of injury
  artery I77.1
    celiac, syndrome I77.4
  brachial plexus G54.0
  brain (stem) G93.5
    due to
      contusion (diffuse) — *see* Injury, intracranial, diffuse
        focal — *see* Injury, intracranial, focal
      injury NEC — *see* Injury, intracranial, diffuse
      traumatic — *see* Injury, intracranial, diffuse
  bronchus J98.09
  cauda equina G83.4
  celiac (artery) (axis) I77.4
  cerebral — *see* Compression, brain
  cervical plexus G54.2

Compression — *continued*
  cord
    spinal — *see* Compression, spinal
    umbilical — *see* Compression, umbilical cord
  cranial nerve G52.9
    eighth H93.3 ☑
    eleventh G52.8
    fifth G50.8
    first G52.0
    fourth — *see* Strabismus, paralytic, fourth nerve
    ninth G52.1
    second — *see* Disorder, nerve, optic
    seventh G51.8
    sixth — *see* Strabismus, paralytic, sixth nerve
    tenth G52.2
    third — *see* Strabismus, paralytic, third nerve
    twelfth G52.3
  diver's squeeze T70.3 ☑
  during birth (newborn) P15.9
  esophagus K22.2
  eustachian tube — *see* Obstruction, eustachian tube, cartilaginous
  facies Q67.1
  fracture
    nontraumatic NOS — *see* Collapse, vertebra
    pathological — *see* Fracture, pathological
    traumatic — *see* Fracture, traumatic
  heart — *see* Disease, heart
  intestine — *see* Obstruction, intestine
  laryngeal nerve, recurrent G52.2
    with paralysis of vocal cords and larynx J38.00
      bilateral J38.02
      unilateral J38.01
  lumbosacral plexus G54.1
  lung J98.4
  lymphatic vessel I89.0
  medulla — *see* Compression, brain
  nerve — *see also* Disorder, nerve G58.9
    arm NEC — *see* Mononeuropathy, upper limb
    axillary G54.0
    cranial — *see* Compression, cranial nerve
    leg NEC — *see* Mononeuropathy, lower limb
    median (in carpal tunnel) — *see* Syndrome, carpal tunnel
    optic — *see* Disorder, nerve, optic
    plantar — *see* Lesion, nerve, plantar
    posterior tibial (in tarsal tunnel) — *see* Syndrome, tarsal tunnel
    root or plexus NOS (in) G54.9
      intervertebral disc disorder NEC — *see* Disorder, disc, with, radiculopathy
        with myelopathy — *see* Disorder, disc, with, myelopathy
      neoplastic disease — *see also* Neoplasm D49.9 *[G55]*
      spondylosis — *see* Spondylosis, with radiculopathy
    sciatic (acute) — *see* Lesion, nerve, sciatic
    sympathetic G90.8
    traumatic — *see* Injury, nerve
    ulnar — *see* Lesion, nerve, ulnar
    upper extremity NEC — *see* Mononeuropathy, upper limb
  spinal (cord) G95.20
    by displacement of intervertebral disc NEC — *see also* Disorder, disc, with, myelopathy
    nerve root NOS G54.9
      due to displacement of intervertebral disc NEC — *see* Disorder, disc, with, radiculopathy
        with myelopathy — *see* Disorder, disc, with, myelopathy
    specified NEC G95.29
    spondylogenic (cervical) (lumbar, lumbosacral) (thoracic) — *see* Spondylosis, with myelopathy NEC
    anterior — *see* Syndrome, anterior, spinal artery, compression
    traumatic — *see* Injury, spinal cord, by region
  subcostal nerve (syndrome) — *see* Mononeuropathy, upper limb, specified NEC
  sympathetic nerve NEC G90.8
  syndrome T79.5 ☑
  trachea J39.8
  ulnar nerve (by scar tissue) — *see* Lesion, nerve, ulnar
  umbilical cord
    complicating delivery O69.2 ☑
      cord around neck O69.1 ☑

Compression — *continued*
  umbilical cord — *continued*
    complicating delivery — *continued*
      prolapse O69.0
      specified NEC O69.2 ☑
  ureter N13.5
  vein I87.1
  vena cava (inferior) (superior) I87.1
Compulsion, compulsive
  gambling F63.0
  neurosis F42.8
  personality F60.5
  states F42.8
  swearing F42.8
    in Gilles de la Tourette's syndrome F95.2
  tics and spasms F95.9
Concato's disease (pericardial polyserositis) A19.9
  nontubercular I31.1
  pleural — *see* Pleurisy, with effusion
Concavity chest wall M95.4
Concealed penis Q55.64
Concern (normal) **about sick person in family** Z63.6
Concrescence (teeth) K00.2
Concretio cordis I31.1
  rheumatic I09.2
Concretion — *see also* Calculus
  appendicular K38.1
  canaliculus — *see* Dacryolith
  clitoris N90.89
  conjunctiva H11.12- ☑
  eyelid — *see* Disorder, eyelid, specified type NEC
  lacrimal passages — *see* Dacryolith
  prepuce (male) N47.8
  salivary gland (any) K11.5
  seminal vesicle N50.89
  tonsil J35.8
Concussion (brain) (cerebral) (current) S06.0X9 ☑
  with
    loss of consciousness of 30 minutes or less S06.0X1 ☑
    loss of consciousness of unspecified duration S06.0X9 ☑
  blast (air) (hydraulic) (immersion) (underwater)
    abdomen or thorax — *see* Injury, blast, by site
    ear with acoustic nerve injury — *see* Injury, nerve, acoustic, specified type NEC
  cauda equina S34.3 ☑
  conus medullaris S34.02 ☑
  ocular S05.8X- ☑
  spinal (cord)
    cervical S14.0 ☑
    lumbar S34.01 ☑
    sacral S34.02 ☑
    thoracic S24.0 ☑
  syndrome F07.81
  without loss of consciousness S06.0X0 ☑
Condition — *see* Disease
Conditions arising in the perinatal period — *see* Newborn, affected by
Conduct disorder — *see* Disorder, conduct
Condyloma A63.0
  acuminatum A63.0
  gonorrheal A54.09
  latum A51.31
  syphilitic A51.31
    congenital A50.07
  venereal, syphilitic A51.31
Conflagration — *see also* Burn
  asphyxia (by inhalation of gases, fumes or vapors) — *see also* Table of Drugs and Chemicals T59.9- ☑
Conflict (with) — *see also* Discord
  family Z73.9
  marital Z63.0
    involving divorce or estrangement Z63.5
  parent-child Z62.820
    parent-adopted child Z62.821
    parent-biological child Z62.820
    parent-foster child Z62.822
  social role NEC Z73.5
Confluent — *see* condition
Confusion, confused R41.0
  epileptic F05
  mental state (psychogenic) F44.89
  psychogenic F44.89
  reactive (from emotional stress, psychological trauma) F44.89
Confusional arousals G47.51

Congelation T69.9 ☑
Congenital — *see also* condition
  aortic septum Q25.49
  intrinsic factor deficiency D51.0
  malformation — *see* Anomaly
Congestion, congestive
  bladder N32.89
  bowel K63.89
  brain G93.89
  breast N64.59
  bronchial J98.09
  catarrhal J31.0
  chest R09.89
  chill, malarial — *see* Malaria
  circulatory NEC I99.8
  duodenum K31.89
  eye — *due see* Hyperemia, conjunctiva
  facial, due to birth injury P15.4
  general R68.89
  glottis J37.0
  heart — *see* Failure, heart, congestive
  hepatic K76.1
  hypostatic (lung) — *see* Edema, lung
  intestine K63.89
  kidney N28.89
  labyrinth H83.8 ☑
  larynx J37.0
  liver K76.1
  lung R09.89
    active or acute — *see* Pneumonia
  malaria, malarial — *see* Malaria
  nasal R09.81
  nose R09.81
  orbit, orbital — *see also* Exophthalmos
    inflammatory (chronic) — *see* Inflammation, orbit
  ovary N83.8
  pancreas K86.89
  pelvic, female N94.89
  pleural J94.8
  prostate (active) N42.1
  pulmonary — *see* Congestion, lung
  renal N28.89
  retina H35.81
  seminal vesicle N50.1
  spinal cord G95.19
  spleen (chronic) D73.2
  stomach K31.89
  trachea — *see* Tracheitis
  urethra N36.8
  uterus N85.8
    with subinvolution N85.3
  venous (passive) I87.8
  viscera R68.89
Congestive — *see* Congestion
Conical
  cervix (hypertrophic elongation) N88.4
  cornea — *see* Keratoconus
  teeth K00.2
Conjoined twins Q89.4
Conjugal maladjustment Z63.0
  involving divorce or estrangement Z63.5
Conjunctiva — *see* condition
Conjunctivitis (staphylococcal) (streptococcal) NOS H10.9
  Acanthamoeba B60.12
  acute H10.3- ☑
    atopic H10.1- ☑
    chemical — *see also* Corrosion, cornea H10.21- ☑
    mucopurulent H10.02- ☑
      follicular H10.01- ☑
    pseudomembranous H10.22- ☑
    serous except viral H10.23- ☑
      viral — *see* Conjunctivitis, viral
    toxic H10.21- ☑
  adenoviral (acute) (follicular) B30.1
  allergic (acute) — *see* Conjunctivitis, acute, atopic
    chronic H10.45
      vernal H10.44
  anaphylactic — *see* Conjunctivitis, acute, atopic
  Apollo B30.3
  atopic (acute) — *see* Conjunctivitis, acute, atopic
  Béal's B30.2
  blennorrhagic (gonococcal) (neonatorum) A54.31
  chemical (acute) — *see also* Corrosion, cornea H10.21- ☑
  chlamydial A74.0
    due to trachoma A71.1
    neonatal P39.1

Conjunctivitis — *continued*
chronic (nodosa) (petrificans) (phlyctenular) H10.40- ☑
allergic H10.45
vernal H10.44
follicular H10.43- ☑
giant papillary H10.41- ☑
simple H10.42- ☑
vernal H10.44
coxsackievirus 24 B30.3
diphtheritic A36.86
due to
dust — *see* Conjunctivitis, acute, atopic
filariasis B74.9
mucocutaneous leishmaniasis B55.2
enterovirus type 70 (hemorrhagic) B30.3
epidemic (viral) B30.9
hemorrhagic B30.3
gonococcal (neonatorum) A54.31
granular (trachomatous) A71.1
sequelae (late effect) B94.0
hemorrhagic (acute) (epidemic) B30.3
herpes zoster B02.31
in (due to)
Acanthamoeba B60.12
adenovirus (acute) (follicular) B30.1
Chlamydia A74.0
coxsackievirus 24 B30.3
diphtheria A36.86
enterovirus type 70 (hemorrhagic) B30.3
filariasis B74.9
gonococci A54.31
herpes (simplex) virus B00.53
zoster B02.31
infectious disease NEC B99 ☑
meningococci A39.89
mucocutaneous leishmaniasis B55.2
rosacea H10.82- ☑
syphilis (late) A52.71
zoster B02.31
inclusion A74.0
infantile P39.1
gonococcal A54.31
Koch-Weeks' — *see* Conjunctivitis, acute, mucopurulent
light — *see* Conjunctivitis, acute, atopic
ligneous — *see* Blepharoconjunctivitis, ligneous
meningococcal A39.89
mucopurulent — *see* Conjunctivitis, acute, mucopurulent
neonatal P39.1
gonococcal A54.31
Newcastle B30.8
of Béal B30.2
parasitic
filariasis B74.9
mucocutaneous leishmaniasis B55.2
Parinaud's H10.89
petrificans H10.89
rosacea H10.82- ☑
specified NEC H10.89
swimming-pool B30.1
trachomatous A71.1
acute A71.0
sequelae (late effect) B94.0
traumatic NEC H10.89
tuberculous A18.59
tularemic A21.1
tularensis A21.1
viral B30.9
due to
adenovirus B30.1
enterovirus B30.3
specified NEC B30.8
Conjunctivochalasis H11.82- ☑
Connective tissue — *see* condition
Conn's syndrome E26.01
Conradi (-Hunermann) **disease** Q77.3
Consanguinity Z84.3
counseling Z71.89
Conscious simulation (of illness) Z76.5
Consecutive — *see* condition
Consolidation lung (base) — *see* Pneumonia, lobar
Constipation (atonic) (neurogenic) (simple) (spastic) K59.00
chronic K59.09
idiopathic K59.04
drug-induced K59.03
functional K59.04
outlet dysfunction K59.02

Constipation — *continued*
psychogenic F45.8
slow transit K59.01
specified NEC K59.09
Constitutional — *see also* condition
substandard F60.7
Constitutionally substandard F60.7
Constriction — *see also* Stricture
auditory canal — *see* Stenosis, external ear canal
bronchial J98.09
duodenum K31.5
esophagus K22.2
external
abdomen, abdominal (wall) S30.841 ☑
alveolar process S00.542 ☑
ankle S90.54- ☑
antecubital space — *see* Constriction, external, forearm
arm (upper) S40.84- ☑
auricle — *see* Constriction, external, ear
axilla — *see* Constriction, external, arm
back, lower S30.840 ☑
breast S20.14- ☑
brow S00.84 ☑
buttock S30.840 ☑
calf — *see* Constriction, external, leg
canthus — *see* Constriction, external, eyelid
cheek S00.84 ☑
internal S00.542 ☑
chest wall — *see* Constriction, external, thorax
chin S00.84 ☑
clitoris S30.844 ☑
costal region — *see* Constriction, external, thorax
digit(s)
foot — *see* Constriction, external, toe
hand — *see* Constriction, external, finger
ear S00.44- ☑
elbow S50.34- ☑
epididymis S30.843 ☑
epigastric region S30.841 ☑
esophagus, cervical S10.14 ☑
eyebrow — *see* Constriction, external, eyelid
eyelid S00.24- ☑
face S00.84 ☑
finger(s) S60.44- ☑
index S60.44- ☑
little S60.44- ☑
middle S60.44- ☑
ring S60.44- ☑
flank S30.841 ☑
foot (except toe(s) alone) S90.84- ☑
toe — *see* Constriction, external, toe
forearm S50.84- ☑
elbow only — *see* Constriction, external, elbow
forehead S00.84 ☑
genital organs, external
female S30.846 ☑
male S30.845 ☑
groin S30.841 ☑
gum S00.542 ☑
hand S60.54- ☑
head S00.94 ☑
ear — *see* Constriction, external, ear
eyelid — *see* Constriction, external, eyelid
lip S00.541 ☑
nose S00.34 ☑
oral cavity S00.542 ☑
scalp S00.04 ☑
specified site NEC S00.84 ☑
heel — *see* Constriction, external, foot
hip S70.24- ☑
inguinal region S30.841 ☑
interscapular region S20.449 ☑
jaw S00.84 ☑
knee S80.24- ☑
labium (majus) (minus) S30.844 ☑
larynx S10.14 ☑
leg (lower) S80.84- ☑
knee — *see* Constriction, external, knee
upper — *see* Constriction, external, thigh
lip S00.541 ☑
lower back S30.840 ☑
lumbar region S30.840 ☑
malar region S00.84 ☑
mammary — *see* Constriction, external, breast
mastoid region S00.84 ☑

Constriction — *continued*
external — *continued*
mouth S00.542 ☑
nail
finger — *see* Constriction, external, finger
toe — *see* Constriction, external, toe
nasal S00.34 ☑
neck S10.94 ☑
specified site NEC S10.84 ☑
throat S10.14 ☑
nose S00.34 ☑
occipital region S00.04 ☑
oral cavity S00.542 ☑
orbital region — *see* Constriction, external, eyelid
palate S00.542 ☑
palm — *see* Constriction, external, hand
parietal region S00.04 ☑
pelvis S30.840 ☑
penis S30.842 ☑
perineum
female S30.844 ☑
male S30.840 ☑
periocular area — *see* Constriction, external, eyelid
phalanges
finger — *see* Constriction, external, finger
toe — *see* Constriction, external, toe
pharynx S10.14 ☑
pinna — *see* Constriction, external, ear
popliteal space — *see* Constriction, external, knee
prepuce S30.842 ☑
pubic region S30.840 ☑
pudendum
female S30.846 ☑
male S30.845 ☑
sacral region S30.840 ☑
scalp S00.04 ☑
scapular region — *see* Constriction, external, shoulder
scrotum S30.843 ☑
shin — *see* Constriction, external, leg
shoulder S40.24- ☑
sternal region S20.349 ☑
submaxillary region S00.84 ☑
submental region S00.84 ☑
subungual
finger(s) — *see* Constriction, external, finger
toe(s) — *see* Constriction, external, toe
supraclavicular fossa S10.84 ☑
supraorbital S00.84 ☑
temple S00.84 ☑
temporal region S00.84 ☑
testis S30.843 ☑
thigh S70.34- ☑
thorax, thoracic (wall) S20.94 ☑
back S20.44- ☑
front S20.34- ☑
throat S10.14 ☑
thumb S60.34- ☑
toe(s) (lesser) S90.44- ☑
great S90.44- ☑
tongue S00.542 ☑
trachea S10.14 ☑
tunica vaginalis S30.843 ☑
uvula S00.542 ☑
vagina S30.844 ☑
vulva S30.844 ☑
wrist S60.84- ☑
gallbladder — *see* Obstruction, gallbladder
intestine — *see* Obstruction, intestine
larynx J38.6
congenital Q31.8
specified NEC Q31.8
subglottic Q31.1
organ or site, congenital NEC — *see* Atresia, by site
prepuce (acquired) (congenital) N47.1
pylorus (adult hypertrophic) K31.1
congenital or infantile Q40.0
newborn Q40.0
ring dystocia (uterus) O62.4
spastic — *see also* Spasm
ureter N13.5
ureter N13.5
with infection N13.6
urethra — *see* Stricture, urethra
visual field (peripheral) (functional) — *see* Defect, visual field

Constrictive — see condition
Consultation
    medical — see Counseling, medical
    religious Z71.81
    specified reason NEC Z71.89
    spiritual Z71.81
    without complaint or sickness Z71.9
        feared complaint unfounded Z71.1
        specified reason NEC Z71.89
Consumption — see Tuberculosis
Contact (with) — see also Exposure (to)
    acariasis Z20.7
    AIDS virus Z20.6
    air pollution Z77.110
    algae and algae toxins Z77.121
    algae bloom Z77.121
    anthrax Z20.810
    aromatic amines Z77.020
    aromatic (hazardous) compounds NEC Z77.028
    aromatic dyes NOS Z77.028
    arsenic Z77.010
    asbestos Z77.090
    bacterial disease NEC Z20.818
    benzene Z77.021
    blue-green algae bloom Z77.121
    body fluids (potentially hazardous) Z77.21
    brown tide Z77.121
    chemicals (chiefly nonmedicinal) (hazardous) NEC
        Z77.098
    cholera Z20.09
    chromium compounds Z77.018
    communicable disease Z20.9
        bacterial NEC Z20.818
        specified NEC Z20.89
        viral NEC Z20.828
        Zika virus Z20.821
    cyanobacteria bloom Z77.121
    dyes Z77.098
    Escherichia coli (E. coli) Z20.01
    fiberglass — see Table of Drugs and Chemicals, fiber-
        glass
    German measles Z20.4
    gonorrhea Z20.2
    hazardous metals NEC Z77.018
    hazardous substances NEC Z77.29
    hazards in the physical environment NEC Z77.128
    hazards to health NEC Z77.9
    HIV Z20.6
    HTLV-III/LAV Z20.6
    human immunodeficiency virus (HIV) Z20.6
    infection Z20.9
        specified NEC Z20.89
    infestation (parasitic) NEC Z20.7
    intestinal infectious disease NEC Z20.09
        Escherichia coli (E. coli) Z20.01
    lead Z77.011
    meningococcus Z20.811
    mold (toxic) Z77.120
    nickel dust Z77.018
    noise Z77.122
    parasitic disease Z20.7
    pediculosis Z20.7
    pfiesteria piscicida Z77.121
    poliomyelitis Z20.89
    pollution
        air Z77.110
        environmental NEC Z77.118
        soil Z77.112
        water Z77.111
    polycyclic aromatic hydrocarbons Z77.028
    rabies Z20.3
    radiation, naturally occurring NEC Z77.123
    radon Z77.123
    red tide (Florida) Z77.121
    rubella Z20.4
    sexually-transmitted disease Z20.2
    smallpox (laboratory) Z20.89
    syphilis Z20.2
    tuberculosis Z20.1
    uranium Z77.012
    varicella Z20.820
    venereal disease Z20.2
    viral disease NEC Z20.828
    viral hepatitis Z20.5
    water pollution Z77.111
    Zika virus Z20.821
Contamination, food see Intoxication, foodborne

Contraception, contraceptive
    advice Z30.09
    counseling Z30.09
    device (intrauterine) (in situ) Z97.5
        causing menorrhagia T83.83 ☑
        checking Z30.431
        complications — see Complications, intrauterine,
            contraceptive device
        in place Z97.5
        initial prescription Z30.014
        reinsertion Z30.433
        removal Z30.432
        replacement Z30.433
    emergency (postcoital) Z30.012
    initial prescription Z30.019
        barrier Z30.018
        diaphragm Z30.018
        injectable Z30.013
        intrauterine device Z30.014
        pills Z30.011
        postcoital (emergency) Z30.012
        specified type NEC Z30.018
        subdermal implantable Z30.017
        transdermal patch hormonal Z30.016
        vaginal ring hormonal Z30.015
    maintenance Z30.40
        barrier Z30.49
        diaphragm Z30.49
        examination Z30.8
        injectable Z30.42
        intrauterine device Z30.431
        pills Z30.41
        specified type NEC Z30.49
        subdermal implantable Z30.46
        transdermal patch hormonal Z30.45
        vaginal ring hormonal Z30.44
    management Z30.9
        specified NEC Z30.8
    postcoital (emergency) Z30.012
    prescription Z30.019
        repeat Z30.40
    sterilization Z30.2
    surveillance (drug) — see Contraception, maintenance
Contraction(s), contracture, contracted
    Achilles tendon — see also Short, tendon, Achilles
        congenital Q66.89
    amputation stump (surgical) (flexion) (late) (next
        proximal joint) T87.89
    anus K59.8
    bile duct (common) (hepatic) K83.8
    bladder N32.89
        neck or sphincter N32.0
    bowel, cecum, colon or intestine, any part — see Ob-
        struction, intestine
    Braxton Hicks — see False, labor
    breast implant, capsular T85.44 ☑
    bronchial J98.09
    burn (old) — see Cicatrix
    cervix — see Stricture, cervix
    cicatricial — see Cicatrix
    conjunctiva, trachomatous, active A71.1
        sequelae (late effect) B94.0
    Dupuytren's M72.0
    eyelid — see Disorder, eyelid function
    fascia (lata) (postural) M72.8
        Dupuytren's M72.0
        palmar M72.0
        plantar M72.2
    finger NEC — see also Deformity, finger
        congenital Q68.1
        joint — see Contraction, joint, hand
    flaccid — see Contraction, paralytic
    gallbladder K82.0
    heart valve — see Endocarditis
    hip — see Contraction, joint, hip
    hourglass
        bladder N32.89
            congenital Q64.79
        gallbladder K82.0
            congenital Q44.1
        stomach K31.89
            congenital Q40.2
            psychogenic F45.8
    uterus (complicating delivery) O62.4
    hysterical F44.4
    internal os — see Stricture, cervix
    joint (abduction) (acquired) (adduction) (flexion) (rota-
        tion) M24.50

Contraction(s), contracture, contracted —
    continued
    joint — continued
        ankle M24.57- ☑
        congenital NEC Q68.8
            hip Q65.89
        elbow M24.52- ☑
        foot joint M24.57- ☑
        hand joint M24.54- ☑
        hip M24.55- ☑
            congenital Q65.89
        hysterical F44.4
        knee M24.56- ☑
        shoulder M24.51- ☑
        wrist M24.53- ☑
    kidney (granular) (secondary) N26.9
        congenital Q63.8
        hydronephritic — see Hydronephrosis
            Page N26.2
        pyelonephritic — see Pyelitis, chronic
        tuberculous A18.11
    ligament — see also Disorder, ligament
        congenital Q79.8
    muscle (postinfective) (postural) NEC M62.40
        with contracture of joint — see Contraction, joint
        ankle M62.47- ☑
        congenital Q79.8
            sternocleidomastoid Q68.0
        extraocular — see Strabismus
        eye (extrinsic) — see Strabismus
        foot M62.47- ☑
        forearm M62.43- ☑
        hand M62.44- ☑
        hysterical F44.4
        ischemic (Volkmann's) T79.6 ☑
        lower leg M62.46- ☑
        multiple sites M62.49
        pelvic region M62.45- ☑
        posttraumatic — see Strabismus, paralytic
        psychogenic F45.8
            conversion reaction F44.4
        shoulder region M62.41- ☑
        specified site NEC M62.48
        thigh M62.45- ☑
        upper arm M62.42- ☑
    neck — see Torticollis
    ocular muscle — see Strabismus
    organ or site, congenital NEC — see Atresia, by site
    outlet (pelvis) — see Contraction, pelvis
    palmar fascia M72.0
    paralytic
        joint — see Contraction, joint
        muscle — see also Contraction, muscle NEC
            ocular — see Strabismus, paralytic
    pelvis (acquired) (general) M95.5
        with disproportion (fetopelvic) O33.1
            causing obstructed labor O65.1
            inlet O33.2
            mid-cavity O33.3 ☑
            outlet O33.3 ☑
    plantar fascia M72.2
    premature
        atrium I49.1
        auriculoventricular I49.49
        heart I49.49
        junctional I49.2
        supraventricular I49.1
        ventricular I49.3
    prostate N42.89
    pylorus NEC — see also Pylorospasm
        psychogenic F45.8
    rectum, rectal (sphincter) K59.8
    ring (Bandl's) (complicating delivery) O62.4
    scar — see Cicatrix
    spine — see Dorsopathy, deforming
    sternocleidomastoid (muscle), congenital Q68.0
    stomach K31.89
        hourglass K31.89
            congenital Q40.2
            psychogenic F45.8
        psychogenic F45.8
    tendon (sheath) M62.40
        with contracture of joint — see Contraction, joint
        Achilles — see Short, tendon, Achilles
        ankle M62.47- ☑
            Achilles — see Short, tendon, Achilles
        foot M62.47- ☑

Contraction(s), contracture, contracted — *continued*
- tendon — *continued*
  - forearm M62.43- ☑
  - hand M62.44- ☑
  - lower leg M62.46- ☑
  - multiple sites M62.49
  - neck M62.48
  - pelvic region M62.45- ☑
  - shoulder region M62.41- ☑
  - specified site NEC M62.48
  - thigh M62.45- ☑
  - thorax M62.48
  - trunk M62.48
  - upper arm M62.42- ☑
- toe — *see* Deformity, toe, specified NEC
- ureterovesical orifice (postinfectional) N13.5
  - with infection N13.6
- urethra — *see also* Stricture, urethra
  - orifice N32.0
- uterus N85.8
  - abnormal NEC O62.9
  - clonic (complicating delivery) O62.4
  - dyscoordinate (complicating delivery) O62.4
  - hourglass (complicating delivery) O62.4
  - hypertonic O62.4
  - hypotonic NEC O62.2
  - inadequate
    - primary O62.0
    - secondary O62.1
  - incoordinate (complicating delivery) O62.4
  - poor O62.2
  - tetanic (complicating delivery) O62.4
- vagina (outlet) N89.5
- vesical N32.89
  - neck or urethral orifice N32.0
- visual field — *see* Defect, visual field, generalized
- Volkmann's (ischemic) T79.6 ☑

Contusion (skin surface intact) T14.8 ☑
- abdomen, abdominal (muscle) (wall) S30.1 ☑
- adnexa, eye NEC S05.8X- ☑
- adrenal gland S37.812 ☑
- alveolar process S00.532 ☑
- ankle S90.0- ☑
- antecubital space — *see* Contusion, forearm
- anus S30.3 ☑
- arm (upper) S40.02- ☑
  - lower (with elbow) — *see* Contusion, forearm
- auditory canal — *see* Contusion, ear
- auricle — *see* Contusion, ear
- axilla — *see* Contusion, arm, upper
- back — *see also* Contusion, thorax, back
  - lower S30.0 ☑
- bile duct S36.13 ☑
- bladder S37.22 ☑
- bone NEC T14.8 ☑
- brain (diffuse) — *see* Injury, intracranial, diffuse
  - focal — *see* Injury, intracranial, focal
- brainstem S06.38- ☑
- breast S20.0- ☑
- broad ligament S37.892 ☑
- brow S00.83 ☑
- buttock S30.0 ☑
- canthus, eye S00.1- ☑
- cauda equina S34.3 ☑
- cerebellar, traumatic S06.37- ☑
- cerebral S06.33- ☑
  - left side S06.32- ☑
  - right side S06.31- ☑
- cheek S00.83 ☑
  - internal S00.532 ☑
- chest (wall) — *see* Contusion, thorax
- chin S00.83 ☑
- clitoris S30.23 ☑
- colon — *see* Injury, intestine, large, contusion
- common bile duct S36.13 ☑
- conjunctiva S05.1- ☑
  - with foreign body (in conjunctival sac) — *see* Foreign body, conjunctival sac
- conus medullaris (spine) S34.139 ☑
- cornea — *see* Contusion, eyeball
  - with foreign body — *see* Foreign body, cornea
- corpus cavernosum S30.21 ☑
- cortex (brain) (cerebral) — *see* Injury, intracranial, diffuse
  - focal — *see* Injury, intracranial, focal
- costal region — *see* Contusion, thorax

Contusion — *continued*
- cystic duct S36.13 ☑
- diaphragm S27.802 ☑
- duodenum S36.420 ☑
- ear S00.43- ☑
- elbow S50.0- ☑
  - with forearm — *see* Contusion, forearm
- epididymis S30.22 ☑
- epigastric region S30.1 ☑
- epiglottis S10.0 ☑
- esophagus (thoracic) S27.812 ☑
  - cervical S10.0 ☑
- eyeball S05.1- ☑
- eyebrow S00.1- ☑
- eyelid (and periocular area) S00.1- ☑
- face NEC S00.83 ☑
- fallopian tube S37.529 ☑
  - bilateral S37.522 ☑
  - unilateral S37.521 ☑
- femoral triangle S30.1 ☑
- finger(s) S60.00 ☑
  - with damage to nail (matrix) S60.10 ☑
  - index S60.02- ☑
    - with damage to nail S60.12- ☑
  - little S60.05- ☑
    - with damage to nail S60.15- ☑
  - middle S60.03- ☑
    - with damage to nail S60.13- ☑
  - ring S60.04- ☑
    - with damage to nail S60.14- ☑
  - thumb — *see* Contusion, thumb
- flank S30.1 ☑
- foot (except toe(s) alone) S90.3- ☑
  - toe — *see* Contusion, toe
- forearm S50.1- ☑
  - elbow only — *see* Contusion, elbow
- forehead S00.83 ☑
- gallbladder S36.122 ☑
- genital organs, external
  - female S30.202 ☑
  - male S30.201 ☑
- globe (eye) — *see* Contusion, eyeball
- groin S30.1 ☑
- gum S00.532 ☑
- hand S60.22- ☑
  - finger(s) — *see* Contusion, finger
  - wrist — *see* Contusion, wrist
- head S00.93 ☑
  - ear — *see* Contusion, ear
  - eyelid — *see* Contusion, eyelid
  - lip S00.531 ☑
  - nose S00.33 ☑
  - oral cavity S00.532 ☑
  - scalp S00.03 ☑
  - specified part NEC S00.83 ☑
- heart — *see also* Injury, heart S26.91 ☑
- heel — *see* Contusion, foot
- hepatic duct S36.13 ☑
- hip S70.0- ☑
- ileum S36.428 ☑
- iliac region S30.1 ☑
- inguinal region S30.1 ☑
- interscapular region S20.229 ☑
- intra-abdominal organ S36.92 ☑
  - colon — *see* Injury, intestine, large, contusion
  - liver S36.112 ☑
  - pancreas — *see* Contusion, pancreas
  - rectum S36.62 ☑
  - small intestine — *see* Injury, intestine, small, contusion
  - specified organ NEC S36.892 ☑
  - spleen — *see* Contusion, spleen
  - stomach S36.32 ☑
- iris (eye) — *see* Contusion, eyeball
- jaw S00.83 ☑
- jejunum S36.428 ☑
- kidney S37.01- ☑
  - major (greater than 2 cm) S37.02- ☑
  - minor (less than 2 cm) S37.01- ☑
- knee S80.0- ☑
- labium (majus) (minus) S30.23 ☑
- lacrimal apparatus, gland or sac S05.8X- ☑
- larynx S10.0 ☑
- leg (lower) S80.1- ☑
  - knee — *see* Contusion, knee
- lens — *see* Contusion, eyeball

Contusion — *continued*
- lip S00.531 ☑
- liver S36.112 ☑
- lower back S30.0 ☑
- lumbar region S30.0 ☑
- lung S27.329 ☑
  - bilateral S27.322 ☑
  - unilateral S27.321 ☑
- malar region S00.83 ☑
- mastoid region S00.83 ☑
- membrane, brain — *see* Injury, intracranial, diffuse
  - focal — *see* Injury, intracranial, focal
- mesentery S36.892 ☑
- mesosalpinx S37.892 ☑
- mouth S00.532 ☑
- muscle — *see* Contusion, by site
- nail
  - finger — *see* Contusion, finger, with damage to nail
  - toe — *see* Contusion, toe, with damage to nail
- nasal S00.33 ☑
- neck S10.93 ☑
  - specified site NEC S10.83 ☑
  - throat S10.0 ☑
- nerve — *see* Injury, nerve
- newborn P54.5
- nose S00.33 ☑
- occipital
  - lobe (brain) — *see* Injury, intracranial, diffuse
    - focal — *see* Injury, intracranial, focal
  - region (scalp) S00.03 ☑
- orbit (region) (tissues) S05.1- ☑
- ovary S37.429 ☑
  - bilateral S37.422 ☑
  - unilateral S37.421 ☑
- palate S00.532 ☑
- pancreas S36.229 ☑
  - body S36.221 ☑
  - head S36.220 ☑
  - tail S36.222 ☑
- parietal
  - lobe (brain) — *see* Injury, intracranial, diffuse
    - focal — *see* Injury, intracranial, focal
  - region (scalp) S00.03 ☑
- pelvic organ S37.92 ☑
  - adrenal gland S37.812 ☑
  - bladder S37.22 ☑
  - fallopian tube — *see* Contusion, fallopian tube
  - kidney — *see* Contusion, kidney
  - ovary — *see* Contusion, ovary
  - prostate S37.822 ☑
  - specified organ NEC S37.892 ☑
  - ureter S37.12 ☑
  - urethra S37.32 ☑
  - uterus S37.62 ☑
- pelvis S30.0 ☑
- penis S30.21 ☑
- perineum
  - female S30.23 ☑
  - male S30.0 ☑
- periocular area S00.1- ☑
- peritoneum S36.81 ☑
- periurethral tissue — *see* Contusion, urethra
- pharynx S10.0 ☑
- pinna — *see* Contusion, ear
- popliteal space — *see* Contusion, knee
- prepuce S30.21 ☑
- prostate S37.822 ☑
- pubic region S30.1 ☑
- pudendum
  - female S30.202 ☑
  - male S30.201 ☑
- quadriceps femoris — *see* Contusion, thigh
- rectum S36.62 ☑
- retroperitoneum S36.892 ☑
- round ligament S37.892 ☑
- sacral region S30.0 ☑
- scalp S00.03 ☑
  - due to birth injury P12.3
- scapular region — *see* Contusion, shoulder
- sclera — *see* Contusion, eyeball
- scrotum S30.22 ☑
- seminal vesicle S37.892 ☑
- shoulder S40.01- ☑
- skin NEC T14.8 ☑
- small intestine — *see* Injury, intestine, small, contusion
- spermatic cord S30.22 ☑

☑ **Additional Character Required** — Refer to the Tabular List for Character Selection   ▼ **Subterms under main terms may continue to next column or page**

Contusion — *continued*
spinal cord — *see* Injury, spinal cord, by region
  cauda equina S34.3 ✔
  conus medullaris S34.139 ✔
spleen S36.029 ✔
  major S36.021 ✔
  minor S36.020 ✔
sternal region S20.219 ✔
stomach S36.32 ✔
subconjunctival S05.1- ✔
subcutaneous NEC T14.8 ✔
submaxillary region S00.83 ✔
submental region S00.83 ✔
subperiosteal NEC T14.8 ✔
subungual
  finger — *see* Contusion, finger, with damage to nail
  toe — *see* Contusion, toe, with damage to nail
supraclavicular fossa S10.83 ✔
supraorbital S00.83 ✔
suprarenal gland S37.812 ✔
temple (region) S00.83 ✔
temporal
  lobe (brain) — *see* Injury, intracranial, diffuse
  focal — *see* Injury, intracranial, focal
  region S00.83 ✔
testis S30.22 ✔
thigh S70.1- ✔
thorax (wall) S20.20 ✔
  back S20.22- ✔
  front S20.21- ✔
throat S10.0 ✔
thumb S60.01- ✔
  with damage to nail S60.11- ✔
toe(s) (lesser) S90.12- ✔
  with damage to nail S90.22- ✔
  great S90.11- ✔
    with damage to nail S90.21- ✔
tongue S00.532 ✔
trachea (cervical) S10.0 ✔
  thoracic S27.52 ✔
tunica vaginalis S30.22 ✔
tympanum, tympanic membrane — *see* Contusion, ear
ureter S37.12 ✔
urethra S37.32 ✔
urinary organ NEC S37.892 ✔
uterus S37.62 ✔
uvula S00.532 ✔
vagina S30.23 ✔
vas deferens S37.892 ✔
vesical S37.22 ✔
vocal cord(s) S10.0 ✔
vulva S30.23 ✔
wrist S60.21- ✔
Conus (congenital) (any type) Q14.8
cornea — *see* Keratoconus
medullaris syndrome G95.81
Conversion hysteria, neurosis or reaction F44.9
Converter, tuberculosis (test reaction) R76.11
Conviction (legal), **anxiety concerning** Z65.0
with imprisonment Z65.1
Convulsions (idiopathic) — *see also* Seizure(s) R56.9
apoplectiform (cerebral ischemia) I67.82
dissociative F44.5
epileptic — *see* Epilepsy
epileptiform, epileptoid — *see* Seizure, epileptiform
ether (anesthetic) — *see* Table of Drugs and Chemicals, by drug
febrile R56.00
  with status epilepticus G40.901
  complex R56.01
    with status epilepticus G40.901
  simple R56.00
hysterical F44.5
infantile P90
  epilepsy — *see* Epilepsy
jacksonian — *see* Epilepsy, localization-related, symptomatic, with simple partial seizures
myoclonic G25.3
newborn P90
obstetrical (nephritic) (uremic) — *see* Eclampsia
paretic A52.17
post traumatic R56.1
psychomotor — *see* Epilepsy, localization-related, symptomatic, with complex partial seizures
recurrent R56.9

Convulsions — *continued*
reflex R25.8
scarlatinal A38.8
tetanus, tetanic — *see* Tetanus
thymic E32.8
Convulsive — *see also* Convulsions
Cooley's anemia D56.1
Coolie itch B76.9
Cooper's
disease — *see* Mastopathy, cystic
hernia — *see* Hernia, abdomen, specified site NEC
Copra itch B88.0
Coprophagy F50.89
Coprophobia F40.298
Coproporphyria, hereditary E80.29
Cor
biloculare Q20.8
bovis, bovinum — *see* Hypertrophy, cardiac
pulmonale (chronic) I27.81
  acute I26.09
triatriatum, triatrium Q24.2
triloculare Q20.8
  biatrium Q20.4
  biventriculare Q21.1
Corbus' disease (gangrenous balanitis) N48.1
Cord — *see also* condition
around neck
  complicating delivery O69.81 ✔
    with compression O69.1 ✔
bladder G95.89
  tabetic A52.19
Cordis ectopia Q24.8
Corditis (spermatic) N49.1
Corectopia Q13.2
Cori's disease (glycogen storage) E74.03
Corkhandler's disease or lung J67.3
Corkscrew esophagus K22.4
Corkworker's disease or lung J67.3
Corn (infected) L84
Cornea — *see also* condition
donor Z52.5
plana Q13.4
Cornelia de Lange syndrome Q87.19
Cornu cutaneum L85.8
Cornual gestation or pregnancy O00.80
with intrauterine pregnancy O00.81
Coronary (artery) — *see* condition
Coronavirus, as cause of disease classified elsewhere
B97.29
SARS-associated B97.21
Corpora — *see also* condition
amylacea, prostate N42.89
cavernosa — *see* condition
Corpulence — *see* Obesity
Corpus — *see* condition
Corrected transposition Q20.5
Corrosion (injury) (acid) (caustic) (chemical) (lime) (external) (internal) T30.4
abdomen, abdominal (muscle) (wall) T21.42 ✔
  first degree T21.52 ✔
  second degree T21.62 ✔
  third degree T21.72 ✔
above elbow T22.439 ✔
  first degree T22.539 ✔
  left T22.432 ✔
    first degree T22.532 ✔
    second degree T22.632 ✔
    third degree T22.732 ✔
  right T22.431 ✔
    first degree T22.531 ✔
    second degree T22.631 ✔
    third degree T22.731 ✔
  second degree T22.639 ✔
  third degree T22.739 ✔
alimentary tract NEC T28.7 ✔
ankle T25.419 ✔
  first degree T25.519 ✔
  left T25.412 ✔
    first degree T25.512 ✔
    second degree T25.612 ✔
    third degree T25.712 ✔
  multiple with foot — *see* Corrosion, lower, limb, multiple, ankle and foot
  right T25.411 ✔
    first degree T25.511 ✔
    second degree T25.611 ✔

Corrosion — *continued*
ankle — *continued*
  right — *continued*
    third degree T25.711 ✔
  second degree T25.619 ✔
  third degree T25.719 ✔
anus — *see* Corrosion, buttock
arm(s) (meaning upper limb(s)) — *see* Corrosion, upper limb
axilla T22.449 ✔
  first degree T22.549 ✔
  left T22.442 ✔
    first degree T22.542 ✔
    second degree T22.642 ✔
    third degree T22.742 ✔
  right T22.441 ✔
    first degree T22.541 ✔
    second degree T22.641 ✔
    third degree T22.741 ✔
  second degree T22.649 ✔
  third degree T22.749 ✔
back (lower) T21.44 ✔
  first degree T21.54 ✔
  second degree T21.64 ✔
  third degree T21.74 ✔
  upper T21.43 ✔
    first degree T21.53 ✔
    second degree T21.63 ✔
    third degree T21.73 ✔
blisters — *code as* Corrosion, second degree, by site
breast(s) — *see* Corrosion, chest wall
buttock(s) T21.45 ✔
  first degree T21.55 ✔
  second degree T21.65 ✔
  third degree T21.75 ✔
calf T24.439 ✔
  first degree T24.539 ✔
  left T24.432 ✔
    first degree T24.532 ✔
    second degree T24.632 ✔
    third degree T24.732 ✔
  right T24.431 ✔
    first degree T24.531 ✔
    second degree T24.631 ✔
    third degree T24.731 ✔
  second degree T24.639 ✔
  third degree T24.739 ✔
canthus (eye) — *see* Corrosion, eyelid
cervix T28.8 ✔
cheek T20.46 ✔
  first degree T20.56 ✔
  second degree T20.66 ✔
  third degree T20.76 ✔
chest wall T21.41 ✔
  first degree T21.51 ✔
  second degree T21.61 ✔
  third degree T21.71 ✔
chin T20.43 ✔
  first degree T20.53 ✔
  second degree T20.63 ✔
  third degree T20.73 ✔
colon T28.7 ✔
conjunctiva (and cornea) — *see* Corrosion, cornea
cornea (and conjunctiva) T26.6- ✔
deep necrosis of underlying tissue — *code as* Corrosion, third degree, by site
dorsum of hand T23.469 ✔
  first degree T23.569 ✔
  left T23.462 ✔
    first degree T23.562 ✔
    second degree T23.662 ✔
    third degree T23.762 ✔
  right T23.461 ✔
    first degree T23.561 ✔
    second degree T23.661 ✔
    third degree T23.761 ✔
  second degree T23.669 ✔
  third degree T23.769 ✔
ear (auricle) (external) (canal) T20.41 ✔
  drum T28.91 ✔
  first degree T20.51 ✔
  second degree T20.61 ✔
  third degree T20.71 ✔
elbow T22.429 ✔
  first degree T22.529 ✔
  left T22.422 ✔

▼ Subterms under main terms may continue to next column or page   ✔ Additional Character Required — Refer to the Tabular List for Character Selection   73

Contusion — Corrosion

Corrosion — *continued*
  elbow — *continued*
    left — *continued*
      first degree T22.522 ☑
      second degree T22.622 ☑
      third degree T22.722 ☑
    right T22.421 ☑
      first degree T22.521 ☑
      second degree T22.621 ☑
      third degree T22.721 ☑
    second degree T22.629 ☑
    third degree T22.729 ☑
  entire body — *see* Corrosion, multiple body regions
  epidermal loss — *code as* Corrosion, second degree, by site
  epiglottis T27.4 ☑
  erythema, erythematous — *code as* Corrosion, first degree, by site
  esophagus T28.6 ☑
  extent (percentage of body surface)
    less than 10 percent T32.0
    10-19 percent (0-9 percent third degree) T32.10
      with 10-19 percent third degree T32.11
    20-29 percent (0-9 percent third degree) T32.20
      with
        10-19 percent third degree T32.21
        20-29 percent third degree T32.22
    30-39 percent (0-9 percent third degree) T32.30
      with
        10-19 percent third degree T32.31
        20-29 percent third degree T32.32
        30-39 percent third degree T32.33
    40-49 percent (0-9 percent third degree) T32.40
      with
        10-19 percent third degree T32.41
        20-29 percent third degree T32.42
        30-39 percent third degree T32.43
        40-49 percent third degree T32.44
    50-59 percent (0-9 percent third degree) T32.50
      with
        10-19 percent third degree T32.51
        20-29 percent third degree T32.52
        30-39 percent third degree T32.53
        40-49 percent third degree T32.54
        50-59 percent third degree T32.55
    60-69 percent (0-9 percent third degree) T32.60
      with
        10-19 percent third degree T32.61
        20-29 percent third degree T32.62
        30-39 percent third degree T32.63
        40-49 percent third degree T32.64
        50-59 percent third degree T32.65
        60-69 percent third degree T32.66
    70-79 percent (0-9 percent third degree) T32.70
      with
        10-19 percent third degree T32.71
        20-29 percent third degree T32.72
        30-39 percent third degree T32.73
        40-49 percent third degree T32.74
        50-59 percent third degree T32.75
        60-69 percent third degree T32.76
        70-79 percent third degree T32.77
    80-89 percent (0-9 percent third degree) T32.80
      with
        10-19 percent third degree T32.81
        20-29 percent third degree T32.82
        30-39 percent third degree T32.83
        40-49 percent third degree T32.84
        50-59 percent third degree T32.85
        60-69 percent third degree T32.86
        70-79 percent third degree T32.87
        80-89 percent third degree T32.88
    90 percent or more (0-9 percent third degree) T32.90
      with
        10-19 percent third degree T32.91
        20-29 percent third degree T32.92
        30-39 percent third degree T32.93
        40-49 percent third degree T32.94
        50-59 percent third degree T32.95
        60-69 percent third degree T32.96
        70-79 percent third degree T32.97
        80-89 percent third degree T32.98
        90-99 percent third degree T32.99
  extremity — *see* Corrosion, limb
  eye(s) and adnexa T26.9- ☑
    with resulting rupture and destruction of eyeball T26.7- ☑
    conjunctival sac — *see* Corrosion, cornea

  eye(s) and adnexa — *continued*
    cornea — *see* Corrosion, cornea
    lid — *see* Corrosion, eyelid
    periocular area — *see* Corrosion eyelid
    specified site NEC T26.8- ☑
  eyeball — *see* Corrosion, eye
  eyelid(s) T26.5- ☑
  face — *see* Corrosion, head
  finger T23.429 ☑
    first degree T23.529 ☑
    left T23.422 ☑
      first degree T23.522 ☑
      second degree T23.622 ☑
      third degree T23.722 ☑
    multiple sites (without thumb) T23.439 ☑
      with thumb T23.449 ☑
        first degree T23.549 ☑
        left T23.442 ☑
          first degree T23.542 ☑
          second degree T23.642 ☑
          third degree T23.742 ☑
        right T23.441 ☑
          first degree T23.541 ☑
          second degree T23.641 ☑
          third degree T23.741 ☑
      second degree T23.649 ☑
      third degree T23.749 ☑
    first degree T23.539 ☑
    left T23.432 ☑
      first degree T23.532 ☑
      second degree T23.632 ☑
      third degree T23.732 ☑
    right T23.431 ☑
      first degree T23.531 ☑
      second degree T23.631 ☑
      third degree T23.731 ☑
    second degree T23.639 ☑
    third degree T23.739 ☑
    right T23.421 ☑
      first degree T23.521 ☑
      second degree T23.621 ☑
      third degree T23.721 ☑
    second degree T23.629 ☑
    third degree T23.729 ☑
  flank — *see* Corrosion, abdomen
  foot T25.429 ☑
    first degree T25.529 ☑
    left T25.422 ☑
      first degree T25.522 ☑
      second degree T25.622 ☑
      third degree T25.722 ☑
    multiple with ankle — *see* Corrosion, lower, limb, multiple, ankle and foot
    right T25.421 ☑
      first degree T25.521 ☑
      second degree T25.621 ☑
      third degree T25.721 ☑
    second degree T25.629 ☑
    third degree T25.729 ☑
  forearm T22.419 ☑
    first degree T22.519 ☑
    left T22.412 ☑
      first degree T22.512 ☑
      second degree T22.612 ☑
      third degree T22.712 ☑
    right T22.411 ☑
      first degree T22.511 ☑
      second degree T22.611 ☑
      third degree T22.711 ☑
    second degree T22.619 ☑
    third degree T22.719 ☑
  forehead T20.46 ☑
    first degree T20.56 ☑
    second degree T20.66 ☑
    third degree T20.76 ☑
  fourth degree — *code as* Corrosion, third degree, by site
  full thickness skin loss — *code as* Corrosion, third degree, by site
  gastrointestinal tract NEC T28.7 ☑
  genital organs
    external
      female T21.47 ☑
        first degree T21.57 ☑
        second degree T21.67 ☑

  genital organs — *continued*
    external — *continued*
      female — *continued*
        third degree T21.77 ☑
      male T21.46 ☑
        first degree T21.56 ☑
        second degree T21.66 ☑
        third degree T21.76 ☑
    internal T28.8 ☑
  groin — *see* Corrosion, abdominal wall
  hand(s) T23.409 ☑
    back — *see* Corrosion, dorsum of hand
    finger — *see* Corrosion, finger
    first degree T23.509 ☑
    left T23.402 ☑
      first degree T23.502 ☑
      second degree T23.602 ☑
      third degree T23.702 ☑
    multiple sites with wrist T23.499 ☑
      first degree T23.599 ☑
      left T23.492 ☑
        first degree T23.592 ☑
        second degree T23.692 ☑
        third degree T23.792 ☑
      right T23.491 ☑
        first degree T23.591 ☑
        second degree T23.691 ☑
        third degree T23.791 ☑
      second degree T23.699 ☑
      third degree T23.799 ☑
    palm — *see* Corrosion, palm
    right T23.401 ☑
      first degree T23.501 ☑
      second degree T23.601 ☑
      third degree T23.701 ☑
    second degree T23.609 ☑
    third degree T23.709 ☑
    thumb — *see* Corrosion, thumb
  head (and face) (and neck) T20.40 ☑
    cheek — *see* Corrosion, cheek
    chin — *see* Corrosion, chin
    ear — *see* Corrosion, ear
    eye(s) only — *see* Corrosion, eye
    first degree T20.50 ☑
    forehead — *see* Corrosion, forehead
    lip — *see* Corrosion, lip
    multiple sites T20.49 ☑
      first degree T20.59 ☑
      second degree T20.69 ☑
      third degree T20.79 ☑
    neck — *see* Corrosion, neck
    nose — *see* Corrosion, nose
    scalp — *see* Corrosion, scalp
    second degree T20.60 ☑
    third degree T20.70 ☑
  hip(s) — *see* Corrosion, lower, limb
  inhalation — *see* Corrosion, respiratory tract
  internal organ(s) — *see also* Corrosion, by site T28.90 ☑
    alimentary tract T28.7 ☑
      esophagus T28.6 ☑
    esophagus T28.6 ☑
    genitourinary T28.8 ☑
    mouth T28.5 ☑
    pharynx T28.5 ☑
    specified organ NEC T28.99 ☑
  interscapular region — *see* Corrosion, back, upper
  intestine (large) (small) T28.7 ☑
  knee T24.429 ☑
    first degree T24.529 ☑
    left T24.422 ☑
      first degree T24.522 ☑
      second degree T24.622 ☑
      third degree T24.722 ☑
    right T24.421 ☑
      first degree T24.521 ☑
      second degree T24.621 ☑
      third degree T24.721 ☑
    second degree T24.629 ☑
    third degree T24.729 ☑
  labium (majus) (minus) — *see* Corrosion, genital organs, external, female
  lacrimal apparatus, duct, gland or sac — *see* Corrosion, eye, specified site NEC
  larynx T27.4 ☑

☑ Additional Character Required — Refer to the Tabular List for Character Selection   ☷ Subterms under main terms may continue to next column or page

Corrosion — Corrosion

Corrosion — *continued*
 larynx — *continued*
  with lung T27.5 ☑
 leg(s) (meaning lower limb(s)) — *see* Corrosion, lower limb
 limb(s)
  lower — *see* Corrosion, lower, limb
  upper — *see* Corrosion, upper limb
 lip(s) T20.42 ☑
  first degree T20.52 ☑
  second degree T20.62 ☑
  third degree T20.72 ☑
 lower
  back — *see* Corrosion, back
  limb T24.409 ☑
   ankle — *see* Corrosion, ankle
   calf — *see* Corrosion, calf
   first degree T24.509 ☑
   foot — *see* Corrosion, foot
   knee — *see* Corrosion, knee
   left T24.402 ☑
    first degree T24.502 ☑
    second degree T24.602 ☑
    third degree T24.702 ☑
   multiple sites, except ankle and foot T24.499 ☑
    ankle and foot T25.499 ☑
     first degree T25.599 ☑
     left T25.492 ☑
      first degree T25.592 ☑
      second degree T25.692 ☑
      third degree T25.792 ☑
     right T25.491 ☑
      first degree T25.591 ☑
      second degree T25.691 ☑
      third degree T25.791 ☑
     second degree T25.699 ☑
     third degree T25.799 ☑
    first degree T24.599 ☑
    left T24.492 ☑
     first degree T24.592 ☑
     second degree T24.692 ☑
     third degree T24.792 ☑
    right T24.491 ☑
     first degree T24.591 ☑
     second degree T24.691 ☑
     third degree T24.791 ☑
    second degree T24.699 ☑
    third degree T24.799 ☑
   right T24.401 ☑
    first degree T24.501 ☑
    second degree T24.601 ☑
    third degree T24.701 ☑
   second degree T24.609 ☑
   thigh — *see* Corrosion, thigh
   third degree T24.709 ☑
 lung (with larynx and trachea) T27.5 ☑
 mouth T28.5 ☑
 neck T20.47 ☑
  first degree T20.57 ☑
  second degree T20.67 ☑
  third degree T20.77 ☑
 nose (septum) T20.44 ☑
  first degree T20.54 ☑
  second degree T20.64 ☑
  third degree T20.74 ☑
 ocular adnexa — *see* Corrosion, eye
 orbit region — *see* Corrosion, eyelid
 palm T23.459 ☑
  first degree T23.559 ☑
  left T23.452 ☑
   first degree T23.552 ☑
   second degree T23.652 ☑
   third degree T23.752 ☑
  right T23.451 ☑
   first degree T23.551 ☑
   second degree T23.651 ☑
   third degree T23.751 ☑
  second degree T23.659 ☑
  third degree T23.759 ☑
 partial thickness — *code as* Corrosion, unspecified degree, by site
 pelvis — *see* Corrosion, trunk
 penis — *see* Corrosion, genital organs, external, male
 perineum
  female — *see* Corrosion, genital organs, external, female

Corrosion — *continued*
 perineum — *continued*
  male — *see* Corrosion, genital organs, external, male
 periocular area — *see* Corrosion, eyelid
 pharynx T28.5 ☑
 rectum T28.7 ☑
 respiratory tract T27.7 ☑
  larynx — *see* Corrosion, larynx
  specified part NEC T27.6 ☑
  trachea — *see* Corrosion, larynx
 sac, lacrimal — *see* Corrosion, eye, specified site NEC
 scalp T20.45 ☑
  first degree T20.55 ☑
  second degree T20.65 ☑
  third degree T20.75 ☑
 scapular region T22.469 ☑
  first degree T22.569 ☑
  left T22.462 ☑
   first degree T22.562 ☑
   second degree T22.662 ☑
   third degree T22.762 ☑
  right T22.461 ☑
   first degree T22.561 ☑
   second degree T22.661 ☑
   third degree T22.761 ☑
  second degree T22.669 ☑
  third degree T22.769 ☑
 sclera — *see* Corrosion, eye, specified site NEC
 scrotum — *see* Corrosion, genital organs, external, male
 shoulder T22.459 ☑
  first degree T22.559 ☑
  left T22.452 ☑
   first degree T22.552 ☑
   second degree T22.652 ☑
   third degree T22.752 ☑
  right T22.451 ☑
   first degree T22.551 ☑
   second degree T22.651 ☑
   third degree T22.751 ☑
  second degree T22.659 ☑
  third degree T22.759 ☑
 stomach T28.7 ☑
 temple — *see* Corrosion, head
 testis — *see* Corrosion, genital organs, external, male
 thigh T24.419 ☑
  first degree T24.519 ☑
  left T24.412 ☑
   first degree T24.512 ☑
   second degree T24.612 ☑
   third degree T24.712 ☑
  right T24.411 ☑
   first degree T24.511 ☑
   second degree T24.611 ☑
   third degree T24.711 ☑
  second degree T24.619 ☑
  third degree T24.719 ☑
 thorax (external) — *see* Corrosion, trunk
 throat (meaning pharynx) T28.5 ☑
 thumb(s) T23.419 ☑
  first degree T23.519 ☑
  left T23.412 ☑
   first degree T23.512 ☑
   second degree T23.612 ☑
   third degree T23.712 ☑
  multiple sites with fingers T23.449 ☑
   first degree T23.549 ☑
   left T23.442 ☑
    first degree T23.542 ☑
    second degree T23.642 ☑
    third degree T23.742 ☑
   right T23.441 ☑
    first degree T23.541 ☑
    second degree T23.641 ☑
    third degree T23.741 ☑
   second degree T23.649 ☑
   third degree T23.749 ☑
  right T23.411 ☑
   first degree T23.511 ☑
   second degree T23.611 ☑
   third degree T23.711 ☑
  second degree T23.619 ☑
  third degree T23.719 ☑
 toe T25.439 ☑
  first degree T25.539 ☑
  left T25.432 ☑

Corrosion — *continued*
 toe — *continued*
  left — *continued*
   first degree T25.532 ☑
   second degree T25.632 ☑
   third degree T25.732 ☑
  right T25.431 ☑
   first degree T25.531 ☑
   second degree T25.631 ☑
   third degree T25.731 ☑
  second degree T25.639 ☑
  third degree T25.739 ☑
 tongue T28.5 ☑
 tonsil(s) T28.5 ☑
 total body — *see* Corrosion, multiple body regions
 trachea T27.4 ☑
  with lung T27.5 ☑
 trunk T21.40 ☑
  abdominal wall — *see* Corrosion, abdominal wall
  anus — *see* Corrosion, buttock
  axilla — *see* Corrosion, upper limb
  back — *see* Corrosion, back
  breast — *see* Corrosion, chest wall
  buttock — *see* Corrosion, buttock
  chest wall — *see* Corrosion, chest wall
  first degree T21.50 ☑
  flank — *see* Corrosion, abdominal wall
  genital
   female — *see* Corrosion, genital organs, external, female
   male — *see* Corrosion, genital organs, external, male
  groin — *see* Corrosion, abdominal wall
  interscapular region — *see* Corrosion, back, upper
  labia — *see* Corrosion, genital organs, external, female
  lower back — *see* Corrosion, back
  penis — *see* Corrosion, genital organs, external, male
  perineum
   female — *see* Corrosion, genital organs, external, female
   male — *see* Corrosion, genital organs, external, male
  scapular region — *see* Corrosion, upper limb
  scrotum — *see* Corrosion, genital organs, external, male
  second degree T21.60 ☑
  shoulder — *see* Corrosion, upper limb
  specified site NEC T21.49 ☑
   first degree T21.59 ☑
   second degree T21.69 ☑
   third degree T21.79 ☑
  testes — *see* Corrosion, genital organs, external, male
  third degree T21.70 ☑
  upper back — *see* Corrosion, back, upper
  vagina T28.8 ☑
  vulva — *see* Corrosion, genital organs, external, female
 unspecified site with extent of body surface involved specified
  less than 10 percent T32.0
  10-19 percent (0-9 percent third degree) T32.10
   with 10-19 percent third degree T32.11
  20-29 percent (0-9 percent third degree) T32.20
   with
    10-19 percent third degree T32.21
    20-29 percent third degree T32.22
  30-39 percent (0-9 percent third degree) T32.30
   with
    10-19 percent third degree T32.31
    20-29 percent third degree T32.32
    30-39 percent third degree T32.33
  40-49 percent (0-9 percent third degree) T32.40
   with
    10-19 percent third degree T32.41
    20-29 percent third degree T32.42
    30-39 percent third degree T32.43
    40-49 percent third degree T32.44
  50-59 percent (0-9 percent third degree) T32.50
   with
    10-19 percent third degree T32.51
    20-29 percent third degree T32.52
    30-39 percent third degree T32.53
    40-49 percent third degree T32.54
    50-59 percent third degree T32.55

Corrosion — *continued*
  unspecified site with extent of body surface involved
      specified — *continued*
      60-69 percent (0-9 percent third degree) T32.60
        with
          10-19 percent third degree T32.61
          20-29 percent third degree T32.62
          30-39 percent third degree T32.63
          40-49 percent third degree T32.64
          50-59 percent third degree T32.65
          60-69 percent third degree T32.66
      70-79 percent (0-9 percent third degree) T32.70
        with
          10-19 percent third degree T32.71
          20-29 percent third degree T32.72
          30-39 percent third degree T32.73
          40-49 percent third degree T32.74
          50-59 percent third degree T32.75
          60-69 percent third degree T32.76
          70-79 percent third degree T32.77
      80-89 percent (0-9 percent third degree) T32.80
        with
          10-19 percent third degree T32.81
          20-29 percent third degree T32.82
          30-39 percent third degree T32.83
          40-49 percent third degree T32.84
          50-59 percent third degree T32.85
          60-69 percent third degree T32.86
          70-79 percent third degree T32.87
          80-89 percent third degree T32.88
      90 percent or more (0-9 percent third degree) T32.90
        with
          10-19 percent third degree T32.91
          20-29 percent third degree T32.92
          30-39 percent third degree T32.93
          40-49 percent third degree T32.94
          50-59 percent third degree T32.95
          60-69 percent third degree T32.96
          70-79 percent third degree T32.97
          80-89 percent third degree T32.98
          90-99 percent third degree T32.99
  upper limb (axilla) (scapular region) T22.40 ☑
    above elbow — *see* Corrosion, above elbow
    axilla — *see* Corrosion, axilla
    elbow — *see* Corrosion, elbow
    first degree T22.50 ☑
    forearm — *see* Corrosion, forearm
    hand — *see* Corrosion, hand
    interscapular region — *see* Corrosion, back, upper
    multiple sites T22.499 ☑
      first degree T22.599 ☑
      left T22.492 ☑
        first degree T22.592 ☑
        second degree T22.692 ☑
        third degree T22.792 ☑
      right T22.491 ☑
        first degree T22.591 ☑
        second degree T22.691 ☑
        third degree T22.791 ☑
      second degree T22.699 ☑
      third degree T22.799 ☑
    scapular region — *see* Corrosion, scapular region
    second degree T22.60 ☑
    shoulder — *see* Corrosion, shoulder
    third degree T22.70 ☑
    wrist — *see* Corrosion, hand
  uterus T28.8 ☑
  vagina T28.8 ☑
  vulva — *see* Corrosion, genital organs, external, female
  wrist T23.479 ☑
    first degree T23.579 ☑
    left T23.472 ☑
      first degree T23.572 ☑
      second degree T23.672 ☑
      third degree T23.772 ☑
    multiple sites with hand T23.499 ☑
      first degree T23.599 ☑
      left T23.492 ☑
        first degree T23.592 ☑
        second degree T23.692 ☑
        third degree T23.792 ☑
      right T23.491 ☑
        first degree T23.591 ☑
        second degree T23.691 ☑
        third degree T23.791 ☑
      second degree T23.699 ☑
      third degree T23.799 ☑

Corrosion — *continued*
  wrist — *continued*
    right T23.471 ☑
      first degree T23.571 ☑
      second degree T23.671 ☑
      third degree T23.771 ☑
    second degree T23.679 ☑
    third degree T23.779 ☑
Corrosive burn — *see* Corrosion
Corsican fever — *see* Malaria
Cortical — *see* condition
Cortico-adrenal — *see* condition
Coryza (acute) J00
  with grippe or influenza — *see* Influenza, with, respiratory manifestations NEC
  syphilitic
    congenital (chronic) A50.05
Costen's syndrome or complex M26.69
Costiveness — *see* Constipation
Costochondritis M94.0
Cot death R99
Cotard's syndrome F22
Cotia virus B08.8
Cotton wool spots (retinal) H35.81
Cotungo's disease — *see* Sciatica
Cough (affected) (chronic) (epidemic) (nervous) R05
  with hemorrhage — *see* Hemoptysis
  bronchial R05
    with grippe or influenza — *see* Influenza, with, respiratory manifestations NEC
  functional F45.8
  hysterical F45.8
  laryngeal, spasmodic R05
  psychogenic F45.8
  smokers' J41.0
  tea taster's B49
Counseling (for) Z71.9
  abuse NEC
    perpetrator Z69.82
    victim Z69.81
  alcohol abuser Z71.41
    family Z71.42
  child abuse
    nonparental
      perpetrator Z69.021
      victim Z69.020
    parental
      perpetrator Z69.011
      victim Z69.010
  consanguinity Z71.89
  contraceptive Z30.09
  dietary Z71.3
  drug abuser Z71.51
    family member Z71.52
  exercise Z71.82
  family Z71.89
  fertility preservation (prior to cancer therapy) (prior to removal of gonads) Z31.62
  for non-attending third party Z71.0
    related to sexual behavior or orientation Z70.2
  genetic
    nonprocreative Z71.83
    procreative NEC Z31.5
  gestational carrier Z31.7
  health (advice) (education) (instruction) — *see* Counseling, medical
    risk for travel (international) Z71.84
  human immunodeficiency virus (HIV) Z71.7
  impotence Z70.1
  insulin pump use Z46.81
  medical (for) Z71.9
    boarding school resident Z59.3
    consanguinity Z71.89
    feared complaint and no disease found Z71.1
    human immunodeficiency virus (HIV) Z71.7
    institutional resident Z59.3
    on behalf of another Z71.0
      related to sexual behavior or orientation Z70.2
    person living alone Z60.2
    specified reason NEC Z71.89
  natural family planning
    procreative Z31.61
    to avoid pregnancy Z30.02
  perpetrator (of)
    abuse NEC Z69.82
    child abuse
      non-parental Z69.021
      parental Z69.011

Counseling — *continued*
  perpetrator — *continued*
    rape NEC Z69.82
    spousal abuse Z69.12
  procreative NEC Z31.69
    fertility preservation (prior to cancer therapy) (prior to removal of gonads) Z31.62
    using natural family planning Z31.61
  promiscuity Z70.1
  rape victim Z69.81
  religious Z71.81
  safety for travel (international) Z71.84
  sex, sexual (related to) Z70.9
    attitude(s) Z70.0
    behavior or orientation Z70.1
    combined concerns Z70.3
    non-responsiveness Z70.1
    on behalf of third party Z70.2
    specified reason NEC Z70.8
  specified reason NEC Z71.89
  spiritual Z71.81
  spousal abuse (perpetrator) Z69.12
    victim Z69.11
  substance abuse Z71.89
    alcohol Z71.41
    drug Z71.51
    tobacco Z71.6
  tobacco use Z71.6
  travel (international) Z71.84
  use (of)
    insulin pump Z46.81
  victim (of)
    abuse Z69.81
    child abuse
      by parent Z69.010
      non-parental Z69.020
    rape NEC Z69.81
Coupled rhythm R00.8
Couvelaire syndrome or uterus (complicating delivery) O45.8X- ☑
Cowperitis — *see* Urethritis
Cowper's gland — *see* condition
Cowpox B08.010
  due to vaccination T88.1 ☑
Coxa
  magna M91.4- ☑
  plana M91.2- ☑
  valga (acquired) — *see also* Deformity, limb, specified type NEC, thigh
    congenital Q65.81
    sequelae (late effect) of rickets E64.3
  vara (acquired) — *see also* Deformity, limb, specified type NEC, thigh
    congenital Q65.82
    sequelae (late effect) of rickets E64.3
Coxalgia, coxalgic (nontuberculous) — *see also* Pain, joint, hip
  tuberculous A18.02
Coxitis — *see* Monoarthritis, hip
Coxsackie (virus) (infection) B34.1
  as cause of disease classified elsewhere B97.11
  carditis B33.20
  central nervous system NEC A88.8
  endocarditis B33.21
  enteritis A08.39
  meningitis (aseptic) A87.0
  myocarditis B33.22
  pericarditis B33.23
  pharyngitis B08.5
  pleurodynia B33.0
  specific disease NEC B33.8
Crabs, meaning pubic lice B85.3
Crack baby P04.41
Cracked nipple N64.0
  associated with
    lactation O92.13
    pregnancy O92.11- ☑
    puerperium O92.12
Cracked tooth K03.81
Cradle cap L21.0
Craft neurosis F48.8
Cramp(s) R25.2
  abdominal — *see* Pain, abdominal
  bathing T75.1 ☑
  colic R10.83
    psychogenic F45.8
  due to immersion T75.1 ☑
  fireman T67.2 ☑

☑ **Additional Character Required** — Refer to the Tabular List for Character Selection   ☑ Subterms under main terms may continue to next column or page

Cramp(s) — *continued*
   heat T67.2 ☑
   immersion T75.1 ☑
   intestinal — *see* Pain, abdominal
      psychogenic F45.8
   leg, sleep related G47.62
   limb (lower) (upper) NEC R25.2
      sleep related G47.62
   linotypist's F48.8
      organic G25.89
   muscle (limb) (general) R25.2
      due to immersion T75.1 ☑
      psychogenic F45.8
   occupational (hand) F48.8
      organic G25.89
   salt-depletion E87.1
   sleep related, leg G47.62
   stoker's T67.2 ☑
   swimmer's T75.1 ☑
   telegrapher's F48.8
      organic G25.89
   typist's F48.8
      organic G25.89
   uterus N94.89
      menstrual — *see* Dysmenorrhea
   writer's F48.8
      organic G25.89
Cranial — *see* condition
Craniocleidodysostosis Q74.0
Craniofenestria (skull) Q75.8
Craniolacunia (skull) Q75.8
Craniopagus Q89.4
Craniopathy, metabolic M85.2
Craniopharyngeal — *see* condition
Craniopharyngioma D44.4
Craniorachischisis (totalis) Q00.1
Cranioschisis Q75.8
Craniostenosis Q75.0
Craniosynostosis Q75.0
Craniotabes (cause unknown) M83.8
   neonatal P96.3
   rachitic E64.3
   syphilitic A50.56
Cranium — *see* condition
Craw-craw — *see* Onchocerciasis
Creaking joint — *see* Derangement, joint, specified type NEC
Creeping
   eruption B76.9
   palsy or paralysis G12.22
Crenated tongue K14.8
Creotoxism A05.9
Crepitus
   caput Q75.8
   joint — *see* Derangement, joint, specified type NEC
Crescent or conus choroid, congenital Q14.3
CREST syndrome M34.1
Cretin, cretinism (congenital) (endemic) (nongoitrous) (sporadic) E00.9
   pelvis
      with disproportion (fetopelvic) O33.0
         causing obstructed labor O65.0
   type
      hypothyroid E00.1
      mixed E00.2
      myxedematous E00.1
      neurological E00.0
Creutzfeldt-Jakob disease or syndrome (with dementia) A81.00
   familial A81.09
   iatrogenic A81.09
   specified NEC A81.09
   sporadic A81.09
   variant (vCJD) A81.01
Crib death R99
Cribriform hymen Q52.3
Cri-du-chat syndrome Q93.4
Crigler-Najjar disease or syndrome E80.5
Crime, victim of Z65.4
Crimean hemorrhagic fever A98.0
Criminalism F60.2
Crisis
   abdomen R10.0
   acute reaction F43.0
   addisonian E27.2
   adrenal (cortical) E27.2
   celiac K90.0

Crisis — *continued*
   Dietl's N13.8
   emotional — *see also* Disorder, adjustment
      acute reaction to stress F43.0
      specific to childhood and adolescence F93.8
   glaucomatocyclitic — *see* Glaucoma, secondary, inflammation
   heart — *see* Failure, heart
   nitritoid I95.2
      correct substance properly administered — *see* Table of Drugs and Chemicals, by drug, adverse effect
      overdose or wrong substance given or taken — *see* Table of Drugs and Chemicals, by drug, poisoning
   oculogyric H51.8
      psychogenic F45.8
   Pel's (tabetic) A52.11
   psychosexual identity F64.2
   renal N28.0
   sickle-cell D57.00
      with
         acute chest syndrome D57.01
         splenic sequestration D57.02
      state (acute reaction) F43.0
   tabetic A52.11
   thyroid — *see* Thyrotoxicosis with thyroid storm
   thyrotoxic — *see* Thyrotoxicosis with thyroid storm
Crocq's disease (acrocyanosis) I73.89
Crohn's disease — *see* Enteritis, regional
Crooked septum, nasal J34.2
Cross syndrome E70.328
Crossbite (anterior) (posterior) M26.24
Cross-eye — *see* Strabismus, convergent concomitant
Croup, croupous (catarrhal) (infectious) (inflammatory) (nondiphtheritic) J05.0
   bronchial J20.9
   diphtheritic A36.2
   false J38.5
   spasmodic J38.5
      diphtheritic A36.2
   stridulous J38.5
      diphtheritic A36.2
Crouzon's disease Q75.1
Crowding, tooth, teeth, fully erupted M26.31
CRST syndrome M34.1
Cruchet's disease A85.8
Cruelty in children — *see also* Disorder, conduct
Crural ulcer — *see* Ulcer, lower limb
Crush, crushed, crushing T14.8
   abdomen S38.1 ☑
   ankle S97.0- ☑
   arm (upper) (and shoulder) S47.- ☑
   axilla — *see* Crush, arm
   back, lower S38.1 ☑
   buttock S38.1 ☑
   cheek S07.0 ☑
   chest S28.0 ☑
   cranium S07.1 ☑
   ear S07.0 ☑
   elbow S57.0- ☑
   extremity
      lower
         ankle — *see* Crush, ankle
         below knee — *see* Crush, leg
         foot — *see* Crush, foot
         hip — *see* Crush, hip
         knee — *see* Crush, knee
         thigh — *see* Crush, thigh
         toe — *see* Crush, toe
      upper
         below elbow S67.9- ☑
         elbow — *see* Crush, elbow
         finger — *see* Crush, finger
         forearm — *see* Crush, forearm
         hand — *see* Crush, hand
         thumb — *see* Crush, thumb
         upper arm — *see* Crush, arm
         wrist — *see* Crush, wrist
   face S07.0 ☑
   finger(s) S67.1- ☑
      with hand (and wrist) — *see* Crush, hand, specified site NEC
      index S67.19- ☑
      little S67.19- ☑
      middle S67.19- ☑
      ring S67.19- ☑

Crush, crushed, crushing — *continued*
   finger(s) — *continued*
      thumb — *see* Crush, thumb
   foot S97.8- ☑
      toe — *see* Crush, toe
   forearm S57.8- ☑
   genitalia, external
      female S38.002 ☑
         vagina S38.03 ☑
         vulva S38.03 ☑
      male S38.001 ☑
         penis S38.01 ☑
         scrotum S38.02 ☑
         testis S38.02 ☑
   hand (except fingers alone) S67.2- ☑
      with wrist S67.4- ☑
   head S07.9 ☑
      specified NEC S07.8 ☑
   heel — *see* Crush, foot
   hip S77.0- ☑
      with thigh S77.2- ☑
   internal organ (abdomen, chest, or pelvis) NEC T14.8 ☑
   knee S87.0- ☑
   labium (majus) (minus) S38.03 ☑
   larynx S17.0 ☑
   leg (lower) S87.8- ☑
      knee — *see* Crush, knee
   lip S07.0 ☑
   lower
      back S38.1 ☑
      leg — *see* Crush, leg
   neck S17.9 ☑
   nerve — *see* Injury, nerve
   nose S07.0 ☑
   pelvis S38.1 ☑
   penis S38.01 ☑
   scalp S07.8 ☑
   scapular region — *see* Crush, arm
   scrotum S38.02 ☑
   severe, unspecified site T14.8 ☑
   shoulder (and upper arm) — *see* Crush, arm
   skull S07.1 ☑
   syndrome (complication of trauma) T79.5 ☑
   testis S38.02 ☑
   thigh S77.1- ☑
      with hip S77.2- ☑
   throat S17.8 ☑
   thumb S67.0- ☑
      with hand (and wrist) — *see* Crush, hand, specified site NEC
   toe(s) S97.10- ☑
      great S97.11- ☑
      lesser S97.12- ☑
   trachea S17.0 ☑
   vagina S38.03 ☑
   vulva S38.03 ☑
   wrist S67.3- ☑
      with hand S67.4- ☑
Crusta lactea L21.0
Crusts R23.4
Crutch paralysis — *see* Injury, brachial plexus
Cruveilhier-Baumgarten cirrhosis, disease or syndrome K74.69
Cruveilhier's atrophy or disease G12.8
Crying (constant) (continuous) (excessive)
   child, adolescent, or adult R45.83
   infant (baby) (newborn) R68.11
Cryofibrinogenemia D89.2
Cryoglobulinemia (essential) (idiopathic) (mixed) (primary) (purpura) (secondary) (vasculitis) D89.1
   with lung involvement D89.1 *[J99]*
Cryptitis (anal) (rectal) K62.89
Cryptococcosis, cryptococcus (infection) (neoformans) B45.9
   bone B45.3
   cerebral B45.1
   cutaneous B45.2
   disseminated B45.7
   generalized B45.7
   meningitis B45.1
   meningocerebralis B45.1
   osseous B45.3
   pulmonary B45.0
   skin B45.2
   specified NEC B45.8
Cryptopapillitis (anus) K62.89

Cryptophthalmos Q11.2
  syndrome Q87.0
Cryptorchid, cryptorchism, cryptorchidism Q53.9
  bilateral Q53.20
    abdominal Q53.211
    perineal Q53.22
  unilateral Q53.10
    abdominal Q53.111
    perineal Q53.12
Cryptosporidiosis A07.2
  hepatobiliary B88.8
  respiratory B88.8
Cryptostromosis J67.6
Crystalluria R82.998
Cubitus
  congenital Q68.8
  valgus (acquired) M21.0- ☑
    congenital Q68.8
    sequelae (late effect) of rickets E64.3
  varus (acquired) M21.1- ☑
    congenital Q68.8
    sequelae (late effect) of rickets E64.3
Cultural deprivation or shock Z60.3
Curling esophagus K22.4
Curling's ulcer — see Ulcer, peptic, acute
Curschmann (-Batten) (-Steinert) **disease or syndrome** G71.11
Curse, Ondine's — see Apnea, sleep
Curvature
  organ or site, congenital NEC — see Distortion
  penis (lateral) Q55.61
  Pott's (spinal) A18.01
  radius, idiopathic, progressive (congenital) Q74.0
  spine (acquired) (angular) (idiopathic) (incorrect) (postural) — see Dorsopathy, deforming
    congenital Q67.5
    due to or associated with
      Charcot-Marie-Tooth disease — see also subcategory M49.8 G60.0
      osteitis
        deformans M88.88
        fibrosa cystica — see also subcategory M49.8 E21.0
      tuberculosis (Pott's curvature) A18.01
    sequelae (late effect) of rickets E64.3
    tuberculous A18.01
Cushingoid due to steroid therapy E24.2
  correct substance properly administered — see Table of Drugs and Chemicals, by drug, adverse effect
  overdose or wrong substance given or taken — see Table of Drugs and Chemicals, by drug, poisoning
Cushing's
  syndrome or disease E24.9
    drug-induced E24.2
    iatrogenic E24.2
    pituitary-dependent E24.0
    specified NEC E24.8
  ulcer — see Ulcer, peptic, acute
Cusp, Carabelli — omit code
Cut (external) — see also Laceration
  muscle — see Injury, muscle
Cutaneous — see also condition
  hemorrhage R23.3
  larva migrans B76.9
Cutis — see also condition
  hyperelastica Q82.8
    acquired L57.4
  laxa (hyperelastica) — see Dermatolysis
  marmorata R23.8
  osteosis L94.2
  pendula — see Dermatolysis
  rhomboidalis nuchae L57.2
  verticis gyrata Q82.8
    acquired L91.8
Cyanosis R23.0
  due to
    patent foramen botalli Q21.1
    persistent foramen ovale Q21.1
  enterogenous D74.8
  paroxysmal digital — see Raynaud's disease
    with gangrene I73.01
  retina, retinal H35.89
Cyanotic heart disease I24.9
  congenital Q24.9
Cycle
  anovulatory N97.0
  menstrual, irregular N92.6
Cyclencephaly Q04.9

Cyclical vomiting, in migraine — see also Vomiting, cyclical G43.A0 (following G43.7)
  psychogenic F50.89
Cyclitis — see also Iridocyclitis H20.9
  chronic — see Iridocyclitis, chronic
  Fuchs' heterochromic H20.81- ☑
  granulomatous — see Iridocyclitis, chronic
  lens-induced — see Iridocyclitis, lens-induced
  posterior H30.2- ☑
Cycloid personality F34.0
Cyclophoria H50.54
Cyclopia, cyclops Q87.0
Cyclopism Q87.0
Cyclosporiasis A07.4
Cyclothymia F34.0
Cyclothymic personality F34.0
Cyclotropia H50.41- ☑
Cylindroma — see also Neoplasm, malignant, by site
  eccrine dermal — see Neoplasm, skin, benign
  skin — see Neoplasm, skin, benign
Cylindruria R82.998
Cynanche
  diphtheritic A36.2
  tonsillaris J36
Cynophobia F40.218
Cynorexia R63.2
Cyphosis — see Kyphosis
Cyprus fever — see Brucellosis
Cyst (colloid) (mucous) (simple) (retention)
  adenoid (infected) J35.8
  adrenal gland E27.8
    congenital Q89.1
  air, lung J98.4
  allantoic Q64.4
  alveolar process (jaw bone) M27.40
  amnion, amniotic O41.8X- ☑
  aneurysmal M27.49
  anterior
    chamber (eye) — see Cyst, iris
    nasopalatine K09.1
  antrum J34.1
  anus K62.89
  apical (tooth) (periodontal) K04.8
  appendix K38.8
  arachnoid, brain (acquired) G93.0
    congenital Q04.6
  arytenoid J38.7
  Baker's M71.2- ☑
    ruptured M66.0
    tuberculous A18.02
  Bartholin's gland N75.0
  bile duct (common) (hepatic) K83.5
  bladder (multiple) (trigone) N32.89
  blue dome (breast) — see Cyst, breast
  bone (local) NEC M85.60
    aneurysmal M85.50
      ankle M85.57- ☑
      foot M85.57- ☑
      forearm M85.53- ☑
      hand M85.54- ☑
      jaw M27.49
      lower leg M85.56- ☑
      multiple site M85.59
      neck M85.58
      rib M85.58
      shoulder M85.51- ☑
      skull M85.58
      specified site NEC M85.58
      thigh M85.55- ☑
      toe M85.57- ☑
      upper arm M85.52- ☑
      vertebra M85.58
    solitary M85.40
      ankle M85.47- ☑
      fibula M85.46- ☑
      foot M85.47- ☑
      hand M85.44- ☑
      humerus M85.42- ☑
      jaw M27.49
      neck M85.48
      pelvis M85.45- ☑
      radius M85.43- ☑
      rib M85.48
      shoulder M85.41- ☑
      skull M85.48
      specified site NEC M85.48
      tibia M85.46- ☑

Cyst — continued
  bone — continued
    solitary — continued
      toe M85.47- ☑
      ulna M85.43- ☑
      vertebra M85.48
    specified type NEC M85.60
      ankle M85.67- ☑
      foot M85.67- ☑
      forearm M85.63- ☑
      hand M85.64- ☑
      jaw M27.40
        developmental (nonodontogenic) K09.1
          odontogenic K09.0
        latent M27.0
      lower leg M85.66- ☑
      multiple site M85.69
      neck M85.68
      rib M85.68
      shoulder M85.61- ☑
      skull M85.68
      specified site NEC M85.68
      thigh M85.65- ☑
      toe M85.67- ☑
      upper arm M85.62- ☑
      vertebra M85.68
  brain (acquired) G93.0
    congenital Q04.6
    hydatid B67.99 [G94]
    third ventricle (colloid), congenital Q04.6
  branchial (cleft) Q18.0
  branchiogenic Q18.0
  breast (benign) (blue dome) (pedunculated) (solitary) N60.0- ☑
    involution — see Dysplasia, mammary, specified type NEC
    sebaceous — see Dysplasia, mammary, specified type NEC
  broad ligament (benign) N83.8
  bronchogenic (mediastinal) (sequestration) J98.4
    congenital Q33.0
  buccal K09.8
  bulbourethral gland N36.8
  bursa, bursal NEC M71.30
    with rupture — see Rupture, synovium
    ankle M71.37- ☑
    elbow M71.32- ☑
    foot M71.37- ☑
    hand M71.34- ☑
    hip M71.35- ☑
    multiple sites M71.39
    pharyngeal J39.2
    popliteal space — see Cyst, Baker's
    shoulder M71.31- ☑
    specified site NEC M71.38
    wrist M71.33- ☑
  calcifying odontogenic D16.5
    upper jaw (bone) (maxilla) D16.4
  canal of Nuck (female) N94.89
    congenital Q52.4
  canthus — see Cyst, conjunctiva
  carcinomatous — see Neoplasm, malignant, by site
  cauda equina G95.89
  cavum septi pellucidi — see Cyst, brain
  celomic (pericardium) Q24.8
  cerebellopontine (angle) — see Cyst, brain
  cerebellum — see Cyst, brain
  cerebral — see Cyst, brain
  cervical lateral Q18.0
  cervix NEC N88.8
    embryonic Q51.6
    nabothian N88.8
  chiasmal optic NEC — see Disorder, optic, chiasm
  chocolate (ovary) N80.1
  choledochus, congenital Q44.4
  chorion O41.8X- ☑
  choroid plexus G93.0
    congenital Q04.6
  ciliary body — see Cyst, iris
  clitoris N90.7
  colon K63.89
  common (bile) duct K83.5
  congenital NEC Q89.8
    adrenal gland Q89.1
    epiglottis Q31.8
    esophagus Q39.8
    fallopian tube Q50.4
    kidney Q61.00

☑ Additional Character Required — Refer to the Tabular List for Character Selection   Ⓦ Subterms under main terms may continue to next column or page

Cyst — *continued*
congenital — *continued*
  kidney — *continued*
    more than one (multiple) Q61.02
      specified as polycystic Q61.3
        adult type Q61.2
        infantile type NEC Q61.19
          collecting duct dilation Q61.11
    solitary Q61.01
  larynx Q31.8
  liver Q44.6
  lung Q33.0
  mediastinum Q34.1
  ovary Q50.1
  oviduct Q50.4
  periurethral (tissue) Q64.79
  prepuce Q55.69
  salivary gland (any) Q38.4
  sublingual Q38.6
  submaxillary gland Q38.6
  thymus (gland) Q89.2
  tongue Q38.3
  ureterovesical orifice Q62.8
  vulva Q52.79
conjunctiva H11.44- ☑
cornea H18.89- ☑
corpora quadrigemina G93.0
corpus
  albicans N83.29- ☑
  luteum (hemorrhagic) (ruptured) N83.1- ☑
Cowper's gland (benign) (infected) N36.8
cranial meninges G93.0
craniobuccal pouch E23.6
craniopharyngeal pouch E23.6
cystic duct K82.8
Cysticercus — *see* Cysticercosis
Dandy-Walker Q03.1
  with spina bifida — *see* Spina bifida
dental (root) K04.8
  developmental K09.0
  eruption K09.0
  primordial K09.0
dentigerous (mandible) (maxilla) K09.0
dermoid — *see* Neoplasm, benign, by site
  with malignant transformation C56.- ☑
  implantation
    external area or site (skin) NEC L72.0
    iris — *see* Cyst, iris, implantation
    vagina N89.8
    vulva N90.7
  mouth K09.8
  oral soft tissue K09.8
  sacrococcygeal — *see* Cyst, pilonidal
developmental K09.1
  odontogenic K09.0
  oral region (nonodontogenic) K09.1
  ovary, ovarian Q50.1
dura (cerebral) G93.0
  spinal G96.19
ear (external) Q18.1
echinococcal — *see* Echinococcus
embryonic
  cervix uteri Q51.6
  fallopian tube Q50.4
  vagina Q52.4
endometrium, endometrial (uterus) N85.8
  ectopic — *see* Endometriosis
enterogenous Q43.8
epidermal, epidermoid (inclusion) (*see also* Cyst, skin) L72.0
  mouth K09.8
  oral soft tissue K09.8
epididymis N50.3
epiglottis J38.7
epiphysis cerebri E34.8
epithelial (inclusion) L72.0
epoophoron Q50.5
eruption K09.0
esophagus K22.8
ethmoid sinus J34.1
external female genital organs NEC N90.7
eyelid (sebaceous) H02.829
  infected — *see* Hordeolum
  left H02.826
    lower H02.825
    upper H02.824
  right H02.823
    lower H02.822

Cyst — *continued*
eyelid — *continued*
  right — *continued*
    upper H02.821
eye NEC H57.89
  congenital Q15.8
fallopian tube N83.8
  congenital Q50.4
fimbrial (twisted) Q50.4
fissural (oral region) K09.1
follicle (graafian) (hemorrhagic) N83.0- ☑
  nabothian N88.8
follicular (atretic) (hemorrhagic) (ovarian) N83.0- ☑
  dentigerous K09.0
  odontogenic K09.0
  skin L72.9
    specified NEC L72.8
frontal sinus J34.1
gallbladder K82.8
ganglion — *see* Ganglion
Gartner's duct Q52.4
gingiva K09.0
gland of Moll — *see* Cyst, eyelid
globulomaxillary K09.1
graafian follicle (hemorrhagic) N83.0- ☑
granulosal lutein (hemorrhagic) N83.1- ☑
hemangiomatous D18.00
  intra-abdominal D18.03
  intracranial D18.02
  skin D18.01
  specified site NEC D18.09
hemorrhagic M27.49
hydatid — *see also* Echinococcus B67.90
  brain B67.99 *[G94]*
  liver — *see also* Cyst, liver, hydatid B67.8
  lung NEC B67.99 *[J99]*
  Morgagni
    female Q50.5
    male (epididymal) Q55.4
      testicular Q55.29
  specified site NEC B67.99
hymen N89.8
  embryonic Q52.4
hypopharynx J39.2
hypophysis, hypophyseal (duct) (recurrent) E23.6
  cerebri E23.6
implantation (dermoid)
  external area or site (skin) NEC L72.0
  iris — *see* Cyst, iris, implantation
  vagina N89.8
  vulva N90.7
incisive canal K09.1
inclusion (epidermal) (epithelial) (epidermoid) (squamous) L72.0
  not of skin — *code under* Cyst, by site
intestine (large) (small) K63.89
intracranial — *see* Cyst, brain
intraligamentous — *see also* Disorder, ligament
  knee — *see* Derangement, knee
intrasellar E23.6
iris H21.309
  exudative H21.31- ☑
  idiopathic H21.30- ☑
  implantation H21.32- ☑
  parasitic H21.33- ☑
  pars plana (primary) H21.34- ☑
    exudative H21.35- ☑
jaw (bone) M27.40
  aneurysmal M27.49
  developmental (odontogenic) K09.0
  fissural K09.1
  hemorrhagic M27.49
  traumatic M27.49
joint NEC — *see* Disorder, joint, specified type NEC
kidney (acquired) N28.1
  calyceal — *see* Hydronephrosis
  congenital Q61.00
  more than one (multiple) Q61.02
    specified as polycystic Q61.3
      adult type (autosomal dominant) Q61.2
      infantile type (autosomal recessive) NEC Q61.19
        collecting duct dilation Q61.11
  pyelogenic — *see* Hydronephrosis
  simple N28.1
  solitary (single) Q61.01
    acquired N28.1
labium (majus) (minus) N90.7

Cyst — *continued*
labium — *continued*
  sebaceous N90.7
lacrimal — *see also* Disorder, lacrimal system, specified NEC
  gland H04.13- ☑
  passages or sac — *see* Disorder, lacrimal system, specified NEC
larynx J38.7
lateral periodontal K09.0
lens H27.8
  congenital Q12.8
lip (gland) K13.0
liver (idiopathic) (simple) K76.89
  congenital Q44.6
  hydatid B67.8
    granulosus B67.0
    multilocularis B67.5
lung J98.4
  congenital Q33.0
  giant bullous J43.9
lutein N83.1- ☑
lymphangiomatous D18.1
lymphoepithelial, oral soft tissue K09.8
macula — *see* Degeneration, macula, hole
malignant — *see* Neoplasm, malignant, by site
mammary gland — *see* Cyst, breast
mandible M27.40
  dentigerous K09.0
  radicular K04.8
maxilla M27.40
  dentigerous K09.0
  radicular K04.8
medial, face and neck Q18.8
median
  anterior maxillary K09.1
  palatal K09.1
mediastinum, congenital Q34.1
meibomian (gland) — *see* Chalazion
  infected — *see* Hordeolum
membrane, brain G93.0
meninges (cerebral) G93.0
  spinal G96.19
meniscus, knee — *see* Derangement, knee, meniscus, cystic
mesentery, mesenteric K66.8
  chyle I89.8
mesonephric duct
  female Q50.5
  male Q55.4
milk N64.89
Morgagni (hydatid)
  female Q50.5
  male (epididymal) Q55.4
    testicular Q55.29
mouth K09.8
Müllerian duct Q50.4
  appendix testis Q55.29
  cervix Q51.6
  fallopian tube Q50.4
  female Q50.4
  male Q55.29
  prostatic utricle Q55.4
  vagina (embryonal) Q52.4
multilocular (ovary) D39.10
  benign — *see* Neoplasm, benign, by site
myometrium N85.8
nabothian (follicle) (ruptured) N88.8
nasoalveolar K09.1
nasolabial K09.1
nasopalatine (anterior) (duct) K09.1
nasopharynx J39.2
neoplastic — *see* Neoplasm, uncertain behavior, by site
  benign — *see* Neoplasm, benign, by site
nervous system NEC G96.8
neuroenteric (congenital) Q06.8
nipple — *see* Cyst, breast
nose (turbinates) J34.1
  sinus J34.1
odontogenic, developmental K09.0
omentum (lesser) K66.8
  congenital Q45.8
ora serrata — *see* Cyst, retina, ora serrata
oral
  region K09.9
    developmental (nonodontogenic) K09.1
    specified NEC K09.8

Cyst — *continued*
oral — *continued*
   soft tissue K09.9
    specified NEC K09.8
orbit H05.81- ☑
ovary, ovarian (twisted) N83.20- ☑
  adherent N83.20- ☑
  chocolate N80.1
  corpus
   albicans N83.29- ☑
   luteum (hemorrhagic) N83.1- ☑
  dermoid D27.9
  developmental Q50.1
  due to failure of involution NEC N83.20- ☑
  endometrial N80.1
  follicular (graafian) (hemorrhagic) N83.0- ☑
  hemorrhagic N83.20- ☑
  in pregnancy or childbirth O34.8- ☑
   with obstructed labor O65.5
  multilocular D39.10
  pseudomucinous D27.9
  retention N83.29- ☑
  serous N83.20- ☑
  specified NEC N83.29- ☑
  theca lutein (hemorrhagic) N83.1- ☑
  tuberculous A18.18
oviduct N83.8
palate (median) (fissural) K09.1
palatine papilla (jaw) K09.1
pancreas, pancreatic (hemorrhagic) (true) K86.2
  congenital Q45.2
  false K86.3
paralabral
  hip M24.85- ☑
  shoulder S43.43- ☑
paramesonephric duct Q50.4
  female Q50.4
  male Q55.29
paranephric N28.1
paraphysis, cerebri, congenital Q04.6
parasitic B89
parathyroid (gland) E21.4
paratubal N83.8
paraurethral duct N36.8
paroophoron Q50.5
parotid gland K11.6
parovarian Q50.5
pelvis, female N94.89
  in pregnancy or childbirth O34.8- ☑
   causing obstructed labor O65.5
penis (sebaceous) N48.89
periapical K04.8
pericardial (congenital) Q24.8
  acquired (secondary) I31.8
pericoronal K09.0
periodontal K04.8
  lateral K09.0
peripelvic (lymphatic) N28.1
peritoneum K66.8
  chylous I89.8
periventricular, acquired, newborn P91.1
pharynx (wall) J39.2
pilar L72.11
pilonidal (infected) (rectum) L05.91
  with abscess L05.01
  malignant C44.59- ☑
pituitary (duct) (gland) E23.6
placenta O43.19- ☑
pleura J94.8
popliteal — *see* Cyst, Baker's
porencephalic Q04.6
  acquired G93.0
postanal (infected) — *see* Cyst, pilonidal
postmastoidectomy cavity (mucosal) — *see* Complications, postmastoidectomy, cyst
preauricular Q18.1
prepuce N47.4
  congenital Q55.69
primordial (jaw) K09.0
prostate N42.83
pseudomucinous (ovary) D27.9
pupillary, miotic H21.27- ☑
radicular (residual) K04.8
radiculodental K04.8
ranular K11.8
Rathke's pouch E23.6
rectum (epithelium) (mucous) K62.89
renal — *see* Cyst, kidney

Cyst — *continued*
residual (radicular) K04.8
retention (ovary) N83.29- ☑
  salivary gland K11.6
retina H33.19- ☑
  ora serrata H33.11- ☑
  parasitic H33.12- ☑
retroperitoneal K68.9
sacrococcygeal (dermoid) — *see* Cyst, pilonidal
salivary gland or duct (mucous extravasation or retention) K11.6
Sampson's N80.1
sclera H15.89
scrotum L72.9
  sebaceous L72.3
sebaceous (duct) (gland) L72.3
  breast — *see* Dysplasia, mammary, specified type NEC
  eyelid — *see* Cyst, eyelid
  genital organ NEC
   female N94.89
   male N50.89
  scrotum L72.3
semilunar cartilage (knee) (multiple) — *see* Derangement, knee, meniscus, cystic
seminal vesicle N50.89
serous (ovary) N83.20- ☑
sinus (accessory) (nasal) J34.1
Skene's gland N36.8
skin L72.9
  breast — *see* Dysplasia, mammary, specified type NEC
  epidermal, epidermoid L72.0
  epithelial L72.0
  eyelid — *see* Cyst, eyelid
  genital organ NEC
   female N90.7
   male N50.89
  inclusion L72.0
  scrotum L72.9
  sebaceous L72.3
  sweat gland or duct L74.8
solitary
  bone — *see* Cyst, bone, solitary
  jaw M27.40
  kidney N28.1
spermatic cord N50.89
sphenoid sinus J34.1
spinal meninges G96.19
spleen NEC D73.4
  congenital Q89.09
  hydatid — *see also* Echinococcus B67.99 *[D77]*
Stafne's M27.0
subarachnoid intrasellar R93.0
subcutaneous, pheomycotic (chromomycotic) B43.2
subdural (cerebral) G93.0
  spinal cord G96.19
sublingual gland K11.6
submandibular gland K11.6
submaxillary gland K11.6
suburethral N36.8
suprarenal gland E27.8
suprasellar — *see* Cyst, brain
sweat gland or duct L74.8
synovial — *see also* Cyst, bursa
  ruptured — *see* Rupture, synovium
tarsal — *see* Chalazion
tendon (sheath) — *see* Disorder, tendon, specified type NEC
testis N44.2
  tunica albuginea N44.1
theca lutein (ovary) N83.1- ☑
Thornwaldt's J39.2
thymus (gland) E32.8
thyroglossal duct (infected) (persistent) Q89.2
thyroid (gland) E04.1
thyrolingual duct (infected) (persistent) Q89.2
tongue K14.8
tonsil J35.8
tooth — *see* Cyst, dental
Tornwaldt's J39.2
trichilemmal (proliferating) L72.12
trichodermal L72.12
tubal (fallopian) N83.8
  inflammatory — *see* Salpingitis, chronic
tubo-ovarian N83.8
  inflammatory N70.13

Cyst — *continued*
tunica
  albuginea testis N44.1
  vaginalis N50.89
turbinate (nose) J34.1
Tyson's gland N48.89
urachus, congenital Q64.4
ureter N28.89
ureterovesical orifice N28.89
urethra, urethral (gland) N36.8
uterine ligament N83.8
uterus (body) (corpus) (recurrent) N85.8
  embryonic Q51.818
   cervix Q51.6
vagina, vaginal (implantation) (inclusion) (squamous cell) (wall) N89.8
  embryonic Q52.4
vallecula, vallecular (epiglottis) J38.7
vesical (orifice) N32.89
vitreous body H43.89
vulva (implantation) (inclusion) N90.7
  congenital Q52.79
  sebaceous gland N90.7
vulvovaginal gland N90.7
wolffian
  female Q50.5
  male Q55.4
Cystadenocarcinoma — *see* Neoplasm, malignant, by site
bile duct C22.1
endometrioid — *see* Neoplasm, malignant, by site
  specified site — *see* Neoplasm, malignant, by site
  unspecified site
   female C56.9
   male C61
mucinous
  papillary
   specified site — *see* Neoplasm, malignant, by site
   unspecified site C56.9
  specified site — *see* Neoplasm, malignant, by site
  unspecified site C56.9
papillary
  mucinous
   specified site — *see* Neoplasm, malignant, by site
   unspecified site C56.9
  pseudomucinous
   specified site — *see* Neoplasm, malignant, by site
   unspecified site C56.9
  serous
   specified site — *see* Neoplasm, malignant, by site
   unspecified site C56.9
  specified site — *see* Neoplasm, malignant, by site
  unspecified site C56.9
pseudomucinous
  papillary
   specified site — *see* Neoplasm, malignant, by site
   unspecified site C56.9
  specified site — *see* Neoplasm, malignant, by site
  unspecified site C56.9
serous
  papillary
   specified site — *see* Neoplasm, malignant, by site
   unspecified site C56.9
  specified site — *see* Neoplasm, malignant, by site
  unspecified site C56.9
Cystadenofibroma
clear cell — *see* Neoplasm, benign, by site
endometrioid D27.9
  borderline malignancy D39.1- ☑
  malignant C56.- ☑
mucinous
  specified site — *see* Neoplasm, benign, by site
  unspecified site D27.9
serous
  specified site — *see* Neoplasm, benign, by site
  unspecified site D27.9
specified site — *see* Neoplasm, benign, by site
unspecified site D27.9
Cystadenoma — *see also* Neoplasm, benign, by site
bile duct D13.4
endometrioid — *see* Neoplasm, benign, by site

☑ **Additional Character Required — Refer to the Tabular List for Character Selection**　　　▼ **Subterms under main terms may continue to next column or page**

Cystadenoma — *continued*
  endometrioid — *see* Neoplasm, benign, by site — *continued*
    borderline malignancy — *see* Neoplasm, uncertain behavior, by site
  malignant — *see* Neoplasm, malignant, by site
  mucinous
    borderline malignancy
      ovary C56.- ☑
      specified site NEC — *see* Neoplasm, uncertain behavior, by site
      unspecified site C56.9
    papillary
      borderline malignancy
        ovary C56.- ☑
        specified site NEC — *see* Neoplasm, uncertain behavior, by site
        unspecified site C56.9
      specified site — *see* Neoplasm, benign, by site
      unspecified site D27.9
    specified site — *see* Neoplasm, benign, by site
    unspecified site D27.9
  papillary
    borderline malignancy
      ovary C56.- ☑
      specified site NEC — *see* Neoplasm, uncertain behavior, by site
      unspecified site C56.9
    lymphomatosum
      specified site — *see* Neoplasm, benign, by site
      unspecified site D11.9
    mucinous
      borderline malignancy
        ovary C56.- ☑
        specified site NEC — *see* Neoplasm, uncertain behavior, by site
        unspecified site C56.9
      specified site — *see* Neoplasm, benign, by site
      unspecified site D27.9
    pseudomucinous
      borderline malignancy
        ovary C56.- ☑
        specified site NEC — *see* Neoplasm, uncertain behavior, by site
        unspecified site C56.9
      specified site — *see* Neoplasm, benign, by site
      unspecified site D27.9
    serous
      borderline malignancy
        ovary C56.- ☑
        specified site NEC — *see* Neoplasm, uncertain behavior, by site
        unspecified site C56.9
      specified site — *see* Neoplasm, benign, by site
      unspecified site D27.9
    specified site — *see* Neoplasm, benign, by site
    unspecified site D27.9
  pseudomucinous
    borderline malignancy
      ovary C56.- ☑
      specified site NEC — *see* Neoplasm, uncertain behavior, by site
      unspecified site C56.9
    papillary
      borderline malignancy
        ovary C56.- ☑
        specified site NEC — *see* Neoplasm, uncertain behavior, by site
        unspecified site C56.9
      specified site — *see* Neoplasm, benign, by site
      unspecified site D27.9
    specified site — *see* Neoplasm, benign, by site
    unspecified site D27.9
  serous
    borderline malignancy
      ovary C56.- ☑
      specified site NEC — *see* Neoplasm, uncertain behavior, by site
      unspecified site C56.9

Cystadenoma — *continued*
  serous — *continued*
    papillary
      borderline malignancy
        ovary C56.- ☑
        specified site NEC — *see* Neoplasm, uncertain behavior, by site
        unspecified site C56.9
      specified site — *see* Neoplasm, benign, by site
      unspecified site D27.9
    specified site — *see* Neoplasm, benign, by site
    unspecified site D27.9
Cystathionine synthase deficiency E72.11
Cystathioninemia E72.19
Cystathioninuria E72.19
Cystic — *see also* condition
  breast (chronic) — *see* Mastopathy, cystic
  corpora lutea (hemorrhagic) N83.1- ☑
  duct — *see* condition
  eyeball (congenital) Q11.0
  fibrosis — *see* Fibrosis, cystic
  kidney (congenital) Q61.9
    adult type Q61.2
    infantile type NEC Q61.19
      collecting duct dilatation Q61.11
    medullary Q61.5
  liver, congenital Q44.6
  lung disease J98.4
    congenital Q33.0
  mastitis, chronic — *see* Mastopathy, cystic
  medullary, kidney Q61.5
  meniscus — *see* Derangement, knee, meniscus, cystic
  ovary N83.20- ☑
Cysticercosis, cysticerciasis B69.9
  with
    epileptiform fits B69.0
    myositis B69.81
  brain B69.0
  central nervous system B69.0
  cerebral B69.0
  ocular B69.1
  specified NEC B69.89
Cysticercus cellulose infestation — *see* Cysticercosis
Cystinosis (malignant) E72.04
Cystinuria E72.01
Cystitis (exudative) (hemorrhagic) (septic) (suppurative) N30.90
  with
    fibrosis — *see* Cystitis, chronic, interstitial
    hematuria N30.91
    leukoplakia — *see* Cystitis, chronic, interstitial
    malakoplakia — *see* Cystitis, chronic, interstitial
    metaplasia — *see* Cystitis, chronic, interstitial
    prostatitis N41.3
  acute N30.00
    with hematuria N30.01
    of trigone N30.30
      with hematuria N30.31
  allergic — *see* Cystitis, specified type NEC
  amebic A06.81
  bilharzial B65.9 *[N33]*
  blennorrhagic (gonococcal) A54.01
  bullous — *see* Cystitis, specified type NEC
  calculous N21.0
  chlamydial A56.01
  chronic N30.20
    with hematuria N30.21
    interstitial N30.10
      with hematuria N30.11
    of trigone N30.30
      with hematuria N30.31
    specified NEC N30.20
      with hematuria N30.21
  cystic (a) — *see* Cystitis, specified type NEC
  diphtheritic A36.85
  echinococcal
    granulosus B67.39
    multilocularis B67.69
  emphysematous — *see* Cystitis, specified type NEC
  encysted — *see* Cystitis, specified type NEC

Cystitis — *continued*
  eosinophilic — *see* Cystitis, specified type NEC
  follicular — *see* Cystitis, of trigone
  gangrenous — *see* Cystitis, specified type NEC
  glandularis — *see* Cystitis, specified type NEC
  gonococcal A54.01
  incrusted — *see* Cystitis, specified type NEC
  interstitial (chronic) — *see* Cystitis, chronic, interstitial
  irradiation N30.40
    with hematuria N30.41
  irritation — *see* Cystitis, specified type NEC
  malignant — *see* Cystitis, specified type NEC
  of trigone N30.30
    with hematuria N30.31
  panmural — *see* Cystitis, chronic, interstitial
  polyposa — *see* Cystitis, specified type NEC
  prostatic N41.3
  puerperal (postpartum) O86.22
  radiation — *see* Cystitis, irradiation
  specified type NEC N30.80
    with hematuria N30.81
  subacute — *see* Cystitis, chronic
  submucous — *see* Cystitis, chronic, interstitial
  syphilitic (late) A52.76
  trichomonal A59.03
  tuberculous A18.12
  ulcerative — *see* Cystitis, chronic, interstitial
Cystocele (-urethrocele)
  female N81.10
    with prolapse of uterus — *see* Prolapse, uterus
    lateral N81.12
    midline N81.11
    paravaginal N81.12
  in pregnancy or childbirth O34.8- ☑
    causing obstructed labor O65.5
  male N32.89
Cystolithiasis N21.0
Cystoma — *see also* Neoplasm, benign, by site
  endometrial, ovary N80.1
  mucinous
    specified site — *see* Neoplasm, benign, by site
    unspecified site D27.9
  serous
    specified site — *see* Neoplasm, benign, by site
    unspecified site D27.9
  simple (ovary) N83.29- ☑
Cystoplegia N31.2
Cystoptosis N32.89
Cystopyelitis — *see* Pyelonephritis
Cystorrhagia N32.89
Cystosarcoma phyllodes D48.6- ☑
  benign D24- ☑
  malignant — *see* Neoplasm, breast, malignant
Cystostomy
  attention to Z43.5
  complication — *see* Complications, cystostomy
  status Z93.50
    appendico-vesicostomy Z93.52
    cutaneous Z93.51
    specified NEC Z93.59
Cystourethritis — *see* Urethritis
Cystourethrocele — *see also* Cystocele
  female N81.10
    with uterine prolapse — *see* Prolapse, uterus
    lateral N81.12
    midline N81.11
    paravaginal N81.12
  male N32.89
Cytomegalic inclusion disease
  congenital P35.1
Cytomegalovirus infection B25.9
Cytomycosis (reticuloendothelial) B39.4
Cytopenia D75.9
  refractory
    with multilineage dysplasia D46.A (*following* D46.2)
      and ring sideroblasts (RCMD RS) D46.B (*following* D46.2)
Czerny's disease (periodic hydrarthrosis of the knee) — *see* Effusion, joint, knee

Subterms under main terms may continue to next column or page   ☑ **Additional Character Required — Refer to the Tabular List for Character Selection**   **81**

Cystadenoma — Czerny's disease

D

Da Costa's syndrome F45.8
Daae (-Finsen) disease (epidemic pleurodynia) B33.0
Dabney's grip B33.0
Dacryoadenitis, dacryadenitis H04.00- ☑
  acute H04.01- ☑
  chronic H04.02- ☑
Dacryocystitis H04.30- ☑
  acute H04.32- ☑
  chronic H04.41- ☑
  neonatal P39.1
  phlegmonous H04.31- ☑
  syphilitic A52.71
    congenital (early) A50.01
  trachomatous, active A71.1
    sequelae (late effect) B94.0
Dacryocystoblenorrhea — see Inflammation, lacrimal, passages, chronic
Dacryocystocele — see Disorder, lacrimal system, changes
Dacryolith, dacryolithiasis H04.51- ☑
Dacryoma — see Disorder, lacrimal system, changes
Dacryopericystitis — see Dacryocystitis
Dacryops H04.11- ☑
Dacryostenosis — see also Stenosis, lacrimal
  congenital Q10.5
Dactylitis
  bone — see Osteomyelitis
  sickle-cell D57.00
    Hb C D57.219
    Hb SS D57.00
    specified NEC D57.819
  skin L08.9
  syphilitic A52.77
  tuberculous A18.03
Dactylolysis spontanea (ainhum) L94.6
Dactylosymphysis Q70.9
  fingers — see Syndactylism, complex, fingers
  toes — see Syndactylism, complex, toes
Damage
  arteriosclerotic — see Arteriosclerosis
  brain (nontraumatic) G93.9
    anoxic, hypoxic G93.1
      resulting from a procedure G97.82
    child NEC G80.9
    due to birth injury P11.2
  cardiorenal (vascular) — see Hypertension, cardiorenal
  cerebral NEC — see Damage, brain
  coccyx, complicating delivery O71.6
  coronary — see Disease, heart, ischemic
  deep tissue, pressure-induced — see also L89 with final character .6
  eye, birth injury P15.3
  liver (nontraumatic) K76.9
    alcoholic K70.9
    due to drugs — see Disease, liver, toxic
    toxic — see Disease, liver, toxic
  medication T88.7 ☑
  pelvic
    joint or ligament, during delivery O71.6
    organ NEC
      during delivery O71.5
      following ectopic or molar pregnancy O08.6
  renal — see Disease, renal
  subendocardium, subendocardial — see Degeneration, myocardial
  vascular I99.9
Dana-Putnam syndrome (subacute combined sclerosis with pernicious anemia) — see Degeneration, combined
Danbolt (-Cross) syndrome (acrodermatitis enteropathica) E83.2
Dandruff L21.0
Dandy-Walker syndrome Q03.1
  with spina bifida — see Spina bifida
Danlos' syndrome — see also Syndrome, Ehlers-Danlos Q79.60
Darier (-White) disease (congenital) Q82.8
  meaning erythema annulare centrifugum L53.1
Darier-Roussy sarcoid D86.3
Darling's disease or histoplasmosis B39.4
Darwin's tubercle Q17.8
Dawson's (inclusion body) encephalitis A81.1
De Beurmann (-Gougerot) disease B42.1
De la Tourette's syndrome F95.2

De Lange's syndrome Q87.19
De Morgan's spots (senile angiomas) I78.1
De Quervain's
  disease (tendon sheath) M65.4
  syndrome E34.51
  thyroiditis (subacute granulomatous thyroiditis) E06.1
De Toni-Fanconi (-Debré) syndrome E72.09
  with cystinosis E72.04
Dead
  fetus, retained (mother) O36.4 ☑
    early pregnancy O02.1
  labyrinth H83.2 ☑
  ovum, retained O02.0
Deaf nonspeaking NEC H91.3
Deafmutism (acquired) (congenital) NEC H91.3
  hysterical F44.6
  syphilitic, congenital — see also subcategory H94.8 A50.09
Deafness (acquired) (complete) (hereditary) (partial) H91.9- ☑
  with blue sclera and fragility of bone Q78.0
  auditory fatigue — see Deafness, specified type NEC
  aviation T70.0 ☑
    nerve injury — see Injury, nerve, acoustic, specified type NEC
  boilermaker's H83.3 ☑
  central — see Deafness, sensorineural
  conductive H90.2
    and sensorineural
      mixed H90.8
        bilateral H90.6
    bilateral H90.0
    unilateral H90.1- ☑
      with restricted hearing on the contralateral side H90.A- ☑
  congenital H90.5
    with blue sclera and fragility of bone Q78.0
  due to toxic agents — see Deafness, ototoxic
  emotional (hysterical) F44.6
  functional (hysterical) F44.6
  high frequency H91.9- ☑
  hysterical F44.6
  low frequency H91.9- ☑
  mental R48.8
  mixed conductive and sensorineural H90.8
    bilateral H90.6
    unilateral H90.7- ☑
  nerve — see Deafness, sensorineural
  neural — see Deafness, sensorineural
  noise-induced — see also subcategory H83.3 ☑
    nerve injury — see Injury, nerve, acoustic, specified type NEC
  nonspeaking H91.3
  ototoxic H91.0 ☑
  perceptive — see Deafness, sensorineural
  psychogenic (hysterical) F44.6
  sensorineural H90.5
    and conductive
      bilateral H90.6
      mixed H90.8
        bilateral H90.6
    bilateral H90.3
    unilateral H90.4- ☑
      with restricted hearing on the contralateral side H90.A- ☑
  sensory — see Deafness, sensorineural
  specified type NEC H91.8 ☑
  sudden (idiopathic) H91.2- ☑
  syphilitic A52.15
  transient ischemic H93.01- ☑
  traumatic — see Injury, nerve, acoustic, specified type NEC
  word (developmental) H93.25
Death (cause unknown) (of) (unexplained) (unspecified cause) R99
  brain G93.82
  cardiac (sudden) (with successful resuscitation) — code to underlying disease
    family history of Z82.41
    personal history of Z86.74
  family member (assumed) Z63.4
Debility (chronic) (general) (nervous) R53.81
  congenital or neonatal NOS P96.9
  nervous R53.81
  old age R54
  senile R54
Débove's disease (splenomegaly) R16.1

Decalcification
  bone — see Osteoporosis
  teeth K03.89
Decapsulation, kidney N28.89
Decay
  dental — see Caries, dental
  senile R54
  tooth, teeth — see Caries, dental
Deciduitis (acute)
  following ectopic or molar pregnancy O08.0
Decline (general) — see Debility
  cognitive, age-associated R41.81
Decompensation
  cardiac (acute) (chronic) — see Disease, heart
  cardiovascular — see Disease, cardiovascular
  heart — see Disease, heart
  hepatic — see Failure, hepatic
  myocardial (acute) (chronic) — see Disease, heart
  respiratory J98.8
Decompression sickness T70.3 ☑
Decrease (d)
  absolute neutrophile count — see Neutropenia
  blood
    platelets — see Thrombocytopenia
    pressure R03.1
      due to shock following
        injury T79.4 ☑
        operation T81.19 ☑
  estrogen E28.39
    postablative E89.40
      asymptomatic E89.40
      symptomatic E89.41
  fragility of erythrocytes D58.8
  function
    lipase (pancreatic) K90.3
    ovary in hypopituitarism E23.0
    parenchyma of pancreas K86.89
    pituitary (gland) (anterior) (lobe) E23.0
      posterior (lobe) E23.0
  functional activity R68.89
  glucose R73.09
  hematocrit R71.0
  hemoglobin R71.0
  leukocytes D72.819
    specified NEC D72.818
  libido R68.82
  lymphocytes D72.810
  platelets D69.6
  respiration, due to shock following injury T79.4 ☑
  sexual desire R68.82
  tear secretion NEC — see Syndrome, dry eye
  tolerance
    fat K90.49
    glucose R73.09
    pancreatic K90.3
    salt and water E87.8
  vision NEC H54.7
  white blood cell count D72.819
    specified NEC D72.818
Decubitus (ulcer) — see Ulcer, pressure, by site
  cervix N86
Deepening acetabulum — see Derangement, joint, specified type NEC, hip
Defect, defective Q89.9
  3-beta-hydroxysteroid dehydrogenase E25.0
  11-hydroxylase E25.0
  21-hydroxylase E25.0
  abdominal wall, congenital Q79.59
  antibody immunodeficiency D80.9
  aorticopulmonary septum Q21.4
  atrial septal (ostium secundum type) Q21.1
    following acute myocardial infarction (current complication) I23.1
    ostium primum type Q21.2
  atrioventricular
    canal Q21.2
    septum Q21.2
  auricular septal Q21.1
  bilirubin excretion NEC E80.6
  biosynthesis, androgen (testicular) E29.1
  bulbar septum Q21.0
  catalase E80.3
  cell membrane receptor complex (CR3) D71
  circulation I99.9
    congenital Q28.9
    newborn Q28.9
  coagulation (factor) — see also Deficiency, factor D68.9

Defect, defective — *continued*
  coagulation — *see also* Deficiency, factor — *continued*
    with
      ectopic pregnancy O08.1
      molar pregnancy O08.1
    acquired D68.4
    antepartum with hemorrhage — *see* Hemorrhage, antepartum, with coagulation defect
    due to
      liver disease D68.4
      vitamin K deficiency D68.4
    hereditary NEC D68.2
    intrapartum O67.0
    newborn, transient P61.6
    postpartum O99.13
      with hemorrhage O72.3
    specified type NEC D68.8
  complement system D84.1
  conduction (heart) I45.9
    bone — *see* Deafness, conductive
  congenital, organ or site not listed — *see* Anomaly, by site
  coronary sinus Q21.1
  cushion, endocardial Q21.2
  degradation, glycoprotein E77.1
  dental bridge, crown, fillings — *see* Defect, dental restoration
  dental restoration K08.50
    specified NEC K08.59
  dentin (hereditary) K00.5
  Descemet's membrane, congenital Q13.89
  developmental — *see also* Anomaly
    cauda equina Q06.3
  diaphragm
    with elevation, eventration or hernia — *see* Hernia, diaphragm
    congenital Q79.1
      with hernia Q79.0
      gross (with hernia) Q79.0
  ectodermal, congenital Q82.9
  Eisenmenger's Q21.8
  enzyme
    catalase E80.3
    peroxidase E80.3
  esophagus, congenital Q39.9
  extensor retinaculum M62.89
  fibrin polymerization D68.2
  filling
    bladder R93.41
    kidney R93.42- ☑
    renal pelvis R93.41
    stomach R93.3
    ureter R93.41
    urinary organs, specified NEC R93.49
  GABA (gamma aminobutyric acid) metabolic E72.81
  Gerbode Q21.0
  glycoprotein degradation E77.1
  Hageman (factor) D68.2
  hearing — *see* Deafness
  high grade F70
  interatrial septal Q21.1
  interauricular septal Q21.1
  interventricular septal Q21.0
    with dextroposition of aorta, pulmonary stenosis and hypertrophy of right ventricle Q21.3
    in tetralogy of Fallot Q21.3
  learning (specific) — *see* Disorder, learning
  lymphocyte function antigen-1 (LFA-1) D84.0
  lysosomal enzyme, post-translational modification E77.0
  major osseous M89.70
    ankle M89.77- ☑
    carpus M89.74- ☑
    clavicle M89.71- ☑
    femur M89.75- ☑
    fibula M89.76- ☑
    fingers M89.74- ☑
    foot M89.77- ☑
    forearm M89.73- ☑
    hand M89.74- ☑
    humerus M89.72- ☑
    lower leg M89.76- ☑
    metacarpus M89.74- ☑
    metatarsus M89.77- ☑
    multiple sites M89.79
    pelvic region M89.75- ☑
    pelvis M89.75- ☑

Defect, defective — *continued*
  major osseous — *continued*
    radius M89.73- ☑
    scapula M89.71- ☑
    shoulder region M89.71- ☑
    specified NEC M89.78
    tarsus M89.77- ☑
    thigh M89.75- ☑
    tibia M89.76- ☑
    toes M89.77- ☑
    ulna M89.73- ☑
  mental — *see* Disability, intellectual
  modification, lysosomal enzymes, post-translational E77.0
  obstructive, congenital
    renal pelvis Q62.39
    ureter Q62.39
      atresia — *see* Atresia, ureter
      cecoureterocele Q62.32
      megaureter Q62.2
      orthotopic ureterocele Q62.31
  osseous, major M89.70
    ankle M89.77- ☑
    carpus M89.74- ☑
    clavicle M89.71- ☑
    femur M89.75- ☑
    fibula M89.76- ☑
    fingers M89.74- ☑
    foot M89.77- ☑
    forearm M89.73- ☑
    hand M89.74- ☑
    humerus M89.72- ☑
    lower leg M89.76- ☑
    metacarpus M89.74- ☑
    metatarsus M89.77- ☑
    multiple sites M89.9
    pelvic region M89.75- ☑
    pelvis M89.75- ☑
    radius M89.73- ☑
    scapula M89.71- ☑
    shoulder region M89.71- ☑
    specified NEC M89.78
    tarsus M89.77- ☑
    thigh M89.75- ☑
    tibia M89.76- ☑
    toes M89.77- ☑
    ulna M89.73- ☑
  osteochondral NEC — *see also* Deformity M95.8
  ostium
    primum Q21.2
    secundum Q21.1
  peroxidase E80.3
  placental blood supply — *see* Insufficiency, placental
  platelets, qualitative D69.1
    constitutional D68.0
  postural NEC, spine — *see* Dorsopathy, deforming
  reduction
    limb Q73.8
      lower Q72.9- ☑
        absence — *see* Agenesis, leg
          foot — *see* Agenesis, foot
        longitudinal
          femur Q72.4- ☑
          fibula Q72.6- ☑
          tibia Q72.5- ☑
        specified type NEC Q72.89- ☑
        split foot Q72.7- ☑
      specified type NEC Q73.8
      upper Q71.9- ☑
        absence — *see* Agenesis, arm
          forearm — *see* Agenesis, forearm
          hand — *see* Agenesis, hand
        lobster-claw hand Q71.6- ☑
        longitudinal
          radius Q71.4- ☑
          ulna Q71.5- ☑
        specified type NEC Q71.89- ☑
  renal pelvis Q63.8
    obstructive Q62.39
  respiratory system, congenital Q34.9
  restoration, dental K08.50
    specified NEC K08.59
  retinal nerve bundle fibers H35.89
  septal (heart) NOS Q21.9
    acquired (atrial) (auricular) (ventricular) (old) I51.0
    atrial Q21.1

Defect, defective — *continued*
  septal — *continued*
    atrial — *continued*
      concurrent with acute myocardial infarction — *see* Infarct, myocardium
      following acute myocardial infarction (current complication) I23.1
      ventricular — *see also* Defect, ventricular septal Q21.0
    sinus venosus Q21.1
  speech R47.9
    developmental F80.9
    specified NEC R47.89
  Taussig-Bing (aortic transposition and overriding pulmonary artery) Q20.1
  teeth, wedge K03.1
  vascular (local) I99.9
    congenital Q27.9
  ventricular septal Q21.0
    concurrent with acute myocardial infarction — *see* Infarct, myocardium
    following acute myocardial infarction (current complication) I23.2
    in tetralogy of Fallot Q21.3
  vision NEC H54.7
  visual field H53.40
    bilateral
      heteronymous H53.47
      homonymous H53.46- ☑
    generalized contraction H53.48- ☑
    localized
      arcuate H53.43- ☑
      scotoma (central area) H53.41- ☑
        blind spot area H53.42- ☑
      sector H53.43- ☑
      specified type NEC H53.45- ☑
  voice R49.9
    specified NEC R49.8
  wedge, tooth, teeth (abrasion) K03.1

Deferentitis N49.1
  gonorrheal (acute) (chronic) A54.23

Defibrination (syndrome) D65
  antepartum — *see* Hemorrhage, antepartum, with coagulation defect, disseminated intravascular coagulation
  following ectopic or molar pregnancy O08.1
  intrapartum O67.0
  newborn P60
  postpartum O72.3

Deficiency, deficient
  3-beta hydroxysteroid dehydrogenase E25.0
  5-alpha reductase (with male pseudohermaphroditism) E29.1
  11-hydroxylase E25.0
  21-hydroxylase E25.0
  abdominal muscle syndrome Q79.4
  AC globulin (congenital) (hereditary) D68.2
    acquired D68.4
  accelerator globulin (Ac G) (blood) D68.2
  acid phosphatase E83.39
  activating factor (blood) D68.2
  ADA2 (adenosine deaminase 2) D81.32
  adenosine deaminase (ADA) D81.30
    with severe combined immunodeficiency (SCID) D81.31
    partial (type 1) D81.39
    specified NEC D81.39
    type 1 (without SCID) (without severe combined immunodeficiency) D81.39
    type 2 D81.32
  aldolase (hereditary) E74.19
  alpha-1-antitrypsin E88.01
  amino-acids E72.9
  anemia — *see* Anemia
  aneurin E51.9
  antibody with
    hyperimmunoglobulinemia D80.6
    near-normal immunoglobins D80.6
  antidiuretic hormone E23.2
  anti-hemophilic
    factor (A) D66
      B D67
      C D68.1
    globulin (AHG) NEC D66
  antithrombin (antithrombin III) D68.59
  ascorbic acid E54
  attention (disorder) (syndrome) F98.8

Deficiency, deficient — *continued*
  attention — *continued*
    with hyperactivity — *see* Disorder, attention-deficit
      hyperactivity
  autoprothrombin
    C D68.2
    I D68.2
    II D67
  beta-glucuronidase E76.29
  biotin E53.8
  biotin-dependent carboxylase D81.819
  biotinidase D81.810
  brancher enzyme (amylopectinosis) E74.03
  C1 esterase inhibitor (C1-INH) D84.1
  calciferol E55.9
    with
      adult osteomalacia M83.8
      rickets — *see* Rickets
  calcium (dietary) E58
  calorie, severe E43
    with marasmus E41
      and kwashiorkor E42
  cardiac — *see* Insufficiency, myocardial
  carnitine E71.40
    due to
      hemodialysis E71.43
      inborn errors of metabolism E71.42
      Valproic acid therapy E71.43
    iatrogenic E71.43
    muscle palmityltransferase E71.314
    primary E71.41
    secondary E71.448
  carotene E50.9
  central nervous system G96.8
  ceruloplasmin (Wilson) E83.01
  choline E53.8
  Christmas factor D67
  chromium E61.4
  clotting (blood) — *see also* Deficiency, coagulation
    factor D68.9
  clotting factor NEC (hereditary) — *see also* Deficiency,
    factor D68.2
  coagulation NOS D68.9
    with
      ectopic pregnancy O08.1
      molar pregnancy O08.1
    acquired (any) D68.4
    antepartum hemorrhage — *see* Hemorrhage, an-
      tepartum, with coagulation defect
    clotting factor NEC — *see also* Deficiency, factor
      D68.2
    due to
      hyperprothrombinemia D68.4
      liver disease D68.4
      vitamin K deficiency D68.4
    newborn, transient P61.6
    postpartum O72.3
    specified NEC D68.8
  cognitive F09
  color vision H53.50
    achromatopsia H53.51
    acquired H53.52
    deuteranomaly H53.53
    protanomaly H53.54
    specified type NEC H53.59
    tritanomaly H53.55
  combined glucocorticoid and mineralocorticoid E27.49
  contact factor D68.2
  copper (nutritional) E61.0
  corticoadrenal E27.40
    primary E27.1
  craniofacial axis Q75.0
  cyanocobalamin E53.8
  debrancher enzyme (limit dextrinosis) E74.03
  dehydrogenase
    long chain/very long chain acyl CoA E71.310
    medium chain acyl CoA E71.311
    short chain acyl CoA E71.312
  diet E63.9
  dihydropyrimidine dehydrogenase (DPD) E88.89
  disaccharidase E73.9
  edema — *see* Malnutrition, severe
  endocrine E34.9
  energy-supply — *see* Malnutrition
  enzymes, circulating NEC E88.09
  ergosterol E55.9
    with
      adult osteomalacia M83.8

Deficiency, deficient — *continued*
  ergosterol — *continued*
    with — *continued*
      rickets — *see* Rickets
  essential fatty acid (EFA) E63.0
  factor — *see also* Deficiency, coagulation
    Hageman D68.2
    I (congenital) (hereditary) D68.2
    II (congenital) (hereditary) D68.2
    IX (congenital) (functional) (hereditary) (with func-
      tional defect) D67
    multiple (congenital) D68.8
      acquired D68.4
    V (congenital) (hereditary) D68.2
    VII (congenital) (hereditary) D68.2
    VIII (congenital) (functional) (hereditary) (with
      functional defect) D66
      with vascular defect D68.0
    X (congenital) (hereditary) D68.2
    XI (congenital) (hereditary) D68.1
    XII (congenital) (hereditary) D68.2
    XIII (congenital) (hereditary) D68.2
  femoral, proximal focal (congenital) — *see* Defect, re-
    duction, lower limb, longitudinal, femur
  fibrinase D68.2
  fibrinogen (congenital) (hereditary) D68.2
    acquired D65
  fibrin-stabilizing factor (congenital) (hereditary) D68.2
    acquired D68.4
  folate E53.8
  folic acid E53.8
  foreskin N47.3
  fructokinase E74.11
  fructose 1,6-diphosphatase E74.19
  fructose-1-phosphate aldolase E74.19
  GABA (gamma aminobutyric acid) transaminase E72.81
  GABA-T (gamma aminobutyric acid transaminase)
    E72.81
  galactokinase E74.29
  galactose-1-phosphate uridyl transferase E74.29
  gammaglobulin in blood D80.1
    hereditary D80.0
  glass factor D68.2
  glucocorticoid E27.49
    mineralocorticoid E27.49
  glucose-6-phosphatase E74.01
  glucose-6-phosphate dehydrogenase
    anemia D55.0
    without anemia D75.A
  glucuronyl transferase E80.5
  glycogen synthetase E74.09
  gonadotropin (isolated) E23.0
  growth hormone (idiopathic) (isolated) E23.0
  Hageman factor D68.2
  hemoglobin D64.9
  hepatophosphorylase E74.09
  homogentisate 1,2-dioxygenase E70.29
  hormone
    anterior pituitary (partial) NEC E23.0
      growth E23.0
    growth (isolated) E23.0
    pituitary E23.0
    testicular E29.1
  hypoxanthine- (guanine)-phosphoribosyltransferase
    (HG- PRT) (total H-PRT) E79.1
  immunity D84.9
    cell-mediated D84.8
      with thrombocytopenia and eczema D82.0
    combined D81.9
    humoral D80.9
    IgA (secretory) D80.2
    IgG D80.3
    IgM D80.4
  immuno — *see* Immunodeficiency
  immunoglobulin, selective
    A (IgA) D80.2
    G (IgG) (subclasses) D80.3
    M (IgM) D80.4
  inositol (B complex) E53.8
  intrinsic
    factor (congenital) D51.0
    sphincter N36.42
      with urethral hypermobility N36.43
  iodine E61.8
    congenital syndrome — *see* Syndrome, iodine-defi-
      ciency, congenital
  iron E61.1
    anemia D50.9
  kalium E87.6

Deficiency, deficient — *continued*
  kappa-light chain D80.8
  labile factor (congenital) (hereditary) D68.2
    acquired D68.4
  lacrimal fluid (acquired) — *see also* Syndrome, dry eye
    congenital Q10.6
  lactase
    congenital E73.0
    secondary E73.1
  Laki-Lorand factor D68.2
  lecithin cholesterol acyltransferase E78.6
  lipocaic K86.89
  lipoprotein (familial) (high density) E78.6
  liver phosphorylase E74.09
  lysosomal alpha-1, 4 glucosidase E74.02
  magnesium E61.2
  major histocompatibility complex
    class I D81.6
    class II D81.7
  manganese E61.3
  menadione (vitamin K) E56.1
    newborn P53
  mental (familial) (hereditary) — *see* Disability, intellec-
    tual
  methylenetetrahydrofolate reductase (MTHFR) E72.12
  mevalonate kinase M04.1
  mineralocorticoid E27.49
    with glucocorticoid E27.49
  mineral NEC E61.8
  molybdenum (nutritional) E61.5
  moral F60.2
  multiple nutrient elements E61.7
  multiple sulfatase (MSD) E75.26
  muscle
    carnitine (palmityltransferase) E71.314
    phosphofructokinase E74.09
  myoadenylate deaminase E79.2
  myocardial — *see* Insufficiency, myocardial
  myophosphorylase E74.04
  NADH diaphorase or reductase (congenital) D74.0
  NADH-methemoglobin reductase (congenital) D74.0
  natrium E87.1
  niacin (amide) (-tryptophan) E52
  nicotinamide E52
  nicotinic acid E52
  number of teeth — *see* Anodontia
  nutrient element E61.9
    multiple E61.7
    specified NEC E61.8
  nutrition, nutritional E63.9
    sequelae — *see* Sequelae, nutritional deficiency
    specified NEC E63.8
  of interleukin 1 receptor antagonist [DIRA] M04.8
  ornithine transcarbamylase E72.4
  ovarian E28.39
  oxygen — *see* Anoxia
  pantothenic acid E53.8
  parathyroid (gland) E20.9
  perineum (female) N81.89
  phenylalanine hydroxylase E70.1
  phosphoenolpyruvate carboxykinase E74.4
  phosphofructokinase E74.19
  phosphomannomutase E74.8
  phosphomannose isomerase E74.8
  phosphomannosyl mutase E74.8
  phosphorylase kinase, liver E74.09
  pituitary hormone (isolated) E23.0
  plasma thromboplastin
    antecedent (PTA) D68.1
    component (PTC) D67
  plasminogen (type 1) (type 2) E88.02
  platelet NEC D69.1
    constitutional D68.0
  polyglandular E31.8
    autoimmune E31.0
  potassium (K) E87.6
  prepuce N47.3
  proaccelerin (congenital) (hereditary) D68.2
    acquired D68.4
  proconvertin factor (congenital) (hereditary) D68.2
    acquired D68.4
  protein — *see also* Malnutrition E46
    anemia D53.0
    C D68.59
    S D68.59
  prothrombin (congenital) (hereditary) D68.2
    acquired D68.4
  Prower factor D68.2

☑ **Additional Character Required** — Refer to the Tabular List for Character Selection   ▽ Subterms under main terms may continue to next column or page

Deficiency, deficient — *continued*
  pseudocholinesterase E88.09
  PTA (plasma thromboplastin antecedent) D68.1
  PTC (plasma thromboplastin component) D67
  purine nucleoside phosphorylase (PNP) D81.5
  pyracin (alpha) (beta) E53.1
  pyridoxal E53.1
  pyridoxamine E53.1
  pyridoxine (derivatives) E53.1
  pyruvate
    carboxylase E74.4
    dehydrogenase E74.4
  riboflavin (vitamin B2) E53.0
  salt E87.1
  secretion
    ovary E28.39
    salivary gland (any) K11.7
    urine R34
  selenium (dietary) E59
  serum antitrypsin, familial E88.01
  short stature homeobox gene (SHOX)
    with
      dyschondrosteosis Q78.8
      short stature (idiopathic) E34.3
      Turner's syndrome Q96.9
  sodium (Na) E87.1
  SPCA (factor VII) D68.2
  sphincter, intrinsic N36.42
    with urethral hypermobility N36.43
  stable factor (congenital) (hereditary) D68.2
    acquired D68.4
  Stuart-Prower (factor X) D68.2
  succinic semialdehyde dehydrogenase E72.81
  sucrase E74.39
  sucrose E74.39
  sulfatase E75.26
  sulfite oxidase E72.19
  thiamin, thiaminic (chloride) E51.9
    beriberi (dry) E51.11
      wet E51.12
  thrombokinase D68.2
    newborn P53
  thyroid (gland) — *see* Hypothyroidism
  tocopherol E56.0
  tooth bud K00.0
  transcobalamine II (anemia) D51.2
  vanadium E61.6
  vascular I99.9
  vasopressin E23.2
  vertical ridge K06.8
  viosterol — *see* Deficiency, calciferol
  vitamin (multiple) NOS E56.9
    A E50.9
      with
        Bitot's spot (corneal) E50.1
        follicular keratosis E50.8
        keratomalacia E50.4
        manifestations NEC E50.8
        night blindness E50.5
        scar of cornea, xerophthalmic E50.6
        xeroderma E50.8
        xerophthalmia E50.7
        xerosis
          conjunctival E50.0
            and Bitot's spot E50.1
          cornea E50.2
            and ulceration E50.3
      sequelae E64.1
    B (complex) NOS E53.9
      with
        beriberi (dry) E51.11
          wet E51.12
        pellagra E52
    B1 NOS E51.9
      beriberi (dry) E51.11
        with circulatory system manifestations E51.11
        wet E51.12
    B12 E53.8
    B2 (riboflavin) E53.0
    B6 E53.1
    C E54
      sequelae E64.2
    D E55.9
      with
        adult osteomalacia M83.8
        rickets — *see* Rickets
        25-hydroxylase E83.32
    E E56.0
    folic acid E53.8
    G E53.0

Deficiency, deficient — *continued*
  vitamin — *continued*
    group B E53.9
      specified NEC E53.8
    H (biotin) E53.8
    K E56.1
      of newborn P53
    nicotinic E52
    P E56.8
    PP (pellagra-preventing) E52
    specified NEC E56.8
    thiamin E51.9
      beriberi — *see* Beriberi
  zinc, dietary E60
Deficit — *see also* Deficiency
  attention and concentration R41.840
    disorder — *see* Attention, deficit
    following
      cerebral infarction I69.310
      cerebrovascular disease I69.910
        specified disease NEC I69.810
      nontraumatic
        intracerebral hemorrhage I69.110
        specified intracranial hemorrhage NEC I69.210
        subarachnoid hemorrhage I69.010
  cognitive
    communication R41.841
    emotional
      following
        cerebral infarction I69.315
        cerebrovascular disease I69.915
          specified disease NEC I69.815
        nontraumatic
          intracerebral hemorrhage I69.115
          specified intracranial hemorrhage NEC I69.215
          subarachnoid hemorrhage I69.015
    following
      cerebral infarction I69.319
      cerebrovascular disease I69.919
        specified disease NEC I69.819
      nontraumatic
        intracerebral hemorrhage I69.119
        specified intracranial hemorrhage NEC I69.219
        subarachnoid hemorrhage I69.019
    social
      following
        cerebral infarction I69.315
        cerebrovascular disease I69.915
          specified disease NEC I69.815
        nontraumatic
          intracerebral hemorrhage I69.115
          specified intracranial hemorrhage NEC I69.215
          subarachnoid hemorrhage I69.015
  cognitive NEC R41.89
    following
      cerebral infarction I69.318
      cerebrovascular disease I69.918
        specified disease NEC I69.818
      nontraumatic
        intracerebral hemorrhage I69.118
        specified intracranial hemorrhage NEC I69.218
        subarachnoid hemorrhage I69.018
  concentration R41.840
  executive function R41.844
    following
      cerebral infarction I69.314
      cerebrovascular disease I69.914
        specified disease NEC I69.814
      nontraumatic
        intracerebral hemorrhage I69.114
        specified intracranial hemorrhage NEC I69.214
        subarachnoid hemorrhage I69.014
  frontal lobe R41.844
    following
      cerebral infarction I69.314
      cerebrovascular disease I69.914
        specified disease NEC I69.814
      nontraumatic
        intracerebral hemorrhage I69.114
        specified intracranial hemorrhage NEC I69.214
        subarachnoid hemorrhage I69.014
  memory
    following
      cerebral infarction I69.311
      cerebrovascular disease I69.911
        specified disease NEC I69.811

Deficit — *continued*
  memory — *continued*
    following — *continued*
      nontraumatic
        intracerebral hemorrhage I69.111
        specified intracranial hemorrhage NEC I69.211
        subarachnoid hemorrhage I69.011
  neurologic NEC R29.818
    ischemic
      reversible (RIND) I63.9
        prolonged (PRIND) I63.9
  oxygen R09.02
  prolonged reversible ischemic neurologic (PRIND) I63.9
  psychomotor R41.843
    following
      cerebral infarction I69.313
      cerebrovascular disease I69.913
        specified disease NEC I69.813
      nontraumatic
        intracerebral hemorrhage I69.113
        specified intracranial hemorrhage NEC I69.213
        subarachnoid hemorrhage I69.013
  visuospatial R41.842
    following
      cerebral infarction I69.312
      cerebrovascular disease I69.912
        specified disease NEC I69.812
      nontraumatic
        intracerebral hemorrhage I69.112
        specified intracranial hemorrhage NEC I69.212
        subarachnoid hemorrhage I69.012
Deflection
  radius — *see* Deformity, limb, specified type NEC, forearm
  septum (acquired) (nasal) (nose) J34.2
  spine — *see* Curvature, spine
  turbinate (nose) J34.2
Defluvium
  capillorum — *see* Alopecia
  ciliorum — *see* Madarosis
  unguium L60.8
Deformity Q89.9
  abdomen, congenital Q89.9
  abdominal wall
    acquired M95.8
    congenital Q79.59
  acquired (unspecified site) M95.9
  adrenal gland Q89.1
  alimentary tract, congenital Q45.9
    upper Q40.9
  ankle (joint) (acquired) — *see also* Deformity, limb, lower leg
    abduction — *see* Contraction, joint, ankle
    congenital Q68.8
    contraction — *see* Contraction, joint, ankle
    specified type NEC — *see* Deformity, limb, foot, specified NEC
  anus (acquired) K62.89
    congenital Q43.9
  aorta (arch) (congenital) Q25.40
    acquired I77.89
  aortic
    arch, acquired I77.89
    cusp or valve (congenital) Q23.8
      acquired — *see also* Endocarditis, aortic I35.8
  arm (acquired) (upper) — *see also* Deformity, limb, upper arm
    congenital Q68.8
    forearm — *see* Deformity, limb, forearm
  artery (congenital) (peripheral) NOS Q27.9
    acquired I77.89
    coronary (acquired) I25.9
      congenital Q24.5
    umbilical Q27.0
  atrial septal Q21.1
  auditory canal (external) (congenital) — *see also* Malformation, ear, external
    acquired — *see* Disorder, ear, external, specified type NEC
  auricle
    ear (congenital) — *see also* Malformation, ear, external
      acquired — *see* Disorder, pinna, deformity
  back — *see* Dorsopathy, deforming
  bile duct (common) (congenital) (hepatic) Q44.5
    acquired K83.8
  biliary duct or passage (congenital) Q44.5
    acquired K83.8

Deformity — *continued*
  bladder (neck) (trigone) (sphincter) (acquired) N32.89
    congenital Q64.79
  bone (acquired) NOS M95.9
    congenital Q79.9
    turbinate M95.0
  brain (congenital) Q04.9
    acquired G93.89
    reduction Q04.3
  breast (acquired) N64.89
    congenital Q83.9
    reconstructed N65.0
  bronchus (congenital) Q32.4
    acquired NEC J98.09
  bursa, congenital Q79.9
  canaliculi (lacrimalis) (acquired) — *see also* Disorder,
      lacrimal system, changes
    congenital Q10.6
  canthus, acquired — *see* Disorder, eyelid, specified
      type NEC
  capillary (acquired) I78.8
  cardiovascular system, congenital Q28.9
  caruncle, lacrimal (acquired) — *see also* Disorder,
      lacrimal system, changes
    congenital Q10.6
  cascade, stomach K31.2
  cecum (congenital) Q43.9
    acquired K63.89
  cerebral, acquired G93.89
    congenital Q04.9
  cervix (uterus) (acquired) NEC N88.8
    congenital Q51.9
  cheek (acquired) M95.2
    congenital Q18.9
  chest (acquired) (wall) M95.4
    congenital Q67.8
    sequelae (late effect) of rickets E64.3
  chin (acquired) M95.2
    congenital Q18.9
  choroid (congenital) Q14.3
    acquired H31.8
    plexus Q07.8
      acquired G96.19
  cicatricial — *see* Cicatrix
  cilia, acquired — *see* Disorder, eyelid, specified type
      NEC
  clavicle (acquired) M95.8
    congenital Q68.8
  clitoris (congenital) Q52.6
    acquired N90.89
  clubfoot — *see* Clubfoot
  coccyx (acquired) — *see* subcategory M43.8 ☑
  colon (congenital) Q43.9
    acquired K63.89
  concha (ear), congenital — *see also* Malformation, ear,
      external
    acquired — *see* Disorder, pinna, deformity
  cornea (acquired) H18.70
    congenital Q13.4
    descemetocele — *see* Descemetocele
    ectasia — *see* Ectasia, cornea
    specified NEC H18.79- ☑
    staphyloma — *see* Staphyloma, cornea
  coronary artery (acquired) I25.9
    congenital Q24.5
  cranium (acquired) — *see* Deformity, skull
  cricoid cartilage (congenital) Q31.8
    acquired J38.7
  cystic duct (congenital) Q44.5
    acquired K82.8
  Dandy-Walker Q03.1
    with spina bifida — *see* Spina bifida
  diaphragm (congenital) Q79.1
    acquired J98.6
  digestive organ NOS Q45.9
  ductus arteriosus Q25.0
  duodenal bulb K31.89
  duodenum (congenital) Q43.9
    acquired K31.89
  dura — *see* Deformity, meninges
  ear (acquired) — *see also* Disorder, pinna, deformity
    congenital (external) Q17.9
      internal Q16.5
      middle Q16.4
        ossicles Q16.3
      ossicles Q16.3
  ectodermal (congenital) NEC Q84.9
  ejaculatory duct (congenital) Q55.4

Deformity — *continued*
  ejaculatory duct — *continued*
    acquired N50.89
  elbow (joint) (acquired) — *see also* Deformity, limb,
      upper arm
    congenital Q68.8
    contraction — *see* Contraction, joint, elbow
  endocrine gland NEC Q89.2
  epididymis (congenital) Q55.4
    acquired N50.89
  epiglottis (congenital) Q31.8
    acquired J38.7
  esophagus (congenital) Q39.9
    acquired K22.8
  eustachian tube (congenital) NEC Q17.8
  eye, congenital Q15.9
  eyebrow (congenital) Q18.8
  eyelid (acquired) — *see also* Disorder, eyelid, specified
      type NEC
    congenital Q10.3
  face (acquired) M95.2
    congenital Q18.9
  fallopian tube, acquired N83.8
  femur (acquired) — *see* Deformity, limb, specified type
      NEC, thigh
  fetal
    with fetopelvic disproportion O33.7 ☑
    causing obstructed labor O66.3
  finger (acquired) M20.00- ☑
    boutonniere M20.02- ☑
    congenital Q68.1
    flexion contracture — *see* Contraction, joint, hand
    mallet finger M20.01- ☑
    specified NEC M20.09- ☑
    swan-neck M20.03- ☑
  flexion (joint) (acquired) — *see also* Deformity, limb,
      flexion M21.20
    congenital NOS Q74.9
    hip Q65.89
  foot (acquired) — *see also* Deformity, limb, lower leg
    cavovarus (congenital) Q66.1- ☑
    congenital NOS Q66.9- ☑
      specified type NEC Q66.89
    specified type NEC — *see* Deformity, limb, foot,
        specified NEC
    valgus (congenital) Q66.6
      acquired — *see* Deformity, valgus, ankle
    varus (congenital) NEC Q66.3- ☑
      acquired — *see* Deformity, varus, ankle
  forearm (acquired) — *see also* Deformity, limb, forearm
    congenital Q68.8
  forehead (acquired) M95.2
    congenital Q75.8
  frontal bone (acquired) M95.2
    congenital Q75.8
  gallbladder (congenital) Q44.1
    acquired K82.8
  gastrointestinal tract (congenital) NOS Q45.9
    acquired K63.89
  genitalia, genital organ(s) or system NEC
    female (congenital) Q52.9
      acquired N94.89
      external Q52.70
    male (congenital) Q55.9
      acquired N50.89
  globe (eye) (congenital) Q15.8
    acquired H44.89
  gum, acquired NEC K06.8
  hand (acquired) — *see* Deformity, limb, hand
    congenital Q68.1
  head (acquired) M95.2
    congenital Q75.8
  heart (congenital) Q24.9
    septum Q21.9
      auricular Q21.1
      ventricular Q21.0
    valve (congenital) NEC Q24.8
      acquired — *see* Endocarditis
  heel — *see* Deformity, foot
  hepatic duct (congenital) Q44.5
    acquired K83.8
  hip (joint) (acquired) (*see also* Deformity, limb, thigh)
    congenital Q65.9
    due to (previous) juvenile osteochondrosis — *see*
        Coxa, plana
    flexion — *see* Contraction, joint, hip
  hourglass — *see* Contraction, hourglass
  humerus (acquired) M21.82- ☑

Deformity — *continued*
  humerus — *continued*
    congenital Q74.0
  hypophyseal (congenital) Q89.2
  ileocecal (coil) (valve) (acquired) K63.89
    congenital Q43.9
  ileum (congenital) Q43.9
    acquired K63.89
  ilium (acquired) M95.5
    congenital Q74.2
  integument (congenital) Q84.9
  intervertebral cartilage or disc (acquired) — *see* Disor-
      der, disc, specified NEC
  intestine (large) (small) (congenital) NOS Q43.9
    acquired K63.89
  intrinsic minus or plus (hand) — *see* Deformity, limb,
      specified type NEC, forearm
  iris (acquired) H21.89
    congenital Q13.2
  ischium (acquired) M95.5
    congenital Q74.2
  jaw (acquired) (congenital) M26.9
  joint (acquired) NEC M21.90
    congenital Q68.8
    elbow M21.92- ☑
    hand M21.94- ☑
    hip M21.95- ☑
    knee M21.96- ☑
    shoulder M21.92- ☑
    wrist M21.93- ☑
  kidney(s) (calyx) (pelvis) (congenital) Q63.9
    acquired N28.89
    artery (congenital) Q27.2
      acquired I77.89
  Klippel-Feil (brevicollis) Q76.1
  knee (acquired) NEC — *see also* Deformity, limb, lower
      leg
    congenital Q68.2
  labium (majus) (minus) (congenital) Q52.79
    acquired N90.89
  lacrimal passages or duct (congenital) NEC Q10.6
    acquired — *see* Disorder, lacrimal system, changes
  larynx (muscle) (congenital) Q31.8
    acquired J38.7
    web (glottic) Q31.0
  leg (upper) (acquired) NEC — *see also* Deformity, limb,
      thigh
    congenital Q68.8
    lower leg — *see* Deformity, limb, lower leg
  lens (acquired) H27.8
    congenital Q12.9
  lid (fold) (acquired) — *see also* Disorder, eyelid, speci-
      fied type NEC
    congenital Q10.3
  ligament (acquired) — *see* Disorder, ligament
    congenital Q79.9
  limb (acquired) M21.90
    clawfoot M21.53- ☑
    clawhand M21.51- ☑
    clubfoot M21.54- ☑
    clubhand M21.52- ☑
    congenital, except reduction deformity Q74.9
    flat foot M21.4- ☑
    flexion M21.20
      ankle M21.27- ☑
      elbow M21.22- ☑
      finger M21.24- ☑
      hip M21.25- ☑
      knee M21.26- ☑
      shoulder M21.21- ☑
      toe M21.27- ☑
      wrist M21.23- ☑
    foot
      claw — *see* Deformity, limb, clawfoot
      club — *see* Deformity, limb, clubfoot
      drop M21.37-0
      flat — *see* Deformity, limb, flat foot
      specified NEC M21.6X- ☑
    forearm M21.93- ☑
    hand M21.94- ☑
    lower leg M21.96- ☑
    specified type NEC M21.80
      forearm M21.83- ☑
      lower leg M21.86- ☑
      thigh M21.85- ☑
      upper arm M21.82- ☑
    thigh M21.95- ☑

Deformity — *continued*
  limb — *continued*
    unequal length M21.70
      short site is
        femur M21.75- ☑
        fibula M21.76- ☑
        humerus M21.72- ☑
        radius M21.73- ☑
        tibia M21.76- ☑
        ulna M21.73- ☑
    upper arm M21.92- ☑
    valgus — *see* Deformity, valgus
    varus — *see* Deformity, varus
    wrist drop M21.33- ☑
  lip (acquired) NEC K13.0
    congenital Q38.0
  liver (congenital) Q44.7
    acquired K76.89
  lumbosacral (congenital) (joint) (region) Q76.49
    acquired — *see* subcategory M43.8 ☑
    kyphosis — *see* Kyphosis, congenital
    lordosis — *see* Lordosis, congenital
  lung (congenital) Q33.9
    acquired J98.4
  lymphatic system, congenital Q89.9
  Madelung's (radius) Q74.0
  mandible (acquired) (congenital) M26.9
  maxilla (acquired) (congenital) M26.9
  meninges or membrane (congenital) Q07.9
    cerebral Q04.8
      acquired G96.19
    spinal cord (congenital) G96.19
      acquired G96.19
  metacarpus (acquired) — *see* Deformity, limb, forearm
    congenital Q74.0
  metatarsus (acquired) — *see* Deformity, foot
    congenital Q66.9- ☑
  middle ear (congenital) Q16.4
    ossicles Q16.3
  mitral (leaflets) (valve) I05.8
    parachute Q23.2
    stenosis, congenital Q23.2
  mouth (acquired) K13.79
    congenital Q38.6
  multiple, congenital NEC Q89.7
  muscle (acquired) M62.89
    congenital Q79.9
      sternocleidomastoid Q68.0
  musculoskeletal system (acquired) M95.9
    congenital Q79.9
    specified NEC M95.8
  nail (acquired) L60.8
    congenital Q84.6
  nasal — *see* Deformity, nose
  neck (acquired) M95.3
    congenital Q18.9
      sternocleidomastoid Q68.0
  nervous system (congenital) Q07.9
  nipple (congenital) Q83.9
    acquired N64.89
  nose (acquired) (cartilage) M95.0
    bone (turbinate) M95.0
    congenital Q30.9
      bent or squashed Q67.4
    saddle M95.0
      syphilitic A50.57
    septum (acquired) J34.2
      congenital Q30.8
    sinus (wall) (congenital) Q30.8
      acquired M95.0
    syphilitic (congenital) A50.57
      late A52.73
  ocular muscle (congenital) Q10.3
    acquired — *see* Strabismus, mechanical
  opticociliary vessels (congenital) Q13.2
  orbit (eye) (acquired) H05.30
    atrophy — *see* Atrophy, orbit
    congenital Q10.7
    due to
      bone disease NEC H05.32- ☑
      trauma or surgery H05.33- ☑
    enlargement — *see* Enlargement, orbit
    exostosis — *see* Exostosis, orbit
  organ of Corti (congenital) Q16.5
  ovary (congenital) Q50.39
    acquired N83.8
  oviduct, acquired N83.8
  palate (congenital) Q38.5

Deformity — *continued*
  palate — *continued*
    acquired M27.8
    cleft (congenital) — *see* Cleft, palate
  pancreas (congenital) Q45.3
    acquired K86.89
  parathyroid (gland) Q89.2
  parotid (gland) (congenital) Q38.4
    acquired K11.8
  patella (acquired) — *see* Disorder, patella, specified NEC
  pelvis, pelvic (acquired) (bony) M95.5
    with disproportion (fetopelvic) O33.0
      causing obstructed labor O65.0
    congenital Q74.2
    rachitic sequelae (late effect) E64.3
  penis (glans) (congenital) Q55.69
    acquired N48.89
  pericardium (congenital) Q24.8
    acquired — *see* Pericarditis
  pharynx (congenital) Q38.8
    acquired J39.2
  pinna, acquired — *see also* Disorder, pinna, deformity
    congenital Q17.9
  pituitary (congenital) Q89.2
  posture — *see* Dorsopathy, deforming
  prepuce (congenital) Q55.69
    acquired N47.8
  prostate (congenital) Q55.4
    acquired N42.89
  pupil (congenital) Q13.2
    acquired — *see* Abnormality, pupillary
  pylorus (congenital) Q40.3
    acquired K31.89
  rachitic (acquired), old or healed E64.3
  radius (acquired) — *see also* Deformity, limb, forearm
    congenital Q68.8
  rectum (congenital) Q43.9
    acquired K62.89
  reduction (extremity) (limb), congenital — *see also* condition and site Q73.8
    brain Q04.3
    lower — *see* Defect, reduction, lower limb
    upper — *see* Defect, reduction, upper limb
  renal — *see* Deformity, kidney
  respiratory system (congenital) Q34.9
  rib (acquired) M95.4
    congenital Q76.6
      cervical Q76.5
  rotation (joint) (acquired) — *see* Deformity, limb, specified site NEC
    congenital Q74.9
    hip — *see* Deformity, limb, specified type NEC, thigh
      congenital Q65.89
  sacroiliac joint (congenital) — *see* subcategory Q74.2
    acquired — *see* subcategory M43.8 ☑
  sacrum (acquired) — *see* subcategory M43.8 ☑
  saddle
    back — *see* Lordosis
    nose M95.0
      syphilitic A50.57
  salivary gland or duct (congenital) Q38.4
    acquired K11.8
  scapula (acquired) M95.8
    congenital Q68.8
  scrotum (congenital) — *see also* Malformation, testis and scrotum
    acquired N50.89
  seminal vesicles (congenital) Q55.4
    acquired N50.89
  septum, nasal (acquired) J34.2
  shoulder (joint) (acquired) — *see* Deformity, limb, upper arm
    congenital Q74.0
    contraction — *see* Contraction, joint, shoulder
  sigmoid (flexure) (congenital) Q43.9
    acquired K63.89
  skin (congenital) Q82.9
  skull (acquired) M95.2
    congenital Q75.8
      with
        anencephaly Q00.0
        encephalocele — *see* Encephalocele
        hydrocephalus Q03.9
          with spina bifida — *see* Spina bifida, by site, with hydrocephalus
        microcephaly Q02

Deformity — *continued*
  soft parts, organs or tissues (of pelvis)
    in pregnancy or childbirth NEC O34.8- ☑
      causing obstructed labor O65.5
  spermatic cord (congenital) Q55.4
    acquired N50.89
      torsion — *see* Torsion, spermatic cord
  spinal — *see* Dorsopathy, deforming
    column (acquired) — *see* Dorsopathy, deforming
      congenital Q67.5
    cord (congenital) Q06.9
      acquired G95.89
    nerve root (congenital) Q07.9
  spine (acquired) — *see also* Dorsopathy, deforming
    congenital Q67.5
    rachitic E64.3
    specified NEC — *see* Dorsopathy, deforming, specified NEC
  spleen
    acquired D73.89
    congenital Q89.09
  Sprengel's (congenital) Q74.0
  sternocleidomastoid (muscle), congenital Q68.0
  sternum (acquired) M95.4
    congenital NEC Q76.7
  stomach (congenital) Q40.3
    acquired K31.89
  submandibular gland (congenital) Q38.4
  submaxillary gland (congenital) Q38.4
    acquired K11.8
  talipes — *see* Talipes
  testis (congenital) — *see also* Malformation, testis and scrotum
    acquired N44.8
    torsion — *see* Torsion, testis
  thigh (acquired) — *see also* Deformity, limb, thigh
    congenital NEC Q68.8
  thorax (acquired) (wall) M95.4
    congenital Q67.8
    sequelae of rickets E64.3
  thumb (acquired) — *see also* Deformity, finger
    congenital NEC Q68.1
  thymus (tissue) (congenital) Q89.2
  thyroid (gland) (congenital) Q89.2
    cartilage Q31.8
      acquired J38.7
  tibia (acquired) — *see also* Deformity, limb, specified type NEC, lower leg
    congenital NEC Q68.8
    saber (syphilitic) A50.56
  toe (acquired) M20.6- ☑
    congenital Q66.9- ☑
    hallux rigidus M20.2- ☑
    hallux valgus M20.1- ☑
    hallux varus M20.3- ☑
    hammer toe M20.4- ☑
    specified NEC M20.5X- ☑
  tongue (congenital) Q38.3
    acquired K14.8
  tooth, teeth K00.2
  trachea (rings) (congenital) Q32.1
    acquired J39.8
  transverse aortic arch (congenital) Q25.49
  tricuspid (leaflets) (valve) I07.8
    atresia or stenosis Q22.4
    Ebstein's Q22.5
  trunk (acquired) M95.8
    congenital Q89.9
  ulna (acquired) — *see also* Deformity, limb, forearm
    congenital NEC Q68.8
  urachus, congenital Q64.4
  ureter (opening) (congenital) Q62.8
    acquired N28.89
  urethra (congenital) Q64.79
    acquired N36.8
  urinary tract (congenital) Q64.9
    urachus Q64.4
  uterus (congenital) Q51.9
    acquired N85.8
  uvula (congenital) Q38.5
  vagina (acquired) N89.8
    congenital Q52.4
  valgus NEC M21.00
    ankle M21.07- ☑
    elbow M21.02- ☑
    hip M21.05- ☑
    knee M21.06- ☑
  valve, valvular (congenital) (heart) Q24.8

Deformity — continued

valve, valvular — *continued*
  acquired — *see* Endocarditis
varus NEC M21.10
  ankle M21.17- ☑
  elbow M21.12- ☑
  hip M21.15 ☑
  knee M21.16- ☑
  tibia — *see* Osteochondrosis, juvenile, tibia
vas deferens (congenital) Q55.4
  acquired N50.89
vein (congenital) Q27.9
  great Q26.9
vertebra — *see* Dorsopathy, deforming
vertical talus (congenital) Q66.80
  left foot Q66.82
  right foot Q66.81
vesicourethral orifice (acquired) N32.89
  congenital NEC Q64.79
vessels of optic papilla (congenital) Q14.2
visual field (contraction) — *see* Defect, visual field
vitreous body, acquired H43.89
vulva (congenital) Q52.79
  acquired N90.89
wrist (joint) (acquired) — *see also* Deformity, limb, forearm
  congenital Q68.8
  contraction — *see* Contraction, joint, wrist

Degeneration, degenerative

adrenal (capsule) (fatty) (gland) (hyaline) (infectional) E27.8
amyloid — *see also* Amyloidosis E85.9
anterior cornua, spinal cord G12.29
anterior labral S43.49- ☑
aorta, aortic I70.0
  fatty I77.89
aortic valve (heart) — *see* Endocarditis, aortic
arteriovascular — *see* Arteriosclerosis
artery, arterial (atheromatous) (calcareous) — *see also* Arteriosclerosis
  cerebral, amyloid E85.4 [I68.0]
  medial — *see* Arteriosclerosis, extremities
articular cartilage NEC — *see* Derangement, joint, articular cartilage, by site
atheromatous — *see* Arteriosclerosis
basal nuclei or ganglia G23.9
  specified NEC G23.8
bone NEC — *see* Disorder, bone, specified type NEC
brachial plexus G54.0
brain (cortical) (progressive) G31.9
  alcoholic G31.2
  arteriosclerotic I67.2
  childhood G31.9
    specified NEC G31.89
  cystic G31.89
    congenital Q04.6
  in
    alcoholism G31.2
    beriberi E51.2
    cerebrovascular disease I67.9
    congenital hydrocephalus Q03.9
      with spina bifida — *see also* Spina bifida
    Fabry-Anderson disease E75.21
    Gaucher's disease E75.22
    Hunter's syndrome E76.1
    lipidosis
      cerebral E75.4
      generalized E75.6
    mucopolysaccharidosis — *see* Mucopolysaccharidosis
    myxedema E03.9 [G32.89]
    neoplastic disease — *see also* Neoplasm D49.6 [G32.89]
    Niemann-Pick disease E75.249 [G32.89]
    sphingolipidosis E75.3 [G32.89]
    vitamin B12 deficiency E53.8 [G32.89]
  senile NEC G31.1
breast N64.89
Bruch's membrane — *see* Degeneration, choroid
capillaries (fatty) I78.8
  amyloid E85.89 [I79.8]
cardiac — *see also* Degeneration, myocardial
  valve, valvular — *see* Endocarditis
cardiorenal — *see* Hypertension, cardiorenal
cardiovascular — *see also* Disease, cardiovascular
  renal — *see* Hypertension, cardiorenal
cerebellar NOS G31.9
  alcoholic G31.2

Degeneration, degenerative — *continued*

cerebellar — *continued*
  primary (hereditary) (sporadic) G11.9
cerebral — *see* Degeneration, brain
cerebrovascular I67.9
  due to hypertension I67.4
cervical plexus G54.2
cervix N88.8
  due to radiation (intended effect) N88.8
    adverse effect or misadventure N99.89
chamber angle H21.21- ☑
changes, spine or vertebra — *see* Spondylosis
chorioretinal — *see also* Degeneration, choroid
  hereditary H31.20
choroid (colloid) (drusen) H31.10- ☑
  atrophy — *see* Atrophy, choroidal
  hereditary — *see* Dystrophy, choroidal, hereditary
ciliary body H21.22- ☑
cochlear — *see* subcategory H83.8 ☑
combined (spinal cord) (subacute) E53.8 [G32.0]
  with anemia (pernicious) D51.0 [G32.0]
    due to dietary vitamin B12 deficiency D51.3 [G32.0]
  in (due to)
    vitamin B12 deficiency E53.8 [G32.0]
      anemia D51.9 [G32.0]
conjunctiva H11.10
  concretions — *see* Concretion, conjunctiva
  deposits — *see* Deposit, conjunctiva
  pigmentations — *see* Pigmentation, conjunctiva
  pinguecula — *see* Pinguecula
  xerosis — *see* Xerosis, conjunctiva
cornea H18.40
  calcerous H18.43
    band keratopathy H18.42- ☑
  familial, hereditary — *see* Dystrophy, cornea
  hyaline (of old scars) H18.49
  keratomalacia — *see* Keratomalacia
  nodular H18.45- ☑
  peripheral H18.46- ☑
  senile H18.41- ☑
  specified type NEC H18.49
cortical (cerebellar) (parenchymatous) G31.89
  alcoholic G31.2
  diffuse, due to arteriopathy I67.2
corticobasal G31.85
cutis L98.8
  amyloid E85.4 [L99]
dental pulp K04.2
disc disease — *see* Degeneration, intervertebral disc NEC
dorsolateral (spinal cord) — *see* Degeneration, combined
extrapyramidal G25.9
eye, macular — *see also* Degeneration, macula
  congenital or hereditary — *see* Dystrophy, retina
facet joints — *see* Spondylosis
fatty
  liver NEC K76.0
    alcoholic K70.0
grey matter (brain) (Alpers') G31.81
heart — *see also* Degeneration, myocardial
  amyloid E85.4 [I43]
  atheromatous — *see* Disease, heart, ischemic, atherosclerotic
  ischemic — *see* Disease, heart, ischemic
hepatolenticular (Wilson's) E83.01
hepatorenal K76.7
hyaline (diffuse) (generalized)
  localized — *see* Degeneration, by site
infrapatellar fat pad M79.4
intervertebral disc NOS
  with
    myelopathy — *see* Disorder, disc, with, myelopathy
    radiculitis or radiculopathy — *see* Disorder, disc, with, radiculopathy
  cervical, cervicothoracic — *see* Disorder, disc, cervical, degeneration
    with
      myelopathy — *see* Disorder, disc, cervical, with myelopathy
      neuritis, radiculitis or radiculopathy — *see* Disorder, disc, cervical, with neuritis
  lumbar region M51.36
    with
      myelopathy M51.06

Degeneration, degenerative — *continued*

intervertebral disc — *continued*
  lumbar region — *continued*
    with — *continued*
      neuritis, radiculitis, radiculopathy or sciatica M51.16
  lumbosacral region M51.37
    with
      neuritis, radiculitis, radiculopathy or sciatica M51.17
  sacrococcygeal region M53.3
  thoracic region M51.34
    with
      myelopathy M51.04
      neuritis, radiculitis, radiculopathy M51.14
  thoracolumbar region M51.35
    with
      myelopathy M51.05
      neuritis, radiculitis, radiculopathy M51.15
intestine, amyloid E85.4
iris (pigmentary) H21.23- ☑
ischemic — *see* Ischemia
joint disease — *see* Osteoarthritis
kidney N28.89
  amyloid E85.4 [N29]
  cystic, congenital Q61.9
  fatty N28.89
  polycystic Q61.3
    adult type (autosomal dominant) Q61.2
    infantile type (autosomal recessive) NEC Q61.19
      collecting duct dilatation Q61.11
Kuhnt-Junius — *see also* Degeneration, macula H35.32- ☑
lens — *see* Cataract
lenticular (familial) (progressive) (Wilson's) (with cirrhosis of liver) E83.01
liver (diffuse) NEC K76.89
  amyloid E85.4 [K77]
  cystic K76.89
    congenital Q44.6
  fatty NEC K76.0
    alcoholic K70.0
  hypertrophic K76.89
  parenchymatous, acute or subacute K72.00
    with coma K72.01
  pigmentary K76.89
  toxic (acute) K71.9
lung J98.4
lymph gland I89.8
  hyaline I89.8
macula, macular (acquired) (age-related) (senile) H35.30
  angioid streaks H35.33
  atrophic age-related H35.31- ☑
  congenital or hereditary — *see* Dystrophy, retina
  cystoid H35.35- ☑
  drusen H35.36- ☑
  dry age-related H35.31- ☑
  exudative H35.32- ☑
  hole H35.34- ☑
  nonexudative H35.31- ☑
  puckering H35.37- ☑
  toxic H35.38- ☑
  wet age-related H35.32- ☑
membranous labyrinth, congenital (causing impairment of hearing) Q16.5
meniscus — *see* Derangement, meniscus
mitral — *see* Insufficiency, mitral
Mönckeberg's — *see* Arteriosclerosis, extremities
motor centers, senile G31.1
multi-system G90.3
mural — *see* Degeneration, myocardial
muscle (fatty) (fibrous) (hyaline) (progressive) M62.89
  heart — *see* Degeneration, myocardial
myelin, central nervous system G37.9
myocardial, myocardium (fatty) (hyaline) (senile) I51.5
  with rheumatic fever (conditions in I00) I09.0
    active, acute or subacute I01.2
      with chorea I02.0
    inactive or quiescent (with chorea) I09.0
  hypertensive — *see* Hypertension, heart
  rheumatic — *see* Degeneration, myocardial, with rheumatic fever
  syphilitic A52.06
nasal sinus (mucosa) J32.9
  frontal J32.1
  maxillary J32.0
nerve — *see* Disorder, nerve

☑ Additional Character Required — Refer to the Tabular List for Character Selection   ⬛ Subterms under main terms may continue to next column or page

Degeneration, degenerative — continued
- nervous system G31.9
  - alcoholic G31.2
  - amyloid E85.4 *[G99.8]*
  - autonomic G90.9
  - fatty G31.89
  - specified NEC G31.89
- nipple N64.89
- olivopontocerebellar (hereditary) (familial) G23.8
- osseous labyrinth — see subcategory H83.8 ☑
- ovary N83.8
  - cystic N83.20- ☑
  - microcystic N83.20- ☑
- pallidal pigmentary (progressive) G23.0
- pancreas K86.89
  - tuberculous A18.83
- penis N48.89
- pigmentary (diffuse) (general)
  - localized — see Degeneration, by site
  - pallidal (progressive) G23.0
- pineal gland E34.8
- pituitary (gland) E23.6
- popliteal fat pad M79.4
- posterolateral (spinal cord) — see Degeneration, combined
- pulmonary valve (heart) I37.8
- pulp (tooth) K04.2
- pupillary margin H21.24- ☑
- renal — see Degeneration, kidney
- retina H35.9
  - hereditary (cerebroretinal) (congenital) (juvenile) (macula) (peripheral) (pigmentary) — see Dystrophy, retina
  - Kuhnt-Junius — see also Degeneration, macula H35.32- ☑
  - macula (cystic) (exudative) (hole) (nonexudative) (pseudohole) (senile) (toxic) — see Degeneration, macula
  - peripheral H35.40
    - lattice H35.41- ☑
    - microcystoid H35.42- ☑
    - paving stone H35.43- ☑
    - secondary
      - pigmentary H35.45- ☑
      - vitreoretinal H35.46- ☑
    - senile reticular H35.44- ☑
  - pigmentary (primary) — see also Dystrophy, retina
    - secondary — see Degeneration, retina, peripheral, secondary
  - posterior pole — see Degeneration, macula
- saccule, congenital (causing impairment of hearing) Q16.5
- senile R54
  - brain G31.1
  - cardiac, heart or myocardium — see Degeneration, myocardial
  - motor centers G31.1
  - vascular — see Arteriosclerosis
- sinus (cystic) — see also Sinusitis
  - polypoid J33.1
- skin L98.8
  - amyloid E85.4 *[L99]*
  - colloid L98.8
- spinal (cord) G31.89
  - amyloid E85.4 *[G32.89]*
  - combined (subacute) — see Degeneration, combined
  - dorsolateral — see Degeneration, combined
  - familial NEC G31.89
  - fatty G31.89
  - funicular — see Degeneration, combined
  - posterolateral — see Degeneration, combined
  - subacute combined — see Degeneration, combined
  - tuberculous A17.81
- spleen D73.0
  - amyloid E85.4 *[D77]*
- stomach K31.89
- striatonigral G23.2
- suprarenal (capsule) (gland) E27.8
- synovial membrane (pulpy) — see Disorder, synovium, specified type NEC
- tapetoretinal — see Dystrophy, retina
- thymus (gland) E32.8
  - fatty E32.8
- thyroid (gland) E07.89
- tricuspid (heart) (valve) I07.9
- tuberculous NEC — see Tuberculosis
- turbinate J34.89

Degeneration, degenerative — continued
- uterus (cystic) N85.8
- vascular (senile) — see Arteriosclerosis
  - hypertensive — see Hypertension
- vitreoretinal, secondary — see Degeneration, retina, peripheral, secondary, vitreoretinal
- vitreous (body) H43.81- ☑
- Wallerian — see Disorder, nerve
- Wilson's hepatolenticular E83.01

Deglutition
- paralysis R13.0
  - hysterical F44.4
- pneumonia J69.0

Degos' disease I77.89

Dehiscence (of)
- amputation stump T87.81
- cesarean wound O90.0
- closure of
  - cornea T81.31 ☑
  - craniotomy T81.32 ☑
  - fascia (muscular) (superficial) T81.32 ☑
  - internal organ or tissue T81.32 ☑
  - laceration (external) (internal) T81.33 ☑
  - ligament T81.32 ☑
  - mucosa T81.31 ☑
  - muscle or muscle flap T81.32 ☑
  - ribs or rib cage T81.32 ☑
  - skin and subcutaneous tissue (full-thickness) (superficial) T81.31 ☑
  - skull T81.32 ☑
  - sternum (sternotomy) T81.32 ☑
  - tendon T81.32 ☑
  - traumatic laceration (external) (internal) T81.33 ☑
- episiotomy O90.1
- operation wound NEC T81.31 ☑
  - external operation wound (superficial) T81.31 ☑
  - internal operation wound (deep) T81.32 ☑
- perineal wound (postpartum) O90.1
- traumatic injury wound repair T81.33 ☑
- wound T81.30 ☑
  - traumatic repair T81.33 ☑

Dehydration E86.0
- newborn P74.1

Déjérine-Roussy syndrome G89.0

Déjérine-Sottas disease or neuropathy (hypertrophic) G60.0

Déjérine-Thomas atrophy G23.8

Delay, delayed
- any plane in pelvis
  - complicating delivery O66.9
- birth or delivery NOS O63.9
- closure, ductus arteriosus (Botalli) P29.38
- coagulation — see Defect, coagulation
- conduction (cardiac) (ventricular) I45.9
- delivery, second twin, triplet, etc O63.2
- development R62.50
  - global F88
  - intellectual (specific) F81.9
  - language F80.9
    - due to hearing loss F80.4
  - learning F81.9
  - pervasive F84.9
  - physiological R62.50
    - specified stage NEC R62.0
  - reading F81.0
  - sexual E30.0
  - speech F80.9
    - due to hearing loss F80.4
  - spelling F81.81
- ejaculation F52.32
- gastric emptying K30
- menarche E30.0
- menstruation (cause unknown) N91.0
- milestone R62.0
- passage of meconium (newborn) P76.0
- primary respiration P28.9
- puberty (constitutional) E30.0
- separation of umbilical cord P96.82
- sexual maturation, female E30.0
- sleep phase syndrome G47.21
- union, fracture — see Fracture, by site
- vaccination Z28.9

Deletion(s)
- autosome Q93.9
  - identified by fluorescence in situ hybridization (FISH) Q93.09
  - identified by in situ hybridization (ISH) Q93.89

Deletion(s) — continued
- chromosome
  - with complex rearrangements NEC Q93.7
  - part of NEC Q93.59
  - seen only at prometaphase Q93.89
  - short arm
    - 22q11.2 Q93.81
    - 4 Q93.3
    - 5p Q93.4
  - specified NEC Q93.89
  - long arm chromosome 18 or 21 Q93.89
  - with complex rearrangements NEC Q93.7
- microdeletions NEC Q93.88

Delhi boil or button B55.1

Delinquency (juvenile) (neurotic) F91.8
- group Z72.810

Delinquent immunization status Z28.3

Delirium, delirious (acute or subacute) (not alcohol- or drug-induced) (with dementia) R41.0
- alcoholic (acute) (tremens) (withdrawal) F10.921
  - with intoxication F10.921
    - in
      - abuse F10.121
      - dependence F10.221
- due to (secondary to)
  - alcohol
    - intoxication F10.921
      - in
        - abuse F10.121
        - dependence F10.221
    - withdrawal F10.231
  - amphetamine intoxication F15.921
    - in
      - abuse F15.121
      - dependence F15.221
  - anxiolytic
    - intoxication F13.921
      - in
        - abuse F13.121
        - dependence F13.221
    - withdrawal F13.231
  - cannabis intoxication (acute) F12.921
    - in
      - abuse F12.121
      - dependence F12.221
  - cocaine intoxication (acute) F14.921
    - in
      - abuse F14.121
      - dependence F14.221
  - general medical condition F05
  - hallucinogen intoxication F16.921
    - in
      - abuse F16.121
      - dependence F16.221
  - hypnotic
    - intoxication F13.921
      - in
        - abuse F13.121
        - dependence F13.221
    - withdrawal F13.231
  - inhalant intoxication (acute) F18.921
    - in
      - abuse F18.121
      - dependence F18.221
  - multiple etiologies F05
  - opioid intoxication (acute) F11.921
    - in
      - abuse F11.121
      - dependence F11.221
  - other (or unknown) substance F19.921
  - phencyclidine intoxication (acute) F16.921
    - in
      - abuse F16.121
      - dependence F16.221
  - psychoactive substance NEC intoxication (acute) F19.921
    - in
      - abuse F19.121
      - dependence F19.221
  - sedative
    - intoxication F13.921
      - in
        - abuse F13.121
        - dependence F13.221
    - withdrawal F13.231
- unknown etiology R41.0
- exhaustion F43.0
- hysterical F44.89
- postprocedural (postoperative) F05

Delirium, delirious — *continued*
 puerperal F05
 thyroid — *see* Thyrotoxicosis with thyroid storm
 traumatic — *see* Injury, intracranial
 tremens (alcohol-induced) F10.231
  sedative-induced F13.231
Delivery (childbirth) (labor)
 arrested active phase O62.1
 cesarean (for)
  abnormal
   pelvis (bony) (deformity) (major) NEC with dispro-
    portion (fetopelvic) O33.0
    with obstructed labor O65.0
   presentation or position O32.9 ☑
  abruptio placentae — *see also* Abruptio placentae
   O45.9- ☑
  acromion presentation O32.2 ☑
  atony, uterus O62.2
  breech presentation O32.1 ☑
   incomplete O32.8 ☑
  brow presentation O32.3 ☑
  cephalopelvic disproportion O33.9
  cerclage O34.3- ☑
  chin presentation O32.3 ☑
  cicatrix of cervix O34.4- ☑
  contracted pelvis (general)
   inlet O33.2
   outlet O33.3 ☑
  cord presentation or prolapse O69.0 ☑
  cystocele O34.8- ☑
  deformity (acquired) (congenital)
   pelvic organs or tissues NEC O34.8- ☑
   pelvis (bony) NEC O33.0
  disproportion NOS O33.9
  eclampsia — *see* Eclampsia
  face presentation O32.3 ☑
  failed
   forceps O66.5
   induction of labor O61.9
    instrumental O61.1
    mechanical O61.1
    medical O61.0
    specified NEC O61.8
    surgical O61.1
   trial of labor NOS O66.40
    following previous cesarean delivery O66.41
   vacuum extraction O66.5
   ventouse O66.5
  fetal-maternal hemorrhage O43.01- ☑
  hemorrhage (intrapartum) O67.9
   with coagulation defect O67.0
   specified cause NEC O67.8
  high head at term O32.4 ☑
  hydrocephalic fetus O33.6
  incarceration of uterus O34.51- ☑
  incoordinate uterine action O62.4
  increased size, fetus O33.5 ☑
  inertia, uterus O62.2
   primary O62.0
   secondary O62.1
  lateroversion, uterus O34.59- ☑
  mal lie O32.9 ☑
  malposition
   fetus O32.9 ☑
   pelvic organs or tissues NEC O34.8- ☑
   uterus NEC O34.59- ☑
  malpresentation NOS O32.9 ☑
  oblique presentation O32.2 ☑
  occurring after 37 completed weeks of gestation
   but before 39 completed weeks gestation due
   to (spontaneous) onset of labor O75.82
  oversize fetus O33.5 ☑
  pelvic tumor NEC O34.8- ☑
  placenta previa O44.0- ☑
   complete O44.0- ☑
    with hemorrhage O44.1- ☑
  placental insufficiency O36.51- ☑
  planned, occurring after 37 completed weeks of
   gestation but before 39 completed weeks
   gestation due to (spontaneous) onset of labor
   O75.82
  polyp, cervix O34.4- ☑
   causing obstructed labor O65.5
  poor dilatation, cervix O62.0
  pre-eclampsia O14.94
   mild O14.04
   moderate O14.04

Delivery — *continued*
 cesarean — *continued*
  pre-eclampsia — *continued*
   severe O14.14
    with hemolysis, elevated liver enzymes and
     low platelet count (HELLP) O14.24
  previous
   cesarean delivery O34.219
    classical (vertical) scar O34.212
    low transverse scar O34.211
   surgery (to)
    cervix O34.4- ☑
    gynecological NEC O34.8- ☑
    rectum O34.7- ☑
    uterus O34.29
    vagina O34.6- ☑
  prolapse
   arm or hand O32.2 ☑
   uterus O34.52- ☑
  prolonged labor NOS O63.9
  rectocele O34.8- ☑
  retroversion
   uterus O34.53- ☑
  rigid
   cervix O34.4- ☑
   pelvic floor O34.8- ☑
   perineum O34.7- ☑
   vagina O34.6- ☑
   vulva O34.7- ☑
  sacculation, pregnant uterus O34.59- ☑
  scar(s)
   cervix O34.4- ☑
   cesarean delivery O34.219
    classical (vertical) O34.212
    low transverse O34.211
   transmural uterine O34.29
   uterus O34.29
  Shirodkar suture in situ O34.3- ☑
  shoulder presentation O32.2 ☑
  stenosis or stricture, cervix O34.4- ☑
  streptococcus group B (GBS) carrier state O99.824
  transmural uterine scar O34.29
  transverse presentation or lie O32.2 ☑
  tumor, pelvic organs or tissues NEC O34.8- ☑
   cervix O34.4- ☑
  umbilical cord presentation or prolapse O69.0 ☑
  without indication O82
 completely normal case O80
 complicated O75.9
  by
   abnormal, abnormality (of)
    forces of labor O62.9
     specified type NEC O62.8
    glucose O99.814
    uterine contractions NOS O62.9
   abruptio placentae — *see also* Abruptio placen-
    tae O45.9- ☑
   abuse
    physical O9A.32 (*following* O99)
    psychological O9A.52 (*following* O99)
    sexual O9A.42 (*following* O99)
   adherent placenta O72.0
    without hemorrhage O73.0
   alcohol use O99.314
   anemia (pre-existing) O99.02
   anesthetic death O74.8
   annular detachment of cervix O71.3
   atony, uterus O62.2
   attempted vacuum extraction and forceps O66.5
   Bandl's ring O62.4
   bariatric surgery status O99.844
   biliary tract disorder O26.62
   bleeding — *see* Delivery, complicated by, hem-
    orrhage
   blood disorder NEC O99.12
   cervical dystocia (hypotonic) O62.2
    primary O62.0
    secondary O62.1
   circulatory system disorder O99.42
   compression of cord (umbilical) NEC O69.2 ☑
   condition NEC O99.89
   contraction, contracted ring O62.4
   cord (umbilical)
    around neck
     with compression O69.1 ☑
     without compression O69.81 ☑
    bruising O69.5 ☑
    complication O69.9 ☑

Delivery — *continued*
 complicated — *continued*
  by — *continued*
   cord — *continued*
    complication — *continued*
     specified NEC O69.89 ☑
    compression NEC O69.2 ☑
    entanglement O69.2 ☑
     without compression O69.82 ☑
    hematoma O69.5 ☑
    presentation O69.0 ☑
    prolapse O69.0 ☑
    short O69.3 ☑
    thrombosis (vessels) O69.5 ☑
    vascular lesion O69.5 ☑
   Couvelaire uterus O45.8X- ☑
   damage to (injury to) NEC
    perineum O71.82
    periurethral tissue O71.82
    vulva O71.82
   delay following rupture of membranes (sponta-
    neous) — *see* Pregnancy, complicated by,
    premature rupture of membranes
   depressed fetal heart tones O76
   diabetes O24.92
    gestational O24.429
     diet controlled O24.420
     insulin controlled O24.424
     oral drug controlled (antidiabetic) (hypo-
      glycemic) O24.425
    pre-existing O24.32
     specified NEC O24.82
     type 1 O24.02
     type 2 O24.12
   diastasis recti (abdominis) O71.89
   dilatation
    bladder O66.8
    cervix incomplete, poor or slow O62.0
   disease NEC O99.89
   disruptio uteri — *see* Delivery, complicated by,
    rupture, uterus
   drug use O99.324
   dysfunction, uterus NOS O62.9
    hypertonic O62.4
    hypotonic O62.2
     primary O62.0
     secondary O62.1
    incoordinate O62.4
   eclampsia O15.1
   embolism (pulmonary) — *see* Embolism, obstet-
    ric
   endocrine, nutritional or metabolic disease NEC
    O99.284
   failed
    attempted vaginal birth after previous cesare-
     an delivery O66.41
    induction of labor O61.9
     instrumental O61.1
     mechanical O61.1
     medical O61.0
     specified NEC O61.8
     surgical O61.1
    trial of labor O66.40
   female genital mutilation O65.5
   fetal
    abnormal acid-base balance O68
    acidemia O68
    acidosis O68
    alkalosis O68
    death, early O02.1
    deformity O66.3
    heart rate or rhythm (abnormal) (non-reassur-
     ing) O76
    hypoxia O77.8
    stress O77.9
     due to drug administration O77.1
     electrocardiographic evidence of O77.8
     specified NEC O77.8
     ultrasound evidence of O77.8
   fever during labor O75.2
   gastric banding status O99.844
   gastric bypass status O99.844
   gastrointestinal disease NEC O99.62
   gestational
    diabetes O24.429
     diet controlled O24.420
     insulin (and diet) controlled O24.424

☑ **Additional Character Required** — Refer to the Tabular List for Character Selection   ▽ **Subterms under main terms may continue to next column or page**

Delivery — *continued*
  complicated — *continued*
    by — *continued*
      gestational — *continued*
        diabetes — *continued*
          oral drug controlled (antidiabetic) (hypo-glycemic) O24.425
        edema O12.04
          with proteinuria O12.24
        proteinuria O12.14
      gonorrhea O98.22
      hematoma O71.7
        ischial spine O71.7
        pelvic O71.7
        vagina O71.7
        vulva or perineum O71.7
      hemorrhage (uterine) O67.9
        associated with
          afibrinogenemia O67.0
          coagulation defect O67.0
          hyperfibrinolysis O67.0
          hypofibrinogenemia O67.0
        due to
          low implantation of placenta O44.5- ☑
          low-lying placenta O44.5- ☑
          placenta previa O44.1- ☑
            marginal O44.3- ☑
            partial O44.3- ☑
          premature separation of placenta (normally implanted) — *see also* Abruptio placentae O45.9- ☑
          retained placenta O72.0
          uterine leiomyoma O67.8
        placenta NEC O67.8
        postpartum NEC (atonic) (immediate) O72.1
          with retained or trapped placenta O72.0
         delayed O72.2
        secondary O72.2
        third stage O72.0
      hourglass contraction, uterus O62.4
      hypertension, hypertensive (pre-existing) — *see* Hypertension, complicated by, childbirth (labor)
      hypotension O26.5- ☑
      incomplete dilatation (cervix) O62.0
      incoordinate uterus contractions O62.4
      inertia, uterus O62.2
        during latent phase of labor O62.0
        primary O62.0
        secondary O62.1
      infection (maternal) O98.92
        carrier state NEC O99.834
        gonorrhea O98.22
        human immunodeficiency virus (HIV) O98.72
        sexually transmitted NEC O98.32
        specified NEC O98.82
        syphilis O98.12
        tuberculosis O98.02
        viral hepatitis O98.42
        viral NEC O98.52
      injury (to mother) — *see also* Delivery, complicated, by, damage to O71.9
        nonobstetric O9A.22 (*following* O99)
          caused by abuse — *see* Delivery, complicated by, abuse
      intrauterine fetal death, early O02.1
      inversion, uterus O71.2
      laceration (perineal) O70.9
        anus (sphincter) O70.4
          with third degree laceration — *see also* Delivery, complicated, by, laceration, perineum, third degree O70.20
            with mucosa O70.3
          without third degree laceration O70.2 ☑
        bladder (urinary) O71.5
        bowel O71.5
        cervix (uteri) O71.3
        fourchette O70.0
        hymen O70.0
        labia O70.0
        pelvic
          floor O70.1
          organ NEC O71.5
        perineum, perineal O70.9
          first degree O70.0
          fourth degree O70.3
          muscles O70.1

Delivery — *continued*
  complicated — *continued*
    by — *continued*
      laceration — *continued*
        perineum, perineal — *continued*
          second degree O70.1
          skin O70.0
          slight O70.0
          third degree O70.20
            with
              both external anal sphincter (EAS) and internal anal sphincter (IAS) torn (IIIc) O70.23
              less than 50% of external anal sphincter (EAS) thickness torn (IIIa) O70.21
              more than 50% external anal sphincter (EAS) thickness torn (IIIb) O70.22
            IIIa O70.21
            IIIb O70.22
            IIIc O70.23
        peritoneum (pelvic) O71.5
        rectovaginal (septum) (without perineal laceration) O71.4
          with perineum — *see also* Delivery, complicated, by, laceration, perineum, third degree O70.20
          with anal or rectal mucosa O70.3
        specified NEC O71.89
        sphincter ani — *see* Delivery, complicated, by, laceration, anus (sphincter)
        urethra O71.5
        uterus O71.81
          before labor O71.81
        vagina, vaginal (deep) (high) (without perineal laceration) O71.4
          with perineum O70.0
            muscles, with perineum O70.1
        vulva O70.0
      liver disorder O26.62
      malignancy O9A.12 (*following* O99)
      malnutrition O25.2
      malposition, malpresentation
        uterus or cervix O65.5
        placenta O44.0- ☑
          with hemorrhage O44.1- ☑
        without obstruction — *see also* Delivery, complicated by, obstruction O32.9 ☑
          breech O32.1 ☑
          compound O32.6 ☑
          face (brow) (chin) O32.3 ☑
          footling O32.8 ☑
          high head O32.4 ☑
          oblique O32.2 ☑
          specified NEC O32.8 ☑
          transverse O32.2 ☑
          unstable lie O32.0 ☑
      meconium in amniotic fluid O77.0
      mental disorder NEC O99.344
      metrorrhexis — *see* Delivery, complicated by, rupture, uterus
      nervous system disorder O99.354
      obesity (pre-existing) O99.214
      obesity surgery status O99.844
      obstetric trauma O71.9
        specified NEC O71.89
      obstructed labor
        due to
          breech (complete) (frank) presentation O64.1 ☑
            incomplete O64.8 ☑
          brow presentation O64.3 ☑
          buttock presentation O64.1 ☑
          chin presentation O64.2 ☑
          compound presentation O64.5 ☑
          contracted pelvis O65.1
          deep transverse arrest O64.0 ☑
          deformed pelvis O65.0
          dystocia (fetal) O66.9
            due to
              conjoined twins O66.3
              fetal
                abnormality NEC O66.3
                ascites O66.3
                hydrops O66.3
                meningomyelocele O66.3
                sacral teratoma O66.3

Delivery — *continued*
  complicated — *continued*
    by — *continued*
      obstructed labor — *continued*
        due to — *continued*
          dystocia — *continued*
            due to — *continued*
              fetal — *continued*
                tumor O66.3
              hydrocephalic fetus O66.3
              shoulder O66.0
          face presentation O64.2 ☑
          fetopelvic disproportion O65.4
          footling presentation O64.8 ☑
          impacted shoulders O66.0
          incomplete rotation of fetal head O64.0 ☑
          large fetus O66.2
          locked twins O66.1
          malposition O64.9 ☑
            specified NEC O64.8 ☑
          malpresentation O64.9 ☑
            specified NEC O64.8 ☑
          multiple fetuses NEC O66.6
          pelvic
            abnormality (maternal) O65.9
              organ O65.5
              specified NEC O65.8
            contraction
              inlet O65.2
              mid-cavity O65.3
              outlet O65.3
          persistent (position)
            occipitoiliac O64.0 ☑
            occipitoposterior O64.0 ☑
            occipitosacral O64.0 ☑
            occipitotransverse O64.0 ☑
          prolapsed arm O64.4 ☑
          shoulder presentation O64.4 ☑
        specified NEC O66.8
      pathological retraction ring, uterus O62.4
      penetration, pregnant uterus by instrument O71.1
      perforation — *see* Delivery, complicated by, laceration
      placenta, placental
        ablatio — *see also* Abruptio placentae O45.9- ☑
        abnormality O43.9- ☑
          specified NEC O43.89- ☑
        abruptio — *see also* Abruptio placentae O45.9- ☑
        accreta O43.21- ☑
        adherent (with hemorrhage) O72.0
          without hemorrhage O73.0
        detachment (premature) — *see also* Abruptio placentae O45.9- ☑
        disorder O43.9- ☑
          specified NEC O43.89- ☑
        hemorrhage NEC O67.8
        increta O43.22- ☑
        low (implantation) (lying) O44.4- ☑
          with hemorrhage O44.5- ☑
        malformation O43.10- ☑
        malposition O44.0- ☑
          without hemorrhage O44.1- ☑
        percreta O43.23- ☑
        previa (central) (complete) (lateral) (total) O44.0- ☑
          with hemorrhage O44.1- ☑
          marginal O44.2- ☑
            with hemorrhage O44.3- ☑
          partial O44.2- ☑
            with hemorrhage O44.3- ☑
        retained (with hemorrhage) O72.0
          without hemorrhage O73.0
        separation (premature) O45.9- ☑
          specified NEC O45.8X- ☑
        vicious insertion O44.1- ☑
      precipitate labor O62.3
      premature rupture, membranes — *see also* Pregnancy, complicated by, premature rupture of membranes O42.90
      prolapse
        arm or hand O32.2 ☑
        cord (umbilical) O69.0 ☑
        foot or leg O32.8 ☑

Delivery — *continued*
complicated — *continued*
  by — *continued*
    prolapse — *continued*
      uterus O34.52- ☑
    prolonged labor O63.9
      first stage O63.0
      second stage O63.1
    protozoal disease (maternal) O98.62
    respiratory disease NEC O99.52
    retained membranes or portions of placenta O72.2
      without hemorrhage O73.1
    retarded birth O63.9
    retention of secundines (with hemorrhage) O72.0
      without hemorrhage O73.0
      partial O72.2
        without hemorrhage O73.1
    rupture
      bladder (urinary) O71.5
      cervix O71.3
      pelvic organ NEC O71.5
      urethra O71.5
      uterus (during or after labor) O71.1
        before labor O71.0- ☑
    separation, pubic bone (symphysis pubis) O71.6
    shock O75.1
    shoulder presentation O64.4 ☑
    skin disorder NEC O99.72
    spasm, cervix O62.4
    stenosis or stricture, cervix O65.5
    streptococcus group B (GBS) carrier state O99.824
    subluxation of symphysis (pubis) O26.72
    syphilis (maternal) O98.12
    tear — *see* Delivery, complicated by, laceration
    tetanic uterus O62.4
    trauma (obstetrical) — *see also* Delivery, complicated, by, damage to O71.9
      non-obstetric O9A.22 (*following* O99)
      periurethral O71.82
      specified NEC O71.89
    tuberculosis (maternal) O98.02
    tumor, pelvic organs or tissues NEC O65.5
    umbilical cord around neck
      with compression O69.1 ☑
      without compression O69.81 ☑
    uterine inertia O62.2
      during latent phase of labor O62.0
      primary O62.0
      secondary O62.1
    vasa previa O69.4 ☑
    velamentous insertion of cord O43.12- ☑
  specified complication NEC O75.89
  delayed NOS O63.9
    •following rupture of membranes
      artificial O75.5
    second twin, triplet, etc. O63.2
  forceps, low following failed vacuum extraction O66.5
  missed (at or near term) O36.4 ☑
  normal O80
  obstructed — *see* Delivery, complicated by, obstructed labor
  precipitate O62.3
  preterm — *see also* Pregnancy, complicated by, preterm labor O60.10 ☑
  spontaneous O80
  term pregnancy NOS O80
  uncomplicated O80
  vaginal, following previous cesarean delivery O34.219
    classical (vertical) scar O34.212
    low transverse scar O34.211
Delusions (paranoid) — *see* Disorder, delusional
Dementia (degenerative (primary)) (old age) (persisting) F03.90
  with
    aggressive behavior F03.91
    behavioral disturbance F03.91
    combative behavior F03.91
    Lewy bodies G31.83 *[F02.80]*
      with behavioral disturbance G31.83 *[F02.81]*
    Parkinsonism G31.83 *[F02.80]*
      with behavioral disturbance G31.83 *[F02.81]*
    Parkinson's disease G20 *[F02.80]*
      with behavioral disturbance G20 *[F02.81]*
    violent behavior F03.91
  alcoholic F10.97
    with dependence F10.27
  Alzheimer's type — *see* Disease, Alzheimer's

Dementia — *continued*
arteriosclerotic — *see* Dementia, vascular
atypical, Alzheimer's type — *see* Disease, Alzheimer's, specified NEC
congenital — *see* Disability, intellectual
frontal (lobe) G31.09 *[F02.80]*
  with behavioral disturbance G31.09 *[F02.81]*
frontotemporal G31.09 *[F02.80]*
  with behavioral disturbance G31.09 *[F02.81]*
  specified NEC G31.09 *[F02.80]*
    with behavioral disturbance G31.09 *[F02.81]*
Huntington's disease or chorea G10
  with dementia G10 *[F02.80]*
in (due to)
  with behavioral disturbance G31.83 *[F02.81]*
  alcohol F10.97
    with dependence F10.27
  Alzheimer's disease — *see* Disease, Alzheimer's
  arteriosclerotic brain disease — *see* Dementia, vascular
  cerebral lipidoses E75.- ☑ *[F02.80]*
    with behavioral disturbance E75.- ☑ *[F02.81]*
  Creutzfeldt-Jakob disease — *see also* Creutzfeldt-Jakob disease or syndrome (with dementia) A81.00
  epilepsy G40.- ☑ *[F02.80]*
    with behavioral disturbance G40.- ☑ *[F02.81]*
  hepatolenticular degeneration E83.01 *[F02.80]*
    with behavioral disturbance E83.01 *[F02.81]*
  human immunodeficiency virus (HIV) disease B20 *[F02.80]*
    with behavioral disturbance B20 *[F02.81]*
  Huntington's disease or chorea G10 *[F02.80]*
    with behavioral disturbance G10 *[F02.81]*
  hypercalcemia E83.52 *[F02.80]*
    with behavioral disturbance E83.52 *[F02.81]*
  hypothyroidism, acquired E03.9 *[F02.80]*
    with behavioral disturbance E03.9 *[F02.81]*
    due to iodine deficiency E01.8 *[F02.80]*
      with behavioral disturbance E01.8 *[F02.81]*
  inhalants F18.97
    with dependence F18.27
  multiple
    etiologies F03 ☑
    sclerosis G35 *[F02.80]*
      with behavioral disturbance G35 *[F02.81]*
  neurosyphilis A52.17 *[F02.80]*
    with behavioral disturbance A52.17 *[F02.81]*
    juvenile A50.49 *[F02.80]*
      with behavioral disturbance A50.49 *[F02.81]*
  niacin deficiency E52 *[F02.80]*
    with behavioral disturbance E52 *[F02.81]*
  paralysis agitans G20 *[F02.80]*
    with behavioral disturbance G20 *[F02.81]*
  Parkinson's disease G20 *[F02.80]*
  pellagra E52 *[F02.80]*
    with behavioral disturbance E52 *[F02.81]*
  Pick's G31.01 *[F02.80]*
    with behavioral disturbance G31.01 *[F02.81]*
  polyarteritis nodosa M30.0 *[F02.80]*
    with behavioral disturbance M30.0 *[F02.81]*
  psychoactive drug F19.97
    with dependence F19.27
    inhalants F18.97
      with dependence F18.27
    sedatives, hypnotics or anxiolytics F13.97
      with dependence F13.27
  sedatives, hypnotics or anxiolytics F13.97
    with dependence F13.27
  systemic lupus erythematosus M32.- ☑ *[F02.80]*
    with behavioral disturbance M32.- ☑ *[F02.81]*
  trypanosomiasis
    African B56.9 *[F02.80]*
      with behavioral disturbance B56.9 *[F02.81]*
  unknown etiology F03 ☑
  vitamin B12 deficiency E53.8 *[F02.80]*
    with behavioral disturbance E53.8 *[F02.81]*
  volatile solvents F18.97
    with dependence F18.27
infantile, infantilis F84.3
Lewy body G31.83 *[F02.80]*
  with behavioral disturbance G31.83 *[F02.81]*
multi-infarct — *see* Dementia, vascular
paralytica, paralytic (syphilitic) A52.17 *[F02.80]*
  with behavioral disturbance A52.17 *[F02.81]*
  juvenilis A50.45
paretic A52.17

Dementia — *continued*
praecox — *see* Schizophrenia
presenile F03 ☑
  Alzheimer's type — *see* Disease, Alzheimer's, early onset
primary degenerative F03 ☑
progressive, syphilitic A52.17
senile F03 ☑
  with acute confusional state F05
  Alzheimer's type — *see* Disease, Alzheimer's, late onset
  depressed or paranoid type F03 ☑
vascular (acute onset) (mixed) (multi-infarct) (subcortical) F01.50
  with behavioral disturbance F01.51
Demineralization, bone — *see* Osteoporosis
Demodex folliculorum (infestation) B88.0
Demophobia F40.248
Demoralization R45.3
Demyelination, demyelinization
  central nervous system G37.9
    specified NEC G37.8
  corpus callosum (central) G37.1
  disseminated, acute G36.9
    specified NEC G36.8
  global G35
  in optic neuritis G36.0
Dengue (classical) (fever) A90
  hemorrhagic A91
  sandfly A93.1
Dennie-Marfan syphilitic syndrome A50.45
Dens evaginatus, in dente or invaginatus K00.2
Dense breasts R92.2
Density
  increased, bone (disseminated) (generalized) (spotted) — *see* Disorder, bone, density and structure, specified type NEC
  lung (nodular) J98.4
Dental — *see also* condition
  examination Z01.20
    with abnormal findings Z01.21
  restoration
    aesthetically inadequate or displeasing K08.56
    defective K08.50
      specified NEC K08.59
    failure of marginal integrity K08.51
    failure of periodontal anatomical integrity K08.54
Dentia praecox K00.6
Denticles (pulp) K04.2
Dentigerous cyst K09.0
Dentin
  irregular (in pulp) K04.3
  opalescent K00.5
  secondary (in pulp) K04.3
  sensitive K03.89
Dentinogenesis imperfecta K00.5
Dentinoma — *see* Cyst, calcifying odontogenic
Dentition (syndrome) K00.7
  delayed K00.6
  difficult K00.7
  precocious K00.6
  premature K00.6
  retarded K00.6
Dependence (on) (syndrome) F19.20
  with remission F19.21
  alcohol (ethyl) (methyl) (without remission) F10.20
    with
      amnestic disorder, persisting F10.26
      anxiety disorder F10.280
      dementia, persisting F10.27
      intoxication F10.229
        with delirium F10.221
        uncomplicated F10.220
      mood disorder F10.24
      psychotic disorder F10.259
        with
          delusions F10.250
          hallucinations F10.251
      remission F10.21
      sexual dysfunction F10.281
      sleep disorder F10.282
      specified disorder NEC F10.288
      withdrawal F10.239
        with
          delirium F10.231
          perceptual disturbance F10.232
        uncomplicated F10.230
    counseling and surveillance Z71.41

Dependence — continued
- amobarbital — see Dependence, drug, sedative
- amphetamine(s) (type) — see Dependence, drug, stimulant NEC
- amytal (sodium) — see Dependence, drug, sedative
- analgesic NEC F55.8
- anesthetic (agent) (gas) (general) (local) NEC — see Dependence, drug, psychoactive NEC
- anxiolytic NEC — see Dependence, drug, sedative
- barbital(s) — see Dependence, drug, sedative
- barbiturate(s) (compounds) (drugs classifiable to T42) — see Dependence, drug, sedative
- benzedrine — see Dependence, drug, stimulant NEC
- bhang — see Dependence, drug, cannabis
- bromide(s) NEC — see Dependence, drug, sedative
- caffeine — see Dependence, drug, stimulant NEC
- cannabis (sativa) (indica) (resin) (derivatives) (type) — see Dependence, drug, cannabis
- chloral (betaine) (hydrate) — see Dependence, drug, sedative
- chlordiazepoxide — see Dependence, drug, sedative
- coca (leaf) (derivatives) — see Dependence, drug, cocaine
- cocaine — see Dependence, drug, cocaine
- codeine — see Dependence, drug, opioid
- combinations of drugs F19.20
- dagga — see Dependence, drug, cannabis
- demerol — see Dependence, drug, opioid
- dexamphetamine — see Dependence, drug, stimulant NEC
- dexedrine — see Dependence, drug, stimulant NEC
- dextromethorphan — see Dependence, drug, opioid
- dextromoramide — see Dependence, drug, opioid
- dextro-nor-pseudo-ephedrine — see Dependence, drug, stimulant NEC
- dextrorphan — see Dependence, drug, opioid
- diazepam — see Dependence, drug, sedative
- dilaudid — see Dependence, drug, opioid
- D-lysergic acid diethylamide — see Dependence, drug, hallucinogen
- drug NEC F19.20
  - with sleep disorder F19.282
  - cannabis F12.20
    - with
      - anxiety disorder F12.280
      - intoxication F12.229
        - with
          - delirium F12.221
          - perceptual disturbance F12.222
        - uncomplicated F12.220
      - other specified disorder F12.288
      - psychosis F12.259
        - delusions F12.250
        - hallucinations F12.251
      - unspecified disorder F12.29
      - withdrawal F12.23
    - in remission F12.21
  - cocaine F14.20
    - with
      - anxiety disorder F14.280
      - intoxication F14.229
        - with
          - delirium F14.221
          - perceptual disturbance F14.222
        - uncomplicated F14.220
      - mood disorder F14.24
      - other specified disorder F14.288
      - psychosis F14.259
        - delusions F14.250
        - hallucinations F14.251
      - sexual dysfunction F14.281
      - sleep disorder F14.282
      - unspecified disorder F14.29
      - withdrawal F14.23
    - in remission F14.21
    - withdrawal symptoms in newborn P96.1
  - counseling and surveillance Z71.51
  - hallucinogen F16.20
    - with
      - anxiety disorder F16.280
      - flashbacks F16.283
      - intoxication F16.229
        - with delirium F16.221
        - uncomplicated F16.220
      - mood disorder F16.24
      - other specified disorder F16.288
      - perception disorder, persisting F16.283
      - psychosis F16.259

Dependence — continued
- drug — continued
  - hallucinogen — continued
    - with — continued
      - psychosis — continued
        - delusions F16.250
        - hallucinations F16.251
      - unspecified disorder F16.29
    - in remission F16.21
  - in remission F19.21
  - inhalant F18.20
    - with
      - anxiety disorder F18.280
      - dementia, persisting F18.27
      - intoxication F18.229
        - with delirium F18.221
        - uncomplicated F18.220
      - mood disorder F18.24
      - other specified disorder F18.288
      - psychosis F18.259
        - delusions F18.250
        - hallucinations F18.251
      - unspecified disorder F18.29
    - in remission F18.21
  - nicotine F17.200
    - with disorder F17.209
      - in remission F17.201
      - specified disorder NEC F17.208
      - withdrawal F17.203
    - chewing tobacco F17.220
      - with disorder F17.229
        - in remission F17.221
        - specified disorder NEC F17.228
        - withdrawal F17.223
    - cigarettes F17.210
      - with disorder F17.219
        - in remission F17.211
        - specified disorder NEC F17.218
        - withdrawal F17.213
    - specified product NEC F17.290
      - with disorder F17.299
        - remission F17.291
        - specified disorder NEC F17.298
        - withdrawal F17.293
  - opioid F11.20
    - with
      - intoxication F11.229
        - with
          - delirium F11.221
          - perceptual disturbance F11.222
        - uncomplicated F11.220
      - mood disorder F11.24
      - other specified disorder F11.288
      - psychosis F11.259
        - delusions F11.250
        - hallucinations F11.251
      - sexual dysfunction F11.281
      - sleep disorder F11.282
      - unspecified disorder F11.29
      - withdrawal F11.23
    - in remission F11.21
  - psychoactive NEC F19.20
    - with
      - amnestic disorder F19.26
      - anxiety disorder F19.280
      - dementia F19.27
      - intoxication F19.229
        - with
          - delirium F19.221
          - perceptual disturbance F19.222
        - uncomplicated F19.220
      - mood disorder F19.24
      - other specified disorder F19.288
      - psychosis F19.259
        - delusions F19.250
        - hallucinations F19.251
      - sexual dysfunction F19.281
      - sleep disorder F19.282
      - unspecified disorder F19.29
      - withdrawal F19.239
        - with
          - delirium F19.231
          - perceptual disturbance F19.232
        - uncomplicated F19.230
  - sedative, hypnotic or anxiolytic F13.20
    - with
      - amnestic disorder F13.26
      - anxiety disorder F13.280
      - dementia, persisting F13.27

Dependence — continued
- drug — continued
  - sedative, hypnotic or anxiolytic — continued
    - with — continued
      - intoxication F13.229
        - with delirium F13.221
        - uncomplicated F13.220
      - mood disorder F13.24
      - other specified disorder F13.288
      - psychosis F13.259
        - delusions F13.250
        - hallucinations F13.251
      - sexual dysfunction F13.281
      - sleep disorder F13.282
      - unspecified disorder F13.29
      - withdrawal F13.239
        - with
          - delirium F13.231
          - perceptual disturbance F13.232
        - uncomplicated F13.230
    - in remission F13.21
  - stimulant NEC F15.20
    - with
      - anxiety disorder F15.280
      - intoxication F15.229
        - with
          - delirium F15.221
          - perceptual disturbance F15.222
        - uncomplicated F15.220
      - mood disorder F15.24
      - other specified disorder F15.288
      - psychosis F15.259
        - delusions F15.250
        - hallucinations F15.251
      - sexual dysfunction F15.281
      - sleep disorder F15.282
      - unspecified disorder F15.29
      - withdrawal F15.23
    - in remission F15.21
- ethyl
  - alcohol (without remission) F10.20
    - with remission F10.21
  - bromide — see Dependence, drug, sedative
  - carbamate F19.20
  - chloride F19.20
  - morphine — see Dependence, drug, opioid
- ganja — see Dependence, drug, cannabis
- glue (airplane) (sniffing) — see Dependence, drug, inhalant
- glutethimide — see Dependence, drug, sedative
- hallucinogenics — see Dependence, drug, hallucinogen
- hashish — see Dependence, drug, cannabis
- hemp — see Dependence, drug, cannabis
- heroin (salt) (any) — see Dependence, drug, opioid
- hypnotic NEC — see Dependence, drug, sedative
- Indian hemp — see Dependence, drug, cannabis
- inhalants — see Dependence, drug, inhalant
- khat — see Dependence, drug, stimulant NEC
- laudanum — see Dependence, drug, opioid
- LSD (-25) (derivatives) — see Dependence, drug, hallucinogen
- luminal — see Dependence, drug, sedative
- lysergic acid — see Dependence, drug, hallucinogen
- maconha — see Dependence, drug, cannabis
- marihuana — see Dependence, drug, cannabis
- meprobamate — see Dependence, drug, sedative
- mescaline — see Dependence, drug, hallucinogen
- methadone — see Dependence, drug, opioid
- methamphetamine(s) — see Dependence, drug, stimulant NEC
- methaqualone — see Dependence, drug, sedative
- methyl
  - alcohol (without remission) F10.20
    - with remission F10.21
  - bromide — see Dependence, drug, sedative
  - morphine — see Dependence, drug, opioid
  - phenidate — see Dependence, drug, stimulant NEC
  - sulfonal — see Dependence, drug, sedative
- morphine (sulfate) (sulfite) (type) — see Dependence, drug, opioid
- narcotic (drug) NEC — see Dependence, drug, opioid
- nembutal — see Dependence, drug, sedative
- neraval — see Dependence, drug, sedative
- neravan — see Dependence, drug, sedative
- neurobarb — see Dependence, drug, sedative
- nicotine — see Dependence, drug, nicotine
- nitrous oxide F19.20

Dependence — *continued*
nonbarbiturate sedatives and tranquilizers with similar effect — *see* Dependence, drug, sedative
on
  artificial heart (fully implantable) (mechanical) Z95.812
  aspirator Z99.0
  care provider (because of) Z74.9
    impaired mobility Z74.09
    need for
      assistance with personal care Z74.1
      continuous supervision Z74.3
    no other household member able to render care Z74.2
    specified reason NEC Z74.8
  machine Z99.89
    enabling NEC Z99.89
    specified type NEC Z99.89
  renal dialysis (hemodialysis) (peritoneal) Z99.2
  respirator Z99.11
  ventilator Z99.11
  wheelchair Z99.3
opiate — *see* Dependence, drug, opioid
opioids — *see* Dependence, drug, opioid
opium (alkaloids) (derivatives) (tincture) — *see* Dependence, drug, opioid
oxygen (long-term) (supplemental) Z99.81
paraldehyde — *see* Dependence, drug, sedative
paregoric — *see* Dependence, drug, opioid
PCP (phencyclidine) (or related substance) — *see* Dependence, drug, hallucinogen
pentobarbital — *see* Dependence, drug, sedative
pentobarbitone (sodium) — *see* Dependence, drug, sedative
pentothal — *see* Dependence, drug, sedative
peyote — *see* Dependence, drug, hallucinogen
phencyclidine (PCP) (or related substance) — *see* Dependence, drug, hallucinogen
phenmetrazine — *see* Dependence, drug, stimulant NEC
phenobarbital — *see* Dependence, drug, sedative
polysubstance F19.20
psilocibin, psilocin, psilocyn, psilocyline — *see* Dependence, drug, hallucinogen
psychostimulant NEC — *see* Dependence, drug, stimulant NEC
secobarbital — *see* Dependence, drug, sedative
seconal — *see* Dependence, drug, sedative
sedative NEC — *see* Dependence, drug, sedative
specified drug NEC — *see* Dependence, drug
stimulant NEC — *see* Dependence, drug, stimulant NEC
substance NEC — *see* Dependence, drug
supplemental oxygen Z99.81
tobacco — *see* Dependence, drug, nicotine
  counseling and surveillance Z71.6
tranquilizer NEC — *see* Dependence, drug, sedative
vitamin B6 E53.1
volatile solvents — *see* Dependence, drug, inhalant

Dependency
care-provider Z74.9
passive F60.7
reactions (persistent) F60.7

Depersonalization (in neurotic state) (neurotic) (syndrome) F48.1

Depletion
extracellular fluid E86.9
plasma E86.1
potassium E87.6
  nephropathy N25.89
salt or sodium E87.1
  causing heat exhaustion or prostration T67.4 ☑
  nephropathy N28.9
volume NOS E86.9

Deployment (current) (military) status Z56.82
in theater or in support of military war, peacekeeping and humanitarian operations Z56.82
personal history of Z91.82
  military war, peacekeeping and humanitarian deployment (current or past conflict) Z91.82
  returned from Z91.82

Depolarization, premature I49.40
atrial I49.1
junctional I49.2
specified NEC I49.49
ventricular I49.3

Deposit
bone in Boeck's sarcoid D86.89
calcareous, calcium — *see* Calcification

Deposit — *continued*
cholesterol
  retina H35.89
  vitreous (body) (humor) — *see* Deposit, crystalline
conjunctiva H11.11- ☑
cornea H18.00- ☑
  argentous H18.02- ☑
  due to metabolic disorder H18.03- ☑
  Kayser-Fleischer ring H18.04- ☑
  pigmentation — *see* Pigmentation, cornea
crystalline, vitreous (body) (humor) H43.2- ☑
hemosiderin in old scars of cornea — *see* Pigmentation, cornea, stromal
metallic in lens — *see* Cataract, specified NEC
skin R23.8
tooth, teeth (betel) (black) (green) (materia alba) (orange) (tobacco) K03.6
urate, kidney — *see* Calculus, kidney

Depraved appetite — *see* Pica

Depressed
HDL cholesterol E78.6

Depression (acute) (mental) F32.9
agitated (single episode) F32.2
anaclitic — *see* Disorder, adjustment
anxiety F41.8
  persistent F34.1
arches — *see also* Deformity, limb, flat foot
atypical (single episode) F32.89
  recurrent episode F33.8
basal metabolic rate R94.8
bone marrow D75.89
central nervous system R09.2
cerebral R29.818
  newborn P91.4
cerebrovascular I67.9
chest wall M95.4
climacteric (single episode) F32.89
  recurrent episode F33.8
endogenous (without psychotic symptoms) F33.2
  with psychotic symptoms F33.3
functional activity R68.89
hysterical F44.89
involutional (single episode) F32.89
  recurrent episode F33.8
major F32.9
  with psychotic symptoms F32.3
  recurrent — *see* Disorder, depressive, recurrent
manic-depressive — *see* Disorder, depressive, recurrent
masked (single episode) F32.89
medullary G93.89
menopausal (single episode) F32.89
  recurrent episode F33.8
metatarsus — *see* Depression, arches
monopolar F33.9
nervous F34.1
neurotic F34.1
nose M95.0
postnatal (NOS) F53.0
postpartum (NOS) F53.0
post-psychotic of schizophrenia F32.89
post-schizophrenic F32.89
psychogenic (reactive) (single episode) F32.9
psychoneurotic F34.1
psychotic (single episode) F32.3
  recurrent F33.3
reactive (psychogenic) (single episode) F32.9
  psychotic (single episode) F32.3
recurrent — *see* Disorder, depressive, recurrent
respiratory center G93.89
seasonal — *see* Disorder, depressive, recurrent
senile F03
severe, single episode F32.2
situational F43.21
skull Q67.4
specified NEC (single episode) F32.89
sternum M95.4
visual field — *see* Defect, visual field
vital (recurrent) (without psychotic symptoms) F33.2
  with psychotic symptoms F33.3
  single episode F32.2

Deprivation
cultural Z60.3
effects NOS T73.9 ☑
  specified NEC T73.8 ☑
emotional NEC Z65.8
  affecting infant or child — *see* Maltreatment, child, psychological
food T73.0 ☑

Deprivation — *continued*
protein — *see* Malnutrition
sleep Z72.820
social Z60.4
  affecting infant or child — *see* Maltreatment, child, psychological
specified NEC T73.8 ☑
vitamins — *see* Deficiency, vitamin
water T73.1 ☑

Derangement
ankle (internal) — *see* Derangement, joint, ankle
cartilage (articular) NEC — *see* Derangement, joint, articular cartilage, by site
  recurrent — *see* Dislocation, recurrent
cruciate ligament, anterior, current injury — *see* Sprain, knee, cruciate, anterior
elbow (internal) — *see* Derangement, joint, elbow
hip (joint) (internal) (old) — *see* Derangement, joint, hip
joint (internal) M24.9
  ankylosis — *see* Ankylosis
  articular cartilage M24.10
    ankle M24.17- ☑
    elbow M24.12- ☑
    foot M24.17- ☑
    hand M24.14- ☑
    hip M24.15- ☑
    knee NEC M23.9- ☑
    loose body — *see* Loose, body
    shoulder M24.11- ☑
    wrist M24.13- ☑
  contracture — *see* Contraction, joint
  current injury — *see also* Dislocation
    knee, meniscus or cartilage — *see* Tear, meniscus
  dislocation
    pathological — *see* Dislocation, pathological
    recurrent — *see* Dislocation, recurrent
  knee — *see* Derangement, knee
  ligament — *see* Disorder, ligament
  loose body — *see* Loose, body
  recurrent — *see* Dislocation, recurrent
  specified type NEC M24.80
    ankle M24.87- ☑
    elbow M24.82- ☑
    foot joint M24.87- ☑
    hand joint M24.84- ☑
    hip M24.85- ☑
    shoulder M24.81- ☑
    wrist M24.83- ☑
  temporomandibular M26.69
knee (recurrent) M23.9- ☑
  ligament disruption, spontaneous M23.60- ☑
    anterior cruciate M23.61- ☑
    capsular M23.67- ☑
    instability, chronic M23.5- ☑
    lateral collateral M23.64- ☑
    medial collateral M23.63- ☑
    posterior cruciate M23.62- ☑
  loose body M23.4- ☑
  meniscus M23.30- ☑
    cystic M23.00- ☑
      lateral M23.002
        anterior horn M23.04- ☑
        posterior horn M23.05- ☑
        specified NEC M23.06- ☑
      medial M23.005
        anterior horn M23.01- ☑
        posterior horn M23.02- ☑
        specified NEC M23.03- ☑
    degenerate — *see* Derangement, knee, meniscus, specified NEC
    detached — *see* Derangement, knee, meniscus specified NEC
    due to old tear or injury M23.20- ☑
      lateral M23.20- ☑
        anterior horn M23.24- ☑
        posterior horn M23.25- ☑
        specified NEC M23.26- ☑
      medial M23.20- ☑
        anterior horn M23.21- ☑
        posterior horn M23.22- ☑
        specified NEC M23.23- ☑
    retained — *see* Derangement, knee, meniscus, specified NEC
    specified NEC M23.30- ☑
      lateral M23.30- ☑

Derangement — continued
- knee — continued
  - meniscus — continued
    - specified — continued
      - lateral — continued
        - anterior horn M23.34- ☑
        - posterior horn M23.35- ☑
        - specified NEC M23.36- ☑
      - medial M23.30- ☑
        - anterior horn M23.31- ☑
        - posterior horn M23.32- ☑
        - specified NEC M23.33- ☑
    - old M23.8X- ☑
    - specified NEC — see subcategory M23.8 ☑
  - low back NEC — see Dorsopathy, specified NEC
  - meniscus — see Derangement, knee, meniscus
  - mental — see Psychosis
  - patella, specified NEC — see Disorder, patella, derangement NEC
  - semilunar cartilage (knee) — see Derangement, knee, meniscus, specified NEC
  - shoulder (internal) — see Derangement, joint, shoulder

Dercum's disease E88.2

Derealization (neurotic) F48.1

Dermal — see condition

Dermaphytid — see Dermatophytosis

Dermatitis (eczematous) L30.9
- ab igne L59.0
- acarine B88.0
- actinic (due to sun) L57.8
  - other than from sun L59.8
- allergic — see Dermatitis, contact, allergic
- ambustionis, due to burn or scald — see Burn
- amebic A06.7
- ammonia L22
- arsenical (ingested) L27.8
- artefacta L98.1
  - psychogenic F54
- atopic L20.9
  - psychogenic F54
  - specified NEC L20.89
- autoimmune progesterone L30.8
- berlock, berloque L56.2
- blastomycotic B40.3
- blister beetle L24.89
- bullous, bullosa L13.9
  - mucosynechial, atrophic L12.1
  - seasonal L30.8
  - specified NEC L13.8
- calorica L59.0
  - due to burn or scald — see Burn
- caterpillar L24.89
- cercarial B65.3
- combustionis L59.0
  - due to burn or scald — see Burn
- congelationis T69.1 ☑
- contact (occupational) L25.9
  - allergic L23.9
    - due to
      - adhesives L23.1
      - cement L23.5
      - chemical products NEC L23.5
      - chromium L23.0
      - cosmetics L23.2
      - dander (cat) (dog) L23.81
      - drugs in contact with skin L23.3
      - dyes L23.4
      - food in contact with skin L23.6
      - hair (cat) (dog) L23.81
      - insecticide L23.5
      - metals L23.0
      - nickel L23.0
      - plants, non-food L23.7
      - plastic L23.5
      - rubber L23.5
      - specified agent NEC L23.89
  - due to
    - cement L25.3
    - chemical products NEC L25.3
    - cosmetics L25.0
    - dander (cat) (dog) L23.81
    - drugs in contact with skin L25.1
    - dyes L25.2
    - food in contact with skin L25.4
    - hair (cat) (dog) L23.81
    - plants, non-food L25.5
    - specified agent NEC L25.8
  - irritant L24.9

Dermatitis — continued
- contact — continued
  - irritant — continued
    - due to
      - cement L24.5
      - chemical products NEC L24.5
      - cosmetics L24.3
      - detergents L24.0
      - drugs in contact with skin L24.4
      - food in contact with skin L24.6
      - oils and greases L24.1
      - plants, non-food L24.7
      - solvents L24.2
      - specified agent NEC L24.89
- contusiformis L52
- diabetic — see E08-E13 with .620
- diaper L22
- diphtheritica A36.3
- dry skin L85.3
- due to
  - acetone (contact) (irritant) L24.2
  - acids (contact) (irritant) L24.5
  - adhesive(s) (allergic) (contact) (plaster) L23.1
    - irritant L24.5
  - alcohol (irritant) (skin contact) (substances in category T51) L24.2
    - taken internally L27.8
  - alkalis (contact) (irritant) L24.5
  - arsenic (ingested) L27.8
  - carbon disulfide (contact) (irritant) L24.2
  - caustics (contact) (irritant) L24.5
  - cement (contact) L25.3
  - cereal (ingested) L27.2
  - chemical(s) NEC L25.3
    - taken internally L27.8
  - chlorocompounds L24.2
  - chromium (contact) (irritant) L24.81
  - coffee (ingested) L27.2
  - cold weather L30.8
  - cosmetics (contact) L25.0
    - allergic L23.2
    - irritant L24.3
  - cyclohexanes L24.2
  - dander (cat) (dog) L23.81
  - Demodex species B88.0
  - Dermanyssus gallinae B88.0
  - detergents (contact) (irritant) L24.0
  - dichromate L24.81
  - drugs and medicaments (generalized) (internal use) L27.0
    - external — see Dermatitis, due to, drugs, in contact with skin
    - in contact with skin L25.1
      - allergic L23.3
      - irritant L24.4
    - localized skin eruption L27.1
    - specified substance — see Table of Drugs and Chemicals
  - dyes (contact) L25.2
    - allergic L23.4
    - irritant L24.89
  - epidermophytosis — see Dermatophytosis
  - esters L24.2
  - external irritant NEC L24.9
  - fish (ingested) L27.2
  - flour (ingested) L27.2
  - food (ingested) L27.2
    - in contact with skin L25.4
  - fruit (ingested) L27.2
  - furs (allergic) (contact) L23.81
  - glues — see Dermatitis, due to, adhesives
  - glycols L24.2
  - greases NEC (contact) (irritant) L24.1
  - hair (cat) (dog) L23.81
  - hot
    - objects and materials — see Burn
    - weather or places L59.0
  - hydrocarbons L24.2
  - infrared rays L59.8
  - ingestion, ingested substance L27.9
    - chemical NEC L27.8
    - drugs and medicaments — see Dermatitis, due to, drugs
    - food L27.2
    - specified NEC L27.8
  - insecticide in contact with skin L24.5
  - internal agent L27.9

Dermatitis — continued
- due to — continued
  - internal agent — continued
    - drugs and medicaments (generalized) — see Dermatitis, due to, drugs
    - food L27.2
  - irradiation — see Dermatitis, due to, radioactive substance
  - ketones L24.2
  - lacquer tree (allergic) (contact) L23.7
  - light (sun) NEC L57.8
    - acute L56.8
    - other L59.8
  - Liponyssoides sanguineus B88.0
  - low temperature L30.8
  - meat (ingested) L27.2
  - metals, metal salts (contact) (irritant) L24.81
  - milk (ingested) L27.2
  - nickel (contact) (irritant) L24.81
  - nylon (contact) (irritant) L24.5
  - oils NEC (contact) (irritant) L24.1
  - paint solvent (contact) (irritant) L24.2
  - petroleum products (contact) (irritant) (substances in T52.0) L24.2
  - plants NEC (contact) L25.5
    - allergic L23.7
    - irritant L24.7
  - plasters (adhesive) (any) (allergic) (contact) L23.1
    - irritant L24.5
  - plastic (contact) L25.3
  - preservatives (contact) — see Dermatitis, due to, chemical, in contact with skin
  - primrose (allergic) (contact) L23.7
  - primula (allergic) (contact) L23.7
  - radiation L59.8
    - nonionizing (chronic exposure) L57.8
    - sun NEC L57.8
      - acute L56.8
  - radioactive substance L58.9
    - acute L58.0
    - chronic L58.1
  - radium L58.9
    - acute L58.0
    - chronic L58.1
  - ragweed (allergic) (contact) L23.7
  - Rhus (allergic) (contact) (diversiloba) (radicans) (toxicodendron) (venenata) (verniciflua) L23.7
  - rubber (contact) L24.5
  - Senecio jacobaea (allergic) (contact) L23.7
  - solvents (contact) (irritant) (substances in category T52) L24.2
  - specified agent NEC (contact) L25.8
    - allergic L23.89
    - irritant L24.89
  - sunshine NEC L57.8
    - acute L56.8
  - tetrachlorethylene (contact) (irritant) L24.2
  - toluene (contact) (irritant) L24.2
  - turpentine (contact) L24.2
  - ultraviolet rays (sun NEC) (chronic exposure) L57.8
    - acute L56.8
  - vaccine or vaccination L27.0
    - specified substance — see Table of Drugs and Chemicals
  - varicose veins — see Varix, leg, with, inflammation
  - X-rays L58.9
    - acute L58.0
    - chronic L58.1
- dyshydrotic L30.1
- dysmenorrheica N94.6
- escharotica — see Burn
- exfoliative, exfoliativa (generalized) L26
  - neonatorum L00
- eyelid — see also Dermatosis, eyelid
  - allergic H01.119
    - left H01.116
      - lower H01.115
      - upper H01.114
    - right H01.113
      - lower H01.112
      - upper H01.111
  - contact — see Dermatitis, eyelid, allergic
  - due to
    - Demodex species B88.0
    - herpes (zoster) B02.39
      - simplex B00.59
  - eczematous H01.139
    - left H01.136

Dermatitis — continued
  eyelid — see also Dermatosis, eyelid — continued
    eczematous — continued
      left — continued
        lower H01.135
        upper H01.134
      right H01.133
        lower H01.132
        upper H01.131
  facta, factitia, factitial L98.1
    psychogenic F54
  flexural NEC L20.82
  friction L30.4
  fungus B36.9
    specified type NEC B36.8
  gangrenosa, gangrenous infantum L08.0
  harvest mite B88.0
  heat L59.0
  herpesviral, vesicular (ear) (lip) B00.1
  herpetiformis (bullous) (erythematous) (pustular)
      (vesicular) L13.0
    juvenile L12.2
    senile L12.0
  hiemalis L30.8
  hypostatic, hypostatica — see Varix, leg, with, inflammation
  infectious eczematoid L30.3
  infective L30.3
  irritant — see Dermatitis, contact, irritant
  Jacquet's (diaper dermatitis) L22
  Leptus B88.0
  lichenified NEC L28.0
  medicamentosa (generalized) (internal use) — see Dermatitis, due to drugs
  mite B88.0
  multiformis L13.0
    juvenile L12.2
  napkin L22
  neurotica L13.0
  nummular L30.0
  papillaris capillitii L73.0
  pellagrous E52
  perioral L71.0
  photocontact L56.2
  polymorpha dolorosa L13.0
  pruriginosa L13.0
  pruritic NEC L30.8
  psychogenic F54
  purulent L08.0
  pustular
    contagious B08.02
    subcorneal L13.1
  pyococcal L08.0
  pyogenica L08.0
  repens L40.2
  Ritter's (exfoliativa) L00
  Schamberg's L81.7
  schistosome B65.3
  seasonal bullous L30.8
  seborrheic L21.9
    infantile L21.1
    specified NEC L21.8
  sensitization NOS L23.9
  septic L08.0
  solare L57.8
  specified NEC L30.8
  stasis I87.2
    with
      varicose ulcer — see Varix, leg, with ulcer, with
          inflammation
      varicose veins — see Varix, leg, with, inflammation
      due to postthrombotic syndrome — see Syndrome,
          postthrombotic
  suppurative L08.0
  traumatic NEC L30.4
  trophoneurotica L13.0
  ultraviolet (sun) (chronic exposure) L57.8
    acute L56.8
  varicose — see Varix, leg, with, inflammation
  vegetans L10.1
  verrucosa B43.0
  vesicular, herpesviral B00.1
Dermatoarthritis, lipoid E78.81
Dermatochalasis, eyelid H02.839
  left H02.836
    lower H02.835
    upper H02.834

Dermatochalasis, eyelid — continued
  right H02.833
    lower H02.832
    upper H02.831
Dermatofibroma (lenticulare) — see Neoplasm, skin,
    benign
  protuberans — see Neoplasm, skin, uncertain behavior
Dermatofibrosarcoma (pigmented) (protuberans) —
    see Neoplasm, skin, malignant
Dermatographia L50.3
Dermatolysis (exfoliativa) (congenital) Q82.8
  acquired L57.4
  eyelids — see Blepharochalasis
  palpebrarum — see Blepharochalasis
  senile L57.4
Dermatomegaly NEC Q82.8
Dermatomucosomyositis M33.10
  with
    myopathy M33.12
    respiratory involvement M33.11
    specified organ involvement NEC M33.19
Dermatomycosis B36.9
  furfuracea B36.0
  specified type NEC B36.8
Dermatomyositis (acute) (chronic) — see also Dermatopolymyositis
  adult — see also Dermatomyositis, specified NEC
      M33.10
  in (due to) neoplastic disease — see also Neoplasm
      D49.9 [M36.0]
  juvenile M33.00
    with
      myopathy M33.02
      respiratory involvement M33.01
      specified organ involvement NEC M33.09
    without myopathy M33.03
  specified NEC M33.10
    with
      myopathy M33.12
      respiratory involvement M33.11
      specified organ involvement NEC M33.19
    without myopathy M33.13
Dermatoneuritis of children — see Poisoning, mercury
Dermatophilosis A48.8
Dermatophytid L30.2
Dermatophytide — see Dermatophytosis
Dermatophytosis (epidermophyton) (infection) (Microsporum) (tinea) (Trichophyton) B35.9
  beard B35.0
  body B35.4
  capitis B35.0
  corporis B35.4
  deep-seated B35.8
  disseminated B35.8
  foot B35.3
  granulomatous B35.8
  groin B35.6
  hand B35.2
  nail B35.1
  perianal (area) B35.6
  scalp B35.0
  specified NEC B35.8
Dermatopolymyositis M33.90
  with
    myopathy M33.92
    respiratory involvement M33.91
    specified organ involvement NEC M33.99
  in neoplastic disease — see also Neoplasm
      D49.9 [M36.0]
  juvenile M33.00
    with
      myopathy M33.02
      respiratory involvement M33.01
      specified organ involvement NEC M33.09
  specified NEC M33.10
    myopathy M33.12
    respiratory involvement M33.11
    specified organ involvement NEC M33.19
  without myopathy M33.93
Dermatopolyneuritis — see Poisoning, mercury
Dermatorrhexis — see also Syndrome, Ehlers-Danlos
    Q79.60
  acquired L57.4
Dermatosclerosis — see also Scleroderma
  localized L94.0
Dermatosis L98.9
  Andrews' L08.89
  Bowen's — see Neoplasm, skin, in situ

Dermatosis — continued
  bullous L13.9
    specified NEC L13.8
  exfoliativa L26
  eyelid (noninfectious)
    dermatitis — see Dermatitis, eyelid
    discoid lupus erythematosus — see Lupus, erythematosus, eyelid
    xeroderma — see Xeroderma, acquired, eyelid
  factitial L98.1
  febrile neutrophilic L98.2
  gonococcal A54.89
  herpetiformis L13.0
    juvenile L12.2
  linear IgA L13.8
  menstrual NEC L98.8
  neutrophilic, febrile L98.2
  occupational — see Dermatitis, contact
  papulosa nigra L82.1
  pigmentary L81.9
    progressive L81.7
    Schamberg's L81.7
  psychogenic F54
  purpuric, pigmented L81.7
  pustular, subcorneal L13.1
  transient acantholytic L11.1
Dermographia, dermographism L50.3
Dermoid (cyst) — see also Neoplasm, benign, by site
  with malignant transformation C56- ☑
  due to radiation (nonionizing) L57.8
Dermopathy
  infiltrative with thyrotoxicosis — see Thyrotoxicosis
  nephrogenic fibrosing L90.8
Dermophytosis — see Dermatophytosis
Descemetocele H18.73- ☑
Descemet's membrane — see condition
Descending — see condition
Descensus uteri — see Prolapse, uterus
Desert
  rheumatism B38.0
  sore — see Ulcer, skin
Desertion (newborn) — see Maltreatment
Desmoid (extra-abdominal) (tumor) — see Neoplasm,
    connective tissue, uncertain behavior
  abdominal D48.1
Despondency F32.9
Desquamation, skin R23.4
Destruction, destructive — see also Damage
  articular facet — see also Derangement, joint, specified
      type NEC
    knee M23.8X- ☑
    vertebra — see Spondylosis
  bone — see also Disorder, bone, specified type NEC
    syphilitic A52.77
  joint — see also Derangement, joint, specified type
      NEC
    sacroiliac M53.3
  rectal sphincter K62.89
  septum (nasal) J34.89
  tuberculous NEC — see Tuberculosis
  tympanum, tympanic membrane (nontraumatic) —
      see Disorder, tympanic membrane, specified NEC
  vertebral disc — see Degeneration, intervertebral disc
Destructiveness — see also Disorder, conduct
  adjustment reaction — see Disorder, adjustment
Desultory labor O62.2
Detachment
  cartilage — see Sprain
  cervix, annular N88.8
    complicating delivery O71.3
  choroid (old) (postinfectional) (simple) (spontaneous)
      H31.40- ☑
    hemorrhagic H31.41- ☑
    serous H31.42- ☑
  ligament — see Sprain
  meniscus (knee) — see also Derangement, knee,
      meniscus, specified NEC
    current injury — see Tear, meniscus
    due to old tear or injury — see Derangement, knee,
        meniscus, due to old tear
  retina (without retinal break) (serous) H33.2- ☑
    with retinal:
      break H33.00- ☑
        giant H33.03- ☑
        multiple H33.02- ☑
        single H33.01- ☑
        dialysis H33.04- ☑

☑ **Additional Character Required** — Refer to the Tabular List for Character Selection   ▼ **Subterms under main terms may continue to next column or page**

Detachment — *continued*
  retina — *continued*
    pigment epithelium — *see* Degeneration, retina,
      separation of layers, pigment epithelium de-
      tachment
    rhegmatogenous — *see* Detachment, retina, with
      retinal, break
    specified NEC H33.8
    total H33.05- ☑
    traction H33.4- ☑
  vitreous (body) H43.81 ☑
Detergent asthma J69.8
Deterioration
  epileptic F06.8
  general physical R53.81
  heart, cardiac — *see* Degeneration, myocardial
  mental — *see* Psychosis
  myocardial, myocardium — *see* Degeneration, myocar-
    dial
  senile (simple) R54
Deuteranomaly (anomalous trichromat) H53.53
Deuteranopia (complete) (incomplete) H53.53
Development
  abnormal, bone Q79.9
  arrested R62.50
    bone — *see* Arrest, development or growth, bone
    child R62.50
    due to malnutrition E45
  defective, congenital — *see also* Anomaly, by site
    cauda equina Q06.3
    left ventricle Q24.8
      in hypoplastic left heart syndrome Q23.4
    valve Q24.8
      pulmonary Q22.3
  delayed — *see also* Delay, development R62.50
    arithmetical skills F81.2
    language (skills) (expressive) F80.1
    learning skill F81.9
    mixed skills F88
    motor coordination F82
    reading F81.0
    specified learning skill NEC F81.89
    speech F80.9
    spelling F81.81
    written expression F81.81
  imperfect, congenital — *see also* Anomaly, by site
    heart Q24.9
    lungs Q33.6
  incomplete
    bronchial tree Q32.4
    organ or site not listed — *see* Hypoplasia, by site
    respiratory system Q34.9
  sexual, precocious NEC E30.1
  tardy, mental — *see also* Disability, intellectual F79
Developmental — *see* condition
  testing, infant or child — *see* Examination, child
Devergie's disease (pityriasis rubra pilaris) L44.0
Deviation (in)
  conjugate palsy (eye) (spastic) H51.0
  esophagus (acquired) K22.8
  eye, skew H51.8
  midline (jaw) (teeth) (dental arch) M26.29
    specified site NEC — *see* Malposition
  nasal septum J34.2
    congenital Q67.4
  opening and closing of the mandible M26.53
  organ or site, congenital NEC — *see* Malposition, con-
    genital
  septum (nasal) (acquired) J34.2
    congenital Q67.4
  sexual F65.9
    bestiality F65.89
    erotomania F52.8
    exhibitionism F65.2
    fetishism, fetishistic F65.0
      transvestism F65.1
    frotteurism F65.81
    masochism F65.51
    multiple F65.89
    necrophilia F65.89
    nymphomania F52.8
    pederosis F65.4
    pedophilia F65.4
    sadism, sadomasochism F65.52
    satyriasis F52.8
    specified type NEC F65.89
    transvestism F64.1
    voyeurism F65.3

Deviation — *continued*
  teeth, midline M26.29
  trachea J39.8
  ureter, congenital Q62.61
Device
  cerebral ventricle (communicating) in situ Z98.2
  contraceptive — *see* Contraceptive, device
  drainage, cerebrospinal fluid, in situ Z98.2
Devic's disease G36.0
Devil's
  grip B33.0
  pinches (purpura simplex) D69.2
Devitalized tooth K04.99
Devonshire colic — *see* Poisoning, lead
Dextraposition, aorta Q20.3
  in tetralogy of Fallot Q21.3
Dextrinosis, limit (debrancher enzyme deficiency) E74.03
Dextrocardia (true) Q24.0
  with
    complete transposition of viscera Q89.3
    situs inversus Q89.3
Dextrotransposition, aorta Q20.3
d-glycericacidemia E72.59
Dhat syndrome F48.8
Dhobi itch B35.6
Di George's syndrome D82.1
Di Guglielmo's disease C94.0- ☑
Diabetes, diabetic (mellitus) (sugar) E11.9
  with
    amyotrophy E11.44
    arthropathy NEC E11.618
    autonomic (poly)neuropathy E11.43
    cataract E11.36
    Charcot's joints E11.610
    chronic kidney disease E11.22
    circulatory complication NEC E11.59
    complication E11.8
      specified NEC E11.69
    dermatitis E11.620
    foot ulcer E11.621
    gangrene E11.52
    gastroparalysis E11.43
    gastroparesis E11.43
    glomerulonephrosis, intracapillary E11.21
    glomerulosclerosis, intercapillary E11.21
    hyperglycemia E11.65
    hyperosmolarity E11.00
      with coma E11.01
    hypoglycemia E11.649
      with coma E11.641
    ketoacidosis E11.10
      with coma E11.11
    kidney complications NEC E11.29
    Kimmelstiel-Wilson disease E11.21
    loss of protective sensation (LOPS) — *see* Diabetes,
      by type, with neuropathy
    mononeuropathy E11.41
    myasthenia E11.44
    necrobiosis lipoidica E11.620
    nephropathy E11.21
    neuralgia E11.42
    neurologic complication NEC E11.49
    neuropathic arthropathy E11.610
    neuropathy E11.40
    ophthalmic complication NEC E11.39
    oral complication NEC E11.638
    osteomyelitis E11.69
    periodontal disease E11.630
    peripheral angiopathy E11.51
      with gangrene E11.52
    polyneuropathy E11.42
    renal complication NEC E11.29
    renal tubular degeneration E11.29
    retinopathy E11.319
      with macular edema E11.311
        resolved following treatment E11.37- ☑
      nonproliferative E11.329 ☑
        with macular edema E11.321 ☑
        mild E11.329 ☑
          with macular edema E11.321 ☑
        moderate E11.339 ☑
          with macular edema E11.331 ☑
        severe E11.349 ☑
          with macular edema E11.341 ☑
      proliferative E11.359 ☑

Diabetes, diabetic — *continued*
  with — *continued*
    retinopathy — *continued*
      proliferative — *continued*
        with
          combined traction retinal detachment
            and rhegmatogenous retinal de-
            tachment E11.354 ☑
          macular edema E11.351 ☑
          stable proliferative diabetic retinopathy
            E11.355 ☑
          traction retinal detachment involving the
            macula E11.352 ☑
          traction retinal detachment not involving
            the macula E11.353 ☑
        resolved following treatment E09.37 ☑
    skin complication NEC E11.628
    skin ulcer NEC E11.622
  brittle — *see* Diabetes, type 1
  bronzed E83.110
  complicating pregnancy — *see* Pregnancy, complicated
    by, diabetes
  dietary counseling and surveillance Z71.3
  due to
    autoimmune process — *see* Diabetes, type 1
    immune mediated pancreatic islet beta-cell destruc-
      tion — *see* Diabetes, type 1
  due to drug or chemical E09.9
    with
      amyotrophy E09.44
      arthropathy NEC E09.618
      autonomic (poly)neuropathy E09.43
      cataract E09.36
      Charcot's joints E09.610
      chronic kidney disease E09.22
      circulatory complication NEC E09.59
      complication E09.8
        specified NEC E09.69
      dermatitis E09.620
      foot ulcer E09.621
      gangrene E09.52
      gastroparalysis E09.43
      gastroparesis E09.43
      glomerulonephrosis, intracapillary E09.21
      glomerulosclerosis, intercapillary E09.21
      hyperglycemia E09.65
      hyperosmolarity E09.00
        with coma E09.01
      hypoglycemia E09.649
        with coma E09.641
      ketoacidosis E09.10
        with coma E09.11
      kidney complications NEC E09.29
      Kimmelstiel-Wilson disease E09.21
      mononeuropathy E09.41
      myasthenia E09.44
      necrobiosis lipoidica E09.620
      nephropathy E09.21
      neuralgia E09.42
      neurologic complication NEC E09.49
      neuropathic arthropathy E09.610
      neuropathy E09.40
      ophthalmic complication NEC E09.39
      oral complication NEC E09.638
      periodontal disease E09.630
      peripheral angiopathy E09.51
        with gangrene E09.52
      polyneuropathy E09.42
      renal complication NEC E09.29
      renal tubular degeneration E09.29
      retinopathy E09.319
        with macular edema E09.311
        resolved following treatment E09.37 ☑
        nonproliferative E09.329 ☑
          with macular edema E09.321 ☑
          mild E09.329 ☑
            with macular edema E09.321 ☑
          moderate E09.339 ☑
            with macular edema E09.331 ☑
          severe E09.349 ☑
            with macular edema E09.341 ☑
        proliferative E09.359 ☑
        with
          combined traction retinal detachment
            and rhegmatogenous retinal
            detachment E09.354 ☑
          macular edema E09.351 ☑

Diabetes, diabetic — *continued*
  due to drug or chemical — *continued*
    with — *continued*
      retinopathy — *continued*
        proliferative — *continued*
          with — *continued*
            stable proliferative diabetic retinopathy E09.355 ☑
            traction retinal detachment involving the macula E09.352 ☑
            traction retinal detachment not involving the macula E09.353 ☑
      skin complication NEC E09.628
      skin ulcer NEC E09.622
  due to underlying condition E08.9
    with
      amyotrophy E08.44
      arthropathy NEC E08.618
      autonomic (poly)neuropathy E08.43
      cataract E08.36
      Charcot's joints E08.610
      chronic kidney disease E08.22
      circulatory complication NEC E08.59
      complication E08.8
        specified NEC E08.69
      dermatitis E08.620
      foot ulcer E08.621
      gangrene E08.52
      gastroparalysis E08.43
      gastroparesis E08.43
      glomerulonephrosis, intracapillary E08.21
      glomerulosclerosis, intercapillary E08.21
      hyperglycemia E08.65
      hyperosmolarity E08.00
        with coma E08.01
      hypoglycemia E08.649
        with coma E08.641
      ketoacidosis E08.10
        with coma E08.11
      kidney complications NEC E08.29
      Kimmelsteil-Wilson disease E08.21
      mononeuropathy E08.41
      myasthenia E08.44
      necrobiosis lipoidica E08.620
      nephropathy E08.21
      neuralgia E08.42
      neurologic complication NEC E08.49
      neuropathic arthropathy E08.610
      neuropathy E08.40
      ophthalmic complication NEC E08.39
      oral complication NEC E08.638
      periodontal disease E08.630
      peripheral angiopathy E08.51
        with gangrene E08.52
      polyneuropathy E08.42
      renal complication NEC E08.29
      renal tubular degeneration E08.29
      retinopathy E08.319
        with macular edema E08.311
        resolved following treatment E08.37 ☑
        nonproliferative E08.329 ☑
          with macular edema E08.321 ☑
          mild E08.329 ☑
            with macular edema E08.321 ☑
          moderate E08.339 ☑
            with macular edema E08.331 ☑
          severe E08.349 ☑
            with macular edema E08.341 ☑
        proliferative E08.359 ☑
          with
            combined traction retinal detachment and rhegmatogenous retinal detachment E08.354 ☑
            macular edema E08.351 ☑
            stable proliferative diabetic retinopathy E08.355 ☑
            traction retinal detachment involving the macula E08.352 ☑
            traction retinal detachment not involving the macula E08.353 ☑
      skin complication NEC E08.628
      skin ulcer NEC E08.622
  gestational (in pregnancy) O24.419
    affecting newborn P70.0
    diet controlled O24.410
    in childbirth O24.429
      diet controlled O24.420
      insulin (and diet) controlled O24.424

Diabetes, diabetic — *continued*
  gestational — *continued*
    in childbirth — *continued*
      oral drug controlled (antidiabetic) (hypoglycemic) O24.425
    insulin (and diet) controlled O24.414
    oral drug controlled (antidiabetic) (hypoglycemic) O24.415
    puerperal O24.439
      diet controlled O24.430
      insulin (and diet) controlled O24.434
      oral drug controlled (antidiabetic) (hypoglycemic) O24.435
  hepatogenous E13.9
  idiopathic — *see* Diabetes, type 1
  inadequately controlled — *code to* Diabetes, by type, with hyperglycemia
  insipidus E23.2
    nephrogenic N25.1
    pituitary E23.2
    vasopressin resistant N25.1
  insulin dependent — *code to* type of diabetes
  juvenile-onset — *see* Diabetes, type 1
  ketosis-prone — *see* Diabetes, type 1
  latent R73.03
  neonatal (transient) P70.2
  non-insulin dependent — *code to* type of diabetes
  out of control — *code to* Diabetes, by type, with hyperglycemia
  phosphate E83.39
  poorly controlled — *code to* Diabetes, by type, with hyperglycemia
  postpancreatectomy — *see* Diabetes, specified type NEC
  postprocedural — *see* Diabetes, specified type NEC
  secondary diabetes mellitus NEC — *see* Diabetes, specified type NEC
  specified type NEC E13.9
    with
      amyotrophy E13.44
      arthropathy NEC E13.618
      autonomic (poly)neuropathy E13.43
      cataract E13.36
      Charcot's joints E13.610
      chronic kidney disease E13.22
      circulatory complication NEC E13.59
      complication E13.8
        specified NEC E13.69
      dermatitis E13.620
      foot ulcer E13.621
      gangrene E13.52
      gastroparalysis E13.43
      gastroparesis E13.43
      glomerulonephrosis, intracapillary E13.21
      glomerulosclerosis, intercapillary E13.21
      hyperglycemia E13.65
      hyperosmolarity E13.00
        with coma E13.01
      hypoglycemia E13.649
        with coma E13.641
      ketoacidosis E13.10
        with coma E13.11
      kidney complications NEC E13.29
      Kimmelsteil-Wilson disease E13.21
      mononeuropathy E13.41
      myasthenia E13.44
      necrobiosis lipoidica E13.620
      nephropathy E13.21
      neuralgia E13.42
      neurologic complication NEC E13.49
      neuropathic arthropathy E13.610
      neuropathy E13.40
      ophthalmic complication NEC E13.39
      oral complication NEC E13.638
      periodontal disease E13.630
      peripheral angiopathy E13.51
        with gangrene E13.52
      polyneuropathy E13.42
      renal complication NEC E13.29
      renal tubular degeneration E13.29
      retinopathy E13.319
        with macular edema E13.311
        resolved following treatment E13.37 ☑
        nonproliferative E13.329 ☑
          with macular edema E13.321 ☑
          mild E13.329 ☑
            with macular edema E13.321 ☑
          moderate E13.339 ☑

Diabetes, diabetic — *continued*
  specified type — *continued*
    with — *continued*
      retinopathy — *continued*
        nonproliferative — *continued*
          moderate — *continued*
            with macular edema E13.331 ☑
          severe E13.349 ☑
            with macular edema E13.341 ☑
        proliferative E13.359 ☑
          with
            combined traction retinal detachment and rhegmatogenous retinal detachment E13.354 ☑
            macular edema E13.351 ☑
            stable proliferative diabetic retinopathy E13.355 ☑
            traction retinal detachment involving the macula E13.352 ☑
            traction retinal detachment not involving the macula E13.353 ☑
      skin complication NEC E13.628
      skin ulcer NEC E13.622
  steroid-induced — *see* Diabetes, due to, drug or chemical
  type 1 E10.9
    with
      amyotrophy E10.44
      arthropathy NEC E10.618
      autonomic (poly)neuropathy E10.43
      cataract E10.36
      Charcot's joints E10.610
      chronic kidney disease E10.22
      circulatory complication NEC E10.59
      complication E10.8
        specified NEC E10.69
      dermatitis E10.620
      foot ulcer E10.621
      gangrene E10.52
      gastroparalysis E10.43
      gastroparesis E10.43
      glomerulonephrosis, intracapillary E10.21
      glomerulosclerosis, intercapillary E10.21
      hyperglycemia E10.65
      hypoglycemia E10.649
        with coma E10.641
      ketoacidosis E10.10
        with coma E10.11
      kidney complications NEC E10.29
      Kimmelsteil-Wilson disease E10.21
      mononeuropathy E10.41
      myasthenia E10.44
      necrobiosis lipoidica E10.620
      nephropathy E10.21
      neuralgia E10.42
      neurologic complication NEC E10.49
      neuropathic arthropathy E10.610
      neuropathy E10.40
      ophthalmic complication NEC E10.39
      oral complication NEC E10.638
      osteomyelitis E10.69
      periodontal disease E10.630
      peripheral angiopathy E10.51
        with gangrene E10.52
      polyneuropathy E10.42
      renal complication NEC E10.29
      renal tubular degeneration E10.29
      retinopathy E10.319
        with macular edema E10.311
        resolved following treatment E10.37 ☑
        nonproliferative E10.329 ☑
          with macular edema E10.321 ☑
          mild E10.329 ☑
            with macular edema E10.321 ☑
          moderate E10.339 ☑
            with macular edema E10.331 ☑
          severe E10.349 ☑
            with macular edema E10.341 ☑
        proliferative E10.359 ☑
          with
            combined traction retinal detachment and rhegmatogenous retinal detachment E10.354 ☑
            macular edema E10.351 ☑
            stable proliferative diabetic retinopathy E10.355 ☑
            traction retinal detachment involving the macula E10.352 ☑

Diabetes, diabetic — *continued*
  type 1 — *continued*
    with — *continued*
      retinopathy — *continued*
        proliferative — *continued*
          with — *continued*
            traction retinal detachment not involv-
              ing the macula E10.353 ☑
      skin complication NEC E10.628
      skin ulcer NEC E10.622
  type 2 E11.9
    with
      amyotrophy E11.44
      arthropathy NEC E11.618
      autonomic (poly)neuropathy E11.43
      cataract E11.36
      Charcot's joints E11.610
      chronic kidney disease E11.22
      circulatory complication NEC E11.59
      complication E11.8
        specified NEC E11.69
      dermatitis E11.620
      foot ulcer E11.621
      gangrene E11.52
      gastroparalysis E11.43
      gastroparesis E11.43
      glomerulonephrosis, intracapillary E11.21
      glomerulosclerosis, intercapillary E11.21
      hyperglycemia E11.65
      hyperosmolarity E11.00
        with coma E11.01
      hypoglycemia E11.649
        with coma E11.641
      ketoacidosis E11.10
        with coma E11.11
      kidney complications NEC E11.29
      Kimmelstiel-Wilson disease E11.21
      mononeuropathy E11.41
      myasthenia E11.44
      necrobiosis lipoidica E11.620
      nephropathy E11.21
      neuralgia E11.42
      neurologic complication NEC E11.49
      neuropathic arthropathy E11.610
      neuropathy E11.40
      ophthalmic complication NEC E11.39
      oral complication NEC E11.638
      osteomyelitis E11.69
      periodontal disease E11.630
      peripheral angiopathy E11.51
        with gangrene E11.52
      polyneuropathy E11.42
      renal complication NEC E11.29
      renal tubular degeneration E11.29
      retinopathy E11.319
        with macular edema E11.311
        resolved following treatment E11.37 ☑
        nonproliferative E11.329 ☑
          with macular edema E11.321 ☑
          mild E11.329 ☑
            with macular edema E11.321 ☑
          moderate E11.339 ☑
            with macular edema E11.331 ☑
          severe E11.349 ☑
            with macular edema E11.341 ☑
        proliferative E11.359 ☑
          with
            combined traction retinal detachment
              and rhegmatogenous retinal
              detachment E11.354 ☑
            macular edema E11.351 ☑
            stable proliferative diabetic retinopa-
              thy E11.355 ☑
            traction retinal detachment involving
              the macula E11.352 ☑
            traction retinal detachment not involv-
              ing the macula E11.353 ☑
      skin complication NEC E11.628
      skin ulcer NEC E11.622
  uncontrolled
    meaning
      hyperglycemia — *see* Diabetes, by type, with,
        hyperglycemia
      hypoglycemia — *see* Diabetes, by type, with,
        hypoglycemia
Diacyclothrombopathia D69.1
Diagnosis deferred R69

Dialysis (intermittent) (treatment)
  noncompliance (with) Z91.15
  renal (hemodialysis) (peritoneal), status Z99.2
  retina, retinal — *see* Detachment, retina, with retinal,
    dialysis
Diamond-Blackfan anemia (congenital hypoplastic)
  D61.01
Diamond-Gardener syndrome (autoerythrocyte sensi-
  tization) D69.2
Diaper rash L22
Diaphoresis (excessive) R61
Diaphragm — *see* condition
Diaphragmalgia R07.1
Diaphragmatitis, diaphragmitis J98.6
Diaphysial aclasis Q78.6
Diaphysitis — *see* Osteomyelitis, specified type NEC
Diarrhea, diarrheal (disease) (infantile) (inflammatory)
  R19.7
  achlorhydric K31.83
  allergic K52.29
    due to
      colitis — *see* Colitis, allergic
      enteritis — *see* Enteritis, allergic
  amebic — *see also* Amebiasis A06.0
    with abscess — *see* Abscess, amebic
    acute A06.0
    chronic A06.1
    nondysenteric A06.2
  bacillary — *see* Dysentery, bacillary
  balantidial A07.0
  cachectic NEC K52.89
  Chilomastix A07.8
  choleriformis A00.1
  chronic (noninfectious) K52.9
  coccidial A07.3
  Cochin-China K90.1
    strongyloidiasis B78.0
  Dientamoeba A07.8
  dietetic — *see also* Diarrhea, allergic K52.29
  drug-induced K52.1
  due to
    bacteria A04.9
      specified NEC A04.8
    Campylobacter A04.5
    Capillaria philippinensis B81.1
    Clostridium difficile
      not specified as recurrent A04.72
      recurrent A04.71
    Clostridium perfringens (C) (F) A04.8
    Cryptosporidium A07.2
    drugs K52.1
    Escherichia coli A04.4
      enteroaggregative A04.4
      enterohemorrhagic A04.3
      enteroinvasive A04.2
      enteropathogenic A04.0
      enterotoxigenic A04.1
      specified NEC A04.4
    food hypersensitivity — *see also* Diarrhea, allergic
      K52.29
    Necator americanus B76.1
    S. japonicum B65.2
    specified organism NEC A08.8
      bacterial A04.8
      viral A08.39
    Staphylococcus A04.8
    Trichuris trichiuria B79
    virus — *see* Enteritis, viral
    Yersinia enterocolitica A04.6
  dysenteric A09
  endemic A09
  epidemic A09
  flagellate A07.9
  Flexner's (ulcerative) A03.1
  functional K59.1
    following gastrointestinal surgery K91.89
    psychogenic F45.8
  Giardia lamblia A07.1
  giardial A07.1
  hill K90.1
  infectious A09
  malarial — *see* Malaria
  mite B88.0
  mycotic NEC B49
  neonatal (noninfectious) P78.3
  nervous F45.8
  neurogenic K59.1
  noninfectious K52.9

Diarrhea, diarrheal — *continued*
  postgastrectomy K91.1
  postvagotomy K91.1
  protozoal A07.9
    specified NEC A07.8
  psychogenic F45.8
  specified
    bacterium NEC A04.8
    virus NEC A08.39
  strongyloidiasis B78.0
  toxic K52.1
  trichomonal A07.8
  tropical K90.1
  tuberculous A18.32
  viral — *see* Enteritis, viral
Diastasis
  cranial bones M84.88
    congenital NEC Q75.8
  joint (traumatic) — *see* Dislocation
  muscle M62.00
    ankle M62.07- ☑
    congenital Q79.8
    foot M62.07- ☑
    forearm M62.03- ☑
    hand M62.04- ☑
    lower leg M62.06- ☑
    pelvic region M62.05- ☑
    shoulder region M62.01- ☑
    specified site NEC M62.08
    thigh M62.05- ☑
    upper arm M62.02- ☑
  recti (abdomen)
    complicating delivery O71.89
    congenital Q79.59
Diastema, tooth, teeth, fully erupted M26.32
Diastematomyelia Q06.2
Diataxia, cerebral G80.4
Diathesis
  allergic — *see* History, allergy
  bleeding (familial) D69.9
  cystine (familial) E72.00
  gouty — *see* Gout
  hemorrhagic (familial) D69.9
    newborn NEC P53
  spasmophilic R29.0
Diaz's disease or osteochondrosis (juvenile) (talus) —
  see Osteochondrosis, juvenile, tarsus
Dibothriocephalus, dibothriocephaliasis (latus) (infection) (infestation) B70.0
  larval B70.1
Dicephalus, dicephaly Q89.4
Dichotomy, teeth K00.2
Dichromat, dichromatopsia (congenital) — *see* Deficiency, color vision
Dichuchwa A65
Dicroceliasis B66.2
Didelphia, didelphys — *see* Double uterus
Didymytis N45.1
  with orchitis N45.3
Dietary
  inadequacy or deficiency E63.9
  surveillance and counseling Z71.3
Dietl's crisis N13.8
Dieulafoy lesion (hemorrhagic)
  duodenum K31.82
  esophagus K22.8
  intestine (colon) K63.81
  stomach K31.82
Difficult, difficulty (in)
  acculturation Z60.3
  feeding R63.3
    newborn P92.9
      breast P92.5
      specified NEC P92.8
    nonorganic (infant or child) F98.29
  intubation, in anesthesia T88.4 ☑
  mechanical, gastroduodenal stoma K91.89
    causing obstruction — *see also* Obstruction, intes-
      tine, postoperative K91.30
  micturition
    need to immediately re-void R39.191
    position dependent R39.192
    specified NEC R39.198
  reading (developmental) F81.0
    secondary to emotional disorders F93.9
  spelling (specific) F81.81
    with reading disorder F81.89
    due to inadequate teaching Z55.8

Difficult, difficulty — *continued*
  swallowing — *see* Dysphagia
  walking R26.2
  work
    conditions NEC Z56.5
    schedule Z56.3
Diffuse — *see* condition
Digestive — *see* condition
Dihydropyrimidine dehydrogenase disease (DPD) E88.89
Diktyoma — *see* Neoplasm, malignant, by site
Dilaceration, tooth K00.4
Dilatation
  anus K59.8
    venule — *see* Hemorrhoids
  aorta (focal) (general) — *see* Ectasia, aorta
    with aneurysm — *see* Aneurysm, aorta
    congenital Q25.44
  artery — *see* Aneurysm
  bladder (sphincter) N32.89
    congenital Q64.79
  blood vessel I99.8
  bronchial J47.9
    with
      exacerbation (acute) J47.1
      lower respiratory infection J47.0
  calyx (due to obstruction) — *see* Hydronephrosis
  capillaries I78.8
  cardiac (acute) (chronic) — *see also* Hypertrophy, cardiac
    congenital Q24.8
      valve NEC Q24.8
        pulmonary Q22.3
    valve — *see* Endocarditis
  cavum septi pellucidi Q06.8
  cervix (uteri) — *see also* Incompetency, cervix
    incomplete, poor, slow complicating delivery O62.0
  colon K59.39
    congenital Q43.1
    psychogenic F45.8
    toxic K59.31
  common duct (acquired) K83.8
    congenital Q44.5
  cystic duct (acquired) K82.8
    congenital Q44.5
  duct, mammary — *see* Ectasia, mammary duct
  duodenum K59.8
  esophagus K22.8
    congenital Q39.5
    due to achalasia K22.0
  eustachian tube, congenital Q17.8
  gallbladder K82.8
  gastric — *see* Dilatation, stomach
  heart (acute) (chronic) — *see also* Hypertrophy, cardiac
    congenital Q24.8
    valve — *see* Endocarditis
  ileum K59.8
    psychogenic F45.8
  jejunum K59.8
    psychogenic F45.8
  kidney (calyx) (collecting structures) (cystic) (parenchyma) (pelvis) (idiopathic) N28.89
  lacrimal passages or duct — *see* Disorder, lacrimal system, changes
  lymphatic vessel I89.0
  mammary duct — *see* Ectasia, mammary duct
  Meckel's diverticulum (congenital) Q43.0
    malignant — *see* Table of Neoplasms, small intestine, malignant
  myocardium (acute) (chronic) — *see* Hypertrophy, cardiac
  organ or site, congenital NEC — *see* Distortion
  pancreatic duct K86.89
  pericardium — *see* Pericarditis
  pharynx J39.2
  prostate N42.89
  pulmonary
    artery (idiopathic) I28.8
    valve, congenital Q22.3
  pupil H57.04
  rectum K59.39
  saccule, congenital Q16.5
  salivary gland (duct) K11.8
  sphincter ani K62.89
  stomach K31.89
    acute K31.0
    psychogenic F45.8
  submaxillary duct K11.8

Dilatation — *continued*
  trachea, congenital Q32.1
  ureter (idiopathic) N28.82
    congenital Q62.2
    due to obstruction N13.4
  urethra (acquired) N36.8
  vasomotor I73.9
  vein I86.8
  ventricular, ventricle (acute) (chronic) — *see also* Hypertrophy, cardiac
    cerebral, congenital Q04.8
  venule NEC I86.8
  vesical orifice N32.89
Dilated, dilation — *see* Dilatation
Diminished, diminution
  hearing (acuity) — *see* Deafness
  sense or sensation (cold) (heat) (tactile) (vibratory) R20.8
  vision NEC H54.7
  vital capacity R94.2
Diminuta taenia B71.0
Dimitri-Sturge-Weber disease Q85.8
Dimple
  congenital sacral Q82.6
  parasacral Q82.6
  pilonidal or postanal — *see* Cyst, pilonidal
Dioctophyme renalis (infection) (infestation) B83.8
Dipetalonemiasis B74.4
Diphallus Q55.69
Diphtheria, diphtheritic (gangrenous) (hemorrhagic) A36.9
  carrier (suspected) Z22.2
  cutaneous A36.3
  faucial A36.0
  infection of wound A36.3
  laryngeal A36.2
  myocarditis A36.81
  nasal, anterior A36.89
  nasopharyngeal A36.1
  neurological complication A36.89
  pharyngeal A36.0
  specified site NEC A36.89
  tonsillar A36.0
Diphyllobothriasis (intestine) B70.0
  larval B70.1
Diplacusis H93.22- ☑
Diplegia (upper limbs) G83.0
  congenital (cerebral) G80.8
  facial G51.0
  lower limbs G82.20
  spastic G80.1
Diplococcus, diplococcal — *see* condition
Diplopia H53.2
Dipsomania F10.20
  with
    psychosis — *see* Psychosis, alcoholic
    remission F10.21
Dipylidiasis B71.1
DIRA (deficiency of interleukin 1 receptor antagonist) M04.8
Direction, teeth, abnormal, fully erupted M26.30
Dirofilariasis B74.8
Dirt-eating child F98.3
Disability, disabilities
  heart — *see* Disease, heart
  intellectual F79
    with
      autistic features F84.9
    mild (I.Q. 50-69) F70
    moderate (I.Q. 35-49) F71
    profound (I.Q. under 20) F73
    severe (I.Q. 20-34) F72
    specified level NEC F78
  knowledge acquisition F81.9
  learning F81.9
  limiting activities Z73.6
  spelling, specific F81.81
Disappearance of family member Z63.4
Disarticulation — *see* Amputation
  meaning traumatic amputation — *see* Amputation, traumatic
Discharge (from)
  abnormal finding in — *see* Abnormal, specimen
  breast (female) (male) N64.52
  diencephalic autonomic idiopathic — *see* Epilepsy, specified NEC
  ear — *see also* Otorrhea
    blood — *see* Otorrhagia

Discharge — *continued*
  excessive urine R35.8
  nipple N64.52
  penile R36.9
  postnasal R09.82
  prison, anxiety concerning Z65.2
  urethral R36.9
    without blood R36.0
    hematospermia R36.1
  vaginal N89.8
Discitis, diskitis M46.40
  cervical region M46.42
  cervicothoracic region M46.43
  lumbar region M46.46
  lumbosacral region M46.47
  multiple sites M46.49
  occipito-atlanto-axial region M46.41
  pyogenic — *see* Infection, intervertebral disc, pyogenic
  sacrococcygeal region M46.48
  thoracic region M46.44
  thoracolumbar region M46.45
Discoid
  meniscus (congenital) Q68.6
  semilunar cartilage (congenital) — *see* Derangement, knee, meniscus, specified NEC
Discoloration
  nails L60.8
  teeth (posteruptive) K03.7
    during formation K00.8
Discomfort
  chest R07.89
  visual H53.14- ☑
Discontinuity, ossicles, ear H74.2- ☑
Discord (with)
  boss Z56.4
  classmates Z55.4
  counselor Z64.4
  employer Z56.4
  family Z63.8
  fellow employees Z56.4
  in-laws Z63.1
  landlord Z59.2
  lodgers Z59.2
  neighbors Z59.2
  probation officer Z64.4
  social worker Z64.4
  teachers Z55.4
  workmates Z56.4
Discordant connection
  atrioventricular (congenital) Q20.5
  ventriculoarterial Q20.3
Discrepancy
  centric occlusion maximum intercuspation M26.55
  leg length (acquired) — *see* Deformity, limb, unequal length
    congenital — *see* Defect, reduction, lower limb
  uterine size date O26.84- ☑
Discrimination
  ethnic Z60.5
  political Z60.5
  racial Z60.5
  religious Z60.5
  sex Z60.5
Disease, diseased — *see also* Syndrome
  absorbent system I87.8
  acid-peptic K30
  Acosta's T70.29 ☑
  Adams-Stokes (-Morgagni) (syncope with heart block) I45.9
  Addison's anemia (pernicious) D51.0
  adenoids (and tonsils) J35.9
  adrenal (capsule) (cortex) (gland) (medullary) E27.9
    hyperfunction E27.0
    specified NEC E27.8
  ainhum L94.6
  airway
    obstructive, chronic J44.9
      due to
        cotton dust J66.0
        specific organic dusts NEC J66.8
    reactive — *see* Asthma
  akamushi (scrub typhus) A75.3
  Albers-Schönberg (marble bones) Q78.2
  Albert's — *see* Tendinitis, Achilles
  alimentary canal K63.9
  alligator-skin Q80.9
    acquired L85.0
  alpha heavy chain C88.3

Disease, diseased — continued
  alpine T70.29 ☑
  altitude T70.20 ☑
  alveolar ridge
    edentulous K06.9
      specified NEC K06.8
  alveoli, teeth K08.9
  Alzheimer's G30.9 [F02.80]
    with behavioral disturbance G30.9 [F02.81]
    early onset G30.0 [F02.80]
      with behavioral disturbance G30.0 [F02.81]
    late onset G30.1 [F02.80]
      with behavioral disturbance G30.1 [F02.81]
    specified NEC G30.8 [F02.80]
      with behavioral disturbance G30.8 [F02.81]
  amyloid — see Amyloidosis
  Andersen's (glycogenosis IV) E74.09
  Andes T70.29 ☑
  Andrews' (bacterid) L08.89
  angiospastic I73.9
    cerebral G45.9
    vein I87.8
  anterior
    chamber H21.9
    horn cell G12.29
  antiglomerular basement membrane (anti- GBM) anti-
      body M31.0
    tubulo-interstitial nephritis N12
  antral — see Sinusitis, maxillary
  anus K62.9
    specified NEC K62.89
  aorta (nonsyphilitic) I77.9
    syphilitic NEC A52.02
  aortic (heart) (valve) I35.9
    rheumatic I06.9
  Apollo B30.3
  aponeuroses — see Enthesopathy
  appendix K38.9
    specified NEC K38.8
  aqueous (chamber) H21.9
  Arnold-Chiari — see Arnold-Chiari disease
  arterial I77.9
    occlusive — see Occlusion, by site
      due to stricture or stenosis I77.1
    peripheral I73.9
  arteriocardiorenal — see Hypertension, cardiorenal
  arteriolar (generalized) (obliterative) I77.9
  arteriorenal — see Hypertension, kidney
  arteriosclerotic — see also Arteriosclerosis
    cardiovascular — see Disease, heart, ischemic,
      atherosclerotic
    coronary (artery) — see Disease, heart, ischemic,
      atherosclerotic
    heart — see Disease, heart, ischemic, atherosclerotic
  artery I77.9
    cerebral I67.9
    coronary I25.10
      with angina pectoris — see Arteriosclerosis,
        coronary (artery)
    peripheral I73.9
  arthropod-borne NOS (viral) A94
    specified type NEC A93.8
  atticoantral, chronic H66.20
    left H66.22
      with right H66.23
    right H66.21
      with left H66.23
  auditory canal — see Disorder, ear, external
  auricle, ear NEC — see Disorder, pinna
  Australian X A83.4
  autoimmune (systemic) NOS M35.9
    hemolytic (cold type) (warm type) D59.1
      drug-induced D59.0
    thyroid E06.3
  autoinflammatory M04.9
    NOD2-associated M04.8
    specified type NEC M04.8
  aviator's — see Effect, adverse, high altitude
  Ayerza's (pulmonary artery sclerosis with pulmonary
      hypertension) I27.0
  Babington's (familial hemorrhagic telangiectasia) I78.0
  bacterial A49.9
    specified NEC A48.8
    zoonotic A28.9
      specified type NEC A28.8
  Baelz's (cheilitis glandularis apostematosa) K13.0
  bagasse J67.1
  balloon — see Effect, adverse, high altitude

Disease, diseased — continued
  Bang's (brucella abortus) A23.1
  Bannister's T78.3 ☑
  barometer makers' — see Poisoning, mercury
  Barraquer (-Simons') (progressive lipodystrophy) E88.1
  Barrett's — see Barrett's, esophagus
  Bartholin's gland N75.9
  basal ganglia G25.9
    degenerative G23.9
      specified NEC G23.8
    specified NEC G25.89
  Basedow's (exophthalmic goiter) — see Hyperthy-
      roidism, with, goiter (diffuse)
  Bateman's B08.1
  Batten-Steinert G71.11
  Battey A31.0
  Beard's (neurasthenia) F48.8
  Becker
    idiopathic mural endomyocardial I42.3
    myotonia congenita G71.12
  Begbie's (exophthalmic goiter) — see Hyperthyroidism,
      with, goiter (diffuse)
  behavioral, organic F07.9
  Beigel's (white piedra) B36.2
  Benson's — see Deposit, crystalline
  Bernard-Soulier (thrombopathy) D69.1
  Bernhardt (-Roth) — see Mononeuropathy, lower limb,
      meralgia paresthetica
  Biermer's (pernicious anemia) D51.0
  bile duct (common) (hepatic) K83.9
    with calculus, stones — see Calculus, bile duct
    specified NEC K83.8
  biliary (tract) K83.9
    specified NEC K83.8
  Billroth's — see Spina bifida
  bird fancier's J67.2
  black lung J60
  bladder N32.9
    in (due to)
      schistosomiasis (bilharziasis) B65.0 [N33]
    specified NEC N32.89
  bleeder's D66
  blood D75.9
    forming organs D75.9
    vessel I99.9
  Bloodgood's — see Mastopathy, cystic
  Bodechtel-Guttmann (subacute sclerosing panen-
      cephalitis) A81.1
  bone — see also Disorder, bone
    aluminum M83.4
    fibrocystic NEC
      jaw M27.49
  bone-marrow D75.9
  Borna A83.9
  Bornholm (epidemic pleurodynia) B33.0
  Bouchard's (myopathic dilatation of the stomach) K31.0
  Bouillaud's (rheumatic heart disease) I01.9
  Bourneville (-Brissaud) (tuberous sclerosis) Q85.1
  Bouveret (-Hoffmann) (paroxysmal tachycardia) I47.9
  bowel K63.9
    functional K59.9
      psychogenic F45.8
  brain G93.9
    arterial, artery I67.9
    arteriosclerotic I67.2
    congenital Q04.9
    degenerative — see Degeneration, brain
    inflammatory — see Encephalitis
    organic G93.9
      arteriosclerotic I67.2
    parasitic NEC B71.9 [G94]
    senile NEC G31.1
    specified NEC G93.89
  breast — see also Disorder, breast N64.9
    cystic (chronic) — see Mastopathy, cystic
    fibrocystic — see Mastopathy, cystic
    Paget's
      female, unspecified side C50.91- ☑
      male, unspecified side C50.92- ☑
    specified NEC N64.89
  Breda's — see Yaws
  Bretonneau's (diphtheritic malignant angina) A36.0
  Bright's — see Nephritis
    arteriosclerotic — see Hypertension, kidney
  Brill's (recrudescent typhus) A75.1
  Brill-Zinsser (recrudescent typhus) A75.1
  Brion-Kayser — see Fever, paratyphoid

Disease, diseased — continued
  broad
    beta E78.2
    ligament (noninflammatory) N83.9
      inflammatory — see Disease, pelvis, inflammato-
        ry
      specified NEC N83.8
  Brocq-Duhring (dermatitis herpetiformis) L13.0
  Brocq's
    meaning
      dermatitis herpetiformis L13.0
      prurigo L28.2
  bronchopulmonary J98.4
  bronchus NEC J98.09
  bronze Addison's E27.1
    tuberculous A18.7
  budgerigar fancier's J67.2
  Buerger's (thromboangiitis obliterans) I73.1
  bullous L13.9
    chronic of childhood L12.2
    specified NEC L13.8
  Bürger-Grütz (essential familial hyperlipemia) E78.3
  bursa — see Bursopathy
  caisson T70.3 ☑
  California — see Coccidioidomycosis
  capillaries I78.9
    specified NEC I78.8
  Carapata A68.0
  cardiac — see Disease, heart
  cardiopulmonary, chronic I27.9
  cardiorenal (hepatic) (hypertensive) (vascular) — see
      Hypertension, cardiorenal
  cardiovascular (atherosclerotic) I25.10
    with angina pectoris — see Arteriosclerosis, coro-
      nary (artery),
    congenital Q28.9
    hypertensive — see Hypertension, heart
    newborn P29.9
      specified NEC P29.89
    renal (hypertensive) — see Hypertension, cardiore-
      nal
    syphilitic (asymptomatic) A52.00
  cartilage — see Disorder, cartilage
  Castellani's A69.8
  Castleman (unicentric) (multicentric) D47.Z2
    HHV-8-associated — see also Herpesvirus, human,
      8 D47.Z2
  cat-scratch A28.1
  Cavare's (familial periodic paralysis) G72.3
  cecum K63.9
  celiac (adult) (infantile) (with steatorrhea) K90.0
  cellular tissue L98.9
  central core G71.2
  cerebellar, cerebellum — see Disease, brain
  cerebral — see also Disease, brain
    degenerative — see Degeneration, brain
  cerebrospinal G96.9
  cerebrovascular I67.9
    acute I67.89
      embolic I63.4- ☑
      thrombotic I63.3- ☑
    arteriosclerotic I67.2
    hereditary NEC I67.858
    specified NEC I67.89
  cervix (uteri) (noninflammatory) N88.9
    inflammatory — see Cervicitis
    specified NEC N88.8
  Chabert's A22.9
  Chandler's (osteochondritis dissecans, hip) — see Os-
      teochondritis, dissecans, hip
  Charlouis — see Yaws
  Chédiak-Steinbrinck (-Higashi) (congenital gigantism
      of peroxidase granules) E70.330
  chest J98.9
  Chiari's (hepatic vein thrombosis) I82.0
  Chicago B40.9
  Chignon B36.8
  chigo, chigoe B88.1
  childhood granulomatous D71
  Chinese liver fluke B66.1
  chlamydial A74.9
    specified NEC A74.89
  cholecystic K82.9
  choroid H31.9
    specified NEC H31.8
  Christmas D67
  chronic bullous of childhood L12.2
  chylomicron retention E78.3

Disease, diseased — continued
ciliary body H21.9
  specified NEC H21.89
circulatory (system) NEC I99.8
  newborn P29.9
  syphilitic A52.00
    congenital A50.54
coagulation factor deficiency (congenital) — see Defect, coagulation
coccidioidal — see Coccidioidomycosis
cold
  agglutinin or hemoglobinuria D59.1
    paroxysmal D59.6
  hemagglutinin (chronic) D59.1
collagen NOS (nonvascular) (vascular) M35.9
  specified NEC M35.8
colon K63.9
  functional K59.9
    congenital Q43.2
  ischemic — see also Ischemia, intestine, acute K55.039
colonic inflammatory bowel, unclassified (IBDU) K52.3
combined system — see Degeneration, combined
compressed air T70.3 ☑
Concato's (pericardial polyserositis) A19.9
  nontubercular I31.1
  pleural — see Pleurisy, with effusion
conjunctiva H11.9
  chlamydial A74.0
  specified NEC H11.89
  viral B30.9
    specified NEC B30.8
connective tissue, systemic (diffuse) M35.9
  in (due to)
    hypogammaglobulinemia D80.1 [M36.8]
    ochronosis E70.29 [M36.8]
  specified NEC M35.8
Conor and Bruch's (boutonneuse fever) A77.1
Cooper's — see Mastopathy, cystic
Cori's (glycogenosis III) E74.03
corkhandler's or corkworker's J67.3
cornea H18.9
  specified NEC H18.89- ☑
coronary (artery) — see Disease, heart, ischemic, atherosclerotic
  congenital Q24.5
  ostial, syphilitic (aortic) (mitral) (pulmonary) A52.03
corpus cavernosum N48.9
  specified NEC N48.89
Cotugno's — see Sciatica
coxsackie (virus) NEC B34.1
cranial nerve NOS G52.9
Creutzfeldt-Jakob — see Creutzfeldt-Jakob disease or syndrome
Crocq's (acrocyanosis) I73.89
Crohn's — see Enteritis, regional
Curschmann G71.11
cystic
  breast (chronic) — see Mastopathy, cystic
  kidney, congenital Q61.9
  liver, congenital Q44.6
  lung J98.4
    congenital Q33.0
cytomegalic inclusion (generalized) B25.9
  with pneumonia B25.0
  congenital P35.1
cytomegaloviral B25.9
  specified NEC B25.8
Czerny's (periodic hydrarthrosis of the knee) — see Effusion, joint, knee
Daae (-Finsen) (epidemic pleurodynia) B33.0
Darling's — see Histoplasmosis capsulati
de Quervain's (tendon sheath) M65.4
  thyroid (subacute granulomatous thyroiditis) E06.1
Débove's (splenomegaly) R16.1
deer fly — see Tularemia
Degos' I77.89
demyelinating, demyelinizating (nervous system) G37.9
  multiple sclerosis G35
  specified NEC G37.8
dense deposit — see also N00-N07 with fourth character .6 N05.6
deposition, hydroxyapatite — see Disease, hydroxyapatite deposition
Devergie's (pityriasis rubra pilaris) L44.0
Devic's G36.0
diaphorase deficiency D74.0
diaphragm J98.6

Disease, diseased — continued
diarrheal, infectious NEC A09
digestive system K92.9
  specified NEC K92.89
disc, degenerative — see Degeneration, intervertebral disc
discogenic — see also Displacement, intervertebral disc NEC
  with myelopathy — see Disorder, disc, with, myelopathy
diverticular — see Diverticula
Dubois (thymus) A50.59 [E35]
Duchenne-Griesinger G71.01
Duchenne's
  muscular dystrophy G71.01
  pseudohypertrophy, muscles G71.01
ductless glands E34.9
Duhring's (dermatitis herpetiformis) L13.0
duodenum K31.9
  specified NEC K31.89
Dupré's (meningism) R29.1
Dupuytren's (muscle contracture) M72.0
Durand-Nicholas-Favre (climatic bubo) A55
Duroziez's (congenital mitral stenosis) Q23.2
ear — see Disorder, ear
Eberth's — see Fever, typhoid
Ebola (virus) A98.4
Ebstein's heart Q22.5
Echinococcus — see Echinococcus
echovirus NEC B34.1
Eddowes' (brittle bones and blue sclera) Q78.0
edentulous (alveolar) ridge K06.9
  specified NEC K06.8
Edsall's T67.2 ☑
Eichstedt's (pityriasis versicolor) B36.0
Eisenmenger's (irreversible) I27.83
Ellis-van Creveld (chondroectodermal dysplasia) Q77.6
end stage renal (ESRD) N18.6
  due to hypertension I12.0
endocrine glands or system NEC E34.9
endomyocardial (eosinophilic) I42.3
English (rickets) E55.0
enteroviral, enterovirus NEC B34.1
  central nervous system NEC A88.8
epidemic B99.9
  specified NEC B99.8
epididymis N50.9
Erb (-Landouzy) G71.02
Erdheim-Chester (ECD) E88.89
esophagus K22.9
  functional K22.4
  psychogenic F45.9
  specified NEC K22.8
Eulenburg's (congenital paramyotonia) G71.19
eustachian tube — see Disorder, eustachian tube
external
  auditory canal — see Disorder, ear, external
  ear — see Disorder, ear, external
extrapyramidal G25.9
  specified NEC G25.89
eye H57.9
  anterior chamber H21.9
  inflammatory NEC H57.89
  muscle (external) — see Strabismus
  specified NEC H57.89
  syphilitic — see Oculopathy, syphilitic
eyeball H44.9
  specified NEC H44.89
eyelid — see Disorder, eyelid
  specified NEC — see Disorder, eyelid, specified type NEC
eyeworm of Africa B74.3
facial nerve (seventh) G51.9
  newborn (birth injury) P11.3
Fahr (of brain) G23.8
Fahr Volhard (of kidney) I12.- ☑
fallopian tube (noninflammatory) N83.9
  inflammatory — see Salpingo-oophoritis
  specified NEC N83.8
familial periodic paralysis G72.3
Fanconi's (congenital pancytopenia) D61.09
fascia NEC — see also Disorder, muscle
  inflammatory — see Myositis
  specified NEC M62.89
Fauchard's (periodontitis) — see Periodontitis
Favre-Durand-Nicolas (climatic bubo) A55
Fede's K14.0
Feer's — see Poisoning, mercury

Disease, diseased — continued
female pelvic inflammatory — see also Disease, pelvis, inflammatory N73.9
  syphilitic (secondary) A51.42
  tuberculous A18.17
Fernels' (aortic aneurysm) I71.9
fibrocaseous of lung — see Tuberculosis, pulmonary
fibrocystic — see Fibrocystic disease
Fiedler's (leptospiral jaundice) A27.0
fifth B08.3
file-cutter's — see Poisoning, lead
fish-skin Q80.9
  acquired L85.0
Flajani (-Basedow) (exophthalmic goiter) — see Hyperthyroidism, with, goiter (diffuse)
flax-dresser's J66.1
fluke — see Infestation, fluke
foot and mouth B08.8
foot process N04.9
Forbes' (glycogenosis III) E74.03
Fordyce-Fox (apocrine miliaria) L75.2
Fordyce's (ectopic sebaceous glands) (mouth) Q38.6
Forestier's (rhizomelic pseudopolyarthritis) M35.3
  meaning ankylosing hyperostosis — see Hyperostosis, ankylosing
Fothergill's
  neuralgia — see Neuralgia, trigeminal
  scarlatina anginosa A38.9
Fournier (gangrene) N49.3
  female N76.89
fourth B08.8
Fox (-Fordyce) (apocrine miliaria) L75.2
Francis' — see Tularemia
Franklin C88.2
Frei's (climatic bubo) A55
Friedreich's
  combined systemic or ataxia G11.1
  myoclonia G25.3
frontal sinus — see Sinusitis, frontal
fungus NEC B49
Gaisböck's (polycythemia hypertonica) D75.1
gallbladder K82.9
  calculus — see Calculus, gallbladder
  cholecystitis — see Cholecystitis
  cholesterolosis K82.4
  fistula — see Fistula, gallbladder
  hydrops K82.1
  obstruction — see Obstruction, gallbladder
  perforation K82.2
  specified NEC K82.8
gamma heavy chain C88.2
Gamna's (siderotic splenomegaly) D73.2
Gamstorp's (adynamia episodica hereditaria) G72.3
Gandy-Nanta (siderotic splenomegaly) D73.2
ganister J62.8
gastric — see Disease, stomach
gastroesophageal reflux (GERD) K21.9
  with esophagitis K21.0
gastrointestinal (tract) K92.9
  amyloid E85.4
  functional K59.9
    psychogenic F45.8
  specified NEC K92.89
Gee (-Herter) (-Heubner) (-Thaysen) (nontropical sprue) K90.0
genital organs
  female N94.9
  male N50.9
Gerhardt's (erythromelalgia) I73.81
Gibert's (pityriasis rosea) L42
Gierke's (glycogenosis I) E74.01
Gilles de la Tourette's (motor-verbal tic) F95.2
gingiva K06.9
  plaque induced K05.00
  specified NEC K06.8
gland (lymph) I89.9
Glanzmann's (hereditary hemorrhagic thrombastheni. D69.1
glass-blower's (cataract) — see Cataract, specified NE
  salivary gland hypertrophy K11.1
Glisson's — see Rickets
globe H44.9
  specified NEC H44.89
glomerular — see also Glomerulonephritis
  with edema — see Nephrosis
  acute — see Nephritis, acute
  chronic — see Nephritis, chronic
  minimal change N05.0

Disease, diseased — *continued*
glomerular — *see also* Glomerulonephritis — *continued*
  rapidly progressive N01.9
glycogen storage E74.00
  Andersen's E74.09
  Cori's E74.03
  Forbes' E74.03
  generalized E74.00
  glucose-6-phosphatase deficiency E74.01
  heart E74.02 *[143]*
  hepatorenal E74.09
  Hers' E74.09
  liver and kidney E74.09
  McArdle's E74.04
  muscle phosphofructokinase E74.09
  myocardium E74.02 *[143]*
  Pompe's E74.02
  Tauri's E74.09
  type 0 E74.09
  type I E74.01
  type II E74.02
  type III E74.03
  type IV E74.09
  type V E74.04
  type VI-XI E74.09
  Von Gierke's E74.01
Goldstein's (familial hemorrhagic telangiectasia) I78.0
gonococcal NOS A54.9
graft-versus-host (GVH) D89.813
  acute D89.810
  acute on chronic D89.812
  chronic D89.811
grainhandler's J67.8
granulomatous (childhood) (chronic) D71
Graves' (exophthalmic goiter) — *see* Hyperthyroidism, with, goiter (diffuse)
Griesinger's — *see* Ancylostomiasis
Grisel's M43.6
Gruby's (tinea tonsurans) B35.0
Guillain-Barré G61.0
Guinon's (motor-verbal tic) F95.2
gum K06.9
gynecological N94.9
H (Hartnup's) E72.02
Haff — *see* Poisoning, mercury
Hageman (congenital factor XII deficiency) D68.2
hair (color) (shaft) L67.9
  follicles L73.9
    specified NEC L73.8
Hamman's (spontaneous mediastinal emphysema) J98.2
hand, foot and mouth B08.4
Hansen's — *see* Leprosy
Hantavirus, with pulmonary manifestations B33.4
  with renal manifestations A98.5
Harada's H30.81- ☑
Hartnup (pellagra-cerebellar ataxia-renal aminoaciduria) E72.02
Hart's (pellagra-cerebellar ataxia-renal aminoaciduria) E72.02
Hashimoto's (struma lymphomatosa) E06.3
Hb — *see* Disease, hemoglobin
heart (organic) I51.9
  with
    pulmonary edema (acute) — *see also* Failure, ventricular, left I50.1
    rheumatic fever (conditions in I00)
      active I01.9
        with chorea I02.0
        specified NEC I01.8
      inactive or quiescent (with chorea) I09.9
        specified NEC I09.89
  amyloid E85.4 *[143]*
  aortic (valve) I35.9
  arteriosclerotic or sclerotic (senile) — *see* Disease, heart, ischemic, atherosclerotic
  artery, arterial — *see* Disease, heart, ischemic, atherosclerotic
  beer drinkers' I42.6
  beriberi (wet) E51.12
  black I27.0
  congenital Q24.9
    cyanotic Q24.9
    specified NEC Q24.8
  coronary — *see* Disease, heart, ischemic
  cryptogenic I51.9
  fibroid — *see* Myocarditis

Disease, diseased — *continued*
heart — *continued*
  functional I51.89
    psychogenic F45.8
  glycogen storage E74.02 *[143]*
  gonococcal A54.83
  hypertensive — *see* Hypertension, heart
  hyperthyroid — *see also* Hyperthyroidism E05.90 *[143]*
    with thyroid storm E05.91 *[143]*
  ischemic (chronic or with a stated duration of over 4 weeks) I25.9
    atherosclerotic (of) I25.10
      with angina pectoris — *see* Arteriosclerosis, coronary (artery)
      coronary artery bypass graft — *see* Arteriosclerosis, coronary (artery),
    cardiomyopathy I25.5
    diagnosed on ECG or other special investigation, but currently presenting no symptoms I25.6
    silent I25.6
    specified form NEC I25.89
  kyphoscoliotic I27.1
  meningococcal A39.50
    endocarditis A39.51
    myocarditis A39.52
    pericarditis A39.53
  mitral I05.9
    specified NEC I05.8
  muscular — *see* Degeneration, myocardial
  psychogenic (functional) F45.8
  pulmonary (chronic) I27.9
    in schistosomiasis B65.9 *[152]*
    specified NEC I27.89
  rheumatic (chronic) (inactive) (old) (quiescent) (with chorea) I09.9
    active or acute I01.9
      with chorea (acute) (rheumatic) (Sydenham's) I02.0
    specified NEC I09.89
  senile — *see* Myocarditis
  syphilitic A52.06
    aortic A52.03
      aneurysm A52.01
    congenital A50.54 *[152]*
  thyrotoxic — *see also* Thyrotoxicosis E05.90 *[143]*
    with thyroid storm E05.91 *[143]*
  valve, valvular (obstructive) (regurgitant) — *see also* Endocarditis
    congenital NEC Q24.8
      pulmonary Q22.3
  vascular — *see* Disease, cardiovascular
heavy chain NEC C88.2
  alpha C88.3
  gamma C88.2
  mu C88.2
Hebra's
  pityriasis
    maculata et circinata L42
    rubra pilaris L44.0
  prurigo L28.2
hematopoietic organs D75.9
hemoglobin or Hb
  abnormal (mixed) NEC D58.2
    with thalassemia D56.9
  AS genotype D57.3
  Bart's D56.0
  C (Hb-C) D58.2
    with other abnormal hemoglobin NEC D58.2
    elliptocytosis D58.1
    Hb-S D57.2- ☑
      sickle-cell D57.2- ☑
    thalassemia D56.8
  Constant Spring D58.2
  D (Hb-D) D58.2
  E (Hb-E) D58.2
  E-beta thalassemia D56.5
  elliptocytosis D58.1
  H (Hb-H) (thalassemia) D56.0
    with other abnormal hemoglobin NEC D56.9
    Constant Spring D56.0
  I thalassemia D56.9
  M D74.0
  S or SS D57.1
  SC D57.2- ☑
  SD D57.8- ☑
  SE D57.8- ☑

Disease, diseased — *continued*
hemoglobin or Hb — *continued*
  spherocytosis D58.0
  unstable, hemolytic D58.2
  hemolytic (newborn) P55.9
  autoimmune (cold type) (warm type) D59.1
  drug-induced D59.0
  due to or with
    incompatibility
      ABO (blood group) P55.1
      blood (group) (Duffy) (K) (Kell) (Kidd) (Lewis) (M) (S) NEC P55.8
      Rh (blood group) (factor) P55.0
    Rh negative mother P55.0
  specified type NEC P55.8
  unstable hemoglobin D58.2
hemorrhagic D69.9
  newborn P53
Henoch (-Schönlein) (purpura nervosa) D69.0
hepatic — *see* Disease, liver
hepatolenticular E83.01
heredodegenerative NEC
  spinal cord G95.89
herpesviral, disseminated B00.7
Hers' (glycogenosis VI) E74.09
Herter (-Gee) (-Heubner) (nontropical sprue) K90.0
Heubner-Herter (nontropical sprue) K90.0
high fetal gene or hemoglobin thalassemia D56.9
Hildenbrand's — *see* Typhus
hip (joint) M25.9
  congenital Q65.89
  suppurative M00.9
  tuberculous A18.02
His (-Werner) (trench fever) A79.0
Hodgson's I71.2
  ruptured I71.1
Holla — *see* Spherocytosis
hookworm B76.9
  specified NEC B76.8
host-versus-graft D89.813
  acute D89.810
  acute on chronic D89.812
  chronic D89.811
human immunodeficiency virus (HIV) B20
Huntington's G10
  with dementia G10 *[F02.80]*
Hutchinson's (cheiropompholyx) — *see* Hutchinson's disease
hyaline (diffuse) (generalized)
  membrane (lung) (newborn) P22.0
    adult J80
hydatid — *see* Echinococcus
hydroxyapatite deposition M11.00
  ankle M11.07- ☑
  elbow M11.02- ☑
  foot joint M11.07- ☑
  hand joint M11.04- ☑
  hip M11.05- ☑
  knee M11.06- ☑
  multiple site M11.09
  shoulder M11.01- ☑
  vertebra M11.08
  wrist M11.03- ☑
hyperkinetic — *see* Hyperkinesia
hypertensive — *see* Hypertension
hypophysis E23.7
Iceland G93.3
I-cell E77.0
immune D89.9
immunoproliferative (malignant) C88.9
  small intestinal C88.3
  specified NEC C88.8
inclusion B25.9
  salivary gland B25.9
infectious, infective B99.9
  congenital P37.9
    specified NEC P37.8
    viral P35.9
      specified type NEC P35.8
  specified NEC B99.8
inflammatory
  penis N48.29
    abscess N48.21
    cellulitis N48.22
  prepuce N47.7
    balanoposthitis N47.6
  tubo-ovarian — *see* Salpingo-oophoritis
intervertebral disc — *see also* Disorder, disc

Disease, diseased — *continued*
- intervertebral disc — *see also* Disorder, disc — *continued*
  - with myelopathy — *see* Disorder, disc, with, myelopathy
  - cervical, cervicothoracic — *see* Disorder, disc, cervical
    - with
      - myelopathy — *see* Disorder, disc, cervical, with myelopathy
      - neuritis, radiculitis or radiculopathy — *see* Disorder, disc, cervical, with neuritis
      - specified NEC — *see* Disorder, disc, cervical, specified type NEC
  - lumbar (with)
    - myelopathy M51.06
    - neuritis, radiculitis, radiculopathy or sciatica M51.16
    - specified NEC M51.86
  - lumbosacral (with)
    - neuritis, radiculitis, radiculopathy or sciatica M51.17
    - specified NEC M51.87
  - specified NEC — *see* Disorder, disc, specified NEC
  - thoracic (with)
    - myelopathy M51.04
    - neuritis, radiculitis or radiculopathy M51.14
    - specified NEC M51.84
  - thoracolumbar (with)
    - myelopathy M51.05
    - neuritis, radiculitis or radiculopathy M51.15
    - specified NEC M51.85
- intestine K63.9
  - functional K59.9
    - psychogenic F45.8
    - specified NEC K59.8
  - organic K63.9
  - protozoal A07.9
  - specified NEC K63.89
- iris H21.9
  - specified NEC H21.89
- iron metabolism or storage E83.10
- island (scrub typhus) A75.3
- itai-itai — *see* Poisoning, cadmium
- Jakob-Creutzfeldt — *see* Creutzfeldt-Jakob disease or syndrome
- jaw M27.9
  - fibrocystic M27.49
  - specified NEC M27.8
- jigger B88.1
- joint — *see also* Disorder, joint
  - Charcot's — *see* Arthropathy, neuropathic (Charcot)
  - degenerative — *see* Osteoarthritis
    - multiple M15.9
    - spine — *see* Spondylosis
  - hypertrophic — *see* Osteoarthritis
  - sacroiliac M53.3
  - specified NEC — *see* Disorder, joint, specified type NEC
  - spine NEC — *see* Dorsopathy
  - suppurative — *see* Arthritis, pyogenic or pyemic
- Jourdain's (acute gingivitis) K05.00
  - nonplaque induced K05.01
  - plaque induced K05.00
- Kaschin-Beck (endemic polyarthritis) M12.10
  - ankle M12.17- ☑
  - elbow M12.12- ☑
  - foot joint M12.17- ☑
  - hand joint M12.14- ☑
  - hip M12.15- ☑
  - knee M12.16- ☑
  - multiple site M12.19
  - shoulder M12.11- ☑
  - vertebra M12.18
  - wrist M12.13- ☑
- Katayama B65.2
- Kedani (scrub typhus) A75.3
- Keshan E59
- kidney (functional) (pelvis) N28.9
  - chronic N18.9
    - hypertensive — *see* Hypertension, kidney
    - stage 1 N18.1
    - stage 2 (mild) N18.2
    - stage 3 (moderate) N18.3
    - stage 4 (severe) N18.4
    - stage 5 N18.5
  - complicating pregnancy — *see* Pregnancy, complicated by, renal disease

Disease, diseased — *continued*
- kidney — *continued*
  - cystic (congenital) Q61.9
  - fibrocystic (congenital) Q61.8
  - hypertensive — *see* Hypertension, kidney
  - in (due to)
    - schistosomiasis (bilharziasis) B65.9 [N29]
  - multicystic Q61.4
  - polycystic Q61.3
    - adult type Q61.2
    - childhood type NEC Q61.19
      - collecting duct dilatation Q61.11
- Kimmelstiel (-Wilson) (intercapillary polycystic (congenital) glomerulosclerosis) — *see* E08-E13 with .21
- Kinnier Wilson's (hepatolenticular degeneration) E83.01
- kissing — *see* Mononucleosis, infectious
- Klebs' — *see also* Glomerulonephritis N05- ☑
- Klippel-Feil (brevicollis) Q76.1
- Köhler-Pellegrini-Stieda (calcification, knee joint) — *see* Bursitis, tibial collateral
- Kok Q89.8
- König's (osteochondritis dissecans) — *see* Osteochondritis, dissecans
- Korsakoff's (nonalcoholic) F04
  - alcoholic F10.96
    - with dependence F10.26
- Kostmann's (infantile genetic agranulocytosis) D70.0
- kuru A81.81
- Kyasanur Forest A98.2
- labyrinth, ear — *see* Disorder, ear, inner
- lacrimal system — *see* Disorder, lacrimal system
- Lafora's — *see* Epilepsy, generalized, idiopathic
- Lancereaux-Mathieu (leptospiral jaundice) A27.0
- Landry's G61.0
- Larrey-Weil (leptospiral jaundice) A27.0
- larynx J38.7
- legionnaires' A48.1
  - nonpneumonic A48.2
- Lenegre's I44.2
- lens H27.9
  - specified NEC H27.8
- Lev's (acquired complete heart block) I44.2
- Lewy body (dementia) G31.83 [F02.80]
  - with behavioral disturbance G31.83 [F02.81]
- Lichtheim's (subacute combined sclerosis with pernicious anemia) D51.0
- Lightwood's (renal tubular acidosis) N25.89
- Lignac's (cystinosis) E72.04
- lip K13.0
- lipid-storage E75.6
  - specified NEC E75.5
- Lipschütz's N76.6
- liver (chronic) (organic) K76.9
  - alcoholic (chronic) K70.9
    - acute — *see* Disease, liver, alcoholic, hepatitis
    - cirrhosis K70.30
      - with ascites K70.31
    - failure K70.40
      - with coma K70.41
    - fatty liver K70.0
    - fibrosis K70.2
    - hepatitis K70.10
      - with ascites K70.11
    - sclerosis K70.2
  - cystic, congenital Q44.6
  - drug-induced (idiosyncratic) (toxic) (predictable) (unpredictable) — *see* Disease, liver, toxic
  - end stage K72.90
    - due to hepatitis — *see* Hepatitis
  - fatty, nonalcoholic (NAFLD) K76.0
    - alcoholic K70.0
  - fibrocystic (congenital) Q44.6
  - fluke
    - Chinese B66.1
    - oriental B66.1
    - sheep B66.3
  - gestational alloimmune (GALD) P78.84
  - glycogen storage E74.09 [K77]
  - in (due to)
    - schistosomiasis (bilharziasis) B65.9 [K77]
  - inflammatory K75.9
    - alcoholic K70.1
    - specified NEC K75.89
  - polycystic (congenital) Q44.6
  - toxic K71.9
    - with
      - cholestasis K71.0
      - cirrhosis (liver) K71.7

Disease, diseased — *continued*
- liver — *continued*
  - toxic — *continued*
    - with — *continued*
      - fibrosis (liver) K71.7
      - focal nodular hyperplasia K71.8
      - hepatic granuloma K71.8
      - hepatic necrosis K71.10
        - with coma K71.11
      - hepatitis NEC K71.6
        - acute K71.2
        - chronic
          - active K71.50
            - with ascites K71.51
          - lobular K71.4
          - persistent K71.3
        - lupoid K71.50
          - with ascites K71.51
      - peliosis hepatis K71.8
  - veno-occlusive disease (VOD) of liver K71.8
  - veno-occlusive K76.5
- Lobo's (keloid blastomycosis) B48.0
- Lobstein's (brittle bones and blue sclera) Q78.0
- Ludwig's (submaxillary cellulitis) K12.2
- lumbosacral region M53.87
- lung J98.4
  - black J60
  - congenital Q33.9
  - cystic J98.4
    - congenital Q33.0
  - fibroid (chronic) — *see* Fibrosis, lung
  - fluke B66.4
    - oriental B66.4
  - in
    - amyloidosis E85.4 [J99]
    - sarcoidosis D86.0
    - Sjögren's syndrome M35.02
    - systemic
      - lupus erythematosus M32.13
      - sclerosis M34.81
  - interstitial J84.9
    - of childhood, specified NEC J84.848
    - respiratory bronchiolitis J84.115
    - specified NEC J84.89
  - obstructive (chronic) J43.9
    - with
      - acute
        - bronchitis J44.0
          - exacerbation NEC J44.1
          - lower respiratory infection J44.0
      - alveolitis, allergic J67.9
      - asthma J44.9
      - bronchiectasis J47.9
        - with
          - exacerbation (acute) J47.1
          - lower respiratory infection J47.0
      - bronchitis J44.9
        - with
          - exacerbation (acute) J44.1
          - lower respiratory infection J44.0
      - emphysema J43.9
      - hypersensitivity pneumonitis J67.9
    - decompensated J44.1
      - with
        - exacerbation (acute) J44.1
  - polycystic J98.4
    - congenital Q33.0
  - rheumatoid (diffuse) (interstitial) — *see* Rheumatoid, lung
- Lutembacher's (atrial septal defect with mitral stenosis) Q21.1
- Lyme A69.20
- lymphatic (gland) (system) (channel) (vessel) I89.9
- lymphoproliferative D47.9
  - specified NEC D47.Z9 (following D47.4)
  - T-gamma D47.Z9 (following D47.4)
  - X-linked D82.3
- Magitot's M27.2
- malarial — *see* Malaria
- malignant — *see also* Neoplasm, malignant, by site
- Manson's B65.1
- maple bark J67.6
- maple-syrup-urine E71.0
- Marburg (virus) A98.3
- Marion's (bladder neck obstruction) N32.0
- Marsh's (exophthalmic goiter) — *see* Hyperthyroidism, with, goiter (diffuse)
- mastoid (process) — *see* Disorder, ear, middle
- Mathieu's (leptospiral jaundice) A27.0

Disease, diseased — *continued*
  Maxcy's A75.2
  McArdle (-Schmid-Pearson) (glycogenosis V) E74.04
  mediastinum J98.59
  medullary center (idiopathic) (respiratory) G93.89
  Meige's (chronic hereditary edema) Q82.0
  meningococcal — *see* Infection, meningococcal
  mental F99
    organic F09
  mesenchymal M35.9
  mesenteric embolic — *see also* Ischemia, intestine,
      acute K55.039
  metabolic, metabolism E88.9
    bilirubin E80.7
  metal-polisher's J62.8
  metastatic — *see also* Neoplasm, secondary, by site
      C79.9
  microvascular - code to condition
  microvillus
    atrophy Q43.8
    inclusion (MVD) Q43.8
  middle ear — *see* Disorder, ear, middle
  Mikulicz' (dryness of mouth, absent or decreased
      lacrimation) K11.8
  Milroy's (chronic hereditary edema) Q82.0
  Minamata — *see* Poisoning, mercury
  minicore G71.2
  Minor's G95.19
  Minot's (hemorrhagic disease, newborn) P53
  Minot-von Willebrand-Jürgens (angiohemophilia) D68.0
  Mitchell's (erythromelalgia) I73.81
  mitral (valve) I05.9
    nonrheumatic I34.9
  mixed connective tissue M35.1
  moldy hay J67.0
  Monge's T70.29 ☑
  Morgagni-Adams-Stokes (syncope with heart block)
      I45.9
  Morgagni's (syndrome) (hyperostosis frontalis interna)
      M85.2
  Morton's (with metatarsalgia) — *see* Lesion, nerve,
      plantar
  Morvan's G60.8
  motor neuron (bulbar) (mixed type) (spinal) G12.20
    amyotrophic lateral sclerosis G12.21
    familial G12.24
    progressive bulbar palsy G12.22
    specified NEC G12.29
  moyamoya I67.5
  mu heavy chain disease C88.2
  multicore G71.2
  muscle — *see also* Disorder, muscle
    inflammatory — *see* Myositis
    ocular (external) — *see* Strabismus
  musculoskeletal system, soft tissue — *see also* Disorder,
      soft tissue
    specified NEC — *see* Disorder, soft tissue, specified
        type NEC
  mushroom workers' J67.5
  mycotic B49
  myelodysplastic, not classified C94.6
  myeloproliferative, not classified C94.6
    chronic D47.1
  myocardium, myocardial — *see also* Degeneration,
      myocardial I51.5
    primary (idiopathic) I42.9
  myoneural G70.9
  Naegeli's D69.1
  nails L60.9
    specified NEC L60.8
  Nairobi (sheep virus) A93.8
  nasal J34.9
  nemaline body G71.2
  nerve — *see* Disorder, nerve
  nervous system G98.8
    autonomic G90.9
    central G96.9
      specified NEC G96.8
    congenital Q07.9
    parasympathetic G90.9
    specified NEC G98.8
    sympathetic G90.9
    vegetative G90.9
  neuromuscular system G70.9
  Newcastle B30.8
  Nicolas (-Durand)-Favre (climatic bubo) A55
  nipple N64.9
    Paget's C50.01 ☑

Disease, diseased — *continued*
  nipple — *continued*
    Paget's — *continued*
      female C50.01- ☑
      male C50.02- ☑
  Nishimoto (-Takeuchi) I67.5
  nonarthropod-borne NOS (viral) B34.9
    enterovirus NEC B34.1
  nonautoimmune hemolytic D59.4
    drug-induced D59.2
  Nonne-Milroy-Meige (chronic hereditary edema) Q82.0
  nose J34.9
  nucleus pulposus — *see* Disorder, disc
  nutritional E63.9
  oast-house-urine E72.19
    ocular
      herpesviral B00.50
      zoster B02.30
  obliterative vascular I77.1
  Ohara's — *see* Tularemia
  Opitz's (congestive splenomegaly) D73.2
  Oppenheim-Urbach (necrobiosis lipoidica diabetico-
      rum) — *see* E08-E13 with .620
  optic nerve NEC — *see* Disorder, nerve, optic
  orbit — *see* Disorder, orbit
  Oriental liver fluke B66.1
  Oriental lung fluke B66.4
  Ormond's N13.5
  Oropouche virus A93.0
  Osler-Rendu (familial hemorrhagic telangiectasia) I78.0
  osteofibrocystic E21.0
  Otto's M24.7
  outer ear — *see* Disorder, ear, external
  ovary (noninflammatory) N83.9
    cystic N83.20- ☑
    inflammatory — *see* Salpingo-oophoritis
    polycystic E28.2
    specified NEC N83.8
  Owren's (congenital) — *see* Defect, coagulation
  pancreas K86.9
    cystic K86.2
    fibrocystic E84.9
    specified NEC K86.89
  panvalvular I08.9
    specified NEC I08.8
  parametrium (noninflammatory) N83.9
  parasitic B89
    cerebral NEC B71.9 *[G94]*
    intestinal NOS B82.9
    mouth B37.0
    skin NOS B88.9
    specified type — *see* Infestation
    tongue B37.0
  parathyroid (gland) E21.5
    specified NEC E21.4
  Parkinson's G20
  parodontal K05.6
  Parrot's (syphilitic osteochondritis) A50.02
  Parry's (exophthalmic goiter) — *see* Hyperthyroidism,
      with, goiter (diffuse)
  Parson's (exophthalmic goiter) — *see* Hyperthyroidism,
      with, goiter (diffuse)
  Paxton's (white piedra) B36.2
  pearl-worker's — *see* Osteomyelitis, specified type NEC
  Pellegrini-Stieda (calcification, knee joint) — *see* Bursi-
      tis, tibial collateral
  pelvis, pelvic
    female NOS N94.9
      specified NEC N94.89
    gonococcal (acute) (chronic) A54.24
    inflammatory (female) N73.9
      acute N73.0
      chlamydial A56.11
      chronic N73.1
      specified NEC N73.8
      syphilitic (secondary) A51.42
        late A52.76
      tuberculous A18.17
    organ, female N94.9
    peritoneum, female NEC N94.89
  penis N48.9
    inflammatory N48.29
      abscess N48.21
      cellulitis N48.22
    specified NEC N48.89
  periapical tissues NOS K04.90
  periodontal K05.6
    specified NEC K05.5

Disease, diseased — *continued*
  periosteum — *see* Disorder, bone, specified type NEC
  peripheral
    arterial I73.9
    autonomic nervous system G90.9
    nerves — *see* Polyneuropathy
    vascular NOS I73.9
  peritoneum K66.9
    pelvic, female NEC N94.89
    specified NEC K66.8
  persistent mucosal (middle ear) H66.20
    left H66.22
      with right H66.23
    right H66.21
      with left H66.23
  Petit's — *see* Hernia, abdomen, specified site NEC
  pharynx J39.2
    specified NEC J39.2
  Phocas' — *see* Mastopathy, cystic
  photochromogenic (acid-fast bacilli) (pulmonary) A31.0
    nonpulmonary A31.9
  Pick's G31.01 *[F02.80]*
    with behavioral disturbance G31.01 *[F02.81]*
    brain G31.01 *[F02.80]*
      with behavioral disturbance G31.01 *[F02.81]*
    of pericardium (pericardial pseudocirrhosis of liver)
        I31.1
  pigeon fancier's J67.2
  pineal gland E34.8
  pink — *see* Poisoning, mercury
  Pinkus' (lichen nitidus) L44.1
  pinworm B80
  Piry virus A93.8
  pituitary (gland) E23.7
  pituitary-snuff-taker's J67.8
  pleura (cavity) J94.9
    specified NEC J94.8
  pneumatic drill (hammer) T75.21 ☑
  Pollitzer's (hidradenitis suppurativa) L73.2
  polycystic
    kidney or renal Q61.3
      adult type Q61.2
      childhood type NEC Q61.19
        collecting duct dilatation Q61.11
    liver or hepatic Q44.6
    lung or pulmonary J98.4
      congenital Q33.0
    ovary, ovaries E28.2
    spleen Q89.09
  polyethylene T84.05- ☑
  Pompe's (glycogenosis II) E74.02
  Posadas-Wernicke B38.9
  Potain's (pulmonary edema) — *see* Edema, lung
  prepuce N47.8
    inflammatory N47.7
    balanoposthitis N47.6
  Pringle's (tuberous sclerosis) Q85.1
  prion, central nervous system A81.9
    specified NEC A81.89
  prostate N42.9
    specified NEC N42.89
  protozoal B64
    acanthamebiasis — *see* Acanthamebiasis
    African trypanosomiasis — *see* African trypanosomi-
        asis
    babesiosis B60.0
    Chagas disease — *see* Chagas disease
    intestine, intestinal A07.9
    leishmaniasis — *see* Leishmaniasis
    malaria — *see* Malaria
    naegleriasis B60.2
    pneumocystosis B59
    specified organism NEC B60.8
    toxoplasmosis — *see* Toxoplasmosis
  pseudo-Hurler's E77.0
  psychiatric F99
  psychotic — *see* Psychosis
  Puente's (simple glandular cheilitis) K13.0
  puerperal — *see also* Puerperal O90.89
  pulmonary — *see also* Disease, lung
    artery I28.9
    chronic obstructive J44.9
      with
        acute bronchitis J44.0
        exacerbation (acute) J44.1
        lower respiratory infection (acute) J44.0
      decompensated J44.1

☞ Subterms under main terms may continue to next column or page   ☑ Additional Character Required — Refer to the Tabular List for Character Selection

Disease, diseased — *continued*
  pulmonary — *see also* Disease, lung — *continued*
    chronic obstructive — *continued*
      decompensated — *continued*
        with
          exacerbation (acute) J44.1
    heart I27.9
      specified NEC I27.89
    hypertensive (vascular) — *see also* Hypertension,
        pulmonary I27.20
      NEC I27.2 ☑
      primary (idiopathic) I27.0
    valve I37.9
      rheumatic I09.89
  pulp (dental) NOS K04.90
  pulseless M31.4
  Putnam's (subacute combined sclerosis with pernicious
      anemia) D51.0
  Pyle (-Cohn) (metaphyseal dysplasia) Q78.5
  ragpicker's or ragsorter's A22.1
  Raynaud's — *see* Raynaud's disease
  reactive airway — *see* Asthma
  Reclus' (cystic) — *see* Mastopathy, cystic
  rectum K62.9
    specified NEC K62.89
  Refsum's (heredopathia atactica polyneuritiformis)
      G60.1
  renal (functional) (pelvis) — *see also* Disease, kidney
      N28.9
    with
      edema — *see* Nephrosis
      glomerular lesion — *see* Glomerulonephritis
        with edema — *see* Nephrosis
      interstitial nephritis N12
    acute N28.9
    chronic — *see also* Disease, kidney, chronic N18.9
    cystic, congenital Q61.9
    diabetic — *see* E08-E13 with .22
    end-stage (failure) N18.6
      due to hypertension I12.0
    fibrocystic (congenital) Q61.8
    hypertensive — *see* Hypertension, kidney
    lupus M32.14
    phosphate-losing (tubular) N25.0
    polycystic (congenital) Q61.3
      adult type Q61.2
      childhood type NEC Q61.19
        collecting duct dilatation Q61.11
    rapidly progressive N01.9
    subacute N01.9
  Rendu-Osler-Weber (familial hemorrhagic telangiecta-
      sia) I78.0
  renovascular (arteriosclerotic) — *see* Hypertension,
      kidney
  respiratory (tract) J98.9
    acute or subacute NOS J06.9
      due to
        chemicals, gases, fumes or vapors (inhalation)
            J68.3
        external agent J70.9
          specified NEC J70.8
        radiation J70.0
        smoke inhalation J70.5
      noninfectious J39.8
    chronic NOS J98.9
      due to
        chemicals, gases, fumes or vapors J68.4
        external agent J70.9
          specified NEC J70.8
        radiation J70.1
      newborn P27.9
        specified NEC P27.8
    due to
      chemicals, gases, fumes or vapors J68.9
        acute or subacute NEC J68.3
        chronic J68.4
      external agent J70.9
        specified NEC J70.8
    newborn P28.9
      specified type NEC P28.89
    upper J39.9
      acute or subacute J06.9
      noninfectious NEC J39.8
      specified NEC J39.8
      streptococcal J06.9
  retina, retinal H35.9
    Batten's or Batten-Mayou E75.4 *[H36]*
    specified NEC H35.89

Disease, diseased — *continued*
  rheumatoid — *see* Arthritis, rheumatoid
  rickettsial NOS A79.9
    specified type NEC A79.89
  Riga (-Fede) (cachectic aphthae) K14.0
  Riggs' (compound periodontitis) — *see* Periodontitis
  Ritter's L00
  Rivalta's (cervicofacial actinomycosis) A42.2
  Robles' (onchocerciasis) B73.01
  Roger's (congenital interventricular septal defect) Q21.0
  Rosenthal's (factor XI deficiency) D68.1
  Ross River B33.1
  Rossbach's (hyperchlorhydria) K31.89
    psychogenic F45.8
  Rotes Quérol — *see* Hyperostosis, ankylosing
  Roth (-Bernhardt) — *see* Mononeuropathy, lower limb,
      meralgia paresthetica
  Runeberg's (progressive pernicious anemia) D51.0
  sacroiliac NEC M53.3
  salivary gland or duct K11.9
    inclusion B25.9
    specified NEC K11.8
    virus B25.9
  sandworm B76.9
  Schimmelbusch's — *see* Mastopathy, cystic
  Schmorl's — *see* Schmorl's disease or nodes
  Schönlein (-Henoch) (purpura rheumatica) D69.0
  Schottmüller's — *see* Fever, paratyphoid
  Schultz's (agranulocytosis) — *see* Agranulocytosis
  Schwalbe-Ziehen-Oppenheim G24.1
  Schwartz-Jampel G71.13
  sclera H15.9
    specified NEC H15.89
  scrofulous (tuberculous) A18.2
  scrotum N50.9
  sebaceous glands L73.9
  semilunar cartilage, cystic — *see also* Derangement,
      knee, meniscus, cystic
  seminal vesicle N50.9
  serum NEC — *see also* Reaction, serum T80.69 ☑
  sexually transmitted A64
    anogenital
      herpesviral infection — *see* Herpes, anogenital
      warts A63.0
    chancroid A57
    chlamydial infection — *see* Chlamydia
    gonorrhea — *see* Gonorrhea
    granuloma inguinale A58
    specified organism NEC A63.8
    syphilis — *see* Syphilis
    trichomoniasis — *see* Trichomoniasis
  Sézary C84.1- ☑
  shimamushi (scrub typhus) A75.3
  shipyard B30.0
  sickle-cell D57.1
    with crisis (vasoocclusive pain) D57.00
      with
        acute chest syndrome D57.01
        splenic sequestration D57.02
    elliptocytosis D57.8- ☑
    Hb-C D57.20
      with crisis (vasoocclusive pain) D57.219
        with
          acute chest syndrome D57.211
          splenic sequestration D57.212
      without crisis D57.20
    Hb-SD D57.80
      with crisis D57.819
        with
          acute chest syndrome D57.811
          splenic sequestration D57.812
    Hb-SE D57.80
      with crisis D57.819
        with
          acute chest syndrome D57.811
          splenic sequestration D57.812
    specified NEC D57.80
      with crisis D57.819
        with
          acute chest syndrome D57.811
          splenic sequestration D57.812
    spherocytosis D57.80
      with crisis D57.819
        with
          acute chest syndrome D57.811
          splenic sequestration D57.812
    thalassemia D57.40
      with crisis (vasoocclusive pain) D57.419

Disease, diseased — *continued*
  sickle-cell — *continued*
    thalassemia — *continued*
      with crisis — *continued*
        with
          acute chest syndrome D57.411
          splenic sequestration D57.412
      without crisis D57.40
  silo-filler's J68.8
    bronchitis J68.0
    pneumonitis J68.0
    pulmonary edema J68.1
  simian B B00.4
  Simons' (progressive lipodystrophy) E88.1
  sin nombre virus B33.4
  sinus — *see* Sinusitis
  Sirkari's B55.9
  sixth B08.20
    due to human herpesvirus 6 B08.21
    due to human herpesvirus 7 B08.22
  skin L98.9
    due to metabolic disorder NEC E88.9 *[L99]*
    specified NEC L98.8
  slim (HIV) B20
  small vessel I73.9
  Sneddon-Wilkinson (subcorneal pustular dermatosis)
      L13.1
  South African creeping B88.0
  spinal (cord) G95.9
    congenital Q06.9
    specified NEC G95.89
  spine — *see also* Spondylopathy
    joint — *see* Dorsopathy
    tuberculous A18.01
  spinocerebellar (hereditary) G11.9
    specified NEC G11.8
  spleen D73.9
    amyloid E85.4 *[D77]*
    organic D73.9
    polycystic Q89.09
    postinfectional D73.89
  sponge-diver's — *see* Toxicity, venom, marine animal,
      sea anemone
  Startle Q89.8
  Steinert's G71.11
  Sticker's (erythema infectiosum) B08.3
  Stieda's (calcification, knee joint) — *see* Bursitis, tibial
      collateral
  Stokes' (exophthalmic goiter) — *see* Hyperthyroidism,
      with, goiter (diffuse)
  Stokes-Adams (syncope with heart block) I45.9
  stomach K31.9
    functional, psychogenic F45.8
    specified NEC K31.89
  stonemason's J62.8
  storage
    glycogen — *see* Disease, glycogen storage
    mucopolysaccharide — *see* Mucopolysaccharidosis
  striatopallidal system NEC G25.89
  Stuart-Prower (congenital factor X deficiency) D68.2
  Stuart's (congenital factor X deficiency) D68.2
  subcutaneous tissue — *see* Disease, skin
  supporting structures of teeth K08.9
    specified NEC K08.89
  suprarenal (capsule) (gland) E27.9
    hyperfunction E27.0
    specified NEC E27.8
  sweat glands L74.9
    specified NEC L74.8
  Sweeley-Klionsky E75.21
  Swift (-Feer) — *see* Poisoning, mercury
  swimming-pool granuloma A31.1
  Sylvest's (epidemic pleurodynia) B33.0
  sympathetic nervous system G90.9
  synovium — *see* Disorder, synovium
  syphilitic — *see* Syphilis
  systemic tissue mast cell D47.02
  tanapox (virus) B08.71
  Tangier E78.6
  Tarral-Besnier (pityriasis rubra pilaris) L44.0
  Tauri's E74.09
  tear duct — *see* Disorder, lacrimal system
  tendon, tendinous — *see also* Disorder, tendon
    nodular — *see* Trigger finger
  terminal vessel I73.9
  testis N50.9
  thalassemia Hb-S — *see* Disease, sickle-cell, thalassemia
  Thaysen-Gee (nontropical sprue) K90.0

☑ **Additional Character Required** — Refer to the Tabular List for Character Selection ⍟ **Subterms under main terms may continue to next column or page**

Dislocation — *continued*
- habitual — *see* Dislocation, recurrent
- hip S73.00- ☑
  - anterior S73.03- ☑
    - obturator S73.02- ☑
  - central S73.04- ☑
  - congenital (total) Q65.2
    - bilateral Q65.1
    - partial Q65.5
      - bilateral Q65.4
      - unilateral Q65.3- ☑
    - unilateral Q65.0- ☑
  - developmental M24.85- ☑
  - pathological — *see* Dislocation, pathological NEC, hip
  - posterior S73.01- ☑
  - recurrent — *see* Dislocation, recurrent, hip
- humerus, proximal end — *see* Dislocation, shoulder
- incomplete — *see* Subluxation, by site
- incus — *see* Discontinuity, ossicles, ear
- infracoracoid — *see* Dislocation, shoulder
- innominate (pubic junction) (sacral junction) S33.39 ☑
  - acetabulum — *see* Dislocation, hip
- interphalangeal (joint(s))
  - finger S63.279
    - distal S63.29- ☑
      - index S63.29- ☑
      - little S63.29- ☑
      - middle S63.29- ☑
      - ring S63.29- ☑
    - index S63.27- ☑
    - little S63.27- ☑
    - middle S63.27- ☑
    - proximal S63.28- ☑
      - index S63.28- ☑
      - little S63.28- ☑
      - middle S63.28- ☑
      - ring S63.28- ☑
    - ring S63.27- ☑
  - foot or toe — *see* Dislocation, toe
  - thumb S63.12- ☑
- jaw (cartilage) (meniscus) S03.0- ☑
- joint prosthesis — *see* Complications, joint prosthesis, mechanical, displacement, by site
- knee S83.106 ☑
  - cap — *see* Dislocation, patella
  - congenital Q68.2
  - old M23.8X- ☑
  - patella — *see* Dislocation, patella
  - pathological — *see* Dislocation, pathological NEC, knee
  - proximal tibia
    - anteriorly S83.11- ☑
    - laterally S83.14- ☑
    - medially S83.13- ☑
    - posteriorly S83.12- ☑
  - recurrent — *see also* Derangement, knee, specified NEC
  - specified type NEC S83.19- ☑
- lacrimal gland H04.16- ☑
- lens (complete) H27.10
  - anterior H27.12- ☑
  - congenital Q12.1
  - ocular implant — *see* Complications, intraocular lens
  - partial H27.11- ☑
  - posterior H27.13- ☑
  - traumatic S05.8X- ☑
- ligament — *code by* site under Dislocation
- lumbar (vertebra) — *see* Dislocation, vertebra, lumbar
- lumbosacral (vertebra) — *see also* Dislocation, vertebra, lumbar
  - congenital Q76.49
- mandible S03.0- ☑
- meniscus (knee) — *see* Tear, meniscus
  - other sites - code by site under Dislocation
- metacarpal (bone)
  - distal end — *see* Dislocation, finger
  - proximal end S63.06- ☑
- metacarpophalangeal (joint)
  - finger S63.26- ☑
    - index S63.26- ☑
    - little S63.26- ☑
    - middle S63.26- ☑
    - ring S63.26- ☑
  - thumb S63.11- ☑

Dislocation — *continued*
- metatarsal (bone) — *see* Dislocation, foot
- metatarsophalangeal (joint(s)) — *see* Dislocation, toe
- midcarpal (joint) S63.03- ☑
- midtarsal (joint) — *see* Dislocation, foot
- neck S13.20 ☑
  - specified site NEC S13.29 ☑
  - vertebra — *see* Dislocation, vertebra, cervical
- nose (septal cartilage) S03.1 ☑
- occipitoatloid S13.111 ☑
- old — *see* Derangement, joint, specified type NEC
- ossicles, ear — *see* Discontinuity, ossicles, ear
- partial — *see* Subluxation, by site
- patella S83.006 ☑
  - congenital Q74.1
  - lateral S83.01- ☑
  - recurrent (nontraumatic) M22.0- ☑
    - incomplete M22.1- ☑
  - specified type NEC S83.09- ☑
- pathological NEC M24.30
  - ankle M24.37- ☑
  - elbow M24.32- ☑
  - foot joint M24.37- ☑
  - hand joint M24.34- ☑
  - hip M24.35- ☑
  - knee M24.36- ☑
  - lumbosacral joint — *see* subcategory M53.2
  - pelvic region — *see* Dislocation, pathological, hip
  - sacroiliac — *see* subcategory M53.2
  - shoulder M24.31- ☑
  - wrist M24.33- ☑
- pelvis NEC S33.30 ☑
  - specified NEC S33.39 ☑
- phalanx
  - finger or hand — *see* Dislocation, finger
  - foot or toe — *see* Dislocation, toe
- prosthesis, internal — *see* Complications, prosthetic device, by site, mechanical
- radial head S53.006 ☑
  - anterior S53.01- ☑
  - posterior S53.02- ☑
  - specified type NEC S53.09- ☑
- radiocarpal (joint) S63.02- ☑
- radiohumeral (joint) — *see* Dislocation, radial head
- radioulnar (joint)
  - distal S63.01- ☑
  - proximal — *see* Dislocation, elbow
- radius
  - distal end — *see* Dislocation, wrist
  - proximal end — *see* Dislocation, radial head
- recurrent M24.40
  - ankle M24.47- ☑
  - elbow M24.42- ☑
  - finger M24.44- ☑
  - foot joint M24.47- ☑
  - hand joint M24.44- ☑
  - hip M24.45- ☑
  - knee M24.46- ☑
    - patella — *see* Dislocation, patella, recurrent
  - patella — *see* Dislocation, patella, recurrent
  - sacroiliac — *see* subcategory M53.2
  - shoulder M24.41- ☑
  - toe M24.47- ☑
  - vertebra — *see also* subcategory M43.5
    - atlantoaxial M43.4
      - with myelopathy M43.3
  - wrist M24.43- ☑
- rib (cartilage) S23.29 ☑
- sacrococcygeal S33.2 ☑
- sacroiliac (joint) (ligament) S33.2 ☑
  - congenital Q74.2
  - recurrent — *see* subcategory M53.2
- sacrum S33.2 ☑
- scaphoid (bone) (hand) (wrist) — *see* Dislocation, wrist
  - foot — *see* Dislocation, foot
- scapula — *see* Dislocation, shoulder, girdle, scapula
- semilunar cartilage, knee — *see* Tear, meniscus
- septal cartilage (nose) S03.1 ☑
- septum (nasal) (old) J34.2
- sesamoid bone — *code by* site under Dislocation
- shoulder (blade) (ligament) (joint) (traumatic) S43.006 ☑
  - acromioclavicular — *see* Dislocation, acromioclavicular
  - chronic — *see* Dislocation, recurrent, shoulder
  - congenital Q68.8

Dislocation — *continued*
- shoulder — *continued*
  - girdle S43.30- ☑
    - scapula S43.31- ☑
    - specified site NEC S43.39- ☑
  - humerus S43.00- ☑
    - anterior S43.01- ☑
    - inferior S43.03- ☑
    - posterior S43.02- ☑
  - pathological — *see* Dislocation, pathological NEC, shoulder
  - recurrent — *see* Dislocation, recurrent, shoulder
  - specified type NEC S43.08- ☑
- spine
  - cervical — *see* Dislocation, vertebra, cervical
  - congenital Q76.49
  - due to birth trauma P11.5
  - lumbar — *see* Dislocation, vertebra, lumbar
  - thoracic — *see* Dislocation, vertebra, thoracic
- spontaneous — *see* Dislocation, pathological
- sternoclavicular (joint) S43.206 ☑
  - anterior S43.21- ☑
  - posterior S43.22- ☑
- sternum S23.29 ☑
- subglenoid — *see* Dislocation, shoulder
- symphysis pubis S33.4 ☑
- talus — *see* Dislocation, ankle
- tarsal (bone(s)) (joint(s)) — *see* Dislocation, foot
- tarsometatarsal (joint(s)) — *see* Dislocation, foot
- temporomandibular (joint) S03.0- ☑
- thigh, proximal end — *see* Dislocation, hip
- thorax S23.20 ☑
  - specified site NEC S23.29 ☑
  - vertebra — *see* Dislocation, vertebra
- thumb S63.10- ☑
  - interphalangeal joint — *see* Dislocation, interphalangeal (joint), thumb
  - metacarpophalangeal joint — *see* Dislocation, metacarpophalangeal (joint), thumb
- thyroid cartilage S13.29 ☑
- tibia
  - distal end — *see* Dislocation, ankle
  - proximal end — *see* Dislocation, knee
- tibiofibular (joint)
  - distal — *see* Dislocation, ankle
  - superior — *see* Dislocation, knee
- toe(s) S93.106 ☑
  - great S93.10- ☑
    - interphalangeal joint S93.11- ☑
    - metatarsophalangeal joint S93.12- ☑
  - interphalangeal joint S93.119 ☑
  - lesser S93.106 ☑
    - interphalangeal joint S93.11- ☑
    - metatarsophalangeal joint S93.12- ☑
  - metatarsophalangeal joint S93.12- ☑
- tooth S03.2 ☑
- trachea S23.29 ☑
- ulna
  - distal end S63.07- ☑
  - proximal end — *see* Dislocation, elbow
- ulnohumeral (joint) — *see* Dislocation, elbow
- vertebra (articular process) (body) (traumatic)
  - cervical S13.101 ☑
    - atlantoaxial joint S13.121 ☑
    - atlantooccipital joint S13.111 ☑
    - atloidooccipital joint S13.111 ☑
    - joint between
      - C0 and C1 S13.111 ☑
      - C1 and C2 S13.121 ☑
      - C2 and C3 S13.131 ☑
      - C3 and C4 S13.141 ☑
      - C4 and C5 S13.151 ☑
      - C5 and C6 S13.161 ☑
      - C6 and C7 S13.171 ☑
      - C7 and T1 S13.181 ☑
    - occipitoatloid joint S13.111 ☑
  - congenital Q76.49
  - lumbar S33.101 ☑
    - joint between
      - L1 and L2 S33.111 ☑
      - L2 and L3 S33.121 ☑
      - L3 and L4 S33.131 ☑
      - L4 and L5 S33.141 ☑
  - nontraumatic — *see* Displacement, intervertebral disc
  - partial — *see* Subluxation, by site

☑ **Additional Character Required** — **Refer to the Tabular List for Character Selection**   ▽ **Subterms under main terms may continue to next column or page**

Dislocation — *continued*
- vertebra — *continued*
  - recurrent NEC — *see* subcategory M43.5 ☑
  - thoracic S23.101 ☑
    - joint between
      - T1 and T2 S23.111 ☑
      - T2 and T3 S23.121 ☑
      - T3 and T4 S23.123 ☑
      - T4 and T5 S23.131 ☑
      - T5 and T6 S23.133 ☑
      - T6 and T7 S23.141 ☑
      - T7 and T8 S23.143 ☑
      - T8 and T9 S23.151 ☑
      - T9 and T10 S23.153 ☑
      - T10 and T11 S23.161 ☑
      - T11 and T12 S23.163 ☑
      - T12 and L1 S23.171 ☑
- wrist (carpal bone) S63.006 ☑
  - carpometacarpal joint — *see* Dislocation, carpometacarpal (joint)
  - distal radioulnar joint — *see* Dislocation, radioulnar (joint), distal
  - metacarpal bone, proximal — *see* Dislocation, metacarpal (bone), proximal end
  - midcarpal — *see* Dislocation, midcarpal (joint)
  - radiocarpal joint — *see* Dislocation, radiocarpal (joint)
  - recurrent — *see* Dislocation, recurrent, wrist
  - specified site NEC S63.09- ☑
  - ulna — *see* Dislocation, ulna, distal end
- xiphoid cartilage S23.29 ☑

Disorder (of) — *see also* Disease
- acantholytic L11.9
  - specified NEC L11.8
- acute
  - psychotic — *see* Psychosis, acute
  - stress F43.0
- adjustment (grief) F43.20
  - with
    - anxiety F43.22
      - with depressed mood F43.23
    - conduct disturbance F43.24
      - with emotional disturbance F43.25
    - depressed mood F43.21
      - with anxiety F43.23
    - other specified symptom F43.29
- adrenal (capsule) (gland) (medullary) E27.9
  - specified NEC E27.8
- adrenogenital E25.9
  - drug-induced E25.8
  - iatrogenic E25.8
  - idiopathic E25.8
- adult personality (and behavior) F69
  - specified NEC F68.8
- affective (mood) — *see* Disorder, mood
- aggressive, unsocialized F91.1
- alcohol use
  - mild F10.10
    - with
      - alcohol intoxication F10.129
        - delirium F10.121
      - alcohol-induced
        - anxiety disorder F10.180
        - bipolar and related disorder F10.14
        - depressive disorder F10.14
        - psychotic disorder F10.159
        - sexual dysfunction F10.181
        - sleep disorder F10.182
    - in remission (early) (sustained) F10.11
  - moderate or severe F10.20
    - with
      - alcohol intoxication F10.229
        - delirium F10.221
      - alcohol-induced
        - anxiety disorder F10.280
        - bipolar and related disorder F10.24
        - depressive disorder F10.24
        - major neurocognitive disorder, amnestic-confabulatory type F10.26
        - major neurocognitive disorder, non-amnestic-confabulatory type F10.27
        - mild neurocognitive disorder F10.288
        - psychotic disorder F10.259
        - sexual dysfunction F10.281
        - sleep disorder F10.282
    - in remission (early) (sustained) F10.21
- alcohol-related F10.99

Disorder — *continued*
- alcohol-related — *continued*
  - with
    - amnestic disorder, persisting F10.96
    - anxiety disorder F10.980
    - dementia, persisting F10.97
    - intoxication F10.929
      - with delirium F10.921
      - uncomplicated F10.920
    - mood disorder F10.94
    - other specified F10.988
    - psychotic disorder F10.959
      - with
        - delusions F10.950
        - hallucinations F10.951
    - sexual dysfunction F10.981
    - sleep disorder F10.982
- allergic — *see* Allergy
- alveolar NEC J84.09
- amino-acid
  - cystathioninuria E72.19
  - cystinosis E72.04
  - cystinuria E72.01
  - glycinuria E72.09
  - homocystinuria E72.11
  - metabolism — *see* Disturbance, metabolism, amino-acid
  - specified NEC E72.89
  - neonatal, transitory P74.8
  - renal transport NEC E72.09
  - transport NEC E72.09
- amnesic, amnestic
  - alcohol-induced F10.96
    - with dependence F10.26
  - due to (secondary to) general medical condition F04
  - psychoactive NEC-induced F19.96
    - with
      - abuse F19.16
      - dependence F19.26
  - sedative, hypnotic or anxiolytic-induced F13.96
    - with dependence F13.26
- amphetamine (or other stimulant) use
  - mild
    - with
      - amphetamine, cocaine, or other stimulant intoxication
        - with perceptual disturbances F15.122
        - without perceptual disturbances F15.129
      - amphetamine (or other stimulant) -induced
        - anxiety disorder F15.180
        - bipolar and related disorder F15.14
        - depressive disorder F15.14
        - obsessive-compulsive and related disorder F15.188
        - psychotic disorder F15.159
        - sexual dysfunction F15.181
      - intoxication delirium F15.121
  - moderate or severe
    - with
      - amphetamine, cocaine, or other stimulant intoxication
        - with perceptual disturbances F15.222
        - without perceptual disturbances F15.229
      - amphetamine (or other stimulant) -induced
        - anxiety disorder F15.280
        - bipolar and related disorder F15.24
        - depressive disorder F15.24
        - obsessive-compulsive and related disorder F15.288
        - psychotic disorder F15.259
        - sexual dysfunction F15.281
      - intoxication delirium F15.221
- amphetamine-type substance use
  - mild F15.10
    - in remission (early) (sustained) F15.11
  - moderate F15.20
    - in remission (early) (sustained) F15.21
  - severe F15.20
    - in remission (early) (sustained) F15.21
- anaerobic glycolysis with anemia D55.2
- anxiety F41.9
  - due to (secondary to)
    - alcohol F10.980
      - in
        - abuse F10.180
        - dependence F10.280
    - amphetamine F15.980
      - in
        - abuse F15.180

Disorder — *continued*
- anxiety — *continued*
  - due to — *continued*
    - amphetamine — *continued*
      - in — *continued*
        - dependence F15.280
    - anxiolytic F13.980
      - in
        - abuse F13.180
        - dependence F13.280
    - caffeine F15.980
      - in
        - abuse F15.180
        - dependence F15.280
    - cannabis F12.980
      - in
        - abuse F12.180
        - dependence F12.280
    - cocaine F14.980
      - in
        - abuse F14.180
        - dependence F14.180
    - general medical condition F06.4
    - hallucinogen F16.980
      - in
        - abuse F16.180
        - dependence F16.280
    - hypnotic F13.980
      - in
        - abuse F13.180
        - dependence F13.280
    - inhalant F18.980
      - in
        - abuse F18.180
        - dependence F18.280
    - phencyclidine F16.980
      - in
        - abuse F16.180
        - dependence F16.280
    - psychoactive substance NEC F19.980
      - in
        - abuse F19.180
        - dependence F19.280
    - sedative F13.980
      - in
        - abuse F13.180
        - dependence F13.280
    - volatile solvents F18.980
      - in
        - abuse F18.180
        - dependence F18.280
  - generalized F41.1
  - illness F45.21
  - mixed
    - with depression (mild) F41.8
    - specified NEC F41.3
  - organic F06.4
  - phobic F40.9
    - of childhood F40.8
  - specified NEC F41.8
- aortic valve — *see* Endocarditis, aortic
- aromatic amino-acid metabolism E70.9
  - specified NEC E70.8
- arteriole NEC I77.89
- artery NEC I77.89
- articulation — *see* Disorder, joint
- attachment (childhood)
  - disinhibited F94.2
  - reactive F94.1
- attention-deficit hyperactivity (adolescent) (adult) (child) F90.9
  - combined
    - presentation F90.2
    - type F90.2
  - hyperactive
    - impulsive presentation F90.1
    - type F90.1
  - inattentive
    - presentation F90.0
    - type F90.0
  - specified type NEC F90.8
- attention-deficit without hyperactivity (adolescent) (adult) (child) F98.8
- auditory processing (central) H93.25
- autism spectrum F84.0
- autistic F84.0
- autoimmune D89.89
- autonomic nervous system G90.9
  - specified NEC G90.8

☟ **Subterms under main terms may continue to next column or page**   ☑ **Additional Character Required — Refer to the Tabular List for Character Selection**

Disorder — continued
  avoidant
    child or adolescent F40.10
    restrictive food intake F50.82
  balance
    acid-base E87.8
      mixed E87.4
    electrolyte E87.8
    fluid NEC E87.8
  behavioral (disruptive) — see Disorder, conduct
  beta-amino-acid metabolism E72.89
  bile acid and cholesterol metabolism E78.70
    Barth syndrome E78.71
    other specified E78.79
    Smith-Lemli-Opitz syndrome E78.72
  bilirubin excretion E80.6
  binge eating F50.81
  binocular
    movement H51.9
      convergence
        excess H51.12
        insufficiency H51.11
      internuclear ophthalmoplegia — see Ophthalmo-
          plegia, internuclear
      palsy of conjugate gaze H51.0
      specified type NEC H51.8
    vision NEC — see Disorder, vision, binocular
  bipolar (I) (type I) F31.9
    and related due to a known physiological condition
      with
        manic features F06.33
        manic- or hypomanic-like episodes F06.33
        mixed features F06.34
    current (or most recent) episode
      depressed F31.9
        with psychotic features F31.5
        without psychotic features F31.30
          mild F31.31
          moderate F31.32
          severe (without psychotic features) F31.4
            with psychotic features F31.5
      hypomanic F31.0
      manic F31.9
        with psychotic features F31.2
        without psychotic features F31.10
          mild F31.11
          moderate F31.12
          severe (without psychotic features)
              F31.13
            with psychotic features F31.2
      mixed F31.60
        mild F31.61
        moderate F31.62
        severe (without psychotic features) F31.63
          with psychotic features F31.64
      severe depression (without psychotic features)
          F31.4
        with psychotic features F31.5
    in remission (currently) F31.70
      in full remission
        most recent episode
          depressed F31.76
          hypomanic F31.72
          manic F31.74
          mixed F31.78
      in partial remission
        most recent episode
          depressed F31.75
          hypomanic F31.71
          manic F31.73
          mixed F31.77
    organic F06.30
    single manic episode F30.9
      mild F30.11
      moderate F30.12
      severe (without psychotic symptoms) F30.13
        with psychotic symptoms F30.2
    specified NEC F31.89
  bipolar II (type 2) F31.81
  bladder N32.9
    functional NEC N31.9
    in schistosomiasis B65.0 [N33]
    specified NEC N32.89
  bleeding D68.9
  blood D75.9
    in congenital early syphilis A50.09 [D77]
  body dysmorphic F45.22
  bone M89.9
    continuity M84.9

Disorder — continued
  bone — continued
    continuity — continued
      specified type NEC M84.80
        ankle M84.87- ☑
        fibula M84.86- ☑
        foot M84.87- ☑
        hand M84.84- ☑
        humerus M84.82- ☑
        neck M84.88
        pelvis M84.859
        radius M84.83- ☑
        rib M84.88
        shoulder M84.81- ☑
        skull M84.88
        thigh M84.85- ☑
        tibia M84.86- ☑
        ulna M84.83- ☑
        vertebra M84.88
    density and structure M85.9
      cyst — see also Cyst, bone, specified type NEC
        aneurysmal — see Cyst, bone, aneurysmal
        solitary — see Cyst, bone, solitary
      diffuse idiopathic skeletal hyperostosis — see
          Hyperostosis, ankylosing
      fibrous dysplasia (monostotic) — see Dysplasia,
          fibrous, bone
      fluorosis — see Fluorosis, skeletal
      hyperostosis of skull M85.2
      osteitis condensans — see Osteitis, condensans
      specified type NEC M85.8- ☑
        ankle M85.87- ☑
        foot M85.87- ☑
        forearm M85.83- ☑
        hand M85.84- ☑
        lower leg M85.86- ☑
        multiple sites M85.89
        neck M85.88
        rib M85.88
        shoulder M85.81- ☑
        skull M85.88
        thigh M85.85- ☑
        upper arm M85.82- ☑
        vertebra M85.88
    development and growth NEC M89.20
      carpus M89.24- ☑
      clavicle M89.21- ☑
      femur M89.25- ☑
      fibula M89.26- ☑
      finger M89.24- ☑
      humerus M89.22- ☑
      ilium M89.259
      ischium M89.259
      metacarpus M89.24- ☑
      metatarsus M89.27- ☑
      multiple sites M89.29
      neck M89.28
      radius M89.23- ☑
      rib M89.28
      scapula M89.21- ☑
      skull M89.28
      tarsus M89.27- ☑
      tibia M89.26- ☑
      toe M89.27- ☑
      ulna M89.23- ☑
      vertebra M89.28
    specified type NEC M89.8X- ☑
  brachial plexus G54.0
  branched-chain amino-acid metabolism E71.2
    specified NEC E71.19
  breast N64.9
    agalactia — see Agalactia
    associated with
      lactation O92.70
        specified NEC O92.79
      pregnancy O92.20
        specified NEC O92.29
      puerperium O92.20
        specified NEC O92.29
    cracked nipple — see Cracked nipple
    galactorrhea — see Galactorrhea
    hypogalactia O92.4
    lactation disorder NEC O92.79
    mastitis — see Mastitis
    nipple infection — see Infection, nipple
    retracted nipple — see Retraction, nipple
    specified type NEC N64.89

Disorder — continued
  Briquet's F45.0
  bullous, in diseases classified elsewhere L14
  caffeine use
    mild
      with
        caffeine-induced
          anxiety disorder F15.180
          sleep disorder F15.182
    moderate or severe
      with
        caffeine-induced
          anxiety disorder F15.280
          sleep disorder F15.282
  cannabis use
    mild F12.10
      with
        cannabis intoxication delirium F12.121
          with perceptual disturbances F12.122
          without perceptual disturbances F12.129
        cannabis-induced
          anxiety disorder F12.180
          psychotic disorder F12.159
          sleep disorder F12.188
      in remission (early) (sustained) F12.11
    moderate or severe F12.20
      with
        cannabis intoxication
          with perceptual disturbances F12.222
          without perceptual disturbances F12.229
        cannabis-induced
          anxiety disorder F12.280
          psychotic disorder F12.259
          sleep disorder F12.288
        delirium F12.221
      in remission (early) (sustained) F12.21
  carbohydrate
    absorption, intestinal NEC E74.39
    metabolism (congenital) E74.9
      specified NEC E74.8
  cardiac, functional I51.89
  carnitine metabolism E71.40
  cartilage M94.9
    articular NEC — see Derangement, joint, articular
        cartilage
    chondrocalcinosis — see Chondrocalcinosis
    specified type NEC M94.8X- ☑
      articular — see Derangement, joint, articular
          cartilage
      multiple sites M94.8X0
  catatonia (due to known physiological condition) (with
      another mental disorder) F06.1
  catatonic
    due to (secondary to) known physiological condition
        F06.1
    organic F06.1
  central auditory processing H93.25
  cervical
    region NEC M53.82
    root (nerve) NEC G54.2
  character NOS F60.9
  childhood disintegrative NEC F84.3
  cholesterol and bile acid metabolism E78.70
    Barth syndrome E78.71
    other specified E78.79
    Smith-Lemli-Opitz syndrome E78.72
  choroid H31.9
    atrophy — see Atrophy, choroid
    degeneration — see Degeneration, choroid
    detachment — see Detachment, choroid
    dystrophy — see Dystrophy, choroid
    hemorrhage — see Hemorrhage, choroid
    rupture — see Rupture, choroid
    scar — see Scar, chorioretinal
    solar retinopathy — see Retinopathy, solar
    specified type NEC H31.8
  ciliary body — see Disorder, iris
    degeneration — see Degeneration, ciliary body
  coagulation (factor) — see also Defect, coagulation
      D68.9
    newborn, transient P61.6
  cocaine use
    mild F14.10
      with
        amphetamine, cocaine, or other stimulant
            intoxication
          with perceptual disturbances F14.122
          without perceptual disturbances F14.129

Disorder — *continued*
cocaine use — *continued*
mild — *continued*
with — *continued*
cocaine intoxication delirium F14.121
cocaine-induced
anxiety disorder F14.180
bipolar and related disorder F14.14
depressive disorder F14.14
obsessive-compulsive and related disorder F14.188
psychotic disorder F14.159
sexual dysfunction F14.181
sleep disorder F14.182
in remission (early) (sustained) F14.11
moderate or severe F14.20
with
amphetamine, cocaine, or other stimulant intoxication
with perceptual disturbances F14.222
without perceptual disturbances F14.229
cocaine intoxication delirium F14.221
cocaine-induced
anxiety disorder F14.280
bipolar and related disorder F14.24
depressive disorder F14.24
obsessive-compulsive and related disorder F14.288
psychotic disorder F14.259
sexual dysfunction F14.281
sleep disorder F14.282
in remission (early) (sustained) F14.21
coccyx NEC M53.3
cognitive F09
due to (secondary to) general medical condition F09
persisting R41.89
due to
alcohol F10.97
with dependence F10.27
anxiolytics F13.97
with dependence F13.27
hypnotics F13.97
with dependence F13.27
sedatives F13.97
with dependence F13.27
specified substance NEC F19.97
with
abuse F19.17
dependence F19.27
communication F80.9
social pragmatic F80.82
conduct (childhood) F91.9
adjustment reaction — *see* Disorder, adjustment
adolescent onset type F91.2
childhood onset type F91.1
compulsive F63.9
confined to family context F91.0
depressive F91.8
group type F91.2
hyperkinetic — *see* Disorder, attention-deficit hyperactivity
oppositional defiance F91.3
socialized F91.2
solitary aggressive type F91.1
specified NEC F91.8
unsocialized (aggressive) F91.1
conduction, heart I45.9
congenital glycosylation (CDG) E74.8
conjunctiva H11.9
infection — *see* Conjunctivitis
connective tissue, localized L94.9
specified NEC L94.8
conversion (functional neurological symptom disorder)
with
abnormal movement F44.4
anesthesia or sensory loss F44.6
attacks or seizures F44.5
mixed symptoms F44.7
special sensory symptoms F44.6
speech symptoms F44.4
swallowing symptoms F44.4
weakness or paralysis F44.4
convulsive (secondary) — *see* Convulsions
cornea H18.9
deformity — *see* Deformity, cornea
degeneration — *see* Degeneration, cornea
deposits — *see* Deposit, cornea
due to contact lens H18.82- ☑

Disorder — *continued*
cornea — *continued*
due to contact lens — *continued*
specified as edema — *see* Edema, cornea
edema — *see* Edema, cornea
keratitis — *see* Keratitis
keratoconjunctivitis — *see* Keratoconjunctivitis
membrane change — *see* Change, corneal membrane
neovascularization — *see* Neovascularization, cornea
scar — *see* Opacity, cornea
specified type NEC H18.89- ☑
ulcer — *see* Ulcer, cornea
corpus cavernosum N48.9
cranial nerve — *see* Disorder, nerve, cranial
cyclothymic F34.0
defiant oppositional F91.3
delusional (persistent) (systematized) F22
induced F24
depersonalization F48.1
depressive F32.9
due to known physiological condition
with
depressive features F06.31
major depressive-like episode F06.32
mixed features F06.34
major F32.9
with psychotic symptoms F32.3
in remission (full) F32.5
partial F32.4
recurrent F33.9
with psychotic features F33.3
single episode F32.9
mild F32.0
moderate F32.1
severe (without psychotic symptoms) F32.2
with psychotic symptoms F32.3
organic F06.31
persistent F34.1
recurrent F33.9
current episode
mild F33.0
moderate F33.1
severe (without psychotic symptoms) F33.2
with psychotic symptoms F33.3
in remission F33.40
full F33.42
partial F33.41
specified NEC F33.8
single episode — *see* Episode, depressive
specified NEC F32.89
developmental F89
arithmetical skills F81.2
coordination (motor) F82
expressive writing F81.81
language F80.9
expressive F80.1
mixed receptive and expressive F80.2
receptive type F80.2
specified NEC F80.89
learning F81.9
arithmetical F81.2
reading F81.0
mixed F88
motor coordination or function F82
pervasive F84.9
specified NEC F84.8
phonological F80.0
reading F81.0
scholastic skills — *see also* Disorder, learning
mixed F81.89
specified NEC F88
speech F80.9
articulation F80.0
specified NEC F80.89
written expression F81.81
diaphragm J98.6
digestive (system) K92.9
newborn P78.9
specified NEC P78.89
postprocedural — *see* Complication, gastrointestinal
psychogenic F45.8
disc (intervertebral) M51.9
with
myelopathy
cervical region M50.00
cervicothoracic region M50.03

Disorder — *continued*
disc — *continued*
with — *continued*
myelopathy — *continued*
high cervical region M50.01
lumbar region M51.06
mid-cervical region M50.020
sacrococcygeal region M53.3
thoracic region M51.04
thoracolumbar region M51.05
radiculopathy
cervical region M50.10
cervicothoracic region M50.13
high cervical region M50.11
lumbar region M51.16
lumbosacral region M51.17
mid-cervical region M50.120
sacrococcygeal region M53.3
thoracic region M51.14
thoracolumbar region M51.15
cervical M50.90
with
myelopathy M50.00
C2-C3 M50.01
C3-C4 M50.01
C4-C5 M50.021
C5-C6 M50.022
C6-C7 M50.023
C7-T1 M50.03
cervicothoracic region M50.03
high cervical region M50.01
mid-cervical region M50.020
neuritis, radiculitis or radiculopathy M50.10
C2-C3 M50.11
C3-C4 M50.11
C4-C5 M50.121
C5-C6 M50.122
C6-C7 M50.123
C7-T1 M50.13
cervicothoracic region M50.13
high cervical region M50.11
mid-cervical region M50.120
C2-C3 M50.91
C3-C4 M50.91
C4-C5 M50.921
C5-C6 M50.922
C6-C7 M50.923
C7-T1 M50.93
cervicothoracic region M50.93
degeneration M50.30
C2-C3 M50.31
C3-C4 M50.31
C4-C5 M50.321
C5-C6 M50.322
C6-C7 M50.323
C7-T1 M50.33
cervicothoracic region M50.33
high cervical region M50.31
mid-cervical region M50.320
displacement M50.20
C2-C3 M50.21
C3-C4 M50.21
C4-C5 M50.221
C5-C6 M50.222
C6-C7 M50.223
C7-T1 M50.23
cervicothoracic region M50.23
high cervical region M50.21
mid-cervical region M50.220
high cervical region M50.91
mid-cervical region M50.920
specified type NEC M50.80
C2-C3 M50.81
C3-C4 M50.81
C4-C5 M50.821
C5-C6 M50.822
C6-C7 M50.823
C7-T1 M50.83
cervicothoracic region M50.83
high cervical region M50.81
mid-cervical region M50.820
specified NEC
lumbar region M51.86
lumbosacral region M51.87
sacrococcygeal region M53.3
thoracic region M51.84
thoracolumbar region M51.85
disinhibited attachment (childhood) F94.2
disintegrative, childhood NEC F84.3

Disorder — *continued*
- disruptive F91.9
  - mood dysregulation F34.81
  - specified NEC F91.8
- disruptive behavior — *see* Disorder, conduct
- dissocial personality F60.2
- dissociative F44.9
  - affecting
    - motor function F44.4
      - and sensation F44.7
    - sensation F44.6
      - and motor function F44.7
  - brief reactive F43.0
  - due to (secondary to) general medical condition F06.8
  - mixed F44.7
  - organic F06.8
  - other specified NEC F44.89
- double heterozygous sickling — *see* Disease, sickle-cell
- dream anxiety F51.5
- drug induced hemorrhagic D68.32
- drug related F19.99
  - abuse — *see* Abuse, drug
  - dependence — *see* Dependence, drug
- dysmorphic body F45.22
- dysthymic F34.1
- ear H93.9- ☑
  - bleeding — *see* Otorrhagia
  - deafness — *see* Deafness
  - degenerative H93.09- ☑
  - discharge — *see* Otorrhea
  - external H61.9- ☑
    - auditory canal stenosis — *see* Stenosis, external ear canal
    - exostosis — *see* Exostosis, external ear canal
    - impacted cerumen — *see* Impaction, cerumen
    - otitis — *see* Otitis, externa
    - perichondritis — *see* Perichondritis, ear
    - pinna — *see* Disorder, pinna
    - specified type NEC H61.89- ☑
  - inner H83.9- ☑
    - vestibular dysfunction — *see* Disorder, vestibular function
  - middle H74.9- ☑
    - adhesive H74.1- ☑
    - ossicle — *see* Abnormal, ear ossicles
    - polyp — *see* Polyp, ear (middle)
    - specified NEC, in diseases classified elsewhere H75.8- ☑
  - postprocedural — *see* Complications, ear, procedure
  - specified NEC, in diseases classified elsewhere H94.8- ☑
- eating (adult) (psychogenic) F50.9
  - anorexia — *see* Anorexia
  - binge F50.81
  - bulimia F50.2
  - child F98.29
    - pica F98.3
    - rumination disorder F98.21
  - pica F50.89
    - childhood F98.3
- electrolyte (balance) NEC E87.8
  - with
    - abortion — *see* Abortion by type complicated by specified condition NEC
    - ectopic pregnancy O08.5
    - molar pregnancy O08.5
  - acidosis (metabolic) (respiratory) E87.2
  - alkalosis (metabolic) (respiratory) E87.3
- elimination, transepidermal L87.9
  - specified NEC L87.8
- emotional (persistent) F34.9
  - of childhood F93.9
    - specified NEC F93.8
- endocrine E34.9
  - postprocedural E89.89
  - specified NEC E89.89
- erectile (male) (organic) — *see also* Dysfunction, sexual, male, erectile N52.9
  - nonorganic F52.21
- erythematous — *see* Erythema
- esophagus K22.9
  - functional K22.4
  - psychogenic F45.8
- eustachian tube H69.9- ☑
  - infection — *see* Salpingitis, eustachian
  - obstruction — *see* Obstruction, eustachian tube
  - patulous — *see* Patulous, eustachian tube

Disorder — *continued*
- eustachian tube — *continued*
  - specified NEC H69.8- ☑
- exhibitionistic F65.2
- extrapyramidal G25.9
  - in deseases classified elsewhere — *see* category G26
  - specified type NEC G25.89
- eye H57.9
  - postprocedural — *see* Complication, postprocedural, eye
- eyelid H02.9
  - cyst — *see* Cyst, eyelid
  - degenerative H02.70
    - chloasma — *see* Chloasma, eyelid
    - madarosis — *see* Madarosis
    - specified type NEC H02.79
    - vitiligo — *see* Vitiligo, eyelid
    - xanthelasma — *see* Xanthelasma
  - dermatochalasis — *see* Dermatochalasis
  - edema — *see* Edema, eyelid
  - elephantiasis — *see* Elephantiasis, eyelid
  - foreign body, retained — *see* Foreign body, retained, eyelid
  - function H02.59
    - abnormal innervation syndrome — *see* Syndrome, abnormal innervation
    - blepharochalasis — *see* Blepharochalasis
    - blepharoclonus — *see* Blepharoclonus
    - blepharophimosis — *see* Blepharophimosis
    - blepharoptosis — *see* Blepharoptosis
    - lagophthalmos — *see* Lagophthalmos
    - lid retraction — *see* Retraction, lid
  - hypertrichosis — *see* Hypertrichosis, eyelid
  - specified type NEC H02.89
  - vascular H02.879
    - left H02.876
      - lower H02.875
      - upper H02.874
    - right H02.873
      - lower H02.872
      - upper H02.871
- factitious
  - by proxy F68.A
  - imposed on another F68.A
  - imposed on self F68.10
    - with predominantly
      - psychological symptoms F68.11
        - with physical symptoms F68.13
      - physical symptoms F68.12
        - with psychological symptoms F68.13
- factor, coagulation — *see* Defect, coagulation
- fatty acid
  - metabolism E71.30
    - specified NEC E71.39
  - oxidation
    - LCAD E71.310
    - MCAD E71.311
    - SCAD E71.312
    - specified deficiency NEC E71.318
- feeding (infant or child) — *see also* Disorder, eating R63.3
  - or eating disorder F50.9
  - specified NEC F50.9
- feigned (with obvious motivation) Z76.5
  - without obvious motivation — *see* Disorder, factitious
- female
  - hypoactive sexual desire F52.0
  - orgasmic F52.31
  - sexual interest/arousal F52.22
- fetishistic F65.0
- fibroblastic M72.9
  - specified NEC M72.8
- fluency
  - adult onset F98.5
  - childhood onset F80.81
  - following
    - cerebral infarction I69.323
    - cerebrovascular disease I69.923
      - specified disease NEC I69.823
    - intracerebral hemorrhage I69.123
    - nontraumatic intracranial hemorrhage NEC I69.223
    - subarachnoid hemorrhage I69.023
  - in conditions classified elsewhere R47.82
- fluid balance E87.8
- follicular (skin) L73.9

Disorder — *continued*
- follicular — *continued*
  - specified NEC L73.8
- frotteuristic F65.81
- fructose metabolism E74.10
  - essential fructosuria E74.11
  - fructokinase deficiency E74.11
  - fructose-1, 6-diphosphatase deficiency E74.19
  - hereditary fructose intolerance E74.12
  - other specified E74.19
- functional polymorphonuclear neutrophils D71
- gallbladder, biliary tract and pancreas in diseases classified elsewhere K87
- gambling F63.0
- gamma aminobutyric acid (GABA) metabolism E72.81
- gamma-glutamyl cycle E72.89
- gastric (functional) K31.9
  - motility K30
  - psychogenic F45.8
  - secretion K30
- gastrointestinal (functional) NOS K92.9
  - newborn P78.9
  - psychogenic F45.8
- gender-identity or -role F64.9
  - childhood F64.2
  - effect on relationship F66
  - of adolescence or adulthood F64.0
    - nontranssexual F64.8
  - specified NEC F64.8
  - uncertainty F66
- genito-pelvic pain penetration F52.6
- genitourinary system
  - female N94.9
  - male N50.9
  - psychogenic F45.8
- globe H44.9
  - degenerated condition H44.50
    - absolute glaucoma H44.51- ☑
    - atrophy H44.52- ☑
    - leucocoria H44.53- ☑
  - degenerative H44.30
    - chalcosis H44.31- ☑
    - myopia — *see also* Myopia, degenerative H44.2- ☑
    - siderosis H44.32- ☑
    - specified type NEC H44.39- ☑
  - endophthalmitis — *see* Endophthalmitis
  - foreign body, retained — *see* Foreign body, intraocular, old, retained
  - hemophthalmos — *see* Hemophthalmos
  - hypotony H44.40
    - due to
      - ocular fistula H44.42- ☑
      - specified disorder NEC H44.43- ☑
    - flat anterior chamber H44.41- ☑
    - primary H44.44- ☑
  - luxation — *see* Luxation, globe
  - specified type NEC H44.89
- glomerular (in) N05.9
  - amyloidosis E85.4 *[N08]*
  - cryoglobulinemia D89.1 *[N08]*
  - disseminated intravascular coagulation D65 *[N08]*
  - Fabry's disease E75.21 *[N08]*
  - familial lecithin cholesterol acyltransferase deficiency E78.6 *[N08]*
  - Goodpasture's syndrome M31.0
  - hemolytic-uremic syndrome D59.3
  - Henoch (-Schönlein) purpura D69.0 *[N08]*
  - malariae malaria B52.0
  - microscopic polyangiitis M31.7 *[N08]*
  - multiple myeloma C90.0- ☑ *[N08]*
  - mumps B26.83
  - schistosomiasis B65.9 *[N08]*
  - sepsis NEC A41.- ☑ *[N08]*
    - streptococcal A40.- ☑ *[N08]*
  - sickle-cell disorders D57.- ☑ *[N08]*
  - strongyloidiasis B78.9 *[N08]*
  - subacute bacterial endocarditis I33.0 *[N08]*
  - syphilis A52.75
  - systemic lupus erythematosus M32.14
  - thrombotic thrombocytopenic purpura M31.1 *[N08]*
  - Waldenström macroglobulinemia C88.0 *[N08]*
  - Wegener's granulomatosis M31.31
- gluconeogenesis E74.4
- glucosaminoglycan metabolism — *see* Disorder, metabolism, glucosaminoglycan
- glycine metabolism E72.50
  - d-glycericacidemia E72.59

Disorder — continued
  glycine metabolism — continued
    hyperhydroxyprolinemia E72.59
    hyperoxaluria R82.992
      primary E72.53
    hyperprolinemia E72.59
    non-ketotic hyperglycinemia E72.51
    oxalosis E72.53
    oxaluria E72.53
    sarcosinemia E72.59
    trimethylaminuria E72.52
  glycoprotein metabolism E77.9
    specified NEC E77.8
  habit (and impulse) F63.9
    involving sexual behavior NEC F65.9
    specified NEC F63.89
  hallucinogen use
    mild F16.10
      with
        hallucinogen intoxication delirium F16.121
        hallucinogen-induced
          anxiety disorder F16.180
          bipolar and related disorder F16.14
          depressive disorder F16.14
          psychotic disorder F16.159
        other hallucinogen intoxication F16.129
      in remission (early) (sustained) F16.11
    moderate or severe F16.20
      with
        hallucinogen intoxication delirium F16.221
        hallucinogen-induced
          anxiety disorder F16.280
          bipolar and related disorder F16.24
          depressive disorder F16.24
          psychotic disorder F16.259
        other hallucinogen intoxication F16.229
      in remission (early) (sustained) F16.21
  heart action I49.9
  hematological D75.9
    newborn (transient) P61.9
      specified NEC P61.8
  hematopoietic organs D75.9
  hemorrhagic NEC D69.9
    drug-induced D68.32
    due to
      extrinsic circulating anticoagulants D68.32
      increase in
        anti-IIa D68.32
        anti-Xa D68.32
      intrinsic
        circulating anticoagulants D68.318
        increase in
          anti-IXa D68.318
          antithrombin D68.318
          anti-VIIIa D68.318
          anti-XIa D68.318
    following childbirth O72.3
  hemostasis — see Defect, coagulation
  histidine metabolism E70.40
    histidinemia E70.41
    other specified E70.49
  hoarding F42.3
  hyperkinetic — see Disorder, attention-deficit hyperactivity
  hyperleucine-isoleucinemia E71.19
  hypervalinemia E71.19
  hypoactive sexual desire F52.0
  hypochondriacal F45.20
    body dysmorphic F45.22
    neurosis F45.21
    other specified F45.29
  identity
    dissociative F44.81
    illness anxiety F45.21
    of childhood F93.8
  immune mechanism (immunity) D89.9
    specified type NEC D89.89
  impaired renal tubular function N25.9
    specified NEC N25.89
  impulse (control) F63.9
  inflammatory
    pelvic, in diseases classified elsewhere — see category N74
    penis N48.29
      abscess N48.21
      cellulitis N48.22
  inhalant use
    mild F18.10

Disorder — continued
  inhalant use — continued
    mild — continued
      with
        inhalant intoxication F18.129
        inhalant intoxication delirium F18.121
        inhalant-induced
          anxiety disorder F18.180
          depressive disorder F18.14
          major neurocognitive disorder F18.17
          mild neurocognitive disorder F18.188
          psychotic disorder F18.159
      in remission (early) (sustained) F18.11
    moderate or severe F18.20
      with
        inhalant intoxication F18.229
        inhalant intoxication delirium F18.221
        inhalant-induced
          anxiety disorder F18.280
          depressive disorder F18.24
          major neurocognitive disorder F18.27
          mild neurocognitive disorder F18.288
          psychotic disorder F18.259
      in remission (early) (sustained) F18.21
  integument, newborn P83.9
    specified NEC P83.88
  intermittent explosive F63.81
  internal secretion pancreas — see Increased, secretion, pancreas, endocrine
  intestine, intestinal
    carbohydrate absorption NEC E74.39
      postoperative K91.2
    functional NEC K59.9
      postoperative K91.89
    psychogenic F45.8
    vascular K55.9
      chronic K55.1
      specified NEC K55.8
  intraoperative (intraprocedural) — see Complications, intraoperative
  involuntary emotional expression (IEED) F07.89
  iris H21.9
    adhesions — see Adhesions, iris
    atrophy — see Atrophy, iris
    chamber angle recession — see Recession, chamber angle
    cyst — see Cyst, iris
    degeneration — see Degeneration, iris
    in diseases classified elsewhere H22
    iridodialysis — see Iridodialysis
    iridoschisis — see Iridoschisis
    miotic pupillary cyst — see Cyst, pupillary
    pupillary
      abnormality — see Abnormality, pupillary
      membrane — see Membrane, pupillary
    specified type NEC H21.89
    vascular NEC H21.1X- ☑
  iron metabolism E83.10
    specified NEC E83.19
  isovaleric acidemia E71.110
  jaw, developmental M27.0
    temporomandibular — see also Anomaly, dentofacial, temporomandibular joint M26.60- ☑
  joint M25.9
    derangement — see Derangement, joint
    effusion — see Effusion, joint
    fistula — see Fistula, joint
    hemarthrosis — see Hemarthrosis
    instability — see Instability, joint
    osteophyte — see Osteophyte
    pain — see Pain, joint
    psychogenic F45.8
    specified type NEC M25.80
      ankle M25.87- ☑
      elbow M25.82- ☑
      foot joint M25.87- ☑
      hand joint M25.84- ☑
      hip M25.85- ☑
      knee M25.86- ☑
      shoulder M25.81- ☑
      wrist M25.83- ☑
    stiffness — see Stiffness, joint
  ketone metabolism E71.32
  kidney N28.9
    functional (tubular) N25.9
    in
      schistosomiasis B65.9 [N29]
    tubular function N25.9

Disorder — continued
  kidney — continued
    tubular function — continued
      specified NEC N25.89
  lacrimal system H04.9
    changes H04.69
      fistula — see Fistula, lacrimal
    gland H04.19
      atrophy — see Atrophy, lacrimal gland
      cyst — see Cyst, lacrimal, gland
      dacryops — see Dacryops
      dislocation — see Dislocation, lacrimal gland
      dry eye syndrome — see Syndrome, dry eye
      infection — see Dacryoadenitis
    granuloma — see Granuloma, lacrimal
    inflammation — see Inflammation, lacrimal
    obstruction — see Obstruction, lacrimal
    specified NEC H04.89
  lactation NEC O92.79
  language (developmental) F80.9
    expressive F80.1
    mixed receptive and expressive F80.2
    receptive F80.2
  late luteal phase dysphoric N94.89
  learning (specific) F81.9
    acalculia R48.8
    alexia R48.0
    mathematics F81.2
    reading F81.0
    specified
      with impairment in
        mathematics F81.2
        reading F81.0
        written expression F81.81
    specified NEC F81.89
    spelling F81.81
    written expression F81.81
  lens H27.9
    aphakia — see Aphakia
    cataract — see Cataract
    dislocation — see Dislocation, lens
    specified type NEC H27.8
  ligament M24.20
    ankle M24.27- ☑
    attachment, spine — see Enthesopathy, spinal
    elbow M24.22- ☑
    foot joint M24.27- ☑
    hand joint M24.24- ☑
    hip M24.25- ☑
    knee — see Derangement, knee, specified NEC
    shoulder M24.21- ☑
    vertebra M24.28
    wrist M24.23- ☑
  ligamentous attachments — see also Enthesopathy
    spine — see Enthesopathy, spinal
  lipid
    metabolism, congenital E78.9
    storage E75.6
      specified NEC E75.5
  lipoprotein
    deficiency (familial) E78.6
    metabolism E78.9
      specified NEC E78.89
  liver K76.9
    malarial B54 [K77]
  low back — see also Dorsopathy, specified NEC
  lumbosacral
    plexus G54.1
    root (nerve) NEC G54.4
  lung, interstitial, drug-induced J70.4
    acute J70.2
    chronic J70.3
  lymphoproliferative, post-transplant (PTLD) D47.Z1
    (following D47.4)
  lysine and hydroxylysine metabolism E72.3
  major neurocognitive — see Dementia, in (due to)
  male
    erectile (organic) — see also Dysfunction, sexual, male, erectile N52.9
      nonorganic F52.21
    hypoactive sexual desire F52.0
    orgasmic F52.32
  manic F30.9
    organic F06.33
  mast cell activation — see Activation, mast cell
  mastoid — see also Disorder, ear, middle
    postprocedural — see Complications, ear, procedure
  meniscus — see Derangement, knee, meniscus

⬃ Subterms under main terms may continue to next column or page   ☑ Additional Character Required — Refer to the Tabular List for Character Selection   113

Disorder — Disorder

Disorder — continued
  menopausal N95.9
    specified NEC N95.8
  menstrual N92.6
    psychogenic F45.8
    specified NEC N92.5
  mental (or behavioral) (nonpsychotic) F99
    due to (secondary to)
      amphetamine
        due to drug abuse — see Abuse, drug, stimulant
        due to drug dependence — see Dependence, drug, stimulant
      brain disease, damage and dysfunction F09
      caffeine use
        due to drug abuse — see Abuse, drug, stimulant
        due to drug dependence — see Dependence, drug, stimulant
      cannabis use
        due to drug abuse — see Abuse, drug, cannabis
        due to drug dependence — see Dependence, drug, cannabis
      general medical condition F09
      sedative or hypnotic use
        due to drug abuse — see Abuse, drug, sedative
        due to drug dependence — see Dependence, drug, sedative
      tobacco (nicotine) use — see Dependence, drug, nicotine
    following organic brain damage F07.9
      frontal lobe syndrome F07.0
      personality change F07.0
      postconcussional syndrome F07.81
      specified NEC F07.89
    infancy, childhood or adolescence F98.9
    neurotic — see Neurosis
    organic or symptomatic F09
    presenile, psychotic F03 ☑
    problem NEC
    psychoneurotic — see Neurosis
    psychotic — see Psychosis
    puerperal F53.0
    senile, psychotic NEC F03 ☑
  metabolic, amino acid, transitory, newborn P74.8
  metabolism NOS E88.9
    amino-acid E72.9
      aromatic E70.9
        albinism — see Albinism
        histidine E70.40
          histidinemia E70.41
          other specified E70.49
        hyperphenylalaninemia E70.1
          classical phenylketonuria E70.0
        other specified E70.8
        tryptophan E70.5
        tyrosine E70.20
          hypertyrosinemia E70.21
          other specified E70.29
      branched chain E71.2
        3-methylglutaconic aciduria E71.111
        hyperleucine-isoleucinemia E71.19
        hypervalinemia E71.19
        isovaleric acidemia E71.110
        maple syrup urine disease E71.0
        methylmalonic acidemia E71.120
        organic aciduria NEC E71.118
        other specified E71.19
        proprionate NEC E71.128
        proprionic acidemia E71.121
      glycine E72.50
        d-glycericacidemia E72.59
        hyperhydroxyprolinemia E72.59
        hyperoxaluria R82.992
          primary E72.53
        hyperprolinemia E72.59
        non-ketotic hyperglycinemia E72.51
        other specified E72.59
        sarcosinemia E72.59
        trimethylaminuria E72.52
      hydroxylysine E72.3
      lysine E72.3
      ornithine E72.4
      other specified E72.89
        beta-amino acid E72.89
        gamma-glutamyl cycle E72.89

Disorder — continued
  metabolism — continued
    amino-acid — continued
      straight-chain E72.89
      sulfur-bearing E72.10
        homocystinuria E72.11
        methylenetetrahydrofolate reductase deficiency E72.12
        other specified E72.19
    bile acid and cholesterol metabolism E78.70
    bilirubin E80.7
      specified NEC E80.6
    calcium E83.50
      hypercalcemia E83.52
      hypocalcemia E83.51
      other specified E83.59
    carbohydrate E74.9
      specified NEC E74.8
    cholesterol and bile acid metabolism E78.70
    congenital E88.9
    copper E83.00
      specified type NEC E83.09
      Wilson's disease E83.01
    cystinuria E72.01
    fructose E74.10
    galactose E74.20
    glucosaminoglycan E76.9
      mucopolysaccharidosis — see Mucopolysaccharidosis
      specified NEC E76.8
    glutamine E72.89
    glycine E72.50
    glycogen storage (hepatorenal) E74.09
    glycoprotein E77.9
      specified NEC E77.8
    glycosaminoglycan E76.9
      specified NEC E76.8
    in labor and delivery O75.89
    iron E83.10
    isoleucine E71.19
    leucine E71.19
    lipoid E78.9
    lipoprotein E78.9
      specified NEC E78.89
    magnesium E83.40
      hypermagnesemia E83.41
      hypomagnesemia E83.42
      other specified E83.49
    mineral E83.9
      specified NEC E83.89
    mitochondrial E88.40
      MELAS syndrome E88.41
      MERRF syndrome (myoclonic epilepsy associated with ragged-red fibers) E88.42
      other specified E88.49
    ornithine E72.4
    phosphatases E83.30
    phosphorus E83.30
      acid phosphatase deficiency E83.39
      hypophosphatasia E83.39
      hypophosphatemia E83.39
        familial E83.31
      other specified E83.39
      pseudovitamin D deficiency E83.32
    plasma protein NEC E88.09
    porphyrin — see Porphyria
    postprocedural E89.89
      specified NEC E89.89
    purine E79.9
      specified NEC E79.8
    pyrimidine E79.9
      specified NEC E79.8
    pyruvate E74.4
    serine E72.89
    sodium E87.8
    specified NEC E88.89
    threonine E72.89
    valine E71.19
    zinc E83.2
  methylmalonic acidemia E71.120
  micturition NEC — see also Difficulty, micturition R39.198
    feeling of incomplete emptying R39.14
    hesitancy R39.11
    poor stream R39.12
    psychogenic F45.8
    split stream R39.13
    straining R39.16
    urgency R39.15

Disorder — continued
  mild neurocognitive G31.84
  mitochondrial metabolism E88.40
  mitral (valve) — see Endocarditis, mitral
  mixed
    anxiety and depressive F41.8
    of scholastic skills (developmental) F81.89
    receptive expressive language F80.2
  mood F39
    bipolar — see Disorder, bipolar
    depressive — see Disorder, depressive
    due to (secondary to)
      alcohol F10.94
      amphetamine F15.94
        in
          abuse F15.14
          dependence F15.24
      anxiolytic F13.94
        in
          abuse F13.14
          dependence F13.24
      cocaine F14.94
        in
          abuse F14.14
          dependence F14.24
      general medical condition F06.30
      hallucinogen F16.94
        in
          abuse F16.14
          dependence F16.24
      hypnotic F13.94
        in
          abuse F13.14
          dependence F13.24
      inhalant F18.94
        in
          abuse F18.14
          dependence F18.24
      opioid F11.94
        in
          abuse F11.14
          dependence F11.24
      phencyclidine (PCP) F16.94
        in
          abuse F16.14
          dependence F16.24
      physiological condition F06.30
        with
          depressive features F06.31
          major depressive-like episode F06.32
          manic features F06.33
          mixed features F06.34
      psychoactive substance NEC F19.94
        in
          abuse F19.14
          dependence F19.24
      sedative F13.94
        in
          abuse F13.14
          dependence F13.24
      volatile solvents F18.94
        in
          abuse F18.14
          dependence F18.24
    manic episode F30.9
      with psychotic symptoms F30.2
      in remission (full) F30.4
        partial F30.3
      specified type NEC F30.8
      without psychotic symptoms F30.10
        mild F30.11
        moderate F30.12
        severe F30.13
    organic F06.30
      right hemisphere F07.89
    persistent F34.9
      cyclothymia F34.0
      dysthymia F34.1
      specified type NEC F34.89
    recurrent F39
    right hemisphere organic F07.89
  movement G25.9
    drug-induced G25.70
      akathisia G25.71
      specified NEC G25.79
    hysterical F44.4
    in diseases classified elsewhere — see category G2
    periodic limb G47.61
      sleep related G47.61

Disorder — *continued*
  movement — *continued*
    sleep related NEC G47.69
    specified NEC G25.89
    stereotyped F98.4
    treatment-induced G25.9
  multiple personality F44.81
  muscle M62.9
    attachment, spine — *see* Enthesopathy, spinal
    in trichinellosis — *see* Trichinellosis, with muscle
      disorder
    psychogenic F45.8
    specified type NEC M62.89
    tone, newborn P94.9
      specified NEC P94.8
  muscular
    attachments — *see also* Enthesopathy
      spine — *see* Enthesopathy, spinal
    urethra N36.44
  musculoskeletal system, soft tissue — *see* Disorder,
    soft tissue
    postprocedural M96.89
    psychogenic F45.8
  myoneural G70.9
    due to lead G70.1
    specified NEC G70.89
    toxic G70.1
  myotonic NEC G71.19
  nail, in diseases classified elsewhere L62
  neck region NEC — *see* Dorsopathy, specified NEC
  neonatal onset multisystemic inflammatory (NOMID)
    M04.2
  nerve G58.9
    abducent NEC — *see* Strabismus, paralytic, sixth
      nerve
    accessory G52.8
    acoustic — *see* subcategory H93.3 ☑
    auditory — *see* subcategory H93.3 ☑
    auriculotemporal G50.8
    axillary G54.0
    cerebral — *see* Disorder, nerve, cranial
    cranial G52.9
      eighth — *see* subcategory H93.3 ☑
      eleventh G52.8
      fifth G50.9
      first G52.0
      fourth NEC — *see* Strabismus, paralytic, fourth
        nerve
      multiple G52.7
      ninth G52.1
      second NEC — *see* Disorder, nerve, optic
      seventh NEC G51.8
      sixth NEC — *see* Strabismus, paralytic, sixth nerve
      specified NEC G52.8
      tenth G52.2
      third NEC — *see* Strabismus, paralytic, third nerve
      twelfth G52.3
    entrapment — *see* Neuropathy, entrapment
    facial G51.9
      specified NEC G51.8
    femoral — *see* Lesion, nerve, femoral
    glossopharyngeal NEC G52.1
    hypoglossal G52.3
    intercostal G58.0
    lateral
      cutaneous of thigh — *see* Mononeuropathy,
        lower limb, meralgia paresthetica
      popliteal — *see* Lesion, nerve, popliteal
    lower limb — *see* Mononeuropathy, lower limb
    medial popliteal — *see* Lesion, nerve, popliteal,
      medial
    median NEC — *see* Lesion, nerve, median
    multiple G58.7
    oculomotor NEC — *see* Strabismus, paralytic, third
      nerve
    olfactory G52.0
    optic NEC H47.09- ☑
      hemorrhage into sheath — *see* Hemorrhage,
        optic nerve
      ischemic H47.01- ☑
    peroneal — *see* Lesion, nerve, popliteal
    phrenic G58.8
    plantar — *see* Lesion, nerve, plantar
    pneumogastric G52.2
    posterior tibial — *see* Syndrome, tarsal tunnel
    radial — *see* Lesion, nerve, radial
    recurrent laryngeal G52.2
    root G54.9

Disorder — *continued*
  nerve — *continued*
    root — *continued*
      cervical G54.2
      lumbosacral G54.1
      specified NEC G54.8
      thoracic G54.3
    sciatic NEC — *see* Lesion, nerve, sciatic
    specified NEC G58.8
      lower limb — *see* Mononeuropathy, lower limb,
        specified NEC
      upper limb — *see* Mononeuropathy, upper limb,
        specified NEC
    sympathetic G90.9
    tibial — *see* Lesion, nerve, popliteal, medial
    trigeminal G50.9
      specified NEC G50.8
    trochlear NEC — *see* Strabismus, paralytic, fourth
      nerve
    ulnar — *see* Lesion, nerve, ulnar
    upper limb — *see* Mononeuropathy, upper limb
    vagus G52.2
  nervous system G98.8
    autonomic (peripheral) G90.9
      specified NEC G90.8
    central G96.9
      specified NEC G96.8
    parasympathetic G90.9
    specified NEC G98.8
    sympathetic G90.9
    vegetative G90.9
  neurocognitive R41.9
    major
      with
        aggressive behavior F01.51
        combative behavior F01.51
        violent behavior F01.51
      due to vascular disease, with behavioral distur-
        bance F01.51
      in (due to) (other diseases classified elsewhere)
        — *see also* Dementia, in (due to) F02.80
        with
          aggressive behavior F02.81
          combative behavior F02.81
          violent behavior F02.81
      without behavioral disturbance F01.50
    mild G31.84
  neurodevelopmental F89
    specified NEC F88
  neurohypophysis NEC E23.3
  neurological NEC R29.818
  neuromuscular G70.9
    hereditary NEC G71.9
    specified NEC G70.89
    toxic G70.1
  neurotic F48.9
    specified NEC F48.8
  neutrophil, polymorphonuclear D71
  nicotine use — *see* Dependence, drug, nicotine
  nightmare F51.5
  non-rapid eye movement sleep arousal
    sleep terror type F51.4
    sleepwalking type F51.3
  nose J34.9
    specified NEC J34.89
  obsessive-compulsive F42.9
    and related disorder due to a known physiological
      condition F06.8
  odontogenesis NOS K00.9
  opioid use
    with
      opioid-induced psychotic disorder F11.959
        with
          delusions F11.950
          hallucinations F11.951
    due to drug abuse — *see* Abuse, drug, opioid
    due to drug dependence — *see* Dependence, drug,
      opioid
    mild F11.10
      with
        opioid-induced
          anxiety disorder F11.188
          depressive disorder F11.14
          sexual dysfunction F11.181
        opioid intoxication
          with perceptual disturbances F11.122
          delirium F11.121
          without perceptual disturbances F11.129

Disorder — *continued*
  opioid use — *continued*
    mild — *continued*
      in remission (early) (sustained) F11.11
    moderate or severe F11.20
      with
        opioid-induced
          anxiety disorder F11.288
          anxiety disorder F11.988
          depressive disorder F11.24
          depressive disorder F11.94
          sexual dysfunction F11.281
          sexual dysfunction F11.981
        opioid intoxication
          with perceptual disturbances F11.222
          delirium F11.221
          without perceptual disturbances F11.229
      in remission (early) (sustained) F11.21
  oppositional defiant F91.3
  optic
    chiasm H47.49
      due to
        inflammatory disorder H47.41
        neoplasm H47.42
        vascular disorder H47.43
    disc H47.39- ☑
      coloboma — *see* Coloboma, optic disc
      drusen — *see* Drusen, optic disc
      pseudopapilledema — *see* Pseudopapilledema
      radiations — *see* Disorder, visual, pathway
      tracts — *see* Disorder, visual, pathway
  orbit H05.9
    cyst — *see* Cyst, orbit
    deformity — *see* Deformity, orbit
    edema — *see* Edema, orbit
    enophthalmos — *see* Enophthalmos
    exophthalmos — *see* Exophthalmos
    hemorrhage — *see* Hemorrhage, orbit
    inflammation — *see* Inflammation, orbit
    myopathy — *see* Myopathy, extraocular muscles
    retained foreign body — *see* Foreign body, orbit,
      old
    specified type NEC H05.89
  organic
    anxiety F06.4
    catatonic F06.1
    delusional F06.2
    dissociative F06.8
    emotionally labile (asthenic) F06.8
    mood (affective) F06.30
    schizophrenia-like F06.2
  orgasmic (female) F52.31
    male F52.32
  ornithine metabolism E72.4
  overanxious F41.1
    of childhood F93.8
  pain
    with related psychological factors F45.42
    exclusively related to psychological factors F45.41
    genito-pelvic penetration disorder F52.6
  pancreatic internal secretion E16.9
    specified NEC E16.8
  panic F41.0
    with agoraphobia F40.01
  papulosquamous L44.9
    in diseases classified elsewhere L45
    specified NEC L44.8
  paranoid F22
    induced F24
    shared F24
  paraphilic F65.9
    specified NEC F65.89
  parathyroid (gland) E21.5
    specified NEC E21.4
  parietoalveolar NEC J84.09
  paroxysmal, mixed R56.9
  patella M22.9-
    chondromalacia — *see* Chondromalacia, patella
    derangement NEC M22.3X- ☑
    recurrent
      dislocation — *see* Dislocation, patella, recurrent
      subluxation — *see* Dislocation, patella, recurrent,
        incomplete
    specified NEC M22.8X- ☑
  patellofemoral M22.2X- ☑
  pedophilic F65.4
  pentose phosphate pathway with anemia D55.1
  perception, due to hallucinogens F16.983

Disorder — continued
  perception, due to hallucinogens — continued
    in
      abuse F16.183
      dependence F16.283
  peripheral nervous system NEC G64
  peroxisomal E71.50
    biogenesis
      neonatal adrenoleukodystrophy E71.511
      specified disorder NEC E71.518
      Zellweger syndrome E71.510
    rhizomelic chondrodysplasia punctata E71.540
    specified form NEC E71.548
      group 1 E71.518
      group 2 E71.53
      group 3 E71.542
    X-linked adrenoleukodystrophy E71.529
      adolescent E71.521
      adrenomyeloneuropathy E71.522
      childhood E71.520
      specified form NEC E71.528
    Zellweger-like syndrome E71.541
  persistent
    (somatoform) pain F45.41
    affective (mood) F34.9
  personality — see also Personality F60.9
    affective F34.0
    aggressive F60.3
    amoral F60.2
    anankastic F60.5
    antisocial F60.2
    anxious F60.6
    asocial F60.2
    asthenic F60.7
    avoidant F60.6
    borderline F60.3
    change (secondary) due to general medical condition F07.0
    compulsive F60.5
    cyclothymic F34.0
    dependent (passive) F60.7
    depressive F34.1
    dissocial F60.2
    emotional instability F60.3
    expansive paranoid F60.0
    explosive F60.3
    following organic brain damage F07.9
    histrionic F60.4
    hyperthymic F34.0
    hypothymic F34.1
    hysterical F60.4
    immature F60.89
    inadequate F60.7
    labile F60.3
    mixed (nonspecific) F60.89
    moral deficiency F60.2
    narcissistic F60.81
    negativistic F60.89
    obsessional F60.5
    obsessive (-compulsive) F60.5
    organic F07.9
    overconscientious F60.5
    paranoid F60.0
    passive (-dependent) F60.7
    passive-aggressive F60.89
    pathological NEC F60.9
    pseudosocial F60.2
    psychopathic F60.2
    schizoid F60.1
    schizotypal F21
    self-defeating F60.7
    specified NEC F60.89
    type A F60.5
    unstable (emotional) F60.3
  pervasive, developmental F84.9
  phencyclidine use
    mild F16.10
      with
        phencyclidine intoxication F16.129
        phencyclidine intoxication delirium F16.121
        phencyclidine-induced
          anxiety disorder F16.180
          bipolar and related disorder F16.14
          depressive disorder F16.14
          psychotic disorder F16.159
      in remission (early) (sustained) F16.11
    moderate or severe F16.20
      with
        phencyclidine intoxication F16.229

Disorder — continued
  phencyclidine use — continued
    moderate or severe — continued
      with — continued
        phencyclidine intoxication delirium F16.221
        phencyclidine-induced
          anxiety disorder F16.280
          bipolar and related disorder F16.14
          depressive disorder F16.24
          psychotic disorder F16.259
      in remission (early) (sustained) F16.21
  phobic anxiety, childhood F40.8
  phosphate-losing tubular N25.0
  pigmentation L81.9
    choroid, congenital Q14.3
    diminished melanin formation L81.6
    iron L81.8
    specified NEC L81.8
  pinna (noninfective) H61.10- ☑
    deformity, acquired H61.11- ☑
    hematoma H61.12- ☑
    perichondritis — see Perichondritis, ear
    specified type NEC H61.19- ☑
  pituitary gland E23.7
    iatrogenic (postprocedural) E89.3
    specified NEC E23.6
  platelets D69.1
  plexus G54.9
    specified NEC G54.8
  polymorphonuclear neutrophils D71
  porphyrin metabolism — see Porphyria
  postconcussional F07.81
  posthallucinogen perception F16.983
    in
      abuse F16.183
      dependence F16.283
  postmenopausal N95.9
    specified NEC N95.8
  postprocedural (postoperative) — see Complications, postprocedural
  post-transplant lymphoproliferative D47.Z1 (following D47.4)
  post-traumatic stress (PTSD) F43.10
    acute F43.11
    chronic F43.12
  premenstrual dysphoric (PMDD) F32.81
  prepuce N47.8
  propionic acidemia E71.121
  prostate N42.9
    specified NEC N42.89
  psychogenic NOS — see also condition F45.9
    anxiety F41.8
    appetite F50.9
    asthenic F48.8
    cardiovascular (system) F45.8
    compulsive F42.8
    cutaneous F54
    depressive F32.9
    digestive (system) F45.8
    dysmenorrheic F45.8
    dyspneic F45.8
    endocrine (system) F54
    eye NEC F45.8
    feeding — see Disorder, eating
    functional NEC F45.8
    gastric F45.8
    gastrointestinal (system) F45.8
    genitourinary (system) F45.8
    heart (function) (rhythm) F45.8
    hyperventilatory F45.8
    hypochondriacal — see Disorder, hypochondriacal
    intestinal F45.8
    joint F45.8
    learning F81.9
    limb F45.8
    lymphatic (system) F45.8
    menstrual F45.8
    micturition F45.8
    monoplegic NEC F44.4
    motor F44.4
    muscle F45.8
    musculoskeletal F45.8
    neurocirculatory F45.8
    obsessive F42.8
    occupational F48.8
    organ or part of body NEC F45.8
    paralytic NEC F44.4
    phobic F40.9

Disorder — continued
  psychogenic — see also condition — continued
    physical NEC F45.8
    rectal F45.8
    respiratory (system) F45.8
    rheumatic F45.8
    sexual (function) F52.9
    skin (allergic) (eczematous) F54
    sleep F51.9
    specified part of body NEC F45.8
    stomach F45.8
  psychological F99
    associated with
      disease classified elsewhere F54
      sexual
        development F66
        relationship F66
      uncertainty about gender identity F64.9
  psychomotor NEC F44.4
    hysterical F44.4
  psychoneurotic — see also Neurosis
    mixed NEC F48.8
  psychophysiologic — see Disorder, somatoform
  psychosexual F65.9
    development F66
    identity of childhood F64.2
  psychosomatic NOS — see Disorder, somatoform
    multiple F45.0
    undifferentiated F45.1
  psychotic — see Psychosis
    transient (acute) F23
  puberty E30.9
    specified NEC E30.8
  pulmonary (valve) — see Endocarditis, pulmonary
  purine metabolism E79.9
  pyrimidine metabolism E79.9
  pyruvate metabolism E74.4
  reactive attachment (childhood) F94.1
  reading R48.0
    developmental (specific) F81.0
  receptive language F80.2
  receptor, hormonal, peripheral — see also Syndrome, androgen insensitivity E34.50
  recurrent brief depressive F33.8
  reflex R29.2
  refraction H52.7
    aniseikonia H52.32
    anisometropia H52.31
    astigmatism — see Astigmatism
    hypermetropia — see Hypermetropia
    myopia — see Myopia
    presbyopia H52.4
    specified NEC H52.6
  relationship F68.8
    due to sexual orientation F66
  REM sleep behavior G47.52
  renal function, impaired (tubular) N25.9
  resonance R49.9
    specified NEC R49.8
  respiratory function, impaired — see also Failure, respiration
    postprocedural — see Complication, postoperative respiratory system
    psychogenic F45.8
  retina H35.9
    angioid streaks H35.33
    changes in vascular appearance H35.01- ☑
    degeneration — see Degeneration, retina
    dystrophy (hereditary) — see Dystrophy, retina
    edema H35.81
    hemorrhage — see Hemorrhage, retina
    ischemia H35.82
    macular degeneration — see Degeneration, macula
    microaneurysms H35.04- ☑
    microvascular abnormality NEC H35.09
    neovascularization — see Neovascularization, retina
    retinopathy — see Retinopathy
    separation of layers H35.70
      central serous chorioretinopathy H35.71- ☑
      pigment epithelium detachment (serous) H35.72- ☑
      hemorrhagic H35.73- ☑
    specified type NEC H35.89
    telangiectasis — see Telangiectasis, retina
    vasculitis — see Vasculitis, retina
  retroperitoneal K68.9
  right hemisphere organic affective F07.89
  rumination (infant or child) F98.21

Disorder — *continued*
  sacrum, sacrococcygeal NEC M53.3
  schizoaffective F25.9
    bipolar type F25.0
    depressive type F25.1
    manic type F25.0
    mixed type F25.0
    specified NEC F25.8
  schizoid of childhood F84.5
  schizophrenia spectrum and other psychotic disorder F29
    specified NEC F28
  schizophreniform F20.81
    brief F23
  schizotypal (personality) F21
  secretion, thyrocalcitonin E07.0
  sedative, hypnotic, or anxiolytic use
    mild F13.10
      with
        sedative, hypnotic, or anxiolytic intoxication F13.129
        sedative, hypnotic, or anxiolytic intoxication delirium F13.121
        sedative, hypnotic, or anxiolytic-induced
          anxiety disorder F13.180
          bipolar and related disorder F13.14
          depressive disorder F13.14
          psychotic disorder F13.159
          sexual dysfunction F13.181
      in remission (early) (sustained) F13.11
    moderate or severe F13.20
      with
        sedative, hypnotic, or anxiolytic intoxication F13.229
        sedative, hypnotic, or anxiolytic intoxication delirium F13.221
        sedative, hypnotic, or anxiolytic-induced
          anxiety disorder F13.280
          bipolar and related disorder F13.24
          depressive disorder F13.24
          major neurocognitive disorder F13.27
          mild neurocognitive disorder F13.288
          psychotic disorder F13.259
          sexual dysfunction F13.281
      in remission (early) (sustained) F13.21
  seizure — *see also* Epilepsy G40.909
    intractable G40.919
      with status epilepticus G40.911
  semantic pragmatic F80.89
    with autism F84.0
  sense of smell R43.1
    psychogenic F45.8
  separation anxiety, of childhood F93.0
  sexual
    aversion F52.1
    function, psychogenic F52.9
    interest/arousal, female F52.22
    masochism F65.51
    maturation F66
    nonorganic F52.9
    preference — *see also* Deviation, sexual F65.9
      fetishistic transvestism F65.1
    relationship F66
    sadism F65.52
  shyness, of childhood and adolescence F40.10
  sibling rivalry F93.8
  sickle-cell (sickling) (homozygous) — *see* Disease, sickle-cell
    heterozygous D57.3
    specified type NEC D57.8- ☑
    trait D57.3
  sinus (nasal) J34.9
    specified NEC J34.89
  skin L98.9
    atrophic L90.9
      specified NEC L90.8
    granulomatous L92.9
      specified NEC L92.8
    hypertrophic L91.9
      specified NEC L91.8
    infiltrative NEC L98.6
    newborn P83.9
      specified NEC P83.88
    picking F42.4
    psychogenic (allergic) (eczematous) F54
  sleep G47.9
    breathing-related — *see* Apnea, sleep
    circadian rhythm G47.20
      advance sleep phase type G47.22

Disorder — *continued*
  sleep — *continued*
    circadian rhythm — *continued*
      delayed sleep phase type G47.21
      due to
        alcohol
          abuse F10.182
          dependence F10.282
          use F10.982
        amphetamines
          abuse F15.182
          dependence F15.282
          use F15.982
        caffeine
          abuse F15.182
          dependence F15.282
          use F15.982
        cocaine
          abuse F14.182
          dependence F14.282
          use F14.982
        drug NEC
          abuse F19.182
          dependence F19.282
          use F19.982
        opioid
          abuse F11.182
          dependence F11.282
          use F11.982
        psychoactive substance NEC
          abuse F19.182
          dependence F19.282
          use F19.982
        sedative, hypnotic, or anxiolytic
          abuse F13.182
          dependence F13.282
          use F13.982
        stimulant NEC
          abuse F15.182
          dependence F15.282
          use F15.982
      free running type G47.24
      in conditions classified elsewhere G47.27
      irregular sleep wake type G47.23
      jet lag type G47.25
      non-24-hour sleep-wake type G47.24
      shift work type G47.26
      specified NEC G47.29
    due to
      alcohol
        abuse F10.182
        dependence F10.282
        use F10.982
      amphetamine
        abuse F15.182
        dependence F15.282
        use F15.982
      anxiolytic
        abuse F13.182
        dependence F13.282
        use F13.982
      caffeine
        abuse F15.182
        dependence F15.282
        use F15.982
      cocaine
        abuse F14.182
        dependence F14.282
        use F14.982
      drug NEC
        abuse F19.182
        dependence F19.282
        use F19.982
      hypnotic
        abuse F13.182
        dependence F13.282
        use F13.982
      opioid
        abuse F11.182
        dependence F11.282
        use F11.982
      psychoactive substance NEC
        abuse F19.182
        dependence F19.282
        use F19.982
      sedative
        abuse F13.182
        dependence F13.282
        use F13.982

Disorder — *continued*
  sleep — *continued*
    due to — *continued*
      stimulant NEC
        abuse F15.182
        dependence F15.282
        use F15.982
      emotional F51.9
      excessive somnolence — *see* Hypersomnia
      hypersomnia type — *see* Hypersomnia
      initiating or maintaining — *see* Insomnia
      nightmares F51.5
      nonorganic F51.9
        specified NEC F51.8
      parasomnia type G47.50
      specified NEC G47.8
      terrors F51.4
      walking F51.3
    sleep-wake pattern or schedule — *see also* Disorder, sleep, circadian rhythm G47.9
      specified NEC G47.8
  social
    anxiety (of childhood) F40.10
      generalized F40.11
    functioning in childhood F94.9
      specified NEC F94.8
    pragmatic F80.82
  soft tissue M79.9
    ankle M79.9
    due to use, overuse and pressure M70.90
      ankle M70.97- ☑
      bursitis — *see* Bursitis
      foot M70.97- ☑
      forearm M70.93- ☑
      hand M70.94- ☑
      lower leg M70.96- ☑
      multiple sites M70.99
      pelvic region M70.95- ☑
      shoulder region M70.91- ☑
      specified site NEC M70.98
      specified type NEC M70.80
        ankle M70.87- ☑
        foot M70.87- ☑
        forearm M70.83- ☑
        hand M70.84- ☑
        lower leg M70.86- ☑
        multiple sites M70.89
        pelvic region M70.85- ☑
        shoulder region M70.81- ☑
        specified site NEC M70.88
        thigh M70.85- ☑
        upper arm M70.82- ☑
      thigh M70.95- ☑
      upper arm M70.92- ☑
    foot M79.9
    forearm M79.9
    hand M79.9
    lower leg M79.9
    multiple sites M79.9
    occupational — *see* Disorder, soft tissue, due to use, overuse and pressure
    pelvic region M79.9
    shoulder region M79.9
    specified type NEC M79.89
    thigh M79.9
    upper arm M79.9
  somatic symptom F45.1
  somatization F45.0
  somatoform F45.9
    pain (persistent) F45.41
    somatization (multiple) (long-lasting) F45.0
    specified NEC F45.8
    undifferentiated F45.1
  somnolence, excessive — *see* Hypersomnia
  specific
    arithmetical F81.2
    developmental, of motor F82
    reading F81.0
    speech and language F80.9
    spelling F81.81
    written expression F81.81
  speech R47.9
    articulation (functional) (specific) F80.0
    developmental F80.9
    specified NEC R47.89
  speech-sound F80.0
  spelling (specific) F81.81
  spine — *see also* Dorsopathy

Disorder — *continued*
  spine — *see also* Dorsopathy — *continued*
    ligamentous or muscular attachments, peripheral
      — *see* Enthesopathy, spinal
    specified NEC — *see* Dorsopathy, specified NEC
  stereotyped, habit or movement F98.4
  stimulant use (other) (unspecified)
    mild F15.10
      in remission (early) (sustained) F15.11
    moderate or severe F15.20
      in remission (early) (sustained) F15.21
  stomach (functional) — *see* Disorder, gastric
  stress F43.9
    acute F43.0
    post-traumatic F43.10
      acute F43.11
      chronic F43.12
  substance use (other) (unknown)
    mild F19.10
      with substance-induced
        anxiety disorder F19.180
        bipolar and related disorder F19.14
        depressive disorder F19.14
        major neurocognitive disorder F19.17
        mild neurocognitive disorder F19.188
        obsessive-compulsive and related disorder
          F19.188
        sexual dysfunction F19.181
      substance intoxication F19.129
      substance intoxication delirium F19.121
    moderate or severe F19.20
      with substance-induced
        anxiety disorder F19.280
        bipolar and related disorder F19.24
        depressive disorder F19.24
        major neurocognitive disorder F19.27
        mild neurocognitive disorder F19.288
        obsessive-compulsive and related disorder
          F19.288
        sexual dysfunction F19.281
      in remission (early) (sustained) F19.21
      substance intoxication F19.229
      substance intoxication delirium F19.221
  sulfur-bearing amino-acid metabolism E72.10
  sweat gland (eccrine) L74.9
    apocrine L75.9
      specified NEC L75.8
    specified NEC L74.8
  synovium M67.90
    acromioclavicular M67.91- ✓
    ankle M67.97- ✓
    elbow M67.92- ✓
    foot M67.97- ✓
    forearm M67.93- ✓
    hand M67.94- ✓
    hip M67.95- ✓
    knee M67.96- ✓
    multiple sites M67.99
    rupture — *see* Rupture, synovium
    shoulder M67.91- ✓
    specified type NEC M67.80
      acromioclavicular M67.81- ✓
      ankle M67.87- ✓
      elbow M67.82- ✓
      foot M67.87- ✓
      hand M67.84- ✓
      hip M67.85- ✓
      knee M67.86- ✓
      multiple sites M67.89
      wrist M67.83- ✓
    synovitis — *see* Synovitis
    upper arm M67.92- ✓
    wrist M67.93- ✓
  temperature regulation, newborn P81.9
    specified NEC P81.8
  temporomandibular joint M26.60- ✓
  tendon M67.90
    acromioclavicular M67.91- ✓
    ankle M67.97- ✓
    contracture — *see* Contracture, tendon
    elbow M67.92- ✓
    foot M67.97- ✓
    forearm M67.93- ✓
    hand M67.94- ✓
    hip M67.95- ✓
    knee M67.96- ✓
    multiple sites M67.99

Disorder — *continued*
  tendon — *continued*
    rupture — *see* Rupture, tendon
    shoulder M67.91- ✓
    specified type NEC M67.80
      acromioclavicular M67.81- ✓
      ankle M67.87- ✓
      elbow M67.82- ✓
      foot M67.87- ✓
      hand M67.84- ✓
      hip M67.85- ✓
      knee M67.86- ✓
      multiple sites M67.89
      trunk M67.88
      wrist M67.83- ✓
    synovitis — *see* Synovitis
    tendinitis — *see* Tendinitis
    tenosynovitis — *see* Tenosynovitis
    trunk M67.98
    upper arm M67.92- ✓
    wrist M67.93- ✓
  thoracic root (nerve) NEC G54.3
  thyrocalcitonin hypersecretion E07.0
  thyroid (gland) E07.9
    function NEC, neonatal, transitory P72.2
    iodine-deficiency related E01.8
    specified NEC E07.89
  tic — *see* Tic
  tobacco use
    chewing tobacco (mild) (moderate) (severe)
      in remission (early) (sustained) F17.221
    cigarettes (mild) (moderate) (severe)
      in remission (early) (sustained) F17.211
    mild F17.200
      in remission (early) (sustained) F17.201
    moderate F17.200
      in remission (early) (sustained) F17.201
    severe F17.200
      in remission (early) (sustained) F17.201
    specified product NEC (mild) (moderate) (severe)
      in remission (early) (sustained) F17.291
  tooth K08.9
    development K00.9
      specified NEC K00.8
    eruption K00.6
  Tourette's F95.2
  trance and possession F44.89
  transvestic F65.1
  trauma and stressor-related F43.9
    other specified F43.8
  tricuspid (valve) — *see* Endocarditis, tricuspid
  tryptophan metabolism E70.5
  tubular, phosphate-losing N25.0
  tubulo-interstitial (in)
    brucellosis A23.9 [N16]
    cystinosis E72.04
    diphtheria A36.84
    glycogen storage disease E74.00 [N16]
    leukemia NEC C95.9- ✓ [N16]
    lymphoma NEC C85.9- ✓ [N16]
    mixed cryoglobulinemia D89.1 [N16]
    multiple myeloma C90.0- ✓ [N16]
    Salmonella infection A02.25
    sarcoidosis D86.84
    sepsis A41.9 [N16]
      streptococcal A40.9 [N16]
    systemic lupus erythematosus M32.15
    toxoplasmosis B58.83
    transplant rejection T86.91 [N16]
    Wilson's disease E83.01 [N16]
  tubulo-renal function, impaired N25.9
    specified NEC N25.89
  tympanic membrane H73.9- ✓
    atrophy — *see* Atrophy, tympanic membrane
    infection — *see* Myringitis
    perforation — *see* Perforation, tympanum
    specified NEC H73.89- ✓
  unsocialized aggressive F91.1
  urea cycle metabolism E72.20
    argininemia E72.21
    arginosuccinic aciduria E72.22
    citrullinemia E72.23
    ornithine transcarbamylase deficiency E72.4
    other specified E72.29
  ureter (in) N28.9
    schistosomiasis B65.0 [N29]
    tuberculosis A18.11
  urethra N36.9

Disorder — *continued*
  urethra — *continued*
    specified NEC N36.8
  urinary system N39.9
    specified NEC N39.8
  valve, heart
    aortic — *see* Endocarditis, aortic
    mitral — *see* Endocarditis, mitral
    pulmonary — *see* Endocarditis, pulmonary
    rheumatic
      aortic — *see* Endocarditis, aortic, rheumatic
      mitral — *see* Endocarditis, mitral
      pulmonary — *see* Endocarditis, pulmonary,
        rheumatic
      tricuspid — *see* Endocarditis, tricuspid
    tricuspid — *see* Endocarditis, tricuspid
  vestibular function H81.9- ✓
    specified NEC — *see* subcategory H81.8 ✓
      in diseases classified elsewhere H82.- ✓
    vertigo — *see* Vertigo
  vision, binocular H53.30
    abnormal retinal correspondence H53.31
    diplopia H53.2
    fusion with defective stereopsis H53.32
    simultaneous perception H53.33
    suppression H53.34
  visual
    cortex
      blindness H47.619
        left brain H47.612
        right brain H47.611
      due to
        inflammatory disorder H47.629
          left brain H47.622
          right brain H47.621
        neoplasm H47.639
          left brain H47.632
          right brain H47.631
        vascular disorder H47.649
          left brain H47.642
          right brain H47.641
    pathway H47.9
      due to
        inflammatory disorder H47.51- ✓
        neoplasm H47.52- ✓
        vascular disorder H47.53- ✓
    optic chiasm — *see* Disorder, optic, chiasm
  vitreous body H43.9
    crystalline deposits — *see* Deposit, crystalline
    degeneration — *see* Degeneration, vitreous
    hemorrhage — *see* Hemorrhage, vitreous
    opacities — *see* Opacity, vitreous
    prolapse — *see* Prolapse, vitreous
    specified type NEC H43.89
  voice R49.9
    specified type NEC R49.8
  volatile solvent use
    due to drug abuse — *see* Abuse, drug, inhalant
    due to drug dependence — *see* Dependence, drug,
      inhalant
  voyeuristic F65.3
  white blood cells D72.9
    specified NEC D72.89
  withdrawing, child or adolescent F40.10
Disorientation R41.0
Displacement, displaced
  acquired traumatic of bone, cartilage, joint, tendon
    NEC — *see* Dislocation
  adrenal gland (congenital) Q89.1
  appendix, retrocecal (congenital) Q43.8
  auricle (congenital) Q17.4
  bladder (acquired) N32.89
    congenital Q64.19
  brachial plexus (congenital) Q07.8
  brain stem, caudal (congenital) Q04.8
  canaliculus (lacrimalis), congenital Q10.6
  cardia through esophageal hiatus (congenital) Q40.1
  cerebellum, caudal (congenital) Q04.8
  cervix — *see* Malposition, uterus
  colon (congenital) Q43.3
  device, implant or graft — *see also* Complications, by
    site and type, mechanical T85.628 ✓
    arterial graft NEC — *see* Complication, cardiovascu-
      lar device, mechanical, vascular
    breast (implant) T85.42 ✓
    catheter NEC T85.628 ✓
      dialysis (renal) T82.42 ✓
        intraperitoneal T85.621 ✓

Displacement, displaced — *continued*
  device, implant or graft — *see also* Complications, by
    site and type, mechanical — *continued*
    catheter — *continued*
      infusion NEC T82.524 ☑
        spinal (epidural) (subdural) T85.620 ☑
      urinary
        cystostomy T83.020 ☑
        Hopkins T83.028 ☑
        ileostomy T83.028 ☑
        indwelling T83.021 ☑
        nephrostomy T83.022 ☑
        specified NEC T83.028 ☑
        urostomy T83.028 ☑
    electronic (electrode) (pulse generator) (stimulator)
      — *see* Complication, electronic stimulator
    fixation, internal (orthopedic) NEC — *see* Complica-
      tion, fixation device, mechanical
    gastrointestinal — *see* Complications, prosthetic
      device, mechanical, gastrointestinal device
    genital NEC T83.428 ☑
      intrauterine contraceptive device (string)
        T83.32 ☑
      penile prosthesis (cylinder) (implanted) (pump)
        (reservoir) T83.420 ☑
      testicular prosthesis T83.421 ☑
    heart NEC — *see* Complication, cardiovascular de-
      vice, mechanical
    joint prosthesis — *see* Complications, joint prosthe-
      sis, mechanical
    ocular — *see* Complications, prosthetic device,
      mechanical, ocular device
    orthopedic NEC — *see* Complication, orthopedic,
      device or graft, mechanical
    specified NEC T85.628 ☑
    urinary NEC T83.128 ☑
      graft T83.22 ☑
      sphincter, implanted T83.121 ☑
      stent (ileal conduit) (nephroureteral) T83.123 ☑
      ureteral indwelling T83.122 ☑
    vascular NEC — *see* Complication, cardiovascular
      device, mechanical
    ventricular intracranial shunt T85.02 ☑
  electronic stimulator
    bone T84.320 ☑
    cardiac — *see* Complications, cardiac device, elec-
      tronic
    nervous system — *see* Complication, prosthetic
      device, mechanical, electronic nervous system
      stimulator
    urinary — *see* Complications, electronic stimulator,
      urinary
  esophageal mucosa into cardia of stomach, congenital
    Q39.8
  esophagus (acquired) K22.8
    congenital Q39.8
  eyeball (acquired) (lateral) (old) — *see* Displacement,
    globe
    congenital Q15.8
    current — *see* Avulsion, eye
  fallopian tube (acquired) N83.4- ☑
    congenital Q50.6
    opening (congenital) Q50.6
  gallbladder (congenital) Q44.1
  gastric mucosa (congenital) Q40.2
  globe (acquired) (old) (lateral) H05.21- ☑
    current — *see* Avulsion, eye
  heart (congenital) Q24.8
    acquired I51.89
  hymen (upward) (congenital) Q52.4
  intervertebral disc NEC
    with myelopathy — *see* Disorder, disc, with,
      myelopathy
    cervical, cervicothoracic (with) M50.20
      myelopathy — *see* Disorder, disc, cervical, with
        myelopathy
      neuritis, radiculitis or radiculopathy — *see* Disor-
        der, disc, cervical, with neuritis
    due to trauma — *see* Dislocation, vertebra
    lumbar region M51.26
      with
        myelopathy M51.06
        neuritis, radiculitis, radiculopathy or sciatica
          M51.16
    lumbosacral region M51.27

Displacement, displaced — *continued*
  intervertebral disc — *continued*
    lumbosacral region — *continued*
      with
        neuritis, radiculitis, radiculopathy or sciatica
          M51.17
    sacrococcygeal region M53.3
    thoracic region M51.24
      with
        myelopathy M51.04
        neuritis, radiculitis, radiculopathy M51.14
    thoracolumbar region M51.25
      with
        myelopathy M51.05
        neuritis, radiculitis, radiculopathy M51.15
  intrauterine device (string) T83.32 ☑
  kidney (acquired) N28.83
    congenital Q63.2
  lachrymal, lacrimal apparatus or duct (congenital) Q10.6
  lens, congenital Q12.1
  macula (congenital) Q14.1
  Meckel's diverticulum Q43.0
    malignant — *see* Table of Neoplasms, small intes-
      tine, malignant
  nail (congenital) Q84.6
    acquired L60.8
  opening of Wharton's duct in mouth Q38.4
  organ or site, congenital NEC — *see* Malposition, con-
    genital
  ovary (acquired) N83.4- ☑
    congenital Q50.39
    free in peritoneal cavity (congenital) Q50.39
    into hernial sac N83.4- ☑
  oviduct (acquired) N83.4- ☑
    congenital Q50.6
  parathyroid (gland) E21.4
  parotid gland (congenital) Q38.4
  punctum lacrimale (congenital) Q10.6
  sacro-iliac (joint) (congenital) Q74.2
    current injury S33.2 ☑
    old — *see* subcategory M53.2 ☑
  salivary gland (any) (congenital) Q38.4
  spleen (congenital) Q89.09
  stomach, congenital Q40.2
  sublingual duct Q38.4
  tongue (downward) (congenital) Q38.3
  tooth, teeth, fully erupted M26.30
    horizontal M26.33
    vertical M26.34
  trachea (congenital) Q32.1
  ureter or ureteric opening or orifice (congenital) Q62.62
  uterine opening of oviducts or fallopian tubes Q50.6
  uterus, uterine — *see* Malposition, uterus
  ventricular septum Q21.0
    with rudimentary ventricle Q20.4

Disproportion
  between native and reconstructed breast N65.1
  fiber-type G71.2

Disruptio uteri — *see* Rupture, uterus
Disruption (of)
  ciliary body NEC H21.89
  closure of
    cornea T81.31 ☑
    craniotomy T81.32 ☑
    fascia (muscular) (superficial) T81.32 ☑
    internal organ or tissue T81.32 ☑
    laceration (external) (internal) T81.33 ☑
    ligament T81.32 ☑
    mucosa T81.31 ☑
    muscle or muscle flap T81.32 ☑
    ribs or rib cage T81.32 ☑
    skin and subcutaneous tissue (full-thickness) (super-
      ficial) T81.31 ☑
    skull T81.32 ☑
    sternum (sternotomy) T81.32 ☑
    tendon T81.32 ☑
    traumatic laceration (external) (internal) T81.33 ☑
  family Z63.8
    due to
      absence of family member due to military deploy-
        ment Z63.31
      absence of family member NEC Z63.32
      alcoholism and drug addiction in family Z63.72
      bereavement Z63.4
      death (assumed) or disappearance of family
        member Z63.4
      divorce or separation Z63.5
      drug addiction in family Z63.72

Disruption — *continued*
  family — *continued*
    due to — *continued*
      return of family member from military deploy-
        ment (current or past conflict) Z63.71
      stressful life events NEC Z63.79
  iris NEC H21.89
  ligament(s) — *see also* Sprain
    knee
      current injury — *see* Dislocation, knee
      old (chronic) — *see* Derangement, knee, instabil-
        ity
      spontaneous NEC — *see* Derangement, knee,
        disruption ligament
  ossicular chain — *see* Discontinuity, ossicles, ear
  pelvic ring (stable) S32.810 ☑
    unstable S32.811 ☑
  traumatic injury wound repair T81.33 ☑
  wound T81.30 ☑
    episiotomy O90.1
    operation T81.31 ☑
      cesarean O90.0
      external operation wound (superficial) T81.31 ☑
      internal operation wound (deep) T81.32 ☑
    perineal (obstetric) O90.1
    traumatic injury repair T81.33 ☑

Dissatisfaction with
  employment Z56.9
  school environment Z55.4
Dissecting — *see* condition
Dissection
  aorta I71.00
    abdominal I71.02
    thoracic I71.01
    thoracoabdominal I71.03
  artery I77.70
    basilar (trunk) I77.75
    carotid I77.71
    cerebral (nonruptured) I67.0
      ruptured — *see* Hemorrhage, intracranial, sub-
        arachnoid
    coronary I25.42
    extremity
      lower I77.77
      upper I77.76
    iliac I77.72
    precerebral
      congenital (nonruptured) Q28.1
      specified site NEC I77.75
    renal I77.73
    specified NEC I77.79
    vertebral I77.74
  precerebral artery, congenital (nonruptured) Q28.1
    Heartland A93.8
  traumatic — *see* Wound, open, by site
  vascular I99.8
  wound — *see* Wound, open
Disseminated — *see* condition
Dissociation
  auriculoventricular or atrioventricular (AV) (any degree)
    (isorhythmic) I45.89
    with heart block I44.2
  interference I45.89
Dissociative reaction, state F44.9
Dissolution, vertebra — *see* Osteoporosis
Distension, distention
  abdomen R14.0
  bladder N32.89
  cecum K63.89
  colon K63.89
  gallbladder K82.8
  intestine K63.89
  kidney N28.89
  liver K76.89
  seminal vesicle N50.89
  stomach K31.89
    acute K31.0
    psychogenic F45.8
  ureter — *see* Dilatation, ureter
  uterus N85.8
Distoma hepaticum infestation B66.3
Distomiasis B66.9
  bile passages B66.3
  hemic B65.9
  hepatic B66.3
    due to Clonorchis sinensis B66.1
  intestinal B66.5
  liver B66.3

Distomiasis — *continued*
  liver — *continued*
    due to Clonorchis sinensis B66.1
  lung B66.4
  pulmonary B66.4
Distomolar (fourth molar) K00.1
Disto-occlusion (Division I) (Division II) M26.212
Distortion(s) (congenital)
  adrenal (gland) Q89.1
  arm NEC Q68.8
  bile duct or passage Q44.5
  bladder Q64.79
  brain Q04.9
  cervix (uteri) Q51.9
  chest (wall) Q67.8
    bones Q76.8
  clavicle Q74.0
  clitoris Q52.6
  coccyx Q76.49
  common duct Q44.5
  coronary Q24.5
  cystic duct Q44.5
  ear (auricle) (external) Q17.3
    inner Q16.5
    middle Q16.4
      ossicles Q16.3
  endocrine NEC Q89.2
  eustachian tube Q17.8
  eye (adnexa) Q15.8
  face bone(s) NEC Q75.8
  fallopian tube Q50.6
  femur NEC Q68.8
  fibula NEC Q68.8
  finger(s) Q68.1
  foot Q66.9- ☑
  genitalia, genital organ(s)
    female Q52.8
      external Q52.79
      internal NEC Q52.8
  gyri Q04.8
  hand bone(s) Q68.1
  heart (auricle) (ventricle) Q24.8
    valve (cusp) Q24.8
  hepatic duct Q44.5
  humerus NEC Q68.8
  hymen Q52.4
  intrafamilial communications Z63.8
  jaw NEC M26.89
  labium (majus) (minus) Q52.79
  leg NEC Q68.8
  lens Q12.8
  liver Q44.7
  lumbar spine Q76.49
    with disproportion O33.8
      causing obstructed labor O65.0
  lumbosacral (joint) (region) Q76.49
    kyphosis — *see* Kyphosis, congenital
    lordosis — *see* Lordosis, congenital
  nerve Q07.8
  nose Q30.8
  organ
    of Corti Q16.5
    or site not listed — *see* Anomaly, by site
  ossicles, ear Q16.3
  oviduct Q50.6
  pancreas Q45.3
  parathyroid (gland) Q89.2
  pituitary (gland) Q89.2
  radius NEC Q68.8
  sacroiliac joint Q74.2
  sacrum Q76.49
  scapula Q74.0
  shoulder girdle Q74.0
  skull bone(s) NEC Q75.8
    with
      anencephalus Q00.0
      encephalocele — *see* Encephalocele
      hydrocephalus Q03.9
        with spina bifida — *see* Spina bifida, with
          hydrocephalus
      microcephaly Q02
  spinal cord Q06.8
  spine Q76.49
    kyphosis — *see* Kyphosis, congenital
    lordosis — *see* Lordosis, congenital
  spleen Q89.09
  sternum NEC Q76.7
  thorax (wall) Q67.8

Distortion(s) — *continued*
  thorax — *continued*
    bony Q76.8
  thymus (gland) Q89.2
  thyroid Q89.2
  tibia NEC Q68.8
  toe(s) Q66.9- ☑
  tongue Q38.3
  trachea (cartilage) Q32.1
  ulna NEC Q68.8
  ureter Q62.8
  urethra Q64.79
    causing obstruction Q64.39
  uterus Q51.9
  vagina Q52.4
  vertebra Q76.49
    kyphosis — *see* Kyphosis, congenital
    lordosis — *see* Lordosis, congenital
  visual — *see also* Disturbance, vision
    shape and size H53.15
  vulva Q52.79
  wrist (bones) (joint) Q68.8
Distress
  abdomen — *see* Pain, abdominal
  acute respiratory R06.03
    syndrome (adult) (child) J80
  epigastric R10.13
  fetal P84
    complicating pregnancy — *see* Stress, fetal
  gastrointestinal (functional) K30
    psychogenic F45.8
  intestinal (functional) NOS K59.9
    psychogenic F45.8
  maternal, during labor and delivery O75.0
  relationship, with spouse or intimate partner Z63.0
  respiratory (adult) (child) R06.03
    newborn P22.9
      specified NEC P22.8
    orthopnea R06.01
    psychogenic F45.8
    shortness of breath R06.02
    specified type NEC R06.09
Distribution vessel, atypical Q27.9
  coronary artery Q24.5
  precerebral Q28.1
Districhiasis L68.8
Disturbance(s) — *see also* Disease
  absorption K90.9
    calcium E58
    carbohydrate K90.49
    fat K90.49
      pancreatic K90.3
    protein K90.49
    starch K90.49
    vitamin — *see* Deficiency, vitamin
  acid-base equilibrium E87.8
    mixed E87.4
  activity and attention (with hyperkinesis) — *see* Disorder, attention-deficit hyperactivity
  amino acid transport E72.00
  assimilation, food K90.9
  auditory nerve, except deafness — *see* subcategory H93.3 ☑
  behavior — *see* Disorder, conduct
  blood clotting (mechanism) — *see also* Defect, coagulation D68.9
  cerebral
    nerve — *see* Disorder, nerve, cranial
    status, newborn P91.9
      specified NEC P91.88
  circulatory I99.9
  conduct — *see also* Disorder, conduct F91.9
    adjustment reaction — *see* Disorder, adjustment
    compulsive F63.9
    disruptive F91.9
    hyperkinetic — *see* Disorder, attention-deficit hyperactivity
    socialized F91.2
    specified NEC F91.8
    unsocialized F91.1
  coordination R27.8
  cranial nerve — *see* Disorder, nerve, cranial
  deep sensibility — *see* Disturbance, sensation
  digestive K30
    psychogenic F45.8
  electrolyte — *see also* Imbalance, electrolyte
    newborn, transitory P74.49
      hyperammonemia P74.6

Disturbance(s) — *continued*
  electrolyte — *see also* Imbalance, electrolyte — *continued*
    newborn, transitory — *continued*
      hyperchloremia P74.421
      hyperchloremic metabolic acidosis P74.421
      hypochloremia P74.422
      potassium balance
        hyperkalemia P74.31
        hypokalemia P74.32
      sodium balance
        hypernatremia P74.21
        hyponatremia P74.22
      specified type NEC P74.49
  emotions specific to childhood and adolescence F93.9
    with
      anxiety and fearfulness NEC F93.8
      elective mutism F94.0
      oppositional disorder F91.3
      sensitivity (withdrawal) F40.10
      shyness F40.10
      social withdrawal F40.10
    involving relationship problems F93.8
    mixed F93.8
    specified NEC F93.8
  endocrine (gland) E34.9
    neonatal, transitory P72.9
      specified NEC P72.8
  equilibrium R42
  fructose metabolism E74.10
  gait — *see* Gait
    hysterical F44.4
    psychogenic F44.4
  gastrointestinal (functional) K30
    psychogenic F45.8
  habit, child F98.9
  hearing, except deafness and tinnitus — *see* Abnormal, auditory perception
  heart, functional (conditions in I44-I50)
    due to presence of (cardiac) prosthesis I97.19- ☑
    postoperative I97.89
      cardiac surgery — *see also* Infarct, myocardium associated with revascularization procedure I97.19- ☑
  hormones E34.9
  innervation uterus (parasympathetic) (sympathetic) N85.8
  keratinization NEC
    gingiva K05.10
      nonplaque induced K05.11
      plaque induced K05.10
    lip K13.0
    oral (mucosa) (soft tissue) K13.29
    tongue K13.29
  learning (specific) — *see* Disorder, learning
  memory — *see* Amnesia
    mild, following organic brain damage F06.8
  mental F99
    associated with diseases classified elsewhere F54
  metabolism E88.9
    with
      abortion — *see* Abortion, by type with other specified complication
      ectopic pregnancy O08.5
      molar pregnancy O08.5
    amino-acid E72.9
      aromatic E70.9
      branched-chain E71.2
      straight-chain E72.89
      sulfur-bearing E72.10
    ammonia E72.20
    arginine E72.21
    arginosuccinic acid E72.22
    carbohydrate E74.9
    cholesterol E78.9
    citrulline E72.23
    cystathionine E72.19
    general E88.9
    glutamine E72.89
    histidine E70.40
    homocystine E72.19
    hydroxylysine E72.3
    in labor or delivery O75.89
    iron E83.10
    lipoid E78.9
    lysine E72.3
    methionine E72.19
    neonatal, transitory P74.9

☑ **Additional Character Required** — Refer to the Tabular List for Character Selection   ▽ **Subterms under main terms may continue to next column or page**

Disturbance(s) — *continued*
metabolism — *continued*
  neonatal, transitory — *continued*
    calcium and magnesium P71.9
      specified type NEC P71.8
    carbohydrate metabolism P70.9
      specified type NEC P70.8
      specified NEC P74.8
    ornithine E72.4
    phosphate E83.39
    sodium NEC E87.8
    threonine E72.89
    tryptophan E70.5
    tyrosine E70.20
    urea cycle E72.20
motor R29.2
nervous, functional R45.0
neuromuscular mechanism (eye), due to syphilis A52.15
nutritional E63.9
  nail L60.3
ocular motion H51.9
  psychogenic F45.8
oculogyric H51.8
  psychogenic F45.8
oculomotor H51.9
  psychogenic F45.8
olfactory nerve R43.1
optic nerve NEC — *see* Disorder, nerve, optic
oral epithelium, including tongue NEC K13.29
perceptual due to
  alcohol withdrawal F10.232
  amphetamine intoxication F15.922
    in
      abuse F15.122
      dependence F15.222
  anxiolytic withdrawal F13.232
  cannabis intoxication (acute) F12.922
    in
      abuse F12.122
      dependence F12.222
  cocaine intoxication (acute) F14.922
    in
      abuse F14.122
      dependence F14.222
  hypnotic withdrawal F13.232
  opioid intoxication (acute) F11.922
    in
      abuse F11.122
      dependence F11.222
  phencyclidine intoxication (acute) F16.122
  sedative withdrawal F13.232
personality (pattern) (trait) — *see also* Disorder, personality F60.9
  following organic brain damage F07.9
polyglandular E31.9
  specified NEC E31.8
potassium balance, newborn
  hyperkalemia P74.31
  hypokalemia P74.32
psychogenic F45.9
psychomotor F44.4
psychophysical visual H53.16
pupillary — *see* Anomaly, pupil, function
reflex R29.2
rhythm, heart I49.9
salivary secretion K11.7
sensation (cold) (heat) (localization) (tactile discrimination) (texture) (vibratory) NEC R20.9
  hysterical F44.6
  skin R20.9
    anesthesia R20.0
    hyperesthesia R20.3
    hypoesthesia R20.1
    paresthesia R20.2
    specified type NEC R20.8
  smell R43.9
    and taste (mixed) R43.8
    anosmia R43.0
    parosmia R43.1
    specified NEC R43.8
  taste R43.9
    and smell (mixed) R43.8
    parageusia R43.2
    specified NEC R43.8
sensory — *see* Disturbance, sensation
situational (transient) — *see also* Disorder, adjustment
  acute F43.0
sleep G47.9
  nonorganic origin F51.9

Disturbance(s) — *continued*
smell — *see* Disturbance, sensation, smell
sociopathic F60.2
sodium balance, newborn
  hypernatremia P74.21
  hyponatremia P74.22
speech R47.9
  developmental F80.9
  specified NEC R47.89
stomach (functional) K31.9
sympathetic (nerve) G90.9
taste — *see* Disturbance, sensation, taste
temperature
  regulation, newborn P81.9
    specified NEC P81.8
  sense R20.8
    hysterical F44.6
tooth
  eruption K00.6
  formation K00.4
  structure, hereditary NEC K00.5
touch — *see* Disturbance, sensation
vascular I99.9
  arteriosclerotic — *see* Arteriosclerosis
vasomotor I73.9
vasospastic I73.9
vision, visual H53.9
  following
    cerebral infarction I69.398
    cerebrovascular disease I69.998
      specified NEC I69.898
    intracerebral hemorrhage I69.198
    nontraumatic intracranial hemorrhage NEC I69.298
    specified disease NEC I69.898
    subarachnoid hemorrhage I69.098
  psychophysical H53.16
  specified NEC H53.8
  subjective H53.10
    day blindness H53.11
    discomfort H53.14- ☑
    distortions of shape and size H53.15
    loss
      sudden H53.13- ☑
      transient H53.12- ☑
    specified type NEC H53.19
voice R49.9
  psychogenic F44.4
  specified NEC R49.8
Diuresis R35.8
Diver's palsy, paralysis or squeeze T70.3 ☑
Diverticulitis (acute) K57.92
bladder — *see* Cystitis
ileum — *see* Diverticulitis, intestine, small
intestine K57.92
  with
    abscess, perforation or peritonitis K57.80
      with bleeding K57.81
    bleeding K57.93
  congenital Q43.8
  large K57.32
    with
      abscess, perforation or peritonitis K57.20
        with bleeding K57.21
      bleeding K57.33
      small intestine K57.52
        with
          abscess, perforation or peritonitis K57.40
            with bleeding K57.41
          bleeding K57.53
  small K57.12
    with
      abscess, perforation or peritonitis K57.00
        with bleeding K57.01
      bleeding K57.13
      large intestine K57.52
        with
          abscess, perforation or peritonitis K57.40
            with bleeding K57.41
          bleeding K57.53
Diverticulosis K57.90
with bleeding K57.91
large intestine K57.30
  with
    bleeding K57.31
    small intestine K57.50

Diverticulosis — *continued*
large intestine — *continued*
  with — *continued*
    small intestine — *continued*
      with bleeding K57.51
  small intestine K57.10
    with
      bleeding K57.11
      large intestine K57.50
        with bleeding K57.51
Diverticulum, diverticula (multiple) K57.90
appendix (noninflammatory) K38.2
bladder (sphincter) N32.3
  congenital Q64.6
bronchus (congenital) Q32.4
  acquired J98.09
calyx, calyceal (kidney) N28.89
cardia (stomach) K31.4
cecum — *see* Diverticulosis, intestine, large
  congenital Q43.8
colon — *see* Diverticulosis, intestine, large
  congenital Q43.8
duodenum — *see* Diverticulosis, intestine, small
  congenital Q43.8
epiphrenic (esophagus) K22.5
esophagus (congenital) Q39.6
  acquired (epiphrenic) (pulsion) (traction) K22.5
eustachian tube — *see* Disorder, eustachian tube, specified NEC
fallopian tube N83.8
gastric K31.4
heart (congenital) Q24.8
ileum — *see* Diverticulosis, intestine, small
jejunum — *see* Diverticulosis, intestine, small
kidney (pelvis) (calyces) N28.89
  with calculus — *see* Calculus, kidney
Meckel's (displaced) (hypertrophic) Q43.0
  malignant — *see* Table of Neoplasms, small intestine, malignant
midthoracic K22.5
organ or site, congenital NEC — *see* Distortion
pericardium (congenital) (cyst) Q24.8
  acquired I31.8
pharyngoesophageal (congenital) Q39.6
  acquired K22.5
pharynx (congenital) Q38.7
rectosigmoid — *see* Diverticulosis, intestine, large
  congenital Q43.8
rectum — *see* Diverticulosis, intestine, large
Rokitansky's K22.5
seminal vesicle N50.89
sigmoid — *see* Diverticulosis, intestine, large
  congenital Q43.8
stomach (acquired) K31.4
  congenital Q40.2
trachea (acquired) J39.8
ureter (acquired) N28.89
  congenital Q62.8
ureterovesical orifice N28.89
urethra (acquired) N36.1
  congenital Q64.79
ventricle, left (congenital) Q24.8
vesical N32.3
  congenital Q64.6
Zenker's (esophagus) K22.5
Division
cervix uteri (acquired) N88.8
glans penis Q55.69
labia minora (congenital) Q52.79
ligament (partial or complete) (current) — *see also* Sprain
  with open wound — *see* Wound, open
muscle (partial or complete) (current) — *see also* Injury, muscle
  with open wound — *see* Wound, open
nerve (traumatic) — *see* Injury, nerve
spinal cord — *see* Injury, spinal cord, by region
vein I87.8
Divorce, causing family disruption Z63.5
Dix-Hallpike neurolabyrinthitis — *see* Neuronitis, vestibular
Dizziness R42
hysterical F44.89
psychogenic F45.8
DMAC (disseminated mycobacterium avium-intracellulare complex) A31.2
DNR (do not resuscitate) Z66

Doan-Wiseman syndrome (primary splenic neutropenia) — *see* Agranulocytosis
Doehle-Heller aortitis A52.02
Dog bite — *see* Bite
Dohle body panmyelopathic syndrome D72.0
Dolichocephaly Q67.2
Dolichocolon Q43.8
Dolichostenomelia — *see* Syndrome, Marfan's
Donohue's syndrome E34.8
Donor (organ or tissue) Z52.9
  blood (whole) Z52.000
    autologous Z52.010
    specified component (lymphocytes) (platelets) NEC Z52.008
      autologous Z52.018
      specified donor NEC Z52.098
    specified donor NEC Z52.090
    stem cells Z52.001
      autologous Z52.011
      specified donor NEC Z52.091
  bone Z52.20
    autologous Z52.21
    marrow Z52.3
    specified type NEC Z52.29
  cornea Z52.5
  egg (Oocyte) Z52.819
    age 35 and over Z52.812
      anonymous recipient Z52.812
      designated recipient Z52.813
    under age 35 Z52.810
      anonymous recipient Z52.810
      designated recipient Z52.811
  kidney Z52.4
  liver Z52.6
  lung Z52.89
  lymphocyte — *see* Donor, blood, specified components NEC
  Oocyte — *see* Donor, egg
  platelets Z52.008
  potential, examination of Z00.5
  semen Z52.89
  skin Z52.10
    autologous Z52.11
    specified type NEC Z52.19
  specified organ or tissue NEC Z52.89
  sperm Z52.89
Donovanosis A58
Dorsalgia M54.9
  psychogenic F45.41
  specified NEC M54.89
Dorsopathy M53.9
  deforming M43.9
    specified NEC — *see* subcategory M43.8 ☑
  specified NEC M53.80
    cervical region M53.82
    cervicothoracic region M53.83
    lumbar region M53.86
    lumbosacral region M53.87
    occipito-atlanto-axial region M53.81
    sacrococcygeal region M53.88
    thoracic region M53.84
    thoracolumbar region M53.85
Double
  albumin E88.09
  aortic arch Q25.45
  auditory canal Q17.8
  auricle (heart) Q20.8
  bladder Q64.79
  cervix Q51.820
    with doubling of uterus (and vagina) Q51.10
      with obstruction Q51.11
  inlet ventricle Q20.4
  kidney with double pelvis (renal) Q63.0
  meatus urinarius Q64.75
  monster Q89.4
  outlet
    left ventricle Q20.2
    right ventricle Q20.1
  pelvis (renal) with double ureter Q62.5
  tongue Q38.3
  ureter (one or both sides) Q62.5
    with double pelvis (renal) Q62.5
  urethra Q64.74
  urinary meatus Q64.75
  uterus Q51.20
    with
      doubling of cervix (and vagina) Q51.10
        with obstruction Q51.11

Double — *continued*
  uterus — *continued*
    complete Q51.21
    in pregnancy or childbirth O34.0- ☑
      causing obstructed labor O65.5
    partial Q51.22
    specified NEC Q51.28
  vagina Q52.10
    with doubling of uterus (and cervix) Q51.10
      with obstruction Q51.11
  vision H53.2
  vulva Q52.79
Douglas' pouch, cul-de-sac — *see* condition
Down syndrome Q90.9
  meiotic nondisjunction Q90.0
  mitotic nondisjunction Q90.1
  mosaicism Q90.1
  translocation Q90.2
DPD (dihydropyrimidine dehydrogenase deficiency) E88.89
Dracontiasis B72
Dracunculiasis, dracunculosis B72
Dream state, hysterical F44.89
Drepanocytic anemia — *see* Disease, sickle-cell
Dresbach's syndrome (elliptocytosis) D58.1
Dreschlera (hawaiiensis) (infection) B43.8
Dressler's syndrome I24.1
Drift, ulnar — *see* Deformity, limb, specified type NEC, forearm
Drinking (alcohol)
  excessive, to excess NEC (without dependence) F10.10
    habitual (continual) (without remission) F10.20
      with remission F10.21
Drip, postnasal (chronic) R09.82
  due to
    allergic rhinitis — *see* Rhinitis, allergic
    common cold J00
    gastroesophageal reflux — *see* Reflux, gastroesophageal
    nasopharyngitis — *see* Nasopharyngitis
    other known condition — *code to* condition
    sinusitis — *see* Sinusitis
Droop
  facial R29.810
    cerebrovascular disease I69.992
      cerebral infarction I69.392
      intracerebral hemorrhage I69.192
      nontraumatic intracranial hemorrhage NEC I69.292
      specified disease NEC I69.892
      subarachnoid hemorrhage I69.092
Drop (in)
  attack NEC R55
  finger — *see* Deformity, finger
  foot — *see* Deformity, limb, foot, drop
  hematocrit (precipitous) R71.0
  hemoglobin R71.0
  toe — *see* Deformity, toe, specified NEC
  wrist — *see* Deformity, limb, wrist drop
Dropped heart beats I45.9
Dropsy, dropsical — *see also* Hydrops
  abdomen R18.8
  brain — *see* Hydrocephalus
  cardiac, heart — *see* Failure, heart, congestive
  gangrenous — *see* Gangrene
  heart — *see* Failure, heart, congestive
  kidney — *see* Nephrosis
  lung — *see* Edema, lung
  newborn due to isoimmunization P56.0
  pericardium — *see* Pericarditis
Drowned, drowning (near) T75.1 ☑
Drowsiness R40.0
Drug
  abuse counseling and surveillance Z71.51
  addiction — *see* Dependence
  dependence — *see* Dependence
  habit — *see* Dependence
  harmful use — *see* Abuse, drug
  induced fever R50.2
  overdose — *see* Table of Drugs and Chemicals, by drug, poisoning
  poisoning — *see* Table of Drugs and Chemicals, by drug, poisoning
  resistant organism infection — *see also* Resistant, organism, to, drug Z16.30

Drug — *continued*
  therapy
    long term (current) (prophylactic) — *see* Therapy, drug long-term (current) (prophylactic)
    short term — *omit code*
  wrong substance given or taken in error — *see* Table of Drugs and Chemicals, by drug, poisoning
Drunkenness (without dependence) F10.129
  acute in alcoholism F10.229
  chronic (without remission) F10.20
    with remission F10.21
  pathological (without dependence) F10.129
    with dependence F10.229
  sleep F51.9
Drusen
  macula (degenerative) (retina) — *see* Degeneration, macula, drusen
  optic disc H47.32- ☑
Dry, dryness — *see also* condition
  larynx J38.7
  mouth R68.2
    due to dehydration E86.0
  nose J34.89
  socket (teeth) M27.3
  throat J39.2
DSAP L56.5
Duane's syndrome H50.81- ☑
Dubin-Johnson disease or syndrome E80.6
Dubois' disease (thymus gland) A50.59 *[E35]*
Dubowitz' syndrome Q87.19
Duchenne-Aran muscular atrophy G12.21
Duchenne-Griesinger disease G71.01
Duchenne's
  disease or syndrome
    motor neuron disease G12.22
    muscular dystrophy G71.01
  locomotor ataxia (syphilitic) A52.11
  paralysis
    birth injury P14.0
    due to or associated with
      motor neuron disease G12.22
      muscular dystrophy G71.01
Ducrey's chancre A57
Duct, ductus — *see* condition
Duhring's disease (dermatitis herpetiformis) L13.0
Dullness, cardiac (decreased) (increased) R01.2
Dumb ague — *see* Malaria
Dumbness — *see* Aphasia
Dumdum fever B55.0
Dumping syndrome (postgastrectomy) K91.1
Duodenitis (nonspecific) (peptic) K29.80
  with bleeding K29.81
Duodenocholangitis — *see* Cholangitis
Duodenum, duodenal — *see* condition
Duplay's bursitis or periarthritis — *see* Tendinitis, calcific, shoulder
Duplication, duplex — *see also* Accessory
  alimentary tract Q45.8
  anus Q43.4
  appendix (and cecum) Q43.4
  biliary duct (any) Q44.5
  bladder Q64.79
  cecum (and appendix) Q43.4
  cervix Q51.820
  chromosome NEC
    with complex rearrangements NEC Q92.5
    seen only at prometaphase Q92.8
  cystic duct Q44.5
  digestive organs Q45.8
  esophagus Q39.8
  frontonasal process Q75.8
  intestine (large) (small) Q43.4
  kidney Q63.0
  liver Q44.7
  pancreas Q45.3
  penis Q55.69
  respiratory organs NEC Q34.8
  salivary duct Q38.4
  spinal cord (incomplete) Q06.2
  stomach Q40.2
Dupré's disease (meningism) R29.1
Dupuytren's contraction or disease M72.0
Durand-Nicolas-Favre disease A55
Durotomy (inadvertent) (incidental) G97.41
Duroziez's disease (congenital mitral stenosis) Q23.2
Dutton's relapsing fever (West African) A68.1
Dwarfism E34.3
  achondroplastic Q77.4

122

☑ Additional Character Required — Refer to the Tabular List for Character Selection   ▽ Subterms under main terms may continue to next column or page

Dwarfism — *continued*
  congenital E34.3
  constitutional E34.3
  hypochondroplastic Q77.4
  hypophyseal E23.0
  infantile E34.3
  Laron-type E34.3
  Lorain (-Levi) type E23.0
  metatropic Q77.8
  nephrotic-glycosuric (with hypophosphatemic rickets) E72.09
  nutritional E45
  pancreatic K86.89
  pituitary E23.0
  renal N25.0
  thanatophoric Q77.1
Dyke-Young anemia (secondary) (symptomatic) D59.1
Dysacusis — *see* Abnormal, auditory perception
Dysadrenocortism E27.9
  hyperfunction E27.0
Dysarthria R47.1
  following
    cerebral infarction I69.322
    cerebrovascular disease I69.922
      specified disease NEC I69.822
    intracerebral hemorrhage I69.122
    nontraumatic intracranial hemorrhage NEC I69.222
    subarachnoid hemorrhage I69.022
Dysautonomia (familial) G90.1
Dysbarism T70.3 ☑
Dysbasia R26.2
  angiosclerotica intermittens I73.9
  hysterical F44.4
  lordotica (progressiva) G24.1
  nonorganic origin F44.4
  psychogenic F44.4
Dysbetalipoproteinemia (familial) E78.2
Dyscalculia R48.8
  developmental F81.2
Dyschezia K59.00
Dyschondroplasia (with hemangiomata) Q78.4
Dyschromia (skin) L81.9
Dyscollagenosis M35.9
Dyscranio-pygo-phalangy Q87.0
Dyscrasia
  blood (with) D75.9
    antepartum hemorrhage — *see* Hemorrhage, antepartum, with coagulation defect
    intrapartum hemorrhage O67.0
    newborn P61.9
      specified type NEC P61.8
    puerperal, postpartum O72.3
  polyglandular, pluriglandular E31.9
Dysendocrinism E34.9
Dysentery, dysenteric (catarrhal) (diarrhea) (epidemic) (hemorrhagic) (infectious) (sporadic) (tropical) A09
  abscess, liver A06.4
  amebic — *see also* Amebiasis A06.0
    with abscess — *see* Abscess, amebic
    acute A06.0
    chronic A06.1
  arthritis — *see also* category M01 A09
    bacillary (*see also* category M01) A03.9
  bacillary A03.9
    arthritis — *see also* category M01 A03.9
    Boyd A03.2
    Flexner A03.1
    Schmitz (-Stutzer) A03.0
    Shiga (-Kruse) A03.0
    Shigella A03.9
      boydii A03.2
      dysenteriae A03.0
      flexneri A03.1
      group A A03.0
      group B A03.1
      group C A03.2
      group D A03.3
      sonnei A03.3
      specified type NEC A03.8
    Sonne A03.3
    specified type NEC A03.8
  balantidial A07.0
  Balantidium coli A07.0
  Boyd's A03.2
  candidal B37.82
  Chilomastix A07.8
  Chinese A03.9
  coccidial A07.3

Dysentery, dysenteric — *continued*
  Dientamoeba (fragilis) A07.8
  Embadomonas A07.8
  Entamoeba, entamebic — *see* Dysentery, amebic
  Flexner-Boyd A03.2
  Flexner's A03.1
  Giardia lamblia A07.1
  Hiss-Russell A03.1
  Lamblia A07.1
  leishmanial B55.0
  malarial — *see* Malaria
  metazoal B82.0
  monilial B37.82
  protozoal A07.9
  Salmonella A02.0
  schistosomal B65.1
  Schmitz (-Stutzer) A03.0
  Shiga (-Kruse) A03.0
  Shigella NOS — *see* Dysentery, bacillary
  Sonne A03.3
  strongyloidiasis B78.0
  trichomonal A07.8
  viral — *see also* Enteritis, viral A08.4
Dysequilibrium R42
Dysesthesia R20.8
  hysterical F44.6
Dysfibrinogenemia (congenital) D68.2
Dysfunction
  adrenal E27.9
    hyperfunction E27.0
  autonomic
    due to alcohol G31.2
    somatoform F45.8
  bladder N31.9
    neurogenic NOS — *see* Dysfunction, bladder, neuromuscular
    neuromuscular NOS N31.9
      atonic (motor) (sensory) N31.2
      autonomous N31.2
      flaccid N31.2
      nonreflex N31.2
      reflex N31.1
      specified NEC N31.8
      uninhibited N31.0
  bleeding, uterus N93.8
  cerebral G93.89
  colon K59.9
    psychogenic F45.8
  colostomy K94.03
  cystic duct K82.8
  cystostomy (stoma) — *see* Complications, cystostomy
  ejaculatory N53.19
    anejaculatory orgasm N53.13
    painful N53.12
    premature F52.4
    retarded N53.11
  endocrine NOS E34.9
  endometrium N85.8
  enterostomy K94.13
  erectile — *see* Dysfunction, sexual, male, erectile
  gallbladder K82.8
  gastrostomy (stoma) K94.23
  gland, glandular NOS E34.9
    meibomian, of eyelid — *see* Dysfunction, meibomian gland
  heart I51.89
  hemoglobin D75.89
  hepatic K76.89
  hypophysis E23.7
  hypothalamic NEC E23.3
  ileostomy (stoma) K94.13
  jejunostomy (stoma) K94.13
  kidney — *see* Disease, renal
  labyrinthine — *see* subcategory H83.2 ☑
  left ventricular, following sudden emotional stress I51.81
  liver K76.89
  male — *see* Dysfunction, sexual, male
  meibomian gland, of eyelid H02.889
    left H02.886
      lower H02.885
      upper H02.884
      upper and lower eyelids H02.88B
    right H02.883
      lower H02.882
      upper H02.881
      upper and lower eyelids H02.88A
  orgasmic (female) F52.31

Dysfunction — *continued*
  orgasmic — *continued*
    male F52.32
  ovary E28.9
    specified NEC E28.8
  papillary muscle I51.89
  parathyroid E21.4
  physiological NEC R68.89
    psychogenic F59
  pineal gland E34.8
  pituitary (gland) E23.3
  platelets D69.1
  polyglandular E31.9
    specified NEC E31.8
  psychophysiologic F59
  psychosexual F52.9
    with
      dyspareunia F52.6
      premature ejaculation F52.4
      vaginismus F52.5
  pylorus K31.9
  rectum K59.9
    psychogenic F45.8
  reflex (sympathetic) — *see* Syndrome, pain, complex regional I
  segmental — *see* Dysfunction, somatic
  senile R54
  sexual (due to) R37
    alcohol F10.981
    amphetamine F15.981
      in
        abuse F15.181
        dependence F15.281
    anxiolytic F13.981
      in
        abuse F13.181
        dependence F13.281
    cocaine F14.981
      in
        abuse F14.181
        dependence F14.281
    excessive sexual drive F52.8
    failure of genital response (male) F52.21
      female F52.22
    female N94.9
      aversion F52.1
      dyspareunia N94.10
        psychogenic F52.6
      frigidity F52.22
      nymphomania F52.8
      orgasmic F52.31
      psychogenic F52.9
        aversion F52.1
        dyspareunia F52.6
        frigidity F52.22
        nymphomania F52.8
        orgasmic F52.31
        vaginismus F52.5
      vaginismus N94.2
        psychogenic F52.5
    hypnotic F13.981
      in
        abuse F13.181
        dependence F13.281
    inhibited orgasm (female) F52.31
      male F52.32
    lack
      of sexual enjoyment F52.1
      or loss of sexual desire F52.0
    male N53.9
      anejaculatory orgasm N53.13
      ejaculatory N53.19
        painful N53.12
        premature F52.4
        retarded N53.11
      erectile N52.9
        drug induced N52.2
        due to
          disease classified elsewhere N52.1
          drug N52.2
        postoperative (postprocedural) N52.39
          following
            cryotherapy N52.37
            interstitial seed therapy N52.36
            prostate ablative therapy N52.37
            prostatectomy N52.34
              radical N52.31
            radiation therapy N52.35
            radical cystectomy N52.32

Dysfunction — *continued*
  sexual — *continued*
    male — *continued*
      erectile — *continued*
        postoperative — *continued*
          following — *continued*
            ultrasound ablative therapy N52.37
            urethral surgery N52.33
        psychogenic F52.21
        specified cause NEC N52.8
        vasculogenic
          arterial insufficiency N52.01
            with corporo-venous occlusive N52.03
          corporo-venous occlusive N52.02
            with arterial insufficiency N52.03
      impotence — *see* Dysfunction, sexual, male, erectile
      psychogenic F52.9
        aversion F52.1
        erectile F52.21
        orgasmic F52.32
        premature ejaculation F52.4
        satyriasis F52.8
        specified type NEC F52.8
      specified type NEC N53.8
    nonorganic F52.9
      specified NEC F52.8
    opioid F11.981
      in
        abuse F11.181
        dependence F11.281
    orgasmic dysfunction (female) F52.31
      male F52.32
    premature ejaculation F52.4
    psychoactive substances NEC F19.981
      in
        abuse F19.181
        dependence F19.281
    psychogenic F52.9
    sedative F13.981
      in
        abuse F13.181
        dependence F13.281
    sexual aversion F52.1
    vaginismus (nonorganic) (psychogenic) F52.5
  sinoatrial node I49.5
  somatic M99.09
    abdomen M99.09
    acromioclavicular M99.07
    cervical region M99.01
    cervicothoracic M99.01
    costochondral M99.08
    costovertebral M99.08
    head region M99.00
    hip M99.05
    lower extremity M99.06
    lumbar region M99.03
    lumbosacral M99.03
    occipitocervical M99.00
    pelvic region M99.05
    pubic M99.05
    rib cage M99.08
    sacral region M99.04
    sacrococcygeal M99.04
    sacroiliac M99.04
    specified NEC M99.09
    sternochondral M99.08
    sternoclavicular M99.07
    thoracic region M99.02
    thoracolumbar M99.02
    upper extremity M99.07
  somatoform autonomic F45.8
  stomach K31.89
    psychogenic F45.8
  suprarenal E27.9
    hyperfunction E27.0
  symbolic R48.9
    specified type NEC R48.8
  temporomandibular (joint) M26.69
    joint-pain syndrome M26.62- ☑
  testicular (endocrine) E29.9
    specified NEC E29.8
  thymus E32.9
  thyroid E07.9
  ureterostomy (stoma) — *see* Complications, stoma, urinary tract
  urethrostomy (stoma) — *see* Complications, stoma, urinary tract
  uterus, complicating delivery O62.9

Dysfunction — *continued*
  uterus, complicating delivery — *continued*
    hypertonic O62.4
    hypotonic O62.2
      primary O62.0
      secondary O62.1
  ventricular I51.9
    with congestive heart failure — *see also* Failure, heart I50.9
    left, reversible, following sudden emotional stress I51.81
Dysgenesis
  gonadal (due to chromosomal anomaly) Q96.9
    pure Q99.1
  renal Q60.5
    bilateral Q60.4
    unilateral Q60.3
  reticular D72.0
  tidal platelet D69.3
Dysgerminoma
  specified site — *see* Neoplasm, malignant, by site
  unspecified site
    female C56.9
    male C62.90
Dysgeusia R43.2
Dysgraphia R27.8
Dyshidrosis, dysidrosis L30.1
Dyskaryotic cervical smear R87.619
Dyskeratosis L85.8
  cervix — *see* Dysplasia, cervix
  congenital Q82.8
  uterus NEC N85.8
Dyskinesia G24.9
  biliary (cystic duct or gallbladder) K82.8
  drug induced
    orofacial G24.01
  esophagus K22.4
  hysterical F44.4
  intestinal K59.8
  nonorganic origin F44.4
  orofacial (idiopathic) G24.4
    drug induced G24.01
  psychogenic F44.4
  subacute, drug induced G24.01
  tardive G24.01
    neuroleptic induced G24.01
  trachea J39.8
  tracheobronchial J98.09
Dyslalia (developmental) F80.0
Dyslexia R48.0
  developmental F81.0
Dyslipidemia E78.5
  depressed HDL cholesterol E78.6
  elevated fasting triglycerides E78.1
Dysmaturity — *see also* Light for dates
  pulmonary (newborn) (Wilson-Mikity) P27.0
Dysmenorrhea (essential) (exfoliative) N94.6
  congestive (syndrome) N94.6
  primary N94.4
  psychogenic F45.8
  secondary N94.5
Dysmetabolic syndrome X E88.81
Dysmetria R27.8
Dysmorphism (due to)
  alcohol Q86.0
  exogenous cause NEC Q86.8
  hydantoin Q86.1
  warfarin Q86.2
Dysmorphophobia (nondelusional) F45.22
  delusional F22
Dysnomia R47.01
Dysorexia R63.0
  psychogenic F50.89
Dysostosis
  cleidocranial, cleidocranialis Q74.0
  craniofacial Q75.1
  Fairbank's (idiopathic familial generalized osteophytosis) Q78.9
  mandibulofacial (incomplete) Q75.4
  multiplex E76.01
  oculomandibular Q75.5
Dyspareunia (female) N94.10
  deep N94.12
  male N53.12
  nonorganic F52.6
  psychogenic F52.6
  secondary N94.19
  specified NEC N94.19

Dyspareunia — *continued*
  superficial (introital) N94.11
Dyspepsia R10.13
  atonic K30
  functional (allergic) (congenital) (gastrointestinal) (occupational) (reflex) K30
  intestinal K59.8
  nervous F45.8
  neurotic F45.8
  psychogenic F45.8
Dysphagia R13.10
  cervical R13.19
  following
    cerebral infarction I69.391
    cerebrovascular disease I69.991
      specified NEC I69.891
    intracerebral hemorrhage I69.191
    nontraumatic intracranial hemorrhage NEC I69.291
    specified disease NEC I69.891
    subarachnoid hemorrhage I69.091
  functional (hysterical) F45.8
  hysterical F45.8
  nervous (hysterical) F45.8
  neurogenic R13.19
  oral phase R13.11
  oropharyngeal phase R13.12
  pharyngeal phase R13.13
  pharyngoesophageal phase R13.14
  psychogenic F45.8
  sideropenic D50.1
  spastica K22.4
  specified NEC R13.19
Dysphagocytosis, congenital D71
Dysphasia R47.02
  developmental
    expressive type F80.1
    receptive type F80.2
  following
    cerebrovascular disease I69.921
      cerebral infarction I69.321
      intracerebral hemorrhage I69.121
      nontraumatic intracranial hemorrhage NEC I69.221
      specified disease NEC I69.821
      subarachnoid hemorrhage I69.021
Dysphonia R49.0
  functional F44.4
  hysterical F44.4
  psychogenic F44.4
  spastica J38.3
Dysphoria
  gender F64.9
    in
      adolescence and adulthood F64.0
      children F64.2
    specified NEC F64.8
  postpartal O90.6
Dyspituitarism E23.3
Dysplasia — *see also* Anomaly
  acetabular, congenital Q65.89
  alveolar capillary, with vein misalignment J84.843
  anus (histologically confirmed) (mild) (moderate) K62.82
    severe D01.3
  arrhythmogenic right ventricular I42.8
  arterial, fibromuscular I77.3
  asphyxiating thoracic (congenital) Q77.2
  brain Q07.9
  bronchopulmonary, perinatal P27.1
  cervix (uteri) N87.9
    mild N87.0
    moderate N87.1
    severe D06.9
  chondroectodermal Q77.6
  colon D12.6
  craniometaphyseal Q78.8
  dentinal K00.5
  diaphyseal, progressive Q78.3
  dystrophic Q77.5
  ectodermal (anhidrotic) (congenital) (hereditary) Q82.4
    hydrotic Q82.8
  epithelial, uterine cervix — *see* Dysplasia, cervix
  eye (congenital) Q11.2
  fibrous
    bone NEC (monostotic) M85.00
      ankle M85.07- ☑
      foot M85.07- ☑
      forearm M85.03- ☑

Dysplasia — *continued*
- fibrous — *continued*
  - bone — *continued*
    - hand M85.04- ☑
    - lower leg M85.06- ☑
    - multiple site M85.09
    - neck M85.08
    - rib M85.08
    - shoulder M85.01- ☑
    - skull M85.08
    - specified site NEC M85.08
    - thigh M85.05- ☑
    - toe M85.07- ☑
    - upper arm M85.02- ☑
    - vertebra M85.08
  - diaphyseal, progressive Q78.3
  - jaw M27.8
  - polyostotic Q78.1
- florid osseous — *see also* Cyst, calcifying odontogenic
- high grade, focal D12.6
- hip, congenital Q65.89
- joint, congenital Q74.8
- kidney Q61.4
  - multicystic Q61.4
- leg Q74.2
- lung, congenital (not associated with short gestation) Q33.6
- mammary (gland) (benign) N60.9- ☑
  - cyst (solitary) — *see* Cyst, breast
  - cystic — *see* Mastopathy, cystic
  - duct ectasia — *see* Ectasia, mammary duct
  - fibroadenosis — *see* Fibroadenosis, breast
  - fibrosclerosis — *see* Fibrosclerosis, breast
  - specified type NEC N60.8- ☑
- metaphyseal Q78.5
- muscle Q79.8
- oculodentodigital Q87.0
- periapical (cemental) (cemento-osseous) — *see* Cyst, calcifying odontogenic
- periosteum — *see* Disorder, bone, specified type NEC
- polyostotic fibrous Q78.1
- prostate — *see also* Neoplasia, intraepithelial, prostate N42.30
  - severe D07.5
  - specified NEC N42.39
- renal Q61.4
  - multicystic Q61.4
- retinal, congenital Q14.1
- right ventricular, arrhythmogenic I42.8
- septo-optic Q04.4
- skin L98.8
- spinal cord Q06.1
- spondyloepiphyseal Q77.7
- thymic, with immunodeficiency D82.1
- vagina N89.3
  - mild N89.0
  - moderate N89.1
  - severe NEC D07.2
- vulva N90.3
  - mild N90.0
  - moderate N90.1
  - severe NEC D07.1

Dysplasminogenemia E88.02
Dyspnea (nocturnal) (paroxysmal) R06.00
- asthmatic (bronchial) J45.909
  - with
    - bronchitis J45.909
      - with
        - exacerbation (acute) J45.901
        - status asthmaticus J45.902
      - chronic J44.9
      - exacerbation (acute) J45.901
      - status asthmaticus J45.902
  - cardiac — *see* Failure, ventricular, left
- cardiac — *see* Failure, ventricular, left
- functional F45.8
- hyperventilation R06.4
- hysterical F45.8
- newborn P28.89
- orthopnea R06.01
- psychogenic F45.8
- shortness of breath R06.02
- specified type NEC R06.09
Dyspraxia R27.8
- developmental (syndrome) F82
Dysproteinemia E88.09
Dysreflexia, autonomic G90.4

Dysrhythmia
- cardiac I49.9
  - newborn
    - bradycardia P29.12
    - occurring before birth P03.819
      - before onset of labor P03.810
      - during labor P03.811
    - tachycardia P29.11
  - postoperative I97.89
- cerebral or cortical — *see* Epilepsy
Dyssomnia — *see* Disorder, sleep
Dyssynergia
- biliary K83.8
- bladder sphincter N36.44
- cerebellaris myoclonica (Hunt's ataxia) G11.1
Dysthymia F34.1
Dysthyroidism E07.9
Dystocia O66.9
- affecting newborn P03.1
- cervical (hypotonic) O62.2
  - affecting newborn P03.6
  - primary O62.0
  - secondary O62.1
- contraction ring O62.4
- fetal O66.9
  - abnormality NEC O66.3
  - conjoined twins O66.3
  - oversize O66.2
- maternal O66.9
- positional O64.9 ☑
- shoulder (girdle) O66.0
  - causing obstructed labor O66.0
- uterine NEC O62.4
Dystonia G24.9
- cervical G24.3
- deformans progressiva G24.1
- drug induced NEC G24.09
  - acute G24.02
  - specified NEC G24.09
- familial G24.1
- idiopathic G24.1
  - familial G24.1
  - nonfamilial G24.2
  - orofacial G24.4
- lenticularis G24.8
- musculorum deformans G24.1
- neuroleptic induced (acute) G24.02
- orofacial (idiopathic) G24.4
- oromandibular G24.4
  - due to drug G24.01
- specified NEC G24.8
- torsion (familial) (idiopathic) G24.1
  - acquired G24.8
  - genetic G24.1
  - symptomatic (nonfamilial) G24.2
Dystonic movements R25.8
Dystrophy, dystrophia
- adiposogenital E23.6
- autosomal recessive, childhood type, muscular dystrophy resembling Duchenne or Becker G71.01
- Becker's type G71.01
- cervical sympathetic G90.2
- choroid (hereditary) H31.20
  - central areolar H31.22
  - choroideremia H31.21
  - gyrate atrophy H31.23
  - specified type NEC H31.29
- cornea (hereditary) H18.50
  - endothelial H18.51
  - epithelial H18.52
  - granular H18.53
  - lattice H18.54
  - macular H18.55
  - specified type NEC H18.59
- Duchenne's type G71.01
- due to malnutrition E45
- Erb's G71.02
- Fuchs' H18.51
- Gower's muscular G71.01
- hair L67.8
- infantile neuraxonal G31.89
- Landouzy-Déjérine G71.02
- Leyden-Möbius G71.09
- muscular G71.00
  - autosomal recessive, childhood type, muscular dystrophy resembling Duchenne or Becker G71.01
  - benign (Becker type) G71.01

Dystrophy, dystrophia — *continued*
- muscular — *continued*
  - benign — *continued*
    - scapuloperoneal with early contractures [Emery-Dreifuss] G71.09
  - congenital (hereditary) (progressive) (with specific morphological abnormalities of the muscle fiber) G71.09
    - myotonic G71.11
  - distal G71.09
  - Duchenne type G71.01
  - Emery-Dreifuss G71.09
  - Erb type G71.02
  - facioscapulohumeral G71.02
  - Gower's G71.01
  - hereditary (progressive) G71.09
  - Landouzy-Déjérine type G71.02
  - limb-girdle G71.09
  - myotonic G71.11
  - progressive (hereditary) G71.09
    - Charcot-Marie (-Tooth) type G60.0
  - pseudohypertrophic (infantile) G71.01
  - scapulohumeral G71.02
  - scapuloperoneal G71.09
  - severe (Duchenne type) G71.01
  - specified type NEC G71.09
- myocardium, myocardial — *see* Degeneration, myocardial
- nail L60.3
  - congenital Q84.6
- nutritional E45
- ocular G71.09
- oculocerebrorenal E72.03
- oculopharyngeal G71.09
- ovarian N83.8
- polyglandular E31.8
- reflex (neuromuscular) (sympathetic) — *see* Syndrome, pain, complex regional I
- retinal (hereditary) H35.50
  - in
    - lipid storage disorders E75.6 *[H36]*
    - systemic lipidoses E75.6 *[H36]*
  - involving
    - pigment epithelium H35.54
    - sensory area H35.53
  - pigmentary H35.52
  - vitreoretinal H35.51
- Salzmann's nodular — *see* Degeneration, cornea, nodular
- scapuloperoneal G71.09
- skin NEC L98.8
- sympathetic (reflex) — *see* Syndrome, pain, complex regional I
  - cervical G90.2
- tapetoretinal H35.54
- thoracic, asphyxiating Q77.2
- unguium L60.3
  - congenital Q84.6
- vitreoretinal H35.51
- vulva N90.4
- yellow (liver) — *see* Failure, hepatic
Dysuria R30.0
- psychogenic F45.8

E

Eales' disease H35.06- ☑
Ear — *see also* condition
- piercing Z41.3
- tropical NEC B36.9 *[H62.40]*
  - in
    - aspergillosis B44.89
    - candidiasis B37.84
    - moniliasis B37.84
- wax (impacted) H61.20
  - left H61.22
    - with right H61.23
  - right H61.21
    - with left H61.23
Earache — *see* subcategory H92.0 ☑
Early satiety R68.81
Eaton-Lambert syndrome — *see* Syndrome, Lambert-Eaton
Eberth's disease (typhoid fever) A01.00
Ebola virus disease A98.4
Ebstein's anomaly or syndrome (heart) Q22.5
Eccentro-osteochondrodysplasia E76.29
Ecchondroma — *see* Neoplasm, bone, benign

Ecchondrosis D48.0
Ecchymosis R58
  conjunctiva — *see* Hemorrhage, conjunctiva
  eye (traumatic) — *see* Contusion, eyeball
  eyelid (traumatic) — *see* Contusion, eyelid
  newborn P54.5
  spontaneous R23.3
  traumatic — *see* Contusion
Echinococciasis — *see* Echinococcus
Echinococcosis — *see* Echinococcus
Echinococcus (infection) B67.90
  granulosus B67.4
    bone B67.2
    liver B67.0
    lung B67.1
    multiple sites B67.32
    specified site NEC B67.39
    thyroid B67.31
  liver NOS B67.8
    granulosus B67.0
    multilocularis B67.5
  lung NEC B67.99
    granulosus B67.1
    multilocularis B67.69
  multilocularis B67.7
    liver B67.5
    multiple sites B67.61
    specified site NEC B67.69
  specified site NEC B67.99
    granulosus B67.39
    multilocularis B67.69
  thyroid NEC B67.99
    granulosus B67.31
    multilocularis B67.69 *[E35]*
Echinorhynchiasis B83.8
Echinostomiasis B66.8
Echolalia R48.8
Echovirus, as cause of disease classified elsewhere
  B97.12
Eclampsia, eclamptic (coma) (convulsions) (delirium)
  (with hypertension) NEC O15.9
  complicating
    labor and delivery O15.1
    postpartum O15.2
    pregnancy O15.0- ☑
    puerperium O15.2
Economic circumstances affecting care Z59.9
Economo's disease A85.8
Ectasia, ectasis
  annuloaortic I35.8
  aorta I77.819
    with aneurysm — *see* Aneurysm, aorta
    abdominal I77.811
    thoracic I77.810
    thoracoabdominal I77.812
  breast — *see* Ectasia, mammary duct
  capillary I78.8
  cornea H18.71- ☑
  gastric antral vascular (GAVE) K31.819
    with hemorrhage K31.811
    without hemorrhage K31.819
  mammary duct N60.4- ☑
  salivary gland (duct) K11.8
  sclera — *see* Sclerectasia
Ecthyma L08.0
  contagiosum B08.02
  gangrenosum L08.0
  infectiosum B08.02
Ectocardia Q24.8
Ectodermal dysplasia (anhidrotic) Q82.4
Ectodermosis erosiva pluriorificialis L51.1
Ectopic, ectopia (congenital)
  abdominal viscera Q45.8
    due to defect in anterior abdominal wall Q79.59
  ACTH syndrome E24.3
  adrenal gland Q89.1
  anus Q43.5
  atrial beats I49.1
  beats I49.49
    atrial I49.1
    ventricular I49.3
  bladder Q64.10
  bone and cartilage in lung Q33.5
  brain Q04.8
  breast tissue Q83.8
  cardiac Q24.8
  cerebral Q04.8
  cordis Q24.8

Ectopic, ectopia — *continued*
  endometrium — *see* Endometriosis
  gastric mucosa Q40.2
  gestation — *see* Pregnancy, by site
  heart Q24.8
  hormone secretion NEC E34.2
  kidney (crossed) (pelvis) Q63.2
  lens, lentis Q12.1
  mole — *see* Pregnancy, by site
  organ or site NEC — *see* Malposition, congenital
  pancreas Q45.3
  pregnancy — *see* Pregnancy, ectopic
  pupil — *see* Abnormality, pupillary
  renal Q63.2
  sebaceous glands of mouth Q38.6
  spleen Q89.09
  testis Q53.00
    bilateral Q53.02
    unilateral Q53.01
  thyroid Q89.2
  tissue in lung Q33.5
  ureter Q62.63
  ventricular beats I49.3
  vesicae Q64.10
Ectromelia Q73.8
  lower limb — *see* Defect, reduction, limb, lower, specified type NEC
  upper limb — *see* Defect, reduction, limb, upper, specified type NEC
Ectropion H02.109
  cervix N86
    with cervicitis N72
  congenital Q10.1
  eyelid H02.109
    cicatricial H02.119
      left H02.116
        lower H02.115
        upper H02.114
      right H02.113
        lower H02.112
        upper H02.111
    congenital Q10.1
    left H02.106
      lower H02.105
      upper H02.104
    mechanical H02.129
      left H02.126
        lower H02.125
        upper H02.124
      right H02.123
        lower H02.122
        upper H02.121
    paralytic H02.159
      left H02.156
        lower H02.155
        upper H02.154
      right H02.153
        lower H02.152
        upper H02.151
    right H02.103
      lower H02.102
      upper H02.101
    senile H02.139
      left H02.136
        lower H02.135
        upper H02.134
      right H02.133
        lower H02.132
        upper H02.131
    spastic H02.149
      left H02.146
        lower H02.145
        upper H02.144
      right H02.143
        lower H02.142
        upper H02.141
  iris H21.89
  lip (acquired) K13.0
    congenital Q38.0
  urethra N36.8
  uvea H21.89
Eczema (acute) (chronic) (erythematous) (fissum)
  (rubrum) (squamous) — *see also* Dermatitis L30.9
  contact — *see* Dermatitis, contact
  dyshidrotic L30.1
  external ear — *see* Otitis, externa, acute, eczematoid
  flexural L20.82
  herpeticum B00.0

Eczema — *continued*
  hypertrophicum L28.0
  hypostatic — *see* Varix, leg, with, inflammation
  impetiginous L01.1
  infantile (due to any substance) L20.83
    intertriginous L21.1
    seborrheic L21.1
  intertriginous NEC L30.4
    infantile L21.1
  intrinsic (allergic) L20.84
  lichenified NEC L28.0
  marginatum (hebrae) B35.6
  pustular L30.3
  stasis I87.2
    with varicose veins — *see* Varix, leg, with, inflammation
  vaccination, vaccinatum T88.1 ☑
  varicose — *see* Varix, leg, with, inflammation
Eczematid L30.2
Eddowes (-Spurway) **syndrome** Q78.0
Edema, edematous (infectious) (pitting) (toxic) R60.9
  with nephritis — *see* Nephrosis
  allergic T78.3 ☑
  amputation stump (surgical) (sequelae (late effect))
    T87.89
  angioneurotic (allergic) (any site) (with urticaria)
    T78.3 ☑
    hereditary D84.1
  angiospastic I73.9
  Berlin's (traumatic) S05.8X- ☑
  brain (cytotoxic) (vasogenic) G93.6
    due to birth injury P11.0
    newborn (anoxia or hypoxia) P52.4
      birth injury P11.0
    traumatic — *see* Injury, intracranial, cerebral edema
  cardiac — *see* Failure, heart, congestive
  cardiovascular — *see* Failure, heart, congestive
  cerebral — *see* Edema, brain
  cerebrospinal — *see* Edema, brain
  cervix (uteri) (acute) N88.8
    puerperal, postpartum O90.89
  chronic hereditary Q82.0
  circumscribed, acute T78.3 ☑
    hereditary D84.1
  conjunctiva H11.42- ☑
  cornea H18.2- ☑
    idiopathic H18.22- ☑
    secondary H18.23- ☑
      due to contact lens H18.21- ☑
  due to
    lymphatic obstruction I89.0
    salt retention E87.0
  epiglottis — *see* Edema, glottis
  essential, acute T78.3 ☑
    hereditary D84.1
  extremities, lower — *see* Edema, legs
  eyelid NEC H02.849
    left H02.846
      lower H02.845
      upper H02.844
    right H02.843
      lower H02.842
      upper H02.841
  familial, hereditary Q82.0
  famine — *see* Malnutrition, severe
  generalized R60.1
  glottis, glottic, glottidis (obstructive) (passive) J38.4
    allergic T78.3 ☑
      hereditary D84.1
  heart — *see* Failure, heart, congestive
  heat T67.7 ☑
  hereditary Q82.0
  inanition — *see* Malnutrition, severe
  intracranial G93.6
  iris H21.89
  joint — *see* Effusion, joint
  larynx — *see* Edema, glottis
  legs R60.0
    due to venous obstruction I87.1
    hereditary Q82.0
  localized R60.0
    due to venous obstruction I87.1
  lower limbs — *see* Edema, legs
  lung J81.1
    with heart condition or failure — *see* Failure, ventricular, left
    acute J81.0
    chemical (acute) J68.1

Edema, edematous — *continued*
　lung — *continued*
　　chemical — *continued*
　　　chronic J68.1
　　chronic J81.1
　　　due to
　　　　chemicals, gases, fumes or vapors (inhalation)
　　　　　J68.1
　　　　external agent J70.9
　　　　　specified NEC J70.8
　　　　radiation J70.1
　　due to
　　　chemicals, fumes or vapors (inhalation) J68.1
　　　external agent J70.9
　　　　specified NEC J70.8
　　　high altitude T70.29 ☑
　　　near drowning T75.1 ☑
　　　radiation J70.0
　　meaning failure, left ventricle I50.1
　lymphatic I89.0
　　due to mastectomy I97.2
　macula H35.81
　　cystoid, following cataract surgery — *see* Complications, postprocedural, following cataract surgery
　　diabetic — *see* Diabetes, by type, with, retinopathy, with macular edema
　malignant — *see* Gangrene, gas
　Milroy's Q82.0
　nasopharynx J39.2
　newborn P83.30
　　hydrops fetalis — *see* Hydrops, fetalis
　　specified NEC P83.39
　nutritional — *see also* Malnutrition, severe
　　with dyspigmentation, skin and hair E40
　optic disc or nerve — *see* Papilledema
　orbit H05.22- ☑
　pancreas K86.89
　papilla, optic — *see* Papilledema
　penis N48.89
　periodic T78.3 ☑
　　hereditary D84.1
　pharynx J39.2
　pulmonary — *see* Edema, lung
　Quincke's T78.3 ☑
　　hereditary D84.1
　renal — *see* Nephrosis
　retina H35.81
　　diabetic — *see* Diabetes, by type, with, retinopathy, with macular edema
　salt E87.0
　scrotum N50.89
　seminal vesicle N50.89
　spermatic cord N50.89
　spinal (cord) (vascular) (nontraumatic) G95.19
　starvation — *see* Malnutrition, severe
　stasis — *see* Hypertension, venous, (chronic)
　subglottic — *see* Edema, glottis
　supraglottic — *see* Edema, glottis
　testis N44.8
　tunica vaginalis N50.89
　vas deferens N50.89
　vulva (acute) N90.89
Edentulism — *see* Absence, teeth, acquired
Edsall's disease T67.2 ☑
Educational handicap Z55.9
　specified NEC Z55.8
Edward's syndrome — *see* Trisomy, 18
Effect(s) (of) (from) — *see* Effect, adverse NEC
Effect, adverse
　abnormal gravitational (G) forces or states T75.81 ☑
　abuse — *see* Maltreatment
　air pressure T70.9 ☑
　　specified NEC T70.8 ☑
　altitude (high) — *see* Effect, adverse, high altitude
　anesthesia — *see also* Anesthesia T88.59 ☑
　　in labor and delivery O74.9
　　local, toxic
　　　in labor and delivery O74.4
　　　in pregnancy NEC O29.3- ☑
　　　postpartum, puerperal O89.3
　　postpartum, puerperal O89.9
　　specified NEC T88.59 ☑
　　　in labor and delivery O74.8
　　　postpartum, puerperal O89.8
　　spinal and epidural T88.59 ☑
　　　headache T88.59 ☑

Effect, adverse — *continued*
　anesthesia — *see also* Anesthesia — *continued*
　　spinal and epidural — *continued*
　　　headache — *continued*
　　　　in labor and delivery O74.5
　　　　postpartum, puerperal O89.4
　　　　specified NEC
　　　　　in labor and delivery O74.6
　　　　　postpartum, puerperal O89.5
　antitoxin — *see* Complications, vaccination
　atmospheric pressure T70.9 ☑
　　due to explosion T70.8 ☑
　　high T70.3 ☑
　　low — *see* Effect, adverse, high altitude
　　specified effect NEC T70.8 ☑
　biological, correct substance properly administered — *see* Effect, adverse, drug
　blood (derivatives) (serum) (transfusion) — *see* Complications, transfusion
　chemical substance — *see* Table of Drugs and Chemicals
　cold (temperature) (weather) T69.9 ☑
　　chilblains T69.1 ☑
　　frostbite — *see* Frostbite
　　specified effect NEC T69.8 ☑
　drugs and medicaments T88.7 ☑
　　specified drug — *see* Table of Drugs and Chemicals, by drug, adverse effect
　　specified effect — *code to* condition
　electric current, electricity (shock) T75.4 ☑
　　burn — *see* Burn
　exertion (excessive) T73.3 ☑
　exposure — *see* Exposure
　external cause NEC T75.89 ☑
　foodstuffs T78.1 ☑
　　allergic reaction — *see* Allergy, food
　　　causing anaphylaxis — *see* Shock, anaphylactic, due to food
　　noxious — *see* Poisoning, food, noxious
　gases, fumes, or vapors T59.9- ☑
　　specified agent — *see* Table of Drugs and Chemicals
　glue (airplane) sniffing
　　due to drug abuse — *see* Abuse, drug, inhalant
　　due to drug dependence — *see* Dependence, drug, inhalant
　heat — *see* Heat
　high altitude NEC T70.29 ☑
　　anoxia T70.29 ☑
　　on
　　　ears T70.0 ☑
　　　sinuses T70.1 ☑
　　polycythemia D75.1
　high pressure fluids T70.4 ☑
　hot weather — *see* Heat
　hunger T73.0 ☑
　immersion, foot — *see* Immersion
　immunization — *see* Complications, vaccination
　immunological agents — *see* Complications, vaccination
　infrared (radiation) (rays) NOS T66 ☑
　　dermatitis or eczema L59.8
　infusion — *see* Complications, infusion
　lack of care of infants — *see* Maltreatment, child
　lightning — *see* Lightning
　medical care T88.9 ☑
　　specified NEC T88.8 ☑
　medicinal substance, correct, properly administered — *see* Effect, adverse, drug
　motion T75.3 ☑
　noise, on inner ear — *see* subcategory H83.3 ☑
　overheated places — *see* Heat
　psychosocial, of work environment Z56.5
　radiation (diagnostic) (infrared) (natural source) (therapeutic) (ultraviolet) (X-ray) NOS T66 ☑
　　dermatitis or eczema — *see* Dermatitis, due to, radiation
　　fibrosis of lung J70.1
　　pneumonitis J70.0
　　pulmonary manifestations
　　　acute J70.0
　　　chronic J70.1
　　skin L59.9
　radioactive substance NOS
　　dermatitis or eczema — *see* Radiodermatitis
　reduced temperature T69.9 ☑
　　immersion foot or hand — *see* Immersion
　　specified effect NEC T69.8 ☑

Effect, adverse — *continued*
　serum NEC — *see also* Reaction, serum T80.69 ☑
　specified NEC T78.8 ☑
　　external cause NEC T75.89 ☑
　strangulation — *see* Asphyxia, traumatic
　submersion T75.1 ☑
　thirst T73.1 ☑
　toxic — *see* Toxicity
　transfusion — *see* Complications, transfusion
　ultraviolet (radiation) (rays) NOS T66 ☑
　　burn — *see* Burn
　　dermatitis or eczema — *see* Dermatitis, due to, ultraviolet rays
　　　acute L56.8
　vaccine (any) — *see* Complications, vaccination
　vibration — *see* Vibration, adverse effects
　water pressure NEC T70.9 ☑
　　specified NEC T70.8 ☑
　weightlessness T75.82 ☑
　whole blood — *see* Complications, transfusion
　work environment Z56.5
Effects, late — *see* Sequelae
Effluvium
　anagen L65.1
　telogen L65.0
Effort syndrome (psychogenic) F45.8
Effusion
　amniotic fluid — *see* Pregnancy, complicated by, premature rupture of membranes
　brain (serous) G93.6
　bronchial — *see* Bronchitis
　cerebral G93.6
　cerebrospinal — *see also* Meningitis
　　vessel G93.6
　chest — *see* Effusion, pleura
　chylous, chyliform (pleura) J94.0
　intracranial G93.6
　joint M25.40
　　ankle M25.47- ☑
　　elbow M25.42- ☑
　　foot joint M25.47- ☑
　　hand joint M25.44- ☑
　　hip M25.45- ☑
　　knee M25.46- ☑
　　shoulder M25.41- ☑
　　specified joint NEC M25.48
　　wrist M25.43- ☑
　malignant pleural J91.0
　meninges — *see* Meningitis
　pericardium, pericardial (noninflammatory) I31.3
　　acute — *see* Pericarditis, acute
　peritoneal (chronic) R18.8
　pleura, pleurisy, pleuritic, pleuropericardial J90
　　chylous, chyliform J94.0
　　due to systemic lupus erythematosis M32.13
　　in conditions classified elsewhere J91.8
　　influenzal — *see* Influenza, with, respiratory manifestations NEC
　　malignant J91.0
　　newborn P28.89
　　tuberculous NEC A15.6
　　　primary (progressive) A15.7
　spinal — *see* Meningitis
　thorax, thoracic — *see* Effusion, pleura
Egg shell nails L60.3
　congenital Q84.6
Egyptian splenomegaly B65.1
Ehlers-Danlos syndrome — *see also* Syndrome, Ehlers-Danlos Q79.60
Ehrlichiosis A77.40
　due to
　　E. chafeensis A77.41
　　E. sennetsu A79.81
　　specified organism NEC A77.49
Eichstedt's disease B36.0
Eisenmenger's
　complex or syndrome I27.83
　defect Q21.8
Ejaculation
　delayed F52.32
　painful N53.12
　premature F52.4
　retarded N53.11
　retrograde N53.14
　semen, painful N53.12
　　psychogenic F52.6
Ekbom's syndrome (restless legs) G25.81

Ekman's syndrome (brittle bones and blue sclera) Q78.0
Elastic skin Q82.8
  acquired L57.4
Elastofibroma — *see* Neoplasm, connective tissue, benign
Elastoma (juvenile) Q82.8
  Miescher's L87.2
Elastomyofibrosis I42.4
Elastosis
  actinic, solar L57.8
  atrophicans (senile) L57.4
  perforans serpiginosa L87.2
  senilis L57.4
Elbow — *see* condition
Electric current, electricity, effects (concussion) (fatal)
    (nonfatal) (shock) T75.4 ☑
  burn — *see* Burn
Electric feet syndrome E53.8
Electrocution T75.4 ☑
  from electroshock gun (taser) T75.4 ☑
Electrolyte imbalance E87.8
  with
    abortion — *see* Abortion by type, complicated by,
        electrolyte imbalance
    ectopic pregnancy O08.5
    molar pregnancy O08.5
Elephantiasis (nonfilarial) I89.0
  arabicum — *see* Infestation, filarial
  bancroftian B74.0
  congenital (any site) (hereditary) Q82.0
  due to
    Brugia (malayi) B74.1
        timori B74.2
    mastectomy I97.2
    Wuchereria (bancrofti) B74.0
  eyelid H02.859
    left H02.856
        lower H02.855
        upper H02.854
    right H02.853
        lower H02.852
        upper H02.851
  filarial, filariensis — *see* Infestation, filarial
  glandular I89.0
  graecorum A30.9
  lymphangiectatic I89.0
  lymphatic vessel I89.0
    due to mastectomy I97.2
  scrotum (nonfilarial) I89.0
  streptococcal I89.0
  surgical I97.89
    postmastectomy I97.2
  telangiectodes I89.0
  vulva (nonfilarial) N90.89
Elevated, elevation
  antibody titer R76.0
  basal metabolic rate R94.8
  blood pressure — *see also* Hypertension
    reading (incidental) (isolated) (nonspecific), no diagnosis of hypertension R03.0
  blood sugar R73.9
  body temperature (of unknown origin) R50.9
  cancer antigen 125 [CA 125] R97.1
  carcinoembryonic antigen [CEA] R97.0
  cholesterol E78.00
    with high triglycerides E78.2
  conjugate, eye H51.0
  C-reactive protein (CRP) R79.82
  diaphragm, congenital Q79.1
  erythrocyte sedimentation rate R70.0
  fasting glucose R73.01
  fasting triglycerides E78.1
  finding on laboratory examination — *see* Findings,
      abnormal, inconclusive, without diagnosis, by
      type of exam
  GFR (glomerular filtration rate) — *see* Findings, abnormal, inconclusive, without diagnosis, by type of
      exam
  glucose tolerance (oral) R73.02
  immunoglobulin level R76.8
  indoleacetic acid R82.5
  lactic acid dehydrogenase (LDH) level R74.0
  leukocytes D72.829
  lipoprotein a (Lp(a)) level E78.41
  liver function
    study R94.5
    test R79.89
        alkaline phosphatase R74.8

Elevated, elevation — *continued*
  liver function — *continued*
    test — *continued*
        aminotransferase R74.0
        bilirubin R17
        hepatic enzyme R74.8
        lactate dehydrogenase R74.0
  Lp(a) (lipoprotein(a)) E78.41
  lymphocytes D72.820
  prostate specific antigen [PSA] R97.20
  Rh titer — *see* Complication(s), transfusion, incompatibility reaction, Rh (factor)
  scapula, congenital Q74.0
  sedimentation rate R70.0
  SGOT R74.0
  SGPT R74.0
  transaminase level R74.0
  triglycerides E78.1
    with high cholesterol E78.2
  tumor associated antigens [TAA] NEC R97.8
  tumor specific antigens [TSA] NEC R97.8
  urine level of
    17-ketosteroids R82.5
    catecholamine R82.5
    indoleacetic acid R82.5
    steroids R82.5
    vanillylmandelic acid (VMA) R82.5
  venous pressure I87.8
  white blood cell count D72.829
    specified NEC D72.828
Elliptocytosis (congenital) (hereditary) D58.1
  Hb C (disease) D58.1
  hemoglobin disease D58.1
  sickle-cell (disease) D57.8- ☑
    trait D57.3
Ellison-Zollinger syndrome E16.4
Ellis-van Creveld syndrome (chondroectodermal dysplasia) Q77.6
Elongated, elongation (congenital) — *see also* Distortion
  bone Q79.9
  cervix (uteri) Q51.828
    acquired N88.4
        hypertrophic N88.4
  colon Q43.8
  common bile duct Q44.5
  cystic duct Q44.5
  frenulum, penis Q55.69
  labia minora (acquired) N90.69
  ligamentum patellae Q74.1
  petiolus (epiglottidis) Q31.8
  tooth, teeth K00.2
  uvula Q38.6
Eltor cholera A00.1
Emaciation (due to malnutrition) E41
Embadomoniasis A07.8
Embedded tooth, teeth K01.0
  root only K08.3
Embolic — *see* condition
Embolism (multiple) (paradoxical) I74.9
  air (any site) (traumatic) T79.0 ☑
    following
        abortion — *see* Abortion by type complicated
            by embolism
        ectopic pregnancy O08.2
    infusion, therapeutic injection or transfusion
        T80.0 ☑
    molar pregnancy O08.2
    procedure NEC
        artery T81.719 ☑
            mesenteric T81.710 ☑
            renal T81.711 ☑
            specified NEC T81.718 ☑
        vein T81.72 ☑
    in pregnancy, childbirth or puerperium — *see* Embolism, obstetric
  amniotic fluid (pulmonary) — *see also* Embolism, obstetric
    following
        abortion — *see* Abortion by type complicated
            by embolism
        ectopic pregnancy O08.2
        molar pregnancy O08.2
  aorta, aortic I74.10
    abdominal I74.09
        saddle I74.01
    bifurcation I74.09
        saddle I74.01

Embolism — *continued*
  aorta, aortic — *continued*
    thoracic I74.11
  artery I74.9
    auditory, internal I65.8
    basilar — *see* Occlusion, artery, basilar
    carotid (common) (internal) — *see* Occlusion, artery, carotid
    cerebellar (anterior inferior) (posterior inferior) (superior) I66.3
    cerebral — *see* Occlusion, artery, cerebral
    choroidal (anterior) I65.8
    communicating posterior I65.8
    coronary — *see also* Infarct, myocardium
        not resulting in infarction I24.0
    extremity I74.4
        lower I74.3
        upper I74.2
    hypophyseal I65.8
    iliac I74.5
    limb I74.4
        lower I74.3
        upper I74.2
    mesenteric (with gangrene) — *see also* Ischemia, intestine, acute K55.059
    ophthalmic — *see* Occlusion, artery, retina
    peripheral I74.4
    pontine I65.8
    precerebral — *see* Occlusion, artery, precerebral
    pulmonary — *see* Embolism, pulmonary
    renal N28.0
    retinal — *see* Occlusion, artery, retina
    septic I76
    specified NEC I74.8
    vertebral — *see* Occlusion, artery, vertebral
  basilar (artery) I65.1
  blood clot
    following
        abortion — *see* Abortion by type complicated
            by embolism
        ectopic or molar pregnancy O08.2
    in pregnancy, childbirth or puerperium — *see* Embolism, obstetric
  brain — *see also* Occlusion, artery, cerebral
    following
        abortion — *see* Abortion by type complicated
            by embolism
        ectopic or molar pregnancy O08.2
    puerperal, postpartum, childbirth — *see* Embolism, obstetric
  capillary I78.8
  cardiac — *see also* Infarct, myocardium
    not resulting in infarction I51.3
  carotid (artery) (common) (internal) — *see* Occlusion, artery, carotid
  cavernous sinus (venous) — *see* Embolism, intracranial venous sinus
  cerebral — *see* Occlusion, artery, cerebral
  cholesterol — *see* Atheroembolism
  coronary (artery or vein) (systemic) — *see* Occlusion, coronary
  due to device, implant or graft — *see also* Complications, by site and type, specified NEC
    arterial graft NEC T82.818 ☑
    breast (implant) T85.818 ☑
    catheter NEC T85.818 ☑
        dialysis (renal) T82.818 ☑
            intraperitoneal T85.818 ☑
        infusion NEC T82.818 ☑
            spinal (epidural) (subdural) T85.810 ☑
        urinary (indwelling) T83.81 ☑
    electronic (electrode) (pulse generator) (stimulator)
        bone T84.81 ☑
        cardiac T82.817 ☑
        nervous system (brain) (peripheral nerve) (spinal)
            T85.810 ☑
        urinary T83.81 ☑
    fixation, internal (orthopedic) NEC T84.81 ☑
    gastrointestinal (bile duct) (esophagus) T85.818 ☑
    genital NEC T83.81 ☑
    heart (graft) (valve) T82.817 ☑
    joint prosthesis T84.81 ☑
    ocular (corneal graft) (orbital implant) T85.818 ☑
    orthopedic (bone graft) NEC T86.838
    specified NEC T85.818 ☑
    urinary (graft) NEC T83.81 ☑
    vascular NEC T82.818 ☑

Embolism — *continued*
- due to device, implant or graft — *see also* Complications, by site and type, specified — *continued*
  - ventricular intracranial shunt T85.810 ☑
- extremities
  - lower — *see* Embolism, vein, lower extremity
    - arterial I74.3
  - upper I74.2
- eye H34.9
- fat (cerebral) (pulmonary) (systemic) T79.1 ☑
  - complicating delivery — *see* Embolism, obstetric
  - following
    - abortion — *see* Abortion by type complicated by embolism
    - ectopic or molar pregnancy O08.2
- following
  - abortion — *see* Abortion by type complicated by embolism
  - ectopic or molar pregnancy O08.2
  - infusion, therapeutic injection or transfusion
    - air T80.0 ☑
- heart (fatty) — *see also* Infarct, myocardium
  - not resulting in infarction I51.3
- hepatic (vein) I82.0
- in pregnancy, childbirth or puerperium — *see* Embolism, obstetric
- intestine (artery) (vein) (with gangrene) — *see also* Ischemia, intestine, acute K55.039
- intracranial — *see also* Occlusion, artery, cerebral
  - venous sinus (any) G08
    - nonpyogenic I67.6
- intraspinal venous sinuses or veins G08
  - nonpyogenic G95.19
- kidney (artery) N28.0
- lateral sinus (venous) — *see* Embolism, intracranial, venous sinus
- leg — *see* Embolism, vein, lower extremity
  - arterial I74.3
- longitudinal sinus (venous) — *see* Embolism, intracranial, venous sinus
- lung (massive) — *see* Embolism, pulmonary
- meninges I66.8
- mesenteric (artery) (vein) (with gangrene) — *see also* Ischemia, intestine, acute K55.059
- obstetric (in) (pulmonary)
  - childbirth O88.22
    - air O88.02
    - amniotic fluid O88.12
    - blood clot O88.22
    - fat O88.82
    - pyemic O88.32
    - septic O88.32
    - specified type NEC O88.82
  - pregnancy O88.21- ☑
    - air O88.01- ☑
    - amniotic fluid O88.11- ☑
    - blood clot O88.21- ☑
    - fat O88.81- ☑
    - pyemic O88.31- ☑
    - septic O88.31- ☑
    - specified type NEC O88.81- ☑
  - puerperal O88.23
    - air O88.03
    - amniotic fluid O88.13
    - blood clot O88.23
    - fat O88.83
    - pyemic O88.33
    - septic O88.33
    - specified type NEC O88.83
- ophthalmic — *see* Occlusion, artery, retina
- penis N48.81
- peripheral artery NOS I74.4
- pituitary E23.6
- popliteal (artery) I74.3
- portal (vein) I81
- postoperative, postprocedural
  - artery T81.719 ☑
    - mesenteric T81.710 ☑
    - renal T81.711 ☑
    - specified NEC T81.718 ☑
  - vein T81.72 ☑
- precerebral artery — *see* Occlusion, artery, precerebral
- puerperal — *see* Embolism, obstetric
- pulmonary (acute) (artery) (vein) I26.99
  - with acute cor pulmonale I26.09
    - chronic I27.82

Embolism — *continued*
- pulmonary — *continued*
  - following
    - abortion — *see* Abortion by type complicated by embolism
    - ectopic or molar pregnancy O08.2
  - healed or old Z86.711
  - in pregnancy, childbirth or puerperium — *see* Embolism, obstetric
  - multiple subsegmental without acute cor pulmonale I26.94
  - personal history of Z86.711
  - saddle I26.92
    - with acute cor pulmonale I26.02
  - septic I26.90
    - with acute cor pulmonale I26.01
  - single subsegmental without acute cor pulmonale I26.93
  - subsegmental NOS I26.93
- pyemic (multiple) I76
  - following
    - abortion — *see* Abortion by type complicated by embolism
    - ectopic or molar pregnancy O08.2
  - Hemophilus influenzae A41.3
  - pneumococcal A40.3
    - with pneumonia J13
  - puerperal, postpartum, childbirth (any organism) — *see* Embolism, obstetric
  - specified organism NEC A41.89
  - staphylococcal A41.2
  - streptococcal A40.9
- renal (artery) N28.0
  - vein I82.3
- retina, retinal — *see* Occlusion, artery, retina
- saddle
  - abdominal aorta I74.01
  - pulmonary artery I26.92
    - with acute cor pulmonale I26.02
- septic (arterial) I76
  - complicating abortion — *see* Abortion, by type, complicated by, embolism
  - sinus — *see* Embolism, intracranial, venous sinus
- soap complicating abortion — *see* Abortion, by type, complicated by, embolism
- spinal cord G95.19
  - pyogenic origin G06.1
- spleen, splenic (artery) I74.8
- upper extremity I74.2
- vein (acute) I82.90
  - antecubital I82.61- ☑
    - chronic I82.71- ☑
  - axillary I82.A1- ☑ (*following* I82.7)
    - chronic I82.A2- ☑ (*following* I82.7)
  - basilic I82.61- ☑
    - chronic I82.71- ☑
  - brachial I82.62- ☑
    - chronic I82.72- ☑
  - brachiocephalic (innominate) I82.290
    - chronic I82.291
  - cephalic I82.61- ☑
    - chronic I82.71- ☑
  - chronic I82.91
  - deep (DVT) I82.40- ☑
    - calf I82.4Z- ☑
      - chronic I82.5Z- ☑
    - lower leg I82.4Z- ☑
      - chronic I82.5Z- ☑
    - thigh I82.4Y- ☑
      - chronic I82.5Y- ☑
    - upper leg I82.4Y ☑
      - chronic I82.5Y-
  - femoral I82.41- ☑
    - chronic I82.51- ☑
  - iliac (iliofemoral) I82.42- ☑
    - chronic I82.52- ☑
  - innominate I82.290
    - chronic I82.291
  - internal jugular I82.C1- ☑ (*following* I82.7)
    - chronic I82.C2- ☑ (*following* I82.7)
  - lower extremity
    - deep I82.40- ☑
      - chronic I82.50- ☑
      - specified NEC I82.49- ☑
        - chronic NEC I82.59- ☑
    - distal
      - deep I82.4Z- ☑

Embolism — *continued*
- vein — *continued*
  - lower extremity — *continued*
    - proximal
      - deep I82.4Y- ☑
        - chronic I82.5Y- ☑
      - superficial I82.81- ☑
    - popliteal I82.43- ☑
      - chronic I82.53- ☑
    - radial I82.62- ☑
      - chronic I82.72- ☑
    - renal I82.3
    - saphenous (greater) (lesser) I82.81- ☑
    - specified NEC I82.890
      - chronic NEC I82.891
    - subclavian I82.B1- ☑ (*following* I82.7)
      - chronic I82.B2- ☑ (*following* I82.7)
    - thoracic NEC I82.290
      - chronic I82.291
    - tibial I82.44- ☑
      - chronic I82.54- ☑
    - ulnar I82.62- ☑
      - chronic I82.72- ☑
    - upper extremity I82.60- ☑
      - chronic I82.70- ☑
      - deep I82.62- ☑
        - chronic I82.72- ☑
      - superficial I82.61- ☑
        - chronic I82.71- ☑
  - vena cava
    - inferior (acute) I82.220
      - chronic I82.221
    - superior (acute) I82.210
      - chronic I82.211
  - venous sinus G08
  - vessels of brain — *see* Occlusion, artery, cerebral
- **Embolus** — *see* Embolism
- **Embryoma** — *see also* Neoplasm, uncertain behavior, by site
  - benign — *see* Neoplasm, benign, by site
  - kidney C64.- ☑
  - liver C22.0
  - malignant — *see also* Neoplasm, malignant, by site
    - kidney C64.- ☑
    - liver C22.0
    - testis C62.9- ☑
      - descended (scrotal) C62.1- ☑
      - undescended C62.0- ☑
  - testis C62.9- ☑
    - descended (scrotal) C62.1- ☑
    - undescended C62.0- ☑
- **Embryonic**
  - circulation Q28.9
  - heart Q28.9
  - vas deferens Q55.4
- **Embryopathia NOS** Q89.9
- **Embryotoxon** Q13.4
- **Emesis** — *see* Vomiting
- **Emotional lability** R45.86
- **Emotionality, pathological** F60.3
- **Emotogenic disease** — *see* Disorder, psychogenic
- **Emphysema** (atrophic) (bullous) (chronic) (interlobular) (lung) (obstructive) (pulmonary) (senile) (vesicular) J43.9
  - cellular tissue (traumatic) T79.7 ☑
    - surgical T81.82 ☑
  - centrilobular J43.2
  - compensatory J98.3
  - congenital (interstitial) P25.0
  - conjunctiva H11.89
  - connective tissue (traumatic) T79.7 ☑
    - surgical T81.82 ☑
  - due to chemicals, gases, fumes or vapors J68.4
  - eyelid(s) — *see* Disorder, eyelid, specified type NEC
    - surgical T81.82 ☑
    - traumatic T79.7 ☑
  - interstitial J98.2
    - congenital P25.0
    - perinatal period P25.0
  - laminated tissue T79.7 ☑
    - surgical T81.82 ☑
  - mediastinal J98.2
    - newborn P25.2
  - orbit, orbital — *see* Disorder, orbit, specified type NEC
  - panacinar J43.1
  - panlobular J43.1
  - specified NEC J43.8

Emphysema — *continued*
  subcutaneous (traumatic) T79.7 ☑
    nontraumatic J98.2
    postprocedural T81.82 ☑
    surgical T81.82 ☑
  surgical T81.82 ☑
  thymus (gland) (congenital) E32.8
  traumatic (subcutaneous) T79.7 ☑
  unilateral J43.0
Empty nest syndrome Z60.0
Empyema (acute) (chest) (double) (pleura) (supradiaphrag-
    matic) (thorax) J86.9
  with fistula J86.0
  accessory sinus (chronic) — *see* Sinusitis
  antrum (chronic) — *see* Sinusitis, maxillary
  brain (any part) — *see* Abscess, brain
  ethmoidal (chronic) (sinus) — *see* Sinusitis, ethmoidal
  extradural — *see* Abscess, extradural
  frontal (chronic) (sinus) — *see* Sinusitis, frontal
  gallbladder K81.0
  mastoid (process) (acute) — *see* Mastoiditis, acute
  maxilla, maxillary M27.2
    sinus (chronic) — *see* Sinusitis, maxillary
  nasal sinus (chronic) — *see* Sinusitis
  sinus (accessory) (chronic) (nasal) — *see* Sinusitis
  sphenoidal (sinus) (chronic) — *see* Sinusitis, sphenoidal
  subarachnoid — *see* Abscess, extradural
  subdural — *see* Abscess, subdural
  tuberculous A15.6
  ureter — *see* Ureteritis
  ventricular — *see* Abscess, brain
En coup de sabre lesion L94.1
Enamel pearls K00.2
Enameloma K00.2
Enanthema, viral B09
Encephalitis (chronic) (hemorrhagic) (idiopathic)
    (nonepidemic) (spurious) (subacute) G04.90
  acute — *see also* Encephalitis, viral A86
    disseminated G04.00
      infectious G04.01
      noninfectious G04.81
      postimmunization (postvaccination) G04.02
      postinfectious G04.01
    inclusion body A85.8
    necrotizing hemorrhagic G04.30
      postimmunization G04.32
      postinfectious G04.31
      specified NEC G04.39
  arboviral, arbovirus NEC A85.2
  arthropod-borne NEC (viral) A85.2
  Australian A83.4
  California (virus) A83.5
  Central European (tick-borne) A84.1
  Czechoslovakian A84.1
  Dawson's (inclusion body) A81.1
  diffuse sclerosing A81.1
  disseminated, acute G04.00
  due to
    cat scratch disease A28.1
    human immunodeficiency virus (HIV) disease
      B20 *[G05.3]*
    malaria — *see* Malaria
    rickettsiosis — *see* Rickettsiosis
    smallpox inoculation G04.02
    typhus — *see* Typhus
  Eastern equine A83.2
  endemic (viral) A86
  epidemic NEC (viral) A86
  equine (acute) (infectious) (viral) A83.9
    Eastern A83.2
    Venezuelan A92.2
    Western A83.1
  Far Eastern (tick-borne) A84.0
  following vaccination or other immunization procedure
    G04.02
  herpes zoster B02.0
  herpesviral B00.4
    due to herpesvirus 6 B10.01
    due to herpesvirus 7 B10.09
    specified NEC B10.09
  Ilheus (virus) A83.8
  in (due to)
    actinomycosis A42.82
    adenovirus A85.1
    African trypanosomiasis B56.9 *[G05.3]*
    Chagas' disease (chronic) B57.42
    cytomegalovirus B25.8
    enterovirus A85.0

Encephalitis — *continued*
  in — *continued*
    herpes (simplex) virus B00.4
      due to herpesvirus 6 B10.01
      due to herpesvirus 7 B10.09
      specified NEC B10.09
    infectious disease NEC B99 ☑ *[G05.3]*
    influenza — *see* Influenza, with, encephalopathy
    listeriosis A32.12
    measles B05.0
    mumps B26.2
    naegleriasis B60.2
    parasitic disease NEC B89 *[G05.3]*
    poliovirus A80.9 *[G05.3]*
    rubella B06.01
    syphilis
      congenital A50.42
      late A52.14
    systemic lupus erythematosus M32.19
    toxoplasmosis (acquired) B58.2
      congenital P37.1
    tuberculosis A17.82
    zoster B02.0
  inclusion body A81.1
  infectious (acute) (virus) NEC A86
  Japanese (B type) A83.0
  La Crosse A83.5
  lead — *see* Poisoning, lead
  lethargica (acute) (infectious) A85.8
  louping ill A84.8
  lupus erythematosus, systemic M32.19
  lymphatica A87.2
  Mengo A85.8
  meningococcal A39.81
  Murray Valley A83.4
  otitic NEC H66.40 *[G05.3]*
  parasitic NOS B71.9
  periaxial G37.0
  periaxialis (concentrica) (diffuse) G37.5
  postchickenpox B01.11
  postexanthematous NEC B09
  postimmunization G04.02
  postinfectious NEC G04.01
  postmeasles B05.0
  postvaccinal G04.02
  postvaricella B01.11
  postviral NEC A86
  Powassan A84.8
  Rasmussen G04.81
  Rio Bravo A85.8
  Russian
    autumnal A83.0
    spring-summer (taiga) A84.0
  saturnine — *see* Poisoning, lead
  specified NEC G04.81
  St. Louis A83.3
  subacute sclerosing A81.1
  summer A83.0
  suppurative G04.81
  tick-borne A84.9
  Torula, torular (cryptococcal) B45.1
  toxic NEC G92
  trichinosis B75 *[G05.3]*
  type
    B A83.0
    C A83.3
  van Bogaert's A81.1
  Venezuelan equine A92.2
  Vienna A85.8
  viral, virus A86
    arthropod-borne NEC A85.2
      mosquito-borne A83.9
        Australian X disease A83.4
        California virus A83.5
        Eastern equine A83.2
        Japanese (B type) A83.0
        Murray Valley A83.4
        specified NEC A83.8
        St. Louis A83.3
        type B A83.0
        type C A83.3
        Western equine A83.1
      tick-borne A84.9
        biundulant A84.1
        central European A84.1
        Czechoslovakian A84.1
        diphasic meningoencephalitis A84.1
        Far Eastern A84.0

Encephalitis — *continued*
  viral, virus — *continued*
    arthropod-borne — *continued*
      tick-borne — *continued*
        Russian spring-summer (taiga) A84.0
        specified NEC A84.8
      specified type NEC A85.8
    Western equine A83.1
Encephalocele Q01.9
  frontal Q01.0
  nasofrontal Q01.1
  occipital Q01.2
  specified NEC Q01.8
Encephalocystocele — *see* Encephalocele
Encephaloduroarteriomyosynangiosis (EDAMS) I67.5
Encephalomalacia (brain) (cerebellar) (cerebral) — *see*
    Softening, brain
Encephalomeningitis — *see* Meningoencephalitis
Encephalomeningocele — *see* Encephalocele
Encephalomeningomyelitis — *see* Meningoencephalitis
Encephalomyelitis — *see also* Encephalitis G04.90
  acute disseminated G04.00
    infectious G04.01
    noninfectious G04.81
    postimmunization G04.02
    postinfectious G04.01
  acute necrotizing hemorrhagic G04.30
    postimmunization G04.32
    postinfectious G04.31
    specified NEC G04.39
  benign myalgic G93.3
  equine A83.9
    Eastern A83.2
    Venezuelan A92.2
    Western A83.1
  in diseases classified elsewhere G05.3
  myalgic, benign G93.3
  postchickenpox B01.11
  postinfectious NEC G04.01
  postmeasles B05.0
  postvaccinal G04.02
  postvaricella B01.11
  rubella B06.01
  specified NEC G04.81
  Venezuelan equine A92.2
Encephalomyelocele — *see* Encephalocele
Encephalomyelomeningitis — *see* Meningoencephalitis
Encephalomyelopathy G96.9
Encephalomyeloradiculitis (acute) G61.0
Encephalomyeloradiculoneuritis (acute) (Guillain-
    Barré) G61.0
Encephalomyeloradiculopathy G96.9
Encephalopathia hyperbilirubinemica, newborn
    P57.9
  due to isoimmunization (conditions in P55) P57.0
Encephalopathy (acute) G93.40
  acute necrotizing hemorrhagic G04.30
    postimmunization G04.32
    postinfectious G04.31
    specified NEC G04.39
  alcoholic G31.2
  anoxic — *see* Damage, brain, anoxic
  arteriosclerotic I67.2
  centrolobar progressive (Schilder) G37.0
  congenital Q07.9
  degenerative, in specified disease NEC G32.89
  demyelinating callosal G37.1
  due to
    drugs — *see also* Table of Drugs and Chemicals G92
  hepatic — *see* Failure, hepatic
  hyperbilirubinemic, newborn P57.9
    due to isoimmunization (conditions in P55) P57.0
  hypertensive I67.4
  hypoglycemic E16.2
  hypoxic — *see* Damage, brain, anoxic
  hypoxic ischemic P91.60
    mild P91.61
    moderate P91.62
    severe P91.63
  in (due to) (with)
    birth injury P11.1
    hyperinsulinism E16.1 *[G94]*
    influenza — *see* Influenza, with, encephalopathy
    lack of vitamin — *see also* Deficiency, vitamin
      E56.9 *[G32.89]*
    neoplastic disease — *see also* Neoplasm
      D49.9 *[G13.1]*
    serum — *see also* Reaction, serum T80.69 ☑

Encephalopathy — *continued*
- in — *continued*
  - syphilis A52.17
  - trauma (postconcussional) F07.81
    - current injury — *see* Injury, intracranial
  - vaccination G04.02
- lead — *see* Poisoning, lead
- metabolic G93.41
  - drug induced G92
  - toxic G92
- myoclonic, early, symptomatic — *see* Epilepsy, generalized, specified NEC
- necrotizing, subacute (Leigh) G31.82
- neonatal P91.819
  - in diseases classified elsewhere P91.811
- pellagrous E52 *[G32.89]*
- portosystemic — *see* Failure, hepatic
- postcontusional F07.81
  - current injury — *see* Injury, intracranial, diffuse
- posthypoglycemic (coma) E16.1 *[G94]*
- postradiation G93.89
- saturnine — *see* Poisoning, lead
- septic G93.41
- specified NEC G93.49
- spongioform, subacute (viral) A81.09
- toxic G92
  - metabolic G92
- traumatic (postconcussional) F07.81
  - current injury — *see* Injury, intracranial
- vitamin B deficiency NEC E53.9 *[G32.89]*
  - vitamin B1 E51.2
- Wernicke's E51.2

Encephalorrhagia — *see* Hemorrhage, intracranial, intracerebral

Encephalosis, posttraumatic F07.81

Enchondroma — *see also* Neoplasm, bone, benign

Enchondromatosis (cartilaginous) (multiple) Q78.4

Encopresis R15.9
- functional F98.1
- nonorganic origin F98.1
- psychogenic F98.1

Encounter (with health service) (for) Z76.89
- adjustment and management (of)
  - breast implant Z45.81 ☑
  - implanted device NEC Z45.89
  - myringotomy device (stent) (tube) Z45.82
  - neurostimulator (brain) (gastric) (peripheral nerve) (sacral nerve) (spinal cord) (vagus nerve) Z45.42
- administrative purpose only Z02.9
  - examination for
    - adoption Z02.82
    - armed forces Z02.3
    - disability determination Z02.71
    - driving license Z02.4
    - employment Z02.1
    - insurance Z02.6
    - medical certificate NEC Z02.79
    - paternity testing Z02.81
    - residential institution admission Z02.2
    - school admission Z02.0
    - sports Z02.5
  - specified reason NEC Z02.89
- aftercare — *see* Aftercare
- antenatal screening Z36.9
  - cervical length Z36.86
  - chromosomal anomalies Z36.0
  - congenital cardiac abnormalities Z36.83
  - elevated maternal serum alphafetoprotein Z36.1
  - fetal growth retardation Z36.4
  - fetal lung maturity Z36.84
  - fetal macrosomia Z36.88
  - hydrops fetalis Z36.81
  - intrauterine growth restriction (IUGR) /small-for-dates Z36.4
  - isoimmunization Z36.5
  - large-for-dates Z36.88
  - malformations Z36.3
  - non-visualized anatomy on a previous scan Z36.2
  - nuchal translucency Z36.82
  - raised alphafetoprotein level Z36.1
  - risk of pre-term labor Z36.86
  - specified follow-up NEC Z36.2
  - specified genetic defects NEC Z36.8A
  - specified type NEC Z36.89
  - Streptococcus B Z36.85
  - suspected anomaly Z36.3
  - uncertain dates Z36.87

Encounter — *continued*
- assisted reproductive fertility procedure cycle Z31.83
- blood typing Z01.83
  - Rh typing Z01.83
- breast augmentation or reduction Z41.1
- breast implant exchange (different material) (different size) Z45.81 ☑
- breast reconstruction following mastectomy Z42.1
- check-up — *see* Examination
- chemotherapy for neoplasm Z51.11
- colonoscopy, screening Z12.11
- counseling — *see* Counseling
- delivery, full-term, uncomplicated O80
  - cesarean, without indication O82
- desensitization to allergens Z51.6
- ear piercing Z41.3
- examination — *see* Examination
- expectant parent(s) (adoptive) pre-birth pediatrician visit Z76.81
- fertility preservation procedure (prior to cancer therapy) (prior to removal of gonads) Z31.84
- fitting (of) — *see* Fitting (and adjustment) (of)
- genetic
  - counseling
    - nonprocreative Z71.83
    - procreative Z31.5
  - testing — *see* Test, genetic
- hearing conservation and treatment Z01.12
- immunotherapy for neoplasm Z51.12
- in vitro fertilization cycle Z31.83
- instruction (in)
  - child care (postpartal) (prenatal) Z32.3
  - childbirth Z32.2
  - natural family planning
    - procreative Z31.61
    - to avoid pregnancy Z30.02
- insulin pump titration Z46.81
- joint prosthesis insertion following prior explantation of joint prosthesis (staged procedure)
  - hip Z47.32
  - knee Z47.33
  - shoulder Z47.31
- laboratory (as part of a general medical examination) Z00.00
  - with abnormal findings Z00.01
- mental health services (for)
  - abuse NEC
    - perpetrator Z69.82
    - victim Z69.81
  - child abuse
    - nonparental
      - perpetrator Z69.021
      - victim Z69.020
    - parental
      - perpetrator Z69.011
      - victim Z69.010
  - child neglect
    - nonparental
      - perpetrator Z69.021
      - victim Z69.020
    - parental
      - perpetrator Z69.011
      - victim Z69.010
  - child psychological abuse
    - nonparental
      - perpetrator Z69.021
      - victim Z69.020
    - parental
      - perpetrator Z69.011
      - victim Z69.010
  - child sexual abuse
    - nonparental
      - perpetrator Z69.021
      - victim Z69.020
    - parental
      - perpetrator Z69.011
      - victim Z69.010
  - non-spousal adult abuse
    - perpetrator Z69.82
    - victim Z69.81
  - spousal or partner
    - abuse
      - perpetrator Z69.12
      - victim Z69.11
    - neglect
      - perpetrator Z69.12
      - victim Z69.11
    - psychological abuse
      - perpetrator Z69.12

Encounter — *continued*
- mental health services — *continued*
  - spousal or partner — *continued*
    - psychological abuse — *continued*
      - victim Z69.11
    - violence
      - perpetrator (physical) (sexual) Z69.12
      - victim (physical) Z69.11
      - sexual Z69.81
- observation (for) (ruled out)
  - exposure to (suspected)
    - anthrax Z03.810
    - biological agent NEC Z03.818
- pediatrician visit, by expectant parent(s) (adoptive) Z76.81
- placental sample (taken vaginally) — *see also* Encounter, antenatal screening Z36.9
- plastic and reconstructive surgery following medical procedure or healed injury NEC Z42.8
- pregnancy
  - supervision of — *see* Pregnancy, supervision of
  - test Z32.00
    - result negative Z32.02
    - result positive Z32.01
- procreative management and counseling for gestational carrier Z31.5
- prophylactic measures Z29.9
  - antivenin Z29.12
  - fluoride administration Z29.3
  - immunotherapy for respiratory syncytial virus (RSV) Z29.11
  - rabies immune globin Z29.14
  - Rho (D) immune globulin Z29.13
  - specified NEC Z29.8
- radiation therapy (antineoplastic) Z51.0
- radiological (as part of a general medical examination) Z00.00
  - with abnormal findings Z00.01
- reconstructive surgery following medical procedure or healed injury NEC Z42.8
- removal (of) — *see also* Removal
  - artificial
    - arm Z44.00- ☑
      - complete Z44.01- ☑
      - partial Z44.02- ☑
    - eye Z44.2- ☑
    - leg Z44.10- ☑
      - complete Z44.11- ☑
      - partial Z44.12- ☑
  - breast implant Z45.81 ☑
    - tissue expander (with or without synchronous insertion of permanent implant) Z45.81 ☑
  - device Z46.9
    - specified NEC Z46.89
  - external
    - fixation device — *code to* fracture with seventh character D
    - prosthesis, prosthetic device Z44.9
      - breast Z44.3- ☑
      - specified NEC Z44.8
  - implanted device NEC Z45.89
  - insulin pump Z46.81
  - internal fixation device Z47.2
  - myringotomy device (stent) (tube) Z45.82
  - nervous system device NEC Z46.2
    - brain neuropacemaker Z46.2
    - visual substitution device Z46.2
      - implanted Z45.31
  - non-vascular catheter Z46.82
  - orthodontic device Z46.4
  - stent
    - ureteral Z46.6
  - urinary device Z46.6
- repeat cervical smear to confirm findings of recent normal smear following initial abnormal smear Z01.42
- respirator [ventilator] use during power failure Z99.12
- Rh typing Z01.83
- screening — *see* Screening
- specified NEC Z76.89
- sterilization Z30.2
- suspected condition, ruled out
  - amniotic cavity and membrane Z03.71
  - cervical shortening Z03.75
  - fetal anomaly Z03.73
  - fetal growth Z03.74
  - maternal and fetal conditions NEC Z03.79
  - oligohydramnios Z03.71

Encounter — *continued*
  suspected condition, ruled out — *continued*
    placental problem Z03.72
    polyhydramnios Z03.71
  suspected exposure (to), ruled out
    anthrax Z03.810
    biological agents NEC Z03.818
  termination of pregnancy, elective Z33.2
  testing — *see* Test
  therapeutic drug level monitoring Z51.81
  titration, insulin pump Z46.81
  to determine fetal viability of pregnancy O36.80 ☑
  training
    insulin pump Z46.81
  X-ray of chest (as part of a general medical examination) Z00.00
    with abnormal findings Z00.01
Encystment — *see* Cyst
Endarteritis (bacterial, subacute) (infective) I77.6
  brain I67.7
  cerebral or cerebrospinal I67.7
  deformans — *see* Arteriosclerosis
  embolic — *see* Embolism
  obliterans — *see also* Arteriosclerosis
    pulmonary I28.8
  pulmonary I28.8
  retina — *see* Vasculitis, retina
  senile — *see* Arteriosclerosis
  syphilitic A52.09
    brain or cerebral A52.04
    congenital A50.54 [I79.8]
  tuberculous A18.89
Endemic — *see* condition
Endocarditis (chronic) (marantic) (nonbacterial) (thrombotic) (valvular) I38
  with rheumatic fever (conditions in I00)
    active — *see* Endocarditis, acute, rheumatic
    inactive or quiescent (with chorea) I09.1
  acute or subacute I33.9
    infective I33.0
    rheumatic (aortic) (mitral) (pulmonary) (tricuspid) I01.1
      with chorea (acute) (rheumatic) (Sydenham's) I02.0
  aortic (heart) (nonrheumatic) (valve) I35.8
    with
      mitral disease I08.0
        with tricuspid (valve) disease I08.3
        active or acute I01.1
          with chorea (acute) (rheumatic) (Sydenham's) I02.0
      rheumatic fever (conditions in I00)
        active — *see* Endocarditis, acute, rheumatic
        inactive or quiescent (with chorea) I06.9
      tricuspid (valve) disease I08.2
        with mitral (valve) disease I08.3
    acute or subacute I33.9
    arteriosclerotic I35.8
    rheumatic I06.9
      with mitral disease I08.0
        with tricuspid (valve) disease I08.3
        active or acute I01.1
          with chorea (acute) (rheumatic) (Sydenham's) I02.0
      active or acute I01.1
        with chorea (acute) (rheumatic) (Sydenham's) I02.0
    specified NEC I06.8
    specified cause NEC I35.8
    syphilitic A52.03
  arteriosclerotic I38
  atypical verrucous (Libman-Sacks) M32.11
  bacterial (acute) (any valve) (subacute) I33.0
  candidal B37.6
  congenital Q24.8
  constrictive I33.0
  Coxiella burnetii A78 [I39]
  Coxsackie B33.21
  due to
    prosthetic cardiac valve T82.6 ☑
    Q fever A78 [I39]
    Serratia marcescens I33.0
    typhoid (fever) A01.02
  gonococcal A54.83
  infectious or infective (acute) (any valve) (subacute) I33.0
  lenta (acute) (any valve) (subacute) I33.0
  Libman-Sacks M32.11

Endocarditis — *continued*
  listerial A32.82
  Löffler's I42.3
  malignant (acute) (any valve) (subacute) I33.0
  meningococcal A39.51
  mitral (chronic) (double) (fibroid) (heart) (inactive) (valve) (with chorea) I05.9
    with
      aortic (valve) disease I08.0
        with tricuspid (valve) disease I08.3
        active or acute I01.1
          with chorea (acute) (rheumatic) (Sydenham's) I02.0
      rheumatic fever (conditions in I00)
        active — *see* Endocarditis, acute, rheumatic
        inactive or quiescent (with chorea) I05.9
      tricuspid (valve) disease I08.1
        with aortic (valve) disease I08.3
    active or acute I01.1
      with chorea (acute) (rheumatic) (Sydenham's) I02.0
    bacterial I33.0
    arteriosclerotic I34.8
    nonrheumatic I34.8
      acute or subacute I33.9
    specified NEC I05.8
  monilial B37.6
  multiple valves I08.9
    specified disorders I08.8
  mycotic (acute) (any valve) (subacute) I33.0
  pneumococcal (acute) (any valve) (subacute) I33.0
  pulmonary (chronic) (heart) (valve) I37.8
    with rheumatic fever (conditions in I00)
      active — *see* Endocarditis, acute, rheumatic
      inactive or quiescent (with chorea) I09.89
        with aortic, mitral or tricuspid disease I08.8
    acute or subacute I33.9
      rheumatic I01.1
        with chorea (acute) (rheumatic) (Sydenham's) I02.0
    arteriosclerotic I37.8
    congenital Q22.2
    rheumatic (chronic) (inactive) (with chorea) I09.89
      active or acute I01.1
        with chorea (acute) (rheumatic) (Sydenham's) I02.0
    syphilitic A52.03
  purulent (acute) (any valve) (subacute) I33.0
  Q fever A78 [I39]
  rheumatic (chronic) (inactive) (with chorea) I09.1
    active or acute (aortic) (mitral) (pulmonary) (tricuspid) I01.1
      with chorea (acute) (rheumatic) (Sydenham's) I02.0
  rheumatoid — *see* Rheumatoid, carditis
  septic (acute) (any valve) (subacute) I33.0
  streptococcal (acute) (any valve) (subacute) I33.0
  subacute — *see* Endocarditis, acute
  suppurative (acute) (any valve) (subacute) I33.0
  syphilitic A52.03
  toxic I33.9
  tricuspid (chronic) (heart) (inactive) (rheumatic) (valve) (with chorea) I07.9
    with
      aortic (valve) disease I08.2
        mitral (valve) disease I08.3
      mitral (valve) disease I08.1
        aortic (valve) disease I08.3
      rheumatic fever (conditions in I00)
        active — *see* Endocarditis, acute, rheumatic
        inactive or quiescent (with chorea) I07.8
    active or acute I01.1
      with chorea (acute) (rheumatic) (Sydenham's) I02.0
    arteriosclerotic I36.8
    nonrheumatic I36.8
      acute or subacute I33.9
    specified cause, except rheumatic I36.8
  tuberculous — *see* Tuberculosis, endocarditis
  typhoid A01.02
  ulcerative (acute) (any valve) (subacute) I33.0
  vegetative (acute) (any valve) (subacute) I33.0
  verrucous (atypical) (nonbacterial) (nonrheumatic) M32.11
Endocardium, endocardial — *see also* condition
  cushion defect Q21.2
Endocervicitis — *see also* Cervicitis
  due to intrauterine (contraceptive) device T83.69 ☑

Endocervicitis — *continued*
  hyperplastic N72
Endocrine — *see* condition
Endocrinopathy, pluriglandular E31.9
Endodontic
  overfill M27.52
  underfill M27.53
Endodontitis K04.01
  irreversible K04.02
  reversible K04.01
Endomastoiditis — *see* Mastoiditis
Endometrioma N80.9
Endometriosis N80.9
  appendix N80.5
  bladder N80.8
  bowel N80.5
  broad ligament N80.3
  cervix N80.0
  colon N80.5
  cul-de-sac (Douglas') N80.3
  exocervix N80.0
  fallopian tube N80.2
  female genital organ NEC N80.8
  gallbladder N80.8
  in scar of skin N80.6
  internal N80.0
  intestine N80.5
  lung N80.8
  myometrium N80.0
  ovary N80.1
  parametrium N80.3
  pelvic peritoneum N80.3
  peritoneal (pelvic) N80.3
  rectovaginal septum N80.4
  rectum N80.5
  round ligament N80.3
  skin (scar) N80.6
  specified site NEC N80.8
  stromal D39.0
  thorax N80.8
  umbilicus N80.8
  uterus (internal) N80.0
  vagina N80.4
  vulva N80.8
Endometritis (decidual) (nonspecific) (purulent) (senile) (atrophic) (suppurative) N71.9
  with ectopic pregnancy O08.0
  acute N71.0
  blenorrhagic (gonococcal) (acute) (chronic) A54.24
  cervix, cervical (with erosion or ectropion) — *see also* Cervicitis
    hyperplastic N72
  chlamydial A56.11
  chronic N71.1
  following
    abortion — *see* Abortion by type complicated by genital infection
    ectopic or molar pregnancy O08.0
  gonococcal, gonorrheal (acute) (chronic) A54.24
  hyperplastic — *see also* Hyperplasia, endometrial N85.00
    cervix N72
  puerperal, postpartum, childbirth O86.12
  subacute N71.0
  tuberculous A18.17
Endometrium — *see* condition
Endomyocardiopathy, South African I42.3
Endomyocarditis — *see* Endocarditis
Endomyofibrosis I42.3
Endomyometritis — *see* Endometritis
Endopericarditis — *see* Endocarditis
Endoperineuritis — *see* Disorder, nerve
Endophlebitis — *see* Phlebitis
Endophthalmia — *see* Endophthalmitis, purulent
Endophthalmitis (acute) (infective) (metastatic) (subacute) H44.009
  bleb associated — *see also* Bleb, inflamed (infected), postprocedural H59.4 ☑
  gonorrheal A54.39
  in (due to)
    cysticercosis B69.1
    onchocerciasis B73.01
    toxocariasis B83.0
  panuveitis — *see* Panuveitis
  parasitic H44.12- ☑
  purulent H44.00- ☑
    panophthalmitis — *see* Panophthalmitis
    vitreous abscess H44.02- ☑

Endophthalmitis — *continued*
    specified NEC H44.19
    sympathetic — *see* Uveitis, sympathetic
Endosalpingioma D28.2
Endosalpingiosis N94.89
Endosteitis — *see* Osteomyelitis
Endothelioma, bone — *see* Neoplasm, bone, malignant
Endotheliosis (hemorrhagic infectional) D69.8
Endotoxemia — code to condition
Endotrachelitis — *see* Cervicitis
Engelmann (-Camurati) **syndrome** Q78.3
English disease — *see* Rickets
Engman's disease L30.3
Engorgement
    breast N64.59
        newborn P83.4
        puerperal, postpartum O92.79
    lung (passive) — *see* Edema, lung
    pulmonary (passive) — *see* Edema, lung
    stomach K31.89
    venous, retina — *see* Occlusion, retina, vein, engorge-
        ment
Enlargement, enlarged — *see also* Hypertrophy
    adenoids J35.2
        with tonsils J35.3
    alveolar ridge K08.89
        congenital — *see* Anomaly, alveolar
    apertures of diaphragm (congenital) Q79.1
    gingival K06.1
    heart, cardiac — *see* Hypertrophy, cardiac
    labium majus, childhood asymmetric (CALME) N90.61
    lacrimal gland, chronic H04.03- ☑
    liver — *see* Hypertrophy, liver
    lymph gland or node R59.9
        generalized R59.1
        localized R59.0
    orbit H05.34- ☑
    organ or site, congenital NEC — *see* Anomaly, by site
    parathyroid (gland) E21.0
    pituitary fossa R93.0
    prostate N40.0
        with lower urinary tract symptoms (LUTS) N40.1
        without lower urinary tract symtpoms (LUTS) N40.0
    sella turcica R93.0
    spleen — *see* Splenomegaly
    thymus (gland) (congenital) E32.0
    thyroid (gland) — *see* Goiter
    tongue K14.8
    tonsils J35.1
        with adenoids J35.3
    uterus N85.2
    vestibular aqueduct Q16.5
Enophthalmos H05.40- ☑
    due to
        orbital tissue atrophy H05.41- ☑
        trauma or surgery H05.42- ☑
Enostosis M27.8
Entamebic, entamebiasis — *see* Amebiasis
Entanglement
    umbilical cord(s) O69.82 ☑
        with compression O69.2 ☑
        around neck (with compression) O69.81 ☑
            with compression O69.1 ☑
            without compression O69.81 ☑
        of twins in monoamniotic sac O69.2 ☑
        without compression O69.82 ☑
Enteralgia — *see* Pain, abdominal
Enteric — *see* condition
Enteritis (acute) (diarrheal) (hemorrhagic) (noninfective)
        K52.9
    adenovirus A08.2
    aertrycke infection A02.0
    allergic K52.29
        with
            eosinophilic gastritis or gastroenteritis K52.81
            food protein-induced enterocolitis syndrome
                K52.21
            food protein-induced enteropathy K52.22
            FPIES K52.21
    amebic (acute) A06.0
        with abscess — *see* Abscess, amebic
        chronic A06.1
            with abscess — *see* Abscess, amebic
            nondysenteric A06.2
        nondysenteric A06.2
    astrovirus A08.32
    bacillary NOS A03.9

Enteritis — *continued*
    bacterial A04.9
        specified NEC A04.8
    calicivirus A08.31
    candidal B37.82
    Chilomastix A07.8
    choleriformis A00.1
    chronic (noninfectious) K52.9
        ulcerative — *see* Colitis, ulcerative
    cicatrizing (chronic) — *see* Enteritis, regional, small in-
        testine
    Clostridium
        botulinum (food poisoning) A05.1
        difficile
            not specified as recurrent A04.72
            recurrent A04.71
    coccidial A07.3
    coxsackie virus A08.39
    dietetic — *see also* Enteritis, allergic K52.29
    drug-induced K52.1
    due to
        astrovirus A08.32
        calicivirus A08.31
        coxsackie virus A08.39
        drugs K52.1
        echovirus A08.39
        enterovirus NEC A08.39
        food hypersensitivity — *see also* Enteritis, allergic
            K52.29
        infectious organism (bacterial) (viral) — *see* Enteritis,
            infectious
        torovirus A08.39
        Yersinia enterocolitica A04.6
    echovirus A08.39
    eltor A00.1
    enterovirus NEC A08.39
    eosinophilic K52.81
    epidemic (infectious) A09
    fulminant — *see also* Ischemia, intestine, acute K55.019
    gangrenous — *see* Enteritis, infectious
    giardial A07.1
    infectious NOS A09
        due to
            adenovirus A08.2
            Aerobacter aerogenes A04.8
            Arizona (bacillus) A02.0
            bacteria NOS A04.9
                specified NEC A04.8
            Campylobacter A04.5
            Clostridium difficile
                not specified as recurrent A04.72
                recurrent A04.71
            Clostridium perfringens A04.8
            Enterobacter aerogenes A04.8
            enterovirus A08.39
            Escherichia coli A04.4
                enteroaggregative A04.4
                enterohemorrhagic A04.3
                enteroinvasive A04.2
                enteropathogenic A04.0
                enterotoxigenic A04.1
                specified NEC A04.4
            specified
                bacteria NEC A04.8
                virus NEC A08.39
            Staphylococcus A04.8
            virus NEC A08.4
                specified type NEC A08.39
            Yersinia enterocolitica A04.6
        specified organism NEC A08.8
    influenzal — *see* Influenza, with, digestive manifesta-
        tions
    ischemic K55.9
        acute — *see also* Ischemia, intestine, acute K55.019
        chronic K55.1
    microsporidial A07.8
    mucomembranous, myxomembranous — *see* Syn-
        drome, irritable bowel
    mucous — *see* Syndrome, irritable bowel
    necroticans A05.2
    necrotizing of newborn — *see* Enterocolitis, necrotiz-
        ing, in newborn
    neurogenic — *see* Syndrome, irritable bowel
    newborn necrotizing — *see* Enterocolitis, necrotizing,
        in newborn
    noninfectious K52.9
    norovirus A08.11
    parasitic NEC B82.9

Enteritis — *continued*
    paratyphoid (fever) — *see* Fever, paratyphoid
    protozoal A07.9
        specified NEC A07.8
    radiation K52.0
    regional (of) K50.90
        with
            complication K50.919
                abscess K50.914
                fistula K50.913
                intestinal obstruction K50.912
                rectal bleeding K50.911
                specified complication NEC K50.918
        colon — *see* Enteritis, regional, large intestine
        duodenum — *see* Enteritis, regional, small intestine
        ileum — *see* Enteritis, regional, small intestine
        jejunum — *see* Enteritis, regional, small intestine
        large bowel — *see* Enteritis, regional, large intestine
        large intestine (colon) (rectum) K50.10
            with
                complication K50.119
                    abscess K50.114
                    fistula K50.113
                    intestinal obstruction K50.112
                    rectal bleeding K50.111
                    small intestine (duodenum) (ileum) (je-
                        junum) involvement K50.80
                        with
                            complication K50.819
                                abscess K50.814
                                fistula K50.813
                                intestinal obstruction K50.812
                                rectal bleeding K50.811
                                specified complication NEC
                                    K50.818
                    specified complication NEC K50.118
        rectum — *see* Enteritis, regional, large intestine
        small intestine (duodenum) (ileum) (jejunum)
            K50.00
            with
                complication K50.019
                    abscess K50.014
                    fistula K50.013
                    intestinal obstruction K50.012
                    large intestine (colon) (rectum) involve-
                        ment K50.80
                        with
                            complication K50.819
                                abscess K50.814
                                fistula K50.813
                                intestinal obstruction K50.812
                                rectal bleeding K50.811
                                specified complication NEC
                                    K50.818
                    rectal bleeding K50.011
                    specified complication NEC K50.018
    rotaviral A08.0
    Salmonella, salmonellosis (arizonae) (cholerae-suis)
        (enteritidis) (typhimurium) A02.0
    segmental — *see* Enteritis, regional
    septic A09
    Shigella — *see* Infection, Shigella
    small round structured NEC A08.19
    spasmodic, spastic — *see* Syndrome, irritable bowel
    staphylococcal A04.8
        due to food A05.0
    torovirus A08.39
    toxic NEC K52.1
        due to Clostridium difficile
            not specified as recurrent A04.72
            recurrent A04.71
    trichomonal A07.8
    tuberculous A18.32
    typhosa A01.00
    ulcerative (chronic) — *see* Colitis, ulcerative
    viral A08.4
        adenovirus A08.2
        enterovirus A08.39
        Rotavirus A08.0
        small round structured NEC A08.19
        specified NEC A08.39
        virus specified NEC A08.39
Enterobiasis B80
Enterobius vermicularis (infection) (infestation) B80
Enterocele — *see also* Hernia, abdomen
    pelvic, pelvis (acquired) (congenital) N81.5
    vagina, vaginal (acquired) (congenital) NEC N81.5
Enterocolitis — *see also* Enteritis K52.9

☑ Subterms under main terms may continue to next column or page   ☑ Additional Character Required — Refer to the Tabular List for Character Selection   133

Endophthalmitis — Enterocolitis

Enterocolitis — *continued*
due to Clostridium difficile
not specified as recurrent A04.72
recurrent A04.71
fulminant ischemic — *see also* Ischemia, intestine, acute K55.059
granulomatous — *see* Enteritis, regional
hemorrhagic (acute) — *see also* Ischemia, intestine, acute K55.059
chronic K55.1
infectious NEC A09
ischemic K55.9
necrotizing K55.30
with
perforation K55.33
pneumatosis K55.32
and perforation K55.33
due to Clostridium difficile
not specified as recurrent A04.72
recurrent A04.71
in non-newborn K55.30
stage 1 (without pneumatosis, without perforation) K55.31
stage 2 (with pneumatosis, without perforation) K55.32
stage 3 (with pneumatosis, with perforation) K55.33
in newborn P77.9
stage 1 (without pneumatosis, without perforation) P77.1
stage 2 (with pneumatosis, without perforation) P77.2
stage 3 (with pneumatosis, with perforation) P77.3
without pneumatosis or perforation K55.31
noninfectious K52.9
newborn — *see* Enterocolitis, necrotizing, in newborn
pseudomembranous (newborn)
not specified as recurrent A04.72
recurrent A04.71
radiation K52.0
newborn — *see* Enterocolitis, necrotizing, in newborn
ulcerative (chronic) — *see* Pancolitis, ulcerative (chronic)
Enterogastritis — *see* Enteritis
Enteropathy K63.9
celiac-gluten-sensitive K90.0
non-celiac K90.41
food protein-induced K52.22
hemorrhagic, terminal — *see also* Ischemia, intestine, acute K55.059
protein-losing K90.49
Enteroperitonitis — *see* Peritonitis
Enteroptosis K63.4
Enterorrhagia K92.2
Enterospasm — *see also* Syndrome, irritable, bowel
psychogenic F45.8
Enterostenosis — *see also* Obstruction, intestine, specified NEC K56.699
Enterostomy
complication — *see* Complication, enterostomy
status Z93.4
Enterovirus, as cause of disease classified elsewhere B97.10
coxsackievirus B97.11
echovirus B97.12
other specified B97.19
Enthesopathy (peripheral) M77.9
Achilles tendinitis — *see* Tendinitis, Achilles
ankle and tarsus M77.5- ☑
specified type NEC — *see* Enthesopathy, foot, specified type NEC
anterior tibial syndrome M76.81- ☑
calcaneal spur — *see* Spur, bone, calcaneal
elbow region M77.8
lateral epicondylitis — *see* Epicondylitis, lateral
medial epicondylitis — *see* Epicondylitis, medial
foot NEC M77.9
metatarsalgia — *see* Metatarsalgia
specified type NEC M77.5- ☑
forearm M77.9
gluteal tendinitis — *see* Tendinitis, gluteal
hand M77.9
hip — *see* Enthesopathy, lower limb, specified type NEC
iliac crest spur — *see* Spur, bone, iliac crest

Enthesopathy — *continued*
iliotibial band syndrome — *see* Syndrome, iliotibial band
knee — *see* Enthesopathy, lower limb, lower leg, specified type NEC
lateral epicondylitis — *see* Epicondylitis, lateral
lower limb (excluding foot) M76.9
Achilles tendinitis — *see* Tendinitis, Achilles
ankle and tarsus M77.5- ☑
specified type NEC — *see* Enthesopathy, foot, specified type NEC
anterior tibial syndrome M76.81- ☑
gluteal tendinitis — *see* Tendinitis, gluteal
iliac crest spur — *see* Spur, bone, iliac crest
iliotibial band syndrome — *see* Syndrome, iliotibial band
patellar tendinitis — *see* Tendinitis, patellar
pelvic region — *see* Enthesopathy, lower limb, specified type NEC
peroneal tendinitis — *see* Tendinitis, peroneal
posterior tibial syndrome M76.82- ☑
psoas tendinitis — *see* Tendinitis, psoas
specified type NEC M76.89- ☑
tibial collateral bursitis — *see* Bursitis, tibial collateral
medial epicondylitis — *see* Epicondylitis, medial
metatarsalgia — *see* Metatarsalgia
multiple sites M77.9
patellar tendinitis — *see* Tendinitis, patellar
pelvis M77.9
periarthritis of wrist — *see* Periarthritis, wrist
peroneal tendinitis — *see* Tendinitis, peroneal
posterior tibial syndrome M76.82- ☑
psoas tendinitis — *see* Tendinitis, psoas
shoulder M77.9
shoulder region — *see* Lesion, shoulder
specified site NEC M77.9
specified type NEC M77.8
spinal M46.00
cervical region M46.02
cervicothoracic region M46.03
lumbar region M46.06
lumbosacral region M46.07
multiple sites M46.09
occipito-atlanto-axial region M46.01
sacrococcygeal region M46.08
thoracic region M46.04
thoracolumbar region M46.05
tibial collateral bursitis — *see* Bursitis, tibial collateral
upper arm M77.9
wrist and carpus NEC M77.8
calcaneal spur — *see* Spur, bone, calcaneal
periarthritis of wrist — *see* Periarthritis, wrist
Entomophobia F40.218
Entomophthoromycosis B46.8
Entrance, air into vein — *see* Embolism, air
Entrapment, nerve — *see* Neuropathy, entrapment
Entropion (eyelid) (paralytic) H02.009
cicatricial H02.019
left H02.016
lower H02.015
upper H02.014
right H02.013
lower H02.012
upper H02.011
congenital Q10.2
left H02.006
lower H02.005
upper H02.004
mechanical H02.029
left H02.026
lower H02.025
upper H02.024
right H02.023
lower H02.022
upper H02.021
right H02.003
lower H02.002
upper H02.001
senile H02.039
left H02.036
lower H02.035
upper H02.034
right H02.033
lower H02.032
upper H02.031
spastic H02.049
left H02.046

Entropion — *continued*
spastic — *continued*
left — *continued*
lower H02.045
upper H02.044
right H02.043
lower H02.042
upper H02.041
Enucleated eye (traumatic, current) S05.7- ☑
Enuresis R32
functional F98.0
habit disturbance F98.0
nocturnal N39.44
psychogenic F98.0
nonorganic origin F98.0
psychogenic F98.0
Eosinopenia — *see* Agranulocytosis
Eosinophilia (allergic) (hereditary) (idiopathic) (secondary) D72.1
with
angiolymphoid hyperplasia (ALHE) D18.01
infiltrative J82
Löffler's J82
peritoneal — *see* Peritonitis, eosinophilic
pulmonary NEC J82
tropical (pulmonary) J82
Eosinophilia-myalgia syndrome M35.8
Ependymitis (acute) (cerebral) (chronic) (granular) — *see* Encephalomyelitis
Ependymoblastoma
specified site — *see* Neoplasm, malignant, by site
unspecified site C71.9
Ependymoma (epithelial) (malignant)
anaplastic
specified site — *see* Neoplasm, malignant, by site
unspecified site C71.9
benign
specified site — *see* Neoplasm, benign, by site
unspecified site D33.2
myxopapillary D43.2
specified site — *see* Neoplasm, uncertain behavior, by site
unspecified site D43.2
papillary D43.2
specified site — *see* Neoplasm, uncertain behavior, by site
unspecified site D43.2
specified site — *see* Neoplasm, malignant, by site
unspecified site C71.9
Ependymopathy G93.89
Ephelis, ephelides L81.2
Epiblepharon (congenital) Q10.3
Epicanthus, epicanthic fold (eyelid) (congenital) Q10.3
Epicondylitis (elbow)
lateral M77.1- ☑
medial M77.0- ☑
Epicystitis — *see* Cystitis
Epidemic — *see* condition
Epidermidalization, cervix — *see* Dysplasia, cervix
Epidermis, epidermal — *see* condition
Epidermodysplasia verruciformis B07.8
Epidermolysis
bullosa (congenital) Q81.9
acquired L12.30
drug-induced L12.31
specified cause NEC L12.35
dystrophica Q81.2
letalis Q81.1
simplex Q81.0
specified NEC Q81.8
necroticans combustiformis L51.2
due to drug — *see* Table of Drugs and Chemicals, by drug
Epidermophytid — *see* Dermatophytosis
Epidermophytosis (infected) — *see* Dermatophytosis
Epididymis — *see* condition
Epididymitis (acute) (nonvenereal) (recurrent) (residual) N45.1
with orchitis N45.3
blennorrhagic (gonococcal) A54.23
caseous (tuberculous) A18.15
chlamydial A56.19
filarial — *see also* Infestation, filarial B74.9 [N51]
gonococcal A54.23
syphilitic A52.76
tuberculous A18.15
Epididymo-orchitis — *see also* Epididymitis N45.3
Epidural — *see* condition

☑ Additional Character Required — Refer to the Tabular List for Character Selection ▽ Subterms under main terms may continue to next column or page

Epigastrium, epigastric — *see* condition
Epigastrocele — *see* Hernia, ventral
Epiglottis — *see* condition
Epiglottitis, epiglottiditis (acute) J05.10
  with obstruction J05.11
  chronic J37.0
Epignathus Q89.4
Epilepsia partialis continua — *see also* Kozhevnikof's epilepsy G40.1- ☑
Epilepsy, epileptic, epilepsia (attack) (cerebral) (convulsion) (fit) (seizure) G40.909

> Note: the following terms are to be considered equivalent to intractable: pharmacoresistant (pharmacologically resistant), treatment resistant, refractory (medically) and poorly controlled

with
  complex partial seizures — *see* Epilepsy, localization-related, symptomatic, with complex partial seizures
  grand mal seizures on awakening — *see* Epilepsy, generalized, specified NEC
  myoclonic absences — *see* Epilepsy, generalized, specified NEC
  myoclonic-astatic seizures — *see* Epilepsy, generalized, specified NEC
  simple partial seizures — *see* Epilepsy, localization-related, symptomatic, with simple partial seizures
akinetic — *see* Epilepsy, generalized, specified NEC
benign childhood with centrotemporal EEG spikes — *see* Epilepsy, localization-related, idiopathic
benign myoclonic in infancy G40.80- ☑
Bravais-jacksonian — *see* Epilepsy, localization-related, symptomatic, with simple partial seizures
childhood
  with occipital EEG paroxysms — *see* Epilepsy, localization-related, idiopathic
  absence G40.A09 (*following* G40.3)
    intractable G40.A19 (*following* G40.3)
      with status epilepticus G40.A11 (*following* G40.3)
      without status epilepticus G40.A19 (*following* G40.3)
    not intractable G40.A09 (*following* G40.3)
      with status epilepticus G40.A01 (*following* G40.3)
      without status epilepticus G40.A09 (*following* G40.3)
climacteric — *see* Epilepsy, specified NEC
cysticercosis B69.0
deterioration (mental) F06.8
due to syphilis A52.19
focal — *see* Epilepsy, localization-related, symptomatic, with simple partial seizures
generalized
  idiopathic G40.309
    intractable G40.319
      with status epilepticus G40.311
      without status epilepticus G40.319
    not intractable G40.309
      with status epilepticus G40.301
      without status epilepticus G40.309
  specified NEC G40.409
    intractable G40.419
      with status epilepticus G40.411
      without status epilepticus G40.419
    not intractable G40.409
      with status epilepticus G40.401
      without status epilepticus G40.409
impulsive petit mal — *see* Epilepsy, juvenile myoclonic
intractable G40.919
  with status epilepticus G40.911
  without status epilepticus G40.919
juvenile absence G40.A09 (*following* G40.3)
  intractable G40.A19 (*following* G40.3)
    with status epilepticus G40.A11 (*following* G40.3)
    without status epilepticus G40.A19 (*following* G40.3)
  not intractable G40.A09 (*following* G40.3)
    with status epilepticus G40.A01 (*following* G40.3)
    without status epilepticus G40.A09 (*following* G40.3)
juvenile myoclonic G40.B09 (*following* G40.3)
  intractable G40.B19 (*following* G40.3)
    with status epilepticus G40.B11 (*following* G40.3)
    without status epilepticus G40.B19 (*following* G40.3)

Epilepsy, epileptic, epilepsia — *continued*
juvenile myoclonic — *continued*
  not intractable G40.B09 (*following* G40.3)
    with status epilepticus G40.B01 (*following* G40.3)
    without status epilepticus G40.B09 (*following* G40.3)
localization-related (focal) (partial)
  idiopathic G40.009
    with seizures of localized onset G40.009
      intractable G40.019
        with status epilepticus G40.011
        without status epilepticus G40.019
      not intractable G40.009
        with status epilepticus G40.001
        without status epilepticus G40.009
  symptomatic
    with complex partial seizures G40.209
      intractable G40.219
        with status epilepticus G40.211
        without status epilepticus G40.219
      not intractable G40.209
        with status epilepticus G40.201
        without status epilepticus G40.209
    with simple partial seizures G40.109
      intractable G40.119
        with status epilepticus G40.111
        without status epilepticus G40.119
      not intractable G40.109
        with status epilepticus G40.101
        without status epilepticus G40.109
myoclonus, myoclonic — *see* Epilepsy, generalized, specified NEC
  progressive — *see* Epilepsy, generalized, idiopathic
not intractable G40.909
  with status epilepticus G40.901
  without status epilepticus G40.909
on awakening — *see* Epilepsy, generalized, specified NEC
parasitic NOS B71.9 [G94]
partialis continua — *see also* Kozhevnikof's epilepsy G40.1- ☑
peripheral — *see* Epilepsy, specified NEC
procursiva — *see* Epilepsy, localization-related, symptomatic, with simple partial seizures
progressive (familial) myoclonic — *see* Epilepsy, generalized, idiopathic
reflex — *see* Epilepsy, specified NEC
related to
  alcohol G40.509
    not intractable G40.509
      with status epilepticus G40.501
      without status epilepticus G40.509
  drugs G40.509
    not intractable G40.509
      with status epilepticus G40.501
      without status epilepticus G40.509
  external causes G40.509
    not intractable G40.509
      with status epilepticus G40.501
      without status epilepticus G40.509
  hormonal changes G40.509
    not intractable G40.509
      with status epilepticus G40.501
      without status epilepticus G40.509
  sleep deprivation G40.509
    not intractable G40.509
      with status epilepticus G40.501
      without status epilepticus G40.509
  stress G40.509
    not intractable G40.509
      with status epilepticus G40.501
      without status epilepticus G40.509
somatomotor — *see* Epilepsy, localization-related, symptomatic, with simple partial seizures
somatosensory — *see* Epilepsy, localization-related, symptomatic, with simple partial seizures
spasms G40.822
  intractable G40.824
    with status epilepticus G40.823
    without status epilepticus G40.824
  not intractable G40.822
    with status epilepticus G40.821
    without status epilepticus G40.822
specified NEC G40.802
  intractable G40.804
    with status epilepticus G40.803
    without status epilepticus G40.804
  not intractable G40.802

Epilepsy, epileptic, epilepsia — *continued*
specified — *continued*
  not intractable — *continued*
    with status epilepticus G40.801
    without status epilepticus G40.802
syndromes
  generalized
    idiopathic G40.309
      intractable G40.319
        with status epilepticus G40.311
        without status epilepticus G40.319
      not intractable G40.309
        with status epilepticus G40.301
        without status epilepticus G40.309
    specified NEC G40.409
      intractable G40.419
        with status epilepticus G40.411
        without status epilepticus G40.419
      not intractable G40.409
        with status epilepticus G40.401
        without status epilepticus G40.409
  localization-related (focal) (partial)
    idiopathic G40.009
      with seizures of localized onset G40.009
        intractable G40.019
          with status epilepticus G40.011
          without status epilepticus G40.019
        not intractable G40.009
          with status epilepticus G40.001
          without status epilepticus G40.009
    symptomatic
      with complex partial seizures G40.209
        intractable G40.219
          with status epilepticus G40.211
          without status epilepticus G40.219
        not intractable G40.209
          with status epilepticus G40.201
          without status epilepticus G40.209
      with simple partial seizures G40.109
        intractable G40.119
          with status epilepticus G40.111
          without status epilepticus G40.119
        not intractable G40.109
          with status epilepticus G40.101
          without status epilepticus G40.109
  specified NEC G40.802
    intractable G40.804
      with status epilepticus G40.803
      without status epilepticus G40.804
    not intractable G40.802
      with status epilepticus G40.801
      without status epilepticus G40.802
tonic (-clonic) — *see* Epilepsy, generalized, specified NEC
twilight F05
uncinate (gyrus) — *see* Epilepsy, localization-related, symptomatic, with complex partial seizures
Unverricht (-Lundborg) (familial myoclonic) — *see* Epilepsy, generalized, idiopathic
visceral — *see* Epilepsy, specified NEC
visual — *see* Epilepsy, specified NEC
Epiloia Q85.1
Epimenorrhea N92.0
Epipharyngitis — *see* Nasopharyngitis
Epiphora H04.20- ☑
  due to
    excess lacrimation H04.21- ☑
    insufficient drainage H04.22- ☑
Epiphyseal arrest — *see* Arrest, epiphyseal
Epiphyseolysis, epiphysiolysis — *see* Osteochondropathy
Epiphysitis — *see also* Osteochondropathy
  juvenile M92.9
  syphilitic (congenital) A50.02
Epiplocele — *see* Hernia, abdomen
Epiploitis — *see* Peritonitis
Epiplosarcomphalocele — *see* Hernia, umbilicus
Episcleritis (suppurative) H15.10- ☑
  in (due to)
    syphilis A52.71
    tuberculosis A18.51
  nodular H15.12- ☑
  periodica fugax H15.11- ☑
    angioneurotic — *see* Edema, angioneurotic
  syphilitic (late) A52.71
  tuberculous A18.51
Episode
affective, mixed F39

Episode — *continued*
  depersonalization (in neurotic state) F48.1
  depressive F32.9
    major F32.9
      mild F32.0
      moderate F32.1
      severe (without psychotic symptoms) F32.2
        with psychotic symptoms F32.3
    recurrent F33.9
      brief F33.8
    specified NEC F32.89
  hypomanic F30.8
  manic F30.9
    with
      psychotic symptoms F30.2
      remission (full) F30.4
        partial F30.3
    other specified F30.8
    recurrent F31.89
    without psychotic symptoms F30.10
      mild F30.11
      moderate F30.12
      severe (without psychotic symptoms) F30.13
        with psychotic symptoms F30.2
  psychotic F23
    organic F06.8
  schizophrenic (acute) NEC, brief F23
Epispadias (female) (male) Q64.0
Episplenitis D73.89
Epistaxis (multiple) R04.0
  hereditary I78.0
  vicarious menstruation N94.89
Epithelioma (malignant) — *see also* Neoplasm, malignant, by site
  adenoides cysticum — *see* Neoplasm, skin, benign
  basal cell — *see* Neoplasm, skin, malignant
  benign — *see* Neoplasm, benign, by site
  Bowen's — *see* Neoplasm, skin, in situ
  calcifying, of Malherbe — *see* Neoplasm, skin, benign
  external site — *see* Neoplasm, skin, malignant
  intraepidermal, Jadassohn — *see* Neoplasm, skin, benign
  squamous cell — *see* Neoplasm, malignant, by site
Epitheliomatosis pigmented Q82.1
Epitheliopathy, multifocal placoid pigment H30.14- ☑
Epithelium, epithelial — *see* condition
Epituberculosis (with atelectasis) (allergic) A15.7
Eponychia Q84.6
Epstein's
  nephrosis or syndrome — *see* Nephrosis
  pearl K09.8
Epulis (gingiva) (fibrous) (giant cell) K06.8
Equinia A24.0
Equinovarus (congenital) (talipes) Q66.0- ☑
  acquired — *see* Deformity, limb, clubfoot
Equivalent
  convulsive (abdominal) — *see* Epilepsy, specified NEC
  epileptic (psychic) — *see* Epilepsy, localization-related, symptomatic, with complex partial seizures
Erb (-Duchenne) **paralysis** (birth injury) (newborn) P14.0
Erb-Goldflam disease or syndrome G70.00
  with exacerbation (acute) G70.01
  in crisis G70.01
Erb's
  disease G71.02
  palsy, paralysis (brachial) (birth) (newborn) P14.0
    spinal (spastic) syphilitic A52.17
  pseudohypertrophic muscular dystrophy G71.02
Erdheim's syndrome (acromegalic macrospondylitis) E22.0
Erection, painful (persistent) — *see* Priapism
Ergosterol deficiency (vitamin D) E55.9
  with
    adult osteomalacia M83.8
    rickets — *see* Rickets
Ergotism — *see also* Poisoning, food, noxious, plant
  from ergot used as drug (migraine therapy) — *see* Table of Drugs and Chemicals
Erosio interdigitalis blastomycetica B37.2
Erosion
  artery I77.2
    without rupture I77.89
  bone — *see* Disorder, bone, density and structure, specified NEC
  bronchus J98.09

Erosion — *continued*
  cartilage (joint) — *see* Disorder, cartilage, specified type NEC
  cervix (uteri) (acquired) (chronic) (congenital) N86
    with cervicitis N72
  cornea (nontraumatic) — *see* Ulcer, cornea
    recurrent H18.83- ☑
    traumatic — *see* Abrasion, cornea
  dental (idiopathic) (occupational) (due to diet, drugs or vomiting) K03.2
  duodenum, postpyloric — *see* Ulcer, duodenum
  esophagus K22.10
    with bleeding K22.11
  gastric — *see* Ulcer, stomach
  gastrojejunal — *see* Ulcer, gastrojejunal
  implanted mesh — *see* Complications, prosthetic device or implant, mesh
  intestine K63.3
  lymphatic vessel I89.8
  pylorus, pyloric (ulcer) — *see* Ulcer, stomach
  spine, aneurysmal A52.09
  stomach — *see* Ulcer, stomach
  subcutaneous device pocket
    nervous system prosthetic device, implant, or graft T85.890 ☑
    other internal prosthetic device, implant, or graft T85.898 ☑
  teeth (idiopathic) (occupational) (due to diet, drugs or vomiting) K03.2
  urethra N36.8
  uterus N85.8
Erotomania F52.8
Error
  metabolism, inborn — *see* Disorder, metabolism
  refractive — *see* Disorder, refraction
Eructation R14.2
  nervous or psychogenic F45.8
Eruption
  creeping B76.9
  drug (generalized) (taken internally) L27.0
    fixed L27.1
    in contact with skin — *see* Dermatitis, due to drugs
    localized L27.1
  Hutchinson, summer L56.4
  Kaposi's varicelliform B00.0
  napkin L22
  polymorphous light (sun) L56.4
  recalcitrant pustular L13.8
  ringed R23.8
  skin (nonspecific) R21
    creeping (meaning hookworm) B76.9
    due to inoculation/vaccination (generalized) — *see also* Dermatitis, due to, vaccine L27.0
      localized L27.1
    erysipeloid A26.0
    feigned L98.1
    Kaposi's varicelliform B00.0
    lichenoid L28.0
    meaning dermatitis — *see* Dermatitis
    toxic NEC L53.0
  tooth, teeth, abnormal (incomplete) (late) (premature) (sequence) K00.6
  vesicular R23.8
Erysipelas (gangrenous) (infantile) (newborn) (phlegmonous) (suppurative) A46
  external ear A46 [H62.40]
  puerperal, postpartum O86.89
Erysipeloid A26.9
  cutaneous (Rosenbach's) A26.0
  disseminated A26.8
  sepsis A26.7
  specified NEC A26.8
Erythema, erythematous (infectional) (inflammation) L53.9
  ab igne L59.0
  annulare (centrifugum) (rheumaticum) L53.1
  arthriticum epidemicum A25.1
  brucellum — *see* Brucellosis
  chronic figurate NEC L53.3
  chronicum migrans (Borrelia burgdorferi) A69.20
  diaper L22
  due to
    chemical NEC L53.0
      in contact with skin L24.5
    drug (internal use) — *see* Dermatitis, due to, drugs
  elevatum diutinum L95.1
  endemic E52
  epidemic, arthritic A25.1

Erythema, erythematous — *continued*
  figuratum perstans L53.3
  gluteal L22
  heat — *code by site under* Burn, first degree
  ichthyosiforme congenitum bullous Q80.3
  in diseases classified elsewhere L54
  induratum (nontuberculous) L52
    tuberculous A18.4
  infectiosum B08.3
  intertrigo L30.4
  iris L51.9
  marginatum L53.2
    in (due to) acute rheumatic fever I00
  medicamentosum — *see* Dermatitis, due to, drugs
  migrans A26.0
    chronicum A69.20
    tongue K14.1
  multiforme (major) (minor) L51.9
    bullous, bullosum L51.1
    conjunctiva L51.1
    nonbullous L51.0
    pemphigoides L12.0
    specified NEC L51.8
  napkin L22
  neonatorum P83.88
    toxic P83.1
  nodosum L52
    tuberculous A18.4
  palmar L53.8
  pernio T69.1 ☑
  rash, newborn P83.88
  scarlatiniform (recurrent) (exfoliative) L53.8
  solare L55.0
  specified NEC L53.8
  toxic, toxicum NEC L53.0
    newborn P83.1
  tuberculous (primary) A18.4
Erythematous, erythematosus — *see* condition
Erythermalgia (primary) I73.81
Erythralgia I73.81
Erythrasma L08.1
Erythredema (polyneuropathy) — *see* Poisoning, mercury
Erythremia (acute) C94.0- ☑
  chronic D45
  secondary D75.1
Erythroblastopenia — *see also* Aplasia, red cell D60.9
  congenital D61.01
Erythroblastophthisis D61.09
Erythroblastosis (fetalis) (newborn) P55.9
  due to
    ABO (antibodies) (incompatibility) (isoimmunization) P55.1
    Rh (antibodies) (incompatibility) (isoimmunization) P55.0
Erythrocyanosis (crurum) I73.89
Erythrocythemia — *see* Erythremia
Erythrocytosis (megalosplenic) (secondary) D75.1
  familial D75.0
  oval, hereditary — *see* Elliptocytosis
  secondary D75.1
  stress D75.1
Erythroderma (secondary) — *see also* Erythema L53.9
  bullous ichthyosiform, congenital Q80.3
  desquamativum L21.1
  ichthyosiform, congenital (bullous) Q80.3
  neonatorum P83.88
  psoriaticum L40.8
Erythrodysesthesia, palmar plantar (PPE) L27.1
Erythrogenesis imperfecta D61.09
Erythroleukemia C94.0- ☑
Erythromelalgia I73.81
Erythrophagocytosis D75.89
Erythrophobia F40.298
Erythroplakia, oral epithelium, and tongue K13.29
Erythroplasia (Queyrat) D07.4
  specified site — *see* Neoplasm, skin, in situ
  unspecified site D07.4
Escherichia coli (E. coli), **as cause of disease classified elsewhere** B96.20
  non-O157 Shiga toxin-producing (with known O group) B96.22
  non-Shiga toxin-producing B96.29
  O157 with confirmation of Shiga toxin when H antigen is unknown, or is not H7 B96.21
  O157:H- (nonmotile) with confirmation of Shiga toxin B96.21

Escherichia coli (E. coli), **as cause of disease classified elsewhere** — *continued*
   O157:H7 with or without confirmation of Shiga toxin-production B96.21
   specified NEC B96.22-
   Shiga toxin-producing (with unspecified O group) (STEC) B96.23
   O157 B96.21
   specified NEC B96.29
Esophagismus K22.4
Esophagitis (acute) (alkaline) (chemical) (chronic) (infectional) (necrotic) (peptic) (postoperative) K20.9
   candidal B37.81
   due to gastrointestinal reflux disease K21.0
   eosinophilic K20.0
   reflux K21.0
   specified NEC K20.8
   tuberculous A18.83
   ulcerative K22.10
      with bleeding K22.11
Esophagocele K22.5
Esophagomalacia K22.8
Esophagospasm K22.4
Esophagostenosis K22.2
Esophagostomiasis B81.8
Esophagotracheal — *see* condition
Esophagus — *see* condition
Esophoria H50.51
   convergence, excess H51.12
   divergence, insufficiency H51.8
Esotropia — *see* Strabismus, convergent concomitant
Espundia B55.2
Essential — *see* condition
Esthesioneuroblastoma C30.0
Esthesioneurocytoma C30.0
Esthesioneuroepithelioma C30.0
Esthiomene A55
Estivo-autumnal malaria (fever) B50.9
Estrangement (marital) Z63.5
   parent-child NEC Z62.890
Estriasis — *see* Myiasis
Ethanolism — *see* Alcoholism
Etherism — *see* Dependence, drug, inhalant
Ethmoid, ethmoidal — *see* condition
Ethmoiditis (chronic) (nonpurulent) (purulent) — *see also* Sinusitis, ethmoidal
   influenzal — *see* Influenza, with, respiratory manifestations NEC
   Woakes' J33.1
Ethylism — *see* Alcoholism
Eulenburg's disease (congenital paramyotonia) G71.19
Eumycetoma B47.0
Eunuchoidism E29.1
   hypogonadotropic E23.0
European blastomycosis — *see* Cryptococcosis
Eustachian — *see* condition
Evaluation (for) (of)
   development state
      adolescent Z00.3
      period of
         delayed growth in childhood Z00.70
            with abnormal findings Z00.71
         rapid growth in childhood Z00.2
      puberty Z00.3
   growth and developmental state (period of rapid growth) Z00.2
      delayed growth Z00.70
         with abnormal findings Z00.71
   mental health (status) Z00.8
      requested by authority Z04.6
   period of
      delayed growth in childhood Z00.70
         with abnormal findings Z00.71
      rapid growth in childhood Z00.2
   suspected condition — *see* Observation
Evans syndrome D69.41
Event
   apparent life threatening in newborn and infant (ALTE) R68.13
   brief resolved unexplained event (BRUE) R68.13
Eventration — *see also* Hernia, ventral
   colon into chest — *see* Hernia, diaphragm
   diaphragm (congenital) Q79.1
Eversion
   bladder N32.89
   cervix (uteri) N86
      with cervicitis N72

Eversion — *continued*
   foot NEC — *see also* Deformity, valgus, ankle
      congenital Q66.6
   punctum lacrimale (postinfectional) (senile) H04.52- ☑
   ureter (meatus) N28.89
   urethra (meatus) N36.8
   uterus N81.4
Evidence
   cytologic
      of malignancy on anal smear R85.614
      of malignancy on cervical smear R87.614
      of malignancy on vaginal smear R87.624
Evisceration
   birth injury P15.8
   traumatic NEC
      eye — *see* Enucleated eye
Evulsion — *see* Avulsion
Ewing's sarcoma or tumor — *see* Neoplasm, bone, malignant
Examination (for) (following) (general) (of) (routine) Z00.00
   with abnormal findings Z00.01
   abuse, physical (alleged), ruled out
      adult Z04.71
      child Z04.72
   adolescent (development state) Z00.3
   alleged rape or sexual assault (victim), ruled out
      adult Z04.41
      child Z04.42
   allergy Z01.82
   annual (adult) (periodic) (physical) Z00.00
      with abnormal findings Z00.01
      gynecological Z01.419
         with abnormal findings Z01.411
   antibody response Z01.84
   blood — *see* Examination, laboratory
   blood pressure Z01.30
      with abnormal findings Z01.31
   cancer staging — *see* Neoplasm, malignant, by site
   cervical Papanicolaou smear Z12.4
      as part of routine gynecological examination Z01.419
         with abnormal findings Z01.411
   child (over 28 days old) Z00.129
      with abnormal findings Z00.121
      under 28 days old — *see* Newborn, examination
   clinical research control or normal comparison (control) (participant) Z00.6
   contraceptive (drug) maintenance (routine) Z30.8
      device (intrauterine) Z30.431
   dental Z01.20
      with abnormal findings Z01.21
   developmental — *see* Examination, child
   donor (potential) Z00.5
   ear Z01.10
      with abnormal findings NEC Z01.118
   eye Z01.00
      with abnormal findings Z01.01
      following failed vision screening Z01.020
         with abnormal findings Z01.021
   follow-up (routine) (following) Z09
      chemotherapy NEC Z09
         malignant neoplasm Z08
      fracture Z09
      malignant neoplasm Z08
      postpartum Z39.2
      psychotherapy Z09
      radiotherapy NEC Z09
         malignant neoplasm Z08
      surgery NEC Z09
         malignant neoplasm Z08
   following
      accident NEC Z04.3
         transport Z04.1
         work Z04.2
      assault, alleged, ruled out
         adult Z04.71
         child Z04.72
      motor vehicle accident Z04.1
      treatment (for) Z09
         combined NEC Z09
            fracture Z09
            malignant neoplasm Z08
         malignant neoplasm Z08
         mental disorder Z09
         specified condition NEC Z09
   forced sexual exploitation Z04.81
   forced labor exploitation Z04.82

Examination — *continued*
   gynecological Z01.419
      with abnormal findings Z01.411
      for contraceptive maintenance Z30.8
   health — *see* Examination, medical
   hearing Z01.10
      with abnormal findings NEC Z01.118
      following failed hearing screening Z01.110
      infant or child (over 28 days old) Z00.129
         with abnormal findings Z00.121
   immunity status testing Z01.84
   laboratory (as part of a general medical examination) Z00.00
      with abnormal findings Z00.01
      preprocedural Z01.812
   lactating mother Z39.1
   medical (adult) (for) (of) Z00.00
      with abnormal findings Z00.01
      administrative purpose only Z02.9
         specified NEC Z02.89
      admission to
         armed forces Z02.3
         old age home Z02.2
         prison Z02.89
         residential institution Z02.2
         school Z02.0
            following illness or medical treatment Z02.0
         summer camp Z02.89
      adoption Z02.82
      blood alcohol or drug level Z02.83
      camp (summer) Z02.89
      clinical research, normal subject (control) (participant) Z00.6
      control subject in clinical research (normal comparison) (participant) Z00.6
      donor (potential) Z00.5
      driving license Z02.4
      general (adult) Z00.00
         with abnormal findings Z00.01
      immigration Z02.89
      insurance purposes Z02.6
      marriage Z02.89
      medicolegal reasons NEC Z04.89
      naturalization Z02.89
      participation in sport Z02.5
      paternity testing Z02.81
      population survey Z00.8
      pre-employment Z02.1
      pre-operative — *see* Examination, pre-procedural
      pre-procedural
         cardiovascular Z01.810
         respiratory Z01.811
         specified NEC Z01.818
      preschool children
         for admission to school Z02.0
      prisoners
         for entrance into prison Z02.89
      recruitment for armed forces Z02.3
      specified NEC Z00.8
      sport competition Z02.5
   medicolegal reason NEC Z04.89
      following
         forced sexual exploitation Z04.81
         forced labor exploitation Z04.82
   newborn — *see* Newborn, examination
   pelvic (annual) (periodic) Z01.419
      with abnormal findings Z01.411
   period of rapid growth in childhood Z00.2
   periodic (adult) (annual) (routine) Z00.00
      with abnormal findings Z00.01
   physical (adult) — *see also* Examination, medical Z00.00
      sports Z02.5
   postpartum
      immediately after delivery Z39.0
      routine follow-up Z39.2
   pre-chemotherapy (antineoplastic) Z01.818
   prenatal (normal pregnancy) — *see also* Pregnancy, normal Z34.9- ☑
   pre-procedural (pre-operative)
      cardiovascular Z01.810
      laboratory Z01.812
      respiratory Z01.811
      specified NEC Z01.818
   prior to chemotherapy (antineoplastic) Z01.818
   psychiatric NEC Z00.8
      follow-up not needing further care Z09
      requested by authority Z04.6
   radiological (as part of a general medical examination) Z00.00

Examination — *continued*
  radiological — *continued*
    with abnormal findings Z00.01
    repeat cervical smear to confirm findings of recent
        normal smear following initial abnormal smear
        Z01.42
  skin (hypersensitivity) Z01.82
  special — *see also* Examination, by type Z01.89
    specified type NEC Z01.89
  specified type or reason NEC Z04.89
  teeth Z01.20
    with abnormal findings Z01.21
  urine — *see* Examination, laboratory
  vision Z01.00
    with abnormal findings Z01.01
    following failed vision screening Z01.020
      with abnormal findings Z01.021
    infant or child (over 28 days old) Z00.129
      with abnormal findings Z00.121
Exanthem, exanthema — *see also* Rash
  with enteroviral vesicular stomatitis B08.4
  Boston A88.0
  epidemic with meningitis A88.0 *[G02]*
  subitum B08.20
    due to human herpesvirus 6 B08.21
    due to human herpesvirus 7 B08.22
  viral, virus B09
    specified type NEC B08.8
Excess, excessive, excessively
  alcohol level in blood R78.0
  androgen (ovarian) E28.1
  attrition, tooth, teeth K03.0
  carotene, carotin (dietary) E67.1
  cold, effects of T69.9 ☑
    specified effect NEC T69.8 ☑
  convergence H51.12
  crying
    in child, adolescent, or adult R45.83
    in infant R68.11
  development, breast N62
  divergence H51.8
  drinking (alcohol) NEC (without dependence) F10.10
    habitual (continual) (without remission) F10.20
  eating R63.2
  estrogen E28.0
  fat — *see also* Obesity
    in heart — *see* Degeneration, myocardial
    localized E65
  foreskin N47.8
  gas R14.0
  glucagon E16.3
  heat — *see* Heat
  intermaxillary vertical dimension of fully erupted teeth
      M26.37
  interocclusal distance of fully erupted teeth M26.37
  kalium E87.5
  large
    colon K59.39
      congenital Q43.8
    infant P08.0
    organ or site, congenital NEC — *see* Anomaly, by
        site
  long
    organ or site, congenital NEC — *see* Anomaly, by
        site
  menstruation (with regular cycle) N92.0
    with irregular cycle N92.1
  napping Z72.821
  natrium E87.0
  number of teeth K00.1
  nutrient (dietary) NEC R63.2
  potassium (K) E87.5
  salivation K11.7
  secretion — *see also* Hypersecretion
    milk O92.6
    sputum R09.3
    sweat R61
  sexual drive F52.8
  short
    organ or site, congenital NEC — *see* Anomaly, by
        site
    umbilical cord in labor or delivery O69.3 ☑
  skin L98.7
    and subcutaneous tissue L98.7
    eyelid (acquired) — *see* Blepharochalasis
      congenital Q10.3
  sodium (Na) E87.0
  spacing of fully erupted teeth M26.32

Excess, excessive, excessively — *continued*
  sputum R09.3
  sweating R61
  thirst R63.1
    due to deprivation of water T73.1 ☑
  tuberosity of jaw M26.07
  vitamin
    A (dietary) E67.0
      administered as drug (prolonged intake) — *see*
          Table of Drugs and Chemicals, vitamins,
          adverse effect
      overdose or wrong substance given or taken —
          see Table of Drugs and Chemicals, vita-
          mins, poisoning
    D (dietary) E67.3
      administered as drug (prolonged intake) — *see*
          Table of Drugs and Chemicals, vitamins,
          adverse effect
      overdose or wrong substance given or taken —
          see Table of Drugs and Chemicals, vita-
          mins, poisoning
  weight
    gain R63.5
    loss R63.4
Excitability, abnormal, under minor stress (personal-
    ity disorder) F60.3
Excitation
  anomalous atrioventricular I45.6
  psychogenic F30.8
  reactive (from emotional stress, psychological trauma)
      F30.8
Excitement
  hypomanic F30.8
  manic F30.8
  mental, reactive (from emotional stress, psychological
      trauma) F30.8
  state, reactive (from emotional stress, psychological
      trauma) F30.8
Excoriation (traumatic) — *see also* Abrasion
  neurotic L98.1
  skin picking disorder F42.4
Exfoliation
  due to erythematous conditions according to extent
      of body surface involved L49.0
    10-19 percent of body surface L49.1
    20-29 percent of body surface L49.2
    30-39 percent of body surface L49.3
    40-49 percent of body surface L49.4
    50-59 percent of body surface L49.5
    60-69 percent of body surface L49.6
    70-79 percent of body surface L49.7
    80-89 percent of body surface L49.8
    90-99 percent of body surface L49.9
    less than 10 percent of body surface L49.0
  teeth, due to systemic causes K08.0
Exfoliative — *see* condition
Exhaustion, exhaustive (physical NEC) R53.83
  battle F43.0
  cardiac — *see* Failure, heart
  delirium F43.0
  due to
    cold T69.8 ☑
    excessive exertion T73.3 ☑
    exposure T73.2 ☑
    neurasthenia F48.8
  heart — *see* Failure, heart
  heat — *see also* Heat, exhaustion T67.5 ☑
    due to
      salt depletion T67.4 ☑
      water depletion T67.3 ☑
  maternal, complicating delivery O75.81
  mental F48.8
  myocardium, myocardial — *see* Failure, heart
  nervous F48.8
  old age R54
  psychogenic F48.8
  psychosis F43.0
  senile R54
  vital NEC Z73.0
Exhibitionism F65.2
Exocervicitis — *see* Cervicitis
Exomphalos Q79.2
  meaning hernia — *see* Hernia, umbilicus
Exophoria H50.52
  convergence, insufficiency H51.11
  divergence, excess H51.8
Exophthalmos H05.2- ☑
  congenital Q15.8

Exophthalmos — *continued*
  constant NEC H05.24- ☑
  displacement, globe — *see* Displacement, globe
  due to thyrotoxicosis (hyperthyroidism) — *see* Hyper-
      thyroidism, with, goiter (diffuse)
  dysthyroid — *see* Hyperthyroidism, with, goiter (dif-
      fuse)
  goiter — *see* Hyperthyroidism, with, goiter (diffuse)
  intermittent NEC H05.25- ☑
  malignant — *see* Hyperthyroidism, with, goiter (diffuse)
  orbital
    edema — *see* Edema, orbit
    hemorrhage — *see* Hemorrhage, orbit
  pulsating NEC H05.26- ☑
  thyrotoxic, thyrotropic — *see* Hyperthyroidism, with,
      goiter (diffuse)
Exostosis — *see also* Disorder, bone
  cartilaginous — *see* Neoplasm, bone, benign
  congenital (multiple) Q78.6
  external ear canal H61.81- ☑
  gonococcal A54.49
  jaw (bone) M27.8
  multiple, congenital Q78.6
  orbit H05.35- ☑
  osteocartilaginous — *see* Neoplasm, bone, benign
  syphilitic A52.77
Exotropia — *see* Strabismus, divergent concomitant
Explanation of
  investigation finding Z71.2
  medication Z71.89
Exposure (to) — *see also* Contact, with T75.89 ☑
  acariasis Z20.7
  AIDS virus Z20.6
  air pollution Z77.110
  algae and algae toxins Z77.121
  algae bloom Z77.121
  anthrax Z20.810
  aromatic amines Z77.020
  aromatic (hazardous) compounds NEC Z77.028
  aromatic dyes NOS Z77.028
  arsenic Z77.010
  asbestos Z77.090
  bacterial disease NEC Z20.818
  benzene Z77.021
  blue-green algae bloom Z77.121
  body fluids (potentially hazardous) Z77.21
  brown tide Z77.121
  chemicals (chiefly nonmedicinal) (hazardous) NEC
      Z77.098
  cholera Z20.09
  chromium compounds Z77.018
  cold, effects of T69.9 ☑
    specified effect NEC T69.8 ☑
  communicable disease Z20.9
    bacterial NEC Z20.818
    specified NEC Z20.89
    viral NEC Z20.828
    Zika virus Z20.821
  cyanobacteria bloom Z77.121
  disaster Z65.5
  discrimination Z60.5
  dyes Z77.098
  effects of T73.9 ☑
  environmental tobacco smoke (acute) (chronic) Z77.22
  Escherichia coli (E. coli) Z20.01
  exhaustion due to T73.2 ☑
  fiberglass — *see* Table of Drugs and Chemicals, fiber-
      glass
  German measles Z20.4
  gonorrhea Z20.2
  hazardous metals NEC Z77.018
  hazardous substances NEC Z77.29
  hazards in the physical environment NEC Z77.128
  hazards to health NEC Z77.9
  human immunodeficiency virus (HIV) Z20.6
  human T-lymphotropic virus type-1 (HTLV-1) Z20.89
  implanted
    mesh — *see* Complications, prosthetic devise or
        implant, mesh
    prosthetic materials NEC — *see* Complications,
        prosthetic materials NEC
  infestation (parasitic) NEC Z20.7
  intestinal infectious disease NEC Z20.09
    Escherichia coli (E. coli) Z20.01
  lead Z77.011
  meningococcus Z20.811
  mold (toxic) Z77.120
  nickel dust Z77.018

Failure, failed — *continued*
  heart — *continued*
    specified NEC I50.89

> *Note: heart failure stages A, B, C, and D are based on the American College of Cardiology and American Heart Association stages of heart failure, which complement and should not be confused with the New York Heart Association Classification of Heart Failure, into Class I, Class II, Class III, and Class IV*

    stage A Z91.89
    stage B — *see also* Failure, heart, by type as diastolic
      or systolic I50.9
    stage C — *see also* Failure, heart, by type as diastolic
      or systolic I50.9
    stage D — *see also* Failure, heart, by type as diastolic
      or systolic, chronic I50.84
    systolic (congestive) (left ventricular) I50.20
      acute (congestive) I50.21
      and (on) chronic (congestive) I50.23
      chronic (congestive) I50.22
      and (on) acute (congestive) I50.23
      combined with diastolic (congestive) I50.40
      acute (congestive) I50.41
        and (on) chronic (congestive) I50.43
      chronic (congestive) I50.42
        and (on) acute (congestive) I50.43
    thyrotoxic — *see also* Thyrotoxicosis E05.90 *[I43]*
      with
        high output — *see also* Thyrotoxicosis I50.83
        thyroid storm E05.91 *[I43]*
          high output — *see also* Thyrotoxicosis
          I50.83
    valvular — *see* Endocarditis
  hepatic K72.90
    with coma K72.91
    acute or subacute K72.00
      with coma K72.01
      due to drugs K71.10
        with coma K71.11
    alcoholic (acute) (chronic) (subacute) K70.40
      with coma K70.41
    chronic K72.10
      with coma K72.11
      due to drugs (acute) (subacute) (chronic) K71.10
        with coma K71.11
    due to drugs (acute) (subacute) (chronic) K71.10
      with coma K71.11
    postprocedural K91.82
  hepatorenal K76.7
  induction (of labor) O61.9
    abortion — *see* Abortion, attempted
    by
      oxytocic drugs O61.0
      prostaglandins O61.0
    instrumental O61.1
    mechanical O61.1
    medical O61.0
    specified NEC O61.8
    surgical O61.1
  intubation during anesthesia T88.4 ☑
    in pregnancy O29.6- ☑
    labor and delivery O74.7
    postpartum, puerperal O89.6
  involution, thymus (gland) E32.0
  kidney — *see also* Disease, kidney, chronic N19
    acute — *see also* Failure, renal, acute N17.9
  lactation (complete) O92.3
    partial O92.4
  Leydig's cell, adult E29.1
  liver — *see* Failure, hepatic
  menstruation at puberty N91.0
  mitral I05.8
  myocardial, myocardium — *see also* Failure, heart I50.9
    chronic — *see also* Failure, heart, congestive I50.9
    congestive — *see also* Failure, heart, congestive
      I50.9
  orgasm (female) (psychogenic) F52.31
    male F52.32
  ovarian (primary) E28.39
    iatrogenic E89.40
      asymptomatic E89.40
      symptomatic E89.41
    postprocedural (postablative) (postirradiation)
      (postsurgical) E89.40
      asymptomatic E89.40
      symptomatic E89.41
  ovulation causing infertility N97.0

Failure, failed — *continued*
  polyglandular, autoimmune E31.0
  prosthetic joint implant — *see* Complications, joint
    prosthesis, mechanical, breakdown, by site
  renal N19
    with
      tubular necrosis (acute) N17.0
    acute N17.9
      with
        cortical necrosis N17.1
        medullary necrosis N17.2
        tubular necrosis N17.0
      specified NEC N17.8
    chronic N18.9
      hypertensive — *see* Hypertension, kidney
    congenital P96.0
    end stage (chronic) N18.6
      due to hypertension I12.0
    following
      abortion — *see* Abortion by type complicated
        by specified condition NEC
      crushing T79.5 ☑
      ectopic or molar pregnancy O08.4
      labor and delivery (acute) O90.4
    hypertensive — *see* Hypertension, kidney
    postprocedural N99.0
  respiration, respiratory J96.90
    with
      hypercapnia J96.92
      hypercarbia J96.92
      hypoxia J96.91
    acute J96.00
      with
        hypercapnia J96.02
        hypercarbia J96.02
        hypoxia J96.01
    center G93.89
    acute and (on) chronic J96.20
      with
        hypercapnia J96.22
        hypercarbia J96.22
        hypoxia J96.21
    chronic J96.10
      with
        hypercapnia J96.12
        hypercarbia J96.12
        hypoxia J96.11
    newborn P28.5
    postprocedural (acute) J95.821
      acute and chronic J95.822
  rotation
    cecum Q43.3
    colon Q43.3
    intestine Q43.3
    kidney Q63.2
  sedation (conscious) (moderate) during procedure
    T88.52 ☑
    history of Z92.83
  segmentation — *see also* Fusion
    fingers — *see* Syndactylism, complex, fingers
    vertebra Q76.49
      with scoliosis Q76.3
  seminiferous tubule, adult E29.1
  senile (general) R54
  sexual arousal (male) F52.21
    female F52.22
  testicular endocrine function E29.1
  to thrive (child over 28 days old) R62.51
    adult R62.7
    newborn P92.6
  transplant T86.92
    bone T86.831
      marrow T86.02
    cornea T86.841
    heart T86.22
      with lung(s) T86.32
    intestine T86.851
    kidney T86.12
    liver T86.42
    lung(s) T86.811
      with heart T86.32
    pancreas T86.891
    skin (allograft) (autograft) T86.821
    specified organ or tissue NEC T86.891
    stem cell (peripheral blood) (umbilical cord) T86.5
  trial of labor (with subsequent cesarean delivery)
    O66.40
    following previous cesarean delivery O66.41

Failure, failed — *continued*
  tubal ligation N99.89
  urinary — *see* Disease, kidney, chronic
  vacuum extraction NOS (with subsequent cesarean
    delivery) O66.5
  vasectomy N99.89
  ventouse NOS (with subsequent cesarean delivery)
    O66.5
  ventricular — *see also* Failure, heart I50.9
    left — *see also* Failure, heart, left I50.1
      with rheumatic fever (conditions in I00)
        active I01.8
          with chorea I02.0
        inactive or quiescent (with chorea) I09.81
        rheumatic (chronic) (inactive) (with chorea)
          I09.81
        active or acute I01.8
          with chorea I02.0
    right — *see* Failure, heart, right
  vital centers, newborn P91.88
Fainting (fit) R55
Fallen arches — *see* Deformity, limb, flat foot
Falling, falls (repeated) R29.6
  any organ or part — *see* Prolapse
Fallopian
  insufflation Z31.41
  tube — *see* condition
Fallot's
  pentalogy Q21.8
  tetrad or tetralogy Q21.3
  triad or trilogy Q22.3
False — *see also* condition
  croup J38.5
  joint — *see* Nonunion, fracture
  labor (pains) O47.9
    at or after 37 completed weeks of gestation O47.1
    before 37 completed weeks of gestation O47.0- ☑
  passage, urethra (prostatic) N36.5
  pregnancy F45.8
Family, familial — *see also* condition
  disruption Z63.8
    involving divorce or separation Z63.5
  Li-Fraumeni (syndrome) Z15.01
  planning advice Z30.09
  problem Z63.9
    specified NEC Z63.8
  retinoblastoma C69.2- ☑
Famine (effects of) T73.0 ☑
  edema — *see* Malnutrition, severe
Fanconi (-de Toni)(-Debré) **syndrome** E72.09
  with cystinosis E72.04
Fanconi's anemia (congenital pancytopenia) D61.09
Farber's disease or syndrome E75.29
Farcy A24.0
Farmer's
  lung J67.0
  skin L57.8
Farsightedness — *see* Hypermetropia
Fascia — *see* condition
Fasciculation R25.3
Fasciitis M72.9
  diffuse (eosinophilic) M35.4
  infective M72.8
    necrotizing M72.6
  necrotizing M72.6
  nodular M72.4
  perirenal (with ureteral obstruction) N13.5
    with infection N13.6
  plantar M72.2
  specified NEC M72.8
  traumatic (old) M72.8
    current — *code by* site under Sprain
Fascioliasis B66.3
Fasciolopsis, fasciolopsiasis (intestinal) B66.5
Fascioscapulohumeral myopathy G71.02
Fast pulse R00.0
Fat
  embolism — *see* Embolism, fat
  excessive — *see also* Obesity
    in heart — *see* Degeneration, myocardial
  in stool R19.5
  localized (pad) E65
    heart — *see* Degeneration, myocardial
    knee M79.4
    retropatellar M79.4
  necrosis
    breast N64.1
    mesentery K65.4

☑ **Additional Character Required** — **Refer to the Tabular List for Character Selection**   ▽ **Subterms under main terms may continue to next column or page**

Fat — *continued*
  necrosis — *continued*
    omentum K65.4
  pad E65
    knee M79.4
Fatigue R53.83
  auditory deafness — *see* Deafness
  chronic R53.82
  combat F43.0
  general R53.83
    psychogenic F48.8
  heat (transient) T67.6 ☑
  muscle M62.89
  myocardium — *see* Failure, heart
  neoplasm-related R53.0
  nervous, neurosis F48.8
  operational F48.8
  psychogenic (general) F48.8
  senile R54
  voice R49.8
Fatness — *see* Obesity
Fatty — *see also* condition
  apron E65
  degeneration — *see* Degeneration, fatty
  heart (enlarged) — *see* Degeneration, myocardial
  liver NEC K76.0
    alcoholic K70.0
    nonalcoholic K76.0
  necrosis — *see* Degeneration, fatty
Fauces — *see* condition
Fauchard's disease (periodontitis) — *see* Periodontitis
Faucitis J02.9
Favism (anemia) D55.0
Fear of — *see* Phobia
Favus — *see* Dermatophytosis
Fazio-Londe disease or syndrome G12.1
Fear complex or reaction F40.9
Fear of — *see* Phobia
Febris, febrile — *see also* Fever
  flava — *see also* Fever, yellow A95.9
  melitensis A23.0
  pestis — *see* Plague
  recurrens — *see* Fever, relapsing
  rubra A38.9
Fecal
  incontinence R15.9
  smearing R15.1
  soiling R15.1
  urgency R15.2
Fecalith (impaction) K56.41
  appendix K38.1
  congenital P76.8
Fede's disease K14.0
Feeble rapid pulse due to shock following injury T79.4 ☑
Feeble-minded F70
Feeding
  difficulties R63.3
  problem R63.3
    newborn P92.9
      specified NEC P92.8
    nonorganic (adult) — *see* Disorder, eating
Feeling (of)
  foreign body in throat R09.89
Feer's disease — *see* Poisoning, mercury
Feet — *see* condition
Feigned illness Z76.5
Feil-Klippel syndrome (brevicollis) Q76.1
Feinmesser's (hidrotic) **ectodermal dysplasia** Q82.4
Felinophobia F40.218
Felon — *see also* Cellulitis, digit
  with lymphangitis — *see* Lymphangitis, acute, digit
Felty's syndrome M05.00
  ankle M05.07- ☑
  elbow M05.02- ☑
  foot joint M05.07- ☑
  hand joint M05.04- ☑
  hip M05.05- ☑
  knee M05.06- ☑
  multiple site M05.09
  shoulder M05.01- ☑
  vertebra — *see* Spondylitis, ankylosing
  wrist M05.03- ☑
Female genital cutting status — *see* Female genital mutilation status (FGM)
Female genital mutilation status (FGM) N90.810
  specified NEC N90.818

Female genital mutilation status — *continued*
  type I (clitorectomy status) N90.811
  type II (clitorectomy with excision of labia minora status) N90.812
  type III (infibulation status) N90.813
  type IV N90.818
Femur, femoral — *see* condition
Fenestration, fenestrated — *see also* Imperfect, closure
  aortico-pulmonary Q21.4
  cusps, heart valve NEC Q24.8
    pulmonary Q22.3
  pulmonic cusps Q22.3
Fernell's disease (aortic aneurysm) I71.9
Fertile eunuch syndrome E23.0
Fetid
  breath R19.6
  sweat L75.0
Fetishism F65.0
  transvestic F65.1
Fetus, fetal — *see also* condition
  alcohol syndrome (dysmorphic) Q86.0
  compressus O31.0- ☑
  hydantoin syndrome Q86.1
  lung tissue P28.0
  papyraceous O31.0- ☑
Fever (inanition) (of unknown origin) (persistent) (with chills) (with rigor) R50.9
  abortus A23.1
  Aden (dengue) A90
  African tick-borne A68.1
  American
    mountain (tick) A93.2
    spotted A77.0
  aphthous B08.8
  arbovirus, arboviral A94
    hemorrhagic A94
    specified NEC A93.8
  Argentinian hemorrhagic A96.0
  Assam B55.0
  Australian Q A78
  Bangkok hemorrhagic A91
  Barmah forest A92.8
  Bartonella A44.0
  bilious, hemoglobinuric B50.8
  blackwater B50.8
  blister B00.1
  Bolivian hemorrhagic A96.1
  Bonvale dam T73.3 ☑
  boutonneuse A77.1
  brain — *see* Encephalitis
  Brazilian purpuric A48.4
  breakbone A90
  Bullis A77.0
  Bunyamwera A92.8
  Burdwan B55.0
  Bwamba A92.8
  Cameroon — *see* Malaria
  Canton A75.9
  catarrhal (acute) J00
    chronic J31.0
  cat-scratch A28.1
  Central Asian hemorrhagic A98.0
  cerebral — *see* Encephalitis
  cerebrospinal meningococcal A39.0
  Chagres B50.9
  Chandipura A92.8
  Changuinola A93.1
  Charcot's (biliary) (hepatic) (intermittent) — *see* Calculus, bile duct
  Chikungunya (viral) (hemorrhagic) A92.0
  Chitral A93.1
  Colombo — *see* Fever, paratyphoid
  Colorado tick (virus) A93.2
  congestive (remittent) — *see* Malaria
  Congo virus A98.0
  continued malarial B50.9
  Corsican — *see* Malaria
  Crimean-Congo hemorrhagic A98.0
  Cyprus — *see* Brucellosis
  dandy A90
  deer fly — *see* Tularemia
  dengue (virus) A90
    hemorrhagic A91
    sandfly A93.1
  desert B38.0
  drug induced R50.2
  due to
    conditions classified elsewhere R50.81

Fever — *continued*
  due to — *continued*
    heat T67.01 ☑
  enteric A01.00
  enteroviral exanthematous (Boston exanthem) A88.0
  ephemeral (of unknown origin) R50.9
  epidemic hemorrhagic A98.5
  erysipelatous — *see* Erysipelas
  estivo-autumnal (malarial) B50.9
  famine A75.0
  five day A79.0
  following delivery O86.4
  Fort Bragg A27.89
  gastroenteric A01.00
  gastromalarial — *see* Malaria
  Gibraltar — *see* Brucellosis
  glandular — *see* Mononucleosis, infectious
  Guama (viral) A92.8
  Haverhill A25.1
  hay (allergic) J30.1
    with asthma (bronchial) J45.909
      with
        exacerbation (acute) J45.901
        status asthmaticus J45.902
    due to
      allergen other than pollen J30.89
      pollen, any plant or tree J30.1
  heat (effects) T67.01 ☑
  hematuric, bilious B50.8
  hemoglobinuric (malarial) (bilious) B50.8
  hemorrhagic (arthropod-borne) NOS A94
    with renal syndrome A98.5
    arenaviral A96.9
      specified NEC A96.8
    Argentinian A96.0
    Bangkok A91
    Bolivian A96.1
    Central Asian A98.0
    Chikungunya A92.0
    Crimean-Congo A98.0
    dengue (virus) A91
    epidemic A98.5
    Junin (virus) A96.0
    Korean A98.5
    Kyasanur forest A98.2
    Machupo (virus) A96.1
    mite-borne A93.8
    mosquito-borne A92.8
    Omsk A98.1
    Philippine A91
    Russian A98.5
    Singapore A91
    Southeast Asia A91
    Thailand A91
    tick-borne NEC A93.8
    viral A99
      specified NEC A98.8
  hepatic — *see* Cholecystitis
  herpetic — *see* Herpes
  icterohemorrhagic A27.0
  Indiana A93.8
  infective B99.9
    specified NEC B99.8
  intermittent (bilious) — *see also* Malaria
    of unknown origin R50.9
    pernicious B50.9
  iodide R50.2
  Japanese river A75.3
  jungle — *see also* Malaria
    yellow A95.0
  Junin (virus) hemorrhagic A96.0
  Katayama B65.2
  kedani A75.3
  Kenya (tick) A77.1
  Kew Garden A79.1
  Korean hemorrhagic A98.5
  Lassa A96.2
  Lone Star A77.0
  Machupo (virus) hemorrhagic A96.1
  malaria, malarial — *see* Malaria
  Malta A23.9
  Marseilles A77.1
  marsh — *see* Malaria
  Mayaro (viral) A92.8
  Mediterranean — *see also* Brucellosis A23.9
    familial M04.1
    tick A77.1
  meningeal — *see* Meningitis

Fever — *continued*
- Meuse A79.Ø
- Mexican A75.2
- mianeh A68.1
- miasmatic — *see* Malaria
- mosquito-borne (viral) A92.9
  - hemorrhagic A92.8
- mountain — *see also* Brucellosis
  - meaning Rocky Mountain spotted fever A77.Ø
  - tick (American) (Colorado) (viral) A93.2
- Mucambo (viral) A92.8
- mud A27.9
- Neapolitan — *see* Brucellosis
- neutropenic D7Ø.9
- newborn P81.9
  - environmental P81.Ø
- Nine-Mile A78
- non-exanthematous tick A93.2
- North Asian tick-borne A77.2
- Omsk hemorrhagic A98.1
- O'nyong-nyong (viral) A92.1
- Oropouche (viral) A93.Ø
- Oroya A44.Ø
- paludal — *see* Malaria
- Panama (malarial) B5Ø.9
- Pappataci A93.1
- paratyphoid A01.4
  - A A01.1
  - B A01.2
  - C A01.3
- parrot A7Ø
- periodic (Mediterranean) MØ4.1
- persistent (of unknown origin) R5Ø.9
- petechial A39.Ø
- pharyngoconjunctival B3Ø.2
- Philippine hemorrhagic A91
- phlebotomus A93.1
- Piry (virus) A93.8
- Pixuna (viral) A92.8
- Plasmodium ovale B53.Ø
- polioviral (nonparalytic) A8Ø.4
- Pontiac A48.2
- postimmunization R5Ø.83
- postoperative R5Ø.82
  - due to infection T81.4Ø ☑
- posttransfusion R5Ø.84
- postvaccination R5Ø.83
- presenting with conditions classified elsewhere R5Ø.81
- pretibial A27.89
- puerperal O86.4
- Q A78
- quadrilateral A78
- quartan (malaria) B52.9
- Queensland (coastal) (tick) A77.3
- quintan A79.Ø
- rabbit — *see* Tularemia
- rat-bite A25.9
  - due to
    - Spirillum A25.Ø
    - Streptobacillus moniliformis A25.1
- recurrent — *see* Fever, relapsing
- relapsing (Borrelia) A68.9
  - Carter's (Asiatic) A68.1
  - Dutton's (West African) A68.1
  - Koch's A68.9
  - louse-borne A68.Ø
  - Novy's
    - louse-borne A68.Ø
    - tick-borne A68.1
  - Obermeyer's (European) A68.Ø
  - tick-borne A68.1
- remittent (bilious) (congestive) (gastric) — *see* Malaria
- rheumatic (active) (acute) (chronic) (subacute) IØØ
  - with central nervous system involvement IØ2.9
  - active with heart involvement — *see* category IØ1 ☑
  - inactive or quiescent with
    - cardiac hypertrophy IØ9.89
    - carditis IØ9.9
    - endocarditis IØ9.1
      - aortic (valve) IØ6.9
        - with mitral (valve) disease IØ8.Ø
      - mitral (valve) IØ5.9
        - with aortic (valve) disease IØ8.Ø
      - pulmonary (valve) IØ9.89
      - tricuspid (valve) IØ7.8
    - heart disease NEC IØ9.89
    - heart failure (congestive) (conditions in category I5Ø.) IØ9.81

Fever — *continued*
- rheumatic — *continued*
  - inactive or quiescent with — *continued*
    - left ventricular failure (conditions in I5Ø.1-I5Ø.4-) IØ9.81
    - myocarditis, myocardial degeneration (conditions in I51.4) IØ9.Ø
    - pancarditis IØ9.9
    - pericarditis IØ9.2
- Rift Valley (viral) A92.4
- Rocky Mountain spotted A77.Ø
- rose J3Ø.1
- Ross River B33.1
- Russian hemorrhagic A98.5
- San Joaquin (Valley) B38.Ø
- sandfly A93.1
- Sao Paulo A77.Ø
- scarlet A38.9
- seven day (leptospirosis) (autumnal) (Japanese) A27.89
  - dengue A9Ø
- shin-bone A79.Ø
- Singapore hemorrhagic A91
- solar A9Ø
- Songo A98.5
- sore BØØ.1
- South African tick-bite A68.1
- Southeast Asia hemorrhagic A91
- spinal — *see* Meningitis
- spirillary A25.Ø
- splenic — *see* Anthrax
- spotted A77.9
  - American A77.Ø
  - Brazilian A77.Ø
  - cerebrospinal meningitis A39.Ø
  - Colombian A77.Ø
  - due to Rickettsia
    - australis A77.3
    - conorii A77.1
    - rickettsii A77.Ø
    - sibirica A77.2
    - specified type NEC A77.8
  - Ehrlichiosis A77.4Ø
    - due to
      - E. chafeensis A77.41
      - specified organism NEC A77.49
  - Rocky Mountain A77.Ø
- steroid R5Ø.2
- streptobacillary A25.1
- subtertian B5Ø.9
- Sumatran mite A75.3
- sun A9Ø
- swamp A27.9
- swine AØ2.8
- sylvatic, yellow A95.Ø
- Tahyna B33.8
- tertian — *see* Malaria, tertian
- Thailand hemorrhagic A91
- thermic T67.Ø1 ☑
- three-day A93.1
- tick
  - American mountain A93.2
  - Colorado A93.2
  - Kemerovo A93.8
  - Mediterranean A77.1
  - mountain A93.2
  - nonexanthematous A93.2
  - Quaranfil A93.8
- tick-bite NEC A93.8
- tick-borne (hemorrhagic) NEC A93.8
- trench A79.Ø
- tsutsugamushi A75.3
- typhogastric AØ1.ØØ
- typhoid (abortive) (hemorrhagic) (intermittent) (malignant) AØ1.ØØ
  - complicated by
    - arthritis AØ1.Ø4
    - heart involvement AØ1.Ø2
    - meningitis AØ1.Ø1
    - osteomyelitis AØ1.Ø5
    - pneumonia AØ1.Ø3
    - specified NEC AØ1.Ø9
- typhomalarial — *see* Malaria
- typhus — *see* Typhus (fever)
- undulant — *see* Brucellosis
- unknown origin R5Ø.9
- uveoparotid D86.89
- valley B38.Ø
- Venezuelan equine A92.2

Fever — *continued*
- vesicular stomatitis A93.8
- viral hemorrhagic — *see* Fever, hemorrhagic, by type of virus
- Volhynian A79.Ø
- Wesselsbron (viral) A92.8
- West
  - African B5Ø.8
  - Nile (viral) A92.3Ø
    - with
      - complications NEC A92.39
      - cranial nerve disorders A92.32
      - encephalitis A92.31
      - encephalomyelitis A92.31
      - neurologic manifestation NEC A92.32
      - optic neuritis A92.32
      - polyradiculitis A92.32
- Whitmore's — *see* Melioidosis
- Wolhynian A79.Ø
- worm B83.9
- yellow A95.9
  - jungle A95.Ø
  - sylvatic A95.Ø
  - urban A95.1
- Zika virus A92.5

Fibrillation
- atrial or auricular (established) I48.91
  - chronic I48.2Ø
    - persistent I48.19
  - paroxysmal I48.Ø
  - permanent I48.21
  - persistent (chronic) (NOS) (other) I48.19
    - longstanding I48.11
- cardiac I49.8
- heart I49.8
- muscular M62.89
- ventricular I49.Ø1

Fibrin
- ball or bodies, pleural (sac) J94.1
- chamber, anterior (eye) (gelatinous exudate) — *see* Iridocyclitis, acute

Fibrinogenolysis — *see* Fibrinolysis
Fibrinogenopenia D68.8
- acquired D65
- congenital D68.2

Fibrinolysis (hemorrhagic) (acquired) D65
- antepartum hemorrhage — *see* Hemorrhage, antepartum, with coagulation defect
- following
  - abortion — *see* Abortion by type complicated by hemorrhage
  - ectopic or molar pregnancy OØ8.1
- intrapartum O67.Ø
- newborn, transient P6Ø
- postpartum O72.3

Fibrinopenia (hereditary) D68.2
- acquired D68.4

Fibrinopurulent — *see* condition
Fibrinous — *see* condition
Fibroadenoma
- cellular intracanalicular D24- ☑
- giant D24- ☑
- intracanalicular
  - cellular D24- ☑
  - giant D24- ☑
  - specified site — *see* Neoplasm, benign, by site
  - unspecified site D24- ☑
- juvenile D24- ☑
- pericanalicular
  - specified site — *see* Neoplasm, benign, by site
  - unspecified site D24- ☑
- phyllodes D24- ☑
- prostate D29.1
- specified site NEC — *see* Neoplasm, benign, by site
- unspecified site D24- ☑

Fibroadenosis, breast (chronic) (cystic) (diffuse) (periodic) (segmental) N6Ø.2- ☑
Fibroangioma — *see also* Neoplasm, benign, by site
- juvenile
  - specified site — *see* Neoplasm, benign, by site
  - unspecified site D1Ø.6
Fibrochondrosarcoma — *see* Neoplasm, cartilage, malignant
Fibrocystic
- disease — *see also* Fibrosis, cystic
  - breast — *see* Mastopathy, cystic
  - jaw M27.49
  - kidney (congenital) Q61.8

Fibrocystic — continued
- disease — see also Fibrosis, cystic — continued
  - liver Q44.6
  - pancreas E84.9
  - kidney (congenital) Q61.8

Fibrodysplasia ossificans progressiva — see Myositis, ossificans, progressiva

Fibroelastosis (cordis) (endocardial) (endomyocardial) I42.4

Fibroid (tumor) — see also Neoplasm, connective tissue, benign
- disease, lung (chronic) — see Fibrosis, lung
- heart (disease) — see Myocarditis
- in pregnancy or childbirth O34.1- ☑
  - causing obstructed labor O65.5
- induration, lung (chronic) — see Fibrosis, lung
- lung — see Fibrosis, lung
- pneumonia (chronic) — see Fibrosis, lung
- uterus — see also Leiomyoma, uterus D25.9

Fibrolipoma — see Lipoma

Fibroliposarcoma — see Neoplasm, connective tissue, malignant

Fibroma — see also Neoplasm, connective tissue, benign
- ameloblastic — see Cyst, calcifying odontogenic
- bone (nonossifying) — see Disorder, bone, specified type NEC
  - ossifying — see Neoplasm, bone, benign
- cementifying — see Neoplasm, bone, benign
- chondromyxoid — see Neoplasm, bone, benign
- desmoplastic — see Neoplasm, connective tissue, uncertain behavior
- durum — see Neoplasm, connective tissue, benign
- fascial — see Neoplasm, connective tissue, benign
- invasive — see Neoplasm, connective tissue, uncertain behavior
- molle — see Lipoma
- myxoid — see Neoplasm, connective tissue, benign
- nasopharynx, nasopharyngeal (juvenile) D10.6
- nonosteogenic (nonossifying) — see Dysplasia, fibrous
- odontogenic (central) — see Cyst, calcifying odontogenic
- ossifying — see Neoplasm, bone, benign
- periosteal — see Neoplasm, bone, benign
- soft — see Lipoma

Fibromatosis M72.9
- abdominal — see Neoplasm, connective tissue, uncertain behavior
- aggressive — see Neoplasm, connective tissue, uncertain behavior
- congenital generalized — see Neoplasm, connective tissue, uncertain behavior
- Dupuytren's M72.0
- gingival K06.1
- palmar (fascial) M72.0
- plantar (fascial) M72.2
- pseudosarcomatous (proliferative) (subcutaneous) M72.4
- retroperitoneal D48.3
- specified NEC M72.8

Fibromyalgia M79.7

Fibromyoma — see also Neoplasm, connective tissue, benign
- uterus (corpus) — see also Leiomyoma, uterus
  - in pregnancy or childbirth — see Fibroid, in pregnancy or childbirth
    - causing obstructed labor O65.5

Fibromyositis M79.7

Fibromyxolipoma D17.9

Fibromyxoma — see Neoplasm, connective tissue, benign

Fibromyxosarcoma — see Neoplasm, connective tissue, malignant

Fibro-odontoma, ameloblastic — see Cyst, calcifying odontogenic

Fibro-osteoma — see Neoplasm, bone, benign

Fibroplasia, retrolental H35.17- ☑

Fibropurulent — see condition

Fibrosarcoma — see also Neoplasm, connective tissue, malignant
- ameloblastic C41.1
  - upper jaw (bone) C41.0
- congenital — see Neoplasm, connective tissue, malignant
- fascial — see Neoplasm, connective tissue, malignant
- infantile — see Neoplasm, connective tissue, malignant
- odontogenic C41.1
  - upper jaw (bone) C41.0

Fibrosarcoma — continued
- periosteal — see Neoplasm, bone, malignant

Fibrosclerosis
- breast N60.3- ☑
- multifocal M35.5
- penis (corpora cavernosa) N48.6

Fibrosis, fibrotic
- adrenal (gland) E27.8
- amnion O41.8X- ☑
- anal papillae K62.89
- arteriocapillary — see Arteriosclerosis
- bladder N32.89
  - interstitial — see Cystitis, chronic, interstitial
  - localized submucosal — see Cystitis, chronic, interstitial
  - panmural — see Cystitis, chronic, interstitial
- breast — see Fibrosclerosis, breast
- capillary — see also Arteriosclerosis I70.90
  - lung (chronic) — see Fibrosis, lung
- cardiac — see Myocarditis
- cervix N88.8
- chorion O41.8X- ☑
- corpus cavernosum (sclerosing) N48.6
- cystic (of pancreas) E84.9
  - with
    - distal intestinal obstruction syndrome E84.19
    - fecal impaction E84.19
    - intestinal manifestations NEC E84.19
    - pulmonary manifestations E84.0
    - specified manifestations NEC E84.8
- due to device, implant or graft — see also Complications, by site and type, specified NEC T85.828 ☑
  - arterial graft NEC T82.828 ☑
  - breast (implant) T85.828 ☑
  - catheter NEC T85.828 ☑
    - dialysis (renal) T82.828 ☑
      - intraperitoneal T85.828 ☑
    - infusion NEC T82.828 ☑
      - spinal (epidural) (subdural) T85.820 ☑
    - urinary (indwelling) T83.82 ☑
  - electronic (electrode) (pulse generator) (stimulator)
    - bone T84.82 ☑
    - cardiac T82.827 ☑
    - nervous system (brain) (peripheral nerve) (spinal) T85.820 ☑
    - urinary T83.82 ☑
  - fixation, internal (orthopedic) NEC T84.82 ☑
  - gastrointestinal (bile duct) (esophagus) T85.828 ☑
  - genital NEC T83.82 ☑
  - heart NEC T82.827 ☑
  - joint prosthesis T84.82 ☑
  - ocular (corneal graft) (orbital implant) NEC T85.828 ☑
  - orthopedic NEC T84.82 ☑
  - specified NEC T85.828 ☑
  - urinary NEC T83.82 ☑
  - vascular NEC T82.828 ☑
  - ventricular intracranial shunt T85.820 ☑
- ejaculatory duct N50.89
- endocardium — see Endocarditis
- endomyocardial (tropical) I42.3
- epididymis N50.89
- eye muscle — see Strabismus, mechanical
- heart — see Myocarditis
- hepatic — see Fibrosis, liver
- hepatolienal (portal hypertension) K76.6
- hepatosplenic (portal hypertension) K76.6
- infrapatellar fat pad M79.4
- intrascrotal N50.89
- kidney N26.9
- liver K74.0
  - with sclerosis K74.2
  - alcoholic K70.2
- lung (atrophic) (chronic) (confluent) (massive) (perialveolar) (peribronchial) J84.10
  - with
    - anthracosilicosis J60
    - anthracosis J60
    - asbestosis J61
    - bagassosis J67.1
    - bauxite J63.1
    - berylliosis J63.2
    - byssinosis J66.0
    - calcicosis J62.8
    - chalicosis J62.8
    - dust reticulation J64
    - farmer's lung J67.0

Fibrosis, fibrotic — continued
- lung — continued
  - with — continued
    - ganister disease J62.8
    - graphite J63.3
    - pneumoconiosis NOS J64
    - siderosis J63.4
    - silicosis J62.8
  - capillary J84.10
  - congenital P27.8
  - diffuse (idiopathic) J84.10
    - chemicals, gases, fumes or vapors (inhalation) J68.4
    - interstitial J84.10
      - acute J84.114
    - talc J62.0
  - following radiation J70.1
  - idiopathic J84.112
  - postinflammatory J84.10
  - silicotic J62.8
  - tuberculous — see Tuberculosis, pulmonary
- lymphatic gland I89.8
- median bar — see Hyperplasia, prostate
- mediastinum (idiopathic) J98.59
- meninges G96.19
- myocardium, myocardial — see Myocarditis
- ovary N83.8
- oviduct N83.8
- pancreas K86.89
- penis NEC N48.6
- pericardium I31.0
- perineum, in pregnancy or childbirth O34.7- ☑
  - causing obstructed labor O65.5
- pleura J94.1
- popliteal fat pad M79.4
- prostate (chronic) — see Hyperplasia, prostate
- pulmonary — see also Fibrosis, lung J84.10
  - congenital P27.8
  - idiopathic J84.112
- rectal sphincter K62.89
- retroperitoneal, idiopathic (with ureteral obstruction) N13.5
  - with infection N13.6
- sclerosing mesenteric (idiopathic) K65.4
- scrotum N50.89
- seminal vesicle N50.89
- senile R54
- skin L90.5
- spermatic cord N50.89
- spleen D73.89
  - in schistosomiasis (bilharziasis) B65.9 [D77]
- subepidermal nodular — see Neoplasm, skin, benign
- submucous (oral) (tongue) K13.5
- testis N44.8
  - chronic, due to syphilis A52.76
- thymus (gland) E32.8
- tongue, submucous K13.5
- tunica vaginalis N50.89
- uterus (non-neoplastic) N85.8
- vagina N89.8
- valve, heart — see Endocarditis
- vas deferens N50.89
- vein I87.8

Fibrositis (periarticular) M79.7
- nodular, chronic (Jaccoud's) (rheumatoid) — see Arthropathy, postrheumatic, chronic

Fibrothorax J94.1

Fibrotic — see Fibrosis

Fibrous — see condition

Fibroxanthoma — see also Neoplasm, connective tissue, benign
- atypical — see Neoplasm, connective tissue, uncertain behavior
- malignant — see Neoplasm, connective tissue, malignant

Fibroxanthosarcoma — see Neoplasm, connective tissue, malignant

Fiedler's
- disease (icterohemorrhagic leptospirosis) A27.0
- myocarditis (acute) I40.1

Fifth disease B08.3
- venereal A55

Filaria, filarial, filariasis — see Infestation, filarial

Filatov's disease — see Mononucleosis, infectious

File-cutter's disease — see Poisoning, lead

Filling defect
- biliary tract R93.2
- bladder R93.41

Filling defect — *continued*
  duodenum R93.3
  gallbladder R93.2
  gastrointestinal tract R93.3
  intestine R93.3
  kidney R93.42- ☑
  stomach R93.3
  ureter R93.41
  urinary organs, specified NEC R93.49
Fimbrial cyst Q50.4
Financial problem affecting care NOS Z59.9
  bankruptcy Z59.8
  foreclosure on loan Z59.8
Findings, abnormal, inconclusive, without diagnosis
    — *see also* Abnormal
  17-ketosteroids, elevated R82.5
  acetonuria R82.4
  alcohol in blood R78.0
  anisocytosis R71.8
  antenatal screening of mother O28.9
    biochemical O28.1
    chromosomal O28.5
    cytological O28.2
    genetic O28.5
    hematological O28.0
    radiological O28.4
    specified NEC O28.8
    ultrasonic O28.3
  antibody titer, elevated R76.0
  anticardiolipin antibody R76.0
  antiphosphatidylglycerol antibody R76.0
  antiphosphatidylinositol antibody R76.0
  antiphosphatidylserine antibody R76.0
  antiphospholipid antibody R76.0
  bacteriuria R82.71
  bicarbonate E87.8
  bile in urine R82.2
  blood sugar R73.09
    high R73.9
    low (transient) E16.2
  body fluid or substance, specified NEC R88.8
  casts, urine R82.998
  catecholamines R82.5
  cells, urine R82.998
  chloride E87.8
  cholesterol E78.9
    high E78.00
      with high triglycerides E78.2
  chyluria R82.0
  cloudy
    dialysis effluent R88.0
    urine R82.90
  creatinine clearance R94.4
  crystals, urine R82.998
  culture
    blood R78.81
    positive — *see* Positive, culture
  echocardiogram R93.1
  electrolyte level, urinary R82.998
  function study NEC R94.8
    bladder R94.8
    endocrine NEC R94.7
      thyroid R94.6
    kidney R94.4
    liver R94.5
    pancreas R94.8
    placenta R94.8
    pulmonary R94.2
    spleen R94.8
  gallbladder, nonvisualization R93.2
  glucose (tolerance test) (non-fasting) R73.09
  glycosuria R81
  heart
    shadow R93.1
    sounds R01.2
  hematinuria R82.3
  hematocrit drop (precipitous) R71.0
  hemoglobinuria R82.3
  human papillomavirus (HPV) DNA test positive
    cervix
      high risk R87.810
      low risk R87.820
    vagina
      high risk R87.811
      low risk R87.821
  in blood (of substance not normally found in blood)
    R78.9
    addictive drug NEC R78.4
    alcohol (excessive level) R78.0

Findings, abnormal, inconclusive, without diagnosis
    — *continued*
  in blood — *continued*
    cocaine R78.2
    hallucinogen R78.3
    heavy metals (abnormal level) R78.79
    lead R78.71
    lithium (abnormal level) R78.89
    opiate drug R78.1
    psychotropic drug R78.5
    specified substance NEC R78.89
    steroid agent R78.6
  indoleacetic acid, elevated R82.5
  ketonuria R82.4
  lactic acid dehydrogenase (LDH) R74.0
  liver function test R79.89
  mammogram NEC R92.8
    calcification (calculus) R92.1
    inconclusive result (due to dense breasts) R92.2
    microcalcification R92.0
  mediastinal shift R93.89
  melanin, urine R82.998
  myoglobinuria R82.1
  neonatal screening P09
  nonvisualization of gallbladder R93.2
  odor of urine NOS R82.90
  Papanicolaou cervix R87.619
    non-atypical endometrial cells R87.618
  pneumoencephalogram R93.0
  poikilocytosis R71.8
  potassium (deficiency) E87.6
    excess E87.5
  PPD R76.11
  radiologic (X-ray) R93.89
    abdomen R93.5
    biliary tract R93.2
    breast R92.8
    gastrointestinal tract R93.3
    genitourinary organs R93.89
    head R93.0
    inconclusive due to excess body fat of patient R93.9
    intrathoracic organs NEC R93.1
    musculoskeletal
      limbs R93.6
      other than limb R93.7
    placenta R93.89
    retroperitoneum R93.5
    skin R93.89
    skull R93.0
    subcutaneous tissue R93.89
    testis R93.81- ☑
  red blood cell (count) (morphology) (sickling) (volume)
    R71.8
  scan NEC R94.8
    bladder R94.8
    bone R94.8
    kidney R94.4
    liver R93.2
    lung R94.2
    pancreas R94.8
    placental R94.8
    spleen R94.8
    thyroid R94.6
  sedimentation rate, elevated R70.0
  SGOT R74.0
  SGPT R74.0
  sodium (deficiency) E87.1
    excess E87.0
  specified body fluid NEC R88.8
  stress test R94.39
  testis R93.81- ☑
  thyroid (function) (metabolic rate) (scan) (uptake) R94.6
  transaminase (level) R74.0
  triglycerides E78.9
    high E78.1
      with high cholesterol E78.2
  tuberculin skin test (without active tuberculosis) R76.11
  urine R82.90
    acetone R82.4
    bacteria R82.71
    bile R82.2
    casts or cells R82.998
    chyle R82.0
    culture positive R82.79
    glucose R81
    hemoglobin R82.3
    ketone R82.4
    sugar R81
  vanillylmandelic acid (VMA), elevated R82.5

Findings, abnormal, inconclusive, without diagnosis
    — *continued*
  vectorcardiogram (VCG) R94.39
  ventriculogram R93.0
  white blood cell (count) (differential) (morphology)
    D72.9
  xerography R92.8
Finger — *see* condition
Fire, Saint Anthony's — *see* Erysipelas
Fire-setting
  pathological (compulsive) F63.1
Fish hook stomach K31.89
Fishmeal-worker's lung J67.8
Fissure, fissured
  anus, anal K60.2
    acute K60.0
    chronic K60.1
    congenital Q43.8
  ear, lobule, congenital Q17.8
  epiglottis (congenital) Q31.8
  larynx J38.7
    congenital Q31.8
  lip K13.0
    congenital — *see* Cleft, lip
  nipple N64.0
    associated with
      lactation O92.13
      pregnancy O92.11- ☑
      puerperium O92.12
  nose Q30.2
  palate (congenital) — *see* Cleft, palate
  skin R23.4
  spine (congenital) — *see also* Spina bifida
    with hydrocephalus — *see* Spina bifida, by site, with
      hydrocephalus
  tongue (acquired) K14.5
    congenital Q38.3
Fistula (cutaneous) L98.8
  abdomen (wall) K63.2
    bladder N32.2
    intestine NEC K63.2
    ureter N28.89
    uterus N82.5
  abdominorectal K63.2
  abdominosigmoidal K63.2
  abdominothoracic J86.0
  abdominouterine N82.5
    congenital Q51.7
  abdominovesical N32.2
  accessory sinuses — *see* Sinusitis
  actinomycotic — *see* Actinomycosis
  alveolar antrum — *see* Sinusitis, maxillary
  alveolar process K04.6
  anorectal K60.5
  antrobuccal — *see* Sinusitis, maxillary
  antrum — *see* Sinusitis, maxillary
  anus, anal (recurrent) (infectional) K60.3
    congenital Q43.6
      with absence, atresia and stenosis Q42.2
    tuberculous A18.32
  aorta-duodenal I77.2
  appendix, appendicular K38.3
  arteriovenous (acquired) (nonruptured) I77.0
    brain I67.1
      congenital Q28.2
        ruptured — *see* Fistula, arteriovenous, brain
          ruptured
      ruptured I60.8
        intracerebral I61.8
        intraparenchymal I61.8
        intraventricular I61.5
        subarachnoid I60.8
    cerebral — *see* Fistula, arteriovenous, brain
    congenital (peripheral) — *see also* Malformation,
      arteriovenous
      brain Q28.2
        ruptured — *see* Fistula, arteriovenous, brain
          ruptured
      coronary Q24.5
      pulmonary Q25.72
    coronary I25.41
      congenital Q24.5
    pulmonary I28.0
      congenital Q25.72
    surgically created (for dialysis) Z99.2
      complication — *see* Complication, arteriovenous
        fistula, surgically created
    traumatic — *see* Injury, blood vessel

Fistula — *continued*
　artery I77.2
　aural (mastoid) — *see* Mastoiditis, chronic
　auricle — *see also* Disorder, pinna, specified type NEC
　　congenital Q18.1
　Bartholin's gland N82.8
　bile duct (common) (hepatic) K83.3
　　with calculus, stones — *see* Calculus, bile duct
　biliary (tract) — *see* Fistula, bile duct
　bladder (sphincter) NEC — *see also* Fistula, vesico-
　　N32.2
　　into seminal vesicle N32.2
　bone — *see also* Disorder, bone, specified type NEC
　　with osteomyelitis, chronic — *see* Osteomyelitis,
　　　chronic, with draining sinus
　brain G93.89
　　arteriovenous (acquired) — *see also* Fistula, arterio-
　　　venous, brain I67.1
　　　congenital Q28.2
　branchial (cleft) Q18.0
　branchiogenous Q18.0
　breast N61.0
　　puerperal, postpartum or gestational, due to mastitis
　　　(purulent) — *see* Mastitis, obstetric, purulent
　bronchial J86.0
　bronchocutaneous, bronchomediastinal, bronchopleu-
　　ral, bronchopleuromediastinal (infective) J86.0
　　tuberculous NEC A15.5
　bronchoesophageal J86.0
　　congenital Q39.2
　　　with atresia of esophagus Q39.1
　bronchovisceral J86.0
　buccal cavity (infective) K12.2
　cecosigmoidal K63.2
　cecum K63.2
　cerebrospinal (fluid) G96.0
　cervical, lateral Q18.1
　cervicoaural Q18.1
　cervicosigmoidal N82.4
　cervicovesical N82.1
　cervix N82.8
　chest (wall) J86.0
　cholecystenteric — *see* Fistula, gallbladder
　cholecystocolic — *see* Fistula, gallbladder
　cholecystocolonic — *see* Fistula, gallbladder
　cholecystoduodenal — *see* Fistula, gallbladder
　cholecystogastric — *see* Fistula, gallbladder
　cholecystointestinal — *see* Fistula, gallbladder
　choledochoduodenal — *see* Fistula, bile duct
　cholocolic K82.3
　coccyx — *see* Sinus, pilonidal
　colon K63.2
　colostomy K94.09
　colovesical N32.1
　common duct — *see* Fistula, bile duct
　congenital, site not listed — *see* Anomaly, by site
　coronary, arteriovenous I25.41
　　congenital Q24.5
　costal region J86.0
　cul-de-sac, Douglas' N82.8
　cystic duct — *see also* Fistula, gallbladder
　　congenital Q44.5
　dental K04.6
　diaphragm J86.0
　duodenum K31.6
　ear (external) (canal) — *see* Disorder, ear, external,
　　specified type NEC
　enterocolic K63.2
　enterocutaneous K63.2
　enterouterine N82.4
　　congenital Q51.7
　enterovaginal N82.4
　　congenital Q52.2
　　large intestine N82.3
　　small intestine N82.2
　enterovesical N32.1
　epididymis N50.89
　　tuberculous A18.15
　esophagobronchial J86.0
　　congenital Q39.2
　　　with atresia of esophagus Q39.1
　esophagocutaneous K22.8
　esophagopleural-cutaneous J86.0
　esophagotracheal J86.0
　　congenital Q39.2
　　　with atresia of esophagus Q39.1
　esophagus K22.8
　　congenital Q39.2

Fistula — *continued*
　esophagus — *continued*
　　congenital — *continued*
　　　with atresia of esophagus Q39.1
　　ethmoid — *see* Sinusitis, ethmoidal
　eyeball (cornea) (sclera) — *see* Disorder, globe, hy-
　　potony
　eyelid H01.8
　fallopian tube, external N82.5
　fecal K63.2
　　congenital Q43.6
　from periapical abscess K04.6
　frontal sinus — *see* Sinusitis, frontal
　gallbladder K82.3
　　with calculus, cholelithiasis, stones — *see* Calculus,
　　　gallbladder
　gastric K31.6
　gastrocolic K31.6
　　congenital Q40.2
　　tuberculous A18.32
　gastroenterocolic K31.6
　gastroesophageal K31.6
　gastrojejunal K31.6
　gastrojejunocolic K31.6
　genital tract (female) N82.9
　　specified NEC N82.8
　　to intestine NEC N82.4
　　to skin N82.5
　hepatic artery-portal vein, congenital Q26.6
　hepatopleural J86.0
　hepatopulmonary J86.0
　ileorectal or ileosigmoidal K63.2
　ileovaginal N82.2
　ileovesical N32.1
　ileum K63.2
　in ano K60.3
　　tuberculous A18.32
　inner ear (labyrinth) — *see* subcategory H83.1 ☑
　intestine NEC K63.2
　intestinocolonic (abdominal) K63.2
　intestinoureteral N28.89
　intestinouterine N82.4
　intestinovaginal N82.4
　　large intestine N82.3
　　small intestine N82.2
　intestinovesical N32.1
　ischiorectal (fossa) K61.39
　jejunum K63.2
　joint M25.10
　　ankle M25.17- ☑
　　elbow M25.12- ☑
　　foot joint M25.17- ☑
　　hand joint M25.14- ☑
　　hip M25.15- ☑
　　knee M25.16- ☑
　　shoulder M25.11- ☑
　　specified joint NEC M25.18
　　tuberculous — *see* Tuberculosis, joint
　　vertebrae M25.18
　　wrist M25.13- ☑
　kidney N28.89
　labium (majus) (minus) N82.8
　labyrinth — *see* subcategory H83.1 ☑
　lacrimal (gland) (sac) H04.61- ☑
　lacrimonasal duct — *see* Fistula, lacrimal
　laryngotracheal, congenital Q34.8
　larynx J38.7
　lip K13.0
　　congenital Q38.0
　lumbar, tuberculous A18.01
　lung J86.0
　lymphatic I89.8
　mammary (gland) N61.0
　mastoid (process) (region) — *see* Mastoiditis, chronic
　maxillary J32.0
　medial, face and neck Q18.8
　mediastinal J86.0
　mediastinobronchial J86.0
　mediastinocutaneous J86.0
　middle ear — *see* subcategory H74.8 ☑
　mouth K12.2
　nasal J34.89
　　sinus — *see* Sinusitis
　nasopharynx J39.2
　nipple N64.0
　nose J34.89
　oral (cutaneous) K12.2
　　maxillary J32.0

Fistula — *continued*
　oral — *continued*
　　nasal (with cleft palate) — *see* Cleft, palate
　orbit, orbital — *see* Disorder, orbit, specified type NEC
　oroantral J32.0
　oviduct, external N82.5
　palate (hard) M27.8
　pancreatic K86.89
　pancreaticoduodenal K86.89
　parotid (gland) K11.4
　　region K12.2
　penis N48.89
　perianal K60.3
　pericardium (pleura) (sac) — *see* Pericarditis
　pericecal K63.2
　perineorectal K60.4
　perineosigmoidal K63.2
　perineum, perineal (with urethral involvement) NEC
　　N36.0
　　tuberculous A18.13
　　ureter N28.89
　perirectal K60.4
　　tuberculous A18.32
　peritoneum K65.9
　pharyngoesophageal J39.2
　pharynx J39.2
　　branchial cleft (congenital) Q18.0
　pilonidal (infected) (rectum) — *see* Sinus, pilonidal
　pleura, pleural, pleurocutaneous, pleuroperitoneal
　　J86.0
　　tuberculous NEC A15.6
　pleuropericardial I31.8
　portal vein-hepatic artery, congenital Q26.6
　postauricular H70.81- ☑
　postoperative, persistent T81.83 ☑
　　specified site — *see* Fistula, by site
　preauricular (congenital) Q18.1
　prostate N42.89
　pulmonary J86.0
　　arteriovenous I28.0
　　　congenital Q25.72
　　tuberculous — *see* Tuberculosis, pulmonary
　pulmonoperitoneal J86.0
　rectolabial N82.4
　rectosigmoid (intercommunicating) K63.2
　rectoureteral N28.89
　rectourethral N36.0
　　congenital Q64.73
　rectouterine N82.4
　　congenital Q51.7
　rectovaginal N82.3
　　congenital Q52.2
　　tuberculous A18.18
　rectovesical N32.1
　　congenital Q64.79
　rectovesicovaginal N82.3
　rectovulval N82.4
　　congenital Q52.79
　rectum (to skin) K60.4
　　congenital Q43.6
　　　with absence, atresia and stenosis Q42.0
　　tuberculous A18.32
　renal N28.89
　retroauricular — *see* Fistula, postauricular
　salivary duct or gland (any) K11.4
　　congenital Q38.4
　scrotum (urinary) N50.89
　　tuberculous A18.15
　semicircular canals — *see* subcategory H83.1 ☑
　sigmoid K63.2
　　to bladder N32.1
　sinus — *see* Sinusitis
　skin L98.8
　　to genital tract (female) N82.5
　splenocolic D73.89
　stercoral K63.2
　stomach K31.6
　sublingual gland K11.4
　submandibular gland K11.4
　submaxillary (gland) K11.4
　　region K12.2
　thoracic J86.0
　　duct I89.8
　thoracoabdominal J86.0
　thoracogastric J86.0
　thoracointestinal J86.0
　thorax J86.0
　thyroglossal duct Q89.2

Fistula — *continued*
- thyroid E07.89
- trachea, congenital (external) (internal) Q32.1
- tracheoesophageal J86.0
  - congenital Q39.2
    - with atresia of esophagus Q39.1
  - following tracheostomy J95.04
- traumatic arteriovenous — *see* Injury, blood vessel, by site
- tuberculous — *code by* site under Tuberculosis
- typhoid A01.09
- umbilicourinary Q64.8
- urachus, congenital Q64.4
- ureter (persistent) N28.89
- ureteroabdominal N28.89
- ureterorectal N28.89
- ureterosigmoido-abdominal N28.89
- ureterovaginal N82.1
- ureterovesical N32.2
- urethra N36.0
  - congenital Q64.79
  - tuberculous A18.13
- urethroperineal N36.0
- urethroperineovesical N32.2
- urethrorectal N36.0
  - congenital Q64.73
- urethroscrotal N50.89
- urethrovaginal N82.1
- urethrovesical N32.2
- urinary (tract) (persistent) (recurrent) N36.0
- uteroabdominal N82.5
  - congenital Q51.7
- uteroenteric, uterointestinal N82.4
  - congenital Q51.7
- uterorectal N82.4
  - congenital Q51.7
- uteroureteric N82.1
- uterourethral Q51.7
- uterovaginal N82.8
- uterovesical N82.1
  - congenital Q51.7
- uterus N82.8
- vagina (postpartal) (wall) N82.8
- vaginocutaneous (postpartal) N82.5
- vaginointestinal NEC N82.4
  - large intestine N82.3
  - small intestine N82.2
- vaginoperineal N82.5
- vasocutaneous, congenital Q55.7
- vesical NEC N32.2
- vesicoabdominal N32.2
- vesicocervicovaginal N82.1
- vesicocolic N32.1
- vesicocutaneous N32.2
- vesicoenteric N32.1
- vesicointestinal N32.1
- vesicometrorectal N82.4
- vesicoperineal N32.2
- vesicorectal N32.1
  - congenital Q64.79
- vesicosigmoidal N32.1
- vesicosigmoidovaginal N82.3
- vesicoureteral N32.2
- vesicoureterovaginal N82.1
- vesicourethral N32.2
- vesicourethrorectal N32.1
- vesicouterine N82.1
  - congenital Q51.7
- vesicovaginal N82.0
- vulvorectal N82.4
  - congenital Q52.79

Fit R56.9
- epileptic — *see* Epilepsy
- fainting R55
- hysterical F44.5
- newborn P90

Fitting (and adjustment) (of)
- artificial
  - arm — *see* Admission, adjustment, artificial, arm
  - breast Z44.3 ☑
  - eye Z44.2 ☑
  - leg — *see* Admission, adjustment, artificial, leg
- automatic implantable cardiac defibrillator (with synchronous cardiac pacemaker) Z45.02
- brain neuropacemaker Z46.2
  - implanted Z45.42
- cardiac defibrillator — *see* Fitting (and adjustment) (of), automatic implantable cardiac defibrillator

Fitting — *continued*
- catheter, non-vascular Z46.82
- colostomy belt Z46.89
- contact lenses Z46.0
- CRT-D (resynchronization therapy defibrillator) Z45.02
- CRT-P (cardiac resynchronization therapy pacemaker) Z45.018
  - pulse generator Z45.010
- cystostomy device Z46.6
- defibrillator, cardiac — *see* Fitting (and adjustment) (of), automatic implantable cardiac defibrillator
- dentures Z46.3
- device NOS Z46.9
  - abdominal Z46.89
  - gastrointestinal NEC Z46.59
  - implanted NEC Z45.89
  - nervous system Z46.2
    - implanted — *see* Admission, adjustment, device, implanted, nervous system
  - orthodontic Z46.4
  - orthoptic Z46.0
  - orthotic Z46.89
  - prosthetic (external) Z44.9
    - breast Z44.3 ☑
    - dental Z46.3
    - eye Z44.2 ☑
    - specified NEC Z44.8
  - specified NEC Z46.89
  - substitution
    - auditory Z46.2
      - implanted — *see* Admission, adjustment, device, implanted, hearing device
    - nervous system Z46.2
      - implanted — *see* Admission, adjustment, device, implanted, nervous system
    - visual Z46.2
      - implanted Z45.31
  - urinary Z46.6
- gastric lap band Z46.51
- gastrointestinal appliance NEC Z46.59
- glasses (reading) Z46.0
- hearing aid Z46.1
- ileostomy device Z46.89
- insulin pump Z46.81
- intestinal appliance NEC Z46.89
- myringotomy device (stent) (tube) Z45.82
- neuropacemaker Z46.2
  - implanted Z45.42
- non-vascular catheter Z46.82
- orthodontic device Z46.4
- orthopedic device (brace) (cast) (corset) (shoes) Z46.89
- pacemaker (cardiac) (cardiac resynchronization therapy (CRT-P)) Z45.018
  - nervous system (brain) (peripheral nerve) (spinal cord) Z46.2
    - implanted Z45.42
  - pulse generator Z45.010
- portacath (port-a-cath) Z45.2
- prosthesis (external) Z44.9
  - arm — *see* Admission, adjustment, artificial, arm
  - breast Z44.3 ☑
  - dental Z46.3
  - eye Z44.2 ☑
  - leg — *see* Admission, adjustment, artificial, leg
  - specified NEC Z44.8
- spectacles Z46.0
- wheelchair Z46.89

Fitzhugh-Curtis syndrome
- due to
  - Chlamydia trachomatis A74.81
  - Neisseria gonorrhorea (gonococcal peritonitis) A54.85

Fitz's syndrome (acute hemorrhagic pancreatitis) — *see also* Pancreatitis, acute K85.80

Fixation
- joint — *see* Ankylosis
- larynx J38.7
- stapes — *see* Ankylosis, ear ossicles
  - deafness — *see* Deafness, conductive
- uterus (acquired) — *see* Malposition, uterus
- vocal cord J38.3

Flabby ridge K06.8

Flaccid — *see also* condition
- palate, congenital Q38.5

Flail
- chest S22.5 ☑
  - newborn (birth injury) P13.8
- joint (paralytic) M25.20

Flail — *continued*
- joint — *continued*
  - ankle M25.27- ☑
  - elbow M25.22- ☑
  - foot joint M25.27- ☑
  - hand joint M25.24- ☑
  - hip M25.25- ☑
  - knee M25.26- ☑
  - shoulder M25.21- ☑
  - specified joint NEC M25.28
  - wrist M25.23- ☑

Flajani's disease — *see* Hyperthyroidism, with, goiter (diffuse)

Flap, liver K71.3

Flashbacks (residual to hallucinogen use) F16.283

Flat
- chamber (eye) — *see* Disorder, globe, hypotony, flat anterior chamber
- chest, congenital Q67.8
- foot (acquired) (fixed type) (painful) (postural) — *see also* Deformity, limb, flat foot
  - congenital (rigid) (spastic (everted)) Q66.5- ☑
  - rachitic sequelae (late effect) E64.3
- organ or site, congenital NEC — *see* Anomaly, by site
- pelvis M95.5
  - with disproportion (fetopelvic) O33.0
    - causing obstructed labor O65.0
  - congenital Q74.2

Flatau-Schilder disease G37.0

Flatback syndrome M40.30
- lumbar region M40.36
- lumbosacral region M40.37
- thoracolumbar region M40.35

Flattening
- head, femur M89.8X5
- hip — *see* Coxa, plana
- lip (congenital) Q18.8
- nose (congenital) Q67.4
  - acquired M95.0

Flatulence R14.3
- psychogenic F45.8

Flatus R14.3
- vaginalis N89.8

Flax-dresser's disease J66.1

Flea bite — *see* Injury, bite, by site, superficial, insect

Flecks, glaucomatous (subcapsular) — *see* Cataract, complicated

Fleischer (-Kayser) **ring** (cornea) H18.04- ☑

Fleshy mole O02.0

Flexibilitas cerea — *see* Catalepsy

Flexion
- amputation stump (surgical) T87.89
- cervix — *see* Malposition, uterus
- contracture, joint — *see* Contraction, joint
- deformity, joint — *see also* Deformity, limb, flexion M21.20
  - hip, congenital Q65.89
- uterus — *see also* Malposition, uterus
  - lateral — *see* Lateroversion, uterus

Flexner-Boyd dysentery A03.2

Flexner's dysentery A03.1

Flexure — *see* Flexion

Flint murmur (aortic insufficiency) I35.1

Floater, vitreous — *see* Opacity, vitreous

Floating
- cartilage (joint) — *see also* Loose, body, joint
  - knee — *see* Derangement, knee, loose body
- gallbladder, congenital Q44.1
- kidney N28.89
  - congenital Q63.8
- spleen D73.89

Flooding N92.0

Floor — *see* condition

Floppy
- baby syndrome (nonspecific) P94.2
- iris syndrome (intraoperative) (IFIS) H21.81
- nonrheumatic mitral valve syndrome I34.1

Flu — *see also* Influenza
- avian — *see also* Influenza, due to, identified novel influenza A virus J09.X2
- bird — *see also* Influenza, due to, identified novel influenza A virus J09.X2
- intestinal NEC A08.4
- swine (viruses that normally cause infections in pigs) — *see also* Influenza, due to, identified novel influenza A virus J09.X2

Fluctuating blood pressure I99.8

Fluid
  abdomen R18.8
  chest J94.8
  heart — *see* Failure, heart, congestive
  joint — *see* Effusion, joint
  loss (acute) E86.9
  lung — *see* Edema, lung
  overload E87.70
    specified NEC E87.79
  peritoneal cavity R18.8
  pleural cavity J94.8
  retention R60.9
Flukes NEC — *see also* Infestation, fluke
  blood NEC — *see* Schistosomiasis
  liver B66.3
Fluor (vaginalis) N89.8
  trichomonal or due to Trichomonas (vaginalis) A59.00
Fluorosis
  dental K00.3
  skeletal M85.10
    ankle M85.17- ☑
    foot M85.17- ☑
    forearm M85.13- ☑
    hand M85.14- ☑
    lower leg M85.16- ☑
    multiple site M85.19
    neck M85.18
    rib M85.18
    shoulder M85.11- ☑
    skull M85.18
    specified site NEC M85.18
    thigh M85.15- ☑
    toe M85.17- ☑
    upper arm M85.12- ☑
    vertebra M85.18
Flush syndrome E34.0
Flushing R23.2
  menopausal N95.1
Flutter
  atrial or auricular I48.92
    atypical I48.4
    type I I48.3
    type II I48.4
    typical I48.3
  heart I49.8
    atrial or auricular I48.92
      atypical I48.4
      type I I48.3
      type II I48.4
      typical I48.3
    ventricular I49.02
  ventricular I49.02
FNHTR (febrile nonhemolytic transfusion reaction) R50.84
Fochier's abscess — *code by* site under Abscess
Focus, Assmann's — *see* Tuberculosis, pulmonary
Fogo selvagem L10.3
Foix-Alajouanine syndrome G95.19
Fold, folds (anomalous) — *see also* Anomaly, by site
  Descemet's membrane — *see* Change, corneal membrane, Descemet's, fold
  epicanthic Q10.3
  heart Q24.8
Folie à deux F24
Follicle
  cervix (nabothian) (ruptured) N88.8
  graafian, ruptured, with hemorrhage N83.0- ☑
  nabothian N88.8
Follicular — *see* condition
Folliculitis (superficial) L73.9
  abscedens et suffodiens L66.3
  cyst N83.0- ☑
  decalvans L66.2
  deep — *see* Furuncle, by site
  gonococcal (acute) (chronic) A54.01
  keloid, keloidalis L73.0
  pustular L01.02
  ulerythematosa reticulata L66.4
Folliculome lipidique
  specified site — *see* Neoplasm, benign, by site
  unspecified site
    female D27.9
    male D29.20
Følling's disease E70.0
Follow-up — *see* Examination, follow-up
Fong's syndrome (hereditary osteo-onychodysplasia)
  Q87.2

Food
  allergy L27.2
  asphyxia (from aspiration or inhalation) — *see* Foreign body, by site
  choked on — *see* Foreign body, by site
  deprivation T73.0
    specified kind of food NEC E63.8
  intoxication — *see* Poisoning, food
  lack of T73.0 ☑
  poisoning — *see* Poisoning, food
  rejection NEC — *see* Disorder, eating
  strangulation or suffocation — *see* Foreign body, by site
  toxemia — *see* Poisoning, food
Foot — *see* condition
Foramen ovale (nonclosure) (patent) (persistent) Q21.1
Forbes' glycogen storage disease E74.03
Fordyce-Fox disease L75.2
Fordyce's disease (mouth) Q38.6
Forearm — *see* condition
Foreign body
  with
    laceration — *see* Laceration, by site, with foreign body
    puncture wound — *see* Puncture, by site, with foreign body
  accidentally left following a procedure T81.509 ☑
    aspiration T81.506 ☑
      resulting in
        adhesions T81.516 ☑
        obstruction T81.526 ☑
        perforation T81.536 ☑
        specified complication NEC T81.596 ☑
    cardiac catheterization T81.505 ☑
      resulting in
        acute reaction T81.60 ☑
          aseptic peritonitis T81.61 ☑
          specified NEC T81.69 ☑
        adhesions T81.515 ☑
        obstruction T81.525 ☑
        perforation T81.535 ☑
        specified complication NEC T81.595 ☑
      causing
        acute reaction T81.60 ☑
          aseptic peritonitis T81.61 ☑
          specified complication NEC T81.69 ☑
        adhesions T81.519 ☑
        aseptic peritonitis T81.61 ☑
        obstruction T81.529 ☑
        perforation T81.539 ☑
        specified complication NEC T81.599 ☑
    endoscopy T81.504 ☑
      resulting in
        adhesions T81.514 ☑
        obstruction T81.524 ☑
        perforation T81.534 ☑
        specified complication NEC T81.594 ☑
    immunization T81.503 ☑
      resulting in
        adhesions T81.513 ☑
        obstruction T81.523 ☑
        perforation T81.533 ☑
        specified complication NEC T81.593 ☑
    infusion T81.501 ☑
      resulting in
        adhesions T81.511 ☑
        obstruction T81.521 ☑
        perforation T81.531 ☑
        specified complication NEC T81.591 ☑
    injection T81.503 ☑
      resulting in
        adhesions T81.513 ☑
        obstruction T81.523 ☑
        perforation T81.533 ☑
        specified complication NEC T81.593 ☑
    kidney dialysis T81.502 ☑
      resulting in
        adhesions T81.512 ☑
        obstruction T81.522 ☑
        perforation T81.532 ☑
        specified complication NEC T81.592 ☑
    packing removal T81.507 ☑
      resulting in
        acute reaction T81.60 ☑
          aseptic peritonitis T81.61 ☑
          specified NEC T81.69 ☑

Foreign body — *continued*
  accidentally left following a procedure — *continued*
    packing removal — *continued*
      resulting in — *continued*
        adhesions T81.517 ☑
        obstruction T81.527 ☑
        perforation T81.537 ☑
        specified complication NEC T81.597 ☑
    puncture T81.506 ☑
      resulting in
        adhesions T81.516 ☑
        obstruction T81.526 ☑
        perforation T81.536 ☑
        specified complication NEC T81.596 ☑
    specified procedure NEC T81.508 ☑
      resulting in
        acute reaction T81.60 ☑
          aseptic peritonitis T81.61 ☑
          specified NEC T81.69 ☑
        adhesions T81.518 ☑
        obstruction T81.528 ☑
        perforation T81.538 ☑
        specified complication NEC T81.598 ☑
    surgical operation T81.500 ☑
      resulting in
        acute reaction T81.60 ☑
          aseptic peritonitis T81.61 ☑
          specified NEC T81.69 ☑
        adhesions T81.510 ☑
        obstruction T81.520 ☑
        perforation T81.530 ☑
        specified complication NEC T81.590 ☑
    transfusion T81.501 ☑
      resulting in
        adhesions T81.511 ☑
        obstruction T81.521 ☑
        perforation T81.531 ☑
        specified complication NEC T81.591 ☑
  alimentary tract T18.9 ☑
    anus T18.5 ☑
    colon T18.4 ☑
    esophagus — *see* Foreign body, esophagus
    mouth T18.0 ☑
    multiple sites T18.8 ☑
    rectosigmoid (junction) T18.5 ☑
    rectum T18.5 ☑
    small intestine T18.3 ☑
    specified site NEC T18.8 ☑
    stomach T18.2 ☑
  anterior chamber (eye) S05.5- ☑
  auditory canal — *see* Foreign body, entering through orifice, ear
  bronchus T17.508 ☑
    causing
      asphyxiation T17.500 ☑
        food (bone) (seed) T17.520 ☑
        gastric contents (vomitus) T17.510 ☑
        specified type NEC T17.590 ☑
      injury NEC T17.508 ☑
        food (bone) (seed) T17.528 ☑
        gastric contents (vomitus) T17.518 ☑
        specified type NEC T17.598 ☑
  canthus — *see* Foreign body, conjunctival sac
  ciliary body (eye) S05.5- ☑
  conjunctival sac T15.1- ☑
  cornea T15.0- ☑
  entering through orifice
    accessory sinus T17.0 ☑
    alimentary canal T18.9 ☑
      multiple parts T18.8 ☑
      specified part NEC T18.8 ☑
    alveolar process T18.0 ☑
    antrum (Highmore's) T17.0 ☑
    anus T18.5 ☑
    appendix T18.4 ☑
    auditory canal — *see* Foreign body, entering through orifice, ear
    auricle — *see* Foreign body, entering through orifice, ear
    bladder T19.1 ☑
    bronchioles — *see* Foreign body, respiratory tract, specified site NEC
    bronchus (main) — *see* Foreign body, bronchus
    buccal cavity T18.0 ☑
    canthus (inner) — *see* Foreign body, conjunctival sac

Foreign body — *continued*
  entering through orifice — *continued*
    cecum T18.4 ☑
    cervix (canal) (uteri) T19.3 ☑
    colon T18.4 ☑
    conjunctival sac — *see* Foreign body, conjunctival sac
    cornea — *see* Foreign body, cornea
    digestive organ or tract NOS T18.9 ☑
      multiple parts T18.8 ☑
      specified part NEC T18.8 ☑
    duodenum T18.3 ☑
    ear (external) T16.- ☑
    esophagus — *see* Foreign body, esophagus
    eye (external) NOS T15.9- ☑
      conjunctival sac — *see* Foreign body, conjunctival sac
      cornea — *see* Foreign body, cornea
      specified part NEC T15.8- ☑
    eyeball — *see also* Foreign body, entering through orifice, eye, specified part NEC
      with penetrating wound — *see* Puncture, eyeball
    eyelid — *see also* Foreign body, conjunctival sac
      with
        laceration — *see* Laceration, eyelid, with foreign body
        puncture — *see* Puncture, eyelid, with foreign body
        superficial injury — *see* Foreign body, superficial, eyelid
    gastrointestinal tract T18.9 ☑
      multiple parts T18.8 ☑
      specified part NEC T18.8 ☑
    genitourinary tract T19.9 ☑
      multiple parts T19.8 ☑
      specified part NEC T19.8 ☑
    globe — *see* Foreign body, entering through orifice, eyeball
    gum T18.0 ☑
    Highmore's antrum T17.0 ☑
    hypopharynx — *see* Foreign body, pharynx
    ileum T18.3 ☑
    intestine (small) T18.3 ☑
      large T18.4 ☑
    lacrimal apparatus (punctum) — *see* Foreign body, entering through orifice, eye, specified part NEC
    large intestine T18.4 ☑
    larynx — *see* Foreign body, larynx
    lung — *see* Foreign body, respiratory tract, specified site NEC
    maxillary sinus T17.0 ☑
    mouth T18.0 ☑
    nasal sinus T17.0 ☑
    nasopharynx — *see* Foreign body, pharynx
    nose (passage) T17.1 ☑
    nostril T17.1 ☑
    oral cavity T18.0 ☑
    palate T18.0 ☑
    penis T19.4 ☑
    pharynx — *see* Foreign body, pharynx
    piriform sinus — *see* Foreign body, pharynx
    rectosigmoid (junction) T18.5 ☑
    rectum T18.5 ☑
    respiratory tract — *see* Foreign body, respiratory tract
    sinus (accessory) (frontal) (maxillary) (nasal) T17.0 ☑
      piriform — *see* Foreign body, pharynx
    small intestine T18.3 ☑
    stomach T18.2 ☑
    suffocation by — *see* Foreign body, by site
    tear ducts or glands — *see* Foreign body, entering through orifice, eye, specified part NEC
    throat — *see* Foreign body, pharynx
    tongue T18.0 ☑
    tonsil, tonsillar (fossa) — *see* Foreign body, pharynx
    trachea — *see* Foreign body, trachea
    ureter T19.8 ☑
    urethra T19.0 ☑
    uterus (any part) T19.3 ☑
    vagina T19.2 ☑
    vulva T19.2 ☑
  esophagus T18.108 ☑
    causing
      injury NEC T18.108 ☑
        food (bone) (seed) T18.128 ☑

Foreign body — *continued*
  esophagus — *continued*
    causing — *continued*
      injury — *continued*
        gastric contents (vomitus) T18.118 ☑
        specified type NEC T18.198 ☑
      tracheal compression T18.100 ☑
        food (bone) (seed) T18.120 ☑
        gastric contents (vomitus) T18.110 ☑
        specified type NEC T18.190 ☑
  feeling of, in throat R09.89
  fragment — *see* Retained, foreign body fragments (type of)
  genitourinary tract T19.9 ☑
    bladder T19.1 ☑
    multiple parts T19.8 ☑
    penis T19.4 ☑
    specified site NEC T19.8 ☑
    urethra T19.0 ☑
    uterus T19.3 ☑
      IUD Z97.5
    vagina T19.2 ☑
      contraceptive device Z97.5
    vulva T19.2 ☑
  granuloma (old) (soft tissue) — *see also* Granuloma, foreign body
    skin L92.3
  in
    laceration — *see* Laceration, by site, with foreign body
    puncture wound — *see* Puncture, by site, with foreign body
    soft tissue (residual) M79.5
  inadvertently left in operation wound — *see* Foreign body, accidentally left during a procedure
  ingestion, ingested NOS T18.9 ☑
  inhalation or inspiration — *see* Foreign body, by site
  internal organ, not entering through a natural orifice — code as specific injury with foreign body
  intraocular S05.5- ☑
    old, retained (nonmagnetic) H44.70- ☑
      anterior chamber H44.71- ☑
      ciliary body H44.72- ☑
      iris H44.72- ☑
      lens H44.73- ☑
      magnetic H44.60- ☑
        anterior chamber H44.61- ☑
        ciliary body H44.62- ☑
        iris H44.62- ☑
        lens H44.63- ☑
        posterior wall H44.64- ☑
        specified site NEC H44.69- ☑
        vitreous body H44.65- ☑
      posterior wall H44.74- ☑
      specified site NEC H44.79- ☑
      vitreous body H44.75- ☑
  iris — *see* Foreign body, intraocular
  lacrimal punctum — *see* Foreign body, entering through orifice, eye, specified part NEC
  larynx T17.308 ☑
    causing
      asphyxiation T17.300 ☑
        food (bone) (seed) T17.320 ☑
        gastric contents (vomitus) T17.310 ☑
        specified type NEC T17.390 ☑
      injury NEC T17.308 ☑
        food (bone) (seed) T17.328 ☑
        gastric contents (vomitus) T17.318 ☑
        specified type NEC T17.398 ☑
  lens — *see* Foreign body, intraocular
  ocular muscle S05.4- ☑
    old, retained — *see* Foreign body, orbit, old
  old or residual
    soft tissue (residual) M79.5
  operation wound, left accidentally — *see* Foreign body, accidentally left during a procedure
  orbit S05.4- ☑
    old, retained H05.5- ☑
  pharynx T17.208 ☑
    causing
      asphyxiation T17.200 ☑
        food (bone) (seed) T17.220 ☑
        gastric contents (vomitus) T17.210 ☑
        specified type NEC T17.290 ☑
      injury NEC T17.208 ☑
        food (bone) (seed) T17.228 ☑

Foreign body — *continued*
  pharynx — *continued*
    causing — *continued*
      injury — *continued*
        gastric contents (vomitus) T17.218 ☑
        specified type NEC T17.298 ☑
  respiratory tract T17.908 ☑
    bronchioles — *see* Foreign body, respiratory tract, specified site NEC
    bronchus — *see* Foreign body, bronchus
    causing
      asphyxiation T17.900 ☑
        food (bone) (seed) T17.920 ☑
        gastric contents (vomitus) T17.910 ☑
        specified type NEC T17.990 ☑
      injury NEC T17.908 ☑
        food (bone) (seed) T17.928 ☑
        gastric contents (vomitus) T17.918 ☑
        specified type NEC T17.998 ☑
    larynx — *see* Foreign body, larynx
    lung — *see* Foreign body, respiratory tract, specified site NEC
    multiple parts — *see* Foreign body, respiratory tract, specified site NEC
    nasal sinus T17.0 ☑
    nasopharynx — *see* Foreign body, pharynx
    nose T17.1 ☑
    nostril T17.1 ☑
    pharynx — *see* Foreign body, pharynx
    specified site NEC T17.808 ☑
      causing
        asphyxiation T17.800 ☑
          food (bone) (seed) T17.820 ☑
          gastric contents (vomitus) T17.810 ☑
          specified type NEC T17.890 ☑
        injury NEC T17.808 ☑
          food (bone) (seed) T17.828 ☑
          gastric contents (vomitus) T17.818 ☑
          specified type NEC T17.898 ☑
    throat — *see* Foreign body, pharynx
    trachea — *see* Foreign body, trachea
  retained (old) (nonmagnetic) (in)
    anterior chamber (eye) — *see* Foreign body, intraocular, old, retained, anterior chamber
      magnetic — *see* Foreign body, intraocular, old, retained, magnetic, anterior chamber
    ciliary body — *see* Foreign body, intraocular, old, retained, ciliary body
      magnetic — *see* Foreign body, intraocular, old, retained, magnetic, ciliary body
    eyelid H02.819
      left H02.816
        lower H02.815
        upper H02.814
      right H02.813
        lower H02.812
        upper H02.811
    fragments — *see* Retained, foreign body fragments (type of)
    globe — *see* Foreign body, intraocular, old, retained
      magnetic — *see* Foreign body, intraocular, old, retained, magnetic
    intraocular — *see* Foreign body, intraocular, old, retained
      magnetic — *see* Foreign body, intraocular, old, retained, magnetic
    iris — *see* Foreign body, intraocular, old, retained, iris
      magnetic — *see* Foreign body, intraocular, old, retained, magnetic, iris
    lens — *see* Foreign body, intraocular, old, retained, lens
      magnetic — *see* Foreign body, intraocular, old, retained, magnetic, lens
    muscle — *see* Foreign body, retained, soft tissue
    orbit — *see* Foreign body, orbit, old
    posterior wall of globe — *see* Foreign body, intraocular, old, retained, posterior wall
      magnetic — *see* Foreign body, intraocular, old, retained, magnetic, posterior wall
    retrobulbar — *see* Foreign body, orbit, old, retrobulbar
    soft tissue M79.5
    vitreous — *see* Foreign body, intraocular, old, retained, vitreous body
      magnetic — *see* Foreign body, intraocular, old, retained, magnetic, vitreous body

☑ Additional Character Required — Refer to the Tabular List for Character Selection   ▽ Subterms under main terms may continue to next column or page

Foreign body — *continued*
retina S05.5- ☑
superficial, without open wound
abdomen, abdominal (wall) S30.851 ☑
alveolar process S00.552 ☑
ankle S90.55- ☑
antecubital space — *see* Foreign body, superficial, forearm
anus S30.857 ☑
arm (upper) S40.85- ☑
auditory canal — *see* Foreign body, superficial, ear
auricle — *see* Foreign body, superficial, ear
axilla — *see* Foreign body, superficial, arm
back, lower S30.850 ☑
breast S20.15- ☑
brow S00.85 ☑
buttock S30.850 ☑
calf — *see* Foreign body, superficial, leg
canthus — *see* Foreign body, superficial, eyelid
cheek S00.85 ☑
internal S00.552 ☑
chest wall — *see* Foreign body, superficial, thorax
chin S00.85 ☑
clitoris S30.854 ☑
costal region — *see* Foreign body, superficial, thorax
digit(s)
foot — *see* Foreign body, superficial, toe
hand — *see* Foreign body, superficial, finger
ear S00.45- ☑
elbow S50.35- ☑
epididymis S30.853 ☑
epigastric region S30.851 ☑
epiglottis S10.15 ☑
esophagus, cervical S10.15 ☑
eyebrow — *see* Foreign body, superficial, eyelid
eyelid S00.25- ☑
face S00.85 ☑
finger(s) S60.459 ☑
index S60.45- ☑
little S60.45- ☑
middle S60.45- ☑
ring S60.45- ☑
flank S30.851 ☑
foot (except toe(s) alone) S90.85- ☑
toe — *see* Foreign body, superficial, toe
forearm S50.85- ☑
elbow only — *see* Foreign body, superficial, elbow
forehead S00.85 ☑
genital organs, external
female S30.856 ☑
male S30.855 ☑
groin S30.851 ☑
gum S00.552 ☑
hand S60.55- ☑
head S00.95 ☑
ear — *see* Foreign body, superficial, ear
eyelid — *see* Foreign body, superficial, eyelid
lip S00.551 ☑
nose S00.35 ☑
oral cavity S00.552 ☑
scalp S00.05 ☑
specified site NEC S00.85 ☑
heel — *see* Foreign body, superficial, foot
hip S70.25- ☑
inguinal region S30.851 ☑
interscapular region S20.459 ☑
jaw S00.85 ☑
knee S80.25- ☑
labium (majus) (minus) S30.854 ☑
larynx S10.15 ☑
leg (lower) S80.85- ☑
knee — *see* Foreign body, superficial, knee
upper — *see* Foreign body, superficial, thigh
lip S00.551 ☑
lower back S30.850 ☑
lumbar region S30.850 ☑
malar region S00.85 ☑
mammary — *see* Foreign body, superficial, breast
mastoid region S00.85 ☑
mouth S00.552 ☑
nail
finger — *see* Foreign body, superficial, finger
toe — *see* Foreign body, superficial, toe
nape S10.85 ☑
nasal S00.35 ☑

Foreign body — *continued*
superficial, without open wound — *continued*
neck S10.95 ☑
specified site NEC S10.85 ☑
throat S10.15 ☑
nose S00.35 ☑
occipital region S00.05 ☑
oral cavity S00.552 ☑
orbital region — *see* Foreign body, superficial, eyelid
palate S00.552 ☑
palm — *see* Foreign body, superficial, hand
parietal region S00.05 ☑
pelvis S30.850 ☑
penis S30.852 ☑
perineum
female S30.854 ☑
male S30.850 ☑
periocular area — *see* Foreign body, superficial, eyelid
phalanges
finger — *see* Foreign body, superficial, finger
toe — *see* Foreign body, superficial, toe
pharynx S10.15 ☑
pinna — *see* Foreign body, superficial, ear
popliteal space — *see* Foreign body, superficial, knee
prepuce S30.852 ☑
pubic region S30.850 ☑
pudendum
female S30.856 ☑
male S30.855 ☑
sacral region S30.850 ☑
scalp S00.05 ☑
scapular region — *see* Foreign body, superficial, shoulder
scrotum S30.853 ☑
shin — *see* Foreign body, superficial, leg
shoulder S40.25- ☑
sternal region S20.359 ☑
submaxillary region S00.85 ☑
submental region S00.85 ☑
subungual
finger(s) — *see* Foreign body, superficial, finger
toe(s) — *see* Foreign body, superficial, toe
supraclavicular fossa S10.85 ☑
supraorbital S00.85 ☑
temple S00.85 ☑
temporal region S00.85 ☑
testis S30.853 ☑
thigh S70.35- ☑
thorax, thoracic (wall) S20.95 ☑
back S20.45- ☑
front S20.35- ☑
throat S10.15 ☑
thumb S60.35- ☑
toe(s) (lesser) S90.456 ☑
great S90.45- ☑
tongue S00.552 ☑
trachea S10.15 ☑
tunica vaginalis S30.853 ☑
tympanum, tympanic membrane — *see* Foreign body, superficial, ear
uvula S00.552 ☑
vagina S30.854 ☑
vocal cords S10.15 ☑
vulva S30.854 ☑
wrist S60.85- ☑
swallowed T18.9 ☑
trachea T17.408 ☑
causing
asphyxiation T17.400 ☑
food (bone) (seed) T17.420 ☑
gastric contents (vomitus) T17.410 ☑
specified type NEC T17.490 ☑
injury NEC T17.408 ☑
food (bone) (seed) T17.428 ☑
gastric contents (vomitus) T17.418 ☑
specified type NEC T17.498 ☑
type of fragment — *see* Retained, foreign body fragments (type of)
vitreous (humor) S05.5- ☑
Forestier's disease (rhizomelic pseudopolyarthritis) M35.3
meaning ankylosing hyperostosis — *see* Hyperostosis, ankylosing

Formation
hyalin in cornea — *see* Degeneration, cornea
sequestrum in bone (due to infection) — *see* Osteomyelitis, chronic
valve
colon, congenital Q43.8
ureter (congenital) Q62.39
Formication R20.2
Fort Bragg fever A27.89
Fossa — *see also* condition
pyriform — *see* condition
Foster-Kennedy syndrome H47.14- ☑
Fothergill's
disease (trigeminal neuralgia) — *see also* Neuralgia, trigeminal
scarlatina anginosa A38.9
Foul breath R19.6
Foundling Z76.1
Fournier disease or gangrene N49.3
female N76.89
Fourth
cranial nerve — *see* condition
molar K00.1
Foville's (peduncular) **disease or syndrome** G46.3
Fox (-Fordyce) disease (apocrine miliaria) L75.2
FPIES (food protein-induced enterocolitis syndrome) K52.21
Fracture, burst — *see* Fracture, traumatic, by site
Fracture, chronic — *see* Fracture, pathological, by site
Fracture, insufficiency — *see* Fracture, pathological, by site
Fracture, nontraumatic, NEC
atypical
femur M84.750- ☑
complete
oblique M84.759 ☑
left side M84.758 ☑
right side M84.757 ☑
transverse M84.756 ☑
left side M84.755 ☑
right side M84.754 ☑
incomplete M84.753 ☑
left side M84.752 ☑
right side M84.751 ☑
Fracture, pathological (pathologic) — *see also* Fracture, traumatic M84.40 ☑
ankle M84.47- ☑
carpus M84.44- ☑
clavicle M84.41- ☑
compression (not due to trauma) — *see also* Collapse, vertebra M48.50- ☑
dental implant M27.63
dental restorative material K08.539
with loss of material K08.531
without loss of material K08.530
due to
neoplastic disease NEC — *see also* Neoplasm M84.50 ☑
ankle M84.57- ☑
carpus M84.54- ☑
clavicle M84.51- ☑
femur M84.55- ☑
fibula M84.56- ☑
finger M84.54- ☑
hip M84.559 ☑
humerus M84.52- ☑
ilium M84.550 ☑
ischium M84.550 ☑
metacarpus M84.54- ☑
metatarsus M84.57- ☑
neck M84.58 ☑
pelvis M84.550 ☑
radius M84.53- ☑
rib M84.58 ☑
scapula M84.51- ☑
skull M84.58 ☑
specified site NEC M84.58 ☑
tarsus M84.57- ☑
tibia M84.56- ☑
toe M84.57- ☑
ulna M84.53- ☑
vertebra M84.58 ☑
osteoporosis M80.00 ☑
disuse — *see* Osteoporosis, specified type NEC, with pathological fracture

Fracture, pathological — *continued*
  due to — *continued*
    osteoporosis — *continued*
      drug-induced — *see* Osteoporosis, drug induced, with pathological fracture
      idiopathic — *see* Osteoporosis, specified type NEC, with pathological fracture
      postmenopausal — *see* Osteoporosis, post-menopausal, with pathological fracture
      postoophorectomy — *see* Osteoporosis, post-toophorectomy, with pathological fracture
      postsurgical malabsorption — *see* Osteoporosis, specified type NEC, with pathological fracture
      specified cause NEC — *see* Osteoporosis, specified type NEC, with pathological fracture
    specified disease NEC M84.60 ☑
      ankle M84.67- ☑
      carpus M84.64- ☑
      clavicle M84.61- ☑
      femur M84.65- ☑
      fibula M84.66- ☑
      finger M84.64- ☑
      hip M84.65- ☑
      humerus M84.62- ☑
      ilium M84.650 ☑
      ischium M84.650 ☑
      metacarpus M84.64- ☑
      metatarsus M84.67- ☑
      neck M84.68 ☑
      radius M84.63- ☑
      rib M84.68 ☑
      scapula M84.61- ☑
      skull M84.68 ☑
      tarsus M84.67- ☑
      tibia M84.66- ☑
      toe M84.67- ☑
      ulna M84.63- ☑
      vertebra M84.68 ☑
  femur M84.45- ☑
  fibula M84.46- ☑
  finger M84.44- ☑
  hip M84.459 ☑
  humerus M84.42- ☑
  ilium M84.454 ☑
  ischium M84.454 ☑
  joint prosthesis — *see* Complications, joint prosthesis, mechanical, breakdown, by site
    periprosthetic — *see* Fracture, pathological, periprosthetic
  metacarpus M84.44- ☑
  metatarsus M84.47- ☑
  neck M84.48 ☑
  pelvis M84.454 ☑
  periprosthetic M97.9 ☑
    ankle M97.2- ☑
    elbow M97.4- ☑
    finger M97.8 ☑
    hip M97.0- ☑
    knee M97.1- ☑
    other specified joint M97.8 ☑
    shoulder M97.3- ☑
    spinal joint M97.8 ☑
    toe joint M97.8 ☑
    wrist joint M97.8 ☑
  radius M84.43- ☑
  restorative material (dental) K08.539
    with loss of material K08.531
    without loss of material K08.530
  rib M84.48 ☑
  scapula M84.41- ☑
  skull M84.48 ☑
  tarsus M84.47- ☑
  tibia M84.46- ☑
  toe M84.47- ☑
  ulna M84.43- ☑
  vertebra M84.48 ☑

Fracture, traumatic (abduction) (adduction) (separation) — *see also* Fracture, pathological T14.8 ☑
  acetabulum S32.40- ☑
    column
      anterior (displaced) (iliopubic) S32.43- ☑
        nondisplaced S32.436
      posterior (displaced) (ilioischial) S32.443 ☑
        nondisplaced S32.44- ☑
    dome (displaced) S32.48- ☑

Fracture, traumatic — *continued*
  acetabulum — *continued*
    dome — *continued*
      nondisplaced S32.48 ☑
      specified NEC S32.49- ☑
      transverse (displaced) S32.45- ☑
        with associated posterior wall fracture (displaced) S32.46- ☑
          nondisplaced S32.46- ☑
        nondisplaced S32.45- ☑
      wall
        anterior (displaced) S32.41- ☑
          nondisplaced S32.41- ☑
        medial (displaced) S32.47- ☑
          nondisplaced S32.47- ☑
        posterior (displaced) S32.42- ☑
          with associated transverse fracture (displaced) S32.46- ☑
            nondisplaced S32.46- ☑
          nondisplaced S32.42- ☑
  acromion — *see* Fracture, scapula, acromial process
  ankle S82.899 ☑
    bimalleolar (displaced) S82.84- ☑
      nondisplaced S82.84- ☑
    lateral malleolus only (displaced) S82.6- ☑
      nondisplaced S82.6- ☑
    medial malleolus (displaced) S82.5- ☑
      associated with Maisonneuve's fracture — *see* Fracture, Maisonneuve's
      nondisplaced S82.5- ☑
    talus — *see* Fracture, tarsal, talus
    trimalleolar (displaced) S82.85- ☑
      nondisplaced S82.85- ☑
  arm (upper) — *see also* Fracture, humerus, shaft
    humerus — *see* Fracture, humerus
    radius — *see* Fracture, radius
    ulna — *see* Fracture, ulna
  astragalus — *see* Fracture, tarsal, talus
  atlas — *see* Fracture, neck, cervical vertebra, first
  axis — *see* Fracture, neck, cervical vertebra, second
  back — *see* Fracture, vertebra
  Barton's — *see* Barton's fracture
  base of skull — *see* Fracture, skull, base
  basicervical (basal) (femoral) S72.0 ☑
  Bennett's — *see* Bennett's fracture
  bimalleolar — *see* Fracture, ankle, bimalleolar
  blow-out S02.3- ☑
  bone NEC T14.8 ☑
    birth injury P13.9
    following insertion of orthopedic implant, joint prosthesis or bone plate — *see* Fracture, following insertion of orthopedic implant, joint prosthesis or bone plate
    in (due to) neoplastic disease NEC — *see* Fracture, pathological, due to, neoplastic disease
    pathological (cause unknown) — *see* Fracture, pathological
  breast bone — *see* Fracture, sternum
  bucket handle (semilunar cartilage) — *see* Tear, meniscus
  burst — *see* Fracture, traumatic, by site
  calcaneus — *see* Fracture, tarsal, calcaneus
  carpal bone(s) S62.10- ☑
    capitate (displaced) S62.13- ☑
      nondisplaced S62.13- ☑
    cuneiform — *see* Fracture, carpal bone, triquetrum
    hamate (body) (displaced) S62.143 ☑
      hook process (displaced) S62.15- ☑
        nondisplaced S62.15- ☑
      nondisplaced S62.14- ☑
    larger multangular — *see* Fracture, carpal bones, trapezium
    lunate (displaced) S62.12- ☑
      nondisplaced S62.12- ☑
    navicular S62.00- ☑
      distal pole (displaced) S62.01- ☑
        nondisplaced S62.01- ☑
      middle third (displaced) S62.02- ☑
        nondisplaced S62.02- ☑
      proximal third (displaced) S62.03- ☑
        nondisplaced S62.03- ☑
      volar tuberosity — *see* Fracture, carpal bones, navicular, distal pole
    os magnum — *see* Fracture, carpal bones, capitate
    pisiform (displaced) S62.16- ☑
      nondisplaced S62.16- ☑

Fracture, traumatic — *continued*
  carpal bone(s) — *continued*
    semilunar — *see* Fracture, carpal bones, lunate
    smaller multangular — *see* Fracture, carpal bones, trapezoid
    trapezium (displaced) S62.17- ☑
      nondisplaced S62.17- ☑
    trapezoid (displaced) S62.18- ☑
      nondisplaced S62.18- ☑
    triquetrum (displaced) S62.11- ☑
      nondisplaced S62.11- ☑
    unciform — *see* Fracture, carpal bones, hamate
  cervical — *see* Fracture, vertebra, cervical
  clavicle S42.00- ☑
    acromial end (displaced) S42.03- ☑
      nondisplaced S42.03- ☑
    birth injury P13.4
    lateral end — *see* Fracture, clavicle, acromial end
    shaft (displaced) S42.02- ☑
      nondisplaced S42.02- ☑
    sternal end (anterior) (displaced) S42.01- ☑
      nondisplaced S42.01- ☑
      posterior S42.01- ☑
  coccyx S32.2 ☑
  collapsed — *see* Collapse, vertebra
  collar bone — *see* Fracture, clavicle
  Colles' — *see* Colles' fracture
  coronoid process — *see* Fracture, ulna, upper end, coronoid process
  corpus cavernosum penis S39.840 ☑
  costochondral cartilage S23.41 ☑
  costochondral, costosternal junction — *see* Fracture, rib
  cranium — *see* Fracture, skull
  cricoid cartilage S12.8 ☑
  cuboid (ankle) — *see* Fracture, tarsal, cuboid
  cuneiform
    foot — *see* Fracture, tarsal, cuneiform
    wrist — *see* Fracture, carpal, triquetrum
  delayed union — *see* Delay, union, fracture
  dental restorative material K08.539
    with loss of material K08.531
    without loss of material K08.530
  due to
    birth injury — *see* Birth, injury, fracture
    osteoporosis — *see* Osteoporosis, with fracture
  Dupuytren's — *see* Fracture, ankle, lateral malleolus
  elbow S42.40- ☑
  ethmoid (bone) (sinus) — *see* Fracture, skull, base
  face bone S02.92 ☑
  fatigue — *see also* Fracture, stress
    vertebra M48.40 ☑
      cervical region M48.42 ☑
      cervicothoracic region M48.43 ☑
      lumbar region M48.46 ☑
      lumbosacral region M48.47 ☑
      occipito-atlanto-axial region M48.41 ☑
      sacrococcygeal region M48.48 ☑
      thoracic region M48.44 ☑
      thoracolumbar region M48.45 ☑
  femur, femoral S72.9- ☑
    basicervical (basal) S72.0 ☑
    birth injury P13.2
    capital epiphyseal S79.01- ☑
    condyles, epicondyles — *see* Fracture, femur, lower end
    distal end — *see* Fracture, femur, lower end
    epiphysis
      head — *see* Fracture, femur, upper end, epiphysis
      lower — *see* Fracture, femur, lower end, epiphysis
      upper — *see* Fracture, femur, upper end, epiphysis
    following insertion of implant, prosthesis or plate M96.66- ☑
    head — *see* Fracture, femur, upper end, head
    intertrochanteric — *see* Fracture, femur, trochanteric
    intratrochanteric — *see* Fracture, femur, trochanteric
    lower end S72.40- ☑
      condyle (displaced) S72.41- ☑
        lateral (displaced) S72.42- ☑
          nondisplaced S72.42- ☑
        medial (displaced) S72.43- ☑
          nondisplaced S72.43- ☑

Fracture, traumatic — *continued*
- humerus — *continued*
  - lower end — *continued*
    - supracondylar (simple) (displaced) S42.41- ☑
      - with intercondylar fracture — *see* Fracture, humerus, lower end
      - comminuted (displaced) S42.42- ☑
        - nondisplaced S42.42- ☑
      - nondisplaced S42.41- ☑
    - torus S42.48- ☑
    - transcondylar (displaced) S42.47- ☑
      - nondisplaced S42.47- ☑
  - proximal end — *see* Fracture, humerus, upper end
  - shaft S42.30- ☑
    - comminuted (displaced) S42.35- ☑
      - nondisplaced S42.35- ☑
    - greenstick S42.31- ☑
    - oblique (displaced) S42.33- ☑
      - nondisplaced S42.33- ☑
    - segmental (displaced) S42.36- ☑
      - nondisplaced S42.36- ☑
    - specified NEC S42.39- ☑
    - spiral (displaced) S42.34- ☑
      - nondisplaced S42.34- ☑
    - transverse (displaced) S42.32- ☑
      - nondisplaced S42.32- ☑
  - supracondylar — *see* Fracture, humerus, lower end
  - surgical neck — *see* Fracture, humerus, upper end, surgical neck
  - trochlea — *see* Fracture, humerus, lower end, condyle, medial
  - tuberosity — *see* Fracture, humerus, upper end
  - upper end S42.20- ☑
    - anatomical neck — *see* Fracture, humerus, upper end, specified NEC
    - articular head — *see* Fracture, humerus, upper end, specified NEC
    - epiphysis — *see* Fracture, humerus, upper end, physeal
    - greater tuberosity (displaced) S42.25- ☑
      - nondisplaced S42.25- ☑
    - lesser tuberosity (displaced) S42.26- ☑
      - nondisplaced S42.26- ☑
    - physeal S49.00- ☑
      - Salter-Harris
        - Type I S49.01- ☑
        - Type II S49.02- ☑
        - Type III S49.03- ☑
        - Type IV S49.04- ☑
      - specified NEC S49.09- ☑
    - specified NEC (displaced) S42.29- ☑
      - nondisplaced S42.29- ☑
    - surgical neck (displaced) S42.21- ☑
      - four-part S42.24- ☑
      - nondisplaced S42.21- ☑
      - three-part S42.23- ☑
      - two-part (displaced) S42.22- ☑
        - nondisplaced S42.22- ☑
    - torus S42.27- ☑
    - transepiphyseal — *see* Fracture, humerus, upper end, physeal
- hyoid bone S12.8 ☑
- ilium S32.30- ☑
  - with disruption of pelvic ring — *see* Disruption, pelvic ring
  - avulsion (displaced) S32.31- ☑
    - nondisplaced S32.31- ☑
  - specified NEC S32.39- ☑
- impaction, impacted — *code as* Fracture, by site
- innominate bone — *see* Fracture, ilium
- instep — *see* Fracture, foot
- ischium S32.60- ☑
  - with disruption of pelvic ring — *see* Disruption, pelvic ring
  - avulsion (displaced) S32.61- ☑
    - nondisplaced S32.61- ☑
  - specified NEC S32.69- ☑
- jaw (bone) (lower) — *see* Fracture, mandible
  - upper — *see* Fracture, maxilla
- joint prosthesis — *see* Complications, joint prosthesis, mechanical, breakdown, by site
  - periprosthetic — *see* Fracture, traumatic, periprosthetic
- knee cap — *see* Fracture, patella
- larynx S12.8 ☑
- late effects — *see* Sequelae, fracture

Fracture, traumatic — *continued*
- leg (lower) S82.9- ☑
  - ankle — *see* Fracture, ankle
  - femur — *see* Fracture, femur
  - fibula — *see* Fracture, fibula
  - malleolus — *see* Fracture, ankle
  - patella — *see* Fracture, patella
  - specified site NEC S82.89- ☑
  - tibia — *see* Fracture, tibia
- lumbar spine — *see* Fracture, vertebra, lumbar
- lumbosacral spine S32.9 ☑
- Maisonneuve's (displaced) S82.86- ☑
  - nondisplaced S82.86- ☑
- malar bone — *see also* Fracture, maxilla S02.400 ☑
  - left side S02.40B ☑
  - right side S02.40A ☑
- malleolus — *see* Fracture, ankle
- malunion — *see* Fracture, by site
- mandible (lower jaw (bone)) S02.609 ☑
  - alveolus S02.67- ☑
  - angle (of jaw) S02.65- ☑
  - body, unspecified S02.600 ☑
    - left side S02.602 ☑
    - right side S02.601 ☑
  - condylar process S02.61- ☑
  - coronoid process S02.63- ☑
  - ramus, unspecified S02.64- ☑
  - specified site NEC S02.69 ☑
  - subcondylar process S02.62- ☑
  - symphysis S02.66 ☑
- manubrium (sterni) S22.21 ☑
  - dissociation from sternum S22.23 ☑
- march — *see* Fracture, traumatic, stress, by site
- maxilla, maxillary (bone) (sinus) (superior) (upper jaw) S02.401 ☑
  - alveolus S02.42 ☑
  - inferior — *see* Fracture, mandible
  - LeFort I S02.411 ☑
  - LeFort II S02.412 ☑
  - LeFort III S02.413 ☑
  - left side S02.40D ☑
  - right side S02.40C ☑
- metacarpal S62.309 ☑
  - base (displaced) S62.319 ☑
    - nondisplaced S62.349 ☑
  - fifth S62.30- ☑
    - base (displaced) S62.31- ☑
      - nondisplaced S62.34- ☑
    - neck (displaced) S62.33- ☑
      - nondisplaced S62.36- ☑
    - shaft (displaced) S62.32- ☑
      - nondisplaced S62.35- ☑
    - specified NEC S62.398 ☑
  - first S62.20- ☑
    - base NEC (displaced) S62.23- ☑
      - nondisplaced S62.23- ☑
    - Bennett's — *see* Bennett's fracture
    - neck (displaced) S62.25- ☑
      - nondisplaced S62.25- ☑
    - shaft (displaced) S62.24- ☑
      - nondisplaced S62.24 ☑
    - specified NEC S62.29- ☑
  - fourth S62.30- ☑
    - base (displaced) S62.31- ☑
      - nondisplaced S62.34- ☑
    - neck (displaced) S62.33- ☑
      - nondisplaced S62.36- ☑
    - shaft (displaced) S62.32- ☑
      - nondisplaced S62.35- ☑
    - specified NEC S62.39- ☑
  - neck (displaced) S62.33- ☑
    - nondisplaced S62.36- ☑
  - Rolando's — *see* Rolando's fracture
  - second S62.30- ☑
    - base (displaced) S62.31- ☑
      - nondisplaced S62.34- ☑
    - neck (displaced) S62.33- ☑
      - nondisplaced S62.36- ☑
    - shaft (displaced) S62.32- ☑
      - nondisplaced S62.35- ☑
    - specified NEC S62.39- ☑
    - shaft (displaced) S62.32- ☑
      - nondisplaced S62.35- ☑
  - specified NEC S62.399 ☑
  - third S62.30- ☑
    - base (displaced) S62.31- ☑

Fracture, traumatic — *continued*
- metacarpal — *continued*
  - third — *continued*
    - base — *continued*
      - nondisplaced S62.34- ☑
    - neck (displaced) S62.33- ☑
      - nondisplaced S62.36- ☑
    - shaft (displaced) S62.32- ☑
      - nondisplaced S62.35- ☑
    - specified NEC S62.39- ☑
- metastatic — *see* Fracture, pathological, due to, neoplastic disease — *see also* Neoplasm
- metatarsal bone S92.30- ☑
  - fifth (displaced) S92.35- ☑
    - nondisplaced S92.35- ☑
  - first (displaced) S92.31- ☑
    - nondisplaced S92.31- ☑
  - fourth (displaced) S92.34- ☑
    - nondisplaced S92.34- ☑
  - physeal S99.10- ☑
    - Salter-Harris
      - Type I S99.11- ☑
      - Type II S99.12- ☑
      - Type III S99.13- ☑
      - Type IV S99.14- ☑
    - specified NEC S99.19- ☑
  - second (displaced) S92.32- ☑
    - nondisplaced S92.32- ☑
  - third (displaced) S92.33- ☑
    - nondisplaced S92.33- ☑
- Monteggia's — *see* Monteggia's fracture
- multiple
  - hand (and wrist) NEC — *see* Fracture, by site
  - ribs — *see* Fracture, rib, multiple
- nasal (bone(s)) S02.2 ☑
- navicular (scaphoid) (foot) — *see also* Fracture, tarsal, navicular
  - hand — *see* Fracture, carpal, navicular
- neck S12.9 ☑
  - cervical vertebra S12.9 ☑
    - fifth (displaced) S12.400 ☑
      - nondisplaced S12.401 ☑
      - specified type NEC (displaced) S12.490 ☑
        - nondisplaced S12.491 ☑
    - first (displaced) S12.000 ☑
      - burst (stable) S12.01 ☑
        - unstable S12.02 ☑
      - lateral mass (displaced) S12.040 ☑
        - nondisplaced S12.041 ☑
      - nondisplaced S12.001 ☑
      - posterior arch (displaced) S12.030 ☑
        - nondisplaced S12.031 ☑
      - specified type NEC (displaced) S12.090 ☑
        - nondisplaced S12.091 ☑
    - fourth (displaced) S12.300 ☑
      - nondisplaced S12.301 ☑
      - specified type NEC (displaced) S12.390 ☑
        - nondisplaced S12.391 ☑
    - second (displaced) S12.100 ☑
      - dens (anterior) (displaced) (type II) S12.110 ☑
        - nondisplaced S12.112 ☑
        - posterior S12.111 ☑
        - specified type NEC (displaced) S12.120 ☑
          - nondisplaced S12.121 ☑
      - nondisplaced S12.101 ☑
      - specified type NEC (displaced) S12.190 ☑
        - nondisplaced S12.191 ☑
    - seventh (displaced) S12.600 ☑
      - nondisplaced S12.601 ☑
      - specified type NEC (displaced) S12.690 ☑
        - nondisplaced S12.691 ☑
    - sixth (displaced) S12.500 ☑
      - nondisplaced S12.501 ☑
      - specified type NEC (displaced) S12.590 ☑
        - nondisplaced S12.591 ☑
    - third (displaced) S12.200 ☑
      - nondisplaced S12.201 ☑
      - specified type NEC (displaced) S12.290 ☑
        - nondisplaced S12.291 ☑
  - hyoid bone S12.8 ☑
  - larynx S12.8 ☑
  - specified site NEC S12.8 ☑
  - thyroid cartilage S12.8 ☑
  - trachea S12.8 ☑
- neoplastic NEC — *see* Fracture, pathological, due to, neoplastic disease

Fracture, traumatic — *continued*
  neural arch — *see* Fracture, vertebra
  newborn — *see* Birth, injury, fracture
  nontraumatic — *see* Fracture, pathological
  nonunion — *see* Nonunion, fracture
  nose, nasal (bone) (septum) S02.2 ☑
  occiput — *see* Fracture, skull, base, occiput
  odontoid process — *see* Fracture, neck, cervical vertebra, second
  olecranon (process) (ulna) — *see* Fracture, ulna, upper end, olecranon process
  orbit, orbital (bone) (region) S02.85 ☑
    floor (blow-out) S02.3- ☑
    roof S02.12- ☑
    wall S02.85 ☑
      lateral S02.84- ☑
      medial S02.83- ☑
  os
    calcis — *see* Fracture, tarsal, calcaneus
    magnum — *see* Fracture, carpal, capitate
    pubis — *see* Fracture, pubis
  palate S02.8- ☑
  parietal bone (skull) S02.0 ☑
  patella S82.00- ☑
    comminuted (displaced) S82.04- ☑
      nondisplaced S82.04- ☑
    longitudinal (displaced) S82.02- ☑
      nondisplaced S82.02- ☑
    osteochondral (displaced) S82.01- ☑
      nondisplaced S82.01- ☑
    specified NEC S82.09- ☑
    transverse (displaced) S82.03- ☑
      nondisplaced S82.03- ☑
  pedicle (of vertebral arch) — *see* Fracture, vertebra
  pelvis, pelvic (bone) S32.9 ☑
    acetabulum — *see* Fracture, acetabulum
    circle — *see* Disruption, pelvic ring
    following insertion of implant, prosthesis or plate M96.65
    ilium — *see* Fracture, ilium
    ischium — *see* Fracture, ischium
    multiple
      with disruption of pelvic ring (circle) — *see* Disruption, pelvic ring
      without disruption of pelvic ring (circle) S32.82 ☑
    pubis — *see* Fracture, pubis
    sacrum — *see* Fracture, sacrum
    specified site NEC S32.89 ☑
  periprosthetic, around internal prosthetic joint M97.9 ☑
    ankle M97.2- ☑
    elbow M97.4- ☑
    finger M97.8 ☑
    hip M97.0- ☑
    knee M97.1- ☑
    shoulder M97.3- ☑
    specified joint NEC M97.8 ☑
    spine M97.8 ☑
    toe M97.8 ☑
    wrist M97.8 ☑
  phalanx
    foot — *see* Fracture, toe
    hand — *see* Fracture, finger
  pisiform — *see* Fracture, carpal, pisiform
  pond — *see* Fracture, skull
  prosthetic device, internal — *see* Complications, prosthetic device, by site, mechanical
  pubis S32.50- ☑
    with disruption of pelvic ring — *see* Disruption, pelvic ring
    specified site NEC S32.59- ☑
    superior rim S32.51- ☑
  radius S52.9- ☑
    distal end — *see* Fracture, radius, lower end
    following insertion of implant, prosthesis or plate M96.63- ☑
    head — *see* Fracture, radius, upper end, head
    lower end S52.50- ☑
      Barton's — *see* Barton's fracture
      Colles' — *see* Colles' fracture
      extraarticular NEC S52.55- ☑
      intraarticular NEC S52.57- ☑
      physeal S59.20- ☑
        Salter-Harris
          Type I S59.21- ☑

Fracture, traumatic — *continued*
  radius — *continued*
    lower end — *continued*
      physeal — *continued*
        Salter-Harris — *continued*
          Type II S59.22- ☑
          Type III S59.23- ☑
          Type IV S59.24- ☑
        specified NEC S59.29- ☑
      Smith's — *see* Smith's fracture
      specified NEC S52.59- ☑
      styloid process (displaced) S52.51- ☑
        nondisplaced S52.51- ☑
      torus S52.52- ☑
    neck — *see* Fracture, radius, upper end
    proximal end — *see* Fracture, radius, upper end
    shaft S52.30- ☑
      bent bone S52.38- ☑
      comminuted (displaced) S52.35- ☑
        nondisplaced S52.35- ☑
      Galeazzi's — *see* Galeazzi's fracture
      greenstick S52.31- ☑
      oblique (displaced) S52.33- ☑
        nondisplaced S52.33- ☑
      segmental (displaced) S52.36- ☑
        nondisplaced S52.36- ☑
      specified NEC S52.39- ☑
      spiral (displaced) S52.34- ☑
        nondisplaced S52.34- ☑
      transverse (displaced) S52.32- ☑
        nondisplaced S52.32- ☑
    upper end S52.10- ☑
      head (displaced) S52.12- ☑
        nondisplaced S52.12- ☑
      neck (displaced) S52.13- ☑
        nondisplaced S52.13- ☑
      physeal S59.10- ☑
        Salter-Harris
          Type I S59.11- ☑
          Type II S59.12- ☑
          Type III S59.13- ☑
          Type IV S59.14- ☑
        specified NEC S59.19- ☑
      specified NEC S52.18- ☑
      torus S52.11- ☑
  ramus
    inferior or superior, pubis — *see* Fracture, pubis
    mandible — *see* Fracture, mandible
  restorative material (dental) K08.539
    with loss of material K08.531
    without loss of material K08.530
  rib S22.3- ☑
    with flail chest — *see* Flail, chest
    multiple S22.4- ☑
      with flail chest — *see* Flail, chest
  root, tooth — *see* Fracture, tooth
  sacrum S32.10 ☑
    specified NEC S32.19 ☑
    Type
      1 S32.14 ☑
      2 S32.15 ☑
      3 S32.16 ☑
      4 S32.17 ☑
    Zone
      I S32.119 ☑
        displaced (minimally) S32.111 ☑
          severely S32.112 ☑
        nondisplaced S32.110 ☑
      II S32.129 ☑
        displaced (minimally) S32.121 ☑
          severely S32.122 ☑
        nondisplaced S32.120 ☑
      III S32.139 ☑
        displaced (minimally) S32.131 ☑
          severely S32.132 ☑
        nondisplaced S32.130 ☑
  scaphoid (hand) — *see also* Fracture, carpal, navicular
    foot — *see* Fracture, tarsal, navicular
  scapula S42.10- ☑
    acromial process (displaced) S42.12- ☑
      nondisplaced S42.12- ☑
    body (displaced) S42.11- ☑
      nondisplaced S42.11- ☑
    coracoid process (displaced) S42.13- ☑
      nondisplaced S42.13- ☑
    glenoid cavity (displaced) S42.14- ☑

Fracture, traumatic — *continued*
  scapula — *continued*
    glenoid cavity — *continued*
      nondisplaced S42.14- ☑
    neck (displaced) S42.15- ☑
      nondisplaced S42.15- ☑
    specified NEC S42.19- ☑
  semilunar bone, wrist — *see* Fracture, carpal, lunate
  sequelae — *see* Sequelae, fracture
  sesamoid bone
    foot S92.81- ☑
    hand — *see* Fracture, carpal
    other — *see* Fracture, traumatic, by site
  shepherd's — *see* Fracture, tarsal, talus
  shoulder (girdle) S42.9- ☑
    blade — *see* Fracture, scapula
  sinus (ethmoid) (frontal) S02.19 ☑
  skull S02.91 ☑
    base S02.10- ☑
      occiput S02.119 ☑
        condyle S02.113 ☑
          specified NEC S02.118 ☑
            left side S02.11H ☑
            right side S02.11G ☑
          type I S02.110 ☑
            left side S02.11B ☑
            right side S02.11A ☑
          type II S02.111 ☑
            left side S02.11D ☑
            right side S02.11C ☑
          type III S02.112 ☑
            left side S02.11F ☑
            right side S02.11E ☑
      specified NEC S02.19 ☑
    birth injury P13.0
    frontal bone S02.0 ☑
    parietal bone S02.0 ☑
    specified site NEC S02.8- ☑
    temporal bone S02.19 ☑
    vault S02.0 ☑
  Smith's — *see* Smith's fracture
  sphenoid (bone) (sinus) S02.19 ☑
  spine — *see* Fracture, vertebra
  spinous process — *see* Fracture, vertebra
  spontaneous (cause unknown) — *see* Fracture, pathological
  stave (of thumb) — *see* Fracture, metacarpal, first
  sternum S22.20 ☑
    with flail chest — *see* Flail, chest
    body S22.22 ☑
    manubrium S22.21 ☑
    xiphoid (process) S22.24 ☑
  stress M84.30 ☑
    ankle M84.37- ☑
    carpus M84.34- ☑
    clavicle M84.31- ☑
    femoral neck M84.359 ☑
    femur M84.35- ☑
    fibula M84.36- ☑
    finger M84.34- ☑
    hip M84.359 ☑
    humerus M84.32- ☑
    ilium M84.350 ☑
    ischium M84.350 ☑
    metacarpus M84.34- ☑
    metatarsus M84.37- ☑
    neck — *see* Fracture, fatigue, vertebra
    pelvis M84.350 ☑
    radius M84.33- ☑
    rib M84.38 ☑
    scapula M84.31- ☑
    skull M84.38 ☑
    tarsus M84.37- ☑
    tibia M84.36- ☑
    toe M84.37- ☑
    ulna M84.33- ☑
    vertebra — *see* Fracture, fatigue, vertebra
  supracondylar, elbow — *see* Fracture, humerus, lower end, supracondylar
  symphysis pubis — *see* Fracture, pubis
  talus (ankle bone) — *see* Fracture, tarsal, talus
  tarsal bone(s) S92.20- ☑
    astragalus — *see* Fracture, tarsal, talus
    calcaneus S92.00- ☑
      anterior process (displaced) S92.02- ☑
        nondisplaced S92.02- ☑

Fracture, traumatic — *continued*
  tarsal bone(s) — *continued*
    calcaneus — *continued*
      body (displaced) S92.01- ☑
        nondisplaced S92.01- ☑
      extraarticular NEC (displaced) S92.05- ☑
        nondisplaced S92.05- ☑
      intraarticular (displaced) S92.06- ☑
        nondisplaced S92.06- ☑
      physeal S99.00- ☑
        Salter-Harris
          Type I S99.01- ☑
          Type II S99.02- ☑
          Type III S99.03- ☑
          Type IV S99.04- ☑
        specified NEC S99.09- ☑
      tuberosity (displaced) S92.04- ☑
        avulsion (displaced) S92.03- ☑
          nondisplaced S92.03- ☑
        nondisplaced S92.04- ☑
    cuboid (displaced) S92.21- ☑
      nondisplaced S92.21- ☑
    cuneiform
      intermediate (displaced) S92.23- ☑
        nondisplaced S92.23- ☑
      lateral (displaced) S92.22- ☑
        nondisplaced S92.22- ☑
      medial (displaced) S92.24- ☑
        nondisplaced S92.24- ☑
    navicular (displaced) S92.25- ☑
      nondisplaced S92.25- ☑
    scaphoid — *see* Fracture, tarsal, navicular
    talus S92.10- ☑
      avulsion (displaced) S92.15- ☑
        nondisplaced S92.15- ☑
      body (displaced) S92.12- ☑
        nondisplaced S92.12- ☑
      dome (displaced) S92.14- ☑
        nondisplaced S92.14- ☑
      head (displaced) S92.12- ☑
        nondisplaced S92.12- ☑
      lateral process (displaced) S92.14- ☑
        nondisplaced S92.14- ☑
      neck (displaced) S92.11- ☑
        nondisplaced S92.11- ☑
      posterior process (displaced) S92.13- ☑
        nondisplaced S92.13- ☑
      specified NEC S92.19- ☑
  temporal bone (styloid) S02.19 ☑
  thorax (bony) S22.9 ☑
    with flail chest — *see* Flail, chest
    rib S22.3- ☑
      multiple S22.4- ☑
        with flail chest — *see* Flail, chest
    sternum S22.20 ☑
      body S22.22 ☑
      manubrium S22.21 ☑
      xiphoid process S22.24 ☑
    vertebra (displaced) S22.009 ☑
      burst (stable) S22.001 ☑
        unstable S22.002 ☑
      eighth S22.069 ☑
        burst (stable) S22.061 ☑
          unstable S22.062 ☑
        specified type NEC S22.068 ☑
        wedge compression S22.060 ☑
      eleventh S22.089 ☑
        burst (stable) S22.081 ☑
          unstable S22.082 ☑
        specified type NEC S22.088 ☑
        wedge compression S22.080 ☑
      fifth S22.059 ☑
        burst (stable) S22.051 ☑
          unstable S22.052 ☑
        specified type NEC S22.058 ☑
        wedge compression S22.050 ☑
      first S22.019 ☑
        burst (stable) S22.011 ☑
          unstable S22.012 ☑
        specified type NEC S22.018 ☑
        wedge compression S22.010 ☑
      fourth S22.049 ☑
        burst (stable) S22.041 ☑
          unstable S22.042 ☑
        specified type NEC S22.048 ☑
        wedge compression S22.040 ☑

Fracture, traumatic — *continued*
  thorax — *continued*
    vertebra — *continued*
      ninth S22.079 ☑
        burst (stable) S22.071 ☑
          unstable S22.072 ☑
        specified type NEC S22.078 ☑
        wedge compression S22.070 ☑
      nondisplaced S22.001 ☑
      second S22.029 ☑
        burst (stable) S22.021 ☑
          unstable S22.022 ☑
        specified type NEC S22.028 ☑
        wedge compression S22.020 ☑
      seventh S22.069 ☑
        burst (stable) S22.061 ☑
          unstable S22.062 ☑
        specified type NEC S22.068 ☑
        wedge compression S22.060 ☑
      sixth S22.059 ☑
        burst (stable) S22.051 ☑
          unstable S22.052 ☑
        specified type NEC S22.058 ☑
        wedge compression S22.050 ☑
      specified type NEC S22.008 ☑
      tenth S22.079 ☑
        burst (stable) S22.071 ☑
          unstable S22.072 ☑
        specified type NEC S22.078 ☑
        wedge compression S22.070 ☑
      third S22.039 ☑
        burst (stable) S22.031 ☑
          unstable S22.032 ☑
        specified type NEC S22.038 ☑
        wedge compression S22.030 ☑
      twelfth S22.089 ☑
        burst (stable) S22.081 ☑
          unstable S22.082 ☑
        specified type NEC S22.088 ☑
        wedge compression S22.080 ☑
      wedge compression S22.000 ☑
  thumb S62.50- ☑
    distal phalanx (displaced) S62.52- ☑
      nondisplaced S62.52- ☑
    proximal phalanx (displaced) S62.51- ☑
      nondisplaced S62.51- ☑
  thyroid cartilage S12.8 ☑
  tibia (shaft) S82.20- ☑
    comminuted (displaced) S82.25- ☑
      nondisplaced S82.25- ☑
    condyles — *see* Fracture, tibia, upper end
    distal end — *see* Fracture, tibia, lower end
    epiphysis
      lower — *see* Fracture, tibia, lower end
      upper — *see* Fracture, tibia, upper end
    following insertion of implant, prosthesis or plate
      M96.67- ☑
    head (involving knee joint) — *see* Fracture, tibia,
      upper end
    intercondyloid eminence — *see* Fracture, tibia, up-
      per end
    involving ankle or malleolus — *see* Fracture, ankle,
      medial malleolus
    lower end S82.30- ☑
      physeal S89.10- ☑
        Salter-Harris
          Type I S89.11- ☑
          Type II S89.12- ☑
          Type III S89.13- ☑
          Type IV S89.14- ☑
        specified NEC S89.19- ☑
      pilon (displaced) S82.87- ☑
        nondisplaced S82.87- ☑
      specified NEC S82.39- ☑
      torus S82.31- ☑
    malleolus — *see* Fracture, ankle, medial malleolus
    oblique (displaced) S82.23- ☑
      nondisplaced S82.23- ☑
    pilon — *see* Fracture, tibia, lower end, pilon
    proximal end — *see* Fracture, tibia, upper end
    segmental (displaced) S82.26- ☑
      nondisplaced S82.26- ☑
    specified NEC S82.29- ☑
    spine — *see* Fracture, tibia, upper end, spine
    spiral (displaced) S82.24- ☑
      nondisplaced S82.24- ☑

Fracture, traumatic — *continued*
  tibia — *continued*
    transverse (displaced) S82.22- ☑
      nondisplaced S82.22- ☑
    tuberosity — *see* Fracture, tibia, upper end,
      tuberosity
    upper end S82.10- ☑
      bicondylar (displaced) S82.14- ☑
        nondisplaced S82.14- ☑
      lateral condyle (displaced) S82.12- ☑
        nondisplaced S82.12- ☑
      medial condyle (displaced) S82.13- ☑
        nondisplaced S82.13- ☑
      physeal S89.00- ☑
        Salter-Harris
          Type I S89.01- ☑
          Type II S89.02- ☑
          Type III S89.03- ☑
          Type IV S89.04- ☑
        specified NEC S89.09- ☑
      plateau — *see* Fracture, tibia, upper end, bicondy-
        lar
      specified NEC S82.19- ☑
      spine (displaced) S82.11- ☑
        nondisplaced S82.11- ☑
      torus S82.16- ☑
      tuberosity (displaced) S82.15- ☑
        nondisplaced S82.15- ☑
  toe S92.91- ☑
    great (displaced) S92.40- ☑
      distal phalanx (displaced) S92.42- ☑
        nondisplaced S92.42- ☑
      nondisplaced S92.40- ☑
      proximal phalanx (displaced) S92.41- ☑
        nondisplaced S92.41- ☑
      specified NEC S92.49- ☑
    lesser (displaced) S92.50- ☑
      distal phalanx (displaced) S92.53- ☑
        nondisplaced S92.53- ☑
      middle phalanx (displaced) S92.52- ☑
        nondisplaced S92.52- ☑
      nondisplaced S92.50- ☑
      proximal phalanx (displaced) S92.51- ☑
        nondisplaced S92.51- ☑
      specified NEC S92.59- ☑
    physeal
      phalanx S99.20- ☑
        Salter-Harris
          Type I S99.21- ☑
          Type II S99.22- ☑
          Type III S99.23- ☑
          Type IV S99.24- ☑
        specified NEC S99.29- ☑
  tooth (root) S02.5 ☑
  trachea (cartilage) S12.8 ☑
  transverse process — *see* Fracture, vertebra
  trapezium or trapezoid bone — *see* Fracture, carpal
  trimalleolar — *see* Fracture, ankle, trimalleolar
  triquetrum (cuneiform of carpus) — *see* Fracture,
    carpal, triquetrum
  trochanter — *see* Fracture, femur, trochanteric
  tuberosity (external) — *see* Fracture, traumatic, by site
  ulna (shaft) S52.20- ☑
    bent bone S52.28- ☑
    coronoid process — *see* Fracture, ulna, upper end,
      coronoid process
    distal end — *see* Fracture, ulna, lower end
    following insertion of implant, prosthesis or plate
      M96.63- ☑
    head S52.60- ☑
    lower end S52.60- ☑
      physeal S59.00- ☑
        Salter-Harris
          Type I S59.01- ☑
          Type II S59.02- ☑
          Type III S59.03- ☑
          Type IV S59.04- ☑
        specified NEC S59.09- ☑
      specified NEC S52.69- ☑
      styloid process (displaced) S52.61- ☑
        nondisplaced S52.61- ☑
      torus S52.62- ☑
    proximal end — *see* Fracture, ulna, upper end
    shaft S52.20- ☑
      comminuted (displaced) S52.25- ☑
        nondisplaced S52.25- ☑

Fracture, traumatic — *continued*
  ulna — *continued*
    shaft — *continued*
      greenstick S52.21-
      Monteggia's — *see* Monteggia's fracture
      oblique (displaced) S52.23- ☑
        nondisplaced S52.23- ☑
      segmental (displaced) S52.26- ☑
        nondisplaced S52.26- ☑
      specified NEC S52.29- ☑
      spiral (displaced) S52.24- ☑
        nondisplaced S52.24- ☑
      transverse (displaced) S52.22- ☑
        nondisplaced S52.22- ☑
    upper end S52.00- ☑
      coronoid process (displaced) S52.04- ☑
        nondisplaced S52.04- ☑
      olecranon process (displaced) S52.02- ☑
        with intraarticular extension S52.03- ☑
        nondisplaced S52.02- ☑
          with intraarticular extension S52.03- ☑
      specified NEC S52.09- ☑
      torus S52.01- ☑
  unciform — *see* Fracture, carpal, hamate
  vault of skull S02.0 ☑
  vertebra, vertebral (arch) (body) (column) (neural arch)
    (pedicle) (spinous process) (transverse process)
    atlas — *see* Fracture, neck, cervical vertebra, first
    axis — *see* Fracture, neck, cervical vertebra, second
    cervical (teardrop) S12.9
      axis — *see* Fracture, neck, cervical vertebra, second
      first (atlas) — *see* Fracture, neck, cervical vertebra, first
      second (axis) — *see* Fracture, neck, cervical vertebra, second
    chronic M84.48 ☑
    coccyx S32.2 ☑
    dorsal — *see* Fracture, thorax, vertebra
    lumbar S32.009 ☑
      burst (stable) S32.001 ☑
        unstable S32.002 ☑
      fifth S32.059 ☑
        burst (stable) S32.051 ☑
          unstable S32.052 ☑
        specified type NEC S32.058 ☑
        wedge compression S32.050 ☑
      first S32.019 ☑
        burst (stable) S32.011 ☑
          unstable S32.012 ☑
        specified type NEC S32.018 ☑
        wedge compression S32.010 ☑
      fourth S32.049 ☑
        burst (stable) S32.041 ☑
          unstable S32.042 ☑
        specified type NEC S32.048 ☑
        wedge compression S32.040 ☑
      second S32.029 ☑
        burst (stable) S32.021 ☑
          unstable S32.022 ☑
        specified type NEC S32.028 ☑
        wedge compression S32.020 ☑
      specified type NEC S32.008 ☑
      third S32.039 ☑
        burst (stable) S32.031 ☑
          unstable S32.032 ☑
        specified type NEC S32.038 ☑
        wedge compression S32.030 ☑
      wedge compression S32.000 ☑
    metastatic — *see* Collapse, vertebra, in, specified
      disease NEC — *see also* Neoplasm
    newborn (birth injury) P11.5
    sacrum S32.10 ☑
      specified NEC S32.19 ☑
      Type
        1 S32.14 ☑
        2 S32.15 ☑
        3 S32.16 ☑
        4 S32.17 ☑
      Zone
        I S32.119 ☑
          displaced (minimally) S32.111 ☑
            severely S32.112 ☑
          nondisplaced S32.110 ☑
        II S32.129 ☑
          displaced (minimally) S32.121 ☑

Fracture, traumatic — *continued*
  vertebra, vertebral — *continued*
    sacrum — *continued*
      Zone — *continued*
        II — *continued*
          displaced — *continued*
            severely S32.122 ☑
          nondisplaced S32.120 ☑
        III S32.139 ☑
          displaced (minimally) S32.131 ☑
            severely S32.132 ☑
          nondisplaced S32.130 ☑
    thoracic — *see* Fracture, thorax, vertebra
  vertex S02.0 ☑
  vomer (bone) S02.2 ☑
  wrist S62.10- ☑
    carpal — *see* Fracture, carpal bone
    navicular (scaphoid) (hand) — *see* Fracture, carpal, navicular
  xiphisternum, xiphoid (process) S22.24 ☑
  zygoma S02.402 ☑
    left side S02.40F ☑
    right side S02.40E ☑
Fragile, fragility
  autosomal site Q95.5
  bone, congenital (with blue sclera) Q78.0
  capillary (hereditary) D69.8
  hair L67.8
  nails L60.3
  non-sex chromosome site Q95.5
  X chromosome Q99.2
Fragilitas
  crinium L67.8
  ossium (with blue sclerae) (hereditary) Q78.0
  unguium L60.3
    congenital Q84.6
Fragments, cataract (lens), **following cataract surgery**
  H59.02- ☑
  retained foreign body — *see* Retained, foreign body fragments (type of)
Frailty (frail) R54
  mental R41.81
Frambesia, frambesial (tropica) — *see also* Yaws
  initial lesion or ulcer A66.0
  primary A66.0
Frambeside
  gummatous A66.4
  of early yaws A66.2
Frambesioma A66.1
Franceschetti-Klein (-Wildervanck) **disease or syndrome** Q75.4
Francis' disease — *see* Tularemia
Franklin disease C88.2
Frank's essential thrombocytopenia D69.3
Fraser's syndrome Q87.0
Freckle(s) L81.2
  malignant melanoma in — *see* Melanoma
  melanotic (Hutchinson's) — *see* Melanoma, in situ
  retinal D49.81
Frederickson's hyperlipoproteinemia, type
  I and V E78.3
  IIA E78.00
  IIB and III E78.2
  IV E78.1
Freeman Sheldon syndrome Q87.0
Freezing — *see also* Effect, adverse, cold T69.9 ☑
Freiberg's disease (infraction of metatarsal head or osteochondrosis) — *see* Osteochondrosis, juvenile, metatarsus
Frei's disease A55
Fremitus, friction, cardiac R01.2
Frenum, frenulum
  external os Q51.828
  tongue (shortening) (congenital) Q38.1
Frequency micturition (nocturnal) R35.0
  psychogenic F45.8
Frey's syndrome
  auriculotemporal G50.8
  hyperhidrosis L74.52
Friction
  burn — *see* Burn, by site
  fremitus, cardiac R01.2
  precordial R01.2
  sounds, chest R09.89
Friderichsen-Waterhouse syndrome or disease A39.1
Friedländer's B (bacillus) **NEC** — *see also* condition A49.8

Friedreich's
  ataxia G11.1
  combined systemic disease G11.1
  facial hemihypertrophy Q67.4
  sclerosis (cerebellum) (spinal cord) G11.1
Frigidity F52.22
Fröhlich's syndrome E23.6
Frontal — *see also* condition
  lobe syndrome F07.0
Frostbite (superficial) T33.90 ☑
  with
    partial thickness skin loss — *see* Frostbite (superficial), by site
    tissue necrosis T34.90 ☑
  abdominal wall T33.3 ☑
    with tissue necrosis T34.3 ☑
  ankle T33.81- ☑
    with tissue necrosis T34.81- ☑
  arm T33.4- ☑
    with tissue necrosis T34.4- ☑
    finger(s) — *see* Frostbite, finger
    hand — *see* Frostbite, hand
    wrist — *see* Frostbite, wrist
  ear T33.01- ☑
    with tissue necrosis T34.01- ☑
  face T33.09 ☑
    with tissue necrosis T34.09 ☑
  finger T33.53- ☑
    with tissue necrosis T34.53- ☑
  foot T33.82- ☑
    with tissue necrosis T34.82- ☑
  hand T33.52- ☑
    with tissue necrosis T34.52- ☑
  head T33.09 ☑
    with tissue necrosis T34.09 ☑
    ear — *see* Frostbite, ear
    nose — *see* Frostbite, nose
  hip (and thigh) T33.6- ☑
    with tissue necrosis T34.6- ☑
  knee T33.7- ☑
    with tissue necrosis T34.7- ☑
  leg T33.9- ☑
    with tissue necrosis T34.9- ☑
    ankle — *see* Frostbite, ankle
    foot — *see* Frostbite, foot
    knee — *see* Frostbite, knee
    lower T33.7- ☑
      with tissue necrosis T34.7- ☑
    thigh — *see* Frostbite, hip
    toe — *see* Frostbite, toe
  limb
    lower T33.99 ☑
      with tissue necrosis T34.99 ☑
    upper — *see* Frostbite, arm
  neck T33.1 ☑
    with tissue necrosis T34.1 ☑
  nose T33.02 ☑
    with tissue necrosis T34.02 ☑
  pelvis T33.3 ☑
    with tissue necrosis T34.3 ☑
  specified site NEC T33.99 ☑
    with tissue necrosis T34.99 ☑
  thigh — *see* Frostbite, hip
  thorax T33.2 ☑
    with tissue necrosis T34.2 ☑
  toes T33.83- ☑
    with tissue necrosis T34.83- ☑
  trunk T33.99 ☑
    with tissue necrosis T34.99 ☑
  wrist T33.51- ☑
    with tissue necrosis T34.51- ☑
Frotteurism F65.81
Frozen — *see also* Effect, adverse, cold T69.9 ☑
  pelvis (female) N94.89
    male K66.8
  shoulder — *see* Capsulitis, adhesive
Fructokinase deficiency E74.11
Fructose 1,6 diphosphatase deficiency E74.19
Fructosemia (benign) (essential) E74.12
Fructosuria (benign) (essential) E74.11
Fuchs'
  black spot (myopic) — *see also* Myopia, degenerative H44.2- ☑
  dystrophy (corneal endothelium) H18.51
  heterochromic cyclitis — *see* Cyclitis, Fuchs' heterochromic

Fucosidosis E77.1
Fugue R68.89
  dissociative F44.1
  hysterical (dissociative) F44.1
  postictal in epilepsy — *see* Epilepsy
  reaction to exceptional stress (transient) F43.0
Fulminant, fulminating — *see* condition
Functional — *see also* condition
  bleeding (uterus) N93.8
Functioning, intellectual, borderline R41.83
Fundus — *see* condition
Fungemia NOS B49
Fungus, fungous
  cerebral G93.89
  disease NOS B49
  infection — *see* Infection, fungus
Funiculitis (acute) (chronic) (endemic) N49.1
  gonococcal (acute) (chronic) A54.23
  tuberculous A18.15
Funnel
  breast (acquired) M95.4
    congenital Q67.6
    sequelae (late effect) of rickets E64.3
  chest (acquired) M95.4
    congenital Q67.6
    sequelae (late effect) of rickets E64.3
  pelvis (acquired) M95.5
    with disproportion (fetopelvic) O33.3 ☑
      causing obstructed labor O65.3
    congenital Q74.2
FUO (fever of unknown origin) R50.9
Furfur L21.0
  microsporon B36.0
Furrier's lung J67.8
Furrowed K14.5
  nail(s) (transverse) L60.4
    congenital Q84.6
  tongue K14.5
    congenital Q38.3
Furuncle L02.92
  abdominal wall L02.221
  ankle — *see* Furuncle, lower limb
  antecubital space — *see* Furuncle, upper limb
  anus K61.0
  arm — *see* Furuncle, upper limb
  auditory canal, external — *see* Abscess, ear, external
  auricle (ear) — *see* Abscess, ear, external
  axilla (region) L02.42- ☑
  back (any part) L02.222
  breast N61.1
  buttock L02.32
  cheek (external) L02.02
  chest wall L02.223
  chin L02.02
  corpus cavernosum N48.21
  ear, external — *see* Abscess, ear, external
  external auditory canal — *see* Abscess, ear, external
  eyelid — *see* Abscess, eyelid
  face L02.02
  femoral (region) — *see* Furuncle, lower limb

Furuncle — *continued*
  finger — *see* Furuncle, hand
  flank L02.221
  foot L02.62- ☑
  forehead L02.02
  gluteal (region) L02.32
  groin L02.224
  hand L02.52- ☑
  head L02.821
    face L02.02
  hip — *see* Furuncle, lower limb
  kidney — *see* Abscess, kidney
  knee — *see* Furuncle, lower limb
  labium (majus) (minus) N76.4
  lacrimal
    gland — *see* Dacryoadenitis
    passages (duct) (sac) — *see* Inflammation, lacrimal,
      passages, acute
  leg (any part) — *see* Furuncle, lower limb
  lower limb L02.42- ☑
  malignant A22.0
  mouth K12.2
  navel L02.226
  neck L02.12
  nose J34.0
  orbit, orbital — *see* Abscess, orbit
  palmar (space) — *see* Furuncle, hand
  partes posteriores L02.32
  pectoral region L02.223
  penis N48.21
  perineum L02.225
  pinna — *see* Abscess, ear, external
  popliteal — *see* Furuncle, lower limb
  prepatellar — *see* Furuncle, lower limb
  scalp L02.821
  seminal vesicle N49.0
  shoulder — *see* Furuncle, upper limb
  specified site NEC L02.828
  submandibular K12.2
  temple (region) L02.02
  thumb — *see* Furuncle, hand
  toe — *see* Furuncle, foot
  trunk L02.229
    abdominal wall L02.221
    back L02.222
    chest wall L02.223
    groin L02.224
    perineum L02.225
    umbilicus L02.226
  umbilicus L02.226
  upper limb L02.42- ☑
  vulva N76.4
Furunculosis — *see* Furuncle
Fused — *see* Fusion, fused
Fusion, fused (congenital)
  astragaloscaphoid Q74.2
  atria Q21.1
  auditory canal Q16.1
  auricles, heart Q21.1
  binocular with defective stereopsis H53.32

Fusion, fused — *continued*
  bone Q79.8
  cervical spine M43.22
  choanal Q30.0
  commissure, mitral valve Q23.2
  cusps, heart valve NEC Q24.8
    mitral Q23.2
    pulmonary Q22.1
    tricuspid Q22.4
  ear ossicles Q16.3
  fingers Q70.0 ☑
  hymen Q52.3
  joint (acquired) — *see also* Ankylosis
    congenital Q74.8
  kidneys (incomplete) Q63.1
  labium (majus) (minus) Q52.5
  larynx and trachea Q34.8
  limb, congenital Q74.8
    lower Q74.2
    upper Q74.0
  lobes, lung Q33.8
  lumbosacral (acquired) M43.27
    arthrodesis status Z98.1
    congenital Q76.49
    postprocedural status Z98.1
  nares, nose, nasal, nostril(s) Q30.0
  organ or site not listed — *see* Anomaly, by site
  ossicles Q79.9
    auditory Q16.3
  pulmonic cusps Q22.1
  ribs Q76.6
  sacroiliac (joint) (acquired) M43.28
    arthrodesis status Z98.1
    congenital Q74.2
    postprocedural status Z98.1
  spine (acquired) NEC M43.20
    arthrodesis status Z98.1
    cervical region M43.22
    cervicothoracic region M43.23
    congenital Q76.49
    lumbar M43.26
    lumbosacral region M43.27
    occipito-atlanto-axial region M43.21
    postoperative status Z98.1
    sacrococcygeal region M43.28
    thoracic region M43.24
    thoracolumbar region M43.25
  sublingual duct with submaxillary duct at opening in
    mouth Q38.4
  testes Q55.1
  toes Q70.2- ☑
  tooth, teeth K00.2
  trachea and esophagus Q39.8
  twins Q89.4
  vagina Q52.4
  ventricles, heart Q21.0
  vertebra (arch) — *see* Fusion, spine
  vulva Q52.5
Fusospirillosis (mouth) (tongue) (tonsil) A69.1
Fussy baby R68.12

☑ **Additional Character Required** — **Refer to the Tabular List for Character Selection**
▽ **Subterms under main terms may continue to next column or page**

G

Gain in weight (abnormal) (excessive) — *see also* Weight, gain
Gaisböck's disease (polycythemia hypertonica) D75.1
Gait abnormality R26.9
  ataxic R26.0
  falling R29.6
  hysterical (ataxic) (staggering) F44.4
  paralytic R26.1
  spastic R26.1
  specified type NEC R26.89
  staggering R26.0
  unsteadiness R26.81
  walking difficulty NEC R26.2
Galactocele (breast) N64.89
  puerperal, postpartum O92.79
Galactokinase deficiency E74.29
Galactophoritis N61.0
  gestational, puerperal, postpartum O91.2- ☑
Galactorrhea O92.6
  not associated with childbirth N64.3
Galactosemia (classic) (congenital) E74.21
Galactosuria E74.29
Galacturia R82.0
  schistosomiasis (bilharziasis) B65.0
GALD (gestational alloimmune liver disease) P78.84
Galeazzi's fracture S52.37- ☑
Galen's vein — *see* condition
Gall duct — *see* condition
Gallbladder — *see also* condition
  acute K81.0
Gallop rhythm R00.8
Gallstone (colic) (cystic duct) (gallbladder) (impacted) (multiple) — *see also* Calculus, gallbladder
  with
    cholecystitis — *see* Calculus, gallbladder, with cholecystitis
  bile duct (common) (hepatic) — *see* Calculus, bile duct
  causing intestinal obstruction K56.3
  specified NEC K80.80
    with obstruction K80.81
Gambling Z72.6
  pathological (compulsive) F63.0
Gammopathy (of undetermined significance [MGUS]) D47.2
  associated with lymphoplasmacytic dyscrasia D47.2
  monoclonal D47.2
  polyclonal D89.0
Gamna's disease (siderotic splenomegaly) D73.1
Gamophobia F40.298
Gampsodactylia (congenital) Q66.7- ☑
Gamstorp's disease (adynamia episodica hereditaria) G72.3
Gandy-Nanta disease (siderotic splenomegaly) D73.1
Gang
  membership offenses Z72.810
Gangliocytoma D36.10
Ganglioglioma — *see* Neoplasm, uncertain behavior, by site
Ganglion (compound) (diffuse) (joint) (tendon (sheath)) M67.40
  ankle M67.47- ☑
  foot M67.47- ☑
  forearm M67.43- ☑
  hand M67.44- ☑
  lower leg M67.46- ☑
  multiple sites M67.49
  of yaws (early) (late) A66.6
  pelvic region M67.45- ☑
  periosteal — *see* Periostitis
  shoulder region M67.41- ☑
  specified site NEC M67.48
  thigh region M67.45- ☑
  tuberculous A18.09
  upper arm M67.42- ☑
  wrist M67.43- ☑
Ganglioneuroblastoma — *see* Neoplasm, nerve, malignant
Ganglioneuroma D36.10
  malignant — *see* Neoplasm, nerve, malignant
Ganglioneuromatosis D36.10
Ganglionitis
  fifth nerve — *see* Neuralgia, trigeminal
  gasserian (postherpetic) (postzoster) B02.21

Ganglionitis — *continued*
  geniculate G51.1
    newborn (birth injury) P11.3
    postherpetic, postzoster B02.21
  herpes zoster B02.21
  postherpetic geniculate B02.21
Gangliosidosis E75.10
  GM1 E75.19
  GM2 E75.00
    other specified E75.09
    Sandhoff disease E75.01
    Tay-Sachs disease E75.02
  GM3 E75.19
  mucolipidosis IV E75.11
Gangosa A66.5
Gangrene, gangrenous (connective tissue) (dropsical) (dry) (moist) (skin) (ulcer) — *see also* Necrosis I96
  with diabetes (mellitus) — *see* Diabetes, gangrene
  abdomen (wall) I96
  alveolar M27.3
  appendix K35.80
    with
      peritonitis, localized — *see also* Appendicitis K35.31
  arteriosclerotic (general) (senile) — *see* Arteriosclerosis, extremities, with, gangrene
  auricle I96
  Bacillus welchii A48.0
  bladder (infectious) — *see* Cystitis, specified type NEC
  bowel, cecum, or colon — *see* Gangrene, intestine
  Clostridium perfringens or welchii A48.0
  cornea H18.89- ☑
  corpora cavernosa N48.29
    noninfective N48.89
  cutaneous, spreading I96
  decubital — *see* Ulcer, pressure, by site
  diabetic (any site) — *see* Diabetes, gangrene
  emphysematous — *see* Gangrene, gas
  epidemic — *see* Poisoning, food, noxious, plant
  epididymis (infectional) N45.1
  erysipelas — *see* Erysipelas
  extremity (lower) (upper) I96
  Fournier N49.3
    female N76.89
  fusospirochetal A69.0
  gallbladder — *see* Cholecystitis, acute
  gas (bacillus) A48.0
    following
      abortion — *see* Abortion by type complicated by infection
      ectopic or molar pregnancy O08.0
  glossitis K14.0
  hernia — *see* Hernia, by site, with gangrene
  intestine, intestinal (hemorrhagic) (massive) — *see also* Infarct, intestine K55.069
    with
      mesenteric embolism — *see also* Infarct, intestine K55.069
      obstruction — *see* Obstruction, intestine
  laryngitis J04.0
  limb (lower) (upper) I96
  lung J85.0
    spirochetal A69.8
  lymphangitis I89.1
  Meleney's (synergistic) — *see* Ulcer, skin
  mesentery — *see also* Infarct, intestine K55.069
    with
      embolism — *see also* Infarct, intestine K55.069
      intestinal obstruction — *see* Obstruction, intestine
  mouth A69.0
  ovary — *see* Oophoritis
  pancreas — *see* Pancreatitis, acute
  penis N48.29
    noninfective N48.89
  perineum I96
  pharynx — *see also* Pharyngitis
    Vincent's A69.1
  presenile I73.1
  progressive synergistic — *see* Ulcer, skin
  pulmonary J85.0
  pulpal (dental) K04.1
  quinsy J36
  Raynaud's (symmetric gangrene) I73.01
  retropharyngeal J39.2
  scrotum N49.3
    noninfective N50.89

Gangrene, gangrenous — *continued*
  senile (atherosclerotic) — *see* Arteriosclerosis, extremities, with, gangrene
  spermatic cord N49.1
    noninfective N50.89
  spine I96
  spirochetal NEC A69.8
  spreading cutaneous I96
  stomatitis A69.0
  symmetrical I73.01
  testis (infectional) N45.2
    noninfective N44.8
  throat — *see also* Pharyngitis
    diphtheritic A36.0
    Vincent's A69.1
  thyroid (gland) E07.89
  tooth (pulp) K04.1
  tuberculous NEC — *see* Tuberculosis
  tunica vaginalis N49.1
    noninfective N50.89
  umbilicus I96
  uterus — *see* Endometritis
  uvulitis K12.2
  vas deferens N49.1
    noninfective N50.89
  vulva N76.89
Ganister disease J62.8
Ganser's syndrome (hysterical) F44.89
Gardner-Diamond syndrome (autoerythrocyte sensitization) D69.2
Gargoylism E76.01
Garré's disease, osteitis (sclerosing), osteomyelitis — *see* Osteomyelitis, specified type NEC
Garrod's pad, knuckle M72.1
Gartner's duct
  cyst Q52.4
  persistent Q50.6
Gas R14.3
  asphyxiation, inhalation, poisoning, suffocation NEC — *see* Table of Drugs and Chemicals
  excessive R14.0
  gangrene A48.0
    following
      abortion — *see* Abortion by type complicated by infection
      ectopic or molar pregnancy O08.0
  on stomach R14.0
  pains R14.1
Gastralgia — *see also* Pain, abdominal
Gastrectasis K31.0
  psychogenic F45.8
Gastric — *see* condition
Gastrinoma
  malignant
    pancreas C25.4
    specified site NEC — *see* Neoplasm, malignant, by site
    unspecified site C25.4
  specified site — *see* Neoplasm, uncertain behavior
  unspecified site D37.9
Gastritis (simple) K29.70
  with bleeding K29.71
  acute (erosive) K29.00
    with bleeding K29.01
  alcoholic K29.20
    with bleeding K29.21
  allergic K29.60
    with bleeding K29.61
  atrophic (chronic) K29.40
    with bleeding K29.41
  chronic (antral) (fundal) K29.50
    with bleeding K29.51
    atrophic K29.40
      with bleeding K29.41
    superficial K29.30
      with bleeding K29.31
  dietary counseling and surveillance Z71.3
  due to diet deficiency E63.9
  eosinophilic K52.81
  giant hypertrophic K29.60
    with bleeding K29.61
  granulomatous K29.60
    with bleeding K29.61
  hypertrophic (mucosa) K29.60
    with bleeding K29.61
  nervous F54
  spastic K29.60
    with bleeding K29.61

Gastritis — *continued*
  specified NEC K29.60
    with bleeding K29.61
  superficial chronic K29.30
    with bleeding K29.31
  tuberculous A18.83
  viral NEC A08.4
Gastrocarcinoma — *see* Neoplasm, malignant, stomach
Gastrocolic — *see* condition
Gastrodisciasis, gastrodiscoidiasis B66.8
Gastroduodenitis K29.90
  with bleeding K29.91
  virus, viral A08.4
    specified type NEC A08.39
Gastrodynia — *see* Pain, abdominal
Gastroenteritis (acute) (chronic) (noninfectious) — *see also* Enteritis K52.9
  allergic K52.29
    with
      eosinophilic gastritis or gastroenteritis K52.81
      food protein-induced enterocolitis syndrome K52.21
      food protein-induced enteropathy K52.22
  dietetic — *see also* Gastroenteritis, allergic K52.29
  drug-induced K52.1
  due to
    Cryptosporidium A07.2
    drugs K52.1
    food poisoning — *see* Intoxication, foodborne
    radiation K52.0
  eosinophilic K52.81
  epidemic (infectious) A09
  food hypersensitivity — *see also* Gastroenteritis, allergic K52.29
  infectious — *see* Enteritis, infectious
  influenzal — *see* Influenza, with gastroenteritis
  noninfectious K52.9
    specified NEC K52.89
  rotaviral A08.0
  Salmonella A02.0
  toxic K52.1
  viral NEC A08.4
    acute infectious A08.39
      type Norwalk A08.11
    infantile (acute) A08.39
    Norwalk agent A08.11
    rotaviral A08.0
    severe of infants A08.39
    specified type NEC A08.39
Gastroenteropathy — *see also* Gastroenteritis K52.9
  acute, due to Norovirus A08.11
  acute, due to Norwalk agent A08.11
  infectious A09
Gastroenteroptosis K63.4
Gastroesophageal laceration- hemorrhage syndrome K22.6
Gastrointestinal — *see* condition
Gastrojejunal — *see* condition
Gastrojejunitis — *see also* Enteritis K52.9
Gastrojejunocolic — *see* condition
Gastroliths K31.89
Gastromalacia K31.89
Gastroparalysis K31.84
  diabetic — *see* Diabetes, gastroparalysis
Gastroparesis K31.84
  diabetic — *see* Diabetes, by type, with gastroparesis
Gastropathy K31.9
  congestive portal K31.89
  erythematous K29.70
  exudative K90.89
  portal hypertensive K31.89
Gastroptosis K31.89
Gastrorrhagia K92.2
  psychogenic F45.8
Gastroschisis (congenital) Q79.3
Gastrospasm (neurogenic) (reflex) K31.89
  neurotic F45.8
  psychogenic F45.8
Gastrostaxis — *see* Gastritis, with bleeding
Gastrostenosis K31.89
Gastrostomy
  attention to Z43.1
  status Z93.1
Gastrosuccorrhea (continuous) (intermittent) K31.89
  neurotic F45.8
  psychogenic F45.8
Gatophobia F40.218

Gaucher's disease or splenomegaly (adult) (infantile) E75.22
Gee (-Herter)(-Thaysen) **disease** (nontropical sprue) K90.0
Gélineau's syndrome G47.419
  with cataplexy G47.411
Gemination, tooth, teeth K00.2
Gemistocytoma
  specified site — *see* Neoplasm, malignant, by site
  unspecified site C71.9
General, generalized — *see* condition
Genetic
  carrier (status)
    cystic fibrosis Z14.1
    hemophilia A (asymptomatic) Z14.01
      symptomatic Z14.02
    specified NEC Z14.8
  susceptibility to disease NEC Z15.89
    malignant neoplasm Z15.09
      breast Z15.01
      endometrium Z15.04
      ovary Z15.02
      prostate Z15.03
      specified NEC Z15.09
    multiple endocrine neoplasia Z15.81
Genital — *see* condition
Genito-anorectal syndrome A55
Genitourinary system — *see* condition
Genu
  congenital Q74.1
  extrorsum (acquired) — *see also* Deformity, varus, knee
    congenital Q74.1
    sequelae (late effect) of rickets E64.3
  introrsum (acquired) — *see also* Deformity, valgus, knee
    congenital Q74.1
    sequelae (late effect) of rickets E64.3
  rachitic (old) E64.3
  recurvatum (acquired) — *see also* Deformity, limb, specified type NEC, lower leg
    congenital Q68.2
    sequelae (late effect) of rickets E64.3
  valgum (acquired) (knock-knee) M21.06- ☑
    congenital Q74.1
    sequelae (late effect) of rickets E64.3
  varum (acquired) (bowleg) M21.16- ☑
    congenital Q74.1
    sequelae (late effect) of rickets E64.3
Geographic tongue K14.1
Geophagia — *see* Pica
Geotrichosis B48.3
  stomatitis B48.3
Gephyrophobia F40.242
Gerbode defect Q21.0
GERD (gastroesophageal reflux disease) K21.9
Gerhardt's
  disease (erythromelalgia) I73.81
  syndrome (vocal cord paralysis) J38.00
    bilateral J38.02
    unilateral J38.01
German measles — *see also* Rubella
  exposure to Z20.4
Germinoblastoma (diffuse) C85.9- ☑
  follicular C82.9- ☑
Germinoma — *see* Neoplasm, malignant, by site
Gerontoxon — *see* Degeneration, cornea, senile
Gerstmann's syndrome R48.8
  developmental F81.2
Gerstmann-Sträussler-Scheinker syndrome (GSS) A81.82
Gestation (period) — *see also* Pregnancy
  ectopic — *see* Pregnancy, by site
  multiple O30.9- ☑
    greater than quadruplets — *see* Pregnancy, multiple (gestation), specified NEC
    specified NEC — *see* Pregnancy, multiple (gestation), specified NEC
Gestational
  mammary abscess O91.11- ☑
  purulent mastitis O91.11- ☑
  subareolar abscess O91.11- ☑
Ghon tubercle, primary infection A15.7
Ghost
  teeth K00.4
  vessels (cornea) H16.41- ☑
Ghoul hand A66.3
Gianotti-Crosti disease L44.4

Giant
  cell
    epulis K06.8
    peripheral granuloma K06.8
  esophagus, congenital Q39.5
  kidney, congenital Q63.3
  urticaria T78.3 ☑
    hereditary D84.1
Giardiasis A07.1
Gibert's disease or pityriasis L42
Giddiness R42
  hysterical F44.89
  psychogenic F45.8
Gierke's disease (glycogenosis I) E74.01
Gigantism (cerebral) (hypophyseal) (pituitary) E22.0
  constitutional E34.4
Gilbert's disease or syndrome E80.4
Gilchrist's disease B40.9
Gilford-Hutchinson disease E34.8
Gilles de la Tourette's disease or syndrome (motor-verbal tic) F95.2
Gingivitis K05.10
  acute (catarrhal) K05.00
    necrotizing A69.1
    nonplaque induced K05.01
    plaque induced K05.00
  chronic (desquamative) (hyperplastic) (simple marginal) (pregnancy associated) (ulcerative) K05.10
    nonplaque induced K05.11
    plaque induced K05.10
  expulsiva — *see* Periodontitis
  necrotizing ulcerative (acute) A69.1
  pellagrous E52
    acute necrotizing A69.1
  Vincent's A69.1
Gingivoglossitis K14.0
Gingivopericementitis — *see* Periodontitis
Gingivosis — *see* Gingivitis, chronic
Gingivostomatitis K05.10
  herpesviral B00.2
  necrotizing ulcerative (acute) A69.1
Gland, glandular — *see* condition
Glanders A24.0
Glanzmann (-Naegeli) **disease or thrombasthenia** D69.1
Glasgow coma scale
  total score
    13-15 R40.241 ☑
    3-8 R40.243 ☑
    9-12 R40.242 ☑
Glass-blower's disease (cataract) — *see* Cataract, specified NEC
Glaucoma H40.9
  with
    increased episcleral venous pressure H40.81- ☑
    pseudoexfoliation of lens — *see* Glaucoma, open angle, primary, capsular
  absolute H44.51- ☑
  angle-closure (primary) H40.20- ☑
    acute (attack) (crisis) H40.21- ☑
    chronic H40.22- ☑
    intermittent H40.23- ☑
    residual stage H40.24- ☑
  borderline H40.00- ☑
  capsular (with pseudoexfoliation of lens) — *see* Glaucoma, open angle, primary, capsular
  childhood Q15.0
  closed angle — *see* Glaucoma, angle-closure
  congenital Q15.0
  corticosteroid-induced — *see* Glaucoma, secondary, drugs
  hypersecretion H40.82- ☑
  in (due to)
    amyloidosis E85.4 *[H42]*
    aniridia Q13.1 *[H42]*
    concussion of globe — *see* Glaucoma, secondary, trauma
    dislocation of lens — *see* Glaucoma, secondary
    disorder of lens NEC — *see* Glaucoma, secondary
    drugs — *see* Glaucoma, secondary, drugs
    endocrine disease NOS E34.9 *[H42]*
    eye
      inflammation — *see* Glaucoma, secondary, inflammation
      trauma — *see* Glaucoma, secondary, trauma
    hypermature cataract — *see* Glaucoma, secondar

☑ Subterms under main terms may continue to next column or page   ☑ Additional Character Required — Refer to the Tabular List for Character Selection   159

Index   Glaucoma — Glycogenosis

Glycopenia E16.2
Glycosuria R81
  renal E74.8
Gnathostoma spinigerum (infection) (infestation),
  gnathostomiasis (wandering swelling) B83.1
Goiter (plunging) (substernal) E04.9
  with
    hyperthyroidism (recurrent) — see Hyperthyroidism,
      with, goiter
    thyrotoxicosis — see Hyperthyroidism, with, goiter
  adenomatous — see Goiter, nodular
  cancerous C73
  congenital (nontoxic) E03.0
    diffuse E03.0
    parenchymatous E03.0
    transitory, with normal functioning P72.0
  cystic E04.2
    due to iodine-deficiency E01.1
  due to
    enzyme defect in synthesis of thyroid hormone
      E07.1
    iodine-deficiency (endemic) E01.2
  dyshormonogenetic (familial) E07.1
  endemic (iodine-deficiency) E01.2
    diffuse E01.0
    multinodular E01.1
  exophthalmic — see Hyperthyroidism, with, goiter
  iodine-deficiency (endemic) E01.2
    diffuse E01.0
    multinodular E01.1
    nodular E01.1
  lingual Q89.2
  lymphadenoid E06.3
  malignant C73
  multinodular (cystic) (nontoxic) E04.2
    toxic or with hyperthyroidism E05.20
      with thyroid storm E05.21
  neonatal NEC P72.0
  nodular (nontoxic) (due to) E04.9
    with
      hyperthyroidism E05.20
        with thyroid storm E05.21
      thyrotoxicosis E05.20
        with thyroid storm E05.21
    endemic E01.1
    iodine-deficiency E01.1
    sporadic E04.9
    toxic E05.20
      with thyroid storm E05.21
    nontoxic E04.9
      diffuse (colloid) E04.0
      multinodular E04.2
      simple E04.0
      specified NEC E04.8
      uninodular E04.1
  simple E04.0
  toxic — see Hyperthyroidism, with, goiter
  uninodular (nontoxic) E04.1
    toxic or with hyperthyroidism E05.10
      with thyroid storm E05.11
Goiter-deafness syndrome E07.1
Goldberg syndrome Q89.8
Goldberg-Maxwell syndrome E34.51
Goldblatt's hypertension or kidney I70.1
Goldenhar (-Gorlin) **syndrome** Q87.0
Goldflam-Erb disease or syndrome G70.00
  with exacerbation (acute) G70.01
  in crisis G70.01
Goldscheider's disease Q81.8
Goldstein's disease (familial hemorrhagic telangiectasia)
  I78.0
Golfer's elbow — see Epicondylitis, medial
Gonadoblastoma
  specified site — see Neoplasm, uncertain behavior, by
    site
  unspecified site
    female D39.10
    male D40.10
Gonecystitis — see Vesiculitis
Gongylonemiasis B83.8
Goniosynechiae — see Adhesions, iris, goniosynechiae
Gonococcemia A54.86
Gonococcus, gonococcal (disease) (infection) — see
  also condition A54.9
  anus A54.6
  bursa, bursitis A54.49
  conjunctiva, conjunctivitis (neonatorum) A54.31
  endocardium A54.83

Gonococcus, gonococcal — continued
  eye A54.30
    conjunctivitis A54.31
    iridocyclitis A54.32
    keratitis A54.33
    newborn A54.31
    other specified A54.39
  fallopian tubes (acute) (chronic) A54.24
  genitourinary (organ) (system) (tract) (acute)
    A54.00
    lower A54.00
      with abscess (accessory gland) (periurethral)
        A54.1
    upper — see also condition A54.29
  heart A54.83
  iridocyclitis A54.32
  joint A54.42
  lymphatic (gland) (node) A54.89
  meninges, meningitis A54.81
  musculoskeletal A54.40
    arthritis A54.42
    osteomyelitis A54.43
    other specified A54.49
    spondylopathy A54.41
  pelviperitonitis A54.24
  pelvis (acute) (chronic) A54.24
  pharynx A54.5
  proctitis A54.6
  pyosalpinx (acute) (chronic) A54.24
  rectum A54.6
  skin A54.89
  specified site NEC A54.89
  tendon sheath A54.49
  throat A54.5
  urethra (acute) (chronic) A54.01
    with abscess (accessory gland) (periurethral) A54.1
  vulva (acute) (chronic) A54.02
Gonocytoma
  specified site — see Neoplasm, uncertain behavior, by
    site
  unspecified site
    female D39.10
    male D40.10
Gonorrhea (acute) (chronic) A54.9
  Bartholin's gland (acute) (chronic) (purulent) A54.02
    with abscess (accessory gland) (periurethral) A54.1
  bladder A54.01
  cervix A54.03
  conjunctiva, conjunctivitis (neonatorum) A54.31
  contact Z20.2
  Cowper's gland (with abscess) A54.1
  exposure to Z20.2
  fallopian tube (acute) (chronic) A54.24
  kidney (acute) (chronic) A54.21
  lower genitourinary tract A54.00
    with abscess (accessory gland) (periurethral) A54.1
  ovary (acute) (chronic) A54.24
  pelvis (acute) (chronic) A54.24
    female pelvic inflammatory disease A54.24
  penis A54.09
  prostate (acute) (chronic) A54.22
  seminal vesicle (acute) (chronic) A54.23
  specified site not listed — see also Gonococcus A54.89
  spermatic cord (acute) (chronic) A54.23
  urethra A54.01
    with abscess (accessory gland) (periurethral) A54.1
  vagina A54.02
  vas deferens (acute) (chronic) A54.23
  vulva A54.02
Goodall's disease A08.19
Goodpasture's syndrome M31.0
Gopalan's syndrome (burning feet) E53.0
Gorlin-Chaudry-Moss syndrome Q87.0
Gottron's papules L94.4
Gougerot-Blum syndrome (pigmented purpuric
  lichenoid dermatitis) L81.7
Gougerot-Carteaud disease or syndrome (confluent
  reticulate papillomatosis) L83
Gougerot's syndrome (trisymptomatic) L81.7
Gouley's syndrome (constrictive pericarditis) I31.1
Goundou A66.6
Gout, chronic — see also Gout, gouty M1A.9 ☑ (following
  M08)
  drug-induced M1A.20 ☑ (following M08)
    ankle M1A.27- ☑ (following M08)
    elbow M1A.22- ☑ (following M08)
    foot joint M1A.27- ☑ (following M08)
    hand joint M1A.24- ☑ (following M08)
    hip M1A.25- ☑ (following M08)

Gout, chronic — continued
  drug-induced — continued
    knee M1A.26- ☑ (following M08)
    multiple site M1A.29- ☑ (following M08)
    shoulder M1A.21- ☑ (following M08)
    vertebrae M1A.28 ☑ (following M08)
    wrist M1A.23- ☑ (following M08)
  idiopathic M1A.00 ☑ (following M08)
    ankle M1A.07- ☑ (following M08)
    elbow M1A.02- ☑ (following M08)
    foot joint M1A.07- ☑ (following M08)
    hand joint M1A.04- ☑ (following M08)
    hip M1A.05- ☑ (following M08)
    knee M1A.06- ☑ (following M08)
    multiple site M1A.09 ☑ (following M08)
    shoulder M1A.01- ☑ (following M08)
    vertebrae M1A.08 ☑ (following M08)
    wrist M1A.03- ☑ (following M08)
  in (due to) renal impairment M1A.30 ☑ (following M08)
    ankle M1A.37- ☑ (following M08)
    elbow M1A.32- ☑ (following M08)
    foot joint M1A.37- ☑ (following M08)
    hand joint M1A.34- ☑ (following M08)
    hip M1A.35- ☑ (following M08)
    knee M1A.36- ☑ (following M08)
    multiple site M1A.39 ☑ (following M08)
    shoulder M1A.31- ☑ (following M08)
    vertebrae M1A.38 ☑ (following M08)
    wrist M1A.33- ☑ (following M08)
  lead-induced M1A.10 ☑ (following M08)
    ankle M1A.17- ☑ (following M08)
    elbow M1A.12- ☑ (following M08)
    foot joint M1A.17- ☑ (following M08)
    hand joint M1A.14- ☑ (following M08)
    hip M1A.15- ☑ (following M08)
    knee M1A.16- ☑ (following M08)
    multiple site M1A.19 ☑ (following M08)
    shoulder M1A.11- ☑ (following M08)
    vertebrae M1A.18 ☑ (following M08)
    wrist M1A.13- ☑ (following M08)
  primary — see Gout, chronic, idiopathic
  saturnine — see Gout, chronic, lead-induced
  secondary NEC M1A.40 ☑ (following M08)
    ankle M1A.47- ☑ (following M08)
    elbow M1A.42- ☑ (following M08)
    foot joint M1A.47- ☑ (following M08)
    hand joint M1A.44- ☑ (following M08)
    hip M1A.45- ☑ (following M08)
    knee M1A.46- ☑ (following M08)
    multiple site M1A.49 ☑ (following M08)
    shoulder M1A.41- ☑ (following M08)
    vertebrae M1A.48 ☑ (following M08)
    wrist M1A.43- ☑ (following M08)
  syphilitic — see also subcategory M14.8- A52.77
  tophi M1A.9 ☑ (following M08)
Gout, gouty (acute) (attack) (flare) — see also Gout,
  chronic M10.9
  drug-induced M10.20
    ankle M10.27- ☑
    elbow M10.22- ☑
    foot joint M10.27- ☑
    hand joint M10.24- ☑
    hip M10.25- ☑
    knee M10.26- ☑
    multiple site M10.29
    shoulder M10.21- ☑
    vertebrae M10.28
    wrist M10.23- ☑
  idiopathic M10.00
    ankle M10.07- ☑
    elbow M10.02- ☑
    foot joint M10.07- ☑
    hand joint M10.04- ☑
    hip M10.05- ☑
    knee M10.06- ☑
    multiple site M10.09
    shoulder M10.01- ☑
    vertebrae M10.08
    wrist M10.03- ☑
  in (due to) renal impairment M10.30
    ankle M10.37- ☑
    elbow M10.32- ☑
    foot joint M10.37- ☑
    hand joint M10.34- ☑
    hip M10.35- ☑
    knee M10.36- ☑

☑ **Additional Character Required** — Refer to the Tabular List for Character Selection   ▽ **Subterms under main terms may continue to next column or page**

Gout, gouty — *continued*
　in renal impairment — *continued*
　　multiple site M10.39
　　shoulder M10.31- ☑
　　vertebrae M10.38
　　wrist M10.33- ☑
　lead-induced M10.10
　　ankle M10.17- ☑
　　elbow M10.12- ☑
　　foot joint M10.17- ☑
　　hand joint M10.14- ☑
　　hip M10.15- ☑
　　knee M10.16- ☑
　　multiple site M10.19
　　shoulder M10.11- ☑
　　vertebrae M10.18
　　wrist M10.13- ☑
　primary — *see* Gout, idiopathic
　saturnine — *see* Gout, lead-induced
　secondary NEC M10.40
　　ankle M10.47- ☑
　　elbow M10.42- ☑
　　foot joint M10.47- ☑
　　hand joint M10.44- ☑
　　hip M10.45- ☑
　　knee M10.46- ☑
　　multiple site M10.49
　　shoulder M10.41- ☑
　　vertebrae M10.48
　　wrist M10.43- ☑
　syphilitic — *see also* subcategory M14.8- A52.77
　tophi — *see* Gout, chronic
Gower's
　muscular dystrophy G71.01
　syndrome (vasovagal attack) R55
Gradenigo's syndrome — *see* Otitis, media, suppurative, acute
Graefe's disease — *see* Strabismus, paralytic, ophthalmoplegia, progressive
Graft-versus-host disease D89.813
　acute D89.810
　acute on chronic D89.812
　chronic D89.811
Grain mite (itch) B88.0
Grainhandler's disease or lung J67.8
Grand mal — *see* Epilepsy, generalized, specified NEC
Grand multipara status only (not pregnant) Z64.1
　pregnant — *see* Pregnancy, complicated by, grand multiparity
Granite worker's lung J62.8
Granular — *see also* condition
　inflammation, pharynx J31.2
　kidney (contracting) — *see* Sclerosis, renal
　liver K74.69
Granulation tissue (abnormal) (excessive) L92.9
　postmastoidectomy cavity — *see* Complications, postmastoidectomy, granulation
Granulocytopenia (primary) (malignant) — *see* Agranulocytosis
Granuloma L92.9
　abdomen K66.8
　　from residual foreign body L92.3
　　pyogenicum L98.0
　actinic L57.5
　annulare (perforating) L92.0
　apical K04.5
　aural — *see* Otitis, externa, specified NEC
　beryllium (skin) L92.3
　bone
　　eosinophilic C96.6
　　from residual foreign body — *see* Osteomyelitis, specified type NEC
　　lung C96.6
　brain (any site) G06.0
　　schistosomiasis B65.9 *[G07]*
　canaliculus lacrimalis — *see* Granuloma, lacrimal
　candidal (cutaneous) B37.2
　cerebral (any site) G06.0
　coccidioidal (primary) (progressive) B38.7
　　lung B38.1
　　meninges B38.4
　colon K63.89
　conjunctiva H11.22- ☑
　dental K04.5
　ear, middle — *see* Cholesteatoma
　eosinophilic C96.6
　　bone C96.6

Granuloma — *continued*
　eosinophilic — *continued*
　　lung C96.6
　　oral mucosa K13.4
　　skin L92.2
　eyelid H01.8
　facial (e) L92.2
　foreign body (in soft tissue) NEC M60.20
　　ankle M60.27- ☑
　　foot M60.27- ☑
　　forearm M60.23- ☑
　　hand M60.24- ☑
　　in operation wound — *see* Foreign body, accidentally left during a procedure
　　lower leg M60.26- ☑
　　pelvic region M60.25- ☑
　　shoulder region M60.21- ☑
　　skin L92.3
　　specified site NEC M60.28
　　subcutaneous tissue L92.3
　　thigh M60.25- ☑
　　upper arm M60.22- ☑
　gangraenescens M31.2
　genito-inguinale A58
　giant cell (central) (reparative) (jaw) M27.1
　　gingiva (peripheral) K06.8
　gland (lymph) I88.8
　hepatic NEC K75.3
　　in (due to)
　　　berylliosis J63.2 *[K77]*
　　　sarcoidosis D86.89
　Hodgkin C81.9 ☑
　ileum K63.89
　infectious B99.9
　　specified NEC B99.8
　inguinale (Donovan) (venereal) A58
　intestine NEC K63.89
　intracranial (any site) G06.0
　intraspinal (any part) G06.1
　iridocyclitis — *see* Iridocyclitis, chronic
　jaw (bone) (central) M27.1
　　reparative giant cell M27.1
　kidney — *see also* Infection, kidney N15.8
　lacrimal H04.81- ☑
　larynx J38.7
　lethal midline (faciale(e)) M31.2
　liver NEC — *see* Granuloma, hepatic
　lung (infectious) — *see also* Fibrosis, lung
　　coccidioidal B38.1
　　eosinophilic C96.6
　Majocchi's B35.8
　malignant (facial(e)) M31.2
　mandible (central) M27.1
　midline (lethal) M31.2
　monilial (cutaneous) B37.2
　nasal sinus — *see* Sinusitis
　operation wound T81.89 ☑
　　foreign body — *see* Foreign body, accidentally left during a procedure
　　stitch T81.89 ☑
　　talc — *see* Foreign body, accidentally left during a procedure
　oral mucosa K13.4
　orbit, orbital H05.11- ☑
　paracoccidioidal B41.8
　penis, venereal A58
　periapical K04.5
　peritoneum K66.8
　　due to ova of helminths NOS — *see also* Helminthiasis B83.9 *[K67]*
　postmastoidectomy cavity — *see* Complications, postmastoidectomy, recurrent cholesteatoma
　prostate N42.89
　pudendi (ulcerating) A58
　pulp, internal (tooth) K04.3
　pyogenic, pyogenicum (of) (skin) L98.0
　　gingiva K06.8
　　maxillary alveolar ridge K04.5
　　oral mucosa K13.4
　rectum K62.89
　reticulohistiocytic D76.3
　rubrum nasi L74.8
　Schistosoma — *see* Schistosomiasis
　septic (skin) L98.0
　silica (skin) L92.3
　sinus (accessory) (infective) (nasal) — *see* Sinusitis
　skin L92.9
　　from residual foreign body L92.3

Granuloma — *continued*
　skin — *continued*
　　pyogenicum L98.0
　spine
　　syphilitic (epidural) A52.19
　　tuberculous A18.01
　stitch (postoperative) T81.89 ☑
　suppurative (skin) L98.0
　swimming pool A31.1
　talc — *see also* Granuloma, foreign body
　　in operation wound — *see* Foreign body, accidentally left during a procedure
　telangiectaticum (skin) L98.0
　tracheostomy J95.09
　trichophyticum B35.8
　tropicum A66.4
　umbilical P83.81
　umbilicus P83.81
　urethra N36.8
　uveitis — *see* Iridocyclitis, chronic
　vagina A58
　venereum A58
　vocal cord J38.3
Granulomatosis L92.9
　lymphoid C83.8- ☑
　miliary (listerial) A32.89
　necrotizing, respiratory M31.30
　progressive septic D71
　specified NEC L92.8
　Wegener's M31.30
　　with renal involvement M31.31
Granulomatous tissue (abnormal) (excessive) L92.9
Granulosis rubra nasi L74.8
Graphite fibrosis (of lung) J63.3
Graphospasm F48.8
　organic G25.89
Grating scapula M89.8X1
Gravel (urinary) — *see* Calculus, urinary
Graves' disease — *see* Hyperthyroidism, with, goiter
Gravis — *see* condition
Grawitz tumor C64.- ☑
Gray syndrome (newborn) P93.0
Grayness, hair (premature) L67.1
　congenital Q84.2
Green sickness D50.8
Greenfield's disease
　meaning
　　concentric sclerosis (encephalitis periaxialis concentrica) G37.5
　　metachromatic leukodystrophy E75.25
Greenstick fracture — *code as* Fracture, by site
Grey syndrome (newborn) P93.0
Grief F43.21
　prolonged F43.29
　reaction — *see also* Disorder, adjustment F43.20
Griesinger's disease B76.0
Grinder's lung or pneumoconiosis J62.8
Grinding, teeth
　psychogenic F45.8
　sleep related G47.63
Grip
　Dabney's B33.0
　devil's B33.0
Grippe, grippal — *see also* Influenza
　Balkan A78
　summer, of Italy A93.1
Grisel's disease M43.6
Groin — *see* condition
Grooved tongue K14.5
Ground itch B76.9
Grover's disease or syndrome L11.1
Growing pains, children R29.898
Growth (fungoid) (neoplastic) (new) — *see also* Neoplasm
　adenoid (vegetative) J35.8
　benign — *see* Neoplasm, benign, by site
　malignant — *see* Neoplasm, malignant, by site
　rapid, childhood Z00.2
　secondary — *see* Neoplasm, secondary, by site
Gruby's disease B35.0
Gubler-Millard paralysis or syndrome G46.3
Guerin-Stern syndrome Q74.3
Guidance, insufficient anterior (occlusal) M26.54
Guillain-Barré disease or syndrome G61.0
　sequelae G65.0
Guinea worms (infection) (infestation) B72
Guinon's disease (motor-verbal tic) F95.2
Gull's disease E03.4

Gum — *see* condition
Gumboil K04.7
  with sinus K04.6
Gumma (syphilitic) A52.79
  artery A52.09
    cerebral A52.04
  bone A52.77
    of yaws (late) A66.6
  brain A52.19
  cauda equina A52.19
  central nervous system A52.3
  ciliary body A52.71
  congenital A50.59
  eyelid A52.71
  heart A52.06
  intracranial A52.19
  iris A52.71
  kidney A52.75
  larynx A52.73
  leptomeninges A52.19
  liver A52.74
  meninges A52.19
  myocardium A52.06
  nasopharynx A52.73
  neurosyphilitic A52.3
  nose A52.73
  orbit A52.71
  palate (soft) A52.79
  penis A52.76
  pericardium A52.06
  pharynx A52.73
  pituitary A52.79
  scrofulous (tuberculous) A18.4
  skin A52.79
  specified site NEC A52.79
  spinal cord A52.19
  tongue A52.79
  tonsil A52.73
  trachea A52.73
  tuberculous A18.4
  ulcerative due to yaws A66.4
  ureter A52.75
  yaws A66.4
    bone A66.6
Gunn's syndrome Q07.8
Gunshot wound — *see also* Wound, open
  fracture — *code as* Fracture, by site
  internal organs — *see* Injury, by site
Gynandrism Q56.0
Gynandroblastoma
  specified site — *see* Neoplasm, uncertain behavior, by site
  unspecified site
    female D39.10
    male D40.10
Gynecological examination (periodic) (routine) Z01.419
  with abnormal findings Z01.411
Gynecomastia N62
Gynephobia F40.291
Gyrate scalp Q82.8

H

H (Hartnup's) **disease** E72.02
Haas' disease or osteochondrosis (juvenile) (head of humerus) — *see* Osteochondrosis, juvenile, humerus
Habit, habituation
  bad sleep Z72.821
  chorea F95.8
  disturbance, child F98.9
  drug — *see* Dependence, drug
  irregular sleep Z72.821
  laxative F55.2
  spasm — *see* Tic
  tic — *see* Tic
Haemophilus (H.) **influenzae, as cause of disease classified elsewhere** B96.3
Haff disease — *see* Poisoning, mercury
Hageman's factor defect, deficiency or disease D68.2
Haglund's disease or osteochondrosis (juvenile) (os tibiale externum) — *see* Osteochondrosis, juvenile, tarsus
Hailey-Hailey disease Q82.8
Hair — *see also* condition
  plucking F63.3
    in stereotyped movement disorder F98.4
  tourniquet syndrome — *see also* Constriction, external, by site

Hair — *continued*
  tourniquet syndrome — *see also* Constriction, external, by site — *continued*
    finger S60.44- ☑
    penis S30.842 ☑
    thumb S60.34- ☑
    toe S90.44- ☑
Hairball in stomach T18.2 ☑
Hair-pulling, pathological (compulsive) F63.3
Hairy black tongue K14.3
Half vertebra Q76.49
Halitosis R19.6
Hallerman-Streiff syndrome Q87.0
Hallervorden-Spatz disease G23.0
Hallopeau's acrodermatitis or disease L40.2
Hallucination R44.3
  auditory R44.0
  gustatory R44.2
  olfactory R44.2
  specified NEC R44.2
  tactile R44.2
  visual R44.1
Hallucinosis (chronic) F28
  alcoholic (acute) F10.951
    in
      abuse F10.151
      dependence F10.251
  drug-induced F19.951
    cannabis F12.951
    cocaine F14.951
    hallucinogen F16.151
    in
      abuse F19.151
        cannabis F12.151
        cocaine F14.151
        hallucinogen F16.151
        inhalant F18.151
        opioid F11.151
        sedative, anxiolytic or hypnotic F13.151
        stimulant NEC F15.151
      dependence F19.251
        cannabis F12.251
        cocaine F14.251
        hallucinogen F16.251
        inhalant F18.251
        opioid F11.251
        sedative, anxiolytic or hypnotic F13.251
        stimulant NEC F15.251
    inhalant F18.951
    opioid F11.951
    sedative, anxiolytic or hypnotic F13.951
    stimulant NEC F15.951
  organic F06.0
Hallux
  deformity (acquired) NEC M20.5X- ☑
  limitus M20.5X- ☑
  malleus (acquired) NEC M20.3- ☑
  rigidus (acquired) M20.2- ☑
    congenital Q74.2
    sequelae (late effect) of rickets E64.3
  valgus (acquired) M20.1- ☑
    congenital Q66.6
  varus (acquired) M20.3- ☑
    congenital Q66.3- ☑
Halo, visual H53.19
Hamartoma, hamartoblastoma Q85.9
  epithelial (gingival), odontogenic, central or peripheral — *see* Cyst, calcifying odontogenic
Hamartosis Q85.9
Hamman-Rich syndrome J84.114
Hammer toe (acquired) NEC — *see also* Deformity, toe, hammer toe
  congenital Q66.89
  sequelae (late effect) of rickets E64.3
Hand — *see* condition
Hand-foot syndrome L27.1
Handicap, handicapped
  educational Z55.9
    specified NEC Z55.8
Hand-Schüller-Christian disease or syndrome C96.5
Hanging (asphyxia) (strangulation) (suffocation) — *see* Asphyxia, traumatic, due to mechanical threat
Hangnail — *see also* Cellulitis, digit
  with lymphangitis — *see* Lymphangitis, acute, digit
Hangover (alcohol) F10.129
Hanhart's syndrome Q87.0
Hanot-Chauffard (-Troisier) **syndrome** E83.19

Hanot's cirrhosis or disease K74.3
Hansen's disease — *see* Leprosy
Hantaan virus disease (Korean hemorrhagic fever) A98.5
Hantavirus disease (with renal manifestations) (Dobrava) (Puumala) (Seoul) A98.5
  with pulmonary manifestations (Andes) (Bayou) (Bermejo) (Black Creek Canal) (Choclo) (Juquitiba) (Laguna negra) (Lechiguanas) (New York) (Oran) (Sin nombre) B33.4
Happy puppet syndrome Q93.51
Harada's disease or syndrome H30.81- ☑
Hardening
  artery — *see* Arteriosclerosis
  brain G93.89
Harelip (complete) (incomplete) — *see* Cleft, lip
Harlequin (newborn) Q80.4
Harley's disease D59.6
Harmful use (of)
  alcohol F10.10
  anxiolytics — *see* Abuse, drug, sedative
  cannabinoids — *see* Abuse, drug, cannabis
  cocaine — *see* Abuse, drug, cocaine
  drug — *see* Abuse, drug
  hallucinogens — *see* Abuse, drug, hallucinogen
  hypnotics — *see* Abuse, drug, sedative
  opioids — *see* Abuse, drug, opioid
  PCP (phencyclidine) — *see* Abuse, drug, hallucinogen
  sedatives — *see* Abuse, drug, sedative
  stimulants NEC — *see* Abuse, drug, stimulant
Harris' lines — *see* Arrest, epiphyseal
Hartnup's disease E72.02
Harvester's lung J67.0
Harvesting ovum for in vitro fertilization Z31.83
Hashimoto's disease or thyroiditis E06.3
Hashitoxicosis (transient) E06.3
Hassal-Henle bodies or warts (cornea) H18.49
Haut mal — *see* Epilepsy, generalized, specified NEC
Haverhill fever A25.1
Hay fever — *see also* Fever, hay J30.1
Hayem-Widal syndrome D59.8
Haygarth's nodes M15.8
Haymaker's lung J67.0
Hb (abnormal)
  Bart's disease D56.0
  disease — *see* Disease, hemoglobin
  trait — *see* Trait
Head — *see* condition
Headache R51
  allergic NEC G44.89
  associated with sexual activity G44.82
  chronic daily R51
  cluster G44.009
    chronic G44.029
      intractable G44.021
      not intractable G44.029
    episodic G44.019
      intractable G44.011
      not intractable G44.019
    intractable G44.001
    not intractable G44.009
  cough (primary) G44.83
  daily chronic R51
  drug-induced NEC G44.40
    intractable G44.41
    not intractable G44.40
  exertional (primary) G44.84
  histamine G44.009
    intractable G44.001
    not intractable G44.009
  hypnic G44.81
  lumbar puncture G97.1
  medication overuse G44.40
    intractable G44.41
    not intractable G44.40
  menstrual — *see* Migraine, menstrual
  migraine (type) — *see also* Migraine G43.909
  nasal septum R51
  neuralgiform, short lasting unilateral, with conjunctival injection and tearing (SUNCT) G44.059
    intractable G44.051
    not intractable G44.059
  new daily persistent (NDPH) G44.52
  orgasmic G44.82
  periodic syndromes in adults and children G43.C0 (*following* G43.7)
    with refractory migraine G43.C1 (*following* G43.7)
    intractable G43.C1 (*following* G43.7)

Headache — *continued*
  periodic syndromes in adults and children — *continued*
    not intractable G43.CØ (*following* G43.7)
    without refractory migraine G43.CØ (*following* G43.7)
  postspinal puncture G97.1
  post-traumatic G44.3Ø9
    acute G44.319
      intractable G44.311
      not intractable G44.319
    chronic G44.329
      intractable G44.321
      not intractable G44.329
    intractable G44.3Ø1
    not intractable G44.3Ø9
  pre-menstrual — *see* Migraine, menstrual
  preorgasmic G44.82
  primary
    cough G44.83
    exertional G44.84
    stabbing G44.85
    thunderclap G44.53
  rebound G44.4Ø
    intractable G44.41
    not intractable G44.4Ø
  short lasting unilateral neuralgiform, with conjunctival injection and tearing (SUNCT) G44.Ø59
    intractable G44.Ø51
    not intractable G44.Ø59
  specified syndrome NEC G44.89
  spinal and epidural anesthesia - induced T88.59 ☑
    in labor and delivery O74.5
    in pregnancy O29.4- ☑
    postpartum, puerperal O89.4
  spinal fluid loss (from puncture) G97.1
  stabbing (primary) G44.85
  tension (-type) G44.2Ø9
    chronic G44.229
      intractable G44.221
      not intractable G44.229
    episodic G44.219
      intractable G44.211
      not intractable G44.219
    intractable G44.2Ø1
    not intractable G44.2Ø9
  thunderclap (primary) G44.53
  vascular NEC G44.1

Healthy
  infant
    accompanying sick mother Z76.3
    receiving care Z76.2
  person accompanying sick person Z76.3

Hearing examination ZØ1.1Ø
  with abnormal findings NEC ZØ1.118
  following failed hearing screening ZØ1.11Ø
  for hearing conservation and treatment ZØ1.12
  infant or child (over 28 days old) ZØØ.129
    with abnormal findings ZØØ.121

Heart — *see* condition
Heart beat
  abnormality RØØ.9
    specified NEC RØØ.8
  awareness RØØ.2
  rapid RØØ.Ø
  slow RØØ.1
Heartburn R12
  psychogenic F45.8
Heartland virus disease A93.8
Heat (effects) T67.9 ☑
  apoplexy T67.Ø1 ☑
  burn — *see also* Burn L55.9
  collapse T67.1 ☑
  cramps T67.2 ☑
  dermatitis or eczema L59.Ø
  edema T67.7 ☑
  erythema — *code by site under* Burn, first degree
  excessive T67.9 ☑
    specified effect NEC T67.8 ☑
  exhaustion T67.5 ☑
    anhydrotic T67.3 ☑
    due to
      salt (and water) depletion T67.4 ☑
      water depletion T67.3 ☑
        with salt depletion T67.4 ☑
  fatigue (transient) T67.6 ☑
  fever T67.Ø1 ☑
  hyperpyrexia T67.Ø1 ☑
  prickly L74.Ø

Heat — *continued*
  prostration — *see* Heat, exhaustion
  pyrexia T67.Ø1 ☑
  rash L74.Ø
  specified effect NEC T67.8 ☑
  stroke T67.Ø1 ☑
    exertional T67.Ø2 ☑
    specified NEC T67.Ø9 ☑
  sunburn — *see* Sunburn
  syncope T67.1 ☑
Heavy-for-dates NEC (infant) (4ØØØg to 4499g) PØ8.1
  exceptionally (45ØØg or more) PØ8.Ø
Hebephrenia, hebephrenic (schizophrenia) F2Ø.1
Heberden's disease or nodes (with arthropathy) M15.1
Hebra's
  pityriasis L26
  prurigo L28.2
Heel — *see* condition
Heerfordt's disease D86.89
Hegglin's anomaly or syndrome D72.Ø
Heilmeyer-Schoner disease D45
Heine-Medin disease A8Ø.9
Heinz body anemia, congenital D58.2
Heliophobia F4Ø.228
Heller's disease or syndrome F84.3
HELLP syndrome (hemolysis, elevated liver enzymes and low platelet count) O14.2- ☑
  complicating
    childbirth O14.24
    puerperium O14.25
Helminthiasis — *see also* Infestation, helminth
  Ancylostoma B76.Ø
  intestinal B82.Ø
    mixed types (types classifiable to more than one of the titles B65.Ø-B81.3 and B81.8) B81.4
    specified type NEC B81.8
  mixed types (intestinal) (types classifiable to more than one of the titles B65.Ø-B81.3 and B81.8) B81.4
  Necator (americanus) B76.1
  specified type NEC B83.8
Heloma L84
Hemangioblastoma — *see* Neoplasm, connective tissue, uncertain behavior
  malignant — *see* Neoplasm, connective tissue, malignant
Hemangioendothelioma — *see also* Neoplasm, uncertain behavior, by site
  benign D18.ØØ
    intra-abdominal D18.Ø3
    intracranial D18.Ø2
    skin D18.Ø1
    specified site NEC D18.Ø9
  bone (diffuse) — *see* Neoplasm, bone, malignant
  epithelioid — *see also* Neoplasm, uncertain behavior, by site
    malignant — *see* Neoplasm, malignant, by site
  malignant — *see* Neoplasm, connective tissue, malignant
Hemangiofibroma — *see* Neoplasm, benign, by site
Hemangiolipoma — *see* Lipoma
Hemangioma D18.ØØ
  arteriovenous D18.ØØ
    intra-abdominal D18.Ø3
    intracranial D18.Ø2
    skin D18.Ø1
    specified site NEC D18.Ø9
  capillary I78.1
    intra-abdominal D18.Ø3
    intracranial D18.Ø2
    skin D18.Ø1
    specified site NEC D18.Ø9
  cavernous D18.ØØ
    intra-abdominal D18.Ø3
    intracranial D18.Ø2
    skin D18.Ø1
    specified site NEC D18.Ø9
  epithelioid D18.ØØ
    intra-abdominal D18.Ø3
    intracranial D18.Ø2
    skin D18.Ø1
    specified site NEC D18.Ø9
  histiocytoid D18.ØØ
    intra-abdominal D18.Ø3
    intracranial D18.Ø2
    skin D18.Ø1
    specified site NEC D18.Ø9
  infantile D18.ØØ
    intra-abdominal D18.Ø3

Hemangioma — *continued*
  infantile — *continued*
    intracranial D18.Ø2
    skin D18.Ø1
    specified site NEC D18.Ø9
  intra-abdominal D18.Ø3
  intracranial D18.Ø2
  intramuscular D18.ØØ
    intra-abdominal D18.Ø3
    intracranial D18.Ø2
    skin D18.Ø1
    specified site NEC D18.Ø9
  intrathoracic structures D18.Ø9
  juvenile D18.ØØ
  malignant — *see* Neoplasm, connective tissue, malignant
  plexiform D18.ØØ
    intra-abdominal D18.Ø3
    intracranial D18.Ø2
    skin D18.Ø1
    specified site NEC D18.Ø9
  racemose D18.ØØ
    intra-abdominal D18.Ø3
    intracranial D18.Ø2
    skin D18.Ø1
    specified site NEC D18.Ø9
  sclerosing — *see* Neoplasm, skin, benign
  simplex D18.ØØ
    intra-abdominal D18.Ø3
    intracranial D18.Ø2
    skin D18.Ø1
    specified site NEC D18.Ø9
  skin D18.Ø1
  specified site NEC D18.Ø9
  venous D18.ØØ
    intra-abdominal D18.Ø3
    intracranial D18.Ø2
    skin D18.Ø1
    specified site NEC D18.Ø9
  verrucous keratotic D18.ØØ
    intra-abdominal D18.Ø3
    intracranial D18.Ø2
    skin D18.Ø1
    specified site NEC D18.Ø9
Hemangiomatosis (systemic) I78.8
  involving single site — *see* Hemangioma
Hemangiopericytoma — *see also* Neoplasm, connective tissue, uncertain behavior
  benign — *see* Neoplasm, connective tissue, benign
  malignant — *see* Neoplasm, connective tissue, malignant
Hemangiosarcoma — *see* Neoplasm, connective tissue, malignant
Hemarthrosis (nontraumatic) M25.ØØ
  ankle M25.Ø7- ☑
  elbow M25.Ø2- ☑
  foot joint M25.Ø7- ☑
  hand joint M25.Ø4- ☑
  hip M25.Ø5- ☑
  in hemophilic arthropathy — *see* Arthropathy, hemophilic
  knee M25.Ø6- ☑
  shoulder M25.Ø1- ☑
  specified joint NEC M25.Ø8
  traumatic — *see* Sprain, by site
  vertebrae M25.Ø8
  wrist M25.Ø3- ☑
Hematemesis K92.Ø
  with ulcer — *code by site under* Ulcer, with hemorrhage K27.4
  newborn, neonatal P54.Ø
    due to swallowed maternal blood P78.2
Hematidrosis L74.8
Hematinuria — *see also* Hemoglobinuria
  malarial B5Ø.8
Hematobilia K83.8
Hematocele
  female NEC N94.89
    with ectopic pregnancy OØØ.9Ø
      with intrauterine pregnancy OØØ.91
    ovary N83.8
  male N5Ø.1
Hematochezia — *see also* Melena K92.1
Hematochyluria — *see also* Infestation, filarial
  schistosomiasis (bilharziasis) B65.Ø
Hematocolpos (with hematometra or hematosalpinx) N89.7
Hematocornea — *see* Pigmentation, cornea, stromal

Hematogenous — see condition
Hematoma (traumatic) (skin surface intact) — see also Contusion
  with
    injury of internal organs — see Injury, by site
    open wound — see Wound, open
  amputation stump (surgical) (late) T87.89
  aorta, dissecting I71.00
    abdominal I71.02
    thoracic I71.01
    thoracoabdominal I71.03
  aortic intramural — see Dissection, aorta
  arterial (complicating trauma) — see Injury, blood vessel, by site
  auricle — see Contusion, ear
    nontraumatic — see Disorder, pinna, hematoma
  birth injury NEC P15.8
  brain (traumatic)
    with
      cerebral laceration or contusion (diffuse) — see Injury, intracranial, diffuse
        focal — see Injury, intracranial, focal
    cerebellar, traumatic S06.37- ✓
    intracerebral, traumatic — see Injury, intracranial, intracerebral hemorrhage
    newborn NEC P52.4
      birth injury P10.1
    nontraumatic — see Hemorrhage, intracranial
    subarachnoid, arachnoid, traumatic — see Injury, intracranial, subarachnoid hemorrhage
    subdural, traumatic — see Injury, intracranial, subdural hemorrhage
  breast (nontraumatic) N64.89
  broad ligament (nontraumatic) N83.7
    traumatic S37.892 ✓
  cerebellar, traumatic S06.37- ✓
  cerebral — see Hematoma, brain
  cerebrum S06.36- ✓
    left S06.35- ✓
    right S06.34- ✓
  cesarean delivery wound O90.2
  complicating delivery (perineal) (pelvic) (vagina) (vulva) O71.7
  corpus cavernosum (nontraumatic) N48.89
  epididymis (nontraumatic) N50.1
  epidural (traumatic) — see Injury, intracranial, epidural hemorrhage
    spinal — see Injury, spinal cord, by region
  episiotomy O90.2
  face, birth injury P15.4
  genital organ NEC (nontraumatic)
    female (nonobstetric) N94.89
      traumatic S30.202 ✓
    male N50.1
      traumatic S30.201 ✓
  internal organs — see Injury, by site
  intracerebral, traumatic — see Injury, intracranial, intracerebral hemorrhage
  intraoperative — see Complications, intraoperative, hemorrhage
  labia (nontraumatic) (nonobstetric) N90.89
  liver (subcapsular) (nontraumatic) K76.89
    birth injury P15.0
  mediastinum — see Injury, intrathoracic
  mesosalpinx (nontraumatic) N83.7
    traumatic S37.898 ✓
  muscle — code by site under Contusion
  nontraumatic
    muscle M79.81
    soft tissue M79.81
  obstetrical surgical wound O90.2
  orbit, orbital (nontraumatic) — see also Hemorrhage, orbit
    traumatic — see Contusion, orbit
  pelvis (female) (nontraumatic) (nonobstetric) N94.89
    obstetric O71.7
    traumatic — see Injury, by site
  penis (nontraumatic) N48.89
    birth injury P15.5
  perianal (nontraumatic) K64.5
  perineal S30.23 ✓
    complicating delivery O71.7
  perirenal — see Injury, kidney
  pinna — see Contusion, ear
    nontraumatic — see Disorder, pinna, hematoma
  placenta O43.89- ✓

Hematoma — continued
  postoperative (postprocedural) — see Complication, postprocedural, hematoma
  retroperitoneal (nontraumatic) K66.1
    traumatic S36.892 ✓
  scrotum, superficial S30.22 ✓
    birth injury P15.5
  seminal vesicle (nontraumatic) N50.1
    traumatic S37.892 ✓
  spermatic cord (traumatic) S37.892 ✓
    nontraumatic N50.1
  spinal (cord) (meninges) — see also Injury, spinal cord, by region
    newborn (birth injury) P11.5
  spleen D73.5
    intraoperative — see Complications, intraoperative, hemorrhage, spleen
    postprocedural (postoperative) — see Complications, postprocedural, hemorrhage, spleen
  sternocleidomastoid, birth injury P15.2
  sternomastoid, birth injury P15.2
  subarachnoid (traumatic) — see Injury, intracranial, subarachnoid hemorrhage
    newborn (nontraumatic) P52.5
      due to birth injury P10.3
    nontraumatic — see Hemorrhage, intracranial, subarachnoid
  subdural (traumatic) — see Injury, intracranial, subdural hemorrhage
    newborn (localized) P52.8
      birth injury P10.0
    nontraumatic — see Hemorrhage, intracranial, subdural
  superficial, newborn P54.5
  testis (nontraumatic) N50.1
    birth injury P15.5
  tunica vaginalis (nontraumatic) N50.1
  umbilical cord, complicating delivery O69.5 ✓
  uterine ligament (broad) (nontraumatic) N83.7
    traumatic S37.892 ✓
  vagina (ruptured) (nontraumatic) N89.8
    complicating delivery O71.7
  vas deferens (nontraumatic) N50.1
    traumatic S37.892 ✓
  vitreous — see Hemorrhage, vitreous
  vulva (nontraumatic) (nonobstetric) N90.89
    complicating delivery O71.7
    newborn (birth injury) P15.5
Hematometra N85.7
  with hematocolpos N89.7
Hematomyelia (central) G95.19
  newborn (birth injury) P11.5
  traumatic T14.8 ✓
Hematomyelitis G04.90
Hematoperitoneum — see Hemoperitoneum
Hematophobia F40.230
Hematopneumothorax (see Hemothorax)
Hematopoiesis, cyclic D70.4
Hematoporphyria — see Porphyria
Hematorachis, hematorrhachis G95.19
  newborn (birth injury) P11.5
Hematosalpinx N83.6
  with
    hematocolpos N89.7
    hematometra N85.7
      with hematocolpos N89.7
  infectional — see Salpingitis
Hematospermia R36.1
Hematothorax (see Hemothorax)
Hematuria R31.9
  benign (familial) (of childhood) — see also Hematuria, idiopathic
    essential microscopic R31.1
  due to sulphonamide, sulfonamide — see Table of Drugs and Chemicals, by drug
  endemic — see also Schistosomiasis B65.0
  gross R31.0
  idiopathic N02.9
    with glomerular lesion
      crescentic (diffuse) glomerulonephritis N02.7
      dense deposit disease N02.6
      endocapillary proliferative glomerulonephritis N02.4
      focal and segmental hyalinosis or sclerosis N02.1
      membranoproliferative (diffuse) N02.5
      membranous (diffuse) N02.2
      mesangial proliferative (diffuse) N02.3
      mesangiocapillary (diffuse) N02.5

Hematuria — continued
  idiopathic — continued
    with glomerular lesion — continued
      minor abnormality N02.0
      proliferative NEC N02.8
      specified pathology NEC N02.8
  intermittent — see Hematuria, idiopathic
  malarial B50.8
  microscopic NEC (with symptoms) R31.29
    asymptomatic R31.21
    benign essential R31.1
  paroxysmal — see also Hematuria, idiopathic
    nocturnal D59.5
  persistent — see Hematuria, idiopathic
  recurrent — see Hematuria, idiopathic
  tropical — see also Schistosomiasis B65.0
  tuberculous A18.13
Hemeralopia (day blindness) H53.11
  vitamin A deficiency E50.5
Hemi-akinesia R41.4
Hemianalgesia R20.0
Hemianencephaly Q00.0
Hemianesthesia R20.0
Hemianopia, hemianopsia (heteronymous) H53.47
  homonymous H53.46- ✓
  syphilitic A52.71
Hemiathetosis R25.8
Hemiatrophy R68.89
  cerebellar G31.9
  face, facial, progressive (Romberg) G51.8
  tongue K14.8
Hemiballism (us) G25.5
Hemicardia Q24.8
Hemicephalus, hemicephaly Q00.0
Hemichorea G25.5
Hemicolitis, left — see Colitis, left sided
Hemicrania
  congenital malformation Q00.0
  continua G44.51
  meaning migraine — see also Migraine G43.909
  paroxysmal G44.039
    chronic G44.049
      intractable G44.041
      not intractable G44.049
    episodic G44.039
      intractable G44.031
      not intractable G44.039
    intractable G44.031
    not intractable G44.039
Hemidystrophy — see Hemiatrophy
Hemiectromelia Q73.8
Hemihypalgesia R20.8
Hemihypesthesia R20.1
Hemi-inattention R41.4
Hemimelia Q73.8
  lower limb — see Defect, reduction, lower limb, specified type NEC
  upper limb — see Defect, reduction, upper limb, specified type NEC
Hemiparalysis — see Hemiplegia
Hemiparesis — see Hemiplegia
Hemiparesthesia R20.2
Hemiparkinsonism G20
Hemiplegia G81.9- ✓
  alternans facialis G83.89
  ascending NEC G81.90
    spinal G95.89
  congenital (cerebral) G80.8
    spastic G80.2
  embolic (current episode) I63.4- ✓
  flaccid G81.0- ✓
  following
    cerebrovascular disease I69.959
      cerebral infarction I69.35- ✓
      intracerebral hemorrhage I69.15- ✓
      nontraumatic intracranial hemorrhage NEC I69.25- ✓
      specified disease NEC I69.85- ✓
      stroke NOS I69.35- ✓
      subarachnoid hemorrhage I69.05- ✓
  hysterical F44.4
  newborn NEC P91.88
    birth injury P11.9
  spastic G81.1- ✓
    congenital G80.2
  thrombotic (current episode) I63.3- ✓

Hemisection, spinal cord — *see* Injury, spinal cord, by region
Hemispasm (facial) R25.2
Hemisporosis B48.8
Hemitremor R25.1
Hemivertebra Q76.49
    failure of segmentation with scoliosis Q76.3
    fusion with scoliosis Q76.3
Hemochromatosis E83.119
    with refractory anemia D46.1
    due to repeated red blood cell transfusion E83.111
    hereditary (primary) E83.110
    neonatal P78.84
    primary E83.110
    specified NEC E83.118
Hemoglobin — *see also* condition
    abnormal (disease) — *see* Disease, hemoglobin
    AS genotype D57.3
    Constant Spring D58.2
    E-beta thalassemia D56.5
    fetal, hereditary persistence (HPFH) D56.4
    H Constant Spring D56.0
    low NOS D64.9
    S (Hb S), heterozygous D57.3
Hemoglobinemia D59.9
    due to blood transfusion T80.89 ☑
    paroxysmal D59.6
        nocturnal D59.5
Hemoglobinopathy (mixed) D58.2
    with thalassemia D56.8
    sickle-cell D57.1
        with thalassemia D57.40
            with crisis (vasoocclusive pain) D57.419
                with
                    acute chest syndrome D57.411
                    splenic sequestration D57.412
            without crisis D57.40
Hemoglobinuria R82.3
    with anemia, hemolytic, acquired (chronic) NEC D59.6
    cold (agglutinin) (paroxysmal) (with Raynaud's syndrome) D59.6
    due to exertion or hemolysis NEC D59.6
    intermittent D59.6
    malarial B50.8
    march D59.6
    nocturnal (paroxysmal) D59.5
    paroxysmal (cold) D59.6
        nocturnal D59.5
Hemolymphangioma D18.1
Hemolysis
    intravascular
        with
            abortion — *see* Abortion, by type, complicated by, hemorrhage
            ectopic or molar pregnancy O08.1
            hemorrhage
                antepartum — *see* Hemorrhage, antepartum, with coagulation defect
                intrapartum — *see also* Hemorrhage, complicating, delivery O67.0
        postpartum O72.3
    neonatal (excessive) P58.9
        specified NEC P58.8
Hemolytic — *see* condition
Hemopericardium I31.2
    following acute myocardial infarction (current complication) I23.0
    newborn P54.8
    traumatic — *see* Injury, heart, with hemopericardium
Hemoperitoneum K66.1
    infectional K65.9
    traumatic S36.899 ☑
        with open wound — *see* Wound, open, with penetration into peritoneal cavity
Hemophilia (classical) (familial) (hereditary) D66
    A D66
    acquired D68.311
    autoimmune D68.311
    B D67
    C D68.1
    calcipriva — *see also* Defect, coagulation D68.4
    nonfamilial — *see also* Defect, coagulation D68.4
    secondary D68.311
    vascular D68.0
Hemophthalmos H44.81- ☑
Hemopneumothorax — *see also* Hemothorax
    traumatic S27.2 ☑
Hemoptysis R04.2

Hemoptysis — *continued*
    newborn P26.9
    tuberculous — *see* Tuberculosis, pulmonary
Hemorrhage, hemorrhagic (concealed) R58
    abdomen R58
    accidental antepartum — *see* Hemorrhage, antepartum
    acute idiopathic pulmonary, in infants R04.81
    adenoid J35.8
    adrenal (capsule) (gland) E27.49
        medulla E27.8
        newborn P54.4
    after delivery — *see* Hemorrhage, postpartum
    alveolar
        lung, newborn P26.8
        process K08.89
    alveolus K08.89
    amputation stump (surgical) T87.89
    anemia (chronic) D50.0
        acute D62
    antepartum (with) O46.90
        with coagulation defect O46.00- ☑
            afibrinogenemia O46.01- ☑
            disseminated intravascular coagulation O46.02- ☑
            hypofibrinogenemia O46.01- ☑
            specified defect NEC O46.09- ☑
        before 20 weeks gestation O20.9
            specified type NEC O20.8
            threatened abortion O20.0
        due to
            abruptio placenta — *see also* Abruptio placentae O45.9- ☑
            leiomyoma, uterus — *see* Hemorrhage, antepartum, specified cause NEC
            placenta previa O44.1- ☑
        specified cause NEC — *see* subcategory O46.8X- ☑
    anus (sphincter) K62.5
    apoplexy (stroke) — *see* Hemorrhage, intracranial, intracerebral
    arachnoid — *see* Hemorrhage, intracranial, subarachnoid
    artery R58
        brain — *see* Hemorrhage, intracranial, intracerebral
    basilar (ganglion) I61.0
    bladder N32.89
    bowel K92.2
        newborn P54.3
    brain (miliary) (nontraumatic) — *see* Hemorrhage, intracranial, intracerebral
        due to
            birth injury P10.1
            syphilis A52.05
        epidural or extradural (traumatic) — *see* Injury, intracranial, epidural hemorrhage
        newborn P52.4
            birth injury P10.1
        subarachnoid — *see* Hemorrhage, intracranial, subarachnoid
        subdural — *see* Hemorrhage, intracranial, subdural
    brainstem (nontraumatic) I61.3
        traumatic S06.38- ☑
    breast N64.59
    bronchial tube — *see* Hemorrhage, lung
    bronchopulmonary — *see* Hemorrhage, lung
    bronchus — *see* Hemorrhage, lung
    bulbar I61.5
    capillary I78.8
        primary D69.8
    cecum K92.2
    cerebellar, cerebellum (nontraumatic) I61.4
        newborn P52.6
        traumatic S06.37- ☑
    cerebral, cerebrum — *see also* Hemorrhage, intracranial, intracerebral
        lobe I61.1
        newborn (anoxic) P52.4
            birth injury P10.1
    cerebromeningeal I61.8
    cerebrospinal — *see* Hemorrhage, intracranial, intracerebral
    cervix (uteri) (stump) NEC N88.8
    chamber, anterior (eye) — *see* Hyphema
    childbirth — *see* Hemorrhage, complicating, delivery
    choroid H31.30- ☑
        expulsive H31.31- ☑
    ciliary body — *see* Hyphema
    cochlea — *see* subcategory H83.8 ☑
    colon K92.2

Hemorrhage, hemorrhagic — *continued*
    complicating
        abortion — *see* Abortion, by type, complicated by, hemorrhage
        delivery O67.9
            associated with coagulation defect (afibrinogenemia) (DIC) (hyperfibrinolysis) O67.0
            specified cause NEC O67.8
            surgical procedure — *see* Hemorrhage, intraoperative
    conjunctiva H11.3- ☑
        newborn P54.8
    cord, newborn (stump) P51.9
    corpus luteum (ruptured) cyst N83.1- ☑
    cortical (brain) I61.1
    cranial — *see* Hemorrhage, intracranial
    cutaneous R23.3
        due to autosensitivity, erythrocyte D69.2
        newborn P54.5
    delayed
        following ectopic or molar pregnancy O08.1
        postpartum O72.2
    diathesis (familial) D69.9
    disease D69.9
        newborn P53
        specified type NEC D69.8
    due to or associated with
        afibrinogenemia or other coagulation defect (conditions in categories D65– D69)
            antepartum — *see* Hemorrhage, antepartum, with coagulation defect
            intrapartum O67.0
        dental implant M27.61
        device, implant or graft — *see also* Complications, by site and type, specified NEC T85.838 ☑
            arterial graft NEC T82.838 ☑
            breast T85.838 ☑
            catheter NEC T85.838 ☑
                dialysis (renal) T82.838 ☑
                    intraperitoneal T85.838 ☑
                infusion NEC T82.838 ☑
                    spinal (epidural) (subdural) T85.830 ☑
                urinary (indwelling) T83.83 ☑
            electronic (electrode) (pulse generator) (stimulator)
                bone T84.83 ☑
                cardiac T82.837 ☑
                nervous system (brain) (peripheral nerve) (spinal) T85.830 ☑
                urinary T83.83 ☑
            fixation, internal (orthopedic) NEC T84.83 ☑
            gastrointestinal (bile duct) (esophagus) T85.838 ☑
            genital NEC T83.83 ☑
            heart NEC T82.837 ☑
            joint prosthesis T84.83 ☑
            ocular (corneal graft) (orbital implant) NEC T85.838 ☑
            orthopedic NEC T84.83 ☑
                bone graft T86.838 ☑
            specified NEC T85.838 ☑
            urinary NEC T83.83 ☑
            vascular NEC T82.838 ☑
            ventricular intracranial shunt T85.830 ☑
    duodenum, duodenal K92.2
        ulcer — *see* Ulcer, duodenum, with hemorrhage
    dura mater — *see* Hemorrhage, intracranial, subdural
    endotracheal — *see* Hemorrhage, lung
    epicranial subaponeurotic (massive), birth injury P12.2
    epidural (traumatic) — *see also* Injury, intracranial, epidural hemorrhage
        nontraumatic I62.1
    esophagus K22.8
        varix I85.01
            secondary I85.11
    excessive, following ectopic gestation (subsequent episode) O08.1
    extradural (traumatic) — *see* Injury, intracranial, epidural hemorrhage
        birth injury P10.8
        newborn (anoxic) (nontraumatic) P52.8
        nontraumatic I62.1
    eye NEC H57.89
        fundus — *see* Hemorrhage, retina
        lid — *see* Disorder, eyelid, specified type NEC
    fallopian tube N83.6
    fibrinogenolysis — *see* Fibrinolysis

Hemorrhage, hemorrhagic — *continued*
  fibrinolytic (acquired) — *see* Fibrinolysis
  from
      ear (nontraumatic) — *see* Otorrhagia
      tracheostomy stoma J95.01
  fundus, eye — *see* Hemorrhage, retina
  funis — *see* Hemorrhage, umbilicus, cord
  gastric — *see* Hemorrhage, stomach
  gastroenteric K92.2
      newborn P54.3
  gastrointestinal (tract) K92.2
      newborn P54.3
  genital organ, male N50.1
  genitourinary (tract) NOS R31.9
  gingiva K06.8
  globe (eye) — *see* Hemophthalmos
  graafian follicle cyst (ruptured) N83.0- ☑
  gum K06.8
  heart I51.89
  hypopharyngeal (throat) R04.1
  intermenstrual (regular) N92.3
      irregular N92.1
  internal (organs) NEC R58
      capsule I61.0
      ear — *see* subcategory H83.8 ☑
      newborn P54.8
  intestine K92.2
      newborn P54.3
  intra-abdominal R58
  intra-alveolar (lung), newborn P26.8
  intracerebral (nontraumatic) — *see* Hemorrhage, in-
          tracranial, intracerebral
  intracranial (nontraumatic) I62.9
      birth injury P10.9
      epidural, nontraumatic I62.1
      extradural, nontraumatic I62.1
      intracerebral (nontraumatic) (in) I61.9
          brain stem I61.3
          cerebellum I61.4
          hemisphere I61.2
              cortical (superficial) I61.1
              subcortical (deep) I61.0
          intraoperative
              during a nervous system procedure G97.31
              during other procedure G97.32
          intraventricular I61.5
          multiple localized I61.6
          newborn P52.4
              birth injury P10.1
          postprocedural
              following a nervous system procedure G97.51
              following other procedure G97.52
          specified NEC I61.8
          superficial I61.1
          traumatic (diffuse) — *see* Injury, intracranial,
              diffuse
          focal — *see* Injury, intracranial, focal
      newborn P52.9
          specified NEC P52.8
      subarachnoid (nontraumatic) (from) I60.9
          intracranial (cerebral) artery I60.7
              anterior communicating I60.2
              basilar I60.4
              carotid siphon and bifurcation I60.0- ☑
              communicating I60.7
                  anterior I60.2
                  posterior I60.3- ☑
              middle cerebral I60.1- ☑
              posterior communicating I60.3- ☑
              specified artery NEC I60.6
              vertebral I60.5- ☑
          newborn P52.5
              birth injury P10.3
          specified NEC I60.8
          traumatic S06.6X- ☑
      subdural (nontraumatic) I62.00
          acute I62.01
          birth injury P10.0
          chronic I62.03
          newborn (anoxic) (hypoxic) P52.8
              birth injury P10.0
          spinal G95.19
          subacute I62.02
          traumatic — *see* Injury, intracranial, subdural
              hemorrhage
      traumatic — *see* Injury, intracranial, focal brain in-
          jury
  intramedullary NEC G95.19

Hemorrhage, hemorrhagic — *continued*
  intraocular — *see* Hemophthalmos
  intraoperative, intraprocedural — *see* Complication,
          hemorrhage (hematoma), intraoperative (in-
          traprocedural), by site
  intrapartum — *see* Hemorrhage, complicating, delivery
  intrapelvic
      female N94.89
      male K66.1
  intraperitoneal K66.1
  intrapontine I61.3
  intraprocedural — *see* Complication, hemorrhage
          (hematoma), intraoperative (intraprocedural),
          by site
  intrauterine N85.7
      complicating delivery — *see also* Hemorrhage,
          complicating, delivery O67.9
      postpartum — *see* Hemorrhage, postpartum
  intraventricular I61.5
      newborn (nontraumatic) — *see also* Newborn, af-
          fected by, hemorrhage P52.3
          due to birth injury P10.2
          grade
              1 P52.0
              2 P52.1
              3 P52.21
              4 P52.22
  intravesical N32.89
  iris (postinfectional) (postinflammatory) (toxic) — *see*
          Hyphema
  joint (nontraumatic) — *see* Hemarthrosis
  kidney N28.89
  knee (joint) (nontraumatic) — *see* Hemarthrosis, knee
  labyrinth — *see* subcategory H83.8 ☑
  lenticular striate artery I61.0
  ligature, vessel — *see* Hemorrhage, postoperative
  liver K76.89
  lung R04.89
      newborn P26.9
          massive P26.1
          specified NEC P26.8
      tuberculous — *see* Tuberculosis, pulmonary
  massive umbilical, newborn P51.0
  mediastinum — *see* Hemorrhage, lung
  medulla I61.3
  membrane (brain) I60.8
      spinal cord — *see* Hemorrhage, spinal cord
  meninges, meningeal (brain) (middle) I60.8
      spinal cord — *see* Hemorrhage, spinal cord
  mesentery K66.1
  metritis — *see* Endometritis
  mouth K13.79
  mucous membrane NEC R58
      newborn P54.8
  muscle M62.89
  nail (subungual) L60.8
  nasal turbinate R04.0
      newborn P54.8
  navel, newborn P51.9
  newborn P54.9
      specified NEC P54.8
  nipple N64.59
  nose R04.0
      newborn P54.8
  omentum K66.1
  optic nerve (sheath) H47.02- ☑
  orbit, orbital H05.23- ☑
  ovary NEC N83.8
  oviduct N83.6
  pancreas K86.89
  parathyroid (gland) (spontaneous) E21.4
  parturition — *see* Hemorrhage, complicating, delivery
  penis N48.89
  pericardium, pericarditis I31.2
  peritoneum, peritoneal K66.1
  peritonsillar tissue J35.8
      due to infection J36
  petechial R23.3
      due to autosensitivity, erythrocyte D69.2
  pituitary (gland) E23.6
  pleura — *see* Hemorrhage, lung
  polioencephalitis, superior E51.2
  polymyositis — *see* Polymyositis
  pons, pontine I61.3
  posterior fossa (nontraumatic) I61.8
      newborn P52.6
  postmenopausal N95.0
  postnasal R04.0

Hemorrhage, hemorrhagic — *continued*
  postoperative — *see* Complications, postprocedural,
          hemorrhage, by site
  postpartum NEC (following delivery of placenta) O72.1
      delayed or secondary O72.2
      retained placenta O72.0
      third stage O72.0
  pregnancy — *see* Hemorrhage, antepartum
  preretinal — *see* Hemorrhage, retina
  prostate N42.1
  puerperal — *see* Hemorrhage, postpartum
      delayed or secondary O72.2
  pulmonary R04.89
      newborn P26.9
          massive P26.1
          specified NEC P26.8
      tuberculous — *see* Tuberculosis, pulmonary
  purpura (primary) D69.3
  rectum (sphincter) K62.5
      newborn P54.2
  recurring, following initial hemorrhage at time of injury
      T79.2 ☑
  renal N28.89
  respiratory passage or tract R04.9
      specified NEC R04.89
  retina, retinal (vessels) H35.6- ☑
      diabetic — *see* Diabetes, retinal, hemorrhage
  retroperitoneal R58
  scalp R58
  scrotum N50.1
  secondary (nontraumatic) R58
      following initial hemorrhage at time of injury
          T79.2 ☑
  seminal vesicle N50.1
  skin R23.3
      newborn P54.5
  slipped umbilical ligature P51.8
  spermatic cord N50.1
  spinal (cord) G95.19
      newborn (birth injury) P11.5
  spleen D73.5
      intraoperative — *see* Complications, intraoperative,
          hemorrhage, spleen
      postprocedural — *see* Complications, postprocedu-
          ral, hemorrhage, spleen
  stomach K92.2
      newborn P54.3
      ulcer — *see* Ulcer, stomach, with hemorrhage
  subarachnoid (nontraumatic) — *see* Hemorrhage, in-
          tracranial, subarachnoid
  subconjunctival — *see also* Hemorrhage, conjunctiva
      birth injury P15.3
  subcortical (brain) I61.0
  subcutaneous R23.3
  subdiaphragmatic R58
  subdural (acute) (nontraumatic) — *see* Hemorrhage,
          intracranial, subdural
  subependymal
      newborn P52.0
          with intraventricular extension P52.1
              and intracerebral extension P52.22
  subgaleal P12.2
  subhyaloid — *see* Hemorrhage, retina
  subperiosteal — *see* Disorder, bone, specified type NEC
  subretinal — *see* Hemorrhage, retina
  subtentorial — *see* Hemorrhage, intracranial, subdural
  subungual L60.8
  suprarenal (capsule) (gland) E27.49
      newborn P54.4
  tentorium (traumatic) NEC — *see* Hemorrhage, brain
      newborn (birth injury) P10.4
  testis N50.1
  third stage (postpartum) O72.0
  thorax — *see* Hemorrhage, lung
  throat R04.1
  thymus (gland) E32.8
  thyroid (cyst) (gland) E07.89
  tongue K14.8
  tonsil J35.8
  trachea — *see* Hemorrhage, lung
  tracheobronchial R04.89
      newborn P26.0
  traumatic — *code to* specific injury
      cerebellar — *see* Hemorrhage, brain
      intracranial — *see* Hemorrhage, brain
      recurring or secondary (following initial hemorrhage
          at time of injury) T79.2 ☑

Hemorrhage, hemorrhagic — *continued*
  tuberculous NEC — *see also* Tuberculosis, pulmonary A15.Ø
  tunica vaginalis N5Ø.1
  ulcer — *code by* site under Ulcer, with hemorrhage K27.4
  umbilicus, umbilical
    cord
      after birth, newborn P51.9
      complicating delivery O69.5 ☑
    newborn P51.9
      massive P51.Ø
      slipped ligature P51.8
    stump P51.9
  urethra (idiopathic) N36.8
  uterus, uterine (abnormal) N93.9
    climacteric N92.4
    complicating delivery — *see* Hemorrhage, complicating, delivery
    dysfunctional or functional N93.8
    intermenstrual (regular) N92.3
      irregular N92.1
    postmenopausal N95.Ø
    postpartum — *see* Hemorrhage, postpartum
    preclimacteric or premenopausal N92.4
    prepubertal N93.8
    pubertal N92.2
  vagina (abnormal) N93.9
    newborn P54.6
  vas deferens N5Ø.1
  vasa previa O69.4 ☑
  ventricular I61.5
  vesical N32.89
  viscera NEC R58
    newborn P54.8
  vitreous (humor) (intraocular) H43.1- ☑
  vulva N9Ø.89
Hemorrhoids (bleeding) (without mention of degree) K64.9
  1st degree (grade/stage I) (without prolapse outside of anal canal) K64.Ø
  2nd degree (grade/stage II) (that prolapse with straining but retract spontaneously) K64.1
  3rd degree (grade/stage III) (that prolapse with straining and require manual replacement back inside anal canal) K64.2
  4th degree (grade/stage IV) (with prolapsed tissue that cannot be manually replaced) K64.3
  complicating
    pregnancy O22.4 ☑
    puerperium O87.2
  external K64.4
    with
      thrombosis K64.5
  internal (without mention of degree) K64.8
  prolapsed K64.8
  skin tags
    anus K64.4
    residual K64.4
  specified NEC K64.8
  strangulated — *see also* Hemorrhoids, by degree K64.8
  thrombosed — *see also* Hemorrhoids, by degree K64.5
  ulcerated — *see also* Hemorrhoids, by degree K64.8
Hemosalpinx N83.6
  with
    hematocolpos N89.7
    hematometra N85.7
      with hematocolpos N89.7
Hemosiderosis (dietary) E83.19
  pulmonary, idiopathic E83.1- ☑ *[J84.Ø3]*
  transfusion T8Ø.89 ☑
Hemothorax (bacterial) (nontuberculous) J94.2
  newborn P54.8
  traumatic S27.1 ☑
    with pneumothorax S27.2 ☑
  tuberculous NEC A15.6
Henoch (-Schönlein) **disease or syndrome** (purpura) D69.Ø
Henpue, henpuye A66.6
Hepar lobatum (syphilitic) A52.74
Hepatalgia K76.89
Hepatitis K75.9
  acute B17.9
    with coma K72.Ø1
    with hepatic failure — *see* Failure, hepatic
    alcoholic — *see* Hepatitis, alcoholic
    infectious B17.9
    non-viral K72.Ø ☑

Hepatitis — *continued*
  acute — *continued*
    viral B17.9
  alcoholic (acute) (chronic) K7Ø.1Ø
    with ascites K7Ø.11
  amebic — *see* Abscess, liver, amebic
  anicteric, (viral) — *see* Hepatitis, viral
  antigen-associated (HAA) — *see* Hepatitis, B
  Australia-antigen (positive) — *see* Hepatitis, B
  autoimmune K75.4
  B B19.1Ø
    with hepatic coma B19.11
    acute B16.9
      with
        delta-agent (coinfection) (without hepatic coma) B16.1
          with hepatic coma B16.Ø
        hepatic coma (without delta-agent coinfection) B16.2
    chronic B18.1
      with delta-agent B18.Ø
  bacterial NEC K75.89
  C (viral) B19.2Ø
    with hepatic coma B19.21
    acute B17.1Ø
      with hepatic coma B17.11
    chronic B18.2
  catarrhal (acute) B15.9
    with hepatic coma B15.Ø
  cholangiolitic K75.89
  cholestatic K75.89
  chronic K73.9
    active NEC K73.2
    lobular NEC K73.1
    persistent NEC K73.Ø
    specified NEC K73.8
  cytomegaloviral B25.1
  due to ethanol (acute) (chronic) — *see* Hepatitis, alcoholic
  epidemic B15.9
    with hepatic coma B15.Ø
  fulminant NEC (viral) — *see* Hepatitis, viral
  granulomatous NEC K75.3
  herpesviral BØØ.81
  history of
    B Z86.19
    C Z86.19
  homologous serum — *see* Hepatitis, viral, type B
  in (due to)
    mumps B26.81
    toxoplasmosis (acquired) B58.1
      congenital (active) P37.1 *[K77]*
  infectious, infective B15.9
    acute (subacute) B17.9
    chronic B18.9
  inoculation — *see* Hepatitis, viral, type B
  interstitial (chronic) K74.69
  lupoid NEC K75.4
  malignant NEC (with hepatic failure) K72.9Ø
    with coma K72.91
  neonatal (idiopathic) (toxic) P59.29
  neonatal giant cell P59.29
  newborn P59.29
  non-viral K72.Ø ☑
  postimmunization — *see* Hepatitis, viral, type B
  post-transfusion — *see* Hepatitis, viral, type B
  reactive, nonspecific K75.2
  serum — *see* Hepatitis, viral, type B
  specified type NEC
    with hepatic failure — *see* Failure, hepatic
  syphilitic (late) A52.74
    congenital (early) A5Ø.Ø8 *[K77]*
      late A5Ø.59 *[K77]*
    secondary A51.45
  toxic — *see also* Disease, liver, toxic K71.6
  tuberculous A18.83
  viral, virus B19.9
    with hepatic coma B19.Ø
    acute B17.9
    chronic B18.9
      specified NEC B18.8
      type
        B B18.1
          with delta-agent B18.Ø
        C B18.2
    congenital P35.3
    coxsackie B33.Ø *[K77]*
    cytomegalic inclusion B25.1

Hepatitis — *continued*
  viral, virus — *continued*
    in remission, any type — *code to* Hepatitis, chronic, by type
    non-A, non-B B17.8
    specified type NEC (with or without coma) B17.8
    type
      A B15.9
        with hepatic coma B15.Ø
      B B19.1Ø
        with hepatic coma B19.11
        acute B16.9
          with
            delta-agent (coinfection) (without hepatic coma) B16.1
              with hepatic coma B16.Ø
            hepatic coma (without delta-agent coinfection) B16.2
        chronic B18.1
          with delta-agent B18.Ø
      C B19.2Ø
        with hepatic coma B19.21
        acute B17.1Ø
          with hepatic coma B17.11
        chronic B18.2
      E B17.2
    non-A, non-B B17.8
Hepatization lung (acute) — *see* Pneumonia, lobar
Hepatoblastoma C22.2
Hepatocarcinoma C22.Ø
Hepatocholangiocarcinoma C22.Ø
Hepatocholangioma, benign D13.4
Hepatocholangitis K75.89
Hepatolenticular degeneration E83.Ø1
Hepatoma (malignant) C22.Ø
  benign D13.4
  embryonal C22.Ø
Hepatomegaly — *see also* Hypertrophy, liver
  with splenomegaly R16.2
  congenital Q44.7
  in mononucleosis
    gammaherpesviral B27.Ø9
    infectious specified NEC B27.89
Hepatoptosis K76.89
Hepatorenal syndrome following labor and delivery O9Ø.4
Hepatosis K76.89
Hepatosplenomegaly R16.2
  hyperlipemic (Bürger-Grütz type) E78.3 *[K77]*
Hereditary — *see* condition
Heredodegeneration, macular — *see* Dystrophy, retina
Heredopathia atactica polyneuritiformis G6Ø.1
Heredosyphilis — *see* Syphilis, congenital
Herlitz' syndrome Q81.1
Hermansky-Pudlak syndrome E7Ø.331
Hermaphrodite, hermaphroditism (true) Q56.Ø
  46,XX with streak gonads Q99.1
  46,XX/46,XY Q99.Ø
  46,XY with streak gonads Q99.1
  chimera 46,XX/46,XY Q99.Ø
Hernia, hernial (acquired) (recurrent) K46.9
  with
    gangrene — *see* Hernia, by site, with, gangrene
    incarceration — *see* Hernia, by site, with, obstruction
    irreducible — *see* Hernia, by site, with, obstruction
    obstruction — *see* Hernia, by site, with, obstruction
    strangulation — *see* Hernia, by site, with, obstruction
  abdomen, abdominal K46.9
    with
      gangrene (and obstruction) K46.1
      obstruction K46.Ø
    femoral — *see* Hernia, femoral
    incisional — *see* Hernia, incisional
    inguinal — *see* Hernia, inguinal
    specified site NEC K45.8
      with
        gangrene (and obstruction) K45.1
        obstruction K45.Ø
    umbilical — *see* Hernia, umbilical
    wall — *see* Hernia, ventral
  appendix — *see* Hernia, abdomen
  bladder (mucosa) (sphincter)
    congenital (female) (male) Q79.51
    female — *see* Cystocele
    male N32.89
  brain, congenital — *see* Encephalocele

Hernia, hernial — *continued*
- cartilage, vertebra — *see* Displacement, intervertebral disc
- cerebral, congenital — *see also* Encephalocele
  - endaural Q01.8
- ciliary body (traumatic) S05.2- ☑
- colon — *see* Hernia, abdomen
- Cooper's — *see* Hernia, abdomen, specified site NEC
- crural — *see* Hernia, femoral
- diaphragm, diaphragmatic K44.9
  - with
    - gangrene (and obstruction) K44.1
    - obstruction K44.0
  - congenital Q79.0
- direct (inguinal) — *see* Hernia, inguinal
- diverticulum, intestine — *see* Hernia, abdomen
- double (inguinal) — *see* Hernia, inguinal, bilateral
- due to adhesions (with obstruction) K56.50
- epigastric — *see also* Hernia, ventral K43.9
- esophageal hiatus — *see* Hernia, hiatal
- external (inguinal) — *see* Hernia, inguinal
- fallopian tube N83.4- ☑
- fascia M62.89
- femoral K41.90
  - with
    - gangrene (and obstruction) K41.40
      - not specified as recurrent K41.40
      - recurrent K41.41
    - obstruction K41.30
      - not specified as recurrent K41.30
      - recurrent K41.31
    - not specified as recurrent K41.90
    - recurrent K41.91
  - bilateral K41.20
    - with
      - gangrene (and obstruction) K41.10
        - not specified as recurrent K41.10
        - recurrent K41.11
      - obstruction K41.00
        - not specified as recurrent K41.00
        - recurrent K41.01
      - not specified as recurrent K41.20
      - recurrent K41.21
  - unilateral K41.90
    - with
      - gangrene (and obstruction) K41.40
        - not specified as recurrent K41.40
        - recurrent K41.41
      - obstruction K41.30
        - not specified as recurrent K41.30
        - recurrent K41.31
      - not specified as recurrent K41.90
      - recurrent K41.91
- foramen magnum G93.5
  - congenital Q01.8
- funicular (umbilical) — *see also* Hernia, umbilicus
  - spermatic (cord) — *see* Hernia, inguinal
- gastrointestinal tract — *see* Hernia, abdomen
- Hesselbach's — *see* Hernia, femoral, specified site NEC
- hiatal (esophageal) (sliding) K44.9
  - with
    - gangrene (and obstruction) K44.1
    - obstruction K44.0
  - congenital Q40.1
- hypogastric — *see* Hernia, ventral
- incarcerated — *see also* Hernia, by site, with obstruction
  - with gangrene — *see* Hernia, by site, with gangrene
- incisional K43.2
  - with
    - gangrene (and obstruction) K43.1
    - obstruction K43.0
- indirect (inguinal) — *see* Hernia, inguinal
- inguinal (direct) (external) (funicular) (indirect) (internal) (oblique) (scrotal) (sliding) K40.90
  - with
    - gangrene (and obstruction) K40.40
      - not specified as recurrent K40.40
      - recurrent K40.41
    - obstruction K40.30
      - not specified as recurrent K40.30
      - recurrent K40.31
    - not specified as recurrent K40.90
    - recurrent K40.91
  - bilateral K40.20
    - with
      - gangrene (and obstruction) K40.10
        - not specified as recurrent K40.10

Hernia, hernial — *continued*
- inguinal — *continued*
  - bilateral — *continued*
    - with — *continued*
      - gangrene — *continued*
        - recurrent K40.11
      - obstruction K40.00
        - not specified as recurrent K40.00
        - recurrent K40.01
    - not specified as recurrent K40.20
    - recurrent K40.21
  - unilateral K40.90
    - with
      - gangrene (and obstruction) K40.40
        - not specified as recurrent K40.40
        - recurrent K40.41
      - obstruction K40.30
        - not specified as recurrent K40.30
        - recurrent K40.31
    - not specified as recurrent K40.90
    - recurrent K40.91
- internal — *see also* Hernia, abdomen
  - inguinal — *see* Hernia, inguinal
- interstitial — *see* Hernia, abdomen
- intervertebral cartilage or disc — *see* Displacement, intervertebral disc
- intestine, intestinal — *see* Hernia, by site
- intra-abdominal — *see* Hernia, abdomen
- iris (traumatic) S05.2- ☑
- irreducible — *see also* Hernia, by site, with obstruction
  - with gangrene — *see* Hernia, by site, with gangrene
- ischiatic — *see* Hernia, abdomen, specified site NEC
- ischiorectal — *see* Hernia, abdomen, specified site NEC
- lens (traumatic) S05.2- ☑
- linea (alba) (semilunaris) — *see* Hernia, ventral
- Littre's — *see* Hernia, abdomen
- lumbar — *see* Hernia, abdomen, specified site NEC
- lung (subcutaneous) J98.4
- mediastinum J98.59
- mesenteric (internal) — *see* Hernia, abdomen
- midline — *see* Hernia, ventral
- muscle (sheath) M62.89
- nucleus pulposus — *see* Displacement, intervertebral disc
- oblique (inguinal) — *see* Hernia, inguinal
- obstructive — *see also* Hernia, by site, with obstruction
  - with gangrene — *see* Hernia, by site, with gangrene
- obturator — *see* Hernia, abdomen, specified site NEC
- omental — *see* Hernia, abdomen
- ovary N83.4- ☑
- oviduct N83.4- ☑
- paraesophageal — *see also* Hernia, diaphragm
  - congenital Q40.1
- parastomal K43.5
  - with
    - gangrene (and obstruction) K43.4
    - obstruction K43.3
- paraumbilical — *see* Hernia, umbilicus
- perineal — *see* Hernia, abdomen, specified site NEC
- Petit's — *see* Hernia, abdomen, specified site NEC
- postoperative — *see* Hernia, incisional
- pregnant uterus — *see* Abnormal, uterus in pregnancy or childbirth
- prevesical N32.89
- properitoneal — *see* Hernia, abdomen, specified site NEC
- pudendal — *see* Hernia, abdomen, specified site NEC
- rectovaginal N81.6
- retroperitoneal — *see* Hernia, abdomen, specified site NEC
- Richter's — *see* Hernia, abdomen, with obstruction
- Rieux's, Riex's — *see* Hernia, abdomen, specified site NEC
- sac condition (adhesion) (dropsy) (inflammation) (laceration) (suppuration) — *code by site under* Hernia
- sciatic — *see* Hernia, abdomen, specified site NEC
- scrotum, scrotal — *see* Hernia, inguinal
- sliding (inguinal) — *see also* Hernia, inguinal
  - hiatus — *see* Hernia, hiatal
- spigelian — *see* Hernia, ventral
- spinal — *see* Spina bifida
- strangulated — *see also* Hernia, by site, with obstruction
  - with gangrene — *see* Hernia, by site, with gangrene
- subxiphoid — *see* Hernia, ventral
- supra-umbilicus — *see* Hernia, ventral

Hernia, hernial — *continued*
- tendon — *see* Disorder, tendon, specified type NEC
- Treitz's (fossa) — *see* Hernia, abdomen, specified site NEC
- tunica vaginalis Q55.29
- umbilicus, umbilical K42.9
  - with
    - gangrene (and obstruction) K42.1
    - obstruction K42.0
- ureter N28.89
- urethra, congenital Q64.79
- urinary meatus, congenital Q64.79
- uterus N81.4
  - pregnant — *see* Abnormal, uterus in pregnancy or childbirth
- vaginal (anterior) (wall) — *see* Cystocele
- Velpeau's — *see* Hernia, femoral
- ventral K43.9
  - with
    - gangrene (and obstruction) K43.7
    - obstruction K43.6
  - incisional K43.2
    - with
      - gangrene (and obstruction) K43.1
      - obstruction K43.0
  - recurrent — *see* Hernia, incisional
  - specified NEC K43.9
    - with
      - gangrene (and obstruction) K43.7
      - obstruction K43.6
- vesical
  - congenital (female) (male) Q79.51
  - female — *see* Cystocele
  - male N32.89
- vitreous (into wound) S05.2- ☑
  - into anterior chamber — *see* Prolapse, vitreous

Herniation — *see also* Hernia
- brain (stem) G93.5
- cerebral G93.5
- mediastinum J98.59
- nucleus pulposus — *see* Displacement, intervertebral disc

Herpangina B08.5
Herpes, herpesvirus, herpetic B00.9
- anogenital A60.9
  - perianal skin A60.1
  - rectum A60.1
  - urogenital tract A60.00
    - cervix A60.03
    - male genital organ NEC A60.02
    - penis A60.01
    - specified site NEC A60.09
    - vagina A60.04
    - vulva A60.04
- blepharitis (zoster) B02.39
  - simplex B00.59
- circinatus B35.4
  - bullosus L12.0
- conjunctivitis (simplex) B00.53
  - zoster B02.31
- cornea B02.33
- encephalitis B00.4
  - due to herpesvirus 6 B10.01
  - due to herpesvirus 7 B10.09
  - specified NEC B10.09
- eye (zoster) B02.30
  - simplex B00.50
- eyelid (zoster) B02.39
  - simplex B00.59
- facialis B00.1
- febrilis B00.1
- geniculate ganglionitis B02.21
- genital, genitalis A60.00
  - female A60.09
  - male A60.02
- gestational, gestationis O26.4- ☑
- gingivostomatitis B00.2
- human B00.9
  - 1 — *see* Herpes, simplex
  - 2 — *see* Herpes, simplex
  - 3 — *see* Varicella
  - 4 — *see* Mononucleosis, Epstein-Barr (virus)
  - 5 — *see* Disease, cytomegalic inclusion (generalized)
  - 6
    - encephalitis B10.01
    - specified NEC B10.81
  - 7
    - encephalitis B10.09

Herpes, herpesvirus, herpetic — *continued*
  human — *continued*
    7 — *continued*
      specified NEC B10.82
      8 B10.89
    infection NEC B10.89
      Kaposi's sarcoma associated B10.89
    iridocyclitis (simplex) B00.51
      zoster B02.32
    iris (vesicular erythema multiforme) L51.9
    iritis (simplex) B00.51
    Kaposi's sarcoma associated B10.89
    keratitis (simplex) (dendritic) (disciform) (interstitial)
      B00.52
      zoster (interstitial) B02.33
    keratoconjunctivitis (simplex) B00.52
      zoster B02.33
    labialis B00.1
    lip B00.1
    meningitis (simplex) B00.3
      zoster B02.1
    ophthalmicus (zoster) NEC B02.30
      simplex B00.50
    penis A60.01
    perianal skin A60.1
    pharyngitis, pharyngotonsillitis B00.2
    rectum A60.1
    scrotum A60.02
    sepsis B00.7
    simplex B00.9
      complicated NEC B00.89
      congenital P35.2
      conjunctivitis B00.53
      external ear B00.1
      eyelid B00.59
      hepatitis B00.81
      keratitis (interstitial) B00.52
      myleitis B00.82
      specified complication NEC B00.89
      visceral B00.89
    stomatitis B00.2
    tonsurans B35.0
    visceral B00.89
    vulva A60.04
    whitlow B00.89
    zoster — *see also* condition B02.9
      auricularis B02.21
      complicated NEC B02.8
      conjunctivitis B02.31
      disseminated B02.7
      encephalitis B02.0
      eye (lid) B02.39
      geniculate ganglionitis B02.21
      keratitis (interstitial) B02.33
      meningitis B02.1
      myelitis B02.24
      neuritis, neuralgia B02.29
      ophthalmicus NEC B02.30
      oticus B02.21
      polyneuropathy B02.23
      specified complication NEC B02.8
      trigeminal neuralgia B02.22
Herpesvirus (human) — *see* Herpes
Herpetophobia F40.218
Herrick's anemia — *see* Disease, sickle-cell
Hers' disease E74.09
Herter-Gee syndrome K90.0
Herxheimer's reaction R68.89
Hesitancy
  of micturition R39.11
  urinary R39.11
Hesselbach's hernia — *see* Hernia, femoral, specified site NEC
Heterochromia (congenital) Q13.2
  cataract — *see* Cataract, complicated
  cyclitis (Fuchs) — *see* Cyclitis, Fuchs' heterochromic
  hair L67.1
  iritis — *see* Cyclitis, Fuchs' heterochromic
  retained metallic foreign body (nonmagnetic) — *see* Foreign body, intraocular, old, retained
    magnetic — *see* Foreign body, intraocular, old, retained, magnetic
  uveitis — *see* Cyclitis, Fuchs' heterochromic
Heterophoria — *see* Strabismus, heterophoria
Heterophyes, heterophyiasis (small intestine) B66.8
Heterotopia, heterotopic — *see also* Malposition, congenital
  cerebralis Q04.8

Heterotropia — *see* Strabismus
Heubner-Herter disease K90.0
Hexadactylism Q69.9
HGSIL (cytology finding) (high grade squamous intraepithelial lesion on cytologic smear) (Pap smear finding)
  anus R85.613
  cervix R87.613
    biopsy (histology) finding — *see* Neoplasia, intraepithelial, cervix, grade II or grade III
  vagina R87.623
    biopsy (histology) finding — *see* Neoplasia, intraepithelial, cervix, grade II or grade III
Hibernoma — *see* Lipoma
Hiccup, hiccough R06.6
  epidemic B33.0
  psychogenic F45.8
Hidden penis (congenital) Q55.64
  acquired N48.83
Hidradenitis (axillaris) (suppurative) L73.2
Hidradenoma (nodular) — *see also* Neoplasm, skin, benign
  clear cell — *see* Neoplasm, skin, benign
  papillary — *see* Neoplasm, skin, benign
Hidrocystoma — *see* Neoplasm, skin, benign
High
  altitude effects T70.20 ☑
    anoxia T70.29 ☑
    on
      ears T70.0 ☑
      sinuses T70.1 ☑
    polycythemia D75.1
  arch
    foot Q66.7- ☑
    palate, congenital Q38.5
  arterial tension — *see* Hypertension
  basal metabolic rate R94.8
  blood pressure — *see also* Hypertension
    borderline R03.0
    reading (incidental) (isolated) (nonspecific), without diagnosis of hypertension R03.0
  cholesterol E78.00
    with high triglycerides E78.2
  diaphragm (congenital) Q79.1
  expressed emotional level within family Z63.8
  head at term O32.4 ☑
  palate, congenital Q38.5
  risk
    infant NEC Z76.2
    sexual behavior (heterosexual) Z72.51
      bisexual Z72.53
      homosexual Z72.52
  scrotal testis, testes
    bilateral Q53.23
    unilateral Q53.13
  temperature (of unknown origin) R50.9
  thoracic rib Q76.6
  triglycerides E78.1
    with high cholesterol E78.2
Hildenbrand's disease A75.0
Hilum — *see* condition
Hip — *see* condition
Hippel's disease Q85.8
Hippophobia F40.218
Hippus H57.09
Hirschsprung's disease or megacolon Q43.1
Hirsutism, hirsuties L68.0
Hirudiniasis
  external B88.3
  internal B83.4
Hiss-Russell dysentery A03.1
Histidinemia, histidinuria E70.41
Histiocytoma — *see also* Neoplasm, skin, benign
  fibrous — *see also* Neoplasm, skin, benign
    atypical — *see* Neoplasm, connective tissue, uncertain behavior
    malignant — *see* Neoplasm, connective tissue, malignant
Histiocytosis D76.3
  acute differentiated progressive C96.0
  Langerhans' cell NEC C96.6
    multifocal X
      multisystemic (disseminated) C96.0
      unisystemic C96.5
    pulmonary, adult (adult PLCH) J84.82
    unifocal (X) C96.6
  lipid, lipoid D76.3

Histiocytosis — *continued*
  lipid, lipoid — *continued*
    essential E75.29
  malignant C96.A (*following* C96.6)
  mononuclear phagocytes NEC D76.1
    Langerhans' cells C96.6
  non-Langerhans cell D76.3
  polyostotic sclerosing D76.3
  sinus, with massive lymphadenopathy D76.3
  syndrome NEC D76.3
  X NEC C96.6
    acute (progressive) C96.0
    chronic C96.6
    multifocal C96.5
    multisystemic C96.0
    unifocal C96.6
Histoplasmosis B39.9
  with pneumonia NEC B39.2
  African B39.5
  American — *see* Histoplasmosis, capsulati
  capsulati B39.4
    disseminated B39.3
    generalized B39.3
    pulmonary B39.2
      acute B39.0
      chronic B39.1
  Darling's B39.4
  duboisii B39.5
  lung NEC B39.2
History
  family (of) — *see also* History, personal (of)
    alcohol abuse Z81.1
    allergy NEC Z84.89
    anemia Z83.2
    arthritis Z82.61
    asthma Z82.5
    blindness Z82.1
    cardiac death (sudden) Z82.41
    carrier of genetic disease Z84.81
    chromosomal anomaly Z82.79
    chronic
      disabling disease NEC Z82.8
      lower respiratory disease Z82.5
    colonic polyps Z83.71
    congenital malformations and deformations Z82.79
      polycystic kidney Z82.71
    consanguinity Z84.3
    deafness Z82.2
    diabetes mellitus Z83.3
    disability NEC Z82.8
    disease or disorder (of)
      allergic NEC Z84.89
      behavioral NEC Z81.8
      blood and blood-forming organs Z83.2
      cardiovascular NEC Z82.49
      chronic disabling NEC Z82.8
      digestive Z83.79
      ear NEC Z83.52
      elevated lipoprotein (a) (Lp(a)) Z83.430
      endocrine NEC Z83.49
      eye NEC Z83.518
        glaucoma Z83.511
      familial hypercholesterolemia Z83.42
      genitourinary NEC Z84.2
      glaucoma Z83.511
      hematological Z83.2
      immune mechanism Z83.2
      infectious NEC Z83.1
      ischemic heart Z82.49
      kidney Z84.1
      lipoprotein metabolism Z83.438
      mental NEC Z81.8
      metabolic Z83.49
      musculoskeletal NEC Z82.69
      neurological NEC Z82.0
      nutritional Z83.49
      parasitic NEC Z83.1
      psychiatric NEC Z81.8
      respiratory NEC Z83.6
      skin and subcutaneous tissue NEC Z84.0
      specified NEC Z84.89
    drug abuse NEC Z81.3
    elevated lipoprotein (a) (Lp(a)) Z83.430
    epilepsy Z82.0
    familial hypercholesterolemia Z83.42
    genetic disease carrier Z84.81
    glaucoma Z83.511
    hearing loss Z82.2
    human immunodeficiency virus (HIV) infection Z83.0

Herpes, herpesvirus, herpetic — History

▼ Subterms under main terms may continue to next column or page   ☑ **Additional Character Required** — Refer to the Tabular List for Character Selection   **169**

History — continued
family — see also History, personal — continued
  Huntington's chorea Z82.0
  hyperlipidemia, familial combined Z83.438
  intellectual disability Z81.0
  leukemia Z80.6
  lipidemia NEC Z83.438
  malignant neoplasm (of) NOS Z80.9
    bladder Z80.52
    breast Z80.3
    bronchus Z80.1
    digestive organ Z80.0
    gastrointestinal tract Z80.0
    genital organ Z80.49
      ovary Z80.41
      prostate Z80.42
      specified organ NEC Z80.49
      testis Z80.43
    hematopoietic NEC Z80.7
    intrathoracic organ NEC Z80.2
    kidney Z80.51
    lung Z80.1
    lymphatic NEC Z80.7
    ovary Z80.41
    prostate Z80.42
    respiratory organ NEC Z80.2
    specified site NEC Z80.8
    testis Z80.43
    trachea Z80.1
    urinary organ or tract Z80.59
      bladder Z80.52
      kidney Z80.51
  mental
    disorder NEC Z81.8
  multiple endocrine neoplasia (MEN) syndrome Z83.41
  osteoporosis Z82.62
  polycystic kidney Z82.71
  polyps (colon) Z83.71
  psychiatric disorder Z81.8
  psychoactive substance abuse NEC Z81.3
  respiratory condition NEC Z83.6
    asthma and other lower respiratory conditions Z82.5
  self-harmful behavior Z81.8
  SIDS (sudden infant death syndrome) Z84.82
  skin condition Z84.0
  specified condition NEC Z84.89
  stroke (cerebrovascular) Z82.3
  substance abuse NEC Z81.4
    alcohol Z81.1
    drug NEC Z81.3
    psychoactive NEC Z81.3
    tobacco Z81.2
  sudden
    cardiac death Z82.41
    infant death syndrome (SIDS) Z84.82
  tobacco abuse Z81.2
  violence, violent behavior Z81.8
  visual loss Z82.1
personal (of) — see also History, family (of)
  abuse
    adult Z91.419
      forced labor or sexual exploitation Z91.42
      physical and sexual Z91.410
      psychological Z91.411
    childhood Z62.819
      forced labor or sexual exploitation in childhood Z62.813
      physical Z62.810
      psychological Z62.811
      sexual Z62.810
  alcohol dependence F10.21
  allergy (to) Z88.9
    analgesic agent NEC Z88.6
    anesthetic Z88.4
    antibiotic agent NEC Z88.1
    anti-infective agent NEC Z88.3
    contrast media Z91.041
    drugs, medicaments and biological substances Z88.9
      specified NEC Z88.8
    food Z91.018
      additives Z91.02
      eggs Z91.012
      milk products Z91.011
      peanuts Z91.010
      seafood Z91.013
      specified food NEC Z91.018

History — continued
personal — see also History, family — continued
  allergy — continued
    insect Z91.038
      bee Z91.030
    latex Z91.040
    medicinal agents Z88.9
      specified NEC Z88.8
    narcotic agent NEC Z88.5
    nonmedicinal agents Z91.048
    penicillin Z88.0
    serum Z88.7
    specified NEC Z91.09
    sulfonamides Z88.2
    vaccine Z88.7
  anaphylactic shock Z87.892
  anaphylaxis Z87.892
  behavioral disorders Z86.59
  benign carcinoid tumor Z86.012
  benign neoplasm Z86.018
    brain Z86.011
    carcinoid Z86.012
    colonic polyps Z86.010
  brain injury (traumatic) Z87.820
  breast implant removal Z98.86
  calculi, renal Z87.442
  cancer — see History, personal (of), malignant neoplasm (of)
  cardiac arrest (death), successfully resuscitated Z86.74
  cerebral infarction without residual deficit Z86.73
  cervical dysplasia Z87.410
  chemotherapy for neoplastic condition Z92.21
  childhood abuse — see History, personal (of), abuse
  cleft lip (corrected) Z87.730
  cleft palate (corrected) Z87.730
  collapsed vertebra (healed) Z87.311
    due to osteoporosis Z87.310
  combat and operational stress reaction Z86.51
  congenital malformation (corrected) Z87.798
    circulatory system (corrected) Z87.74
    digestive system (corrected) NEC Z87.738
    ear (corrected) Z87.721
    eye (corrected) Z87.720
    face and neck (corrected) Z87.790
    genitourinary system (corrected) NEC Z87.718
    heart (corrected) Z87.74
    integument (corrected) Z87.76
    limb(s) (corrected) Z87.76
    musculoskeletal system (corrected) Z87.76
    neck (corrected) Z87.790
    nervous system (corrected) NEC Z87.728
    respiratory system (corrected) Z87.75
    sense organs (corrected) NEC Z87.728
    specified NEC Z87.798
  contraception Z92.0
  deployment (military) Z91.82
  diabetic foot ulcer Z86.31
  disease or disorder (of) Z87.898
    anaphylaxis Z87.892
    blood and blood-forming organs Z86.2
    circulatory system Z86.79
      specified condition NEC Z86.79
    connective tissue Z87.39
    digestive system Z87.19
      colonic polyp Z86.010
      peptic ulcer disease Z87.11
      specified condition NEC Z87.19
    ear Z86.69
    endocrine Z86.39
      diabetic foot ulcer Z86.31
      gestational diabetes Z86.32
      specified type NEC Z86.39
    eye Z86.69
    genital (track) system NEC
      female Z87.42
      male Z87.438
    hematological Z86.2
    Hodgkin Z85.71
    immune mechanism Z86.2
    infectious Z86.19
      malaria Z86.13
      Methicillin resistant Staphylococcus aureus (MRSA) Z86.14
      poliomyelitis Z86.12
      specified NEC Z86.19
      tuberculosis Z86.11
    mental NEC Z86.59
    metabolic Z86.39

History — continued
personal — see also History, family — continued
  disease or disorder — continued
    metabolic — continued
      diabetic foot ulcer Z86.31
      gestational diabetes Z86.32
      specified type NEC Z86.39
    musculoskeletal NEC Z87.39
    nervous system Z86.69
    nutritional Z86.39
    parasitic Z86.19
    respiratory system NEC Z87.09
    sense organs Z86.69
    skin Z87.2
    specified site or type NEC Z87.898
    subcutaneous tissue Z87.2
    trophoblastic Z87.59
    urinary system NEC Z87.448
  drug dependence — see Dependence, drug, by type, in remission
  drug therapy
    antineoplastic chemotherapy Z92.21
    estrogen Z92.23
    immunosupression Z92.25
    inhaled steroids Z92.240
    monoclonal drug Z92.22
    specified NEC Z92.29
    steroid Z92.241
    systemic steroids Z92.241
  dysplasia
    cervical (mild) (moderate) Z87.410
      severe (grade III) Z86.001
    prostatic Z87.430
    vaginal (mild) (moderate) Z87.411
      severe (grade III) Z86.002
    vulvar (mild) (moderate) Z87.412
      severe (grade III) Z86.002
  embolism (venous) Z86.718
    pulmonary Z86.711
  encephalitis Z86.61
  estrogen therapy Z92.23
  extracorporeal membrane oxygenation (ECMO) Z92.81
  failed conscious sedation Z92.83
  failed moderate sedation Z92.83
  fall, falling Z91.81
  forced labor or sexual exploitation Z91.42
    in childhood Z62.813
  fracture (healed)
    fatigue Z87.312
    fragility Z87.310
    osteoporosis Z87.310
    pathological NEC Z87.311
    stress Z87.312
    traumatic Z87.81
  gestational diabetes Z86.32
  hepatitis
    B Z86.19
    C Z86.19
  Hodgkin disease Z85.71
  hyperthermia, malignant Z88.4
  hypospadias (corrected) Z87.710
  hysterectomy Z90.710
  immunosupression therapy Z92.25
  in situ neoplasm
    breast Z86.000
    cervix uteri Z86.001
    digestive organs, specified NEC Z86.004
    esophagus Z86.003
    genital organs, specified NEC Z86.002
    melanoma Z86.006
    middle ear Z86.005
    oral cavity Z86.003
    respiratory system Z86.005
    skin Z86.007
    specified NEC Z86.008
    stomach Z86.003
  in utero procedure during pregnancy Z98.870
  in utero procedure while a fetus Z98.871
  infection NEC Z86.19
    central nervous system Z86.61
    latent tuberculosis Z86.15
    Methicillin resistant Staphylococcus aureus (MRSA) Z86.14
    urinary (recurrent) (tract) Z87.440
  injury NEC Z87.828
  irradiation Z92.3
  kidney stones Z87.442
  latent tuberculosis infection Z86.15

☑ Additional Character Required — Refer to the Tabular List for Character Selection   ▽ Subterms under main terms may continue to next column or page

History — *continued*
  personal — *see also* History, family — *continued*
    leukemia Z85.6
    lymphoma (non-Hodgkin) Z85.72
    malignant melanoma (skin) Z85.820
    malignant neoplasm (of) Z85.9
      accessory sinuses Z85.22
      anus NEC Z85.048
        carcinoid Z85.040
      bladder Z85.51
      bone Z85.830
      brain Z85.841
      breast Z85.3
      bronchus NEC Z85.118
        carcinoid Z85.110
      carcinoid — *see* History, personal (of), malignant neoplasm, by site, carcinioid
      cervix Z85.41
      colon NEC Z85.038
        carcinoid Z85.030
      digestive organ Z85.00
        specified NEC Z85.09
      endocrine gland NEC Z85.858
      epididymis Z85.48
      esophagus Z85.01
      eye Z85.840
      gastrointestinal tract — *see* History, malignant neoplasm, digestive organ
      genital organ
        female Z85.40
          specified NEC Z85.44
        male Z85.45
          specified NEC Z85.49
      hematopoietic NEC Z85.79
      intrathoracic organ Z85.20
      kidney NEC Z85.528
        carcinoid Z85.520
      large intestine NEC Z85.038
        carcinoid Z85.030
      larynx Z85.21
      liver Z85.05
      lung NEC Z85.118
        carcinoid Z85.110
      mediastinum Z85.29
      Merkel cell Z85.821
      middle ear Z85.22
      nasal cavities Z85.22
      nervous system NEC Z85.848
      oral cavity Z85.819
        specified site NEC Z85.818
      ovary Z85.43
      pancreas Z85.07
      pelvis Z85.53
      pharynx Z85.819
        specified site NEC Z85.818
      pleura Z85.29
      prostate Z85.46
      rectosigmoid junction NEC Z85.048
        carcinoid Z85.040
      rectum NEC Z85.048
        carcinoid Z85.040
      respiratory organ Z85.20
      sinuses, accessory Z85.22
      skin NEC Z85.828
        melanoma Z85.820
        Merkel cell Z85.821
      small intestine NEC Z85.068
        carcinoid Z85.060
      soft tissue Z85.831
      specified site NEC Z85.89
      stomach NEC Z85.028
        carcinoid Z85.020
      testis Z85.47
      thymus NEC Z85.238
        carcinoid Z85.230
      thyroid Z85.850
      tongue Z85.810
      trachea Z85.12
      urinary organ or tract Z85.50
        specified NEC Z85.59
      uterus Z85.42
    maltreatment Z91.89
    medical treatment NEC Z92.89
    melanoma Z85.820
      in situ Z86.006
      malignant (skin) Z85.820
    meningitis Z86.61
    mental disorder Z86.59
    Merkel cell carcinoma (skin) Z85.821

History — *continued*
  personal — *see also* History, family — *continued*
    Methicillin resistant Staphylococcus aureus (MRSA) Z86.14
    military deployment Z91.82
    military war, peacekeeping and humanitarian deployment (current or past conflict) Z91.82
    myocardial infarction (old) I25.2
    neglect (in)
      adult Z91.412
      childhood Z62.812
    neoplasia
      anal intraepithelial, III [AIN III] Z86.004
      high-grade prostatic intraepithelial, III [HGPIN III] Z86.002
      vaginal intraepithelial, III [VAIN III] Z86.002
      vulvar intraepithelial, III [VIN III] Z86.002
    neoplasm
      benign Z86.018
        brain Z86.011
        colon polyp Z86.010
      in situ
        breast Z86.000
        cervix uteri Z86.001
        digestive organs, specified NEC Z86.004
        esophagus Z86.003
        genital organs, specified NEC Z86.002
        melanoma Z86.006
        middle ear Z86.005
        oral cavity Z86.003
        respiratory system Z86.005
        skin Z86.007
        specified NEC Z86.008
        stomach Z86.003
      malignant — *see* History of, malignant neoplasm
      uncertain behavior Z86.03
    nephrotic syndrome Z87.441
    nicotine dependence Z87.891
    noncompliance with medical treatment or regimen — *see* Noncompliance
    nutritional deficiency Z86.39
    obstetric complications Z87.59
      childbirth Z87.59
      pregnancy Z87.59
      pre-term labor Z87.51
      puerperium Z87.59
    osteoporosis fractures Z87.31 ☑
    parasuicide (attempt) Z91.5
    physical trauma NEC Z87.828
      self-harm or suicide attempt Z91.5
    pneumonia (recurrent) Z87.01
    poisoning NEC Z91.89
      self-harm or suicide attempt Z91.5
    poor personal hygiene Z91.89
    preterm labor Z87.51
    procedure during pregnancy Z98.870
    procedure while a fetus Z98.871
    prolonged reversible ischemic neurologic deficit (PRIND) Z86.73
    prostatic dysplasia Z87.430
    psychological
      abuse
        adult Z91.411
        child Z62.811
      trauma, specified NEC Z91.49
    radiation therapy Z92.3
    removal
      implant
        breast Z98.86
    renal calculi Z87.442
    respiratory condition NEC Z87.09
    retained foreign body fully removed Z87.821
    risk factors NEC Z91.89
    self-harm Z91.5
    self-poisoning attempt Z91.5
    sex reassignment Z87.890
    sleep-wake cycle problem Z72.821
    specified NEC Z87.898
    steroid therapy (systemic) Z92.241
      inhaled Z92.240
    stroke without residual deficits Z86.73
    substance abuse NEC F10-F19
    sudden cardiac arrest Z86.74
    sudden cardiac death successfully resuscitated Z86.74
    suicide attempt Z91.5
    surgery NEC Z98.890
      with uterine scar Z98.891
      sex reassignment Z87.890

History — *continued*
  personal — *see also* History, family — *continued*
    surgery — *continued*
      transplant — *see* Transplant
    thrombophlebitis Z86.72
    thrombosis (venous) Z86.718
      pulmonary Z86.711
    tobacco dependence Z87.891
    transient ischemic attack (TIA) without residual deficits Z86.73
    trauma (physical) NEC Z87.828
      psychological NEC Z91.49
      self-harm Z91.5
    traumatic brain injury Z87.820
    tuberculosis, latent infection Z86.15
    unhealthy sleep-wake cycle Z72.821
    unintended awareness under general anesthesia Z92.84
    urinary calculi Z87.442
    urinary (recurrent) (tract) infection(s) Z87.440
    uterine scar from previous surgery Z98.891
    vaginal dysplasia Z87.411
    venous thrombosis or embolism Z86.718
      pulmonary Z86.711
    vulvar dysplasia Z87.412
His-Werner disease A79.0
HIV — *see also* Human, immunodeficiency virus B20
  laboratory evidence (nonconclusive) R75
  nonconclusive test (in infants) R75
  positive, seropositive Z21
Hives (bold) — *see* Urticaria
Hoarseness R49.0
Hobo Z59.0
Hodgkin disease — *see* Lymphoma, Hodgkin
Hodgson's disease I71.2
  ruptured I71.1
Hoffa-Kastert disease E88.89
Hoffa's disease E88.89
Hoffmann-Bouveret syndrome I47.9
Hoffmann's syndrome E03.9 *[G73.7]*
Hole (round)
  macula H35.34- ☑
  retina (without detachment) — *see* Break, retina, round hole
    with detachment — *see* Detachment, retina, with retinal, break
Holiday relief care Z75.5
Hollenhorst's plaque — *see* Occlusion, artery, retina
Hollow foot (congenital) Q66.7- ☑
  acquired — *see* Deformity, limb, foot, specified NEC
Holoprosencephaly Q04.2
Holt-Oram syndrome Q87.2
Homelessness Z59.0
Homesickness — *see* Disorder, adjustment
Homocystinemia, homocystinuria E72.11
Homogentisate 1,2-dioxygenase deficiency E70.29
Homologous serum hepatitis (prophylactic) (therapeutic) — *see* Hepatitis, viral, type B
Honeycomb lung J98.4
  congenital Q33.0
Hooded
  clitoris Q52.6
  penis Q55.69
Hookworm (disease) (infection) (infestation) B76.9
  with anemia B76.9 *[D63.8]*
  specified NEC B76.8
Hordeolum (eyelid) (externum) (recurrent) H00.019
  internum H00.029
    left H00.026
      lower H00.025
      upper H00.024
    right H00.023
      lower H00.022
      upper H00.021
  left H00.016
    lower H00.015
    upper H00.014
  right H00.013
    lower H00.012
    upper H00.011
Horn
  cutaneous L85.8
  nail L60.2
    congenital Q84.6
Horner (-Claude Bernard) **syndrome** G90.2
  traumatic — *see* Injury, nerve, cervical sympathetic
Horseshoe kidney (congenital) Q63.1

Horton's headache or neuralgia G44.099
  intractable G44.091
  not intractable G44.099
Hospital hopper syndrome — *see* Disorder, factitious
Hospitalism in children — *see* Disorder, adjustment
Hostility R45.5
  towards child Z62.3
Hot flashes
  menopausal N95.1
Hourglass (contracture) — *see also* Contraction, hourglass
  stomach K31.89
    congenital Q40.2
    stricture K31.2
Household, housing circumstance affecting care Z59.9
  specified NEC Z59.8
Housemaid's knee — *see* Bursitis, prepatellar
Hudson (-Stähli) **line** (cornea) — *see* Pigmentation, cornea, anterior
Human
  bite (open wound) — *see also* Bite
    intact skin surface — *see* Bite, superficial
  herpesvirus — *see* Herpes
  immunodeficiency virus (HIV) disease (infection) B20
    asymptomatic status Z21
    contact Z20.6
    counseling Z71.7
    dementia B20 [F02.80]
      with behavioral disturbance B20 [F02.81]
    exposure to Z20.6
    laboratory evidence R75
    type-2 (HIV 2) as cause of disease classified elsewhere B97.35
  papillomavirus (HPV)
    DNA test positive
      high risk
        cervix R87.810
        vagina R87.811
      low risk
        cervix R87.820
        vagina R87.821
    screening for Z11.51
  T-cell lymphotropic virus
    type-1 (HTLV-I) infection B33.3
      as cause of disease classified elsewhere B97.33
      carrier Z22.6
    type-2 (HTLV-II) as cause of disease classified elsewhere B97.34
Humidifier lung or pneumonitis J67.7
Humiliation (experience) **in childhood** Z62.898
Humpback (acquired) — *see* Kyphosis
Hunchback (acquired) — *see* Kyphosis
Hunger T73.0 ☑
  air, psychogenic F45.8
Hungry bone syndrome E83.81
Hunner's ulcer — *see* Cystitis, chronic, interstitial
Hunter's
  glossitis D51.0
  syndrome E76.1
Huntington's disease or chorea G10
  with dementia G10 [F02.80]
    with behavioral disturbance G10 [F02.81]
Hunt's
  disease or syndrome (herpetic geniculate ganglionitis) B02.21
    dyssynergia cerebellaris myoclonica G11.1
  neuralgia B02.21
Hurler (-Scheie) **disease or syndrome** E76.02
Hurst's disease G36.1
Hurthle cell
  adenocarcinoma C73
  adenoma D34
  carcinoma C73
  tumor D34
Hutchinson-Boeck disease or syndrome — *see* Sarcoidosis
Hutchinson-Gilford disease or syndrome E34.8
Hutchinson's
  disease, meaning
    angioma serpiginosum L81.7
    pompholyx (cheiropompholyx) L30.1
    prurigo estivalis L56.4
    summer eruption or summer prurigo L56.4
  melanotic freckle — *see* Melanoma, in situ
    malignant melanoma in — *see* Melanoma
  teeth or incisors (congenital syphilis) A50.52
  triad (congenital syphilis) A50.53

Hyalin plaque, sclera, senile H15.89
Hyaline membrane (disease) (lung) (pulmonary) (newborn) P22.0
Hyalinosis
  cutis (et mucosae) E78.89
  focal and segmental (glomerular) — *see also* N00-N07
    with fourth character .1 N05.1
Hyalitis, hyalosis, asteroid — *see also* Deposit, crystalline
  syphilitic (late) A52.71
Hydatid
  cyst or tumor — *see* Echinococcus
  mole — *see* Hydatidiform mole
  Morgagni
    female Q50.5
    male (epididymal) Q55.4
      testicular Q55.29
Hydatidiform mole (benign) (complicating pregnancy) (delivered) (undelivered) O01.9
  classical O01.0
  complete O01.0
  incomplete O01.1
  invasive D39.2
  malignant D39.2
  partial O01.1
Hydatidosis — *see* Echinococcus
Hydradenitis (axillaris) (suppurative) L73.2
Hydradenoma — *see* Hidradenoma
Hydramnios O40.- ☑
Hydrancephaly, hydranencephaly Q04.3
  with spina bifida — *see* Spina bifida, with hydrocephalus
Hydrargyrism NEC — *see* Poisoning, mercury
Hydrarthrosis — *see also* Effusion, joint
  gonococcal A54.42
  intermittent M12.40
    ankle M12.47- ☑
    elbow M12.42- ☑
    foot joint M12.47- ☑
    hand joint M12.44- ☑
    hip M12.45- ☑
    knee M12.46- ☑
    multiple site M12.49
    shoulder M12.41- ☑
    specified joint NEC M12.48
    wrist M12.43- ☑
  of yaws (early) (late) — *see also* subcategory M14.8- A66.6
  syphilitic (late) A52.77
    congenital A50.55 [M12.80]
Hydremia D64.89
Hydrencephalocele (congenital) — *see* Encephalocele
Hydrencephalomeningocele (congenital) — *see* Encephalocele
Hydroa R23.8
  aestivale L56.4
  vacciniforme L56.4
Hydroadenitis (axillaris) (suppurative) L73.2
Hydrocalycosis — *see* Hydronephrosis
Hydrocele (spermatic cord) (testis) (tunica vaginalis) N43.3
  canal of Nuck N94.89
  communicating N43.2
    congenital P83.5
  congenital P83.5
  encysted N43.0
  female NEC N94.89
  infected N43.1
  newborn P83.5
  round ligament N94.89
  specified NEC N43.2
  spinalis — *see* Spina bifida
  vulva N90.89
Hydrocephalus (acquired) (external) (internal) (malignant) (recurrent) G91.9
  aqueduct Sylvius stricture Q03.0
  causing disproportion O33.6 ☑
    with obstructed labor O66.3
  communicating G91.0
  congenital (external) (internal) Q03.9
    with spina bifida Q05.4
      cervical Q05.0
      dorsal Q05.1
      lumbar Q05.2
      lumbosacral Q05.2
      sacral Q05.3
      thoracic Q05.1

Hydrocephalus — *continued*
  congenital — *continued*
    with spina bifida — *continued*
      thoracolumbar Q05.1
    specified NEC Q03.8
  due to toxoplasmosis (congenital) P37.1
  foramen Magendie block (acquired) G91.1
    congenital — *see also* Hydrocephalus, congenital Q03.1
  in (due to)
    infectious disease NEC B89 [G91.4]
    neoplastic disease NEC — *see also* Neoplasm G91.4
    parasitic disease B89 [G91.4]
  newborn Q03.9
    with spina bifida — *see* Spina bifida, with hydrocephalus
  noncommunicating G91.1
  normal pressure G91.2
    secondary G91.0
  obstructive G91.1
  otitic G93.2
  post-traumatic NEC G91.3
  secondary G91.4
    post-traumatic G91.3
  specified NEC G91.8
  syphilitic, congenital A50.49
Hydrocolpos (congenital) N89.8
Hydrocystoma — *see* Neoplasm, skin, benign
Hydroencephalocele (congenital) — *see* Encephalocele
Hydroencephalomeningocele (congenital) — *see* Encephalocele
Hydrohematopneumothorax — *see* Hemothorax
Hydromeningitis — *see* Meningitis
Hydromeningocele (spinal) — *see also* Spina bifida
  cranial — *see* Encephalocele
Hydrometra N85.8
Hydrometrocolpos N89.8
Hydromicrocephaly Q02
Hydromphalos (since birth) Q45.8
Hydromyelia Q06.4
Hydromyelocele — *see* Spina bifida
Hydronephrosis (atrophic) (early) (functionless) (intermittent) (primary) (secondary) NEC N13.30
  with
    infection N13.6
    obstruction (by) (of)
      renal calculus N13.2
        with infection N13.6
      ureteral NEC N13.1
        with infection N13.6
        calculus N13.2
          with infection N13.6
      ureteropelvic junction (congenital) Q62.11
        acquired N13.0
          with infection N13.6
    ureteral stricture NEC N13.1
      with infection N13.6
  congenital Q62.0
  due to acquired occlusion of ureteropelvic junction N13.0
  specified type NEC N13.39
  tuberculous A18.11
Hydropericarditis — *see* Pericarditis
Hydropericardium — *see* Pericarditis
Hydroperitoneum R18.8
Hydrophobia — *see* Rabies
Hydrophthalmos Q15.0
Hydropneumohemothorax — *see* Hemothorax
Hydropneumopericarditis — *see* Pericarditis
Hydropneumopericardium — *see* Pericarditis
Hydropneumothorax J94.8
  traumatic — *see* Injury, intrathoracic, lung
  tuberculous NEC A15.6
Hydrops R60.9
  abdominis R18.8
  articulorum intermittens — *see* Hydrarthrosis, intermittent
  cardiac — *see* Failure, heart, congestive
  causing obstructed labor (mother) O66.3
  endolymphatic H81.0- ☑
  fetal — *see* Pregnancy, complicated by, hydrops, fetalis
  fetalis P83.2
    due to
      ABO isoimmunization P56.0
      alpha thalassemia D56.0
      hemolytic disease P56.90
        specified NEC P56.99
      isoimmunization (ABO) (Rh) P56.0

Hydrops — *continued*
  fetalis — *continued*
    due to — *continued*
      other specified nonhemolytic disease NEC P83.2
      Rh incompatibility P56.0
    during pregnancy — *see* Pregnancy, complicated
      by, hydrops, fetalis
  gallbladder K82.1
  joint — *see* Effusion, joint
  labyrinth H81.0- ☑
  newborn (idiopathic) P83.2
    due to
      ABO isoimmunization P56.0
      alpha thalassemia P83.2
      hemolytic disease P56.90
        specified NEC P56.99
      isoimmunization (ABO) (Rh) P56.0
      Rh incompatibility P56.0
  nutritional — *see* Malnutrition, severe
  pericardium — *see* Pericarditis
  pleura — *see* Hydrothorax
  spermatic cord — *see* Hydrocele
Hydropyonephrosis N13.6
Hydrorachis Q06.4
Hydrorrhea (nasal) J34.89
  pregnancy — *see* Rupture, membranes, premature
Hydrosadenitis (axillaris) (suppurative) L73.2
Hydrosalpinx (fallopian tube) (follicularis) N70.11
Hydrothorax (double) (pleura) J94.8
  chylous (nonfilarial) I89.8
    filarial — *see also* Infestation, filarial B74.9 *[J91.8]*
  traumatic — *see* Injury, intrathoracic
  tuberculous NEC (non primary) A15.6
Hydroureter — *see also* Hydronephrosis N13.4
  with infection N13.6
  congenital Q62.39
Hydroureteronephrosis — *see* Hydronephrosis
Hydrourethra N36.8
Hydroxykynureninuria E70.8
Hydroxylysinemia E72.3
Hydroxyprolinemia E72.59
Hygiene, sleep
  abuse Z72.821
  inadequate Z72.821
  poor Z72.821
Hygroma (congenital) (cystic) D18.1
  praepatellare, prepatellar — *see* Bursitis, prepatellar
Hymen — *see* condition
Hymenolepis, hymenolepiasis (diminuta) (infection)
  (infestation) (nana) B71.0
Hypalgesia R20.8
Hyperacidity (gastric) K31.89
  psychogenic F45.8
Hyperactive, hyperactivity F90.9
  basal cell, uterine cervix — *see* Dysplasia, cervix
  bowel sounds R19.12
  cervix epithelial (basal) — *see* Dysplasia, cervix
  child F90.9
    attention deficit — *see* Disorder, attention-deficit
      hyperactivity
  detrusor muscle N32.81
  gastrointestinal K31.89
    psychogenic F45.8
  nasal mucous membrane J34.3
  stomach K31.89
  thyroid (gland) — *see* Hyperthyroidism
Hyperacusis H93.23- ☑
Hyperadrenalism E27.5
Hyperadrenocorticism E24.9
  congenital E25.0
  iatrogenic E24.2
    correct substance properly administered — *see* Ta-
      ble of Drugs and Chemicals, by drug, adverse
      effect
    overdose or wrong substance given or taken — *see*
      Table of Drugs and Chemicals, by drug, poi-
      soning
  not associated with Cushing's syndrome E27.0
  pituitary-dependent E24.0
Hyperaldosteronism E26.9
  familial (type I) E26.02
  glucocorticoid-remediable E26.02
  primary (due to (bilateral) adrenal hyperplasia) E26.09
  primary NEC E26.09
  secondary E26.1
  specified NEC E26.09
Hyperalgesia R20.8

Hyperalimentation R63.2
  carotene, carotin E67.1
  specified NEC E67.8
  vitamin
    A E67.0
    D E67.3
Hyperaminoaciduria
  arginine E72.21
  cystine E72.01
  lysine E72.3
  ornithine E72.4
Hyperammonemia (congenital) E72.20
Hyperazotemia — *see* Uremia
Hyperbetalipoproteinemia (familial) E78.00
  with prebetalipoproteinemia E78.2
Hyperbicarbonatemia P74.41
Hyperbilirubinemia
  constitutional E80.6
  familial conjugated E80.6
  neonatal (transient) — *see* Jaundice, newborn
Hypercalcemia, hypocalciuric, familial E83.52
Hypercalciuria, idiopathic R82.994
Hypercapnia R06.89
  newborn P84
Hypercarotenemia (dietary) E67.1
Hypercementosis K03.4
Hyperchloremia E87.8
Hyperchlorhydria K31.89
  neurotic F45.8
  psychogenic F45.8
Hypercholesterinemia — *see* Hypercholesterolemia
Hypercholesterolemia (essential) (primary) (pure) E78.00
  with hyperglyceridemia, endogenous E78.2
  dietary counseling and surveillance Z71.3
  familial E78.01
  hereditary E78.01
Hyperchylia gastrica, psychogenic F45.8
Hyperchylomicronemia (familial) (primary) E78.3
  with hyperbetalipoproteinemia E78.3
Hypercoagulable (state) D68.59
  activated protein C resistance D68.51
  antithrombin (III) deficiency D68.59
  factor V Leiden mutation D68.51
  primary NEC D68.59
  protein C deficiency D68.59
  protein S deficiency D68.59
  prothrombin gene mutation D68.52
  secondary D68.69
  specified NEC D68.69
Hypercoagulation (state) D68.59
Hypercorticalism, pituitary-dependent E24.0
Hypercorticosolism — *see* Cushing's, syndrome
Hypercorticosteronism E24.2
  correct substance properly administered — *see* Table
    of Drugs and Chemicals, by drug, adverse effect
  overdose or wrong substance given or taken — *see*
    Table of Drugs and Chemicals, by drug, poisoning
Hypercortisonism E24.2
  correct substance properly administered — *see* Table
    of Drugs and Chemicals, by drug, adverse effect
  overdose or wrong substance given or taken — *see*
    Table of Drugs and Chemicals, by drug, poisoning
Hyperekplexia Q89.8
Hyperelectrolytemia E87.8
Hyperemesis R11.10
  with nausea R11.2
  gravidarum (mild) O21.0
    with
      carbohydrate depletion O21.1
      dehydration O21.1
      electrolyte imbalance O21.1
      metabolic disturbance O21.1
    severe (with metabolic disturbance) O21.1
  projectile R11.12
  psychogenic F45.8
Hyperemia (acute) (passive) R68.89
  anal mucosa K62.89
  bladder N32.89
  cerebral I67.89
  conjunctiva H11.43- ☑
  ear internal, acute — *see* subcategory H83.0 ☑
  enteric K59.8
  eye — *see* Hyperemia, conjunctiva
  eyelid (active) (passive) — *see* Disorder, eyelid, speci-
    fied type NEC
  intestine K59.8
  iris — *see* Disorder, iris, vascular
  kidney N28.89

Hyperemia — *continued*
  labyrinth — *see* subcategory H83.0 ☑
  liver (active) K76.89
  lung (passive) — *see* Edema, lung
  pulmonary (passive) — *see* Edema, lung
  renal N28.89
  retina H35.89
  stomach K31.89
Hyperesthesia (body surface) R20.3
  larynx (reflex) J38.7
    hysterical F44.89
  pharynx (reflex) J39.2
    hysterical F44.89
Hyperestrogenism (drug-induced) (iatrogenic) E28.0
Hyperexplexia Q89.8
Hyperfibrinolysis — *see* Fibrinolysis
Hyperfructosemia E74.19
Hyperfunction
  adrenal cortex, not associated with Cushing's syndrome
    E27.0
    medulla E27.5
      adrenomedullary E27.5
    virilism E25.9
      congenital E25.0
  ovarian E28.8
  pancreas K86.89
  parathyroid (gland) E21.3
  pituitary (gland) (anterior) E22.9
    specified NEC E22.8
  polyglandular E31.1
  testicular E29.0
Hypergammaglobulinemia D89.2
  polyclonal D89.0
  Waldenström D89.0
Hypergastrinemia E16.4
Hyperglobulinemia R77.1
Hyperglycemia, hyperglycemic (transient) R73.9
  coma — *see* Diabetes, by type, with coma
  postpancreatectomy E89.1
Hyperglyceridemia (endogenous) (essential) (familial)
  (hereditary) (pure) E78.1
  mixed E78.3
Hyperglycinemia (non-ketotic) E72.51
Hypergonadism
  ovarian E28.8
  testicular (primary) (infantile) E29.0
Hyperheparinemia D68.32
Hyperhidrosis, hyperidrosis R61
  focal
    primary L74.519
      axilla L74.510
      face L74.511
      palms L74.512
      soles L74.513
    secondary L74.52
  generalized R61
  localized
    primary L74.519
      axilla L74.510
      face L74.511
      palms L74.512
      soles L74.513
    secondary L74.52
  psychogenic F45.8
  secondary R61
    focal L74.52
Hyperhistidinemia E70.41
Hyperhomocysteinemia E72.11
Hyperhydroxyprolinemia E72.59
Hyperinsulinism (functional) E16.1
  with
    coma (hypoglycemic) E15
    encephalopathy E16.1 *[G94]*
  ectopic E16.1
  therapeutic misadventure (from administration of in-
    sulin) — *see* subcategory T38.3 ☑
Hyperkalemia E87.5
Hyperkeratosis — *see also* Keratosis L85.9
  cervix N88.0
  due to yaws (early) (late) (palmar or plantar) A66.3
  follicularis Q82.8
    penetrans (in cutem) L87.0
  palmoplantaris climacterica L85.1
  pinta A67.1
  senile (with pruritus) L57.0
  universalis congenita Q80.8
  vocal cord J38.3
  vulva N90.4

Hyperkinesia, hyperkinetic (disease) (reaction) (syndrome) (childhood) (adolescence) — *see also* Disorder, attention-deficit hyperactivity
heart I51.89
Hyperleucine-isoleucinemia E71.19
Hyperlipemia, hyperlipidemia E78.5
combined E78.2
familial E78.49
group
A E78.00
B E78.1
C E78.2
D E78.3
mixed E78.2
specified NEC E78.49
Hyperlipidosis E75.6
hereditary NEC E75.5
Hyperlipoproteinemia E78.5
Fredrickson's type
I E78.3
IIa E78.00
IIb E78.2
III E78.2
IV E78.1
V E78.3
low-density-lipoprotein-type (LDL) E78.00
very-low-density-lipoprotein-type (VLDL) E78.1
Hyperlucent lung, unilateral J43.0
Hyperlysinemia E72.3
Hypermagnesemia E83.41
neonatal P71.8
Hypermenorrhea N92.0
Hypermethioninemia E72.19
Hypermetropia (congenital) H52.0- ☑
Hypermobility, hypermotility
cecum — *see* Syndrome, irritable bowel
coccyx — *see* subcategory M53.2 ☑
colon — *see* Syndrome, irritable bowel
psychogenic F45.8
ileum K58.9
intestine — *see also* Syndrome, irritable bowel K58.9
psychogenic F45.8
meniscus (knee) — *see* Derangement, knee, meniscus
scapula — *see* Instability, joint, shoulder
stomach K31.89
psychogenic F45.8
syndrome M35.7
urethra N36.41
with intrinsic sphincter deficiency N36.43
Hypernasality R49.21
Hypernatremia E87.0
Hypernephroma C64.- ☑
Hyperopia — *see* Hypermetropia
Hyperorexia nervosa F50.2
Hyperornithinemia E72.4
Hyperosmia R43.1
Hyperosmolality E87.0
Hyperostosis (monomelic) — *see also* Disorder, bone, density and structure, specified NEC
ankylosing (spine) M48.10
cervical region M48.12
cervicothoracic region M48.13
lumbar region M48.16
lumbosacral region M48.17
multiple sites M48.19
occipito-atlanto-axial region M48.11
sacrococcygeal region M48.18
thoracic region M48.14
thoracolumbar region M48.15
cortical (skull) M85.2
infantile M89.8X- ☑
frontal, internal of skull M85.2
interna frontalis M85.2
skeletal, diffuse idiopathic — *see* Hyperostosis, ankylosing
skull M85.2
congenital Q75.8
vertebral, ankylosing — *see* Hyperostosis, ankylosing
Hyperovarism E28.8
Hyperoxaluria R82.992
primary E72.53
Hyperparathyroidism E21.3
primary E21.0
secondary (renal) N25.81
non-renal E21.1
specified NEC E21.2
tertiary E21.2
Hyperpathia R20.8

Hyperperistalsis R19.2
psychogenic F45.8
Hyperpermeability, capillary I78.8
Hyperphagia R63.2
Hyperphenylalaninemia NEC E70.1
Hyperphoria (alternating) H50.53
Hyperphosphatemia E83.39
Hyperpiesis, hyperpiesia — *see* Hypertension
Hyperpigmentation — *see also* Pigmentation
melanin NEC L81.4
postinflammatory L81.0
Hyperpinealism E34.8
Hyperpituitarism E22.9
Hyperplasia, hyperplastic
adenoids J35.2
adrenal (capsule) (cortex) (gland) E27.8
with
sexual precocity (male) E25.9
congenital E25.0
virilism, adrenal E25.9
congenital E25.0
virilization (female) E25.9
congenital E25.0
congenital E25.0
salt-losing E25.0
adrenomedullary E27.5
angiolymphoid, eosinophilia (ALHE) D18.01
appendix (lymphoid) K38.0
artery, fibromuscular I77.3
bone — *see also* Hypertrophy, bone
marrow D75.89
breast — *see also* Hypertrophy, breast
atypical, atypia N60.9- ☑
ductal N60.9- ☑
lobular N60.9- ☑
C-cell, thyroid E07.0
cementation (tooth) (teeth) K03.4
cervical gland R59.0
cervix (uteri) (basal cell) (endometrium) (polypoid) — *see also* Dysplasia, cervix
congenital Q51.828
clitoris, congenital Q52.6
denture K06.2
endocervicitis N72
endometrium, endometrial (adenomatous) (cystic) (glandular) (glandular-cystic) (polypoid) N85.00
with atypia N85.02
benign N85.01
cervix — *see* Dysplasia, cervix
complex (without atypia) N85.01
simple (without atypia) N85.01
epithelial L85.9
focal, oral, including tongue K13.29
nipple N62
skin L85.9
tongue K13.29
vaginal wall N89.3
erythroid D75.89
fibromuscular of artery (carotid) (renal) I77.3
genital
female NEC N94.89
male N50.89
glnglva K06.1
glandularis cystica uteri (interstitialis) — *see also* Hyperplasia, endometrial N85.00
gum K06.1
hymen, congenital Q52.4
irritative, edentulous (alveolar) K06.2
jaw M26.09
alveolar M26.79
lower M26.03
alveolar M26.72
upper M26.01
alveolar M26.71
kidney (congenital) Q63.3
labia N90.69
epithelial N90.3
liver (congenital) Q44.7
nodular, focal K76.89
lymph gland or node R59.9
mandible, mandibular M26.03
alveolar M26.72
unilateral condylar M27.8
maxilla, maxillary M26.01
alveolar M26.71
myometrium, myometrial N85.2
neuroendocrine cell, of infancy J84.841

Hyperplasia, hyperplastic — *continued*
nose
lymphoid J34.89
polypoid J33.9
oral mucosa (irritative) K13.6
organ or site, congenital NEC — *see* Anomaly, by site
ovary N83.8
palate, papillary (irritative) K13.6
pancreatic islet cells E16.9
alpha E16.8
with excess
gastrin E16.4
glucagon E16.3
beta E16.1
parathyroid (gland) E21.0
pharynx (lymphoid) J39.2
prostate (adenofibromatous) (nodular) N40.0
with lower urinary tract symptoms (LUTS) N40.1
without lower urinary tract symptoms (LUTS) N40.0
renal artery I77.89
reticulo-endothelial (cell) D75.89
salivary gland (any) K11.1
Schimmelbusch's — *see* Mastopathy, cystic
suprarenal capsule (gland) E27.8
thymus (gland) (persistent) E32.0
thyroid (gland) — *see* Goiter
tonsils (faucial) (infective) (lingual) (lymphoid) J35.1
with adenoids J35.3
unilateral condylar M27.8
uterus, uterine N85.2
endometrium (glandular) — *see also* Hyperplasia, endometrial N85.00
vulva N90.69
epithelial N90.3
Hyperpnea — *see* Hyperventilation
Hyperpotassemia E87.5
Hyperprebetalipoproteinemia (familial) E78.1
Hyperprolactinemia E22.1
Hyperprolinemia (type I) (type II) E72.59
Hyperproteinemia E88.09
Hyperprothrombinemia, causing coagulation factor deficiency D68.4
Hyperpyrexia R50.9
heat (effects) T67.01 ☑
malignant, due to anesthetic T88.3 ☑
rheumatic — *see* Fever, rheumatic
unknown origin R50.9
Hyper-reflexia R29.2
Hypersalivation K11.7
Hypersecretion
ACTH (not associated with Cushing's syndrome) E27.0
pituitary E24.0
adrenaline E27.5
adrenomedullary E27.5
androgen (testicular) E29.0
ovarian (drug-induced) (iatrogenic) E28.1
calcitonin E07.0
catecholamine E27.5
corticoadrenal E24.9
cortisol E24.9
epinephrine E27.5
estrogen E28.0
gastric K31.89
psychogenic F45.8
gastrin E16.4
glucagon E16.3
hormone(s)
ACTH (not associated with Cushing's syndrome) E27.0
pituitary E24.0
antidiuretic E22.2
growth E22.0
intestinal NEC E34.1
ovarian androgen E28.1
pituitary E22.9
testicular E29.0
thyroid stimulating E05.80
with thyroid storm E05.81
insulin — *see* Hyperinsulinism
lacrimal glands — *see* Epiphora
medulloadrenal E27.5
milk O92.6
ovarian androgens E28.1
salivary gland (any) K11.7
thyrocalcitonin E07.0
upper respiratory J39.8
Hypersegmentation, leukocytic, hereditary D72.0

☑ Additional Character Required — Refer to the Tabular List for Character Selection   ▽ Subterms under main terms may continue to next column or page

Hypersensitive, hypersensitiveness, hypersensitivity
— see also Allergy
  carotid sinus G90.01
  colon — see Irritable, colon
  drug T88.7 ☑
  gastrointestinal K52.29
    immediate K52.29
    psychogenic F45.8
  labyrinth — see subcategory H83.2 ☑
  pain R20.8
  pneumonitis — see Pneumonitis, allergic
  reaction T78.40 ☑
    upper respiratory tract NEC J39.3
Hypersomnia (organic) G47.10
  due to
    alcohol
      abuse F10.182
      dependence F10.282
      use F10.982
    amphetamines
      abuse F15.182
      dependence F15.282
      use F15.982
    caffeine
      abuse F15.182
      dependence F15.282
      use F15.982
    cocaine
      abuse F14.182
      dependence F14.282
      use F14.982
    drug NEC
      abuse F19.182
      dependence F19.282
      use F19.982
    medical condition G47.14
    mental disorder F51.13
    opioid
      abuse F11.182
      dependence F11.282
      use F11.982
    psychoactive substance NEC
      abuse F19.182
      dependence F19.282
      use F19.982
    sedative, hypnotic, or anxiolytic
      abuse F13.182
      dependence F13.282
      use F13.982
    stimulant NEC
      abuse F15.182
      dependence F15.282
      use F15.982
  idiopathic G47.11
    with long sleep time G47.11
    without long sleep time G47.12
  menstrual related G47.13
  nonorganic origin F51.11
    specified NEC F51.19
  not due to a substance or known physiological condition F51.11
    specified NEC F51.19
  primary F51.11
  recurrent G47.13
  specified NEC G47.19
Hypersplenia, hypersplenism D73.1
Hyperstimulation, ovaries (associated with induced ovulation) N98.1
Hypersusceptibility — see Allergy
Hypertelorism (ocular) (orbital) Q75.2
Hypertension, hypertensive (accelerated) (benign) (essential) (idiopathic) (malignant) (systemic) I10
  with
    heart failure (congestive) I11.0
    heart involvement (conditions in I50.-, I51.4- I51.9 due to hypertension) — see Hypertension, heart
    kidney involvement — see Hypertension, kidney
  benign, intracranial G93.2
  borderline R03.0
  cardiorenal (disease) I13.10
    with heart failure I13.0
      with stage 1 through stage 4 chronic kidney disease I13.0
      with stage 5 or end stage renal disease I13.2
    without heart failure I13.10
      with stage 1 through stage 4 chronic kidney disease I13.10

Hypertension, hypertensive — continued
  cardiorenal — continued
    without heart failure — continued
      with stage 5 or end stage renal disease I13.11
  cardiovascular
    disease (arteriosclerotic) (sclerotic) — see Hypertension, heart
    renal (disease) — see Hypertension, cardiorenal
  chronic venous — see Hypertension, venous (chronic)
  complicating
    childbirth (labor) O16.4
      pre-existing O10.92
        with
          heart disease O10.12
            with renal disease O10.32
          pre-eclampsia O11.4
          renal disease O10.22
            with heart disease O10.32
        essential O10.02
      secondary O10.42
    pregnancy O16.- ☑
      with edema — see also Pre-eclampsia O14.9- ☑
      gestational (pregnancy induced) (without proteinuria) O13.- ☑
        with proteinuria O14.9- ☑
          mild pre-eclampsia O14.0- ☑
          moderate pre-eclampsia O14.0- ☑
          severe pre-eclampsia O14.1- ☑
            with hemolysis, elevated liver enzymes and low platelet count (HELLP) O14.2- ☑
      pre-existing O10.91- ☑
        with
          heart disease O10.11- ☑
            with renal disease O10.31- ☑
          pre-eclampsia — see category O11
          renal disease O10.21- ☑
            with heart disease O10.31- ☑
        essential O10.01- ☑
        secondary O10.41- ☑
      transient O13- ☑
    puerperium, pre-existing O16.5
      pre-existing
        with
          heart disease O10.13
            with renal disease O10.33
          pre-eclampsia O11.5
          renal disease O10.23
            with heart disease O10.33
        essential O10.03
      pregnancy-induced O13.9
      secondary O10.43
  crisis I16.9
  due to
    endocrine disorders I15.2
    pheochromocytoma I15.2
    renal disorders NEC I15.1
      arterial I15.0
    renovascular disorders I15.0
    specified disease NEC I15.8
  emergency I16.1
  encephalopathy I67.4
  gestational (without significant proteinuria) (pregnancy-induced) (transient) O13.- ☑
    with significant proteinuria — see Pre-eclampsia
    complicating
      delivery O13.4
      puerperium O13.5
  Goldblatt's I70.1
  heart (disease) (conditions in I51.4-I51.9 due to hypertension) I11.9
    with
      heart failure (congestive) I11.0
      kidney disease (chronic) — see Hypertension, cardiorenal
  intracranial (benign) G93.2
  kidney I12.9
    with
      heart disease — see Hypertension, cardiorenal
      stage 1 through stage 4 chronic kidney disease I12.9
      stage 5 chronic kidney disease (CKD) or end stage renal disease (ESRD) I12.0
  lesser circulation I27.0
  maternal O16- ☑
  newborn P29.2
    pulmonary (persistent) P29.30
  ocular H40.05- ☑

Hypertension, hypertensive — continued
  pancreatic duct — code to underlying condition
    with chronic pancreatitis K86.1
  portal (due to chronic liver disease) (idiopathic) K76.6
    gastropathy K31.89
    in (due to) schistosomiasis (bilharziasis) B65.9 [K77]
  postoperative I97.3
  psychogenic F45.8
  pulmonary I27.20
    with
      cor pulmonale (chronic) I27.29
        acute I26.09
      right heart ventricular strain/failure I27.29
        acute I26.09
      right to left shunt related to congenital heart disease I27.83
      unclear multifactorial mechanisms I27.29
    arterial (associated) (drug-induced) (toxin-induced) I27.21
    chronic thromboembolic I27.24
    due to
      hematologic disorders I27.29
      left heart disease I27.22
      lung diseases and hypoxia I27.23
      metabolic disorders I27.29
      specified systemic disorders I27.29
    group 1 (associated) (drug-induced) (toxin-induced) I27.21
    group 2 I27.22
    group 3 I27.23
    group 4 I27.24
    group 5 I27.29
    of newborn (persistent) P29.30
    primary (idiopathic) I27.0
    secondary
      arterial I27.21
      specified NEC I27.29
  renal — see Hypertension, kidney
  renovascular I15.0
  secondary NEC I15.9
    due to
      endocrine disorders I15.2
      pheochromocytoma I15.2
      renal disorders NEC I15.1
        arterial I15.0
      renovascular disorders I15.0
    specified NEC I15.8
  transient R03.0
    of pregnancy O13.- ☑
  urgency I16.0
  venous (chronic)
    due to
      deep vein thrombosis — see Syndrome, postthrombotic
    idiopathic I87.309
      with
        inflammation I87.32- ☑
          with ulcer I87.33- ☑
        specified complication NEC I87.39- ☑
        ulcer I87.31- ☑
          with inflammation I87.33- ☑
      asymptomatic I87.30- ☑
Hypertensive urgency — see Hypertension
Hyperthecosis ovary E28.8
Hyperthermia (of unknown origin) — see also Hyperpyrexia
  malignant, due to anesthesia T88.3 ☑
  newborn P81.9
    environmental P81.0
Hyperthyroid (recurrent) — see Hyperthyroidism
Hyperthyroidism (latent) (pre-adult) (recurrent) E05.90
  with
    goiter (diffuse) E05.00
      with thyroid storm E05.01
      nodular (multinodular) E05.20
        with thyroid storm E05.21
        uninodular E05.10
          with thyroid storm E05.11
    storm E05.91
  due to ectopic thyroid tissue E05.30
    with thyroid storm E05.31
  neonatal, transitory P72.1
  specified NEC E05.80
    with thyroid storm E05.81
Hypertony, hypertonia, hypertonicity
  bladder N31.8
  congenital P94.1
  stomach K31.89

Hypertony, hypertonia, hypertonicity — *continued*
  stomach — *continued*
    psychogenic F45.8
  uterus, uterine (contractions) (complicating delivery) O62.4
Hypertrichosis L68.9
  congenital Q84.2
  eyelid H02.869
    left H02.866
      lower H02.865
      upper H02.864
    right H02.863
      lower H02.862
      upper H02.861
  lanuginosa Q84.2
    acquired L68.1
  localized L68.2
  specified NEC L68.8
Hypertriglyceridemia, essential E78.1
Hypertrophy, hypertrophic
  adenofibromatous, prostate — *see* Enlargement, enlarged, prostate
  adenoids (infective) J35.2
    with tonsils J35.3
  adrenal cortex E27.8
  alveolar process or ridge — *see* Anomaly, alveolar
  anal papillae K62.89
  artery I77.89
    congenital NEC Q27.8
      digestive system Q27.8
      lower limb Q27.8
      specified site NEC Q27.8
      upper limb Q27.8
  auricular — *see* Hypertrophy, cardiac
  Bartholin's gland N75.8
  bile duct (common) (hepatic) K83.8
  bladder (sphincter) (trigone) N32.89
  bone M89.30
    carpus M89.34- ☑
    clavicle M89.31- ☑
    femur M89.35- ☑
    fibula M89.36- ☑
    finger M89.34- ☑
    humerus M89.32- ☑
    ilium M89.359
    ischium M89.359
    metacarpus M89.34- ☑
    metatarsus M89.37- ☑
    multiple sites M89.39
    neck M89.38
    radius M89.33- ☑
    rib M89.38
    scapula M89.31- ☑
    skull M89.38
    tarsus M89.37- ☑
    tibia M89.36- ☑
    toe M89.37- ☑
    ulna M89.33- ☑
    vertebra M89.38
  brain G93.89
  breast N62
    cystic — *see* Mastopathy, cystic
    newborn P83.4
    pubertal, massive N62
    puerperal, postpartum — *see* Disorder, breast, specified type NEC
    senile (parenchymatous) N62
  cardiac (chronic) (idiopathic) I51.7
    with rheumatic fever (conditions in I00)
      active I01.8
      inactive or quiescent (with chorea) I09.89
    congenital NEC Q24.8
    fatty — *see* Degeneration, myocardial
    hypertensive — *see* Hypertension, heart
    rheumatic (with chorea) I09.89
      active or acute I01.8
        with chorea I02.0
    valve — *see* Endocarditis
  cartilage — *see* Disorder, cartilage, specified type NEC
  cecum — *see* Megacolon
  cervix (uteri) N88.8
    congenital Q51.828
    elongation N88.4
  clitoris (cirrhotic) N90.89
    congenital Q52.6
  colon — *see also* Megacolon
    congenital Q43.2

Hypertrophy, hypertrophic — *continued*
  conjunctiva, lymphoid H11.89
  corpora cavernosa N48.89
  cystic duct K82.8
  duodenum K31.89
  endometrium (glandular) — *see also* Hyperplasia, endometrial N85.00
    cervix N88.8
  epididymis N50.89
  esophageal hiatus (congenital) Q79.1
    with hernia — *see* Hernia, hiatal
  eyelid — *see* Disorder, eyelid, specified type NEC
  fat pad E65
    knee (infrapatellar) (popliteal) (prepatellar) (retropatellar) M79.4
  foot (congenital) Q74.2
  frenulum, frenum (tongue) K14.8
    lip K13.0
  gallbladder K82.8
  gastric mucosa K29.60
    with bleeding K29.61
  gland, glandular R59.9
    generalized R59.1
    localized R59.0
  gum (mucous membrane) K06.1
  heart (idiopathic) — *see also* Hypertrophy, cardiac
    valve — *see also* Endocarditis I38
  hemifacial Q67.4
  hepatic — *see* Hypertrophy, liver
  hiatus (esophageal) Q79.1
  hilus gland R59.0
  hymen, congenital Q52.4
  ileum K63.89
  intestine NEC K63.89
  jejunum K63.89
  kidney (compensatory) N28.81
    congenital Q63.3
  labium (majus) (minus) N90.60
  ligament — *see* Disorder, ligament
  lingual tonsil (infective) J35.1
    with adenoids J35.3
  lip K13.0
    congenital Q18.6
  liver R16.0
    acute K76.89
    cirrhotic — *see* Cirrhosis, liver
    congenital Q44.7
    fatty — *see* Fatty, liver
  lymph, lymphatic gland R59.9
    generalized R59.1
    localized R59.0
    tuberculous — *see* Tuberculosis, lymph gland
  mammary gland — *see* Hypertrophy, breast
  Meckel's diverticulum (congenital) Q43.0
    malignant — *see* Table of Neoplasms, small intestine, malignant
  median bar — *see* Hyperplasia, prostate
  meibomian gland — *see* Chalazion
  meniscus, knee, congenital Q74.1
  metatarsal head — *see* Hypertrophy, bone, metatarsus
  metatarsus — *see* Hypertrophy, bone, metatarsus
  mucous membrane
    alveolar ridge K06.2
    gum K06.1
    nose (turbinate) J34.3
  muscle M62.89
  muscular coat, artery I77.89
  myocardium — *see also* Hypertrophy, cardiac
    idiopathic I42.2
  myometrium N85.2
  nail L60.2
    congenital Q84.5
  nasal J34.89
    alae J34.89
    bone J34.89
    cartilage J34.89
    mucous membrane (septum) J34.3
    sinus J34.89
    turbinate J34.3
  nasopharynx, lymphoid (infectional) (tissue) (wall) J35.2
  nipple N62
  organ or site, congenital NEC — *see* Anomaly, by site
  ovary N83.8
  palate (hard) M27.8
    soft K13.79
  pancreas, congenital Q45.3
  parathyroid (gland) E21.0
  parotid gland K11.1

Hypertrophy, hypertrophic — *continued*
  penis N48.89
  pharyngeal tonsil J35.2
  pharynx J39.2
    lymphoid (infectional) (tissue) (wall) J35.2
  pituitary (anterior) (fossa) (gland) E23.6
  prepuce (congenital) N47.8
    female N90.89
  prostate — *see* Enlargement, enlarged, prostate
    congenital Q55.4
  pseudomuscular G71.09
  pylorus (adult) (muscle) (sphincter) K31.1
    congenital or infantile Q40.0
  rectal, rectum (sphincter) K62.89
  rhinitis (turbinate) J31.0
  salivary gland (any) K11.1
    congenital Q38.4
  scaphoid (tarsal) — *see* Hypertrophy, bone, tarsus
  scar L91.0
  scrotum N50.89
  seminal vesicle N50.89
  sigmoid — *see* Megacolon
  skin L91.9
    specified NEC L91.8
  spermatic cord N50.89
  spleen — *see* Splenomegaly
  spondylitis — *see* Spondylosis
  stomach K31.89
  sublingual gland K11.1
  submandibular gland K11.1
  suprarenal cortex (gland) E27.8
  synovial NEC M67.20
    acromioclavicular M67.21- ☑
    ankle M67.27- ☑
    elbow M67.22- ☑
    foot M67.27- ☑
    hand M67.24- ☑
    hip M67.25- ☑
    knee M67.26- ☑
    multiple sites M67.29
    specified site NEC M67.28
    wrist M67.23- ☑
  tendon — *see* Disorder, tendon, specified type NEC
  testis N44.8
    congenital Q55.29
  thymic, thymus (gland) (congenital) E32.0
  thyroid (gland) — *see* Goiter
  toe (congenital) Q74.2
    acquired — *see also* Deformity, toe, specified NEC
  tongue K14.8
    congenital Q38.2
    papillae (foliate) K14.3
  tonsils (faucial) (infective) (lingual) (lymphoid) J35.1
    with adenoids J35.3
  tunica vaginalis N50.89
  ureter N28.89
  urethra N36.8
  uterus N85.2
    neck (with elongation) N88.4
    puerperal O90.89
  uvula K13.79
  vagina N89.8
  vas deferens N50.89
  vein I87.8
  ventricle, ventricular (heart) — *see also* Hypertrophy, cardiac
    congenital Q24.8
    in tetralogy of Fallot Q21.3
  verumontanum N36.8
  vocal cord J38.3
  vulva N90.60
    stasis (nonfilarial) N90.69
Hypertropia H50.2- ☑
Hypertyrosinemia E70.21
Hyperuricemia (asymptomatic) E79.0
Hyperuricosuria R82.993
Hypervalinemia E71.19
Hyperventilation (tetany) R06.4
  hysterical F45.8
  psychogenic F45.8
  syndrome F45.8
Hypervitaminosis (dietary) NEC E67.8
  A E67.0
    administered as drug (prolonged intake) — *see* Table of Drugs and Chemicals, vitamins, adverse effect

Hypervitaminosis — *continued*
A — *continued*
overdose or wrong substance given or taken — *see* Table of Drugs and Chemicals, vitamins, poisoning
B6 E67.2
D E67.3
administered as drug (prolonged intake) — *see* Table of Drugs and Chemicals, vitamins, adverse effect
overdose or wrong substance given or taken — *see* Table of Drugs and Chemicals, vitamins, poisoning
K E67.8
administered as drug (prolonged intake) — *see* Table of Drugs and Chemicals, vitamins, adverse effect
overdose or wrong substance given or taken — *see* Table of Drugs and Chemicals, vitamins, poisoning
Hypervolemia E87.70
specified NEC E87.79
Hypesthesia R20.1
cornea — *see* Anesthesia, cornea
Hyphema H21.0- ☑
traumatic S05.1- ☑
Hypoacidity, gastric K31.89
psychogenic F45.8
Hypoadrenalism, hypoadrenia E27.40
primary E27.1
tuberculous A18.7
Hypoadrenocorticism E27.40
pituitary E23.0
primary E27.1
Hypoalbuminemia E88.09
Hypoaldosteronism E27.40
Hypoalphalipoproteinemia E78.6
Hypobarism T70.29 ☑
Hypobaropathy T70.29 ☑
Hypobetalipoproteinemia (familial) E78.6
Hypocalcemia E83.51
dietary E58
neonatal P71.1
due to cow's milk P71.0
phosphate-loading (newborn) P71.1
Hypochloremia E87.8
Hypochlorhydria K31.89
neurotic F45.8
psychogenic F45.8
Hypochondria, hypochondriac, hypochondriasis (reaction) F45.21
sleep F51.03
Hypochondrogenesis Q77.0
Hypochondroplasia Q77.4
Hypochromasia, blood cells D50.8
Hypocitraturia R82.991
Hypodontia — *see* Anodontia
Hypoeosinophilia D72.89
Hypoesthesia R20.1
Hypofibrinogenemia D68.8
acquired D65
congenital (hereditary) D68.2
Hypofunction
adrenocortical E27.40
drug-induced E27.3
postprocedural E89.6
primary E27.1
adrenomedullary, postprocedural E89.6
cerebral R29.818
corticoadrenal NEC E27.40
intestinal K59.8
labyrinth — *see* subcategory H83.2 ☑
ovary E28.39
pituitary (gland) (anterior) E23.0
testicular E29.1
postprocedural (postsurgical) (postirradiation) (iatrogenic) E89.5
Hypogalactia O92.4
Hypogammaglobulinemia — *see also* Agammaglobulinemia D80.1
hereditary D80.0
nonfamilial D80.1
transient, of infancy D80.7
Hypogenitalism (congenital) — *see* Hypogonadism
Hypoglossia Q38.3
Hypoglycemia (spontaneous) E16.2
coma E15

Hypoglycemia — *continued*
coma — *continued*
diabetic — *see* Diabetes, by type, with hypoglycemia, with coma
diabetic — *see* Diabetes, hypoglycemia
dietary counseling and surveillance Z71.3
drug-induced E16.0
with coma (nondiabetic) E15
due to insulin E16.0
with coma (nondiabetic) E15
therapeutic misadventure — *see* subcategory T38.3 ☑
functional, nonhyperinsulinemic E16.1
iatrogenic E16.0
with coma (nondiabetic) E15
in infant of diabetic mother P70.1
gestational diabetes P70.0
infantile E16.1
leucine-induced E71.19
neonatal (transitory) P70.4
iatrogenic P70.3
reactive (not drug-induced) E16.1
transitory neonatal P70.4
Hypogonadism
female E28.39
hypogonadotropic E23.0
male E29.1
ovarian (primary) E28.39
pituitary E23.0
testicular (primary) E29.1
Hypohidrosis, hypoidrosis L74.4
Hypoinsulinemia, postprocedural E89.1
Hypokalemia E87.6
Hypoleukocytosis — *see* Agranulocytosis
Hypolipoproteinemia (alpha) (beta) E78.6
Hypomagnesemia E83.42
neonatal P71.2
Hypomania, hypomanic reaction F30.8
Hypomenorrhea — *see* Oligomenorrhea
Hypometabolism R63.8
Hypomotility
gastrointestinal (tract) K31.89
psychogenic F45.8
intestine K59.8
psychogenic F45.8
stomach K31.89
psychogenic F45.8
Hyponasality R49.22
Hyponatremia E87.1
Hypo-osmolality E87.1
Hypo-ovarianism, hypo-ovarism E28.39
Hypoparathyroidism E20.9
familial E20.8
idiopathic E20.0
neonatal, transitory P71.4
postprocedural E89.2
specified NEC E20.8
Hypoperfusion (in)
newborn P96.89
Hypopharyngitis — *see* Laryngopharyngitis
Hypophoria H50.53
Hypophosphatemia, hypophosphatasia (acquired) (congenital) (renal) E83.39
familial E83.31
Hypophyseal, hypophysis — *see also* condition
dwarfism E23.0
gigantism E22.0
Hypopiesis — *see* Hypotension
Hypopinealism E34.8
Hypopituitarism (juvenile) E23.0
drug-induced E23.1
due to
hypophysectomy E89.3
radiotherapy E89.3
iatrogenic NEC E23.1
postirradiation E89.3
postpartum O99.285
postprocedural E89.3
Hypoplasia, hypoplastic
adrenal (gland), congenital Q89.1
alimentary tract, congenital Q45.8
upper Q40.8
anus, anal (canal) Q42.3
with fistula Q42.2 *
aorta, aortic Q25.42
ascending, in hypoplastic left heart syndrome Q23.4
valve Q23.1
in hypoplastic left heart syndrome Q23.4

Hypoplasia, hypoplastic — *continued*
areola, congenital Q83.8
arm (congenital) — *see* Defect, reduction, upper limb
artery (peripheral) Q27.8
brain (congenital) Q28.3
coronary Q24.5
digestive system Q27.8
lower limb Q27.8
pulmonary Q25.79
functional, unilateral J43.0
retinal (congenital) Q14.1
specified site NEC Q27.8
umbilical Q27.0
upper limb Q27.8
auditory canal Q17.8
causing impairment of hearing Q16.9
biliary duct or passage Q44.5
bone NOS Q79.9
face Q75.8
marrow D61.9
megakaryocytic D69.49
skull — *see* Hypoplasia, skull
brain Q02
gyri Q04.3
part of Q04.3
breast (areola) N64.82
bronchus Q32.4
cardiac Q24.8
carpus — *see* Defect, reduction, upper limb, specified type NEC
cartilage hair Q78.8
cecum Q42.8
cementum K00.4
cephalic Q02
cerebellum Q04.3
cervix (uteri), congenital Q51.821
clavicle (congenital) Q74.0
coccyx Q76.49
colon Q42.9
specified NEC Q42.8
corpus callosum Q04.0
cricoid cartilage Q31.2
digestive organ(s) or tract NEC Q45.8
upper (congenital) Q40.8
ear (auricle) (lobe) Q17.2
middle Q16.4
enamel of teeth (neonatal) (postnatal) (prenatal) K00.4
endocrine (gland) NEC Q89.2
endometrium N85.8
epididymis (congenital) Q55.4
epiglottis Q31.2
erythroid, congenital D61.01
esophagus (congenital) Q39.8
eustachian tube Q17.8
eye Q11.2
eyelid (congenital) Q10.3
face Q18.8
bone(s) Q75.8
femur (congenital) — *see* Defect, reduction, lower limb, specified type NEC
fibula (congenital) — *see* Defect, reduction, lower limb, specified type NEC
finger (congenital) — *see* Defect, reduction, upper limb, specified type NEC
focal dermal Q82.8
foot — *see* Defect, reduction, lower limb, specified type NEC
gallbladder Q44.0
genitalia, genital organ(s)
female Q52.8
external Q52.79
internal NEC Q52.8
in adiposogenital dystrophy E23.6
glottis Q31.2
hair Q84.2
hand (congenital) — *see* Defect, reduction, upper limb, specified type NEC
heart Q24.8
humerus (congenital) — *see* Defect, reduction, upper limb, specified type NEC
intestine (small) Q41.9
large Q42.9
specified NEC Q42.8
jaw M26.09
alveolar M26.79
lower M26.04
alveolar M26.74
upper M26.02

Hypoplasia, hypoplastic — *continued*
  jaw — *continued*
    upper — *continued*
      alveolar M26.73
  kidney(s) Q60.5
    bilateral Q60.4
    unilateral Q60.3
  labium (majus) (minus), congenital Q52.79
  larynx Q31.2
  left heart syndrome Q23.4
  leg (congenital) — *see* Defect, reduction, lower limb
  limb Q73.8
    lower (congenital) — *see* Defect, reduction, lower
      limb
    upper (congenital) — *see* Defect, reduction, upper
      limb
  liver Q44.7
  lung (lobe) (not associated with short gestation) Q33.6
    associated with immaturity, low birth weight, pre-
      maturity, or short gestation P28.0
  mammary (areola), congenital Q83.8
  mandible, mandibular M26.04
    alveolar M26.74
    unilateral condylar M27.8
  maxillary M26.02
    alveolar M26.73
  medullary D61.9
  megakaryocytic D69.49
  metacarpus — *see* Defect, reduction, upper limb,
    specified type NEC
  metatarsus — *see* Defect, reduction, lower limb, spec-
    ified type NEC
  muscle Q79.8
  nail(s) Q84.6
  nose, nasal Q30.1
  optic nerve H47.03- ☑
  osseous meatus (ear) Q17.8
  ovary, congenital Q50.39
  pancreas Q45.0
  parathyroid (gland) Q89.2
  parotid gland Q38.4
  patella Q74.1
  pelvis, pelvic girdle Q74.2
  penis (congenital) Q55.62
  peripheral vascular system Q27.8
    digestive system Q27.8
    lower limb Q27.8
    specified site NEC Q27.8
    upper limb Q27.8
  pituitary (gland) (congenital) Q89.2
  pulmonary (not associated with short gestation) Q33.6
    artery, functional J43.0
    associated with short gestation P28.0
  radioulnar — *see* Defect, reduction, upper limb, speci-
    fied type NEC
  radius — *see* Defect, reduction, upper limb
  rectum Q42.1
    with fistula Q42.0
  respiratory system NEC Q34.8
  rib Q76.6
  right heart syndrome Q22.6
  sacrum Q76.49
  scapula Q74.0
  scrotum Q55.1
  shoulder girdle Q74.0
  skin Q82.8
  skull (bone) Q75.8
    with
      anencephaly Q00.0
      encephalocele — *see* Encephalocele
      hydrocephalus Q03.9
        with spina bifida — *see* Spina bifida, by site,
          with hydrocephalus
      microcephaly Q02
  spinal (cord) (ventral horn cell) Q06.1
  spine Q76.49
  sternum Q76.7
  tarsus — *see* Defect, reduction, lower limb, specified
    type NEC
  testis Q55.1
  thymic, with immunodeficiency D82.1
  thymus (gland) Q89.2
    with immunodeficiency D82.1
  thyroid (gland) E03.1
    cartilage Q31.2
  tibiofibular (congenital) — *see* Defect, reduction, lower
    limb, specified type NEC

Hypoplasia, hypoplastic — *continued*
  toe — *see* Defect, reduction, lower limb, specified type
    NEC
  tongue Q38.3
  Turner's K00.4
  ulna (congenital) — *see* Defect, reduction, upper limb
  umbilical artery Q27.0
  unilateral condylar M27.8
  ureter Q62.8
  uterus, congenital Q51.811
  vagina Q52.4
  vascular NEC peripheral Q27.8
    brain Q28.3
    digestive system Q27.8
    lower limb Q27.8
    specified site NEC Q27.8
    upper limb Q27.8
  vein(s) (peripheral) Q27.8
    brain Q28.3
    digestive system Q27.8
    great Q26.8
    lower limb Q27.8
    specified site NEC Q27.8
    upper limb Q27.8
  vena cava (inferior) (superior) Q26.8
  vertebra Q76.49
  vulva, congenital Q52.79
  zonule (ciliary) Q12.8
Hypoplasminogenemia E88.02
Hypopnea, obstructive sleep apnea G47.33
Hypopotassemia E87.6
Hypoproconvertinemia, congenital (hereditary) D68.2
Hypoproteinemia E77.8
Hypoprothrombinemia (congenital) (hereditary) (idiopathic) D68.2
  acquired D68.4
  newborn, transient P61.6
Hypoptyalism K11.7
Hypopyon (eye) (anterior chamber) — *see* Iridocyclitis,
  acute, hypopyon
Hypopyrexia R68.0
Hyporeflexia R29.2
Hyposecretion
  ACTH E23.0
  antidiuretic hormone E23.2
  ovary E28.39
  salivary gland (any) K11.7
  vasopressin E23.2
Hyposegmentation, leukocytic, hereditary D72.0
Hyposiderinemia D50.9
Hypospadias Q54.9
  balanic Q54.0
  coronal Q54.0
  glandular Q54.0
  penile Q54.1
  penoscrotal Q54.2
  perineal Q54.3
  specified NEC Q54.8
Hypospermatogenesis — *see* Oligospermia
Hyposplenism D73.0
Hypostasis pulmonary, passive — *see* Edema, lung
Hypostatic — *see* condition
Hyposthenuria N28.89
Hypotension (arterial) (constitutional) I95.9
  chronic I95.89
  due to (of) hemodialysis I95.3
  drug-induced I95.2
  iatrogenic I95.89
  idiopathic (permanent) I95.0
  intracranial, following ventricular shunting (ventricu-
    lostomy) G97.2
  intra-dialytic I95.3
  maternal, syndrome (following labor and delivery)
    O26.5- ☑
  neurogenic, orthostatic G90.3
  orthostatic (chronic) I95.1
    due to drugs I95.2
    neurogenic G90.3
  postoperative I95.81
  postural I95.1
  specified NEC I95.89
Hypothermia (accidental) T68 ☑
  due to anesthesia, anesthetic T88.51 ☑
  low environmental temperature T68 ☑
  neonatal P80.9
    environmental (mild) NEC P80.8
    mild P80.8
    severe (chronic) (cold injury syndrome) P80.0

Hypothermia — *continued*
  neonatal — *continued*
    specified NEC P80.8
  not associated with low environmental temperature
    R68.0
Hypothyroidism (acquired) E03.9
  autoimmune — *see* Thyroiditis, autoimmune
  congenital (without goiter) E03.1
    with goiter (diffuse) E03.0
  due to
    exogenous substance NEC E03.2
    iodine-deficiency, acquired E01.8
      subclinical E02
    irradiation therapy E89.0
    medicament NEC E03.2
    P-aminosalicylic acid (PAS) E03.2
    phenylbutazone E03.2
    resorcinol E03.2
    sulfonamide E03.2
    surgery E89.0
    thiourea group drugs E03.2
  iatrogenic NEC E03.2
  iodine-deficiency (acquired) E01.8
    congenital — *see* Syndrome, iodine- deficiency,
      congenital
    subclinical E02
  neonatal, transitory P72.2
  postinfectious E03.3
  postirradiation E89.0
  postprocedural E89.0
  postsurgical E89.0
  specified NEC E03.8
  subclinical, iodine-deficiency related E02
Hypotonia, hypotonicity, hypotony
  bladder N31.2
  congenital (benign) P94.2
  eye — *see* Disorder, globe, hypotony
Hypotrichosis — *see* Alopecia
Hypotropia H50.2- ☑
Hypoventilation R06.89
  congenital central alveolar G47.35
  sleep related
    idiopathic nonobstructive alveolar G47.34
    in conditions classified elsewhere G47.36
Hypovitaminosis — *see* Deficiency, vitamin
Hypovolemia E86.1
  surgical shock T81.19 ☑
  traumatic (shock) T79.4 ☑
Hypoxemia R09.02
  newborn P84
  sleep related, in conditions classified elsewhere G47.3
Hypoxia — *see also* Anoxia R09.02
  cerebral, during a procedure NEC G97.81
    postprocedural NEC G97.82
  intrauterine P84
  myocardial — *see* Insufficiency, coronary
  newborn P84
  sleep-related G47.34
Hypsarhythmia — *see* Epilepsy, generalized, specifiec
  NEC
Hysteralgia, pregnant uterus O26.89- ☑
Hysteria, hysterical (conversion) (dissociative state)
  F44.9
  anxiety F41.8
  convulsions F44.5
  psychosis, acute F44.9
Hysteroepilepsy F44.5

I

IBDU (colonic inflammatory bowel dissease unclassifie●
  K52.3
Ichthyoparasitism due to Vandellia cirrhosa B88.8
Ichthyosis (congenital) Q80.9
  acquired L85.0
  fetalis Q80.4
  hystrix Q80.8
  lamellar Q80.2
  lingual K13.29
  palmaris and plantaris Q82.8
  simplex Q80.0
  vera Q80.8
  vulgaris Q80.0
  X-linked Q80.1
Ichthyotoxism — *see* Poisoning, fish
  bacterial — *see* Intoxication, foodborne
Icteroanemia, hemolytic (acquired) D59.9
  congenital — *see* Spherocytosis

   ☑ **Additional Character Required** — Refer to the Tabular List for Character Selection   ▽ Subterms under main terms may continue to next column or pag

Icterus — *see also* Jaundice
  conjunctiva R17
  gravis, newborn P55.0
  hematogenous (acquired) D59.9
  hemolytic (acquired) D59.9
    congenital — *see* Spherocytosis
  hemorrhagic (acute) (leptospiral) (spirochetal) A27.0
    newborn P53
  infectious B15.9
    with hepatic coma B15.0
    leptospiral A27.0
    spirochetal A27.0
  neonatorum — *see* Jaundice, newborn
  newborn P59.9
  spirochetal A27.0
Ictus solaris, solis T67.01 ☑
Id reaction (due to bacteria) L30.2
Ideation
  homicidal R45.850
  suicidal R45.851
Identity disorder (child) F64.9
  gender role F64.2
  psychosexual F64.2
Idioglossia F80.0
Idiopathic — *see* condition
Idiot, idiocy (congenital) F73
  amaurotic (Bielschowsky(-Jansky)) (family) (infantile
    (late)) (juvenile (late)) (Vogt-Spielmeyer) E75.4
  microcephalic Q02
IgE asthma J45.909
IIAC (idiopathic infantile arterial calcification) Q28.8
Ileitis (chronic) (noninfectious) — *see also* Enteritis K52.9
  backwash — *see* Pancolitis, ulcerative (chronic)
  infectious A09
  regional (ulcerative) — *see* Enteritis, regional, small
    intestine
  segmental — *see* Enteritis, regional
  terminal (ulcerative) — *see* Enteritis, regional, small
    intestine
Ileocolitis — *see also* Enteritis K52.9
  infectious A09
  regional — *see* Enteritis, regional
  ulcerative K51.0- ☑
Ileostomy
  attention to Z43.2
  malfunctioning K94.13
  status Z93.2
    with complication — *see* Complications, enterosto-
      my
Ileotyphus — *see* Typhoid
Ileum — *see* condition
Ileus (bowel) (colon) (inhibitory) (intestine) K56.7
  adynamic K56.0
  due to gallstone (in intestine) K56.3
  duodenal (chronic) K31.5
  gallstone K56.3
  mechanical NEC — *see also* Obstruction, intestine,
    specified NEC K56.699
  meconium P76.0
    in cystic fibrosis E84.11
    meaning meconium plug (without cystic fibrosis)
      P76.0
  myxedema K59.8
  neurogenic K56.0
    Hirschsprung's disease or megacolon Q43.1
  newborn
    due to meconium P76.0
      in cystic fibrosis E84.11
      meaning meconium plug (without cystic fibrosis)
        P76.0
    transitory P76.1
  obstructive — *see also* Obstruction, intestine, specified
    NEC K56.699
  paralytic K56.0
  postoperative K91.89
Iliac — *see* condition
Iliotibial band syndrome M76.3- ☑
Illiteracy Z55.0
Illness — *see also* Disease R69
  manic-depressive — *see* Disorder, bipolar
Imbalance R26.89
  autonomic G90.8
  constituents of food intake E63.1
  electrolyte E87.8
    with
      abortion — *see* Abortion by type, complicated
        by, electrolyte imbalance
      molar pregnancy O08.5

Imbalance — *continued*
  electrolyte — *continued*
    due to hyperemesis gravidarum O21.1
    following ectopic or molar pregnancy O08.5
    neonatal, transitory NEC P74.49
      potassium
        hyperkalemia P74.31
        hypokalemia P74.32
      sodium
        hypernatremia P74.21
        hyponatremia P74.22
  endocrine E34.9
  eye muscle NOS H50.9
  hormone E34.9
  hysterical F44.4
  labyrinth — *see* subcategory H83.2 ☑
  posture R29.3
  protein-energy — *see* Malnutrition
  sympathetic G90.8
Imbecile, imbecility (I.Q. 35-49) F71
Imbedding, intrauterine device T83.39 ☑
Imbibition, cholesterol (gallbladder) K82.4
Imbrication, teeth,, fully erupted M26.30
Imerslund (-Gräsbeck) **syndrome** D51.1
Immature — *see also* Immaturity
  birth (less than 37 completed weeks) — *see* Preterm,
    newborn
  extremely (less than 28 completed weeks) — *see*
    Immaturity, extreme
  personality F60.89
Immaturity (less than 37 completed weeks) — *see also*
    Preterm, newborn
  extreme of newborn (less than 28 completed weeks of
    gestation) (less than 196 completed days of
    gestation) (unspecified weeks of gestation)
    P07.20
    gestational age
      23 completed weeks (23 weeks, 0 days through
        23 weeks, 6 days) P07.22
      24 completed weeks (24 weeks, 0 days through
        24 weeks, 6 days) P07.23
      25 completed weeks (25 weeks, 0 days through
        25 weeks, 6 days) P07.24
      26 completed weeks (26 weeks, 0 days through
        26 weeks, 6 days) P07.25
      27 completed weeks (27 weeks, 0 days through
        27 weeks, 6 days) P07.26
      less than 23 completed weeks P07.21
  fetus or infant light-for-dates — *see* Light-for-dates
  lung, newborn P28.0
  organ or site NEC — *see* Hypoplasia
  pulmonary, newborn P28.0
  reaction F60.89
  sexual (female) (male), after puberty E30.0
Immersion T75.1 ☑
  foot T69.02- ☑
  hand T69.01- ☑
Immobile, immobility
  complete, due to severe physical disability or frailty
    R53.2
  intestine K59.8
  syndrome (paraplegic) M62.3
Immune reconstitution (inflammatory) syndrome [IRIS]
    D89.3
Immunization — *see also* Vaccination
  ABO — *see* Incompatibility, ABO
    in newborn P55.1
  appropriate for age
    child (over 28 days old) Z00.129
      with abnormal findings Z00.121
  complication — *see* Complications, vaccination
  encounter for Z23
  not done (not carried out) Z28.9
    because (of)
      acute illness of patient Z28.01
      allergy to vaccine (or component) Z28.04
      caregiver refusal Z28.82
      chronic illness of patient Z28.02
      contraindication NEC Z28.09
      delay in delivery of vaccine Z28.83
      group pressure Z28.1
      guardian refusal Z28.82
      immune compromised state of patient Z28.03
      lack of availability of vaccine Z28.83
      manufacturer delay of vaccine Z28.83
      parent refusal Z28.82
      patient had disease being vaccinated against
        Z28.81

Immunization — *continued*
  not done — *continued*
    because — *continued*
      patient refusal Z28.21
      patient's belief Z28.1
      religious beliefs of patient Z28.1
      specified reason NEC Z28.89
        of patient Z28.29
      unavailability of vaccine Z28.83
      unspecified patient reason Z28.20
  Rh factor
    affecting management of pregnancy NEC O36.09- ☑
    anti-D antibody O36.01- ☑
  from transfusion — *see* Complication(s), transfusion,
    incompatibility reaction, Rh (factor)
Immunocytoma C83.0- ☑
Immunodeficiency D84.9
  with
    adenosine-deaminase deficiency — *see also* Defi-
      ciency, adenosine deaminase D81.30
    antibody defects D80.9
      specified type NEC D80.8
    hyperimmunoglobulinemia D80.6
    increased immunoglobulin M (IgM) D80.5
    major defect D82.9
      specified type NEC D82.8
    partial albinism D82.8
    short-limbed stature D82.2
    thrombocytopenia and eczema D82.0
  antibody with
    hyperimmunoglobulinemia D80.6
    near-normal immunoglobulins D80.6
  autosomal recessive, Swiss type D80.0
  combined D81.9
    biotin-dependent carboxylase D81.819
      biotinidase D81.810
      holocarboxylase synthetase D81.818
      specified type NEC D81.818
    severe (SCID) D81.9
      with
        low or normal B-cell numbers D81.2
        low T- and B-cell numbers D81.1
        reticular dysgenesis D81.0
    specified type NEC D81.89
  common variable D83.9
    with
      abnormalities of B-cell numbers and function
        D83.0
      autoantibodies to B- or T-cells D83.2
      immunoregulatory T-cell disorders D83.1
    specified type NEC D83.8
  following hereditary defective response to Epstein-Barr
    virus (EBV) D82.3
  selective, immunoglobulin
    A (IgA) D80.2
    G (IgG) (subclasses) D80.3
    M (IgM) D80.4
  severe combined (SCID) D81.9
    due to adenosine deaminase deficiency D81.31
  specified type NEC D84.8
  X-linked, with increased IgM D80.5
Immunotherapy (encounter for)
  antineoplastic Z51.12
Impaction, impacted
  bowel, colon, rectum — *see also* Impaction, fecal
    K56.49
    by gallstone K56.3
  calculus — *see* Calculus
  cerumen (ear) (external) H61.2- ☑
  cuspid — *see* Impaction, tooth
  dental (same or adjacent tooth) K01.1
  fecal, feces K56.41
  fracture — *see* Fracture, by site
  gallbladder — *see* Calculus, gallbladder
  gallstone(s) — *see* Calculus, gallbladder
    bile duct (common) (hepatic) — *see* Calculus, bile
      duct
    cystic duct — *see* Calculus, gallbladder
    in intestine, with obstruction (any part) K56.3
  intestine (calculous) NEC — *see also* Impaction, fecal
    K56.49
    gallstone, with ileus K56.3
  intrauterine device (IUD) T83.39 ☑
  molar — *see* Impaction, tooth
  shoulder, causing obstructed labor O66.0
  tooth, teeth K01.1
  turbinate J34.89

Impaired, impairment (function)
- auditory discrimination — *see* Abnormal, auditory perception
- cognitive, mild, so stated G31.84
- dual sensory Z73.82
- fasting glucose R73.01
- glucose tolerance (oral) R73.02
- hearing — *see* Deafness
- heart — *see* Disease, heart
- kidney N28.9
  - disorder resulting from N25.9
    - specified NEC N25.89
- liver K72.90
  - with coma K72.91
- mastication K08.89
- mild cognitive, so stated G31.84
- mobility
  - ear ossicles — *see* Ankylosis, ear ossicles
  - requiring care provider Z74.09
- myocardium, myocardial — *see* Insufficiency, myocardial
- rectal sphincter R19.8
- renal (acute) (chronic) N28.9
  - disorder resulting from N25.9
    - specified NEC N25.89
- vision NEC H54.7
  - both eyes H54.3

Impediment, speech R47.9
- psychogenic (childhood) F98.8
- slurring R47.81
- specified NEC R47.89

Impending
- coronary syndrome I20.0
- delirium tremens F10.239
- myocardial infarction I20.0

Imperception auditory (acquired) — *see also* Deafness
- congenital H93.25

Imperfect
- aeration, lung (newborn) NEC — *see* Atelectasis
- closure (congenital)
  - alimentary tract NEC Q45.8
    - lower Q43.8
    - upper Q40.8
  - atrioventricular ostium Q21.2
  - atrium (secundum) Q21.1
  - branchial cleft NOS Q18.2
    - cyst Q18.0
    - fistula Q18.0
    - sinus Q18.0
  - choroid Q14.3
  - cricoid cartilage Q31.8
  - cusps, heart valve NEC Q24.8
    - pulmonary Q22.3
  - ductus
    - arteriosus Q25.0
    - Botalli Q25.0
  - ear drum (causing impairment of hearing) Q16.4
  - esophagus with communication to bronchus or trachea Q39.1
  - eyelid Q10.3
  - foramen
    - botalli Q21.1
    - ovale Q21.1
  - genitalia, genital organ(s) or system
    - female Q52.8
      - external Q52.79
      - internal NEC Q52.8
    - male Q55.8
  - glottis Q31.8
  - interatrial ostium or septum Q21.1
  - interauricular ostium or septum Q21.1
  - interventricular ostium or septum Q21.0
  - larynx Q31.8
  - lip — *see* Cleft, lip
  - nasal septum Q30.3
  - nose Q30.2
  - omphalomesenteric duct Q43.0
  - optic nerve entry Q14.2
  - organ or site not listed — *see* Anomaly, by site
  - ostium
    - interatrial Q21.1
    - interauricular Q21.1
    - interventricular Q21.0
  - palate — *see* Cleft, palate
  - preauricular sinus Q18.1
  - retina Q14.1
  - roof of orbit Q75.8
  - sclera Q13.5

Imperfect — *continued*
- closure — *continued*
  - septum
    - aorticopulmonary Q21.4
    - atrial (secundum) Q21.1
    - between aorta and pulmonary artery Q21.4
    - heart Q21.9
    - interatrial (secundum) Q21.1
    - interauricular (secundum) Q21.1
    - interventricular Q21.0
      - in tetralogy of Fallot Q21.3
    - nasal Q30.3
    - ventricular Q21.0
      - with pulmonary stenosis or atresia, dextraposition of aorta, and hypertrophy of right ventricle Q21.3
      - in tetralogy of Fallot Q21.3
  - skull Q75.0
    - with
      - anencephaly Q00.0
      - encephalocele — *see* Encephalocele
      - hydrocephalus Q03.9
        - with spina bifida — *see* Spina bifida, by site, with hydrocephalus
      - microcephaly Q02
  - spine (with meningocele) — *see* Spina bifida
  - trachea Q32.1
  - tympanic membrane (causing impairment of hearing) Q16.4
  - uterus Q51.818
  - vitelline duct Q43.0
- erection — *see* Dysfunction, sexual, male, erectile
- fusion — *see* Imperfect, closure
- inflation, lung (newborn) — *see* Atelectasis
- posture R29.3
- rotation, intestine Q43.3
- septum, ventricular Q21.0

Imperfectly descended testis — *see* Cryptorchid
Imperforate (congenital) — *see also* Atresia
- anus Q42.3
  - with fistula Q42.2
- cervix (uteri) Q51.828
- esophagus Q39.0
  - with tracheoesophageal fistula Q39.1
- hymen Q52.3
- jejunum Q41.1
- pharynx Q38.8
- rectum Q42.1
  - with fistula Q42.0
- urethra Q64.39
- vagina Q52.4

Impervious (congenital) — *see also* Atresia
- anus Q42.3
  - with fistula Q42.2
- bile duct Q44.2
- esophagus Q39.0
  - with tracheoesophageal fistula Q39.1
- intestine (small) Q41.9
  - large Q42.9
    - specified NEC Q42.8
- rectum Q42.1
  - with fistula Q42.0
- ureter — *see* Atresia, ureter
- urethra Q64.39

Impetiginization of dermatoses L01.1
Impetigo (any organism) (any site) (circinate) (contagiosa) (simplex) (vulgaris) L01.00
- Bockhart's L01.02
- bullous, bullosa L01.03
- external ear L01.00 [H62.40]
- follicularis L01.02
- furfuracea L30.5
- herpetiformis L40.1
  - nonobstetrical L40.1
- neonatorum L01.03
- nonbullous L01.01
- specified type NEC L01.09
- ulcerative L01.09

Impingement (on teeth)
- joint — *see* Disorder, joint, specified type NEC
- soft tissue
  - anterior M26.81
  - posterior M26.82

Implant, endometrial N80.9
Implantation
- anomalous — *see* Anomaly, by site
  - ureter Q62.63

Implantation — *continued*
- cyst
  - external area or site (skin) NEC L72.0
  - iris — *see* Cyst, iris, implantation
  - vagina N89.8
  - vulva N90.7
- dermoid (cyst) — *see* Implantation, cyst

Impotence (sexual) N52.9
- counseling Z70.1
- organic origin — *see also* Dysfunction, sexual, male, erectile N52.9
- psychogenic F52.21

Impression, basilar Q75.8
Imprisonment, anxiety concerning Z65.1
Improper care (child) (newborn) — *see* Maltreatment
Improperly tied umbilical cord (causing hemorrhage) P51.8
Impulsiveness (impulsive) R45.87
Inability to swallow — *see* Aphagia
Inaccessible, inaccessibility
- health care NEC Z75.3
  - due to
    - waiting period Z75.2
      - for admission to facility elsewhere Z75.1
  - other helping agencies Z75.4

Inactive — *see* condition
Inadequate, inadequacy
- aesthetics of dental restoration K08.56
- biologic, constitutional, functional, or social F60.7
- development
  - child R62.50
  - genitalia
    - after puberty NEC E30.0
    - congenital
      - female Q52.8
        - external Q52.79
        - internal Q52.8
      - male Q55.8
  - lungs Q33.6
    - associated with short gestation P28.0
  - organ or site not listed — *see* Anomaly, by site
- diet (causing nutritional deficiency) E63.9
- eating habits Z72.4
- environment, household Z59.1
- family support Z63.8
- food (supply) NEC Z59.4
  - hunger effects T73.0 ☑
- functional F60.7
- household care, due to
  - family member
    - handicapped or ill Z74.2
    - on vacation Z75.5
    - temporarily away from home Z74.2
  - technical defects in home Z59.1
  - temporary absence from home of person rendering care Z74.2
- housing (heating) (space) Z59.1
- income (financial) Z59.6
- intrafamilial communication Z63.8
- material resources Z59.9
- mental — *see* Disability, intellectual
- parental supervision or control of child Z62.0
- personality F60.7
- pulmonary
  - function R06.89
    - newborn P28.5
  - ventilation, newborn P28.5
- sample of cytologic smear
  - anus R85.615
  - cervix R87.615
  - vagina R87.625
- social F60.7
  - insurance Z59.7
  - skills NEC Z73.4
- supervision of child by parent Z62.0
- teaching affecting education Z55.8
- welfare support Z59.7

Inanition R64
- with edema — *see* Malnutrition, severe
- due to
  - deprivation of food T73.0 ☑
  - malnutrition — *see* Malnutrition
- fever R50.9

Inappropriate
- change in quantitative human chorionic gonadotropin (hCG) in early pregnancy O02.81
- diet or eating habits Z72.4

☑ Additional Character Required — Refer to the Tabular List for Character Selection   ▽ Subterms under main terms may continue to next column or page

Inappropriate — *continued*
  level of quantitative human chorionic gonadotropin
    (hCG) for gestational age in early pregnancy
    O02.81
  secretion
    antidiuretic hormone (ADH) (excessive) E22.2
      deficiency E23.2
    pituitary (posterior) E22.2
Inattention at or after birth — *see* Neglect
Incarceration, incarcerated
  enterocele K46.0
    gangrenous K46.1
  epiplocele K46.0
    gangrenous K46.1
  exomphalos K42.0
    gangrenous K42.1
  hernia — *see also* Hernia, by site, with obstruction
    with gangrene — *see* Hernia, by site, with gangrene
  iris, in wound — *see* Injury, eye, laceration, with pro-
    lapse
  lens, in wound — *see* Injury, eye, laceration, with pro-
    lapse
  omphalocele K42.0
  prison, anxiety concerning Z65.1
  rupture — *see* Hernia, by site
  sarcoepiplocele K46.0
    gangrenous K46.1
  sarcoepiplomphalocele K42.0
    with gangrene K42.1
  uterus N85.8
    gravid O34.51- ☑
      causing obstructed labor O65.5
Incised wound
  external — *see* Laceration
  internal organs — *see* Injury, by site
Incision, incisional
  hernia K43.2
    with
      gangrene (and obstruction) K43.1
      obstruction K43.0
  surgical, complication — *see* Complications, surgical
    procedure
  traumatic
    external — *see* Laceration
    internal organs — *see* Injury, by site
Inclusion
  azurophilic leukocytic D72.0
  blennorrhea (neonatal) (newborn) P39.1
  gallbladder in liver (congenital) Q44.1
Incompatibility
  ABO
    affecting management of pregnancy O36.11- ☑
      anti-A sensitization O36.11- ☑
      anti-B sensitization O36.19- ☑
      specified NEC O36.19- ☑
    infusion or transfusion reaction — *see* Complica-
      tion(s), transfusion, incompatibility reaction,
      ABO
    newborn P55.1
  blood (group) (Duffy) (K) (Kell) (Kidd) (Lewis) (M) (S)
    NEC
    affecting management of pregnancy O36.11- ☑
      anti-A sensitization O36.11- ☑
      anti-B sensitization O36.19- ☑
    infusion or transfusion reaction T80.89 ☑
    newborn P55.8
  divorce or estrangement Z63.5
  Rh (blood group) (factor) Z31.82
    affecting management of pregnancy NEC O36.09- ☑
      anti-D antibody O36.01- ☑
    infusion or transfusion reaction — *see* Complica-
      tion(s), transfusion, incompatibility reaction,
      Rh (factor)
    newborn P55.0
  rhesus — *see* Incompatibility, Rh
Incompetency, incompetent, incompetence
  annular
    aortic (valve) — *see* Insufficiency, aortic
    mitral (valve) I34.0
    pulmonary valve (heart) I37.1
  aortic (valve) — *see* Insufficiency, aortic
  cardiac valve — *see* Endocarditis
  cervix, cervical (os) N88.3
    in pregnancy O34.3- ☑
  chronotropic I45.89
    with
      autonomic dysfunction G90.8
      ischemic heart disease I25.89

Incompetency, incompetent, incompetence —
  continued
  chronotropic — *continued*
    with — *continued*
      left ventricular dysfunction I51.89
      sinus node dysfunction I49.8
  esophagogastric (junction) (sphincter) K22.0
  mitral (valve) — *see* Insufficiency, mitral
  pelvic fundus N81.89
  pubocervical tissue N81.82
  pulmonary valve (heart) I37.1
    congenital Q22.3
  rectovaginal tissue N81.83
  tricuspid (annular) (valve) — *see* Insufficiency, tricuspid
  valvular — *see* Endocarditis
    congenital Q24.8
  vein, venous (saphenous) (varicose) — *see* Varix, leg
Incomplete — *see also* condition
  bladder, emptying R33.9
  defecation R15.0
  expansion lungs (newborn) NEC — *see* Atelectasis
  rotation, intestine Q43.3
Inconclusive
  diagnostic imaging due to excess body fat of patient
    R93.9
  findings on diagnostic imaging of breast NEC R92.8
  mammogram (due to dense breasts) R92.2
Incontinence R32
  anal sphincter R15.9
  coital N39.491
  feces R15.9
    nonorganic origin F98.1
  insensible (urinary) N39.42
  overflow N39.490
  postural (urinary) N39.492
  psychogenic F45.8
  rectal R15.9
  reflex N39.498
  stress (female) (male) N39.3
    and urge N39.46
  urethral sphincter R32
  urge N39.41
    and stress (female) (male) N39.46
  urine (urinary) R32
    continuous N39.45
    due to cognitive impairment, or severe physical
      disability or immobility R39.81
    functional R39.81
    insensible N39.42
    mixed (stress and urge) N39.46
    nocturnal N39.44
    nonorganic origin F98.0
    overflow N39.490
    post dribbling N39.43
    postural N39.492
    reflex N39.498
    specified NEC N39.498
    stress (female) (male) N39.3
      and urge N39.46
    total N39.498
    unaware N39.42
    urge N39.41
      and stress (female) (male) N39.46
Incontinentia pigmenti Q82.3
Incoordinate, incoordination
  esophageal-pharyngeal (newborn) — *see* Dysphagia
  muscular R27.8
  uterus (action) (contractions) (complicating delivery)
    O62.4
Increase, increased
  abnormal, in development R63.8
  androgens (ovarian) E28.1
  anticoagulants (antithrombin) (anti-VIIIa) (anti-IXa)
    (anti-Xa) (anti-XIa) — *see* Circulating anticoagu-
    lants
  cold sense R20.8
  estrogen E28.0
  function
    adrenal
      cortex — *see* Cushing's, syndrome
      medulla E27.5
    pituitary (gland) (anterior) (lobe) E22.9
      posterior E22.2
  heat sense R20.8
  intracranial pressure (benign) G93.2
  permeability, capillaries I78.8
  pressure, intracranial G93.2

Increase, increased — *continued*
  secretion
    gastrin E16.4
    glucagon E16.3
    pancreas, endocrine E16.9
      growth hormone-releasing hormone E16.8
      pancreatic polypeptide E16.8
      somatostatin E16.8
      vasoactive-intestinal polypeptide E16.8
    sphericity, lens Q12.4
    splenic activity D73.1
    venous pressure I87.8
      portal K76.6
Increta placenta O43.22- ☑
Incrustation, cornea, foreign body (lead)(zinc) — *see*
  Foreign body, cornea
Incyclophoria H50.54
Incyclotropia — *see* Cyclotropia
Indeterminate sex Q56.4
India rubber skin Q82.8
Indigestion (acid) (bilious) (functional) K30
  catarrhal K31.89
  due to decomposed food NOS A05.9
  nervous F45.8
  psychogenic F45.8
Indirect — *see* condition
Induratio penis plastica N48.6
Induration, indurated
  brain G93.89
  breast (fibrous) N64.51
    puerperal, postpartum O92.29
  broad ligament N83.8
  chancre
    anus A51.1
    congenital A50.07
    extragenital NEC A51.2
  corpora cavernosa (penis) (plastic) N48.6
  liver (chronic) K76.89
  lung (black) (chronic) (fibroid) — *see also* Fibrosis, lung
    J84.10
    essential brown J84.03
  penile (plastic) N48.6
  phlebitic — *see* Phlebitis
  skin R23.4
Inebriety (without dependence) — *see* Alcohol, intoxication
Inefficiency, kidney N28.9
Inelasticity, skin R23.4
Inequality, leg (length) (acquired) — *see also* Deformity,
  limb, unequal length
  congenital — *see* Defect, reduction, lower limb
  lower leg — *see* Deformity, limb, unequal length
Inertia
  bladder (neurogenic) N31.2
  stomach K31.89
    psychogenic F45.8
  uterus, uterine during labor O62.2
    during latent phase of labor O62.0
    primary O62.0
    secondary O62.1
  vesical (neurogenic) N31.2
Infancy, infantile, infantilism — *see also* condition
  celiac K90.0
  genitalia, genitals (after puberty) E30.0
  Herter's (nontropical sprue) K90.0
  intestinal K90.0
  Lorain E23.0
  pancreatic K86.89
  pelvis M95.5
    with disproportion (fetopelvic) O33.1
      causing obstructed labor O65.1
  pituitary E23.0
  renal N25.0
  uterus — *see* Infantile, genitalia
Infant(s) — *see also* Infancy
  excessive crying R68.11
  irritable child R68.12
  lack of care — *see* Neglect
  liveborn (singleton) Z38.2
    born in hospital Z38.00
      by cesarean Z38.01
    born outside hospital Z38.1
    multiple NEC Z38.8
      born in hospital Z38.68
        by cesarean Z38.69
      born outside hospital Z38.7
    quadruplet Z38.8
      born in hospital Z38.63

Infant(s) — *continued*
  liveborn — *continued*
    quadruplet — *continued*
      born in hospital — *continued*
        by cesarean Z38.64
      born outside hospital Z38.7
    quintuplet Z38.8
      born in hospital Z38.65
        by cesarean Z38.66
      born outside hospital Z38.7
    triplet Z38.8
      born in hospital Z38.61
        by cesarean Z38.62
      born outside hospital Z38.7
    twin Z38.5
      born in hospital Z38.30
        by cesarean Z38.31
      born outside hospital Z38.4
  of diabetic mother (syndrome of) P70.1
    gestational diabetes P70.0
Infantile — *see also* condition
  genitalia, genitals E30.0
  os, uterine E30.0
  penis E30.0
  testis E29.1
  uterus E30.0
Infantilism — *see* Infancy
Infarct, infarction
  adrenal (capsule) (gland) E27.49
  appendices epiploicae — *see also* Infarct, intestine K55.069
  bowel — *see also* Infarct, intestine K55.069
  brain (stem) — *see* Infarct, cerebral
  breast N64.89
  brewer's (kidney) N28.0
  cardiac — *see* Infarct, myocardium
  cerebellar — *see* Infarct, cerebral
  cerebral (acute) (chronic) — *see also* Occlusion, artery cerebral or precerebral, with infarction I63.9
    aborted I63.9
    cortical I63.9
    due to
      cerebral venous thrombosis, nonpyogenic I63.6
      embolism
        cerebral arteries I63.4- ☑
        precerebral arteries I63.1- ☑
      occlusion NEC
        cerebral arteries I63.5- ☑
        precerebral arteries I63.2- ☑
        small artery I63.81
      stenosis NEC
        cerebral arteries I63.5- ☑
        precerebral arteries I63.2- ☑
        small artery I63.81
      thrombosis
        cerebral artery I63.3- ☑
        precerebral artery I63.0- ☑
    intraoperative
      during cardiac surgery I97.810
      during other surgery I97.811
    postprocedural
      following cardiac surgery I97.820
      following other surgery I97.821
    specified NEC I63.89
  colon (acute) (agnogenic) (embolic) (hemorrhagic) (nonocclusive) (nonthrombotic) (occlusive) (segmental) (thrombotic) (with gangrene) — *see also* Infarct, intestine K55.049
  coronary artery — *see* Infarct, myocardium
  embolic — *see* Embolism
  fallopian tube N83.8
  gallbladder K82.8
  heart — *see* Infarct, myocardium
  hepatic K76.3
  hypophysis (anterior lobe) E23.6
  impending (myocardium) I20.0
  intestine (acute) (agnogenic) (embolic) (hemorrhagic) (nonocclusive) (nonthrombotic) (occlusive) (thrombotic) (with gangrene) K55.069
    diffuse K55.062
    focal K55.061
    large K55.049
      diffuse K55.042
      focal K55.041
    small K55.029
      diffuse K55.022
      focal K55.021
  kidney N28.0

Infarct, infarction — *continued*
  lacunar I63.81
  liver K76.3
  lung (embolic) (thrombotic) — *see* Embolism, pulmonary
  lymph node I89.8
  mesentery, mesenteric (embolic) (thrombotic) (with gangrene) — *see also* Infarct, intestine K55.069
  muscle (ischemic) M62.20
    ankle M62.27- ☑
    foot M62.27- ☑
    forearm M62.23- ☑
    hand M62.24- ☑
    lower leg M62.26- ☑
    pelvic region M62.25- ☑
    shoulder region M62.21- ☑
    specified site NEC M62.28
    thigh M62.25- ☑
    upper arm M62.22- ☑
  myocardium, myocardial (acute) (with stated duration of 4 weeks or less) I21.9
    associated with revascularization procedure I21.A9
    diagnosed on ECG, but presenting no symptoms I25.2
    due to
      demand ischemia I21.A1
      ischemic imbalance I21.A1
    healed or old I25.2
    intraoperative — *see also* Infarct, myocardium, associated with revascularization procedure
      during cardiac surgery I97.790
      during other surgery I97.791
    non-Q wave I21.4
    non-ST elevation (NSTEMI) I21.4
      subsequent I22.2
    nontransmural I21.4
    past (diagnosed on ECG or other investigation, but currently presenting no symptoms) I25.2
    postprocedural — *see also* Infarct, myocardium, associated with revascularization procedure
      following cardiac surgery — *see also* Infarct, myocardium, type 4 or type 5 I97.190
      following other surgery I97.191
    Q wave (*see also* Infarct, myocardium, by site) I21.3
    secondary to
      demand ischemia I21.A1
      ischemic imbalance I21.A1
    ST elevation (STEMI) I21.3
      anterior (anteroapical) (anterolateral) (anteroseptal) (Q wave) (wall) I21.09
        subsequent I22.0
      inferior (diaphragmatic) (inferolateral) (inferoposterior) (wall) NEC I21.19
        subsequent I22.1
      inferoposterior transmural (Q wave) I21.11
      involving
        coronary artery of anterior wall NEC I21.09
        coronary artery of inferior wall NEC I21.19
        diagonal coronary artery I21.02
        left anterior descending coronary artery I21.02
        left circumflex coronary artery I21.21
        left main coronary artery I21.01
        oblique marginal coronary artery I21.21
        right coronary artery I21.11
      lateral (apical-lateral) (basal-lateral) (high) I21.29
        subsequent I22.8
      posterior (posterobasal) (posterolateral) (posteroseptal) (true) I21.29
        subsequent I22.8
      septal I21.29
        subsequent I22.8
      specified NEC I21.29
        subsequent I22.8
    subsequent I22.9
    subsequent (recurrent) (reinfarction) I22.9
      anterior (anteroapical) (anterolateral) (anteroseptal) (wall) I22.0
      diaphragmatic (wall) I22.1
      inferior (diaphragmatic) (inferolateral) (inferoposterior) (wall) I22.1
      lateral (apical-lateral) (basal-lateral) (high) I22.8
      non-ST elevation (NSTEMI) I22.2
      posterior (posterobasal) (posterolateral) (posteroseptal) (true) I22.8
      septal I22.8
      specified NEC I22.8
      ST elevation I22.9

Infarct, infarction — *continued*
  myocardium, myocardial — *continued*
    subsequent — *continued*
      ST elevation — *continued*
        anterior (anteroapical) (anterolateral) (anteroseptal) (wall) I22.0
        inferior (diaphragmatic) (inferolateral) (inferoposterior) (wall) I22.1
        specified NEC I22.8
      subendocardial I22.2
      transmural I22.9
        anterior (anteroapical) (anterolateral) (anteroseptal) (wall) I22.0
        diaphragmatic (wall) I22.1
        inferior (diaphragmatic) (inferolateral) (inferoposterior) (wall) I22.1
        lateral (apical-lateral) (basal-lateral) (high) I22.8
        posterior (posterobasal) (posterolateral) (posteroseptal) (true) I22.8
        specified NEC I22.8
      type 1 — *see also* Infarction, myocardial, subsequent, by site, or by ST elevation or non-ST elevation I22.9
      type 2 I21.A1
      type 3 I21.A9
      type 4 I21.A9
      type 5 I21.A9
    syphilitic A52.06
    transmural I21.9
      anterior (anteroapical) (anterolateral) (anteroseptal) (Q wave) (wall) NEC I21.09
      inferior (diaphragmatic) (inferolateral) (inferoposterior) (Q wave) (wall) NEC I21.19
      inferoposterior (Q wave) I21.11
      lateral (apical-lateral) (basal-lateral) (high) NEC I21.29
      posterior (posterobasal) (posterolateral) (posteroseptal) (true) NEC I21.29
      septal NEC I21.29
      specified NEC I21.29
      type 1 — *see also* Infarction, myocardial, by site, or by ST elevation or non-ST elevation I21.9
      type 2 I21.A1
      type 3 I21.A9
      type 4 (a) (b) (c) I21.A9
      type 5 I21.A9
    nontransmural I21.4
  omentum — *see also* Infarct, intestine K55.069
  ovary N83.8
  pancreas K86.89
  papillary muscle — *see* Infarct, myocardium
  parathyroid gland E21.4
  pituitary (gland) E23.6
  placenta O43.81- ☑
  prostate N42.89
  pulmonary (artery) (vein) (hemorrhagic) — *see* Embolism, pulmonary
  renal (embolic) (thrombotic) N28.0
  retina, retinal (artery) — *see* Occlusion, artery, retina
  spinal (cord) (acute) (embolic) (nonembolic) G95.11
  spleen D73.5
    embolic or thrombotic I74.8
  subendocardial (acute) (nontransmural) I21.4
  suprarenal (capsule) (gland) E27.49
  testis N50.1
  thrombotic — *see also* Thrombosis
    artery, arterial — *see* Embolism
  thyroid (gland) E07.89
  ventricle (heart) — *see* Infarct, myocardium
Infecting — *see* condition
Infection, infected, infective (opportunistic) B99.9
  with
    drug resistant organism — *see* Resistance (to), drug — *see also* specific organism
    lymphangitis — *see* Lymphangitis
    organ dysfunction (acute) R65.20
      with septic shock R65.21
  abscess (skin) — *code by* site under Abscess
  Absidia — *see* Mucormycosis
  Acanthamoeba — *see* Acanthamebiasis
  Acanthocheilonema (perstans) (streptocerca) B74.4
  accessory sinus (chronic) — *see* Sinusitis
  achorion — *see* Dermatophytosis
  Acremonium falciforme B47.0
  acromioclavicular M00.9
  Actinobacillus (actinomycetem-comitans) A28.8
    mallei A24.0

☑ **Additional Character Required** — Refer to the Tabular List for Character Selection   ▽ Subterms under main terms may continue to next column or page

Infection, infected, infective — *continued*
  Actinobacillus — *continued*
    muris A25.1
  Actinomadura B47.1
  Actinomyces (israelii) — *see also* Actinomycosis A42.9
  Actinomycetales — *see* Actinomycosis
  actinomycotic NOS — *see* Actinomycosis
  adenoid (and tonsil) J03.90
    chronic J35.02
  adenovirus NEC
    as cause of disease classified elsewhere B97.0
    unspecified nature or site B34.0
  aerogenes capsulatus A48.0
  aertrycke — *see* Infection, salmonella
  alimentary canal NOS — *see* Enteritis, infectious
  Allescheria boydii B48.2
  Alternaria B48.8
  alveolus, alveolar (process) K04.7
  Ameba, amebic (histolytica) — *see* Amebiasis
  amniotic fluid, sac or cavity O41.10- ☑
    chorioamnionitis O41.12- ☑
    placentitis O41.14- ☑
  amputation stump (surgical) — *see* Complication, amputation stump, infection
  Ancylostoma (duodenalis) B76.0
  Anisakiasis, Anisakis larvae B81.0
  anthrax — *see* Anthrax
  antrum (chronic) — *see* Sinusitis, maxillary
  anus, anal (papillae) (sphincter) K62.89
  arbovirus (arbor virus) A94
    specified type NEC A93.8
  artificial insemination N98.0
  Ascaris lumbricoides — *see* Ascariasis
  Ascomycetes B47.0
  Aspergillus (flavus) (fumigatus) (terreus) — *see* Aspergillosis
  atypical
    acid-fast (bacilli) — *see* Mycobacterium, atypical
    mycobacteria — *see* Mycobacterium, atypical
    virus A81.9
      specified type NEC A81.89
  auditory meatus (external) — *see* Otitis, externa, infective
  auricle (ear) — *see* Otitis, externa, infective
  axillary gland (lymph) L04.2
  Bacillus A49.9
    abortus A23.1
    anthracis — *see* Anthrax
    Ducrey's (any location) A57
    Flexner's A03.1
    Friedländer's NEC A49.8
    gas (gangrene) A48.0
    mallei A24.0
    melitensis A23.0
    paratyphoid, paratyphosus A01.4
      A A01.1
      B A01.2
      C A01.3
    Shiga (-Kruse) A03.0
    suipestifer — *see* Infection, salmonella
    swimming pool A31.1
    typhosa A01.00
    welchii — *see* Gangrene, gas
  bacterial NOS A49.9
    as cause of disease classified elsewhere B96.89
      Bacteroides fragilis [B. fragilis] B96.6
      Clostridium perfringens [C. perfringens] B96.7
      Enterobacter sakazakii B96.89
      Enterococcus B95.2
      Escherichia coli [E. coli] — *see also* Escherichia coli B96.20
      Helicobacter pylori [H.pylori] B96.81
      Hemophilus influenzae [H. influenzae] B96.3
      Klebsiella pneumoniae [K. pneumoniae] B96.1
      Mycoplasma pneumoniae [M. pneumoniae] B96.0
      Proteus (mirabilis) (morganii) B96.4
      Pseudomonas (aeruginosa) (mallei) (pseudomallei) B96.5
      Staphylococcus B95.8
        aureus (methicillin susceptible) (MSSA) B95.61
          methicillin resistant (MRSA) B95.62
        specified NEC B95.7
      Streptococcus B95.5
        group A B95.0
        group B B95.1
        pneumoniae B95.3
        specified NEC B95.4

Infection, infected, infective — *continued*
  bacterial — *continued*
    as cause of disease classified elsewhere — *continued*
      Vibrio vulnificus B96.82
    specified NEC A48.8
  Bacterium
    paratyphosum A01.4
      A A01.1
      B A01.2
      C A01.3
    typhosum A01.00
  Bacteroides NEC A49.8
    fragilis, as cause of disease classified elsewhere B96.6
  Balantidium coli A07.0
  Bartholin's gland N75.8
  Basidiobolus B46.8
  bile duct (common) (hepatic) — *see* Cholangitis
  bladder — *see* Cystitis
  Blastomyces, blastomycotic — *see also* Blastomycosis
    brasiliensis — *see* Paracoccidioidomycosis
    dermatitidis — *see* Blastomycosis
    European — *see* Cryptococcosis
    Loboi B48.0
    North American B40.9
    South American — *see* Paracoccidioidomycosis
  bleb, postprocedure — *see* Blebitis
  bone — *see* Osteomyelitis
  Bordetella — *see* Whooping cough
  Borrelia bergdorfi A69.20
  brain — *see also* Encephalitis G04.90
    membranes — *see* Meningitis
    septic G06.0
      meninges — *see* Meningitis, bacterial
  branchial cyst Q18.0
  breast — *see* Mastitis
  bronchus — *see* Bronchitis
  Brucella A23.9
    abortus A23.1
    canis A23.3
    melitensis A23.0
    mixed A23.8
    specified NEC A23.8
    suis A23.2
  Brugia (malayi) B74.1
    timori B74.2
  bursa — *see* Bursitis, infective
  buttocks (skin) L08.9
  Campylobacter, intestinal A04.5
    as cause of disease classified elsewhere B96.81
  Candida (albicans) (tropicalis) — *see* Candidiasis
  candiru B88.8
  Capillaria (intestinal) B81.1
    hepatica B83.8
    philippinensis B81.1
  cartilage — *see* Disorder, cartilage, specified type NEC
  cat liver fluke B66.0
  catheter-related bloodstream (CRBSI) T80.211 ☑
  cellulitis — *code by* site under Cellulitis
  central line-associated T80.219 ☑
    bloodstream (CLABSI) T80.211 ☑
    specified NEC T80.218 ☑
  Cephalosporium falciforme B47.0
  cerebrospinal — *see* Meningitis
  cervical gland (lymph) L04.0
  cervix — *see* Cervicitis
  cesarean delivery wound (puerperal) O86.00
  cestodes — *see* Infestation, cestodes
  chest J22
  Chilomastix (intestinal) A07.8
  Chlamydia, chlamydial A74.9
    anus A56.3
    genitourinary tract A56.2
      lower A56.00
      specified NEC A56.19
    lymphogranuloma A55
    pharynx A56.4
    psittaci A70
    rectum A56.3
    sexually transmitted NEC A56.8
  cholera — *see* Cholera
  Cladosporium
    bantianum (brain abscess) B43.1
    carrionii B43.0
    castellanii B36.1
    trichoides (brain abscess) B43.1
    werneckii B36.1

Infection, infected, infective — *continued*
  Clonorchis (sinensis) (liver) B66.1
  Clostridium NEC
    bifermentans A48.0
    botulinum (food poisoning) A05.1
      infant A48.51
      wound A48.52
    difficile
      as cause of disease classified elsewhere B96.89
      foodborne (disease)
        not specified as recurrent A04.72
        recurrent A04.71
      gas gangrene A48.0
      necrotizing enterocolitis
        not specified as recurrent A04.72
        recurrent A04.71
      sepsis A41.4
    gas-forming NEC A48.0
    histolyticum A48.0
    novyi, causing gas gangrene A48.0
    oedematiens A48.0
    perfringens
      as cause of disease classified elsewhere B96.7
      due to food A05.2
      foodborne (disease) A05.2
      gas gangrene A48.0
      sepsis A41.4
    septicum, causing gas gangrene A48.0
    sordellii, causing gas gangrene A48.0
    welchii
      as cause of disease classified elsewhere B96.7
      foodborne (disease) A05.2
      gas gangrene A48.0
      necrotizing enteritis A05.2
      sepsis A41.4
  Coccidioides (immitis) — *see* Coccidioidomycosis
  colon — *see* Enteritis, infectious
  colostomy K94.02
  common duct — *see* Cholangitis
  congenital P39.9
    Candida (albicans) P37.5
    cytomegalovirus P35.1
    hepatitis, viral P35.3
    herpes simplex P35.2
    infectious or parasitic disease P37.9
      specified NEC P37.8
    listeriosis (disseminated) P37.2
    malaria NEC P37.4
      falciparum P37.3
    Plasmodium falciparum P37.3
    poliomyelitis P35.8
    rubella P35.0
    skin P39.4
    toxoplasmosis (acute) (subacute) (chronic) P37.1
    tuberculosis P37.0
    urinary (tract) P39.3
    vaccinia P35.8
    virus P35.9
      specified type NEC P35.8
  Conidiobolus B46.8
  coronavirus NEC B34.2
    as cause of disease classified elsewhere B97.29
    severe acute respiratory syndrome (SARS associated) B97.21
  corpus luteum — *see* Salpingo-oophoritis
  Corynebacterium diphtheriae — *see* Diphtheria
  cotia virus B08.8
  Coxiella burnetii A78
  coxsackie — *see* Coxsackie
  Cryptococcus neoformans — *see* Cryptococcosis
  Cryptosporidium A07.2
  Cunninghamella — *see* Mucormycosis
  cyst — *see* Cyst
  cystic duct — *see also* Cholecystitis K81.9
  Cysticercus cellulosae — *see* Cysticercosis
  cytomegalovirus, cytomegaloviral B25.9
    congenital P35.1
    maternal, maternal care for (suspected) damage to fetus O35.3 ☑
    mononucleosis B27.10
      with
        complication NEC B27.19
        meningitis B27.12
        polyneuropathy B27.11
  delta-agent (acute), in hepatitis B carrier B17.0
  dental (pulpal origin) K04.7
  Deuteromycetes B47.0
  Dicrocoelium dendriticum B66.2

Infection, infected, infective — *continued*
Dipetalonema (perstans) (streptocerca) B74.4
diphtherial — *see* Diphtheria
Diphyllobothrium (adult) (latum) (pacificum) B70.0
  larval B70.1
Diplogonoporus (grandis) B71.8
Dipylidium caninum B67.4
Dirofilaria B74.8
Dracunculus medinensis B72
Drechslera (hawaiiensis) B43.8
Ducrey Haemophilus (any location) A57
due to or resulting from
  artificial insemination N98.0
  central venous catheter T80.219 ☑
    bloodstream T80.211 ☑
    exit or insertion site T80.212 ☑
    localized T80.212 ☑
    port or reservoir T80.212 ☑
    specified NEC T80.218 ☑
    tunnel T80.212 ☑
  device, implant or graft — *see also* Complications,
    by site and type, infection or inflammation
    T85.79 ☑
    arterial graft NEC T82.7 ☑
    breast (implant) T85.79 ☑
    catheter NEC T85.79 ☑
      dialysis (renal) T82.7 ☑
        intraperitoneal T85.71 ☑
      infusion NEC T82.7 ☑
        cranial T85.735 ☑
        intrathecal T85.735 ☑
        spinal (epidural) (subdural) T85.735 ☑
        subarachnoid T85.735 ☑
      urinary T83.518 ☑
        cystostomy T83.510 ☑
        Hopkins T83.518 ☑
        ileostomy T83.518 ☑
        nephrostomy T83.512 ☑
        specified NEC T83.518 ☑
        urethral indwelling T83.511 ☑
        urostomy T83.518 ☑
    electronic (electrode) (pulse generator) (stimula-
      tor)
      bone T84.7 ☑
      cardiac T82.7 ☑
      nervous system T85.738 ☑
        brain T85.731 ☑
        cranial nerve T85.732 ☑
        gastric nerve T85.732 ☑
        generator pocket T85.734 ☑
        neurostimulator generator T85.734 ☑
        peripheral nerve T85.732 ☑
        sacral nerve T85.732 ☑
        spinal cord T85.733 ☑
        vagal nerve T85.732 ☑
      urinary (indwelling) T83.51 ☑
    fixation, internal (orthopedic) NEC — *see* Compli-
      cation, fixation device, infection
    gastrointestinal (bile duct) (esophagus) T85.79 ☑
      neurostimulator electrode (lead) T85.732 ☑
    genital NEC T83.69 ☑
    heart NEC T82.7 ☑
      valve (prosthesis) T82.6 ☑
        graft T82.7 ☑
    joint prosthesis — *see* Complication, joint pros-
      thesis, infection
    ocular (corneal graft) (orbital implant) NEC
      T85.79 ☑
    orthopedic NEC T84.7 ☑
    penile (cylinder) (pump) (resevoir) T83.61 ☑
    specified NEC T85.79 ☑
    testicular T83.62 ☑
    urinary NEC T83.598 ☑
      ileal conduit stent T83.593 ☑
      implanted neurostimulation T83.590 ☑
      implanted sphincter T83.591 ☑
      indwelling ureteral stent T83.592 ☑
      nephroureteral stent T83.593 ☑
      specified stent NEC T83.593 ☑
    vascular NEC T82.7 ☑
    ventricular intracranial (communicating) shunt
      T85.730 ☑
  Hickman catheter T80.219 ☑
    bloodstream T80.211 ☑
    localized T80.212 ☑
    specified NEC T80.218 ☑

Infection, infected, infective — *continued*
due to or resulting from — *continued*
  immunization or vaccination T88.0 ☑
  infusion, injection or transfusion NEC T80.29 ☑
  injury NEC — *code by* site under Wound, open
  peripherally inserted central catheter (PICC)
    T80.219 ☑
    bloodstream T80.211 ☑
    localized T80.212 ☑
    specified NEC T80.218 ☑
  portacath (port-a-cath) T80.219 ☑
    bloodstream T80.211 ☑
    localized T80.212 ☑
    specified NEC T80.218 ☑
  pulmonary artery catheter — *see* Infection, due to
    or resulting from, central venous catheter
  surgery T81.40 ☑
  Swan Ganz catheter — *see* Infection, due to or re-
    sulting from, central venous catheter
  triple lumen catheter T80.219 ☑
    bloodstream T80.211 ☑
    localized T80.212 ☑
    specified NEC T80.218 ☑
  umbilical venous catheter T80.219 ☑
    bloodstream T80.211 ☑
    localized T80.212 ☑
    specified NEC T80.218 ☑
during labor NEC O75.3
ear (middle) — *see also* Otitis media
  external — *see* Otitis, externa, infective
  inner — *see* subcategory H83.0 ☑
Eberthella typhosa A01.00
Echinococcus — *see* Echinococcus
echovirus
  as cause of disease classified elsewhere B97.12
  unspecified nature or site B34.1
endocardium I33.0
endocervix — *see* Cervicitis
Entamoeba — *see* Amebiasis
enteric — *see* Enteritis, infectious
Enterobacter sakazakii B96.89
Enterobius vermicularis B80
enterostomy K94.12
enterovirus B34.1
  as cause of disease classified elsewhere B97.10
    coxsackievirus B97.11
    echovirus B97.12
    specified NEC B97.19
Entomophthora B46.8
Epidermophyton — *see* Dermatophytosis
epididymis — *see* Epididymitis
episiotomy (puerperal) O86.09
Erysipelothrix (insidiosa) (rhusiopathiae) — *see*
  Erysipeloid
erythema infectiosum B08.3
Escherichia (E.) coli NEC A49.8
  as cause of disease classified elsewhere — *see also*
    Escherichia coli B96.20
  congenital P39.8
    sepsis P36.4
  generalized A41.51
  intestinal — *see* Enteritis, infectious, due to, Es-
    cherichia coli
ethmoidal (chronic) (sinus) — *see* Sinusitis, ethmoidal
eustachian tube (ear) — *see* Salpingitis, eustachian
external auditory canal (meatus) NEC — *see* Otitis, externa, infective
eye (purulent) — *see* Endophthalmitis, purulent
eyelid — *see* Inflammation, eyelid
fallopian tube — *see* Salpingo-oophoritis
Fasciola (gigantica) (hepatica) (indica) B66.3
Fasciolopsis (buski) B66.5
filarial — *see* Infestation, filarial
finger (skin) L08.9
  nail L03.01- ☑
    fungus B35.1
fish tapeworm B70.0
  larval B70.1
flagellate, intestinal A07.9
fluke — *see* Infestation, fluke
focal
  teeth (pulpal origin) K04.7
  tonsils J35.01
Fonsecaea (compactum) (pedrosoi) B43.0
food — *see* Intoxication, foodborne
foot (skin) L08.9
  dermatophytic fungus B35.3

Infection, infected, infective — *continued*
Francisella tularensis — *see* Tularemia
frontal (sinus) (chronic) — *see* Sinusitis, frontal
fungus NOS B49
  beard B35.0
  dermatophytic — *see* Dermatophytosis
  foot B35.3
  groin B35.6
  hand B35.2
  nail B35.1
  pathogenic to compromised host only B48.8
  perianal (area) B35.6
  scalp B35.0
  skin B36.9
    foot B35.3
    hand B35.2
    toenails B35.1
Fusarium B48.8
gallbladder — *see* Cholecystitis
gas bacillus — *see* Gangrene, gas
gastrointestinal — *see* Enteritis, infectious
generalized NEC — *see* Sepsis
generator pocket, implanted electronic neurostimulator
  T85.734 ☑
genital organ or tract
  female — *see* Disease, pelvis, inflammatory
  male N49.9
    multiple sites N49.8
    specified NEC N49.8
Ghon tubercle, primary A15.7
Giardia lamblia A07.1
gingiva (chronic) K05.10
  acute K05.00
    nonplaque induced K05.01
    plaque induced K05.00
  nonplaque induced K05.11
  plaque induced K05.10
glanders A24.0
glenosporopsis B48.0
Gnathostoma (spinigerum) B83.1
Gongylonema B83.8
gonococcal — *see* Gonococcus
gram-negative bacilli NOS A49.9
guinea worm B72
gum (chronic) K05.10
  acute K05.00
    nonplaque induced K05.01
    plaque induced K05.00
  nonplaque induced K05.11
  plaque induced K05.10
Haemophilus — *see* Infection, Hemophilus
heart — *see* Carditis
Helicobacter pylori A04.8
  as cause of disease classified elsewhere B96.81
helminths B83.9
  intestinal B82.0
    mixed (types classifiable to more than one of the
      titles B65.0-B81.3 and B81.8) B81.4
    specified type NEC B81.8
  specified type NEC B83.8
Hemophilus
  aegyptius, systemic A48.4
  ducrey (any location) A57
  generalized A41.3
  influenzae NEC A49.2
    as cause of disease classified elsewhere B96.3
herpes (simplex) — *see also* Herpes
  congenital P35.2
  disseminated B00.7
  zoster B02.9
herpesvirus, herpesviral — *see* Herpes
Heterophyes (heterophyes) B66.8
hip (joint) NEC M00.9
  due to internal joint prosthesis
    left T84.52 ☑
    right T84.51 ☑
  skin NEC L08.9
Histoplasma — *see* Histoplasmosis
  American B39.4
  capsulatum B39.4
hookworm B76.9
human
  papilloma virus A63.0
  T-cell lymphotropic virus type-1 (HTLV-1) B33.3
hydrocele N43.0
Hymenolepis B71.0
hypopharynx — *see* Pharyngitis
inguinal (lymph) glands L04.1

☑ **Additional Character Required** — Refer to the Tabular List for Character Selection   Subterms under main terms may continue to next column or page

Infection, infected, infective — *continued*
  inguinal glands — *continued*
    due to soft chancre A57
  intervertebral disc, pyogenic M46.30
    cervical region M46.32
    cervicothoracic region M46.33
    lumbar region M46.36
    lumbosacral region M46.37
    multiple sites M46.39
    occipito-atlanto-axial region M46.31
    sacrococcygeal region M46.38
    thoracic region M46.34
    thoracolumbar region M46.35
  intestine, intestinal — *see* Enteritis, infectious
    specified NEC A08.8
  intra-amniotic affecting newborn NEC P39.2
  Isospora belli or hominis A07.3
  Japanese B encephalitis A83.0
  jaw (bone) (lower) (upper) M27.2
  joint NEC M00.9
    due to internal joint prosthesis T84.50 ☑
  kidney (cortex) (hematogenous) N15.9
    with calculus N20.0
      with hydronephrosis N13.6
    following ectopic gestation O08.83
    pelvis and ureter (cystic) N28.85
    puerperal (postpartum) O86.21
    specified NEC N15.8
  Klebsiella (K.) pneumoniae NEC A49.8
    as cause of disease classified elsewhere B96.1
  knee (joint) NEC M00.9
    joint M00.9
    due to internal joint prosthesis
      left T84.54 ☑
      right T84.53 ☑
    skin L08.9
  Koch's — *see* Tuberculosis
  labia (majora) (minora) (acute) — *see* Vulvitis
  lacrimal
    gland — *see* Dacryoadenitis
    passages (duct) (sac) — *see* Inflammation, lacrimal, passages
  lancet fluke B66.2
  larynx NEC J38.7
  leg (skin) NOS L08.9
  Legionella pneumophila A48.1
    nonpneumonic A48.2
  Leishmania — *see also* Leishmaniasis
    aethiopica B55.1
    braziliensis B55.2
    chagasi B55.0
    donovani B55.0
    infantum B55.0
    major B55.1
    mexicana B55.1
    tropica B55.1
  lentivirus, as cause of disease classified elsewhere B97.31
  Leptosphaeria senegalensis B47.0
  Leptospira interrogans A27.9
    autumnalis A27.89
    canicola A27.89
    hebdomadis A27.89
    icterohaemorrhagiae A27.0
    pomona A27.89
    specified type NEC A27.89
  leptospirochetal NEC — *see* Leptospirosis
  Listeria monocytogenes — *see also* Listeriosis
    congenital P37.2
  Loa loa B74.3
    with conjunctival infestation B74.3
    eyelid B74.3
  Loboa loboi B48.0
  local, skin (staphylococcal) (streptococcal) L08.9
    abscess — *code by* site under Abscess
    cellulitis — *code by* site under Cellulitis
    specified NEC L08.89
    ulcer — *see* Ulcer, skin
  Loefflerella mallei A24.0
  lung — *see also* Pneumonia J18.9
    atypical Mycobacterium A31.0
    spirochetal A69.8
    tuberculous — *see* Tuberculosis, pulmonary
    virus — *see* Pneumonia, viral
  lymph gland — *see also* Lymphadenitis, acute
    mesenteric I88.0
  lymphoid tissue, base of tongue or posterior pharynx, NEC (chronic) J35.03

Infection, infected, infective — *continued*
  Madurella (grisea) (mycetomii) B47.0
  major
    following ectopic or molar pregnancy O08.0
    puerperal, postpartum, childbirth O85
  Malassezia furfur B36.0
  Malleomyces
    mallei A24.0
    pseudomallei (whitmori) — *see* Melioidosis
  mammary gland N61.0
  Mansonella (ozzardi) (perstans) (streptocerca) B74.4
  mastoid — *see* Mastoiditis
  maxilla, maxillary M27.2
    sinus (chronic) — *see* Sinusitis, maxillary
  mediastinum J98.51
  Medina (worm) B72
  meibomian cyst or gland — *see* Hordeolum
  meninges — *see* Meningitis, bacterial
  meningococcal — *see also* condition A39.9
    adrenals A39.1
    brain A39.81
    cerebrospinal A39.0
    conjunctiva A39.89
    endocardium A39.51
    heart A39.50
      endocardium A39.51
      myocardium A39.52
      pericardium A39.53
    joint A39.83
    meninges A39.0
    meningococcemia A39.4
      acute A39.2
      chronic A39.3
    myocardium A39.52
    pericardium A39.53
    retrobulbar neuritis A39.82
    specified site NEC A39.89
  mesenteric lymph nodes or glands NEC I88.0
  Metagonimus B66.8
  metatarsophalangeal M00.9
  methicillin
    resistant Staphylococcus aureus (MRSA) A49.02
    susceptible Staphylococcus aureus (MSSA) A49.01
  Microsporum, microsporic — *see* Dermatophytosis
  mixed flora (bacterial) NEC A49.8
  Monilia — *see* Candidiasis
  Monosporium apiospermum B48.2
  mouth, parasitic B37.0
  Mucor — *see* Mucormycosis
  muscle NEC — *see* Myositis, infective
  mycelium NOS B49
  mycetoma B47.9
    actinomycotic NEC B47.1
    mycotic NEC B47.0
  Mycobacterium, mycobacterial — *see* Mycobacterium
  Mycoplasma NEC A49.3
    pneumoniae, as cause of disease classified elsewhere B96.0
  mycotic NOS B49
    pathogenic to compromised host only B48.8
    skin NOS B36.9
  myocardium NEC I40.0
  nail (chronic)
    with lymphangitis — *see* Lymphangitis, acute, digit
    finger L03.01- ☑
      fungus B35.1
    ingrowing L60.0
    toe L03.03- ☑
      fungus B35.1
  nasal sinus (chronic) — *see* Sinusitis
  nasopharynx — *see* Nasopharyngitis
  navel L08.82
  Necator americanus B76.1
  Neisseria — *see* Gonococcus
  Neotestudina rosatii B47.0
  newborn P39.9
    intra-amniotic NEC P39.2
    skin P39.4
    specified type NEC P39.8
  nipple N61.0
    associated with
      lactation O91.03
      pregnancy O91.01- ☑
      puerperium O91.02
  Nocardia — *see* Nocardiosis
  obstetrical surgical wound (puerperal) O86.00
    incisional site
      deep O86.02

Infection, infected, infective — *continued*
  obstetrical surgical wound — *continued*
    incisional site — *continued*
      superficial O86.01
    organ and space site O86.03
    surgical site specified NEC O86.09
  Oesophagostomum (apiostomum) B81.8
  Oestrus ovis — *see* Myiasis
  Oidium albicans B37.9
  Onchocerca (volvulus) — *see* Onchocerciasis
  oncovirus, as cause of disease classified elsewhere B97.32
  operation wound T81.49 ☑
  Opisthorchis (felineus) (viverrini) B66.0
  orbit, orbital — *see* Inflammation, orbit
  orthopoxvirus NEC B08.09
  ovary — *see* Salpingo-oophoritis
  Oxyuris vermicularis B80
  pancreas (acute) — *see* Pancreatitis, acute
    abscess — *see* Pancreatitis, acute
    specified NEC — *see also* Pancreatitis, acute K85.80
  papillomavirus, as cause of disease classified elsewhere B97.7
  papovavirus NEC B34.4
  Paracoccidioides brasiliensis — *see* Paracoccidioidomycosis
  Paragonimus (westermani) B66.4
  parainfluenza virus B34.8
  parameningococcus NOS A39.9
  parapoxvirus B08.60
    specified NEC B08.69
  parasitic B89
  Parastrongylus
    cantonensis B83.2
    costaricensis B81.3
    paratyphoid A01.4
      Type A A01.1
      Type B A01.2
      Type C A01.3
  paraurethral ducts N34.2
  parotid gland — *see* Sialoadenitis
  parvovirus NEC B34.3
    as cause of disease classified elsewhere B97.6
  Pasteurella NEC A28.0
    multocida A28.0
    pestis — *see* Plague
    pseudotuberculosis A28.0
    septica (cat bite) (dog bite) A28.0
    tularensis — *see* Tularemia
  pelvic, female — *see* Disease, pelvis, inflammatory
  Penicillium (marneffei) B48.4
  penis (glans) (retention) NEC N48.29
  periapical K04.5
  peridental, periodontal K05.20
    generalized — *see* Periodontitis, aggressive, generalized
    localized — *see* Periodontitis, aggressive, localized
  perinatal period P39.9
    specified type NEC P39.8
  perineal repair (puerperal) O86.09
  periorbital — *see* Inflammation, orbit
  perirectal K62.89
  perirenal — *see* Infection, kidney
  peritoneal — *see* Peritonitis
  periureteral N28.89
  Petriellidium boydii B48.2
  pharynx — *see also* Pharyngitis
    coxsackievirus B08.5
    posterior, lymphoid (chronic) J35.03
  Phialophora
    gougerotii (subcutaneous abscess or cyst) B43.2
    jeanselmei (subcutaneous abscess or cyst) B43.2
    verrucosa (skin) B43.0
  Piedraia hortae B36.3
  pinta A67.9
    intermediate A67.1
    late A67.2
    mixed A67.3
    primary A67.0
  pinworm B80
  pityrosporum furfur B36.0
  pleuro-pneumonia-like organism (PPLO) NEC A49.3
    as cause of disease classified elsewhere B96.0
  pneumococcus, pneumococcal NEC A49.1
    as cause of disease classified elsewhere B95.3
    generalized (purulent) A40.3
      with pneumonia J13
  Pneumocystis carinii (pneumonia) B59

Infection, infected, infective — *continued*
Pneumocystis jiroveci (pneumonia) B59
port or reservoir T80.212 ☑
postoperative T81.40 ☑
postoperative wound T81.49 ☑
surgical site
deep incisional T81.42 ☑
organ and space T81.43 ☑
specified NEC T81.49 ☑
superficial incisional T81.41 ☑
postprocedural T81.40 ☑
postvaccinal T88.0 ☑
prepuce NEC N47.7
with penile inflammation N47.6
prion — *see* Disease, prion, central nervous system
prostate (capsule) — *see* Prostatitis
Proteus (mirabilis) (morganii) (vulgaris) NEC A49.8
as cause of disease classified elsewhere B96.4
protozoal NEC B64
intestinal A07.9
specified NEC A07.8
specified NEC B60.8
Pseudoallescheria boydii B48.2
Pseudomonas NEC A49.8
as cause of disease classified elsewhere B96.5
mallei A24.0
pneumonia J15.1
pseudomallei — *see* Melioidosis
puerperal O86.4
genitourinary tract NEC O86.89
major or generalized O85
minor O86.4
specified NEC O86.89
pulmonary — *see* Infection, lung
purulent — *see* Abscess
Pyrenochaeta romeroi B47.0
Q fever A78
rectum (sphincter) K62.89
renal — *see also* Infection, kidney
pelvis and ureter (cystic) N28.85
reovirus, as cause of disease classified elsewhere B97.5
respiratory (tract) NEC J98.8
acute J22
chronic J98.8
influenzal (upper) (acute) — *see* Influenza, with, respiratory manifestations NEC
lower (acute) J22
chronic — *see* Bronchitis, chronic
rhinovirus J00
syncytial virus (RSV) — *see* Infection, virus, respiratory syncytial (RSV)
upper (acute) NOS J06.9
chronic J39.8
streptococcal J06.9
viral NOS J06.9
due to respiratory syncytial virus (RSV) J06.9 [B97.4]
resulting from
presence of internal prosthesis, implant, graft — *see* Complications, by site and type, infection
retortamoniasis A07.8
retroperitoneal NEC K68.9
retrovirus B33.3
as cause of disease classified elsewhere B97.30
human
immunodeficiency, type 2 (HIV 2) B97.35
T-cell lymphotropic
type I (HTLV-I) B97.33
type II (HTLV-II) B97.34
lentivirus B97.31
oncovirus B97.32
specified NEC B97.39
Rhinosporidium (seeberi) B48.1
rhinovirus
as cause of disease classified elsewhere B97.89
unspecified nature or site B34.8
Rhizopus — *see* Mucormycosis
rickettsial NOS A79.9
roundworm (large) NEC B82.0
Ascariasis — *see also* Ascariasis B77.9
rubella — *see* Rubella
Saccharomyces — *see* Candidiasis
salivary duct or gland (any) — *see* Sialoadenitis
Salmonella (aertrycke) (arizonae) (callinarum) (choleraesuis) (enteritidis) (suipestifer) (typhimurium) A02.9
with
(gastro)enteritis A02.0

Infection, infected, infective — *continued*
Salmonella — *continued*
with — *continued*
sepsis A02.1
specified manifestation NEC A02.8
due to food (poisoning) A02.9
hirschfeldii A01.3
localized A02.20
arthritis A02.23
meningitis A02.21
osteomyelitis A02.24
pneumonia A02.22
pyelonephritis A02.25
specified NEC A02.29
paratyphi A01.4
A A01.1
B A01.2
C A01.3
schottmuelleri A01.2
typhi, typhosa — *see* Typhoid
Sarcocystis A07.8
scabies B86
Schistosoma — *see* Infestation, Schistosoma
scrotum (acute) NEC N49.2
seminal vesicle — *see* Vesiculitis
septic
localized, skin — *see* Abscess
sheep liver fluke B66.3
Shigella A03.9
boydii A03.2
dysenteriae A03.0
flexneri A03.1
group
A A03.0
B A03.1
C A03.2
D A03.3
Schmitz (-Stutzer) A03.0
schmitzii A03.0
shigae A03.0
sonnei A03.3
specified NEC A03.8
shoulder (joint) NEC M00.9
due to internal joint prosthesis T84.59 ☑
skin NEC L08.9
sinus (accessory) (chronic) (nasal) — *see also* Sinusitis
pilonidal — *see* Sinus, pilonidal
skin NEC L08.89
Skene's duct or gland — *see* Urethritis
skin (local) (staphylococcal) (streptococcal) L08.9
abscess — *code by* site under Abscess
cellulitis — *code by* site under Cellulitis
due to fungus B36.9
specified type NEC B36.8
mycotic B36.9
specified type NEC B36.8
newborn P39.4
ulcer — *see* Ulcer, skin
slow virus A81.9
specified NEC A81.89
Sparganum (mansoni) (proliferum) (baxteri) B70.1
specific — *see also* Syphilis
to perinatal period — *see* Infection, congenital
specified NEC B99.8
spermatic cord NEC N49.1
sphenoidal (sinus) — *see* Sinusitis, sphenoidal
spinal cord NOS — *see also* Myelitis G04.91
abscess G06.1
meninges — *see* Meningitis
streptococcal G04.89
Spirillum A25.1
spirochetal NOS A69.9
lung A69.8
specified NEC A69.8
Spirometra larvae B70.1
spleen D73.89
Sporotrichum, Sporothrix (schenckii) — *see* Sporotrichosis
staphylococcal, unspecified site
as cause of disease classified elsewhere B95.8
aureus (methicillin susceptible) (MSSA) B95.61
methicillin resistant (MRSA) B95.62
specified NEC B95.7
aureus (methicillin susceptible) (MSSA) A49.01
methicillin resistant (MRSA) A49.02
food poisoning A05.0
generalized (purulent) A41.2
pneumonia — *see* Pneumonia, staphylococcal

Infection, infected, infective — *continued*
Stellantchasmus falcatus B66.8
streptobacillus moniliformis A25.1
streptococcal NEC A49.1
as cause of disease classified elsewhere B95.5
B genitourinary complicating
childbirth O98.82
pregnancy O98.81- ☑
puerperium O98.83
congenital
sepsis P36.10
group B P36.0
specified NEC P36.19
generalized (purulent) A40.9
Streptomyces B47.1
Strongyloides (stercoralis) — *see* Strongyloidiasis
stump (amputation) (surgical) — *see* Complication, amputation stump, infection
subcutaneous tissue, local L08.9
suipestifer — *see* Infection, salmonella
swimming pool bacillus A31.1
Taenia — *see* Infestation, Taenia
Taeniarhynchus saginatus B68.1
tapeworm — *see* Infestation, tapeworm
tendon (sheath) — *see* Tenosynovitis, infective NEC
Ternidens diminutus B81.8
testis — *see* Orchitis
threadworm B80
throat — *see* Pharyngitis
thyroglossal duct K14.8
toe (skin) L08.9
cellulitis L03.03- ☑
fungus B35.1
nail L03.03- ☑
fungus B35.1
tongue NEC K14.0
parasitic B37.0
tonsil (and adenoid) (faucial) (lingual) (pharyngeal) — *see* Tonsillitis
tooth, teeth K04.7
periapical K04.7
peridental, periodontal K05.20
generalized — *see* Periodontitis, aggressive, generalized
localized — *see* Periodontitis, aggressive, localized
pulp K04.01
irreversible K04.02
reversible K04.01
socket M27.3
TORCH — *see* Infection, congenital
without active infection P00.2
Torula histolytica — *see* Cryptococcosis
Toxocara (canis) (cati) (felis) B83.0
Toxoplasma gondii — *see* Toxoplasma
trachea, chronic J42
trematode NEC — *see* Infestation, fluke
trench fever A79.0
Treponema pallidum — *see* Syphilis
Trichinella (spiralis) B75
Trichomonas A59.9
cervix A59.09
intestine A07.8
prostate A59.02
specified site NEC A59.8
urethra A59.03
urogenitalis A59.00
vagina A59.01
vulva A59.01
Trichophyton, trichophytic — *see* Dermatophytosis
Trichosporon (beigelii) cutaneum B36.2
Trichostrongylus B81.2
Trichuris (trichiura) B79
Trombicula (irritans) B88.0
Trypanosoma
brucei
gambiense B56.0
rhodesiense B56.1
cruzi — *see* Chagas' disease
tubal — *see* Salpingo-oophoritis
tuberculous
latent (LTBI) Z22.7
NEC — *see* Tuberculosis
tubo-ovarian — *see* Salpingo-oophoritis
tunica vaginalis N49.1
tunnel T80.212 ☑
tympanic membrane NEC — *see* Myringitis
typhoid (abortive) (ambulant) (bacillus) — *see* Typho

☑ Additional Character Required — Refer to the Tabular List for Character Selection   Subterms under main terms may continue to next column or pag

Infection, infected, infective — *continued*
  typhus A75.9
    flea-borne A75.2
    mite-borne A75.3
    recrudescent A75.1
    tick-borne A77.9
      African A77.1
      North Asian A77.2
  umbilicus L08.82
  ureter — *see* Ureteritis
  urethra — *see* Urethritis
  urinary (tract) N39.0
    bladder — *see* Cystitis
    complicating
      pregnancy O23.4- ☑
        specified type NEC O23.3- ☑
    kidney — *see* Infection, kidney
    newborn P39.3
    puerperal (postpartum) O86.20
    tuberculous A18.13
    urethra — *see* Urethritis
  uterus, uterine — *see* Endometritis
  vaccination T88.0 ☑
  vaccinia not from vaccination B08.011
  vagina (acute) — *see* Vaginitis
  varicella B01.9
  varicose veins — *see* Varix
  vas deferens NEC N49.1
  vesical — *see* Cystitis
  Vibrio
    cholerae A00.0
      El Tor A00.1
    parahaemolyticus (food poisoning) A05.3
    vulnificus
      as cause of disease classified elsewhere B96.82
      foodborne intoxication A05.5
  Vincent's (gum) (mouth) (tonsil) A69.1
  virus, viral NOS B34.9
    adenovirus
      as cause of disease classified elsewhere B97.0
      unspecified nature or site B34.0
    arborvirus, arbovirus arthropod-borne A94
    as cause of disease classified elsewhere B97.89
      adenovirus B97.0
      coronavirus B97.29
        SARS-associated B97.21
      coxsackievirus B97.11
      echovirus B97.12
      enterovirus B97.10
        coxsackievirus B97.11
        echovirus B97.12
        specified NEC B97.19
      human
        immunodeficiency, type 2 (HIV 2) B97.35
        metapneumovirus B97.81
        T-cell lymphotropic,
          type I (HTLV-I) B97.33
          type II (HTLV-II) B97.34
      papillomavirus B97.7
      parvovirus B97.6
      reovirus B97.5
      respiratory syncytial (RSV) — *see* Infection, virus,
        respiratory syncytial (RSV)
      retrovirus B97.30
        human
          immunodeficiency, type 2 (HIV 2) B97.35
          T-cell lymphotropic,
            type I (HTLV-I) B97.33
            type II (HTLV-II) B97.34
        lentivirus B97.31
        oncovirus B97.32
        specified NEC B97.39
      specified NEC B97.89
    central nervous system A89
      atypical A81.9
        specified NEC A81.89
      enterovirus NEC A88.8
        meningitis A87.0
      slow virus A81.9
        specified NEC A81.89
      specified NEC A88.8
    chest J98.8
    cotia B08.8
    coxsackie — *see also* Infection, coxsackie B34.1
      as cause of disease classified elsewhere B97.11
    ECHO
      as cause of disease classified elsewhere B97.12
      unspecified nature or site B34.1

Infection, infected, infective — *continued*
  virus, viral — *continued*
    encephalitis, tick-borne A84.9
    enterovirus, as cause of disease classified elsewhere
      B97.10
      coxsackievirus B97.11
      echovirus B97.12
      specified NEC B97.19
    exanthem NOS B09
    human metapneumovirus as cause of disease clas-
      sified elsewhere B97.81
    human papilloma as cause of disease classified
      elsewhere B97.7
    intestine — *see* Enteritis, viral
    respiratory syncytial (RSV)
      as cause of disease classified elsewhere B97.4
      bronchiolitis J21.0
      bronchitis J20.5
      bronchopneumonia J12.1
      otitis media H65- ☑ *[B97.4]*
      pneumonia J12.1
      upper respiratory infection J06.9 *[B97.4]*
    rhinovirus
      as cause of disease classified elsewhere B97.89
      unspecified nature or site B34.8
    slow A81.9
      specified NEC A81.89
    specified type NEC B33.8
      as cause of disease classified elsewhere B97.89
      unspecified nature or site B34.8
    unspecified nature or site B34.9
    West Nile — *see* Virus, West Nile
  vulva (acute) — *see* Vulvitis
  West Nile — *see* Virus, West Nile
  whipworm B79
  worms B83.9
    specified type NEC B83.8
  Wuchereria (bancrofti) B74.0
    malayi B74.1
  yatapoxvirus B08.70
    specified NEC B08.79
  yeast — *see also* Candidiasis B37.9
  yellow fever — *see* Fever, yellow
  Yersinia
    enterocolitica (intestinal) A04.6
    pestis — *see* Plague
    pseudotuberculosis A28.2
  Zeis' gland — *see* Hordeolum
  Zika virus A92.5
    congenital P35.4
  zoonotic bacterial NOS A28.9
  Zopfia senegalensis B47.0
Infective, infectious — *see* condition
Infertility
  female N97.9
    age-related N97.8
    associated with
      anovulation N97.0
      cervical (mucus) disease or anomaly N88.3
      congenital anomaly
        cervix N88.3
        fallopian tube N97.1
        uterus N97.2
        vagina N97.8
      dysmucorrhea N88.3
      fallopian tube disease or anomaly N97.1
      pituitary-hypothalamic origin E23.0
      specified origin NEC N97.8
      Stein-Leventhal syndrome E28.2
      uterine disease or anomaly N97.2
      vaginal disease or anomaly N97.8
    due to
      cervical anomaly N88.3
      fallopian tube anomaly N97.1
      ovarian failure E28.39
      Stein-Leventhal syndrome E28.2
      uterine anomaly N97.2
      vaginal anomaly N97.8
    nonimplantation N97.2
    origin
      cervical N88.3
      tubal (block) (occlusion) (stenosis) N97.1
      uterine N97.2
      vaginal N97.8
  male N46.9
    azoospermia N46.01
      extratesticular cause N46.029
        drug therapy N46.021

Infertility — *continued*
  male — *continued*
    azoospermia — *continued*
      extratesticular cause — *continued*
        efferent duct obstruction N46.023
        infection N46.022
        radiation N46.024
        specified cause NEC N46.029
        systemic disease N46.025
    oligospermia N46.11
      extratesticular cause N46.129
        drug therapy N46.121
        efferent duct obstruction N46.123
        infection N46.122
        radiation N46.124
        specified cause NEC N46.129
        systemic disease N46.125
    specified type NEC N46.8
Infestation B88.9
  Acanthocheilonema (perstans) (streptocerca) B74.4
  Acariasis B88.0
    demodex folliculorum B88.0
    sarcoptes scabiei B86
    trombiculae B88.0
  Agamofilaria streptocerca B74.4
  Ancylostoma, ankylostoma (braziliense) (caninum)
    (ceylanicum) (duodenale) B76.0
    americanum B76.1
    new world B76.1
  Anisakis larvae, anisakiasis B81.0
  arthropod NEC B88.2
  Ascaris lumbricoides — *see* Ascariasis
  Balantidium coli A07.0
  beef tapeworm B68.1
  Bothriocephalus (latus) B70.0
    larval B70.1
  broad tapeworm B70.0
    larval B70.1
  Brugia (malayi) B74.1
    timori B74.2
  candiru B88.8
  Capillaria
    hepatica B83.8
    philippinensis B81.1
  cat liver fluke B66.0
  cestodes B71.9
    diphyllobothrium — *see* Infestation, diphyllobothe-
      rium
    dipylidiasis B71.1
    hymenolepiasis B71.0
    specified type NEC B71.8
  chigger B88.0
  chigo, chigoe B88.1
  Clonorchis (sinensis) (liver) B66.1
  coccidial A07.3
  crab-lice B85.3
  Cysticercus cellulosae — *see* Cysticercosis
  Demodex (folliculorum) B88.0
  Dermanyssus gallinae B88.0
  Dermatobia (hominis) — *see* Myiasis
  Dibothriocephalus (latus) B70.0
    larval B70.1
  Dicrocoelium dendriticum B66.2
  Diphyllobothrium (adult) (latum) (intestinal) (pacificum)
    B70.0
    larval B70.1
  Diplogonoporus (grandis) B71.8
  Dipylidium caninum B67.4
  Distoma hepaticum B66.3
  dog tapeworm B67.4
  Dracunculus medinensis B72
  dragon worm B72
  dwarf tapeworm B71.0
  Echinococcus — *see* Echinococcus
  Echinostomum ilocanum B66.8
  Entamoeba (histolytica) — *see* Infection, Ameba
  Enterobius vermicularis B80
  eyelid
    in (due to)
      leishmaniasis B55.1
      loiasis B74.3
      onchocerciasis B73.09
      phthiriasis B85.3
    parasitic NOS B89
  eyeworm B74.3
  Fasciola (gigantica) (hepatica) (indica) B66.3
  Fasciolopsis (buski) (intestine) B66.5
  filarial B74.9

Infestation — *continued*
filarial — *continued*
  bancroftian B74.0
  conjunctiva B74.9
  due to
    Acanthocheilonema (perstans) (streptocerca)
        B74.4
    Brugia (malayi) B74.1
      timori B74.2
    Dracunculus medinensis B72
    guinea worm B72
    loa loa B74.3
    Mansonella (ozzardi) (perstans) (streptocerca)
        B74.4
    Onchocerca volvulus B73.00
      eye B73.00
      eyelid B73.09
    Wuchereria (bancrofti) B74.0
  Malayan B74.1
  ozzardi B74.4
  specified type NEC B74.8
fish tapeworm B70.0
  larval B70.1
fluke B66.9
  blood NOS — *see* Schistosomiasis
  cat liver B66.0
  intestinal B66.5
  lancet B66.2
  liver (sheep) B66.3
    cat B66.0
    Chinese B66.1
    due to clonorchiasis B66.1
    oriental B66.1
  lung (oriental) B66.4
  sheep liver B66.3
  specified type NEC B66.8
fly larvae — *see* Myiasis
Gasterophilus (intestinalis) — *see* Myiasis
Gastrodiscoides hominis B66.8
Giardia lamblia A07.1
Gnathostoma (spinigerum) B83.1
Gongylonema B83.8
guinea worm B72
helminth B83.9
  angiostrongyliasis B83.2
    intestinal B81.3
  gnathostomiasis B83.1
  hirudiniasis, internal B83.4
  intestinal B82.0
    angiostrongyliasis B81.3
    anisakiasis B81.0
    ascariasis — *see* Ascariasis
    capillariasis B81.1
    cysticercosis — *see* Cysticercosis
    diphyllobothriasis — *see* Infestation, diphyl-
        lobothriasis
    dracunculiasis B72
    echinococcus — *see* Echinococcosis
    enterobiasis B80
    filariasis — *see* Infestation, filarial
    fluke — *see* Infestation, fluke
    hookworm — *see* Infestation, hookworm
    mixed (types classifiable to more than one of the
        titles B65.0-B81.3 and B81.8) B81.4
    onchocerciasis — *see* Onchocerciasis
    schistosomiasis — *see* Infestation, schistosoma
    specified
      cestode NEC — *see* Infestation, cestode
        type NEC B81.8
      strongyloidiasis — *see* Strongyloidiasis
      taenia — *see* Infestation, taenia
      trichinellosis B75
      trichostrongyliasis B81.2
      trichuriasis B79
  specified type NEC B83.8
  syngamiasis B83.3
  visceral larva migrans B83.0
Heterophyes (heterophyes) B66.8
hookworm B76.9
  ancylostomiasis B76.0
  necatoriasis B76.1
  specified type NEC B76.8
Hymenolepis (diminuta) (nana) B71.0
intestinal NEC B82.9
leeches (aquatic) (land) — *see* Hirudiniasis
Leishmania — *see* Leishmaniasis
lice, louse — *see* Infestation, Pediculus
Linguatula B88.8

Infestation — *continued*
Liponyssoides sanguineus B88.0
Loa loa B74.3
  conjunctival B74.3
  eyelid B74.3
louse — *see* Infestation, Pediculus
maggots — *see* Myiasis
Mansonella (ozzardi) (perstans) (streptocerca) B74.4
Medina (worm) B72
Metagonimus (yokogawai) B66.8
microfilaria streptocerca — *see* Onchocerciasis
  eye B73.00
  eyelid B73.09
mites B88.9
  scabic B86
Monilia (albicans) — *see* Candidiasis
mouth B37.0
Necator americanus B76.1
nematode NEC (intestinal) B82.0
  Ancylostoma B76.0
  conjunctiva NEC B83.9
  Enterobius vermicularis B80
  Gnathostoma spinigerum B83.1
  physaloptera B80
  specified NEC B81.8
  trichostrongylus B81.2
  trichuris (trichuria) B79
Oesophagostomum (apiostomum) B81.8
Oestrus ovis — *see also* Myiasis B87.9
Onchocerca (volvulus) — *see* Onchocerciasis
Opisthorchis (felineus) (viverrini) B66.0
orbit, parasitic NOS B89
Oxyuris vermicularis B80
Paragonimus (westermani) B66.4
parasite, parasitic B89
  eyelid B89
  intestinal NOS B82.9
  mouth B37.0
  skin B88.9
  tongue B37.0
Parastrongylus
  cantonensis B83.2
  costaricensis B81.3
Pediculus B85.2
  body B85.1
  capitis (humanus) (any site) B85.0
  corporis (humanus) (any site) B85.1
  head B85.0
  mixed (classifiable to more than one of the titles
      B85.0 - B85.3) B85.4
  pubis (any site) B85.3
Pentastoma B88.8
Phthirus (pubis) (any site) B85.3
  with any infestation classifiable to B85.0 - B85.2
      B85.4
pinworm B80
pork tapeworm (adult) B68.0
protozoal NEC B64
  intestinal A07.9
    specified NEC A07.8
  specified NEC B60.8
pubic, louse B85.3
rat tapeworm B71.0
red bug B88.0
roundworm (large) NEC B82.0
  Ascariasis — *see also* Ascariasis B77.9
sandflea B88.1
Sarcoptes scabiei B86
scabies B86
Schistosoma B65.9
  bovis B65.8
  cercariae B65.3
  haematobium B65.0
  intercalatum B65.8
  japonicum B65.2
  mansoni B65.1
  mattheei B65.8
  mekongi B65.8
  specified type NEC B65.8
  spindale B65.8
screw worms — *see* Myiasis
skin NOS B88.9
Sparganum (mansoni) (proliferum) (baxteri) B70.1
  larval B70.1
specified type NEC B88.8
Spirometra larvae B70.1
Stellantchasmus falcatus B66.8
Strongyloides stercoralis — *see* Strongyloidiasis

Infestation — *continued*
Taenia B68.9
  diminuta B71.0
  echinococcus — *see* Echinococcus
  mediocanellata B68.1
  nana B71.0
  saginata B68.1
  solium (intestinal form) B68.0
    larval form — *see* Cysticercosis
Taeniarhynchus saginatus B68.1
tapeworm B71.9
  beef B68.1
  broad B70.0
    larval B70.1
  dog B67.4
  dwarf B71.0
  fish B70.0
    larval B70.1
  pork B68.0
  rat B71.0
Ternidens diminutus B81.8
Tetranychus molestissimus B88.0
threadworm B80
tongue B37.0
Toxocara (canis) (cati) (felis) B83.0
trematode(s) NEC — *see* Infestation, fluke
Trichinella (spiralis) B75
Trichocephalus B79
Trichomonas — *see* Trichomoniasis
Trichostrongylus B81.2
Trichuris (trichiura) B79
Trombicula (irritans) B88.0
Tunga penetrans B88.1
Uncinaria americana B76.1
Vandellia cirrhosa B88.8
whipworm B79
worms B83.9
  intestinal B82.0
Wuchereria (bancrofti) B74.0

Infiltrate, infiltration
amyloid (generalized) (localized) — *see* Amyloidosis
calcareous NEC R89.7
  localized — *see* Degeneration, by site
calcium salt R89.7
cardiac
  fatty — *see* Degeneration, myocardial
  glycogenic E74.02 *[I43]*
corneal — *see* Edema, cornea
eyelid — *see* Inflammation, eyelid
glycogen, glycogenic — *see* Disease, glycogen storage
heart, cardiac
  fatty — *see* Degeneration, myocardial
  glycogenic E74.02 *[I43]*
inflammatory in vitreous H43.89
kidney N28.89
leukemic — *see* Leukemia
liver K76.89
  fatty — *see* Fatty, liver NEC
  glycogen — *see also* Disease, glycogen storage
      E74.03 *[K77]*
lung R91.8
  eosinophilic J82
lymphatic — *see also* Leukemia, lymphatic C91.9-
  gland I88.9
muscle, fatty M62.89
myocardium, myocardial
  fatty — *see* Degeneration, myocardial
  glycogenic E74.02 *[I43]*
on chest x-ray R91.8
pulmonary R91.8
  with eosinophilia J82
skin (lymphocytic) L98.6
thymus (gland) (fatty) E32.8
urine R39.0
vesicant agent
  antineoplastic chemotherapy T80.810 ☑
  other agent NEC T80.818 ☑
vitreous body H43.89

Infirmity R68.89
senile R54

Inflammation, inflamed, inflammatory (with exuda-
tion)
abducent (nerve) — *see* Strabismus, paralytic, sixth
    nerve
accessory sinus (chronic) — *see* Sinusitis
adrenal (gland) E27.8
alveoli, teeth M27.3
  scorbutic E54

☑ **Additional Character Required** — Refer to the Tabular List for Character Selection   ▽ **Subterms under main terms may continue to next column or pa**

Inflammation, inflamed, inflammatory —
continued
- anal canal, anus K62.89
- antrum (chronic) — *see* Sinusitis, maxillary
- appendix — *see* Appendicitis
- arachnoid — *see* Meningitis
- areola N61.0
  - puerperal, postpartum or gestational — *see* Infection, nipple
- areolar tissue NOS L08.9
- artery — *see* Arteritis
- auditory meatus (external) — *see* Otitis, externa
- Bartholin's gland N75.8
- bile duct (common) (hepatic) or passage — *see* Cholangitis
- bladder — *see* Cystitis
- bone — *see* Osteomyelitis
- brain — *see also* Encephalitis
  - membrane — *see* Meningitis
- breast N61.0
  - puerperal, postpartum, gestational — *see* Mastitis, obstetric
- broad ligament — *see* Disease, pelvis, inflammatory
- bronchi — *see* Bronchitis
- catarrhal J00
- cecum — *see* Appendicitis
- cerebral — *see also* Encephalitis
  - membrane — *see* Meningitis
- cerebrospinal
  - meningococcal A39.0
- cervix (uteri) — *see* Cervicitis
- chest J98.8
- chorioretinal H30.9- ☑
  - cyclitis — *see* Cyclitis
  - disseminated H30.10- ☑
    - generalized H30.13- ☑
    - peripheral H30.12- ☑
    - posterior pole H30.11- ☑
  - epitheliopathy — *see* Epitheliopathy
  - focal H30.00- ☑
    - juxtapapillary H30.01- ☑
    - macular H30.04- ☑
    - paramacular — *see* Inflammation, chorioretinal, focal, macular
    - peripheral H30.03- ☑
    - posterior pole H30.02- ☑
  - specified type NEC H30.89- ☑
- choroid — *see* Inflammation, chorioretinal
- chronic, postmastoidectomy cavity — *see* Complications, postmastoidectomy, inflammation
- colon — *see* Enteritis
- connective tissue (diffuse) NEC — *see* Disorder, soft tissue, specified type NEC
- cornea — *see* Keratitis
- corpora cavernosa N48.29
- cranial nerve — *see* Disorder, nerve, cranial
- Douglas' cul-de-sac or pouch (chronic) N73.0
- due to device, implant or graft — *see also* Complications, by site and type, infection or inflammation
  - arterial graft T82.7 ☑
  - breast (implant) T85.79 ☑
  - catheter T85.79 ☑
    - dialysis (renal) T82.7 ☑
      - intraperitoneal T85.71 ☑
    - infusion T82.7 ☑
      - cranial T85.735 ☑
      - intrathecal T85.735 ☑
      - spinal (epidural) (subdural) T85.735 ☑
      - subarachnoid T85.735 ☑
    - urinary T83.518 ☑
      - cystostomy T83.510 ☑
      - Hopkins T83.518 ☑
      - ileostomy T83.518 ☑
      - nephrostomy T83.512 ☑
      - specified NEC T83.518 ☑
      - urethral indwelling T83.511 ☑
      - urostomy T83.518 ☑
  - electronic (electrode) (pulse generator) (stimulator)
    - bone T84.7 ☑
    - cardiac T82.7 ☑
    - nervous system T85.738 ☑
      - brain T85.731 ☑
      - cranial nerve T85.732 ☑
      - gastric nerve T85.732 ☑
      - neurostimulator generator T85.734 ☑
      - peripheral nerve T85.732 ☑

Inflammation, inflamed, inflammatory —
continued
- due to device, implant or graft — *see also* Complications, by site and type, infection or inflammation
  — *continued*
  - electronic — *continued*
    - nervous system — *continued*
      - sacral nerve T85.732 ☑
      - spinal cord T85.733 ☑
      - vagal nerve T85.732 ☑
    - urinary T83.590 ☑
  - fixation, internal (orthopedic) NEC — *see* Complication, fixation device, infection
  - gastrointestinal (bile duct) (esophagus) T85.79 ☑
    - neurostimulator electrode (lead) T85.732 ☑
  - genital NEC T83.69 ☑
  - heart NEC T82.7 ☑
    - valve (prosthesis) T82.6 ☑
      - graft T82.7 ☑
  - joint prosthesis — *see* Complication, joint prosthesis, infection
  - ocular (corneal graft) (orbital implant) NEC T85.79 ☑
  - orthopedic NEC T84.7 ☑
  - penile (cylinder) (pump) (resevoir) T83.61 ☑
  - specified NEC T85.79 ☑
  - testicular T83.62 ☑
  - urinary NEC T83.598 ☑
    - ileal conduit stent T83.593 ☑
    - implanted neurostimulation T83.590 ☑
    - implanted sphincter T83.591 ☑
    - indwelling ureteral stent T83.592 ☑
    - nephroureteral stent T83.593 ☑
    - specified stent NEC T83.593 ☑
  - vascular NEC T82.7 ☑
  - ventricular intracranial (communicating) shunt T85.730 ☑
- duodenum K29.80
  - with bleeding K29.81
- dura mater — *see* Meningitis
- ear (middle) — *see also* Otitis, media
  - external — *see* Otitis, externa
  - inner — *see* subcategory H83.0 ☑
- epididymis — *see* Epididymitis
- esophagus K20.9
- ethmoidal (sinus) (chronic) — *see* Sinusitis, ethmoidal
- eustachian tube (catarrhal) — *see* Salpingitis, eustachian
- eyelid H01.9
  - abscess — *see* Abscess, eyelid
  - blepharitis — *see* Blepharitis
  - chalazion — *see* Chalazion
  - dermatosis (noninfectious) — *see* Dermatosis, eyelid
  - hordeolum — *see* Hordeolum
  - specified NEC H01.8
- fallopian tube — *see* Salpingo-oophoritis
- fascia — *see* Myositis
- follicular, pharynx J31.2
- frontal (sinus) (chronic) — *see* Sinusitis, frontal
- gallbladder — *see* Cholecystitis
- gastric — *see* Gastritis
- gastrointestinal — *see* Enteritis
- genital organ (internal) (diffuse)
  - female — *see* Disease, pelvis, inflammatory
  - male N49.9
    - multiple sites N49.8
    - specified NEC N49.8
- gland (lymph) — *see* Lymphadenitis
- glottis — *see* Laryngitis
- granular, pharynx J31.2
- gum K05.10
  - nonplaque induced K05.11
  - plaque induced K05.10
- heart — *see* Carditis
- hepatic duct — *see* Cholangitis
- ileoanal (internal) pouch K91.850
- ileum — *see also* Enteritis
  - regional or terminal — *see* Enteritis, regional
- intestinal pouch K91.850
- intestine (any part) — *see* Enteritis
- jaw (acute) (bone) (chronic) (lower) (suppurative) (upper) M27.2
- joint NEC — *see* Arthritis
  - sacroiliac M46.1
- kidney — *see* Nephritis
- knee (joint) M13.169
  - tuberculous A18.02
- labium (majus) (minus) — *see* Vulvitis

Inflammation, inflamed, inflammatory —
continued
- lacrimal
  - gland — *see* Dacryoadenitis
  - passages (duct) (sac) — *see also* Dacryocystitis
    - canaliculitis — *see* Canaliculitis, lacrimal
- larynx — *see* Laryngitis
- leg NOS L08.9
- lip K13.0
- liver (capsule) — *see also* Hepatitis
  - chronic K73.9
  - suppurative K75.0
- lung (acute) — *see also* Pneumonia
  - chronic J98.4
- lymph gland or node — *see* Lymphadenitis
- lymphatic vessel — *see* Lymphangitis
- maxilla, maxillary M27.2
  - sinus (chronic) — *see* Sinusitis, maxillary
- membranes of brain or spinal cord — *see* Meningitis
- meninges — *see* Meningitis
- mouth K12.1
- muscle — *see* Myositis
- myocardium — *see* Myocarditis
- nasal sinus (chronic) — *see* Sinusitis
- nasopharynx — *see* Nasopharyngitis
- navel L08.82
- nerve NEC — *see* Neuralgia
- nipple N61.0
  - puerperal, postpartum or gestational — *see* Infection, nipple
- nose — *see* Rhinitis
- oculomotor (nerve) — *see* Strabismus, paralytic, third nerve
- optic nerve — *see* Neuritis, optic
- orbit (chronic) H05.10
  - acute H05.00
    - abscess — *see* Abscess, orbit
    - cellulitis — *see* Cellulitis, orbit
    - osteomyelitis — *see* Osteomyelitis, orbit
    - periostitis — *see* Periostitis, orbital
    - tenonitis — *see* Tenonitis, eye
    - granuloma — *see* Granuloma, orbit
    - myositis — *see* Myositis, orbital
- ovary — *see* Salpingo-oophoritis
- oviduct — *see* Salpingo-oophoritis
- pancreas (acute) — *see* Pancreatitis
- parametrium N73.0
- parotid region L08.9
- pelvis, female — *see* Disease, pelvis, inflammatory
- penis (corpora cavernosa) N48.29
- perianal K62.89
- pericardium — *see* Pericarditis
- perineum (female) (male) L08.9
- perirectal K62.89
- peritoneum — *see* Peritonitis
- periuterine — *see* Disease, pelvis, inflammatory
- perivesical — *see* Cystitis
- petrous bone (acute) (chronic) — *see* Petrositis
- pharynx (acute) — *see* Pharyngitis
- pia mater — *see* Meningitis
- pleura — *see* Pleurisy
- polyp, colon — *see also* Polyp, colon, inflammatory K51.40
- prostate — *see also* Prostatitis
  - specified type NEC N41.8
- rectosigmoid — *see* Rectosigmoiditis
- rectum — *see also* Proctitis K62.89
- respiratory, upper — *see also* Infection, respiratory, upper J06.9
  - acute, due to radiation J70.0
  - chronic, due to external agent — *see* condition, respiratory, chronic, due to
  - due to
    - chemicals, gases, fumes or vapors (inhalation) J68.2
    - radiation J70.1
- retina — *see* Chorioretinitis
- retrocecal — *see* Appendicitis
- retroperitoneal — *see* Peritonitis
- salivary duct or gland (any) (suppurative) — *see* Sialoadenitis
- scorbutic, alveoli, teeth E54
- scrotum N49.2
- seminal vesicle — *see* Vesiculitis
- sigmoid — *see* Enteritis
- sinus — *see* Sinusitis
- Skene's duct or gland — *see* Urethritis

Inflammation, inflamed, inflammatory — *continued*
 skin L08.9
 spermatic cord N49.1
 sphenoidal (sinus) — *see* Sinusitis, sphenoidal
 spinal
  cord — *see* Encephalitis
  membrane — *see* Meningitis
  nerve — *see* Disorder, nerve
 spine — *see* Spondylopathy, inflammatory
 spleen (capsule) D73.89
 stomach — *see* Gastritis
 subcutaneous tissue L08.9
 suprarenal (gland) E27.8
 synovial — *see* Tenosynovitis
 tendon (sheath) NEC — *see* Tenosynovitis
 testis — *see* Orchitis
 throat (acute) — *see* Pharyngitis
 thymus (gland) E32.8
 thyroid (gland) — *see* Thyroiditis
 tongue K14.0
 tonsil — *see* Tonsillitis
 trachea — *see* Tracheitis
 trochlear (nerve) — *see* Strabismus, paralytic, fourth
   nerve
 tubal — *see* Salpingo-oophoritis
 tuberculous NEC — *see* Tuberculosis
 tubo-ovarian — *see* Salpingo-oophoritis
 tunica vaginalis N49.1
 tympanic membrane — *see* Tympanitis
 umbilicus, umbilical L08.82
 uterine ligament — *see* Disease, pelvis, inflammatory
 uterus (catarrhal) — *see* Endometritis
 uveal tract (anterior) NOS — *see also* Iridocyclitis
  posterior — *see* Chorioretinitis
 vagina — *see* Vaginitis
 vas deferens N49.1
 vein — *see also* Phlebitis
  intracranial or intraspinal (septic) G08
  thrombotic I80.9
   leg — *see* Phlebitis, leg
   lower extremity — *see* Phlebitis, leg
 vocal cord J38.3
 vulva — *see* Vulvitis
 Wharton's duct (suppurative) — *see* Sialoadenitis
Inflation, lung, imperfect (newborn) — *see* Atelectasis
Influenza (bronchial) (epidemic) (respiratory (upper))
   (unidentified influenza virus) J11.1
 with
  digestive manifestations J11.2
  encephalopathy J11.81
  enteritis J11.2
  gastroenteritis J11.2
  gastrointestinal manifestations J11.2
  laryngitis J11.1
  myocarditis J11.82
  otitis media J11.83
  pharyngitis J11.1
  pneumonia J11.00
   specified type J11.08
  respiratory manifestations NEC J11.1
  specified manifestation NEC J11.89
 A/H5N1 — *see also* Influenza, due to, identified novel
    influenza A virus J09.X2
 avian — *see also* Influenza, due to, identified novel in-
    fluenza A virus J09.X2
 bird — *see also* Influenza, due to, identified novel in-
    fluenza A virus J09.X2
 novel (2009) H1N1 influenza — *see also* Influenza, due
    to, identified influenza virus NEC J10.1
 novel influenza A/H1N1 — *see also* Influenza, due to,
    identified influenza virus NEC J10.1
 due to
  avian — *see also* Influenza, due to, identified novel
    influenza A virus J09.X2
  identified influenza virus NEC J10.1
   with
    digestive manifestations J10.2
    encephalopathy J10.81
    enteritis J10.2
    gastroenteritis J10.2
    gastrointestinal manifestations J10.2
    laryngitis J10.1
    myocarditis J10.82
    otitis media J10.83
    pharyngitis J10.1
    pneumonia (unspecified type) J10.00

Influenza — *continued*
 due to — *continued*
  identified influenza virus — *continued*
   with — *continued*
    pneumonia — *continued*
     with same identified influenza virus
      J10.01
     specified type NEC J10.08
    respiratory manifestations NEC J10.1
    specified manifestation NEC J10.89
  identified novel influenza A virus J09.X2
   with
    digestive manifestations J09.X3
    encephalopathy J09.X9
    enteritis J09.X3
    gastroenteritis J09.X3
    gastrointestinal manifestations J09.X3
    laryngitis J09.X2
    myocarditis J09.X9
    otitis media J09.X9
    pharyngitis J09.X2
    pneumonia J09.X1
    respiratory manifestations NEC J09.X2
    specified manifestation NEC J09.X9
    upper respiratory symptoms J09.X2
  of other animal origin, not bird or swine — *see also*
    Influenza, due to, identified novel influenza A
    virus J09.X2
  swine (viruses that normally cause infections in pigs)
    — *see also* Influenza, due to, identified novel
    influenza A virus J09.X2
Influenzal — *see* Influenza
Influenza-like disease — *see* Influenza
Infraction, Freiberg's (metatarsal head) — *see* Osteochondrosis, juvenile, metatarsus
Infraeruption of tooth (teeth) M26.34
Infusion complication, misadventure, or reaction —
   see Complications, infusion
Ingestion
 chemical — *see* Table of Drugs and Chemicals, by
    substance, poisoning
 drug or medicament
  correct substance properly administered — *see* Ta-
    ble of Drugs and Chemicals, by drug, adverse
    effect
  overdose or wrong substance given or taken — *see*
    Table of Drugs and Chemicals, by drug, poi-
    soning
 foreign body — *see* Foreign body, alimentary tract
 multiple drug — *see* Table of Drugs and Chemicals,
    multiple
 tularemia A21.3
Ingrowing
 hair (beard) L73.1
 nail (finger) (toe) L60.0
Inguinal — *see also* condition
 testicle Q53.9
  bilateral Q53.212
  unilateral Q53.112
Inhalant-induced
 anxiety disorder F18.980
 depressive disorder F18.94
 major neurocognitive disorder F18.97
 mild neurocognitive disorder F18.988
 psychotic disorder F18.959
Inhalation
 anthrax A22.1
 flame T27.3 ☑
 food or foreign body — *see* Foreign body, by site
 gases, fumes, or vapors NEC T59.9- ☑
  specified agent — *see* Table of Drugs and Chemicals,
    by substance
 liquid or vomitus — *see* Asphyxia
 meconium (newborn) P24.00
  with
   with respiratory symptoms P24.01
   pneumonia (pneumonitis) P24.01
 mucus — *see* Asphyxia, mucus
 oil or gasoline (causing suffocation) — *see* Foreign
    body, by site
 smoke J70.5
  due to chemicals, gases, fumes and vapors J68.9
 steam — *see* Toxicity, vapors
 stomach contents or secretions — *see* Foreign body,
    by site
  due to anesthesia (general) (local) or other sedation
    T88.59 ☑
   in labor and delivery O74.0

Inhalation — *continued*
 stomach contents or secretions — *see* Foreign body,
    by site — *continued*
  due to anesthesia or other sedation — *continued*
   in pregnancy O29.01- ☑
   postpartum, puerperal O89.01
Inhibition, orgasm
 female F52.31
 male F52.32
Inhibitor, systemic lupus erythematosus (presence
   of) D68.62
Iniencephalus, iniencephaly Q00.2
Injection, traumatic jet (air) (industrial) (water) (paint
   or dye) T70.4 ☑
Injury — *see also* specified injury type T14.90 ☑
 abdomen, abdominal S39.91 ☑
  blood vessel — *see* Injury, blood vessel, abdomen
  cavity — *see* Injury, intra-abdominal
  contusion S30.1 ☑
  internal — *see* Injury, intra-abdominal
  intra-abdominal organ — *see* Injury, intra-abdomi-
    nal
  nerve — *see* Injury, nerve, abdomen
  open — *see* Wound, open, abdomen
  specified NEC S39.81 ☑
  superficial — *see* Injury, superficial, abdomen
 Achilles tendon S86.00- ☑
  laceration S86.02- ☑
  specified type NEC S86.09- ☑
  strain S86.01- ☑
 acoustic, resulting in deafness — *see* Injury, nerve,
    acoustic
 adrenal (gland) S37.819 ☑
  contusion S37.812 ☑
  laceration S37.813 ☑
  specified type NEC S37.818 ☑
 alveolar (process) S09.93 ☑
 ankle S99.91- ☑
  contusion — *see* Contusion, ankle
  dislocation — *see* Dislocation, ankle
  fracture — *see* Fracture, ankle
  nerve — *see* Injury, nerve, ankle
  open — *see* Wound, open, ankle
  specified type NEC S99.81- ☑
  sprain — *see* Sprain, ankle
  superficial — *see* Injury, superficial, ankle
 anterior chamber, eye — *see* Injury, eye, specified site
    NEC
 anus — *see* Injury, abdomen
 aorta (thoracic) S25.00 ☑
  abdominal S35.00 ☑
   laceration (minor) (superficial) S35.01 ☑
    major S35.02 ☑
   specified type NEC S35.09 ☑
  laceration (minor) (superficial) S25.01 ☑
   major S25.02 ☑
  specified type NEC S25.09 ☑
 arm (upper) S49.9- ☑
  blood vessel — *see* Injury, blood vessel, arm
  contusion — *see* Contusion, arm, upper
  fracture — *see* Fracture, humerus
  lower — *see* Injury, forearm
  muscle — *see* Injury, muscle, shoulder
  nerve — *see* Injury, nerve, arm
  open — *see* Wound, open, arm
  specified type NEC S49.8- ☑
  superficial — *see* Injury, superficial, arm
 artery (complicating trauma) — *see also* Injury, blood
    vessel, by site
  cerebral or meningeal — *see* Injury, intracranial
 auditory canal (external) (meatus) S09.91 ☑
 auricle, auris, ear S09.91 ☑
 axilla — *see* Injury, shoulder
 back — *see* Injury, back, lower
 bile duct S36.13 ☑
 birth — *see also* Birth, injury P15.9
 bladder (sphincter) S37.20 ☑
  at delivery O71.5
  contusion S37.22 ☑
  laceration S37.23 ☑
  obstetrical trauma O71.5
  specified type NEC S37.29 ☑
 blast (air) (hydraulic) (immersion) (underwater) NEC
    T14.8 ☑
  acoustic nerve trauma — *see* Injury, nerve, acous-
  bladder — *see* Injury, bladder

Injury — continued
  blast — continued
    brain — see Concussion
    colon — see Injury, intestine, large
    ear (primary) S09.31- ☑
      secondary S09.39- ☑
    generalized T70.8 ☑
    lung — see Injury, intrathoracic, lung
    multiple body organs T70.8 ☑
    peritoneum S36.81 ☑
    rectum S36.61 ☑
    retroperitoneum S36.898 ☑
    small intestine S36.419 ☑
      duodenum S36.410 ☑
      specified site NEC S36.418 ☑
    specified
      intra-abdominal organ NEC S36.898 ☑
      pelvic organ NEC S37.899 ☑
  blood vessel NEC T14.8 ☑
    abdomen S35.9 ☑
      aorta — see Injury, aorta, abdominal
      celiac artery — see Injury, blood vessel, celiac artery
      iliac vessel — see Injury, blood vessel, iliac
      laceration S35.91 ☑
      mesenteric vessel — see Injury, mesenteric
      portal vein — see Injury, blood vessel, portal vein
      renal vessel — see Injury, blood vessel, renal
      specified vessel NEC S35.8X- ☑
      splenic vessel — see Injury, blood vessel, splenic
      vena cava — see Injury, vena cava, inferior
    ankle — see Injury, blood vessel, foot
    aorta (abdominal) (thoracic) — see Injury, aorta
    arm (upper) NEC S45.90- ☑
      forearm — see Injury, blood vessel, forearm
      laceration S45.91- ☑
      specified
        site NEC S45.80- ☑
          laceration S45.81- ☑
          specified type NEC S45.89- ☑
        type NEC S45.99- ☑
      superficial vein S45.30- ☑
        laceration S45.31- ☑
        specified type NEC S45.39- ☑
    axillary
      artery S45.00- ☑
        laceration S45.01- ☑
        specified type NEC S45.09- ☑
      vein S45.20- ☑
        laceration S45.21- ☑
        specified type NEC S45.29- ☑
    azygos vein — see Injury, blood vessel, thoracic, specified site NEC
    brachial
      artery S45.10- ☑
        laceration S45.11- ☑
        specified type NEC S45.19- ☑
      vein S45.20- ☑
        laceration S45.219 ☑
        specified type NEC S45.29- ☑
    carotid artery (common) (external) (internal, extracranial) S15.00- ☑
      internal, intracranial S06.8- ☑
      laceration (minor) (superficial) S15.01- ☑
        major S15.02- ☑
      specified type NEC S15.09- ☑
    celiac artery S35.219 ☑
      branch S35.299 ☑
        laceration (minor) (superficial) S35.291 ☑
          major S35.292 ☑
        specified NEC S35.298 ☑
      laceration (minor) (superficial) S35.211 ☑
        major S35.212 ☑
      specified type NEC S35.218 ☑
    cerebral — see Injury, intracranial
    deep plantar — see Injury, blood vessel, plantar artery
    digital (hand) — see Injury, blood vessel, finger
    dorsal
      artery (foot) S95.00- ☑
        laceration S95.01- ☑
        specified type NEC S95.09- ☑
      vein (foot) S95.20- ☑
        laceration S95.21- ☑
        specified type NEC S95.29- ☑

Injury — continued
  blood vessel — continued
    due to accidental laceration during procedure — see Laceration, accidental complicating surgery
    extremity — see Injury, blood vessel, limb
    femoral
      artery (common) (superficial) S75.00- ☑
        laceration (minor) (superficial) S75.01- ☑
          major S75.02- ☑
        specified type NEC S75.09- ☑
      vein (hip level) (thigh level) S75.10- ☑
        laceration (minor) (superficial) S75.11- ☑
          major S75.12- ☑
        specified type NEC S75.19- ☑
    finger S65.50- ☑
      index S65.50- ☑
        laceration S65.51- ☑
        specified type NEC S65.59- ☑
      laceration S65.51- ☑
      little S65.50- ☑
        laceration S65.51- ☑
        specified type NEC S65.59- ☑
      middle S65.50- ☑
        laceration S65.51- ☑
        specified type NEC S65.59- ☑
      specified type NEC S65.59- ☑
      thumb — see Injury, blood vessel, thumb
    foot S95.90- ☑
      dorsal
        artery — see Injury, blood vessel, dorsal, artery
        vein — see Injury, blood vessel, dorsal, vein
      laceration S95.91- ☑
      plantar artery — see Injury, blood vessel, plantar artery
      specified
        site NEC S95.80- ☑
          laceration S95.81- ☑
          specified type NEC S95.89- ☑
        specified type NEC S95.99- ☑
    forearm S55.90- ☑
      laceration S55.91- ☑
      radial artery — see Injury, blood vessel, radial artery
      specified
        site NEC S55.80- ☑
          laceration S55.81- ☑
          specified type NEC S55.89- ☑
        type NEC S55.99- ☑
      ulnar artery — see Injury, blood vessel, ulnar artery
      vein S55.20- ☑
        laceration S55.21- ☑
        specified type NEC S55.29- ☑
    gastric
      artery — see Injury, mesenteric, artery, branch
      vein — see Injury, blood vessel, abdomen
    gastroduodenal artery — see Injury, mesenteric, artery, branch
    greater saphenous vein (lower leg level) S85.30- ☑
      hip (and thigh) level S75.20- ☑
        laceration (minor) (superficial) S75.21- ☑
          major S75.22- ☑
        specified type NEC S75.29- ☑
      laceration S85.31- ☑
      specified type NEC S85.39- ☑
    hand (level) S65.90- ☑
      finger — see Injury, blood vessel, finger
      laceration S65.91- ☑
      palmar arch — see Injury, blood vessel, palmar arch
      radial artery — see Injury, blood vessel, radial artery, hand
      specified
        site NEC S65.80- ☑
          laceration S65.81- ☑
          specified type NEC S65.89- ☑
        type NEC S65.99- ☑
      thumb — see Injury, blood vessel, thumb
      ulnar artery — see Injury, blood vessel, ulnar artery, hand
    head S09.0 ☑
      intracranial — see Injury, intracranial
      multiple S09.0 ☑

Injury — continued
  blood vessel — continued
    hepatic
      artery — see Injury, mesenteric, artery
      vein — see Injury, vena cava, inferior
    hip S75.90- ☑
      femoral artery — see Injury, blood vessel, femoral, artery
      femoral vein — see Injury, blood vessel, femoral, vein
      greater saphenous vein — see Injury, blood vessel, greater saphenous, hip level
      laceration S75.91- ☑
      specified
        site NEC S75.80- ☑
          laceration S75.81- ☑
          specified type NEC S75.89- ☑
        type NEC S75.99- ☑
    hypogastric (artery) (vein) — see Injury, blood vessel, iliac
    iliac S35.5- ☑
      artery S35.51- ☑
      specified vessel NEC S35.5- ☑
      uterine vessel — see Injury, blood vessel, uterine
      vein S35.51- ☑
    innominate — see Injury, blood vessel, thoracic, innominate
    intercostal (artery) (vein) — see Injury, blood vessel, thoracic, intercostal
    jugular vein (external) S15.20- ☑
      internal S15.30- ☑
        laceration (minor) (superficial) S15.31- ☑
          major S15.32- ☑
        specified type NEC S15.39- ☑
      laceration (minor) (superficial) S15.21- ☑
        major S15.22- ☑
      specified type NEC S15.29- ☑
    leg (level) (lower) S85.90- ☑
      greater saphenous — see Injury, blood vessel, greater saphenous
      laceration S85.91- ☑
      lesser saphenous — see Injury, blood vessel, lesser saphenous
      peroneal artery — see Injury, blood vessel, peroneal artery
      popliteal
        artery — see Injury, blood vessel, popliteal, artery
        vein — see Injury, blood vessel, popliteal, vein
      specified
        site NEC S85.80- ☑
          laceration S85.81- ☑
          specified type NEC S85.89- ☑
        type NEC S85.99- ☑
      thigh — see Injury, blood vessel, hip
      tibial artery — see Injury, blood vessel, tibial artery
    lesser saphenous vein (lower leg level) S85.40- ☑
      laceration S85.41- ☑
      specified type NEC S85.49- ☑
    limb
      lower — see Injury, blood vessel, leg
      upper — see Injury, blood vessel, arm
    lower back — see Injury, blood vessel, abdomen
      specified NEC — see Injury, blood vessel, abdomen, specified, site NEC
    mammary (artery) (vein) — see Injury, blood vessel, thoracic, specified site NEC
    mesenteric (inferior) (superior)
      artery — see Injury, mesenteric, artery
      vein — see Injury, blood vessel, mesenteric, vein
    neck S15.9 ☑
      specified site NEC S15.8 ☑
    ovarian (artery) (vein) — see subcategory S35.8 ☑
    palmar arch (superficial) S65.20- ☑
      deep S65.30- ☑
        laceration S65.31- ☑
        specified type NEC S65.39- ☑
      laceration S65.21- ☑
      specified type NEC S65.29- ☑
    pelvis — see Injury, blood vessel, abdomen
      specified NEC — see Injury, blood vessel, abdomen, specified, site NEC
    peroneal artery S85.20- ☑
      laceration S05.21- ☑
      specified type NEC S85.29- ☑

Injury — *continued*
- blood vessel — *continued*
  - plantar artery (deep) (foot) S95.10- ☑
    - laceration S95.11- ☑
    - specified type NEC S95.19- ☑
  - popliteal
    - artery S85.00- ☑
      - laceration S85.01- ☑
      - specified type NEC S85.09- ☑
    - vein S85.50- ☑
      - laceration S85.51- ☑
      - specified type NEC S85.59- ☑
  - portal vein S35.319 ☑
    - laceration S35.311 ☑
    - specified type NEC S35.318 ☑
  - precerebral — *see* Injury, blood vessel, neck
  - pulmonary (artery) (vein) — *see* Injury, blood vessel, thoracic, pulmonary
  - radial artery (forearm level) S55.10- ☑
    - hand and wrist (level) S65.10- ☑
      - laceration S65.11- ☑
      - specified type NEC S65.19- ☑
    - laceration S55.11- ☑
    - specified type NEC S55.19- ☑
  - renal
    - artery S35.40- ☑
      - laceration S35.41- ☑
      - specified NEC S35.49- ☑
    - vein S35.40- ☑
      - laceration S35.41- ☑
      - specified NEC S35.49- ☑
  - saphenous vein (greater) (lower leg level) — *see* Injury, blood vessel, greater saphenous
    - hip and thigh level — *see* Injury, blood vessel, greater saphenous, hip level
    - lesser — *see* Injury, blood vessel, lesser saphenous
  - shoulder
    - specified NEC — *see* Injury, blood vessel, arm, specified site NEC
    - superficial vein — *see* Injury, blood vessel, arm, superficial vein
  - specified NEC T14.8 ☑
  - splenic
    - artery — *see* Injury, blood vessel, celiac artery, branch
    - vein S35.329 ☑
      - laceration S35.321 ☑
      - specified NEC S35.328 ☑
  - subclavian — *see* Injury, blood vessel, thoracic, innominate
  - thigh — *see* Injury, blood vessel, hip
  - thoracic S25.90 ☑
    - aorta S25.00 ☑
      - laceration (minor) (superficial) S25.01 ☑
        - major S25.02 ☑
      - specified type NEC S25.09 ☑
    - azygos vein — *see* Injury, blood vessel, thoracic, specified, site NEC
    - innominate
      - artery S25.10- ☑
        - laceration (minor) (superficial) S25.11- ☑
          - major S25.12- ☑
        - specified type NEC S25.19- ☑
      - vein S25.30- ☑
        - laceration (minor) (superficial) S25.31- ☑
          - major S25.32- ☑
        - specified type NEC S25.39- ☑
    - intercostal S25.50- ☑
      - laceration S25.51- ☑
      - specified type NEC S25.59- ☑
    - laceration S25.91 ☑
    - mammary vessel — *see* Injury, blood vessel, thoracic, specified, site NEC
    - pulmonary S25.40- ☑
      - laceration (minor) (superficial) S25.41- ☑
        - major S25.42- ☑
      - specified type NEC S25.49- ☑
    - specified
      - site NEC S25.80- ☑
        - laceration S25.81 ☑
        - specified type NEC S25.89 ☑
      - type NEC S25.99 ☑
    - subclavian — *see* Injury, blood vessel, thoracic, innominate
    - vena cava (superior) S25.20 ☑

Injury — *continued*
- blood vessel — *continued*
  - thoracic — *continued*
    - vena cava — *continued*
      - laceration (minor) (superficial) S25.21 ☑
        - major S25.22 ☑
      - specified type NEC S25.29 ☑
    - thumb S65.40- ☑
      - laceration S65.41- ☑
      - specified type NEC S65.49- ☑
    - tibial artery S85.10- ☑
      - anterior S85.13- ☑
        - laceration S85.14- ☑
        - specified injury NEC S85.15- ☑
      - laceration S85.11- ☑
      - posterior S85.16- ☑
        - laceration S85.17- ☑
        - specified injury NEC S85.18- ☑
      - specified injury NEC S85.12- ☑
    - ulnar artery (forearm level) S55.00- ☑
      - hand and wrist (level) S65.00- ☑
        - laceration S65.01- ☑
        - specified type NEC S65.09- ☑
      - laceration S55.01- ☑
      - specified type NEC S55.09- ☑
    - upper arm (level) — *see* Injury, blood vessel, arm
      - superficial vein — *see* Injury, blood vessel, arm, superficial vein
    - uterine S35.5- ☑
      - artery S35.53- ☑
      - vein S35.53- ☑
    - vena cava — *see* Injury, vena cava
    - vertebral artery S15.10- ☑
      - laceration (minor) (superficial) S15.11- ☑
        - major S15.12- ☑
      - specified type NEC S15.19- ☑
    - wrist (level) — *see* Injury, blood vessel, hand
  - brachial plexus S14.3 ☑
    - newborn P14.3
  - brain (traumatic) S06.9- ☑
    - diffuse (axonal) S06.2X- ☑
    - focal S06.30- ☑
    - brainstem S06.38- ☑
  - breast NOS S29.9 ☑
  - broad ligament — *see* Injury, pelvic organ, specified site NEC
  - bronchus, bronchi — *see* Injury, intrathoracic, bronchus
  - brow S09.90 ☑
  - buttock S39.92 ☑
  - canthus, eye S05.90 ☑
  - cardiac plexus — *see* Injury, nerve, thorax, sympathetic
  - cauda equina S34.3 ☑
  - cavernous sinus — *see* Injury, intracranial
  - cecum — *see* Injury, colon
  - celiac ganglion or plexus — *see* Injury, nerve, lumbosacral, sympathetic
  - cerebellum — *see* Injury, intracranial
  - cerebral — *see* Injury, intracranial
  - cervix (uteri) — *see* Injury, uterus
  - cheek (wall) S09.93 ☑
  - chest — *see* Injury, thorax
  - childbirth (newborn) — *see also* Birth, injury
    - maternal NEC O71.9
  - chin S09.93 ☑
  - choroid (eye) — *see* Injury, eye, specified site NEC
  - clitoris S39.94 ☑
  - coccyx — *see also* Injury, back, lower
    - complicating delivery O71.6
  - colon — *see* Injury, intestine, large
  - common bile duct — *see* Injury, liver
  - conjunctiva (superficial) — *see* Injury, eye, conjunctiva
  - conus medullaris — *see* Injury, spinal, sacral
  - cord
    - spermatic (pelvic region) S37.898 ☑
      - scrotal region S39.848 ☑
    - spinal — *see* Injury, spinal cord, by region
  - cornea — *see* Injury, eye, specified site NEC
    - abrasion — *see* Injury, eye, cornea, abrasion
  - cortex (cerebral) — *see also* Injury, intracranial
    - visual — *see* Injury, nerve, optic
  - costal region NEC S29.9 ☑
  - costochondral NEC S29.9 ☑
  - cranial
    - cavity — *see* Injury, intracranial
    - nerve — *see* Injury, nerve, cranial
  - crushing — *see* Crush

Injury — *continued*
- cutaneous sensory nerve
- cystic duct — *see* Injury, liver
- deep tissue — *see* Contusion, by site
  - meaning pressure ulcer — *see* Ulcer, pressure, unstageable, by site
- delivery (newborn) P15.9
  - maternal NEC O71.9
- Descemet's membrane — *see* Injury, eyeball, penetrating
- diaphragm — *see* Injury, intrathoracic, diaphragm
- duodenum — *see* Injury, intestine, small, duodenum
- ear (auricle) (external) (canal) S09.91 ☑
  - abrasion — *see* Abrasion, ear
  - bite — *see* Bite, ear
  - blister — *see* Blister, ear
  - bruise — *see* Contusion, ear
  - contusion — *see* Contusion, ear
  - external constriction — *see* Constriction, external, ear
  - hematoma — *see* Hematoma, ear
  - inner — *see* Injury, ear, middle
  - laceration — *see* Laceration, ear
  - middle S09.30- ☑
    - blast — *see* Injury, blast, ear
    - specified NEC S09.39- ☑
  - puncture — *see* Puncture, ear
  - superficial — *see* Injury, superficial, ear
- eighth cranial nerve (acoustic or auditory) — *see* Injury, nerve, acoustic
- elbow S59.90- ☑
  - contusion — *see* Contusion, elbow
  - dislocation — *see* Dislocation, elbow
  - fracture — *see* Fracture, ulna, upper end
  - open — *see* Wound, open, elbow
  - specified NEC S59.80- ☑
  - sprain — *see* Sprain, elbow
  - superficial — *see* Injury, superficial, elbow
- eleventh cranial nerve (accessory) — *see* Injury, nerve, accessory
- epididymis S39.94 ☑
- epigastric region S39.91 ☑
- epiglottis NEC S19.89 ☑
- esophageal plexus — *see* Injury, nerve, thorax, sympathetic
- esophagus (thoracic part) — *see also* Injury, intrathoracic, esophagus
  - cervical NEC S19.85 ☑
- eustachian tube S09.30 ☑
- eye S05.9- ☑
  - avulsion S05.7- ☑
  - ball — *see* Injury, eyeball
  - conjunctiva S05.0- ☑
  - cornea
    - abrasion S05.0- ☑
    - laceration S05.3- ☑
      - with prolapse S05.2- ☑
  - lacrimal apparatus S05.8X- ☑
  - orbit penetration S05.4- ☑
  - specified site NEC S05.8X- ☑
- eyeball S05.8X- ☑
  - contusion S05.1- ☑
  - penetrating S05.6- ☑
    - with
      - foreign body S05.5- ☑
      - prolapse or loss of intraocular tissue S05.2-
    - without prolapse or loss of intraocular tissue S05.3- ☑
  - specified type NEC S05.8- ☑
- eyebrow S09.93 ☑
- eyelid S09.93 ☑
  - abrasion — *see* Abrasion, eyelid
  - contusion — *see* Contusion, eyelid
  - open — *see* Wound, open, eyelid
- face S09.93 ☑
- fallopian tube S37.509 ☑
  - bilateral S37.502 ☑
    - blast injury S37.512 ☑
    - contusion S37.522 ☑
    - laceration S37.532 ☑
    - specified type NEC S37.592 ☑
  - blast injury (primary) S37.519 ☑
    - bilateral S37.512 ☑
    - secondary — *see* Injury, fallopian tube, specified type NEC
  - unilateral S37.511 ☑

Injury — *continued*
  fallopian tube — *continued*
    contusion S37.529 ☑
      bilateral S37.522 ☑
      unilateral S37.521 ☑
    laceration S37.539 ☑
      bilateral S37.532 ☑
      unilateral S37.531 ☑
    specified type NEC S37.599 ☑
      bilateral S37.592 ☑
      unilateral S37.591 ☑
    unilateral S37.501 ☑
      blast injury S37.511 ☑
      contusion S37.521 ☑
      laceration S37.531 ☑
      specified type NEC S37.591 ☑
  fascia — *see* Injury, muscle
  fifth cranial nerve (trigeminal) — *see* Injury, nerve, trigeminal
  finger (nail) S69.9- ☑
    blood vessel — *see* Injury, blood vessel, finger
    contusion — *see* Contusion, finger
    dislocation — *see* Dislocation, finger
    fracture — *see* Fracture, finger
    muscle — *see* Injury, muscle, finger
    nerve — *see* Injury, nerve, digital, finger
    open — *see* Wound, open, finger
    specified NEC S69.8- ☑
    sprain — *see* Sprain, finger
    superficial — *see* Injury, superficial, finger
  first cranial nerve (olfactory) — *see* Injury, nerve, olfactory
  flank — *see* Injury, abdomen
  foot S99.92- ☑
    blood vessel — *see* Injury, blood vessel, foot
    contusion — *see* Contusion, foot
    dislocation — *see* Dislocation, foot
    fracture — *see* Fracture, foot
    muscle — *see* Injury, muscle, foot
    open — *see* Wound, open, foot
    specified type NEC S99.82- ☑
    sprain — *see* Sprain, foot
    superficial — *see* Injury, superficial, foot
  forceps NOS P15.9
  forearm S59.91- ☑
    blood vessel — *see* Injury, blood vessel, forearm
    contusion — *see* Contusion, forearm
    fracture — *see* Fracture, forearm
    muscle — *see* Injury, muscle, forearm
    nerve — *see* Injury, nerve, forearm
    open — *see* Wound, open, forearm
    specified NEC S59.81- ☑
    superficial — *see* Injury, superficial, forearm
  forehead S09.90 ☑
  fourth cranial nerve (trochlear) — *see* Injury, nerve, trochlear
  gallbladder S36.129 ☑
    contusion S36.122 ☑
    laceration S36.123 ☑
    specified NEC S36.128 ☑
  ganglion
    celiac, coeliac — *see* Injury, nerve, lumbosacral, sympathetic
    gasserian — *see* Injury, nerve, trigeminal
    stellate — *see* Injury, nerve, thorax, sympathetic
    thoracic sympathetic — *see* Injury, nerve, thorax, sympathetic
  gasserian ganglion — *see* Injury, nerve, trigeminal
  gastric artery — *see* Injury, blood vessel, celiac artery, branch
  gastroduodenal artery — *see* Injury, blood vessel, celiac artery, branch
  gastrointestinal tract — *see* Injury, intra-abdominal
    with open wound into abdominal cavity — *see* Wound, open, with penetration into peritoneal cavity
    colon — *see* Injury, intestine, large
    rectum — *see* Injury, intestine, large, rectum
      with open wound into abdominal cavity S36.61
    small intestine — *see* Injury, intestine, small
    specified site NEC — *see* Injury, intra-abdominal, specified, site NEC
    stomach — *see* Injury, stomach
  genital organ(s)
    external S39.94 ☑

Injury — *continued*
  genital organ(s) — *continued*
    external — *continued*
      specified NEC S39.848 ☑
    internal S37.90 ☑
      fallopian tube — *see* Injury, fallopian tube
      ovary — *see* Injury, ovary
      prostate — *see* Injury, prostate
      seminal vesicle — *see* Injury, pelvis, organ, specified site NEC
      uterus — *see* Injury, uterus
      vas deferens — *see* Injury, pelvis, organ, specified site NEC
    obstetrical trauma O71.9
  gland
    lacrimal laceration — *see* Injury, eye, specified site NEC
    salivary S09.93 ☑
    thyroid NEC S19.84 ☑
  globe (eye) S05.90 ☑
    specified NEC S05.8X- ☑
  groin — *see* Injury, abdomen
  gum S09.90 ☑
  hand S69.9- ☑
    blood vessel — *see* Injury, blood vessel, hand
    contusion — *see* Contusion, hand
    fracture — *see* Fracture, hand
    muscle — *see* Injury, muscle, hand
    nerve — *see* Injury, nerve, hand
    open — *see* Wound, open, hand
    specified NEC S69.8- ☑
    sprain — *see* Sprain, hand
    superficial — *see* Injury, superficial, hand
  head S09.90 ☑
    with loss of consciousness S06.9- ☑
    specified NEC S09.8 ☑
  heart S26.90 ☑
    with hemopericardium S26.00 ☑
      contusion S26.01 ☑
      laceration (mild) S26.020 ☑
        major S26.022 ☑
        moderate S26.021 ☑
      specified type NEC S26.09 ☑
    contusion S26.91 ☑
    laceration S26.92 ☑
    specified type NEC S26.99 ☑
    without hemopericardium S26.10 ☑
      contusion S26.11 ☑
      laceration S26.12 ☑
      specified type NEC S26.19 ☑
  heel — *see* Injury, foot
  hepatic
    artery — *see* Injury, blood vessel, celiac artery, branch
    duct — *see* Injury, liver
    vein — *see* Injury, vena cava, inferior
  hip S79.91- ☑
    blood vessel — *see* Injury, blood vessel, hip
    contusion — *see* Contusion, hip
    dislocation — *see* Dislocation, hip
    fracture — *see* Fracture, femur, neck
    muscle — *see* Injury, muscle, hip
    nerve — *see* Injury, nerve, hip
    open — *see* Wound, open, hip
    specified NEC S79.81- ☑
    sprain — *see* Sprain, hip
    superficial — *see* Injury, superficial, hip
  hymen S39.94 ☑
  hypogastric
    blood vessel — *see* Injury, blood vessel, iliac
    plexus — *see* Injury, nerve, lumbosacral, sympathetic
  ileum — *see* Injury, intestine, small
  iliac region S39.91 ☑
  instrumental (during surgery) — *see* Laceration, accidental complicating surgery
    birth injury — *see* Birth, injury
    nonsurgical — *see* Injury, by site
    obstetrical O71.9
      bladder O71.5
      cervix O71.3
      high vaginal O71.4
      perineal NOS O70.9
      urethra O71.5
      uterus O71.5
        with rupture or perforation O71.1

Injury — *continued*
  internal T14.8 ☑
    aorta — *see* Injury, aorta
    bladder (sphincter) — *see* Injury, bladder
      with
        ectopic or molar pregnancy O08.6
        following ectopic or molar pregnancy O08.6
        obstetrical trauma O71.5
    bronchus, bronchi — *see* Injury, intrathoracic, bronchus
    cecum — *see* Injury, intestine, large
    cervix (uteri) — *see also* Injury, uterus
      with ectopic or molar pregnancy O08.6
      following ectopic or molar pregnancy O08.6
      obstetrical trauma O71.3
    chest — *see* Injury, intrathoracic
    gastrointestinal tract — *see* Injury, intra-abdominal
    heart — *see* Injury, heart
    intestine NEC — *see* Injury, intestine
    intrauterine — *see* Injury, uterus
    mesentery — *see* Injury, intra-abdominal, specified, site NEC
    pelvis, pelvic (organ) S37.90 ☑
      following ectopic or molar pregnancy (subsequent episode) O08.6
      obstetrical trauma NEC O71.5
        rupture or perforation O71.1
      specified NEC S39.83 ☑
    rectum — *see* Injury, intestine, large, rectum
    stomach — *see* Injury, stomach
    ureter — *see* Injury, ureter
    urethra (sphincter) following ectopic or molar pregnancy O08.6
    uterus — *see* Injury, uterus
  interscapular area — *see* Injury, thorax
  intestine
    large S36.509 ☑
      ascending (right) S36.500 ☑
        blast injury (primary) S36.510 ☑
          secondary S36.590 ☑
        contusion S36.520 ☑
        laceration S36.530 ☑
        specified type NEC S36.590 ☑
      blast injury (primary) S36.519 ☑
        ascending (right) S36.510 ☑
        descending (left) S36.512 ☑
        rectum S36.61 ☑
        sigmoid S36.513 ☑
        specified site NEC S36.518 ☑
        transverse S36.511 ☑
      contusion S36.529 ☑
        ascending (right) S36.520 ☑
        descending (left) S36.522 ☑
        rectum S36.62 ☑
        sigmoid S36.523 ☑
        specified site NEC S36.528 ☑
        transverse S36.521 ☑
      descending (left) S36.502 ☑
        blast injury (primary) S36.512 ☑
          secondary S36.592 ☑
        contusion S36.522 ☑
        laceration S36.532 ☑
        specified type NEC S36.592 ☑
      laceration S36.539 ☑
        ascending (right) S36.530 ☑
        descending (left) S36.532 ☑
        rectum S36.63 ☑
        sigmoid S36.533 ☑
        specified site NEC S36.538 ☑
        transverse S36.531 ☑
      rectum S36.60 ☑
        blast injury (primary) S36.61 ☑
          secondary S36.69 ☑
        contusion S36.62 ☑
        laceration S36.63 ☑
        specified type NEC S36.69 ☑
      sigmoid S36.503 ☑
        blast injury (primary) S36.513 ☑
          secondary S36.593 ☑
        contusion S36.523 ☑
        laceration S36.533 ☑
        specified type NEC S36.593 ☑
      specified
        site NEC S36.508 ☑
          blast injury (primary) S36.518 ☑
            secondary S36.598 ☑

☑ Subterms under main terms may continue to next column or page   ☑ Additional Character Required — Refer to the Tabular List for Character Selection   193

Injury — Injury

Injury — *continued*
  intestine — *continued*
    large — *continued*
      specified — *continued*
        site — *continued*
          contusion S36.528 ☑
          laceration S36.538 ☑
          specified type NEC S36.598 ☑
        type NEC S36.599 ☑
          ascending (right) S36.590 ☑
          descending (left) S36.592 ☑
          rectum S36.69 ☑
          sigmoid S36.593 ☑
          specified site NEC S36.598 ☑
          transverse S36.591 ☑
      transverse S36.501 ☑
        blast injury (primary) S36.511 ☑
          secondary S36.591 ☑
        contusion S36.521 ☑
        laceration S36.531 ☑
        specified type NEC S36.591 ☑
    small S36.409 ☑
      blast injury (primary) S36.419 ☑
        duodenum S36.410 ☑
        secondary S36.499 ☑
          duodenum S36.490 ☑
          specified site NEC S36.498 ☑
        specified site NEC S36.418 ☑
      contusion S36.429 ☑
        duodenum S36.420 ☑
        specified site NEC S36.428 ☑
      duodenum S36.400 ☑
        blast injury (primary) S36.410 ☑
          secondary S36.490 ☑
        contusion S36.420 ☑
        laceration S36.430 ☑
        specified NEC S36.490 ☑
      laceration S36.439 ☑
        duodenum S36.430 ☑
        specified site NEC S36.438 ☑
      specified
        site NEC S36.408 ☑
        type NEC S36.499 ☑
          duodenum S36.490 ☑
          specified site NEC S36.498 ☑
  intra-abdominal S36.90 ☑
    adrenal gland — *see* Injury, adrenal gland
    bladder — *see* Injury, bladder
    colon — *see* Injury, intestine, large
    contusion S36.92 ☑
    fallopian tube — *see* Injury, fallopian tube
    gallbladder — *see* Injury, gallbladder
    intestine — *see* Injury, intestine
    kidney — *see* Injury, kidney
    laceration S36.93 ☑
    liver — *see* Injury, liver
    ovary — *see* Injury, ovary
    pancreas — *see* Injury, pancreas
    pelvic NOS S37.90 ☑
    peritoneum — *see* Injury, intra-abdominal, specified, site NEC
    prostate — *see* Injury, prostate
    rectum — *see* Injury, intestine, large, rectum
    retroperitoneum — *see* Injury, intra-abdominal, specified, site NEC
    seminal vesicle — *see* Injury, pelvis, organ, specified site NEC
    small intestine — *see* Injury, intestine, small
    specified
      pelvic S37.90 ☑
        specified
          site NEC S37.899 ☑
            specified type NEC S37.898 ☑
          type NEC S37.99 ☑
      site NEC S36.899 ☑
        contusion S36.892 ☑
        laceration S36.893 ☑
        specified type NEC S36.898 ☑
      type NEC S36.99 ☑
    spleen — *see* Injury, spleen
    stomach — *see* Injury, stomach
    ureter — *see* Injury, ureter
    urethra — *see* Injury, urethra
    uterus — *see* Injury, uterus
    vas deferens — *see* Injury, pelvis, organ, specified site NEC

Injury — *continued*
  intracranial (traumatic) S06.9- ☑
    cerebellar hemorrhage, traumatic — *see* Injury, intracranial, focal
    cerebral edema, traumatic S06.1X- ☑
      diffuse S06.1X- ☑
      focal S06.1X- ☑
    diffuse (axonal) S06.2X- ☑
    epidural hemorrhage (traumatic) S06.4X- ☑
    focal brain injury S06.30- ☑
      contusion — *see* Contusion, cerebral
      laceration — *see* Laceration, cerebral
    intracerebral hemorrhage, traumatic S06.36- ☑
      left side S06.35- ☑
      right side S06.34- ☑
    subarachnoid hemorrhage, traumatic S06.6X- ☑
    subdural hemorrhage, traumatic S06.5X- ☑
  intraocular — *see* Injury, eyeball, penetrating
  intrathoracic S27.9 ☑
    bronchus S27.409 ☑
      bilateral S27.402 ☑
      blast injury (primary) S27.419 ☑
        bilateral S27.412 ☑
        secondary — *see* Injury, intrathoracic, bronchus, specified type NEC
        unilateral S27.411 ☑
      contusion S27.429 ☑
        bilateral S27.422 ☑
        unilateral S27.421 ☑
      laceration S27.439 ☑
        bilateral S27.432 ☑
        unilateral S27.431 ☑
      specified type NEC S27.499 ☑
        bilateral S27.492 ☑
        unilateral S27.491 ☑
      unilateral S27.401 ☑
    diaphragm S27.809 ☑
      contusion S27.802 ☑
      laceration S27.803 ☑
      specified type NEC S27.808 ☑
    esophagus (thoracic) S27.819 ☑
      contusion S27.812 ☑
      laceration S27.813 ☑
      specified type NEC S27.818 ☑
    heart — *see* Injury, heart
    hemopneumothorax S27.2 ☑
    hemothorax S27.1 ☑
    lung S27.309 ☑
      aspiration J69.0
      bilateral S27.302 ☑
      blast injury (primary) S27.319 ☑
        bilateral S27.312 ☑
        secondary — *see* Injury, intrathoracic, lung, specified type NEC
        unilateral S27.311 ☑
      contusion S27.329 ☑
        bilateral S27.322 ☑
        unilateral S27.321 ☑
      laceration S27.339 ☑
        bilateral S27.332 ☑
        unilateral S27.331 ☑
      specified type NEC S27.399 ☑
        bilateral S27.392 ☑
        unilateral S27.391 ☑
      unilateral S27.301 ☑
    pleura S27.60 ☑
      laceration S27.63 ☑
      specified type NEC S27.69 ☑
    pneumothorax S27.0 ☑
    specified organ NEC S27.899 ☑
      contusion S27.892 ☑
      laceration S27.893 ☑
      specified type NEC S27.898 ☑
    thoracic duct — *see* Injury, intrathoracic, specified organ NEC
    thymus gland — *see* Injury, intrathoracic, specified organ NEC
    trachea, thoracic S27.50 ☑
      blast (primary) S27.51 ☑
      contusion S27.52 ☑
      laceration S27.53 ☑
      specified type NEC S27.59 ☑
  iris — *see* Injury, eye, specified site NEC
    penetrating — *see* Injury, eyeball, penetrating
  jaw S09.93 ☑
  jejunum — *see* Injury, intestine, small

Injury — *continued*
  joint NOS T14.8 ☑
    old or residual — *see* Disorder, joint, specified type NEC
  kidney S37.00- ☑
    acute (nontraumatic) N17.9
    contusion — *see* Contusion, kidney
    laceration — *see* Laceration, kidney
    specified NEC S37.09- ☑
  knee S89.9- ☑
    contusion — *see* Contusion, knee
    dislocation — *see* Dislocation, knee
    meniscus (lateral) (medial) — *see* Sprain, knee, specified site NEC
      old injury or tear — *see* Derangement, knee, meniscus, due to old injury
    open — *see* Wound, open, knee
    specified NEC S89.8- ☑
    sprain — *see* Sprain, knee
    superficial — *see* Injury, superficial, knee
  labium (majus) (minus) S39.94 ☑
  labyrinth, ear S09.30- ☑
  lacrimal apparatus, duct, gland, or sac — *see* Injury, eye, specified site NEC
  larynx NEC S19.81 ☑
  leg (lower) S89.9- ☑
    blood vessel — *see* Injury, blood vessel, leg
    contusion — *see* Contusion, leg
    fracture — *see* Fracture, leg
    muscle — *see* Injury, muscle, leg
    nerve — *see* Injury, nerve, leg
    open — *see* Wound, open, leg
    specified NEC S89.8- ☑
    superficial — *see* Injury, superficial, leg
  lens, eye — *see* Injury, eye, specified site NEC
    penetrating — *see* Injury, eyeball, penetrating
  limb NEC T14.8 ☑
  lip S09.93 ☑
  liver S36.119 ☑
    contusion S36.112 ☑
    laceration S36.113 ☑
      major (stellate) S36.116 ☑
      minor S36.114 ☑
      moderate S36.115 ☑
    specified NEC S36.118 ☑
  lower back S39.92 ☑
    specified NEC S39.82 ☑
  lumbar, lumbosacral (region) S39.92 ☑
    plexus — *see* Injury, lumbosacral plexus
  lumbosacral plexus S34.4 ☑
  lung — *see also* Injury, intrathoracic, lung
    aspiration J69.0
    transfusion-related (TRALI) J95.84
  lymphatic thoracic duct — *see* Injury, intrathoracic, specified organ NEC
  malar region S09.93 ☑
  mastoid region S09.90 ☑
  maxilla S09.93 ☑
  mediastinum — *see* Injury, intrathoracic, specified organ NEC
  membrane, brain — *see* Injury, intracranial
  meningeal artery — *see* Injury, intracranial, subdural hemorrhage
  meninges (cerebral) — *see* Injury, intracranial
  mesenteric
    artery
      branch S35.299 ☑
        laceration (minor) (superficial) S35.291 ☑
          major S35.292 ☑
        specified NEC S35.298 ☑
      inferior S35.239 ☑
        laceration (minor) (superficial) S35.231 ☑
          major S35.232 ☑
        specified NEC S35.238 ☑
      superior S35.229 ☑
        laceration (minor) (superficial) S35.221 ☑
          major S35.222 ☑
        specified NEC S35.228 ☑
    plexus (inferior) (superior) — *see* Injury, nerve, lumbosacral, sympathetic
    vein
      inferior S35.349 ☑
        laceration S35.341 ☑
        specified NEC S35.348 ☑
      superior S35.339 ☑
        laceration S35.331 ☑

Injury — *continued*
  mesenteric — *continued*
    vein — *continued*
      superior — *continued*
        specified NEC S35.338 ☑
  mesentery — *see* Injury, intra-abdominal, specified site NEC
  mesosalpinx — *see* Injury, pelvic organ, specified site NEC
  middle ear S09.30- ☑
  midthoracic region NOS S29.9 ☑
  mouth S09.93 ☑
  multiple NOS T07 ☑
  muscle (and fascia) (and tendon)
    abdomen S39.001 ☑
      laceration S39.021 ☑
      specified type NEC S39.091 ☑
      strain S39.011 ☑
    abductor
      thumb, forearm level — *see* Injury, muscle, thumb, abductor
    adductor
      thigh S76.20- ☑
        laceration S76.22- ☑
        specified type NEC S76.29- ☑
        strain S76.21- ☑
    ankle — *see* Injury, muscle, foot
    anterior muscle group, at leg level (lower) S86.20- ☑
      laceration S86.22- ☑
      specified type NEC S86.29- ☑
      strain S86.21- ☑
    arm (upper) — *see* Injury, muscle, shoulder
    biceps (parts NEC) S46.20- ☑
      laceration S46.22- ☑
      long head S46.10- ☑
        laceration S46.12- ☑
        specified type NEC S46.19- ☑
        strain S46.11- ☑
      specified type NEC S46.29- ☑
      strain S46.21- ☑
    extensor
      finger(s) (other than thumb) — *see* Injury, muscle, finger by site, extensor
      forearm level, specified NEC — *see* Injury, muscle, forearm, extensor
      thumb — *see* Injury, muscle, thumb, extensor
      toe (large) (ankle level) (foot level) — *see* Injury, muscle, toe, extensor
    finger
      extensor (forearm level) S56.40- ☑
        hand level S66.309 ☑
          laceration S66.329 ☑
          specified type NEC S66.399 ☑
          strain S66.319 ☑
        laceration S56.429 ☑
        specified type NEC S56.499 ☑
        strain S56.419 ☑
      flexor (forearm level) S56.10- ☑
        hand level S66.109 ☑
          laceration S66.129 ☑
          specified type NEC S66.199 ☑
          strain S66.119 ☑
        laceration S56.129 ☑
        specified type NEC S56.199 ☑
        strain S56.119 ☑
      index
        extensor (forearm level)
          hand level S66.308 ☑
            laceration S66.32- ☑
            specified type NEC S66.39- ☑
            strain S66.31- ☑
          specified type NEC S56.492- ☑
        flexor (forearm level)
          hand level S66.108 ☑
            laceration S66.12- ☑
            specified type NEC S66.19- ☑
            strain S66.11- ☑
          specified type NEC S56.19- ☑
          strain S56.11- ☑
        intrinsic S66.50- ☑
          laceration S66.52- ☑
          specified type NEC S66.59- ☑
          strain S66.51- ☑
      intrinsic S66.509 ☑
        laceration S66.529 ☑
        specified type NEC S66.599 ☑

Injury — *continued*
  muscle — *continued*
    finger — *continued*
      intrinsic — *continued*
        strain S66.519 ☑
      little
        extensor (forearm level)
          hand level S66.30- ☑
            laceration S66.32- ☑
            specified type NEC S66.39- ☑
            strain S66.31- ☑
          laceration S56.42- ☑
          specified type NEC S56.49- ☑
          strain S56.41- ☑
        flexor (forearm level)
          hand level S66.10- ☑
            laceration S66.12- ☑
            specified type NEC S66.19- ☑
            strain S66.11- ☑
          laceration S56.12- ☑
          specified type NEC S56.19- ☑
          strain S56.11- ☑
        intrinsic S66.50- ☑
          laceration S66.52- ☑
          specified type NEC S66.59- ☑
          strain S66.51- ☑
      middle
        extensor (forearm level)
          hand level S66.30- ☑
            laceration S66.32- ☑
            specified type NEC S66.39- ☑
            strain S66.31- ☑
          laceration S56.42- ☑
          specified type NEC S56.49- ☑
          strain S56.41- ☑
        flexor (forearm level)
          hand level S66.10- ☑
            laceration S66.12- ☑
            specified type NEC S66.19- ☑
            strain S66.11- ☑
          laceration S56.12- ☑
          specified type NEC S56.19- ☑
          strain S56.11- ☑
        intrinsic S66.50- ☑
          laceration S66.52- ☑
          specified type NEC S66.59- ☑
          strain S66.51- ☑
      ring
        extensor (forearm level)
          hand level S66.30- ☑
            laceration S66.32- ☑
            specified type NEC S66.39- ☑
            strain S66.31- ☑
          laceration S56.42- ☑
          specified type NEC S56.49- ☑
          strain S56.41- ☑
        flexor (forearm level)
          hand level S66.10- ☑
            laceration S66.12- ☑
            specified type NEC S66.19- ☑
            strain S66.11- ☑
          laceration S56.12- ☑
          specified type NEC S56.19- ☑
          strain S56.11- ☑
        intrinsic S66.50- ☑
          laceration S66.52- ☑
          specified type NEC S66.59- ☑
          strain S66.51- ☑
    flexor
      finger(s) (other than thumb) — *see* Injury, muscle, finger
      forearm level, specified NEC — *see* Injury, muscle, forearm, flexor
      thumb — *see* Injury, muscle, thumb, flexor
      toe (long) (ankle level) (foot level) — *see* Injury, muscle, toe, flexor
    foot S96.90- ☑
      intrinsic S96.20- ☑
        laceration S96.22- ☑
        specified type NEC S96.29- ☑
        strain S96.21- ☑
      laceration S96.92- ☑
      long extensor, toe — *see* Injury, muscle, toe, extensor
      long flexor, toe — *see* Injury, muscle, toe, flexor

Injury — *continued*
  muscle — *continued*
    foot — *continued*
      specified
        site NEC S96.80- ☑
          laceration S96.82- ☑
          specified type NEC S96.89- ☑
          strain S96.81- ☑
        type S96.99- ☑
      strain S96.91- ☑
    forearm (level) S56.90- ☑
      extensor S56.50- ☑
        laceration S56.52- ☑
        specified type NEC S56.59- ☑
        strain S56.51- ☑
      flexor S56.20- ☑
        laceration S56.22- ☑
        specified type NEC S56.29- ☑
        strain S56.21- ☑
      laceration S56.92- ☑
      specified S56.99- ☑
        site NEC S56.80- ☑
          laceration S56.82- ☑
          strain S56.81- ☑
          type NEC S56.89- ☑
      strain S56.91- ☑
    hand (level) S66.90- ☑
      laceration S66.92- ☑
      specified
        site NEC S66.80- ☑
          laceration S66.82- ☑
          specified type NEC S66.89- ☑
          strain S66.81- ☑
        type NEC S66.99- ☑
      strain S66.91- ☑
    head S09.10 ☑
      laceration S09.12 ☑
      specified type NEC S09.19 ☑
      strain S09.11 ☑
    hip NEC S76.00- ☑
      laceration S76.02- ☑
      specified type NEC S76.09- ☑
      strain S76.01- ☑
    intrinsic
      ankle and foot level — *see* Injury, muscle, foot, intrinsic
      finger (other than thumb) — *see* Injury, muscle, finger by site, intrinsic
      foot (level) — *see* Injury, muscle, foot, intrinsic
      thumb — *see* Injury, muscle, thumb, intrinsic
    leg (level) (lower) S86.90- ☑
      Achilles tendon — *see* Injury, Achilles tendon
      anterior muscle group — *see* Injury, muscle, anterior muscle group
      laceration S86.92- ☑
      peroneal muscle group — *see* Injury, muscle, peroneal muscle group
      posterior muscle group — *see* Injury, muscle, posterior muscle group, leg level
      specified
        site NEC S86.80- ☑
          laceration S86.82- ☑
          specified type NEC S86.89- ☑
          strain S86.81- ☑
        type NEC S86.99- ☑
      strain S86.91- ☑
    long
      extensor toe, at ankle and foot level — *see* Injury, muscle, toe, extensor
      flexor, toe, at ankle and foot level — *see* Injury, muscle, toe, flexor
      head, biceps — *see* Injury, muscle, biceps, long head
    lower back S39.002 ☑
      laceration S39.022 ☑
      specified type NEC S39.092 ☑
      strain S39.012 ☑
    neck (level) S16.9 ☑
      laceration S16.2 ☑
      specified type NEC S16.8 ☑
      strain S16.1 ☑
    pelvis S39.003 ☑
      laceration S39.023 ☑
      specified type NEC S39.093 ☑
      strain S39.013 ☑

Injury — continued
  muscle — continued
    peroneal muscle group, at leg level (lower)
      S86.30- ☑
      laceration S86.32- ☑
      specified type NEC S86.39- ☑
      strain S86.31- ☑
    posterior muscle (group)
      leg level (lower) S86.10- ☑
        laceration S86.12- ☑
        specified type NEC S86.19- ☑
        strain S86.11- ☑
      thigh level S76.30- ☑
        laceration S76.32- ☑
        specified type NEC S76.39- ☑
        strain S76.31- ☑
    quadriceps (thigh) S76.10- ☑
      laceration S76.12- ☑
      specified type NEC S76.19- ☑
      strain S76.11- ☑
    shoulder S46.90- ☑
      laceration S46.92- ☑
      rotator cuff — see Injury, rotator cuff
      specified site NEC S46.80- ☑
        laceration S46.82- ☑
        specified type NEC S46.89- ☑
        strain S46.81- ☑
      specified type NEC S46.99- ☑
      strain S46.91- ☑
    thigh NEC (level) S76.90- ☑
      adductor — see Injury, muscle, adductor, thigh
      laceration S76.92- ☑
      posterior muscle (group) — see Injury, muscle,
        posterior muscle, thigh level
      quadriceps — see Injury, muscle, quadriceps
      specified
        site NEC S76.80- ☑
          laceration S76.82- ☑
          specified type NEC S76.89- ☑
          strain S76.81- ☑
        type NEC S76.99- ☑
      strain S76.91- ☑
    thorax (level) S29.009 ☑
      back wall S29.002 ☑
      front wall S29.001 ☑
      laceration S29.029 ☑
        back wall S29.022 ☑
        front wall S29.021 ☑
      specified type NEC S29.099 ☑
        back wall S29.092 ☑
        front wall S29.091 ☑
      strain S29.019 ☑
        back wall S29.012 ☑
        front wall S29.011 ☑
    thumb
      abductor (forearm level) S56.30- ☑
        laceration S56.32- ☑
        specified type NEC S56.39- ☑
        strain S56.31- ☑
      extensor (forearm level) S56.30- ☑
        hand level S66.20- ☑
          laceration S66.22- ☑
          specified type NEC S66.29- ☑
          strain S66.21- ☑
        laceration S56.32- ☑
        specified type NEC S56.39- ☑
        strain S56.31- ☑
      flexor (forearm level) S56.00- ☑
        hand level S66.00- ☑
          laceration S66.02- ☑
          specified type NEC S66.09- ☑
          strain S66.01- ☑
        laceration S56.02- ☑
        specified type NEC S56.09- ☑
        strain S56.01- ☑
        wrist level — see Injury, muscle, thumb, flex-
          or, hand level
      intrinsic S66.40- ☑
        laceration S66.42- ☑
        specified type NEC S66.49- ☑
        strain S66.41- ☑
    toe — see also Injury, muscle, foot
      extensor, long S96.10- ☑
        laceration S96.12- ☑
        specified type NEC S96.19- ☑
        strain S96.11- ☑

Injury — continued
  muscle — continued
    toe — see also Injury, muscle, foot — continued
      flexor, long S96.00- ☑
        laceration S96.02- ☑
        specified type NEC S96.09- ☑
        strain S96.01- ☑
    triceps S46.30- ☑
      laceration S46.32- ☑
      specified type NEC S46.39- ☑
      strain S46.31- ☑
    wrist (and hand) level — see Injury, muscle, hand
  musculocutaneous nerve — see Injury, nerve, muscu-
    locutaneous
  myocardium — see Injury, heart
  nape — see Injury, neck
  nasal (septum) (sinus) S09.92 ☑
  nasopharynx S09.92 ☑
  neck S19.9 ☑
    specified NEC S19.80 ☑
      specified site NEC S19.89 ☑
  nerve NEC T14.8 ☑
    abdomen S34.9 ☑
      peripheral S34.6 ☑
      specified site NEC S34.8 ☑
    abducens S04.4- ☑
      contusion S04.4- ☑
      laceration S04.4- ☑
      specified type NEC S04.4- ☑
    abducent — see Injury, nerve, abducens
    accessory S04.7- ☑
      contusion S04.7- ☑
      laceration S04.7- ☑
      specified type NEC S04.7- ☑
    acoustic S04.6- ☑
      contusion S04.6- ☑
      laceration S04.6- ☑
      specified type NEC S04.6- ☑
    ankle S94.9- ☑
      cutaneous sensory S94.3- ☑
      specified site NEC — see subcategory S94.8 ☑
    anterior crural, femoral — see Injury, nerve, femoral
    arm (upper) S44.9- ☑
      axillary — see Injury, nerve, axillary
      cutaneous — see Injury, nerve, cutaneous, arm
      median — see Injury, nerve, median, upper arm
      musculocutaneous — see Injury, nerve, muscu-
        locutaneous
      radial — see Injury, nerve, radial, upper arm
      specified site NEC — see subcategory S44.8 ☑
      ulnar — see Injury, nerve, ulnar, arm
    auditory — see Injury, nerve, acoustic
    axillary S44.3- ☑
    brachial plexus — see Injury, brachial plexus
    cervical sympathetic S14.5 ☑
    cranial S04.9 ☑
      contusion S04.9 ☑
      eighth (acoustic or auditory) — see Injury, nerve,
        acoustic
      eleventh (accessory) — see Injury, nerve, acces-
        sory
      fifth (trigeminal) — see Injury, nerve, trigeminal
      first (olfactory) — see Injury, nerve, olfactory
      fourth (trochlear) — see Injury, nerve, trochlear
      laceration S04.9 ☑
      ninth (glossopharyngeal) — see Injury, nerve,
        glossopharyngeal
      second (optic) — see Injury, nerve, optic
      seventh (facial) — see Injury, nerve, facial
      sixth (abducent) — see Injury, nerve, abducens
      specified
        nerve NEC S04.89- ☑
          contusion S04.89- ☑
          laceration S04.89- ☑
          specified type NEC S04.89- ☑
        type NEC S04.9 ☑
      tenth (pneumogastric or vagus) — see Injury,
        nerve, vagus
      third (oculomotor) — see Injury, nerve, oculomo-
        tor
      twelfth (hypoglossal) — see Injury, nerve, hy-
        poglossal
    cutaneous sensory
      ankle (level) S94.3- ☑
      arm (upper) (level) S44.5- ☑

Injury — continued
  nerve — continued
    cutaneous sensory — continued
      foot (level) — see Injury, nerve, cutaneous senso-
        ry, ankle
      forearm (level) S54.3- ☑
      hip (level) S74.2- ☑
      leg (lower level) S84.2- ☑
      shoulder (level) — see Injury, nerve, cutaneous
        sensory, arm
      thigh (level) — see Injury, nerve, cutaneous
        sensory, hip
    deep peroneal — see Injury, nerve, peroneal, foot
    digital
      finger S64.4- ☑
        index S64.49- ☑
        little S64.49- ☑
        middle S64.49- ☑
        ring S64.49- ☑
      thumb S64.3- ☑
      toe — see Injury, nerve, ankle, specified site NEC
    eighth cranial (acoustic or auditory) — see Injury,
      nerve, acoustic
    eleventh cranial (accessory) — see Injury, nerve,
      accessory
    facial S04.5- ☑
      contusion S04.5- ☑
      laceration S04.5- ☑
      newborn P11.3
      specified type NEC S04.5- ☑
    femoral (hip level) (thigh level) S74.1- ☑
    fifth cranial (trigeminal) — see Injury, nerve,
      trigeminal
    finger (digital) — see Injury, nerve, digital, finger
    first cranial (olfactory) — see Injury, nerve, olfactory
    foot S94.9- ☑
      cutaneous sensory S94.3- ☑
      deep peroneal S94.2- ☑
      lateral plantar S94.0- ☑
      medial plantar S94.1- ☑
      specified site NEC — see subcategory S94.8 ☑
    forearm (level) S54.9- ☑
      cutaneous sensory — see Injury, nerve, cuta-
        neous sensory, forearm
      median — see Injury, nerve, median
      radial — see Injury, nerve, radial
      specified site NEC — see subcategory S54.8 ☑
      ulnar — see Injury, nerve, ulnar
    fourth cranial (trochlear) — see Injury, nerve,
      trochlear
    glossopharyngeal S04.89- ☑
      specified type NEC S04.89- ☑
    hand S64.9- ☑
      median — see Injury, nerve, median, hand
      radial — see Injury, nerve, radial, hand
      specified NEC — see subcategory S64.8 ☑
      ulnar — see Injury, nerve, ulnar, hand
    hip (level) S74.9- ☑
      cutaneous sensory — see Injury, nerve, cuta-
        neous sensory, hip
      femoral — see Injury, nerve, femoral
      sciatic — see Injury, nerve, sciatic
      specified site NEC — see subcategory S74.8 ☑
    hypoglossal S04.89- ☑
      specified type NEC S04.89- ☑
    lateral plantar S94.0- ☑
    leg (lower) S84.9- ☑
      cutaneous sensory — see Injury, nerve, cuta-
        neous sensory, leg
      peroneal — see Injury, nerve, peroneal
      specified site NEC — see subcategory S84.8 ☑
      tibial — see Injury, nerve, tibial
      upper — see Injury, nerve, thigh
    lower
      back — see Injury, nerve, abdomen, specified
        site NEC
        peripheral — see Injury, nerve, abdomen,
          peripheral
      limb — see Injury, nerve, leg
    lumbar plexus — see Injury, nerve, lumbosacral,
      sympathetic
    lumbar spinal — see Injury, nerve, spinal, lumbar
    lumbosacral
      plexus — see Injury, nerve, lumbosacral, sympa-
        thetic
      sympathetic S34.5 ☑

☑ Additional Character Required — Refer to the Tabular List for Character Selection   ▼ Subterms under main terms may continue to next column or page

Injury — *continued*
  nerve — *continued*
    medial plantar S94.1- ☑
    median (forearm level) S54.1- ☑
      hand (level) S64.1- ☑
      upper arm (level) S44.1- ☑
      wrist (level) — *see* Injury, nerve, median, hand
    musculocutaneous S44.4- ☑
    musculospiral (upper arm level) — *see* Injury, nerve, radial, upper arm
    neck S14.9
      peripheral S14.4 ☑
      specified site NEC S14.8 ☑
      sympathetic S14.5 ☑
    ninth cranial (glossopharyngeal) — *see* Injury, nerve, glossopharyngeal
    oculomotor S04.1- ☑
      contusion S04.1- ☑
      ·laceration S04.1- ☑
      specified type NEC S04.1- ☑
    olfactory S04.81- ☑
      specified type NEC S04.81- ☑
    optic S04.01- ☑
      contusion S04.01- ☑
      laceration S04.01- ☑
      specified type NEC S04.01- ☑
    pelvic girdle — *see* Injury, nerve, hip
    pelvis — *see* Injury, nerve, abdomen, specified site NEC
    peripheral — *see* Injury, nerve, abdomen, peripheral
    peripheral NEC T14.8 ☑
      abdomen — *see* Injury, nerve, abdomen, peripheral
      lower back — *see* Injury, nerve, abdomen, peripheral
      neck — *see* Injury, nerve, neck, peripheral
      pelvis — *see* Injury, nerve, abdomen, peripheral
      specified NEC T14.8 ☑
    peroneal (lower leg level) S84.1- ☑
      foot S94.2- ☑
    plexus
      brachial — *see* Injury, brachial plexus
      celiac, coeliac — *see* Injury, nerve, lumbosacral, sympathetic
      mesenteric, inferior — *see* Injury, nerve, lumbosacral, sympathetic
      sacral — *see* Injury, lumbosacral plexus
      spinal
        brachial — *see* Injury, brachial plexus
        lumbosacral — *see* Injury, lumbosacral plexus
    pneumogastric — *see* Injury, nerve, vagus
    radial (forearm level) S54.2- ☑
      hand (level) S64.2- ☑
      upper arm (level) S44.2- ☑
      wrist (level) — *see* Injury, nerve, radial, hand
    root — *see* Injury, nerve, spinal, root
    sacral plexus — *see* Injury, lumbosacral plexus
    sacral spinal — *see* Injury, nerve, spinal, sacral
    sciatic (hip level) (thigh level) S74.0- ☑
    second cranial (optic) — *see* Injury, nerve, optic
    seventh cranial (facial) — *see* Injury, nerve, facial
    shoulder — *see* Injury, nerve, arm
    sixth cranial (abducent) — *see* Injury, nerve, abducens
    spinal
      plexus — *see* Injury, nerve, plexus, spinal
      root
        cervical S14.2 ☑
        dorsal S24.2 ☑
        lumbar S34.21 ☑
        sacral S34.22 ☑
        thoracic — *see* Injury, nerve, spinal, root, dorsal
    splanchnic — *see* Injury, nerve, lumbosacral, sympathetic
    sympathetic NEC — *see* Injury, nerve, lumbosacral, sympathetic
      cervical — *see* Injury, nerve, cervical sympathetic
    tenth cranial (pneumogastric or vagus) — *see* Injury, nerve, vagus
    thigh (level) — *see* Injury, nerve, hip
      cutaneous sensory — *see* Injury, nerve, cutaneous sensory, hip
      femoral — *see* Injury, nerve, femoral
      sciatic — *see* Injury, nerve, sciatic

Injury — *continued*
  nerve — *continued*
    thigh — *see* Injury, nerve, hip — *continued*
      specified NEC — *see* Injury, nerve, hip
    third cranial (oculomotor) — *see* Injury, nerve, oculomotor
    thorax S24.9 ☑
      peripheral S24.3 ☑
      specified site NEC S24.8 ☑
      sympathetic S24.4 ☑
    thumb, digital — *see* Injury, nerve, digital, thumb
    tibial (lower leg level) (posterior) S84.0- ☑
    toe — *see* Injury, nerve, ankle
    trigeminal S04.3- ☑
      contusion S04.3- ☑
      laceration S04.3- ☑
      specified type NEC S04.3- ☑
    trochlear S04.2- ☑
      contusion S04.2- ☑
      laceration S04.2- ☑
      specified type NEC S04.2- ☑
    twelfth cranial (hypoglossal) — *see* Injury, nerve, hypoglossal
    ulnar (forearm level) S54.0- ☑
      arm (upper) (level) S44.0- ☑
      hand (level) S64.0- ☑
      wrist (level) — *see* Injury, nerve, ulnar, hand
    vagus S04.89- ☑
      specified type NEC S04.89- ☑
    wrist (level) — *see* Injury, nerve, hand
  ninth cranial nerve (glossopharyngeal) — *see* Injury, nerve, glossopharyngeal
  nose (septum) S09.92 ☑
  obstetrical O71.9
    specified NEC O71.89
  occipital (region) (scalp) S09.90 ☑
    lobe — *see* Injury, intracranial
  optic chiasm S04.02 ☑
  optic radiation S04.03- ☑
  optic tract and pathways S04.03- ☑
  orbit, orbital (region) — *see* Injury, eye
    penetrating (with foreign body) — *see* Injury, eye, orbit, penetrating
    specified NEC — *see* Injury, eye, specified site NEC
  ovary, ovarian S37.409 ☑
    bilateral S37.402 ☑
      contusion S37.422 ☑
      laceration S37.432 ☑
      specified type NEC S37.492 ☑
    blood vessel — *see* Injury, blood vessel, ovarian
    contusion S37.429 ☑
      bilateral S37.422 ☑
      unilateral S37.421 ☑
    laceration S37.439 ☑
      bilateral S37.432 ☑
      unilateral S37.431 ☑
    specified type NEC S37.499 ☑
      bilateral S37.492 ☑
      unilateral S37.491 ☑
    unilateral S37.401 ☑
      contusion S37.421 ☑
      laceration S37.431 ☑
      specified type NEC S37.491 ☑
  palate (hard) (soft) S09.93 ☑
  pancreas S36.209 ☑
    body S36.201 ☑
      contusion S36.221 ☑
      laceration S36.231 ☑
        major S36.261 ☑
        minor S36.241 ☑
        moderate S36.251 ☑
      specified type NEC S36.291 ☑
    contusion S36.229 ☑
    head S36.200 ☑
      contusion S36.220 ☑
      laceration S36.230 ☑
        major S36.260 ☑
        minor S36.240 ☑
        moderate S36.250 ☑
      specified type NEC S36.290 ☑
    laceration S36.239 ☑
      major S36.269 ☑
      minor S36.249 ☑
      moderate S36.259 ☑
    specified type NEC S36.299 ☑
    tail S36.202 ☑

Injury — *continued*
  pancreas — *continued*
    tail — *continued*
      contusion S36.222 ☑
      laceration S36.232 ☑
        major S36.262 ☑
        minor S36.242 ☑
        moderate S36.252 ☑
      specified type NEC S36.292 ☑
  parietal (region) (scalp) S09.90 ☑
    lobe — *see* Injury, intracranial
  patellar ligament (tendon) S76.10- ☑
    laceration S76.12- ☑
    specified NEC S76.19- ☑
    strain S76.11- ☑
  pelvis, pelvic (floor) S39.93 ☑
    complicating delivery O70.1
    joint or ligament, complicating delivery O71.6
    organ S37.90 ☑
      with ectopic or molar pregnancy O08.6
      complication of abortion — *see* Abortion
      contusion S37.92 ☑
      following ectopic or molar pregnancy O08.6
      laceration S37.93 ☑
      obstetrical trauma NEC O71.5
      specified
        site NEC S37.899 ☑
          contusion S37.892 ☑
          laceration S37.893 ☑
          specified type NEC S37.898 ☑
        type NEC S37.99 ☑
    specified NEC S39.83 ☑
  penis S39.94 ☑
  perineum S39.94 ☑
  peritoneum S36.81 ☑
    laceration S36.893 ☑
  periurethral tissue — *see* Injury, urethra
    complicating delivery O71.82
  phalanges
    foot — *see* Injury, foot
    hand — *see* Injury, hand
  pharynx NEC S19.85 ☑
  pleura — *see* Injury, intrathoracic, pleura
  plexus
    brachial — *see* Injury, brachial plexus
    cardiac — *see* Injury, nerve, thorax, sympathetic
    celiac, coeliac — *see* Injury, nerve, lumbosacral, sympathetic
    esophageal — *see* Injury, nerve, thorax, sympathetic
    hypogastric — *see* Injury, nerve, lumbosacral, sympathetic
    lumbar, lumbosacral — *see* Injury, lumbosacral plexus
    mesenteric — *see* Injury, nerve, lumbosacral, sympathetic
    pulmonary — *see* Injury, nerve, thorax, sympathetic
  postcardiac surgery (syndrome) I97.0
  prepuce S39.94 ☑
  pressure
    injury — *see* Ulcer, pressure, by site
  prostate S37.829 ☑
    contusion S37.822 ☑
    laceration S37.823 ☑
    specified type NEC S37.828 ☑
  pubic region S39.94 ☑
  pudendum S39.94 ☑
  pulmonary plexus — *see* Injury, nerve, thorax, sympathetic
  rectovaginal septum NEC S39.83 ☑
  rectum — *see* Injury, intestine, large, rectum
  retina — *see* Injury, eye, specified site NEC
    penetrating — *see* Injury, eyeball, penetrating
  retroperitoneal — *see* Injury, intra-abdominal, specified site NEC
  rotator cuff (muscle(s)) (tendon(s)) S46.00- ☑
    laceration S46.02- ☑
    specified type NEC S46.09- ☑
    strain S46.01- ☑
  round ligament — *see* Injury, pelvic organ, specified site NEC
  sacral plexus — *see* Injury, lumbosacral plexus
  salivary duct or gland S09.93 ☑
  scalp S09.90 ☑
    newborn (birth injury) P12.9
      due to monitoring (electrode) (sampling incision) P12.4

Injury — *continued*
scalp — *continued*
  newborn — *continued*
    specified NEC P12.89
      caput succedaneum P12.81
scapular region — *see* Injury, shoulder
sclera — *see* Injury, eye, specified site NEC
  penetrating — *see* Injury, eyeball, penetrating
scrotum S39.94 ☑
second cranial nerve (optic) — *see* Injury, nerve, optic
seminal vesicle — *see* Injury, pelvic organ, specified
  site NEC
seventh cranial nerve (facial) — *see* Injury, nerve, facial
shoulder S49.9- ☑
  blood vessel — *see* Injury, blood vessel, arm
  contusion — *see* Contusion, shoulder
  dislocation — *see* Dislocation, shoulder
  fracture — *see* Fracture, shoulder
  muscle — *see* Injury, muscle, shoulder
  nerve — *see* Injury, nerve, shoulder
  open — *see* Wound, open, shoulder
  specified type NEC S49.8- ☑
  sprain — *see* Sprain, shoulder girdle
  superficial — *see* Injury, superficial, shoulder
sinus
  cavernous — *see* Injury, intracranial
  nasal S09.92 ☑
sixth cranial nerve (abducent) — *see* Injury, nerve, abducens
skeleton, birth injury P13.9
  specified part NEC P13.8
skin NEC T14.8 ☑
  surface intact — *see* Injury, superficial
skull NEC S09.90 ☑
specified NEC T14.8 ☑
spermatic cord (pelvic region) S37.898 ☑
  scrotal region S39.848 ☑
spinal (cord)
  cervical (neck) S14.109 ☑
    anterior cord syndrome S14.139 ☑
      C1 level S14.131 ☑
      C2 level S14.132 ☑
      C3 level S14.133 ☑
      C4 level S14.134 ☑
      C5 level S14.135 ☑
      C6 level S14.136 ☑
      C7 level S14.137 ☑
      C8 level S14.138 ☑
    Brown-Séquard syndrome S14.149 ☑
      C1 level S14.141 ☑
      C2 level S14.142 ☑
      C3 level S14.143 ☑
      C4 level S14.144 ☑
      C5 level S14.145 ☑
      C6 level S14.146 ☑
      C7 level S14.147 ☑
      C8 level S14.148 ☑
    C1 level S14.101 ☑
    C2 level S14.102 ☑
    C3 level S14.103 ☑
    C4 level S14.104 ☑
    C5 level S14.105 ☑
    C6 level S14.106 ☑
    C7 level S14.107 ☑
    C8 level S14.108 ☑
    central cord syndrome S14.129 ☑
      C1 level S14.121 ☑
      C2 level S14.122 ☑
      C3 level S14.123 ☑
      C4 level S14.124 ☑
      C5 level S14.125 ☑
      C6 level S14.126 ☑
      C7 level S14.127 ☑
      C8 level S14.128 ☑
    complete lesion S14.119 ☑
      C1 level S14.111 ☑
      C2 level S14.112 ☑
      C3 level S14.113 ☑
      C4 level S14.114 ☑
      C5 level S14.115 ☑
      C6 level S14.116 ☑
      C7 level S14.117 ☑
      C8 level S14.118 ☑
    concussion S14.0 ☑
    edema S14.0 ☑
    incomplete lesion specified NEC S14.159 ☑

Injury — *continued*
spinal — *continued*
  cervical — *continued*
    incomplete lesion specified — *continued*
      C1 level S14.151 ☑
      C2 level S14.152 ☑
      C3 level S14.153 ☑
      C4 level S14.154 ☑
      C5 level S14.155 ☑
      C6 level S14.156 ☑
      C7 level S14.157 ☑
      C8 level S14.158 ☑
    posterior cord syndrome S14.159 ☑
      C1 level S14.151 ☑
      C2 level S14.152 ☑
      C3 level S14.153 ☑
      C4 level S14.154 ☑
      C5 level S14.155 ☑
      C6 level S14.156 ☑
      C7 level S14.157 ☑
      C8 level S14.158 ☑
  dorsal — *see* Injury, spinal, thoracic
  lumbar S34.109 ☑
    complete lesion S34.119 ☑
      L1 level S34.111 ☑
      L2 level S34.112 ☑
      L3 level S34.113 ☑
      L4 level S34.114 ☑
      L5 level S34.115 ☑
    concussion S34.01 ☑
    edema S34.01 ☑
    incomplete lesion S34.129 ☑
      L1 level S34.121 ☑
      L2 level S34.122 ☑
      L3 level S34.123 ☑
      L4 level S34.124 ☑
      L5 level S34.125 ☑
    L1 level S34.101 ☑
    L2 level S34.102 ☑
    L3 level S34.103 ☑
    L4 level S34.104 ☑
    L5 level S34.105 ☑
  nerve root NEC
    cervical — *see* Injury, nerve, spinal, root, cervical
    dorsal — *see* Injury, nerve, spinal, root, dorsal
    lumbar S34.21 ☑
    sacral S34.22 ☑
    thoracic — *see* Injury, nerve, spinal, root, dorsal
  plexus
    brachial — *see* Injury, brachial plexus
    lumbosacral — *see* Injury, lumbosacral plexus
  sacral S34.139 ☑
    complete lesion S34.131 ☑
    incomplete lesion S34.132 ☑
  thoracic S24.109 ☑
    anterior cord syndrome S24.139 ☑
      T1 level S24.131 ☑
      T2-T6 level S24.132 ☑
      T7-T10 level S24.133 ☑
      T11-T12 level S24.134 ☑
    Brown-Séquard syndrome S24.149 ☑
      T1 level S24.141 ☑
      T2-T6 level S24.142 ☑
      T7-T10 level S24.143 ☑
      T11-T12 level S24.144 ☑
    complete lesion S24.119 ☑
      T1 level S24.111 ☑
      T2-T6 level S24.112 ☑
      T7-T10 level S24.113 ☑
      T11-T12 level S24.114 ☑
    concussion S24.0 ☑
    edema S24.0 ☑
    incomplete lesion specified NEC S24.159 ☑
      T1 level S24.151 ☑
      T2-T6 level S24.152 ☑
      T7-T10 level S24.153 ☑
      T11-T12 level S24.154 ☑
    posterior cord syndrome S24.159 ☑
      T1 level S24.151 ☑
      T2-T6 level S24.152 ☑
      T7-T10 level S24.153 ☑
      T11-T12 level S24.154 ☑
    T1 level S24.101 ☑
    T2-T6 level S24.102 ☑
    T7-T10 level S24.103 ☑
    T11-T12 level S24.104 ☑

Injury — *continued*
splanchnic nerve — *see* Injury, nerve, lumbosacral,
  sympathetic
spleen S36.00 ☑
  contusion S36.029 ☑
    major S36.021 ☑
    minor S36.020 ☑
  laceration S36.039 ☑
    major (massive) (stellate) S36.032 ☑
    moderate S36.031 ☑
    superficial (capsular) (minor) S36.030 ☑
  specified type NEC S36.09 ☑
splenic artery — *see* Injury, blood vessel, celiac artery,
  branch
stellate ganglion — *see* Injury, nerve, thorax, sympathetic
sternal region S29.9 ☑
stomach S36.30 ☑
  contusion S36.32 ☑
  laceration S36.33 ☑
  specified type NEC S36.39 ☑
subconjunctival — *see* Injury, eye, conjunctiva
subcutaneous NEC T14.8 ☑
submaxillary region S09.93 ☑
submental region S09.93 ☑
subungual
  fingers — *see* Injury, hand
  toes — *see* Injury, foot
superficial NEC T14.8 ☑
  abdomen, abdominal (wall) S30.92 ☑
    abrasion S30.811 ☑
    bite S30.871 ☑
      insect S30.861 ☑
    contusion S30.1 ☑
    external constriction S30.841 ☑
    foreign body S30.851 ☑
  abrasion — *see* Abrasion, by site
  adnexa, eye NEC — *see* Injury, eye, specified site
    NEC
  alveolar process — *see* Injury, superficial, oral cavity
  ankle S90.91- ☑
    abrasion — *see* Abrasion, ankle
    bite — *see* Bite, ankle
    blister — *see* Blister, ankle
    contusion — *see* Contusion, ankle
    external constriction — *see* Constriction, exter-
      nal, ankle
    foreign body — *see* Foreign body, superficial,
      ankle
  anus S30.98 ☑
  arm (upper) S40.92- ☑
    abrasion — *see* Abrasion, arm
    bite — *see* Bite, superficial, arm
    blister — *see* Blister, arm (upper)
    contusion — *see* Contusion, arm
    external constriction — *see* Constriction, exter-
      nal, arm
    foreign body — *see* Foreign body, superficial,
      arm
  auditory canal (external) (meatus) — *see* Injury, su-
    perficial, ear
  auricle — *see* Injury, superficial, ear
  axilla — *see* Injury, superficial, arm
  back — *see also* Injury, superficial, thorax, back
    lower S30.91 ☑
      abrasion S30.810 ☑
      contusion S30.0 ☑
      external constriction S30.840 ☑
      superficial
        bite NEC S30.870 ☑
          insect S30.860 ☑
        foreign body S30.850 ☑
  bite NEC — *see* Bite, superficial NEC, by site
  blister — *see* Blister, by site
  breast S20.10- ☑
    abrasion — *see* Abrasion, breast
    bite — *see* Bite, superficial, breast
    contusion — *see* Contusion, breast
    external constriction — *see* Constriction, exter-
      nal, breast
    foreign body — *see* Foreign body, superficial,
      breast
  brow — *see* Injury, superficial, head, specified NEC
  buttock S30.91 ☑
  calf — *see* Injury, superficial, leg

Injury — *continued*
  superficial — *continued*
    canthus, eye — *see* Injury, superficial, periocular area
    cheek (external) — *see* Injury, superficial, head, specified NEC
      internal — *see* Injury, superficial, oral cavity
    chest wall — *see* Injury, superficial, thorax
    chin — *see* Injury, superficial, head NEC
    clitoris S30.95 ☑
    conjunctiva — *see* Injury, eye, conjunctiva
      with foreign body (in conjunctival sac) — *see* Foreign body, conjunctival sac
    contusion — *see* Contusion, by site
    costal region — *see* Injury, superficial, thorax
    digit(s)
      hand — *see* Injury, superficial, finger
    ear (auricle) (canal) (external) S00.40- ☑
      abrasion — *see* Abrasion, ear
      bite — *see* Bite, superficial, ear
      contusion — *see* Contusion, ear
      external constriction — *see* Constriction, external, ear
      foreign body — *see* Foreign body, superficial, ear
    elbow S50.90- ☑
      abrasion — *see* Abrasion, elbow
      bite — *see* Bite, superficial, elbow
      blister — *see* Blister, elbow
      contusion — *see* Contusion, elbow
      external constriction — *see* Constriction, external, elbow
      foreign body — *see* Foreign body, superficial, elbow
    epididymis S30.94 ☑
    epigastric region S30.92 ☑
    epiglottis — *see* Injury, superficial, throat
    esophagus
      cervical — *see* Injury, superficial, throat
    external constriction — *see* Constriction, external, by site
    extremity NEC T14.8 ☑
    eyeball NEC — *see* Injury, eye, specified site NEC
    eyebrow — *see* Injury, superficial, periocular area
    eyelid S00.20- ☑
      abrasion — *see* Abrasion, eyelid
      bite — *see* Bite, superficial, eyelid
      contusion — *see* Contusion, eyelid
      external constriction — *see* Constriction, external, eyelid
      foreign body — *see* Foreign body, superficial, eyelid
    face NEC — *see* Injury, superficial, head, specified NEC
    finger(s) S60.949 ☑
      abrasion — *see* Abrasion, finger
      bite — *see* Bite, superficial, finger
      blister — *see* Blister, finger
      contusion — *see* Contusion, finger
      external constriction — *see* Constriction, external, finger
      foreign body — *see* Foreign body, superficial, finger
      index S60.94- ☑
      insect bite — *see* Bite, by site, superficial, insect
      little S60.94- ☑
      middle S60.94- ☑
      ring S60.94- ☑
    flank S30.92 ☑
    foot S90.92- ☑
      abrasion — *see* Abrasion, foot
      bite — *see* Bite, foot
      blister — *see* Blister, foot
      contusion — *see* Contusion, foot
      external constriction — *see* Constriction, external, foot
      foreign body — *see* Foreign body, superficial, foot
    forearm S50.91- ☑
      abrasion — *see* Abrasion, forearm
      bite — *see* Bite, forearm, superficial
      blister — *see* Blister, forearm
      contusion — *see* Contusion, forearm
      elbow only — *see* Injury, superficial, elbow
      external constriction — *see* Constriction, external, forearm

Injury — *continued*
  superficial — *continued*
    forearm — *continued*
      foreign body — *see* Foreign body, superficial, forearm
    forehead — *see* Injury, superficial, head NEC
    foreign body — *see* Foreign body, superficial
    genital organs, external
      female S30.97 ☑
      male S30.96 ☑
    globe (eye) — *see* Injury, eye, specified site NEC
    groin S30.92 ☑
    gum — *see* Injury, superficial, oral cavity
    hand S60.92- ☑
      abrasion — *see* Abrasion, hand
      bite — *see* Bite, superficial, hand
      contusion — *see* Contusion, hand
      external constriction — *see* Constriction, external, hand
      foreign body — *see* Foreign body, superficial, hand
    head S00.90 ☑
      ear — *see* Injury, superficial, ear
      eyelid — *see* Injury, superficial, eyelid
      nose S00.30 ☑
      oral cavity S00.502 ☑
      scalp S00.00 ☑
      specified site NEC S00.80 ☑
    heel — *see* Injury, superficial, foot
    hip S70.91- ☑
      abrasion — *see* Abrasion, hip
      bite — *see* Bite, superficial, hip
      blister — *see* Blister, hip
      contusion — *see* Contusion, hip
      external constriction — *see* Constriction, external, hip
      foreign body — *see* Foreign body, superficial, hip
    iliac region — *see* Injury, superficial, abdomen
    inguinal region — *see* Injury, superficial, abdomen
    insect bite — *see* Bite, by site, superficial, insect
    interscapular region — *see* Injury, superficial, thorax, back
    jaw — *see* Injury, superficial, head, specified NEC
    knee S80.91- ☑
      abrasion — *see* Abrasion, knee
      bite — *see* Bite, superficial, knee
      blister — *see* Blister, knee
      contusion — *see* Contusion, knee
      external constriction — *see* Constriction, external, knee
      foreign body — *see* Foreign body, superficial, knee
    labium (majus) (minus) S30.95 ☑
    lacrimal (apparatus) (gland) (sac) — *see* Injury, eye, specified site NEC
    larynx — *see* Injury, superficial, throat
    leg (lower) S80.92- ☑
      abrasion — *see* Abrasion, leg
      bite — *see* Bite, superficial, leg
      contusion — *see* Contusion, leg
      external constriction — *see* Constriction, external, leg
      foreign body — *see* Foreign body, superficial, leg
      knee — *see* Injury, superficial, knee
    limb NEC T14.8 ☑
    lip S00.501 ☑
    lower back S30.91 ☑
    lumbar region S30.91 ☑
    malar region — *see* Injury, superficial, head, specified NEC
    mammary — *see* Injury, superficial, breast
    mastoid region — *see* Injury, superficial, head, specified NEC
    mouth — *see* Injury, superficial, oral cavity
    muscle NEC T14.8 ☑
    nail NEC T14.8 ☑
      finger — *see* Injury, superficial, finger
      toe — *see* Injury, superficial, toe
    nasal (septum) — *see* Injury, superficial, nose
    neck S10.90 ☑
      specified site NEC S10.80 ☑
    nose (septum) S00.30 ☑
    occipital region — *see* Injury, superficial, scalp
    oral cavity S00.502 ☑

Injury — *continued*
  superficial — *continued*
    orbital region — *see* Injury, superficial, periocular area
    palate — *see* Injury, superficial, oral cavity
    palm — *see* Injury, superficial, hand
    parietal region — *see* Injury, superficial, scalp
    pelvis S30.91 ☑
      girdle — *see* Injury, superficial, hip
    penis S30.93 ☑
    perineum
      female S30.95 ☑
      male S30.91 ☑
    periocular area S00.20- ☑
      abrasion — *see* Abrasion, eyelid
      bite — *see* Bite, superficial, eyelid
      contusion — *see* Contusion, eyelid
      external constriction — *see* Constriction, external, eyelid
      foreign body — *see* Foreign body, superficial, eyelid
    phalanges
      finger — *see* Injury, superficial, finger
      toe — *see* Injury, superficial, toe
    pharynx — *see* Injury, superficial, throat
    pinna — *see* Injury, superficial, ear
    popliteal space — *see* Injury, superficial, knee
    prepuce S30.93 ☑
    pubic region S30.91 ☑
    pudendum
      female S30.97 ☑
      male S30.96 ☑
    sacral region S30.91 ☑
    scalp S00.00 ☑
    scapular region — *see* Injury, superficial, shoulder
    sclera — *see* Injury, eye, specified site NEC
    scrotum S30.94 ☑
    shin — *see* Injury, superficial, leg
    shoulder S40.91- ☑
      abrasion — *see* Abrasion, shoulder
      bite — *see* Bite, superficial, shoulder
      blister — *see* Blister, shoulder
      contusion — *see* Contusion, shoulder
      external constriction — *see* Constriction, external, shoulder
      foreign body — *see* Foreign body, superficial, shoulder
    skin NEC T14.8 ☑
    sternal region — *see* Injury, superficial, thorax, front
    subconjunctival — *see* Injury, eye, specified site NEC
    subcutaneous NEC T14.8 ☑
    submaxillary region — *see* Injury, superficial, head, specified NEC
    submental region — *see* Injury, superficial, head, specified NEC
    subungual
      finger(s) — *see* Injury, superficial, finger
      toe(s) — *see* Injury, superficial, toe
    supraclavicular fossa — *see* Injury, superficial, neck
    supraorbital — *see* Injury, superficial, head, specified NEC
    temple — *see* Injury, superficial, head, specified NEC
    temporal region — *see* Injury, superficial, head, specified NEC
    testis S30.94 ☑
    thigh S70.92- ☑
      abrasion — *see* Abrasion, thigh
      bite — *see* Bite, superficial, thigh
      blister — *see* Blister, thigh
      contusion — *see* Contusion, thigh
      external constriction — *see* Constriction, external, thigh
      foreign body — *see* Foreign body, superficial, thigh
    thorax, thoracic (wall) S20.90 ☑
      abrasion — *see* Abrasion, thorax
      back S20.40- ☑
      bite — *see* Bite, thorax, superficial
      blister — *see* Blister, thorax
      contusion — *see* Contusion, thorax
      external constriction — *see* Constriction, external, thorax
      foreign body — *see* Foreign body, superficial, thorax
      front S20.30- ☑
    throat S10.10 ☑

⛳ Subterms under main terms may continue to next column or page   ☑ Additional Character Required — Refer to the Tabular List for Character Selection   199

Injury — Injury

Injury — *continued*
  superficial — *continued*
    throat — *continued*
      abrasion S10.11 ☑
      bite S10.17 ☑
        insect S10.16 ☑
      blister S10.12 ☑
      contusion S10.0 ☑
      external constriction S10.14 ☑
      foreign body S10.15 ☑
    thumb S60.93- ☑
      abrasion — *see* Abrasion, thumb
      bite — *see* Bite, superficial, thumb
      blister — *see* Blister, thumb
      contusion — *see* Contusion, thumb
      external constriction — *see* Constriction, external, thumb
      foreign body — *see* Foreign body, superficial, thumb
      insect bite — *see* Bite, by site, superficial, insect
      specified type NEC S60.39 ☑
    toe(s) S90.93- ☑
      abrasion — *see* Abrasion, toe
      bite — *see* Bite, toe
      blister — *see* Blister, toe
      contusion — *see* Contusion, toe
      external constriction — *see* Constriction, external, toe
      foreign body — *see* Foreign body, superficial, toe
      great S90.93- ☑
    tongue — *see* Injury, superficial, oral cavity
    tooth, teeth — *see* Injury, superficial, oral cavity
    trachea S10.10 ☑
    tunica vaginalis S30.94 ☑
    tympanum, tympanic membrane — *see* Injury, superficial, ear
    uvula — *see* Injury, superficial, oral cavity
    vagina S30.95 ☑
    vocal cords — *see* Injury, superficial, throat
    vulva S30.95 ☑
    wrist S60.91- ☑
  supraclavicular region — *see* Injury, neck
  supraorbital S09.93 ☑
  suprarenal gland (multiple) — *see* Injury, adrenal
  surgical complication (external or internal site) — *see* Laceration, accidental complicating surgery
  temple S09.90 ☑
  temporal region S09.90 ☑
  tendon — *see also* Injury, muscle, by site
    abdomen — *see* Injury, muscle, abdomen
    Achilles — *see* Injury, Achilles tendon
    lower back — *see* Injury, muscle, lower back
    pelvic organs — *see* Injury, muscle, pelvis
  tenth cranial nerve (pneumogastric or vagus) — *see* Injury, nerve, vagus
  testis S39.94 ☑
  thigh S79.92- ☑
    blood vessel — *see* Injury, blood vessel, hip
    contusion — *see* Contusion, thigh
    fracture — *see* Fracture, femur
    muscle — *see* Injury, muscle, thigh
    nerve — *see* Injury, nerve, thigh
    open — *see* Wound, open, thigh
    specified NEC S79.82- ☑
    superficial — *see* Injury, superficial, thigh
  third cranial nerve (oculomotor) — *see* Injury, nerve, oculomotor
  thorax, thoracic S29.9 ☑
    blood vessel — *see* Injury, blood vessel, thorax
    cavity — *see* Injury, intrathoracic
    dislocation — *see* Dislocation, thorax
    external (wall) S29.9 ☑
      contusion — *see* Contusion, thorax
      nerve — *see* Injury, nerve, thorax
      open — *see* Wound, open, thorax
      specified NEC S29.8 ☑
      sprain — *see* Sprain, thorax
      superficial — *see* Injury, superficial, thorax
    fracture — *see* Fracture, thorax
    internal — *see* Injury, intrathoracic
    intrathoracic organ — *see* Injury, intrathoracic
    sympathetic ganglion — *see* Injury, nerve, thorax, sympathetic
  throat — *see also* Injury, neck S19.9 ☑
  thumb S69.9- ☑

Injury — *continued*
  thumb — *continued*
    blood vessel — *see* Injury, blood vessel, thumb
    contusion — *see* Contusion, thumb
    dislocation — *see* Dislocation, thumb
    fracture — *see* Fracture, thumb
    muscle — *see* Injury, muscle, thumb
    nerve — *see* Injury, nerve, digital, thumb
    open — *see* Wound, open, thumb
    specified NEC S69.8- ☑
    sprain — *see* Sprain, thumb
    superficial — *see* Injury, superficial, thumb
  thymus (gland) — *see* Injury, Intrathoracic, specified organ NEC
  thyroid (gland) NEC S19.84 ☑
  toe S99.92- ☑
    contusion — *see* Contusion, toe
    dislocation — *see* Dislocation, toe
    fracture — *see* Fracture, toe
    muscle — *see* Injury, muscle, toe
    open — *see* Wound, open, toe
    specified type NEC S99.82- ☑
    sprain — *see* Sprain, toe
    superficial — *see* Injury, superficial, toe
  tongue S09.93 ☑
  tonsil S09.93 ☑
  tooth S09.93 ☑
  trachea (cervical) NEC S19.82 ☑
    thoracic — *see* Injury, intrathoracic, trachea, thoracic
  transfusion-related acute lung (TRALI) J95.84
  tunica vaginalis S39.94 ☑
  twelfth cranial nerve (hypoglossal) — *see* Injury, nerve, hypoglossal
  ureter S37.10 ☑
    contusion S37.12 ☑
    laceration S37.13 ☑
    specified type NEC S37.19 ☑
  urethra (sphincter) S37.30 ☑
    at delivery O71.5
    contusion S37.32 ☑
    laceration S37.33 ☑
    specified type NEC S37.39 ☑
  urinary organ S37.90 ☑
    contusion S37.92 ☑
    laceration S37.93 ☑
    specified
      site NEC S37.899 ☑
        contusion S37.892 ☑
        laceration S37.893 ☑
        specified type NEC S37.898 ☑
      type NEC S37.99 ☑
  uterus, uterine S37.60 ☑
    with ectopic or molar pregnancy O08.6
    blood vessel — *see* Injury, blood vessel, iliac
    contusion S37.62 ☑
    laceration S37.63 ☑
      cervix at delivery O71.3
    rupture associated with obstetrics — *see* Rupture, uterus
    specified type NEC S37.69 ☑
  uvula S09.93 ☑
  vagina S39.93 ☑
    abrasion S30.814 ☑
    bite S31.45 ☑
      insect S30.864 ☑
      superficial NEC S30.874 ☑
    contusion S30.23 ☑
    crush S38.03 ☑
    during delivery — *see* Laceration, vagina, during delivery
    external constriction S30.844 ☑
    insect bite S30.864 ☑
    laceration S31.41 ☑
      with foreign body S31.42 ☑
    open wound S31.40 ☑
    puncture S31.43 ☑
      with foreign body S31.44 ☑
    superficial S30.95 ☑
      foreign body S30.854 ☑
  vas deferens — *see* Injury, pelvic organ, specified site NEC
  vascular NEC T14.8 ☑
  vein — *see* Injury, blood vessel
  vena cava (superior) S25.20 ☑
    inferior S35.10 ☑
      laceration (minor) (superficial) S35.11 ☑

Injury — *continued*
  vena cava — *continued*
    inferior — *continued*
      laceration — *continued*
        major S35.12 ☑
      specified type NEC S35.19 ☑
    laceration (minor) (superficial) S25.21 ☑
      major S25.22 ☑
    specified type NEC S25.29 ☑
  vesical (sphincter) — *see* Injury, bladder
  visual cortex S04.04- ☑
  vitreous (humor) S05.90 ☑
    specified NEC S05.8X- ☑
  vocal cord NEC S19.83 ☑
  vulva S39.94 ☑
    abrasion S30.814 ☑
    bite S31.45 ☑
      insect S30.864 ☑
      superficial NEC S30.874 ☑
    contusion S30.23 ☑
    crush S38.03 ☑
    during delivery — *see* Laceration, perineum, female, during delivery
    external constriction S30.844 ☑
    insect bite S30.864 ☑
    laceration S31.41 ☑
      with foreign body S31.42 ☑
    open wound S31.40 ☑
    puncture S31.43 ☑
      with foreign body S31.44 ☑
    superficial S30.95 ☑
      foreign body S30.854 ☑
  whiplash (cervical spine) S13.4 ☑
  wrist S69.9- ☑
    blood vessel — *see* Injury, blood vessel, hand
    contusion — *see* Contusion, wrist
    dislocation — *see* Dislocation, wrist
    fracture — *see* Fracture, wrist
    muscle — *see* Injury, muscle, hand
    nerve — *see* Injury, nerve, hand
    open — *see* Wound, open, wrist
    specified NEC S69.8- ☑
    sprain — *see* Sprain, wrist
    superficial — *see* Injury, superficial, wrist
Inoculation — *see also* Vaccination
  complication or reaction — *see* Complications, vaccination
Insanity, insane — *see also* Psychosis
  adolescent — *See* Schizophrenia
  confusional F28
    acute or subacute F05
  delusional F22
  senile F03 ☑
Insect
  bite — *see* Bite, by site, superficial, insect
  venomous, poisoning NEC (by) — *see* Venom, arthropod
Insensitivity
  adrenocorticotropin hormone (ACTH) E27.49
  androgen E34.50
    complete E34.51
    partial E34.52
Insertion
  cord (umbilical) lateral or velamentous O43.12- ☑
  intrauterine contraceptive device (encounter for) — *see* Intrauterine contraceptive device
Insolation (sunstroke) T67.01 ☑
Insomnia (organic) G47.00
  adjustment F51.02
  adjustment disorder F51.02
  behavioral, of childhood Z73.819
    combined type Z73.812
    limit setting type Z73.811
    sleep-onset association type Z73.810
  childhood Z73.819
  chronic F51.04
    somatized tension F51.04
  conditioned F51.04
  due to
    alcohol
      abuse F10.182
      dependence F10.282
      use F10.982
    amphetamines
      abuse F15.182
      dependence F15.282
      use F15.982

Insomnia — continued
  due to — continued
    anxiety disorder F51.05
    caffeine
      abuse F15.182
      dependence F15.282
      use F15.982
    cocaine
      abuse F14.182
      dependence F14.282
      use F14.982
    depression F51.05
    drug NEC
      abuse F19.182
      dependence F19.282
      use F19.982
    medical condition G47.01
    mental disorder NEC F51.05
    opioid
      abuse F11.182
      dependence F11.282
      use F11.982
    psychoactive substance NEC
      abuse F19.182
      dependence F19.182
      use F19.982
    sedative, hypnotic, or anxiolytic
      abuse F13.182
      dependence F13.282
      use F13.982
    stimulant NEC
      abuse F15.182
      dependence F15.282
      use F15.982
  fatal familial (FFI) A81.83
  idiopathic F51.01
  learned F51.3
  nonorganic origin F51.01
  not due to a substance or known physiological condition F51.01
    specified NEC F51.09
  paradoxical F51.03
  primary F51.01
  psychiatric F51.05
  psychophysiologic F51.04
  related to psychopathology F51.05
  short-term F51.02
  specified NEC G47.09
  stress-related F51.02
  transient F51.02
  without objective findings F51.02

Inspiration
  food or foreign body — see Foreign body, by site
  mucus — see Asphyxia, mucus

Inspissated bile syndrome (newborn) P59.1

Instability
  emotional (excessive) F60.3
  joint (post-traumatic) M25.30
    ankle M25.37- ☑
    due to old ligament injury — see Disorder, ligament
    elbow M25.32- ☑
    flail — see Flail, joint
    foot M25.37- ☑
    hand M25.34- ☑
    hip M25.35- ☑
    knee M25.36- ☑
    lumbosacral — see subcategory M53.2 ☑
    prosthesis — see Complications, joint prosthesis, mechanical, displacement, by site
    sacroiliac — see subcategory M53.2 ☑
    secondary to
      old ligament injury — see Disorder, ligament
      removal of joint prosthesis M96.89
    shoulder (region) M25.31- ☑
    spine — see subcategory M53.2 ☑
    wrist M25.33- ☑
  knee (chronic) M23.5- ☑
  lumbosacral — see subcategory M53.2 ☑
  nervous F48.8
  personality (emotional) F60.3
  spine — see Instability, joint, spine
  vasomotor R55

Institutional syndrome (childhood) F94.2

Institutionalization, affecting child Z62.22
  disinhibited attachment F94.2

Insufficiency, insufficient
  accommodation, old age H52.4
  adrenal (gland) E27.40

Insufficiency, insufficient — continued
  adrenal — continued
    primary E27.1
  adrenocortical E27.40
    drug-induced E27.3
    iatrogenic E27.3
    primary E27.1
  anatomic crown height K08.89
  anterior (occlusal) guidance M26.54
  anus K62.89
  aortic (valve) I35.1
    with
      mitral (valve) disease I08.0
        with tricuspid (valve) disease I08.3
      stenosis I35.2
      tricuspid (valve) disease I08.2
        with mitral (valve) disease I08.3
    congenital Q23.1
    rheumatic I06.1
      with
        mitral (valve) disease I08.0
          with tricuspid (valve) disease I08.3
        stenosis I06.2
          with mitral (valve) disease I08.0
            with tricuspid (valve) disease I08.3
        tricuspid (valve) disease I08.2
          with mitral (valve) disease I08.3
    specified cause NEC I35.1
    syphilitic A52.03
  arterial I77.1
    basilar G45.0
    carotid (hemispheric) G45.1
    cerebral I67.81
    coronary (acute or subacute) I24.8
    mesenteric K55.1
    peripheral I73.9
    precerebral (multiple) (bilateral) G45.2
    vertebral G45.0
  arteriovenous I99.8
  biliary K83.8
  cardiac — see also Insufficiency, myocardial
    due to presence of (cardiac) prosthesis I97.11- ☑
    postprocedural I97.11- ☑
  cardiorenal, hypertensive I13.2
  cardiovascular — see Disease, cardiovascular
  cerebrovascular (acute) I67.81
    with transient focal neurological signs and symptoms G45.8
  circulatory NEC I99.8
    newborn P29.89
  clinical crown length K08.89
  convergence H51.11
  coronary (acute or subacute) I24.8
    chronic or with a stated duration of over 4 weeks I25.89
  corticoadrenal E27.40
    primary E27.1
  dietary E63.9
  divergence H51.8
  food T73.0 ☑
  gastroesophageal K22.8
  gonadal
    ovary E28.39
    testis E29.1
  heart — see also Insufficiency, myocardial
    newborn P29.0
    valve — see Endocarditis
  hepatic — see Failure, hepatic
  idiopathic autonomic G90.09
  interocclusal distance of fully erupted teeth (ridge) M26.36
  kidney N28.9
    acute N28.9
    chronic N18.9
  lacrimal (secretion) H04.12- ☑
    passages — see Stenosis, lacrimal
  liver — see Failure, hepatic
  lung — see Insufficiency, pulmonary
  mental (congenital) — see Disability, intellectual
  mesenteric K55.1
  mitral (valve) I34.0
    with
      aortic valve disease I08.0
        with tricuspid (valve) disease I08.3
      obstruction or stenosis I05.2
        with aortic valve disease I08.0
      tricuspid (valve) disease I08.1
        with aortic (valve) disease I08.3

Insufficiency, insufficient — continued
  mitral — continued
    congenital Q23.3
    rheumatic I05.1
      with
        aortic valve disease I08.0
          with tricuspid (valve) disease I08.3
        obstruction or stenosis I05.2
          with aortic valve disease I08.0
            with tricuspid (valve) disease I08.3
        tricuspid (valve) disease I08.1
          with aortic (valve) disease I08.3
    active or acute I01.1
      with chorea, rheumatic (Sydenham's) I02.0
    specified cause, except rheumatic I34.0
  muscle — see also Disease, muscle
    heart — see Insufficiency, myocardial
    ocular NEC H50.9
  myocardial, myocardium (with arteriosclerosis) — see also Failure, heart I50.9
    with
      rheumatic fever (conditions in I00) I09.0
        active, acute or subacute I01.2
          with chorea I02.0
        inactive or quiescent (with chorea) I09.0
    congenital Q24.8
    hypertensive — see Hypertension, heart
    newborn P29.0
    rheumatic I09.0
      active, acute, or subacute I01.2
    syphilitic A52.06
  nourishment T73.0 ☑
  pancreatic K86.89
    exocrine K86.81
  parathyroid (gland) E20.9
  peripheral vascular (arterial) I73.9
  pituitary E23.0
  placental (mother) O36.51- ☑
  platelets D69.6
  prenatal care affecting management of pregnancy O09.3- ☑
  progressive pluriglandular E31.0
  pulmonary J98.4
    acute, following surgery (nonthoracic) J95.2
      thoracic J95.1
    chronic, following surgery J95.3
    following
      shock J98.4
      trauma J98.4
    newborn P28.89
    valve I37.1
      with stenosis I37.2
      congenital Q22.2
      rheumatic I09.89
        with aortic, mitral or tricuspid (valve) disease I08.8
  pyloric K31.89
  renal (acute) N28.9
    chronic N18.9
  respiratory R06.89
    newborn P28.5
  rotation — see Malrotation
  sleep syndrome F51.12
  social insurance Z59.7
  suprarenal E27.40
    primary E27.1
  tarso-orbital fascia, congenital Q10.3
  testis E29.1
  thyroid (gland) (acquired) E03.9
    congenital E03.1
  tricuspid (valve) (rheumatic) I07.1
    with
      aortic (valve) disease I08.2
        with mitral (valve) disease I08.3
      mitral (valve) disease I08.1
        with aortic (valve) disease I08.3
      obstruction or stenosis I07.2
        with aortic (valve) disease I08.2
          with mitral (valve) disease I08.3
    congenital Q22.8
    nonrheumatic I36.1
      with stenosis I36.2
  urethral sphincter R32
  valve, valvular (heart) I38
    aortic — see Insufficiency, aortic (valve)
    congenital Q24.8
    mitral — see Insufficiency, mitral (valve)
    pulmonary — see Insufficiency, pulmonary, valve

Insufficiency, insufficient — *continued*
  valve, valvular — *continued*
    tricuspid — *see* Insufficiency, tricuspid (valve)
  vascular I99.8
    intestine K55.9
      acute — *see also* Ischemia, intestine, acute
        K55.059
    mesenteric K55.1
    peripheral I73.9
    renal — *see* Hypertension, kidney
  velopharyngeal
    acquired K13.79
    congenital Q38.8
  venous (chronic) (peripheral) I87.2
  ventricular — *see* Insufficiency, myocardial
  welfare support Z59.7
Insufflation, fallopian Z31.41
Insular — *see* condition
Insulinoma
  pancreas
    benign D13.7
    malignant C25.4
    uncertain behavior D37.8
  specified site
    benign — *see* Neoplasm, by site, benign
    malignant — *see* Neoplasm, by site, malignant
    uncertain behavior — *see* Neoplasm, by site, uncertain behavior
  unspecified site
    benign D13.7
    malignant C25.4
    uncertain behavior D37.8
Insuloma — *see* Insulinoma
Interference
  balancing side M26.56
  non-working side M26.56
Intermenstrual — *see* condition
Intermittent — *see* condition
Internal — *see* condition
Interrogation
  cardiac defibrillator (automatic) (implantable) Z45.02
  cardiac pacemaker Z45.018
  cardiac (event) (loop) recorder Z45.09
  infusion pump (implanted) (intrathecal) Z45.1
  neurostimulator Z46.2
Interruption
  aortic arch Q25.21
  bundle of His I44.30
  phase-shift, sleep cycle — *see* Disorder, sleep, circadian rhythm
  sleep phase-shift, or 24 hour sleep-wake cycle — *see* Disorder, sleep, circadian rhythm
Interstitial — *see* condition
Intertrigo L30.4
  labialis K13.0
Intervertebral disc — *see* condition
Intestine, intestinal — *see* condition
Intolerance
  carbohydrate K90.49
  disaccharide, hereditary E73.0
  fat NEC K90.49
    pancreatic K90.3
  food K90.49
    dietary counseling and surveillance Z71.3
  fructose E74.10
    hereditary E74.12
  glucose (-galactose) E74.39
  gluten K90.41
  lactose E73.9
    specified NEC E73.8
  lysine E72.3
  milk NEC K90.49
    lactose E73.9
  protein K90.49
  starch NEC K90.49
  sucrose (-isomaltose) E74.31
Intoxicated NEC (without dependence) — *see* Alcohol, intoxication
Intoxication
  acid E87.2
  alcoholic (acute) (without dependence) — *see* Alcohol, intoxication
  alimentary canal K52.1
  amphetamine (without dependence) — *see also* Abuse, drug, stimulant, with intoxication
    with dependence — *see* Dependence, drug, stimulant, with intoxication
      stimulant NEC F15.10

Intoxication — *continued*
  amphetamine — *see also* Abuse, drug, stimulant, with intoxication — *continued*
    stimulant — *continued*
      with
        anxiety disorder F15.180
        intoxication F15.129
          with
            delirium F15.121
            perceptual disturbance F15.122
  anxiolytic (acute) (without dependence) — *see* Abuse, drug, sedative, with intoxication
    with dependence — *see* Dependence, drug, sedative, with intoxication
  caffeine F15.929
    with dependence — *see* Dependence, drug, stimulant, with intoxication
  cannabinoids (acute) (without dependence) — *see* Use, cannabis, with intoxication
    with
      abuse — *see* Abuse, drug, cannabis, with intoxication
      dependence — *see* Dependence, drug, cannabis, with intoxication
  chemical — *see* Table of Drugs and Chemicals
    via placenta or breast milk — *see* - Absorption, chemical, through placenta
  cocaine (acute) (without dependence) — *see* Abuse, drug, cocaine, with intoxication
    with dependence — *see* Dependence, drug, cocaine, with intoxication
  drug
    acute (without dependence) — *see* Abuse, drug, by type with intoxication
      with dependence — *see* Dependence, drug, by type with intoxication
    addictive
      via placenta or breast milk — *see* Absorption, drug, addictive, through placenta
    newborn P93.8
      gray baby syndrome P93.0
    overdose or wrong substance given or taken — *see* Table of Drugs and Chemicals, by drug, poisoning
  enteric K52.1
  foodborne A05.9
    bacterial A05.9
    classical (Clostridium botulinum) A05.1
    due to
      Bacillus cereus A05.4
      bacterium A05.9
        specified NEC A05.8
      Clostridium
        botulinum A05.1
        perfringens A05.2
        welchii A05.2
      Salmonella A02.9
        with
          (gastro)enteritis A02.0
          localized infection(s) A02.20
            arthritis A02.23
            meningitis A02.21
            osteomyelitis A02.24
            pneumonia A02.22
            pyelonephritis A02.25
            specified NEC A02.29
          sepsis A02.1
          specified manifestation NEC A02.8
      Staphylococcus A05.0
      Vibrio
        parahaemolyticus A05.3
        vulnificus A05.5
    enterotoxin, staphylococcal A05.0
    noxious — *see* Poisoning, food, noxious
  gastrointestinal K52.1
  hallucinogenic (without dependence) — *see* Abuse, drug, hallucinogen, with intoxication
    with dependence — *see* Dependence, drug, hallucinogen, with intoxication
  hypnotic (acute) (without dependence) — *see* Abuse, drug, sedative, with intoxication
    with dependence — *see* Dependence, drug, sedative, with intoxication
  inhalant (acute) (without dependence) — *see* Abuse, drug, inhalant, with intoxication
    with dependence — *see* Dependence, drug, inhalant, with intoxication

Intoxication — *continued*
  meaning
    inebriation — *see* category F10 ☑
    poisoning — *see* Table of Drugs and Chemicals
  methyl alcohol (acute) (without dependence) — *see* Alcohol, intoxication
  opioid (acute) (without dependence) — *see* Abuse, drug, opioid, with intoxication
    with dependence — *see* Dependence, drug, opioid, with intoxication
  pathologic NEC (without dependence) — *see* Alcohol, intoxication
  phencyclidine (without dependence) — *see* Abuse, drug, hallucinogen, with intoxication
    with dependence — *see* Dependence, drug, hallucinogen, with intoxication
  potassium (K) E87.5
  psychoactive substance NEC (without dependence) — *see* Abuse, drug, psychoactive NEC, with intoxication
    with dependence — *see* Dependence, drug, psychoactive NEC, with intoxication
  sedative (acute) (without dependence) — *see* Abuse, drug, sedative, with intoxication
    with dependence — *see* Dependence, drug, sedative, with intoxication
  serum — *see also* Reaction, serum T80.69 ☑
  uremic — *see* Uremia
  volatile solvents (acute) (without dependence) — *see* Abuse, drug, inhalant, with intoxication
    with dependence — *see* Dependence, drug, inhalant, with intoxication
  water E87.79
Intraabdominal testis, testes
  bilateral Q53.211
  unilateral Q53.111
Intracranial — *see* condition
Intrahepatic gallbladder Q44.1
Intraligamentous — *see* condition
Intrathoracic — *see also* condition
  kidney Q63.2
Intrauterine contraceptive device
  checking Z30.431
  in situ Z97.5
  insertion Z30.430
    immediately following removal Z30.433
  management Z30.431
  reinsertion Z30.433
  removal Z30.432
  replacement Z30.433
  retention in pregnancy O26.3- ☑
Intraventricular — *see* condition
Intrinsic deformity — *see* Deformity
Intubation, difficult or failed T88.4 ☑
Intumescence, lens (eye) (cataract) — *see* Cataract
Intussusception (bowel) (colon) (enteric) (ileocecal) (ileocolic) (intestine) (rectum) K56.1
  appendix K38.8
  congenital Q43.8
  ureter (with obstruction) N13.5
Invagination (bowel, colon, intestine or rectum) K56.1
Inversion
  albumin-globulin (A-G) ratio E88.09
  bladder N32.89
  cecum — *see* Intussusception
  cervix N88.8
  chromosome in normal individual Q95.1
  circadian rhythm — *see* Disorder, sleep, circadian rhythm
  nipple N64.59
    congenital Q83.8
    gestational — *see* Retraction, nipple
    puerperal, postpartum — *see* Retraction, nipple
  nyctohemeral rhythm — *see* Disorder, sleep, circadian rhythm
  optic papilla Q14.2
  organ or site, congenital NEC — *see* Anomaly, by site
  sleep rhythm — *see* Disorder, sleep, circadian rhythm
  testis (congenital) Q55.29
  uterus (chronic) (postinfectional) (postpartal, old) N85.5
    postpartum O71.2
  vagina (posthysterectomy) N99.3
  ventricular Q20.5
Investigation — *see also* Examination Z04.9
  clinical research subject (control) (normal comparison) (participant) Z00.6
Involuntary movement, abnormal R25.9

☑ **Additional Character Required — Refer to the Tabular List for Character Selection**   ▽ **Subterms under main terms may continue to next column or page**

Involution, involutional — see also condition
  breast, cystic — see Dysplasia, mammary, specified
      type NEC
  depression (single episode) F32.89
    recurrent episode F33.9
  melancholia (single episode) F32.89
    recurrent episode F33.8
  ovary, senile — see Atrophy, ovary
  thymus failure E32.8
I.Q.
  20-34 F72
  35-49 F71
  50-69 F70
  under 20 F73
IRDS (type I) P22.0
  type II P22.1
Irideremia Q13.1
Iridis rubeosis — see Disorder, iris, vascular
Iridochoroiditis (panuveitis) — see Panuveitis
Iridocyclitis H20.9
  acute H20.0- ☑
    hypopyon H20.05- ☑
    primary H20.01- ☑
    recurrent H20.02- ☑
    secondary (noninfectious) H20.04- ☑
      infectious H20.03- ☑
  chronic H20.1- ☑
  due to allergy — see Iridocyclitis, acute, secondary
  endogenous — see Iridocyclitis, acute, primary
  Fuchs' — see Cyclitis, Fuchs' heterochromic
  gonococcal A54.32
  granulomatous — see Iridocyclitis, chronic
  herpes, herpetic (simplex) B00.51
    zoster B02.32
  hypopyon — see Iridocyclitis, acute, hypopyon
  in (due to)
    ankylosing spondylitis M45.9
    gonococcal infection A54.32
    herpes (simplex) virus B00.51
      zoster B02.32
    infectious disease NOS B99 ☑
    parasitic disease NOS B89 [H22]
    sarcoidosis D86.83
    syphilis A51.43
    tuberculosis A18.54
    zoster B02.32
  lens-induced H20.2- ☑
  nongranulomatous — see Iridocyclitis, acute
  recurrent — see Iridocyclitis, acute, recurrent
  rheumatic — see Iridocyclitis, chronic
  subacute — see Iridocyclitis, acute
  sympathetic — see Uveitis, sympathetic
  syphilitic (secondary) A51.43
  tuberculous (chronic) A18.54
  Vogt-Koyanagi H20.82- ☑
Iridocyclochoroiditis (panuveitis) — see Panuveitis
Iridodialysis H21.53- ☑
Iridodonesis H21.89
Iridoplegia (complete) (partial) (reflex) H57.09
Iridoschisis H21.25- ☑
Iris — see also condition
  bombé — see Membrane, pupillary
Iritis — see also Iridocyclitis
  chronic — see Iridocyclitis, chronic
  diabetic — see E08-E13 with .39
  due to
    herpes simplex B00.51
    leprosy A30.9 [H22]
  gonococcal A54.32
  gouty — see also Gout, by type M10.9 [H22]
  granulomatous — see Iridocyclitis, chronic
  lens induced — see Iridocyclitis, lens-induced
  papulosa (syphilitic) A52.71
  rheumatic — see Iridocyclitis, chronic
  syphilitic (secondary) A51.43
    congenital (early) A50.01
    late A52.71
  tuberculous A18.54
Iron — see condition
Iron-miner's lung J63.4
Irradiated enamel (tooth, teeth) K03.89
Irradiation effects, adverse T66 ☑
Irreducible, irreducibility — see condition
Irregular, irregularity
  action, heart I49.9
  alveolar process K08.89
  bleeding N92.6

Irregular, irregularity — continued
  breathing R06.89
  contour of cornea (acquired) — see Deformity, cornea
    congenital Q13.4
  contour, reconstructed breast N65.0
  dentin (in pulp) K04.3
  eye movements H55.89
    nystagmus — see Nystagmus
    saccadic H55.81
  labor O62.2
  menstruation (cause unknown) N92.6
  periods N92.6
  prostate N42.9
  pupil — see Abnormality, pupillary
  reconstructed breast N65.0
  respiratory R06.89
  septum (nasal) J34.2
  shape, organ or site, congenital NEC — see Distortion
  sleep-wake pattern (rhythm) G47.23
Irritable, irritability R45.4
  bladder N32.89
  bowel (syndrome) K58.9
    with
      constipation K58.1
      diarrhea K58.0
      mixed K58.2
      psychogenic F45.8
      specified NEC K58.8
  bronchial — see Bronchitis
  cerebral, in newborn P91.3
  colon — see also Irritable, bowel K58.9
    with diarrhea K58.0
    psychogenic F45.8
  duodenum K59.8
  heart (psychogenic) F45.8
  hip — see Derangement, joint, specified type NEC, hip
  ileum K59.8
  infant R68.12
  jejunum K59.8
  rectum K59.8
  stomach K31.89
    psychogenic F45.8
  sympathetic G90.8
  urethra N36.8
Irritation
  anus K62.89
  axillary nerve G54.0
  bladder N32.89
  brachial plexus G54.0
  bronchial — see Bronchitis
  cervical plexus G54.2
  cervix — see Cervicitis
  choroid, sympathetic — see Endophthalmitis
  cranial nerve — see Disorder, nerve, cranial
  gastric K31.89
    psychogenic F45.8
  globe, sympathetic — see Uveitis, sympathetic
  labyrinth — see subcategory H83.2 ☑
  lumbosacral plexus G54.1
  meninges (traumatic) — see Injury, intracranial
    nontraumatic — see Meningismus
  nerve — see Disorder, nerve
  nervous R45.0
  penis N48.89
  perineum NEC L29.3
  peripheral autonomic nervous system G90.8
  peritoneum — see Peritonitis
  pharynx J39.2
  plantar nerve — see Lesion, nerve, plantar
  spinal (cord) (traumatic) — see also Injury, spinal cord,
    by region
    nerve G58.9
      root NEC — see Radiculopathy
    nontraumatic — see Myelopathy
  stomach K31.89
    psychogenic F45.8
  sympathetic nerve NEC G90.8
  ulnar nerve — see Lesion, nerve, ulnar
  vagina N89.8
Ischemia, ischemic I99.8
  bowel (transient)
    acute — see also Ischemia, intestine, acute K55.059
    chronic K55.1
    due to mesenteric artery insufficiency K55.1
  brain — see Ischemia, cerebral
  cardiac (see Disease, heart, ischemic)
  cardiomyopathy I25.5
  cerebral (chronic) (generalized) I67.82

Ischemia, ischemic — continued
  cerebral — continued
    arteriosclerotic I67.2
    intermittent G45.9
    newborn P91.0
    recurrent focal G45.8
    transient G45.9
  colon chronic (due to mesenteric artery insufficiency)
    K55.1
  coronary — see Disease, heart, ischemic
  demand (coronary) — see also Angina I24.8
    with myocardial infarction I21.A1
    resulting in myocardial infarction I21.A1
  heart (chronic or with a stated duration of over 4 weeks)
    I25.9
    acute or with a stated duration of 4 weeks or less
      I24.9
    subacute I24.9
  infarction, muscle — see Infarct, muscle
  intestine (large) (small) (transient) K55.9
    acute K55.059
      diffuse K55.052
      focal K55.051
      large K55.039
        diffuse K55.032
        focal K55.031
      small K55.019
        diffuse K55.012
        focal K55.011
    chronic K55.1
    due to mesenteric artery insufficiency K55.1
  kidney N28.0
  mesenteric, acute — see also Ischemia, intestine, acute
    K55.059
  muscle, traumatic T79.6 ☑
  myocardium, myocardial (chronic or with a stated du-
    ration of over 4 weeks) I25.9
    acute, without myocardial infarction I51.3
    silent (asymptomatic) I25.6
    transient of newborn P29.4
  renal N28.0
  retina, retinal — see Occlusion, artery, retina
  small bowel
    acute K55.019
      diffuse K55.012
      focal K55.011
    chronic K55.1
    due to mesenteric artery insufficiency K55.1
  spinal cord G95.11
  subendocardial — see Insufficiency, coronary
  supply (coronary) — see also Angina I25.9
    due to vasospasm I20.1
Ischial spine — see condition
Ischialgia — see Sciatica
Ischiopagus Q89.4
Ischium, ischial — see condition
Ischuria R34
Iselin's disease or osteochondrosis — see Osteochon-
  drosis, juvenile, metatarsus
Islands of
  parotid tissue in
    lymph nodes Q38.6
    neck structures Q38.6
  submaxillary glands in
    fascia Q38.6
    lymph nodes Q38.6
    neck muscles Q38.6
Islet cell tumor, pancreas D13.7
Isoimmunization NEC — see also Incompatibility
  affecting management of pregnancy (ABO) (with hy-
    drops fetalis) O36.11- ☑
    anti-A sensitization O36.11- ☑
    anti-B sensitization O36.19- ☑
    anti-c sensitization O36.09- ☑
    anti-C sensitization O36.09- ☑
    anti-e sensitization O36.09- ☑
    anti-E sensitization O36.09- ☑
    Rh NEC O36.09- ☑
      anti-D antibody O36.01- ☑
    specified NEC O36.19- ☑
  newborn P55.9
    with
      hydrops fetalis P56.0
      kernicterus P57.0
    ABO (blood groups) P55.1
    Rhesus (Rh) factor P55.0
    specified type NEC P55.8

Isolation, isolated
- dwelling Z59.8
- family Z63.79
- social Z60.4

Isoleucinosis E71.19

Isomerism atrial appendages (with asplenia or polysplenia) Q20.6

Isosporiasis, isosporosis A07.3

Isovaleric acidemia E71.110

Issue of
- medical certificate Z02.79
  - for disability determination Z02.71
- repeat prescription (appliance) (glasses) (medicinal substance, medicament, medicine) Z76.0
  - contraception — see Contraception

Itch, itching — see also Pruritus
- baker's L23.6
- barber's B35.0
- bricklayer's L24.5
- cheese B88.0
- clam digger's B65.3
- coolie B76.9
- copra B88.0
- dew B76.9
- dhobi B35.6
- filarial — see Infestation, filarial
- grain B88.0
- grocer's B88.0
- ground B76.9
- harvest B88.0
- jock B35.6
- Malabar B35.5
  - beard B35.0
  - foot B35.3
  - scalp B35.0
- meaning scabies B86
- Norwegian B86
- perianal L29.0
- poultrymen's B88.0
- sarcoptic B86
- scabies B86
- scrub B88.0
- straw B88.0
- swimmer's B65.3
- water B76.9
- winter L29.8

Ivemark's syndrome (asplenia with congenital heart disease) Q89.01

Ivory bones Q78.2

Ixodiasis NEC B88.8

J

Jaccoud's syndrome — see Arthropathy, postrheumatic, chronic

Jackson's
- membrane Q43.3
- paralysis or syndrome G83.89
- veil Q43.3

Jacquet's dermatitis (diaper dermatitis) L22

Jadassohn-Pellizari's disease or anetoderma L90.2

Jadassohn's
- blue nevus — see Nevus
- intraepidermal epithelioma — see Neoplasm, skin, benign

Jaffe-Lichtenstein (-Uehlinger) **syndrome** — see Dysplasia, fibrous, bone NEC

Jakob-Creutzfeldt disease or syndrome — see Creutzfeldt-Jakob disease or syndrome

Jaksch-Luzet disease D64.89

Jamaican
- neuropathy G92
- paraplegic tropical ataxic-spastic syndrome G92

Janet's disease F48.8

Janiceps Q89.4

Jansky-Bielschowsky amaurotic idiocy E75.4

Japanese
- B-type encephalitis A83.0
- river fever A75.3

Jaundice (yellow) R17
- acholuric (familial) (splenomegalic) — see also Spherocytosis
  - acquired D59.8
- breast-milk (inhibitor) P59.3
- catarrhal (acute) B15.9
  - with hepatic coma B15.0
- cholestatic (benign) R17

Jaundice — continued
- due to or associated with
  - delayed conjugation P59.8
    - associated with (due to) preterm delivery P59.0
  - preterm delivery P59.0
- epidemic (catarrhal) B15.9
  - with hepatic coma B15.0
  - leptospiral A27.0
  - spirochetal A27.0
- familial nonhemolytic (congenital) (Gilbert) E80.4
  - Crigler-Najjar E80.5
- febrile (acute) B15.9
  - with hepatic coma B15.0
  - leptospiral A27.0
  - spirochetal A27.0
- hematogenous D59.9
- hemolytic (acquired) D59.9
  - congenital — see Spherocytosis
- hemorrhagic (acute) (leptospiral) (spirochetal) A27.0
- infectious (acute) (subacute) B15.9
  - with hepatic coma B15.0
  - leptospiral A27.0
  - spirochetal A27.0
- leptospiral (hemorrhagic) A27.0
- malignant (without coma) K72.90
  - with coma K72.91
- neonatal — see Jaundice, newborn
- newborn P59.9
  - due to or associated with
    - ABO
      - antibodies P55.1
      - incompatibility, maternal/fetal P55.1
      - isoimmunization P55.1
    - absence or deficiency of enzyme system for bilirubin conjugation (congenital) P59.8
    - bleeding P58.1
    - breast milk inhibitors to conjugation P59.3
      - associated with preterm delivery P59.0
    - bruising P58.0
    - Crigler-Najjar syndrome E80.5
    - delayed conjugation P59.8
      - associated with preterm delivery P59.0
    - drugs or toxins
      - given to newborn P58.42
      - transmitted from mother P58.41
    - excessive hemolysis P58.9
      - due to
        - bleeding P58.1
        - bruising P58.0
        - drugs or toxins
          - given to newborn P58.42
          - transmitted from mother P58.41
        - infection P58.2
        - polycythemia P58.3
        - swallowed maternal blood P58.5
      - specified type NEC P58.8
    - galactosemia E74.21
    - Gilbert syndrome E80.4
    - hemolytic disease P55.9
      - ABO isoimmunization P55.1
      - Rh isoimmunization P55.0
      - specified NEC P55.8
    - hepatocellular damage P59.20
      - specified NEC P59.29
    - hereditary hemolytic anemia P58.8
    - hypothyroidism, congenital E03.1
    - incompatibility, maternal/fetal NOS P55.9
    - infection P58.2
    - inspissated bile syndrome P59.1
    - isoimmunization NOS P55.9
    - mucoviscidosis E84.9
    - polycythemia P58.3
    - preterm delivery P59.0
    - Rh
      - antibodies P55.0
      - incompatibility, maternal/fetal P55.0
      - isoimmunization P55.0
    - specified cause NEC P59.8
    - swallowed maternal blood P58.5
  - spherocytosis (congenital) D58.0
- nonhemolytic congenital familial (Gilbert) E80.4
- nuclear, newborn — see also Kernicterus of newborn P57.9
- obstructive — see also Obstruction, bile duct K83.1
- post-immunization — see Hepatitis, viral, type, B
- post-transfusion — see Hepatitis, viral, type, B
- regurgitation — see also Obstruction, bile duct K83.1

Jaundice — continued
- serum (homologous) (prophylactic) (therapeutic) — see Hepatitis, viral, type, B
- spirochetal (hemorrhagic) A27.0
- symptomatic R17
  - newborn P59.9

Jaw — see condition

Jaw-winking phenomenon or syndrome Q07.8

Jealousy
- alcoholic F10.988
- childhood F93.8
- sibling F93.8

Jejunitis — see Enteritis

Jejunostomy status Z93.4

Jejunum, jejunal — see condition

Jensen's disease — see Inflammation, chorioretinal, focal, juxtapapillary

Jerks, myoclonic G25.3

Jervell-Lange-Nielsen syndrome I45.81

Jeune's disease Q77.2

Jigger disease B88.1

Job's syndrome (chronic granulomatous disease) D71

Joint — see also condition
- mice — see Loose, body, joint
  - knee M23.4- ☑

Jordan's anomaly or syndrome D72.0

Joseph-Diamond-Blackfan anemia (congenital hypoplastic) D61.01

Jungle yellow fever A95.0

Jüngling's disease — see Sarcoidosis

Juvenile — see condition

K

Kahler's disease C90.0- ☑

Kakke E51.11

Kala-azar B55.0

Kallmann's syndrome E23.0

Kanner's syndrome (autism) — see Psychosis, childhood

Kaposi's
- dermatosis (xeroderma pigmentosum) Q82.1
- lichen ruber L44.0
  - acuminatus L44.0
- sarcoma
  - colon C46.4
  - connective tissue C46.1
  - gastrointestinal organ C46.4
  - lung C46.5- ☑
  - lymph node (multiple) C46.3
  - palate (hard) (soft) C46.2
  - rectum C46.4
  - skin (multiple sites) C46.0
  - specified site NEC C46.7
  - stomach C46.4
  - unspecified site C46.9
- varicelliform eruption B00.0
  - vaccinia T88.1 ☑

Kartagener's syndrome or triad (sinusitis, bronchiectasis, situs inversus) Q89.3

Karyotype
- with abnormality except iso (Xq) Q96.2
- 45,X Q96.0
- 46,X
  - iso (Xq) Q96.1
- 46,XX Q98.3
  - with streak gonads Q50.32
  - hermaphrodite (true) Q99.1
  - male Q98.3
- 46,XY
  - with streak gonads Q56.1
  - female Q97.3
  - hermaphrodite (true) Q99.1
- 47,XXX Q97.0
- 47,XXY Q98.0
- 47,XYY Q98.5

Kaschin-Beck disease — see Disease, Kaschin-Beck

Katayama's disease or fever B65.2

Kawasaki's syndrome M30.3

Kayser-Fleischer ring (cornea) (pseudosclerosis) H18.04- ☑

Kaznelson's syndrome (congenital hypoplastic anemia) D61.01

Kearns-Sayre syndrome H49.81- ☑

Kedani fever A75.3

Kelis L91.0

Kelly (-Patterson) **syndrome** (sideropenic dysphagia) D50.1

Keloid, cheloid L91.0
  acne L73.0
  Addison's L94.0
  cornea — see Opacity, cornea
  Hawkin's L91.0
  scar L91.0
Keloma L91.0
Kenya fever A77.1
Keratectasia — see also Ectasia, cornea
  congenital Q13.4
Keratinization of alveolar ridge mucosa
  excessive K13.23
  minimal K13.22
Keratinized residual ridge mucosa
  excessive K13.23
  minimal K13.22
Keratitis (nodular) (nonulcerative) (simple) (zonular) H16.9
  with ulceration (central) (marginal) (perforated) (ring) — see Ulcer, cornea
  actinic — see Photokeratitis
  arborescens (herpes simplex) B00.52
  areolar H16.1- ☑
  bullosa H16.8
  deep H16.309
    specified type NEC H16.399
  dendritic (a) (herpes simplex) B00.52
  disciform (is) (herpes simplex) B00.52
    varicella B01.81
  filamentary H16.12- ☑
  gonococcal (congenital or prenatal) A54.33
  herpes, herpetic (simplex) B00.52
    zoster B02.33
  in (due to)
    acanthamebiasis B60.13
    adenovirus B30.0
    exanthema — see also Exanthem B09
    herpes (simplex) virus B00.52
    measles B05.81
    syphilis A50.31
    tuberculosis A18.52
    zoster B02.33
  interstitial (nonsyphilitic) H16.30- ☑
    diffuse H16.32- ☑
    herpes, herpetic (simplex) B00.52
      zoster B02.33
    sclerosing H16.33- ☑
    specified type NEC H16.39- ☑
    syphilitic (congenital) (late) A50.31
    tuberculous A18.52
  macular H16.11- ☑
  nummular H16.11- ☑
  oyster shuckers' H16.8
  parenchymatous — see Keratitis, interstitial
  petrificans H16.8
  postmeasles B05.81
  punctata
    leprosa A30.9 [H16.14-] ☑
    syphilitic (profunda) A50.31
  punctate H16.14- ☑
  purulent H16.8
  rosacea L71.8
  sclerosing H16.33- ☑
  specified type NEC H16.8
  stellate H16.11- ☑
  striate H16.11- ☑
  superficial H16.10- ☑
    with conjunctivitis — see Keratoconjunctivitis
    due to light — see Photokeratitis
  suppurative H16.8
  syphilitic (congenital) (prenatal) A50.31
  trachomatous A71.1
    sequelae B94.0
  tuberculous A18.52
  vesicular H16.8
  xerotic — see also Keratomalacia H16.8
    vitamin A deficiency E50.4
Keratoacanthoma L85.8
Keratocele — see Descemetocele
Keratoconjunctivitis H16.20- ☑
  Acanthamoeba B60.13
  adenoviral B30.0
  epidemic B30.0
  exposure H16.21- ☑
  herpes, herpetic (simplex) B00.52
    zoster B02.33
  in exanthema — see also Exanthem B09
  infectious B30.0

Keratoconjunctivitis — continued
  lagophthalmic — see Keratoconjunctivitis, specified type NEC
  neurotrophic H16.23- ☑
  phlyctenular H16.25- ☑
  postmeasles B05.81
  shipyard B30.0
  sicca (Sjogren's) M35.0- ☑
    not Sjogren's H16.22- ☑
  specified type NEC H16.29- ☑
  tuberculous (phlyctenular) A18.52
  vernal H16.26- ☑
Keratoconus H18.60- ☑
  congenital Q13.4
  stable H18.61- ☑
  unstable H18.62- ☑
Keratocyst (dental) (odontogenic) — see Cyst, calcifying odontogenic
Keratoderma, keratodermia (congenital) (palmaris et plantaris) (symmetrical) Q82.8
  acquired L85.1
    in diseases classified elsewhere L86
  climactericum L85.1
  gonococcal A54.89
  gonorrheal A54.89
  punctata L85.2
  Reiter's — see Reiter's disease
Keratodermatocele — see Descemetocele
Keratoglobus H18.79 ☑
  congenital Q15.8
    with glaucoma Q15.0
Keratohemia — see Pigmentation, cornea, stromal
Keratoiritis — see also Iridocyclitis
  syphilitic A50.39
  tuberculous A18.54
Keratoma L57.0
  palmaris and plantaris hereditarium Q82.8
  senile L57.0
Keratomalacia H18.44- ☑
  vitamin A deficiency E50.4
Keratomegaly Q13.4
Keratomycosis B49
  nigrans, nigricans (palmaris) B36.1
Keratopathy H18.9
  band H18.42- ☑
  bullous (aphakic), following cataract surgery H59.01- ☑
  bullous H18.1- ☑
Keratoscleritis, tuberculous A18.52
Keratosis L57.0
  actinic L57.0
  arsenical L85.8
  congenital, specified NEC Q80.8
  female genital NEC N94.89
  follicularis Q82.8
    acquired L11.0
    congenita Q82.8
    et parafollicularis in cutem penetrans L87.0
    spinulosa (decalvans) Q82.8
    vitamin A deficiency E50.8
  gonococcal A54.89
  male genital (external) N50.89
  nigricans L83
  obturans, external ear (canal) — see Cholesteatoma, external ear
  palmaris et plantaris (inherited) (symmetrical) Q82.8
    acquired L85.1
  penile N48.89
  pharynx J39.2
  pilaris, acquired L85.8
  punctata (palmaris et plantaris) L85.2
  scrotal N50.89
  seborrheic L82.1
    inflamed L82.0
  senile L57.0
  solar L57.0
  tonsillaris J35.8
  vagina N89.4
  vegetans Q82.8
  vitamin A deficiency E50.8
  vocal cord J38.3
Kerato-uveitis — see Iridocyclitis
Kerion (celsi) B35.0
Kernicterus of newborn (not due to isoimmunization) P57.9
  due to isoimmunization (conditions in P55.0-P55.9) P57.0
  specified type NEC P57.8
Kerunoparalysis T75.09 ☑

Keshan disease E59
Ketoacidosis E87.2
  diabetic — see Diabetes, by type, with ketoacidosis
Ketonuria R82.4
Ketosis NEC E88.89
  diabetic — see Diabetes, by type, with ketoacidosis
Kew Garden fever A79.1
Kidney — see condition
Kienböck's disease — see also Osteochondrosis, juvenile, hand, carpal lunate
  adult M93.1
Kimmelstiel (-Wilson) disease — see Diabetes, Kimmelstiel (-Wilson) disease
Kink, kinking
  artery I77.1
  hair (acquired) L67.8
  ileum or intestine — see Obstruction, intestine
  Lane's — see Obstruction, intestine
  organ or site, congenital NEC — see Anomaly, by site
  ureter (pelvic junction) N13.5
    with
      hydronephrosis N13.1
        with infection N13.6
      pyelonephritis (chronic) N11.1
    congenital Q62.39
  vein(s) I87.8
    caval I87.1
    peripheral I87.1
Kinnier Wilson's disease (hepatolenticular degeneration) E83.01
Kissing spine M48.20
  cervical region M48.22
  cervicothoracic region M48.23
  lumbar region M48.26
  lumbosacral region M48.27
  occipito-atlanto-axial region M48.21
  thoracic region M48.24
  thoracolumbar region M48.25
Klatskin's tumor C22.1
Klauder's disease A26.8
Klebs' disease — see also Glomerulonephritis N05- ☑
Klebsiella (K.) pneumoniae, as cause of disease classified elsewhere B96.1
Klein (e)-Levin syndrome G47.13
Kleptomania F63.2
Klinefelter's syndrome Q98.4
  karyotype 47,XXY Q98.0
  male with more than two X chromosomes Q98.1
Klippel-Feil deficiency, disease, or syndrome (brevicollis) Q76.1
Klippel's disease I67.2
Klippel-Trenaunay (-Weber) syndrome Q87.2
Klumpke (-Déjerine) palsy, paralysis (birth) (newborn) P14.1
Knee — see condition
Knock knee (acquired) M21.06- ☑
  congenital Q74.1
Knot(s)
  intestinal, syndrome (volvulus) K56.2
  surfer S89.8- ☑
  umbilical cord (true) O69.2 ☑
Knotting (of)
  hair L67.8
  intestine K56.2
Knuckle pad (Garrod's) M72.1
Koch's
  infection — see Tuberculosis
  relapsing fever A68.9
Koch-Weeks' conjunctivitis — see Conjunctivitis, acute, mucopurulent
Köebner's syndrome Q81.8
Köenig's disease (osteochondritis dissecans) — see Osteochondritis, dissecans
Köhler-Pellegrini-Steida disease or syndrome (calcification, knee joint) — see Bursitis, tibial collateral
Köhler's disease
  patellar — see Osteochondrosis, juvenile, patella
  tarsal navicular — see Osteochondrosis, juvenile, tarsus
Koilonychia L60.3
  congenital Q84.6
Kojevnikov's, epilepsy — see Kozhevnikof's epilepsy
Koplik's spots B05.9
Kopp's asthma E32.8
Korsakoff's (Wernicke) disease, psychosis or syndrome (alcoholic) F10.96
  with dependence F10.26

Korsakoff's (Wernicke) **disease, psychosis or syndrome** — *continued*
  drug-induced
    due to drug abuse — *see* Abuse, drug, by type, with amnestic disorder
    due to drug dependence — *see* Dependence, drug, by type, with amnestic disorder
  nonalcoholic F04
Korsakov's disease, psychosis or syndrome — *see* Korsakoff's disease
Korsakow's disease, psychosis or syndrome — *see* Korsakoff's disease
Kostmann's disease or syndrome (infantile genetic agranulocytosis) — *see* Agranulocytosis
Kozhevnikof's epilepsy G40.109
  intractable G40.119
    with status epilepticus G40.111
    without status epilepticus G40.119
  not intractable G40.109
    with status epilepticus G40.101
    without status epilepticus G40.109
Krabbe's
  disease E75.23
  syndrome, congenital muscle hypoplasia Q79.8
Kraepelin-Morel disease — *see* Schizophrenia
Kraft-Weber-Dimitri disease Q85.8
Kraurosis
  ani K62.89
  penis N48.0
  vagina N89.8
  vulva N90.4
Kreotoxism A05.9
Krukenberg's
  spindle — *see* Pigmentation, cornea, posterior
  tumor C79.6- ☑
Kufs' disease E75.4
Kugelberg-Welander disease G12.1
Kuhnt-Junius degeneration — *see also* Degeneration, macula H35.32- ☑
Kümmell's disease or spondylitis — *see* Spondylopathy, traumatic
Kupffer cell sarcoma C22.3
Kuru A81.81
Kussmaul's
  disease M30.0
  respiration E87.2
    in diabetic acidosis — *see* Diabetes, by type, with ketoacidosis
Kwashiorkor E40
  marasmic, marasmus type E42
Kyasanur Forest disease A98.2
Kyphoscoliosis, kyphoscoliotic (acquired) — *see also* Scoliosis M41.9
  congenital Q67.5
  heart (disease) I27.1
  sequelae of rickets E64.3
  tuberculous A18.01
Kyphosis, kyphotic (acquired) M40.209
  cervical region M40.202
  cervicothoracic region M40.203
  congenital Q76.419
    cervical region Q76.412
    cervicothoracic region Q76.413
    occipito-atlanto-axial region Q76.411
    thoracic region Q76.414
    thoracolumbar region Q76.415
  Morquio-Brailsford type (spinal) — *see also* subcategory M49.8 E76.219
  postlaminectomy M96.3
  postradiation therapy M96.2
  postural (adolescent) M40.00
    cervicothoracic region M40.03
    thoracic region M40.04
    thoracolumbar region M40.05
  secondary NEC M40.10
    cervical region M40.12
    cervicothoracic region M40.13
    thoracic region M40.14
    thoracolumbar region M40.15
  sequelae of rickets E64.3
  specified type NEC M40.299
    cervical region M40.292
    cervicothoracic region M40.293
    thoracic region M40.294
    thoracolumbar region M40.295
  syphilitic, congenital A50.56
  thoracic region M40.204
  thoracolumbar region M40.205

Kyphosis, kyphotic — *continued*
  tuberculous A18.01
Kyrle disease L87.0

L

Labia, labium — *see* condition
Labile
  blood pressure R09.89
  vasomotor system I73.9
Labioglossal paralysis G12.29
Labium leporinum — *see* Cleft, lip
Labor — *see* Delivery
Labored breathing — *see* Hyperventilation
Labyrinthitis (circumscribed) (destructive) (diffuse) (inner ear) (latent) (purulent) (suppurative) — *see also* subcategory H83.0 ☑
  syphilitic A52.79
Laceration
  with abortion — *see* Abortion, by type, complicated by laceration of pelvic organs
  abdomen, abdominal
    wall S31.119 ☑
      with
        foreign body S31.129 ☑
        penetration into peritoneal cavity S31.619 ☑
          with foreign body S31.629 ☑
      epigastric region S31.112 ☑
        with
          foreign body S31.122 ☑
          penetration into peritoneal cavity S31.612 ☑
            with foreign body S31.622 ☑
      left
        lower quadrant S31.114 ☑
          with
            foreign body S31.124 ☑
            penetration into peritoneal cavity S31.614 ☑
              with foreign body S31.624 ☑
        upper quadrant S31.111 ☑
          with
            foreign body S31.121 ☑
            penetration into peritoneal cavity S31.611 ☑
              with foreign body S31.621 ☑
      periumbilic region S31.115 ☑
        with
          foreign body S31.125 ☑
          penetration into peritoneal cavity S31.615 ☑
            with foreign body S31.625 ☑
      right
        lower quadrant S31.113 ☑
          with
            foreign body S31.123 ☑
            penetration into peritoneal cavity S31.613 ☑
              with foreign body S31.623 ☑
        upper quadrant S31.110 ☑
          with
            foreign body S31.120 ☑
            penetration into peritoneal cavity S31.610 ☑
              with foreign body S31.620 ☑
  accidental, complicating surgery — *see* Complications, surgical, accidental puncture or laceration
  Achilles tendon S86.02- ☑
  adrenal gland S37.813 ☑
  alveolar (process) — *see* Laceration, oral cavity
  ankle S91.01- ☑
    with
      foreign body S91.02- ☑
  antecubital space — *see* Laceration, elbow
  anus (sphincter) S31.831 ☑
    with
      ectopic or molar pregnancy O08.6
      foreign body S31.832 ☑
    complicating delivery — *see* Delivery, complicated, by, laceration, anus (sphincter)
    following ectopic or molar pregnancy O08.6
    nontraumatic, nonpuerperal — *see* Fissure, anus
  arm (upper) S41.11- ☑
    with foreign body S41.12- ☑
    lower — *see* Laceration, forearm

Laceration — *continued*
  auditory canal (external) (meatus) — *see* Laceration, ear
  auricle, ear — *see* Laceration, ear
  axilla — *see* Laceration, arm
  back — *see also* Laceration, thorax, back
    lower S31.010 ☑
      with
        foreign body S31.020 ☑
          with penetration into retroperitoneal space S31.021 ☑
        penetration into retroperitoneal space S31.011 ☑
  bile duct S36.13 ☑
  bladder S37.23 ☑
    with ectopic or molar pregnancy O08.6
    following ectopic or molar pregnancy O08.6
    obstetrical trauma O71.5
  blood vessel — *see* Injury, blood vessel
  bowel — *see also* Laceration, intestine
    with ectopic or molar pregnancy O08.6
    complicating abortion — *see* Abortion, by type, complicated by, specified condition NEC
    following ectopic or molar pregnancy O08.6
    obstetrical trauma O71.5
  brain (any part) (cortex) (diffuse) (membrane) — *see also* Injury, intracranial, diffuse
    during birth P10.8
      with hemorrhage P10.1
    focal — *see* Injury, intracranial, focal brain injury
  brainstem S06.38- ☑
  breast S21.01- ☑
    with foreign body S21.02- ☑
  broad ligament S37.893 ☑
    with ectopic or molar pregnancy O08.6
    following ectopic or molar pregnancy O08.6
    laceration syndrome N83.8
    obstetrical trauma O71.6
    syndrome (laceration) N83.8
  buttock S31.801 ☑
    with foreign body S31.802 ☑
    left S31.821 ☑
      with foreign body S31.822 ☑
    right S31.811 ☑
      with foreign body S31.812 ☑
  calf — *see* Laceration, leg
  canaliculus lacrimalis — *see* Laceration, eyelid
  canthus, eye — *see* Laceration, eyelid
  capsule, joint — *see* Sprain
  causing eversion of cervix uteri (old) N86
  central (perineal), complicating delivery O70.9
  cerebellum, traumatic S06.37- ☑
  cerebral S06.33- ☑
    during birth P10.8
      with hemorrhage P10.1
    left side S06.32- ☑
    right side S06.31- ☑
  cervix (uteri)
    with ectopic or molar pregnancy O08.6
    following ectopic or molar pregnancy O08.6
    nonpuerperal, nontraumatic N88.1
    obstetrical trauma (current) O71.3
    old (postpartal) N88.1
    traumatic S37.63 ☑
  cheek (external) S01.41- ☑
    with foreign body S01.42- ☑
    internal — *see* Laceration, oral cavity
  chest wall — *see* Laceration, thorax
  chin — *see* Laceration, head, specified site NEC
  chordae tendinae NEC I51.1
    concurrent with acute myocardial infarction — *see* Infarct, myocardium
    following acute myocardial infarction (current complication) I23.4
  clitoris — *see* Laceration, vulva
  colon — *see* Laceration, intestine, large, colon
  common bile duct S36.13 ☑
  cortex (cerebral) — *see* Injury, intracranial, diffuse
  costal region — *see* Laceration, thorax
  cystic duct S36.13 ☑
  diaphragm S27.803 ☑
  digit(s)
    foot — *see* Laceration, toe
    hand — *see* Laceration, finger
  duodenum S36.430 ☑
  ear (canal) (external) S01.31- ☑
    with foreign body S01.32- ☑

☑ Additional Character Required — Refer to the Tabular List for Character Selection
Subterms under main terms may continue to next column or page

Laceration — *continued*
  ear — *continued*
    drum S09.2- ☑
  elbow S51.01- ☑
    with
      foreign body S51.02- ☑
  epididymis — *see* Laceration, testis
  epigastric region — *see* Laceration, abdomen, wall,
      epigastric region
  esophagus K22.8
    traumatic
      cervical S11.21 ☑
        with foreign body S11.22 ☑
      thoracic S27.813 ☑
  eye (ball) S05.3- ☑
    with prolapse or loss of intraocular tissue S05.2- ☑
    penetrating S05.6- ☑
  eyebrow — *see* Laceration, eyelid
  eyelid S01.11- ☑
    with foreign body S01.12- ☑
  face NEC — *see* Laceration, head, specified site NEC
  fallopian tube S37.539 ☑
    bilateral S37.532 ☑
    unilateral S37.531 ☑
  finger(s) S61.219 ☑
    with
      damage to nail S61.319 ☑
        with
          foreign body S61.329 ☑
      foreign body S61.229 ☑
    index S61.218 ☑
      with
        damage to nail S61.318 ☑
          with
            foreign body S61.328 ☑
        foreign body S61.228 ☑
      left S61.211 ☑
        with
          damage to nail S61.311 ☑
            with
              foreign body S61.321 ☑
          foreign body S61.221 ☑
      right S61.210 ☑
        with
          damage to nail S61.310 ☑
            with
              foreign body S61.320 ☑
          foreign body S61.220 ☑
    little S61.218 ☑
      with
        damage to nail S61.318 ☑
          with
            foreign body S61.328 ☑
        foreign body S61.228 ☑
      left S61.217 ☑
        with
          damage to nail S61.317 ☑
            with
              foreign body S61.327 ☑
          foreign body S61.227 ☑
      right S61.216 ☑
        with
          damage to nail S61.316 ☑
            with
              foreign body S61.326 ☑
          foreign body S61.226 ☑
    middle S61.218 ☑
      with
        damage to nail S61.318 ☑
          with
            foreign body S61.328 ☑
        foreign body S61.228 ☑
      left S61.213 ☑
        with
          damage to nail S61.313 ☑
            with
              foreign body S61.323 ☑
          foreign body S61.223 ☑
      right S61.212 ☑
        with
          damage to nail S61.312 ☑
            with
              foreign body S61.322 ☑
          foreign body S61.222 ☑
    ring S61.218 ☑

Laceration — *continued*
  finger(s) — *continued*
    ring — *continued*
      with
        damage to nail S61.318 ☑
          with
            foreign body S61.328 ☑
        foreign body S61.228 ☑
      left S61.215 ☑
        with
          damage to nail S61.315 ☑
            with
              foreign body S61.325 ☑
        foreign body S61.225 ☑
      right S61.214 ☑
        with
          damage to nail S61.314 ☑
            with
              foreign body S61.324 ☑
        foreign body S61.224 ☑
  flank S31.119 ☑
    with foreign body S31.129 ☑
  foot (except toe(s) alone) S91.319 ☑
    with foreign body S91.329 ☑
    left S91.312 ☑
      with foreign body S91.322 ☑
    right S91.311 ☑
      with foreign body S91.321 ☑
    toe — *see* Laceration, toe
  forearm S51.819 ☑
    with
      foreign body S51.829 ☑
    elbow only — *see* Laceration, elbow
    left S51.812 ☑
      with
        foreign body S51.822 ☑
    right S51.811 ☑
      with
        foreign body S51.821 ☑
  forehead S01.81 ☑
    with foreign body S01.82 ☑
  fourchette O70.0
    with ectopic or molar pregnancy O08.6
    complicating delivery O70.0
    following ectopic or molar pregnancy O08.6
  gallbladder S36.123 ☑
  genital organs, external
    female S31.512 ☑
      with foreign body S31.522 ☑
      vagina — *see* Laceration, vagina
      vulva — *see* Laceration, vulva
    male S31.511 ☑
      with foreign body S31.521 ☑
      penis — *see* Laceration, penis
      scrotum — *see* Laceration, scrotum
      testis — *see* Laceration, testis
  groin — *see* Laceration, abdomen, wall
  gum — *see* Laceration, oral cavity
  hand S61.419 ☑
    with
      foreign body S61.429 ☑
    finger — *see* Laceration, finger
    left S61.412 ☑
      with
        foreign body S61.422 ☑
    right S61.411 ☑
      with
        foreign body S61.421 ☑
    thumb — *see* Laceration, thumb
  head S01.91 ☑
    with foreign body S01.92 ☑
    cheek — *see* Laceration, cheek
    ear — *see* Laceration, ear
    eyelid — *see* Laceration, eyelid
    lip — *see* Laceration, lip
    nose — *see* Laceration, nose
    oral cavity — *see* Laceration, oral cavity
    scalp S01.01 ☑
      with foreign body S01.02 ☑
    specified site NEC S01.81 ☑
      with foreign body S01.82 ☑
    temporomandibular area — *see* Laceration, cheek
  heart — *see* Injury, heart, laceration
  heel — *see* Laceration, foot
  hepatic duct S36.13 ☑
  hip S71.019 ☑

Laceration — *continued*
  hip — *continued*
    with foreign body S71.029 ☑
    left S71.012 ☑
      with foreign body S71.022 ☑
    right S71.011 ☑
      with foreign body S71.021 ☑
  hymen — *see* Laceration, vagina
  hypochondrium — *see* Laceration, abdomen, wall
  hypogastric region — *see* Laceration, abdomen, wall
  ileum S36.438 ☑
  inguinal region — *see* Laceration, abdomen, wall
  instep — *see* Laceration, foot
  internal organ — *see* Injury, by site
  interscapular region — *see* Laceration, thorax, back
  intestine
    large
      colon S36.539 ☑
        ascending S36.530 ☑
        descending S36.532 ☑
        sigmoid S36.533 ☑
        specified site NEC S36.538 ☑
      rectum S36.63 ☑
      transverse S36.531 ☑
    small S36.439 ☑
      duodenum S36.430 ☑
      specified site NEC S36.438 ☑
  intra-abdominal organ S36.93 ☑
    intestine — *see* Laceration, intestine
    liver — *see* Laceration, liver
    pancreas — *see* Laceration, pancreas
    peritoneum S36.81 ☑
    specified site NEC S36.893 ☑
    spleen — *see* Laceration, spleen
    stomach — *see* Laceration, stomach
  intracranial NEC — *see also* Injury, intracranial, diffuse
    birth injury P10.9
  jaw — *see* Laceration, head, specified site NEC
  jejunum S36.438 ☑
  joint capsule — *see* Sprain, by site
  kidney S37.03- ☑
    major (greater than 3 cm) (massive) (stellate)
        S37.06- ☑
    minor (less than 1 cm) S37.04- ☑
    moderate (1 to 3 cm) S37.05- ☑
    multiple S37.06- ☑
  knee S81.01- ☑
    with foreign body S81.02- ☑
  labium (majus) (minus) — *see* Laceration, vulva
  lacrimal duct — *see* Laceration, eyelid
  large intestine — *see* Laceration, intestine, large
  larynx S11.011 ☑
    with foreign body S11.012 ☑
  leg (lower) S81.819 ☑
    with foreign body S81.829 ☑
    foot — *see* Laceration, foot
    knee — *see* Laceration, knee
    left S81.812 ☑
      with foreign body S81.822 ☑
    right S81.811 ☑
      with foreign body S81.821 ☑
    upper — *see* Laceration, thigh
  ligament — *see* Sprain
  lip S01.511 ☑
    with foreign body S01.521 ☑
  liver S36.113 ☑
    major (stellate) S36.116 ☑
    minor S36.114 ☑
    moderate S36.115 ☑
  loin — *see* Laceration, abdomen, wall
  lower back — *see* Laceration, back, lower
  lumbar region — *see* Laceration, back, lower
  lung S27.339 ☑
    bilateral S27.332 ☑
    unilateral S27.331 ☑
  malar region — *see* Laceration, head, specified site NEC
  mammary — *see* Laceration, breast
  mastoid region — *see* Laceration, head, specified site
      NEC
  meninges — *see* Injury, intracranial, diffuse
  meniscus — *see* Tear, meniscus
  mesentery S36.893 ☑
  mesosalpinx S37.893 ☑
  mouth — *see* Laceration, oral cavity
  muscle — *see* Injury, muscle, by site, laceration

Laceration — *continued*
nail
finger — *see* Laceration, finger, with damage to nail
toe — *see* Laceration, toe, with damage to nail
nasal (septum) (sinus) — *see* Laceration, nose
nasopharynx — *see* Laceration, head, specified site
NEC
neck S11.91 ☑
with foreign body S11.92 ☑
involving
cervical esophagus S11.21 ☑
with foreign body S11.22 ☑
larynx — *see* Laceration, larynx
pharynx — *see* Laceration, pharynx
thyroid gland — *see* Laceration, thyroid gland
trachea — *see* Laceration, trachea
specified site NEC S11.81 ☑
with foreign body S11.82 ☑
nerve — *see* Injury, nerve
nose (septum) (sinus) S01.21 ☑
with foreign body S01.22 ☑
ocular NOS S05.3- ☑
adnexa NOS S01.11- ☑
oral cavity S01.512 ☑
with foreign body S01.522 ☑
orbit (eye) — *see* Wound, open, ocular, orbit
ovary S37.439 ☑
bilateral S37.432 ☑
unilateral S37.431 ☑
palate — *see* Laceration, oral cavity
palm — *see* Laceration, hand
pancreas S36.239 ☑
pelvic S31.010 ☑
with
foreign body S31.020 ☑
penetration into retroperitoneal cavity
S31.021 ☑
penetration into retroperitoneal cavity
S31.011 ☑
floor — *see also* Laceration, back, lower
with ectopic or molar pregnancy O08.6
complicating delivery O70.1
following ectopic or molar pregnancy O08.6
old (postpartal) N81.89
organ S37.93 ☑
penis S31.21 ☑
with foreign body S31.22 ☑
perineum
female S31.41 ☑
with
ectopic or molar pregnancy O08.6
foreign body S31.42 ☑
during delivery O70.9
first degree O70.0
fourth degree O70.3
second degree O70.1
third degree — *see also* Delivery, complicated, by, laceration, perineum, third degree O70.20
old (postpartal) N81.89
postpartal N81.89
secondary (postpartal) O90.1
male S31.119 ☑
with foreign body S31.129 ☑
periocular area (with or without lacrimal passages) —
see Laceration, eyelid
peritoneum S36.893 ☑
periumbilic region — *see* Laceration, abdomen, wall,
periumbilic
periurethral tissue — *see* Laceration, urethra
phalanges
finger — *see* Laceration, finger
toe — *see* Laceration, toe
pharynx S11.21 ☑
with foreign body S11.22 ☑
pinna — *see* Laceration, ear
popliteal space — *see* Laceration, knee
prepuce — *see* Laceration, penis
prostate S37.823 ☑
pubic region S31.119 ☑
with foreign body S31.129 ☑
pudendum — *see* Laceration, genital organs, external
rectovaginal septum — *see* Laceration, vagina
rectum S36.63 ☑
retroperitoneum S36.893 ☑
round ligament S37.893 ☑
sacral region — *see* Laceration, back, lower

Laceration — *continued*
sacroiliac region — *see* Laceration, back, lower
salivary gland — *see* Laceration, oral cavity
scalp S01.01 ☑
with foreign body S01.02 ☑
scapular region — *see* Laceration, shoulder
scrotum S31.31 ☑
with foreign body S31.32 ☑
seminal vesicle S37.893 ☑
shin — *see* Laceration, leg
shoulder S41.019 ☑
with foreign body S41.029 ☑
left S41.012 ☑ •
with foreign body S41.022 ☑
right S41.011 ☑
with foreign body S41.021 ☑
small intestine — *see* Laceration, intestine, small
spermatic cord — *see* Laceration, testis
spinal cord (meninges) — *see also* Injury, spinal cord,
by region
due to injury at birth P11.5
newborn (birth injury) P11.5
spleen S36.039 ☑
major (massive) (stellate) S36.032 ☑
moderate S36.031 ☑
superficial (minor) S36.030 ☑
sternal region — *see* Laceration, thorax, front
stomach S36.33 ☑
submaxillary region — *see* Laceration, head, specified
site NEC
submental region — *see* Laceration, head, specified
site NEC
subungual
finger(s) — *see* Laceration, finger, with damage to
nail
toe(s) — *see* Laceration, toe, with damage to nail
suprarenal gland — *see* Laceration, adrenal gland
temple, temporal region — *see* Laceration, head,
specified site NEC
temporomandibular area — *see* Laceration, cheek
tendon — *see* Injury, muscle, by site, laceration
Achilles S86.02- ☑
tentorium cerebelli — *see* Injury, intracranial, diffuse
testis S31.31 ☑
with foreign body S31.32 ☑
thigh S71.11- ☑
with foreign body S71.12- ☑
thorax, thoracic (wall) S21.91 ☑
with foreign body S21.92 ☑
back S21.22- ☑
with penetration into thoracic cavity
S21.42- ☑
front S21.12- ☑
with penetration into thoracic cavity
S21.32- ☑
back S21.21- ☑
with
foreign body S21.22- ☑
with penetration into thoracic cavity
S21.42- ☑
penetration into thoracic cavity S21.41- ☑
breast — *see* Laceration, breast
front S21.11- ☑
with
foreign body S21.12- ☑
with penetration into thoracic cavity
S21.32- ☑
penetration into thoracic cavity S21.31- ☑
thumb S61.019 ☑
with
damage to nail S61.119 ☑
with
foreign body S61.129 ☑
foreign body S61.029 ☑
left S61.012 ☑
with
damage to nail S61.112 ☑
with
foreign body S61.122 ☑
foreign body S61.022 ☑
right S61.011 ☑
with
damage to nail S61.111 ☑
with
foreign body S61.121 ☑
foreign body S61.021 ☑

Laceration — *continued*
thyroid gland S11.11 ☑
with foreign body S11.12 ☑
toe(s) S91.119 ☑
with
damage to nail S91.219 ☑
with
foreign body S91.229 ☑
foreign body S91.129 ☑
great S91.113 ☑
with
damage to nail S91.213 ☑
with
foreign body S91.223 ☑
foreign body S91.123 ☑
left S91.112 ☑
with
damage to nail S91.212 ☑
with
foreign body S91.222 ☑
foreign body S91.122 ☑
right S91.111 ☑
with
damage to nail S91.211 ☑
with
foreign body S91.221 ☑
foreign body S91.121 ☑
lesser S91.116 ☑
with
damage to nail S91.216 ☑
with
foreign body S91.226 ☑
foreign body S91.126 ☑
left S91.115 ☑
with
damage to nail S91.215 ☑
with
foreign body S91.225 ☑
foreign body S91.125 ☑
right S91.114 ☑
with
damage to nail S91.214 ☑
with
foreign body S91.224 ☑
foreign body S91.124 ☑
tongue — *see* Laceration, oral cavity
trachea S11.021 ☑
with foreign body S11.022 ☑
tunica vaginalis — *see* Laceration, testis
tympanum, tympanic membrane — *see* Laceration,
ear, drum
umbilical region S31.115 ☑
with foreign body S31.125 ☑
ureter S37.13 ☑
urethra S37.33 ☑
with or following ectopic or molar pregnancy O08.6
obstetrical trauma O71.5
urinary organ NEC S37.893 ☑
uterus S37.63 ☑
with ectopic or molar pregnancy O08.6
following ectopic or molar pregnancy O08.6
nonpuerperal, nontraumatic N85.8
obstetrical trauma NEC O71.81
old (postpartal) N85.8
uvula — *see* Laceration, oral cavity
vagina S31.41 ☑
with
ectopic or molar pregnancy O08.6
foreign body S31.42 ☑
during delivery O71.4
with perineal laceration — *see* Laceration, perineum, female, during delivery
following ectopic or molar pregnancy O08.6
nonpuerperal, nontraumatic N89.8
old (postpartal) N89.8
vas deferens S37.893 ☑
vesical — *see* Laceration, bladder
vocal cords S11.031 ☑
with foreign body S11.032 ☑
vulva S31.41 ☑
with
ectopic or molar pregnancy O08.6
foreign body S31.42 ☑
complicating delivery O70.0
following ectopic or molar pregnancy O08.6
nonpuerperal, nontraumatic N90.89
old (postpartal) N90.89

☑ **Additional Character Required — Refer to the Tabular List for Character Selection**   ▽ **Subterms under main terms may continue to next column or page**

Laceration — *continued*
  wrist S61.519 ☑
    with
      foreign body S61.529 ☑
    left S61.512 ☑
      with
        foreign body S61.522 ☑
    right S61.511 ☑
      with
        foreign body S61.521 ☑
Lack of
  achievement in school Z55.3
  adequate
    food Z59.4
    intermaxillary vertical dimension of fully erupted
      teeth M26.36
    sleep Z72.820
  appetite (see Anorexia) R63.0
  awareness R41.9
  care
    in home Z74.2
    of infant (at or after birth) T76.02 ☑
      confirmed T74.02 ☑
  cognitive functions R41.9
  coordination R27.9
    ataxia R27.0
    specified type NEC R27.8
  development (physiological) R62.50
    failure to thrive (child over 28 days old) R62.51
      adult R62.7
      newborn P92.6
    short stature R62.52
    specified type NEC R62.59
  energy R53.83
  financial resources Z59.6
  food T73.0 ☑
  growth R62.52
  heating Z59.1
  housing (permanent) (temporary) Z59.0
    adequate Z59.1
  learning experiences in childhood Z62.898
  leisure time (affecting life-style) Z73.2
  material resources Z59.9
  memory — *see also* Amnesia
    mild, following organic brain damage F06.8
  ovulation N97.0
  parental supervision or control of child Z62.0
  person able to render necessary care Z74.2
  physical exercise Z72.3
  play experience in childhood Z62.898
  posterior occlusal support M26.57
  relaxation (affecting life-style) Z73.2
  sexual
    desire F52.0
    enjoyment F52.1
  shelter Z59.0
  sleep (adequate) Z72.820
  supervision of child by parent Z62.0
  support, posterior occlusal M26.57
  water T73.1 ☑
Lacrimal — *see* condition
Lacrimation, abnormal — *see* Epiphora
Lacrimonasal duct — *see* condition
Lactation, lactating (breast) (puerperal, postpartum)
  associated
    cracked nipple O92.13
    retracted nipple O92.03
  defective O92.4
  disorder NEC O92.79
  excessive O92.6
  failed (complete) O92.3
    partial O92.4
  mastitis NEC — *see* Mastitis, obstetric
  mother (care and/or examination) Z39.1
  nonpuerperal N64.3
Lacticemia, excessive E87.2
Lacunar skull Q75.8
Laennec's cirrhosis K70.30
  with ascites K70.31
  nonalcoholic K74.69
Lafora's disease — *see* Epilepsy, generalized, idiopathic
Lag, lid (nervous) — *see* Retraction, lid
Lagophthalmos (eyelid) (nervous) H02.209
  bilateral, upper and lower eyelids H02.20C
  cicatricial H02.219
    bilateral, upper and lower eyelids H02.21C
    left H02.216
      lower H02.215

Lagophthalmos — *continued*
  cicatricial — *continued*
    left — *continued*
      upper H02.214
      upper and lower eyelids H02.21B
    right H02.213
      lower H02.212
      upper H02.211
      upper and lower eyelids H02.21A
  keratoconjunctivitis — *see* Keratoconjunctivitis
  left H02.206
    lower H02.205
    upper H02.204
    upper and lower eyelids H02.20B
  mechanical H02.229
    bilateral, upper and lower eyelids H02.22C
    left H02.226
      lower H02.225
      upper H02.224
      upper and lower eyelids H02.22B
    right H02.223
      lower H02.222
      upper H02.221
      upper and lower eyelids H02.22A
  paralytic H02.239
    bilateral, upper and lower eyelids H02.23C
    left H02.236
      lower H02.235
      upper H02.234
      upper and lower eyelids H02.23B
    right H02.233
      lower H02.232
      upper H02.231
      upper and lower eyelids H02.23A
  right H02.203
    lower H02.202
    upper H02.201
    upper and lower eyelids H02.20A
Laki-Lorand factor deficiency — *see* Defect, coagulation, specified type NEC
Lalling F80.0
Lambert-Eaton syndrome — *see* Syndrome, Lambert-Eaton
Lambliasis, lambliosis A07.1
Landau-Kleffner syndrome — *see* Epilepsy, specified NEC
Landouzy-Déjérine dystrophy or facioscapulohumeral atrophy G71.02
Landouzy's disease (icterohemorrhagic leptospirosis) A27.0
Landry-Guillain-Barré, syndrome or paralysis G61.0
Landry's disease or paralysis G61.0
Lane's
  band Q43.3
  kink — *see* Obstruction, intestine
  syndrome K90.2
Langdon Down syndrome — *see* Trisomy, 21
Lapsed immunization schedule status Z28.3
Large
  baby (regardless of gestational age) (4000g to 4499g) P08.1
  ear, congenital Q17.1
  physiological cup Q14.2
  stature R68.89
Large-for-dates NEC (infant) (4000g to 4499g) P08.1
  affecting management of pregnancy O36.6- ☑
  exceptionally (4500g or more) P08.0
Larsen-Johansson disease orosteochondrosis — *see* Osteochondrosis, juvenile, patella
Larsen's syndrome (flattened facies and multiple congenital dislocations) Q74.8
Larva migrans
  cutaneous B76.9
    Ancylostoma B76.0
  visceral B83.0
Laryngeal — *see* condition
Laryngismus (stridulus) J38.5
  congenital P28.89
  diphtheritic A36.2
Laryngitis (acute) (edematous) (fibrinous) (infective) (infiltrative) (malignant) (membranous) (phlegmonous) (pneumococcal) (pseudomembranous) (septic) (subglottic) (suppurative) (ulcerative) J04.0
  with
    influenza, flu, or grippe — *see* Influenza, with, laryngitis
    tracheitis (acute) — *see* Laryngotracheitis
  atrophic J37.0

Laryngitis — *continued*
  catarrhal J37.0
  chronic J37.0
    with tracheitis (chronic) J37.1
  diphtheritic A36.2
  due to external agent — *see* Inflammation, respiratory, upper, due to
  H. influenzae J04.0
  Hemophilus influenzae J04.0
  hypertrophic J37.0
  influenzal — *see* Influenza, with, respiratory manifestations NEC
  obstructive J05.0
  sicca J37.0
  spasmodic J05.0
    acute J04.0
  streptococcal J04.0
  stridulous J05.0
  syphilitic (late) A52.73
    congenital A50.59 *[J99]*
      early A50.03 *[J99]*
  tuberculous A15.5
  Vincent's A69.1
Laryngocele (congenital) (ventricular) Q31.3
Laryngofissure J38.7
  congenital Q31.8
Laryngomalacia (congenital) Q31.5
Laryngopharyngitis (acute) J06.0
  chronic J37.0
  due to external agent — *see* Inflammation, respiratory, upper, due to
Laryngoplegia J38.00
  bilateral J38.02
  unilateral J38.01
Laryngoptosis J38.7
Laryngospasm J38.5
Laryngostenosis J38.6
Laryngotracheitis (acute) (Infectional) (infective) (viral) J04.2
  atrophic J37.1
  catarrhal J37.1
  chronic J37.1
  diphtheritic A36.2
  due to external agent — *see* Inflammation, respiratory, upper, due to
  Hemophilus influenzae J04.2
  hypertrophic J37.1
  influenzal — *see* Influenza, with, respiratory manifestations NEC
  pachydermic J38.7
  sicca J37.1
  spasmodic J38.5
    acute J05.0
  streptococcal J04.2
  stridulous J38.5
  syphilitic (late) A52.73
    congenital A50.59 *[J99]*
      early A50.03 *[J99]*
  tuberculous A15.5
  Vincent's A69.1
Laryngotracheobronchitis — *see* Bronchitis
Larynx, laryngeal — *see* condition
Lassa fever A96.2
Lassitude — *see* Weakness
Late
  talker R62.0
  walker R62.0
Late effect(s) — *see* Sequelae
Latent — *see* condition
Laterocession — *see* Lateroversion
Lateroflexion — *see* Lateroversion
Lateroversion
  cervix — *see* Lateroversion, uterus
  uterus, uterine (cervix) (postinfectional) (postpartal, old) N85.4
    congenital Q51.818
    in pregnancy or childbirth O34.59- ☑
Lathyrism — *see* Poisoning, food, noxious, plant
Launois' syndrome (pituitary gigantism) E22.0
Launois-Bensaude adenolipomatosis E88.89
Laurence-Moon (-Bardet)-**Biedl syndrome** Q87.89
Lax, laxity — *see also* Relaxation
  ligament (ous) — *see also* Disorder, ligament
    familial M35.7
    knee — *see* Derangement, knee
  skin (acquired) L57.4
    congenital Q82.8
Laxative habit F55.2

Lazy leukocyte syndrome D70.8
Lead miner's lung J63.6
Leak, leakage
- air NEC J93.82
  - postprocedural J95.812
- amniotic fluid — see Rupture, membranes, premature
- blood (microscopic), fetal, into maternal circulation affecting management of pregnancy — see Pregnancy, complicated by
- cerebrospinal fluid G96.0
  - from spinal (lumbar) puncture G97.0
- device, implant or graft — see also Complications, by site and type, mechanical
  - arterial graft NEC — see Complication, cardiovascular device, mechanical, vascular
    - breast (implant) T85.43 ☑
    - catheter NEC T85.638 ☑
      - dialysis (renal) T82.43 ☑
        - intraperitoneal T85.631 ☑
      - infusion NEC T82.534 ☑
        - spinal (epidural) (subdural) T85.630 ☑
      - urinary T83.038 ☑
        - cystostomy T83.030 ☑
        - Hopkins T83.038 ☑
        - ileostomy T83.038 ☑
        - indwelling T83.031 ☑
        - nephrostomy T83.032 ☑
        - specified T83.038 ☑
        - urostomy T83.038 ☑
    - gastrointestinal — see Complications, prosthetic device, mechanical, gastrointestinal device
    - genital NEC T83.498 ☑
      - penile prosthesis (cylinder) (implanted) (pump) (reservoir) T83.490 ☑
      - testicular prosthesis T83.491 ☑
    - heart NEC — see Complication, cardiovascular device, mechanical
    - joint prosthesis — see Complications, joint prosthesis, mechanical, specified NEC, by site
    - ocular NEC — see Complications, prosthetic device, mechanical, ocular device
    - orthopedic NEC — see Complication, orthopedic, device, mechanical
    - persistent air J93.82
    - specified NEC T85.638 ☑
    - urinary NEC — see also Complication, genitourinary, device, urinary, mechanical
      - graft T83.23 ☑
    - vascular NEC — see Complication, cardiovascular device, mechanical
    - ventricular intracranial shunt T85.03 ☑
  - urine — see Incontinence
Leaky heart — see Endocarditis
Learning defect (specific) F81.9
Leather bottle stomach C16.9
Leber's
- congenital amaurosis H35.50
- optic atrophy (hereditary) H47.22
Lederer's anemia D59.1
Leeches (external) — see Hirudiniasis
Leg — see condition
Legg (-Calvé)-**Perthes disease, syndrome or osteochondrosis** M91.1- ☑
Legionellosis A48.1
- nonpneumonic A48.2
Legionnaires'
- disease A48.1
  - nonpneumonic A48.2
  - pneumonia A48.1
Leigh's disease G31.82
Leiner's disease L21.1
Leiofibromyoma — see Leiomyoma
Leiomyoblastoma — see Neoplasm, connective tissue, benign
Leiomyofibroma — see also Neoplasm, connective tissue, benign
- uterus (cervix) (corpus) D25.9
Leiomyoma — see also Neoplasm, connective tissue, benign
- bizarre — see Neoplasm, connective tissue, benign
- cellular — see Neoplasm, connective tissue, benign
- epithelioid — see Neoplasm, connective tissue, benign
- uterus (cervix) (corpus) D25.9
  - intramural D25.1
  - submucous D25.0
  - subserosal D25.2
- vascular — see Neoplasm, connective tissue, benign

Leiomyoma, leiomyomatosis (intravascular) — see Neoplasm, connective tissue, uncertain behavior
Leiomyosarcoma — see also Neoplasm, connective tissue, malignant
- epithelioid — see Neoplasm, connective tissue, malignant
- myxoid — see Neoplasm, connective tissue, malignant
Leishmaniasis B55.9
- American (mucocutaneous) B55.2
  - cutaneous B55.1
- Asian Desert B55.1
- Brazilian B55.2
- cutaneous (any type) B55.1
- dermal — see also Leishmaniasis, cutaneous
  - post-kala-azar B55.0
- eyelid B55.1
- infantile B55.0
- Mediterranean B55.0
- mucocutaneous (American) (New World) B55.2
- naso-oral B55.2
- nasopharyngeal B55.2
- old world B55.1
- tegumentaria diffusa B55.1
- visceral B55.0
Leishmanoid, dermal — see also Leishmaniasis, cutaneous
- post-kala-azar B55.0
Lenegre's disease I44.2
Lengthening, leg — see Deformity, limb, unequal length
Lennert's lymphoma — see Lymphoma, Lennert's
Lennox-Gastaut syndrome G40.812
- intractable G40.814
  - with status epilepticus G40.813
  - without status epilepticus G40.814
- not intractable G40.812
  - with status epilepticus G40.811
  - without status epilepticus G40.812
Lens — see condition
Lenticonus (anterior) (posterior) (congenital) Q12.8
Lenticular degeneration, progressive E83.01
Lentiglobus (posterior) (congenital) Q12.8
Lentigo (congenital) L81.4
- maligna — see also Melanoma, in situ
  - melanoma — see Melanoma
Lentivirus, as cause of disease classified elsewhere B97.31
Leontiasis
- ossium M85.2
- syphilitic (late) A52.78
  - congenital A50.59
Lepothrix A48.8
Lepra — see Leprosy
Leprechaunism E34.8
Leprosy A30.- ☑
- with muscle disorder A30.9 [M63.80]
  - ankle A30.9 [M63.87-] ☑
  - foot A30.9 [M63.87-] ☑
  - forearm A30.9 [M63.83-] ☑
  - hand A30.9 [M63.84-] ☑
  - lower leg A30.9 [M63.86-] ☑
  - multiple sites A30.9 [M63.89]
  - pelvic region A30.9 [M63.85-] ☑
  - shoulder region A30.9 [M63.81-] ☑
  - specified site NEC A30.9 [M63.88]
  - thigh A30.9 [M63.85-] ☑
  - upper arm A30.9 [M63.82-] ☑
- anesthetic A30.9
- BB A30.3
- BL A30.4
- borderline (infiltrated) (neuritic) A30.3
  - lepromatous A30.4
  - tuberculoid A30.2
- BT A30.2
- dimorphous (infiltrated) (neuritic) A30.3
- I A30.0
- indeterminate (macular) (neuritic) A30.0
- lepromatous (diffuse) (infiltrated) (macular) (neuritic) (nodular) A30.5
- LL A30.5
- macular (early) (neuritic) (simple) A30.9
- maculoanesthetic A30.9
- mixed A30.3
- neural A30.9
- nodular A30.5
- primary neuritic A30.3
- specified type NEC A30.8
- TT A30.1

Leprosy — continued
- tuberculoid (major) (minor) A30.1
Leptocytosis, hereditary D56.9
Leptomeningitis (chronic) (circumscribed) (hemorrhagic) (nonsuppurative) — see Meningitis
Leptomeningopathy G96.19
Leptospiral — see condition
Leptospirochetal — see condition
Leptospirosis A27.9
- canicola A27.89
- due to Leptospira interrogans serovar icterohaemorrhagiae A27.0
- icterohemorrhagica A27.0
- pomona A27.89
- Weil's disease A27.0
Leptus dermatitis B88.0
Leriche's syndrome (aortic bifurcation occlusion) I74.09
Leri's pleonosteosis Q78.8
Leri-Weill syndrome Q77.8
Lermoyez' syndrome — see Vertigo, peripheral NEC
Lesch-Nyhan syndrome E79.1
Leser-Trélat disease L82.1
- inflamed L82.0
Lesion(s) (nontraumatic)
- abducens nerve — see Strabismus, paralytic, sixth nerve
- alveolar process K08.9
- angiocentric immunoproliferative D47.Z9 (following D47.4)
- anorectal K62.9
- aortic (valve) I35.9
- auditory nerve — see subcategory H93.3 ☑
- basal ganglion G25.9
- bile duct — see Disease, bile duct
- biomechanical M99.9
  - specified type NEC M99.89
    - abdomen M99.89
    - acromioclavicular M99.87
    - cervical region M99.81
    - cervicothoracic M99.81
    - costochondral M99.88
    - costovertebral M99.88
    - head region M99.80
    - hip M99.85
    - lower extremity M99.86
    - lumbar region M99.83
    - lumbosacral M99.83
    - occipitocervical M99.80
    - pelvic region M99.85
    - pubic M99.85
    - rib cage M99.88
    - sacral region M99.84
    - sacrococcygeal M99.84
    - sacroiliac M99.84
    - specified NEC M99.89
    - sternochondral M99.88
    - sternoclavicular M99.87
    - thoracic region M99.82
    - thoracolumbar M99.82
    - upper extremity M99.87
- bladder N32.9
- bone — see Disorder, bone
- brachial plexus G54.0
- brain G93.9
  - congenital Q04.9
  - vascular I67.9
    - degenerative I67.9
    - hypertensive I67.4
- buccal cavity K13.79
- calcified — see Calcification
- canthus — see Disorder, eyelid
- carate — see Pinta, lesions
- cardia K31.9
- cardiac — see also Disease, heart I51.9
  - congenital Q24.9
  - valvular — see Endocarditis
- cauda equina G83.4
- cecum K63.9
- cerebral — see Lesion, brain
- cerebrovascular I67.9
  - degenerative I67.9
  - hypertensive I67.4
- cervical (nerve) root NEC G54.2
- chiasmal — see Disorder, optic, chiasm
- chorda tympani G51.8
- coin, lung R91.1
- colon K63.9
- combined periodontic - endodontic K05.5
- congenital — see Anomaly, by site

Lesion(s) — *continued*
  conjunctiva H11.9
  conus medullaris — *see* Injury, conus medullaris
  coronary artery — *see* Ischemia, heart
  cranial nerve G52.9
    eighth — *see* Disorder, ear
    eleventh G52.9
    fifth G50.9
    first G52.0
    fourth — *see* Strabismus, paralytic, fourth nerve
    seventh G51.9
    sixth — *see* Strabismus, paralytic, sixth nerve
    tenth G52.2
    twelfth G52.3
  cystic — *see* Cyst
  degenerative — *see* Degeneration
  duodenum K31.9
  edentulous (alveolar) ridge, associated with trauma, due to traumatic occlusion K06.2
  en coup de sabre L94.1
  eyelid — *see* Disorder, eyelid
  gasserian ganglion G50.8
  gastric K31.9
  gastroduodenal K31.9
  gastrointestinal K63.9
  gingiva, associated with trauma K06.2
  glomerular
    focal and segmental — *see also* N00-N07 with fourth character .1 N05.1
    minimal change — *see also* N00-N07 with fourth character .0 N05.0
  heart (organic) — *see* Disease, heart
  hyperchromic, due to pinta (carate) A67.1
  hyperkeratotic — *see* Hyperkeratosis
  hypothalamic E23.7
  ileocecal K63.9
  ileum K63.9
  iliohypogastric nerve G57.8- ☑
  inflammatory — *see* Inflammation
  intestine K63.9
  intracerebral — *see* Lesion, brain
  intrachiasmal (optic) — *see* Disorder, optic, chiasm
  intracranial, space-occupying R90.0
  joint — *see* Disorder, joint
    sacroiliac (old) M53.3
  keratotic — *see* Keratosis
  kidney — *see* Disease, renal
  laryngeal nerve (recurrent) G52.2
  lip K13.0
  liver K76.9
  lumbosacral
    plexus G54.1
    root (nerve) NEC G54.4
  lung (coin) R91.1
  maxillary sinus J32.0
  mitral I05.9
  Morel-Lavallée — *see* Hematoma, by site
  motor cortex NEC G93.89
  mouth K13.79
  nerve G58.9
    femoral G57.2- ☑
    median G56.1- ☑
      carpal tunnel syndrome — *see* Syndrome, carpal tunnel
    plantar G57.6- ☑
    popliteal (lateral) G57.3- ☑
      medial G57.4- ☑
    radial G56.3- ☑
    sciatic G57.0- ☑
    spinal — *see* Injury, nerve, spinal
    ulnar G56.2- ☑
  nervous system, congenital Q07.9
  nonallopathic — *see* Lesion, biomechanical
  nose (internal) J34.89
  obstructive — *see* Obstruction
  obturator nerve G57.8- ☑
  oral mucosa K13.70
  organ or site NEC — *see* Disease, by site
  osteolytic — *see* Osteolysis
  peptic K27.9
  periodontal, due to traumatic occlusion K05.5
  pharynx J39.2
  pigment, pigmented (skin) L81.9
  pinta — *see* Pinta, lesions
  polypoid — *see* Polyp
  prechiasmal (optic) — *see* Disorder, optic, chiasm
  primary — *see also* Syphilis, primary A51.0

Lesion(s) — *continued*
  primary — *see also* Syphilis, primary — *continued*
    carate A67.0
    pinta A67.0
    yaws A66.0
  pulmonary J98.4
    valve I37.9
  pylorus K31.9
  rectosigmoid K63.9
  retina, retinal H35.9
  sacroiliac (joint) (old) M53.3
  salivary gland K11.9
    benign lymphoepithelial K11.8
  saphenous nerve G57.8- ☑
  sciatic nerve G57.0- ☑
  secondary — *see* Syphilis, secondary
  shoulder (region) M75.9- ☑
    specified NEC M75.8- ☑
  sigmoid K63.9
  sinus (accessory) (nasal) J34.89
  skin L98.9
    suppurative L08.0
  SLAP S43.43- ☑
  spinal cord G95.9
    congenital Q06.9
  spleen D73.89
  stomach K31.9
  superior glenoid labrum S43.43- ☑
  syphilitic — *see* Syphilis
  tertiary — *see* Syphilis, tertiary
  thoracic root (nerve) NEC G54.3
  tonsillar fossa J35.9
  tooth, teeth K08.9
    white spot
      chewing surface K02.51
      pit and fissure surface K02.51
      smooth surface K02.61
  traumatic — *see* specific type of injury by site
  tricuspid (valve) I07.9
    nonrheumatic I36.9
  trigeminal nerve G50.9
  ulcerated or ulcerative — *see* Ulcer, skin
  uterus N85.9
  vagina N89.8
  vagus nerve G52.2
  valvular — *see* Endocarditis
  vascular I99.9
    affecting central nervous system I67.9
    following trauma NEC T14.8 ☑
    umbilical cord, complicating delivery O69.5 ☑
  vulva N90.89
  warty — *see* Verruca
  white spot (tooth)
    chewing surface K02.51
    pit and fissure surface K02.51
    smooth surface K02.61
Lethargic — *see* condition
Lethargy R53.83
Letterer-Siwe's disease C96.0
Leukemia, leukemic C95.9- ☑
  acute basophilic C94.8- ☑
  acute bilineal C95.0- ☑
  acute erythroid C94.0- ☑
  acute lymphoblastic C91.0- ☑
  acute megakaryoblastic C94.2- ☑
  acute megakaryocytic C94.2- ☑
  acute mixed lineage C95.0- ☑
  acute monoblastic (monoblastic/monocytic) C93.0- ☑
  acute monocytic (monoblastic/monocytic) C93.0- ☑
  acute myeloblastic (minimal differentiation) (with maturation) C92.0- ☑
  acute myeloid, NOS C92.0- ☑
    with
      11q23-abnormality C92.6- ☑
      dysplasia of remaining hematopoesis and/or myelodysplastic disease in its history C92.A- ☑ (*following* C92.6)
      multilineage dysplasia C92.A- ☑ (*following* C92.6)
      variation of MLL-gene C92.6- ☑
    M6 (a)(b) C94.0- ☑
    M7 C94.2- ☑
  acute myelomonocytic C92.5- ☑
  acute promyelocytic C92.4- ☑
  adult T-cell (HTLV-1-associated) (acute variant) (chronic variant) (lymphomatoid variant) (smouldering variant) C91.5- ☑

Leukemia, leukemic — *continued*
  aggressive NK-cell C94.8- ☑
  AML (1/ETO) (M0) (M1) (M2) (without a FAB classification) C92.0- ☑
  AML M3 C92.4- ☑
  AML M4 (Eo with inv(16) or t(16;16)) C92.5- ☑
  AML M5 C93.0- ☑
  AML M5a C93.0- ☑
  AML M5b C93.0- ☑
  AML Me with t (15;17) and variants C92.4- ☑
  atypical chronic myeloid, BCR/ABL-negative C92.2- ☑
  biphenotypic acute C95.0- ☑
  blast cell C95.0- ☑
  Burkitt-type, mature B-cell C91.A- ☑ (*following* C91.6)
  chronic lymphocytic, of B-cell type C91.1- ☑
  chronic monocytic C93.1- ☑
  chronic myelogenous (Philadelphia chromosome (Ph1) positive) (t(9;22)) (q34;q11) (with crisis of blast cells) C92.1- ☑
  chronic myeloid, BCR/ABL-positive C92.1- ☑
    atypical, BCR/ABL-negative C92.2- ☑
  chronic myelomonocytic C93.1- ☑
  chronic neutrophilic D47.1
  CMML (-1) (-2) (with eosinophilia) C93.1- ☑
  granulocytic — *see also* Category C92 C92.9- ☑
  hairy cell C91.4- ☑
  juvenile myelomonocytic C93.3- ☑
  lymphoid C91.9- ☑
    specified NEC C91.Z- ☑ (*following* C91.6)
  mast cell C94.3- ☑
  mature B-cell, Burkitt-type C91.A- ☑ (*following* C91.6)
  monocytic (subacute) C93.9- ☑
    specified NEC C93.Z- ☑ (*following* C93.3)
  myelogenous — *see also* Category C92 C92.9- ☑
  myeloid C92.9- ☑
    specified NEC C92.Z- ☑ (*following* C92.6)
  plasma cell C90.1- ☑
  plasmacytic C90.1- ☑
  prolymphocytic
    of B-cell type C91.3- ☑
    of T-cell type C91.6- ☑
  specified NEC C94.8- ☑
  stem cell, of unclear lineage C95.0- ☑
  subacute lymphocytic C91.9- ☑
  T-cell large granular lymphocytic C91.Z- ☑ (*following* C91.6)
  unspecified cell type C95.9- ☑
    acute C95.0- ☑
    chronic C95.1- ☑
Leukemoid reaction — *see also* Reaction, leukemoid D72.823
Leukoaraiosis (hypertensive) I67.81
Leukoariosis — *see* Leukoaraiosis
Leukocoria — *see* Disorder, globe, degenerated condition, leucocoria
Leukocytopenia D72.819
Leukocytosis D72.829
  eosinophilic D72.1
Leukoderma, leukodermia NEC L81.5
  syphilitic A51.39
    late A52.79
Leukodystrophy E75.29
Leukoedema, oral epithelium K13.29
Leukoencephalitis G04.81
  acute (subacute) hemorrhagic G36.1
    postimmunization or postvaccinal G04.02
  postinfectious G04.01
  subacute sclerosing A81.1
  van Bogaert's (sclerosing) A81.1
Leukoencephalopathy — *see also* Encephalopathy G93.49
  Binswanger's I67.3
  heroin vapor G92
  metachromatic E75.25
  multifocal (progressive) A81.2
  postimmunization and postvaccinal G04.02
  progressive multifocal A81.2
  reversible, posterior G93.6
  van Bogaert's (sclerosing) A81.1
  vascular, progressive I67.3
Leukoerythroblastosis D75.9
Leukokeratosis — *see also* Leukoplakia
  mouth K13.21
  nicotina palati K13.24
  oral mucosa K13.21
  tongue K13.21
  vocal cord J38.3

Leukokraurosis vulva (e) N90.4
Leukoma (cornea) — *see also* Opacity, cornea
  adherent H17.0- ☑
  interfering with central vision — *see* Opacity, cornea, central
Leukomalacia, cerebral, newborn P91.2
  periventricular P91.2
Leukomelanopathy, hereditary D72.0
Leukonychia (punctata) (striata) L60.8
  congenital Q84.4
Leukopathia unguium L60.8
  congenital Q84.4
Leukopenia D72.819
  basophilic D72.818
  chemotherapy (cancer) induced D70.1
  congenital D70.0
  cyclic D70.0
  drug induced NEC D70.2
    due to cytoreductive cancer chemotherapy D70.1
  eosinophilic D72.818
  familial D70.0
  infantile genetic D70.0
  malignant D70.9
  periodic D70.0
  transitory neonatal P61.5
Leukopenic — *see* condition
Leukoplakia
  anus K62.89
  bladder (postinfectional) N32.89
  buccal K13.21
  cervix (uteri) N88.0
  esophagus K22.8
  gingiva K13.21
  hairy (oral mucosa) (tongue) K13.3
  kidney (pelvis) N28.89
  larynx J38.7
  lip K13.21
  mouth K13.21
  oral epithelium, including tongue (mucosa) K13.21
  palate K13.21
  pelvis (kidney) N28.89
  penis (infectional) N48.0
  rectum K62.89
  syphilitic (late) A52.79
  tongue K13.21
  ureter (postinfectional) N28.89
  urethra (postinfectional) N36.8
  uterus N85.8
  vagina N89.4
  vocal cord J38.3
  vulva N90.4
Leukorrhea N89.8
  due to Trichomonas (vaginalis) A59.00
  trichomonal A59.00
Leukosarcoma C85.9- ☑
Levocardia (isolated) Q24.1
  with situs inversus Q89.3
Levotransposition Q20.5
Lev's disease or syndrome (acquired complete heart block) I44.2
Levulosuria — *see* Fructosuria
Levurid L30.2
Lewy body (ies) (dementia) (disease) G31.83
Leyden-Moebius dystrophy G71.09
Leydig cell
  carcinoma
    specified site — *see* Neoplasm, malignant, by site
    unspecified site
      female C56.9
      male C62.9- ☑
  tumor
    benign
      specified site — *see* Neoplasm, benign, by site
      unspecified site
        female D27.- ☑
        male D29.2- ☑
    malignant
      specified site — *see* Neoplasm, malignant, by site
      unspecified site
        female C56.- ☑
        male C62.9- ☑
    specified site — *see* Neoplasm, uncertain behavior, by site
    unspecified site
      female D39.1- ☑
      male D40.1- ☑

Leydig-Sertoli cell tumor
  specified site — *see* Neoplasm, benign, by site
  unspecified site
    female D27.- ☑
    male D29.2- ☑
LGSIL (Low grade squamous intraepithelial lesion on cytologic smear of)
  anus R85.612
  cervix R87.612
  vagina R87.622
Liar, pathologic F60.2
Libido
  decreased R68.82
Libman-Sacks disease M32.11
Lice (infestation) B85.2
  body (Pediculus corporis) B85.1
  crab B85.3
  head (Pediculus capitis) B85.0
  mixed (classifiable to more than one of the titles B85.0-B85.3) B85.4
  pubic (Phthirus pubis) B85.3
Lichen L28.0
  albus L90.0
    penis N48.0
    vulva N90.4
  amyloidosis E85.4 *[L99]*
  atrophicus L90.0
    penis N48.0
    vulva N90.4
  congenital Q82.8
  myxedematosus L98.5
  nitidus L44.1
  pilaris Q82.8
    acquired L85.8
  planopilaris L66.1
  planus (chronicus) L43.9
    annularis L43.8
    bullous L43.1
    follicular L66.1
    hypertrophic L43.0
    moniliformis L44.3
    of Wilson L43.9
    specified NEC L43.8
    subacute (active) L43.3
    tropicus L43.3
  ruber
    acuminatus L44.0
    moniliformis L44.3
    planus L43.9
  sclerosus (et atrophicus) L90.0
    penis N48.0
    vulva N90.4
  scrofulosus (primary) (tuberculous) A18.4
  simplex (chronicus) (circumscriptus) L28.0
  striatus L44.2
  urticatus L28.2
Lichenification L28.0
Lichenoides tuberculosis (primary) A18.4
Lichtheim's disease or syndrome D51.0
Lien migrans D73.89
Ligament — *see* condition
Light
  for gestational age — *see* Light for dates
  headedness R42
Light-for-dates (infant) P05.00
  with weight of
    499 grams or less P05.01
    500-749 grams P05.02
    750-999 grams P05.03
    1000-1249 grams P05.04
    1250-1499 grams P05.05
    1500-1749 grams P05.06
    1750-1999 grams P05.07
    2000-2499 grams P05.08
    2500 grams and over P05.09
  affecting management of pregnancy O36.59- ☑
  and small-for-dates — *see* Small for dates
  specified NEC P05.09
Lightning (effects) (stroke) (struck by) T75.00 ☑
  burn — *see* Burn
  foot E53.8
  shock T75.01 ☑
  specified effect NEC T75.09 ☑
Lightwood-Albright syndrome N25.89
Lightwood's disease or syndrome (renal tubular acidosis) N25.89
Lignac (-de Toni) (-Fanconi) (-Debré) **disease or syndrome** E72.09

Lignac (-de Toni) (-Fanconi) (-Debré) **disease or syndrome** — *continued*
  with cystinosis E72.04
Ligneous thyroiditis E06.5
Likoff's syndrome I20.8
Limb — *see* condition
Limbic epilepsy personality syndrome F07.0
Limitation, limited
  activities due to disability Z73.6
  cardiac reserve — *see* Disease, heart
  eye muscle duction, traumatic — *see* Strabismus, mechanical
  mandibular range of motion M26.52
Lindau (-von Hippel) **disease** Q85.8
Line(s)
  Beau's L60.4
  Harris' — *see* Arrest, epiphyseal
  Hudson's (cornea) — *see* Pigmentation, cornea, anterior
  Stähli's (cornea) — *see* Pigmentation, cornea, anterior
Linea corneae senilis — *see* Change, cornea, senile
Lingua
  geographica K14.1
  nigra (villosa) K14.3
  plicata K14.5
  tylosis K13.29
Lingual — *see* condition
Linguatulosis B88.8
Linitis (gastric) **plastica** C16.9
Lip — *see* condition
Lipedema — *see* Edema
Lipemia — *see also* Hyperlipidemia
  retina, retinalis E78.3
Lipidosis E75.6
  cerebral (infantile) (juvenile) (late) E75.4
  cerebroretinal E75.4
  cerebroside E75.22
  cholesterol (cerebral) E75.5
  glycolipid E75.21
  hepatosplenomegalic E78.3
  sphingomyelin — *see* Niemann-Pick disease or syndrome
  sulfatide E75.29
Lipoadenoma — *see* Neoplasm, benign, by site
Lipoblastoma — *see* Lipoma
Lipoblastomatosis — *see* Lipoma
Lipochondrodystrophy E76.01
Lipochrome histiocytosis (familial) D71
Lipodermatosclerosis — *see* Varix, leg, with, inflammation
  ulcerated — *see* Varix, leg, with, ulcer, with inflammation by site
Lipodystrophia progressiva E88.1
Lipodystrophy (progressive) E88.1
  insulin E88.1
  intestinal K90.81
  mesenteric K65.4
Lipofibroma — *see* Lipoma
Lipofuscinosis, neuronal (with ceroidosis) E75.4
Lipogranuloma, sclerosing L92.8
Lipogranulomatosis E78.89
Lipoid — *see also* condition
  histiocytosis D76.3
    essential E75.29
  nephrosis N04.9
  proteinosis of Urbach E78.89
Lipoidemia — *see* Hyperlipidemia
Lipoidosis — *see* Lipidosis
Lipoma D17.9
  fetal D17.9
    fat cell D17.9
  infiltrating D17.9
  intramuscular D17.9
  pleomorphic D17.9
  site classification
    arms (skin) (subcutaneous) D17.2- ☑
    connective tissue D17.30
      intra-abdominal D17.5
      intrathoracic D17.4
      peritoneum D17.79
      retroperitoneum D17.79
      specified site NEC D17.39
      spermatic cord D17.6
    face (skin) (subcutaneous) D17.0
    genitourinary organ NEC D17.72
    head (skin) (subcutaneous) D17.0
    intra-abdominal D17.5
    intrathoracic D17.4

Lipoma — *continued*
  site classification — *continued*
    kidney D17.71
    legs (skin) (subcutaneous) D17.2- ☑
    neck (skin) (subcutaneous) D17.0
    peritoneum D17.79
    retroperitoneum D17.79
    skin D17.30
      specified site NEC D17.39
    specified site NEC D17.79
    spermatic cord D17.6
    subcutaneous D17.30
      specified site NEC D17.39
    trunk (skin) (subcutaneous) D17.1
    unspecified D17.9
  spindle cell D17.9
Lipomatosis E88.2
  dolorosa (Dercum) E88.2
  fetal — *see* Lipoma
  Launois-Bensaude E88.89
Lipomyoma — *see* Lipoma
Lipomyxoma — *see* Lipoma
Lipomyxosarcoma — *see* Neoplasm, connective tissue, malignant
Lipoprotein metabolism disorder E78.9
Lipoproteinemia E78.5
  broad-beta E78.2
  floating-beta E78.2
  hyper-pre-beta E78.1
Liposarcoma — *see also* Neoplasm, connective tissue, malignant
  dedifferentiated — *see* Neoplasm, connective tissue, malignant
  differentiated type — *see* Neoplasm, connective tissue, malignant
  embryonal — *see* Neoplasm, connective tissue, malignant
  mixed type — *see* Neoplasm, connective tissue, malignant
  myxoid — *see* Neoplasm, connective tissue, malignant
  pleomorphic — *see* Neoplasm, connective tissue, malignant
  round cell — *see* Neoplasm, connective tissue, malignant
  well differentiated type — *see* Neoplasm, connective tissue, malignant
Liposynovitis prepatellaris E88.89
Lipping, cervix N86
Lipschütz disease or ulcer N76.6
Lipuria R82.0
  schistosomiasis (bilharziasis) B65.0
Lisping F80.0
Lissauer's paralysis A52.17
Lissencephalia, lissencephaly Q04.3
Listeriosis, listerellosis A32.9
  congenital (disseminated) P37.2
  cutaneous A32.0
  neonatal, newborn (disseminated) P37.2
  oculoglandular A32.81
  specified NEC A32.89
Lithemia E79.0
Lithiasis — *see* Calculus
Lithosis J62.8
Lithuria R82.998
Litigation, anxiety concerning Z65.3
Little leaguer's elbow — *see* Epicondylitis, medial
Little's disease G80.9
Littre's
  gland — *see* condition
  hernia — *see* Hernia, abdomen
Littritis — *see* Urethritis
Livedo (annularis) (racemosa) (reticularis) R23.1
Liver — *see* condition
Living alone (problems with) Z60.2
  with handicapped person Z74.2
Lloyd's syndrome — *see* Adenomatosis, endocrine
Loa loa, loaiasis, loasis B74.3
Lobar — *see* condition
Lobomycosis B48.0
Lobo's disease B48.0
Lobotomy syndrome F07.0
Lobstein (-Ekman) **disease or syndrome** Q78.0
Lobster-claw hand Q71.6- ☑
Lobulation (congenital) — *see also* Anomaly, by site
  kidney, Q63.1
  liver, abnormal Q44.7
  spleen Q89.09

Lobule, lobular — *see* condition
Local, localized — *see* condition
Locked twins causing obstructed labor O66.1
Locked-in state G83.5
Locking
  joint — *see* Derangement, joint, specified type NEC
  knee — *see* Derangement, knee
Lockjaw — *see* Tetanus
Löffler's
  endocarditis I42.3
  eosinophilia J82
  pneumonia J82
  syndrome (eosinophilic pneumonitis) J82
Loiasis (with conjunctival infestation) (eyelid) B74.3
Lone Star fever A77.0
Long
  labor O63.9
    first stage O63.0
    second stage O63.1
  QT syndrome I45.81
Longitudinal stripes or grooves, nails L60.8
  congenital Q84.6
Long-term (current) (prophylactic) **drug therapy** (use of)
  agents affecting estrogen receptors and estrogen levels NEC Z79.818
  anastrozole (Arimidex) Z79.811
  antibiotics Z79.2
    short-term use — *omit code*
  anticoagulants Z79.01
  anti-inflammatory, non-steroidal (NSAID) Z79.1
  antiplatelet Z79.02
  antithrombotics Z79.02
  aromatase inhibitors Z79.811
  aspirin Z79.82
  birth control pill or patch Z79.3
  bisphosphonates Z79.83
  contraceptive, oral Z79.3
  drug, specified NEC Z79.899
  estrogen receptor downregulators Z79.818
  Evista Z79.810
  exemestane (Aromasin) Z79.811
  Fareston Z79.810
  fulvestrant (Faslodex) Z79.818
  gonadotropin-releasing hormone (GnRH) agonist Z79.818
  goserelin acetate (Zoladex) Z79.818
  hormone replacement Z79.890
  insulin Z79.4
  letrozole (Femara) Z79.811
  leuprolide acetate (leuprorelin) (Lupron) Z79.818
  megestrol acetate (Megace) Z79.818
  methadone for pain management Z79.891
  Nolvadex Z79.810
  non-steroidal anti-inflammatories (NSAID) Z79.1
  opiate analgesic Z79.891
  oral
    antidiabetic Z79.84
    contraceptive Z79.3
    hypoglycemic Z79.84
  raloxifene (Evista) Z79.810
  selective estrogen receptor modulators (SERMs) Z79.810
  steroids
    inhaled Z79.51
    systemic Z79.52
  tamoxifen (Nolvadex) Z79.810
  toremifene (Fareston) Z79.810
Loop
  intestine — *see* Volvulus
  vascular on papilla (optic) Q14.2
Loose — *see also* condition
  body
    joint M24.00
      ankle M24.07- ☑
      elbow M24.02- ☑
      hand M24.04- ☑
      hip M24.05- ☑
      knee M23.4- ☑
      shoulder (region) M24.01- ☑
      specified site NEC M24.08
      toe M24.07- ☑
      vertebra M24.08
      wrist M24.03- ☑
    knee M23.4- ☑
    sheath, tendon — *see* Disorder, tendon, specified type NEC
  cartilage — *see* Loose, body, joint

Loose — *continued*
  skin and subcutaneous tissue (following bariatric surgery weight loss) (following dietary weight loss) L98.7
  tooth, teeth K08.89
Loosening
  aseptic
    joint prosthesis — *see* Complications, joint prosthesis, mechanical, loosening, by site
  epiphysis — *see* Osteochondropathy
  mechanical
    joint prosthesis — *see* Complications, joint prosthesis, mechanical, loosening, by site
Looser-Milkman (-Debray) **syndrome** M83.8
Lop ear (deformity) Q17.3
Lorain (-Levi) **short stature syndrome** E23.0
Lordosis M40.50
  acquired — *see* Lordosis, specified type NEC
  congenital Q76.429
    lumbar region Q76.426
    lumbosacral region Q76.427
    sacral region Q76.428
    sacrococcygeal region Q76.428
    thoracolumbar region Q76.425
  lumbar region M40.56
  lumbosacral region M40.57
  postsurgical M96.4
  postural — *see* Lordosis, specified type NEC
  rachitic (late effect) (sequelae) E64.3
  sequelae of rickets E64.3
  specified type NEC M40.40
    lumbar region M40.46
    lumbosacral region M40.47
    thoracolumbar region M40.45
  thoracolumbar region M40.55
  tuberculous A18.01
Loss (of)
  appetite — *see also* Anorexia R63.0
    hysterical F50.89
    nonorganic origin F50.89
    psychogenic F50.89
  blood — *see* Hemorrhage
  bone —*see* Loss, substance of, bone
  consciousness, transient R55
    traumatic — *see* Injury, intracranial
  control, sphincter, rectum R15.9
    nonorganic origin F98.1
  elasticity, skin R23.4
  family (member) in childhood Z62.898
  fluid (acute) E86.9
  function of labyrinth — *see* subcategory H83.2 ☑
  hair, nonscarring — *see* Alopecia
  hearing — *see also* Deafness
    central NOS H90.5
    conductive H90.2
      bilateral H90.0
      unilateral
        with
          restricted hearing on the contralateral side H90.A1- ☑
          unrestricted hearing on the contralateral side H90.1- ☑
    mixed conductive and sensorineural hearing loss H90.8
      bilateral H90.6
      unilateral
        with
          restricted hearing on the contralateral side H90.A3- ☑
          unrestricted hearing on the contralateral side H90.7- ☑
    neural NOS H90.5
    perceptive NOS H90.5
    sensorineural NOS H90.5
      bilateral H90.3
      unilateral
        with
          restricted hearing on the contralateral side H90.A2- ☑
          unrestricted hearing on the contralateral side H90.4- ☑
    sensory NOS H90.5
  height R29.890
  limb or member, traumatic, current — *see* Amputation, traumatic
  love relationship in childhood Z62.898
  memory — *see also* Amnesia
    mild, following organic brain damage F06.8

▽ Subterms under main terms may continue to next column or page   ☑ Additional Character Required — Refer to the Tabular List for Character Selection   213

Lipoma — Loss

Loss — *continued*
  mind — *see* Psychosis
  occlusal vertical dimension of fully erupted teeth M26.37
  organ or part — *see* Absence, by site, acquired
  ossicles, ear (partial) H74.32- ☑
  parent in childhood Z63.4
  pregnancy, recurrent N96
    care in current pregnancy O26.2- ☑
    without current pregnancy N96
  recurrent pregnancy — *see* Loss, pregnancy, recurrent
  self-esteem, in childhood Z62.898
  sense of
    smell — *see* Disturbance, sensation, smell
    taste — *see* Disturbance, sensation, taste
    touch R20.8
  sensory R44.9
    dissociative F44.6
  sexual desire F52.0
  sight (acquired) (complete) (congenital) — *see* Blindness
  substance of
    bone — *see* Disorder, bone, density and structure, specified NEC
      horizontal alveolar K06.3
    cartilage — *see* Disorder, cartilage, specified type NEC
      auricle (ear) — *see* Disorder, pinna, specified type NEC
    vitreous (humor) H15.89
  tooth, teeth — *see* Absence, teeth, acquired
  vision, visual H54.7
    both eyes H54.3
    one eye H54.60
      left (normal vision on right) H54.62
      right (normal vision on left) H54.61
    specified as blindness — *see* Blindness
    subjective
      sudden H53.13- ☑
      transient H53.12- ☑
  vitreous — *see* Prolapse, vitreous
  voice — *see* Aphonia
  weight (abnormal) (cause unknown) R63.4
Louis-Bar syndrome (ataxia-telangiectasia) G11.3
Louping ill (encephalitis) A84.8
Louse, lousiness — *see* Lice
Low
  achiever, school Z55.3
  back syndrome M54.5
  basal metabolic rate R94.8
  birthweight (2499 grams or less) P07.10
    with weight of
      1000-1249 grams P07.14
      1250-1499 grams P07.15
      1500-1749 grams P07.16
      1750-1999 grams P07.17
      2000-2499 grams P07.18
    extreme (999 grams or less) P07.00
      with weight of
        499 grams or less P07.01
        500-749 grams P07.02
        750-999 grams P07.03
    for gestational age — *see* Light for dates
  blood pressure — *see also* Hypotension
    reading (incidental) (isolated) (nonspecific) R03.1
  cardiac reserve — *see* Disease, heart
  function — *see also* Hypofunction
    kidney N28.9
  hematocrit D64.9
  hemoglobin D64.9
  income Z59.6
  level of literacy Z55.0
  lying
    kidney N28.89
    organ or site, congenital — *see* Malposition, congenital
  output syndrome (cardiac) — *see* Failure, heart
  platelets (blood) — *see* Thrombocytopenia
  reserve, kidney N28.89
  salt syndrome E87.1
  self esteem R45.81
  set ears Q17.4
  vision H54.2X- ☑
    one eye (other eye normal) H54.50
      left (normal vision on right) H54.52A- ☑
      other eye blind — *see* Blindness
      right (normal vision on left) H54.511- ☑

Low-density-lipoprotein-type (LDL) **hyperlipoproteinemia** E78.00
Lowe's syndrome E72.03
Lown-Ganong-Levine syndrome I45.6
LSD reaction (acute) (without dependence) F16.90
  with dependence F16.20
L-shaped kidney Q63.8
LTBI (latent tuberculosis infection) Z22.7
Ludwig's angina or disease K12.2
Lues (venerea), **luetic** — *see* Syphilis
Luetscher's syndrome (dehydration) E86.0
Lumbago, lumbalgia M54.5
  with sciatica M54.4- ☑
    due to intervertebral disc disorder M51.17
  due to displacement, intervertebral disc M51.27
    with sciatica M51.17
Lumbar — *see* condition
Lumbarization, vertebra, congenital Q76.49
Lumbermen's itch B88.0
Lump — *see also* Mass
  breast N63.0
    axillary tail
      left N63.32
      right N63.31
    left
      lower inner quadrant N63.24
      lower outer quadrant N63.23
      overlapping quadrants N63.25
      unspecified quadrant N63.20
      upper inner quadrant N63.22
      upper outer quadrant N63.21
    right
      lower inner quadrant N63.14
      lower outer quadrant N63.13
      overlapping quadrants N63.15
      unspecified quadrant N63.10
      upper inner quadrant N63.12
      upper outer quadrant N63.11
    subareolar
      left N63.42
      right N63.41
Lunacy — *see* Psychosis
Lung — *see* condition
Lupoid (miliary) **of Boeck** D86.3
Lupus
  anticoagulant D68.62
    with
      hemorrhagic disorder D68.312
      hypercoagulable state D68.62
    finding without diagnosis R76.0
  discoid (local) L93.0
  erythematosus (discoid) (local) L93.0
    disseminated — *see* Lupus, erythematosus, systemic
    eyelid H01.129
      left H01.126
        lower H01.125
        upper H01.124
      right H01.123
        lower H01.122
        upper H01.121
    profundus L93.2
    specified NEC L93.2
    subacute cutaneous L93.1
    systemic M32.9
      with organ or system involvement M32.10
        endocarditis M32.11
        lung M32.13
        pericarditis M32.12
        renal (glomerular) M32.14
          tubulo-interstitial M32.15
        specified organ or system NEC M32.19
      drug-induced M32.0
      inhibitor (presence of) D68.62
        with
          hemorrhagic disorder D68.312
          hypercoagulable state D68.62
        finding without diagnosis R76.0
      specified NEC M32.8
  exedens A18.4
  hydralazine M32.0
    correct substance properly administered — *see* Table of Drugs and Chemicals, by drug, adverse effect
    overdose or wrong substance given or taken — *see* Table of Drugs and Chemicals, by drug, poisoning
  nephritis (chronic) M32.14
  nontuberculous, not disseminated L93.0

Lupus — *continued*
  panniculitis L93.2
  pernio (Besnier) D86.3
  systemic — *see* Lupus, erythematosus, systemic
  tuberculous A18.4
    eyelid A18.4
  vulgaris A18.4
    eyelid A18.4
Luteinoma D27.- ☑
Lutembacher's disease or syndrome (atrial septal defect with mitral stenosis) Q21.1
Luteoma D27.- ☑
Lutz (-Splendore-de Almeida) **disease** — *see* Paracoccidioidomycosis
Luxation — *see also* Dislocation
  eyeball (nontraumatic) — *see* Luxation, globe
    birth injury P15.3
  globe, nontraumatic H44.82- ☑
  lacrimal gland — *see* Dislocation, lacrimal gland
  lens (old) (partial) (spontaneous)
    congenital Q12.1
    syphilitic A50.39
Lycanthropy F22
Lyell's syndrome L51.2
  due to drug L51.2
    correct substance properly administered — *see* Table of Drugs and Chemicals, by drug, adverse effect
    overdose or wrong substance given or taken — *see* Table of Drugs and Chemicals, by drug, poisoning
Lyme disease A69.20
Lymph
  gland or node — *see* condition
  scrotum — *see* Infestation, filarial
Lymphadenitis I88.9
  with ectopic or molar pregnancy O08.0
  acute L04.9
    axilla L04.2
    face L04.0
    head L04.0
    hip L04.3
    limb
      lower L04.3
      upper L04.2
    neck L04.0
    shoulder L04.2
    specified site NEC L04.8
    trunk L04.1
  anthracosis (occupational) J60
  any site, except mesenteric I88.9
    chronic I88.1
    subacute I88.1
  breast
    gestational — *see* Mastitis, obstetric
    puerperal, postpartum (nonpurulent) O91.22
  chancroidal (congenital) A57
  chronic I88.1
    mesenteric I88.0
  due to
    Brugia (malayi) B74.1
      timori B74.2
    chlamydial lymphogranuloma A55
    diphtheria (toxin) A36.89
    lymphogranuloma venereum A55
    Wuchereria bancrofti B74.0
  following ectopic or molar pregnancy O08.0
  gonorrheal A54.89
  infective — *see* Lymphadenitis, acute
  mesenteric (acute) (chronic) (nonspecific) (subacute) I88.0
    due to Salmonella typhi A01.09
    tuberculous A18.39
  mycobacterial A31.8
  purulent — *see* Lymphadenitis, acute
  pyogenic — *see* Lymphadenitis, acute
  regional, nonbacterial I88.8
  septic — *see* Lymphadenitis, acute
  subacute, unspecified site I88.1
  suppurative — *see* Lymphadenitis, acute
  syphilitic (early) (secondary) A51.49
    late A52.79
  tuberculous — *see* Tuberculosis, lymph gland
  venereal (chlamydial) A55
Lymphadenoid goiter E06.3
Lymphadenopathy (generalized) R59.1
  angioimmunoblastic, with dysproteinemia (AILD) C86.5
  due to toxoplasmosis (acquired) B58.89

Lymphadenopathy — continued
  due to toxoplasmosis — continued
    congenital (acute) (subacute) (chronic) P37.1
  localized R59.Ø
  syphilitic (early) (secondary) A51.49
Lymphadenosis R59.1
Lymphangiectasis I89.Ø
  conjunctiva H11.89
  postinfectional I89.Ø
  scrotum I89.Ø
Lymphangiectatic elephantiasis, nonfilarial I89.Ø
Lymphangioendothelioma D18.1
  malignant — see Neoplasm, connective tissue, malignant
Lymphangioleiomyomatosis J84.81
Lymphangioma D18.1
  capillary D18.1
  cavernous D18.1
  cystic D18.1
  malignant — see Neoplasm, connective tissue, malignant
Lymphangiomyoma D18.1
Lymphangiomyomatosis J84.81
Lymphangiosarcoma — see Neoplasm, connective tissue, malignant
Lymphangitis I89.1
  with
    abscess — code by site under Abscess
    cellulitis — code by site under Cellulitis
    ectopic or molar pregnancy OØ8.Ø
  acute LØ3.91
    abdominal wall LØ3.321
    ankle — see Lymphangitis, acute, lower limb
    arm — see Lymphangitis, acute, upper limb
    auricle (ear) — see Lymphangitis, acute, ear
    axilla LØ3.12- ☑
    back (any part) LØ3.322
    buttock LØ3.327
    cervical (meaning neck) LØ3.222
    cheek (external) LØ3.212
    chest wall LØ3.323
    digit
      finger — see Lymphangitis, acute, finger
      toe — see Lymphangitis, acute, toe
    ear (external) H6Ø.1- ☑
    external auditory canal — see Lymphangitis, acute, ear
    eyelid — see Abscess, eyelid
    face NEC LØ3.212
    finger (intrathecal) (periosteal) (subcutaneous) (subcuticular) LØ3.Ø2- ☑
    foot — see Lymphangitis, acute, lower limb
    gluteal (region) LØ3.327
    groin LØ3.324
    hand — see Lymphangitis, acute, upper limb
    head NEC LØ3.891
      face (any part, except ear, eye and nose) LØ3.212
    heel — see Lymphangitis, acute, lower limb
    hip — see Lymphangitis, acute, lower limb
    jaw (region) LØ3.212
    knee — see Lymphangitis, acute, lower limb
    leg — see Lymphangitis, acute, lower limb
    lower limb LØ3.12- ☑
      toe — see Lymphangitis, acute, toe
    navel LØ3.326
    neck (region) LØ3.222
    orbit, orbital — see Cellulitis, orbit
    pectoral (region) LØ3.323
    perineal, perineum LØ3.325
    scalp (any part) LØ3.891
    shoulder — see Lymphangitis, acute, upper limb
    specified site NEC LØ3.898
    thigh — see Lymphangitis, acute, lower limb
    thumb (intrathecal) (periosteal) (subcutaneous) (subcuticular) — see Lymphangitis, acute, finger
    toe (intrathecal) (periosteal) (subcutaneous) (subcuticular) LØ3.Ø4- ☑
    trunk LØ3.329
      abdominal wall LØ3.321
      back (any part) LØ3.322
      buttock LØ3.327
      chest wall LØ3.323
      groin LØ3.324
      perineal, perineum LØ3.325
      umbilicus LØ3.326
    umbilicus LØ3.326

Lymphangitis — continued
  acute — continued
    upper limb LØ3.12- ☑
      axilla — see Lymphangitis, acute, axilla
      finger — see Lymphangitis, acute, finger
      thumb — see Lymphangitis, acute, finger
      wrist — see Lymphangitis, acute, upper limb
  breast
    gestational — see Mastitis, obstetric
  chancroidal A57
  chronic (any site) I89.1
  due to
    Brugia (malayi) B74.1
      timori B74.2
    Wuchereria bancrofti B74.Ø
  following ectopic or molar pregnancy OØ8.89
  penis
    acute N48.29
    gonococcal (acute) (chronic) A54.Ø9
  puerperal, postpartum, childbirth O86.89
  strumous, tuberculous A18.2
  subacute (any site) I89.1
  tuberculous — see Tuberculosis, lymph gland
Lymphatic (vessel) — see condition
Lymphatism E32.8
Lymphectasia I89.Ø
Lymphedema (acquired) — see also Elephantiasis
  congenital Q82.Ø
  hereditary (chronic) (idiopathic) Q82.Ø
  postmastectomy I97.2
  praecox I89.Ø
  secondary I89.Ø
  surgical NEC I97.89
    postmastectomy (syndrome) I97.2
Lymphoblastic — see condition
Lymphoblastoma (diffuse) — see Lymphoma, lymphoblastic (diffuse)
  giant follicular — see Lymphoma, lymphoblastic (diffuse)
  macrofollicular — see Lymphoma, lymphoblastic (diffuse)
Lymphocele I89.8
Lymphocytic
  chorioencephalitis (acute) (serous) A87.2
  choriomeningitis (acute) (serous) A87.2
  meningoencephalitis A87.2
Lymphocytoma, benign cutis L98.8
Lymphocytopenia D72.81Ø
Lymphocytosis (symptomatic) D72.82Ø
  infectious (acute) B33.8
Lymphoepithelioma — see Neoplasm, malignant, by site
Lymphogranuloma (malignant) — see also Lymphoma, Hodgkin
  chlamydial A55
  inguinale A55
  venereum (any site) (chlamydial) (with stricture of rectum) A55
Lymphogranulomatosis (malignant) — see also Lymphoma, Hodgkin
  benign (Boeck's sarcoid) (Schaumann's) D86.1
Lymphohistiocytosis, hemophagocytic (familial) D76.1
Lymphoid — see condition
Lymphoma (of) (malignant) C85.9Ø
  adult T-cell (HTLV-1-associated) (acute variant) (chronic variant) (lymphomatoid variant) (smouldering variant) C91.5- ☑
  anaplastic large cell
    ALK-negative C84.7- ☑
    ALK-positive C84.6- ☑
    CD3Ø-positive C84.6- ☑
    primary cutaneous C86.6
  angioimmunoblastic T-cell C86.5
  BALT C88.4
  B-cell C85.1- ☑
  blastic NK-cell C86.4
  blastic plasmacytoid dendritic cell neoplasm (BPDCN) C86.4
  B-precursor C83.5- ☑
  bronchial-associated lymphoid tissue [BALT-lymphoma] C88.4
  Burkitt (atypical) C83.7- ☑
  Burkitt-like C83.7- ☑
  centrocytic C83.1- ☑
  cutaneous follicle center C82.6- ☑
  cutaneous T-cell C84.A- ☑ (following C84.7)
  diffuse follicle center C82.5- ☑

Lymphoma — continued
  diffuse large cell C83.3- ☑
    anaplastic C83.3- ☑
    B-cell C83.3- ☑
    CD3Ø-positive C83.3- ☑
    centroblastic C83.3- ☑
    immunoblastic C83.3- ☑
    plasmablastic C83.3- ☑
    subtype not specified C83.3- ☑
    T-cell rich C83.3- ☑
  enteropathy-type (associated) (intestinal) T-cell C86.2
  extranodal marginal zone B-cell lymphoma of mucosa-associated lymphoid tissue [MALT-lymphoma] C88.4
  extranodal NK/T-cell, nasal type C86.Ø
  follicular C82.9- ☑
    grade
      I C82.Ø- ☑
      II C82.1- ☑
      III C82.2- ☑
      IIIa C82.3- ☑
      IIIb C82.4- ☑
    specified NEC C82.8- ☑
  hepatosplenic T-cell (alpha-beta) (gamma-delta) C86.1
  histiocytic C85.9- ☑
    true C96.A (following C96.6)
  Hodgkin C81.9 ☑
    lymphocyte depleted (classical) C81.3- ☑
    lymphocyte-rich (classical) C81.4- ☑
    mixed cellularity (classical) C81.2- ☑
    nodular
      lymphocyte predominant C81.Ø- ☑
      sclerosis (classical) C81.1- ☑
    nodular sclerosis (classical) C81.1- ☑
    specified NEC (classical) C81.7- ☑
  intravascular large B-cell C83.8- ☑
  Lennert's C84.4- ☑
  lymphoblastic (diffuse) C83.5- ☑
  lymphoblastic B-cell C83.5- ☑
  lymphoblastic T-cell C83.5- ☑
  lymphoepithelioid C84.4- ☑
  lymphoplasmacytic C83.Ø- ☑
    with IgM-production C88.Ø
  MALT C88.4
  mantle cell C83.1- ☑
  mature T-cell NEC C84.4- ☑
  mature T/NK-cell C84.9- ☑
    specified NEC C84.Z- ☑ (following C84.7)
  mediastinal (thymic) large B-cell C85.2- ☑
  Mediterranean C88.3
  mucosa-associated lymphoid tissue [MALT-lymphoma] C88.4
  NK/T cell C84.9- ☑
  nodal marginal zone C83.Ø- ☑
  non-follicular (diffuse) C83.9- ☑
    specified NEC C83.8- ☑
  non-Hodgkin — see also Lymphoma, by type C85.9- ☑
    specified NEC C85.8- ☑
  non-leukemic variant of B-CLL C83.Ø- ☑
  peripheral T-cell, not classified C84.4- ☑
  primary cutaneous
    anaplastic large cell C86.6
    CD3Ø-positive large T-cell C86.6
  primary effusion B-cell C83.8- ☑
  SALT C88.4
  skin-associated lymphoid tissue [SALT-lymphoma] C88.4
  small cell B-cell C83.Ø- ☑
  splenic marginal zone C83.Ø- ☑
  subcutaneous panniculitis-like T-cell C86.3
  T-precursor C83.5- ☑
  true histiocytic C96.A (following C96.6)
Lymphomatosis — see Lymphoma
Lymphopathia venereum, veneris A55
Lymphopenia D72.81Ø
Lymphoplasmacytic leukemia — see Leukemia, chronic lymphocytic, B-cell type
Lymphoproliferation, X-linked disease D82.3
Lymphoreticulosis, benign (of inoculation) A28.1
Lymphorrhea I89.8
Lymphosarcoma (diffuse) — see also Lymphoma C85.9- ☑
Lymphostasis I89.8
Lypemania — see Melancholia
Lysine and hydroxylysine metabolism disorder E72.3
Lyssa — see Rabies

▽ Subterms under main terms may continue to next column or page   ☑ Additional Character Required — Refer to the Tabular List for Character Selection   215

Lymphadenopathy — Lyssa

M

Macacus ear Q17.3
Maceration, wet feet, tropical (syndrome) T69.02- ☑
MacLeod's syndrome J43.0
Macrocephalia, macrocephaly Q75.3
Macrocheilia, macrochilia (congenital) Q18.6
Macrocolon — see also Megacolon Q43.1
Macrocornea Q15.8
  with glaucoma Q15.0
Macrocytic — see condition
Macrocytosis D75.89
Macrodactylia, macrodactylism (fingers) (thumbs)
    Q74.0
  toes Q74.2
Macrodontia K00.2
Macrogenia M26.05
Macrogenitosomia (adrenal) (male) (praecox) E25.9
  congenital E25.0
Macroglobulinemia (idiopathic) (primary) C88.0
  monoclonal (essential) D47.2
  Waldenström C88.0
Macroglossia (congenital) Q38.2
  acquired K14.8
Macrognathia, macrognathism (congenital)
    (mandibular) (maxillary) M26.09
Macrogyria (congenital) Q04.8
Macrohydrocephalus — see Hydrocephalus
Macromastia — see Hypertrophy, breast
Macrophthalmos Q11.3
  in congenital glaucoma Q15.0
Macropsia H53.15
Macrosigmoid K59.39
  congenital Q43.2
Macrospondylitis , acromegalic E22.0
Macrostomia (congenital) Q18.4
Macrotia (external ear) (congenital) Q17.1
Macula
  cornea, corneal — see Opacity, cornea
  degeneration (atrophic) (exudative) (senile) — see also
      Degeneration, macula
    hereditary — see Dystrophy, retina
Maculae ceruleae B85.1
Maculopathy, toxic — see Degeneration, macula, toxic
Madarosis (eyelid) H02.729
  left H02.726
    lower H02.725
    upper H02.724
  right H02.723
    lower H02.722
    upper H02.721
Madelung's
  deformity (radius) Q74.0
  disease
    radial deformity Q74.0
    symmetrical lipomas, neck E88.89
Madness — see Psychosis
Madura
  foot B47.9
    actinomycotic B47.1
    mycotic B47.0
Maduromycosis B47.0
Maffucci's syndrome Q78.4
Magnesium metabolism disorder — see Disorder,
    metabolism, magnesium
Main en griffe (acquired) — see also Deformity, limb,
    clawhand
  congenital Q74.0
Maintenance (encounter for)
  antineoplastic chemotherapy Z51.11
  antineoplastic radiation therapy Z51.0
  methadone F11.20
Majocchi's
  disease L81.7
  granuloma B35.8
Major — see condition
Mal de los pintos — see Pinta
Mal de mer T75.3 ☑
Malabar itch (any site) B35.5
Malabsorption K90.9
  calcium K90.89
  carbohydrate K90.49
  disaccharide E73.9
  fat K90.49
  galactose E74.20
  glucose (-galactose) E74.39

Malabsorption — continued
  intestinal K90.9
    specified NEC K90.89
  isomaltose E74.31
  lactose E73.9
  methionine E72.19
  monosaccharide E74.39
  postgastrectomy K91.2
  postsurgical K91.2
  protein K90.49
  starch K90.49
  sucrose E74.39
  syndrome K90.9
    postsurgical K91.2
Malacia, bone (adult) M83.9
  juvenile — see Rickets
Malacoplakia
  bladder N32.89
  pelvis (kidney) N28.89
  ureter N28.89
  urethra N36.8
Malacosteon, juvenile — see Rickets
Maladaptation — see Maladjustment
Maladie de Roger Q21.0
Maladjustment
  conjugal Z63.0
    involving divorce or estrangement Z63.5
  educational Z55.4
  family Z63.9
  marital Z63.0
    involving divorce or estrangement Z63.5
  occupational NEC Z56.89
  simple, adult — see Disorder, adjustment
  situational — see Disorder, adjustment
  social Z60.9
    due to
      acculturation difficulty Z60.3
      discrimination and persecution (perceived) Z60.5
      exclusion and isolation Z60.4
      life-cycle (phase of life) transition Z60.0
      rejection Z60.4
      specified reason NEC Z60.8
Malaise R53.81
Malakoplakia — see Malacoplakia
Malaria, malarial (fever) B54
  with
    blackwater fever B50.8
      hemoglobinuric (bilious) B50.8
    hemoglobinuria B50.8
  accidentally induced (therapeutically) — code by type
      under Malaria
  algid B50.9
  cerebral B50.0 [G94]
  clinically diagnosed (without parasitological confirmation) B54
  congenital NEC P37.4
    falciparum P37.3
  congestion, congestive B54
  continued (fever) B50.9
  estivo-autumnal B50.9
  falciparum B50.9
    with complications NEC B50.8
      cerebral B50.0 [G94]
    severe B50.8
  hemorrhagic B54
  malariae B52.9
    with
      complications NEC B52.8
      glomerular disorder B52.0
  malignant (tertian) — see Malaria, falciparum
  mixed infections — code to first listed type in B50-B53
  ovale B53.0
  parasitologically confirmed NEC B53.8
  pernicious, acute — see Malaria, falciparum
  Plasmodium (P.)
    falciparum NEC — see Malaria, falciparum
    malariae NEC B52.9
      with Plasmodium
        falciparum (and or vivax) — see Malaria, falci-
            parum
        vivax — see also Malaria, vivax
          and falciparum — see Malaria, falciparum
    ovale B53.0
      with Plasmodium malariae — see also Malaria,
          malariae
        and vivax — see also Malaria, vivax
          and falciparum — see Malaria, falciparum
    simian B53.1

Malaria, malarial — continued
  Plasmodium — continued
    simian — continued
      with Plasmodium malariae — see also Malaria,
          malariae
        and vivax — see also Malaria, vivax
          and falciparum — see Malaria, falciparum
      vivax NEC B51.9
        with Plasmodium falciparum — see Malaria, fal-
            ciparum
    quartan — see Malaria, malariae
    quotidian — see Malaria, falciparum
    recurrent B54
    remittent B54
    specified type NEC (parasitologically confirmed) B53.8
    spleen B54
    subtertian (fever) — see Malaria, falciparum
    tertian (benign) — see also Malaria, vivax
      malignant B50.9
    tropical B50.9
    typhoid B54
    vivax B51.9
      with
        complications NEC B51.8
        ruptured spleen B51.0
Malassez's disease (cystic) N50.89
Malassimilation K90.9
Maldescent, testis Q53.9
  bilateral Q53.20
    abdominal Q53.211
    perineal Q53.22
  unilateral Q53.10
    abdominal Q53.111
    perineal Q53.12
Maldevelopment — see also Anomaly
  brain Q07.9
  colon Q43.9
  hip Q74.2
    congenital dislocation Q65.2
      bilateral Q65.1
      unilateral Q65.0- ☑
  mastoid process Q75.8
  middle ear Q16.4
    except ossicles Q16.4
    ossicles Q16.3
  ossicles Q16.3
  spine Q76.49
  toe Q74.2
Male type pelvis Q74.2
  with disproportion (fetopelvic) O33.3 ☑
    causing obstructed labor O65.3
Malformation (congenital) — see also Anomaly
  adrenal gland Q89.1
  affecting multiple systems with skeletal changes NEC
      Q87.5
  alimentary tract Q45.9
    specified type NEC Q45.8
    upper Q40.9
      specified type NEC Q40.8
  aorta Q25.40
    absence Q25.41
    aneurysm, congenital Q25.43
    aplasia Q25.41
    atresia Q25.29
      aortic arch Q25.21
    coarctation (preductal) (postductal) Q25.1
    dilatation, congenital Q25.44
    hypoplasia Q25.42
    patent ductus arteriosus Q25.0
    specified type NEC Q25.49
    stenosis Q25.1
    supravalvular Q25.3
  aortic valve Q23.9
    specified NEC Q23.8
  arteriovenous, aneurysmatic (congenital) Q27.30
    brain Q28.2
      ruptured I60.8
        intracerebral I61.8
        intraparenchymal I61.8
        intraventricular I61.5
        subarachnoid I60.8
    cerebral — see also Malformation, arteriovenous,
        brain Q28.2
    peripheral Q27.30
      digestive system — see Angiodysplasia
        congenital Q27.33
        lower limb Q27.32
        other specified site Q27.39

Malformation — *continued*
  arteriovenous, aneurysmatic — *continued*
    peripheral — *continued*
      renal vessel Q27.34
      upper limb Q27.31
    precerebral vessels (nonruptured) Q28.0
  auricle
    ear (congenital) Q17.3
      acquired H61.119
        left H61.112
          with right H61.113
        right H61.111
          with left H61.113
  bile duct Q44.5
  bladder Q64.79
    aplasia Q64.5
    diverticulum Q64.6
    exstrophy — *see* Exstrophy, bladder
    neck obstruction Q64.31
  bone Q79.9
    face Q75.9
      specified type NEC Q75.8
    skull Q75.9
      specified type NEC Q75.8
  brain (multiple) Q04.9
    arteriovenous Q28.2
    specified type NEC Q04.8
  branchial cleft Q18.2
  breast Q83.9
    specified type NEC Q83.8
  broad ligament Q50.6
  bronchus Q32.4
  bursa Q79.9
  cardiac
    chambers Q20.9
      specified type NEC Q20.8
    septum Q21.9
      specified type NEC Q21.8
  cerebral Q04.9
    vessels Q28.3
  cervix uteri Q51.9
    specified type NEC Q51.828
  Chiari
    Type I G93.5
    Type II Q07.01
  choroid (congenital) Q14.3
    plexus Q07.8
  circulatory system Q28.9
  cochlea Q16.5
  cornea Q13.4
  coronary vessels Q24.5
  corpus callosum (congenital) Q04.0
  diaphragm Q79.1
  digestive system NEC, specified type NEC Q45.8
  dura Q07.9
    brain Q04.9
    spinal Q06.9
  ear Q17.9
    causing impairment of hearing Q16.9
    external Q17.9
      accessory auricle Q17.0
      causing impairment of hearing Q16.9
        absence of
          auditory canal Q16.1
          auricle Q16.0
      macrotia Q17.1
      microtia Q17.2
      misplacement Q17.4
      misshapen NEC Q17.3
      prominence Q17.5
      specified type NEC Q17.8
    inner Q16.5
    middle Q16.4
      absence of eustachian tube Q16.2
      ossicles (fusion) Q16.3
    ossicles Q16.3
    specified type NEC Q17.8
  epididymis Q55.4
  esophagus Q39.9
    specified type NEC Q39.8
  eye Q15.9
    lid Q10.3
    specified NEC Q15.8
  fallopian tube Q50.6
  genital organ — *see* Anomaly, genitalia
  great
    artery Q25.9
      aorta — *see* Malformation, aorta

Malformation — *continued*
  great — *continued*
    artery — *continued*
      pulmonary artery — *see* Malformation, pulmonary, artery
      specified type NEC Q25.8
    vein Q26.9
      anomalous
        portal venous connection Q26.5
        pulmonary venous connection Q26.4
          partial Q26.3
          total Q26.2
      persistent left superior vena cava Q26.1
      portal vein-hepatic artery fistula Q26.6
      specified type NEC Q26.8
      vena cava stenosis, congenital Q26.0
  gum Q38.6
  hair Q84.2
  heart Q24.9
    specified type NEC Q24.8
  integument Q84.9
    specified type NEC Q84.8
  internal ear Q16.5
  intestine Q43.9
    specified type NEC Q43.8
  iris Q13.2
  joint Q74.9
    ankle Q74.2
    lumbosacral Q76.49
    sacroiliac Q74.2
    specified type NEC Q74.8
  kidney Q63.9
    accessory Q63.0
    giant Q63.3
    horseshoe Q63.1
    hydronephrosis Q62.0
    malposition Q63.2
    specified type NEC Q63.8
  lacrimal apparatus Q10.6
  lingual Q38.3
  lip Q38.0
  liver Q44.7
  lung Q33.9
  meninges or membrane (congenital) Q07.9
    cerebral Q04.8
    spinal (cord) Q06.9
  middle ear Q16.4
    ossicles Q16.3
  mitral valve Q23.9
    specified NEC Q23.8
  Mondini's (congenital) (malformation, cochlea) Q16.5
  mouth (congenital) Q38.6
  multiple types NEC Q89.7
  musculoskeletal system Q79.9
  myocardium Q24.8
  nail Q84.6
  nervous system (central) Q07.9
  nose Q30.9
    specified type NEC Q30.8
  optic disc Q14.2
  orbit Q10.7
  ovary Q50.39
  palate Q38.5
  parathyroid gland Q89.2
  pelvic organs or tissues NEC
    in pregnancy or childbirth O34.8- ☑
      causing obstructed labor O65.5
  penis Q55.69
    aplasia Q55.5
    curvature (lateral) Q55.61
    hypoplasia Q55.62
  pericardium Q24.8
  peripheral vascular system Q27.9
    specified type NEC Q27.8
  pharynx Q38.8
  precerebral vessels Q28.1
  prostate Q55.4
  pulmonary
    arteriovenous Q25.72
    artery Q25.9
      atresia Q25.5
      specified type NEC Q25.79
      stenosis Q25.6
    valve Q22.3
  renal artery Q27.2
  respiratory system Q34.9
  retina Q14.1
  scrotum — *see* Malformation, testis and scrotum
  seminal vesicles Q55.4

Malformation — *continued*
  sense organs NEC Q07.9
  skin Q82.9
  specified NEC Q89.8
  spinal
    cord Q06.9
    nerve root Q07.8
  spine Q76.49
    kyphosis — *see* Kyphosis, congenital
    lordosis — *see* Lordosis, congenital
  spleen Q89.09
  stomach Q40.3
    specified type NEC Q40.2
  teeth, tooth K00.9
  tendon Q79.9
  testis and scrotum Q55.20
    aplasia Q55.0
    hypoplasia Q55.1
    polyorchism Q55.21
    retractile testis Q55.22
    scrotal transposition Q55.23
    specified NEC Q55.29
  thorax, bony Q76.9
  throat Q38.8
  thyroid gland Q89.2
  tongue (congenital) Q38.3
    hypertrophy Q38.2
    tie Q38.1
  trachea Q32.1
  tricuspid valve Q22.9
    specified type NEC Q22.8
  umbilical cord NEC (complicating delivery) O69.89 ☑
  umbilicus Q89.9
  ureter Q62.8
    agenesis Q62.4
    duplication Q62.5
    malposition — *see* Malposition, congenital, ureter
    obstructive defect — *see* Defect, obstructive, ureter
    vesico-uretero-renal reflux Q62.7
  urethra Q64.79
    aplasia Q64.5
    duplication Q64.74
    posterior valves Q64.2
    prolapse Q64.71
    stricture Q64.32
  urinary system Q64.9
  uterus Q51.9
    specified type NEC Q51.818
  vagina Q52.4
  vas deferens Q55.4
    atresia Q55.3
  vascular system, peripheral Q27.9
  venous — *see* Anomaly, vein(s)
  vulva Q52.70
Malfunction — *see also* Dysfunction
  cardiac electronic device T82.119 ☑
    electrode T82.110 ☑
    pulse generator T82.111 ☑
    specified type NEC T82.118 ☑
  catheter device NEC T85.618 ☑
    cystostomy T83.010 ☑
    dialysis (renal) (vascular) T82.41 ☑
      intraperitoneal T85.611 ☑
    infusion NEC T82.514 ☑
      cranial T85.610 ☑
      epidural T85.610 ☑
      intrathecal T85.610 ☑
      spinal T85.610 ☑
      subarachnoid T85.610 ☑
      subdural T85.610 ☑
    urinary — *see also* Breakdown, device, catheter T83.018 ☑
  colostomy K94.03
    valve K94.03
  cystostomy (stoma) N99.512
    catheter T83.010 ☑
  enteric stoma K94.13
  enterostomy K94.13
  esophagostomy K94.33
  gastroenteric K31.89
  gastrostomy K94.23
  ileostomy K94.13
    valve K94.13
  intrathecal infusion pump T85.615 ☑
  jejunostomy K94.13
  nervous system device, implant or graft, specified NEC T85.615 ☑

Malfunction — *continued*
   pacemaker — *see* Malfunction, cardiac electronic device
   prosthetic device, internal — *see* Complications, prosthetic device, by site, mechanical
   tracheostomy J95.03
   urinary device NEC — *see* Complication, genitourinary, device, urinary, mechanical
   valve
      colostomy K94.03
      heart T82.09 ☑
      ileostomy K94.13
   vascular graft or shunt NEC — *see* Complication, cardiovascular device, mechanical, vascular
   ventricular (communicating shunt) T85.01 ☑
Malherbe's tumor — *see* Neoplasm, skin, benign
Malibu disease L98.8
Malignancy — *see also* Neoplasm, malignant, by site
   unspecified site (primary) C80.1
Malignant — *see* condition
Malingerer, malingering Z76.5
Mallet finger (acquired) — *see* Deformity, finger, mallet
   finger
   congenital Q74.0
   sequelae of rickets E64.3
Malleus A24.0
Mallory's bodies R89.7
Mallory-Weiss syndrome K22.6
Malnutrition E46
   degree
      first E44.1
      mild (protein) E44.1
      moderate (protein) E44.0
      second E44.0
      severe (protein-energy) E43
         intermediate form E42
            with
               kwashiorkor (and marasmus) E42
               marasmus E41
      third E43
   following gastrointestinal surgery K91.2
   intrauterine
      light-for-dates — *see* Light for dates
      small-for-dates — *see* Small for dates
   lack of care, or neglect (child) (infant) T76.02 ☑
      confirmed T74.02 ☑
   malignant E40
   protein E46
      calorie E46
         mild E44.1
         moderate E44.0
         severe E43
            intermediate form E42
               with
                  kwashiorkor (and marasmus) E42
                  marasmus E41
      energy E46
         mild E44.1
         moderate E44.0
         severe E43
            intermediate form E42
               with
                  kwashiorkor (and marasmus) E42
                  marasmus E41
   severe (protein-energy) E43
      with
         kwashiorkor (and marasmus) E42
         marasmus E41
Malocclusion (teeth) M26.4
   Angle's M26.219
      class I M26.211
      class II M26.212
      class III M26.213
   due to
      abnormal swallowing M26.59
      mouth breathing M26.59
      tongue, lip or finger habits M26.59
   temporomandibular (joint) M26.69
Malposition
   cervix — *see* Malposition, uterus
   congenital
      adrenal (gland) Q89.1
      alimentary tract Q45.8
         lower Q43.8
         upper Q40.8
      aorta Q25.49
      appendix Q43.8
      arterial trunk Q20.0

Malposition — *continued*
   congenital — *continued*
      artery (peripheral) Q27.8
         coronary Q24.5
         digestive system Q27.8
         lower limb Q27.8
         pulmonary Q25.79
         specified site NEC Q27.8
         upper limb Q27.8
      auditory canal Q17.8
         causing impairment of hearing Q16.9
      auricle (ear) Q17.4
         causing impairment of hearing Q16.9
         cervical Q18.2
      biliary duct or passage Q44.5
      bladder (mucosa) — *see* Exstrophy, bladder
      brachial plexus Q07.8
      brain tissue Q04.8
      breast Q83.8
      bronchus Q32.4
      cecum Q43.8
      clavicle Q74.0
      colon Q43.8
      digestive organ or tract NEC Q45.8
         lower Q43.8
         upper Q40.8
      ear (auricle) (external) Q17.4
         ossicles Q16.3
      endocrine (gland) NEC Q89.2
      epiglottis Q31.8
      eustachian tube Q17.8
      eye Q15.8
      facial features Q18.8
      fallopian tube Q50.6
      finger(s) Q68.1
         supernumerary Q69.0
      foot Q66.9- ☑
      gallbladder Q44.1
      gastrointestinal tract Q45.8
      genitalia, genital organ(s) or tract
         female Q52.8
            external Q52.79
            internal NEC Q52.8
         male Q55.8
      glottis Q31.8
      hand Q68.1
      heart Q24.8
         dextrocardia Q24.0
            with complete transposition of viscera Q89.3
      hepatic duct Q44.5
      hip (joint) Q65.89
      intestine (large) (small) Q43.8
         with anomalous adhesions, fixation or malrotation Q43.3
      joint NEC Q68.8
      kidney Q63.2
      larynx Q31.8
      limb Q68.8
         lower Q68.8
         upper Q68.8
      liver Q44.7
      lung (lobe) Q33.8
      nail(s) Q84.6
      nerve Q07.8
      nervous system NEC Q07.8
      nose, nasal (septum) Q30.8
      organ or site not listed — *see* Anomaly, by site
      ovary Q50.39
      pancreas Q45.3
      parathyroid (gland) Q89.2
      patella Q74.1
      peripheral vascular system Q27.8
      pituitary (gland) Q89.2
      respiratory organ or system NEC Q34.8
      rib (cage) Q76.6
         supernumerary in cervical region Q76.5
      scapula Q74.0
      shoulder Q74.0
      spinal cord Q06.8
      spleen Q89.09
      sternum NEC Q76.7
      stomach Q40.2
      symphysis pubis Q74.2
      thymus (gland) Q89.2
      thyroid (gland) (tissue) Q89.2
         cartilage Q31.8
      toe(s) Q66.9- ☑
         supernumerary Q69.2
      tongue Q38.3

Malposition — *continued*
   congenital — *continued*
      trachea Q32.1
      ureter Q62.60
         deviation Q62.61
         displacement Q62.62
         ectopia Q62.63
         specified type NEC Q62.69
      uterus Q51.818
      vein(s) (peripheral) Q27.8
         great Q26.8
      vena cava (inferior) (superior) Q26.8
   device, implant or graft — *see also* Complications, by site and type, mechanical T85.628 ☑
      arterial graft NEC — *see* Complication, cardiovascular device, mechanical, vascular
      breast (implant) T85.42 ☑
      catheter NEC T85.628 ☑
         cystostomy T83.020 ☑
         dialysis (renal) T82.42 ☑
            intraperitoneal T85.621 ☑
         infusion NEC T82.524 ☑
            spinal (epidural) (subdural) T85.620 ☑
         urinary — *see also* Displacement, device, catheter, urinary T83.028 ☑
      electronic (electrode) (pulse generator) (stimulator)
         bone T84.320 ☑
         cardiac T82.129 ☑
            electrode T82.120 ☑
            pulse generator T82.121 ☑
            specified type NEC T82.128 ☑
         nervous system — *see* Complication, prosthetic device, mechanical, electronic nervous system stimulator
         urinary — *see* Complication, genitourinary, device, urinary, mechanical
      fixation, internal (orthopedic) NEC — *see* Complication, fixation device, mechanical
      gastrointestinal — *see* Complications, prosthetic device, mechanical, gastrointestinal device
      genital NEC T83.428 ☑
         intrauterine contraceptive device (string) T83.32 ☑
         penile prosthesis (cylinder) (implanted) (pump) (reservoir) T83.420 ☑
         testicular prosthesis T83.421 ☑
      heart NEC — *see* Complication, cardiovascular device, mechanical
      joint prosthesis — *see* Complication, joint prosthesis, mechanical
      ocular NEC — *see* Complications, prosthetic device mechanical, ocular device
      orthopedic NEC — *see* Complication, orthopedic, device, mechanical
      specified NEC T85.628 ☑
      urinary NEC — *see also* Complication, genitourinary device, urinary, mechanical
         graft T83.22 ☑
      vascular NEC — *see* Complication, cardiovascular device, mechanical
      ventricular intracranial shunt T85.02 ☑
   fetus — *see* Pregnancy, complicated by (management affected by), presentation, fetal
   gallbladder K82.8
   gastrointestinal tract, congenital Q45.8
   heart, congenital NEC Q24.8
   joint prosthesis — *see* Complications, joint prosthesis mechanical, displacement, by site
   stomach K31.89
      congenital Q40.2
   tooth, teeth, fully erupted M26.30
   uterus (acute) (acquired) (adherent) (asymptomatic) (postinfectional) (postpartal, old) N85.4
      anteflexion or anteversion N85.4
         congenital Q51.818
      flexion N85.4
         lateral — *see* Lateroversion, uterus
      inversion N85.5
      lateral (flexion) (version) — *see* Lateroversion, uteru
         in pregnancy or childbirth — *see* subcategory O34.5 ☑
      retroflexion or retroversion — *see* Retroversion, uterus
Malposture R29.3
Malrotation
   cecum Q43.3
   colon Q43.3

Malrotation — *continued*
   intestine Q43.3
   kidney Q63.2
Malta fever — *see* Brucellosis
Maltreatment
   adult
      abandonment
         confirmed T74.01 ☑
         suspected T76.01 ☑
      bullying
         confirmed T74.31 ☑
         suspected T76.31 ☑
      confirmed T74.91 ☑
      history of Z91.419
      intimidation (through social media)
         confirmed T74.31 ☑
         suspected T76.31 ☑
      neglect
         confirmed T74.01 ☑
         suspected T76.01 ☑
      physical abuse
         confirmed T74.11 ☑
         suspected T76.11 ☑
      psychological abuse
         confirmed T74.31 ☑
         history of Z91.411
         suspected T76.31 ☑
      sexual abuse
         confirmed T74.21 ☑
         suspected T76.21 ☑
      suspected T76.91 ☑
   child
      abandonment
         confirmed T74.02 ☑
         suspected T76.02 ☑
      bullying
         confirmed T74.32 ☑
         suspected T76.32 ☑
      confirmed T74.92 ☑
      history of — *see* History, personal (of), abuse
      intimidation (through social media)
         confirmed T74.32 ☑
         suspected T76.32 ☑
      neglect
         confirmed T74.02 ☑
         history of — *see* History, personal (of), abuse
         suspected T76.02 ☑
      physical abuse
         confirmed T74.12 ☑
         history of — *see* History, personal (of), abuse
         suspected T76.12 ☑
      psychological abuse
         confirmed T74.32 ☑
         history of — *see* History, personal (of), abuse
         suspected T76.32 ☑
      sexual abuse
         confirmed T74.22 ☑
         history of — *see* History, personal (of), abuse
         suspected T76.22 ☑
      suspected T76.92 ☑
   personal history of Z91.89
Maltworker's lung J67.4
Malunion, fracture — *see* Fracture, by site
Mammillitis N61.0
   puerperal, postpartum O91.02
Mammitis — *see* Mastitis
Mammogram (examination) Z12.39
   routine Z12.31
Mammoplasia N62
Management (of)
   bone conduction hearing device (implanted) Z45.320
   cardiac pacemaker NEC Z45.018
   cerebrospinal fluid drainage device Z45.41
   cochlear device (implanted) Z45.321
   contraceptive Z30.9
      specified NEC Z30.8
   implanted device Z45.9
      specified NEC Z45.89
   infusion pump Z45.1
   procreative Z31.9
      male factor infertility in female Z31.81
      specified NEC Z31.89
   prosthesis (external) — *see also* Fitting Z44.9
      implanted Z45.9
         specified NEC Z45.89
   renal dialysis catheter Z49.01
   vascular access device Z45.2

Mangled — *see* specified injury by site
Mania (monopolar) — *see also* Disorder, mood, manic
      episode
   with psychotic symptoms F30.2
   without psychotic symptoms F30.10
      mild F30.11
      moderate F30.12
      severe F30.13
   Bell's F30.8
   chronic (recurrent) F31.89
   hysterical F44.89
   puerperal F30.8
   recurrent F31.89
Manic depression F31.9
Manic-depressive insanity, psychosis, or syndrome
      — *see* Disorder, bipolar
Mannosidosis E77.1
Mansonelliasis, mansonellosis B74.4
Manson's
   disease B65.1
   schistosomiasis B65.1
Manual — *see* condition
Maple-bark-stripper's lung (disease) J67.6
Maple-syrup-urine disease E71.0
Marable's syndrome (celiac artery compression) I77.4
Marasmus E41
   due to malnutrition E41
   intestinal E41
   nutritional E41
   senile R54
   tuberculous NEC — *see* Tuberculosis
Marble
   bones Q78.2
   skin R23.8
Marburg virus disease A98.3
March
   fracture — *see* Fracture, traumatic, stress, by site
   hemoglobinuria D59.6
Marchesani (-Weill) **syndrome** Q87.0
Marchiafava (-Bignami) **syndrome or disease** G37.1
Marchiafava-Micheli syndrome D59.5
Marcus Gunn's syndrome Q07.8
Marfan's syndrome — *see* Syndrome, Marfan's
Marie-Bamberger disease — *see* Osteoarthropathy,
      hypertrophic, specified NEC
Marie-Charcot-Tooth neuropathic muscular atrophy
      G60.0
Marie's
   cerebellar ataxia (late-onset) G11.2
   disease or syndrome (acromegaly) E22.0
Marie-Strümpell arthritis, disease or spondylitis —
      see Spondylitis, ankylosing
Marion's disease (bladder neck obstruction) N32.0
Marital conflict Z63.0
Mark
   port wine Q82.5
   raspberry Q82.5
   strawberry Q82.5
   stretch L90.6
   tattoo L81.8
Marker heterochromatin — *see* Extra, marker chromo-
      somes
Maroteaux-Lamy syndrome (mild) (severe) E76.29
Marrow (bone)
   arrest D61.9
   poor function D75.89
Marseilles fever A77.1
Marsh fever — *see* Malaria
Marshall's (hidrotic) **ectodermal dysplasia** Q82.4
Marsh's disease (exophthalmic goiter) E05.00
   with storm E05.01
Masculinization (female) **with adrenal hyperplasia**
      E25.9
   congenital E25.0
Masculinovoblastoma D27.- ☑
Masochism (sexual) F65.51
Mason's lung J62.8
Mass
   abdominal R19.00
      epigastric R19.06
      generalized R19.07
      left lower quadrant R19.04
      left upper quadrant R19.02
      periumbilic R19.05
      right lower quadrant R19.03
      right upper quadrant R19.01
      specified site NEC R19.09

Mass — *continued*
   breast — *see also* Lump, breast N63.0
   chest R22.2
   cystic — *see* Cyst
   ear H93.8- ☑
   head R22.0
   intra-abdominal (diffuse) (generalized) — *see* Mass,
      abdominal
   kidney N28.89
   liver R16.0
   localized (skin) R22.9
      chest R22.2
      head R22.0
      limb
         lower R22.4- ☑
         upper R22.3- ☑
      neck R22.1
      trunk R22.2
   lung R91.8
   malignant — *see* Neoplasm, malignant, by site
   neck R22.1
   pelvic (diffuse) (generalized) — *see* Mass, abdominal
   specified organ NEC — *see* Disease, by site
   splenic R16.1
   substernal thyroid — *see* Goiter
   superficial (localized) R22.9
   umbilical (diffuse) (generalized) R19.09
Massive — *see* condition
Mast cell
   disease, systemic tissue D47.02
   leukemia C94.3- ☑
   neoplasm
      malignant C96.20
         specified type NEC C96.29
      of uncertain behavior NEC D47.09
   sarcoma C96.22
   tumor D47.09
Mastalgia N64.4
Masters-Allen syndrome N83.8
Mastitis (acute) (diffuse) (nonpuerperal) (subacute) N61.0
   with abscess N61.1
   chronic (cystic) — *see* Mastopathy, cystic
   cystic (Schimmelbusch's type) — *see* Mastopathy, cystic
   fibrocystic — *see* Mastopathy, cystic
   infective N61.0
      newborn P39.0
   interstitial, gestational or puerperal — *see* Mastitis,
      obstetric
   neonatal (noninfective) P83.4
      infective P39.0
   obstetric (interstitial) (nonpurulent)
      associated with
         lactation O91.23
         pregnancy O91.21- ☑
         puerperium O91.22
      purulent
         associated with
            lactation O91.13
            pregnancy O91.11- ☑
            puerperium O91.12
   periductal — *see* Ectasia, mammary duct
   phlegmonous — *see* Mastopathy, cystic
   plasma cell — *see* Ectasia, mammary duct
   without abscess N61.0
Mastocytoma (extracutaneous) D47.09
   malignant C96.29
   solitary D47.01
Mastocytosis D47.09
   aggressive systemic C96.21
   cutaneous (diffuse) (maculopapular) D47.01
      congenital Q82.2
      of neonatal onset Q82.2
      of newborn onset Q82.2
   indolent systemic D47.02
   isolated bone marrow D47.02
   malignant C96.29
   systemic (indolent) (smoldering)
      with an associated hematological non-mast cell
         lineage disease (SM-AHNMD) D47.02
Mastodynia N64.4
Mastoid — *see* condition
Mastoidalgia — *see* subcategory H92.0 ☑
Mastoiditis (coalescent) (hemorrhagic) (suppurative)
      H70.9- ☑
   acute, subacute H70.00- ☑
      complicated NEC H70.09- ☑
      subperiosteal H70.01- ☑

Mastoiditis — *continued*
- chronic (necrotic) (recurrent) H70.1- ☑
- in (due to)
  - infectious disease NEC B99 ☑ *[H75.0-]* ☑
  - parasitic disease NEC B89 *[H75.0-]* ☑
  - tuberculosis A18.03
- petrositis — *see* Petrositis
- postauricular fistula — *see* Fistula, postauricular
- specified NEC H70.89- ☑
- tuberculous A18.03

Mastopathy, mastopathia N64.9
- chronica cystica — *see* Mastopathy, cystic
- cystic (chronic) (diffuse) N60.1- ☑
  - with epithelial proliferation N60.3- ☑
- diffuse cystic — *see* Mastopathy, cystic
- estrogenic, oestrogenica N64.89
- ovarian origin N64.89

Mastoplasia, mastoplastia N62

Masturbation (excessive) F98.8

Maternal care (for) — *see* Pregnancy (complicated by) (management affected by)

Matheiu's disease (leptospiral jaundice) A27.0

Mauclaire's disease or osteochondrosis — *see* Osteochondrosis, juvenile, hand, metacarpal

Maxcy's disease A75.2

Maxilla, maxillary — *see* condition

May (-Hegglin) **anomaly or syndrome** D72.0

McArdle (-Schmid)(-Pearson) **disease** (glycogen storage) E74.04

McCune-Albright syndrome Q78.1

McQuarrie's syndrome (idiopathic familial hypoglycemia) E16.2

Meadow's syndrome Q86.1

Measles (black) (hemorrhagic) (suppressed) B05.9
- with
  - complications NEC B05.89
  - encephalitis B05.0
  - intestinal complications B05.4
  - keratitis (keratoconjunctivitis) B05.81
  - meningitis B05.1
  - otitis media B05.3
  - pneumonia B05.2
- French — *see* Rubella
- German — *see* Rubella
- Liberty — *see* Rubella

Meatitis, urethral — *see* Urethritis

Meatus, meatal — *see* condition

Meat-wrappers' asthma J68.9

Meckel-Gruber syndrome Q61.9

Meckel's diverticulitis, diverticulum (displaced) (hypertrophic) Q43.0
- malignant — *see* Table of Neoplasms, small intestine, malignant

Meconium
- ileus, newborn P76.0
  - in cystic fibrosis E84.11
  - meaning meconium plug (without cystic fibrosis) P76.0
- obstruction, newborn P76.0
  - due to fecaliths P76.0
  - in mucoviscidosis E84.11
- peritonitis P78.0
- plug syndrome (newborn) NEC P76.0

Median — *see also* condition
- arcuate ligament syndrome I77.4
- bar (prostate) (vesical orifice) — *see* Hyperplasia, prostate
- rhomboid glossitis K14.2

Mediastinal shift R93.89

Mediastinitis (acute) (chronic) J98.51
- syphilitic A52.73
- tuberculous A15.8

Mediastinopericarditis — *see also* Pericarditis
- acute I30.9
- adhesive I31.0
- chronic I31.8
  - rheumatic I09.2

Mediastinum, mediastinal — *see* condition

Medicine poisoning — *see* Table of Drugs and Chemicals, by drug, poisoning

Mediterranean
- fever — *see* Brucellosis
  - familial M04.1
    - tick A77.1
  - kala-azar B55.0
  - leishmaniasis B55.0
  - tick fever A77.1

Medulla — *see* condition

Medullary cystic kidney Q61.5

Medullated fibers
- optic (nerve) Q14.8
- retina Q14.1

Medulloblastoma
- desmoplastic C71.6
- specified site — *see* Neoplasm, malignant, by site
- unspecified site C71.6

Medulloepithelioma — *see also* Neoplasm, malignant, by site
- teratoid — *see* Neoplasm, malignant, by site

Medullomyoblastoma
- specified site — *see* Neoplasm, malignant, by site
- unspecified site C71.6

Meekeren-Ehlers-Danlos syndrome — *see also* Syndrome, Ehlers-Danlos Q79.69

Megacolon (acquired) (functional) (not Hirschsprung's disease) (in) K59.39
- Chagas' disease B57.32
- congenital, congenitum (aganglionic) Q43.1
- Hirschsprung's (disease) Q43.1
- toxic NEC K59.31
  - due to Clostridium difficile
    - not specified as recurrent A04.72
    - recurrent A04.71

Megaesophagus (functional) K22.0
- congenital Q39.5
- in (due to) Chagas' disease B57.31

Megalencephaly Q04.5

Megalerythema (epidemic) B08.3

Megaloappendix Q43.8

Megalocephalus, megalocephaly NEC Q75.3

Megalocornea Q15.8
- with glaucoma Q15.0

Megalocytic anemia D53.1

Megalodactylia (fingers) (thumbs) (congenital) Q74.0
- toes Q74.2

Megaloduodenum Q43.8

Megaloesophagus (functional) K22.0
- congenital Q39.5

Megalogastria (acquired) K31.89
- congenital Q40.2

Megalophthalmos Q11.3

Megalopsia H53.15

Megalosplenia — *see* Splenomegaly

Megaloureter N28.82
- congenital Q62.2

Megarectum K62.89

Megasigmoid K59.39
- congenital Q43.8

Megaureter N28.82
- congenital Q62.2

Megavitamin-B6 syndrome E67.2

Megrim — *see* Migraine

Meibomian
- cyst, infected — *see* Hordeolum
- gland — *see* condition
- sty, stye — *see* Hordeolum

Meibomitis — *see* Hordeolum

Meige-Milroy disease (chronic hereditary edema) Q82.0

Meige's syndrome Q82.0

Melalgia, nutritional E53.8

Melancholia F32.9
- climacteric (single episode) F32.89
  - recurrent episode F33.8
- hypochondriac F45.29
- intermittent (single episode) F32.89
  - recurrent episode F33.8
- involutional (single episode) F32.89
  - recurrent episode F33.8
- menopausal (single episode) F32.89
  - recurrent episode F33.8
- puerperal F32.89
- reactive (emotional stress or trauma) F32.3
- recurrent F33.9
- senile F03 ☑
- stuporous (single episode) F32.89
  - recurrent episode F33.8

Melanemia R79.89

Melanoameloblastoma — *see* Neoplasm, bone, benign

Melanoblastoma — *see* Melanoma

Melanocarcinoma — *see* Melanoma

Melanocytoma, eyeball D31.9- ☑

Melanocytosis, neurocutaneous Q82.8

Melanoderma, melanodermia L81.4

Melanodontia, infantile K03.89

Melanodontoclasia K03.89

Melanoepithelioma — *see* Melanoma

Melanoma (malignant) C43.9
- acral lentiginous, malignant — *see* Melanoma, skin, by site
- amelanotic — *see* Melanoma, skin, by site
- balloon cell — *see* Melanoma, skin, by site
- benign — *see* Nevus
- desmoplastic, malignant — *see* Melanoma, skin, by site
- epithelioid cell — *see* Melanoma, skin, by site
  - with spindle cell, mixed — *see* Melanoma, skin, by site
- in
  - giant pigmented nevus — *see* Melanoma, skin, by site
  - Hutchinson's melanotic freckle — *see* Melanoma, skin, by site
  - junctional nevus — *see* Melanoma, skin, by site
  - precancerous melanosis — *see* Melanoma, skin, by site
- in situ D03.9
  - abdominal wall D03.59
  - ala nasi D03.39
  - ankle D03.7- ☑
  - anus, anal (margin) (skin) D03.51
  - arm D03.6- ☑
  - auditory canal D03.2- ☑
  - auricle (ear) D03.2- ☑
  - auricular canal (external) D03.2- ☑
  - axilla, axillary fold D03.59
  - back D03.59
  - breast D03.52
  - brow D03.39
  - buttock D03.59
  - canthus (eye) D03.1- ☑
  - cheek (external) D03.39
  - chest wall D03.59
  - chin D03.39
  - choroid D03.8
  - conjunctiva D03.8
  - ear (external) D03.2- ☑
  - external meatus (ear) D03.2- ☑
  - eye D03.8
  - eyebrow D03.39
  - eyelid (lower) (upper) D03.1- ☑
  - face D03.30
    - specified NEC D03.39
  - female genital organ (external) NEC D03.8
  - finger D03.6- ☑
  - flank D03.59
  - foot D03.7- ☑
  - forearm D03.6- ☑
  - forehead D03.39
  - foreskin D03.8
  - gluteal region D03.59
  - groin D03.59
  - hand D03.6- ☑
  - heel D03.7- ☑
  - helix D03.2- ☑
  - hip D03.7- ☑
  - interscapular region D03.59
  - iris D03.8
  - jaw D03.39
  - knee D03.7- ☑
  - labium (majus) (minus) D03.8
  - lacrimal gland D03.8
  - leg D03.7- ☑
  - lip (lower) (upper) D03.0
  - lower limb NEC D03.7- ☑
  - male genital organ (external) NEC D03.8
  - nail D03.9
    - finger D03.6- ☑
    - toe D03.7- ☑
  - neck D03.4
  - nose (external) D03.39
  - orbit D03.8
  - penis D03.8
  - perianal skin D03.51
  - perineum D03.51
  - pinna D03.2- ☑
  - popliteal fossa or space D03.7- ☑
  - prepuce D03.8
  - pudendum D03.8
  - retina D03.8
  - retrobulbar D03.8
  - scalp D03.4

Melanoma — *continued*
  in situ — *continued*
    scrotum D03.8
    shoulder D03.6- ☑
    specified site NEC D03.8
    submammary fold D03.52
    temple D03.39
    thigh D03.7- ☑
    toe D03.7- ☑
    trunk NEC D03.59
    umbilicus D03.59
    upper limb NEC D03.6- ☑
    vulva D03.8
  juvenile — *see* Nevus
  malignant, of soft parts except skin — *see* Neoplasm,
    connective tissue, malignant
  metastatic
    breast C79.81
    genital organ C79.82
    specified site NEC C79.89
  neurotropic, malignant — *see* Melanoma, skin, by site
  nodular — *see* Melanoma, skin, by site
  regressing, malignant — *see* Melanoma, skin, by site
  skin C43.9
    abdominal wall C43.59
    ala nasi C43.31
    ankle C43.7- ☑
    anus, anal (skin) C43.51
    arm C43.6- ☑
    auditory canal (external) C43.2- ☑
    auricle (ear) C43.2- ☑
    auricular canal (external) C43.2- ☑
    axilla, axillary fold C43.59
    back C43.59
    breast (female) (male) C43.52
    brow C43.39
    buttock C43.59
    canthus (eye) C43.1- ☑
    cheek (external) C43.39
    chest wall C43.59
    chin C43.39
    ear (external) C43.2- ☑
    elbow C43.6- ☑
    external meatus (ear) C43.2- ☑
    eyebrow C43.39
    eyelid (lower) (upper) C43.1- ☑
    face C43.30
      specified NEC C43.39
    female genital organ (external) NEC C51.9
    finger C43.6- ☑
    flank C43.59
    foot C43.7- ☑
    forearm C43.6- ☑
    forehead C43.39
    foreskin C60.0
    glabella C43.39
    gluteal region C43.59
    groin C43.59
    hand C43.6- ☑
    heel C43.7- ☑
    helix C43.2- ☑
    hip C43.7- ☑
    interscapular region C43.59
    jaw (external) C43.39
    knee C43.7- ☑
    labium C51.9
      majus C51.0
      minus C51.1
    leg C43.7- ☑
    lip (lower) (upper) C43.0
    lower limb NEC C43.7- ☑
    male genital organ (external) NEC C63.9
    nail
      finger C43.6- ☑
      toe C43.7- ☑
    nasolabial groove C43.39
    nates C43.59
    neck C43.4
    nose (external) C43.31
    overlapping site C43.8
    palpebra C43.1- ☑
    penis C60.9
    perianal skin C43.51
    perineum C43.51
    pinna C43.2- ☑
    popliteal fossa or space C43.7- ☑
    prepuce C60.0

Melanoma — *continued*
  skin — *continued*
    pudendum C51.9
    scalp C43.4
    scrotum C63.2
    shoulder C43.6- ☑
    skin NEC C43.9
    submammary fold C43.52
    temple C43.39
    thigh C43.7- ☑
    toe C43.7- ☑
    trunk NEC C43.59
    umbilicus C43.59
    upper limb NEC C43.6- ☑
    vulva C51.9
      overlapping sites C51.8
  spindle cell
    with epithelioid, mixed — *see* Melanoma, skin, by
      site
    type A C69.4- ☑
    type B C69.4- ☑
  superficial spreading — *see* Melanoma, skin, by site
Melanosarcoma — *see also* Melanoma
  epithelioid cell — *see* Melanoma
Melanosis L81.4
  addisonian E27.1
    tuberculous A18.7
  adrenal E27.1
  colon K63.89
  conjunctiva — *see* Pigmentation, conjunctiva
    congenital Q13.89
  cornea (presenile) (senile) — *see also* Pigmentation,
    cornea
    congenital Q13.4
  eye NEC H57.89
    congenital Q15.8
  lenticularis progressiva Q82.1
  liver K76.89
  precancerous — *see also* Melanoma, in situ
    malignant melanoma in — *see* Melanoma
  Riehl's L81.4
  sclera H15.89
    congenital Q13.89
  suprarenal E27.1
  tar L81.4
  toxic L81.4
Melanuria R82.998
MELAS syndrome E88.41
Melasma L81.1
  adrenal (gland) E27.1
  suprarenal (gland) E27.1
Melena K92.1
  with ulcer — *code by* site under Ulcer, with hemorrhage
    K27.4
  due to swallowed maternal blood P78.2
  newborn, neonatal P54.1
    due to swallowed maternal blood P78.2
Meleney's
  gangrene (cutaneous) — *see* Ulcer, skin
  ulcer (chronic undermining) — *see* Ulcer, skin
Melioidosis A24.9
  acute A24.1
  chronic A24.2
  fulminating A24.1
  pneumonia A24.1
  pulmonary (chronic) A24.2
    acute A24.1
    subacute A24.2
  sepsis A24.1
  specified NEC A24.3
  subacute A24.2
Melitensis, febris A23.0
Melkersson (-Rosenthal) **syndrome** G51.2
Mellitus, diabetes — *see* Diabetes
Melorheostosis (bone) — *see* Disorder, bone, density
  and structure, specified NEC
Meloschisis Q18.4
Melotia Q17.4
Membrana
  capsularis lentis posterior Q13.89
  epipapillaris Q14.2
Membranacea placenta O43.19- ☑
Membranaceous uterus N85.8
Membrane(s), membranous — *see also* condition
  cyclitic — *see* Membrane, pupillary
  folds, congenital — *see* Web
  Jackson's Q43.3
  over face of newborn P28.9

Membrane(s), membranous — *continued*
  premature rupture — *see* Rupture, membranes, prema-
    ture
  pupillary H21.4- ☑
    persistent Q13.89
  retained (with hemorrhage) (complicating delivery)
    O72.2
    without hemorrhage O73.1
  secondary cataract — *see* Cataract, secondary
  unruptured (causing asphyxia) — *see* Asphyxia, new-
    born
  vitreous — *see* Opacity, vitreous, membranes and
    strands
Membranitis — *see* Chorioamnionitis
Memory disturbance, lack or loss — *see also* Amnesia
  mild, following organic brain damage F06.8
Menadione deficiency E56.1
Menarche
  delayed E30.0
  precocious E30.1
Mendacity, pathologic F60.2
Mendelson's syndrome (due to anesthesia) J95.4
  in labor and delivery O74.0
  in pregnancy O29.01- ☑
  obstetric O74.0
  postpartum, puerperal O89.01
Ménétrier's disease or syndrome K29.60
  with bleeding K29.61
Ménière's disease, syndrome or vertigo H81.0- ☑
Meninges, meningeal — *see* condition
Meningioma — *see also* Neoplasm, meninges, benign
  angioblastic — *see* Neoplasm, meninges, benign
  angiomatous — *see* Neoplasm, meninges, benign
  endotheliomatous — *see* Neoplasm, meninges, benign
  fibroblastic — *see* Neoplasm, meninges, benign
  fibrous — *see* Neoplasm, meninges, benign
  hemangioblastic — *see* Neoplasm, meninges, benign
  hemangiopericytic — *see* Neoplasm, meninges, benign
  malignant — *see* Neoplasm, meninges, malignant
  meningiothelial — *see* Neoplasm, meninges, benign
  meningotheliomatous — *see* Neoplasm, meninges,
    benign
  mixed — *see* Neoplasm, meninges, benign
  multiple — *see* Neoplasm, meninges, uncertain behav-
    ior
  papillary — *see* Neoplasm, meninges, uncertain behav-
    ior
  psammomatous — *see* Neoplasm, meninges, benign
  syncytial — *see* Neoplasm, meninges, benign
  transitional — *see* Neoplasm, meninges, benign
Meningiomatosis (diffuse) — *see* Neoplasm, meninges,
  uncertain behavior
Meningism — *see* Meningismus
Meningismus (infectional) (pneumococcal) R29.1
  due to serum or vaccine R29.1
  influenzal — *see* Influenza, with, manifestations NEC
Meningitis (basal) (basic) (brain) (cerebral) (cervical)
  (congestive) (diffuse) (hemorrhagic) (infantile)
  (membranous) (metastatic) (nonspecific) (pontine)
  (progressive) (simple) (spinal) (subacute) (sympathetic) (toxic) G03.9
  abacterial G03.0
  actinomycotic A42.81
  adenoviral A87.1
  arbovirus A87.8
  aseptic (acute) G03.0
  bacterial G00.9
    Escherichia coli (E. coli) G00.8
    Friedländer (bacillus) G00.8
    gram-negative G00.9
    H. influenzae G00.0
    Klebsiella G00.8
    pneumococcal G00.1
    specified organism NEC G00.8
    staphylococcal G00.3
    streptococcal (acute) G00.2
  benign recurrent (Mollaret) G03.2
  candidal B37.5
  caseous (tuberculous) A17.0
  cerebrospinal A39.0
  chronic NEC G03.1
  clear cerebrospinal fluid NEC G03.0
  coxsackievirus A87.0
  cryptococcal B45.1
  diplococcal (gram positive) A39.0
  echovirus A87.0
  enteroviral A87.0
  eosinophilic B83.2

Meningitis — *continued*
epidemic NEC A39.0
Escherichia coli (E. coli) G00.8
fibrinopurulent G00.9
    specified organism NEC G00.8
Friedländer (bacillus) G00.8
gonococcal A54.81
gram-negative cocci G00.9
gram-positive cocci G00.9
H. influenzae G00.0
Haemophilus (influenzae) G00.0
in (due to)
    adenovirus A87.1
    African trypanosomiasis B56.9 [G02]
    anthrax A22.8
    bacterial disease NEC A48.8 [G01]
    Chagas' disease (chronic) B57.41
    chickenpox B01.0
    coccidioidomycosis B38.4
    Diplococcus pneumoniae G00.1
    enterovirus A87.0
    herpes (simplex) virus B00.3
        zoster B02.1
    infectious mononucleosis B27.92
    leptospirosis A27.81
    Listeria monocytogenes A32.11
    Lyme disease A69.21
    measles B05.1
    mumps (virus) B26.1
    neurosyphilis (late) A52.13
    parasitic disease NEC B89 [G02]
    poliovirus A80.9 [G02]
    preventive immunization, inoculation or vaccination
        G03.8
    rubella B06.02
    Salmonella infection A02.21
    specified cause NEC G03.8
    Streptococcal pneumoniae G00.1
    typhoid fever A01.01
    varicella B01.0
    viral disease NEC A87.8
    whooping cough A37.90
    zoster B02.1
infectious G00.9
influenzal (H. influenzae) G00.0
Klebsiella G00.8
leptospiral (aseptic) A27.81
lymphocytic (acute) (benign) (serous) A87.2
meningococcal A39.0
Mima polymorpha G00.8
Mollaret (benign recurrent) G03.2
monilial B37.5
mycotic NEC B49 [G02]
Neisseria A39.0
nonbacterial G03.0
nonpyogenic NEC G03.0
ossificans G96.19
pneumococcal streptococcus pneumoniae G00.1
poliovirus A80.9 [G02]
postmeasles B05.1
purulent G00.9
    specified organism NEC G00.8
pyogenic G00.9
    specified organism NEC G00.8
Salmonella (arizonae) (Cholerae-Suis) (enteritidis) (ty-
    phimurium) A02.21
septic G00.9
    specified organism NEC G00.8
serosa circumscripta NEC G03.0
serous NEC G93.2
specified organism NEC G00.8
sporotrichosis B42.81
staphylococcal G00.3
sterile G03.0
Streptococcal (acute) G00.2
    pneumoniae G00.1
suppurative G00.9
    specified organism NEC G00.8
syphilitic (late) (tertiary) A52.13
    acute A51.41
    congenital A50.41
    secondary A51.41
Torula histolytica (cryptococcal) B45.1
traumatic (complication of injury) T79.8 ☑
tuberculous A17.0
typhoid A01.01
viral NEC A87.9
Yersinia pestis A20.3

Meningocele (spinal) — *see also* Spina bifida
with hydrocephalus — *see* Spina bifida, by site, with
    hydrocephalus
acquired (traumatic) G96.19
cerebral — *see* Encephalocele
Meningocerebritis — *see* Meningoencephalitis
Meningococcemia A39.4
acute A39.2
chronic A39.3
Meningococcus, meningococcal — *see also* condition
    A39.9
adrenalitis, hemorrhagic A39.1
carrier (suspected) of Z22.31
meningitis (cerebrospinal) A39.0
Meningoencephalitis — *see also* Encephalitis G04.90
acute NEC — *see also* Encephalitis, viral A86
bacterial NEC G04.2
California A83.5
diphasic A84.1
eosinophilic B83.2
epidemic A39.81
herpesviral, herpetic B00.4
    due to herpesvirus 6 B10.01
    due to herpesvirus 7 B10.09
    specified NEC B10.09
in (due to)
    blastomycosis NEC B40.81
    diseases classified elsewhere G05.3
    free-living amebae B60.2
    H. influenzae G00.0
    Hemophilus influenzae (H .influenzae) G00.0
    herpes B00.4
        due to herpesvirus 6 B10.01
        due to herpesvirus 7 B10.09
        specified NEC B10.09
    Lyme disease A69.22
    mercury — *see* subcategory T56.1 ☑
    mumps B26.2
    Naegleria (amebae) (organisms) (fowleri) B60.2
    Parastrongylus cantonensis B83.2
    toxoplasmosis (acquired) B58.2
        congenital P37.1
infectious (acute) (viral) A86
influenzal (H. influenzae) G00.0
Listeria monocytogenes A32.12
lymphocytic (serous) A87.2
mumps B26.2
parasitic NEC B89 [G05.3]
pneumococcal G04.2
primary amebic B60.2
specific (syphilitic) A52.14
specified organism NEC G04.81
staphylococcal G04.2
streptococcal G04.2
syphilitic A52.14
toxic NEC G92
    due to mercury — *see* subcategory T56.1 ☑
tuberculous A17.82
virus NEC A86
Meningoencephalocele — *see also* Encephalocele
syphilitic A52.19
congenital A50.49
Meningoencephalomyelitis — *see also* Meningoen-
    cephalitis
acute NEC (viral) A86
    disseminated G04.00
        postimmunization or postvaccination G04.02
        postinfectious G04.01
    due to
        actinomycosis A42.82
        Torula B45.1
        Toxoplasma or toxoplasmosis (acquired) B58.2
            congenital P37.1
    postimmunization or postvaccination G04.02
Meningoencephalomyelopathy G96.9
Meningoencephalopathy G96.9
Meningomyelitis — *see also* Meningoencephalitis
    bacterial NEC G04.2
    blastomycotic NEC B40.81
    cryptococcal B45.1
    in diseases classified elsewhere G05.4
    meningococcal A39.81
    syphilitic A52.14
    tuberculous A17.82
Meningomyelocele — *see also* Spina bifida
    syphilitic A52.19
Meningomyeloneuritis — *see* Meningoencephalitis
Meningoradiculitis — *see* Meningitis

Meningovascular — *see* condition
Menkes' disease or syndrome E83.09
    meaning maple-syrup-urine disease E71.0
Menometrorrhagia N92.1
Menopause, menopausal (asymptomatic) (state) Z78.0
    arthritis (any site) NEC — *see* Arthritis, specified form
        NEC
    bleeding N92.4
    depression (single episode) F32.89
        agitated (single episode) F32.2
            recurrent episode F33.9
        psychotic (single episode) F32.89
            recurrent episode F33.9
        recurrent episode F33.8
    melancholia (single episode) F32.89
        recurrent episode F33.8
    paranoid state F22
    premature E28.319
        asymptomatic E28.319
            postirradiation E89.40
            postsurgical E89.40
        symptomatic E28.310
            postirradiation E89.41
            postsurgical E89.41
    psychosis NEC F28
    symptomatic N95.1
    toxic polyarthritis NEC — *see* Arthritis, specified form
        NEC
Menorrhagia (primary) N92.0
    climacteric N92.4
        menopausal N92.4
    menopausal N92.4
    perimenopausal N92.4
    postclimacteric N95.0
    postmenopausal N95.0
    preclimacteric or premenopausal N92.4
    pubertal (menses retained) N92.2
Menostaxis N92.0
Menses, retention N94.89
Menstrual — *see* Menstruation
Menstruation
    absent — *see* Amenorrhea
    anovulatory N97.0
    cycle, irregular N92.6
    delayed N91.0
    disorder N93.9
        psychogenic F45.8
    during pregnancy O20.8
    excessive (with regular cycle) N92.0
        with irregular cycle N92.1
        at puberty N92.2
    frequent N92.0
    infrequent — *see* Oligomenorrhea
    irregular N92.6
        specified NEC N92.5
    latent N92.5
    membranous N92.5
    painful — *see also* Dysmenorrhea N94.6
        primary N94.4
        psychogenic F45.8
        secondary N94.5
    passage of clots N92.0
    precocious E30.1
    protracted N92.5
    rare — *see* Oligomenorrhea
    retained N94.89
    retrograde N92.5
    scanty — *see* Oligomenorrhea
    suppression N94.89
    vicarious (nasal) N94.89
Mental — *see also* condition
    deficiency — *see* Disability, intellectual
    deterioration — *see* Psychosis
    disorder — *see* Disorder, mental
    exhaustion F48.8
    insufficiency (congenital) — *see* Disability, intellectual
    observation without need for further medical care
        Z03.89
    retardation — *see* Disability, intellectual
    subnormality — *see* Disability, intellectuall
    upset — *see* Disorder, mental
Meralgia paresthetica G57.1- ☑
Mercurial — *see* condition
Mercurialism — *see* subcategory T56.1 ☑
Merkel cell tumor — *see* Carcinoma, Merkel cell
Merocele — *see* Hernia, femoral
Meromelia
    lower limb — *see* Defect, reduction, lower limb

☑ **Additional Character Required** — Refer to the Tabular List for Character Selection   ▽ᵉ Subterms under main terms may continue to next column or page

Meromelia — *continued*
  lower limb — *see* Defect, reduction, lower limb — *continued*
    intercalary
      femur — *see* Defect, reduction, lower limb, specified type NEC
      tibiofibular (complete) (incomplete) — *see* Defect, reduction, lower limb
  upper limb — *see* Defect, reduction, upper limb
    intercalary, humeral, radioulnar — *see* Agenesis, arm, with hand present
MERRF syndrome (myoclonic epilepsy associated with ragged-red fiber) E88.42
Merzbacher-Pelizaeus disease E75.29
Mesaortitis — *see* Aortitis
Mesarteritis — *see* Arteritis
Mesencephalitis — *see* Encephalitis
Mesenchymoma — *see also* Neoplasm, connective tissue, uncertain behavior
  benign — *see* Neoplasm, connective tissue, benign
  malignant — *see* Neoplasm, connective tissue, malignant
Mesenteritis
  retractile K65.4
  sclerosing K65.4
Mesentery, mesenteric — *see* condition
Mesiodens, mesiodentes K00.1
Mesio-occlusion M26.213
Mesocolon — *see* condition
Mesonephroma (malignant) — *see* Neoplasm, malignant, by site
  benign — *see* Neoplasm, benign, by site
Mesophlebitis — *see* Phlebitis
Mesostromal dysgenesia Q13.89
Mesothelioma (malignant) C45.9
  benign
    mesentery D19.1
    mesocolon D19.1
    omentum D19.1
    peritoneum D19.1
    pleura D19.0
    specified site NEC D19.7
    unspecified site D19.9
  biphasic C45.9
    benign
      mesentery D19.1
      mesocolon D19.1
      omentum D19.1
      peritoneum D19.1
      pleura D19.0
      specified site NEC D19.7
      unspecified site D19.9
  cystic D48.4
  epithelioid C45.9
    benign
      mesentery D19.1
      mesocolon D19.1
      omentum D19.1
      peritoneum D19.1
      pleura D19.0
      specified site NEC D19.7
      unspecified site D19.9
  fibrous C45.9
    benign
      mesentery D19.1
      mesocolon D19.1
      omentum D19.1
      peritoneum D19.1
      pleura D19.0
      specified site NEC D19.7
      unspecified site D19.9
  site classification
    liver C45.7
    lung C45.7
    mediastinum C45.7
    mesentery C45.1
    mesocolon C45.1
    omentum C45.1
    pericardium C45.2
    peritoneum C45.1
    pleura C45.0
      parietal C45.0
    retroperitoneum C45.7
    specified site NEC C45.7
    unspecified C45.9
Metabolic syndrome E00.01
Metagonimiasis B66.8
Metagonimus infestation (intestine) B66.8

Metal
  pigmentation L81.8
  polisher's disease J62.8
Metamorphopsia H53.15
Metaplasia
  apocrine (breast) — *see* Dysplasia, mammary, specified type NEC
  cervix (squamous) — *see* Dysplasia, cervix
  endometrium (squamous) (uterus) N85.8
  esophagus K22.7- ☑
  kidney (pelvis) (squamous) N28.89
  myelogenous D73.1
  myeloid (agnogenic) (megakaryocytic) D73.1
  spleen D73.1
  squamous cell, bladder N32.89
Metastasis, metastatic
  abscess — *see* Abscess
  calcification E83.59
  cancer
    from specified site — *see* Neoplasm, malignant, by site
    to specified site — *see* Neoplasm, secondary, by site
  deposits (in) — *see* Neoplasm, secondary, by site
  disease — *see also* Neoplasm, secondary, by site C79.9
  spread (to) — *see* Neoplasm, secondary, by site
Metastrongyliasis B83.8
Metatarsalgia M77.4- ☑
  anterior G57.6- ☑
  Morton's G57.6- ☑
Metatarsus, metatarsal — *see also* condition
  adductus, congenital Q66.22- ☑
  valgus (abductus), congenital Q66.6
  varus (congenital) Q66.22- ☑
    primus Q66.21- ☑
Methadone use — *see* Use, opioid
Methemoglobinemia D74.9
  acquired (with sulfhemoglobinemia) D74.8
  congenital D74.0
  enzymatic (congenital) D74.0
  Hb M disease D74.0
  hereditary D74.0
  toxic D74.8
Methemoglobinuria — *see* Hemoglobinuria
Methioninemia E72.19
Methylmalonic acidemia E71.120
Metritis (catarrhal) (hemorrhagic) (septic) (suppurative) — *see also* Endometritis
  cervical — *see* Cervicitis
Metropathia hemorrhagica N93.8
Metroperitonitis — *see* Peritonitis, pelvic, female
Metrorrhagia N92.1
  climacteric N92.4
  menopausal N92.4
  perimenopausal N92.4
  postpartum NEC (atonic) (following delivery of placenta) O72.1
    delayed or secondary O72.2
  preclimacteric or premenopausal N92.4
  psychogenic F45.8
Metrorrhexis — *see* Rupture, uterus
Metrosalpingitis N70.91
Metrostaxis N93.8
Metrovaginitis — *see* Endometritis
Meyer-Schwickerath and Weyers syndrome Q87.0
Meynert's amentia (nonalcoholic) F04
  alcoholic F10.96
    with dependence F10.26
Mibelli's disease (porokeratosis) Q82.8
Mice, joint — *see* Loose, body, joint
  knee M23.4- ☑
Micrencephalon, micrencephaly Q02
Microalbuminuria R80.9
Microaneurysm, retinal — *see also* Disorder, retina, microaneurysms
  diabetic — *see* E08-E13 with .31
Microangiopathy (peripheral) I73.9
  thrombotic M31.1
Microcalcifications, breast R92.0
Microcephalus, microcephalic, microcephaly Q02
  due to toxoplasmosis (congenital) P37.1
Microcheilia Q18.7
Microcolon (congenital) Q43.8
Microcornea (congenital) Q13.4
Microcytic — *see* condition
Microdeletions NEC Q93.88
Microdontia K00.2
Microdrepanocytosis D57.40

Microdrepanocytosis — *continued*
  with crisis (vasoocclusive pain) D57.419
    with
      acute chest syndrome D57.411
      splenic sequestration D57.412
Microembolism
  atherothrombotic — *see* Atheroembolism
  retinal — *see* Occlusion, artery, retina
Microencephalon Q02
Microfilaria streptocerca infestation — *see* Onchocerciasis
Microgastria (congenital) Q40.2
Microgenia M26.06
Microgenitalia, congenital
  female Q52.8
  male Q55.8
Microglioma — *see* Lymphoma, non-Hodgkin, specified NEC
Microglossia (congenital) Q38.3
Micrognathia, micrognathism (congenital) (mandibular) (maxillary) M26.09
Microgyria (congenital) Q04.3
Microinfarct of heart — *see* Insufficiency, coronary
Microlentia (congenital) Q12.8
Microlithiasis, alveolar, pulmonary J84.02
Micromastia N64.82
Micromyelia (congenital) Q06.8
Micropenis Q55.62
Microphakia (congenital) Q12.8
Microphthalmos, microphthalmia (congenital) Q11.2
  due to toxoplasmosis P37.1
Micropsia H53.15
Microscopic polyangiitis (polyarteritis) M31.7
Microsporidiosis B60.8
  intestinal A07.8
Microsporon furfur infestation B36.0
Microsporosis — *see also* Dermatophytosis
  nigra B36.1
Microstomia (congenital) Q18.5
Microtia (congenital) (external ear) Q17.2
Microtropia H50.40
Microvillus inclusion disease (MVD) (MVID) Q43.8
Micturition
  disorder NEC — *see also* Difficulty, micturition R39.198
    psychogenic F45.8
  frequency R35.0
    psychogenic F45.8
  hesitancy R39.11
  incomplete emptying R39.14
  nocturnal R35.1
  painful R30.9
    dysuria R30.0
      psychogenic F45.8
    tenesmus R30.1
  poor stream R39.12
  position dependent R39.192
  split stream R39.13
  straining R39.16
  urgency R39.15
Mid plane — *see* condition
Middle
  ear — *see* condition
  lobe (right) syndrome J98.19
Miescher's elastoma L87.2
Mietens' syndrome Q87.2
Migraine (idiopathic) G43.909
  with refractory migraine G43.919
    with status migrainosus G43.911
    without status migrainosus G43.919
  with aura (acute-onset) (prolonged) (typical) (without headache) G43.109
    with refractory migraine G43.119
      with status migrainosus G43.111
      without status migrainosus G43.119
    intractable G43.119
      with status migrainosus G43.111
      without status migrainosus G43.119
    not intractable G43.109
      with status migrainosus G43.101
      without status migrainosus G43.109
    persistent G43.509
      with cerebral infarction G43.609
        with refractory migraine G43.619
          with status migrainosus G43.611
          without status migrainosus G43.619
        intractable G43.619
          with status migrainosus G43.611
          without status migrainosus G43.619

▽ Subterms under main terms may continue to next column or page   ☑ Additional Character Required — Refer to the Tabular List for Character Selection   **223**

Meromelia — Migraine

Migraine — *continued*
with aura — *continued*
persistent — *continued*
with cerebral infarction — *continued*
not intractable G43.609
with status migrainosus G43.601
without status migrainosus G43.609
without refractory migraine G43.609
with status migrainosus G43.601
without status migrainosus G43.609
without cerebral infarction G43.509
with refractory migraine G43.519
with status migrainosus G43.511
without status migrainosus G43.519
intractable G43.519
with status migrainosus G43.511
without status migrainosus G43.519
not intractable G43.509
with status migrainosus G43.501
without status migrainosus G43.509
without refractory migraine G43.509
with status migrainosus G43.501
without status migrainosus G43.509
without mention of refractory migraine G43.109
with status migrainosus G43.101
without status migrainosus G43.109
abdominal G43.D0 (*following* G43.7)
with refractory migraine G43.D1 (*following* G43.7)
intractable G43.D1 (*following* G43.7)
not intractable G43.D0 (*following* G43.7)
without refractory migraine G43.D0 (*following* G43.7)
basilar — *see* Migraine, with aura
classical — *see* Migraine, with aura
common — *see* Migraine, without aura
complicated G43.109
equivalents — *see* Migraine, with aura
familiar — *see* Migraine, hemiplegic
hemiplegic G43.409
with refractory migraine G43.419
with status migrainosus G43.411
without status migrainosus G43.419
intractable G43.419
with status migrainosus G43.411
without status migrainosus G43.419
not intractable G43.409
with status migrainosus G43.401
without status migrainosus G43.409
without refractory migraine G43.409
with status migrainosus G43.401
without status migrainosus G43.409
intractable G43.919
with status migrainosus G43.911
without status migrainosus G43.919
menstrual G43.829
with refractory migraine G43.839
with status migrainosus G43.831
without status migrainosus G43.839
intractable G43.839
with status migrainosus G43.831
without status migrainosus G43.839
not intractable 4G43.829
with status migrainosus G43.821
without status migrainosus G43.829
without refractory migraine G43.829
with status migrainosus G43.821
without status migrainosus G43.829
menstrually related — *see* Migraine, menstrual
not intractable G43.909
with status migrainosus G43.901
without status migrainosus G43.919
ophthalmoplegic G43.B0 (*following* G43.7)
with refractory migraine G43.B1 (*following* G43.7)
intractable G43.B1 (*following* G43.7)
not intractable G43.B0 (*following* G43.7)
without refractory migraine G43.B0 (*following* G43.7)
persistent aura (with, without) cerebral infarction — *see* Migraine, with aura, persistent
preceded or accompanied by transient focal neurological phenomena — *see* Migraine, with aura
pre-menstrual — *see* Migraine, menstrual
pure menstrual — *see* Migraine, menstrual
retinal — *see* Migraine, with aura
specified NEC G43.809
intractable G43.819
with status migrainosus G43.811
without status migrainosus G43.819
not intractable G43.809
with status migrainosus G43.801

Migraine — *continued*
specified — *continued*
not intractable — *continued*
without status migrainosus G43.809
sporadic — *see* Migraine, hemiplegic
transformed — *see* Migraine, without aura, chronic
triggered seizures — *see* Migraine, with aura
without aura G43.009
with refractory migraine G43.019
with status migrainosus G43.011
without status migrainosus G43.019
chronic G43.709
with refractory migraine G43.719
with status migrainosus G43.711
without status migrainosus G43.719
intractable
with status migrainosus G43.711
without status migrainosus G43.719
not intractable
with status migrainosus G43.701
without status migrainosus G43.709
without refractory migraine G43.709
with status migrainosus G43.701
without status migrainosus G43.709
intractable
with status migrainosus G43.011
without status migrainosus G43.019
not intractable
with status migrainosus G43.001
without status migrainosus G43.009
without mention of refractory migraine G43.009
with status migrainosus G43.001
without status migrainosus G43.009
without refractory migraine G43.909
with status migrainosus G43.901
without status migrainosus G43.919
Migrant, social Z59.0
Migration, anxiety concerning Z60.3
Migratory, migrating — *see also* condition
person Z59.0
testis Q55.29
Mikity-Wilson disease or syndrome P27.0
Mikulicz' disease or syndrome K11.8
Miliaria L74.3
alba L74.1
apocrine L75.2
crystallina L74.1
profunda L74.2
rubra L74.0
tropicalis L74.2
Miliary — *see* condition
Milium L72.0
colloid L57.8
Milk
crust L21.0
excessive secretion O92.6
poisoning — *see* Poisoning, food, noxious
retention O92.79
sickness — *see* Poisoning, food, noxious
spots I31.0
Milk-alkali disease or syndrome E83.52
Milk-leg (deep vessels) (nonpuerperal) — *see* Embolism, vein, lower extremity
complicating pregnancy O22.3- ☑
puerperal, postpartum, childbirth O87.1
Milkman's disease or syndrome M83.8
Milky urine — *see* Chyluria
Millard-Gubler (-Foville) **paralysis or syndrome** G46.3
Millar's asthma J38.5
Miller Fisher syndrome G61.0
Mills' disease — *see* Hemiplegia
Millstone maker's pneumoconiosis J62.8
Milroy's disease (chronic hereditary edema) Q82.0
Minamata disease T56.1 ☑
Miners' asthma or lung J60
Minkowski-Chauffard syndrome — *see* Spherocytosis
Minor — *see* condition
Minor's disease (hematomyelia) G95.19
Minot's disease (hemorrhagic disease), newborn P53
Minot-von Willebrand-Jurgens disease or syndrome (angiohemophilia) D68.0
Minus (and plus) **hand** (intrinsic) — *see* Deformity, limb, specified type NEC, forearm
Miosis (pupil) H57.03
Mirizzi's syndrome (hepatic duct stenosis) K83.1
Mirror writing F81.0

Misadventure (of) (prophylactic) (therapeutic) — *see also* Complications T88.9 ☑
administration of insulin (by accident) — *see* subcategory T38.3 ☑
infusion — *see* Complications, infusion
local applications (of fomentations, plasters, etc.) T88.9 ☑
burn or scald — *see* Burn
specified NEC T88.8 ☑
medical care (early) (late) T88.9 ☑
adverse effect of drugs or chemicals — *see* Table of Drugs and Chemicals
burn or scald — *see* Burn
specified NEC T88.8 ☑
specified NEC T88.8 ☑
surgical procedure (early) (late) — *see* Complications, surgical procedure
transfusion — *see* Complications, transfusion
vaccination or other immunological procedure — *see* Complications, vaccination
Miscarriage O03.9
Misdirection, aqueous H40.83- ☑
Misperception, sleep state F51.02
Misplaced, misplacement
ear Q17.4
kidney (acquired) N28.89
congenital Q63.2
organ or site, congenital NEC — *see* Malposition, congenital
Missed
abortion O02.1
delivery O36.4 ☑
Missing — *see also* Absence
string of intrauterine contraceptive device T83.32- ☑
Misuse of drugs F19.99
Mitchell's disease (erythromelalgia) I73.81
Mite(s) (infestation) B88.9
diarrhea B88.0
grain (itch) B88.0
hair follicle (itch) B88.0
in sputum B88.0
Mitral — *see* condition
Mittelschmerz N94.0
Mixed — *see* condition
MMN (multifocal motor neuropathy) G61.82
MNGIE (Mitochondrial Neurogastrointestinal Encephalopathy) **syndrome** E88.49
Mobile, mobility
cecum Q43.3
excessive — *see* Hypermobility
gallbladder, congenital Q44.1
kidney N28.89
organ or site, congenital NEC — *see* Malposition, congenital
Mobitz heart block (atrioventricular) I44.1
Moebius, Möbius
disease (ophthalmoplegic migraine) — *see* Migraine, ophthalmoplegic
syndrome Q87.0
congenital oculofacial paralysis (with other anomalies) Q87.0
ophthalmoplegic migraine — *see* Migraine, ophthalmoplegic
Moeller's glossitis K14.0
Mohr's syndrome (Types I and II) Q87.0
Mola destruens D39.2
Molar pregnancy O02.0
Molarization of premolars K00.2
Molding, head (during birth) — *omit code*
Mole (pigmented) — *see also* Nevus
blood O02.0
Breus' O02.0
cancerous — *see* Melanoma
carneous O02.0
destructive D39.2
fleshy O02.0
hydatid, hydatidiform (benign) (complicating pregnancy) (delivered) (undelivered) O01.9
classical O01.0
complete O01.0
incomplete O01.1
invasive D39.2
malignant D39.2
partial O01.1
intrauterine O02.0
invasive (hydatidiform) D39.2

☑ **Additional Character Required** — Refer to the Tabular List for Character Selection
▽ Subterms under main terms may continue to next column or page

Mole — *continued*
  malignant
    meaning
      malignant hydatidiform mole D39.2
      melanoma — *see* Melanoma
  nonhydatidiform O02.0
  nonpigmented — *see* Nevus
  pregnancy NEC O02.0
  skin — *see* Nevus
  tubal O00.10- ☑
    with intrauterine pregnancy O00.11- ☑
  vesicular — *see* Mole, hydatidiform
Molimen, molimina (menstrual) N94.3
Molluscum contagiosum (epitheliale) B08.1
Mönckeberg's arteriosclerosis, disease, or sclerosis
  — *see* Arteriosclerosis, extremities
Mondini's malformation (cochlea) Q16.5
Mondor's disease I80.8
Monge's disease T70.29 ☑
Monilethrix (congenital) Q84.1
Moniliasis — *see also* Candidiasis B37.9
  neonatal P37.5
Monitoring (encounter for)
  therapeutic drug level Z51.81
Monkey malaria B53.1
Monkeypox B04
Monoarthritis M13.10
  ankle M13.17- ☑
  elbow M13.12- ☑
  foot joint M13.17- ☑
  hand joint M13.14- ☑
  hip M13.15- ☑
  knee M13.16- ☑
  shoulder M13.11- ☑
  wrist M13.13- ☑
Monoblastic — *see* condition
Monochromat (ism), monochromatopsia (acquired)
  (congenital) H53.51
Monocytic — *see* condition
Monocytopenia D72.818
Monocytosis (symptomatic) D72.821
Monomania — *see* Psychosis
Mononeuritis G58.9
  cranial nerve — *see* Disorder, nerve, cranial
  femoral nerve G57.2- ☑
  lateral
    cutaneous nerve of thigh G57.1- ☑
    popliteal nerve G57.3- ☑
  lower limb G57.9- ☑
    specified nerve NEC G57.8- ☑
  medial popliteal nerve G57.4- ☑
  median nerve G56.1- ☑
  multiplex G58.7
  plantar nerve G57.6- ☑
  posterior tibial nerve G57.5- ☑
  radial nerve G56.3- ☑
  sciatic nerve G57.0- ☑
  specified NEC G58.8
  tibial nerve G57.4- ☑
  ulnar nerve G56.2- ☑
  upper limb G56.9- ☑
    specified nerve NEC G56.8- ☑
  vestibular — *see* subcategory H93.3 ☑
Mononeuropathy G58.9
  carpal tunnel syndrome — *see* Syndrome, carpal tunnel
  diabetic NEC — *see* E08-E13 with .41
  femoral nerve — *see* Lesion, nerve, femoral
  ilioinguinal nerve G57.8- ☑
  in diseases classified elsewhere — *see* category G59
  intercostal G58.0
  lower limb G57.9- ☑
    causalgia — *see* Causalgia, lower limb
    femoral nerve — *see* Lesion, nerve, femoral
    meralgia paresthetica G57.1- ☑
    plantar nerve — *see* Lesion, nerve, plantar
    popliteal nerve — *see* Lesion, nerve, popliteal
    sciatic nerve — *see* Lesion, nerve, sciatic
    specified NEC G57.8- ☑
    tarsal tunnel syndrome — *see* Syndrome, tarsal
      tunnel
  median nerve — *see* Lesion, nerve, median
  multiplex G58.7
  obturator nerve G57.8- ☑
  popliteal nerve — *see* Lesion, nerve, popliteal
  radial nerve — *see* Lesion, nerve, radial
  saphenous nerve G57.8- ☑

Mononeuropathy — *continued*
  specified NEC G58.8
  tarsal tunnel syndrome — *see* Syndrome, tarsal tunnel
  tuberculous A17.83
  ulnar nerve — *see* Lesion, nerve, ulnar
  upper limb G56.9- ☑
    carpal tunnel syndrome — *see* Syndrome, carpal
      tunnel
    causalgia — *see* Causalgia
    median nerve — *see* Lesion, nerve, median
    radial nerve — *see* Lesion, nerve, radial
    specified site NEC G56.8- ☑
    ulnar nerve — *see* Lesion, nerve, ulnar
Mononucleosis, infectious B27.90
  with
    complication NEC B27.99
    meningitis B27.92
    polyneuropathy B27.91
  cytomegaloviral B27.10
    with
      complication NEC B27.19
      meningitis B27.12
      polyneuropathy B27.11
  Epstein-Barr (virus) B27.00
    with
      complication NEC B27.09
      meningitis B27.02
      polyneuropathy B27.01
  gammaherpesviral B27.00
    with
      complication NEC B27.09
      meningitis B27.02
      polyneuropathy B27.01
  specified NEC B27.80
    with
      complication NEC B27.89
      meningitis B27.82
      polyneuropathy B27.81
Monoplegia G83.3- ☑
  congenital (cerebral) G80.8
    spastic G80.1
  embolic (current episode) I63.4- ☑
  following
    cerebrovascular disease
      cerebral infarction
        lower limb I69.34- ☑
        upper limb I69.33- ☑
      intracerebral hemorrhage
        lower limb I69.14- ☑
        upper limb I69.13- ☑
      lower limb I69.94- ☑
      nontraumatic intracranial hemorrhage NEC
        lower limb I69.24- ☑
        upper limb I69.23- ☑
      specified disease NEC
        lower limb I69.84- ☑
        upper limb I69.83- ☑
      stroke NOS
        lower limb I69.34- ☑
        upper limb I69.33- ☑
      subarachnoid hemorrhage
        lower limb I69.04- ☑
        upper limb I69.03- ☑
      upper limb I69.93- ☑
  hysterical (transient) F44.4
  lower limb G83.1- ☑
  psychogenic (conversion reaction) F44.4
  thrombotic (current episode) I63.3- ☑
  transient R29.818
  upper limb G83.2- ☑
Monorchism, monorchidism Q55.0
Monosomy — *see also* Deletion, chromosome Q93.9
  specified NEC Q93.89
  whole chromosome
    meiotic nondisjunction Q93.0
    mitotic nondisjunction Q93.1
    mosaicism Q93.1
  X Q96.9
Monster, monstrosity (single) Q89.7
  acephalic Q00.0
  twin Q89.4
Monteggia's fracture (-dislocation) S52.27- ☑
Mooren's ulcer (cornea) — *see* Ulcer, cornea, Mooren's
Moore's syndrome — *see* Epilepsy, specified NEC
Mooser-Neill reaction A75.2
Mooser's bodies A75.2
Morbidity not stated or unknown R69

Morbilli — *see* Measles
Morbus — *see also* Disease
  angelicus, anglorum E55.0
  Beigel B36.2
  caducus — *see* Epilepsy
  celiacus K90.0
  comitialis — *see* Epilepsy
  cordis — *see also* Disease, heart I51.9
    valvulorum — *see* Endocarditis
  coxae senilis M16.9
    tuberculous A18.02
  hemorrhagicus neonatorum P53
  maculosus neonatorum P54.5
Morel (-Stewart)(-Morgagni) **syndrome** M85.2
Morel-Kraepelin disease — *see* Schizophrenia
Morel-Moore syndrome M85.2
Morgagni's
  cyst, organ, hydatid, or appendage
    female Q50.5
    male (epididymal) Q55.4
      testicular Q55.29
  syndrome M85.2
Morgagni-Stewart-Morel syndrome M85.2
Morgagni-Stokes-Adams syndrome I45.9
Morgagni-Turner (-Albright) **syndrome** Q96.9
Moria F07.0
Moron (I.Q. 50-69) F70
Morphea L94.0
Morphinism (without remission) F11.20
  with remission F11.21
Morphinomania (without remission) F11.20
  with remission F11.21
Morquio (-Ullrich)(-Brailsford) **disease or syndrome** —
  see Mucopolysaccharidosis
Mortification (dry) (moist) — *see* Gangrene
Morton's metatarsalgia (neuralgia)(neuroma) (syn-
  drome) G57.6- ☑
Morvan's disease or syndrome G60.8
Mosaicism, mosaic (autosomal) (chromosomal)
  45,X/46,XX Q96.3
  45,X/other cell lines NEC with abnormal sex chromo-
    some Q96.4
  sex chromosome
    female Q97.8
    lines with various numbers of X chromosomes Q97.2
    male Q98.7
  XY Q96.3
Moschowitz' disease M31.1
Mother yaw A66.0
Motion sickness (from travel, any vehicle) (from round-
  abouts or swings) T75.3 ☑
Mottled, mottling, teeth (enamel) (endemic) (nonen-
  demic) K00.3
Mounier-Kuhn syndrome Q32.4
  with bronchiectasis J47.9
    exacerbation (acute) J47.1
    lower respiratory infection J47.0
  acquired J98.09
    with bronchiectasis J47.9
      with
        exacerbation (acute) J47.1
        lower respiratory infection J47.0
Mountain
  sickness T70.29 ☑
    with polycythemia , acquired (acute) D75.1
  tick fever A93.2
Mouse, joint — *see* Loose, body, joint
  knee M23.4- ☑
Mouth — *see* condition
Movable
  coccyx — *see* subcategory M53.2 ☑
  kidney N28.89
    congenital Q63.8
  spleen D73.89
Movements, dystonic R25.8
Moyamoya disease I67.5
MRSA (Methicillin resistant Staphylococcus aureus)
  infection A49.02
    as the cause of diseases classified elsewhere B95.62
  sepsis A41.02
MSD (multiple sulfatase deficiency) E75.26
MSSA (Methicillin susceptible Staphylococcus aureus)
  infection A49.01
    as the cause of diseases classified elsewhere B95.61
  sepsis A41.01
Mucha-Habermann disease L41.0
Mucinosis (cutaneous) (focal) (papular) (skin) L98.5

Mole — Mucinosis

▼ Subterms under main terms may continue to next column or page   ☑ Additional Character Required — Refer to the Tabular List for Character Selection   225

Mucinosis — *continued*
  oral K13.79
Mucocele
  appendix K38.8
  buccal cavity K13.79
  gallbladder K82.1
  lacrimal sac, chronic H04.43- ☑
  nasal sinus J34.1
  nose J34.1
  salivary gland (any) K11.6
  sinus (accessory) (nasal) J34.1
  turbinate (bone) (middle) (nasal) J34.1
  uterus N85.8
Mucolipidosis
  I E77.1
  II, III E77.0
  IV E75.11
Mucopolysaccharidosis E76.3
  beta-gluduronidase deficiency E76.29
  cardiopathy E76.3 *[I52]*
  Hunter's syndrome E76.1
  Hurler's syndrome E76.01
  Hurler-Scheie syndrome E76.02
  Maroteaux-Lamy syndrome E76.29
  Morquio syndrome E76.219
    A E76.210
    B E76.211
    classic E76.210
  Sanfilippo syndrome E76.22
  Scheie's syndrome E76.03
  specified NEC E76.29
  type
    I
      Hurler's syndrome E76.01
      Hurler-Scheie syndrome E76.02
      Scheie's syndrome E76.03
    II E76.1
    III E76.22
    IV E76.219
    IVA E76.210
    IVB E76.211
    VI E76.29
    VII E76.29
Mucormycosis B46.5
  cutaneous B46.3
  disseminated B46.4
  gastrointestinal B46.2
  generalized B46.4
  pulmonary B46.0
  rhinocerebral B46.1
  skin B46.3
  subcutaneous B46.3
Mucositis (ulcerative) K12.30
  due to drugs NEC K12.32
  gastrointestinal K92.81
  mouth (oral) (oropharyngeal) K12.30
    due to antineoplastic therapy K12.31
    due to drugs NEC K12.32
    due to radiation K12.33
    specified NEC K12.39
    viral K12.39
  nasal J34.81
  oral cavity — *see* Mucositis, mouth
  oral soft tissues — *see* Mucositis, mouth
  vagina and vulva N76.81
Mucositis necroticans agranulocytica — *see* Agranulocytosis
Mucous — *see also* condition
  patches (syphilitic) A51.39
    congenital A50.07
Mucoviscidosis E84.9
  with meconium obstruction E84.11
Mucus
  asphyxia or suffocation — *see* Asphyxia, mucus
  in stool R19.5
  plug — *see* Asphyxia, mucus
Muguet B37.0
Mulberry molars (congenital syphilis) A50.52
Müllerian mixed tumor
  specified site — *see* Neoplasm, malignant, by site
  unspecified site C54.9
Multicystic kidney (development) Q61.4
Multiparity (grand) Z64.1
  affecting management of pregnancy, labor and delivery (supervision only) O09.4- ☑
  requiring contraceptive management — *see* Contraception
Multipartita placenta O43.19- ☑

Multiple, multiplex — *see also* condition
  digits (congenital) Q69.9
  endocrine neoplasia — *see* Neoplasia, endocrine, multiple (MEN)
  personality F44.81
Mumps B26.9
  arthritis B26.85
  complication NEC B26.89
  encephalitis B26.2
  hepatitis B26.81
  meningitis (aseptic) B26.1
  meningoencephalitis B26.2
  myocarditis B26.82
  oophoritis B26.89
  orchitis B26.0
  pancreatitis B26.3
  polyneuropathy B26.84
Mumu — *see also* Infestation, filarial B74.9 *[N51]*
Münchhausen's syndrome — *see* Disorder, factitious
Münchmeyer's syndrome — *see* Myositis, ossificans, progressiva
Mural — *see* condition
Murmur (cardiac) (heart) (organic) R01.1
  abdominal R19.15
  aortic (valve) — *see* Endocarditis, aortic
  benign R01.0
  diastolic — *see* Endocarditis
  Flint I35.1
  functional R01.0
  Graham Steell I37.1
  innocent R01.0
  mitral (valve) — *see* Insufficiency, mitral
  nonorganic R01.0
  presystolic, mitral — *see* Insufficiency, mitral
  pulmonic (valve) I37.8
  systolic R01.1
  tricuspid (valve) I07.9
  valvular — *see* Endocarditis
Murri's disease (intermittent hemoglobinuria) D59.6
Muscle, muscular — *see also* condition
  carnitine (palmityltransferase) deficiency E71.314
Musculoneuralgia — *see* Neuralgia
Mushrooming hip — *see* Derangement, joint, specified NEC, hip
Mushroom-workers' (pickers') **disease or lung** J67.5
Mutation(s)
  factor V Leiden D68.51
  prothrombin gene D68.52
  surfactant, of lung J84.83
Mutism — *see also* Aphasia
  deaf (acquired) (congenital) NEC H91.3
  elective (adjustment reaction) (childhood) F94.0
  hysterical F44.4
  selective (childhood) F94.0
MVD (microvillus inclusion disease) Q43.8
MVID (microvillus inclusion disease) Q43.8
Myalgia M79.10
  auxiliary muscles, head and neck M79.12
  epidemic (cervical) B33.0
  mastication muscle M79.11
  site specified NEC M79.18
  traumatic NEC T14.8 ☑
Myasthenia G70.9
  congenital G70.2
  cordis — *see* Failure, heart
  developmental G70.2
  gravis G70.00
    with exacerbation (acute) G70.01
    in crisis G70.01
    neonatal, transient P94.0
    pseudoparalytica G70.00
      with exacerbation (acute) G70.01
      in crisis G70.01
  stomach, psychogenic F45.8
  syndrome
    in
      diabetes mellitus — *see* E08-E13 with .44
      neoplastic disease — *see also* Neoplasm D49.9 *[G73.3]*
      pernicious anemia D51.0 *[G73.3]*
      thyrotoxicosis E05.90 *[G73.3]*
        with thyroid storm E05.91 *[G73.3]*
Myasthenic M62.81
Mycelium infection B49
Mycetismus — *see* Poisoning, food, noxious, mushroom
Mycetoma B47.9
  actinomycotic B47.1
  bone (mycotic) B47.9 *[M90.80]*

Mycetoma — *continued*
  eumycotic B47.0
  foot B47.9
    actinomycotic B47.1
    mycotic B47.0
  madurae NEC B47.9
    mycotic B47.0
  maduromycotic B47.0
  mycotic B47.0
  nocardial B47.1
Mycobacteriosis — *see* Mycobacterium
Mycobacterium, mycobacterial (infection) A31.9
  anonymous A31.9
  atypical A31.9
    cutaneous A31.1
    pulmonary A31.0
      tuberculous — *see* Tuberculosis, pulmonary
    specified site NEC A31.8
  avium (intracellulare complex) A31.0
  balnei A31.1
  Battey A31.0
  chelonei A31.8
  cutaneous A31.1
  extrapulmonary systemic A31.8
  fortuitum A31.8
  intracellulare (Battey bacillus) A31.0
  kakaferifu A31.8
  kansasii (yellow bacillus) A31.0
  kasongo A31.8
  leprae — *see also* Leprosy A30.9
  luciflavum A31.1
  marinum (M. balnei) A31.1
  nonspecific — *see* Mycobacterium, atypical
  pulmonary (atypical) A31.0
    tuberculous — *see* Tuberculosis, pulmonary
  scrofulaceum A31.8
  simiae A31.8
  systemic, extrapulmonary A31.8
  szulgai A31.8
  terrae A31.8
  triviale A31.8
  tuberculosis (human, bovine) — *see* Tuberculosis
  ulcerans A31.1
  xenopi A31.8
Mycoplasma (M.) **pneumoniae, as cause of disease classified elsewhere** B96.0
Mycosis, mycotic B49
  cutaneous NEC B36.9
  ear B36.9
    in
      aspergillosis B44.89
      candidiasis B37.84
      moniliasis B37.84
  fungoides (extranodal) (solid organ) C84.0- ☑
  mouth B37.0
  nails B35.1
  opportunistic B48.8
  skin NEC B36.9
  specified NEC B48.8
  stomatitis B37.0
  vagina, vaginitis (candidal) B37.3
Mydriasis (pupil) H57.04
Myelatelia Q06.1
Myelinolysis, pontine, central G37.2
Myelitis (acute) (ascending) (childhood) (chronic) (descending) (diffuse) (disseminated) (idiopathic) (pressure) (progressive) (spinal cord) (subacute) — *see also* Encephalitis G04.91
  herpes simplex B00.82
  herpes zoster B02.24
  in diseases classified elsewhere G05.4
  necrotizing, subacute G37.4
  optic neuritis in G36.0
  postchickenpox B01.12
  postherpetic B02.24
  postimmunization G04.02
  postinfectious NEC G04.89
  postvaccinal G04.02
  specified NEC G04.89
  syphilitic (transverse) A52.14
  toxic G92
  transverse (in demyelinating diseases of central nervous system) G37.3
  tuberculous A17.82
  varicella B01.12
Myeloblastic — *see* condition
Myeloblastoma
  granular cell — *see also* Neoplasm, connective tissu

Myeloblastoma — *continued*
  granular cell — *see also* Neoplasm, connective tissue
    — *continued*
      malignant — *see* Neoplasm, connective tissue, malignant
    tongue D10.1
Myelocele — *see* Spina bifida
Myelocystocele — *see* Spina bifida
Myelocytic — *see* condition
Myelodysplasia D46.9
  specified NEC D46.Z (*following* D46.4)
  spinal cord (congenital) Q06.1
Myelodysplastic syndrome D46.9
  with
    5q deletion D46.C (*following* D46.2)
    isolated del (5q) chromosomal abnormality D46.C (*following* D46.2)
  specified NEC D46.Z (*following* D46.4)
Myeloencephalitis — *see* Encephalitis
Myelofibrosis D75.81
  with myeloid metaplasia D47.4
  acute C94.4- ☑
  idiopathic (chronic) D47.4
  primary D47.1
  secondary D75.81
    in myeloproliferative disease D47.4
Myelogenous — *see* condition
Myeloid — *see* condition
Myelokathexis D70.9
Myeloleukodystrophy E75.29
Myelolipoma — *see* Lipoma
Myeloma (multiple) C90.0- ☑
  monostotic C90.3 ☑
    plasma cell C90.0- ☑
  plasma cell C90.0- ☑
  solitary — *see also* Plasmacytoma, solitary C90.3- ☑
Myelomalacia G95.89
Myelomatosis C90.0- ☑
Myelomeningitis — *see* Meningoencephalitis
Myelomeningocele (spinal cord) — *see* Spina bifida
Myelo-osteo-musculodysplasia hereditaria Q79.8
Myelopathic
  anemia D64.89
  muscle atrophy — *see* Atrophy, muscle, spinal
  pain syndrome G89.0
Myelopathy (spinal cord) G95.9
  drug-induced G95.89
  in (due to)
    degeneration or displacement, intervertebral disc NEC — *see* Disorder, disc, with, myelopathy
    infection — *see* Encephalitis
    intervertebral disc disorder — *see also* Disorder, disc, with, myelopathy
    mercury — *see* subcategory T56.1 ☑
    neoplastic disease — *see also* Neoplasm D49.9 [G99.2]
    pernicious anemia D51.0 [G99.2]
    spondylosis — *see* Spondylosis, with myelopathy NEC
  necrotic (subacute) (vascular) G95.19
  radiation-induced G95.89
  spondylogenic NEC — *see* Spondylosis, with myelopathy NEC
  toxic G95.89
  transverse, acute G37.3
  vascular G95.19
  vitamin B12 E53.8 [G32.0]
Myelophthisis D61.82
Myeloradiculitis G04.91
Myeloradiculodysplasia (spinal) Q06.1
Myelosarcoma C92.3- ☑
Myelosclerosis D75.89
  with myeloid metaplasia D47.4
  disseminated, of nervous system G35
  megakaryocytic D47.4
    with myeloid metaplasia D47.4
Myelosis
  acute C92.0- ☑
  aleukemic C92.9- ☑
  chronic D47.1
  erythremic (acute) C94.0- ☑
  megakaryocytic C94.2- ☑
  nonleukemic D72.828
  subacute C92.9- ☑
Myiasis (cavernous) B87.9
  aural B87.4
  creeping B87.0

Myiasis — *continued*
  cutaneous B87.0
  dermal B87.0
  ear (external) (middle) B87.4
  eye B87.2
  genitourinary B87.81
  intestinal B87.82
  laryngeal B87.3
  nasopharyngeal B87.3
  ocular B87.2
  orbit B87.2
  skin B87.0
  specified site NEC B87.89
  traumatic B87.1
  wound B87.1
Myoadenoma, prostate — *see* Hyperplasia, prostate
Myoblastoma
  granular cell — *see also* Neoplasm, connective tissue, benign
    malignant — *see* Neoplasm, connective tissue, malignant
  tongue D10.1
Myocardial — *see* condition
Myocardiopathy (congestive) (constrictive) (familial) (hypertrophic nonobstructive) (idiopathic) (infiltrative) (obstructive) (primary) (restrictive) (sporadic) — *see also* Cardiomyopathy I42.9
  alcoholic I42.6
  cobalt-beer I42.6
  glycogen storage E74.02 [I43]
  hypertrophic obstructive I42.1
  in (due to)
    beriberi E51.12
    cardiac glycogenosis E74.02 [I43]
    Friedreich's ataxia G11.1 [I43]
    myotonia atrophica G71.11 [I43]
    progressive muscular dystrophy G71.09 [I43]
  obscure (African) I42.8
  secondary I42.9
  thyrotoxic E05.90 [I43]
    with storm E05.91 [I43]
  toxic NEC I42.7
Myocarditis (with arteriosclerosis)(chronic)(fibroid) (interstitial) (old) (progressive) (senile) I51.4
  with
    rheumatic fever (conditions in I00) I09.0
      active — *see* Myocarditis, acute, rheumatic
      inactive or quiescent (with chorea) I09.0
  active I40.9
    rheumatic I01.2
      with chorea (acute) (rheumatic) (Sydenham's) I02.0
  acute or subacute (interstitial) I40.9
    due to
      streptococcus (beta-hemolytic) I01.2
    idiopathic I40.1
    rheumatic I01.2
      with chorea (acute) (rheumatic) (Sydenham's) I02.0
    specified NEC I40.8
  aseptic of newborn B33.22
  bacterial (acute) I40.0
  Coxsackie (virus) B33.22
  diphtheritic A36.81
  eosinophilic I40.1
  epidemic of newborn (Coxsackie) B33.22
  Fiedler's (acute) (isolated) I40.1
  giant cell (acute) (subacute) I40.1
  gonococcal A54.83
  granulomatous (idiopathic) (isolated) (nonspecific) I40.1
  hypertensive — *see* Hypertension, heart
  idiopathic (granulomatous) I40.1
  in (due to)
    diphtheria A36.81
    epidemic louse-borne typhus A75.0 [I41]
    Lyme disease A69.29
    sarcoidosis D86.85
    scarlet fever A38.1
    toxoplasmosis (acquired) B58.81
    typhoid A01.02
    typhus NEC A75.9 [I41]
  infective I40.0
  influenzal — *see* Influenza, with, myocarditis
  isolated (acute) I40.1
  meningococcal A39.52
  mumps B26.82
  nonrheumatic, active I40.9
  parenchymatous I40.9

Myocarditis — *continued*
  pneumococcal I40.0
  rheumatic (chronic) (inactive) (with chorea) I09.0
    active or acute I01.2
      with chorea (acute) (rheumatic) (Sydenham's) I02.0
  rheumatoid — *see* Rheumatoid, carditis
  septic I40.0
  staphylococcal I40.0
  suppurative I40.0
  syphilitic (chronic) A52.06
  toxic I40.8
    rheumatic — *see* Myocarditis, acute, rheumatic
  tuberculous A18.84
  typhoid A01.02
  valvular — *see* Endocarditis
  virus, viral I40.0
    of newborn (Coxsackie) B33.22
Myocardium, myocardial — *see* condition
Myocardosis — *see* Cardiomyopathy
Myoclonus, myoclonic, myoclonia (familial) (essential) (multifocal) (simplex) G25.3
  drug-induced G25.3
  epilepsy — *see also* Epilepsy, generalized, specified NEC G40.4- ☑
  familial (progressive) G25.3
  epileptica G40.409
    with status epilepticus G40.401
  facial G51.3- ☑
  familial progressive G25.3
  Friedreich's G25.3
  jerks G25.3
  massive G25.3
  palatal G25.3
  pharyngeal G25.3
Myocytolysis I51.5
Myodiastasis — *see* Diastasis, muscle
Myoendocarditis — *see* Endocarditis
Myoepithelioma — *see* Neoplasm, benign, by site
Myofasciitis (acute) — *see* Myositis
Myofibroma — *see also* Neoplasm, connective tissue, benign
  uterus (cervix) (corpus) — *see* Leiomyoma
Myofibromatosis D48.1
  infantile Q89.8
Myofibrosis M62.89
  heart — *see* Myocarditis
  scapulohumeral — *see* Lesion, shoulder, specified NEC
Myofibrositis M79.7
  scapulohumeral — *see* Lesion, shoulder, specified NEC
Myoglobulinuria, myoglobinuria (primary) R82.1
Myokymia, facial G51.4
Myolipoma — *see* Lipoma
Myoma — *see also* Neoplasm, connective tissue, benign
  malignant — *see* Neoplasm, connective tissue, malignant
  prostate D29.1
  uterus (cervix) (corpus) — *see* Leiomyoma
Myomalacia M62.89
Myometritis — *see* Endometritis
Myometrium — *see* condition
Myonecrosis, clostridial A48.0
Myopathy G72.9
  acute
    necrotizing G72.81
    quadriplegic G72.81
  alcoholic G72.1
  benign congenital G71.2
  central core G71.2
  centronuclear G71.2
  congenital (benign) G71.2
  critical illness G72.81
  distal G71.09
  drug-induced G72.0
  endocrine NEC E34.9 [G73.7]
  extraocular muscles H05.82- ☑
  facioscapulohumeral G71.02
  hereditary G71.9
    specified NEC G71.8
  immune NEC G72.49
  in (due to)
    Addison's disease E27.1 [G73.7]
    alcohol G72.1
    amyloidosis E85.0 [G73.7]
    cretinism E00.9 [G73.7]
    Cushing's syndrome E24.9 [G73.7]
    drugs G72.0

Myeloblastoma — Myopathy

▽ Subterms under main terms may continue to next column or page   ☑ Additional Character Required — Refer to the Tabular List for Character Selection   227

Myopathy — continued
  in — continued
    endocrine disease NEC E34.9 [G73.7]
    giant cell arteritis M31.6 [G73.7]
    glycogen storage disease E74.00 [G73.7]
    hyperadrenocorticism E24.9 [G73.7]
    hyperparathyroidism NEC E21.3 [G73.7]
    hypoparathyroidism E20.9 [G73.7]
    hypopituitarism E23.0 [G73.7]
    hypothyroidism E03.9 [G73.7]
    infectious disease NEC B99 ☑ [G73.7]
    lipid storage disease E75.6 [G73.7]
    metabolic disease NEC E88.9 [G73.7]
    myxedema E03.9 [G73.7]
    parasitic disease NEC B89 [G73.7]
    polyarteritis nodosa M30.0 [G73.7]
    rheumatoid arthritis — see Rheumatoid, myopathy
    sarcoidosis D86.87
    scleroderma M34.82
    sicca syndrome M35.03
    Sjögren's syndrome M35.03
    systemic lupus erythematosus M32.19
    thyrotoxicosis (hyperthyroidism) E05.90 [G73.7]
      with thyroid storm E05.91 [G73.7]
    toxic agent NEC G72.2
  inflammatory NEC G72.49
  intensive care (ICU) G72.81
  limb-girdle G71.09
  mitochondrial NEC G71.3
  myotubular G71.2
  mytonic, proximal (PROMM) G71.11
  nemaline G71.2
  ocular G71.09
  oculopharyngeal G71.09
  of critical illness G72.81
  primary G71.9
    specified NEC G71.8
  progressive NEC G72.89
  proximal myotonic (PROMM) G71.11
  rod G71.2
  scapulohumeral G71.02
  specified NEC G72.89
  toxic G72.2

Myopericarditis — see also Pericarditis
  chronic rheumatic I09.2

Myopia (axial) (congenital) H52.1- ☑
  degenerative (malignant) H44.20
    with
      choroidal neovascularization H44.2A- ☑
      foveoschisis H44.2D- ☑
      macular hole H44.2B- ☑
      retinal detachment H44.2C- ☑
      specified maculopathy NEC H44.2E- ☑
    bilateral H44.23
    left eye H44.22
    right eye H44.21
  malignant — see also Myopia, degenerative H44.2- ☑
  pernicious — see also Myopia, degenerative H44.2- ☑
  progressive high (degenerative) — see also Myopia, degenerative H44.2- ☑

Myosarcoma — see Neoplasm, connective tissue, malignant

Myosis (pupil) H57.03
  stromal (endolymphatic) D39.0

Myositis M60.9
  clostridial A48.0
  due to posture — see Myositis, specified type NEC
  epidemic B33.0
  fibrosa or fibrous (chronic), Volkmann's T79.6 ☑
  foreign body granuloma — see Granuloma, foreign body
  in (due to)
    bilharziasis B65.9 [M63.8-] ☑
    cysticercosis B69.81
    leprosy A30.9 [M63.8-] ☑
    mycosis B49 [M63.8-] ☑
    sarcoidosis D86.87
    schistosomiasis B65.9 [M63.8-] ☑
    syphilis
      late A52.78
      secondary A51.49
    toxoplasmosis (acquired) B58.82

Myositis — continued
  in — continued
    trichinellosis B75 [M63.8-] ☑
    tuberculosis A18.09
  inclusion body [IBM] G72.41
  infective M60.009
    arm M60.002
      left M60.001
      right M60.000
    leg M60.005
      left M60.004
      right M60.003
    lower limb M60.005
      ankle M60.07- ☑
      foot M60.07- ☑
      lower leg M60.06- ☑
      thigh M60.05- ☑
      toe M60.07- ☑
    multiple sites M60.09
    specified site NEC M60.08
    upper limb M60.002
      finger M60.04- ☑
      forearm M60.03- ☑
      hand M60.04- ☑
      shoulder region M60.01- ☑
      upper arm M60.02- ☑
  interstitial M60.10
    ankle M60.17- ☑
    foot M60.17- ☑
    forearm M60.13- ☑
    hand M60.14- ☑
    lower leg M60.16- ☑
    multiple sites M60.19
    shoulder region M60.11- ☑
    specified site NEC M60.18
    thigh M60.15- ☑
    upper arm M60.12- ☑
  mycotic B49 [M63.8-] ☑
  orbital, chronic H05.12- ☑
  ossificans or ossifying (circumscripta) — see also Ossification, muscle, specified NEC
    in (due to)
      burns M61.30
        ankle M61.37- ☑
        foot M61.37- ☑
        forearm M61.33- ☑
        hand M61.34- ☑
        lower leg M61.36- ☑
        multiple sites M61.39
        pelvic region M61.35- ☑
        shoulder region M61.31- ☑
        specified site NEC M61.38
        thigh M61.35- ☑
        upper arm M61.32- ☑
      quadriplegia or paraplegia M61.20
        ankle M61.27- ☑
        foot M61.27- ☑
        forearm M61.23- ☑
        hand M61.24- ☑
        lower leg M61.26- ☑
        multiple sites M61.29
        pelvic region M61.25- ☑
        shoulder region M61.21- ☑
        specified site NEC M61.28
        thigh M61.25- ☑
        upper arm M61.22- ☑
      progressiva M61.10
        ankle M61.17- ☑
        finger M61.14- ☑
        foot M61.17- ☑
        forearm M61.13- ☑
        hand M61.14- ☑
        lower leg M61.16- ☑
        multiple sites M61.19
        pelvic region M61.15- ☑
        shoulder region M61.11- ☑
        specified site NEC M61.18
        thigh M61.15- ☑
        toe M61.17- ☑
        upper arm M61.12- ☑
    traumatica M61.00

Myositis — continued
  ossificans or ossifying — see also Ossification, muscle, specified — continued
    traumatica — continued
      ankle M61.07- ☑
      foot M61.07- ☑
      forearm M61.03- ☑
      hand M61.04- ☑
      lower leg M61.06- ☑
      multiple sites M61.09
      pelvic region M61.05- ☑
      shoulder region M61.01- ☑
      specified site NEC M61.08
      thigh M61.05- ☑
      upper arm M61.02- ☑
  purulent — see Myositis, infective
  specified type NEC M60.80
    ankle M60.87- ☑
    foot M60.87- ☑
    forearm M60.83- ☑
    hand M60.84- ☑
    lower leg M60.86- ☑
    multiple sites M60.89
    pelvic region M60.85- ☑
    shoulder region M60.81- ☑
    specified site NEC M60.88
    thigh M60.85- ☑
    upper arm M60.82- ☑
  suppurative — see Myositis, infective
  traumatic (old) — see Myositis, specified type NEC

Myospasia impulsiva F95.2

Myotonia (acquisita) (intermittens) M62.89
  atrophica G71.11
  chondrodystrophic G71.13
  congenita (acetazolamide responsive) (dominant) (recessive) G71.12
  drug-induced G71.14
  dystrophica G71.11
  fluctuans G71.19
  levior G71.12
  permanens G71.19
  symptomatic G71.19

Myotonic pupil — see Anomaly, pupil, function, tonic pupil

Myriapodiasis B88.2

Myringitis H73.2- ☑
  with otitis media — see Otitis, media
  acute H73.00- ☑
    bullous H73.01- ☑
    specified NEC H73.09- ☑
  bullous — see Myringitis, acute, bullous
  chronic H73.1- ☑

Mysophobia F40.228

Mytilotoxism — see Poisoning, fish

Myxadenitis labialis K13.0

Myxedema (adult) (idiocy) (infantile) (juvenile) — see also Hypothyroidism E03.9
  circumscribed E05.90
    with storm E05.91
  coma E03.5
  congenital E00.1
  cutis L98.5
  localized (pretibial) E05.90
    with storm E05.91
  papular L98.5

Myxochondrosarcoma — see Neoplasm, cartilage, malignant

Myxofibroma — see Neoplasm, connective tissue, benign
  odontogenic — see Cyst, calcifying odontogenic

Myxofibrosarcoma — see Neoplasm, connective tissue, malignant

Myxolipoma D17.9

Myxoliposarcoma — see Neoplasm, connective tissue, malignant

Myxoma — see also Neoplasm, connective tissue, benign
  nerve sheath — see Neoplasm, nerve, benign
  odontogenic — see Cyst, calcifying odontogenic

Myxosarcoma — see Neoplasm, connective tissue, malignant

N

Naegeli's
- disease Q82.8
- leukemia, monocytic C93.1- ☑

Nageleriasis (with meningoencephalitis) B60.2
Naffziger's syndrome G54.0
Naga sore — *see* Ulcer, skin
Nägele's pelvis M95.5
- with disproportion (fetopelvic) O33.0
  - causing obstructed labor O65.0

Nail — *see also* condition
- biting F98.8
- patella syndrome Q87.2

Nanism, nanosomia — *see* Dwarfism
Nanophyetiasis B66.8
Nanukayami A27.89
Napkin rash L22
Narcolepsy G47.419
- with cataplexy G47.411
- in conditions classified elsewhere G47.429
  - with cataplexy G47.421

Narcosis R06.89
Narcotism — *see* Dependence
NARP (Neuropathy, Ataxia and Retinitis pigmentosa)
- syndrome E88.49

Narrow
- anterior chamber angle H40.03- ☑
- gingival width (of periodontal soft tissue) K05.5
- pelvis — *see* Contraction, pelvis

Narrowing — *see also* Stenosis
- artery I77.1
  - auditory, internal I65.8
  - basilar — *see* Occlusion, artery, basilar
  - carotid — *see* Occlusion, artery, carotid
  - cerebellar — *see* Occlusion, artery, cerebellar
  - cerebral — *see* Occlusion artery, cerebral
  - choroidal — *see* Occlusion, artery, precerebral, specified NEC
  - communicating posterior — *see* Occlusion, artery, precerebral, specified NEC
  - coronary — *see also* Disease, heart, ischemic, atherosclerotic
    - congenital Q24.5
      - syphilitic A50.54 *[I52]*
    - due to syphilis NEC A52.06
  - hypophyseal — *see* Occlusion, artery, precerebral, specified NEC
  - pontine — *see* Occlusion, artery, precerebral, specified NEC
  - precerebral — *see* Occlusion, artery, precerebral
  - vertebral — *see* Occlusion, artery, vertebral
- auditory canal (external) — *see* Stenosis, external ear canal
- eustachian tube — *see* Obstruction, eustachian tube
- eyelid — *see* Disorder, eyelid function
- larynx J38.6
- mesenteric artery — *see also* Ischemia, intestine, acute K55.059
- palate M26.89
- palpebral fissure — *see* Disorder, eyelid function
- ureter N13.5
  - with infection N13.6
- urethra — *see* Stricture, urethra

Narrowness, abnormal, eyelid Q10.3
Nasal — *see* condition
Nasolachrymal, nasolacrimal — *see* condition
Nasopharyngeal — *see also* condition
- pituitary gland Q89.2
- torticollis M43.6

Nasopharyngitis (acute) (infective) (streptococcal) (subacute) J00
- chronic (suppurative) (ulcerative) J31.1

Nasopharynx, nasopharyngeal — *see* condition
Natal tooth, teeth K00.6
Nausea (without vomiting) R11.0
- with vomiting R11.2
- gravidarum — *see* Hyperemesis, gravidarum
- marina T75.3 ☑
- navalis T75.3 ☑

Navel — *see* condition
Neapolitan fever — *see* Brucellosis
Near drowning T75.1 ☑
Nearsightedness — *see* Myopia
Near-syncope R55
Nebula, cornea — *see* Opacity, cornea

Necator americanus infestation B76.1
Necatoriasis B76.1
Neck — *see* condition
Necrobiosis R68.89
- lipoidica NEC L92.1
  - with diabetes — *see* E08-E13 with .620

Necrolysis, toxic epidermal L51.2
- due to drug
  - correct substance properly administered — *see* Table of Drugs and Chemicals, by drug, adverse effect
  - overdose or wrong substance given or taken — *see* Table of Drugs and Chemicals, by drug, poisoning

Necrophilia F65.89
Necrosis, necrotic (ischemic) — *see also* Gangrene
- adrenal (capsule) (gland) E27.49
- amputation stump (surgical) (late) T87.50
  - arm T87.5- ☑
  - leg T87.5- ☑
- antrum J32.0
- aorta (hyaline) — *see also* Aneurysm, aorta
  - cystic medial — *see* Dissection, aorta
- artery I77.5
- bladder (aseptic) (sphincter) N32.89
- bone — *see also* Osteonecrosis M87.9
  - aseptic or avascular — *see* Osteonecrosis
    - idiopathic M87.00
  - ethmoid J32.2
  - jaw M27.2
  - tuberculous — *see* Tuberculosis, bone
- brain I67.89
- breast (aseptic) (fat) (segmental) N64.1
- bronchus J98.09
- central nervous system NEC I67.89
- cerebellar I67.89
- cerebral I67.89
- colon — *see also* Infarct, intestine K55.049
- cornea H18.89- ☑
- cortical (acute) (renal) N17.1
- cystic medial (aorta) — *see* Dissection, aorta
- dental pulp K04.1
- esophagus K22.8
- ethmoid (bone) J32.2
- eyelid — *see* Disorder, eyelid, degenerative
- fat, fatty (generalized) — *see also* Disorder, soft tissue, specified type NEC
  - abdominal wall K65.4
  - breast (aseptic) (segmental) N64.1
  - localized — *see* Degeneration, by site, fatty
  - mesentery K65.4
  - omentum K65.4
  - pancreas K86.89
  - peritoneum K65.4
  - skin (subcutaneous), newborn P83.0
  - subcutaneous, due to birth injury P15.6
- gallbladder — *see* Cholecystitis, acute
- heart — *see* Infarct, myocardium
- hip, aseptic or avascular — *see* Osteonecrosis, by type, femur
- intestine (acute) (hemorrhagic) (massive) — *see also* Infarct, intestine K55.069
- jaw M27.2
- kidney (bilateral) N28.0
  - acute N17.9
  - cortical (acute) (bilateral) N17.1
    - with ectopic or molar pregnancy O08.4
  - medullary (bilateral) (in acute renal failure) (papillary) N17.2
  - papillary (bilateral) (in acute renal failure) N17.2
  - tubular N17.0
    - with ectopic or molar pregnancy O08.4
    - complicating
      - abortion — *see* Abortion, by type, complicated by, tubular necrosis
      - ectopic or molar pregnancy O08.4
      - pregnancy — *see* Pregnancy, complicated by, diseases of, specified type or system NEC
    - following ectopic or molar pregnancy O08.4
    - traumatic T79.5 ☑
- larynx J38.7
- liver (with hepatic failure) (cell) — *see* Failure, hepatic
  - hemorrhagic, central K76.2
- lung J85.0
- lymphatic gland — *see* Lymphadenitis, acute
- mammary gland (fat) (segmental) N64.1
- mastoid (chronic) — *see* Mastoiditis, chronic

Necrosis, necrotic — *continued*
- medullary (acute) (renal) N17.2
- mesentery — *see also* Infarct, intestine K55.069
  - fat K65.4
- mitral valve — *see* Insufficiency, mitral
- myocardium, myocardial — *see* Infarct, myocardium
- nose J34.0
- omentum (with mesenteric infarction) — *see also* Infarct, intestine K55.069
  - fat K65.4
- orbit, orbital — *see* Osteomyelitis, orbit
- ossicles, ear — *see* Abnormal, ear ossicles
- ovary N70.92
- pancreas (aseptic) (duct) (fat) K86.89
  - acute (infective) — *see* Pancreatitis, acute
  - infective — *see* Pancreatitis, acute
- papillary (acute) (renal) N17.2
- perineum N90.89
- peritoneum (with mesenteric infarction) — *see also* Infarct, intestine K55.069
  - fat K65.4
- pharynx J02.9
  - in granulocytopenia — *see* Neutropenia
  - Vincent's A69.1
- phosphorus — *see* subcategory T54.2 ☑
- pituitary (gland) E23.0
  - postpartum O99.285
  - Sheehan O99.285
- pressure — *see* Ulcer, pressure, by site
- pulmonary J85.0
- pulp (dental) K04.1
- radiation — *see* Necrosis, by site
- radium — *see* Necrosis, by site
- renal — *see* Necrosis, kidney
- sclera H15.89
- scrotum N50.89
- skin or subcutaneous tissue NEC I96
- spine, spinal (column) — *see also* Osteonecrosis, by type, vertebra
  - cord G95.19
- spleen D73.5
- stomach K31.89
- stomatitis (ulcerative) A69.0
- subcutaneous fat, newborn P83.88
- subendocardial (acute) I21.4
  - chronic I25.89
- suprarenal (capsule) (gland) E27.49
- testis N50.89
- thymus (gland) E32.8
- tonsil J35.8
- trachea J39.8
- tuberculous NEC — *see* Tuberculosis
- tubular (acute) (anoxic) (renal) (toxic) N17.0
  - postprocedural N99.0
- vagina N89.8
- vertebra — *see also* Osteonecrosis, by type, vertebra
  - tuberculous A18.01
- vulva N90.89
- X-ray — *see* Necrosis, by site

Necrospermia — *see* Infertility, male
Need (for)
- care provider because (of)
  - assistance with personal care Z74.1
  - continuous supervision required Z74.3
  - impaired mobility Z74.09
  - no other household member able to render care Z74.2
  - specified reason NEC Z74.8
- immunization — *see* Vaccination
- vaccination — *see* Vaccination

Neglect
- adult
  - confirmed T74.01 ☑
  - history of Z91.412
  - suspected T76.01 ☑
- child (childhood)
  - confirmed T74.02 ☑
  - history of Z62.812
  - suspected T76.02 ☑
- emotional, in childhood Z62.898
- hemispatial R41.4
- left-sided R41.4
- sensory R41.4
- visuospatial R41.4

Neisserian infection NEC — *see* Gonococcus
Nelaton's syndrome G60.8
Nelson's syndrome E24.1
Nematodiasis (intestinal) B82.0

Nematodiasis — continued
  Ancylostoma B76.0
Neonatal — see also Newborn
  acne L70.4
  bradycardia P29.12
  screening, abnormal findings on P09
  tachycardia P29.11
  tooth, teeth K00.6
Neonatorum — see condition
Neoplasia
  endocrine, multiple (MEN) E31.20
    type I E31.21
    type IIA E31.22
    type IIB E31.23
  intraepithelial (histologically confirmed)
    anal (AIN) (histologically confirmed) K62.82
      grade I K62.82
      grade II K62.82
      severe D01.3
    cervical glandular (histologically confirmed) D06.9
    cervix (uteri) (CIN) (histologically confirmed) N87.9
      glandular D06.9
      grade I N87.0
      grade II N87.1
      grade III (severe dysplasia) — see also Carcinoma,
        cervix uteri, in situ D06.9
    prostate (histologically confirmed) (PIN) N42.31
      grade I N42.31
      grade II N42.31
      grade III (severe dysplasia) D07.5
    vagina (histologically confirmed) (VAIN) N89.3
      grade I N89.0
      grade II N89.1
      grade III (severe dysplasia) D07.2
    vulva (histologically confirmed) (VIN) N90.3
      grade I N90.0
      grade II N90.1
      grade III (severe dysplasia) D07.1
Neoplasm, neoplastic — see also Table of Neoplasms
  lipomatous, benign — see Lipoma
  malignant mast cell C96.20
    specified type NEC C96.29
  mast cell, of uncertain behavior NEC D47.09
Neovascularization
  ciliary body — see Disorder, iris, vascular
  cornea H16.40- ☑
    deep H16.44- ☑
    ghost vessels — see Ghost, vessels
    localized H16.43- ☑
    pannus — see Pannus
  iris — see Disorder, iris, vascular
  retina H35.05- ☑
Nephralgia N23
Nephritis, nephritic (albuminuric) (azotemic) (congenital) (disseminated) (epithelial) (familial) (focal) (granulomatous) (hemorrhagic) (infantile) (nonsuppurative, excretory) (uremic) N05.9
  with
    dense deposit disease N05.6
    diffuse
      crescentic glomerulonephritis N05.7
      endocapillary proliferative glomerulonephritis N05.4
      membranous glomerulonephritis N05.2
      mesangial proliferative glomerulonephritis N05.3
      mesangiocapillary glomerulonephritis N05.5
    edema — see Nephrosis
    focal and segmental glomerular lesions N05.1
    foot process disease N04.9
    glomerular lesion
      diffuse sclerosing N05.8
      hypocomplementemic — see Nephritis, membranoproliferative
      IgA — see Nephropathy, IgA
      lobular, lobulonodular — see Nephritis, membranoproliferative
      nodular — see Nephritis, membranoproliferative
    lesion of
      glomerulonephritis, proliferative N05.8
      renal necrosis N05.9
    minor glomerular abnormality N05.0
    specified morphological changes NEC N05.8
  acute N00.9
    with
      dense deposit disease N00.6
      diffuse
        crescentic glomerulonephritis N00.7

Nephritis, nephritic — continued
  acute — continued
    with — continued
      diffuse — continued
        endocapillary proliferative glomerulonephritis N00.4
        membranous glomerulonephritis N00.2
        mesangial proliferative glomerulonephritis N00.3
        mesangiocapillary glomerulonephritis N00.5
      focal and segmental glomerular lesions N00.1
      minor glomerular abnormality N00.0
      specified morphological changes NEC N00.8
  amyloid E85.4 [N08]
  antiglomerular basement membrane (anti-GBM) antibody NEC
    in Goodpasture's syndrome M31.0
  antitubular basement membrane (tubulo-interstitial) NEC N12
    toxic — see Nephropathy, toxic
  arteriolar — see Hypertension, kidney
  arteriosclerotic — see Hypertension, kidney
  ascending — see Nephritis, tubulo-interstitial
  atrophic N03.9
  Balkan (endemic) N15.0
  calculous, calculus — see Calculus, kidney
  cardiac — see Hypertension, kidney
  cardiovascular — see Hypertension, kidney
  chronic N03.9
    with
      dense deposit disease N03.6
      diffuse
        crescentic glomerulonephritis N03.7
        endocapillary proliferative glomerulonephritis N03.4
        membranous glomerulonephritis N03.2
        mesangial proliferative glomerulonephritis N03.3
        mesangiocapillary glomerulonephritis N03.5
      focal and segmental glomerular lesions N03.1
      minor glomerular abnormality N03.0
      specified morphological changes NEC N03.8
    arteriosclerotic — see Hypertension, kidney
  cirrhotic N26.9
  complicating pregnancy O26.83- ☑
  croupous N00.9
  degenerative — see Nephrosis
  diffuse sclerosing N05.8
  due to
    diabetes mellitus — see E08-E13 with .21
    subacute bacterial endocarditis I33.0
    systemic lupus erythematosus (chronic) M32.14
    typhoid fever A01.09
  gonococcal (acute) (chronic) A54.21
  hypocomplementemic — see Nephritis, membranoproliferative
  IgA — see Nephropathy, IgA
  immune complex (circulating) NEC N05.8
  infective — see Nephritis, tubulo-interstitial
  interstitial — see Nephritis, tubulo-interstitial
  lead N14.3
  membranoproliferative (diffuse) (type 1 or 3) — see also N00-N07 with fourth character .5 N05.5
    type 2 — see also N00-N07 with fourth character .6 N05.6
  minimal change N05.0
  necrotic, necrotizing NEC — see also N00-N07 with fourth character .8 N05.8
  nephrotic — see Nephrosis
  nodular — see Nephritis, membranoproliferative
  polycystic Q61.3
    adult type Q61.2
    autosomal
      dominant Q61.2
      recessive NEC Q61.19
    childhood type NEC Q61.19
    infantile type NEC Q61.19
  poststreptococcal N05.9
    acute N00.9
    chronic N03.9
    rapidly progressive N01.9
  proliferative NEC — see also N00-N07 with fourth character .8 N05.8
  purulent — see Nephritis, tubulo-interstitial
  rapidly progressive N01.9
    with
      dense deposit disease N01.6

Nephritis, nephritic — continued
  rapidly progressive — continued
    with — continued
      diffuse
        crescentic glomerulonephritis N01.7
        endocapillary proliferative glomerulonephritis N01.4
        membranous glomerulonephritis N01.2
        mesangial proliferative glomerulonephritis N01.3
        mesangiocapillary glomerulonephritis N01.5
      focal and segmental glomerular lesions N01.1
      minor glomerular abnormality N01.0
      specified morphological changes NEC N01.8
  salt losing or wasting NEC N28.89
  saturnine N14.3
  sclerosing, diffuse N05.8
  septic — see Nephritis, tubulo-interstitial
  specified pathology NEC — see also N00-N07 with fourth character .8 N05.8
  subacute N01.9
  suppurative — see Nephritis, tubulo-interstitial
  syphilitic (late) A52.75
    congenital A50.59 [N08]
    early (secondary) A51.44
  toxic — see Nephropathy, toxic
  tubal, tubular — see Nephritis, tubulo-interstitial
  tuberculous A18.11
  tubulo-interstitial (in) N12
    acute (infectious) N10
    chronic (infectious) N11.9
      nonobstructive N11.8
        reflux-associated N11.0
      obstructive N11.1
      specified NEC N11.8
    due to
      brucellosis A23.9 [N16]
      cryoglobulinemia D89.1 [N16]
      glycogen storage disease E74.00 [N16]
    Sjögren's syndrome M35.04
  vascular — see Hypertension, kidney
  war N00.9
Nephroblastoma (epithelial) (mesenchymal) C64- ☑
Nephrocalcinosis E83.59 [N29]
Nephrocystitis, pustular — see Nephritis, tubulo-interstitial
Nephrolithiasis (congenital) (pelvis) (recurrent) — see also Calculus, kidney
Nephroma C64- ☑
  mesoblastic D41.0- ☑
Nephronephritis — see Nephrosis
Nephronophthisis Q61.5
Nephropathia epidemica A98.5
Nephropathy — see also Nephritis N28.9
  with
    edema — see Nephrosis
    glomerular lesion — see Glomerulonephritis
  amyloid, hereditary E85.0
  analgesic N14.0
    with medullary necrosis, acute N17.2
  Balkan (endemic) N15.0
  chemical — see Nephropathy, toxic
  diabetic — see E08-E13 with .21
  drug-induced N14.2
    specified NEC N14.1
  focal and segmental hyalinosis or sclerosis N02.1
  heavy metal-induced N14.3
  hereditary NEC N07.9
    with
      dense deposit disease N07.6
      diffuse
        crescentic glomerulonephritis N07.7
        endocapillary proliferative glomerulonephrit N07.4
        membranous glomerulonephritis N07.2
        mesangial proliferative glomerulonephritis N07.3
        mesangiocapillary glomerulonephritis N07
      focal and segmental glomerular lesions N07.1
      minor glomerular abnormality N07.0
      specified morphological changes NEC N07.8
  hypercalcemic N25.89
  hypertensive — see Hypertension, kidney
  hypokalemic (vacuolar) N25.89
  IgA N02.8
    with glomerular lesion N02.9
      focal and segmental hyalinosis or sclerosis N02
      membranoproliferative (diffuse) N02.5

☑ Additional Character Required — Refer to the Tabular List for Character Selection   Subterms under main terms may continue to next column or page

Nephropathy — *continued*
  IgA — *continued*
    with glomerular lesion — *continued*
      membranous (diffuse) N02.2
      mesangial proliferative (diffuse) N02.3
      mesangiocapillary (diffuse) N02.5
      proliferative NEC N02.8
      specified pathology NEC N02.8
  lead N14.3
  membranoproliferative (diffuse) N02.5
  membranous (diffuse) N02.2
  mesangial (IgA/IgG) — *see* Nephropathy, IgA
    proliferative (diffuse) N02.3
  mesangiocapillary (diffuse) N02.5
  obstructive N13.8
  phenacetin N17.2
  phosphate-losing N25.0
  potassium depletion N25.89
  pregnancy-related O26.83- ☑
  proliferative NEC — *see also* N00-N07 with fourth
    character .8 N05.8
  protein-losing N25.89
  saturnine N14.3
  sickle-cell D57.- ☑ *[N08]*
  toxic NEC N14.4
    due to
      drugs N14.2
        analgesic N14.0
        specified NEC N14.1
      heavy metals N14.3
  vasomotor N17.0
  water-losing N25.89
Nephroptosis N28.83
Nephropyosis — *see* Abscess, kidney
Nephrorrhagia N28.89
Nephrosclerosis (arteriolar)(arteriosclerotic) (chronic)
  (hyaline) — *see also* Hypertension, kidney
  hyperplastic — *see* Hypertension, kidney
  senile N26.9
Nephrosis, nephrotic (Epstein's) (syndrome) (congenital)
  N04.9
  with
    foot process disease N04.9
    glomerular lesion N04.1
    hypocomplementemic N04.5
  acute N04.9
  anoxic — *see* Nephrosis, tubular
  chemical — *see* Nephrosis, tubular
  cholemic K76.7
  diabetic — *see* E08-E13 with .21
  Finnish type (congenital) Q89.8
  hemoglobin N10
  hemoglobinuric — *see* Nephrosis, tubular
  in
    amyloidosis E85.4 *[N08]*
    diabetes mellitus — *see* E08-E13 with .21
    epidemic hemorrhagic fever A98.5
    malaria (malariae) B52.0
  ischemic — *see* Nephrosis, tubular
  lipoid N04.9
  lower nephron — *see* Nephrosis, tubular
  malarial (malariae) B52.0
  minimal change N04.0
  myoglobin N10
  necrotizing — *see* Nephrosis, tubular
  osmotic (sucrose) N25.89
  radiation N04.9
  syphilitic (late) A52.75
  toxic — *see* Nephrosis, tubular
  tubular (acute) N17.0
    postprocedural N99.0
    radiation N04.9
Nephrosonephritis, hemorrhagic (endemic) A98.5
Nephrostomy
  attention to Z43.6
  status Z93.6
Nerve — *see also* condition
  injury — *see* Injury, nerve, by body site
Nerves R45.0
Nervous — *see also* condition R45.0
  heart F45.8
  stomach F45.8
  tension R45.0
Nervousness R45.0
Nesidioblastoma
  pancreas D13.7
  specified site NEC — *see* Neoplasm, benign, by site
  unspecified site D13.7

Nettleship's syndrome — *see* Urticaria pigmentosa
Neumann's disease or syndrome L10.1
Neuralgia, neuralgic (acute) M79.2
  accessory (nerve) G52.8
  acoustic (nerve) — *see* subcategory H93.3 ☑
  auditory (nerve) — *see* subcategory H93.3 ☑
  ciliary G44.009
    intractable G44.001
    not intractable G44.009
  cranial
    nerve — *see also* Disorder, nerve, cranial
      fifth or trigeminal — *see* Neuralgia, trigeminal
    postherpetic, postzoster B02.29
  ear — *see* subcategory H92.0 ☑
  facialis vera G51.1
  Fothergill's — *see* Neuralgia, trigeminal
  glossopharyngeal (nerve) G52.1
  Horton's G44.009
    intractable G44.001
    not intractable G44.009
  Hunt's B02.21
  hypoglossal (nerve) G52.3
  infraorbital — *see* Neuralgia, trigeminal
  malarial — *see* Malaria
  migrainous G44.009
    intractable G44.001
    not intractable G44.009
  Morton's G57.6- ☑
  nerve, cranial — *see* Disorder, nerve, cranial
  nose G52.0
  occipital M54.81
  olfactory G52.0
  penis N48.9
  perineum R10.2
  postherpetic NEC B02.29
    trigeminal B02.22
  pubic region R10.2
  scrotum R10.2
  Sluder's G44.89
  specified nerve NEC G58.8
  spermatic cord R10.2
  sphenopalatine (ganglion) G90.09
  trifacial — *see* Neuralgia, trigeminal
  trigeminal G50.0
    postherpetic, postzoster B02.22
  vagus (nerve) G52.2
  writer's F48.8
    organic G25.89
Neurapraxia — *see* Injury, nerve
Neurasthenia F48.8
  cardiac F45.8
  gastric F45.8
  heart F45.8
Neurilemmoma — *see also* Neoplasm, nerve, benign
  acoustic (nerve) D33.3
  malignant — *see also* Neoplasm, nerve, malignant
    acoustic (nerve) C72.4- ☑
Neurilemmosarcoma — *see* Neoplasm, nerve, malignant
Neurinoma — *see* Neoplasm, nerve, benign
Neurinomatosis — *see* Neoplasm, nerve, uncertain behavior
Neuritis (rheumatoid) M79.2
  abducens (nerve) — *see* Strabismus, paralytic, sixth
    nerve
  accessory (nerve) G52.8
  acoustic (nerve) — *see also* subcategory H93.3 ☑
    in (due to)
      infectious disease NEC B99 ☑ *[H94.0-]* ☑
      parasitic disease NEC B89 *[H94.0-]* ☑
    syphilitic A52.15
  alcoholic G62.1
    with psychosis — *see* Psychosis, alcoholic
  amyloid, any site E85.4 *[G63]*
  auditory (nerve) — *see* subcategory H93.3 ☑
  brachial — *see* Radiculopathy
    due to displacement, intervertebral disc — *see* Dis-
      order, disc, cervical, with neuritis
  cranial nerve
    due to Lyme disease A69.22
    eighth or acoustic or auditory — *see* subcategory
      H93.3 ☑
    eleventh or accessory G52.8
    fifth or trigeminal G51.0
    first or olfactory G52.0
    fourth or trochlear — *see* Strabismus, paralytic,
      fourth nerve
    second or optic — *see* Neuritis, optic

Neuritis — *continued*
  cranial nerve — *continued*
    seventh or facial G51.8
      newborn (birth injury) P11.3
    sixth or abducent — *see* Strabismus, paralytic, sixth
      nerve
    tenth or vagus G52.2
    third or oculomotor — *see* Strabismus, paralytic,
      third nerve
    twelfth or hypoglossal G52.3
  Déjérine-Sottas G60.0
  diabetic (mononeuropathy) — *see* E08-E13 with .41
    polyneuropathy — *see* E08-E13 with .42
  due to
    beriberi E51.11
    displacement, prolapse or rupture, intervertebral
      disc — *see* Disorder, disc, with, radiculopathy
    herniation, nucleus pulposus M51.9 *[G55]*
  endemic E51.11
  facial G51.8
    newborn (birth injury) P11.3
  general — *see* Polyneuropathy
  geniculate ganglion G51.1
    due to herpes (zoster) B02.21
  gouty — *see also* Gout, by type M10.9 *[G63]*
  hypoglossal (nerve) G52.3
  ilioinguinal (nerve) G57.9- ☑
  infectious (multiple) NEC G61.0
  interstitial hypertrophic progressive G60.0
  lumbar M54.16
  lumbosacral M54.17
  multiple — *see also* Polyneuropathy
    endemic E51.11
    infective, acute G61.0
  multiplex endemica E51.11
  nerve root — *see* Radiculopathy
  oculomotor (nerve) — *see* Strabismus, paralytic, third
    nerve
  olfactory nerve G52.0
  optic (nerve) (hereditary) (sympathetic) H46.9
    with demyelination G36.0
    in myelitis G36.0
    nutritional H46.2
    papillitis — *see* Papillitis, optic
    retrobulbar H46.1- ☑
    specified type NEC H46.8
    toxic H46.3
  peripheral (nerve) G62.9
    multiple — *see* Polyneuropathy
    single — *see* Mononeuritis
  pneumogastric (nerve) G52.2
  postherpetic, postzoster B02.29
  progressive hypertrophic interstitial G60.0
  retrobulbar — *see also* Neuritis, optic, retrobulbar
    in (due to)
      late syphilis A52.15
      meningococcal infection A39.82
    meningococcal A39.82
    syphilitic A52.15
  sciatic (nerve) — *see also* Sciatica
    due to displacement of intervertebral disc — *see*
      Disorder, disc, with, radiculopathy
  serum — *see also* Reaction, serum T80.69 ☑
  shoulder-girdle G54.5
  specified nerve NEC G58.8
  spinal (nerve) root — *see* Radiculopathy
  syphilitic A52.15
  thenar (median) G56.1- ☑
  thoracic M54.14
  toxic NEC G62.2
  trochlear (nerve) — *see* Strabismus, paralytic, fourth
    nerve
  vagus (nerve) G52.2
Neuroastrocytoma — *see* Neoplasm, uncertain behavior,
  by site
Neuroavitaminosis E56.9 *[G99.8]*
Neuroblastoma
  olfactory C30.0
  specified site — *see* Neoplasm, malignant, by site
  unspecified site C74.90
Neurochorioretinitis — *see* Chorioretinitis
Neurocirculatory asthenia F45.8
Neurocysticercosis B69.0
Neurocytoma — *see* Neoplasm, benign, by site
Neurodermatitis (circumscribed) (circumscripta) (local)
  L20.0
  atopic L20.81
  diffuse (Brocq) L20.81

◄ Subterms under main terms may continue to next column or page   ☑ Additional Character Required — Refer to the Tabular List for Character Selection   231

Nephropathy — Neurodermatitis

Neurodermatitis — *continued*
  disseminated L20.81
Neuroencephalomyelopathy, optic G36.0
Neuroepithelioma — *see also* Neoplasm, malignant, by site
  olfactory C30.0
Neurofibroma — *see also* Neoplasm, nerve, benign
  melanotic — *see* Neoplasm, nerve, benign
  multiple — *see* Neurofibromatosis
  plexiform — *see* Neoplasm, nerve, benign
Neurofibromatosis (multiple) (nonmalignant) Q85.00
  acoustic Q85.02
  malignant — *see* Neoplasm, nerve, malignant
  specified NEC Q85.09
  type 1 (von Recklinghausen) Q85.01
  type 2 Q85.02
Neurofibrosarcoma — *see* Neoplasm, nerve, malignant
Neurogenic — *see also* condition
  bladder — *see also* Dysfunction, bladder, neuromuscular N31.9
    cauda equina syndrome G83.4
  bowel NEC K59.2
  heart F45.8
Neuroglioma — *see* Neoplasm, uncertain behavior, by site
Neurolabyrinthitis (of Dix and Hallpike) — *see* Neuronitis, vestibular
Neurolathyrism — *see* Poisoning, food, noxious, plant
Neuroleprosy A30.9
Neuroma — *see also* Neoplasm, nerve, benign
  acoustic (nerve) D33.3
  amputation (stump) (traumatic) (surgical complication) (late) T87.3- ☑
    arm T87.3- ☑
    leg T87.3- ☑
  digital (toe) G57.6- ☑
  interdigital G58.8
    lower limb (toe) G57.8- ☑
    upper limb G56.8- ☑
  intermetatarsal G57.8- ☑
  Morton's G57.6- ☑
  nonneoplastic
    arm G56.9- ☑
    leg G57.9- ☑
    lower extremity G57.9- ☑
    upper extremity G56.9- ☑
  optic (nerve) D33.3
  plantar G57.6- ☑
  plexiform — *see* Neoplasm, nerve, benign
  surgical (nonneoplastic)
    arm G56.9- ☑
    leg G57.9- ☑
    lower extremity G57.9- ☑
    upper extremity G56.9- ☑
Neuromyalgia — *see* Neuralgia
Neuromyasthenia (epidemic) (postinfectious) G93.3
Neuromyelitis G36.9
  ascending G61.0
  optica G36.0
Neuromyopathy G70.9
  paraneoplastic D49.9 [G13.0]
Neuromyotonia (Isaacs) G71.19
Neuronevus — *see* Nevus
Neuronitis G58.9
  ascending (acute) G57.2- ☑
  vestibular H81.2- ☑
Neuroparalytic — *see* condition
Neuropathy, neuropathic G62.9
  acute motor G62.81
  alcoholic G62.1
    with psychosis — *see* Psychosis, alcoholic
  arm G56.9- ☑
  autonomic, peripheral — *see* Neuropathy, peripheral, autonomic
  axillary G56.9- ☑
  bladder N31.9
    atonic (motor) (sensory) N31.2
    autonomous N31.2
    flaccid N31.2
    nonreflex N31.2
    reflex N31.1
    uninhibited N31.0
  brachial plexus G54.0
  cervical plexus G54.2
  chronic
    progressive segmentally demyelinating G62.89
    relapsing demyelinating G62.89

Neuropathy, neuropathic — *continued*
  Déjérine-Sottas G60.0
  diabetic — *see* E08-E13 with .40
    mononeuropathy — *see* E08-E13 with .41
    polyneuropathy — *see* E08-E13 with .42
  entrapment G58.9
    iliohypogastric nerve G57.8- ☑
    ilioinguinal nerve G57.8- ☑
    lateral cutaneous nerve of thigh G57.1- ☑
    median nerve G56.0- ☑
    obturator nerve G57.8- ☑
    peroneal nerve G57.3- ☑
    posterior tibial nerve G57.5- ☑
    saphenous nerve G57.8- ☑
    ulnar nerve G56.2- ☑
  facial nerve G51.9
  hereditary G60.9
    motor and sensory (types I-IV) G60.0
    sensory G60.8
    specified NEC G60.8
  hypertrophic G60.0
    Charcot-Marie-Tooth G60.0
    Déjérine-Sottas G60.0
    interstitial progressive G60.0
    of infancy G60.0
    Refsum G60.1
  idiopathic G60.9
    progressive G60.3
    specified NEC G60.8
  in association with hereditary ataxia G60.2
  intercostal G58.0
  ischemic — *see* Disorder, nerve
  Jamaica (ginger) G62.2
  leg NEC G57.9- ☑
  lower extremity G57.9- ☑
  lumbar plexus G54.1
  median nerve G56.1- ☑
  motor and sensory — *see also* Polyneuropathy
    hereditary (types I-IV) G60.0
  multifocal motor (MMN) G61.82
  multiple (acute) (chronic) — *see* Polyneuropathy
  optic (nerve) — *see also* Neuritis, optic
    ischemic H47.01- ☑
  paraneoplastic (sensorial) (Denny Brown) D49.9 [G13.0]
  peripheral (nerve) — *see also* Polyneuropathy G62.9
    autonomic G90.9
      idiopathic G90.09
      in (due to)
        amyloidosis E85.4 [G99.0]
        diabetes mellitus — *see* E08-E13 with .43
        endocrine disease NEC E34.9 [G99.0]
        gout M10.00 [G99.0]
        hyperthyroidism E05.90 [G99.0]
          with thyroid storm E05.91 [G99.0]
        metabolic disease NEC E88.9 [G99.0]
    idiopathic G60.9
      progressive G60.3
    in (due to)
      antitetanus serum G62.0
      arsenic G62.2
      drugs NEC G62.0
      lead G62.2
      organophosphate compounds G62.2
      toxic agent NEC G62.2
  plantar nerves G57.6- ☑
  progressive
    hypertrophic interstitial G60.0
    inflammatory G62.81
  radicular NEC — *see* Radiculopathy
  sacral plexus G54.1
  sciatic G57.0- ☑
  serum G61.1
  toxic NEC G62.2
  trigeminal sensory G50.8
  ulnar nerve G56.2- ☑
  uremic N18.9 [G63]
  vitamin B12 E53.8 [G63]
    with anemia (pernicious) D51.0 [G63]
    due to dietary deficiency D51.3 [G63]
Neurophthisis — *see also* Disorder, nerve
  peripheral, diabetic — *see* E08-E13 with .42
Neuroretinitis — *see* Chorioretinitis
Neuroretinopathy, hereditary optic H47.22
Neurosarcoma — *see* Neoplasm, nerve, malignant
Neurosclerosis — *see* Disorder, nerve
Neurosis, neurotic F48.9
  anankastic F42.8

Neurosis, neurotic — *continued*
  anxiety (state) F41.1
    panic type F41.0
  asthenic F48.8
  bladder F45.8
  cardiac (reflex) F45.8
  cardiovascular F45.8
  character F60.9
  colon F45.8
  compensation F68.10
  compulsive, compulsion F42.8
  conversion F44.9
  craft F48.8
  cutaneous F45.8
  depersonalization F48.1
  depressive (reaction) (type) F34.1
  environmental F48.8
  excoriation L98.1
  fatigue F48.8
  functional — *see* Disorder, somatoform
  gastric F45.8
  gastrointestinal F45.8
  heart F45.8
  hypochondriacal F45.21
  hysterical F44.9
  incoordination F45.8
    larynx F45.8
    vocal cord F45.8
  intestine F45.8
  larynx (sensory) F45.8
    hysterical F44.4
  mixed NEC F48.8
  musculoskeletal F45.8
  obsessional F42.8
  obsessive-compulsive F42.8
  occupational F48.8
  ocular NEC F45.8
  organ — *see* Disorder, somatoform
  pharynx F45.8
  phobic F40.9
  posttraumatic (situational) F43.10
    acute F43.11
    chronic F43.12
  psychasthenic (type) F48.8
  railroad F48.8
  rectum F45.8
  respiratory F45.8
  rumination F45.8
  sexual F65.9
  situational F48.8
  social F40.10
    generalized F40.11
  specified type NEC F48.8
  state F48.9
    with depersonalization episode F48.1
  stomach F45.8
  traumatic F43.10
    acute F43.11
    chronic F43.12
  vasomotor F45.8
  visceral F45.8
  war F48.8
Neurospongioblastosis diffusa Q85.1
Neurosyphilis (arrested) (early) (gumma) (late) (latent) (recurrent) (relapse) A52.3
  with ataxia (cerebellar) (locomotor) (spastic) (spinal) A52.19
  aneurysm (cerebral) A52.05
  arachnoid (adhesive) A52.13
  arteritis (any artery) (cerebral) A52.04
  asymptomatic A52.2
  congenital A50.40
  dura (mater) A52.13
  general paresis A52.17
  hemorrhagic A52.05
  juvenile (asymptomatic) (meningeal) A50.40
  leptomeninges (aseptic) A52.13
  meningeal, meninges (adhesive) A52.13
  meningitis A52.13
  meningovascular (diffuse) A52.13
  optic atrophy A52.15
  parenchymatous (degenerative) A52.19
  paresis, paretic A52.17
    juvenile A50.45
  remission in (sustained) A52.3
  serological (without symptoms) A52.2
  specified nature or site NEC A52.19
  tabes, tabetic (dorsalis) A52.11
    juvenile A50.45

☑ **Additional Character Required — Refer to the Tabular List for Character Selection**   ▽ Subterms under main terms may continue to next column or page

Neurosyphilis — *continued*
  taboparesis A52.17
    juvenile A50.45
  thrombosis (cerebral) A52.05
  vascular (cerebral) NEC A52.05
Neurothekeoma — *see* Neoplasm, nerve, benign
Neurotic — *see* Neurosis
Neurotoxemia — *see* Toxemia
Neutroclusion M26.211
Neutropenia, neutropenic (chronic) (genetic) (idiopathic) (immune) (infantile) (malignant) (pernicious) (splenic) D70.9
  congenital (primary) D70.0
  cyclic D70.4
  cytoreductive cancer chemotherapy sequela D70.1
  drug-induced D70.2
    due to cytoreductive cancer chemotherapy D70.1
  due to infection D70.3
  fever D70.9
  neonatal, transitory (isoimmune) (maternal transfer) P61.5
  periodic D70.4
  secondary (cyclic) (periodic) (splenic) D70.4
    drug-induced D70.2
      due to cytoreductive cancer chemotherapy D70.1
  toxic D70.8
Neutrophilia, hereditary giant D72.0
Nevocarcinoma — *see* Melanoma
Nevus D22.9
  achromic — *see* Neoplasm, skin, benign
  amelanotic — *see* Neoplasm, skin, benign
  angiomatous D18.00
    intra-abdominal D18.03
    intracranial D18.02
    skin D18.01
    specified site NEC D18.09
  araneus I78.1
  balloon cell — *see* Neoplasm, skin, benign
  bathing trunk D48.5
  blue — *see* Neoplasm, skin, benign
    cellular — *see* Neoplasm, skin, benign
    giant — *see* Neoplasm, skin, benign
    Jadassohn's — *see* Neoplasm, skin, benign
    malignant — *see* Melanoma
  capillary D18.00
    intra-abdominal D18.03
    intracranial D18.02
    skin D18.01
    specified site NEC D18.09
  cavernous D18.00
    intra-abdominal D18.03
    intracranial D18.02
    skin D18.01
    specified site NEC D18.09
  cellular — *see* Neoplasm, skin, benign
    blue — *see* Neoplasm, skin, benign
  choroid D31.3- ☑
  comedonicus Q82.5
  conjunctiva D31.0- ☑
  dermal — *see* Neoplasm, skin, benign
    with epidermal nevus — *see* Neoplasm, skin, benign
  dysplastic — *see* Neoplasm, skin, benign
  eye D31.9- ☑
  flammeus Q82.5
  hemangiomatous D18.00
    intra-abdominal D18.03
    intracranial D18.02
    skin D18.01
    specified site NEC D18.09
  iris D31.4- ☑
  lacrimal gland D31.5- ☑
  lymphatic D18.1
  magnocellular
    specified site — *see* Neoplasm, benign, by site
    unspecified site D31.40
  malignant — *see* Melanoma
  meaning hemangioma D18.00
    intra-abdominal D18.03
    intracranial D18.02
    skin D18.01
    specified site NEC D18.09
  mouth (mucosa) D10.30
    specified site NEC D10.39
    white sponge Q38.6
  multiplex Q85.1
  non neoplastic I78.1
  oral mucosa D10.30
    specified site NEC D10.39

Nevus — *continued*
  oral mucosa — *continued*
    white sponge Q38.6
  orbit D31.6- ☑
  pigmented
    giant — *see also* Neoplasm, skin, uncertain behavior D48.5
      malignant melanoma in — *see* Melanoma
  portwine Q82.5
  retina D31.2- ☑
  retrobulbar D31.6- ☑
  sanguineous Q82.5
  senile I78.1
  skin D22.9
    abdominal wall D22.5
    ala nasi D22.39
    ankle D22.7- ☑
    anus, anal D22.5
    arm D22.6- ☑
    auditory canal (external) D22.2- ☑
    auricle (ear) D22.2- ☑
    auricular canal (external) D22.2- ☑
    axilla, axillary fold D22.5
    back D22.5
    breast D22.5
    brow D22.39
    buttock D22.5
    canthus (eye) D22.1- ☑
    cheek (external) D22.39
    chest wall D22.5
    chin D22.39
    ear (external) D22.2- ☑
    external meatus (ear) D22.2- ☑
    eyebrow D22.39
    eyelid (lower) (upper) D22.1- ☑
    face D22.30
      specified NEC D22.39
    female genital organ (external) NEC D28.0
    finger D22.6- ☑
    flank D22.5
    foot D22.7- ☑
    forearm D22.6- ☑
    forehead D22.39
    foreskin D29.0
    genital organ (external) NEC
      female D28.0
      male D29.9
    gluteal region D22.5
    groin D22.5
    hand D22.6- ☑
    heel D22.7- ☑
    helix D22.2- ☑
    hip D22.7- ☑
    interscapular region D22.5
    jaw D22.39
    knee D22.7- ☑
    labium (majus) (minus) D28.0
    leg D22.7- ☑
    lip (lower) (upper) D22.0
    lower limb D22.7- ☑
    male genital organ (external) D29.9
    nail D22.9
      finger D22.6- ☑
      toe D22.7- ☑
    nasolabial groove D22.39
    nates D22.5
    neck D22.4
    nose (external) D22.39
    palpebra D22.1- ☑
    penis D29.0
    perianal skin D22.5
    perineum D22.5
    pinna D22.2- ☑
    popliteal fossa or space D22.7- ☑
    prepuce D29.0
    pudendum D28.0
    scalp D22.4
    scrotum D29.4
    shoulder D22.6- ☑
    submammary fold D22.5
    temple D22.39
    thigh D22.7- ☑
    toe D22.7- ☑
    trunk NEC D22.5
    umbilicus D22.5
    upper limb D22.6- ☑
    vulva D28.0

Nevus — *continued*
  specified site NEC — *see* Neoplasm, by site, benign
  spider I78.1
  stellar I78.1
  strawberry Q82.5
  Sutton's benign D22.9
  unius lateris Q82.5
  Unna's Q82.5
  vascular Q82.5
  verrucous Q82.5
Newborn (infant) (liveborn) (singleton) Z38.2
  abstinence syndrome P96.1
  acne L70.4
  affected by
    abnormalities of membranes P02.9
      specified NEC P02.8
    abruptio placenta P02.1
    amino-acid metabolic disorder, transitory P74.8
    amniocentesis (while in utero) P00.6
    amnionitis P02.78
    apparent life threatening event (ALTE) R68.13
    bleeding (into)
      cerebral cortex P52.22
      germinal matrix P52.0
      ventricles P52.1
    breech delivery P03.0
    cardiac arrest P29.81
    cardiomyopathy I42.8
      congenital I42.4
    cerebral ischemia P91.0
    Cesarean delivery P03.4
    chemotherapy agents P04.11
    chorioamnionitis P02.78
    cocaine (crack) P04.41
    complications of labor and delivery P03.9
      specified NEC P03.89
    compression of umbilical cord NEC P02.5
    contracted pelvis P03.1
    cyanosis P28.2
    delivery P03.9
      Cesarean P03.4
      forceps P03.2
      vacuum extractor P03.3
    drugs of addiction P04.40
      cocaine P04.41
      hallucinogens P04.42
      specified drug NEC P04.49
    entanglement (knot) in umbilical cord P02.5
    environmental chemicals P04.6
    fetal (intrauterine)
      growth retardation P05.9
      inflammatory response syndrome (FIRS) P02.70
      malnutrition not light or small for gestational age P05.2
    FIRS (fetal inflammatory response syndrome) P02.70
    forceps delivery P03.2
    heart rate abnormalities
      bradycardia P29.12
      intrauterine P03.819
        before onset of labor P03.810
        during labor P03.811
      tachycardia P29.11
    hemorrhage (antepartum) P02.1
      cerebellar (nontraumatic) P52.6
      intracerebral (nontraumatic) P52.4
      intracranial (nontraumatic) P52.9
        specified NEC P52.8
      intraventricular (nontraumatic) P52.3
        grade 1 P52.0
        grade 2 P52.1
        grade 3 P52.21
        grade 4 P52.22
      posterior fossa (nontraumatic) P52.6
      subarachnoid (nontraumatic) P52.5
      subependymal P52.0
        with intracerebral extension P52.22
        with intraventricular extension P52.1
          with enlargment of ventricles P52.21
          without intraventricular extension P52.0
    hypoxic ischemic encephalopathy [HIE] P91.60
      mild P91.61
      moderate P91.62
      severe P91.63
    induction of labor P03.89
    intestinal perforation P78.0
    intrauterine (fetal) blood loss P50.9
      due to (from)
        cut end of co-twin cord P50.5

↳ **Subterms under main terms may continue to next column or page**   ☑ **Additional Character Required — Refer to the Tabular List for Character Selection**   **233**

Neurosyphilis — Newborn

Newborn — *continued*
affected by — *continued*
  intrauterine blood loss — *continued*
    due to — *continued*
      hemorrhage into
        co-twin P50.3
          maternal circulation P50.4
        placenta P50.2
        ruptured cord blood P50.1
        vasa previa P50.0
      specified NEC P50.8
  intrauterine (fetal) hemorrhage P50.9
  intrauterine (in utero) procedure P96.5
  malpresentation (malposition) NEC P03.1
  maternal (complication of) (use of)
    alcohol P04.3
    amphetamines P04.16
    analgesia (maternal) P04.0
    anesthesia (maternal) P04.0
    anticonvulsants P04.13
    antidepressants P04.15
    antineoplastic chemotherapy P04.11
    anxiolytics P04.1A
    blood loss P02.1
    cannabis P04.81
    circulatory disease P00.3
    condition P00.9
      specified NEC P00.89
    cytotoxic drugs P04.12
    delivery P03.9
      Cesarean P03.4
      forceps P03.2
      vacuum extractor P03.3
    diabetes mellitus (pre-existing) P70.1
    disorder P00.9
      specified NEC P00.89
    drugs (addictive) (illegal) NEC P04.49
    ectopic pregnancy P01.4
    gestational diabetes P70.0
    hemorrhage P02.1
    hypertensive disorder P00.0
    incompetent cervix P01.0
    infectious disease P00.2
    injury P00.5
    labor and delivery P03.9
    malpresentation before labor P01.7
    maternal death P01.6
    medical procedure P00.7
    medication P04.19
      specified type NEC P04.18
    multiple pregnancy P01.5
    nutritional disorder P00.4
    oligohydramnios P01.2
    opiates P04.14
      administered for procedures during pregnancy or labor and delivery P04.0
    parasitic disease P00.2
    periodontal disease P00.81
    placenta previa P02.0
    polyhydramnios P01.3
    precipitate delivery P03.5
    pregnancy P01.9
      specified P01.8
    premature rupture of membranes P01.1
    renal disease P00.1
    respiratory disease P00.3
    sedative-hypnotics P04.17
    surgical procedure P00.6
    tranquilizers administered for procedures during pregnancy or labor and delivery P04.0
    urinary tract disease P00.1
    uterine contraction (abnormal) P03.6
  meconium peritonitis P78.0
  medication (legal) (maternal use) (prescribed) P04.19
  membrane abnormalities P02.9
    specified NEC P02.8
  membranitis P02.78
  methamphetamine(s) P04.49
  mixed metabolic and respiratory acidosis P84
  neonatal abstinence syndrome P96.1
  noxious substances transmitted via placenta or breast milk P04.9
    cannabis P04.81
    specified NEC P04.89
  nutritional supplements P04.5
  placenta previa P02.0
  placental
    abnormality (functional) (morphological) P02.20

Newborn — *continued*
affected by — *continued*
  placental — *continued*
    abnormality — *continued*
      specified NEC P02.29
    dysfunction P02.29
    infarction P02.29
    insufficiency P02.29
    separation NEC P02.1
    transfusion syndromes P02.3
  placentitis P02.78
  precipitate delivery P03.5
  prolapsed cord P02.4
  respiratory arrest P28.81
  slow intrauterine growth P05.9
  tobacco P04.2
  twin to twin transplacental transfusion P02.3
  umbilical cord (tightly) around neck P02.5
  umbilical cord condition P02.60
    short cord P02.69
    specified NEC P02.69
  uterine contractions (abnormal) P03.6
  vasa previa P02.69
    from intrauterine blood loss P50.0
apnea P28.4
  obstructive P28.4
  primary P28.3
  sleep (central) (obstructive) (primary) P28.3
born in hospital Z38.00
  by cesarean Z38.01
born outside hospital Z38.1
breast buds P96.89
breast engorgement P83.4
check-up — *see* Newborn, examination
convulsion P90
dehydration P74.1
examination
  8 to 28 days old Z00.111
  under 8 days old Z00.110
fever P81.9
  environmentally-induced P81.0
hyperbilirubinemia P59.9
  of prematurity P59.0
hypernatremia P74.21
hyponatremia P74.22
infection P39.9
  candidal P37.5
  specified NEC P39.8
  urinary tract P39.3
jaundice P59.9
  due to
    breast milk inhibitor P59.3
    hepatocellular damage P59.20
      specified NEC P59.29
    preterm delivery P59.0
  of prematurity P59.0
  specified NEC P59.8
late metabolic acidosis P74.0
mastitis P39.0
  infective P39.0
  noninfective P83.4
multiple born NEC Z38.8
  born in hospital Z38.68
    by cesarean Z38.69
  born outside hospital Z38.7
omphalitis P38.9
  with mild hemorrhage P38.1
  without hemorrhage P38.9
post-term P08.21
prolonged gestation (over 42 completed weeks) P08.22
quadruplet Z38.8
  born in hospital Z38.63
    by cesarean Z38.64
  born outside hospital Z38.7
quintuplet Z38.8
  born in hospital Z38.65
    by cesarean Z38.66
  born outside hospital Z38.7
seizure P90
sepsis (congenital) P36.9
  due to
    anaerobes NEC P36.5
    Escherichia coli P36.4
    Staphylococcus P36.30
      aureus P36.2
      specified NEC P36.39
    Streptococcus P36.10
      group B P36.0
      specified NEC P36.19

Newborn — *continued*
sepsis — *continued*
  specified NEC P36.8
triplet Z38.8
  born in hospital Z38.61
    by cesarean Z38.62
  born outside hospital Z38.7
twin Z38.5
  born in hospital Z38.30
    by cesarean Z38.31
  born outside hospital Z38.4
vomiting P92.09
  bilious P92.01
weight check Z00.111
Newcastle conjunctivitis or disease B30.8
Nezelof's syndrome (pure alymphocytosis) D81.4
Niacin (amide) **deficiency** E52
Nicolas (-Durand)-**Favre disease** A55
Nicotine — *see* Tobacco
Nicotinic acid deficiency E52
Niemann-Pick disease or syndrome E75.249
  specified NEC E75.248
  type
    A E75.240
    B E75.241
    C E75.242
    D E75.243
Night
  blindness — *see* Blindness, night
  sweats R61
  terrors (child) F51.4
Nightmares (REM sleep type) F51.5
NIHSS (National Institutes of Health Stroke Scale) **score** R29.7- ☑
Nipple — *see* condition
Nisbet's chancre A57
Nishimoto (-Takeuchi) **disease** I67.5
Nitritoid crisis or reaction — *see* Crisis, nitritoid
Nitrosohemoglobinemia D74.8
Njovera A65
Nocardiosis, nocardiasis A43.9
  cutaneous A43.1
  lung A43.0
  pneumonia A43.0
  pulmonary A43.0
  specified site NEC A43.8
Nocturia R35.1
  psychogenic F45.8
Nocturnal — *see* condition
Nodal rhythm I49.8
Node(s) — *see also* Nodule
  Bouchard's (with arthropathy) M15.2
  Haygarth's M15.8
  Heberden's (with arthropathy) M15.1
  larynx J38.7
  lymph — *see* condition
  milker's B08.03
  Osler's I33.0
  Schmorl's — *see* Schmorl's disease
  singer's J38.2
  teacher's J38.2
  tuberculous — *see* Tuberculosis, lymph gland
  vocal cord J38.2
Nodule(s), nodular
  actinomycotic — *see* Actinomycosis
  breast NEC — *see also* Lump, breast N63.0
  colloid (cystic), thyroid E04.1
  cutaneous — *see* Swelling, localized
  endometrial (stromal) D26.1
  Haygarth's M15.8
  inflammatory — *see* Inflammation
  juxta-articular
    syphilitic A52.77
    yaws A66.7
  larynx J38.7
  lung, solitary (subsegmental branch of the bronchial tree) R91.1
    multiple R91.8
  milker's B08.03
  prostate N40.2
    with lower urinary tract symptoms (LUTS) N40.3
    without lower urinary tract symtpoms (LUTS) N40
  pulmonary, solitary (subsegmental branch of the bronchial tree) R91.1
  retrocardiac R09.89
  rheumatoid M06.30
    ankle M06.37- ☑
    elbow M06.32- ☑

☑ Additional Character Required — Refer to the Tabular List for Character Selection   ▽ Subterms under main terms may continue to next column or page

odule(s), nodular — *continued*
  rheumatoid — *continued*
    foot joint M06.37- ☑
    hand joint M06.34- ☑
    hip M06.35- ☑
    knee M06.36- ☑
    multiple site M06.39
    shoulder M06.31- ☑
    vertebra M06.38
    wrist M06.33- ☑
  scrotum (inflammatory) N49.2
  singer's J38.2
  solitary, lung (subsegmental branch of the bronchial tree) R91.1
    multiple R91.8
  subcutaneous — *see* Swelling, localized
  teacher's J38.2
  thyroid (cold) (gland) (nontoxic) E04.1
    with thyrotoxicosis E05.20
      with thyroid storm E05.21
    toxic or with hyperthyroidism E05.20
      with thyroid storm E05.21
  vocal cord J38.2
oma (gangrenous) (hospital) (infective) A69.0
  auricle I96
  mouth A69.0
  pudendi N76.89
  vulvae N76.89
omad, nomadism Z59.0
OMID (neonatal onset multisystemic inflammatory disorder) M04.2
onadherence to medical treatment Z91.19
onautoimmune hemolytic anemia D59.4
  drug-induced D59.2
onclosure — *see also* Imperfect, closure
  ductus arteriosus (Botallo's) Q25.0
  foramen
    botalli Q21.1
    ovale Q21.1
oncompliance Z91.19
  with
    dialysis Z91.15
    dietary regimen Z91.11
    medical treatment Z91.19
    medication regimen NEC Z91.14
      underdosing — *see also* Table of Drugs and Chemicals, categories T36-T50, with final character 6 Z91.14
        intentional NEC Z91.128
          due to financial hardship of patient Z91.120
        unintentional NEC Z91.138
          due to patient's age related debility Z91.130
    renal dialysis Z91.15
ondescent (congenital) — *see also* Malposition, congenital
  cecum Q43.3
  colon Q43.3
  testicle Q53.9
    bilateral Q53.20
      abdominal Q53.211
      perineal Q53.22
    unilateral Q53.10
      abdominal Q53.111
      perineal Q53.12
ondevelopment
  brain Q02
    part of Q04.3
  heart Q24.8
  organ or site, congenital NEC — *see* Hypoplasia
onengagement
  head NEC O32.4 ☑
    in labor, causing obstructed labor O64.8 ☑
onexanthematous tick fever A93.2
onexpansion, lung (newborn) P28.0
onfunctioning
  cystic duct — *see also* Disease, gallbladder K82.8
  gallbladder — *see also* Disease, gallbladder K82.8
  kidney N28.9
  labyrinth — *see* subcategory H83.2 ☑
on-Hodgkin lymphoma NEC — *see* Lymphoma, non-Hodgkin
onimplantation, ovum N97.2
oninsufflation, fallopian tube N97.1
on-ketotic hyperglycinemia E72.51
onne-Milroy syndrome Q82.0
onovulation N97.0

Non-palpable testicle(s)
  bilateral R39.84
  unilateral R39.83
Nonpatent fallopian tube N97.1
Nonpneumatization, lung NEC P28.0
Nonrotation — *see* Malrotation
Nonsecretion, urine — *see* Anuria
Nonunion
  fracture — *see* Fracture, by site
  joint, following fusion or arthrodesis M96.0
  organ or site, congenital NEC — *see* Imperfect, closure
  symphysis pubis, congenital Q74.2
Nonvisualization, gallbladder R93.2
Nonvital, nonvitalized tooth K04.99
Non-working side interference M26.56
Noonan's syndrome Q87.19
Normocytic anemia (infectional) due to blood loss (chronic) D50.0
  acute D62
Norrie's disease (congenital) Q15.8
North American blastomycosis B40.9
Norwegian itch B86
Nose, nasal — *see* condition
Nosebleed R04.0
Nose-picking F98.8
Nosomania F45.21
Nosophobia F45.22
Nostalgia F43.20
Notch of iris Q13.2
Notching nose, congenital (tip) Q30.2
Nothnagel's
  syndrome — *see* Strabismus, paralytic, third nerve
  vasomotor acroparesthesia I73.89
Novy's relapsing fever A68.9
  louse-borne A68.0
  tick-borne A68.1
Noxious
  foodstuffs, poisoning by — *see* Poisoning, food, noxious, plant
  substances transmitted through placenta or breast milk P04.9
Nucleus pulposus — *see* condition
Numbness R20.0
Nuns' knee — *see* Bursitis, prepatellar
Nursemaid's elbow S53.03- ☑
Nutcracker esophagus K22.4
Nutmeg liver K76.1
Nutrient element deficiency E61.9
  specified NEC E61.8
Nutrition deficient or insufficient — *see also* Malnutrition E46
  due to
    insufficient food T73.0 ☑
    lack of
      care (child) T76.02 ☑
        adult T76.01 ☑
      food T73.0 ☑
Nutritional stunting E45
Nyctalopia (night blindness) — *see* Blindness, night
Nycturia R35.1
  psychogenic F45.8
Nymphomania F52.8
Nystagmus H55.00
  benign paroxysmal — *see* Vertigo, benign paroxysmal
  central positional H81.4
  congenital H55.01
  dissociated H55.04
  latent H55.02
  miners' H55.09
  positional
    benign paroxysmal H81.4
    central H81.4
  specified form NEC H55.09
  visual deprivation H55.03

O

Obermeyer's relapsing fever (European) A68.0
Obesity E66.9
  with alveolar hypoventilation E66.2
  adrenal E27.8
  complicating
    childbirth O99.214
    pregnancy O99.21- ☑
    puerperium O99.215
  constitutional E66.8
  dietary counseling and surveillance Z71.3

Obesity — *continued*
  drug-induced E66.1
  due to
    drug E66.1
    excess calories E66.09
      morbid E66.01
      severe E66.01
  endocrine E66.8
  endogenous E66.8
  exogenous E66.09
  familial E66.8
  glandular E66.8
  hypothyroid — *see* Hypothyroidism
  hypoventilation syndrome (OHS) E66.2
  morbid E66.01
    with
      alveolar hypoventilation E66.2
      obesity hypoventilation syndrome (OHS) E66.2
    due to excess calories E66.01
  nutritional E66.09
  pituitary E23.6
  severe E66.01
  specified type NEC E66.8
Oblique — *see* condition
Obliteration
  appendix (lumen) K38.8
  artery I77.1
  bile duct (noncalculous) K83.1
  common duct (noncalculous) K83.1
  cystic duct — *see* Obstruction, gallbladder
  disease, arteriolar I77.1
  endometrium N85.8
  eye, anterior chamber — *see* Disorder, globe, hypotony
  fallopian tube N97.1
  lymphatic vessel I89.0
    due to mastectomy I97.2
  organ or site, congenital NEC — *see* Atresia, by site
  ureter N13.5
    with infection N13.6
  urethra — *see* Stricture, urethra
  vein I87.8
  vestibule (oral) K08.89
Observation (following) (for) (without need for further medical care) Z04.9
  accident NEC Z04.3
    at work Z04.2
    transport Z04.1
  adverse effect of drug Z03.6
  alleged rape or sexual assault (victim), ruled out
    adult Z04.41
    child Z04.42
  criminal assault Z04.89
  development state
    adolescent Z00.3
    period of rapid growth in childhood Z00.2
    puberty Z00.3
  disease, specified NEC Z03.89
  following work accident Z04.2
  forced sexual exploitation Z04.81
  forced labor exploitation Z04.82
  growth and development state — *see* Observation, development state
  injuries (accidental) NEC — *see also* Observation, accident
  newborn (for)
    suspected condition, related to exposure from the mother or birth process — *see* Newborn, affected by, maternal
    ruled out Z05.9
      cardiac Z05.0
      connective tissue Z05.73
      gastrointestinal Z05.5
      genetic Z05.41
      genitourinary Z05.6
      immunologic Z05.43
      infectious Z05.1
      metabolic Z05.42
      musculoskeletal Z05.72
      neurological Z05.2
      respiratory Z05.3
      skin and subcutaneous tissue Z05.71
      specified condition NEC Z05.8
  postpartum
    immediately after delivery Z39.0
    routine follow-up Z39.2
  pregnancy (normal) (without complication) Z34.9- ☑
    high risk O09.9- ☑
  suicide attempt, alleged NEC Z03.89

Nodule — Observation

Subterms under main terms may continue to next column or page   ☑ Additional Character Required — Refer to the Tabular List for Character Selection   235

Observation — *continued*
  suicide attempt, alleged — *continued*
    self-poisoning Z03.6
  suspected, ruled out — *see also* Suspected condition, ruled out
    abuse, physical
      adult Z04.71
      child Z04.72
    accident at work Z04.2
    adult battering victim Z04.71
    child battering victim Z04.72
    condition NEC Z03.89
      newborn — *see also* Observation, newborn (for), suspected condition, ruled out Z05.9
    drug poisoning or adverse effect Z03.6
    exposure (to)
      anthrax Z03.810
      biological agent NEC Z03.818
    inflicted injury NEC Z04.89
    suicide attempt, alleged Z03.89
      self-poisoning Z03.6
    toxic effects from ingested substance (drug) (poison) Z03.6
  toxic effects from ingested substance (drug) (poison) Z03.6

Obsession, obsessional state F42.8
  mixed thoughts and acts F42.2
Obsessive-compulsive neurosis or reaction F42.8
Obstetric embolism, septic — *see* Embolism, obstetric, septic
Obstetrical trauma (complicating delivery) O71.9
  with or following ectopic or molar pregnancy O08.6
  specified type NEC O71.89
Obstipation — *see* Constipation
Obstruction, obstructed, obstructive
  airway J98.8
    with
      allergic alveolitis J67.9
      asthma J45.909
        with
          exacerbation (acute) J45.901
          status asthmaticus J45.902
      bronchiectasis J47.9
        with
          exacerbation (acute) J47.1
          lower respiratory infection J47.0
      bronchitis (chronic) J44.9
      emphysema J43.9
    chronic J44.9
      with
        allergic alveolitis — *see* Pneumonitis, hypersensitivity
        bronchiectasis J47.9
          with
            exacerbation (acute) J47.1
            lower respiratory infection J47.0
    due to
      foreign body — *see* Foreign body, by site, causing asphyxia
      inhalation of fumes or vapors J68.9
      laryngospasm J38.5
  ampulla of Vater K83.1
  aortic (heart) (valve) — *see* Stenosis, aortic
  aortoiliac I74.09
  aqueduct of Sylvius G91.1
    congenital Q03.0
      with spina bifida — *see* Spina bifida, by site, with hydrocephalus
  Arnold-Chiari — *see* Arnold-Chiari disease
  artery — *see also* Atherosclerosis, artery I70.9 ☑
    basilar (complete) (partial) — *see* Occlusion, artery, basilar
    carotid (complete) (partial) — *see* Occlusion, artery, carotid
    cerebellar — *see* Occlusion, artery, cerebellar
    cerebral (anterior) (middle) (posterior) — *see* Occlusion, artery, cerebral
    precerebral — *see* Occlusion, artery, precerebral
    renal N28.0
    retinal NEC — *see* Occlusion, artery, retina
    stent — *see* Restenosis, stent
    vertebral (complete) (partial) — *see* Occlusion, artery, vertebral
  band (intestinal) — *see also* Obstruction, intestine, specified NEC K56.699
  bile duct or passage (common) (hepatic) (noncalculous) K83.1
    with calculus K80.51

Obstruction, obstructed, obstructive — *continued*
  bile duct or passage — *continued*
    congenital (causing jaundice) Q44.3
  biliary (duct) (tract) K83.1
    gallbladder K82.0
  bladder-neck (acquired) N32.0
    congenital Q64.31
    due to hyperplasia (hypertrophy) of prostate — *see* Hyperplasia, prostate
  bowel — *see* Obstruction, intestine
  bronchus J98.09
  canal, ear — *see* Stenosis, external ear canal
  cardia K22.2
  caval veins (inferior) (superior) I87.1
  cecum — *see* Obstruction, intestine
  circulatory I99.8
  colon — *see* Obstruction, intestine
  common duct (noncalculous) K83.1
  coronary (artery) — *see* Occlusion, coronary
  cystic duct — *see also* Obstruction, gallbladder
    with calculus K80.21
  device, implant or graft — *see also* Complications, by site and type, mechanical T85.698 ☑
    arterial graft NEC — *see* Complication, cardiovascular device, mechanical, vascular
    catheter NEC T85.628 ☑
      cystostomy T83.090 ☑
      dialysis (renal) T82.49 ☑
        intraperitoneal T85.691 ☑
      Hopkins T83.098 ☑
      ileostomy T83.098 ☑
      infusion NEC T82.594 ☑
        spinal (epidural) (subdural) T85.690 ☑
      nephrostomy T83.092 ☑
      urethral indwelling T83.091 ☑
      urinary T83.098 ☑
      urostomy T83.098 ☑
    due to infection T85.79 ☑
    gastrointestinal — *see* Complications, prosthetic device, mechanical, gastrointestinal device
    genital NEC T83.498 ☑
      intrauterine contraceptive device T83.39 ☑
      penile prosthesis (cylinder) (implanted) (pump) (resevoir) T83.490 ☑
      testicular prosthesis T83.491 ☑
    heart NEC — *see* Complication, cardiovascular device, mechanical
    joint prosthesis — *see* Complications, joint prosthesis, mechanical, specified NEC, by site
    orthopedic NEC — *see* Complication, orthopedic, device, mechanical
    specified NEC T85.628 ☑
    urinary NEC — *see also* Complication, genitourinary, device, urinary, mechanical
      graft T83.29 ☑
    vascular NEC — *see* Complication, cardiovascular device, mechanical
    ventricular intracranial shunt T85.09 ☑
  due to foreign body accidentally left in operative wound T81.529 ☑
  duodenum K31.5
  ejaculatory duct N50.89
  esophagus K22.2
  eustachian tube (complete) (partial) H68.10- ☑
    cartilagenous (extrinsic) H68.13- ☑
      intrinsic H68.12- ☑
    osseous H68.11- ☑
  fallopian tube (bilateral) N97.1
  fecal K56.41
    with hernia — *see* Hernia, by site, with obstruction
  foramen of Monro (congenital) Q03.8
    with spina bifida — *see* Spina bifida, by site, with hydrocephalus
  foreign body — *see* Foreign body
  gallbladder K82.0
    with calculus, stones K80.21
    congenital Q44.1
  gastric outlet K31.1
  gastrointestinal — *see* Obstruction, intestine
  hepatic K76.89
    duct (noncalculous) K83.1
  ileum — *see* Obstruction, intestine
  iliofemoral (artery) I74.5
  intestine K56.609
    with
      adhesions (intestinal) (peritoneal) K56.50
        complete K56.52

Obstruction, obstructed, obstructive — *continued*
  intestine — *continued*
    with — *continued*
      adhesions — *continued*
        incomplete K56.51
        partial K56.51
    adynamic K56.0
    by gallstone K56.3
    complete K56.601
    congenital (small) Q41.9
      large Q42.9
        specified part NEC Q42.8
    incomplete K56.600
    neurogenic K56.0
      Hirschsprung's disease or megacolon Q43.1
    newborn P76.9
      due to
        fecaliths P76.8
        inspissated milk P76.2
        meconium (plug) P76.0
          in mucoviscidosis E84.11
      specified NEC P76.8
    partial K56.600
    postoperative K91.30
      complete K91.32
      incomplete K91.31
      partial K91.31
    reflex K56.0
    specified NEC K56.699
      complete K56.691
      incomplete K56.690
      partial K56.690
    volvulus K56.2
  intracardiac ball valve prosthesis T82.09 ☑
  jejunum — *see* Obstruction, intestine
  joint prosthesis — *see* Complications, joint prosthesis mechanical, specified NEC, by site
  kidney (calices) N28.89
  labor — *see* Delivery
  lacrimal (passages) (duct)
    by
      dacryolith — *see* Dacryolith
      stenosis — *see* Stenosis, lacrimal
    congenital Q10.5
    neonatal H04.53- ☑
  lacrimonasal duct — *see* Obstruction, lacrimal
  lacteal, with steatorrhea K90.2
  laryngitis — *see* Laryngitis
  larynx NEC J38.6
    congenital Q31.8
  lung J98.4
    disease, chronic J44.9
  lymphatic I89.0
  meconium (plug)
    newborn P76.0
      due to fecaliths P76.0
      in mucoviscidosis E84.11
  mitral — *see* Stenosis, mitral
  nasal J34.89
  nasolacrimal duct — *see also* Obstruction, lacrimal
    congenital Q10.5
  nasopharynx J39.2
  nose J34.89
  organ or site, congenital NEC — *see* Atresia, by site
  pancreatic duct K86.89
  parotid duct or gland K11.8
  pelviureteral junction N13.5
    with hydronephrosis N13.0
    congenital Q62.39
  pharynx J39.2
  portal (circulation) (vein) I81
  prostate — *see also* Hyperplasia, prostate
    valve (urinary) N32.0
  pulmonary valve (heart) I37.0
  pyelonephritis (chronic) N11.1
  pylorus
    adult K31.1
    congenital or infantile Q40.0
  rectosigmoid — *see* Obstruction, intestine
  rectum K62.4
  renal N28.89
    outflow N13.8
    pelvis, congenital Q62.39
  respiratory J98.8
    chronic J44.9
  retinal (vessels) H34.9
  salivary duct (any) K11.8
    with calculus K11.5

Obstruction, obstructed, obstructive — *continued*
  sigmoid — *see* Obstruction, intestine
  sinus (accessory) (nasal) J34.89
  Stensen's duct K11.8
  stomach NEC K31.89
    acute K31.0
    congenital Q40.2
    due to pylorospasm K31.3
  submandibular duct K11.8
  submaxillary gland K11.8
    with calculus K11.5
  thoracic duct I89.0
  thrombotic — *see* Thrombosis
  trachea J39.8
  tracheostomy airway J95.03
  tricuspid (valve) — *see* Stenosis, tricuspid
  upper respiratory, congenital Q34.8
  ureter (functional) (pelvic junction) NEC N13.5
    with
      hydronephrosis N13.1
        with infection N13.6
        pyelonephritis (chronic) N11.1
      congenital Q62.39
      due to calculus — *see* Calculus, ureter
  urethra NEC N36.8
    congenital Q64.39
  urinary (moderate) N13.9
    due to hyperplasia (hypertrophy) of prostate — *see* Hyperplasia, prostate
    organ or tract (lower) N13.9
    prostatic valve N32.0
    specified NEC N13.8
  uropathy N13.9
  uterus N85.8
  vagina N89.5
  valvular — *see* Endocarditis
  vein, venous I87.1
    caval (inferior) (superior) I87.1
    thrombotic — *see* Thrombosis
  vena cava (inferior) (superior) I87.1
  vesical NEC N32.0
  vesicourethral orifice N32.0
    congenital Q64.31
  vessel NEC I99.8
    stent — *see* Restenosis, stent
Obturator — *see* condition
Occlusal wear, teeth K03.0
Occlusio pupillae — *see* Membrane, pupillary
Occlusion, occluded
  anus K62.4
    congenital Q42.3
      with fistula Q42.2
  aortoiliac (chronic) I74.09
  aqueduct of Sylvius G91.1
    congenital Q03.0
      with spina bifida — *see* Spina bifida, by site, with hydrocephalus
  artery — *see also* Atherosclerosis, artery I70.9 ☑
    auditory, internal I65.8
    basilar I65.1
      with
        infarction I63.22
          due to
            embolism I63.12
            thrombosis I63.02
    brain or cerebral I66.9
      with infarction (due to) I63.5- ☑
        embolism I63.4- ☑
        thrombosis I63.3- ☑
    carotid I65.2- ☑
      with
        infarction I63.23- ☑
          due to
            embolism I63.13- ☑
            thrombosis I63.03- ☑
    cerebellar (anterior inferior) (posterior inferior) (superior) I66.3
      with infarction I63.54- ☑
        due to
          embolism I63.44- ☑
          thrombosis I63.34- ☑
    cerebral I66.9
      with infarction I63.50
        due to
          embolism I63.40
            specified NEC I63.49
          thrombosis I63.30
            specified NEC I63.39

Occlusion, occluded — *continued*
  artery — *see also* Atherosclerosis, artery — *continued*
    cerebral — *continued*
      anterior I66.1- ☑
        with infarction I63.52- ☑
          due to
            embolism I63.42- ☑
            thrombosis I63.32- ☑
      middle I66.0- ☑
        with infarction I63.51- ☑
          due to
            embolism I63.41- ☑
            thrombosis I63.31- ☑
      posterior I66.2- ☑
        with infarction I63.53- ☑
          due to
            embolism I63.43- ☑
            thrombosis I63.33- ☑
      specified NEC I66.8
        with infarction I63.59
          due to
            embolism I63.4- ☑
            thrombosis I63.3- ☑
    choroidal (anterior) — *see* Occlusion, artery, precerebral, specified NEC
    communicating posterior — *see* Occlusion, artery, precerebral, specified NEC
    complete
      coronary I25.82
      extremities I70.92
    coronary (acute) (thrombotic) (without myocardial infarction) I24.0
      with myocardial infarction — *see* Infarction, myocardium
      chronic total I25.82
      complete I25.82
      healed or old I25.2
      total (chronic) I25.82
    hypophyseal — *see* Occlusion, artery, precerebral, specified NEC
    iliac I74.5
    lower extremities due to stenosis or stricture I77.1
    mesenteric (embolic) (thrombotic) — *see also* Infarct, intestine K55.069
    perforating — *see* Occlusion, artery, cerebral, specified NEC
    peripheral I77.9
      thrombotic or embolic I74.4
    pontine — *see* Occlusion, artery, precerebral, specified NEC
    precerebral I65.9
      with infarction I63.20
        specified NEC I63.29
        due to
          embolism I63.10
            specified NEC I63.19
          thrombosis I63.00
            specified NEC I63.09
      basilar — *see* Occlusion, artery, basilar
      carotid — *see* Occlusion, artery, carotid
      puerperal O88.23
      specified NEC I65.8
        with infarction I63.29
          due to
            embolism I63.19
            thrombosis I63.09
      vertebral — *see* Occlusion, artery, vertebral
    renal N28.0
    retinal
      branch H34.23- ☑
      central H34.1- ☑
      partial H34.21- ☑
      transient H34.0- ☑
    spinal — *see* Occlusion, artery, precerebral, vertebral
    total (chronic)
      coronary I25.82
      extremities I70.92
    vertebral I65.0- ☑
      with
        infarction I63.21- ☑
          due to
            embolism I63.11- ☑
            thrombosis I63.01- ☑
  basilar artery — *see* Occlusion, artery, basilar
  bile duct (common) (hepatic) (noncalculous) K83.1
  bowel — *see* Obstruction, intestine

Occlusion, occluded — *continued*
  carotid (artery) (common) (internal) — *see* Occlusion, artery, carotid
  centric (of teeth) M26.59
    maximum intercuspation discrepancy M26.55
  cerebellar (artery) — *see* Occlusion, artery, cerebellar
  cerebral (artery) — *see* Occlusion, artery, cerebral
  cerebrovascular — *see also* Occlusion, artery, cerebral
    with infarction I63.5- ☑
  cervical canal — *see* Stricture, cervix
  cervix (uteri) — *see* Stricture, cervix
  choanal Q30.0
  choroidal (artery) — *see* Occlusion, artery, precerebral, specified NEC
  colon — *see* Obstruction, intestine
  communicating posterior artery — *see* Occlusion, artery, precerebral, specified NEC
  coronary (artery) (vein) (thrombotic) — *see also* Infarct, myocardium
    chronic total I25.82
    healed or old I25.2
    not resulting in infarction I24.0
    total (chronic) I25.82
  cystic duct — *see* Obstruction, gallbladder
  embolic — *see* Embolism
  fallopian tube N97.1
    congenital Q50.6
  gallbladder — *see also* Obstruction, gallbladder
    congenital (causing jaundice) Q44.1
  gingiva, traumatic K06.2
  hymen N89.6
    congenital Q52.3
  hypophyseal (artery) — *see* Occlusion, artery, precerebral, specified NEC
  iliac artery I74.5
  intestine — *see* Obstruction, intestine
  lacrimal passages — *see* Obstruction, lacrimal
  lung J98.4
  lymph or lymphatic channel I89.0
  mammary duct N64.89
  mesenteric artery (embolic) (thrombotic) — *see also* Infarct, intestine K55.069
  nose J34.89
    congenital Q30.0
  organ or site, congenital NEC — *see* Atresia, by site
  oviduct N97.1
    congenital Q50.6
  peripheral arteries
    due to stricture or stenosis I77.1
    upper extremity I74.2
  pontine (artery) — *see* Occlusion, artery, precerebral, specified NEC
  posterior lingual, of mandibular teeth M26.29
  precerebral artery — *see* Occlusion, artery, precerebral
  punctum lacrimale — *see* Obstruction, lacrimal
  pupil — *see* Membrane, pupillary
  pylorus, adult — *see also* Stricture, pylorus K31.1
  renal artery N28.0
  retina, retinal
    artery — *see* Occlusion, artery, retinal
    vein (central) H34.81- ☑
      engorgement H34.82- ☑
      tributary H34.83- ☑
    vessels H34.9
  spinal artery — *see* Occlusion, artery, precerebral, vertebral
  teeth (mandibular) (posterior lingual) M26.29
  thoracic duct I89.0
  thrombotic — *see* Thrombosis, artery
  traumatic
    edentulous (alveolar) ridge K06.2
    gingiva K06.2
    periodontal K05.5
  tubal N97.1
  ureter (complete) (partial) N13.5
    congenital Q62.10
  ureteropelvic junction N13.5
    congenital Q62.11
  ureterovesical orifice N13.5
    congenital Q62.12
  urethra — *see* Stricture, urethra
  uterus N85.8
  vagina N89.5
  vascular NEC I99.8
  vein — *see* Thrombosis
    retinal — *see* Occlusion, retinal, vein
  vena cava (inferior) (superior) — *see* Embolism, vena cava

Occlusion, occluded — *continued*
ventricle (brain) NEC G91.1
vertebral (artery) — *see* Occlusion, artery, vertebral
vessel (blood) I99.8
vulva N90.5
Occult
blood in feces (stools) R19.5
Occupational
problems NEC Z56.89
Ochlophobia — *see* Agoraphobia
Ochronosis (endogenous) E70.29
Ocular muscle — *see* condition
Oculogyric crisis or disturbance H51.8
psychogenic F45.8
Oculomotor syndrome H51.9
Oculopathy
syphilitic NEC A52.71
congenital
early A50.01
late A50.30
early (secondary) A51.43
late A52.71
Oddi's sphincter spasm K83.4
Odontalgia K08.89
Odontoameloblastoma — *see* Cyst, calcifying odontogenic
Odontoclasia K03.89
Odontodysplasia, regional K00.4
Odontogenesis imperfecta K00.5
Odontoma (ameloblastic) (complex) (compound) (fibroameloblastic) — *see* Cyst, calcifying odontogenic
Odontomyelitis (closed) (open) K04.01
irreversible K04.02
reversible K04.01
Odontorrhagia K08.89
Odontosarcoma, ameloblastic C41.1
upper jaw (bone) C41.0
Oestriasis — *see* Myiasis
Oguchi's disease H53.63
Ohara's disease — *see* Tularemia
OHS (obesity hypoventilation syndrome) E66.2
Oidiomycosis — *see* Candidiasis
Oidium albicans infection — *see* Candidiasis
Old age (without mention of debility) R54
dementia F03 ☑
Old (previous) **myocardial infarction** I25.2
Olfactory — *see* condition
Oligemia — *see* Anemia
Oligoastrocytoma
specified site — *see* Neoplasm, malignant, by site
unspecified site C71.9
Oligocythemia D64.9
Oligodendroblastoma
specified site — *see* Neoplasm, malignant
unspecified site C71.9
Oligodendroglioma
anaplastic type
specified site — *see* Neoplasm, malignant, by site
unspecified site C71.9
specified site — *see* Neoplasm, malignant, by site
unspecified site C71.9
Oligodontia — *see* Anodontia
Oligoencephalon Q02
Oligohidrosis L74.4
Oligohydramnios O41.0- ☑
Oligohydrosis L74.4
Oligomenorrhea N91.5
primary N91.3
secondary N91.4
Oligophrenia — *see also* Disability, intellectual
phenylpyruvic E70.0
Oligospermia N46.11
due to
drug therapy N46.121
efferent duct obstruction N46.123
infection N46.122
radiation N46.124
specified cause NEC N46.129
systemic disease N46.125
Oligotrichia — *see* Alopecia
Oliguria R34
with, complicating or following ectopic or molar pregnancy O08.4
postprocedural N99.0
Ollier's disease Q78.4
Omenotocele — *see* Hernia, abdomen, specified site NEC
Omentitis — *see* Peritonitis

Omentum, omental — *see* condition
Omphalitis (congenital) (newborn) P38.9
with mild hemorrhage P38.1
without hemorrhage P38.9
not of newborn L08.82
tetanus A33
Omphalocele Q79.2
Omphalomesenteric duct, persistent Q43.0
Omphalorrhagia, newborn P51.9
Omsk hemorrhagic fever A98.1
Onanism (excessive) F98.8
Onchocerciasis, onchocercosis B73.1
with
eye disease B73.00
endophthalmitis B73.01
eyelid B73.09
glaucoma B73.02
specified NEC B73.09
eyelid B73.09
eye NEC B73.00
Oncocytoma — *see* Neoplasm, benign, by site
Oncovirus, as cause of disease classified elsewhere B97.32
Ondine's curse — *see* Apnea, sleep
Oneirophrenia F23
Onychauxis L60.2
congenital Q84.5
Onychia — *see also* Cellulitis, digit
with lymphangitis — *see* Lymphangitis, acute, digit
candidal B37.2
dermatophytic B35.1
Onychitis — *see also* Cellulitis, digit
with lymphangitis — *see* Lymphangitis, acute, digit
Onychocryptosis L60.0
Onychodystrophy L60.3
congenital Q84.6
Onychogryphosis, onychogryposis L60.2
Onycholysis L60.1
Onychomadesis L60.8
Onychomalacia L60.3
Onychomycosis (finger) (toe) B35.1
Onycho-osteodysplasia Q87.2
Onychophagia F98.8
Onychophosis L60.8
Onychoptosis L60.8
Onychorrhexis L60.3
congenital Q84.6
Onychoschizia L60.3
Onyxis (finger) (toe) L60.0
Onyxitis — *see also* Cellulitis, digit
with lymphangitis — *see* Lymphangitis, acute, digit
Oophoritis (cystic) (infectional) (interstitial) N70.92
with salpingitis N70.93
acute N70.02
with salpingitis N70.03
chronic N70.12
with salpingitis N70.13
complicating abortion — *see* Abortion, by type, complicated by, oophoritis
Oophorocele N83.4- ☑
Opacity, opacities
cornea H17.- ☑
central H17.1- ☑
congenital Q13.3
degenerative — *see* Degeneration, cornea
hereditary — *see* Dystrophy, cornea
inflammatory — *see* Keratitis
minor H17.81- ☑
peripheral H17.82- ☑
sequelae of trachoma (healed) B94.0
specified NEC H17.89
enamel (teeth) (fluoride) (nonfluoride) K00.3
lens — *see* Cataract
snowball — *see* Deposit, crystalline
vitreous (humor) NEC H43.39- ☑
congenital Q14.0
membranes and strands H43.31- ☑
Opalescent dentin (hereditary) K00.5
Open, opening
abnormal, organ or site, congenital — *see* Imperfect, closure
angle with
borderline
findings
high risk H40.02- ☑
low risk H40.01- ☑
intraocular pressure H40.00- ☑

Open, opening — *continued*
angle with — *continued*
cupping of discs H40.01- ☑
glaucoma (primary) — *see* Glaucoma, open angle
bite
anterior M26.220
posterior M26.221
false — *see* Imperfect, closure
margin on tooth restoration K08.51
restoration margins of tooth K08.51
wound — *see* Wound, open
Operational fatigue F48.8
Operative — *see* condition
Operculitis — *see* Periodontitis
Operculum — *see* Break, retina
Ophiasis L63.2
Ophthalmia — *see also* Conjunctivitis H10.9
actinic rays — *see* Photokeratitis
allergic (acute) — *see* Conjunctivitis, acute, atopic
blennorrhagic (gonococcal) (neonatorum) A54.31
diphtheritic A36.86
Egyptian A71.1
electrica — *see* Photokeratitis
gonococcal (neonatorum) A54.31
metastatic — *see* Endophthalmitis, purulent
migraine — *see* Migraine, ophthalmoplegic
neonatorum, newborn P39.1
gonococcal A54.31
nodosa H16.24- ☑
purulent — *see* Conjunctivitis, acute, mucopurulent
spring — *see* Conjunctivitis, acute, atopic
sympathetic — *see* Uveitis, sympathetic
Ophthalmitis — *see* Ophthalmia
Ophthalmocele (congenital) Q15.8
Ophthalmoneuromyelitis G36.0
Ophthalmoplegia — *see also* Strabismus, paralytic
anterior internuclear — *see* Ophthalmoplegia, internuclear
ataxia-areflexia G61.0
diabetic — *see* E08-E13 with .39
exophthalmic E05.00
with thyroid storm E05.01
external H49.88- ☑
progressive H49.4- ☑
with pigmentary retinopathy — *see* Kearns-Sayre syndrome
total H49.3- ☑
internal (complete) (total) H52.51- ☑
internuclear H51.2- ☑
migraine — *see* Migraine, ophthalmoplegic
Parinaud's H49.88- ☑
progressive external — *see* Ophthalmoplegia, external, progressive
supranuclear, progressive G23.1
total (external) — *see* Ophthalmoplegia, external, total
Opioid(s)
abuse — *see* Abuse, drug, opioids
dependence — *see* Dependence, drug, opioids
induced, without use disorder
anxiety disorder F11.988
delirium F11.921
depressive disorder F11.94
sexual dysfunction F11.981
sleep disorder F11.982
Opisthognathism M26.09
Opisthorchiasis (felineus) (viverrini) B66.0
Opitz' disease D73.2
Opiumism — *see* Dependence, drug, opioid
Oppenheim's disease G70.2
Oppenheim-Urbach disease (necrobiosis lipoidica diabeticorum) — *see* E08-E13 with .620
Optic nerve — *see* condition
Orbit — *see* condition
Orchioblastoma C62.9- ☑
Orchitis (gangrenous) (nonspecific) (septic) (suppurative) N45.2
blennorrhagic (gonococcal) (acute) (chronic) A54.23
chlamydial A56.19
filarial — *see also* Infestation, filarial B74.9 [N51]
gonococcal (acute) (chronic) A54.23
mumps B26.0
syphilitic A52.76
tuberculous A18.15
Orf (virus disease) B08.02
Organic — *see also* condition
brain syndrome F09
heart — *see* Disease, heart

☑ **Additional Character Required** — Refer to the Tabular List for Character Selection   ▼ Subterms under main terms may continue to next column or page

Organic — *continued*
  mental disorder F09
  psychosis F09
Orgasm
  anejaculatory N53.13
Oriental
  bilharziasis B65.2
  schistosomiasis B65.2
Orifice — *see* condition
Origin of both great vessels from right ventricle
  Q20.1
Ormond's disease (with ureteral obstruction) N13.5
  with infection N13.6
Ornithine metabolism disorder E72.4
Ornithinemia (Type I) (Type II) E72.4
Ornithosis A70
Orotaciduria, oroticaciduria (congenital) (hereditary)
  (pyrimidine deficiency) E79.8
  anemia D53.0
Orthodontics
  adjustment Z46.4
  fitting Z46.4
Orthopnea R06.01
Orthopoxvirus B08.09
Os, uterus — *see* condition
Osgood-Schlatter disease or osteochondrosis — *see* Osteochondrosis, juvenile, tibia
Osler (-Weber)-**Rendu disease** I78.0
Osler's nodes I33.0
Osmidrosis L75.0
Osseous — *see* condition
Ossification
  artery — *see* Arteriosclerosis
  auricle (ear) — *see* Disorder, pinna, specified type NEC
  bronchial J98.09
  cardiac — *see* Degeneration, myocardial
  cartilage (senile) — *see* Disorder, cartilage, specified type NEC
  coronary (artery) — *see* Disease, heart, ischemic, atherosclerotic
  diaphragm J98.6
  ear, middle — *see* Otosclerosis
  falx cerebri G96.19
  fontanel, premature Q75.0
  heart — *see also* Degeneration, myocardial
    valve — *see* Endocarditis
  larynx J38.7
  ligament — *see* Disorder, tendon, specified type NEC
    posterior longitudinal — *see* Spondylopathy, specified NEC
  meninges (cerebral) (spinal) G96.19
  multiple, eccentric centers — *see* Disorder, bone, development or growth
  muscle — *see also* Calcification, muscle
    due to burns — *see* Myositis, ossificans, in, burns
    paralytic — *see* Myositis, ossificans, in, quadriplegia
    progressive — *see* Myositis, ossificans, progressiva
    specified NEC M61.50
      ankle M61.57- ☑
      foot M61.57- ☑
      forearm M61.53- ☑
      hand M61.54- ☑
      lower leg M61.56- ☑
      multiple sites M61.59
      pelvic region M61.55- ☑
      shoulder region M61.51- ☑
      specified site NEC M61.58
      thigh M61.55- ☑
      upper arm M61.52- ☑
    traumatic — *see* Myositis, ossificans, traumatica
  myocardium, myocardial — *see* Degeneration, myocardial
  penis N48.89
  periarticular — *see* Disorder, joint, specified type NEC
  pinna — *see* Disorder, pinna, specified type NEC
  rider's bone — *see* Ossification, muscle, specified NEC
  sclera H15.89
  subperiosteal, post-traumatic M89.8X- ☑
  tendon — *see* Disorder, tendon, specified type NEC
  trachea J39.8
  tympanic membrane — *see* Disorder, tympanic membrane, specified NEC
  vitreous (humor) — *see* Deposit, crystalline
Osteitis — *see also* Osteomyelitis
  alveolar M27.3
  condensans M85.30
    ankle M85.37- ☑

Osteitis — *continued*
  condensans — *continued*
    foot M85.37- ☑
    forearm M85.33- ☑
    hand M85.34- ☑
    lower leg M85.36- ☑
    multiple site M85.39
    neck M85.38
    rib M85.38
    shoulder M85.31- ☑
    skull M85.38
    specified site NEC M85.38
    thigh M85.35- ☑
    toe M85.37- ☑
    upper arm M85.32- ☑
    vertebra M85.38
  deformans M88.9
    in (due to)
      malignant neoplasm of bone C41.9 *[M90.60]*
      neoplastic disease — *see also* Neoplasm
        D49.9 *[M90.60]*
        carpus D49.9 *[M90.64-]* ☑
        clavicle D49.9 *[M90.61-]* ☑
        femur D49.9 *[M90.65-]* ☑
        fibula D49.9 *[M90.66-]* ☑
        finger D49.9 *[M90.64-]* ☑
        humerus D49.9 *[M90.62-]* ☑
        ilium D49.9 *[M90.65-]* ☑
        ischium D49.9 *[M90.65-]* ☑
        metacarpus D49.9 *[M90.64-]* ☑
        metatarsus D49.9 *[M90.67-]* ☑
        multiple sites D49.9 *[M90.69]*
        neck D49.9 *[M90.68]*
        radius D49.9 *[M90.63-]* ☑
        rib D49.9 *[M90.68]*
        scapula D49.9 *[M90.61-]* ☑
        skull D49.9 *[M90.68]*
        tarsus D49.9 *[M90.67-]* ☑
        tibia D49.9 *[M90.66-]* ☑
        toe D49.9 *[M90.67-]* ☑
        ulna D49.9 *[M90.63-]* ☑
        vertebra D49.9 *[M90.68]*
    skull M88.0
    specified NEC — *see* Paget's disease, bone, by site
    vertebra M88.1
  due to yaws A66.6
  fibrosa NEC — *see* Cyst, bone, by site
    circumscripta — *see* Dysplasia, fibrous, bone NEC
    cystica (generalisata) E21.0
    disseminata Q78.1
    osteoplastica E21.0
  fragilitans Q78.0
  Garr's (sclerosing) — *see* Osteomyelitis, specified type NEC
  jaw (acute) (chronic) (lower) (suppurative) (upper) M27.2
  parathyroid E21.0
  petrous bone (acute) (chronic) — *see* Petrositis
  sclerotic, nonsuppurative — *see* Osteomyelitis, specified type NEC
  tuberculosa A18.09
    cystica D86.89
    multiplex cystoides D86.89
Osteoarthritis M19.90
  ankle M19.07- ☑
  elbow M19.02- ☑
  foot joint M19.07- ☑
  generalized M15.9
    erosive M15.4
    primary M15.0
    specified NEC M15.8
  hand joint M19.04- ☑
    first carpometacarpal joint M18.9
  hip M16.1- ☑
    bilateral M16.0
    due to hip dysplasia (unilateral) M16.3- ☑
      bilateral M16.2
  interphalangeal
    distal (Heberden) M15.1
    proximal (Bouchard) M15.2
  knee M17.1- ☑
    bilateral M17.0
  post-traumatic NEC M19.92
    ankle M19.17- ☑
    elbow M19.12- ☑
    foot joint M19.17- ☑
    hand joint M19.14- ☑

Osteoarthritis — *continued*
  post-traumatic — *continued*
    hand joint — *continued*
      first carpometacarpal joint M18.3- ☑
        bilateral M18.2
    hip M16.5- ☑
      bilateral M16.4
    knee M17.3- ☑
      bilateral M17.2
    shoulder M19.11- ☑
    wrist M19.13- ☑
  primary M19.91
    ankle M19.07- ☑
    elbow M19.02- ☑
    foot joint M19.07- ☑
    hand joint M19.04- ☑
      first carpometacarpal joint M18.1- ☑
        bilateral M18.0
    hip M16.1- ☑
      bilateral M16.0
    knee M17.1- ☑
      bilateral M17.0
    multiple sites M89.49
    shoulder M19.01- ☑
    spine — *see* Spondylosis
    wrist M19.03- ☑
  secondary M19.93
    ankle M19.27- ☑
    elbow M19.22- ☑
    foot joint M19.27- ☑
    hand joint M19.24- ☑
      first carpometacarpal joint M18.5- ☑
        bilateral M18.4
    hip M16.7
      bilateral M16.6
    knee M17.5
      bilateral M17.4
    multiple M15.3
    shoulder M19.21- ☑
    spine — *see* Spondylosis
    wrist M19.23- ☑
  shoulder M19.01- ☑
  spine — *see* Spondylosis
  wrist M19.03- ☑
Osteoarthropathy (hypertrophic) M19.90
  ankle — *see* Osteoarthritis, primary, ankle
  elbow — *see* Osteoarthritis, primary, elbow
  foot joint — *see* Osteoarthritis, primary, foot
  hand joint — *see* Osteoarthritis, primary, hand joint
  knee joint — *see* Osteoarthritis, primary, knee
  multiple site — *see* Osteoarthritis, primary, multiple joint
  pulmonary — *see also* Osteoarthropathy, specified type NEC
    hypertrophic — *see* Osteoarthropathy, hypertrophic, specified type NEC
  secondary — *see* Osteoarthropathy, specified type NEC
  secondary hypertrophic — *see* Osteoarthropathy, specified type NEC
  shoulder — *see* Osteoarthritis, primary, shoulder
  specified joint NEC — *see* Osteoarthritis, primary, specified joint NEC
  specified type NEC M89.40
    carpus M89.44- ☑
    clavicle M89.41- ☑
    femur M89.45- ☑
    fibula M89.46- ☑
    finger M89.44- ☑
    humerus M89.42- ☑
    ilium M89.459
    ischium M89.459
    metacarpus M89.44- ☑
    metatarsus M89.47- ☑
    multiple sites M89.49
    neck M89.48
    radius M89.43- ☑
    rib M89.48
    scapula M89.41- ☑
    skull M89.48
    tarsus M89.47- ☑
    tibia M89.46- ☑
    toe M89.47- ☑
    ulna M89.43- ☑
    vertebra M89.48
  spine — *see* Spondylosis
  wrist — *see* Osteoarthritis, primary, wrist

Osteoarthrosis (degenerative) (hypertrophic) (joint) —
see also Osteoarthritis
- deformans alkaptonurica E70.29 *[M36.8]*
- erosive M15.4
- generalized M15.9
  - primary M15.0
- polyarticular M15.9
- spine — see Spondylosis

Osteoblastoma — see Neoplasm, bone, benign
- aggressive — see Neoplasm, bone, uncertain behavior

Osteochondritis — see also Osteochondropathy, by site
- Brailsford's — see Osteochondrosis, juvenile, radius
- dissecans M93.20
  - ankle M93.27- ☑
  - elbow M93.22- ☑
  - foot M93.27- ☑
  - hand M93.24- ☑
  - hip M93.25- ☑
  - knee M93.26- ☑
  - multiple sites M93.29
  - shoulder joint M93.21- ☑
  - specified site NEC M93.28
  - wrist M93.23- ☑
- juvenile M92.9
  - patellar — see Osteochondrosis, juvenile, patella
- syphilitic (congenital) (early) A50.02 *[M90.80]*
  - ankle A50.02 *[M90.87-]* ☑
  - elbow A50.02 *[M90.82-]* ☑
  - foot A50.02 *[M90.87-]* ☑
  - forearm A50.02 *[M90.83-]* ☑
  - hand A50.02 *[M90.84-]* ☑
  - hip A50.02 *[M90.85-]* ☑
  - knee A50.02 *[M90.86-]* ☑
  - multiple sites A50.02 *[M90.89]*
  - shoulder joint A50.02 *[M90.81-]* ☑
  - specified site NEC A50.02 *[M90.88]*

Osteochondroarthrosis deformans endemica — see
Disease, Kaschin-Beck

Osteochondrodysplasia Q78.9
- with defects of growth of tubular bones and spine
  Q77.9
  - specified NEC Q77.8
- specified NEC Q78.8

Osteochondrodystrophy E78.9

Osteochondrolysis — see Osteochondritis, dissecans

Osteochondroma — see Neoplasm, bone, benign

Osteochondromatosis D48.0
- syndrome Q78.4

Osteochondromyxosarcoma — see Neoplasm, bone,
malignant

Osteochondropathy M93.90
- ankle M93.97- ☑
- elbow M93.92- ☑
- foot M93.97- ☑
- hand M93.94- ☑
- hip M93.95- ☑
- Kienböck's disease of adults M93.1
- knee M93.96- ☑
- multiple joints M93.99
- osteochondritis dissecans — see Osteochondritis, dissecans
- osteochondrosis — see Osteochondrosis
- shoulder region M93.91- ☑
- slipped upper femoral epiphysis — see Slipped, epiphysis, upper femoral
- specified joint NEC M93.98
- specified type NEC M93.80
  - ankle M93.87- ☑
  - elbow M93.82- ☑
  - foot M93.87- ☑
  - hand M93.84- ☑
  - hip M93.85- ☑
  - knee M93.86- ☑
  - multiple joints M93.89
  - shoulder region M93.81- ☑
  - specified joint NEC M93.88
  - wrist M93.83- ☑
- syphilitic, congenital
  - early A50.02 *[M90.80]*
  - late A50.56 *[M90.80]*
- wrist M93.93- ☑

Osteochondrosarcoma — see Neoplasm, bone, malignant

Osteochondrosis — see also Osteochondropathy, by
site
- acetabulum (juvenile) M91.0

Osteochondrosis — continued
- adult — see Osteochondropathy, specified type NEC,
  by site
- astragalus (juvenile) — see Osteochondrosis, juvenile,
  tarsus
- Blount's — see Osteochondrosis, juvenile, tibia
- Buchanan's M91.0
- Burns' — see Osteochondrosis, juvenile, ulna
- calcaneus (juvenile) — see Osteochondrosis, juvenile,
  tarsus
- capitular epiphysis (femur) (juvenile) — see Legg-Calvé-
  Perthes disease
- carpal (juvenile) (lunate) (scaphoid) — see Osteochondrosis, juvenile, hand, carpal lunate
  - adult M93.1
- coxae juvenilis — see Legg-Calvé-Perthes disease
- deformans juvenilis, coxae — see Legg-Calvé-Perthes
  disease
- Diaz's — see Osteochondrosis, juvenile, tarsus
- dissecans (knee) (shoulder) — see Osteochondritis,
  dissecans
- femoral capital epiphysis (juvenile) — see Legg-Calvé-
  Perthes disease
- femur (head), juvenile — see Legg-Calvé-Perthes disease
- fibula (juvenile) — see Osteochondrosis, juvenile,
  fibula
- foot NEC (juvenile) M92.8
- Freiberg's — see Osteochondrosis, juvenile, metatarsus
- Haas' (juvenile) — see Osteochondrosis, juvenile,
  humerus
- Haglund's — see Osteochondrosis, juvenile, tarsus
- hip (juvenile) — see Legg-Calvé-Perthes disease
- humerus (capitulum) (head) (juvenile) — see Osteochondrosis, juvenile, humerus
- ilium, iliac crest (juvenile) M91.0
- ischiopubic synchondrosis M91.0
- Iselin's — see Osteochondrosis, juvenile, metatarsus
- juvenile, juvenilis M92.9
  - after congenital dislocation of hip reduction — see
    Osteochondrosis, juvenile, hip, specified NEC
  - arm — see Osteochondrosis, juvenile, upper limb
    NEC
  - capitular epiphysis (femur) — see Legg-Calvé-
    Perthes disease
  - clavicle, sternal epiphysis — see Osteochondrosis,
    juvenile, upper limb NEC
  - coxae — see Legg-Calvé-Perthes disease
  - deformans M92.9
  - fibula M92.5- ☑
  - foot NEC M92.8
  - hand M92.20- ☑
    - carpal lunate M92.21- ☑
    - metacarpal head M92.22- ☑
    - specified site NEC M92.29- ☑
  - head of femur — see Legg-Calvé-Perthes disease
  - hip and pelvis M91.9- ☑
    - coxa plana — see Coxa, plana
    - femoral head — see Legg-Calvé-Perthes disease
    - pelvis M91.0
    - pseudocoxalgia — see Pseudocoxalgia
    - specified NEC M91.8- ☑
  - humerus M92.0- ☑
  - limb
    - lower NEC M92.8
    - upper NEC — see Osteochondrosis, juvenile,
      upper limb NEC
  - medial cuneiform bone — see Osteochondrosis,
    juvenile, tarsus
  - metatarsus M92.7- ☑
  - patella M92.4- ☑
  - radius M92.1- ☑
  - specified site NEC M92.8
  - spine M42.00
    - cervical region M42.02
    - cervicothoracic region M42.03
    - lumbar region M42.06
    - lumbosacral region M42.07
    - multiple sites M42.09
    - occipito-atlanto-axial region M42.01
    - sacrococcygeal region M42.08
    - thoracic region M42.04
    - thoracolumbar region M42.05
  - tarsus M92.6- ☑
  - tibia M92.5- ☑
  - ulna M92.1- ☑
  - upper limb NEC M92.3- ☑

Osteochondrosis — continued
- juvenile, juvenilis — continued
  - vertebra (body) (epiphyseal plates) (Calvé's)
    (Scheuermann's) — see Osteochondrosis, ju-
    venile, spine
  - Kienböck's — see Osteochondrosis, juvenile, hand,
    carpal lunate
    - adult M93.1
  - Köhler's
    - patellar — see Osteochondrosis, juvenile, patella
    - tarsal navicular — see Osteochondrosis, juvenile,
      tarsus
  - Legg-Perthes (-Calvé)(-Waldenström) — see Legg-
    Calvé-Perthes disease
  - limb
    - lower NEC (juvenile) M92.8
    - upper NEC (juvenile) — see Osteochondrosis, juve-
      nile, upper limb NEC
  - lunate bone (carpal) (juvenile) — see also Osteochon-
    drosis, juvenile, hand, carpal lunate
    - adult M93.1
  - Mauclaire's — see Osteochondrosis, juvenile, hand,
    metacarpal
  - metacarpal (head) (juvenile) — see Osteochondrosis,
    juvenile, hand, metacarpal
  - metatarsus (fifth) (head) (juvenile) (second) — see Os-
    teochondrosis, juvenile, metatarsus
  - navicular (juvenile) — see Osteochondrosis, juvenile,
    tarsus
  - os
    - calcis (juvenile) — see Osteochondrosis, juvenile,
      tarsus
    - tibiale externum (juvenile) — see Osteochondrosis,
      juvenile, tarsus
  - Osgood-Schlatter — see Osteochondrosis, juvenile,
    tibia
  - Panner's — see Osteochondrosis, juvenile, humerus
  - patellar center (juvenile) (primary) (secondary) — see
    Osteochondrosis, juvenile, patella
  - pelvis (juvenile) M91.0
  - Pierson's M91.0
  - radius (head) (juvenile) — see Osteochondrosis, juve-
    nile, radius
  - Scheuermann's — see Osteochondrosis, juvenile, spine
  - Sever's — see Osteochondrosis, juvenile, tarsus
  - Sinding-Larsen — see Osteochondrosis, juvenile,
    patella
  - spine M42.9
    - adult M42.10
      - cervical region M42.12
      - cervicothoracic region M42.13
      - lumbar region M42.16
      - lumbosacral region M42.17
      - multiple sites M42.19
      - occipito-atlanto-axial region M42.11
      - sacrococcygeal region M42.18
      - thoracic region M42.14
      - thoracolumbar region M42.15
    - juvenile — see Osteochondrosis, juvenile, spine
  - symphysis pubis (juvenile) M91.0
  - syphilitic (congenital) A50.02
  - talus (juvenile) — see Osteochondrosis, juvenile, tarsus
  - tarsus (navicular) (juvenile) — see Osteochondrosis,
    juvenile, tarsus
  - tibia (proximal) (tubercle) (juvenile) — see Osteochon-
    drosis, juvenile, tibia
  - tuberculous — see Tuberculosis, bone
  - ulna (lower) (juvenile) — Osteochondrosis, juvenile,
    ulna
  - van Neck's M91.0
  - vertebral — see Osteochondrosis, spine

Osteoclastoma D48.0
- malignant — see Neoplasm, bone, malignant

Osteodynia — see Disorder, bone, specified type NEC

Osteodystrophy Q78.9
- azotemic N25.0
- congenital Q78.9
- parathyroid, secondary E21.1
- renal N25.0

Osteofibroma — see Neoplasm, bone, benign

Osteofibrosarcoma — see Neoplasm, bone, maligna

Osteogenesis imperfecta Q78.0

Osteogenic — see condition

Osteolysis M89.50
- carpus M89.54- ☑
- clavicle M89.51- ☑
- femur M89.55- ☑

☑ Additional Character Required — Refer to the Tabular List for Character Selection   ⬇ Subterms under main terms may continue to next column or page

Osteolysis — *continued*
  fibula M89.56- ☑
  finger M89.54- ☑
  humerus M89.52- ☑
  ilium M89.559
  ischium M89.559
  joint prosthesis (periprosthetic) — *see* Complications,
      joint prosthesis, mechanical, periprosthetic, oste-
      olysis, by site
  metacarpus M89.54- ☑
  metatarsus M89.57- ☑
  multiple sites M89.59
  neck M89.58
  periprosthetic — *see* Complications, joint prosthesis,
      mechanical, periprosthetic, osteolysis, by site
  radius M89.53- ☑
  rib M89.58
  scapula M89.51- ☑
  skull M89.58
  tarsus M89.57- ☑
  tibia M89.56- ☑
  toe M89.57- ☑
  ulna M89.53- ☑
  vertebra M89.58
Osteoma — *see also* Neoplasm, bone, benign
  osteoid — *see also* Neoplasm, bone, benign
    giant — *see* Neoplasm, bone, benign
Osteomalacia M83.9
  adult M83.9
    drug-induced NEC M83.5
    due to
      malabsorption (postsurgical) M83.2
      malnutrition M83.3
    specified NEC M83.8
  aluminium-induced M83.4
  infantile — *see* Rickets
  juvenile — *see* Rickets
  oncogenic E83.89
  pelvis M83.8
  puerperal M83.0
  senile M83.1
  vitamin-D-resistant in adults E83.31 *[M90.8-]* ☑
    carpus E83.31 *[M90.84-]* ☑
    clavicle E83.31 *[M90.81-]* ☑
    femur E83.31 *[M90.85-]* ☑
    fibula E83.31 *[M90.86-]* ☑
    finger E83.31 *[M90.84-]* ☑
    humerus E83.31 *[M90.82-]* ☑
    ilium E83.31 *[M90.859]*
    ischium E83.31 *[M90.859]*
    metacarpus E83.31 *[M90.84-]* ☑
    metatarsus E83.31 *[M90.87-]* ☑
    multiple sites E83.31 *[M90.89]*
    neck E83.31 *[M90.88]*
    radius E83.31 *[M90.83-]* ☑
    rib E83.31 *[M90.88]*
    scapula E83.31 *[M90.819]*
    skull E83.31 *[M90.88]*
    tarsus E83.31 *[M90.879]*
    tibia E83.31 *[M90.869]*
    toe E83.31 *[M90.879]*
    ulna E83.31 *[M90.839]*
    vertebra E83.31 *[M90.88]*
Osteomyelitis (general) (infective) (localized) (neonatal)
      (purulent) (septic) (staphylococcal) (streptococcal)
      (suppurative) (with periostitis) M86.9
  acute M86.10
    carpus M86.14- ☑
    clavicle M86.11- ☑
    femur M86.15- ☑
    fibula M86.16- ☑
    finger M86.14- ☑
    hematogenous M86.00
      carpus M86.04- ☑
      clavicle M86.01- ☑
      femur M86.05- ☑
      fibula M86.06- ☑
      finger M86.04- ☑
      humerus M86.02- ☑
      ilium M86.059
      ischium M86.059
      mandible M27.2
      metacarpus M86.04- ☑
      metatarsus M86.07- ☑
      multiple sites M86.09
      neck M86.08
      orbit H05.02- ☑

Osteomyelitis — *continued*
  acute — *continued*
    hematogenous — *continued*
      petrous bone — *see* Petrositis
      radius M86.03- ☑
      rib M86.08
      scapula M86.01- ☑
      skull M86.08
      tarsus M86.07- ☑
      tibia M86.06- ☑
      toe M86.07- ☑
      ulna M86.03- ☑
      vertebra — *see* Osteomyelitis, vertebra
    humerus M86.12- ☑
    ilium M86.18
    ischium M86.18
    mandible M27.2
    metacarpus M86.14- ☑
    metatarsus M86.17- ☑
    multiple sites M86.19
    neck M86.18
    orbit H05.02- ☑
    petrous bone — *see* Petrositis
    radius M86.13- ☑
    rib M86.18
    scapula M86.11- ☑
    skull M86.18
    tarsus M86.17- ☑
    tibia M86.16- ☑
    toe M86.17- ☑
    ulna M86.13- ☑
    vertebra — *see* Osteomyelitis, vertebra
  chronic (or old) M86.60
    with draining sinus M86.40
      carpus M86.44- ☑
      clavicle M86.41- ☑
      femur M86.45- ☑
      fibula M86.46- ☑
      finger M86.44- ☑
      humerus M86.42- ☑
      ilium M86.459
      ischium M86.459
      mandible M27.2
      metacarpus M86.44- ☑
      metatarsus M86.47- ☑
      multiple sites M86.49
      neck M86.48
      orbit H05.02- ☑
      petrous bone — *see* Petrositis
      radius M86.43- ☑
      rib M86.48
      scapula M86.41- ☑
      skull M86.48
      tarsus M86.47- ☑
      tibia M86.46- ☑
      toe M86.47- ☑
      ulna M86.43- ☑
      vertebra — *see* Osteomyelitis, vertebra
    carpus M86.64- ☑
    clavicle M86.61- ☑
    femur M86.65- ☑
    fibula M86.66- ☑
    finger M86.64- ☑
    hematogenous NEC M86.50
      carpus M86.54- ☑
      clavicle M86.51- ☑
      femur M86.55- ☑
      fibula M86.56- ☑
      finger M86.54- ☑
      humerus M86.52- ☑
      ilium M86.559
      ischium M86.559
      mandible M27.2
      metacarpus M86.54- ☑
      metatarsus M86.57- ☑
      multifocal M86.30
        carpus M86.34- ☑
        clavicle M86.31- ☑
        femur M86.35- ☑
        fibula M86.36- ☑
        finger M86.34- ☑
        humerus M86.32- ☑
        ilium M86.359
        ischium M86.359
        metacarpus M86.34- ☑
        metatarsus M86.37- ☑

Osteomyelitis — *continued*
  chronic — *continued*
    hematogenous — *continued*
      multifocal — *continued*
        multiple sites M86.39
        neck M86.38
        radius M86.33- ☑
        rib M86.38
        scapula M86.31- ☑
        skull M86.38
        tarsus M86.37- ☑
        tibia M86.36- ☑
        toe M86.37- ☑
        ulna M86.33- ☑
        vertebra — *see* Osteomyelitis, vertebra
      multiple sites M86.59
      neck M86.58
      orbit H05.02- ☑
      petrous bone — *see* Petrositis
      radius M86.53- ☑
      rib M86.58
      scapula M86.51- ☑
      skull M86.58
      tarsus M86.57- ☑
      tibia M86.56- ☑
      toe M86.57- ☑
      ulna M86.53- ☑
      vertebra — *see* Osteomyelitis, vertebra
    humerus M86.62- ☑
    ilium M86.659
    ischium M86.659
    mandible M27.2
    metacarpus M86.64- ☑
    metatarsus M86.67- ☑
    multifocal — *see* Osteomyelitis, chronic,
        hematogenous, multifocal
    multiple sites M86.69
    neck M86.68
    orbit H05.02- ☑
    petrous bone — *see* Petrositis
    radius M86.63- ☑
    rib M86.68
    scapula M86.61- ☑
    skull M86.68
    tarsus M86.67- ☑
    tibia M86.66- ☑
    toe M86.67- ☑
    ulna M86.63- ☑
    vertebra — *see* Osteomyelitis, vertebra
  echinococcal B67.2
  Garr's — *see* Osteomyelitis, specified type NEC
  in diabetes mellitus — *see* E08-E13 with .69
  jaw (acute) (chronic) (lower) (neonatal) (suppurative)
      (upper) M27.2
  nonsuppurating — *see* Osteomyelitis, specified type
      NEC
  orbit H05.02- ☑
  petrous bone — *see* Petrositis
  Salmonella (arizonae) (cholerae-suis) (enteritidis) (ty-
      phimurium) A02.24
  sclerosing, nonsuppurative — *see* Osteomyelitis,
      specified type NEC
  specified type NEC — *see also* subcategory M86.8X- ☑
    mandible M27.2
    orbit H05.02- ☑
    petrous bone — *see* Petrositis
    vertebra — *see* Osteomyelitis, vertebra
  subacute M86.20
    carpus M86.24- ☑
    clavicle M86.21- ☑
    femur M86.25- ☑
    fibula M86.26- ☑
    finger M86.24- ☑
    humerus M86.22- ☑
    mandible M27.2
    metacarpus M86.24- ☑
    metatarsus M86.27- ☑
    multiple sites M86.29
    neck M86.28
    orbit H05.02- ☑
    petrous bone — *see* Petrositis
    radius M86.23- ☑
    rib M86.28
    scapula M86.21- ☑
    skull M86.28
    tarsus M86.27- ☑
    tibia M86.26- ☑

Osteomyelitis — *continued*
  subacute — *continued*
    toe M86.27- ☑
    ulna M86.23- ☑
    vertebra — *see* Osteomyelitis, vertebra
  syphilitic A52.77
    congenital (early) A50.02 *[M90.80]*
  tuberculous — *see* Tuberculosis, bone
  typhoid A01.05
  vertebra M46.20
    cervical region M46.22
    cervicothoracic region M46.23
    lumbar region M16.26
    lumbosacral region M46.27
    occipito-atlanto-axial region M46.21
    sacrococcygeal region M46.28
    thoracic region M46.24
    thoracolumbar region M46.25
Osteomyelofibrosis D47.4
Osteomyelosclerosis D75.89
Osteonecrosis M87.9
  due to
    drugs — *see* Osteonecrosis, secondary, due to, drugs
    trauma — *see* Osteonecrosis, secondary, due to, trauma
  idiopathic aseptic M87.00
    ankle M87.07- ☑
    carpus M87.03- ☑
    clavicle M87.01- ☑
    femur M87.05- ☑
    fibula M87.06- ☑
    finger M87.04- ☑
    humerus M87.02- ☑
    ilium M87.050
    ischium M87.050
    metacarpus M87.04- ☑
    metatarsus M87.07- ☑
    multiple sites M87.09
    neck M87.08
    pelvis M87.050
    radius M87.03- ☑
    rib M87.08
    scapula M87.01- ☑
    skull M87.08
    tarsus M87.07- ☑
    tibia M87.06- ☑
    toe M87.07- ☑
    ulna M87.03- ☑
    vertebra M87.08
  secondary NEC M87.30
    carpus M87.33- ☑
    clavicle M87.31- ☑
    due to
      drugs M87.10
        carpus M87.13- ☑
        clavicle M87.11- ☑
        femur M87.15- ☑
        fibula M87.16- ☑
        finger M87.14- ☑
        humerus M87.12- ☑
        ilium M87.159
        ischium M87.159
        jaw M87.180
        metacarpus M87.14- ☑
        metatarsus M87.17- ☑
        multiple sites M87.19
        neck M87.18 ☑
        radius M87.13- ☑
        rib M87.18 ☑
        scapula M87.11- ☑
        skull M87.18 ☑
        tarsus M87.17- ☑
        tibia M87.16- ☑
        toe M87.17- ☑
        ulna M87.13- ☑
        vertebra M87.18 ☑
      hemoglobinopathy NEC D58.2 *[M90.50]*
        carpus D58.2 *[M90.54-]*
        clavicle D58.2 *[M90.51-]*
        femur D58.2 *[M90.55-]*
        fibula D58.2 *[M90.56-]*
        finger D58.2 *[M90.54-]*
        humerus D58.2 *[M90.52-]*
        ilium D58.2 *[M90.55-]*
        ischium D58.2 *[M90.55-]*
        metacarpus D58.2 *[M90.54-]*
        metatarsus D58.2 *[M90.57-]*

Osteonecrosis — *continued*
  secondary — *continued*
    due to — *continued*
      hemoglobinopathy — *continued*
        multiple sites D58.2 *[M90.58]*
        neck D58.2 *[M90.58]*
        radius D58.2 *[M90.53-]*
        rib D58.2 *[M90.58]*
        scapula D58.2 *[M90.51-]*
        skull D58.2 *[M90.58]*
        tarsus D58.2 *[M90.57-]*
        tibia D58.2 *[M90.56-]*
        toe D58.2 *[M90.57-]*
        ulna D58.2 *[M90.53-]*
        vertebra D58.2 *[M90.58]*
      trauma (previous) M87.20
        carpus M87.23- ☑
        clavicle M87.21- ☑
        femur M87.25- ☑
        fibula M87.26- ☑
        finger M87.24- ☑
        humerus M87.22- ☑
        ilium M87.25- ☑
        ischium M87.25- ☑
        metacarpus M87.24- ☑
        metatarsus M87.27- ☑
        multiple sites M87.29
        neck M87.28
        radius M87.23- ☑
        rib M87.28
        scapula M87.21- ☑
        skull M87.28
        tarsus M87.27- ☑
        tibia M87.26- ☑
        toe M87.27- ☑
        ulna M87.23- ☑
        vertebra M87.28
    femur M87.35- ☑
    fibula M87.36- ☑
    finger M87.34- ☑
    humerus M87.32- ☑
    ilium M87.350
    in
      caisson disease T70.3 ☑ *[M90.50]*
        carpus T70.3 ☑ *[M90.54-]*
        clavicle T70.3 ☑ *[M90.51-]*
        femur T70.3 ☑ *[M90.55-]*
        fibula T70.3 ☑ *[M90.56-]*
        finger T70.3 ☑ *[M90.54-]*
        humerus T70.3 ☑ *[M90.52-]*
        ilium T70.3 ☑ *[M90.55-]*
        ischium T70.3 ☑ *[M90.55-]*
        metacarpus T70.3 ☑ *[M90.54-]*
        metatarsus T70.3 ☑ *[M90.57-]*
        multiple sites T70.3 ☑ *[M90.59]*
        neck T70.3 ☑ *[M90.58]*
        radius T70.3 ☑ *[M90.53-]*
        rib T70.3 ☑ *[M90.58]*
        scapula T70.3 ☑ *[M90.51-]*
        skull T70.3 ☑ *[M90.58]*
        tarsus T70.3 ☑ *[M90.57-]*
        tibia T70.3 ☑ *[M90.56-]*
        toe T70.3 ☑ *[M90.57-]*
        ulna T70.3 ☑ *[M90.53-]*
        vertebra T70.3 ☑ *[M90.58]*
    ischium M87.350
    metacarpus M87.34- ☑
    metatarsus M87.37- ☑
    multiple site M87.39
    neck M87.38
    radius M87.33- ☑
    rib M87.38
    scapula M87.319
    skull M87.38
    tarsus M87.379
    tibia M87.366
    toe M87.379
    ulna M87.33- ☑
    vertebra M87.38
  specified type NEC M87.80
    carpus M87.83- ☑
    clavicle M87.81- ☑
    femur M87.85- ☑
    fibula M87.86- ☑
    finger M87.84- ☑
    humerus M87.82- ☑

Osteonecrosis — *continued*
  specified type — *continued*
    ilium M87.85- ☑
    ischium M87.85- ☑
    metacarpus M87.84- ☑
    metatarsus M87.87- ☑
    multiple sites M87.89
    neck M87.88
    radius M87.83- ☑
    rib M87.88
    scapula M87.81- ☑
    skull M87.88
    tarsus M87.87- ☑
    tibia M87.86- ☑
    toe M87.87- ☑
    ulna M87.83- ☑
    vertebra M87.88
Osteo-onycho-arthro-dysplasia Q87.2
Osteo-onychodysplasia, hereditary Q87.2
Osteopathia condensans disseminata Q78.8
Osteopathy — *see also* Osteomyelitis, Osteonecrosis, Osteoporosis
  after poliomyelitis M89.60
    carpus M89.64- ☑
    clavicle M89.61- ☑
    femur M89.65- ☑
    fibula M89.66- ☑
    finger M89.64- ☑
    humerus M89.62- ☑
    ilium M89.659
    ischium M89.659
    metacarpus M89.64- ☑
    metatarsus M89.67- ☑
    multiple sites M89.69
    neck M89.68
    radius M89.63- ☑
    rib M89.68
    scapula M89.61- ☑
    skull M89.68
    tarsus M89.67- ☑
    tibia M89.66- ☑
    toe M89.67- ☑
    ulna M89.63- ☑
    vertebra M89.68
  in (due to)
    renal osteodystrophy N25.0
    specified diseases classified elsewhere — *see* subcategory M90.8 ☑
Osteopenia M85.8- ☑
  borderline M85.8- ☑
Osteoperiostitis — *see* Osteomyelitis, specified type NEC
Osteopetrosis (familial) Q78.2
Osteophyte M25.70
  ankle M25.77- ☑
  elbow M25.72- ☑
  foot joint M25.77- ☑
  hand joint M25.74- ☑
  hip M25.75- ☑
  knee M25.76- ☑
  shoulder M25.71- ☑
  spine M25.78
  vertebrae M25.78
  wrist M25.73- ☑
Osteopoikilosis Q78.8
Osteoporosis (female) (male) M81.0
  with current pathological fracture M80.00 ☑
  age-related M81.0
    with current pathologic fracture M80.00 ☑
      carpus M80.04- ☑
      clavicle M80.01- ☑
      fibula M80.06- ☑
      finger M80.04- ☑
      humerus M80.02- ☑
      ilium M80.05- ☑
      ischium M80.05- ☑
      metacarpus M80.04- ☑
      metatarsus M80.07- ☑
      pelvis M80.05- ☑
      radius M80.03- ☑
      scapula M80.01- ☑
      tarsus M80.07- ☑
      tibia M80.06- ☑
      toe M80.07- ☑
      ulna M80.03- ☑
      vertebra M80.08 ☑

Osteoporosis — *continued*
  disuse M81.8
    with current pathological fracture M80.80 ☑
      carpus M80.84- ☑
      clavicle M80.81- ☑
      fibula M80.86- ☑
      finger M80.84- ☑
      humerus M80.82- ☑
      ilium M80.85- ☑
      ischium M80.85- ☑
      metacarpus M80.84- ☑
      metatarsus M80.87- ☑
      pelvis M80.85- ☑
      radius M80.83- ☑
      scapula M80.81- ☑
      tarsus M80.87- ☑
      tibia M80.86- ☑
      toe M80.87- ☑
      ulna M80.83- ☑
      vertebra M80.88 ☑
  drug-induced — *see* Osteoporosis, specified type NEC
  idiopathic — *see* Osteoporosis, specified type NEC
  involutional — *see* Osteoporosis, age-related
  Lequesne M81.6
  localized M81.6
  postmenopausal M81.0
    with pathological fracture M80.00 ☑
      carpus M80.04- ☑
      clavicle M80.01- ☑
      fibula M80.06- ☑
      finger M80.04- ☑
      humerus M80.02- ☑
      ilium M80.05- ☑
      ischium M80.05- ☑
      metacarpus M80.04- ☑
      metatarsus M80.07- ☑
      pelvis M80.05- ☑
      radius M80.03- ☑
      scapula M80.01- ☑
      tarsus M80.07- ☑
      tibia M80.06- ☑
      toe M80.07- ☑
      ulna M80.03- ☑
      vertebra M80.08 ☑
  postoophorectomy — *see* Osteoporosis, specified type NEC
  postsurgical malabsorption — *see* Osteoporosis, specified type NEC
  post-traumatic — *see* Osteoporosis, specified type NEC
  senile — *see* Osteoporosis, age-related
  specified type NEC M81.8
    with pathological fracture M80.80 ☑
      carpus M80.84- ☑
      clavicle M80.81- ☑
      fibula M80.86- ☑
      finger M80.84- ☑
      humerus M80.82- ☑
      ilium M80.85- ☑
      ischium M80.85- ☑
      metacarpus M80.84- ☑
      metatarsus M80.87- ☑
      pelvis M80.85- ☑
      radius M80.83- ☑
      scapula M80.81- ☑
      tarsus M80.87- ☑
      tibia M80.86- ☑
      toe M80.87- ☑
      ulna M80.83- ☑
      vertebra M80.88 ☑
Osteopsathyrosis (idiopathica) Q78.0
Osteoradionecrosis, jaw (acute) (chronic) (lower) (suppurative) (upper) M27.2
Osteosarcoma (any form) — *see* Neoplasm, bone, malignant
Osteosclerosis Q78.2
  acquired M85.8- ☑
  congenita Q77.4
  fragilitas (generalisata) Q78.2
  myelofibrosis D75.81
Osteosclerotic anemia D64.89
Osteosis
  cutis L94.2
  renal fibrocystic N25.0
Osterreicher-Turner syndrome Q87.2
Ostium
  atrioventriculare commune Q21.2

Ostium — *continued*
  primum (arteriosum) (defect) (persistent) Q21.2
  secundum (arteriosum) (defect) (patent) (persistent) Q21.1
Ostrum-Furst syndrome Q75.8
Otalgia H92.0
Otitis (acute) H66.90
  with effusion — *see also* Otitis, media, nonsuppurative
    purulent — *see* Otitis, media, suppurative
  adhesive — *see* subcategory H74.1
  chronic — *see also* Otitis, media, chronic
    with effusion — *see also* Otitis, media, nonsuppurative, chronic
  externa H60.9-
    abscess — *see* Abscess, ear, external
    acute (noninfective) H60.50- ☑
      actinic H60.51- ☑
      chemical H60.52- ☑
      contact H60.53- ☑
      eczematoid H60.54- ☑
      infective — *see* Otitis, externa, infective
      reactive H60.55- ☑
      specified NEC H60.59- ☑
    cellulitis — *see* Cellulitis, ear
    chronic H60.6- ☑
    diffuse — *see* Otitis, externa, infective, diffuse
    hemorrhagic — *see* Otitis, externa, infective, hemorrhagic
    in (due to)
      aspergillosis B44.89
      candidiasis B37.84
      erysipelas A46 *[H62.40]*
      herpes (simplex) virus infection B00.1
        zoster B02.8
      impetigo L01.00 *[H62.40]*
      infectious disease NEC B99 ☑ *[H62.4-]* ☑
      mycosis NEC B36.9 *[H62.40]*
      parasitic disease NEC B89 *[H62.40]*
      viral disease NEC B34.9 *[H62.40]*
      zoster B02.8
    infective NEC H60.39- ☑
      abscess — *see* Abscess, ear, external
      cellulitis — *see* Cellulitis, ear
      diffuse H60.31- ☑
      hemorrhagic H60.32- ☑
      swimmer's ear — *see* Swimmer's, ear
    malignant H60.2- ☑
    mycotic NEC B36.9 *[H62.40]*
      in
        aspergillosis B44.89
        candidiasis B37.84
        moniliasis B37.84
    necrotizing — *see* Otitis, externa, malignant
    Pseudomonas aeruginosa — *see* Otitis, externa, malignant
    reactive — *see* Otitis, externa, acute, reactive
    specified NEC — *see* subcategory H60.8 ☑
    tropical NEC B36.9 *[H62.40]*
      in
        aspergillosis B44.89
        candidiasis B37.84
        moniliasis B37.84
  insidiosa — *see* Otosclerosis
  interna H83.0 ☑
  media (hemorrhagic) (staphylococcal) (streptococcal) H66.9- ☑
    with effusion (nonpurulent) — *see* Otitis, media, nonsuppurative
    acute, subacute H66.90
      allergic — *see* Otitis, media, nonsuppurative, acute, allergic
      exudative — *see* Otitis, media, suppurative, acute
      mucoid — *see* Otitis, media, nonsuppurative, acute
      necrotizing — *see also* Otitis, media, suppurative, acute
        in
          measles B05.3
          scarlet fever A38.0
      nonsuppurative NEC — *see* Otitis, media, nonsuppurative, acute
      purulent — *see* Otitis, media, suppurative, acute
      sanguinous — *see* Otitis, media, nonsuppurative, acute
      secretory — *see* Otitis, media, nonsuppurative, acute, serous

Otitis — *continued*
  media — *continued*
    acute, subacute — *continued*
      seromucinous — *see* Otitis, media, nonsuppurative, acute
      serous — *see* Otitis, media, nonsuppurative, acute, serous
      suppurative — *see* Otitis, media, suppurative, acute
    allergic — *see* Otitis, media, nonsuppurative
    catarrhal — *see* Otitis, media, nonsuppurative
    chronic H66.90
      with effusion (nonpurulent) — *see* Otitis, media, nonsuppurative, chronic
      allergic — *see* Otitis, media, nonsuppurative, chronic, allergic
      benign suppurative — *see* Otitis, media, suppurative, chronic, tubotympanic
      catarrhal — *see* Otitis, media, nonsuppurative, chronic, serous
      exudative — *see* Otitis, media, nonsuppurative, chronic
      mucinous — *see* Otitis, media, nonsuppurative, chronic, mucoid
      mucoid — *see* Otitis, media, nonsuppurative, chronic, mucoid
      nonsuppurative NEC — *see* Otitis, media, nonsuppurative, chronic
      purulent — *see* Otitis, media, suppurative, chronic
      secretory — *see* Otitis, media, nonsuppurative, chronic, mucoid
      seromucinous — *see* Otitis, media, nonsuppurative, chronic
      serous — *see* Otitis, media, nonsuppurative, chronic, serous
      suppurative — *see* Otitis, media, suppurative, chronic
      transudative — *see* Otitis, media, nonsuppurative, chronic, mucoid
    exudative — *see* Otitis, media, suppurative
    in (due to) (with)
      influenza — *see* Influenza, with, otitis media
      measles B05.3
      scarlet fever A38.0
      tuberculosis A18.6
      viral disease NEC B34.- ☑ *[H67.-]* ☑
    mucoid — *see* Otitis, media, nonsuppurative
    nonsuppurative H65.9- ☑
      acute or subacute NEC H65.19- ☑
        allergic H65.11- ☑
          recurrent H65.11- ☑
        recurrent H65.19- ☑
        secretory — *see* Otitis, media, nonsuppurative, serous
        serous H65.0- ☑
          recurrent H65.0- ☑
      chronic H65.49- ☑
        allergic H65.41- ☑
        mucoid H65.3- ☑
        serous H65.2- ☑
    postmeasles B05.3
    purulent — *see* Otitis, media, suppurative
    secretory — *see* Otitis, media, nonsuppurative
    seromucinous — *see* Otitis, media, nonsuppurative
    serous — *see* Otitis, media, nonsuppurative
    suppurative H66.4- ☑
      acute H66.00- ☑
        with rupture of ear drum H66.01- ☑
        recurrent H66.00- ☑
          with rupture of ear drum H66.01- ☑
      chronic — *see also* subcategory H66.3 ☑
        atticoantral H66.2- ☑
        benign — *see* Otitis, media, suppurative, chronic, tubotympanic
        tubotympanic H66.1- ☑
      transudative — *see* Otitis, media, nonsuppurative
      tuberculous A18.6
Otocephaly Q18.2
Otolith syndrome — *see* subcategory H81.8 ☑
Otomycosis (diffuse) **NEC** B36.9 *[H62.40]*
  in
    aspergillosis B44.89
    candidiasis B37.84
    moniliasis B37.84
Otoporosis — *see* Otosclerosis
Otorrhagia (nontraumatic) H92.2- ☑

✎ **Subterms under main terms may continue to next column or page**   ☑ **Additional Character Required — Refer to the Tabular List for Character Selection**   243

Osteoporosis — Otorrhagia

Otorrhagia — *continued*
  traumatic — *code by* Type of injury
Otorrhea H92.1- ☑
  cerebrospinal G96.0
Otosclerosis (general) H80.9- ☑
  cochlear (endosteal) H80.2- ☑
  involving
    otic capsule — *see* Otosclerosis, cochlear
    oval window
      nonobliterative H80.0- ☑
      obliterative H80.1- ☑
    round window — *see* Otosclerosis, cochlear
    nonobliterative — *see* Otosclerosis, involving, oval
      window, nonobliterative
    obliterative — *see* Otosclerosis, involving, oval window,
      obliterative
  specified NEC H80.8- ☑
Otospongiosis — *see* Otosclerosis
Otto's disease or pelvis M24.7
Outcome of delivery Z37.9
  multiple births Z37.9
    all liveborn Z37.50
      quadruplets Z37.52
      quintuplets Z37.53
      sextuplets Z37.54
      specified number NEC Z37.59
      triplets Z37.51
    all stillborn Z37.7
    some liveborn Z37.60
      quadruplets Z37.62
      quintuplets Z37.63
      sextuplets Z37.64
      specified number NEC Z37.69
      triplets Z37.61
  single NEC Z37.9
    liveborn Z37.0
    stillborn Z37.1
  twins NEC Z37.9
    both liveborn Z37.2
    both stillborn Z37.4
    one liveborn, one stillborn Z37.3
Outlet — *see* condition
Ovalocytosis (congenital) (hereditary) — *see* Elliptocytosis
Ovarian — *see* Condition
Ovariocele N83.4- ☑
Ovaritis (cystic) — *see* Oophoritis
Ovary, ovarian — *see also* condition
  resistant syndrome E28.39
  vein syndrome N13.8
Overactive — *see also* Hyperfunction
  adrenal cortex NEC E27.0
  bladder N32.81
  hypothalamus E23.3
  thyroid — *see* Hyperthyroidism
Overactivity R46.3
  child — *see* Disorder, attention-deficit hyperactivity
Overbite (deep) (excessive) (horizontal) (vertical) M26.29
Overbreathing — *see* Hyperventilation
Overconscientious personality F60.5
Overdevelopment — *see* Hypertrophy
Overdistension — *see* Distension
Overdose, overdosage (drug) — *see* Table of Drugs and
  Chemicals, by drug, poisoning
Overeating R63.2
  nonorganic origin F50.89
  psychogenic F50.89
Overexertion (effects) (exhaustion) T73.3 ☑
Overexposure (effects) T73.9 ☑
  exhaustion T73.2 ☑
Overfeeding — *see* Overeating
  newborn P92.4
Overfill, endodontic M27.52
Overgrowth, bone — *see* Hypertrophy, bone
Overhanging of dental restorative material (unre-
  pairable) K08.52
Overheated (places) (effects) — *see* Heat
Overjet (excessive horizontal) M26.23
Overlaid, overlying (suffocation) — *see* Asphyxia, trau-
  matic, due to mechanical threat
Overlap, excessive horizontal (teeth) M26.23
Overlapping toe (acquired) — *see also* Deformity, toe,
  specified NEC
  congenital (fifth toe) Q66.89
Overload
  circulatory, due to transfusion (blood) (blood compo-
    nents) (TACO) E87.71

Overload — *continued*
  fluid E87.70
    due to transfusion (blood) (blood components)
      E87.71
    specified NEC E87.79
  iron, due to repeated red blood cell transfusions
    E83.111
  potassium (K) E87.5
  sodium (Na) E87.0
Overnutrition — *see* Hyperalimentation
Overproduction — *see also* Hypersecretion
  ACTH E27.0
  catecholamine E27.5
  growth hormone E22.0
Overprotection, child by parent Z62.1
Overriding
  aorta Q25.49
  finger (acquired) — *see* Deformity, finger
    congenital Q68.1
  toe (acquired) — *see also* Deformity, toe, specified NEC
    congenital Q66.89
Overstrained R53.83
  heart — *see* Hypertrophy, cardiac
Overuse, muscle NEC M70.8- ☑
Overweight E66.3
Overworked R53.83
Oviduct — *see* condition
Ovotestis Q56.0
Ovulation (cycle)
  failure or lack of N97.0
  pain N94.0
Ovum — *see* condition
Owren's disease or syndrome (parahemophilia) D68.2
Ox heart — *see* Hypertrophy, cardiac
Oxalosis E72.53
Oxaluria E72.53
Oxycephaly, oxycephalic Q75.0
  syphilitic, congenital A50.02
Oxyuriasis B80
Oxyuris vermicularis (infestation) B80
Ozena J31.0

P

Pachyderma, pachydermia L85.9
  larynx (verrucosa) J38.7
Pachydermatocele (congenital) Q82.8
Pachydermoperiostosis — *see also* Osteoarthropathy,
  hypertrophic, specified type NEC
  clubbed nail M89.40 *[L62]*
Pachygyria Q04.3
Pachymeningitis (adhesive) (basal) (brain) (cervical)
  (chronic)(circumscribed) (external) (fibrous) (hemorrhagic) (hypertrophic) (internal) (purulent) (spinal)
  (suppurative) — *see* Meningitis
Pachyonychia (congenital) Q84.5
Pacinian tumor — *see* Neoplasm, skin, benign
Pad, knuckle or Garrod's M72.1
Paget's disease
  with infiltrating duct carcinoma — *see* Neoplasm,
    breast, malignant
  bone M88.9
    carpus M88.84- ☑
    clavicle M88.81- ☑
    femur M88.85- ☑
    fibula M88.86- ☑
    finger M88.84- ☑
    humerus M88.82- ☑
    ilium M88.85- ☑
    in neoplastic disease — *see* Osteitis, deformans, in
      neoplastic disease
    ischium M88.85- ☑
    metacarpus M88.84- ☑
    metatarsus M88.87- ☑
    multiple sites M88.89
    neck M88.88
    radius M88.83- ☑
    rib M88.88
    scapula M88.81- ☑
    skull M88.0
    specified NEC M88.88
    tarsus M88.87- ☑
    tibia M88.86- ☑
    toe M88.87- ☑
    ulna M88.83- ☑
    vertebra M88.1
  breast (female) C50.01- ☑

Paget's disease — *continued*
  breast — *continued*
    male C50.02- ☑
  extramammary — *see also* Neoplasm, skin, malignant
    anus C21.0
    margin C44.590
    skin C44.590
  intraductal carcinoma — *see* Neoplasm, breast, malig-
    nant
  malignant — *see* Neoplasm, skin, malignant
    breast (female) C50.01- ☑
      male C50.02- ☑
    unspecified site (female) C50.01- ☑
      male C50.02- ☑
  mammary — *see* Paget's disease, breast
  nipple — *see* Paget's disease, breast
  osteitis deformans — *see* Paget's disease, bone
Paget-Schroetter syndrome I82.890
Pain(s) — *see also* Painful R52
  abdominal R10.9
    colic R10.83
    generalized R10.84
      with acute abdomen R10.0
    lower R10.30
      left quadrant R10.32
      pelvic or perineal R10.2
      periumbilical R10.33
      right quadrant R10.31
    rebound — *see* Tenderness, abdominal, rebound
    severe with abdominal rigidity R10.0
    tenderness — *see* Tenderness, abdominal
    upper R10.10
      epigastric R10.13
      left quadrant R10.12
      right quadrant R10.11
  acute R52
    due to trauma G89.11
    neoplasm related G89.3
    postprocedural NEC G89.18
    post-thoracotomy G89.12
    specified by site — *code to* Pain, by site
  adnexa (uteri) R10.2
  anginoid — *see* Pain, precordial
  anus K62.89
  arm — *see* Pain, limb, upper
  axillary (axilla) M79.62- ☑
  back (postural) M54.9
  bladder R39.89
    associated with micturition — *see* Micturition,
      painful
    chronic R39.82
  bone — *see* Disorder, bone, specified type NEC
  breast N64.4
  broad ligament R10.2
  cancer associated (acute) (chronic) G89.3
  cecum — *see* Pain, abdominal
  cervicobrachial M53.1
  chest (central) R07.9
    anterior wall R07.89
    atypical R07.89
    ischemic I20.9
    musculoskeletal R07.89
    non-cardiac R07.89
    on breathing R07.1
    pleurodynia R07.81
    precordial R07.2
    wall (anterior) R07.89
  chronic G89.29
    associated with significant psychosocial dysfunction
      G89.4
    due to trauma G89.21
    neoplasm related G89.3
    postoperative NEC G89.28
    postprocedural NEC G89.28
    post-thoracotomy G89.22
    specified NEC G89.29
  coccyx M53.3
  colon — *see* Pain, abdominal
  coronary — *see* Angina
  costochondral R07.1
  diaphragm R07.1
  due to cancer G89.3
  due to device, implant or graft — *see also* Complica-
    tions, by site and type, specified NEC T85.848 ☑
    arterial graft NEC T82.848 ☑
    breast (implant) T85.848 ☑
    catheter NEC T85.848 ☑
      dialysis (renal) T82.848 ☑

Pain(s) — *continued*
  due to device, implant or graft — *see also* Complications, by site and type, specified — *continued*
    catheter — *continued*
      dialysis — *continued*
        intraperitoneal T85.848 ☑
      infusion NEC T82.848 ☑
        spinal (epidural) (subdural) T85.840 ☑
      urinary (indwelling) T83.84 ☑
    electronic (electrode) (pulse generator) (stimulator)
      bone T85.840 ☑
      cardiac T82.847 ☑
      nervous system (brain) (peripheral nerve) (spinal) T85.84 ☑
      urinary T83.84 ☑
    fixation, internal (orthopedic) NEC T84.84 ☑
    gastrointestinal (bile duct) (esophagus) T85.848 ☑
    genital NEC T83.84 ☑
    heart NEC T82.847 ☑
    infusion NEC T85.848 ☑
    joint prosthesis T84.84 ☑
    ocular (corneal graft) (orbital implant) NEC T85.848 ☑
    orthopedic NEC T84.84 ☑
    specified NEC T85.848 ☑
    urinary NEC T83.84 ☑
    vascular NEC T82.848 ☑
    ventricular intracranial shunt T85.840 ☑
  due to malignancy (primary) (secondary) G89.3
  ear — *see* subcategory H92.0 ☑
  epigastric, epigastrium R10.13
  eye — *see* Pain, ocular
  face, facial R51
    atypical G50.1
  female genital organs NEC N94.89
  finger — *see* Pain, limb, upper
  flank — *see* Pain, abdominal
  foot — *see* Pain, limb, lower
  gallbladder K82.9
  gas (intestinal) R14.1
  gastric — *see* Pain, abdominal
  generalized NOS R52
  genital organ
    female N94.89
    male N50.89
  groin — *see* Pain, abdominal, lower
  hand — *see* Pain, limb, upper
  head — *see* Headache
  heart — *see* Pain, precordial
  infra-orbital — *see* Neuralgia, trigeminal
  intercostal R07.82
  intermenstrual N94.0
  jaw R68.84
  joint M25.50
    ankle M25.57- ☑
    elbow M25.52- ☑
    finger M25.54- ☑
    foot M25.57- ☑
    hand M25.54- ☑
    hip M25.55- ☑
    knee M25.56- ☑
    shoulder M25.51- ☑
    toe M25.57- ☑
    wrist M25.53- ☑
  kidney N23
  laryngeal R07.0
  leg — *see* Pain, limb, lower
  limb M79.609
    lower M79.60- ☑
      foot M79.67- ☑
      lower leg M79.66- ☑
      thigh M79.65- ☑
      toe M79.67- ☑
    upper M79.60- ☑
      axilla M79.62- ☑
      finger M79.64- ☑
      forearm M79.63- ☑
      hand M79.64- ☑
      upper arm M79.62- ☑
  loin M54.5
  low back M54.5
  lumbar region M54.5
  mandibular R68.84
  mastoid — *see* subcategory H92.0 ☑
  maxilla R68.84
  menstrual — *see also* Dysmenorrhea N94.6
  metacarpophalangeal (joint) — *see* Pain, joint, hand

Pain(s) — *continued*
  metatarsophalangeal (joint) — *see* Pain, joint, foot
  mouth K13.79
  muscle — *see* Myalgia
  musculoskeletal — *see also* Pain, by site M79.18
  myofascial M79.18
  nasal J34.89
  nasopharynx J39.2
  neck NEC M54.2
  nerve NEC — *see* Neuralgia
  neuromuscular — *see* Neuralgia
  nose J34.89
  ocular H57.1- ☑
  ophthalmic — *see* Pain, ocular
  orbital region — *see* Pain, ocular
  ovary N94.89
  over heart — *see* Pain, precordial
  ovulation N94.0
  pelvic (female) R10.2
  penis N48.89
  pericardial — *see* Pain, precordial
  perineal, perineum R10.2
  pharynx J39.2
  pleura, pleural, pleuritic R07.81
  postoperative NOS G89.18
  postprocedural NOS G89.18
  post-thoracotomy G89.12
  precordial (region) R07.2
  premenstrual N94.3
  psychogenic (persistent) (any site) F45.41
  radicular (spinal) — *see* Radiculopathy
  rectum K62.89
  respiration R07.1
  retrosternal R07.2
  rheumatoid, muscular — *see* Myalgia
  rib R07.81
  root (spinal) — *see* Radiculopathy
  round ligament (stretch) R10.2
  sacroiliac M53.3
  sciatic — *see* Sciatica
  scrotum N50.82
  seminal vesicle N50.89
  shoulder M25.51- ☑
  spermatic cord N50.89
  spinal root — *see* Radiculopathy
  spine M54.9
    cervical M54.2
    low back M54.5
      with sciatica M54.4- ☑
    thoracic M54.6
  stomach — *see* Pain, abdominal
  substernal R07.2
  temporomandibular (joint) M26.62- ☑
  testis N50.81- ☑
  thoracic spine M54.6
    with radicular and visceral pain M54.14
  throat R07.0
  tibia — *see* Pain, limb, lower
  toe — *see* Pain, limb, lower
  tongue K14.6
  tooth K08.89
  trigeminal — *see* Neuralgia, trigeminal
  tumor associated G89.3
  ureter N23
  urinary (organ) (system) N23
  uterus NEC N94.89
  vagina R10.2
  vertebrogenic (syndrome) M54.89
  vesical R39.89
    associated with micturition — *see* Micturition, painful
  vulva R10.2
Painful — *see also* Pain
  coitus
    female N94.10
    male N53.12
    psychogenic F52.6
  ejaculation (semen) N53.12
    psychogenic F52.6
  erection — *see* Priapism
  feet syndrome E53.8
  joint replacement (hip) (knee) T84.84 ☑
  menstruation — *see* Dysmenorrhea
    psychogenic F45.8
  micturition — *see* Micturition, painful
  respiration R07.1
  scar NEC L90.5
  wire sutures T81.89 ☑

Painter's colic — *see* subcategory T56.0 ☑
Palate — *see* condition
Palatoplegia K13.79
Palatoschisis — *see* Cleft, palate
Palilalia R48.8
Palliative care Z51.5
Pallor R23.1
  optic disc, temporal — *see* Atrophy, optic
Palmar — *see also* condition
  fascia — *see* condition
Palpable
  cecum K63.89
  kidney N28.89
  ovary N83.8
  prostate N42.9
  spleen — *see* Splenomegaly
Palpitations (heart) R00.2
  psychogenic F45.8
Palsy — *see also* Paralysis G83.9
  atrophic diffuse (progressive) G12.22
  Bell's — *see also* Palsy, facial
    newborn P11.3
  brachial plexus NEC G54.0
    newborn (birth injury) P14.3
  brain — *see* Palsy, cerebral
  bulbar (progressive) (chronic) G12.22
    of childhood (Fazio-Londe) G12.1
    pseudo NEC G12.29
    supranuclear (progressive) G23.1
  cerebral (congenital) G80.9
    ataxic G80.4
    athetoid G80.3
    choreathetoid G80.3
    diplegic G80.8
      spastic G80.1
    dyskinetic G80.3
      athetoid G80.3
      choreathetoid G80.3
      distonic G80.3
    dystonic G80.3
    hemiplegic G80.8
      spastic G80.2
    mixed G80.8
    monoplegic G80.8
      spastic G80.1
    paraplegic G80.8
      spastic G80.1
    quadriplegic G80.8
      spastic G80.0
    spastic G80.1
      diplegic G80.1
      hemiplegic G80.2
      monoplegic G80.1
      quadriplegic G80.0
      specified NEC G80.1
      tetrapelgic G80.0
    specified NEC G80.8
    syphilitic A52.12
      congenital A50.49
    tetraplegic G80.8
      spastic G80.0
  cranial nerve — *see also* Disorder, nerve, cranial
    multiple G52.7
      in
        infectious disease B99 ☑ *[G53]*
        neoplastic disease — *see also* Neoplasm D49.9 *[G53]*
        parasitic disease B89 *[G53]*
        sarcoidosis D86.82
  creeping G12.22
  diver's T70.3 ☑
  Erb's P14.0
  facial G51.0
    newborn (birth injury) P11.3
  glossopharyngeal G52.1
  Klumpke (-Déjérine) P14.1
  lead — *see* subcategory T56.0 ☑
  median nerve (tardy) G56.1- ☑
  nerve G58.9
    specified NEC G58.8
  peroneal nerve (acute) (tardy) G57.3- ☑
  progressive supranuclear G23.1
  pseudobulbar NEC G12.29
  radial nerve (acute) G56.3- ☑
  seventh nerve — *see also* Palsy, facial
    newborn P11.3
  shaking — *see* Parkinsonism
  spastic (cerebral) (spinal) G80.1

Palsy — *continued*
  ulnar nerve (tardy) G56.2- ☑
  wasting G12.29
Paludism — *see* Malaria
Panangiitis M30.0
Panaris, panaritium — *see also* Cellulitis, digit
  with lymphangitis — *see* Lymphangitis, acute, digit
Panarteritis nodosa M30.0
  brain or cerebral I67.7
Pancake heart R93.1
  with cor pulmonale (chronic) I27.81
Pancarditis (acute) (chronic) I51.89
  rheumatic I09.89
    active or acute I01.8
Pancoast's syndrome or tumor C34.1- ☑
Pancolitis, ulcerative (chronic) K51.00
  with
    abscess K51.014
    complication K51.019
    fistula K51.013
    obstruction K51.012
    rectal bleeding K51.011
    specified complication NEC K51.018
Pancreas, pancreatic — *see* condition
Pancreatitis (annular) (apoplectic) (calcareous) (edematous) (hemorrhagic) (malignant) (recurrent) (subacute) (suppurative) K85.90
  with necrosis (uninfected) K85.91
    infected K85.92
  acute (without necrosis or infection) K85.90
    with necrosis (uninfected) K85.91
      infected K85.92
    alcohol induced (without necrosis or infection) K85.20
      with necrosis (uninfected) K85.21
        infected K85.22
    biliary (without necrosis or infection) K85.10
      with necrosis (uninfected) K85.11
        infected K85.12
    drug induced (without necrosis or infection) K85.30
      with necrosis (uninfected) K85.31
        infected K85.32
    gallstone (without necrosis or infection) K85.10
      with necrosis (uninfected) K85.11
        infected K85.12
    idiopathic (without necrosis or infection) K85.00
      with necrosis (uninfected) K85.01
        infected K85.02
    specified NEC (without necrosis or infection) K85.80
      with necrosis (uninfected) K85.81
        infected K85.82
  chronic (infectious) K86.1
    alcohol-induced K86.0
    recurrent K86.1
    relapsing K86.1
  cystic (chronic) K86.1
  cytomegaloviral B25.2
  fibrous (chronic) K86.1
  gallstone (without necrosis or infection) K85.10
    with necrosis (uninfected) K85.11
      infected K85.12
  gangrenous — *see* Pancreatitis, acute
  interstitial (chronic) K86.1
    acute — *see also* Pancreatitis, acute K85.80
  mumps B26.3
  recurrent (chronic) K86.1
  relapsing, chronic K86.1
  syphilitic A52.74
Pancreatoblastoma — *see* Neoplasm, pancreas, malignant
Pancreolithiasis K86.89
Pancytolysis D75.89
Pancytopenia (acquired) D61.818
  with
    malformations D61.09
    myelodysplastic syndrome — *see* Syndrome, myelodysplastic
  antineoplastic chemotherapy induced D61.810
  congenital D61.09
  drug-induced NEC D61.811
PANDAS (pediatric autoimmune neuropsychiatric disorders associated with streptococcal infections syndrome) D89.89
Panencephalitis, subacute, sclerosing A81.1
Panhematopenia D61.9
  congenital D61.09
  constitutional D61.09
  splenic, primary D73.1

Panhemocytopenia D61.9
  congenital D61.09
  constitutional D61.09
Panhypogonadism E29.1
Panhypopituitarism E23.0
  prepubertal E23.0
Panic (attack) (state) F41.0
  reaction to exceptional stress (transient) F43.0
Panmyelopathy, familial, constitutional D61.09
Panmyelophthisis D61.82
  congenital D61.09
Panmyelosis (acute) (with myelofibrosis) C94.4- ☑
Panner's disease — *see* Osteochondrosis, juvenile, humerus
Panneuritis endemica E51.11
Panniculitis (nodular) (nonsuppurative) M79.3
  back M54.00
    cervical region M54.02
    cervicothoracic region M54.03
    lumbar region M54.06
    lumbosacral region M54.07
    multiple sites M54.09
    occipito-atlanto-axial region M54.01
    sacrococcygeal region M54.08
    thoracic region M54.04
    thoracolumbar region M54.05
  lupus L93.2
  mesenteric K65.4
  neck M54.02
    cervicothoracic region M54.03
    occipito-atlanto-axial region M54.01
  relapsing M35.6
Panniculus adiposus (abdominal) E65
Pannus (allergic) (cornea) (degenerativus) (keratic) H16.42- ☑
  abdominal (symptomatic) E65
  trachomatosus, trachomatous (active) A71.1
Panophthalmitis H44.01- ☑
Pansinusitis (chronic) (hyperplastic) (nonpurulent) (purulent) J32.4
  acute J01.40
    recurrent J01.41
  tuberculous A15.8
Panuveitis (sympathetic) H44.11- ☑
Panvalvular disease I08.9
  specified NEC I08.8
PAPA (pyogenic arthritis, pyoderma gangrenosum, and acne syndrome) M04.8
Papanicolaou smear, cervix Z12.4
  as part of routine gynecological examination Z01.419
    with abnormal findings Z01.411
  for suspected neoplasm Z12.4
  nonspecific abnormal finding R87.619
  routine Z01.419
    with abnormal findings Z01.411
Papilledema (choked disc) H47.10
  associated with
    decreased ocular pressure H47.12
    increased intracranial pressure H47.11
    retinal disorder H47.13
  Foster-Kennedy syndrome H47.14- ☑
Papillitis H46.00
  anus K62.89
  chronic lingual K14.4
  necrotizing, kidney N17.2
  optic H46.0- ☑
  rectum K62.89
  renal, necrotizing N17.2
  tongue K14.0
Papilloma — *see also* Neoplasm, benign, by site
  acuminatum (female) (male) (anogenital) A63.0
  basal cell L82.1
    inflamed L82.0
  benign pinta (primary) A67.0
  bladder (urinary) (transitional cell) D41.4
  choroid plexus (lateral ventricle) (third ventricle) D33.0
    anaplastic C71.5
    fourth ventricle D33.1
    malignant C71.5
  renal pelvis (transitional cell) D41.1- ☑
    benign D30.1- ☑
  Schneiderian
    specified site — *see* Neoplasm, benign, by site
    unspecified site D14.0
  serous surface
    borderline malignancy
      specified site — *see* Neoplasm, uncertain behavior, by site

Papilloma — *continued*
  serous surface — *continued*
    borderline malignancy — *continued*
      unspecified site D39.10
    specified site — *see* Neoplasm, benign, by site
    unspecified site D27.9
  transitional (cell)
    bladder (urinary) D41.4
    inverted type — *see* Neoplasm, uncertain behavior, by site
    renal pelvis D41.1- ☑
    ureter D41.2- ☑
  ureter (transitional cell) D41.2- ☑
    benign D30.2- ☑
  urothelial — *see* Neoplasm, uncertain behavior, by site
  villous — *see* Neoplasm, uncertain behavior, by site
    adenocarcinoma in — *see* Neoplasm, malignant, by site
    in situ — *see* Neoplasm, in situ
  yaws, plantar or palmar A66.1
Papillomata, multiple, of yaws A66.1
Papillomatosis — *see also* Neoplasm, benign, by site
  confluent and reticulated L83
  cystic, breast — *see* Mastopathy, cystic
  ductal, breast — *see* Mastopathy, cystic
  intraductal (diffuse) — *see* Neoplasm, benign, by site
  subareolar duct D24- ☑
Papillomavirus, as cause of disease classified elsewhere B97.7
Papillon-Léage and Psaume syndrome Q87.0
Papule(s) R23.8
  carate (primary) A67.0
  fibrous, of nose D22.39
  Gottron's L94.4
  pinta (primary) A67.0
Papulosis
  lymphomatoid C86.6
  malignant I77.89
Papyraceous fetus O31.0- ☑
Para-albuminemia E88.09
Paracephalus Q89.7
Parachute mitral valve Q23.2
Paracoccidioidomycosis B41.9
  disseminated B41.7
  generalized B41.7
  mucocutaneous-lymphangitic B41.8
  pulmonary B41.0
  specified NEC B41.8
  visceral B41.8
Paradentosis K05.4
Paraffinoma T88.8 ☑
Paraganglioma D44.7
  adrenal D35.0- ☑
    malignant C74.1- ☑
  aortic body D44.7
    malignant C75.5
  carotid body D44.6
    malignant C75.4
  chromaffin — *see also* Neoplasm, benign, by site
    malignant — *see* Neoplasm, malignant, by site
  extra-adrenal D44.7
    malignant C75.5
      specified site — *see* Neoplasm, malignant, by site
      unspecified site C75.5
    specified site — *see* Neoplasm, uncertain behavior, by site
    unspecified site D44.7
  gangliocytic D13.2
    specified site — *see* Neoplasm, benign, by site
    unspecified site D13.2
  glomus jugulare D44.7
    malignant C75.5
  jugular D44.7
  malignant C75.5
    specified site — *see* Neoplasm, malignant, by site
    unspecified site C75.5
  nonchromaffin D44.7
    malignant C75.5
      specified site — *see* Neoplasm, malignant, by site
      unspecified site C75.5
    specified site — *see* Neoplasm, uncertain behavior, by site
    unspecified site D44.7
  parasympathetic D44.7

☑ **Additional Character Required — Refer to the Tabular List for Character Selection**   🔺 **Subterms under main terms may continue to next column or page**

Paraganglioma — *continued*
  parasympathetic — *continued*
    specified site — *see* Neoplasm, uncertain behavior, by site
    unspecified site D44.7
  specified site — *see* Neoplasm, uncertain behavior, by site
  sympathetic D44.7
    specified site — *see* Neoplasm, uncertain behavior, by site
    unspecified site D44.7
  unspecified site D44.7
Parageusia R43.2
  psychogenic F45.8
Paragonimiasis B66.4
Paragranuloma, Hodgkin — *see* Lymphoma, Hodgkin, specified NEC
Parahemophilia — *see also* Defect, coagulation D68.2
Parakeratosis R23.4
  variegata L41.0
Paralysis, paralytic (complete) (incomplete) G83.9
  with
    syphilis A52.17
  abducens, abducent (nerve) — *see* Strabismus, paralytic, sixth nerve
  abductor, lower extremity G57.9- ☑
  accessory nerve G52.8
  accommodation — *see also* Paresis, of accommodation
    hysterical F44.89
  acoustic nerve (except Deafness) H93.3 ☑
  agitans — *see also* Parkinsonism G20
    arteriosclerotic G21.4
  alternating (oculomotor) G83.89
  amyotrophic G12.21
  ankle G57.9- ☑
  anus (sphincter) K62.89
  arm — *see* Monoplegia, upper limb
  ascending (spinal), acute G61.0
  association G12.29
  asthenic bulbar G70.00
    with exacerbation (acute) G70.01
    in crisis G70.01
  ataxic (hereditary) G11.9
    general (syphilitic) A52.17
  atrophic G58.9
    infantile, acute — *see* Poliomyelitis, paralytic
    progressive G12.22
    spinal (acute) — *see* Poliomyelitis, paralytic
  axillary G54.0
  Babinski-Nageotte's G83.89
  Bell's G51.0
    newborn P11.3
  Benedikt's G46.3
  birth injury P14.9
    spinal cord P11.5
  bladder (neurogenic) (sphincter) N31.2
  bowel, colon or intestine K56.0
  brachial plexus G54.0
    birth injury P14.3
    newborn (birth injury) P14.3
  brain G83.9
    diplegia G83.0
    triplegia G83.89
  bronchial J98.09
  Brown-Séquard G83.81
  bulbar (chronic) (progressive) G12.22
    infantile — *see* Poliomyelitis, paralytic
    poliomyelitic — *see* Poliomyelitis, paralytic
    pseudo G12.29
  bulbospinal G70.00
    with exacerbation (acute) G70.01
    in crisis G70.01
  cardiac — *see also* Failure, heart I50.9
  cerebrocerebellar, diplegic G80.1
  cervical
    plexus G54.2
    sympathetic G90.09
  Céstan-Chenais G46.3
  Charcot-Marie-Tooth type G60.0
  Clark's G80.9
  colon K56.0
  compressed air T70.3 ☑
  compression
    arm G56.9- ☑
    leg G57.9- ☑
    lower extremity G57.9- ☑
    upper extremity G56.9- ☑
  congenital (cerebral) — *see* Palsy, cerebral

Paralysis, paralytic — *continued*
  conjugate movement (gaze) (of eye) H51.0
    cortical (nuclear) (supranuclear) H51.0
  cordis — *see* Failure, heart
  cranial or cerebral nerve G52.9
  creeping G12.22
  crossed leg G83.89
  crutch — *see* Injury, brachial plexus
  deglutition R13.0
    hysterical F44.4
  dementia A52.17
  descending (spinal) NEC G12.29
  diaphragm (flaccid) J98.6
    due to accidental dissection of phrenic nerve during procedure — *see* Puncture, accidental complicating surgery
  digestive organs NEC K59.8
  diplegic — *see* Diplegia
  divergence (nuclear) H51.8
  diver's T70.3 ☑
  Duchenne's
    birth injury P14.0
    due to or associated with
      motor neuron disease G12.22
      muscular dystrophy G71.01
  due to intracranial or spinal birth injury — *see* Palsy, cerebral
  embolic (current episode) I63.4- ☑
  Erb (-Duchenne) (birth) (newborn) P14.0
  Erb's syphilitic spastic spinal A52.17
  esophagus K22.8
  eye muscle (extrinsic) H49.9
    intrinsic — *see also* Paresis, of accommodation
  facial (nerve) G51.0
    birth injury P11.3
    congenital P11.3
    following operation NEC — *see* Puncture, accidental complicating surgery
    newborn (birth injury) P11.3
  familial (recurrent) (periodic) G72.3
    spastic G11.4
  fauces J39.2
  finger G56.9- ☑
  gait R26.1
  gastric nerve (nondiabetic) G52.2
  gaze, conjugate H51.0
  general (progressive) (syphilitic) A52.17
    juvenile A50.45
  glottis J38.00
    bilateral J38.02
    unilateral J38.01
  gluteal G54.1
  Gubler (-Millard) G46.3
  hand — *see* Monoplegia, upper limb
  heart — *see* Arrest, cardiac
  hemiplegic — *see* Hemiplegia
  hyperkalemic periodic (familial) G72.3
  hypoglossal (nerve) G52.3
  hypokalemic periodic G72.3
  hysterical F44.4
  ileus K56.0
  infantile — *see also* Poliomyelitis, paralytic A80.30
    bulbar — *see* Poliomyelitis, paralytic
    cerebral — *see* Palsy, cerebral
    spastic — *see* Palsy, cerebral, spastic
  infective — *see* Poliomyelitis, paralytic
  inferior nuclear G83.9
  internuclear — *see* Ophthalmoplegia, internuclear
  intestine K56.0
  iris H57.09
    due to diphtheria (toxin) A36.89
  ischemic, Volkmann's (complicating trauma) T79.6 ☑
  Jackson's G83.89
  jake — *see* Poisoning, food, noxious, plant
  Jamaica ginger (jake) G62.2
  juvenile general A50.45
  Klumpke (-Déjérine) (birth) (newborn) P14.1
  labioglossal (laryngeal) (pharyngeal) G12.29
  Landry's G61.0
  laryngeal nerve (recurrent) (superior) (unilateral) J38.00
    bilateral J38.02
    unilateral J38.01
  larynx J38.00
    bilateral J38.02
    due to diphtheria (toxin) A36.2
    unilateral J38.01
  lateral G12.23
  lead T56.0 ☑

Paralysis, paralytic — *continued*
  left side — *see* Hemiplegia
  leg G83.1- ☑
    both — *see* Paraplegia
    crossed G83.89
    hysterical F44.4
    psychogenic F44.4
    transient or transitory R29.818
      traumatic NEC — *see* Injury, nerve, leg
  levator palpebrae superioris — *see* Blepharoptosis, paralytic
  limb — *see* Monoplegia
  lip K13.0
  Lissauer's A52.17
  lower limb — *see* Monoplegia, lower limb
    both — *see* Paraplegia
  lung J98.4
  median nerve G56.1- ☑
  medullary (tegmental) G83.89
  mesencephalic NEC G83.89
    tegmental G83.89
  middle alternating G83.89
  Millard-Gubler-Foville G46.3
  monoplegic — *see* Monoplegia
  motor G83.9
  muscle, muscular NEC G72.89
    due to nerve lesion G58.9
    eye (extrinsic) H49.9
      intrinsic — *see* Paresis, of accommodation
      oblique — *see* Strabismus, paralytic, fourth nerve
    iris sphincter H21.9
    ischemic (Volkmann's) (complicating trauma) T79.6 ☑
    progressive G12.21
    progressive, spinal G12.25
    pseudohypertrophic G71.02
    spinal progressive G12.25
  musculocutaneous nerve G56.9- ☑
  musculospiral G56.9- ☑
  nerve — *see also* Disorder, nerve
    abducent — *see* Strabismus, paralytic, sixth nerve
    accessory G52.8
    auditory (except Deafness) H93.3 ☑
    birth injury P14.9
    cranial or cerebral G52.9
    facial G51.0
      birth injury P11.3
      congenital P11.3
      newborn (birth injury) P11.3
    fourth or trochlear — *see* Strabismus, paralytic, fourth nerve
    newborn (birth injury) P14.9
    oculomotor — *see* Strabismus, paralytic, third nerve
    phrenic (birth injury) P14.2
    radial G56.3- ☑
    seventh or facial G51.0
      newborn (birth injury) P11.3
    sixth or abducent — *see* Strabismus, paralytic, sixth nerve
    syphilitic A52.15
    third or oculomotor — *see* Strabismus, paralytic, third nerve
    trigeminal G50.9
    trochlear — *see* Strabismus, paralytic, fourth nerve
    ulnar G56.2- ☑
  normokalemic periodic G72.3
  ocular H49.9
    alternating G83.89
  oculofacial, congenital (Moebius) Q87.0
  oculomotor (external bilateral) (nerve) — *see* Strabismus, paralytic, third nerve
  palate (soft) K13.79
  paratrigeminal G50.9
  periodic (familial) (hyperkalemic) (hypokalemic) (myotonic) (normokalemic) (potassium sensitive) (secondary) G72.3
  peripheral autonomic nervous system — *see* Neuropathy, peripheral, autonomic
  peroneal (nerve) G57.3- ☑
  pharynx J39.2
  phrenic nerve G56.8- ☑
  plantar nerve(s) G57.6- ☑
  pneumogastric nerve G52.2
  poliomyelitis (current) — *see* Poliomyelitis, paralytic
  popliteal nerve G57.3- ☑
  postepileptic transitory G83.84
  progressive (atrophic) (bulbar) (spinal) G12.22
    general A52.17

Paralysis, paralytic — *continued*
- progressive — *continued*
  - infantile acute — *see* Poliomyelitis, paralytic
  - supranuclear G23.1
- pseudobulbar G12.29
- pseudohypertrophic (muscle) G71.09
- psychogenic F44.4
- quadriceps G57.9- ☑
- quadriplegic — *see* Tetraplegia
- radial nerve G56.3- ☑
- rectus muscle (eye) H49.9
- recurrent isolated sleep G47.53
- respiratory (muscle) (system) (tract) R06.81
  - center NEC G93.89
  - congenital P28.89
  - newborn P28.89
- right side — *see* Hemiplegia
- saturnine T56.0 ☑
- sciatic nerve G57.0- ☑
- senile G83.9
- shaking — *see* Parkinsonism
- shoulder G56.9- ☑
- sleep, recurrent isolated G47.53
- spastic G83.9
  - cerebral — *see* Palsy, cerebral, spastic
  - congenital (cerebral) — *see* Palsy, cerebral, spastic
  - familial G11.4
  - hereditary G11.4
  - quadriplegic G80.0
  - syphilitic (spinal) A52.17
- sphincter, bladder — *see* Paralysis, bladder
- spinal (cord) G83.9
  - accessory nerve G52.8
  - acute — *see* Poliomyelitis, paralytic
  - ascending acute G61.0
  - atrophic (acute) — *see also* Poliomyelitis, paralytic
    - spastic, syphilitic A52.17
  - congenital NEC — *see* Palsy, cerebral
  - hereditary G95.89
  - infantile — *see* Poliomyelitis, paralytic
  - progressive G12.21
    - muscle G12.25
  - sequelae NEC G83.89
- sternomastoid G52.8
- stomach K31.84
  - diabetic — *see* Diabetes, by type, with gastroparesis
  - nerve G52.2
    - diabetic — *see* Diabetes, by type, with gastro-paresis
- stroke — *see* Infarct, brain
- subcapsularis G56.8- ☑
- supranuclear (progressive) G23.1
- sympathetic G90.8
  - cervical G90.09
  - nervous system — *see* Neuropathy, peripheral, autonomic
- syndrome G83.9
  - specified NEC G83.89
- syphilitic spastic spinal (Erb's) A52.17
- thigh G57.9- ☑
- throat J39.2
  - diphtheritic A36.0
  - muscle J39.2
- thrombotic (current episode) I63.3- ☑
- thumb G56.9- ☑
- tick — *see* Toxicity, venom, arthropod, specified NEC
- Todd's (postepileptic transitory paralysis) G83.84
- toe G57.6- ☑
- tongue K14.8
- transient R29.5
  - arm or leg NEC R29.818
  - traumatic NEC — *see* Injury, nerve
- trapezius G52.8
- traumatic, transient NEC — *see* Injury, nerve
- trembling — *see* Parkinsonism
- triceps brachii G56.9- ☑
- trigeminal nerve G50.9
- trochlear (nerve) — *see* Strabismus, paralytic, fourth nerve
- ulnar nerve G56.2- ☑
- upper limb — *see* Monoplegia, upper limb
- uremic N18.9 *[G99.8]*
- uveoparotitic D86.89
- uvula K13.79
  - postdiphtheritic A36.0
- vagus nerve G52.2
- vasomotor NEC G90.8
- velum palati K13.79

Paralysis, paralytic — *continued*
- vesical — *see* Paralysis, bladder
- vestibular nerve (except Vertigo) H93.3 ☑
- vocal cords J38.00
  - bilateral J38.02
  - unilateral J38.01
- Volkmann's (complicating trauma) T79.6 ☑
- wasting G12.29
- Weber's G46.3
- wrist G56.9- ☑

Paramedial urethrovesical orifice Q64.79
Paramenia N92.6
Parametritis — *see also* Disease, pelvis, inflammatory N73.2
- acute N73.0
- complicating abortion — *see* Abortion, by type, complicated by, parametritis

Parametrium, parametric — *see* condition
Paramnesia — *see* Amnesia
Paramolar K00.1
Paramyloidosis E85.89
Paramyoclonus multiplex G25.3
Paramyotonia (congenita) G71.19
Parangi — *see* Yaws
Paranoia (querulans) F22
- senile F03 ☑

Paranoid
- dementia (senile) F03 ☑
  - praecox — *see* Schizophrenia
- personality F60.0
- psychosis (climacteric) (involutional) (menopausal) F22
  - psychogenic (acute) F23
  - senile F03 ☑
- reaction (acute) F23
  - chronic F22
- schizophrenia F20.0
- state (climacteric) (involutional) (menopausal) (simple) F22
  - senile F03 ☑
- tendencies F60.0
- traits F60.0
- trends F60.0
- type, psychopathic personality F60.0

Paraparesis — *see* Paraplegia
Paraphasia R47.02
Paraphilia F65.9
Paraphimosis (congenital) N47.2
- chancroidal A57
Paraphrenia, paraphrenic (late) F22
- schizophrenia F20.0
Paraplegia (lower) G82.20
- ataxic — *see* Degeneration, combined, spinal cord
- complete G82.21
- congenital (cerebral) G80.8
  - spastic G80.1
- familial spastic G11.4
- functional (hysterical) F44.4
- hereditary, spastic G11.4
- hysterical F44.4
- incomplete G82.22
- Pott's A18.01
- psychogenic F44.4
- spastic
  - Erb's spinal, syphilitic A52.17
  - hereditary G11.4
  - tropical G04.1
- syphilitic (spastic) A52.17
- traumatic
  - current injury — code to injury with seventh character A
  - sequela of previous injury — code to injury with seventh character S
  - tropical spastic G04.1
Parapoxvirus B08.60
- specified NEC B08.69
Paraproteinemia D89.2
- benign (familial) D89.2
- monoclonal D47.2
- secondary to malignant disease D47.2
Parapsoriasis L41.9
- en plaques L41.4
- guttata L41.1
- large plaque L41.4
- retiform, retiformis L41.5
- small plaque L41.3
- specified NEC L41.8
- varioliformis (acuta) L41.0
Parasitic — *see also* condition

Parasitic — *continued*
- disease NEC B89
- stomatitis B37.0
- sycosis (beard) (scalp) B35.0
- twin Q89.4
Parasitism B89
- intestinal B82.9
- skin B88.9
- specified — *see* Infestation
Parasitophobia F40.218
Parasomnia G47.50
- due to
  - alcohol
    - abuse F10.182
    - dependence F10.282
    - use F10.982
  - amphetamines
    - abuse F15.182
    - dependence F15.282
    - use F15.982
  - caffeine
    - abuse F15.182
    - dependence F15.282
    - use F15.982
  - cocaine
    - abuse F14.182
    - dependence F14.282
    - use F14.982
  - drug NEC
    - abuse F19.182
    - dependence F19.282
    - use F19.982
  - opioid
    - abuse F11.182
    - dependence F11.282
    - use F11.982
  - psychoactive substance NEC
    - abuse F19.182
    - dependence F19.282
    - use F19.982
  - sedative, hypnotic, or anxiolytic
    - abuse F13.182
    - dependence F13.282
    - use F13.982
  - stimulant NEC
    - abuse F15.182
    - dependence F15.282
    - use F15.982
- in conditions classified elsewhere G47.54
- nonorganic origin F51.8
- organic G47.50
- specified NEC G47.59
Paraspadias Q54.9
Paraspasmus facialis G51.8
Parasuicide (attempt)
- history of (personal) Z91.5
  - in family Z81.8
Parathyroid gland — *see* condition
Parathyroid tetany E20.9
Paratrachoma A74.0
Paratyphilitis — *see* Appendicitis
Paratyphoid (fever) — *see* Fever, paratyphoid
Paratyphus — *see* Fever, paratyphoid
Paraurethral duct Q64.79
Paraurethritis — *see also* Urethritis
- gonococcal (acute) (chronic) (with abscess) A54.1
Paravaccinia NEC B08.04
Paravaginitis — *see* Vaginitis
Parencephalitis — *see also* Encephalitis
- sequelae G09
Parent-child conflict — *see* Conflict, parent-child
- estrangement NEC Z62.890
Paresis — *see also* Paralysis
- accommodation — *see* Paresis, of accommodation
- Bernhardt's G57.1- ☑
- bladder (sphincter) — *see also* Paralysis, bladder
  - tabetic A52.17
- bowel, colon or intestine K56.0
- extrinsic muscle, eye H49.9
- general (progressive) (syphilitic) A52.17
  - juvenile A50.45
- heart — *see* Failure, heart
- insane (syphilitic) A52.17
- juvenile (general) A50.45
- of accommodation H52.52- ☑
- peripheral progressive (idiopathic) G60.3
- pseudohypertrophic G71.09
- senile G83.9

Paresis — *continued*
  syphilitic (general) A52.17
    congenital A50.45
  vesical NEC N31.2
Paresthesia — *see also* Disturbance, sensation, skin R20.2
  Bernhardt G57.1- ☑
Paretic — *see* condition
Parinaud's
  conjunctivitis H10.89
  oculoglandular syndrome H10.89
  ophthalmoplegia H49.88- ☑
Parkinsonism (idiopathic) (primary) G20
  with neurogenic orthostatic hypotension (symptomatic) G90.3
  arteriosclerotic G21.4
  dementia G31.83 *[F02.80]*
    with behavioral disturbance G31.83 *[F02.81]*
  due to
    drugs NEC G21.19
      neuroleptic G21.11
    medication-induced NEC G21.19
    neuroleptic induced G21.11
    postencephalitic G21.3
  secondary G21.9
    due to
      arteriosclerosis G21.4
      drugs NEC G21.19
        neuroleptic G21.11
      encephalitis G21.3
      external agents NEC G21.2
      syphilis A52.19
    specified NEC G21.8
  syphilitic A52.19
  treatment-induced NEC G21.19
  vascular G21.4
Parkinson's disease, syndrome or tremor — *see* Parkinsonism
Parodontitis — *see* Periodontitis
Parodontosis K05.4
Paronychia — *see also* Cellulitis, digit
  with lymphangitis — *see* Lymphangitis, acute, digit
  candidal (chronic) B37.2
  tuberculous (primary) A18.4
Parorexia (psychogenic) F50.89
Parosmia R43.1
  psychogenic F45.8
Parotid gland — *see* condition
Parotitis, parotiditis (allergic)(nonspecific toxic) (purulent) (septic) (suppurative) — *see also* Sialoadenitis
  epidemic — *see* Mumps
  infectious — *see* Mumps
  postoperative K91.89
  surgical K91.89
Parrot fever A70
Parrot's disease (early congenital syphilitic pseudoparalysis) A50.02
Parry-Romberg syndrome G51.8
Parry's disease or syndrome E05.00
  with thyroid storm E05.01
Pars planitis — *see* Cyclitis
Parsonage (-Aldren)-**Turner syndrome** G54.5
Parson's disease (exophthalmic goiter) E05.00
  with thyroid storm E05.01
Particolored infant Q82.8
Parturition — *see* Delivery
Parulis K04.7
  with sinus K04.6
Parvovirus, as cause of disease classified elsewhere B97.6
Pasini and Pierini's atrophoderma L90.3
Passage
  false, urethra N36.5
  meconium (newborn) during delivery P03.82
  of sounds or bougies — *see* Attention to, artificial, opening
Passive — *see* condition
  smoking Z77.22
Pasteurella septica A28.0
Pasteurellosis — *see* Infection, Pasteurella
PAT (paroxysmal atrial tachycardia) I47.1
Patau's syndrome — *see* Trisomy, 13
Patches
  mucous (syphilitic) A51.39
    congenital A50.07
  smokers' (mouth) K13.24
Patellar — *see* condition
Patent — *see also* Imperfect, closure

Patent — *continued*
  canal of Nuck Q52.4
  cervix N88.3
  ductus arteriosus or Botallo's Q25.0
  foramen
    botalli Q21.1
    ovale Q21.1
  interauricular septum Q21.1
  interventricular septum Q21.0
  omphalomesenteric duct Q43.0
  os (uteri) — *see* Patent, cervix
  ostium secundum Q21.1
  urachus Q64.4
  vitelline duct Q43.0
Paterson (-Brown)(-Kelly) **syndrome or web** D50.1
Pathologic, pathological — *see also* condition
  asphyxia R09.01
  fire-setting F63.1
  gambling F63.0
  ovum O02.0
  resorption, tooth K03.3
  stealing F63.2
Pathology (of) — *see* Disease
  periradicular, associated with previous endodontic treatment NEC M27.59
Pattern, sleep-wake, irregular G47.23
Patulous — *see also* Imperfect, closure (congenital)
  alimentary tract Q45.8
    lower Q43.8
    upper Q40.8
  eustachian tube H69.0- ☑
Pause, sinoatrial I49.5
Paxton's disease B36.2
Pearl(s)
  enamel K00.2
  Epstein's K09.8
Pearl-worker's disease — *see* Osteomyelitis, specified type NEC
Pectenosis K62.4
Pectoral — *see* condition
Pectus
  carinatum (congenital) Q67.7
    acquired M95.4
    rachitic sequelae (late effect) E64.3
  excavatum (congenital) Q67.6
    acquired M95.4
    rachitic sequelae (late effect) E64.3
  recurvatum (congenital) Q67.6
Pedatrophia E41
Pederosis F65.4
Pediculosis (infestation) B85.2
  capitis (head-louse) (any site) B85.0
  corporis (body-louse) (any site) B85.1
  eyelid B85.0
  mixed (classifiable to more than one of the titles B85.0-B85.3) B85.4
  pubis (pubic louse) (any site) B85.3
  vestimenti B85.1
  vulvae B85.3
Pediculus (infestation) — *see* Pediculosis
Pedophilia F65.4
Peg-shaped teeth K00.2
Pelade — *see* Alopecia, areata
Pelger-Huët anomaly or syndrome D72.0
Peliosis (rheumatica) D69.0
  hepatis K76.4
    with toxic liver disease K71.8
Pelizaeus-Merzbacher disease E75.29
Pellagra (alcoholic) (with polyneuropathy) E52
Pellagra-cerebellar-ataxia-renal aminoaciduria syndrome E72.02
Pellegrini (-Stieda) **disease or syndrome** — *see* Bursitis, tibial collateral
Pellizzi's syndrome E34.8
Pel's crisis A52.11
Pelvic — *see also* condition
  examination (periodic) (routine) Z01.419
    with abnormal findings Z01.411
  kidney, congenital Q63.2
Pelviolithiasis — *see* Calculus, kidney
Pelviperitonitis — *see also* Peritonitis, pelvic
  gonococcal A54.24
  puerperal O85
Pelvis — *see* condition or type
Pemphigoid L12.9
  benign, mucous membrane L12.1
  bullous L12.0
  cicatricial L12.1

Pemphigoid — *continued*
  juvenile L12.2
  ocular L12.1
  specified NEC L12.8
Pemphigus L10.9
  benign familial (chronic) Q82.8
  Brazilian L10.3
  circinatus L13.0
  conjunctiva L12.1
  drug-induced L10.5
  erythematosus L10.4
  foliaceous L10.2
  gangrenous — *see* Gangrene
  neonatorum L01.03
  ocular L12.1
  paraneoplastic L10.81
  specified NEC L10.89
  syphilitic (congenital) A50.06
  vegetans L10.1
  vulgaris L10.0
  wildfire L10.3
Pendred's syndrome E07.1
Pendulous
  abdomen, in pregnancy — *see* Pregnancy, complicated by, abnormal, pelvic organs or tissues NEC
  breast N64.89
Penetrating wound — *see also* Puncture
  with internal injury — *see* Injury, by site
  eyeball — *see* Puncture, eyeball
  orbit (with or without foreign body) — *see* Puncture, orbit
  uterus by instrument with or following ectopic or molar pregnancy O08.6
Penicillosis B48.4
Penis — *see* condition
Penitis N48.29
Pentalogy of Fallot Q21.8
Pentasomy X syndrome Q97.1
Pentosuria (essential) E74.8
Percreta placenta - O43.23 ☑
Peregrinating patient — *see* Disorder, factitious
Perforation, perforated (nontraumatic) (of)
  accidental during procedure (blood vessel) (nerve) (organ) — *see* Complication, accidental puncture or laceration
  antrum — *see* Sinusitis, maxillary
  appendix K35.32
    with localized peritonitis K35.32
  atrial septum, multiple Q21.1
  attic, ear — *see* Perforation, tympanum, attic
  bile duct (common) (hepatic) K83.2
    cystic K82.2
  bladder (urinary)
    with following ectopic or molar pregnancy O08.6
    obstetrical trauma O71.5
    traumatic S37.29 ☑
      at delivery O71.5
  bowel K63.1
    with or following ectopic or molar pregnancy O08.6
    newborn P78.0
    obstetrical trauma O71.5
    traumatic — *see* Laceration, intestine
  broad ligament N83.8
    with or following ectopic or molar pregnancy O08.6
    obstetrical trauma O71.6
  by
    device, implant or graft — *see also* Complications, by site and type, mechanical T85.628 ☑
      arterial graft NEC — *see* Complication, cardiovascular device, mechanical, vascular
      breast (implant) T85.49 ☑
      catheter NEC T85.698 ☑
        cystostomy T83.090 ☑
        dialysis (renal) T82.49 ☑
          intraperitoneal T85.691 ☑
        infusion NEC T82.594 ☑
          spinal (epidural) (subdural) T85.690 ☑
        urinary — *see also* Complications, catheter, urinary T83.098 ☑
      electronic (electrode) (pulse generator) (stimulator)
        bone T84.390 ☑
        cardiac T82.199 ☑
          electrode T82.190 ☑
          pulse generator T82.191 ☑
          specified type NEC T82.198 ☑

Perforation, perforated — *continued*
  by — *continued*
    device, implant or graft — *see also* Complications, by site and type, mechanical — *continued*
      electronic — *continued*
        nervous system — *see* Complication, prosthetic device, mechanical, electronic nervous system stimulator
        urinary — *see* Complication, genitourinary, device, urinary, mechanical
      fixation, internal (orthopedic) NEC — *see* Complication, fixation device, mechanical
      gastrointestinal — *see* Complications, prosthetic device, mechanical, gastrointestinal device
      genital NEC T83.498 ☑
        intrauterine contraceptive device T83.39 ☑
        penile prosthesis T83.490 ☑
      heart NEC — *see* Complication, cardiovascular device, mechanical
      joint prosthesis — *see* Complications, joint prosthesis, mechanical, specified NEC, by site
      ocular NEC — *see* Complication, prosthetic device, mechanical, ocular device
      orthopedic NEC — *see* Complication, orthopedic, device, mechanical
      specified NEC T85.628 ☑
      urinary NEC — *see also* Complication, genitourinary, device, urinary, mechanical
        graft T83.29 ☑
      vascular NEC — *see* Complication, cardiovascular device, mechanical
      ventricular intracranial shunt T85.09 ☑
    foreign body left accidentally in operative wound T81.539 ☑
    instrument (any) during a procedure, accidental — *see* Puncture, accidental complicating surgery
  cecum K35.32
    with localized peritonitis K35.32
  cervix (uteri) N88.8
    with or following ectopic or molar pregnancy O08.6
    obstetrical trauma O71.3
  colon K63.1
    newborn P78.0
    obstetrical trauma O71.5
    traumatic — *see* Laceration, intestine, large
  common duct (bile) K83.2
  cornea (due to ulceration) — *see* Ulcer, cornea, perforated
  cystic duct K82.2
  diverticulum (intestine) K57.80
    with bleeding K57.81
    large intestine K57.20
      with
        bleeding K57.21
        small intestine K57.40
          with bleeding K57.41
    small intestine K57.00
      with
        bleeding K57.01
        large intestine K57.40
          with bleeding K57.41
  ear drum — *see* Perforation, tympanum
  esophagus K22.3
  ethmoidal sinus — *see* Sinusitis, ethmoidal
  frontal sinus — *see* Sinusitis, frontal
  gallbladder K82.2
  heart valve — *see* Endocarditis
  ileum K63.1
    newborn P78.0
    obstetrical trauma O71.5
    traumatic — *see* Laceration, intestine, small
  instrumental, surgical (accidental) (blood vessel) (nerve) (organ) — *see* Puncture, accidental complicating surgery
  intestine NEC K63.1
    with ectopic or molar pregnancy O08.6
    newborn P78.0
    obstetrical trauma O71.5
    traumatic — *see* Laceration, intestine
    ulcerative NEC K63.1
      newborn P78.0
  jejunum, jejunal K63.1
    obstetrical trauma O71.5
    traumatic — *see* Laceration, intestine, small
    ulcer — *see* Ulcer, gastrojejunal, with perforation
  joint prosthesis — *see* Complications, joint prosthesis, mechanical, specified NEC, by site

Perforation, perforated — *continued*
  mastoid (antrum) (cell) — *see* Disorder, mastoid, specified NEC
  maxillary sinus — *see* Sinusitis, maxillary
  membrana tympani — *see* Perforation, tympanum
  nasal
    septum J34.89
      congenital Q30.3
      syphilitic A52.73
    sinus J34.89
      congenital Q30.8
      due to sinusitis — *see* Sinusitis
  palate — *see also* Cleft, palate Q35.9
    syphilitic A52.79
  palatine vault — *see also* Cleft, palate, hard Q35.1
    syphilitic A52.79
    congenital A50.59
  pars flaccida (ear drum) — *see* Perforation, tympanum, attic
  pelvic
    floor S31.030 ☑
      with
        ectopic or molar pregnancy O08.6
        penetration into retroperitoneal space S31.031 ☑
        retained foreign body S31.040 ☑
          with penetration into retroperitoneal space S31.041 ☑
      following ectopic or molar pregnancy O08.6
      obstetrical trauma O70.1
    organ S37.99 ☑
      adrenal gland S37.818 ☑
      bladder — *see* Perforation, bladder
      fallopian tube S37.599 ☑
        bilateral S37.592 ☑
        unilateral S37.591 ☑
      kidney S37.09- ☑
      obstetrical trauma O71.5
      ovary S37.499 ☑
        bilateral S37.492 ☑
        unilateral S37.491 ☑
      prostate S37.828 ☑
      specified organ NEC S37.898 ☑
      ureter — *see* Perforation, ureter
      urethra — *see* Perforation, urethra
      uterus — *see* Perforation, uterus
  perineum — *see* Laceration, perineum
  pharynx J39.2
  rectum K63.1
    newborn P78.0
    obstetrical trauma O71.5
    traumatic S36.63 ☑
  root canal space due to endodontic treatment M27.51
  sigmoid K63.1
    newborn P78.0
    obstetrical trauma O71.5
    traumatic S36.533 ☑
  sinus (accessory) (chronic) (nasal) J34.89
  sphenoidal sinus — *see* Sinusitis, sphenoidal
  surgical (accidental) (by instrument) (blood vessel) (nerve) (organ) — *see* Puncture, accidental complicating surgery
  traumatic
    external — *see* Puncture
    eye — *see* Puncture, eyeball
    internal organ — *see* Injury, by site
  tympanum, tympanic (membrane) (persistent post-traumatic) (postinflammatory) H72.9- ☑
    attic H72.1- ☑
      multiple — *see* Perforation, tympanum, multiple
      total — *see* Perforation, tympanum, total
    central H72.0- ☑
      multiple — *see* Perforation, tympanum, multiple
      total — *see* Perforation, tympanum, total
    marginal NEC — *see* subcategory H72.2 ☑
    multiple H72.81- ☑
    pars flaccida — *see* Perforation, tympanum, attic
    total H72.82- ☑
    traumatic, current episode S09.2- ☑
  typhoid, gastrointestinal — *see* Typhoid
  ulcer — *see* Ulcer, by site, with perforation
  ureter N28.89
    traumatic S37.19 ☑
  urethra N36.8
    with ectopic or molar pregnancy O08.6
    following ectopic or molar pregnancy O08.6
    obstetrical trauma O71.5

Perforation, perforated — *continued*
  urethra — *continued*
    traumatic S37.39 ☑
      at delivery O71.5
  uterus
    with ectopic or molar pregnancy O08.6
    by intrauterine contraceptive device T83.39 ☑
    following ectopic or molar pregnancy O08.6
    obstetrical trauma O71.1
    traumatic S37.69 ☑
      obstetric O71.1
  uvula K13.79
    syphilitic A52.79
  vagina O71.4
    obstetrical trauma O71.4
    other trauma — *see* Puncture, vagina
Periadenitis mucosa necrotica recurrens K12.0
Periappendicitis (acute) — *see* Appendicitis
Periarteritis nodosa (disseminated) (infectious) (necrotizing) M30.0
Periarthritis (joint) — *see also* Enthesopathy
  Duplay's M75.0- ☑
  gonococcal A54.42
  humeroscapularis — *see* Capsulitis, adhesive
  scapulohumeral — *see* Capsulitis, adhesive
  shoulder — *see* Capsulitis, adhesive
  wrist M77.2-
Periarthrosis (angioneural) — *see* Enthesopathy
Pericapsulitis, adhesive (shoulder) — *see* Capsulitis, adhesive
Pericarditis (with decompensation) (with effusion) I31.9
  with rheumatic fever (conditions in I00)
    active — *see* Pericarditis, rheumatic
    inactive or quiescent I09.2
  acute (hemorrhagic) (nonrheumatic) (Sicca) I30.9
    with chorea (acute) (rheumatic) (Sydenham's) I02.0
    benign I30.8
    nonspecific I30.0
    rheumatic I01.0
      with chorea (acute) (Sydenham's) I02.0
  adhesive or adherent (chronic) (external) (internal) I31.0
    acute — *see* Pericarditis, acute
    rheumatic I09.2
  bacterial (acute) (subacute) (with serous or seropurulent effusion) I30.1
  calcareous I31.1
  cholesterol (chronic) I31.8
    acute I30.9
  chronic (nonrheumatic) I31.9
    rheumatic I09.2
  constrictive (chronic) I31.1
  coxsackie B33.23
  fibrinocaseous (tuberculous) A18.84
  fibrinopurulent I30.1
  fibrinous I30.8
  fibrous I31.0
  gonococcal A54.83
  idiopathic I30.0
  in systemic lupus erythematosus M32.12
  infective I30.1
  meningococcal A39.53
  neoplastic (chronic) I31.8
    acute I30.9
  obliterans, obliterating I31.0
  plastic I31.0
  pneumococcal I30.1
  postinfarction I24.1
  purulent I30.1
  rheumatic (active) (acute) (with effusion) (with pneumonia) I01.0
    with chorea (acute) (rheumatic) (Sydenham's) I02.0
    chronic or inactive (with chorea) I09.2
  rheumatoid — *see* Rheumatoid, carditis
  septic I30.1
  serofibrinous I30.8
  staphylococcal I30.1
  streptococcal I30.1
  suppurative I30.1
  syphilitic A52.06
  tuberculous A18.84
  uremic N18.9 *[I32]*
  viral I30.0
Pericardium, pericardial — *see* condition
Pericellulitis — *see* Cellulitis
Pericementitis (chronic) (suppurative) — *see also* Periodontitis
  acute K05.20

☑ Additional Character Required — Refer to the Tabular List for Character Selection   ▽ Subterms under main terms may continue to next column or page

Pericementitis — *continued*
  acute — *continued*
    generalized — *see* Periodontitis, aggressive, generalized
    localized — *see* Periodontitis, aggressive, localized
Perichondritis
  auricle — *see* Perichondritis, ear
  bronchus J98.09
  ear (external) H61.00- ☑
    acute H61.01- ☑
    chronic H61.02- ☑
  external auditory canal — *see* Perichondritis, ear
  larynx J38.7
    syphilitic A52.73
    typhoid A01.09
  nose J34.89
  pinna — *see* Perichondritis, ear
  trachea J39.8
Periclasia K05.4
Pericoronitis — *see* Periodontitis
Pericystitis N30.90
  with hematuria N30.91
Peridiverticulitis (intestine) K57.92
  cecum — *see* Diverticulitis, intestine, large
  colon — *see* Diverticulitis, intestine, large
  duodenum — *see* Diverticulitis, intestine, small
  intestine — *see* Diverticulitis, intestine
  jejunum — *see* Diverticulitis, intestine, small
  rectosigmoid — *see* Diverticulitis, intestine, large
  rectum — *see* Diverticulitis, intestine, large
  sigmoid — *see* Diverticulitis, intestine, large
Periendocarditis — *see* Endocarditis
Periepididymitis N45.1
Perifolliculitis L01.02
  abscedens, caput, scalp L66.3
  capitis, abscedens (et suffodiens) L66.3
  superficial pustular L01.02
Perihepatitis K65.8
Perilabyrinthitis (acute) — *see* subcategory H83.0 ☑
Perimeningitis — *see* Meningitis
Perimetritis — *see* Endometritis
Perimetrosalpingitis — *see* Salpingo-oophoritis
Perineocele N81.81
Perinephric, perinephritic — *see* condition
Perinephritis — *see also* Infection, kidney
  purulent — *see* Abscess, kidney
Perineum, perineal — *see* condition
Perineuritis NEC — *see* Neuralgia
Periodic — *see* condition
Periodontitis (chronic) (complex) (compound) (local) (simplex) K05.30
  acute K05.20
    generalized K05.229
      moderate K05.222
      severe K05.223
      slight K05.221
    localized K05.219
      moderate K05.212
      severe K05.213
      slight K05.211
  apical K04.5
    acute (pulpal origin) K04.4
  generalized K05.329
    moderate K05.322
    severe K05.323
    slight K05.321
  localized K05.319
    moderate K05.312
    severe K05.313
    slight K05.311
Periodontoclasia K05.4
Periodontosis (juvenile) K05.4
Periods — *see also* Menstruation
  heavy N92.0
  irregular N92.6
  shortened intervals (irregular) N92.1
Perionychia — *see also* Cellulitis, digit
  with lymphangitis — *see* Lymphangitis, acute, digit
Perioophoritis — *see* Salpingo-oophoritis
Periorchitis N45.2
Periosteum, periosteal — *see* condition
Periostitis (albuminosa) (circumscribed) (diffuse) (infective) (monomelic) — *see also* Osteomyelitis
  alveolar M27.3
  alveolodental M27.3
  dental M27.3
  gonorrheal A54.43

Periostitis — *continued*
  jaw (lower) (upper) M27.2
  orbit H05.03- ☑
  syphilitic A52.77
    congenital (early) A50.02 *[M90.80]*
    secondary A51.46
  tuberculous — *see* Tuberculosis, bone
  yaws (hypertrophic) (early) (late) A66.6 *[M90.80]*
Periostosis (hyperplastic) — *see also* Disorder, bone, specified type NEC
  with osteomyelitis — *see* Osteomyelitis, specified type NEC
Peripartum
  cardiomyopathy O90.3
Periphlebitis — *see* Phlebitis
Periproctitis K62.89
Periprostatitis — *see* Prostatitis
Perirectal — *see* condition
Perirenal — *see* condition
Perisalpingitis — *see* Salpingo-oophoritis
Perisplenitis (infectional) D73.89
Peristalsis, visible or reversed R19.2
Peritendinitis — *see* Enthesopathy
Peritoneum, peritoneal — *see* condition
Peritonitis (adhesive) (bacterial) (fibrinous) (hemorrhagic) (idiopathic) (localized) (perforative) (primary) (with adhesions) (with effusion) K65.9
  with or following
    abscess K65.1
    appendicitis
      with perforation or rupture K35.32
      generalized — *see also* Appendicitis K35.20
      localized — *see also* Appendicitis K35.30
    diverticular disease (intestine) K57.80
      with bleeding K57.81
    ectopic or molar pregnancy O08.0
    large intestine K57.20
      with
        bleeding K57.21
        small intestine K57.40
          with bleeding K57.41
    small intestine K57.00
      with
        bleeding K57.01
        large intestine K57.40
          with bleeding K57.41
  acute (generalized) K65.0
  aseptic T81.61 ☑
  bile, biliary K65.3
  chemical T81.61 ☑
  chlamydial A74.81
  chronic proliferative K65.8
  complicating abortion — *see* Abortion, by type, complicated by, pelvic peritonitis
  congenital P78.1
  diaphragmatic K65.0
  diffuse K65.0
  diphtheritic A36.89
  disseminated K65.0
  due to
    bile K65.3
    foreign
      body or object accidentally left during a procedure (instrument) (sponge) (swab) T81.599 ☑
      substance accidentally left during a procedure (chemical) (powder) (talc) T81.61 ☑
    talc T81.61 ☑
    urine K65.8
  eosinophilic K65.8
    acute K65.0
  fibrocaseous (tuberculous) A18.31
  fibropurulent K65.0
  following ectopic or molar pregnancy O08.0
  general (ized) K65.0
  gonococcal A54.85
  meconium (newborn) P78.0
  neonatal P78.1
    meconium P78.0
  pancreatic K65.0
  paroxysmal, familial E85.0
    benign E85.0
  pelvic
    female N73.5
      acute N73.3
      chronic N73.4
        with adhesions N73.6
    male K65.0- ☑

Peritonitis — *continued*
  periodic, familial E85.0
  proliferative, chronic K65.8
  puerperal, postpartum, childbirth O85
  purulent K65.0
  septic K65.0
  specified NEC K65.8
  spontaneous bacterial K65.2
  subdiaphragmatic K65.0
  subphrenic K65.0
  suppurative K65.0
  syphilitic A52.74
    congenital (early) A50.08 *[K67]*
  talc T81.61 ☑
  tuberculous A18.31
  urine K65.8
Peritonsillar — *see* condition
Peritonsillitis J36
Perityphlitis K37
Periureteritis N28.89
Periurethral — *see* condition
Periurethritis (gangrenous) — *see* Urethritis
Periuterine — *see* condition
Perivaginitis — *see* Vaginitis
Perivasculitis, retinal H35.06- ☑
Perivasitis (chronic) N49.1
Perivesiculitis (seminal) — *see* Vesiculitis
Perlèche NEC K13.0
  due to
    candidiasis B37.83
    moniliasis B37.83
    riboflavin deficiency E53.0
    vitamin B2 (riboflavin) deficiency E53.0
Pernicious — *see* condition
Pernio, perniosis T69.1 ☑
Perpetrator (of abuse) — *see* Index to External Causes of Injury, Perpetrator
Persecution
  delusion F22
  social Z60.5
Perseveration (tonic) R48.8
Persistence, persistent (congenital)
  anal membrane Q42.3
    with fistula Q42.2
  arteria stapedia Q16.3
  atrioventricular canal Q21.2
  branchial cleft NOS Q18.2
    cyst Q18.0
    fistula Q18.0
    sinus Q18.0
  bulbus cordis in left ventricle Q21.8
  canal of Cloquet Q14.0
  capsule (opaque) Q12.8
  cilioretinal artery or vein Q14.8
  cloaca Q43.7
  communication — *see* Fistula, congenital
  convolutions
    aortic arch Q25.46
    fallopian tube Q50.6
    oviduct Q50.6
    uterine tube Q50.6
  double aortic arch Q25.45
  ductus arteriosus (Botalli) Q25.0
  fetal
    circulation P29.38
    form of cervix (uteri) Q51.828
    hemoglobin, hereditary (HPFH) D56.4
  foramen
    Botalli Q21.1
    ovale Q21.1
  Gartner's duct Q52.4
  hemoglobin, fetal (hereditary) (HPFH) D56.4
  hyaloid
    artery (generally incomplete) Q14.0
    system Q14.8
  hymen, in pregnancy or childbirth — *see* Pregnancy, complicated by, abnormal, vulva
  lanugo Q84.2
  left
    posterior cardinal vein Q26.8
    root with right arch of aorta Q25.49
    superior vena cava Q26.1
  Meckel's diverticulum Q43.0
    malignant — *see* Table of Neoplasms, small intestine, malignant
  mucosal disease (middle ear) — *see* Otitis, media, suppurative, chronic, tubotympanic
  nail(s), anomalous Q84.6

Persistence, persistent — *continued*
  omphalomesenteric duct Q43.0
  organ or site not listed — *see* Anomaly, by site
  ostium
    atrioventriculare commune Q21.2
      primum Q21.2
      secundum Q21.1
  ovarian rests in fallopian tube Q50.6
  pancreatic tissue in intestinal tract Q43.8
  primary (deciduous)
    teeth K00.6
    vitreous hyperplasia Q14.0
  pupillary membrane Q13.89
  rhesus (Rh) titer — *see* Complication(s), transfusion,
      incompatibility reaction, Rh (factor)
  right aortic arch Q25.47
  sinus
    urogenitalis
      female Q52.8
      male Q55.8
    venosus with imperfect incorporation in right auricle
        Q26.8
  thymus (gland) (hyperplasia) E32.0
  thyroglossal duct Q89.2
  thyrolingual duct Q89.2
  truncus arteriosus or communis Q20.0
  tunica vasculosa lentis Q12.2
  umbilical sinus Q64.4
  urachus Q64.4
  vitelline duct Q43.0
Person (with)
  admitted for clinical research, as a control subject
      (normal comparison) (participant) Z00.6
  awaiting admission to adequate facility elsewhere
      Z75.1
  concern (normal) about sick person in family Z63.6
  consulting on behalf of another Z71.0
  feigning illness Z76.5
  living (in)
    alone Z60.2
    boarding school Z59.3
    residential institution Z59.3
    without
      adequate housing (heating) (space) Z59.1
      housing (permanent) (temporary) Z59.0
      person able to render necessary care Z74.2
      shelter Z59.0
  on waiting list Z75.1
  sick or handicapped in family Z63.6
Personality (disorder) F60.9
  accentuation of traits (type A pattern) Z73.1
  affective F34.0
  aggressive F60.3
  amoral F60.2
  anacastic, anankastic F60.5
  antisocial F60.2
  anxious F60.6
  asocial F60.2
  asthenic F60.7
  avoidant F60.6
  borderline F60.3
  change due to organic condition (enduring) F07.0
  compulsive F60.5
  cycloid F34.0
  cyclothymic F34.0
  dependent F60.7
  depressive F34.1
  dissocial F60.2
  dual F44.81
  eccentric F60.89
  emotionally unstable F60.3
  expansive paranoid F60.0
  explosive F60.3
  fanatic F60.0
  haltlose type F60.89
  histrionic F60.4
  hyperthymic F34.0
  hypothymic F34.1
  hysterical F60.4
  immature F60.89
  inadequate F60.7
  labile (emotional) F60.3
  mixed (nonspecific) F60.89
  morally defective F60.2
  multiple F44.81
  narcissistic F60.81
  obsessional F60.5
  obsessive (-compulsive) F60.5
  organic F07.0

Personality — *continued*
  overconscientious F60.5
  paranoid F60.0
  passive (-dependent) F60.7
  passive-aggressive F60.89
  pathologic F60.9
  pattern defect or disturbance F60.9
  pseudopsychopathic (organic) F07.0
  pseudoretarded (organic) F07.0
  psychoinfantile F60.4
  psychoneurotic NEC F60.89
  psychopathic F60.2
  querulant F60.0
  sadistic F60.89
  schizoid F60.1
  self-defeating F60.89
  sensitive paranoid F60.0
  sociopathic (amoral) (antisocial) (asocial) (dissocial)
      F60.2
  specified NEC F60.89
  type A Z73.1
  unstable (emotional) F60.3
Perthes' disease — *see* Legg-Calvé-Perthes disease
Pertussis — *see also* Whooping cough A37.90
Perversion, perverted
  appetite F50.89
    psychogenic F50.89
  function
    pituitary gland E23.2
      posterior lobe E22.2
  sense of smell and taste R43.8
    psychogenic F45.8
  sexual — *see* Deviation, sexual
Pervious, congenital — *see also* Imperfect, closure
  ductus arteriosus Q25.0
Pes (congenital) — *see also* Talipes
  acquired — *see also* Deformity, limb, foot, specified
      NEC
    planus — *see* Deformity, limb, flat foot
  adductus Q66.89
  cavus Q66.7- ☑
  deformity NEC, acquired — *see* Deformity, limb, foot,
      specified NEC
  planus (acquired) (any degree) — *see also* Deformity,
      limb, flat foot
    rachitic sequelae (late effect) E64.3
  valgus Q66.6
Pest, pestis — *see* Plague
Petechia, petechiae R23.3
  newborn P54.5
Petechial typhus A75.9
Peter's anomaly Q13.4
Petit mal seizure — *see* Epilepsy, childhood, absence
Petit's hernia — *see* Hernia, abdomen, specified site NEC
Petrellidosis B48.2
Petrositis H70.20- ☑
  acute H70.21- ☑
  chronic H70.22- ☑
Peutz-Jeghers disease or syndrome Q85.8
Peyronie's disease N48.6
PFAPA (periodic fever, aphthous stomatitis, pharyngitis,
    and adenopathy syndrome) M04.8
Pfeiffer's disease — *see* Mononucleosis, infectious
Phagedena (dry) (moist) (sloughing) — *see also* Gan-
    grene
  geometric L88
  penis N48.29
  tropical — *see* Ulcer, skin
  vulva N76.6
Phagedenic — *see* condition
Phakoma H35.89
Phakomatosis — *see also* specific eponymous syndromes
    Q85.9
  Bourneville's Q85.1
  specified NEC Q85.8
Phantom limb syndrome (without pain) G54.7
  with pain G54.6
Pharyngeal pouch syndrome D82.1
Pharyngitis (acute) (catarrhal)(gangrenous) (infective)
    (malignant) (membranous) (phlegmonous) (pseu-
    domembranous) (simple) (subacute) (suppurative)
    (ulcerative) (viral) J02.9
  with influenza, flu, or grippe — *see* Influenza, with,
      pharyngitis
  aphthous B08.5
  atrophic J31.2
  chlamydial A56.4
  chronic (atrophic) (granular) (hypertrophic) J31.2

Pharyngitis — *continued*
  coxsackievirus B08.5
  diphtheritic A36.0
  enteroviral vesicular B08.5
  follicular (chronic) J31.2
  fusospirochetal A69.1
  gonococcal A54.5
  granular (chronic) J31.2
  herpesviral B00.2
  hypertrophic J31.2
  infectional, chronic J31.2
  influenzal — *see* Influenza, with, respiratory manifesta-
      tions NEC
  lymphonodular, acute (enteroviral) B08.8
  pneumococcal J02.8
  purulent J02.9
  putrid J02.9
  septic J02.0
  sicca J31.2
  specified organism NEC J02.8
  staphylococcal J02.8
  streptococcal J02.0
  syphilitic, congenital (early) A50.03
  tuberculous A15.8
  vesicular, enteroviral B08.5
  viral NEC J02.8
Pharyngoconjunctivitis, viral B30.2
Pharyngolaryngitis (acute) J06.0
  chronic J37.0
Pharyngoplegia J39.2
Pharyngotonsillitis, herpesviral B00.2
Pharyngotracheitis, chronic J42
Pharynx, pharyngeal — *see* condition
Phencyclidine-induced
  anxiety disorder F16.980
  bipolar and related disorder F16.94
  depressive disorder F16.94
  psychotic disorder F16.959
Phenomenon
  Arthus' — *see* Arthus' phenomenon
  jaw-winking Q07.8
  lupus erythematosus (LE) cell M32.9
  Raynaud's (secondary) I73.00
    with gangrene I73.01
  vasomotor R55
  vasospastic I73.9
  vasovagal R55
  Wenckebach's I44.1
Phenylketonuria E70.1
  classical E70.0
  maternal E70.1
Pheochromoblastoma
  specified site — *see* Neoplasm, malignant, by site
  unspecified site C74.10
Pheochromocytoma
  malignant
    specified site — *see* Neoplasm, malignant, by site
    unspecified site C74.10
  specified site — *see* Neoplasm, benign, by site
  unspecified site D35.00
Pheohyphomycosis — *see* Chromomycosis
Pheomycosis — *see* Chromomycosis
Phimosis (congenital) (due to infection) N47.1
  chancroidal A57
Phlebectasia — *see also* Varix
  congenital Q27.4
Phlebitis (infective) (pyemic) (septic) (suppurative) I80.9☑
  antepartum — *see* Thrombophlebitis, antepartum
  blue — *see* Phlebitis, leg, deep
  breast, superficial I80.8
  calf muscular vein (NOS) I80.25- ☑
  cavernous (venous) sinus — *see* Phlebitis, intracrania
      (venous) sinus
  cerebral (venous) sinus — *see* Phlebitis, intracranial
      (venous) sinus
  chest wall, superficial I80.8
  cranial (venous) sinus — *see* Phlebitis, intracranial
      (venous) sinus
  deep (vessels) — *see* Phlebitis, leg, deep
  due to implanted device — *see* Complications, by site
      and type, specified NEC
  during or resulting from a procedure T81.72 ☑
  femoral vein (superficial) I80.1- ☑
  femoropopliteal vein I80.0- ☑
  gastrocnemial vein I80.25- ☑
  gestational — *see* Phlebopathy, gestational
  hepatic veins I80.8
  iliac vein (common) (external) (internal) I80.21- ☑

☑ **Additional Character Required** — **Refer to the Tabular List for Character Selection**   ⍌ **Subterms under main terms may continue to next column or page**

Phlebitis — *continued*
iliofemoral — *see* Phlebitis, femoral vein
intracranial (venous) sinus (any) G08
nonpyogenic I67.6
intraspinal venous sinuses and veins G08
nonpyogenic G95.19
lateral (venous) sinus — *see* Phlebitis, intracranial (venous) sinus
leg I80.3
antepartum — *see* Thrombophlebitis, antepartum
deep (vessels) NEC I80.20- ☑
iliac I80.21- ☑
popliteal vein I80.22- ☑
specified vessel NEC I80.29- ☑
tibial vein (anterior) (posterior) I80.23- ☑
femoral vein (superficial) I80.1- ☑
superficial (vessels) I80.0- ☑
longitudinal sinus — *see* Phlebitis, intracranial (venous) sinus
lower limb — *see* Phlebitis, leg
migrans, migrating (superficial) I82.1
pelvic
with ectopic or molar pregnancy O08.0
following ectopic or molar pregnancy O08.0
puerperal, postpartum O87.1
peroneal vein I80.24- ☑
popliteal vein — *see* Phlebitis, leg, deep, popliteal
portal (vein) K75.1
postoperative T81.72 ☑
pregnancy — *see* Thrombophlebitis, antepartum
puerperal, postpartum, childbirth O87.0
deep O87.1
pelvic O87.1
superficial O87.0
retina — *see* Vasculitis, retina
saphenous (accessory) (great) (long) (small) — *see* Phlebitis, leg, superficial
sinus (meninges) — *see* Phlebitis, intracranial (venous) sinus
soleal vein I80.25- ☑
specified site NEC I80.8
syphilitic A52.09
tibial vein — *see* Phlebitis, leg, deep, tibial
ulcerative I80.9
leg — *see* Phlebitis, leg
umbilicus I80.8
uterus (septic) — *see* Endometritis
varicose (leg) (lower limb) — *see* Varix, leg, with, inflammation
Phlebofibrosis I87.8
Phleboliths I87.8
Phlebopathy,
gestational O22.9- ☑
puerperal O87.9
Phlebosclerosis I87.8
Phlebothrombosis — *see also* Thrombosis
antepartum — *see* Thrombophlebitis, antepartum
pregnancy — *see* Thrombophlebitis, antepartum
puerperal — *see* Thrombophlebitis, puerperal
Phlebotomus fever A93.1
Phlegmasia
alba dolens O87.1
nonpuerperal — *see* Phlebitis, femoral vein
cerulea dolens — *see* Phlebitis, leg, deep
Phlegmon — *see* Abscess
Phlegmonous — *see* condition
Phlyctenulosis (allergic) (keratoconjunctivitis) (nontuberculous) — *see also* Keratoconjunctivitis
cornea — *see* Keratoconjunctivitis
tuberculous A18.52
Phobia, phobic F40.9
animal F40.218
spiders F40.210
examination F40.298
reaction F40.9
simple F40.298
social F40.10
generalized F40.11
specific (isolated) F40.298
animal F40.218
spiders F40.210
blood F40.230
injection F40.231
injury F40.233
men F40.290
natural environment F40.228
thunderstorms F40.220

Phobia, phobic — *continued*
specific — *continued*
situational F40.248
bridges F40.242
closed in spaces F40.240
flying F40.243
heights F40.241
specified focus NEC F40.298
transfusion F40.231
women F40.291
specified NEC F40.8
medical care NEC F40.232
state F40.9
Phocas' disease — *see* Mastopathy, cystic
Phocomelia Q73.1
lower limb — *see* Agenesis, leg, with foot present
upper limb — *see* Agenesis, arm, with hand present
Phoria H50.50
Phosphate-losing tubular disorder N25.0
Phosphatemia E83.39
Phosphaturia E83.39
Photodermatitis (sun) L56.8
chronic L57.8
due to drug L56.8
light other than sun L59.8
Photokeratitis H16.13- ☑
Photophobia H53.14- ☑
Photophthalmia — *see* Photokeratitis
Photopsia H53.19
Photoretinitis — *see* Retinopathy, solar
Photosensitivity, photosensitization (sun) skin L56.8
light other than sun L59.8
Phrenitis — *see* Encephalitis
Phrynoderma (vitamin A deficiency) E50.8
Phthiriasis (pubis) B85.3
with any infestation classifiable to B85.0-B85.2 B85.4
Phthirus infestation — *see* Phthiriasis
Phthisis — *see also* Tuberculosis
bulbi (infectional) — *see* Disorder, globe, degenerated condition, atrophy
eyeball (due to infection) — *see* Disorder, globe, degenerated condition, atrophy
Phycomycosis — *see* Zygomycosis
Physalopteriasis B81.8
Physical restraint status Z78.1
Phytobezoar T18.9 ☑
intestine T18.3 ☑
stomach T18.2 ☑
Pian — *see* Yaws
Pianoma A66.1
Pica F50.89
in adults F50.89
infant or child F98.3
Picking, nose F98.8
Pick-Niemann disease — *see* Niemann-Pick disease or syndrome
Pick's
cerebral atrophy G31.01 *[F02.80]*
with behavioral disturbance G31.01 *[F02.81]*
disease or syndrome (brain) G31.01 *[F02.80]*
with behavioral disturbance G31.01 *[F02.81]*
brain G31.01 *[F02.80]*
with behavioral disturbance G31.01 *[F02.81]*
pericardium (pericardial pseudocirrhosis of liver) I31.1
syndrome
brain G31.01 *[F02.80]*
with behavioral disturbance G31.01 *[F02.81]*
of heart (pericardial pseudocirrhosis of liver) I31.1
Pickwickian syndrome E66.2
Piebaldism E70.39
Piedra (beard) (scalp) B36.8
black B36.3
white B36.2
Pierre Robin deformity or syndrome Q87.0
Pierson's disease or osteochondrosis M91.0
Pig-bel A05.2
Pigeon
breast or chest (acquired) M95.4
congenital Q67.7
rachitic sequelae (late effect) E64.3
breeder's disease or lung J67.2
fancier's disease or lung J67.2
toe — *see* Deformity, toe, specified NEC
Pigmentation (abnormal) (anomaly) L81.9
conjunctiva H11.13- ☑
cornea (anterior) H18.01- ☑

Pigmentation — *continued*
cornea — *continued*
posterior H18.05- ☑
stromal H18.06- ☑
diminished melanin formation NEC L81.6
iron L81.8
lids, congenital Q82.8
limbus corneae — *see* Pigmentation, cornea
metals L81.8
optic papilla, congenital Q14.2
retina, congenital (grouped) (nevoid) Q14.1
scrotum, congenital Q82.8
tattoo L81.8
Piles — *see also* Hemorrhoids K64.9
Pili
annulati or torti (congenital) Q84.1
incarnati L73.1
Pill roller hand (intrinsic) — *see* Parkinsonism
Pilomatrixoma — *see* Neoplasm, skin, benign
malignant — *see* Neoplasm, skin, malignant
Pilonidal — *see* condition
Pimple R23.8
PIN — *see* Neoplasia, intraepithelial, prostate
Pinched nerve — *see* Neuropathy, entrapment
Pindborg tumor — *see* Cyst, calcifying odontogenic
Pineal body or gland — *see* condition
Pinealoblastoma C75.3
Pinealoma D44.5
malignant C75.3
Pineoblastoma C75.3
Pineocytoma D44.5
Pinguecula H11.15- ☑
Pingueculitis H10.81- ☑
Pinhole meatus — *see also* Stricture, urethra N35.919
Pink
disease — *see* subcategory T56.1 ☑
eye — *see* Conjunctivitis, acute, mucopurulent
Pinkus' disease (lichen nitidus) L44.1
Pinpoint
meatus — *see* Stricture, urethra
os (uteri) — *see* Stricture, cervix
Pins and needles R20.2
Pinta A67.9
cardiovascular lesions A67.2
chancre (primary) A67.0
erythematous plaques A67.1
hyperchromic lesions A67.1
hyperkeratosis A67.1
lesions A67.9
cardiovascular A67.2
hyperchromic A67.1
intermediate A67.1
late A67.2
mixed A67.3
primary A67.0
skin (achromic) (cicatricial) (dyschromic) A67.2
hyperchromic A67.1
mixed (achromic and hyperchromic) A67.3
papule (primary) A67.0
skin lesions (achromic) (cicatricial) (dyschromic) A67.2
hyperchromic A67.1
mixed (achromic and hyperchromic) A67.3
vitiligo A67.2
Pintids A67.1
Pinworm (disease) (infection) (infestation) B80
Piroplasmosis B60.0
Pistol wound — *see* Gunshot wound
Pitchers' elbow — *see* Derangement, joint, specified type NEC, elbow
Pithecoid pelvis Q74.2
with disproportion (fetopelvic) O33.0
causing obstructed labor O65.0
Pithiatism F48.8
Pitted — *see* Pitting
Pitting — *see also* Edema R60.9
lip R60.0
nail L60.8
teeth K00.4
Pituitary gland — *see* condition
Pituitary-snuff-taker's disease J67.8
Pityriasis (capitis) L21.0
alba L30.5
circinata (et maculata) L42
furfuracea L21.0
Hebra's L26
lichenoides L41.0
chronica L41.1

Pityriasis — *continued*
 lichenoides — *continued*
  et varioliformis (acuta) L41.0
 maculata (et circinata) L30.5
 nigra B36.1
 pilaris, Hebra's L44.0
 rosea L42
 rotunda L44.8
 rubra (Hebra) pilaris L44.0
 simplex L30.5
 specified type NEC L30.5
 streptogenes L30.5
 versicolor (scrotal) B36.0
Placenta, placental — *see* Pregnancy, complicated by (care of) (management affected by), specified condition
Placentitis O41.14- ☑
Plagiocephaly Q67.3
Plague A20.9
 abortive A20.8
 ambulatory A20.8
 asymptomatic A20.8
 bubonic A20.0
 cellulocutaneous A20.1
 cutaneobubonic A20.1
 lymphatic gland A20.0
 meningitis A20.3
 pharyngeal A20.8
 pneumonic (primary) (secondary) A20.2
 pulmonary, pulmonic A20.2
 septicemic A20.7
 tonsillar A20.8
  septicemic A20.7
Planning, family
 contraception Z30.9
 procreation Z31.69
Plaque(s)
 artery, arterial — *see* Arteriosclerosis
 calcareous — *see* Calcification
 coronary, lipid rich I25.83
 epicardial I31.8
 erythematous, of pinta A67.1
 Hollenhorst's — *see* Occlusion, artery, retina
 lipid rich, coronary I25.83
 pleural (without asbestos) J92.9
  with asbestos J92.0
 tongue K13.29
Plasmacytoma C90.3- ☑
 extramedullary C90.2- ☑
 medullary C90.0- ☑
 solitary C90.3- ☑
Plasmacytopenia D72.818
Plasmacytosis D72.822
Plaster ulcer — *see* Ulcer, pressure, by site
Plateau iris syndrome (post-iridectomy) (postprocedural) (without glaucoma) H21.82
 with glaucoma H40.22- ☑
Platybasia Q75.8
Platyonychia (congenital) Q84.6
 acquired L60.8
Platypelloid pelvis M95.5
 with disproportion (fetopelvic) O33.0
  causing obstructed labor O65.0
 congenital Q74.2
Platyspondylisis Q76.49
Plaut (-Vincent) **disease** — *see also* Vincent's A69.1
Plethora R23.2
 newborn P61.1
Pleura, pleural — *see* condition
Pleuralgia R07.81
Pleurisy (acute) (adhesive) (chronic) (costal) (diaphragmatic) (double) (dry) (fibrinous) (fibrous) (interlobar) (latent) (plastic) (primary) (residual) (sicca) (sterile) (subacute) (unresolved) R09.1
 with
  adherent pleura J86.0
  effusion J90
   chylous, chyliform J94.0
   tuberculous (non primary) A15.6
    primary (progressive) A15.7
  tuberculosis — *see* Pleurisy, tuberculous (non primary)
 encysted — *see* Pleurisy, with effusion
 exudative — *see* Pleurisy, with effusion
 fibrinopurulent, fibropurulent — *see* Pyothorax
 hemorrhagic — *see* Hemothorax
 pneumococcal J90
 purulent — *see* Pyothorax

Pleurisy — *continued*
 septic — *see* Pyothorax
 serofibrinous — *see* Pleurisy, with effusion
 seropurulent — *see* Pyothorax
 serous — *see* Pleurisy, with effusion
 staphylococcal J86.9
 streptococcal J90
 suppurative — *see* Pyothorax
 traumatic (post) (current) — *see* Injury, intrathoracic, pleura
 tuberculous (with effusion) (non primary) A15.6
  primary (progressive) A15.7
Pleuritis sicca — *see* Pleurisy
Pleurobronchopneumonia — *see* Pneumonia, broncho-
Pleurodynia R07.81
 epidemic B33.0
 viral B33.0
Pleuropericarditis — *see also* Pericarditis
 acute I30.9
Pleuropneumonia (acute) (bilateral) (double) (septic) — *see also* Pneumonia J18.8
 chronic — *see* Fibrosis, lung
Pleuro-pneumonia-like-organism (PPLO), as cause of disease classified elsewhere B96.0
Pleurorrhea — *see* Pleurisy, with effusion
Plexitis, brachial G54.0
Plica
 polonica B85.0
 syndrome, knee M67.5- ☑
 tonsil J35.8
Plicated tongue K14.5
Plug
 bronchus NEC J98.09
 meconium (newborn) NEC syndrome P76.0
 mucus — *see* Asphyxia, mucus
Plumbism — *see* subcategory T56.0 ☑
Plummer's disease E05.20
 with thyroid storm E05.21
Plummer-Vinson syndrome D50.1
Pluricarential syndrome of infancy E40
Plus (and minus) **hand** (intrinsic) — *see* Deformity, limb, specified type NEC, forearm
Pneumathemia — *see* Air, embolism
Pneumatic hammer (drill) syndrome T75.21 ☑
Pneumatocele (lung) J98.4
 intracranial G93.89
 tension J44.9
Pneumatosis
 cystoides intestinalis K63.89
 intestinalis K63.89
 peritonei K66.8
Pneumaturia R39.89
Pneumoblastoma — *see* Neoplasm, lung, malignant
Pneumocephalus G93.89
Pneumococcemia A40.3
Pneumococcus, pneumococcal — *see* condition
Pneumoconiosis (due to) (inhalation of) J64
 with tuberculosis (any type in A15) J65
 aluminum J63.0
 asbestos J61
 bagasse, bagassosis J67.1
 bauxite J63.1
 beryllium J63.2
 coal miners' (simple) J60
 coalworkers' (simple) J60
 collier's J60
 cotton dust J66.0
 diatomite (diatomaceous earth) J62.8
 dust
  inorganic NEC J63.6
  lime J62.8
  marble J62.8
  organic NEC J66.8
 fumes or vapors (from silo) J68.9
 graphite J63.3
 grinder's J62.8
 kaolin J62.8
 mica J62.8
 millstone maker's J62.8
 mineral fibers NEC J61
 miner's J60
 moldy hay J67.0
 potter's J62.8
 rheumatoid — *see* Rheumatoid, lung
 sandblaster's J62.8
 silica, silicate NEC J62.8
  with carbon J60
 stonemason's J62.8

Pneumoconiosis — *continued*
 talc (dust) J62.0
Pneumocystis carinii pneumonia B59
Pneumocystis jiroveci (pneumonia) B59
Pneumocystosis (with pneumonia) B59
Pneumohemopericardium I31.2
Pneumohemothorax J94.2
 traumatic S27.2 ☑
Pneumohydropericardium — *see* Pericarditis
Pneumohydrothorax — *see* Hydrothorax
Pneumomediastinum J98.2
 congenital or perinatal P25.2
Pneumomycosis B49 *[J99]*
Pneumonia (acute) (double) (migratory) (purulent) (septic) (unresolved) J18.9
 with
  influenza — *see* Influenza, with, pneumonia
  lung abscess J85.1
   due to specified organism — *see* Pneumonia, in (due to)
 adenoviral J12.0
 adynamic J18.2
 alba A50.04
 allergic (eosinophilic) J82
 alveolar — *see* Pneumonia, lobar
 anaerobes J15.8
 anthrax A22.1
 apex, apical — *see* Pneumonia, lobar
 Ascaris B77.81
 aspiration J69.0
  due to
   aspiration of microorganisms
    bacterial J15.9
    viral J12.9
   food (regurgitated) J69.0
   gastric secretions J69.0
   milk (regurgitated) J69.0
   oils, essences J69.1
   solids, liquids NEC J69.8
   vomitus J69.0
  newborn P24.81
   amniotic fluid (clear) P24.11
   blood P24.21
   food (regurgitated) P24.31
   liquor (amnii) P24.11
   meconium P24.01
   milk P24.31
   mucus P24.11
   specified NEC P24.81
   stomach contents P24.31
  postprocedural J95.4
 atypical NEC J18.9
 bacillus J15.9
  specified NEC J15.8
 bacterial J15.9
  specified NEC J15.8
 Bacteroides (fragilis) (oralis) (melaninogenicus) J15.8
 basal, basic, basilar — *see* Pneumonia, by type
 bronchiolitis obliterans organized (BOOP) J84.89
 broncho-, bronchial (confluent) (croupous) (diffuse) (disseminated) (hemorrhagic) (involving lobes) (lobar) (terminal) J18.0
  allergic (eosinophilic) J82
  aspiration — *see* Pneumonia, aspiration
  bacterial J15.9
   specified NEC J15.8
  chronic — *see* Fibrosis, lung
  diplococcal J13
  Eaton's agent J15.7
  Escherichia coli (E. coli) J15.5
  Friedländer's bacillus J15.0
  Hemophilus influenzae J14
  hypostatic J18.2
  inhalation — *see also* Pneumonia, aspiration
   due to fumes or vapors (chemical) J68.0
   of oils or essences J69.1
  Klebsiella (pneumoniae) J15.0
  lipid, lipoid J69.1
   endogenous J84.89
  Mycoplasma (pneumoniae) J15.7
  pleuro-pneumonia-like-organisms (PPLO) J15.7
  pneumococcal J13
  Proteus J15.6
  Pseudomonas J15.1
  Serratia marcescens J15.6
  specified organism NEC J16.8
  staphylococcal — *see* Pneumonia, staphylococca
  streptococcal NEC J15.4

☑ Additional Character Required — Refer to the Tabular List for Character Selection   ▽ Subterms under main terms may continue to next column or page

Pneumonia — *continued*
  broncho-, bronchial — *continued*
    streptococcal — *continued*
      group B J15.3
      pneumoniae J13
    viral, virus — *see* Pneumonia, viral
  Butyrivibrio (fibriosolvens) J15.8
  Candida B37.1
  caseous — *see* Tuberculosis, pulmonary
  catarrhal — *see* Pneumonia, broncho
  chlamydial J16.0
    congenital P23.1
  cholesterol J84.89
  cirrhotic (chronic) — *see* Fibrosis, lung
  Clostridium (haemolyticum) (novyi) J15.8
  confluent — *see* Pneumonia, broncho
  congenital (infective) P23.9
    due to
      bacterium NEC P23.6
      Chlamydia P23.1
      Escherichia coli P23.4
      Haemophilus influenzae P23.6
      infective organism NEC P23.8
      Klebsiella pneumoniae P23.6
      Mycoplasma P23.6
      Pseudomonas P23.5
      Staphylococcus P23.2
      Streptococcus (except group B) P23.6
        group B P23.3
      viral agent P23.0
    specified NEC P23.8
  croupous — *see* Pneumonia, lobar
  cryptogenic organizing J84.116
  cytomegalic inclusion B25.0
  cytomegaloviral B25.0
  deglutition — *see* Pneumonia, aspiration
  desquamative interstitial J84.117
  diffuse — *see* Pneumonia, broncho
  diplococcal, diplococcus (broncho-) (lobar) J13
  disseminated (focal) — *see* Pneumonia, broncho
  Eaton's agent J15.7
  embolic, embolism — *see* Embolism, pulmonary
  Enterobacter J15.6
  eosinophilic J82
  Escherichia coli (E. coli) J15.5
  Eubacterium J15.8
  fibrinous — *see* Pneumonia, lobar
  fibroid, fibrous (chronic) — *see* Fibrosis, lung
  Friedländer's bacillus J15.0
  Fusobacterium (nucleatum) J15.8
  gangrenous J85.0
  giant cell (measles) B05.2
  gonococcal A54.84
  gram-negative bacteria NEC J15.6
    anaerobic J15.8
  Hemophilus influenzae (broncho) (lobar) J14
  human metapneumovirus J12.3
  hypostatic (broncho) (lobar) J18.2
  in (due to)
    actinomycosis A42.0
    adenovirus J12.0
    anthrax A22.1
    ascariasis B77.81
    aspergillosis B44.9
    Bacillus anthracis A22.1
    Bacterium anitratum J15.6
    candidiasis B37.1
    chickenpox B01.2
    Chlamydia J16.0
      neonatal P23.1
    coccidioidomycosis B38.2
      acute B38.0
      chronic B38.1
    cytomegalovirus disease B25.0
    Diplococcus (pneumoniae) J13
    Eaton's agent J15.7
    Enterobacter J15.6
    Escherichia coli (E. coli) J15.5
    Friedländer's bacillus J15.0
    fumes and vapors (chemical) (inhalation) J68.0
    gonorrhea A54.84
    Hemophilus influenzae (H. influenzae) J14
    Herellea J15.6
    histoplasmosis B39.2
      acute B39.0
      chronic B39.1
    human metapneumovirus J12.3
    Klebsiella (pneumoniae) J15.0

Pneumonia — *continued*
  in — *continued*
    measles B05.2
    Mycoplasma (pneumoniae) J15.7
    nocardiosis, nocardiasis A43.0
    ornithosis A70
    parainfluenza virus J12.2
    pleuro-pneumonia-like-organism (PPLO) J15.7
    pneumococcus J13
    pneumocystosis (Pneumocystis carinii) (Pneumocys-
      tis jiroveci) B59
    Proteus J15.6
    Pseudomonas NEC J15.1
      pseudomallei A24.1
    psittacosis A70
    Q fever A78
    respiratory syncytial virus (RSV) J12.1
    rheumatic fever I00 *[J17]*
    rubella B06.81
    Salmonella (infection) A02.22
      typhi A01.03
    schistosomiasis B65.9 *[J17]*
    Serratia marcescens J15.6
    specified
      bacterium NEC J15.8
      organism NEC J16.8
    spirochetal NEC A69.8
    Staphylococcus J15.20
      aureus (methicillin susceptible) (MSSA) J15.211
        methicillin resistant (MRSA) J15.212
      specified NEC J15.29
    Streptococcus J15.4
      group B J15.3
      pneumoniae J13
      specified NEC J15.4
    toxoplasmosis B58.3
    tularemia A21.2
    typhoid (fever) A01.03
    varicella B01.2
    virus — *see* Pneumonia, viral
    whooping cough A37.91
      due to
        Bordetella parapertussis A37.11
        Bordetella pertussis A37.01
        specified NEC A37.81
    Yersinia pestis A20.2
  inhalation of food or vomit — *see* Pneumonia, aspira-
    tion
  interstitial J84.9
    chronic J84.111
    desquamative J84.117
    due to
      collagen vascular disease J84.17
      known underlying cause J84.17
    idiopathic NOS J84.111
    in disease classified elsewhere J84.17
    lymphocytic (due to collagen vascular disease) (in
      diseases classified elsewhere) J84.17
    lymphoid J84.2
    non-specific J84.89
      due to
        collagen vascular disease J84.17
        known underlying cause J84.17
      idiopathic J84.113
      in diseases classified elsewhere J84.17
    plasma cell B59
    pseudomonas J15.1
    usual J84.112
      due to collagen vascular disease J84.17
      idiopathic J84.112
      in diseases classified elsewhere J84.17
  Klebsiella (pneumoniae) J15.0
  lipid, lipoid (exogenous) J69.1
    endogenous J84.89
  lobar (disseminated) (double) (interstitial) J18.1
    bacterial J15.9
      specified NEC J15.8
    chronic — *see* Fibrosis, lung
    Escherichia coli (E. coli) J15.5
    Friedländer's bacillus J15.0
    Hemophilus influenzae J14
    hypostatic J18.2
    Klebsiella (pneumoniae) J15.0
    pneumococcal J13
    Proteus J15.6
    Pseudomonas J15.1
    specified organism NEC J16.8
    staphylococcal — *see* Pneumonia, staphylococcal
    streptococcal NEC J15.4

Pneumonia — *continued*
  lobar — *continued*
    Streptococcus pneumoniae J13
    viral, virus — *see* Pneumonia, viral
  lobular — *see* Pneumonia, broncho
  Löffler's J82
  lymphoid interstitial J84.2
  massive — *see* Pneumonia, lobar
  meconium P24.01
  MRSA (methicillin resistant Staphylococcus aureus)
    J15.212
  MSSA (methicillin susceptible Staphylococcus aureus)
    J15.211
  multilobar — *see* Pneumonia, by type
  Mycoplasma (pneumoniae) J15.7
  necrotic J85.0
  neonatal P23.9
    aspiration — *see* Aspiration, by substance, with
      pneumonia
  nitrogen dioxide J68.0
  organizing J84.89
    due to
      collagen vascular disease J84.17
      known underlying cause J84.17
    in diseases classified elsewhere J84.17
  orthostatic J18.2
  parainfluenza virus J12.2
  parenchymatous — *see* Fibrosis, lung
  passive J18.2
  patchy — *see* Pneumonia, broncho
  Peptococcus J15.8
  Peptostreptococcus J15.8
  plasma cell (of infants) B59
  pleurolobar — *see* Pneumonia, lobar
  pleuro-pneumonia-like organism (PPLO) J15.7
  pneumococcal (broncho) (lobar) J13
  Pneumocystis (carinii) (jiroveci) B59
  postinfectional NEC B99 ☑ *[J17]*
  postmeasles B05.2
  Proteus J15.6
  Pseudomonas J15.1
  psittacosis A70
  radiation J70.0
  respiratory syncytial virus (RSV) J12.1
  resulting from a procedure J95.89
  rheumatic I00 *[J17]*
  Salmonella (arizonae) (cholerae-suis) (enteritidis) (ty-
    phimurium) A02.22
    typhi A01.03
    typhoid fever A01.03
  SARS-associated coronavirus J12.81
  segmented, segmental — *see* Pneumonia, broncho-
  Serratia marcescens J15.6
  specified NEC J18.8
    bacterium NEC J15.8
    organism NEC J16.8
    virus NEC J12.89
  spirochetal NEC A69.8
  staphylococcal (broncho) (lobar) J15.20
    aureus (methicillin susceptible) (MSSA) J15.211
      methicillin resistant (MRSA) J15.212
    specified NEC J15.29
  static, stasis J18.2
  streptococcal NEC (broncho) (lobar) J15.4
    group
      A J15.4
      B J15.3
      specified NEC J15.4
  Streptococcus pneumoniae J13
  syphilitic, congenital (early) A50.04
  traumatic (complication) (early) (secondary) T79.8 ☑
  tuberculous (any) — *see* Tuberculosis, pulmonary
  tularemic A21.2
  varicella B01.2
  Veillonella J15.8
  ventilator associated J95.851
  viral, virus (broncho) (interstitial) (lobar) J12.9
    adenoviral J12.0
    congenital P23.0
    human metapneumovirus J12.3
    parainfluenza J12.2
    respiratory syncytial (RSV) J12.1
    SARS-associated coronavirus J12.81
    specified NEC J12.89
  white (congenital) A50.04
Pneumonic — *see* condition
Pneumonitis (acute) (primary) — *see also* Pneumonia
  air-conditioner J67.7

Pneumonitis — *continued*
  allergic (due to) J67.9
    organic dust NEC J67.8
    red cedar dust J67.8
    sequoiosis J67.8
    wood dust J67.8
  aspiration J69.0
    due to
      anesthesia J95.4
        during
          labor and delivery O74.0
          pregnancy O29.01- ☑
          puerperium O89.01
      fumes or gases J68.0
      obstetric O74.0
  chemical (due to gases, fumes or vapors) (inhalation) J68.0
    due to anesthesia J95.4
  cholesterol J84.89
  chronic — *see* Fibrosis, lung
  congenital rubella P35.0
  crack (cocaine) J68.0
  due to
    beryllium J68.0
    cadmium J68.0
    crack (cocaine) J68.0
    detergent J69.8
    fluorocarbon-polymer J68.0
    food, vomit (aspiration) J69.0
    fumes or vapors J68.0
    gases, fumes or vapors (inhalation) J68.0
    inhalation
      blood J69.8
      essences J69.1
      food (regurgitated), milk, vomit J69.0
      oils, essences J69.1
      saliva J69.0
      solids, liquids NEC J69.8
    manganese J68.0
    nitrogen dioxide J68.0
    oils, essences J69.1
    solids, liquids NEC J69.8
    toxoplasmosis (acquired) B58.3
      congenital P37.1
    vanadium J68.0
    ventilator J95.851
  eosinophilic J82
  hypersensitivity J67.9
    air conditioner lung J67.7
    bagassosis J67.1
    bird fancier's lung J67.2
    farmer's lung J67.0
    maltworker's lung J67.4
    maple bark-stripper's lung J67.6
    mushroom worker's lung J67.5
    specified organic dust NEC J67.8
    suberosis J67.3
  interstitial (chronic) J84.89
    acute J84.114
    lymphoid J84.2
    non-specific J84.89
      idiopathic J84.113
  lymphoid, interstitial J84.2
  meconium P24.01
  postanesthetic J95.4
    correct substance properly administered — *see* Table of Drugs and Chemicals, by drug, adverse effect
    in labor and delivery O74.0
    in pregnancy O29.01- ☑
    obstetric O74.0
    overdose or wrong substance given or taken (by accident) — *see* Table of Drugs and Chemicals, by drug, poisoning
    postpartum, puerperal O89.01
  postoperative J95.4
    obstetric O74.0
  radiation J70.0
  rubella, congenital P35.0
  ventilation (air-conditioning) J67.7
  ventilator associated J95.851
  wood-dust J67.8
Pneumonoconiosis — *see* Pneumoconiosis
Pneumoparotid K11.8
Pneumopathy NEC J98.4
  alveolar J84.09
  due to organic dust NEC J66.8
  parietoalveolar J84.09

Pneumopericarditis — *see also* Pericarditis
  acute I30.9
Pneumopericardium — *see also* Pericarditis
  congenital P25.3
  newborn P25.3
  traumatic (post) — *see* Injury, heart
Pneumophagia (psychogenic) F45.8
Pneumopleurisy, pneumopleuritis — *see also* Pneumonia J18.8
Pneumopyopericardium I30.1
Pneumopyothorax — *see* Pyopneumothorax
  with fistula J86.0
Pneumorrhagia — *see also* Hemorrhage, lung
  tuberculous — *see* Tuberculosis, pulmonary
Pneumothorax NOS J93.9
  acute J93.83
  chronic J93.81
  congenital P25.1
    perinatal period P25.1
  postprocedural J95.811
  specified NEC J93.83
  spontaneous NOS J93.83
    newborn P25.1
    primary J93.11
    secondary J93.12
    tension J93.0
  tense valvular, infectional J93.0
  tension (spontaneous) J93.0
  traumatic S27.0 ☑
    with hemothorax S27.2 ☑
  tuberculous — *see* Tuberculosis, pulmonary
Podagra — *see also* Gout M10.9
Podencephalus Q01.9
Poikilocytosis R71.8
Poikiloderma L81.6
  Civatte's L57.3
  congenital Q82.8
  vasculare atrophicans L94.5
Poikilodermatomyositis M33.10
  with
    myopathy M33.12
    respiratory involvement M33.11
    specified organ involvement NEC M33.19
Pointed ear (congenital) Q17.3
Poison ivy, oak, sumac or other plant dermatitis (allergic) (contact) L23.7
Poisoning (acute) — *see also* Table of Drugs and Chemicals
  algae and toxins T65.82- ☑
  Bacillus B (aertrycke) (cholerae (suis)) (paratyphosus) (suipestifer) A02.9
    botulinus A05.1
  bacterial toxins A05.9
  berries, noxious — *see* Poisoning, food, noxious, berries
  botulism A05.1
  ciguatera fish T61.0- ☑
  Clostridium botulinum A05.1
  death-cap (Amanita phalloides) (Amanita verna) — *see* Poisoning, food, noxious, mushrooms
  drug — *see* Table of Drugs and Chemicals, by drug, poisoning
  epidemic, fish (noxious) — *see* Poisoning, seafood
    bacterial A05.9
  fava bean D55.0
  fish (noxious) T61.9- ☑
    bacterial — *see* Intoxication, foodborne, by agent
    ciguatera fish — *see* Poisoning, ciguatera fish
    scombroid fish — *see* Poisoning, scombroid fish
    specified type NEC T61.77- ☑
  food NEC A05.9
    bacterial — *see* Intoxication, foodborne, by agent
    due to
      Bacillus (aertrycke) (choleraesuis) (paratyphosus) (suipestifer) A02.9
        botulinus A05.1
      Clostridium (perfringens) (Welchii) A05.2
      salmonella (aertrycke) (callinarum) (choleraesuis) (enteritidis) (paratyphi) (suipestifer) A02.9
        with
          gastroenteritis A02.0
          sepsis A02.1
      staphylococcus A05.0
      Vibrio
        parahaemolyticus A05.3
        vulnificus A05.5
    noxious or naturally toxic T62.9- ☑
      berries — *see* subcategory T62.1 ☑
      fish — *see* Poisoning, seafood

Poisoning — *continued*
  food — *continued*
    noxious or naturally toxic — *continued*
      mushrooms — *see* subcategory T62.0X ☑
      plants NEC — *see* subcategory T62.2X ☑
      seafood — *see* Poisoning, seafood
      specified NEC — *see* subcategory T62.8X ☑
  ichthyotoxism — *see* Poisoning, seafood
  kreotoxism, food A05.9
  latex T65.81- ☑
  lead T56.0- ☑
  mushroom — *see* Poisoning, food, noxious, mushroom
  mussels — *see also* Poisoning, shellfish
    bacterial — *see* Intoxication, foodborne, by agent
  nicotine (tobacco) T65.2- ☑
  noxious foodstuffs — *see* Poisoning, food, noxious
  plants, noxious — *see* Poisoning, food, noxious, plants NEC
  ptomaine — *see* Poisoning, food
  radiation J70.0
  Salmonella (arizonae) (cholerae-suis) (enteritidis) (typhimurium) A02.9
  scombroid fish T61.1- ☑
  seafood (noxious) T61.9- ☑
    bacterial — *see* Intoxication, foodborne, by agent
    fish — *see* Poisoning, fish
    shellfish — *see* Poisoning, shellfish
    specified NEC — *see* subcategory T61.8X ☑
  shellfish (amnesic) (azaspiracid) (diarrheic) (neurotoxic) (noxious) (paralytic) T61.78- ☑
    bacterial — *see* Intoxication, foodborne, by agent
    ciguatera mollusk — *see* Poisoning, ciguatera fish
  specified substance NEC T65.891 ☑
  Staphylococcus, food A05.0
  tobacco (nicotine) T65.2- ☑
  water E87.79
Poker spine — *see* Spondylitis, ankylosing
Poland syndrome Q79.8
Polioencephalitis (acute) (bulbar) A80.9
  inferior G12.22
  influenzal — *see* Influenza, with, encephalopathy
  superior hemorrhagic (acute) (Wernicke's) E51.2
  Wernicke's E51.2
Polioencephalomyelitis (acute) (anterior) A80.9
  with beriberi E51.2
Polioencephalopathy, superior hemorrhagic E51.2
  with
    beriberi E51.11
    pellagra E52
Poliomeningoencephalitis — *see* Meningoencephalitis
Poliomyelitis (acute) (anterior) (epidemic) A80.9
  with paralysis (bulbar) — *see* Poliomyelitis, paralytic
  abortive A80.4
  ascending (progressive) — *see* Poliomyelitis, paralytic
  bulbar (paralytic) — *see* Poliomyelitis, paralytic
  congenital P35.8
  nonepidemic A80.9
  nonparalytic A80.4
  paralytic A80.30
    specified NEC A80.39
    vaccine-associated A80.0
    wild virus
      imported A80.1
      indigenous A80.2
  spinal, acute A80.9
Poliosis (eyebrow) (eyelashes) L67.1
  circumscripta, acquired L67.1
Pollakiuria R35.0
  psychogenic F45.8
Pollinosis J30.1
Pollitzer's disease L73.2
Polyadenitis — *see also* Lymphadenitis
  malignant A20.0
Polyalgia M79.89
Polyangiitis M30.0
  microscopic M31.7
  overlap syndrome M30.8
Polyarteritis
  microscopic M31.7
  nodosa M30.0
    with lung involvement M30.1
    juvenile M30.2
    related condition NEC M30.8
Polyarthralgia — *see* Pain, joint
Polyarthritis, polyarthropathy — *see also* Arthritis M13.0

☑ Additional Character Required — Refer to the Tabular List for Character Selection
Ⓥ Subterms under main terms may continue to next column or page

Polyarthritis, polyarthropathy — *continued*
   due to or associated with other specified conditions — *see* Arthritis
   epidemic (Australian) (with exanthema) B33.1
   infective — *see* Arthritis, pyogenic or pyemic
   Inflammatory M06.4
   juvenile (chronic) (seronegative) M08.3
   migratory M13.8- ☑
   rheumatic, acute — *see* Fever, rheumatic
Polyarthrosis M15.9
   post-traumatic M15.3
   primary M15.0
   specified NEC M15.8
Polycarential syndrome of infancy E40
Polychondritis (atrophic) (chronic) — *see also* Disorder, cartilage, specified type NEC
   relapsing M94.1
Polycoria Q13.2
Polycystic (disease)
   degeneration, kidney Q61.3
      autosomal dominant (adult type) Q61.2
      autosomal recessive (infantile type) NEC Q61.19
   kidney Q61.3
      autosomal
         dominant Q61.2
         recessive NEC Q61.19
      autosomal dominant (adult type) Q61.2
      autosomal recessive (childhood type) NEC Q61.19
      infantile type NEC Q61.19
   liver Q44.6
   lung J98.4
      congenital Q33.0
   ovary, ovaries E28.2
   spleen Q89.09
Polycythemia (secondary) D75.1
   acquired D75.1
   benign (familial) D75.0
   due to
      donor twin P61.1
      erythropoietin D75.1
      fall in plasma volume D75.1
      high altitude D75.1
      maternal-fetal transfusion P61.1
      stress D75.1
   emotional D75.1
   erythropoietin D75.1
   familial (benign) D75.0
   Gaisböck's (hypertonica) D75.1
   high altitude D75.1
   hypertonica D75.1
   hypoxemic D75.1
   neonatorum P61.1
   nephrogenous D75.1
   relative D75.1
   secondary D75.1
   spurious D75.1
   stress D75.1
   vera D45
Polycytosis cryptogenica D75.1
Polydactylism, polydactyly Q69.9
   toes Q69.2
Polydipsia R63.1
Polydystrophy, pseudo-Hurler E77.0
Polyembryoma — *see* Neoplasm, malignant, by site
Polyglandular
   deficiency E31.0
   dyscrasia E31.9
   dysfunction E31.9
   syndrome E31.8
Polyhydramnios O40.- ☑
Polymastia Q83.1
Polymenorrhea N92.0
Polymyalgia M35.3
   arteritica, giant cell M31.5
   rheumatica M35.3
      with giant cell arteritis M31.5
Polymyositis (acute) (chronic) (hemorrhagic) M33.20
   with
      myopathy M33.22
      respiratory involvement M33.21
      skin involvement — *see* Dermatopolymyositis
      specified organ involvement NEC M33.29
   ossificans (generalisata) (progressiva) — *see* Myositis, ossificans, progressiva
Polyneuritis, polyneuritic — *see also* Polyneuropathy
   acute (post-)infective G61.0
   alcoholic G62.1
   cranialis G52.7

Polyneuritis, polyneuritic — *continued*
   demyelinating, chronic inflammatory (CIDP) G61.81
   diabetic — *see* Diabetes, polyneuropathy
   diphtheritic A36.83
   due to lack of vitamin NEC E56.9 *[G63]*
   endemic E51.11
   erythredema — *see* subcategory T56.1 ☑
   febrile, acute G61.0
   hereditary ataxic G60.1
   idiopathic, acute G61.0
   infective (acute) G61.0
   inflammatory, chronic demyelinating (CIDP) G61.81
   nutritional E63.9 *[G63]*
   postinfective (acute) G61.0
   specified NEC G62.89
Polyneuropathy (peripheral) G62.9
   alcoholic G62.1
   amyloid (Portuguese) E85.1 *[G63]*
      transthyretin-related (ATTR) familial E85.1 *[G63]*
   arsenical G62.2
   critical illness G62.81
   demyelinating, chronic inflammatory (CIDP) G61.81
   diabetic — *see* Diabetes, polyneuropathy
   drug-induced G62.0
   hereditary G60.9
      specified NEC G60.8
   idiopathic G60.9
      progressive G60.3
   in (due to)
      alcohol G62.1
         sequelae G65.2
      amyloidosis, familial (Portuguese) E85.1 *[G63]*
      antitetanus serum G61.1
      arsenic G62.2
         sequelae G65.2
      avitaminosis NEC E56.9 *[G63]*
      beriberi E51.11
      collagen vascular disease NEC M35.9 *[G63]*
      deficiency (of)
         B (-complex) vitamins E53.9 *[G63]*
         vitamin B6 E53.1 *[G63]*
      diabetes — *see* Diabetes, polyneuropathy
      diphtheria A36.83
      drug or medicament G62.0
         correct substance properly administered — *see* Table of Drugs and Chemicals, by drug, adverse effect
         overdose or wrong substance given or taken — *see* Table of Drugs and Chemicals, by drug, poisoning
      endocrine disease NEC E34.9 *[G63]*
      herpes zoster B02.23
      hypoglycemia E16.2 *[G63]*
      infectious
         disease NEC B99 ☑ *[G63]*
         mononucleosis B27.91
      lack of vitamin NEC E56.9 *[G63]*
      lead G62.2
         sequelae G65.2
      leprosy A30.9 *[G63]*
      Lyme disease A69.22
      metabolic disease NEC E88.9 *[G63]*
      microscopic polyangiitis M31.7 *[G63]*
      mumps B26.84
      neoplastic disease — *see also* Neoplasm D49.9 *[G63]*
      nutritional deficiency NEC E63.9 *[G63]*
      organophosphate compounds G62.2
         sequelae G65.2
      parasitic disease NEC B89 *[G63]*
      pellagra E52 *[G63]*
      polyarteritis nodosa M30.0
      porphyria E80.20 *[G63]*
      radiation G62.82
      rheumatoid arthritis — *see* Rheumatoid, polyneuropathy
      sarcoidosis D86.89
      serum G61.1
      syphilis (late) A52.15
         congenital A50.43
      systemic
         connective tissue disorder M35.9 *[G63]*
         lupus erythematosus M32.19
      toxic agent NEC G62.2
         sequelae G65.2
   inflammatory G61.9
      chronic demyelinating (CIDP) G61.81
      sequelae G65.1
      specified NEC G61.89

Polyneuropathy — *continued*
   lead G62.2
      sequelae G65.2
   nutritional NEC E63.9 *[G63]*
   postherpetic (zoster) B02.23
   progressive G60.3
   radiation-induced G62.82
   sensory (hereditary) (idiopathic) G60.8
   specified NEC G62.89
   syphilitic (late) A52.15
      congenital A50.43
   transthyretin-related (ATTR) familial amyloid E85.1
      triorthocresyl phosphate G62.2
         sequelae G65.2
      tuberculosis A17.89
      uremia N18.9 *[G63]*
      vitamin B12 deficiency E53.8 *[G63]*
         with anemia (pernicious) D51.0 *[G63]*
         due to dietary deficiency D51.3 *[G63]*
      zoster B02.23
Polyopia H53.8
Polyorchism, polyorchidism Q55.21
Polyosteoarthritis — *see also* Osteoarthritis, generalized M15.9
   post-traumatic M15.3
   specified NEC M15.8
Polyostotic fibrous dysplasia Q78.1
Polyotia Q17.0
Polyp, polypus
   accessory sinus J33.8
   adenocarcinoma in — *see* Neoplasm, malignant, by site
   adenocarcinoma in situ in — *see* Neoplasm, in situ, by site
   adenoid tissue J33.0
   adenomatous — *see also* Neoplasm, benign, by site
      adenocarcinoma in — *see* Neoplasm, malignant, by site
      adenocarcinoma in situ in — *see* Neoplasm, in situ, by site
      carcinoma in — *see* Neoplasm, malignant, by site
      carcinoma in situ in — *see* Neoplasm, in situ, by site
      multiple — *see* Neoplasm, benign
         adenocarcinoma in — *see* Neoplasm, malignant, by site
         adenocarcinoma in situ in — *see* Neoplasm, in situ, by site
   antrum J33.8
   anus, anal (canal) K62.0
   Bartholin's gland N84.3
   bladder D41.4
   carcinoma in — *see* Neoplasm, malignant, by site
   carcinoma in situ in — *see* Neoplasm, in situ, by site
   cecum D12.0
   cervix (uteri) N84.1
      in pregnancy or childbirth — *see* Pregnancy, complicated by, abnormal, cervix
      mucous N84.1
      nonneoplastic N84.1
   choanal J33.0
   cholesterol K82.4
   clitoris N84.3
   colon K63.5
      adenomatous D12.6
         ascending D12.2
         cecum D12.0
         descending D12.4
      hyperplastic, (any site) K63.5
      inflammatory K51.40
         with
            abscess K51.414
            complication K51.419
               specified NEC K51.418
            fistula K51.413
            intestinal obstruction K51.412
            rectal bleeding K51.411
      sigmoid D12.5
      transverse D12.3
   corpus uteri N84.0
   dental K04.01
      irreversible K04.02
      reversible K04.01
   duodenum K31.7
   ear (middle) H74.4- ☑
   endometrium N84.0
   ethmoidal (sinus) J33.8
   fallopian tube N84.8
   female genital tract N84.9

Polyp, polypus — *continued*
- female genital tract — *continued*
  - specified NEC N84.8
- frontal (sinus) J33.8
- gallbladder K82.4
- gingiva, gum K06.8
- labia, labium (majus) (minus) N84.3
- larynx (mucous) J38.1
  - adenomatous D14.1
- malignant — *see* Neoplasm, malignant, by site
- maxillary (sinus) J33.8
- middle ear — *see* Polyp, ear (middle)
- myometrium N84.0
- nares
  - anterior J33.9
  - posterior J33.0
- nasal (mucous) J33.9
  - cavity J33.0
  - septum J33.0
- nasopharyngeal J33.0
- nose (mucous) J33.9
- oviduct N84.8
- pharynx J39.2
- placenta O90.89
- prostate — *see* Enlargement, enlarged, prostate
- pudenda, pudendum N84.3
- pulpal (dental) K04.01
  - irreversible K04.02
  - reversible K04.01
- rectum (nonadenomatous) K62.1
  - adenomatous — *see* Polyp, adenomatous
- septum (nasal) J33.0
- sinus (accessory) (ethmoidal) (frontal) (maxillary) (sphenoidal) J33.8
- sphenoidal (sinus) J33.8
- stomach K31.7
  - adenomatous D13.1
- tube, fallopian N84.8
- turbinate, mucous membrane J33.8
- umbilical, newborn P83.6
- ureter N28.89
- urethra N36.2
- uterus (body) (corpus) (mucous) N84.0
  - cervix N84.1
  - in pregnancy or childbirth — *see* Pregnancy, complicated by, tumor, uterus
- vagina N84.2
- vocal cord (mucous) J38.1
- vulva N84.3

Polyphagia R63.2
Polyploidy Q92.7
Polypoid — *see* condition
Polyposis — *see also* Polyp
- coli (adenomatous) D12.6
  - adenocarcinoma in C18.9
  - adenocarcinoma in situ in — *see* Neoplasm, in situ, by site
  - carcinoma in C18.9
- colon (adenomatous) D12.6
- familial D12.6
  - adenocarcinoma in situ in — *see* Neoplasm, in situ, by site
- intestinal (adenomatous) D12.6
- malignant lymphomatous C83.1- ☑
- multiple, adenomatous — *see also* Neoplasm, benign D36.9

Polyradiculitis — *see* Polyneuropathy
Polyradiculoneuropathy (acute) (postinfective) (segmentally demyelinating) G61.0
Polyserositis
- due to pericarditis I31.1
- pericardial I31.1
- periodic, familial E85.0
- tuberculous A19.9
  - acute A19.1
  - chronic A19.8

Polysplenia syndrome Q89.09
Polysyndactyly — *see also* Syndactylism, syndactyly Q70.4
Polytrichia L68.3
Polyunguia Q84.6
Polyuria R35.8
- nocturnal R35.1
- psychogenic F45.8

Pompe's disease (glycogen storage) E74.02
Pompholyx L30.1
Poncet's disease (tuberculous rheumatism) A18.09
Pond fracture — *see* Fracture, skull

Ponos B55.0
Pons, pontine — *see* condition
Poor
- aesthetic of existing restoration of tooth K08.56
- contractions, labor O62.2
- gingival margin to tooth restoration K08.51
- personal hygiene R46.0
- prenatal care, affecting management of pregnancy — *see* Pregnancy, complicated by, insufficient, prenatal care
- sucking reflex (newborn) R29.2
- urinary stream R39.12
- vision NEC H54.7

Poradenitis, nostras inguinalis or venerea A55
Porencephaly (congenital) (developmental) (true) Q04.6
- acquired G93.0
- nondevelopmental G93.0
- traumatic (post) F07.89

Porocephaliasis B88.8
Porokeratosis Q82.8
Poroma, eccrine — *see* Neoplasm, skin, benign
Porphyria (South African) E80.20
- acquired E80.20
- acute intermittent (hepatic) (Swedish) E80.21
- cutanea tarda (hereditary) (symptomatic) E80.1
- due to drugs E80.20
  - correct substance properly administered — *see* Table of Drugs and Chemicals, by drug, adverse effect
  - overdose or wrong substance given or taken — *see* Table of Drugs and Chemicals, by drug, poisoning
- erythropoietic (congenital) (hereditary) E80.0
- hepatocutaneous type E80.1
- secondary E80.20
- toxic NEC E80.20
- variegata E80.20

Porphyrinuria — *see* Porphyria
Porphyruria — *see* Porphyria
Port wine nevus, mark, or stain Q82.5
Portal — *see* condition
Posadas-Wernicke disease B38.9
Positive
- culture (nonspecific)
  - blood R78.81
  - bronchial washings R84.5
  - cerebrospinal fluid R83.5
  - cervix uteri R87.5
  - nasal secretions R84.5
  - nipple discharge R89.5
  - nose R84.5
    - staphylococcus (Methicillin susceptible) Z22.321
      - Methicillin resistant Z22.322
  - peritoneal fluid R85.5
  - pleural fluid R84.5
  - prostatic secretions R86.5
  - saliva R85.5
  - seminal fluid R86.5
  - sputum R84.5
  - synovial fluid R89.5
  - throat scrapings R84.5
  - urine R82.79
  - vagina R87.5
  - vulva R87.5
  - wound secretions R89.5
- PPD (skin test) R76.11
- serology for syphilis A53.0
  - false R76.8
  - with signs or symptoms — *code as* Syphilis, by site and stage
- skin test, tuberculin (without active tuberculosis) R76.11
- test, human immunodeficiency virus (HIV) R75
- VDRL A53.0
  - with signs or symptoms — *code by* site and stage under Syphilis A53.9
- Wassermann reaction A53.0

Postcardiotomy syndrome I97.0
Postcaval ureter Q62.62
Postcholecystectomy syndrome K91.5
Postclimacteric bleeding N95.0
Postcommissurotomy syndrome I97.0
Postconcussional syndrome F07.81
Postcontusional syndrome F07.81
Postcricoid region — *see* condition
Post-dates (40-42 weeks) (pregnancy) (mother) O48.0
- more than 42 weeks gestation O48.1
Postencephalitic syndrome F07.89
Posterior — *see* condition

Posterolateral sclerosis (spinal cord) — *see* Degeneration, combined
Postexanthematous — *see* condition
Postfebrile — *see* condition
Postgastrectomy dumping syndrome K91.1
Posthemiplegic chorea — *see* Monoplegia
Posthemorrhagic anemia (chronic) D50.0
- acute D62
- newborn P61.3
Postherpetic neuralgia (zoster) B02.29
- trigeminal B02.22
Posthitis N47.7
Postimmunization complication or reaction — *see* Complications, vaccination
Postinfectious — *see* condition
Postlaminectomy syndrome NEC M96.1
Postleukotomy syndrome F07.0
Postmastectomy lymphedema (syndrome) I97.2
Postmaturity, postmature (over 42 weeks)
- maternal (over 42 weeks gestation) O48.1
- newborn P08.22
Postmeasles complication NEC — *see also* condition B05.89
Postmenopausal
- endometrium (atrophic) N95.8
  - suppurative — *see also* Endometritis N71.9
- osteoporosis — *see* Osteoporosis, postmenopausal
Postnasal drip R09.82
- due to
  - allergic rhinitis — *see* Rhinitis, allergic
  - common cold J00
  - gastroesophageal reflux — *see* Reflux, gastroesophageal
  - nasopharyngitis — *see* Nasopharyngitis
  - other known condition — *code to* condition
  - sinusitis — *see* Sinusitis
Postnatal — *see* condition
Postoperative (postprocedural) — *see* Complication, postoperative
- pneumothorax, therapeutic Z98.3
- state NEC Z98.890
Postpancreatectomy hyperglycemia E89.1
Postpartum — *see* Puerperal
Postphlebitic syndrome — *see* Syndrome, postthrombotic
Postpolio (myelitic) **syndrome** G14
Postpoliomyelitic — *see also* condition
- osteopathy — *see* Osteopathy, after poliomyelitis
Postprocedural — *see also* Postoperative
- hypoinsulinemia E89.1
Postschizophrenic depression F32.89
Postsurgery status — *see also* Status (post)
- pneumothorax, therapeutic Z98.3
Post-term (40-42 weeks) (pregnancy) (mother) O48.0
- infant P08.21
- more than 42 weeks gestation (mother) O48.1
Post-traumatic brain syndrome, nonpsychotic F07.81
Post-typhoid abscess A01.09
Postures, hysterical F44.2
Postvaccinal reaction or complication — *see* Complications, vaccination
Postvalvulotomy syndrome I97.0
Potain's
- disease (pulmonary edema) — *see* Edema, lung
- syndrome (gastrectasis with dyspepsia) K31.0
Potter's
- asthma J62.8
- facies Q60.6
- lung J62.8
- syndrome (with renal agenesis) Q60.6
Pott's
- curvature (spinal) A18.01
- disease or paraplegia A18.01
- spinal curvature A18.01
- tumor, puffy — *see* Osteomyelitis, specified type NEC
Pouch
- bronchus Q32.4
- Douglas' — *see* condition
- esophagus, esophageal, congenital Q39.6
  - acquired K22.5
- gastric K31.4
- Hartmann's K82.8
- pharynx, pharyngeal (congenital) Q38.7
Pouchitis K91.850
Poultrymen's itch B88.0
Poverty NEC Z59.6
- extreme Z59.5

☑ **Additional Character Required** — Refer to the Tabular List for Character Selection   ▽ Subterms under main terms may continue to next column or page

Poxvirus NEC B08.8
Prader-Willi syndrome Q87.11
Prader-Willi-like syndrome Q87.19
Preauricular appendage or tag Q17.0
Prebetalipoproteinemia (acquired) (essential) (familial)
    (hereditary) (primary) (secondary) E78.1
    with chylomicronemia E78.3
Precipitate labor or delivery O62.3
Preclimacteric bleeding (menorrhagia) N92.4
Precocious
    adrenarche E30.1
    menarche E30.1
    menstruation E30.1
    pubarche E30.1
    puberty E30.1
        central E22.8
    sexual development NEC E30.1
    thelarche E30.8
Precocity, sexual (constitutional) (cryptogenic) (female)
    (idiopathic) (male) E30.1
    with adrenal hyperplasia E25.9
        congenital E25.0
Precordial pain R07.2
Predeciduous teeth K00.2
Prediabetes, prediabetic R73.03
    complicating
        pregnancy — see Pregnancy, complicated by, dis-
            eases of, specified type or system NEC
        puerperium O99.89
Predislocation status of hip at birth Q65.6
Pre-eclampsia O14.9- ☑
    with pre-existing hypertension — see Hypertension,
        complicating pregnancy, pre-existing, with, pre-
        eclampsia
    complicating
        childbirth O14.94
        puerperium O14.95
    mild O14.0- ☑
        complicating
            childbirth O14.04
            puerperium O14.05
    moderate O14.0- ☑
        complicating
            childbirth O14.04
            puerperium O14.05
    severe O14.1- ☑
        with hemolysis, elevated liver enzymes and low
            platelet count (HELLP) O14.2- ☑
            complicating
                childbirth O14.24
                puerperium O14.25
        complicating
            childbirth O14.14
            puerperium O14.15
Pre-eruptive color change, teeth, tooth K00.8
Pre-excitation atrioventricular conduction I45.6
Preglaucoma H40.00- ☑
Pregnancy (single) (uterine) — see also Delivery and
    Puerperal

> Note: The Tabular must be reviewed for assign-
> ment of appropriate seventh character for mul-
> tiple gestation codes in Chapter 15

> Note: The Tabular must be reviewed for assign-
> ment of the appropriate character indicating the
> trimester of the pregnancy

    abdominal (ectopic) O00.00
        with intrauterine pregnancy O00.01
        with viable fetus O36.7- ☑
    ampullar O00.10- ☑
        with intrauterine pregnancy O00.11- ☑
    biochemical O02.81
    broad ligament O00.80
        with intrauterine pregnancy O00.81
    cervical O00.8
        with intrauterine pregnancy O00.81
    chemical O02.81
    complicated by (care of) (management affected by)
        abnormal, abnormality
            cervix O34.4- ☑
                causing obstructed labor O65.5
            cord (umbilical) O69.9 ☑
            fetal heart rate or rhythm O36.83- ☑
            findings on antenatal screening of mother O28.9
                biochemical O28.1
                chromosomal O28.5

Pregnancy — continued
    complicated by — continued
        abnormal, abnormality — continued
            findings on antenatal screening of mother —
                continued
                cytological O28.2
                genetic O28.5
                hematological O28.0
                radiological O28.4
                specified NEC O28.8
                ultrasonic O28.3
            glucose (tolerance) NEC O99.810
            pelvic organs O34.9- ☑
                specified NEC O34.8- ☑
                    causing obstructed labor O65.5
            pelvis (bony) (major) NEC O33.0
            perineum O34.7- ☑
            position
                placenta O44.0- ☑
                    with hemorrhage O44.1- ☑
                uterus O34.59- ☑
            uterus O34.59- ☑
                causing obstructed labor O65.5
                congenital O34.0- ☑
            vagina O34.6- ☑
                causing obstructed labor O65.5
            vulva O34.7- ☑
                causing obstructed labor O65.5
        abruptio placentae — see Abruptio placentae
        abscess or cellulitis
            bladder O23.1- ☑
            breast O91.11- ☑
            genital organ or tract O23.9- ☑
        abuse
            physical O9A.31 ☑ (following O99)
            psychological O9A.51 ☑ (following O99)
            sexual O9A.41 ☑ (following O99)
        adverse effect anesthesia O29.9- ☑
            aspiration pneumonitis O29.01- ☑
            cardiac arrest O29.11- ☑
            cardiac complication NEC O29.19- ☑
            cardiac failure O29.12- ☑
            central nervous system complication NEC
                O29.29- ☑
            cerebral anoxia O29.21- ☑
            failed or difficult intubation O29.6- ☑
            inhalation of stomach contents or secretions NOS
                O29.01- ☑
            local, toxic reaction O29.3X ☑
            Mendelson's syndrome O29.01- ☑
            pressure collapse of lung O29.02- ☑
            pulmonary complications NEC O29.09- ☑
            specified NEC O29.8X- ☑
            spinal and epidural type NEC O29.5X ☑
                induced headache O29.4- ☑
        albuminuria — see also Proteinuria, gestational
            O12.1- ☑
        alcohol use O99.31- ☑
        amnionitis O41.12- ☑
        anaphylactoid syndrome of pregnancy O88.01- ☑
        anemia (conditions in D50-D64) (pre-existing)
            O99.01- ☑
            complicating the puerperium O99.03
        antepartum hemorrhage O46.9- ☑
            with coagulation defect — see Hemorrhage,
                antepartum, with coagulation defect
            specified NEC O46.8X- ☑
        appendicitis O99.61- ☑
        atrophy (yellow) (acute) liver (subacute) O26.61- ☑
        bariatric surgery status O99.84- ☑
        bicornis or bicornuate uterus O34.0- ☑
        biliary tract problems O26.61- ☑
        breech presentation O32.1 ☑
        cardiovascular diseases (conditions in I00-I09, I20-
            I52, I70-I99) O99.41- ☑
        cerebrovascular disorders (conditions in I60-I69)
            O99.41- ☑
        cervical shortening O26.87- ☑
        cervicitis O23.51- ☑
        chloasma (gravidarum) O26.89- ☑
        cholecystitis O99.61- ☑
        cholestasis (intrahepatic) O26.61- ☑
        chorioamnionitis O41.12- ☑
        circulatory system disorder (conditions in I00-I09,
            I20-I99, O99.41)
        compound presentation O32.6 ☑

Pregnancy — continued
    complicated by — continued
        conjoined twins O30.02- ☑
        connective system disorders (conditions in M00-
            M99) O99.89
        contracted pelvis (general) O33.1
            inlet O33.2
            outlet O33.3 ☑
        convulsions (eclamptic) (uremic) — see also
            Eclampsia O15.9
        cracked nipple O92.11- ☑
        cystitis O23.1- ☑
        cystocele O34.8- ☑
        death of fetus (near term) O36.4 ☑
            early pregnancy O02.1
            of one fetus or more in multiple gestation
                O31.2- ☑
        deciduitis O41.14- ☑
        decreased fetal movement O36.81- ☑
        dental problems O99.61- ☑
        diabetes (mellitus) O24.91- ☑
            gestational (pregnancy induced) — see Diabetes,
                gestational
            pre-existing O24.31- ☑
                specified NEC O24.81- ☑
                type 1 O24.01- ☑
                type 2 O24.11- ☑
        digestive system disorders (conditions in K00-K93)
            O99.61- ☑
        diseases of — see Pregnancy, complicated by,
            specified body system disease
            biliary tract O26.61- ☑
            blood NEC (conditions in D65-D77) O99.11- ☑
            liver O26.61- ☑
            specified NEC O99.89
        disorders of — see Pregnancy, complicated by,
            specified body system disorder
            amniotic fluid and membranes O41.9- ☑
                specified NEC O41.8X- ☑
            biliary tract O26.61- ☑
            ear and mastoid process (conditions in H60-H95)
                O99.89
            eye and adnexa (conditions in H00-H59) O99.89
            liver O26.61- ☑
            skin (conditions in L00-L99) O99.71- ☑
            specified NEC O99.89
        displacement, uterus NEC O34.59- ☑
            causing obstructed labor O65.5
        disproportion (due to) O33.9
            fetal (ascites) (hydrops) (meningomyelocele)
                (sacral teratoma) (tumor) deformities NEC
                O33.7 ☑
            generally contracted pelvis O33.1
            hydrocephalic fetus O33.6 ☑
            inlet contraction of pelvis O33.2
            mixed maternal and fetal origin O33.4 ☑
            specified NEC O33.8
        double uterus O34.0- ☑
            causing obstructed labor O65.5
        drug use (conditions in F11-F19) O99.32- ☑
        eclampsia, eclamptic (coma) (convulsions) (delirium)
            (nephritis) (uremia) — see also Eclampsia
            O15.- ☑
        ectopic pregnancy — see Pregnancy, ectopic
        edema O12.0- ☑
            with
                gestational hypertension, mild — see also
                    Pre-eclampsia O14.0- ☑
                proteinuria O12.2- ☑
        effusion, amniotic fluid — see Pregnancy, compli-
            cated by, premature rupture of membranes
        elderly
            multigravida O09.52- ☑
            primigravida O09.51- ☑
        embolism — see also Embolism, obstetric, pregnan-
            cy O88.- ☑
        endocrine diseases NEC O99.28- ☑
        endometritis O86.12
        excessive weight gain O26.0- ☑
        exhaustion O26.81- ☑
            during labor and delivery O75.81
        face presentation O32.3 ☑
        failed induction of labor O61.9
            instrumental O61.1
            mechanical O61.1
            medical O61.0
            specified NEC O61.8

Pregnancy — *continued*
  complicated by — *continued*
    failed induction of labor — *continued*
      surgical O61.1
    failed or difficult intubation for anesthesia O29.6- ☑
    false labor (pains) O47.9
      at or after 37 completed weeks of pregnancy O47.1
      before 37 completed weeks of pregnancy O47.0- ☑
    fatigue O26.81- ☑
      during labor and delivery O75.81
    fatty metamorphosis of liver O26.61- ☑
    female genital mutilation O34.8- *[N90.81-]* ☑
    fetal (maternal care for)
      abnormality or damage O35.9 ☑
        acid-base balance O68
        specified type NEC O35.8 ☑
      acidemia O68
      acidosis O68
      alkalosis O68
      anemia and thrombocytopenia O36.82- ☑
      anencephaly O35.0 ☑
      bradycardia O36.83- ☑
      chromosomal abnormality (conditions in Q90-Q99) O35.1 ☑
      conjoined twins O30.02- ☑
      damage from
        amniocentesis O35.7 ☑
        biopsy procedures O35.7 ☑
        drug addiction O35.5 ☑
        hematological investigation O35.7 ☑
        intrauterine contraceptive device O35.7 ☑
        maternal
          alcohol addiction O35.4 ☑
          cytomegalovirus infection O35.3 ☑
          disease NEC O35.8 ☑
          drug addiction O35.5 ☑
          listeriosis O35.8 ☑
          rubella O35.3 ☑
          toxoplasmosis O35.8 ☑
          viral infection O35.3 ☑
        medical procedure NEC O35.7 ☑
        radiation O35.6 ☑
      death (near term) O36.4 ☑
        early pregnancy O02.1
      decreased movement O36.81- ☑
      depressed heart rate tones O36.83- ☑
      disproportion due to deformity (fetal) O33.7 ☑
      excessive growth (large for dates) O36.6- ☑
      growth retardation O36.59- ☑
        light for dates O36.59- ☑
        small for dates O36.59- ☑
      heart rate irregularity (abnormal variability) (bradycardia) (decelerations) (tachycardia) O36.83- ☑
      hereditary disease O35.2 ☑
      hydrocephalus O35.0 ☑
      intrauterine death O36.4 ☑
      non-reassuring heart rate or rhythm O36.83- ☑
      poor growth O36.59- ☑
        light for dates O36.59- ☑
        small for dates O36.59- ☑
      problem O36.9- ☑
        specified NEC O36.89- ☑
      reduction (elective) O31.3- ☑
      selective termination O31.3- ☑
      spina bifida O35.0 ☑
      thrombocytopenia O36.82- ☑
    fibroid (tumor) (uterus) O34.1- ☑
    fissure of nipple O92.11- ☑
    gallstones O99.61- ☑
    gastric banding status O99.84- ☑
    gastric bypass status O99.84- ☑
    genital herpes (asymptomatic) (history of) (inactive) O98.3- ☑
    genital tract infection O23.9- ☑
    glomerular diseases (conditions in N00-N07) O26.83- ☑
      with hypertension, pre-existing — *see* Hypertension, complicating, pregnancy, pre-existing, with, renal disease
    gonorrhea O98.21- ☑
    grand multiparity O09.4 ☑
    habitual aborter — *see* Pregnancy, complicated by, recurrent pregnancy loss

Pregnancy — *continued*
  complicated by — *continued*
    HELLP syndrome (hemolysis, elevated liver enzymes and low platelet count) O14.2- ☑
    hemorrhage
      antepartum — *see* Hemorrhage, antepartum
      before 20 completed weeks gestation O20.9
        specified NEC O20.8
      due to premature separation, placenta — *see also* Abruptio placentae O45.9- ☑
      early O20.9
        specified NEC O20.8
      threatened abortion O20.0
    hemorrhoids O22.4- ☑
    hepatitis (viral) O98.41- ☑
    herniation of uterus O34.59- ☑
    high
      head at term O32.4 ☑
      risk — *see* Supervision (of) (for), high-risk
    history of in utero procedure during previous pregnancy O09.82- ☑
    HIV O98.71- ☑
    human immunodeficiency virus (HIV) disease O98.71- ☑
    hydatidiform mole — *see also* Mole, hydatidiform O01.9
    hydramnios O40.- ☑
    hydrocephalic fetus (disproportion) O33.6 ☑
    hydrops
      amnii O40.- ☑
      fetalis O36.2- ☑
        associated with isoimmunization — *see also* Pregnancy, complicated by, isoimmunization O36.11- ☑
    hydrorrhea O42.90
    hyperemesis (gravidarum) (mild) — *see also* Hyperemesis, gravidarum O21.0
    hypertension — *see* Hypertension, complicating pregnancy
    hypertensive
      heart and renal disease, pre-existing — *see* Hypertension, complicating, pregnancy, pre-existing, with, heart disease, with renal disease
      heart disease, pre-existing — *see* Hypertension, complicating, pregnancy, pre-existing, with, heart disease
      renal disease, pre-existing — *see* Hypertension, complicating, pregnancy, pre-existing, with, renal disease
    hypotension O26.5- ☑
    immune disorders NEC (conditions in D80-D89) O99.11- ☑
    incarceration, uterus O34.51- ☑
    incompetent cervix O34.3- ☑
    inconclusive fetal viability O36.80 ☑
    infection(s) O98.91- ☑
      amniotic fluid or sac O41.10- ☑
      bladder O23.1- ☑
      carrier state NEC O99.830
        streptococcus B O99.820
      genital organ or tract O23.9- ☑
        specified NEC O23.59- ☑
      genitourinary tract O23.9- ☑
      gonorrhea O98.21- ☑
      hepatitis (viral) O98.41- ☑
      HIV O98.71- ☑
      human immunodeficiency virus (HIV) O98.71- ☑
      kidney O23.0- ☑
      nipple O91.01- ☑
      parasitic disease O98.91- ☑
        specified NEC O98.81- ☑
      protozoal disease O98.61- ☑
      sexually transmitted NEC O98.31- ☑
      specified type NEC O98.81- ☑
      syphilis O98.11- ☑
      tuberculosis O98.01- ☑
      urethra O23.2- ☑
      urinary (tract) O23.4- ☑
        specified NEC O23.3- ☑
      viral disease O98.51- ☑
    injury or poisoning (conditions in S00-T88) O9A.21- ☑ (*following* O99)
      due to abuse
        physical O9A.31- ☑ (*following* O99)
        psychological O9A.51- ☑ (*following* O99)
        sexual O9A.41- ☑ (*following* O99)

Pregnancy — *continued*
  complicated by — *continued*
    insufficient
      prenatal care O09.3- ☑
      weight gain O26.1- ☑
    insulin resistance O26.89
    intrauterine fetal death (near term) O36.4
      early pregnancy O02.1
      multiple gestation (one fetus or more) O31.2- ☑
    isoimmunization O36.11- ☑
      anti-A sensitization O36.11- ☑
      anti-B sensitization O36.19- ☑
      Rh O36.09- ☑
        anti-D antibody O36.01- ☑
      specified NEC O36.19- ☑
    laceration of uterus NEC O71.81
    malformation
      placenta, placental (vessel) O43.10- ☑
        specified NEC O43.19- ☑
      uterus (congenital) O34.0- ☑
    malnutrition (conditions in E40-E46) O25.1- ☑
    maternal hypotension syndrome O26.5- ☑
    mental disorders (conditions in F01-F09, F20-F99) O99.34- ☑
      alcohol use O99.31- ☑
      drug use O99.32- ☑
      smoking O99.33- ☑
    mentum presentation O32.3 ☑
    metabolic disorders O99.28- ☑
    missed
      abortion O02.1
      delivery O36.4 ☑
    multiple gestations O30.9- ☑
      conjoined twins O30.02- ☑
      quadruplet — *see* Pregnancy, quadruplet
      specified complication NEC O31.8X- ☑
      specified number of multiples NEC — *see* Pregnancy, multiple (gestation), specified NEC
      triplet — *see* Pregnancy, triplet
      twin — *see* Pregnancy, twin
    musculoskeletal condition (conditions is M00-M99) O99.89
    necrosis, liver (conditions in K72) O26.61- ☑
    neoplasm
      benign
        cervix O34.4- ☑
        corpus uteri O34.1- ☑
        uterus O34.1- ☑
      malignant O9A.11- ☑ (*following* O99)
    nephropathy NEC O26.83- ☑
    nervous system condition (conditions in G00-G99) O99.35- ☑
    nutritional diseases NEC O99.28- ☑
    obesity (pre-existing) O99.21- ☑
    obesity surgery status O99.84- ☑
    oblique lie or presentation O32.2 ☑
    older mother — *see* Pregnancy, complicated by, elderly
    oligohydramnios O41.0- ☑
      with premature rupture of membranes — *see also* Pregnancy, complicated by, premature rupture of membranes O42.- ☑
    onset (spontaneous) of labor after 37 completed weeks of gestation but before 39 completed weeks gestation, with delivery by (planned) cesarean section O75.82
    oophoritis O23.52- ☑
    overdose, drug — *see also* Table of Drugs and Chemicals, by drug, poisoning O9A.21- ☑ (*following* O99)
    oversize fetus O33.5 ☑
    papyraceous fetus O31.0- ☑
    pelvic inflammatory disease O99.89
    periodontal disease O99.61- ☑
    peripheral neuritis O26.82- ☑
    peritoneal (pelvic) adhesions O99.89
    phlebitis O22.9- ☑
    phlebopathy O22.9- ☑
    phlebothrombosis (superficial) O22.2- ☑
      deep O22.3- ☑
    placenta accreta O43.21- ☑
    placenta increta O43.22- ☑
    placenta percreta O43.23- ☑
    placenta previa O44.0- ☑
      complete O44.0- ☑
        with hemorrhage O44.1- ☑

Pregnancy — *continued*
  complicated by — *continued*
    placenta previa — *continued*
      marginal O44.2- ☑
        with hemorrhage O44.3- ☑
      partial O44.2- ☑
        with hemorrhage O44.3- ☑
    placental disorder O43.9- ☑
      specified NEC O43.89- ☑
    placental dysfunction O43.89- ☑
    placental infarction O43.81- ☑
    placental insufficiency O36.51- ☑
    placental transfusion syndromes
      fetomaternal O43.01- ☑
      fetus to fetus O43.02- ☑
      maternofetal O43.01- ☑
    placentitis O41.14- ☑
    pneumonia O99.51- ☑
    poisoning — *see also* Table of Drugs and Chemicals
      O9A.21 (*following* O99)
    polyhydramnios O40- ☑
    polymorphic eruption of pregnancy O26.86
    poor obstetric history NEC O09.29- ☑
    postmaturity (post-term) (40 to 42 weeks) O48.0
      more than 42 completed weeks gestation (pro-
        longed) O48.1
    pre-eclampsia O14.9- ☑
      mild O14.0- ☑
      moderate O14.0- ☑
      severe O14.1- ☑
        with hemolysis, elevated liver enzymes and
          low platelet count (HELLP) O14.2- ☑
    premature labor — *see* Pregnancy, complicated by,
      preterm labor
    premature rupture of membranes O42.90
      with onset of labor
        within 24 hours O42.00
          at or after 37 weeks gestation, onset of
            labor within 24 hours of rupture
            O42.02
          pre-term (before 37 completed weeks of
            gestation) O42.01- ☑
        after 24 hours O42.10
          at or after 37 weeks gestation, onset of
            labor more than 24 hours following
            rupture O42.12
          pre-term (before 37 completed weeks of
            gestation) O42.11- ☑
      at or after 37 weeks gestation, unspecified as to
        length of time between rupture and onset
        of labor O42.92
      full-term, unspecified as to length of time be-
        tween rupture and onset of labor O42.92
      pre-term (before 37 completed weeks of gesta-
        tion) O42.91- ☑
    premature separation of placenta — *see also*
      Abruptio placentae O45.9- ☑
    presentation, fetal — *see* Delivery, complicated by,
      malposition
    preterm delivery O60.10 ☑
    preterm labor
      with delivery O60.10 ☑
        preterm O60.10 ☑
        term O60.20 ☑
      second trimester
        with term delivery O60.22 ☑
        without delivery O60.02
        with preterm delivery
          second trimester O60.12 ☑
          third trimester O60.13 ☑
      third trimester
        with term delivery O60.23 ☑
        without delivery O60.03
        with third trimester preterm delivery
          O60.14 ☑
      without delivery O60.00
        second trimester O60.02
        third trimester O60.03
    previous history of — *see* Pregnancy, supervision
      of, high-risk
    prolapse, uterus O34.52- ☑
    proteinuria (gestational) — *see also* Proteinuria,
      gestational O12.1- ☑
      with edema O12.2- ☑
    pruritic urticarial papules and plaques of pregnancy
      (PUPPP) O26.86
    pruritus (neurogenic) O26.89- ☑

Pregnancy — *continued*
  complicated by — *continued*
    psychosis or psychoneurosis (puerperal) F53.1
    ptyalism O26.89- ☑
    PUPPP (pruritic urticarial papules and plaques of
      pregnancy) O26.86
    pyelitis O23.0- ☑
    recurrent pregnancy loss O26.2- ☑
    renal disease or failure NEC O26.83- ☑
      with secondary hypertension, pre-existing —
        see Hypertension, complicating, pregnan-
        cy, pre-existing, secondary
      hypertensive, pre-existing — *see* Hypertension,
        complicating, pregnancy, pre-existing,
        with, renal disease
    respiratory condition (conditions in J00-J99)
      O99.51- ☑
    retained, retention
      dead ovum O02.0
      intrauterine contraceptive device O26.3- ☑
    retroversion, uterus O34.53- ☑
    Rh immunization, incompatibility or sensitization
      NEC O36.09- ☑
      anti-D antibody O36.01- ☑
    rupture
      amnion (premature) — *see also* Pregnancy,
        complicated by, premature rupture of
        membranes O42- ☑
      membranes (premature) — *see also* Pregnancy,
        complicated by, premature rupture of
        membranes O42- ☑
      uterus (during labor) O71.1
        before onset of labor O71.0- ☑
    salivation (excessive) O26.89- ☑
    salpingitis O23.52- ☑
    salpingo-oophoritis O23.52- ☑
    sepsis (conditions in A40, A41) O98.81- ☑
    size date discrepancy (uterine) O26.84- ☑
    skin condition (conditions in L00-L99) O99.71- ☑
    smoking (tobacco) O99.33- ☑
    social problem O09.7- ☑
    specified condition NEC O26.89- ☑
    spotting O26.85- ☑
    streptococcus group B (GBS) carrier state O99.820
    subluxation of symphysis (pubis) O26.71- ☑
    syphilis (conditions in A50-A53) O98.11- ☑
    threatened
      abortion O20.0
      labor O47.9
        at or after 37 completed weeks of gestation
          O47.1
        before 37 completed weeks of gestation
          O47.0- ☑
    thrombophlebitis (superficial) O22.2- ☑
    thrombosis O22.9- ☑
      cerebral venous O22.5- ☑
      cerebrovenous sinus O22.5- ☑
      deep O22.3- ☑
    tobacco use disorder (smoking) O99.33- ☑
    torsion of uterus O34.59- ☑
    toxemia O14.9- ☑
    transverse lie or presentation O32.2 ☑
    tuberculosis (conditions in A15-A19) O98.01- ☑
    tumor (benign)
      cervix O34.4- ☑
      malignant O9A.11- ☑ (*following* O99)
      uterus O34.1- ☑
    unstable lie O32.0 ☑
    upper respiratory infection O99.51- ☑
    urethritis O23.2- ☑
    uterine size date discrepancy O26.84- ☑
    vaginitis or vulvitis O23.59- ☑
    varicose veins (lower extremities) O22.0- ☑
      genitals O22.1- ☑
      legs O22.0- ☑
      perineal O22.1- ☑
      vaginal or vulval O22.1- ☑
    venereal disease NEC (conditions in A63.8)
      O98.31- ☑
    venous disorders O22.9- ☑
      specified NEC O22.8X- ☑
    very young mother — *see* Pregnancy, complicated
      by, young mother
    viral diseases (conditions in A80-B09, B25-B34)
      O98.51 ☑
    vomiting O21.9
      due to diseases classified elsewhere O21.8

Pregnancy — *continued*
  complicated by — *continued*
    vomiting — *continued*
      hyperemesis gravidarum (mild) — *see also* Hy-
        peremesis, gravidarum O21.0
      late (occurring after 20 weeks of gestation) O21.2
    young mother
      multigravida O09.62- ☑
      primigravida O09.61- ☑
  complicated NOS O26.9- ☑
  concealed O09.3- ☑
  continuing following
    elective fetal reduction of one or more fetus
      O31.3- ☑
    intrauterine death of one or more fetus O31.2- ☑
    spontaneous abortion of one or more fetus
      O31.1- ☑
  cornual O00.80
    with intrauterine pregnancy O00.81
  ectopic (ruptured) O00.90
    with intrauterine pregnancy O00.91
    abdominal O00.00
      with
        intrauterine pregnancy O00.01
        viable fetus O36.7- ☑
    cervical O00.80
      with intrauterine pregnancy O00.81
    complicated (by) O08.9
      afibrinogenemia O08.1
      cardiac arrest O08.81
      chemical damage of pelvic organ(s) O08.6
      circulatory collapse O08.3
      defibrination syndrome O08.1
      electrolyte imbalance O08.5
      embolism (amniotic fluid) (blood clot) (pul-
        monary) (septic) O08.2
      endometritis O08.0
      genital tract and pelvic infection O08.0
      hemorrhage (delayed) (excessive) O08.1
      infection
        genital tract or pelvic O08.0
        kidney O08.83
        urinary tract O08.3
      intravascular coagulation O08.1
      laceration of pelvic organ(s) O08.6
      metabolic disorder O08.5
      oliguria O08.4
      oophoritis O08.0
      parametritis O08.0
      pelvic peritonitis O08.0
      perforation of pelvic organ(s) O08.6
      renal failure or shutdown O08.4
      salpingitis or salpingo-oophoritis O08.0
      sepsis O08.82
      shock O08.83
        septic O08.82
      specified condition NEC O08.89
      tubular necrosis (renal) O08.4
      uremia O08.4
      urinary infection O08.83
      venous complication NEC O08.7
        embolism O08.2
    cornual O00.80
      with intrauterine pregnancy O00.81
    intraligamentous O00.80
      with intrauterine pregnancy O00.81
    mural O00.80
      with intrauterine pregnancy O00.81
    ovarian O00.20- ☑
      with intrauterine pregnancy O00.21- ☑
    specified site NEC O00.80
      with intrauterine pregnancy O00.81
    tubal (ruptured) O00.10- ☑
      with intrauterine pregnancy O00.11- ☑
  examination (normal) Z34.9- ☑
    first Z34.0- ☑
    high-risk — *see* Pregnancy, supervision of, high-risk
    specified Z34.8- ☑
  extrauterine — *see* Pregnancy, ectopic
  fallopian O00.10- ☑
    with intrauterine pregnancy O00.11- ☑
  false F45.8
  gestational carrier Z33.3
  heptachorionic, hepta-amniotic (septuplets) O30.83- ☑
  hexachorionic, hexa-amniotic (sextuplets) O30.83- ☑
  hidden O09.3- ☑
  high-risk — *see* Pregnancy, supervision of, high-risk
  incidental finding Z33.1

Pregnancy — *continued*
interstitial O00.80
  with intrauterine pregnancy O00.81
intraligamentous O00.80
  with intrauterine pregnancy O00.81
intramural O00.80
  with intrauterine pregnancy O00.81
intraperitoneal O00.00
  with intrauterine pregnancy O00.01
isthmian O00.10- ☑
  with intrauterine pregnancy O00.11- ☑
mesometric (mural) O00.80
  with intrauterine pregnancy O00.81
molar NEC O02.0
  complicated (by) O08.9
    afibrinogenemia O08.1
    cardiac arrest O08.81
    chemical damage of pelvic organ(s) O08.6
    circulatory collapse O08.3
    defibrination syndrome O08.1
    electrolyte imbalance O08.5
    embolism (amniotic fluid) (blood clot) (pulmonary) (septic) O08.2
    endometritis O08.0
    genital tract and pelvic infection O08.0
    hemorrhage (delayed) (excessive) O08.1
    infection
      genital tract or pelvic O08.0
      kidney O08.83
      urinary tract O08.83
    intravascular coagulation O08.1
    laceration of pelvic organ(s) O08.6
    metabolic disorder O08.5
    oliguria O08.4
    oophoritis O08.0
    parametritis O08.0
    pelvic peritonitis O08.0
    perforation of pelvic organ(s) O08.6
    renal failure or shutdown O08.4
    salpingitis or salpingo-oophoritis O08.0
    sepsis O08.82
    shock O08.3
      septic O08.82
    specified condition NEC O08.89
    tubular necrosis (renal) O08.4
    uremia O08.4
    urinary infection O08.83
    venous complication NEC O08.7
      embolism O08.2
hydatidiform — *see also* Mole, hydatidiform O01.9
multiple (gestation) O30.9- ☑
  greater than quadruplets — *see* Pregnancy, multiple (gestation), specified NEC
  specified NEC O30.80- ☑
    with
      two or more monoamniotic fetuses O30.82-
      two or more monochorionic fetuses O30.81- ☑
      number of chorions and amnions are both equal to the number of fetuses O30.83- ☑
      two or more monoamniotic fetuses O30.82- ☑
      two or more monochorionic fetuses O30.81- ☑
      unable to determine number of placenta and number of amniotic sacs O30.89- ☑
      unspecified number of placenta and unspecified number of amniotic sacs O30.80- ☑
  mural O00.80
    with intrauterine pregnancy O00.81
  normal (supervision of) Z34.9- ☑
    first Z34.0- ☑
    high-risk — *see* Pregnancy, supervision of, high-risk
    specified Z34.8- ☑
  ovarian O00.20- ☑
    with intrauterine pregnancy O00.21- ☑
  pentachorionic, penta-amniotic (quintuplets) O30.83- ☑
  postmature (40 to 42 weeks) O48.0
    more than 42 weeks gestation O48.1
  post-term (40 to 42 weeks) O48.0
  prenatal care only Z34.9- ☑
    first Z34.0- ☑
    high-risk — *see* Pregnancy, supervision of, high-risk
    specified Z34.8- ☑
  prolonged (more than 42 weeks gestation) O48.1
  quadruplet O30.20- ☑
    with
      two or more monoamniotic fetuses O30.22- ☑

Pregnancy — *continued*
quadruplet — *continued*
  with — *continued*
    two or more monochorionic fetuses O30.21- ☑
    quadrachorionic/quadra-amniotic O30.23- ☑
  two or more monoamniotic fetuses O30.22- ☑
  two or more monochorionic fetuses O30.21- ☑
  unable to determine number of placenta and number of amniotic sacs O30.29- ☑
  unspecified number of placenta and unspecified number of amniotic sacs O30.20- ☑
quintuplet — *see* Pregnancy, multiple (gestation), specified NEC
sextuplet — *see* Pregnancy, multiple (gestation), specified NEC
supervision of
  concealed pregnancy O09.3- ☑
  elderly mother
    multigravida O09.52- ☑
    primigravida O09.51- ☑
  hidden pregnancy O09.3- ☑
  high-risk O09.9- ☑
    due to (history of)
      ectopic pregnancy O09.1- ☑
      elderly — *see* Pregnancy, supervision, elderly mother
      grand multiparity O09.4 ☑
      in utero procedure during previous pregnancy O09.82- ☑
      in vitro fertilization O09.81- ☑
      infertility O09.0- ☑
      insufficient prenatal care O09.3- ☑
      molar pregnancy O09.A- ☑
      multiple previous pregnancies O09.4- ☑
      older mother — *see* Pregnancy, supervision of, elderly mother
      poor reproductive or obstetric history NEC O09.29- ☑
      pre-term labor O09.21- ☑
      previous
        neonatal death O09.29- ☑
      social problems O09.7- ☑
      specified NEC O09.89- ☑
      very young mother — *see* Pregnancy, supervision, young mother
  resulting from in vitro fertilization O09.81- ☑
  normal Z34.9- ☑
    first Z34.0- ☑
    specified NEC Z34.8- ☑
  young mother
    multigravida O09.62- ☑
    primigravida O09.61- ☑
triplet O30.10- ☑
  with
    two or more monoamniotic fetuses O30.12- ☑
    two or more monochorionic fetuses O30.11- ☑
  trichorionic/triamniotic O30.13- ☑
  two or more monoamniotic fetuses O30.12- ☑
  two or more monochorionic fetuses O30.11- ☑
  unable to determine number of placenta and number of amniotic sacs O30.19- ☑
  unspecified number of placenta and unspecified number of amniotic sacs O30.10- ☑
tubal (with abortion) (with rupture) O00.10- ☑
  with intrauterine pregnancy O00.11- ☑
twin O30.00- ☑
  conjoined O30.02- ☑
  dichorionic/diamniotic (two placenta, two amniotic sacs) O30.04- ☑
  monochorionic/diamniotic (one placenta, two amniotic sacs) O30.03- ☑
  monochorionic/monoamniotic (one placenta, one amniotic sac) O30.01- ☑
  unable to determine number of placenta and number of amniotic sacs O30.09- ☑
  unspecified number of placenta and unspecified number of amniotic sacs O30.00- ☑
unwanted Z64.0
weeks of gestation
  8 weeks Z3A.08 (*following* Z36)
  9 weeks Z3A.09 (*following* Z36)
  10 weeks Z3A.10 (*following* Z36)
  11 weeks Z3A.11 (*following* Z36)
  12 weeks Z3A.12 (*following* Z36)
  13 weeks Z3A.13 (*following* Z36)
  14 weeks Z3A.14 (*following* Z36)
  15 weeks Z3A.15 (*following* Z36)

Pregnancy — *continued*
weeks of gestation — *continued*
  16 weeks Z3A.16 (*following* Z36)
  17 weeks Z3A.17 (*following* Z36)
  18 weeks Z3A.18 (*following* Z36)
  19 weeks Z3A.19 (*following* Z36)
  20 weeks Z3A.20 (*following* Z36)
  21 weeks Z3A.21 (*following* Z36)
  22 weeks Z3A.22 (*following* Z36)
  23 weeks Z3A.23 (*following* Z36)
  24 weeks Z3A.24 (*following* Z36)
  25 weeks Z3A.25 (*following* Z36)
  26 weeks Z3A.26 (*following* Z36)
  27 weeks Z3A.27 (*following* Z36)
  28 weeks Z3A.28 (*following* Z36)
  29 weeks Z3A.29 (*following* Z36)
  30 weeks Z3A.30 (*following* Z36)
  31 weeks Z3A.31 (*following* Z36)
  32 weeks Z3A.32 (*following* Z36)
  33 weeks Z3A.33 (*following* Z36)
  34 weeks Z3A.34 (*following* Z36)
  35 weeks Z3A.35 (*following* Z36)
  36 weeks Z3A.36 (*following* Z36)
  37 weeks Z3A.37 (*following* Z36)
  38 weeks Z3A.38 (*following* Z36)
  39 weeks Z3A.39 (*following* Z36)
  40 weeks Z3A.40 (*following* Z36)
  41 weeks Z3A.41 (*following* Z36)
  42 weeks Z3A.42 (*following* Z36)
  greater than 42 weeks Z3A.49 (*following* Z36)
  less than 8 weeks Z3A.01 (*following* Z36)
  not specified Z3A.00 (*following* Z36)
Preiser's disease — *see* Osteonecrosis, secondary, due to, trauma, metacarpus
Pre-kwashiorkor — *see* Malnutrition, severe
Preleukemia (syndrome) D46.9
Preluxation, hip, congenital Q65.6
Premature — *see also* condition
adrenarche E27.0
aging E34.8
beats I49.40
  atrial I49.1
  auricular I49.1
  supraventricular I49.1
birth NEC — *see* Preterm, newborn
closure, foramen ovale Q21.8
contraction
  atrial I49.1
  atrioventricular I49.2
  auricular I49.1
  auriculoventricular I49.49
  heart (extrasystole) I49.49
  junctional I49.2
  ventricular I49.3
delivery — *see also* Pregnancy, complicated by, preterm labor O60.10 ☑
ejaculation F52.4
infant NEC — *see* Preterm, newborn
  light-for-dates — *see* Light for dates
labor — *see* Pregnancy, complicated by, preterm labor
lungs P28.0
menopause E28.319
  asymptomatic E28.319
  symptomatic E28.310
newborn
  extreme (less than 28 completed weeks) — *see* Immaturity, extreme
  less than 37 completed weeks — *see* Preterm, newborn
puberty E30.1
rupture membranes or amnion — *see* Pregnancy, complicated by, premature rupture of membranes
senility E34.8
thelarche E30.8
ventricular systole I49.3
Prematurity NEC (less than 37 completed weeks) — *see* Preterm, newborn
extreme (less than 28 completed weeks) — *see* Immaturity, extreme
Premenstrual
dysphoric disorder (PMDD) F32.81
tension (syndrome) N94.3
Premolarization, cuspids K00.2
Prenatal
care, normal pregnancy — *see* Pregnancy, normal
screening of mother — *see also* Encounter, antenatal screening Z36.9

Prenatal — *continued*
  teeth K00.6
Preparatory care for subsequent treatment NEC
  for dialysis Z49.01
    peritoneal Z49.02
Prepartum — *see* condition
Preponderance, left or right ventricular I51.7
Prepuce — *see* condition
PRES (posterior reversible encephalopathy syndrome)
  I67.83
Presbycardia R54
Presbycusis, presbyacusia H91.1- ☑
Presbyesophagus K22.8
Presbyophrenia F03 ☑
Presbyopia H52.4
Prescription of contraceptives (initial) Z30.019
  barrier Z30.018
  diaphragm Z30.018
  emergency (postcoital) Z30.012
  implantable subdermal Z30.017
  injectable Z30.013
  intrauterine contraceptive device Z30.014
  pills Z30.011
  postcoital (emergency) Z30.012
  repeat Z30.40
    barrier Z30.49
    diaphragm Z30.49
    implantable subdermal Z30.46
    injectable Z30.42
    pills Z30.41
    specified type NEC Z30.49
    transdermal patch hormonal Z30.45
    vaginal ring hormonal Z30.44
  specified type NEC Z30.018
    transdermal patch hormonal Z30.016
    vaginal ring hormonal Z30.015
Presence (of)
  ankle-joint implant (functional) (prosthesis) Z96.66- ☑
  aortocoronary (bypass) graft Z95.1
  arterial-venous shunt (dialysis) Z99.2
  artificial
    eye (globe) Z97.0
    heart (fully implantable) (mechanical) Z95.812
      valve Z95.2
    larynx Z96.3
    lens (intraocular) Z96.1
    limb (complete) (partial) Z97.1- ☑
      arm Z97.1- ☑
        bilateral Z97.15
      leg Z97.1- ☑
        bilateral Z97.16
  audiological implant (functional) Z96.29
  bladder implant (functional) Z96.0
  bone
    conduction hearing device Z96.29
    implant (functional) NEC Z96.7
    joint (prosthesis) — *see* Presence, joint implant
  cardiac
    defibrillator (functional) (with synchronous cardiac
      pacemaker) Z95.810
    implant or graft Z95.9
      specified type NEC Z95.818
    pacemaker Z95.0
    resynchronization therapy
      defibrillator Z95.810
      pacemaker Z95.0
  cardioverter-defibrillator (ICD) Z95.810
  cerebrospinal fluid drainage device Z98.2
  cochlear implant (functional) Z96.21
  contact lens (es) Z97.3
  coronary artery graft or prosthesis Z95.5
  CRT-D (cardiac resynchronization therapy defibrillator)
    Z95.810
  CRT-P (cardiac resynchronization therapy pacemaker)
    Z95.0
  CSF shunt Z98.2
  dental prosthesis device Z97.2
  dentures Z97.2
  device (external) NEC Z97.8
    cardiac NEC Z95.818
    heart assist Z95.811
    implanted (functional) Z96.9
      specified NEC Z96.89
    prosthetic Z97.8
  ear implant Z96.20
    cochlear implant Z96.21
    myringotomy tube Z96.22
    specified type NEC Z96.29

Presence — *continued*
  elbow-joint implant (functional) (prosthesis) Z96.62- ☑
  endocrine implant (functional) NEC Z96.49
  eustachian tube stent or device (functional) Z96.29
  external hearing-aid or device Z97.4
  finger-joint implant (functional) (prosthetic) Z96.69- ☑
  functional implant Z96.9
    specified NEC Z96.89
  graft
    cardiac NEC Z95.818
    vascular NEC Z95.828
  hearing-aid or device (external) Z97.4
    implant (bone) (cochlear) (functional) Z96.21
  heart assist device Z95.811
  heart valve implant (functional) Z95.2
    prosthetic Z95.2
    specified type NEC Z95.4
    xenogenic Z95.3
  hip-joint implant (functional) (prosthesis) Z96.64- ☑
  ICD (cardioverter-defibrillator) Z95.810
  implanted device (artificial) (functional) (prosthetic)
    Z96.9
    automatic cardiac defibrillator (with synchronous
      cardiac pacemaker) Z95.810
    cardiac pacemaker Z95.0
    cochlear Z96.21
    dental Z96.5
    heart Z95.812
    heart valve Z95.2
      prosthetic Z95.2
      specified NEC Z95.4
      xenogenic Z95.3
    insulin pump Z96.41
    intraocular lens Z96.1
    joint Z96.60
      ankle Z96.66- ☑
      elbow Z96.62- ☑
      finger Z96.69- ☑
      hip Z96.64- ☑
      knee Z96.65- ☑
      shoulder Z96.61- ☑
      specified NEC Z96.698
      wrist Z96.63- ☑
    larynx Z96.3
    myringotomy tube Z96.22
    otological Z96.20
      cochlear Z96.21
      eustachian stent Z96.29
      myringotomy Z96.22
      specified NEC Z96.29
      stapes Z96.29
    skin Z96.81
    skull plate Z96.7
    specified NEC Z96.89
    urogenital Z96.0
  insulin pump (functional) Z96.41
  intestinal bypass or anastomosis Z98.0
  intraocular lens (functional) Z96.1
  intrauterine contraceptive device (IUD) Z97.5
  intravascular implant (functional) (prosthetic) NEC
    Z95.9
    coronary artery Z95.5
    defibrillator (with synchronous cardiac pacemaker)
      Z95.810
    peripheral vessel (with angioplasty) Z95.820
  joint implant (prosthetic) (any) Z96.60
    ankle — *see* Presence, ankle joint implant
    elbow — *see* Presence, elbow joint implant
    finger — *see* Presence, finger joint implant
    hip — *see* Presence, hip joint implant
    knee — *see* Presence, knee joint implant
    shoulder — *see* Presence, shoulder joint implant
    specified joint NEC Z96.698
    wrist — *see* Presence, wrist joint implant
  knee-joint implant (functional) (prosthesis) Z96.65- ☑
  laryngeal implant (functional) Z96.3
  mandibular implant (dental) Z96.5
  myringotomy tube(s) Z96.22
  neurostimulator (brain) (gastric) (peripheral nerve)
    (sacral nerve) (spinal cord) (vagus nerve) Z96.82
  orthopedic-joint implant (prosthetic) (any) — *see*
    Presence, joint implant
  otological implant (functional) Z96.29
  shoulder-joint implant (functional) (prosthesis)
    Z96.61- ☑
  skull-plate implant Z96.7
  spectacles Z97.3
  stapes implant (functional) Z96.29

Presence — *continued*
  systemic lupus erythematosus [SLE] inhibitor D68.62
  tendon implant (functional) (graft) Z96.7
  tooth root(s) implant Z96.5
  ureteral stent Z96.0
  urethral stent Z96.0
  urogenital implant (functional) Z96.0
  vascular implant or device Z95.9
    access port device Z95.828
    specified type NEC Z95.828
  wrist-joint implant (functional) (prosthesis) Z96.63- ☑
Presenile — *see also* condition
  dementia F03 ☑
  premature aging E34.8
Presentation, fetal — *see* Delivery, complicated by,
  malposition
Prespondylolisthesis (congenital) Q76.2
Pressure
  area, skin — *see* Ulcer, pressure, by site
  brachial plexus G54.0
  brain G93.5
    injury at birth NEC P11.1
  cerebral — *see* Pressure, brain
  chest R07.89
  cone, tentorial G93.5
  hyposystolic — *see also* Hypotension
    incidental reading, without diagnosis of hypoten-
      sion R03.1
  increased
    intracranial (benign) G93.2
      injury at birth P11.0
    intraocular H40.05- ☑
  injury — *see* Ulcer, pressure, by site
  lumbosacral plexus G54.1
  mediastinum J98.59
  necrosis (chronic) — *see* Ulcer, pressure, by site
  parental, inappropriate (excessive) Z62.6
  sore (chronic) — *see* Ulcer, pressure, by site
  spinal cord G95.20
  ulcer (chronic) — *see* Ulcer, pressure, by site
  venous, increased I87.8
Pre-syncope R55
Preterm
  delivery — *see also* Pregnancy, complicated by,
    preterm labor O60.10 ☑
  labor — *see* Pregnancy, complicated by, preterm labor
  newborn (infant) P07.30
    gestational age
      28 completed weeks (28 weeks, 0 days through
        28 weeks, 6 days) P07.31
      29 completed weeks (29 weeks, 0 days through
        29 weeks, 6 days) P07.32
      30 completed weeks (30 weeks, 0 days through
        30 weeks, 6 days) P07.33
      31 completed weeks (31 weeks, 0 days through
        31 weeks, 6 days) P07.34
      32 completed weeks (32 weeks, 0 days through
        32 weeks, 6 days) P07.35
      33 completed weeks (33 weeks, 0 days through
        33 weeks, 6 days) P07.36
      34 completed weeks (34 weeks, 0 days through
        34 weeks, 6 days) P07.37
      35 completed weeks (35 weeks, 0 days through
        35 weeks, 6 days) P07.38
      36 completed weeks (36 weeks, 0 days through
        36 weeks, 6 days) P07.39
Previa
  placenta (total) (without hemorrhage) O44.0- ☑
    with hemorrhage O44.1- ☑
    complete O44.0- ☑
      with hemorrhage O44.1- ☑
    low — *see also* Delivery, complicated, by, placenta,
      low O44.4- ☑
      with hemorrhage O44.5- ☑
    marginal O44.2- ☑
      with hemorrhage O44.3- ☑
    partial O44.2- ☑
      with hemorrhage O44.3- ☑
  vasa O69.4 ☑
Priapism N48.30
  due to
    disease classified elsewhere N48.32
    drug N48.33
    specified cause NEC N48.39
    trauma N48.31
Prickling sensation (skin) R20.2
Prickly heat L74.0

Primary — *see* condition
Primigravida
  elderly, affecting management of pregnancy, labor and delivery (supervision only) — *see* Pregnancy, complicated by, elderly, primigravida
  older, affecting management of pregnancy, labor and delivery (supervision only) — *see* Pregnancy, complicated by, elderly, primigravida
  very young, affecting management of pregnancy, labor and delivery (supervision only) — *see* Pregnancy, complicated by, young mother, primigravida
Primipara
  elderly, affecting management of pregnancy, labor and delivery (supervision only) — *see* Pregnancy, complicated by, elderly, primigravida
  older, affecting management of pregnancy, labor and delivery (supervision only) — *see* Pregnancy, complicated by, elderly, primigravida
  very young, affecting management of pregnancy, labor and delivery (supervision only) — *see* Pregnancy, complicated by, young mother, primigravida
Primus varus Q66.21- ☑
PRIND (Prolonged reversible ischemic neurologic deficit) I63.9
Pringle's disease (tuberous sclerosis) Q85.1
Prinzmetal angina I20.1
Prizefighter ear — *see* Cauliflower ear
Problem (with) (related to)
  academic Z55.8
  acculturation Z60.3
  adjustment (to)
    change of job Z56.1
    life-cycle transition Z60.0
    pension Z60.0
    retirement Z60.0
  adopted child Z62.821
  alcoholism in family Z63.72
  atypical parenting situation Z62.9
  bankruptcy Z59.8
  behavioral (adult) F69
    drug seeking Z76.5
  birth of sibling affecting child Z62.898
  care (of)
    provider dependency Z74.9
      specified NEC Z74.8
    sick or handicapped person in family or household Z63.6
  child
    abuse (affecting the child) — *see* Maltreatment, child
    custody or support proceedings Z65.3
    in care of non-parental family member Z62.21
    in foster care Z62.21
    in welfare custody Z62.21
    living in orphanage or group home Z62.22
  child-rearing Z62.9
    specified NEC Z62.898
  communication (developmental) F80.9
  conflict or discord (with)
    boss Z56.4
    classmates Z55.4
    counselor Z64.4
    employer Z56.4
    family Z63.9
      specified NEC Z63.8
    probation officer Z64.4
    social worker Z64.4
    teachers Z55.4
    workmates Z56.4
  conviction in legal proceedings Z65.0
    with imprisonment Z65.1
  counselor Z64.4
  creditors Z59.8
  digestive K92.9
  drug addict in family Z63.72
  ear — *see* Disorder, ear
  economic Z59.9
    affecting care Z59.9
    specified NEC Z59.8
  education Z55.9
    specified NEC Z55.8
  employment Z56.9
    change of job Z56.1
    discord Z56.4
    environment Z56.5
    sexual harassment Z56.81
    specified NEC Z56.89
    stressful schedule Z56.3

Problem — *continued*
  employment — *continued*
    stress NEC Z56.6
    threat of job loss Z56.2
    unemployment Z56.0
  enuresis, child F98.0
  eye H57.9
  failed examinations (school) Z55.2
  falling Z91.81
  family — *see also* Disruption, family Z63.9
    specified NEC Z63.8
  feeding (elderly) (infant) R63.3
    newborn P92.9
      breast P92.5
      overfeeding P92.4
      slow P92.2
      specified NEC P92.8
      underfeeding P92.3
    nonorganic F50.89
  finance Z59.9
    specified NEC Z59.8
  foreclosure on loan Z59.8
  foster child Z62.822
  frightening experience(s) in childhood Z62.898
  genital NEC
    female N94.9
    male N50.9
  health care Z75.9
    specified NEC Z75.8
  hearing — *see* Deafness
  homelessness Z59.0
  housing Z59.9
    inadequate Z59.1
    isolated Z59.8
    specified NEC Z59.8
  identity (of childhood) F93.8
  illegitimate pregnancy (unwanted) Z64.0
  illiteracy Z55.0
  impaired mobility Z74.09
  imprisonment or incarceration Z65.1
  inadequate teaching affecting education Z55.8
  inappropriate (excessive) parental pressure Z62.6
  influencing health status NEC Z78.9
  in-law Z63.1
  institutionalization, affecting child Z62.22
  intrafamilial communication Z63.8
  jealousy, child F93.8
  landlord Z59.2
  language (developmental) F80.9
  learning (developmental) F81.9
  legal Z65.3
    conviction without imprisonment Z65.0
    imprisonment Z65.1
    release from prison Z65.2
  life-management Z73.9
    specified NEC Z73.89
  life-style Z72.9
    gambling Z72.6
    high-risk sexual behavior (heterosexual) Z72.51
      bisexual Z72.53
      homosexual Z72.52
    inappropriate eating habits Z72.4
    self-damaging behavior NEC Z72.89
    specified NEC Z72.89
    tobacco use Z72.0
  literacy Z55.9
    low level Z55.0
    specified NEC Z55.8
  living alone Z60.2
  lodgers Z59.2
  loss of love relationship in childhood Z62.898
  marital Z63.0
    involving
      divorce Z63.5
      estrangement Z63.5
      gender identity F66
  mastication K08.89
  medical
    care, within family Z63.6
    facilities Z75.9
      specified NEC Z75.8
  mental F48.9
  multiparity Z64.1
  negative life events in childhood Z62.9
    altered pattern of family relationships Z62.898
    frightening experience Z62.898
    loss of
      love relationship Z62.898
      self-esteem Z62.898

Problem — *continued*
  negative life events in childhood — *continued*
    physical abuse (alleged) — *see* Maltreatment, child
    removal from home Z62.29
    specified event NEC Z62.898
  neighbor Z59.2
  neurological NEC R29.818
  new step-parent affecting child Z62.898
  none (feared complaint unfounded) Z71.1
  occupational NEC Z56.89
  parent-child — *see* Conflict, parent-child
  personal hygiene Z91.89
  personality F69
  phase-of-life transition, adjustment Z60.0
  presence of sick or disabled person in family or household Z63.79
    needing care Z63.6
  primary support group (family) Z63.9
    specified NEC Z63.8
  probation officer Z64.4
  psychiatric F99
  psychosexual (development) F66
  psychosocial Z65.9
    religious or spiritual Z65.8
    specified NEC Z65.8
  relationship Z63.9
    childhood F93.8
  release from prison Z65.2
    religious or spiritual Z65.8
  removal from home affecting child Z62.29
  seeking and accepting known hazardous and harmful behavioral or psychological interventions Z65.8
    chemical, nutritional or physical interventions Z65.8
  sexual function (nonorganic) F52.9
  sight H54.7
  sleep disorder, child F51.9
  smell — *see* Disturbance, sensation, smell
  social
    environment Z60.9
      specified NEC Z60.8
    exclusion and rejection Z60.4
    worker Z64.4
  speech R47.9
    developmental F80.9
    specified NEC R47.89
  swallowing — *see* Dysphagia
  taste — *see* Disturbance, sensation, taste
  tic, child F95.0
  underachievement in school Z55.3
  unemployment Z56.0
    threatened Z56.2
  unwanted pregnancy Z64.0
  upbringing Z62.9
    specified NEC Z62.898
  urinary N39.9
  voice production R47.89
  work schedule (stressful) Z56.3
Procedure (surgical)
  converted
    arthroscopic to open Z53.33
    laparoscopic to open Z53.31
    specified procedure NEC to open Z53.39
    thoracoscopic to open Z53.32
  for purpose other than remedying health state Z41.9
    specified NEC Z41.8
  not done Z53.9
    because of
      administrative reasons Z53.8
      contraindication Z53.09
        smoking Z53.01
      patient's decision Z53.20
        for reasons of belief or group pressure Z53.1
        left against medical advice (AMA) Z53.21
        specified reason NEC Z53.29
      specified reason NEC Z53.8
Procidentia (uteri) N81.3
Proctalgia K62.89
  fugax K59.4
  spasmodic K59.4
Proctitis K62.89
  amebic (acute) A06.0
  chlamydial A56.3
  gonococcal A54.6
  granulomatous — *see* Enteritis, regional, large intestine
  herpetic A60.1
  radiation K62.7
  tuberculous A18.32
  ulcerative (chronic) K51.20

Proctitis — *continued*
  ulcerative — *continued*
    with
      complication K51.219
        abscess K51.214
        fistula K51.213
        obstruction K51.212
        rectal bleeding K51.211
        specified NEC K51.218
Proctocele
  female (without uterine prolapse) N81.6
    with uterine prolapse N81.2
      complete N81.3
  male K62.3
Proctocolitis
  food protein-induced K52.82
  food-induced eosinophilic K52.82
  milk protein-induced K52.82
  mucosal — *see* Rectosigmoiditis, ulcerative
Proctoptosis K62.3
Proctorrhagia K62.5
Proctosigmoiditis K63.89
  ulcerative (chronic) — *see* Rectosigmoiditis, ulcerative
Proctospasm N59.4
  psychogenic F45.8
Profichet's disease — *see* Disorder, soft tissue, specified type NEC
Progeria E34.8
Prognathism (mandibular) (maxillary) M26.19
Progonoma (melanotic) — *see* Neoplasm, benign, by site
Progressive — *see* condition
Prolactinoma
  specified site — *see* Neoplasm, benign, by site
  unspecified site D35.2
Prolapse, prolapsed
  anus, anal (canal) (sphincter) K62.2
  arm or hand O32.2 ☑
    causing obstructed labor O64.4 ☑
  bladder (mucosa) (sphincter) (acquired)
    congenital Q79.4
    female — *see* Cystocele
    male N32.89
  breast implant (prosthetic) T85.49 ☑
  cecostomy K94.09
  cecum K63.4
  cervix, cervical (hypertrophied) N81.2
    anterior lip, obstructing labor O65.5
    congenital Q51.828
    postpartal, old N81.2
    stump N81.85
  ciliary body (traumatic) — *see* Laceration, eye(ball), with prolapse or loss of interocular tissue
  colon (pedunculated) K63.4
  colostomy K94.09
  disc (intervertebral) — *see* Displacement, intervertebral disc
  eye implant (orbital) T85.398 ☑
    lens (ocular) — *see* Complications, intraocular lens
  fallopian tube N83.4- ☑
  gastric (mucosa) K31.89
  genital, female N81.9
    specified NEC N81.89
  globe, nontraumatic — *see* Luxation, globe
  ileostomy bud K94.19
  intervertebral disc — *see* Displacement, intervertebral disc
  intestine (small) K63.4
  iris (traumatic) — *see* Laceration, eye(ball), with prolapse or loss of interocular tissue
    nontraumatic H21.89
  kidney N28.83
    congenital Q63.2
  laryngeal muscles or ventricle J38.7
  liver K76.89
  meatus urinarius N36.8
  mitral (valve) I34.1
  ocular lens implant — *see* Complications, intraocular lens
  organ or site, congenital NEC — *see* Malposition, congenital
  ovary N83.4- ☑
  pelvic floor, female N81.89
  perineum, female N81.89
  rectum (mucosa) (sphincter) K62.3
    due to trichuris trichuria B79
  spleen D73.89
  stomach K31.89

Prolapse, prolapsed — *continued*
  umbilical cord
    complicating delivery O69.0 ☑
  urachus, congenital Q64.4
  ureter N28.89
    with obstruction N13.5
    with infection N13.6
  ureterovesical orifice N28.89
  urethra (acquired) (infected) (mucosa) N36.8
    congenital Q64.71
  urinary meatus N36.8
    congenital Q64.72
  uterovaginal N81.4
    complete N81.3
    incomplete N81.2
  uterus (with prolapse of vagina) N81.4
    complete N81.3
    congenital Q51.818
    first degree N81.2
    in pregnancy or childbirth — *see* Pregnancy, complicated by, abnormal, uterus
    incomplete N81.2
    postpartal (old) N81.4
    second degree N81.2
    third degree N81.3
  uveal (traumatic) — *see* Laceration, eye(ball), with prolapse or loss of interocular tissue
  vagina (anterior) (wall) — *see* Cystocele
    with prolapse of uterus N81.4
      complete N81.3
      incomplete N81.2
    posterior wall N81.6
    posthysterectomy N99.3
  vitreous (humor) H43.0- ☑
    in wound — *see* Laceration, eye(ball), with prolapse or loss of interocular tissue
  womb — *see* Prolapse, uterus
Prolapsus, female N81.9
  specified NEC N81.89
Proliferation(s)
  primary cutaneous CD30-positive large T-cell C86.6
  prostate, atypical small acinar N42.32
Proliferative — *see* condition
Prolonged, prolongation (of)
  bleeding (time) (idiopathic) R79.1
  coagulation (time) R79.1
  gestation (over 42 completed weeks)
    mother O48.1
    newborn P08.22
  interval I44.0
  labor O63.9
    first stage O63.0
    second stage O63.1
  partial thromboplastin time (PTT) R79.1
  pregnancy (more than 42 weeks gestation) O48.1
  prothrombin time R79.1
  QT interval R94.31
  uterine contractions in labor O62.4
Prominence, prominent
  auricle (congenital) (ear) Q17.5
  ischial spine or sacral promontory with disproportion (fetopelvic)
    with disproportion (fetopelvic) O33.0
      causing obstructed labor O65.0-
  nose (congenital) acquired M95.0
Promiscuity — *see* High, risk, sexual behavior
Pronation
  ankle — *see* Deformity, limb, foot, specified NEC
  foot — *see also* Deformity, limb, foot, specified NEC
    congenital Q74.2
Prophylactic
  administration of
    antibiotics, long-term Z79.2
      short-term use — *omit code*
    drug — *see also* Long-term (current) drug therapy (use of) Z79.899
  medication Z79.899
  organ removal (for neoplasia management) Z40.00
    breast Z40.01
    fallopian tube(s) Z40.03
      with ovary(s) Z40.02
    ovary(s) Z40.02
    specified site NEC Z40.09
  surgery Z40.9
    for risk factors related to malignant neoplasm — *see* Prophylactic, organ removal
    specified NEC Z40.8
  vaccination Z23

Propionic acidemia E71.121
Proptosis (ocular) — *see also* Exophthalmos
  thyroid — *see* Hyperthyroidism, with goiter
Prosecution, anxiety concerning Z65.3
Prosopagnosia R48.3
Prostadynia N42.81
Prostate, prostatic — *see* condition
Prostatism — *see* Hyperplasia, prostate
Prostatitis (congestive) (suppurative) (with cystitis) N41.9
  acute N41.0
  cavitary N41.8
  chronic N41.1
  diverticular N41.8
  due to Trichomonas (vaginalis) A59.02
  fibrous N41.1
  gonococcal (acute) (chronic) A54.22
  granulomatous N41.4
  hypertrophic N41.1
  subacute N41.1
  trichomonal A59.02
  tuberculous A18.14
Prostatocystitis N41.3
Prostatorrhea N42.89
Prostatosis N42.82
Prostration R53.83
  heat — *see also* Heat, exhaustion
    anhydrotic T67.3 ☑
    due to
      salt (and water) depletion T67.4 ☑
      water depletion T67.3 ☑
  nervous F48.8
  senile R54
Protanomaly (anomalous trichromat) H53.54
Protanopia (complete) (incomplete) H53.54
Protection (against) (from) — *see* Prophylactic
Protein
  deficiency NEC — *see* Malnutrition
  malnutrition — *see* Malnutrition
  sickness — *see also* Reaction, serum T80.69 ☑
Proteinemia R77.9
Proteinosis
  alveolar (pulmonary) J84.01
  lipid or lipoid (of Urbach) E78.89
Proteinuria R80.9
  Bence Jones R80.3
  complicating pregnancy — *see* Proteinuria, gestational
  gestational
    complicating
      childbirth O12.14
      pregnancy O12.1- ☑
        with edema O12.2- ☑
      puerperium O12.15
  idiopathic R80.0
  isolated R80.0
    with glomerular lesion N06.9
      dense deposit disease N06.6
      diffuse
        crescentic glomerulonephritis N06.7
        endocapillary proliferative glomerulonephritis N06.4
        mesangiocapillary glomerulonephritis N06.5
      focal and segmental hyalinosis or sclerosis N06.1
      membranous (diffuse) N06.2
      mesangial proliferative (diffuse) N06.3
      minimal change N06.0
      specified pathology NEC N06.8
  orthostatic R80.2
    with glomerular lesion — *see* Proteinuria, isolated, with glomerular lesion
  persistent R80.1
    with glomerular lesion — *see* Proteinuria, isolated, with glomerular lesion
  postural R80.2
    with glomerular lesion — *see* Proteinuria, isolated, with glomerular lesion
  pre-eclamptic — *see* Pre-eclampsia
  puerperal O12.15
  specified type NEC R80.8
Proteolysis, pathologic D65
Proteus (mirabilis) (morganii), **as cause of disease classified elsewhere** B96.4
Prothrombin gene mutation D68.52
Protoporphyria, erythropoietic E80.0
Protozoal — *see also* condition
  disease B64
    specified NEC B60.8

Protrusion, protrusio
- acetabuli M24.7
- acetabulum (into pelvis) M24.7
- device, implant or graft — *see also* Complications, by site and type, mechanical T85.698 ☑
  - arterial graft NEC — *see* Complication, cardiovascular device, mechanical, vascular
  - breast (implant) T85.49 ☑
  - catheter NEC T85.698 ☑
    - cystostomy T83.090 ☑
    - dialysis (renal) T82.49 ☑
      - intraperitoneal T85.691 ☑
    - infusion NEC T82.594 ☑
      - spinal (epidural) (subdural) T85.690 ☑
    - urinary — *see also* Complications, catheter, urinary T83.098 ☑
  - electronic (electrode) (pulse generator) (stimulator)
    - bone T84.390 ☑
    - nervous system — *see* Complication, prosthetic device, mechanical, electronic nervous system stimulator
  - fixation, internal (orthopedic) NEC — *see* Complication, fixation device, mechanical
  - gastrointestinal — *see* Complications, prosthetic device, mechanical, gastrointestinal device
  - genital NEC T83.498 ☑
    - intrauterine contraceptive device T83.39 ☑
    - penile prosthesis (cylinder) (implanted) (pump) (resevoir) T83.490 ☑
    - testicular prosthesis T83.491 ☑
  - heart NEC — *see* Complication, cardiovascular device, mechanical
  - joint prosthesis — *see* Complications, joint prosthesis, mechanical, specified NEC, by site
  - ocular NEC — *see* Complications, prosthetic device, mechanical, ocular device
  - orthopedic NEC — *see* Complication, orthopedic, device, mechanical
  - specified NEC T85.628 ☑
  - urinary NEC — *see also* Complication, genitourinary, device, urinary, mechanical
    - graft T83.29 ☑
  - vascular NEC — *see* Complication, cardiovascular device, mechanical
  - ventricular intracranial shunt T85.09 ☑
- intervertebral disc — *see* Displacement, intervertebral disc
- joint prosthesis — *see* Complications, joint prosthesis, mechanical, specified NEC, by site
- nucleus pulposus — *see* Displacement, intervertebral disc
Prune belly (syndrome) Q79.4
Prurigo (ferox) (gravis) (Hebrae) (Hebra's) (mitis) (simplex) L28.2
- Besnier's L20.0
- estivalis L56.4
- nodularis L28.1
- psychogenic F45.8
Pruritus, pruritic (essential) L29.9
- ani, anus L29.0
  - psychogenic F45.8
- anogenital L29.3
  - psychogenic F45.8
- due to onchocerca volvulus B73.1
- gravidarum — *see* Pregnancy, complicated by, specified pregnancy-related condition NEC
- hiemalis L29.8
- neurogenic (any site) F45.8
- perianal L29.0
- psychogenic (any site) F45.8
- scroti, scrotum L29.1
  - psychogenic F45.8
- senile, senilis L29.8
- specified NEC L29.8
  - psychogenic F45.8
- Trichomonas A59.9
- vulva, vulvae L29.2
  - psychogenic F45.8
Pseudarthrosis, pseudoarthrosis (bone) — *see* Nonunion, fracture
- clavicle, congenital Q74.0
- joint, following fusion or arthrodesis M96.0
Pseudoaneurysm — *see* Aneurysm
Pseudoangina (pectoris) — *see* Angina
Pseudoangioma I81
Pseudoarteriosus Q28.8
Pseudoarthrosis — *see* Pseudarthrosis

Pseudobulbar affect (PBA) F48.2
Pseudochromhidrosis L67.8
Pseudocirrhosis, liver, pericardial I31.1
Pseudocowpox B08.03
Pseudocoxalgia M91.3- ☑
Pseudocroup J38.5
Pseudo-Cushing's syndrome, alcohol-induced E24.4
Pseudocyesis F45.8
Pseudocyst
- lung J98.4
- pancreas K86.3
- retina — *see* Cyst, retina
Pseudoelephantiasis neuroarthritica Q82.0
Pseudoexfoliation, capsule (lens) — *see* Cataract, specified NEC
Pseudofolliculitis barbae L73.1
Pseudoglioma H44.89
Pseudohemophilia (Bernuth's) (hereditary) (type B) D68.0
- Type A D69.8
- vascular D69.8
Pseudohermaphroditism Q56.3
- adrenal E25.8
- female Q56.2
  - with adrenocortical disorder E25.8
  - without adrenocortical disorder Q56.2
  - adrenal (congenital) E25.0
  - unspecified E25.9
- male Q56.1
  - with
    - 5-alpha-reductase deficiency E29.1
    - adrenocortical disorder E25.8
    - androgen resistance E34.51
    - cleft scrotum Q56.1
    - feminizing testis E34.51
  - without gonadal disorder Q56.1
  - adrenal E25.8
  - unspecified E25.9
Pseudo-Hurler's polydystrophy E77.0
Pseudohydrocephalus G93.2
Pseudohypertrophic muscular dystrophy (Erb's) G71.02
Pseudohypertrophy, muscle G71.09
Pseudohypoparathyroidism E20.1
Pseudoinsomnia F51.03
Pseudoleukemia, infantile D64.89
Pseudomembranous — *see* condition
Pseudomeningocele (cerebral) (infective) (post-traumatic) G96.19
- postprocedural (spinal) G97.82
Pseudomenses (newborn) P54.6
Pseudomenstruation (newborn) P54.6
Pseudomonas
- aeruginosa, as cause of disease classified elsewhere B96.5
- mallei infection A24.0
  - as cause of disease classified elsewhere B96.5
  - pseudomallei, as cause of disease classified elsewhere B96.5
Pseudomyotonia G71.19
Pseudomyxoma peritonei C78.6
Pseudoneuritis, optic (nerve) (disc) (papilla), **congenital** Q14.2
Pseudo-obstruction intestine (acute) (chronic) (idiopathic) (intermittent secondary) (primary) K59.8
Pseudopapilledema H47.33- ☑
- congenital Q14.2
Pseudoparalysis
- arm or leg R29.818
- atonic, congenital P94.2
Pseudopelade L66.0
Pseudophakia Z96.1
Pseudopolyarthritis, rhizomelic M35.3
Pseudopolycythemia D75.1
Pseudopseudohypoparathyroidism E20.1
Pseudopterygium H11.81- ☑
Pseudoptosis (eyelid) — *see* Blepharochalasis
Pseudopuberty, precocious
- female heterosexual E25.8
- male isosexual E25.8
Pseudorickets (renal) N25.0
Pseudorubella B08.20
Pseudoscrema, newborn P83.88
Pseudosclerosis (brain)
- Jakob's — *see* Creutzfeldt-Jakob disease or syndrome
- of Westphal (Strümpell) E83.01
- spastic — *see* Creutzfeldt-Jakob disease or syndrome

Pseudotetanus — *see* Convulsions
Pseudotetany R29.0
- hysterical F44.5
Pseudotruncus arteriosus Q25.49
Pseudotuberculosis A28.2
- enterocolitis A04.8
- pasteurella (infection) A28.0
Pseudotumor
- cerebri G93.2
- orbital H05.11 ☑
Pseudoxanthoma elasticum Q82.8
Psilosis (sprue) (tropical) K90.1
- nontropical K90.0
Psittacosis A70
Psoitis M60.88
Psoriasis L40.9
- arthropathic L40.50
  - arthritis mutilans L40.52
  - distal interphalangeal L40.51
  - juvenile L40.54
  - other specified L40.59
  - spondylitis L40.53
- buccal K13.29
- flexural L40.8
- guttate L40.4
- mouth K13.29
- nummular L40.0
- plaque L40.0
- psychogenic F54
- pustular (generalized) L40.1
  - palmaris et plantaris L40.3
- specified NEC L40.8
- vulgaris L40.0
Psychasthenia F48.8
Psychiatric disorder or problem F99
Psychogenic — *see also* condition
- factors associated with physical conditions F54
Psychological and behavioral factors affecting medical condition F59
Psychoneurosis, psychoneurotic — *see also* Neurosis
- anxiety (state) F41.1
- depersonalization F48.1
- hypochondriacal F45.21
- hysteria F44.9
- neurasthenia F48.8
- personality NEC F60.89
Psychopathy, psychopathic
- affectionless F94.2
- autistic F84.5
- constitution, post-traumatic F07.81
- personality — *see* Disorder, personality
- sexual — *see* Deviation, sexual
- state F60.2
Psychosexual identity disorder of childhood F64.2
Psychosis, psychotic F29
- acute (transient) F23
  - hysterical F44.9
- affective — *see* Disorder, mood
- alcoholic F10.959
  - with
    - abuse F10.159
    - anxiety disorder F10.980
      - with
        - abuse F10.180
        - dependence F10.280
    - delirium tremens F10.231
    - delusions F10.950
      - with
        - abuse F10.150
        - dependence F10.250
    - dementia F10.97
      - with dependence F10.27
    - dependence F10.259
    - hallucinosis F10.951
      - with
        - abuse F10.151
        - dependence F10.251
    - mood disorder F10.94
      - with
        - abuse F10.14
        - dependence F10.24
    - paranoia F10.950
      - with
        - abuse F10.150
        - dependence F10.250
    - persisting amnesia F10.96
      - with dependence F10.26
    - amnestic confabulatory F10.96

☑ Additional Character Required — Refer to the Tabular List for Character Selection   Subterms under main terms may continue to next column or page

Psychosis, psychotic — *continued*
  alcoholic — *continued*
    amnestic confabulatory — *continued*
      with dependence F10.26
    delirium tremens F10.231
    Korsakoff's, Korsakov's, Korsakow's F10.26
    paranoid type F10.950
      with
        abuse F10.150
        dependence F10.250
  anergastic — *see* Psychosis, organic
  arteriosclerotic (simple type) (uncomplicated) F01.50
    with behavioral disturbance F01.51
  childhood F84.0
    atypical F84.8
  climacteric — *see* Psychosis, involutional
  confusional F29
    acute or subacute F05
    reactive F23
  cycloid F23
  depressive — *see* Disorder, depressive
  disintegrative (childhood) F84.3
  drug-induced — *see* F11-F19 with .X59
    paranoid and hallucinatory states — *see* F11-F19
      with .X50 or .X51
  due to or associated with
    addiction, drug — *see* F11-F19 with .X59
    dependence
      alcohol F10.259
      drug — *see* F11-F19 with .X59
    epilepsy F06.8
    Huntington's chorea F06.8
    ischemia, cerebrovascular (generalized) F06.8
    multiple sclerosis F06.8
    physical disease F06.8
    presenile dementia F03 ☑
    senile dementia F03 ☑
    vascular disease (arteriosclerotic) (cerebral) F01.50
      with behavioral disturbance F01.51
  epileptic F06.8
  episode F23
    due to or associated with physical condition F06.8
  exhaustive F43.0
  hallucinatory, chronic F28
  hypomanic F30.8
  hysterical (acute) F44.9
  induced F24
  infantile F84.0
    atypical F84.8
  infective (acute) (subacute) F05
  involutional F28
    depressive — *see* Disorder, depressive
    melancholic — *see* Disorder, depressive
    paranoid (state) F22
  Korsakoff's, Korsakov's, Korsakow's (nonalcoholic) F04
    alcoholic F10.96
      in dependence F10.26
    induced by other psychoactive substance — *see*
      categories F11-F19 with .X5X
  mania, manic (single episode) F30.2
    recurrent type F31.89
  manic-depressive — *see* Disorder, bipolar
  menopausal — *see* Psychosis, involutional
  mixed schizophrenic and affective F25.8
  multi-infarct (cerebrovascular) F01.50
    with behavioral disturbance F01.51
  nonorganic F29
    specified NEC F28
  organic F09
    due to or associated with
      arteriosclerosis (cerebral) — *see* Psychosis, arteriosclerotic
      cerebrovascular disease, arteriosclerotic — *see* Psychosis, arteriosclerotic
      childbirth — *see* Psychosis, puerperal
      Creutzfeldt-Jakob disease or syndrome — *see* Creutzfeldt-Jakob disease or syndrome
      dependence, alcohol F10.259
      disease
        alcoholic liver F10.259
        brain, arteriosclerotic — *see* Psychosis, arteriosclerotic
        cerebrovascular F01.50
          with behavioral disturbance F01.51
        Creutzfeldt-Jakob — *see* Creutzfeldt-Jakob disease or syndrome
        endocrine or metabolic F06.8
          acute or subacute F05

Psychosis, psychotic — *continued*
  organic — *continued*
    due to or associated with — *continued*
      disease — *continued*
        liver, alcoholic F10.259
      epilepsy transient (acute) F05
      infection
        brain (intracranial) F06.8
          acute or subacute F05
      intoxication
        alcoholic (acute) F10.259
        drug F11-F19 with .x59
      ischemia, cerebrovascular (generalized) — *see* Psychosis, arteriosclerotic
      puerperium — *see* Psychosis, puerperal
      trauma, brain (birth) (from electric current) (surgical) F06.8
        acute or subacute F05
  infective F06.8
    acute or subacute F05
  post-traumatic F06.8
    acute or subacute F05
  paranoiac F22
  paranoid (climacteric) (involutional) (menopausal) F22
    psychogenic (acute) F23
    schizophrenic F20.0
    senile F03 ☑
  postpartum (NOS) F53.1
  presbyophrenic (type) F03 ☑
  presenile F03 ☑
  psychogenic (paranoid) F23
    depressive F32.3
  puerperal (NOS) F53.1
    specified type — *see* Psychosis, by type
  reactive (brief) (transient) (emotional stress) (psychological trauma) F23
    depressive F32.3
      recurrent F33.3
    excitative type F30.8
  schizoaffective F25.9
    depressive type F25.1
    manic type F25.0
  schizophrenia, schizophrenic — *see* Schizophrenia
  schizophrenia-like, in epilepsy F06.2
  schizophreniform F20.81
    affective type F25.9
    brief F23
    confusional type F23
    mixed type F25.0
  senile NEC F03 ☑
    depressed or paranoid type F03 ☑
    simple deterioration F03 ☑
    specified type — *code to* condition
  shared F24
  situational (reactive) F23
  symbiotic (childhood) F84.3
  symptomatic F09
Psychosomatic — *see* Disorder, psychosomatic
Psychosyndrome, organic F07.9
Psychotic episode due to or associated with physical condition F06.8
Pterygium (eye) H11.00- ☑
  amyloid H11.01- ☑
  central H11.02- ☑
  colli Q18.3
  double H11.03- ☑
  peripheral
    progressive H11.05- ☑
    stationary H11.04- ☑
  recurrent H11.06- ☑
Ptilosis (eyelid) — *see* Madarosis
Ptomaine (poisoning) — *see* Poisoning, food
Ptosis — *see also* Blepharoptosis
  adiposa (false) — *see* Blepharoptosis
  breast N64.81-
  brow H57.81- ☑
  cecum K63.4
  colon K63.4
  congenital (eyelid) Q10.0
    specified site NEC — *see* Anomaly, by site
  eyebrow H57.81- ☑
  eyelid — *see* Blepharoptosis
    congenital Q10.0
  gastric K31.89
  intestine K63.4
  kidney N20.03
  liver K76.89
  renal N28.83

Ptosis — *continued*
  splanchnic K63.4
  spleen D73.89
  stomach K31.89
  viscera K63.4
PTP D69.51
Ptyalism (periodic) K11.7
  hysterical F45.8
  pregnancy — *see* Pregnancy, complicated by, specified pregnancy-related condition NEC
  psychogenic F45.8
Ptyalolithiasis K11.5
Pubarche, precocious E30.1
Pubertas praecox E30.1
Puberty (development state) Z00.3
  bleeding (excessive) N92.2
  delayed E30.0
  precocious (constitutional) (cryptogenic) (idiopathic) E30.1
    central E22.8
    due to
      ovarian hyperfunction E28.1
        estrogen E28.0
      testicular hyperfunction E29.0
  premature E30.1
    due to
      adrenal cortical hyperfunction E25.8
      pineal tumor E34.8
      pituitary (anterior) hyperfunction E22.8
Puckering, macula — *see* Degeneration, macula, puckering
Pudenda, pudendum — *see* condition
Puente's disease (simple glandular cheilitis) K13.0
Puerperal, puerperium (complicated by, complications)
  abnormal glucose (tolerance test) O99.815
  abscess
    areola O91.02
      associated with lactation O91.03
    Bartholin's gland O86.19
    breast O91.12
      associated with lactation O91.13
    cervix (uteri) O86.11
    genital organ NEC O86.19
    kidney O86.21
    mammary O91.12
      associated with lactation O91.13
    nipple O91.02
      associated with lactation O91.03
    peritoneum O85
    subareolar O91.12
      associated with lactation O91.13
    urinary tract — *see* Puerperal, infection, urinary
    uterus O86.12
    vagina (wall) O86.13
    vaginorectal O86.13
    vulvovaginal gland O86.13
  adnexitis O86.19
  afibrinogenemia, or other coagulation defect O72.3
  albuminuria (acute) (subacute) — *see* Proteinuria, gestational
  alcohol use O99.315
  anemia O90.81
    pre-existing (pre-pregnancy) O99.03
  anesthetic death O89.8
  apoplexy O99.43
  bariatric surgery status O99.845
  blood disorder NEC O99.13
  blood dyscrasia O72.3
  cardiomyopathy O90.3
  cerebrovascular disorder (conditions in I60-I69) O99.43
  cervicitis O86.11
  circulatory system disorder O99.43
  coagulopathy (any) O99.13
    with hemorrhage O72.3
  complications O90.9
    specified NEC O90.89
  convulsions — *see* Eclampsia
  cystitis O86.22
  cystopyelitis O86.29
  delirium NEC F05
  diabetes O24.93
    gestational — *see* Puerperal, gestational diabetes
    pre-existing O24.33
      specified NEC O24.83
      type 1 O24.03
      type 2 O24.13
  digestive system disorder O99.63
  disease O90.9

Puerperal, puerperium — *continued*
- disease — *continued*
  - breast NEC O92.29
  - cerebrovascular (acute) O99.43
  - nonobstetric NEC O99.89
  - tubo-ovarian O86.19
  - Valsuani's O99.03
- disorder O90.9
  - biliary tract O26.63
  - lactation O92.70
  - liver O26.63
  - nonobstetric NEC O99.89
- disruption
  - cesarean wound O90.0
  - episiotomy wound O90.1
  - perineal laceration wound O90.1
- drug use O99.325
- eclampsia (with pre-existing hypertension) O15.2
- embolism (pulmonary) (blood clot) — *see* Embolism, obstetric, puerperal
- endocrine, nutritional or metabolic disease NEC O99.285
- endophlebitis — *see* Puerperal, phlebitis
- endotrachelitis O86.11
- failure
  - lactation (complete) O92.3
    - partial O92.4
  - renal, acute O90.4
- fever (of unknown origin) O86.4
  - septic O85
- fissure, nipple O92.12
  - associated with lactation O92.13
- fistula
  - breast (due to mastitis) O91.12
    - associated with lactation O91.13
  - nipple O91.02
    - associated with lactation O91.03
- galactophoritis O91.22
  - associated with lactation O91.23
- galactorrhea O92.6
- gastric banding status O99.845
- gastric bypass status O99.845
- gastrointestinal disease NEC O99.63
- gestational
  - diabetes O24.439
    - diet controlled O24.430
    - insulin (and diet) controlled O24.434
    - oral drug controlled (antidiabetic) (hypoglycemic) O24.435
  - edema O12.05
    - with proteinuria O12.25
  - proteinuria O12.15
- gonorrhea O98.23
- hematoma, subdural O99.43
- hemiplegia, cerebral O99.355
  - due to cerbrovascular disorder O99.43
- hemorrhage O72.1
  - brain O99.43
  - bulbar O99.43
  - cerebellar O99.43
  - cerebral O99.43
  - cortical O99.43
  - delayed or secondary O72.2
  - extradural O99.43
  - internal capsule O99.43
  - intracranial O99.43
  - intrapontine O99.43
  - meningeal O99.43
  - pontine O99.43
  - retained placenta O72.0
  - subarachnoid O99.43
  - subcortical O99.43
  - subdural O99.43
  - third stage O72.0
  - uterine, delayed O72.2
  - ventricular O99.43
- hemorrhoids O87.2
- hepatorenal syndrome O90.4
- hypertension — *see* Hypertension, complicating, puerperium
- hypertrophy, breast O92.29
- induration breast (fibrous) O92.29
- infection O86.4
  - cervix O86.11
  - generalized O85
  - genital tract NEC O86.19
    - obstetric surgical wound O86.09
  - kidney (bacillus coli) O86.21
  - maternal O98.93

Puerperal, puerperium — *continued*
- infection — *continued*
  - maternal — *continued*
    - carrier state NEC O99.835
    - gonorrhea O98.23
    - human immunodeficiency virus (HIV) O98.73
    - protozoal O98.63
    - sexually transmitted NEC O98.33
    - specified NEC O98.83
    - streptococcus group B (GBS) carrier state O99.825
    - syphilis O98.13
    - tuberculosis O98.03
    - viral hepatitis O98.43
    - viral NEC O98.53
  - nipple O91.02
    - associated with lactation O91.03
  - peritoneum O85
  - renal O86.21
  - specified NEC O86.89
  - urinary (asymptomatic) (tract) NEC O86.20
    - bladder O86.22
    - kidney O86.21
    - specified site NEC O86.29
    - urethra O86.22
  - vagina O86.13
  - vein — *see* Puerperal, phlebitis
- ischemia, cerebral O99.43
- lymphangitis O86.89
  - breast O91.22
    - associated with lactation O91.23
- malignancy O9A.13 (*following* O99)
- malnutrition O25.3
- mammillitis O91.02
  - associated with lactation O91.03
- mammitis O91.22
  - associated with lactation O91.23
- mania F30.8
- mastitis O91.22
  - associated with lactation O91.23
  - purulent O91.12
    - associated with lactation O91.13
- melancholia — *see* Disorder, depressive
- mental disorder NEC O99.345
- metroperitonitis O85
- metrorrhagia — *see* Hemorrhage, postpartum
- metrosalpingitis O86.19
- metrovaginitis O86.13
- milk leg O87.1
- monoplegia, cerebral O99.43
- mood disturbance O90.6
- necrosis, liver (acute) (subacute) (conditions in subcategory K72.0) O26.63
  - with renal failure O90.4
- nervous system disorder O99.355
- obesity (pre-existing prior to pregnancy) O99.215
- obesity surgery status O99.845
- occlusion, precerebral artery O99.43
- paralysis
  - bladder (sphincter) O90.89
  - cerebral O99.43
- paralytic stroke O99.43
- parametritis O85
- paravaginitis O86.13
- pelviperitonitis O85
- perimetritis O86.12
- perimetrosalpingitis O86.19
- perinephritis O86.21
- periphlebitis — *see* Puerperal phlebitis
- peritoneal infection O85
- peritonitis (pelvic) O85
- perivaginitis O86.13
- phlebitis O87.0
  - deep O87.1
  - pelvic O87.1
  - superficial O87.0
- phlebothrombosis, deep O87.1
- phlegmasia alba dolens O87.1
- placental polyp O90.89
- pneumonia, embolic — *see* Embolism, obstetric, puerperal
- pre-eclampsia — *see* Pre-eclampsia
- psychosis (NOS) F53.1
- pyelitis O86.21
- pyelocystitis O86.29
- pyelonephritis O86.21
- pyelonephrosis O86.21
- pyemia O85
- pyocystitis O86.29
- pyohemia O85

Puerperal, puerperium — *continued*
- pyometra O86.12
- pyonephritis O86.21
- pyosalpingitis O86.19
- pyrexia (of unknown origin) O86.4
- renal
  - disease NEC O90.89
  - failure O90.4
- respiratory disease NEC O99.53
- retention
  - decidua — *see* Retention, decidua
  - placenta O72.0
  - secundines — *see* Retention, secundines
- retrated nipple O92.02
- salpingo-ovaritis O86.19
- salpingoperitonitis O85
- secondary perineal tear O90.1
- sepsis (pelvic) O85
- sepsis O85
- septic thrombophlebitis O86.81
- skin disorder NEC O99.73
- specified condition NEC O99.89
- stroke O99.43
- subinvolution (uterus) O90.89
- subluxation of symphysis (pubis) O26.73
- suppuration — *see* Puerperal, abscess
- tetanus A34
- thelitis O91.02
  - associated with lactation O91.03
- thrombocytopenia O72.3
- thrombophlebitis (superficial) O87.0
  - deep O87.1
  - pelvic O87.1
  - septic O86.81
- thrombosis (venous) — *see* Thrombosis, puerperal
- thyroiditis O90.5
- toxemia (eclamptic) (pre-eclamptic) (with convulsions) O15.2
- trauma, non-obstetric O9A.23 (*following* O99)
- caused by abuse (physical) (suspected) O9A.33 (*following* O99)
  - confirmed O9A.33 (*following* O99)
  - psychological (suspected) O9A.53 (*following* O99)
    - confirmed O9A.53 (*following* O99)
  - sexual (suspected) O9A.43 (*following* O99)
    - confirmed O9A.43 (*following* O99)
- uremia (due to renal failure) O90.4
- urethritis O86.22
- vaginitis O86.13
- varicose veins (legs) O87.4
  - vulva or perineum O87.8
- venous O87.9
- vulvitis O86.19
- vulvovaginitis O86.13
- white leg O87.1

Puerperium — *see* Puerperal
Pulmolithiasis J98.4
Pulmonary — *see* condition
Pulpitis (acute) (anachoretic) (chronic) (hyperplastic) (putrescent) (suppurative) (ulcerative) K04.01
- irreversible K04.02
- reversible K04.01
Pulpless tooth K04.99
Pulse
- alternating R00.8
- bigeminal R00.8
- fast R00.0
- feeble, rapid due to shock following injury T79.4 ☑
- rapid R00.0
- weak R09.89
Pulsus alternans or trigeminus R00.8
Punch drunk F07.81
Punctum lacrimale occlusion — *see* Obstruction, lacrimal
Puncture
- abdomen, abdominal
  - wall S31.139 ☑
    - with
      - foreign body S31.149 ☑
      - penetration into peritoneal cavity S31.639
        - with foreign body S31.649 ☑
    - epigastric region S31.132 ☑
      - with
        - foreign body S31.142 ☑
        - penetration into peritoneal cavity S31.632 ☑
          - with foreign body S31.642 ☑

Puncture — *continued*
  abdomen, abdominal — *continued*
    wall — *continued*
      left
        lower quadrant S31.134 ☑
          with
            foreign body S31.144 ☑
            penetration into peritoneal cavity
              S31.634 ☑
              with foreign body S31.644 ☑
        upper quadrant S31.131 ☑
          with
            foreign body S31.141 ☑
            penetration into peritoneal cavity
              S31.631 ☑
              with foreign body S31.641 ☑
      periumbilic region S31.135 ☑
        with
          foreign body S31.145 ☑
          penetration into peritoneal cavity
            S31.635 ☑
            with foreign body S31.645 ☑
      right
        lower quadrant S31.133 ☑
          with
            foreign body S31.143 ☑
            penetration into peritoneal cavity
              S31.633 ☑
              with foreign body S31.643 ☑
        upper quadrant S31.130 ☑
          with
            foreign body S31.140 ☑
            penetration into peritoneal cavity
              S31.630 ☑
              with foreign body S31.640 ☑
  accidental, complicating surgery — *see* Complication, accidental puncture or laceration
  alveolar (process) — *see* Puncture, oral cavity
  ankle S91.039 ☑
    with
      foreign body S91.049 ☑
    left S91.032 ☑
      with
        foreign body S91.042 ☑
    right S91.031 ☑
      with
        foreign body S91.041 ☑
  anus S31.833 ☑
    with foreign body S31.834 ☑
  arm (upper) S41.139 ☑
    with foreign body S41.149 ☑
    left S41.132 ☑
      with foreign body S41.142 ☑
    lower — *see* Puncture, forearm
    right S41.131 ☑
      with foreign body S41.141 ☑
  auditory canal (external) (meatus) — *see* Puncture, ear
  auricle, ear — *see* Puncture, ear
  axilla — *see* Puncture, arm
  back — *see also* Puncture, thorax, back
    lower S31.030 ☑
      with
        foreign body S31.040 ☑
          with penetration into retroperitoneal space S31.041 ☑
        penetration into retroperitoneal space S31.031 ☑
  bladder (traumatic) S37.29 ☑
    nontraumatic N32.89
  breast S21.039 ☑
    with foreign body S21.049 ☑
    left S21.032 ☑
      with foreign body S21.042 ☑
    right S21.031 ☑
      with foreign body S21.041 ☑
  buttock S31.803 ☑
    with foreign body S31.804 ☑
    left S31.823 ☑
      with foreign body S31.824 ☑
    right S31.813 ☑
      with foreign body S31.814 ☑
  by
    device, implant or graft — *see* Complications, by site and type, mechanical
    foreign body left accidentally in operative wound T81.539 ☑

Puncture — *continued*
  by — *continued*
    instrument (any) during a procedure, accidental — *see* Puncture, accidental complicating surgery
  calf — *see* Puncture, leg
  canaliculus lacrimalis — *see* Puncture, eyelid
  canthus, eye — *see* Puncture, eyelid
  cervical esophagus S11.23 ☑
    with foreign body S11.24 ☑
  cheek (external) S01.439 ☑
    with foreign body S01.449 ☑
    internal — *see* Puncture, oral cavity
    left S01.432 ☑
      with foreign body S01.442 ☑
    right S01.431 ☑
      with foreign body S01.441 ☑
  chest wall — *see* Puncture, thorax
  chin — *see* Puncture, head, specified site NEC
  clitoris — *see* Puncture, vulva
  costal region — *see* Puncture, thorax
  digit(s)
    foot — *see* Puncture, toe
    hand — *see* Puncture, finger
  ear (canal) (external) S01.339 ☑
    with foreign body S01.349 ☑
    drum S09.2- ☑
    left S01.332 ☑
      with foreign body S01.342 ☑
    right S01.331 ☑
      with foreign body S01.341 ☑
  elbow S51.039 ☑
    with
      foreign body S51.049 ☑
    left S51.032 ☑
      with
        foreign body S51.042 ☑
    right S51.031 ☑
      with
        foreign body S51.041 ☑
  epididymis — *see* Puncture, testis
  epigastric region — *see* Puncture, abdomen, wall, epigastric
  epiglottis S11.83 ☑
    with foreign body S11.84 ☑
  esophagus
    cervical S11.23 ☑
      with foreign body S11.24 ☑
    thoracic S27.818 ☑
  eyeball S05.6- ☑
    with foreign body S05.5- ☑
  eyebrow — *see* Puncture, eyelid
  eyelid S01.13- ☑
    with foreign body S01.14- ☑
    left S01.132 ☑
      with foreign body S01.142 ☑
    right S01.131 ☑
      with foreign body S01.141 ☑
  face NEC — *see* Puncture, head, specified site NEC
  finger(s) S61.239 ☑
    with
      damage to nail S61.339 ☑
        with
          foreign body S61.349 ☑
      foreign body S61.249 ☑
    index S61.238 ☑
      with
        damage to nail S61.338 ☑
          with
            foreign body S61.348 ☑
        foreign body S61.248 ☑
      left S61.231 ☑
        with
          damage to nail S61.331 ☑
            with
              foreign body S61.341 ☑
          foreign body S61.241 ☑
      right S61.230 ☑
        with
          damage to nail S61.330 ☑
            with
              foreign body S61.340 ☑
          foreign body S61.240 ☑
    little S61.238 ☑
      with
        damage to nail S61.338 ☑

Puncture — *continued*
  finger(s) — *continued*
    little — *continued*
      with — *continued*
        damage to nail — *continued*
          with
            foreign body S61.348 ☑
        foreign body S61.248 ☑
      left S61.237 ☑
        with
          damage to nail S61.337 ☑
            with
              foreign body S61.347 ☑
          foreign body S61.247 ☑
      right S61.236 ☑
        with
          damage to nail S61.336 ☑
            with
              foreign body S61.346 ☑
          foreign body S61.246 ☑
    middle S61.238 ☑
      with
        damage to nail S61.338 ☑
          with
            foreign body S61.348 ☑
        foreign body S61.248 ☑
      left S61.233 ☑
        with
          damage to nail S61.333 ☑
            with
              foreign body S61.343 ☑
          foreign body S61.243 ☑
      right S61.232 ☑
        with
          damage to nail S61.332 ☑
            with
              foreign body S61.342 ☑
          foreign body S61.242 ☑
    ring S61.238 ☑
      with
        damage to nail S61.338 ☑
          with
            foreign body S61.348 ☑
        foreign body S61.248 ☑
      left S61.235 ☑
        with
          damage to nail S61.335 ☑
            with
              foreign body S61.345 ☑
          foreign body S61.245 ☑
      right S61.234 ☑
        with
          damage to nail S61.334 ☑
            with
              foreign body S61.344 ☑
          foreign body S61.244 ☑
  flank S31.139 ☑
    with foreign body S31.149 ☑
  foot (except toe(s) alone) S91.339 ☑
    with foreign body S91.349 ☑
    left S91.332 ☑
      with foreign body S91.342 ☑
    right S91.331 ☑
      with foreign body S91.341 ☑
    toe — *see* Puncture, toe
  forearm S51.839 ☑
    with
      foreign body S51.849 ☑
    elbow only — *see* Puncture, elbow
    left S51.832 ☑
      with
        foreign body S51.842 ☑
    right S51.831 ☑
      with
        foreign body S51.841 ☑
  forehead — *see* Puncture, head, specified site NEC
  genital organs, external
    female S31.532 ☑
      with foreign body S31.542 ☑
      vagina — *see* Puncture, vagina
      vulva — *see* Puncture, vulva
    male S31.531 ☑
      with foreign body S31.541 ☑
      penis — *see* Puncture, penis
      scrotum — *see* Puncture, scrotum
      testis — *see* Puncture, testis

Ⓥ Subterms under main terms may continue to next column or page   ☑ Additional Character Required — Refer to the Tabular List for Character Selection   269

Puncture — Puncture

Puncture — *continued*

groin — *see* Puncture, abdomen, wall
gum — *see* Puncture, oral cavity
hand S61.439 ☑
   with
      foreign body S61.449 ☑
   finger — *see* Puncture, finger
   left S61.432 ☑
      with
         foreign body S61.442 ☑
   right S61.431 ☑
      with
         foreign body S61.441 ☑
   thumb — *see* Puncture, thumb
head S01.93 ☑
   with foreign body S01.94 ☑
   cheek — *see* Puncture, cheek
   ear — *see* Puncture, ear
   eyelid — *see* Puncture, eyelid
   lip — *see* Puncture, oral cavity
   nose — *see* Puncture, nose
   oral cavity — *see* Puncture, oral cavity
   scalp S01.03 ☑
      with foreign body S01.04 ☑
   specified site NEC S01.83 ☑
      with foreign body S01.84 ☑
   temporomandibular area — *see* Puncture, cheek
heart S26.99 ☑
   with hemopericardium S26.09 ☑
   without hemopericardium S26.19 ☑
heel — *see* Puncture, foot
hip S71.039 ☑
   with foreign body S71.049 ☑
   left S71.032 ☑
      with foreign body S71.042 ☑
   right S71.031 ☑
      with foreign body S71.041 ☑
hymen — *see* Puncture, vagina
hypochondrium — *see* Puncture, abdomen, wall
hypogastric region — *see* Puncture, abdomen, wall
inguinal region — *see* Puncture, abdomen, wall
instep — *see* Puncture, foot
internal organs — *see* Injury, by site
interscapular region — *see* Puncture, thorax, back
intestine
   large
      colon S36.599 ☑
         ascending S36.590 ☑
         descending S36.592 ☑
         sigmoid S36.593 ☑
         specified site NEC S36.598 ☑
         transverse S36.591 ☑
      rectum S36.69 ☑
   small S36.499 ☑
      duodenum S36.490 ☑
      specified site NEC S36.498 ☑
intra-abdominal organ S36.99 ☑
   gallbladder S36.128 ☑
   intestine — *see* Puncture, intestine
   liver S36.118 ☑
   pancreas — *see* Puncture, pancreas
   peritoneum S36.81 ☑
   specified site NEC S36.898 ☑
   spleen S36.09 ☑
   stomach S36.39 ☑
jaw — *see* Puncture, head, specified site NEC
knee S81.039 ☑
   with foreign body S81.049 ☑
   left S81.032 ☑
      with foreign body S81.042 ☑
   right S81.031 ☑
      with foreign body S81.041 ☑
labium (majus) (minus) — *see* Puncture, vulva
lacrimal duct — *see* Puncture, eyelid
larynx S11.013 ☑
   with foreign body S11.014 ☑
leg (lower) S81.839 ☑
   with foreign body S81.849 ☑
   foot — *see* Puncture, foot
   knee — *see* Puncture, knee
   left S81.832 ☑
      with foreign body S81.842 ☑
   right S81.831 ☑
      with foreign body S81.841 ☑
   upper — *see* Puncture, thigh
lip S01.531 ☑

Puncture — *continued*

lip — *continued*
   with foreign body S01.541 ☑
loin — *see* Puncture, abdomen, wall
lower back — *see* Puncture, back, lower
lumbar region — *see* Puncture, back, lower
malar region — *see* Puncture, head, specified site NEC
mammary — *see* Puncture, breast
mastoid region — *see* Puncture, head, specified site NEC
mouth — *see* Puncture, oral cavity
nail
   finger — *see* Puncture, finger, with damage to nail
   toe — *see* Puncture, toe, with damage to nail
nasal (septum) (sinus) — *see* Puncture, nose
nasopharynx — *see* Puncture, head, specified site NEC
neck S11.93 ☑
   with foreign body S11.94 ☑
   involving
      cervical esophagus — *see* Puncture, cervical
         esophagus
      larynx — *see* Puncture, larynx
      pharynx — *see* Puncture, pharynx
      thyroid gland — *see* Puncture, thyroid gland
      trachea — *see* Puncture, trachea
   specified site NEC S11.83 ☑
      with foreign body S11.84 ☑
nose (septum) (sinus) S01.23 ☑
   with foreign body S01.24 ☑
ocular — *see* Puncture, eyeball
oral cavity S01.532 ☑
   with foreign body S01.542 ☑
orbit S05.4- ☑
palate — *see* Puncture, oral cavity
palm — *see* Puncture, hand
pancreas S36.299 ☑
   body S36.291 ☑
   head S36.290 ☑
   tail S36.292 ☑
pelvis — *see* Puncture, back, lower
penis S31.23 ☑
   with foreign body S31.24 ☑
perineum
   female S31.43 ☑
      with foreign body S31.44 ☑
   male S31.139 ☑
      with foreign body S31.149 ☑
periocular area (with or without lacrimal passages) — *see* Puncture, eyelid
phalanges
   finger — *see* Puncture, finger
   toe — *see* Puncture, toe
pharynx S11.23 ☑
   with foreign body S11.24 ☑
pinna — *see* Puncture, ear
popliteal space — *see* Puncture, knee
prepuce — *see* Puncture, penis
pubic region S31.139 ☑
   with foreign body S31.149 ☑
pudendum — *see* Puncture, genital organs, external
rectovaginal septum — *see* Puncture, vagina
sacral region — *see* Puncture, back, lower
sacroiliac region — *see* Puncture, back, lower
salivary gland — *see* Puncture, oral cavity
scalp S01.03 ☑
   with foreign body S01.04 ☑
scapular region — *see* Puncture, shoulder
scrotum S31.33 ☑
   with foreign body S31.34 ☑
shin — *see* Puncture, leg
shoulder S41.039 ☑
   with foreign body S41.049 ☑
   left S41.032 ☑
      with foreign body S41.042 ☑
   right S41.031 ☑
      with foreign body S41.041 ☑
spermatic cord — *see* Puncture, testis
sternal region — *see* Puncture, thorax, front
submaxillary region — *see* Puncture, head, specified site NEC
submental region — *see* Puncture, head, specified site NEC
subungual
   finger(s) — *see* Puncture, finger, with damage to nail
   toe — *see* Puncture, toe, with damage to nail

Puncture — *continued*

supraclavicular fossa — *see* Puncture, neck, specified site NEC
temple, temporal region — *see* Puncture, head, specified site NEC
temporomandibular area — *see* Puncture, cheek
testis S31.33 ☑
   with foreign body S31.34 ☑
thigh S71.139 ☑
   with foreign body S71.149 ☑
   left S71.132 ☑
      with foreign body S71.142 ☑
   right S71.131 ☑
      with foreign body S71.141 ☑
thorax, thoracic (wall) S21.93 ☑
   with foreign body S21.94 ☑
   back S21.23- ☑
      with
         foreign body S21.24- ☑
            with penetration S21.44 ☑
         penetration S21.43 ☑
   breast — *see* Puncture, breast
   front S21.13- ☑
      with
         foreign body S21.14- ☑
            with penetration S21.34 ☑
         penetration S21.33 ☑
throat — *see* Puncture, neck
thumb S61.039 ☑
   with
      damage to nail S61.139 ☑
         with
            foreign body S61.149 ☑
      foreign body S61.049 ☑
   left S61.032 ☑
      with
         damage to nail S61.132 ☑
           with
              foreign body S61.142 ☑
         foreign body S61.042 ☑
   right S61.031 ☑
      with
         damage to nail S61.131 ☑
           with
              foreign body S61.141 ☑
         foreign body S61.041 ☑
thyroid gland S11.13 ☑
   with foreign body S11.14 ☑
toe(s) S91.139 ☑
   with
      damage to nail S91.239 ☑
         with
            foreign body S91.249 ☑
      foreign body S91.149 ☑
   great S91.133 ☑
      with
         damage to nail S91.233 ☑
           with
              foreign body S91.243 ☑
         foreign body S91.143 ☑
      left S91.132 ☑
         with
           damage to nail S91.232 ☑
             with
                foreign body S91.242 ☑
           foreign body S91.142 ☑
      right S91.131 ☑
         with
           damage to nail S91.231 ☑
             with
                foreign body S91.241 ☑
           foreign body S91.141 ☑
   lesser S91.136 ☑
      with
         damage to nail S91.236 ☑
           with
              foreign body S91.246 ☑
         foreign body S91.146 ☑
      left S91.135 ☑
         with
           damage to nail S91.235 ☑
             with
                foreign body S91.245 ☑
           foreign body S91.145 ☑
      right S91.134 ☑

☑ Additional Character Required — Refer to the Tabular List for Character Selection   ▼ Subterms under main terms may continue to next column or page

Puncture — *continued*
 toe(s) — *continued*
  lesser — *continued*
   right — *continued*
    with
     damage to nail S91.234 ☑
      with
       foreign body S91.244 ☑
      foreign body S91.144 ☑
  tongue — *see* Puncture, oral cavity
  trachea S11.023 ☑
   with foreign body S11.024 ☑
  tunica vaginalis — *see* Puncture, testis
  tympanum, tympanic membrane S09.2- ☑
  umbilical region S31.135 ☑
   with foreign body S31.145 ☑
  uvula — *see* Puncture, oral cavity
  vagina S31.43 ☑
   with foreign body S31.44 ☑
  vocal cords S11.033 ☑
   with foreign body S11.034 ☑
  vulva S31.43 ☑
   with foreign body S31.44 ☑
  wrist S61.539 ☑
   with
    foreign body S61.549 ☑
   left S61.532 ☑
    with
     foreign body S61.542 ☑
   right S61.531 ☑
    with
     foreign body S61.541 ☑
PUO (pyrexia of unknown origin) R50.9
Pupillary membrane (persistent) Q13.89
Pupillotonia — *see* Anomaly, pupil, function, tonic pupil
Purpura D69.2
 abdominal D69.0
 allergic D69.0
 anaphylactoid D69.0
 annularis telangiectodes L81.7
 arthritic D69.0
 autoerythrocyte sensitization D69.2
 autoimmune D69.0
 bacterial D69.0
 Bateman's (senile) D69.2
 capillary fragility (hereditary) (idiopathic) D69.8
 cryoglobulinemic D89.1
 Devil's pinches D69.2
 fibrinolytic — *see* Fibrinolysis
 fulminans, fulminous D65
 gangrenous D65
 hemorrhagic, hemorrhagica D69.3
  not due to thrombocytopenia D69.0
 Henoch (-Schönlein) (allergic) D69.0
 hypergammaglobulinemic (benign) (Waldenström) D89.0
 idiopathic (thrombocytopenic) D69.3
  nonthrombocytopenic D69.0
 immune thrombocytopenic D69.3
 infectious D69.0
 malignant D69.0
 neonatorum P54.5
 nervosa D69.0
 newborn P54.5
 nonthrombocytopenic D69.2
  hemorrhagic D69.0
  idiopathic D69.0
 nonthrombopenic D69.2
 peliosis rheumatica D69.0
 posttransfusion (post-transfusion) (from (fresh) whole blood or blood products) D69.51
 primary D69.49
 red cell membrane sensitivity D69.2
 rheumatica D69.0
 Schönlein (-Henoch) (allergic) D69.0
 scorbutic E54 [D77]
 senile D69.2
 simplex D69.2
 symptomatica D69.0
 telangiectasia annularis L81.7
 thrombocytopenic D69.49
  congenital D69.42
  hemorrhagic D69.3
  hereditary D69.42
  idiopathic D69.3
  immune D69.3
  neonatal, transitory P61.0
  thrombotic M31.1

Purpura — *continued*
 thrombohemolytic — *see* Fibrinolysis
 thrombolytic — *see* Fibrinolysis
 thrombopenic D69.49
 thrombotic, thrombocytopenic M31.1
 toxic D69.0
 vascular D69.0
 visceral symptoms D69.0
Purpuric spots R23.3
Purulent — *see* condition
Pus
 in
  stool R19.5
  urine N39.0
 tube (rupture) — *see* Salpingo-oophoritis
Pustular rash L08.0
Pustule (nonmalignant) L08.9
 malignant A22.0
Pustulosis palmaris et plantaris L40.3
Putnam (-Dana) disease or syndrome — *see* Degeneration, combined
Putrescent pulp (dental) K04.1
Pyarthritis, pyarthrosis — *see* Arthritis, pyogenic or pyemic
 tuberculous — *see* Tuberculosis, joint
Pyelectasis — *see* Hydronephrosis
Pyelitis (congenital) (uremic) — *see also* Pyelonephritis
 with
  calculus — *see* category N20 ☑
   with hydronephrosis N13.6
  contracted kidney N11.9
 acute N10
 chronic N11.9
  with calculus — *see* category N20 ☑
   with hydronephrosis N13.6
 cystica N28.84
 puerperal (postpartum) O86.21
 tuberculous A18.11
Pyelocystitis — *see* Pyelonephritis
Pyelonephritis — *see also* Nephritis, tubulo-interstitial
 with
  calculus — *see* category N20 ☑
   with hydronephrosis N13.6
  contracted kidney N11.9
 acute N10
 calculous — *see* category N20 ☑
  with hydronephrosis N13.6
 chronic N11.9
  with calculus — *see* category N20 ☑
   with hydronephrosis N13.6
  associated with ureteral obstruction or stricture N11.1
  nonobstructive N11.8
   with reflux (vesicoureteral) N11.0
  obstructive N11.1
  specified NEC N11.8
 in (due to)
  brucellosis A23.9 [N16]
  cryoglobulinemia (mixed) D89.1 [N16]
  cystinosis E72.04
  diphtheria A36.84
  glycogen storage disease E74.09 [N16]
  leukemia NEC C95.9- ☑ [N16]
  lymphoma NEC C85.90 [N16]
  multiple myeloma C90.0- ☑ [N16]
  obstruction N11.1
  Salmonella infection A02.25
  sarcoidosis D86.84
  sepsis A41.9 [N16]
  Sjögren's disease M35.04
  toxoplasmosis B58.83
  transplant rejection T86.91 [N16]
  Wilson's disease E83.01 [N16]
 nonobstructive N12
  with reflux (vesicoureteral) N11.0
  chronic N11.8
 syphilitic A52.75
Pyelonephrosis (obstructive) N11.1
 chronic N11.9
Pyelophlebitis I80.8
Pyeloureteritis cystica N28.85
Pyemia, pyemic (fever) (infection) (purulent) — *see also* Sepsis
 joint — *see* Arthritis, pyogenic or pyemic
 liver K75.1
 pneumococcal A40.3
 portal K75.1

Pyemia, pyemic — *continued*
 postvaccinal T88.0 ☑
 puerperal, postpartum, childbirth O85
 specified organism NEC A41.89
 tuberculous — *see* Tuberculosis, miliary
Pygopagus Q89.4
Pyknoepilepsy (idiopathic) — *see* Pyknolepsy
Pyknolepsy G40.A09 (*following* G40.3)
 intractable G40.A19 (*following* G40.3)
  with status epilepticus G40.A11 (*following* G40.3)
  without status epilepticus G40.A19 (*following* G40.3)
 not intractable G40.A09 (*following* G40.3)
  with status epilepticus G40.A01 (*following* G40.3)
  without status epilepticus G40.A09 (*following* G40.3)
Pylephlebitis K75.1
Pyle's syndrome Q78.5
Pylethrombophlebitis K75.1
Pylethrombosis K75.1
Pyloritis K29.90
 with bleeding K29.91
Pylorospasm (reflex) **NEC** K31.3
 congenital or infantile Q40.0
 neurotic F45.8
 newborn Q40.0
 psychogenic F45.8
Pylorus, pyloric — *see* condition
Pyoarthrosis — *see* Arthritis, pyogenic or pyemic
Pyocele
 mastoid — *see* Mastoiditis, acute
 sinus (accessory) — *see* Sinusitis
 turbinate (bone) J32.9
 urethra — *see also* Urethritis N34.0
Pyocolpos — *see* Vaginitis
Pyocystitis N30.80
 with hematuria N30.81
Pyoderma, pyodermia L08.0
 gangrenosum L88
 newborn P39.4
 phagedenic L88
 vegetans L08.81
Pyodermatitis L08.0
 vegetans L08.81
Pyogenic — *see* condition
Pyohydronephrosis N13.6
Pyometra, pyometrium, pyometritis — *see* Endometritis
Pyomyositis (tropical) — *see* Myositis, infective
Pyonephritis N12
Pyonephrosis N13.6
 tuberculous A18.11
Pyo-oophoritis — *see* Salpingo-oophoritis
Pyo-ovarium — *see* Salpingo-oophoritis
Pyopericarditis, pyopericardium I30.1
Pyophlebitis — *see* Phlebitis
Pyopneumopericardium I30.1
Pyopneumothorax (infective) J86.9
 with fistula J86.0
 tuberculous NEC A15.6
Pyosalpinx, pyosalpingitis — *see also* Salpingo-oophoritis
Pyothorax J86.9
 with fistula J86.0
 tuberculous NEC A15.6
Pyoureter N28.89
 tuberculous A18.11
Pyramidopallidonigral syndrome G20
Pyrexia (of unknown origin) R50.9
 atmospheric T67.01 ☑
 during labor NEC O75.2
 heat T67.01 ☑
 newborn P81.9
  environmentally-induced P81.0
 persistent R50.9
 puerperal O86.4
Pyroglobulinemia NEC E88.09
Pyromania F63.1
Pyrosis R12
Pyuria (bacterial) (sterile) R82.81

Q

Q fever A78
 with pneumonia A78
Quadricuspid aortic valve Q23.8
Quadrilateral fever A78
Quadriparesis — *see* Quadriplegia
 meaning muscle weakness M62.81

⬙ Subterms under main terms may continue to next column or page   ☑ Additional Character Required — Refer to the Tabular List for Character Selection   271

Puncture — Quadriparesis

Quadriplegia G82.50
  complete
    C1-C4 level G82.51
    C5-C7 level G82.53
  congenital (cerebral) (spinal) G80.8
    spastic G80.0
  embolic (current episode) I63.4- ☑
  functional R53.2
  incomplete
    C1-C4 level G82.52
    C5-C7 level G82.54
  thrombotic (current episode) I63.3- ☑
  traumatic — *code to* injury with seventh character S
    current episode — *see* Injury, spinal (cord), cervical
Quadruplet, pregnancy — *see* Pregnancy, quadruplet
Quarrelsomeness F60.3
Queensland fever A77.3
Quervain's disease M65.4
  thyroid E06.1
Queyrat's erythroplasia D07.4
  penis D07.4
  specified site — *see* Neoplasm, skin, in situ
  unspecified site D07.4
Quincke's disease or edema T78.3 ☑
  hereditary D84.1
Quinsy (gangrenous) J36
Quintan fever A79.0
Quintuplet, pregnancy — *see* Pregnancy, quintuplet

R

Rabbit fever — *see* Tularemia
Rabies A82.9
  contact Z20.3
  exposure to Z20.3
  inoculation reaction — *see* Complications, vaccination
  sylvatic A82.0
  urban A82.1
Rachischisis — *see* Spina bifida
Rachitic — *see also* condition
  deformities of spine (late effect) (sequelae) E64.3
  pelvis (late effect) (sequelae) E64.3
    with disproportion (fetopelvic) O33.0
      causing obstructed labor O65.0
Rachitis, rachitism (acute) (tarda) — *see also* Rickets
  renalis N25.0
  sequelae E64.3
Radial nerve — *see* condition
Radiation
  burn — *see* Burn
  effects NOS T66 ☑
  sickness NOS T66 ☑
  therapy, encounter for Z51.0
Radiculitis (pressure) (vertebrogenic) — *see* Radiculopathy
Radiculomyelitis — *see also* Encephalitis
  toxic, due to
    Clostridium tetani A35
    Corynebacterium diphtheriae A36.82
Radiculopathy M54.10
  cervical region M54.12
  cervicothoracic region M54.13
  due to
    disc disorder
      C3 M50.11
      C4 M50.11
      C5 M50.121
      C6 M50.122
      C7 M50.123
    displacement of intervertebral disc — *see* Disorder, disc, with, radiculopathy
  leg M54.1- ☑
  lumbar region M54.16
  lumbosacral region M54.17
  occipito-atlanto-axial region M54.11
  postherpetic B02.29
  sacrococcygeal region M54.18
  syphilitic A52.11
  thoracic region (with visceral pain) M54.14
  thoracolumbar region M54.15
Radiodermal burns (acute, chronic, or occupational) — *see* Burn
Radiodermatitis L58.9
  acute L58.0
  chronic L58.1
Radiotherapy session Z51.0
RAEB (refractory anemia with excess blasts) D46.2- ☑

Rage, meaning rabies — *see* Rabies
Ragpicker's disease A22.1
Ragsorter's disease A22.1
Raillietiniasis B71.8
Railroad neurosis F48.8
Railway spine F48.8
Raised — *see also* Elevated
  antibody titer R76.0
Rake teeth, tooth M26.39
Rales R09.89
Ramifying renal pelvis Q63.8
Ramsay-Hunt disease or syndrome — *see also* Hunt's disease B02.21
  meaning dyssynergia cerebellaris myoclonica G11.1
Ranula K11.6
  congenital Q38.4
Rape
  adult
    confirmed T74.21 ☑
    suspected T76.21 ☑
  alleged, observation or examination, ruled out
    adult Z04.41
    child Z04.42
  child
    confirmed T74.22 ☑
    suspected T76.22 ☑
Rapid
  feeble pulse, due to shock, following injury T79.4 ☑
  heart (beat) R00.0
    psychogenic F45.8
  second stage (delivery) O62.3
  time-zone change syndrome G47.25
Rarefaction, bone — *see* Disorder, bone, density and structure, specified NEC
Rash (toxic) R21
  canker A38.9
  diaper L22
  drug (internal use) L27.0
    contact — *see also* Dermatitis, due to, drugs, external L25.1
  following immunization T88.1 ☑
  food — *see* Dermatitis, due to, food
  heat L74.0
  napkin (psoriasiform) L22
  nettle — *see* Urticaria
  pustular L08.0
  rose R21
    epidemic B06.9
  scarlet A38.9
  serum — *see also* Reaction, serum T80.69 ☑
  wandering tongue K14.1
Rasmussen aneurysm — *see* Tuberculosis, pulmonary
Rasmussen encephalitis G04.81
Rat-bite fever A25.9
  due to Streptobacillus moniliformis A25.1
  spirochetal (morsus muris) A25.0
Rathke's pouch tumor D44.3
Raymond (-Céstan) **syndrome** I65.8
Raynaud's disease, phenomenon or syndrome (secondary) I73.00
  with gangrene (symmetric) I73.01
RDS (newborn) (type I) P22.0
  type II P22.1
Reaction — *see also* Disorder
  withdrawing, child or adolescent F93.8
  adaptation — *see* Disorder, adjustment
  adjustment (anxiety) (conduct disorder) (depressiveness) (distress) — *see* Disorder, adjustment
    with
      mutism, elective (child) (adolescent) F94.0
  adverse
    food (any) (ingested) NEC T78.1 ☑
      anaphylactic — *see* Shock, anaphylactic, due to food
  affective — *see* Disorder, mood
  allergic — *see* Allergy
  anaphylactic — *see* Shock, anaphylactic
  anaphylactoid — *see* Shock, anaphylactic
  anesthesia — *see* Anesthesia, complication
  antitoxin (prophylactic) (therapeutic) — *see* Complications, vaccination
  anxiety F41.1
  Arthus — *see* Arthus' phenomenon
  asthenic F48.8
  combat and operational stress F43.0
  compulsive F42.8
  conversion F44.9

Reaction — *continued*
  crisis, acute F43.0
  deoxyribonuclease (DNA) (DNase) hypersensitivity D69.2
  depressive (single episode) F32.9
    affective (single episode) F31.4
      recurrent episode F33.9
    neurotic F34.1
    psychoneurotic F34.1
    psychotic F32.3
    recurrent — *see* Disorder, depressive, recurrent
  dissociative F44.9
  drug NEC T88.7 ☑
    addictive — *see* Dependence, drug
      transmitted via placenta or breast milk — *see* Absorption, drug, addictive, through placenta
    allergic — *see* Allergy, drug
    lichenoid L43.2
    newborn P93.8
      gray baby syndrome P93.0
    overdose or poisoning (by accident) — *see* Table of Drugs and Chemicals, by drug, poisoning
    photoallergic L56.1
    phototoxic L56.0
    withdrawal — *see* Dependence, by drug, with, withdrawal
      infant of dependent mother P96.1
      newborn P96.1
    wrong substance given or taken (by accident) — *see* Table of Drugs and Chemicals, by drug, poisoning
  fear F40.9
    child (abnormal) F93.8
  febrile nonhemolytic transfusion (FNHTR) R50.84
  fluid loss, cerebrospinal G97.1
  foreign
    body NEC — *see* Granuloma, foreign body
      in operative wound (inadvertently left) — *see* Foreign body, accidentally left during a procedure
    substance accidentally left during a procedure (chemical) (powder) (talc) T81.60 ☑
      aseptic peritonitis T81.61 ☑
      body or object (instrument) (sponge) (swab) — *see* Foreign body, accidentally left during a procedure
      specified reaction NEC T81.69 ☑
  grief — *see* Disorder, adjustment
  Herxheimer's R68.89
  hyperkinetic — *see* Hyperkinesia
  hypochondriacal F45.20
  hypoglycemic, due to insulin E16.0
    with coma (diabetic) — *see* Diabetes, coma nondiabetic E15
    therapeutic misadventure — *see* subcategory T38.3 ☑
  hypomanic F30.8
  hysterical F44.9
  immunization — *see* Complications, vaccination
  incompatibility
    ABO blood group (infusion) (transfusion) — *see* Complication(s), transfusion, incompatibility reaction, ABO
    delayed serologic T80.39 ☑
    minor blood group (Duffy) (E) (K) (Kell) (Kidd) (Lewis) (M) (N) (P) (S) T80.89 ☑
    Rh (factor) (infusion) (transfusion) — *see* Complication(s), transfusion, incompatibility reaction, Rh (factor)
  inflammatory — *see* Infection
  infusion — *see* Complications, infusion
  inoculation (immune serum) — *see* Complications, vaccination
  insulin T38.3- ☑
  involutional psychotic — *see* Disorder, depressive
  leukemoid D72.823
    basophilic D72.823
    lymphocytic D72.823
    monocytic D72.823
    myelocytic D72.823
    neutrophilic D72.823
  LSD (acute)
    due to drug abuse — *see* Abuse, drug, hallucinogen
    due to drug dependence — *see* Dependence, drug, hallucinogen
  lumbar puncture G97.1
  manic-depressive — *see* Disorder, bipolar

☑ **Additional Character Required** — Refer to the Tabular List for Character Selection   Subterms under main terms may continue to next column or page

Reaction — *continued*
  neurasthenic F48.8
  neurogenic — *see* Neurosis
  neurotic F48.9
  neurotic-depressive F34.1
  nitritoid — *see* Crisis, nitritoid
  nonspecific
    to
      cell mediated immunity measurement of gamma
        interferon antigen response without active
        tuberculosis R76.12
      QuantiFERON-TB test (QFT) without active tuber-
        culosis R76.12
      tuberculin test — *see also* Reaction, tuberculin
        skin test R76.11
  obsessive-compulsive F42.8
  organic, acute or subacute — *see* Delirium
  paranoid (acute) F23
    chronic F22
    senile F03 ☑
  passive dependency F60.7
  phobic F40.9
  post-traumatic stress, uncomplicated Z73.3
  psychogenic F99
  psychoneurotic — *see also* Neurosis
    compulsive F42.8
    depersonalization F48.1
    depressive F34.1
    hypochondriacal F45.20
    neurasthenic F48.8
    obsessive F42.8
  psychophysiologic — *see* Disorder, somatoform
  psychosomatic — *see* Disorder, somatoform
  psychotic — *see* Psychosis
  scarlet fever toxin — *see* Complications, vaccination
  schizophrenic F23
    acute (brief) (undifferentiated) F23
    latent F21
    undifferentiated (acute) (brief) F23
  serological for syphilis — *see* Serology for syphilis
  serum T80.69 ☑
    anaphylactic (immediate) — *see also* Shock, anaphy-
      lactic T80.59 ☑
    specified reaction NEC
      due to
        administration of blood and blood products
          T80.61 ☑
        immunization T80.62 ☑
        serum specified NEC T80.69 ☑
        vaccination T80.62 ☑
  situational — *see* Disorder, adjustment
  somatization — *see* Disorder, somatoform
  spinal puncture G97.1
  stress (severe) F43.9
    acute (agitation) ("daze") (disorientation) (distur-
      bance of consciousness) (flight reaction)
      (fugue) F43.0
    specified NEC F43.8
  surgical procedure — *see* Complications, surgical pro-
    cedure
  tetanus antitoxin — *see* Complications, vaccination
  toxic, to local anesthesia T88.59 ☑
    in labor and delivery O74.4
    in pregnancy O29.3X- ☑
    postpartum, puerperal O89.3
  toxin-antitoxin — *see* Complications, vaccination
  transfusion (blood) (bone marrow) (lymphocytes) (al-
    lergic) — *see* Complications, transfusion
  tuberculin skin test, abnormal R76.11
  vaccination (any) — *see* Complications, vaccination
Reactive airway disease — *see* Asthma
Reactive depression — *see* Reaction, depressive
Rearrangement
  chromosomal
    balanced (in) Q95.9
      abnormal individual (autosomal) Q95.2
        non-sex (autosomal) chromosomes Q95.2
        sex/non-sex chromosomes Q95.3
      specified NEC Q95.8
Recalcitrant patient — *see* Noncompliance
Recanalization, thrombus — *see* Thrombosis
Recession, receding
  chamber angle (eye) H21.55- ☑
  chin M26.09
  gingival (postinfective) (postoperative)
    generalized K06.020
      minimal K06.021
      moderate K06.022

Recession, receding — *continued*
  gingival — *continued*
    generalized — *continued*
      severe K06.023
    localized K06.010
      minimal K06.011
      moderate K06.012
      severe K06.013
Recklinghausen disease Q85.01
  bones E21.0
Reclus' disease (cystic) — *see* Mastopathy, cystic
Recrudescent typhus (fever) A75.1
Recruitment, auditory H93.21- ☑
Rectalgia K62.89
Rectitis K62.89
Rectocele
  female (without uterine prolapse) N81.6
    with uterine prolapse N81.4
      incomplete N81.2
  in pregnancy — *see* Pregnancy, complicated by, abnor-
    mal, pelvic organs or tissues NEC
  male K62.3
Rectosigmoid junction — *see* condition
Rectosigmoiditis K63.89
  ulcerative (chronic) K51.30
    with
      complication K51.319
        abscess K51.314
        fistula K51.313
        obstruction K51.312
        rectal bleeding K51.311
        specified NEC K51.318
Rectourethral — *see* condition
Rectovaginal — *see* condition
Rectovesical — *see* condition
Rectum, rectal — *see* condition
Recurrent — *see* condition
  pregnancy loss — *see* Loss (of), pregnancy, recurrent
Red bugs B88.0
Red tide — *see also* Table of Drugs and Chemicals
  T65.82- ☑
Red-cedar lung or pneumonitis J67.8
Reduced
  mobility Z74.09
  ventilatory or vital capacity R94.2
Redundant, redundancy
  anus (congenital) Q43.8
  clitoris N90.89
  colon (congenital) Q43.8
  foreskin (congenital) N47.8
  intestine (congenital) Q43.8
  labia N90.69
  organ or site, congenital NEC — *see* Accessory
  panniculus (abdominal) E65
  prepuce (congenital) N47.8
  pylorus K31.89
  rectum (congenital) Q43.8
  scrotum N50.89
  sigmoid (congenital) Q43.8
  skin L98.7
    and subcutaneous tissue L98.7
    of face L57.4
      eyelids — *see* Blepharochalasis
  stomach K31.89
Reduplication — *see* Duplication
Reflex R29.2
  hyperactive gag J39.2
  pupillary, abnormal — *see* Anomaly, pupil, function
  vasoconstriction I73.9
  vasovagal R55
Reflux K21.9
  acid K21.9
  esophageal K21.9
    with esophagitis K21.0
    newborn P78.83
  gastroesophageal K21.9
    with esophagitis K21.0
  mitral — *see* Insufficiency, mitral
  ureteral — *see* Reflux, vesicoureteral
  vesicoureteral (with scarring) N13.70
    with
      nephropathy N13.729
        with hydroureter N13.739
          bilateral N13.732
          unilateral N13.731
        bilateral N13.722
        unilateral N13.721
        without hydroureter N13.729

Reflux — *continued*
  vesicoureteral — *continued*
    with — *continued*
      nephropathy — *continued*
        without hydroureter — *continued*
          bilateral N13.722
          unilateral N13.721
      pyelonephritis (chronic) N11.0
    congenital Q62.7
    without nephropathy N13.71
Reforming, artificial openings — *see* Attention to, artificial, opening
Refractive error — *see* Disorder, refraction
Refsum's disease or syndrome G60.1
Refusal of
  food, psychogenic F50.89
  treatment (because of) Z53.20
    left against medical advice (AMA) Z53.21
    patient's decision NEC Z53.29
    reasons of belief or group pressure Z53.1
Regional — *see* condition
Regurgitation R11.10
  aortic (valve) — *see* Insufficiency, aortic
  food — *see also* Vomiting
    with reswallowing — *see* Rumination
    newborn P92.1
  gastric contents — *see* Vomiting
  heart — *see* Endocarditis
  mitral (valve) — *see* Insufficiency, mitral
    congenital Q23.3
  myocardial — *see* Endocarditis
  pulmonary (valve) (heart) I37.1
    congenital Q22.2
    syphilitic A52.03
  tricuspid — *see* Insufficiency, tricuspid
  valve, valvular — *see* Endocarditis
    congenital Q24.8
  vesicoureteral — *see* Reflux, vesicoureteral
Reichmann's disease or syndrome K31.89
Reifenstein syndrome E34.52
Reinsertion
  implantable subdermal contraceptive Z30.46
  intrauterine contraceptive device Z30.433
Reiter's disease, syndrome, or urethritis M02.30
  ankle M02.37- ☑
  elbow M02.32- ☑
  foot joint M02.37- ☑
  hand joint M02.34- ☑
  hip M02.35- ☑
  knee M02.36- ☑
  multiple site M02.39
  shoulder M02.31- ☑
  vertebra M02.38
  wrist M02.33- ☑
Rejection
  food, psychogenic F50.89
  transplant T86.91
    bone T86.830
      marrow T86.01
    cornea T86.840
    heart T86.21
      with lung(s) T86.31
    intestine T86.850
    kidney T86.11
    liver T86.41
    lung(s) T86.810
      with heart T86.31
    organ (immune or nonimmune cause) T86.91
    pancreas T86.890
    skin (allograft) (autograft) T86.820
    specified NEC T86.890
    stem cell (peripheral blood) (umbilical cord) T86.5
Relapsing fever A68.9
  Carter's (Asiatic) A68.1
  Dutton's (West African) A68.1
  Koch's A68.9
  louse-borne (epidemic) A68.0
  Novy's (American) A68.1
  Obermeyers's (European) A68.0
  Spirillum A68.9
  tick-borne (endemic) A68.1
Relationship
  occlusal
    open anterior M26.220
    open posterior M26.221
Relaxation
  anus (sphincter) K62.89
    psychogenic F45.8

Relaxation — *continued*
  arch (foot) — *see also* Deformity, limb, flat foot
  back ligaments — *see* Instability, joint, spine
  bladder (sphincter) N31.2
  cardioesophageal K21.9
  cervix — *see* Incompetency, cervix
  diaphragm J98.6
  joint (capsule) (ligament) (paralytic) — *see* Flail, joint
    congenital NEC Q74.8
  lumbosacral (joint) — *see* subcategory M53.2 ☑
  pelvic floor N81.89
  perineum N81.89
  posture R29.3
  rectum (sphincter) K62.89
  sacroiliac (joint) — *see* subcategory M53.2 ☑
  scrotum N50.89
  urethra (sphincter) N36.44
  vesical N31.2
Release from prison, anxiety concerning Z65.2
Remains
  canal of Cloquet Q14.0
  capsule (opaque) Q14.8
Remittent fever (malarial) B54
Remnant
  canal of Cloquet Q14.0
  capsule (opaque) Q14.8
  cervix, cervical stump (acquired) (postoperative) N88.8
  cystic duct, postcholecystectomy K91.5
  fingernail L60.8
    congenital Q84.6
  meniscus, knee — *see* Derangement, knee, meniscus,
    specified NEC
  thyroglossal duct Q89.2
  tonsil J35.8
    infected (chronic) J35.01
  urachus Q64.4
Removal (from) (of)
  artificial
    arm Z44.00- ☑
      complete Z44.01- ☑
      partial Z44.02- ☑
    eye Z44.2- ☑
    leg Z44.10- ☑
      complete Z44.11- ☑
      partial Z44.12- ☑
  breast implant Z45.81 ☑
  cardiac pulse generator (battery) (end-of-life) Z45.010
  catheter (urinary) (indwelling) Z46.6
    from artificial opening — *see* Attention to, artificial,
      opening
    non-vascular Z46.82
    vascular NEC Z45.2
  device Z46.9
    contraceptive Z30.432
      implantable subdermal Z30.46
    implanted NEC Z45.89
    specified NEC Z46.89
  drains Z48.03
  dressing (nonsurgical) Z48.00
    surgical Z48.01
  external
    fixation device — *code to* fracture with seventh
      character D
    prosthesis, prosthetic device Z44.9
      breast Z44.3- ☑
      specified NEC Z44.8
  home in childhood (to foster home or institution)
    Z62.29
  ileostomy Z43.2
  insulin pump Z46.81
  myringotomy device (stent) (tube) Z45.82
  nervous system device NEC Z46.2
    brain neuropacemaker Z46.2
    visual substitution device Z46.2
      implanted Z45.31
  non-vascular catheter Z46.82
  organ, prophylactic (for neoplasia management) —
    see Prophylactic, organ removal
  orthodontic device Z46.4
  staples Z48.02
  stent
    ureteral Z46.6
  suture Z48.02
  urinary device Z46.6
  vascular access device or catheter Z45.2
Ren
  arcuatus Q63.1
  mobile, mobilis N28.89

Ren — *continued*
  mobile, mobilis — *continued*
    congenital Q63.8
  unguliformis Q63.1
Renal — *see* condition
Rendu-Osler-Weber disease or syndrome I78.0
Reninoma D41.0- ☑
Renon-Delille syndrome E23.3
Reovirus, as cause of disease classified elsewhere
  B97.5
Repeated falls NEC R29.6
Replaced chromosome by dicentric ring Q93.2
Replacement by artificial or mechanical device or
  prosthesis of
  bladder Z96.0
  blood vessel NEC Z95.828
  bone NEC Z96.7
  cochlea Z96.21
  coronary artery Z95.5
  eustachian tube Z96.29
  eye globe Z97.0
  heart Z95.812
    valve Z95.2
      prosthetic Z95.2
      specified NEC Z95.4
      xenogenic Z95.3
  intestine Z96.89
  joint Z96.60
    hip — *see* Presence, hip joint implant
    knee — *see* Presence, knee joint implant
    specified site NEC Z96.698
  larynx Z96.3
  lens Z96.1
  limb(s) — *see* Presence, artificial, limb
  mandible NEC (for tooth root implant(s)) Z96.5
  organ NEC Z96.89
  peripheral vessel NEC Z95.828
  stapes Z96.29
  teeth Z97.2
  tendon Z96.7
  tissue NEC Z96.89
  tooth root(s) Z96.5
  vessel NEC Z95.828
    coronary (artery) Z95.5
Request for expert evidence Z04.89
Reserve, decreased or low
  cardiac — *see* Disease, heart
  kidney N28.89
Residual — *see also* condition
  ovary syndrome N99.83
  state, schizophrenic F20.5
  urine R39.198
Resistance, resistant (to)
  activated protein C D68.51
  complicating pregnancy O26.89 ☑
  insulin E88.81
  organism(s)
    to
      drug Z16.30
        aminoglycosides Z16.29
        amoxicillin Z16.11
        ampicillin Z16.11
        antibiotic(s) Z16.20
          multiple Z16.24
          specified NEC Z16.29
        antifungal Z16.32
        antimicrobial (single) Z16.30
          multiple Z16.35
          specified NEC Z16.39
        antimycobacterial (single) Z16.341
          multiple Z16.342
        antiparasitic Z16.31
        antiviral Z16.33
        beta lactam antibiotics Z16.10
          specified NEC Z16.19
        cephalosporins Z16.19
        extended beta lactamase (ESBL) Z16.12
        fluoroquinolones Z16.23
        macrolides Z16.29
        methicillin — *see* MRSA
        multiple drugs (MDRO)
          antibiotics Z16.24
          antimicrobial Z16.35
          antimycobacterials Z16.342
        penicillins Z16.11
        quinine (and related compounds) Z16.31
        quinolones Z16.23
        sulfonamides Z16.29

Resistance, resistant — *continued*
  organism(s) — *continued*
    to — *continued*
      drug — *continued*
        tetracyclines Z16.29
        tuberculostatics (single) Z16.341
          multiple Z16.342
        vancomycin Z16.21
          related antibiotics Z16.22
  thyroid hormone E07.89
Resorption
  dental (roots) K03.3
    alveoli M26.79
  teeth (external) (internal) (pathological) (roots) K03.3
Respiration
  Cheyne-Stokes R06.3
  decreased due to shock, following injury T79.4 ☑
  disorder of, psychogenic F45.8
  insufficient, or poor R06.89
    newborn P28.5
  painful R07.1
  sighing, psychogenic F45.8
Respiratory — *see also* condition
  distress syndrome (newborn) (type I) P22.0
    type II P22.1
  syncytial virus, as cause of disease classified elsewhere
    — *see also* Virus, respiratory syncytial (RSV) B97.4
Respite care Z75.5
Response (drug)
  photoallergic L56.1
  phototoxic L56.0
Restenosis
  stent
    vascular
      end stent
        adjacent to stent — *see* Arteriosclerosis
        within the stent
          coronary T82.855 ☑
          peripheral T82.856 ☑
      in stent
        coronary vessel T82.855 ☑
        peripheral vessel T82.856 ☑
Restless legs (syndrome) G25.81
Restlessness R45.1
Restoration (of)
  dental
    aesthetically inadequate or displeasing K08.56
      defective K08.50
        specified NEC K08.59
    failure of marginal integrity K08.51
    failure of periodontal anatomical intergrity K08.54
    organ continuity from previous sterilization (tuboplas
      ty) (vasoplasty) Z31.0
      aftercare Z31.42
    tooth (existing)
      contours biologically incompatible with oral health
        K08.54
      open margins K08.51
      overhanging K08.52
      poor aesthetic K08.56
      poor gingival margins K08.51
    unsatisfactory, of tooth K08.50
      specified NEC K08.59
Restorative material (dental)
  allergy to K08.55
  fractured K08.539
    with loss of material K08.531
    without loss of material K08.530
  unrepairable overhanging of K08.52
Restriction of housing space Z59.1
Rests, ovarian, in fallopian tube Q50.6
Restzustand (schizophrenic) F20.5
Retained — *see also* Retention
  cholelithiasis following cholecystectomy K91.86
  foreign body fragments (type of) Z18.9
    acrylics Z18.2
    animal quill(s) or spines Z18.31
    cement Z18.83
    concrete Z18.83
    crystalline Z18.83
    depleted isotope Z18.09
    depleted uranium Z18.01
    diethylhexyl phthalates Z18.2
    glass Z18.81
    isocyanate Z18.2
    magnetic metal Z18.11
    metal Z18.10
    nonmagnectic metal Z18.12

☑ **Additional Character Required** — Refer to the Tabular List for Character Selection   ▽ Subterms under main terms may continue to next column or pag

Retained — *continued*
  foreign body fragments — *continued*
    nontherapeutic radioactive Z18.09
    organic NEC Z18.39
    plastic Z18.2
    quill(s) (animal) Z18.31
    radioactive (nontherapeutic) NEC Z18.09
    specified NEC Z18.89
    spine(s) (animal) Z18.31
    stone Z18.83
    tooth (teeth) Z18.32
    wood Z18.33
  fragments (type of) Z18.9
    acrylics Z18.2
    animal quill(s) or spines Z18.31
    cement Z18.83
    concrete Z18.83
    crystalline Z18.83
    depleted isotope Z18.09
    depleted uranium Z18.01
    diethylhexyl phthalates Z18.2
    glass Z18.81
    isocyanate Z18.2
    magnetic metal Z18.11
    metal Z18.10
    nonmagnectic metal Z18.12
    nontherapeutic radioactive Z18.09
    organic NEC Z18.39
    plastic Z18.2
    quill(s) (animal) Z18.31
    radioactive (nontherapeutic) NEC Z18.09
    specified NEC Z18.89
    spine(s) (animal) Z18.31
    stone Z18.83
    tooth (teeth) Z18.32
    wood Z18.33
  gallstones, following cholecystectomy K91.86
Retardation
  development, developmental, specific — *see* Disorder,
    developmental
  endochondral bone growth — *see* Disorder, bone, de-
    velopment or growth
  growth R62.50
    due to malnutrition E45
  mental — *see* Disability, intellectual
  motor function, specific F82
  physical (child) R62.52
    due to malnutrition E45
  reading (specific) F81.0
  spelling (specific) (without reading disorder) F81.81
Retching — *see* Vomiting
Retention — *see also* Retained
  bladder — *see* Retention, urine
  carbon dioxide E87.2
  cholelithiasis following cholecystectomy K91.86
  cyst — *see* Cyst
  dead
    fetus (at or near term) (mother) O36.4 ☑
      early fetal death O02.1
    ovum O02.0
  decidua (fragments) (following delivery) (with hemor-
    rhage) O72.2
    without hemorrhage O73.1
  deciduous tooth K00.6
  dental root K08.3
  fecal — *see* Constipation
  fetus
    dead O36.4 ☑
      early O02.1
  fluid R60.9
  foreign body — *see also* Foreign body, retained
    current trauma — *code as* Foreign body, by site or
      type
  gallstones, following cholecystectomy K91.86
  gastric K31.89
  intrauterine contraceptive device, in pregnancy — *see*
    Pregnancy, complicated by, retention, intrauter-
    ine device
  membranes (complicating delivery) (with hemorrhage)
    O72.2
    with abortion — *see* Abortion, by type
    without hemorrhage O73.1
  meniscus — *see* Derangement, meniscus
  menses N94.89
  milk (puerperal, postpartum) O92.79
  nitrogen, extrarenal R39.2
  ovary syndrome N99.83
  placenta (total) (with hemorrhage) O72.0

Retention — *continued*
  placenta — *continued*
    without hemorrhage O73.0
    portions or fragments (with hemorrhage) O72.2
      without hemorrhage O73.1
  products of conception
    early pregnancy (dead fetus) O02.1
    following
      delivery (with hemorrhage) O72.2
        without hemorrhage O73.1
    secundines (following delivery) (with hemorrhage)
      O72.0
      without hemorrhage O73.0
    complicating puerperium (delayed hemorrhage)
      O72.2
    partial O72.2
      without hemorrhage O73.1
  smegma, clitoris N90.89
  urine R33.9
    due to hyperplasia (hypertrophy) of prostate — *see*
      Hyperplasia, prostate
    drug-induced R33.0
    organic R33.8
      drug-induced R33.0
    psychogenic F45.8
    specified NEC R33.8
  water (in tissues) — *see* Edema
Reticulation, dust — *see* Pneumoconiosis
Reticulocytosis R70.1
Reticuloendotheliosis
  acute infantile C96.0
  leukemic C91.4- ☑
  nonlipid C96.0
Reticulohistiocytoma (giant-cell) D76.3
Reticuloid, actinic L57.1
Reticulosis (skin)
  acute of infancy C96.0
  hemophagocytic, familial D76.1
  histiocytic medullary C96.A (*following* C96.6)
  lipomelanotic I89.8
  malignant (midline) C86.0
  polymorphic C83.8- ☑
  Sézary — *see* Sézary disease
Retina, retinal — *see also* condition
  dark area D49.81
Retinitis — *see also* Inflammation, chorioretinal
  albuminurica N18.9 *[H32]*
  diabetic — *see* Diabetes, retinitis
  disciformis — *see* Degeneration, macula
  focal — *see* Inflammation, chorioretinal, focal
  gravidarum — *see* Pregnancy, complicated by, speci-
    fied pregnancy-related condition NEC
  juxtapapillaris — *see* Inflammation, chorioretinal, focal,
    juxtapapillary
  luetic — *see* Retinitis, syphilitic
  pigmentosa H35.52
  proliferans — *see* Disorder, globe, degenerative, spec-
    ified type NEC
  proliferating — *see* Disorder, globe, degenerative,
    specified type NEC
  renal N18.9 *[H32]*
  syphilitic (early) (secondary) A51.43
    central, recurrent A52.71
    congenital (early) A50.01 *[H32]*
    late A52.71
  tuberculous A18.53
Retinoblastoma C69.2- ☑
  differentiated C69.2- ☑
  undifferentiated C69.2- ☑
Retinochoroiditis — *see also* Inflammation, chorioretinal
  disseminated — *see* Inflammation, chorioretinal, dis-
    seminated
    syphilitic A52.71
  focal — *see* Inflammation, chorioretinal
  juxtapapillaris — *see* Inflammation, chorioretinal, focal,
    juxtapapillary
Retinopathy (background) H35.00
  arteriosclerotic I70.8 *[H35.0-]* ☑
  atherosclerotic I70.8 *[H35.0-]* ☑
  central serous — *see* Chorioretinopathy, central serous
  Coats H35.02- ☑
  diabetic — *see* Diabetes, retinopathy
  exudative H35.02- ☑
  hypertensive H35.03- ☑
  in (due to)
    diabetes — *see* Diabetes, retinopathy
    sickle-cell disorders D57.- ☑ *[H36]*

Retinopathy — *continued*
  of prematurity H35.10- ☑
    stage 0 H35.11- ☑
    stage 1 H35.12- ☑
    stage 2 H35.13- ☑
    stage 3 H35.14- ☑
    stage 4 H35.15- ☑
    stage 5 H35.16- ☑
  pigmentary, congenital — *see* Dystrophy, retina
  proliferative NEC H35.2- ☑
    diabetic — *see* Diabetes, retinopathy, proliferative
    sickle-cell D57.- ☑ *[H36]*
  solar H31.02- ☑
Retinoschisis H33.10- ☑
  congenital Q14.1
  specified type NEC H33.19- ☑
Retortamoniasis A07.8
Retractile testis Q55.22
Retraction
  cervix — *see* Retroversion, uterus
  drum (membrane) — *see* Disorder, tympanic mem-
    brane, specified NEC
  finger — *see* Deformity, finger
  lid H02.539
    left H02.536
      lower H02.535
      upper H02.534
    right H02.533
      lower H02.532
      upper H02.531
  lung J98.4
  mediastinum J98.59
  nipple N64.53
    associated with
      lactation O92.03
      pregnancy O92.01- ☑
      puerperium O92.02
    congenital Q83.8
  palmar fascia M72.0
  pleura — *see* Pleurisy
  ring, uterus (Bandl's) (pathological) O62.4
  sternum (congenital) Q76.7
    acquired M95.4
  uterus — *see* Retroversion, uterus
  valve (heart) — *see* Endocarditis
Retrobulbar — *see* condition
Retrocecal — *see* condition
Retrocession — *see* Retroversion
Retrodisplacement — *see* Retroversion
Retroflection, retroflexion — *see* Retroversion
Retrognathia, retrognathism (mandibular) (maxillary)
  M26.19
Retrograde menstruation N92.5
Retroperineal — *see* condition
Retroperitoneal — *see* condition
Retroperitonitis K68.9
Retropharyngeal — *see* condition
Retroplacental — *see* condition
Retroposition — *see* Retroversion
Retroprosthetic membrane T85.398 ☑
Retrosternal thyroid (congenital) Q89.2
Retroversion, retroverted
  cervix — *see* Retroversion, uterus
  female NEC — *see* Retroversion, uterus
  iris H21.89
  testis (congenital) Q55.29
  uterus (acquired) (acute) (any degree) (asymptomatic)
    (cervix) (postinfectional) (postpartal, old) N85.4
    congenital Q51.818
    in pregnancy O34.53- ☑
Retrovirus, as cause of disease classified elsewhere
  B97.30
  human
    immunodeficiency, type 2 (HIV 2) B97.35
    T-cell lymphotropic
      type I (HTLV-I) B97.33
      type II (HTLV-II) B97.34
  lentivirus B97.31
  oncovirus B97.32
  specified NEC B97.39
Retrusion, premaxilla (developmental) M26.09
Rett's disease or syndrome F84.2
Reverse peristalsis R19.2
Reye's syndrome G93.7
Rh (factor)
  hemolytic disease (newborn) P55.0

▽ Subterms under main terms may continue to next column or page   ☑ **Additional Character Required** — Refer to the Tabular List for Character Selection   275

Retained — Rh

Rh — *continued*
incompatibility, immunization or sensitization
affecting management of pregnancy NEC O36.09- ☑
anti-D antibody O36.01- ☑
newborn P55.0
transfusion reaction — *see* Complication(s), transfusion, incompatibility reaction, Rh (factor)
negative mother affecting newborn P55.0
titer elevated — *see* Complication(s), transfusion, incompatibility reaction, Rh (factor)
transfusion reaction — *see* Complication(s), transfusion, incompatibility reaction, Rh (factor)

Rhabdomyolysis (idiopathic) NEC M62.82
traumatic T79.6 ☑

Rhabdomyoma — *see also* Neoplasm, connective tissue, benign
adult — *see* Neoplasm, connective tissue, benign
fetal — *see* Neoplasm, connective tissue, benign
glycogenic — *see* Neoplasm, connective tissue, benign

Rhabdomyosarcoma (any type) — *see* Neoplasm, connective tissue, malignant

Rhabdosarcoma — *see* Rhabdomyosarcoma

Rhesus (factor) **incompatibility** — *see* Rh, incompatibility

Rheumatic (acute) (subacute)
adherent pericardium I09.2
chronic I09.89
coronary arteritis I01.8
degeneration, myocardium I09.0
fever (acute) — *see* Fever, rheumatic
heart — *see* Disease, heart, rheumatic
myocardial degeneration — *see* Degeneration, myocardium
myocarditis (chronic) (inactive) (with chorea) I09.0
active or acute I01.2
with chorea (acute) (rheumatic) (Sydenham's) I02.0
pancarditis, acute I01.8
with chorea (acute (rheumatic) Sydenham's) I02.0
pericarditis (active) (acute) (with effusion) (with pneumonia) I01.0
with chorea (acute) (rheumatic) (Sydenham's) I02.0
chronic or inactive I09.2
pneumonia I00 *[J17]*
torticollis M43.6
typhoid fever A01.09

Rheumatism (articular) (neuralgic) (nonarticular) M79.0
gout — *see* Arthritis, rheumatoid
intercostal, meaning Tietze's disease M94.0
palindromic (any site) M12.30
ankle M12.37- ☑
elbow M12.32- ☑
foot joint M12.37- ☑
hand joint M12.34- ☑
hip M12.35- ☑
knee M12.36- ☑
multiple site M12.39
shoulder M12.31- ☑
specified joint NEC M12.38
vertebrae M12.38
wrist M12.33- ☑
sciatic M54.4- ☑

Rheumatoid — *see also* condition
arthritis — *see also* Arthritis, rheumatoid
with involvement of organs NEC M05.60
ankle M05.67- ☑
elbow M05.62- ☑
foot joint M05.67- ☑
hand joint M05.64- ☑
hip M05.65- ☑
knee M05.66- ☑
multiple site M05.69
shoulder M05.61- ☑
vertebra — *see* Spondylitis, ankylosing
wrist M05.63- ☑
seronegative — *see* Arthritis, rheumatoid, seronegative
seropositive — *see* Arthritis, rheumatoid, seropositive
carditis M05.30
ankle M05.37- ☑
elbow M05.32- ☑
foot joint M05.37- ☑
hand joint M05.34- ☑
hip M05.35- ☑
knee M05.36- ☑
multiple site M05.39
shoulder M05.31- ☑

Rheumatoid — *continued*
carditis — *continued*
vertebra — *see* Spondylitis, ankylosing
wrist M05.33- ☑
endocarditis — *see* Rheumatoid, carditis
lung (disease) M05.10
ankle M05.17- ☑
elbow M05.12- ☑
foot joint M05.17- ☑
hand joint M05.14- ☑
hip M05.15- ☑
knee M05.16- ☑
multiple site M05.19
shoulder M05.11- ☑
vertebra — *see* Spondylitis, ankylosing
wrist M05.13- ☑
myocarditis — *see* Rheumatoid, carditis
myopathy M05.40
ankle M05.47- ☑
elbow M05.42- ☑
foot joint M05.47- ☑
hand joint M05.44- ☑
hip M05.45- ☑
knee M05.46- ☑
multiple site M05.49
shoulder M05.41- ☑
vertebra — *see* Spondylitis, ankylosing
wrist M05.43- ☑
pericarditis — *see* Rheumatoid, carditis
polyarthritis — *see* Arthritis, rheumatoid
polyneuropathy M05.50
ankle M05.57- ☑
elbow M05.52- ☑
foot joint M05.57- ☑
hand joint M05.54- ☑
hip M05.55- ☑
knee M05.56- ☑
multiple site M05.59
shoulder M05.51- ☑
vertebra — *see* Spondylitis, ankylosing
wrist M05.53- ☑
vasculitis M05.20
ankle M05.27- ☑
elbow M05.22- ☑
foot joint M05.27- ☑
hand joint M05.24- ☑
hip M05.25- ☑
knee M05.26- ☑
multiple site M05.29
shoulder M05.21- ☑
vertebra — *see* Spondylitis, ankylosing
wrist M05.23- ☑

Rhinitis (atrophic) (catarrhal) (chronic) (croupous) (fibrinous) (granulomatous) (hyperplastic) (hypertrophic) (membranous) (obstructive) (purulent) (suppurative) (ulcerative) J31.0
with
sore throat — *see* Nasopharyngitis
acute J00
allergic J30.9
with asthma J45.909
with
exacerbation (acute) J45.901
status asthmaticus J45.902
due to
food J30.5
pollen J30.1
nonseasonal J30.89
perennial J30.89
seasonal NEC J30.2
specified NEC J30.89
infective J00
pneumococcal J00
syphilitic A52.73
congenital A50.05 *[J99]*
tuberculous A15.8
vasomotor J30.0

Rhinoantritis (chronic) — *see* Sinusitis, maxillary

Rhinodacryolith — *see* Dacryolith

Rhinolith (nasal sinus) J34.89

Rhinomegaly J34.89

Rhinopharyngitis (acute) (subacute) — *see also* Nasopharyngitis
chronic J31.1
destructive ulcerating A66.5
mutilans A66.5

Rhinophyma L71.1

Rhinorrhea J34.89
cerebrospinal (fluid) G96.0
paroxysmal — *see* Rhinitis, allergic
spasmodic — *see* Rhinitis, allergic

Rhinosalpingitis — *see* Salpingitis, eustachian

Rhinoscleroma A48.8

Rhinosporidiosis B48.1

Rhinovirus infection NEC B34.8

Rhizomelic chondrodysplasia punctata E71.540

Rhythm
atrioventricular nodal I49.8
disorder I49.9
coronary sinus I49.8
ectopic I49.8
nodal I49.8
escape I49.9
heart, abnormal I49.9
idioventricular I44.2
nodal I49.8
sleep, inversion G47.2- ☑
nonorganic origin — *see* Disorder, sleep, circadian rhythm, psychogenic

Rhytidosis facialis L98.8

Rib — *see also* condition
cervical Q76.5

Riboflavin deficiency E53.0

Rice bodies — *see also* Loose, body, joint
knee M23.4- ☑

Richter syndrome — *see* Leukemia, chronic lymphocytic, B-cell type

Richter's hernia — *see* Hernia, abdomen, with obstruction

Ricinism — *see* Poisoning, food, noxious, plant

Rickets (active) (acute) (adolescent) (chest wall) (congenital) (current) (infantile) (intestinal) E55.0
adult — *see* Osteomalacia
celiac K90.0
hypophosphatemic with nephrotic-glycosuric dwarfism E72.09
inactive E64.3
kidney N25.0
renal N25.0
sequelae, any E64.3
vitamin-D-resistant E83.31 *[M90.80]*

Rickettsial disease A79.9
specified type NEC A79.89

Rickettsialpox (Rickettsia akari) A79.1

Rickettsiosis A79.9
due to
Ehrlichia sennetsu A79.81
Rickettsia akari (rickettsialpox) A79.1
specified type NEC A79.89
tick-borne A77.9
vesicular A79.1

Rider's bone — *see* Ossification, muscle, specified NEC

Ridge, alveolus — *see also* condition
flabby K06.8

Ridged ear, congenital Q17.3

Riedel's
lobe, liver Q44.7
struma, thyroiditis or disease E06.5

Rieger's anomaly or syndrome Q13.81

Riehl's melanosis L81.4

Rietti-Greppi-Micheli anemia D56.9

Rieux's hernia — *see* Hernia, abdomen, specified site NEC

Riga (-Fede) **disease** K14.0

Riggs' disease — *see* Periodontitis

Right aortic arch Q25.47

Right middle lobe syndrome J98.11

Rigid, rigidity — *see also* condition
abdominal R19.30
with severe abdominal pain R10.0
epigastric R19.36
generalized R19.37
left lower quadrant R19.34
left upper quadrant R19.32
periumbilic R19.35
right lower quadrant R19.33
right upper quadrant R19.31
articular, multiple, congenital Q68.8
cervix (uteri) in pregnancy — *see* Pregnancy, complicated by, abnormal, cervix
hymen (acquired) (congenital) N89.6
nuchal R29.1
pelvic floor in pregnancy — *see* Pregnancy, complicated by, abnormal, pelvic organs or tissues NEC

Rigid, rigidity — *continued*
  perineum or vulva in pregnancy — *see* Pregnancy, complicated by, abnormal, vulva
  spine — *see* Dorsopathy, specified NEC
  vagina in pregnancy — *see* Pregnancy, complicated by, abnormal, vagina
Rigors R68.89
  with fever R50.9
Riley-Day syndrome G90.1
RIND (reversible ischemic neurologic deficit) I63.9
Ring(s)
  aorta (vascular) Q25.45
  Bandl's O62.4
  contraction, complicating delivery O62.4
  esophageal, lower (muscular) K22.2
  Fleischer's (cornea) H18.04- ☑
  hymenal, tight (acquired) (congenital) N89.6
  Kayser-Fleischer (cornea) H18.04- ☑
  retraction, uterus, pathological O62.4
  Schatzki's (esophagus) (lower) K22.2
    congenital Q39.3
  Soemmerring's — *see* Cataract, secondary
  vascular (congenital) Q25.8
    aorta Q25.45
Ringed hair (congenital) Q84.1
Ringworm B35.9
  beard B35.0
  black dot B35.0
  body B35.4
  Burmese B35.5
  corporeal B35.4
  foot B35.3
  groin B35.6
  hand B35.2
  honeycomb B35.0
  nails B35.1
  perianal (area) B35.6
  scalp B35.0
  specified NEC B35.8
  Tokelau B35.5
Rise, venous pressure I87.8
Rising, PSA following treatment for malignant neoplasm of prostate R97.21
Risk
  for
    dental caries Z91.849
      high Z91.843
      low Z91.841
      moderate Z91.842
  suicidal
    meaning personal history of attempted suicide Z91.5
    meaning suicidal ideation — *see* Ideation, suicidal
Ritter's disease L00
Rivalry, sibling Z62.891
Rivalta's disease A42.2
River blindness B73.01
Robert's pelvis Q74.2
  with disproportion (fetopelvic) O33.0
    causing obstructed labor O65.0
Robin (-Pierre) **syndrome** Q87.0
Robinow-Silvermann-Smith syndrome Q87.19
Robinson's (hidrotic) **ectodermal dysplasia or syndrome** Q82.4
Robles' disease B73.01
Rocky Mountain (spotted) **fever** A77.0
Roetheln — *see* Rubella
Roger's disease Q21.0
Rokitansky-Aschoff sinuses (gallbladder) K82.8
Rolando's fracture (displaced) S62.22- ☑
  nondisplaced S62.22- ☑
Romano-Ward (prolonged QT interval) **syndrome** I45.81
Romberg's disease or syndrome G51.8
Roof, mouth — *see* condition
Rosacea L71.9
  acne L71.9
  keratitis L71.8
  specified NEC L71.8
Rosary, rachitic E55.0
Rose
  cold J30.1
  fever J30.1
  rash R21
    epidemic B06.9
Rosenbach's erysipeloid A26.0
Rosenthal's disease or syndrome D68.1
Roseola B09
  infantum B08.20

Roseola — *continued*
  infantum — *continued*
    due to human herpesvirus 6 B08.21
    due to human herpesvirus 7 B08.22
Ross River disease or fever B33.1
Rossbach's disease K31.89
  psychogenic F45.8
Rostan's asthma (cardiac) — *see* Failure, ventricular, left
Rotation
  anomalous, incomplete or insufficient, intestine Q43.3
  cecum (congenital) Q43.3
  colon (congenital) Q43.3
  spine, incomplete or insufficient — *see* Dorsopathy, deforming, specified NEC
  tooth, teeth, fully erupted M26.35
  vertebra, incomplete or insufficient — *see* Dorsopathy, deforming, specified NEC
Rotes Quérol disease or syndrome — *see* Hyperostosis, ankylosing
Roth (-Bernhardt) **disease or syndrome** — *see* Meralgia paraesthetica
Rothmund (-Thomson) **syndrome** Q82.8
Rotor's disease or syndrome E80.6
Round
  back (with wedging of vertebrae) — *see* Kyphosis
    sequelae (late effect) of rickets E64.3
  worms (large) (infestation) NEC B82.0
    Ascariasis — *see also* Ascariasis B77.9
Roussy-Lévy syndrome G60.0
Rubella (German measles) B06.9
  complication NEC B06.09
    neurological B06.00
  congenital P35.0
  contact Z20.4
  exposure to Z20.4
  maternal
    care for (suspected) damage to fetus O35.3 ☑
    manifest rubella in infant P35.0
    suspected damage to fetus affecting management of pregnancy O35.3 ☑
  specified complications NEC B06.09
Rubeola (meaning measles) — *see* Measles
  meaning rubella — *see* Rubella
Rubeosis, iris — *see* Disorder, iris, vascular
Rubinstein-Taybi syndrome Q87.2
Rudimentary (congenital) — *see also* Agenesis
  arm — *see* Defect, reduction, upper limb
  bone Q79.9
  cervix uteri Q51.828
  eye Q11.2
  lobule of ear Q17.3
  patella Q74.1
  respiratory organs in thoracopagus Q89.4
  tracheal bronchus Q32.4
  uterus Q51.818
    in male Q56.1
  vagina Q52.0
Ruled out condition — *see* Observation, suspected
Rumination R11.10
  with nausea R11.2
  disorder of infancy F98.21
  neurotic F42.8
  newborn P92.1
  obsessional F42.8
  psychogenic F42.8
Runeberg's disease D51.0
Runny nose R09.89
Rupia (syphilitic) A51.39
  congenital A50.06
  tertiary A52.79
Rupture, ruptured
  abscess (spontaneous) — *code by* site under Abscess
  aneurysm — *see* Aneurysm
  anus (sphincter) — *see* Laceration, anus
  aorta, aortic I71.8
    abdominal I71.3
    arch I71.1
    ascending I71.1
    descending I71.8
      abdominal I71.3
      thoracic I71.1
    syphilitic A52.01
    thoracoabdominal I71.5
    thorax, thoracic I71.1
    transverse I71.1
    traumatic — *see* Injury, aorta, laceration, major
  valve or cusp — *see also* Endocarditis, aortic I35.8

Rupture, ruptured — *continued*
  appendix (with peritonitis) — *see also* Appendicitis K35.32
    with localized peritonitis — *see also* Appendicitis K35.32
  arteriovenous fistula, brain — *see* Fistula, arteriovenous, brain, ruptured
  artery I77.2
    brain — *see* Hemorrhage, intracranial, intracerebral
    coronary — *see* Infarct, myocardium
    heart — *see* Infarct, myocardium
    pulmonary I28.8
    traumatic (complication) — *see* Injury, blood vessel
  bile duct (common) (hepatic) K83.2
    cystic K82.8
  bladder (sphincter) (nontraumatic) (spontaneous) N32.89
    following ectopic or molar pregnancy O08.6
    obstetrical trauma O71.5
    traumatic S37.29 ☑
  blood vessel — *see also* Hemorrhage
    brain — *see* Hemorrhage, intracranial, intracerebral
    heart — *see* Infarct, myocardium
    traumatic (complication) — *see* Injury, blood vessel, laceration, major, by site
  bone — *see* Fracture
  bowel (nontraumatic) K63.1
  brain
    aneurysm (congenital) — *see also* Hemorrhage, intracranial, subarachnoid
      syphilitic A52.05
    hemorrhagic — *see* Hemorrhage, intracranial, intracerebral
  capillaries I78.8
  cardiac (auricle) (ventricle) (wall) I23.3
    with hemopericardium I23.0
    infectional I40.9
    traumatic — *see* Injury, heart
  cartilage (articular) (current) — *see also* Sprain
    knee S83.3- ☑
    semilunar — *see* Tear, meniscus
  cecum (with peritonitis) K65.0
    with peritoneal abscess K35.33
    traumatic S36.598 ☑
  celiac artery, traumatic — *see* Injury, blood vessel, celiac artery, laceration, major
  cerebral aneurysm (congenital) (see Hemorrhage, intracranial, subarachnoid)
  cervix (uteri)
    with ectopic or molar pregnancy O08.6
    following ectopic or molar pregnancy O08.6
    obstetrical trauma O71.3
    traumatic S37.69 ☑
  chordae tendineae NEC I51.1
    concurrent with acute myocardial infarction — *see* Infarct, myocardium
    following acute myocardial infarction (current complication) I23.4
  choroid (direct) (indirect) (traumatic) H31.32- ☑
  circle of Willis I60.6
  colon (nontraumatic) K63.1
    traumatic — *see* Injury, intestine, large
  cornea (traumatic) — *see* Injury, eye, laceration
  coronary (artery) (thrombotic) — *see* Infarct, myocardium
  corpus luteum (infected) (ovary) N83.1- ☑
  cyst — *see* Cyst
  cystic duct K82.2
  Descemet's membrane — *see* Change, corneal membrane, Descemet's, rupture
    traumatic — *see* Injury, eye, laceration
  diaphragm, traumatic — *see* Injury, intrathoracic, diaphragm
  disc — *see* Rupture, intervertebral disc
  diverticulum (intestine) K57.80
    with bleeding K57.81
    bladder N32.3
    large intestine K57.20
      with
        bleeding K57.21
        small intestine K57.40
          with bleeding K57.41
    small intestine K57.00
      with
        bleeding K57.01
        large intestine K57.40
          with bleeding K57.41
  duodenal stump K31.89

Rupture, ruptured — *continued*
  ear drum (nontraumatic) — *see also* Perforation, tympanum
    traumatic S09.2- ☑
      due to blast injury — *see* Injury, blast, ear
  esophagus K22.3
  eye (without prolapse or loss of intraocular tissue) — *see* Injury, eye, laceration
  fallopian tube NEC (nonobstetric) (nontraumatic) N83.8
    due to pregnancy O00.10- ☑
      with intrauterine pregnancy O00.11- ☑
  fontanel P13.1
  gallbladder K82.2
    traumatic S36.128 ☑
  gastric — *see also* Rupture, stomach
    vessel K92.2
  globe (eye) (traumatic) — *see* Injury, eye, laceration
  graafian follicle (hematoma) N83.0- ☑
  heart — *see* Rupture, cardiac
  hymen (nontraumatic) (nonintentional) N89.8
  internal organ, traumatic — *see* Injury, by site
  intervertebral disc — *see* Displacement, intervertebral disc
    traumatic — *see* Rupture, traumatic, intervertebral disc
  intestine NEC (nontraumatic) K63.1
    traumatic — *see* Injury, intestine
  iris — *see also* Abnormality, pupillary
    traumatic — *see* Injury, eye, laceration
  joint capsule, traumatic — *see* Sprain
  kidney (traumatic) S37.06- ☑
    birth injury P15.8
    nontraumatic N28.89
  lacrimal duct (traumatic) — *see* Injury, eye, specified site NEC
  lens (cataract) (traumatic) — *see* Cataract, traumatic
  ligament, traumatic — *see* Rupture, traumatic, ligament, by site
  liver S36.116 ☑
    birth injury P15.0
  lymphatic vessel I89.8
  marginal sinus (placental) (with hemorrhage) — *see* Hemorrhage, antepartum, specified cause NEC
  membrana tympani (nontraumatic) — *see* Perforation, tympanum
  membranes (spontaneous)
    artificial
      delayed delivery following O75.5
    delayed delivery following — *see* Pregnancy, complicated by, premature rupture of membranes
  meningeal artery I60.8
  meniscus (knee) — *see also* Tear, meniscus
    old — *see* Derangement, meniscus
    site other than knee — *code as* Sprain
  mesenteric artery, traumatic — *see* Injury, mesenteric, artery, laceration, major
  mesentery (nontraumatic) K66.8
    traumatic — *see* Injury, intra-abdominal, specified, site NEC
  mitral (valve) I34.8
  muscle (traumatic) — *see also* Strain
    diastasis — *see* Diastasis, muscle
    nontraumatic M62.10
      ankle M62.17- ☑
      foot M62.17- ☑
      forearm M62.13- ☑
      hand M62.14- ☑
      lower leg M62.16- ☑
      pelvic region M62.15- ☑
      shoulder region M62.11- ☑
      specified site NEC M62.18
      thigh M62.15- ☑
      upper arm M62.12- ☑
    traumatic — *see* Strain, by site
  musculotendinous junction NEC, nontraumatic — *see* Rupture, tendon, spontaneous
  mycotic aneurysm causing cerebral hemorrhage — *see* Hemorrhage, intracranial, subarachnoid
  myocardium, myocardial — *see* Rupture, cardiac
    traumatic — *see* Injury, heart
  nontraumatic, meaning hernia — *see* Hernia
  obstructed — *see* Hernia, by site, obstructed
  operation wound — *see* Disruption, wound, operation
  ovary, ovarian N83.8
    corpus luteum cyst N83.1- ☑
    follicle (graafian) N83.0- ☑
  oviduct (nonobstetric) (nontraumatic) N83.8

Rupture, ruptured — *continued*
  oviduct — *continued*
    due to pregnancy O00.10- ☑
      with intrauterine pregnancy O00.11- ☑
  pancreas (nontraumatic) K86.89
    traumatic S36.299 ☑
  papillary muscle NEC I51.2
    following acute myocardial infarction (current complication) I23.5
  pelvic
    floor, complicating delivery O70.1
    organ NEC, obstetrical trauma O71.5
  perineum (nonobstetric) (nontraumatic) N90.89
    complicating delivery — *see* Delivery, complicated, by, laceration, anus (sphincter)
  postoperative wound — *see* Disruption, wound, operation
  prostate (traumatic) S37.828 ☑
  pulmonary
    artery I28.8
    valve (heart) I37.8
    vein I28.8
    vessel I28.8
  pus tube — *see* Salpingitis
  pyosalpinx — *see* Salpingitis
  rectum (nontraumatic) K63.1
    traumatic S36.69 ☑
  retina, retinal (traumatic) (without detachment) — *see also* Break, retina
    with detachment — *see* Detachment, retina, with retinal, break
  rotator cuff (nontraumatic) M75.10- ☑
    complete M75.12- ☑
    incomplete M75.11- ☑
  sclera — *see* Injury, eye, laceration
  sigmoid (nontraumatic) K63.1
    traumatic S36.593 ☑
  spinal cord — *see also* Injury, spinal cord, by region
    due to injury at birth P11.5
    newborn (birth injury) P11.5
  spleen (traumatic) S36.09 ☑
    birth injury P15.1
    congenital (birth injury) P15.1
    due to P. vivax malaria B51.0
    nontraumatic D73.5
    spontaneous D73.5
  splenic vein R58
    traumatic — *see* Injury, blood vessel, splenic vein
  stomach (nontraumatic) (spontaneous) K31.89
    traumatic S36.39 ☑
  supraspinatus (complete) (incomplete) (nontraumatic) — *see* Tear, rotator cuff
  symphysis pubis
    obstetric O71.6
    traumatic S33.4 ☑
  synovium (cyst) M66.10
    ankle M66.17- ☑
    elbow M66.12- ☑
    finger M66.14- ☑
    foot M66.17- ☑
    forearm M66.13- ☑
    hand M66.14- ☑
    pelvic region M66.15- ☑
    shoulder region M66.11- ☑
    specified site NEC M66.18
    thigh M66.15- ☑
    toe M66.17- ☑
    upper arm M66.12- ☑
    wrist M66.13- ☑
  tendon (traumatic) — *see* Strain
    nontraumatic (spontaneous) M66.9
      ankle M66.87- ☑
      extensor M66.20
        ankle M66.27- ☑
        foot M66.27- ☑
        forearm M66.23- ☑
        hand M66.24- ☑
        lower leg M66.26- ☑
        multiple sites M66.29
        pelvic region M66.25- ☑
        shoulder region M66.21- ☑
        specified site NEC M66.28
        thigh M66.25- ☑
        upper arm M66.22- ☑
      flexor M66.30
        ankle M66.37- ☑
        foot M66.37- ☑

Rupture, ruptured — *continued*
  tendon — *see* Strain — *continued*
    nontraumatic — *continued*
      flexor — *continued*
        forearm M66.33- ☑
        hand M66.34- ☑
        lower leg M66.36- ☑
        multiple sites M66.39
        pelvic region M66.35- ☑
        shoulder region M66.31- ☑
        specified site NEC M66.38
        thigh M66.35- ☑
        upper arm M66.32- ☑
      foot M66.87- ☑
      forearm M66.83- ☑
      hand M66.84- ☑
      lower leg M66.86- ☑
      multiple sites M66.89
      pelvic region M66.85- ☑
      shoulder region M66.81- ☑
      specified
        site NEC M66.88
        tendon M66.80
      thigh M66.85- ☑
      upper arm M66.82- ☑
  thoracic duct I89.8
  tonsil J35.8
  traumatic
    aorta — *see* Injury, aorta, laceration, major
    diaphragm — *see* Injury, intrathoracic, diaphragm
    external site — *see* Wound, open, by site
    eye — *see* Injury, eye, laceration
    internal organ — *see* Injury, by site
    intervertebral disc
      cervical S13.0 ☑
      lumbar S33.0 ☑
      thoracic S23.0 ☑
    kidney S37.06- ☑
    ligament — *see also* Sprain
      ankle — *see* Sprain, ankle
      carpus — *see* Rupture, traumatic, ligament, wrist
      collateral (hand) — *see* Rupture, traumatic, ligament, finger, collateral
      finger (metacarpophalangeal) (interphalangeal) S63.40- ☑
        collateral S63.41- ☑
          index S63.41- ☑
          little S63.41- ☑
          middle S63.41- ☑
          ring S63.41- ☑
        index S63.40- ☑
        little S63.40- ☑
        middle S63.40- ☑
        palmar S63.42- ☑
          index S63.42- ☑
          little S63.42- ☑
          middle S63.42- ☑
          ring S63.42- ☑
        ring S63.40- ☑
        specified site NEC S63.499 ☑
          index S63.49- ☑
          little S63.49- ☑
          middle S63.49- ☑
          ring S63.49- ☑
        volar plate S63.43- ☑
          index S63.43- ☑
          little S63.43- ☑
          middle S63.43- ☑
          ring S63.43- ☑
      foot — *see* Sprain, foot
      radial collateral S53.2- ☑
      radiocarpal — *see* Rupture, traumatic, ligament, wrist, radiocarpal
      ulnar collateral S53.3- ☑
      ulnocarpal — *see* Rupture, traumatic, ligament, wrist, ulnocarpal
      wrist S63.30- ☑
        collateral S63.31- ☑
        radiocarpal S63.32- ☑
        specified site NEC S63.39- ☑
        ulnocarpal (palmar) S63.33- ☑
    liver S36.116 ☑
    membrana tympani — *see* Rupture, ear drum, traumatic
    muscle or tendon — *see* Strain
    myocardium — *see* Injury, heart

☑ **Additional Character Required** — **Refer to the Tabular List for Character Selection** ▽ **Subterms under main terms may continue to next column or page**

Rupture, ruptured — *continued*
  traumatic — *continued*
    pancreas S36.299 ☑
    rectum S36.69 ☑
    sigmoid S36.593 ☑
    spleen S36.09 ☑
    stomach S36.39 ☑
    symphysis pubis S33.4 ☑
    tympanum, tympanic (membrane) — *see* Rupture, ear drum, traumatic
    ureter S37.19 ☑
    uterus S37.69 ☑
    vagina — *see* Injury, vagina
    vena cava — *see* Injury, vena cava, laceration, major
  tricuspid (heart) (valve) I07.8
  tube, tubal (nonobstetric) (nontraumatic) N83.8
    abscess — *see* Salpingitis
    due to pregnancy O00.10- ☑
      with intrauterine pregnancy O00.11- ☑
  tympanum, tympanic (membrane) (nontraumatic) — *see also* Perforation, tympanic membrane H72.9- ☑
    traumatic — *see* Rupture, ear drum, traumatic
  umbilical cord, complicating delivery O69.89 ☑
  ureter (traumatic) S37.19 ☑
    nontraumatic N28.89
  urethra (nontraumatic) N36.8
    with ectopic or molar pregnancy O08.6
    following ectopic or molar pregnancy O08.6
    obstetrical trauma O71.5
    traumatic S37.39 ☑
  uterosacral ligament (nonobstetric) (nontraumatic) N83.8
  uterus (traumatic) S37.69 ☑
    before labor O71.0- ☑
    during or after labor O71.1
    nonpuerperal, nontraumatic N85.8
    pregnant (during labor) O71.1
      before labor O71.0- ☑
  vagina — *see* Injury, vagina
  valve, valvular (heart) — *see* Endocarditis
  varicose vein — *see* Varix
  varix — *see* Varix
  vena cava R58
    traumatic — *see* Injury, vena cava, laceration, major
  vesical (urinary) N32.89
  vessel (blood) R58
    pulmonary I28.8
    traumatic — *see* Injury, blood vessel
  viscus R19.8
  vulva complicating delivery O70.0
Russell-Silver syndrome Q87.19
Russian spring-summer type encephalitis A84.0
Rust's disease (tuberculous cervical spondylitis) A18.01
Ruvalcaba-Myhre-Smith syndrome E71.440
Rytand-Lipsitch syndrome I44.2

S

Saber, sabre shin or tibia (syphilitic) A50.56 *[M90.8-]* ☑
Sac lacrimal — *see* condition
Saccharomyces infection B37.9
Saccharopinuria E72.3
Saccular — *see* condition
Sacculation
  aorta (nonsyphilitic) — *see* Aneurysm, aorta
  bladder N32.3
  intralaryngeal (congenital) (ventricular) Q31.3
  larynx (congenital) (ventricular) Q31.3
  organ or site, congenital — *see* Distortion
  pregnant uterus — *see* Pregnancy, complicated by, abnormal, uterus
  ureter N28.89
  urethra N36.1
  vesical N32.3
Sachs' amaurotic familial idiocy or disease E75.02
Sachs-Tay disease E75.02
Sacks-Libman disease M32.11
Sacralgia M53.3
Sacralization Q76.49
Sacrodynia M53.3
Sacroiliac joint — *see* condition
Sacroiliitis NEC M46.1
Sacrum — *see* condition
Saddle
  back — *see* Lordosis

Saddle — *continued*
  embolus
    abdominal aorta I74.01
    pulmonary artery I26.92
      with acute cor pulmonale I26.02
  injury — *code to* condition
  nose M95.0
    due to syphilis A50.57
Sadism (sexual) F65.52
Sadness, postpartal O90.6
Sadomasochism F65.50
Saemisch's ulcer (cornea) — *see* Ulcer, cornea, central
Sagging
  skin and subcutaneous tissue (following bariatric surgery weight loss) (following dietary weight loss) L98.7
Sahib disease B55.0
Sailors' skin L57.8
Saint
  Anthony's fire — *see* Erysipelas
  triad — *see* Hernia, diaphragm
  Vitus' dance — *see* Chorea, Sydenham's
Salaam
  attack(s) — *see* Epilepsy, spasms
  tic R25.8
Salicylism
  abuse F55.8
  overdose or wrong substance given — *see* Table of Drugs and Chemicals, by drug, poisoning
Salivary duct or gland — *see* condition
Salivation, excessive K11.7
Salmonella — *see* Infection, Salmonella
Salmonellosis A02.0
Salpingitis (catarrhal) (fallopian tube) (nodular) (pseudofollicular) (purulent) (septic) N70.91
  with oophoritis N70.93
  acute N70.01
    with oophoritis N70.03
  chlamydial A56.11
  chronic N70.11
    with oophoritis N70.13
  complicating abortion — *see* Abortion, by type, complicated by, salpingitis
  ear — *see* Salpingitis, eustachian
  eustachian (tube) H68.00- ☑
    acute H68.01- ☑
    chronic H68.02- ☑
  follicularis N70.11
    with oophoritis N70.13
  gonococcal (acute) (chronic) A54.24
  interstitial, chronic N70.11
    with oophoritis N70.13
  isthmica nodosa N70.11
    with oophoritis N70.13
  specific (gonococcal) (acute) (chronic) A54.24
  tuberculous (acute) (chronic) A18.17
  venereal (gonococcal) (acute) (chronic) A54.24
Salpingocele N83.4- ☑
Salpingo-oophoritis (catarrhal) (purulent) (ruptured) (septic) (suppurative) N70.93
  acute N70.03
    with ectopic or molar pregnancy O08.0
    following ectopic or molar pregnancy O08.0
    gonococcal A54.24
  chronic N70.13
  following ectopic or molar pregnancy O08.0
  gonococcal (acute) (chronic) A54.24
  puerperal O86.19
  specific (gonococcal) (acute) (chronic) A54.24
  subacute N70.03
  tuberculous (acute) (chronic) A18.17
  venereal (gonococcal) (acute) (chronic) A54.24
Salpingo-ovaritis — *see* Salpingo-oophoritis
Salpingoperitonitis — *see* Salpingo-oophoritis
Salzmann's nodular dystrophy — *see* Degeneration, cornea, nodular
Sampson's cyst or tumor N80.1
San Joaquin (Valley) **fever** B38.0
Sandblaster's asthma, lung or pneumoconiosis J62.8
Sander's disease (paranoia) F22
Sandfly fever A93.1
Sandhoff's disease E75.01
Sanfilippo (Type B) (Type C) (Type D) **syndrome** E76.22
Sanger-Brown ataxia G11.2
Sao Paulo fever or typhus A77.0
Saponification, mesenteric K65.8

Sarcocele (benign)
  syphilitic A52.76
    congenital A50.59
Sarcocystosis A07.8
Sarcoepiplocele — *see* Hernia
Sarcoepiplomphalocele Q79.2
Sarcoid — *see also* Sarcoidosis
  arthropathy D86.86
  Boeck's D86.9
  Darier-Roussy D86.3
  iridocyclitis D86.83
  meningitis D86.81
  myocarditis D86.85
  myositis D86.87
  pyelonephritis D86.84
  Spiegler-Fendt L08.89
Sarcoidosis D86.9
  with
    cranial nerve palsies D86.82
    hepatic granuloma D86.89
    polyarthritis D86.86
    tubulo-interstitial nephropathy D86.84
  combined sites NEC D86.89
  lung D86.0
    and lymph nodes D86.2
  lymph nodes D86.1
    and lung D86.2
  meninges D86.81
  skin D86.3
  specified type NEC D86.89
Sarcoma (of) — *see also* Neoplasm, connective tissue, malignant
  alveolar soft part — *see* Neoplasm, connective tissue, malignant
  ameloblastic C41.1
    upper jaw (bone) C41.0
  botryoid — *see* Neoplasm, connective tissue, malignant
  botryoides — *see* Neoplasm, connective tissue, malignant
  cerebellar C71.6
    circumscribed (arachnoidal) C71.6
  circumscribed (arachnoidal) cerebellar C71.6
  clear cell — *see also* Neoplasm, connective tissue, malignant
    kidney C64.- ☑
  dendritic cells (accessory cells) C96.4
  embryonal — *see* Neoplasm, connective tissue, malignant
  endometrial (stromal) C54.1
    isthmus C54.0
  epithelioid (cell) — *see* Neoplasm, connective tissue, malignant
  Ewing's — *see* Neoplasm, bone, malignant
  follicular dendritic cell C96.4
  germinoblastic (diffuse) — *see* Lymphoma, diffuse large cell
    follicular — *see* Lymphoma, follicular, specified NEC
  giant cell (except of bone) — *see also* Neoplasm, connective tissue, malignant
    bone — *see* Neoplasm, bone, malignant
  glomoid — *see* Neoplasm, connective tissue, malignant
  granulocytic C92.3- ☑
  hemangioendothelial — *see* Neoplasm, connective tissue, malignant
  hemorrhagic, multiple — *see* Sarcoma, Kaposi's
  histiocytic C96.A (following C96.6)
  Hodgkin — *see* Lymphoma, Hodgkin
  immunoblastic (diffuse) — *see* Lymphoma, diffuse large cell
  interdigitating dendritic cell C96.4
  Kaposi's
    colon C46.4
    connective tissue C46.1
    gastrointestinal organ C46.4
    lung C46.5- ☑
    lymph node(s) C46.3
    palate (hard) (soft) C46.2
    rectum C46.4
    skin C46.0
    specified site NEC C46.7
    stomach C46.4
    unspecified site C46.9
  Kupffer cell C22.3
  Langerhans cell C96.4
  leptomeningeal — *see* Neoplasm, meninges, malignant
  liver NEC C22.4
  lymphangioendothelial — *see* Neoplasm, connective tissue, malignant

Sarcoma — *continued*
  lymphoblastic — *see* Lymphoma, lymphoblastic (diffuse)
  lymphocytic — *see* Lymphoma, small cell B-cell
  mast cell C96.22
  melanotic — *see* Melanoma
  meningeal — *see* Neoplasm, meninges, malignant
  meningothelial — *see* Neoplasm, meninges, malignant
  mesenchymal — *see also* Neoplasm, connective tissue, malignant
    mixed — *see* Neoplasm, connective tissue, malignant
  mesothelial — *see* Mesothelioma
  monstrocellular
    specified site — *see* Neoplasm, malignant, by site
    unspecified site C71.9
  myeloid C92.3- ☑
  neurogenic — *see* Neoplasm, nerve, malignant
  odontogenic C41.1
    upper jaw (bone) C41.0
  osteoblastic — *see* Neoplasm, bone, malignant
  osteogenic — *see also* Neoplasm, bone, malignant
    juxtacortical — *see* Neoplasm, bone, malignant
    periosteal — *see* Neoplasm, bone, malignant
  periosteal — *see also* Neoplasm, bone, malignant
    osteogenic — *see* Neoplasm, bone, malignant
  pleomorphic cell — *see* Neoplasm, connective tissue, malignant
  reticulum cell (diffuse) — *see* Lymphoma, diffuse large cell
    nodular — *see* Lymphoma, follicular
    pleomorphic cell type — *see* Lymphoma, diffuse large cell
  rhabdoid — *see* Neoplasm, malignant, by site
  round cell — *see* Neoplasm, connective tissue, malignant
  small cell — *see* Neoplasm, connective tissue, malignant
  soft tissue — *see* Neoplasm, connective tissue, malignant
  spindle cell — *see* Neoplasm, connective tissue, malignant
  stromal (endometrial) C54.1
    isthmus C54.0
  synovial — *see also* Neoplasm, connective tissue, malignant
    biphasic — *see* Neoplasm, connective tissue, malignant
    epithelioid cell — *see* Neoplasm, connective tissue, malignant
    spindle cell — *see* Neoplasm, connective tissue, malignant
Sarcomatosis
  meningeal — *see* Neoplasm, meninges, malignant
  specified site NEC — *see* Neoplasm, connective tissue, malignant
  unspecified site C80.1
Sarcopenia (age-related) M62.84
Sarcosinemia E72.59
Sarcosporidiosis (intestinal) A07.8
Satiety, early R68.81
Saturnine — *see* condition
Saturnism
  overdose or wrong substance given or taken — *see* Table of Drugs and Chemicals, by drug, poisoning
Satyriasis F52.8
Sauriasis — *see* Ichthyosis
SBE (subacute bacterial endocarditis) I33.0
Scabies (any site) B86
Scaglietti-Dagnini syndrome E22.0
Scald — *see* Burn
Scalenus anticus (anterior) **syndrome** G54.0
Scales R23.4
Scaling, skin R23.4
Scalp — *see* condition
Scapegoating affecting child Z62.3
Scaphocephaly Q75.0
Scapulalgia M89.8X1
Scapulohumeral myopathy G71.02
Scar, scarring — *see also* Cicatrix L90.5
  adherent L90.5
  atrophic L90.5
  cervix
    in pregnancy or childbirth — *see* Pregnancy, complicated by, abnormal cervix
  cheloid L91.0

Scar, scarring — *continued*
  chorioretinal H31.00- ☑
    posterior pole macula H31.01- ☑
    postsurgical H59.81- ☑
    solar retinopathy H31.02- ☑
    specified type NEC H31.09- ☑
  choroid — *see* Scar, chorioretinal
  conjunctiva H11.24- ☑
  cornea H17.9
    xerophthalmic — *see also* Opacity, cornea
      vitamin A deficiency E50.6
  duodenum, obstructive K31.5
  hypertrophic L91.0
  keloid L91.0
  labia N90.89
  lung (base) J98.4
  macula — *see* Scar, chorioretinal, posterior pole
  muscle M62.89
  myocardium, myocardial I25.2
  painful L90.5
  posterior pole (eye) — *see* Scar, chorioretinal, posterior pole
  retina — *see* Scar, chorioretinal
  trachea J39.8
  transmural uterine, in pregnancy O34.29
  uterus N85.8
    in pregnancy O34.29
  vagina N89.8
    postoperative N99.2
  vulva N90.89
Scarabiasis B88.2
Scarlatina (anginosa) (maligna) A38.9
  myocarditis (acute) A38.1
    old — *see* Myocarditis
  otitis media A38.0
  ulcerosa A38.8
Scarlet fever (albuminuria) (angina) A38.9
Schamberg's disease (progressive pigmentary dermatosis) L81.7
Schatzki's ring (acquired) (esophagus) (lower) K22.2
  congenital Q39.3
Schaufenster krankheit I20.8
Schaumann's
  benign lymphogranulomatosis D86.1
  disease or syndrome — *see* Sarcoidosis
Scheie's syndrome E76.03
Schenck's disease B42.1
Scheuermann's disease or osteochondrosis — *see* Osteochondrosis, juvenile, spine
Schilder (-Flatau) **disease** G37.0
Schilling-type monocytic leukemia C93.0- ☑
Schimmelbusch's disease, cystic mastitis, or hyperplasia — *see* Mastopathy, cystic
Schistosoma infestation — *see* Infestation, Schistosoma
Schistosomiasis B65.9
  with muscle disorder B65.9 *[M63.80]*
    ankle B65.9 *[M63.87-]* ☑
    foot B65.9 *[M63.87-]* ☑
    forearm B65.9 *[M63.83-]* ☑
    hand B65.9 *[M63.84-]* ☑
    lower leg B65.9 *[M63.86-]* ☑
    multiple sites B65.9 *[M63.89]*
    pelvic region B65.9 *[M63.85-]* ☑
    shoulder region B65.9 *[M63.81-]* ☑
    specified site NEC B65.9 *[M63.88]*
    thigh B65.9 *[M63.85-]* ☑
    upper arm B65.9 *[M63.82-]* ☑
  Asiatic B65.2
  bladder B65.0
  chestermani B65.8
  colon B65.1
  cutaneous B65.3
  due to
    S. haematobium B65.0
    S. japonicum B65.2
    S. mansoni B65.1
    S. mattheii B65.8
  Eastern B65.2
  genitourinary tract B65.0
  intestinal B65.1
  lung NEC B65.9 *[J99]*
    pneumonia B65.9 *[J17]*
  Manson's (intestinal) B65.1
  oriental B65.2
  pulmonary NEC B65.9 *[J99]*
    pneumonia B65.9

Schistosomiasis — *continued*
  Schistosoma
    haematobium B65.0
    japonicum B65.2
    mansoni B65.1
  specified type NEC B65.8
  urinary B65.0
  vesical B65.0
Schizencephaly Q04.6
Schizoaffective psychosis F25.9
Schizodontia K00.2
Schizoid personality F60.1
Schizophrenia, schizophrenic F20.9
  acute (brief) (undifferentiated) F23
  atypical (form) F20.3
  borderline F21
  catalepsy F20.2
  catatonic (type) (excited) (withdrawn) F20.2
  cenesthopathic, cenesthesiopathic F20.89
  childhood type F84.5
  chronic undifferentiated F20.5
  cyclic F25.0
  disorganized (type) F20.1
  flexibilitas cerea F20.2
  hebephrenic (type) F20.1
  incipient F21
  latent F21
  negative type F20.5
  paranoid (type) F20.0
  paraphrenic F20.0
  post-psychotic depression F32.89
  prepsychotic F21
  prodromal F21
  pseudoneurotic F21
  pseudopsychopathic F21
  reaction F23
  residual (state) (type) F20.5
  restzustand F20.5
  schizoaffective (type) — *see* Psychosis, schizoaffective
  simple (type) F20.89
  simplex F20.89
  specified type NEC F20.89
  spectrum and other psychotic disorder F29
    specified NEC F28
  stupor F20.2
  syndrome of childhood F84.5
  undifferentiated (type) F20.3
    chronic F20.5
Schizothymia (persistent) F60.1
Schlatter-Osgood disease or osteochondrosis — *see* Osteochondrosis, juvenile, tibia
Schlatter's tibia — *see* Osteochondrosis, juvenile, tibia
Schmidt's syndrome (polyglandular, autoimmune) E31.0
Schmincke's carcinoma or tumor — *see* Neoplasm, nasopharynx, malignant
Schmitz (-Stutzer) **dysentery** A03.0
Schmorl's disease or nodes
  lumbar region M51.46
  lumbosacral region M51.47
  sacrococcygeal region M53.3
  thoracic region M51.44
  thoracolumbar region M51.45
Schneiderian
  papilloma — *see* Neoplasm, nasopharynx, benign
    specified site — *see* Neoplasm, benign, by site
    unspecified site D14.0
  specified site — *see* Neoplasm, malignant, by site
    unspecified site C30.0
Scholte's syndrome (malignant carcinoid) E34.0
Scholz (-Bielchowsky-Henneberg) **disease or syndrome** E75.25
Schönlein (-Henoch) disease or purpura (primary) (rheumatic) D69.0
Schottmuller's disease A01.4
Schroeder's syndrome (endocrine hypertensive) E27
Schüller-Christian disease or syndrome C96.5
Schultze's type acroparesthesia, simple I73.89
Schultz's disease or syndrome — *see* Agranulocytosis
Schwalbe-Ziehen-Oppenheim disease G24.1
Schwannoma — *see also* Neoplasm, nerve, benign
  malignant — *see also* Neoplasm, nerve, malignant
    with rhabdomyoblastic differentiation — *see* Neoplasm, nerve, malignant
  melanocytic — *see* Neoplasm, nerve, benign
  pigmented — *see* Neoplasm, nerve, benign
Schwannomatosis Q85.03
Schwartz (-Jampel) **syndrome** G71.13
Schwartz-Bartter syndrome E22.2

☑ **Additional Character Required** — Refer to the Tabular List for Character Selection   ◣ Subterms under main terms may continue to next column or page

Schweniger-Buzzi anetoderma L90.1
Sciatic — *see* condition
Sciatica (infective)
  with lumbago M54.4- ☑
    due to intervertebral disc disorder — *see* Disorder, disc, with, radiculopathy
    due to displacement of intervertebral disc (with lumbago) — *see* Disorder, disc, with, radiculopathy
  wallet M54.3- ☑
Scimitar syndrome Q26.8
Sclera — *see* condition
Sclerectasia H15.84- ☑
Scleredema
  adultorum — *see* Sclerosis, systemic
  Buschke's — *see* Sclerosis, systemic
  newborn P83.0
Sclerema (adiposum) (edematosum) (neonatorum) (newborn) P83.0
  adultorum — *see* Sclerosis, systemic
Scleriasis — *see* Scleroderma
Scleritis H15.00- ☑
  with corneal involvement H15.04- ☑
  anterior H15.01- ☑
  brawny H15.02- ☑
  in (due to) zoster B02.34
  posterior H15.03- ☑
  specified type NEC H15.09- ☑
  syphilitic A52.71
  tuberculous (nodular) A18.51
Sclerochoroiditis H31.8
Scleroconjunctivitis — *see* Scleritis
Sclerocystic ovary syndrome E28.2
Sclerodactyly, sclerodactylia L94.3
Scleroderma, sclerodermia (acrosclerotic) (diffuse) (generalized) (progressive) (pulmonary) — *see also* Sclerosis, systemic M34.9
  circumscribed L94.0
  linear L94.1
  localized L94.0
  newborn P83.88
  systemic M34.9
Sclerokeratitis H16.8
  tuberculous A18.52
Scleroma nasi A48.8
Scleromalacia (perforans) H15.05- ☑
Scleromyxedema L98.5
Sclérose en plaques G35
Sclerosis, sclerotic
  adrenal (gland) E27.8
  Alzheimer's — *see* Disease, Alzheimer's
  amyotrophic (lateral) G12.21
  aorta, aortic I70.0
    valve — *see* Endocarditis, aortic
  artery, arterial, arteriolar, arteriovascular — *see* Arteriosclerosis
  ascending multiple G35
  brain (generalized) (lobular) G37.9
    artery, arterial I67.2
    diffuse G37.0
    disseminated G35
    insular G35
    Krabbe's E75.23
    miliary G35
    multiple G35
    presenile (Alzheimer's) — *see* Disease, Alzheimer's, early onset
    senile (arteriosclerotic) I67.2
    stem, multiple G35
    tuberous Q85.1
  bulbar, multiple G35
  bundle of His I44.39
  cardiac — *see* Disease, heart, ischemic, atherosclerotic
  cardiorenal — *see* Hypertension, cardiorenal
  cardiovascular — *see also* Disease, cardiovascular
    renal — *see* Hypertension, cardiorenal
  cerebellar — *see* Sclerosis, brain
  cerebral — *see* Sclerosis, brain
  cerebrospinal (disseminated) (multiple) G35
  cerebrovascular I67.2
  choroid — *see* Degeneration, choroid
  combined (spinal cord) — *see also* Degeneration, combined
    multiple G35
  concentric (Balo) G37.5
  cornea — *see* Opacity, cornea
  coronary (artery) I25.10

Sclerosis, sclerotic — *continued*
  coronary — *continued*
    with angina pectoris — *see* Arteriosclerosis, coronary (artery),
  corpus cavernosum
    female N90.89
    male N48.6
  diffuse (brain) (spinal cord) G37.0
  disseminated G35
  dorsal G35
  dorsolateral (spinal cord) — *see* Degeneration, combined
  endometrium N85.5
  extrapyramidal G25.9
  eye, nuclear (senile) — *see* Cataract, senile, nuclear
  focal and segmental (glomerular) — *see also* N00-N07
    with fourth character .1 N05.1
  Friedreich's (spinal cord) G11.1
  funicular (spermatic cord) N50.89
  general (vascular) — *see* Arteriosclerosis
  gland (lymphatic) I89.8
  hepatic K74.1
    alcoholic K70.2
  hereditary
    cerebellar G11.9
    spinal (Friedreich's ataxia) G11.1
  hippocampal G93.81
  insular G35
  kidney — *see* Sclerosis, renal
  larynx J38.7
  lateral (amyotrophic) (descending) (spinal) G12.21
    primary G12.23
  lens, senile nuclear — *see* Cataract, senile, nuclear
  liver K74.1
    with fibrosis K74.2
      alcoholic K70.2
    alcoholic K70.2
    cardiac K76.1
  lung — *see* Fibrosis, lung
  mastoid — *see* Mastoiditis, chronic
  mesial temporal G93.81
  mitral I05.8
  Mönckeberg's (medial) — *see* Arteriosclerosis, extremities
  multiple (brain stem) (cerebral) (generalized) (spinal cord) G35
  myocardium, myocardial — *see* Disease, heart, ischemic, atherosclerotic
  nuclear (senile), eye — *see* Cataract, senile, nuclear
  ovary N83.8
  pancreas K86.89
  penis N48.6
  peripheral arteries — *see* Arteriosclerosis, extremities
  plaques G35
  pluriglandular E31.8
  polyglandular E31.8
  posterolateral (spinal cord) — *see* Degeneration, combined
  presenile (Alzheimer's) — *see* Disease, Alzheimer's, early onset
  primary, lateral G12.23
  progressive, systemic M34.0
  pulmonary — *see* Fibrosis, lung
    artery I27.0
    valve (heart) — *see* Endocarditis, pulmonary
  renal N26.9
    with
      cystine storage disease E72.09
      hypertensive heart disease (conditions in I11) — *see* Hypertension, cardiorenal
    arteriolar (hyaline) (hyperplastic) — *see* Hypertension, kidney
  retina (senile) (vascular) H35.00
  senile (vascular) — *see* Arteriosclerosis
  spinal (cord) (progressive) G95.89
    ascending G61.0
    combined — *see also* Degeneration, combined
      multiple G35
      syphilitic A52.11
    disseminated G35
    dorsolateral — *see* Degeneration, combined
    hereditary (Friedreich's) (mixed form) G11.1
    lateral (amyotrophic) G12.21
      progressive G12.23
    multiple G35
    posterior (syphilitic) A52.11
  stomach K31.89
  subendocardial, congenital I42.4

Sclerosis, sclerotic — *continued*
  systemic M34.9
    with
      lung involvement M34.81
      myopathy M34.82
      polyneuropathy M34.83
    drug-induced M34.2
    due to chemicals NEC M34.2
    progressive M34.0
    specified NEC M34.89
  temporal (mesial) G93.81
  tricuspid (heart) (valve) I07.8
  tuberous (brain) Q85.1
  tympanic membrane — *see* Disorder, tympanic membrane, specified NEC
  valve, valvular (heart) — *see* Endocarditis
  vascular — *see* Arteriosclerosis
  vein I87.8
Scoliosis (acquired) (postural) M41.9
  adolescent (idiopathic) — *see* Scoliosis, idiopathic, adolescent
  congenital Q67.5
    due to bony malformation Q76.3
    failure of segmentation (hemivertebra) Q76.3
    hemivertebra fusion Q76.3
    postural Q67.5
  idiopathic M41.20
    adolescent M41.129
      cervical region M41.122
      cervicothoracic region M41.123
      lumbar region M41.126
      lumbosacral region M41.127
      thoracic region M41.124
      thoracolumbar region M41.125
    cervical region M41.22
    cervicothoracic region M41.23
    infantile M41.00
      cervical region M41.02
      cervicothoracic region M41.03
      lumbar region M41.06
      lumbosacral region M41.07
      sacrococcygeal region M41.08
      thoracic region M41.04
      thoracolumbar region M41.05
    juvenile M41.119
      cervical region M41.112
      cervicothoracic region M41.113
      lumbar region M41.116
      lumbosacral region M41.117
      thoracic region M41.114
      thoracolumbar region M41.115
    lumbar region M41.26
    lumbosacral region M41.27
    thoracic region M41.24
    thoracolumbar region M41.25
  infantile — *see* Scoliosis, idiopathic, infantile
  neuromuscular M41.40
    cervical region M41.42
    cervicothoracic region M41.43
    lumbar region M41.46
    lumbosacral region M41.47
    occipito-atlanto-axial region M41.41
    thoracic region M41.44
    thoracolumbar region M41.45
  paralytic — *see* Scoliosis, neuromuscular
  postradiation therapy M96.5
  rachitic (late effect or sequelae) E64.3 [M49.80]
    cervical region E64.3 [M49.82]
    cervicothoracic region E64.3 [M49.83]
    lumbar region E64.3 [M49.86]
    lumbosacral region E64.3 [M49.87]
    multiple sites E64.3 [M49.89]
    occipito-atlanto-axial region E64.3 [M49.81]
    sacrococcygeal region E64.3 [M49.88]
    thoracic region E64.3 [M49.84]
    thoracolumbar region E64.3 [M49.85]
  sciatic M54.4- ☑
  secondary (to) NEC M41.50
    cerebral palsy, Friedreich's ataxia, poliomyelitis, neuromuscular disorders — *see* Scoliosis, neuromuscular
    cervical region M41.52
    cervicothoracic region M41.53
    lumbar region M41.56
    lumbosacral region M41.57
    thoracic region M41.54
    thoracolumbar region M41.55
  specified form NEC M41.80

Subterms under main terms may continue to next column or page   ☑ Additional Character Required — Refer to the Tabular List for Character Selection   281

Schweniger-Buzzi anetoderma — Scoliosis

Scoliosis — *continued*
- specified form — *continued*
  - cervical region M41.82
  - cervicothoracic region M41.83
  - lumbar region M41.86
  - lumbosacral region M41.87
  - thoracic region M41.84
  - thoracolumbar region M41.85
  - thoracogenic M41.30
    - thoracic region M41.34
    - thoracolumbar region M41.35
  - tuberculous A18.01

Scoliotic pelvis
- with disproportion (fetopelvic) O33.0
  - causing obstructed labor O65.0

Scorbutus, scorbutic — *see also* Scurvy
- anemia D53.2

Score, NIHSS (National Institutes of Health Stroke Scale) R29.7- ☑

Scotoma (arcuate) (Bjerrum) (central) (ring) — *see also* Defect, visual field, localized, scotoma
- scintillating H53.19

Scratch — *see* Abrasion

Scratchy throat R09.89

Screening (for) Z13.9
- alcoholism Z13.39
- anemia Z13.0
- anomaly, congenital Z13.89
- antenatal, of mother — *see also* Encounter, antenatal screening Z36.9
- arterial hypertension Z13.6
- arthropod-borne viral disease NEC Z11.59
- autism Z13.41
- bacteriuria, asymptomatic Z13.89
- behavioral disorder Z13.30
  - specified NEC Z13.39
- brain injury, traumatic Z13.850
- bronchitis, chronic Z13.83
- brucellosis Z11.2
- cardiovascular disorder Z13.6
- cataract Z13.5
- chlamydial diseases Z11.8
- cholera Z11.0
- chromosomal abnormalities (nonprocreative) NEC Z13.79
- colonoscopy Z12.11
- congenital
  - dislocation of hip Z13.89
  - eye disorder Z13.5
  - malformation or deformation Z13.89
- contamination NEC Z13.88
- cystic fibrosis Z13.228
- dengue fever Z11.59
- dental disorder Z13.84
- depression (adult) (adolescent) (child) Z13.31
  - maternal Z13.32
  - perinatal Z13.32
- developmental
  - delays Z13.40
    - global (milestones) Z13.42
    - specified NEC Z13.49
  - handicap Z13.42
    - in early childhood Z13.42
- diabetes mellitus Z13.1
- diphtheria Z11.2
- disability, intellectual Z13.39
- disease or disorder Z13.9
  - bacterial NEC Z11.2
    - intestinal infectious Z11.0
    - respiratory tuberculosis Z11.1
  - behavioral Z13.30
    - specified NEC Z13.39
  - blood or blood-forming organ Z13.0
  - cardiovascular Z13.6
  - Chagas' Z11.6
  - chlamydial Z11.8
  - dental Z13.89
  - developmental delays Z13.40
    - global (milestones) Z13.42
    - specified NEC Z13.49
  - digestive tract NEC Z13.818
    - lower GI Z13.811
    - upper GI Z13.810
  - ear Z13.5
  - endocrine Z13.29
  - eye Z13.5
  - genitourinary Z13.89
  - heart Z13.6

Screening — *continued*
- disease or disorder — *continued*
  - human immunodeficiency virus (HIV) infection Z11.4
  - immunity Z13.0
  - infection
    - intestinal Z11.0
      - specified NEC Z11.6
  - infectious Z11.9
  - mental health and behavioral Z13.30
    - specified NEC Z13.39
  - metabolic Z13.228
  - neurological Z13.89
  - nutritional Z13.21
    - metabolic Z13.228
      - lipid disorders Z13.220
  - protozoal Z11.6
    - intestinal Z11.0
  - respiratory Z13.83
  - rheumatic Z13.828
  - rickettsial Z11.8
  - sexually-transmitted NEC Z11.3
    - human immunodeficiency virus (HIV) Z11.4
  - sickle-cell (trait) Z13.0
  - skin Z13.89
  - specified NEC Z13.89
  - spirochetal Z11.8
  - thyroid Z13.29
  - vascular Z13.6
  - venereal Z11.3
  - viral NEC Z11.59
    - human immunodeficiency virus (HIV) Z11.4
    - intestinal Z11.0
- elevated titer Z13.89
- emphysema Z13.83
- encephalitis, viral (mosquito- or tick-borne) Z11.59
- exposure to contaminants (toxic) Z13.88
- fever
  - dengue Z11.59
  - hemorrhagic Z11.59
  - yellow Z11.59
- filariasis Z11.6
- galactosemia Z13.228
- gastrointestinal condition Z13.818
- genetic (nonprocreative) - for procreative management — *see* Testing, genetic, for procreative management
  - disease carrier status (nonprocreative) Z13.71
  - specified NEC (nonprocreative) Z13.79
- genitourinary condition Z13.89
- glaucoma Z13.5
- gonorrhea Z11.3
- gout Z13.89
- helminthiasis (intestinal) Z11.6
- hematopoietic malignancy Z12.89
- hemoglobinopathies NEC Z13.0
- hemorrhagic fever Z11.59
- Hodgkin disease Z12.89
- human immunodeficiency virus (HIV) Z11.4
- human papillomavirus Z11.51
- hypertension Z13.6
- immunity disorders Z13.0
- infant or child (over 28 days old) Z00.129
  - with abnormal findings Z00.121
- infection
  - mycotic Z11.8
  - parasitic Z11.8
- ingestion of radioactive substance Z13.88
- intellectual disability Z13.39
- intestinal
  - helminthiasis Z11.6
  - infectious disease Z11.0
- leishmaniasis Z11.6
- leprosy Z11.2
- leptospirosis Z11.8
- leukemia Z12.89
- lymphoma Z12.89
- malaria Z11.6
- malnutrition Z13.29
  - metabolic Z13.228
  - nutritional Z13.21
- measles Z11.59
- mental health disorder Z13.30
  - specified NEC Z13.39
- metabolic errors, inborn Z13.228
- multiphasic Z13.89
- musculoskeletal disorder Z13.828
  - osteoporosis Z13.820
- mycoses Z11.8
- myocardial infarction (acute) Z13.6

Screening — *continued*
- neoplasm (malignant) (of) Z12.9
  - bladder Z12.6
  - blood Z12.89
  - breast Z12.39
    - routine mammogram Z12.31
  - cervix Z12.4
  - colon Z12.11
  - genitourinary organs NEC Z12.79
    - bladder Z12.6
    - cervix Z12.4
    - ovary Z12.73
    - prostate Z12.5
    - testis Z12.71
    - vagina Z12.72
  - hematopoietic system Z12.89
  - intestinal tract Z12.10
    - colon Z12.11
    - rectum Z12.12
    - small intestine Z12.13
  - lung Z12.2
  - lymph (glands) Z12.89
  - nervous system Z12.82
  - oral cavity Z12.81
  - prostate Z12.5
  - rectum Z12.12
  - respiratory organs Z12.2
  - skin Z12.83
  - small intestine Z12.13
  - specified site NEC Z12.89
  - stomach Z12.89
- nephropathy Z13.89
- nervous system disorders NEC Z13.858
- neurological condition Z13.89
- osteoporosis Z13.820
- parasitic infestation Z11.9
  - specified NEC Z11.8
- phenylketonuria Z13.228
- plague Z11.2
- poisoning (chemical) (heavy metal) Z13.88
- poliomyelitis Z11.59
- postnatal, chromosomal abnormalities Z13.89
- prenatal, of mother — *see also* Encounter, antenatal screening Z36.9
- protozoal disease Z11.6
  - intestinal Z11.0
- pulmonary tuberculosis Z11.1
- radiation exposure Z13.88
- respiratory condition Z13.83
- respiratory tuberculosis Z11.1
- rheumatoid arthritis Z13.828
- rubella Z11.59
- schistosomiasis Z11.6
- sexually-transmitted disease NEC Z11.3
  - human immunodeficiency virus (HIV) Z11.4
- sickle-cell disease or trait Z13.0
- skin condition Z13.89
- sleeping sickness Z11.6
- special Z13.9
  - specified NEC Z13.89
- syphilis Z11.3
- tetanus Z11.2
- trachoma Z11.8
- traumatic brain injury Z13.850
- trypanosomiasis Z11.6
- tuberculosis, respiratory Z11.1
  - active Z11.1
  - latent Z11.7
- venereal disease Z11.3
- viral encephalitis (mosquito- or tick-borne) Z11.59
- whooping cough Z11.2
- worms, intestinal Z11.6
- yaws Z11.8
- yellow fever Z11.59

Scrofula, scrofulosis (tuberculosis of cervical lymph glands) A18.2

Scrofulide (primary) (tuberculous) A18.4

Scrofuloderma, scrofulodermia (any site) (primary) A18.4

Scrofulosus lichen (primary) (tuberculous) A18.4

Scrofulous — *see* condition

Scrotal tongue K14.5

Scrotum — *see* condition

Scurvy, scorbutic E54
- anemia D53.2
- gum E54
- infantile E54
- rickets E55.0 [M90.80]

Sealpox B08.62

Seasickness T75.3 ☑

Seatworm (infection) (infestation) B80

Sebaceous — see also condition
 cyst — see Cyst, sebaceous

Seborrhea, seborrheic L21.9
 capillitii R23.8
 capitis L21.0
 dermatitis L21.9
  infantile L21.1
 eczema L21.9
  infantile L21.1
 sicca L21.0

Seckel's syndrome Q87.19

Seclusion, pupil — see Membrane, pupillary

Second hand tobacco smoke exposure (acute)
  (chronic) Z77.22
 in the perinatal period P96.81

Secondary
 dentin (in pulp) K04.3
 neoplasm, secondaries — see Table of Neoplasms,
  secondary

Secretion
 antidiuretic hormone, inappropriate E22.2
 catecholamine, by pheochromocytoma E27.5
 hormone
  antidiuretic, inappropriate (syndrome) E22.2
  by
   carcinoid tumor E34.0
   pheochromocytoma E27.5
  ectopic NEC E34.2
 urinary
  excessive R35.8
  suppression R34

Section
 nerve, traumatic — see Injury, nerve

Sedative, hypnotic, or anxiolytic-induced
 anxiety disorder F13.980
 bipolar and related disorder F13.94
 delirium F13.921
 depressive disorder F13.94
 major neurocognitive disorder F13.97
 mild neurocognitive disorder F13.988
 psychotic disorder F13.959
 sexual dysfunction F13.981
 sleep disorder F13.982

Segmentation, incomplete (congenital) — see also
  Fusion
 bone NEC Q78.8
 lumbosacral (joint) (vertebra) Q76.49

Seitelberger's syndrome (infantile neuraxonal dystrophy) G31.89

Seizure(s) — see also Convulsions R56.9
 absence G40.A- ☑ (following G40.3)
 akinetic — see Epilepsy, generalized, specified NEC
 atonic — see Epilepsy, generalized, specified NEC
 autonomic (hysterical) F44.5
 convulsive — see Convulsions
 cortical (focal) (motor) — see Epilepsy, localization-related, symptomatic, with simple partial seizures
 disorder — see also Epilepsy G40.909
 due to stroke — see Sequelae (of), disease, cerebrovascular, by type, specified NEC
 epileptic — see Epilepsy
 febrile (simple) R56.00
  with status epilepticus G40.901
  complex (atypical) (complicated) R56.01
   with status epilepticus G40.901
 grand mal G40.409
  intractable G40.419
   with status epilepticus G40.411
   without status epilepticus G40.419
  not intractable G40.409
   with status epilepticus G40.401
   without status epilepticus G40.409
 heart — see Disease, heart
 hysterical F44.5
 intractable G40.919
  with status epilepticus G40.911
 Jacksonian (focal) (motor type) (sensory type) — see
  Epilepsy, localization-related, symptomatic, with
  simple partial seizures
 newborn P90
 nonspecific epileptic
  atonic — see Epilepsy, generalized, specified NEC
  clonic — see Epilepsy, generalized, specified NEC
  myoclonic — see Epilepsy, generalized, specified
   NEC

Seizure(s) — continued
 nonspecific epileptic — continued
  tonic — see Epilepsy, generalized, specified NEC
  tonic-clonic — see Epilepsy, generalized, specified
   NEC
 partial, developing into secondarily generalized
  seizures
  complex — see Epilepsy, localization-related,
   symptomatic, with complex partial seizures
  simple — see Epilepsy, localization-related, symptomatic, with simple partial seizures
 petit mal G40.A- ☑ (following G40.3)
  intractable G40.419
   with status epilepticus G40.411
   without status epilepticus G40.419
  not intractable G40.409
   with status epilepticus G40.401
   without status epilepticus G40.409
 post traumatic R56.1
 recurrent G40.909
 specified NEC G40.89
 uncinate — see Epilepsy, localization-related, symptomatic, with complex partial seizures

Selenium deficiency, dietary E59

Self-damaging behavior (life-style) Z72.89

Self-harm (attempted)
 history (personal) Z91.5
  in family Z81.8

Self-mutilation (attempted)
 history (personal) Z91.5
  in family Z81.8

Self-poisoning
 history (personal) Z91.5
  in family Z81.8
 observation following (alleged) attempt Z03.6

Semicoma R40.1

Seminal vesiculitis N49.0

Seminoma C62.9- ☑
 specified site — see Neoplasm, malignant, by site

Senear-Usher disease or syndrome L10.4

Senectus R54

Senescence (without mention of psychosis) R54

Senile, senility — see also condition R41.81
 with
  acute confusional state F05
  mental changes NOS F03 ☑
  psychosis NEC — see Psychosis, senile
 asthenia R54
 cervix (atrophic) N88.8
 debility R54
 endometrium (atrophic) N85.8
 fallopian tube (atrophic) — see Atrophy, fallopian tube
 heart (failure) R54
 ovary (atrophic) — see Atrophy, ovary
 premature E34.8
 vagina, vaginitis (atrophic) N95.2
 wart L82.1

Sensation
 burning (skin) R20.8
  tongue K14.6
 loss of R20.8
 prickling (skin) R20.2
 tingling (skin) R20.2

Sense loss
 smell — see Disturbance, sensation, smell
 taste — see Disturbance, sensation, taste
 touch R20.8

Sensibility disturbance (cortical) (deep) (vibratory) R20.9

Sensitive, sensitivity — see also Allergy
 carotid sinus G90.01
 child (excessive) F93.8
 cold, autoimmune D59.1
 dentin K03.89
 gluten (non-celiac) K90.41
 latex Z91.040
 methemoglobin D74.8
 tuberculin, without clinical or radiological symptoms
  R76.11
 visual
  glare H53.71
  impaired contrast H53.72

Sensitiver Beziehungswahn F22

Sensitization, auto-erythrocytic D69.2

Separation
 anxiety, abnormal (of childhood) F93.0
 apophysis, traumatic — code as Fracture, by site
 choroid — see Detachment, choroid

Separation — continued
 epiphysis, epiphyseal
  nontraumatic — see also Osteochondropathy,
   specified type NEC
   upper femoral — see Slipped, epiphysis, upper
    femoral
  traumatic — code as Fracture, by site
 fracture — see Fracture
 infundibulum cardiac from right ventricle by a partition
  Q24.3
 joint (traumatic) (current) — code by site under Dislocation
 muscle (nontraumatic) — see Diastasis, muscle
 pubic bone, obstetrical trauma O71.6
 retina, retinal — see Detachment, retina
 symphysis pubis, obstetrical trauma O71.6
 tracheal ring, incomplete, congenital Q32.1

Sepsis (generalized) (unspecified organism) A41.9
 with
  organ dysfunction (acute) (multiple) R65.20
   with septic shock R65.21
 actinomycotic A42.7
 adrenal hemorrhage syndrome (meningococcal) A39.1
 anaerobic A41.4
 Bacillus anthracis A22.7
 Brucella — see also Brucellosis A23.9
 candidal B37.7
 cryptogenic A41.9
 due to device, implant or graft T85.79 ☑
  arterial graft NEC T82.7 ☑
  breast (implant) T85.79 ☑
  catheter NEC T85.79 ☑
   dialysis (renal) T82.7 ☑
    intraperitoneal T85.71 ☑
   infusion NEC T82.7 ☑
    spinal (cranial) (epidural) (intrathecal) (spinal)
     (subarachnoid) (subdural) T85.735 ☑
   urethral indwelling T83.511 ☑
   urinary T83.518 ☑
  ectopic or molar pregnancy O08.82
  electronic (electrode) (pulse generator) (stimulator)
   bone T84.7 ☑
   cardiac T82.7 ☑
   nervous system T85.738 ☑
    brain T85.731 ☑
    neurostimulator generator T85.734 ☑
    peripheral nerve T85.732 ☑
    spinal cord T85.733 ☑
   urinary T83.590 ☑
  fixation, internal (orthopedic) — see Complication,
   fixation device, infection
  gastrointestinal (bile duct) (esophagus) T85.79 ☑
   neurostimulator electrode (lead) T85.732 ☑
  genital T83.69 ☑
  heart NEC T82.7 ☑
   valve (prosthesis) T82.6 ☑
    graft T82.7 ☑
  joint prosthesis — see Complication, joint prosthesis, infection
  ocular (corneal graft) (orbital implant) T85.79 ☑
  orthopedic NEC T84.7 ☑
   fixation device, internal — see Complication,
    fixation device, infection
  specified NEC T85.79 ☑
  vascular T82.7 ☑
  ventricular intracranial (communicating) shunt
   T85.730 ☑
 during labor O75.3
 Enterococcus A41.81
 Erysipelothrix (rhusiopathiae) (erysipeloid) A26.7
 Escherichia coli (E. coli) A41.5 ☑
 extraintestinal yersiniosis A28.2
 following
  abortion (subsequent episode) O08.0
   current episode — see Abortion
  ectopic or molar pregnancy O08.82
  immunization T88.0 ☑
  infusion, therapeutic injection or transfusion NEC
   T80.29 ☑
  obstetrical procedure O86.04
 gangrenous A41.9
 gonococcal A54.86
 Gram-negative (organism) A41.5 ☑
  anaerobic A41.4
 Haemophilus influenzae A41.3
 herpesviral B00.7
 intra-abdominal K65.1

Sepsis — *continued*
intraocular — *see* Endophthalmitis, purulent
Listeria monocytogenes A32.7
localized — *code to* specific localized infection
　　in operation wound T81.49 ☑
　　skin — *see* Abscess
malleus A24.0
melioidosis A24.1
meningeal — *see* Meningitis
meningococcal A39.4
　acute A39.2
　chronic A39.3
MSSA (Methicillin susceptible Staphylococcus aureus)
　　A41.01
newborn P36.9
　due to
　　anaerobes NEC P36.5
　　Escherichia coli P36.4
　　Staphylococcus P36.30
　　　aureus P36.2
　　　specified NEC P36.39
　　Streptococcus P36.10
　　　group B P36.0
　　　specified NEC P36.19
　　specified NEC P36.8
Pasteurella multocida A28.0
pelvic, puerperal, postpartum, childbirth O85
pneumococcal A40.3
postprocedural T81.44 ☑
puerperal, postpartum, childbirth (pelvic) O85
Salmonella (arizonae) (cholerae-suis) (enteritidis) (ty-
　　phimurium) A02.1
severe R65.20
　with septic shock R65.21
Shigella — *see also* Dysentery, bacillary A03.9
skin, localized — *see* Abscess
specified organism NEC A41.89
Staphylococcus, staphylococcal A41.2
　aureus (methicillin susceptible) (MSSA) A41.01
　　methicillin resistant (MRSA) A41.02
　coagulase-negative A41.1
　specified NEC A41.1
Streptococcus, streptococcal A40.9
　agalactiae A40.1
　group
　　A A40.0
　　B A40.1
　　D A41.81
　neonatal P36.10
　　group B P36.0
　　specified NEC P36.19
　pneumoniae A40.3
　pyogenes A40.0
　specified NEC A40.8
tracheostomy stoma J95.02
tularemic A21.7
umbilical, umbilical cord (newborn) — *see* Sepsis,
　　newborn
Yersinia pestis A20.7
Septate — *see* Septum
Septic — *see* condition
arm — *see* Cellulitis, upper limb
　with lymphangitis — *see* Lymphangitis, acute, upper
　　　limb
embolus — *see* Embolism
finger — *see* Cellulitis, digit
　with lymphangitis — *see* Lymphangitis, acute, digit
foot — *see* Cellulitis, lower limb
　with lymphangitis — *see* Lymphangitis, acute,
　　　lower limb
gallbladder (acute) K81.0
hand — *see* Cellulitis, upper limb
　with lymphangitis — *see* Lymphangitis, acute, upper
　　　limb
joint — *see* Arthritis, pyogenic or pyemic
leg — *see* Cellulitis, lower limb
　with lymphangitis — *see* Lymphangitis, acute,
　　　lower limb
nail — *see also* Cellulitis, digit
　with lymphangitis — *see* Lymphangitis, acute, digit
sore — *see also* Abscess
　throat J02.0
　　streptococcal J02.0
spleen (acute) D73.89
teeth, tooth (pulpal origin) K04.4
throat — *see* Pharyngitis
thrombus — *see* Thrombosis
toe — *see* Cellulitis, digit

Septic — *continued*
toe — *see* Cellulitis, digit — *continued*
　with lymphangitis — *see* Lymphangitis, acute, digit
tonsils, chronic J35.01
　with adenoiditis J35.03
uterus — *see* Endometritis
Septicemia A41.9
meaning sepsis — *see* Sepsis
Septum, septate (congenital) — *see also* Anomaly, by
　site
anal Q42.3
　with fistula Q42.2
aqueduct of Sylvius Q03.0
　with spina bifida — *see* Spina bifida, by site, with
　　　hydrocephalus
uterus Q51.20
　complete Q51.21
　partial Q51.22
　specified NEC Q51.28
vagina Q52.10
　in pregnancy — *see* Pregnancy, complicated by,
　　　abnormal vagina
　　causing obstructed labor O65.5
　longitudinal Q52.129
　　microperforate
　　　left side Q52.124
　　　right side Q52.123
　　nonobstruction Q52.120
　　obstructing Q52.129
　　　left side Q52.122
　　　right side Q52.121
　transverse Q52.11
Sequelae (of) — *see also* condition
abscess, intracranial or intraspinal (conditions in G06)
　　G09
amputation — *code to* injury with seventh character
　　S
burn and corrosion — *code to* injury with seventh
　　character S
calcium deficiency E64.8
cerebrovascular disease — *see* Sequelae, disease,
　　cerebrovascular
childbirth O94
contusion — *code to* injury with seventh character S
corrosion — *see* Sequelae, burn and corrosion
crushing injury — *code to* injury with seventh character
　　S
disease
　cerebrovascular I69.90
　　alteration of sensation I69.998
　　aphasia I69.920
　　apraxia I69.990
　　ataxia I69.993
　　cognitive deficits I69.91 ☑
　　disturbance of vision I69.998
　　dysarthria I69.922
　　dysphagia I69.991
　　dysphasia I69.921
　　facial droop I69.992
　　facial weakness I69.992
　　fluency disorder I69.923
　　hemiplegia I69.95- ☑
　　hemorrhage
　　　intracerebral — *see* Sequelae, hemorrhage,
　　　　intracerebral
　　　intracranial, nontraumatic NEC — *see* Seque-
　　　　lae, hemorrhage, intracranial, nontrau-
　　　　matic
　　　subarachnoid — *see* Sequelae, hemorrhage,
　　　　subarachnoid
　　language deficit I69.928
　　monoplegia
　　　lower limb I69.94- ☑
　　　upper limb I69.93- ☑
　　paralytic syndrome I69.96- ☑
　　specified effect NEC I69.998
　　specified type NEC I69.80
　　　alteration of sensation I69.898
　　　aphasia I69.820
　　　apraxia I69.890
　　　ataxia I69.893
　　　cognitive deficits I69.81 ☑
　　　disturbance of vision I69.898
　　　dysarthria I69.822
　　　dysphagia I69.891
　　　dysphasia I69.821
　　　facial droop I69.892
　　　facial weakness I69.892

Sequelae — *continued*
disease — *continued*
　cerebrovascular — *continued*
　　specified type — *continued*
　　　fluency disorder I69.823
　　　hemiplegia I69.85- ☑
　　　language deficit I69.828
　　　monoplegia
　　　　lower limb I69.84- ☑
　　　　upper limb I69.83- ☑
　　　paralytic syndrome I69.86- ☑
　　　specified effect NEC I69.898
　　　speech deficit I69.928
　　　speech deficit I69.828
　　　stroke NOS — *see* Sequelae, stroke NOS
dislocation — *code to* injury with seventh character S
encephalitis or encephalomyelitis (conditions in G04)
　　G09
　in infectious disease NEC B94.8
　viral B94.1
external cause — *code to* injury with seventh character
　　S
foreign body entering natural orifice — *code to* injury
　　with seventh character S
fracture — *code to* injury with seventh character S
frostbite — *code to* injury with seventh character S
Hansen's disease B92
hemorrhage
　intracerebral I69.10
　　alteration of sensation I69.198
　　aphasia I69.120
　　apraxia I69.190
　　ataxia I69.193
　　cognitive deficits I69.11 ☑
　　disturbance of vision I69.198
　　dysarthria I69.122
　　dysphagia I69.191
　　dysphasia I69.121
　　facial droop I69.192
　　facial weakness I69.192
　　fluency disorder I69.123
　　hemiplegia I69.15- ☑
　　language deficit NEC I69.128
　　monoplegia
　　　lower limb I69.14- ☑
　　　upper limb I69.13- ☑
　　paralytic syndrome I69.16- ☑
　　specified effect NEC I69.198
　　speech deficit NEC I69.128
　intracranial, nontraumatic NEC I69.20
　　alteration of sensation I69.298
　　aphasia I69.220
　　apraxia I69.290
　　ataxia I69.293
　　cognitive deficits I69.21 ☑
　　disturbance of vision I69.298
　　dysarthria I69.222
　　dysphagia I69.291
　　dysphasia I69.221
　　facial droop I69.292
　　facial weakness I69.292
　　fluency disorder I69.223
　　hemiplegia I69.25- ☑
　　language deficit NEC I69.228
　　monoplegia
　　　lower limb I69.24- ☑
　　　upper limb I69.23- ☑
　　paralytic syndrome I69.26- ☑
　　specified effect NEC I69.298
　　speech deficit NEC I69.228
　subarachnoid I69.00
　　alteration of sensation I69.098
　　aphasia I69.020
　　apraxia I69.090
　　ataxia I69.093
　　cognitive deficits — *see* subcategory I69.01- ▶
　　disturbance of vision I69.098
　　dysarthria I69.022
　　dysphagia I69.091
　　dysphasia I69.021
　　facial droop I69.092
　　facial weakness I69.092
　　fluency disorder I69.023
　　hemiplegia I69.05- ☑
　　language deficit NEC I69.028
　　monoplegia
　　　lower limb I69.04- ☑
　　　upper limb I69.03- ☑

　　☑ **Additional Character Required** — Refer to the Tabular List for Character Selection　　▽ Subterms under main terms may continue to next column or pag

Sequelae — *continued*
  hemorrhage — *continued*
    subarachnoid — *continued*
      paralytic syndrome I69.06- ☑
      specified effect NEC I69.098
      speech deficit NEC I69.028
  hepatitis, viral B94.2
  hyperalimentation E68
  infarction
    cerebral I69.30
      alteration of sensation I69.398
      aphasia I69.320
      apraxia I69.390
      ataxia I69.393
      cognitive deficits I69.31 ☑
      disturbance of vision I69.398
      dysarthria I69.322
      dysphagia I69.391
      dysphasia I69.321
      facial droop I69.392
      facial weakness I69.392
      fluency disorder I69.323
      hemiplegia I69.35- ☑
      language deficit NEC I69.328
      monoplegia
        lower limb I69.34- ☑
        upper limb I69.33- ☑
      paralytic syndrome I69.36- ☑
      specified effect NEC I69.398
      speech deficit NEC I69.328
  infection, pyogenic, intracranial or intraspinal G09
  infectious disease B94.9
    specified NEC B94.8
  injury — *code to* injury with seventh character S
  leprosy B92
  meningitis
    bacterial (conditions in G00) G09
    other or unspecified cause (conditions in G03) G09
  muscle (and tendon) injury — *code to* injury with seventh character S
  myelitis — *see* Sequelae, encephalitis
  niacin deficiency E64.8
  nutritional deficiency E64.9
    specified NEC E64.8
  obstetrical condition O94
  parasitic disease B94.9
  phlebitis or thrombophlebitis of intracranial or intraspinal venous sinuses and veins (conditions in G08) G09
  poisoning — *code to* poisoning with seventh character S
    nonmedicinal substance — *see* Sequelae, toxic effect, nonmedicinal substance
  poliomyelitis (acute) B91
  pregnancy O94
  protein-energy malnutrition E64.0
  puerperium O94
  rickets E64.3
  selenium deficiency E64.8
  sprain and strain — *code to* injury with seventh character S
  stroke NOS I69.30
    alteration in sensation I69.398
    aphasia I69.320
    apraxia I69.390
    ataxia I69.393
    cognitive deficits I69.31 ☑
    disturbance of vision I69.398
    dysarthria I69.322
    dysphagia I69.391
    dysphasia I69.321
    facial droop I69.392
    facial weakness I69.392
    hemiplegia I69.35- ☑
    language deficit NEC I69.328
    monoplegia
      lower limb I69.34- ☑
      upper limb I69.33- ☑
    paralytic syndrome I69.36- ☑
    specified effect NEC I69.398
    speech deficit NEC I69.328
  tendon and muscle injury — *code to* injury with seventh character S
  thiamine deficiency E64.8
  trachoma B94.0
  tuberculosis B90.9
    bones and joints B90.2
    central nervous system B90.0

Sequelae — *continued*
  tuberculosis — *continued*
    genitourinary B90.1
    pulmonary (respiratory) B90.9
    specified organs NEC B90.8
  viral
    encephalitis B94.1
    hepatitis B94.2
  vitamin deficiency NEC E64.8
    A E64.1
    B E64.8
    C E64.2
  wound, open — *code to* injury with seventh character S
Sequestration — *see also* Sequestrum
  disk — *see* Displacement, intervertebral disk
  lung, congenital Q33.2
Sequestrum
  bone — *see* Osteomyelitis, chronic
  dental M27.2
  jaw bone M27.2
  orbit — *see* Osteomyelitis, orbit
  sinus (accessory) (nasal) — *see* Sinusitis
Sequoiosis lung or pneumonitis J67.8
Serology for syphilis
  doubtful
    with signs or symptoms — *code by* site and stage under Syphilis
    follow-up of latent syphilis — *see* Syphilis, latent
  negative, with signs or symptoms — *code by* site and stage under Syphilis
  positive A53.0
    with signs or symptoms — *code by* site and stage under Syphilis
  reactivated A53.0
Seroma — *see also* Hematoma
  postprocedural — *see* Complication, postprocedural, seroma
  traumatic, secondary and recurrent T79.2 ☑
Seropurulent — *see* condition
Serositis, multiple K65.8
  pericardial I31.1
  peritoneal K65.8
Serous — *see* condition
Sertoli cell
  adenoma
    specified site — *see* Neoplasm, benign, by site
    unspecified site
      female D27.9
      male D29.20
  carcinoma
    specified site — *see* Neoplasm, malignant, by site
    unspecified site (male) C62.9- ☑
      female C56.9
  tumor
    with lipid storage
      specified site — *see* Neoplasm, benign, by site
      unspecified site
        female D27.9
        male D29.20
    specified site — *see* Neoplasm, benign, by site
    unspecified site
      female D27.9
      male D29.20
Sertoli-Leydig cell tumor — *see* Neoplasm, benign, by site
  specified site — *see* Neoplasm, benign, by site
  unspecified site
    female D27.9
    male D29.20
Serum
  allergy, allergic reaction — *see also* Reaction, serum T80.69 ☑
    shock — *see also* Shock, anaphylactic T80.59 ☑
  arthritis — *see also* Reaction, serum T80.69 ☑
  complication or reaction NEC — *see also* Reaction, serum T80.69 ☑
  disease NEC — *see also* Reaction, serum T80.69 ☑
  hepatitis — *see also* Hepatitis, viral, type B
    carrier (suspected) of B18.1
  intoxication — *see also* Reaction, serum T80.69 ☑
  neuritis — *see also* Reaction, serum T80.69 ☑
  neuropathy G61.1
  poisoning NEC — *see also* Reaction, serum T80.69 ☑
  rash NEC — *see also* Reaction, serum T80.69 ☑
  reaction NEC — *see also* Reaction, serum T80.69 ☑
  sickness NEC — *see also* Reaction, serum T80.69 ☑

Serum — *continued*
  urticaria — *see also* Reaction, serum T80.69 ☑
Sesamoiditis M25.8- ☑
Severe sepsis R65.20
  with septic shock R65.21
Sever's disease or osteochondrosis — *see* Osteochondrosis, juvenile, tarsus
Sex
  chromosome mosaics Q97.8
    lines with various numbers of X chromosomes Q97.2
  education Z70.8
  reassignment surgery status Z87.890
Sextuplet pregnancy — *see* Pregnancy, sextuplet
Sexual
  function, disorder of (psychogenic) F52.9
  immaturity (female) (male) E30.0
  impotence (psychogenic) organic origin NEC — *see* Dysfunction, sexual, male
  precocity (constitutional) (cryptogenic)(female) (idiopathic) (male) E30.1
Sexuality, pathologic — *see* Deviation, sexual
Sézary disease C84.1- ☑
Shadow, lung R91.8
Shaking palsy or paralysis — *see* Parkinsonism
Shallowness, acetabulum — *see* Derangement, joint, specified type NEC, hip
Shaver's disease J63.1
Sheath (tendon) — *see* condition
Sheathing, retinal vessels H35.01- ☑
Shedding
  nail L60.8
  premature, primary (deciduous) teeth K00.6
Sheehan's disease or syndrome E23.0
Shelf, rectal K62.89
Shell teeth K00.5
Shellshock (current) F43.0
  lasting state — *see* Disorder, post-traumatic stress
Shield kidney Q63.1
Shift
  auditory threshold (temporary) H93.24- ☑
  mediastinal R93.89
Shifting sleep-work schedule (affecting sleep) G47.26
Shiga (-Kruse) **dysentery** A03.0
Shiga's bacillus A03.0
Shigella (dysentery) — *see* Dysentery, bacillary
Shigellosis A03.9
  Group A A03.0
  Group B A03.1
  Group C A03.2
  Group D A03.3
Shin splints S86.89- ☑
Shingles — *see* Herpes, zoster
Shipyard disease or eye B30.0
Shirodkar suture, in pregnancy — *see* Pregnancy, complicated by, incompetent cervix
Shock R57.9
  with ectopic or molar pregnancy O08.3
  adrenal (cortical) (Addisonian) E27.2
  adverse food reaction (anaphylactic) — *see* Shock, anaphylactic, due to food
  allergic — *see* Shock, anaphylactic
  anaphylactic T78.2 ☑
    chemical — *see* Table of Drugs and Chemicals
    due to drug or medicinal substance
      correct substance properly administered T88.6 ☑
      overdose or wrong substance given (by accident) — *see* Table of Drugs and Chemicals, by drug, poisoning
    due to food (nonpoisonous) T78.00 ☑
      additives T78.06 ☑
      dairy products T78.07 ☑
      eggs T78.08 ☑
      fish T78.03 ☑
        shellfish T78.02 ☑
      fruit T78.04 ☑
      milk T78.07 ☑
      nuts T78.05 ☑
        multiple types T78.05 ☑
        peanuts T78.01 ☑
      peanuts T78.01 ☑
      seeds T78.05 ☑
      specified type NEC T78.09 ☑
      vegetable T78.04 ☑
    following sting(s) — *see* Venom
    immunization T80.52 ☑
    serum T80.59 ☑
      blood and blood products T80.51 ☑

☝ Subterms under main terms may continue to next column or page   ☑ Additional Character Required — Refer to the Tabular List for Character Selection   285

Sequelae — Shock

Shock — *continued*
  anaphylactic — *continued*
    serum — *continued*
      immunization T80.52 ✓
      specified NEC T80.59 ✓
      vaccination T80.52 ✓
  anaphylactoid — *see* Shock, anaphylactic
  anesthetic
    correct substance properly administered T88.2 ✓
    overdose or wrong substance given or taken — *see* Table of Drugs and Chemicals, by drug, poisoning
      specified anesthetic — *see* Table of Drugs and Chemicals, by drug, poisoning
  cardiogenic R57.0
  chemical substance — *see* Table of Drugs and Chemicals
  complicating ectopic or molar pregnancy O08.3
  culture — *see* Disorder, adjustment
  drug
    due to correct substance properly administered T88.6 ✓
    overdose or wrong substance given or taken (by accident) — *see* Table of Drugs and Chemicals, by drug, poisoning
  during or after labor and delivery O75.1
  electric T75.4 ✓
    (taser) T75.4 ✓
  endotoxic R65.21
    postprocedural (resulting from a procedure, not elsewhere classified) T81.12 ✓
  following
    ectopic or molar pregnancy O08.3
    injury (immediate) (delayed) T79.4 ✓
    labor and delivery O75.1
  food (anaphylactic) — *see* Shock, anaphylactic, due to food
  from electroshock gun (taser) T75.4 ✓
  gram-negative R65.21
    postprocedural (resulting from a procedure, not elsewhere classified) T81.12 ✓
  hematologic R57.8
  hemorrhagic R57.8
    surgery (intraoperative) (postoperative) T81.19 ✓
    trauma T79.4 ✓
  hypovolemic R57.1
    surgical T81.19 ✓
    traumatic T79.4 ✓
  insulin E15
    therapeutic misadventure — *see* subcategory T38.3 ✓
  kidney N17.0
    traumatic (following crushing) T79.5 ✓
  lightning T75.01 ✓
  liver K72.00
  lung J80
  obstetric O75.1
    with ectopic or molar pregnancy O08.3
    following ectopic or molar pregnancy O08.3
  pleural (surgical) T81.19 ✓
    due to trauma T79.4 ✓
  postprocedural (postoperative) T81.10 ✓
    with ectopic or molar pregnancy O08.3
    cardiogenic T81.11 ✓
    endotoxic T81.12 ✓
    following ectopic or molar pregnancy O08.3
    gram-negative T81.12 ✓
    hypovolemic T81.19 ✓
    septic T81.12 ✓
    specified type NEC T81.19 ✓
  psychic F43.0
  septic (due to severe sepsis) R65.21
  specified NEC R57.8
  surgical T81.10 ✓
  taser gun (taser) T75.4 ✓
  therapeutic misadventure NEC T81.10 ✓
  thyroxin
    overdose or wrong substance given or taken — *see* Table of Drugs and Chemicals, by drug, poisoning
  toxic, syndrome A48.3
  transfusion — *see* Complications, transfusion
  traumatic (immediate) (delayed) T79.4 ✓
Shoemaker's chest M95.4
Short, shortening, shortness
  arm (acquired) — *see also* Deformity, limb, unequal length

Short, shortening, shortness — *continued*
  arm — *see also* Deformity, limb, unequal length — *continued*
    congenital Q71.81- ✓
    forearm — *see* Deformity, limb, unequal length
  bowel syndrome K91.2
  breath R06.02
  cervical (complicating pregnancy) O26.87- ✓
    non-gravid uterus N88.3
  common bile duct, congenital Q44.5
  cord (umbilical), complicating delivery O69.3 ✓
  cystic duct, congenital Q44.5
  esophagus (congenital) Q39.8
  femur (acquired) — *see* Deformity, limb, unequal length, femur
    congenital — *see* Defect, reduction, lower limb, longitudinal, femur
  frenum, frenulum, linguae (congenital) Q38.1
  hip (acquired) — *see also* Deformity, limb, unequal length
    congenital Q65.89
  leg (acquired) — *see also* Deformity, limb, unequal length
    congenital Q72.81- ✓
    lower leg — *see also* Deformity, limb, unequal length
  limbed stature, with immunodeficiency D82.2
  lower limb (acquired) — *see also* Deformity, limb, unequal length
    congenital Q72.81- ✓
  organ or site, congenital NEC — *see* Distortion
  palate, congenital Q38.5
  radius (acquired) — *see also* Deformity, limb, unequal length
    congenital — *see* Defect, reduction, upper limb, longitudinal, radius
  rib syndrome Q77.2
  stature (child) (hereditary) (idiopathic) NEC R62.52
    constitutional E34.3
    due to endocrine disorder E34.3
    Laron-type E34.3
  tendon — *see also* Contraction, tendon
    with contracture of joint — *see* Contraction, joint
    Achilles (acquired) M67.0- ✓
      congenital Q66.89
    congenital Q79.8
  thigh (acquired) — *see also* Deformity, limb, unequal length, femur
    congenital — *see* Defect, reduction, lower limb, longitudinal, femur
  tibialis anterior (tendon) — *see* Contraction, tendon
  umbilical cord
    complicating delivery O69.3 ✓
  upper limb, congenital — *see* Defect, reduction, upper limb, specified type NEC
  urethra N36.8
  uvula, congenital Q38.5
  vagina (congenital) Q52.4
Shortsightedness — *see* Myopia
Shoshin (acute fulminating beriberi) E51.11
Shoulder — *see* condition
Shovel-shaped incisors K00.2
Shower, thromboembolic — *see* Embolism
Shunt
  arterial-venous (dialysis) Z99.2
  arteriovenous, pulmonary (acquired) I28.0
    congenital Q25.72
  cerebral ventricle (communicating) in situ Z98.2
  surgical, prosthetic, with complications — *see* Complications, cardiovascular, device or implant
Shutdown, renal N28.9
Shy-Drager syndrome G90.3
Sialadenitis, sialadenosis (any gland) (chronic) (periodic) (suppurative) — *see* Sialoadenitis
Sialectasia K11.8
Sialidosis E77.1
Sialitis, silitis (any gland) (chronic) (suppurative) — *see* Sialoadenitis
Sialoadenitis (any gland) (periodic) (suppurative) K11.20
  acute K11.21
    recurrent K11.22
  chronic K11.23
Sialoadenopathy K11.9
Sialoangitis — *see* Sialoadenitis
Sialodochitis (fibrinosa) — *see* Sialoadenitis
Sialodocholithiasis K11.5
Sialolithiasis K11.5

Sialometaplasia, necrotizing K11.8
Sialorrhea — *see also* Ptyalism
  periodic — *see* Sialoadenitis
Sialosis K11.7
Siamese twin Q89.4
Sibling rivalry Z62.891
Sicard's syndrome G52.7
Sicca syndrome M35.00
  with
    keratoconjunctivitis M35.01
    lung involvement M35.02
    myopathy M35.03
    renal tubulo-interstitial disorders M35.04
    specified organ involvement NEC M35.09
Sick R69
  or handicapped person in family Z63.79
    needing care at home Z63.6
  sinus (syndrome) I49.5
Sick-euthyroid syndrome E07.81
Sickle-cell
  anemia — *see* Disease, sickle-cell
  trait D57.3
Sicklemia — *see also* Disease, sickle-cell
  trait D57.3
Sickness
  air (travel) T75.3 ✓
  airplane T75.3 ✓
  alpine T70.29 ✓
  altitude T70.20 ✓
  Andes T70.29 ✓
  aviator's T70.29 ✓
  balloon T70.29 ✓
  car T75.3 ✓
  compressed air T70.3 ✓
  decompression T70.3 ✓
  green D50.8
  milk — *see* Poisoning, food, noxious
  motion T75.3 ✓
  mountain T70.29 ✓
    acute D75.1
  protein — *see also* Reaction, serum T80.69 ✓
  radiation T66 ✓
  roundabout (motion) T75.3 ✓
  sea T75.3 ✓
  serum NEC — *see also* Reaction, serum T80.69 ✓
  sleeping (African) B56.9
    by Trypanosoma B56.9
      brucei
        gambiense B56.0
        rhodesiense B56.1
      East African B56.1
      Gambian B56.0
      Rhodesian B56.1
      West African B56.0
  swing (motion) T75.3 ✓
  train (railway) (travel) T75.3 ✓
  travel (any vehicle) T75.3 ✓
Sideropenia — *see* Anemia, iron deficiency
Siderosilicosis J62.8
Siderosis (lung) J63.4
  eye (globe) — *see* Disorder, globe, degenerative, siderosis
Siemens' syndrome (ectodermal dysplasia) Q82.8
Sighing R06.89
  psychogenic F45.8
Sigmoid — *see also* condition
  flexure — *see* condition
  kidney Q63.1
Sigmoiditis — *see also* Enteritis K52.9
  infectious A09
  noninfectious K52.9
Silfversköld's syndrome Q78.9
Silicosiderosis J62.8
Silicosis, silicotic (simple) (complicated) J62.8
  with tuberculosis J65
Silicotuberculosis J65
Silo-fillers' disease J68.8
  bronchitis J68.0
  pneumonitis J68.0
  pulmonary edema J68.1
Silver's syndrome Q87.19
Simian malaria B53.1
Simmonds' cachexia or disease E23.0
Simons' disease or syndrome (progressive lipodystrophy) E88.1
Simple, simplex — *see* condition
Simulation, conscious (of illness) Z76.5

✓ Additional Character Required — Refer to the Tabular List for Character Selection ▽ Subterms under main terms may continue to next column or page

Simultanagnosia (asimultagnosia) R48.3
Sin Nombre virus disease (Hantavirus) (cardio)-pulmonary syndrome) B33.4
Sinding-Larsen disease or osteochondrosis — see Osteochondrosis, juvenile, patella
Singapore hemorrhagic fever A91
Singer's node or nodule J38.2
Single
  atrium Q21.2
  coronary artery Q24.5
  umbilical artery Q27.0
  ventricle Q20.4
Singultus R06.6
  epidemicus B33.0
Sinus — see also Fistula
  abdominal K63.89
  arrest I45.5
  arrhythmia I49.8
  bradycardia R00.1
  branchial cleft (internal) (external) Q18.0
  coccygeal — see Sinus, pilonidal
  dental K04.6
  dermal (congenital) Q06.8
    with abscess Q06.8
    coccygeal, pilonidal — see Sinus, coccygeal
  infected, skin NEC L08.89
  marginal, ruptured or bleeding — see Hemorrhage, antepartum, specified cause NEC
  medial, face and neck Q18.8
  pause I45.5
  pericranii Q01.9
  pilonidal (infected) (rectum) L05.92
    with abscess L05.02
  preauricular Q18.1
  rectovaginal N82.3
  Rokitansky-Aschoff (gallbladder) K82.8
  sacrococcygeal (dermoid) (infected) — see Sinus, pilonidal
  tachycardia R00.0
    paroxysmal I47.1
  tarsi syndrome M25.57- ☑
  testis N50.89
  tract (postinfective) — see Fistula
  urachus Q64.4
Sinusitis (accessory) (chronic) (hyperplastic) (nasal) (nonpurulent) (purulent) J32.9
  acute J01.90
    ethmoidal J01.20
      recurrent J01.21
    frontal J01.10
      recurrent J01.11
    involving more than one sinus, other than pansinusitis J01.80
      recurrent J01.81
    maxillary J01.00
      recurrent J01.01
    pansinusitis J01.40
      recurrent J01.41
      recurrent J01.91
    specified NEC J01.80
      recurrent J01.81
    sphenoidal J01.30
      recurrent J01.31
  allergic — see Rhinitis, allergic
  due to high altitude T70.1 ☑
  ethmoidal J32.2
    acute J01.20
      recurrent J01.21
  frontal J32.1
    acute J01.10
      recurrent J01.11
  influenzal — see Influenza, with, respiratory manifestations NEC
  involving more than one sinus but not pansinusitis J32.8
    acute J01.80
      recurrent J01.81
  maxillary J32.0
    acute J01.00
      recurrent J01.01
  sphenoidal J32.3
    acute J01.30
      recurrent J01.31
  tuberculous, any sinus A15.8
Sinusitis-bronchiectasis-situs inversus (syndrome) (triad) Q89.3
Sipple's syndrome E31.22
Sirenomelia (syndrome) Q87.2

Siriasis T67.01 ☑
Sirkari's disease B55.0
Siti A65
Situation, psychiatric F99
Situational
  disturbance (transient) — see Disorder, adjustment
    acute F43.0
  maladjustment — see Disorder, adjustment
  reaction — see Disorder, adjustment
    acute F43.0
Situs inversus or transversus (abdominalis) (thoracis) Q89.3
Sixth disease B08.20
  due to human herpesvirus 6 B08.21
  due to human herpesvirus 7 B08.22
Sjögren-Larsson syndrome Q87.19
Sjögren's syndrome or disease — see Sicca syndrome
Skeletal — see condition
Skene's gland — see condition
Skenitis — see Urethritis
Skerljevo A65
Skevas-Zerfus disease — see Toxicity, venom, marine animal, sea anemone
Skin — see also condition
  clammy R23.1
  donor — see Donor, skin
  hidebound M35.9
Slate-dressers' or slate-miners' lung J62.8
Sleep
  apnea — see Apnea, sleep
  deprivation Z72.820
  disorder or disturbance G47.9
    child F51.9
      nonorganic origin F51.9
      specified NEC G47.8
  disturbance G47.9
    nonorganic origin F51.9
  drunkenness F51.9
  rhythm inversion G47.2- ☑
  terrors F51.4
  walking F51.3
    hysterical F44.89
Sleep hygiene
  abuse Z72.821
  inadequate Z72.821
  poor Z72.821
Sleeping sickness — see Sickness, sleeping
Sleeplessness — see Insomnia
  menopausal N95.1
Sleep-wake schedule disorder G47.20
Slim disease (in HIV infection) B20
Slipped, slipping
  epiphysis (traumatic) — see also Osteochondropathy, specified type NEC
    capital femoral (traumatic)
      acute (on chronic) S79.01- ☑
    current traumatic — code as Fracture, by site
    upper femoral (nontraumatic) M93.00- ☑
      acute M93.01- ☑
        on chronic M93.03- ☑
      chronic M93.02- ☑
  intervertebral disc — see Displacement, intervertebral disc
  ligature, umbilical P51.8
  patella — see Disorder, patella, derangement NEC
  rib M89.8X8
  sacroiliac joint — see subcategory M53.2 ☑
  tendon — see Disorder, tendon
  ulnar nerve, nontraumatic — see Lesion, nerve, ulnar
  vertebra NEC — see Spondylolisthesis
Slocumb's syndrome E27.0
Sloughing (multiple) (phagedena) (skin) — see also Gangrene
  abscess — see Abscess
  appendix K38.8
  fascia — see Disorder, soft tissue, specified type NEC
  scrotum N50.89
  tendon — see Disorder, tendon
  transplanted organ — see Rejection, transplant
  ulcer — see Ulcer, skin
Slow
  feeding, newborn P92.2
  flow syndrome, coronary I20.8
  heart (beat) R00.1
Slowing, urinary stream R39.198
Sluder's neuralgia (syndrome) G44.89
Slurred, slurring speech R47.81

Small (ness)
  for gestational age — see Small for dates
  introitus, vagina N89.6
  kidney (unknown cause) N27.9
    bilateral N27.1
    unilateral N27.0
  ovary (congenital) Q50.39
  pelvis
    with disproportion (fetopelvic) O33.1
      causing obstructed labor O65.1
  uterus N85.8
  white kidney N03.9
Small-and-light-for-dates — see Small for dates
Small-for-dates (infant) P05.10
  with weight of
    499 grams or less P05.11
    500-749 grams P05.12
    750-999 grams P05.13
    1000-1249 grams P05.14
    1250-1499 grams P05.15
    1500-1749 grams P05.16
    1750-1999 grams P05.17
    2000-2499 grams P05.18
    2500 grams and over P05.19
  specified NEC P05.19
Smallpox B03
Smearing, fecal R15.1
Smith-Lemli-Opitz syndrome E78.72
Smith's fracture S52.54- ☑
Smoker — see Dependence, drug, nicotine
Smoker's
  bronchitis J41.0
  cough J41.0
  palate K13.24
  throat J31.2
  tongue K13.24
Smoking
  passive Z77.22
Smothering spells R06.81
Snaggle teeth, tooth M26.39
Snapping
  finger — see Trigger finger
  hip — see Derangement, joint, specified type NEC, hip
    involving the iliotiblial band M76.3- ☑
  knee — see Derangement, knee
    involving the iliotiblial band M76.3- ☑
Sneddon-Wilkinson disease or syndrome (sub-corneal pustular dermatosis) L13.1
Sneezing (intractable) R06.7
Sniffing
  cocaine
    abuse — see Abuse, drug, cocaine
    dependence — see Dependence, drug, cocaine
  gasoline
    abuse — see Abuse, drug, inhalant
    dependence — see Dependence, drug, inhalant
  glue (airplane)
    abuse — see Abuse, drug, inhalant
    drug dependence — see Dependence, drug, inhalant
Sniffles
  newborn P28.89
Snoring R06.83
Snow blindness — see Photokeratitis
Snuffles (non-syphilitic) R06.5
  newborn P28.89
  syphilitic (infant) A50.05 [J99]
Social
  exclusion Z60.4
    due to discrimination or persecution (perceived) Z60.5
  migrant Z59.0
    acculturation difficulty Z60.3
  rejection Z60.4
    due to discrimination or persecution Z60.5
  role conflict NEC Z73.5
  skills inadequacy NEC Z73.4
  transplantation Z60.3
Sodoku A25.0
Soemmerring's ring — see Cataract, secondary
Soft — see also condition
  nails L60.3
Softening
  bone — see Osteomalacia
  brain (necrotic) (progressive) G93.89
    congenital Q04.0
    embolic I63.4- ☑

Subterms under main terms may continue to next column or page   ☑ Additional Character Required — Refer to the Tabular List for Character Selection   **287**

Simultanagnosia — Softening

Softening — continued
- brain — continued
  - hemorrhagic — see Hemorrhage, intracranial, intracerebral
    - occlusive I63.5- ☑
    - thrombotic I63.3- ☑
  - cartilage M94.2- ☑
    - patella M22.4- ☑
  - cerebellar — see Softening, brain
  - cerebral — see Softening, brain
  - cerebrospinal — see Softening, brain
  - myocardial, heart — see Degeneration, myocardial
  - spinal cord G95.89
  - stomach K31.89
- **Soldier's**
  - heart F45.8
  - patches I31.0
- **Solitary**
  - cyst, kidney N28.1
  - kidney, congenital Q60.0
- **Solvent abuse** — see Abuse, drug, inhalant
  - dependence — see Dependence, drug, inhalant
- **Somatization reaction, somatic reaction** — see Disorder, somatoform
- **Somnambulism** F51.3
  - hysterical F44.89
- **Somnolence** R40.0
  - nonorganic origin F51.11
- **Sonne dysentery** A03.3
- **Soor** B37.0
- **Sore**
  - bed — see Ulcer, pressure, by site
  - chiclero B55.1
  - Delhi B55.1
  - desert — see Ulcer, skin
  - eye H57.1- ☑
  - Lahore B55.1
  - mouth K13.79
    - canker K12.0
  - muscle M79.10
  - Naga — see Ulcer, skin
  - of skin — see Ulcer, skin
  - oriental B55.1
  - pressure — see Ulcer, pressure, by site
  - skin L98.9
  - soft A57
  - throat (acute) — see also Pharyngitis
    - with influenza, flu, or grippe — see Influenza, with, respiratory manifestations NEC
    - chronic J31.2
    - coxsackie (virus) B08.5
    - diphtheritic A36.0
    - herpesviral B00.2
    - influenzal — see Influenza, with, respiratory manifestations NEC
    - septic J02.0
    - streptococcal (ulcerative) J02.0
    - viral NEC J02.8
      - coxsackie B08.5
  - tropical — see Ulcer, skin
  - veldt — see Ulcer, skin
- **Soto's syndrome** (cerebral gigantism) Q87.3
- **South African cardiomyopathy syndrome** I42.8
- **Southeast Asian hemorrhagic fever** A91
- **Spacing**
  - abnormal, tooth, teeth, fully erupted M26.30
  - excessive, tooth, fully erupted M26.32
- **Spade-like hand** (congenital) Q68.1
- **Spading nail** L60.8
  - congenital Q84.6
- **Spanish collar** N47.1
- **Sparganosis** B70.1
- **Spasm**(s), **spastic, spasticity** — see also condition R25.2
  - accommodation — see Spasm, of accommodation
  - ampulla of Vater K83.4
  - anus, ani (sphincter) (reflex) K59.4
    - psychogenic F45.8
  - artery I73.9
    - cerebral G45.9
  - Bell's G51.3- ☑
  - bladder (sphincter, external or internal) N32.89
    - psychogenic F45.8
  - bronchus, bronchiole J98.01
  - cardia K22.0
  - cardiac I20.1
  - carpopedal — see Tetany
  - cerebral (arteries) (vascular) G45.9

Spasm(s), **spastic, spasticity** — continued
- cervix, complicating delivery O62.4
- ciliary body (of accommodation) — see Spasm, of accommodation
- colon — see also Irritable, bowel K58.9
  - with diarrhea K58.0
  - psychogenic F45.8
- common duct K83.8
- compulsive — see Tic
- conjugate H51.8
- coronary (artery) I20.1
- diaphragm (reflex) R06.6
  - epidemic B33.0
  - psychogenic F45.8
- duodenum K59.8
- epidemic diaphragmatic (transient) B33.0
- esophagus (diffuse) K22.4
  - psychogenic F45.8
- facial G51.3- ☑
- fallopian tube N83.8
- gastrointestinal (tract) K31.89
  - psychogenic F45.8
- glottis J38.5
  - hysterical F44.4
  - psychogenic F45.8
    - conversion reaction F44.4
  - reflex through recurrent laryngeal nerve J38.5
- habit — see Tic
- heart I20.1
- hemifacial (clonic) G51.3- ☑
- hourglass — see Contraction, hourglass
- hysterical F44.4
- infantile — see Epilepsy, spasms
- inferior oblique, eye H51.8
- intestinal — see also Syndrome, irritable bowel K58.9
  - psychogenic F45.8
- larynx, laryngeal J38.5
  - hysterical F44.4
  - psychogenic F45.8
    - conversion reaction F44.4
- levator palpebrae superioris — see Disorder, eyelid function
- muscle NEC M62.838
  - back M62.830
- nerve, trigeminal G51.0
- nervous F45.8
- nodding F98.4
- occupational F48.8
- oculogyric H51.8
  - psychogenic F45.8
- of accommodation H52.53- ☑
- ophthalmic artery — see Occlusion, artery, retina
- perineal, female N94.89
- peroneo-extensor — see also Deformity, limb, flat foot
- pharynx (reflex) J39.2
  - hysterical F45.8
  - psychogenic F45.8
- psychogenic F45.8
- pylorus NEC K31.3
  - adult hypertrophic K31.89
  - congenital or infantile Q40.0
  - psychogenic F45.8
- rectum (sphincter) K59.4
  - psychogenic F45.8
- retinal (artery) — see Occlusion, artery, retina
- sigmoid — see also Syndrome, irritable bowel K58.9
  - psychogenic F45.8
- sphincter of Oddi K83.4
- stomach K31.89
  - neurotic F45.8
- throat J39.2
  - hysterical F45.8
  - psychogenic F45.8
- tic F95.9
  - chronic F95.1
  - transient of childhood F95.0
- tongue K14.8
- torsion (progressive) G24.1
- trigeminal nerve — see Neuralgia, trigeminal
- ureter N13.5
- urethra (sphincter) N35.919
- uterus N85.8
  - complicating labor O62.4
- vagina N94.2
  - psychogenic F52.5
- vascular I73.9
- vasomotor I73.9
- vein NEC I87.8

Spasm(s), **spastic, spasticity** — continued
- viscera — see Pain, abdominal
- **Spasmodic** — see condition
- **Spasmophilia** — see Tetany
- **Spasmus nutans** F98.4
- **Spastic, spasticity** — see also Spasm
  - child (cerebral) (congenital) (paralysis) G80.1
- **Speaker's throat** R49.8
- **Specific, specified** — see condition
- **Speech**
  - defect, disorder, disturbance, impediment R47.9
    - psychogenic, in childhood and adolescence F98.8
    - slurring R47.81
    - specified NEC R47.89
- **Spencer's disease** A08.19
- **Spens' syndrome** (syncope with heart block) I45.9
- **Sperm counts** (fertility testing) Z31.41
  - postvasectomy Z30.8
  - reversal Z31.42
- **Spermatic cord** — see condition
- **Spermatocele** N43.40
  - congenital Q55.4
  - multiple N43.42
  - single N43.41
- **Spermatocystitis** N49.0
- **Spermatocytoma** C62.9- ☑
  - specified site — see Neoplasm, malignant, by site
- **Spermatorrhea** N50.89
- **Sphacelus** — see Gangrene
- **Sphenoidal** — see condition
- **Sphenoiditis** (chronic) — see Sinusitis, sphenoidal
- **Sphenopalatine ganglion neuralgia** G90.09
- **Sphericity, increased, lens** (congenital) Q12.4
- **Spherocytosis** (congenital) (familial) (hereditary) D58.0
  - hemoglobin disease D58.0
  - sickle-cell (disease) D57.8- ☑
- **Spherophakia** Q12.4
- **Sphincter** — see condition
- **Sphincteritis, sphincter of Oddi** — see Cholangitis
- **Sphingolipidosis** E75.3
  - specified NEC E75.29
- **Sphingomyelinosis** E75.3
- **Spicule tooth** K00.2
- **Spider**
  - bite — see Toxicity, venom, spider
  - fingers — see Syndrome, Marfan's
  - nevus I78.1
  - toes — see Syndrome, Marfan's
  - vascular I78.1
- **Spiegler-Fendt**
  - benign lymphocytoma L98.8
  - sarcoid L08.89
- **Spielmeyer-Vogt disease** E75.4
- **Spina bifida** (aperta) Q05.9
  - with hydrocephalus NEC Q05.4
  - cervical Q05.5
    - with hydrocephalus Q05.0
  - dorsal Q05.6
    - with hydrocephalus Q05.1
  - lumbar Q05.7
    - with hydrocephalus Q05.2
  - lumbosacral Q05.7
    - with hydrocephalus Q05.2
  - occulta Q76.0
  - sacral Q05.8
    - with hydrocephalus Q05.3
  - thoracic Q05.6
    - with hydrocephalus Q05.1
  - thoracolumbar Q05.6
    - with hydrocephalus Q05.1
- **Spindle, Krukenberg's** — see Pigmentation, cornea, posterior
- **Spine, spinal** — see condition
- **Spiradenoma** (eccrine) — see Neoplasm, skin, benign
- **Spirillosis** A25.0
- **Spirillum**
  - minus A25.0
  - obermeieri infection A68.0
- **Spirochetal** — see condition
- **Spirochetosis** A69.9
  - arthritic, arthritica A69.9
  - bronchopulmonary A69.8
  - icterohemorrhagic A27.0
  - lung A69.8
- **Spirometrosis** B70.1
- **Spitting blood** — see Hemoptysis
- **Splanchnoptosis** K63.4

Spleen, splenic — *see* condition
Splenectasis — *see* Splenomegaly
Splenitis (interstitial) (malignant) (nonspecific) D73.89
  malarial — *see also* Malaria B54 *[D77]*
  tuberculous A18.85
Splenocele D73.89
Splenomegaly, splenomegalia (Bengal) (cryptogenic)
    (idiopathic) (tropical) R16.1
  with hepatomegaly R16.2
  cirrhotic D73.2
  congenital Q89.09
  congestive, chronic D73.2
  Egyptian B65.1
  Gaucher's E75.22
  malarial — *see also* Malaria B54 *[D77]*
  neutropenic D73.81
  Niemann-Pick — *see* Niemann-Pick disease or syndrome
  sideritic D73.2
  syphilitic A52.79
    congenital (early) A50.08 *[D77]*
Splenopathy D73.9
Splenoptosis D73.89
Splenosis D73.89
Splinter — *see* Foreign body, superficial, by site
Split, splitting
  foot Q72.7- ☑
  hand Q71.6 ☑
  heart sounds R01.2
  lip, congenital — *see* Cleft, lip
  nails L60.3
  urinary stream R39.13
Spondylarthrosis — *see* Spondylosis
Spondylitis (chronic) — *see also* Spondylopathy, inflammatory
  ankylopoietica — *see* Spondylitis, ankylosing
  ankylosing (chronic) M45.9
    with lung involvement M45.9 *[J99]*
    cervical region M45.2
    cervicothoracic region M45.3
    juvenile M08.1
    lumbar region M45.6
    lumbosacral region M45.7
    multiple sites M45.0
    occipito-atlanto-axial region M45.1
    sacrococcygeal region M45.8
    thoracic region M45.4
    thoracolumbar region M45.5
  atrophic (ligamentous) — *see* Spondylitis, ankylosing
  deformans (chronic) — *see* Spondylosis
  gonococcal A54.41
  gouty — *see also* Gout, by type, vertebrae M10.08
  in (due to)
    brucellosis A23.9 *[M49.80]*
      cervical region A23.9 *[M49.82]*
      cervicothoracic region A23.9 *[M49.83]*
      lumbar region A23.9 *[M49.86]*
      lumbosacral region A23.9 *[M49.87]*
      multiple sites A23.9 *[M49.89]*
      occipito-atlanto-axial region A23.9 *[M49.81]*
      sacrococcygeal region A23.9 *[M49.88]*
      thoracic region A23.9 *[M49.84]*
      thoracolumbar region A23.9 *[M49.85]*
    enterobacteria — *see also* subcategory M49.8 A04.9
    tuberculosis A18.01
  infectious NEC — *see* Spondylopathy, infective
  juvenile ankylosing (chronic) M08.1
  Kümmell's — *see* Spondylopathy, traumatic
  Marie-Strümpell — *see* Spondylitis, ankylosing
  muscularis — *see* Spondylopathy, specified NEC
  psoriatic L40.53
  rheumatoid — *see* Spondylitis, ankylosing
  rhizomelica — *see* Spondylitis, ankylosing
  sacroiliac NEC M46.1
  senescent, senile — *see* Spondylosis
  traumatic (chronic) or post-traumatic — *see* Spondylopathy, traumatic
  tuberculous A18.01
  typhosa A01.05
Spondylolisthesis (acquired) (degenerative) M43.10
  with disproportion (fetopelvic) O33.0
    causing obstructed labor O65.0
  cervical region M43.12
  cervicothoracic region M43.13
  congenital Q76.2
  lumbar region M43.16
  lumbosacral region M43.17

Spondylolisthesis — *continued*
  multiple sites M43.19
  occipito-atlanto-axial region M43.11
  sacrococcygeal region M43.18
  thoracic region M43.14
  thoracolumbar region M43.15
  traumatic (old) M43.10
    acute
      fifth cervical (displaced) S12.430 ☑
        nondisplaced S12.431 ☑
        specified type NEC (displaced) S12.450 ☑
          nondisplaced S12.451 ☑
        type III S12.44 ☑
      fourth cervical (displaced) S12.330 ☑
        nondisplaced S12.331 ☑
        specified type NEC (displaced) S12.350 ☑
          nondisplaced S12.351 ☑
        type III S12.34 ☑
      second cervical (displaced) S12.130 ☑
        nondisplaced S12.131 ☑
        specified type NEC (displaced) S12.150 ☑
          nondisplaced S12.151 ☑
        type III S12.14 ☑
      seventh cervical (displaced) S12.630 ☑
        nondisplaced S12.631 ☑
        specified type NEC (displaced) S12.650 ☑
          nondisplaced S12.651 ☑
        type III S12.64 ☑
      sixth cervical (displaced) S12.530 ☑
        nondisplaced S12.531 ☑
        specified type NEC (displaced) S12.550 ☑
          nondisplaced S12.551 ☑
        type III S12.54 ☑
      third cervical (displaced) S12.230 ☑
        nondisplaced S12.231 ☑
        specified type NEC (displaced) S12.250 ☑
          nondisplaced S12.251 ☑
        type III S12.24 ☑
Spondylolysis (acquired) M43.00
  cervical region M43.02
  cervicothoracic region M43.03
  congenital Q76.2
  lumbar region M43.06
  lumbosacral region M43.07
    with disproportion (fetopelvic) O33.0
      causing obstructed labor O65.8
  multiple sites M43.09
  occipito-atlanto-axial region M43.01
  sacrococcygeal region M43.08
  thoracic region M43.04
  thoracolumbar region M43.05
Spondylopathy M48.9
  infective NEC M46.50
    cervical region M46.52
    cervicothoracic region M46.53
    lumbar region M46.56
    lumbosacral region M46.57
    multiple sites M46.59
    occipito-atlanto-axial region M46.51
    sacrococcygeal region M46.58
    thoracic region M46.54
    thoracolumbar region M46.55
  inflammatory M46.90
    cervical region M46.92
    cervicothoracic region M46.93
    lumbar region M46.96
    lumbosacral region M46.97
    multiple sites M46.99
    occipito-atlanto-axial region M46.91
    sacrococcygeal region M46.98
    specified type NEC M46.80
      cervical region M46.82
      cervicothoracic region M46.83
      lumbar region M46.86
      lumbosacral region M46.87
      multiple sites M46.89
      occipito-atlanto-axial region M46.81
      sacrococcygeal region M46.88
      thoracic region M46.84
      thoracolumbar region M46.85
    thoracic region M46.94
    thoracolumbar region M46.95
  neuropathic, in
    syringomyelia and syringobulbia G95.0
    tabes dorsalis A52.11
  specified NEC — *see* subcategory M48.8 ☑
  traumatic M48.30

Spondylopathy — *continued*
  traumatic — *continued*
    cervical region M48.32
    cervicothoracic region M48.33
    lumbar region M48.36
    lumbosacral region M48.37
    occipito-atlanto-axial region M48.31
    sacrococcygeal region M48.38
    thoracic region M48.34
    thoracolumbar region M48.35
Spondylosis M47.9
  with
    disproportion (fetopelvic) O33.0
      causing obstructed labor O65.0
    myelopathy NEC M47.10
      cervical region M47.12
      cervicothoracic region M47.13
      lumbar region M47.16
      occipito-atlanto-axial region M47.11
      thoracic region M47.14
      thoracolumbar region M47.15
    radiculopathy M47.20
      cervical region M47.22
      cervicothoracic region M47.23
      lumbar region M47.26
      lumbosacral region M47.27
      occipito-atlanto-axial region M47.21
      sacrococcygeal region M47.28
      thoracic region M47.24
      thoracolumbar region M47.25
  specified NEC M47.899
    cervical region M47.892
    cervicothoracic region M47.893
    lumbar region M47.896
    lumbosacral region M47.897
    occipito-atlanto-axial region M47.891
    sacrococcygeal region M47.898
    thoracic region M47.894
    thoracolumbar region M47.895
  traumatic — *see* Spondylopathy, traumatic
  without myelopathy or radiculopathy M47.819
    cervical region M47.812
    cervicothoracic region M47.813
    lumbar region M47.816
    lumbosacral region M47.817
    occipito-atlanto-axial region M47.811
    sacrococcygeal region M47.818
    thoracic region M47.814
    thoracolumbar region M47.815
Sponge
  inadvertently left in operation wound — *see* Foreign body, accidentally left during a procedure
  kidney (medullary) Q61.5
Sponge-diver's disease — *see* Toxicity, venom, marine animal, sea anemone
Spongioblastoma (any type) — *see* Neoplasm, malignant, by site
  specified site — *see* Neoplasm, malignant, by site
  unspecified site C71.9
Spongioneuroblastoma — *see* Neoplasm, malignant, by site
Spontaneous — *see also* condition
  fracture (cause unknown) — *see* Fracture, pathological
Spoon nail L60.3
  congenital Q84.6
Sporadic — *see* condition
Sporothrix schenckii infection — *see* Sporotrichosis
Sporotrichosis B42.9
  arthritis B42.82
  disseminated B42.7
  generalized B42.7
  lymphocutaneous (fixed) (progressive) B42.1
  pulmonary B42.0
  specified NEC B42.89
Spots, spotting (in) (of)
  Bitot's — *see also* Pigmentation, conjunctiva
    in the young child E50.1
    vitamin A deficiency E50.1
  café, au lait L81.3
  Cayenne pepper I78.1
  cotton wool, retina — *see* Occlusion, artery, retina
  de Morgan's (senile angiomas) I78.1
  Fuchs' black (myopic) — *see also* Myopia, degenerative H44.2- ☑
  intermenstrual (regular) N92.0
    irregular N92.1
  Koplik's B05.9
  liver L81.4

Spots, spotting — *continued*
   pregnancy O26.85- ☑
   purpuric R23.3
   ruby I78.1
Spotted fever — *see* Fever, spotted N92.3
Sprain (joint) (ligament)
   acromioclavicular joint or ligament S43.5- ☑
   ankle S93.40- ☑
     calcaneofibular ligament S93.41- ☑
     deltoid ligament S93.42- ☑
     internal collateral ligament — *see* Sprain, ankle, specified ligament NEC
     specified ligament NEC S93.49- ☑
     talofibular ligament — *see* Sprain, ankle, specified ligament NEC
     tibiofibular ligament S93.43- ☑
   anterior longitudinal, cervical S13.4 ☑
   atlas, atlanto-axial, atlanto-occipital S13.4 ☑
   breast bone — *see* Sprain, sternum
   calcaneofibular — *see* Sprain, ankle
   carpal — *see* Sprain, wrist
   carpometacarpal — *see* Sprain, hand, specified site NEC
   cartilage
     costal S23.41 ☑
     semilunar (knee) — *see* Sprain, knee, specified site NEC
       with current tear — *see* Tear, meniscus
     thyroid region S13.5 ☑
     xiphoid — *see* Sprain, sternum
   cervical, cervicodorsal, cervicothoracic S13.4 ☑
   chondrosternal S23.421 ☑
   coracoclavicular S43.8- ☑
   coracohumeral S43.41- ☑
   coronary, knee — *see* Sprain, knee, specified site NEC
   costal cartilage S23.41 ☑
   cricoarytenoid articulation or ligament S13.5 ☑
   cricothyroid articulation S13.5 ☑
   cruciate, knee — *see* Sprain, knee, cruciate
   deltoid, ankle — *see* Sprain, ankle
   dorsal (spine) S23.3 ☑
   elbow S53.40- ☑
     radial collateral ligament S53.43- ☑
     radiohumeral S53.41- ☑
     rupture
       radial collateral ligament — *see* Rupture, traumatic, ligament, radial collateral
       ulnar collateral ligament — *see* Rupture, traumatic, ligament, ulnar collateral
     specified type NEC S53.49- ☑
     ulnar collateral ligament S53.44- ☑
     ulnohumeral S53.42- ☑
   femur, head — *see* Sprain, hip
   fibular collateral, knee — *see* Sprain, knee, collateral
   fibulocalcaneal — *see* Sprain, ankle
   finger(s) S63.61- ☑
     index S63.61- ☑
     interphalangeal (joint) S63.63- ☑
       index S63.63- ☑
       little S63.63- ☑
       middle S63.63- ☑
       ring S63.63- ☑
     little S63.61- ☑
     metacarpophalangeal (joint) S63.65- ☑
     middle S63.61- ☑
     ring S63.61- ☑
     specified site NEC S63.69- ☑
       index S63.69- ☑
       little S63.69- ☑
       middle S63.69- ☑
       ring S63.69- ☑
   foot S93.60- ☑
     specified ligament NEC S93.69- ☑
     tarsal ligament S93.61- ☑
     tarsometatarsal ligament S93.62- ☑
     toe — *see* Sprain, toe
   hand S63.9- ☑
     finger — *see* Sprain, finger
     specified site NEC — *see* subcategory S63.8 ☑
     thumb — *see* Sprain, thumb
   head S03.9 ☑
   hip S73.10- ☑
     iliofemoral ligament S73.11- ☑
     ischiocapsular (ligament) S73.12- ☑
     specified NEC S73.19- ☑
   iliofemoral — *see* Sprain, hip

Sprain — *continued*
   innominate
     acetabulum — *see* Sprain, hip
     sacral junction S33.6 ☑
   internal
     collateral, ankle — *see* Sprain, ankle
     semilunar cartilage — *see* Sprain, knee, specified site NEC
   interphalangeal
     finger — *see* Sprain, finger, interphalangeal (joint)
     toe — *see* Sprain, toe, interphalangeal joint
   ischiocapsular — *see* Sprain, hip
   ischiofemoral — *see* Sprain, hip
   jaw (articular disc) (cartilage) (meniscus) S03.4- ☑
     old M26.69
   knee S83.9- ☑
     collateral ligament S83.40- ☑
       lateral (fibular) S83.42- ☑
       medial (tibial) S83.41- ☑
     cruciate ligament S83.50- ☑
       anterior S83.51- ☑
       posterior S83.52- ☑
     lateral (fibular) collateral ligament S83.42- ☑
     medial (tibial) collateral ligament S83.41- ☑
     patellar ligament S76.11- ☑
     specified site NEC S83.8X- ☑
     superior tibiofibular joint (ligament) S83.6- ☑
   lateral collateral, knee — *see* Sprain, knee, collateral
   lumbar (spine) S33.5 ☑
   lumbosacral S33.9 ☑
   mandible (articular disc) S03.4- ☑
     old M26.69
   medial collateral, knee — *see* Sprain, knee, collateral
   meniscus
     jaw S03.4- ☑
       old M26.69
     knee — *see* Sprain, knee, specified site NEC
       with current tear — *see* Tear, meniscus
         old — *see* Derangement, knee, meniscus, due to old tear
     mandible S03.4- ☑
       old M26.69
   metacarpal (distal) (proximal) — *see* Sprain, hand, specified site NEC
   metacarpophalangeal — *see* Sprain, finger, metacarpophalangeal (joint)
   metatarsophalangeal — *see* Sprain, toe, metatarsophalangeal joint
   midcarpal — *see* Sprain, hand, specified site NEC
   midtarsal — *see* Sprain, foot, specified site NEC
   neck S13.9 ☑
     anterior longitudinal cervical ligament S13.4 ☑
     atlanto-axial joint S13.4 ☑
     atlanto-occipital joint S13.4 ☑
     cervical spine S13.4 ☑
     cricoarytenoid ligament S13.5 ☑
     cricothyroid ligament S13.5 ☑
     specified site NEC S13.8 ☑
     thyroid region (cartilage) S13.5 ☑
   nose S03.8 ☑
   orbicular, hip — *see* Sprain, hip
   patella — *see* Sprain, knee, specified site NEC
   patellar ligament S76.11- ☑
   pelvis NEC S33.8 ☑
   phalanx
     finger — *see* Sprain, finger
     toe — *see* Sprain, toe
   pubofemoral — *see* Sprain, hip
   radiocarpal — *see* Sprain, wrist
   radiohumeral — *see* Sprain, elbow
   radius, collateral — *see* Rupture, traumatic, ligament, radial collateral
   rib (cage) S23.41 ☑
   rotator cuff (capsule) S43.42- ☑
   sacroiliac (region)
     chronic or old — *see* subcategory M53.2 ☑
     joint S33.6 ☑
   scaphoid (hand) — *see* Sprain, hand, specified site NEC
   scapula (r) — *see* Sprain, shoulder girdle, specified site NEC
   semilunar cartilage (knee) — *see* Sprain, knee, specified site NEC
     with current tear — *see* Tear, meniscus
       old — *see* Derangement, knee, meniscus, due to old tear
   shoulder joint S43.40- ☑

Sprain — *continued*
   shoulder joint — *continued*
     acromioclavicular joint (ligament) — *see* Sprain, acromioclavicular joint
     blade — *see* Sprain, shoulder, girdle, specified site NEC
     coracoclavicular joint (ligament) — *see* Sprain, coracoclavicular joint
     coracohumeral ligament — *see* Sprain, coracohumeral joint
     girdle S43.9- ☑
       specified site NEC S43.8- ☑
     rotator cuff — *see* Sprain, rotator cuff
     specified site NEC S43.49- ☑
     sternoclavicular joint (ligament) — *see* Sprain, sternoclavicular joint
   spine
     cervical S13.4 ☑
     lumbar S33.5 ☑
     thoracic S23.3 ☑
   sternoclavicular joint S43.6- ☑
   sternum S23.429 ☑
     chondrosternal joint S23.421 ☑
     specified site NEC S23.428 ☑
     sternoclavicular (joint) (ligament) S23.420 ☑
   symphysis
     jaw S03.4- ☑
       old M26.69
     mandibular S03.4- ☑
       old M26.69
   talofibular — *see* Sprain, ankle
   tarsal — *see* Sprain, foot, specified site NEC
   tarsometatarsal — *see* Sprain, foot, specified site NEC
   temporomandibular S03.4- ☑
     old M26.69
   thorax S23.9 ☑
     ribs S23.41 ☑
     specified site NEC S23.8 ☑
     spine S23.3 ☑
     sternum — *see* Sprain, sternum
   thumb S63.60- ☑
     interphalangeal (joint) S63.62- ☑
     metacarpophalangeal (joint) S63.64- ☑
     specified site NEC S63.68- ☑
   thyroid cartilage or region S13.5 ☑
   tibia (proximal end) — *see* Sprain, knee, specified site NEC
   tibial collateral, knee — *see* Sprain, knee, collateral
   tibiofibular
     distal — *see* Sprain, ankle
     superior — *see* Sprain, knee, specified site NEC
   toe(s) S93.50- ☑
     great S93.50- ☑
     interphalangeal joint S93.51- ☑
       great S93.51- ☑
       lesser S93.51- ☑
     lesser S93.50- ☑
     metatarsophalangeal joint S93.52- ☑
       great S93.52- ☑
       lesser S93.52- ☑
   ulna, collateral — *see* Rupture, traumatic, ligament, ulnar collateral
   ulnohumeral — *see* Sprain, elbow
   wrist S63.50- ☑
     carpal S63.51- ☑
     radiocarpal S63.52- ☑
     specified site NEC S63.59- ☑
   xiphoid cartilage — *see* Sprain, sternum
Sprengel's deformity (congenital) Q74.0
Sprue (tropical) K90.1
   celiac K90.0
   idiopathic K90.49
   meaning thrush B37.0
   nontropical K90.0
Spur, bone — *see also* Enthesopathy
   calcaneal M77.3- ☑
   iliac crest M76.2- ☑
   nose (septum) J34.89
Spurway's syndrome Q78.0
Sputum
   abnormal (amount) (color) (odor) (purulent) R09.3
   blood-stained R04.2
   excessive (cause unknown) R09.3
Squamous — *see also* condition
   epithelium in
     cervical canal (congenital) Q51.828

Squamous — *continued*
  epithelium in — *continued*
    uterine mucosa (congenital) Q51.818
Squashed nose M95.Ø
  congenital Q67.4
Squeeze, diver's T70.3 ☑
Squint — *see also* Strabismus
  accommodative — *see* Strabismus, convergent concomitant
SSADHD (succinic semialdehyde dehydrogenase deficiency) E72.81
St. Hubert's disease A82.9
Stab — *see also* Laceration
  internal organs — *see* Injury, by site
Stafne's cyst or cavity M27.Ø
Staggering gait R26.Ø
  hysterical F44.4
Staghorn calculus — *see* Calculus, kidney
Stähli's line (cornea) (pigment) — *see* Pigmentation, cornea, anterior
Stain, staining
  meconium (newborn) P96.83
  port wine Q82.5
  tooth, teeth (hard tissues) (extrinsic) KØ3.6
    due to
      accretions KØ3.6
      deposits (betel) (black) (green) (materia alba) (orange) (soft) (tobacco) KØ3.6
      metals (copper) (silver) KØ3.7
      nicotine KØ3.6
      pulpal bleeding KØ3.7
      tobacco KØ3.6
    intrinsic KØØ.8
Stammering — *see also* Disorder, fluency F8Ø.81
Standstill
  auricular I45.5
  cardiac — *see* Arrest, cardiac
  sinoatrial I45.5
  ventricular — *see* Arrest, cardiac
Stannosis J63.5
Stanton's disease — *see* Melioidosis
Staphylitis (acute) (catarrhal) (chronic) (gangrenous) (membranous) (suppurative) (ulcerative) K12.2
Staphylococcal scalded skin syndrome LØØ
Staphylococcemia A41.2
Staphylococcus, staphylococcal — *see also* condition
  as cause of disease classified elsewhere B95.8
    aureus (methicillin susceptible) (MSSA) B95.61
      methicillin resistant (MRSA) B95.62
  specified NEC, as cause of disease classified elsewhere B95.7
Staphyloma (sclera)
  cornea H18.72- ☑
  equatorial H15.81- ☑
  localized (anterior) H15.82- ☑
  posticum H15.83- ☑
  ring H15.85- ☑
Stargardt's disease — *see* Dystrophy, retina
Starvation (inanition) (due to lack of food) T73.Ø ☑
  edema — *see* Malnutrition, severe
Stasis
  bile (noncalculous) K83.1
  bronchus J98.Ø9
    with infection — *see* Bronchitis
  cardiac — *see* Failure, heart, congestive
  cecum K59.8
  colon K59.8
  dermatitis I87.2
    with
      varicose ulcer — *see* Varix, leg, with ulcer, with inflammation
      varicose veins — *see* Varix, leg, with, inflammation
      due to postthrombotic syndrome — *see* Syndrome, postthrombotic
  duodenal K31.5
  eczema — *see* Varix, leg, with, inflammation
  edema — *see* Hypertension, venous (chronic), idiopathic
  foot T69.Ø- ☑
  ileocecal coil K59.8
  ileum K59.8
  intestinal K59.8
  jejunum K59.8
  kidney N19
  liver (cirrhotic) K76.1
  lymphatic I89.8

Stasis — *continued*
  pneumonia J18.2
  pulmonary — *see* Edema, lung
  rectal K59.8
  renal N19
    tubular N17.Ø
  ulcer — *see* Varix, leg, with, ulcer
    without varicose veins I87.2
  urine — *see* Retention, urine
  venous I87.8
State (of)
  affective and paranoid, mixed, organic psychotic FØ6.8
  agitated R45.1
    acute reaction to stress F43.Ø
  anxiety (neurotic) F41.1
  apprehension F41.1
  burn-out Z73.Ø
  climacteric, female Z78.Ø
    symptomatic N95.1
  compulsive F42.8
    mixed with obsessional thoughts F42.2
  confusional (psychogenic) F44.89
    acute — *see also* Delirium
      with
        arteriosclerotic dementia FØ1.5Ø
          with behavioral disturbance FØ1.51
        senility or dementia FØ5
      alcoholic F1Ø.231
      epileptic FØ5
      reactive (from emotional stress, psychological trauma) F44.89
      subacute — *see* Delirium
  convulsive — *see* Convulsions
  crisis F43.Ø
  depressive F32.9
    neurotic F34.1
  dissociative F44.9
  emotional shock (stress) R45.7
  hypercoagulation — *see* Hypercoagulable
  locked-in G83.5
  menopausal Z78.Ø
    symptomatic N95.1
  neurotic F48.9
    with depersonalization F48.1
  obsessional F42.8
  oneiroid (schizophrenia-like) F23
  organic
    hallucinatory (nonalcoholic) FØ6.Ø
    paranoid (-hallucinatory) FØ6.2
  panic F41.Ø
  paranoid F22
    climacteric F22
    involutional F22
    menopausal F22
    organic FØ6.2
    senile FØ3 ☑
    simple F22
  persistent vegetative R4Ø.3
  phobic F4Ø.9
  postleukotomy FØ7.Ø
  pregnant
    gestational carrier Z33.3
    incidental Z33.1
  psychogenic, twilight F44.89
  psychopathic (constitutional) F6Ø.2
  psychotic, organic — *see also* Psychosis, organic
    mixed paranoid and affective FØ6.8
    senile or presenile FØ3 ☑
    transient NEC FØ6.8
      with
        depression FØ6.31
        hallucinations FØ6.Ø
  residual schizophrenic F2Ø.5
  restlessness R45.1
  stress (emotional) R45.7
  tension (mental) F48.9
    specified NEC F48.8
  transient organic psychotic NEC FØ6.8
    depressive type FØ6.31
    hallucinatory type FØ6.Ø
  twilight
    epileptic FØ5
    psychogenic F44.89
  vegetative, persistent R4Ø.3
  vital exhaustion Z73.Ø
  withdrawal, — *see* Withdrawal, state
Status (post) — *see also* Presence (of)

Status — *continued*
  absence, epileptic — *see* Epilepsy, by type, with status epilepticus
  administration of tPA (rtPA) in a different facility within the last 24 hours prior to admission to current facility Z92.82
  adrenalectomy (unilateral) (bilateral) E89.6
  anastomosis Z98.Ø
  anginosus I2Ø.9
  angioplasty (peripheral) Z98.62
    with implant Z95.82Ø
    coronary artery Z98.61
      with implant Z95.5
  aortocoronary bypass Z95.1
  arthrodesis Z98.1
  artificial opening (of) Z93.9
    gastrointestinal tract Z93.4
    specified NEC Z93.8
    urinary tract Z93.6
    vagina Z93.8
  asthmaticus — *see* Asthma, by type, with status asthmaticus
  awaiting organ transplant Z76.82
  bariatric surgery Z98.84
  bed confinement Z74.Ø1
  bleb, filtering (vitreous), after glaucoma surgery Z98.83
  breast implant Z98.82
    removal Z98.86
  cataract extraction Z98.4- ☑
  cholecystectomy Z9Ø.49
  clitorectomy N9Ø.811
    with excision of labia minora N9Ø.812
  colectomy (complete) (partial) Z9Ø.49
  colonization — *see* Carrier (suspected) of
  colostomy Z93.3
  convulsivus idiopathicus — *see* Epilepsy, by type, with status epilepticus
  coronary artery angioplasty — *see* Status, angioplasty, coronary artery
  coronary artery bypass graft Z95.1
  cystectomy (urinary bladder) Z9Ø.6
  cystostomy Z93.5Ø
    appendico-vesicostomy Z93.52
    cutaneous Z93.51
    specified NEC Z93.59
  delinquent immunization Z28.3
  dental Z98.818
    crown Z98.811
    fillings Z98.811
    restoration Z98.811
    sealant Z98.81Ø
    specified NEC Z98.818
  deployment (current) (military) Z56.82
  dialysis (hemodialysis) (peritoneal) Z99.2
  do not resuscitate (DNR) Z66
  donor — *see* Donor
  embedded fragments — *see* Retained, foreign body fragments (type of)
  embedded splinter — *see* Retained, foreign body fragments (type of)
  enterostomy Z93.4
  epileptic, epilepticus — *see also* Epilepsy, by type, with status epilepticus G4Ø.9Ø1
  estrogen receptor
    negative Z17.1
    positive Z17.Ø
  female genital cutting — *see* Female genital mutilation status
  female genital mutilation — *see* Female genital mutilation status
  filtering (vitreous) bleb after glaucoma surgery Z98.83
  gastrectomy (complete) (partial) Z9Ø.3
  gastric banding Z98.84
  gastric bypass for obesity Z98.84
  gastrostomy Z93.1
  human immunodeficiency virus (HIV) infection, asymptomatic Z21
  hysterectomy (complete) (total) Z9Ø.71Ø
    partial (with remaining cervial stump) Z9Ø.711
  ileostomy Z93.2
  implant
    breast Z98.82
  infibulation N9Ø.813
  intestinal bypass Z98.Ø
  jejunostomy Z93.4
  lapsed immunization schedule Z28.3
  laryngectomy Z9Ø.Ø2
  lymphaticus E32.8

Status — *continued*
malignancy
castrate resistant prostate Z19.2
hormone resistant Z19.2
hormone sensitive Z19.1
marmoratus G80.3
mastectomy (unilateral) (bilateral) Z90.1- ☑
military deployment status (current) Z56.82
in theater or in support of military war, peacekeeping and humanitarian operations Z56.82
nephrectomy (unilateral) (bilateral) Z90.5
nephrostomy Z93.6
obesity surgery Z98.84
oophorectomy
bilateral Z90.722
unilateral Z90.721
organ replacement
by artificial or mechanical device or prosthesis of
artery Z95.828
bladder Z96.0
blood vessel Z95.828
breast Z97.8
eye globe Z97.0
heart Z95.812
valve Z95.2
intestine Z97.8
joint Z96.60
hip — *see* Presence, hip joint implant
knee — *see* Presence, knee joint implant
specified site NEC Z96.698
kidney Z97.8
larynx Z96.3
lens Z96.1
limbs — *see* Presence, artificial, limb
liver Z97.8
lung Z97.8
pancreas Z97.8
by organ transplant (heterologous)(homologous) — *see* Transplant
pacemaker
brain Z96.89
cardiac Z95.0
specified NEC Z96.89
pancreatectomy Z90.410
complete Z90.410
partial Z90.411
total Z90.410
physical restraint Z78.1
pneumonectomy (complete) (partial) Z90.2
pneumothorax, therapeutic Z98.3
postcommotio cerebri F07.81
postoperative (postprocedural) NEC Z98.890
breast implant Z98.82
dental Z98.818
crown Z98.811
fillings Z98.811
restoration Z98.811
sealant Z98.810
specified NEC Z98.818
pneumothorax, therapeutic Z98.3
uterine scar Z98.891
postpartum (routine follow-up) Z39.2
care immediately after delivery Z39.0
postsurgical (postprocedural) NEC Z98.890
pneumothorax, therapeutic Z98.3
pregnancy, incidental Z33.1
prosthesis coronary angioplasty Z95.5
pseudophakia Z96.1
renal dialysis (hemodialysis) (peritoneal) Z99.2
retained foreign body — *see* Retained, foreign body fragments (type of)
reversed jejunal transposition (for bypass) Z98.0
salpingo-oophorectomy
bilateral Z90.722
unilateral Z90.721
sex reassignment surgery status Z87.890
shunt
arteriovenous (for dialysis) Z99.2
cerebrospinal fluid Z98.2
ventricular (communicating) (for drainage) Z98.2
splenectomy Z90.81
thymicolymphaticus E32.8
thymicus E32.8
thymolymphaticus E32.8
thyroidectomy (hypothyroidism) E89.0
tooth (teeth) extraction — *see also* Absence, teeth, acquired K08.409

Status — *continued*
tPA (rtPA) administration in a different facility within the last 24 hours prior to admission to current facility Z92.82
tracheostomy Z93.0
transplant — *see* Transplant
organ removed Z98.85
tubal ligation Z98.51
underimmunization Z28.3
ureterostomy Z93.6
urethrostomy Z93.6
vagina, artificial Z93.8
vasectomy Z98.52
wheelchair confinement Z99.3
Stealing
child problem F91.8
in company with others Z72.810
pathological (compulsive) F63.2
Steam burn — *see* Burn
Steatocystoma multiplex L72.2
Steatohepatitis (nonalcoholic) (NASH) K75.81
Steatoma L72.3
eyelid (cystic) — *see* Dermatosis, eyelid
infected — *see* Hordeolum
Steatorrhea (chronic) K90.9
with lacteal obstruction K90.2
idiopathic (adult) (infantile) K90.9
pancreatic K90.3
primary K90.0
tropical K90.1
Steatosis E88.89
heart — *see* Degeneration, myocardial
kidney N28.89
liver NEC K76.0
Steele-Richardson-Olszewski disease or syndrome G23.1
Steinbrocker's syndrome G90.8
Steinert's disease G71.11
Stein-Leventhal syndrome E28.2
Stein's syndrome E28.2
STEMI — *see also* Infarct, myocardium, ST elevation I21.3
Stenocardia I20.8
Stenocephaly Q75.8
Stenosis, stenotic (cicatricial) — *see also* Stricture
ampulla of Vater K83.1
anus, anal (canal) (sphincter) K62.4
and rectum K62.4
congenital Q42.3
with fistula Q42.2
aorta (ascending) (supraventricular) (congenital) Q25.1
arteriosclerotic I70.0
calcified I70.0
supravalvular Q25.3
aortic (valve) I35.0
with insufficiency I35.2
congenital Q23.0
rheumatic I06.0
with
incompetency, insufficiency or regurgitation I06.2
with mitral (valve) disease I08.0
with tricuspid (valve) disease I08.3
mitral (valve) disease I08.0
with tricuspid (valve) disease I08.3
tricuspid (valve) disease I08.2
with mitral (valve) disease I08.3
specified cause NEC I35.0
syphilitic A52.03
aqueduct of Sylvius (congenital) Q03.0
with spina bifida — *see* Spina bifida, by site, with hydrocephalus
acquired G91.1
artery NEC — *see also* Arteriosclerosis I77.1
celiac I77.4
cerebral — *see* Occlusion, artery, cerebral
extremities — *see* Arteriosclerosis, extremities
precerebral — *see* Occlusion, artery, precerebral
pulmonary (congenital) Q25.6
acquired I28.8
renal I70.1
stent
coronary T82.855 ☑
peripheral T82.856 ☑
bile duct (common) (hepatic) K83.1
congenital Q44.3
bladder-neck (acquired) N32.0
congenital Q64.31
brain G93.89

Stenosis, stenotic — *continued*
bronchus J98.09
congenital Q32.3
syphilitic A52.72
cardia (stomach) K22.2
congenital Q39.3
cardiovascular — *see* Disease, cardiovascular
caudal M48.08
cervix, cervical (canal) N88.2
congenital Q51.828
in pregnancy or childbirth — *see* Pregnancy, complicated by, abnormal cervix
colon — *see also* Obstruction, intestine
congenital Q42.9
specified NEC Q42.8
colostomy K94.03
common (bile) duct K83.1
congenital Q44.3
coronary (artery) — *see* Disease, heart, ischemic, atherosclerotic
cystic duct — *see* Obstruction, gallbladder
due to presence of device, implant or graft — *see also* Complications, by site and type, specified NEC T85.858 ☑
arterial graft NEC T82.858 ☑
breast (implant) T85.858 ☑
catheter T85.858 ☑
dialysis (renal) T82.858 ☑
intraperitoneal T85.858 ☑
infusion NEC T82.858 ☑
spinal (epidural) (subdural) T85.850 ☑
urinary (indwelling) T83.85 ☑
fixation, internal (orthopedic) NEC T84.85 ☑
gastrointestinal (bile duct) (esophagus) T85.858 ☑
genital NEC T83.85 ☑
heart NEC T82.857 ☑
joint prosthesis T84.85 ☑
ocular (corneal graft) (orbital implant) NEC T85.858 ☑
orthopedic NEC T84.85 ☑
specified NEC T85.858 ☑
urinary NEC T83.85 ☑
vascular NEC T82.858 ☑
ventricular intracranial shunt T85.850 ☑
duodenum K31.5
congenital Q41.0
ejaculatory duct NEC N50.89
stent
vascular
end stent
adjacent to stent — *see* Arteriosclerosis
within the stent
coronary T82.855 ☑
peripheral T82.856 ☑
in stent
coronary vessel T82.855 ☑
peripheral vessel T82.856 ☑
endocervical os — *see* Stenosis, cervix
enterostomy K94.13
esophagus K22.2
congenital Q39.3
syphilitic A52.79
congenital A50.59 *[K23]*
eustachian tube — *see* Obstruction, eustachian tube
external ear canal (acquired) H61.30- ☑
congenital Q16.1
due to
inflammation H61.32- ☑
trauma H61.31- ☑
postprocedural H95.81- ☑
specified cause NEC H61.39- ☑
gallbladder — *see* Obstruction, gallbladder
glottis J38.6
heart valve (congenital) Q24.8
aortic Q23.0
mitral Q23.2
pulmonary Q22.1
tricuspid Q22.4
hepatic duct K83.1
hymen N89.6
hypertrophic subaortic (idiopathic) I42.1
ileum — *see also* Obstruction, intestine, specified NEC K56.699
congenital Q41.2
infundibulum cardia Q24.3
intervertebral foramina — *see also* Lesion, biomechanical, specified NEC

☑ **Additional Character Required** — **Refer to the Tabular List for Character Selection**   ▽ **Subterms under main terms may continue to next column or page**

Stenosis, stenotic — *continued*
  intervertebral foramina — *see also* Lesion, biomechan-
    ical, specified — *continued*
    connective tissue M99.79
      abdomen M99.79
      cervical region M99.71
      cervicothoracic M99.71
      head region M99.70
      lumbar region M99.73
      lumbosacral M99.73
      occipitocervical M99.70
      sacral region M99.74
      sacrococcygeal M99.74
      sacroiliac M99.74
      specified NEC M99.79
      thoracic region M99.72
      thoracolumbar M99.72
    disc M99.79
      abdomen M99.79
      cervical region M99.71
      cervicothoracic M99.71
      head region M99.70
      lower extremity M99.76
      lumbar region M99.73
      lumbosacral M99.73
      occipitocervical M99.70
      pelvic M99.75
      rib cage M99.78
      sacral region M99.74
      sacrococcygeal M99.74
      sacroiliac M99.74
      specified NEC M99.79
      thoracic region M99.72
      thoracolumbar M99.72
      upper extremity M99.77
    osseous M99.69
      abdomen M99.69
      cervical region M99.61
      cervicothoracic M99.61
      head region M99.60
      lower extremity M99.66
      lumbar region M99.63
      lumbosacral M99.63
      occipitocervical M99.60
      pelvic M99.65
      rib cage M99.68
      sacral region M99.64
      sacrococcygeal M99.64
      sacroiliac M99.64
      specified NEC M99.69
      thoracic region M99.62
      thoracolumbar M99.62
      upper extremity M99.67
    subluxation — *see* Stenosis, intervertebral foramina,
      osseous
  intestine — *see also* Obstruction, intestine
    congenital (small) Q41.9
      large Q42.9
        specified NEC Q42.8
      specified NEC Q41.8
  jejunum — *see also* Obstruction, intestine, specified
    NEC K56.699
    congenital Q41.1
  lacrimal (passage)
    canaliculi H04.54- ☑
    congenital Q10.5
    duct H04.55- ☑
    punctum H04.56- ☑
    sac H04.57- ☑
  lacrimonasal duct — *see* Stenosis, lacrimal, duct
    congenital Q10.5
  larynx J38.6
    congenital NEC Q31.8
      subglottic Q31.1
    syphilitic A52.73
      congenital A50.59 [J99]
  mitral (chronic) (inactive) (valve) I05.0
    with
      aortic valve disease I08.0
      incompetency, insufficiency or regurgitation
        I05.2
    active or acute I01.1
      with rheumatic or Sydenham's chorea I02.0
    congenital Q23.2
    specified cause, except rheumatic I34.2
    syphilitic A52.03
  myocardium, myocardial — *see also* Degeneration,
    myocardial

Stenosis, stenotic — *continued*
  myocardium, myocardial — *see also* Degeneration,
    myocardial — *continued*
    hypertrophic subaortic (idiopathic) I42.1
  nares (anterior) (posterior) J34.89
    congenital Q30.0
  nasal duct — *see also* Stenosis, lacrimal, duct
    congenital Q10.5
  nasolacrimal duct — *see also* Stenosis, lacrimal, duct
    congenital Q10.5
  neural canal — *see also* Lesion, biomechanical, speci-
    fied NEC
    connective tissue M99.49
      abdomen M99.49
      cervical region M99.41
      cervicothoracic M99.41
      head region M99.40
      lower extremity M99.46
      lumbar region M99.43
      lumbosacral M99.43
      occipitocervical M99.40
      pelvic M99.45
      rib cage M99.48
      sacral region M99.44
      sacrococcygeal M99.44
      sacroiliac M99.44
      specified NEC M99.49
      thoracic region M99.42
      thoracolumbar M99.42
      upper extremity M99.47
    intervertebral disc M99.59
      abdomen M99.59
      cervical region M99.51
      cervicothoracic M99.51
      head region M99.50
      lower extremity M99.56
      lumbar region M99.53
      lumbosacral M99.53
      occipitocervical M99.50
      pelvic M99.55
      rib cage M99.58
      sacral region M99.54
      sacrococcygeal M99.54
      sacroiliac M99.54
      specified NEC M99.59
      thoracic region M99.52
      thoracolumbar M99.52
      upper extremity M99.57
    osseous M99.39
      abdomen M99.39
      cervical region M99.31
      cervicothoracic M99.31
      head region M99.30
      lower extremity M99.36
      lumbar region M99.33
      lumbosacral M99.33
      occipitocervical M99.30
      pelvic M99.35
      rib cage M99.38
      sacral region M99.34
      sacrococcygeal M99.34
      sacroiliac M99.34
      specified NEC M99.39
      thoracic region M99.32
      thoracolumbar M99.32
      upper extremity M99.37
    subluxation M99.29
      cervical region M99.21
      cervicothoracic M99.21
      head region M99.20
      lower extremity M99.26
      lumbar region M99.23
      lumbosacral M99.23
      occipitocervical M99.20
      pelvic M99.25
      rib cage M99.28
      sacral region M99.24
      sacrococcygeal M99.24
      sacroiliac M99.24
      specified NEC M99.29
      thoracic region M99.22
      thoracolumbar M99.22
      upper extremity M99.27
  organ or site, congenital NEC — *see* Atresia, by site
  papilla of Vater K83.1
  pulmonary (artery) (congenital) Q25.6
    with ventricular septal defect, transposition of aorta,
      and hypertrophy of right ventricle Q21.3
    acquired I28.8

Stenosis, stenotic — *continued*
  pulmonary — *continued*
    in tetralogy of Fallot Q21.3
    infundibular Q24.3
    subvalvular Q24.3
    supravalvular Q25.6
    valve I37.0
      with insufficiency I37.2
      congenital Q22.1
      rheumatic I09.89
        with aortic, mitral or tricuspid (valve) disease
          I08.8
    vein, acquired I28.8
    vessel NEC I28.8
  pulmonic (congenital) Q22.1
    infundibular Q24.3
    subvalvular Q24.3
  pylorus (hypertrophic) (acquired) K31.1
    adult K31.1
    congenital Q40.0
    infantile Q40.0
  rectum (sphincter) — *see* Stricture, rectum
  renal artery I70.1
    congenital Q27.1
  salivary duct (any) K11.8
  sphincter of Oddi K83.1
  spinal M48.00
    cervical region M48.02
    cervicothoracic region M48.03
    lumbar region (NOS) (without neurogenic claudica-
      tion) M48.061
      with neurogenic claudication M48.062
    lumbosacral region M48.07
    occipito-atlanto-axial region M48.01
    sacrococcygeal region M48.08
    thoracic region M48.04
    thoracolumbar region M48.05
  stomach, hourglass K31.2
  subaortic (congenital) Q24.4
    hypertrophic (idiopathic) I42.1
  subglottic J38.6
    congenital Q31.1
    postprocedural J95.5
  trachea J39.8
    congenital Q32.1
    syphilitic A52.73
    tuberculous NEC A15.5
  tracheostomy J95.03
  tricuspid (valve) I07.0
    with
      aortic (valve) disease I08.2
      incompetency, insufficiency or regurgitation
        I07.2
        with aortic (valve) disease I08.2
          with mitral (valve) disease I08.3
      mitral (valve) disease I08.1
        with aortic (valve) disease I08.3
    congenital Q22.4
    nonrheumatic I36.0
      with insufficiency I36.2
  tubal N97.1
  ureter — *see* Atresia, ureter
  ureteropelvic junction, congenital Q62.11
  ureterovesical orifice, congenital Q62.12
  urethra (valve) *see also* Stricture, urethra
    congenital Q64.32
  urinary meatus, congenital Q64.33
  vagina N89.5
    congenital Q52.4
    in pregnancy — *see* Pregnancy, complicated by,
      abnormal vagina
      causing obstructed labor O65.5
  valve (cardiac) (heart) — *see also* Endocarditis I38
    congenital Q24.8
      aortic Q23.0
      mitral Q23.2
      pulmonary Q22.1
      tricuspid Q22.4
  vena cava (inferior) (superior) I87.1
    congenital Q26.0
  vesicourethral orifice Q64.31
  vulva N90.5
Stent jail T82.897 ☑
Stercolith (impaction) K56.41
  appendix K38.1
Stercoraceous, stercoral ulcer K63.3
  anus or rectum K62.6
Stereotypies NEC F98.4

▽ Subterms under main terms may continue to next column or page   ☑ Additional Character Required — Refer to the Tabular List for Character Selection   293

Stenosis, stenotic — Stereotypies NEC

Sterility — *see* Infertility
Sterilization — *see* Encounter (for), sterilization
Sternalgia — *see* Angina
Sternopagus Q89.4
Sternum bifidum Q76.7
Steroid
  effects (adverse) (adrenocortical) (iatrogenic)
    cushingoid E24.2
      correct substance properly administered — *see*
        Table of Drugs and Chemicals, by drug,
        adverse effect
      overdose or wrong substance given or taken —
        see Table of Drugs and Chemicals, by drug,
        poisoning
    diabetes — *see* subcategory E09 ☑
      correct substance properly administered — *see*
        Table of Drugs and Chemicals, by drug,
        adverse effect
      overdose or wrong substance given or taken —
        see Table of Drugs and Chemicals, by drug,
        poisoning
    fever R50.2
    insufficiency E27.3
      correct substance properly administered — *see*
        Table of Drugs and Chemicals, by drug,
        adverse effect
      overdose or wrong substance given or taken —
        see Table of Drugs and Chemicals, by drug,
        poisoning
  responder H40.04- ☑
Stevens-Johnson disease or syndrome L51.1
  toxic epidermal necrolysis overlap L51.3
Stewart-Morel syndrome M85.2
Sticker's disease B08.3
Sticky eye — *see* Conjunctivitis, acute, mucopurulent
Stieda's disease — *see* Bursitis, tibial collateral
Stiff neck — *see* Torticollis
Stiff-man syndrome G25.82
Stiffness, joint NEC M25.60
  ankle M25.67- ☑
  ankylosis — *see* Ankylosis, joint
  contracture — *see* Contraction, joint
  elbow M25.62- ☑
  foot M25.67- ☑
  hand M25.64- ☑
  hip M25.65- ☑
  knee M25.66- ☑
  shoulder M25.61- ☑
  wrist M25.63- ☑
Stigmata congenital syphilis A50.59
Stillbirth P95
Still-Felty syndrome — *see* Felty's syndrome
Still's disease or syndrome (juvenile) M08.20
  adult-onset M06.1
  ankle M08.27- ☑
  elbow M08.22- ☑
  foot joint M08.27- ☑
  hand joint M08.24- ☑
  hip M08.25- ☑
  knee M08.26- ☑
  multiple site M08.29
  shoulder M08.21- ☑
  vertebra M08.28
  wrist M08.23- ☑
Stimulation, ovary E28.1
Sting (venomous) (with allergic or anaphylactic shock)
    — *see* Table of Drugs and Chemicals, by animal or
    substance, poisoning
Stippled epiphyses Q78.8
Stitch
  abscess T81.41 ☑
  burst (in operation wound) — *see* Disruption, wound,
    operation
Stokes' disease E05.00
  with thyroid storm E05.01
Stokes-Adams disease or syndrome I45.9
Stokvis (-Talma) **disease** D74.8
Stoma malfunction
  colostomy K94.03
  enterostomy K94.13
  gastrostomy K94.23
  ileostomy K94.13
  tracheostomy J95.03
Stomach — *see* condition
Stomatitis (denture) (ulcerative) K12.1
  angular K13.0
    due to dietary or vitamin deficiency E53.0

Stomatitis — *continued*
  aphthous K12.0
  bovine B08.61
  candidal B37.0
  catarrhal K12.1
  diphtheritic A36.89
  due to
    dietary deficiency E53.0
    thrush B37.0
    vitamin deficiency
      B group NEC E53.9
      B2 (riboflavin) E53.0
  epidemic B08.8
  epizootic B08.8
  follicular K12.1
  gangrenous A69.0
  Geotrichum B48.3
  herpesviral, herpetic B00.2
  herpetiformis K12.0
  malignant K12.1
  membranous acute K12.1
  monilial B37.0
  mycotic B37.0
  necrotizing ulcerative A69.0
  parasitic B37.0
  septic K12.1
  spirochetal A69.1
  suppurative (acute) K12.2
  ulceromembranous A69.1
  vesicular K12.1
    with exanthem (enteroviral) B08.4
    virus disease A93.8
  Vincent's A69.1
Stomatocytosis D58.8
Stomatomycosis B37.0
Stomatorrhagia K13.79
Stone(s) — *see also* Calculus
  bladder (diverticulum) N21.0
  cystine E72.09
  heart syndrome I50.1
  kidney N20.0
  prostate N42.0
  pulpal (dental) K04.2
  renal N20.0
  salivary gland or duct (any) K11.5
  urethra (impacted) N21.1
  urinary (duct) (impacted) (passage) N20.9
    bladder (diverticulum) N21.0
    lower tract N21.9
    specified NEC N21.8
  xanthine E79.8 *[N22]*
Stonecutter's lung J62.8
**Stonemason's asthma, disease, lung or pneumoco-
  niosis** J62.8
Stoppage
  heart — *see* Arrest, cardiac
  urine — *see* Retention, urine
Storm, thyroid — *see* Thyrotoxicosis
Strabismus (congenital) (nonparalytic) H50.9
  concomitant H50.40
    convergent — *see* Strabismus, convergent concomi-
      tant
    divergent — *see* Strabismus, divergent concomitant
  convergent concomitant H50.00
    accommodative component H50.43
    alternating H50.05
      with
        A pattern H50.06
        specified nonconcomitances NEC H50.08
        V pattern H50.07
    monocular H50.01- ☑
      with
        A pattern H50.02- ☑
        specified nonconcomitances NEC H50.04- ☑
        V pattern H50.03- ☑
    intermittent H50.31- ☑
      alternating H50.32
  cyclotropia H50.41 ☑
  divergent concomitant H50.10
    alternating H50.15
      with
        A pattern H50.16
        specified nonconcomitances NEC H50.18
        V pattern H50.17
    monocular H50.11- ☑
      with
        A pattern H50.12- ☑
        specified nonconcomitances NEC H50.14- ☑

Strabismus — *continued*
  divergent concomitant — *continued*
    monocular — *continued*
      with — *continued*
        V pattern H50.13- ☑
      intermittent H50.33 ☑
        alternating H50.34
  Duane's syndrome H50.81- ☑
  due to adhesions, scars H50.69
  heterophoria H50.50
    alternating H50.55
    cyclophoria H50.54
    esophoria H50.51
    exophoria H50.52
    vertical H50.53
  heterotropia H50.40
    intermittent H50.30
  hypertropia H50.2- ☑
  hypotropia — *see* Hypertropia
  latent H50.50
  mechanical H50.60
    Brown's sheath syndrome H50.61- ☑
    specified type NEC H50.69
  monofixation syndrome H50.42
  paralytic H49.9
    abducens nerve H49.2- ☑
    fourth nerve H49.1- ☑
    Kearns-Sayre syndrome H49.81- ☑
    ophthalmoplegia (external)
      progressive H49.4- ☑
        with pigmentary retinopathy H49.81- ☑
      total H49.3- ☑
    sixth nerve H49.2- ☑
    specified type NEC H49.88- ☑
    third nerve H49.0- ☑
    trochlear nerve H49.1- ☑
  specified type NEC H50.89
  vertical H50.2- ☑
Strain
  back S39.012 ☑
  cervical S16.1 ☑
  eye NEC — *see* Disturbance, vision, subjective
  heart — *see* Disease, heart
  low back S39.012 ☑
  mental NOS Z73.3
    work-related Z56.6
  muscle (tendon) — *see* Injury, muscle, by site, strain
  neck S16.1 ☑
  physical NOS Z73.3
    work-related Z56.6
  postural — *see also* Disorder, soft tissue, due to use
  psychological NEC Z73.3
  tendon — *see* Injury, muscle, by site, strain
Straining, on urination R39.16
Strand, vitreous — *see* Opacity, vitreous, membranes
  and strands
Strangulation, strangulated — *see also* Asphyxia,
  traumatic
  appendix K38.8
  bladder-neck N32.0
  bowel or colon K56.2
  food or foreign body — *see* Foreign body, by site
  hemorrhoids — *see* Hemorrhoids, with complication
  hernia — *see also* Hernia, by site, with obstruction
    with gangrene — *see* Hernia, by site, with gangrene
  intestine (large) (small) K56.2
    with hernia — *see also* Hernia, by site, with obstruc-
      tion
      with gangrene — *see* Hernia, by site, with gan-
        grene
  mesentery K56.2
  mucus — *see* Asphyxia, mucus
  omentum K56.2
  organ or site, congenital NEC — *see* Atresia, by site
  ovary — *see* Torsion, ovary
  penis N48.89
    foreign body T19.4 ☑
  rupture — *see* Hernia, by site, with obstruction
  stomach due to hernia — *see also* Hernia, by site, with
    obstruction
    with gangrene — *see* Hernia, by site, with gangrene
  vesicourethral orifice N32.0
Strangury R30.0
Straw itch B88.0
Strawberry
  gallbladder K82.4
  mark Q82.5

Strawberry — continued
tongue (red) (white) K14.3
Streak(s)
macula, angioid H35.33
ovarian Q50.32
Strephosymbolia F81.0
secondary to organic lesion R48.8
Streptobacillary fever A25.1
Streptobacillosis A25.1
Streptobacillus moniliformis A25.1
Streptococcus, streptococcal — see also condition
as cause of disease classified elsewhere B95.5
group
A, as cause of disease classified elsewhere B95.0
B, as cause of disease classified elsewhere B95.1
D, as cause of disease classified elsewhere B95.2
pneumoniae, as cause of disease classified elsewhere
B95.3
specified NEC, as cause of disease classified elsewhere
B95.4
Streptomycosis B47.1
Streptotrichosis A48.8
Stress F43.9
family — see Disruption, family
fetal P84
complicating pregnancy O77.9
due to drug administration O77.1
mental NEC Z73.3
work-related Z56.6
physical NEC Z73.3
work-related Z56.6
polycythemia D75.1
reaction — see also Reaction, stress F43.9
work schedule Z56.3
Stretching, nerve — see Injury, nerve
Striae albicantes, atrophicae or distensae (cutis) L90.6
Stricture — see also Stenosis
ampulla of Vater K83.1
anus (sphincter) K62.4
congenital Q42.3
with fistula Q42.2
infantile Q42.3
with fistula Q42.2
aorta (ascending) (congenital) Q25.1
arteriosclerotic I70.0
calcified I70.0
supravalvular, congenital Q25.3
aortic (valve) — see Stenosis, aortic
aqueduct of Sylvius (congenital) Q03.0
with spina bifida — see Spina bifida, by site, with
hydrocephalus
acquired G91.1
artery I77.1
basilar — see Occlusion, artery, basilar
carotid — see Occlusion, artery, carotid
celiac I77.4
congenital (peripheral) Q27.8
cerebral Q28.3
coronary Q24.5
digestive system Q27.8
lower limb Q27.8
retinal Q14.1
specified site NEC Q27.8
umbilical Q27.0
upper limb Q27.8
coronary — see Disease, heart, ischemic,
atherosclerotic
congenital Q24.5
precerebral — see Occlusion, artery, precerebral
pulmonary (congenital) Q25.6
acquired I28.8
renal I70.1
vertebral — see Occlusion, artery, vertebral
auditory canal (external) (congenital)
acquired — see Stenosis, external ear canal
bile duct (common) (hepatic) K83.1
congenital Q44.3
postoperative K91.89
bladder N32.89
neck N32.0
bowel — see Obstruction, intestine
brain G93.89
bronchus J98.09
congenital Q32.3
syphilitic A52.72
cardia (stomach) K22.2
congenital Q39.3
cardiac — see also Disease, heart

Stricture — continued
cardiac — see also Disease, heart — continued
orifice (stomach) K22.2
cecum — see Obstruction, intestine
cervix, cervical (canal) N88.2
congenital Q51.828
in pregnancy — see Pregnancy, complicated by,
abnormal cervix
causing obstructed labor O65.5
colon — see also Obstruction, intestine
congenital Q42.9
specified NEC Q42.8
colostomy K94.03
common (bile) duct K83.1
coronary (artery) — see Disease, heart, ischemic,
atherosclerotic
cystic duct — see Obstruction, gallbladder
digestive organs NEC, congenital Q45.8
duodenum K31.5
congenital Q41.0
ear canal (external) (congenital) Q16.1
acquired — see Stricture, auditory canal, acquired
ejaculatory duct N50.89
enterostomy K94.13
esophagus K22.2
congenital Q39.3
syphilitic A52.79
congenital A50.59 [K23]
eustachian tube — see also Obstruction, eustachian
tube
congenital Q17.8
fallopian tube N97.1
gonococcal A54.24
tuberculous A18.17
gallbladder — see Obstruction, gallbladder
glottis J38.6
heart — see also Disease, heart
valve — see also Endocarditis I38
aortic Q23.0
mitral Q23.2
pulmonary Q22.1
tricuspid Q22.4
hepatic duct K83.1
hourglass, of stomach K31.2
hymen N89.6
hypopharynx J39.2
ileum — see also Obstruction, intestine, specified NEC
K56.699
congenital Q41.2
intestine — see also Obstruction, intestine
congenital (small) Q41.9
large Q42.9
specified NEC Q42.8
specified NEC Q41.8
ischemic K55.1
jejunum — see also Obstruction, intestine, specified
NEC K56.699
congenital Q41.1
lacrimal passages — see also Stenosis, lacrimal
congenital Q10.5
larynx J38.6
congenital NEC Q31.8
subglottic Q31.1
syphilitic A52.73
congenital A50.59 [J99]
meatus
ear (congenital) Q16.1
acquired — see Stricture, auditory canal, acquired
osseous (ear) (congenital) Q16.1
acquired — see Stricture, auditory canal, acquired
urinarius — see also Stricture, urethra
congenital Q64.33
mitral (valve) — see Stenosis, mitral
myocardium, myocardial I51.5
hypertrophic subaortic (idiopathic) I42.1
nares (anterior) (posterior) J34.89
congenital Q30.0
nasal duct — see also Stenosis, lacrimal, duct
congenital Q10.5
nasolacrimal duct — see also Stenosis, lacrimal, duct
congenital Q10.5
nasopharynx J39.2
syphilitic A52.73
nose J34.89
congenital Q30.0
nostril (anterior) (posterior) J34.89

Stricture — continued
nostril — continued
congenital Q30.0
syphilitic A52.73
congenital A50.59 [J99]
organ or site, congenital NEC — see Atresia, by site
os uteri — see Stricture, cervix
osseous meatus (ear) (congenital) Q16.1
acquired — see Stricture, auditory canal, acquired
oviduct — see Stricture, fallopian tube
pelviureteric junction (congenital) Q62.11
acquired, with hydronephrosis N13.0
penis, by foreign body T19.4 ☑
pharynx J39.2
prostate N42.89
pulmonary, pulmonic
artery (congenital) Q25.6
acquired I28.8
noncongenital I28.8
infundibulum (congenital) Q24.3
valve I37.0
congenital Q22.1
vein, acquired I28.8
vessel NEC I28.8
punctum lacrimale — see also Stenosis, lacrimal,
punctum
congenital Q10.5
pylorus (hypertrophic) K31.1
adult K31.1
congenital Q40.0
infantile Q40.0
rectosigmoid — see also Obstruction, intestine, specified NEC K56.699
rectum (sphincter) K62.4
congenital Q42.1
with fistula Q42.0
due to
chlamydial lymphogranuloma A55
irradiation K91.89
lymphogranuloma venereum A55
gonococcal A54.6
inflammatory (chlamydial) A55
syphilitic A52.74
tuberculous A18.32
renal artery I70.1
congenital Q27.1
salivary duct or gland (any) K11.8
sigmoid (flexure) — see Obstruction, intestine
spermatic cord N50.89
stoma (following) (of)
colostomy K94.03
enterostomy K94.13
gastrostomy K94.23
ileostomy K94.13
tracheostomy J95.03
stomach K31.89
congenital Q40.2
hourglass K31.2
subaortic Q24.4
hypertrophic (acquired) (idiopathic) I42.1
subglottic J38.6
syphilitic NEC A52.79
trachea J39.8
congenital Q32.1
syphilitic A52.73
tuberculous NEC A15.5
tracheostomy J95.03
tricuspid (valve) — see Stenosis, tricuspid
tunica vaginalis N50.89
ureter (postoperative) N13.5
with
hydronephrosis N13.1
with infection N13.6
pyelonephritis (chronic) N11.1
congenital — see Atresia, ureter
tuberculous A18.11
ureteropelvic junction (congenital) Q62.11
acquired, with hydronephrosis N13.0
ureterovesical orifice N13.5
with infection N13.6
urethra (organic) (spasmodic) — see also Stricture,
urethra, male N35.919
associated with schistosomiasis B65.0 [N37]
congenital Q64.39
valvular (posterior) Q64.2
due to
infection — see Stricture, urethra, postinfective
trauma — see Stricture, urethra, post-traumatic

▽ Subterms under main terms may continue to next column or page   ☑ Additional Character Required — Refer to the Tabular List for Character Selection   295

Strawberry — Stricture

Stricture — continued
  urethra — see also Stricture, urethra, male — continued
    female N35.92
    gonococcal, gonorrheal A54.01
    infective NEC — see Stricture, urethra, postinfective
    late effect (sequelae) of injury — see Stricture, urethra, post-traumatic
    male N35.919
      anterior urethra N35.914
      bulbous urethra N35.912
      meatal N35.911
      membranous urethra N35.913
      overlapping sites N35.916
    postcatheterization — see Stricture, urethra, postprocedural
    postinfective NEC
      female N35.12
      male N35.119
        anterior urethra N35.114
        bulbous urethra N35.112
        meatal N35.111
        membranous urethra N35.113
        overlapping sites N35.116
    postobstetric N35.021
    postoperative — see Stricture, urethra, postprocedural
    postprocedural
      female N99.12
      male N99.114
        anterior bulbous urethra N99.113
        bulbous urethra N99.111
        fossa navicularis N99.115
        meatal N99.110
        membranous urethra N99.112
        overlapping sites N99.116
    post-traumatic
      female N35.028
        due to childbirth N35.021
      male N35.014
        anterior urethra N35.013
        bulbous urethra N35.011
        meatal N35.010
        membranous urethra N35.012
        overlapping sites N35.016
    sequela (late effect) of
      childbirth N35.021
      injury — see Stricture, urethra, post-traumatic
    specified cause NEC
      female N35.82
      male N35.819
        anterior urethra N35.814
        bulbous urethra N35.812
        meatal N35.811
        membranous urethra N35.813
        overlapping sites N35.816
    syphilitic A52.76
    traumatic — see Stricture, urethra, post-traumatic
    valvular (posterior), congenital Q64.2
  urinary meatus — see Stricture, urethra
  uterus, uterine (synechiae) N85.6
    os (external) (internal) — see Stricture, cervix
  vagina (outlet) — see Stenosis, vagina
  valve (cardiac) (heart) — see also Endocarditis
    congenital
      aortic Q23.0
      mitral Q23.2
      pulmonary Q22.1
      tricuspid Q22.4
  vas deferens N50.89
    congenital Q55.4
  vein I87.1
  vena cava (inferior) (superior) NEC I87.1
    congenital Q26.0
  vesicourethral orifice N32.0
    congenital Q64.31
  vulva (acquired) N90.5
Stridor R06.1
  congenital (larynx) P28.89
Stridulous — see condition
Stroke (apoplectic) (brain) (embolic) (ischemic) (paralytic) (thrombotic) I63.9
  cryptogenic — see also infarction, cerebral I63.9
  epileptic — see Epilepsy
  heat T67.01 ☑
    exertional T67.02 ☑
    specified NEC T67.09 ☑
  in evolution I63.9

Stroke — continued
  intraoperative
    during cardiac surgery I97.810
    during other surgery I97.811
  lightning — see Lightning
  meaning
    cerebral hemorrhage — code to Hemorrhage, intracranial
    cerebral infarction — code to Infarction, cerebral
  postprocedural
    following cardiac surgery I97.820
    following other surgery I97.821
  sun T67.01 ☑
    specified NEC T67.09 ☑
  unspecified (NOS) I63.9
Stromatosis, endometrial D39.0
Strongyloidiasis, strongyloidosis B78.9
  cutaneous B78.1
  disseminated B78.7
  intestinal B78.0
Strophulus pruriginosus L28.2
Struck by lightning — see Lightning
Struma — see also Goiter
  Hashimoto E06.3
  lymphomatosa E06.3
  nodosa (simplex) E04.9
    endemic E01.2
      multinodular E01.1
    multinodular E04.2
      iodine-deficiency related E01.1
    toxic or with hyperthyroidism E05.20
      with thyroid storm E05.21
      multinodular E05.20
        with thyroid storm E05.21
      uninodular E05.10
        with thyroid storm E05.11
    toxicosa E05.20
      with thyroid storm E05.21
      multinodular E05.20
        with thyroid storm E05.21
      uninodular E05.10
        with thyroid storm E05.11
    uninodular E04.1
  ovarii D27.- ☑
  Riedel's E06.5
Strumipriva cachexia E03.4
Strümpell-Marie spine — see Spondylitis, ankylosing
Strümpell-Westphal pseudosclerosis E83.01
Stuart deficiency disease (factor X) D68.2
Stuart-Prower factor deficiency (factor X) D68.2
Student's elbow — see Bursitis, elbow, olecranon
Stump — see Amputation
Stunting, nutritional E45
Stupor (catatonic) R40.1
  depressive (single episode) F32.89
    recurrent episode F33.8
  dissociative F44.2
  manic F30.2
  manic-depressive F31.89
  psychogenic (anergic) F44.2
  reaction to exceptional stress (transient) F43.0
Sturge (-Weber) (-Dimitri) (-Kalischer) **disease or syndrome** Q85.8
Stuttering F80.81
  adult onset F98.5
  childhood onset F80.81
  following cerebrovascular disease — see Disorder, fluency. following cerebrovascular disease
  in conditions classified elsewhere R47.82
Sty, stye (external) (internal) (meibomian) (zeisian) — see Hordeolum
Subacidity, gastric K31.89
  psychogenic F45.8
Subacute — see condition
Subarachnoid — see condition
Subcortical — see condition
Subcostal syndrome, nerve compression — see Mononeuropathy, upper limb, specified site NEC
Subcutaneous, subcuticular — see condition
Subdural — see condition
Subendocardium — see condition
Subependymoma
  specified site — see Neoplasm, uncertain behavior, by site
  unspecified site D43.2
Suberosis J67.3
Subglossitis — see Glossitis

Subhemophilia D66
Subinvolution
  breast (postlactational) (postpuerperal) N64.89
  puerperal O90.89
  uterus (chronic) (nonpuerperal) N85.3
    puerperal O90.89
Sublingual — see condition
Sublinguitis — see Sialoadenitis
Subluxatable hip Q65.6
Subluxation — see also Dislocation
  acromioclavicular S43.11- ☑
  ankle S93.0- ☑
  atlantoaxial, recurrent M43.4
    with myelopathy M43.3
  carpometacarpal (joint) NEC S63.05- ☑
    thumb S63.04- ☑
  complex, vertebral — see Complex, subluxation
  congenital — see also Malposition, congenital
    hip — see Dislocation, hip, congenital, partial
    joint (excluding hip)
      lower limb Q68.8
      shoulder Q68.8
      upper limb Q68.8
  elbow (traumatic) S53.10- ☑
    anterior S53.11- ☑
    lateral S53.14- ☑
    medial S53.13- ☑
    posterior S53.12- ☑
    specified type NEC S53.19- ☑
  finger S63.20- ☑
    index S63.20- ☑
    interphalangeal S63.22- ☑
      distal S63.24- ☑
        index S63.24- ☑
        little S63.24- ☑
        middle S63.24- ☑
        ring S63.24- ☑
      index S63.22- ☑
      little S63.22- ☑
      middle S63.22- ☑
      proximal S63.23- ☑
        index S63.23- ☑
        little S63.23- ☑
        middle S63.23- ☑
        ring S63.23- ☑
    little S63.20- ☑
    metacarpophalangeal S63.21- ☑
      index S63.21- ☑
      little S63.21- ☑
      middle S63.21- ☑
      ring S63.21- ☑
    middle S63.20- ☑
    ring S63.20- ☑
  foot S93.30- ☑
    specified site NEC S93.33- ☑
    tarsal joint S93.31- ☑
    tarsometatarsal joint S93.32- ☑
    toe — see Subluxation, toe
  hip S73.00- ☑
    anterior S73.03- ☑
      obturator S73.02- ☑
    central S73.04- ☑
    posterior S73.01- ☑
  interphalangeal (joint)
    finger S63.22- ☑
      distal joint S63.24- ☑
        index S63.24- ☑
        little S63.24- ☑
        middle S63.24- ☑
        ring S63.24- ☑
      index S63.22- ☑
      little S63.22- ☑
      middle S63.22- ☑
      proximal joint S63.23- ☑
        index S63.23- ☑
        little S63.23- ☑
        middle S63.23- ☑
        ring S63.23- ☑
      ring S63.22- ☑
    thumb S63.12- ☑
    toe S93.13- ☑
      great S93.13- ☑
      lesser S93.13- ☑
  joint prosthesis — see Complications, joint prosthesis, mechanical, displacement, by site

☑ Additional Character Required — Refer to the Tabular List for Character Selection   ▽ Subterms under main terms may continue to next column or page

Subluxation — *continued*
  knee S83.10- ☑
    cap — *see* Subluxation, patella
    patella — *see* Subluxation, patella
    proximal tibia
      anteriorly S83.11- ☑
      laterally S83.14- ☑
      medially S83.13- ☑
      posteriorly S83.12- ☑
    specified type NEC S83.19- ☑
  lens — *see* Dislocation, lens, partial
  ligament, traumatic — *see* Sprain, by site
  metacarpal (bone)
    proximal end S63.06- ☑
  metacarpophalangeal (joint)
    finger S63.21- ☑
      index S63.21- ☑
      little S63.21- ☑
      middle S63.21- ☑
      ring S63.21- ☑
    thumb S63.11- ☑
  metatarsophalangeal joint S93.14- ☑
    great toe S93.14- ☑
    lesser toe S93.14- ☑
  midcarpal (joint) S63.03- ☑
  patella S83.00- ☑
    lateral S83.01- ☑
    recurrent (nontraumatic) — *see* Dislocation, patella, recurrent, incomplete
    specified type NEC S83.09- ☑
  pathological — *see* Dislocation, pathological
  radial head S53.00- ☑
    anterior S53.01- ☑
    nursemaid's elbow S53.03- ☑
    posterior S53.02- ☑
    specified type NEC S53.09- ☑
  radiocarpal (joint) S63.02- ☑
  radioulnar (joint)
    distal S63.01- ☑
    proximal — *see* Subluxation, elbow
  shoulder
    congenital Q68.8
    girdle S43.30- ☑
      scapula S43.31- ☑
      specified site NEC S43.39- ☑
    traumatic S43.00- ☑
      anterior S43.01- ☑
      inferior S43.03- ☑
      posterior S43.02- ☑
      specified type NEC S43.08- ☑
  sternoclavicular (joint) S43.20- ☑
    anterior S43.21- ☑
    posterior S43.22- ☑
  symphysis (pubis)
  thumb S63.103 ☑
    interphalangeal joint — *see* Subluxation, interphalangeal (joint), thumb
    metacarpophalangeal joint — *see* Subluxation, metacarpophalangeal (joint), thumb
  toe(s) S93.10- ☑
    great S93.10- ☑
      interphalangeal joint S93.13- ☑
      metatarsophalangeal joint S93.14- ☑
    interphalangeal joint S93.13- ☑
    lesser S93.10- ☑
      interphalangeal joint S93.13- ☑
      metatarsophalangeal joint S93.14- ☑
    metatarsophalangeal joint S93.149 ☑
  ulna
    distal end S63.07- ☑
    proximal end — *see* Subluxation, elbow
  ulnohumeral joint — *see* Subluxation, elbow
  vertebral
    recurrent NEC — *see* subcategory M43.5 ☑
    traumatic
      cervical S13.100 ☑
        atlantoaxial joint S13.120 ☑
        atlantooccipital joint S13.110 ☑
        atloidooccipital joint S13.110 ☑
        joint between
          C0 and C1 S13.110 ☑
          C1 and C2 S13.120 ☑
          C2 and C3 S13.130 ☑
          C3 and C4 S13.140 ☑
          C4 and C5 S13.150 ☑
          C5 and C6 S13.160 ☑

Subluxation — *continued*
  vertebral — *continued*
    traumatic — *continued*
      cervical — *continued*
        joint between — *continued*
          C6 and C7 S13.170 ☑
          C7 and T1 S13.180 ☑
        occipitoatloid joint S13.110 ☑
      lumbar S33.100 ☑
        joint between
          L1 and L2 S33.110 ☑
          L2 and L3 S33.120 ☑
          L3 and L4 S33.130 ☑
          L4 and L5 S33.140 ☑
      thoracic S23.100 ☑
        joint between
          T1 and T2 S23.110 ☑
          T2 and T3 S23.120 ☑
          T3 and T4 S23.122 ☑
          T4 and T5 S23.130 ☑
          T5 and T6 S23.132 ☑
          T6 and T7 S23.140 ☑
          T7 and T8 S23.142 ☑
          T8 and T9 S23.150 ☑
          T9 and T10 S23.152 ☑
          T10 and T11 S23.160 ☑
          T11 and T12 S23.162 ☑
          T12 and L1 S23.170 ☑
  wrist (carpal bone) S63.00- ☑
    carpometacarpal joint — *see* Subluxation, carpometacarpal (joint)
    distal radioulnar joint — *see* Subluxation, radioulnar (joint), distal
    metacarpal bone, proximal — *see* Subluxation, metacarpal (bone), proximal end
    midcarpal — *see* Subluxation, midcarpal (joint)
    radiocarpal joint — *see* Subluxation, radiocarpal (joint)
    recurrent — *see* Dislocation, recurrent, wrist
    specified site NEC S63.09- ☑
    ulna — *see* Subluxation, ulna, distal end
Submaxillary — *see* condition
Submersion (fatal) (nonfatal) T75.1 ☑
Submucous — *see* condition
Subnormal, subnormality
  accommodation (old age) H52.4
  mental — *see* Disability, intellectual
  temperature (accidental) T68 ☑
Subphrenic — *see* condition
Subscapular nerve — *see* condition
Subseptus uterus Q51.28
Subsiding appendicitis K36
Substance (other psychoactive) **-induced**
  anxiety disorder F19.980
  bipolar and related disorder F19.94
  delirium F19.921
  depressive disorder F19.94
  major neurocognitive disorder F19.97
  mild neurocognitive disorder F19.988
  obsessive-compulsive and related disorder F19.988
  psychotic disorder F19.959
  sexual dysfunction F19.981
  sleep disorder F19.982
Substernal thyroid E04.9
  congenital Q89.2
Substitution disorder F44.9
Subtentorial — *see* condition
Subthyroidism (acquired) — *see also* Hypothyroidism
  congenital E03.1
Succenturiate placenta O43.19- ☑
Sucking thumb, child (excessive) F98.8
Sudamen, sudamina L74.1
Sudanese kala-azar B55.0
Sudden
  hearing loss — *see* Deafness, sudden
  heart failure — *see* Failure, heart
Sudeck's atrophy, disease, or syndrome — *see* Algoneurodystrophy
Suffocation — *see* Asphyxia, traumatic
Sugar
  blood
    high (transient) R73.9
    low (transient) E16.2
  in urine R81
Suicide, suicidal (attempted) T14.91 ☑
  by poisoning — *see* Table of Drugs and Chemicals
  history of (personal) Z91.5

Suicide, suicidal — *continued*
  history of — *continued*
    in family Z81.8
  ideation — *see* Ideation, suicidal
  risk
    meaning personal history of attempted suicide Z91.5
    meaning suicidal ideation — *see* Ideation, suicidal
  tendencies
    meaning personal history of attempted suicide Z91.5
    meaning suicidal ideation — *see* Ideation, suicidal
  trauma — *see* nature of injury by site
Suipestifer infection — *see* Infection, salmonella
Sulfhemoglobinemia, sulphemoglobinemia (acquired) (with methemoglobinemia) D74.8
Sumatran mite fever A75.3
Summer — *see* condition
Sunburn L55.9
  due to
    tanning bed (acute) L56.8
      chronic L57.8
    ultraviolet radiation (acute) L56.8
      chronic L57.8
  first degree L55.0
  second degree L55.1
  third degree L55.2
SUNCT (short lasting unilateral neuralgiform headache with conjunctival injection and tearing) G44.059
  intractable G44.051
  not intractable G44.059
Sundowning F05
Sunken acetabulum — *see* Derangement, joint, specified type NEC, hip
Sunstroke T67.01 ☑
  specified NEC T67.09 ☑
Superfecundation — *see* Pregnancy, multiple
Superfetation — *see* Pregnancy, multiple
Superinvolution (uterus) N85.8
Supernumerary (congenital)
  aortic cusps Q23.8
  auditory ossicles Q16.3
  bone Q79.8
  breast Q83.1
  carpal bones Q74.0
  cusps, heart valve NEC Q24.8
    aortic Q23.8
    mitral Q23.2
    pulmonary Q22.3
  digit(s) Q69.9
  ear (lobule) Q17.0
  fallopian tube Q50.6
  finger Q69.0
  hymen Q52.4
  kidney Q63.0
  lacrimonasal duct Q10.6
  lobule (ear) Q17.0
  mitral cusps Q23.2
  muscle Q79.8
  nipple(s) Q83.3
  organ or site not listed — *see* Accessory
  ossicles, auditory Q16.3
  ovary Q50.31
  oviduct Q50.6
  pulmonary, pulmonic cusps Q22.3
  rib Q76.6
    cervical or first (syndrome) Q76.5
  roots (of teeth) K00.2
  spleen Q89.09
  tarsal bones Q74.2
  teeth K00.1
  testis Q55.29
  thumb Q69.1
  toe Q69.2
  uterus Q51.28
  vagina Q52.1 ☑
  vertebra Q76.49
Supervision (of)
  contraceptive — *see* Prescription, contraceptives
  dietary (for) Z71.3
    allergy (food) Z71.3
    colitis Z71.3
    diabetes mellitus Z71.3
    food allergy or intolerance Z71.3
    gastritis Z71.3
    hypercholesterolemia Z71.3
    hypoglycemia Z71.3
    intolerance (food) Z71.3
    obesity Z71.3
    specified NEC Z71.3

Supervision — *continued*
  healthy infant or child Z76.2
    foundling Z76.1
  high-risk pregnancy — *see* Pregnancy, complicated
    by, high, risk
  lactation Z39.1
  pregnancy — *see* Pregnancy, supervision of
Supplemental teeth K00.1
Suppression
  binocular vision H53.34
  lactation O92.5
  menstruation N94.89
  ovarian secretion E28.39
  renal N28.9
  urine, urinary secretion R34
Suppuration, suppurative — *see also* condition
  accessory sinus (chronic) — *see* Sinusitis
  adrenal gland
  antrum (chronic) — *see* Sinusitis, maxillary
  bladder — *see* Cystitis
  brain G06.0
    sequelae G09
  breast N61.1
    puerperal, postpartum or gestational — *see* Mastitis,
      obstetric, purulent
  dental periosteum M27.3
  ear (middle) — *see* Otitis, media
    external NEC — *see* Otitis, externa, infective
    internal — *see* subcategory H83.0 ☑
  ethmoidal (chronic) (sinus) — *see* Sinusitis, ethmoidal
  fallopian tube — *see* Salpingo-oophoritis
  frontal (chronic) (sinus) — *see* Sinusitis, frontal
  gallbladder (acute) K81.0
  gum K05.20
    generalized — *see* Periodontitis, aggressive, gener-
      alized
    localized — *see* Periodontitis, aggressive, localized
  intracranial G06.0
  joint — *see* Arthritis, pyogenic or pyemic
  labyrinthine — *see* subcategory H83.0 ☑
  lung — *see* Abscess, lung
  mammary gland N61.1
    puerperal, postpartum O91.12
      associated with lactation O91.13
  maxilla, maxillary M27.2
    sinus (chronic) — *see* Sinusitis, maxillary
  muscle — *see* Myositis, infective
  nasal sinus (chronic) — *see* Sinusitis
  pancreas, acute — *see also* Pancreatitis, acute K85.80
  parotid gland — *see* Sialoadenitis
  pelvis, pelvic
    female — *see* Disease, pelvis, inflammatory
    male K65.0
  pericranial — *see* Osteomyelitis
  salivary duct or gland (any) — *see* Sialoadenitis
  sinus (accessory) (chronic) (nasal) — *see* Sinusitis
  sphenoidal sinus (chronic) — *see* Sinusitis, sphenoidal
  thymus (gland) E32.1
  thyroid (gland) E06.0
  tonsil — *see* Tonsillitis
  uterus — *see* Endometritis
Supraeruption of tooth (teeth) M26.34
Supraglottitis J04.30
  with obstruction J04.31
Suprarenal (gland) — *see* condition
Suprascapular nerve — *see* condition
Suprasellar — *see* condition
Surfer's knots or nodules S89.8- ☑
Surgical
  emphysema T81.82 ☑
  procedures, complication or misadventure — *see*
    Complications, surgical procedures
  shock T81.10 ☑
Surveillance (of) (for) — *see also* Observation
  alcohol abuse Z71.41
  contraceptive — *see* Prescription, contraceptives
  dietary Z71.3
  drug abuse Z71.51
Susceptibility to disease, genetic Z15.89
  malignant neoplasm Z15.09
    breast Z15.01
    endometrium Z15.04
    ovary Z15.02
    prostate Z15.03
    specified NEC Z15.09
  multiple endocrine neoplasia Z15.81

Suspected condition, ruled out — *see also* Observation, suspected
  amniotic cavity and membrane Z03.71
  cervical shortening Z03.75
  fetal anomaly Z03.73
  fetal growth Z03.74
  maternal and fetal conditions NEC Z03.79
  newborn — *see also* Observation, newborn, suspected
    condition ruled out Z05.9
  oligohydramnios Z03.71
  placental problem Z03.72
  polyhydramnios Z03.71
Suspended uterus
  in pregnancy or childbirth — *see* Pregnancy, compli-
    cated by, abnormal uterus
Sutton's nevus D22.9
Suture
  burst (in operation wound) T81.31 ☑
    external operation wound T81.31 ☑
    internal operation wound T81.32 ☑
  inadvertently left in operation wound — *see* Foreign
    body, accidentally left during a procedure
  removal Z48.02
Swab inadvertently left in operation wound — *see*
  Foreign body, accidentally left during a procedure
Swallowed, swallowing
  difficulty — *see* Dysphagia
  foreign body — *see* Foreign body, alimentary tract
Swan-neck deformity (finger) — *see* Deformity, finger,
  swan-neck
Swearing, compulsive F42.8
  in Gilles de la Tourette's syndrome F95.2
Sweat, sweats
  fetid L75.0
  night R61
Sweating, excessive R61
Sweeley-Klionsky disease E75.21
Sweet's disease or dermatosis L98.2
Swelling (of) R60.9
  abdomen, abdominal (not referable to any particular
    organ) — *see* Mass, abdominal
  ankle — *see* Effusion, joint, ankle
  arm M79.89
    forearm M79.89
  breast — *see also* Lump, breast N63.0
  Calabar B74.3
  cervical gland R59.0
  chest, localized R22.2
  ear H93.8- ☑
  extremity (lower) (upper) — *see* Disorder, soft tissue,
    specified type NEC
  finger M79.89
  foot M79.89
  glands R59.9
    generalized R59.1
    localized R59.0
  hand M79.89
  head (localized) R22.0
  inflammatory — *see* Inflammation
  intra-abdominal — *see* Mass, abdominal
  joint — *see* Effusion, joint
  leg M79.89
    lower M79.89
  limb — *see* Disorder, soft tissue, specified type NEC
  localized (skin) R22.9
    chest R22.2
    head R22.0
    limb
      lower — *see* Mass, localized, limb, lower
      upper — *see* Mass, localized, limb, upper
    neck R22.1
    trunk R22.2
  neck (localized) R22.1
  pelvic — *see* Mass, abdominal
  scrotum N50.89
  splenic — *see* Splenomegaly
  testis N50.89
  toe M79.89
  umbilical R19.09
  wandering, due to Gnathostoma (spinigerum) B83.1
  white — *see* Tuberculosis, arthritis
Swift (-Feer) disease
  overdose or wrong substance given or taken — *see*
    Table of Drugs and Chemicals, by drug, poisoning
Swimmer's
  cramp T75.1 ☑
  ear H60.33- ☑

Swimmer's — *continued*
  itch B65.3
Swimming in the head R42
Swollen — *see* Swelling
Swyer syndrome Q99.1
Sycosis L73.8
  barbae (not parasitic) L73.8
  contagiosa (mycotic) B35.0
  lupoides L73.8
  mycotic B35.0
  parasitic B35.0
  vulgaris L73.8
Sydenham's chorea — *see* Chorea, Sydenham's
Sylvatic yellow fever A95.0
Sylvest's disease B33.0
Symblepharon H11.23- ☑
  congenital Q10.3
Symond's syndrome G93.2
Sympathetic — *see* condition
Sympatheticotonia G90.8
Sympathicoblastoma
  specified site — *see* Neoplasm, malignant, by site
  unspecified site C74.90
Sympathogonioma — *see* Sympathicoblastoma
Symphalangy (fingers) (toes) Q70.9
Symptoms NEC R68.89
  breast NEC N64.59
  cold J00
  development NEC R63.8
  factitious, self-induced — *see* Disorder, factitious
  genital organs, female R10.2
  involving
    abdomen NEC R19.8
    appearance NEC R46.89
    awareness R41.9
      altered mental status R41.82
      amnesia — *see* Amnesia
      borderline intellectual functioning R41.83
      coma — *see* Coma
      disorientation R41.0
      neurologic neglect syndrome R41.4
      senile cognitive decline R41.81
      specified symptom NEC R41.89
    behavior NEC R46.89
    cardiovascular system NEC R09.89
    chest NEC R09.89
    circulatory system NEC R09.89
    cognitive functions R41.9
      altered mental status R41.82
      amnesia — *see* Amnesia
      borderline intellectual functioning R41.83
      coma — *see* Coma
      disorientation R41.0
      neurologic neglect syndrome R41.4
      senile cognitive decline R41.81
      specified symptom NEC R41.89
    development NEC R62.50
    digestive system NEC R19.8
    emotional state NEC R45.89
      emotional lability R45.86
    food and fluid intake R63.8
    general perceptions and sensations R44.9
      specified NEC R44.8
    musculoskeletal system R29.91
      specified NEC R29.898
    nervous system R29.90
      specified NEC R29.818
    pelvis NEC R19.8
    respiratory system NEC R09.89
    skin and integument R23.9
    urinary system R39.9
  menopausal N95.1
  metabolism NEC R63.8
  neurotic F48.8
  of infancy R68.19
  pelvis NEC, female R10.2
  skin and integument NEC R23.9
  subcutaneous tissue NEC R23.9
  viral cold J00
Sympus Q74.2
Syncephalus Q89.4
Synchondrosis
  abnormal (congenital) Q78.8
  ischiopubic M91.0
Synchysis (scintillans) (senile) (vitreous body) H43.89
Syncope (near) (pre-) R55
  anginosa I20.8
  bradycardia R00.1

Syncope — *continued*
  cardiac R55
  carotid sinus G90.Ø1
  due to spinal (lumbar) puncture G97.1
  heart R55
  heat T67.1 ☑
  laryngeal RØ5
  psychogenic F48.8
  tussive RØ5
  vasoconstriction R55
  vasodepressor R55
  vasomotor R55
  vasovagal R55
Syndactylism, syndactyly Q7Ø.9
  complex (with synostosis)
    fingers Q7Ø.Ø- ☑
    toes Q7Ø.2- ☑
  simple (without synostosis)
    fingers Q7Ø.1- ☑
    toes Q7Ø.3- ☑
Syndrome — *see also* Disease
  5q minus NOS D46.C (*following* D46.2)
  48,XXXX Q97.1
  49,XXXXX Q97.1
  abdominal
    acute R1Ø.Ø
    muscle deficiency Q79.4
  abnormal innervation HØ2.519
    left HØ2.516
      lower HØ2.515
      upper HØ2.514
    right HØ2.513
      lower HØ2.512
      upper HØ2.511
  abstinence, neonatal P96.1
  acid pulmonary aspiration, obstetric O74.Ø
  acquired immunodeficiency — *see* Human, immunod-
    eficiency virus (HIV) disease
  acute abdominal R1Ø.Ø
  acute respiratory distress (adult) (child) J80
    idiopathic J84.114
  Adair-Dighton Q78.Ø
  Adams-Stokes (-Morgagni) I45.9
  adiposogenital E23.6
  adrenal
    hemorrhage (meningococcal) A39.1
    meningococcic A39.1
  adrenocortical — *see* Cushing's, syndrome
  adrenogenital E25.9
    congenital, associated with enzyme deficiency E25.Ø
  afferent loop NEC K91.89
  Alagille's Q44.7
  alcohol withdrawal (without convulsions) — *see* De-
    pendence, alcohol, with, withdrawal
  Alder's D72.Ø
  Aldrich (-Wiskott) D82.Ø
  alien hand R41.4
  Alport Q87.81
  alveolar hypoventilation E66.2
  alveolocapillary block J84.1Ø
  amnesic, amnestic (confabulatory) (due to) — *see* Dis-
    order, amnesic
  amyostatic (Wilson's disease) E83.Ø1
  androgen insensitivity E34.5Ø
    complete E34.51
    partial E34.52
  androgen resistance — *see also* Syndrome, androgen
    insensitivity E34.5Ø
  Angelman Q93.51
  anginal — *see* Angina
  ankyloglossia superior Q38.1
  anterior
    chest wall RØ7.89
    cord G83.82
    spinal artery G95.19
      compression M47.Ø19
        cervical region M47.Ø12
        cervicothoracic region M47.Ø13
        lumbar region M47.Ø16
        occipito-atlanto-axial region M47.Ø11
        thoracic region M47.Ø14
        thoracolumbar region M47.Ø15
    tibial M76.81- ☑
  antibody deficiency D8Ø.9
    agammaglobulinemic D8Ø.1
      hereditary D8Ø.Ø
    congenital D8Ø.Ø
    hypogammaglobulinemic D8Ø.1

Syndrome — *continued*
  antibody deficiency — *continued*
    hypogammaglobulinemic — *continued*
      hereditary D8Ø.Ø
  anticardiolipin (-antibody) D68.61
  antidepressant discontinuation T43.2Ø5 ☑
  antiphospholipid (-antibody) D68.61
  aortic
    arch M31.4
    bifurcation I74.Ø9
  aortomesenteric duodenum occlusion K31.5
  apical ballooning (transient left ventricular) I51.81
  arcuate ligament I77.4
  argentaffin, argintaffinoma E34.Ø
  Arnold-Chiari — *see* Arnold-Chiari disease
  Arrillaga-Ayerza I27.Ø
  arterial tortuosity Q87.82
  arteriovenous steal T82.898- ☑
  Asherman's N85.6
  aspiration, of newborn — *see* Aspiration, by substance,
    with pneumonia
    meconium P24.Ø1
  ataxia-telangiectasia G11.3
  auriculotemporal G5Ø.8
  autoerythrocyte sensitization (Gardner-Diamond) D69.2
  autoimmune lymphoproliferative [ALPS] D89.82
  autoimmune polyglandular E31.Ø
  autoinflammatory MØ4.9
    specified type NEC MØ4.8
  autosomal — *see* Abnormal, autosomes
  Avellis' G46.8
  Ayerza (-Arrillaga) I27.Ø
  Babinski-Nageotte G83.89
  Bakwin-Krida Q78.5
  bare lymphocyte D81.6
  Barré-Guillain G61.Ø
  Barré-Liéou M53.Ø
  Barrett's — *see* Barrett's, esophagus
  Barsony-Polgar K22.4
  Bársony-Teschendorf K22.4
  Barth E78.71
  Bartter's E26.81
  basal cell nevus Q87.89
  Basedow's EØ5.ØØ
    with thyroid storm EØ5.Ø1
  basilar artery G45.Ø
  Batten-Steinert G71.11
  battered
    baby or child — *see* Maltreatment, child, physical
      abuse
    spouse — *see* Maltreatment, adult, physical abuse
  Beals Q87.4Ø
  Beau's I51.5
  Beck's I65.8
  Benedikt's G46.3
  Béquez César (-Steinbrinck-Chédiak-Higashi) E7Ø.33Ø
  Bernhardt-Roth — *see* Meralgia paresthetica
  Bernheim's — *see* Failure, heart, right
  big spleen D73.1
  bilateral polycystic ovarian E28.2
  Bing-Horton's — *see* Horton's headache
  Birt-Hogg-Dube syndrome Q87.89
  Björck (-Thorsen) E34.Ø
  black
    lung J6Ø
    widow spider bite — *see* Toxicity, venom, spider,
      black widow
  Blackfan-Diamond D61.Ø1
  Blau MØ4.8
  blind loop K9Ø.2
    congenital Q43.8
    postsurgical K91.2
  blue sclera Q78.Ø
  blue toe I75.Ø2- ☑
  Boder-Sedgewick G11.3
  Boerhaave's K22.3
  Borjeson Forssman Lehmann Q89.8
  Bouillaud's IØ1.9
  Bourneville (-Pringle) Q85.1
  Bouveret (-Hoffman) I47.9
  brachial plexus G54.Ø
  bradycardia-tachycardia I49.5
  brain (nonpsychotic) FØ9
    with psychosis, psychotic reaction FØ9
    acute or subacute — *see* Delirium
    congenital — *see* Disability, intellectual
    organic FØ9
      post-traumatic (nonpsychotic) FØ7.81

Syndrome — *continued*
  brain — *continued*
    organic — *continued*
      post-traumatic — *continued*
        psychotic FØ9
    personality change FØ7.Ø
    postcontusional FØ7.81
    post-traumatic, nonpsychotic FØ7.81
    psycho-organic FØ9
    psychotic FØ6.8
  brain stem stroke G46.3
  Brandt's (acrodermatitis enteropathica) E83.2
  broad ligament laceration N83.8
  Brock's J98.11
  bronze baby P83.88
  Brown-Sequard G83.81
  Brugada I49.8
  bubbly lung P27.Ø
  Buchem's M85.2
  Budd-Chiari I82.Ø
  bulbar (progressive) G12.22
  Bürger-Grütz E78.3
  Burke's K86.89
  Burnett's (milk-alkali) E83.52
  burning feet E53.9
  Bywaters' T79.5 ☑
  Call-Fleming I67.841
  carbohydrate-deficient glycoprotein (CDGS) E77.8
  carcinogenic thrombophlebitis I82.1
  carcinoid E34.Ø
  cardiac asthma I5Ø.1
  cardiacos negros I27.Ø
  cardiofaciocutaneous Q87.89
  cardiopulmonary-obesity E66.2
  cardiorenal — *see* Hypertension, cardiorenal
  cardiorespiratory distress (idiopathic), newborn P22.Ø
  cardiovascular renal — *see* Hypertension, cardiorenal
  carotid
    artery (hemispheric) (internal) G45.1
    body G9Ø.Ø1
    sinus G9Ø.Ø1
  carpal tunnel G56.Ø- ☑
  Cassidy (-Scholte) E34.Ø
  cat cry Q93.4
  cat eye Q92.8
  cauda equina G83.4
  causalgia — *see* Causalgia
  celiac K9Ø.Ø
    artery compression I77.4
    axis I77.4
  central pain G89.Ø
  cerebellar
    hereditary G11.9
    stroke G46.4
  cerebellomedullary malformation — *see* Spina bifida
  cerebral
    artery
      anterior G46.1
      middle G46.Ø
      posterior G46.2
    gigantism E22.Ø
  cervical (root) M53.1
    disc — *see* Disorder, disc, cervical, with neuritis
    fusion Q76.1
    posterior, sympathicus M53.Ø
    rib Q76.5
    sympathetic paralysis G9Ø.2
  cervicobrachial (diffuse) M53.1
  cervicocranial M53.Ø
  cervicodorsal outlet G54.2
  cervicothoracic outlet G54.Ø
  Céstan (-Raymond) I65.8
  Charcot's (angina cruris) (intermittent claudication)
    I73.9
  Charcot-Weiss-Baker G9Ø.Ø9
  CHARGE Q89.8
  Chédiak-Higashi (-Steinbrinck) E7Ø.33Ø
  chest wall RØ7.1
  Chiari's (hepatic vein thrombosis) I82.Ø
  Chilaiditi's Q43.3
  child maltreatment — *see* Maltreatment, child
  chondrocostal junction M94.Ø
  chondroectodermal dysplasia Q77.6
  chromosome 4 short arm deletion Q93.3
  chromosome 5 short arm deletion Q93.4
  chronic
    infantile neurological, cutaneous and articular
      (CINCA) MØ4.2

Syndrome — *continued*
  chronic — *continued*
    pain G89.4
      personality F68.8
  Churg-Strauss M30.1
  Clarke-Hadfield K86.89
  Clerambault's automatism G93.89
  Clouston's (hidrotic ectodermal dysplasia) Q82.4
  clumsiness, clumsy child F82
  cluster headache G44.009
    intractable G44.001
    not intractable G44.009
  Coffin-Lowry Q89.8
  cold injury (newborn) P80.0
  combined immunity deficiency D81.9
  compartment (deep) (posterior) (traumatic) T79.A0 ☑
    (*following* T79.7)
    abdomen T79.A3 ☑ (*following* T79.7)
    lower extremity (hip, buttock, thigh, leg, foot, toes) T79.A2 ☑ (*following* T79.7)
    nontraumatic
      abdomen M79.A3 (*following* M79.7)
      lower extremity (hip, buttock, thigh, leg, foot, toes) M79.A2- ☑ (*following* M79.7)
      specified site NEC M79.A9 (*following* M79.7)
      upper extremity (shoulder, arm, forearm, wrist, hand, fingers) M79.A1- ☑ (*following* M79.7)
    postprocedural — *see* Syndrome, compartment, nontraumatic
    specified site NEC T79.A9 ☑ (*following* T79.7)
    upper extremity (shoulder, arm, forearm, wrist, hand, fingers) T79.A1 ☑ (*following* T79.7)
  complex regional pain — *see* Syndrome, pain, complex regional
  compression T79.5 ☑
    anterior spinal — *see* Syndrome, anterior, spinal artery, compression
    cauda equina G83.4
    celiac artery I77.4
    vertebral artery M47.029
      cervical region M47.022
      occipito-atlanto-axial region M47.021
  concussion F07.81
  congenital
    affecting multiple systems NEC Q87.89
    central alveolar hypoventilation G47.35
    facial diplegia Q87.0
    muscular hypertrophy-cerebral Q87.89
    oculo-auriculovertebral Q87.0
    oculofacial diplegia (Moebius) Q87.0
    rubella (manifest) P35.0
  congestion-fibrosis (pelvic), female N94.89
  congestive dysmenorrhea N94.6
  connective tissue M35.9
    overlap NEC M35.1
  Conn's E26.01
  conus medullaris G95.81
  cord
    anterior G83.82
    posterior G83.83
  coronary
    acute NEC I24.9
    insufficiency or intermediate I20.0
    slow flow I20.8
  Costen's (complex) M26.69
  costochondral junction M94.0
  costoclavicular G54.0
  costovertebral E22.0
  Cowden Q85.8
  craniovertebral M53.0
  Creutzfeldt-Jakob — *see* Creutzfeldt-Jakob disease or syndrome
  crib death R99
  cricopharyngeal — *see* Dysphagia
  cri-du-chat Q93.4
  croup J05.0
  CRPS I — *see* Syndrome, pain, complex regional I
  crush T79.5 ☑
  cryopyrin-associated perodic M04.2
  cryptophthalmos Q87.0
  cubital tunnel — *see* Lesion, nerve, ulnar
  Curschmann (-Batten) (-Steinert) G71.11
  Cushing's E24.9
    alcohol-induced E24.4
    due to
      alcohol
      drugs E24.2

Syndrome — *continued*
  Cushing's — *continued*
    due to — *continued*
      ectopic ACTH E24.3
      overproduction of pituitary ACTH E24.0
    drug-induced E24.2
    overdose or wrong substance given or taken — *see* Table of Drugs and Chemicals, by drug, poisoning
    pituitary-dependent E24.0
    specified type NEC E24.8
  cystic duct stump K91.5
  Dana-Putnam D51.0
  Danbolt (-Cross) (acrodermatitis enteropathica) E83.2
  Dandy-Walker Q03.1
    with spina bifida Q07.01
  Danlos' — *see also* Syndrome, Ehlers-Danlos Q79.60
  De Quervain E34.51
  de Toni-Fanconi (-Debré) E72.09
    with cystinosis E72.04
  defibrination — *see also* Fibrinolysis
    with
      antepartum hemorrhage — *see* Hemorrhage, antepartum, with coagulation defect
      intrapartum hemorrhage — *see* Hemorrhage, complicating, delivery
    newborn P60
    postpartum O72.3
  Degos' I77.89
  Déjérine-Roussy G89.0
  delayed sleep phase G47.21
  demyelinating G37.9
  dependence — *see* F10-F19 with fourth character .2
  depersonalization (-derealization) F48.1
  di George's D82.1
  diabetes mellitus in newborn infant P70.2
  diabetes mellitus-hypertension-nephrosis — *see* Diabetes, nephrosis
  diabetes-nephrosis — *see* Diabetes, nephrosis
  diabetic amyotrophy — *see* Diabetes, amyotrophy
  dialysis associated steal T82.898- ☑
  Diamond-Blackfan D61.01
  Diamond-Gardener D69.2
  DIC (diffuse or disseminated intravascular coagulopathy) D65
  Dighton's Q78.0
  disequilibrium E87.8
  Döhle body-panmyelopathic D72.0
  dorsolateral medullary G46.4
  double athetosis G80.3
  Down — *see also* Down syndrome Q90.9
  Dresbach's (elliptocytosis) D58.1
  Dressler's (postmyocardial infarction) I24.1
    postcardiotomy I97.0
  drug withdrawal, infant of dependent mother P96.1
  dry eye H04.12- ☑
  due to abnormality
    chromosomal Q99.9
      sex
        female phenotype Q97.9
        male phenotype Q98.9
      specified NEC Q99.8
  dumping (postgastrectomy) K91.1
    nonsurgical K31.89
  Dupré's (meningism) R29.1
  dysmetabolic X E88.81
  dyspraxia, developmental F82
  Eagle-Barrett Q79.4
  Eaton-Lambert — *see* Syndrome, Lambert-Eaton
  Ebstein's Q22.5
  ectopic ACTH E24.3
  eczema-thrombocytopenia D82.0
  Eddowes' Q78.0
  effort (psychogenic) F45.8
  Ehlers-Danlos Q79.60
    classical (cEDS) (classical EDS) Q79.61
    hypermobile (hEDS) (hypermobile EDS) Q79.62
    specified NEC Q79.69
    vascular (vascular EDS) (vEDS) Q79.63
  Eisenmenger's I27.83
  Ekman's Q78.0
  electric feet E53.8
  Ellis-van Creveld Q77.6
  empty nest Z60.0
  endocrine-hypertensive E27.0
  entrapment — *see* Neuropathy, entrapment
  eosinophilia-myalgia M35.8
  epileptic — *see also* Epilepsy, by type

Syndrome — *continued*
  epileptic — *see also* Epilepsy, by type — *continued*
    absence G40.A09 (*following* G40.3)
      intractable G40.A19 (*following* G40.3)
        with status epilepticus G40.A11 (*following* G40.3)
        without status epilepticus G40.A19 (*following* G40.3)
      not intractable G40.A09 (*following* G40.3)
        with status epilepticus G40.A01 (*following* G40.3)
        without status epilepticus G40.A09 (*following* G40.3)
  Erdheim-Chester (ECD) E88.89
  Erdheim's E22.0
  erythrocyte fragmentation D59.4
  Evans D69.41
  exhaustion F48.8
  extrapyramidal G25.9
    specified NEC G25.89
  eye retraction — *see* Strabismus
  eyelid-malar-mandible Q87.0
  Faber's D50.9
  facial pain, paroxysmal G50.0
  Fallot's Q21.3
  familial cold autoinflammatory M04.2
  familial eczema-thrombocytopenia (Wiskott-Aldrich) D82.0
  Fanconi (-de Toni) (-Debré) E72.09
    with cystinosis E72.04
  Fanconi's (anemia) (congenital pancytopenia) D61.09
  fatigue
    chronic R53.82
    psychogenic F48.8
  faulty bowel habit K59.39
  Feil-Klippel (brevicollis) Q76.1
  Felty's — *see* Felty's syndrome
  fertile eunuch E23.0
  fetal
    alcohol (dysmorphic) Q86.0
    hydantoin Q86.1
  Fiedler's I40.1
  first arch Q87.0
  fish odor E72.89
  Fisher's G61.0
  Fitzhugh-Curtis
    due to
      Chlamydia trachomatis A74.81
      Neisseria gonorrhorea (gonococcal peritonitis) A54.85
  Fitz's — *see also* Pancreatitis, acute K85.80
  Flajani (-Basedow) E05.00
    with thyroid storm E05.01
  flatback — *see* Flatback syndrome
  floppy
    baby P94.2
    iris (intraoeprative) (IFIS) H21.81
    mitral valve I34.1
  flush E34.0
  Foix-Alajouanine G95.19
  Fong's Q87.2
  food protein-induced enterocolitis (FPIES) K52.21
  foramen magnum G93.5
  Foster-Kennedy H47.14- ☑
  Foville's (peduncular) G46.3
  fragile X Q99.2
  Franceschetti Q75.4
  Frey's
    auriculotemporal G50.8
    hyperhidrosis L74.52
  Friderichsen-Waterhouse A39.1
  Froin's G95.89
  frontal lobe F07.0
  Fukuhara E88.49
  functional
    bowel K59.9
    prepubertal castrate E29.1
  Gaisböck's D75.1
  ganglion (basal ganglia brain) G25.9
    geniculi G51.1
  Gardner-Diamond D69.2
  gastroesophageal
    junction K22.0
    laceration-hemorrhage K22.6
  gastrojejunal loop obstruction K91.89
  Gee-Herter-Heubner K90.0
  Gelineau's G47.419
    with cataplexy G47.411
  genito-anorectal A55

☑ Additional Character Required — Refer to the Tabular List for Character Selection   ▽ Subterms under main terms may continue to next column or page

Syndrome — *continued*
  Gerstmann-Sträussler-Scheinker (GSS) A81.82
  Gianotti-Crosti L44.4
  giant platelet (Bernard-Soulier) D69.1
  Gilles de la Tourette's F95.2
  Glass Q87.89
  goiter-deafness E07.1
  Goldberg Q89.8
  Goldberg-Maxwell E34.51
  Good's D83.8
  Gopalan' (burning feet) E53.8
  Gorlin's Q87.89
  Gougerot-Blum L81.7
  Gouley's I31.1
  Gower's R55
  gray or grey (newborn) P93.0
    platelet D69.1
  Gubler-Millard G46.3
  Guillain-Barré (-Strohl) G61.0
  gustatory sweating G50.8
  Hadfield-Clarke K86.89
  hair tourniquet — *see* Constriction, external, by site
  Hamman's J98.19
  hand-foot L27.1
  hand-shoulder G90.8
  hantavirus (cardio)-pulmonary (HPS) (HCPS) B33.4
  happy puppet Q93.51
  Harada's H30.81- ☑
  Hayem-Faber D50.9
  headache NEC G44.89
    complicated NEC G44.59
  Heberden's I20.8
  Hedinger's E34.0
  Hegglin's D72.0
  HELLP (hemolysis, elevated liver enzymes and low
    platelet count) O14.2- ☑
    complicating
      childbirth O14.24
      puerperium O14.25
  hemolytic-uremic D59.3
  hemophagocytic, infection-associated D76.2
  Henoch-Schönlein D69.0
  hepatic flexure K59.8
  hepatopulmonary K76.81
  hepatorenal K76.7
    following delivery O90.4
    postoperative or postprocedural K91.83
    postpartum, puerperal O90.4
  hepatourologic K76.7
  Herter (-Gee) (nontropical sprue) K90.0
  Heubner-Herter K90.0
  Heyd's K76.7
  Hilger's G90.09
  histamine-like (fish poisoning) — *see* Poisoning, fish
  histiocytic D76.3
  histiocytosis NEC D76.3
  HIV infection, acute B20
  Hoffmann-Werdnig G12.0
  Hollander-Simons E88.1
  Hoppe-Goldflam G70.00
    with exacerbation (acute) G70.01
    in crisis G70.01
  Horner's G90.2
  hungry bone E83.81
  hunterian glossitis D51.0
  Hutchinson's triad A50.53
  hyperabduction G54.0
  hyperammonemia-hyperornithinemia-homocitrulline-
    mia E72.4
  hypereosinophilic (idiopathic) D72.1
  hyperimmunoglobulin D M04.1
  hyperimmunoglobulin E (IgE) D82.4
  hyperkalemic E87.5
  hyperkinetic — *see* Hyperkinesia
  hypermobility M35.7
  hypernatremia E87.0
  hyperosmolarity E87.0
  hyperperfusion G97.82
  hypersplenic D73.1
  hypertransfusion, newborn P61.1
  hyperventilation F45.8
  hyperviscosity (of serum)
    polycythemic D75.1
    sclerothymic D58.8
  hypoglycemic (familial) (neonatal) E16.2
  hypokalemic E87.6
  hyponatremic E87.1
  hypopituitarism E23.0
  hypoplastic left-heart Q23.4

Syndrome — *continued*
  hypopotassemia E87.6
  hyposmolality E87.1
  hypotension, maternal O26.5- ☑
  hypothenar hammer I73.89
  hypoventilation, obesity (OHS) E66.2
  ICF (intravascular coagulation-fibrinolysis) D65
  idiopathic
    cardiorespiratory distress, newborn P22.0
    nephrotic (infantile) N04.9
  iliotibial band M76.3- ☑
  immobility, immobilization (paraplegic) M62.3
  immune reconstitution D89.3
  immune reconstitution inflammatory [IRIS] D89.3
  immunity deficiency, combined D81.9
  immunodeficiency
    acquired — *see* Human, immunodeficiency virus
      (HIV) disease
    combined D81.9
  impending coronary I20.0
  impingement, shoulder M75.4- ☑
  inappropriate secretion of antidiuretic hormone E22.2
  infant
    gestational diabetes P70.0
    of diabetic mother P70.1
  infantilism (pituitary) E23.0
  inferior vena cava I87.1
  inspissated bile (newborn) P59.1
  institutional (childhood) F94.2
  insufficient sleep F51.12
  intermediate coronary (artery) I20.0
  interspinous ligament — *see* Spondylopathy, specified
    NEC
  intestinal
    carcinoid E34.0
    knot K56.2
  intravascular coagulation-fibrinolysis (ICF) D65
  iodine-deficiency, congenital E00.9
    type
      mixed E00.2
      myxedematous E00.1
      neurological E00.0
  IRDS (idiopathic respiratory distress, newborn) P22.0
  irritable
    bowel K58.9
      with
        constipation K58.1
        diarrhea K58.0
      mixed K58.2
      psychogenic F45.8
      specified NEC K58.8
    heart (psychogenic) F45.8
    weakness F48.8
  ischemic
    bowel (transient) K55.9
      chronic K55.1
      due to mesenteric artery insufficiency K55.1
    steal T82.898 ☑
  IVC (intravascular coagulopathy) D65
  Ivemark's Q89.01
  Jaccoud's — *see* Arthropathy, postrheumatic, chronic
  Jackson's G83.89
  Jakob-Creutzfeldt — *see* Creutzfeldt-Jakob disease or
    syndrome
  jaw-winking Q07.8
  Jervell-Lange-Nielsen I45.81
  jet lag G47.25
  Job's D71
  Joseph-Diamond-Blackfan D61.01
  jugular foramen G52.7
  Kabuki Q89.8
  Kanner's (autism) F84.0
  Kartagener's Q89.3
  Kelly's D50.1
  Kimmelstiel-Wilson — *see* Diabetes, specified type,
    with Kimmelstiel-Wilson disease
  Klein (e)-Levine G47.13
  Klippel-Feil (brevicollis) Q76.1
  Köhler-Pellegrini-Steida — *see* Bursitis, tibial collateral
  König's K59.8
  Korsakoff (-Wernicke) (nonalcoholic) F04
    alcoholic F10.26
  Kostmann's D70.0
  Krabbe's congenital muscle hypoplasia Q79.8
  labyrinthine — *see* subcategory H83.2 ☑
  lacunar NEC G46.7
  Lambert-Eaton G70.80

Syndrome — *continued*
  Lambert-Eaton — *continued*
    in
      neoplastic disease G73.1
      specified disease NEC G70.81
  Landau-Kleffner — *see* Epilepsy, specified NEC
  Larsen's Q74.8
  lateral
    cutaneous nerve of thigh G57.1- ☑
    medullary G46.4
  Launois' E22.0
  lazy
    leukocyte D70.8
    posture M62.3
  Lemiere I80.8
  Lennox-Gastaut G40.812
    intractable G40.814
      with status epilepticus G40.813
      without status epilepticus G40.814
    not intractable G40.812
      with status epilepticus G40.811
      without status epilepticus G40.812
  lenticular, progressive E83.01
  Leopold-Levi's E05.90
  Lev's I44.2
  Lichtheim's D51.0
  Li-Fraumeni Z15.01
  Lightwood's N25.89
  Lignac (de Toni) (-Fanconi) (-Debré) E72.09
    with cystinosis E72.04
  Likoff's I20.8
  limbic epilepsy personality F07.0
  liver-kidney K76.7
  lobotomy F07.0
  Loffler's J82
  long arm 18 or 21 deletion Q93.89
  long QT I45.81
  Louis-Barré G11.3
  low
    atmospheric pressure T70.29 ☑
    back M54.5
    output (cardiac) I50.9
  lower radicular, newborn (birth injury) P14.8
  Luetscher's (dehydration) E86.0
  Lupus anticoagulant D68.62
  Lutembacher's Q21.1
  macrophage activation D76.1
    due to infection D76.2
  magnesium-deficiency R29.0
  Majeed M04.8
  Mal de Debarquement R42
  malabsorption K90.9
    postsurgical K91.2
  malformation, congenital, due to
    alcohol Q86.0
    exogenous cause NEC Q86.8
    hydantoin Q86.1
    warfarin Q86.2
  malignant
    carcinoid E34.0
    neuroleptic G21.0
  Mallory-Weiss K22.6
  mandibulofacial dysostosis Q75.4
  manic-depressive — *see* Disorder, bipolar
  maple-syrup-urine E71.0
  Marable's I77.4
  Marfan's Q87.40
    with
      cardiovascular manifestations Q87.418
        aortic dilation Q87.410
      ocular manifestations Q87.42
      skeletal manifestations Q87.43
  Marie's (acromegaly) E22.0
  mast cell activation — *see* Activation, mast cell
  maternal hypotension — *see* Syndrome, hypotension,
    maternal
  May (-Hegglin) D72.0
  McArdle (-Schmidt) (-Pearson) E74.04
  McQuarrie's E16.2
  meconium plug (newborn) P76.0
  median arcuate ligament I77.4
  Meekeren-Ehlers-Danlos Q79.6 ☑
  megavitamin-B6 E67.2
  Meige G24.4
  MELAS E88.41
  Mendelson's O74.0
  MERRF (myoclonic epilepsy associated with ragged-
    red fibers) E88.42

Syndrome — continued

mesenteric
    artery (superior) K55.1
    vascular insufficiency K55.1
metabolic E88.81
metastatic carcinoid E34.0
micrognathia-glossoptosis Q87.0
midbrain NEC G93.89
middle lobe (lung) J98.19
middle radicular G54.0
migraine — see also Migraine G43.909
Mikulicz' K11.8
milk-alkali E83.52
Millard-Gubler G46.3
Miller-Dieker Q93.88
Miller-Fisher G61.0
Minkowski-Chauffard D58.0
Mirizzi's K83.1
MNGIE (Mitochondrial Neurogastrointestinal En-
    cephalopathy) E88.49
Möbius, ophthalmoplegic migraine — see Migraine,
    ophthalmoplegic
monofixation H50.42
Morel-Moore M85.2
Morel-Morgagni M85.2
Morgagni (-Morel) (-Stewart) M85.2
Morgagni-Adams-Stokes I45.9
Mounier-Kuhn Q32.4
    with bronchiectasis J47.9
        with
            exacerbation (acute) J47.1
            lower respiratory infection J47.0
    acquired J98.09
        with bronchiectasis J47.9
            with
                exacerbation (acute) J47.1
                lower respiratory infection J47.0
Muckle-Wells M04.2
mucocutaneous lymph node (acute febrile) (MCLS)
    M30.3
multiple endocrine neoplasia (MEN) — see Neoplasia,
    endocrine, multiple (MEN)
multiple operations — see Disorder, factitious
myasthenic G70.9
    in
        diabetes mellitus — see Diabetes, amyotrophy
        endocrine disease NEC E34.9 [G73.3]
        neoplastic disease — see also Neoplasm
            D49.9 [G73.3]
        thyrotoxicosis (hyperthyroidism) E05.90 [G73.3]
            with thyroid storm E05.91 [G73.3]
myelodysplastic D46.9
    with
        5q deletion D46.C (following D46.2)
        isolated del (5q) chromosomal abnormality D46.C
            (following D46.2)
        lesions, low grade D46.20
        specified NEC D46.Z (following D46.4)
myelopathic pain G89.0
myeloproliferative (chronic) D47.1
myofascial pain M79.18
Naffziger's G54.0
nail patella Q87.2
NARP (Neuropathy, Ataxia and Retinitis pigmentosa)
    E88.49
neonatal abstinence P96.1
nephritic — see also Nephritis
    with edema — see Nephrosis
    acute N00.9
    chronic N03.9
    rapidly progressive N01.9
nephrotic (congenital) — see also Nephrosis N04.9
    with
        dense deposit disease N04.6
        diffuse
            crescentic glomerulonephritis N04.7
            endocapillary proliferative glomerulonephritis
                N04.4
            membranous glomerulonephritis N04.2
            mesangial proliferative glomerulonephritis
                N04.3
            mesangiocapillary glomerulonephritis N04.5
        focal and segmental glomerular lesions N04.1
        minor glomerular abnormality N04.0
        specified morphological changes NEC N04.8
    diabetic — see Diabetes, nephrosis
neurologic neglect R41.4
Nezelof's D81.4

Nonne-Milroy-Meige Q82.0
Nothnagel's vasomotor acroparesthesia I73.89
obesity hypoventilation (OHS) E66.2
oculomotor H51.9
ophthalmoplegia-cerebellar ataxia — see Strabismus,
    paralytic, third nerve
oral allergy T78.1 ☑
oral-facial-digital Q87.0
organic
    affective F06.30
    amnesic (not alcohol- or drug-induced) F04
    brain F09
    depressive F06.31
    hallucinosis F06.0
    personality F07.0
Ormond's N13.5
oro-facial-digital Q87.0
os trigonum Q68.8
Osler-Weber-Rendu I78.0
osteoporosis-osteomalacia M83.8
Osterreicher-Turner Q87.2
otolith — see subcategory H81.8 ☑
oto-palatal-digital Q87.0
outlet (thoracic) G54.0
ovary
    polycystic E28.2
    resistant E28.39
    sclerocystic E28.2
Owren's D68.2
Paget-Schroetter I82.890
pain — see also Pain
    complex regional I G90.50
        lower limb G90.52- ☑
        specified site NEC G90.59
        upper limb G90.51- ☑
    complex regional II — see Causalgia
painful
    bruising D69.2
    feet E53.8
    prostate N42.81
paralysis agitans — see Parkinsonism
paralytic G83.9
    specified NEC G83.89
Parinaud's H51.0
parkinsonian — see Parkinsonism
Parkinson's — see Parkinsonism
paroxysmal facial pain G50.0
Parry's E05.00
    with thyroid storm E05.01
Parsonage (-Aldren)-Turner G54.5
patella clunk M25.86- ☑
Paterson (-Brown) (-Kelly) D50.1
pectoral girdle I77.89
pectoralis minor I77.89
pediatric autoimmune neuropsychiatric disorders asso-
    ciated with streptococcal infections (PANDAS)
    D89.89
Pelger-Huet D72.0
pellagra-cerebellar ataxia-renal aminoaciduria E72.02
pellagroid E52
Pellegrini-Stieda — see Bursitis, tibial collateral
pelvic congestion-fibrosis, female N94.89
penta X Q97.1
peptic ulcer — see Ulcer, peptic
perabduction I77.89
periodic fever M04.1
periodic fever, aphthous stomatitis, pharyngitis, and
    adenopathy [PFAPA] M04.8
periodic headache, in adults and children — see
    Headache, periodic syndromes in adults and
    children
periurethral fibrosis N13.5
phantom limb (without pain) G54.7
    with pain G54.6
pharyngeal pouch D82.1
Pick's — see Disease, Pick's
Pickwickian E66.2
PIE (pulmonary infiltration with eosinophilia) J82
pigmentary pallidal degeneration (progressive) G23.0
pineal E34.8
pituitary E22.0
placental transfusion — see Pregnancy, complicated
    by, placental transfusion syndromes
plantar fascia M72.2
plateau iris (post-iridectomy) (postprocedural) H21.82
Plummer-Vinson D50.1
pluricarential of infancy E40

plurideficiency E40
pluriglandular (compensatory) E31.8
    autoimmune E31.0
pneumatic hammer T75.21 ☑
polyangiitis overlap M30.8
polycarential of infancy E40
polyglandular E31.8
    autoimmune E31.0
polysplenia Q89.09
pontine NEC G93.89
popliteal
    artery entrapment I77.89
    post endometrial ablation N99.85
    web Q87.89
post chemoembolization — code to associated condi-
    tions
postcardiac injury
    postcardiotomy I97.0
    postmyocardial infarction I24.1
postcardiotomy I97.0
postcholecystectomy K91.5
postcommissurotomy I97.0
postconcussional F07.81
postcontusional F07.81
postencephalitic F07.89
posterior
    cervical sympathetic M53.0
    cord G83.83
    fossa compression G93.5
    reversible encephalopathy (PRES) I67.83
postgastrectomy (dumping) K91.1
postgastric surgery K91.1
postinfarction I24.1
postlaminectomy NEC M96.1
postleukotomy F07.0
postmastectomy lymphedema I97.2
postmyocardial infarction I24.1
postoperative NEC T81.9 ☑
    blind loop K90.2
postpartum panhypopituitary (Sheehan) E23.0
postpolio (myelitic) G14
postthrombotic I87.009
    with
        inflammation I87.02- ☑
            with ulcer I87.03- ☑
        specified complication NEC I87.09- ☑
        ulcer I87.01- ☑
            with inflammation I87.03- ☑
    asymptomatic I87.00- ☑
postvagotomy K91.1
postvalvulotomy I97.0
postviral NEC G93.3
    fatigue G93.3
Potain's K31.0
potassium intoxication E87.5
Prader-Willi Q87.11
Prader-Willi-like Q87.19
precerebral artery (multiple) (bilateral) G45.2
preinfarction I20.0
preleukemic D46.9
premature senility E34.8
premenstrual dysphoric F32.81
premenstrual tension N94.3
Prinzmetal-Massumi R07.1
prune belly Q79.4
pseudo -Turner's Q87.19
pseudocarpal tunnel (sublimis) — see Syndrome, carpa
    tunnel
pseudoparalytica G70.00
    with exacerbation (acute) G70.01
    in crisis G70.01
psycho-organic (nonpsychotic severity) F07.9
    acute or subacute F05
    depressive type F06.31
    hallucinatory type F06.0
    nonpsychotic severity F07.0
    specified NEC F07.89
pulmonary
    arteriosclerosis I27.0
    dysmaturity (Wilson-Mikity) P27.0
    hypoperfusion (idiopathic) P22.0
    renal (hemorrhagic) (Goodpasture's) M31.0
pure
    motor lacunar G46.5
    sensory lacunar G46.6
Putnam-Dana D51.0

☑ Additional Character Required — Refer to the Tabular List for Character Selection   ▽ Subterms under main terms may continue to next column or page

Syndrome — continued
pyogenic arthritis, pyoderma gangrenosum, and acne [PAPA] M04.8
pyramidopallidonigral G20
pyriformis — see Lesion, nerve, sciatic
QT interval prolongation I45.81
radicular NEC — see Radiculopathy
   upper limbs, newborn (birth injury) P14.3
rapid time-zone change G47.25
Rasmussen G04.81
Raymond (-Céstan) I65.8
Raynaud's I73.00
   with gangrene I73.01
RDS (respiratory distress syndrome, newborn) P22.0
reactive airways dysfunction J68.3
Refsum's G60.1
Reifenstein E34.52
renal glomerulohyalinosis-diabetic — see Diabetes, nephrosis
Rendu-Osler-Weber I78.0
residual ovary N99.83
resistant ovary E28.39
respiratory
   distress
     acute J80
      adult J80
      child J80
      idiopathic J84.114
      newborn (idiopathic) (type I) P22.0
        type II P22.1
restless legs G25.81
retinoblastoma (familial) C69.2 ☑
retroperitoneal fibrosis N13.5
retroviral seroconversion (acute) Z21
Reye's G93.7
Richter — see Leukemia, chronic lymphocytic, B-cell type
Ridley's I50.1
right
   heart, hypoplastic Q22.6
   ventricular obstruction — see Failure, heart, right
Romano-Ward (prolonged QT interval) I45.81
rotator cuff, shoulder — see also Tear, rotator cuff M75.10- ☑
Rotes Quérol — see Hyperostosis, ankylosing
Roth — see Meralgia paresthetica
rubella (congenital) P35.0
Ruvalcaba-Myhre-Smith E71.440
Rytand-Lipsitch I44.2
salt
   depletion E87.1
     due to heat NEC T67.8 ☑
      causing heat exhaustion or prostration T67.4 ☑
   low E87.1
salt-losing N28.89
SATB2-associated Q87.89
Scaglietti-Dagnini E22.0
scalenus anticus (anterior) G54.0
scapulocostal — see Mononeuropathy, upper limb, specified site NEC
scapuloperoneal G71.09
schizophrenic, of childhood NEC F84.5
Schnitzler D47.2
Scholte's E34.0
Schroeder's E27.0
Schüller-Christian C96.5
Schwachman's — see Syndrome, Shwachman's
Schwartz (-Jampel) G71.13
Schwartz-Bartter E22.2
scimitar Q26.8
sclerocystic ovary E28.2
Seitelberger's G31.89
septicemic adrenal hemorrhage A39.1
seroconversion, retroviral (acute) Z21
serous meningitis G93.2
severe acute respiratory (SARS) J12.81
shaken infant T74.4 ☑
shock (traumatic) T79.4 ☑
   kidney N17.0
     following crush injury T79.5 ☑
   toxic A48.3
shock-lung J80
Shone's — code to specific anomalies
short
   bowel K91.2
   rib Q77.2
shoulder-hand — see Algoneurodystrophy

Syndrome — continued
Shwachman's D70.4
sicca — see Sicca syndrome
sick
   cell E87.1
   sinus I49.5
sick-euthyroid E07.81
sideropenic D50.1
Siemens' ectodermal dysplasia Q82.4
Silfversköld's Q78.9
Simons' E88.1
sinus tarsi M25.57- ☑
sinusitis-bronchiectasis-situs inversus Q89.3
Sipple's E31.22
sirenomelia Q87.2
Slocumb's E27.0
slow flow, coronary I20.8
Sluder's G44.89
Smith-Magenis Q93.88
Sneddon-Wilkinson L13.1
Sotos' Q87.3
South African cardiomyopathy I42.8
spasmodic
   upward movement, eyes H51.8
   winking F95.8
Spen's I45.9
splenic
   agenesis Q89.01
   flexure K59.8
   neutropenia D73.81
Spurway's Q78.0
staphylococcal scalded skin L00
steal
   arteriovenous T82.898- ☑
   ischemic T82.898- ☑
   subclavian G45.8
Stein-Leventhal E28.2
Stein's E28.2
Stevens-Johnson syndrome L51.1
   toxic epidermal necrolysis overlap L51.3
Stewart-Morel M85.2
Stickler Q89.8
stiff baby Q89.8
stiff man G25.82
Still-Felty — see Felty's syndrome
Stokes (-Adams) I45.9
stone heart I50.1
straight back, congenital Q76.49
subclavian steal G45.8
subcoracoid-pectoralis minor G54.0
subcostal nerve compression I77.89
subphrenic interposition Q43.3
superior
   cerebellar artery I63.89
   mesenteric artery K55.1
   semi-circular canal dehiscence H83.8X- ☑
   vena cava I87.1
supine hypotensive (maternal) — see Syndrome, hypotension, maternal
suprarenal cortical E27.0
supraspinatus — see also Tear, rotator cuff M75.10- ☑
Susac G93.49
swallowed blood P78.2
sweat retention L74.0
Swyer Q99.1
Symond's G93.2
sympathetic
   cervical paralysis G90.2
   pelvic, female N94.89
systemic inflammatory response (SIRS), of non-infectious origin (without organ dysfunction) R65.10
   with acute organ dysfunction R65.11
tachycardia-bradycardia I49.5
takotsubo I51.81
TAR (thrombocytopenia with absent radius) Q87.2
tarsal tunnel G57.5- ☑
teething K00.7
tegmental G93.89
telangiectasic-pigmentation-cataract Q82.8
temporal pyramidal apex — see Otitis, media, suppurative, acute
temporomandibular joint-pain-dysfunction M26.62- ☑
Terry's — see also Myopia, degenerative H44.2- ☑
testicular feminization — see also Syndrome, androgen insensitivity E34.51
thalamic pain (hyperesthetic) G89.0
thoracic outlet (compression) G54.0
Thorson-Björck E34.0

Syndrome — continued
thrombocytopenia with absent radius (TAR) Q87.2
thyroid-adrenocortical insufficiency E31.0
tibial
   anterior M76.81- ☑
   posterior M76.82- ☑
Tietze's M94.0
time-zone (rapid) G47.25
Toni-Fanconi E72.09
   with cystinosis E72.04
Touraine's Q79.8
tourniquet — see Constriction, external, by site
toxic shock A48.3
transient left ventricular apical ballooning I51.81
traumatic vasospastic T75.22 ☑
Treacher Collins Q75.4
triple X, female Q97.0
trisomy Q92.9
   13 Q91.7
     meiotic nondisjunction Q91.4
     mitotic nondisjunction Q91.5
     mosaicism Q91.5
     translocation Q91.6
   18 Q91.3
     meiotic nondisjunction Q91.0
     mitotic nondisjunction Q91.1
     mosaicism Q91.1
     translocation Q91.2
   20 (q)(p) Q92.8
   21 Q90.9
     meiotic nondisjunction Q90.0
     mitotic nondisjunction Q90.1
     mosaicism Q90.1
     translocation Q90.2
   22 Q92.8
tropical wet feet T69.0- ☑
Trousseau's I82.1
tumor lysis (following antineoplastic chemotherapy) (spontaneous) NEC E88.3
tumor necrosis factor receptor associated periodic (TRAPS) M04.1
Twiddler's (due to)
   automatic implantable defibrillator T82.198 ☑
   cardiac pacemaker T82.198 ☑
Unverricht (-Lundborg) — see Epilepsy, generalized, idiopathic
upward gaze H51.8
uremia, chronic — see also Disease, kidney, chronic N18.9
urethral N34.3
urethro-oculo-articular — see Reiter's disease
urohepatic K76.7
vago-hypoglossal G52.7
van Buchem's M85.2
van der Hoeve's Q78.0
vascular NEC in cerebrovascular disease G46.8
vasoconstriction, reversible cerebrovascular I67.841
vasomotor I73.9
vasospastic (traumatic) T75.22 ☑
vasovagal R55
VATER Q87.2
velo-cardio-facial Q93.81
vena cava (inferior) (superior) (obstruction) I87.1
vertebral
   artery G45.0
     compression — see Syndrome, anterior, spinal artery, compression
   steal G45.0
vertebro-basilar artery G45.0
vertebrogenic (pain) M54.89
vertiginous — see Disorder, vestibular function
Vinson-Plummer D50.1
virus B34.9
visceral larva migrans B83.0
visual disorientation H53.8
vitamin B6 deficiency E53.1
vitreal corneal H59.01- ☑
vitreous (touch) H59.01- ☑
Vogt-Koyanagi H20.82- ☑
Volkmann's T79.6 ☑
von Schroetter's I82.890
von Willebrand (-Jürgen) D68.0
Waldenström-Kjellberg D50.1
Wallenberg's G46.3
water retention E87.79
Waterhouse (-Friderichsen) A39.1
Weber-Gubler G46.3
Weber-Leyden G46.3

Syndrome — continued
Weber's G46.3
Wegener's M31.30
    with
        kidney involvement M31.31
        lung involvement M31.30
            with kidney involvement M31.31
Weingarten's (tropical eosinophilia) J82
Weiss-Baker G90.09
Werdnig-Hoffman G12.0
Wermer's E31.21
Werner's E34.8
Wernicke-Korsakoff (nonalcoholic) F04
    alcoholic F10.26
Westphal-Strümpell E83.01
West's — see Epilepsy, spasms
wet
    feet (maceration) (tropical) T69.0- ☑
    lung, newborn P22.1
whiplash S13.4 ☑
whistling face Q87.0
Wilkie's K55.1
Wilkinson-Sneddon L13.1
Willebrand (-Jürgens) D68.0
Williams Q93.82
Wilson's (hepatolenticular degeneration) E83.01
Wiskott-Aldrich D82.0
withdrawal — see Withdrawal, state
    drug
        infant of dependent mother P96.1
        therapeutic use, newborn P96.2
Woakes' (ethmoiditis) J33.1
Wright's (hyperabduction) G54.0
X I20.9
XXXX Q97.1
XXXXX Q97.1
XXXXY Q98.1
XXY Q98.0
Yao M04.8
yellow nail L60.5
Zahorsky's B08.5
Zellweger syndrome E71.510
Zellweger-like syndrome E71.541
Synechia (anterior) (iris) (posterior) (pupil) — see also
    Adhesions, iris
    intra-uterine (traumatic) N85.6
Synesthesia R20.8
Syngamiasis, syngamosis B83.3
Synodontia K00.2
Synorchidism, synorchism Q55.1
Synostosis (congenital) Q78.8
    astragalo-scaphoid Q74.2
    radioulnar Q74.0
Synovial sarcoma — see Neoplasm, connective tissue,
    malignant
Synovioma (malignant) — see also Neoplasm, connective
    tissue, malignant
    benign — see Neoplasm, connective tissue, benign
Synoviosarcoma — see Neoplasm, connective tissue,
    malignant
Synovitis — see also Tenosynovitis M65.9
    crepitant
        hand M70.0- ☑
        wrist M70.03- ☑
    gonococcal A54.49
    gouty — see Gout
    in (due to)
        crystals M65.8- ☑
        gonorrhea A54.49
        syphilis (late) A52.78
        use, overuse, pressure — see Disorder, soft tissue,
            due to use
    infective NEC — see Tenosynovitis, infective NEC
    specified NEC — see Tenosynovitis, specified type NEC
    syphilitic A52.78
        congenital (early) A50.02
    toxic — see Synovitis, transient
    transient M67.3- ☑
        ankle M67.37- ☑
        elbow M67.32- ☑
        foot joint M67.37- ☑
        hand joint M67.34- ☑
        hip M67.35- ☑
        knee M67.36- ☑
        multiple site M67.39
        pelvic region M67.35- ☑
        shoulder M67.31- ☑
        specified joint NEC M67.38

Synovitis — continued
    transient — continued
        wrist M67.33- ☑
    traumatic, current — see Sprain
    tuberculous — see Tuberculosis, synovitis
    villonodular (pigmented) M12.2- ☑
        ankle M12.27- ☑
        elbow M12.22- ☑
        foot joint M12.27- ☑
        hand joint M12.24- ☑
        hip M12.25- ☑
        knee M12.26- ☑
        multiple site M12.29
        pelvic region M12.25- ☑
        shoulder M12.21- ☑
        specified joint NEC M12.28
        vertebrae M12.28
        wrist M12.23- ☑
Syphilid A51.39
    congenital A50.06
    newborn A50.06
    tubercular (late) A52.79
Syphilis, syphilitic (acquired) A53.9
    abdomen (late) A52.79
    acoustic nerve A52.15
    adenopathy (secondary) A51.49
    adrenal (gland) (with cortical hypofunction) A52.79
    age under 2 years NOS — see also Syphilis, congenital,
        early
        acquired A51.9
    alopecia (secondary) A51.32
    anemia (late) A52.79 [D63.8]
    aneurysm (aorta) (ruptured) A52.01
        central nervous system A52.05
        congenital A50.54 [I79.0]
    anus (late) A52.74
        primary A51.1
        secondary A51.39
    aorta (arch) (abdominal) (thoracic) A52.02
        aneurysm A52.01
    aortic (insufficiency) (regurgitation) (stenosis) A52.03
        aneurysm A52.01
    arachnoid (adhesive) (cerebral) (spinal) A52.13
    asymptomatic — see Syphilis, latent
    ataxia (locomotor) A52.11
    atrophoderma maculatum A51.39
    auricular fibrillation A52.06
    bladder (late) A52.76
    bone A52.77
        secondary A51.46
    brain A52.17
    breast (late) A52.79
    bronchus (late) A52.72
    bubo (primary) A51.0
    bulbar palsy A52.19
    bursa (late) A52.78
    cardiac decompensation A52.06
    cardiovascular A52.00
    central nervous system (late) (recurrent) (relapse) (ter-
        tiary) A52.3
        with
            ataxia A52.11
            general paralysis A52.17
                juvenile A50.45
            paresis (general) A52.17
                juvenile A50.45
            tabes (dorsalis) A52.11
                juvenile A50.45
            taboparesis A52.17
                juvenile A50.45
        aneurysm A52.05
        congenital A50.40
        juvenile A50.40
        remission in (sustained) A52.3
        serology doubtful, negative, or positive A52.3
        specified nature or site NEC A52.19
        vascular A52.05
    cerebral A52.17
        meningovascular A52.13
        nerves (multiple palsies) A52.15
        sclerosis A52.17
        thrombosis A52.05
    cerebrospinal (tabetic type) A52.12
    cerebrovascular A52.05
    cervix (late) A52.76
    chancre (multiple) A51.0
        extragenital A51.2
        Rollet's A51.0

Syphilis, syphilitic — continued
    Charcot's joint A52.16
    chorioretinitis A51.43
        congenital A50.01
        late A52.71
        prenatal A50.01
    choroiditis — see Syphilitic chorioretinitis
    choroidoretinitis — see Syphilitic chorioretinitis
    ciliary body (secondary) A51.43
        late A52.71
    colon (late) A52.74
    combined spinal sclerosis A52.11
    condyloma (latum) A51.31
    congenital A50.9
        with
            paresis (general) A50.45
            tabes (dorsalis) A50.45
            taboparesis A50.45
        chorioretinitis, choroiditis A50.01 [H32]
        early, or less than 2 years after birth NEC A50.2
            with manifestations — see Syphilis, congenital,
                early, symptomatic
            latent (without manifestations) A50.1
                negative spinal fluid test A50.1
                serology positive A50.1
            symptomatic A50.09
                cutaneous A50.06
                mucocutaneous A50.07
                oculopathy A50.01
                osteochondropathy A50.02
                pharyngitis A50.03
                pneumonia A50.04
                rhinitis A50.05
                visceral A50.08
            interstitial keratitis A50.31
            juvenile neurosyphilis A50.45
        late, or 2 years or more after birth NEC A50.7
            chorioretinitis, choroiditis A50.32
            interstitial keratitis A50.31
            juvenile neurosyphilis A50.45
            latent (without manifestations) A50.6
                negative spinal fluid test A50.6
                serology positive A50.6
            symptomatic or with manifestations NEC A50.59
                arthropathy A50.55
                cardiovascular A50.54
                Clutton's joints A50.51
                Hutchinson's teeth A50.52
                Hutchinson's triad A50.53
                osteochondropathy A50.56
                saddle nose A50.57
    conjugal A53.9
        tabes A52.11
    conjunctiva (late) A52.71
    contact Z20.2
    cord bladder A52.19
    cornea, late A52.71
    coronary (artery) (sclerosis) A52.06
    coryza, congenital A50.05
    cranial nerve A52.15
        multiple palsies A52.15
    cutaneous — see Syphilis, skin
    dacryocystitis (late) A52.71
    degeneration, spinal cord A52.12
    dementia paralytica A52.17
        juvenilis A50.45
    destruction of bone A52.77
    dilatation, aorta A52.01
    due to blood transfusion A53.9
    dura mater A52.13
    ear A52.79
        inner A52.79
            nerve (eighth) A52.15
            neurorecurrence A52.15
    early A51.9
        cardiovascular A52.00
        central nervous system A52.3
        latent (without manifestations) (less than 2 years
            after infection) A51.5
            negative spinal fluid test A51.5
            serological relapse after treatment A51.5
            serology positive A51.5
        relapse (treated, untreated) A51.9
        skin A51.39
        symptomatic A51.9
            extragenital chancre A51.2
            primary, except extragenital chancre A51.0
            secondary — see also Syphilis, secondary A51.3◀
                relapse (treated, untreated) A51.49

Syphilis, syphilitic — *continued*
 early — *continued*
  ulcer A51.39
 eighth nerve (neuritis) A52.15
 endemic A65
 endocarditis A52.03
  aortic A52.03
  pulmonary A52.03
 epididymis (late) A52.76
 epiglottis (late) A52.73
 epiphysitis (congenital) (early) A50.02
 episcleritis (late) A52.71
 esophagus A52.79
 eustachian tube A52.73
 exposure to Z20.2
 eye A52.71
 eyelid (late) (with gumma) A52.71
 fallopian tube (late) A52.76
 fracture A52.77
 gallbladder (late) A52.74
 gastric (polyposis) (late) A52.74
 general A53.9
  paralysis A52.17
   juvenile A50.45
 genital (primary) A51.0
 glaucoma A52.71
 gumma NEC A52.79
  cardiovascular system A52.00
  central nervous system A52.3
  congenital A50.59
 heart (block) (decompensation) (disease) (failure)
   A52.06 *[I52]*
  valve NEC A52.03
 hemianesthesia A52.19
 hemianopsia A52.71
 hemiparesis A52.17
 hemiplegia A52.17
 hepatic artery A52.09
 hepatis A52.74
 hepatomegaly, congenital A50.08
 hereditaria tarda — *see* Syphilis, congenital, late
 hereditary — *see* Syphilis, congenital
 Hutchinson's teeth A50.52
 hyalitis A52.71
 inactive — *see* Syphilis, latent
 infantum — *see* Syphilis, congenital
 inherited — *see* Syphilis, congenital
 internal ear A52.79
 intestine (late) A52.74
 iris, iritis (secondary) A51.43
  late A52.71
 joint (late) A52.77
 keratitis (congenital) (interstitial) (late) A50.31
 kidney (late) A52.75
 lacrimal passages (late) A52.71
 larynx (late) A52.73
 late A52.9
  cardiovascular A52.00
  central nervous system A52.3
  kidney A52.75
  latent or 2 years or more after infection (without
    manifestations) A52.8
   negative spinal fluid test A52.8
   serology positive A52.8
  paresis A52.17
  specified site NEC A52.79
  symptomatic or with manifestations A52.79
  tabes A52.11
 latent A53.0
  with signs or symptoms — *code by* site and stage
    under Syphilis
  central nervous system A52.2
  date of infection unspecified A53.0
  early, or less than 2 years after infection A51.5
  follow-up of latent syphilis A53.0
   date of infection unspecified A53.0
   late, or 2 years or more after infection A52.8
   positive serology (only finding) A53.0
   date of infection unspecified A53.0
   early, or less than 2 years after infection A51.5
   late, or 2 years or more after infection A52.8
 lens (late) A52.71
 leukoderma A51.39
  late A52.79
 lienitis A52.79
 lip A51.39
  chancre (primary) A51.2

Syphilis, syphilitic — *continued*
 lip — *continued*
  late A52.79
 Lissauer's paralysis A52.17
 liver A52.74
 locomotor ataxia A52.11
 lung A52.72
 lymph gland (early) (secondary) A51.49
  late A52.79
 lymphadenitis (secondary) A51.49
 macular atrophy of skin A51.39
  striated A52.79
 mediastinum (late) A52.73
 meninges (adhesive) (brain) (spinal cord) A52.13
 meningitis A52.13
  acute (secondary) A51.41
  congenital A50.41
 meningoencephalitis A52.14
 meningovascular A52.13
  congenital A50.41
 mesarteritis A52.09
  brain A52.04
 middle ear A52.77
 mitral stenosis A52.03
 monoplegia A52.17
 mouth (secondary) A51.39
  late A52.79
 mucocutaneous (secondary) A51.39
  late A52.79
 mucous
  membrane (secondary) A51.39
   late A52.79
  patches A51.39
   congenital A50.07
 mulberry molars A50.52
 muscle A52.78
 myocardium A52.06
 nasal sinus (late) A52.73
 neonatorum — *see* Syphilis, congenital
 nephrotic syndrome (secondary) A51.44
 nerve palsy (any cranial nerve) A52.15
  multiple A52.15
 nervous system, central A52.3
 neuritis A52.15
  acoustic A52.15
 neurorecidive of retina A52.19
 neuroretinitis A52.19
 newborn — *see* Syphilis, congenital
 nodular superficial (late) A52.79
 nonvenereal A65
 nose (late) A52.73
  saddle back deformity A50.57
 occlusive arterial disease A52.09
 oculopathy A52.71
 ophthalmic (late) A52.71
 optic nerve (atrophy) (neuritis) (papilla) A52.15
 orbit (late) A52.71
 organic A53.9
 osseous (late) A52.77
 osteochondritis (congenital) (early) A50.02 *[M90.80]*
 osteoporosis A52.77
 ovary (late) A52.76
 oviduct (late) A52.76
 palate (late) A52.79
 pancreas (late) A52.74
 paralysis A52.17
  general A52.17
   juvenile A50.45
 paresis (general) A52.17
  juvenile A50.45
 paresthesia A52.19
 Parkinson's disease or syndrome A52.19
 paroxysmal tachycardia A52.06
 pemphigus (congenital) A50.06
 penis (chancre) A51.0
  late A52.76
 pericardium A52.06
 perichondritis, larynx (late) A52.73
 periosteum (late) A52.77
  congenital (early) A50.02 *[M90.80]*
  early (secondary) A51.46
 peripheral nerve A52.79
 petrous bone (late) A52.77
 pharynx (late) A52.73
  secondary A51.39
 pituitary (gland) A52.79
 pleura (late) A52.73
 pneumonia, white A50.04
 pontine lesion A52.17

Syphilis, syphilitic — *continued*
 portal vein A52.09
 primary A51.0
  anal A51.1
  and secondary — *see* Syphilis, secondary
  central nervous system A52.3
  extragenital chancre NEC A51.2
  fingers A51.2
  genital A51.0
  lip A51.2
  specified site NEC A51.2
  tonsils A51.2
 prostate (late) A52.76
 ptosis (eyelid) A52.71
 pulmonary (late) A52.72
  artery A52.09
 pyelonephritis (late) A52.75
 recently acquired, symptomatic A51.9
 rectum (late) A52.74
 respiratory tract (late) A52.73
 retina, late A52.71
 retrobulbar neuritis A52.15
 salpingitis A52.76
 sclera (late) A52.71
 sclerosis
  cerebral A52.17
  coronary A52.06
  multiple A52.11
 scotoma (central) A52.71
 scrotum (late) A52.76
 secondary (and primary) A51.49
  adenopathy A51.49
  anus A51.39
  bone A51.46
  chorioretinitis, choroiditis A51.43
  hepatitis A51.45
  liver A51.45
  lymphadenitis A51.49
  meningitis (acute) A51.41
  mouth A51.39
  mucous membranes A51.39
  periosteum, periostitis A51.46
  pharynx A51.39
  relapse (treated, untreated) A51.49
  skin A51.39
  specified form NEC A51.49
  tonsil A51.39
  ulcer A51.39
  viscera NEC A51.49
  vulva A51.39
 seminal vesicle (late) A52.76
 seronegative with signs or symptoms — *code by* site
   and stage under Syphilis
 seropositive
  with signs or symptoms — *code by* site and stage
    under Syphilis
  follow-up of latent syphilis — *see* Syphilis, latent
  only finding — *see* Syphilis, latent
 seventh nerve (paralysis) A52.15
 sinus, sinusitis (late) A52.73
 skeletal system A52.77
 skin (with ulceration) (early) (secondary) A51.39
  late or tertiary A52.79
 small intestine A52.74
 spastic spinal paralysis A52.17
 spermatic cord (late) A52.76
 spinal (cord) A52.12
 spleen A52.79
 splenomegaly A52.79
 spondylitis A52.77
 staphyloma A52.71
 stigmata (congenital) A50.59
 stomach A52.74
 synovium A52.78
 tabes dorsalis (late) A52.11
  juvenile A50.45
 tabetic type A52.11
  juvenile A50.45
 taboparesis A52.17
  juvenile A50.45
 tachycardia A52.06
 tendon (late) A52.78
 tertiary A52.9
  with symptoms NEC A52.79
  cardiovascular A52.00
  central nervous system A52.3
  multiple NEC A52.79
  specified site NEC A52.79
 testis A52.76

Syphilis, syphilitic — *continued*
  thorax A52.73
  throat A52.73
  thymus (gland) (late) A52.79
  thyroid (late) A52.79
  tongue (late) A52.79
  tonsil (lingual) (late) A52.73
    primary A51.2
    secondary A51.39
  trachea (late) A52.73
  tunica vaginalis (late) A52.76
  ulcer (any site) (early) (secondary) A51.39
    late A52.79
    perforating A52.79
      foot A52.11
  urethra (late) A52.76
  urogenital (late) A52.76
  uterus (late) A52.76
  uveal tract (secondary) A51.43
    late A52.71
  uveitis (secondary) A51.43
    late A52.71

Syphilis, syphilitic — *continued*
  uvula (late) (perforated) A52.79
  vagina A51.0
    late A52.76
  valvulitis NEC A52.03
  vascular A52.00
    brain (cerebral) A52.05
  ventriculi A52.74
  vesicae urinariae (late) A52.76
  viscera (abdominal) (late) A52.74
    secondary A51.49
  vitreous (opacities) (late) A52.71
    hemorrhage A52.71
  vulva A51.0
    late A52.76
    secondary A51.39
Syphiloma A52.79
  cardiovascular system A52.00
  central nervous system A52.3
  circulatory system A52.00
  congenital A50.59
Syphilophobia F45.29

Syringadenoma — *see also* Neoplasm, skin, benign
  papillary — *see* Neoplasm, skin, benign
Syringobulbia G95.0
Syringocystadenoma — *see* Neoplasm, skin, benign
  papillary — *see* Neoplasm, skin, benign
Syringoma — *see also* Neoplasm, skin, benign
  chondroid — *see* Neoplasm, skin, benign
Syringomyelia G95.0
Syringomyelitis — *see* Encephalitis
Syringomyelocele — *see* Spina bifida
Syringopontia G95.0
System, systemic — *see also* condition
  disease, combined — *see* Degeneration, combined
  inflammatory response syndrome (SIRS) of non-infectious origin (without organ dysfunction) R65.10
    with acute organ dysfunction R65.11
  lupus erythematosus M32.9
    inhibitor present D68.62

T

Tabacism, tabacosis, tabagism — *see also* Poisoning, tobacco
  meaning dependence (without remission) F17.200
    with
      disorder F17.299
        in remission F17.211
        specified disorder NEC F17.298
        withdrawal F17.203
Tabardillo A75.9
  flea-borne A75.2
  louse-borne A75.0
Tabes, tabetic A52.10
  with
    central nervous system syphilis A52.10
    Charcot's joint A52.16
    cord bladder A52.19
    crisis, viscera (any) A52.19
    paralysis, general A52.17
    paresis (general) A52.17
    perforating ulcer (foot) A52.19
  arthropathy (Charcot) A52.16
  bladder A52.19
  bone A52.11
  cerebrospinal A52.12
  congenital A50.45
  conjugal A52.10
  dorsalis A52.11
    juvenile A50.49
  juvenile A50.49
  latent A52.19
  mesenterica A18.39
  paralysis, insane, general A52.17
  spasmodic A52.17
  syphilis (cerebrospinal) A52.12
Taboparalysis A52.17
Taboparesis (remission) A52.17
  juvenile A50.45
TAC (trigeminal autonomic cephalgia) **NEC** G44.099
  intractable G44.091
  not intractable G44.099
Tache noir S60.22- ☑
Tachyalimentation K91.2
Tachyarrhythmia, tachyrhythmia — *see* Tachycardia
Tachycardia R00.0
  atrial (paroxysmal) I47.1
  auricular I47.1
  AV nodal re-entry (re-entrant) I47.1
  junctional (paroxysmal) I47.1
  newborn P29.11
  nodal (paroxysmal) I47.1
  non-paroxysmal AV nodal I45.89
  paroxysmal (sustained) (nonsustained) I47.9
    with sinus bradycardia I49.5
    atrial (PAT) I47.1
    atrioventricular (AV) (re-entrant) I47.1
      psychogenic F54
    junctional I47.1
      ectopic I47.1
    nodal I47.1
    psychogenic (atrial) (supraventricular) (ventricular) F54
    supraventricular (sustained) I47.1
      psychogenic F54
    ventricular I47.2
      psychogenic F54
  psychogenic F45.8
  sick sinus I49.5
  sinoauricular NOS R00.0
    paroxysmal I47.1
  sinus [sinusal] NOS R00.0
    paroxysmal I47.1
  supraventricular I47.1
  ventricular (paroxysmal) (sustained) I47.2
    psychogenic F54
Tachygastria K31.89
Tachypnea R06.82
  hysterical F45.8
  newborn (idiopathic) (transitory) P22.1
  psychogenic F45.8
  transitory, of newborn P22.1
TACO (transfusion associated circulatory overload) E87.71
Taenia (infection) (infestation) B68.9
  diminuta B71.0
  echinococcal infestation B67.90
  mediocanellata B68.1

Taenia — *continued*
  nana B71.0
  saginata B68.1
  solium (intestinal form) B68.0
    larval form — *see* Cysticercosis
Taeniasis (intestine) — *see* Taenia
Tag (hypertrophied skin) (infected) L91.8
  adenoid J35.8
  anus K64.4
  hemorrhoidal K64.4
  hymen N89.8
  perineal N90.89
  preauricular Q17.0
  sentinel K64.4
  skin L91.8
    accessory (congenital) Q82.8
    anus K64.4
    congenital Q82.8
    preauricular Q17.0
  tonsil J35.8
  urethra, urethral N36.8
  vulva N90.89
Tahyna fever B33.8
Takahara's disease E80.3
Takayasu's disease or syndrome M31.4
Talcosis (pulmonary) J62.0
Talipes (congenital) Q66.89
  acquired, planus — *see* Deformity, limb, flat foot
  asymmetric Q66.89
  calcaneovalgus Q66.4- ☑
  calcaneovarus Q66.1- ☑
  calcaneus Q66.89
  cavus Q66.7- ☑
  equinovalgus Q66.6
  equinovarus Q66.0- ☑
  equinus Q66.89
  percavus Q66.7- ☑
  planovalgus Q66.6
  planus (acquired) (any degree) — *see also* Deformity, limb, flat foot
    congenital Q66.5- ☑
    due to rickets (sequelae) E64.3
  valgus Q66.6
  varus Q66.3- ☑
Tall stature, constitutional E34.4
Talma's disease M62.89
Talon noir S90.3- ☑
  hand S60.22- ☑
  heel S90.3- ☑
  toe S90.1- ☑
Tamponade, heart I31.4
Tanapox (virus disease) B08.71
Tangier disease E78.6
Tantrum, child problem F91.8
Tapeworm (infection) (infestation) — *see* Infestation, tapeworm
Tapia's syndrome G52.7
TAR (thrombocytopenia with absent radius) **syndrome** Q87.2
Tarral-Besnier disease L44.0
Tarsal tunnel syndrome — *see* Syndrome, tarsal tunnel
Tarsalgia — *see* Pain, limb, lower
Tarsitis (eyelid) H01.8
  syphilitic A52.71
  tuberculous A18.4
Tartar (teeth) (dental calculus) K03.6
Tattoo (mark) L81.8
Tauri's disease E74.09
Taurodontism K00.2
Taussig-Bing syndrome Q20.1
Taybi's syndrome Q87.2
Tay-Sachs amaurotic familial idiocy or disease E75.02
TBI (traumatic brain injury) S06.9 ☑
Teacher's node or nodule J38.2
Tear, torn (traumatic) — *see also* Laceration
  with abortion — *see* Abortion
  annular fibrosis M51.35
  anus, anal (sphincter) S31.831 ☑
    complicating delivery
      with third degree perineal laceration — *see also* Delivery, complicated, by, laceration, perineum, third degree O70.20
        with mucosa O70.3
      without third degree perineal laceration O70.4
    nontraumatic (healed) (old) K62.81
  articular cartilage, old — *see* Derangement, joint, articular cartilage, by site

Tear, torn — *continued*
  bladder
    with ectopic or molar pregnancy O08.6
    following ectopic or molar pregnancy O08.6
    obstetrical O71.5
    traumatic — *see* Injury, bladder
  bowel
    with ectopic or molar pregnancy O08.6
    following ectopic or molar pregnancy O08.6
    obstetrical trauma O71.5
  broad ligament
    with ectopic or molar pregnancy O08.6
    following ectopic or molar pregnancy O08.6
    obstetrical trauma O71.6
  bucket handle (knee) (meniscus) — *see* Tear, meniscus
  capsule, joint — *see* Sprain
  cartilage — *see also* Sprain
    articular, old — *see* Derangement, joint, articular cartilage, by site
  cervix
    with ectopic or molar pregnancy O08.6
    following ectopic or molar pregnancy O08.6
    obstetrical trauma (current) O71.3
    old N88.1
    traumatic — *see* Injury, uterus
  dural G97.41
    nontraumatic G96.11
  internal organ — *see* Injury, by site
  knee cartilage
    articular (current) S83.3- ☑
    old — *see* Derangement, knee, meniscus, due to old tear
  ligament — *see* Sprain
  meniscus (knee) (current injury) S83.209 ☑
    bucket-handle S83.20- ☑
    lateral
      bucket-handle S83.25- ☑
      complex S83.27- ☑
      peripheral S83.26- ☑
      specified type NEC S83.28- ☑
    medial
      bucket-handle S83.21- ☑
      complex S83.23- ☑
      peripheral S83.22- ☑
      specified type NEC S83.24- ☑
    old — *see* Derangement, knee, meniscus, due to old tear
    site other than knee — *code as* Sprain
    specified type NEC S83.20- ☑
  muscle — *see* Strain
  pelvic
    floor, complicating delivery O70.1
    organ NEC, obstetrical trauma O71.5
      with ectopic or molar pregnancy O08.6
      following ectopic or molar pregnancy O08.6
  perineal, secondary O90.1
  periurethral tissue, obstetrical trauma O71.82
    with ectopic or molar pregnancy O08.6
    following ectopic or molar pregnancy O08.6
  rectovaginal septum — *see* Laceration, vagina
  retina, retinal (without detachment) (horseshoe) — *see also* Break, retina, horseshoe
    with detachment — *see* Detachment, retina, with retinal, break
  rotator cuff (nontraumatic) M75.10- ☑
    complete M75.12- ☑
    incomplete M75.11- ☑
    traumatic S46.01- ☑
      capsule S43.42- ☑
  semilunar cartilage, knee — *see* Tear, meniscus
  supraspinatus (complete) (incomplete) (nontraumatic) — *see also* Tear, rotator cuff M75.10- ☑
  tendon — *see* Strain
  tentorial, at birth P10.4
  umbilical cord
    complicating delivery O69.89 ☑
  urethra
    with ectopic or molar pregnancy O08.6
    following ectopic or molar pregnancy O08.6
    obstetrical trauma O71.5
  uterus — *see* Injury, uterus
  vagina — *see* Laceration, vagina
  vessel, from catheter — *see* Puncture, accidental complicating surgery
  vulva, complicating delivery O70.0
Tear-stone — *see* Dacryolith
Teeth — *see also* condition

Teeth — *continued*
  grinding
    psychogenic F45.8
    sleep related G47.63
Teething (syndrome) K00.7
Telangiectasia, telangiectasis (verrucous) I78.1
  ataxic (cerebellar) (Louis-Bar) G11.3
  familial I78.0
  hemorrhagic, hereditary (congenital) (senile) I78.0
  hereditary, hemorrhagic (congenital) (senile) I78.0
  juxtafoveal H35.07- ☑
  macular H35.07- ☑
  macularis eruptiva perstans D47.01
  parafoveal H35.07- ☑
  retinal (idiopathic) (juxtafoveal) (macular) (parafoveal) H35.07- ☑
  spider I78.1
Telephone scatologia F65.89
Telescoped bowel or intestine K56.1
  congenital Q43.8
Temperature
  body, high (of unknown origin) R50.9
  cold, trauma from T69.9 ☑
    newborn P80.0
    specified effect NEC T69.8 ☑
Temple — *see* condition
Temporal — *see* condition
Temporomandibular joint pain-dysfunction syndrome M26.62-
Temporosphenoidal — *see* condition
Tendency
  bleeding — *see* Defect, coagulation
  suicide
    meaning personal history of attempted suicide Z91.5
    meaning suicidal ideation — *see* Ideation, suicidal
  to fall R29.6
Tenderness, abdominal R10.819
  epigastric R10.816
  generalized R10.817
  left lower quadrant R10.814
  left upper quadrant R10.812
  periumbilic R10.815
  rebound R10.829
    epigastric R10.826
    generalized R10.827
    left lower quadrant R10.824
    left upper quadrant R10.822
    periumbilic R10.825
    right lower quadrant R10.823
    right upper quadrant R10.821
  right lower quadrant R10.813
  right upper quadrant R10.811
Tendinitis, tendonitis — *see also* Enthesopathy
  Achilles M76.6- ☑
  adhesive — *see* Tenosynovitis, specified type NEC
    shoulder — *see* Capsulitis, adhesive
  bicipital M75.2- ☑
  calcific M65.2- ☑
    ankle M65.27- ☑
    foot M65.27- ☑
    forearm M65.23- ☑
    hand M65.24- ☑
    lower leg M65.26- ☑
    multiple sites M65.29
    pelvic region M65.25- ☑
    shoulder M75.3- ☑
    specified site NEC M65.28
    thigh M65.25- ☑
    upper arm M65.22- ☑
  due to use, overuse, pressure — *see also* Disorder, soft tissue, due to use
    specified NEC — *see* Disorder, soft tissue, due to use, specified NEC
  gluteal M76.0- ☑
  patellar M76.5- ☑
  peroneal M76.7- ☑
  psoas M76.1- ☑
  tibial (posterior) M76.82- ☑
    anterior M76.81- ☑
  trochanteric — *see* Bursitis, hip, trochanteric
Tendon — *see* condition
Tendosynovitis — *see* Tenosynovitis
Tenesmus (rectal) R19.8
  vesical R30.1
Tennis elbow — *see* Epicondylitis, lateral
Tenonitis — *see also* Tenosynovitis
  eye (capsule) H05.04- ☑

Tenontosynovitis — *see* Tenosynovitis
Tenonthothecitis — *see* Tenosynovitis
Tenophyte — *see* Disorder, synovium, specified type NEC
Tenosynovitis — *see also* Synovitis M65.9
  adhesive — *see* Tenosynovitis, specified type NEC
    shoulder — *see* Capsulitis, adhesive
  bicipital (calcifying) — *see* Tendinitis, bicipital
  gonococcal A54.49
  in (due to)
    crystals M65.8- ☑
    gonorrhea A54.49
    syphilis (late) A52.78
    use, overuse, pressure — *see also* Disorder, soft tissue, due to use
      specified NEC — *see* Disorder, soft tissue, due to use, specified NEC
  infective NEC M65.1- ☑
    ankle M65.17- ☑
    foot M65.17- ☑
    forearm M65.13- ☑
    hand M65.14- ☑
    lower leg M65.16- ☑
    multiple sites M65.19
    pelvic region M65.15- ☑
    shoulder region M65.11- ☑
    specified site NEC M65.18
    thigh M65.15- ☑
    upper arm M65.12- ☑
  radial styloid M65.4
  shoulder region M65.81- ☑
    adhesive — *see* Capsulitis, adhesive
  specified type NEC M65.88
    ankle M65.87- ☑
    foot M65.87- ☑
    forearm M65.83- ☑
    hand M65.84- ☑
    lower leg M65.86- ☑
    multiple sites M65.89
    pelvic region M65.85- ☑
    shoulder region M65.81- ☑
    specified site NEC M65.88
    thigh M65.85- ☑
    upper arm M65.82- ☑
  tuberculous — *see* Tuberculosis, tenosynovitis
Tenovaginitis — *see* Tenosynovitis
Tension
  arterial, high — *see also* Hypertension
    without diagnosis of hypertension R03.0
  headache G44.209
    intractable G44.201
    not intractable G44.209
  nervous R45.0
  pneumothorax J93.0
  premenstrual N94.3
  state (mental) F48.9
Tentorium — *see* condition
Teratencephalus Q89.8
Teratism Q89.7
Teratoblastoma (malignant) — *see* Neoplasm, malignant, by site
Teratocarcinoma — *see also* Neoplasm, malignant, by site
  liver C22.7
Teratoma (solid) — *see also* Neoplasm, uncertain behavior, by site
  with embryonal carcinoma, mixed — *see* Neoplasm, malignant, by site
  with malignant transformation — *see* Neoplasm, malignant, by site
  adult (cystic) — *see* Neoplasm, benign, by site
  benign — *see* Neoplasm, benign, by site
  combined with choriocarcinoma — *see* Neoplasm, malignant, by site
  cystic (adult) — *see* Neoplasm, benign, by site
  differentiated — *see* Neoplasm, benign, by site
  embryonal — *see also* Neoplasm, malignant, by site
    liver C22.7
  immature — *see* Neoplasm, malignant, by site
  liver C22.7
    adult, benign, cystic, differentiated type or mature D13.4
  malignant — *see also* Neoplasm, malignant, by site
    anaplastic — *see* Neoplasm, malignant, by site
    intermediate — *see* Neoplasm, malignant, by site
      specified site — *see* Neoplasm, malignant, by site
      unspecified site C62.90

Teratoma — *continued*
  malignant — *see also* Neoplasm, malignant, by site — *continued*
    undifferentiated — *see* Neoplasm, malignant, by site
  mature — *see* Neoplasm, uncertain behavior, by site
    malignant — *see* Neoplasm, by site, malignant, by site
  ovary D27.- ☑
    embryonal, immature or malignant C56- ☑
  solid — *see* Neoplasm, uncertain behavior, by site
  testis C62.9- ☑
    adult, benign, cystic, differentiated type or mature D29.2- ☑
    scrotal C62.1- ☑
    undescended C62.0- ☑
Termination
  anomalous — *see also* Malposition, congenital
    right pulmonary vein Q26.3
  pregnancy, elective Z33.2
Ternidens diminutus infestation B81.8
Ternidensiasis B81.8
Terror(s) night (child) F51.4
Terrorism, victim of Z65.4
Terry's syndrome — *see also* Myopia, degenerative H44.2- ☑
Tertiary — *see* condition
Test, tests, testing (for)
  adequacy (for dialysis)
    hemodialysis Z49.31
    peritoneal Z49.32
  blood pressure Z01.30
    abnormal reading — *see* Blood, pressure
  blood typing Z01.83
    Rh typing Z01.83
  blood-alcohol Z04.89
    positive — *see* Findings, abnormal, in blood
  blood-drug Z04.89
    positive — *see* Findings, abnormal, in blood
  cardiac pulse generator (battery) Z45.010
  fertility Z31.41
  genetic
    disease carrier status for procreative management
      female Z31.430
      male Z31.440
    male partner of patient with recurrent pregnancy loss Z31.441
    procreative management NEC
      female Z31.438
      male Z31.448
  hearing Z01.10
    with abnormal findings NEC Z01.118
    infant or child (over 28 days old) Z00.129
      with abnormal findings Z00.121
  HIV (human immunodeficiency virus)
    nonconclusive (in infants) R75
    positive Z21
    seropositive Z21
  immunity status Z01.84
  intelligence NEC Z01.89
  laboratory (as part of a general medical examination) Z00.00
    with abnormal finding Z00.01
    for medicolegal reason NEC Z04.89
  male partner of patient with recurrent pregnancy loss Z31.441
  Mantoux (for tuberculosis) Z11.1
    abnormal result R76.11
  pregnancy, positive first pregnancy — *see* Pregnancy, normal, first
  procreative Z31.49
    fertility Z31.41
  skin, diagnostic
    allergy Z01.82
      special screening examination — *see* Screening by name of disease
    Mantoux Z11.1
    tuberculin Z11.1
  specified NEC Z01.89
  tuberculin Z11.1
    abnormal result R76.11
  vision Z01.00
    with abnormal findings Z01.01
    following failed vision screening Z01.020
      with abnormal findings Z01.021
    infant or child (over 28 days old) Z00.129
      with abnormal findings Z00.121
  Wassermann Z11.3

Test, tests, testing — *continued*
Wassermann — *continued*
positive — *see* Serology for syphilis, positive
Testicle, testicular, testis — *see also* condition
feminization syndrome — *see also* Syndrome, androgen insensitivity E34.51
migrans Q55.29
Tetanus, tetanic (cephalic) (convulsions) A35
with
abortion A34
ectopic or molar pregnancy O08.0
following ectopic or molar pregnancy O08.0
inoculation reaction (due to serum) — *see* Complications, vaccination
neonatorum A33
obstetrical A34
puerperal, postpartum, childbirth A34
Tetany (due to) R29.0
alkalosis E87.3
associated with rickets E55.0
convulsions R29.0
hysterical F44.5
functional (hysterical) F44.5
hyperkinetic R29.0
hysterical F44.5
hyperpnea R06.4
hysterical F44.5
psychogenic F45.8
hyperventilation — *see also* Hyperventilation R06.4
hysterical F44.5
neonatal (without calcium or magnesium deficiency) P71.3
parathyroid (gland) E20.9
parathyroprival E89.2
post- (para)thyroidectomy E89.2
postoperative E89.2
pseudotetany R29.0
psychogenic (conversion reaction) F44.5
Tetralogy of Fallot Q21.3
Tetraplegia (chronic) — *see also* Quadriplegia G82.50
Thailand hemorrhagic fever A91
Thalassanemia — *see* Thalassemia
Thalassemia (anemia) (disease) D56.9
with other hemoglobinopathy D56.8
alpha (major) (severe) (triple gene defect) D56.0
minor D56.3
silent carrier D56.3
trait D56.3
beta (severe) D56.1
homozygous D56.1
major D56.1
minor D56.3
trait D56.3
delta-beta (homozygous) D56.2
minor D56.3
trait D56.3
dominant D56.8
hemoglobin
C D56.8
E-beta D56.5
intermedia D56.1
major D56.1
minor D56.3
mixed D56.8
sickle-cell — *see* Disease, sickle-cell, thalassemia
specified type NEC D56.8
trait D56.3
variants D56.8
Thanatophoric dwarfism or short stature Q77.1
Thaysen-Gee disease (nontropical sprue) K90.0
Thaysen's disease K90.0
Thecoma D27- ☑
luteinized D27- ☑
malignant C56- ☑
Thelarche, premature E30.8
Thelaziasis B83.8
Thelitis N61.0
puerperal, postpartum or gestational — *see* Infection, nipple
Therapeutic — *see* condition
Therapy
drug, long-term (current) (prophylactic)
agents affecting estrogen receptors and estrogen levels NEC Z79.818
anastrozole (Arimidex) Z79.811
antibiotics Z79.2
short-term use — *omit code*
anticoagulants Z79.01

Therapy — *continued*
drug, long-term — *continued*
anti-inflammatory Z79.1
antiplatelet Z79.02
antithrombotics Z79.02
aromatase inhibitors Z79.811
aspirin Z79.82
birth control pill or patch Z79.3
bisphosphonates Z79.83
contraceptive, oral Z79.3
drug, specified NEC Z79.899
estrogen receptor downregulators Z79.818
Evista Z79.810
exemestane (Aromasin) Z79.811
Fareston Z79.810
fulvestrant (Faslodex) Z79.818
gonadotropin-releasing hormone (GnRH) agonist Z79.818
goserelin acetate (Zoladex) Z79.818
hormone replacement Z79.890
insulin Z79.4
letrozole (Femara) Z79.811
leuprolide acetate (leuprorelin) (Lupron) Z79.818
megestrol acetate (Megace) Z79.818
methadone
for pain management Z79.891
maintenance therapy F11.20
Nolvadex Z79.810
opiate analgesic Z79.891
oral contraceptive Z79.3
raloxifene (Evista) Z79.810
selective estrogen receptor modulators (SERMs) Z79.810
short term — *omit code*
steroids
inhaled Z79.51
systemic Z79.52
tamoxifen (Nolvadex) Z79.810
toremifene (Fareston) Z79.810
Thermic — *see* condition
Thermography (abnormal) — *see also* Abnormal, diagnostic imaging R93.89
breast R92.8
Thermoplegia T67.01 ☑
Thesaurismosis, glycogen — *see* Disease, glycogen storage
Thiamin deficiency E51.9
specified NEC E51.8
Thiaminic deficiency with beriberi E51.11
Thibierge-Weissenbach syndrome — *see* Sclerosis, systemic
Thickening
bone — *see* Hypertrophy, bone
breast N64.59
endometrium R93.89
epidermal L85.9
specified NEC L85.8
hymen N89.6
larynx J38.7
nail L60.2
congenital Q84.5
periosteal — *see* Hypertrophy, bone
pleura J92.9
with asbestos J92.0
skin R23.4
subepiglottic J38.7
tongue K14.8
valve, heart — *see* Endocarditis
Thigh — *see* condition
Thinning vertebra — *see* Spondylopathy, specified NEC
Thirst, excessive R63.1
due to deprivation of water T73.1 ☑
Thomsen disease G71.12
Thoracic — *see also* condition
kidney Q63.2
outlet syndrome G54.0
Thoracogastroschisis (congenital) Q79.8
Thoracopagus Q89.4
Thorax — *see* condition
Thorn's syndrome N28.89
Thorson-Björck syndrome E34.0
Threadworm (infection) (infestation) B80
Threatened
abortion O20.0
with subsequent abortion O03.9
job loss, anxiety concerning Z56.2
labor (without delivery) O47.9
at or after 37 completed weeks of gestation O47.1

Threatened — *continued*
labor — *continued*
before 37 completed weeks of gestation O47.0- ☑
loss of job, anxiety concerning Z56.2
miscarriage O20.0
unemployment, anxiety concerning Z56.2
Three-day fever A93.1
Threshers' lung J67.0
Thrix annulata (congenital) Q84.1
Throat — *see* condition
Thrombasthenia (Glanzmann) (hemorrhagic) (hereditary) D69.1
Thromboangiitis I73.1
obliterans (general) I73.1
cerebral I67.89
vessels
brain I67.89
spinal cord I67.89
Thromboarteritis — *see* Arteritis
Thromboasthenia (Glanzmann) (hemorrhagic) (hereditary) D69.1
Thrombocytasthenia (Glanzmann) D69.1
Thrombocythemia (essential) (hemorrhagic) (idiopathic) (primary) D47.3
Thrombocytopathy (dystrophic) (granulopenic) D69.1
Thrombocytopenia, thrombocytopenic D69.6
with absent radius (TAR) Q87.2
congenital D69.42
dilutional D69.59
due to
(massive) blood transfusion D69.59
drugs D69.59
extracorporeal circulation of blood D69.59
platelet alloimmunization D69.59
essential D69.3
heparin induced (HIT) D75.82
hereditary D69.42
idiopathic D69.3
neonatal, transitory P61.0
due to
exchange transfusion P61.0
idiopathic maternal thrombocytopenia P61.0
isoimmunization P61.0
primary NEC D69.49
idiopathic D69.3
puerperal, postpartum O72.3
secondary D69.59
transient neonatal P61.0
Thrombocytosis, essential D47.3
primary D47.3
Thromboembolism — *see* Embolism
Thrombopathy (Bernard-Soulier) D69.1
constitutional D68.0
Willebrand-Jurgens D68.0
Thrombopenia — *see* Thrombocytopenia
Thrombophilia D68.59
primary NEC D68.59
secondary NEC D68.69
specified NEC D68.69
Thrombophlebitis I80.9
antepartum O22.2- ☑
deep O22.3- ☑
superficial O22.2- ☑
calf muscular vein (NOS) I80.25- ☑
cavernous (venous) sinus G08
complicating pregnancy O22.5- ☑
nonpyogenic I67.6
cerebral (sinus) (vein) G08
nonpyogenic I67.6
sequelae G09
due to implanted device — *see* Complications, by site and type, specified NEC
during or resulting from a procedure NEC T81.72 ☑
femoral vein (superficial) I80.1- ☑
femoropopliteal vein I80.0- ☑
gastrocnemial vein I80.25- ☑
hepatic (vein) I80.8
idiopathic, recurrent I82.1
iliac vein (common) (external) (internal) I80.21- ☑
iliofemoral I80.1- ☑
intracranial venous sinus (any) G08
nonpyogenic I67.6
sequelae G09
intraspinal venous sinuses and veins G08
nonpyogenic G95.19
lateral (venous) sinus G08
nonpyogenic I67.6
leg I80.3

▽ Subterms under main terms may continue to next column or page   ☑ Additional Character Required — Refer to the Tabular List for Character Selection   309

Test, tests, testing — Thrombophlebitis

Thrombophlebitis — *continued*
- leg — *continued*
  - superficial I80.0- ☑
- longitudinal (venous) sinus G08
  - nonpyogenic I67.6
- lower extremity I80.299
- migrans, migrating I82.1
- pelvic
  - with ectopic or molar pregnancy O08.0
  - following ectopic or molar pregnancy O08.0
  - puerperal O87.1
- peroneal vein I80.24- ☑
- popliteal vein — *see* Phlebitis, leg, deep, popliteal
- portal (vein) K75.1
- postoperative T81.72 ☑
- pregnancy — *see* Thrombophlebitis, antepartum
- puerperal, postpartum, childbirth O87.0
  - deep O87.1
  - pelvic O87.1
  - septic O86.81
  - superficial O87.0
- saphenous (greater) (lesser) I80.0- ☑
- sinus (intracranial) G08
  - nonpyogenic I67.6
- soleal vein I80.25- ☑
- specified site NEC I80.8
- tibial vein (anterior) (posterior) I80.23- ☑

Thrombosis, thrombotic (bland) (multiple) (progressive) (silent) (vessel) I82.90
- anal K64.5
- antepartum — *see* Thrombophlebitis, antepartum
- aorta, aortic I74.10
  - abdominal I74.09
    - saddle I74.01
  - bifurcation I74.09
  - saddle I74.01
  - specified site NEC I74.19
  - terminal I74.09
  - thoracic I74.11
  - valve — *see* Endocarditis, aortic
- apoplexy I63.3- ☑
- artery, arteries (postinfectional) I74.9
  - auditory, internal — *see* Occlusion, artery, precerebral, specified NEC
  - basilar — *see* Occlusion, artery, basilar
  - carotid (common) (internal) — *see* Occlusion, artery, carotid
  - cerebellar (anterior inferior) (posterior inferior) (superior) — *see* Occlusion, artery, cerebellar
  - cerebral — *see* Occlusion, artery, cerebral
  - choroidal (anterior) — *see* Occlusion, artery, precerebral, specified NEC
  - communicating, posterior — *see* Occlusion, artery, precerebral, specified NEC
  - coronary — *see also* Infarct, myocardium
    - not resulting in infarction I24.0
  - hepatic I74.8
  - hypophyseal — *see* Occlusion, artery, precerebral, specified NEC
  - iliac I74.5
  - limb I74.4
    - lower I74.3
    - upper I74.2
  - meningeal, anterior or posterior — *see* Occlusion, artery, cerebral, specified NEC
  - mesenteric (with gangrene) — *see also* Infarct, intestine K55.069
  - ophthalmic — *see* Occlusion, artery, retina
  - pontine — *see* Occlusion, artery, precerebral, specified NEC
  - precerebral — *see* Occlusion, artery, precerebral
  - pulmonary (iatrogenic) — *see* Embolism, pulmonary
  - renal N28.0
  - retinal — *see* Occlusion, artery, retina
  - spinal, anterior or posterior G95.11
  - traumatic NEC T14.8 ☑
  - vertebral — *see* Occlusion, artery, vertebral
- atrium, auricular — *see also* Infarct, myocardium
  - following acute myocardial infarction (current complication) I23.6
  - not resulting in infarction I51.3
  - old I51.3
- basilar (artery) — *see* Occlusion, artery, basilar
- brain (artery) (stem) — *see also* Occlusion, artery, cerebral
  - due to syphilis A52.05
  - puerperal O99.43
  - sinus — *see* Thrombosis, intracranial venous sinus

Thrombosis, thrombotic — *continued*
- capillary I78.8
- cardiac — *see also* Infarct, myocardium
  - not resulting in infarction I51.3
  - old I51.3
  - valve — *see* Endocarditis
- carotid (artery) (common) (internal) — *see* Occlusion, artery, carotid
- cavernous (venous) sinus — *see* Thrombosis, intracranial venous sinus
- cerebellar artery (anterior inferior) (posterior inferior) (superior) I66.3
- cerebral (artery) — *see* Occlusion, artery, cerebral
- cerebrovenous sinus — *see also* Thrombosis, intracranial venous sinus
  - puerperium O87.3
- chronic I82.91
- coronary (artery) (vein) — *see also* Infarct, myocardium
  - not resulting in infarction I24.0
- corpus cavernosum N48.89
- cortical I66.9
- deep — *see* Embolism, vein, lower extremity
- due to device, implant or graft — *see also* Complications, by site and type, specified NEC T85.868 ☑
  - arterial graft NEC T82.868 ☑
  - breast (implant) T85.868 ☑
  - catheter NEC T85.868 ☑
    - dialysis (renal) T82.868 ☑
      - intraperitoneal T85.868 ☑
    - infusion NEC T82.868 ☑
      - spinal (epidural) (subdural) T85.860 ☑
    - urinary (indwelling) T83.86 ☑
  - electronic (electrode) (pulse generator) (stimulator)
    - bone T84.86 ☑
    - cardiac T82.867 ☑
    - nervous system (brain) (peripheral nerve) (spinal) T85.860 ☑
    - urinary T83.86 ☑
  - fixation, internal (orthopedic) NEC T84.86 ☑
  - gastrointestinal (bile duct) (esophagus) T85.868 ☑
  - genital NEC T83.86 ☑
  - heart T82.867 ☑
  - joint prosthesis T84.86 ☑
  - ocular (corneal graft) (orbital implant) NEC T85.868 ☑
  - orthopedic NEC T84.86 ☑
  - specified NEC T85.868 ☑
  - urinary NEC T83.86 ☑
  - vascular NEC T82.868 ☑
  - ventricular intracranial shunt T85.860 ☑
- during the puerperium — *see* Thrombosis, puerperal
- endocardial — *see also* Infarct, myocardium
  - not resulting in infarction I51.3
- eye — *see* Occlusion, retina
- genital organ
  - female NEC N94.89
    - pregnancy — *see* Thrombophlebitis, antepartum
  - male N50.1
- gestational — *see* Phlebopathy, gestational
- heart (chamber) — *see also* Infarct, myocardium
  - not resulting in infarction I51.3
  - old I51.3
- hepatic (vein) I82.0
  - artery I74.8
- history (of) Z86.718
- intestine (with gangrene) — *see also* Infarct, intestine K55.069
- intracardiac NEC (apical) (atrial) (auricular) (ventricular) (old) I51.3
- intracranial (arterial) I66.9
  - venous sinus (any) G08
    - nonpyogenic origin I67.6
    - puerperium O87.3
- intramural — *see also* Infarct, myocardium
  - not resulting in infarction I51.3
  - old I51.3
- intraspinal venous sinuses and veins G08
  - nonpyogenic G95.19
- kidney (artery) N28.0
- lateral (venous) sinus — *see* Thrombosis, intracranial venous sinus
- leg — *see* Thrombosis, vein, lower extremity
  - arterial I74.3
- liver (venous) I82.0
  - artery I74.8
  - portal vein I81

Thrombosis, thrombotic — *continued*
- longitudinal (venous) sinus — *see* Thrombosis, intracranial venous sinus
- lower limb — *see* Thrombosis, vein, lower extremity
- lung (iatrogenic) (postoperative) — *see* Embolism, pulmonary
- meninges (brain) (arterial) I66.8
- mesenteric (artery) (with gangrene) — *see also* Infarct, intestine K55.069
  - vein (inferior) (superior) K55.0 ☑
- mitral I34.8
- mural — *see also* Infarct, myocardium
  - due to syphilis A52.06
  - not resulting in infarction I51.3
  - old I51.3
- omentum (with gangrene) — *see also* Infarct, intestine K55.069
- ophthalmic — *see* Occlusion, retina
- pampiniform plexus (male) N50.1
- parietal — *see* Infarct, myocardium
  - not resulting in infarction I24.0
- penis, superficial vein N48.81
- perianal venous K64.5
- peripheral arteries I74.4
  - upper I74.2
- personal history (of) Z86.718
- portal I81
  - due to syphilis A52.09
- precerebral artery — *see* Occlusion, artery, precerebral
- puerperal, postpartum O87.0
  - brain (artery) O99.43
    - venous (sinus) O87.3
  - cardiac O99.43
  - cerebral (artery) O99.43
    - venous (sinus) O87.3
  - superficial O87.0
- pulmonary (artery) (iatrogenic) (postoperative) (vein) — *see* Embolism, pulmonary
- renal (artery) N28.0
  - vein I82.3
- resulting from presence of device, implant or graft — *see* Complications, by site and type, specified NEC
- retina, retinal — *see* Occlusion, retina
- scrotum N50.1
- seminal vesicle N50.1
- sigmoid (venous) sinus — *see* Thrombosis, intracranial venous sinus
- sinus, intracranial (any) — *see* Thrombosis, intracranial venous sinus
- specified site NEC I82.890
  - chronic I82.891
- spermatic cord N50.1
- spinal cord (arterial) G95.11
  - due to syphilis A52.09
  - pyogenic origin G06.1
- spleen, splenic D73.5
  - artery I74.8
- testis N50.1
- traumatic NEC T14.8 ☑
- tricuspid I07.8
- tumor — *see* Neoplasm, unspecified behavior, by site
- tunica vaginalis N50.1
- umbilical cord (vessels), complicating delivery O69.5 ☑
- vas deferens N50.1
- vein (acute) I82.90
  - antecubital I82.61- ☑
    - chronic I82.71- ☑
  - axillary I82.A1- ☑ (*following* I82.7)
    - chronic I82.A2- ☑ (*following* I82.7)
  - basilic I82.61- ☑
    - chronic I82.71- ☑
  - brachial I82.62- ☑
    - chronic I82.72- ☑
  - brachiocephalic (innominate) I82.290
    - chronic I82.291
  - cephalic I82.61- ☑
    - chronic I82.71- ☑
  - cerebral, nonpyogenic I67.6
  - chronic I82.91
  - deep (DVT) I82.40- ☑
    - calf I82.4Z- ☑
      - chronic I82.5Z- ☑
    - lower leg I82.4Z- ☑
      - chronic I82.5Z- ☑
    - thigh I82.4Y- ☑
      - chronic I82.5Y- ☑

Thrombosis, thrombotic — *continued*
 vein — *continued*
  deep — *continued*
   upper leg I82.4Y ☑
    chronic I82.5Y- ☑
   femoral I82.41- ☑
    chronic I82.51- ☑
   iliac (iliofemoral) I82.42- ☑
    chronic I82.52- ☑
   innominate I82.290
    chronic I82.291
   internal jugular I82.C1- ☑ (*following* I82.7)
    chronic I82.C2- ☑ (*following* I82.7)
   lower extremity
    deep I82.40- ☑
     chronic I82.50- ☑
     specified NEC I82.49- ☑
      chronic NEC I82.59- ☑
    distal
     deep I82.4Z- ☑
    proximal
     deep I82.4Y- ☑
      chronic I82.5Y- ☑
    superficial I82.81- ☑
   perianal K64.5
   popliteal I82.43- ☑
    chronic I82.53- ☑
   radial I82.62- ☑
    chronic I82.72- ☑
   renal I82.3
   saphenous (greater) (lesser) I82.81- ☑
   specified NEC I82.890
    chronic NEC I82.891
   subclavian I82.B1- ☑ (*following* I82.7)
    chronic I82.B2- ☑ (*following* I82.7)
   thoracic NEC I82.290
    chronic I82.291
   tibial I82.44- ☑
    chronic I82.54- ☑
   ulnar I82.62- ☑
    chronic I82.72- ☑
   upper extremity I82.60- ☑
    chronic I82.70- ☑
    deep I82.62- ☑
     chronic I82.72- ☑
    superficial I82.61- ☑
     chronic I82.71- ☑
  vena cava
   inferior I82.220
    chronic I82.221
   superior I82.210
    chronic I82.211
  venous, perianal K64.5
  ventricle — *see also* Infarct, myocardium
   following acute myocardial infarction (current complication) I23.6
   not resulting in infarction I24.0
   old I51.3
Thrombus — *see* Thrombosis
Thrush — *see also* Candidiasis
 newborn P37.5
 oral B37.0
 vaginal B37.3
Thumb — *see also* condition
 sucking (child problem) F98.8
Thymitis E32.8
Thymoma (benign) D15.0
 malignant C37
Thymus, thymic (gland) — *see* condition
Thyrocele — *see* Goiter
Thyroglossal — *see also* condition
 cyst Q89.2
 duct, persistent Q89.2
Thyroid (gland) (body) — *see also* condition
 hormone resistance E07.89
 lingual Q89.2
 nodule (cystic) (nontoxic) (single) E04.1
Thyroiditis E06.9
 acute (nonsuppurative) (pyogenic) (suppurative) E06.0
 autoimmune E06.3
 chronic (nonspecific) (sclerosing) E06.5
  with thyrotoxicosis, transient E06.2
  fibrous E06.5
  lymphadenoid E06.3
  lymphocytic E06.3
  lymphoid E06.3
 de Quervain's E06.1

Thyroiditis — *continued*
 drug-induced E06.4
 fibrous (chronic) E06.5
 giant-cell (follicular) E06.1
 granulomatous (de Quervain) (subacute) E06.1
 Hashimoto's (struma lymphomatosa) E06.3
 iatrogenic E06.4
 ligneous E06.5
 lymphocytic (chronic) E06.3
 lymphoid E06.3
 lymphomatous E06.3
 nonsuppurative E06.1
 postpartum, puerperal O90.5
 pseudotuberculous E06.1
 pyogenic E06.0
 radiation E06.4
 Riedel's E06.5
 subacute (granulomatous) E06.1
 suppurative E06.0
 tuberculous A18.81
 viral E06.1
 woody E06.5
Thyrolingual duct, persistent Q89.2
Thyromegaly E01.0
Thyrotoxic
 crisis — *see* Thyrotoxicosis
 heart disease or failure — *see also* Thyrotoxicosis E05.90 [143]
  with thyroid storm E05.91 [143]
 storm — *see* Thyrotoxicosis
Thyrotoxicosis (recurrent) E05.90
 with
  goiter (diffuse) E05.00
   with thyroid storm E05.01
   adenomatous uninodular E05.10
    with thyroid storm E05.11
   multinodular E05.20
    with thyroid storm E05.21
   nodular E05.20
    with thyroid storm E05.21
   uninodular E05.10
    with thyroid storm E05.11
  infiltrative
   dermopathy E05.00
    with thyroid storm E05.01
   ophthalmopathy E05.00
    with thyroid storm E05.01
  single thyroid nodule E05.10
   with thyroid storm E05.11
  thyroid storm E05.91
 due to
  ectopic thyroid nodule or tissue E05.30
   with thyroid storm E05.31
  ingestion of (excessive) thyroid material E05.40
   with thyroid storm E05.41
  overproduction of thyroid-stimulating hormone E05.80
   with thyroid storm E05.81
  specified cause NEC E05.80
   with thyroid storm E05.81
 factitia E05.40
  with thyroid storm E05.41
 heart — *see also* Failure, heart, high-output E05.90 [143]
  with thyroid storm — *see also* Failure, heart, high-output E05.91 [143]
  failure — *see also* Failure, heart, high-output E05.90 [143]
 neonatal (transient) P72.1
 transient with chronic thyroiditis E06.2
Tibia vara — *see* Osteochondrosis, juvenile, tibia
Tic (disorder) F95.9
 breathing F95.8
 child problem F95.0
 compulsive F95.1
 de la Tourette F95.2
 degenerative (generalized) (localized) G25.69
  facial G25.69
 disorder
  chronic
   motor F95.1
   vocal F95.1
  combined vocal and multiple motor F95.2
  transient F95.0
 douloureux G50.0
  atypical G50.1
  postherpetic, postzoster B02.22
 drug-induced G25.61
 eyelid F95.8

Tic — *continued*
 habit F95.9
  chronic F95.1
  transient of childhood F95.0
 lid, transient of childhood F95.0
 motor-verbal F95.2
 occupational F48.8
 orbicularis F95.8
  transient of childhood F95.0
 organic origin G25.69
 postchoreic G25.69
 provisional F95.0
 psychogenic, compulsive F95.1
 salaam R25.8
 spasm (motor or vocal) F95.9
  chronic F95.1
  transient of childhood F95.0
 specified NEC F95.8
Tick-borne — *see* condition
Tietze's disease or syndrome M94.0
Tight, tightness
 anus K62.89
 chest R07.89
 fascia (lata) M62.89
 foreskin (congenital) N47.1
 hymen, hymenal ring N89.6
 introitus (acquired) (congenital) N89.6
 rectal sphincter K62.89
 tendon — *see* Short, tendon
 urethral sphincter N35.919
Tilting vertebra — *see* Dorsopathy, deforming, specified NEC
Timidity, child F93.8
Tinea (intersecta) (tarsi) B35.9
 amiantacea L44.8
 asbestina B35.0
 barbae B35.0
 beard B35.0
 black dot B35.0
 blanca B36.2
 capitis B35.0
 corporis B35.4
 cruris B35.6
 flava B36.0
 foot B35.3
 furfuracea B36.0
 imbricata (Tokelau) B35.5
 kerion B35.0
 manuum B35.2
 microsporic — *see* Dermatophytosis
 nigra B36.1
 nodosa — *see* Piedra
 pedis B35.3
 scalp B35.0
 specified NEC B35.8
 sycosis B35.0
 tonsurans B35.0
 trichophytic — *see* Dermatophytosis
 unguium B35.1
 versicolor B36.0
Tingling sensation (skin) R20.2
Tin-miner's lung J63.5
Tinnitus NOS H93.1- ☑
 audible H93.1- ☑
 aurium H93.1- ☑
 pulsatile H93.A- ☑
 subjective H93.1- ☑
Tipped tooth (teeth) M26.33
Tipping
 pelvis M95.5
  with disproportion (fetopelvic) O33.0
   causing obstructed labor O65.0
 tooth (teeth), fully erupted M26.33
Tiredness R53.83
Tissue — *see* condition
Tobacco (nicotine)
 abuse — *see* Tobacco, use
 dependence — *see* Dependence, drug, nicotine
 harmful use Z72.0
 heart — *see* Tobacco, toxic effect
 maternal use, affecting newborn P04.2
 toxic effect — *see* Table of Drugs and Chemicals, by substance, poisoning
  chewing tobacco — *see* Table of Drugs and Chemicals, by substance, poisoning
  cigarettes — *see* Table of Drugs and Chemicals, by substance, poisoning
 use Z72.0

Tobacco — *continued*
  use — *continued*
    complicating
      childbirth O99.334
      pregnancy O99.33- ☑
      puerperium O99.335
    counseling and surveillance Z71.6
    history Z87.891
    withdrawal state — *see also* Dependence, drug, nicotine F17.203
Tocopherol deficiency E56.0
Todd's
  cirrhosis K74.3
  paralysis (postepileptic) (transitory) G83.84
Toe — *see* condition
Toilet, artificial opening — *see* Attention to, artificial, opening
Tokelau (ringworm) B35.5
Tollwut — *see* Rabies
Tommaselli's disease R31.9
  correct substance properly administered — *see* Table of Drugs and Chemicals, by drug, adverse effect
  overdose or wrong substance given or taken — *see* Table of Drugs and Chemicals, by drug, poisoning
Tongue — *see also* condition
  tie Q38.1
Tonic pupil — *see* Anomaly, pupil, function, tonic pupil
Toni-Fanconi syndrome (cystinosis) E72.09
  with cystinosis E72.04
Tonsil — *see* condition
Tonsillitis (acute) (catarrhal) (croupous) (follicular) (gangrenous) (infective) (lacunar) (lingual) (malignant) (membranous) (parenchymatous) (phlegmonous) (pseudomembranous) (purulent) (septic) (subacute) (suppurative) (toxic) (ulcerative) (vesicular) (viral) J03.90
  chronic J35.01
    with adenoiditis J35.03
  diphtheritic A36.0
  hypertrophic J35.01
    with adenoiditis J35.03
  recurrent J03.91
  specified organism NEC J03.80
    recurrent J03.81
  staphylococcal J03.80
    recurrent J03.81
  streptococcal J03.00
    recurrent J03.01
  tuberculous A15.8
  Vincent's A69.1
Tooth, teeth — *see* condition
Toothache K08.89
Topagnosis R20.8
Tophi — *see* Gout, chronic
TORCH infection — *see* Infection, congenital
  without active infection P00.2
Torn — *see* Tear
Tornwaldt's cyst or disease J39.2
Torsion
  accessory tube — *see* Torsion, fallopian tube
  adnexa (female) — *see* Torsion, fallopian tube
  aorta, acquired I77.1
  appendix epididymis N44.04
  appendix testis N44.03
  bile duct (common) (hepatic) K83.8
    congenital Q44.5
  bowel, colon or intestine K56.2
  cervix — *see* Malposition, uterus
  cystic duct K82.8
  dystonia — *see* Dystonia, torsion
  epididymis (appendix) N44.04
  fallopian tube N83.52- ☑
    with ovary N83.53
  gallbladder K82.8
    congenital Q44.1
  hydatid of Morgagni
    female N83.52- ☑
    male N44.03
  kidney (pedicle) (leading to infarction) N28.0
  Meckel's diverticulum (congenital) Q43.0
    malignant — *see* Table of Neoplasms, small intestine, malignant
  mesentery K56.2
  omentum K56.2
  organ or site, congenital NEC — *see* Anomaly, by site
  ovary (pedicle) N83.51- ☑
    with fallopian tube N83.53
    congenital Q50.2

Torsion — *continued*
  oviduct — *see* Torsion, fallopian tube
  penis (acquired) N48.82
    congenital Q55.63
  spasm — *see* Dystonia, torsion
  spermatic cord N44.02
    extravaginal N44.01
    intravaginal N44.02
  spleen D73.5
  testis, testicle N44.00
    appendix N44.03
  tibia — *see* Deformity, limb, specified type NEC, lower leg
  uterus — *see* Malposition, uterus
Torticollis (intermittent) (spastic) M43.6
  congenital (sternomastoid) Q68.0
  due to birth injury P15.8
  hysterical F44.4
  ocular R29.891
  psychogenic F45.8
    conversion reaction F44.4
  rheumatic M43.6
  rheumatoid M06.88
  spasmodic G24.3
  traumatic, current S13.4 ☑
Tortipelvis G24.1
Tortuous
  aortic arch Q25.46
  artery I77.1
  organ or site, congenital NEC — *see* Distortion
  retinal vessel, congenital Q14.1
  ureter N13.8
  urethra N36.8
  vein — *see* Varix
Torture, victim of Z65.4
Torula, torular (histolytica) (infection) — *see* Cryptococcosis
Torulosis — *see* Cryptococcosis
Torus (mandibularis) (palatinus) M27.0
  fracture — *see* Fracture, by site, torus
Touraine's syndrome Q79.8
Tourette's syndrome F95.2
Tourniquet syndrome — *see* Constriction, external, by site
Tower skull Q75.0
  with exophthalmos Q87.0
Toxemia R68.89
  bacterial — *see* Sepsis
  burn — *see* Burn
  eclamptic (with pre-existing hypertension) — *see* Eclampsia
  erysipelatous — *see* Erysipelas
  fatigue R68.89
  food — *see* Poisoning, food
  gastrointestinal K52.1
  intestinal K52.1
  kidney — *see* Uremia
  malarial — *see* Malaria
  myocardial — *see* Myocarditis, toxic
  of pregnancy — *see* Pre-eclampsia
  pre-eclamptic — *see* Pre-eclampsia
  small intestine K52.1
  staphylococcal, due to food A05.0
  stasis R68.89
  uremic — *see* Uremia
  urinary — *see* Uremia
Toxemica cerebropathia psychica (nonalcoholic) F04
  alcoholic — *see* Alcohol, amnestic disorder
Toxic (poisoning) — *see also* condition T65.91 ☑
  effect — *see* Table of Drugs and Chemicals, by substance, poisoning
  shock syndrome A48.3
  thyroid (gland) — *see* Thyrotoxicosis
Toxicemia — *see* Toxemia
Toxicity — *see* Table of Drugs and Chemicals, by substance, poisoning
  fava bean D55.0
  food, noxious — *see* Poisoning, food
  from drug or nonmedicinal substance — *see* Table of Drugs and Chemicals, by drug
Toxicosis — *see also* Toxemia
  capillary, hemorrhagic D69.0
Toxinfection, gastrointestinal K52.1
Toxocariasis B83.0
Toxoplasma, toxoplasmosis (acquired) B58.9
  with
    hepatitis B58.1

Toxoplasma, toxoplasmosis — *continued*
  with — *continued*
    meningoencephalitis B58.2
    ocular involvement B58.00
    other organ involvement B58.89
    pneumonia, pneumonitis B58.3
  congenital (acute) (subacute) (chronic) P37.1
  maternal, manifest toxoplasmosis in infant (acute) (subacute) (chronic) P37.1
tPA (rtPA) administration in a different facility within the last 24 hours prior to admission to current facility Z92.82
Trabeculation, bladder N32.89
Trachea — *see* condition
Tracheitis (catarrhal) (infantile) (membranous) (plastic) (septal) (suppurative) (viral) J04.10
  with
    bronchitis (15 years of age and above) J40
      acute or subacute — *see* Bronchitis, acute
      chronic J42
      tuberculous NEC A15.5
      under 15 years of age J20.9
    laryngitis (acute) J04.2
      chronic J37.1
      tuberculous NEC A15.5
  acute J04.10
    with obstruction J04.11
  chronic J42
    with
      bronchitis (chronic) J42
      laryngitis (chronic) J37.1
  diphtheritic (membranous) A36.89
  due to external agent — *see* Inflammation, respiratory, upper, due to
  syphilitic A52.73
  tuberculous A15.5
Trachelitis (nonvenereal) — *see* Cervicitis
Tracheobronchial — *see* condition
Tracheobronchitis (15 years of age and above) — *see also* Bronchitis
  due to
    Bordetella bronchiseptica A37.80
      with pneumonia A37.81
    Francisella tularensis A21.8
Tracheobronchomegaly Q32.4
  with bronchiectasis J47.9
    with
      exacerbation (acute) J47.1
      lower respiratory infection J47.0
  acquired J98.09
    with bronchiectasis J47.9
      with
        exacerbation (acute) J47.1
        lower respiratory infection J47.0
Tracheobronchopneumonitis — *see* Pneumonia, broncho-
Tracheocele (external) (internal) J39.8
  congenital Q32.1
Tracheomalacia J39.8
  congenital Q32.0
Tracheopharyngitis (acute) J06.9
  chronic J42
  due to external agent — *see* Inflammation, respiratory, upper, due to
Tracheostenosis J39.8
Tracheostomy
  complication — *see* Complication, tracheostomy
  status Z93.0
    attention to Z43.0
    malfunctioning J95.03
Trachoma, trachomatous A71.9
  active (stage) A71.1
  contraction of conjunctiva A71.1
  dubium A71.0
  healed or sequelae B94.0
  initial (stage) A71.0
  pannus A71.1
  Türck's J37.0
Traction, vitreomacular H43.82- ☑
Train sickness T75.3 ☑
Trait(s)
  Hb-S D57.3
  hemoglobin
    abnormal NEC D58.2
      with thalassemia D56.3
    C — *see* Disease, hemoglobin C
    S (Hb-S) D57.3
  Lepore D56.3

☑ **Additional Character Required — Refer to the Tabular List for Character Selection**   ▽ **Subterms under main terms may continue to next column or page**

Trait(s) — *continued*
  personality, accentuated Z73.1
  sickle-cell D57.3
    with elliptocytosis or spherocytosis D57.3
  type A personality Z73.1
Tramp Z59.0
Trance R41.89
  hysterical F44.89
Transaminasemia R74.0
Transection
  abdomen (partial) S38.3 ☑
  aorta (incomplete) — *see also* Injury, aorta
    complete — *see* Injury, aorta, laceration, major
  carotid artery (incomplete) — *see also* Injury, blood
    vessel, carotid, laceration
    complete — *see* Injury, blood vessel, carotid, lacer-
      ation, major
  celiac artery (incomplete) S35.211 ☑
    branch (incomplete) S35.291 ☑
      complete S35.292 ☑
    complete S35.212 ☑
  innominate
    artery (incomplete) — *see also* Injury, blood vessel,
      thoracic, innominate, artery, laceration
      complete — *see* Injury, blood vessel, thoracic,
        innominate, artery, laceration, major
    vein (incomplete) — *see also* Injury, blood vessel,
      thoracic, innominate, vein, laceration
      complete — *see* Injury, blood vessel, thoracic,
        innominate, vein, laceration, major
  jugular vein (external) (incomplete) — *see also* Injury,
    blood vessel, jugular vein, laceration
    complete — *see* Injury, blood vessel, jugular vein,
      laceration, major
    internal (incomplete) — *see also* Injury, blood vessel,
      jugular vein, internal, laceration
      complete — *see* Injury, blood vessel, jugular vein,
        internal, laceration, major
  mesenteric artery (incomplete) — *see also* Injury,
    mesenteric, artery, laceration
    complete — *see* Injury, mesenteric artery, laceration,
      major
  pulmonary vessel (incomplete) — *see also* Injury, blood
    vessel, thoracic, pulmonary, laceration
    complete — *see* Injury, blood vessel, thoracic, pul-
      monary, laceration, major
  subclavian — *see* Transection, innominate
  vena cava (incomplete) — *see also* Injury, vena cava
    complete — *see* Injury, vena cava, laceration, major
  vertebral artery (incomplete) — *see also* Injury, blood
    vessel, vertebral, laceration
    complete — *see* Injury, blood vessel, vertebral, lac-
      eration, major
Transfusion
  associated (red blood cell) hemochromatosis E83.111
  blood
    ABO incompatible — *see* Complication(s), transfu-
      sion, incompatibility reaction, ABO
    minor blood group (Duffy) (E) (K) (Kell) (Kidd) (Lewis)
      (M) (N) (P) (S) T80.89 ☑
    reaction or complication — *see* Complications,
      transfusion
  fetomaternal (mother) — *see* Pregnancy, complicated
    by, placenta, transfusion syndrome
  maternofetal (mother) — *see* Pregnancy, complicated
    by, placenta, transfusion syndrome
  placental (syndrome) (mother) — *see* Pregnancy,
    complicated by, placenta, transfusion syndrome
  reaction (adverse) — *see* Complications, transfusion
  related acute lung injury (TRALI) J95.84
  twin-to-twin — *see* Pregnancy, complicated by, placen-
    ta, transfusion syndrome, fetus to fetus
Transient (meaning homeless) — *see also* condition Z59.0
Translocation
  balanced autosomal Q95.9
    in normal individual Q95.0
  chromosomes NEC Q99.8
    balanced and insertion in normal individual Q95.0
  Down syndrome Q90.2
  trisomy
    13 Q91.6
    18 Q91.2
    21 Q90.2
Translucency, iris — *see* Degeneration, iris
Transmission of chemical substances through the
  placenta — *see* Absorption, chemical, through
  placenta

Transparency, lung, unilateral J43.0
Transplant (ed) (status) Z94.9
  awaiting organ Z76.82
  bone Z94.6
    marrow Z94.81
  candidate Z76.82
  complication — *see* Complication, transplant
  cornea Z94.7
  heart Z94.1
    and lung(s) Z94.3
    valve Z95.2
      prosthetic Z95.2
      specified NEC Z95.4
      xenogenic Z95.3
  intestine Z94.82
  kidney Z94.0
  liver Z94.4
  lung(s) Z94.2
    and heart Z94.3
  organ (failure) (infection) (rejection) Z94.9
    removal status Z98.85
  pancreas Z94.83
  skin Z94.5
  social Z60.3
  specified organ or tissue NEC Z94.89
  stem cells Z94.84
  tissue Z94.9
Transplants, ovarian, endometrial N80.1
Transposed — *see* Transposition
Transposition (congenital) — *see also* Malposition,
  congenital
  abdominal viscera Q89.3
  aorta (dextra) Q20.3
  appendix Q43.8
  colon Q43.8
  corrected Q20.5
  great vessels (complete) (partial) Q20.3
  heart Q24.0
    with complete transposition of viscera Q89.3
  intestine (large) (small) Q43.8
  reversed jejunal (for bypass) (status) Z98.0
  scrotum Q55.23
  stomach Q40.2
    with general transposition of viscera Q89.3
  tooth, teeth, fully erupted M26.30
  vessels, great (complete) (partial) Q20.3
  viscera (abdominal) (thoracic) Q89.3
Transsexualism F64.0
Transverse — *see also* condition
  arrest (deep), in labor O64.0 ☑
  lie (mother) O32.2 ☑
    causing obstructed labor O64.8 ☑
Transvestism, transvestitism (dual-role) F64.1
  fetishistic F65.1
Trapped placenta (with hemorrhage) O72.0
  without hemorrhage O73.0
TRAPS (tumor necrosis factor receptor associated periodic
  syndrome) M04.1
Trauma, traumatism — *see also* Injury
  acoustic — *see* subcategory H83.3 ☑
  birth — *see* Birth, injury
  complicating ectopic or molar pregnancy O08.6
  during delivery O71.9
  following ectopic or molar pregnancy O08.6
  obstetric O71.9
    specified NEC O71.89
  occusal
    primary K08.81
    secondary K08.82
Traumatic — *see also* condition
  brain injury S06.9 ☑
Treacher Collins syndrome Q75.4
Treitz's hernia — *see* Hernia, abdomen, specified site
  NEC
Trematode infestation — *see* Infestation, fluke
Trematodiasis — *see* Infestation, fluke
Trembling paralysis — *see* Parkinsonism
Tremor(s) R25.1
  drug induced G25.1
  essential (benign) G25.0
  familial G25.0
  hereditary G25.0
  hysterical F44.4
  intention G25.2
  medication induced postural G25.1
  mercurial — *see* subcategory T56.1 ☑
  Parkinson's — *see* Parkinsonism
  psychogenic (conversion reaction) F44.4

Tremor(s) — *continued*
  senilis R54
  specified type NEC G25.2
Trench
  fever A79.0
  foot — *see* Immersion, foot
  mouth A69.1
Treponema pallidum infection — *see* Syphilis
Treponematosis
  due to
    T. pallidum — *see* Syphilis
    T. pertenue — *see* Yaws
Triad
  Hutchinson's (congenital syphilis) A50.53
  Kartagener's Q89.3
  Saint's — *see* Hernia, diaphragm
Trichiasis (eyelid) H02.059
  with entropion — *see* Entropion
  left H02.056
    lower H02.055
    upper H02.054
  right H02.053
    lower H02.052
    upper H02.051
Trichinella spiralis (infection) (infestation) B75
Trichinellosis, trichiniasis, trichinelliasis, trichinosis
  B75
  with muscle disorder B75 *[M63.80]*
    ankle B75 *[M63.87-]* ☑
    foot B75 *[M63.87-]* ☑
    forearm B75 *[M63.83-]* ☑
    hand B75 *[M63.84-]* ☑
    lower leg B75 *[M63.86-]* ☑
    multiple sites B75 *[M63.89]*
    pelvic region B75 *[M63.85-]* ☑
    shoulder region B75 *[M63.81-]* ☑
    specified site NEC B75 *[M63.88]*
    thigh B75 *[M63.85-]* ☑
    upper arm B75 *[M63.82-]* ☑
Trichobezoar T18.9 ☑
  intestine T18.3 ☑
  stomach T18.2 ☑
Trichocephaliasis, trichocephalosis B79
Trichocephalus infestation B79
Trichoclasis L67.8
Trichoepithelioma — *see also* Neoplasm, skin, benign
  malignant — *see* Neoplasm, skin, malignant
Trichofolliculoma — *see* Neoplasm, skin, benign
Tricholemmoma — *see* Neoplasm, skin, benign
Trichomoniasis A59.9
  bladder A59.03
  cervix A59.09
  intestinal A07.8
  prostate A59.02
  seminal vesicles A59.09
  specified site NEC A59.8
  urethra A59.03
  urogenitalis A59.00
  vagina A59.01
  vulva A59.01
Trichomycosis
  axillaris A48.8
  nodosa, nodularis B36.8
Trichonodosis L67.8
Trichophytid, trichophyton infection — *see* Dermato-
  phytosis
Trichophytobezoar T18.9 ☑
  intestine T18.3 ☑
  stomach T18.2 ☑
Trichophytosis — *see* Dermatophytosis
Trichoptilosis L67.8
Trichorrhexis (nodosa) (invaginata) L67.0
Trichosis axillaris A48.8
Trichosporosis nodosa B36.2
Trichostasis spinulosa (congenital) Q84.1
Trichostrongyliasis, trichostrongylosis (small intes-
  tine) B81.2
Trichostrongylus infection B81.2
Trichotillomania F63.3
Trichromat, trichromatopsia, anomalous (congenital)
  H53.55
Trichuriasis B79
Trichuris trichiura (infection) (infestation) (any site) B79
Tricuspid (valve) — *see* condition
Trifid — *see also* Accessory
  kidney (pelvis) Q63.8
  tongue Q38.3

Trigeminal neuralgia — see Neuralgia, trigeminal
Trigeminy R00.8
Trigger finger (acquired) M65.30
  congenital Q74.0
  index finger M65.32- ☑
  little finger M65.35- ☑
  middle finger M65.33- ☑
  ring finger M65.34- ☑
  thumb M65.31- ☑
Trigonitis (bladder) (chronic) (pseudomembranous)
  N30.30
  with hematuria N30.31
Trigonocephaly Q75.0
Trilocular heart — see Cor triloculare
Trimethylaminuria E72.52
Tripartite placenta O43.19- ☑
Triphalangeal thumb Q74.0
Triple — see also Accessory
  kidneys Q63.0
  uteri Q51.818
  X, female Q97.0
Triplegia G83.89
  congenital G80.8
Triplet (newborn) — see also Newborn, triplet
  complicating pregnancy — see Pregnancy, triplet
Triplication — see Accessory
Triploidy Q92.7
Trismus R25.2
  neonatorum A33
  newborn A33
Trisomy (syndrome) Q92.9
  13 (partial) Q91.7
    meiotic nondisjunction Q91.4
    mitotic nondisjunction Q91.5
    mosaicism Q91.5
    translocation Q91.6
  18 (partial) Q91.3
    meiotic nondisjunction Q91.0
    mitotic nondisjunction Q91.1
    mosaicism Q91.1
    translocation Q91.2
  20 Q92.8
  21 (partial) Q90.9
    meiotic nondisjunction Q90.0
    mitotic nondisjunction Q90.1
    mosaicism Q90.1
    translocation Q90.2
  22 Q92.8
  autosomes Q92.9
  chromosome specified NEC Q92.8
    partial Q92.2
      due to unbalanced translocation Q92.5
    specified NEC Q92.8
    whole (nonsex chromosome)
      meiotic nondisjunction Q92.0
      mitotic nondisjunction Q92.1
      mosaicism Q92.1
  due to
    dicentrics — see Extra, marker chromosomes
    extra rings — see Extra, marker chromosomes
    isochromosomes — see Extra, marker chromosomes
  specified NEC Q92.8
  whole chromosome Q92.9
    meiotic nondisjunction Q92.0
    mitotic nondisjunction Q92.1
    mosaicism Q92.1
    partial Q92.9
    specified NEC Q92.8
Tritanomaly, tritanopia H53.55
Trombiculosis, trombiculiasis, trombidiosis B88.0
Trophedema (congenital) (hereditary) Q82.0
Trophoblastic disease — see also Mole, hydatidiform
  O01.9
Tropholymphedema Q82.0
Trophoneurosis NEC G96.8
  disseminated M34.9
Tropical — see condition
Trouble — see also Disease
  heart — see Disease, heart
  kidney — see Disease, renal
  nervous R45.0
  sinus — see Sinusitis
Trousseau's syndrome (thrombophlebitis migrans) I82.1
Truancy, childhood
  from school Z72.810
Truncus
  arteriosus (persistent) Q20.0

Truncus — continued
  communis Q20.0
Trunk — see condition
Trypanosomiasis
  African B56.9
    by Trypanosoma brucei
      gambiense B56.0
      rhodesiense B56.1
  American — see Chagas' disease
  Brazilian — see Chagas' disease
  by Trypanosoma
    brucei gambiense B56.0
    brucei rhodesiense B56.1
    cruzi — see Chagas' disease
  gambiensis, Gambian B56.0
  rhodesiensis, Rhodesian B56.1
  South American — see Chagas' disease
  where
    African trypanosomiasis is prevalent B56.9
    Chagas' disease is prevalent B57.2
T-shaped incisors K00.2
Tsutsugamushi (disease) (fever) A75.3
Tube, tubal, tubular — see condition
Tubercle — see also Tuberculosis
  brain, solitary A17.81
  Darwin's Q17.8
  Ghon, primary infection A15.7
Tuberculid, tuberculide (indurating, subcutaneous)
  (lichenoid) (miliary) (papulonecrotic) (primary) (skin)
  A18.4
Tuberculoma — see also Tuberculosis
  brain A17.81
  meninges (cerebral) (spinal) A17.1
  spinal cord A17.81
Tuberculosis, tubercular, tuberculous (calcification)
  (calcified) (caseous) (chromogenic acid-fast bacilli)
  (degeneration) (fibrocaseous) (fistula) (interstitial)
  (isolated circumscribed lesions) (necrosis)
  (parenchymatous) (ulcerative) A15.9
  with pneumoconiosis (any condition in J60-J64) J65
  abdomen (lymph gland) A18.39
  abscess (respiratory) A15.9
    bone A18.03
      hip A18.02
      knee A18.02
      sacrum A18.01
      specified site NEC A18.03
      spinal A18.01
      vertebra A18.01
    brain A17.81
    breast A18.89
    Cowper's gland A18.15
    dura (mater) (cerebral) (spinal) A17.81
    epidural (cerebral) (spinal) A17.81
    female pelvis A18.17
    frontal sinus A15.8
    genital organs NEC A18.10
    genitourinary A18.10
    gland (lymphatic) — see Tuberculosis, lymph gland
    hip A18.02
    intestine A18.32
    ischiorectal A18.32
    joint NEC A18.02
      hip A18.02
      knee A18.02
      specified NEC A18.02
      vertebral A18.01
    kidney A18.11
    knee A18.02
    latent Z22.7
    lumbar (spine) A18.01
    lung — see Tuberculosis, pulmonary
    meninges (cerebral) (spinal) A17.0
    muscle A18.09
    perianal (fistula) A18.32
    perinephritic A18.11
    perirectal A18.32
    rectum A18.32
    retropharyngeal A15.8
    sacrum A18.01
    scrofulous A18.2
    scrotum A18.15
    skin (primary) A18.4
    spinal cord A17.81
    spine or vertebra (column) A18.01
    subdiaphragmatic A18.31
    testis A18.15
    urinary A18.13

Tuberculosis, tubercular, tuberculous — continued
  abscess — continued
    uterus A18.17
  accessory sinus — see Tuberculosis, sinus
  Addison's disease A18.7
  adenitis — see Tuberculosis, lymph gland
  adenoids A15.8
  adenopathy — see Tuberculosis, lymph gland
  adherent pericardium A18.84
  adnexa (uteri) A18.17
  adrenal (capsule) (gland) A18.7
  alimentary canal A18.32
  anemia A18.89
  ankle (joint) (bone) A18.02
  anus A18.32
  apex, apical — see Tuberculosis, pulmonary
  appendicitis, appendix A18.32
  arachnoid A17.0
  artery, arteritis A18.89
    cerebral A18.89
  arthritis (chronic) (synovial) A18.02
    spine or vertebra (column) A18.01
  articular — see Tuberculosis, joint
  ascites A18.31
  asthma — see Tuberculosis, pulmonary
  axilla, axillary (gland) A18.2
  bladder A18.12
  bone A18.03
    hip A18.02
    knee A18.02
    limb NEC A18.03
    sacrum A18.01
    spine or vertebral column A18.01
  bowel (miliary) A18.32
  brain A17.81
  breast A18.89
  broad ligament A18.17
  bronchi, bronchial, bronchus A15.5
    ectasia, ectasis (bronchiectasis) — see Tuberculosis,
      pulmonary
    fistula A15.5
      primary (progressive) A15.7
    gland or node A15.4
      primary (progressive) A15.7
    lymph gland or node A15.4
      primary (progressive) A15.7
  bronchiectasis — see Tuberculosis, pulmonary
  bronchitis A15.5
  bronchopleural A15.6
  bronchopneumonia, bronchopneumonic — see Tuber-
    culosis, pulmonary
  bronchorrhagia A15.5
  bronchotracheal A15.5
  bronze disease A18.7
  buccal cavity A18.83
  bulbourethral gland A18.15
  bursa A18.09
  cachexia A15.9
  cardiomyopathy A18.84
  caries — see Tuberculosis, bone
  cartilage A18.02
    intervertebral A18.01
  catarrhal — see Tuberculosis, respiratory
  cecum A18.32
  cellulitis (primary) A18.4
  cerebellum A17.81
  cerebral, cerebrum A17.81
  cerebrospinal A17.81
    meninges A17.0
  cervical (lymph gland or node) A18.2
  cervicitis, cervix (uteri) A18.16
  chest — see Tuberculosis, respiratory
  chorioretinitis A18.53
  choroid, choroiditis A18.53
  ciliary body A18.54
  colitis A18.32
  collier's J65
  colliquativa (primary) A18.4
  colon A18.32
  complex, primary A15.7
  congenital P37.0
  conjunctiva A18.59
  connective tissue (systemic) A18.89
  contact Z20.1
  cornea (ulcer) A18.52
  Cowper's gland A18.15
  coxae A18.02
  coxalgia A18.02

☑ **Additional Character Required** — Refer to the Tabular List for Character Selection   ▽ Subterms under main terms may continue to next column or page

Tuberculosis, tubercular, tuberculous — *continued*
- cul-de-sac of Douglas A18.17
- curvature, spine A18.01
- cutis (colliquativa) (primary) A18.4
- cyst, ovary A18.18
- cystitis A18.12
- dactylitis A18.03
- diarrhea A18.32
- diffuse — *see* Tuberculosis, miliary
- digestive tract A18.32
- disseminated — *see* Tuberculosis, miliary
- duodenum A18.32
- dura (mater) (cerebral) (spinal) A17.0
  - abscess (cerebral) (spinal) A17.81
- dysentery A18.32
- ear (inner) (middle) A18.6
  - bone A18.03
  - external (primary) A18.4
  - skin (primary) A18.4
- elbow A18.02
- emphysema — *see* Tuberculosis, pulmonary
- empyema A15.6
- encephalitis A17.82
- endarteritis A18.89
- endocarditis A18.84
  - aortic A18.84
  - mitral A18.84
  - pulmonary A18.84
  - tricuspid A18.84
- endocrine glands NEC A18.82
- endometrium A18.17
- enteric, enterica, enteritis A18.32
- enterocolitis A18.32
- epididymis, epididymitis A18.15
- epidural abscess (cerebral) (spinal) A17.81
- epiglottis A15.5
- episcleritis A18.51
- erythema (induratum) (nodosum) (primary) A18.4
- esophagus A18.83
- eustachian tube A18.6
- exposure (to) Z20.1
- exudative — *see* Tuberculosis, pulmonary
- eye A18.50
- eyelid (primary) (lupus) A18.4
- fallopian tube (acute) (chronic) A18.17
- fascia A18.09
- fauces A15.8
- female pelvic inflammatory disease A18.17
- finger A18.03
- first infection A15.7
- gallbladder A18.83
- ganglion A18.09
- gastritis A18.83
- gastrocolic fistula A18.32
- gastroenteritis A18.32
- gastrointestinal tract A18.32
- general, generalized — *see* Tuberculosis, miliary
- genital organs A18.10
- genitourinary A18.10
- genu A18.02
- glandula suprarenalis A18.7
- glandular, general A18.2
- glottis A15.5
- grinder's J65
- gum A18.83
- hand A18.03
- heart A18.84
- hematogenous — *see* Tuberculosis, miliary
- hemoptysis — *see* Tuberculosis, pulmonary
- hemorrhage NEC — *see* Tuberculosis, pulmonary
- hemothorax A15.6
- hepatitis A18.83
- hilar lymph nodes A15.4
  - primary (progressive) A15.7
- hip (joint) (disease) (bone) A18.02
- hydropneumothorax A15.6
- hydrothorax A15.6
- hypoadrenalism A18.7
- hypopharynx A15.8
- ileocecal (hyperplastic) A18.32
- ileocolitis A18.32
- ileum A18.32
- iliac spine (superior) A18.03
- immunological findings only A15.7
- indurativa (primary) A18.4
- infantile A15.7
- infection A15.9
  - without clinical manifestations A15.7

Tuberculosis, tubercular, tuberculous — *continued*
- infraclavicular gland A18.2
- inguinal gland A18.2
- inguinalis A18.2
- intestine (any part) A18.32
- iridocyclitis A18.54
- iris, iritis A18.54
- ischiorectal A18.32
- jaw A18.03
- jejunum A18.32
- joint A18.02
  - vertebral A18.01
- keratitis (interstitial) A18.52
- keratoconjunctivitis A18.52
- kidney A18.11
- knee (joint) A18.02
- kyphosis, kyphoscoliosis A18.01
- laryngitis A15.5
- larynx A15.5
- latent Z22.7
- leptomeninges, leptomeningitis (cerebral) (spinal) A17.0
- lichenoides (primary) A18.4
- linguae A18.83
- lip A18.83
- liver A18.83
- lordosis A18.01
- lung — *see* Tuberculosis, pulmonary
- lupus vulgaris A18.4
- lymph gland or node (peripheral) A18.2
  - abdomen A18.39
  - bronchial A15.4
    - primary (progressive) A15.7
  - cervical A18.2
  - hilar A15.4
    - primary (progressive) A15.7
  - intrathoracic A15.4
    - primary (progressive) A15.7
  - mediastinal A15.4
    - primary (progressive) A15.7
  - mesenteric A18.39
  - retroperitoneal A18.39
  - tracheobronchial A15.4
    - primary (progressive) A15.7
- lymphadenitis — *see* Tuberculosis, lymph gland
- lymphangitis — *see* Tuberculosis, lymph gland
- lymphatic (gland) (vessel) — *see* Tuberculosis, lymph gland
- mammary gland A18.89
- marasmus A15.9
- mastoiditis A18.03
- mediastinal lymph gland or node A15.4
  - primary (progressive) A15.7
- mediastinitis A15.8
  - primary (progressive) A15.7
- mediastinum A15.8
  - primary (progressive) A15.7
- medulla A17.81
- melanosis, Addisonian A18.7
- meninges, meningitis (basilar) (cerebral) (cerebrospinal) (spinal) A17.0
- meningoencephalitis A17.82
- mesentery, mesenteric (gland or node) A18.39
- miliary A19.9
  - acute A19.2
    - multiple sites A19.1
    - single specified site A19.0
  - chronic A19.8
  - specified NEC A19.8
- millstone makers' J65
- miner's J65
- molder's J65
- mouth A18.83
- multiple A19.9
  - acute A19.1
  - chronic A19.8
- muscle A18.09
- myelitis A17.82
- myocardium, myocarditis A18.84
- nasal (passage) (sinus) A15.8
- nasopharynx A15.8
- neck gland A18.2
- nephritis A18.11
- nerve (mononeuropathy) A17.83
- nervous system A17.9
- nose (septum) A15.8
- ocular A18.50
- omentum A18.31
- oophoritis (acute) (chronic) A18.17

Tuberculosis, tubercular, tuberculous — *continued*
- optic (nerve trunk) (papilla) A18.59
- orbit A18.59
- orchitis A18.15
- organ, specified NEC A18.89
- osseous — *see* Tuberculosis, bone
- osteitis — *see* Tuberculosis, bone
- osteomyelitis — *see* Tuberculosis, bone
- otitis media A18.6
- ovary, ovaritis (acute) (chronic) A18.17
- oviduct (acute) (chronic) A18.17
- pachymeningitis A17.0
- palate (soft) A18.83
- pancreas A18.83
- papulonecrotic (a) (primary) A18.4
- parathyroid glands A18.82
- paronychia (primary) A18.4
- parotid gland or region A18.83
- pelvis (bony) A18.03
- penis A18.15
- peribronchitis A15.5
- pericardium, pericarditis A18.84
- perichondritis, larynx A15.5
- periostitis — *see* Tuberculosis, bone
- perirectal fistula A18.32
- peritoneum NEC A18.31
- peritonitis A18.31
- pharynx, pharyngitis A15.8
- phlyctenulosis (keratoconjunctivitis) A18.52
- phthisis NEC — *see* Tuberculosis, pulmonary
- pituitary gland A18.82
- pleura, pleural, pleurisy, pleuritis (fibrinous) (obliterative) (purulent) (simple plastic) (with effusion) A15.6
  - primary (progressive) A15.7
- pneumonia, pneumonic — *see* Tuberculosis, pulmonary
- pneumothorax (spontaneous) (tense valvular) — *see* Tuberculosis, pulmonary
- polyneuropathy A17.89
- polyserositis A19.9
  - acute A19.1
  - chronic A19.8
- potter's J65
- prepuce A18.15
- primary (complex) A15.7
- proctitis A18.32
- prostate, prostatitis A18.14
- pulmonalis — *see* Tuberculosis, pulmonary
- pulmonary (cavitated) (fibrotic) (infiltrative) (nodular) A15.0
  - childhood type or first infection A15.7
  - primary (complex) A15.7
- pyelitis A18.11
- pyelonephritis A18.11
- pyemia — *see* Tuberculosis, miliary
- pyonephrosis A18.11
- pyopneumothorax A15.6
- pyothorax A15.6
- rectum (fistula) (with abscess) A18.32
- reinfection stage — *see* Tuberculosis, pulmonary
- renal A18.11
- renis A18.11
- respiratory A15.9
  - primary A15.7
  - specified site NEC A15.8
- retina, retinitis A18.53
- retroperitoneal (lymph gland or node) A18.39
- rheumatism NEC A18.09
- rhinitis A15.8
- sacroiliac (joint) A18.01
- sacrum A18.01
- salivary gland A18.83
- salpingitis (acute) (chronic) A18.17
- sandblaster's J65
- sclera A18.51
- scoliosis A18.01
- scrofulous A18.2
- scrotum A18.15
- seminal tract or vesicle A18.15
- senile A15.9
- septic — *see* Tuberculosis, miliary
- shoulder (joint) A18.02
  - blade A18.03
- sigmoid A18.32
- sinus (any nasal) A15.8
  - bone A18.03
  - epididymis A18.15

Tuberculosis, tubercular, tuberculous — *continued*
  skeletal NEC A18.03
  skin (any site) (primary) A18.4
  small intestine A18.32
  soft palate A18.83
  spermatic cord A18.15
  spine, spinal (column) A18.01
    cord A17.81
    medulla A17.81
    membrane A17.0
    meninges A17.0
  spleen, splenitis A18.85
  spondylitis A18.01
  sternoclavicular joint A18.02
  stomach A18.83
  stonemason's J65
  subcutaneous tissue (cellular) (primary) A18.4
  subcutis (primary) A18.4
  subdeltoid bursa A18.83
  submaxillary (region) A18.83
  supraclavicular gland A18.2
  suprarenal (capsule) (gland) A18.7
  swelling, joint (*see also* category M01) — *see also* Tuberculosis, joint A18.02
  symphysis pubis A18.02
  synovitis A18.09
    articular A18.02
    spine or vertebra A18.01
  systemic — *see* Tuberculosis, miliary
  tarsitis A18.4
  tendon (sheath) — *see* Tuberculosis, tenosynovitis
  tenosynovitis A18.09
    spine or vertebra A18.01
  testis A18.15
  throat A15.8
  thymus gland A18.82
  thyroid gland A18.81
  tongue A18.83
  tonsil, tonsillitis A15.8
  trachea, tracheal A15.5
    lymph gland or node A15.4
      primary (progressive) A15.7
  tracheobronchial A15.5
    lymph gland or node A15.4
      primary (progressive) A15.7
  tubal (acute) (chronic) A18.17
  tunica vaginalis A18.15
  ulcer (skin) (primary) A18.4
    bowel or intestine A18.32
    specified NEC — *see* Tuberculosis, by site
  unspecified site A15.9
  ureter A18.11
  urethra, urethral (gland) A18.13
  urinary organ or tract A18.13
  uterus A18.17
  uveal tract A18.54
  uvula A18.83
  vagina A18.18
  vas deferens A18.15
  verruca, verrucosa (cutis) (primary) A18.4
  vertebra (column) A18.01
  vesiculitis A18.15
  vulva A18.18
  wrist (joint) A18.02
Tuberculum
  Carabelli — *see* Excludes Note at K00.2
  occlusal — *see* Excludes Note at K00.2
  paramolare K00.2
Tuberosity, enitre maxillary M26.07
Tuberous sclerosis (brain) Q85.1
Tubo-ovarian — *see* condition
Tuboplasty, after previous sterilization Z31.0
  aftercare Z31.42
Tubotympanitis, catarrhal (chronic) — *see* Otitis, media, nonsuppurative, chronic, serous
Tularemia A21.9
  with
    conjunctivitis A21.1
    pneumonia A21.2
  abdominal A21.3
  bronchopneumonic A21.2
  conjunctivitis A21.1
  cryptogenic A21.3
  enteric A21.3
  gastrointestinal A21.3
  generalized A21.7
  ingestion A21.3
  intestinal A21.3

Tularemia — *continued*
  oculoglandular A21.1
  ophthalmic A21.1
  pneumonia (any), pneumonic A21.2
  pulmonary A21.2
  sepsis A21.7
  specified NEC A21.8
  typhoidal A21.7
  ulceroglandular A21.0
Tularensis conjunctivitis A21.1
Tumefaction — *see also* Swelling
  liver — *see* Hypertrophy, liver
Tumor — *see also* Neoplasm, unspecified behavior, by site
  acinar cell — *see* Neoplasm, uncertain behavior, by site
  acinic cell — *see* Neoplasm, uncertain behavior, by site
  adenocarcinoid — *see* Neoplasm, malignant, by site
  adenomatoid — *see also* Neoplasm, benign, by site
    odontogenic — *see* Cyst, calcifying odontogenic
  adnexal (skin) — *see* Neoplasm, skin, benign, by site
  adrenal
    cortical (benign) D35.0- ☑
      malignant C74.0- ☑
    rest — *see* Neoplasm, benign, by site
  alpha-cell
    malignant
      pancreas C25.4
      specified site NEC — *see* Neoplasm, malignant, by site
      unspecified site C25.4
    pancreas D13.7
    specified site NEC — *see* Neoplasm, benign, by site
    unspecified site D13.7
  aneurysmal — *see* Aneurysm
  aortic body D44.7
    malignant C75.5
  Askin's — *see* Neoplasm, connective tissue, malignant
  basal cell — *see also* Neoplasm, skin, uncertain behavior D48.5
  Bednar — *see* Neoplasm, skin, malignant
  benign (unclassified) — *see* Neoplasm, benign, by site
  beta-cell
    malignant
      pancreas C25.4
      specified site NEC — *see* Neoplasm, malignant, by site
      unspecified site C25.4
    pancreas D13.7
    specified site NEC — *see* Neoplasm, benign, by site
    unspecified site D13.7
  Brenner D27.9
    borderline malignancy D39.1- ☑
    malignant C56- ☑
    proliferating D39.1- ☑
  bronchial alveolar, intravascular D38.1
  Brooke's — *see* Neoplasm, skin, benign
  brown fat — *see* Lipoma
  Burkitt — *see* Lymphoma, Burkitt
  calcifying epithelial odontogenic — *see* Cyst, calcifying odontogenic
  carcinoid D3A.00 (*following* D36)
    benign D3A.00 (*following* D36)
      appendix D3A.020 (*following* D36)
      ascending colon D3A.022 (*following* D36)
      bronchus (lung) D3A.090 (*following* D36)
      cecum D3A.021 (*following* D36)
      colon D3A.029 (*following* D36)
      descending colon D3A.024 (*following* D36)
      duodenum D3A.010 (*following* D36)
      foregut NOS D3A.094 (*following* D36)
      hindgut NOS D3A.096 (*following* D36)
      ileum D3A.012 (*following* D36)
      jejunum D3A.011 (*following* D36)
      kidney D3A.093 (*following* D36)
      large intestine D3A.029 (*following* D36)
      lung (bronchus) D3A.090 (*following* D36)
      midgut NOS D3A.095 (*following* D36)
      rectum D3A.026 (*following* D36)
      sigmoid colon D3A.025 (*following* D36)
      small intestine D3A.019 (*following* D36)
      specified NEC D3A.098 (*following* D36)
      stomach D3A.092 (*following* D36)
      thymus D3A.091 (*following* D36)
      transverse colon D3A.023 (*following* D36)
    malignant C7A.00 (*following* C75)
      appendix C7A.020 (*following* C75)
      ascending colon C7A.022 (*following* C75)
      bronchus (lung) C7A.090 (*following* C75)

Tumor — *continued*
  carcinoid — *continued*
    malignant — *continued*
      cecum C7A.021 (*following* C75)
      colon C7A.029 (*following* C75)
      descending colon C7A.024 (*following* C75)
      duodenum C7A.010 (*following* C75)
      foregut NOS C7A.094 (*following* C75)
      hindgut NOS C7A.096 (*following* C75)
      ileum C7A.012 (*following* C75)
      jejunum C7A.011 (*following* C75)
      kidney C7A.093 (*following* C75)
      large intestine C7A.029 (*following* C75)
      lung (bronchus) C7A.090 (*following* C75)
      midgut NOS C7A.095 (*following* C75)
      rectum C7A.026 (*following* C75)
      sigmoid colon C7A.025 (*following* C75)
      small intestine C7A.019 (*following* C75)
      specified NEC C7A.098 (*following* C75)
      stomach C7A.092 (*following* C75)
      thymus C7A.091 (*following* C75)
      transverse colon C7A.023 (*following* C75)
    mesentery metastasis C7B.04 (*following* C75)
    secondary C7B.00 (*following* C75)
      bone C7B.03 (*following* C75)
      distant lymph nodes C7B.01 (*following* C75)
      liver C7B.02 (*following* C75)
      peritoneum C7B.04 (*following* C75)
      specified NEC C7B.09 (*following* C75)
  carotid body D44.6
    malignant C75.4
  cells — *see also* Neoplasm, unspecified behavior, by site
    benign — *see* Neoplasm, benign, by site
    malignant — *see* Neoplasm, malignant, by site
    uncertain whether benign or malignant — *see* Neoplasm, uncertain behavior, by site
  cervix, in pregnancy or childbirth — *see* Pregnancy, complicated by, tumor, cervix
  chondromatous giant cell — *see* Neoplasm, bone, benign
  chromaffin — *see also* Neoplasm, benign, by site
    malignant — *see* Neoplasm, malignant, by site
  Cock's peculiar L72.3
  Codman's — *see* Neoplasm, bone, benign
  dentigerous, mixed — *see* Cyst, calcifying odontogenic
  dermoid — *see* Neoplasm, benign, by site
    with malignant transformation C56- ☑
  desmoid (extra-abdominal) — *see also* Neoplasm, connective tissue, uncertain behavior
    abdominal — *see* Neoplasm, connective tissue, uncertain behavior
  embolus — *see* Neoplasm, secondary, by site
  embryonal (mixed) — *see also* Neoplasm, uncertain behavior, by site
    liver C22.7
  endodermal sinus
    specified site — *see* Neoplasm, malignant, by site
    unspecified site
      female C56.- ☑
      male C62.90
  epithelial
    benign — *see* Neoplasm, benign, by site
    malignant — *see* Neoplasm, malignant, by site
  Ewing's — *see* Neoplasm, bone, malignant, by site
  fatty — *see* Lipoma
  fibroid — *see* Leiomyoma
  G cell
    malignant
      pancreas C25.4
      specified site NEC — *see* Neoplasm, malignant by site
      unspecified site C25.4
    specified site — *see* Neoplasm, uncertain behavior by site
    unspecified site D37.8
  germ cell — *see also* Neoplasm, malignant, by site
    mixed — *see* Neoplasm, malignant, by site
  ghost cell, odontogenic — *see* Cyst, calcifying odontogenic
  giant cell — *see also* Neoplasm, uncertain behavior, by site
    bone D48.0
      malignant — *see* Neoplasm, bone, malignant
    chondromatous — *see* Neoplasm, bone, benign
    malignant — *see* Neoplasm, malignant, by site
    soft parts — *see* Neoplasm, connective tissue, uncertain behavior

☑ **Additional Character Required** — **Refer to the Tabular List for Character Selection**   ᴹᴰ **Subterms under main terms may continue to next column or page**

Tumor — *continued*
  giant cell — *see also* Neoplasm, uncertain behavior,
    by site — *continued*
    soft parts — *see* Neoplasm, connective tissue, un-
      certain behavior — *continued*
      malignant — *see* Neoplasm, connective tissue,
        malignant
  glomus D18.00
    intra-abdominal D18.03
    intracranial D18.02
    jugulare D44.7
      malignant C75.5
    skin D18.01
    specified site NEC D18.09
  gonadal stromal — *see* Neoplasm, uncertain behavior,
    by site
  granular cell — *see also* Neoplasm, connective tissue,
    benign
    malignant — *see* Neoplasm, connective tissue, ma-
      lignant
  granulosa cell D39.1- ☑
    juvenile D39.1- ☑
    malignant C56- ☑
  granulosa cell-theca cell D39.1- ☑
    malignant C56- ☑
  Grawitz's C64- ☑
  hemorrhoidal — *see* Hemorrhoids
  hilar cell D27- ☑
  hilus cell D27- ☑
  Hurthle cell (benign) D34
    malignant C73
  hydatid — *see* Echinococcus
  hypernephroid — *see also* Neoplasm, uncertain behav-
    ior, by site
  interstitial cell — *see also* Neoplasm, uncertain behav-
    ior, by site
    benign — *see* Neoplasm, benign, by site
    malignant — *see* Neoplasm, malignant, by site
  intravascular bronchial alveolar D38.1
  islet cell — *see* Neoplasm, benign, by site
    malignant — *see* Neoplasm, malignant, by site
      pancreas C25.4
      specified site NEC — *see* Neoplasm, malignant,
        by site
      unspecified site C25.4
    pancreas D13.7
    specified site NEC — *see* Neoplasm, benign, by site
    unspecified site D13.7
  juxtaglomerular D41.0- ☑
  Klatskin's C22.1
  Krukenberg's C79.6- ☑
  Leydig cell — *see* Neoplasm, uncertain behavior, by
    site
    benign — *see* Neoplasm, benign, by site
      specified site — *see* Neoplasm, benign, by site
      unspecified site
        female D27.9
        male D29.20
    malignant — *see* Neoplasm, malignant, by site
      specified site — *see* Neoplasm, malignant, by
        site
      unspecified site
        female C56.9
        male C62.90
    specified site — *see* Neoplasm, uncertain behavior,
      by site
    unspecified site
      female D39.10
      male D40.10
  lipid cell, ovary D27- ☑
  lipoid cell, ovary D27- ☑
  malignant — *see also* Neoplasm, malignant, by site
    C80.1
    fusiform cell (type) C80.1
    giant cell (type) C80.1
    localized, plasma cell — *see* Plasmacytoma, solitary
    mixed NEC C80.1
    small cell (type) C80.1
    spindle cell (type) C80.1
    unclassified C80.1
  mast cell D47.09
  melanotic, neuroectodermal — *see* Neoplasm, benign,
    by site
  Merkel cell — *see* Carcinoma, Merkel cell
  mesenchymal
    malignant — *see* Neoplasm, connective tissue, ma-
      lignant

Tumor — *continued*
  mesenchymal — *continued*
    mixed — *see* Neoplasm, connective tissue, uncertain
      behavior
  mesodermal, mixed — *see also* Neoplasm, malignant,
    by site
    liver C22.4
  mesonephric — *see also* Neoplasm, uncertain behavior,
    by site
    malignant — *see* Neoplasm, malignant, by site
  metastatic
    from specified site — *see* Neoplasm, malignant, by
      site
    of specified site — *see* Neoplasm, malignant, by site
    to specified site — *see* Neoplasm, secondary, by site
  mixed NEC — *see also* Neoplasm, benign, by site
    malignant — *see* Neoplasm, malignant, by site
  mucinous of low malignant potential
    specified site — *see* Neoplasm, malignant, by site
    unspecified site C56.9
  mucocarcinoid
    specified site — *see* Neoplasm, malignant, by site
    unspecified site C18.1
  mucoepidermoid — *see* Neoplasm, uncertain behavior,
    by site
  Müllerian, mixed
    specified site — *see* Neoplasm, malignant, by site
    unspecified site C54.9
  myoepithelial — *see* Neoplasm, benign, by site
  neuroectodermal (peripheral) — *see* Neoplasm, malig-
    nant, by site
    primitive
      specified site — *see* Neoplasm, malignant, by
        site
      unspecified site C71.9
  neuroendocrine D3A.8 (*following* D36)
    malignant poorly differentiated C7A.1 (*following*
      C75)
    secondary NEC C7B.8 (*following* C75)
    specified NEC C7A.8 (*following* C75)
  neurogenic olfactory C30.0
  nonencapsulated sclerosing C73
  odontogenic (adenomatoid) (benign) (calcifying epithe-
    lial) (keratocystic) (squamous) — *see* Cyst, calci-
    fying odontogenic
    malignant C41.1
      upper jaw (bone) C41.0
  ovarian stromal D39.1- ☑
  ovary, in pregnancy — *see* Pregnancy, complicated by
  pacinian — *see* Neoplasm, skin, benign
  Pancoast's — *see* Pancoast's syndrome
  papillary — *see also* Papilloma
    cystic D37.9
    mucinous of low malignant potential C56- ☑
      specified site — *see* Neoplasm, malignant, by
        site
      unspecified site C56.9
    serous of low malignant potential
      specified site — *see* Neoplasm, malignant, by
        site
      unspecified site C56.9
  pelvic, in pregnancy or childbirth — *see* Pregnancy,
    complicated by
  phantom F45.8
  phyllodes D48.6- ☑
    benign D24- ☑
    malignant — *see* Neoplasm, breast, malignant
  Pindborg — *see* Cyst, calcifying odontogenic
  placental site trophoblastic D39.2
  plasma cell (malignant) (localized) — *see* Plasmacy-
    toma, solitary
  polyvesicular vitelline
    specified site — *see* Neoplasm, malignant, by site
    unspecified site
      female C56.9
      male C62.90
  Pott's puffy — *see* Osteomyelitis, specified NEC
  Rathke's pouch D44.3
  retinal anlage — *see* Neoplasm, benign, by site
  salivary gland type, mixed — *see* Neoplasm, salivary
    gland, benign
    malignant — *see* Neoplasm, salivary gland, malig-
      nant
  Sampson's N80.1
  Schmincke's — *see* Neoplasm, nasopharynx, malignant
  sclerosing stromal D27 ☑
  sebaceous — *see* Cyst, sebaceous

Tumor — *continued*
  secondary — *see* Neoplasm, secondary, by site
    carcinoid C7B.00 (*following* C75)
      bone C7B.03 (*following* C75)
      distant lymph nodes C7B.01 (*following* C75)
      liver C7B.02 (*following* C75)
      peritoneum C7B.04 (*following* C75)
      specified NEC C7B.09 (*following* C75)
    neuroendocrine NEC C7B.8 (*following* C75)
  serous of low malignant potential
    specified site — *see* Neoplasm, malignant, by site
    unspecified site C56.9
  Sertoli cell — *see* Neoplasm, benign, by site
    with lipid storage
      specified site — *see* Neoplasm, benign, by site
      unspecified site
        female D27.9
        male D29.20
    specified site — *see* Neoplasm, benign, by site
    unspecified site
      female D27.9
      male D29.20
  Sertoli-Leydig cell — *see* Neoplasm, benign, by site
    specified site — *see* Neoplasm, benign, by site
    unspecified site
      female D27.9
      male D29.20
  sex cord (-stromal) — *see* Neoplasm, uncertain behav-
    ior, by site
    with annular tubules D39.1- ☑
  skin appendage — *see* Neoplasm, skin, benign
  smooth muscle — *see* Neoplasm, connective tissue,
    uncertain behavior
  soft tissue
    benign — *see* Neoplasm, connective tissue, benign
    malignant — *see* Neoplasm, connective tissue, ma-
      lignant
  sternomastoid (congenital) Q68.0
  stromal
    endometrial D39.0
    gastric D48.1
      benign D21.4
      malignant C16.9
      uncertain behavior D48.1
    gastrointestinal C49.A- ☑
      benign D21.4
      esophagus C49.A1
      malignant C49.A0
        colon C49.A4
        duodenum C49.A3
        esophagus C49.A1
        ileum C49.A3
        jejunum C49.A3
        large intestine C49.A4
        Meckel diverticulum C49.A3
        omentum C49.A9
        peritoneum C49.A9
        rectum C49.A5
        small intestine C49.A3
        specified site NEC C49.A9
        stomach C49.A2
      rectum C49.A5
      small intestine C49.A3
      specified site NEC C49.A9
      stomach C49.A2
      uncertain behavior D48.1
    intestine
      benign D21.4
      malignant
        large C49.A4
        small C49.A3
      uncertain behavior D48.1
    ovarian D39.1- ☑
    stomach C49.A2
      benign D21.4
      malignant C49.A2
      uncertain behavior D48.1
  sweat gland — *see also* Neoplasm, skin, uncertain be-
    havior
    benign — *see* Neoplasm, skin, benign
    malignant — *see* Neoplasm, skin, malignant
  syphilitic, brain A52.17
  testicular D40.10
  testicular stromal D40.1- ☑
  theca cell D27.- ☑
  theca cell-granulosa cell D39.1- ☑
  Triton, malignant — *see* Neoplasm, nerve, malignant
  trophoblastic, placental site D39.2

Tumor — *continued*
  turban D23.4
  uterus (body), in pregnancy or childbirth — *see* Pregnancy, complicated by, tumor, uterus
  vagina, in pregnancy or childbirth — *see* Pregnancy, complicated by
  varicose — *see* Varix
  von Recklinghausen's — *see* Neurofibromatosis
  vulva or perineum, in pregnancy or childbirth — *see* Pregnancy, complicated by
    causing obstructed labor O65.5
  Warthin's — *see* Neoplasm, salivary gland, benign
  Wilms' C64- ☑
  yolk sac — *see* Neoplasm, malignant, by site
    specified site — *see* Neoplasm, malignant, by site
    unspecified site
      female C56.9
      male C62.90
Tumor lysis syndrome (following antineoplastic chemotherapy) (spontaneous) NEC E88.3
Tumorlet — *see* Neoplasm, uncertain behavior, by site
Tungiasis B88.1
Tunica vasculosa lentis Q12.2
Turban tumor D23.4
Türck's trachoma J37.0
Turner-Kieser syndrome Q87.2
Turner-like syndrome Q87.19
Turner's
  hypoplasia (tooth) K00.4
  syndrome Q96.9
    specified NEC Q96.8
  tooth K00.4
Turner-Ullrich syndrome Q96.9
Tussis convulsiva — *see* Whooping cough
Twiddler's syndrome (due to)
  automatic implantable defibrillator T82.198
  cardiac pacemaker T82.198 ☑
Twilight state
  epileptic F05
  psychogenic F44.89
Twin (newborn) — *see also* Newborn, twin
  conjoined Q89.4
  pregnancy — *see* Pregnancy, twin
Twinning, teeth K00.2
Twist, twisted
  bowel, colon or intestine K56.2
  hair (congenital) Q84.1
  mesentery K56.2
  omentum K56.2
  organ or site, congenital NEC — *see* Anomaly, by site
  ovarian pedicle — *see* Torsion, ovary
Twitching R25.3
Tylosis (acquired) L84
  buccalis K13.29
  linguae K13.29
  palmaris et plantaris (congenital) (inherited) Q82.8
    acquired L85.1
Tympanism R14.0
Tympanites (abdominal) (intestinal) R14.0
Tympanitis — *see* Myringitis
Tympanosclerosis H74.0 ☑
Tympanum — *see* condition
Tympany
  abdomen R14.0
  chest R09.89
Type A behavior pattern Z73.1
Typhlitis — *see* Appendicitis
Typhoenteritis — *see* Typhoid
Typhoid (abortive) (ambulant) (any site) (clinical) (fever) (hemorrhagic) (infection) (intermittent) (malignant) (rheumatic) (Widal negative) A01.00
  with pneumonia A01.03
  abdominal A01.09
  arthritis A01.04
  carrier (suspected) of Z22.0
  cholecystitis (current) A01.09
  endocarditis A01.02
  heart involvement A01.02
  inoculation reaction — *see* Complications, vaccination
  meningitis A01.01
  mesenteric lymph nodes A01.09
  myocarditis A01.02
  osteomyelitis A01.05
  perichondritis, larynx A01.09
  pneumonia A01.03
  specified NEC A01.09
  spine A01.05

Typhoid — *continued*
  ulcer (perforating) A01.09
Typhomalaria (fever) — *see* Malaria
Typhomania A01.00
Typhoperitonitis A01.09
Typhus (fever) A75.9
  abdominal, abdominalis — *see* Typhoid
  African tick A77.1
  amarillic A95.9
  brain A75.9 *[G94]*
  cerebral A75.9 *[G94]*
  classical A75.0
  due to Rickettsia
    prowazekii A75.0
      recrudescent A75.1
    tsutsugamushi A75.3
    typhi A75.2
  endemic (flea-borne) A75.2
  epidemic (louse-borne) A75.0
  exanthematous SAI A75.0
    brillii SAI A75.1
    mexicanus SAI A75.2
    typhus murinus A75.2
  exanthematic NEC A75.0
  flea-borne A75.2
  India tick A77.1
  Kenya (tick) A77.1
  louse-borne A75.0
  Mexican A75.2
  mite-borne A75.3
  murine A75.2
  North Asian tick-borne A77.2
  petechial A75.9
  Queensland tick A77.3
  rat A75.2
  recrudescent A75.1
  recurrens — *see* Fever, relapsing
  Sao Paulo A77.0
  scrub (China) (India) (Malaysia) (New Guinea) A75.3
  shop (of Malaysia) A75.2
  Siberian tick A77.2
  tick-borne A77.9
  tropical (mite-borne) A75.3
Tyrosinemia E70.21
  newborn, transitory P74.5
Tyrosinosis E70.21
Tyrosinuria E70.29

U

Uhl's anomaly or disease Q24.8
Ulcer, ulcerated, ulcerating, ulceration, ulcerative
  alveolar process M27.3
  amebic (intestine) A06.1
    skin A06.7
  anastomotic — *see* Ulcer, gastrojejunal
  anorectal K62.6
  antral — *see* Ulcer, stomach
  anus (sphincter) (solitary) K62.6
  aorta — *see* Aneurysm
  aphthous (oral) (recurrent) K12.0
    genital organ(s)
      female N76.6
      male N50.89
  artery I77.2
  atrophic — *see* Ulcer, skin
    decubitus — *see* Ulcer, pressure, by site
  back L98.429
    with
      bone involvement without evidence of necrosis L98.426
      bone necrosis L98.424
      exposed fat layer L98.422
      muscle involvement without evidence of necrosis L98.425
      muscle necrosis L98.423
      skin breakdown only L98.421
      specified severity NEC L98.428
  Barrett's (esophagus) K22.10
    with bleeding K22.11
  bile duct (common) (hepatic) K83.8
  bladder (solitary) (sphincter) NEC N32.89
    bilharzial B65.9 *[N33]*
    in schistosomiasis (bilharzial) B65.9 *[N33]*
    submucosal — *see* Cystitis, interstitial
    tuberculous A18.12
  bleeding K27.4
  bone — *see* Osteomyelitis, specified type NEC

Ulcer, ulcerated, ulcerating, ulceration, ulcerative — *continued*
  bowel — *see* Ulcer, intestine
  breast N61.1
  bronchus J98.09
  buccal (cavity) (traumatic) K12.1
  Buruli A31.1
  buttock L98.419
    with
      bone involvement without evidence of necrosis L98.416
      bone necrosis L98.414
      exposed fat layer L98.412
      muscle involvement without evidence of necrosis L98.415
      muscle necrosis L98.413
      skin breakdown only L98.411
      specified severity NEC L98.418
  cancerous — *see* Neoplasm, malignant, by site
  cardia K22.10
    with bleeding K22.11
  cardioesophageal (peptic) K22.10
    with bleeding K22.11
  cecum — *see* Ulcer, intestine
  cervix (uteri) (decubitus) (trophic) N86
    with cervicitis N72
  chancroidal A57
  chiclero B55.1
  chronic (cause unknown) — *see* Ulcer, skin
  Cochin-China B55.1
  colon — *see* Ulcer, intestine
  conjunctiva H10.89
  cornea H16.00- ☑
    with hypopyon H16.03- ☑
      central H16.01- ☑
      dendritic (herpes simplex) B00.52
      marginal H16.04- ☑
      Mooren's H16.05- ☑
      mycotic H16.06- ☑
      perforated H16.07- ☑
      ring H16.02- ☑
    tuberculous (phlyctenular) A18.52
  corpus cavernosum (chronic) N48.5
  crural — *see* Ulcer, lower limb
  Curling's — *see* Ulcer, peptic, acute
  Cushing's — *see* Ulcer, peptic, acute
  cystic duct K82.8
  cystitis (interstitial) — *see* Cystitis, interstitial
  decubitus — *see* Ulcer, pressure, by site
  dendritic, cornea (herpes simplex) B00.52
  diabetes, diabetic — *see* Diabetes, ulcer
  Dieulafoy's K25.0
  due to
    infection NEC — *see* Ulcer, skin
    radiation NEC L59.8
    trophic disturbance (any region) — *see* Ulcer, skin
    X-ray L58.1
  duodenum, duodenal (eroded) (peptic) K26.9
    with
      hemorrhage K26.4
        and perforation K26.6
      perforation K26.5
    acute K26.3
      with
        hemorrhage K26.0
          and perforation K26.2
        perforation K26.1
    chronic K26.7
      with
        hemorrhage K26.4
          and perforation K26.6
        perforation K26.5
  dysenteric A09
  elusive — *see* Cystitis, interstitial
  endocarditis (acute) (chronic) (subacute) I28.8
  epiglottis J38.7
  esophagus (peptic) K22.10
    with bleeding K22.11
    due to
      aspirin K22.10
        with bleeding K22.11
      gastrointestinal reflux disease K21.0
      ingestion of chemical or medicament K22.10
        with bleeding K22.11
    fungal K22.10
      with bleeding K22.11
    infective K22.10
      with bleeding K22.11

Ulcer, ulcerated, ulcerating, ulceration, ulcerative
— *continued*
esophagus — *continued*
  varicose — *see* Varix, esophagus
eyelid (region) H01.8
fauces J39.2
Fenwick (-Hunner) (solitary) — *see* Cystitis, interstitial
fistulous — *see* Ulcer, skin
foot (indolent) (trophic) — *see* Ulcer, lower limb
frambesial, initial A66.0
frenum (tongue) K14.0
gallbladder or duct K82.8
gangrenous — *see* Gangrene
gastric — *see* Ulcer, stomach
gastrocolic — *see* Ulcer, gastrojejunal
gastroduodenal — *see* Ulcer, peptic
gastroesophageal — *see* Ulcer, stomach
gastrointestinal — *see* Ulcer, gastrojejunal
gastrojejunal (peptic) K28.9
  with
    hemorrhage K28.4
      and perforation K28.6
    perforation K28.5
  acute K28.3
    with
      hemorrhage K28.0
        and perforation K28.2
      perforation K28.1
  chronic K28.7
    with
      hemorrhage K28.4
        and perforation K28.6
      perforation K28.5
gastrojejunocolic — *see* Ulcer, gastrojejunal
gingiva K06.8
gingivitis K05.10
  nonplaque induced K05.11
  plaque induced K05.10
glottis J38.7
granuloma of pudenda A58
gum K06.8
gumma, due to yaws A66.4
heel — *see* Ulcer, lower limb
hemorrhoid — *see also* Hemorrhoids, by degree K64.8
Hunner's — *see* Cystitis, interstitial
hypopharynx J39.2
hypopyon (chronic) (subacute) — *see* Ulcer, cornea, with hypopyon
hypostaticum — *see* Ulcer, varicose
ileum — *see* Ulcer, intestine
intestine, intestinal K63.3
  with perforation K63.1
  amebic A06.1
  duodenal — *see* Ulcer, duodenum
  granulocytopenic (with hemorrhage) — *see* Neutropenia
  marginal — *see* Ulcer, gastrojejunal
  perforating K63.1
    newborn P78.0
  primary, small intestine K63.3
  rectum K62.6
  stercoraceous, stercoral K63.3
  tuberculous A18.32
  typhoid (fever) — *see* Typhoid
  varicose I86.8
jejunum, jejunal — *see* Ulcer, gastrojejunal
keratitis — *see* Ulcer, cornea
knee — *see* Ulcer, lower limb
labium (majus) (minus) N76.6
laryngitis — *see* Laryngitis
larynx (aphthous) (contact) J38.7
  diphtheritic A36.2
leg — *see* Ulcer, lower limb
lip K13.0
Lipschütz's N76.6
lower limb (atrophic) (chronic) (neurogenic) (perforating) (pyogenic) (trophic) (tropical) L97.909
  with
    bone involvement without evidence of necrosis L97.906
    bone necrosis L97.904
    exposed fat layer L97.902
    muscle involvement without evidence of necrosis L97.905
    muscle necrosis L97.903
    skin breakdown only L97.901
    specified severity NEC L97.908
  ankle L97.309

Ulcer, ulcerated, ulcerating, ulceration, ulcerative
— *continued*
lower limb — *continued*
  ankle — *continued*
    with
      bone involvement without evidence of necrosis L97.306
      bone necrosis L97.304
      exposed fat layer L97.302
      muscle involvement without evidence of necrosis L97.305
      muscle necrosis L97.303
      skin breakdown only L97.301
      specified severity NEC L97.308
    left L97.329
      with
        bone involvement without evidence of necrosis L97.326
        bone necrosis L97.324
        exposed fat layer L97.322
        muscle involvement without evidence of necrosis L97.325
        muscle necrosis L97.323
        skin breakdown only L97.321
        specified severity NEC L97.328
    right L97.319
      with
        bone involvement without evidence of necrosis L97.316
        bone necrosis L97.314
        exposed fat layer L97.312
        muscle involvement without evidence of necrosis L97.315
        muscle necrosis L97.313
        skin breakdown only L97.311
        specified severity NEC L97.318
  calf L97.209
    with
      bone involvement without evidence of necrosis L97.206
      bone necrosis L97.204
      exposed fat layer L97.202
      muscle involvement without evidence of necrosis L97.205
      muscle necrosis L97.203
      skin breakdown only L97.201
      specified severity NEC L97.208
    left L97.229
      with
        bone involvement without evidence of necrosis L97.226
        bone necrosis L97.224
        exposed fat layer L97.222
        muscle involvement without evidence of necrosis L97.225
        muscle necrosis L97.223
        skin breakdown only L97.221
        specified severity NEC L97.228
    right L97.219
      with
        bone involvement without evidence of necrosis L97.216
        bone necrosis L97.214
        exposed fat layer L97.212
        muscle involvement without evidence of necrosis L97.215
        muscle necrosis L97.213
        skin breakdown only L97.211
        specified severity NEC L97.218
  decubitus — *see* Ulcer, pressure, by site
  foot specified NEC L97.509
    with
      bone involvement without evidence of necrosis L97.506
      bone necrosis L97.504
      exposed fat layer L97.502
      muscle involvement without evidence of necrosis L97.505
      muscle necrosis L97.503
      skin breakdown only L97.501
      specified severity NEC L97.508
    left L97.529
      with
        bone involvement without evidence of necrosis L97.526
        bone necrosis L97.524
        exposed fat layer L97.522
        muscle involvement without evidence of necrosis L97.525

Ulcer, ulcerated, ulcerating, ulceration, ulcerative
— *continued*
lower limb — *continued*
  foot specified — *continued*
    left — *continued*
      with — *continued*
        muscle necrosis L97.523
        skin breakdown only L97.521
        specified severity NEC L97.528
    right L97.519
      with
        bone involvement without evidence of necrosis L97.516
        bone necrosis L97.514
        exposed fat layer L97.512
        muscle involvement without evidence of necrosis L97.515
        muscle necrosis L97.513
        skin breakdown only L97.511
        specified severity NEC L97.518
  heel L97.409
    with
      bone involvement without evidence of necrosis L97.406
      bone necrosis L97.404
      exposed fat layer L97.402
      muscle involvement without evidence of necrosis L97.405
      muscle necrosis L97.403
      skin breakdown only L97.401
      specified severity NEC L97.408
    left L97.429
      with
        bone involvement without evidence of necrosis L97.426
        bone necrosis L97.424
        exposed fat layer L97.422
        muscle involvement without evidence of necrosis L97.425
        muscle necrosis L97.423
        skin breakdown only L97.421
        specified severity NEC L97.428
    right L97.419
      with
        bone involvement without evidence of necrosis L97.416
        bone necrosis L97.414
        exposed fat layer L97.412
        muscle involvement without evidence of necrosis L97.415
        muscle necrosis L97.413
        skin breakdown only L97.411
        specified severity NEC L97.418
  left L97.929
    with
      bone involvement without evidence of necrosis L97.926
      bone necrosis L97.924
      exposed fat layer L97.922
      muscle involvement without evidence of necrosis L97.925
      muscle necrosis L97.923
      skin breakdown only L97.921
      specified severity NEC L97.928
  leprous A30.1
  lower leg NOS L97.909
    with
      bone involvement without evidence of necrosis L97.906
      bone necrosis L97.904
      exposed fat layer L97.902
      muscle involvement without evidence of necrosis L97.905
      muscle necrosis L97.903
      skin breakdown only L97.901
      specified severity NEC L97.908
    left L97.929
      with
        bone involvement without evidence of necrosis L97.926
        bone necrosis L97.924
        exposed fat layer L97.922
        muscle involvement without evidence of necrosis L97.925
        muscle necrosis L97.923
        skin breakdown only L97.921
        specified severity NEC L97.928
    right L97.919

Ulcer, ulcerated, ulcerating, ulceration, ulcerative

— *continued*
lower limb — *continued*
  lower leg — *continued*
    right — *continued*
      with
        bone involvement without evidence of necrosis L97.916
        bone necrosis L97.914
        exposed fat layer L97.912
        muscle involvement without necrosis L97.915
        muscle necrosis L97.913
        skin breakdown only L97.911
        specified severity NEC L97.918
    specified site NEC L97.809
      with
        bone involvement without evidence of necrosis L97.806
        bone necrosis L97.804
        exposed fat layer L97.802
        muscle involvement without necrosis L97.805
        muscle necrosis L97.803
        skin breakdown only L97.801
        specified severity NEC L97.808
    left L97.829
      with
        bone involvement without evidence of necrosis L97.826
        bone necrosis L97.824
        exposed fat layer L97.822
        muscle involvement without evidence of necrosis L97.825
        muscle necrosis L97.823
        skin breakdown only L97.821
        specified severity NEC L97.828
    right L97.819
      with
        bone involvement without evidence of necrosis L97.816
        bone necrosis L97.814
        exposed fat layer L97.812
        muscle involvement without evidence of necrosis L97.815
        muscle necrosis L97.813
        skin breakdown only L97.811
        specified severity NEC L97.818
  midfoot L97.409
    with
      bone involvement without evidence of necrosis L97.406
      bone necrosis L97.404
      exposed fat layer L97.402
      muscle involvement without evidence of necrosis L97.405
      muscle necrosis L97.403
      skin breakdown only L97.401
      specified severity NEC L97.408
    left L97.429
      with
        bone involvement without evidence of necrosis L97.426
        bone necrosis L97.424
        exposed fat layer L97.422
        muscle involvement without evidence of necrosis L97.425
        muscle necrosis L97.423
        skin breakdown only L97.421
        specified severity NEC L97.428
    right L97.419
      with
        bone involvement without evidence of necrosis L97.416
        bone necrosis L97.414
        exposed fat layer L97.412
        muscle involvement without evidence of necrosis L97.415
        muscle necrosis L97.413
        skin breakdown only L97.411
        specified severity NEC L97.418
    right L97.919
      with
        bone involvement without evidence of necrosis L97.916
        bone necrosis L97.914
        exposed fat layer L97.912
        muscle involvement without evidence of necrosis L97.915

Ulcer, ulcerated, ulcerating, ulceration, ulcerative

— *continued*
lower limb — *continued*
  right — *continued*
    with
      muscle necrosis L97.913
      skin breakdown only L97.911
      specified severity NEC L97.918
  syphilitic A52.19
  thigh L97.109
    with
      bone involvement without evidence of necrosis L97.106
      bone necrosis L97.104
      exposed fat layer L97.102
      muscle involvement without evidence of necrosis L97.105
      muscle necrosis L97.103
      skin breakdown only L97.101
      specified severity NEC L97.108
    left L97.129
      with
        bone involvement without evidence of necrosis L97.126
        bone necrosis L97.124
        exposed fat layer L97.122
        muscle involvement without evidence of necrosis L97.125
        muscle necrosis L97.123
        skin breakdown only L97.121
        specified severity NEC L97.128
    right L97.119
      with
        bone involvement without evidence of necrosis L97.116
        bone necrosis L97.114
        exposed fat layer L97.112
        muscle involvement without evidence of necrosis L97.115
        muscle necrosis L97.113
        skin breakdown only L97.111
        specified severity NEC L97.118
  toe L97.509
    with
      bone involvement without evidence of necrosis L97.506
      bone necrosis L97.504
      exposed fat layer L97.502
      muscle involvement without evidence of necrosis L97.505
      muscle necrosis L97.503
      skin breakdown only L97.501
      specified severity NEC L97.508
    left L97.529
      with
        bone involvement without evidence of necrosis L97.526
        bone necrosis L97.524
        exposed fat layer L97.522
        muscle involvement without evidence of necrosis L97.525
        muscle necrosis L97.523
        skin breakdown only L97.521
        specified severity NEC L97.528
    right L97.519
      with
        bone involvement without evidence of necrosis L97.516
        bone necrosis L97.514
        exposed fat layer L97.512
        muscle involvement without evidence of necrosis L97.515
        muscle necrosis L97.513
        skin breakdown only L97.511
        specified severity NEC L97.518
  varicose — *see* Varix, leg, with, ulcer
luetic — *see* Ulcer, syphilitic
lung J98.4
  tuberculous — *see* Tuberculosis, pulmonary
malignant — *see* Neoplasm, malignant, by site
marginal NEC — *see* Ulcer, gastrojejunal
meatus (urinarius) N34.2
Meckel's diverticulum Q43.0
  malignant — *see* Table of Neoplasms, small intestine, malignant
Meleney's (chronic undermining) — *see* Ulcer, skin
Mooren's (cornea) — *see* Ulcer, cornea, Mooren's
mycobacterial (skin) A31.1

Ulcer, ulcerated, ulcerating, ulceration, ulcerative

— *continued*
nasopharynx J39.2
neck, uterus N86
neurogenic NEC — *see* Ulcer, skin
nose, nasal (passage) (infective) (septum) J34.0
  skin — *see* Ulcer, skin
  spirochetal A69.8
  varicose (bleeding) I86.8
oral mucosa (traumatic) K12.1
palate (soft) K12.1
penis (chronic) N48.5
peptic (site unspecified) K27.9
  with
    hemorrhage K27.4
      and perforation K27.6
    perforation K27.5
  acute K27.3
    with
      hemorrhage K27.0
        and perforation K27.2
      perforation K27.1
  chronic K27.7
    with
      hemorrhage K27.4
        and perforation K27.6
      perforation K27.5
  esophagus K22.10
    with bleeding K22.11
  newborn P78.82
  perforating K27.5
  skin — *see* Ulcer, skin
peritonsillar J35.8
phagedenic (tropical) — *see* Ulcer, skin
pharynx J39.2
phlebitis — *see* Phlebitis
plaster — *see* Ulcer, pressure, by site
popliteal space — *see* Ulcer, lower limb
postpyloric — *see* Ulcer, duodenum
prepuce N47.7
prepyloric — *see* Ulcer, stomach
pressure (pressure area) L89.9- ☑
  ankle L89.5- ☑
  back L89.1- ☑
  buttock L89.3- ☑
  coccyx L89.15- ☑
  contiguous site of back, buttock, hip L89.4- ☑
  elbow L89.0- ☑
  face L89.81- ☑
  head L89.81- ☑
  heel L89.6- ☑
  hip L89.2- ☑
  sacral region (tailbone) L89.15- ☑
  specified site NEC L89.89- ☑
  stage 1 (healing) (pre-ulcer skin changes limited to persistent focal edema)
    ankle L89.5- ☑
    back L89.1- ☑
    buttock L89.3- ☑
    coccyx L89.15- ☑
    contiguous site of back, buttock, hip L89.4- ☑
    elbow L89.0- ☑
    face L89.81- ☑
    head L89.81- ☑
    heel L89.6- ☑
    hip L89.2- ☑
    sacral region (tailbone) L89.15- ☑
    specified site NEC L89.89- ☑
  stage 2 (healing) (abrasion, blister, partial thickness skin loss involving epidermis and/or dermis)
    ankle L89.5- ☑
    back L89.1- ☑
    buttock L89.3- ☑
    coccyx L89.15- ☑
    contiguous site of back, buttock, hip L89.4- ☑
    elbow L89.0- ☑
    face L89.81- ☑
    head L89.81- ☑
    heel L89.6- ☑
    hip L89.2- ☑
    sacral region (tailbone) L89.15- ☑
    specified site NEC L89.89- ☑
  stage 3 (healing) (full thickness skin loss involving damage or necrosis of subcutaneous tissue)
    ankle L89.5- ☑
    back L89.1- ☑
    buttock L89.3- ☑

Ulcer, ulcerated, ulcerating, ulceration, ulcerative
— *continued*
pressure — *continued*
  stage 3 — *continued*
    coccyx L89.15- ☑
    contiguous site of back, buttock, hip L89.4- ☑
    elbow L89.0- ☑
    face L89.81- ☑
    head L89.81- ☑
    heel L89.6- ☑
    hip L89.2- ☑
    sacral region (tailbone) L89.15- ☑
    specified site NEC L89.89- ☑
  stage 4 (healing) (necrosis of soft tissues through
    to underlying muscle, tendon, or bone)
    ankle L89.5- ☑
    back L89.1- ☑
    buttock L89.3- ☑
    coccyx L89.15- ☑
    contiguous site of back, buttock, hip L89.4- ☑
    elbow L89.0- ☑
    face L89.81- ☑
    head L89.81- ☑
    heel L89.6- ☑
    hip L89.2- ☑
    sacral region (tailbone) L89.15- ☑
    specified site NEC L89.89- ☑
  unspecified stage
    ankle L89.5- ☑
    back L89.1- ☑
    buttock L89.3- ☑
    coccyx L89.15- ☑
    contiguous site of back, buttock, hip L89.4- ☑
    elbow L89.0- ☑
    face L89.81- ☑
    head L89.81- ☑
    heel L89.6- ☑
    hip L89.2- ☑
    sacral region (tailbone) L89.15- ☑
    specified site NEC L89.89- ☑
  unstageable
    ankle L89.5- ☑
    back L89.1- ☑
    buttock L89.3- ☑
    coccyx L89.15- ☑
    contiguous site of back, buttock, hip L89.4- ☑
    elbow L89.0- ☑
    face L89.81- ☑
    head L89.81- ☑
    heel L89.6- ☑
    hip L89.2- ☑
    sacral region (tailbone) L89.15- ☑
    specified site NEC L89.89- ☑
primary of intestine K63.3
  with perforation K63.1
prostate N41.9
pyloric — *see* Ulcer, stomach
rectosigmoid K63.3
  with perforation K63.1
rectum (sphincter) (solitary) K62.6
  stercoraceous, stercoral K62.6
retina — *see* Inflammation, chorioretinal
rodent — *see also* Neoplasm, skin, malignant
sclera — *see* Scleritis
scrofulous (tuberculous) A18.2
scrotum N50.89
  tuberculous A18.15
  varicose I86.1
seminal vesicle N50.89
sigmoid — *see* Ulcer, intestine
skin (atrophic) (chronic) (neurogenic) (non-healing)
  (perforating) (pyogenic) (trophic) (tropical)
  L98.499
  with gangrene — *see* Gangrene
  amebic A06.7
  back — *see* Ulcer, back
  buttock — *see* Ulcer, buttock
  decubitus — *see* Ulcer, pressure
  lower limb — *see* Ulcer, lower limb
  mycobacterial A31.1
  specified site NEC L98.499
    with
      bone involvement without evidence of
        necrosis L98.496
      bone necrosis L98.494
      exposed fat layer L98.492

Ulcer, ulcerated, ulcerating, ulceration, ulcerative
— *continued*
skin — *continued*
  specified site — *continued*
    with — *continued*
      muscle involvement without evidence of
        necrosis L98.495
      muscle necrosis L98.493
      skin breakdown only L98.491
      specified severity NEC L98.498
  tuberculous (primary) A18.4
  varicose — *see* Ulcer, varicose
sloughing — *see* Ulcer, skin
solitary, anus or rectum (sphincter) K62.6
sore throat J02.9
  streptococcal J02.0
spermatic cord N50.89
spine (tuberculous) A18.01
stasis (venous) — *see* Varix, leg, with, ulcer
  without varicose veins I87.2
stercoraceous, stercoral K63.3
  with perforation K63.1
  anus or rectum K62.6
stoma, stomal — *see* Ulcer, gastrojejunal
stomach (eroded) (peptic) (round) K25.9
  with
    hemorrhage K25.4
      and perforation K25.6
    perforation K25.5
  acute K25.3
    with
      hemorrhage K25.0
        and perforation K25.2
      perforation K25.1
  chronic K25.7
    with
      hemorrhage K25.4
        and perforation K25.6
      perforation K25.5
stomal — *see* Ulcer, gastrojejunal
stomatitis K12.1
stress — *see* Ulcer, peptic
strumous (tuberculous) A18.2
submucosal, bladder — *see* Cystitis, interstitial
syphilitic (any site) (early) (secondary) A51.39
  late A52.79
  perforating A52.79
    foot A52.11
testis N50.89
thigh — *see* Ulcer, lower limb
throat J39.2
  diphtheritic A36.0
toe — *see* Ulcer, lower limb
tongue (traumatic) K14.0
tonsil J35.8
  diphtheritic A36.0
trachea J39.8
trophic — *see* Ulcer, skin
tropical — *see* Ulcer, skin
tuberculous — *see* Tuberculosis, ulcer
tunica vaginalis N50.89
turbinate J34.89
typhoid (perforating) — *see* Typhoid
unspecified site — *see* Ulcer, skin
urethra (meatus) — *see* Urethritis
uterus N85.8
  cervix N86
    with cervicitis N72
  neck N86
    with cervicitis N72
vagina N76.5
  in Behçet's disease M35.2 *[N77.0]*
  pessary N89.8
valve, heart I33.0
varicose (lower limb, any part) — *see also* Varix, leg,
  with, ulcer
  broad ligament I86.2
  esophagus — *see* Varix, esophagus
  inflamed or infected — *see* Varix, leg, with ulcer,
    with inflammation
  nasal septum I86.8
  perineum I86.3
  scrotum I86.1
  specified site NEC I86.8
  sublingual I86.0
  vulva I86.3
vas deferens N50.89
vulva (acute) (infectional) N76.6

Ulcer, ulcerated, ulcerating, ulceration, ulcerative
— *continued*
vulva — *continued*
  in (due to)
    Behçet's disease M35.2 *[N77.0]*
    herpesviral (herpes simplex) infection A60.04
    tuberculosis A18.18
  vulvobuccal, recurring N76.6
  X-ray L58.1
  yaws A66.4
Ulcerosa scarlatina A38.8
Ulcus — *see also* Ulcer
  cutis tuberculosum A18.4
  duodeni — *see* Ulcer, duodenum
  durum (syphilitic) A51.0
    extragenital A51.2
  gastrojejunale — *see* Ulcer, gastrojejunal
  hypostaticum — *see* Ulcer, varicose
  molle (cutis) (skin) A57
  serpens corneae — *see* Ulcer, cornea, central
  ventriculi — *see* Ulcer, stomach
Ulegyria Q04.8
Ulerythema
  ophryogenes, congenital Q84.2
  sycosiforme L73.8
Ullrich (-Bonnevie)(-Turner) **syndrome** — *see also*
  Turner's syndrome Q87.19
Ullrich-Feichtiger syndrome Q87.0
Ulnar — *see* condition
Ulorrhagia, ulorrhea K06.8
Umbilicus, umbilical — *see* condition
Unacceptable
  contours of tooth K08.54
  morphology of tooth K08.54
Unavailability (of)
  bed at medical facility Z75.1
  health service-related agencies Z75.4
  medical facilities (at) Z75.3
    due to
      investigation by social service agency Z75.2
      lack of services at home Z75.0
      remoteness from facility Z75.3
      waiting list Z75.1
    home Z75.0
    outpatient clinic Z75.3
  schooling Z55.1
  social service agencies Z75.4
Uncinaria americana infestation B76.1
Uncinariasis B76.9
Uncongenial work Z56.5
Unconscious (ness) — *see* Coma
Under observation — *see* Observation
Underachievement in school Z55.3
Underdevelopment — *see also* Undeveloped
  nose Q30.1
  sexual E30.0
Underdosing — *see also* Table of Drugs and Chemicals,
  categories T36-T50, with final character 6 Z91.14
  intentional NEC Z91.128
    due to financial hardship of patient Z91.120
  unintentional NEC Z91.138
    due to patient's age related debility Z91.130
Underfeeding, newborn P92.3
Underfill, endodontic M27.53
Underimmunization status Z28.3
Undernourishment — *see* Malnutrition
Undernutrition — *see* Malnutrition
Underweight R63.6
  for gestational age — *see* Light for dates
Underwood's disease P83.0
Undescended — *see also* Malposition, congenital
  cecum Q43.3
  colon Q43.3
  testicle — *see* Cryptorchid
Undeveloped, undevelopment — *see also* Hypoplasia
  brain (congenital) Q02
  cerebral (congenital) Q02
  heart Q24.8
  lung Q33.6
  testis E29.1
  uterus E30.0
Undiagnosed (disease) R69
Undulant fever — *see* Brucellosis
Unemployment, anxiety concerning Z56.0
  threatened Z56.2
Unequal length (acquired) (limb)   *see also* Deformity,
  limb, unequal length

Unequal length — *continued*
 leg — *see also* Deformity, limb, unequal length
  congenital Q72.9- ☑
Unextracted dental root K08.3
Unguis incarnatus L60.0
Unhappiness R45.2
Unicornate uterus Q51.4
 in pregnancy or childbirth O34.00
Unilateral — *see also* condition
 development, breast N64.89
 organ or site, congenital NEC — *see* Agenesis, by site
Unilocular heart Q20.8
Union, abnormal — *see also* Fusion
 larynx and trachea Q34.8
Universal mesentery Q43.3
Unrepairable overhanging of dental restorative materials K08.52
Unsatisfactory
 restoration of tooth K08.50
  specified NEC K08.59
 sample of cytologic smear
  anus R85.615
  cervix R87.615
  vagina R87.625
 surroundings Z59.1
 work Z56.5
Unsoundness of mind — *see* Psychosis
Unstable
 back NEC — *see* Instability, joint, spine
 hip (congenital) Q65.6
  acquired — *see* Derangement, joint, specified type NEC, hip
 joint — *see* Instability, joint
  secondary to removal of joint prosthesis M96.89
 lie (mother) O32.0 ☑
 lumbosacral joint (congenital) — *see* subcategory M53.2
 sacroiliac — *see* subcategory M53.2 ☑
 spine NEC — *see* Instability, joint, spine
Unsteadiness on feet R26.81
Untruthfulness, child problem F91.8
Unverricht (-Lundborg) **disease or epilepsy** — *see* Epilepsy, generalized, idiopathic
Unwanted pregnancy Z64.0
Upbringing, institutional Z62.22
 away from parents NEC Z62.29
 in care of non-parental family member Z62.21
 in foster care Z62.21
 in orphanage or group home Z62.22
 in welfare custody Z62.21
Upper respiratory — *see* condition
Upset
 gastric K30
 gastrointestinal K30
  psychogenic F45.8
 intestinal (large) (small) K59.9
  psychogenic F45.8
 menstruation N93.9
 mental F48.9
 stomach K30
  psychogenic F45.8
Urachus — *see also* condition
 patent or persistent Q64.4
Urbach-Oppenheim disease (necrobiosis lipoidica diabeticorum) — *see* E08-E13 with .620
Urbach's lipoid proteinosis E78.89
Urbach-Wiethe disease E78.89
Urban yellow fever A95.1
Urea
 blood, high — *see* Uremia
 cycle metabolism disorder — *see* Disorder, urea cycle metabolism
Uremia, uremic N19
 with
  ectopic or molar pregnancy O08.4
  polyneuropathy N18.9 *[G63]*
 chronic NOS — *see also* Disease, kidney, chronic N18.9
  due to hypertension — *see* Hypertensive, kidney
 complicating
  ectopic or molar pregnancy O08.4
 congenital P96.0
 extrarenal R39.2
 following ectopic or molar pregnancy O08.4
 newborn P96.0
 prerenal R39.2
Ureter, ureteral — *see* condition
Ureteralgia N23

Ureterectasis — *see* Hydroureter
Ureteritis N28.89
 cystica N28.86
 due to calculus N20.1
  with calculus, kidney N20.2
   with hydronephrosis N13.2
 gonococcal (acute) (chronic) A54.21
 nonspecific N28.89
Ureterocele N28.89
 congenital (orthotopic) Q62.31
  ectopic Q62.32
Ureterolith, ureterolithiasis — *see* Calculus, ureter
Ureterostomy
 attention to Z43.6
 status Z93.6
Urethra, urethral — *see* condition
Urethralgia R39.89
Urethritis (anterior) (posterior) N34.2
 calculous N21.1
 candidal B37.41
 chlamydial A56.01
 diplococcal (gonococcal) A54.01
  with abscess (accessory gland) (periurethral) A54.1
 gonococcal A54.01
  with abscess (accessory gland) (periurethral) A54.1
 nongonococcal N34.1
  Reiter's — *see* Reiter's disease
 nonspecific N34.1
 nonvenereal N34.1
 postmenopausal N34.2
 puerperal O86.22
 Reiter's — *see* Reiter's disease
 specified NEC N34.2
 trichomonal or due to Trichomonas (vaginalis) A59.03
Urethrocele N81.0
 with
  cystocele — *see* Cystocele
  prolapse of uterus — *see* Prolapse, uterus
Urethrolithiasis (with colic or infection) N21.1
Urethrorectal — *see* condition
Urethrorrhagia N36.8
Urethrorrhea R36.9
Urethrostomy
 attention to Z43.6
 status Z93.6
Urethrotrigonitis — *see* Trigonitis
Urethrovaginal — *see* condition
Urgency
 fecal R15.2
 hypertensive — *see* Hypertension
 urinary R39.15
Urhidrosis, uridrosis L74.8
Uric acid in blood (increased) E79.0
Uricacidemia (asymptomatic) E79.0
Uricemia (asymptomatic) E79.0
Uricosuria R82.998
Urinary — *see* condition
Urination
 frequent R35.0
 painful R30.9
Urine
 blood in — *see* Hematuria
 discharge, excessive R35.8
 enuresis, nonorganic origin F98.0
 extravasation R39.0
 frequency R35.0
 incontinence R32
  nonorganic origin F98.0
 intermittent stream R39.198
 pus in N39.0
 retention or stasis R33.9
  organic R33.8
   drug-induced R33.0
  psychogenic F45.8
 secretion
  deficient R34
  excessive R35.8
  frequency R35.0
 stream
  intermittent R39.198
  slowing R39.198
  splitting R39.13
  weak R39.12
Urinemia — *see* Uremia
Urinoma, urethra N36.8
Uroarthritis, infectious (Reiter's) — *see* Reiter's disease
Urodialysis R34
Urolithiasis — *see* Calculus, urinary

Uronephrosis — *see* Hydronephrosis
Uropathy N39.9
 obstructive N13.9
  specified NEC N13.8
 reflux N13.9
  specified NEC N13.8
 vesicoureteral reflux-associated — *see* Reflux, vesicoureteral
Urosepsis — *code to* condition
Urticaria L50.9
 with angioneurotic edema T78.3 ☑
  hereditary D84.1
 allergic L50.0
 cholinergic L50.5
 chronic L50.8
 cold, familial L50.2
 contact L50.6
 dermatographic L50.3
 due to
  cold or heat L50.2
  drugs L50.0
  food L50.0
  inhalants L50.0
  plants L50.6
  serum — *see also* Reaction, serum T80.69 ☑
 factitial L50.3
 familial cold M04.2
 giant T78.3 ☑
  hereditary D84.1
 gigantea T78.3 ☑
 idiopathic L50.1
 larynx T78.3 ☑
  hereditary D84.1
 neonatorum P83.88
 nonallergic L50.1
 papulosa (Hebra) L28.2
 pigmentosa D47.01
  congenital Q82.2
  of neonatal onset Q82.2
  of newborn onset Q82.2
 recurrent periodic L50.8
 serum — *see also* Reaction, serum T80.69 ☑
 solar L56.3
 specified type NEC L50.8
 thermal (cold) (heat) L50.2
 vibratory L50.4
 xanthelasmoidea — *see* Urticaria pigmentosa
Use (of)
 alcohol Z72.89
  with
   intoxication F10.929
   sleep disorder F10.982
  harmful — *see* Abuse, alcohol
 amphetamines — *see* Use, stimulant NEC
 caffeine — *see* Use, stimulant NEC
 cannabis F12.90
  with
   anxiety disorder F12.980
   intoxication F12.929
    with
     delirium F12.921
     perceptual disturbance F12.922
    uncomplicated F12.920
   other specified disorder F12.988
   psychosis F12.959
    delusions F12.950
    hallucinations F12.951
   unspecified disorder F12.99
   withdrawal F12.93
 cocaine F14.90
  with
   anxiety disorder F14.980
   intoxication F14.929
    with
     delirium F14.921
     perceptual disturbance F14.922
    uncomplicated F14.920
   other specified disorder F14.988
   psychosis F14.959
    delusions F14.950
    hallucinations F14.951
   sexual dysfunction F14.981
   sleep disorder F14.982
   unspecified disorder F14.99
  harmful — *see* Abuse, drug, cocaine
 drug(s) NEC F19.90
  with sleep disorder F19.982
  harmful — *see* Abuse, drug, by type

☑ **Additional Character Required — Refer to the Tabular List for Character Selection** ▽ Subterms under main terms may continue to next column or page

Use — *continued*
  hallucinogen NEC F16.90
    with
      anxiety disorder F16.980
      intoxication F16.929
        with
          delirium F16.921
        uncomplicated F16.920
      mood disorder F16.94
      other specified disorder F16.988
      perception disorder (flashbacks) F16.983
      psychosis F16.959
        delusions F16.950
        hallucinations F16.951
      unspecified disorder F16.99
    harmful — *see* Abuse, drug, hallucinogen NEC
  inhalants F18.90
    with
      anxiety disorder F18.980
      intoxication F18.929
        with delirium F18.921
        uncomplicated F18.920
      mood disorder F18.94
      other specified disorder F18.988
      persisting dementia F18.97
      psychosis F18.959
        delusions F18.950
        hallucinations F18.951
      unspecified disorder F18.99
    harmful — *see* Abuse, drug, inhalant
  methadone — *see* Use, opioid
  nonprescribed drugs F19.90
    harmful — *see* Abuse, non-psychoactive substance
  opioid F11.90
    with
      disorder F11.99
        mood F11.94
        sleep F11.982
        specified type NEC F11.988
      intoxication F11.929
        with
          delirium F11.921
          perceptual disturbance F11.922
        uncomplicated F11.920
      withdrawal F11.93
    harmful — *see* Abuse, drug, opioid
  patent medicines F19.90
    harmful — *see* Abuse, non-psychoactive substance
  psychoactive drug NEC F19.90
    with
      anxiety disorder F19.980
      intoxication F19.929
        with
          delirium F19.921
          perceptual disturbance F19.922
        uncomplicated F19.920
      mood disorder F19.94
      other specified disorder F19.988
      persisting
        amnestic disorder F19.96
        dementia F19.97
      psychosis F19.959
        delusions F19.950
        hallucinations F19.951
      sexual dysfunction F19.981
      sleep disorder F19.982
      unspecified disorder F19.99
      withdrawal F19.939
        with
          delirium F19.931
          perceptual disturbance F19.932
        uncomplicated F19.930
    harmful — *see* Abuse, drug NEC, psychoactive NEC
  sedative, hypnotic, or anxiolytic F13.90
    with
      anxiety disorder F13.980
      intoxication F13.929
        with
          delirium F13.921
        uncomplicated F13.920
      other specified disorder F13.988
      persisting
        amnestic disorder F13.96
        dementia F13.97
      psychosis F13.959
        delusions F13.950
        hallucinations F13.951
      sexual dysfunction F13.981

Use — *continued*
  sedative, hypnotic, or anxiolytic — *continued*
    with — *continued*
      sleep disorder F13.982
      unspecified disorder F13.99
    harmful — *see* Abuse, drug, sedative, hypnotic, or
      anxiolytic
  stimulant NEC F15.90
    with
      anxiety disorder F15.980
      intoxication F15.929
        with
          delirium F15.921
          perceptual disturbance F15.922
        uncomplicated F15.920
      mood disorder F15.94
      other specified disorder F15.988
      psychosis F15.959
        delusions F15.950
        hallucinations F15.951
      sexual dysfunction F15.981
      sleep disorder F15.982
      unspecified disorder F15.99
      withdrawal F15.93
    harmful — *see* Abuse, drug, stimulant NEC
  tobacco Z72.0
    with dependence — *see* Dependence, drug, nicotine
  volatile solvents — *see also* Use, inhalant F18.90
    harmful — *see* Abuse, drug, inhalant
Usher-Senear disease or syndrome L10.4
Uta B55.1
Uteromegaly N85.2
Uterovaginal — *see* condition
Uterovesical — *see* condition
Uveal — *see* condition
Uveitis (anterior) — *see also* Iridocyclitis
  acute — *see* Iridocyclitis, acute
  chronic — *see* Iridocyclitis, chronic
  due to toxoplasmosis (acquired) B58.09
    congenital P37.1
  granulomatous — *see* Iridocyclitis, chronic
  heterochromic — *see* Cyclitis, Fuchs' heterochromic
  lens-induced — *see* Iridocyclitis, lens-induced
  posterior — *see* Chorioretinitis
  sympathetic H44.13- ☑
  syphilitic (secondary) A51.43
    congenital (early) A50.01
    late A52.71
  tuberculous A18.54
Uveoencephalitis — *see* Inflammation, chorioretinal
Uveokeratitis — *see* Iridocyclitis
Uveoparotitis D86.89
Uvula — *see* condition
Uvulitis (acute) (catarrhal) (chronic) (membranous)
  (suppurative) (ulcerative) K12.2

V

Vaccination (prophylactic)
  complication or reaction — *see* Complications, vacci-
    nation
  delayed Z28.9
  encounter for Z23
  not done — *see* Immunization, not done, because of)
Vaccinia (generalized) (localized) T88.1 ☑
  congenital P35.8
  without vaccination B08.011
Vacuum, in sinus (accessory) (nasal) J34.89
Vagabond, vagabondage Z59.0
Vagabond's disease B85.1
Vagina, vaginal — *see* condition
Vaginalitis (tunica) (testis) N49.1
Vaginismus (reflex) N94.2
  functional F52.5
  nonorganic F52.5
  psychogenic F52.5
  secondary N94.2
Vaginitis (acute) (circumscribed) (diffuse) (emphysematous) (nonvenereal) (ulcerative) N76.0
  with ectopic or molar pregnancy O08.0
  amebic A06.82
  atrophic, postmenopausal N95.2
  bacterial N76.0
  blennorrhagic (gonococcal) A54.02
  candidal B37.3
  chlamydial A56.02
  chronic N76.1

Vaginitis — *continued*
  due to Trichomonas (vaginalis) A59.01
  following ectopic or molar pregnancy O08.0
  gonococcal A54.02
    with abscess (accessory gland) (periurethral) A54.1
  granuloma A58
  in (due to)
    candidiasis B37.3
    herpesviral (herpes simplex) infection A60.04
    pinworm infection B80 *[N77.1]*
  monilial B37.3
  mycotic (candidal) B37.3
  postmenopausal atrophic N95.2
  puerperal (postpartum) O86.13
  senile (atrophic) N95.2
  subacute or chronic N76.1
  syphilitic (early) A51.0
    late A52.76
  trichomonal A59.01
  tuberculous A18.18
Vaginosis — *see* Vaginitis
Vagotonia G52.2
Vagrancy Z59.0
VAIN — *see* Neoplasia, intraepithelial, vagina
Vallecula — *see* condition
Valley fever B38.0
Valsuani's disease — *see* Anemia, obstetric
Valve, valvular (formation) — *see also* condition
  cerebral ventricle (communicating) in situ Z98.2
  cervix, internal os Q51.828
  congenital NEC — *see* Atresia, by site
  ureter (pelvic junction) (vesical orifice) Q62.39
  urethra (congenital) (posterior) Q64.2
Valvulitis (chronic) — *see* Endocarditis
Valvulopathy — *see* Endocarditis
Van Bogaert's leukoencephalopathy (sclerosing)
  (subacute) A81.1
Van Bogaert-Scherer-Epstein disease or syndrome
  E75.5
Van Buchem's syndrome M85.2
Van Creveld-von Gierke disease E74.01
Van der Hoeve (-de Kleyn) **syndrome** Q78.0
Van der Woude's syndrome Q38.0
Van Neck's disease or osteochondrosis M91.0
Vanishing lung J44.9
Vapor asphyxia or suffocation T59.9 ☑
  specified agent — *see* Table of Drugs and Chemicals
Variance, lethal ball, prosthetic heart valve T82.09 ☑
Variants, thalassemic D56.8
Variations in hair color L67.1
Varicella B01.9
  with
    complications NEC B01.89
    encephalitis B01.11
    encephalomyelitis B01.11
    meningitis B01.0
    myelitis B01.12
    pneumonia B01.2
  congenital P35.8
Varices — *see* Varix
Varicocele (scrotum) (thrombosed) I86.1
  ovary I86.2
  perineum I86.3
  spermatic cord (ulcerated) I86.1
Varicose
  aneurysm (ruptured) I77.0
  dermatitis — *see* Varix, leg, with, inflammation
  eczema — *see* Varix, leg, with, inflammation
  phlebitis — *see* Varix, with, inflammation
  tumor — *see* Varix
  ulcer (lower limb, any part) — *see also* Varix, leg, with,
    ulcer
    anus — *see also* Hemorrhoids K64.8
    esophagus — *see* Varix, esophagus
    inflamed or infected — *see* Varix, leg, with ulcer,
      with inflammation
    nasal septum I86.8
    perineum I86.3
    scrotum I86.1
    specified site NEC I86.8
  vein — *see* Varix
  vessel — *see* Varix, leg
Varicosis, varicosities, varicosity — *see* Varix
Variola (major) (minor) B03
Varioloid B03
Varix (lower limb) I83.90

Varix — *continued*
with
  bleeding I83.899
  edema I83.899
  inflammation I83.10
    with ulcer (venous) I83.209
  pain I83.819
  rupture I83.899
  specified complication NEC I83.899
  stasis dermatitis I83.10
    with ulcer (venous) I83.209
  swelling I83.899
  ulcer I83.009
    with inflammation I83.209
aneurysmal I77.0
asymptomatic I83.9- ☑
bladder I86.2
broad ligament I86.2
complicating
  childbirth (lower extremity) O87.4
    anus or rectum O87.2
    genital (vagina, vulva or perineum) O87.8
  pregnancy (lower extremity) O22.0- ☑
    anus or rectum O22.4- ☑
    genital (vagina, vulva or perineum) O22.1- ☑
  puerperium (lower extremity) O87.4
    anus or rectum O87.2
    genital (vagina, vulva, perineum) O87.8
congenital (any site) Q27.8
esophagus (idiopathic) (primary) (ulcerated) I85.00
  bleeding I85.01
  congenital Q27.8
  in (due to)
    alcoholic liver disease I85.10
      bleeding I85.11
    cirrhosis of liver I85.10
      bleeding I85.11
    portal hypertension I85.10
      bleeding I85.11
    schistosomiasis I85.10
      bleeding I85.11
    toxic liver disease I85.10
      bleeding I85.11
  secondary I85.10
    bleeding I85.11
gastric I86.4
inflamed or infected I83.10
  ulcerated I83.209
labia (majora) I86.3
leg (asymptomatic) I83.90
  with
    edema I83.899
    inflammation I83.10
      with ulcer — *see* Varix, leg, with, ulcer, with
        inflammation by site
    pain I83.819
    specified complication NEC I83.899
    swelling I83.899
    ulcer I83.009
      with inflammation I83.209
      ankle I83.003
        with inflammation I83.203
      calf I83.002
        with inflammation I83.202
      foot NEC I83.005
        with inflammation I83.205
      heel I83.004
        with inflammation I83.204
      lower leg NEC I83.008
        with inflammation I83.208
      midfoot I83.004
        with inflammation I83.204
      thigh I83.001
        with inflammation I83.201
  bilateral (asymptomatic) I83.93
    with
      edema I83.893
      pain I83.813
      specified complication NEC I83.893
      swelling I83.893
      ulcer I83.0- ☑
        with inflammation I83.209
  left (asymptomatic) I83.92
    with
      edema I83.892
      inflammation I83.12
        with ulcer — *see* Varix, leg, with, ulcer, with inflammation by site

Varix — *continued*
leg — *continued*
  left — *continued*
    with — *continued*
      pain I83.812
      specified complication NEC I83.892
      swelling I83.892
      ulcer I83.029
        with inflammation I83.229
        ankle I83.023
          with inflammation I83.223
        calf I83.022
          with inflammation I83.222
        foot NEC I83.025
          with inflammation I83.225
        heel I83.024
          with inflammation I83.224
        lower leg NEC I83.028
          with inflammation I83.228
        midfoot I83.024
          with inflammation I83.224
        thigh I83.021
          with inflammation I83.221
  right (asymptomatic) I83.91
    with
      edema I83.891
      inflammation I83.11
        with ulcer — *see* Varix, leg, with, ulcer, with inflammation by site
      pain I83.811
      specified complication NEC I83.891
      swelling I83.891
      ulcer I83.019
        with inflammation I83.219
        ankle I83.013
          with inflammation I83.213
        calf I83.012
          with inflammation I83.212
        foot NEC I83.015
          with inflammation I83.215
        heel I83.014
          with inflammation I83.214
        lower leg NEC I83.018
          with inflammation I83.218
        midfoot I83.014
          with inflammation I83.214
        thigh I83.011
          with inflammation I83.211
nasal septum I86.8
orbit I86.8
  congenital Q27.8
ovary I86.2
papillary I78.1
pelvis I86.2
perineum I86.3
pharynx I86.8
placenta O43.89- ☑
renal papilla I86.8
retina H35.09
scrotum (ulcerated) I86.1
sigmoid colon I86.8
specified site NEC I86.8
spinal (cord) (vessels) I86.8
spleen, splenic (vein) (with phlebolith) I86.8
stomach I86.4
sublingual I86.0
ulcerated I83.009
  inflamed or infected I83.209
uterine ligament I86.2
vagina I86.8
vocal cord I86.8
vulva I86.3
Vas deferens — *see* condition
Vas deferentitis N49.1
Vasa previa O69.4 ☑
  hemorrhage from, affecting newborn P50.0
Vascular — *see also* condition
  loop on optic papilla Q14.2
  spasm I73.9
  spider I78.1
Vascularization, cornea — *see* Neovascularization, cornea
Vasculitis I77.6
  allergic D69.0
  cryoglobulinemic D89.1
  disseminated I77.6
  hypocomplementemic M31.8
  kidney I77.89

Vasculitis — *continued*
  livedoid L95.0
  nodular L95.8
  retina H35.06- ☑
  rheumatic — *see* Fever, rheumatic
  rheumatoid — *see* Rheumatoid, vasculitis
  skin (limited to) L95.9
    specified NEC L95.8
  systemic M31.8
Vasculopathy, necrotizing M31.9
  cardiac allograft T86.290
  specified NEC M31.8
Vasitis (nodosa) N49.1
  tuberculous A18.15
Vasodilation I73.9
Vasomotor — *see* condition
Vasoplasty, after previous sterilization Z31.0
  aftercare Z31.42
Vasospasm (vasoconstriction) I73.9
  cerebral (cerebrovascular) (artery) I67.848
    reversible I67.841
  coronary I20.1
  nerve
    arm — *see* Mononeuropathy, upper limb
    brachial plexus G54.0
    cervical plexus G54.2
    leg — *see* Mononeuropathy, lower limb
  peripheral NOS I73.9
  retina (artery) — *see* Occlusion, artery, retina
Vasospastic — *see* condition
Vasovagal attack (paroxysmal) R55
  psychogenic F45.8
VATER syndrome Q87.2
Vater's ampulla — *see* condition
Vegetation, vegetative
  adenoid (nasal fossa) J35.8
  endocarditis (acute) (any valve) (subacute) I33.0
  heart (mycotic) (valve) I33.0
Veil
  Jackson's Q43.3
Vein, venous — *see* condition
Veldt sore — *see* Ulcer, skin
Velpeau's hernia — *see* Hernia, femoral
Venereal
  bubo A55
  disease A64
  granuloma inguinale A58
  lymphogranuloma (Durand-Nicolas-Favre) A55
Venofibrosis I87.8
Venom, venomous — *see* Table of Drugs and Chemicals, by animal or substance, poisoning
Venous — *see* condition
Ventilator lung, newborn P27.8
Ventral — *see* condition
Ventricle, ventricular — *see also* condition
  escape I49.3
  inversion Q20.5
Ventriculitis (cerebral) — *see also* Encephalitis G04.90
Ventriculostomy status Z98.2
Vernet's syndrome G52.7
Verneuil's disease (syphilitic bursitis) A52.78
Verruca (due to HPV) (filiformis) (simplex) (viral) (vulgaris) B07.9
  acuminata A63.0
  necrogenica (primary) (tuberculosa) A18.4
  plana B07.8
  plantaris B07.0
  seborrheica L82.1
    inflamed L82.0
  senile (seborrheic) L82.1
    inflamed L82.0
  tuberculosa (primary) A18.4
  venereal A63.0
Verrucosities — *see* Verruca
Verruga peruana, peruviana A44.1
Version
  with extraction
  cervix — *see* Malposition, uterus
  uterus (postinfectional) (postpartal, old) — *see* Malposition, uterus
Vertebra, vertebral — *see* condition
Vertical talus (congenital) Q66.80
  left foot Q66.82
  right foot Q66.81
Vertigo R42
  auditory — *see* Vertigo, aural
  aural H81.31- ☑

☑ **Additional Character Required** — Refer to the Tabular List for Character Selection   ▽ **Subterms under main terms may continue to next column or page**

Vertigo — *continued*
　benign paroxysmal (positional) H81.1- ☑
　central (origin) H81.4
　cerebral H81.4
　Dix and Hallpike (epidemic) — *see* Neuronitis,
　　vestibular
　due to infrasound T75.23 ☑
　epidemic A88.1
　　Dix and Hallpike — *see* Neuronitis, vestibular
　　Pedersen's — *see* Neuronitis, vestibular
　　vestibular neuronitis — *see* Neuronitis, vestibular
　hysterical F44.89
　infrasound T75.23 ☑
　labyrinthine — *see* subcategory H81.0 ☑
　laryngeal R05
　malignant positional H81.4
　Ménière's — *see* subcategory H81.0 ☑
　menopausal N95.1
　otogenic — *see* Vertigo, aural
　paroxysmal positional, benign — *see* Vertigo, benign
　　paroxysmal
　Pedersen's (epidemic) — *see* Neuronitis, vestibular
　peripheral NEC H81.39- ☑
　positional
　　benign paroxysmal — *see* Vertigo, benign paroxys-
　　　mal
　　malignant H81.4
Very-low-density-lipoprotein-type (VLDL) **hyper-**
　lipoproteinemia E78.1
Vesania — *see* Psychosis
Vesical — *see* condition
Vesicle
　cutaneous R23.8
　seminal — *see* condition
　skin R23.8
Vesicocolic — *see* condition
Vesicoperineal — *see* condition
Vesicorectal — *see* condition
Vesicourethrorectal — *see* condition
Vesicovaginal — *see* condition
Vesicular — *see* condition
Vesiculitis (seminal) N49.0
　amebic A06.82
　gonorrheal (acute) (chronic) A54.23
　trichomonal A59.09
　tuberculous A18.15
Vestibulitis (ear) — *see also* subcategory H83.0 ☑
　nose (external) J34.89
　vulvar N94.810
Vestibulopathy , acute peripheral (recurrent) — *see*
　Neuronitis, vestibular
Vestige, vestigial — *see also* Persistence
　branchial Q18.0
　structures in vitreous Q14.0
Vibration
　adverse effects T75.20 ☑
　　pneumatic hammer syndrome T75.21 ☑
　　specified effect NEC T75.29 ☑
　　vasospastic syndrome T75.22 ☑
　　vertigo from infrasound T75.23 ☑
　exposure (occupational) Z57.7
　vertigo T75.23 ☑
Vibriosis A28.9
Victim (of)
　crime Z65.4
　disaster Z65.5
　terrorism Z65.4
　torture Z65.4
　war Z65.5
Vidal's disease L28.0
Villaret's syndrome G52.7
Villous — *see* condition
VIN — *see* Neoplasia, intraepithelial, vulva
Vincent's infection (angina) (gingivitis) A69.1
　stomatitis NEC A69.1
Vinson-Plummer syndrome D50.1
Violence, physical R45.6
Viosterol deficiency — *see* Deficiency, calciferol
Vipoma — *see* Neoplasm, malignant, by site
Viremia B34.9
Virilism (adrenal) E25.9
　congenital E25.0
Virilization (female) (suprarenal) E25.9
　congenital E25.0
　isosexual E28.2
Virulent bubo A57
Virus, viral — *see also* condition

Virus, viral — *continued*
　as cause of disease classified elsewhere B97.89
　　respiratory syncytial virus (RSV) — *see* Virus, infec-
　　　tion, respiratory syncytial (RSV)
　cytomegalovirus B25.9
　human immunodeficiency (HIV) — *see* Human, immun-
　　odeficiency virus (HIV) disease
　infection — *see* Infection, virus
　respiratory syncytial (RSV)
　　as cause of disease classified elsewhere B97.4
　　bronchiolitis J21.0
　　bronchitis J20.5
　　bronchopneumonia J12.1
　　otitis media H65.- ☑ [B97.4]
　　pneumonia J12.1
　　upper respiratory infection J06.9 [B97.4]
　specified NEC B34.8
　swine influenza (viruses that normally cause infections
　　in pigs) — *see also* Influenza, due to, identified
　　novel influenza A virus J09.X2
　West Nile (fever) A92.30
　　with
　　　complications NEC A92.39
　　　cranial nerve disorders A92.32
　　　encephalitis A92.31
　　　encephalomyelitis A92.31
　　　neurologic manifestation NEC A92.32
　　　optic neuritis A92.32
　　　polyradiculitis A92.32
Viscera, visceral — *see* condition
Visceroptosis K63.4
Visible peristalsis R19.2
Vision, visual
　binocular, suppression H53.34
　blurred, blurring H53.8
　　hysterical F44.6
　defect, defective NEC H54.7
　disorientation (syndrome) H53.8
　disturbance H53.9
　　hysterical F44.6
　double H53.2
　examination Z01.00
　　with abnormal findings Z01.01
　　following failed vision screening Z01.020
　　　with abnormal findings Z01.021
　field, limitation (defect) — *see* Defect, visual field
　hallucinations R44.1
　halos H53.19
　loss — *see* Loss, vision
　　sudden — *see* Disturbance, vision, subjective, loss,
　　　sudden
　low (both eyes) — *see* Low, vision
　perception, simultaneous without fusion H53.33
Vitality, lack or want of R53.83
　newborn P96.89
Vitamin deficiency — *see* Deficiency, vitamin
Vitelline duct, persistent Q43.0
Vitiligo L80
　eyelid H02.739
　　left H02.736
　　　lower H02.735
　　　upper H02.734
　　right H02.733
　　　lower H02.732
　　　upper H02.731
　pinta A67.2
　vulva N90.89
Vitreal corneal syndrome H59.01- ☑
Vitreoretinopathy, proliferative — *see also*
　Retinopathy, proliferative
　with retinal detachment — *see* Detachment, retina,
　　traction
Vitreous — *see also* condition
　touch syndrome — *see* Complication, postprocedural,
　　following cataract surgery
Vocal cord — *see* condition
Vogt-Koyanagi syndrome H20.82- ☑
Vogt's disease or syndrome G80.3
Vogt-Spielmeyer amaurotic idiocy or disease E75.4
Voice
　change R49.9
　　specified NEC R49.8
　loss — *see* Aphonia
Volhynian fever A79.0
Volkmann's ischemic contracture or paralysis (com-
　plicating trauma) T79.6 ☑
Volvulus (bowel) (colon) (intestine) K56.2
　with perforation K56.2

Volvulus — *continued*
　congenital Q43.8
　duodenum K31.5
　fallopian tube — *see* Torsion, fallopian tube
　oviduct — *see* Torsion, fallopian tube
　stomach (due to absence of gastrocolic ligament)
　　K31.89
Vomiting R11.10
　with nausea R11.2
　asphyxia — *see* Foreign body, by site, causing asphyxia,
　　gastric contents
　bilious (cause unknown) R11.14
　　following gastro-intestinal surgery K91.0
　　in newborn P92.01
　blood — *see* Hematemesis
　causing asphyxia, choking, or suffocation — *see* For-
　　eign body, by site
　cyclical, in migraine G43.A0 (*following* G43.7)
　　with refractory migraine G43.A1 (*following* G43.7)
　　intractable G43.A1 (*following* G43.7)
　　not intractable G43.A0 (*following* G43.7)
　　psychogenic F50.89
　　without refractory migraine G43.A0 (*following* G43.7)
　cyclical syndrome NOS (unrelated to migraine) R11.15
　fecal mater R11.13
　following gastrointestinal surgery K91.0
　　psychogenic F50.89
　functional K31.89
　hysterical F50.89
　nervous F50.89
　neurotic F50.89
　newborn NEC P92.09
　　bilious P92.01
　periodic R11.10
　　psychogenic F50.89
　persistent R11.15
　projectile R11.12
　psychogenic F50.89
　uremic — *see* Uremia
　without nausea R11.11
Vomito negro — *see* Fever, yellow
Von Bezold's abscess — *see* Mastoiditis, acute
Von Economo-Cruchet disease A85.8
Von Eulenburg's disease G71.19
Von Gierke's disease E74.01
Von Hippel (-Lindau) **disease or syndrome** Q85.8
Von Jaksch's anemia or disease D64.89
Von Recklinghausen
　disease (neurofibromatosis) Q85.01
　　bones E21.0
Von Schroetter's syndrome I82.890
Von Willebrand (-Jurgens)(-Minot) **disease or syn-**
　drome D68.0
Von Zumbusch's disease L40.1
Voyeurism F65.3
Vrolik's disease Q78.0
Vulva — *see* condition
Vulvismus N94.2
Vulvitis (acute) (allergic) (atrophic) (hypertrophic) (inter-
　triginous) (senile) N76.2
　with ectopic or molar pregnancy O08.0
　adhesive, congenital Q52.79
　blennorrhagic (gonococcal) A54.02
　candidal B37.3
　chlamydial A56.02
　due to Haemophilus ducreyi A57
　following ectopic or molar pregnancy O08.0
　gonococcal A54.02
　　with abscess (accessory gland) (periurethral) A54.1
　herpesviral A60.04
　leukoplakic N90.4
　monilial B37.3
　puerperal (postpartum) O86.19
　subacute or chronic N76.3
　syphilitic (early) A51.0
　　late A52.76
　trichomonal A59.01
　tuberculous A18.18
Vulvodynia N94.819
　specified NEC N94.818
Vulvorectal — *see* condition
Vulvovaginitis (acute) — *see* Vaginitis

W

Waiting list, person on Z75.1
　for organ transplant Z76.82
　undergoing social agency investigation Z75.2

Waldenström
  hypergammaglobulinemia D89.0
  syndrome or macroglobulinemia C88.0
Waldenström-Kjellberg syndrome D50.1
Walking
  difficulty R26.2
    psychogenic F44.4
  sleep F51.3
    hysterical F44.89
Wall, abdominal — see condition
Wallenberg's disease or syndrome G46.3
Wallgren's disease I87.8
Wandering
  gallbladder, congenital Q44.1
  in diseases classified elsewhere Z91.83
  kidney, congenital Q63.8
  organ or site, congenital NEC — see Malposition, congenital, by site
  pacemaker (heart) I49.8
  spleen D73.89
War neurosis F48.8
Wart (due to HPV) (filiform) (infectious) (viral) B07.9
  anogenital region (venereal) A63.0
  common B07.8
  external genital organs (venereal) A63.0
  flat B07.8
  Hassal-Henle's (of cornea) H18.49
  Peruvian A44.1
  plantar B07.0
  prosector (tuberculous) A18.4
  seborrheic L82.1
    inflamed L82.0
  senile (seborrheic) L82.1
    inflamed L82.0
  tuberculous A18.4
  venereal A63.0
Warthin's tumor — see Neoplasm, salivary gland, benign
Wassilieff's disease A27.0
Wasting
  disease R64
    due to malnutrition E41
  extreme (due to malnutrition) E41
  muscle NEC — see Atrophy, muscle
Water
  clefts (senile cataract) — see Cataract, senile, incipient
  deprivation of T73.1 ☑
  intoxication E87.79
  itch B76.9
  lack of T73.1 ☑
  loading E87.70
  on
    brain — see Hydrocephalus
    chest J94.8
  poisoning E87.79
Waterbrash R12
Waterhouse (-Friderichsen) **syndrome or disease** (meningococcal) A39.1
Water-losing nephritis N25.89
Watermelon stomach K31.819
  with hemorrhage K31.811
  without hemorrhage K31.819
Watsoniasis B66.8
Wax in ear — see Impaction, cerumen
Weak, weakening, weakness (generalized) R53.1
  arches (acquired) — see also Deformity, limb, flat foot
  bladder (sphincter) R32
  facial R29.810
    following
      cerebrovascular disease I69.992
        cerebral infarction I69.392
        intracerebral hemorrhage I69.192
        nontraumatic intracranial hemorrhage NEC I69.292
        specified disease NEC I69.892
        stroke I69.392
        subarachnoid hemorrhage I69.092
  foot (double) — see also Weak, arches
  heart, cardiac — see Failure, heart
  mind F70
  muscle M62.81
  myocardium — see Failure, heart
  newborn P96.89
  pelvic fundus N81.89
  pubocervical tissue N81.82
  rectovaginal tissue N81.83
  senile R54
  urinary stream R39.12
  valvular — see Endocarditis

Wear, worn (with normal or routine use)
  articular bearing surface of internal joint prosthesis — see Complications, joint prosthesis, mechanical, wear of articular bearing surfaces, by site
  device, implant or graft — see Complications, by site, mechanical complication
  tooth, teeth (approximal) (hard tissues) (interproximal) (occlusal) K03.0
Weather, weathered
  effects of
    cold T69.9 ☑
      specified effect NEC T69.8 ☑
    hot — see Heat
  skin L57.8
Weaver's syndrome Q87.3
Web, webbed (congenital)
  duodenal Q43.8
  esophagus Q39.4
  fingers Q70.1- ☑
  larynx (glottic) (subglottic) Q31.0
  neck (pterygium colli) Q18.3
  Paterson-Kelly D50.1
  popliteal syndrome Q87.89
  toes Q70.3- ☑
Weber-Christian disease M35.6
Weber-Cockayne syndrome (epidermolysis bullosa) Q81.8
Weber-Gubler syndrome G46.3
Weber-Leyden syndrome G46.3
Weber-Osler syndrome I78.0
Weber's paralysis or syndrome G46.3
Wedge-shaped or wedging vertebra — see Collapse, vertebra NEC
Wegener's granulomatosis or syndrome M31.30
  with
    kidney involvement M31.31
    lung involvement M31.30
      with kidney involvement M31.31
Wegner's disease A50.02
Weight
  1000-2499 grams at birth (low) — see Low, birthweight
  999 grams or less at birth (extremely low) — see Low, birthweight, extreme
  and length below 10th percentile for gestational age P05.1- ☑
  below but length above 10th percentile for gestational age P05.0- ☑
  gain (abnormal) (excessive) R63.5
    in pregnancy — see Pregnancy, complicated by, excessive weight gain
    low — see Pregnancy, complicated by, insufficient, weight gain
  loss (abnormal) (cause unknown) R63.4
Weightlessness (effect of) T75.82 ☑
Weil (l)-**Marchesani syndrome** Q87.19
Weil's disease A27.0
Weingarten's syndrome J82
Weir Mitchell's disease I73.81
Weiss-Baker syndrome G90.09
Wells' disease L98.3
Wen — see Cyst, sebaceous
Wenckebach's block or phenomenon I44.1
Werdnig-Hoffmann syndrome (muscular atrophy) G12.0
Werlhof's disease D69.3
Wermer's disease or syndrome E31.21
Werner-His disease A79.0
Werner's disease or syndrome E34.8
Wernicke-Korsakoff's syndrome or psychosis (alcoholic) F10.96
  with dependence F10.26
  drug-induced
    due to drug abuse — see Abuse, drug, by type, with amnestic disorder
    due to drug dependence — see Dependence, drug, by type, with amnestic disorder
  nonalcoholic F04
Wernicke-Posadas disease B38.9
Wernicke's
  developmental aphasia F80.2
  disease or syndrome E51.2
  encephalopathy E51.2
  polioencephalitis, superior E51.2
West African fever B50.8
Westphal-Strümpell syndrome E83.01
West's syndrome — see Epilepsy, spasms

Wet
  feet, tropical (maceration) (syndrome) — see Immersion, foot
  lung (syndrome), newborn P22.1
Wharton's duct — see condition
Wheal — see Urticaria
Wheezing R06.2
Whiplash injury S13.4 ☑
Whipple's disease — see also subcategory M14.8- K90.81
Whipworm (disease) (infection) (infestation) B79
Whistling face Q87.0
White — see also condition
  kidney, small N03.9
  leg, puerperal, postpartum, childbirth O87.1
  mouth B37.0
  patches of mouth K13.29
  spot lesions, teeth
    chewing surface K02.51
    pit and fissure surface K02.51
    smooth surface K02.61
Whitehead L70.0
Whitlow — see also Cellulitis, digit
  with lymphangitis — see Lymphangitis, acute, digit
  herpesviral B00.89
Whitmore's disease or fever — see Melioidosis
Whooping cough A37.90
  with pneumonia A37.91
    due to Bordetella
      bronchiseptica A37.81
      parapertussis A37.11
      pertussis A37.01
    specified organism NEC A37.81
  due to
    Bordetella
      bronchiseptica A37.80
        with pneumonia A37.81
      parapertussis A37.10
        with pneumonia A37.11
      pertussis A37.00
        with pneumonia A37.01
    specified NEC A37.80
      with pneumonia A37.81
Wichman's asthma J38.5
Wide cranial sutures, newborn P96.3
Widening aorta — see Ectasia, aorta
  with aneurysm — see Aneurysm, aorta
Wilkie's disease or syndrome K55.1
Wilkinson-Sneddon disease or syndrome L13.1
Willebrand (-Jürgens) **thrombopathy** D68.0
Williams syndrome Q93.82
Willige-Hunt disease or syndrome G23.1
Wilms' tumor C64- ☑
Wilson-Mikity syndrome P27.0
Wilson's
  disease or syndrome E83.01
  hepatolenticular degeneration E83.01
  lichen ruber L43.9
Window — see also Imperfect, closure
  aorticopulmonary Q21.4
Winter — see condition
Wiskott-Aldrich syndrome D82.0
Withdrawal state — see also Dependence, drug by type
  with withdrawal
  alcohol
    with perceptual disturbances F10.232
    without perceptual disturbances F10.239
  caffeine F15.93
  cannabis F12.23
  newborn
    correct therapeutic substance properly administered P96.2
    infant of dependent mother P96.1
  therapeutic substance, neonatal P96.2
Witts' anemia D50.8
Witzelsucht F07.0
Woakes' ethmoiditis or syndrome J33.1
Wolff-Hirschorn syndrome Q93.3
Wolff-Parkinson-White syndrome I45.6
Wolhynian fever A79.0
Wolman's disease E75.5
Wood lung or pneumonitis J67.8
Woolly, wooly hair (congenital) (nevus) Q84.1
Woolsorter's disease A22.1
Word
  blindness (congenital) (developmental) F81.0
  deafness (congenital) (developmental) H93.25

Worm(s) (infection) (infestation) — *see also* Infestation, helminth
  guinea B72
  in intestine NEC B82.Ø
Worm-eaten soles A66.3
Worn out — *see* Exhaustion
  cardiac
    defibrillator (with synchronous cardiac pacemaker) Z45.Ø2
    pacemaker
      battery Z45.Ø1Ø
      lead Z45.Ø18
  device, implant or graft — *see* Complications, by site, mechanical
Worried well Z71.1
Worries R45.82
Wound check Z48.Ø- ☑
  due to injury — *code to* Injury, by site, using appropriate seventh character for subsequent encounter
Wound, open T14.8- ☑
  abdomen, abdominal
    wall S31.1Ø9 ☑
      with penetration into peritoneal cavity S31.6Ø9 ☑
      bite — *see* Bite, abdomen, wall
      epigastric region S31.1Ø2 ☑
        with penetration into peritoneal cavity S31.6Ø2 ☑
        bite — *see* Bite, abdomen, wall, epigastric region
        laceration — *see* Laceration, abdomen, wall, epigastric region
        puncture — *see* Puncture, abdomen, wall, epigastric region
      laceration — *see* Laceration, abdomen, wall
      left
        lower quadrant S31.1Ø4 ☑
          with penetration into peritoneal cavity S31.6Ø4 ☑
          bite — *see* Bite, abdomen, wall, left, lower quadrant
          laceration — *see* Laceration, abdomen, wall, left, lower quadrant
          puncture — *see* Puncture, abdomen, wall, left, lower quadrant
        upper quadrant S31.1Ø1 ☑
          with penetration into peritoneal cavity S31.6Ø1 ☑
          bite — *see* Bite, abdomen, wall, left, upper quadrant
          laceration — *see* Laceration, abdomen, wall, left, upper quadrant
          puncture — *see* Puncture, abdomen, wall, left, upper quadrant
      periumbilic region S31.1Ø5 ☑
        with penetration into peritoneal cavity S31.6Ø5 ☑
        bite — *see* Bite, abdomen, wall, periumbilic region
        laceration — *see* Laceration, abdomen, wall, periumbilic region
        puncture — *see* Puncture, abdomen, wall, periumbilic region
      puncture — *see* Puncture, abdomen, wall
      right
        lower quadrant S31.1Ø3 ☑
          with penetration into peritoneal cavity S31.6Ø3 ☑
          bite — *see* Bite, abdomen, wall, right, lower quadrant
          laceration — *see* Laceration, abdomen, wall, right, lower quadrant
          puncture — *see* Puncture, abdomen, wall, right, lower quadrant
        upper quadrant S31.1ØØ ☑
          with penetration into peritoneal cavity S31.6ØØ ☑
          bite — *see* Bite, abdomen, wall, right, upper quadrant
          laceration — *see* Laceration, abdomen, wall, right, upper quadrant
          puncture — *see* Puncture, abdomen, wall, right, upper quadrant
  alveolar (process) — *see* Wound, open, oral cavity
  ankle S91.ØØ- ☑
    bite — *see* Bite, ankle
    laceration — *see* Laceration, ankle

Wound, open — *continued*
  ankle — *continued*
    puncture — *see* Puncture, ankle
  antecubital space — *see* Wound, open, elbow
  anterior chamber, eye — *see* Wound, open, ocular
  anus S31.839 ☑
    bite S31.835 ☑
    laceration — *see* Laceration, anus
    puncture — *see* Puncture, anus
  arm (upper) S41.1Ø- ☑
    with amputation — *see* Amputation, traumatic, arm
    bite — *see* Bite, arm
    forearm — *see* Wound, open, forearm
    laceration — *see* Laceration, arm
    puncture — *see* Puncture, arm
  auditory canal (external) (meatus) — *see* Wound, open, ear
  auricle, ear — *see* Wound, open, ear
  axilla — *see* Wound, open, arm
  back — *see also* Wound, open, thorax, back
    lower S31.ØØØ ☑
      with penetration into retroperitoneal space S31.ØØ1 ☑
      bite — *see* Bite, back, lower
      laceration — *see* Laceration, back, lower
      puncture — *see* Puncture, back, lower
  bite — *see* Bite
  blood vessel — *see* Injury, blood vessel
  breast S21.ØØ- ☑
    with amputation — *see* Amputation, traumatic, breast
    bite — *see* Bite, breast
    laceration — *see* Laceration, breast
    puncture — *see* Puncture, breast
  buttock S31.8Ø9 ☑
    bite — *see* Bite, buttock
    laceration — *see* Laceration, buttock
    left S31.829 ☑
    puncture — *see* Puncture, buttock
    right S31.819 ☑
  calf — *see* Wound, open, leg
  canaliculus lacrimalis — *see* Wound, open, eyelid
  canthus, eye — *see* Wound, open, eyelid
  cervical esophagus S11.2Ø ☑
    bite S11.25 ☑
    laceration — *see* Laceration, esophagus, traumatic, cervical
    puncture — *see* Puncture, cervical esophagus
  cheek (external) SØ1.4Ø- ☑
    bite — *see* Bite, cheek
    internal — *see* Wound, open, oral cavity
    laceration — *see* Laceration, cheek
    puncture — *see* Puncture, cheek
  chest wall — *see* Wound, open, thorax
  chin — *see* Wound, open, head, specified site NEC
  choroid — *see* Wound, open, ocular
  ciliary body (eye) — *see* Wound, open, ocular
  clitoris S31.4Ø ☑
    with amputation — *see* Amputation, traumatic, clitoris
    bite S31.45 ☑
    laceration — *see* Laceration, vulva
    puncture — *see* Puncture, vulva
  conjunctiva — *see* Wound, open, ocular
  cornea — *see* Wound, open, ocular
  costal region — *see* Wound, open, thorax
  Descemet's membrane — *see* Wound, open, ocular
  digit(s)
    foot — *see* Wound, open, toe
    hand — *see* Wound, open, finger
  ear (canal) (external) SØ1.3Ø- ☑
    with amputation — *see* Amputation, traumatic, ear
    bite — *see* Bite, ear
    drum SØ9.2- ☑
    laceration — *see* Laceration, ear
    puncture — *see* Puncture, ear
  elbow S51.ØØ- ☑
    bite — *see* Bite, elbow
    laceration — *see* Laceration, elbow
    puncture — *see* Puncture, elbow
  epididymis — *see* Wound, open, testis
  epigastric region S31.1Ø2 ☑
    with penetration into peritoneal cavity S31.6Ø2 ☑
    bite — *see* Bite, abdomen, wall, epigastric region
    laceration — *see* Laceration, abdomen, wall, epigastric region

Wound, open — *continued*
  epigastric region — *continued*
    puncture — *see* Puncture, abdomen, wall, epigastric region
  epiglottis — *see* Wound, open, neck, specified site NEC
  esophagus (thoracic) S27.819 ☑
    cervical — *see* Wound, open, cervical esophagus
    laceration S27.813 ☑
    specified type NEC S27.818 ☑
  eye — *see* Wound, open, ocular
  eyeball — *see* Wound, open, ocular
  eyebrow — *see* Wound, open, eyelid
  eyelid SØ1.1Ø- ☑
    bite — *see* Bite, eyelid
    laceration — *see* Laceration, eyelid
    puncture — *see* Puncture, eyelid
  face NEC — *see* Wound, open, head, specified site NEC
  finger(s) S61.2Ø9 ☑
    with
      amputation — *see* Amputation, traumatic, finger
      damage to nail S61.3Ø9 ☑
    bite — *see* Bite, finger
    index S61.2Ø8 ☑
      with
        damage to nail S61.3Ø8 ☑
      left S61.2Ø1 ☑
        with
          damage to nail S61.3Ø1 ☑
      right S61.2ØØ ☑
        with
          damage to nail S61.3ØØ ☑
    laceration — *see* Laceration, finger
    little S61.2Ø8 ☑
      with
        damage to nail S61.3Ø8 ☑
      left S61.2Ø7 ☑
        with damage to nail S61.3Ø7 ☑
      right S61.2Ø6 ☑
        with damage to nail S61.3Ø6 ☑
    middle S61.2Ø8 ☑
      with
        damage to nail S61.3Ø8 ☑
      left S61.2Ø3 ☑
        with damage to nail S61.3Ø3 ☑
      right S61.2Ø2 ☑
        with damage to nail S61.3Ø2 ☑
    puncture — *see* Puncture, finger
    ring S61.2Ø8 ☑
      with
        damage to nail S61.3Ø8 ☑
      left S61.2Ø5 ☑
        with damage to nail S61.3Ø5 ☑
      right S61.2Ø4 ☑
        with damage to nail S61.3Ø4 ☑
  flank — *see* Wound, open, abdomen, wall
  foot (except toe(s) alone) S91.3Ø- ☑
    with amputation — *see* Amputation, traumatic, foot
    bite — *see* Bite, foot
    laceration — *see* Laceration, foot
    puncture — *see* Puncture, foot
    toe — *see* Wound, open, toe
  forearm S51.8Ø- ☑
    with
      amputation — *see* Amputation, traumatic, forearm
    bite — *see* Bite, forearm
    elbow only — *see* Wound, open, elbow
    laceration — *see* Laceration, forearm
    puncture — *see* Puncture, forearm
  forehead — *see* Wound, open, head, specified site NEC
  genital organs, external
    with amputation — *see* Amputation, traumatic, genital organs
    bite — *see* Bite, genital organ
    female S31.5Ø2 ☑
      vagina S31.4Ø ☑
      vulva S31.4Ø ☑
    laceration — *see* Laceration, genital organ
    male S31.5Ø1 ☑
      penis S31.2Ø ☑
      scrotum S31.3Ø ☑
      testes S31.3Ø ☑
    puncture — *see* Puncture, genital organ
  globe (eye) — *see* Wound, open, ocular
  groin — *see* Wound, open, abdomen, wall
  gum — *see* Wound, open, oral cavity

Wound, open — *continued*
 thigh S71.10- ☑
  with amputation — *see* Amputation, traumatic, hip
  bite — *see* Bite, thigh
  laceration — *see* Laceration, thigh
  puncture — *see* Puncture, thigh
 thorax, thoracic (wall) S21.90 ☑
  back S21.20- ☑
   with penetration S21.40 ☑
  bite — *see* Bite, thorax
  breast — *see* Wound, open, breast
  front S21.10- ☑
   with penetration S21.30 ☑
  laceration — *see* Laceration, thorax
  puncture — *see* Puncture, thorax
 throat — *see* Wound, open, neck
 thumb S61.009 ☑
  with
   amputation — *see* Amputation, traumatic, thumb
   damage to nail S61.109 ☑
  bite — *see* Bite, thumb
  laceration — *see* Laceration, thumb
  left S61.002 ☑
   with
    damage to nail S61.102 ☑
   puncture — *see* Puncture, thumb
  right S61.001 ☑
   with
    damage to nail S61.101 ☑
 thyroid (gland) — *see* Wound, open, neck, thyroid
 toe(s) S91.109 ☑
  with
   amputation — *see* Amputation, traumatic, toe
   damage to nail S91.209 ☑
  bite — *see* Bite, toe
  great S91.103 ☑
   with
    damage to nail S91.203 ☑
   left S91.102 ☑
    with
     damage to nail S91.202 ☑
   right S91.101 ☑
    with
     damage to nail S91.201 ☑
   laceration — *see* Laceration, toe
  lesser S91.106 ☑
   with
    damage to nail S91.206 ☑
   left S91.105 ☑
    with
     damage to nail S91.205 ☑
   right S91.104 ☑
    with
     damage to nail S91.204 ☑
  puncture — *see* Puncture, toe
 tongue — *see* Wound, open, oral cavity
 trachea (cervical region) — *see* Wound, open, neck, trachea
 tunica vaginalis — *see* Wound, open, testis
 tympanum, tympanic membrane S09.2- ☑
  laceration — *see* Laceration, ear, drum
  puncture — *see* Puncture, tympanum
 umbilical region — *see* Wound, open, abdomen, wall, periumbilic region
 uvula — *see* Wound, open, oral cavity
 vagina S31.40 ☑
  bite S31.45 ☑
  laceration — *see* Laceration, vagina
  puncture — *see* Puncture, vagina
 vitreous (humor) — *see* Wound, open, ocular
 vocal cord S11.039 ☑
  bite — *see* Bite, vocal cord
  laceration S11.031 ☑
   with foreign body S11.032 ☑
  puncture S11.033 ☑
   with foreign body S11.034 ☑
 vulva S31.40 ☑
  with amputation — *see* Amputation, traumatic, vulva
  bite S31.45 ☑
  laceration — *see* Laceration, vulva
  puncture — *see* Puncture, vulva
 wrist S61.50- ☑
  bite — *see* Bite, wrist

Wound, open — *continued*
 wrist — *continued*
  laceration — *see* Laceration, wrist
  puncture — *see* Puncture, wrist
Wound, superficial — *see* Injury — *see also* specified injury type
Wright's syndrome G54.0
Wrist — *see* condition
Wrong drug (by accident) (given in error) — *see* Table of Drugs and Chemicals, by drug, poisoning
Wry neck — *see* Torticollis
Wuchereria (bancrofti) **infestation** B74.0
Wuchereriasis B74.0
Wuchernde Struma Langhans C73

X

Xanthelasma (eyelid) (palpebrarum) H02.60
 left H02.66
  lower H02.65
  upper H02.64
 right H02.63
  lower H02.62
  upper H02.61
Xanthelasmatosis (essential) E78.2
Xanthinuria, hereditary E79.8
Xanthoastrocytoma
 specified site — *see* Neoplasm, malignant, by site
 unspecified site C71.9
Xanthofibroma — *see* Neoplasm, connective tissue, benign
Xanthogranuloma D76.3
Xanthoma(s), xanthomatosis (primary) (familial) (hereditary) E75.5
 with
  hyperlipoproteinemia
   Type I E78.3
   Type III E78.2
   Type IV E78.1
   Type V E78.3
 bone (generalisata) C96.5
 cerebrotendinous E75.5
 cutaneotendinous E75.5
 disseminatum (skin) E78.2
 eruptive E78.2
 hypercholesterinemic E78.00
 hypercholesterolemic E78.00
 hyperlipidemic E78.5
 joint E75.5
 multiple (skin) E78.2
 tendon (sheath) E75.5
 tuberosum E78.2
 tuberous E78.2
 tubo-eruptive E78.2
 verrucous, oral mucosa K13.4
Xanthosis R23.8
Xenophobia F40.10
Xeroderma — *see also* Ichthyosis
 acquired L85.0
 eyelid H01.149
  left H01.146
   lower H01.145
   upper H01.144
  right H01.143
   lower H01.142
   upper H01.141
 pigmentosum Q82.1
 vitamin A deficiency E50.8
Xerophthalmia (vitamin A deficiency) E50.7
 unrelated to vitamin A deficiency — *see* Keratoconjunctivitis
Xerosis
 conjunctiva H11.14- ☑
  with Bitot's spots — *see also* Pigmentation, conjunctiva
   vitamin A deficiency E50.1
  vitamin A deficiency E50.0
 cornea H18.89- ☑
  with ulceration — *see* Ulcer, cornea
   vitamin A deficiency E50.3
  vitamin A deficiency E50.2
 cutis L85.3
 skin L85.3
Xerostomia K11.7
Xiphopagus Q89.4
XO syndrome Q96.9

X-ray (of)
 abnormal findings — *see* Abnormal, diagnostic imaging
 breast (mammogram) (routine) Z12.31
 chest
  routine (as part of a general medical examination) Z00.00
   with abnormal findings Z00.01
  routine (as part of a general medical examination) Z00.00
   with abnormal findings Z00.01
XXXXY syndrome Q98.1
XXY syndrome Q98.0

Y

Yaba pox (virus disease) B08.72
Yatapoxvirus B08.70
 specified NEC B08.79
Yawning R06.89
 psychogenic F45.8
Yaws A66.9
 bone lesions A66.6
 butter A66.1
 chancre A66.0
 cutaneous, less than five years after infection A66.2
 early (cutaneous) (macular) (maculopapular) (micropapular) (papular) A66.2
  frambeside A66.2
  skin lesions NEC A66.2
 eyelid A66.6
 ganglion A66.6
 gangosis, gangosa A66.5
 gumma, gummata A66.4
  bone A66.6
 gummatous
  frambeside A66.4
  osteitis A66.6
  periostitis A66.6
 hydrarthrosis — *see also* subcategory M14.8- A66.6
 hyperkeratosis (early) (late) A66.3
 initial lesions A66.0
 joint lesions — *see also* subcategory M14.8- A66.6
 juxta-articular nodules A66.7
 late nodular (ulcerated) A66.4
 latent (without clinical manifestations) (with positive serology) A66.8
 mother A66.0
 mucosal A66.7
 multiple papillomata A66.1
 nodular, late (ulcerated) A66.4
 osteitis A66.6
 papilloma, plantar or palmar A66.1
 periostitis (hypertrophic) A66.6
 specified NEC A66.7
 ulcers A66.4
 wet crab A66.1
Yeast infection — *see also* Candidiasis B37.9
Yellow
 atrophy (liver) — *see* Failure, hepatic
 fever — *see* Fever, yellow
 jack — *see* Fever, yellow
 jaundice — *see* Jaundice
 nail syndrome L60.5
Yersiniosis — *see also* Infection, Yersinia
 extraintestinal A28.2
 intestinal A04.6

Z

Zahorsky's syndrome (herpangina) B08.5
Zellweger's syndrome E71.510
Zenker's diverticulum (esophagus) K22.5
Ziehen-Oppenheim disease G24.1
Zieve's syndrome K70.0
Zika NOS A92.5
 congenital P35.4
Zinc
 deficiency, dietary E60
 metabolism disorder E83.2
Zollinger-Ellison syndrome E16.4
Zona — *see* Herpes, zoster
Zoophobia F40.218
Zoster (herpes) — *see* Herpes, zoster
Zygomycosis B46.9
 specified NEC B46.8
Zymotic — *see* condition

Neoplasm, abdomen, abdominal — Neoplasm, bile or biliary

Handwritten note: Mal neoplasm transplanted organ C80.2

Note: The list below gives the code number for neoplasms by anatomical site. For each site there are six possible code numbers according to whether the neoplasm in question is malignant, benign, in situ, of uncertain behavior, or of unspecified nature. The description of the neoplasm will often indicate which of the six columns is appropriate; e.g., malignant melanoma of skin, benign fibroadenoma of breast, carcinoma in situ of cervix uteri. Where such descriptors are not present, the remainder of the Index should be consulted where guidance is given to the appropriate column for each morphological (histological) variety listed; e.g., Mesonephroma – see Neoplasm, malignant; Embryoma — see also Neoplasm, uncertain behavior; Disease, Bowen's – see Neoplasm, skin, in situ. However, the guidance in the Index can be overridden if one of the descriptors mentioned above is present; e.g., malignant adenoma of colon is coded to C18.9 and not to D12.6 as the adjective "malignant" overrides the Index entry "Adenoma — see also Neoplasm, benign, by site." Codes listed with a dash -, following the code have a required additional character for laterality. The tabular list must be reviewed for the complete code.

	Malignant Primary	Malignant Secondary	Ca in situ	Benign	Uncertain Behavior	Unspecified Behavior
Neoplasm, neoplastic	C80.1	C79.9	D09.9	D36.9	D48.9	D49.9
abdomen, abdominal	C76.2	C79.8-☑	D09.8	D36.7	D48.7	D49.89
cavity	C76.2	C79.8-☑	D09.8	D36.7	D48.7	D49.89
organ	C76.2	C79.8-☑	D09.8	D36.7	D48.7	D49.89
viscera	C76.2	C79.8-☑	D09.8	D36.7	D48.7	D49.89
wall — *see also* Neoplasm, abdomen, wall, skin	C44.509	C79.2	D04.5	D23.5	D48.5	D49.2
connective tissue	C49.4	C79.8-☑	—	D21.4	D48.1	D49.2
skin	C44.509	—	—	—	—	—
basal cell carcinoma	C44.519	—	—	—	—	—
specified type NEC	C44.599	—	—	—	—	—
squamous cell carcinoma	C44.529	—	—	—	—	—
abdominopelvic	C76.8	C79.8-☑	—	D36.7	D48.7	D49.89
accessory sinus — *see* Neoplasm, sinus						
acoustic nerve	C72.4-☑	C79.49	—	D33.3	D43.3	D49.7
adenoid (pharynx) (tissue)	C11.1	C79.89	D00.08	D10.6	D37.05	D49.0
adipose tissue — *see also* Neoplasm, connective tissue	C49.4	C79.89	—	D21.9	D48.1	D49.2
adnexa (uterine)	C57.4	C79.89	D07.39	D28.7	D39.8	D49.59
adrenal	C74.9-☑	C79.7-☑	D09.3	D35.0-☑	D44.1-☑	D49.7
capsule	C74.9-☑	C79.7-☑	D09.3	D35.0-☑	D44.1-☑	D49.7
cortex	C74.0-☑	C79.7-☑	D09.3	D35.0-☑	D44.1-☑	D49.7
gland	C74.9-☑	C79.7-☑	D09.3	D35.0-☑	D44.1-☑	D49.7
medulla	C74.1-☑	C79.7-☑	D09.3	D35.0-☑	D44.1-☑	D49.7
ala nasi (external) — *see also* Neoplasm, skin, nose	C44.301	C79.2	D04.39	D23.39	D48.5	D49.2
alimentary canal or tract NEC	C26.9	C78.80	D01.9	D13.9	D37.9	D49.0
alveolar	C03.9	C79.89	D00.03	D10.39	D37.09	D49.0
mucosa	C03.9	C79.89	D00.03	D10.39	D37.09	D49.0
lower	C03.1	C79.89	D00.03	D10.39	D37.09	D49.0
upper	C03.0	C79.89	D00.03	D10.39	D37.09	D49.0
ridge or process	C41.1	C79.51	—	D16.5	D48.0	D49.2
carcinoma	C03.9	C79.8-☑	—	—	—	—
lower	C03.1	C79.8-☑	—	—	—	—
upper	C03.0	C79.8-☑	—	—	—	—
lower	C41.1	C79.51	—	D16.5	D48.0	D49.2
mucosa	C03.9	C79.89	D00.03	D10.39	D37.09	D49.0
lower	C03.1	C79.89	D00.03	D10.39	D37.09	D49.0
upper	C03.0	C79.89	D00.03	D10.39	D37.09	D49.0
upper	C41.0	C79.51	—	D16.4	D48.0	D49.2
sulcus	C06.1	C79.89	D00.02	D10.39	D37.09	D49.0
alveolus	C03.9	C79.89	D00.03	D10.39	D37.09	D49.0
lower	C03.1	C79.89	D00.03	D10.39	D37.09	D49.0
upper	C03.0	C79.89	D00.03	D10.39	D37.09	D49.0
ampulla of Vater	C24.1	C78.89	D01.5	D13.5	D37.6	D49.0
ankle NEC	C76.5-☑	C79.89	D04.7-☑	D36.7	D48.7	D49.89
anorectum, anorectal (junction)	C21.8	C78.5	D01.3	D12.9	D37.8	D49.0
antecubital fossa or space	C76.4-☑	C79.89	D04.6-☑	D36.7	D48.7	D49.89

	Malignant Primary	Malignant Secondary	Ca in situ	Benign	Uncertain Behavior	Unspecified Behavior
Neoplasm, neoplastic — *continued*						
antrum (Highmore) (maxillary)	C31.0	C78.39	D02.3	D14.0	D38.5	D49.1
pyloric	C16.3	C78.89	D00.2	D13.1	D37.1	D49.0
tympanicum	C30.1	C78.39	D02.3	D14.0	D38.5	D49.1
anus, anal	C21.0	C78.5	D01.3	D12.9	D37.8	D49.0
canal	C21.1	C78.5	D01.3	D12.9	D37.8	D49.0
cloacogenic zone	C21.2	C78.5	D01.3	D12.9	D37.8	D49.0
margin — *see also* Neoplasm, anus, skin	C44.500	C79.2	D04.5	D23.5	D48.5	D49.2
overlapping lesion with rectosigmoid junction or rectum	C21.8	—	—	—	—	—
skin	C44.500	C79.2	D04.5	D23.5	D48.5	D49.2
basal cell carcinoma	C44.510	—	—	—	—	—
specified type NEC	C44.590	—	—	—	—	—
squamous cell carcinoma	C44.520	—	—	—	—	—
sphincter	C21.1	C78.5	D01.3	D12.9	D37.8	D49.0
aorta (thoracic)	C49.3	C79.89	—	D21.3	D48.1	D49.2
abdominal	C49.4	C79.89	—	D21.4	D48.1	D49.2
aortic body	C75.5	C79.89	—	D35.6	D44.7	D49.7
aponeurosis	C49.9	C79.89	—	D21.9	D48.1	D49.2
palmar	C49.1-☑	C79.89	—	D21.1-☑	D48.1	D49.2
plantar	C49.2-☑	C79.89	—	D21.2-☑	D48.1	D49.2
appendix	C18.1	C78.5	D01.0	D12.1	D37.3	D49.0
arachnoid	C70.9	C79.49	—	D32.9	D42.9	D49.7
cerebral	C70.0	C79.32	—	D32.0	D42.0	D49.7
spinal	C70.1	C79.49	—	D32.1	D42.1	D49.7
areola	C50.0-☑	C79.81	D05-☑	D24-☑	D48.6-☑	D49.3
arm NEC	C76.4-☑	C79.89	D04.6-☑	D36.7	D48.7	D49.89
artery — *see* Neoplasm, connective tissue						
aryepiglottic fold	C13.1	C79.89	D00.08	D10.7	D37.05	D49.0
hypopharyngeal aspect	C13.1	C79.89	D00.08	D10.7	D37.05	D49.0
laryngeal aspect	C32.1	C78.39	D02.0	D14.1	D38.0	D49.1
marginal zone	C13.1	C79.89	D00.08	D10.7	D37.05	D49.0
arytenoid (cartilage)	C32.3	C78.39	D02.0	D14.1	D38.0	D49.1
fold — *see* Neoplasm, aryepiglottic						
associated with transplanted organ	C80.2	—	—	—	—	—
atlas	C41.2	C79.51	—	D16.6	D48.0	D49.2
atrium, cardiac	C38.0	C79.89	—	D15.1	D48.7	D49.89
auditory						
canal (external) (skin)	C44.20-☑	C79.2	D04.2-☑	D23.2-☑	D48.5	D49.2
internal	C30.1	C78.39	D02.3	D14.0	D38.5	D49.1
nerve	C72.4-☑	C79.49	—	D33.3	D43.3	D49.7
tube	C30.1	C78.39	D02.3	D14.0	D38.5	D49.1
opening	C11.2	C79.89	D00.08	D10.6	D37.05	D49.0
auricle, ear — *see also* Neoplasm, skin, ear	C44.20-☑	C79.2	D04.2-☑	D23.2-☑	D48.5	D49.2
auricular canal (external) — *see also* Neoplasm, skin, ear	C44.20-☑	C79.2	D04.2-☑	D23.2-☑	D48.5	D49.2
internal	C30.1	C78.39	D02.3	D14.0	D38.5	D49.2
autonomic nerve or nervous system NEC (*see* Neoplasm, nerve, peripheral)						
axilla, axillary	C76.1	C79.89	D09.8	D36.7	D48.7	D49.89
fold — *see also* Neoplasm, skin, trunk	C44.509	C79.2	D04.5	D23.5	D48.5	D49.2
back NEC	C76.8	C79.89	D04.5	D36.7	D48.7	D49.89
Bartholin's gland	C51.0	C79.82	D07.1	D28.0	D39.8	D49.59
basal ganglia	C71.0	C79.31	—	D33.0	D43.0	D49.6
basis pedunculi	C71.7	C79.31	—	D33.1	D43.1	D49.6
bile or biliary (tract)	C24.9	C78.89	D01.5	D13.5	D37.6	D49.0

	Malignant Primary	Malignant Secondary	Ca in situ	Benign	Uncertain Behavior	Unspecified Behavior
Neoplasm, neoplastic — *continued*						
bile or biliary — *continued*						
canaliculi (biliferi) (intrahepatic)	C22.1	C78.7	D01.5	D13.4	D37.6	D49.0
canals, interlobular	C22.1	C78.89	D01.5	D13.4	D37.6	D49.0
duct or passage (common) (cystic) (extrahepatic)	C24.0	C78.89	D01.5	D13.5	D37.6	D49.0
interlobular	C22.1	C78.89	D01.5	D13.4	D37.6	D49.0
intrahepatic	C22.1	C78.7	D01.5	D13.4	D37.6	D49.0
and extrahepatic	C24.8	C78.89	D01.5	D13.5	D37.6	D49.0
bladder (urinary)	C67.9	C79.11	D09.0	D30.3	D41.4	D49.4
dome	C67.1	C79.11	D09.0	D30.3	D41.4	D49.4
neck	C67.5	C79.11	D09.0	D30.3	D41.4	D49.4
orifice	C67.9	C79.11	D09.0	D30.3	D41.4	D49.4
ureteric	C67.6	C79.11	D09.0	D30.3	D41.4	D49.4
urethral	C67.5	C79.11	D09.0	D30.3	D41.4	D49.4
overlapping lesion	C67.8	—	—	—	—	—
sphincter	C67.8	C79.11	D09.0	D30.3	D41.4	D49.4
trigone	C67.0	C79.11	D09.0	D30.3	D41.4	D49.4
urachus	C67.7	C79.11	D09.0	D30.3	D41.4	D49.4
wall	C67.9	C79.11	D09.0	D30.3	D41.4	D49.4
anterior	C67.3	C79.11	D09.0	D30.3	D41.4	D49.4
lateral	C67.2	C79.11	D09.0	D30.3	D41.4	D49.4
posterior	C67.4	C79.11	D09.0	D30.3	D41.4	D49.4
blood vessel — *see* Neoplasm, connective tissue						
bone (periosteum)	C41.9	C79.51	—	D16.9-	D48.0	D49.2
acetabulum						
ankle	C40.3-☑	C79.51	—	D16.3-☑	—	—
arm NEC	C40.0-☑	C79.51	—	D16.0-☑	—	—
astragalus	C40.3-☑	C79.51	—	D16.3-☑	—	—
atlas	C41.2	C79.51	—	D16.6	D48.0	D49.2
axis	C41.2	C79.51	—	D16.6	D48.0	D49.2
back NEC	C41.2	C79.51	—	D16.6	D48.0	D49.2
calcaneus	C40.3-☑	C79.51	—	D16.3-☑	—	—
calvarium	C41.0	C79.51	—	D16.4	D48.0	D49.2
carpus (any)	C40.1-☑	C79.51	—	D16.1-☑	—	—
cartilage NEC	C41.9	C79.51	—	D16.9	D48.0	D49.2
clavicle	C41.3	C79.51	—	D16.7	D48.0	D49.2
clivus	C41.0	C79.51	—	D16.4	D48.0	D49.2
coccygeal vertebra	C41.4	C79.51	—	D16.8	D48.0	D49.2
coccyx	C41.4	C79.51	—	D16.8	D48.0	D49.2
costal cartilage	C41.3	C79.51	—	D16.7	D48.0	D49.2
costovertebral joint	C41.3	C79.51	—	D16.7	D48.0	D49.2
cranial	C41.0	C79.51	—	D16.4	D48.0	D49.2
cuboid	C40.3-☑	C79.51	—	D16.3-☑	—	—
cuneiform	C41.9	C79.51	—	D16.9	D48.0	D49.2
elbow	C40.0-☑	C79.51	—	D16.0-☑	—	—
ethmoid (labyrinth)	C41.0	C79.51	—	D16.4	D48.0	D49.2
face	C41.0	C79.51	—	D16.4	D48.0	D49.2
femur (any part)	C40.2-☑	C79.51	—	D16.2-☑	—	—
fibula (any part)	C40.2-☑	C79.51	—	D16.2-☑	—	—
finger (any)	C40.1-☑	C79.51	—	D16.1-☑	—	—
foot	C40.3-☑	C79.51	—	D16.3-☑	—	—
forearm	C40.0-☑	C79.51	—	D16.0-☑	—	—
frontal	C41.0	C79.51	—	D16.4	D48.0	D49.2
hand	C40.1-☑	C79.51	—	D16.1-☑	—	—
heel	C40.3-☑	C79.51	—	D16.3-☑	—	—
hip	C41.4	C79.51	—	D16.8	D48.0	D49.2
humerus (any part)	C40.0-☑	C79.51	—	D16.0-☑	—	—
hyoid	C41.0	C79.51	—	D16.4	D48.0	D49.2
ilium	C41.4	C79.51	—	D16.8	D48.0	D49.2
innominate	C41.4	C79.51	—	D16.8	D48.0	D49.2
intervertebral cartilage or disc	C41.2	C79.51	—	D16.6	D48.0	D49.2
ischium	C41.4	C79.51	—	D16.8	D48.0	D49.2
jaw (lower)	C41.1	C79.51	—	D16.5	D48.0	D49.2
knee	C40.2-☑	C79.51	—	D16.2-☑	—	—
leg NEC	C40.2-☑	C79.51	—	D16.2-☑	—	—
limb NEC	C40.9-☑	C79.51	—	D16.9	—	—

	Malignant Primary	Malignant Secondary	Ca in situ	Benign	Uncertain Behavior	Unspecified Behavior
Neoplasm, neoplastic — *continued*						
bone — *continued*						
limb — *continued*						
lower (long bones)	C40.2-☑	C79.51	—	D16.2-☑	—	—
short bones	C40.3-☑	C79.51	—	D16.3-☑	—	—
upper (long bones)	C40.0-☑	C79.51	—	D16.0-☑	—	—
short bones	C40.1-☑	C79.51	—	D16.1-☑	—	—
malar	C41.0	C79.51	—	D16.4	D48.0	D49.2
mandible	C41.1	C79.51	—	D16.5	D48.0	D49.2
marrow NEC (any bone)	C96.9	C79.52	—	—	D47.9	D49.89
mastoid	C41.0	C79.51	—	D16.4	D48.0	D49.2
maxilla, maxillary (superior)	C41.0	C79.51	—	D16.4	D48.0	D49.2
inferior	C41.1	C79.51	—	D16.5	D48.0	D49.2
metacarpus (any)	C40.1-☑	C79.51	—	D16.1-☑	—	—
metatarsus (any)	C40.3-☑	C79.51	—	D16.3-☑	—	—
navicular						
ankle	C40.3-☑	C79.51	—	—	—	—
hand	C40.1-☑	C79.51	—	—	—	—
nose, nasal	C41.0	C79.51	—	D16.4	D48.0	D49.2
occipital	C41.0	C79.51	—	D16.4	D48.0	D49.2
orbit	C41.0	C79.51	—	D16.4	D48.0	D49.2
overlapping sites	C40.8-☑	—	—	—	—	—
parietal	C41.0	C79.51	—	D16.4	D48.0	D49.2
patella	C40.2-☑	C79.51	—	—	—	—
pelvic	C41.4	C79.51	—	D16.8	D48.0	D49.2
phalanges						
foot	C40.3-☑	C79.51	—	—	—	—
hand	C40.1-☑	C79.51	—	—	—	—
pubic	C41.4	C79.51	—	D16.8	D48.0	D49.2
radius (any part)	C40.0-☑	C79.51	—	D16.0-☑	—	—
rib	C41.3	C79.51	—	D16.7	D48.0	D49.2
sacral vertebra	C41.4	C79.51	—	D16.8	D48.0	D49.2
sacrum	C41.4	C79.51	—	D16.8	D48.0	D49.2
scaphoid						
of ankle	C40.3-☑	C79.51	—	—	—	—
of hand	C40.1-☑	C79.51	—	—	—	—
scapula (any part)	C40.0-☑	C79.51	—	D16.0-☑	—	—
sella turcica	C41.0	C79.51	—	D16.4	D48.0	D49.2
shoulder	C40.0-☑	C79.51	—	D16.0-☑	—	—
skull	C41.0	C79.51	—	D16.4	D48.0	D49.2
sphenoid	C41.0	C79.51	—	D16.4	D48.0	D49.2
spine, spinal (column)	C41.2	C79.51	—	D16.6	D48.0	D49.2
coccyx	C41.4	C79.51	—	D16.8	D48.0	D49.2
sacrum	C41.4	C79.51	—	D16.8	D48.0	D49.2
sternum	C41.3	C79.51	—	D16.7	D48.0	D49.2
tarsus (any)	C40.3-☑	C79.51	—	—	—	—
temporal	C41.0	C79.51	—	D16.4	D48.0	D49.2
thumb	C40.1-☑	C79.51	—	—	—	—
tibia (any part)	C40.2-☑	C79.51	—	—	—	—
toe (any)	C40.3-☑	C79.51	—	—	—	—
trapezium	C40.1-☑	C79.51	—	—	—	—
trapezoid	C40.1-☑	C79.51	—	—	—	—
turbinate	C41.0	C79.51	—	D16.4	D48.0	D49.2
ulna (any part)	C40.0-☑	C79.51	—	D16.0-☑	—	—
unciform	C40.1-☑	C79.51	—	—	—	—
vertebra (column)	C41.2	C79.51	—	D16.6	D48.0	D49.2
coccyx	C41.4	C79.51	—	D16.8	D48.0	D49.2
sacrum	C41.4	C79.51	—	D16.8	D48.0	D49.2
vomer	C41.0	C79.51	—	D16.4	D48.0	D49.2
wrist	C40.1-☑	C79.51	—	—	—	—
xiphoid process	C41.3	C79.51	—	D16.7	D48.0	D49.2
zygomatic	C41.0	C79.51	—	D16.4	D48.0	D49.2
book-leaf (mouth) — *ventral surface of tongue and floor of mouth*	C06.89	C79.89	D00.00	D10.39	D37.09	D49.0
bowel — *see* Neoplasm, intestine						
brachial plexus	C47.1-☑	C79.89	—	D36.12	D48.2	D49.2
brain NEC	C71.9	C79.31	—	D33.2	D43.2	D49.6

Neoplasm, neoplastic — continued

	Malignant Primary	Malignant Secondary	Ca in situ	Benign	Uncertain Behavior	Unspecified Behavior
brain — *continued*						
basal ganglia	C71.0	C79.31	—	D33.0	D43.0	D49.6
cerebellopontine angle	C71.6	C79.31	—	D33.1	D43.1	D49.6
cerebellum NOS	C71.6	C79.31	—	D33.1	D43.1	D49.6
cerebrum	C71.0	C79.31	—	D33.0	D43.0	D49.6
choroid plexus	C71.7	C79.31	—	D33.1	D43.1	D49.6
corpus callosum	C71.8	C79.31	—	D33.2	D43.2	D49.6
corpus striatum	C71.0	C79.31	—	D33.0	D43.0	D49.6
cortex (cerebral)	C71.0	C79.31	—	D33.0	D43.0	D49.6
frontal lobe	C71.1	C79.31	—	D33.0	D43.0	D49.6
globus pallidus	C71.0	C79.31	—	D33.0	D43.0	D49.6
hippocampus	C71.2	C79.31	—	D33.0	D43.0	D49.6
hypothalamus	C71.0	C79.31	—	D33.0	D43.0	D49.6
internal capsule	C71.0	C79.31	—	D33.0	D43.0	D49.6
medulla oblongata	C71.7	C79.31	—	D33.1	D43.1	D49.6
meninges	C70.0	C79.32	—	D32.0	D42.0	D49.7
midbrain	C71.7	C79.31	—	D33.1	D43.1	D49.6
occipital lobe	C71.4	C79.31	—	D33.0	D43.0	D49.6
overlapping lesion	C71.8	C79.31	—	—	—	—
parietal lobe	C71.3	C79.31	—	D33.0	D43.0	D49.6
peduncle	C71.7	C79.31	—	D33.1	D43.1	D49.6
pons	C71.7	C79.31	—	D33.1	D43.1	D49.6
stem	C71.7	C79.31	—	D33.1	D43.1	D49.6
tapetum	C71.8	C79.31	—	D33.2	D43.2	D49.6
temporal lobe	C71.2	C79.31	—	D33.0	D43.0	D49.6
thalamus	C71.0	C79.31	—	D33.0	D43.0	D49.6
uncus	C71.2	C79.31	—	D33.0	D43.0	D49.6
ventricle (floor)	C71.5	C79.31	—	D33.0	D43.0	D49.6
fourth	C71.7	C79.31	—	D33.1	D43.1	D49.6
branchial (cleft) (cyst) (vestiges)	C10.4	C79.89	D00.08	D10.5	D37.05	D49.0
breast (connective tissue) (glandular tissue) (soft parts)	C50.9-✓	C79.81	D05.-✓	D24.-✓	D48.6-✓	D49.3
areola	C50.0-✓	C79.81	D05.-✓	D24.-✓	D48.6-✓	D49.3
axillary tail	C50.6-✓	C79.81	D05.-✓	D24.-✓	D48.6-✓	D49.3
central portion	C50.1-✓	C79.81	D05.-✓	D24.-✓	D48.6-✓	D49.3
inner	C50.8-✓	C79.81	D05.-✓	D24.-✓	D48.6-✓	D49.3
lower	C50.8-✓	C79.81	D05.-✓	D24.-✓	D48.6-✓	D49.3
lower-inner quadrant	C50.3-✓	C79.81	D05.-✓	D24.-✓	D48.6-✓	D49.3
lower-outer quadrant	C50.5-✓	C79.81	D05.-✓	D24.-✓	D48.6-✓	D49.3
mastectomy site (skin) — *see also* Neoplasm, breast, skin	C44.501	C79.2	—	—	—	—
specified as breast tissue	C50.8-✓	C79.81	—	—	—	—
midline	C50.8-✓	C79.81	D05.-✓	D24.-✓	D48.6-✓	D49.3
nipple	C50.0-✓	C79.81	D05.-✓	D24.-✓	D48.6-✓	D49.3
outer	C50.8-✓	C79.81	D05.-✓	D24.-✓	D48.6-✓	D49.3
overlapping lesion	C50.8-✓	—	—	—	—	—
skin	C44.501	C79.2	D04.5	D23.5	D48.5	D49.2
basal cell carcinoma	C44.511	—	—	—	—	—
specified type NEC	C44.591	—	—	—	—	—
squamous cell carcinoma	C44.521	—	—	—	—	—
tail (axillary)	C50.6-✓	C79.81	D05.-✓	D24.-✓	D48.6-✓	D49.3
upper	C50.8-✓	C79.81	D05.-✓	D24.-✓	D48.6-✓	D49.3
upper-inner quadrant	C50.2-✓	C79.81	D05.-✓	D24.-✓	D48.6-✓	D49.3
upper-outer quadrant	C50.4-✓	C79.81	D05.-✓	D24.-✓	D48.6-✓	D49.3
broad ligament	C57.1-✓	C79.82	D07.39	D28.2	D39.8	D49.59
bronchiogenic, bronchogenic (lung)	C34.9-✓	C78.0-✓	D02.2-✓	D14.3-✓	D38.1	D49.1
bronchiole	C34.9-✓	C78.0-✓	D02.2-✓	D14.3-✓	D38.1	D49.1
bronchus	C34.9-✓	C78.0-✓	D02.2-✓	D14.3-✓	D38.1	D49.1
carina	C34.0-✓	C78.0-✓	D02.2-✓	D14.3-✓	D38.1	D49.1
lower lobe of lung	C34.3-✓	C78.0-✓	D02.2-✓	D14.3-✓	D38.1	D49.1

Neoplasm, neoplastic — continued

	Malignant Primary	Malignant Secondary	Ca in situ	Benign	Uncertain Behavior	Unspecified Behavior
bronchus — *continued*						
main	C34.0-✓	C78.0-✓	D02.2-✓	D14.3-✓	D38.1	D49.1
middle lobe of lung	C34.2	C78.0-✓	D02.21	D14.31	D38.1	D49.1
overlapping lesion	C34.8-✓	—	—	—	—	—
upper lobe of lung	C34.1-✓	C78.0-✓	D02.2-✓	D14.3-✓	D38.1	D49.1
brow	C44.309	C79.2	D04.39	D23.39	D48.5	D49.2
basal cell carcinoma	C44.319	—	—	—	—	—
specified type NEC	C44.399	—	—	—	—	—
squamous cell carcinoma	C44.329	—	—	—	—	—
buccal (cavity)	C06.9	C79.89	D00.00	D10.39	D37.09	D49.0
commissure	C06.0	C79.89	D00.02	D10.39	D37.09	D49.0
groove (lower) (upper)	C06.1	C79.89	D00.02	D10.39	D37.09	D49.0
mucosa	C06.0	C79.89	D00.02	D10.39	D37.09	D49.0
sulcus (lower) (upper)	C06.1	C79.89	D00.02	D10.39	D37.09	D49.0
bulbourethral gland	C68.0	C79.19	D09.19	D30.4	D41.3	D49.59
bursa — *see* Neoplasm, connective tissue						
buttock NEC	C76.3	C79.89	D04.5	D36.7	D48.7	D49.89
calf	C76.5-✓	C79.89	D04.7-✓	D36.7	D48.7	D49.89
calvarium	C41.0	C79.51	—	D16.4	D48.0	D49.2
calyx, renal	C65.-✓	C79.0-✓	D09.19	D30.1-✓	D41.1-✓	D49.51-✓
canal						
anal	C21.1	C78.5	D01.3	D12.9	D37.8	D49.0
auditory (external) — *see also* Neoplasm, skin, ear	C44.20-✓	C79.2	D04.2-✓	D23.2-✓	D48.5	D49.2
auricular (external) — *see also* Neoplasm, skin, ear	C44.20-✓	C79.2	D04.2-✓	D23.2-✓	D48.5	D49.2
canaliculi, biliary (biliferi) (intrahepatic)	C22.1	C78.7	D01.5	D13.4	D37.6	D49.0
canthus (eye) (inner) (outer)	C44.10-✓	C79.2	D04.1-✓	D23.1-✓	D48.5	D49.2
basal cell carcinoma	C44.11-✓	—	—	—	—	—
sebaceous cell	C44.13-✓	—	—	—	—	—
specified type NEC	C44.19-✓	—	—	—	—	—
squamous cell carcinoma	C44.12-✓	—	—	—	—	—
capillary — *see* Neoplasm, connective tissue						
caput coli	C18.0	C78.5	D01.0	D12.0	D37.4	D49.0
carcinoid — *see* Tumor, carcinoid						
cardia (gastric)	C16.0	C78.89	D00.2	D13.1	D37.1	D49.0
cardiac orifice (stomach)	C16.0	C78.89	D00.2	D13.1	D37.1	D49.0
cardio-esophageal junction	C16.0	C78.89	D00.2	D13.1	D37.1	D49.0
cardio-esophagus	C16.0	C78.89	D00.2	D13.1	D37.1	D49.0
carina (bronchus)	C34.0-✓	C78.0-✓	D02.2-✓	D14.3-✓	D38.1	D49.1
carotid (artery)	C49.0	C79.89	—	D21.0	D48.1	D49.2
body	C75.4	C79.89	—	D35.5	D44.6	D49.7
carpus (any bone)	C40.1-✓	C79.51	—	D16.1-✓	—	—
cartilage (articular) (joint) NEC — *see also* Neoplasm, bone,	C41.9	C79.51	—	D16.9	D48.0	D49.2
arytenoid	C32.3	C78.39	D02.0	D14.1	D38.0	D49.1
auricular	C49.0	C79.89	—	D21.0	D48.1	D49.2
bronchi	C34.0-✓	C78.39	—	D14.3-✓	D38.1	D49.1
costal	C41.3	C79.51	—	D16.7	D48.0	D49.2
cricoid	C32.3	C78.39	D02.0	D14.1	D38.0	D49.1
cuneiform	C32.3	C78.39	D02.0	D14.1	D38.0	D49.1
ear (external)	C49.0	C79.89	—	D21.0	D48.1	D49.2
ensiform	C41.3	C79.51	—	D16.7	D48.0	D49.2
epiglottis	C32.1	C78.39	D02.0	D14.1	D38.0	D49.1

✓ **Additional Character Required — Refer to the Tabular List for Character Selection**   ▽ Subterms under main terms may continue to next column or page

Neoplasm, neoplastic — continued	Malignant Primary	Malignant Secondary	Ca in situ	Benign	Uncertain Behavior	Unspecified Behavior
cartilage — see also Neoplasm, bone — continued						
epiglottis — continued						
anterior surface	C10.1	C79.89	D00.08	D10.5	D37.05	D49.0
eyelid	C49.0	C79.89	—	D21.0	D48.1	D49.2
intervertebral	C41.2	C79.51	—	D16.6	D48.0	D49.2
larynx, laryngeal	C32.3	C78.39	D02.0	D14.1	D38.0	D49.1
nose, nasal	C30.0	C78.39	D02.3	D14.0	D38.5	D49.1
pinna	C49.0	C79.89	—	D21.0	D48.1	D49.2
rib	C41.3	C79.51	—	D16.7	D48.0	D49.2
semilunar (knee)	C40.2-☑	C79.51	—	D16.2-☑	D48.0	D49.2
thyroid	C32.3	C78.39	D02.0	D14.1	D38.0	D49.1
trachea	C33	C78.39	D02.1	D14.2	D38.1	D49.1
cauda equina	C72.1	C79.49	—	D33.4	D43.4	D49.7
cavity						
buccal	C06.9	C79.89	D00.00	D10.30	D37.09	D49.0
nasal	C30.0	C78.39	D02.3	D14.0	D38.5	D49.1
oral	C06.9	C79.89	D00.00	D10.30	D37.09	D49.0
peritoneal	C48.2	C78.6	—	D20.1	D48.4	D49.0
tympanic	C30.1	C78.39	D02.3	D14.0	D38.5	D49.1
cecum	C18.0	C78.5	D01.0	D12.0	D37.4	D49.0
central nervous system	C72.9	C79.40	—	—	—	—
cerebellopontine (angle)	C71.6	C79.31		D33.1	D43.1	D49.6
cerebellum, cerebellar	C71.6	C79.31		D33.1	D43.1	D49.6
cerebrum, cerebra (cortex) (hemisphere) (white matter)	C71.0	C79.31	—	D33.0	D43.0	D49.6
meninges	C70.0	C79.32	—	D32.0	D42.0	D49.7
peduncle	C71.7	C79.31	—	D33.1	D43.1	D49.6
ventricle	C71.5	C79.31	—	D33.0	D43.0	D49.6
fourth	C71.7	C79.31	—	D33.1	D43.1	D49.6
cervical region	C76.0	C79.89	D09.8	D36.7	D48.7	D49.89
cervix (cervical) (uteri) (uterus)	C53.9	C79.82	D06.9	D26.0	D39.0	D49.59
canal	C53.0	C79.82	D06.0	D26.0	D39.0	D49.59
endocervix (canal) (gland)	C53.0	C79.82	D06.0	D26.0	D39.0	D49.59
exocervix	C53.1	C79.82	D06.1	D26.0	D39.0	D49.59
external os	C53.1	C79.82	D06.1	D26.0	D39.0	D49.59
internal os	C53.0	C79.82	D06.0	D26.0	D39.0	D49.59
nabothian gland	C53.0	C79.82	D06.0	D26.0	D39.0	D49.59
overlapping lesion	C53.8	—	—	—	—	—
squamocolumnar junction	C53.8	C79.82	D06.7	D26.0	D39.0	D49.59
stump	C53.8	C79.82	D06.7	D26.0	D39.0	D49.59
cheek	C76.0	C79.89	D09.8	D36.7	D48.7	D49.89
external	C44.309	C79.2	D04.39	D23.39	D48.5	D49.2
basal cell carcinoma	C44.319	—	—	—	—	—
specified type NEC	C44.399	—	—	—	—	—
squamous cell carcinoma	C44.329	—	—	—	—	—
inner aspect	C06.0	C79.89	D00.02	D10.39	D37.09	D49.0
internal	C06.0	C79.89	D00.02	D10.39	D37.09	D49.0
mucosa	C06.0	C79.89	D00.02	D10.39	D37.09	D49.0
chest (wall) NEC	C76.1	C79.89	D09.8	D36.7	D48.7	D49.89
chiasma opticum	C72.3-☑	C79.49	—	D33.3	D43.3	D49.7
chin	C44.309	C79.2	D04.39	D23.39	D48.5	D49.2
basal cell carcinoma	C44.319	—	—	—	—	—
specified type NEC	C44.399	—	—	—	—	—
squamous cell carcinoma	C44.329	—	—	—	—	—
choana	C11.3	C79.89	D00.08	D10.6	D37.05	D49.0
cholangiole	C22.1	C78.89	D01.5	D13.4	D37.6	D49.0
choledochal duct	C24.0	C78.89	D01.5	D13.5	D37.6	D49.0
choroid	C69.3-☑	C79.49	D09.2-☑	D31.3-☑	D48.7	D49.81
plexus	C71.5	C79.31	—	D33.0	D43.0	D49.6
ciliary body	C69.4-☑	C79.49	D09.2-☑	D31.4-☑	D48.7	D49.89
clavicle	C41.3	C79.51	—	D16.7	D48.0	D49.2

Neoplasm, neoplastic — continued	Malignant Primary	Malignant Secondary	Ca in situ	Benign	Uncertain Behavior	Unspecified Behavior
clitoris	C51.2	C79.82	D07.1	D28.0	D39.8	D49.59
clivus	C41.0	C79.51	—	D16.4	D48.0	D49.2
cloacogenic zone	C21.2	C78.5	D01.3	D12.9	D37.8	D49.0
coccygeal body or glomus	C49.5	C79.89	—	D21.5	D48.1	D49.2
vertebra	C41.4	C79.51	—	D16.8	D48.0	D49.2
coccyx	C41.4	C79.51	—	D16.8	D48.0	D49.2
colon — see also Neoplasm, intestine, large	C18.9	C78.5		—	—	—
with rectum	C19	C78.5	D01.1	D12.7	D37.5	D49.0
columnella — see also Neoplasm, skin, face	C44.390	C79.2	D04.39	D23.39	D48.5	D49.2
column, spinal — see Neoplasm, spine						
commissure						
labial, lip	C00.6	C79.89	D00.01	D10.39	D37.01	D49.0
laryngeal	C32.0	C78.39	D02.0	D14.1	D38.0	D49.1
common (bile) duct	C24.0	C78.89	D01.5	D13.5	D37.6	D49.0
concha — see also Neoplasm, skin, ear	C44.20-☑	C79.2	D04.2-☑	D23.2-☑	D48.5	D49.2
nose	C30.0	C78.39	D02.3	D14.0	D38.5	D49.1
conjunctiva	C69.0-☑	C79.49	D09.2-☑	D31.0-☑	D48.7	D49.89
connective tissue NEC	C49.9	C79.89	—	D21.9	D48.1	D49.2

Note: For neoplasms of connective tissue (blood vessel, bursa, fascia, ligament, muscle, peripheral nerves, sympathetic and parasympathetic nerves and ganglia, synovia, tendon, etc.) or of morphological types that indicate connective tissue, code according to the list under "Neoplasm, connective tissue". For sites that do not appear in this list, code to neoplasm of that site; e.g., fibrosarcoma, pancreas (C25.9)

Note: Morphological types that indicate connective tissue appear in their proper place in the alphabetic index with the instruction "see Neoplasm, connective tissue ...."

	Malignant Primary	Malignant Secondary	Ca in situ	Benign	Uncertain Behavior	Unspecified Behavior
abdomen	C49.4	C79.89	—	D21.4	D48.1	D49.2
abdominal wall	C49.4	C79.89	—	D21.4	D48.1	D49.2
ankle	C49.2-☑	C79.89	—	D21.2-☑	D48.1	D49.2
antecubital fossa or space	C49.1-☑	C79.89	—	D21.1-☑	D48.1	D49.2
arm	C49.0	C79.89	—	D21.0	D48.1	D49.2
auricle (ear)	C49.0	C79.89	—	D21.0	D48.1	D49.2
axilla	C49.3	C79.89	—	D21.3	D48.1	D49.2
back	C49.6	C79.89	—	D21.6	D48.1	D49.2
breast — see Neoplasm, breast						
buttock	C49.5	C79.89	—	D21.5	D48.1	D49.2
calf	C49.2-☑	C79.89	—	D21.2-☑	D48.1	D49.2
cervical region	C49.0	C79.89	—	D21.0	D48.1	D49.2
cheek	C49.0	C79.89	—	D21.0	D48.1	D49.2
chest (wall)	C49.3	C79.89	—	D21.3	D48.1	D49.2
chin	C49.0	C79.89	—	D21.0	D48.1	D49.2
diaphragm	C49.3	C79.89	—	D21.3	D48.1	D49.2
ear (external)	C49.0	C79.89	—	D21.0	D48.1	D49.2
elbow	C49.1-☑	C79.89	—	D21.1-☑	D48.1	D49.2
extrarectal	C49.5	C79.89	—	D21.5	D48.1	D49.2
extremity	C49.9	C79.89	—	D21.9	D48.1	D49.2
lower	C49.2-☑	C79.89	—	D21.2-☑	D48.1	D49.2
upper	C49.1-☑	C79.89	—	D21.1-☑	D48.1	D49.2
eyelid	C49.0	C79.89	—	D21.0	D48.1	D49.2
face	C49.0	C79.89	—	D21.0	D48.1	D49.2
finger	C49.1-☑	C79.89	—	D21.1-☑	D48.1	D49.2
flank	C49.6	C79.89	—	D21.6	D48.1	D49.2
foot	C49.2-☑	C79.89	—	D21.2-☑	D48.1	D49.2
forearm	C49.1-☑	C79.89	—	D21.1-☑	D48.1	D49.2
forehead	C49.0	C79.89	—	D21.0	D48.1	D49.2
gastric	C49.4	C79.89	—	D21.4	D48.1	D49.2
gastrointestinal	C49.4	C79.89	—	D21.4	D48.1	D49.2
gluteal region	C49.5	C79.89	—	D21.5	D48.1	D49.2
great vessels NEC	C49.3	C79.89	—	D21.3	D48.1	D49.2
groin	C49.5	C79.89	—	D21.5	D48.1	D49.2
hand	C49.1-☑	C79.89	—	D21.1-☑	D48.1	D49.2
head	C49.0	C79.89	—	D21.0	D48.1	D49.2

	Malignant Primary	Malignant Secondary	Ca in situ	Benign	Uncertain Behavior	Unspecified Behavior
Neoplasm, neoplastic						
— continued						
connective tissue —						
continued						
heel	C49.2-☑	C79.89	—	D21.2-☑	D48.1	D49.2
hip	C49.2-☑	C79.89	—	D21.2-☑	D48.1	D49.2
hypochondrium	C49.4	C79.89	—	D21.4	D48.1	D49.2
iliopsoas muscle	C49.5	C79.89	—	D21.5	D48.1	D49.2
infraclavicular						
region	C49.3	C79.89	—	D21.3	D48.1	D49.2
inguinal (canal)						
(region)	C49.5	C79.89	—	D21.5	D48.1	D49.2
intestinal	C49.4	C79.89	—	D21.4	D48.1	D49.2
intrathoracic	C49.3	C79.89	—	D21.3	D48.1	D49.2
ischiorectal						
fossa	C49.5	C79.89	—	D21.5	D48.1	D49.2
jaw	C03.9	C79.89	D00.03	D10.39	D48.1	D49.0
knee	C49.2-☑	C79.89	—	D21.2-☑	D48.1	D49.2
leg	C49.2-☑	C79.89	—	D21.2-☑	D48.1	D49.2
limb NEC	C49.9	C79.89	—	D21.9	D48.1	D49.2
lower	C49.2-☑	C79.89	—	D21.2-☑	D48.1	D49.2
upper	C49.1-☑	C79.89	—	D21.1-☑	D48.1	D49.2
nates	C49.5	C79.89	—	D21.5	D48.1	D49.2
neck	C49.0	C79.89	—	D21.0	D48.1	D49.2
orbit	C69.6-☑	C79.49	D09.2-☑	D31.6-☑	D48.1	D49.89
overlapping						
lesion	C49.8	—	—	—	—	—
pararectal	C49.5	C79.89	—	D21.5	D48.1	D49.2
para-urethral	C49.5	C79.89	—	D21.5	D48.1	D49.2
paravaginal	C49.5	C79.89	—	D21.5	D48.1	D49.2
pelvis (floor)	C49.5	C79.89	—	D21.5	D48.1	D49.2
pelvo-abdominal	C49.8	C79.89	—	D21.6	D48.1	D49.2
perineum	C49.5	C79.89	—	D21.5	D48.1	D49.2
perirectal						
(tissue)	C49.5	C79.89	—	D21.5	D48.1	D49.2
periurethral						
(tissue)	C49.5	C79.89	—	D21.5	D48.1	D49.2
popliteal fossa or						
space	C49.2-☑	C79.89	—	D21.2-☑	D48.1	D49.2
presacral	C49.5	C79.89	—	D21.5	D48.1	D49.2
psoas muscle	C49.4	C79.89	—	D21.4	D48.1	D49.2
pterygoid fossa	C49.0	C79.89	—	D21.0	D48.1	D49.2
rectovaginal septum						
or wall	C49.5	C79.89	—	D21.5	D48.1	D49.2
rectovesical	C49.5	C79.89	—	D21.5	D48.1	D49.2
retroperitoneum	C48.0	C78.6	—	D20.0	D48.3	D49.0
sacrococcygeal						
region	C49.5	C79.89	—	D21.5	D48.1	D49.2
scalp	C49.0	C79.89	—	D21.0	D48.1	D49.2
scapular region	C49.3	C79.89	—	D21.3	D48.1	D49.2
shoulder	C49.1-☑	C79.89	—	D21.1-☑	D48.1	D49.2
skin (dermis) NEC —						
see also						
Neoplasm, skin,						
by site	C44.90	C79.2	D04.9	D23.9	D48.5	D49.2
stomach	C49.4	C79.89	—	D21.4	D48.1	D49.2
submental	C49.0	C79.89	—	D21.0	D48.1	D49.2
supraclavicular						
region	C49.0	C79.89	—	D21.0	D48.1	D49.2
temple	C49.0	C79.89	—	D21.0	D48.1	D49.2
temporal region	C49.0	C79.89	—	D21.0	D48.1	D49.2
thigh	C49.2-☑	C79.89	—	D21.2-☑	D48.1	D49.2
thoracic (duct)						
(wall)	C49.3	C79.89	—	D21.3	D48.1	D49.2
thorax	C49.3	C79.89	—	D21.3	D48.1	D49.2
thumb	C49.1-☑	C79.89	—	D21.1-☑	D48.1	D49.2
toe	C49.2-☑	C79.89	—	D21.2-☑	D48.1	D49.2
trunk	C49.6	C79.89	—	D21.6	D48.1	D49.2
umbilicus	C49.4	C79.89	—	D21.4	D48.1	D49.2
vesicorectal	C49.5	C79.89	—	D21.5	D48.1	D49.2
wrist	C49.1-☑	C79.89	—	D21.1-☑	D48.1	D49.2
conus medullaris	C72.0	C79.49	—	D33.4	D43.4	D49.7
cord (true) (vocal)	C32.0	C78.39	D02.0	D14.1	D38.0	D49.1
false	C32.1	C78.39	D02.0	D14.1	D38.0	D49.1
spermatic	C63.1-☑	C79.82	D07.69	D29.8	D40.8	D49.59
spinal (cervical)						
(lumbar)						
(thoracic)	C72.0	C79.49	—	D33.4	D43.4	D49.7
cornea (limbus)	C69.1-☑	C79.49	D09.2-☑	D31.1-☑	D48.7	D49.89
corpus						
albicans	C56.-☑	C79.6-☑	D07.39	D27.-☑	D39.1-☑	D49.59
callosum, brain	C71.0	C79.31	—	D33.2	D43.2	D49.6

	Malignant Primary	Malignant Secondary	Ca in situ	Benign	Uncertain Behavior	Unspecified Behavior
Neoplasm, neoplastic						
— continued						
corpus — continued						
cavernosum	C60.2	C79.82	D07.4	D29.0	D40.8	D49.59
gastric	C16.2	C78.89	D00.2	D13.1	D37.1	D49.0
overlapping						
sites	C54.8	—	—	—	—	—
penis	C60.2	C79.82	D07.4	D29.0	D40.8	D49.59
striatum,						
cerebrum	C71.0	C79.31	—	D33.0	D43.0	D49.6
uteri	C54.9	C79.82	D07.0	D26.1	D39.0	D49.59
isthmus	C54.0	C79.82	D07.0	D26.1	D39.0	D49.59
cortex						
adrenal	C74.0-☑	C79.7-☑	D09.3	D35.0-☑	D44.1-☑	D49.7
cerebral	C71.0	C79.31	—	D33.0	D43.0	D49.6
costal cartilage	C41.3	C79.51	—	D16.7	D48.0	D49.2
costovertebral						
joint	C41.3	C79.51	—	D16.7	D48.0	D49.2
Cowper's gland	C68.0	C79.19	D09.19	D30.4	D41.3	D49.59
cranial (fossa, any)	C71.9	C79.31	—	D33.2	D43.2	D49.6
meninges	C70.0	C79.32	—	D32.0	D42.0	D49.7
nerve	C72.50	C79.49	—	D33.3	D43.3	D49.7
specified NEC	C72.59	C79.49	—	D33.3	D43.3	D49.7
craniobuccal						
pouch	C75.2	C79.89	D09.3	D35.2	D44.3	D49.7
craniopharyngeal (duct)						
(pouch)	C75.2	C79.89	D09.3	D35.3	D44.4	D49.7
cricoid	C13.0	C79.89	D00.08	D10.7	D37.05	D49.0
cartilage	C32.3	C78.39	D02.0	D14.1	D38.0	D49.1
cricopharynx	C13.0	C79.89	D00.08	D10.7	D37.05	D49.0
crypt of Morgagni	C21.8	C78.5	D01.3	D12.9	D37.8	D49.0
crystalline lens	C69.4-☑	C79.49	D09.2-☑	D31.4-☑	D48.7	D49.89
cul-de-sac						
(Douglas')	C48.1	C78.6	—	D20.1	D48.4	D49.0
cuneiform						
cartilage	C32.3	C78.39	D02.0	D14.1	D38.0	D49.1
cutaneous — see						
Neoplasm, skin						
cutis — see Neoplasm,						
skin						
cystic (bile) duct						
(common)	C24.0	C78.89	D01.5	D13.5	D37.6	D49.0
dermis — see						
Neoplasm, skin						
diaphragm	C49.3	C79.89	—	D21.3	D48.1	D49.2
digestive organs,						
system, tube, or						
tract NEC	C26.9	C78.89	D01.9	D13.9	D37.9	D49.0
disc,						
intervertebral	C41.2	C79.51	—	D16.6	D48.0	D49.2
disease,						
generalized	C80.0	—	—	—	—	—
disseminated	C80.0	—	—	—	—	—
Douglas' cul-de-sac or						
pouch	C48.1	C78.6	—	D20.1	D48.4	D49.0
duodenojejunal						
junction	C17.8	C78.4	D01.49	D13.39	D37.2	D49.0
duodenum	C17.0	C78.4	D01.49	D13.2	D37.2	D49.0
dura (cranial)						
(mater)	C70.9	C79.49	—	D32.9	D42.9	D49.7
cerebral	C70.0	C79.32	—	D32.0	D42.0	D49.7
spinal	C70.1	C79.49	—	D32.1	D42.1	D49.7
ear (external) — see						
also Neoplasm, skin,						
ear	C44.20-☑	C79.2	D04.2-☑	D23.2-☑	D48.5	D49.2
auricle or auris — see						
also Neoplasm,						
skin, ear	C44.20-☑	C79.2	D04.2-☑	D23.2-☑	D48.5	D49.2
canal, external — see						
also Neoplasm,						
skin, ear	C44.20-☑	C79.2	D04.2-☑	D23.2-☑	D48.5	D49.2
cartilage	C49.0	C79.89	—	D21.0	D48.1	D49.2
external meatus —						
see also						
Neoplasm, skin,						
ear	C44.20-☑	C79.2	D04.2-☑	D23.2-☑	D48.5	D49.2
inner	C30.1	C78.39	D02.3	D14.0	D38.5	D49.1
lobule — see also						
Neoplasm, skin,						
ear	C44.20-☑	C79.2	D04.2-☑	D23.2-☑	D48.5	D49.2
middle	C30.1	C78.39	D02.3	D14.0	D38.5	D49.1
overlapping lesion						
with accessory						
sinuses	C31.8	—	—	—	—	—

☑ **Additional Character Required — Refer to the Tabular List for Character Selection**   ⬇ Subterms under main terms may continue to next column or page

Neoplasm, neoplastic	Malignant Primary	Malignant Secondary	Ca in situ	Benign	Uncertain Behavior	Unspecified Behavior
— continued						
ear — see also						
Neoplasm, skin, ear						
— continued						
skin	C44.20-☑	C79.2	D04.2-☑	D23.2-☑	D48.5	D49.2
basal cell						
carcinoma	C44.21-☑	—	—	—	—	—
specified type						
NEC	C44.29-☑	—	—	—	—	—
squamous cell						
carcinoma	C44.22-☑	—	—	—	—	—
earlobe	C44.20-☑	C79.2	D04.2-☑	D23.2-☑	D48.5	D49.2
basal cell						
carcinoma	C44.21-☑	—	—	—	—	—
specified type						
NEC	C44.29-☑	—	—	—	—	—
squamous cell						
carcinoma	C44.22-☑	—	—	—	—	—
ejaculatory duct	C63.7	C79.82	D07.69	D29.8	D40.8	D49.59
elbow NEC	C76.4-☑	C79.89	D04.6-☑	D36.7	D48.7	D49.89
endocardium	C38.0	C79.89	—	D15.1	D48.7	D49.89
endocervix (canal)						
(gland)	C53.0	C79.82	D06.0	D26.0	D39.0	D49.59
endocrine gland						
NEC	C75.9	C79.89	D09.3	D35.9	D44.9	D49.7
pluriglandular	C75.8	C79.89	D09.3	D35.7	D44.9	D49.7
endometrium (gland)						
(stroma)	C54.1	C79.82	D07.0	D26.1	D39.0	D49.59
ensiform cartilage	C41.3	C79.51	—	D16.7	D48.0	D49.2
enteric — see						
Neoplasm,						
intestine						
ependyma (brain)	C71.5	C79.31	—	D33.0	D43.0	D49.6
fourth ventricle	C71.7	C79.31	—	D33.1	D43.1	D49.6
epicardium	C38.0	C79.89	—	D15.1	D48.7	D49.89
epididymis	C63.0-☑	C79.82	D07.69	D29.3-☑	D40.8	D49.59
epidural	C72.9	C79.49	—	D33.9	D43.9	D49.7
epiglottis	C32.1	C78.39	D02.0	D14.1	D38.0	D49.1
anterior aspect or						
surface	C10.1	C79.89	D00.08	D10.5	D37.05	D49.0
cartilage	C32.3	C78.39	D02.0	D14.1	D38.0	D49.1
free border						
(margin)	C10.1	C79.89	D00.08	D10.5	D37.05	D49.0
junctional						
region	C10.8	C79.89	D00.08	D10.5	D37.05	D49.0
posterior (laryngeal)						
surface	C32.1	C78.39	D02.0	D14.1	D38.0	D49.1
suprahyoid						
portion	C32.1	C78.39	D02.0	D14.1	D38.0	D49.1
esophagogastric						
junction	C16.0	C78.89	D00.2	D13.1	D37.1	D49.0
esophagus	C15.9	C78.89	D00.1	D13.0	D37.8	D49.0
abdominal	C15.5	C78.89	D00.1	D13.0	D37.8	D49.0
cervical	C15.3	C78.89	D00.1	D13.0	D37.8	D49.0
distal (third)	C15.5	C78.89	D00.1	D13.0	D37.8	D49.0
lower (third)	C15.5	C78.89	D00.1	D13.0	D37.8	D49.0
middle (third)	C15.4	C78.89	D00.1	D13.0	D37.8	D49.0
overlapping						
lesion	C15.8	—	—	—	—	—
proximal (third)	C15.3	C78.89	D00.1	D13.0	D37.8	D49.0
thoracic	C15.4	C78.89	D00.1	D13.0	D37.8	D49.0
upper (third)	C15.3	C78.89	D00.1	D13.0	D37.8	D49.0
ethmoid (sinus)	C31.1	C78.39	D02.3	D14.0	D38.5	D49.1
bone or						
labyrinth	C41.0	C79.51	—	D16.4	D48.0	D49.2
eustachian tube	C30.1	C78.39	D02.3	D14.0	D38.5	D49.1
exocervix	C53.1	C79.82	D06.1	D26.0	D39.0	D49.59
external						
meatus (ear) — see						
also Neoplasm,						
skin, ear	C44.20-☑	C79.2	D04.2-☑	D23.2-☑	D48.5	D49.2
os, cervix uteri	C53.1	C79.82	D06.1	D26.0	D39.0	D49.59
extradural	C72.9	C79.49	—	D33.9	D43.9	D49.7
extrahepatic (bile)						
duct	C24.0	C78.89	D01.5	D13.5	D37.6	D49.0
overlapping lesion						
with						
gallbladder	C24.8	—	—	—	—	—
extraocular						
muscle	C69.6-☑	C79.49	D09.2-☑	D31.6-☑	D48.7	D49.89
extrarectal	C76.3	C79.89	D09.8	D36.7	D48.7	D49.89
extremity	C76.8	C79.89	D04.8	D36.7	D48.7	D49.89

Neoplasm, neoplastic	Malignant Primary	Malignant Secondary	Ca in situ	Benign	Uncertain Behavior	Unspecified Behavior
— continued						
extremity — continued						
lower	C76.5-☑	C79.89	D04.7-☑	D36.7	D48.7	D49.89
upper	C76.4-☑	C79.89	D04.6-☑	D36.7	D48.7	D49.89
eyeball	C69.9-☑	C79.49	D09.2-☑	D31.9-☑	D48.7	D49.89
eyebrow	C44.309	C79.2	D04.39	D23.39	D48.5	D49.2
basal cell						
carcinoma	C44.319	—	—	—	—	—
specified type						
NEC	C44.399	—	—	—	—	—
squamous cell						
carcinoma	C44.329	—	—	—	—	—
eyelid (lower) (skin)						
(upper)	C44.10-☑	—	—	—	—	—
basal cell						
carcinoma	C44.11-☑	—	—	—	—	—
cartilage	C49.0	C79.89	—	D21.0	D48.1	D49.2
sebaceous cell	C44.13-☑	—	—	—	—	—
specified type						
NEC	C44.19-☑	—	—	—	—	—
squamous cell						
carcinoma	C44.12-☑	—	—	—	—	—
eye NEC	C69.9-☑	C79.49	D09.2-☑	D31.9-☑	D48.7	D49.89
overlapping						
sites	C69.8-☑	—	—	—	—	—
face NEC	C76.0	C79.89	D04.39	D36.7	D48.7	D49.89
fallopian tube						
(accessory)	C57.0-☑	C79.82	D07.39	D28.2	D39.8	D49.59
falx (cerebella)						
(cerebri)	C70.0	C79.32	—	D32.0	D42.0	D49.7
fascia — see also						
Neoplasm,						
connective tissue						
palmar	C49.1-☑	C79.89	—	D21.1-☑	D48.1	D49.2
plantar	C49.2-☑	C79.89	—	D21.2-☑	D48.1	D49.2
fatty tissue — see						
Neoplasm,						
connective tissue						
fauces, faucial NEC	C10.9	C79.89	D00.08	D10.5	D37.05	D49.0
pillars	C09.1	C79.89	D00.08	D10.5	D37.05	D49.0
tonsil	C09.9	C79.89	D00.08	D10.4	D37.05	D49.0
femur (any part)	C40.2-☑	—	—	D16.2-☑	—	—
fetal membrane	C58	C79.82	D07.0	D26.7	D39.2	D49.59
fibrous tissue — see						
Neoplasm,						
connective tissue						
fibula (any part)	C40.2-☑	C79.51	—	D16.2-☑	—	—
filum terminale	C72.0	C79.49	—	D33.4	D43.4	D49.7
finger NEC	C76.4-☑	C79.89	D04.6-☑	D36.7	D48.7	D49.89
flank NEC	C76.8	C79.89	D04.5	D36.7	D48.7	D49.89
follicle, nabothian	C53.0	C79.82	D06.0	D26.0	D39.0	D49.59
foot NEC	C76.5-☑	C79.89	D04.7-☑	D36.7	D48.7	D49.89
forearm NEC	C76.4-☑	C79.89	D04.6-☑	D36.7	D48.7	D49.89
forehead (skin)	C44.309	C79.2	D04.39	D23.39	D48.5	D49.2
basal cell						
carcinoma	C44.319	—	—	—	—	—
specified type						
NEC	C44.399	—	—	—	—	—
squamous cell						
carcinoma	C44.329	—	—	—	—	—
foreskin	C60.0	C79.82	D07.4	D29.0	D40.8	D49.59
fornix						
pharyngeal	C11.3	C79.89	D00.08	D10.6	D37.05	D49.0
vagina	C52	C79.82	D07.2	D28.1	D39.8	D49.59
fossa (of)						
anterior (cranial)	C71.9	C79.31	—	D33.2	D43.2	D49.6
cranial	C71.9	C79.31	—	D33.2	D43.2	D49.6
ischiorectal	C76.3	C79.89	D09.8	D36.7	D48.7	D49.89
middle (cranial)	C71.9	C79.31	—	D33.2	D43.2	D49.6
piriform	C12	C79.89	D00.08	D10.7	D37.05	D49.0
pituitary	C75.1	C79.89	D09.3	D35.2	D44.3	D49.7
posterior						
(cranial)	C71.9	C79.31	—	D33.2	D43.2	D49.6
pterygoid	C49.0	C79.89	—	D21.0	D48.1	D49.2
pyriform	C12	C79.89	D00.08	D10.7	D37.05	D49.0
Rosenmuller	C11.2	C79.89	D00.08	D10.6	D37.05	D49.0
tonsillar	C09.0	C79.89	D00.08	D10.5	D37.05	D49.0
fourchette	C51.9	C79.82	D07.1	D28.0	D39.8	D49.59
frenulum						
labii — see						
Neoplasm, lip,						
internal						

Neoplasm Table

Neoplasm, frenulum — Neoplasm, intestine, intestinal

Neoplasm, neoplastic — continued	Malignant Primary	Malignant Secondary	Ca in situ	Benign	Uncertain Behavior	Unspecified Behavior
frenulum — continued						
linguae	C02.2	C79.89	D00.07	D10.1	D37.02	D49.0
frontal						
bone	C41.0	C79.51	—	D16.4	D48.0	D49.2
lobe, brain	C71.1	C79.31	—	D33.0	D43.0	D49.6
pole	C71.1	C79.31	—	D33.0	D43.0	D49.6
sinus	C31.2	C78.39	D02.3	D14.0	D38.5	D49.1
fundus						
stomach	C16.1	C78.89	D00.2	D13.1	D37.1	D49.0
uterus	C54.3	C79.82	D07.0	D26.1	D39.0	D49.59
gallbladder	C23	C78.89	D01.5	D13.5	D37.6	D49.0
overlapping lesion with extrahepatic bile ducts	C24.8	—	—	—	—	—
gall duct						
(extrahepatic)	C24.0	C78.89	D01.5	D13.5	D37.6	D49.0
intrahepatic	C22.1	C78.7	D01.5	D13.4	D37.6	D49.0
ganglia — see also Neoplasm, nerve, peripheral	C47.9	C79.89	—	D36.10	D48.2	D49.2
basal	C71.0	C79.31	—	D33.0	D43.0	D49.6
cranial nerve	C72.50	C79.49	—	D33.3	D43.3	D49.7
Gartner's duct	C52	C79.82	D07.2	D28.1	D39.8	D49.59
gastric — see Neoplasm, stomach						
gastrocolic	C26.9	C78.89	D01.9	D13.9	D37.9	D49.0
gastroesophageal junction	C16.0	C78.89	D00.2	D13.1	D37.1	D49.0
gastrointestinal (tract) NEC	C26.9	C78.89	D01.9	D13.9	D37.9	D49.0
generalized	C80.0	—	—	—	—	—
genital organ or tract						
female NEC	C57.9	C79.82	D07.30	D28.9	D39.9	D49.59
overlapping lesion	C57.8	—	—	—	—	—
specified site NEC	C57.7	C79.82	D07.39	D28.7	D39.8	D49.59
male NEC	C63.9	C79.82	D07.60	D29.9	D40.9	D49.59
overlapping lesion	C63.8	—	—	—	—	—
specified site NEC	C63.7	C79.82	D07.69	D29.8	D40.8	D49.59
genitourinary tract						
female	C57.9	C79.82	D07.30	D28.9	D39.9	D49.59
male	C63.9	C79.82	D07.60	D29.9	D40.9	D49.59
gingiva (alveolar) (marginal)	C03.9	C79.89	D00.03	D10.39	D37.09	D49.0
lower	C03.1	C79.89	D00.03	D10.39	D37.09	D49.0
mandibular	C03.1	C79.89	D00.03	D10.39	D37.09	D49.0
maxillary	C03.0	C79.89	D00.03	D10.39	D37.09	D49.0
upper	C03.0	C79.89	D00.03	D10.39	D37.09	D49.0
gland, glandular (lymphatic) (system) — see also Neoplasm, lymph gland						
endocrine NEC	C75.9	C79.89	D09.3	D35.9	D44.9	D49.7
salivary — see Neoplasm, salivary gland						
glans penis	C60.1	C79.82	D07.4	D29.0	D40.8	D49.59
globus pallidus	C71.0	C79.31	—	D33.0	D43.0	D49.6
glomus						
coccygeal	C49.5	C79.89	—	D21.5	D48.1	D49.2
jugularis	C75.5	C79.89	—	D35.6	D44.7	D49.7
glosso-epiglottic fold(s)	C10.1	C79.89	D00.08	D10.5	D37.05	D49.0
glossopalatine fold	C09.1	C79.89	D00.08	D10.5	D37.05	D49.0
glossopharyngeal sulcus	C09.0	C79.89	D00.08	D10.5	D37.05	D49.0
glottis	C32.0	C78.39	D02.0	D14.1	D38.0	D49.1
gluteal region	C76.3	C79.89	D04.5	D36.7	D48.7	D49.89
great vessels NEC	C49.3	C79.89	—	D21.3	D48.1	D49.2
groin NEC	C76.3	C79.89	D04.5	D36.7	D48.7	D49.89
gum	C03.9	C79.89	D00.03	D10.39	D37.09	D49.0
lower	C03.1	C79.89	D00.03	D10.39	D37.09	D49.0
upper	C03.0	C79.89	D00.03	D10.39	D37.09	D49.0
hand NEC	C76.4-✓	C79.89	D04.6-✓	D36.7	D48.7	D49.89
head NEC	C76.0	C79.89	D04.4	D36.7	D48.7	D49.89
heart	C38.0	C79.89	—	D15.1	D48.7	D49.89

Neoplasm, neoplastic — continued	Malignant Primary	Malignant Secondary	Ca in situ	Benign	Uncertain Behavior	Unspecified Behavior
heel NEC	C76.5-✓	C79.89	D04.7-✓	D36.7	D48.7	D49.89
helix — see also Neoplasm, skin, ear	C44.20-✓	C79.2	D04.2-✓	D23.2-✓	D48.5	D49.2
hematopoietic, hemopoietic tissue NEC	C96.9	—	—	—	—	—
specified NEC	C96.Z	—	—	—	—	—
hemisphere, cerebral	C71.0	C79.31	—	D33.0	D43.0	D49.6
hemorrhoidal zone	C21.1	C78.5	D01.3	D12.9	D37.8	D49.0
hepatic — see also Index to disease, by histology	C22.9	C78.7	D01.5	D13.4	D37.6	D49.0
duct (bile)	C24.0	C78.89	D01.5	D13.5	D37.6	D49.0
flexure (colon)	C18.3	C78.5	D01.0	D12.3	D37.4	D49.0
primary	C22.8	C78.7	D01.5	D13.4	D37.6	D49.0
hepatobiliary	C24.9	C78.89	D01.5	D13.5	D37.6	D49.0
hepatoblastoma	C22.2	C78.7	D01.5	D13.4	D37.6	D49.0
hepatoma	C22.0	C78.7	D01.5	D13.4	D37.6	D49.0
hilus of lung	C34.0-✓	C78.0-✓	D02.2-✓	D14.3-✓	D38.1	D49.1
hippocampus, brain	C71.2	C79.31	—	D33.0	D43.0	D49.6
hip NEC	C76.5-✓	C79.89	D04.7-✓	D36.7	D48.7	D49.89
humerus (any part)	C40.0-✓	C79.51	—	D16.0-✓	—	—
hymen	C52	C79.82	D07.2	D28.1	D39.8	D49.59
hypopharynx, hypopharyngeal NEC	C13.9	C79.89	D00.08	D10.7	D37.05	D49.0
overlapping lesion	C13.8	—	—	—	—	—
postcricoid region	C13.0	C79.89	D00.08	D10.7	D37.05	D49.0
posterior wall	C13.2	C79.89	D00.08	D10.7	D37.05	D49.0
pyriform fossa (sinus)	C12	C79.89	D00.08	D10.7	D37.05	D49.0
hypophysis	C75.1	C79.89	D09.3	D35.2	D44.3	D49.7
hypothalamus	C71.0	C79.31	—	D33.0	D43.0	D49.6
ileocecum, ileocecal (coil) (junction) (valve)	C18.0	C78.5	D01.0	D12.0	D37.4	D49.0
ileum	C17.2	C78.4	D01.49	D13.39	D37.2	D49.0
ilium	C41.4	C79.51	—	D16.8	D48.0	D49.2
immunoproliferative NEC	C88.9	—	—	—	—	—
infraclavicular (region)	C76.1	C79.89	D04.5	D36.7	D48.7	D49.89
inguinal (region)	C76.3	C79.89	D04.5	D36.7	D48.7	D49.89
insula	C71.0	C79.31	—	D33.0	D43.0	D49.6
insular tissue (pancreas)	C25.4	C78.89	D01.7	D13.7	D37.8	D49.0
brain	C71.0	C79.31	—	D33.0	D43.0	D49.6
interarytenoid fold	C13.1	C78.39	D00.08	D10.7	D37.05	D49.0
hypopharyngeal aspect	C13.1	C79.89	D00.08	D10.7	D37.05	D49.0
laryngeal aspect	C32.1	C78.39	D02.0	D14.1	D38.0	D49.1
marginal zone	C13.1	C79.89	D00.08	D10.7	D37.05	D49.0
interdental papillae	C03.9	C79.89	D00.03	D10.39	D37.09	D49.0
lower	C03.1	C79.89	D00.03	D10.39	D37.09	D49.0
upper	C03.0	C79.89	D00.03	D10.39	D37.09	D49.0
internal						
capsule	C71.0	C79.31	—	D33.0	D43.0	D49.6
os (cervix)	C53.0	C79.82	D06.0	D26.0	D39.0	D49.59
intervertebral cartilage or disc	C41.2	C79.51	—	D16.6	D48.0	D49.2
intestine, intestinal	C26.0	C78.80	D01.40	D13.9	D37.8	D49.0
large	C18.9	C78.5	D01.0	D12.6	D37.4	D49.0
appendix	C18.1	C78.5	D01.0	D12.1	D37.3	D49.0
caput coli	C18.0	C78.5	D01.0	D12.0	D37.4	D49.0
cecum	C18.0	C78.5	D01.0	D12.0	D37.4	D49.0
colon	C18.9	C78.5	D01.0	D12.6	D37.4	D49.0
and rectum	C19	C78.5	D01.1	D12.7	D37.5	D49.0
ascending	C18.2	C78.5	D01.0	D12.2	D37.4	D49.0
caput	C18.0	C78.5	D01.0	D12.0	D37.4	D49.0
descending	C18.6	C78.5	D01.0	D12.4	D37.4	D49.0
distal	C18.6	C78.5	D01.0	D12.4	D37.4	D49.0

✓ Additional Character Required — Refer to the Tabular List for Character Selection   ▽ Subterms under main terms may continue to next column or page

Neoplasm, neoplastic — continued	Malignant Primary	Malignant Secondary	Ca in situ	Benign	Uncertain Behavior	Unspecified Behavior
intestine, intestinal — continued						
large — continued						
colon — continued						
left	C18.6	C78.5	D01.0	D12.4	D37.4	D49.0
overlapping lesion	C18.8	—	—	—	—	—
pelvic	C18.7	C78.5	D01.0	D12.5	D37.4	D49.0
right	C18.2	C78.5	D01.0	D12.2	D37.4	D49.0
sigmoid (flexure)	C18.7	C78.5	D01.0	D12.5	D37.4	D49.0
transverse	C18.4	C78.5	D01.0	D12.3	D37.4	D49.0
hepatic flexure	C18.3	C78.5	D01.0	D12.3	D37.4	D49.0
ileocecum, ileocecal (coil) (valve)	C18.0	C78.5	D01.0	D12.0	D37.4	D49.0
overlapping lesion	C18.8	—	—	—	—	—
sigmoid flexure (lower) (upper)	C18.7	C78.5	D01.0	D12.5	D37.4	D49.0
splenic flexure	C18.5	C78.5	D01.0	D12.3	D37.4	D49.0
small	C17.9	C78.4	D01.40	D13.30	D37.2	D49.0
duodenum	C17.0	C78.4	D01.49	D13.2	D37.2	D49.0
ileum	C17.2	C78.4	D01.49	D13.39	D37.2	D49.0
jejunum	C17.1	C78.4	D01.49	D13.39	D37.2	D49.0
overlapping lesion	C17.8	—	—	—	—	—
tract NEC	C26.0	C78.89	D01.40	D13.9	D37.8	D49.0
intra-abdominal	C76.2	C79.89	D09.8	D36.7	D48.7	D49.89
intracranial NEC	C71.9	C79.31	—	D33.2	D43.2	D49.6
intrahepatic (bile) duct	C22.1	C78.7	D01.5	D13.4	D37.6	D49.0
intraocular	C69.9-✓	C79.49	D09.2-✓	D31.9-✓	D48.7	D49.89
intraorbital	C69.6-✓	C79.49	D09.2-✓	D31.6-✓	D48.7	D49.89
intrasellar	C75.1	C79.89	D09.3	D35.2	D44.3	D49.7
intrathoracic (cavity) (organs)	C76.1	C79.89	D09.8	D15.9	D48.7	D49.89
specified NEC	C76.1	C79.89	D09.8	D15.7	—	—
iris	C69.4-✓	C79.49	D09.2-✓	D31.4-✓	D48.7	D49.89
ischiorectal (fossa)	C76.3	C79.89	D09.8	D36.7	D48.7	D49.89
ischium	C41.4	C79.51	—	D16.8	D48.0	D49.2
island of Reil	C71.0	C79.31	—	D33.0	D43.0	D49.6
islands or islets of Langerhans	C25.4	C78.89	D01.7	D13.7	D37.8	D49.0
isthmus uteri	C54.0	C79.82	D07.0	D26.1	D39.0	D49.59
jaw	C76.0	C79.89	D09.8	D36.7	D48.7	D49.89
bone	C41.1	C79.51	—	D16.5	D48.0	D49.2
lower	C41.1	C79.51	—	D16.5	—	—
upper	C41.0	C79.51	—	D16.4	—	—
carcinoma (any type) (lower) (upper)	C76.0	C79.89	—	—	—	—
skin — see also Neoplasm, skin, face	C44.309	C79.2	D04.39	D23.39	D48.5	D49.2
soft tissues	C03.9	C79.89	D00.03	D10.39	D37.09	D49.0
lower	C03.1	C79.89	D00.03	D10.39	D37.09	D49.0
upper	C03.0	C79.89	D00.03	D10.39	D37.09	D49.0
jejunum	C17.1	C78.4	D01.49	D13.39	D37.2	D49.0
joint NEC — see also Neoplasm, bone	C41.9	C79.51	—	D16.9	D48.0	D49.2
acromioclavicular	C40.0-✓	C79.51	—	D16.0-✓	—	—
bursa or synovial membrane — see Neoplasm, connective tissue						
costovertebral	C41.3	C79.51	—	D16.7	D48.0	D49.2
sternocostal	C41.3	C79.51	—	D16.7	D48.0	D49.2
temporomandibular	C41.1	C79.51	—	D16.5	D48.0	D49.2
junction						
anorectal	C21.8	C78.5	D01.3	D12.9	D37.8	D49.0
cardioesophageal	C16.0	C78.89	D00.2	D13.1	D37.1	D49.0
esophagogastric	C16.0	C78.89	D00.2	D13.1	D37.1	D49.0
gastroesophageal	C16.0	C78.89	D00.2	D13.1	D37.1	D49.0
hard and soft palate	C05.9	C79.89	D00.00	D10.39	D37.09	D49.0
ileocecal	C18.0	C78.5	D01.0	D12.0	D37.4	D49.0

Neoplasm, neoplastic — continued	Malignant Primary	Malignant Secondary	Ca in situ	Benign	Uncertain Behavior	Unspecified Behavior
junction — continued						
pelvirectal	C19	C78.5	D01.1	D12.7	D37.5	D49.0
pelviureteric	C65.-✓	C79.0-✓	D09.19	D30.1-✓	D41.1-✓	D49.59
rectosigmoid	C19	C78.5	D01.1	D12.7	D37.5	D49.0
squamocolumnar, of cervix	C53.8	C79.82	D06.7	D26.0	D39.0	D49.59
Kaposi's sarcoma — see Kaposi's, sarcoma						
kidney (parenchymal)	C64.-✓	C79.0-✓	D09.19	D30.0-✓	D41.0-✓	D49.51-✓
calyx	C65.-✓	C79.0-✓	D09.19	D30.1-✓	D41.1-✓	D49.51-✓
hilus	C65.-✓	C79.0-✓	D09.19	D30.1-✓	D41.1-✓	D49.51-✓
pelvis	C65.-✓	C79.0-✓	D09.19	D30.1-✓	D41.1-✓	D49.51-✓
knee NEC	C76.5-✓	C79.89	D04.7-✓	D36.7	D48.7	D49.89
labia (skin)	C51.9	C79.82	D07.1	D28.0	D39.8	D49.59
majora	C51.0	C79.82	D07.1	D28.0	D39.8	D49.59
minora	C51.1	C79.82	D07.1	D28.0	D39.8	D49.59
labial — see also Neoplasm, lip	C00.9	C79.89	D00.01	D10.0	D37.01	D49.0
sulcus (lower) (upper)	C06.1	C79.89	D00.02	D10.39	D37.09	D49.0
labium (skin)	C51.9	C79.82	D07.1	D28.0	D39.8	D49.59
majus	C51.0	C79.82	D07.1	D28.0	D39.8	D49.59
minus	C51.1	C79.82	D07.1	D28.0	D39.8	D49.59
lacrimal						
canaliculi	C69.5-✓	C79.49	D09.2-✓	D31.5-✓	D48.7	D49.89
duct (nasal)	C69.5-✓	C79.49	D09.2-✓	D31.5-✓	D48.7	D49.89
gland	C69.5-✓	C79.49	D09.2-✓	D31.5-✓	D48.7	D49.89
punctum	C69.5-✓	C79.49	D09.2-✓	D31.5-✓	D48.7	D49.89
sac	C69.5-✓	C79.49	D09.2-✓	D31.5-✓	D48.7	D49.89
Langerhans, islands or islets	C25.4	C78.89	D01.7	D13.7	D37.8	D49.0
laryngopharynx	C13.9	C79.89	D00.08	D10.7	D37.05	D49.0
larynx, laryngeal NEC	C32.9	C78.39	D02.0	D14.1	D38.0	D49.1
aryepiglottic fold	C32.1	C78.39	D02.0	D14.1	D38.0	D49.1
cartilage (arytenoid) (cricoid) (cuneiform) (thyroid)	C32.3	C78.39	D02.0	D14.1	D38.0	D49.1
commissure (anterior) (posterior)	C32.0	C78.39	D02.0	D14.1	D38.0	D49.1
extrinsic NEC	C32.1	C78.39	D02.0	D14.1	D38.0	D49.1
meaning hypopharynx	C13.9	C79.89	D00.08	D10.7	D37.05	D49.0
interarytenoid fold	C32.1	C78.39	D02.0	D14.1	D38.0	D49.1
intrinsic	C32.0	C78.39	D02.0	D14.1	D38.0	D49.1
overlapping lesion	C32.8	—	—	—	—	—
ventricular band	C32.1	C78.39	D02.0	D14.1	D38.0	D49.1
leg NEC	C76.5-✓	C79.89	D04.7-✓	D36.7	D48.7	D49.89
lens, crystalline	C69.4-✓	C79.49	D09.2-✓	D31.4-✓	D48.7	D49.89
lid (lower) (upper)	C44.10-✓	C79.2	D04.1-✓	D23.1-✓	D48.5	D49.2
basal cell carcinoma	C44.11-✓	—	—	—	—	—
sebaceous cell	C44.13-✓	—	—	—	—	—
specified type NEC	C44.19-✓	—	—	—	—	—
squamous cell carcinoma	C44.12-✓	—	—	—	—	—
ligament — see also Neoplasm, connective tissue						
broad	C57.1-✓	C79.82	D07.39	D28.2	D39.8	D49.59
Mackenrodt's	C57.7	C79.82	D07.39	D28.7	D39.8	D49.59
non-uterine — see Neoplasm, connective tissue						
round	C57.2-✓	C79.82	—	D28.2	D39.8	D49.59
sacro-uterine	C57.3	C79.82	—	D28.2	D39.8	D49.59
uterine	C57.3	C79.82	—	D28.2	D39.8	D49.59
utero-ovarian	C57.7	C79.82	D07.39	D28.2	D39.8	D49.59
uterosacral	C57.3	C79.82	—	D28.2	D39.8	D49.59
limb	C76.8	C79.89	D04.8	D36.7	D48.7	D49.89
lower	C76.5-✓	C79.89	D04.7-✓	D36.7	D48.7	D49.89
upper	C76.4-✓	C79.89	D04.6-✓	D36.7	D48.7	D49.89
limbus of cornea	C69.1-✓	C79.49	D09.2-✓	D31.1-✓	D48.7	D49.89

Neoplasm Table

Neoplasm, intestine, intestinal — Neoplasm, limbus of cornea

Neoplasm, neoplastic — continued

	Malignant Primary	Malignant Secondary	Ca in situ	Benign	Uncertain Behavior	Unspecified Behavior
lingual NEC — *see also* Neoplasm, tongue	C02.9	C79.89	D00.07	D10.1	D37.02	D49.0
lingula, lung	C34.1-☑	C78.0-☑	D02.2-☑	D14.3-☑	D38.1	D49.1
lip	C00.9	C79.89	D00.01	D10.0	D37.01	D49.0
buccal aspect — *see* Neoplasm, lip, internal						
commissure	C00.6	C79.89	D00.01	D10.0	D37.01	D49.0
external	C00.2	C79.89	D00.01	D10.0	D37.01	D49.0
lower	C00.1	C79.89	D00.01	D10.0	D37.01	D49.0
upper	C00.0	C79.89	D00.01	D10.0	D37.01	D49.0
frenulum — *see* Neoplasm, lip, internal						
inner aspect — *see* Neoplasm, lip, internal						
internal	C00.5	C79.89	D00.01	D10.0	D37.01	D49.0
lower	C00.4	C79.89	D00.01	D10.0	D37.01	D49.0
upper	C00.3	C79.89	D00.01	D10.0	D37.01	D49.0
lipstick area	C00.2	C79.89	D00.01	D10.0	D37.01	D49.0
lower	C00.1	C79.89	D00.01	D10.0	D37.01	D49.0
upper	C00.0	C79.89	D00.01	D10.0	D37.01	D49.0
lower	C00.1	C79.89	D00.01	D10.0	D37.01	D49.0
internal	C00.4	C79.89	D00.01	D10.0	D37.01	D49.0
mucosa — *see* Neoplasm, lip, internal						
oral aspect — *see* Neoplasm, lip, internal						
overlapping lesion	C00.8	—	—	—	—	—
with oral cavity or pharynx	C14.8	—	—	—	—	—
skin (commissure) (lower)						
(upper)	C44.00	C79.2	D04.0	D23.0	D48.5	D49.2
basal cell carcinoma	C44.01	—	—	—	—	—
specified type NEC	C44.09	—	—	—	—	—
squamous cell carcinoma	C44.02	—	—	—	—	—
upper	C00.0	C79.89	D00.01	D10.0	D37.01	D49.0
internal	C00.3	C79.89	D00.01	D10.0	D37.01	D49.0
vermilion border	C00.2	C79.89	D00.01	D10.0	D37.01	D49.0
lower	C00.1	C79.89	D00.01	D10.0	D37.01	D49.0
upper	C00.0	C79.89	D00.01	D10.0	D37.01	D49.0
lipomatous — *see* Lipoma, by site						
liver — *see also* Index to disease, by histology	C22.9	C78.7	D01.5	D13.4	D37.6	D49.0
primary	C22.8	C78.7	D01.5	D13.4	D37.6	D49.0
lumbosacral plexus	C47.5	C79.89	—	D36.16	D48.2	D49.2
lung	C34.9-☑	C78.0-☑	D02.2-☑	D14.3-☑	D38.1	D49.1
azygos lobe	C34.1-☑	C78.0-☑	D02.2-☑	D14.3-☑	D38.1	D49.1
carina	C34.0-☑	C78.0-☑	D02.2-☑	D14.3-☑	D38.1	D49.1
hilus	C34.0-☑	C78.0-☑	D02.2-☑	D14.3-☑	D38.1	D49.1
linqula	C34.1-☑	C78.0-☑	D02.2-☑	D14.3-☑	D38.1	D49.1
lobe NEC	C34.9-☑	C78.0-☑	D02.2-☑	D14.3-☑	D38.1	D49.1
lower lobe	C34.3-☑	C78.0-☑	D02.2-☑	D14.3-☑	D38.1	D49.1
main bronchus	C34.0-☑	C78.0-☑	D02.2-☑	D14.3-☑	D38.1	D49.1
mesothelioma — *see* Mesothelioma						
middle lobe	C34.2	C78.0-☑	D02.21	D14.31	D38.1	D49.1
overlapping lesion	C34.8-☑	—	—	—	—	—
upper lobe	C34.1-☑	C78.0-☑	D02.2-☑	D14.3-☑	D38.1	D49.1
lymph, lymphatic channel NEC	C49.9	C79.89	—	D21.9	D48.1	D49.2
gland						
(secondary)	—	C77.9	—	D36.0	D48.7	D49.89
abdominal	—	C77.2	—	D36.0	D48.7	D49.89
aortic	—	C77.2	—	D36.0	D48.7	D49.89
arm	—	C77.3	—	D36.0	D48.7	D49.89

Neoplasm, neoplastic — continued
lymph, lymphatic channel — continued
gland — continued

	Malignant Primary	Malignant Secondary	Ca in situ	Benign	Uncertain Behavior	Unspecified Behavior
auricular (anterior) (posterior)	—	C77.0	—	D36.0	D48.7	D49.89
axilla, axillary	—	C77.3	—	D36.0	D48.7	D49.89
brachial	—	C77.3	—	D36.0	D48.7	D49.89
bronchial	—	C77.1	—	D36.0	D48.7	D49.89
bronchopulmonary	—	C77.1	—	D36.0	D48.7	D49.89
celiac	—	C77.2	—	D36.0	D48.7	D49.89
cervical	—	C77.0	—	D36.0	D48.7	D49.89
cervicofacial	—	C77.0	—	D36.0	D48.7	D49.89
Cloquet	—	C77.4	—	D36.0	D48.7	D49.89
colic	—	C77.2	—	D36.0	D48.7	D49.89
common duct	—	C77.2	—	D36.0	D48.7	D49.89
cubital	—	C77.3	—	D36.0	D48.7	D49.89
diaphragmatic	—	C77.1	—	D36.0	D48.7	D49.89
epigastric, inferior	—	C77.1	—	D36.0	D48.7	D49.89
epitrochlear	—	C77.3	—	D36.0	D48.7	D49.89
esophageal	—	C77.1	—	D36.0	D48.7	D49.89
face	—	C77.0	—	D36.0	D48.7	D49.89
femoral	—	C77.4	—	D36.0	D48.7	D49.89
gastric	—	C77.2	—	D36.0	D48.7	D49.89
groin	—	C77.4	—	D36.0	D48.7	D49.89
head	—	C77.0	—	D36.0	D48.7	D49.89
hepatic	—	C77.2	—	D36.0	D48.7	D49.89
hilar (pulmonary)	—	C77.1	—	D36.0	D48.7	D49.89
splenic	—	C77.2	—	D36.0	D48.7	D49.89
hypogastric	—	C77.5	—	D36.0	D48.7	D49.89
ileocolic	—	C77.2	—	D36.0	D48.7	D49.89
iliac	—	C77.5	—	D36.0	D48.7	D49.89
infraclavicular	—	C77.3	—	D36.0	D48.7	D49.89
inguina, inguinal	—	C77.4	—	D36.0	D48.7	D49.89
innominate	—	C77.1	—	D36.0	D48.7	D49.89
intercostal	—	C77.1	—	D36.0	D48.7	D49.89
intestinal	—	C77.2	—	D36.0	D48.7	D49.89
intrabdominal	—	C77.2	—	D36.0	D48.7	D49.89
intrapelvic	—	C77.5	—	D36.0	D48.7	D49.89
intrathoracic	—	C77.1	—	D36.0	D48.7	D49.89
jugular	—	C77.0	—	D36.0	D48.7	D49.89
leg	—	C77.4	—	D36.0	D48.7	D49.89
limb lower	—	C77.4	—	D36.0	D48.7	D49.89
upper	—	C77.3	—	D36.0	D48.7	D49.89
lower limb	—	C77.4	—	D36.0	D48.7	D49.89
lumbar	—	C77.2	—	D36.0	D48.7	D49.89
mandibular	—	C77.0	—	D36.0	D48.7	D49.89
mediastinal	—	C77.1	—	D36.0	D48.7	D49.89
mesenteric (inferior) (superior)	—	C77.2	—	D36.0	D48.7	D49.89
midcolic	—	C77.2	—	D36.0	D48.7	D49.89
multiple sites in categories C77.0 - C77.5	—	C77.8	—	D36.0	D48.7	D49.89
neck	—	C77.0	—	D36.0	D48.7	D49.89
obturator	—	C77.5	—	D36.0	D48.7	D49.89
occipital	—	C77.0	—	D36.0	D48.7	D49.89
pancreatic	—	C77.2	—	D36.0	D48.7	D49.89
para-aortic	—	C77.2	—	D36.0	D48.7	D49.89
paracervical	—	C77.5	—	D36.0	D48.7	D49.89
parametrial	—	C77.5	—	D36.0	D48.7	D49.89
parasternal	—	C77.1	—	D36.0	D48.7	D49.89
parotid	—	C77.0	—	D36.0	D48.7	D49.89
pectoral	—	C77.3	—	D36.0	D48.7	D49.89
pelvic	—	C77.5	—	D36.0	D48.7	D49.89
peri-aortic	—	C77.2	—	D36.0	D48.7	D49.89
peripancreatic	—	C77.2	—	D36.0	D48.7	D49.89
popliteal	—	C77.4	—	D36.0	D48.7	D49.89
porta hepatis	—	C77.2	—	D36.0	D48.7	D49.89
portal	—	C77.2	—	D36.0	D48.7	D49.89
preauricular	—	C77.0	—	D36.0	D48.7	D49.89
prelaryngeal	—	C77.0	—	D36.0	D48.7	D49.89
presymphysial	—	C77.5	—	D36.0	D48.7	D49.89
pretracheal	—	C77.0	—	D36.0	D48.7	D49.89
primary (any site) NEC	C96.9	—	—	—	—	—

Neoplasm, neoplastic	Malignant Primary	Malignant Secondary	Ca in situ	Benign	Uncertain Behavior	Unspecified Behavior
— continued						
lymph, lymphatic						
channel —						
continued						
gland — continued						
pulmonary						
(hiler)	—	C77.1	—	D36.0	D48.7	D49.89
pyloric	—	C77.2	—	D36.0	D48.7	D49.89
retroperitoneal	—	C77.2	—	D36.0	D48.7	D49.89
retropharyngeal	—	C77.0	—	D36.0	D48.7	D49.89
Rosenmuller's	—	C77.4	—	D36.0	D48.7	D49.89
sacral	—	C77.5	—	D36.0	D48.7	D49.89
scalene	—	C77.0	—	D36.0	D48.7	D49.89
site NEC	—	C77.9	—	D36.0	D48.7	D49.89
splenic (hilar)	—	C77.2	—	D36.0	D48.7	D49.89
subclavicular	—	C77.3	—	D36.0	D48.7	D49.89
subinguinal	—	C77.4	—	D36.0	D48.7	D49.89
sublingual	—	C77.0	—	D36.0	D48.7	D49.89
submandibular	—	C77.0	—	D36.0	D48.7	D49.89
submaxillary	—	C77.0	—	D36.0	D48.7	D49.89
submental	—	C77.0	—	D36.0	D48.7	D49.89
subscapular	—	C77.3	—	D36.0	D48.7	D49.89
supraclavicular	—	C77.0	—	D36.0	D48.7	D49.89
thoracic	—	C77.1	—	D36.0	D48.7	D49.89
tibial	—	C77.4	—	D36.0	D48.7	D49.89
tracheal	—	C77.1	—	D36.0	D48.7	D49.89
tracheobronchial	—	C77.1	—	D36.0	D48.7	D49.89
upper limb	—	C77.3	—	D36.0	D48.7	D49.89
Virchow's	—	C77.0	—	D36.0	D48.7	D49.89
node — see also						
Neoplasm, lymph						
gland						
primary NEC	C96.9	—	—	—	—	—
vessel — see also						
Neoplasm,						
connective						
tissue	C49.9	C79.89	—	D21.9	D48.1	D49.2
Mackenrodt's						
ligament	C57.7	C79.82	D07.39	D28.7	D39.8	D49.59
malar	C41.0	C79.51	—	D16.4	D48.0	D49.2
region — see						
Neoplasm, cheek						
mammary gland — see						
Neoplasm, breast						
mandible	C41.1	C79.51	—	D16.5	D48.0	D49.2
alveolar						
mucosa						
(carcinoma)	C03.1	C79.89	D00.03	D10.39	D37.09	D49.0
ridge or						
process	C41.1	C79.51	—	D16.5	D48.0	D49.2
marrow (bone)						
NEC	C96.9	C79.52	—	—	D47.9	D49.89
mastectomy site (skin)						
— see also						
Neoplasm, breast,						
skin	C44.501	C79.2	—	—	—	—
specified as breast						
tissue	C50.8-☑	C79.81	—	—	—	—
mastoid (air cells)						
(antrum)						
(cavity)	C30.1	C78.39	D02.3	D14.0	D38.5	D49.1
bone or process	C41.0	C79.51	—	D16.4	D48.0	D49.2
maxilla, maxillary						
(superior)	C41.0	C79.51	—	D16.4	D48.0	D49.2
alveolar						
mucosa	C03.0	C79.89	D00.03	D10.39	D37.09	D49.0
ridge or process						
(carcinoma)	C41.0	C79.51	—	D16.4	D48.0	D49.2
antrum	C31.0	C78.39	D02.3	D14.0	D38.5	D49.1
carcinoma	C03.0	C79.51	—	—	—	—
inferior — see						
Neoplasm,						
mandible						
sinus	C31.0	C78.39	D02.3	D14.0	D38.5	D49.1
meatus external (ear)						
— see also						
Neoplasm, skin,						
ear	C44.20-☑	C79.2	D04.2-☑	D23.2-☑	D48.5	D49.2
Meckel diverticulum,						
malignant	C17.3	C78.4	D01.49	D13.39	D37.2	D49.0
mediastinum,						
mediastinal	C38.3	C78.1	—	D15.2	D38.3	D49.89
anterior	C38.1	C78.1	—	D15.2	D38.3	D49.89

Neoplasm, neoplastic	Malignant Primary	Malignant Secondary	Ca in situ	Benign	Uncertain Behavior	Unspecified Behavior
— continued						
mediastinum,						
mediastinal —						
continued						
posterior	C38.2	C78.1	—	D15.2	D38.3	D49.89
medulla						
adrenal	C74.1-☑	C79.7-☑	D09.3	D35.0-☑	D44.1-☑	D49.7
oblongata	C71.7	C79.31	—	D33.1	D43.1	D49.6
meibomian gland	C44.10-☑	C79.2	D04.1-☑	D23.1-☑	D48.5	D49.2
basal cell						
carcinoma	C44.11-☑	—	—	—	—	—
sebaceous cell	C44.13-☑	—	—	—	—	—
specified type						
NEC	C44.19-☑	—	—	—	—	—
squamous cell						
carcinoma	C44.12-☑	—	—	—	—	—
melanoma — see						
Melanoma						
meninges	C70.9	C79.49	—	D32.9	D42.9	D49.7
brain	C70.0	C79.32	—	D32.0	D42.0	D49.7
cerebral	C70.0	C79.32	—	D32.0	D42.0	D49.7
crainial	C70.0	C79.32	—	D32.0	D42.0	D49.7
intracranial	C70.0	C79.32	—	D32.0	D42.0	D49.7
spinal (cord)	C70.1	C79.49	—	D32.1	D42.1	D49.7
meniscus, knee joint						
(lateral)						
(medial)	C40.2-☑	C79.51	—	D16.2-☑	D48.0	D49.2
Merkel cell — see						
Carcinoma, Merkel						
cell						
mesentery,						
mesenteric	C48.1	C78.6	—	D20.1	D48.4	D49.0
mesoappendix	C48.1	C78.6	—	D20.1	D48.4	D49.0
mesocolon	C48.1	C78.6	—	D20.1	D48.4	D49.0
mesopharynx — see						
Neoplasm,						
oropharynx						
mesosalpinx	C57.1-☑	C79.82	D07.39	D28.2	D39.8	D49.59
mesothelial tissue —						
see Mesothelioma						
mesothelioma — see						
Mesothelioma						
mesovarium	C57.1-☑	C79.82	D07.39	D28.2	D39.8	D49.59
metacarpus (any						
bone)	C40.1-☑	C79.51	—	D16.1-☑	—	—
metastatic NEC — see						
also Neoplasm, by						
site,						
secondary	—	C79.9	—	—	—	—
metatarsus (any						
bone)	C40.3-☑	C79.51	—	D16.3-☑	—	—
midbrain	C71.7	C79.31	—	D33.1	D43.1	D49.6
milk duct — see						
Neoplasm, breast						
mons						
pubis	C51.9	C79.82	D07.1	D28.0	D39.8	D49.59
veneris	C51.9	C79.82	D07.1	D28.0	D39.8	D49.59
motor tract	C72.9	C79.49	—	D33.9	D43.9	D49.7
brain	C71.9	C79.31	—	D33.2	D43.2	D49.6
cauda equina	C72.1	C79.49	—	D33.4	D43.4	D49.7
spinal	C72.0	C79.49	—	D33.4	D43.4	D49.7
mouth	C06.9	C79.89	D00.00	D10.30	D37.09	D49.0
book-leaf	C06.89	C79.89	—	—	—	—
floor	C04.9	C79.89	D00.06	D10.2	D37.09	D49.0
anterior						
portion	C04.0	C79.89	D00.06	D10.2	D37.09	D49.0
lateral portion	C04.1	C79.89	D00.06	D10.2	D37.09	D49.0
overlapping						
lesion	C04.8	—	—	—	—	—
overlapping						
NEC	C06.80	—	—	—	—	—
roof	C05.9	C79.89	D00.00	D10.39	D37.09	D49.0
specified part						
NEC	C06.89	C79.89	D00.00	D10.39	D37.09	D49.0
vestibule	C06.1	C79.89	D00.00	D10.39	D37.09	D49.0
mucosa						
alveolar (ridge or						
process)	C03.9	C79.89	D00.03	D10.39	D37.09	D49.0
lower	C03.1	C79.89	D00.03	D10.39	D37.09	D49.0
upper	C03.0	C79.89	D00.03	D10.39	D37.09	D49.0
buccal	C06.0	C79.89	D00.02	D10.39	D37.09	D49.0
cheek	C06.0	C79.89	D00.02	D10.39	D37.09	D49.0

Neoplasm, neoplastic — continued	Malignant Primary	Malignant Secondary	Ca in situ	Benign	Uncertain Behavior	Unspecified Behavior
mucosa — continued						
lip — see Neoplasm, lip, internal						
nasal	C30.0	C78.39	D02.3	D14.0	D38.5	D49.1
oral	C06.0	C79.89	D00.02	D10.39	D37.09	D49.0
Mullerian duct						
female	C57.7	C79.82	D07.39	D28.7	D39.8	D49.59
male	C63.7	C79.82	D07.69	D29.8	D40.8	D49.59
muscle — see also Neoplasm, connective tissue						
extraocular	C69.6-✓	C79.49	D09.2-✓	D31.6-✓	D48.7	D49.89
myocardium	C38.0	C79.89	—	D15.1	D48.7	D49.89
myometrium	C54.2	C79.82	D07.0	D26.1	D39.0	D49.59
myopericardium	C38.0	C79.89	—	D15.1	D48.7	D49.89
nabothian gland (follicle)	C53.0	C79.82	D06.0	D26.0	D39.0	D49.59
nail — see also Neoplasm, skin, limb	C44.90	C79.2	D04.9	D23.9	D48.5	D49.2
finger — see also Neoplasm, skin, limb, upper	C44.60-✓	C79.2	D04.6-✓	D23.6-✓	D48.5	D49.2
toe — see also Neoplasm, skin, limb, lower	C44.70-✓	C79.2	D04.7-✓	D23.7-✓	D48.5	D49.2
nares, naris (anterior) (posterior)	C30.0	C78.39	D02.3	D14.0	D38.5	D49.1
nasal — see Neoplasm, nose						
nasolabial groove — see also Neoplasm, skin, face	C44.309	C79.2	D04.39	D23.39	D48.5	D49.2
nasolacrimal duct	C69.5-✓	C79.49	D09.2-✓	D31.5-✓	D48.7	D49.89
nasopharynx, nasopharyngeal	C11.9	C79.89	D00.08	D10.6	D37.05	D49.0
floor	C11.3	C79.89	D00.08	D10.6	D37.05	D49.0
overlapping lesion	C11.8	—	—	—	—	—
roof	C11.0	C79.89	D00.08	D10.6	D37.05	D49.0
wall	C11.9	C79.89	D00.08	D10.6	D37.05	D49.0
anterior	C11.3	C79.89	D00.08	D10.6	D37.05	D49.0
lateral	C11.2	C79.89	D00.08	D10.6	D37.05	D49.0
posterior	C11.1	C79.89	D00.08	D10.6	D37.05	D49.0
superior	C11.0	C79.89	D00.08	D10.6	D37.05	D49.0
nates — see also Neoplasm, skin, trunk	C44.509	C79.2	D04.5	D23.5	D48.5	D49.2
neck NEC	C76.0	C79.89	D09.8	D36.7	D48.7	D49.89
skin	C44.40	—	—	—	—	—
basal cell carcinoma	C44.41	—	—	—	—	—
specified type NEC	C44.49	—	—	—	—	—
squamous cell carcinoma	C44.42	—	—	—	—	—
nerve (ganglion)	C47.9	C79.89	—	D36.10	D48.2	D49.2
abducens	C72.59	C79.49	—	D33.3	D43.3	D49.7
accessory (spinal)	C72.59	C79.49	—	D33.3	D43.3	D49.7
acoustic	C72.4-✓	C79.49	—	D33.3	D43.3	D49.7
auditory	C72.4-✓	C79.49	—	D33.3	D43.3	D49.7
autonomic NEC — see also Neoplasm, nerve, peripheral	C47.9	C79.89	—	D36.10	D48.2	D49.2
brachial	C47.1-✓	C79.89	—	D36.12	D48.2	D49.2
cranial	C72.50	C79.49	—	D33.3	D43.3	D49.7
specified NEC	C72.59	C79.49	—	D33.3	D43.3	D49.7
facial	C72.59	C79.49	—	D33.3	D43.3	D49.7
femoral	C47.2-✓	C79.89	—	D36.13	D48.2	D49.2
ganglion NEC — see also Neoplasm, nerve, peripheral	C47.9	C79.89	—	D36.10	D48.2	D49.2
glossopharyngeal	C72.59	C79.49	—	D33.3	D43.3	D49.7
hypoglossal	C72.59	C79.49	—	D33.3	D43.3	D49.7
intercostal	C47.3	C79.89	—	D36.14	D48.2	D49.2
lumbar	C47.6	C79.89	—	D36.17	D48.2	D49.2
median	C47.1-✓	C79.89	—	D36.12	D48.2	D49.2
obturator	C47.2-✓	C79.89	—	D36.13	D48.2	D49.2

Neoplasm, neoplastic — continued	Malignant Primary	Malignant Secondary	Ca in situ	Benign	Uncertain Behavior	Unspecified Behavior
nerve — continued						
oculomotor	C72.59	C79.49	—	D33.3	D43.3	D49.7
olfactory	C47.2-✓	C79.49	—	D33.3	D43.3	D49.7
optic	C72.3-✓	C79.49	—	D33.3	D43.3	D49.7
parasympathetic NEC	C47.9	C79.89	—	D36.10	D48.2	D49.2
peripheral NEC	C47.9	C79.89	—	D36.10	D48.2	D49.2
abdomen	C47.4	C79.89	—	D36.15	D48.2	D49.2
abdominal wall	C47.4	C79.89	—	D36.15	D48.2	D49.2
ankle	C47.2-✓	C79.89	—	D36.13	D48.2	D49.2
antecubital fossa or space	C47.1-✓	C79.89	—	D36.12	D48.2	D49.2
arm	C47.1-✓	C79.89	—	D36.12	D48.2	D49.2
auricle (ear)	C47.0	C79.89	—	D36.11	D48.2	D49.2
axilla	C47.3	C79.89	—	D36.12	D48.2	D49.2
back	C47.6	C79.89	—	D36.17	D48.2	D49.2
buttock	C47.5	C79.89	—	D36.16	D48.2	D49.2
calf	C47.2-✓	C79.89	—	D36.13	D48.2	D49.2
cervical region	C47.0	C79.89	—	D36.11	D48.2	D49.2
cheek	C47.0	C79.89	—	D36.11	D48.2	D49.2
chest (wall)	C47.3	C79.89	—	D36.14	D48.2	D49.2
chin	C47.0	C79.89	—	D36.11	D48.2	D49.2
ear (external)	C47.0	C79.89	—	D36.11	D48.2	D49.2
elbow	C47.1-✓	C79.89	—	D36.12	D48.2	D49.2
extrarectal	C47.5	C79.89	—	D36.16	D48.2	D49.2
extremity	C47.9	C79.89	—	D36.10	D48.2	D49.2
lower	C47.2-✓	C79.89	—	D36.13	D48.2	D49.2
upper	C47.1-✓	C79.89	—	D36.12	D48.2	D49.2
eyelid	C47.0	C79.89	—	D36.11	D48.2	D49.2
face	C47.0	C79.89	—	D36.11	D48.2	D49.2
finger	C47.1-✓	C79.89	—	D36.12	D48.2	D49.2
flank	C47.6	C79.89	—	D36.17	D48.2	D49.2
foot	C47.2-✓	C79.89	—	D36.13	D48.2	D49.2
forearm	C47.1-✓	C79.89	—	D36.12	D48.2	D49.2
forehead	C47.0	C79.89	—	D36.11	D48.2	D49.2
gluteal region	C47.5	C79.89	—	D36.16	D48.2	D49.2
groin	C47.5	C79.89	—	D36.16	D48.2	D49.2
hand	C47.1-✓	C79.89	—	D36.12	D48.2	D49.2
head	C47.0	C79.89	—	D36.11	D48.2	D49.2
heel	C47.2-✓	C79.89	—	D36.13	D48.2	D49.2
hip	C47.2-✓	C79.89	—	D36.13	D48.2	D49.2
infraclavicular region	C47.3	C79.89	—	D36.14	D48.2	D49.2
inguinal (canal) (region)	C47.5	C79.89	—	D36.16	D48.2	D49.2
intrathoracic	C47.3	C79.89	—	D36.14	D48.2	D49.2
ischiorectal fossa	C47.5	C79.89	—	D36.16	D48.2	D49.2
knee	C47.2-✓	C79.89	—	D36.13	D48.2	D49.2
leg	C47.2-✓	C79.89	—	D36.13	D48.2	D49.2
limb NEC	C47.9	C79.89	—	D36.10	D48.2	D49.2
lower	C47.2-✓	C79.89	—	D36.13	D48.2	D49.2
upper	C47.1-✓	C79.89	—	D36.12	D48.2	D49.2
nates	C47.5	C79.89	—	D36.16	D48.2	D49.2
neck	C47.0	C79.89	—	D36.11	D48.2	D49.2
orbit	C69.6-✓	C79.49	—	D31.6-✓	D48.7	D49.2
pararectal	C47.5	C79.89	—	D36.16	D48.2	D49.2
paraurethral	C47.5	C79.89	—	D36.16	D48.2	D49.2
paravaginal	C47.5	C79.89	—	D36.16	D48.2	D49.2
pelvis (floor)	C47.5	C79.89	—	D36.16	D48.2	D49.2
pelvoabdominal	C47.8	C79.89	—	D36.17	D48.2	D49.2
perineum	C47.5	C79.89	—	D36.16	D48.2	D49.2
perirectal (tissue)	C47.5	C79.89	—	D36.16	D48.2	D49.2
periurethral (tissue)	C47.5	C79.89	—	D36.16	D48.2	D49.2
popliteal fossa or space	C47.2-✓	C79.89	—	D36.13	D48.2	D49.2
presacral	C47.5	C79.89	—	D36.16	D48.2	D49.2
pterygoid fossa	C47.0	C79.89	—	D36.11	D48.2	D49.2
rectovaginal septum or wall	C47.5	C79.89	—	D36.16	D48.2	D49.2
rectovesical	C47.5	C79.89	—	D36.16	D48.2	D49.2
sacrococcygeal region	C47.5	C79.89	—	D36.16	D48.2	D49.2
scalp	C47.0	C79.89	—	D36.11	D48.2	D49.2

✓ Additional Character Required — Refer to the Tabular List for Character Selection   ▼ Subterms under main terms may continue to next column or page

Neoplasm Table

Neoplasm, mucosa — Neoplasm, nerve

Neoplasm, neoplastic	Malignant Primary	Malignant Secondary	Ca in situ	Benign	Uncertain Behavior	Unspecified Behavior
— continued						
nerve — continued						
peripheral — continued						
scapular region	C47.3	C79.89	—	D36.14	D48.2	D49.2
shoulder	C47.1-✓	C79.89	—	D36.12	D48.2	D49.2
submental	C47.0	C79.89	—	D36.11	D48.2	D49.2
supraclavicular region	C47.0	C79.89	—	D36.11	D48.2	D49.2
temple	C47.0	C79.89	—	D36.11	D48.2	D49.2
temporal region	C47.0	C79.89	—	D36.11	D48.2	D49.2
thigh	C47.2-✓	C79.89	—	D36.13	D48.2	D49.2
thoracic (duct) (wall)	C47.3	C79.89	—	D36.14	D48.2	D49.2
thorax	C47.3	C79.89	—	D36.14	D48.2	D49.2
thumb	C47.1-✓	C79.89	—	D36.12	D48.2	D49.2
toe	C47.2-✓	C79.89	—	D36.13	D48.2	D49.2
trunk	C47.6	C79.89	—	D36.17	D48.2	D49.2
umbilicus	C47.4	C79.89	—	D36.15	D48.2	D49.2
vesicorectal	C47.5	C79.89	—	D36.16	D48.2	D49.2
wrist	C47.1-✓	C79.89	—	D36.12	D48.2	D49.2
radial	C47.1-✓	C79.89	—	D36.12	D48.2	D49.2
sacral	C47.5	C79.89	—	D36.16	D48.2	D49.2
sciatic	C47.2-✓	C79.89	—	D36.13	D48.2	D49.2
spinal NEC	C47.9	C79.89	—	D36.10	D48.2	D49.2
accessory	C72.59	C79.49	—	D33.3	D43.3	D49.7
sympathetic NEC — see also Neoplasm, nerve, peripheral	C47.9	C79.89	—	D36.10	D48.2	D49.2
trigeminal	C72.59	C79.49	—	D33.3	D43.3	D49.7
trochlear	C72.59	C79.49	—	D33.3	D43.3	D49.7
ulnar	C47.1-✓	C79.89	—	D36.12	D48.2	D49.2
vagus	C72.59	C79.49	—	D33.3	D43.3	D49.7
nervous system (central)	C72.9	C79.40	—	D33.9	D43.9	D49.7
autonomic — see Neoplasm, nerve, peripheral						
parasympathetic — see Neoplasm, nerve, peripheral						
specified site NEC	—	C79.49	—	D33.7	D43.8	—
sympathetic — see Neoplasm, nerve, peripheral						
nevus — see Nevus						
nipple	C50.0-✓	C79.81	D05.-✓	D24.-✓	—	—
nose, nasal	C76.0	C79.89	D09.8	D36.7	D48.7	D49.89
ala (external) (nasi) — see also Neoplasm, nose, skin						
skin	C44.301	C79.2	D04.39	D23.39	D48.5	D49.2
bone	C41.0	C79.51	—	D16.4	D48.0	D49.2
cartilage	C30.0	C78.39	D02.3	D14.0	D38.5	D49.1
cavity	C30.0	C78.39	D02.3	D14.0	D38.5	D49.1
choana	C11.3	C79.89	D00.08	D10.6	D37.05	D49.0
external (skin) — see also Neoplasm, nose, skin						
fossa	C30.0	C78.39	D02.3	D14.0	D38.5	D49.1
internal	C30.0	C78.39	D02.3	D14.0	D38.5	D49.1
mucosa	C30.0	C78.39	D02.3	D14.0	D38.5	D49.1
septum	C30.0	C78.39	D02.3	D14.0	D38.5	D49.1
posterior margin	C11.3	C79.89	D00.08	D10.6	D37.05	D49.0
sinus — see Neoplasm, sinus						
skin	C44.301	C79.2	D04.39	D23.39	D48.5	D49.2
basal cell carcinoma	C44.311	—	—	—	—	—
specified type NEC	C44.391	—	—	—	—	—
squamous cell carcinoma	C44.321	—	—	—	—	—
turbinate (mucosa)	C30.0	C78.39	D02.3	D14.0	D38.5	D49.1
bone	C41.0	C79.51	—	D16.4	D48.0	D49.2
vestibule	C30.0	C78.39	D02.3	D14.0	D38.5	D49.1

Neoplasm, neoplastic	Malignant Primary	Malignant Secondary	Ca in situ	Benign	Uncertain Behavior	Unspecified Behavior
— continued						
nostril	C30.0	C78.39	D02.3	D14.0	D38.5	D49.1
nucleus pulposus	C41.2	C79.51	—	D16.6	D48.0	D49.2
occipital bone	C41.0	C79.51	—	D16.4	D48.0	D49.2
lobe or pole, brain	C71.4	C79.31	—	D33.0	D43.0	D49.6
odontogenic — see Neoplasm, jaw bone						
olfactory nerve or bulb	C72.2-✓	C79.49	—	D33.3	D43.3	D49.7
olive (brain)	C71.7	C79.31	—	D33.1	D43.1	D49.6
omentum	C48.1	C78.6	—	D20.1	D48.4	D49.0
operculum (brain)	C71.0	C79.31	—	D33.0	D43.0	D49.6
optic nerve, chiasm, or tract	C72.3-✓	C79.49	—	D33.3	D43.3	D49.7
oral (cavity)	C06.9	C79.89	D00.00	D10.30	D37.09	D49.0
ill-defined	C14.8	C79.89	D00.00	D10.30	D37.09	D49.0
mucosa	C06.0	C79.89	D00.02	D10.39	D37.09	D49.0
orbit	C69.6-✓	C79.49	D09.2-✓	D31.6-✓	D48.7	D49.89
autonomic nerve	C69.6-✓	C79.49	—	D31.6-✓	D48.7	D49.2
bone	C41.0	C79.51	—	D16.4	D48.0	D49.2
eye	C69.6-✓	C79.49	D09.2-✓	D31.6-✓	D48.7	D49.89
peripheral nerves	C69.6-✓	C79.49	—	D31.6-✓	D48.7	D49.2
soft parts	C69.6-✓	C79.49	D09.2-✓	D31.6-✓	D48.7	D49.89
organ of Zuckerkandl	C75.5	C79.89	—	D35.6	D44.7	D49.7
oropharynx	C10.9	C79.89	D00.08	D10.5	D37.05	D49.0
branchial cleft (vestige)	C10.4	C79.89	D00.08	D10.5	D37.05	D49.0
junctional region	C10.8	C79.89	D00.08	D10.5	D37.05	D49.0
lateral wall	C10.2	C79.89	D00.08	D10.5	D37.05	D49.0
overlapping lesion	C10.8	—	—	—	—	—
pillars or fauces	C09.1	C79.89	D00.08	D10.5	D37.05	D49.0
posterior wall	C10.3	C79.89	D00.08	D10.5	D37.05	D49.0
vallecula	C10.0	C79.89	D00.08	D10.5	D37.05	D49.0
os						
external	C53.1	C79.82	D06.1	D26.0	D39.0	D49.59
internal	C53.0	C79.82	D06.0	D26.0	D39.0	D49.59
ovary	C56.-✓	C79.6-✓	D07.39	D27.-✓	D39.1-✓	D49.59
oviduct	C57.0-✓	C79.82	D07.39	D28.2	D39.8	D49.59
palate	C05.9	C79.89	D00.00	D10.39	D37.09	D49.0
hard	C05.0	C79.89	D00.05	D10.39	D37.09	D49.0
junction of hard and soft palate	C05.9	C79.89	D00.00	D10.39	D37.09	D49.0
overlapping lesions	C05.8	—	—	—	—	—
soft	C05.1	C79.89	D00.04	D10.39	D37.09	D49.0
nasopharyngeal surface	C11.3	C79.89	D00.08	D10.6	D37.05	D49.0
posterior surface	C11.3	C79.89	D00.08	D10.6	D37.05	D49.0
superior surface	C11.3	C79.89	D00.08	D10.6	D37.05	D49.0
palatoglossal arch	C09.1	C79.89	D00.00	D10.5	D37.09	D49.0
palatopharyngeal arch	C09.1	C79.89	D00.00	D10.5	D37.09	D49.0
pallium	C71.0	C79.31	—	D33.0	D43.0	D49.6
palpebra	C44.10-✓	C79.2	D04.1-✓	D23.1-✓	D48.5	D49.2
basal cell carcinoma	C44.11-✓	—	—	—	—	—
sebaceous cell	C44.13-✓	—	—	—	—	—
specified type NEC	C44.19-✓	—	—	—	—	—
squamous cell carcinoma	C44.12-✓	—	—	—	—	—
pancreas	C25.9	C78.89	D01.7	D13.6	D37.8	D49.0
body	C25.1	C78.89	D01.7	D13.6	D37.8	D49.0
duct (of Santorini) (of Wirsung)	C25.3	C78.89	D01.7	D13.6	D37.8	D49.0
ectopic tissue	C25.7	C78.89	—	D13.6	D37.8	D49.0
head	C25.0	C78.89	D01.7	D13.6	D37.8	D49.0
islet cells	C25.4	C78.89	D01.7	D13.7	D37.8	D49.0
neck	C25.7	C78.89	D01.7	D13.6	D37.8	D49.0
overlapping lesion	C25.8	—	—	—	—	—
tail	C25.2	C78.89	D01.7	D13.6	D37.8	D49.0

Neoplasm, neoplastic
— *continued*

	Malignant Primary	Malignant Secondary	Ca in situ	Benign	Uncertain Behavior	Unspecified Behavior
para-aortic body	C75.5	C79.89	—	D35.6	D44.7	D49.7
paraganglion NEC	C75.5	C79.89	—	D35.6	D44.7	D49.7
parametrium	C57.3	C79.82	—	D28.2	D39.8	D49.59
paranephric	C48.0	C78.6	—	D20.0	D48.3	D49.0
pararectal	C76.3	C79.89	—	D36.7	D48.7	D49.89
parasagittal (region)	C76.0	C79.89	D09.8	D36.7	D48.7	D49.89
parasellar	C72.9	C79.49		D33.9	D43.8	D49.7
parathyroid (gland)	C75.0	C79.89	D09.3	D35.1	D44.2	D49.7
paraurethral	C76.3	C79.89		D36.7	D48.7	D49.89
gland	C68.1	C79.19	D09.19	D30.8	D41.8	D49.59
paravaginal	C76.3	C79.89		D36.7	D48.7	D49.89
parenchyma, kidney	C64.-☑	C79.0-☑	D09.19	D30.0-☑	D41.0-☑	D49.51-☑
parietal						
bone	C41.0	C79.51	—	D16.4	D48.0	D49.2
lobe, brain	C71.3	C79.31	—	D33.0	D43.0	D49.6
paroophoron	C57.1-☑	C79.82	D07.39	D28.2	D39.8	D49.59
parotid (duct) (gland)	C07	C79.89	D00.00	D11.0	D37.030	D49.0
parovarium	C57.1-☑	C79.82	D07.39	D28.2	D39.8	D49.59
patella	C40.20	C79.51		—	—	—
peduncle, cerebral	C71.7	C79.31	—	D33.1	D43.1	D49.6
pelvirectal junction	C19	C78.5	D01.1	D12.7	D37.5	D49.0
pelvis, pelvic	C76.3	C79.89	D09.8	D36.7	D48.7	D49.89
bone	C41.4	C79.51	—	D16.8	D48.0	D49.2
floor	C76.3	C79.89	D09.8	D36.7	D48.7	D49.89
renal	C65.-☑	C79.0-☑	D09.19	D30.1-☑	D41.1-☑	D49.51-☑
viscera	C76.3	C79.89	D09.8	D36.7	D48.7	D49.89
wall	C76.3	C79.89	D09.8	D36.7	D48.7	D49.89
pelvo-abdominal	C76.8	C79.89	D09.8	D36.7	D48.7	D49.89
penis	C60.9	C79.82	D07.4	D29.0	D40.8	D49.59
body	C60.2	C79.82	D07.4	D29.0	D40.8	D49.59
corpus (cavernosum)	C60.2	C79.82	D07.4	D29.0	D40.8	D49.59
glans	C60.1	C79.82	D07.4	D29.0	D40.8	D49.59
overlapping sites	C60.8	—	—	—	—	—
skin NEC	C60.9	C79.82	D07.4	D29.0	D40.8	D49.59
periadrenal (tissue)	C48.0	C78.6	—	D20.0	D48.3	D49.0
perianal (skin) — *see also* Neoplasm, anus, skin	C44.500	C79.2	D04.5	D23.5	D48.5	D49.2
pericardium	C38.0	C79.89	—	D15.1	D48.7	D49.89
perinephric	C48.0	C78.6	—	D20.0	D48.3	D49.0
perineum	C76.3	C79.89	D09.8	D36.7	D48.7	D49.89
periodontal tissue NEC	C03.9	C79.89	D00.03	D10.39	D37.09	D49.0
periosteum — *see* Neoplasm, bone						
peripancreatic	C48.0	C78.6	—	D20.0	D48.3	D49.0
peripheral nerve NEC	C47.9	C79.89		D36.10	D48.2	D49.2
perirectal (tissue)	C76.3	C79.89	—	D36.7	D48.7	D49.89
perirenal (tissue)	C48.0	C78.6	—	D20.0	D48.3	D49.0
peritoneum, peritoneal (cavity)	C48.2	C78.6	—	D20.1	D48.4	D49.0
benign mesothelial tissue — *see* Mesothelioma, benign						
overlapping lesion	C48.8	—	—	—	—	—
with digestive organs	C26.9	—	—	—	—	—
parietal	C48.1	C78.6	—	D20.1	D48.4	D49.0
pelvic	C48.1	C78.6	—	D20.1	D48.4	D49.0
specified part NEC	C48.1	C78.6	—	D20.1	D48.4	D49.0
peritonsillar (tissue)	C76.0	C79.89	D09.8	D36.7	D48.7	D49.89
periurethral tissue	C76.3	C79.89		D36.7	D48.7	D49.89
phalanges						
foot	C40.3-☑	C79.51		D16.3-☑	—	—
hand	C40.1-☑	C79.51	—	D16.1-☑	—	—
pharynx, pharyngeal	C14.0	C79.89	D00.08	D10.9	D37.05	D49.0
bursa	C11.1	C79.89	D00.08	D10.6	D37.05	D49.0

Neoplasm, neoplastic
— *continued*

pharynx, pharyngeal
  — *continued*

	Malignant Primary	Malignant Secondary	Ca in situ	Benign	Uncertain Behavior	Unspecified Behavior
fornix	C11.3	C79.89	D00.08	D10.6	D37.05	D49.0
recess	C11.2	C79.89	D00.08	D10.6	D37.05	D49.0
region	C14.0	C79.89	D00.08	D10.9	D37.05	D49.0
tonsil	C11.1	C79.89	D00.08	D10.6	D37.05	D49.0
wall (lateral) (posterior)	C14.0	C79.89	D00.08	D10.9	D37.05	D49.0
pia mater	C70.9	C79.40	—	D32.9	D42.9	D49.7
cerebral	C70.0	C79.32	—	D32.0	D42.0	D49.7
cranial	C70.0	C79.32	—	D32.0	D42.0	D49.7
spinal	C70.1	C79.49	—	D32.1	D42.1	D49.7
pillars of fauces	C09.1	C79.89	D00.08	D10.5	D37.05	D49.0
pineal (body) (gland)	C75.3	C79.89	D09.3	D35.4	D44.5	D49.7
pinna (ear) NEC — *see also* Neoplasm, skin, ear	C44.20-☑	C79.2	D04.2-☑	D23.2-☑	D48.5	D49.2
piriform fossa or sinus	C12	C79.89	D00.08	D10.7	D37.05	D49.0
pituitary (body) (fossa) (gland) (lobe)	C75.1	C79.89	D09.3	D35.2	D44.3	D49.7
placenta	C58	C79.82	D07.0	D26.7	D39.2	D49.59
pleura, pleural (cavity)	C38.4	C78.2	—	D19.0	D38.2	D49.1
overlapping lesion with heart or mediastinum	C38.8	—	—	—	—	—
parietal	C38.4	C78.2	—	D19.0	D38.2	D49.1
visceral	C38.4	C78.2	—	D19.0	D38.2	D49.1
plexus						
brachial	C47.1-☑	C79.89	—	D36.12	D48.2	D49.2
cervical	C47.0	C79.89	—	D36.11	D48.2	D49.2
choroid	C71.5	C79.31	—	D33.0	D43.0	D49.6
lumbosacral	C47.5	C79.89	—	D36.16	D48.2	D49.2
sacral	C47.5	C79.89	—	D36.16	D48.2	D49.2
pluriendocrine	C75.8	C79.89	D09.3	D35.7	D44.9	D49.7
pole						
frontal	C71.1	C79.31	—	D33.0	D43.0	D49.6
occipital	C71.4	C79.31	—	D33.0	D43.0	D49.6
pons (varolii)	C71.7	C79.31	—	D33.1	D43.1	D49.6
popliteal fossa or space	C76.5-☑	C79.89	D04.7-☑	D36.7	D48.7	D49.89
postcricoid (region)	C13.0	C79.89	D00.08	D10.7	D37.05	D49.0
posterior fossa (cranial)	C71.9	C79.31	—	D33.2	D43.2	D49.6
postnasal space	C11.9	C79.89	D00.08	D10.6	D37.05	D49.0
prepuce	C60.0	C79.82	D07.4	D29.0	D40.8	D49.59
prepylorus	C16.4	C78.89	D00.2	D13.1	D37.1	D49.0
presacral (region)	C76.3	C79.89	—	D36.7	D48.7	D49.89
prostate (gland)	C61	C79.82	D07.5	D29.1	D40.0	D49.59
utricle	C68.0	C79.19	D09.19	D30.4	D41.3	D49.59
pterygoid fossa	C49.0	C79.89	—	D21.0	D48.1	D49.2
pubic bone	C41.4	C79.51	—	D16.8	D48.0	D49.2
pudenda, pudendum (female)	C51.9	C79.82	D07.1	D28.0	D39.8	D49.59
pulmonary — *see also* Neoplasm, lung	C34.9-☑	C78.0-☑	D02.2-☑	D14.3-☑	D38.1	D49.1
putamen	C71.0	C79.31	—	D33.0	D43.0	D49.6
pyloric						
antrum	C16.3	C78.89	D00.2	D13.1	D37.1	D49.0
canal	C16.4	C78.89	D00.2	D13.1	D37.1	D49.0
pylorus	C16.4	C78.89	D00.2	D13.1	D37.1	D49.0
pyramid (brain)	C71.7	C79.31	—	D33.1	D43.1	D49.6
pyriform fossa or sinus	C12	C79.89	D00.08	D10.7	D37.05	D49.0
radius (any part)	C40.0-☑	C79.51	—	D16.0-☑	—	—
Rathke's pouch	C75.1	C79.89	D09.3	D35.2	D44.3	D49.7
rectosigmoid (junction)	C19	C78.5	D01.1	D12.7	D37.5	D49.0
overlapping lesion with anus or rectum	C21.8	—	—	—	—	—
rectouterine pouch	C48.1	C78.6	—	D20.1	D48.4	D49.0
rectovaginal septum or wall	C76.3	C79.89	D09.8	D36.7	D48.7	D49.89
rectovesical septum	C76.3	C79.89	D09.8	D36.7	D48.7	D49.89
rectum (ampulla)	C20	C78.5	D01.2	D12.8	D37.5	D49.0

☑ Additional Character Required — Refer to the Tabular List for Character Selection   ▽ Subterms under main terms may continue to next column or page

Neoplasm, neoplastic

	Malignant Primary	Malignant Secondary	Ca in situ	Benign	Uncertain Behavior	Unspecified Behavior
— *continued*						
rectum — *continued*						
and colon	C19	C78.5	D01.1	D12.7	D37.5	D49.0
overlapping lesion						
with anus or						
rectosigmoid						
junction	C21.8	—	—	—	—	—
renal	C64.-☑	C79.0-☑	D09.19	D30.0-☑	D41.0-☑	D49.51-☑
calyx	C65.-☑	C79.0-☑	D09.19	D30.1-☑	D41.1-☑	D49.51-☑
hilus	C65.-☑	C79.0-☑	D09.19	D30.1-☑	D41.1-☑	D49.51-☑
parenchyma	C64.-☑	C79.0-☑	D09.19	D30.0-☑	D41.0-☑	D49.51-☑
pelvis	C65.-☑	C79.0-☑	D09.19	D30.1-☑	D41.1-☑	D49.51-☑
respiratory						
organs or system						
NEC	C39.9	C78.30	D02.4	D14.4	D38.6	D49.1
tract NEC	C39.9	C78.30	D02.4	D14.4	D38.5	D49.1
upper	C39.0	C78.30	D02.4	D14.4	D38.5	D49.1
retina	C69.2-☑	C79.49	D09.2-☑	D31.2-☑	D48.7	D49.81
retrobulbar	C69.6-☑	C79.49	—	D31.6-☑	D48.7	D49.89
retrocecal	C48.0	C78.6	—	D20.0	D48.3	D49.0
retromolar (area)						
(triangle)						
(trigone)	C06.2	C79.89	D00.00	D10.39	D37.09	D49.0
retro-orbital	C76.0	C79.89	D09.8	D36.7	D48.7	D49.89
retroperitoneal (space)						
(tissue)	C48.0	C78.6	—	D20.0	D48.3	D49.0
retroperitoneum	C48.0	C78.6	—	D20.0	D48.3	D49.0
retropharyngeal	C14.0	C79.89	D00.08	D10.9	D37.05	D49.0
retrovesical						
(septum)	C76.3	C79.89	D09.8	D36.7	D48.7	D49.89
rhinencephalon	C71.0	C79.31	—	D33.0	D43.0	D49.6
rib	C41.3	C79.51	—	D16.7	D48.0	D49.2
Rosenmuller's						
fossa	C11.2	C79.89	D00.08	D10.6	D37.05	D49.0
round ligament	C57.2-☑	C79.82	—	D28.2	D39.8	D49.59
sacrococcyx,						
sacrococcygeal	C41.4	C79.51	—	D16.8	D48.0	D49.2
region	C76.3	C79.89	D09.8	D36.7	D48.7	D49.89
sacrouterine						
ligament	C57.3	C79.82	—	D28.2	D39.8	D49.59
sacrum, sacral						
(vertebra)	C41.4	C79.51	—	D16.8	D48.0	D49.2
salivary gland or duct						
(major)	C08.9	C79.89	D00.00	D11.9	D37.039	D49.0
minor NEC	C06.9	C79.89	D00.00	D10.39	D37.04	D49.0
overlapping						
lesion	C08.9	—	—	—	—	—
parotid	C07	C79.89	D00.00	D11.0	D37.030	D49.0
pluriglandular	C08.9	C79.89	D00.00	D11.9	D37.039	D49.0
sublingual	C08.1	C79.89	D00.00	D11.7	D37.031	D49.0
submandibular	C08.0	C79.89	D00.00	D11.7	D37.032	D49.0
submaxillary	C08.0	C79.89	D00.00	D11.7	D37.032	D49.0
salpinx (uterine)	C57.0-☑	C79.82	D07.39	D28.2	D39.8	D49.59
Santorini's duct	C25.3	C78.89	D01.7	D13.6	D37.8	D49.0
scalp	C44.40	C79.2	D04.4	D23.4	D48.5	D49.2
basal cell						
carcinoma	C44.41	—	—	—	—	—
specified type						
NEC	C44.49	—	—	—	—	—
squamous cell						
carcinoma	C44.42	—	—	—	—	—
scapula (any part)	C40.0-☑	C79.51	—	D16.0-☑	—	—
scapular region	C76.1	C79.89	D09.8	D36.7	D48.7	D49.89
scar NEC — *see also*						
Neoplasm, skin, by						
site	C44.90	C79.2	D04.9	D23.9	D48.5	D49.2
sciatic nerve	C47.2-☑	C79.89	—	D36.13	D48.2	D49.2
sclera	C69.4-☑	C79.49	D09.2-☑	D31.4-☑	D48.7	D49.89
scrotum (skin)	C63.2	C79.82	D07.61	D29.4	D40.8	D49.59
sebaceous gland — *see*						
Neoplasm, skin						
sella turcica	C75.1	C79.89	D09.3	D35.2	D44.3	D49.7
bone	C41.0	C79.51	—	D16.4	D48.0	D49.2
semilunar cartilage						
(knee)	C40.2-☑	C79.51	—	D16.2-☑	D48.0	D49.2
seminal vesicle	C63.7	C79.82	D07.69	D29.8	D40.8	D49.59
septum						
nasal	C30.0	C78.39	D02.3	D14.0	D38.5	D49.1
posterior						
margin	C11.3	C79.89	D00.08	D10.6	D37.05	D49.0
rectovaginal	C76.3	C79.89	D09.8	D36.7	D48.7	D49.89
rectovesical	C76.3	C79.89	D09.8	D36.7	D48.7	D49.89

Neoplasm, neoplastic

	Malignant Primary	Malignant Secondary	Ca in situ	Benign	Uncertain Behavior	Unspecified Behavior
— *continued*						
septum — *continued*						
urethrovaginal	C57.9	C79.82	D07.30	D28.9	D39.9	D49.59
vesicovaginal	C57.9	C79.82	D07.30	D28.9	D39.9	D49.59
shoulder NEC	C76.4-☑	C79.89	D04.6-☑	D36.7	D48.7	D49.89
sigmoid flexure (lower)						
(upper)	C18.7	C78.5	D01.0	D12.5	D37.4	D49.0
sinus (accessory)	C31.9	C78.39	D02.3	D14.0	D38.5	D49.1
bone (any)	C41.0	C79.51	—	D16.4	D48.0	D49.2
ethmoidal	C31.1	C78.39	D02.3	D14.0	D38.5	D49.1
frontal	C31.2	C78.39	D02.3	D14.0	D38.5	D49.1
maxillary	C31.0	C78.39	D02.3	D14.0	D38.5	D49.1
nasal, paranasal						
NEC	C31.9	C78.39	D02.3	D14.0	D38.5	D49.1
overlapping						
lesion	C31.8	—	—	—	—	—
pyriform	C12	C79.89	D00.08	D10.7	D37.05	D49.0
sphenoid	C31.3	C78.39	D02.3	D14.0	D38.5	D49.1
skeleton, skeletal						
NEC	C41.9	C79.51	—	D16.9	D48.0	D49.2
Skene's gland	C68.1	C79.19	D09.19	D30.8	D41.8	D49.59
skin NOS	C44.90	C79.2	D04.9	D23.9	D48.5	D49.2
abdominal wall	C44.509	C79.2	D04.5	D23.5	D48.5	D49.2
basal cell						
carcinoma	C44.519	—	—	—	—	—
specified type						
NEC	C44.599	—	—	—	—	—
squamous cell						
carcinoma	C44.529	—	—	—	—	—
ala nasi — *see also*						
Neoplasm, nose,						
skin	C44.301	C79.2	D04.39	D23.39	D48.5	D49.2
ankle — *see also*						
Neoplasm, skin,						
limb, lower	C44.70-☑	C79.2	D04.7-☑	D23.7-☑	D48.5	D49.2
antecubital space —						
see also						
Neoplasm, skin,						
limb, upper	C44.60-☑	C79.2	D04.6-☑	D23.6-☑	D48.5	D49.2
anus	C44.500	C79.2	D04.5	D23.5	D48.5	D49.2
basal cell						
carcinoma	C44.510	—	—	—	—	—
specified type						
NEC	C44.590	—	—	—	—	—
squamous cell						
carcinoma	C44.520	—	—	—	—	—
arm — *see also*						
Neoplasm, skin,						
limb, upper	C44.60-☑	C79.2	D04.6-☑	D23.6-☑	D48.5	D49.2
auditory canal						
(external) — *see*						
also Neoplasm,						
skin, ear	C44.20-☑	C79.2	D04.2-☑	D23.2-☑	D48.5	D49.2
auricle (ear) — *see*						
also Neoplasm,						
skin, ear	C44.20-☑	C79.2	D04.2-☑	D23.2-☑	D48.5	D49.2
auricular canal						
(external) — *see*						
also Neoplasm,						
skin, ear	C44.20-☑	C79.2	D04.2-☑	D23.2-☑	D48.5	D49.2
axilla, axillary fold —						
see also						
Neoplasm, skin,						
trunk	C44.509	C79.2	D04.5	D23.5	D48.5	D49.2
back — *see also*						
Neoplasm, skin,						
trunk	C44.509	C79.2	D04.5	D23.5	D48.5	D49.2
basal cell						
carcinoma	C44.91	—	—	—	—	—
breast	C44.501	C79.2	D04.5	D23.5	D48.5	D49.2
basal cell						
carcinoma	C44.511	—	—	—	—	—
specified type						
NEC	C44.591	—	—	—	—	—
squamous cell						
carcinoma	C44.521	—	—	—	—	—
brow — *see also*						
Neoplasm, skin,						
face	C44.309	C79.2	D04.39	D23.39	D48.5	D49.2
buttock — *see also*						
Neoplasm, skin,						
trunk	C44.509	C79.2	D04.5	D23.5	D48.5	D49.2

Neoplasm, neoplastic — continued skin — continued	Malignant Primary	Malignant Secondary	Ca in situ	Benign	Uncertain Behavior	Unspecified Behavior
calf — see also Neoplasm, skin, limb, lower	C44.70-☑	C79.2	D04.7-☑	D23.7-☑	D48.5	D49.2
canthus (eye) (inner) (outer)	C44.10-☑	C79.2	D04.1-☑	D23.1-☑	D48.5	D49.2
basal cell carcinoma	C44.11-☑	—	—	—	—	—
sebaceous cell	C44.13-☑	—	—	—	—	—
specified type NEC	C44.19-☑	—	—	—	—	—
squamous cell carcinoma	C44.12-☑	—	—	—	—	—
cervical region — see also Neoplasm, skin, neck	C44.40	C79.2	D04.4	D23.4	D48.5	D49.2
cheek (external) — see also Neoplasm, skin, face	C44.309	C79.2	D04.39	D23.39	D48.5	D49.2
chest (wall) — see also Neoplasm, skin, trunk	C44.509	C79.2	D04.5	D23.5	D48.5	D49.2
chin — see also Neoplasm, skin, face	C44.309	C79.2	D04.39	D23.39	D48.5	D49.2
clavicular area — see also Neoplasm, skin, trunk	C44.509	C79.2	D04.5	D23.5	D48.5	D49.2
clitoris	C51.2	C79.82	D07.1	D28.0	D39.8	D49.59
columnella — see also Neoplasm, skin, face	C44.309	C79.2	D04.39	D23.39	D48.5	D49.2
concha — see also Neoplasm, skin, ear	C44.20-☑	C79.2	D04.2-☑	D23.2-☑	D48.5	D49.2
ear (external)	C44.20-☑	C79.2	D04.2-☑	D23.2-☑	D48.5	D49.2
basal cell carcinoma	C44.21-☑	—	—	—	—	—
specified type NEC	C44.29-☑	—	—	—	—	—
squamous cell carcinoma	C44.22-☑	—	—	—	—	—
elbow — see also Neoplasm, skin, limb, upper	C44.60-☑	C79.2	D04.6-☑	D23.6-☑	D48.5	D49.2
eyebrow — see also Neoplasm, skin, face	C44.309	C79.2	D04.39	D23.39	D48.5	D49.2
eyelid	C44.10-☑	C79.2	D04.1-☑	D23.1-☑	D48.5	D49.2
basal cell carcinoma	C44.11-☑	—	—	—	—	—
sebaceous cell	C44.13-☑	—	—	—	—	—
specified type NEC	C44.19-☑	—	—	—	—	—
squamous cell carcinoma	C44.12-☑	—	—	—	—	—
face NOS	C44.300	C79.2	D04.30	D23.30	D48.5	D49.2
basal cell carcinoma	C44.310	—	—	—	—	—
specified type NEC	C44.390	—	—	—	—	—
squamous cell carcinoma	C44.320	—	—	—	—	—
female genital organs (external)	C51.9	C79.82	D07.1	D28.0	D39.8	D49.59
clitoris	C51.2	C79.82	D07.1	D28.0	D39.8	D49.59
labium NEC	C51.9	C79.82	D07.1	D28.0	D39.8	D49.59
majus	C51.0	C79.82	D07.1	D28.0	D39.8	D49.59
minus	C51.1	C79.82	D07.1	D28.0	D39.8	D49.59
pudendum	C51.9	C79.82	D07.1	D28.0	D39.8	D49.59
vulva	C51.9	C79.82	D07.1	D28.0	D39.8	D49.59
finger — see also Neoplasm, skin, limb, upper	C44.60-☑	C79.2	D04.6-☑	D23.6-☑	D48.5	D49.2
flank — see also Neoplasm, skin, trunk	C44.509	C79.2	D04.5	D23.5	D48.5	D49.2
foot — see also Neoplasm, skin, limb, lower	C44.70-☑	C79.2	D04.7-☑	D23.7-☑	D48.5	D49.2

Neoplasm, neoplastic — continued skin — continued	Malignant Primary	Malignant Secondary	Ca in situ	Benign	Uncertain Behavior	Unspecified Behavior
forearm — see also Neoplasm, skin, limb, upper	C44.60-☑	C79.2	D04.6-☑	D23.6-☑	D48.5	D49.2
forehead — see also Neoplasm, skin, face	C44.309	C79.2	D04.39	D23.39	D48.5	D49.2
glabella — see also Neoplasm, skin, face	C44.309	C79.2	D04.39	D23.39	D48.5	D49.2
gluteal region — see also Neoplasm, skin, trunk	C44.509	C79.2	D04.5	D23.5	D48.5	D49.2
groin — see also Neoplasm, skin, trunk	C44.509	C79.2	D04.5	D23.5	D48.5	D49.2
hand — see also Neoplasm, skin, limb, upper	C44.60-☑	C79.2	D04.6-☑	D23.6-☑	D48.5	D49.2
head NEC — see also Neoplasm, skin, scalp	C44.40	C79.2	D04.4	D23.4	D48.5	D49.2
heel — see also Neoplasm, skin, limb, lower	C44.70-☑	C79.2	D04.7-☑	D23.7-☑	D48.5	D49.2
helix — see also Neoplasm, skin, ear	C44.20-☑	C79.2	D04.2-☑	D23.2-☑	D48.5	D49.2
hip — see also Neoplasm, skin, limb, lower	C44.70-☑	C79.2	D04.7-☑	D23.7-☑	D48.5	D49.2
infraclavicular region — see also Neoplasm, skin, trunk	C44.509	C79.2	D04.5	D23.5	D48.5	D49.2
inguinal region — see also Neoplasm, skin, trunk	C44.509	C79.2	D04.5	D23.5	D48.5	D49.2
jaw — see also Neoplasm, skin, face	C44.309	C79.2	D04.39	D23.39	D48.5	D49.2
Kaposi's sarcoma — see Kaposi's, sarcoma, skin						
knee — see also Neoplasm, skin, limb, lower	C44.70-☑	C79.2	D04.7-☑	D23.7-☑	D48.5	D49.2
labia						
majora	C51.0	C79.82	D07.1	D28.0	D39.8	D49.59
minora	C51.1	C79.82	D07.1	D28.0	D39.8	D49.59
leg — see also Neoplasm, skin, limb, lower	C44.70-☑	C79.2	D04.7-☑	D23.7-☑	D48.5	D49.2
lid (lower) (upper)	C44.10-☑	C79.2	D04.1-☑	D23.1-☑	D48.5	D49.2
basal cell carcinoma	C44.11-☑	—	—	—	—	—
sebaceous cell	C44.13-☑	—	—	—	—	—
specified type NEC	C44.19-☑	—	—	—	—	—
squamous cell carcinoma	C44.12-☑	—	—	—	—	—
limb NEC	C44.90	C79.2	D04.9	D23.9	D48.5	D49.2
basal cell carcinoma	C44.91					
lower	C44.70-☑	C79.2	D04.7-☑	D23.7-☑	D48.5	D49.2
basal cell carcinoma	C44.71-☑	—	—	—	—	—
specified type NEC	C44.79-☑	—	—	—	—	—
squamous cell carcinoma	C44.72-☑	—	—	—	—	—
upper	C44.60-☑	C79.2	D04.6-☑	D23.6-☑	D48.5	D49.2
basal cell carcinoma	C44.61-☑	—	—	—	—	—
specified type NEC	C44.69-☑	—	—	—	—	—
squamous cell carcinoma	C44.62-☑	—	—	—	—	—
lip (lower) (upper)	C44.00	C79.2	D04.0	D23.0	D48.5	D49.2

☑ Additional Character Required — Refer to the Tabular List for Character Selection   ▽ Subterms under main terms may continue to next column or page

Neoplasm, neoplastic — continued	Malignant Primary	Malignant Secondary	Ca in situ	Benign	Uncertain Behavior	Unspecified Behavior
skin — *continued*						
lip — *continued*						
basal cell carcinoma	C44.01	—	—	—	—	—
specified type NEC	C44.09	—	—	—	—	—
squamous cell carcinoma	C44.02	—	—	—	—	—
male genital organs	C63.9	C79.82	D07.60	D29.9	D40.8	D49.59
penis	C60.9	C79.82	D07.4	D29.0	D40.8	D49.59
prepuce	C60.0	C79.82	D07.4	D29.0	D40.8	D49.59
scrotum	C63.2	C79.82	D07.61	D29.4	D40.8	D49.59
mastectomy site (skin) — *see also* Neoplasm, skin, breast	C44.501	C79.2	—	—	—	—
specified as breast tissue	C50.8-☑	C79.81	—	—	—	—
meatus, acoustic (external) — *see also* Neoplasm, skin, ear	C44.20-☑	C79.2	D04.2-☑	D23.2-☑	D48.5	D49.2
melanotic — *see* Melanoma						
Merkel cell — *see* Carcinoma, Merkel cell						
nates — *see also* Neoplasm, skin, trunk	C44.509	C79.2	D04.5	D23.5	D48.5	D49.2
neck	C44.40	C79.2	D04.4	D23.4	D48.5	D49.2
basal cell carcinoma	C44.41	—	—	—	—	—
specified type NEC	C44.49	—	—	—	—	—
squamous cell carcinoma	C44.42	—	—	—	—	—
nevus — *see* Nevus, skin						
nose (external) — *see also* Neoplasm, nose, skin	C44.301	C79.2	D04.39	D23.39	D48.5	D49.2
overlapping lesion	C44.80					
basal cell carcinoma	C44.81	—	—	—	—	—
specified type NEC	C44.89	—	—	—	—	—
squamous cell carcinoma	C44.82	—	—	—	—	—
palm — *see also* Neoplasm, skin, limb, upper	C44.60-☑	C79.2	D04.6-☑	D23.6-☑	D48.5	D49.2
palpebra	C44.10-☑	C79.2	D04.1-☑	D23.1-☑	D48.5	D49.2
basal cell carcinoma	C44.11-☑	—	—	—	—	—
sebaceous cell	C44.13-☑	—	—	—	—	—
specified type NEC	C44.19-☑	—	—	—	—	—
squamous cell carcinoma	C44.12-☑	—	—	—	—	—
penis NEC	C60.9	C79.82	D07.4	D29.0	D40.8	D49.59
perianal — *see also* Neoplasm, skin, anus	C44.500	C79.2	D04.5	D23.5	D48.5	D49.2
perineum — *see also* Neoplasm, skin, anus	C44.500	C79.2	D04.5	D23.5	D48.5	D49.2
pinna — *see also* Neoplasm, skin, ear	C44.20-☑	C79.2	D04.2-☑	D23.2-☑	D48.5	D49.2
plantar — *see also* Neoplasm, skin, limb, lower	C44.70-☑	C79.2	D04.7-☑	D23.7-☑	D48.5	D49.2
popliteal fossa or space — *see also* Neoplasm, skin, limb, lower	C44.70-☑	C79.2	D04.7-☑	D23.7-☑	D48.5	D49.2
prepuce	C60.0	C79.82	D07.4	D29.0	D40.8	D49.59

Neoplasm, neoplastic — continued	Malignant Primary	Malignant Secondary	Ca in situ	Benign	Uncertain Behavior	Unspecified Behavior
skin — *continued*						
pubes — *see also* Neoplasm, skin, trunk	C44.509	C79.2	D04.5	D23.5	D48.5	D49.2
sacrococcygeal region — *see also* Neoplasm, skin, trunk	C44.509	C79.2	D04.5	D23.5	D48.5	D49.2
scalp	C44.40	C79.2	D04.4	D23.4	D48.5	D49.2
basal cell carcinoma	C44.41	—	—	—	—	—
specified type NEC	C44.49	—	—	—	—	—
squamous cell carcinoma	C44.42	—	—	—	—	—
scapular region — *see also* Neoplasm, skin, trunk	C44.509	C79.2	D04.5	D23.5	D48.5	D49.2
scrotum	C63.2	C79.82	D07.61	D29.4	D40.8	D49.59
shoulder — *see also* Neoplasm, skin, limb, upper	C44.60-☑	C79.2	D04.6-☑	D23.6-☑	D48.5	D49.2
sole (foot) — *see also* Neoplasm, skin, limb, lower	C44.70-☑	C79.2	D04.7-☑	D23.7-☑	D48.5	D49.2
specified sites NEC	C44.80	C79.2	D04.8	D23.9	D48.5	D49.2
basal cell carcinoma	C44.81	—	—	—	—	—
specified type NEC	C44.89	—	—	—	—	—
squamous cell carcinoma	C44.82	—	—	—	—	—
specified type NEC	C44.99	—	—	—	—	—
squamous cell carcinoma	C44.92	—	—	—	—	—
submammary fold — *see also* Neoplasm, skin, trunk	C44.509	C79.2	D04.5	D23.5	D48.5	D49.2
supraclavicular region — *see also* Neoplasm, skin, neck	C44.40	C79.2	D04.4	D23.4	D48.5	D49.2
temple — *see also* Neoplasm, skin, face	C44.309	C79.2	D04.39	D23.39	D48.5	D49.2
thigh — *see also* Neoplasm, skin, limb, lower	C44.70-☑	C79.2	D04.7-☑	D23.7-☑	D48.5	D49.2
thoracic wall — *see also* Neoplasm, skin, trunk	C44.509	C79.2	D04.5	D23.5	D48.5	D49.2
thumb — *see also* Neoplasm, skin, limb, upper	C44.60-☑	C79.2	D04.6-☑	D23.6-☑	D48.5	D49.2
toe — *see also* Neoplasm, skin, limb, lower	C44.70-☑	C79.2	D04.7-☑	D23.7-☑	D48.5	D49.2
tragus — *see also* Neoplasm, skin, ear	C44.20-☑	C79.2	D04.2-☑	D23.2-☑	D48.5	D49.2
trunk	C44.509	C79.2	D04.5	D23.5	D48.5	D49.2
basal cell carcinoma	C44.519	—	—	—	—	—
specified type NEC	C44.599	—	—	—	—	—
squamous cell carcinoma	C44.529	—	—	—	—	—
umbilicus — *see also* Neoplasm, skin, trunk	C44.509	C79.2	D04.5	D23.5	D48.5	D49.2
vulva	C51.9	C79.82	D07.1	D28.0	D39.8	D49.59
overlapping lesion	C51.8	—		—	—	—
wrist — *see also* Neoplasm, skin, limb, upper	C44.60-☑	C79.2	D04.6-☑	D23.6-☑	D48.5	D49.2
skull	C41.0	C79.51	—	D16.4	D48.0	D49.2

Neoplasm, soft parts or tissues — Neoplasm, tongue

Neoplasm, neoplastic	Malignant Primary	Malignant Secondary	Ca in situ	Benign	Uncertain Behavior	Unspecified Behavior
— continued						
soft parts or tissues —						
see Neoplasm, connective tissue						
specified site NEC	C76.8	C79.89	D09.8	D36.7	D48.7	D49.89
spermatic cord	C63.1-☑	C79.82	D07.69	D29.8	D40.8	D49.59
sphenoid	C31.3	C78.39	D02.3	D14.0	D38.5	D49.1
bone	C41.0	C79.51	—	D16.4	D48.0	D49.2
sinus	C31.3	C78.39	D02.3	D14.0	D38.5	D49.1
sphincter						
anal	C21.1	C78.5	D01.3	D12.9	D37.8	D49.0
of Oddi	C24.0	C78.89	D01.5	D13.5	D37.6	D49.0
spine, spinal						
(column)	C41.2	C79.51	—	D16.6	D48.0	D49.2
bulb	C71.7	C79.31	—	D33.1	D43.1	D49.6
coccyx	C41.4	C79.51	—	D16.8	D48.0	D49.2
cord (cervical) (lumbar) (sacral) (thoracic)	C72.0	C79.49	—	D33.4	D43.4	D49.7
dura mater	C70.1	C79.49	—	D32.1	D42.1	D49.7
lumbosacral	C41.2	C79.51	—	D16.6	D48.0	D49.2
marrow NEC	C96.9	C79.52	—	—	D47.9	D49.89
membrane	C70.1	C79.49	—	D32.1	D42.1	D49.7
meninges	C70.1	C79.49	—	D32.1	D42.1	D49.7
nerve (root)	C47.9	C79.89	—	D36.10	D48.2	D49.2
pia mater	C70.1	C79.49	—	D32.1	D42.1	D49.7
root	C47.9	C79.89	—	D36.10	D48.2	D49.2
sacrum	C41.4	C79.51	—	D16.8	D48.0	D49.2
spleen, splenic NEC	C26.1	C78.89	D01.7	D13.9	D37.8	D49.0
flexure (colon)	C18.5	C78.5	D01.0	D12.3	D37.4	D49.0
stem, brain	C71.7	C79.31	—	D33.1	D43.1	D49.6
Stensen's duct	C07	C79.89	D00.00	D11.0	D37.030	D49.0
sternum	C41.3	C79.51	—	D16.7	D48.0	D49.2
stomach	C16.9	C78.89	D00.2	D13.1	D37.1	D49.0
antrum (pyloric)	C16.3	C78.89	D00.2	D13.1	D37.1	D49.0
body	C16.2	C78.89	D00.2	D13.1	D37.1	D49.0
cardia	C16.0	C78.89	D00.2	D13.1	D37.1	D49.0
cardiac orifice	C16.0	C78.89	D00.2	D13.1	D37.1	D49.0
corpus	C16.2	C78.89	D00.2	D13.1	D37.1	D49.0
fundus	C16.1	C78.89	D00.2	D13.1	D37.1	D49.0
greater curvature NEC	C16.6	C78.89	D00.2	D13.1	D37.1	D49.0
lesser curvature NEC	C16.5	C78.89	D00.2	D13.1	D37.1	D49.0
overlapping lesion	C16.8	—	—	—	—	—
prepylorus	C16.4	C78.89	D00.2	D13.1	D37.1	D49.0
pylorus	C16.4	C78.89	D00.2	D13.1	D37.1	D49.0
wall NEC	C16.9	C78.89	D00.2	D13.1	D37.1	D49.0
anterior NEC	C16.8	C78.89	D00.2	D13.1	D37.1	D49.0
posterior NEC	C16.8	C78.89	D00.2	D13.1	D37.1	D49.0
stroma, endometrial	C54.1	C79.82	D07.0	D26.1	D39.0	D49.59
stump, cervical	C53.8	C79.82	D06.7	D26.0	D39.0	D49.59
subcutaneous (nodule) (tissue) NEC — see Neoplasm, connective tissue						
subdural	C70.9	C79.32	—	D32.9	D42.9	D49.7
subglottis, subglottic	C32.2	C78.39	D02.0	D14.1	D38.0	D49.1
sublingual	C04.9	C79.89	D00.06	D10.2	D37.09	D49.0
gland or duct	C08.1	C79.89	D00.00	D11.7	D37.031	D49.0
submandibular gland	C08.0	C79.89	D00.00	D11.7	D37.032	D49.0
submaxillary gland or duct	C08.0	C79.89	D00.00	D11.7	D37.032	D49.0
submental	C76.0	C79.89	D09.8	D36.7	D48.7	D49.89
subpleural	C34.9-☑	C78.0-☑	D02.2-☑	D14.3-☑	D38.1	D49.1
substernal	C38.1	C78.1	—	D15.2	D38.3	D49.89
sudoriferous, sudoriparous gland, site unspecified	C44.90	C79.2	D04.9	D23.9	D48.5	D49.2
specified site — see Neoplasm, skin						
supraclavicular region	C76.0	C79.89	D09.8	D36.7	D48.7	D49.89
supraglottis	C32.1	C78.39	D02.0	D14.1	D38.0	D49.1
suprarenal	C74.9-☑	C79.7-☑	D09.3	D35.0-☑	D44.1-☑	D49.7
capsule	C74.9-☑	C79.7-☑	D09.3	D35.0-☑	D44.1-☑	D49.7
— continued						
suprarenal — continued						
cortex	C74.0-☑	C79.7-☑	D09.3	D35.0-☑	D44.1-☑	D49.7
gland	C74.9-☑	C79.7-☑	D09.3	D35.0-☑	D44.1-☑	D49.7
medulla	C74.1-☑	C79.7-☑	D09.3	D35.0-☑	D44.1-☑	D49.7
suprasellar (region)	C71.9	C79.31	—	D33.2	D43.2	D49.6
supratentorial (brain) NEC	C71.0	C79.31	—	D33.0	D43.0	D49.6
sweat gland (apocrine) (eccrine), site unspecified	C44.90	C79.2	D04.9	D23.9	D48.5	D49.2
specified site — see Neoplasm, skin						
sympathetic nerve or nervous system NEC	C47.9	C79.89	—	D36.10	D48.2	D49.2
symphysis pubis	C41.4	C79.51	—	D16.8	D48.0	D49.2
synovial membrane — see Neoplasm, connective tissue						
tapetum, brain	C71.8	C79.31	—	D33.2	D43.2	D49.6
tarsus (any bone)	C40.3-☑	C79.51	—	D16.3-☑	—	—
temple (skin) — see also Neoplasm, skin, face	C44.309	C79.2	D04.39	D23.39	D48.5	D49.2
temporal						
bone	C41.0	C79.51	—	D16.4	D48.0	D49.2
lobe or pole	C71.2	C79.31	—	D33.0	D43.0	D49.6
region	C76.0	C79.89	D09.8	D36.7	D48.7	D49.89
skin — see also Neoplasm, skin, face	C44.309	C79.2	D04.39	D23.39	D48.5	D49.2
tendon (sheath) — see Neoplasm, connective tissue						
tentorium (cerebelli)	C70.0	C79.32	—	D32.0	D42.0	D49.7
testis, testes	C62.9-☑	C79.82	D07.69	D29.2-☑	D40.1-☑	D49.59
descended	C62.1-☑	C79.82	D07.69	D29.2-☑	D40.1-☑	D49.59
ectopic	C62.0-☑	C79.82	D07.69	D29.2-☑	D40.1-☑	D49.59
retained	C62.0-☑	C79.82	D07.69	D29.2-☑	D40.1-☑	D49.59
scrotal	C62.1-☑	C79.82	D07.69	D29.2-☑	D40.1-☑	D49.59
undescended	C62.0-☑	C79.82	D07.69	D29.2-☑	D40.1-☑	D49.59
unspecified whether descended or undescended	C62.9-☑	C79.82	D07.69	D29.2-☑	D40.1-☑	D49.59
thalamus	C71.0	C79.31	—	D33.0	D43.0	D49.6
thigh NEC	C76.5-☑	C79.89	D04.7-☑	D36.7	D48.7	D49.89
thorax, thoracic (cavity) (organs NEC)	C76.1	C79.89	D09.8	D36.7	D48.7	D49.89
duct	C49.3	C79.89	—	D21.3	D48.1	D49.2
wall NEC	C76.1	C79.89	D09.8	D36.7	D48.7	D49.89
throat	C14.0	C79.89	D00.08	D10.9	D37.05	D49.0
thumb NEC	C76.4-☑	C79.89	D04.6-☑	D36.7	D48.7	D49.89
thymus (gland)	C37	C79.89	D09.3	D15.0	D38.4	D49.89
thyroglossal duct	C73	C79.89	D09.3	D34	D44.0	D49.7
thyroid (gland)	C73	C79.89	D09.3	D34	D44.0	D49.7
cartilage	C32.3	C78.39	D02.0	D14.1	D38.0	D49.1
tibia (any part)	C40.2-☑	C79.51	—	D16.2-☑	—	—
toe NEC	C76.5-☑	C79.89	D04.7-☑	D36.7	D48.7	D49.89
tongue	C02.9	C79.89	D00.07	D10.1	D37.02	D49.0
anterior (two-thirds) NEC	C02.3	C79.89	D00.07	D10.1	D37.02	D49.0
dorsal surface	C02.0	C79.89	D00.07	D10.1	D37.02	D49.0
ventral surface	C02.2	C79.89	D00.07	D10.1	D37.02	D49.0
base (dorsal surface)	C01	C79.89	D00.07	D10.1	D37.02	D49.0
border (lateral)	C02.1	C79.89	D00.07	D10.1	D37.02	D49.0
dorsal surface NEC	C02.0	C79.89	D00.07	D10.1	D37.02	D49.0
fixed part NEC	C01	C79.89	D00.07	D10.1	D37.02	D49.0
foreamen cecum	C02.0	C79.89	D00.07	D10.1	D37.02	D49.0
frenulum linguae	C02.2	C79.89	D00.07	D10.1	D37.02	D49.0
junctional zone	C02.8	C79.89	D00.07	D10.1	D37.02	D49.0
margin (lateral)	C02.1	C79.89	D00.07	D10.1	D37.02	D49.0
midline NEC	C02.0	C79.89	D00.07	D10.1	D37.02	D49.0
mobile part NEC	C02.3	C79.89	D00.07	D10.1	D37.02	D49.0

☑ Additional Character Required — Refer to the Tabular List for Character Selection ▽ Subterms under main terms may continue to next column or page

Neoplasm, neoplastic	Malignant Primary	Malignant Secondary	Ca in situ	Benign	Uncertain Behavior	Unspecified Behavior
— continued						
tongue — continued						
overlapping lesion	C02.8	—	—	—	—	—
posterior (third)	C01	C79.89	D00.07	D10.1	D37.02	D49.0
root	C01	C79.89	D00.07	D10.1	D37.02	D49.0
surface (dorsal)	C02.0	C79.89	D00.07	D10.1	D37.02	D49.0
base	C01	C79.89	D00.07	D10.1	D37.02	D49.0
ventral	C02.2	C79.89	D00.07	D10.1	D37.02	D49.0
tip	C02.1	C79.89	D00.07	D10.1	D37.02	D49.0
tonsil	C02.4	C79.89	D00.07	D10.1	D37.02	D49.0
tonsil	C09.9	C79.89	D00.08	D10.4	D37.05	D49.0
fauces, faucial	C09.9	C79.89	D00.08	D10.4	D37.05	D49.0
lingual	C02.4	C79.89	D00.07	D10.1	D37.02	D49.0
overlapping sites	C09.8	—	—	—	—	—
palatine	C09.9	C79.89	D00.08	D10.4	D37.05	D49.0
pharyngeal	C11.1	C79.89	D00.08	D10.6	D37.05	D49.0
pillar (anterior)	C09.1	C79.89	D00.08	D10.5	D37.05	D49.0
(posterior)	C09.0	C79.89	D00.08	D10.5	D37.05	D49.0
tonsillar fossa	C09.0	C79.89	D00.08	D10.5	D37.05	D49.0
tooth socket NEC	C03.9	C79.89	D00.03	D10.39	D37.09	D49.0
trachea (cartilage) (mucosa)	C33	C78.39	D02.1	D14.2	D38.1	D49.1
overlapping lesion with bronchus or lung	C34.8-☑	—	—	—	—	—
tracheobronchial	C34.8-☑	C78.39	D02.1	D14.2	D38.1	D49.1
overlapping lesion with lung	C34.8-☑					
tragus — see also Neoplasm, skin, ear	C44.20-☑	C79.2	D04.2-☑	D23.2-☑	D48.5	D49.2
trunk NEC	C76.8	C79.89	D04.5	D36.7	D48.7	D49.89
tubo-ovarian	C57.8	C79.82	D07.39	D28.7	D39.8	D49.59
tunica vaginalis	C63.7	C79.82	D07.69	D29.8	D40.8	D49.59
turbinate (bone)	C41.0	C79.51	—	D16.4	D48.0	D49.2
nasal	C30.0	C78.39	D02.3	D14.0	D38.5	D49.1
tympanic cavity	C30.1	C78.39	D02.3	D14.0	D38.5	D49.1
ulna (any part)	C40.0-☑	C79.51	—	D16.0-☑	—	—
umbilicus, umbilical — see also Neoplasm, skin, trunk	C44.509	C79.2	D04.5	D23.5	D48.5	D49.2
uncus, brain	C71.2	C79.31	—	D33.0	D43.0	D49.6
unknown site or unspecified	C80.1	C79.9	D09.9	D36.9	D48.9	D49.9
urachus	C67.7	C79.11	D09.0	D30.3	D41.4	D49.4
ureter-bladder (junction)	C67.6	C79.11	D09.0	D30.3	D41.4	D49.4
ureter, ureteral	C66.-☑	C79.19	D09.19	D30.2-☑	D41.2-☑	D49.59
orifice (bladder)	C67.6	C79.11	D09.0	D30.3	D41.4	D49.4
urethra, urethral (gland)	C68.0	C79.19	D09.19	D30.4	D41.3	D49.59
orifice, internal	C67.5	C79.11	D09.0	D30.3	D41.4	D49.4
urethrovaginal (septum)	C57.9	C79.82	D07.30	D28.9	D39.8	D49.59
urinary organ or system	C68.9	C79.10	D09.10	D30.9	D41.9	D49.59
bladder — see Neoplasm, bladder						
overlapping lesion	C68.8	—	—	—	—	—
specified sites NEC	C68.8	C79.19	D09.19	D30.8	D41.8	D49.59
utero-ovarian	C57.8	C79.82	D07.39	D28.7	D39.8	D49.59
ligament	C57.1-☑	C79.82	D07.39	D28.2	D39.8	D49.59
uterosacral ligament	C57.3	C79.82	—	D28.2	D39.8	D49.59
uterus, uteri, uterine	C55	C79.82	D07.0	D26.9	D39.0	D49.59
adnexa NEC	C57.4	C79.82	D07.39	D28.7	D39.8	D49.59
body	C54.9	C79.82	D07.0	D26.1	D39.0	D49.59
cervix	C53.9	C79.82	D06.9	D26.0	D39.0	D49.59
cornu	C54.9	C79.82	D07.0	D26.1	D39.0	D49.59
corpus	C54.9	C79.82	D07.0	D26.1	D39.0	D49.59
endocervix (canal) (gland)	C53.0	C79.82	D06.0	D26.0	D39.0	D49.59
endometrium	C54.1	C79.82	D07.0	D26.1	D39.0	D49.59
exocervix	C53.1	C79.82	D06.1	D26.0	D39.0	D49.59
external os	C53.1	C79.82	D06.1	D26.0	D39.0	D49.59
fundus	C54.3	C79.82	D07.0	D26.1	D39.0	D49.59

Neoplasm, neoplastic	Malignant Primary	Malignant Secondary	Ca in situ	Benign	Uncertain Behavior	Unspecified Behavior
— continued						
uterus, uteri, uterine — continued						
internal os	C53.0	C79.82	D06.0	D26.0	D39.0	D49.59
isthmus	C54.0	C79.82	D07.0	D26.1	D39.0	D49.59
ligament	C57.3	C79.82	—	D28.2	D39.8	D49.59
broad	C57.1-☑	C79.82	D07.39	D28.2	D39.8	D49.59
round	C57.2-☑	C79.82	—	D28.2	D39.8	D49.59
lower segment	C54.0	C79.82	D07.0	D26.1	D39.0	D49.59
myometrium	C54.2	C79.82	D07.0	D26.1	D39.0	D49.59
overlapping sites	C54.8	—	—	—	—	—
squamocolumnar junction	C53.8	C79.82	D06.7	D26.0	D39.0	D49.59
tube	C57.0-☑	C79.82	D07.39	D28.2	D39.8	D49.59
utricle, prostatic	C68.0	C79.19	D09.19	D30.4	D41.3	D49.59
uveal tract	C69.4-☑	C79.49	D09.2-☑	D31.4-☑	D48.7	D49.89
uvula	C05.2	C79.89	D00.04	D10.39	D37.09	D49.0
vagina, vaginal (fornix) (vault) (wall)	C52	C79.82	D07.2	D28.1	D39.8	D49.59
vaginovesical	C57.9	C79.82	D07.30	D28.9	D39.9	D49.59
septum	C57.9	C79.82	D07.30	D28.9	D39.9	D49.59
vallecula (epigiottis)	C10.0	C79.89	D00.08	D10.5	D37.05	D49.0
vascular — see Neoplasm, connective tissue						
vas deferens	C63.1-☑	C79.82	D07.69	D29.8	D40.8	D49.59
Vater's ampulla	C24.1	C78.89	D01.5	D13.5	D37.6	D49.0
vein, venous — see Neoplasm, connective tissue						
vena cava (abdominal) (inferior)	C49.4	C79.89	—	D21.4	D48.1	D49.2
superior	C49.3	C79.89	—	D21.3	D48.1	D49.2
ventricle (cerebral) (floor) (lateral) (third)	C71.5	C79.31	—	D33.0	D43.0	D49.6
cardiac (left) (right)	C38.0	C79.89	—	D15.1	D48.7	D49.89
fourth	C71.7	C79.31	—	D33.1	D43.1	D49.6
ventricular band of larynx	C32.1	C78.39	D02.0	D14.1	D38.0	D49.1
ventriculus — see Neoplasm, stomach						
vermillion border — see Neoplasm, lip						
vermis, cerebellum	C71.6	C79.31	—	D33.1	D43.1	D49.6
vertebra (column)	C41.2	C79.51	—	D16.6	D48.0	D49.2
coccyx	C41.4	C79.51	—	D16.8	D48.0	D49.2
marrow NEC	C96.9	C79.52	—	—	D47.9	D49.89
sacrum	C41.4	C79.51	—	D16.8	D48.0	D49.2
vesical — see Neoplasm, bladder						
vesicle, seminal	C63.7	C79.82	D07.69	D29.8	D40.8	D49.59
vesicocervical tissue	C57.9	C79.82	D07.30	D28.9	D39.9	D49.59
vesicorectal	C76.3	C79.82	D09.8	D36.7	D48.7	D49.89
vesicovaginal	C57.9	C79.82	D07.30	D28.9	D39.9	D49.59
septum	C57.9	C79.82	D07.30	D28.9	D39.8	D49.59
vessel (blood) — see Neoplasm, connective tissue						
vestibular gland, greater	C51.0	C79.82	D07.1	D28.0	D39.8	D49.59
vestibule mouth	C06.1	C79.89	D00.00	D10.39	D37.09	D49.0
nose	C30.0	C78.39	D02.3	D14.0	D38.5	D49.1
Virchow's gland	C77.0	C77.0	—	D36.0	D48.7	D49.89
viscera NEC	C76.8	C79.89	D09.8	D36.7	D48.7	D49.89
vocal cords (true)	C32.0	C78.39	D02.0	D14.1	D38.0	D49.1
false	C32.1	C78.39	D02.0	D14.1	D38.0	D49.1
vomer	C41.0	C79.51	—	D16.4	D48.0	D49.2
vulva	C51.9	C79.82	D07.1	D28.0	D39.8	D49.59
vulvovaginal gland	C51.0	C79.82	D07.1	D28.0	D39.8	D49.59
Waldeyer's ring	C14.2	C79.89	D00.08	D10.9	D37.05	D49.0
Wharton's duct	C08.0	C79.89	D00.00	D11.7	D37.032	D49.0
white matter (central) (cerebral)	C71.0	C79.31	—	D33.0	D43.0	D49.6

	Malignant Primary	Malignant Secondary	Ca in situ	Benign	Uncertain Behavior	Unspecified Behavior
Neoplasm, neoplastic						
— *continued*						
windpipe	C33	C78.39	D02.1	D14.2	D38.1	D49.1
Wirsung's duct	C25.3	C78.89	D01.7	D13.6	D37.8	D49.0
wolffian (body) (duct)						
female	C57.7	C79.82	D07.39	D28.7	D39.8	D49.59
male	C63.7	C79.82	D07.69	D29.8	D40.8	D49.59
womb — *see*						
Neoplasm, uterus						
wrist NEC	C76.4-☑	C79.89	D04.6-☑	D36.7	D48.7	D49.89
xiphoid process	C41.3	C79.51	—	D16.7	D48.0	D49.2
Zuckerkandl						
organ	C75.5	C79.89	—	D35.6	D44.7	D49.7

☑ Additional Character Required — Refer to the Tabular List for Character Selection   ▽ Subterms under main terms may continue to next column or page

Substance	Poisoning, Accidental (unintentional)	Poisoning, Intentional Self-harm	Poisoning, Assault	Poisoning, Undetermined	Adverse Effect	Under-dosing
14-Hydroxydihydromorphinone	T40.2X1	T40.2X2	T40.2X3	T40.2X4	T40.2X5	T40.2X6
1-Propanol	T51.3X1	T51.3X2	T51.3X3	T51.3X4	—	—
2,3,7,8-Tetrachlorodibenzo-p-dioxin	T53.7X1	T53.7X2	T53.7X3	T53.7X4	—	—
2,4,5-T (trichlorophenoxyacetic acid)	T60.1X1	T60.1X2	T60.1X3	T60.1X4	—	—
2,4,5-Trichlorophenoxyacetic acid	T60.3X1	T60.3X2	T60.3X3	T60.3X4	—	—
2,4-D (dichlorophenoxyacetic acid)	T60.3X1	T60.3X2	T60.3X3	T60.3X4	—	—
2,4-Toluene diisocyanate	T65.0X1	T65.0X2	T65.0X3	T65.0X4	—	—
2-Deoxy-5-fluorouridine	T45.1X1	T45.1X2	T45.1X3	T45.1X4	T45.1X5	T45.1X6
2-Ethoxyethanol	T52.3X1	T52.3X2	T52.3X3	T52.3X4	—	—
2-Methoxyethanol	T52.3X1	T52.3X2	T52.3X3	T52.3X4	—	—
2-Propanol	T51.2X1	T51.2X2	T51.2X3	T51.2X4	—	—
3,4-methylenedioxymeth-amphetamine	T43.641	T43.642	T43.643	T43.644	—	—
4-Aminobutyric acid	T43.8X1	T43.8X2	T43.8X3	T43.8X4	T43.8X5	T43.8X6
4-Aminophenol derivatives	T39.1X1	T39.1X2	T39.1X3	T39.1X4	T39.1X5	T39.1X6
5-Deoxy-5-fluorouridine	T45.1X1	T45.1X2	T45.1X3	T45.1X4	T45.1X5	T45.1X6
5-Methoxypsoralen (5-MOP)	T50.991	T50.992	T50.993	T50.994	T50.995	T50.996
8-Aminoquinoline drugs	T37.2X1	T37.2X2	T37.2X3	T37.2X4	T37.2X5	T37.2X6
8-Methoxypsoralen (8-MOP)	T50.991	T50.992	T50.993	T50.994	T50.995	T50.996
ABOB	T37.5X1	T37.5X2	T37.5X3	T37.5X4	T37.5X5	T37.5X6
Abrine	T62.2X1	T62.2X2	T62.2X3	T62.2X4	—	—
Abrus (seed)	T62.2X1	T62.2X2	T62.2X3	T62.2X4	—	—
Absinthe	T51.0X1	T51.0X2	T51.0X3	T51.0X4	—	—
beverage	T51.0X1	T51.0X2	T51.0X3	T51.0X4	—	—
Acaricide	T60.8X1	T60.8X2	T60.8X3	T60.8X4	—	—
Acebutolol	T44.7X1	T44.7X2	T44.7X3	T44.7X4	T44.7X5	T44.7X6
Acecarbromal	T42.6X1	T42.6X2	T42.6X3	T42.6X4	T42.6X5	T42.6X6
Aceclidine	T44.1X1	T44.1X2	T44.1X3	T44.1X4	T44.1X5	T44.1X6
Acedapsone	T37.0X1	T37.0X2	T37.0X3	T37.0X4	T37.0X5	T37.0X6
Acefylline piperazine	T48.6X1	T48.6X2	T48.6X3	T48.6X4	T48.6X5	T48.6X6
Acemorphan	T40.2X1	T40.2X2	T40.2X3	T40.2X4	T40.2X5	T40.2X6
Acenocoumarin	T45.511	T45.512	T45.513	T45.514	T45.515	T45.516
Acenocoumarol	T45.511	T45.512	T45.513	T45.514	T45.515	T45.516
Acepifylline	T48.6X1	T48.6X2	T48.6X3	T48.6X4	T48.6X5	T48.6X6
Acepromazine	T43.3X1	T43.3X2	T43.3X3	T43.3X4	T43.3X5	T43.3X6
Acesulfamethoxypyridazine	T37.0X1	T37.0X2	T37.0X3	T37.0X4	T37.0X5	T37.0X6
Acetal	T52.8X1	T52.8X2	T52.8X3	T52.8X4	—	—
Acetaldehyde (vapor)	T52.8X1	T52.8X2	T52.8X3	T52.8X4	—	—
liquid	T65.891	T65.892	T65.893	T65.894	—	—
Acetaminophen	T39.1X1	T39.1X2	T39.1X3	T39.1X4	T39.1X5	T39.1X6
Acetaminosalol	T39.1X1	T39.1X2	T39.1X3	T39.1X4	T39.1X5	T39.1X6
Acetanilide	T39.1X1	T39.1X2	T39.1X3	T39.1X4	T39.1X5	T39.1X6
Acetarsol	T37.3X1	T37.3X2	T37.3X3	T37.3X4	T37.3X5	T37.3X6
Acetazolamide	T50.2X1	T50.2X2	T50.2X3	T50.2X4	T50.2X5	T50.2X6
Acetiamine	T45.2X1	T45.2X2	T45.2X3	T45.2X4	T45.2X5	T45.2X6
Acetic						
acid	T54.2X1	T54.2X2	T54.2X3	T54.2X4	—	—
with sodium acetate (ointment)	T49.3X1	T49.3X2	T49.3X3	T49.3X4	T49.3X5	T49.3X6
ester (solvent)(vapor)	T52.8X1	T52.8X2	T52.8X3	T52.8X4	—	—
irrigating solution	T50.3X1	T50.3X2	T50.3X3	T50.3X4	T50.3X5	T50.3X6
medicinal (lotion)	T49.2X1	T49.2X2	T49.2X3	T49.2X4	T49.2X5	T49.2X6
anhydride	T65.891	T65.892	T65.893	T65.894	—	—
ether (vapor)	T52.8X1	T52.8X2	T52.8X3	T52.8X4	—	—
Acetohexamide	T38.3X1	T38.3X2	T38.3X3	T38.3X4	T38.3X5	T38.3X6
Acetohydroxamic acid	T50.991	T50.992	T50.993	T50.994	T50.995	T50.996
Acetomenaphthone	T45.7X1	T45.7X2	T45.7X3	T45.7X4	T45.7X5	T45.7X6
Acetomorphine	T40.1X1	T40.1X2	T40.1X3	T40.1X4	—	—
Acetone (oils)	T52.4X1	T52.4X2	T52.4X3	T52.4X4	—	—
chlorinated	T52.4X1	T52.4X2	T52.4X3	T52.4X4	—	—
vapor	T52.4X1	T52.4X2	T52.4X3	T52.4X4	—	—
Acetonitrile	T52.8X1	T52.8X2	T52.8X3	T52.8X4	—	—
Acetophenazine	T43.3X1	T43.3X2	T43.3X3	T43.3X4	T43.3X5	T43.3X6
Acetophenetedin	T39.1X1	T39.1X2	T39.1X3	T39.1X4	T39.1X5	T39.1X6
Acetophenone	T52.4X1	T52.4X2	T52.4X3	T52.4X4	—	—
Acetorphine	T40.2X1	T40.2X2	T40.2X3	T40.2X4	—	—
Acetosulfone (sodium)	T37.1X1	T37.1X2	T37.1X3	T37.1X4	T37.1X5	T37.1X6
Acetrizoate (sodium)	T50.8X1	T50.8X2	T50.8X3	T50.8X4	T50.8X5	T50.8X6
Acetrizoic acid	T50.8X1	T50.8X2	T50.8X3	T50.8X4	T50.8X5	T50.8X6
Acetyl						
bromide	T53.6X1	T53.6X2	T53.6X3	T53.6X4	—	—
chloride	T53.6X1	T53.6X2	T53.6X3	T53.6X4	—	—
Acetylcarbromal	T42.6X1	T42.6X2	T42.6X3	T42.6X4	T42.6X5	T42.6X6
Acetylcholine						
chloride	T44.1X1	T44.1X2	T44.1X3	T44.1X4	T44.1X5	T44.1X6
derivative	T44.1X1	T44.1X2	T44.1X3	T44.1X4	T44.1X5	T44.1X6
Acetylcysteine	T48.4X1	T48.4X2	T48.4X3	T48.4X4	T48.4X5	T48.4X6
Acetyldigitoxin	T46.0X1	T46.0X2	T46.0X3	T46.0X4	T46.0X5	T46.0X6
Acetyldigoxin	T46.0X1	T46.0X2	T46.0X3	T46.0X4	T46.0X5	T46.0X6
Acetyldihydrocodeine	T40.2X1	T40.2X2	T40.2X3	T40.2X4	—	—
Acetyldihydrocodeinone	T40.2X1	T40.2X2	T40.2X3	T40.2X4	—	—
Acetylene (gas)	T59.891	T59.892	T59.893	T59.894	—	—
dichloride	T53.6X1	T53.6X2	T53.6X3	T53.6X4	—	—
incomplete combustion of	T58.11	T58.12	T58.13	T58.14	—	—
industrial	T59.891	T59.892	T59.893	T59.894	—	—
tetrachloride	T53.6X1	T53.6X2	T53.6X3	T53.6X4	—	—
vapor	T53.6X1	T53.6X2	T53.6X3	T53.6X4	—	—
Acetylphenturide	T42.6X1	T42.6X2	T42.6X3	T42.6X4	T42.6X5	T42.6X6
Acetylphenylhydrazine	T39.8X1	T39.8X2	T39.8X3	T39.8X4	T39.8X5	T39.8X6
Acetylsalicylic acid (salts)	T39.011	T39.012	T39.013	T39.014	T39.015	T39.016
enteric coated	T39.011	T39.012	T39.013	T39.014	T39.015	T39.016
Acetylsulfamethoxypyridazine	T37.0X1	T37.0X2	T37.0X3	T37.0X4	T37.0X5	T37.0X6
Achromycin	T36.4X1	T36.4X2	T36.4X3	T36.4X4	T36.4X5	T36.4X6
ophthalmic preparation	T49.5X1	T49.5X2	T49.5X3	T49.5X4	T49.5X5	T49.5X6
topical NEC	T49.0X1	T49.0X2	T49.0X3	T49.0X4	T49.0X5	T49.0X6
Aciclovir	T37.5X1	T37.5X2	T37.5X3	T37.5X4	T37.5X5	T37.5X6
Acidifying agent NEC	T50.901	T50.902	T50.903	T50.904	T50.905	T50.906
Acid (corrosive) NEC	T54.2X1	T54.2X2	T54.2X3	T54.2X4	—	—
Acipimox	T46.6X1	T46.6X2	T46.6X3	T46.6X4	T46.6X5	T46.6X6
Acitretin	T50.991	T50.992	T50.993	T50.994	T50.995	T50.996
Aclarubicin	T45.1X1	T45.1X2	T45.1X3	T45.1X4	T45.1X5	T45.1X6
Aclatonium napadisilate	T48.1X1	T48.1X2	T48.1X3	T48.1X4	T48.1X5	T48.1X6
Aconite (wild)	T46.991	T46.992	T46.993	T46.994	T46.995	T46.996
Aconitine	T46.991	T46.992	T46.993	T46.994	T46.995	T46.996
Aconitum ferox	T46.991	T46.992	T46.993	T46.994	T46.995	T46.996
Acridine	T65.6X1	T65.6X2	T65.6X3	T65.6X4	—	—
vapor	T59.891	T59.892	T59.893	T59.894	—	—
Acriflavine	T37.91	T37.92	T37.93	T37.94	T37.95	T37.96
Acriflavinium chloride	T49.0X1	T49.0X2	T49.0X3	T49.0X4	T49.0X5	T49.0X6
Acrinol	T49.0X1	T49.0X2	T49.0X3	T49.0X4	T49.0X5	T49.0X6
Acrisorcin	T49.0X1	T49.0X2	T49.0X3	T49.0X4	T49.0X5	T49.0X6
Acrivastine	T45.0X1	T45.0X2	T45.0X3	T45.0X4	T45.0X5	T45.0X6
Acrolein (gas)	T59.891	T59.892	T59.893	T59.894	—	—
liquid	T54.1X1	T54.1X2	T54.1X3	T54.1X4	—	—
Acrylamide	T65.891	T65.892	T65.893	T65.894	—	—
Acrylic resin	T49.3X1	T49.3X2	T49.3X3	T49.3X4	T49.3X5	T49.3X6
Acrylonitrile	T65.891	T65.892	T65.893	T65.894	—	—
Actaea spicata	T62.2X1	T62.2X2	T62.2X3	T62.2X4	—	—
berry	T62.1X1	T62.1X2	T62.1X3	T62.1X4	—	—
Acterol	T37.3X1	T37.3X2	T37.3X3	T37.3X4	T37.3X5	T37.3X6
ACTH	T38.811	T38.812	T38.813	T38.814	T38.815	T38.816
Actinomycin C	T45.1X1	T45.1X2	T45.1X3	T45.1X4	T45.1X5	T45.1X6
Actinomycin D	T45.1X1	T45.1X2	T45.1X3	T45.1X4	T45.1X5	T45.1X6
Activated charcoal — see also Charcoal, medicinal	T47.6X1	T47.6X2	T47.6X3	T47.6X4	T47.6X5	T47.6X6
Acyclovir	T37.5X1	T37.5X2	T37.5X3	T37.5X4	T37.5X5	T37.5X6
Adenine	T45.2X1	T45.2X2	T45.2X3	T45.2X4	T45.2X5	T45.2X6
arabinoside	T37.5X1	T37.5X2	T37.5X3	T37.5X4	T37.5X5	T37.5X6
Adenosine (phosphate)	T46.2X1	T46.2X2	T46.2X3	T46.2X4	T46.2X5	T46.2X6
ADH	T38.891	T38.892	T38.893	T38.894	T38.895	T38.896
Adhesive NEC	T65.891	T65.892	T65.893	T65.894	—	—
Adicillin	T36.0X1	T36.0X2	T36.0X3	T36.0X4	T36.0X5	T36.0X6
Adiphenine	T44.3X1	T44.3X2	T44.3X3	T44.3X4	T44.3X5	T44.3X6
Adipiodone	T50.8X1	T50.8X2	T50.8X3	T50.8X4	T50.8X5	T50.8X6
Adjunct, pharmaceutical	T50.901	T50.902	T50.903	T50.904	T50.905	T50.906
Adrenal (extract, cortex or medulla) (glucocorticoids) (hormones) (mineralocorticoids)	T38.0X1	T38.0X2	T38.0X3	T38.0X4	T38.0X5	T38.0X6
ENT agent	T49.6X1	T49.6X2	T49.6X3	T49.6X4	T49.6X5	T49.6X6
ophthalmic preparation	T49.5X1	T49.5X2	T49.5X3	T49.5X4	T49.5X5	T49.5X6
topical NEC	T49.0X1	T49.0X2	T49.0X3	T49.0X4	T49.0X5	T49.0X6
Adrenalin — see Adrenaline						
Adrenaline	T44.5X1	T44.5X2	T44.5X3	T44.5X4	T44.5X5	T44.5X6
Adrenergic NEC	T44.901	T44.902	T44.903	T44.904	T44.905	T44.906
blocking agent NEC	T44.8X1	T44.8X2	T44.8X3	T44.8X4	T44.8X5	T44.8X6
beta, heart	T44.7X1	T44.7X2	T44.7X3	T44.7X4	T44.7X5	T44.7X6
specified NEC	T44.991	T44.992	T44.993	T44.994	T44.995	T44.996
Adrenochrome						
derivative	T46.991	T46.992	T46.993	T46.994	T46.995	T46.996
(mono) semicarbazone	T46.991	T46.992	T46.993	T46.994	T46.995	T46.996
Adrenocorticotrophic hormone	T38.811	T38.812	T38.813	T38.814	T38.815	T38.816
Adrenocorticotrophin	T38.811	T38.812	T38.813	T38.814	T38.815	T38.816
Adriamycin	T45.1X1	T45.1X2	T45.1X3	T45.1X4	T45.1X5	T45.1X6
Aerosol spray NEC	T65.91	T65.92	T65.93	T65.94	—	—
Aerosporin	T36.8X1	T36.8X2	T36.8X3	T36.8X4	T36.8X5	T36.8X6
ENT agent	T49.6X1	T49.6X2	T49.6X3	T49.6X4	T49.6X5	T49.6X6
ophthalmic preparation	T49.5X1	T49.5X2	T49.5X3	T49.5X4	T49.5X5	T49.5X6

14-Hydroxydihydromorphinone — Aerosporin

Substance	Poisoning, Accidental (unintentional)	Poisoning, Intentional Self-harm	Poisoning, Assault	Poisoning, Undetermined	Adverse Effect	Under-dosing
Aerosporin — continued						
topical NEC	T49.0X1	T49.0X2	T49.0X3	T49.0X4	T49.0X5	T49.0X6
Aethusa cynapium	T62.2X1	T62.2X2	T62.2X3	T62.2X4	—	—
Afghanistan black	T40.7X1	T40.7X2	T40.7X3	T40.7X4	T40.7X5	T40.7X6
Aflatoxin	T64.01	T64.02	T64.03	T64.04	—	—
Afloqualone	T42.8X1	T42.8X2	T42.8X3	T42.8X4	T42.8X5	T42.8X6
African boxwood	T62.2X1	T62.2X2	T62.2X3	T62.2X4	—	—
Agar	T47.4X1	T47.4X2	T47.4X3	T47.4X4	T47.4X5	T47.4X6
Agonist						
predominantly						
alpha-adrenoreceptor	T44.4X1	T44.4X2	T44.4X3	T44.4X4	T44.4X5	T44.4X6
beta-adrenoreceptor	T44.5X1	T44.5X2	T44.5X3	T44.5X4	T44.5X5	T44.5X6
Agricultural agent NEC	T65.91	T65.92	T65.93	T65.94	—	—
Agrypnal	T42.3X1	T42.3X2	T42.3X3	T42.3X4	T42.3X5	T42.3X6
AHLG	T50.Z11	T50.Z12	T50.Z13	T50.Z14	T50.Z15	T50.Z16
Air contaminant(s), **source/type NOS**	T65.91	T65.92	T65.93	T65.94	—	—
Ajmaline	T46.2X1	T46.2X2	T46.2X3	T46.2X4	T46.2X5	T46.2X6
Akee	T62.1X1	T62.1X2	T62.1X3	T62.1X4	—	—
Akrinol	T49.0X1	T49.0X2	T49.0X3	T49.0X4	T49.0X5	T49.0X6
Akritoin	T37.8X1	T37.8X2	T37.8X3	T37.8X4	T37.8X5	T37.8X6
Alacepril	T46.4X1	T46.4X2	T46.4X3	T46.4X4	T46.4X5	T46.4X6
Alantolactone	T37.4X1	T37.4X2	T37.4X3	T37.4X4	T37.4X5	T37.4X6
Albamycin	T36.8X1	T36.8X2	T36.8X3	T36.8X4	T36.8X5	T36.8X6
Albendazole	T37.4X1	T37.4X2	T37.4X3	T37.4X4	T37.4X5	T37.4X6
Albumin						
bovine	T45.8X1	T45.8X2	T45.8X3	T45.8X4	T45.8X5	T45.8X6
human serum	T45.8X1	T45.8X2	T45.8X3	T45.8X4	T45.8X5	T45.8X6
salt-poor	T45.8X1	T45.8X2	T45.8X3	T45.8X4	T45.8X5	T45.8X6
normal human serum	T45.8X1	T45.8X2	T45.8X3	T45.8X4	T45.8X5	T45.8X6
Albuterol	T48.6X1	T48.6X2	T48.6X3	T48.6X4	T48.6X5	T48.6X6
Albutoin	T42.0X1	T42.0X2	T42.0X3	T42.0X4	T42.0X5	T42.0X6
Alclometasone	T49.0X1	T49.0X2	T49.0X3	T49.0X4	T49.0X5	T49.0X6
Alcohol	T51.91	T51.92	T51.93	T51.94	—	—
absolute	T51.0X1	T51.0X2	T51.0X3	T51.0X4	—	—
beverage	T51.0X1	T51.0X2	T51.0X3	T51.0X4	—	—
allyl	T51.8X1	T51.8X2	T51.8X3	T51.8X4	—	—
amyl	T51.3X1	T51.3X2	T51.3X3	T51.3X4	—	—
antifreeze	T51.1X1	T51.1X2	T51.1X3	T51.1X4	—	—
beverage	T51.0X1	T51.0X2	T51.0X3	T51.0X4	—	—
butyl	T51.3X1	T51.3X2	T51.3X3	T51.3X4	—	—
dehydrated	T51.0X1	T51.0X2	T51.0X3	T51.0X4	—	—
beverage	T51.0X1	T51.0X2	T51.0X3	T51.0X4	—	—
denatured	T51.0X1	T51.0X2	T51.0X3	T51.0X4	—	—
deterrent NEC	T50.6X1	T50.6X2	T50.6X3	T50.6X4	T50.6X5	T50.6X6
diagnostic (gastric function)	T50.8X1	T50.8X2	T50.8X3	T50.8X4	T50.8X5	T50.8X6
ethyl	T51.0X1	T51.0X2	T51.0X3	T51.0X4	—	—
beverage	T51.0X1	T51.0X2	T51.0X3	T51.0X4	—	—
grain	T51.0X1	T51.0X2	T51.0X3	T51.0X4	—	—
beverage	T51.0X1	T51.0X2	T51.0X3	T51.0X4	—	—
industrial	T51.0X1	T51.0X2	T51.0X3	T51.0X4	—	—
isopropyl	T51.2X1	T51.2X2	T51.2X3	T51.2X4	—	—
methyl	T51.1X1	T51.1X2	T51.1X3	T51.1X4	—	—
preparation for consumption	T51.0X1	T51.0X2	T51.0X3	T51.0X4	—	—
propyl	T51.3X1	T51.3X2	T51.3X3	T51.3X4	—	—
secondary	T51.2X1	T51.2X2	T51.2X3	T51.2X4	—	—
radiator	T51.1X1	T51.1X2	T51.1X3	T51.1X4	—	—
rubbing	T51.2X1	T51.2X2	T51.2X3	T51.2X4	—	—
specified type NEC	T51.8X1	T51.8X2	T51.8X3	T51.8X4	—	—
surgical	T51.0X1	T51.0X2	T51.0X3	T51.0X4	—	—
vapor (from any type of Alcohol)	T59.891	T59.892	T59.893	T59.894	—	—
wood	T51.1X1	T51.1X2	T51.1X3	T51.1X4	—	—
Alcuronium (chloride)	T48.1X1	T48.1X2	T48.1X3	T48.1X4	T48.1X5	T48.1X6
Aldactone	T50.0X1	T50.0X2	T50.0X3	T50.0X4	T50.0X5	T50.0X6
Aldesulfone sodium	T37.1X1	T37.1X2	T37.1X3	T37.1X4	T37.1X5	T37.1X6
Aldicarb	T60.0X1	T60.0X2	T60.0X3	T60.0X4	—	—
Aldomet	T46.5X1	T46.5X2	T46.5X3	T46.5X4	T46.5X5	T46.5X6
Aldosterone	T50.0X1	T50.0X2	T50.0X3	T50.0X4	T50.0X5	T50.0X6
Aldrin (dust)	T60.1X1	T60.1X2	T60.1X3	T60.1X4	—	—
Aleve — see Naproxen						
Alexitol sodium	T47.1X1	T47.1X2	T47.1X3	T47.1X4	T47.1X5	T47.1X6
Alfacalcidol	T45.2X1	T45.2X2	T45.2X3	T45.2X4	T45.2X5	T45.2X6
Alfadolone	T41.1X1	T41.1X2	T41.1X3	T41.1X4	T41.1X5	T41.1X6
Alfaxalone	T41.1X1	T41.1X2	T41.1X3	T41.1X4	T41.1X5	T41.1X6
Alfentanil	T40.4X1	T40.4X2	T40.4X3	T40.4X4	T40.4X5	T40.4X6
Alfuzosin (hydrochloride)	T44.8X1	T44.8X2	T44.8X3	T44.8X4	T44.8X5	T44.8X6
Algae (harmful) (toxin)	T65.821	T65.822	T65.823	T65.824	—	—
Algeldrate	T47.1X1	T47.1X2	T47.1X3	T47.1X4	T47.1X5	T47.1X6
Algin	T47.8X1	T47.8X2	T47.8X3	T47.8X4	T47.8X5	T47.8X6
Alglucerase	T45.3X1	T45.3X2	T45.3X3	T45.3X4	T45.3X5	T45.3X6

Substance	Poisoning, Accidental (unintentional)	Poisoning, Intentional Self-harm	Poisoning, Assault	Poisoning, Undetermined	Adverse Effect	Under-dosing
Alidase	T45.3X1	T45.3X2	T45.3X3	T45.3X4	T45.3X5	T45.3X6
Alimemazine	T43.3X1	T43.3X2	T43.3X3	T43.3X4	T43.3X5	T43.3X6
Aliphatic thiocyanates	T65.0X1	T65.0X2	T65.0X3	T65.0X4	—	—
Alizapride	T45.0X1	T45.0X2	T45.0X3	T45.0X4	T45.0X5	T45.0X6
Alkali (caustic)	T54.3X1	T54.3X2	T54.3X3	T54.3X4	—	—
Alkaline antiseptic solution (aromatic)	T49.6X1	T49.6X2	T49.6X3	T49.6X4	T49.6X5	T49.6X6
Alkalinizing agents (medicinal)	T50.901	T50.902	T50.903	T50.904	T50.905	T50.906
Alkalizing agent NEC	T50.901	T50.902	T50.903	T50.904	T50.905	T50.906
Alka-seltzer	T39.011	T39.012	T39.013	T39.014	T39.015	T39.016
Alkavervir	T46.5X1	T46.5X2	T46.5X3	T46.5X4	T46.5X5	T46.5X6
Alkonium (bromide)	T49.0X1	T49.0X2	T49.0X3	T49.0X4	T49.0X5	T49.0X6
Alkylating drug NEC	T45.1X1	T45.1X2	T45.1X3	T45.1X4	T45.1X5	T45.1X6
antimyeloproliferative	T45.1X1	T45.1X2	T45.1X3	T45.1X4	T45.1X5	T45.1X6
lymphatic	T45.1X1	T45.1X2	T45.1X3	T45.1X4	T45.1X5	T45.1X6
Alkylisocyanate	T65.0X1	T65.0X2	T65.0X3	T65.0X4	—	—
Allantoin	T49.4X1	T49.4X2	T49.4X3	T49.4X4	T49.4X5	T49.4X6
Allegron	T43.011	T43.012	T43.013	T43.014	T43.015	T43.016
Allethrin	T49.0X1	T49.0X2	T49.0X3	T49.0X4	T49.0X5	T49.0X6
Allobarbital	T42.3X1	T42.3X2	T42.3X3	T42.3X4	T42.3X5	T42.3X6
Allopurinol	T50.4X1	T50.4X2	T50.4X3	T50.4X4	T50.4X5	T50.4X6
Allyl						
alcohol	T51.8X1	T51.8X2	T51.8X3	T51.8X4	—	—
disulfide	T46.6X1	T46.6X2	T46.6X3	T46.6X4	T46.6X5	T46.6X6
Allylestrenol	T38.5X1	T38.5X2	T38.5X3	T38.5X4	T38.5X5	T38.5X6
Allylisopropylacetylurea	T42.6X1	T42.6X2	T42.6X3	T42.6X4	T42.6X5	T42.6X6
Allylisopropylmalonylurea	T42.3X1	T42.3X2	T42.3X3	T42.3X4	T42.3X5	T42.3X6
Allylthiourea	T49.3X1	T49.3X2	T49.3X3	T49.3X4	T49.3X5	T49.3X6
Allyltribromide	T42.6X1	T42.6X2	T42.6X3	T42.6X4	T42.6X5	T42.6X6
Allypropymal	T42.3X1	T42.3X2	T42.3X3	T42.3X4	T42.3X5	T42.3X6
Almagate	T47.1X1	T47.1X2	T47.1X3	T47.1X4	T47.1X5	T47.1X6
Almasilate	T47.1X1	T47.1X2	T47.1X3	T47.1X4	T47.1X5	T47.1X6
Almitrine	T50.7X1	T50.7X2	T50.7X3	T50.7X4	T50.7X5	T50.7X6
Aloes	T47.2X1	T47.2X2	T47.2X3	T47.2X4	T47.2X5	T47.2X6
Aloglutamol	T47.1X1	T47.1X2	T47.1X3	T47.1X4	T47.1X5	T47.1X6
Aloin	T47.2X1	T47.2X2	T47.2X3	T47.2X4	T47.2X5	T47.2X6
Aloxidone	T42.2X1	T42.2X2	T42.2X3	T42.2X4	T42.2X5	T42.2X6
Alpha						
acetyldigoxin	T46.0X1	T46.0X2	T46.0X3	T46.0X4	T46.0X5	T46.0X6
adrenergic blocking drug	T44.6X1	T44.6X2	T44.6X3	T44.6X4	T44.6X5	T44.6X6
amylase	T45.3X1	T45.3X2	T45.3X3	T45.3X4	T45.3X5	T45.3X6
tocoferol (acetate)	T45.2X1	T45.2X2	T45.2X3	T45.2X4	T45.2X5	T45.2X6
tocopherol	T45.2X1	T45.2X2	T45.2X3	T45.2X4	T45.2X5	T45.2X6
Alphadolone	T41.1X1	T41.1X2	T41.1X3	T41.1X4	T41.1X5	T41.1X6
Alphaprodine	T40.4X1	T40.4X2	T40.4X3	T40.4X4	T40.4X5	T40.4X6
Alphaxalone	T41.1X1	T41.1X2	T41.1X3	T41.1X4	T41.1X5	T41.1X6
Alprazolam	T42.4X1	T42.4X2	T42.4X3	T42.4X4	T42.4X5	T42.4X6
Alprenolol	T44.7X1	T44.7X2	T44.7X3	T44.7X4	T44.7X5	T44.7X6
Alprostadil	T46.7X1	T46.7X2	T46.7X3	T46.7X4	T46.7X5	T46.7X6
Alsactide	T38.811	T38.812	T38.813	T38.814	T38.815	T38.816
Alseroxylon	T46.5X1	T46.5X2	T46.5X3	T46.5X4	T46.5X5	T46.5X6
Alteplase	T45.611	T45.612	T45.613	T45.614	T45.615	T45.616
Altizide	T50.2X1	T50.2X2	T50.2X3	T50.2X4	T50.2X5	T50.2X6
Altretamine	T45.1X1	T45.1X2	T45.1X3	T45.1X4	T45.1X5	T45.1X6
Alum (medicinal)	T49.4X1	T49.4X2	T49.4X3	T49.4X4	T49.4X5	T49.4X6
nonmedicinal (ammonium) (potassium)	T56.891	T56.892	T56.893	T56.894	—	—
Aluminium, aluminum						
acetate	T49.2X1	T49.2X2	T49.2X3	T49.2X4	T49.2X5	T49.2X6
solution	T49.0X1	T49.0X2	T49.0X3	T49.0X4	T49.0X5	T49.0X6
aspirin	T39.011	T39.012	T39.013	T39.014	T39.015	T39.016
bis (acetylsalicylate)	T39.011	T39.012	T39.013	T39.014	T39.015	T39.016
carbonate (gel, basic)	T47.1X1	T47.1X2	T47.1X3	T47.1X4	T47.1X5	T47.1X6
chlorhydroxide-complex	T47.1X1	T47.1X2	T47.1X3	T47.1X4	T47.1X5	T47.1X6
chloride	T49.2X1	T49.2X2	T49.2X3	T49.2X4	T49.2X5	T49.2X6
clofibrate	T46.6X1	T46.6X2	T46.6X3	T46.6X4	T46.6X5	T46.6X6
diacetate	T49.2X1	T49.2X2	T49.2X3	T49.2X4	T49.2X5	T49.2X6
glycinate	T47.1X1	T47.1X2	T47.1X3	T47.1X4	T47.1X5	T47.1X6
hydroxide (gel)	T47.1X1	T47.1X2	T47.1X3	T47.1X4	T47.1X5	T47.1X6
hydroxide-magnesium carb. gel	T47.1X1	T47.1X2	T47.1X3	T47.1X4	T47.1X5	T47.1X6
magnesium silicate	T47.1X1	T47.1X2	T47.1X3	T47.1X4	T47.1X5	T47.1X6
nicotinate	T46.7X1	T46.7X2	T46.7X3	T46.7X4	T46.7X5	T46.7X6
ointment (surgical) (topical)	T49.3X1	T49.3X2	T49.3X3	T49.3X4	T49.3X5	T49.3X6
phosphate	T47.1X1	T47.1X2	T47.1X3	T47.1X4	T47.1X5	T47.1X6
salicylate	T39.091	T39.092	T39.093	T39.094	T39.095	T39.096
silicate	T47.1X1	T47.1X2	T47.1X3	T47.1X4	T47.1X5	T47.1X6
sodium silicate	T47.1X1	T47.1X2	T47.1X3	T47.1X4	T47.1X5	T47.1X6
subacetate	T49.2X1	T49.2X2	T49.2X3	T49.2X4	T49.2X5	T49.2X6
sulfate	T49.0X1	T49.0X2	T49.0X3	T49.0X4	T49.0X5	T49.0X6
tannate	T47.6X1	T47.6X2	T47.6X3	T47.6X4	T47.6X5	T47.6X6

Table of Drugs and Chemicals — Aerosporin — Aluminium, aluminum

Substance	Poisoning, Accidental (unintentional)	Poisoning, Intentional Self-harm	Poisoning, Assault	Poisoning, Undetermined	Adverse Effect	Under-dosing
Aluminium, aluminum — *continued*						
topical NEC	T49.3X1	T49.3X2	T49.3X3	T49.3X4	T49.3X5	T49.3X6
Alurate	T42.3X1	T42.3X2	T42.3X3	T42.3X4	T42.3X5	T42.3X6
Alverine	T44.3X1	T44.3X2	T44.3X3	T44.3X4	T44.3X5	T44.3X6
Alvodine	T40.2X1	T40.2X2	T40.2X3	T40.2X4	T40.2X5	T40.2X6
Amanita phalloides	T62.0X1	T62.0X2	T62.0X3	T62.0X4	—	—
Amanitine	T62.0X1	T62.0X2	T62.0X3	T62.0X4	—	—
Amantadine	T42.8X1	T42.8X2	T42.8X3	T42.8X4	T42.8X5	T42.8X6
Ambazone	T49.6X1	T49.6X2	T49.6X3	T49.6X4	T49.6X5	T49.6X6
Ambenonium (chloride)	T44.0X1	T44.0X2	T44.0X3	T44.0X4	T44.0X5	T44.0X6
Ambroxol	T48.4X1	T48.4X2	T48.4X3	T48.4X4	T48.4X5	T48.4X6
Ambuphylline	T48.6X1	T48.6X2	T48.6X3	T48.6X4	T48.6X5	T48.6X6
Ambutonium bromide	T44.3X1	T44.3X2	T44.3X3	T44.3X4	T44.3X5	T44.3X6
Amcinonide	T49.0X1	T49.0X2	T49.0X3	T49.0X4	T49.0X5	T49.0X6
Amdinocilline	T36.0X1	T36.0X2	T36.0X3	T36.0X4	T36.0X5	T36.0X6
Ametazole	T50.8X1	T50.8X2	T50.8X3	T50.8X4	T50.8X5	T50.8X6
Amethocaine	T41.3X1	T41.3X2	T41.3X3	T41.3X4	T41.3X5	T41.3X6
regional	T41.3X1	T41.3X2	T41.3X3	T41.3X4	T41.3X5	T41.3X6
spinal	T41.3X1	T41.3X2	T41.3X3	T41.3X4	T41.3X5	T41.3X6
Amethopterin	T45.1X1	T45.1X2	T45.1X3	T45.1X4	T45.1X5	T45.1X6
Amezinium metilsulfate	T44.991	T44.992	T44.993	T44.994	T44.995	T44.996
Amfebutamone	T43.291	T43.292	T43.293	T43.294	T43.295	T43.296
Amfepramone	T50.5X1	T50.5X2	T50.5X3	T50.5X4	T50.5X5	T50.5X6
Amfetamine	T43.621	T43.622	T43.623	T43.624	T43.625	T43.626
Amfetaminil	T43.621	T43.622	T43.623	T43.624	T43.625	T43.626
Amfomycin	T36.8X1	T36.8X2	T36.8X3	T36.8X4	T36.8X5	T36.8X6
Amidefrine mesilate	T48.5X1	T48.5X2	T48.5X3	T48.5X4	T48.5X5	T48.5X6
Amidone	T40.3X1	T40.3X2	T40.3X3	T40.3X4	T40.3X5	T40.3X6
Amidopyrine	T39.2X1	T39.2X2	T39.2X3	T39.2X4	T39.2X5	T39.2X6
Amidotrizoate	T50.8X1	T50.8X2	T50.8X3	T50.8X4	T50.8X5	T50.8X6
Amiflamine	T43.1X1	T43.1X2	T43.1X3	T43.1X4	T43.1X5	T43.1X6
Amikacin	T36.5X1	T36.5X2	T36.5X3	T36.5X4	T36.5X5	T36.5X6
Amikhelline	T46.3X1	T46.3X2	T46.3X3	T46.3X4	T46.3X5	T46.3X6
Amiloride	T50.2X1	T50.2X2	T50.2X3	T50.2X4	T50.2X5	T50.2X6
Aminacrine	T49.0X1	T49.0X2	T49.0X3	T49.0X4	T49.0X5	T49.0X6
Amineptine	T43.011	T43.012	T43.013	T43.014	T43.015	T43.016
Aminitrozole	T37.3X1	T37.3X2	T37.3X3	T37.3X4	T37.3X5	T37.3X6
Aminoacetic acid (derivatives)	T50.3X1	T50.3X2	T50.3X3	T50.3X4	T50.3X5	T50.3X6
Amino acids	T50.3X1	T50.3X2	T50.3X3	T50.3X4	T50.3X5	T50.3X6
Aminoacridine	T49.0X1	T49.0X2	T49.0X3	T49.0X4	T49.0X5	T49.0X6
Aminobenzoic acid (-p)	T49.3X1	T49.3X2	T49.3X3	T49.3X4	T49.3X5	T49.3X6
Aminocaproic acid	T45.621	T45.622	T45.623	T45.624	T45.625	T45.626
Aminoethylisothiourium	T45.8X1	T45.8X2	T45.8X3	T45.8X4	T45.8X5	T45.8X6
Aminofenazone	T39.2X1	T39.2X2	T39.2X3	T39.2X4	T39.2X5	T39.2X6
Aminoglutethimide	T45.1X1	T45.1X2	T45.1X3	T45.1X4	T45.1X5	T45.1X6
Aminohippuric acid	T50.8X1	T50.8X2	T50.8X3	T50.8X4	T50.8X5	T50.8X6
Aminomethylbenzoic acid	T45.691	T45.692	T45.693	T45.694	T45.695	T45.696
Aminometradine	T50.2X1	T50.2X2	T50.2X3	T50.2X4	T50.2X5	T50.2X6
Aminopentamide	T44.3X1	T44.3X2	T44.3X3	T44.3X4	T44.3X5	T44.3X6
Aminophenazone	T39.2X1	T39.2X2	T39.2X3	T39.2X4	T39.2X5	T39.2X6
Aminophenol	T54.0X1	T54.0X2	T54.0X3	T54.0X4	—	—
Aminophenylpyridone	T43.591	T43.592	T43.593	T43.594	T43.595	T43.596
Aminophylline	T48.6X1	T48.6X2	T48.6X3	T48.6X4	T48.6X5	T48.6X6
Aminopterin sodium	T45.1X1	T45.1X2	T45.1X3	T45.1X4	T45.1X5	T45.1X6
Aminopyrine	T39.2X1	T39.2X2	T39.2X3	T39.2X4	T39.2X5	T39.2X6
Aminorex	T50.5X1	T50.5X2	T50.5X3	T50.5X4	T50.5X5	T50.5X6
Aminosalicylic acid	T37.1X1	T37.1X2	T37.1X3	T37.1X4	T37.1X5	T37.1X6
Aminosalylum	T37.1X1	T37.1X2	T37.1X3	T37.1X4	T37.1X5	T37.1X6
Amiodarone	T46.2X1	T46.2X2	T46.2X3	T46.2X4	T46.2X5	T46.2X6
Amiphenazole	T50.7X1	T50.7X2	T50.7X3	T50.7X4	T50.7X5	T50.7X6
Amiquinsin	T46.5X1	T46.5X2	T46.5X3	T46.5X4	T46.5X5	T46.5X6
Amisometradine	T50.2X1	T50.2X2	T50.2X3	T50.2X4	T50.2X5	T50.2X6
Amisulpride	T43.591	T43.592	T43.593	T43.594	T43.595	T43.596
Amitriptyline	T43.011	T43.012	T43.013	T43.014	T43.015	T43.016
Amitriptylinoxide	T43.011	T43.012	T43.013	T43.014	T43.015	T43.016
Amlexanox	T48.6X1	T48.6X2	T48.6X3	T48.6X4	T48.6X5	T48.6X6
Ammonia (fumes) (gas) (vapor)	T59.891	T59.892	T59.893	T59.894	—	—
aromatic spirit	T48.991	T48.992	T48.993	T48.994	T48.995	T48.996
liquid (household)	T54.3X1	T54.3X2	T54.3X3	T54.3X4	—	—
Ammoniated mercury	T49.0X1	T49.0X2	T49.0X3	T49.0X4	T49.0X5	T49.0X6
Ammonium						
acid tartrate	T49.5X1	T49.5X2	T49.5X3	T49.5X4	T49.5X5	T49.5X6
bromide	T42.6X1	T42.6X2	T42.6X3	T42.6X4	T42.6X5	T42.6X6
carbonate	T54.3X1	T54.3X2	T54.3X3	T54.3X4	—	—
chloride	T50.991	T50.992	T50.993	T50.994	T50.995	T50.996
expectorant	T48.4X1	T48.4X2	T48.4X3	T48.4X4	T48.4X5	T48.4X6
compounds (household) NEC	T54.3X1	T54.3X2	T54.3X3	T54.3X4	—	—
fumes (any usage)	T59.891	T59.892	T59.893	T59.894	—	—
industrial	T54.3X1	T54.3X2	T54.3X3	T54.3X4	—	—
Ammonium — *continued*						
ichthyosulronate	T49.4X1	T49.4X2	T49.4X3	T49.4X4	T49.4X5	T49.4X6
mandelate	T37.91	T37.92	T37.93	T37.94	T37.95	T37.96
sulfamate	T60.3X1	T60.3X2	T60.3X3	T60.3X4	—	—
sulfonate resin	T47.8X1	T47.8X2	T47.8X3	T47.8X4	T47.8X5	T47.8X6
Amobarbital (sodium)	T42.3X1	T42.3X2	T42.3X3	T42.3X4	T42.3X5	T42.3X6
Amodiaquine	T37.2X1	T37.2X2	T37.2X3	T37.2X4	T37.2X5	T37.2X6
Amopyroquin (e)	T37.2X1	T37.2X2	T37.2X3	T37.2X4	T37.2X5	T37.2X6
Amoxapine	T43.011	T43.012	T43.013	T43.014	T43.015	T43.016
Amoxicillin	T36.0X1	T36.0X2	T36.0X3	T36.0X4	T36.0X5	T36.0X6
Amperozide	T43.591	T43.592	T43.593	T43.594	T43.595	T43.596
Amphenidone	T43.591	T43.592	T43.593	T43.594	T43.595	T43.596
Amphetamine NEC	T43.621	T43.622	T43.623	T43.624	T43.625	T43.626
Amphomycin	T36.8X1	T36.8X2	T36.8X3	T36.8X4	T36.8X5	T36.8X6
Amphotalide	T37.4X1	T37.4X2	T37.4X3	T37.4X4	T37.4X5	T37.4X6
Amphotericin B	T36.7X1	T36.7X2	T36.7X3	T36.7X4	T36.7X5	T36.7X6
topical	T49.0X1	T49.0X2	T49.0X3	T49.0X4	T49.0X5	T49.0X6
Ampicillin	T36.0X1	T36.0X2	T36.0X3	T36.0X4	T36.0X5	T36.0X6
Amprotropine	T44.3X1	T44.3X2	T44.3X3	T44.3X4	T44.3X5	T44.3X6
Amsacrine	T45.1X1	T45.1X2	T45.1X3	T45.1X4	T45.1X5	T45.1X6
Amygdaline	T62.2X1	T62.2X2	T62.2X3	T62.2X4	—	—
Amyl						
acetate	T52.8X1	T52.8X2	T52.8X3	T52.8X4	—	—
vapor	T59.891	T59.892	T59.893	T59.894	—	—
alcohol	T51.3X1	T51.3X2	T51.3X3	T51.3X4	—	—
chloride	T53.6X1	T53.6X2	T53.6X3	T53.6X4	—	—
formate	T52.8X1	T52.8X2	T52.8X3	T52.8X4	—	—
nitrite	T46.3X1	T46.3X2	T46.3X3	T46.3X4	T46.3X5	T46.3X6
propionate	T65.891	T65.892	T65.893	T65.894	—	—
Amylase	T47.5X1	T47.5X2	T47.5X3	T47.5X4	T47.5X5	T47.5X6
Amyleine, regional	T41.3X1	T41.3X2	T41.3X3	T41.3X4	T41.3X5	T41.3X6
Amylene						
dichloride	T53.6X1	T53.6X2	T53.6X3	T53.6X4	—	—
hydrate	T51.3X1	T51.3X2	T51.3X3	T51.3X4	—	—
Amylmetacresol	T49.6X1	T49.6X2	T49.6X3	T49.6X4	T49.6X5	T49.6X6
Amylobarbitone	T42.3X1	T42.3X2	T42.3X3	T42.3X4	T42.3X5	T42.3X6
Amylocaine, regional	T41.3X1	T41.3X2	T41.3X3	T41.3X4	T41.3X5	T41.3X6
infiltration (subcutaneous)	T41.3X1	T41.3X2	T41.3X3	T41.3X4	T41.3X5	T41.3X6
nerve block (peripheral) (plexus)	T41.3X1	T41.3X2	T41.3X3	T41.3X4	T41.3X5	T41.3X6
spinal	T41.3X1	T41.3X2	T41.3X3	T41.3X4	T41.3X5	T41.3X6
topical (surface)	T41.3X1	T41.3X2	T41.3X3	T41.3X4	T41.3X5	T41.3X6
Amylopectin	T47.6X1	T47.6X2	T47.6X3	T47.6X4	T47.6X5	T47.6X6
Amytal (sodium)	T42.3X1	T42.3X2	T42.3X3	T42.3X4	T42.3X5	T42.3X6
Anabolic steroid	T38.7X1	T38.7X2	T38.7X3	T38.7X4	T38.7X5	T38.7X6
Analeptic NEC	T50.7X1	T50.7X2	T50.7X3	T50.7X4	T50.7X5	T50.7X6
Analgesic	T39.91	T39.92	T39.93	T39.94	T39.95	T39.96
anti-inflammatory NEC	T39.91	T39.92	T39.93	T39.94	T39.95	T39.96
propionic acid derivative	T39.311	T39.312	T39.313	T39.314	T39.315	T39.316
antirheumatic NEC	T39.4X1	T39.4X2	T39.4X3	T39.4X4	T39.4X5	T39.4X6
aromatic NEC	T39.1X1	T39.1X2	T39.1X3	T39.1X4	T39.1X5	T39.1X6
narcotic NEC	T40.601	T40.602	T40.603	T40.604	T40.605	T40.606
combination	T40.601	T40.602	T40.603	T40.604	T40.605	T40.606
obstetric	T40.601	T40.602	T40.603	T40.604	T40.605	T40.606
non-narcotic NEC	T39.91	T39.92	T39.93	T39.94	T39.95	T39.96
combination	T39.91	T39.92	T39.93	T39.94	T39.95	T39.96
pyrazole	T39.2X1	T39.2X2	T39.2X3	T39.2X4	T39.2X5	T39.2X6
specified NEC	T39.8X1	T39.8X2	T39.8X3	T39.8X4	T39.8X5	T39.8X6
Analgin	T39.2X1	T39.2X2	T39.2X3	T39.2X4	T39.2X5	T39.2X6
Anamirta cocculus	T62.1X1	T62.1X2	T62.1X3	T62.1X4	—	—
Ancillin	T36.0X1	T36.0X2	T36.0X3	T36.0X4	T36.0X5	T36.0X6
Ancrod	T45.691	T45.692	T45.693	T45.694	T45.695	T45.696
Androgen	T38.7X1	T38.7X2	T38.7X3	T38.7X4	T38.7X5	T38.7X6
Androgen-estrogen mixture	T38.7X1	T38.7X2	T38.7X3	T38.7X4	T38.7X5	T38.7X6
Androstalone	T38.7X1	T38.7X2	T38.7X3	T38.7X4	T38.7X5	T38.7X6
Androstanolone	T38.7X1	T38.7X2	T38.7X3	T38.7X4	T38.7X5	T38.7X6
Androsterone	T38.7X1	T38.7X2	T38.7X3	T38.7X4	T38.7X5	T38.7X6
Anemone pulsatilla	T62.2X1	T62.2X2	T62.2X3	T62.2X4	—	—
Anesthesia						
caudal	T41.3X1	T41.3X2	T41.3X3	T41.3X4	T41.3X5	T41.3X6
endotracheal	T41.0X1	T41.0X2	T41.0X3	T41.0X4	T41.0X5	T41.0X6
epidural	T41.3X1	T41.3X2	T41.3X3	T41.3X4	T41.3X5	T41.3X6
inhalation	T41.0X1	T41.0X2	T41.0X3	T41.0X4	T41.0X5	T41.0X6
local	T41.3X1	T41.3X2	T41.3X3	T41.3X4	T41.3X5	T41.3X6
mucosal	T41.3X1	T41.3X2	T41.3X3	T41.3X4	T41.3X5	T41.3X6
muscle relaxation	T48.1X1	T48.1X2	T48.1X3	T48.1X4	T48.1X5	T48.1X6
nerve blocking	T41.3X1	T41.3X2	T41.3X3	T41.3X4	T41.3X5	T41.3X6
plexus blocking	T41.3X1	T41.3X2	T41.3X3	T41.3X4	T41.3X5	T41.3X6
potentiated	T41.201	T41.202	T41.203	T41.204	T41.205	T41.206
rectal	T41.201	T41.202	T41.203	T41.204	T41.205	T41.206
general	T41.201	T41.202	T41.203	T41.204	T41.205	T41.206
local	T41.3X1	T41.3X2	T41.3X3	T41.3X4	T41.3X5	T41.3X6

Substance	Poisoning, Accidental (unintentional)	Poisoning, Intentional Self-harm	Poisoning, Assault	Poisoning, Undetermined	Adverse Effect	Under-dosing
Anesthesia — *continued*						
regional	T41.3X1	T41.3X2	T41.3X3	T41.3X4	T41.3X5	T41.3X6
surface	T41.3X1	T41.3X2	T41.3X3	T41.3X4	T41.3X5	T41.3X6
Anesthetic NEC — *see also*	T41.41	T41.42	T41.43	T41.44	T41.45	T41.46
Anesthesia						
with muscle relaxant	T41.201	T41.202	T41.203	T41.204	T41.205	T41.206
general	T41.201	T41.202	T41.203	T41.204	T41.205	T41.206
local	T41.3X1	T41.3X2	T41.3X3	T41.3X4	T41.3X5	T41.3X6
gaseous NEC	T41.0X1	T41.0X2	T41.0X3	T41.0X4	T41.0X5	T41.0X6
general NEC	T41.201	T41.202	T41.203	T41.204	T41.205	T41.206
halogenated hydrocarbon	T41.0X1	T41.0X2	T41.0X3	T41.0X4	T41.0X5	T41.0X6
derivatives NEC						
infiltration NEC	T41.3X1	T41.3X2	T41.3X3	T41.3X4	T41.3X5	T41.3X6
intravenous NEC	T41.1X1	T41.1X2	T41.1X3	T41.1X4	T41.1X5	T41.1X6
local NEC	T41.3X1	T41.3X2	T41.3X3	T41.3X4	T41.3X5	T41.3X6
rectal	T41.201	T41.202	T41.203	T41.204	T41.205	T41.206
general	T41.201	T41.202	T41.203	T41.204	T41.205	T41.206
local	T41.3X1	T41.3X2	T41.3X3	T41.3X4	T41.3X5	T41.3X6
regional NEC	T41.3X1	T41.3X2	T41.3X3	T41.3X4	T41.3X5	T41.3X6
spinal NEC	T41.3X1	T41.3X2	T41.3X3	T41.3X4	T41.3X5	T41.3X6
thiobarbiturate	T41.1X1	T41.1X2	T41.1X3	T41.1X4	T41.1X5	T41.1X6
topical	T41.3X1	T41.3X2	T41.3X3	T41.3X4	T41.3X5	T41.3X6
Aneurine	T45.2X1	T45.2X2	T45.2X3	T45.2X4	T45.2X5	T45.2X6
Angio-Conray	T50.8X1	T50.8X2	T50.8X3	T50.8X4	T50.8X5	T50.8X6
Angiotensin	T44.5X1	T44.5X2	T44.5X3	T44.5X4	T44.5X5	T44.5X6
Angiotensinamide	T44.991	T44.992	T44.993	T44.994	T44.995	T44.996
Anhydrohydroxy-progesterone	T38.5X1	T38.5X2	T38.5X3	T38.5X4	T38.5X5	T38.5X6
Anhydron	T50.2X1	T50.2X2	T50.2X3	T50.2X4	T50.2X5	T50.2X6
Anileridine	T40.4X1	T40.4X2	T40.4X3	T40.4X4	T40.4X5	T40.4X6
Aniline (dye) (liquid)	T65.3X1	T65.3X2	T65.3X3	T65.3X4	—	—
analgesic	T39.1X1	T39.1X2	T39.1X3	T39.1X4	T39.1X5	T39.1X6
derivatives, therapeutic NEC	T39.1X1	T39.1X2	T39.1X3	T39.1X4	T39.1X5	T39.1X6
vapor	T65.3X1	T65.3X2	T65.3X3	T65.3X4	—	—
Aniscoropine	T44.3X1	T44.3X2	T44.3X3	T44.3X4	T44.3X5	T44.3X6
Anise oil	T47.5X1	T47.5X2	T47.5X3	T47.5X4	T47.5X5	T47.5X6
Anisidine	T65.3X1	T65.3X2	T65.3X3	T65.3X4	—	—
Anisindione	T45.511	T45.512	T45.513	T45.514	T45.515	T45.516
Anisotropine	T44.3X1	T44.3X2	T44.3X3	T44.3X4	T44.3X5	T44.3X6
methyl-bromide						
Anistreplase	T45.611	T45.612	T45.613	T45.614	T45.615	T45.616
Anorexiant (central)	T50.5X1	T50.5X2	T50.5X3	T50.5X4	T50.5X5	T50.5X6
Anorexic agents	T50.5X1	T50.5X2	T50.5X3	T50.5X4	T50.5X5	T50.5X6
Ansamycin	T36.6X1	T36.6X2	T36.6X3	T36.6X4	T36.6X5	T36.6X6
Ant (bite) (sting)	T63.421	T63.422	T63.423	T63.424		
Antabuse	T50.6X1	T50.6X2	T50.6X3	T50.6X4	T50.6X5	T50.6X6
Antacid NEC	T47.1X1	T47.1X2	T47.1X3	T47.1X4	T47.1X5	T47.1X6
Antagonist						
Aldosterone	T50.0X1	T50.0X2	T50.0X3	T50.0X4	T50.0X5	T50.0X6
alpha-adrenoreceptor	T44.6X1	T44.6X2	T44.6X3	T44.6X4	T44.6X5	T44.6X6
anticoagulant	T45.7X1	T45.7X2	T45.7X3	T45.7X4	T45.7X5	T45.7X6
beta-adrenoreceptor	T44.7X1	T44.7X2	T44.7X3	T44.7X4	T44.7X5	T44.7X6
extrapyramidal NEC	T44.3X1	T44.3X2	T44.3X3	T44.3X4	T44.3X5	T44.3X6
folic acid	T45.1X1	T45.1X2	T45.1X3	T45.1X4	T45.1X5	T45.1X6
H2 receptor	T47.0X1	T47.0X2	T47.0X3	T47.0X4	T47.0X5	T47.0X6
heavy metal	T45.8X1	T45.8X2	T45.8X3	T45.8X4	T45.8X5	T45.8X6
narcotic analgesic	T50.7X1	T50.7X2	T50.7X3	T50.7X4	T50.7X5	T50.7X6
opiate	T50.7X1	T50.7X2	T50.7X3	T50.7X4	T50.7X5	T50.7X6
pyrimidine	T45.1X1	T45.1X2	T45.1X3	T45.1X4	T45.1X5	T45.1X6
serotonin	T46.5X1	T46.5X2	T46.5X3	T46.5X4	T46.5X5	T46.5X6
Antazolin (e)	T45.0X1	T45.0X2	T45.0X3	T45.0X4	T45.0X5	T45.0X6
Anterior pituitary hormone NEC	T38.811	T38.812	T38.813	T38.814	T38.815	T38.816
Anthelmintic NEC	T37.4X1	T37.4X2	T37.4X3	T37.4X4	T37.4X5	T37.4X6
Anthiolimine	T37.4X1	T37.4X2	T37.4X3	T37.4X4	T37.4X5	T37.4X6
Anthralin	T49.4X1	T49.4X2	T49.4X3	T49.4X4	T49.4X5	T49.4X6
Anthramycin	T45.1X1	T45.1X2	T45.1X3	T45.1X4	T45.1X5	T45.1X6
Antiadrenergic NEC	T44.8X1	T44.8X2	T44.8X3	T44.8X4	T44.8X5	T44.8X6
Antiallergic NEC	T45.0X1	T45.0X2	T45.0X3	T45.0X4	T45.0X5	T45.0X6
Antiandrogen NEC	T38.6X1	T38.6X2	T38.6X3	T38.6X4	T38.6X5	T38.6X6
Anti-anemic (drug) (preparation)	T45.8X1	T45.8X2	T45.8X3	T45.8X4	T45.8X5	T45.8X6
Antianxiety drug NEC	T43.501	T43.502	T43.503	T43.504	T43.505	T43.506
Antiaris toxicaria	T65.891	T65.892	T65.893	T65.894		
Antiarteriosclerotic drug	T46.6X1	T46.6X2	T46.6X3	T46.6X4	T46.6X5	T46.6X6
Antiasthmatic drug NEC	T48.6X1	T48.6X2	T48.6X3	T48.6X4	T48.6X5	T48.6X6
Antibiotic NEC	T36.91	T36.92	T36.93	T36.94	T36.95	T36.96
aminoglycoside	T36.5X1	T36.5X2	T36.5X3	T36.5X4	T36.5X5	T36.5X6
anticancer	T45.1X1	T45.1X2	T45.1X3	T45.1X4	T45.1X5	T45.1X6
antifungal	T36.7X1	T36.7X2	T36.7X3	T36.7X4	T36.7X5	T36.7X6
antimycobacterial	T36.5X1	T36.5X2	T36.5X3	T36.5X4	T36.5X5	T36.5X6
antineoplastic	T45.1X1	T45.1X2	T45.1X3	T45.1X4	T45.1X5	T45.1X6
b-lactam NEC	T36.1X1	T36.1X2	T36.1X3	T36.1X4	T36.1X5	T36.1X6

Substance	Poisoning, Accidental (unintentional)	Poisoning, Intentional Self-harm	Poisoning, Assault	Poisoning, Undetermined	Adverse Effect	Under-dosing
Antibiotic — *continued*						
cephalosporin (group)	T36.1X1	T36.1X2	T36.1X3	T36.1X4	T36.1X5	T36.1X6
chloramphenicol (group)	T36.2X1	T36.2X2	T36.2X3	T36.2X4	T36.2X5	T36.2X6
ENT	T49.6X1	T49.6X2	T49.6X3	T49.6X4	T49.6X5	T49.6X6
eye	T49.5X1	T49.5X2	T49.5X3	T49.5X4	T49.5X5	T49.5X6
fungicidal (local)	T49.0X1	T49.0X2	T49.0X3	T49.0X4	T49.0X5	T49.0X6
intestinal	T36.8X1	T36.8X2	T36.8X3	T36.8X4	T36.8X5	T36.8X6
local	T49.0X1	T49.0X2	T49.0X3	T49.0X4	T49.0X5	T49.0X6
macrolides	T36.3X1	T36.3X2	T36.3X3	T36.3X4	T36.3X5	T36.3X6
polypeptide	T36.8X1	T36.8X2	T36.8X3	T36.8X4	T36.8X5	T36.8X6
specified NEC	T36.8X1	T36.8X2	T36.8X3	T36.8X4	T36.8X5	T36.8X6
tetracycline (group)	T36.4X1	T36.4X2	T36.4X3	T36.4X4	T36.4X5	T36.4X6
throat	T49.6X1	T49.6X2	T49.6X3	T49.6X4	T49.6X5	T49.6X6
Anticancer agents NEC	T45.1X1	T45.1X2	T45.1X3	T45.1X4	T45.1X5	T45.1X6
Anticholesterolemic drug NEC	T46.6X1	T46.6X2	T46.6X3	T46.6X4	T46.6X5	T46.6X6
Anticholinergic NEC	T44.3X1	T44.3X2	T44.3X3	T44.3X4	T44.3X5	T44.3X6
Anticholinesterase	T44.0X1	T44.0X2	T44.0X3	T44.0X4	T44.0X5	T44.0X6
organophosphorus	T44.0X1	T44.0X2	T44.0X3	T44.0X4	T44.0X5	T44.0X6
insecticide	T60.0X1	T60.0X2	T60.0X3	T60.0X4	—	—
nerve gas	T59.891	T59.892	T59.893	T59.894	—	—
reversible	T44.0X1	T44.0X2	T44.0X3	T44.0X4	T44.0X5	T44.0X6
ophthalmological	T49.5X1	T49.5X2	T49.5X3	T49.5X4	T49.5X5	T49.5X6
Anticoagulant NEC	T45.511	T45.512	T45.513	T45.514	T45.515	T45.516
Antagonist	T45.7X1	T45.7X2	T45.7X3	T45.7X4	T45.7X5	T45.7X6
Anti-common-cold drug NEC	T48.5X1	T48.5X2	T48.5X3	T48.5X4	T48.5X5	T48.5X6
Anticonvulsant	T42.71	T42.72	T42.73	T42.74	T42.75	T42.76
barbiturate	T42.3X1	T42.3X2	T42.3X3	T42.3X4	T42.3X5	T42.3X6
combination (with barbiturate)	T42.3X1	T42.3X2	T42.3X3	T42.3X4	T42.3X5	T42.3X6
hydantoin	T42.0X1	T42.0X2	T42.0X3	T42.0X4	T42.0X5	T42.0X6
hypnotic NEC	T42.6X1	T42.6X2	T42.6X3	T42.6X4	T42.6X5	T42.6X6
oxazolidinedione	T42.2X1	T42.2X2	T42.2X3	T42.2X4	T42.2X5	T42.2X6
pyrimidinedione	T42.6X1	T42.6X2	T42.6X3	T42.6X4	T42.6X5	T42.6X6
specified NEC	T42.6X1	T42.6X2	T42.6X3	T42.6X4	T42.6X5	T42.6X6
succinimide	T42.2X1	T42.2X2	T42.2X3	T42.2X4	T42.2X5	T42.2X6
Antidepressant	T43.201	T43.202	T43.203	T43.204	T43.205	T43.206
monoamine oxidase inhibitor	T43.1X1	T43.1X2	T43.1X3	T43.1X4	T43.1X5	T43.1X6
selective serotonin norepinephrine reuptake inhibitor	T43.211	T43.212	T43.213	T43.214	T43.215	T43.216
selective serotonin reuptake inhibitor	T43.221	T43.222	T43.223	T43.224	T43.225	T43.226
specified NEC	T43.291	T43.292	T43.293	T43.294	T43.295	T43.296
tetracyclic	T43.021	T43.022	T43.023	T43.024	T43.025	T43.026
triazolopyridine	T43.211	T43.212	T43.213	T43.214	T43.215	T43.216
tricyclic	T43.011	T43.012	T43.013	T43.014	T43.015	T43.016
Antidiabetic NEC	T38.3X1	T38.3X2	T38.3X3	T38.3X4	T38.3X5	T38.3X6
biguanide	T38.3X1	T38.3X2	T38.3X3	T38.3X4	T38.3X5	T38.3X6
and sulfonyl combined	T38.3X1	T38.3X2	T38.3X3	T38.3X4	T38.3X5	T38.3X6
combined	T38.3X1	T38.3X2	T38.3X3	T38.3X4	T38.3X5	T38.3X6
sulfonylurea	T38.3X1	T38.3X2	T38.3X3	T38.3X4	T38.3X5	T38.3X6
Antidiarrheal drug NEC	T47.6X1	T47.6X2	T47.6X3	T47.6X4	T47.6X5	T47.6X6
absorbent	T47.6X1	T47.6X2	T47.6X3	T47.6X4	T47.6X5	T47.6X6
Anti-D immunoglobulin (human)	T50.Z11	T50.Z12	T50.Z13	T50.Z14	T50.Z15	T50.Z16
Antidiphtheria serum	T50.Z11	T50.Z12	T50.Z13	T50.Z14	T50.Z15	T50.Z16
Antidiuretic hormone	T38.891	T38.892	T38.893	T38.894	T38.895	T38.896
Antidote NEC	T50.6X1	T50.6X2	T50.6X3	T50.6X4	T50.6X5	T50.6X6
heavy metal	T45.8X1	T45.8X2	T45.8X3	T45.8X4	T45.8X5	T45.8X6
Antidysrhythmic NEC	T46.2X1	T46.2X2	T46.2X3	T46.2X4	T46.2X5	T46.2X6
Antiemetic drug	T45.0X1	T45.0X2	T45.0X3	T45.0X4	T45.0X5	T45.0X6
Antiepilepsy agent	T42.71	T42.72	T42.73	T42.74	T42.75	T42.76
combination	T42.5X1	T42.5X2	T42.5X3	T42.5X4	T42.5X5	T42.5X6
mixed	T42.5X1	T42.5X2	T42.5X3	T42.5X4	T42.5X5	T42.5X6
specified, NEC	T42.6X1	T42.6X2	T42.6X3	T42.6X4	T42.6X5	T42.6X6
Antiestrogen NEC	T38.6X1	T38.6X2	T38.6X3	T38.6X4	T38.6X5	T38.6X6
Antifertility pill	T38.4X1	T38.4X2	T38.4X3	T38.4X4	T38.4X5	T38.4X6
Antifibrinolytic drug	T45.621	T45.622	T45.623	T45.624	T45.625	T45.626
Antifilarial drug	T37.4X1	T37.4X2	T37.4X3	T37.4X4	T37.4X5	T37.4X6
Antiflatulent	T47.5X1	T47.5X2	T47.5X3	T47.5X4	T47.5X5	T47.5X6
Antifreeze	T65.91	T65.92	T65.93	T65.94	—	—
alcohol	T51.1X1	T51.1X2	T51.1X3	T51.1X4	—	—
ethylene glycol	T51.8X1	T51.8X2	T51.8X3	T51.8X4	—	—
Antifungal						
antibiotic (systemic)	T36.7X1	T36.7X2	T36.7X3	T36.7X4	T36.7X5	T36.7X6
anti-infective NEC	T37.91	T37.92	T37.93	T37.94	T37.95	T37.96
disinfectant, local	T49.0X1	T49.0X2	T49.0X3	T49.0X4	T49.0X5	T49.0X6
nonmedicinal (spray)	T60.3X1	T60.3X2	T60.3X3	T60.3X4	—	—
topical	T49.0X1	T49.0X2	T49.0X3	T49.0X4	T49.0X5	T49.0X6

Substance	Poisoning, Accidental (unintentional)	Poisoning, Intentional Self-harm	Poisoning, Assault	Poisoning, Undetermined	Adverse Effect	Under-dosing
Anti-gastric-secretion drug NEC	T47.1X1	T47.1X2	T47.1X3	T47.1X4	T47.1X5	T47.1X6
Antigonadotrophin NEC	T38.6X1	T38.6X2	T38.6X3	T38.6X4	T38.6X5	T38.6X6
Antihallucinogen	T43.501	T43.502	T43.503	T43.504	T43.505	T43.506
Antihelmintics	T37.4X1	T37.4X2	T37.4X3	T37.4X4	T37.4X5	T37.4X6
Antihemophilic						
factor	T45.8X1	T45.8X2	T45.8X3	T45.8X4	T45.8X5	T45.8X6
fraction	T45.8X1	T45.8X2	T45.8X3	T45.8X4	T45.8X5	T45.8X6
globulin concentrate	T45.7X1	T45.7X2	T45.7X3	T45.7X4	T45.7X5	T45.7X6
human plasma	T45.8X1	T45.8X2	T45.8X3	T45.8X4	T45.8X5	T45.8X6
plasma, dried	T45.7X1	T45.7X2	T45.7X3	T45.7X4	T45.7X5	T45.7X6
Antihemorrhoidal preparation	T49.2X1	T49.2X2	T49.2X3	T49.2X4	T49.2X5	T49.2X6
Antiheparin drug	T45.7X1	T45.7X2	T45.7X3	T45.7X4	T45.7X5	T45.7X6
Antihistamine	T45.0X1	T45.0X2	T45.0X3	T45.0X4	T45.0X5	T45.0X6
Antihookworm drug	T37.4X1	T37.4X2	T37.4X3	T37.4X4	T37.4X5	T37.4X6
Anti-human lymphocytic globulin	T50.Z11	T50.Z12	T50.Z13	T50.Z14	T50.Z15	T50.Z16
Antihyperlipidemic drug	T46.6X1	T46.6X2	T46.6X3	T46.6X4	T46.6X5	T46.6X6
Antihypertensive drug NEC	T46.5X1	T46.5X2	T46.5X3	T46.5X4	T46.5X5	T46.5X6
Anti-infective NEC	T37.91	T37.92	T37.93	T37.94	T37.95	T37.96
anthelmintic	T37.4X1	T37.4X2	T37.4X3	T37.4X4	T37.4X5	T37.4X6
antibiotics	T36.91	T36.92	T36.93	T36.94	T36.95	T36.96
specified NEC	T36.8X1	T36.8X2	T36.8X3	T36.8X4	T36.8X5	T36.8X6
antimalarial	T37.2X1	T37.2X2	T37.2X3	T37.2X4	T37.2X5	T37.2X6
antimycobacterial NEC	T37.1X1	T37.1X2	T37.1X3	T37.1X4	T37.1X5	T37.1X6
antibiotics	T36.5X1	T36.5X2	T36.5X3	T36.5X4	T36.5X5	T36.5X6
antiprotozoal NEC	T37.3X1	T37.3X2	T37.3X3	T37.3X4	T37.3X5	T37.3X6
blood	T37.2X1	T37.2X2	T37.2X3	T37.2X4	T37.2X5	T37.2X6
antiviral	T37.5X1	T37.5X2	T37.5X3	T37.5X4	T37.5X5	T37.5X6
arsenical	T37.8X1	T37.8X2	T37.8X3	T37.8X4	T37.8X5	T37.8X6
bismuth, local	T49.0X1	T49.0X2	T49.0X3	T49.0X4	T49.0X5	T49.0X6
ENT	T49.6X1	T49.6X2	T49.6X3	T49.6X4	T49.6X5	T49.6X6
eye NEC	T49.5X1	T49.5X2	T49.5X3	T49.5X4	T49.5X5	T49.5X6
heavy metals NEC	T37.8X1	T37.8X2	T37.8X3	T37.8X4	T37.8X5	T37.8X6
local NEC	T49.0X1	T49.0X2	T49.0X3	T49.0X4	T49.0X5	T49.0X6
specified NEC	T49.0X1	T49.0X2	T49.0X3	T49.0X4	T49.0X5	T49.0X6
mixed	T37.91	T37.92	T37.93	T37.94	T37.95	T37.96
ophthalmic preparation	T49.5X1	T49.5X2	T49.5X3	T49.5X4	T49.5X5	T49.5X6
topical NEC	T49.0X1	T49.0X2	T49.0X3	T49.0X4	T49.0X5	T49.0X6
Anti-inflammatory drug NEC	T39.391	T39.392	T39.393	T39.394	T39.395	T39.396
local	T49.0X1	T49.0X2	T49.0X3	T49.0X4	T49.0X5	T49.0X6
nonsteroidal NEC	T39.391	T39.392	T39.393	T39.394	T39.395	T39.396
propionic acid derivative	T39.311	T39.312	T39.313	T39.314	T39.315	T39.316
specified NEC	T39.391	T39.392	T39.393	T39.394	T39.395	T39.396
Antikaluretic	T50.3X1	T50.3X2	T50.3X3	T50.3X4	T50.3X5	T50.3X6
Antiknock (tetraethyl lead)	T56.0X1	T56.0X2	T56.0X3	T56.0X4	—	—
Antilipemic drug NEC	T46.6X1	T46.6X2	T46.6X3	T46.6X4	T46.6X5	T46.6X6
Antimalarial	T37.2X1	T37.2X2	T37.2X3	T37.2X4	T37.2X5	T37.2X6
prophylactic NEC	T37.2X1	T37.2X2	T37.2X3	T37.2X4	T37.2X5	T37.2X6
pyrimidine derivative	T37.2X1	T37.2X2	T37.2X3	T37.2X4	T37.2X5	T37.2X6
Antimetabolite	T45.1X1	T45.1X2	T45.1X3	T45.1X4	T45.1X5	T45.1X6
Antimitotic agent	T45.1X1	T45.1X2	T45.1X3	T45.1X4	T45.1X5	T45.1X6
Antimony (compounds) (vapor) NEC	T56.891	T56.892	T56.893	T56.894	—	—
anti-infectives	T37.8X1	T37.8X2	T37.8X3	T37.8X4	T37.8X5	T37.8X6
dimercaptosuccinate	T37.3X1	T37.3X2	T37.3X3	T37.3X4	T37.3X5	T37.3X6
hydride	T56.891	T56.892	T56.893	T56.894	—	—
pesticide (vapor)	T60.8X1	T60.8X2	T60.8X3	T60.8X4	—	—
potassium (sodium) tartrate	T37.8X1	T37.8X2	T37.8X3	T37.8X4	T37.8X5	T37.8X6
sodium dimercaptosuccinate	T37.3X1	T37.3X2	T37.3X3	T37.3X4	T37.3X5	T37.3X6
tartrated	T37.8X1	T37.8X2	T37.8X3	T37.8X4	T37.8X5	T37.8X6
Antimuscarinic NEC	T44.3X1	T44.3X2	T44.3X3	T44.3X4	T44.3X5	T44.3X6
Antimycobacterial drug NEC	T37.1X1	T37.1X2	T37.1X3	T37.1X4	T37.1X5	T37.1X6
antibiotics	T36.5X1	T36.5X2	T36.5X3	T36.5X4	T36.5X5	T36.5X6
combination	T37.1X1	T37.1X2	T37.1X3	T37.1X4	T37.1X5	T37.1X6
Antinausea drug	T45.0X1	T45.0X2	T45.0X3	T45.0X4	T45.0X5	T45.0X6
Antinematode drug	T37.4X1	T37.4X2	T37.4X3	T37.4X4	T37.4X5	T37.4X6
Antineoplastic NEC	T45.1X1	T45.1X2	T45.1X3	T45.1X4	T45.1X5	T45.1X6
alkaloidal	T45.1X1	T45.1X2	T45.1X3	T45.1X4	T45.1X5	T45.1X6
antibiotics	T45.1X1	T45.1X2	T45.1X3	T45.1X4	T45.1X5	T45.1X6
combination	T45.1X1	T45.1X2	T45.1X3	T45.1X4	T45.1X5	T45.1X6
estrogen	T38.5X1	T38.5X2	T38.5X3	T38.5X4	T38.5X5	T38.5X6
steroid	T38.7X1	T38.7X2	T38.7X3	T38.7X4	T38.7X5	T38.7X6
Antiparasitic drug (systemic)	T37.91	T37.92	T37.93	T37.94	T37.95	T37.96
local	T49.0X1	T49.0X2	T49.0X3	T49.0X4	T49.0X5	T49.0X6
specified NEC	T37.8X1	T37.8X2	T37.8X3	T37.8X4	T37.8X5	T37.8X6

Substance	Poisoning, Accidental (unintentional)	Poisoning, Intentional Self-harm	Poisoning, Assault	Poisoning, Undetermined	Adverse Effect	Under-dosing
Antiparkinsonism drug NEC	T42.8X1	T42.8X2	T42.8X3	T42.8X4	T42.8X5	T42.8X6
Antiperspirant NEC	T49.2X1	T49.2X2	T49.2X3	T49.2X4	T49.2X5	T49.2X6
Antiphlogistic NEC	T39.4X1	T39.4X2	T39.4X3	T39.4X4	T39.4X5	T39.4X6
Antiplatyhelmintic drug	T37.4X1	T37.4X2	T37.4X3	T37.4X4	T37.4X5	T37.4X6
Antiprotozoal drug NEC	T37.3X1	T37.3X2	T37.3X3	T37.3X4	T37.3X5	T37.3X6
blood	T37.2X1	T37.2X2	T37.2X3	T37.2X4	T37.2X5	T37.2X6
local	T49.0X1	T49.0X2	T49.0X3	T49.0X4	T49.0X5	T49.0X6
Antipruritic drug NEC	T49.1X1	T49.1X2	T49.1X3	T49.1X4	T49.1X5	T49.1X6
Antipsychotic drug	T43.501	T43.502	T43.503	T43.504	T43.505	T43.506
specified NEC	T43.591	T43.592	T43.593	T43.594	T43.595	T43.596
Antipyretic	T39.91	T39.92	T39.93	T39.94	T39.95	T39.96
specified NEC	T39.8X1	T39.8X2	T39.8X3	T39.8X4	T39.8X5	T39.8X6
Antipyrine	T39.2X1	T39.2X2	T39.2X3	T39.2X4	T39.2X5	T39.2X6
Antirabies hyperimmune serum	T50.Z11	T50.Z12	T50.Z13	T50.Z14	T50.Z15	T50.Z16
Antirheumatic NEC	T39.4X1	T39.4X2	T39.4X3	T39.4X4	T39.4X5	T39.4X6
Antirigidity drug NEC	T42.8X1	T42.8X2	T42.8X3	T42.8X4	T42.8X5	T42.8X6
Antischistosomal drug	T37.4X1	T37.4X2	T37.4X3	T37.4X4	T37.4X5	T37.4X6
Antiscorpion sera	T50.Z11	T50.Z12	T50.Z13	T50.Z14	T50.Z15	T50.Z16
Antiseborrheics	T49.4X1	T49.4X2	T49.4X3	T49.4X4	T49.4X5	T49.4X6
Antiseptics (external) (medicinal)	T49.0X1	T49.0X2	T49.0X3	T49.0X4	T49.0X5	T49.0X6
Antistine	T45.0X1	T45.0X2	T45.0X3	T45.0X4	T45.0X5	T45.0X6
Antitapeworm drug	T37.4X1	T37.4X2	T37.4X3	T37.4X4	T37.4X5	T37.4X6
Antitetanus immunoglobulin	T50.Z11	T50.Z12	T50.Z13	T50.Z14	T50.Z15	T50.Z16
Antithrombotic	T45.521	T45.522	T45.523	T45.524	T45.525	T45.526
Antithyroid drug NEC	T38.2X1	T38.2X2	T38.2X3	T38.2X4	T38.2X5	T38.2X6
Antitoxin	T50.Z11	T50.Z12	T50.Z13	T50.Z14	T50.Z15	T50.Z16
diphtheria	T50.Z11	T50.Z12	T50.Z13	T50.Z14	T50.Z15	T50.Z16
gas gangrene	T50.Z11	T50.Z12	T50.Z13	T50.Z14	T50.Z15	T50.Z16
tetanus	T50.Z11	T50.Z12	T50.Z13	T50.Z14	T50.Z15	T50.Z16
Antitrichomonal drug	T37.3X1	T37.3X2	T37.3X3	T37.3X4	T37.3X5	T37.3X6
Antituberculars	T37.1X1	T37.1X2	T37.1X3	T37.1X4	T37.1X5	T37.1X6
antibiotics	T36.5X1	T36.5X2	T36.5X3	T36.5X4	T36.5X5	T36.5X6
Antitussive NEC	T48.3X1	T48.3X2	T48.3X3	T48.3X4	T48.3X5	T48.3X6
codeine mixture	T40.2X1	T40.2X2	T40.2X3	T40.2X4	T40.2X5	T40.2X6
opiate	T40.2X1	T40.2X2	T40.2X3	T40.2X4	T40.2X5	T40.2X6
Antivaricose drug	T46.8X1	T46.8X2	T46.8X3	T46.8X4	T46.8X5	T46.8X6
Antivenin, antivenom (sera)	T50.Z11	T50.Z12	T50.Z13	T50.Z14	T50.Z15	T50.Z16
crotaline	T50.Z11	T50.Z12	T50.Z13	T50.Z14	T50.Z15	T50.Z16
spider bite	T50.Z11	T50.Z12	T50.Z13	T50.Z14	T50.Z15	T50.Z16
Antivertigo drug	T45.0X1	T45.0X2	T45.0X3	T45.0X4	T45.0X5	T45.0X6
Antiviral drug NEC	T37.5X1	T37.5X2	T37.5X3	T37.5X4	T37.5X5	T37.5X6
eye	T49.5X1	T49.5X2	T49.5X3	T49.5X4	T49.5X5	T49.5X6
Antiwhipworm drug	T37.4X1	T37.4X2	T37.4X3	T37.4X4	T37.4X5	T37.4X6
Ant poison — see Insecticide						
Antrol — see also by specific chemical substance	T60.91	T60.92	T60.93	T60.94		
fungicide	T60.91	T60.92	T60.93	T60.94	—	—
ANTU (alpha naphthylthiourea)	T60.4X1	T60.4X2	T60.4X3	T60.4X4	—	—
Apalcillin	T36.0X1	T36.0X2	T36.0X3	T36.0X4	T36.0X5	T36.0X6
APC	T48.5X1	T48.5X2	T48.5X3	T48.5X4	T48.5X5	T48.5X6
Aplonidine	T44.4X1	T44.4X2	T44.4X3	T44.4X4	T44.4X5	T44.4X6
Apomorphine	T47.7X1	T47.7X2	T47.7X3	T47.7X4	T47.7X5	T47.7X6
Appetite depressants, central	T50.5X1	T50.5X2	T50.5X3	T50.5X4	T50.5X5	T50.5X6
Apraclonidine (hydrochloride)	T44.4X1	T44.4X2	T44.4X3	T44.4X4	T44.4X5	T44.4X6
Apresoline	T46.5X1	T46.5X2	T46.5X3	T46.5X4	T46.5X5	T46.5X6
Aprindine	T46.2X1	T46.2X2	T46.2X3	T46.2X4	T46.2X5	T46.2X6
Aprobarbital	T42.3X1	T42.3X2	T42.3X3	T42.3X4	T42.3X5	T42.3X6
Apronalide	T42.6X1	T42.6X2	T42.6X3	T42.6X4	T42.6X5	T42.6X6
Aprotinin	T45.621	T45.622	T45.623	T45.624	T45.625	T45.626
Aptocaine	T41.3X1	T41.3X2	T41.3X3	T41.3X4	T41.3X5	T41.3X6
Aqua fortis	T54.2X1	T54.2X2	T54.2X3	T54.2X4	—	—
Ara-A	T37.5X1	T37.5X2	T37.5X3	T37.5X4	T37.5X5	T37.5X6
Ara-C	T45.1X1	T45.1X2	T45.1X3	T45.1X4	T45.1X5	T45.1X6
Arachis oil	T49.3X1	T49.3X2	T49.3X3	T49.3X4	T49.3X5	T49.3X6
cathartic	T47.4X1	T47.4X2	T47.4X3	T47.4X4	T47.4X5	T47.4X6
Aralen	T37.2X1	T37.2X2	T37.2X3	T37.2X4	T37.2X5	T37.2X6
Arecoline	T44.1X1	T44.1X2	T44.1X3	T44.1X4	T44.1X5	T44.1X6
Arginine	T50.991	T50.992	T50.993	T50.994	T50.995	T50.996
glutamate	T50.991	T50.992	T50.993	T50.994	T50.995	T50.996
Argyrol	T49.0X1	T49.0X2	T49.0X3	T49.0X4	T49.0X5	T49.0X6
ENT agent	T49.6X1	T49.6X2	T49.6X3	T49.6X4	T49.6X5	T49.6X6
ophthalmic preparation	T49.5X1	T49.5X2	T49.5X3	T49.5X4	T49.5X5	T49.5X6
Aristocort	T38.0X1	T38.0X2	T38.0X3	T38.0X4	T38.0X5	T38.0X6
ENT agent	T49.6X1	T49.6X2	T49.6X3	T49.6X4	T49.6X5	T49.6X6
ophthalmic preparation	T49.5X1	T49.5X2	T49.5X3	T49.5X4	T49.5X5	T49.5X6

Substance	Poisoning, Accidental (unintentional)	Poisoning, Intentional Self-harm	Poisoning, Assault	Poisoning, Undetermined	Adverse Effect	Under-dosing
Aristocort — *continued*						
topical NEC	T49.0X1	T49.0X2	T49.0X3	T49.0X4	T49.0X5	T49.0X6
Aromatics, corrosive	T54.1X1	T54.1X2	T54.1X3	T54.1X4	—	—
disinfectants	T54.1X1	T54.1X2	T54.1X3	T54.1X4	—	—
Arsenate of lead	T57.0X1	T57.0X2	T57.0X3	T57.0X4	—	—
herbicide	T57.0X1	T57.0X2	T57.0X3	T57.0X4	—	—
Arsenic, arsenicals (compounds) (dust) (vapor) **NEC**	T57.0X1	T57.0X2	T57.0X3	T57.0X4	—	—
anti-infectives	T37.8X1	T37.8X2	T37.8X3	T37.8X4	T37.8X5	T37.8X6
pesticide (dust) (fumes)	T57.0X1	T57.0X2	T57.0X3	T57.0X4	—	—
Arsine (gas)	T57.0X1	T57.0X2	T57.0X3	T57.0X4	—	—
Arsphenamine (silver)	T37.8X1	T37.8X2	T37.8X3	T37.8X4	T37.8X5	T37.8X6
Arsthinol	T37.3X1	T37.3X2	T37.3X3	T37.3X4	T37.3X5	T37.3X6
Artane	T44.3X1	T44.3X2	T44.3X3	T44.3X4	T44.3X5	T44.3X6
Arthropod (venomous) **NEC**	T63.481	T63.482	T63.483	T63.484	—	—
Articaine	T41.3X1	T41.3X2	T41.3X3	T41.3X4	T41.3X5	T41.3X6
Asbestos	T57.8X1	T57.8X2	T57.8X3	T57.8X4	—	—
Ascaridole	T37.4X1	T37.4X2	T37.4X3	T37.4X4	T37.4X5	T37.4X6
Ascorbic acid	T45.2X1	T45.2X2	T45.2X3	T45.2X4	T45.2X5	T45.2X6
Asiaticoside	T49.0X1	T49.0X2	T49.0X3	T49.0X4	T49.0X5	T49.0X6
Asparaginase	T45.1X1	T45.1X2	T45.1X3	T45.1X4	T45.1X5	T45.1X6
Aspidium (oleoresin)	T37.4X1	T37.4X2	T37.4X3	T37.4X4	T37.4X5	T37.4X6
Aspirin (aluminum) (soluble)	T39.011	T39.012	T39.013	T39.014	T39.015	T39.016
Aspoxicillin	T36.0X1	T36.0X2	T36.0X3	T36.0X4	T36.0X5	T36.0X6
Astemizole	T45.0X1	T45.0X2	T45.0X3	T45.0X4	T45.0X5	T45.0X6
Astringent (local)	T49.2X1	T49.2X2	T49.2X3	T49.2X4	T49.2X5	T49.2X6
specified NEC	T49.2X1	T49.2X2	T49.2X3	T49.2X4	T49.2X5	T49.2X6
Astromicin	T36.5X1	T36.5X2	T36.5X3	T36.5X4	T36.5X5	T36.5X6
Ataractic drug NEC	T43.501	T43.502	T43.503	T43.504	T43.505	T43.506
Atenolol	T44.7X1	T44.7X2	T44.7X3	T44.7X4	T44.7X5	T44.7X6
Atonia drug, intestinal	T47.4X1	T47.4X2	T47.4X3	T47.4X4	T47.4X5	T47.4X6
Atophan	T50.4X1	T50.4X2	T50.4X3	T50.4X4	T50.4X5	T50.4X6
Atracurium besilate	T48.1X1	T48.1X2	T48.1X3	T48.1X4	T48.1X5	T48.1X6
Atropine	T44.3X1	T44.3X2	T44.3X3	T44.3X4	T44.3X5	T44.3X6
derivative	T44.3X1	T44.3X2	T44.3X3	T44.3X4	T44.3X5	T44.3X6
methonitrate	T44.3X1	T44.3X2	T44.3X3	T44.3X4	T44.3X5	T44.3X6
Attapulgite	T47.6X1	T47.6X2	T47.6X3	T47.6X4	T47.6X5	T47.6X6
Auramine	T65.891	T65.892	T65.893	T65.894	—	—
dye	T65.6X1	T65.6X2	T65.6X3	T65.6X4	—	—
fungicide	T60.3X1	T60.3X2	T60.3X3	T60.3X4	—	—
Auranofin	T39.4X1	T39.4X2	T39.4X3	T39.4X4	T39.4X5	T39.4X6
Aurantiin	T46.991	T46.992	T46.993	T46.994	T46.995	T46.996
Aureomycin	T36.4X1	T36.4X2	T36.4X3	T36.4X4	T36.4X5	T36.4X6
ophthalmic preparation	T49.5X1	T49.5X2	T49.5X3	T49.5X4	T49.5X5	T49.5X6
topical NEC	T49.0X1	T49.0X2	T49.0X3	T49.0X4	T49.0X5	T49.0X6
Aurothioglucose	T39.4X1	T39.4X2	T39.4X3	T39.4X4	T39.4X5	T39.4X6
Aurothioglycanide	T39.4X1	T39.4X2	T39.4X3	T39.4X4	T39.4X5	T39.4X6
Aurothiomalate sodium	T39.4X1	T39.4X2	T39.4X3	T39.4X4	T39.4X5	T39.4X6
Aurotioprol	T39.4X1	T39.4X2	T39.4X3	T39.4X4	T39.4X5	T39.4X6
Automobile fuel	T52.0X1	T52.0X2	T52.0X3	T52.0X4	—	—
Autonomic nervous system agent NEC	T44.901	T44.902	T44.903	T44.904	T44.905	T44.906
Avlosulfon	T37.1X1	T37.1X2	T37.1X3	T37.1X4	T37.1X5	T37.1X6
Avomine	T42.6X1	T42.6X2	T42.6X3	T42.6X4	T42.6X5	T42.6X6
Axerophthol	T45.2X1	T45.2X2	T45.2X3	T45.2X4	T45.2X5	T45.2X6
Azacitidine	T45.1X1	T45.1X2	T45.1X3	T45.1X4	T45.1X5	T45.1X6
Azacyclonol	T43.591	T43.592	T43.593	T43.594	T43.595	T43.596
Azadirachta	T60.2X1	T60.2X2	T60.2X3	T60.2X4	—	—
Azanidazole	T37.3X1	T37.3X2	T37.3X3	T37.3X4	T37.3X5	T37.3X6
Azapetine	T46.7X1	T46.7X2	T46.7X3	T46.7X4	T46.7X5	T46.7X6
Azapropazone	T39.2X1	T39.2X2	T39.2X3	T39.2X4	T39.2X5	T39.2X6
Azaribine	T45.1X1	T45.1X2	T45.1X3	T45.1X4	T45.1X5	T45.1X6
Azaserine	T45.1X1	T45.1X2	T45.1X3	T45.1X4	T45.1X5	T45.1X6
Azatadine	T45.0X1	T45.0X2	T45.0X3	T45.0X4	T45.0X5	T45.0X6
Azatepa	T45.1X1	T45.1X2	T45.1X3	T45.1X4	T45.1X5	T45.1X6
Azathioprine	T45.1X1	T45.1X2	T45.1X3	T45.1X4	T45.1X5	T45.1X6
Azelaic acid	T49.0X1	T49.0X2	T49.0X3	T49.0X4	T49.0X5	T49.0X6
Azelastine	T45.0X1	T45.0X2	T45.0X3	T45.0X4	T45.0X5	T45.0X6
Azidocillin	T36.0X1	T36.0X2	T36.0X3	T36.0X4	T36.0X5	T36.0X6
Azidothymidine	T37.5X1	T37.5X2	T37.5X3	T37.5X4	T37.5X5	T37.5X6
Azinphos (ethyl) (methyl)	T60.0X1	T60.0X2	T60.0X3	T60.0X4	—	—
Aziridine (chelating)	T54.1X1	T54.1X2	T54.1X3	T54.1X4	—	—
Azithromycin	T36.3X1	T36.3X2	T36.3X3	T36.3X4	T36.3X5	T36.3X6
Azlocillin	T36.0X1	T36.0X2	T36.0X3	T36.0X4	T36.0X5	T36.0X6
Azobenzene smoke	T65.3X1	T65.3X2	T65.3X3	T65.3X4	—	—
acaricide	T60.8X1	T60.8X2	T60.8X3	T60.8X4	—	—
Azosulfamide	T37.0X1	T37.0X2	T37.0X3	T37.0X4	T37.0X5	T37.0X6
AZT	T37.5X1	T37.5X2	T37.5X3	T37.5X4	T37.5X5	T37.5X6
Aztreonam	T36.1X1	T36.1X2	T36.1X3	T36.1X4	T36.1X5	T36.1X6
Azulfidine	T37.0X1	T37.0X2	T37.0X3	T37.0X4	T37.0X5	T37.0X6
Azuresin	T50.8X1	T50.8X2	T50.8X3	T50.8X4	T50.8X5	T50.8X6
b-acetyldigoxin	T46.0X1	T46.0X2	T46.0X3	T46.0X4	T46.0X5	T46.0X6
P-Acetamidophenol	T39.1X1	T39.1X2	T39.1X3	T39.1X4	T39.1X5	T39.1X6
Bacampicillin	T36.0X1	T36.0X2	T36.0X3	T36.0X4	T36.0X5	T36.0X6
Bacillus						
lactobacillus	T47.8X1	T47.8X2	T47.8X3	T47.8X4	T47.8X5	T47.8X6
subtilis	T47.6X1	T47.6X2	T47.6X3	T47.6X4	T47.6X5	T47.6X6
Bacimycin	T49.0X1	T49.0X2	T49.0X3	T49.0X4	T49.0X5	T49.0X6
ophthalmic preparation	T49.5X1	T49.5X2	T49.5X3	T49.5X4	T49.5X5	T49.5X6
Bacitracin zinc	T49.0X1	T49.0X2	T49.0X3	T49.0X4	T49.0X5	T49.0X6
with neomycin	T49.0X1	T49.0X2	T49.0X3	T49.0X4	T49.0X5	T49.0X6
ENT agent	T49.6X1	T49.6X2	T49.6X3	T49.6X4	T49.6X5	T49.6X6
ophthalmic preparation	T49.5X1	T49.5X2	T49.5X3	T49.5X4	T49.5X5	T49.5X6
topical NEC	T49.0X1	T49.0X2	T49.0X3	T49.0X4	T49.0X5	T49.0X6
Baclofen	T42.8X1	T42.8X2	T42.8X3	T42.8X4	T42.8X5	T42.8X6
Baking soda	T50.991	T50.992	T50.993	T50.994	T50.995	T50.996
BAL	T45.8X1	T45.8X2	T45.8X3	T45.8X4	T45.8X5	T45.8X6
Bambuterol	T48.6X1	T48.6X2	T48.6X3	T48.6X4	T48.6X5	T48.6X6
Bamethan (sulfate)	T46.7X1	T46.7X2	T46.7X3	T46.7X4	T46.7X5	T46.7X6
Bamifylline	T48.6X1	T48.6X2	T48.6X3	T48.6X4	T48.6X5	T48.6X6
Bamipine	T45.0X1	T45.0X2	T45.0X3	T45.0X4	T45.0X5	T45.0X6
Baneberry — *see* Actaea spicata						
Banewort — *see* Belladonna						
Barbenyl	T42.3X1	T42.3X2	T42.3X3	T42.3X4	T42.3X5	T42.3X6
Barbexaclone	T42.6X1	T42.6X2	T42.6X3	T42.6X4	T42.6X5	T42.6X6
Barbital	T42.3X1	T42.3X2	T42.3X3	T42.3X4	T42.3X5	T42.3X6
sodium	T42.3X1	T42.3X2	T42.3X3	T42.3X4	T42.3X5	T42.3X6
Barbitone	T42.3X1	T42.3X2	T42.3X3	T42.3X4	T42.3X5	T42.3X6
Barbiturate NEC	T42.3X1	T42.3X2	T42.3X3	T42.3X4	T42.3X5	T42.3X6
with tranquilizer	T42.3X1	T42.3X2	T42.3X3	T42.3X4	T42.3X5	T42.3X6
anesthetic (intravenous)	T41.1X1	T41.1X2	T41.1X3	T41.1X4	T41.1X5	T41.1X6
Barium (carbonate) (chloride) (sulfite)	T57.8X1	T57.8X2	T57.8X3	T57.8X4	—	—
diagnostic agent	T50.8X1	T50.8X2	T50.8X3	T50.8X4	T50.8X5	T50.8X6
pesticide	T60.4X1	T60.4X2	T60.4X3	T60.4X4	—	—
rodenticide	T60.4X1	T60.4X2	T60.4X3	T60.4X4	—	—
sulfate (medicinal)	T50.8X1	T50.8X2	T50.8X3	T50.8X4	T50.8X5	T50.8X6
Barrier cream	T49.3X1	T49.3X2	T49.3X3	T49.3X4	T49.3X5	T49.3X6
Basic fuchsin	T49.0X1	T49.0X2	T49.0X3	T49.0X4	T49.0X5	T49.0X6
Battery acid or fluid	T54.2X1	T54.2X2	T54.2X3	T54.2X4	—	—
Bay rum	T51.8X1	T51.8X2	T51.8X3	T51.8X4	—	—
b-benzalbutyramide	T46.6X1	T46.6X2	T46.6X3	T46.6X4	T46.6X5	T46.6X6
BCG (vaccine)	T50.A91	T50.A92	T50.A93	T50.A94	T50.A95	T50.A96
BCNU	T45.1X1	T45.1X2	T45.1X3	T45.1X4	T45.1X5	T45.1X6
Bearsfoot	T62.2X1	T62.2X2	T62.2X3	T62.2X4	—	—
Beclamide	T42.6X1	T42.6X2	T42.6X3	T42.6X4	T42.6X5	T42.6X6
Beclomethasone	T44.5X1	T44.5X2	T44.5X3	T44.5X4	T44.5X5	T44.5X6
Bee (sting) (venom)	T63.441	T63.442	T63.443	T63.444	—	—
Befunolol	T49.5X1	T49.5X2	T49.5X3	T49.5X4	T49.5X5	T49.5X6
Bekanamycin	T36.5X1	T36.5X2	T36.5X3	T36.5X4	T36.5X5	T36.5X6
Belladonna — *see also* Nightshade						
alkaloids	T44.3X1	T44.3X2	T44.3X3	T44.3X4	T44.3X5	T44.3X6
extract	T44.3X1	T44.3X2	T44.3X3	T44.3X4	T44.3X5	T44.3X6
herb	T44.3X1	T44.3X2	T44.3X3	T44.3X4	T44.3X5	T44.3X6
Bemegride	T50.7X1	T50.7X2	T50.7X3	T50.7X4	T50.7X5	T50.7X6
Benactyzine	T44.3X1	T44.3X2	T44.3X3	T44.3X4	T44.3X5	T44.3X6
Benadryl	T45.0X1	T45.0X2	T45.0X3	T45.0X4	T45.0X5	T45.0X6
Benaprizine	T44.3X1	T44.3X2	T44.3X3	T44.3X4	T44.3X5	T44.3X6
Benazepril	T46.4X1	T46.4X2	T46.4X3	T46.4X4	T46.4X5	T46.4X6
Bencyclane	T46.7X1	T46.7X2	T46.7X3	T46.7X4	T46.7X5	T46.7X6
Bendazol	T46.3X1	T46.3X2	T46.3X3	T46.3X4	T46.3X5	T46.3X6
Bendrofluazide	T50.2X1	T50.2X2	T50.2X3	T50.2X4	T50.2X5	T50.2X6
Bendroflumethiazide	T50.2X1	T50.2X2	T50.2X3	T50.2X4	T50.2X5	T50.2X6
Benemid	T50.4X1	T50.4X2	T50.4X3	T50.4X4	T50.4X5	T50.4X6
Benethamine penicillin	T36.0X1	T36.0X2	T36.0X3	T36.0X4	T36.0X5	T36.0X6
Benexate	T47.1X1	T47.1X2	T47.1X3	T47.1X4	T47.1X5	T47.1X6
Benfluorex	T46.6X1	T46.6X2	T46.6X3	T46.6X4	T46.6X5	T46.6X6
Benfotiamine	T45.2X1	T45.2X2	T45.2X3	T45.2X4	T45.2X5	T45.2X6
Benisone	T49.0X1	T49.0X2	T49.0X3	T49.0X4	T49.0X5	T49.0X6
Benomyl	T60.0X1	T60.0X2	T60.0X3	T60.0X4	—	—
Benoquin	T49.8X1	T49.8X2	T49.8X3	T49.8X4	T49.8X5	T49.8X6
Benoxinate	T41.3X1	T41.3X2	T41.3X3	T41.3X4	T41.3X5	T41.3X6
Benperidol	T43.4X1	T43.4X2	T43.4X3	T43.4X4	T43.4X5	T43.4X6
Benproperine	T48.3X1	T48.3X2	T48.3X3	T48.3X4	T48.3X5	T48.3X6
Benserazide	T42.8X1	T42.8X2	T42.8X3	T42.8X4	T42.8X5	T42.8X6
Bentazepam	T42.4X1	T42.4X2	T42.4X3	T42.4X4	T42.4X5	T42.4X6
Bentiromide	T50.8X1	T50.8X2	T50.8X3	T50.8X4	T50.8X5	T50.8X6
Bentonite	T49.3X1	T49.3X2	T49.3X3	T49.3X4	T49.3X5	T49.3X6
Benzalbutyramide	T46.6X1	T46.6X2	T46.6X3	T46.6X4	T46.6X5	T46.6X6
Benzalkonium (chloride)	T49.0X1	T49.0X2	T49.0X3	T49.0X4	T49.0X5	T49.0X6
ophthalmic preparation	T49.5X1	T49.5X2	T49.5X3	T49.5X4	T49.5X5	T49.5X6
Benzamidosalicylate (calcium)	T37.1X1	T37.1X2	T37.1X3	T37.1X4	T37.1X5	T37.1X6
Benzamine	T41.3X1	T41.3X2	T41.3X3	T41.3X4	T41.3X5	T41.3X6

Substance	Poisoning, Accidental (unintentional)	Poisoning, Intentional Self-harm	Poisoning, Assault	Poisoning, Undetermined	Adverse Effect	Under-dosing
Benzamine — *continued*						
lactate	T49.1X1	T49.1X2	T49.1X3	T49.1X4	T49.1X5	T49.1X6
Benzamphetamine	T50.5X1	T50.5X2	T50.5X3	T50.5X4	T50.5X5	T50.5X6
Benzapril hydrochloride	T46.5X1	T46.5X2	T46.5X3	T46.5X4	T46.5X5	T46.5X6
Benzathine benzylpenicillin	T36.0X1	T36.0X2	T36.0X3	T36.0X4	T36.0X5	T36.0X6
Benzathine penicillin	T36.0X1	T36.0X2	T36.0X3	T36.0X4	T36.0X5	T36.0X6
Benzatropine	T42.8X1	T42.8X2	T42.8X3	T42.8X4	T42.8X5	T42.8X6
Benzbromarone	T50.4X1	T50.4X2	T50.4X3	T50.4X4	T50.4X5	T50.4X6
Benzcarbimine	T45.1X1	T45.1X2	T45.1X3	T45.1X4	T45.1X5	T45.1X6
Benzedrex	T44.991	T44.992	T44.993	T44.994	T44.995	T44.996
Benzedrine (amphetamine)	T43.621	T43.622	T43.623	T43.624	T43.625	T43.626
Benzenamine	T65.3X1	T65.3X2	T65.3X3	T65.3X4	—	—
Benzene	T52.1X1	T52.1X2	T52.1X3	T52.1X4	—	—
homologues (acetyl) (dimethyl) (methyl) (solvent)	T52.2X1	T52.2X2	T52.2X3	T52.2X4	—	—
Benzethonium (chloride)	T49.0X1	T49.0X2	T49.0X3	T49.0X4	T49.0X5	T49.0X6
Benzfetamine	T50.5X1	T50.5X2	T50.5X3	T50.5X4	T50.5X5	T50.5X6
Benzhexol	T44.3X1	T44.3X2	T44.3X3	T44.3X4	T44.3X5	T44.3X6
Benzhydramine (chloride)	T45.0X1	T45.0X2	T45.0X3	T45.0X4	T45.0X5	T45.0X6
Benzidine	T65.891	T65.892	T65.893	T65.894	—	—
Benzilonium bromide	T44.3X1	T44.3X2	T44.3X3	T44.3X4	T44.3X5	T44.3X6
Benzimidazole	T60.3X1	T60.3X2	T60.3X3	T60.3X4	—	—
Benzin (e) — *see* Ligroin						
Benziodarone	T46.3X1	T46.3X2	T46.3X3	T46.3X4	T46.3X5	T46.3X6
Benznidazole	T37.3X1	T37.3X2	T37.3X3	T37.3X4	T37.3X5	T37.3X6
Benzocaine	T41.3X1	T41.3X2	T41.3X3	T41.3X4	T41.3X5	T41.3X6
Benzodiapin	T42.4X1	T42.4X2	T42.4X3	T42.4X4	T42.4X5	T42.4X6
Benzodiazepine NEC	T42.4X1	T42.4X2	T42.4X3	T42.4X4	T42.4X5	T42.4X6
Benzoic acid	T49.0X1	T49.0X2	T49.0X3	T49.0X4	T49.0X5	T49.0X6
with salicylic acid	T49.0X1	T49.0X2	T49.0X3	T49.0X4	T49.0X5	T49.0X6
Benzoin (tincture)	T48.5X1	T48.5X2	T48.5X3	T48.5X4	T48.5X5	T48.5X6
Benzol (benzene)	T52.1X1	T52.1X2	T52.1X3	T52.1X4	—	—
vapor	T52.0X1	T52.0X2	T52.0X3	T52.0X4	—	—
Benzomorphan	T40.2X1	T40.2X2	T40.2X3	T40.2X4	T40.2X5	T40.2X6
Benzonatate	T48.3X1	T48.3X2	T48.3X3	T48.3X4	T48.3X5	T48.3X6
Benzophenones	T49.3X1	T49.3X2	T49.3X3	T49.3X4	T49.3X5	T49.3X6
Benzopyrone	T46.991	T46.992	T46.993	T46.994	T46.995	T46.996
Benzothiadiazides	T50.2X1	T50.2X2	T50.2X3	T50.2X4	T50.2X5	T50.2X6
Benzoxonium chloride	T49.0X1	T49.0X2	T49.0X3	T49.0X4	T49.0X5	T49.0X6
Benzoylpas calcium	T37.1X1	T37.1X2	T37.1X3	T37.1X4	T37.1X5	T37.1X6
Benzoyl peroxide	T49.0X1	T49.0X2	T49.0X3	T49.0X4	T49.0X5	T49.0X6
Benzperidin	T43.591	T43.592	T43.593	T43.594	T43.595	T43.596
Benzperidol	T43.591	T43.592	T43.593	T43.594	T43.595	T43.596
Benzphetamine	T50.5X1	T50.5X2	T50.5X3	T50.5X4	T50.5X5	T50.5X6
Benzpyrinium bromide	T44.1X1	T44.1X2	T44.1X3	T44.1X4	T44.1X5	T44.1X6
Benzquinamide	T45.0X1	T45.0X2	T45.0X3	T45.0X4	T45.0X5	T45.0X6
Benzthiazide	T50.2X1	T50.2X2	T50.2X3	T50.2X4	T50.2X5	T50.2X6
Benztropine						
anticholinergic	T44.3X1	T44.3X2	T44.3X3	T44.3X4	T44.3X5	T44.3X6
antiparkinson	T42.8X1	T42.8X2	T42.8X3	T42.8X4	T42.8X5	T42.8X6
Benzydamine	T49.0X1	T49.0X2	T49.0X3	T49.0X4	T49.0X5	T49.0X6
Benzyl						
acetate	T52.8X1	T52.8X2	T52.8X3	T52.8X4	—	—
alcohol	T49.0X1	T49.0X2	T49.0X3	T49.0X4	T49.0X5	T49.0X6
benzoate	T49.0X1	T49.0X2	T49.0X3	T49.0X4	T49.0X5	T49.0X6
Benzoic acid	T49.0X1	T49.0X2	T49.0X3	T49.0X4	T49.0X5	T49.0X6
morphine	T40.2X1	T40.2X2	T40.2X3	T40.2X4	—	—
nicotinate	T46.6X1	T46.6X2	T46.6X3	T46.6X4	T46.6X5	T46.6X6
penicillin	T36.0X1	T36.0X2	T36.0X3	T36.0X4	T36.0X5	T36.0X6
Benzylhydrochlorthiazide	T50.2X1	T50.2X2	T50.2X3	T50.2X4	T50.2X5	T50.2X6
Benzylpenicillin	T36.0X1	T36.0X2	T36.0X3	T36.0X4	T36.0X5	T36.0X6
Benzylthiouracil	T38.2X1	T38.2X2	T38.2X3	T38.2X4	T38.2X5	T38.2X6
Bephenium hydroxynaphthoate	T37.4X1	T37.4X2	T37.4X3	T37.4X4	T37.4X5	T37.4X6
Bepridil	T46.1X1	T46.1X2	T46.1X3	T46.1X4	T46.1X5	T46.1X6
Bergamot oil	T65.891	T65.892	T65.893	T65.894	—	—
Bergapten	T50.991	T50.992	T50.993	T50.994	T50.995	T50.996
Berries, poisonous	T62.1X1	T62.1X2	T62.1X3	T62.1X4	—	—
Beryllium (compounds)	T56.7X1	T56.7X2	T56.7X3	T56.7X4	—	—
beta adrenergic blocking agent, heart	T44.7X1	T44.7X2	T44.7X3	T44.7X4	T44.7X5	T44.7X6
Betacarotene	T45.2X1	T45.2X2	T45.2X3	T45.2X4	T45.2X5	T45.2X6
Beta-Chlor	T42.6X1	T42.6X2	T42.6X3	T42.6X4	T42.6X5	T42.6X6
Betahistine	T46.7X1	T46.7X2	T46.7X3	T46.7X4	T46.7X5	T46.7X6
Betaine	T47.5X1	T47.5X2	T47.5X3	T47.5X4	T47.5X5	T47.5X6
Betamethasone	T49.0X1	T49.0X2	T49.0X3	T49.0X4	T49.0X5	T49.0X6
topical	T49.0X1	T49.0X2	T49.0X3	T49.0X4	T49.0X5	T49.0X6
Betamicin	T36.8X1	T36.8X2	T36.8X3	T36.8X4	T36.8X5	T36.8X6
Betanidine	T46.5X1	T46.5X2	T46.5X3	T46.5X4	T46.5X5	T46.5X6
Betaxolol	T44.7X1	T44.7X2	T44.7X3	T44.7X4	T44.7X5	T44.7X6
Betazole	T50.8X1	T50.8X2	T50.8X3	T50.8X4	T50.8X5	T50.8X6
Bethanechol	T44.1X1	T44.1X2	T44.1X3	T44.1X4	T44.1X5	T44.1X6

Substance	Poisoning, Accidental (unintentional)	Poisoning, Intentional Self-harm	Poisoning, Assault	Poisoning, Undetermined	Adverse Effect	Under-dosing
Bethanechol — *continued*						
chloride	T44.1X1	T44.1X2	T44.1X3	T44.1X4	T44.1X5	T44.1X6
Bethanidine	T46.5X1	T46.5X2	T46.5X3	T46.5X4	T46.5X5	T46.5X6
Betoxycaine	T41.3X1	T41.3X2	T41.3X3	T41.3X4	T41.3X5	T41.3X6
Betula oil	T49.3X1	T49.3X2	T49.3X3	T49.3X4	T49.3X5	T49.3X6
Bevantolol	T44.7X1	T44.7X2	T44.7X3	T44.7X4	T44.7X5	T44.7X6
Bevonium metilsulfate	T44.3X1	T44.3X2	T44.3X3	T44.3X4	T44.3X5	T44.3X6
Bezafibrate	T46.6X1	T46.6X2	T46.6X3	T46.6X4	T46.6X5	T46.6X6
Bezitramide	T40.4X1	T40.4X2	T40.4X3	T40.4X4	T40.4X5	T40.4X6
BHA	T50.991	T50.992	T50.993	T50.994	T50.995	T50.996
Bhang	T40.7X1	T40.7X2	T40.7X3	T40.7X4	T40.7X5	T40.7X6
BHC (medicinal)	T49.0X1	T49.0X2	T49.0X3	T49.0X4	T49.0X5	T49.0X6
nonmedicinal (vapor)	T53.6X1	T53.6X2	T53.6X3	T53.6X4	—	—
Bialamicol	T37.3X1	T37.3X2	T37.3X3	T37.3X4	T37.3X5	T37.3X6
Bibenzonium bromide	T48.3X1	T48.3X2	T48.3X3	T48.3X4	T48.3X5	T48.3X6
Bibrocathol	T49.5X1	T49.5X2	T49.5X3	T49.5X4	T49.5X5	T49.5X6
Bichloride of mercury — *see* Mercury, chloride						
Bichromates (calcium) (potassium) (sodium) (crystals)	T57.8X1	T57.8X2	T57.8X3	T57.8X4		
fumes	T56.2X1	T56.2X2	T56.2X3	T56.2X4	—	—
Biclotymol	T49.6X1	T49.6X2	T49.6X3	T49.6X4	T49.6X5	T49.6X6
Bicucculine	T50.7X1	T50.7X2	T50.7X3	T50.7X4	T50.7X5	T50.7X6
Bifemelane	T43.291	T43.292	T43.293	T43.294	T43.295	T43.296
Biguanide derivatives, oral	T38.3X1	T38.3X2	T38.3X3	T38.3X4	T38.3X5	T38.3X6
Bile salts	T47.5X1	T47.5X2	T47.5X3	T47.5X4	T47.5X5	T47.5X6
Biligrafin	T50.8X1	T50.8X2	T50.8X3	T50.8X4	T50.8X5	T50.8X6
Bilopaque	T50.8X1	T50.8X2	T50.8X3	T50.8X4	T50.8X5	T50.8X6
Binifibrate	T46.6X1	T46.6X2	T46.6X3	T46.6X4	T46.6X5	T46.6X6
Binitrobenzol	T65.3X1	T65.3X2	T65.3X3	T65.3X4	—	—
Bioflavonoid(s)	T46.991	T46.992	T46.993	T46.994	T46.995	T46.996
Biological substance NEC	T50.901	T50.902	T50.903	T50.904	T50.905	T50.906
Biotin	T45.2X1	T45.2X2	T45.2X3	T45.2X4	T45.2X5	T45.2X6
Biperiden	T44.3X1	T44.3X2	T44.3X3	T44.3X4	T44.3X5	T44.3X6
Bisacodyl	T47.2X1	T47.2X2	T47.2X3	T47.2X4	T47.2X5	T47.2X6
Bisbentiamine	T45.2X1	T45.2X2	T45.2X3	T45.2X4	T45.2X5	T45.2X6
Bisbutiamine	T45.2X1	T45.2X2	T45.2X3	T45.2X4	T45.2X5	T45.2X6
Bisdequalinium (salts) (diacetate)	T49.6X1	T49.6X2	T49.6X3	T49.6X4	T49.6X5	T49.6X6
Bishydroxycoumarin	T45.511	T45.512	T45.513	T45.514	T45.515	T45.516
Bismarsen	T37.8X1	T37.8X2	T37.8X3	T37.8X4	T37.8X5	T37.8X6
Bismuth salts	T47.6X1	T47.6X2	T47.6X3	T47.6X4	T47.6X5	T47.6X6
aluminate	T47.1X1	T47.1X2	T47.1X3	T47.1X4	T47.1X5	T47.1X6
anti-infectives	T37.8X1	T37.8X2	T37.8X3	T37.8X4	T37.8X5	T37.8X6
formic iodide	T49.0X1	T49.0X2	T49.0X3	T49.0X4	T49.0X5	T49.0X6
glycolylarsenate	T49.0X1	T49.0X2	T49.0X3	T49.0X4	T49.0X5	T49.0X6
nonmedicinal (compounds) NEC	T65.91	T65.92	T65.93	T65.94	—	—
subcarbonate	T47.6X1	T47.6X2	T47.6X3	T47.6X4	T47.6X5	T47.6X6
subsalicylate	T37.8X1	T37.8X2	T37.8X3	T37.8X4	T37.8X5	T37.8X6
sulfarsphenamine	T37.8X1	T37.8X2	T37.8X3	T37.8X4	T37.8X5	T37.8X6
Bisoprolol	T44.7X1	T44.7X2	T44.7X3	T44.7X4	T44.7X5	T44.7X6
Bisoxatin	T47.2X1	T47.2X2	T47.2X3	T47.2X4	T47.2X5	T47.2X6
Bisulepin (hydrochloride)	T45.0X1	T45.0X2	T45.0X3	T45.0X4	T45.0X5	T45.0X6
Bithionol	T37.8X1	T37.8X2	T37.8X3	T37.8X4	T37.8X5	T37.8X6
anthelminthic	T37.4X1	T37.4X2	T37.4X3	T37.4X4	T37.4X5	T37.4X6
Bitolterol	T48.6X1	T48.6X2	T48.6X3	T48.6X4	T48.6X5	T48.6X6
Bitoscanate	T37.4X1	T37.4X2	T37.4X3	T37.4X4	T37.4X5	T37.4X6
Bitter almond oil	T62.8X1	T62.8X2	T62.8X3	T62.8X4	—	—
Bittersweet	T62.2X1	T62.2X2	T62.2X3	T62.2X4	—	—
Black						
flag	T60.91	T60.92	T60.93	T60.94	—	—
henbane	T62.2X1	T62.2X2	T62.2X3	T62.2X4	—	—
leaf (40)	T60.91	T60.92	T60.93	T60.94	—	—
widow spider (bite)	T63.311	T63.312	T63.313	T63.314	—	—
antivenin	T50.Z11	T50.Z12	T50.Z13	T50.Z14	T50.Z15	T50.Z16
Blast furnace gas (carbon monoxide from)	T58.8X1	T58.8X2	T58.8X3	T58.8X4	—	—
Bleach	T54.91	T54.92	T54.93	T54.94	—	—
Bleaching agent (medicinal)	T49.4X1	T49.4X2	T49.4X3	T49.4X4	T49.4X5	T49.4X6
Bleomycin	T45.1X1	T45.1X2	T45.1X3	T45.1X4	T45.1X5	T45.1X6
Blockain	T41.3X1	T41.3X2	T41.3X3	T41.3X4	T41.3X5	T41.3X6
infiltration (subcutaneous)	T41.3X1	T41.3X2	T41.3X3	T41.3X4	T41.3X5	T41.3X6
nerve block (peripheral) (plexus)	T41.3X1	T41.3X2	T41.3X3	T41.3X4	T41.3X5	T41.3X6
topical (surface)	T41.3X1	T41.3X2	T41.3X3	T41.3X4	T41.3X5	T41.3X6
Blockers, calcium channel	T46.1X1	T46.1X2	T46.1X3	T46.1X4	T46.1X5	T46.1X6
Blood (derivatives) (natural) (plasma) (whole)	T45.8X1	T45.8X2	T45.8X3	T45.8X4	T45.8X5	T45.8X6
dried	T45.8X1	T45.8X2	T45.8X3	T45.8X4	T45.8X5	T45.8X6

Benzamine — Blood

Substance	Poisoning, Accidental (unintentional)	Poisoning, Intentional Self-harm	Poisoning, Assault	Poisoning, Undetermined	Adverse Effect	Under-dosing
Blood — *continued*						
drug affecting NEC	T45.91	T45.92	T45.93	T45.94	T45.95	T45.96
expander NEC	T45.8X1	T45.8X2	T45.8X3	T45.8X4	T45.8X5	T45.8X6
fraction NEC	T45.8X1	T45.8X2	T45.8X3	T45.8X4	T45.8X5	T45.8X6
substitute (macromolecular)	T45.8X1	T45.8X2	T45.8X3	T45.8X4	T45.8X5	T45.8X6
Blue velvet	T40.2X1	T40.2X2	T40.2X3	T40.2X4	—	—
Bone meal	T62.8X1	T62.8X2	T62.8X3	T62.8X4	—	—
Bonine	T45.0X1	T45.0X2	T45.0X3	T45.0X4	T45.0X5	T45.0X6
Bopindolol	T44.7X1	T44.7X2	T44.7X3	T44.7X4	T44.7X5	T44.7X6
Boracic acid	T49.0X1	T49.0X2	T49.0X3	T49.0X4	T49.0X5	T49.0X6
ENT agent	T49.6X1	T49.6X2	T49.6X3	T49.6X4	T49.6X5	T49.6X6
ophthalmic preparation	T49.5X1	T49.5X2	T49.5X3	T49.5X4	T49.5X5	T49.5X6
Borane complex	T57.8X1	T57.8X2	T57.8X3	T57.8X4	—	—
Borate(s)	T57.8X1	T57.8X2	T57.8X3	T57.8X4	—	—
buffer	T50.991	T50.992	T50.993	T50.994	T50.995	T50.996
cleanser	T54.91	T54.92	T54.93	T54.94	—	—
sodium	T57.8X1	T57.8X2	T57.8X3	T57.8X4	—	—
Borax (cleanser)	T54.91	T54.92	T54.93	T54.94	—	—
Bordeaux mixture	T60.3X1	T60.3X2	T60.3X3	T60.3X4	—	—
Boric acid	T49.0X1	T49.0X2	T49.0X3	T49.0X4	T49.0X5	T49.0X6
ENT agent	T49.6X1	T49.6X2	T49.6X3	T49.6X4	T49.6X5	T49.6X6
ophthalmic preparation	T49.5X1	T49.5X2	T49.5X3	T49.5X4	T49.5X5	T49.5X6
Bornaprine	T44.3X1	T44.3X2	T44.3X3	T44.3X4	T44.3X5	T44.3X6
Boron	T57.8X1	T57.8X2	T57.8X3	T57.8X4	—	—
hydride NEC	T57.8X1	T57.8X2	T57.8X3	T57.8X4	—	—
fumes or gas	T57.8X1	T57.8X2	T57.8X3	T57.8X4	—	—
trifluoride	T59.891	T59.892	T59.893	T59.894	—	—
Botox	T48.291	T48.292	T48.293	T48.294	T48.295	T48.296
Botulinus anti-toxin (type A, B)	T50.Z11	T50.Z12	T50.Z13	T50.Z14	T50.Z15	T50.Z16
Brake fluid vapor	T59.891	T59.892	T59.893	T59.894	—	—
Brallobarbital	T42.3X1	T42.3X2	T42.3X3	T42.3X4	T42.3X5	T42.3X6
Bran (wheat)	T47.4X1	T47.4X2	T47.4X3	T47.4X4	T47.4X5	T47.4X6
Brass (fumes)	T56.891	T56.892	T56.893	T56.894	—	—
Brasso	T52.0X1	T52.0X2	T52.0X3	T52.0X4	—	—
Bretylium tosilate	T46.2X1	T46.2X2	T46.2X3	T46.2X4	T46.2X5	T46.2X6
Brevital (sodium)	T41.1X1	T41.1X2	T41.1X3	T41.1X4	T41.1X5	T41.1X6
Brinase	T45.3X1	T45.3X2	T45.3X3	T45.3X4	T45.3X5	T45.3X6
British antilewisite	T45.8X1	T45.8X2	T45.8X3	T45.8X4	T45.8X5	T45.8X6
Brodifacoum	T60.4X1	T60.4X2	T60.4X3	T60.4X4	—	—
Bromal (hydrate)	T42.6X1	T42.6X2	T42.6X3	T42.6X4	T42.6X5	T42.6X6
Bromazepam	T42.4X1	T42.4X2	T42.4X3	T42.4X4	T42.4X5	T42.4X6
Bromazine	T45.0X1	T45.0X2	T45.0X3	T45.0X4	T45.0X5	T45.0X6
Brombenzylcyanide	T59.3X1	T59.3X2	T59.3X3	T59.3X4	—	—
Bromelains	T45.3X1	T45.3X2	T45.3X3	T45.3X4	T45.3X5	T45.3X6
Bromethalin	T60.4X1	T60.4X2	T60.4X3	T60.4X4	—	—
Bromhexine	T48.4X1	T48.4X2	T48.4X3	T48.4X4	T48.4X5	T48.4X6
Bromide salts	T42.6X1	T42.6X2	T42.6X3	T42.6X4	T42.6X5	T42.6X6
Bromindione	T45.511	T45.512	T45.513	T45.514	T45.515	T45.516
Bromine						
compounds (medicinal)	T42.6X1	T42.6X2	T42.6X3	T42.6X4	T42.6X5	T42.6X6
sedative	T42.6X1	T42.6X2	T42.6X3	T42.6X4	T42.6X5	T42.6X6
vapor	T59.891	T59.892	T59.893	T59.894	—	—
Bromisoval	T42.6X1	T42.6X2	T42.6X3	T42.6X4	T42.6X5	T42.6X6
Bromisovalum	T42.6X1	T42.6X2	T42.6X3	T42.6X4	T42.6X5	T42.6X6
Bromobenzylcyanide	T59.3X1	T59.3X2	T59.3X3	T59.3X4	—	—
Bromochlorosalicylani-lide	T49.0X1	T49.0X2	T49.0X3	T49.0X4	T49.0X5	T49.0X6
Bromocriptine	T42.8X1	T42.8X2	T42.8X3	T42.8X4	T42.8X5	T42.8X6
Bromodiphenhydramine	T45.0X1	T45.0X2	T45.0X3	T45.0X4	T45.0X5	T45.0X6
Bromoform	T42.6X1	T42.6X2	T42.6X3	T42.6X4	T42.6X5	T42.6X6
Bromophenol blue reagent	T50.991	T50.992	T50.993	T50.994	T50.995	T50.996
Bromopride	T47.8X1	T47.8X2	T47.8X3	T47.8X4	T47.8X5	T47.8X6
Bromosalicylchloranitide	T49.0X1	T49.0X2	T49.0X3	T49.0X4	T49.0X5	T49.0X6
Bromosalicylhydroxamic acid	T37.1X1	T37.1X2	T37.1X3	T37.1X4	T37.1X5	T37.1X6
Bromo-seltzer	T39.1X1	T39.1X2	T39.1X3	T39.1X4	T39.1X5	T39.1X6
Bromoxynil	T60.3X1	T60.3X2	T60.3X3	T60.3X4	—	—
Bromperidol	T43.4X1	T43.4X2	T43.4X3	T43.4X4	T43.4X5	T43.4X6
Brompheniramine	T45.0X1	T45.0X2	T45.0X3	T45.0X4	T45.0X5	T45.0X6
Bromsulphthalein	T50.8X1	T50.8X2	T50.8X3	T50.8X4	T50.8X5	T50.8X6
Bromural	T42.6X1	T42.6X2	T42.6X3	T42.6X4	T42.6X5	T42.6X6
Bromvaletone	T42.6X1	T42.6X2	T42.6X3	T42.6X4	T42.6X5	T42.6X6
Bronchodilator NEC	T48.6X1	T48.6X2	T48.6X3	T48.6X4	T48.6X5	T48.6X6
Brotizolam	T42.4X1	T42.4X2	T42.4X3	T42.4X4	T42.4X5	T42.4X6
Brovincamine	T46.7X1	T46.7X2	T46.7X3	T46.7X4	T46.7X5	T46.7X6
Brown recluse spider (bite) (venom)	T63.331	T63.332	T63.333	T63.334	—	—
Brown spider (bite) (venom)	T63.391	T63.392	T63.393	T63.394	—	—
Broxaterol	T48.6X1	T48.6X2	T48.6X3	T48.6X4	T48.6X5	T48.6X6
Broxuridine	T45.1X1	T45.1X2	T45.1X3	T45.1X4	T45.1X5	T45.1X6
Broxyquinoline	T37.8X1	T37.8X2	T37.8X3	T37.8X4	T37.8X5	T37.8X6
Bruceine	T48.291	T48.292	T48.293	T48.294	T48.295	T48.296
Brucia	T62.2X1	T62.2X2	T62.2X3	T62.2X4	—	—
Brucine	T65.1X1	T65.1X2	T65.1X3	T65.1X4	—	—
Brunswick green — *see* Copper						
Bruten — *see* Ibuprofen						
Bryonia	T47.2X1	T47.2X2	T47.2X3	T47.2X4	T47.2X5	T47.2X6
Buclizine	T45.0X1	T45.0X2	T45.0X3	T45.0X4	T45.0X5	T45.0X6
Buclosamide	T49.0X1	T49.0X2	T49.0X3	T49.0X4	T49.0X5	T49.0X6
Budesonide	T44.5X1	T44.5X2	T44.5X3	T44.5X4	T44.5X5	T44.5X6
Budralazine	T46.5X1	T46.5X2	T46.5X3	T46.5X4	T46.5X5	T46.5X6
Bufferin	T39.011	T39.012	T39.013	T39.014	T39.015	T39.016
Buflomedil	T46.7X1	T46.7X2	T46.7X3	T46.7X4	T46.7X5	T46.7X6
Buformin	T38.3X1	T38.3X2	T38.3X3	T38.3X4	T38.3X5	T38.3X6
Bufotenine	T40.991	T40.992	T40.993	T40.994	—	—
Bufrolin	T48.6X1	T48.6X2	T48.6X3	T48.6X4	T48.6X5	T48.6X6
Bufylline	T48.6X1	T48.6X2	T48.6X3	T48.6X4	T48.6X5	T48.6X6
Bulk filler	T50.5X1	T50.5X2	T50.5X3	T50.5X4	T50.5X5	T50.5X6
cathartic	T47.4X1	T47.4X2	T47.4X3	T47.4X4	T47.4X5	T47.4X6
Bumetanide	T50.1X1	T50.1X2	T50.1X3	T50.1X4	T50.1X5	T50.1X6
Bunaftine	T46.2X1	T46.2X2	T46.2X3	T46.2X4	T46.2X5	T46.2X6
Bunamiodyl	T50.8X1	T50.8X2	T50.8X3	T50.8X4	T50.8X5	T50.8X6
Bunazosin	T44.6X1	T44.6X2	T44.6X3	T44.6X4	T44.6X5	T44.6X6
Bunitrolol	T44.7X1	T44.7X2	T44.7X3	T44.7X4	T44.7X5	T44.7X6
Buphenine	T46.7X1	T46.7X2	T46.7X3	T46.7X4	T46.7X5	T46.7X6
Bupivacaine	T41.3X1	T41.3X2	T41.3X3	T41.3X4	T41.3X5	T41.3X6
infiltration (subcutaneous)	T41.3X1	T41.3X2	T41.3X3	T41.3X4	T41.3X5	T41.3X6
nerve block (peripheral) (plexus)	T41.3X1	T41.3X2	T41.3X3	T41.3X4	T41.3X5	T41.3X6
spinal	T41.3X1	T41.3X2	T41.3X3	T41.3X4	T41.3X5	T41.3X6
Bupranolol	T44.7X1	T44.7X2	T44.7X3	T44.7X4	T44.7X5	T44.7X6
Buprenorphine	T40.4X1	T40.4X2	T40.4X3	T40.4X4	T40.4X5	T40.4X6
Bupropion	T43.291	T43.292	T43.293	T43.294	T43.295	T43.296
Burimamide	T47.1X1	T47.1X2	T47.1X3	T47.1X4	T47.1X5	T47.1X6
Buserelin	T38.891	T38.892	T38.893	T38.894	T38.895	T38.896
Buspirone	T43.591	T43.592	T43.593	T43.594	T43.595	T43.596
Busulfan, busulphan	T45.1X1	T45.1X2	T45.1X3	T45.1X4	T45.1X5	T45.1X6
Butabarbital (sodium)	T42.3X1	T42.3X2	T42.3X3	T42.3X4	T42.3X5	T42.3X6
Butabarbitone	T42.3X1	T42.3X2	T42.3X3	T42.3X4	T42.3X5	T42.3X6
Butabarpal	T42.3X1	T42.3X2	T42.3X3	T42.3X4	T42.3X5	T42.3X6
Butacaine	T41.3X1	T41.3X2	T41.3X3	T41.3X4	T41.3X5	T41.3X6
Butalamine	T46.7X1	T46.7X2	T46.7X3	T46.7X4	T46.7X5	T46.7X6
Butalbital	T42.3X1	T42.3X2	T42.3X3	T42.3X4	T42.3X5	T42.3X6
Butallylonal	T42.3X1	T42.3X2	T42.3X3	T42.3X4	T42.3X5	T42.3X6
Butamben	T41.3X1	T41.3X2	T41.3X3	T41.3X4	T41.3X5	T41.3X6
Butamirate	T48.3X1	T48.3X2	T48.3X3	T48.3X4	T48.3X5	T48.3X6
Butane (distributed in mobile container)	T59.891	T59.892	T59.893	T59.894	—	—
distributed through pipes	T59.891	T59.892	T59.893	T59.894	—	—
incomplete combustion	T58.11	T58.12	T58.13	T58.14	—	—
Butanilicaine	T41.3X1	T41.3X2	T41.3X3	T41.3X4	T41.3X5	T41.3X6
Butanol	T51.3X1	T51.3X2	T51.3X3	T51.3X4	—	—
Butanone, 2-butanone	T52.4X1	T52.4X2	T52.4X3	T52.4X4	—	—
Butantrone	T49.4X1	T49.4X2	T49.4X3	T49.4X4	T49.4X5	T49.4X6
Butaperazine	T43.3X1	T43.3X2	T43.3X3	T43.3X4	T43.3X5	T43.3X6
Butazolidin	T39.2X1	T39.2X2	T39.2X3	T39.2X4	T39.2X5	T39.2X6
Butetamate	T48.6X1	T48.6X2	T48.6X3	T48.6X4	T48.6X5	T48.6X6
Butethal	T42.3X1	T42.3X2	T42.3X3	T42.3X4	T42.3X5	T42.3X6
Butethamate	T44.3X1	T44.3X2	T44.3X3	T44.3X4	T44.3X5	T44.3X6
Buthalitone (sodium)	T41.1X1	T41.1X2	T41.1X3	T41.1X4	T41.1X5	T41.1X6
Butisol (sodium)	T42.3X1	T42.3X2	T42.3X3	T42.3X4	T42.3X5	T42.3X6
Butizide	T50.2X1	T50.2X2	T50.2X3	T50.2X4	T50.2X5	T50.2X6
Butobarbital	T42.3X1	T42.3X2	T42.3X3	T42.3X4	T42.3X5	T42.3X6
sodium	T42.3X1	T42.3X2	T42.3X3	T42.3X4	T42.3X5	T42.3X6
Butobarbitone	T42.3X1	T42.3X2	T42.3X3	T42.3X4	T42.3X5	T42.3X6
Butoconazole (nitrate)	T49.0X1	T49.0X2	T49.0X3	T49.0X4	T49.0X5	T49.0X6
Butorphanol	T40.4X1	T40.4X2	T40.4X3	T40.4X4	T40.4X5	T40.4X6
Butriptyline	T43.011	T43.012	T43.013	T43.014	T43.015	T43.016
Butropium bromide	T44.3X1	T44.3X2	T44.3X3	T44.3X4	T44.3X5	T44.3X6
Buttercups	T62.2X1	T62.2X2	T62.2X3	T62.2X4	—	—
Butter of antimony — *see* Antimony						
Butyl						
acetate (secondary)	T52.8X1	T52.8X2	T52.8X3	T52.8X4	—	—
alcohol	T51.3X1	T51.3X2	T51.3X3	T51.3X4	—	—
aminobenzoate	T41.3X1	T41.3X2	T41.3X3	T41.3X4	T41.3X5	T41.3X6
butyrate	T52.8X1	T52.8X2	T52.8X3	T52.8X4	—	—
carbinol	T51.3X1	T51.3X2	T51.3X3	T51.3X4	—	—
carbitol	T52.3X1	T52.3X2	T52.3X3	T52.3X4	—	—
cellosolve	T52.3X1	T52.3X2	T52.3X3	T52.3X4	—	—
chloral (hydrate)	T42.6X1	T42.6X2	T42.6X3	T42.6X4	T42.6X5	T42.6X6
formate	T52.8X1	T52.8X2	T52.8X3	T52.8X4	—	—
lactate	T52.8X1	T52.8X2	T52.8X3	T52.8X4	—	—

Substance	Poisoning, Accidental (unintentional)	Poisoning, Intentional Self-harm	Poisoning, Assault	Poisoning, Undetermined	Adverse Effect	Under-dosing
Butyl — *continued*						
propionate	T52.8X1	T52.8X2	T52.8X3	T52.8X4	—	—
scopolamine bromide	T44.3X1	T44.3X2	T44.3X3	T44.3X4	T44.3X5	T44.3X6
thiobarbital sodium	T41.1X1	T41.1X2	T41.1X3	T41.1X4	T41.1X5	T41.1X6
Butylated hydroxanisole	T50.991	T50.992	T50.993	T50.994	T50.995	T50.996
Butylchloral hydrate	T42.6X1	T42.6X2	T42.6X3	T42.6X4	T42.6X5	T42.6X6
Butyltoluene	T52.2X1	T52.2X2	T52.2X3	T52.2X4	—	—
Butyn	T41.3X1	T41.3X2	T41.3X3	T41.3X4	T41.3X5	T41.3X6
Butyrophenone (-based tranquilizers)	T43.4X1	T43.4X2	T43.4X3	T43.4X4	T43.4X5	T43.4X6
Cabergoline	T42.8X1	T42.8X2	T42.8X3	T42.8X4	T42.8X5	T42.8X6
Cacodyl, cacodylic acid	T57.0X1	T57.0X2	T57.0X3	T57.0X4	—	—
Cactinomycin	T45.1X1	T45.1X2	T45.1X3	T45.1X4	T45.1X5	T45.1X6
Cade oil	T49.4X1	T49.4X2	T49.4X3	T49.4X4	T49.4X5	T49.4X6
Cadexomer iodine	T49.0X1	T49.0X2	T49.0X3	T49.0X4	T49.0X5	T49.0X6
Cadmium (chloride) (fumes) (oxide)	T56.3X1	T56.3X2	T56.3X3	T56.3X4	—	—
sulfide (medicinal) NEC	T49.4X1	T49.4X2	T49.4X3	T49.4X4	T49.4X5	T49.4X6
Cadralazine	T46.5X1	T46.5X2	T46.5X3	T46.5X4	T46.5X5	T46.5X6
Caffeine	T43.611	T43.612	T43.613	T43.614	T43.615	T43.616
Calabar bean	T62.2X1	T62.2X2	T62.2X3	T62.2X4	—	—
Caladium seguinum	T62.2X1	T62.2X2	T62.2X3	T62.2X4	—	—
Calamine (lotion)	T49.3X1	T49.3X2	T49.3X3	T49.3X4	T49.3X5	T49.3X6
Calcifediol	T45.2X1	T45.2X2	T45.2X3	T45.2X4	T45.2X5	T45.2X6
Calciferol	T45.2X1	T45.2X2	T45.2X3	T45.2X4	T45.2X5	T45.2X6
Calcitonin	T50.991	T50.992	T50.993	T50.994	T50.995	T50.996
Calcitriol	T45.2X1	T45.2X2	T45.2X3	T45.2X4	T45.2X5	T45.2X6
Calcium	T50.3X1	T50.3X2	T50.3X3	T50.3X4	T50.3X5	T50.3X6
actylsalicylate	T39.011	T39.012	T39.013	T39.014	T39.015	T39.016
benzamidosalicylate	T37.1X1	T37.1X2	T37.1X3	T37.1X4	T37.1X5	T37.1X6
bromide	T42.6X1	T42.6X2	T42.6X3	T42.6X4	T42.6X5	T42.6X6
bromolactobionate	T42.6X1	T42.6X2	T42.6X3	T42.6X4	T42.6X5	T42.6X6
carbaspirin	T39.011	T39.012	T39.013	T39.014	T39.015	T39.016
carbimide	T50.6X1	T50.6X2	T50.6X3	T50.6X4	T50.6X5	T50.6X6
carbonate	T47.1X1	T47.1X2	T47.1X3	T47.1X4	T47.1X5	T47.1X6
chloride	T50.991	T50.992	T50.993	T50.994	T50.995	T50.996
anhydrous	T50.991	T50.992	T50.993	T50.994	T50.995	T50.996
cyanide	T57.8X1	T57.8X2	T57.8X3	T57.8X4	—	—
dioctyl sulfosuccinate	T47.4X1	T47.4X2	T47.4X3	T47.4X4	T47.4X5	T47.4X6
disodium edathamil	T45.8X1	T45.8X2	T45.8X3	T45.8X4	T45.8X5	T45.8X6
disodium edetate	T45.8X1	T45.8X2	T45.8X3	T45.8X4	T45.8X5	T45.8X6
dobesilate	T46.991	T46.992	T46.993	T46.994	T46.995	T46.996
EDTA	T45.8X1	T45.8X2	T45.8X3	T45.8X4	T45.8X5	T45.8X6
ferrous citrate	T45.4X1	T45.4X2	T45.4X3	T45.4X4	T45.4X5	T45.4X6
folinate	T45.8X1	T45.8X2	T45.8X3	T45.8X4	T45.8X5	T45.8X6
glubionate	T50.3X1	T50.3X2	T50.3X3	T50.3X4	T50.3X5	T50.3X6
gluconate	T50.3X1	T50.3X2	T50.3X3	T50.3X4	T50.3X5	T50.3X6
gluconogalactogluconate	T50.3X1	T50.3X2	T50.3X3	T50.3X4	T50.3X5	T50.3X6
hydrate, hydroxide	T54.3X1	T54.3X2	T54.3X3	T54.3X4	—	—
hypochlorite	T54.3X1	T54.3X2	T54.3X3	T54.3X4	—	—
iodide	T48.4X1	T48.4X2	T48.4X3	T48.4X4	T48.4X5	T48.4X6
ipodate	T50.8X1	T50.8X2	T50.8X3	T50.8X4	T50.8X5	T50.8X6
lactate	T50.3X1	T50.3X2	T50.3X3	T50.3X4	T50.3X5	T50.3X6
leucovorin	T45.8X1	T45.8X2	T45.8X3	T45.8X4	T45.8X5	T45.8X6
mandelate	T37.91	T37.92	T37.93	T37.94	T37.95	T37.96
oxide	T54.3X1	T54.3X2	T54.3X3	T54.3X4	—	—
pantothenate	T45.2X1	T45.2X2	T45.2X3	T45.2X4	T45.2X5	T45.2X6
phosphate	T50.3X1	T50.3X2	T50.3X3	T50.3X4	T50.3X5	T50.3X6
salicylate	T39.091	T39.092	T39.093	T39.094	T39.095	T39.096
salts	T50.3X1	T50.3X2	T50.3X3	T50.3X4	T50.3X5	T50.3X6
Calculus-dissolving drug	T50.991	T50.992	T50.993	T50.994	T50.995	T50.996
Calomel	T49.0X1	T49.0X2	T49.0X3	T49.0X4	T49.0X5	T49.0X6
Caloric agent	T50.3X1	T50.3X2	T50.3X3	T50.3X4	T50.3X5	T50.3X6
Calusterone	T38.7X1	T38.7X2	T38.7X3	T38.7X4	T38.7X5	T38.7X6
Camazepam	T42.4X1	T42.4X2	T42.4X3	T42.4X4	T42.4X5	T42.4X6
Camomile	T49.0X1	T49.0X2	T49.0X3	T49.0X4	T49.0X5	T49.0X6
Camoquin	T37.2X1	T37.2X2	T37.2X3	T37.2X4	T37.2X5	T37.2X6
Camphor						
insecticide	T60.2X1	T60.2X2	T60.2X3	T60.2X4	—	—
medicinal	T49.8X1	T49.8X2	T49.8X3	T49.8X4	T49.8X5	T49.8X6
Camylofin	T44.3X1	T44.3X2	T44.3X3	T44.3X4	T44.3X5	T44.3X6
Cancer chemotherapy drug regimen	T45.1X1	T45.1X2	T45.1X3	T45.1X4	T45.1X5	T45.1X6
Candeptin	T49.0X1	T49.0X2	T49.0X3	T49.0X4	T49.0X5	T49.0X6
Candicidin	T49.0X1	T49.0X2	T49.0X3	T49.0X4	T49.0X5	T49.0X6
Cannabinol	T40.7X1	T40.7X2	T40.7X3	T40.7X4	T40.7X5	T40.7X6
Cannabis (derivatives)	T40.7X1	T40.7X2	T40.7X3	T40.7X4	T40.7X5	T40.7X6
Canned heat	T51.1X1	T51.1X2	T51.1X3	T51.1X4	—	—
Canrenoic acid	T50.0X1	T50.0X2	T50.0X3	T50.0X4	T50.0X5	T50.0X6
Canrenone	T50.0X1	T50.0X2	T50.0X3	T50.0X4	T50.0X5	T50.0X6
Cantharides, cantharidin, cantharis	T49.8X1	T49.8X2	T49.8X3	T49.8X4	T49.8X5	T49.8X6
Canthaxanthin	T50.991	T50.992	T50.993	T50.994	T50.995	T50.996

Substance	Poisoning, Accidental (unintentional)	Poisoning, Intentional Self-harm	Poisoning, Assault	Poisoning, Undetermined	Adverse Effect	Under-dosing
Capillary-active drug NEC	T46.901	T46.902	T46.903	T46.904	T46.905	T46.906
Capreomycin	T36.8X1	T36.8X2	T36.8X3	T36.8X4	T36.8X5	T36.8X6
Capsicum	T49.4X1	T49.4X2	T49.4X3	T49.4X4	T49.4X5	T49.4X6
Captafol	T60.3X1	T60.3X2	T60.3X3	T60.3X4	—	—
Captan	T60.3X1	T60.3X2	T60.3X3	T60.3X4	—	—
Captodiame, captodiamine	T43.591	T43.592	T43.593	T43.594	T43.595	T43.596
Captopril	T46.4X1	T46.4X2	T46.4X3	T46.4X4	T46.4X5	T46.4X6
Caramiphen	T44.3X1	T44.3X2	T44.3X3	T44.3X4	T44.3X5	T44.3X6
Carazolol	T44.7X1	T44.7X2	T44.7X3	T44.7X4	T44.7X5	T44.7X6
Carbachol	T44.1X1	T44.1X2	T44.1X3	T44.1X4	T44.1X5	T44.1X6
Carbacrylamine (resin)	T50.3X1	T50.3X2	T50.3X3	T50.3X4	T50.3X5	T50.3X6
Carbamate (insecticide)	T60.0X1	T60.0X2	T60.0X3	T60.0X4	—	—
Carbamate (sedative)	T42.6X1	T42.6X2	T42.6X3	T42.6X4	T42.6X5	T42.6X6
herbicide	T60.0X1	T60.0X2	T60.0X3	T60.0X4	—	—
insecticide	T60.0X1	T60.0X2	T60.0X3	T60.0X4	—	—
Carbamazepine	T42.1X1	T42.1X2	T42.1X3	T42.1X4	T42.1X5	T42.1X6
Carbamide	T47.3X1	T47.3X2	T47.3X3	T47.3X4	T47.3X5	T47.3X6
peroxide	T49.0X1	T49.0X2	T49.0X3	T49.0X4	T49.0X5	T49.0X6
topical	T49.8X1	T49.8X2	T49.8X3	T49.8X4	T49.8X5	T49.8X6
Carbamylcholine chloride	T44.1X1	T44.1X2	T44.1X3	T44.1X4	T44.1X5	T44.1X6
Carbaril	T60.0X1	T60.0X2	T60.0X3	T60.0X4	—	—
Carbarsone	T37.3X1	T37.3X2	T37.3X3	T37.3X4	T37.3X5	T37.3X6
Carbaryl	T60.0X1	T60.0X2	T60.0X3	T60.0X4	—	—
Carbaspirin	T39.011	T39.012	T39.013	T39.014	T39.015	T39.016
Carbazochrome (salicylate) (sodium sulfonate)	T49.4X1	T49.4X2	T49.4X3	T49.4X4	T49.4X5	T49.4X6
Carbenicillin	T36.0X1	T36.0X2	T36.0X3	T36.0X4	T36.0X5	T36.0X6
Carbenoxolone	T47.1X1	T47.1X2	T47.1X3	T47.1X4	T47.1X5	T47.1X6
Carbetapentane	T48.3X1	T48.3X2	T48.3X3	T48.3X4	T48.3X5	T48.3X6
Carbethyl salicylate	T39.091	T39.092	T39.093	T39.094	T39.095	T39.096
Carbidopa (with levodopa)	T42.8X1	T42.8X2	T42.8X3	T42.8X4	T42.8X5	T42.8X6
Carbimazole	T38.2X1	T38.2X2	T38.2X3	T38.2X4	T38.2X5	T38.2X6
Carbinol	T51.1X1	T51.1X2	T51.1X3	T51.1X4	—	—
Carbinoxamine	T45.0X1	T45.0X2	T45.0X3	T45.0X4	T45.0X5	T45.0X6
Carbiphene	T39.8X1	T39.8X2	T39.8X3	T39.8X4	T39.8X5	T39.8X6
Carbitol	T52.3X1	T52.3X2	T52.3X3	T52.3X4	—	—
Carbocaine	T41.3X1	T41.3X2	T41.3X3	T41.3X4	T41.3X5	T41.3X6
infiltration (subcutaneous)	T41.3X1	T41.3X2	T41.3X3	T41.3X4	T41.3X5	T41.3X6
nerve block (peripheral) (plexus)	T41.3X1	T41.3X2	T41.3X3	T41.3X4	T41.3X5	T41.3X6
topical (surface)	T41.3X1	T41.3X2	T41.3X3	T41.3X4	T41.3X5	T41.3X6
Carbocisteine	T48.4X1	T48.4X2	T48.4X3	T48.4X4	T48.4X5	T48.4X6
Carbocromen	T46.3X1	T46.3X2	T46.3X3	T46.3X4	T46.3X5	T46.3X6
Carbol fuchsin	T49.0X1	T49.0X2	T49.0X3	T49.0X4	T49.0X5	T49.0X6
Carbolic acid — *see also* Phenol	T54.0X1	T54.0X2	T54.0X3	T54.0X4		
Carbolonium (bromide)	T48.1X1	T48.1X2	T48.1X3	T48.1X4	T48.1X5	T48.1X6
Carbo medicinalis	T47.6X1	T47.6X2	T47.6X3	T47.6X4	T47.6X5	T47.6X6
Carbomycin	T36.8X1	T36.8X2	T36.8X3	T36.8X4	T36.8X5	T36.8X6
Carbon						
bisulfide (liquid)	T65.4X1	T65.4X2	T65.4X3	T65.4X4	—	—
vapor	T65.4X1	T65.4X2	T65.4X3	T65.4X4	—	—
dioxide (gas)	T59.7X1	T59.7X2	T59.7X3	T59.7X4	—	—
medicinal	T41.5X1	T41.5X2	T41.5X3	T41.5X4	T41.5X5	T41.5X6
nonmedicinal	T59.7X1	T59.7X2	T59.7X3	T59.7X4	—	—
snow	T49.4X1	T49.4X2	T49.4X3	T49.4X4	T49.4X5	T49.4X6
disulfide (liquid)	T65.4X1	T65.4X2	T65.4X3	T65.4X4	—	—
vapor	T65.4X1	T65.4X2	T65.4X3	T65.4X4	—	—
monoxide (from incomplete combustion)	T58.91	T58.92	T58.93	T58.94		
blast furnace gas	T58.8X1	T58.8X2	T58.8X3	T58.8X4		
butane (distributed in mobile container)	T58.11	T58.12	T58.13	T58.14		
distributed through pipes	T58.11	T58.12	T58.13	T58.14		
charcoal fumes	T58.2X1	T58.2X2	T58.2X3	T58.2X4		
coal	T58.2X1	T58.2X2	T58.2X3	T58.2X4		
coke (in domestic stoves, fireplaces)	T58.2X1	T58.2X2	T58.2X3	T58.2X4		
exhaust gas (motor) not in transit	T58.01	T58.02	T58.03	T58.04		
combustion engine, any not in watercraft	T58.01	T58.02	T58.03	T58.04		
farm tractor, not in transit	T58.01	T58.02	T58.03	T58.04		
gas engine	T58.01	T58.02	T58.03	T58.04		
motor pump	T58.01	T58.02	T58.03	T58.04		
motor vehicle, not in transit	T58.01	T58.02	T58.03	T58.04		
fuel (in domestic use)	T58.2X1	T58.2X2	T58.2X3	T58.2X4		
gas (piped)	T58.11	T58.12	T58.13	T58.14		
in mobile container	T58.11	T58.12	T58.13	T58.14		

Substance	Poisoning, Accidental (unintentional)	Poisoning, Intentional Self-harm	Poisoning, Assault	Poisoning, Undetermined	Adverse Effect	Under-dosing
Carbon — *continued*						
monoxide — *continued*						
fuel — *continued*						
piped (natural)	T58.11	T58.12	T58.13	T58.14	—	—
utility	T58.11	T58.12	T58.13	T58.14	—	—
in mobile container	T58.11	T58.12	T58.13	T58.14	—	—
gas (piped)	T58.11	T58.12	T58.13	T58.14	—	—
illuminating gas	T58.11	T58.12	T58.13	T58.14	—	—
industrial fuels or gases, any	T58.8X1	T58.8X2	T58.8X3	T58.8X4	—	—
kerosene (in domestic stoves, fireplaces)	T58.2X1	T58.2X2	T58.2X3	T58.2X4	—	—
kiln gas or vapor	T58.8X1	T58.8X2	T58.8X3	T58.8X4	—	—
motor exhaust gas, not in transit	T58.01	T58.02	T58.03	T58.04	—	—
piped gas (manufactured) (natural)	T58.11	T58.12	T58.13	T58.14	—	—
producer gas	T58.8X1	T58.8X2	T58.8X3	T58.8X4	—	—
propane (distributed in mobile container)	T58.11	T58.12	T58.13	T58.14	—	—
distributed through pipes	T58.11	T58.12	T58.13	T58.14	—	—
solid (in domestic stoves, fireplaces)	T58.2X1	T58.2X2	T58.2X3	T58.2X4	—	—
specified source NEC	T58.8X1	T58.8X2	T58.8X3	T58.8X4	—	—
stove gas	T58.11	T58.12	T58.13	T58.14	—	—
piped	T58.11	T58.12	T58.13	T58.14	—	—
utility gas	T58.11	T58.12	T58.13	T58.14	—	—
piped	T58.11	T58.12	T58.13	T58.14	—	—
water gas	T58.11	T58.12	T58.13	T58.14	—	—
wood (in domestic stoves, fireplaces)	T58.2X1	T58.2X2	T58.2X3	T58.2X4	—	—
tetrachloride (vapor) NEC	T53.0X1	T53.0X2	T53.0X3	T53.0X4	—	—
liquid (cleansing agent) NEC	T53.0X1	T53.0X2	T53.0X3	T53.0X4	—	—
solvent	T53.0X1	T53.0X2	T53.0X3	T53.0X4	—	—
Carbonic acid gas	T59.7X1	T59.7X2	T59.7X3	T59.7X4	—	—
anhydrase inhibitor NEC	T50.2X1	T50.2X2	T50.2X3	T50.2X4	T50.2X5	T50.2X6
Carbophenothion	T60.0X1	T60.0X2	T60.0X3	T60.0X4	—	—
Carboplatin	T45.1X1	T45.1X2	T45.1X3	T45.1X4	T45.1X5	T45.1X6
Carboprost	T48.0X1	T48.0X2	T48.0X3	T48.0X4	T48.0X5	T48.0X6
Carboquone	T45.1X1	T45.1X2	T45.1X3	T45.1X4	T45.1X5	T45.1X6
Carbowax	T49.3X1	T49.3X2	T49.3X3	T49.3X4	T49.3X5	T49.3X6
Carboxymethylcellulose	T47.4X1	T47.4X2	T47.4X3	T47.4X4	T47.4X5	T47.4X6
Carbrital	T42.3X1	T42.3X2	T42.3X3	T42.3X4	T42.3X5	T42.3X6
Carbromal	T42.6X1	T42.6X2	T42.6X3	T42.6X4	T42.6X5	T42.6X6
Carbutamide	T38.3X1	T38.3X2	T38.3X3	T38.3X4	T38.3X5	T38.3X6
Carbuterol	T48.6X1	T48.6X2	T48.6X3	T48.6X4	T48.6X5	T48.6X6
Cardiac						
depressants	T46.2X1	T46.2X2	T46.2X3	T46.2X4	T46.2X5	T46.2X6
rhythm regulator	T46.2X1	T46.2X2	T46.2X3	T46.2X4	T46.2X5	T46.2X6
specified NEC	T46.2X1	T46.2X2	T46.2X3	T46.2X4	T46.2X5	T46.2X6
Cardiografin	T50.8X1	T50.8X2	T50.8X3	T50.8X4	T50.8X5	T50.8X6
Cardiogreen	T50.8X1	T50.8X2	T50.8X3	T50.8X4	T50.8X5	T50.8X6
Cardiotonic (glycoside) **NEC**	T46.0X1	T46.0X2	T46.0X3	T46.0X4	T46.0X5	T46.0X6
Cardiovascular drug NEC	T46.901	T46.902	T46.903	T46.904	T46.905	T46.906
Cardrase	T50.2X1	T50.2X2	T50.2X3	T50.2X4	T50.2X5	T50.2X6
Carfecillin	T36.0X1	T36.0X2	T36.0X3	T36.0X4	T36.0X5	T36.0X6
Carfenazine	T43.3X1	T43.3X2	T43.3X3	T43.3X4	T43.3X5	T43.3X6
Carfusin	T49.0X1	T49.0X2	T49.0X3	T49.0X4	T49.0X5	T49.0X6
Carindacillin	T36.0X1	T36.0X2	T36.0X3	T36.0X4	T36.0X5	T36.0X6
Carisoprodol	T42.8X1	T42.8X2	T42.8X3	T42.8X4	T42.8X5	T42.8X6
Carmellose	T47.4X1	T47.4X2	T47.4X3	T47.4X4	T47.4X5	T47.4X6
Carminative	T47.5X1	T47.5X2	T47.5X3	T47.5X4	T47.5X5	T47.5X6
Carmofur	T45.1X1	T45.1X2	T45.1X3	T45.1X4	T45.1X5	T45.1X6
Carmustine	T45.1X1	T45.1X2	T45.1X3	T45.1X4	T45.1X5	T45.1X6
Carotene	T45.2X1	T45.2X2	T45.2X3	T45.2X4	T45.2X5	T45.2X6
Carphenazine	T43.3X1	T43.3X2	T43.3X3	T43.3X4	T43.3X5	T43.3X6
Carpipramine	T42.4X1	T42.4X2	T42.4X3	T42.4X4	T42.4X5	T42.4X6
Carprofen	T39.311	T39.312	T39.313	T39.314	T39.315	T39.316
Carpronium chloride	T44.3X1	T44.3X2	T44.3X3	T44.3X4	T44.3X5	T44.3X6
Carrageenan	T47.8X1	T47.8X2	T47.8X3	T47.8X4	T47.8X5	T47.8X6
Carteolol	T44.7X1	T44.7X2	T44.7X3	T44.7X4	T44.7X5	T44.7X6
Carter's Little Pills	T47.2X1	T47.2X2	T47.2X3	T47.2X4	T47.2X5	T47.2X6
Cascara (sagrada)	T47.2X1	T47.2X2	T47.2X3	T47.2X4	T47.2X5	T47.2X6
Cassava	T62.2X1	T62.2X2	T62.2X3	T62.2X4	—	—
Castellani's paint	T49.0X1	T49.0X2	T49.0X3	T49.0X4	T49.0X5	T49.0X6
Castor						
bean	T62.2X1	T62.2X2	T62.2X3	T62.2X4	—	—
oil	T47.2X1	T47.2X2	T47.2X3	T47.2X4	T47.2X5	T47.2X6
Catalase	T45.3X1	T45.3X2	T45.3X3	T45.3X4	T45.3X5	T45.3X6
Caterpillar (sting)	T63.431	T63.432	T63.433	T63.434	—	—
Catha (edulis) (tea)	T43.691	T43.692	T43.693	T43.694	—	—

Substance	Poisoning, Accidental (unintentional)	Poisoning, Intentional Self-harm	Poisoning, Assault	Poisoning, Undetermined	Adverse Effect	Under-dosing
Cathartic NEC	T47.4X1	T47.4X2	T47.4X3	T47.4X4	T47.4X5	T47.4X6
anthacene derivative	T47.2X1	T47.2X2	T47.2X3	T47.2X4	T47.2X5	T47.2X6
bulk	T47.4X1	T47.4X2	T47.4X3	T47.4X4	T47.4X5	T47.4X6
contact	T47.2X1	T47.2X2	T47.2X3	T47.2X4	T47.2X5	T47.2X6
emollient NEC	T47.4X1	T47.4X2	T47.4X3	T47.4X4	T47.4X5	T47.4X6
irritant NEC	T47.2X1	T47.2X2	T47.2X3	T47.2X4	T47.2X5	T47.2X6
mucilage	T47.4X1	T47.4X2	T47.4X3	T47.4X4	T47.4X5	T47.4X6
saline	T47.3X1	T47.3X2	T47.3X3	T47.3X4	T47.3X5	T47.3X6
vegetable	T47.2X1	T47.2X2	T47.2X3	T47.2X4	T47.2X5	T47.2X6
Cathine	T50.5X1	T50.5X2	T50.5X3	T50.5X4	T50.5X5	T50.5X6
Cathomycin	T36.8X1	T36.8X2	T36.8X3	T36.8X4	T36.8X5	T36.8X6
Cation exchange resin	T50.3X1	T50.3X2	T50.3X3	T50.3X4	T50.3X5	T50.3X6
Caustic(s) NEC	T54.91	T54.92	T54.93	T54.94	—	—
alkali	T54.3X1	T54.3X2	T54.3X3	T54.3X4	—	—
hydroxide	T54.3X1	T54.3X2	T54.3X3	T54.3X4	—	—
potash	T54.3X1	T54.3X2	T54.3X3	T54.3X4	—	—
soda	T54.3X1	T54.3X2	T54.3X3	T54.3X4	—	—
specified NEC	T54.91	T54.92	T54.93	T54.94	—	—
Ceepryn	T49.0X1	T49.0X2	T49.0X3	T49.0X4	T49.0X5	T49.0X6
ENT agent	T49.6X1	T49.6X2	T49.6X3	T49.6X4	T49.6X5	T49.6X6
lozenges	T49.6X1	T49.6X2	T49.6X3	T49.6X4	T49.6X5	T49.6X6
Cefacetrile	T36.1X1	T36.1X2	T36.1X3	T36.1X4	T36.1X5	T36.1X6
Cefaclor	T36.1X1	T36.1X2	T36.1X3	T36.1X4	T36.1X5	T36.1X6
Cefadroxil	T36.1X1	T36.1X2	T36.1X3	T36.1X4	T36.1X5	T36.1X6
Cefalexin	T36.1X1	T36.1X2	T36.1X3	T36.1X4	T36.1X5	T36.1X6
Cefaloglycin	T36.1X1	T36.1X2	T36.1X3	T36.1X4	T36.1X5	T36.1X6
Cefaloridine	T36.1X1	T36.1X2	T36.1X3	T36.1X4	T36.1X5	T36.1X6
Cefalosporins	T36.1X1	T36.1X2	T36.1X3	T36.1X4	T36.1X5	T36.1X6
Cefalotin	T36.1X1	T36.1X2	T36.1X3	T36.1X4	T36.1X5	T36.1X6
Cefamandole	T36.1X1	T36.1X2	T36.1X3	T36.1X4	T36.1X5	T36.1X6
Cefamycin antibiotic	T36.1X1	T36.1X2	T36.1X3	T36.1X4	T36.1X5	T36.1X6
Cefapirin	T36.1X1	T36.1X2	T36.1X3	T36.1X4	T36.1X5	T36.1X6
Cefatrizine	T36.1X1	T36.1X2	T36.1X3	T36.1X4	T36.1X5	T36.1X6
Cefazedone	T36.1X1	T36.1X2	T36.1X3	T36.1X4	T36.1X5	T36.1X6
Cefazolin	T36.1X1	T36.1X2	T36.1X3	T36.1X4	T36.1X5	T36.1X6
Cefbuperazone	T36.1X1	T36.1X2	T36.1X3	T36.1X4	T36.1X5	T36.1X6
Cefetamet	T36.1X1	T36.1X2	T36.1X3	T36.1X4	T36.1X5	T36.1X6
Cefixime	T36.1X1	T36.1X2	T36.1X3	T36.1X4	T36.1X5	T36.1X6
Cefmenoxime	T36.1X1	T36.1X2	T36.1X3	T36.1X4	T36.1X5	T36.1X6
Cefmetazole	T36.1X1	T36.1X2	T36.1X3	T36.1X4	T36.1X5	T36.1X6
Cefminox	T36.1X1	T36.1X2	T36.1X3	T36.1X4	T36.1X5	T36.1X6
Cefonicid	T36.1X1	T36.1X2	T36.1X3	T36.1X4	T36.1X5	T36.1X6
Cefoperazone	T36.1X1	T36.1X2	T36.1X3	T36.1X4	T36.1X5	T36.1X6
Ceforanide	T36.1X1	T36.1X2	T36.1X3	T36.1X4	T36.1X5	T36.1X6
Cefotaxime	T36.1X1	T36.1X2	T36.1X3	T36.1X4	T36.1X5	T36.1X6
Cefotetan	T36.1X1	T36.1X2	T36.1X3	T36.1X4	T36.1X5	T36.1X6
Cefotiam	T36.1X1	T36.1X2	T36.1X3	T36.1X4	T36.1X5	T36.1X6
Cefoxitin	T36.1X1	T36.1X2	T36.1X3	T36.1X4	T36.1X5	T36.1X6
Cefpimizole	T36.1X1	T36.1X2	T36.1X3	T36.1X4	T36.1X5	T36.1X6
Cefpiramide	T36.1X1	T36.1X2	T36.1X3	T36.1X4	T36.1X5	T36.1X6
Cefradine	T36.1X1	T36.1X2	T36.1X3	T36.1X4	T36.1X5	T36.1X6
Cefroxadine	T36.1X1	T36.1X2	T36.1X3	T36.1X4	T36.1X5	T36.1X6
Cefsulodin	T36.1X1	T36.1X2	T36.1X3	T36.1X4	T36.1X5	T36.1X6
Ceftazidime	T36.1X1	T36.1X2	T36.1X3	T36.1X4	T36.1X5	T36.1X6
Cefteram	T36.1X1	T36.1X2	T36.1X3	T36.1X4	T36.1X5	T36.1X6
Ceftezole	T36.1X1	T36.1X2	T36.1X3	T36.1X4	T36.1X5	T36.1X6
Ceftizoxime	T36.1X1	T36.1X2	T36.1X3	T36.1X4	T36.1X5	T36.1X6
Ceftriaxone	T36.1X1	T36.1X2	T36.1X3	T36.1X4	T36.1X5	T36.1X6
Cefuroxime	T36.1X1	T36.1X2	T36.1X3	T36.1X4	T36.1X5	T36.1X6
Cefuzonam	T36.1X1	T36.1X2	T36.1X3	T36.1X4	T36.1X5	T36.1X6
Celestone	T38.0X1	T38.0X2	T38.0X3	T38.0X4	T38.0X5	T38.0X
topical	T49.0X1	T49.0X2	T49.0X3	T49.0X4	T49.0X5	T49.0X
Celiprolol	T44.7X1	T44.7X2	T44.7X3	T44.7X4	T44.7X5	T44.7X
Cellosolve	T52.91	T52.92	T52.93	T52.94	—	—
Cell stimulants and proliferants	T49.8X1	T49.8X2	T49.8X3	T49.8X4	T49.8X5	T49.8X
Cellulose						
cathartic	T47.4X1	T47.4X2	T47.4X3	T47.4X4	T47.4X5	T47.4X
hydroxyethyl	T47.4X1	T47.4X2	T47.4X3	T47.4X4	T47.4X5	T47.4X
nitrates (topical)	T49.3X1	T49.3X2	T49.3X3	T49.3X4	T49.3X5	T49.3X
oxidized	T49.4X1	T49.4X2	T49.4X3	T49.4X4	T49.4X5	T49.4X
Centipede (bite)	T63.411	T63.412	T63.413	T63.414	—	—
Central nervous system						
depressants	T42.71	T42.72	T42.73	T42.74	T42.75	T42.7
anesthetic (general) NEC	T41.201	T41.202	T41.203	T41.204	T41.205	T41.20
gases NEC	T41.0X1	T41.0X2	T41.0X3	T41.0X4	T41.0X5	T41.0X
intravenous	T41.1X1	T41.1X2	T41.1X3	T41.1X4	T41.1X5	T41.1X
barbiturates	T42.3X1	T42.3X2	T42.3X3	T42.3X4	T42.3X5	T42.3X
benzodiazepines	T42.4X1	T42.4X2	T42.4X3	T42.4X4	T42.4X5	T42.4X
bromides	T42.6X1	T42.6X2	T42.6X3	T42.6X4	T42.6X5	T42.6X
cannabis sativa	T40.7X1	T40.7X2	T40.7X3	T40.7X4	T40.7X5	T40.7X
chloral hydrate	T42.6X1	T42.6X2	T42.6X3	T42.6X4	T42.6X5	T42.6X
ethanol	T51.0X1	T51.0X2	T51.0X3	T51.0X4	—	—

Substance	Poisoning, Accidental (unintentional)	Poisoning, Intentional Self-harm	Poisoning, Assault	Poisoning, Undetermined	Adverse Effect	Under-dosing
Central nervous system — *continued*						
depressants — *continued*						
hallucinogenics	T40.901	T40.902	T40.903	T40.904	T40.905	T40.906
hypnotics	T42.71	T42.72	T42.73	T42.74	T42.75	T42.76
specified NEC	T42.6X1	T42.6X2	T42.6X3	T42.6X4	T42.6X5	T42.6X6
muscle relaxants	T42.8X1	T42.8X2	T42.8X3	T42.8X4	T42.8X5	T42.8X6
paraldehyde	T42.6X1	T42.6X2	T42.6X3	T42.6X4	T42.6X5	T42.6X6
sedatives;	T42.71	T42.72	T42.73	T42.74	T42.75	T42.76
sedative-hypnotics						
mixed NEC	T42.6X1	T42.6X2	T42.6X3	T42.6X4	T42.6X5	T42.6X6
specified NEC	T42.6X1	T42.6X2	T42.6X3	T42.6X4	T42.6X5	T42.6X6
muscle-tone depressants	T42.8X1	T42.8X2	T42.8X3	T42.8X4	T42.8X5	T42.8X6
stimulants	T43.601	T43.602	T43.603	T43.604	T43.605	T43.606
amphetamines	T43.621	T43.622	T43.623	T43.624	T43.625	T43.626
analeptics	T50.7X1	T50.7X2	T50.7X3	T50.7X4	T50.7X5	T50.7X6
antidepressants	T43.201	T43.202	T43.203	T43.204	T43.205	T43.206
opiate antagonists	T50.7X1	T50.7X2	T50.7X3	T50.7X4	T50.7X5	T50.7X6
specified NEC	T43.691	T43.692	T43.693	T43.694	T43.695	T43.696
Cephalexin	T36.1X1	T36.1X2	T36.1X3	T36.1X4	T36.1X5	T36.1X6
Cephaloglycin	T36.1X1	T36.1X2	T36.1X3	T36.1X4	T36.1X5	T36.1X6
Cephaloridine	T36.1X1	T36.1X2	T36.1X3	T36.1X4	T36.1X5	T36.1X6
Cephalosporins	T36.1X1	T36.1X2	T36.1X3	T36.1X4	T36.1X5	T36.1X6
N (adicillin)	T36.0X1	T36.0X2	T36.0X3	T36.0X4	T36.0X5	T36.0X6
Cephalothin	T36.1X1	T36.1X2	T36.1X3	T36.1X4	T36.1X5	T36.1X6
Cephalotin	T36.1X1	T36.1X2	T36.1X3	T36.1X4	T36.1X5	T36.1X6
Cephradine	T36.1X1	T36.1X2	T36.1X3	T36.1X4	T36.1X5	T36.1X6
Cerbera (odallam)	T62.2X1	T62.2X2	T62.2X3	T62.2X4	—	—
Cerberin	T46.0X1	T46.0X2	T46.0X3	T46.0X4	T46.0X5	T46.0X6
Cerebral stimulants	T43.601	T43.602	T43.603	T43.604	T43.605	T43.606
psychotherapeutic	T43.601	T43.602	T43.603	T43.604	T43.605	T43.606
specified NEC	T43.691	T43.692	T43.693	T43.694	T43.695	T43.696
Cerium oxalate	T45.0X1	T45.0X2	T45.0X3	T45.0X4	T45.0X5	T45.0X6
Cerous oxalate	T45.0X1	T45.0X2	T45.0X3	T45.0X4	T45.0X5	T45.0X6
Ceruletide	T50.8X1	T50.8X2	T50.8X3	T50.8X4	T50.8X5	T50.8X6
Cetalkonium (chloride)	T49.0X1	T49.0X2	T49.0X3	T49.0X4	T49.0X5	T49.0X6
Cethexonium chloride	T49.0X1	T49.0X2	T49.0X3	T49.0X4	T49.0X5	T49.0X6
Cetiedil	T46.7X1	T46.7X2	T46.7X3	T46.7X4	T46.7X5	T46.7X6
Cetirizine	T45.0X1	T45.0X2	T45.0X3	T45.0X4	T45.0X5	T45.0X6
Cetomacrogol	T50.991	T50.992	T50.993	T50.994	T50.995	T50.996
Cetotiamine	T45.2X1	T45.2X2	T45.2X3	T45.2X4	T45.2X5	T45.2X6
Cetoxime	T45.0X1	T45.0X2	T45.0X3	T45.0X4	T45.0X5	T45.0X6
Cetraxate	T47.1X1	T47.1X2	T47.1X3	T47.1X4	T47.1X5	T47.1X6
Cetrimide	T49.0X1	T49.0X2	T49.0X3	T49.0X4	T49.0X5	T49.0X6
Cetrimonium (bromide)	T49.0X1	T49.0X2	T49.0X3	T49.0X4	T49.0X5	T49.0X6
Cetylpyridinium chloride	T49.0X1	T49.0X2	T49.0X3	T49.0X4	T49.0X5	T49.0X6
ENT agent	T49.6X1	T49.6X2	T49.6X3	T49.6X4	T49.6X5	T49.6X6
lozenges	T49.6X1	T49.6X2	T49.6X3	T49.6X4	T49.6X5	T49.6X6
Cevadilla — *see* Sabadilla						
Cevitamic acid	T45.2X1	T45.2X2	T45.2X3	T45.2X4	T45.2X5	T45.2X6
Chalk, precipitated	T47.1X1	T47.1X2	T47.1X3	T47.1X4	T47.1X5	T47.1X6
Chamomile	T49.0X1	T49.0X2	T49.0X3	T49.0X4	T49.0X5	T49.0X6
Ch'an su	T46.0X1	T46.0X2	T46.0X3	T46.0X4	T46.0X5	T46.0X6
Charcoal	T47.6X1	T47.6X2	T47.6X3	T47.6X4	T47.6X5	T47.6X6
activated — *see also* Charcoal, medicinal	T47.6X1	T47.6X2	T47.6X3	T47.6X4	T47.6X5	T47.6X6
fumes (Carbon monoxide)	T58.2X1	T58.2X2	T58.2X3	T58.2X4	—	—
industrial	T58.8X1	T58.8X2	T58.8X3	T58.8X4	—	—
medicinal (activated)	T47.6X1	T47.6X2	T47.6X3	T47.6X4	T47.6X5	T47.6X6
antidiarrheal	T47.6X1	T47.6X2	T47.6X3	T47.6X4	T47.6X5	T47.6X6
poison control	T47.8X1	T47.8X2	T47.8X3	T47.8X4	T47.8X5	T47.8X6
specified use other than for diarrhea	T47.8X1	T47.8X2	T47.8X3	T47.8X4	T47.8X5	T47.8X6
topical	T49.8X1	T49.8X2	T49.8X3	T49.8X4	T49.8X5	T49.8X6
Chaulmosulfone	T37.1X1	T37.1X2	T37.1X3	T37.1X4	T37.1X5	T37.1X6
Chelating agent NEC	T50.6X1	T50.6X2	T50.6X3	T50.6X4	T50.6X5	T50.6X6
Chelidonium majus	T62.2X1	T62.2X2	T62.2X3	T62.2X4	—	—
Chemical substance NEC	T65.91	T65.92	T65.93	T65.94	—	—
Chenodeoxycholic acid	T47.5X1	T47.5X2	T47.5X3	T47.5X4	T47.5X5	T47.5X6
Chenodiol	T47.5X1	T47.5X2	T47.5X3	T47.5X4	T47.5X5	T47.5X6
Chenopodium	T37.4X1	T37.4X2	T37.4X3	T37.4X4	T37.4X5	T37.4X6
Cherry laurel	T62.2X1	T62.2X2	T62.2X3	T62.2X4	—	—
Chinidin (e)	T46.2X1	T46.2X2	T46.2X3	T46.2X4	T46.2X5	T46.2X6
Chiniofon	T37.8X1	T37.8X2	T37.8X3	T37.8X4	T37.8X5	T37.8X6
Chlophedianol	T48.3X1	T48.3X2	T48.3X3	T48.3X4	T48.3X5	T48.3X6
Chloral	T42.6X1	T42.6X2	T42.6X3	T42.6X4	T42.6X5	T42.6X6
derivative	T42.6X1	T42.6X2	T42.6X3	T42.6X4	T42.6X5	T42.6X6
hydrate	T42.6X1	T42.6X2	T42.6X3	T42.6X4	T42.6X5	T42.6X6
Chloralamide	T42.6X1	T42.6X2	T42.6X3	T42.6X4	T42.6X5	T42.6X6
Chloralodol	T42.6X1	T42.6X2	T42.6X3	T42.6X4	T42.6X5	T42.6X6
Chloralose	T60.4X1	T60.4X2	T60.4X3	T60.4X4	—	—
Chlorambucil	T45.1X1	T45.1X2	T45.1X3	T45.1X4	T45.1X5	T45.1X6
Chloramine	T57.8X1	T57.8X2	T57.8X3	T57.8X4	—	—

Substance	Poisoning, Accidental (unintentional)	Poisoning, Intentional Self-harm	Poisoning, Assault	Poisoning, Undetermined	Adverse Effect	Under-dosing
Chloramine — *continued*						
T	T49.0X1	T49.0X2	T49.0X3	T49.0X4	T49.0X5	T49.0X6
topical	T49.0X1	T49.0X2	T49.0X3	T49.0X4	T49.0X5	T49.0X6
Chloramphenicol	T36.2X1	T36.2X2	T36.2X3	T36.2X4	T36.2X5	T36.2X6
ENT agent	T49.6X1	T49.6X2	T49.6X3	T49.6X4	T49.6X5	T49.6X6
ophthalmic preparation	T49.5X1	T49.5X2	T49.5X3	T49.5X4	T49.5X5	T49.5X6
topical NEC	T49.0X1	T49.0X2	T49.0X3	T49.0X4	T49.0X5	T49.0X6
Chlorate (potassium) (sodium) NEC	T60.3X1	T60.3X2	T60.3X3	T60.3X4	—	—
herbicide	T60.3X1	T60.3X2	T60.3X3	T60.3X4	—	—
Chlorazanil	T50.2X1	T50.2X2	T50.2X3	T50.2X4	T50.2X5	T50.2X6
Chlorbenzene, chlorbenzol	T53.7X1	T53.7X2	T53.7X3	T53.7X4	—	—
Chlorbenzoxamine	T44.3X1	T44.3X2	T44.3X3	T44.3X4	T44.3X5	T44.3X6
Chlorbutol	T42.6X1	T42.6X2	T42.6X3	T42.6X4	T42.6X5	T42.6X6
Chlorcyclizine	T45.0X1	T45.0X2	T45.0X3	T45.0X4	T45.0X5	T45.0X6
Chlordan (e) (dust)	T60.1X1	T60.1X2	T60.1X3	T60.1X4	—	—
Chlordantoin	T49.0X1	T49.0X2	T49.0X3	T49.0X4	T49.0X5	T49.0X6
Chlordiazepoxide	T42.4X1	T42.4X2	T42.4X3	T42.4X4	T42.4X5	T42.4X6
Chlordiethyl benzamide	T49.3X1	T49.3X2	T49.3X3	T49.3X4	T49.3X5	T49.3X6
Chloresium	T49.8X1	T49.8X2	T49.8X3	T49.8X4	T49.8X5	T49.8X6
Chlorethiazol	T42.6X1	T42.6X2	T42.6X3	T42.6X4	T42.6X5	T42.6X6
Chlorethyl — *see* Ethyl chloride						
Chloretone	T42.6X1	T42.6X2	T42.6X3	T42.6X4	T42.6X5	T42.6X6
Chlorex	T53.6X1	T53.6X2	T53.6X3	T53.6X4	—	—
insecticide	T60.1X1	T60.1X2	T60.1X3	T60.1X4	—	—
Chlorfenvinphos	T60.0X1	T60.0X2	T60.0X3	T60.0X4	—	—
Chlorhexadol	T42.6X1	T42.6X2	T42.6X3	T42.6X4	T42.6X5	T42.6X6
Chlorhexamide	T45.1X1	T45.1X2	T45.1X3	T45.1X4	T45.1X5	T45.1X6
Chlorhexidine	T49.0X1	T49.0X2	T49.0X3	T49.0X4	T49.0X5	T49.0X6
Chlorhydroxyquinolin	T49.0X1	T49.0X2	T49.0X3	T49.0X4	T49.0X5	T49.0X6
Chloride of lime (bleach)	T54.3X1	T54.3X2	T54.3X3	T54.3X4	—	—
Chlorimipramine	T43.011	T43.012	T43.013	T43.014	T43.015	T43.016
Chlorinated						
camphene	T53.6X1	T53.6X2	T53.6X3	T53.6X4	—	—
diphenyl	T53.7X1	T53.7X2	T53.7X3	T53.7X4	—	—
hydrocarbons NEC	T53.91	T53.92	T53.93	T53.94	—	—
solvents	T53.91	T53.92	T53.93	T53.94	—	—
lime (bleach)	T54.3X1	T54.3X2	T54.3X3	T54.3X4	—	—
and boric acid solution	T49.0X1	T49.0X2	T49.0X3	T49.0X4	T49.0X5	T49.0X6
naphthalene (insecticide)	T60.1X1	T60.1X2	T60.1X3	T60.1X4	—	—
industrial (non-pesticide)	T53.7X1	T53.7X2	T53.7X3	T53.7X4	—	—
pesticide NEC	T60.8X1	T60.8X2	T60.8X3	T60.8X4	—	—
soda — *see also* sodium hypochlorite						
solution	T49.0X1	T49.0X2	T49.0X3	T49.0X4	T49.0X5	T49.0X6
Chlorine (fumes) (gas)	T59.4X1	T59.4X2	T59.4X3	T59.4X4	—	—
bleach	T54.3X1	T54.3X2	T54.3X3	T54.3X4	—	—
compound gas NEC	T59.4X1	T59.4X2	T59.4X3	T59.4X4	—	—
disinfectant	T59.4X1	T59.4X2	T59.4X3	T59.4X4	—	—
releasing agents NEC	T59.4X1	T59.4X2	T59.4X3	T59.4X4	—	—
Chlorisondamine chloride	T46.991	T46.992	T46.993	T46.994	T46.995	T46.996
Chlormadinone	T38.5X1	T38.5X2	T38.5X3	T38.5X4	T38.5X5	T38.5X6
Chlormephos	T60.0X1	T60.0X2	T60.0X3	T60.0X4	—	—
Chlormerodrin	T50.2X1	T50.2X2	T50.2X3	T50.2X4	T50.2X5	T50.2X6
Chlormethiazole	T42.6X1	T42.6X2	T42.6X3	T42.6X4	T42.6X5	T42.6X6
Chlormethine	T45.1X1	T45.1X2	T45.1X3	T45.1X4	T45.1X5	T45.1X6
Chlormethylenecycline	T36.4X1	T36.4X2	T36.4X3	T36.4X4	T36.4X5	T36.4X6
Chlormezanone	T42.6X1	T42.6X2	T42.6X3	T42.6X4	T42.6X5	T42.6X6
Chloroacetic acid	T60.3X1	T60.3X2	T60.3X3	T60.3X4	—	—
Chloroacetone	T59.3X1	T59.3X2	T59.3X3	T59.3X4	—	—
Chloroacetophenone	T59.3X1	T59.3X2	T59.3X3	T59.3X4	—	—
Chloroaniline	T53.7X1	T53.7X2	T53.7X3	T53.7X4	—	—
Chlorobenzene, chlorbenzol	T53.7X1	T53.7X2	T53.7X3	T53.7X4	—	—
Chlorobromomethane (fire extinguisher)	T53.6X1	T53.6X2	T53.6X3	T53.6X4	—	—
Chlorobutanol	T49.0X1	T49.0X2	T49.0X3	T49.0X4	T49.0X5	T49.0X6
Chlorocresol	T49.0X1	T49.0X2	T49.0X3	T49.0X4	T49.0X5	T49.0X6
Chlorodehydromethyltestosterone	T38.7X1	T38.7X2	T38.7X3	T38.7X4	T38.7X5	T38.7X6
Chlorodinitrobenzene	T53.7X1	T53.7X2	T53.7X3	T53.7X4	—	—
dust or vapor	T53.7X1	T53.7X2	T53.7X3	T53.7X4	—	—
Chlorodiphenyl	T53.7X1	T53.7X2	T53.7X3	T53.7X4	—	—
Chloroethane — *see* Ethyl chloride						
Chloroethylene	T53.6X1	T53.6X2	T53.6X3	T53.6X4	—	—
Chlorofluorocarbons	T53.5X1	T53.5X2	T53.5X3	T53.5X4	—	—
Chloroform (fumes) (vapor)	T53.1X1	T53.1X2	T53.1X3	T53.1X4	—	—
anesthetic	T41.0X1	T41.0X2	T41.0X3	T41.0X4	T41.0X5	T41.0X6
solvent	T53.1X1	T53.1X2	T53.1X3	T53.1X4	—	—
water, concentrated	T41.0X1	T41.0X2	T41.0X3	T41.0X4	T41.0X5	T41.0X6
Chloroguanide	T37.2X1	T37.2X2	T37.2X3	T37.2X4	T37.2X5	T37.2X6

Substance	Poisoning, Accidental (unintentional)	Poisoning, Intentional Self-harm	Poisoning, Assault	Poisoning, Undetermined	Adverse Effect	Under-dosing
Chloromycetin	T36.2X1	T36.2X2	T36.2X3	T36.2X4	T36.2X5	T36.2X6
ENT agent	T49.6X1	T49.6X2	T49.6X3	T49.6X4	T49.6X5	T49.6X6
ophthalmic preparation	T49.5X1	T49.5X2	T49.5X3	T49.5X4	T49.5X5	T49.5X6
otic solution	T49.6X1	T49.6X2	T49.6X3	T49.6X4	T49.6X5	T49.6X6
topical NEC	T49.0X1	T49.0X2	T49.0X3	T49.0X4	T49.0X5	T49.0X6
Chloronitrobenzene	T53.7X1	T53.7X2	T53.7X3	T53.7X4	—	—
dust or vapor	T53.7X1	T53.7X2	T53.7X3	T53.7X4	—	—
Chlorophacinone	T60.4X1	T60.4X2	T60.4X3	T60.4X4	—	—
Chlorophenol	T53.7X1	T53.7X2	T53.7X3	T53.7X4	—	—
Chlorophenothane	T60.1X1	T60.1X2	T60.1X3	T60.1X4	—	—
Chlorophyll	T50.991	T50.992	T50.993	T50.994	T50.995	T50.996
Chloropicrin (fumes)	T53.6X1	T53.6X2	T53.6X3	T53.6X4	—	—
fumigant	T60.8X1	T60.8X2	T60.8X3	T60.8X4	—	—
fungicide	T60.3X1	T60.3X2	T60.3X3	T60.3X4	—	—
pesticide	T60.8X1	T60.8X2	T60.8X3	T60.8X4	—	—
Chloroprocaine	T41.3X1	T41.3X2	T41.3X3	T41.3X4	T41.3X5	T41.3X6
infiltration (subcutaneous)	T41.3X1	T41.3X2	T41.3X3	T41.3X4	T41.3X5	T41.3X6
nerve block (peripheral) (plexus)	T41.3X1	T41.3X2	T41.3X3	T41.3X4	T41.3X5	T41.3X6
spinal	T41.3X1	T41.3X2	T41.3X3	T41.3X4	T41.3X5	T41.3X6
Chloroptic	T49.5X1	T49.5X2	T49.5X3	T49.5X4	T49.5X5	T49.5X6
Chloropurine	T45.1X1	T45.1X2	T45.1X3	T45.1X4	T45.1X5	T45.1X6
Chloropyramine	T45.0X1	T45.0X2	T45.0X3	T45.0X4	T45.0X5	T45.0X6
Chloropyrifos	T60.0X1	T60.0X2	T60.0X3	T60.0X4	—	—
Chloropyrilene	T45.0X1	T45.0X2	T45.0X3	T45.0X4	T45.0X5	T45.0X6
Chloroquine	T37.2X1	T37.2X2	T37.2X3	T37.2X4	T37.2X5	T37.2X6
Chlorothalonil	T60.3X1	T60.3X2	T60.3X3	T60.3X4	—	—
Chlorothen	T45.0X1	T45.0X2	T45.0X3	T45.0X4	T45.0X5	T45.0X6
Chlorothiazide	T50.2X1	T50.2X2	T50.2X3	T50.2X4	T50.2X5	T50.2X6
Chlorothymol	T49.4X1	T49.4X2	T49.4X3	T49.4X4	T49.4X5	T49.4X6
Chlorotrianisene	T38.5X1	T38.5X2	T38.5X3	T38.5X4	T38.5X5	T38.5X6
Chlorovinyldichloroarsine, not in war	T57.0X1	T57.0X2	T57.0X3	T57.0X4	—	—
Chloroxine	T49.4X1	T49.4X2	T49.4X3	T49.4X4	T49.4X5	T49.4X6
Chloroxylenol	T49.0X1	T49.0X2	T49.0X3	T49.0X4	T49.0X5	T49.0X6
Chlorphenamine	T45.0X1	T45.0X2	T45.0X3	T45.0X4	T45.0X5	T45.0X6
Chlorphenesin	T42.8X1	T42.8X2	T42.8X3	T42.8X4	T42.8X5	T42.8X6
topical (antifungal)	T49.0X1	T49.0X2	T49.0X3	T49.0X4	T49.0X5	T49.0X6
Chlorpheniramine	T45.0X1	T45.0X2	T45.0X3	T45.0X4	T45.0X5	T45.0X6
Chlorphenoxamine	T45.0X1	T45.0X2	T45.0X3	T45.0X4	T45.0X5	T45.0X6
Chlorphentermine	T50.5X1	T50.5X2	T50.5X3	T50.5X4	T50.5X5	T50.5X6
Chlorprocaine — see Chloroprocaine						
Chlorproguanil	T37.2X1	T37.2X2	T37.2X3	T37.2X4	T37.2X5	T37.2X6
Chlorpromazine	T43.3X1	T43.3X2	T43.3X3	T43.3X4	T43.3X5	T43.3X6
Chlorpropamide	T38.3X1	T38.3X2	T38.3X3	T38.3X4	T38.3X5	T38.3X6
Chlorprothixene	T43.4X1	T43.4X2	T43.4X3	T43.4X4	T43.4X5	T43.4X6
Chlorquinaldol	T49.0X1	T49.0X2	T49.0X3	T49.0X4	T49.0X5	T49.0X6
Chlorquinol	T49.0X1	T49.0X2	T49.0X3	T49.0X4	T49.0X5	T49.0X6
Chlortalidone	T50.2X1	T50.2X2	T50.2X3	T50.2X4	T50.2X5	T50.2X6
Chlortetracycline	T36.4X1	T36.4X2	T36.4X3	T36.4X4	T36.4X5	T36.4X6
Chlorthalidone	T50.2X1	T50.2X2	T50.2X3	T50.2X4	T50.2X5	T50.2X6
Chlorthion	T60.0X1	T60.0X2	T60.0X3	T60.0X4	—	—
Chlorthiophos	T60.0X1	T60.0X2	T60.0X3	T60.0X4	—	—
Chlortrianisene	T38.5X1	T38.5X2	T38.5X3	T38.5X4	T38.5X5	T38.5X6
Chlor-Trimeton	T45.0X1	T45.0X2	T45.0X3	T45.0X4	T45.0X5	T45.0X6
Chlorzoxazone	T42.8X1	T42.8X2	T42.8X3	T42.8X4	T42.8X5	T42.8X6
Choke damp	T59.7X1	T59.7X2	T59.7X3	T59.7X4	—	—
Cholagogues	T47.5X1	T47.5X2	T47.5X3	T47.5X4	T47.5X5	T47.5X6
Cholebrine	T50.8X1	T50.8X2	T50.8X3	T50.8X4	T50.8X5	T50.8X6
Cholecalciferol	T45.2X1	T45.2X2	T45.2X3	T45.2X4	T45.2X5	T45.2X6
Cholecystokinin	T50.8X1	T50.8X2	T50.8X3	T50.8X4	T50.8X5	T50.8X6
Cholera vaccine	T50.A91	T50.A92	T50.A93	T50.A94	T50.A95	T50.A96
Choleretic	T47.5X1	T47.5X2	T47.5X3	T47.5X4	T47.5X5	T47.5X6
Cholesterol-lowering agents	T46.6X1	T46.6X2	T46.6X3	T46.6X4	T46.6X5	T46.6X6
Cholestyramine (resin)	T46.6X1	T46.6X2	T46.6X3	T46.6X4	T46.6X5	T46.6X6
Cholic acid	T47.5X1	T47.5X2	T47.5X3	T47.5X4	T47.5X5	T47.5X6
Choline	T48.6X1	T48.6X2	T48.6X3	T48.6X4	T48.6X5	T48.6X6
chloride	T50.991	T50.992	T50.993	T50.994	T50.995	T50.996
dihydrogen citrate	T50.991	T50.992	T50.993	T50.994	T50.995	T50.996
salicylate	T39.091	T39.092	T39.093	T39.094	T39.095	T39.096
theophyllinate	T48.6X1	T48.6X2	T48.6X3	T48.6X4	T48.6X5	T48.6X6
Cholinergic (drug) NEC	T44.1X1	T44.1X2	T44.1X3	T44.1X4	T44.1X5	T44.1X6
muscle tone enhancer	T44.1X1	T44.1X2	T44.1X3	T44.1X4	T44.1X5	T44.1X6
organophosphorus	T44.0X1	T44.0X2	T44.0X3	T44.0X4	T44.0X5	T44.0X6
insecticide	T60.0X1	T60.0X2	T60.0X3	T60.0X4	—	—
nerve gas	T59.891	T59.892	T59.893	T59.894	—	—
trimethyl ammonium propanediol	T44.1X1	T44.1X2	T44.1X3	T44.1X4	T44.1X5	T44.1X6
Cholinesterase reactivator	T50.6X1	T50.6X2	T50.6X3	T50.6X4	T50.6X5	T50.6X6
Cholografin	T50.8X1	T50.8X2	T50.8X3	T50.8X4	T50.8X5	T50.8X6
Chorionic gonadotropin	T38.891	T38.892	T38.893	T38.894	T38.895	T38.896
Chromate	T56.2X1	T56.2X2	T56.2X3	T56.2X4	—	—
dust or mist	T56.2X1	T56.2X2	T56.2X3	T56.2X4	—	—
lead — see also lead	T56.0X1	T56.0X2	T56.0X3	T56.0X4	—	—
paint	T56.0X1	T56.0X2	T56.0X3	T56.0X4	—	—
Chromic						
acid	T56.2X1	T56.2X2	T56.2X3	T56.2X4	—	—
dust or mist	T56.2X1	T56.2X2	T56.2X3	T56.2X4	—	—
phosphate 32P	T45.1X1	T45.1X2	T45.1X3	T45.1X4	T45.1X5	T45.1X6
Chromium	T56.2X1	T56.2X2	T56.2X3	T56.2X4	—	—
compounds — see Chromate						
sesquioxide	T50.8X1	T50.8X2	T50.8X3	T50.8X4	T50.8X5	T50.8X6
Chromomycin A3	T45.1X1	T45.1X2	T45.1X3	T45.1X4	T45.1X5	T45.1X6
Chromonar	T46.3X1	T46.3X2	T46.3X3	T46.3X4	T46.3X5	T46.3X6
Chromyl chloride	T56.2X1	T56.2X2	T56.2X3	T56.2X4	—	—
Chrysarobin	T49.4X1	T49.4X2	T49.4X3	T49.4X4	T49.4X5	T49.4X6
Chrysazin	T47.2X1	T47.2X2	T47.2X3	T47.2X4	T47.2X5	T47.2X6
Chymar	T45.3X1	T45.3X2	T45.3X3	T45.3X4	T45.3X5	T45.3X6
ophthalmic preparation	T49.5X1	T49.5X2	T49.5X3	T49.5X4	T49.5X5	T49.5X6
Chymopapain	T45.3X1	T45.3X2	T45.3X3	T45.3X4	T45.3X5	T45.3X6
Chymotrypsin	T45.3X1	T45.3X2	T45.3X3	T45.3X4	T45.3X5	T45.3X6
ophthalmic preparation	T49.5X1	T49.5X2	T49.5X3	T49.5X4	T49.5X5	T49.5X6
Cianidanol	T50.991	T50.992	T50.993	T50.994	T50.995	T50.996
Cianopramine	T43.011	T43.012	T43.013	T43.014	T43.015	T43.016
Cibenzoline	T46.2X1	T46.2X2	T46.2X3	T46.2X4	T46.2X5	T46.2X6
Ciclacillin	T36.0X1	T36.0X2	T36.0X3	T36.0X4	T36.0X5	T36.0X6
Ciclobarbital — see Hexobarbital						
Ciclonicate	T46.7X1	T46.7X2	T46.7X3	T46.7X4	T46.7X5	T46.7X6
Ciclopirox (olamine)	T49.0X1	T49.0X2	T49.0X3	T49.0X4	T49.0X5	T49.0X6
Ciclosporin	T45.1X1	T45.1X2	T45.1X3	T45.1X4	T45.1X5	T45.1X6
Cicuta maculata or virosa	T62.2X1	T62.2X2	T62.2X3	T62.2X4	—	—
Cicutoxin	T62.2X1	T62.2X2	T62.2X3	T62.2X4	—	—
Cigarette lighter fluid	T52.0X1	T52.0X2	T52.0X3	T52.0X4	—	—
Cigarettes (tobacco)	T65.221	T65.222	T65.223	T65.224	—	—
Ciguatoxin	T61.01	T61.02	T61.03	T61.04	—	—
Cilazapril	T46.4X1	T46.4X2	T46.4X3	T46.4X4	T46.4X5	T46.4X6
Cimetidine	T47.0X1	T47.0X2	T47.0X3	T47.0X4	T47.0X5	T47.0X6
Cimetropium bromide	T44.3X1	T44.3X2	T44.3X3	T44.3X4	T44.3X5	T44.3X6
Cinchocaine	T41.3X1	T41.3X2	T41.3X3	T41.3X4	T41.3X5	T41.3X6
topical (surface)	T41.3X1	T41.3X2	T41.3X3	T41.3X4	T41.3X5	T41.3X6
Cinchona	T37.2X1	T37.2X2	T37.2X3	T37.2X4	T37.2X5	T37.2X6
Cinchonine alkaloids	T37.2X1	T37.2X2	T37.2X3	T37.2X4	T37.2X5	T37.2X6
Cinchophen	T50.4X1	T50.4X2	T50.4X3	T50.4X4	T50.4X5	T50.4X6
Cinepazide	T46.7X1	T46.7X2	T46.7X3	T46.7X4	T46.7X5	T46.7X6
Cinnamedrine	T48.5X1	T48.5X2	T48.5X3	T48.5X4	T48.5X5	T48.5X6
Cinnarizine	T45.0X1	T45.0X2	T45.0X3	T45.0X4	T45.0X5	T45.0X6
Cinoxacin	T37.8X1	T37.8X2	T37.8X3	T37.8X4	T37.8X5	T37.8X6
Ciprofibrate	T46.6X1	T46.6X2	T46.6X3	T46.6X4	T46.6X5	T46.6X6
Ciprofloxacin	T36.8X1	T36.8X2	T36.8X3	T36.8X4	T36.8X5	T36.8X6
Cisapride	T47.8X1	T47.8X2	T47.8X3	T47.8X4	T47.8X5	T47.8X6
Cisplatin	T45.1X1	T45.1X2	T45.1X3	T45.1X4	T45.1X5	T45.1X6
Citalopram	T43.221	T43.222	T43.223	T43.224	T43.225	T43.226
Citanest	T41.3X1	T41.3X2	T41.3X3	T41.3X4	T41.3X5	T41.3X6
infiltration (subcutaneous)	T41.3X1	T41.3X2	T41.3X3	T41.3X4	T41.3X5	T41.3X6
nerve block (peripheral) (plexus)	T41.3X1	T41.3X2	T41.3X3	T41.3X4	T41.3X5	T41.3X6
Citric acid	T47.5X1	T47.5X2	T47.5X3	T47.5X4	T47.5X5	T47.5X6
Citrovorum (factor)	T45.8X1	T45.8X2	T45.8X3	T45.8X4	T45.8X5	T45.8X6
Claviceps purpurea	T62.2X1	T62.2X2	T62.2X3	T62.2X4	—	—
Clavulanic acid	T36.1X1	T36.1X2	T36.1X3	T36.1X4	T36.1X5	T36.1X6
Cleaner, cleansing agent, type not specified	T65.891	T65.892	T65.893	T65.894	—	—
of paint or varnish	T52.91	T52.92	T52.93	T52.94	—	—
specified type NEC	T65.891	T65.892	T65.893	T65.894	—	—
Clebopride	T47.8X1	T47.8X2	T47.8X3	T47.8X4	T47.8X5	T47.8X6
Clefamide	T37.3X1	T37.3X2	T37.3X3	T37.3X4	T37.3X5	T37.3X6
Clemastine	T45.0X1	T45.0X2	T45.0X3	T45.0X4	T45.0X5	T45.0X6
Clematis vitalba	T62.2X1	T62.2X2	T62.2X3	T62.2X4	—	—
Clemizole	T45.0X1	T45.0X2	T45.0X3	T45.0X4	T45.0X5	T45.0X6
penicillin	T36.0X1	T36.0X2	T36.0X3	T36.0X4	T36.0X5	T36.0X6
Clenbuterol	T48.6X1	T48.6X2	T48.6X3	T48.6X4	T48.6X5	T48.6X6
Clidinium bromide	T44.3X1	T44.3X2	T44.3X3	T44.3X4	T44.3X5	T44.3X6
Clindamycin	T36.8X1	T36.8X2	T36.8X3	T36.8X4	T36.8X5	T36.8X6
Clinofibrate	T46.6X1	T46.6X2	T46.6X3	T46.6X4	T46.6X5	T46.6X6
Clioquinol	T37.8X1	T37.8X2	T37.8X3	T37.8X4	T37.8X5	T37.8X6
Cliradon	T40.2X1	T40.2X2	T40.2X3	T40.2X4	—	—
Clobazam	T42.4X1	T42.4X2	T42.4X3	T42.4X4	T42.4X5	T42.4X6
Clobenzorex	T50.5X1	T50.5X2	T50.5X3	T50.5X4	T50.5X5	T50.5X6
Clobetasol	T49.0X1	T49.0X2	T49.0X3	T49.0X4	T49.0X5	T49.0X6
Clobetasone	T49.0X1	T49.0X2	T49.0X3	T49.0X4	T49.0X5	T49.0X6
Clobutinol	T48.3X1	T48.3X2	T48.3X3	T48.3X4	T48.3X5	T48.3X6
Clocortolone	T38.0X1	T38.0X2	T38.0X3	T38.0X4	T38.0X5	T38.0X6
Clodantoin	T49.0X1	T49.0X2	T49.0X3	T49.0X4	T49.0X5	T49.0X6

Substance	Poisoning, Accidental (unintentional)	Poisoning, Intentional Self-harm	Poisoning, Assault	Poisoning, Undetermined	Adverse Effect	Under-dosing
Clodronic acid	T50.991	T50.992	T50.993	T50.994	T50.995	T50.996
Clofazimine	T37.1X1	T37.1X2	T37.1X3	T37.1X4	T37.1X5	T37.1X6
Clofedanol	T48.3X1	T48.3X2	T48.3X3	T48.3X4	T48.3X5	T48.3X6
Clofenamide	T50.2X1	T50.2X2	T50.2X3	T50.2X4	T50.2X5	T50.2X6
Clofenotane	T49.0X1	T49.0X2	T49.0X3	T49.0X4	T49.0X5	T49.0X6
Clofezone	T39.2X1	T39.2X2	T39.2X3	T39.2X4	T39.2X5	T39.2X6
Clofibrate	T46.6X1	T46.6X2	T46.6X3	T46.6X4	T46.6X5	T46.6X6
Clofibride	T46.6X1	T46.6X2	T46.6X3	T46.6X4	T46.6X5	T46.6X6
Cloforex	T50.5X1	T50.5X2	T50.5X3	T50.5X4	T50.5X5	T50.5X6
Clomethiazole	T42.6X1	T42.6X2	T42.6X3	T42.6X4	T42.6X5	T42.6X6
Clometocillin	T36.0X1	T36.0X2	T36.0X3	T36.0X4	T36.0X5	T36.0X6
Clomifene	T38.5X1	T38.5X2	T38.5X3	T38.5X4	T38.5X5	T38.5X6
Clomiphene	T38.5X1	T38.5X2	T38.5X3	T38.5X4	T38.5X5	T38.5X6
Clomipramine	T43.011	T43.012	T43.013	T43.014	T43.015	T43.016
Clomocycline	T36.4X1	T36.4X2	T36.4X3	T36.4X4	T36.4X5	T36.4X6
Clonazepam	T42.4X1	T42.4X2	T42.4X3	T42.4X4	T42.4X5	T42.4X6
Clonidine	T46.5X1	T46.5X2	T46.5X3	T46.5X4	T46.5X5	T46.5X6
Clonixin	T39.8X1	T39.8X2	T39.8X3	T39.8X4	T39.8X5	T39.8X6
Clopamide	T50.2X1	T50.2X2	T50.2X3	T50.2X4	T50.2X5	T50.2X6
Clopenthixol	T43.4X1	T43.4X2	T43.4X3	T43.4X4	T43.4X5	T43.4X6
Cloperastine	T48.3X1	T48.3X2	T48.3X3	T48.3X4	T48.3X5	T48.3X6
Clophedianol	T48.3X1	T48.3X2	T48.3X3	T48.3X4	T48.3X5	T48.3X6
Cloponone	T36.2X1	T36.2X2	T36.2X3	T36.2X4	T36.2X5	T36.2X6
Cloprednol	T38.0X1	T38.0X2	T38.0X3	T38.0X4	T38.0X5	T38.0X6
Cloral betaine	T42.6X1	T42.6X2	T42.6X3	T42.6X4	T42.6X5	T42.6X6
Cloramfenicol	T36.2X1	T36.2X2	T36.2X3	T36.2X4	T36.2X5	T36.2X6
Clorazepate (dipotassium)	T42.4X1	T42.4X2	T42.4X3	T42.4X4	T42.4X5	T42.4X6
Clorexolone	T50.2X1	T50.2X2	T50.2X3	T50.2X4	T50.2X5	T50.2X6
Clorfenamine	T45.0X1	T45.0X2	T45.0X3	T45.0X4	T45.0X5	T45.0X6
Clorgiline	T43.1X1	T43.1X2	T43.1X3	T43.1X4	T43.1X5	T43.1X6
Clorotepine	T44.3X1	T44.3X2	T44.3X3	T44.3X4	T44.3X5	T44.3X6
Clorox (bleach)	T54.91	T54.92	T54.93	T54.94	—	—
Clorprenaline	T48.6X1	T48.6X2	T48.6X3	T48.6X4	T48.6X5	T48.6X6
Clortermine	T50.5X1	T50.5X2	T50.5X3	T50.5X4	T50.5X5	T50.5X6
Clotiapine	T43.591	T43.592	T43.593	T43.594	T43.595	T43.596
Clotiazepam	T42.4X1	T42.4X2	T42.4X3	T42.4X4	T42.4X5	T42.4X6
Clotibric acid	T46.6X1	T46.6X2	T46.6X3	T46.6X4	T46.6X5	T46.6X6
Clotrimazole	T49.0X1	T49.0X2	T49.0X3	T49.0X4	T49.0X5	T49.0X6
Cloxacillin	T36.0X1	T36.0X2	T36.0X3	T36.0X4	T36.0X5	T36.0X6
Cloxazolam	T42.4X1	T42.4X2	T42.4X3	T42.4X4	T42.4X5	T42.4X6
Cloxiquine	T49.0X1	T49.0X2	T49.0X3	T49.0X4	T49.0X5	T49.0X6
Clozapine	T42.4X1	T42.4X2	T42.4X3	T42.4X4	T42.4X5	T42.4X6
Coagulant NEC	T45.7X1	T45.7X2	T45.7X3	T45.7X4	T45.7X5	T45.7X6
Coal (carbon monoxide from) — see also Carbon, monoxide, coal	T58.2X1	T58.2X2	T58.2X3	T58.2X4		
oil — see Kerosene						
tar	T49.1X1	T49.1X2	T49.1X3	T49.1X4	T49.1X5	T49.1X6
fumes	T59.891	T59.892	T59.893	T59.894		
medicinal (ointment)	T49.4X1	T49.4X2	T49.4X3	T49.4X4	T49.4X5	T49.4X6
analgesics NEC	T39.2X1	T39.2X2	T39.2X3	T39.2X4	T39.2X5	T39.2X6
naphtha (solvent)	T52.0X1	T52.0X2	T52.0X3	T52.0X4		
Cobalamine	T45.2X1	T45.2X2	T45.2X3	T45.2X4	T45.2X5	T45.2X6
Cobalt (nonmedicinal) (fumes) (industrial)	T56.891	T56.892	T56.893	T56.894	—	—
medicinal (trace) (chloride)	T45.8X1	T45.8X2	T45.8X3	T45.8X4	T45.8X5	T45.8X6
Cobra (venom)	T63.041	T63.042	T63.043	T63.044	—	—
Coca (leaf)	T40.5X1	T40.5X2	T40.5X3	T40.5X4	T40.5X5	T40.5X6
Cocaine	T40.5X1	T40.5X2	T40.5X3	T40.5X4	T40.5X5	T40.5X6
topical anesthetic	T41.3X1	T41.3X2	T41.3X3	T41.3X4	T41.3X5	T41.3X6
Cocarboxylase	T45.3X1	T45.3X2	T45.3X3	T45.3X4	T45.3X5	T45.3X6
Coccidioidin	T50.8X1	T50.8X2	T50.8X3	T50.8X4	T50.8X5	T50.8X6
Cocculus indicus	T62.1X1	T62.1X2	T62.1X3	T62.1X4	—	—
Cochineal	T65.6X1	T65.6X2	T65.6X3	T65.6X4	—	—
medicinal products	T50.991	T50.992	T50.993	T50.994	T50.995	T50.996
Codeine	T40.2X1	T40.2X2	T40.2X3	T40.2X4	T40.2X5	T40.2X6
Cod-liver oil	T45.2X1	T45.2X2	T45.2X3	T45.2X4	T45.2X5	T45.2X6
Coenzyme A	T50.991	T50.992	T50.993	T50.994	T50.995	T50.996
Coffee	T62.8X1	T62.8X2	T62.8X3	T62.8X4	—	—
Cogalactoisomerase	T50.991	T50.992	T50.993	T50.994	T50.995	T50.996
Cogentin	T44.3X1	T44.3X2	T44.3X3	T44.3X4	T44.3X5	T44.3X6
Coke fumes or gas (carbon monoxide)	T58.2X1	T58.2X2	T58.2X3	T58.2X4		
industrial use	T58.8X1	T58.8X2	T58.8X3	T58.8X4		
Colace	T47.4X1	T47.4X2	T47.4X3	T47.4X4	T47.4X5	T47.4X6
Colaspase	T45.1X1	T45.1X2	T45.1X3	T45.1X4	T45.1X5	T45.1X6
Colchicine	T50.4X1	T50.4X2	T50.4X3	T50.4X4	T50.4X5	T50.4X6
Colchicum	T62.2X1	T62.2X2	T62.2X3	T62.2X4	—	—
Cold cream	T49.3X1	T49.3X2	T49.3X3	T49.3X4	T49.3X5	T49.3X6
Colecalciferol	T45.2X1	T45.2X2	T45.2X3	T45.2X4	T45.2X5	T45.2X6
Colestipol	T46.6X1	T46.6X2	T46.6X3	T46.6X4	T46.6X5	T46.6X6
Colestyramine	T46.6X1	T46.6X2	T46.6X3	T46.6X4	T46.6X5	T46.6X6
Colimycin	T36.8X1	T36.8X2	T36.8X3	T36.8X4	T36.8X5	T36.8X6

Substance	Poisoning, Accidental (unintentional)	Poisoning, Intentional Self-harm	Poisoning, Assault	Poisoning, Undetermined	Adverse Effect	Under-dosing
Colistimethate	T36.8X1	T36.8X2	T36.8X3	T36.8X4	T36.8X5	T36.8X6
Colistin	T36.8X1	T36.8X2	T36.8X3	T36.8X4	T36.8X5	T36.8X6
sulfate (eye preparation)	T49.5X1	T49.5X2	T49.5X3	T49.5X4	T49.5X5	T49.5X6
Collagen	T50.991	T50.992	T50.993	T50.994	T50.995	T50.996
Collagenase	T49.4X1	T49.4X2	T49.4X3	T49.4X4	T49.4X5	T49.4X6
Collodion	T49.3X1	T49.3X2	T49.3X3	T49.3X4	T49.3X5	T49.3X6
Colocynth	T47.2X1	T47.2X2	T47.2X3	T47.2X4	T47.2X5	T47.2X6
Colophony adhesive	T49.3X1	T49.3X2	T49.3X3	T49.3X4	T49.3X5	T49.3X6
Colorant — see also Dye	T50.991	T50.992	T50.993	T50.994	T50.995	T50.996
Coloring matter — see Dye(s)						
Combustion gas (after combustion) — see Carbon, monoxide						
prior to combustion	T59.891	T59.892	T59.893	T59.894	—	—
Compazine	T43.3X1	T43.3X2	T43.3X3	T43.3X4	T43.3X5	T43.3X6
Compound						
1080 (sodium fluoroacetate)	T60.4X1	T60.4X2	T60.4X3	T60.4X4		
269 (endrin)	T60.1X1	T60.1X2	T60.1X3	T60.1X4		
3422 (parathion)	T60.0X1	T60.0X2	T60.0X3	T60.0X4		
3911 (phorate)	T60.0X1	T60.0X2	T60.0X3	T60.0X4		
3956 (toxaphene)	T60.1X1	T60.1X2	T60.1X3	T60.1X4		
4049 (malathion)	T60.0X1	T60.0X2	T60.0X3	T60.0X4		
4069 (malathion)	T60.0X1	T60.0X2	T60.0X3	T60.0X4		
4124 (dicapthon)	T60.0X1	T60.0X2	T60.0X3	T60.0X4		
42 (warfarin)	T60.4X1	T60.4X2	T60.4X3	T60.4X4		
497 (dieldrin)	T60.1X1	T60.1X2	T60.1X3	T60.1X4		
E (cortisone)	T38.0X1	T38.0X2	T38.0X3	T38.0X4	T38.0X5	T38.0X6
F (hydrocortisone)	T38.0X1	T38.0X2	T38.0X3	T38.0X4	T38.0X5	T38.0X6
Congener, anabolic	T38.7X1	T38.7X2	T38.7X3	T38.7X4	T38.7X5	T38.7X6
Congo red	T50.8X1	T50.8X2	T50.8X3	T50.8X4	T50.8X5	T50.8X6
Coniine, conine	T62.2X1	T62.2X2	T62.2X3	T62.2X4	—	—
Conium (maculatum)	T62.2X1	T62.2X2	T62.2X3	T62.2X4	—	—
Conjugated estrogenic substances	T38.5X1	T38.5X2	T38.5X3	T38.5X4	T38.5X5	T38.5X6
Contac	T48.5X1	T48.5X2	T48.5X3	T48.5X4	T48.5X5	T48.5X6
Contact lens solution	T49.5X1	T49.5X2	T49.5X3	T49.5X4	T49.5X5	T49.5X6
Contraceptive (oral)	T38.4X1	T38.4X2	T38.4X3	T38.4X4	T38.4X5	T38.4X6
vaginal	T49.8X1	T49.8X2	T49.8X3	T49.8X4	T49.8X5	T49.8X6
Contrast medium, radiography	T50.8X1	T50.8X2	T50.8X3	T50.8X4	T50.8X5	T50.8X6
Convallaria glycosides	T46.0X1	T46.0X2	T46.0X3	T46.0X4	T46.0X5	T46.0X6
Convallaria majalis	T62.2X1	T62.2X2	T62.2X3	T62.2X4	—	—
berry	T62.1X1	T62.1X2	T62.1X3	T62.1X4	—	—
Copperhead snake (bite) (venom)	T63.061	T63.062	T63.063	T63.064	—	—
Copper (dust) (fumes) (nonmedicinal) NEC	T56.4X1	T56.4X2	T56.4X3	T56.4X4	—	—
arsenate, arsenite	T57.0X1	T57.0X2	T57.0X3	T57.0X4		
insecticide	T60.2X1	T60.2X2	T60.2X3	T60.2X4		
emetic	T47.7X1	T47.7X2	T47.7X3	T47.7X4	T47.7X5	T47.7X6
fungicide	T60.3X1	T60.3X2	T60.3X3	T60.3X4	—	—
gluconate	T49.0X1	T49.0X2	T49.0X3	T49.0X4	T49.0X5	T49.0X6
insecticide	T60.2X1	T60.2X2	T60.2X3	T60.2X4	—	—
medicinal (trace)	T45.8X1	T45.8X2	T45.8X3	T45.8X4	T45.8X5	T45.8X6
oleate	T49.0X1	T49.0X2	T49.0X3	T49.0X4	T49.0X5	T49.0X6
sulfate	T56.4X1	T56.4X2	T56.4X3	T56.4X4	—	—
cupric	T56.4X1	T56.4X2	T56.4X3	T56.4X4	—	—
fungicide	T60.3X1	T60.3X2	T60.3X3	T60.3X4	—	—
medicinal						
ear	T49.6X1	T49.6X2	T49.6X3	T49.6X4	T49.6X5	T49.6X6
emetic	T47.7X1	T47.7X2	T47.7X3	T47.7X4	T47.7X5	T47.7X6
eye	T49.5X1	T49.5X2	T49.5X3	T49.5X4	T49.5X5	T49.5X6
cuprous	T56.4X1	T56.4X2	T56.4X3	T56.4X4	—	—
fungicide	T60.3X1	T60.3X2	T60.3X3	T60.3X4	—	—
medicinal						
ear	T49.6X1	T49.6X2	T49.6X3	T49.6X4	T49.6X5	T49.6X6
emetic	T47.7X1	T47.7X2	T47.7X3	T47.7X4	T47.7X5	T47.7X6
eye	T49.5X1	T49.5X2	T49.5X3	T49.5X4	T49.5X5	T49.5X6
Coral (sting)	T63.691	T63.692	T63.693	T63.694	—	—
snake (bite) (venom)	T63.021	T63.022	T63.023	T63.024	—	—
Corbadrine	T49.6X1	T49.6X2	T49.6X3	T49.6X4	T49.6X5	T49.6X6
Cordite	T65.891	T65.892	T65.893	T65.894	—	—
vapor	T59.891	T59.892	T59.893	T59.894	—	—
Cordran	T49.0X1	T49.0X2	T49.0X3	T49.0X4	T49.0X5	T49.0X6
Corn cures	T49.4X1	T49.4X2	T49.4X3	T49.4X4	T49.4X5	T49.4X6
Cornhusker's lotion	T49.3X1	T49.3X2	T49.3X3	T49.3X4	T49.3X5	T49.3X6
Corn starch	T49.3X1	T49.3X2	T49.3X3	T49.3X4	T49.3X5	T49.3X6
Coronary vasodilator NEC	T46.3X1	T46.3X2	T46.3X3	T46.3X4	T46.3X5	T46.3X6
Corrosive NEC	T54.91	T54.92	T54.93	T54.94	—	—
acid NEC	T54.2X1	T54.2X2	T54.2X3	T54.2X4	—	—
aromatics	T54.1X1	T54.1X2	T54.1X3	T54.1X4	—	—
disinfectant	T54.1X1	T54.1X2	T54.1X3	T54.1X4	—	—

Substance	Poisoning, Accidental (unintentional)	Poisoning, Intentional Self-harm	Poisoning, Assault	Poisoning, Undetermined	Adverse Effect	Under-dosing
Corrosive — continued						
fumes NEC	T54.91	T54.92	T54.93	T54.94	—	—
specified NEC	T54.91	T54.92	T54.93	T54.94	—	—
sublimate	T56.1X1	T56.1X2	T56.1X3	T56.1X4	—	—
Cortate	T38.0X1	T38.0X2	T38.0X3	T38.0X4	T38.0X5	T38.0X6
Cort-Dome	T38.0X1	T38.0X2	T38.0X3	T38.0X4	T38.0X5	T38.0X6
ENT agent	T49.6X1	T49.6X2	T49.6X3	T49.6X4	T49.6X5	T49.6X6
ophthalmic preparation	T49.5X1	T49.5X2	T49.5X3	T49.5X4	T49.5X5	T49.5X6
topical NEC	T49.0X1	T49.0X2	T49.0X3	T49.0X4	T49.0X5	T49.0X6
Cortef	T38.0X1	T38.0X2	T38.0X3	T38.0X4	T38.0X5	T38.0X6
ENT agent	T49.6X1	T49.6X2	T49.6X3	T49.6X4	T49.6X5	T49.6X6
ophthalmic preparation	T49.5X1	T49.5X2	T49.5X3	T49.5X4	T49.5X5	T49.5X6
topical NEC	T49.0X1	T49.0X2	T49.0X3	T49.0X4	T49.0X5	T49.0X6
Corticosteroid	T38.0X1	T38.0X2	T38.0X3	T38.0X4	T38.0X5	T38.0X6
ENT agent	T49.6X1	T49.6X2	T49.6X3	T49.6X4	T49.6X5	T49.6X6
mineral	T50.0X1	T50.0X2	T50.0X3	T50.0X4	T50.0X5	T50.0X6
ophthalmic	T49.5X1	T49.5X2	T49.5X3	T49.5X4	T49.5X5	T49.5X6
topical NEC	T49.0X1	T49.0X2	T49.0X3	T49.0X4	T49.0X5	T49.0X6
Corticotropin	T38.811	T38.812	T38.813	T38.814	T38.815	T38.816
Cortisol	T49.0X1	T49.0X2	T49.0X3	T49.0X4	T49.0X5	T49.0X6
ENT agent	T49.6X1	T49.6X2	T49.6X3	T49.6X4	T49.6X5	T49.6X6
ophthalmic preparation	T49.5X1	T49.5X2	T49.5X3	T49.5X4	T49.5X5	T49.5X6
topical NEC	T49.0X1	T49.0X2	T49.0X3	T49.0X4	T49.0X5	T49.0X6
Cortisone (acetate)	T38.0X1	T38.0X2	T38.0X3	T38.0X4	T38.0X5	T38.0X6
ENT agent	T49.6X1	T49.6X2	T49.6X3	T49.6X4	T49.6X5	T49.6X6
ophthalmic preparation	T49.5X1	T49.5X2	T49.5X3	T49.5X4	T49.5X5	T49.5X6
topical NEC	T49.0X1	T49.0X2	T49.0X3	T49.0X4	T49.0X5	T49.0X6
Cortivazol	T38.0X1	T38.0X2	T38.0X3	T38.0X4	T38.0X5	T38.0X6
Cortogen	T38.0X1	T38.0X2	T38.0X3	T38.0X4	T38.0X5	T38.0X6
ENT agent	T49.6X1	T49.6X2	T49.6X3	T49.6X4	T49.6X5	T49.6X6
ophthalmic preparation	T49.5X1	T49.5X2	T49.5X3	T49.5X4	T49.5X5	T49.5X6
Cortone	T38.0X1	T38.0X2	T38.0X3	T38.0X4	T38.0X5	T38.0X6
ENT agent	T49.6X1	T49.6X2	T49.6X3	T49.6X4	T49.6X5	T49.6X6
ophthalmic preparation	T49.5X1	T49.5X2	T49.5X3	T49.5X4	T49.5X5	T49.5X6
Cortril	T38.0X1	T38.0X2	T38.0X3	T38.0X4	T38.0X5	T38.0X6
ENT agent	T49.6X1	T49.6X2	T49.6X3	T49.6X4	T49.6X5	T49.6X6
ophthalmic preparation	T49.5X1	T49.5X2	T49.5X3	T49.5X4	T49.5X5	T49.5X6
topical NEC	T49.0X1	T49.0X2	T49.0X3	T49.0X4	T49.0X5	T49.0X6
Corynebacterium parvum	T45.1X1	T45.1X2	T45.1X3	T45.1X4	T45.1X5	T45.1X6
Cosmetic preparation	T49.8X1	T49.8X2	T49.8X3	T49.8X4	T49.8X5	T49.8X6
Cosmetics	T49.8X1	T49.8X2	T49.8X3	T49.8X4	T49.8X5	T49.8X6
Cosyntropin	T38.811	T38.812	T38.813	T38.814	T38.815	T38.816
Cotarnine	T45.7X1	T45.7X2	T45.7X3	T45.7X4	T45.7X5	T45.7X6
Co-trimoxazole	T36.8X1	T36.8X2	T36.8X3	T36.8X4	T36.8X5	T36.8X6
Cottonseed oil	T49.3X1	T49.3X2	T49.3X3	T49.3X4	T49.3X5	T49.3X6
Cough mixture (syrup)	T48.4X1	T48.4X2	T48.4X3	T48.4X4	T48.4X5	T48.4X6
containing opiates	T40.2X1	T40.2X2	T40.2X3	T40.2X4	T40.2X5	T40.2X6
expectorants	T48.4X1	T48.4X2	T48.4X3	T48.4X4	T48.4X5	T48.4X6
Coumadin	T45.511	T45.512	T45.513	T45.514	T45.515	T45.516
rodenticide	T60.4X1	T60.4X2	T60.4X3	T60.4X4	—	—
Coumaphos	T60.0X1	T60.0X2	T60.0X3	T60.0X4	—	—
Coumarin	T45.511	T45.512	T45.513	T45.514	T45.515	T45.516
Coumetarol	T45.511	T45.512	T45.513	T45.514	T45.515	T45.516
Cowbane	T62.2X1	T62.2X2	T62.2X3	T62.2X4	—	—
Cozyme	T45.2X1	T45.2X2	T45.2X3	T45.2X4	T45.2X5	T45.2X6
Crack	T40.5X1	T40.5X2	T40.5X3	T40.5X4	—	—
Crataegus extract	T46.0X1	T46.0X2	T46.0X3	T46.0X4	T46.0X5	T46.0X6
Creolin	T54.1X1	T54.1X2	T54.1X3	T54.1X4	—	—
disinfectant	T54.1X1	T54.1X2	T54.1X3	T54.1X4	—	—
Creosol (compound)	T49.0X1	T49.0X2	T49.0X3	T49.0X4	T49.0X5	T49.0X6
Creosote (coal tar)	T49.0X1	T49.0X2	T49.0X3	T49.0X4	T49.0X5	T49.0X6
(beechwood)						
medicinal (expectorant)	T48.4X1	T48.4X2	T48.4X3	T48.4X4	T48.4X5	T48.4X6
syrup	T48.4X1	T48.4X2	T48.4X3	T48.4X4	T48.4X5	T48.4X6
Cresol(s)	T49.0X1	T49.0X2	T49.0X3	T49.0X4	T49.0X5	T49.0X6
and soap solution	T49.0X1	T49.0X2	T49.0X3	T49.0X4	T49.0X5	T49.0X6
Cresyl acetate	T49.0X1	T49.0X2	T49.0X3	T49.0X4	T49.0X5	T49.0X6
Cresylic acid	T49.0X1	T49.0X2	T49.0X3	T49.0X4	T49.0X5	T49.0X6
Crimidine	T60.4X1	T60.4X2	T60.4X3	T60.4X4	—	—
Croconazole	T37.8X1	T37.8X2	T37.8X3	T37.8X4	T37.8X5	T37.8X6
Cromoglicic acid	T48.6X1	T48.6X2	T48.6X3	T48.6X4	T48.6X5	T48.6X6
Cromolyn	T48.6X1	T48.6X2	T48.6X3	T48.6X4	T48.6X5	T48.6X6
Cromonar	T46.3X1	T46.3X2	T46.3X3	T46.3X4	T46.3X5	T46.3X6
Cropropamide	T39.8X1	T39.8X2	T39.8X3	T39.8X4	T39.8X5	T39.8X6
with crotethamide	T50.7X1	T50.7X2	T50.7X3	T50.7X4	T50.7X5	T50.7X6
Crotamiton	T49.0X1	T49.0X2	T49.0X3	T49.0X4	T49.0X5	T49.0X6
Crotethamide	T39.8X1	T39.8X2	T39.8X3	T39.8X4	T39.8X5	T39.8X6
with cropropamide	T50.7X1	T50.7X2	T50.7X3	T50.7X4	T50.7X5	T50.7X6
Croton (oil)	T47.2X1	T47.2X2	T47.2X3	T47.2X4	T47.2X5	T47.2X6
chloral	T42.6X1	T42.6X2	T42.6X3	T42.6X4	T42.6X5	T42.6X6
Crude oil	T52.0X1	T52.0X2	T52.0X3	T52.0X4	—	—
Cryogenine	T39.8X1	T39.8X2	T39.8X3	T39.8X4	T39.8X5	T39.8X6
Cryolite (vapor)	T60.1X1	T60.1X2	T60.1X3	T60.1X4	—	—

Substance	Poisoning, Accidental (unintentional)	Poisoning, Intentional Self-harm	Poisoning, Assault	Poisoning, Undetermined	Adverse Effect	Under-dosing
Cryolite — continued						
insecticide	T60.1X1	T60.1X2	T60.1X3	T60.1X4	—	—
Cryptenamine (tannates)	T46.5X1	T46.5X2	T46.5X3	T46.5X4	T46.5X5	T46.5X6
Crystal violet	T49.0X1	T49.0X2	T49.0X3	T49.0X4	T49.0X5	T49.0X6
Cuckoopint	T62.2X1	T62.2X2	T62.2X3	T62.2X4	—	—
Cumetharol	T45.511	T45.512	T45.513	T45.514	T45.515	T45.516
Cupric						
acetate	T60.3X1	T60.3X2	T60.3X3	T60.3X4	—	—
acetoarsenite	T57.0X1	T57.0X2	T57.0X3	T57.0X4	—	—
arsenate	T57.0X1	T57.0X2	T57.0X3	T57.0X4	—	—
gluconate	T49.0X1	T49.0X2	T49.0X3	T49.0X4	T49.0X5	T49.0X6
oleate	T49.0X1	T49.0X2	T49.0X3	T49.0X4	T49.0X5	T49.0X6
sulfate	T56.4X1	T56.4X2	T56.4X3	T56.4X4	—	—
Cuprous sulfate — see also	T56.4X1	T56.4X2	T56.4X3	T56.4X4	—	—
Copper sulfate						
Curare, curarine	T48.1X1	T48.1X2	T48.1X3	T48.1X4	T48.1X5	T48.1X6
Cyamemazine	T43.3X1	T43.3X2	T43.3X3	T43.3X4	T43.3X5	T43.3X6
Cyamopsis tetragonoloba	T46.6X1	T46.6X2	T46.6X3	T46.6X4	T46.6X5	T46.6X6
Cyanacetyl hydrazide	T37.1X1	T37.1X2	T37.1X3	T37.1X4	T37.1X5	T37.1X6
Cyanic acid (gas)	T59.891	T59.892	T59.893	T59.894	—	—
Cyanide(s) (compounds) (potassium) (sodium) NEC	T65.0X1	T65.0X2	T65.0X3	T65.0X4	—	—
dust or gas (inhalation) NEC	T57.3X1	T57.3X2	T57.3X3	T57.3X4	—	—
fumigant	T65.0X1	T65.0X2	T65.0X3	T65.0X4	—	—
hydrogen	T57.3X1	T57.3X2	T57.3X3	T57.3X4	—	—
mercuric — see Mercury						
pesticide (dust) (fumes)	T65.0X1	T65.0X2	T65.0X3	T65.0X4	—	—
Cyanoacrylate adhesive	T49.3X1	T49.3X2	T49.3X3	T49.3X4	T49.3X5	T49.3X6
Cyanocobalamin	T45.8X1	T45.8X2	T45.8X3	T45.8X4	T45.8X5	T45.8X6
Cyanogen (chloride) (gas) NEC	T59.891	T59.892	T59.893	T59.894	—	—
Cyclacillin	T36.0X1	T36.0X2	T36.0X3	T36.0X4	T36.0X5	T36.0X6
Cyclaine	T41.3X1	T41.3X2	T41.3X3	T41.3X4	T41.3X5	T41.3X6
Cyclamate	T50.991	T50.992	T50.993	T50.994	T50.995	T50.996
Cyclamen europaeum	T62.2X1	T62.2X2	T62.2X3	T62.2X4	—	—
Cyclandelate	T46.7X1	T46.7X2	T46.7X3	T46.7X4	T46.7X5	T46.7X6
Cyclazocine	T50.7X1	T50.7X2	T50.7X3	T50.7X4	T50.7X5	T50.7X6
Cyclizine	T45.0X1	T45.0X2	T45.0X3	T45.0X4	T45.0X5	T45.0X6
Cyclobarbital	T42.3X1	T42.3X2	T42.3X3	T42.3X4	T42.3X5	T42.3X6
Cyclobarbitone	T42.3X1	T42.3X2	T42.3X3	T42.3X4	T42.3X5	T42.3X6
Cyclobenzaprine	T48.1X1	T48.1X2	T48.1X3	T48.1X4	T48.1X5	T48.1X6
Cyclodrine	T44.3X1	T44.3X2	T44.3X3	T44.3X4	T44.3X5	T44.3X6
Cycloguanil embonate	T37.2X1	T37.2X2	T37.2X3	T37.2X4	T37.2X5	T37.2X6
Cyclohexane	T52.8X1	T52.8X2	T52.8X3	T52.8X4	—	—
Cyclohexanol	T51.8X1	T51.8X2	T51.8X3	T51.8X4	—	—
Cyclohexanone	T52.4X1	T52.4X2	T52.4X3	T52.4X4	—	—
Cycloheximide	T60.3X1	T60.3X2	T60.3X3	T60.3X4	—	—
Cyclohexyl acetate	T52.8X1	T52.8X2	T52.8X3	T52.8X4	—	—
Cycloleucin	T45.1X1	T45.1X2	T45.1X3	T45.1X4	T45.1X5	T45.1X6
Cyclomethycaine	T41.3X1	T41.3X2	T41.3X3	T41.3X4	T41.3X5	T41.3X6
Cyclopentamine	T44.4X1	T44.4X2	T44.4X3	T44.4X4	T44.4X5	T44.4X6
Cyclopenthiazide	T50.2X1	T50.2X2	T50.2X3	T50.2X4	T50.2X5	T50.2X6
Cyclopentolate	T44.3X1	T44.3X2	T44.3X3	T44.3X4	T44.3X5	T44.3X6
Cyclophosphamide	T45.1X1	T45.1X2	T45.1X3	T45.1X4	T45.1X5	T45.1X6
Cycloplegic drug	T49.5X1	T49.5X2	T49.5X3	T49.5X4	T49.5X5	T49.5X6
Cyclopropane	T41.291	T41.292	T41.293	T41.294	T41.295	T41.296
Cyclopyrabital	T39.8X1	T39.8X2	T39.8X3	T39.8X4	T39.8X5	T39.8X6
Cycloserine	T37.1X1	T37.1X2	T37.1X3	T37.1X4	T37.1X5	T37.1X6
Cyclosporin	T45.1X1	T45.1X2	T45.1X3	T45.1X4	T45.1X5	T45.1X6
Cyclothiazide	T50.2X1	T50.2X2	T50.2X3	T50.2X4	T50.2X5	T50.2X6
Cycrimine	T44.3X1	T44.3X2	T44.3X3	T44.3X4	T44.3X5	T44.3X6
Cyhalothrin	T60.1X1	T60.1X2	T60.1X3	T60.1X4	—	—
Cymarin	T46.0X1	T46.0X2	T46.0X3	T46.0X4	T46.0X5	T46.0X6
Cypermethrin	T60.1X1	T60.1X2	T60.1X3	T60.1X4	—	—
Cyphenothrin	T60.2X1	T60.2X2	T60.2X3	T60.2X4	—	—
Cyproheptadine	T45.0X1	T45.0X2	T45.0X3	T45.0X4	T45.0X5	T45.0X6
Cyproterone	T38.6X1	T38.6X2	T38.6X3	T38.6X4	T38.6X5	T38.6X6
Cysteamine	T50.6X1	T50.6X2	T50.6X3	T50.6X4	T50.6X5	T50.6X6
Cytarabine	T45.1X1	T45.1X2	T45.1X3	T45.1X4	T45.1X5	T45.1X6
Cytisus						
laburnum	T62.2X1	T62.2X2	T62.2X3	T62.2X4	—	—
scoparius	T62.2X1	T62.2X2	T62.2X3	T62.2X4	—	—
Cytochrome C	T47.5X1	T47.5X2	T47.5X3	T47.5X4	T47.5X5	T47.5X6
Cytomel	T38.1X1	T38.1X2	T38.1X3	T38.1X4	T38.1X5	T38.1X6
Cytosine arabinoside	T45.1X1	T45.1X2	T45.1X3	T45.1X4	T45.1X5	T45.1X6
Cytoxan	T45.1X1	T45.1X2	T45.1X3	T45.1X4	T45.1X5	T45.1X6
Cytozyme	T45.7X1	T45.7X2	T45.7X3	T45.7X4	T45.7X5	T45.7X6
S-Carboxymethylcysteine	T48.4X1	T48.4X2	T48.4X3	T48.4X4	T48.4X5	T48.4X6
Dacarbazine	T45.1X1	T45.1X2	T45.1X3	T45.1X4	T45.1X5	T45.1X6
Dactinomycin	T45.1X1	T45.1X2	T45.1X3	T45.1X4	T45.1X5	T45.1X6
DADPS	T37.1X1	T37.1X2	T37.1X3	T37.1X4	T37.1X5	T37.1X6

Substance	Poisoning, Accidental (unintentional)	Poisoning, Intentional Self-harm	Poisoning, Assault	Poisoning, Undetermined	Adverse Effect	Under-dosing
Dakin's solution	T49.0X1	T49.0X2	T49.0X3	T49.0X4	T49.0X5	T49.0X6
Dalapon (sodium)	T60.3X1	T60.3X2	T60.3X3	T60.3X4	—	—
Dalmane	T42.4X1	T42.4X2	T42.4X3	T42.4X4	T42.4X5	T42.4X6
Danazol	T38.6X1	T38.6X2	T38.6X3	T38.6X4	T38.6X5	T38.6X6
Danilone	T45.511	T45.512	T45.513	T45.514	T45.515	T45.516
Danthron	T47.2X1	T47.2X2	T47.2X3	T47.2X4	T47.2X5	T47.2X6
Dantrolene	T42.8X1	T42.8X2	T42.8X3	T42.8X4	T42.8X5	T42.8X6
Dantron	T47.2X1	T47.2X2	T47.2X3	T47.2X4	T47.2X5	T47.2X6
Daphne (gnidium) (mezereum)	T62.2X1	T62.2X2	T62.2X3	T62.2X4	—	—
berry	T62.1X1	T62.1X2	T62.1X3	T62.1X4	—	—
Dapsone	T37.1X1	T37.1X2	T37.1X3	T37.1X4	T37.1X5	T37.1X6
Daraprim	T37.2X1	T37.2X2	T37.2X3	T37.2X4	T37.2X5	T37.2X6
Darnel	T62.2X1	T62.2X2	T62.2X3	T62.2X4	—	—
Darvon	T39.8X1	T39.8X2	T39.8X3	T39.8X4	T39.8X5	T39.8X6
Daunomycin	T45.1X1	T45.1X2	T45.1X3	T45.1X4	T45.1X5	T45.1X6
Daunorubicin	T45.1X1	T45.1X2	T45.1X3	T45.1X4	T45.1X5	T45.1X6
DBI	T38.3X1	T38.3X2	T38.3X3	T38.3X4	T38.3X5	T38.3X6
D-Con	T60.91	T60.92	T60.93	T60.94	—	—
insecticide	T60.2X1	T60.2X2	T60.2X3	T60.2X4	—	—
rodenticide	T60.4X1	T60.4X2	T60.4X3	T60.4X4	—	—
DDAVP	T38.891	T38.892	T38.893	T38.894	T38.895	T38.896
DDE (bis(chlorophenyl)-dichloroethylene)	T60.2X1	T60.2X2	T60.2X3	T60.2X4	—	—
DDS	T37.1X1	T37.1X2	T37.1X3	T37.1X4	T37.1X5	T37.1X6
DDT (dust)	T60.1X1	T60.1X2	T60.1X3	T60.1X4	—	—
Deadly nightshade — see also Belladonna	T62.2X1	T62.2X2	T62.2X3	T62.2X4	—	—
berry	T62.1X1	T62.1X2	T62.1X3	T62.1X4	—	—
Deamino-D-arginine vasopressin	T38.891	T38.892	T38.893	T38.894	T38.895	T38.896
Deanol (aceglumate)	T50.991	T50.992	T50.993	T50.994	T50.995	T50.996
Debrisoquine	T46.5X1	T46.5X2	T46.5X3	T46.5X4	T46.5X5	T46.5X6
Decaborane	T57.8X1	T57.8X2	T57.8X3	T57.8X4	—	—
fumes	T59.891	T59.892	T59.893	T59.894	—	—
Decadron	T38.0X1	T38.0X2	T38.0X3	T38.0X4	T38.0X5	T38.0X6
ENT agent	T49.6X1	T49.6X2	T49.6X3	T49.6X4	T49.6X5	T49.6X6
ophthalmic preparation	T49.5X1	T49.5X2	T49.5X3	T49.5X4	T49.5X5	T49.5X6
topical NEC	T49.0X1	T49.0X2	T49.0X3	T49.0X4	T49.0X5	T49.0X6
Decahydronaphthalene	T52.8X1	T52.8X2	T52.8X3	T52.8X4	—	—
Decalin	T52.8X1	T52.8X2	T52.8X3	T52.8X4	—	—
Decamethonium (bromide)	T48.1X1	T48.1X2	T48.1X3	T48.1X4	T48.1X5	T48.1X6
Decholin	T47.5X1	T47.5X2	T47.5X3	T47.5X4	T47.5X5	T47.5X6
Declomycin	T36.4X1	T36.4X2	T36.4X3	T36.4X4	T36.4X5	T36.4X6
Decongestant, nasal (mucosa)	T48.5X1	T48.5X2	T48.5X3	T48.5X4	T48.5X5	T48.5X6
combination	T48.5X1	T48.5X2	T48.5X3	T48.5X4	T48.5X5	T48.5X6
Deet	T60.8X1	T60.8X2	T60.8X3	T60.8X4	—	—
Deferoxamine	T45.8X1	T45.8X2	T45.8X3	T45.8X4	T45.8X5	T45.8X6
Deflazacort	T38.0X1	T38.0X2	T38.0X3	T38.0X4	T38.0X5	T38.0X6
Deglycyrrhizinized extract of licorice	T48.4X1	T48.4X2	T48.4X3	T48.4X4	T48.4X5	T48.4X6
Dehydrocholic acid	T47.5X1	T47.5X2	T47.5X3	T47.5X4	T47.5X5	T47.5X6
Dehydroemetine	T37.3X1	T37.3X2	T37.3X3	T37.3X4	T37.3X5	T37.3X6
Dekalin	T52.8X1	T52.8X2	T52.8X3	T52.8X4	—	—
Delalutin	T38.5X1	T38.5X2	T38.5X3	T38.5X4	T38.5X5	T38.5X6
Delorazepam	T42.4X1	T42.4X2	T42.4X3	T42.4X4	T42.4X5	T42.4X6
Delphinium	T62.2X1	T62.2X2	T62.2X3	T62.2X4	—	—
Deltamethrin	T60.1X1	T60.1X2	T60.1X3	T60.1X4	—	—
Deltasone	T38.0X1	T38.0X2	T38.0X3	T38.0X4	T38.0X5	T38.0X6
Deltra	T38.0X1	T38.0X2	T38.0X3	T38.0X4	T38.0X5	T38.0X6
Delvinal	T42.3X1	T42.3X2	T42.3X3	T42.3X4	T42.3X5	T42.3X6
Demecarium (bromide)	T49.5X1	T49.5X2	T49.5X3	T49.5X4	T49.5X5	T49.5X6
Demeclocycline	T36.4X1	T36.4X2	T36.4X3	T36.4X4	T36.4X5	T36.4X6
Demecolcine	T45.1X1	T45.1X2	T45.1X3	T45.1X4	T45.1X5	T45.1X6
Demegestone	T38.5X1	T38.5X2	T38.5X3	T38.5X4	T38.5X5	T38.5X6
Demelanizing agents	T49.8X1	T49.8X2	T49.8X3	T49.8X4	T49.8X5	T49.8X6
Demephion -O and -S	T60.0X1	T60.0X2	T60.0X3	T60.0X4	—	—
Demerol	T40.2X1	T40.2X2	T40.2X3	T40.2X4	T40.2X5	T40.2X6
Demethylchlortetracycline	T36.4X1	T36.4X2	T36.4X3	T36.4X4	T36.4X5	T36.4X6
Demethyltetracycline	T36.4X1	T36.4X2	T36.4X3	T36.4X4	T36.4X5	T36.4X6
Demeton -O and -S	T60.0X1	T60.0X2	T60.0X3	T60.0X4	—	—
Demulcent (external)	T49.3X1	T49.3X2	T49.3X3	T49.3X4	T49.3X5	T49.3X6
specified NEC	T49.3X1	T49.3X2	T49.3X3	T49.3X4	T49.3X5	T49.3X6
Demulen	T38.4X1	T38.4X2	T38.4X3	T38.4X4	T38.4X5	T38.4X6
Denatured alcohol	T51.0X1	T51.0X2	T51.0X3	T51.0X4	—	—
Dendrid	T49.5X1	T49.5X2	T49.5X3	T49.5X4	T49.5X5	T49.5X6
Dental drug, topical application NEC	T49.7X1	T49.7X2	T49.7X3	T49.7X4	T49.7X5	T49.7X6
Dentifrice	T49.7X1	T49.7X2	T49.7X3	T49.7X4	T49.7X5	T49.7X6
Deodorant spray (feminine hygiene)	T49.8X1	T49.8X2	T49.8X3	T49.8X4	T49.8X5	T49.8X6
Deoxycortone	T50.0X1	T50.0X2	T50.0X3	T50.0X4	T50.0X5	T50.0X6

Substance	Poisoning, Accidental (unintentional)	Poisoning, Intentional Self-harm	Poisoning, Assault	Poisoning, Undetermined	Adverse Effect	Under-dosing
Deoxyribonuclease (pancreatic)	T45.3X1	T45.3X2	T45.3X3	T45.3X4	T45.3X5	T45.3X6
Depilatory	T49.4X1	T49.4X2	T49.4X3	T49.4X4	T49.4X5	T49.4X6
Deprenalin	T42.8X1	T42.8X2	T42.8X3	T42.8X4	T42.8X5	T42.8X6
Deprenyl	T42.8X1	T42.8X2	T42.8X3	T42.8X4	T42.8X5	T42.8X6
Depressant						
appetite (central)	T50.5X1	T50.5X2	T50.5X3	T50.5X4	T50.5X5	T50.5X6
cardiac	T46.2X1	T46.2X2	T46.2X3	T46.2X4	T46.2X5	T46.2X6
central nervous system (anesthetic) — see also Central nervous system, depressants	T42.71	T42.72	T42.73	T42.74	T42.75	T42.76
general anesthetic	T41.201	T41.202	T41.203	T41.204	T41.205	T41.206
muscle tone	T42.8X1	T42.8X2	T42.8X3	T42.8X4	T42.8X5	T42.8X6
muscle tone, central	T42.8X1	T42.8X2	T42.8X3	T42.8X4	T42.8X5	T42.8X6
psychotherapeutic	T43.501	T43.502	T43.503	T43.504	T43.505	T43.506
Depressant, appetite	T50.5X1	T50.5X2	T50.5X3	T50.5X4	T50.5X5	T50.5X6
Deptropine	T45.0X1	T45.0X2	T45.0X3	T45.0X4	T45.0X5	T45.0X6
Dequalinium (chloride)	T49.0X1	T49.0X2	T49.0X3	T49.0X4	T49.0X5	T49.0X6
Derris root	T60.2X1	T60.2X2	T60.2X3	T60.2X4	—	—
Deserpidine	T46.5X1	T46.5X2	T46.5X3	T46.5X4	T46.5X5	T46.5X6
Desferrioxamine	T45.8X1	T45.8X2	T45.8X3	T45.8X4	T45.8X5	T45.8X6
Desipramine	T43.011	T43.012	T43.013	T43.014	T43.015	T43.016
Deslanoside	T46.0X1	T46.0X2	T46.0X3	T46.0X4	T46.0X5	T46.0X6
Desloughing agent	T49.4X1	T49.4X2	T49.4X3	T49.4X4	T49.4X5	T49.4X6
Desmethylimipramine	T43.011	T43.012	T43.013	T43.014	T43.015	T43.016
Desmopressin	T38.891	T38.892	T38.893	T38.894	T38.895	T38.896
Desocodeine	T40.2X1	T40.2X2	T40.2X3	T40.2X4	T40.2X5	T40.2X6
Desogestrel	T38.5X1	T38.5X2	T38.5X3	T38.5X4	T38.5X5	T38.5X6
Desomorphine	T40.2X1	T40.2X2	T40.2X3	T40.2X4	—	—
Desonide	T49.0X1	T49.0X2	T49.0X3	T49.0X4	T49.0X5	T49.0X6
Desoximetasone	T49.0X1	T49.0X2	T49.0X3	T49.0X4	T49.0X5	T49.0X6
Desoxycorticosteroid	T50.0X1	T50.0X2	T50.0X3	T50.0X4	T50.0X5	T50.0X6
Desoxycortone	T50.0X1	T50.0X2	T50.0X3	T50.0X4	T50.0X5	T50.0X6
Desoxyephedrine	T43.621	T43.622	T43.623	T43.624	T43.625	T43.626
Detaxtran	T46.6X1	T46.6X2	T46.6X3	T46.6X4	T46.6X5	T46.6X6
Detergent	T49.2X1	T49.2X2	T49.2X3	T49.2X4	T49.2X5	T49.2X6
external medication	T49.2X1	T49.2X2	T49.2X3	T49.2X4	T49.2X5	T49.2X6
local	T49.2X1	T49.2X2	T49.2X3	T49.2X4	T49.2X5	T49.2X6
medicinal	T49.2X1	T49.2X2	T49.2X3	T49.2X4	T49.2X5	T49.2X6
nonmedicinal	T55.1X1	T55.1X2	T55.1X3	T55.1X4	—	—
specified NEC	T55.1X1	T55.1X2	T55.1X3	T55.1X4	—	—
Deterrent, alcohol	T50.6X1	T50.6X2	T50.6X3	T50.6X4	T50.6X5	T50.6X6
Detoxifying agent	T50.6X1	T50.6X2	T50.6X3	T50.6X4	T50.6X5	T50.6X6
Detrothyronine	T38.1X1	T38.1X2	T38.1X3	T38.1X4	T38.1X5	T38.1X6
Dettol (external medication)	T49.0X1	T49.0X2	T49.0X3	T49.0X4	T49.0X5	T49.0X6
Dexamethasone	T38.0X1	T38.0X2	T38.0X3	T38.0X4	T38.0X5	T38.0X6
ENT agent	T49.6X1	T49.6X2	T49.6X3	T49.6X4	T49.6X5	T49.6X6
ophthalmic preparation	T49.5X1	T49.5X2	T49.5X3	T49.5X4	T49.5X5	T49.5X6
topical NEC	T49.0X1	T49.0X2	T49.0X3	T49.0X4	T49.0X5	T49.0X6
Dexamfetamine	T43.621	T43.622	T43.623	T43.624	T43.625	T43.626
Dexamphetamine	T43.621	T43.622	T43.623	T43.624	T43.625	T43.626
Dexbrompheniramine	T45.0X1	T45.0X2	T45.0X3	T45.0X4	T45.0X5	T45.0X6
Dexchlorpheniramine	T45.0X1	T45.0X2	T45.0X3	T45.0X4	T45.0X5	T45.0X6
Dexedrine	T43.621	T43.622	T43.623	T43.624	T43.625	T43.626
Dexetimide	T44.3X1	T44.3X2	T44.3X3	T44.3X4	T44.3X5	T44.3X6
Dexfenfluramine	T50.5X1	T50.5X2	T50.5X3	T50.5X4	T50.5X5	T50.5X6
Dexpanthenol	T45.2X1	T45.2X2	T45.2X3	T45.2X4	T45.2X5	T45.2X6
Dextran (40) (70) (150)	T45.8X1	T45.8X2	T45.8X3	T45.8X4	T45.8X5	T45.8X6
Dextriferron	T45.4X1	T45.4X2	T45.4X3	T45.4X4	T45.4X5	T45.4X6
Dextroamphetamine	T43.621	T43.622	T43.623	T43.624	T43.625	T43.626
Dextro calcium pantothenate	T45.2X1	T45.2X2	T45.2X3	T45.2X4	T45.2X5	T45.2X6
Dextromethorphan	T48.3X1	T48.3X2	T48.3X3	T48.3X4	T48.3X5	T48.3X6
Dextromoramide	T40.4X1	T40.4X2	T40.4X3	T40.4X4	—	—
topical	T49.8X1	T49.8X2	T49.8X3	T49.8X4	T49.8X5	T49.8X6
Dextro pantothenyl alcohol	T45.2X1	T45.2X2	T45.2X3	T45.2X4	T45.2X5	T45.2X6
Dextropropoxyphene	T40.4X1	T40.4X2	T40.4X3	T40.4X4	T40.4X5	T40.4X6
Dextrorphan	T40.2X1	T40.2X2	T40.2X3	T40.2X4	T40.2X5	T40.2X6
Dextrose	T50.3X1	T50.3X2	T50.3X3	T50.3X4	T50.3X5	T50.3X6
concentrated solution, intravenous	T46.8X1	T46.8X2	T46.8X3	T46.8X4	T46.8X5	T46.8X6
Dextrothyroxin	T38.1X1	T38.1X2	T38.1X3	T38.1X4	T38.1X5	T38.1X6
Dextrothyroxine sodium	T38.1X1	T38.1X2	T38.1X3	T38.1X4	T38.1X5	T38.1X6
DFP	T44.0X1	T44.0X2	T44.0X3	T44.0X4	T44.0X5	T44.0X6
DHE	T37.3X1	T37.3X2	T37.3X3	T37.3X4	T37.3X5	T37.3X6
45	T46.5X1	T46.5X2	T46.5X3	T46.5X4	T46.5X5	T46.5X6
Diabinese	T38.3X1	T38.3X2	T38.3X3	T38.3X4	T38.3X5	T38.3X6
Diacetone alcohol	T52.4X1	T52.4X2	T52.4X3	T52.4X4	—	—
Diacetyl monoxime	T50.991	T50.992	T50.993	T50.994	—	—
Diacetylmorphine	T40.1X1	T40.1X2	T40.1X3	T40.1X4	—	—
Diachylon plaster	T49.4X1	T49.4X2	T49.4X3	T49.4X4	T49.4X5	T49.4X6

Substance	Poisoning, Accidental (unintentional)	Poisoning, Intentional Self-harm	Poisoning, Assault	Poisoning, Undetermined	Adverse Effect	Under-dosing
Diaethylstilboestrolum	T38.5X1	T38.5X2	T38.5X3	T38.5X4	T38.5X5	T38.5X6
Diagnostic agent NEC	T50.8X1	T50.8X2	T50.8X3	T50.8X4	T50.8X5	T50.8X6
Dial (soap)	T49.2X1	T49.2X2	T49.2X3	T49.2X4	T49.2X5	T49.2X6
sedative	T42.3X1	T42.3X2	T42.3X3	T42.3X4	T42.3X5	T42.3X6
Dialkyl carbonate	T52.91	T52.92	T52.93	T52.94	—	—
Diallylbarbituric acid	T42.3X1	T42.3X2	T42.3X3	T42.3X4	T42.3X5	T42.3X6
Diallymal	T42.3X1	T42.3X2	T42.3X3	T42.3X4	T42.3X5	T42.3X6
Dialysis solution	T50.3X1	T50.3X2	T50.3X3	T50.3X4	T50.3X5	T50.3X6
(intraperitoneal)						
Diaminodiphenylsulfone	T37.1X1	T37.1X2	T37.1X3	T37.1X4	T37.1X5	T37.1X6
Diamorphine	T40.1X1	T40.1X2	T40.1X3	T40.1X4	—	—
Diamox	T50.2X1	T50.2X2	T50.2X3	T50.2X4	T50.2X5	T50.2X6
Diamthazole	T49.0X1	T49.0X2	T49.0X3	T49.0X4	T49.0X5	T49.0X6
Dianthone	T47.2X1	T47.2X2	T47.2X3	T47.2X4	T47.2X5	T47.2X6
Diaphenylsulfone	T37.0X1	T37.0X2	T37.0X3	T37.0X4	T37.0X5	T37.0X6
Diasone (sodium)	T37.1X1	T37.1X2	T37.1X3	T37.1X4	T37.1X5	T37.1X6
Diastase	T47.5X1	T47.5X2	T47.5X3	T47.5X4	T47.5X5	T47.5X6
Diatrizoate	T50.8X1	T50.8X2	T50.8X3	T50.8X4	T50.8X5	T50.8X6
Diazepam	T42.4X1	T42.4X2	T42.4X3	T42.4X4	T42.4X5	T42.4X6
Diazinon	T60.0X1	T60.0X2	T60.0X3	T60.0X4	—	—
Diazomethane (gas)	T59.891	T59.892	T59.893	T59.894	—	—
Diazoxide	T46.5X1	T46.5X2	T46.5X3	T46.5X4	T46.5X5	T46.5X6
Dibekacin	T36.5X1	T36.5X2	T36.5X3	T36.5X4	T36.5X5	T36.5X6
Dibenamine	T44.6X1	T44.6X2	T44.6X3	T44.6X4	T44.6X5	T44.6X6
Dibenzepin	T43.011	T43.012	T43.013	T43.014	T43.015	T43.016
Dibenzheptropine	T45.0X1	T45.0X2	T45.0X3	T45.0X4	T45.0X5	T45.0X6
Dibenzyline	T44.6X1	T44.6X2	T44.6X3	T44.6X4	T44.6X5	T44.6X6
Diborane (gas)	T59.891	T59.892	T59.893	T59.894	—	—
Dibromochloropropane	T60.8X1	T60.8X2	T60.8X3	T60.8X4	—	—
Dibromodulcitol	T45.1X1	T45.1X2	T45.1X3	T45.1X4	T45.1X5	T45.1X6
Dibromoethane	T53.6X1	T53.6X2	T53.6X3	T53.6X4	—	—
Dibromomannitol	T45.1X1	T45.1X2	T45.1X3	T45.1X4	T45.1X5	T45.1X6
Dibromopropamidine isethionate	T49.0X1	T49.0X2	T49.0X3	T49.0X4	T49.0X5	T49.0X6
Dibrompropamidine	T49.0X1	T49.0X2	T49.0X3	T49.0X4	T49.0X5	T49.0X6
Dibucaine	T41.3X1	T41.3X2	T41.3X3	T41.3X4	T41.3X5	T41.3X6
topical (surface)	T41.3X1	T41.3X2	T41.3X3	T41.3X4	T41.3X5	T41.3X6
Dibunate sodium	T48.3X1	T48.3X2	T48.3X3	T48.3X4	T48.3X5	T48.3X6
Dibutoline sulfate	T44.3X1	T44.3X2	T44.3X3	T44.3X4	T44.3X5	T44.3X6
Dicamba	T60.3X1	T60.3X2	T60.3X3	T60.3X4	—	—
Dicapthon	T60.0X1	T60.0X2	T60.0X3	T60.0X4	—	—
Dichlobenil	T60.3X1	T60.3X2	T60.3X3	T60.3X4	—	—
Dichlone	T60.3X1	T60.3X2	T60.3X3	T60.3X4	—	—
Dichloralphenazone	T42.6X1	T42.6X2	T42.6X3	T42.6X4	T42.6X5	T42.6X6
Dichlorbenzidine	T65.3X1	T65.3X2	T65.3X3	T65.3X4	—	—
Dichlorhydrin	T52.8X1	T52.8X2	T52.8X3	T52.8X4	—	—
Dichlorhydroxyquinoline	T37.8X1	T37.8X2	T37.8X3	T37.8X4	T37.8X5	T37.8X6
Dichlorobenzene	T53.7X1	T53.7X2	T53.7X3	T53.7X4	—	—
Dichlorobenzyl alcohol	T49.6X1	T49.6X2	T49.6X3	T49.6X4	T49.6X5	T49.6X6
Dichlorodifluoromethane	T53.5X1	T53.5X2	T53.5X3	T53.5X4	—	—
Dichloroethane	T52.8X1	T52.8X2	T52.8X3	T52.8X4	—	—
Dichloroethylene	T53.6X1	T53.6X2	T53.6X3	T53.6X4	—	—
Dichloroethyl sulfide, not in war	T59.891	T59.892	T59.893	T59.894	—	—
Dichloroformoxine, not in war	T59.891	T59.892	T59.893	T59.894	—	—
Dichlorohydrin, alpha-dichlorohydrin	T52.8X1	T52.8X2	T52.8X3	T52.8X4	—	—
Dichloromethane (solvent)	T53.4X1	T53.4X2	T53.4X3	T53.4X4	—	—
vapor	T53.4X1	T53.4X2	T53.4X3	T53.4X4	—	—
Dichloronaphthoquinone	T60.3X1	T60.3X2	T60.3X3	T60.3X4	—	—
Dichlorophen	T37.4X1	T37.4X2	T37.4X3	T37.4X4	T37.4X5	T37.4X6
Dichloropropene	T60.3X1	T60.3X2	T60.3X3	T60.3X4	—	—
Dichloropropionic acid	T60.3X1	T60.3X2	T60.3X3	T60.3X4	—	—
Dichlorphenamide	T50.2X1	T50.2X2	T50.2X3	T50.2X4	T50.2X5	T50.2X6
Dichlorvos	T60.0X1	T60.0X2	T60.0X3	T60.0X4	—	—
Diclofenac	T39.391	T39.392	T39.393	T39.394	T39.395	T39.396
Diclofenamide	T50.2X1	T50.2X2	T50.2X3	T50.2X4	T50.2X5	T50.2X6
Diclofensine	T43.291	T43.292	T43.293	T43.294	T43.295	T43.296
Diclonixine	T39.8X1	T39.8X2	T39.8X3	T39.8X4	T39.8X5	T39.8X6
Dicloxacillin	T36.0X1	T36.0X2	T36.0X3	T36.0X4	T36.0X5	T36.0X6
Dicophane	T49.0X1	T49.0X2	T49.0X3	T49.0X4	T49.0X5	T49.0X6
Dicoumarol, dicoumarin, dicumarol	T45.511	T45.512	T45.513	T45.514	T45.515	T45.516
Dicrotophos	T60.0X1	T60.0X2	T60.0X3	T60.0X4	—	—
Dicyanogen (gas)	T65.0X1	T65.0X2	T65.0X3	T65.0X4	—	—
Dicyclomine	T44.3X1	T44.3X2	T44.3X3	T44.3X4	T44.3X5	T44.3X6
Dicycloverine	T44.3X1	T44.3X2	T44.3X3	T44.3X4	T44.3X5	T44.3X6
Dideoxycytidine	T37.5X1	T37.5X2	T37.5X3	T37.5X4	T37.5X5	T37.5X6
Dideoxyinosine	T37.5X1	T37.5X2	T37.5X3	T37.5X4	T37.5X5	T37.5X6
Dieldrin (vapor)	T60.1X1	T60.1X2	T60.1X3	T60.1X4	—	—
Diemal	T42.3X1	T42.3X2	T42.3X3	T42.3X4	T42.3X5	T42.3X6
Dienestrol	T38.5X1	T38.5X2	T38.5X3	T38.5X4	T38.5X5	T38.5X6

Substance	Poisoning, Accidental (unintentional)	Poisoning, Intentional Self-harm	Poisoning, Assault	Poisoning, Undetermined	Adverse Effect	Under-dosing
Dienoestrol	T38.5X1	T38.5X2	T38.5X3	T38.5X4	T38.5X5	T38.5X6
Dietetic drug NEC	T50.901	T50.902	T50.903	T50.904	T50.905	T50.906
Diethazine	T42.8X1	T42.8X2	T42.8X3	T42.8X4	T42.8X5	T42.8X6
Diethyl						
barbituric acid	T42.3X1	T42.3X2	T42.3X3	T42.3X4	T42.3X5	T42.3X6
carbamazine	T37.4X1	T37.4X2	T37.4X3	T37.4X4	T37.4X5	T37.4X6
carbinol	T51.3X1	T51.3X2	T51.3X3	T51.3X4	—	—
carbonate	T52.8X1	T52.8X2	T52.8X3	T52.8X4	—	—
ether (vapor) — see also ether	T41.0X1	T41.0X2	T41.0X3	T41.0X4	T41.0X5	T41.0X6
oxide	T52.8X1	T52.8X2	T52.8X3	T52.8X4	—	—
propion	T50.5X1	T50.5X2	T50.5X3	T50.5X4	T50.5X5	T50.5X6
stilbestrol	T38.5X1	T38.5X2	T38.5X3	T38.5X4	T38.5X5	T38.5X6
toluamide (nonmedicinal)	T60.8X1	T60.8X2	T60.8X3	T60.8X4	—	—
medicinal	T49.3X1	T49.3X2	T49.3X3	T49.3X4	T49.3X5	T49.3X6
Diethylcarbamazine	T37.4X1	T37.4X2	T37.4X3	T37.4X4	T37.4X5	T37.4X6
Diethylene						
dioxide	T52.8X1	T52.8X2	T52.8X3	T52.8X4	—	—
glycol (monoacetate) (monobutyl ether) (monoethyl ether)	T52.3X1	T52.3X2	T52.3X3	T52.3X4	—	—
Diethylhexylphthalate	T65.891	T65.892	T65.893	T65.894	—	—
Diethylpropion	T50.5X1	T50.5X2	T50.5X3	T50.5X4	T50.5X5	T50.5X6
Diethylstilbestrol	T38.5X1	T38.5X2	T38.5X3	T38.5X4	T38.5X5	T38.5X6
Diethylstilboestrol	T38.5X1	T38.5X2	T38.5X3	T38.5X4	T38.5X5	T38.5X6
Diethylsulfone-diethylmethane	T42.6X1	T42.6X2	T42.6X3	T42.6X4	T42.6X5	T42.6X6
Diethyltoluamide	T49.0X1	T49.0X2	T49.0X3	T49.0X4	T49.0X5	T49.0X6
Diethyltryptamine (DET)	T40.991	T40.992	T40.993	T40.994	—	—
Difebarbamate	T42.3X1	T42.3X2	T42.3X3	T42.3X4	T42.3X5	T42.3X6
Difencloxazine	T40.2X1	T40.2X2	T40.2X3	T40.2X4	T40.2X5	T40.2X6
Difenidol	T45.0X1	T45.0X2	T45.0X3	T45.0X4	T45.0X5	T45.0X6
Difenoxin	T47.6X1	T47.6X2	T47.6X3	T47.6X4	T47.6X5	T47.6X6
Difetarsone	T37.3X1	T37.3X2	T37.3X3	T37.3X4	T37.3X5	T37.3X6
Diffusin	T45.3X1	T45.3X2	T45.3X3	T45.3X4	T45.3X5	T45.3X6
Diflorasone	T49.0X1	T49.0X2	T49.0X3	T49.0X4	T49.0X5	T49.0X6
Diflos	T44.0X1	T44.0X2	T44.0X3	T44.0X4	T44.0X5	T44.0X6
Diflubenzuron	T60.1X1	T60.1X2	T60.1X3	T60.1X4	—	—
Diflucortolone	T49.0X1	T49.0X2	T49.0X3	T49.0X4	T49.0X5	T49.0X6
Diflunisal	T39.091	T39.092	T39.093	T39.094	T39.095	T39.096
Difluoromethyldopa	T42.8X1	T42.8X2	T42.8X3	T42.8X4	T42.8X5	T42.8X6
Difluorophate	T44.0X1	T44.0X2	T44.0X3	T44.0X4	T44.0X5	T44.0X6
Digestant NEC	T47.5X1	T47.5X2	T47.5X3	T47.5X4	T47.5X5	T47.5X6
Digitalin (e)	T46.0X1	T46.0X2	T46.0X3	T46.0X4	T46.0X5	T46.0X6
Digitalis (leaf)(glycoside)	T46.0X1	T46.0X2	T46.0X3	T46.0X4	T46.0X5	T46.0X6
lanata	T46.0X1	T46.0X2	T46.0X3	T46.0X4	T46.0X5	T46.0X6
purpurea	T46.0X1	T46.0X2	T46.0X3	T46.0X4	T46.0X5	T46.0X6
Digitoxin	T46.0X1	T46.0X2	T46.0X3	T46.0X4	T46.0X5	T46.0X6
Digitoxose	T46.0X1	T46.0X2	T46.0X3	T46.0X4	T46.0X5	T46.0X6
Digoxin	T46.0X1	T46.0X2	T46.0X3	T46.0X4	T46.0X5	T46.0X6
Digoxine	T46.0X1	T46.0X2	T46.0X3	T46.0X4	T46.0X5	T46.0X6
Dihydralazine	T46.5X1	T46.5X2	T46.5X3	T46.5X4	T46.5X5	T46.5X6
Dihydrazine	T46.5X1	T46.5X2	T46.5X3	T46.5X4	T46.5X5	T46.5X6
Dihydrocodeine	T40.2X1	T40.2X2	T40.2X3	T40.2X4	T40.2X5	T40.2X6
Dihydrocodeinone	T40.2X1	T40.2X2	T40.2X3	T40.2X4	T40.2X5	T40.2X6
Dihydroergocornine	T46.7X1	T46.7X2	T46.7X3	T46.7X4	T46.7X5	T46.7X6
Dihydroergocristine (mesilate)	T46.7X1	T46.7X2	T46.7X3	T46.7X4	T46.7X5	T46.7X6
Dihydroergokryptine	T46.7X1	T46.7X2	T46.7X3	T46.7X4	T46.7X5	T46.7X6
Dihydroergotamine	T46.5X1	T46.5X2	T46.5X3	T46.5X4	T46.5X5	T46.5X6
Dihydroergotoxine	T46.7X1	T46.7X2	T46.7X3	T46.7X4	T46.7X5	T46.7X6
mesilate	T46.7X1	T46.7X2	T46.7X3	T46.7X4	T46.7X5	T46.7X6
Dihydrohydroxycodeinone	T40.2X1	T40.2X2	T40.2X3	T40.2X4	T40.2X5	T40.2X6
Dihydrohydroxymorphinone	T40.2X1	T40.2X2	T40.2X3	T40.2X4	T40.2X5	T40.2X6
Dihydroisocodeine	T40.2X1	T40.2X2	T40.2X3	T40.2X4	T40.2X5	T40.2X6
Dihydromorphine	T40.2X1	T40.2X2	T40.2X3	T40.2X4	—	T40.2X6
Dihydromorphinone	T40.2X1	T40.2X2	T40.2X3	T40.2X4	T40.2X5	T40.2X6
Dihydrostreptomycin	T36.5X1	T36.5X2	T36.5X3	T36.5X4	T36.5X5	T36.5X6
Dihydrotachysterol	T45.2X1	T45.2X2	T45.2X3	T45.2X4	T45.2X5	T45.2X6
Dihydroxyaluminum aminoacetate	T47.1X1	T47.1X2	T47.1X3	T47.1X4	T47.1X5	T47.1X6
Dihydroxyaluminum sodium carbonate	T47.1X1	T47.1X2	T47.1X3	T47.1X4	T47.1X5	T47.1X6
Dihydroxyanthraquinone	T47.2X1	T47.2X2	T47.2X3	T47.2X4	T47.2X5	T47.2X6
Dihydroxycodeinone	T40.2X1	T40.2X2	T40.2X3	T40.2X4	T40.2X5	T40.2X6
Dihydroxypropyl theophylline	T50.2X1	T50.2X2	T50.2X3	T50.2X4	T50.2X5	T50.2X6
Diiodohydroxyquin	T37.8X1	T37.8X2	T37.8X3	T37.8X4	T37.8X5	T37.8X6
topical	T49.0X1	T49.0X2	T49.0X3	T49.0X4	T49.0X5	T49.0X6
Diiodohydroxyquinoline	T37.8X1	T37.8X2	T37.8X3	T37.8X4	T37.8X5	T37.8X6
Diiodotyrosine	T38.2X1	T38.2X2	T38.2X3	T38.2X4	T38.2X5	T38.2X6
Diisopromine	T44.3X1	T44.3X2	T44.3X3	T44.3X4	T44.3X5	T44.3X6
Diisopropylamine	T46.3X1	T46.3X2	T46.3X3	T46.3X4	T46.3X5	T46.3X6
Diisopropylfluorophosphonate	T44.0X1	T44.0X2	T44.0X3	T44.0X4	T44.0X5	T44.0X6

Additional Character May Be Required — Refer to the Tabular List for Character Selection ▽ Subterms under main terms may continue to next column or page

Substance	Poisoning, Accidental (unintentional)	Poisoning, Intentional Self-harm	Poisoning, Assault	Poisoning, Undetermined	Adverse Effect	Under-dosing
Dilantin	T42.0X1	T42.0X2	T42.0X3	T42.0X4	T42.0X5	T42.0X6
Dilaudid	T40.2X1	T40.2X2	T40.2X3	T40.2X4	T40.2X5	T40.2X6
Dilazep	T46.3X1	T46.3X2	T46.3X3	T46.3X4	T46.3X5	T46.3X6
Dill	T47.5X1	T47.5X2	T47.5X3	T47.5X4	T47.5X5	T47.5X6
Diloxanide	T37.3X1	T37.3X2	T37.3X3	T37.3X4	T37.3X5	T37.3X6
Diltiazem	T46.1X1	T46.1X2	T46.1X3	T46.1X4	T46.1X5	T46.1X6
Dimazole	T49.0X1	T49.0X2	T49.0X3	T49.0X4	T49.0X5	T49.0X6
Dimefline	T50.7X1	T50.7X2	T50.7X3	T50.7X4	T50.7X5	T50.7X6
Dimemorfan	T48.3X1	T48.3X2	T48.3X3	T48.3X4	T48.3X5	T48.3X6
Dimenhydrinate	T45.0X1	T45.0X2	T45.0X3	T45.0X4	T45.0X5	T45.0X6
Dimercaprol (British anti-lewisite)	T45.8X1	T45.8X2	T45.8X3	T45.8X4	T45.8X5	T45.8X6
Dimercaptopropanol	T45.8X1	T45.8X2	T45.8X3	T45.8X4	T45.8X5	T45.8X6
Dimestrol	T38.5X1	T38.5X2	T38.5X3	T38.5X4	T38.5X5	T38.5X6
Dimetane	T45.0X1	T45.0X2	T45.0X3	T45.0X4	T45.0X5	T45.0X6
Dimethicone	T47.1X1	T47.1X2	T47.1X3	T47.1X4	T47.1X5	T47.1X6
Dimethindene	T45.0X1	T45.0X2	T45.0X3	T45.0X4	T45.0X5	T45.0X6
Dimethisoquin	T49.1X1	T49.1X2	T49.1X3	T49.1X4	T49.1X5	T49.1X6
Dimethisterone	T38.5X1	T38.5X2	T38.5X3	T38.5X4	T38.5X5	T38.5X6
Dimethoate	T60.0X1	T60.0X2	T60.0X3	T60.0X4	—	—
Dimethocaine	T41.3X1	T41.3X2	T41.3X3	T41.3X4	T41.3X5	T41.3X6
Dimethoxanate	T48.3X1	T48.3X2	T48.3X3	T48.3X4	T48.3X5	T48.3X6
Dimethyl						
arsine, arsinic acid	T57.0X1	T57.0X2	T57.0X3	T57.0X4	—	—
carbinol	T51.2X1	T51.2X2	T51.2X3	T51.2X4	—	—
carbonate	T52.8X1	T52.8X2	T52.8X3	T52.8X4	—	—
diguanide	T38.3X1	T38.3X2	T38.3X3	T38.3X4	T38.3X5	T38.3X6
ketone	T52.4X1	T52.4X2	T52.4X3	T52.4X4	—	—
vapor	T52.4X1	T52.4X2	T52.4X3	T52.4X4	—	—
meperidine	T40.2X1	T40.2X2	T40.2X3	T40.2X4	T40.2X5	T40.2X6
parathion	T60.0X1	T60.0X2	T60.0X3	T60.0X4	—	—
phthlate	T49.3X1	T49.3X2	T49.3X3	T49.3X4	T49.3X5	T49.3X6
polysiloxane	T47.8X1	T47.8X2	T47.8X3	T47.8X4	T47.8X5	T47.8X6
sulfate (fumes)	T59.891	T59.892	T59.893	T59.894	—	—
liquid	T65.891	T65.892	T65.893	T65.894	—	—
sulfoxide (nonmedicinal)	T52.8X1	T52.8X2	T52.8X3	T52.8X4	—	—
medicinal	T49.4X1	T49.4X2	T49.4X3	T49.4X4	T49.4X5	T49.4X6
tryptamine	T40.991	T40.992	T40.993	T40.994	—	—
tubocurarine	T48.1X1	T48.1X2	T48.1X3	T48.1X4	T48.1X5	T48.1X6
Dimethylamine sulfate	T49.4X1	T49.4X2	T49.4X3	T49.4X4	T49.4X5	T49.4X6
Dimethylformamide	T52.8X1	T52.8X2	T52.8X3	T52.8X4	—	—
Dimethyltubocurarinium chloride	T48.1X1	T48.1X2	T48.1X3	T48.1X4	T48.1X5	T48.1X6
Dimeticone	T47.1X1	T47.1X2	T47.1X3	T47.1X4	T47.1X5	T47.1X6
Dimetilan	T60.0X1	T60.0X2	T60.0X3	T60.0X4	—	—
Dimetindene	T45.0X1	T45.0X2	T45.0X3	T45.0X4	T45.0X5	T45.0X6
Dimetotiazine	T43.3X1	T43.3X2	T43.3X3	T43.3X4	T43.3X5	T43.3X6
Dimorpholamine	T50.7X1	T50.7X2	T50.7X3	T50.7X4	T50.7X5	T50.7X6
Dimoxyline	T46.3X1	T46.3X2	T46.3X3	T46.3X4	T46.3X5	T46.3X6
Dinitrobenzene	T65.3X1	T65.3X2	T65.3X3	T65.3X4	—	—
vapor	T59.891	T59.892	T59.893	T59.894	—	—
Dinitrobenzol	T65.3X1	T65.3X2	T65.3X3	T65.3X4	—	—
vapor	T59.891	T59.892	T59.893	T59.894	—	—
Dinitrobutylphenol	T65.3X1	T65.3X2	T65.3X3	T65.3X4	—	—
Dinitro (-ortho-)cresol (pesticide) (spray)	T65.3X1	T65.3X2	T65.3X3	T65.3X4	—	—
Dinitrocyclohexylphenol	T65.3X1	T65.3X2	T65.3X3	T65.3X4	—	—
Dinitrophenol	T65.3X1	T65.3X2	T65.3X3	T65.3X4	—	—
Dinoprost	T48.0X1	T48.0X2	T48.0X3	T48.0X4	T48.0X5	T48.0X6
Dinoprostone	T48.0X1	T48.0X2	T48.0X3	T48.0X4	T48.0X5	T48.0X6
Dinoseb	T60.3X1	T60.3X2	T60.3X3	T60.3X4	—	—
Dioctyl sulfosuccinate (calcium) (sodium)	T47.4X1	T47.4X2	T47.4X3	T47.4X4	T47.4X5	T47.4X6
Diodone	T50.8X1	T50.8X2	T50.8X3	T50.8X4	T50.8X5	T50.8X6
Diodoquin	T37.8X1	T37.8X2	T37.8X3	T37.8X4	T37.8X5	T37.8X6
Dionin	T40.2X1	T40.2X2	T40.2X3	T40.2X4	T40.2X5	T40.2X6
Diosmin	T46.991	T46.992	T46.993	T46.994	T46.995	T46.996
Dioxane	T52.8X1	T52.8X2	T52.8X3	T52.8X4	—	—
Dioxathion	T60.0X1	T60.0X2	T60.0X3	T60.0X4	—	—
Dioxin	T53.7X1	T53.7X2	T53.7X3	T53.7X4	—	—
Dioxopromethazine	T43.3X1	T43.3X2	T43.3X3	T43.3X4	T43.3X5	T43.3X6
Dioxyline	T46.3X1	T46.3X2	T46.3X3	T46.3X4	T46.3X5	T46.3X6
Dipentene	T52.8X1	T52.8X2	T52.8X3	T52.8X4	—	—
Diperodon	T41.3X1	T41.3X2	T41.3X3	T41.3X4	T41.3X5	T41.3X6
Diphacinone	T60.4X1	T60.4X2	T60.4X3	T60.4X4	—	—
Diphemanil	T44.3X1	T44.3X2	T44.3X3	T44.3X4	T44.3X5	T44.3X6
metilsulfate	T44.3X1	T44.3X2	T44.3X3	T44.3X4	T44.3X5	T44.3X6
Diphenadione	T45.511	T45.512	T45.513	T45.514	T45.515	T45.516
rodenticide	T60.4X1	T60.4X2	T60.4X3	T60.4X4	—	—
Diphenhydramine	T45.0X1	T45.0X2	T45.0X3	T45.0X4	T45.0X5	T45.0X6
Diphenidol	T45.0X1	T45.0X2	T45.0X3	T45.0X4	T45.0X5	T45.0X6
Diphenoxylate	T47.6X1	T47.6X2	T47.6X3	T47.6X4	T47.6X5	T47.6X6

Substance	Poisoning, Accidental (unintentional)	Poisoning, Intentional Self-harm	Poisoning, Assault	Poisoning, Undetermined	Adverse Effect	Under-dosing
Diphenylamine	T65.3X1	T65.3X2	T65.3X3	T65.3X4	—	—
Diphenylbutazone	T39.2X1	T39.2X2	T39.2X3	T39.2X4	T39.2X5	T39.2X6
Diphenylchloroarsine, not in war	T57.0X1	T57.0X2	T57.0X3	T57.0X4	—	—
Diphenylhydantoin	T42.0X1	T42.0X2	T42.0X3	T42.0X4	T42.0X5	T42.0X6
Diphenylmethane dye	T52.1X1	T52.1X2	T52.1X3	T52.1X4	—	—
Diphenylpyraline	T45.0X1	T45.0X2	T45.0X3	T45.0X4	T45.0X5	T45.0X6
Diphtheria						
antitoxin	T50.Z11	T50.Z12	T50.Z13	T50.Z14	T50.Z15	T50.Z16
toxoid	T50.A91	T50.A92	T50.A93	T50.A94	T50.A95	T50.A96
with tetanus toxoid	T50.A21	T50.A22	T50.A23	T50.A24	T50.A25	T50.A26
with pertussis component	T50.A11	T50.A12	T50.A13	T50.A14	T50.A15	T50.A16
vaccine	T50.A91	T50.A92	T50.A93	T50.A94	T50.A95	T50.A96
combination						
without pertussis	T50.A21	T50.A22	T50.A23	T50.A24	T50.A25	T50.A26
including pertussis	T50.A11	T50.A12	T50.A13	T50.A14	T50.A15	T50.A16
Diphylline	T50.2X1	T50.2X2	T50.2X3	T50.2X4	T50.2X5	T50.2X6
Dipipanone	T40.4X1	T40.4X2	T40.4X3	T40.4X4	—	—
Dipivefrine	T49.5X1	T49.5X2	T49.5X3	T49.5X4	T49.5X5	T49.5X6
Diplovax	T50.B91	T50.B92	T50.B93	T50.B94	T50.B95	T50.B96
Diprophylline	T50.2X1	T50.2X2	T50.2X3	T50.2X4	T50.2X5	T50.2X6
Dipropyline	T48.291	T48.292	T48.293	T48.294	T48.295	T48.296
Dipyridamole	T46.3X1	T46.3X2	T46.3X3	T46.3X4	T46.3X5	T46.3X6
Dipyrone	T39.2X1	T39.2X2	T39.2X3	T39.2X4	T39.2X5	T39.2X6
Diquat (dibromide)	T60.3X1	T60.3X2	T60.3X3	T60.3X4	—	—
Disinfectant	T65.891	T65.892	T65.893	T65.894	—	—
alkaline	T54.3X1	T54.3X2	T54.3X3	T54.3X4	—	—
aromatic	T54.1X1	T54.1X2	T54.1X3	T54.1X4	—	—
intestinal	T37.8X1	T37.8X2	T37.8X3	T37.8X4	T37.8X5	T37.8X6
Disipal	T42.8X1	T42.8X2	T42.8X3	T42.8X4	T42.8X5	T42.8X6
Disodium edetate	T50.6X1	T50.6X2	T50.6X3	T50.6X4	T50.6X5	T50.6X6
Disoprofol	T41.291	T41.292	T41.293	T41.294	T41.295	T41.296
Disopyramide	T46.2X1	T46.2X2	T46.2X3	T46.2X4	T46.2X5	T46.2X6
Distigmine (bromide)	T44.0X1	T44.0X2	T44.0X3	T44.0X4	T44.0X5	T44.0X6
Disulfamide	T50.2X1	T50.2X2	T50.2X3	T50.2X4	T50.2X5	T50.2X6
Disulfanilamide	T37.0X1	T37.0X2	T37.0X3	T37.0X4	T37.0X5	T37.0X6
Disulfiram	T50.6X1	T50.6X2	T50.6X3	T50.6X4	T50.6X5	T50.6X6
Disulfoton	T60.0X1	T60.0X2	T60.0X3	T60.0X4	—	—
Dithiazanine iodide	T37.4X1	T37.4X2	T37.4X3	T37.4X4	T37.4X5	T37.4X6
Dithiocarbamate	T60.0X1	T60.0X2	T60.0X3	T60.0X4	—	—
Dithranol	T49.4X1	T49.4X2	T49.4X3	T49.4X4	T49.4X5	T49.4X6
Diucardin	T50.2X1	T50.2X2	T50.2X3	T50.2X4	T50.2X5	T50.2X6
Diupres	T50.2X1	T50.2X2	T50.2X3	T50.2X4	T50.2X5	T50.2X6
Diuretic NEC	T50.2X1	T50.2X2	T50.2X3	T50.2X4	T50.2X5	T50.2X6
benzothiadiazine	T50.2X1	T50.2X2	T50.2X3	T50.2X4	T50.2X5	T50.2X6
carbonic acid anhydrase inhibitors	T50.2X1	T50.2X2	T50.2X3	T50.2X4	T50.2X5	T50.2X6
furfuryl NEC	T50.2X1	T50.2X2	T50.2X3	T50.2X4	T50.2X5	T50.2X6
loop (high-ceiling)	T50.1X1	T50.1X2	T50.1X3	T50.1X4	T50.1X5	T50.1X6
mercurial NEC	T50.2X1	T50.2X2	T50.2X3	T50.2X4	T50.2X5	T50.2X6
osmotic	T50.2X1	T50.2X2	T50.2X3	T50.2X4	T50.2X5	T50.2X6
purine NEC	T50.2X1	T50.2X2	T50.2X3	T50.2X4	T50.2X5	T50.2X6
saluretic NEC	T50.2X1	T50.2X2	T50.2X3	T50.2X4	T50.2X5	T50.2X6
sulfonamide	T50.2X1	T50.2X2	T50.2X3	T50.2X4	T50.2X5	T50.2X6
thiazide NEC	T50.2X1	T50.2X2	T50.2X3	T50.2X4	T50.2X5	T50.2X6
xanthine	T50.2X1	T50.2X2	T50.2X3	T50.2X4	T50.2X5	T50.2X6
Diurgin	T50.2X1	T50.2X2	T50.2X3	T50.2X4	T50.2X5	T50.2X6
Diuril	T50.2X1	T50.2X2	T50.2X3	T50.2X4	T50.2X5	T50.2X6
Diuron	T60.3X1	T60.3X2	T60.3X3	T60.3X4	—	—
Divalproex	T42.6X1	T42.6X2	T42.6X3	T42.6X4	T42.6X5	T42.6X6
Divinyl ether	T41.0X1	T41.0X2	T41.0X3	T41.0X4	T41.0X5	T41.0X6
Dixanthogen	T49.0X1	T49.0X2	T49.0X3	T49.0X4	T49.0X5	T49.0X6
Dixyrazine	T43.3X1	T43.3X2	T43.3X3	T43.3X4	T43.3X5	T43.3X6
D-lysergic acid diethylamide	T40.8X1	T40.8X2	T40.8X3	T40.8X4	—	—
DMCT	T36.4X1	T36.4X2	T36.4X3	T36.4X4	T36.4X5	T36.4X6
DMSO — see Dimethyl sulfoxide						
DNBP	T60.3X1	T60.3X2	T60.3X3	T60.3X4	—	—
DNOC	T65.3X1	T65.3X2	T65.3X3	T65.3X4	—	—
Dobutamine	T44.5X1	T44.5X2	T44.5X3	T44.5X4	T44.5X5	T44.5X6
DOCA	T38.0X1	T38.0X2	T38.0X3	T38.0X4	T38.0X5	T38.0X6
Docusate sodium	T47.4X1	T47.4X2	T47.4X3	T47.4X4	T47.4X5	T47.4X6
Dodicin	T49.0X1	T49.0X2	T49.0X3	T49.0X4	T49.0X5	T49.0X6
Dofamium chloride	T49.0X1	T49.0X2	T49.0X3	T49.0X4	T49.0X5	T49.0X6
Dolophine	T40.3X1	T40.3X2	T40.3X3	T40.3X4	T40.3X5	T40.3X6
Doloxene	T39.8X1	T39.8X2	T39.8X3	T39.8X4	T39.8X5	T39.8X6
Domestic gas (after combustion) — see Gas, utility						
prior to combustion	T59.891	T59.892	T59.893	T59.894	—	—
Domiodol	T48.4X1	T48.4X2	T48.4X3	T48.4X4	T48.4X5	T48.4X6
Domiphen (bromide)	T49.0X1	T49.0X2	T49.0X3	T49.0X4	T49.0X5	T49.0X6
Domperidone	T45.0X1	T45.0X2	T45.0X3	T45.0X4	T45.0X5	T45.0X6

Substance	Poisoning, Accidental (unintentional)	Poisoning, Intentional Self-harm	Poisoning, Assault	Poisoning, Undetermined	Adverse Effect	Under-dosing
Dopa	T42.8X1	T42.8X2	T42.8X3	T42.8X4	T42.8X5	T42.8X6
Dopamine	T44.991	T44.992	T44.993	T44.994	T44.995	T44.996
Doriden	T42.6X1	T42.6X2	T42.6X3	T42.6X4	T42.6X5	T42.6X6
Dormiral	T42.3X1	T42.3X2	T42.3X3	T42.3X4	T42.3X5	T42.3X6
Dormison	T42.6X1	T42.6X2	T42.6X3	T42.6X4	T42.6X5	T42.6X6
Dornase	T48.4X1	T48.4X2	T48.4X3	T48.4X4	T48.4X5	T48.4X6
Dorsacaine	T41.3X1	T41.3X2	T41.3X3	T41.3X4	T41.3X5	T41.3X6
Dosulepin	T43.011	T43.012	T43.013	T43.014	T43.015	T43.016
Dothiepin	T43.011	T43.012	T43.013	T43.014	T43.015	T43.016
Doxantrazole	T48.6X1	T48.6X2	T48.6X3	T48.6X4	T48.6X5	T48.6X6
Doxapram	T50.7X1	T50.7X2	T50.7X3	T50.7X4	T50.7X5	T50.7X6
Doxazosin	T44.6X1	T44.6X2	T44.6X3	T44.6X4	T44.6X5	T44.6X6
Doxepin	T43.011	T43.012	T43.013	T43.014	T43.015	T43.016
Doxifluridine	T45.1X1	T45.1X2	T45.1X3	T45.1X4	T45.1X5	T45.1X6
Doxorubicin	T45.1X1	T45.1X2	T45.1X3	T45.1X4	T45.1X5	T45.1X6
Doxycycline	T36.4X1	T36.4X2	T36.4X3	T36.4X4	T36.4X5	T36.4X6
Doxylamine	T45.0X1	T45.0X2	T45.0X3	T45.0X4	T45.0X5	T45.0X6
Dramamine	T45.0X1	T45.0X2	T45.0X3	T45.0X4	T45.0X5	T45.0X6
Drano (drain cleaner)	T54.3X1	T54.3X2	T54.3X3	T54.3X4		
Dressing, live pulp	T49.7X1	T49.7X2	T49.7X3	T49.7X4	T49.7X5	T49.7X6
Drocode	T40.2X1	T40.2X2	T40.2X3	T40.2X4	T40.2X5	T40.2X6
Dromoran	T40.2X1	T40.2X2	T40.2X3	T40.2X4	T40.2X5	T40.2X6
Dromostanolone	T38.7X1	T38.7X2	T38.7X3	T38.7X4	T38.7X5	T38.7X6
Dronabinol	T40.7X1	T40.7X2	T40.7X3	T40.7X4	T40.7X5	T40.7X6
Droperidol	T43.591	T43.592	T43.593	T43.594	T43.595	T43.596
Dropropizine	T48.3X1	T48.3X2	T48.3X3	T48.3X4	T48.3X5	T48.3X6
Drostanolone	T38.7X1	T38.7X2	T38.7X3	T38.7X4	T38.7X5	T38.7X6
Drotaverine	T44.3X1	T44.3X2	T44.3X3	T44.3X4	T44.3X5	T44.3X6
Drotrecogin alfa	T45.511	T45.512	T45.513	T45.514	T45.515	T45.516
Drug NEC	T50.901	T50.902	T50.903	T50.904	T50.905	T50.906
specified NEC	T50.991	T50.992	T50.993	T50.994	T50.995	T50.996
DTIC	T45.1X1	T45.1X2	T45.1X3	T45.1X4	T45.1X5	T45.1X6
Duboisine	T44.3X1	T44.3X2	T44.3X3	T44.3X4	T44.3X5	T44.3X6
Dulcolax	T47.2X1	T47.2X2	T47.2X3	T47.2X4	T47.2X5	T47.2X6
Duponol (C) (EP)	T49.2X1	T49.2X2	T49.2X3	T49.2X4	T49.2X5	T49.2X6
Durabolin	T38.7X1	T38.7X2	T38.7X3	T38.7X4	T38.7X5	T38.7X6
Dyclone	T41.3X1	T41.3X2	T41.3X3	T41.3X4	T41.3X5	T41.3X6
Dyclonine	T41.3X1	T41.3X2	T41.3X3	T41.3X4	T41.3X5	T41.3X6
Dydrogesterone	T38.5X1	T38.5X2	T38.5X3	T38.5X4	T38.5X5	T38.5X6
Dye NEC	T65.6X1	T65.6X2	T65.6X3	T65.6X4	—	—
antiseptic	T49.0X1	T49.0X2	T49.0X3	T49.0X4	T49.0X5	T49.0X6
diagnostic agents	T50.8X1	T50.8X2	T50.8X3	T50.8X4	T50.8X5	T50.8X6
pharmaceutical NEC	T50.901	T50.902	T50.903	T50.904	T50.905	T50.906
Dyflos	T44.0X1	T44.0X2	T44.0X3	T44.0X4	T44.0X5	T44.0X6
Dymelor	T38.3X1	T38.3X2	T38.3X3	T38.3X4	T38.3X5	T38.3X6
Dynamite	T65.3X1	T65.3X2	T65.3X3	T65.3X4	—	—
fumes	T59.891	T59.892	T59.893	T59.894	—	—
Dyphylline	T44.3X1	T44.3X2	T44.3X3	T44.3X4	T44.3X5	T44.3X6
b-eucaine	T49.1X1	T49.1X2	T49.1X3	T49.1X4	T49.1X5	T49.1X6
Ear drug NEC	T49.6X1	T49.6X2	T49.6X3	T49.6X4	T49.6X5	T49.6X6
Ear preparations	T49.6X1	T49.6X2	T49.6X3	T49.6X4	T49.6X5	T49.6X6
Echothiophate, echothiopate, ecothiopate	T49.5X1	T49.5X2	T49.5X3	T49.5X4	T49.5X5	T49.5X6
Econazole	T49.0X1	T49.0X2	T49.0X3	T49.0X4	T49.0X5	T49.0X6
Ecothiopate iodide	T49.5X1	T49.5X2	T49.5X3	T49.5X4	T49.5X5	T49.5X6
Ecstasy	T43.641	T43.642	T43.643	T43.644	—	—
Ectylurea	T42.6X1	T42.6X2	T42.6X3	T42.6X4	T42.6X5	T42.6X6
Edathamil disodium	T45.8X1	T45.8X2	T45.8X3	T45.8X4	T45.8X5	T45.8X6
Edecrin	T50.1X1	T50.1X2	T50.1X3	T50.1X4	T50.1X5	T50.1X6
Edetate, disodium (calcium)	T45.8X1	T45.8X2	T45.8X3	T45.8X4	T45.8X5	T45.8X6
Edoxudine	T49.5X1	T49.5X2	T49.5X3	T49.5X4	T49.5X5	T49.5X6
Edrophonium	T44.0X1	T44.0X2	T44.0X3	T44.0X4	T44.0X5	T44.0X6
chloride	T44.0X1	T44.0X2	T44.0X3	T44.0X4	T44.0X5	T44.0X6
EDTA	T50.6X1	T50.6X2	T50.6X3	T50.6X4	T50.6X5	T50.6X6
Eflornithine	T37.2X1	T37.2X2	T37.2X3	T37.2X4	T37.2X5	T37.2X6
Efloxate	T46.3X1	T46.3X2	T46.3X3	T46.3X4	T46.3X5	T46.3X6
Elase	T49.8X1	T49.8X2	T49.8X3	T49.8X4	T49.8X5	T49.8X6
Elastase	T47.5X1	T47.5X2	T47.5X3	T47.5X4	T47.5X5	T47.5X6
Elaterium	T47.2X1	T47.2X2	T47.2X3	T47.2X4	T47.2X5	T47.2X6
Elcatonin	T50.991	T50.992	T50.993	T50.994	T50.995	T50.996
Elder	T62.2X1	T62.2X2	T62.2X3	T62.2X4	—	—
berry, (unripe)	T62.1X1	T62.1X2	T62.1X3	T62.1X4	—	—
Electrolyte balance drug	T50.3X1	T50.3X2	T50.3X3	T50.3X4	T50.3X5	T50.3X6
Electrolytes NEC	T50.3X1	T50.3X2	T50.3X3	T50.3X4	T50.3X5	T50.3X6
Electrolytic agent NEC	T50.3X1	T50.3X2	T50.3X3	T50.3X4	T50.3X5	T50.3X6
Elemental diet	T50.901	T50.902	T50.903	T50.904	T50.905	T50.906
Elliptinium acetate	T45.1X1	T45.1X2	T45.1X3	T45.1X4	T45.1X5	T45.1X6
Embramine	T45.0X1	T45.0X2	T45.0X3	T45.0X4	T45.0X5	T45.0X6
Emepronium (salts)	T44.3X1	T44.3X2	T44.3X3	T44.3X4	T44.3X5	T44.3X6
bromide	T44.3X1	T44.3X2	T44.3X3	T44.3X4	T44.3X5	T44.3X6
Emetic NEC	T47.7X1	T47.7X2	T47.7X3	T47.7X4	T47.7X5	T47.7X6
Emetine	T37.3X1	T37.3X2	T37.3X3	T37.3X4	T37.3X5	T37.3X6
Emollient NEC	T49.3X1	T49.3X2	T49.3X3	T49.3X4	T49.3X5	T49.3X6
Emorfazone	T39.8X1	T39.8X2	T39.8X3	T39.8X4	T39.8X5	T39.8X6
Emylcamate	T43.591	T43.592	T43.593	T43.594	T43.595	T43.596
Enalapril	T46.4X1	T46.4X2	T46.4X3	T46.4X4	T46.4X5	T46.4X6
Enalaprilat	T46.4X1	T46.4X2	T46.4X3	T46.4X4	T46.4X5	T46.4X6
Encainide	T46.2X1	T46.2X2	T46.2X3	T46.2X4	T46.2X5	T46.2X6
Endocaine	T41.3X1	T41.3X2	T41.3X3	T41.3X4	T41.3X5	T41.3X6
Endosulfan	T60.2X1	T60.2X2	T60.2X3	T60.2X4		
Endothall	T60.3X1	T60.3X2	T60.3X3	T60.3X4	—	—
Endralazine	T46.5X1	T46.5X2	T46.5X3	T46.5X4	T46.5X5	T46.5X6
Endrin	T60.1X1	T60.1X2	T60.1X3	T60.1X4	—	—
Enflurane	T41.0X1	T41.0X2	T41.0X3	T41.0X4	T41.0X5	T41.0X6
Enhexymal	T42.3X1	T42.3X2	T42.3X3	T42.3X4	T42.3X5	T42.3X6
Enocitabine	T45.1X1	T45.1X2	T45.1X3	T45.1X4	T45.1X5	T45.1X6
Enovid	T38.4X1	T38.4X2	T38.4X3	T38.4X4	T38.4X5	T38.4X6
Enoxacin	T36.8X1	T36.8X2	T36.8X3	T36.8X4	T36.8X5	T36.8X6
Enoxaparin (sodium)	T45.511	T45.512	T45.513	T45.514	T45.515	T45.516
Enpiprazole	T43.591	T43.592	T43.593	T43.594	T43.595	T43.596
Enprofylline	T48.6X1	T48.6X2	T48.6X3	T48.6X4	T48.6X5	T48.6X6
Enprostil	T47.1X1	T47.1X2	T47.1X3	T47.1X4	T47.1X5	T47.1X6
Enterogastrone	T38.891	T38.892	T38.893	T38.894	T38.895	T38.896
ENT preparations (anti-infectives)	T49.6X1	T49.6X2	T49.6X3	T49.6X4	T49.6X5	T49.6X6
Enviomycin	T36.8X1	T36.8X2	T36.8X3	T36.8X4	T36.8X5	T36.8X6
Enzodase	T45.3X1	T45.3X2	T45.3X3	T45.3X4	T45.3X5	T45.3X6
Enzyme NEC	T45.3X1	T45.3X2	T45.3X3	T45.3X4	T45.3X5	T45.3X6
depolymerizing	T49.8X1	T49.8X2	T49.8X3	T49.8X4	T49.8X5	T49.8X6
fibrolytic	T45.3X1	T45.3X2	T45.3X3	T45.3X4	T45.3X5	T45.3X6
gastric	T47.5X1	T47.5X2	T47.5X3	T47.5X4	T47.5X5	T47.5X6
intestinal	T47.5X1	T47.5X2	T47.5X3	T47.5X4	T47.5X5	T47.5X6
local action	T49.4X1	T49.4X2	T49.4X3	T49.4X4	T49.4X5	T49.4X6
proteolytic	T49.4X1	T49.4X2	T49.4X3	T49.4X4	T49.4X5	T49.4X6
thrombolytic	T45.3X1	T45.3X2	T45.3X3	T45.3X4	T45.3X5	T45.3X6
EPAB	T41.3X1	T41.3X2	T41.3X3	T41.3X4	T41.3X5	T41.3X6
Epanutin	T42.0X1	T42.0X2	T42.0X3	T42.0X4	T42.0X5	T42.0X6
Ephedra	T44.991	T44.992	T44.993	T44.994	T44.995	T44.996
Ephedrine	T44.991	T44.992	T44.993	T44.994	T44.995	T44.996
Epichlorhydrin, epichlorohydrin	T52.8X1	T52.8X2	T52.8X3	T52.8X4		
Epicillin	T36.0X1	T36.0X2	T36.0X3	T36.0X4	T36.0X5	T36.0X6
Epiestriol	T38.5X1	T38.5X2	T38.5X3	T38.5X4	T38.5X5	T38.5X6
Epilim — *see* Sodium valproate						
Epimestrol	T38.5X1	T38.5X2	T38.5X3	T38.5X4	T38.5X5	T38.5X6
Epinephrine	T44.5X1	T44.5X2	T44.5X3	T44.5X4	T44.5X5	T44.5X6
Epirubicin	T45.1X1	T45.1X2	T45.1X3	T45.1X4	T45.1X5	T45.1X6
Epitiostanol	T38.7X1	T38.7X2	T38.7X3	T38.7X4	T38.7X5	T38.7X6
Epitizide	T50.2X1	T50.2X2	T50.2X3	T50.2X4	T50.2X5	T50.2X6
EPN	T60.0X1	T60.0X2	T60.0X3	T60.0X4	—	—
EPO	T45.8X1	T45.8X2	T45.8X3	T45.8X4	T45.8X5	T45.8X6
Epoetin alpha	T45.8X1	T45.8X2	T45.8X3	T45.8X4	T45.8X5	T45.8X6
Epomediol	T50.991	T50.992	T50.993	T50.994	T50.995	T50.996
Epoprostenol	T45.521	T45.522	T45.523	T45.524	T45.525	T45.526
Epoxy resin	T65.891	T65.892	T65.893	T65.894	—	—
Eprazinone	T48.4X1	T48.4X2	T48.4X3	T48.4X4	T48.4X5	T48.4X6
Epsilon aminocaproic acid	T45.621	T45.622	T45.623	T45.624	T45.625	T45.626
Epsom salt	T47.3X1	T47.3X2	T47.3X3	T47.3X4	T47.3X5	T47.3X6
Eptazocine	T40.4X1	T40.4X2	T40.4X3	T40.4X4	T40.4X5	T40.4X6
Equanil	T43.591	T43.592	T43.593	T43.594	T43.595	T43.596
Equisetum	T62.2X1	T62.2X2	T62.2X3	T62.2X4	—	—
diuretic	T50.2X1	T50.2X2	T50.2X3	T50.2X4	T50.2X5	T50.2X6
Ergobasine	T48.0X1	T48.0X2	T48.0X3	T48.0X4	T48.0X5	T48.0X6
Ergocalciferol	T45.2X1	T45.2X2	T45.2X3	T45.2X4	T45.2X5	T45.2X6
Ergoloid mesylates	T46.7X1	T46.7X2	T46.7X3	T46.7X4	T46.7X5	T46.7X6
Ergometrine	T48.0X1	T48.0X2	T48.0X3	T48.0X4	T48.0X5	T48.0X6
Ergonovine	T48.0X1	T48.0X2	T48.0X3	T48.0X4	T48.0X5	T48.0X6
Ergotamine	T46.5X1	T46.5X2	T46.5X3	T46.5X4	T46.5X5	T46.5X6
Ergotocine	T48.0X1	T48.0X2	T48.0X3	T48.0X4	T48.0X5	T48.0X6
Ergotrate	T48.0X1	T48.0X2	T48.0X3	T48.0X4	T48.0X5	T48.0X6
Ergot NEC	T64.81	T64.82	T64.83	T64.84	—	—
derivative	T48.0X1	T48.0X2	T48.0X3	T48.0X4	T48.0X5	T48.0X6
medicinal (alkaloids)	T48.0X1	T48.0X2	T48.0X3	T48.0X4	T48.0X5	T48.0X6
prepared	T48.0X1	T48.0X2	T48.0X3	T48.0X4	T48.0X5	T48.0X6
Eritrityl tetranitrate	T46.3X1	T46.3X2	T46.3X3	T46.3X4	T46.3X5	T46.3X6
Erythrityl tetranitrate	T46.3X1	T46.3X2	T46.3X3	T46.3X4	T46.3X5	T46.3X6
Erythrol tetranitrate	T46.3X1	T46.3X2	T46.3X3	T46.3X4	T46.3X5	T46.3X6
Erythromycin (salts)	T36.3X1	T36.3X2	T36.3X3	T36.3X4	T36.3X5	T36.3X6
ophthalmic preparation	T49.5X1	T49.5X2	T49.5X3	T49.5X4	T49.5X5	T49.5X6
topical NEC	T49.0X1	T49.0X2	T49.0X3	T49.0X4	T49.0X5	T49.0X6
Erythropoietin	T45.8X1	T45.8X2	T45.8X3	T45.8X4	T45.8X5	T45.8X6
human	T45.8X1	T45.8X2	T45.8X3	T45.8X4	T45.8X5	T45.8X6
Escin	T46.991	T46.992	T46.993	T46.994	T46.995	T46.996
Esculin	T45.2X1	T45.2X2	T45.2X3	T45.2X4	T45.2X5	T45.2X6
Esculoside	T45.2X1	T45.2X2	T45.2X3	T45.2X4	T45.2X5	T45.2X6

Substance	Poisoning, Accidental (unintentional)	Poisoning, Intentional Self-harm	Poisoning, Assault	Poisoning, Undetermined	Adverse Effect	Under-dosing
ESDT (ether-soluble tar distillate)	T49.1X1	T49.1X2	T49.1X3	T49.1X4	T49.1X5	T49.1X6
Eserine	T49.5X1	T49.5X2	T49.5X3	T49.5X4	T49.5X5	T49.5X6
Esflurbiprofen	T39.311	T39.312	T39.313	T39.314	T39.315	T39.316
Eskabarb	T42.3X1	T42.3X2	T42.3X3	T42.3X4	T42.3X5	T42.3X6
Eskalith	T43.8X1	T43.8X2	T43.8X3	T43.8X4	T43.8X5	T43.8X6
Esmolol	T44.7X1	T44.7X2	T44.7X3	T44.7X4	T44.7X5	T44.7X6
Estanozolol	T38.7X1	T38.7X2	T38.7X3	T38.7X4	T38.7X5	T38.7X6
Estazolam	T42.4X1	T42.4X2	T42.4X3	T42.4X4	T42.4X5	T42.4X6
Estradiol	T38.5X1	T38.5X2	T38.5X3	T38.5X4	T38.5X5	T38.5X6
with testosterone	T38.7X1	T38.7X2	T38.7X3	T38.7X4	T38.7X5	T38.7X6
benzoate	T38.5X1	T38.5X2	T38.5X3	T38.5X4	T38.5X5	T38.5X6
Estramustine	T45.1X1	T45.1X2	T45.1X3	T45.1X4	T45.1X5	T45.1X6
Estriol	T38.5X1	T38.5X2	T38.5X3	T38.5X4	T38.5X5	T38.5X6
Estrogen	T38.5X1	T38.5X2	T38.5X3	T38.5X4	T38.5X5	T38.5X6
with progesterone	T38.5X1	T38.5X2	T38.5X3	T38.5X4	T38.5X5	T38.5X6
conjugated	T38.5X1	T38.5X2	T38.5X3	T38.5X4	T38.5X5	T38.5X6
Estrone	T38.5X1	T38.5X2	T38.5X3	T38.5X4	T38.5X5	T38.5X6
Estropipate	T38.5X1	T38.5X2	T38.5X3	T38.5X4	T38.5X5	T38.5X6
Etacrynate sodium	T50.1X1	T50.1X2	T50.1X3	T50.1X4	T50.1X5	T50.1X6
Etacrynic acid	T50.1X1	T50.1X2	T50.1X3	T50.1X4	T50.1X5	T50.1X6
Etafedrine	T48.6X1	T48.6X2	T48.6X3	T48.6X4	T48.6X5	T48.6X6
Etafenone	T46.3X1	T46.3X2	T46.3X3	T46.3X4	T46.3X5	T46.3X6
Etambutol	T37.1X1	T37.1X2	T37.1X3	T37.1X4	T37.1X5	T37.1X6
Etamiphyllin	T48.6X1	T48.6X2	T48.6X3	T48.6X4	T48.6X5	T48.6X6
Etamivan	T50.7X1	T50.7X2	T50.7X3	T50.7X4	T50.7X5	T50.7X6
Etamsylate	T45.7X1	T45.7X2	T45.7X3	T45.7X4	T45.7X5	T45.7X6
Etebenecid	T50.4X1	T50.4X2	T50.4X3	T50.4X4	T50.4X5	T50.4X6
Ethacridine	T49.0X1	T49.0X2	T49.0X3	T49.0X4	T49.0X5	T49.0X6
Ethacrynic acid	T50.1X1	T50.1X2	T50.1X3	T50.1X4	T50.1X5	T50.1X6
Ethadione	T42.2X1	T42.2X2	T42.2X3	T42.2X4	T42.2X5	T42.2X6
Ethambutol	T37.1X1	T37.1X2	T37.1X3	T37.1X4	T37.1X5	T37.1X6
Ethamide	T50.2X1	T50.2X2	T50.2X3	T50.2X4	T50.2X5	T50.2X6
Ethamivan	T50.7X1	T50.7X2	T50.7X3	T50.7X4	T50.7X5	T50.7X6
Ethamsylate	T45.7X1	T45.7X2	T45.7X3	T45.7X4	T45.7X5	T45.7X6
Ethanol	T51.0X1	T51.0X2	T51.0X3	T51.0X4	—	—
beverage	T51.0X1	T51.0X2	T51.0X3	T51.0X4	—	—
Ethanolamine oleate	T46.8X1	T46.8X2	T46.8X3	T46.8X4	T46.8X5	T46.8X6
Ethaverine	T44.3X1	T44.3X2	T44.3X3	T44.3X4	T44.3X5	T44.3X6
Ethchlorvynol	T42.6X1	T42.6X2	T42.6X3	T42.6X4	T42.6X5	T42.6X6
Ethebenecid	T50.4X1	T50.4X2	T50.4X3	T50.4X4	T50.4X5	T50.4X6
Ether (vapor)	T41.0X1	T41.0X2	T41.0X3	T41.0X4	T41.0X5	T41.0X6
anesthetic	T41.0X1	T41.0X2	T41.0X3	T41.0X4	T41.0X5	T41.0X6
divinyl	T41.0X1	T41.0X2	T41.0X3	T41.0X4	T41.0X5	T41.0X6
ethyl (medicinal)	T41.0X1	T41.0X2	T41.0X3	T41.0X4	T41.0X5	T41.0X6
nonmedicinal	T52.8X1	T52.8X2	T52.8X3	T52.8X4		
petroleum — see Ligroin						
solvent	T52.8X1	T52.8X2	T52.8X3	T52.8X4	—	—
Ethiazide	T50.2X1	T50.2X2	T50.2X3	T50.2X4	T50.2X5	T50.2X6
Ethidium chloride (vapor)	T59.891	T59.892	T59.893	T59.894		
Ethinamate	T42.6X1	T42.6X2	T42.6X3	T42.6X4	T42.6X5	T42.6X6
Ethinylestradiol, ethinyloestradiol	T38.5X1	T38.5X2	T38.5X3	T38.5X4	T38.5X5	T38.5X6
with						
levonorgestrel	T38.4X1	T38.4X2	T38.4X3	T38.4X4	T38.4X5	T38.4X6
norethisterone	T38.4X1	T38.4X2	T38.4X3	T38.4X4	T38.4X5	T38.4X6
Ethiodized oil (131 I)	T50.8X1	T50.8X2	T50.8X3	T50.8X4	T50.8X5	T50.8X6
Ethion	T60.0X1	T60.0X2	T60.0X3	T60.0X4	—	—
Ethionamide	T37.1X1	T37.1X2	T37.1X3	T37.1X4	T37.1X5	T37.1X6
Ethioniamide	T37.1X1	T37.1X2	T37.1X3	T37.1X4	T37.1X5	T37.1X6
Ethisterone	T38.5X1	T38.5X2	T38.5X3	T38.5X4	T38.5X5	T38.5X6
Ethobral	T42.3X1	T42.3X2	T42.3X3	T42.3X4	T42.3X5	T42.3X6
Ethocaine (infiltration) (topical)	T41.3X1	T41.3X2	T41.3X3	T41.3X4	T41.3X5	T41.3X6
nerve block (peripheral) (plexus)	T41.3X1	T41.3X2	T41.3X3	T41.3X4	T41.3X5	T41.3X6
spinal	T41.3X1	T41.3X2	T41.3X3	T41.3X4	T41.3X5	T41.3X6
Ethoheptazine	T40.4X1	T40.4X2	T40.4X3	T40.4X4	T40.4X5	T40.4X6
Ethopropazine	T44.3X1	T44.3X2	T44.3X3	T44.3X4	T44.3X5	T44.3X6
Ethosuximide	T42.2X1	T42.2X2	T42.2X3	T42.2X4	T42.2X5	T42.2X6
Ethotoin	T42.0X1	T42.0X2	T42.0X3	T42.0X4	T42.0X5	T42.0X6
Ethoxazene	T37.91	T37.92	T37.93	T37.94	T37.95	T37.96
Ethoxazorutoside	T46.991	T46.992	T46.993	T46.994	T46.995	T46.996
Ethoxzolamide	T50.2X1	T50.2X2	T50.2X3	T50.2X4	T50.2X5	T50.2X6
Ethyl						
acetate	T52.8X1	T52.8X2	T52.8X3	T52.8X4	—	—
alcohol	T51.0X1	T51.0X2	T51.0X3	T51.0X4	—	—
beverage	T51.0X1	T51.0X2	T51.0X3	T51.0X4	—	—
aldehyde (vapor)	T59.891	T59.892	T59.893	T59.894		
liquid	T52.8X1	T52.8X2	T52.8X3	T52.8X4	—	—
aminobenzoate	T41.3X1	T41.3X2	T41.3X3	T41.3X4	T41.3X5	T41.3X6
aminophenothiazine	T43.3X1	T43.3X2	T43.3X3	T43.3X4	T43.3X5	T43.3X6
benzoate	T52.8X1	T52.8X2	T52.8X3	T52.8X4	—	—

Substance	Poisoning, Accidental (unintentional)	Poisoning, Intentional Self-harm	Poisoning, Assault	Poisoning, Undetermined	Adverse Effect	Under-dosing
Ethyl — continued						
biscoumacetate	T45.511	T45.512	T45.513	T45.514	T45.515	T45.516
bromide (anesthetic)	T41.0X1	T41.0X2	T41.0X3	T41.0X4	T41.0X5	T41.0X6
carbamate	T45.1X1	T45.1X2	T45.1X3	T45.1X4	T45.1X5	T45.1X6
carbinol	T51.3X1	T51.3X2	T51.3X3	T51.3X4	—	—
carbonate	T52.8X1	T52.8X2	T52.8X3	T52.8X4	—	—
chaulmoograte	T37.1X1	T37.1X2	T37.1X3	T37.1X4	T37.1X5	T37.1X6
chloride (anesthetic)	T41.0X1	T41.0X2	T41.0X3	T41.0X4	T41.0X5	T41.0X6
anesthetic (local)	T41.3X1	T41.3X2	T41.3X3	T41.3X4	T41.3X5	T41.3X6
inhaled	T41.0X1	T41.0X2	T41.0X3	T41.0X4	T41.0X5	T41.0X6
local	T49.4X1	T49.4X2	T49.4X3	T49.4X4	T49.4X5	T49.4X6
solvent	T53.6X1	T53.6X2	T53.6X3	T53.6X4	—	—
dibunate	T48.3X1	T48.3X2	T48.3X3	T48.3X4	T48.3X5	T48.3X6
dichloroarsine (vapor)	T57.0X1	T57.0X2	T57.0X3	T57.0X4	—	—
estranol	T38.7X1	T38.7X2	T38.7X3	T38.7X4	T38.7X5	T38.7X6
ether — see also ether						
formate NEC (solvent)	T52.0X1	T52.0X2	T52.0X3	T52.0X4	—	—
fumarate	T49.4X1	T49.4X2	T49.4X3	T49.4X4	T49.4X5	T49.4X6
hydroxyisobutyrate NEC (solvent)	T52.8X1	T52.8X2	T52.8X3	T52.8X4	—	—
iodoacetate	T59.3X1	T59.3X2	T59.3X3	T59.3X4	—	—
lactate NEC (solvent)	T52.8X1	T52.8X2	T52.8X3	T52.8X4	—	—
loflazepate	T42.4X1	T42.4X2	T42.4X3	T42.4X4	T42.4X5	T42.4X6
mercuric chloride	T56.1X1	T56.1X2	T56.1X3	T56.1X4	—	—
methylcarbinol	T51.8X1	T51.8X2	T51.8X3	T51.8X4	—	—
morphine	T40.2X1	T40.2X2	T40.2X3	T40.2X4	T40.2X5	T40.2X6
noradrenaline	T48.6X1	T48.6X2	T48.6X3	T48.6X4	T48.6X5	T48.6X6
oxybutyrate NEC (solvent)	T52.8X1	T52.8X2	T52.8X3	T52.8X4	—	—
Ethylene (gas)	T59.891	T59.892	T59.893	T59.894		
anesthetic (general)	T41.0X1	T41.0X2	T41.0X3	T41.0X4	T41.0X5	T41.0X6
chlorohydrin	T52.8X1	T52.8X2	T52.8X3	T52.8X4	—	—
vapor	T53.6X1	T53.6X2	T53.6X3	T53.6X4	—	—
dichloride	T52.8X1	T52.8X2	T52.8X3	T52.8X4	—	—
vapor	T53.6X1	T53.6X2	T53.6X3	T53.6X4	—	—
dinitrate	T52.3X1	T52.3X2	T52.3X3	T52.3X4	—	—
glycol(s)	T52.8X1	T52.8X2	T52.8X3	T52.8X4	—	—
dinitrate	T52.3X1	T52.3X2	T52.3X3	T52.3X4	—	—
monobutyl ether	T52.3X1	T52.3X2	T52.3X3	T52.3X4	—	—
imine	T54.1X1	T54.1X2	T54.1X3	T54.1X4	—	—
oxide (fumigant) (nonmedicinal)	T59.891	T59.892	T59.893	T59.894		
medicinal	T49.0X1	T49.0X2	T49.0X3	T49.0X4	T49.0X5	T49.0X6
Ethylenediaminetetra-acetic acid	T50.6X1	T50.6X2	T50.6X3	T50.6X4	T50.6X5	T50.6X6
Ethylenediamine theophylline	T48.6X1	T48.6X2	T48.6X3	T48.6X4	T48.6X5	T48.6X6
Ethylenedinitrilotetra-acetate	T50.6X1	T50.6X2	T50.6X3	T50.6X4	T50.6X5	T50.6X6
Ethylestrenol	T38.7X1	T38.7X2	T38.7X3	T38.7X4	T38.7X5	T38.7X6
Ethylhydroxycellulose	T47.4X1	T47.4X2	T47.4X3	T47.4X4	T47.4X5	T47.4X6
Ethylidene						
chloride NEC	T53.6X1	T53.6X2	T53.6X3	T53.6X4	—	—
diacetate	T60.3X1	T60.3X2	T60.3X3	T60.3X4	—	—
dicoumarin	T45.511	T45.512	T45.513	T45.514	T45.515	T45.516
dicoumarol	T45.511	T45.512	T45.513	T45.514	T45.515	T45.516
diethyl ether	T52.0X1	T52.0X2	T52.0X3	T52.0X4	—	—
Ethylmorphine	T40.2X1	T40.2X2	T40.2X3	T40.2X4	T40.2X5	T40.2X6
Ethylnorepinephrine	T48.6X1	T48.6X2	T48.6X3	T48.6X4	T48.6X5	T48.6X6
Ethylparachlorophen-oxyisobutyrate	T46.6X1	T46.6X2	T46.6X3	T46.6X4	T46.6X5	T46.6X6
Ethynodiol	T38.4X1	T38.4X2	T38.4X3	T38.4X4	T38.4X5	T38.4X6
with mestranol diacetate	T38.4X1	T38.4X2	T38.4X3	T38.4X4	T38.4X5	T38.4X6
Etidocaine	T41.3X1	T41.3X2	T41.3X3	T41.3X4	T41.3X5	T41.3X6
infiltration (subcutaneous)	T41.3X1	T41.3X2	T41.3X3	T41.3X4	T41.3X5	T41.3X6
nerve (peripheral) (plexus)	T41.3X1	T41.3X2	T41.3X3	T41.3X4	T41.3X5	T41.3X6
Etidronate	T50.991	T50.992	T50.993	T50.994	T50.995	T50.996
Etidronic acid (disodium salt)	T50.991	T50.992	T50.993	T50.994	T50.995	T50.996
Etifoxine	T42.6X1	T42.6X2	T42.6X3	T42.6X4	T42.6X5	T42.6X6
Etilefrine	T44.4X1	T44.4X2	T44.4X3	T44.4X4	T44.4X5	T44.4X6
Etilfen	T42.3X1	T42.3X2	T42.3X3	T42.3X4	T42.3X5	T42.3X6
Etinodiol	T38.4X1	T38.4X2	T38.4X3	T38.4X4	T38.4X5	T38.4X6
Etiroxate	T46.6X1	T46.6X2	T46.6X3	T46.6X4	T46.6X5	T46.6X6
Etizolam	T42.4X1	T42.4X2	T42.4X3	T42.4X4	T42.4X5	T42.4X6
Etodolac	T39.391	T39.392	T39.393	T39.394	T39.395	T39.396
Etofamide	T37.3X1	T37.3X2	T37.3X3	T37.3X4	T37.3X5	T37.3X6
Etofibrate	T46.6X1	T46.6X2	T46.6X3	T46.6X4	T46.6X5	T46.6X6
Etofylline	T46.7X1	T46.7X2	T46.7X3	T46.7X4	T46.7X5	T46.7X6
clofibrate	T46.6X1	T46.6X2	T46.6X3	T46.6X4	T46.6X5	T46.6X6
Etoglucid	T45.1X1	T45.1X2	T45.1X3	T45.1X4	T45.1X5	T45.1X6
Etomidate	T41.1X1	T41.1X2	T41.1X3	T41.1X4	T41.1X5	T41.1X6
Etomide	T39.8X1	T39.8X2	T39.8X3	T39.8X4	T39.8X5	T39.8X6
Etomidoline	T44.3X1	T44.3X2	T44.3X3	T44.3X4	T44.3X5	T44.3X6
Etoposide	T45.1X1	T45.1X2	T45.1X3	T45.1X4	T45.1X5	T45.1X6

Substance	Poisoning, Accidental (unintentional)	Poisoning, Intentional Self-harm	Poisoning, Assault	Poisoning, Undetermined	Adverse Effect	Under-dosing
Etorphine	T40.2X1	T40.2X2	T40.2X3	T40.2X4	T40.2X5	T40.2X6
Etoval	T42.3X1	T42.3X2	T42.3X3	T42.3X4	T42.3X5	T42.3X6
Etozolin	T50.1X1	T50.1X2	T50.1X3	T50.1X4	T50.1X5	T50.1X6
Etretinate	T50.991	T50.992	T50.993	T50.994	T50.995	T50.996
Etryptamine	T43.691	T43.692	T43.693	T43.694	T43.695	T43.696
Etybenzatropine	T44.3X1	T44.3X2	T44.3X3	T44.3X4	T44.3X5	T44.3X6
Etynodiol	T38.4X1	T38.4X2	T38.4X3	T38.4X4	T38.4X5	T38.4X6
Eucaine	T41.3X1	T41.3X2	T41.3X3	T41.3X4	T41.3X5	T41.3X6
Eucalyptus oil	T49.7X1	T49.7X2	T49.7X3	T49.7X4	T49.7X5	T49.7X6
Eucatropine	T49.5X1	T49.5X2	T49.5X3	T49.5X4	T49.5X5	T49.5X6
Eucodal	T40.2X1	T40.2X2	T40.2X3	T40.2X4	T40.2X5	T40.2X6
Euneryl	T42.3X1	T42.3X2	T42.3X3	T42.3X4	T42.3X5	T42.3X6
Euphthalmine	T44.3X1	T44.3X2	T44.3X3	T44.3X4	T44.3X5	T44.3X6
Eurax	T49.0X1	T49.0X2	T49.0X3	T49.0X4	T49.0X5	T49.0X6
Euresol	T49.4X1	T49.4X2	T49.4X3	T49.4X4	T49.4X5	T49.4X6
Euthroid	T38.1X1	T38.1X2	T38.1X3	T38.1X4	T38.1X5	T38.1X6
Evans blue	T50.8X1	T50.8X2	T50.8X3	T50.8X4	T50.8X5	T50.8X6
Evipal	T42.3X1	T42.3X2	T42.3X3	T42.3X4	T42.3X5	T42.3X6
sodium	T41.1X1	T41.1X2	T41.1X3	T41.1X4	T41.1X5	T41.1X6
Evipan	T42.3X1	T42.3X2	T42.3X3	T42.3X4	T42.3X5	T42.3X6
sodium	T41.1X1	T41.1X2	T41.1X3	T41.1X4	T41.1X5	T41.1X6
Exalamide	T49.0X1	T49.0X2	T49.0X3	T49.0X4	T49.0X5	T49.0X6
Exalgin	T39.1X1	T39.1X2	T39.1X3	T39.1X4	T39.1X5	T39.1X6
Excipients, pharmaceutical	T50.901	T50.902	T50.903	T50.904	T50.905	T50.906
Exhaust gas (engine) (motor vehicle)	T58.01	T58.02	T58.03	T58.04	—	—
Ex-Lax (phenolphthalein)	T47.2X1	T47.2X2	T47.2X3	T47.2X4	T47.2X5	T47.2X6
Expectorant NEC	T48.4X1	T48.4X2	T48.4X3	T48.4X4	T48.4X5	T48.4X6
Extended insulin zinc suspension	T38.3X1	T38.3X2	T38.3X3	T38.3X4	T38.3X5	T38.3X6
External medications (skin) (mucous membrane)	T49.91	T49.92	T49.93	T49.94	T49.95	T49.96
dental agent	T49.7X1	T49.7X2	T49.7X3	T49.7X4	T49.7X5	T49.7X6
ENT agent	T49.6X1	T49.6X2	T49.6X3	T49.6X4	T49.6X5	T49.6X6
ophthalmic preparation	T49.5X1	T49.5X2	T49.5X3	T49.5X4	T49.5X5	T49.5X6
specified NEC	T49.8X1	T49.8X2	T49.8X3	T49.8X4	T49.8X5	T49.8X6
Extrapyramidal antagonist NEC	T44.3X1	T44.3X2	T44.3X3	T44.3X4	T44.3X5	T44.3X6
Eye agents (anti-infective)	T49.5X1	T49.5X2	T49.5X3	T49.5X4	T49.5X5	T49.5X6
Eye drug NEC	T49.5X1	T49.5X2	T49.5X3	T49.5X4	T49.5X5	T49.5X6
FAC (fluorouracil + doxorubicin + cyclophosphamide)	T45.1X1	T45.1X2	T45.1X3	T45.1X4	T45.1X5	T45.1X6
Factor						
I (fibrinogen)	T45.8X1	T45.8X2	T45.8X3	T45.8X4	T45.8X5	T45.8X6
III (thromboplastin)	T45.8X1	T45.8X2	T45.8X3	T45.8X4	T45.8X5	T45.8X6
IX complex	T45.7X1	T45.7X2	T45.7X3	T45.7X4	T45.7X5	T45.7X6
human	T45.8X1	T45.8X2	T45.8X3	T45.8X4	T45.8X5	T45.8X6
VIII (antihemophilic Factor) (concentrate)	T45.8X1	T45.8X2	T45.8X3	T45.8X4	T45.8X5	T45.8X6
Famotidine	T47.0X1	T47.0X2	T47.0X3	T47.0X4	T47.0X5	T47.0X6
Fat suspension, intravenous	T50.991	T50.992	T50.993	T50.994	T50.995	T50.996
Fazadinium bromide	T48.1X1	T48.1X2	T48.1X3	T48.1X4	T48.1X5	T48.1X6
Febarbamate	T42.3X1	T42.3X2	T42.3X3	T42.3X4	T42.3X5	T42.3X6
Fecal softener	T47.4X1	T47.4X2	T47.4X3	T47.4X4	T47.4X5	T47.4X6
Fedrilate	T48.3X1	T48.3X2	T48.3X3	T48.3X4	T48.3X5	T48.3X6
Felodipine	T46.1X1	T46.1X2	T46.1X3	T46.1X4	T46.1X5	T46.1X6
Felypressin	T38.891	T38.892	T38.893	T38.894	T38.895	T38.896
Femoxetine	T43.221	T43.222	T43.223	T43.224	T43.225	T43.226
Fenalcomine	T46.3X1	T46.3X2	T46.3X3	T46.3X4	T46.3X5	T46.3X6
Fenamisal	T37.1X1	T37.1X2	T37.1X3	T37.1X4	T37.1X5	T37.1X6
Fenazone	T39.2X1	T39.2X2	T39.2X3	T39.2X4	T39.2X5	T39.2X6
Fenbendazole	T37.4X1	T37.4X2	T37.4X3	T37.4X4	T37.4X5	T37.4X6
Fenbutrazate	T50.5X1	T50.5X2	T50.5X3	T50.5X4	T50.5X5	T50.5X6
Fencamfamine	T43.691	T43.692	T43.693	T43.694	T43.695	T43.696
Fendiline	T46.1X1	T46.1X2	T46.1X3	T46.1X4	T46.1X5	T46.1X6
Fenetylline	T43.691	T43.692	T43.693	T43.694	T43.695	T43.696
Fenflumizole	T39.391	T39.392	T39.393	T39.394	T39.395	T39.396
Fenfluramine	T50.5X1	T50.5X2	T50.5X3	T50.5X4	T50.5X5	T50.5X6
Fenobarbital	T42.3X1	T42.3X2	T42.3X3	T42.3X4	T42.3X5	T42.3X6
Fenofibrate	T46.6X1	T46.6X2	T46.6X3	T46.6X4	T46.6X5	T46.6X6
Fenoprofen	T39.311	T39.312	T39.313	T39.314	T39.315	T39.316
Fenoterol	T48.6X1	T48.6X2	T48.6X3	T48.6X4	T48.6X5	T48.6X6
Fenoverine	T44.3X1	T44.3X2	T44.3X3	T44.3X4	T44.3X5	T44.3X6
Fenoxazoline	T48.5X1	T48.5X2	T48.5X3	T48.5X4	T48.5X5	T48.5X6
Fenproporex	T50.5X1	T50.5X2	T50.5X3	T50.5X4	T50.5X5	T50.5X6
Fenquizone	T50.2X1	T50.2X2	T50.2X3	T50.2X4	T50.2X5	T50.2X6
Fentanyl	T40.4X1	T40.4X2	T40.4X3	T40.4X4	T40.4X5	T40.4X6
Fentazin	T43.3X1	T43.3X2	T43.3X3	T43.3X4	T43.3X5	T43.3X6
Fenthion	T60.0X1	T60.0X2	T60.0X3	T60.0X4	—	—
Fenticlor	T49.0X1	T49.0X2	T49.0X3	T49.0X4	T49.0X5	T49.0X6
Fenylbutazone	T39.2X1	T39.2X2	T39.2X3	T39.2X4	T39.2X5	T39.2X6

Substance	Poisoning, Accidental (unintentional)	Poisoning, Intentional Self-harm	Poisoning, Assault	Poisoning, Undetermined	Adverse Effect	Under-dosing
Feprazone	T39.2X1	T39.2X2	T39.2X3	T39.2X4	T39.2X5	T39.2X6
Fer de lance (bite) (venom)	T63.061	T63.062	T63.063	T63.064	—	—
Ferric — see also Iron						
chloride	T45.4X1	T45.4X2	T45.4X3	T45.4X4	T45.4X5	T45.4X6
citrate	T45.4X1	T45.4X2	T45.4X3	T45.4X4	T45.4X5	T45.4X6
hydroxide						
colloidal	T45.4X1	T45.4X2	T45.4X3	T45.4X4	T45.4X5	T45.4X6
polymaltose	T45.4X1	T45.4X2	T45.4X3	T45.4X4	T45.4X5	T45.4X6
pyrophosphate	T45.4X1	T45.4X2	T45.4X3	T45.4X4	T45.4X5	T45.4X6
Ferritin	T45.4X1	T45.4X2	T45.4X3	T45.4X4	T45.4X5	T45.4X6
Ferrocholinate	T45.4X1	T45.4X2	T45.4X3	T45.4X4	T45.4X5	T45.4X6
Ferrodextrane	T45.4X1	T45.4X2	T45.4X3	T45.4X4	T45.4X5	T45.4X6
Ferropolimaler	T45.4X1	T45.4X2	T45.4X3	T45.4X4	T45.4X5	T45.4X6
Ferrous — see also Iron						
phosphate	T45.4X1	T45.4X2	T45.4X3	T45.4X4	T45.4X5	T45.4X6
salt	T45.4X1	T45.4X2	T45.4X3	T45.4X4	T45.4X5	T45.4X6
with folic acid	T45.4X1	T45.4X2	T45.4X3	T45.4X4	T45.4X5	T45.4X6
Ferrous fumerate, gluconate, lactate, salt NEC, sulfate (medicinal)	T45.4X1	T45.4X2	T45.4X3	T45.4X4	T45.4X5	T45.4X6
Ferrovanadium (fumes)	T59.891	T59.892	T59.893	T59.894	—	—
Ferrum — see Iron						
Fertilizers NEC	T65.891	T65.892	T65.893	T65.894	—	—
with herbicide mixture	T60.3X1	T60.3X2	T60.3X3	T60.3X4	—	—
Fetoxilate	T47.6X1	T47.6X2	T47.6X3	T47.6X4	T47.6X5	T47.6X6
Fiber, dietary	T47.4X1	T47.4X2	T47.4X3	T47.4X4	T47.4X5	T47.4X6
Fiberglass	T65.831	T65.832	T65.833	T65.834	—	—
Fibrinogen (human)	T45.8X1	T45.8X2	T45.8X3	T45.8X4	T45.8X5	T45.8X6
Fibrinolysin (human)	T45.691	T45.692	T45.693	T45.694	T45.695	T45.696
Fibrinolysis						
affecting drug	T45.601	T45.602	T45.603	T45.604	T45.605	T45.606
inhibitor NEC	T45.621	T45.622	T45.623	T45.624	T45.625	T45.626
Fibrinolytic drug	T45.611	T45.612	T45.613	T45.614	T45.615	T45.616
Filix mas	T37.4X1	T37.4X2	T37.4X3	T37.4X4	T37.4X5	T37.4X6
Filtering cream	T49.3X1	T49.3X2	T49.3X3	T49.3X4	T49.3X5	T49.3X6
Fiorinal	T39.011	T39.012	T39.013	T39.014	T39.015	T39.016
Firedamp	T59.891	T59.892	T59.893	T59.894	—	—
Fish, noxious, nonbacterial	T61.91	T61.92	T61.93	T61.94	—	—
ciguatera	T61.01	T61.02	T61.03	T61.04	—	—
scombroid	T61.11	T61.12	T61.13	T61.14	—	—
shell	T61.781	T61.782	T61.783	T61.784	—	—
specified NEC	T61.771	T61.772	T61.773	T61.774	—	—
Flagyl	T37.3X1	T37.3X2	T37.3X3	T37.3X4	T37.3X5	T37.3X6
Flavine adenine dinucleotide	T45.2X1	T45.2X2	T45.2X3	T45.2X4	T45.2X5	T45.2X6
Flavodic acid	T46.991	T46.992	T46.993	T46.994	T46.995	T46.996
Flavoxate	T44.3X1	T44.3X2	T44.3X3	T44.3X4	T44.3X5	T44.3X6
Flaxedil	T48.1X1	T48.1X2	T48.1X3	T48.1X4	T48.1X5	T48.1X6
Flaxseed (medicinal)	T49.3X1	T49.3X2	T49.3X3	T49.3X4	T49.3X5	T49.3X6
Flecainide	T46.2X1	T46.2X2	T46.2X3	T46.2X4	T46.2X5	T46.2X6
Fleroxacin	T36.8X1	T36.8X2	T36.8X3	T36.8X4	T36.8X5	T36.8X6
Floctafenine	T39.8X1	T39.8X2	T39.8X3	T39.8X4	T39.8X5	T39.8X6
Flomax	T44.6X1	T44.6X2	T44.6X3	T44.6X4	T44.6X5	T44.6X6
Flomoxef	T36.1X1	T36.1X2	T36.1X3	T36.1X4	T36.1X5	T36.1X6
Flopropione	T44.3X1	T44.3X2	T44.3X3	T44.3X4	T44.3X5	T44.3X6
Florantyrone	T47.5X1	T47.5X2	T47.5X3	T47.5X4	T47.5X5	T47.5X6
Floraquin	T37.8X1	T37.8X2	T37.8X3	T37.8X4	T37.8X5	T37.8X6
Florinef	T38.0X1	T38.0X2	T38.0X3	T38.0X4	T38.0X5	T38.0X6
ENT agent	T49.6X1	T49.6X2	T49.6X3	T49.6X4	T49.6X5	T49.6X6
ophthalmic preparation	T49.5X1	T49.5X2	T49.5X3	T49.5X4	T49.5X5	T49.5X6
topical NEC	T49.0X1	T49.0X2	T49.0X3	T49.0X4	T49.0X5	T49.0X6
Flowers of sulfur	T49.4X1	T49.4X2	T49.4X3	T49.4X4	T49.4X5	T49.4X6
Floxuridine	T45.1X1	T45.1X2	T45.1X3	T45.1X4	T45.1X5	T45.1X6
Fluanisone	T43.4X1	T43.4X2	T43.4X3	T43.4X4	T43.4X5	T43.4X6
Flubendazole	T37.4X1	T37.4X2	T37.4X3	T37.4X4	T37.4X5	T37.4X6
Fluclorolone acetonide	T49.0X1	T49.0X2	T49.0X3	T49.0X4	T49.0X5	T49.0X6
Flucloxacillin	T36.0X1	T36.0X2	T36.0X3	T36.0X4	T36.0X5	T36.0X6
Fluconazole	T37.8X1	T37.8X2	T37.8X3	T37.8X4	T37.8X5	T37.8X6
Flucytosine	T37.8X1	T37.8X2	T37.8X3	T37.8X4	T37.8X5	T37.8X6
Fludeoxyglucose (18F)	T50.8X1	T50.8X2	T50.8X3	T50.8X4	T50.8X5	T50.8X6
Fludiazepam	T42.4X1	T42.4X2	T42.4X3	T42.4X4	T42.4X5	T42.4X6
Fludrocortisone	T50.0X1	T50.0X2	T50.0X3	T50.0X4	T50.0X5	T50.0X6
ENT agent	T49.6X1	T49.6X2	T49.6X3	T49.6X4	T49.6X5	T49.6X6
ophthalmic preparation	T49.5X1	T49.5X2	T49.5X3	T49.5X4	T49.5X5	T49.5X6
topical NEC	T49.0X1	T49.0X2	T49.0X3	T49.0X4	T49.0X5	T49.0X6
Fludroxycortide	T49.0X1	T49.0X2	T49.0X3	T49.0X4	T49.0X5	T49.0X6
Flufenamic acid	T39.391	T39.392	T39.393	T39.394	T39.395	T39.396
Fluindione	T45.511	T45.512	T45.513	T45.514	T45.515	T45.51
Flumequine	T37.8X1	T37.8X2	T37.8X3	T37.8X4	T37.8X5	T37.8X
Flumethasone	T49.0X1	T49.0X2	T49.0X3	T49.0X4	T49.0X5	T49.0X
Flumethiazide	T50.2X1	T50.2X2	T50.2X3	T50.2X4	T50.2X5	T50.2X
Flumidin	T37.5X1	T37.5X2	T37.5X3	T37.5X4	T37.5X5	T37.5X

Additional Character May Be Required — Refer to the Tabular List for Character Selection

▽ Subterms under main terms may continue to next column or page

Substance	Poisoning, Accidental (unintentional)	Poisoning, Intentional Self-harm	Poisoning, Assault	Poisoning, Undetermined	Adverse Effect	Under-dosing
Flunarizine	T46.7X1	T46.7X2	T46.7X3	T46.7X4	T46.7X5	T46.7X6
Flunidazole	T37.8X1	T37.8X2	T37.8X3	T37.8X4	T37.8X5	T37.8X6
Flunisolide	T48.6X1	T48.6X2	T48.6X3	T48.6X4	T48.6X5	T48.6X6
Flunitrazepam	T42.4X1	T42.4X2	T42.4X3	T42.4X4	T42.4X5	T42.4X6
Fluocinolone (acetonide)	T49.0X1	T49.0X2	T49.0X3	T49.0X4	T49.0X5	T49.0X6
Fluocinonide	T49.0X1	T49.0X2	T49.0X3	T49.0X4	T49.0X5	T49.0X6
Fluocortin (butyl)	T49.0X1	T49.0X2	T49.0X3	T49.0X4	T49.0X5	T49.0X6
Fluocortolone	T49.0X1	T49.0X2	T49.0X3	T49.0X4	T49.0X5	T49.0X6
Fluohydrocortisone	T38.0X1	T38.0X2	T38.0X3	T38.0X4	T38.0X5	T38.0X6
ENT agent	T49.6X1	T49.6X2	T49.6X3	T49.6X4	T49.6X5	T49.6X6
ophthalmic preparation	T49.5X1	T49.5X2	T49.5X3	T49.5X4	T49.5X5	T49.5X6
topical NEC	T49.0X1	T49.0X2	T49.0X3	T49.0X4	T49.0X5	T49.0X6
Fluonid	T49.0X1	T49.0X2	T49.0X3	T49.0X4	T49.0X5	T49.0X6
Fluopromazine	T43.3X1	T43.3X2	T43.3X3	T43.3X4	T43.3X5	T43.3X6
Fluoracetate	T60.8X1	T60.8X2	T60.8X3	T60.8X4	—	—
Fluorescein	T50.8X1	T50.8X2	T50.8X3	T50.8X4	T50.8X5	T50.8X6
Fluorhydrocortisone	T50.0X1	T50.0X2	T50.0X3	T50.0X4	T50.0X5	T50.0X6
Fluoride (nonmedicinal) (pesticide) (sodium) NEC	T60.8X1	T60.8X2	T60.8X3	T60.8X4	—	—
hydrogen — see Hydrofluoric acid						
medicinal NEC	T50.991	T50.992	T50.993	T50.994	T50.995	T50.996
dental use	T49.7X1	T49.7X2	T49.7X3	T49.7X4	T49.7X5	T49.7X6
not pesticide NEC	T54.91	T54.92	T54.93	T54.94		
stannous	T49.7X1	T49.7X2	T49.7X3	T49.7X4	T49.7X5	T49.7X6
Fluorinated corticosteroids	T38.0X1	T38.0X2	T38.0X3	T38.0X4	T38.0X5	T38.0X6
Fluorine (gas)	T59.5X1	T59.5X2	T59.5X3	T59.5X4		
salt — see Fluoride(s)						
Fluoristan	T49.7X1	T49.7X2	T49.7X3	T49.7X4	T49.7X5	T49.7X6
Fluormetholone	T49.0X1	T49.0X2	T49.0X3	T49.0X4	T49.0X5	T49.0X6
Fluoroacetate	T60.8X1	T60.8X2	T60.8X3	T60.8X4	—	—
Fluorocarbon monomer	T53.6X1	T53.6X2	T53.6X3	T53.6X4		
Fluorocytosine	T37.8X1	T37.8X2	T37.8X3	T37.8X4	T37.8X5	T37.8X6
Fluorodeoxyuridine	T45.1X1	T45.1X2	T45.1X3	T45.1X4	T45.1X5	T45.1X6
Fluorometholone	T49.0X1	T49.0X2	T49.0X3	T49.0X4	T49.0X5	T49.0X6
ophthalmic preparation	T49.5X1	T49.5X2	T49.5X3	T49.5X4	T49.5X5	T49.5X6
Fluorophosphate insecticide	T60.0X1	T60.0X2	T60.0X3	T60.0X4	—	
Fluorosol	T46.3X1	T46.3X2	T46.3X3	T46.3X4	T46.3X5	T46.3X6
Fluorouracil	T45.1X1	T45.1X2	T45.1X3	T45.1X4	T45.1X5	T45.1X6
Fluorphenylalanine	T49.5X1	T49.5X2	T49.5X3	T49.5X4	T49.5X5	T49.5X6
Fluothane	T41.0X1	T41.0X2	T41.0X3	T41.0X4	T41.0X5	T41.0X6
Fluoxetine	T43.221	T43.222	T43.223	T43.224	T43.225	T43.226
Fluoxymesterone	T38.7X1	T38.7X2	T38.7X3	T38.7X4	T38.7X5	T38.7X6
Flupenthixol	T43.4X1	T43.4X2	T43.4X3	T43.4X4	T43.4X5	T43.4X6
Flupentixol	T43.4X1	T43.4X2	T43.4X3	T43.4X4	T43.4X5	T43.4X6
Fluphenazine	T43.3X1	T43.3X2	T43.3X3	T43.3X4	T43.3X5	T43.3X6
Fluprednidene	T49.0X1	T49.0X2	T49.0X3	T49.0X4	T49.0X5	T49.0X6
Fluprednisolone	T38.0X1	T38.0X2	T38.0X3	T38.0X4	T38.0X5	T38.0X6
Fluradoline	T39.8X1	T39.8X2	T39.8X3	T39.8X4	T39.8X5	T39.8X6
Flurandrenolide	T49.0X1	T49.0X2	T49.0X3	T49.0X4	T49.0X5	T49.0X6
Flurandrenolone	T49.0X1	T49.0X2	T49.0X3	T49.0X4	T49.0X5	T49.0X6
Flurazepam	T42.4X1	T42.4X2	T42.4X3	T42.4X4	T42.4X5	T42.4X6
Flurbiprofen	T39.311	T39.312	T39.313	T39.314	T39.315	T39.316
Flurobate	T49.0X1	T49.0X2	T49.0X3	T49.0X4	T49.0X5	T49.0X6
Fluroxene	T41.0X1	T41.0X2	T41.0X3	T41.0X4	T41.0X5	T41.0X6
Fluspirilene	T43.591	T43.592	T43.593	T43.594	T43.595	T43.596
Flutamide	T38.6X1	T38.6X2	T38.6X3	T38.6X4	T38.6X5	T38.6X6
Flutazolam	T38.0X1	T38.0X2	T38.0X3	T38.0X4	T38.0X5	T38.0X6
Fluticasone propionate	T38.0X1	T38.0X2	T38.0X3	T38.0X4	T38.0X5	T38.0X6
Flutoprazepam	T42.4X1	T42.4X2	T42.4X3	T42.4X4	T42.4X5	T42.4X6
Flutropium bromide	T48.6X1	T48.6X2	T48.6X3	T48.6X4	T48.6X5	T48.6X6
Fluvoxamine	T43.221	T43.222	T43.223	T43.224	T43.225	T43.226
Folacin	T45.8X1	T45.8X2	T45.8X3	T45.8X4	T45.8X5	T45.8X6
Folic acid	T45.8X1	T45.8X2	T45.8X3	T45.8X4	T45.8X5	T45.8X6
with ferrous salt	T45.2X1	T45.2X2	T45.2X3	T45.2X4	T45.2X5	T45.2X6
antagonist	T45.1X1	T45.1X2	T45.1X3	T45.1X4	T45.1X5	T45.1X6
Folinic acid	T45.8X1	T45.8X2	T45.8X3	T45.8X4	T45.8X5	T45.8X6
Folium stramoniae	T48.6X1	T48.6X2	T48.6X3	T48.6X4	T48.6X5	T48.6X6
Follicle-stimulating hormone, human	T38.811	T38.812	T38.813	T38.814	T38.815	T38.816
Folpet	T60.3X1	T60.3X2	T60.3X3	T60.3X4	—	—
Fominoben	T48.3X1	T48.3X2	T48.3X3	T48.3X4	T48.3X5	T48.3X6
Food, foodstuffs, noxious, nonbacterial, NEC	T62.91	T62.92	T62.93	T62.94	—	—
berries	T62.1X1	T62.1X2	T62.1X3	T62.1X4	—	—
fish — see also Fish	T61.91	T61.92	T61.93	T61.94	—	—
mushrooms	T62.0X1	T62.0X2	T62.0X3	T62.0X4	—	—
plants	T62.2X1	T62.2X2	T62.2X3	T62.2X4	—	—
seafood	T61.91	T61.92	T61.93	T61.94	—	—
specified NEC	T61.8X1	T61.8X2	T61.8X3	T61.8X4	—	—
seeds	T62.2X1	T62.2X2	T62.2X3	T62.2X4	—	—
Food, foodstuffs, noxious, nonbacterial, — continued						
shellfish	T61.781	T61.782	T61.783	T61.784	—	—
specified NEC	T62.8X1	T62.8X2	T62.8X3	T62.8X4	—	—
Fool's parsley	T62.2X1	T62.2X2	T62.2X3	T62.2X4	—	—
Formaldehyde (solution), gas or vapor	T59.2X1	T59.2X2	T59.2X3	T59.2X4	—	—
fungicide	T60.3X1	T60.3X2	T60.3X3	T60.3X4	—	—
Formalin	T59.2X1	T59.2X2	T59.2X3	T59.2X4	—	—
fungicide	T60.3X1	T60.3X2	T60.3X3	T60.3X4	—	—
vapor	T59.2X1	T59.2X2	T59.2X3	T59.2X4	—	—
Formic acid	T54.2X1	T54.2X2	T54.2X3	T54.2X4	—	—
vapor	T59.891	T59.892	T59.893	T59.894	—	—
Foscarnet sodium	T37.5X1	T37.5X2	T37.5X3	T37.5X4	T37.5X5	T37.5X6
Fosfestrol	T38.5X1	T38.5X2	T38.5X3	T38.5X4	T38.5X5	T38.5X6
Fosfomycin	T36.8X1	T36.8X2	T36.8X3	T36.8X4	T36.8X5	T36.8X6
Fosfonet sodium	T37.5X1	T37.5X2	T37.5X3	T37.5X4	T37.5X5	T37.5X6
Fosinopril	T46.4X1	T46.4X2	T46.4X3	T46.4X4	T46.4X5	T46.4X6
sodium	T46.4X1	T46.4X2	T46.4X3	T46.4X4	T46.4X5	T46.4X6
Fowler's solution	T57.0X1	T57.0X2	T57.0X3	T57.0X4	—	—
Foxglove	T62.2X1	T62.2X2	T62.2X3	T62.2X4		
Framycetin	T36.5X1	T36.5X2	T36.5X3	T36.5X4	T36.5X5	T36.5X6
Frangula	T47.2X1	T47.2X2	T47.2X3	T47.2X4	T47.2X5	T47.2X6
extract	T47.2X1	T47.2X2	T47.2X3	T47.2X4	T47.2X5	T47.2X6
Frei antigen	T50.8X1	T50.8X2	T50.8X3	T50.8X4	T50.8X5	T50.8X6
Freon	T53.5X1	T53.5X2	T53.5X3	T53.5X4	—	—
Fructose	T50.3X1	T50.3X2	T50.3X3	T50.3X4	T50.3X5	T50.3X6
Frusemide	T50.1X1	T50.1X2	T50.1X3	T50.1X4	T50.1X5	T50.1X6
FSH	T38.811	T38.812	T38.813	T38.814	T38.815	T38.816
Ftorafur	T45.1X1	T45.1X2	T45.1X3	T45.1X4	T45.1X5	T45.1X6
Fuel						
automobile	T52.0X1	T52.0X2	T52.0X3	T52.0X4	—	—
exhaust gas, not in transit	T58.01	T58.02	T58.03	T58.04	—	—
vapor NEC	T52.0X1	T52.0X2	T52.0X3	T52.0X4	—	—
gas (domestic use) — see also Carbon, monoxide, fuel, utility						
utility	T59.891	T59.892	T59.893	T59.894	—	—
incomplete combustion of — see Carbon, monoxide, fuel, utility						
in mobile container	T59.891	T59.892	T59.893	T59.894	—	—
piped (natural)	T59.891	T59.892	T59.893	T59.894	—	—
industrial, incomplete combustion	T58.8X1	T58.8X2	T58.8X3	T58.8X4	—	—
Fugillin	T36.8X1	T36.8X2	T36.8X3	T36.8X4	T36.8X5	T36.8X6
Fulminate of mercury	T56.1X1	T56.1X2	T56.1X3	T56.1X4	—	—
Fulvicin	T36.7X1	T36.7X2	T36.7X3	T36.7X4	T36.7X5	T36.7X6
Fumadil	T36.8X1	T36.8X2	T36.8X3	T36.8X4	T36.8X5	T36.8X6
Fumagillin	T36.8X1	T36.8X2	T36.8X3	T36.8X4	T36.8X5	T36.8X6
Fumaric acid	T49.4X1	T49.4X2	T49.4X3	T49.4X4	T49.4X5	T49.4X6
Fumes (from)	T59.91	T59.92	T59.93	T59.94	—	—
carbon monoxide — see Carbon, monoxide						
charcoal (domestic use) — see Charcoal, fumes						
chloroform — see Chloroform						
coke (in domestic stoves, fireplaces) — see Coke fumes						
corrosive NEC	T54.91	T54.92	T54.93	T54.94		
ether — see ether						
freons	T53.5X1	T53.5X2	T53.5X3	T53.5X4	—	—
hydrocarbons	T59.891	T59.892	T59.893	T59.894	—	—
petroleum (liquefied)	T59.891	T59.892	T59.893	T59.894	—	—
distributed through pipes (pure or mixed with air)	T59.891	T59.892	T59.893	T59.894	—	—
lead — see lead						
metal — see Metals, or the specified metal						
nitrogen dioxide	T59.0X1	T59.0X2	T59.0X3	T59.0X4	—	—
pesticides — see Pesticides						
petroleum (liquefied)	T59.891	T59.892	T59.893	T59.894	—	—
distributed through pipes (pure or mixed with air)	T59.891	T59.892	T59.893	T59.894	—	—
polyester	T59.891	T59.892	T59.893	T59.894	—	—
specified source NEC — see also substance specified	T59.891	T59.892	T59.893	T59.894	—	—
sulfur dioxide	T59.1X1	T59.1X2	T59.1X3	T59.1X4	—	—
Fumigant NEC	T60.91	T60.92	T60.93	T60.94	—	—

Flunarizine — Fuel

Substance	Poisoning, Accidental (unintentional)	Poisoning, Intentional Self-harm	Poisoning, Assault	Poisoning, Undetermined	Adverse Effect	Under-dosing
Fungicide NEC (nonmedicinal)	T60.3X1	T60.3X2	T60.3X3	T60.3X4	—	—
Fungi, noxious, used as food	T62.0X1	T62.0X2	T62.0X3	T62.0X4	—	—
Fungizone	T36.7X1	T36.7X2	T36.7X3	T36.7X4	T36.7X5	T36.7X6
topical	T49.0X1	T49.0X2	T49.0X3	T49.0X4	T49.0X5	T49.0X6
Furacin	T49.0X1	T49.0X2	T49.0X3	T49.0X4	T49.0X5	T49.0X6
Furadantin	T37.91	T37.92	T37.93	T37.94	T37.95	T37.96
Furazolidone	T37.8X1	T37.8X2	T37.8X3	T37.8X4	T37.8X5	T37.8X6
Furazolium chloride	T49.0X1	T49.0X2	T49.0X3	T49.0X4	T49.0X5	T49.0X6
Furfural	T52.8X1	T52.8X2	T52.8X3	T52.8X4	—	—
Furnace (coal burning) (domestic), gas from	T58.2X1	T58.2X2	T58.2X3	T58.2X4	—	—
industrial	T58.8X1	T58.8X2	T58.8X3	T58.8X4	—	—
Furniture polish	T65.891	T65.892	T65.893	T65.894	—	—
Furosemide	T50.1X1	T50.1X2	T50.1X3	T50.1X4	T50.1X5	T50.1X6
Furoxone	T37.91	T37.92	T37.93	T37.94	T37.95	T37.96
Fursultiamine	T45.2X1	T45.2X2	T45.2X3	T45.2X4	T45.2X5	T45.2X6
Fusafungine	T36.8X1	T36.8X2	T36.8X3	T36.8X4	T36.8X5	T36.8X6
Fusel oil (any) (amyl) (butyl) (propyl), vapor	T51.3X1	T51.3X2	T51.3X3	T51.3X4	—	—
Fusidate (ethanolamine) (sodium)	T36.8X1	T36.8X2	T36.8X3	T36.8X4	T36.8X5	T36.8X6
Fusidic acid	T36.8X1	T36.8X2	T36.8X3	T36.8X4	T36.8X5	T36.8X6
Fytic acid, nonasodium	T50.6X1	T50.6X2	T50.6X3	T50.6X4	T50.6X5	T50.6X6
b-Galactosidase	T47.5X1	T47.5X2	T47.5X3	T47.5X4	T47.5X5	T47.5X6
GABA	T43.8X1	T43.8X2	T43.8X3	T43.8X4	T43.8X5	T43.8X6
Gadopentetic acid	T50.8X1	T50.8X2	T50.8X3	T50.8X4	T50.8X5	T50.8X6
Galactose	T50.3X1	T50.3X2	T50.3X3	T50.3X4	T50.3X5	T50.3X6
Galantamine	T44.0X1	T44.0X2	T44.0X3	T44.0X4	T44.0X5	T44.0X6
Gallamine (triethiodide)	T48.1X1	T48.1X2	T48.1X3	T48.1X4	T48.1X5	T48.1X6
Gallium citrate	T50.991	T50.992	T50.993	T50.994	T50.995	T50.996
Gallopamil	T46.1X1	T46.1X2	T46.1X3	T46.1X4	T46.1X5	T46.1X6
Gamboge	T47.2X1	T47.2X2	T47.2X3	T47.2X4	T47.2X5	T47.2X6
Gamimune	T50.Z11	T50.Z12	T50.Z13	T50.Z14	T50.Z15	T50.Z16
Gamma-aminobutyric acid	T43.8X1	T43.8X2	T43.8X3	T43.8X4	T43.8X5	T43.8X6
Gamma-benzene hexachloride (medicinal)	T49.0X1	T49.0X2	T49.0X3	T49.0X4	T49.0X5	T49.0X6
nonmedicinal, vapor	T53.6X1	T53.6X2	T53.6X3	T53.6X4	—	—
Gamma-BHC (medicinal) — see also Gamma-benzene hexachloride	T49.0X1	T49.0X2	T49.0X3	T49.0X4	T49.0X5	T49.0X6
Gamma globulin	T50.Z11	T50.Z12	T50.Z13	T50.Z14	T50.Z15	T50.Z16
Gamulin	T50.Z11	T50.Z12	T50.Z13	T50.Z14	T50.Z15	T50.Z16
Ganciclovir (sodium)	T37.5X1	T37.5X2	T37.5X3	T37.5X4	T37.5X5	T37.5X6
Ganglionic blocking drug NEC	T44.2X1	T44.2X2	T44.2X3	T44.2X4	T44.2X5	T44.2X6
specified NEC	T44.2X1	T44.2X2	T44.2X3	T44.2X4	T44.2X5	T44.2X6
Ganja	T40.7X1	T40.7X2	T40.7X3	T40.7X4	T40.7X5	T40.7X6
Garamycin	T36.5X1	T36.5X2	T36.5X3	T36.5X4	T36.5X5	T36.5X6
ophthalmic preparation	T49.5X1	T49.5X2	T49.5X3	T49.5X4	T49.5X5	T49.5X6
topical NEC	T49.0X1	T49.0X2	T49.0X3	T49.0X4	T49.0X5	T49.0X6
Gardenal	T42.3X1	T42.3X2	T42.3X3	T42.3X4	T42.3X5	T42.3X6
Gardepanyl	T42.3X1	T42.3X2	T42.3X3	T42.3X4	T42.3X5	T42.3X6
Gaseous substance — see Gas						
Gasoline	T52.0X1	T52.0X2	T52.0X3	T52.0X4	—	—
vapor	T52.0X1	T52.0X2	T52.0X3	T52.0X4	—	—
Gastric enzymes	T47.5X1	T47.5X2	T47.5X3	T47.5X4	T47.5X5	T47.5X6
Gastrografin	T50.8X1	T50.8X2	T50.8X3	T50.8X4	T50.8X5	T50.8X6
Gastrointestinal drug	T47.91	T47.92	T47.93	T47.94	T47.95	T47.96
biological	T47.8X1	T47.8X2	T47.8X3	T47.8X4	T47.8X5	T47.8X6
specified NEC	T47.8X1	T47.8X2	T47.8X3	T47.8X4	T47.8X5	T47.8X6
Gas NEC	T59.91	T59.92	T59.93	T59.94	—	—
acetylene	T59.891	T59.892	T59.893	T59.894	—	—
incomplete combustion of	T58.11	T58.12	T58.13	T58.14	—	—
air contaminants, source or type not specified	T59.91	T59.92	T59.93	T59.94	—	—
anesthetic	T41.0X1	T41.0X2	T41.0X3	T41.0X4	T41.0X5	T41.0X6
blast furnace	T58.8X1	T58.8X2	T58.8X3	T58.8X4	—	—
butane — see butane						
carbon monoxide — see Carbon, monoxide						
chlorine	T59.4X1	T59.4X2	T59.4X3	T59.4X4	—	—
coal	T58.2X1	T58.2X2	T58.2X3	T58.2X4	—	—
cyanide	T57.3X1	T57.3X2	T57.3X3	T57.3X4	—	—
dicyanogen	T65.0X1	T65.0X2	T65.0X3	T65.0X4	—	—
domestic — see Domestic gas						
exhaust	T58.01	T58.02	T58.03	T58.04	—	—
from utility (for cooking, heating, or lighting) (after combustion) — see Carbon, monoxide, fuel, utility						

Substance	Poisoning, Accidental (unintentional)	Poisoning, Intentional Self-harm	Poisoning, Assault	Poisoning, Undetermined	Adverse Effect	Under-dosing
Gas — continued						
from utility — see Carbon, monoxide, fuel, utility — continued						
prior to combustion	T59.891	T59.892	T59.893	T59.894	—	—
from wood- or coal-burning stove or fireplace	T58.2X1	T58.2X2	T58.2X3	T58.2X4	—	—
fuel (domestic use) (after combustion) — see also Carbon, monoxide, fuel						
industrial use	T58.8X1	T58.8X2	T58.8X3	T58.8X4	—	—
prior to combustion	T59.891	T59.892	T59.893	T59.894	—	—
utility	T59.891	T59.892	T59.893	T59.894	—	—
incomplete combustion of — see Carbon, monoxide, fuel, utility						
in mobile container	T59.891	T59.892	T59.893	T59.894	—	—
piped (natural)	T59.891	T59.892	T59.893	T59.894	—	—
garage	T58.01	T58.02	T58.03	T58.04	—	—
hydrocarbon NEC	T59.891	T59.892	T59.893	T59.894	—	—
incomplete combustion of — see Carbon, monoxide, fuel, utility						
liquefied — see butane						
piped	T59.891	T59.892	T59.893	T59.894	—	—
hydrocyanic acid	T65.0X1	T65.0X2	T65.0X3	T65.0X4	—	—
illuminating (after combustion)	T58.11	T58.12	T58.13	T58.14	—	—
prior to combustion	T59.891	T59.892	T59.893	T59.894	—	—
incomplete combustion, any — see Carbon, monoxide						
kiln	T58.8X1	T58.8X2	T58.8X3	T58.8X4	—	—
lacrimogenic	T59.3X1	T59.3X2	T59.3X3	T59.3X4	—	—
liquefied petroleum — see butane						
marsh	T59.891	T59.892	T59.893	T59.894	—	—
motor exhaust, not in transit	T58.01	T58.02	T58.03	T58.04	—	—
mustard, not in war	T59.891	T59.892	T59.893	T59.894	—	—
natural	T59.891	T59.892	T59.893	T59.894	—	—
nerve, not in war	T59.91	T59.92	T59.93	T59.94	—	—
oil	T52.0X1	T52.0X2	T52.0X3	T52.0X4	—	—
petroleum (liquefied) (distributed in mobile containers)	T59.891	T59.892	T59.893	T59.894	—	—
piped (pure or mixed with air)	T59.891	T59.892	T59.893	T59.894	—	—
piped (manufactured) (natural) NEC	T59.891	T59.892	T59.893	T59.894	—	—
producer	T58.8X1	T58.8X2	T58.8X3	T58.8X4	—	—
propane — see propane						
refrigerant (chlorofluoro-carbon)	T53.5X1	T53.5X2	T53.5X3	T53.5X4	—	—
not chlorofluoro-carbon	T59.891	T59.892	T59.893	T59.894	—	—
sewer	T59.91	T59.92	T59.93	T59.94	—	—
specified source NEC	T59.91	T59.92	T59.93	T59.94	—	—
stove (after combustion)	T58.11	T58.12	T58.13	T58.14	—	—
prior to combustion	T59.891	T59.892	T59.893	T59.894	—	—
tear	T59.3X1	T59.3X2	T59.3X3	T59.3X4	—	—
therapeutic	T41.5X1	T41.5X2	T41.5X3	T41.5X4	T41.5X5	T41.5X6
utility (for cooking, heating, or lighting) (piped) NEC	T59.891	T59.892	T59.893	T59.894	—	—
incomplete combustion of — see Carbon, monoxide, fuel, utilty						
in mobile container	T59.891	T59.892	T59.893	T59.894	—	—
piped (natural)	T59.891	T59.892	T59.893	T59.894	—	—
water	T58.11	T58.12	T58.13	T58.14	—	—
incomplete combustion of — see Carbon, monoxide, fuel, utility						
Gaultheria procumbens	T62.2X1	T62.2X2	T62.2X3	T62.2X4	—	—
Gefarnate	T44.3X1	T44.3X2	T44.3X3	T44.3X4	T44.3X5	T44.3X6
Gelatin (intravenous)	T45.8X1	T45.8X2	T45.8X3	T45.8X4	T45.8X5	T45.8X6
absorbable (sponge)	T45.7X1	T45.7X2	T45.7X3	T45.7X4	T45.7X5	T45.7X6
Gelfilm	T49.8X1	T49.8X2	T49.8X3	T49.8X4	T49.8X5	T49.8X6
Gelfoam	T45.7X1	T45.7X2	T45.7X3	T45.7X4	T45.7X5	T45.7X6
Gelsemine	T50.991	T50.992	T50.993	T50.994	T50.995	T50.996
Gelsemium (sempervirens)	T62.2X1	T62.2X2	T62.2X3	T62.2X4	—	—
Gemeprost	T48.0X1	T48.0X2	T48.0X3	T48.0X4	T48.0X5	T48.0X6
Gemfibrozil	T46.6X1	T46.6X2	T46.6X3	T46.6X4	T46.6X5	T46.6X6
Gemonil	T42.3X1	T42.3X2	T42.3X3	T42.3X4	T42.3X5	T42.3X6
Gentamicin	T36.5X1	T36.5X2	T36.5X3	T36.5X4	T36.5X5	T36.5X6

Substance	Poisoning, Accidental (unintentional)	Poisoning, Intentional Self-harm	Poisoning, Assault	Poisoning, Undetermined	Adverse Effect	Under-dosing
Gentamicin — continued						
ophthalmic preparation	T49.5X1	T49.5X2	T49.5X3	T49.5X4	T49.5X5	T49.5X6
topical NEC	T49.0X1	T49.0X2	T49.0X3	T49.0X4	T49.0X5	T49.0X6
Gentian	T47.5X1	T47.5X2	T47.5X3	T47.5X4	T47.5X5	T47.5X6
violet	T49.0X1	T49.0X2	T49.0X3	T49.0X4	T49.0X5	T49.0X6
Gepefrine	T44.4X1	T44.4X2	T44.4X3	T44.4X4	T44.4X5	T44.4X6
Gestonorone caproate	T38.5X1	T38.5X2	T38.5X3	T38.5X4	T38.5X5	T38.5X6
Gexane	T49.0X1	T49.0X2	T49.0X3	T49.0X4	T49.0X5	T49.0X6
Gila monster (venom)	T63.111	T63.112	T63.113	T63.114	—	—
Ginger	T47.5X1	T47.5X2	T47.5X3	T47.5X4	T47.5X5	T47.5X6
Jamaica — see Jamaica, ginger						
Gitalin	T46.0X1	T46.0X2	T46.0X3	T46.0X4	T46.0X5	T46.0X6
amorphous	T46.0X1	T46.0X2	T46.0X3	T46.0X4	T46.0X5	T46.0X6
Gitaloxin	T46.0X1	T46.0X2	T46.0X3	T46.0X4	T46.0X5	T46.0X6
Gitoxin	T46.0X1	T46.0X2	T46.0X3	T46.0X4	T46.0X5	T46.0X6
Glafenine	T39.8X1	T39.8X2	T39.8X3	T39.8X4	T39.8X5	T39.8X6
Glandular extract (medicinal) NEC	T50.Z91	T50.Z92	T50.Z93	T50.Z94	T50.Z95	T50.Z96
Glaucarubin	T37.3X1	T37.3X2	T37.3X3	T37.3X4	T37.3X5	T37.3X6
Glibenclamide	T38.3X1	T38.3X2	T38.3X3	T38.3X4	T38.3X5	T38.3X6
Glibornuride	T38.3X1	T38.3X2	T38.3X3	T38.3X4	T38.3X5	T38.3X6
Gliclazide	T38.3X1	T38.3X2	T38.3X3	T38.3X4	T38.3X5	T38.3X6
Glimidine	T38.3X1	T38.3X2	T38.3X3	T38.3X4	T38.3X5	T38.3X6
Glipizide	T38.3X1	T38.3X2	T38.3X3	T38.3X4	T38.3X5	T38.3X6
Gliquidone	T38.3X1	T38.3X2	T38.3X3	T38.3X4	T38.3X5	T38.3X6
Glisolamide	T38.3X1	T38.3X2	T38.3X3	T38.3X4	T38.3X5	T38.3X6
Glisoxepide	T38.3X1	T38.3X2	T38.3X3	T38.3X4	T38.3X5	T38.3X6
Globin zinc insulin	T38.3X1	T38.3X2	T38.3X3	T38.3X4	T38.3X5	T38.3X6
Globulin						
antilymphocytic	T50.Z11	T50.Z12	T50.Z13	T50.Z14	T50.Z15	T50.Z16
antirhesus	T50.Z11	T50.Z12	T50.Z13	T50.Z14	T50.Z15	T50.Z16
antivenin	T50.Z11	T50.Z12	T50.Z13	T50.Z14	T50.Z15	T50.Z16
antiviral	T50.Z11	T50.Z12	T50.Z13	T50.Z14	T50.Z15	T50.Z16
Glucagon	T38.3X1	T38.3X2	T38.3X3	T38.3X4	T38.3X5	T38.3X6
Glucocorticoids	T38.0X1	T38.0X2	T38.0X3	T38.0X4	T38.0X5	T38.0X6
Glucocorticosteroid	T38.0X1	T38.0X2	T38.0X3	T38.0X4	T38.0X5	T38.0X6
Gluconic acid	T50.991	T50.992	T50.993	T50.994	T50.995	T50.996
Glucosamine sulfate	T39.4X1	T39.4X2	T39.4X3	T39.4X4	T39.4X5	T39.4X6
Glucose	T50.3X1	T50.3X2	T50.3X3	T50.3X4	T50.3X5	T50.3X6
with sodium chloride	T50.3X1	T50.3X2	T50.3X3	T50.3X4	T50.3X5	T50.3X6
Glucosulfone sodium	T37.1X1	T37.1X2	T37.1X3	T37.1X4	T37.1X5	T37.1X6
Glucurolactone	T47.8X1	T47.8X2	T47.8X3	T47.8X4	T47.8X5	T47.8X6
Glue NEC	T52.8X1	T52.8X2	T52.8X3	T52.8X4	—	—
Glutamic acid	T47.5X1	T47.5X2	T47.5X3	T47.5X4	T47.5X5	T47.5X6
Glutaral (medicinal)	T49.0X1	T49.0X2	T49.0X3	T49.0X4	T49.0X5	T49.0X6
nonmedicinal	T65.891	T65.892	T65.893	T65.894	—	—
Glutaraldehyde	T65.891	T65.892	T65.893	T65.894	—	—
(nonmedicinal)						
medicinal	T49.0X1	T49.0X2	T49.0X3	T49.0X4	T49.0X5	T49.0X6
Glutathione	T50.6X1	T50.6X2	T50.6X3	T50.6X4	T50.6X5	T50.6X6
Glutethimide	T42.6X1	T42.6X2	T42.6X3	T42.6X4	T42.6X5	T42.6X6
Glyburide	T38.3X1	T38.3X2	T38.3X3	T38.3X4	T38.3X5	T38.3X6
Glycerin	T47.4X1	T47.4X2	T47.4X3	T47.4X4	T47.4X5	T47.4X6
Glycerol	T47.4X1	T47.4X2	T47.4X3	T47.4X4	T47.4X5	T47.4X6
borax	T49.6X1	T49.6X2	T49.6X3	T49.6X4	T49.6X5	T49.6X6
intravenous	T50.3X1	T50.3X2	T50.3X3	T50.3X4	T50.3X5	T50.3X6
iodinated	T48.4X1	T48.4X2	T48.4X3	T48.4X4	T48.4X5	T48.4X6
Glycerophosphate	T50.991	T50.992	T50.993	T50.994	T50.995	T50.996
Glyceryl						
gualacolate	T48.4X1	T48.4X2	T48.4X3	T48.4X4	T48.4X5	T48.4X6
nitrate	T46.3X1	T46.3X2	T46.3X3	T46.3X4	T46.3X5	T46.3X6
triacetate (topical)	T49.0X1	T49.0X2	T49.0X3	T49.0X4	T49.0X5	T49.0X6
trinitrate	T46.3X1	T46.3X2	T46.3X3	T46.3X4	T46.3X5	T46.3X6
Glycine	T50.3X1	T50.3X2	T50.3X3	T50.3X4	T50.3X5	T50.3X6
Glyclopyramide	T38.3X1	T38.3X2	T38.3X3	T38.3X4	T38.3X5	T38.3X6
Glycobiarsol	T37.3X1	T37.3X2	T37.3X3	T37.3X4	T37.3X5	T37.3X6
Glycols (ether)	T52.3X1	T52.3X2	T52.3X3	T52.3X4	—	—
Glyconiazide	T37.1X1	T37.1X2	T37.1X3	T37.1X4	T37.1X5	T37.1X6
Glycopyrrolate	T44.3X1	T44.3X2	T44.3X3	T44.3X4	T44.3X5	T44.3X6
Glycopyrronium	T44.3X1	T44.3X2	T44.3X3	T44.3X4	T44.3X5	T44.3X6
bromide	T44.3X1	T44.3X2	T44.3X3	T44.3X4	T44.3X5	T44.3X6
Glycoside, cardiac (stimulant)	T46.0X1	T46.0X2	T46.0X3	T46.0X4	T46.0X5	T46.0X6
Glycyclamide	T38.3X1	T38.3X2	T38.3X3	T38.3X4	T38.3X5	T38.3X6
Glycyrrhiza extract	T48.4X1	T48.4X2	T48.4X3	T48.4X4	T48.4X5	T48.4X6
Glycyrrhizic acid	T48.4X1	T48.4X2	T48.4X3	T48.4X4	T48.4X5	T48.4X6
Glycyrrhizinate potassium	T48.4X1	T48.4X2	T48.4X3	T48.4X4	T48.4X5	T48.4X6
Glymidine sodium	T38.3X1	T38.3X2	T38.3X3	T38.3X4	T38.3X5	T38.3X6
Glyphosate	T60.3X1	T60.3X2	T60.3X3	T60.3X4	—	—
Glyphylline	T48.6X1	T48.6X2	T48.6X3	T48.6X4	T48.6X5	T48.6X6
Gold						
colloidal (l98Au)	T45.1X1	T45.1X2	T45.1X3	T45.1X4	T45.1X5	T45.1X6
salts	T39.4X1	T39.4X2	T39.4X3	T39.4X4	T39.4X5	T39.4X6

Substance	Poisoning, Accidental (unintentional)	Poisoning, Intentional Self-harm	Poisoning, Assault	Poisoning, Undetermined	Adverse Effect	Under-dosing
Golden sulfide of antimony	T56.891	T56.892	T56.893	T56.894	—	—
Goldylocks	T62.2X1	T62.2X2	T62.2X3	T62.2X4	—	—
Gonadal tissue extract	T38.901	T38.902	T38.903	T38.904	T38.905	T38.906
female	T38.5X1	T38.5X2	T38.5X3	T38.5X4	T38.5X5	T38.5X6
male	T38.7X1	T38.7X2	T38.7X3	T38.7X4	T38.7X5	T38.7X6
Gonadorelin	T38.891	T38.892	T38.893	T38.894	T38.895	T38.896
Gonadotropin	T38.891	T38.892	T38.893	T38.894	T38.895	T38.896
chorionic	T38.891	T38.892	T38.893	T38.894	T38.895	T38.896
pituitary	T38.811	T38.812	T38.813	T38.814	T38.815	T38.816
Goserelin	T45.1X1	T45.1X2	T45.1X3	T45.1X4	T45.1X5	T45.1X6
Grain alcohol	T51.0X1	T51.0X2	T51.0X3	T51.0X4	—	—
Gramicidin	T49.0X1	T49.0X2	T49.0X3	T49.0X4	T49.0X5	T49.0X6
Granisetron	T45.0X1	T45.0X2	T45.0X3	T45.0X4	T45.0X5	T45.0X6
Gratiola officinalis	T62.2X1	T62.2X2	T62.2X3	T62.2X4	—	—
Grease	T65.891	T65.892	T65.893	T65.894	—	—
Green hellebore	T62.2X1	T62.2X2	T62.2X3	T62.2X4	—	—
Green soap	T49.2X1	T49.2X2	T49.2X3	T49.2X4	T49.2X5	T49.2X6
Grifulvin	T36.7X1	T36.7X2	T36.7X3	T36.7X4	T36.7X5	T36.7X6
Griseofulvin	T36.7X1	T36.7X2	T36.7X3	T36.7X4	T36.7X5	T36.7X6
Growth hormone	T38.811	T38.812	T38.813	T38.814	T38.815	T38.816
Guaiacol derivatives	T48.4X1	T48.4X2	T48.4X3	T48.4X4	T48.4X5	T48.4X6
Guaiac reagent	T50.991	T50.992	T50.993	T50.994	T50.995	T50.996
Guaifenesin	T48.4X1	T48.4X2	T48.4X3	T48.4X4	T48.4X5	T48.4X6
Guaimesal	T48.4X1	T48.4X2	T48.4X3	T48.4X4	T48.4X5	T48.4X6
Guaiphenesin	T48.4X1	T48.4X2	T48.4X3	T48.4X4	T48.4X5	T48.4X6
Guamecycline	T36.4X1	T36.4X2	T36.4X3	T36.4X4	T36.4X5	T36.4X6
Guanabenz	T46.5X1	T46.5X2	T46.5X3	T46.5X4	T46.5X5	T46.5X6
Guanacline	T46.5X1	T46.5X2	T46.5X3	T46.5X4	T46.5X5	T46.5X6
Guanadrel	T46.5X1	T46.5X2	T46.5X3	T46.5X4	T46.5X5	T46.5X6
Guanatol	T37.2X1	T37.2X2	T37.2X3	T37.2X4	T37.2X5	T37.2X6
Guanethidine	T46.5X1	T46.5X2	T46.5X3	T46.5X4	T46.5X5	T46.5X6
Guanfacine	T46.5X1	T46.5X2	T46.5X3	T46.5X4	T46.5X5	T46.5X6
Guano	T65.891	T65.892	T65.893	T65.894	—	—
Guanochlor	T46.5X1	T46.5X2	T46.5X3	T46.5X4	T46.5X5	T46.5X6
Guanoclor	T46.5X1	T46.5X2	T46.5X3	T46.5X4	T46.5X5	T46.5X6
Guanoctine	T46.5X1	T46.5X2	T46.5X3	T46.5X4	T46.5X5	T46.5X6
Guanoxabenz	T46.5X1	T46.5X2	T46.5X3	T46.5X4	T46.5X5	T46.5X6
Guanoxan	T46.5X1	T46.5X2	T46.5X3	T46.5X4	T46.5X5	T46.5X6
Guar gum (medicinal)	T46.6X1	T46.6X2	T46.6X3	T46.6X4	T46.6X5	T46.6X6
Hachimycin	T36.7X1	T36.7X2	T36.7X3	T36.7X4	T36.7X5	T36.7X6
Hair						
dye	T49.4X1	T49.4X2	T49.4X3	T49.4X4	T49.4X5	T49.4X6
preparation NEC	T49.4X1	T49.4X2	T49.4X3	T49.4X4	T49.4X5	T49.4X6
Halazepam	T42.4X1	T42.4X2	T42.4X3	T42.4X4	T42.4X5	T42.4X6
Halcinolone	T49.0X1	T49.0X2	T49.0X3	T49.0X4	T49.0X5	T49.0X6
Halcinonide	T49.0X1	T49.0X2	T49.0X3	T49.0X4	T49.0X5	T49.0X6
Halethazole	T49.0X1	T49.0X2	T49.0X3	T49.0X4	T49.0X5	T49.0X6
Hallucinogen NOS	T40.901	T40.902	T40.903	T40.904	T40.905	T40.906
specified NEC	T40.991	T40.992	T40.993	T40.994	T40.995	T40.996
Halofantrine	T37.2X1	T37.2X2	T37.2X3	T37.2X4	T37.2X5	T37.2X6
Halofenate	T46.6X1	T46.6X2	T46.6X3	T46.6X4	T46.6X5	T46.6X6
Halometasone	T49.0X1	T49.0X2	T49.0X3	T49.0X4	T49.0X5	T49.0X6
Haloperidol	T43.4X1	T43.4X2	T43.4X3	T43.4X4	T43.4X5	T43.4X6
Haloprogin	T49.0X1	T49.0X2	T49.0X3	T49.0X4	T49.0X5	T49.0X6
Halotex	T49.0X1	T49.0X2	T49.0X3	T49.0X4	T49.0X5	T49.0X6
Halothane	T41.0X1	T41.0X2	T41.0X3	T41.0X4	T41.0X5	T41.0X6
Haloxazolam	T42.4X1	T42.4X2	T42.4X3	T42.4X4	T42.4X5	T42.4X6
Halquinols	T49.0X1	T49.0X2	T49.0X3	T49.0X4	T49.0X5	T49.0X6
Hamamelis	T49.2X1	T49.2X2	T49.2X3	T49.2X4	T49.2X5	T49.2X6
Haptendextran	T45.8X1	T45.8X2	T45.8X3	T45.8X4	T45.8X5	T45.8X6
Harmonyl	T46.5X1	T46.5X2	T46.5X3	T46.5X4	T46.5X5	T46.5X6
Hartmann's solution	T50.3X1	T50.3X2	T50.3X3	T50.3X4	T50.3X5	T50.3X6
Hashish	T40.7X1	T40.7X2	T40.7X3	T40.7X4	T40.7X5	T40.7X6
Hawaiian Woodrose seeds	T40.991	T40.992	T40.993	T40.994	—	—
HCB	T60.3X1	T60.3X2	T60.3X3	T60.3X4	—	—
HCH	T53.6X1	T53.6X2	T53.6X3	T53.6X4	—	—
medicinal	T49.0X1	T49.0X2	T49.0X3	T49.0X4	T49.0X5	T49.0X6
HCN	T57.3X1	T57.3X2	T57.3X3	T57.3X4	—	—
Headache cures, drugs, powders NEC	T50.901	T50.902	T50.903	T50.904	T50.905	T50.906
Heavenly Blue (morning glory)	T40.991	T40.992	T40.993	T40.994	—	—
Heavy metal antidote	T45.8X1	T45.8X2	T45.8X3	T45.8X4	T45.8X5	T45.8X6
Hedaquinium	T49.0X1	T49.0X2	T49.0X3	T49.0X4	T49.0X5	T49.0X6
Hedge hyssop	T62.2X1	T62.2X2	T62.2X3	T62.2X4	—	—
Heet	T49.8X1	T49.8X2	T49.8X3	T49.8X4	T49.8X5	T49.8X6
Helenin	T37.4X1	T37.4X2	T37.4X3	T37.4X4	T37.4X5	T37.4X6
Helium (nonmedicinal) NEC	T59.891	T59.892	T59.893	T59.894	—	—
medicinal	T48.991	T48.992	T48.993	T48.994	T48.995	T48.996
Hellebore (black) (green) (white)	T62.2X1	T62.2X2	T62.2X3	T62.2X4	—	—
Hematin	T45.8X1	T45.8X2	T45.8X3	T45.8X4	T45.8X5	T45.8X6

▽ Subterms under main terms may continue to next column or page   Additional Character May Be Required — Refer to the Tabular List for Character Selection

Substance	Poisoning, Accidental (unintentional)	Poisoning, Intentional Self-harm	Poisoning, Assault	Poisoning, Undetermined	Adverse Effect	Under-dosing
Hematinic preparation	T45.8X1	T45.8X2	T45.8X3	T45.8X4	T45.8X5	T45.8X6
Hematological agent	T45.91	T45.92	T45.93	T45.94	T45.95	T45.96
specified NEC	T45.8X1	T45.8X2	T45.8X3	T45.8X4	T45.8X5	T45.8X6
Hemlock	T62.2X1	T62.2X2	T62.2X3	T62.2X4	—	—
Hemostatic	T45.621	T45.622	T45.623	T45.624	T45.625	T45.626
drug, systemic	T45.621	T45.622	T45.623	T45.624	T45.625	T45.626
Hemostyptic	T49.4X1	T49.4X2	T49.4X3	T49.4X4	T49.4X5	T49.4X6
Henbane	T62.2X1	T62.2X2	T62.2X3	T62.2X4	—	—
Heparin (sodium)	T45.511	T45.512	T45.513	T45.514	T45.515	T45.516
action reverser	T45.7X1	T45.7X2	T45.7X3	T45.7X4	T45.7X5	T45.7X6
Heparin-fraction	T45.511	T45.512	T45.513	T45.514	T45.515	T45.516
Heparinoid (systemic)	T45.511	T45.512	T45.513	T45.514	T45.515	T45.516
Hepatic secretion stimulant	T47.8X1	T47.8X2	T47.8X3	T47.8X4	T47.8X5	T47.8X6
Hepatitis B						
immune globulin	T50.Z11	T50.Z12	T50.Z13	T50.Z14	T50.Z15	T50.Z16
vaccine	T50.B91	T50.B92	T50.B93	T50.B94	T50.B95	T50.B96
Hepronicate	T46.7X1	T46.7X2	T46.7X3	T46.7X4	T46.7X5	T46.7X6
Heptabarb	T42.3X1	T42.3X2	T42.3X3	T42.3X4	T42.3X5	T42.3X6
Heptabarbital	T42.3X1	T42.3X2	T42.3X3	T42.3X4	T42.3X5	T42.3X6
Heptabarbitone	T42.3X1	T42.3X2	T42.3X3	T42.3X4	T42.3X5	T42.3X6
Heptachlor	T60.1X1	T60.1X2	T60.1X3	T60.1X4	—	—
Heptalgin	T40.2X1	T40.2X2	T40.2X3	T40.2X4	T40.2X5	T40.2X6
Heptaminol	T46.3X1	T46.3X2	T46.3X3	T46.3X4	T46.3X5	T46.3X6
Herbicide NEC	T60.3X1	T60.3X2	T60.3X3	T60.3X4	—	—
Heroin	T40.1X1	T40.1X2	T40.1X3	T40.1X4	—	—
Herplex	T49.5X1	T49.5X2	T49.5X3	T49.5X4	T49.5X5	T49.5X6
HES	T45.8X1	T45.8X2	T45.8X3	T45.8X4	T45.8X5	T45.8X6
Hesperidin	T46.991	T46.992	T46.993	T46.994	T46.995	T46.996
Hetacillin	T36.0X1	T36.0X2	T36.0X3	T36.0X4	T36.0X5	T36.0X6
Hetastarch	T45.8X1	T45.8X2	T45.8X3	T45.8X4	T45.8X5	T45.8X6
HETP	T60.0X1	T60.0X2	T60.0X3	T60.0X4	—	—
Hexachlorobenzene (vapor)	T60.3X1	T60.3X2	T60.3X3	T60.3X4	—	—
Hexachlorocyclohexane	T53.6X1	T53.6X2	T53.6X3	T53.6X4	—	—
Hexachlorophene	T49.0X1	T49.0X2	T49.0X3	T49.0X4	T49.0X5	T49.0X6
Hexadiline	T46.3X1	T46.3X2	T46.3X3	T46.3X4	T46.3X5	T46.3X6
Hexadimethrine (bromide)	T45.7X1	T45.7X2	T45.7X3	T45.7X4	T45.7X5	T45.7X6
Hexadylamine	T46.3X1	T46.3X2	T46.3X3	T46.3X4	T46.3X5	T46.3X6
Hexaethyl tetraphosphate	T60.0X1	T60.0X2	T60.0X3	T60.0X4	—	—
Hexafluorenium bromide	T48.1X1	T48.1X2	T48.1X3	T48.1X4	T48.1X5	T48.1X6
Hexafluronium (bromide)	T48.1X1	T48.1X2	T48.1X3	T48.1X4	T48.1X5	T48.1X6
Hexa-germ	T49.2X1	T49.2X2	T49.2X3	T49.2X4	T49.2X5	T49.2X6
Hexahydrobenzol	T52.8X1	T52.8X2	T52.8X3	T52.8X4	—	—
Hexahydrocresol(s)	T51.8X1	T51.8X2	T51.8X3	T51.8X4	—	—
arsenide	T57.0X1	T57.0X2	T57.0X3	T57.0X4	—	—
arseniurated	T57.0X1	T57.0X2	T57.0X3	T57.0X4	—	—
cyanide	T57.3X1	T57.3X2	T57.3X3	T57.3X4	—	—
gas	T59.891	T59.892	T59.893	T59.894	—	—
Fluoride (liquid)	T57.8X1	T57.8X2	T57.8X3	T57.8X4	—	—
vapor	T59.891	T59.892	T59.893	T59.894	—	—
phophorated	T60.0X1	T60.0X2	T60.0X3	T60.0X4	—	—
sulfate	T57.8X1	T57.8X2	T57.8X3	T57.8X4	—	—
sulfide (gas)	T59.6X1	T59.6X2	T59.6X3	T59.6X4	—	—
arseniurated	T57.0X1	T57.0X2	T57.0X3	T57.0X4	—	—
sulfurated	T57.8X1	T57.8X2	T57.8X3	T57.8X4	—	—
Hexahydrophenol	T51.8X1	T51.8X2	T51.8X3	T51.8X4	—	—
Hexalen	T51.8X1	T51.8X2	T51.8X3	T51.8X4	—	—
Hexamethonium bromide	T44.2X1	T44.2X2	T44.2X3	T44.2X4	T44.2X5	T44.2X6
Hexamethylene	T52.8X1	T52.8X2	T52.8X3	T52.8X4	—	—
Hexamethylmelamine	T45.1X1	T45.1X2	T45.1X3	T45.1X4	T45.1X5	T45.1X6
Hexamidine	T49.0X1	T49.0X2	T49.0X3	T49.0X4	T49.0X5	T49.0X6
Hexamine (mandelate)	T37.8X1	T37.8X2	T37.8X3	T37.8X4	T37.8X5	T37.8X6
Hexanone, 2-hexanone	T52.4X1	T52.4X2	T52.4X3	T52.4X4	—	—
Hexanuorenium	T48.1X1	T48.1X2	T48.1X3	T48.1X4	T48.1X5	T48.1X6
Hexapropymate	T42.6X1	T42.6X2	T42.6X3	T42.6X4	T42.6X5	T42.6X6
Hexasonium iodide	T44.3X1	T44.3X2	T44.3X3	T44.3X4	T44.3X5	T44.3X6
Hexcarbacholine bromide	T48.1X1	T48.1X2	T48.1X3	T48.1X4	T48.1X5	T48.1X6
Hexemal	T42.3X1	T42.3X2	T42.3X3	T42.3X4	T42.3X5	T42.3X6
Hexestrol	T38.5X1	T38.5X2	T38.5X3	T38.5X4	T38.5X5	T38.5X6
Hexethal (sodium)	T42.3X1	T42.3X2	T42.3X3	T42.3X4	T42.3X5	T42.3X6
Hexetidine	T37.8X1	T37.8X2	T37.8X3	T37.8X4	T37.8X5	T37.8X6
Hexobarbital	T42.3X1	T42.3X2	T42.3X3	T42.3X4	T42.3X5	T42.3X6
rectal	T41.291	T41.292	T41.293	T41.294	T41.295	T41.296
sodium	T41.1X1	T41.1X2	T41.1X3	T41.1X4	T41.1X5	T41.1X6
Hexobendine	T46.3X1	T46.3X2	T46.3X3	T46.3X4	T46.3X5	T46.3X6
Hexocyclium	T44.3X1	T44.3X2	T44.3X3	T44.3X4	T44.3X5	T44.3X6
metilsulfate	T44.3X1	T44.3X2	T44.3X3	T44.3X4	T44.3X5	T44.3X6
Hexoestrol	T38.5X1	T38.5X2	T38.5X3	T38.5X4	T38.5X5	T38.5X6
Hexone	T52.4X1	T52.4X2	T52.4X3	T52.4X4	—	—
Hexoprenaline	T48.6X1	T48.6X2	T48.6X3	T48.6X4	T48.6X5	T48.6X6
Hexylcaine	T41.3X1	T41.3X2	T41.3X3	T41.3X4	T41.3X5	T41.3X6
Hexylresorcinol	T52.2X1	T52.2X2	T52.2X3	T52.2X4	—	—

Substance	Poisoning, Accidental (unintentional)	Poisoning, Intentional Self-harm	Poisoning, Assault	Poisoning, Undetermined	Adverse Effect	Under-dosing
HGH (human growth hormone)	T38.811	T38.812	T38.813	T38.814	T38.815	T38.816
Hinkle's pills	T47.2X1	T47.2X2	T47.2X3	T47.2X4	T47.2X5	T47.2X6
Histalog	T50.8X1	T50.8X2	T50.8X3	T50.8X4	T50.8X5	T50.8X6
Histamine (phosphate)	T50.8X1	T50.8X2	T50.8X3	T50.8X4	T50.8X5	T50.8X6
Histoplasmin	T50.8X1	T50.8X2	T50.8X3	T50.8X4	T50.8X5	T50.8X6
Holly berries	T62.2X1	T62.2X2	T62.2X3	T62.2X4	—	—
Homatropine	T44.3X1	T44.3X2	T44.3X3	T44.3X4	T44.3X5	T44.3X6
methylbromide	T44.3X1	T44.3X2	T44.3X3	T44.3X4	T44.3X5	T44.3X6
Homochlorcyclizine	T45.0X1	T45.0X2	T45.0X3	T45.0X4	T45.0X5	T45.0X6
Homosalate	T49.3X1	T49.3X2	T49.3X3	T49.3X4	T49.3X5	T49.3X6
Homo-tet	T50.Z11	T50.Z12	T50.Z13	T50.Z14	T50.Z15	T50.Z16
Hormone	T38.801	T38.802	T38.803	T38.804	T38.805	T38.806
adrenal cortical steroids	T38.0X1	T38.0X2	T38.0X3	T38.0X4	T38.0X5	T38.0X6
androgenic	T38.7X1	T38.7X2	T38.7X3	T38.7X4	T38.7X5	T38.7X6
anterior pituitary NEC	T38.811	T38.812	T38.813	T38.814	T38.815	T38.816
antidiabetic agents	T38.3X1	T38.3X2	T38.3X3	T38.3X4	T38.3X5	T38.3X6
antidiuretic	T38.891	T38.892	T38.893	T38.894	T38.895	T38.896
cancer therapy	T45.1X1	T45.1X2	T45.1X3	T45.1X4	T45.1X5	T45.1X6
follicle stimulating	T38.811	T38.812	T38.813	T38.814	T38.815	T38.816
gonadotropic	T38.891	T38.892	T38.893	T38.894	T38.895	T38.896
pituitary	T38.811	T38.812	T38.813	T38.814	T38.815	T38.816
growth	T38.811	T38.812	T38.813	T38.814	T38.815	T38.816
luteinizing	T38.811	T38.812	T38.813	T38.814	T38.815	T38.816
ovarian	T38.5X1	T38.5X2	T38.5X3	T38.5X4	T38.5X5	T38.5X6
oxytocic	T48.0X1	T48.0X2	T48.0X3	T48.0X4	T48.0X5	T48.0X6
parathyroid (derivatives)	T50.991	T50.992	T50.993	T50.994	T50.995	T50.996
pituitary (posterior) NEC	T38.891	T38.892	T38.893	T38.894	T38.895	T38.896
anterior	T38.811	T38.812	T38.813	T38.814	T38.815	T38.816
specified, NEC	T38.891	T38.892	T38.893	T38.894	T38.895	T38.896
thyroid	T38.1X1	T38.1X2	T38.1X3	T38.1X4	T38.1X5	T38.1X6
Hornet (sting)	T63.451	T63.452	T63.453	T63.454	—	—
Horse anti-human lymphocytic serum	T50.Z11	T50.Z12	T50.Z13	T50.Z14	T50.Z15	T50.Z16
Horticulture agent NEC	T65.91	T65.92	T65.93	T65.94	—	—
with pesticide	T60.91	T60.92	T60.93	T60.94	—	—
Human						
albumin	T45.8X1	T45.8X2	T45.8X3	T45.8X4	T45.8X5	T45.8X6
growth hormone (HGH)	T38.811	T38.812	T38.813	T38.814	T38.815	T38.816
immune serum	T50.Z11	T50.Z12	T50.Z13	T50.Z14	T50.Z15	T50.Z16
Hyaluronidase	T45.3X1	T45.3X2	T45.3X3	T45.3X4	T45.3X5	T45.3X6
Hyazyme	T45.3X1	T45.3X2	T45.3X3	T45.3X4	T45.3X5	T45.3X6
Hycodan	T40.2X1	T40.2X2	T40.2X3	T40.2X4	T40.2X5	T40.2X6
Hydantoin derivative NEC	T42.0X1	T42.0X2	T42.0X3	T42.0X4	T42.0X5	T42.0X6
Hydeltra	T38.0X1	T38.0X2	T38.0X3	T38.0X4	T38.0X5	T38.0X6
Hydergine	T44.6X1	T44.6X2	T44.6X3	T44.6X4	T44.6X5	T44.6X6
Hydrabamine penicillin	T36.0X1	T36.0X2	T36.0X3	T36.0X4	T36.0X5	T36.0X6
Hydralazine	T46.5X1	T46.5X2	T46.5X3	T46.5X4	T46.5X5	T46.5X6
Hydrargaphen	T49.0X1	T49.0X2	T49.0X3	T49.0X4	T49.0X5	T49.0X6
Hydrargyri aminochloridum	T49.0X1	T49.0X2	T49.0X3	T49.0X4	T49.0X5	T49.0X6
Hydrastine	T48.291	T48.292	T48.293	T48.294	T48.295	T48.296
Hydrazine	T54.1X1	T54.1X2	T54.1X3	T54.1X4	—	—
monoamine oxidase inhibitors	T43.1X1	T43.1X2	T43.1X3	T43.1X4	T43.1X5	T43.1X6
Hydrazoic acid, azides	T54.2X1	T54.2X2	T54.2X3	T54.2X4	—	—
Hydriodic acid	T48.4X1	T48.4X2	T48.4X3	T48.4X4	T48.4X5	T48.4X6
Hydrocarbon gas	T59.891	T59.892	T59.893	T59.894	—	—
incomplete combustion of — *see* Carbon, monoxide, fuel, utility						
liquefied (mobile container)	T59.891	T59.892	T59.893	T59.894	—	—
piped (natural)	T59.891	T59.892	T59.893	T59.894	—	—
Hydrochloric acid (liquid)	T54.2X1	T54.2X2	T54.2X3	T54.2X4	—	—
medicinal (digestant)	T47.5X1	T47.5X2	T47.5X3	T47.5X4	T47.5X5	T47.5X6
vapor	T59.891	T59.892	T59.893	T59.894	—	—
Hydrochlorothiazide	T50.2X1	T50.2X2	T50.2X3	T50.2X4	T50.2X5	T50.2X6
Hydrocodone	T40.2X1	T40.2X2	T40.2X3	T40.2X4	T40.2X5	T40.2X6
Hydrocortisone (derivatives)	T38.0X1	T38.0X2	T38.0X3	T38.0X4	T38.0X5	T38.0X6
aceponate	T49.0X1	T49.0X2	T49.0X3	T49.0X4	T49.0X5	T49.0X6
ENT agent	T49.6X1	T49.6X2	T49.6X3	T49.6X4	T49.6X5	T49.6X6
ophthalmic preparation	T49.5X1	T49.5X2	T49.5X3	T49.5X4	T49.5X5	T49.5X6
topical NEC	T49.0X1	T49.0X2	T49.0X3	T49.0X4	T49.0X5	T49.0X6
Hydrocortone	T38.0X1	T38.0X2	T38.0X3	T38.0X4	T38.0X5	T38.0X6
ENT agent	T49.6X1	T49.6X2	T49.6X3	T49.6X4	T49.6X5	T49.6X6
ophthalmic preparation	T49.5X1	T49.5X2	T49.5X3	T49.5X4	T49.5X5	T49.5X6
topical NEC	T49.0X1	T49.0X2	T49.0X3	T49.0X4	T49.0X5	T49.0X6
Hydrocyanic acid (liquid)	T57.3X1	T57.3X2	T57.3X3	T57.3X4	—	—
gas	T65.0X1	T65.0X2	T65.0X3	T65.0X4	—	—
Hydroflumethiazide	T50.2X1	T50.2X2	T50.2X3	T50.2X4	T50.2X5	T50.2X6
Hydrofluoric acid (liquid)	T54.2X1	T54.2X2	T54.2X3	T54.2X4	—	—

Additional Character May Be Required — Refer to the Tabular List for Character Selection   ▽ Subterms under main terms may continue to next column or page

Substance	Poisoning, Accidental (unintentional)	Poisoning, Intentional Self-harm	Poisoning, Assault	Poisoning, Undetermined	Adverse Effect	Under-dosing
Hydrofluoric acid — *continued*						
vapor	T59.891	T59.892	T59.893	T59.894	—	—
Hydrogen	T59.891	T59.892	T59.893	T59.894	—	—
arsenide	T57.0X1	T57.0X2	T57.0X3	T57.0X4	—	—
arseniureted	T57.0X1	T57.0X2	T57.0X3	T57.0X4	—	—
chloride	T57.8X1	T57.8X2	T57.8X3	T57.8X4	—	—
cyanide (salts)	T57.3X1	T57.3X2	T57.3X3	T57.3X4	—	—
gas	T57.3X1	T57.3X2	T57.3X3	T57.3X4	—	—
Fluoride	T59.5X1	T59.5X2	T59.5X3	T59.5X4	—	—
vapor	T59.5X1	T59.5X2	T59.5X3	T59.5X4	—	—
peroxide	T49.0X1	T49.0X2	T49.0X3	T49.0X4	T49.0X5	T49.0X6
phosphureted	T57.1X1	T57.1X2	T57.1X3	T57.1X4	—	—
sulfide	T59.6X1	T59.6X2	T59.6X3	T59.6X4	—	—
arseniureted	T57.0X1	T57.0X2	T57.0X3	T57.0X4	—	—
sulfureted	T59.6X1	T59.6X2	T59.6X3	T59.6X4	—	—
Hydromethylpyridine	T46.7X1	T46.7X2	T46.7X3	T46.7X4	T46.7X5	T46.7X6
Hydromorphinol	T40.2X1	T40.2X2	T40.2X3	T40.2X4		
Hydromorphinone	T40.2X1	T40.2X2	T40.2X3	T40.2X4	T40.2X5	T40.2X6
Hydromorphone	T40.2X1	T40.2X2	T40.2X3	T40.2X4	T40.2X5	T40.2X6
Hydromox	T50.2X1	T50.2X2	T50.2X3	T50.2X4	T50.2X5	T50.2X6
Hydrophilic lotion	T49.3X1	T49.3X2	T49.3X3	T49.3X4	T49.3X5	T49.3X6
Hydroquinidine	T46.2X1	T46.2X2	T46.2X3	T46.2X4	T46.2X5	T46.2X6
Hydroquinone	T52.2X1	T52.2X2	T52.2X3	T52.2X4	—	—
vapor	T59.891	T59.892	T59.893	T59.894		
Hydrosulfuric acid (gas)	T59.6X1	T59.6X2	T59.6X3	T59.6X4	—	—
Hydrotalcite	T47.1X1	T47.1X2	T47.1X3	T47.1X4	T47.1X5	T47.1X6
Hydrous wool fat	T49.3X1	T49.3X2	T49.3X3	T49.3X4	T49.3X5	T49.3X6
Hydroxide, caustic	T54.3X1	T54.3X2	T54.3X3	T54.3X4	—	—
Hydroxocobalamin	T45.8X1	T45.8X2	T45.8X3	T45.8X4	T45.8X5	T45.8X6
Hydroxyamphetamine	T49.5X1	T49.5X2	T49.5X3	T49.5X4	T49.5X5	T49.5X6
Hydroxycarbamide	T45.1X1	T45.1X2	T45.1X3	T45.1X4	T45.1X5	T45.1X6
Hydroxychloroquine	T37.8X1	T37.8X2	T37.8X3	T37.8X4	T37.8X5	T37.8X6
Hydroxydihydrocodeinone	T40.2X1	T40.2X2	T40.2X3	T40.2X4	T40.2X5	T40.2X6
Hydroxyestrone	T38.5X1	T38.5X2	T38.5X3	T38.5X4	T38.5X5	T38.5X6
Hydroxyethyl starch	T45.8X1	T45.8X2	T45.8X3	T45.8X4	T45.8X5	T45.8X6
Hydroxymethylpentanone	T52.4X1	T52.4X2	T52.4X3	T52.4X4	—	—
Hydroxyphenamate	T43.591	T43.592	T43.593	T43.594	T43.595	T43.596
Hydroxyphenylbutazone	T39.2X1	T39.2X2	T39.2X3	T39.2X4	T39.2X5	T39.2X6
Hydroxyprogesterone	T38.5X1	T38.5X2	T38.5X3	T38.5X4	T38.5X5	T38.5X6
caproate	T38.5X1	T38.5X2	T38.5X3	T38.5X4	T38.5X5	T38.5X6
Hydroxyquinoline (derivatives) NEC	T37.8X1	T37.8X2	T37.8X3	T37.8X4	T37.8X5	T37.8X6
Hydroxystilbamidine	T37.3X1	T37.3X2	T37.3X3	T37.3X4	T37.3X5	T37.3X6
Hydroxytoluene (nonmedicinal)	T54.0X1	T54.0X2	T54.0X3	T54.0X4	—	—
medicinal	T49.0X1	T49.0X2	T49.0X3	T49.0X4	T49.0X5	T49.0X6
Hydroxyurea	T45.1X1	T45.1X2	T45.1X3	T45.1X4	T45.1X5	T45.1X6
Hydroxyzine	T43.591	T43.592	T43.593	T43.594	T43.595	T43.596
Hyoscine	T44.3X1	T44.3X2	T44.3X3	T44.3X4	T44.3X5	T44.3X6
Hyoscyamine	T44.3X1	T44.3X2	T44.3X3	T44.3X4	T44.3X5	T44.3X6
Hyoscyamus	T44.3X1	T44.3X2	T44.3X3	T44.3X4	T44.3X5	T44.3X6
dry extract	T44.3X1	T44.3X2	T44.3X3	T44.3X4	T44.3X5	T44.3X6
Hypaque	T50.8X1	T50.8X2	T50.8X3	T50.8X4	T50.8X5	T50.8X6
Hypertussis	T50.Z11	T50.Z12	T50.Z13	T50.Z14	T50.Z15	T50.Z16
Hypnotic	T42.71	T42.72	T42.73	T42.74	T42.75	T42.76
anticonvulsant	T42.71	T42.72	T42.73	T42.74	T42.75	T42.76
specified NEC	T42.6X1	T42.6X2	T42.6X3	T42.6X4	T42.6X5	T42.6X6
Hypochlorite	T49.0X1	T49.0X2	T49.0X3	T49.0X4	T49.0X5	T49.0X6
Hypophysis, posterior	T38.891	T38.892	T38.893	T38.894	T38.895	T38.896
Hypotensive NEC	T46.5X1	T46.5X2	T46.5X3	T46.5X4	T46.5X5	T46.5X6
Hypromellose	T49.5X1	T49.5X2	T49.5X3	T49.5X4	T49.5X5	T49.5X6
Ibacitabine	T37.5X1	T37.5X2	T37.5X3	T37.5X4	T37.5X5	T37.5X6
Ibopamine	T44.991	T44.992	T44.993	T44.994	T44.995	T44.996
Ibufenac	T39.311	T39.312	T39.313	T39.314	T39.315	T39.316
Ibuprofen	T39.311	T39.312	T39.313	T39.314	T39.315	T39.316
Ibuproxam	T39.311	T39.312	T39.313	T39.314	T39.315	T39.316
Ibuterol	T48.6X1	T48.6X2	T48.6X3	T48.6X4	T48.6X5	T48.6X6
Ichthammol	T49.0X1	T49.0X2	T49.0X3	T49.0X4	T49.0X5	T49.0X6
Ichthyol	T49.4X1	T49.4X2	T49.4X3	T49.4X4	T49.4X5	T49.4X6
Idarubicin	T45.1X1	T45.1X2	T45.1X3	T45.1X4	T45.1X5	T45.1X6
Idrocilamide	T42.8X1	T42.8X2	T42.8X3	T42.8X4	T42.8X5	T42.8X6
Ifenprodil	T46.7X1	T46.7X2	T46.7X3	T46.7X4	T46.7X5	T46.7X6
Ifosfamide	T45.1X1	T45.1X2	T45.1X3	T45.1X4	T45.1X5	T45.1X6
Iletin	T38.3X1	T38.3X2	T38.3X3	T38.3X4	T38.3X5	T38.3X6
Ilex	T62.2X1	T62.2X2	T62.2X3	T62.2X4	—	—
Illuminating gas (after combustion)	T58.11	T58.12	T58.13	T58.14		
prior to combustion	T59.891	T59.892	T59.893	T59.894		
Ilopan	T45.2X1	T45.2X2	T45.2X3	T45.2X4	T45.2X5	T45.2X6
Iloprost	T46.7X1	T46.7X2	T46.7X3	T46.7X4	T46.7X5	T46.7X6
Ilotycin	T36.3X1	T36.3X2	T36.3X3	T36.3X4	T36.3X5	T36.3X6
ophthalmic preparation	T49.5X1	T49.5X2	T49.5X3	T49.5X4	T49.5X5	T49.5X6
topical NEC	T49.0X1	T49.0X2	T49.0X3	T49.0X4	T49.0X5	T49.0X6

Substance	Poisoning, Accidental (unintentional)	Poisoning, Intentional Self-harm	Poisoning, Assault	Poisoning, Undetermined	Adverse Effect	Under-dosing
Imidazole-4-carboxamide	T45.1X1	T45.1X2	T45.1X3	T45.1X4	T45.1X5	T45.1X6
Iminostilbene	T42.1X1	T42.1X2	T42.1X3	T42.1X4	T42.1X5	T42.1X6
Imipenem	T36.0X1	T36.0X2	T36.0X3	T36.0X4	T36.0X5	T36.0X6
Imipramine	T43.011	T43.012	T43.013	T43.014	T43.015	T43.016
Immu-G	T50.Z11	T50.Z12	T50.Z13	T50.Z14	T50.Z15	T50.Z16
Immuglobin	T50.Z11	T50.Z12	T50.Z13	T50.Z14	T50.Z15	T50.Z16
Immune						
globulin	T50.Z11	T50.Z12	T50.Z13	T50.Z14	T50.Z15	T50.Z16
serum globulin	T50.Z11	T50.Z12	T50.Z13	T50.Z14	T50.Z15	T50.Z16
Immunoglobin human (intravenous) (normal)	T50.Z11	T50.Z12	T50.Z13	T50.Z14	T50.Z15	T50.Z16
unmodified	T50.Z11	T50.Z12	T50.Z13	T50.Z14	T50.Z15	T50.Z16
Immunosuppressive drug	T45.1X1	T45.1X2	T45.1X3	T45.1X4	T45.1X5	T45.1X6
Immu-tetanus	T50.Z11	T50.Z12	T50.Z13	T50.Z14	T50.Z15	T50.Z16
Indalpine	T43.221	T43.222	T43.223	T43.224	T43.225	T43.226
Indanazoline	T48.5X1	T48.5X2	T48.5X3	T48.5X4	T48.5X5	T48.5X6
Indandione (derivatives)	T45.511	T45.512	T45.513	T45.514	T45.515	T45.516
Indapamide	T46.5X1	T46.5X2	T46.5X3	T46.5X4	T46.5X5	T46.5X6
Indendione (derivatives)	T45.511	T45.512	T45.513	T45.514	T45.515	T45.516
Indenolol	T44.7X1	T44.7X2	T44.7X3	T44.7X4	T44.7X5	T44.7X6
Inderal	T44.7X1	T44.7X2	T44.7X3	T44.7X4	T44.7X5	T44.7X6
Indian						
hemp	T40.7X1	T40.7X2	T40.7X3	T40.7X4	T40.7X5	T40.7X6
tobacco	T62.2X1	T62.2X2	T62.2X3	T62.2X4	—	—
Indigo carmine	T50.8X1	T50.8X2	T50.8X3	T50.8X4	T50.8X5	T50.8X6
Indobufen	T45.521	T45.522	T45.523	T45.524	T45.525	T45.526
Indocin	T39.2X1	T39.2X2	T39.2X3	T39.2X4	T39.2X5	T39.2X6
Indocyanine green	T50.8X1	T50.8X2	T50.8X3	T50.8X4	T50.8X5	T50.8X6
Indometacin	T39.391	T39.392	T39.393	T39.394	T39.395	T39.396
Indomethacin	T39.391	T39.392	T39.393	T39.394	T39.395	T39.396
farnesil	T39.4X1	T39.4X2	T39.4X3	T39.4X4	T39.4X5	T39.4X6
Indoramin	T44.6X1	T44.6X2	T44.6X3	T44.6X4	T44.6X5	T44.6X6
Industrial						
alcohol	T51.0X1	T51.0X2	T51.0X3	T51.0X4	—	—
fumes	T59.891	T59.892	T59.893	T59.894	—	—
solvents (fumes) (vapors)	T52.91	T52.92	T52.93	T52.94	—	—
Influenza vaccine	T50.B91	T50.B92	T50.B93	T50.B94	T50.B95	T50.B96
Ingested substance NEC	T65.91	T65.92	T65.93	T65.94	—	—
INH	T37.1X1	T37.1X2	T37.1X3	T37.1X4	T37.1X5	T37.1X6
Inhalation, gas (noxious) — *see* Gas						
Inhibitor						
angiotensin-converting enzyme	T46.4X1	T46.4X2	T46.4X3	T46.4X4	T46.4X5	T46.4X6
carbonic anhydrase	T50.2X1	T50.2X2	T50.2X3	T50.2X4	T50.2X5	T50.2X6
fibrinolysis	T45.621	T45.622	T45.623	T45.624	T45.625	T45.626
monoamine oxidase NEC	T43.1X1	T43.1X2	T43.1X3	T43.1X4	T43.1X5	T43.1X6
hydrazine	T43.1X1	T43.1X2	T43.1X3	T43.1X4	T43.1X5	T43.1X6
postsynaptic	T43.8X1	T43.8X2	T43.8X3	T43.8X4	T43.8X5	T43.8X6
prothrombin synthesis	T45.511	T45.512	T45.513	T45.514	T45.515	T45.516
Ink	T65.891	T65.892	T65.893	T65.894	—	—
Inorganic substance NEC	T57.91	T57.92	T57.93	T57.94	—	—
Inosine pranobex	T37.5X1	T37.5X2	T37.5X3	T37.5X4	T37.5X5	T37.5X6
Inositol	T50.991	T50.992	T50.993	T50.994	T50.995	T50.996
nicotinate	T46.7X1	T46.7X2	T46.7X3	T46.7X4	T46.7X5	T46.7X6
Inproquone	T45.1X1	T45.1X2	T45.1X3	T45.1X4	T45.1X5	T45.1X6
Insecticide NEC	T60.91	T60.92	T60.93	T60.94	—	—
carbamate	T60.0X1	T60.0X2	T60.0X3	T60.0X4	—	—
chlorinated	T60.1X1	T60.1X2	T60.1X3	T60.1X4	—	—
mixed	T60.91	T60.92	T60.93	T60.94	—	—
organochlorine	T60.1X1	T60.1X2	T60.1X3	T60.1X4	—	—
organophosphorus	T60.0X1	T60.0X2	T60.0X3	T60.0X4	—	—
Insect (sting), venomous	T63.481	T63.482	T63.483	T63.484	—	—
ant	T63.421	T63.422	T63.423	T63.424	—	—
bee	T63.441	T63.442	T63.443	T63.444	—	—
caterpillar	T63.431	T63.432	T63.433	T63.434	—	—
hornet	T63.451	T63.452	T63.453	T63.454	—	—
wasp	T63.461	T63.462	T63.463	T63.464	—	—
Insular tissue extract	T38.3X1	T38.3X2	T38.3X3	T38.3X4	T38.3X5	T38.3X6
Insulin (amorphous) (globin) (isophane) (Lente) (NPH) (Semilente) (Ultralente)	T38.3X1	T38.3X2	T38.3X3	T38.3X4	T38.3X5	T38.3X6
defalan	T38.3X1	T38.3X2	T38.3X3	T38.3X4	T38.3X5	T38.3X6
human	T38.3X1	T38.3X2	T38.3X3	T38.3X4	T38.3X5	T38.3X6
injection, soluble	T38.3X1	T38.3X2	T38.3X3	T38.3X4	T38.3X5	T38.3X6
biphasic	T38.3X1	T38.3X2	T38.3X3	T38.3X4	T38.3X5	T38.3X6
intermediate acting	T38.3X1	T38.3X2	T38.3X3	T38.3X4	T38.3X5	T38.3X6
protamine zinc	T38.3X1	T38.3X2	T38.3X3	T38.3X4	T38.3X5	T38.3X6
slow acting	T38.3X1	T38.3X2	T38.3X3	T38.3X4	T38.3X5	T38.3X6
zinc						
protamine injection	T38.3X1	T38.3X2	T38.3X3	T38.3X4	T38.3X5	T38.3X6
suspension (amorphous) (crystalline)	T38.3X1	T38.3X2	T38.3X3	T38.3X4	T38.3X5	T38.3X6

Substance	Poisoning, Accidental (unintentional)	Poisoning, Intentional Self-harm	Poisoning, Assault	Poisoning, Undetermined	Adverse Effect	Under-dosing
Interferon (alpha) (beta) (gamma)	T37.5X1	T37.5X2	T37.5X3	T37.5X4	T37.5X5	T37.5X6
Intestinal motility control drug	T47.6X1	T47.6X2	T47.6X3	T47.6X4	T47.6X5	T47.6X6
biological	T47.8X1	T47.8X2	T47.8X3	T47.8X4	T47.8X5	T47.8X6
Intranarcon	T41.1X1	T41.1X2	T41.1X3	T41.1X4	T41.1X5	T41.1X6
Intravenous						
amino acids	T50.991	T50.992	T50.993	T50.994	T50.995	T50.996
fat suspension	T50.991	T50.992	T50.993	T50.994	T50.995	T50.996
Inulin	T50.8X1	T50.8X2	T50.8X3	T50.8X4	T50.8X5	T50.8X6
Invert sugar	T50.3X1	T50.3X2	T50.3X3	T50.3X4	T50.3X5	T50.3X6
Inza — see Naproxen						
Iobenzamic acid	T50.8X1	T50.8X2	T50.8X3	T50.8X4	T50.8X5	T50.8X6
Iocarmic acid	T50.8X1	T50.8X2	T50.8X3	T50.8X4	T50.8X5	T50.8X6
Iocetamic acid	T50.8X1	T50.8X2	T50.8X3	T50.8X4	T50.8X5	T50.8X6
Iodamide	T50.8X1	T50.8X2	T50.8X3	T50.8X4	T50.8X5	T50.8X6
Iodide NEC — see also Iodine	T49.0X1	T49.0X2	T49.0X3	T49.0X4	T49.0X5	T49.0X6
mercury (ointment)	T49.0X1	T49.0X2	T49.0X3	T49.0X4	T49.0X5	T49.0X6
methylate	T49.0X1	T49.0X2	T49.0X3	T49.0X4	T49.0X5	T49.0X6
potassium (expectorant) NEC	T48.4X1	T48.4X2	T48.4X3	T48.4X4	T48.4X5	T48.4X6
Iodinated						
contrast medium	T50.8X1	T50.8X2	T50.8X3	T50.8X4	T50.8X5	T50.8X6
glycerol	T48.4X1	T48.4X2	T48.4X3	T48.4X4	T48.4X5	T48.4X6
human serum albumin (131I)	T50.8X1	T50.8X2	T50.8X3	T50.8X4	T50.8X5	T50.8X6
Iodine (antiseptic, external) (tincture) **NEC**	T49.0X1	T49.0X2	T49.0X3	T49.0X4	T49.0X5	T49.0X6
125 — see also Radiation sickness, and Exposure to radioactivce isotopes	T50.8X1	T50.8X2	T50.8X3	T50.8X4	T50.8X5	T50.8X6
therapeutic	T50.991	T50.992	T50.993	T50.994	T50.995	T50.996
131 — see also Radiation sickness, and Exposure to radioactivce isotopes	T50.8X1	T50.8X2	T50.8X3	T50.8X4	T50.8X5	T50.8X6
therapeutic	T38.2X1	T38.2X2	T38.2X3	T38.2X4	T38.2X5	T38.2X6
diagnostic	T50.8X1	T50.8X2	T50.8X3	T50.8X4	T50.8X5	T50.8X6
for thyroid conditions (antithyroid)	T38.2X1	T38.2X2	T38.2X3	T38.2X4	T38.2X5	T38.2X6
solution	T49.0X1	T49.0X2	T49.0X3	T49.0X4	T49.0X5	T49.0X6
vapor	T59.891	T59.892	T59.893	T59.894	—	—
Iodipamide	T50.8X1	T50.8X2	T50.8X3	T50.8X4	T50.8X5	T50.8X6
Iodized (poppy seed) oil	T50.8X1	T50.8X2	T50.8X3	T50.8X4	T50.8X5	T50.8X6
Iodobismitol	T37.8X1	T37.8X2	T37.8X3	T37.8X4	T37.8X5	T37.8X6
Iodochlorhydroxyquin	T37.8X1	T37.8X2	T37.8X3	T37.8X4	T37.8X5	T37.8X6
topical	T49.0X1	T49.0X2	T49.0X3	T49.0X4	T49.0X5	T49.0X6
Iodochlorhydroxyquinoline	T37.8X1	T37.8X2	T37.8X3	T37.8X4	T37.8X5	T37.8X6
Iodocholesterol (131I)	T50.8X1	T50.8X2	T50.8X3	T50.8X4	T50.8X5	T50.8X6
Iodoform	T49.0X1	T49.0X2	T49.0X3	T49.0X4	T49.0X5	T49.0X6
Iodohippuric acid	T50.8X1	T50.8X2	T50.8X3	T50.8X4	T50.8X5	T50.8X6
Iodopanoic acid	T50.8X1	T50.8X2	T50.8X3	T50.8X4	T50.8X5	T50.8X6
Iodophthalein (sodium)	T50.8X1	T50.8X2	T50.8X3	T50.8X4	T50.8X5	T50.8X6
Iodopyracet	T50.8X1	T50.8X2	T50.8X3	T50.8X4	T50.8X5	T50.8X6
Iodoquinol	T37.8X1	T37.8X2	T37.8X3	T37.8X4	T37.8X5	T37.8X6
Iodoxamic acid	T50.8X1	T50.8X2	T50.8X3	T50.8X4	T50.8X5	T50.8X6
Iofendylate	T50.8X1	T50.8X2	T50.8X3	T50.8X4	T50.8X5	T50.8X6
Ioglycamic acid	T50.8X1	T50.8X2	T50.8X3	T50.8X4	T50.8X5	T50.8X6
Iohexol	T50.8X1	T50.8X2	T50.8X3	T50.8X4	T50.8X5	T50.8X6
Ion exchange resin						
anion	T47.8X1	T47.8X2	T47.8X3	T47.8X4	T47.8X5	T47.8X6
cation	T50.3X1	T50.3X2	T50.3X3	T50.3X4	T50.3X5	T50.3X6
cholestyramine	T46.6X1	T46.6X2	T46.6X3	T46.6X4	T46.6X5	T46.6X6
intestinal	T47.8X1	T47.8X2	T47.8X3	T47.8X4	T47.8X5	T47.8X6
Iopamidol	T50.8X1	T50.8X2	T50.8X3	T50.8X4	T50.8X5	T50.8X6
Iopanoic acid	T50.8X1	T50.8X2	T50.8X3	T50.8X4	T50.8X5	T50.8X6
Iophenoic acid	T50.8X1	T50.8X2	T50.8X3	T50.8X4	T50.8X5	T50.8X6
Iopodate, sodium	T50.8X1	T50.8X2	T50.8X3	T50.8X4	T50.8X5	T50.8X6
Iopodic acid	T50.8X1	T50.8X2	T50.8X3	T50.8X4	T50.8X5	T50.8X6
Iopromide	T50.8X1	T50.8X2	T50.8X3	T50.8X4	T50.8X5	T50.8X6
Iopydol	T50.8X1	T50.8X2	T50.8X3	T50.8X4	T50.8X5	T50.8X6
Iotalamic acid	T50.8X1	T50.8X2	T50.8X3	T50.8X4	T50.8X5	T50.8X6
Iothalamate	T50.8X1	T50.8X2	T50.8X3	T50.8X4	T50.8X5	T50.8X6
Iothiouracil	T38.2X1	T38.2X2	T38.2X3	T38.2X4	T38.2X5	T38.2X6
Iotrol	T50.8X1	T50.8X2	T50.8X3	T50.8X4	T50.8X5	T50.8X6
Iotrolan	T50.8X1	T50.8X2	T50.8X3	T50.8X4	T50.8X5	T50.8X6
Iotroxate	T50.8X1	T50.8X2	T50.8X3	T50.8X4	T50.8X5	T50.8X6
Iotroxic acid	T50.8X1	T50.8X2	T50.8X3	T50.8X4	T50.8X5	T50.8X6
Ioversol	T50.8X1	T50.8X2	T50.8X3	T50.8X4	T50.8X5	T50.8X6
Ioxaglate	T50.8X1	T50.8X2	T50.8X3	T50.8X4	T50.8X5	T50.8X6
Ioxaglic acid	T50.8X1	T50.8X2	T50.8X3	T50.8X4	T50.8X5	T50.8X6
Ioxitalamic acid	T50.8X1	T50.8X2	T50.8X3	T50.8X4	T50.8X5	T50.8X6
Ipecac	T47.7X1	T47.7X2	T47.7X3	T47.7X4	T47.7X5	T47.7X6
Ipecacuanha	T48.4X1	T48.4X2	T48.4X3	T48.4X4	T48.4X5	T48.4X6
Ipodate, calcium	T50.8X1	T50.8X2	T50.8X3	T50.8X4	T50.8X5	T50.8X6
Ipral	T42.3X1	T42.3X2	T42.3X3	T42.3X4	T42.3X5	T42.3X6
Ipratropium (bromide)	T48.6X1	T48.6X2	T48.6X3	T48.6X4	T48.6X5	T48.6X6
Ipriflavone	T46.3X1	T46.3X2	T46.3X3	T46.3X4	T46.3X5	T46.3X6
Iprindole	T43.011	T43.012	T43.013	T43.014	T43.015	T43.016
Iproclozide	T43.1X1	T43.1X2	T43.1X3	T43.1X4	T43.1X5	T43.1X6
Iprofenin	T50.8X1	T50.8X2	T50.8X3	T50.8X4	T50.8X5	T50.8X6
Iproheptine	T49.2X1	T49.2X2	T49.2X3	T49.2X4	T49.2X5	T49.2X6
Iproniazid	T43.1X1	T43.1X2	T43.1X3	T43.1X4	T43.1X5	T43.1X6
Iproplatin	T45.1X1	T45.1X2	T45.1X3	T45.1X4	T45.1X5	T45.1X6
Iproveratril	T46.1X1	T46.1X2	T46.1X3	T46.1X4	T46.1X5	T46.1X6
Iron (compounds) (medicinal) **NEC**	T45.4X1	T45.4X2	T45.4X3	T45.4X4	T45.4X5	T45.4X6
ammonium	T45.4X1	T45.4X2	T45.4X3	T45.4X4	T45.4X5	T45.4X6
dextran injection	T45.4X1	T45.4X2	T45.4X3	T45.4X4	T45.4X5	T45.4X6
nonmedicinal	T56.891	T56.892	T56.893	T56.894	—	—
salts	T45.4X1	T45.4X2	T45.4X3	T45.4X4	T45.4X5	T45.4X6
sorbitex	T45.4X1	T45.4X2	T45.4X3	T45.4X4	T45.4X5	T45.4X6
sorbitol citric acid complex	T45.4X1	T45.4X2	T45.4X3	T45.4X4	T45.4X5	T45.4X6
Irrigating fluid (vaginal)	T49.8X1	T49.8X2	T49.8X3	T49.8X4	T49.8X5	T49.8X6
eye	T49.5X1	T49.5X2	T49.5X3	T49.5X4	T49.5X5	T49.5X6
Isepamicin	T36.5X1	T36.5X2	T36.5X3	T36.5X4	T36.5X5	T36.5X6
Isoaminile (citrate)	T48.3X1	T48.3X2	T48.3X3	T48.3X4	T48.3X5	T48.3X6
Isoamyl nitrite	T46.3X1	T46.3X2	T46.3X3	T46.3X4	T46.3X5	T46.3X6
Isobenzan	T60.1X1	T60.1X2	T60.1X3	T60.1X4	—	—
Isobutyl acetate	T52.8X1	T52.8X2	T52.8X3	T52.8X4	—	—
Isocarboxazid	T43.1X1	T43.1X2	T43.1X3	T43.1X4	T43.1X5	T43.1X6
Isoconazole	T49.0X1	T49.0X2	T49.0X3	T49.0X4	T49.0X5	T49.0X6
Isocyanate	T65.0X1	T65.0X2	T65.0X3	T65.0X4	—	—
Isoephedrine	T44.991	T44.992	T44.993	T44.994	T44.995	T44.996
Isoetarine	T48.6X1	T48.6X2	T48.6X3	T48.6X4	T48.6X5	T48.6X6
Isoethadione	T42.2X1	T42.2X2	T42.2X3	T42.2X4	T42.2X5	T42.2X6
Isoetharine	T44.5X1	T44.5X2	T44.5X3	T44.5X4	T44.5X5	T44.5X6
Isoflurane	T41.0X1	T41.0X2	T41.0X3	T41.0X4	T41.0X5	T41.0X6
Isoflurophate	T44.0X1	T44.0X2	T44.0X3	T44.0X4	T44.0X5	T44.0X6
Isomaltose, ferric complex	T45.4X1	T45.4X2	T45.4X3	T45.4X4	T45.4X5	T45.4X6
Isometheptene	T44.3X1	T44.3X2	T44.3X3	T44.3X4	T44.3X5	T44.3X6
Isoniazid	T37.1X1	T37.1X2	T37.1X3	T37.1X4	T37.1X5	T37.1X6
with						
rifampicin	T36.6X1	T36.6X2	T36.6X3	T36.6X4	T36.6X5	T36.6X6
thioacetazone	T37.1X1	T37.1X2	T37.1X3	T37.1X4	T37.1X5	T37.1X6
Isonicotinic acid hydrazide	T37.1X1	T37.1X2	T37.1X3	T37.1X4	T37.1X5	T37.1X6
Isonipecaine	T40.4X1	T40.4X2	T40.4X3	T40.4X4	T40.4X5	T40.4X6
Isopentaquine	T37.2X1	T37.2X2	T37.2X3	T37.2X4	T37.2X5	T37.2X6
Isophane insulin	T38.3X1	T38.3X2	T38.3X3	T38.3X4	T38.3X5	T38.3X6
Isophorone	T65.891	T65.892	T65.893	T65.894	—	—
Isophosphamide	T45.1X1	T45.1X2	T45.1X3	T45.1X4	T45.1X5	T45.1X6
Isopregnenone	T38.5X1	T38.5X2	T38.5X3	T38.5X4	T38.5X5	T38.5X6
Isoprenaline	T48.6X1	T48.6X2	T48.6X3	T48.6X4	T48.6X5	T48.6X6
Isopromethazine	T43.3X1	T43.3X2	T43.3X3	T43.3X4	T43.3X5	T43.3X6
Isopropamide	T44.3X1	T44.3X2	T44.3X3	T44.3X4	T44.3X5	T44.3X6
iodide	T44.3X1	T44.3X2	T44.3X3	T44.3X4	T44.3X5	T44.3X6
Isopropanol	T51.2X1	T51.2X2	T51.2X3	T51.2X4	—	—
Isopropyl						
acetate	T52.8X1	T52.8X2	T52.8X3	T52.8X4	—	—
alcohol	T51.2X1	T51.2X2	T51.2X3	T51.2X4	—	—
medicinal	T49.4X1	T49.4X2	T49.4X3	T49.4X4	T49.4X5	T49.4X6
ether	T52.8X1	T52.8X2	T52.8X3	T52.8X4	—	—
Isopropylaminophenazone	T39.2X1	T39.2X2	T39.2X3	T39.2X4	T39.2X5	T39.2X6
Isoproterenol	T48.6X1	T48.6X2	T48.6X3	T48.6X4	T48.6X5	T48.6X6
Isosorbide dinitrate	T46.3X1	T46.3X2	T46.3X3	T46.3X4	T46.3X5	T46.3X6
Isothipendyl	T45.0X1	T45.0X2	T45.0X3	T45.0X4	T45.0X5	T45.0X6
Isotretinoin	T50.991	T50.992	T50.993	T50.994	T50.995	T50.996
Isoxazolyl penicillin	T36.0X1	T36.0X2	T36.0X3	T36.0X4	T36.0X5	T36.0X6
Isoxicam	T39.391	T39.392	T39.393	T39.394	T39.395	T39.396
Isoxsuprine	T46.7X1	T46.7X2	T46.7X3	T46.7X4	T46.7X5	T46.7X6
Ispagula	T47.4X1	T47.4X2	T47.4X3	T47.4X4	T47.4X5	T47.4X6
husk	T47.4X1	T47.4X2	T47.4X3	T47.4X4	T47.4X5	T47.4X6
Isradipine	T46.1X1	T46.1X2	T46.1X3	T46.1X4	T46.1X5	T46.1X6
I-thyroxine sodium	T38.1X1	T38.1X2	T38.1X3	T38.1X4	T38.1X5	T38.1X6
Itraconazole	T37.8X1	T37.8X2	T37.8X3	T37.8X4	T37.8X5	T37.8X6
Itramin tosilate	T46.3X1	T46.3X2	T46.3X3	T46.3X4	T46.3X5	T46.3X6
Ivermectin	T37.4X1	T37.4X2	T37.4X3	T37.4X4	T37.4X5	T37.4X6
Izoniazid	T37.1X1	T37.1X2	T37.1X3	T37.1X4	T37.1X5	T37.1X6
with thioacetazone	T37.1X1	T37.1X2	T37.1X3	T37.1X4	T37.1X5	T37.1X6
Jalap	T47.2X1	T47.2X2	T47.2X3	T47.2X4	T47.2X5	T47.2X6
Jamaica						
dogwood (bark)	T39.8X1	T39.8X2	T39.8X3	T39.8X4	T39.8X5	T39.8X6
ginger	T65.891	T65.892	T65.893	T65.894	—	—
root	T62.2X1	T62.2X2	T62.2X3	T62.2X4	—	—
Jatropha						
curcas	T62.2X1	T62.2X2	T62.2X3	T62.2X4	—	—

Substance	Poisoning, Accidental (unintentional)	Poisoning, Intentional Self-harm	Poisoning, Assault	Poisoning, Undetermined	Adverse Effect	Under-dosing
Jectofer	T45.4X1	T45.4X2	T45.4X3	T45.4X4	T45.4X5	T45.4X6
Jellyfish (sting)	T63.621	T63.622	T63.623	T63.624	—	—
Jequirity (bean)	T62.2X1	T62.2X2	T62.2X3	T62.2X4	—	—
Jimson weed (stramonium)	T62.2X1	T62.2X2	T62.2X3	T62.2X4	—	—
seeds	T62.2X1	T62.2X2	T62.2X3	T62.2X4	—	—
Josamycin	T36.3X1	T36.3X2	T36.3X3	T36.3X4	T36.3X5	T36.3X6
Juniper tar	T49.1X1	T49.1X2	T49.1X3	T49.1X4	T49.1X5	T49.1X6
Kallidinogenase	T46.7X1	T46.7X2	T46.7X3	T46.7X4	T46.7X5	T46.7X6
Kallikrein	T46.7X1	T46.7X2	T46.7X3	T46.7X4	T46.7X5	T46.7X6
Kanamycin	T36.5X1	T36.5X2	T36.5X3	T36.5X4	T36.5X5	T36.5X6
Kantrex	T36.5X1	T36.5X2	T36.5X3	T36.5X4	T36.5X5	T36.5X6
Kaolin	T47.6X1	T47.6X2	T47.6X3	T47.6X4	T47.6X5	T47.6X6
light	T47.6X1	T47.6X2	T47.6X3	T47.6X4	T47.6X5	T47.6X6
Karaya (gum)	T47.4X1	T47.4X2	T47.4X3	T47.4X4	T47.4X5	T47.4X6
Kebuzone	T39.2X1	T39.2X2	T39.2X3	T39.2X4	T39.2X5	T39.2X6
Kelevan	T60.1X1	T60.1X2	T60.1X3	T60.1X4	—	—
Kemithal	T41.1X1	T41.1X2	T41.1X3	T41.1X4	T41.1X5	T41.1X6
Kenacort	T38.0X1	T38.0X2	T38.0X3	T38.0X4	T38.0X5	T38.0X6
Keratolytic drug NEC	T49.4X1	T49.4X2	T49.4X3	T49.4X4	T49.4X5	T49.4X6
anthracene	T49.4X1	T49.4X2	T49.4X3	T49.4X4	T49.4X5	T49.4X6
Keratoplastic NEC	T49.4X1	T49.4X2	T49.4X3	T49.4X4	T49.4X5	T49.4X6
Kerosene, kerosine (fuel) (solvent) NEC	T52.0X1	T52.0X2	T52.0X3	T52.0X4	—	—
insecticide	T52.0X1	T52.0X2	T52.0X3	T52.0X4	—	—
vapor	T52.0X1	T52.0X2	T52.0X3	T52.0X4	—	—
Ketamine	T41.291	T41.292	T41.293	T41.294	T41.295	T41.296
Ketazolam	T42.4X1	T42.4X2	T42.4X3	T42.4X4	T42.4X5	T42.4X6
Ketazon	T39.2X1	T39.2X2	T39.2X3	T39.2X4	T39.2X5	T39.2X6
Ketobemidone	T40.4X1	T40.4X2	T40.4X3	T40.4X4	—	—
Ketoconazole	T49.0X1	T49.0X2	T49.0X3	T49.0X4	T49.0X5	T49.0X6
Ketols	T52.4X1	T52.4X2	T52.4X3	T52.4X4	—	—
Ketone oils	T52.4X1	T52.4X2	T52.4X3	T52.4X4	—	—
Ketoprofen	T39.311	T39.312	T39.313	T39.314	T39.315	T39.316
Ketorolac	T39.8X1	T39.8X2	T39.8X3	T39.8X4	T39.8X5	T39.8X6
Ketotifen	T45.0X1	T45.0X2	T45.0X3	T45.0X4	T45.0X5	T45.0X6
Khat	T43.691	T43.692	T43.693	T43.694	—	—
Khellin	T46.3X1	T46.3X2	T46.3X3	T46.3X4	T46.3X5	T46.3X6
Khelloside	T46.3X1	T46.3X2	T46.3X3	T46.3X4	T46.3X5	T46.3X6
Kiln gas or vapor (carbon monoxide)	T58.8X1	T58.8X2	T58.8X3	T58.8X4	—	—
Kitasamycin	T36.3X1	T36.3X2	T36.3X3	T36.3X4	T36.3X5	T36.3X6
Konsyl	T47.4X1	T47.4X2	T47.4X3	T47.4X4	T47.4X5	T47.4X6
Kosam seed	T62.2X1	T62.2X2	T62.2X3	T62.2X4	—	—
Krait (venom)	T63.091	T63.092	T63.093	T63.094	—	—
Kwell (insecticide)	T60.1X1	T60.1X2	T60.1X3	T60.1X4	—	—
anti-infective (topical)	T49.0X1	T49.0X2	T49.0X3	T49.0X4	T49.0X5	T49.0X6
Labetalol	T44.8X1	T44.8X2	T44.8X3	T44.8X4	T44.8X5	T44.8X6
Laburnum (seeds)	T62.2X1	T62.2X2	T62.2X3	T62.2X4	—	—
leaves	T62.2X1	T62.2X2	T62.2X3	T62.2X4	—	—
Lachesine	T49.5X1	T49.5X2	T49.5X3	T49.5X4	T49.5X5	T49.5X6
Lacidipine	T46.5X1	T46.5X2	T46.5X3	T46.5X4	T46.5X5	T46.5X6
Lacquer	T65.6X1	T65.6X2	T65.6X3	T65.6X4	—	—
Lacrimogenic gas	T59.3X1	T59.3X2	T59.3X3	T59.3X4	—	—
Lactated potassic saline	T50.3X1	T50.3X2	T50.3X3	T50.3X4	T50.3X5	T50.3X6
Lactic acid	T49.8X1	T49.8X2	T49.8X3	T49.8X4	T49.8X5	T49.8X6
Lactobacillus						
acidophilus	T47.6X1	T47.6X2	T47.6X3	T47.6X4	T47.6X5	T47.6X6
compound	T47.6X1	T47.6X2	T47.6X3	T47.6X4	T47.6X5	T47.6X6
bifidus, lyophilized	T47.6X1	T47.6X2	T47.6X3	T47.6X4	T47.6X5	T47.6X6
bulgaricus	T47.6X1	T47.6X2	T47.6X3	T47.6X4	T47.6X5	T47.6X6
sporogenes	T47.6X1	T47.6X2	T47.6X3	T47.6X4	T47.6X5	T47.6X6
Lactoflavin	T45.2X1	T45.2X2	T45.2X3	T45.2X4	T45.2X5	T45.2X6
Lactose (as excipient)	T50.901	T50.902	T50.903	T50.904	T50.905	T50.906
Lactuca (virosa) (extract)	T42.6X1	T42.6X2	T42.6X3	T42.6X4	T42.6X5	T42.6X6
Lactucarium	T42.6X1	T42.6X2	T42.6X3	T42.6X4	T42.6X5	T42.6X6
Lactulose	T47.3X1	T47.3X2	T47.3X3	T47.3X4	T47.3X5	T47.3X6
Laevo — see Levo-						
Lanatosides	T46.0X1	T46.0X2	T46.0X3	T46.0X4	T46.0X5	T46.0X6
Lanolin	T49.3X1	T49.3X2	T49.3X3	T49.3X4	T49.3X5	T49.3X6
Largactil	T43.3X1	T43.3X2	T43.3X3	T43.3X4	T43.3X5	T43.3X6
Larkspur	T62.2X1	T62.2X2	T62.2X3	T62.2X4	—	—
Laroxyl	T43.011	T43.012	T43.013	T43.014	T43.015	T43.016
Lasix	T50.1X1	T50.1X2	T50.1X3	T50.1X4	T50.1X5	T50.1X6
Lassar's paste	T49.4X1	T49.4X2	T49.4X3	T49.4X4	T49.4X5	T49.4X6
Latamoxef	T36.1X1	T36.1X2	T36.1X3	T36.1X4	T36.1X5	T36.1X6
Latex	T65.811	T65.812	T65.813	T65.814	—	—
Lathyrus (seed)	T62.2X1	T62.2X2	T62.2X3	T62.2X4	—	—
Laudanum	T40.0X1	T40.0X2	T40.0X3	T40.0X4	T40.0X5	T40.0X6
Laudexium	T48.1X1	T48.1X2	T48.1X3	T48.1X4	T48.1X5	T48.1X6
Laughing gas	T41.0X1	T41.0X2	T41.0X3	T41.0X4	T41.0X5	T41.0X6
Laurel, black or cherry	T62.2X1	T62.2X2	T62.2X3	T62.2X4	—	—
Laurolinium	T49.0X1	T49.0X2	T49.0X3	T49.0X4	T49.0X5	T49.0X6
Lauryl sulfoacetate	T49.2X1	T49.2X2	T49.2X3	T49.2X4	T49.2X5	T49.2X6

Substance	Poisoning, Accidental (unintentional)	Poisoning, Intentional Self-harm	Poisoning, Assault	Poisoning, Undetermined	Adverse Effect	Under-dosing
Laxative NEC	T47.4X1	T47.4X2	T47.4X3	T47.4X4	T47.4X5	T47.4X6
osmotic	T47.3X1	T47.3X2	T47.3X3	T47.3X4	T47.3X5	T47.3X6
saline	T47.3X1	T47.3X2	T47.3X3	T47.3X4	T47.3X5	T47.3X6
stimulant	T47.2X1	T47.2X2	T47.2X3	T47.2X4	T47.2X5	T47.2X6
L-dopa	T42.8X1	T42.8X2	T42.8X3	T42.8X4	T42.8X5	T42.8X6
Lead (dust) (fumes) (vapor)	T56.0X1	T56.0X2	T56.0X3	T56.0X4	—	—
NEC						
acetate	T49.2X1	T49.2X2	T49.2X3	T49.2X4	T49.2X5	T49.2X6
alkyl (fuel additive)	T56.0X1	T56.0X2	T56.0X3	T56.0X4	—	—
anti-infectives	T37.8X1	T37.8X2	T37.8X3	T37.8X4	T37.8X5	T37.8X6
antiknock compound (tetraethyl)	T56.0X1	T56.0X2	T56.0X3	T56.0X4	—	—
arsenate, arsenite (dust)(herbicide) (insecticide) (vapor)	T57.0X1	T57.0X2	T57.0X3	T57.0X4	—	—
carbonate	T56.0X1	T56.0X2	T56.0X3	T56.0X4	—	—
paint	T56.0X1	T56.0X2	T56.0X3	T56.0X4	—	—
chromate	T56.0X1	T56.0X2	T56.0X3	T56.0X4	—	—
paint	T56.0X1	T56.0X2	T56.0X3	T56.0X4	—	—
dioxide	T56.0X1	T56.0X2	T56.0X3	T56.0X4	—	—
inorganic	T56.0X1	T56.0X2	T56.0X3	T56.0X4	—	—
iodide	T56.0X1	T56.0X2	T56.0X3	T56.0X4	—	—
pigment (paint)	T56.0X1	T56.0X2	T56.0X3	T56.0X4	—	—
monoxide (dust)	T56.0X1	T56.0X2	T56.0X3	T56.0X4	—	—
paint	T56.0X1	T56.0X2	T56.0X3	T56.0X4	—	—
organic	T56.0X1	T56.0X2	T56.0X3	T56.0X4	—	—
oxide	T56.0X1	T56.0X2	T56.0X3	T56.0X4	—	—
paint	T56.0X1	T56.0X2	T56.0X3	T56.0X4	—	—
paint	T56.0X1	T56.0X2	T56.0X3	T56.0X4	—	—
salts	T56.0X1	T56.0X2	T56.0X3	T56.0X4	—	—
specified compound NEC	T56.0X1	T56.0X2	T56.0X3	T56.0X4	—	—
tetra-ethyl	T56.0X1	T56.0X2	T56.0X3	T56.0X4	—	—
Lebanese red	T40.7X1	T40.7X2	T40.7X3	T40.7X4	T40.7X5	T40.7X6
Lefetamine	T39.8X1	T39.8X2	T39.8X3	T39.8X4	T39.8X5	T39.8X6
Lenperone	T43.4X1	T43.4X2	T43.4X3	T43.4X4	T43.4X5	T43.4X6
Lente lietin (insulin)	T38.3X1	T38.3X2	T38.3X3	T38.3X4	T38.3X5	T38.3X6
Leptazol	T50.7X1	T50.7X2	T50.7X3	T50.7X4	T50.7X5	T50.7X6
Leptophos	T60.0X1	T60.0X2	T60.0X3	T60.0X4	—	—
Leritine	T40.2X1	T40.2X2	T40.2X3	T40.2X4	T40.2X5	T40.2X6
Letosteine	T48.4X1	T48.4X2	T48.4X3	T48.4X4	T48.4X5	T48.4X6
Letter	T38.1X1	T38.1X2	T38.1X3	T38.1X4	T38.1X5	T38.1X6
Lettuce opium	T42.6X1	T42.6X2	T42.6X3	T42.6X4	T42.6X5	T42.6X6
Leucinocaine	T41.3X1	T41.3X2	T41.3X3	T41.3X4	T41.3X5	T41.3X6
Leucocianidol	T46.991	T46.992	T46.993	T46.994	T46.995	T46.996
Leucovorin (factor)	T45.8X1	T45.8X2	T45.8X3	T45.8X4	T45.8X5	T45.8X6
Leukeran	T45.1X1	T45.1X2	T45.1X3	T45.1X4	T45.1X5	T45.1X6
Leuprolide	T38.891	T38.892	T38.893	T38.894	T38.895	T38.896
Levalbuterol	T48.6X1	T48.6X2	T48.6X3	T48.6X4	T48.6X5	T48.6X6
Levallorphan	T50.7X1	T50.7X2	T50.7X3	T50.7X4	T50.7X5	T50.7X6
Levamisole	T37.4X1	T37.4X2	T37.4X3	T37.4X4	T37.4X5	T37.4X6
Levanil	T42.6X1	T42.6X2	T42.6X3	T42.6X4	T42.6X5	T42.6X6
Levarterenol	T44.4X1	T44.4X2	T44.4X3	T44.4X4	T44.4X5	T44.4X6
Levdropropizine	T48.3X1	T48.3X2	T48.3X3	T48.3X4	T48.3X5	T48.3X6
Levobunolol	T49.5X1	T49.5X2	T49.5X3	T49.5X4	T49.5X5	T49.5X6
Levocabastine (hydrochloride)	T45.0X1	T45.0X2	T45.0X3	T45.0X4	T45.0X5	T45.0X6
Levocarnitine	T50.991	T50.992	T50.993	T50.994	T50.995	T50.996
Levodopa	T42.8X1	T42.8X2	T42.8X3	T42.8X4	T42.8X5	T42.8X6
with carbidopa	T42.8X1	T42.8X2	T42.8X3	T42.8X4	T42.8X5	T42.8X6
Levo-dromoran	T40.2X1	T40.2X2	T40.2X3	T40.2X4	T40.2X5	T40.2X6
Levoglutamide	T50.991	T50.992	T50.993	T50.994	T50.995	T50.996
Levoid	T38.1X1	T38.1X2	T38.1X3	T38.1X4	T38.1X5	T38.1X6
Levo-isomethadone	T40.3X1	T40.3X2	T40.3X3	T40.3X4	T40.3X5	T40.3X6
Levomepromazine	T43.3X1	T43.3X2	T43.3X3	T43.3X4	T43.3X5	T43.3X6
Levonordefrin	T49.6X1	T49.6X2	T49.6X3	T49.6X4	T49.6X5	T49.6X6
Levonorgestrel	T38.4X1	T38.4X2	T38.4X3	T38.4X4	T38.4X5	T38.4X6
with ethinylestradiol	T38.5X1	T38.5X2	T38.5X3	T38.5X4	T38.5X5	T38.5X6
Levopromazine	T43.3X1	T43.3X2	T43.3X3	T43.3X4	T43.3X5	T43.3X6
Levoprome	T42.6X1	T42.6X2	T42.6X3	T42.6X4	T42.6X5	T42.6X6
Levopropoxyphene	T40.4X1	T40.4X2	T40.4X3	T40.4X4	T40.4X5	T40.4X6
Levopropylhexedrine	T50.5X1	T50.5X2	T50.5X3	T50.5X4	T50.5X5	T50.5X6
Levoproxyphylline	T48.6X1	T48.6X2	T48.6X3	T48.6X4	T48.6X5	T48.6X6
Levorphanol	T40.4X1	T40.4X2	T40.4X3	T40.4X4	T40.4X5	T40.4X6
Levothyroxine	T38.1X1	T38.1X2	T38.1X3	T38.1X4	T38.1X5	T38.1X6
sodium	T38.1X1	T38.1X2	T38.1X3	T38.1X4	T38.1X5	T38.1X6
Levsin	T44.3X1	T44.3X2	T44.3X3	T44.3X4	T44.3X5	T44.3X6
Levulose	T50.3X1	T50.3X2	T50.3X3	T50.3X4	T50.3X5	T50.3X6
Lewisite (gas), not in war	T57.0X1	T57.0X2	T57.0X3	T57.0X4	—	—
Librium	T42.4X1	T42.4X2	T42.4X3	T42.4X4	T42.4X5	T42.4X6
Lidex	T49.0X1	T49.0X2	T49.0X3	T49.0X4	T49.0X5	T49.0X6
Lidocaine	T41.3X1	T41.3X2	T41.3X3	T41.3X4	T41.3X5	T41.3X6
regional	T41.3X1	T41.3X2	T41.3X3	T41.3X4	T41.3X5	T41.3X6
spinal	T41.3X1	T41.3X2	T41.3X3	T41.3X4	T41.3X5	T41.3X6

▼ Subterms under main terms may continue to next column or page   Additional Character May Be Required — Refer to the Tabular List for Character Selection   375

Jectofer — Lidocaine

Substance	Poisoning, Accidental (unintentional)	Poisoning, Intentional Self-harm	Poisoning, Assault	Poisoning, Undetermined	Adverse Effect	Under-dosing
Lidofenin	T50.8X1	T50.8X2	T50.8X3	T50.8X4	T50.8X5	T50.8X6
Lidoflazine	T46.1X1	T46.1X2	T46.1X3	T46.1X4	T46.1X5	T46.1X6
Lighter fluid	T52.0X1	T52.0X2	T52.0X3	T52.0X4	—	—
Lignin hemicellulose	T47.6X1	T47.6X2	T47.6X3	T47.6X4	T47.6X5	T47.6X6
Lignocaine	T41.3X1	T41.3X2	T41.3X3	T41.3X4	T41.3X5	T41.3X6
regional	T41.3X1	T41.3X2	T41.3X3	T41.3X4	T41.3X5	T41.3X6
spinal	T41.3X1	T41.3X2	T41.3X3	T41.3X4	T41.3X5	T41.3X6
Ligroin (e) (solvent)	T52.0X1	T52.0X2	T52.0X3	T52.0X4	—	—
vapor	T59.891	T59.892	T59.893	T59.894		
Ligustrum vulgare	T62.2X1	T62.2X2	T62.2X3	T62.2X4	—	—
Lily of the valley	T62.2X1	T62.2X2	T62.2X3	T62.2X4	—	—
Lime (chloride)	T54.3X1	T54.3X2	T54.3X3	T54.3X4	—	—
Limonene	T52.8X1	T52.8X2	T52.8X3	T52.8X4	—	—
Lincomycin	T36.8X1	T36.8X2	T36.8X3	T36.8X4	T36.8X5	T36.8X6
Lindane (insecticide) (nonmedicinal) (vapor)	T53.6X1	T53.6X2	T53.6X3	T53.6X4	—	—
medicinal	T49.0X1	T49.0X2	T49.0X3	T49.0X4	T49.0X5	T49.0X6
Liniments NEC	T49.91	T49.92	T49.93	T49.94	T49.95	T49.96
Linoleic acid	T46.6X1	T46.6X2	T46.6X3	T46.6X4	T46.6X5	T46.6X6
Linolenic acid	T46.6X1	T46.6X2	T46.6X3	T46.6X4	T46.6X5	T46.6X6
Linseed	T47.4X1	T47.4X2	T47.4X3	T47.4X4	T47.4X5	T47.4X6
Liothyronine	T38.1X1	T38.1X2	T38.1X3	T38.1X4	T38.1X5	T38.1X6
Liotrix	T38.1X1	T38.1X2	T38.1X3	T38.1X4	T38.1X5	T38.1X6
Lipancreatin	T47.5X1	T47.5X2	T47.5X3	T47.5X4	T47.5X5	T47.5X6
Lipo-alprostadil	T46.7X1	T46.7X2	T46.7X3	T46.7X4	T46.7X5	T46.7X6
Lipo-Lutin	T38.5X1	T38.5X2	T38.5X3	T38.5X4	T38.5X5	T38.5X6
Lipotropic drug NEC	T50.901	T50.902	T50.903	T50.904	T50.905	T50.906
Liquefied petroleum gases	T59.891	T59.892	T59.893	T59.894	—	—
piped (pure or mixed with air)	T59.891	T59.892	T59.893	T59.894		
Liquid						
paraffin	T47.4X1	T47.4X2	T47.4X3	T47.4X4	T47.4X5	T47.4X6
petrolatum	T47.4X1	T47.4X2	T47.4X3	T47.4X4	T47.4X5	T47.4X6
topical	T49.3X1	T49.3X2	T49.3X3	T49.3X4	T49.3X5	T49.3X6
specified NEC	T65.891	T65.892	T65.893	T65.894	—	—
substance	T65.91	T65.92	T65.93	T65.94	—	—
Liquor creosolis compositus	T65.891	T65.892	T65.893	T65.894	—	—
Liquorice	T48.4X1	T48.4X2	T48.4X3	T48.4X4	T48.4X5	T48.4X6
extract	T47.8X1	T47.8X2	T47.8X3	T47.8X4	T47.8X5	T47.8X6
Lisinopril	T46.4X1	T46.4X2	T46.4X3	T46.4X4	T46.4X5	T46.4X6
Lisuride	T42.8X1	T42.8X2	T42.8X3	T42.8X4	T42.8X5	T42.8X6
Lithane	T43.8X1	T43.8X2	T43.8X3	T43.8X4	T43.8X5	T43.8X6
Lithium	T56.891	T56.892	T56.893	T56.894	—	—
gluconate	T43.591	T43.592	T43.593	T43.594	T43.595	T43.596
salts (carbonate)	T43.591	T43.592	T43.593	T43.594	T43.595	T43.596
Lithonate	T43.8X1	T43.8X2	T43.8X3	T43.8X4	T43.8X5	T43.8X6
Liver						
extract	T45.8X1	T45.8X2	T45.8X3	T45.8X4	T45.8X5	T45.8X6
for parenteral use	T45.8X1	T45.8X2	T45.8X3	T45.8X4	T45.8X5	T45.8X6
fraction 1	T45.8X1	T45.8X2	T45.8X3	T45.8X4	T45.8X5	T45.8X6
hydrolysate	T45.8X1	T45.8X2	T45.8X3	T45.8X4	T45.8X5	T45.8X6
Lizard (bite) (venom)	T63.121	T63.122	T63.123	T63.124	—	—
LMD	T45.8X1	T45.8X2	T45.8X3	T45.8X4	T45.8X5	T45.8X6
Lobelia	T62.2X1	T62.2X2	T62.2X3	T62.2X4	—	—
Lobeline	T50.7X1	T50.7X2	T50.7X3	T50.7X4	T50.7X5	T50.7X6
Local action drug NEC	T49.8X1	T49.8X2	T49.8X3	T49.8X4	T49.8X5	T49.8X6
Locorten	T49.0X1	T49.0X2	T49.0X3	T49.0X4	T49.0X5	T49.0X6
Lofepramine	T43.011	T43.012	T43.013	T43.014	T43.015	T43.016
Lolium temulentum	T62.2X1	T62.2X2	T62.2X3	T62.2X4	—	—
Lomotil	T47.6X1	T47.6X2	T47.6X3	T47.6X4	T47.6X5	T47.6X6
Lomustine	T45.1X1	T45.1X2	T45.1X3	T45.1X4	T45.1X5	T45.1X6
Lonidamine	T45.1X1	T45.1X2	T45.1X3	T45.1X4	T45.1X5	T45.1X6
Loperamide	T47.6X1	T47.6X2	T47.6X3	T47.6X4	T47.6X5	T47.6X6
Loprazolam	T42.4X1	T42.4X2	T42.4X3	T42.4X4	T42.4X5	T42.4X6
Lorajmine	T46.2X1	T46.2X2	T46.2X3	T46.2X4	T46.2X5	T46.2X6
Loratidine	T45.0X1	T45.0X2	T45.0X3	T45.0X4	T45.0X5	T45.0X6
Lorazepam	T42.4X1	T42.4X2	T42.4X3	T42.4X4	T42.4X5	T42.4X6
Lorcainide	T46.2X1	T46.2X2	T46.2X3	T46.2X4	T46.2X5	T46.2X6
Lormetazepam	T42.4X1	T42.4X2	T42.4X3	T42.4X4	T42.4X5	T42.4X6
Lotions NEC	T49.91	T49.92	T49.93	T49.94	T49.95	T49.96
Lotusate	T42.3X1	T42.3X2	T42.3X3	T42.3X4	T42.3X5	T42.3X6
Lovastatin	T46.6X1	T46.6X2	T46.6X3	T46.6X4	T46.6X5	T46.6X6
Lowila	T49.2X1	T49.2X2	T49.2X3	T49.2X4	T49.2X5	T49.2X6
Loxapine	T43.591	T43.592	T43.593	T43.594	T43.595	T43.596
Lozenges (throat)	T49.6X1	T49.6X2	T49.6X3	T49.6X4	T49.6X5	T49.6X6
LSD	T40.8X1	T40.8X2	T40.8X3	T40.8X4	—	—
L-Tryptophan — see amino acid						
Lubricant, eye	T49.5X1	T49.5X2	T49.5X3	T49.5X4	T49.5X5	T49.5X6
Lubricating oil NEC	T52.0X1	T52.0X2	T52.0X3	T52.0X4	—	—
Lucanthone	T37.4X1	T37.4X2	T37.4X3	T37.4X4	T37.4X5	T37.4X6
Luminal	T42.3X1	T42.3X2	T42.3X3	T42.3X4	T42.3X5	T42.3X6
Lung irritant (gas) NEC	T59.91	T59.92	T59.93	T59.94	—	—

Substance	Poisoning, Accidental (unintentional)	Poisoning, Intentional Self-harm	Poisoning, Assault	Poisoning, Undetermined	Adverse Effect	Under-dosing
Luteinizing hormone	T38.811	T38.812	T38.813	T38.814	T38.815	T38.816
Lutocylol	T38.5X1	T38.5X2	T38.5X3	T38.5X4	T38.5X5	T38.5X6
Lutromone	T38.5X1	T38.5X2	T38.5X3	T38.5X4	T38.5X5	T38.5X6
Lututrin	T48.291	T48.292	T48.293	T48.294	T48.295	T48.296
Lye (concentrated)	T54.3X1	T54.3X2	T54.3X3	T54.3X4		
Lygranum (skin test)	T50.8X1	T50.8X2	T50.8X3	T50.8X4	T50.8X5	T50.8X6
Lymecycline	T36.4X1	T36.4X2	T36.4X3	T36.4X4	T36.4X5	T36.4X6
Lymphogranuloma venereum antigen	T50.8X1	T50.8X2	T50.8X3	T50.8X4	T50.8X5	T50.8X6
Lynestrenol	T38.4X1	T38.4X2	T38.4X3	T38.4X4	T38.4X5	T38.4X6
Lyovac Sodium Edecrin	T50.1X1	T50.1X2	T50.1X3	T50.1X4	T50.1X5	T50.1X6
Lypressin	T38.891	T38.892	T38.893	T38.894	T38.895	T38.896
Lysergic acid diethylamide	T40.8X1	T40.8X2	T40.8X3	T40.8X4	—	—
Lysergide	T40.8X1	T40.8X2	T40.8X3	T40.8X4	—	—
Lysine vasopressin	T38.891	T38.892	T38.893	T38.894	T38.895	T38.896
Lysol	T54.1X1	T54.1X2	T54.1X3	T54.1X4	—	—
Lysozyme	T49.0X1	T49.0X2	T49.0X3	T49.0X4	T49.0X5	T49.0X6
Lytta (vitatta)	T49.8X1	T49.8X2	T49.8X3	T49.8X4	T49.8X5	T49.8X6
Mace	T59.3X1	T59.3X2	T59.3X3	T59.3X4	—	—
Macrogol	T50.991	T50.992	T50.993	T50.994	T50.995	T50.996
Macrolide						
anabolic drug	T38.7X1	T38.7X2	T38.7X3	T38.7X4	T38.7X5	T38.7X6
antibiotic	T36.3X1	T36.3X2	T36.3X3	T36.3X4	T36.3X5	T36.3X6
Mafenide	T49.0X1	T49.0X2	T49.0X3	T49.0X4	T49.0X5	T49.0X6
Magaldrate	T47.1X1	T47.1X2	T47.1X3	T47.1X4	T47.1X5	T47.1X6
Magic mushroom	T40.991	T40.992	T40.993	T40.994	—	—
Magnamycin	T36.8X1	T36.8X2	T36.8X3	T36.8X4	T36.8X5	T36.8X6
Magnesia magma	T47.1X1	T47.1X2	T47.1X3	T47.1X4	T47.1X5	T47.1X6
Magnesium NEC	T56.891	T56.892	T56.893	T56.894		
carbonate	T47.1X1	T47.1X2	T47.1X3	T47.1X4	T47.1X5	T47.1X6
citrate	T47.4X1	T47.4X2	T47.4X3	T47.4X4	T47.4X5	T47.4X6
hydroxide	T47.1X1	T47.1X2	T47.1X3	T47.1X4	T47.1X5	T47.1X6
oxide	T47.1X1	T47.1X2	T47.1X3	T47.1X4	T47.1X5	T47.1X6
peroxide	T49.0X1	T49.0X2	T49.0X3	T49.0X4	T49.0X5	T49.0X6
salicylate	T39.091	T39.092	T39.093	T39.094	T39.095	T39.096
silicofluoride	T50.3X1	T50.3X2	T50.3X3	T50.3X4	T50.3X5	T50.3X6
sulfate	T47.4X1	T47.4X2	T47.4X3	T47.4X4	T47.4X5	T47.4X6
thiosulfate	T45.0X1	T45.0X2	T45.0X3	T45.0X4	T45.0X5	T45.0X6
trisilicate	T47.1X1	T47.1X2	T47.1X3	T47.1X4	T47.1X5	T47.1X6
Malathion (medicinal)	T49.0X1	T49.0X2	T49.0X3	T49.0X4	T49.0X5	T49.0X6
insecticide	T60.0X1	T60.0X2	T60.0X3	T60.0X4	—	—
Male fern extract	T37.4X1	T37.4X2	T37.4X3	T37.4X4	T37.4X5	T37.4X6
M-AMSA	T45.1X1	T45.1X2	T45.1X3	T45.1X4	T45.1X5	T45.1X6
Mandelic acid	T37.8X1	T37.8X2	T37.8X3	T37.8X4	T37.8X5	T37.8X6
Manganese (dioxide) (salts)	T57.2X1	T57.2X2	T57.2X3	T57.2X4		
medicinal	T50.991	T50.992	T50.993	T50.994	T50.995	T50.996
Mannitol	T47.3X1	T47.3X2	T47.3X3	T47.3X4	T47.3X5	T47.3X6
hexanitrate	T46.3X1	T46.3X2	T46.3X3	T46.3X4	T46.3X5	T46.3X6
Mannomustine	T45.1X1	T45.1X2	T45.1X3	T45.1X4	T45.1X5	T45.1X6
MAO inhibitors	T43.1X1	T43.1X2	T43.1X3	T43.1X4	T43.1X5	T43.1X6
Mapharsen	T37.8X1	T37.8X2	T37.8X3	T37.8X4	T37.8X5	T37.8X6
Maphenide	T49.0X1	T49.0X2	T49.0X3	T49.0X4	T49.0X5	T49.0X6
Maprotiline	T43.021	T43.022	T43.023	T43.024	T43.025	T43.026
Marcaine	T41.3X1	T41.3X2	T41.3X3	T41.3X4	T41.3X5	T41.3X6
infiltration (subcutaneous)	T41.3X1	T41.3X2	T41.3X3	T41.3X4	T41.3X5	T41.3X6
nerve block (peripheral) (plexus)	T41.3X1	T41.3X2	T41.3X3	T41.3X4	T41.3X5	T41.3X6
Marezine	T45.0X1	T45.0X2	T45.0X3	T45.0X4	T45.0X5	T45.0X6
Marihuana	T40.7X1	T40.7X2	T40.7X3	T40.7X4	T40.7X5	T40.7X6
Marijuana	T40.7X1	T40.7X2	T40.7X3	T40.7X4	T40.7X5	T40.7X6
Marine (sting)	T63.691	T63.692	T63.693	T63.694	—	—
animals (sting)	T63.691	T63.692	T63.693	T63.694	—	—
plants (sting)	T63.711	T63.712	T63.713	T63.714	—	—
Marplan	T43.1X1	T43.1X2	T43.1X3	T43.1X4	T43.1X5	T43.1X6
Marsh gas	T59.891	T59.892	T59.893	T59.894	—	—
Marsilid	T43.1X1	T43.1X2	T43.1X3	T43.1X4	T43.1X5	T43.1X6
Matulane	T45.1X1	T45.1X2	T45.1X3	T45.1X4	T45.1X5	T45.1X6
Mazindol	T50.5X1	T50.5X2	T50.5X3	T50.5X4	T50.5X5	T50.5X6
MCPA	T60.3X1	T60.3X2	T60.3X3	T60.3X4	—	—
MDMA	T43.641	T43.642	T43.643	T43.644	—	—
Meadow saffron	T62.2X1	T62.2X2	T62.2X3	T62.2X4	—	—
Measles virus vaccine (attenuated)	T50.B91	T50.B92	T50.B93	T50.B94	T50.B95	T50.B96
Meat, noxious	T62.8X1	T62.8X2	T62.8X3	T62.8X4	—	—
Meballymal	T42.3X1	T42.3X2	T42.3X3	T42.3X4	T42.3X5	T42.3X6
Mebanazine	T43.1X1	T43.1X2	T43.1X3	T43.1X4	T43.1X5	T43.1X6
Mebaral	T42.3X1	T42.3X2	T42.3X3	T42.3X4	T42.3X5	T42.3X6
Mebendazole	T37.4X1	T37.4X2	T37.4X3	T37.4X4	T37.4X5	T37.4X6
Mebeverine	T44.3X1	T44.3X2	T44.3X3	T44.3X4	T44.3X5	T44.3X6
Mebhydrolin	T45.0X1	T45.0X2	T45.0X3	T45.0X4	T45.0X5	T45.0X6
Mebumal	T42.3X1	T42.3X2	T42.3X3	T42.3X4	T42.3X5	T42.3X6
Mebutamate	T43.591	T43.592	T43.593	T43.594	T43.595	T43.596
Mecamylamine	T44.2X1	T44.2X2	T44.2X3	T44.2X4	T44.2X5	T44.2X6

Substance	Poisoning, Accidental (unintentional)	Poisoning, Intentional Self-harm	Poisoning, Assault	Poisoning, Undetermined	Adverse Effect	Under-dosing
Mechlorethamine	T45.1X1	T45.1X2	T45.1X3	T45.1X4	T45.1X5	T45.1X6
Mecillinam	T36.0X1	T36.0X2	T36.0X3	T36.0X4	T36.0X5	T36.0X6
Meclizine (hydrochloride)	T45.0X1	T45.0X2	T45.0X3	T45.0X4	T45.0X5	T45.0X6
Meclocycline	T36.4X1	T36.4X2	T36.4X3	T36.4X4	T36.4X5	T36.4X6
Meclofenamate	T39.391	T39.392	T39.393	T39.394	T39.395	T39.396
Meclofenamic acid	T39.391	T39.392	T39.393	T39.394	T39.395	T39.396
Meclofenoxate	T43.691	T43.692	T43.693	T43.694	T43.695	T43.696
Meclozine	T45.0X1	T45.0X2	T45.0X3	T45.0X4	T45.0X5	T45.0X6
Mecobalamin	T45.8X1	T45.8X2	T45.8X3	T45.8X4	T45.8X5	T45.8X6
Mecoprop	T60.3X1	T60.3X2	T60.3X3	T60.3X4	—	—
Mecrilate	T49.3X1	T49.3X2	T49.3X3	T49.3X4	T49.3X5	T49.3X6
Mecysteine	T48.4X1	T48.4X2	T48.4X3	T48.4X4	T48.4X5	T48.4X6
Medazepam	T42.4X1	T42.4X2	T42.4X3	T42.4X4	T42.4X5	T42.4X6
Medicament NEC	T50.901	T50.902	T50.903	T50.904	T50.905	T50.906
Medinal	T42.3X1	T42.3X2	T42.3X3	T42.3X4	T42.3X5	T42.3X6
Medomin	T42.3X1	T42.3X2	T42.3X3	T42.3X4	T42.3X5	T42.3X6
Medrogestone	T38.5X1	T38.5X2	T38.5X3	T38.5X4	T38.5X5	T38.5X6
Medroxalol	T44.8X1	T44.8X2	T44.8X3	T44.8X4	T44.8X5	T44.8X6
Medroxyprogesterone acetate (depot)	T38.5X1	T38.5X2	T38.5X3	T38.5X4	T38.5X5	T38.5X6
Medrysone	T49.0X1	T49.0X2	T49.0X3	T49.0X4	T49.0X5	T49.0X6
Mefenamic acid	T39.391	T39.392	T39.393	T39.394	T39.395	T39.396
Mefenorex	T50.5X1	T50.5X2	T50.5X3	T50.5X4	T50.5X5	T50.5X6
Mefloquine	T37.2X1	T37.2X2	T37.2X3	T37.2X4	T37.2X5	T37.2X6
Mefruside	T50.2X1	T50.2X2	T50.2X3	T50.2X4	T50.2X5	T50.2X6
Megahallucinogen	T40.901	T40.902	T40.903	T40.904	T40.905	T40.906
Megestrol	T38.5X1	T38.5X2	T38.5X3	T38.5X4	T38.5X5	T38.5X6
Meglumine						
antimoniate	T37.8X1	T37.8X2	T37.8X3	T37.8X4	T37.8X5	T37.8X6
diatrizoate	T50.8X1	T50.8X2	T50.8X3	T50.8X4	T50.8X5	T50.8X6
iodipamide	T50.8X1	T50.8X2	T50.8X3	T50.8X4	T50.8X5	T50.8X6
iotroxate	T50.8X1	T50.8X2	T50.8X3	T50.8X4	T50.8X5	T50.8X6
MEK (methyl ethyl ketone)	T52.4X1	T52.4X2	T52.4X3	T52.4X4	—	—
Meladinin	T49.3X1	T49.3X2	T49.3X3	T49.3X4	T49.3X5	T49.3X6
Meladrazine	T44.3X1	T44.3X2	T44.3X3	T44.3X4	T44.3X5	T44.3X6
Melaleuca alternifolia oil	T49.0X1	T49.0X2	T49.0X3	T49.0X4	T49.0X5	T49.0X6
Melanizing agents	T49.3X1	T49.3X2	T49.3X3	T49.3X4	T49.3X5	T49.3X6
Melanocyte-stimulating hormone	T38.891	T38.892	T38.893	T38.894	T38.895	T38.896
Melarsonyl potassium	T37.3X1	T37.3X2	T37.3X3	T37.3X4	T37.3X5	T37.3X6
Melarsoprol	T37.3X1	T37.3X2	T37.3X3	T37.3X4	T37.3X5	T37.3X6
Melia azedarach	T62.2X1	T62.2X2	T62.2X3	T62.2X4	—	—
Melitracen	T43.011	T43.012	T43.013	T43.014	T43.015	T43.016
Mellaril	T43.3X1	T43.3X2	T43.3X3	T43.3X4	T43.3X5	T43.3X6
Meloxine	T49.3X1	T49.3X2	T49.3X3	T49.3X4	T49.3X5	T49.3X6
Melperone	T43.4X1	T43.4X2	T43.4X3	T43.4X4	T43.4X5	T43.4X6
Melphalan	T45.1X1	T45.1X2	T45.1X3	T45.1X4	T45.1X5	T45.1X6
Memantine	T43.8X1	T43.8X2	T43.8X3	T43.8X4	T43.8X5	T43.8X6
Menadiol	T45.7X1	T45.7X2	T45.7X3	T45.7X4	T45.7X5	T45.7X6
sodium sulfate	T45.7X1	T45.7X2	T45.7X3	T45.7X4	T45.7X5	T45.7X6
Menadione	T45.7X1	T45.7X2	T45.7X3	T45.7X4	T45.7X5	T45.7X6
sodium bisulfite	T45.7X1	T45.7X2	T45.7X3	T45.7X4	T45.7X5	T45.7X6
Menaphthone	T45.7X1	T45.7X2	T45.7X3	T45.7X4	T45.7X5	T45.7X6
Menaquinone	T45.7X1	T45.7X2	T45.7X3	T45.7X4	T45.7X5	T45.7X6
Menatetrenone	T45.7X1	T45.7X2	T45.7X3	T45.7X4	T45.7X5	T45.7X6
Meningococcal vaccine	T50.A91	T50.A92	T50.A93	T50.A94	T50.A95	T50.A96
Menningovax (-AC) (-C)	T50.A91	T50.A92	T50.A93	T50.A94	T50.A95	T50.A96
Menotropins	T38.811	T38.812	T38.813	T38.814	T38.815	T38.816
Menthol	T48.5X1	T48.5X2	T48.5X3	T48.5X4	T48.5X5	T48.5X6
Mepacrine	T37.2X1	T37.2X2	T37.2X3	T37.2X4	T37.2X5	T37.2X6
Meparfynol	T42.6X1	T42.6X2	T42.6X3	T42.6X4	T42.6X5	T42.6X6
Mepartricin	T36.7X1	T36.7X2	T36.7X3	T36.7X4	T36.7X5	T36.7X6
Mepazine	T43.3X1	T43.3X2	T43.3X3	T43.3X4	T43.3X5	T43.3X6
Mepenzolate	T44.3X1	T44.3X2	T44.3X3	T44.3X4	T44.3X5	T44.3X6
bromide	T44.3X1	T44.3X2	T44.3X3	T44.3X4	T44.3X5	T44.3X6
Meperidine	T40.4X1	T40.4X2	T40.4X3	T40.4X4	T40.4X5	T40.4X6
Mephebarbital	T42.3X1	T42.3X2	T42.3X3	T42.3X4	T42.3X5	T42.3X6
Mephenamin (e)	T42.8X1	T42.8X2	T42.8X3	T42.8X4	T42.8X5	T42.8X6
Mephenesin	T42.8X1	T42.8X2	T42.8X3	T42.8X4	T42.8X5	T42.8X6
Mephenhydramine	T45.0X1	T45.0X2	T45.0X3	T45.0X4	T45.0X5	T45.0X6
Mephenoxalone	T42.8X1	T42.8X2	T42.8X3	T42.8X4	T42.8X5	T42.8X6
Mephentermine	T44.991	T44.992	T44.993	T44.994	T44.995	T44.996
Mephenytoin	T42.0X1	T42.0X2	T42.0X3	T42.0X4	T42.0X5	T42.0X6
with phenobarbital	T42.3X1	T42.3X2	T42.3X3	T42.3X4	T42.3X5	T42.3X6
Mephobarbital	T42.3X1	T42.3X2	T42.3X3	T42.3X4	T42.3X5	T42.3X6
Mephosfolan	T60.0X1	T60.0X2	T60.0X3	T60.0X4	—	—
Mepindolol	T44.7X1	T44.7X2	T44.7X3	T44.7X4	T44.7X5	T44.7X6
Mepiperphenidol	T44.3X1	T44.3X2	T44.3X3	T44.3X4	T44.3X5	T44.3X6
Mepitiostane	T38.7X1	T38.7X2	T38.7X3	T38.7X4	T38.7X5	T38.7X6
Mepivacaine	T41.3X1	T41.3X2	T41.3X3	T41.3X4	T41.3X5	T41.3X6
epidural	T41.3X1	T41.3X2	T41.3X3	T41.3X4	T41.3X5	T41.3X6
Meprednisone	T38.0X1	T38.0X2	T38.0X3	T38.0X4	T38.0X5	T38.0X6
Meprobam	T43.591	T43.592	T43.593	T43.594	T43.595	T43.596
Meprobamate	T43.591	T43.592	T43.593	T43.594	T43.595	T43.596
Meproscillarin	T46.0X1	T46.0X2	T46.0X3	T46.0X4	T46.0X5	T46.0X6
Meprylcaine	T41.3X1	T41.3X2	T41.3X3	T41.3X4	T41.3X5	T41.3X6
Meptazinol	T39.8X1	T39.8X2	T39.8X3	T39.8X4	T39.8X5	T39.8X6
Mepyramine	T45.0X1	T45.0X2	T45.0X3	T45.0X4	T45.0X5	T45.0X6
Mequitazine	T43.3X1	T43.3X2	T43.3X3	T43.3X4	T43.3X5	T43.3X6
Meralluride	T50.2X1	T50.2X2	T50.2X3	T50.2X4	T50.2X5	T50.2X6
Merbaphen	T50.2X1	T50.2X2	T50.2X3	T50.2X4	T50.2X5	T50.2X6
Merbromin	T49.0X1	T49.0X2	T49.0X3	T49.0X4	T49.0X5	T49.0X6
Mercaptobenzothiazole salts	T49.0X1	T49.0X2	T49.0X3	T49.0X4	T49.0X5	T49.0X6
Mercaptomerin	T50.2X1	T50.2X2	T50.2X3	T50.2X4	T50.2X5	T50.2X6
Mercaptopurine	T45.1X1	T45.1X2	T45.1X3	T45.1X4	T45.1X5	T45.1X6
Mercumatilin	T50.2X1	T50.2X2	T50.2X3	T50.2X4	T50.2X5	T50.2X6
Mercuramide	T50.2X1	T50.2X2	T50.2X3	T50.2X4	T50.2X5	T50.2X6
Mercurochrome	T49.0X1	T49.0X2	T49.0X3	T49.0X4	T49.0X5	T49.0X6
Mercurophylline	T50.2X1	T50.2X2	T50.2X3	T50.2X4	T50.2X5	T50.2X6
Mercury, mercurial, mercuric, mercurous (compounds) (cyanide) (fumes) (nonmedicinal) (vapor) NEC	T56.1X1	T56.1X2	T56.1X3	T56.1X4	—	—
ammoniated	T49.0X1	T49.0X2	T49.0X3	T49.0X4	T49.0X5	T49.0X6
anti-infective						
local	T49.0X1	T49.0X2	T49.0X3	T49.0X4	T49.0X5	T49.0X6
systemic	T37.8X1	T37.8X2	T37.8X3	T37.8X4	T37.8X5	T37.8X6
topical	T49.0X1	T49.0X2	T49.0X3	T49.0X4	T49.0X5	T49.0X6
chloride (ammoniated)	T49.0X1	T49.0X2	T49.0X3	T49.0X4	T49.0X5	T49.0X6
fungicide	T56.1X1	T56.1X2	T56.1X3	T56.1X4	—	—
diuretic NEC	T50.2X1	T50.2X2	T50.2X3	T50.2X4	T50.2X5	T50.2X6
fungicide	T56.1X1	T56.1X2	T56.1X3	T56.1X4	—	—
organic (fungicide)	T56.1X1	T56.1X2	T56.1X3	T56.1X4	—	—
oxide, yellow	T49.0X1	T49.0X2	T49.0X3	T49.0X4	T49.0X5	T49.0X6
Mersalyl	T50.2X1	T50.2X2	T50.2X3	T50.2X4	T50.2X5	T50.2X6
Merthiolate	T49.0X1	T49.0X2	T49.0X3	T49.0X4	T49.0X5	T49.0X6
ophthalmic preparation	T49.5X1	T49.5X2	T49.5X3	T49.5X4	T49.5X5	T49.5X6
Meruvax	T50.B91	T50.B92	T50.B93	T50.B94	T50.B95	T50.B96
Mesalazine	T47.8X1	T47.8X2	T47.8X3	T47.8X4	T47.8X5	T47.8X6
Mescal buttons	T40.991	T40.992	T40.993	T40.994	—	—
Mescaline	T40.991	T40.992	T40.993	T40.994	—	—
Mesna	T48.4X1	T48.4X2	T48.4X3	T48.4X4	T48.4X5	T48.4X6
Mesoglycan	T46.6X1	T46.6X2	T46.6X3	T46.6X4	T46.6X5	T46.6X6
Mesoridazine	T43.3X1	T43.3X2	T43.3X3	T43.3X4	T43.3X5	T43.3X6
Mestanolone	T38.7X1	T38.7X2	T38.7X3	T38.7X4	T38.7X5	T38.7X6
Mesterolone	T38.7X1	T38.7X2	T38.7X3	T38.7X4	T38.7X5	T38.7X6
Mestranol	T38.5X1	T38.5X2	T38.5X3	T38.5X4	T38.5X5	T38.5X6
Mesulergine	T42.8X1	T42.8X2	T42.8X3	T42.8X4	T42.8X5	T42.8X6
Mesulfen	T49.0X1	T49.0X2	T49.0X3	T49.0X4	T49.0X5	T49.0X6
Mesuximide	T42.2X1	T42.2X2	T42.2X3	T42.2X4	T42.2X5	T42.2X6
Metabutethamine	T41.3X1	T41.3X2	T41.3X3	T41.3X4	T41.3X5	T41.3X6
Metactesylacetate	T49.0X1	T49.0X2	T49.0X3	T49.0X4	T49.0X5	T49.0X6
Metacycline	T36.4X1	T36.4X2	T36.4X3	T36.4X4	T36.4X5	T36.4X6
Metaldehyde (snail killer) NEC	T60.8X1	T60.8X2	T60.8X3	T60.8X4	—	—
Metals (heavy) (nonmedicinal)	T56.91	T56.92	T56.93	T56.94	—	—
dust, fumes, or vapor NEC	T56.91	T56.92	T56.93	T56.94	—	—
light NEC	T56.91	T56.92	T56.93	T56.94	—	—
dust, fumes, or vapor NEC	T56.91	T56.92	T56.93	T56.94	—	—
specified NEC	T56.891	T56.892	T56.893	T56.894	—	—
thallium	T56.811	T56.812	T56.813	T56.814	—	—
Metamfetamine	T43.621	T43.622	T43.623	T43.624	T43.625	T43.626
Metamizole sodium	T39.2X1	T39.2X2	T39.2X3	T39.2X4	T39.2X5	T39.2X6
Metampicillin	T36.0X1	T36.0X2	T36.0X3	T36.0X4	T36.0X5	T36.0X6
Metamucil	T47.4X1	T47.4X2	T47.4X3	T47.4X4	T47.4X5	T47.4X6
Metandienone	T38.7X1	T38.7X2	T38.7X3	T38.7X4	T38.7X5	T38.7X6
Metandrostenolone	T38.7X1	T38.7X2	T38.7X3	T38.7X4	T38.7X5	T38.7X6
Metaphen	T49.0X1	T49.0X2	T49.0X3	T49.0X4	T49.0X5	T49.0X6
Metaphos	T60.0X1	T60.0X2	T60.0X3	T60.0X4	—	—
Metapramine	T43.011	T43.012	T43.013	T43.014	T43.015	T43.016
Metaproterenol	T48.291	T48.292	T48.293	T48.294	T48.295	T48.296
Metaraminol	T44.4X1	T44.4X2	T44.4X3	T44.4X4	T44.4X5	T44.4X6
Metaxalone	T42.8X1	T42.8X2	T42.8X3	T42.8X4	T42.8X5	T42.8X6
Metenolone	T38.7X1	T38.7X2	T38.7X3	T38.7X4	T38.7X5	T38.7X6
Metergoline	T42.8X1	T42.8X2	T42.8X3	T42.8X4	T42.8X5	T42.8X6
Metescufylline	T46.991	T46.992	T46.993	T46.994	T46.995	T46.996
Metetoin	T42.0X1	T42.0X2	T42.0X3	T42.0X4	T42.0X5	T42.0X6
Metformin	T38.3X1	T38.3X2	T38.3X3	T38.3X4	T38.3X5	T38.3X6
Methacholine	T44.1X1	T44.1X2	T44.1X3	T44.1X4	T44.1X5	T44.1X6
Methacycline	T36.4X1	T36.4X2	T36.4X3	T36.4X4	T36.4X5	T36.4X6
Methadone	T40.3X1	T40.3X2	T40.3X3	T40.3X4	T40.3X5	T40.3X6
Methallenestril	T38.5X1	T38.5X2	T38.5X3	T38.5X4	T38.5X5	T38.5X6

Mechlorethamine — Methallenestril

Substance	Poisoning, Accidental (unintentional)	Poisoning, Intentional Self-harm	Poisoning, Assault	Poisoning, Undetermined	Adverse Effect	Under-dosing
Methallenoestril	T38.5X1	T38.5X2	T38.5X3	T38.5X4	T38.5X5	T38.5X6
Methamphetamine	T43.621	T43.622	T43.623	T43.624	T43.625	T43.626
Methampyrone	T39.2X1	T39.2X2	T39.2X3	T39.2X4	T39.2X5	T39.2X6
Methandienone	T38.7X1	T38.7X2	T38.7X3	T38.7X4	T38.7X5	T38.7X6
Methandriol	T38.7X1	T38.7X2	T38.7X3	T38.7X4	T38.7X5	T38.7X6
Methandrostenolone	T38.7X1	T38.7X2	T38.7X3	T38.7X4	T38.7X5	T38.7X6
Methane	T59.891	T59.892	T59.893	T59.894	—	—
Methanethiol	T59.891	T59.892	T59.893	T59.894	—	—
Methaniazide	T37.1X1	T37.1X2	T37.1X3	T37.1X4	T37.1X5	T37.1X6
Methanol (vapor)	T51.1X1	T51.1X2	T51.1X3	T51.1X4	—	—
Methantheline	T44.3X1	T44.3X2	T44.3X3	T44.3X4	T44.3X5	T44.3X6
Methanthelinium bromide	T44.3X1	T44.3X2	T44.3X3	T44.3X4	T44.3X5	T44.3X6
Methaphenilene	T45.0X1	T45.0X2	T45.0X3	T45.0X4	T45.0X5	T45.0X6
Methapyrilene	T45.0X1	T45.0X2	T45.0X3	T45.0X4	T45.0X5	T45.0X6
Methaqualone (compound)	T42.6X1	T42.6X2	T42.6X3	T42.6X4	T42.6X5	T42.6X6
Metharbital	T42.3X1	T42.3X2	T42.3X3	T42.3X4	T42.3X5	T42.3X6
Methazolamide	T50.2X1	T50.2X2	T50.2X3	T50.2X4	T50.2X5	T50.2X6
Methdilazine	T43.3X1	T43.3X2	T43.3X3	T43.3X4	T43.3X5	T43.3X6
Methedrine	T43.621	T43.622	T43.623	T43.624	T43.625	T43.626
Methenamine (mandelate)	T37.8X1	T37.8X2	T37.8X3	T37.8X4	T37.8X5	T37.8X6
Methenolone	T38.7X1	T38.7X2	T38.7X3	T38.7X4	T38.7X5	T38.7X6
Methergine	T48.0X1	T48.0X2	T48.0X3	T48.0X4	T48.0X5	T48.0X6
Methetoin	T42.0X1	T42.0X2	T42.0X3	T42.0X4	T42.0X5	T42.0X6
Methiacil	T38.2X1	T38.2X2	T38.2X3	T38.2X4	T38.2X5	T38.2X6
Methicillin	T36.0X1	T36.0X2	T36.0X3	T36.0X4	T36.0X5	T36.0X6
Methimazole	T38.2X1	T38.2X2	T38.2X3	T38.2X4	T38.2X5	T38.2X6
Methiodal sodium	T50.8X1	T50.8X2	T50.8X3	T50.8X4	T50.8X5	T50.8X6
Methionine	T50.991	T50.992	T50.993	T50.994	T50.995	T50.996
Methisazone	T37.5X1	T37.5X2	T37.5X3	T37.5X4	T37.5X5	T37.5X6
Methisoprinol	T37.5X1	T37.5X2	T37.5X3	T37.5X4	T37.5X5	T37.5X6
Methitural	T42.3X1	T42.3X2	T42.3X3	T42.3X4	T42.3X5	T42.3X6
Methixene	T44.3X1	T44.3X2	T44.3X3	T44.3X4	T44.3X5	T44.3X6
Methobarbital, methobarbitone	T42.3X1	T42.3X2	T42.3X3	T42.3X4	T42.3X5	T42.3X6
Methocarbamol	T42.8X1	T42.8X2	T42.8X3	T42.8X4	T42.8X5	T42.8X6
skeletal muscle relaxant	T48.1X1	T48.1X2	T48.1X3	T48.1X4	T48.1X5	T48.1X6
Methohexital	T41.1X1	T41.1X2	T41.1X3	T41.1X4	T41.1X5	T41.1X6
Methohexitone	T41.1X1	T41.1X2	T41.1X3	T41.1X4	T41.1X5	T41.1X6
Methoin	T42.0X1	T42.0X2	T42.0X3	T42.0X4	T42.0X5	T42.0X6
Methopholine	T39.8X1	T39.8X2	T39.8X3	T39.8X4	T39.8X5	T39.8X6
Methopromazine	T43.3X1	T43.3X2	T43.3X3	T43.3X4	T43.3X5	T43.3X6
Methorate	T48.3X1	T48.3X2	T48.3X3	T48.3X4	T48.3X5	T48.3X6
Methoserpidine	T46.5X1	T46.5X2	T46.5X3	T46.5X4	T46.5X5	T46.5X6
Methotrexate	T45.1X1	T45.1X2	T45.1X3	T45.1X4	T45.1X5	T45.1X6
Methotrimeprazine	T43.3X1	T43.3X2	T43.3X3	T43.3X4	T43.3X5	T43.3X6
Methoxa-Dome	T49.3X1	T49.3X2	T49.3X3	T49.3X4	T49.3X5	T49.3X6
Methoxamine	T44.4X1	T44.4X2	T44.4X3	T44.4X4	T44.4X5	T44.4X6
Methoxsalen	T50.991	T50.992	T50.993	T50.994	T50.995	T50.996
Methoxyaniline	T65.3X1	T65.3X2	T65.3X3	T65.3X4	—	—
Methoxybenzyl penicillin	T36.0X1	T36.0X2	T36.0X3	T36.0X4	T36.0X5	T36.0X6
Methoxychlor	T53.7X1	T53.7X2	T53.7X3	T53.7X4	—	—
Methoxy-DDT	T53.7X1	T53.7X2	T53.7X3	T53.7X4	—	—
Methoxyflurane	T41.0X1	T41.0X2	T41.0X3	T41.0X4	T41.0X5	T41.0X6
Methoxyphenamine	T48.6X1	T48.6X2	T48.6X3	T48.6X4	T48.6X5	T48.6X6
Methoxypromazine	T43.3X1	T43.3X2	T43.3X3	T43.3X4	T43.3X5	T43.3X6
Methscopolamine bromide	T44.3X1	T44.3X2	T44.3X3	T44.3X4	T44.3X5	T44.3X6
Methsuximide	T42.2X1	T42.2X2	T42.2X3	T42.2X4	T42.2X5	T42.2X6
Methyclothiazide	T50.2X1	T50.2X2	T50.2X3	T50.2X4	T50.2X5	T50.2X6
Methyl						
acetate	T52.4X1	T52.4X2	T52.4X3	T52.4X4	—	—
acetone	T52.4X1	T52.4X2	T52.4X3	T52.4X4	—	—
acrylate	T65.891	T65.892	T65.893	T65.894	—	—
alcohol	T51.1X1	T51.1X2	T51.1X3	T51.1X4	—	—
aminophenol	T65.3X1	T65.3X2	T65.3X3	T65.3X4	—	—
amphetamine	T43.621	T43.622	T43.623	T43.624	T43.625	T43.626
androstanolone	T38.7X1	T38.7X2	T38.7X3	T38.7X4	T38.7X5	T38.7X6
atropine	T44.3X1	T44.3X2	T44.3X3	T44.3X4	T44.3X5	T44.3X6
benzene	T52.2X1	T52.2X2	T52.2X3	T52.2X4	—	—
benzoate	T52.8X1	T52.8X2	T52.8X3	T52.8X4	—	—
benzol	T52.2X1	T52.2X2	T52.2X3	T52.2X4	—	—
bromide (gas)	T59.891	T59.892	T59.893	T59.894	—	—
fumigant	T60.8X1	T60.8X2	T60.8X3	T60.8X4	—	—
butanol	T51.3X1	T51.3X2	T51.3X3	T51.3X4	—	—
carbinol	T51.1X1	T51.1X2	T51.1X3	T51.1X4	—	—
carbonate	T52.8X1	T52.8X2	T52.8X3	T52.8X4	—	—
CCNU	T45.1X1	T45.1X2	T45.1X3	T45.1X4	T45.1X5	T45.1X6
cellosolve	T52.91	T52.92	T52.93	T52.94	—	—
cellulose	T47.4X1	T47.4X2	T47.4X3	T47.4X4	T47.4X5	T47.4X6
chloride (gas)	T59.891	T59.892	T59.893	T59.894	—	—
chloroformate	T59.3X1	T59.3X2	T59.3X3	T59.3X4	—	—
cyclohexane	T52.8X1	T52.8X2	T52.8X3	T52.8X4	—	—
cyclohexanol	T51.8X1	T51.8X2	T51.8X3	T51.8X4	—	—

Substance	Poisoning, Accidental (unintentional)	Poisoning, Intentional Self-harm	Poisoning, Assault	Poisoning, Undetermined	Adverse Effect	Under-dosing
Methyl — continued						
cyclohexanone	T52.8X1	T52.8X2	T52.8X3	T52.8X4	—	—
cyclohexyl acetate	T52.8X1	T52.8X2	T52.8X3	T52.8X4	—	—
demeton	T60.0X1	T60.0X2	T60.0X3	T60.0X4	—	—
dihydromorphinone	T40.2X1	T40.2X2	T40.2X3	T40.2X4	T40.2X5	T40.2X6
ergometrine	T48.0X1	T48.0X2	T48.0X3	T48.0X4	T48.0X5	T48.0X6
ergonovine	T48.0X1	T48.0X2	T48.0X3	T48.0X4	T48.0X5	T48.0X6
ethyl ketone	T52.4X1	T52.4X2	T52.4X3	T52.4X4	—	—
glucamine antimonate	T37.8X1	T37.8X2	T37.8X3	T37.8X4	T37.8X5	T37.8X6
hydrazine	T65.891	T65.892	T65.893	T65.894	—	—
iodide	T65.891	T65.892	T65.893	T65.894	—	—
isobutyl ketone	T52.4X1	T52.4X2	T52.4X3	T52.4X4	—	—
isothiocyanate	T60.3X1	T60.3X2	T60.3X3	T60.3X4	—	—
mercaptan	T59.891	T59.892	T59.893	T59.894	—	—
morphine NEC	T40.2X1	T40.2X2	T40.2X3	T40.2X4	T40.2X5	T40.2X6
nicotinate	T49.4X1	T49.4X2	T49.4X3	T49.4X4	T49.4X5	T49.4X6
paraben	T49.0X1	T49.0X2	T49.0X3	T49.0X4	T49.0X5	T49.0X6
parafynol	T42.6X1	T42.6X2	T42.6X3	T42.6X4	T42.6X5	T42.6X6
parathion	T60.0X1	T60.0X2	T60.0X3	T60.0X4	—	—
peridol	T43.4X1	T43.4X2	T43.4X3	T43.4X4	T43.4X5	T43.4X6
phenidate	T43.631	T43.632	T43.633	T43.634	T43.635	T43.636
prednisolone	T38.0X1	T38.0X2	T38.0X3	T38.0X4	T38.0X5	T38.0X6
ENT agent	T49.6X1	T49.6X2	T49.6X3	T49.6X4	T49.6X5	T49.6X6
ophthalmic preparation	T49.5X1	T49.5X2	T49.5X3	T49.5X4	T49.5X5	T49.5X6
topical NEC	T49.0X1	T49.0X2	T49.0X3	T49.0X4	T49.0X5	T49.0X6
propylcarbinol	T51.3X1	T51.3X2	T51.3X3	T51.3X4	—	—
rosaniline NEC	T49.0X1	T49.0X2	T49.0X3	T49.0X4	T49.0X5	T49.0X6
salicylate	T49.2X1	T49.2X2	T49.2X3	T49.2X4	T49.2X5	T49.2X6
sulfate (fumes)	T59.891	T59.892	T59.893	T59.894	—	—
liquid	T52.8X1	T52.8X2	T52.8X3	T52.8X4	—	—
sulfonal	T42.6X1	T42.6X2	T42.6X3	T42.6X4	T42.6X5	T42.6X6
testosterone	T38.7X1	T38.7X2	T38.7X3	T38.7X4	T38.7X5	T38.7X6
thiouracil	T38.2X1	T38.2X2	T38.2X3	T38.2X4	T38.2X5	T38.2X6
Methylamphetamine	T43.621	T43.622	T43.623	T43.624	T43.625	T43.626
Methylated spirit	T51.1X1	T51.1X2	T51.1X3	T51.1X4	—	—
Methylatropine nitrate	T44.3X1	T44.3X2	T44.3X3	T44.3X4	T44.3X5	T44.3X6
Methylbenactyzium bromide	T44.3X1	T44.3X2	T44.3X3	T44.3X4	T44.3X5	T44.3X6
Methylbenzethonium chloride	T49.0X1	T49.0X2	T49.0X3	T49.0X4	T49.0X5	T49.0X6
Methylcellulose	T47.4X1	T47.4X2	T47.4X3	T47.4X4	T47.4X5	T47.4X6
laxative	T47.4X1	T47.4X2	T47.4X3	T47.4X4	T47.4X5	T47.4X6
Methylchlorophenoxyacetic acid	T60.3X1	T60.3X2	T60.3X3	T60.3X4	—	—
Methyldopa	T46.5X1	T46.5X2	T46.5X3	T46.5X4	T46.5X5	T46.5X6
Methyldopate	T46.5X1	T46.5X2	T46.5X3	T46.5X4	T46.5X5	T46.5X6
Methylene						
blue	T50.6X1	T50.6X2	T50.6X3	T50.6X4	T50.6X5	T50.6X6
chloride or dichloride (solvent) NEC	T53.4X1	T53.4X2	T53.4X3	T53.4X4	—	—
Methylenedioxyamphetamine	T43.621	T43.622	T43.623	T43.624	T43.625	T43.626
Methylenedioxymeth-amphetamine	T43.641	T43.642	T43.643	T43.644	—	—
Methylergometrine	T48.0X1	T48.0X2	T48.0X3	T48.0X4	T48.0X5	T48.0X6
Methylergonovine	T48.0X1	T48.0X2	T48.0X3	T48.0X4	T48.0X5	T48.0X6
Methylestrenolone	T38.5X1	T38.5X2	T38.5X3	T38.5X4	T38.5X5	T38.5X6
Methylethyl cellulose	T50.991	T50.992	T50.993	T50.994	T50.995	T50.996
Methylhexabital	T42.3X1	T42.3X2	T42.3X3	T42.3X4	T42.3X5	T42.3X6
Methylmorphine	T40.2X1	T40.2X2	T40.2X3	T40.2X4	T40.2X5	T40.2X6
Methylparaben (ophthalmic)	T49.5X1	T49.5X2	T49.5X3	T49.5X4	T49.5X5	T49.5X6
Methylparafynol	T42.6X1	T42.6X2	T42.6X3	T42.6X4	T42.6X5	T42.6X6
Methylpentynol, methylpenthynol	T43.631	T43.632	T43.633	T43.634	T43.635	T43.636
Methylphenidate	T42.3X1	T42.3X2	T42.3X3	T42.3X4	T42.3X5	T42.3X6
Methylphenobarbital	T47.1X1	T47.1X2	T47.1X3	T47.1X4	T47.1X5	T47.1X6
Methylpolysiloxane						
Methylprednisolone — see Methyl, prednisolone						
Methylrosaniline	T49.0X1	T49.0X2	T49.0X3	T49.0X4	T49.0X5	T49.0X6
Methylrosanilinium chloride	T49.0X1	T49.0X2	T49.0X3	T49.0X4	T49.0X5	T49.0X6
Methyltestosterone	T38.7X1	T38.7X2	T38.7X3	T38.7X4	T38.7X5	T38.7X6
Methylthionine chloride	T50.6X1	T50.6X2	T50.6X3	T50.6X4	T50.6X5	T50.6X6
Methylthioninium chloride	T50.6X1	T50.6X2	T50.6X3	T50.6X4	T50.6X5	T50.6X6
Methylthiouracil	T38.2X1	T38.2X2	T38.2X3	T38.2X4	T38.2X5	T38.2X6
Methyprylon	T42.6X1	T42.6X2	T42.6X3	T42.6X4	T42.6X5	T42.6X6
Methysergide	T46.5X1	T46.5X2	T46.5X3	T46.5X4	T46.5X5	T46.5X6
Metiamide	T47.1X1	T47.1X2	T47.1X3	T47.1X4	T47.1X5	T47.1X6
Meticillin	T36.0X1	T36.0X2	T36.0X3	T36.0X4	T36.0X5	T36.0X6
Meticrane	T50.2X1	T50.2X2	T50.2X3	T50.2X4	T50.2X5	T50.2X6
Metildigoxin	T46.0X1	T46.0X2	T46.0X3	T46.0X4	T46.0X5	T46.0X6

Substance	Poisoning, Accidental (unintentional)	Poisoning, Intentional Self-harm	Poisoning, Assault	Poisoning, Undetermined	Adverse Effect	Under-dosing
Metipranolol	T49.5X1	T49.5X2	T49.5X3	T49.5X4	T49.5X5	T49.5X6
Metirosine	T46.5X1	T46.5X2	T46.5X3	T46.5X4	T46.5X5	T46.5X6
Metisazone	T37.5X1	T37.5X2	T37.5X3	T37.5X4	T37.5X5	T37.5X6
Metixene	T44.3X1	T44.3X2	T44.3X3	T44.3X4	T44.3X5	T44.3X6
Metizoline	T48.5X1	T48.5X2	T48.5X3	T48.5X4	T48.5X5	T48.5X6
Metoclopramide	T45.0X1	T45.0X2	T45.0X3	T45.0X4	T45.0X5	T45.0X6
Metofenazate	T43.3X1	T43.3X2	T43.3X3	T43.3X4	T43.3X5	T43.3X6
Metofoline	T39.8X1	T39.8X2	T39.8X3	T39.8X4	T39.8X5	T39.8X6
Metolazone	T50.2X1	T50.2X2	T50.2X3	T50.2X4	T50.2X5	T50.2X6
Metopon	T40.2X1	T40.2X2	T40.2X3	T40.2X4	T40.2X5	T40.2X6
Metoprine	T45.1X1	T45.1X2	T45.1X3	T45.1X4	T45.1X5	T45.1X6
Metoprolol	T44.7X1	T44.7X2	T44.7X3	T44.7X4	T44.7X5	T44.7X6
Metrifonate	T60.0X1	T60.0X2	T60.0X3	T60.0X4	—	—
Metrizamide	T50.8X1	T50.8X2	T50.8X3	T50.8X4	T50.8X5	T50.8X6
Metrizoic acid	T50.8X1	T50.8X2	T50.8X3	T50.8X4	T50.8X5	T50.8X6
Metronidazole	T37.8X1	T37.8X2	T37.8X3	T37.8X4	T37.8X5	T37.8X6
Metycaine	T41.3X1	T41.3X2	T41.3X3	T41.3X4	T41.3X5	T41.3X6
infiltration (subcutaneous)	T41.3X1	T41.3X2	T41.3X3	T41.3X4	T41.3X5	T41.3X6
nerve block (peripheral) (plexus)	T41.3X1	T41.3X2	T41.3X3	T41.3X4	T41.3X5	T41.3X6
topical (surface)	T41.3X1	T41.3X2	T41.3X3	T41.3X4	T41.3X5	T41.3X6
Metyrapone	T50.8X1	T50.8X2	T50.8X3	T50.8X4	T50.8X5	T50.8X6
Mevinphos	T60.0X1	T60.0X2	T60.0X3	T60.0X4	—	—
Mexazolam	T42.4X1	T42.4X2	T42.4X3	T42.4X4	T42.4X5	T42.4X6
Mexenone	T49.3X1	T49.3X2	T49.3X3	T49.3X4	T49.3X5	T49.3X6
Mexiletine	T46.2X1	T46.2X2	T46.2X3	T46.2X4	T46.2X5	T46.2X6
Mezereon	T62.2X1	T62.2X2	T62.2X3	T62.2X4	—	—
berries	T62.1X1	T62.1X2	T62.1X3	T62.1X4	—	—
Mezlocillin	T36.0X1	T36.0X2	T36.0X3	T36.0X4	T36.0X5	T36.0X6
Mianserin	T43.021	T43.022	T43.023	T43.024	T43.025	T43.026
Micatin	T49.0X1	T49.0X2	T49.0X3	T49.0X4	T49.0X5	T49.0X6
Miconazole	T49.0X1	T49.0X2	T49.0X3	T49.0X4	T49.0X5	T49.0X6
Micronomicin	T36.5X1	T36.5X2	T36.5X3	T36.5X4	T36.5X5	T36.5X6
Midazolam	T42.4X1	T42.4X2	T42.4X3	T42.4X4	T42.4X5	T42.4X6
Midecamycin	T36.3X1	T36.3X2	T36.3X3	T36.3X4	T36.3X5	T36.3X6
Mifepristone	T38.6X1	T38.6X2	T38.6X3	T38.6X4	T38.6X5	T38.6X6
Milk of magnesia	T47.1X1	T47.1X2	T47.1X3	T47.1X4	T47.1X5	T47.1X6
Millipede (tropical) (venomous)	T63.411	T63.412	T63.413	T63.414	—	—
Miltown	T43.591	T43.592	T43.593	T43.594	T43.595	T43.596
Milverine	T44.3X1	T44.3X2	T44.3X3	T44.3X4	T44.3X5	T44.3X6
Minaprine	T43.291	T43.292	T43.293	T43.294	T43.295	T43.296
Minaxolone	T41.291	T41.292	T41.293	T41.294	T41.295	T41.296
Mineral						
acids	T54.2X1	T54.2X2	T54.2X3	T54.2X4	—	—
oil (laxative)(medicinal)	T47.4X1	T47.4X2	T47.4X3	T47.4X4	T47.4X5	T47.4X6
emulsion	T47.2X1	T47.2X2	T47.2X3	T47.2X4	T47.2X5	T47.2X6
nonmedicinal	T52.0X1	T52.0X2	T52.0X3	T52.0X4	—	—
topical	T49.3X1	T49.3X2	T49.3X3	T49.3X4	T49.3X5	T49.3X6
salt NEC	T50.3X1	T50.3X2	T50.3X3	T50.3X4	T50.3X5	T50.3X6
spirits	T52.0X1	T52.0X2	T52.0X3	T52.0X4	—	—
Mineralocorticosteroid	T50.0X1	T50.0X2	T50.0X3	T50.0X4	T50.0X5	T50.0X6
Minocycline	T36.4X1	T36.4X2	T36.4X3	T36.4X4	T36.4X5	T36.4X6
Minoxidil	T46.7X1	T46.7X2	T46.7X3	T46.7X4	T46.7X5	T46.7X6
Miokamycin	T36.3X1	T36.3X2	T36.3X3	T36.3X4	T36.3X5	T36.3X6
Miotic drug	T49.5X1	T49.5X2	T49.5X3	T49.5X4	T49.5X5	T49.5X6
Mipafox	T60.0X1	T60.0X2	T60.0X3	T60.0X4	—	—
Mirex	T60.1X1	T60.1X2	T60.1X3	T60.1X4	—	—
Mirtazapine	T43.021	T43.022	T43.023	T43.024	T43.025	T43.026
Misonidazole	T37.3X1	T37.3X2	T37.3X3	T37.3X4	T37.3X5	T37.3X6
Misoprostol	T47.1X1	T47.1X2	T47.1X3	T47.1X4	T47.1X5	T47.1X6
Mithramycin	T45.1X1	T45.1X2	T45.1X3	T45.1X4	T45.1X5	T45.1X6
Mitobronitol	T45.1X1	T45.1X2	T45.1X3	T45.1X4	T45.1X5	T45.1X6
Mitoguazone	T45.1X1	T45.1X2	T45.1X3	T45.1X4	T45.1X5	T45.1X6
Mitolactol	T45.1X1	T45.1X2	T45.1X3	T45.1X4	T45.1X5	T45.1X6
Mitomycin	T45.1X1	T45.1X2	T45.1X3	T45.1X4	T45.1X5	T45.1X6
Mitopodozide	T45.1X1	T45.1X2	T45.1X3	T45.1X4	T45.1X5	T45.1X6
Mitotane	T45.1X1	T45.1X2	T45.1X3	T45.1X4	T45.1X5	T45.1X6
Mitoxantrone	T45.1X1	T45.1X2	T45.1X3	T45.1X4	T45.1X5	T45.1X6
Mivacurium chloride	T48.1X1	T48.1X2	T48.1X3	T48.1X4	T48.1X5	T48.1X6
Miyari bacteria	T47.6X1	T47.6X2	T47.6X3	T47.6X4	T47.6X5	T47.6X6
Moclobemide	T43.1X1	T43.1X2	T43.1X3	T43.1X4	T43.1X5	T43.1X6
Moderil	T46.5X1	T46.5X2	T46.5X3	T46.5X4	T46.5X5	T46.5X6
Mofebutazone	T39.2X1	T39.2X2	T39.2X3	T39.2X4	T39.2X5	T39.2X6
Mogadon — see Nitrazepam						
Molindone	T43.591	T43.592	T43.593	T43.594	T43.595	T43.596
Molsidomine	T46.3X1	T46.3X2	T46.3X3	T46.3X4	T46.3X5	T46.3X6
Mometasone	T49.0X1	T49.0X2	T49.0X3	T49.0X4	T49.0X5	T49.0X6
Monistat	T49.0X1	T49.0X2	T49.0X3	T49.0X4	T49.0X5	T49.0X6
Monkshood	T62.2X1	T62.2X2	T62.2X3	T62.2X4	—	—
Monoamine oxidase inhibitor NEC	T43.1X1	T43.1X2	T43.1X3	T43.1X4	T43.1X5	T43.1X6
hydrazine	T43.1X1	T43.1X2	T43.1X3	T43.1X4	T43.1X5	T43.1X6

Substance	Poisoning, Accidental (unintentional)	Poisoning, Intentional Self-harm	Poisoning, Assault	Poisoning, Undetermined	Adverse Effect	Under-dosing
Monobenzone	T49.4X1	T49.4X2	T49.4X3	T49.4X4	T49.4X5	T49.4X6
Monochloroacetic acid	T60.3X1	T60.3X2	T60.3X3	T60.3X4	—	—
Monochlorobenzene	T53.7X1	T53.7X2	T53.7X3	T53.7X4	—	—
Monoethanolamine	T46.8X1	T46.8X2	T46.8X3	T46.8X4	T46.8X5	T46.8X6
oleate	T46.8X1	T46.8X2	T46.8X3	T46.8X4	T46.8X5	T46.8X6
Monooctanoin	T50.991	T50.992	T50.993	T50.994	T50.995	T50.996
Monophenylbutazone	T39.2X1	T39.2X2	T39.2X3	T39.2X4	T39.2X5	T39.2X6
Monosodium glutamate	T65.891	T65.892	T65.893	T65.894	—	—
Monosulfiram	T49.0X1	T49.0X2	T49.0X3	T49.0X4	T49.0X5	T49.0X6
Monoxide, carbon — see Carbon, monoxide						
Monoxidine hydrochloride	T46.1X1	T46.1X2	T46.1X3	T46.1X4	T46.1X5	T46.1X6
Monuron	T60.3X1	T60.3X2	T60.3X3	T60.3X4	—	—
Moperone	T43.4X1	T43.4X2	T43.4X3	T43.4X4	T43.4X5	T43.4X6
Mopidamol	T45.1X1	T45.1X2	T45.1X3	T45.1X4	T45.1X5	T45.1X6
MOPP (mechloreth-amine + vincristine + prednisone + procarba-zine)	T45.1X1	T45.1X2	T45.1X3	T45.1X4	T45.1X5	T45.1X6
Morfin	T40.2X1	T40.2X2	T40.2X3	T40.2X4	T40.2X5	T40.2X6
Morinamide	T37.1X1	T37.1X2	T37.1X3	T37.1X4	T37.1X5	T37.1X6
Morning glory seeds	T40.991	T40.992	T40.993	T40.994	—	—
Moroxydine	T37.5X1	T37.5X2	T37.5X3	T37.5X4	T37.5X5	T37.5X6
Morphazinamide	T37.1X1	T37.1X2	T37.1X3	T37.1X4	T37.1X5	T37.1X6
Morphine	T40.2X1	T40.2X2	T40.2X3	T40.2X4	T40.2X5	T40.2X6
antagonist	T50.7X1	T50.7X2	T50.7X3	T50.7X4	T50.7X5	T50.7X6
Morpholinylethylmorphine	T40.2X1	T40.2X2	T40.2X3	T40.2X4		
Morsuximide	T42.2X1	T42.2X2	T42.2X3	T42.2X4	T42.2X5	T42.2X6
Mosapramine	T43.591	T43.592	T43.593	T43.594	T43.595	T43.596
Moth balls — see also Pesticides	T60.2X1	T60.2X2	T60.2X3	T60.2X4	—	—
naphthalene	T60.2X1	T60.2X2	T60.2X3	T60.2X4	—	—
paradichlorobenzene	T60.1X1	T60.1X2	T60.1X3	T60.1X4	—	—
Motor exhaust gas	T58.01	T58.02	T58.03	T58.04	—	—
Mouthwash (antiseptic) (zinc chloride)	T49.6X1	T49.6X2	T49.6X3	T49.6X4	T49.6X5	T49.6X6
Moxastine	T45.0X1	T45.0X2	T45.0X3	T45.0X4	T45.0X5	T45.0X6
Moxaverine	T44.3X1	T44.3X2	T44.3X3	T44.3X4	T44.3X5	T44.3X6
Moxisylyte	T46.7X1	T46.7X2	T46.7X3	T46.7X4	T46.7X5	T46.7X6
Mucilage, plant	T47.4X1	T47.4X2	T47.4X3	T47.4X4	T47.4X5	T47.4X6
Mucolytic drug	T48.4X1	T48.4X2	T48.4X3	T48.4X4	T48.4X5	T48.4X6
Mucomyst	T48.4X1	T48.4X2	T48.4X3	T48.4X4	T48.4X5	T48.4X6
Mucous membrane agents (external)	T49.91	T49.92	T49.93	T49.94	T49.95	T49.96
specified NEC	T49.8X1	T49.8X2	T49.8X3	T49.8X4	T49.8X5	T49.8X6
Multiple unspecified drugs, medicaments and biological substances	T50.911	T50.912	T50.913	T50.914	T50.915	T50.916
Mumps						
immune globulin (human)	T50.Z11	T50.Z12	T50.Z13	T50.Z14	T50.Z15	T50.Z16
skin test antigen	T50.8X1	T50.8X2	T50.8X4	T50.8X5	T50.8X6	
vaccine	T50.B91	T50.B92	T50.B93	T50.B95	T50.B96	
Mumpsvax	T50.B91	T50.B92	T50.B93	T50.B94	T50.B95	T50.B96
Mupirocin	T49.0X1	T49.0X2	T49.0X3	T49.0X4	T49.0X5	T49.0X6
Muriatic acid — see Hydrochloric acid						
Muromonab-CD3	T45.1X1	T45.1X2	T45.1X3	T45.1X4	T45.1X5	T45.1X6
Muscle-action drug NEC	T48.201	T48.202	T48.203	T48.204	T48.205	T48.206
Muscle affecting agents NEC	T48.201	T48.202	T48.203	T48.204	T48.205	T48.206
oxytocic	T48.0X1	T48.0X2	T48.0X3	T48.0X4	T48.0X5	T48.0X6
relaxants	T48.201	T48.202	T48.203	T48.204	T48.205	T48.206
central nervous system	T42.8X1	T42.8X2	T42.8X3	T42.8X4	T42.8X5	T42.8X6
skeletal	T48.1X1	T48.1X2	T48.1X3	T48.1X4	T48.1X5	T48.1X6
smooth	T44.3X1	T44.3X2	T44.3X3	T44.3X4	T44.3X5	T44.3X6
Muscle relaxant — see Relaxant, muscle						
Muscle-tone depressant, central NEC	T42.8X1	T42.8X2	T42.8X3	T42.8X4	T42.8X5	T42.8X6
specified NEC	T42.8X1	T42.8X2	T42.8X3	T42.8X4	T42.8X5	T42.8X6
Mushroom, noxious	T62.0X1	T62.0X2	T62.0X3	T62.0X4	—	—
Mussel, noxious	T61.781	T61.782	T61.783	T61.784	—	—
Mustard (emetic)	T47.7X1	T47.7X2	T47.7X3	T47.7X4	T47.7X5	T47.7X6
black	T47.7X1	T47.7X2	T47.7X3	T47.7X4	T47.7X5	T47.7X6
gas, not in war	T59.91	T59.92	T59.93	T59.94	—	—
nitrogen	T45.1X1	T45.1X2	T45.1X3	T45.1X4	T45.1X5	T45.1X6
Mustine	T45.1X1	T45.1X2	T45.1X3	T45.1X4	T45.1X5	T45.1X6
M-vac	T45.1X1	T45.1X2	T45.1X3	T45.1X4	T45.1X5	T45.1X6
Mycifradin	T36.5X1	T36.5X2	T36.5X3	T36.5X4	T36.5X5	T36.5X6
topical	T49.0X1	T49.0X2	T49.0X3	T49.0X4	T49.0X5	T49.0X6
Mycitracin	T36.8X1	T36.8X2	T36.8X3	T36.8X4	T36.8X5	T36.8X6
ophthalmic preparation	T49.5X1	T49.5X2	T49.5X3	T49.5X4	T49.5X5	T49.5X6
Mycostatin	T36.7X1	T36.7X2	T36.7X3	T36.7X4	T36.7X5	T36.7X6
topical	T49.0X1	T49.0X2	T49.0X3	T49.0X4	T49.0X5	T49.0X6

Substance	Poisoning, Accidental (unintentional)	Poisoning, Intentional Self-harm	Poisoning, Assault	Poisoning, Undetermined	Adverse Effect	Under-dosing
Mycotoxins	T64.81	T64.82	T64.83	T64.84	—	—
aflatoxin	T64.01	T64.02	T64.03	T64.04	—	—
specified NEC	T64.81	T64.82	T64.83	T64.84	—	—
Mydriacyl	T44.3X1	T44.3X2	T44.3X3	T44.3X4	T44.3X5	T44.3X6
Mydriatic drug	T49.5X1	T49.5X2	T49.5X3	T49.5X4	T49.5X5	T49.5X6
Myelobromal	T45.1X1	T45.1X2	T45.1X3	T45.1X4	T45.1X5	T45.1X6
Myleran	T45.1X1	T45.1X2	T45.1X3	T45.1X4	T45.1X5	T45.1X6
Myochrysin (e)	T39.2X1	T39.2X2	T39.2X3	T39.2X4	T39.2X5	T39.2X6
Myoneural blocking agents	T48.1X1	T48.1X2	T48.1X3	T48.1X4	T48.1X5	T48.1X6
Myralact	T49.0X1	T49.0X2	T49.0X3	T49.0X4	T49.0X5	T49.0X6
Myristica fragrans	T62.2X1	T62.2X2	T62.2X3	T62.2X4	—	—
Myristicin	T65.891	T65.892	T65.893	T65.894	—	—
Mysoline	T42.3X1	T42.3X2	T42.3X3	T42.3X4	T42.3X5	T42.3X6
Nabilone	T40.7X1	T40.7X2	T40.7X3	T40.7X4	T40.7X5	T40.7X6
Nabumetone	T39.391	T39.392	T39.393	T39.394	T39.395	T39.396
Nadolol	T44.7X1	T44.7X2	T44.7X3	T44.7X4	T44.7X5	T44.7X6
Nafcillin	T36.0X1	T36.0X2	T36.0X3	T36.0X4	T36.0X5	T36.0X6
Nafoxidine	T38.6X1	T38.6X2	T38.6X3	T38.6X4	T38.6X5	T38.6X6
Naftazone	T46.991	T46.992	T46.993	T46.994	T46.995	T46.996
Naftidrofuryl (oxalate)	T46.7X1	T46.7X2	T46.7X3	T46.7X4	T46.7X5	T46.7X6
Naftifine	T49.0X1	T49.0X2	T49.0X3	T49.0X4	T49.0X5	T49.0X6
Nail polish remover	T52.91	T52.92	T52.93	T52.94	—	—
Nalbuphine	T40.4X1	T40.4X2	T40.4X3	T40.4X4	T40.4X5	T40.4X6
Naled	T60.0X1	T60.0X2	T60.0X3	T60.0X4	—	—
Nalidixic acid	T37.8X1	T37.8X2	T37.8X3	T37.8X4	T37.8X5	T37.8X6
Nalorphine	T50.7X1	T50.7X2	T50.7X3	T50.7X4	T50.7X5	T50.7X6
Naloxone	T50.7X1	T50.7X2	T50.7X3	T50.7X4	T50.7X5	T50.7X6
Naltrexone	T43.8X1	T43.8X2	T43.8X3	T43.8X4	T43.8X5	T43.8X6
Namenda	T43.8X1	T43.8X2	T43.8X3	T43.8X4	T43.8X5	T43.8X6
Nandrolone	T38.7X1	T38.7X2	T38.7X3	T38.7X4	T38.7X5	T38.7X6
Naphazoline	T48.5X1	T48.5X2	T48.5X3	T48.5X4	T48.5X5	T48.5X6
Naphtha (painters') (petroleum)	T52.0X1	T52.0X2	T52.0X3	T52.0X4	—	—
solvent	T52.0X1	T52.0X2	T52.0X3	T52.0X4	—	—
vapor	T52.0X1	T52.0X2	T52.0X3	T52.0X4	—	—
Naphthalene (non-chlorinated)	T60.2X1	T60.2X2	T60.2X3	T60.2X4	—	—
chlorinated	T60.1X1	T60.1X2	T60.1X3	T60.1X4	—	—
vapor	T60.1X1	T60.1X2	T60.1X3	T60.1X4	—	—
insecticide or moth repellent	T60.2X1	T60.2X2	T60.2X3	T60.2X4	—	—
chlorinated	T60.1X1	T60.1X2	T60.1X3	T60.1X4	—	—
vapor	T60.2X1	T60.2X2	T60.2X3	T60.2X4	—	—
chlorinated	T60.1X1	T60.1X2	T60.1X3	T60.1X4	—	—
Naphthol	T65.891	T65.892	T65.893	T65.894	—	—
Naphthylamine	T65.891	T65.892	T65.893	T65.894	—	—
Naphthylthiourea (ANTU)	T60.4X1	T60.4X2	T60.4X3	T60.4X4	—	—
Naprosyn — *see* Naproxen						
Naproxen	T39.311	T39.312	T39.313	T39.314	T39.315	T39.316
Narcotic (drug)	T40.601	T40.602	T40.603	T40.604	T40.605	T40.606
analgesic NEC	T40.601	T40.602	T40.603	T40.604	T40.605	T40.606
antagonist	T50.7X1	T50.7X2	T50.7X3	T50.7X4	T50.7X5	T50.7X6
specified NEC	T40.691	T40.692	T40.693	T40.694	T40.695	T40.696
synthetic	T40.4X1	T40.4X2	T40.4X3	T40.4X4	T40.4X5	T40.4X6
Narcotine	T48.3X1	T48.3X2	T48.3X3	T48.3X4	T48.3X5	T48.3X6
Nardil	T43.1X1	T43.1X2	T43.1X3	T43.1X4	T43.1X5	T43.1X6
Nasal drug NEC	T49.6X1	T49.6X2	T49.6X3	T49.6X4	T49.6X5	T49.6X6
Natamycin	T49.0X1	T49.0X2	T49.0X3	T49.0X4	T49.0X5	T49.0X6
Natrium cyanide — *see* Cyanide(s)						
Natural						
blood (product)	T45.8X1	T45.8X2	T45.8X3	T45.8X4	T45.8X5	T45.8X6
gas (piped)	T59.891	T59.892	T59.893	T59.894	—	—
incomplete combustion	T58.11	T58.12	T58.13	T58.14	—	—
Nealbarbital	T42.3X1	T42.3X2	T42.3X3	T42.3X4	T42.3X5	T42.3X6
Nectadon	T48.3X1	T48.3X2	T48.3X3	T48.3X4	T48.3X5	T48.3X6
Nedocromil	T48.6X1	T48.6X2	T48.6X3	T48.6X4	T48.6X5	T48.6X6
Nefopam	T39.8X1	T39.8X2	T39.8X3	T39.8X4	T39.8X5	T39.8X6
Nematocyst (sting)	T63.691	T63.692	T63.693	T63.694	—	—
Nembutal	T42.3X1	T42.3X2	T42.3X3	T42.3X4	T42.3X5	T42.3X6
Nemonapride	T43.591	T43.592	T43.593	T43.594	T43.595	T43.596
Neoarsphenamine	T37.8X1	T37.8X2	T37.8X3	T37.8X4	T37.8X5	T37.8X6
Neocinchophen	T50.4X1	T50.4X2	T50.4X3	T50.4X4	T50.4X5	T50.4X6
Neomycin (derivatives)	T36.5X1	T36.5X2	T36.5X3	T36.5X4	T36.5X5	T36.5X6
with						
bacitracin	T49.0X1	T49.0X2	T49.0X3	T49.0X4	T49.0X5	T49.0X6
neostigmine	T44.0X1	T44.0X2	T44.0X3	T44.0X4	T44.0X5	T44.0X6
ENT agent	T49.6X1	T49.6X2	T49.6X3	T49.6X4	T49.6X5	T49.6X6
ophthalmic preparation	T49.5X1	T49.5X2	T49.5X3	T49.5X4	T49.5X5	T49.5X6
topical NEC	T49.0X1	T49.0X2	T49.0X3	T49.0X4	T49.0X5	T49.0X6
Neonal	T42.3X1	T42.3X2	T42.3X3	T42.3X4	T42.3X5	T42.3X6
Neoprontosil	T37.0X1	T37.0X2	T37.0X3	T37.0X4	T37.0X5	T37.0X6
Neosalvarsan	T37.8X1	T37.8X2	T37.8X3	T37.8X4	T37.8X5	T37.8X6
Neosilversalvarsan	T37.8X1	T37.8X2	T37.8X3	T37.8X4	T37.8X5	T37.8X6
Neosporin	T36.8X1	T36.8X2	T36.8X3	T36.8X4	T36.8X5	T36.8X6
ENT agent	T49.6X1	T49.6X2	T49.6X3	T49.6X4	T49.6X5	T49.6X6
opthalmic preparation	T49.5X1	T49.5X2	T49.5X3	T49.5X4	T49.5X5	T49.5X6
topical NEC	T49.0X1	T49.0X2	T49.0X3	T49.0X4	T49.0X5	T49.0X6
Neostigmine bromide	T44.0X1	T44.0X2	T44.0X3	T44.0X4	T44.0X5	T44.0X6
Neraval	T42.3X1	T42.3X2	T42.3X3	T42.3X4	T42.3X5	T42.3X6
Neravan	T42.3X1	T42.3X2	T42.3X3	T42.3X4	T42.3X5	T42.3X6
Nerium oleander	T62.2X1	T62.2X2	T62.2X3	T62.2X4	—	—
Nerve gas, not in war	T59.91	T59.92	T59.93	T59.94	—	—
Nesacaine	T41.3X1	T41.3X2	T41.3X3	T41.3X4	T41.3X5	T41.3X6
infiltration (subcutaneous)	T41.3X1	T41.3X2	T41.3X3	T41.3X4	T41.3X5	T41.3X6
nerve block (peripheral) (plexus)	T41.3X1	T41.3X2	T41.3X3	T41.3X4	T41.3X5	T41.3X6
Netilmicin	T36.5X1	T36.5X2	T36.5X3	T36.5X4	T36.5X5	T36.5X6
Neurobarb	T42.3X1	T42.3X2	T42.3X3	T42.3X4	T42.3X5	T42.3X6
Neuroleptic drug NEC	T43.501	T43.502	T43.503	T43.504	T43.505	T43.506
Neuromuscular blocking drug	T48.1X1	T48.1X2	T48.1X3	T48.1X4	T48.1X5	T48.1X6
Neutral insulin injection	T38.3X1	T38.3X2	T38.3X3	T38.3X4	T38.3X5	T38.3X6
Neutral spirits	T51.0X1	T51.0X2	T51.0X3	T51.0X4	—	—
beverage	T51.0X1	T51.0X2	T51.0X3	T51.0X4	—	—
Niacin	T46.7X1	T46.7X2	T46.7X3	T46.7X4	T46.7X5	T46.7X6
Niacinamide	T45.2X1	T45.2X2	T45.2X3	T45.2X4	T45.2X5	T45.2X6
Nialamide	T43.1X1	T43.1X2	T43.1X3	T43.1X4	T43.1X5	T43.1X6
Niaprazine	T42.6X1	T42.6X2	T42.6X3	T42.6X4	T42.6X5	T42.6X6
Nicametate	T46.7X1	T46.7X2	T46.7X3	T46.7X4	T46.7X5	T46.7X6
Nicardipine	T46.1X1	T46.1X2	T46.1X3	T46.1X4	T46.1X5	T46.1X6
Nicergoline	T46.7X1	T46.7X2	T46.7X3	T46.7X4	T46.7X5	T46.7X6
Nickel (carbonyl) (tetra-carbonyl) (fumes) (vapor)	T56.891	T56.892	T56.893	T56.894	—	—
Nickelocene	T56.891	T56.892	T56.893	T56.894	—	—
Niclosamide	T37.4X1	T37.4X2	T37.4X3	T37.4X4	T37.4X5	T37.4X6
Nicofuranose	T46.7X1	T46.7X2	T46.7X3	T46.7X4	T46.7X5	T46.7X6
Nicomorphine	T40.2X1	T40.2X2	T40.2X3	T40.2X4	—	—
Nicorandil	T46.3X1	T46.3X2	T46.3X3	T46.3X4	T46.3X5	T46.3X6
Nicotiana (plant)	T62.2X1	T62.2X2	T62.2X3	T62.2X4	—	—
Nicotinamide	T45.2X1	T45.2X2	T45.2X3	T45.2X4	T45.2X5	T45.2X6
Nicotine (insecticide) (spray) (sulfate) **NEC**	T60.2X1	T60.2X2	T60.2X3	T60.2X4	—	—
from tobacco	T65.291	T65.292	T65.293	T65.294	—	—
cigarettes	T65.221	T65.222	T65.223	T65.224	—	—
not insecticide	T65.291	T65.292	T65.293	T65.294	—	—
Nicotinic acid	T46.7X1	T46.7X2	T46.7X3	T46.7X4	T46.7X5	T46.7X6
Nicotinyl alcohol	T46.7X1	T46.7X2	T46.7X3	T46.7X4	T46.7X5	T46.7X6
Nicoumalone	T45.511	T45.512	T45.513	T45.514	T45.515	T45.516
Nifedipine	T46.1X1	T46.1X2	T46.1X3	T46.1X4	T46.1X5	T46.1X6
Nifenazone	T39.2X1	T39.2X2	T39.2X3	T39.2X4	T39.2X5	T39.2X6
Nifuraldezone	T37.91	T37.92	T37.93	T37.94	T37.95	T37.96
Nifuratel	T37.8X1	T37.8X2	T37.8X3	T37.8X4	T37.8X5	T37.8X6
Nifurtimox	T37.3X1	T37.3X2	T37.3X3	T37.3X4	T37.3X5	T37.3X6
Nifurtoinol	T37.8X1	T37.8X2	T37.8X3	T37.8X4	T37.8X5	T37.8X6
Nightshade, deadly (solanum) — *see also* Belladonna	T62.2X1	T62.2X2	T62.2X3	T62.2X4	—	—
berry	T62.1X1	T62.1X2	T62.1X3	T62.1X4	—	—
Nikethamide	T50.7X1	T50.7X2	T50.7X3	T50.7X4	T50.7X5	T50.7X6
Nilstat	T36.7X1	T36.7X2	T36.7X3	T36.7X4	T36.7X5	T36.7X6
topical	T49.0X1	T49.0X2	T49.0X3	T49.0X4	T49.0X5	T49.0X6
Nilutamide	T38.6X1	T38.6X2	T38.6X3	T38.6X4	T38.6X5	T38.6X6
Nimesulide	T39.391	T39.392	T39.393	T39.394	T39.395	T39.396
Nimetazepam	T42.4X1	T42.4X2	T42.4X3	T42.4X4	T42.4X5	T42.4X6
Nimodipine	T46.1X1	T46.1X2	T46.1X3	T46.1X4	T46.1X5	T46.1X6
Nimorazole	T37.3X1	T37.3X2	T37.3X3	T37.3X4	T37.3X5	T37.3X6
Nimustine	T45.1X1	T45.1X2	T45.1X3	T45.1X4	T45.1X5	T45.1X6
Niridazole	T37.4X1	T37.4X2	T37.4X3	T37.4X4	T37.4X5	T37.4X6
Nisentil	T40.2X1	T40.2X2	T40.2X3	T40.2X4	T40.2X5	T40.2X6
Nisoldipine	T46.1X1	T46.1X2	T46.1X3	T46.1X4	T46.1X5	T46.1X6
Nitramine	T65.3X1	T65.3X2	T65.3X3	T65.3X4	—	—
Nitrate, organic	T46.3X1	T46.3X2	T46.3X3	T46.3X4	T46.3X5	T46.3X6
Nitrazepam	T42.4X1	T42.4X2	T42.4X3	T42.4X4	T42.4X5	T42.4X6
Nitrefazole	T50.6X1	T50.6X2	T50.6X3	T50.6X4	T50.6X5	T50.6X6
Nitrendipine	T46.1X1	T46.1X2	T46.1X3	T46.1X4	T46.1X5	T46.1X6
Nitric						
acid (liquid)	T54.2X1	T54.2X2	T54.2X3	T54.2X4	—	—
vapor	T59.891	T59.892	T59.893	T59.894	—	—
oxide (gas)	T59.0X1	T59.0X2	T59.0X3	T59.0X4	—	—
Nitrimidazine	T37.3X1	T37.3X2	T37.3X3	T37.3X4	T37.3X5	T37.3X6
Nitrite, amyl (medicinal) (vapor)	T46.3X1	T46.3X2	T46.3X3	T46.3X4	T46.3X5	T46.3X6
Nitroaniline	T65.3X1	T65.3X2	T65.3X3	T65.3X4	—	—
vapor	T59.891	T59.892	T59.893	T59.894	—	—
Nitrobenzene, nitrobenzol	T65.3X1	T65.3X2	T65.3X3	T65.3X4	—	—

Additional Character May Be Required — Refer to the Tabular List for Character Selection   ▽ Subterms under main terms may continue to next column or page

Substance	Poisoning, Accidental (unintentional)	Poisoning, Intentional Self-harm	Poisoning, Assault	Poisoning, Undetermined	Adverse Effect	Under-dosing
Nitrobenzene, nitrobenzol — *continued*						
vapor	T65.3X1	T65.3X2	T65.3X3	T65.3X4	—	—
Nitrocellulose	T65.891	T65.892	T65.893	T65.894	—	—
lacquer	T65.891	T65.892	T65.893	T65.894	—	—
Nitrodiphenyl	T65.3X1	T65.3X2	T65.3X3	T65.3X4	—	—
Nitrofural	T49.0X1	T49.0X2	T49.0X3	T49.0X4	T49.0X5	T49.0X6
Nitrofurantoin	T37.8X1	T37.8X2	T37.8X3	T37.8X4	T37.8X5	T37.8X6
Nitrofurazone	T49.0X1	T49.0X2	T49.0X3	T49.0X4	T49.0X5	T49.0X6
Nitrogen	T59.0X1	T59.0X2	T59.0X3	T59.0X4	—	—
mustard	T45.1X1	T45.1X2	T45.1X3	T45.1X4	T45.1X5	T45.1X6
Nitroglycerin, nitroglycerol (medicinal)	T46.3X1	T46.3X2	T46.3X3	T46.3X4	T46.3X5	T46.3X6
nonmedicinal	T65.5X1	T65.5X2	T65.5X3	T65.5X4	—	—
fumes	T65.5X1	T65.5X2	T65.5X3	T65.5X4	—	—
Nitroglycol	T52.3X1	T52.3X2	T52.3X3	T52.3X4	—	—
Nitrohydrochloric acid	T54.2X1	T54.2X2	T54.2X3	T54.2X4	—	—
Nitromersol	T49.0X1	T49.0X2	T49.0X3	T49.0X4	T49.0X5	T49.0X6
Nitronaphthalene	T65.891	T65.892	T65.893	T65.894	—	—
Nitrophenol	T54.0X1	T54.0X2	T54.0X3	T54.0X4	—	—
Nitropropane	T52.8X1	T52.8X2	T52.8X3	T52.8X4	—	—
Nitroprusside	T46.5X1	T46.5X2	T46.5X3	T46.5X4	T46.5X5	T46.5X6
Nitrosodimethylamine	T65.3X1	T65.3X2	T65.3X3	T65.3X4	—	—
Nitrothiazol	T37.4X1	T37.4X2	T37.4X3	T37.4X4	T37.4X5	T37.4X6
Nitrotoluene, nitrotoluol	T65.3X1	T65.3X2	T65.3X3	T65.3X4	—	—
vapor	T65.3X1	T65.3X2	T65.3X3	T65.3X4	—	—
Nitrous						
acid (liquid)	T54.2X1	T54.2X2	T54.2X3	T54.2X4	—	—
fumes	T59.891	T59.892	T59.893	T59.894	—	—
ether spirit	T46.3X1	T46.3X2	T46.3X3	T46.3X4	T46.3X5	T46.3X6
oxide	T41.0X1	T41.0X2	T41.0X3	T41.0X4	T41.0X5	T41.0X6
Nitroxoline	T37.8X1	T37.8X2	T37.8X3	T37.8X4	T37.8X5	T37.8X6
Nitrozone	T49.0X1	T49.0X2	T49.0X3	T49.0X4	T49.0X5	T49.0X6
Nizatidine	T47.0X1	T47.0X2	T47.0X3	T47.0X4	T47.0X5	T47.0X6
Nizofenone	T43.8X1	T43.8X2	T43.8X3	T43.8X4	T43.8X5	T43.8X6
Noctec	T42.6X1	T42.6X2	T42.6X3	T42.6X4	T42.6X5	T42.6X6
Noludar	T42.6X1	T42.6X2	T42.6X3	T42.6X4	T42.6X5	T42.6X6
Nomegestrol	T38.5X1	T38.5X2	T38.5X3	T38.5X4	T38.5X5	T38.5X6
Nomifensine	T43.291	T43.292	T43.293	T43.294	T43.295	T43.296
Nonoxinol	T49.8X1	T49.8X2	T49.8X3	T49.8X4	T49.8X5	T49.8X6
Nonylphenoxy (polyethoxyethanol)	T49.8X1	T49.8X2	T49.8X3	T49.8X4	T49.8X5	T49.8X6
Noptil	T42.3X1	T42.3X2	T42.3X3	T42.3X4	T42.3X5	T42.3X6
Noradrenaline	T44.4X1	T44.4X2	T44.4X3	T44.4X4	T44.4X5	T44.4X6
Noramidopyrine	T39.2X1	T39.2X2	T39.2X3	T39.2X4	T39.2X5	T39.2X6
methanesulfonate sodium	T39.2X1	T39.2X2	T39.2X3	T39.2X4	T39.2X5	T39.2X6
Norbormide	T60.4X1	T60.4X2	T60.4X3	T60.4X4	—	—
Nordazepam	T42.4X1	T42.4X2	T42.4X3	T42.4X4	T42.4X5	T42.4X6
Norepinephrine	T44.4X1	T44.4X2	T44.4X3	T44.4X4	T44.4X5	T44.4X6
Norethandrolone	T38.7X1	T38.7X2	T38.7X3	T38.7X4	T38.7X5	T38.7X6
Norethindrone	T38.4X1	T38.4X2	T38.4X3	T38.4X4	T38.4X5	T38.4X6
Norethisterone (acetate) (enantate)	T38.4X1	T38.4X2	T38.4X3	T38.4X4	T38.4X5	T38.4X6
with ethinylestradiol	T38.5X1	T38.5X2	T38.5X3	T38.5X4	T38.5X5	T38.5X6
Noretynodrel	T38.5X1	T38.5X2	T38.5X3	T38.5X4	T38.5X5	T38.5X6
Norfenefrine	T44.4X1	T44.4X2	T44.4X3	T44.4X4	T44.4X5	T44.4X6
Norfloxacin	T36.8X1	T36.8X2	T36.8X3	T36.8X4	T36.8X5	T36.8X6
Norgestrel	T38.4X1	T38.4X2	T38.4X3	T38.4X4	T38.4X5	T38.4X6
Norgestrienone	T38.4X1	T38.4X2	T38.4X3	T38.4X4	T38.4X5	T38.4X6
Norlestrin	T38.4X1	T38.4X2	T38.4X3	T38.4X4	T38.4X5	T38.4X6
Norlutin	T38.4X1	T38.4X2	T38.4X3	T38.4X4	T38.4X5	T38.4X6
Normal serum albumin (human), salt-poor	T45.8X1	T45.8X2	T45.8X3	T45.8X4	T45.8X5	T45.8X6
Normethandrone	T38.5X1	T38.5X2	T38.5X3	T38.5X4	T38.5X5	T38.5X6
Normison — *see* Benzodiazepines						
Normorphine	T40.2X1	T40.2X2	T40.2X3	T40.2X4	—	—
Norpseudoephedrine	T50.5X1	T50.5X2	T50.5X3	T50.5X4	T50.5X5	T50.5X6
Nortestosterone (furanpropionate)	T38.7X1	T38.7X2	T38.7X3	T38.7X4	T38.7X5	T38.7X6
Nortriptyline	T43.011	T43.012	T43.013	T43.014	T43.015	T43.016
Noscapine	T48.3X1	T48.3X2	T48.3X3	T48.3X4	T48.3X5	T48.3X6
Nose preparations	T49.6X1	T49.6X2	T49.6X3	T49.6X4	T49.6X5	T49.6X6
Novobiocin	T36.5X1	T36.5X2	T36.5X3	T36.5X4	T36.5X5	T36.5X6
Novocain (infiltration)	T41.3X1	T41.3X2	T41.3X3	T41.3X4	T41.3X5	T41.3X6
(topical)						
nerve block (peripheral) (plexus)	T41.3X1	T41.3X2	T41.3X3	T41.3X4	T41.3X5	T41.3X6
spinal	T41.3X1	T41.3X2	T41.3X3	T41.3X4	T41.3X5	T41.3X6
Noxious foodstuff	T62.91	T62.92	T62.93	T62.94	—	—
specified NEC	T62.8X1	T62.8X2	T62.8X3	T62.8X4	—	—
Noxiptiline	T43.011	T43.012	T43.013	T43.014	T43.015	T43.016
Noxytiolin	T49.0X1	T49.0X2	T49.0X3	T49.0X4	T49.0X5	T49.0X6

Substance	Poisoning, Accidental (unintentional)	Poisoning, Intentional Self-harm	Poisoning, Assault	Poisoning, Undetermined	Adverse Effect	Under-dosing
NPH Iletin (insulin)	T38.3X1	T38.3X2	T38.3X3	T38.3X4	T38.3X5	T38.3X6
Numorphan	T40.2X1	T40.2X2	T40.2X3	T40.2X4	T40.2X5	T40.2X6
Nunol	T42.3X1	T42.3X2	T42.3X3	T42.3X4	T42.3X5	T42.3X6
Nupercaine (spinal anesthetic)	T41.3X1	T41.3X2	T41.3X3	T41.3X4	T41.3X5	T41.3X6
topical (surface)	T41.3X1	T41.3X2	T41.3X3	T41.3X4	T41.3X5	T41.3X6
Nutmeg oil (liniment)	T49.3X1	T49.3X2	T49.3X3	T49.3X4	T49.3X5	T49.3X6
Nutritional supplement	T50.901	T50.902	T50.903	T50.904	T50.905	T50.906
Nux vomica	T65.1X1	T65.1X2	T65.1X3	T65.1X4	—	—
Nydrazid	T37.1X1	T37.1X2	T37.1X3	T37.1X4	T37.1X5	T37.1X6
Nylidrin	T46.7X1	T46.7X2	T46.7X3	T46.7X4	T46.7X5	T46.7X6
Nystatin	T36.7X1	T36.7X2	T36.7X3	T36.7X4	T36.7X5	T36.7X6
topical	T49.0X1	T49.0X2	T49.0X3	T49.0X4	T49.0X5	T49.0X6
Nytol	T45.0X1	T45.0X2	T45.0X3	T45.0X4	T45.0X5	T45.0X6
Obidoxime chloride	T50.6X1	T50.6X2	T50.6X3	T50.6X4	T50.6X5	T50.6X6
Octafonium (chloride)	T49.3X1	T49.3X2	T49.3X3	T49.3X4	T49.3X5	T49.3X6
Octamethyl pyrophosphoramide	T60.0X1	T60.0X2	T60.0X3	T60.0X4	—	—
Octanoin	T50.991	T50.992	T50.993	T50.994	T50.995	T50.996
Octatropine methylbromide	T44.3X1	T44.3X2	T44.3X3	T44.3X4	T44.3X5	T44.3X6
Octotiamine	T45.2X1	T45.2X2	T45.2X3	T45.2X4	T45.2X5	T45.2X6
Octoxinol (9)	T49.8X1	T49.8X2	T49.8X3	T49.8X4	T49.8X5	T49.8X6
Octreotide	T38.991	T38.992	T38.993	T38.994	T38.995	T38.996
Octyl nitrite	T46.3X1	T46.3X2	T46.3X3	T46.3X4	T46.3X5	T46.3X6
Oestradiol	T38.5X1	T38.5X2	T38.5X3	T38.5X4	T38.5X5	T38.5X6
Oestriol	T38.5X1	T38.5X2	T38.5X3	T38.5X4	T38.5X5	T38.5X6
Oestrogen	T38.5X1	T38.5X2	T38.5X3	T38.5X4	T38.5X5	T38.5X6
Oestrone	T38.5X1	T38.5X2	T38.5X3	T38.5X4	T38.5X5	T38.5X6
Ofloxacin	T36.8X1	T36.8X2	T36.8X3	T36.8X4	T36.8X5	T36.8X6
Oil (of)	T65.891	T65.892	T65.893	T65.894	—	—
bitter almond	T62.8X1	T62.8X2	T62.8X3	T62.8X4	—	—
cloves	T49.7X1	T49.7X2	T49.7X3	T49.7X4	T49.7X5	T49.7X6
colors	T65.6X1	T65.6X2	T65.6X3	T65.6X4	—	—
fumes	T59.891	T59.892	T59.893	T59.894	—	—
lubricating	T52.0X1	T52.0X2	T52.0X3	T52.0X4	—	—
Niobe	T52.8X1	T52.8X2	T52.8X3	T52.8X4	—	—
vitriol (liquid)	T54.2X1	T54.2X2	T54.2X3	T54.2X4	—	—
fumes	T54.2X1	T54.2X2	T54.2X3	T54.2X4	—	—
wintergreen (bitter) NEC	T49.3X1	T49.3X2	T49.3X3	T49.3X4	T49.3X5	T49.3X6
Oily preparation (for skin)	T49.3X1	T49.3X2	T49.3X3	T49.3X4	T49.3X5	T49.3X6
Ointment NEC	T49.3X1	T49.3X2	T49.3X3	T49.3X4	T49.3X5	T49.3X6
Olanzapine	T43.591	T43.592	T43.593	T43.594	T43.595	T43.596
Oleander	T62.2X1	T62.2X2	T62.2X3	T62.2X4	—	—
Oleandomycin	T36.3X1	T36.3X2	T36.3X3	T36.3X4	T36.3X5	T36.3X6
Oleandrin	T46.0X1	T46.0X2	T46.0X3	T46.0X4	T46.0X5	T46.0X6
Oleic acid	T46.6X1	T46.6X2	T46.6X3	T46.6X4	T46.6X5	T46.6X6
Oleovitamin A	T45.2X1	T45.2X2	T45.2X3	T45.2X4	T45.2X5	T45.2X6
Oleum ricini	T47.2X1	T47.2X2	T47.2X3	T47.2X4	T47.2X5	T47.2X6
Olive oil (medicinal) **NEC**	T47.4X1	T47.4X2	T47.4X3	T47.4X4	T47.4X5	T47.4X6
Olivomycin	T45.1X1	T45.1X2	T45.1X3	T45.1X4	T45.1X5	T45.1X6
Olsalazine	T47.8X1	T47.8X2	T47.8X3	T47.8X4	T47.8X5	T47.8X6
Omeprazole	T47.1X1	T47.1X2	T47.1X3	T47.1X4	T47.1X5	T47.1X6
OMPA	T60.0X1	T60.0X2	T60.0X3	T60.0X4	—	—
Oncovin	T45.1X1	T45.1X2	T45.1X3	T45.1X4	T45.1X5	T45.1X6
Ondansetron	T45.0X1	T45.0X2	T45.0X3	T45.0X4	T45.0X5	T45.0X6
Ophthaine	T41.3X1	T41.3X2	T41.3X3	T41.3X4	T41.3X5	T41.3X6
Ophthetic	T41.3X1	T41.3X2	T41.3X3	T41.3X4	T41.3X5	T41.3X6
Opiate NEC	T40.601	T40.602	T40.603	T40.604	T40.605	T40.606
antagonists	T50.7X1	T50.7X2	T50.7X3	T50.7X4	T50.7X5	T50.7X6
Opioid NEC	T40.2X1	T40.2X2	T40.2X3	T40.2X4	T40.2X5	T40.2X6
Opipramol	T43.011	T43.012	T43.013	T43.014	T43.015	T43.016
Opium alkaloids (total)	T40.0X1	T40.0X2	T40.0X3	T40.0X4	T40.0X5	T40.0X6
standardized powdered	T40.0X1	T40.0X2	T40.0X3	T40.0X4	T40.0X5	T40.0X6
tincture (camphorated)	T40.0X1	T40.0X2	T40.0X3	T40.0X4	T40.0X5	T40.0X6
Oracon	T38.4X1	T38.4X2	T38.4X3	T38.4X4	T38.4X5	T38.4X6
Oragrafin	T50.8X1	T50.8X2	T50.8X3	T50.8X4	T50.8X5	T50.8X6
Oral contraceptives	T38.4X1	T38.4X2	T38.4X3	T38.4X4	T38.4X5	T38.4X6
Oral rehydration salts	T50.3X1	T50.3X2	T50.3X3	T50.3X4	T50.3X5	T50.3X6
Orazamide	T50.991	T50.992	T50.993	T50.994	T50.995	T50.996
Orciprenaline	T48.291	T48.292	T48.293	T48.294	T48.295	T48.296
Organidin	T48.4X1	T48.4X2	T48.4X3	T48.4X4	T48.4X5	T48.4X6
Organonitrate NEC	T46.3X1	T46.3X2	T46.3X3	T46.3X4	T46.3X5	T46.3X6
Organophosphates	T60.0X1	T60.0X2	T60.0X3	T60.0X4	—	—
Orimune	T50.B91	T50.B92	T50.B93	T50.B94	T50.B95	T50.B96
Orinase	T38.3X1	T38.3X2	T38.3X3	T38.3X4	T38.3X5	T38.3X6
Ormeloxifene	T38.6X1	T38.6X2	T38.6X3	T38.6X4	T38.6X5	T38.6X6
Ornidazole	T37.3X1	T37.3X2	T37.3X3	T37.3X4	T37.3X5	T37.3X6
Ornithine aspartate	T50.991	T50.992	T50.993	T50.994	T50.995	T50.996
Ornoprostil	T47.1X1	T47.1X2	T47.1X3	T47.1X4	T47.1X5	T47.1X6
Orphenadrine (hydrochloride)	T42.0X1	T42.0X2	T42.0X3	T42.0X4	T42.0X5	T42.0X6
Ortal (sodium)	T42.3X1	T42.3X2	T42.3X3	T42.3X4	T42.3X5	T42.3X6

▼ Subterms under main terms may continue to next column or page — Additional Character May Be Required — Refer to the Tabular List for Character Selection — 381

Nitrobenzene, nitrobenzol — Ortal

Substance	Poisoning, Accidental (unintentional)	Poisoning, Intentional Self-harm	Poisoning, Assault	Poisoning, Undetermined	Adverse Effect	Under-dosing
Orthoboric acid	T49.0X1	T49.0X2	T49.0X3	T49.0X4	T49.0X5	T49.0X6
ENT agent	T49.6X1	T49.6X2	T49.6X3	T49.6X4	T49.6X5	T49.6X6
ophthalmic preparation	T49.5X1	T49.5X2	T49.5X3	T49.5X4	T49.5X5	T49.5X6
Orthocaine	T41.3X1	T41.3X2	T41.3X3	T41.3X4	T41.3X5	T41.3X6
Orthodichlorobenzene	T53.7X1	T53.7X2	T53.7X3	T53.7X4	—	—
Ortho-Novum	T38.4X1	T38.4X2	T38.4X3	T38.4X4	T38.4X5	T38.4X6
Orthotolidine (reagent)	T54.2X1	T54.2X2	T54.2X3	T54.2X4	—	—
Osmic acid (liquid)	T54.2X1	T54.2X2	T54.2X3	T54.2X4	—	—
fumes	T54.2X1	T54.2X2	T54.2X3	T54.2X4	—	—
Osmotic diuretics	T50.2X1	T50.2X2	T50.2X3	T50.2X4	T50.2X5	T50.2X6
Otilonium bromide	T44.3X1	T44.3X2	T44.3X3	T44.3X4	T44.3X5	T44.3X6
Otorhinolaryngological drug NEC	T49.6X1	T49.6X2	T49.6X3	T49.6X4	T49.6X5	T49.6X6
Ouabain (e)	T46.0X1	T46.0X2	T46.0X3	T46.0X4	T46.0X5	T46.0X6
Ovarian						
hormone	T38.5X1	T38.5X2	T38.5X3	T38.5X4	T38.5X5	T38.5X6
stimulant	T38.5X1	T38.5X2	T38.5X3	T38.5X4	T38.5X5	T38.5X6
Ovral	T38.4X1	T38.4X2	T38.4X3	T38.4X4	T38.4X5	T38.4X6
Ovulen	T38.4X1	T38.4X2	T38.4X3	T38.4X4	T38.4X5	T38.4X6
Oxacillin	T36.0X1	T36.0X2	T36.0X3	T36.0X4	T36.0X5	T36.0X6
Oxalic acid	T54.2X1	T54.2X2	T54.2X3	T54.2X4	—	—
ammonium salt	T50.991	T50.992	T50.993	T50.994	T50.995	T50.996
Oxamniquine	T37.4X1	T37.4X2	T37.4X3	T37.4X4	T37.4X5	T37.4X6
Oxanamide	T43.591	T43.592	T43.593	T43.594	T43.595	T43.596
Oxandrolone	T38.7X1	T38.7X2	T38.7X3	T38.7X4	T38.7X5	T38.7X6
Oxantel	T37.4X1	T37.4X2	T37.4X3	T37.4X4	T37.4X5	T37.4X6
Oxapium iodide	T44.3X1	T44.3X2	T44.3X3	T44.3X4	T44.3X5	T44.3X6
Oxaprotiline	T43.021	T43.022	T43.023	T43.024	T43.025	T43.026
Oxaprozin	T39.311	T39.312	T39.313	T39.314	T39.315	T39.316
Oxatomide	T45.0X1	T45.0X2	T45.0X3	T45.0X4	T45.0X5	T45.0X6
Oxazepam	T42.4X1	T42.4X2	T42.4X3	T42.4X4	T42.4X5	T42.4X6
Oxazimedrine	T50.5X1	T50.5X2	T50.5X3	T50.5X4	T50.5X5	T50.5X6
Oxazolam	T42.4X1	T42.4X2	T42.4X3	T42.4X4	T42.4X5	T42.4X6
Oxazolidine derivatives	T42.2X1	T42.2X2	T42.2X3	T42.2X4	T42.2X5	T42.2X6
Oxazolidinedione (derivative)	T42.2X1	T42.2X2	T42.2X3	T42.2X4	T42.2X5	T42.2X6
Ox bile extract	T47.5X1	T47.5X2	T47.5X3	T47.5X4	T47.5X5	T47.5X6
Oxcarbazepine	T42.1X1	T42.1X2	T42.1X3	T42.1X4	T42.1X5	T42.1X6
Oxedrine	T44.4X1	T44.4X2	T44.4X3	T44.4X4	T44.4X5	T44.4X6
Oxeladin (citrate)	T48.3X1	T48.3X2	T48.3X3	T48.3X4	T48.3X5	T48.3X6
Oxendolone	T38.5X1	T38.5X2	T38.5X3	T38.5X4	T38.5X5	T38.5X6
Oxetacaine	T41.3X1	T41.3X2	T41.3X3	T41.3X4	T41.3X5	T41.3X6
Oxethazine	T41.3X1	T41.3X2	T41.3X3	T41.3X4	T41.3X5	T41.3X6
Oxetorone	T39.8X1	T39.8X2	T39.8X3	T39.8X4	T39.8X5	T39.8X6
Oxiconazole	T49.0X1	T49.0X2	T49.0X3	T49.0X4	T49.0X5	T49.0X6
Oxidizing agent NEC	T54.91	T54.92	T54.93	T54.94	—	—
Oxipurinol	T50.4X1	T50.4X2	T50.4X3	T50.4X4	T50.4X5	T50.4X6
Oxitriptan	T43.291	T43.292	T43.293	T43.294	T43.295	T43.296
Oxitropium bromide	T48.6X1	T48.6X2	T48.6X3	T48.6X4	T48.6X5	T48.6X6
Oxodipine	T46.1X1	T46.1X2	T46.1X3	T46.1X4	T46.1X5	T46.1X6
Oxolamine	T48.3X1	T48.3X2	T48.3X3	T48.3X4	T48.3X5	T48.3X6
Oxolinic acid	T37.8X1	T37.8X2	T37.8X3	T37.8X4	T37.8X5	T37.8X6
Oxomemazine	T43.3X1	T43.3X2	T43.3X3	T43.3X4	T43.3X5	T43.3X6
Oxophenarsine	T37.3X1	T37.3X2	T37.3X3	T37.3X4	T37.3X5	T37.3X6
Oxprenolol	T44.7X1	T44.7X2	T44.7X3	T44.7X4	T44.7X5	T44.7X6
Oxsoralen	T49.3X1	T49.3X2	T49.3X3	T49.3X4	T49.3X5	T49.3X6
Oxtriphylline	T48.6X1	T48.6X2	T48.6X3	T48.6X4	T48.6X5	T48.6X6
Oxybate sodium	T41.291	T41.292	T41.293	T41.294	T41.295	T41.296
Oxybuprocaine	T41.3X1	T41.3X2	T41.3X3	T41.3X4	T41.3X5	T41.3X6
Oxybutynin	T44.3X1	T44.3X2	T44.3X3	T44.3X4	T44.3X5	T44.3X6
Oxychlorosene	T49.0X1	T49.0X2	T49.0X3	T49.0X4	T49.0X5	T49.0X6
Oxycodone	T40.2X1	T40.2X2	T40.2X3	T40.2X4	T40.2X5	T40.2X6
Oxyfedrine	T46.3X1	T46.3X2	T46.3X3	T46.3X4	T46.3X5	T46.3X6
Oxygen	T41.5X1	T41.5X2	T41.5X3	T41.5X4	T41.5X5	T41.5X6
Oxylone	T49.0X1	T49.0X2	T49.0X3	T49.0X4	T49.0X5	T49.0X6
ophthalmic preparation	T49.5X1	T49.5X2	T49.5X3	T49.5X4	T49.5X5	T49.5X6
Oxymesterone	T38.7X1	T38.7X2	T38.7X3	T38.7X4	T38.7X5	T38.7X6
Oxymetazoline	T48.5X1	T48.5X2	T48.5X3	T48.5X4	T48.5X5	T48.5X6
Oxymetholone	T38.7X1	T38.7X2	T38.7X3	T38.7X4	T38.7X5	T38.7X6
Oxymorphone	T40.2X1	T40.2X2	T40.2X3	T40.2X4	T40.2X5	T40.2X6
Oxypertine	T43.591	T43.592	T43.593	T43.594	T43.595	T43.596
Oxyphenbutazone	T39.2X1	T39.2X2	T39.2X3	T39.2X4	T39.2X5	T39.2X6
Oxyphencyclimine	T44.3X1	T44.3X2	T44.3X3	T44.3X4	T44.3X5	T44.3X6
Oxyphenisatine	T47.2X1	T47.2X2	T47.2X3	T47.2X4	T47.2X5	T47.2X6
Oxyphenonium bromide	T44.3X1	T44.3X2	T44.3X3	T44.3X4	T44.3X5	T44.3X6
Oxypolygelatin	T45.8X1	T45.8X2	T45.8X3	T45.8X4	T45.8X5	T45.8X6
Oxyquinoline (derivatives)	T37.8X1	T37.8X2	T37.8X3	T37.8X4	T37.8X5	T37.8X6
Oxytetracycline	T36.4X1	T36.4X2	T36.4X3	T36.4X4	T36.4X5	T36.4X6
Oxytocic drug NEC	T48.0X1	T48.0X2	T48.0X3	T48.0X4	T48.0X5	T48.0X6
Oxytocin (synthetic)	T48.0X1	T48.0X2	T48.0X3	T48.0X4	T48.0X5	T48.0X6
Ozone	T59.891	T59.892	T59.893	T59.894	—	—
PABA	T49.3X1	T49.3X2	T49.3X3	T49.3X4	T49.3X5	T49.3X6
Packed red cells	T45.8X1	T45.8X2	T45.8X3	T45.8X4	T45.8X5	T45.8X6

Substance	Poisoning, Accidental (unintentional)	Poisoning, Intentional Self-harm	Poisoning, Assault	Poisoning, Undetermined	Adverse Effect	Under-dosing
Padimate	T49.3X1	T49.3X2	T49.3X3	T49.3X4	T49.3X5	T49.3X6
Paint NEC	T65.6X1	T65.6X2	T65.6X3	T65.6X4	—	—
cleaner	T52.91	T52.92	T52.93	T52.94	—	—
fumes NEC	T59.891	T59.892	T59.893	T59.894	—	—
lead (fumes)	T56.0X1	T56.0X2	T56.0X3	T56.0X4	—	—
solvent NEC	T52.8X1	T52.8X2	T52.8X3	T52.8X4	—	—
stripper	T52.8X1	T52.8X2	T52.8X3	T52.8X4	—	—
Palfium	T40.2X1	T40.2X2	T40.2X3	T40.2X4	—	—
Palm kernel oil	T50.991	T50.992	T50.993	T50.994	T50.995	T50.996
Paludrine	T37.2X1	T37.2X2	T37.2X3	T37.2X4	T37.2X5	T37.2X6
PAM (pralidoxime)	T50.6X1	T50.6X2	T50.6X3	T50.6X4	T50.6X5	T50.6X6
Pamaquine (naphthoute)	T37.2X1	T37.2X2	T37.2X3	T37.2X4	T37.2X5	T37.2X6
Panadol	T39.1X1	T39.1X2	T39.1X3	T39.1X4	T39.1X5	T39.1X6
Pancreatic						
digestive secretion stimulant	T47.8X1	T47.8X2	T47.8X3	T47.8X4	T47.8X5	T47.8X6
dornase	T45.3X1	T45.3X2	T45.3X3	T45.3X4	T45.3X5	T45.3X6
Pancreatin	T47.5X1	T47.5X2	T47.5X3	T47.5X4	T47.5X5	T47.5X6
Pancrelipase	T47.5X1	T47.5X2	T47.5X3	T47.5X4	T47.5X5	T47.5X6
Pancuronium (bromide)	T48.1X1	T48.1X2	T48.1X3	T48.1X4	T48.1X5	T48.1X6
Pangamic acid	T45.2X1	T45.2X2	T45.2X3	T45.2X4	T45.2X5	T45.2X6
Panthenol	T45.2X1	T45.2X2	T45.2X3	T45.2X4	T45.2X5	T45.2X6
topical	T49.8X1	T49.8X2	T49.8X3	T49.8X4	T49.8X5	T49.8X6
Pantopon	T40.0X1	T40.0X2	T40.0X3	T40.0X4	T40.0X5	T40.0X6
Pantothenic acid	T45.2X1	T45.2X2	T45.2X3	T45.2X4	T45.2X5	T45.2X6
Panwarfin	T45.511	T45.512	T45.513	T45.514	T45.515	T45.516
Papain	T47.5X1	T47.5X2	T47.5X3	T47.5X4	T47.5X5	T47.5X6
digestant	T47.5X1	T47.5X2	T47.5X3	T47.5X4	T47.5X5	T47.5X6
Papaveretum	T40.0X1	T40.0X2	T40.0X3	T40.0X4	T40.0X5	T40.0X6
Papaverine	T44.3X1	T44.3X2	T44.3X3	T44.3X4	T44.3X5	T44.3X6
Para-acetamidophenol	T39.1X1	T39.1X2	T39.1X3	T39.1X4	T39.1X5	T39.1X6
Para-aminobenzoic acid	T49.3X1	T49.3X2	T49.3X3	T49.3X4	T49.3X5	T49.3X6
Para-aminophenol derivatives	T39.1X1	T39.1X2	T39.1X3	T39.1X4	T39.1X5	T39.1X6
Para-aminosalicylic acid	T37.1X1	T37.1X2	T37.1X3	T37.1X4	T37.1X5	T37.1X6
Paracetaldehyde	T42.6X1	T42.6X2	T42.6X3	T42.6X4	T42.6X5	T42.6X6
Paracetamol	T39.1X1	T39.1X2	T39.1X3	T39.1X4	T39.1X5	T39.1X6
Parachlorophenol (camphorated)	T49.0X1	T49.0X2	T49.0X3	T49.0X4	T49.0X5	T49.0X6
Paracodin	T40.2X1	T40.2X2	T40.2X3	T40.2X4	T40.2X5	T40.2X6
Paradione	T42.2X1	T42.2X2	T42.2X3	T42.2X4	T42.2X5	T42.2X6
Paraffin(s) (wax)	T52.0X1	T52.0X2	T52.0X3	T52.0X4	—	—
liquid (medicinal)	T47.4X1	T47.4X2	T47.4X3	T47.4X4	T47.4X5	T47.4X6
nonmedicinal	T52.0X1	T52.0X2	T52.0X3	T52.0X4	—	—
Paraformaldehyde	T60.3X1	T60.3X2	T60.3X3	T60.3X4	—	—
Paraldehyde	T42.6X1	T42.6X2	T42.6X3	T42.6X4	T42.6X5	T42.6X6
Paramethadione	T42.2X1	T42.2X2	T42.2X3	T42.2X4	T42.2X5	T42.2X6
Paramethasone	T38.0X1	T38.0X2	T38.0X3	T38.0X4	T38.0X5	T38.0X6
acetate	T49.0X1	T49.0X2	T49.0X3	T49.0X4	T49.0X5	T49.0X6
Paraoxon	T60.0X1	T60.0X2	T60.0X3	T60.0X4	—	—
Paraquat	T60.3X1	T60.3X2	T60.3X3	T60.3X4	—	—
Parasympatholytic NEC	T44.3X1	T44.3X2	T44.3X3	T44.3X4	T44.3X5	T44.3X6
Parasympathomimetic drug NEC	T44.1X1	T44.1X2	T44.1X3	T44.1X4	T44.1X5	T44.1X6
Parathion	T60.0X1	T60.0X2	T60.0X3	T60.0X4	—	—
Parathormone	T50.991	T50.992	T50.993	T50.994	T50.995	T50.996
Parathyroid extract	T50.991	T50.992	T50.993	T50.994	T50.995	T50.996
Paratyphoid vaccine	T50.A91	T50.A92	T50.A93	T50.A94	T50.A95	T50.A96
Paredrine	T44.4X1	T44.4X2	T44.4X3	T44.4X4	T44.4X5	T44.4X6
Paregoric	T40.0X1	T40.0X2	T40.0X3	T40.0X4	T40.0X5	T40.0X6
Pargyline	T46.5X1	T46.5X2	T46.5X3	T46.5X4	T46.5X5	T46.5X6
Paris green	T57.0X1	T57.0X2	T57.0X3	T57.0X4	—	—
insecticide	T57.0X1	T57.0X2	T57.0X3	T57.0X4	—	—
Parnate	T43.1X1	T43.1X2	T43.1X3	T43.1X4	T43.1X5	T43.1X6
Paromomycin	T36.5X1	T36.5X2	T36.5X3	T36.5X4	T36.5X5	T36.5X6
Paroxypropione	T45.1X1	T45.1X2	T45.1X3	T45.1X4	T45.1X5	T45.1X6
Parzone	T40.2X1	T40.2X2	T40.2X3	T40.2X4	T40.2X5	T40.2X6
PAS	T37.1X1	T37.1X2	T37.1X3	T37.1X4	T37.1X5	T37.1X6
Pasiniazid	T37.1X1	T37.1X2	T37.1X3	T37.1X4	T37.1X5	T37.1X6
PBB (polybrominated biphenyls)	T65.891	T65.892	T65.893	T65.894	—	—
PCB	T65.891	T65.892	T65.893	T65.894	—	—
PCP						
meaning pentachlorophenol	T60.1X1	T60.1X2	T60.1X3	T60.1X4	—	—
fungicide	T60.3X1	T60.3X2	T60.3X3	T60.3X4	—	—
herbicide	T60.3X1	T60.3X2	T60.3X3	T60.3X4	—	—
insecticide	T60.1X1	T60.1X2	T60.1X3	T60.1X4	—	—
meaning phencyclidine	T40.991	T40.992	T40.993	T40.994	—	—
Peach kernel oil (emulsion)	T47.4X1	T47.4X2	T47.4X3	T47.4X4	T47.4X5	T47.4X6
Peanut oil (emulsion) NEC	T47.4X1	T47.4X2	T47.4X3	T47.4X4	T47.4X5	T47.4X6
topical	T49.3X1	T49.3X2	T49.3X3	T49.3X4	T49.3X5	T49.3X6

Additional Character May Be Required — Refer to the Tabular List for Character Selection ⬥ Subterms under main terms may continue to next column or page

Substance	Poisoning, Accidental (unintentional)	Poisoning, Intentional Self-harm	Poisoning, Assault	Poisoning, Undetermined	Adverse Effect	Under-dosing
Pearly Gates (morning glory seeds)	T40.991	T40.992	T40.993	T40.994	—	—
Pecazine	T43.3X1	T43.3X2	T43.3X3	T43.3X4	T43.3X5	T43.3X6
Pectin	T47.6X1	T47.6X2	T47.6X3	T47.6X4	T47.6X5	T47.6X6
Pefloxacin	T37.8X1	T37.8X2	T37.8X3	T37.8X4	T37.8X5	T37.8X6
Pegademase, bovine	T50.Z91	T50.Z92	T50.Z93	T50.Z94	T50.Z95	T50.Z96
Pelletierine tannate	T37.4X1	T37.4X2	T37.4X3	T37.4X4	T37.4X5	T37.4X6
Pemirolast (potassium)	T48.6X1	T48.6X2	T48.6X3	T48.6X4	T48.6X5	T48.6X6
Pemoline	T50.7X1	T50.7X2	T50.7X3	T50.7X4	T50.7X5	T50.7X6
Pempidine	T44.2X1	T44.2X2	T44.2X3	T44.2X4	T44.2X5	T44.2X6
Penamecillin	T36.0X1	T36.0X2	T36.0X3	T36.0X4	T36.0X5	T36.0X6
Penbutolol	T44.7X1	T44.7X2	T44.7X3	T44.7X4	T44.7X5	T44.7X6
Penethamate	T36.0X1	T36.0X2	T36.0X3	T36.0X4	T36.0X5	T36.0X6
Penfluridol	T43.591	T43.592	T43.593	T43.594	T43.595	T43.596
Penflutizide	T50.2X1	T50.2X2	T50.2X3	T50.2X4	T50.2X5	T50.2X6
Pengitoxin	T46.0X1	T46.0X2	T46.0X3	T46.0X4	T46.0X5	T46.0X6
Penicillamine	T50.6X1	T50.6X2	T50.6X3	T50.6X4	T50.6X5	T50.6X6
Penicillin (any)	T36.0X1	T36.0X2	T36.0X3	T36.0X4	T36.0X5	T36.0X6
Penicillinase	T45.3X1	T45.3X2	T45.3X3	T45.3X4	T45.3X5	T45.3X6
Penicilloyl polylysine	T50.8X1	T50.8X2	T50.8X3	T50.8X4	T50.8X5	T50.8X6
Penimepicycline	T36.4X1	T36.4X2	T36.4X3	T36.4X4	T36.4X5	T36.4X6
Pentachloroethane	T53.6X1	T53.6X2	T53.6X3	T53.6X4	—	—
Pentachloronaphthalene	T53.7X1	T53.7X2	T53.7X3	T53.7X4	—	—
Pentachlorophenol (pesticide)	T60.1X1	T60.1X2	T60.1X3	T60.1X4	—	—
fungicide	T60.3X1	T60.3X2	T60.3X3	T60.3X4	—	—
herbicide	T60.3X1	T60.3X2	T60.3X3	T60.3X4	—	—
insecticide	T60.1X1	T60.1X2	T60.1X3	T60.1X4	—	—
Pentaerythritol	T46.3X1	T46.3X2	T46.3X3	T46.3X4	T46.3X5	T46.3X6
chloral	T42.6X1	T42.6X2	T42.6X3	T42.6X4	T42.6X5	T42.6X6
tetranitrate NEC	T46.3X1	T46.3X2	T46.3X3	T46.3X4	T46.3X5	T46.3X6
Pentaerythrityl tetranitrate	T46.3X1	T46.3X2	T46.3X3	T46.3X4	T46.3X5	T46.3X6
Pentagastrin	T50.8X1	T50.8X2	T50.8X3	T50.8X4	T50.8X5	T50.8X6
Pentalin	T53.6X1	T53.6X2	T53.6X3	T53.6X4	—	—
Pentamethonium bromide	T44.2X1	T44.2X2	T44.2X3	T44.2X4	T44.2X5	T44.2X6
Pentamidine	T37.3X1	T37.3X2	T37.3X3	T37.3X4	T37.3X5	T37.3X6
Pentanol	T51.3X1	T51.3X2	T51.3X3	T51.3X4	—	—
Pentapyrrolinium (bitartrate)	T44.2X1	T44.2X2	T44.2X3	T44.2X4	T44.2X5	T44.2X6
Pentaquine	T37.2X1	T37.2X2	T37.2X3	T37.2X4	T37.2X5	T37.2X6
Pentazocine	T40.4X1	T40.4X2	T40.4X3	T40.4X4	T40.4X5	T40.4X6
Pentetrazole	T50.7X1	T50.7X2	T50.7X3	T50.7X4	T50.7X5	T50.7X6
Penthienate bromide	T44.3X1	T44.3X2	T44.3X3	T44.3X4	T44.3X5	T44.3X6
Pentifylline	T46.7X1	T46.7X2	T46.7X3	T46.7X4	T46.7X5	T46.7X6
Pentobarbital	T42.3X1	T42.3X2	T42.3X3	T42.3X4	T42.3X5	T42.3X6
sodium	T42.3X1	T42.3X2	T42.3X3	T42.3X4	T42.3X5	T42.3X6
Pentobarbitone	T42.3X1	T42.3X2	T42.3X3	T42.3X4	T42.3X5	T42.3X6
Pentolonium tartrate	T44.2X1	T44.2X2	T44.2X3	T44.2X4	T44.2X5	T44.2X6
Pentosan polysulfate (sodium)	T39.8X1	T39.8X2	T39.8X3	T39.8X4	T39.8X5	T39.8X6
Pentostatin	T45.1X1	T45.1X2	T45.1X3	T45.1X4	T45.1X5	T45.1X6
Pentothal	T41.1X1	T41.1X2	T41.1X3	T41.1X4	T41.1X5	T41.1X6
Pentoxifylline	T46.7X1	T46.7X2	T46.7X3	T46.7X4	T46.7X5	T46.7X6
Pentoxyverine	T48.3X1	T48.3X2	T48.3X3	T48.3X4	T48.3X5	T48.3X6
Pentrinat	T46.3X1	T46.3X2	T46.3X3	T46.3X4	T46.3X5	T46.3X6
Pentylenetetrazole	T50.7X1	T50.7X2	T50.7X3	T50.7X4	T50.7X5	T50.7X6
Pentylsalicylamide	T37.1X1	T37.1X2	T37.1X3	T37.1X4	T37.1X5	T37.1X6
Pentymal	T42.3X1	T42.3X2	T42.3X3	T42.3X4	T42.3X5	T42.3X6
Peplomycin	T45.1X1	T45.1X2	T45.1X3	T45.1X4	T45.1X5	T45.1X6
Peppermint (oil)	T47.5X1	T47.5X2	T47.5X3	T47.5X4	T47.5X5	T47.5X6
Pepsin	T47.5X1	T47.5X2	T47.5X3	T47.5X4	T47.5X5	T47.5X6
digestant	T47.5X1	T47.5X2	T47.5X3	T47.5X4	T47.5X5	T47.5X6
Pepstatin	T47.1X1	T47.1X2	T47.1X3	T47.1X4	T47.1X5	T47.1X6
Peptavlon	T50.8X1	T50.8X2	T50.8X3	T50.8X4	T50.8X5	T50.8X6
Perazine	T43.3X1	T43.3X2	T43.3X3	T43.3X4	T43.3X5	T43.3X6
Percaine (spinal)	T41.3X1	T41.3X2	T41.3X3	T41.3X4	T41.3X5	T41.3X6
topical (surface)	T41.3X1	T41.3X2	T41.3X3	T41.3X4	T41.3X5	T41.3X6
Perchloroethylene	T53.3X1	T53.3X2	T53.3X3	T53.3X4	—	—
medicinal	T37.4X1	T37.4X2	T37.4X3	T37.4X4	T37.4X5	T37.4X6
vapor	T53.3X1	T53.3X2	T53.3X3	T53.3X4	—	—
Percodan	T40.2X1	T40.2X2	T40.2X3	T40.2X4	T40.2X5	T40.2X6
Percogesic — see also acetaminophen	T45.0X1	T45.0X2	T45.0X3	T45.0X4	T45.0X5	T45.0X6
Percorten	T38.0X1	T38.0X2	T38.0X3	T38.0X4	T38.0X5	T38.0X6
Pergolide	T42.8X1	T42.8X2	T42.8X3	T42.8X4	T42.8X5	T42.8X6
Pergonal	T38.811	T38.812	T38.813	T38.814	T38.815	T38.816
Perhexilene	T46.3X1	T46.3X2	T46.3X3	T46.3X4	T46.3X5	T46.3X6
Perhexiline (maleate)	T46.3X1	T46.3X2	T46.3X3	T46.3X4	T46.3X5	T46.3X6
Periactin	T45.0X1	T45.0X2	T45.0X3	T45.0X4	T45.0X5	T45.0X6
Periciazine	T43.3X1	T43.3X2	T43.3X3	T43.3X4	T43.3X5	T43.3X6
Periclor	T42.6X1	T42.6X2	T42.6X3	T42.6X4	T42.6X5	T42.6X6
Perindopril	T46.4X1	T46.4X2	T46.4X3	T46.4X4	T46.4X5	T46.4X6
Perisoxal	T39.8X1	T39.8X2	T39.8X3	T39.8X4	T39.8X5	T39.8X6
Peritoneal dialysis solution	T50.3X1	T50.3X2	T50.3X3	T50.3X4	T50.3X5	T50.3X6
Peritrate	T46.3X1	T46.3X2	T46.3X3	T46.3X4	T46.3X5	T46.3X6
Perlapine	T42.4X1	T42.4X2	T42.4X3	T42.4X4	T42.4X5	T42.4X6
Permanganate	T65.891	T65.892	T65.893	T65.894	—	—
Permethrin	T60.1X1	T60.1X2	T60.1X3	T60.1X4	—	—
Pernocton	T42.3X1	T42.3X2	T42.3X3	T42.3X4	T42.3X5	T42.3X6
Pernoston	T42.3X1	T42.3X2	T42.3X3	T42.3X4	T42.3X5	T42.3X6
Peronine	T40.2X1	T40.2X2	T40.2X3	T40.2X4	—	—
Perphenazine	T43.3X1	T43.3X2	T43.3X3	T43.3X4	T43.3X5	T43.3X6
Pertofrane	T43.011	T43.012	T43.013	T43.014	T43.015	T43.016
Pertussis						
immune serum (human)	T50.Z11	T50.Z12	T50.Z13	T50.Z14	T50.Z15	T50.Z16
vaccine (with diphtheria toxoid) (with tetanus toxoid)	T50.A11	T50.A12	T50.A13	T50.A14	T50.A15	T50.A16
Peruvian balsam	T49.0X1	T49.0X2	T49.0X3	T49.0X4	T49.0X5	T49.0X6
Peruvoside	T46.0X1	T46.0X2	T46.0X3	T46.0X4	T46.0X5	T46.0X6
Pesticide (dust) (fumes) (vapor)	T60.91	T60.92	T60.93	T60.94	—	—
NEC						
arsenic	T57.0X1	T57.0X2	T57.0X3	T57.0X4	—	—
chlorinated	T60.1X1	T60.1X2	T60.1X3	T60.1X4	—	—
cyanide	T65.0X1	T65.0X2	T65.0X3	T65.0X4	—	—
kerosene	T52.0X1	T52.0X2	T52.0X3	T52.0X4	—	—
mixture (of compounds)	T60.91	T60.92	T60.93	T60.94	—	—
naphthalene	T60.2X1	T60.2X2	T60.2X3	T60.2X4	—	—
organochlorine (compounds)	T60.1X1	T60.1X2	T60.1X3	T60.1X4	—	—
petroleum (distillate) (products) NEC	T60.8X1	T60.8X2	T60.8X3	T60.8X4	—	—
specified ingredient NEC	T60.8X1	T60.8X2	T60.8X3	T60.8X4	—	—
strychnine	T65.1X1	T65.1X2	T65.1X3	T65.1X4	—	—
thallium	T60.4X1	T60.4X2	T60.4X3	T60.4X4	—	—
Pethidine	T40.4X1	T40.4X2	T40.4X3	T40.4X4	T40.4X5	T40.4X6
Petrichloral	T42.6X1	T42.6X2	T42.6X3	T42.6X4	T42.6X5	T42.6X6
Petrol	T52.0X1	T52.0X2	T52.0X3	T52.0X4	—	—
vapor	T52.0X1	T52.0X2	T52.0X3	T52.0X4	—	—
Petrolatum	T49.3X1	T49.3X2	T49.3X3	T49.3X4	T49.3X5	T49.3X6
hydrophilic	T49.3X1	T49.3X2	T49.3X3	T49.3X4	T49.3X5	T49.3X6
liquid	T47.4X1	T47.4X2	T47.4X3	T47.4X4	T47.4X5	T47.4X6
topical	T49.3X1	T49.3X2	T49.3X3	T49.3X4	T49.3X5	T49.3X6
nonmedicinal	T52.0X1	T52.0X2	T52.0X3	T52.0X4	—	—
red veterinary	T49.3X1	T49.3X2	T49.3X3	T49.3X4	T49.3X5	T49.3X6
white	T49.3X1	T49.3X2	T49.3X3	T49.3X4	T49.3X5	T49.3X6
Petroleum (products) **NEC**	T52.0X1	T52.0X2	T52.0X3	T52.0X4	—	—
benzine(s) — see Ligroin						
ether — see Ligroin						
jelly — see Petrolatum						
naphtha — see Ligroin						
pesticide	T60.8X1	T60.8X2	T60.8X3	T60.8X4	—	—
solids	T52.0X1	T52.0X2	T52.0X3	T52.0X4	—	—
solvents	T52.0X1	T52.0X2	T52.0X3	T52.0X4	—	—
vapor	T52.0X1	T52.0X2	T52.0X3	T52.0X4	—	—
Peyote	T40.991	T40.992	T40.993	T40.994	—	—
Phanodorm, phanodorn	T42.3X1	T42.3X2	T42.3X3	T42.3X4	T42.3X5	T42.3X6
Phanquinone	T37.3X1	T37.3X2	T37.3X3	T37.3X4	T37.3X5	T37.3X6
Phanquone	T37.3X1	T37.3X2	T37.3X3	T37.3X4	T37.3X5	T37.3X6
Pharmaceutical						
adjunct NEC	T50.901	T50.902	T50.903	T50.904	T50.905	T50.906
excipient NEC	T50.901	T50.902	T50.903	T50.904	T50.905	T50.906
sweetener	T50.901	T50.902	T50.903	T50.904	T50.905	T50.906
viscous agent	T50.901	T50.902	T50.903	T50.904	T50.905	T50.906
Phemitone	T42.3X1	T42.3X2	T42.3X3	T42.3X4	T42.3X5	T42.3X6
Phenacaine	T41.3X1	T41.3X2	T41.3X3	T41.3X4	T41.3X5	T41.3X6
Phenacemide	T42.6X1	T42.6X2	T42.6X3	T42.6X4	T42.6X5	T42.6X6
Phenacetin	T39.1X1	T39.1X2	T39.1X3	T39.1X4	T39.1X5	T39.1X6
Phenadoxone	T40.2X1	T40.2X2	T40.2X3	T40.2X4	—	—
Phenaglycodol	T43.591	T43.592	T43.593	T43.594	T43.595	T43.596
Phenantoin	T42.0X1	T42.0X2	T42.0X3	T42.0X4	T42.0X5	T42.0X6
Phenaphthazine reagent	T50.991	T50.992	T50.993	T50.994	T50.995	T50.996
Phenazocine	T40.4X1	T40.4X2	T40.4X3	T40.4X4	T40.4X5	T40.4X6
Phenazone	T39.2X1	T39.2X2	T39.2X3	T39.2X4	T39.2X5	T39.2X6
Phenazopyridine	T39.8X1	T39.8X2	T39.8X3	T39.8X4	T39.8X5	T39.8X6
Phenbenicillin	T36.0X1	T36.0X2	T36.0X3	T36.0X4	T36.0X5	T36.0X6
Phenbutrazate	T50.5X1	T50.5X2	T50.5X3	T50.5X4	T50.5X5	T50.5X6
Phencyclidine	T40.991	T40.992	T40.993	T40.994	T40.995	T40.996
Phendimetrazine	T50.5X1	T50.5X2	T50.5X3	T50.5X4	T50.5X5	T50.5X6
Phenelzine	T43.1X1	T43.1X2	T43.1X3	T43.1X4	T43.1X5	T43.1X6
Phenemal	T42.3X1	T42.3X2	T42.3X3	T42.3X4	T42.3X5	T42.3X6
Phenergan	T42.6X1	T42.6X2	T42.6X3	T42.6X4	T42.6X5	T42.6X6
Pheneticillin	T36.0X1	T36.0X2	T36.0X3	T36.0X4	T36.0X5	T36.0X6
Pheneturide	T42.6X1	T42.6X2	T42.6X3	T42.6X4	T42.6X5	T42.6X6
Phenformin	T38.3X1	T38.3X2	T38.3X3	T38.3X4	T38.3X5	T38.3X6

Substance	Poisoning, Accidental (unintentional)	Poisoning, Intentional Self-harm	Poisoning, Assault	Poisoning, Undetermined	Adverse Effect	Under-dosing
Phenglutarimide	T44.3X1	T44.3X2	T44.3X3	T44.3X4	T44.3X5	T44.3X6
Phenicarbazide	T39.8X1	T39.8X2	T39.8X3	T39.8X4	T39.8X5	T39.8X6
Phenindamine	T45.0X1	T45.0X2	T45.0X3	T45.0X4	T45.0X5	T45.0X6
Phenindione	T45.511	T45.512	T45.513	T45.514	T45.515	T45.516
Pheniprazine	T43.1X1	T43.1X2	T43.1X3	T43.1X4	T43.1X5	T43.1X6
Pheniramine	T45.0X1	T45.0X2	T45.0X3	T45.0X4	T45.0X5	T45.0X6
Phenisatin	T47.2X1	T47.2X2	T47.2X3	T47.2X4	T47.2X5	T47.2X6
Phenmetrazine	T50.5X1	T50.5X2	T50.5X3	T50.5X4	T50.5X5	T50.5X6
Phenobal	T42.3X1	T42.3X2	T42.3X3	T42.3X4	T42.3X5	T42.3X6
Phenobarbital	T42.3X1	T42.3X2	T42.3X3	T42.3X4	T42.3X5	T42.3X6
with						
mephenytoin	T42.3X1	T42.3X2	T42.3X3	T42.3X4	T42.3X5	T42.3X6
phenytoin	T42.3X1	T42.3X2	T42.3X3	T42.3X4	T42.3X5	T42.3X6
sodium	T42.3X1	T42.3X2	T42.3X3	T42.3X4	T42.3X5	T42.3X6
Phenobarbitone	T42.3X1	T42.3X2	T42.3X3	T42.3X4	T42.3X5	T42.3X6
Phenobutiodil	T50.8X1	T50.8X2	T50.8X3	T50.8X4	T50.8X5	T50.8X6
Phenoctide	T49.0X1	T49.0X2	T49.0X3	T49.0X4	T49.0X5	T49.0X6
Phenol	T49.0X1	T49.0X2	T49.0X3	T49.0X4	T49.0X5	T49.0X6
disinfectant	T54.0X1	T54.0X2	T54.0X3	T54.0X4	—	—
in oil injection	T46.8X1	T46.8X2	T46.8X3	T46.8X4	T46.8X5	T46.8X6
medicinal	T49.1X1	T49.1X2	T49.1X3	T49.1X4	T49.1X5	T49.1X6
nonmedicinal NEC	T54.0X1	T54.0X2	T54.0X3	T54.0X4	—	—
pesticide	T60.8X1	T60.8X2	T60.8X3	T60.8X4	—	—
red	T50.8X1	T50.8X2	T50.8X3	T50.8X4	T50.8X5	T50.8X6
Phenolic preparation	T49.1X1	T49.1X2	T49.1X3	T49.1X4	T49.1X5	T49.1X6
Phenolphthalein	T47.2X1	T47.2X2	T47.2X3	T47.2X4	T47.2X5	T47.2X6
Phenolsulfonphthalein	T50.8X1	T50.8X2	T50.8X3	T50.8X4	T50.8X5	T50.8X6
Phenomorphan	T40.2X1	T40.2X2	T40.2X3	T40.2X4	—	—
Phenonyl	T42.3X1	T42.3X2	T42.3X3	T42.3X4	T42.3X5	T42.3X6
Phenoperidine	T40.4X1	T40.4X2	T40.4X3	T40.4X4	—	—
Phenopyrazone	T46.991	T46.992	T46.993	T46.994	T46.995	T46.996
Phenoquin	T50.4X1	T50.4X2	T50.4X3	T50.4X4	T50.4X5	T50.4X6
Phenothiazine (psychotropic)	T43.3X1	T43.3X2	T43.3X3	T43.3X4	T43.3X5	T43.3X6
NEC						
insecticide	T60.2X1	T60.2X2	T60.2X3	T60.2X4	—	—
Phenothrin	T49.0X1	T49.0X2	T49.0X3	T49.0X4	T49.0X5	T49.0X6
Phenoxybenzamine	T46.7X1	T46.7X2	T46.7X3	T46.7X4	T46.7X5	T46.7X6
Phenoxyethanol	T49.0X1	T49.0X2	T49.0X3	T49.0X4	T49.0X5	T49.0X6
Phenoxymethyl penicillin	T36.0X1	T36.0X2	T36.0X3	T36.0X4	T36.0X5	T36.0X6
Phenprobamate	T42.8X1	T42.8X2	T42.8X3	T42.8X4	T42.8X5	T42.8X6
Phenprocoumon	T45.511	T45.512	T45.513	T45.514	T45.515	T45.516
Phensuximide	T42.2X1	T42.2X2	T42.2X3	T42.2X4	T42.2X5	T42.2X6
Phentermine	T50.5X1	T50.5X2	T50.5X3	T50.5X4	T50.5X5	T50.5X6
Phenthicillin	T36.0X1	T36.0X2	T36.0X3	T36.0X4	T36.0X5	T36.0X6
Phentolamine	T46.7X1	T46.7X2	T46.7X3	T46.7X4	T46.7X5	T46.7X6
Phenyl						
butazone	T39.2X1	T39.2X2	T39.2X3	T39.2X4	T39.2X5	T39.2X6
enediamine	T65.3X1	T65.3X2	T65.3X3	T65.3X4	—	—
hydrazine	T65.3X1	T65.3X2	T65.3X3	T65.3X4	—	—
antineoplastic	T45.1X1	T45.1X2	T45.1X3	T45.1X4	T45.1X5	T45.1X6
mercuric compounds — see Mercury						
salicylate	T49.3X1	T49.3X2	T49.3X3	T49.3X4	T49.3X5	T49.3X6
Phenylalanine mustard	T45.1X1	T45.1X2	T45.1X3	T45.1X4	T45.1X5	T45.1X6
Phenylbutazone	T39.2X1	T39.2X2	T39.2X3	T39.2X4	T39.2X5	T39.2X6
Phenylenediamine	T65.3X1	T65.3X2	T65.3X3	T65.3X4	—	—
Phenylephrine	T44.4X1	T44.4X2	T44.4X3	T44.4X4	T44.4X5	T44.4X6
Phenylethylbiguanide	T38.3X1	T38.3X2	T38.3X3	T38.3X4	T38.3X5	T38.3X6
Phenylmercuric						
acetate	T49.0X1	T49.0X2	T49.0X3	T49.0X4	T49.0X5	T49.0X6
borate	T49.0X1	T49.0X2	T49.0X3	T49.0X4	T49.0X5	T49.0X6
nitrate	T49.0X1	T49.0X2	T49.0X3	T49.0X4	T49.0X5	T49.0X6
Phenylmethylbarbitone	T42.3X1	T42.3X2	T42.3X3	T42.3X4	T42.3X5	T42.3X6
Phenylpropanol	T47.5X1	T47.5X2	T47.5X3	T47.5X4	T47.5X5	T47.5X6
Phenylpropanolamine	T44.991	T44.992	T44.993	T44.994	T44.995	T44.996
Phenylsulfthion	T60.0X1	T60.0X2	T60.0X3	T60.0X4	—	—
Phenyltoloxamine	T45.0X1	T45.0X2	T45.0X3	T45.0X4	T45.0X5	T45.0X6
Phenyramidol, phenyramidon	T39.8X1	T39.8X2	T39.8X3	T39.8X4	T39.8X5	T39.8X6
Phenytoin	T42.0X1	T42.0X2	T42.0X3	T42.0X4	T42.0X5	T42.0X6
with Phenobarbital	T42.3X1	T42.3X2	T42.3X3	T42.3X4	T42.3X5	T42.3X6
pHisoHex	T49.2X1	T49.2X2	T49.2X3	T49.2X4	T49.2X5	T49.2X6
Pholcodine	T48.3X1	T48.3X2	T48.3X3	T48.3X4	T48.3X5	T48.3X6
Pholedrine	T46.991	T46.992	T46.993	T46.994	T46.995	T46.996
Phorate	T60.0X1	T60.0X2	T60.0X3	T60.0X4	—	—
Phosdrin	T60.0X1	T60.0X2	T60.0X3	T60.0X4	—	—
Phosfolan	T60.0X1	T60.0X2	T60.0X3	T60.0X4	—	—
Phosgene (gas)	T59.891	T59.892	T59.893	T59.894	—	—
Phosphamidon	T60.0X1	T60.0X2	T60.0X3	T60.0X4	—	—
Phosphate	T65.891	T65.892	T65.893	T65.894	—	—
laxative	T47.4X1	T47.4X2	T47.4X3	T47.4X4	T47.4X5	T47.4X6
organic	T60.0X1	T60.0X2	T60.0X3	T60.0X4	—	—
solvent	T52.91	T52.92	T52.93	T52.94	—	—
Phosphate — continued						
tricresyl	T65.891	T65.892	T65.893	T65.894	—	—
Phosphine	T57.1X1	T57.1X2	T57.1X3	T57.1X4	—	—
fumigant	T57.1X1	T57.1X2	T57.1X3	T57.1X4	—	—
Pholine	T49.5X1	T49.5X2	T49.5X3	T49.5X4	T49.5X5	T49.5X6
Phosphoric acid	T54.2X1	T54.2X2	T54.2X3	T54.2X4	—	—
Phosphorus (compound)	T57.1X1	T57.1X2	T57.1X3	T57.1X4	—	—
NEC						
pesticide	T60.0X1	T60.0X2	T60.0X3	T60.0X4	—	—
Phthalates	T65.891	T65.892	T65.893	T65.894	—	—
Phthalic anhydride	T65.891	T65.892	T65.893	T65.894	—	—
Phthalimidoglutarimide	T42.6X1	T42.6X2	T42.6X3	T42.6X4	T42.6X5	T42.6X6
Phthalylsulfathiazole	T37.0X1	T37.0X2	T37.0X3	T37.0X4	T37.0X5	T37.0X6
Phylloquinone	T45.7X1	T45.7X2	T45.7X3	T45.7X4	T45.7X5	T45.7X6
Physeptone	T40.3X1	T40.3X2	T40.3X3	T40.3X4	T40.3X5	T40.3X6
Physostigma venenosum	T62.2X1	T62.2X2	T62.2X3	T62.2X4	—	—
Physostigmine	T49.5X1	T49.5X2	T49.5X3	T49.5X4	T49.5X5	T49.5X6
Phytolacca decandra	T62.2X1	T62.2X2	T62.2X3	T62.2X4	—	—
berries	T62.1X1	T62.1X2	T62.1X3	T62.1X4	—	—
Phytomenadione	T45.7X1	T45.7X2	T45.7X3	T45.7X4	T45.7X5	T45.7X6
Phytonadione	T45.7X1	T45.7X2	T45.7X3	T45.7X4	T45.7X5	T45.7X6
Picoperine	T48.3X1	T48.3X2	T48.3X3	T48.3X4	T48.3X5	T48.3X6
Picosulfate (sodium)	T47.2X1	T47.2X2	T47.2X3	T47.2X4	T47.2X5	T47.2X6
Picric (acid)	T54.2X1	T54.2X2	T54.2X3	T54.2X4	—	—
Picrotoxin	T50.7X1	T50.7X2	T50.7X3	T50.7X4	T50.7X5	T50.7X6
Piketoprofen	T49.0X1	T49.0X2	T49.0X3	T49.0X4	T49.0X5	T49.0X6
Pilocarpine	T44.1X1	T44.1X2	T44.1X3	T44.1X4	T44.1X5	T44.1X6
Pilocarpus (jaborandi) extract	T44.1X1	T44.1X2	T44.1X3	T44.1X4	T44.1X5	T44.1X6
Pilsicainide (hydrochloride)	T46.2X1	T46.2X2	T46.2X3	T46.2X4	T46.2X5	T46.2X6
Pimaricin	T36.7X1	T36.7X2	T36.7X3	T36.7X4	T36.7X5	T36.7X6
Pimeclone	T50.7X1	T50.7X2	T50.7X3	T50.7X4	T50.7X5	T50.7X6
Pimelic ketone	T52.8X1	T52.8X2	T52.8X3	T52.8X4	—	—
Pimethixene	T45.0X1	T45.0X2	T45.0X3	T45.0X4	T45.0X5	T45.0X6
Piminodine	T40.2X1	T40.2X2	T40.2X3	T40.2X4	T40.2X5	T40.2X6
Pimozide	T43.591	T43.592	T43.593	T43.594	T43.595	T43.596
Pinacidil	T46.5X1	T46.5X2	T46.5X3	T46.5X4	T46.5X5	T46.5X6
Pinaverium bromide	T44.3X1	T44.3X2	T44.3X3	T44.3X4	T44.3X5	T44.3X6
Pinazepam	T42.4X1	T42.4X2	T42.4X3	T42.4X4	T42.4X5	T42.4X6
Pindolol	T44.7X1	T44.7X2	T44.7X3	T44.7X4	T44.7X5	T44.7X6
Pindone	T60.4X1	T60.4X2	T60.4X3	T60.4X4	—	—
Pine oil (disinfectant)	T65.891	T65.892	T65.893	T65.894	—	—
Pinkroot	T37.4X1	T37.4X2	T37.4X3	T37.4X4	T37.4X5	T37.4X6
Pipadone	T40.2X1	T40.2X2	T40.2X3	T40.2X4	—	—
Pipamazine	T45.0X1	T45.0X2	T45.0X3	T45.0X4	T45.0X5	T45.0X6
Pipamperone	T43.4X1	T43.4X2	T43.4X3	T43.4X4	T43.4X5	T43.4X6
Pipazetate	T48.3X1	T48.3X2	T48.3X3	T48.3X4	T48.3X5	T48.3X6
Pipemidic acid	T37.8X1	T37.8X2	T37.8X3	T37.8X4	T37.8X5	T37.8X6
Pipenzolate bromide	T44.3X1	T44.3X2	T44.3X3	T44.3X4	T44.3X5	T44.3X6
Piperacetazine	T43.3X1	T43.3X2	T43.3X3	T43.3X4	T43.3X5	T43.3X6
Piperacillin	T36.0X1	T36.0X2	T36.0X3	T36.0X4	T36.0X5	T36.0X6
Piperazine	T37.4X1	T37.4X2	T37.4X3	T37.4X4	T37.4X5	T37.4X6
estrone sulfate	T38.5X1	T38.5X2	T38.5X3	T38.5X4	T38.5X5	T38.5X6
Piper cubeba	T62.2X1	T62.2X2	T62.2X3	T62.2X4	—	—
Piperidione	T48.3X1	T48.3X2	T48.3X3	T48.3X4	T48.3X5	T48.3X6
Piperidolate	T44.3X1	T44.3X2	T44.3X3	T44.3X4	T44.3X5	T44.3X6
Piperocaine	T41.3X1	T41.3X2	T41.3X3	T41.3X4	T41.3X5	T41.3X6
infiltration (subcutaneous)	T41.3X1	T41.3X2	T41.3X3	T41.3X4	T41.3X5	T41.3X6
nerve block (peripheral) (plexus)	T41.3X1	T41.3X2	T41.3X3	T41.3X4	T41.3X5	T41.3X6
topical (surface)	T41.3X1	T41.3X2	T41.3X3	T41.3X4	T41.3X5	T41.3X6
Piperonyl butoxide	T60.8X1	T60.8X2	T60.8X3	T60.8X4	—	—
Pipethanate	T44.3X1	T44.3X2	T44.3X3	T44.3X4	T44.3X5	T44.3X6
Pipobroman	T45.1X1	T45.1X2	T45.1X3	T45.1X4	T45.1X5	T45.1X6
Pipotiazine	T43.3X1	T43.3X2	T43.3X3	T43.3X4	T43.3X5	T43.3X6
Pipoxizine	T45.0X1	T45.0X2	T45.0X3	T45.0X4	T45.0X5	T45.0X6
Pipradrol	T43.691	T43.692	T43.693	T43.694	T43.695	T43.696
Piprinhydrinate	T45.0X1	T45.0X2	T45.0X3	T45.0X4	T45.0X5	T45.0X6
Pirarubicin	T45.1X1	T45.1X2	T45.1X3	T45.1X4	T45.1X5	T45.1X6
Pirazinamide	T37.1X1	T37.1X2	T37.1X3	T37.1X4	T37.1X5	T37.1X6
Pirbuterol	T48.6X1	T48.6X2	T48.6X3	T48.6X4	T48.6X5	T48.6X6
Pirenzepine	T47.1X1	T47.1X2	T47.1X3	T47.1X4	T47.1X5	T47.1X6
Piretanide	T50.1X1	T50.1X2	T50.1X3	T50.1X4	T50.1X5	T50.1X6
Piribedil	T42.8X1	T42.8X2	T42.8X3	T42.8X4	T42.8X5	T42.8X6
Piridoxilate	T46.3X1	T46.3X2	T46.3X3	T46.3X4	T46.3X5	T46.3X6
Piritramide	T40.4X1	T40.4X2	T40.4X3	T40.4X4	—	—
Piromidic acid	T37.8X1	T37.8X2	T37.8X3	T37.8X4	T37.8X5	T37.8X6
Piroxicam	T39.391	T39.392	T39.393	T39.394	T39.395	T39.396
beta-cyclodextrin complex	T39.8X1	T39.8X2	T39.8X3	T39.8X4	T39.8X5	T39.8X6
Pirozadil	T46.6X1	T46.6X2	T46.6X3	T46.6X4	T46.6X5	T46.6X6
Piscidia (bark) (erythrina)	T39.8X1	T39.8X2	T39.8X3	T39.8X4	T39.8X5	T39.8X6
Pitch	T65.891	T65.892	T65.893	T65.894	—	—
Pitkin's solution	T41.3X1	T41.3X2	T41.3X3	T41.3X4	T41.3X5	T41.3X6

Additional Character May Be Required — Refer to the Tabular List for Character Selection   Subterms under main terms may continue to next column or page

Substance	Poisoning, Accidental (unintentional)	Poisoning, Intentional Self-harm	Poisoning, Assault	Poisoning, Undetermined	Adverse Effect	Under-dosing
Pitocin	T48.0X1	T48.0X2	T48.0X3	T48.0X4	T48.0X5	T48.0X6
Pitressin (tannate)	T38.891	T38.892	T38.893	T38.894	T38.895	T38.896
Pituitary extracts	T38.891	T38.892	T38.893	T38.894	T38.895	T38.896
(posterior)						
anterior	T38.811	T38.812	T38.813	T38.814	T38.815	T38.816
Pituitrin	T38.891	T38.892	T38.893	T38.894	T38.895	T38.896
Pivampicillin	T36.0X1	T36.0X2	T36.0X3	T36.0X4	T36.0X5	T36.0X6
Pivmecillinam	T36.0X1	T36.0X2	T36.0X3	T36.0X4	T36.0X5	T36.0X6
Placental hormone	T38.891	T38.892	T38.893	T38.894	T38.895	T38.896
Placidyl	T42.6X1	T42.6X2	T42.6X3	T42.6X4	T42.6X5	T42.6X6
Plague vaccine	T50.A91	T50.A92	T50.A93	T50.A94	T50.A95	T50.A96
Plant						
food or fertilizer NEC	T65.891	T65.892	T65.893	T65.894	—	—
containing herbicide	T60.3X1	T60.3X2	T60.3X3	T60.3X4	—	—
noxious, used as food	T62.2X1	T62.2X2	T62.2X3	T62.2X4	—	—
berries	T62.1X1	T62.1X2	T62.1X3	T62.1X4	—	—
seeds	T62.2X1	T62.2X2	T62.2X3	T62.2X4	—	—
specified type NEC	T62.2X1	T62.2X2	T62.2X3	T62.2X4	—	—
Plasma	T45.8X1	T45.8X2	T45.8X3	T45.8X4	T45.8X5	T45.8X6
expander NEC	T45.8X1	T45.8X2	T45.8X3	T45.8X4	T45.8X5	T45.8X6
protein fraction (human)	T45.8X1	T45.8X2	T45.8X3	T45.8X4	T45.8X5	T45.8X6
Plasmanate	T45.8X1	T45.8X2	T45.8X3	T45.8X4	T45.8X5	T45.8X6
Plasminogen (tissue)	T45.611	T45.612	T45.613	T45.614	T45.615	T45.616
activator						
Plaster dressing	T49.3X1	T49.3X2	T49.3X3	T49.3X4	T49.3X5	T49.3X6
Plastic dressing	T49.3X1	T49.3X2	T49.3X3	T49.3X4	T49.3X5	T49.3X6
Plegicil	T43.3X1	T43.3X2	T43.3X3	T43.3X4	T43.3X5	T43.3X6
Plicamycin	T45.1X1	T45.1X2	T45.1X3	T45.1X4	T45.1X5	T45.1X6
Podophyllotoxin	T49.8X1	T49.8X2	T49.8X3	T49.8X4	T49.8X5	T49.8X6
Podophyllum (resin)	T49.4X1	T49.4X2	T49.4X3	T49.4X4	T49.4X5	T49.4X6
Poisonous berries	T62.1X1	T62.1X2	T62.1X3	T62.1X4	—	—
Poison NEC	T65.91	T65.92	T65.93	T65.94	—	—
Pokeweed (any part)	T62.2X1	T62.2X2	T62.2X3	T62.2X4	—	—
Poldine metilsulfate	T44.3X1	T44.3X2	T44.3X3	T44.3X4	T44.3X5	T44.3X6
Polidexide (sulfate)	T46.6X1	T46.6X2	T46.6X3	T46.6X4	T46.6X5	T46.6X6
Polidocanol	T46.8X1	T46.8X2	T46.8X3	T46.8X4	T46.8X5	T46.8X6
Poliomyelitis vaccine	T50.B91	T50.B92	T50.B93	T50.B94	T50.B95	T50.B96
Polish (car) (floor) (furniture)	T65.891	T65.892	T65.893	T65.894	—	—
(metal) (porcelain)						
(silver)						
abrasive	T65.891	T65.892	T65.893	T65.894	—	—
porcelain	T65.891	T65.892	T65.893	T65.894	—	—
Poloxalkol	T47.4X1	T47.4X2	T47.4X3	T47.4X4	T47.4X5	T47.4X6
Poloxamer	T47.4X1	T47.4X2	T47.4X3	T47.4X4	T47.4X5	T47.4X6
Polyaminostyrene resins	T50.3X1	T50.3X2	T50.3X3	T50.3X4	T50.3X5	T50.3X6
Polycarbophil	T47.4X1	T47.4X2	T47.4X3	T47.4X4	T47.4X5	T47.4X6
Polychlorinated biphenyl	T65.891	T65.892	T65.893	T65.894	—	—
Polycycline	T36.4X1	T36.4X2	T36.4X3	T36.4X4	T36.4X5	T36.4X6
Polyester fumes	T59.891	T59.892	T59.893	T59.894	—	—
Polyester resin hardener	T52.91	T52.92	T52.93	T52.94	—	—
fumes	T59.891	T59.892	T59.893	T59.894	—	—
Polyestradiol phosphate	T38.5X1	T38.5X2	T38.5X3	T38.5X4	T38.5X5	T38.5X6
Polyethanolamine alkyl sulfate	T49.2X1	T49.2X2	T49.2X3	T49.2X4	T49.2X5	T49.2X6
Polyethylene adhesive	T49.3X1	T49.3X2	T49.3X3	T49.3X4	T49.3X5	T49.3X6
Polyferose	T45.4X1	T45.4X2	T45.4X3	T45.4X4	T45.4X5	T45.4X6
Polygeline	T45.8X1	T45.8X2	T45.8X3	T45.8X4	T45.8X5	T45.8X6
Polymyxin	T36.8X1	T36.8X2	T36.8X3	T36.8X4	T36.8X5	T36.8X6
B	T36.8X1	T36.8X2	T36.8X3	T36.8X4	T36.8X5	T36.8X6
ENT agent	T49.6X1	T49.6X2	T49.6X3	T49.6X4	T49.6X5	T49.6X6
ophthalmic preparation	T49.5X1	T49.5X2	T49.5X3	T49.5X4	T49.5X5	T49.5X6
topical NEC	T49.0X1	T49.0X2	T49.0X3	T49.0X4	T49.0X5	T49.0X6
E sulfate (eye preparation)	T49.5X1	T49.5X2	T49.5X3	T49.5X4	T49.5X5	T49.5X6
Polynoxylin	T49.0X1	T49.0X2	T49.0X3	T49.0X4	T49.0X5	T49.0X6
Polyoestradiol phosphate	T38.5X1	T38.5X2	T38.5X3	T38.5X4	T38.5X5	T38.5X6
Polyoxymethyleneurea	T49.0X1	T49.0X2	T49.0X3	T49.0X4	T49.0X5	T49.0X6
Polysilane	T47.8X1	T47.8X2	T47.8X3	T47.8X4	T47.8X5	T47.8X6
Polytetrafluoroethylene (inhaled)	T59.891	T59.892	T59.893	T59.894	—	—
Polythiazide	T50.2X1	T50.2X2	T50.2X3	T50.2X4	T50.2X5	T50.2X6
Polyvidone	T45.8X1	T45.8X2	T45.8X3	T45.8X4	T45.8X5	T45.8X6
Polyvinylpyrrolidone	T45.8X1	T45.8X2	T45.8X3	T45.8X4	T45.8X5	T45.8X6
Pontocaine (hydrochloride)	T41.3X1	T41.3X2	T41.3X3	T41.3X4	T41.3X5	T41.3X6
(infiltration) (topical)						
nerve block (peripheral) (plexus)	T41.3X1	T41.3X2	T41.3X3	T41.3X4	T41.3X5	T41.3X6
spinal	T41.3X1	T41.3X2	T41.3X3	T41.3X4	T41.3X5	T41.3X6
Porfiromycin	T45.1X1	T45.1X2	T45.1X3	T45.1X4	T45.1X5	T45.1X6
Posterior pituitary hormone NEC	T38.891	T38.892	T38.893	T38.894	T38.895	T38.896
Pot	T40.7X1	T40.7X2	T40.7X3	T40.7X4	T40.7X5	T40.7X6
Potash (caustic)	T54.3X1	T54.3X2	T54.3X3	T54.3X4	—	—
Potassic saline injection (lactated)	T50.3X1	T50.3X2	T50.3X3	T50.3X4	T50.3X5	T50.3X6
Potassium (salts) NEC	T50.3X1	T50.3X2	T50.3X3	T50.3X4	T50.3X5	T50.3X6
aminobenzoate	T45.8X1	T45.8X2	T45.8X3	T45.8X4	T45.8X5	T45.8X6
aminosalicylate	T37.1X1	T37.1X2	T37.1X3	T37.1X4	T37.1X5	T37.1X6
antimony ' tartrate'	T37.8X1	T37.8X2	T37.8X3	T37.8X4	T37.8X5	T37.8X6
arsenite (solution)	T57.0X1	T57.0X2	T57.0X3	T57.0X4	—	—
bichromate	T56.2X1	T56.2X2	T56.2X3	T56.2X4	—	—
bisulfate	T47.3X1	T47.3X2	T47.3X3	T47.3X4	T47.3X5	T47.3X6
bromide	T42.6X1	T42.6X2	T42.6X3	T42.6X4	T42.6X5	T42.6X6
canrenoate	T50.0X1	T50.0X2	T50.0X3	T50.0X4	T50.0X5	T50.0X6
carbonate	T54.3X1	T54.3X2	T54.3X3	T54.3X4	—	—
chlorate NEC	T65.891	T65.892	T65.893	T65.894	—	—
chloride	T50.3X1	T50.3X2	T50.3X3	T50.3X4	T50.3X5	T50.3X6
citrate	T50.991	T50.992	T50.993	T50.994	T50.995	T50.996
cyanide	T65.0X1	T65.0X2	T65.0X3	T65.0X4	—	—
ferric hexacyanoferrate (medicinal)	T50.6X1	T50.6X2	T50.6X3	T50.6X4	T50.6X5	T50.6X6
nonmedicinal	T65.891	T65.892	T65.893	T65.894	—	—
Fluoride	T57.8X1	T57.8X2	T57.8X3	T57.8X4	—	—
glucaldrate	T47.1X1	T47.1X2	T47.1X3	T47.1X4	T47.1X5	T47.1X6
hydroxide	T54.3X1	T54.3X2	T54.3X3	T54.3X4	—	—
iodate	T49.0X1	T49.0X2	T49.0X3	T49.0X4	T49.0X5	T49.0X6
iodide	T48.4X1	T48.4X2	T48.4X3	T48.4X4	T48.4X5	T48.4X6
nitrate	T57.8X1	T57.8X2	T57.8X3	T57.8X4	—	—
oxalate	T65.891	T65.892	T65.893	T65.894	—	—
perchlorate (nonmedicinal) NEC	T65.891	T65.892	T65.893	T65.894	—	—
antithyroid	T38.2X1	T38.2X2	T38.2X3	T38.2X4	T38.2X5	T38.2X6
medicinal	T38.2X1	T38.2X2	T38.2X3	T38.2X4	T38.2X5	T38.2X6
Permanganate (nonmedicinal)	T65.891	T65.892	T65.893	T65.894	—	—
medicinal	T49.0X1	T49.0X2	T49.0X3	T49.0X4	T49.0X5	T49.0X6
sulfate	T47.2X1	T47.2X2	T47.2X3	T47.2X4	T47.2X5	T47.2X6
Potassium-removing resin	T50.3X1	T50.3X2	T50.3X3	T50.3X4	T50.3X5	T50.3X6
Potassium-retaining drug	T50.3X1	T50.3X2	T50.3X3	T50.3X4	T50.3X5	T50.3X6
Povidone	T45.8X1	T45.8X2	T45.8X3	T45.8X4	T45.8X5	T45.8X6
iodine	T49.0X1	T49.0X2	T49.0X3	T49.0X4	T49.0X5	T49.0X6
Practolol	T44.7X1	T44.7X2	T44.7X3	T44.7X4	T44.7X5	T44.7X6
Prajmalium bitartrate	T46.2X1	T46.2X2	T46.2X3	T46.2X4	T46.2X5	T46.2X6
Pralidoxime (iodide)	T50.6X1	T50.6X2	T50.6X3	T50.6X4	T50.6X5	T50.6X6
chloride	T50.6X1	T50.6X2	T50.6X3	T50.6X4	T50.6X5	T50.6X6
Pramiverine	T44.3X1	T44.3X2	T44.3X3	T44.3X4	T44.3X5	T44.3X6
Pramocaine	T49.1X1	T49.1X2	T49.1X3	T49.1X4	T49.1X5	T49.1X6
Pramoxine	T49.1X1	T49.1X2	T49.1X3	T49.1X4	T49.1X5	T49.1X6
Prasterone	T38.7X1	T38.7X2	T38.7X3	T38.7X4	T38.7X5	T38.7X6
Pravastatin	T46.6X1	T46.6X2	T46.6X3	T46.6X4	T46.6X5	T46.6X6
Prazepam	T42.4X1	T42.4X2	T42.4X3	T42.4X4	T42.4X5	T42.4X6
Praziquantel	T37.4X1	T37.4X2	T37.4X3	T37.4X4	T37.4X5	T37.4X6
Prazitone	T43.291	T43.292	T43.293	T43.294	T43.295	T43.296
Prazosin	T44.6X1	T44.6X2	T44.6X3	T44.6X4	T44.6X5	T44.6X6
Prednicarbate	T49.0X1	T49.0X2	T49.0X3	T49.0X4	T49.0X5	T49.0X6
Prednimustine	T45.1X1	T45.1X2	T45.1X3	T45.1X4	T45.1X5	T45.1X6
Prednisolone	T38.0X1	T38.0X2	T38.0X3	T38.0X4	T38.0X5	T38.0X6
ENT agent	T49.6X1	T49.6X2	T49.6X3	T49.6X4	T49.6X5	T49.6X6
ophthalmic preparation	T49.5X1	T49.5X2	T49.5X3	T49.5X4	T49.5X5	T49.5X6
steaglate	T49.0X1	T49.0X2	T49.0X3	T49.0X4	T49.0X5	T49.0X6
topical NEC	T49.0X1	T49.0X2	T49.0X3	T49.0X4	T49.0X5	T49.0X6
Prednisone	T38.0X1	T38.0X2	T38.0X3	T38.0X4	T38.0X5	T38.0X6
Prednylidene	T38.0X1	T38.0X2	T38.0X3	T38.0X4	T38.0X5	T38.0X6
Pregnandiol	T38.5X1	T38.5X2	T38.5X3	T38.5X4	T38.5X5	T38.5X6
Pregneninolone	T38.5X1	T38.5X2	T38.5X3	T38.5X4	T38.5X5	T38.5X6
Preludin	T43.691	T43.692	T43.693	T43.694	T43.695	T43.696
Premarin	T38.5X1	T38.5X2	T38.5X3	T38.5X4	T38.5X5	T38.5X6
Premedication anesthetic	T41.201	T41.202	T41.203	T41.204	T41.205	T41.206
Prenalterol	T44.5X1	T44.5X2	T44.5X3	T44.5X4	T44.5X5	T44.5X6
Prenoxdiazine	T48.3X1	T48.3X2	T48.3X3	T48.3X4	T48.3X5	T48.3X6
Prenylamine	T46.3X1	T46.3X2	T46.3X3	T46.3X4	T46.3X5	T46.3X6
Preparation H	T49.8X1	T49.8X2	T49.8X3	T49.8X4	T49.8X5	T49.8X6
Preparation, local	T49.4X1	T49.4X2	T49.4X3	T49.4X4	T49.4X5	T49.4X6
Preservative (nonmedicinal)	T65.891	T65.892	T65.893	T65.894	—	—
medicinal	T50.901	T50.902	T50.903	T50.904	T50.905	T50.906
wood	T60.91	T60.92	T60.93	T60.94	—	—
Prethcamide	T50.7X1	T50.7X2	T50.7X3	T50.7X4	T50.7X5	T50.7X6
Pride of China	T62.2X1	T62.2X2	T62.2X3	T62.2X4	—	—
Pridinol	T44.3X1	T44.3X2	T44.3X3	T44.3X4	T44.3X5	T44.3X6
Prifinium bromide	T44.3X1	T44.3X2	T44.3X3	T44.3X4	T44.3X5	T44.3X6
Prilocaine	T41.3X1	T41.3X2	T41.3X3	T41.3X4	T41.3X5	T41.3X6
infiltration (subcutaneous)	T41.3X1	T41.3X2	T41.3X3	T41.3X4	T41.3X5	T41.3X6
nerve block (peripheral) (plexus)	T41.3X1	T41.3X2	T41.3X3	T41.3X4	T41.3X5	T41.3X6
regional	T41.3X1	T41.3X2	T41.3X3	T41.3X4	T41.3X5	T41.3X6

Subterms under main terms may continue to next column or page   Additional Character May Be Required — Refer to the Tabular List for Character Selection   385

Pitocin — Prilocaine

Substance	Poisoning, Accidental (unintentional)	Poisoning, Intentional Self-harm	Poisoning, Assault	Poisoning, Undetermined	Adverse Effect	Under-dosing
Primaquine	T37.2X1	T37.2X2	T37.2X3	T37.2X4	T37.2X5	T37.2X6
Primidone	T42.6X1	T42.6X2	T42.6X3	T42.6X4	T42.6X5	T42.6X6
Primula (veris)	T62.2X1	T62.2X2	T62.2X3	T62.2X4	—	—
Prinadol	T40.2X1	T40.2X2	T40.2X3	T40.2X4	T40.2X5	T40.2X6
Priscol, Priscoline	T46.6X1	T46.6X2	T46.6X3	T46.6X4	T46.6X5	T46.6X6
Pristinamycin	T36.3X1	T36.3X2	T36.3X3	T36.3X4	T36.3X5	T36.3X6
Privet	T62.2X1	T62.2X2	T62.2X3	T62.2X4	—	—
berries	T62.1X1	T62.1X2	T62.1X3	T62.1X4	—	—
Privine	T44.4X1	T44.4X2	T44.4X3	T44.4X4	T44.4X5	T44.4X6
Pro-Banthine	T44.3X1	T44.3X2	T44.3X3	T44.3X4	T44.3X5	T44.3X6
Probarbital	T42.3X1	T42.3X2	T42.3X3	T42.3X4	T42.3X5	T42.3X6
Probenecid	T50.4X1	T50.4X2	T50.4X3	T50.4X4	T50.4X5	T50.4X6
Probucol	T46.6X1	T46.6X2	T46.6X3	T46.6X4	T46.6X5	T46.6X6
Procainamide	T46.2X1	T46.2X2	T46.2X3	T46.2X4	T46.2X5	T46.2X6
Procaine	T41.3X1	T41.3X2	T41.3X3	T41.3X4	T41.3X5	T41.3X6
benzylpenicillin	T36.0X1	T36.0X2	T36.0X3	T36.0X4	T36.0X5	T36.0X6
nerve block (periphreal) (plexus)	T41.3X1	T41.3X2	T41.3X3	T41.3X4	T41.3X5	T41.3X6
penicillin G	T36.0X1	T36.0X2	T36.0X3	T36.0X4	T36.0X5	T36.0X6
regional	T41.3X1	T41.3X2	T41.3X3	T41.3X4	T41.3X5	T41.3X6
spinal	T41.3X1	T41.3X2	T41.3X3	T41.3X4	T41.3X5	T41.3X6
Procalmidol	T43.591	T43.592	T43.593	T43.594	T43.595	T43.596
Procarbazine	T45.1X1	T45.1X2	T45.1X3	T45.1X4	T45.1X5	T45.1X6
Procaterol	T44.5X1	T44.5X2	T44.5X3	T44.5X4	T44.5X5	T44.5X6
Prochlorperazine	T43.3X1	T43.3X2	T43.3X3	T43.3X4	T43.3X5	T43.3X6
Procyclidine	T44.3X1	T44.3X2	T44.3X3	T44.3X4	T44.3X5	T44.3X6
Producer gas	T58.8X1	T58.8X2	T58.8X3	T58.8X4	—	—
Profadol	T40.4X1	T40.4X2	T40.4X3	T40.4X4	T40.4X5	T40.4X6
Profenamine	T44.3X1	T44.3X2	T44.3X3	T44.3X4	T44.3X5	T44.3X6
Profenil	T44.3X1	T44.3X2	T44.3X3	T44.3X4	T44.3X5	T44.3X6
Proflavine	T49.0X1	T49.0X2	T49.0X3	T49.0X4	T49.0X5	T49.0X6
Progabide	T42.6X1	T42.6X2	T42.6X3	T42.6X4	T42.6X5	T42.6X6
Progesterone	T38.5X1	T38.5X2	T38.5X3	T38.5X4	T38.5X5	T38.5X6
Progestin	T38.5X1	T38.5X2	T38.5X3	T38.5X4	T38.5X5	T38.5X6
oral contraceptive	T38.4X1	T38.4X2	T38.4X3	T38.4X4	T38.4X5	T38.4X6
Progestogen NEC	T38.5X1	T38.5X2	T38.5X3	T38.5X4	T38.5X5	T38.5X6
Progestone	T38.5X1	T38.5X2	T38.5X3	T38.5X4	T38.5X5	T38.5X6
Proglumide	T47.1X1	T47.1X2	T47.1X3	T47.1X4	T47.1X5	T47.1X6
Proguanil	T37.2X1	T37.2X2	T37.2X3	T37.2X4	T37.2X5	T37.2X6
Prolactin	T38.811	T38.812	T38.813	T38.814	T38.815	T38.816
Prolintane	T43.691	T43.692	T43.693	T43.694	T43.695	T43.696
Proloid	T38.1X1	T38.1X2	T38.1X3	T38.1X4	T38.1X5	T38.1X6
Proluton	T38.5X1	T38.5X2	T38.5X3	T38.5X4	T38.5X5	T38.5X6
Promacetin	T37.1X1	T37.1X2	T37.1X3	T37.1X4	T37.1X5	T37.1X6
Promazine	T43.3X1	T43.3X2	T43.3X3	T43.3X4	T43.3X5	T43.3X6
Promedol	T40.2X1	T40.2X2	T40.2X3	T40.2X4	—	—
Promegestone	T38.5X1	T38.5X2	T38.5X3	T38.5X4	T38.5X5	T38.5X6
Promethazine (teoclate)	T43.3X1	T43.3X2	T43.3X3	T43.3X4	T43.3X5	T43.3X6
Promin	T37.1X1	T37.1X2	T37.1X3	T37.1X4	T37.1X5	T37.1X6
Pronase	T45.3X1	T45.3X2	T45.3X3	T45.3X4	T45.3X5	T45.3X6
Pronestyl (hydrochloride)	T46.2X1	T46.2X2	T46.2X3	T46.2X4	T46.2X5	T46.2X6
Pronetalol	T44.7X1	T44.7X2	T44.7X3	T44.7X4	T44.7X5	T44.7X6
Prontosil	T37.0X1	T37.0X2	T37.0X3	T37.0X4	T37.0X5	T37.0X6
Propachlor	T60.3X1	T60.3X2	T60.3X3	T60.3X4	—	—
Propafenone	T46.2X1	T46.2X2	T46.2X3	T46.2X4	T46.2X5	T46.2X6
Propallylonal	T42.3X1	T42.3X2	T42.3X3	T42.3X4	T42.3X5	T42.3X6
Propamidine	T49.0X1	T49.0X2	T49.0X3	T49.0X4	T49.0X5	T49.0X6
Propane (distributed in mobile container)	T59.891	T59.892	T59.893	T59.894	—	—
distributed through pipes	T59.891	T59.892	T59.893	T59.894	—	—
incomplete combustion	T58.11	T58.12	T58.13	T58.14	—	—
Propanidid	T41.291	T41.292	T41.293	T41.294	T41.295	T41.296
Propanil	T60.3X1	T60.3X2	T60.3X3	T60.3X4	—	—
Propantheline	T44.3X1	T44.3X2	T44.3X3	T44.3X4	T44.3X5	T44.3X6
bromide	T44.3X1	T44.3X2	T44.3X3	T44.3X4	T44.3X5	T44.3X6
Proparacaine	T41.3X1	T41.3X2	T41.3X3	T41.3X4	T41.3X5	T41.3X6
Propatylnitrate	T46.3X1	T46.3X2	T46.3X3	T46.3X4	T46.3X5	T46.3X6
Propicillin	T36.0X1	T36.0X2	T36.0X3	T36.0X4	T36.0X5	T36.0X6
Propiolactone	T49.0X1	T49.0X2	T49.0X3	T49.0X4	T49.0X5	T49.0X6
Propiomazine	T45.0X1	T45.0X2	T45.0X3	T45.0X4	T45.0X5	T45.0X6
Propionaldehyde (medicinal)	T42.6X1	T42.6X2	T42.6X3	T42.6X4	T42.6X5	T42.6X6
Propionate (calcium) (sodium)	T49.0X1	T49.0X2	T49.0X3	T49.0X4	T49.0X5	T49.0X6
Propion gel	T49.0X1	T49.0X2	T49.0X3	T49.0X4	T49.0X5	T49.0X6
Propitocaine	T41.3X1	T41.3X2	T41.3X3	T41.3X4	T41.3X5	T41.3X6
infiltration (subcutaneous)	T41.3X1	T41.3X2	T41.3X3	T41.3X4	T41.3X5	T41.3X6
nerve block (peripheral) (plexus)	T41.3X1	T41.3X2	T41.3X3	T41.3X4	T41.3X5	T41.3X6
Propofol	T41.291	T41.292	T41.293	T41.294	T41.295	T41.296
Propoxur	T60.0X1	T60.0X2	T60.0X3	T60.0X4	—	—
Propoxycaine	T41.3X1	T41.3X2	T41.3X3	T41.3X4	T41.3X5	T41.3X6
infiltration (subcutaneous)	T41.3X1	T41.3X2	T41.3X3	T41.3X4	T41.3X5	T41.3X6

Substance	Poisoning, Accidental (unintentional)	Poisoning, Intentional Self-harm	Poisoning, Assault	Poisoning, Undetermined	Adverse Effect	Under-dosing
Propoxycaine — continued						
nerve block (peripheral) (plexus)	T41.3X1	T41.3X2	T41.3X3	T41.3X4	T41.3X5	T41.3X6
topical (surface)	T41.3X1	T41.3X2	T41.3X3	T41.3X4	T41.3X5	T41.3X6
Propoxyphene	T40.4X1	T40.4X2	T40.4X3	T40.4X4	T40.4X5	T40.4X6
Propranolol	T44.7X1	T44.7X2	T44.7X3	T44.7X4	T44.7X5	T44.7X6
Propyl						
alcohol	T51.3X1	T51.3X2	T51.3X3	T51.3X4	—	—
carbinol	T51.3X1	T51.3X2	T51.3X3	T51.3X4	—	—
hexadrine	T44.4X1	T44.4X2	T44.4X3	T44.4X4	T44.4X5	T44.4X6
iodone	T50.8X1	T50.8X2	T50.8X3	T50.8X4	T50.8X5	T50.8X6
thiouracil	T38.2X1	T38.2X2	T38.2X3	T38.2X4	T38.2X5	T38.2X6
Propylaminophenothiazine	T43.3X1	T43.3X2	T43.3X3	T43.3X4	T43.3X5	T43.3X6
Propylene	T59.891	T59.892	T59.893	T59.894	—	—
Propylhexedrine	T48.5X1	T48.5X2	T48.5X3	T48.5X4	T48.5X5	T48.5X6
Propyliodone	T50.8X1	T50.8X2	T50.8X3	T50.8X4	T50.8X5	T50.8X6
Propylparaben (ophthalmic)	T49.5X1	T49.5X2	T49.5X3	T49.5X4	T49.5X5	T49.5X6
Propylthiouracil	T38.2X1	T38.2X2	T38.2X3	T38.2X4	T38.2X5	T38.2X6
Propyphenazone	T39.2X1	T39.2X2	T39.2X3	T39.2X4	T39.2X5	T39.2X6
Proquazone	T39.391	T39.392	T39.393	T39.394	T39.395	T39.396
Proscillaridin	T46.0X1	T46.0X2	T46.0X3	T46.0X4	T46.0X5	T46.0X6
Prostacyclin	T45.521	T45.522	T45.523	T45.524	T45.525	T45.526
Prostaglandin (I2)	T45.521	T45.522	T45.523	T45.524	T45.525	T45.526
E1	T46.7X1	T46.7X2	T46.7X3	T46.7X4	T46.7X5	T46.7X6
E2	T48.0X1	T48.0X2	T48.0X3	T48.0X4	T48.0X5	T48.0X6
F2 alpha	T48.0X1	T48.0X2	T48.0X3	T48.0X4	T48.0X5	T48.0X6
Prostigmin	T44.0X1	T44.0X2	T44.0X3	T44.0X4	T44.0X5	T44.0X6
Prosultiamine	T45.2X1	T45.2X2	T45.2X3	T45.2X4	T45.2X5	T45.2X6
Protamine sulfate	T45.7X1	T45.7X2	T45.7X3	T45.7X4	T45.7X5	T45.7X6
zinc insulin	T38.3X1	T38.3X2	T38.3X3	T38.3X4	T38.3X5	T38.3X6
Protease	T45.5X1	T45.5X2	T45.5X3	T45.5X4	T45.5X5	T45.5X6
Protectant, skin NEC	T49.3X1	T49.3X2	T49.3X3	T49.3X4	T49.3X5	T49.3X6
Protein hydrolysate	T50.991	T50.992	T50.993	T50.994	T50.995	T50.996
Prothiaden — see Dothiepin hydrochloride						
Prothionamide	T37.1X1	T37.1X2	T37.1X3	T37.1X4	T37.1X5	T37.1X6
Prothipendyl	T43.591	T43.592	T43.593	T43.594	T43.595	T43.596
Prothoate	T60.0X1	T60.0X2	T60.0X3	T60.0X4	—	—
Prothrombin						
activator	T45.7X1	T45.7X2	T45.7X3	T45.7X4	T45.7X5	T45.7X6
synthesis inhibitor	T45.511	T45.512	T45.513	T45.514	T45.515	T45.516
Protionamide	T37.1X1	T37.1X2	T37.1X3	T37.1X4	T37.1X5	T37.1X6
Protirelin	T38.891	T38.892	T38.893	T38.894	T38.895	T38.896
Protokylol	T48.6X1	T48.6X2	T48.6X3	T48.6X4	T48.6X5	T48.6X6
Protopam	T50.6X1	T50.6X2	T50.6X3	T50.6X4	T50.6X5	T50.6X6
Protoveratrine(s) (A) (B)	T46.5X1	T46.5X2	T46.5X3	T46.5X4	T46.5X5	T46.5X6
Protriptyline	T43.011	T43.012	T43.013	T43.014	T43.015	T43.016
Provera	T38.5X1	T38.5X2	T38.5X3	T38.5X4	T38.5X5	T38.5X6
Provitamin A	T45.2X1	T45.2X2	T45.2X3	T45.2X4	T45.2X5	T45.2X6
Proxibarbal	T42.3X1	T42.3X2	T42.3X3	T42.3X4	T42.3X5	T42.3X6
Proxymetacaine	T41.3X1	T41.3X2	T41.3X3	T41.3X4	T41.3X5	T41.3X6
Proxyphylline	T48.6X1	T48.6X2	T48.6X3	T48.6X4	T48.6X5	T48.6X6
Prozac — see Fluoxetine hydrochloride						
Prunus						
laurocerasus	T62.2X1	T62.2X2	T62.2X3	T62.2X4	—	—
virginiana	T62.2X1	T62.2X2	T62.2X3	T62.2X4	—	—
Prussian blue						
commercial	T65.891	T65.892	T65.893	T65.894	—	—
therapeutic	T50.6X1	T50.6X2	T50.6X3	T50.6X4	T50.6X5	T50.6X6
Prussic acid	T65.0X1	T65.0X2	T65.0X3	T65.0X4	—	—
vapor	T57.3X1	T57.3X2	T57.3X3	T57.3X4	—	—
Pseudoephedrine	T44.991	T44.992	T44.993	T44.994	T44.995	T44.996
Psilocin	T40.991	T40.992	T40.993	T40.994	—	—
Psilocybin	T40.991	T40.992	T40.993	T40.994	—	—
Psilocybine	T40.991	T40.992	T40.993	T40.994	—	—
Psoralene (nonmedicinal)	T65.891	T65.892	T65.893	T65.894	—	—
Psoralens (medicinal)	T50.991	T50.992	T50.993	T50.994	T50.995	T50.996
PSP (phenolsulfonphthalein)	T50.8X1	T50.8X2	T50.8X3	T50.8X4	T50.8X5	T50.8X6
Psychodysleptic drug NOS	T40.901	T40.902	T40.903	T40.904	T40.905	T40.906
specified NEC	T40.991	T40.992	T40.993	T40.994	T40.995	T40.996
Psychostimulant	T43.601	T43.602	T43.603	T43.604	T43.605	T43.606
amphetamine	T43.621	T43.622	T43.623	T43.624	T43.625	T43.626
caffeine	T43.611	T43.612	T43.613	T43.614	T43.615	T43.616
methylphenidate	T43.631	T43.632	T43.633	T43.634	T43.635	T43.636
specified NEC	T43.691	T43.692	T43.693	T43.694	T43.695	T43.696
Psychotherapeutic drug NEC	T43.91	T43.92	T43.93	T43.94	T43.95	T43.96
antidepressants — see also Antidepressant	T43.201	T43.202	T43.203	T43.204	T43.205	T43.206
specified NEC	T43.8X1	T43.8X2	T43.8X3	T43.8X4	T43.8X5	T43.8X6

Primaquine — Psychotherapeutic drug NEC

Substance	Poisoning, Accidental (unintentional)	Poisoning, Intentional Self-harm	Poisoning, Assault	Poisoning, Undetermined	Adverse Effect	Under-dosing
Psychotherapeutic drug — *continued*						
tranquilizers NEC	T43.501	T43.502	T43.503	T43.504	T43.505	T43.506
Psychotomimetic agents	T40.901	T40.902	T40.903	T40.904	T40.905	T40.906
Psychotropic drug NEC	T43.91	T43.92	T43.93	T43.94	T43.95	T43.96
specified NEC	T43.8X1	T43.8X2	T43.8X3	T43.8X4	T43.8X5	T43.8X6
Psyllium hydrophilic mucilloid	T47.4X1	T47.4X2	T47.4X3	T47.4X4	T47.4X5	T47.4X6
Pteroylglutamic acid	T45.8X1	T45.8X2	T45.8X3	T45.8X4	T45.8X5	T45.8X6
Pteroyltriglutamate	T45.1X1	T45.1X2	T45.1X3	T45.1X4	T45.1X5	T45.1X6
PTFE — *see* Polytetrafluoroethylene						
Pulp						
devitalizing paste	T49.7X1	T49.7X2	T49.7X3	T49.7X4	T49.7X5	T49.7X6
dressing	T49.7X1	T49.7X2	T49.7X3	T49.7X4	T49.7X5	T49.7X6
Pulsatilla	T62.2X1	T62.2X2	T62.2X3	T62.2X4	—	—
Pumpkin seed extract	T37.4X1	T37.4X2	T37.4X3	T37.4X4	T37.4X5	T37.4X6
Purex (bleach)	T54.91	T54.92	T54.93	T54.94	—	—
Purgative NEC — *see also* Cathartic	T47.4X1	T47.4X2	T47.4X3	T47.4X4	T47.4X5	T47.4X6
Purine analogue (antineoplastic)	T45.1X1	T45.1X2	T45.1X3	T45.1X4	T45.1X5	T45.1X6
Purine diuretics	T50.2X1	T50.2X2	T50.2X3	T50.2X4	T50.2X5	T50.2X6
Purinethol	T45.1X1	T45.1X2	T45.1X3	T45.1X4	T45.1X5	T45.1X6
PVP	T45.8X1	T45.8X2	T45.8X3	T45.8X4	T45.8X5	T45.8X6
Pyrabital	T39.8X1	T39.8X2	T39.8X3	T39.8X4	T39.8X5	T39.8X6
Pyramidon	T39.2X1	T39.2X2	T39.2X3	T39.2X4	T39.2X5	T39.2X6
Pyrantel	T37.4X1	T37.4X2	T37.4X3	T37.4X4	T37.4X5	T37.4X6
Pyrathiazine	T45.0X1	T45.0X2	T45.0X3	T45.0X4	T45.0X5	T45.0X6
Pyrazinamide	T37.1X1	T37.1X2	T37.1X3	T37.1X4	T37.1X5	T37.1X6
Pyrazinoic acid (amide)	T37.1X1	T37.1X2	T37.1X3	T37.1X4	T37.1X5	T37.1X6
Pyrazole (derivatives)	T39.2X1	T39.2X2	T39.2X3	T39.2X4	T39.2X5	T39.2X6
Pyrazolone analgesic NEC	T39.2X1	T39.2X2	T39.2X3	T39.2X4	T39.2X5	T39.2X6
Pyrethrin, pyrethrum (nonmedicinal)	T60.2X1	T60.2X2	T60.2X3	T60.2X4	—	—
Pyrethrum extract	T49.0X1	T49.0X2	T49.0X3	T49.0X4	T49.0X5	T49.0X6
Pyribenzamine	T45.0X1	T45.0X2	T45.0X3	T45.0X4	T45.0X5	T45.0X6
Pyridine	T52.8X1	T52.8X2	T52.8X3	T52.8X4	—	—
aldoxime methiodide	T50.6X1	T50.6X2	T50.6X3	T50.6X4	T50.6X5	T50.6X6
aldoxime methyl chloride	T50.6X1	T50.6X2	T50.6X3	T50.6X4	T50.6X5	T50.6X6
vapor	T59.891	T59.892	T59.893	T59.894	—	—
Pyridium	T39.8X1	T39.8X2	T39.8X3	T39.8X4	T39.8X5	T39.8X6
Pyridostigmine bromide	T44.0X1	T44.0X2	T44.0X3	T44.0X4	T44.0X5	T44.0X6
Pyridoxal phosphate	T45.2X1	T45.2X2	T45.2X3	T45.2X4	T45.2X5	T45.2X6
Pyridoxine	T45.2X1	T45.2X2	T45.2X3	T45.2X4	T45.2X5	T45.2X6
Pyrilamine	T45.0X1	T45.0X2	T45.0X3	T45.0X4	T45.0X5	T45.0X6
Pyrimethamine	T37.2X1	T37.2X2	T37.2X3	T37.2X4	T37.2X5	T37.2X6
with sulfadoxine	T37.2X1	T37.2X2	T37.2X3	T37.2X4	T37.2X5	T37.2X6
Pyrimidine antagonist	T45.1X1	T45.1X2	T45.1X3	T45.1X4	T45.1X5	T45.1X6
Pyriminil	T60.4X1	T60.4X2	T60.4X3	T60.4X4	—	—
Pyrithione zinc	T49.4X1	T49.4X2	T49.4X3	T49.4X4	T49.4X5	T49.4X6
Pyrithyldione	T42.6X1	T42.6X2	T42.6X3	T42.6X4	T42.6X5	T42.6X6
Pyrogallic acid	T49.0X1	T49.0X2	T49.0X3	T49.0X4	T49.0X5	T49.0X6
Pyrogallol	T49.0X1	T49.0X2	T49.0X3	T49.0X4	T49.0X5	T49.0X6
Pyroxylin	T49.3X1	T49.3X2	T49.3X3	T49.3X4	T49.3X5	T49.3X6
Pyrrobutamine	T45.0X1	T45.0X2	T45.0X3	T45.0X4	T45.0X5	T45.0X6
Pyrrolizidine alkaloids	T62.8X1	T62.8X2	T62.8X3	T62.8X4	—	—
Pyrvinium chloride	T37.4X1	T37.4X2	T37.4X3	T37.4X4	T37.4X5	T37.4X6
PZI	T38.3X1	T38.3X2	T38.3X3	T38.3X4	T38.3X5	T38.3X6
Quaalude	T42.6X1	T42.6X2	T42.6X3	T42.6X4	T42.6X5	T42.6X6
Quarternary ammonium						
anti-infective	T49.0X1	T49.0X2	T49.0X3	T49.0X4	T49.0X5	T49.0X6
ganglion blocking	T44.2X1	T44.2X2	T44.2X3	T44.2X4	T44.2X5	T44.2X6
parasympatholytic	T44.3X1	T44.3X2	T44.3X3	T44.3X4	T44.3X5	T44.3X6
Quazepam	T42.4X1	T42.4X2	T42.4X3	T42.4X4	T42.4X5	T42.4X6
Quicklime	T54.3X1	T54.3X2	T54.3X3	T54.3X4	—	—
Quillaja extract	T48.4X1	T48.4X2	T48.4X3	T48.4X4	T48.4X5	T48.4X6
Quinacrine	T37.2X1	T37.2X2	T37.2X3	T37.2X4	T37.2X5	T37.2X6
Quinaglute	T46.2X1	T46.2X2	T46.2X3	T46.2X4	T46.2X5	T46.2X6
Quinalbarbital	T42.3X1	T42.3X2	T42.3X3	T42.3X4	T42.3X5	T42.3X6
Quinalbarbitone sodium	T42.3X1	T42.3X2	T42.3X3	T42.3X4	T42.3X5	T42.3X6
Quinalphos	T60.0X1	T60.0X2	T60.0X3	T60.0X4	—	—
Quinapril	T46.4X1	T46.4X2	T46.4X3	T46.4X4	T46.4X5	T46.4X6
Quinestradiol	T38.5X1	T38.5X2	T38.5X3	T38.5X4	T38.5X5	T38.5X6
Quinestradol	T38.5X1	T38.5X2	T38.5X3	T38.5X4	T38.5X5	T38.5X6
Quinestrol	T38.5X1	T38.5X2	T38.5X3	T38.5X4	T38.5X5	T38.5X6
Quinethazone	T50.2X1	T50.2X2	T50.2X3	T50.2X4	T50.2X5	T50.2X6
Quingestanol	T38.4X1	T38.4X2	T38.4X3	T38.4X4	T38.4X5	T38.4X6
Quinidine	T46.2X1	T46.2X2	T46.2X3	T46.2X4	T46.2X5	T46.2X6
Quinine	T37.2X1	T37.2X2	T37.2X3	T37.2X4	T37.2X5	T37.2X6
Quiniobine	T37.8X1	T37.8X2	T37.8X3	T37.8X4	T37.8X5	T37.8X6
Quinisocaine	T49.1X1	T49.1X2	T49.1X3	T49.1X4	T49.1X5	T49.1X6
Quinocide	T37.2X1	T37.2X2	T37.2X3	T37.2X4	T37.2X5	T37.2X6
Quinoline (derivatives) NEC	T37.8X1	T37.8X2	T37.8X3	T37.8X4	T37.8X5	T37.8X6
Quinupramine	T43.011	T43.012	T43.013	T43.014	T43.015	T43.016
Quotane	T41.3X1	T41.3X2	T41.3X3	T41.3X4	T41.3X5	T41.3X6
Rabies						
immune globulin (human)	T50.Z11	T50.Z12	T50.Z13	T50.Z14	T50.Z15	T50.Z16
vaccine	T50.B91	T50.B92	T50.B93	T50.B94	T50.B95	T50.B96
Racemoramide	T40.2X1	T40.2X2	T40.2X3	T40.2X4	—	—
Racemorphan	T40.2X1	T40.2X2	T40.2X3	T40.2X4	T40.2X5	T40.2X6
Racepinefrin	T44.5X1	T44.5X2	T44.5X3	T44.5X4	T44.5X5	T44.5X6
Raclopride	T43.591	T43.592	T43.593	T43.594	T43.595	T43.596
Radiator alcohol	T51.1X1	T51.1X2	T51.1X3	T51.1X4	—	—
Radioactive drug NEC	T50.8X1	T50.8X2	T50.8X3	T50.8X4	T50.8X5	T50.8X6
Radio-opaque (drugs) (materials)	T50.8X1	T50.8X2	T50.8X3	T50.8X4	T50.8X5	T50.8X6
Ramifenazone	T39.2X1	T39.2X2	T39.2X3	T39.2X4	T39.2X5	T39.2X6
Ramipril	T46.4X1	T46.4X2	T46.4X3	T46.4X4	T46.4X5	T46.4X6
Ranitidine	T47.0X1	T47.0X2	T47.0X3	T47.0X4	T47.0X5	T47.0X6
Ranunculus	T62.2X1	T62.2X2	T62.2X3	T62.2X4	—	—
Rat poison NEC	T60.4X1	T60.4X2	T60.4X3	T60.4X4	—	—
Rattlesnake (venom)	T63.011	T63.012	T63.013	T63.014	—	—
Raubasine	T46.7X1	T46.7X2	T46.7X3	T46.7X4	T46.7X5	T46.7X6
Raudixin	T46.5X1	T46.5X2	T46.5X3	T46.5X4	T46.5X5	T46.5X6
Rautensin	T46.5X1	T46.5X2	T46.5X3	T46.5X4	T46.5X5	T46.5X6
Rautina	T46.5X1	T46.5X2	T46.5X3	T46.5X4	T46.5X5	T46.5X6
Rautotal	T46.5X1	T46.5X2	T46.5X3	T46.5X4	T46.5X5	T46.5X6
Rauwiloid	T46.5X1	T46.5X2	T46.5X3	T46.5X4	T46.5X5	T46.5X6
Rauwoldin	T46.5X1	T46.5X2	T46.5X3	T46.5X4	T46.5X5	T46.5X6
Rauwolfia (alkaloids)	T46.5X1	T46.5X2	T46.5X3	T46.5X4	T46.5X5	T46.5X6
Razoxane	T45.1X1	T45.1X2	T45.1X3	T45.1X4	T45.1X5	T45.1X6
Realgar	T57.0X1	T57.0X2	T57.0X3	T57.0X4	—	—
Recombinant (R) — *see* specific protein						
Red blood cells, packed	T45.8X1	T45.8X2	T45.8X3	T45.8X4	T45.8X5	T45.8X6
Red squill (scilliroside)	T60.4X1	T60.4X2	T60.4X3	T60.4X4	—	—
Reducing agent, industrial NEC	T65.891	T65.892	T65.893	T65.894	—	—
Refrigerant gas (chlorofluorocarbon)	T53.5X1	T53.5X2	T53.5X3	T53.5X4	—	—
not chlorofluorocarbon	T59.891	T59.892	T59.893	T59.894	—	—
Regroton	T50.2X1	T50.2X2	T50.2X3	T50.2X4	T50.2X5	T50.2X6
Rehydration salts (oral)	T50.3X1	T50.3X2	T50.3X3	T50.3X4	T50.3X5	T50.3X6
Rela	T42.8X1	T42.8X2	T42.8X3	T42.8X4	T42.8X5	T42.8X6
Relaxant, muscle						
anesthetic	T48.1X1	T48.1X2	T48.1X3	T48.1X4	T48.1X5	T48.1X6
central nervous system	T42.8X1	T42.8X2	T42.8X3	T42.8X4	T42.8X5	T42.8X6
skeletal NEC	T48.1X1	T48.1X2	T48.1X3	T48.1X4	T48.1X5	T48.1X6
smooth NEC	T44.3X1	T44.3X2	T44.3X3	T44.3X4	T44.3X5	T44.3X6
Remoxipride	T43.591	T43.592	T43.593	T43.594	T43.595	T43.596
Renese	T50.2X1	T50.2X2	T50.2X3	T50.2X4	T50.2X5	T50.2X6
Renografin	T50.8X1	T50.8X2	T50.8X3	T50.8X4	T50.8X5	T50.8X6
Replacement solution	T50.3X1	T50.3X2	T50.3X3	T50.3X4	T50.3X5	T50.3X6
Reproterol	T48.6X1	T48.6X2	T48.6X3	T48.6X4	T48.6X5	T48.6X6
Rescinnamine	T46.5X1	T46.5X2	T46.5X3	T46.5X4	T46.5X5	T46.5X6
Reserpin (e)	T46.5X1	T46.5X2	T46.5X3	T46.5X4	T46.5X5	T46.5X6
Resorcin, resorcinol (nonmedicinal)	T65.891	T65.892	T65.893	T65.894	—	—
medicinal	T49.4X1	T49.4X2	T49.4X3	T49.4X4	T49.4X5	T49.4X6
Respaire	T48.4X1	T48.4X2	T48.4X3	T48.4X4	T48.4X5	T48.4X6
Respiratory drug NEC	T48.901	T48.902	T48.903	T48.904	T48.905	T48.906
antiasthmatic NEC	T48.6X1	T48.6X2	T48.6X3	T48.6X4	T48.6X5	T48.6X6
anti-common-cold NEC	T48.5X1	T48.5X2	T48.5X3	T48.5X4	T48.5X5	T48.5X6
expectorant NEC	T48.4X1	T48.4X2	T48.4X3	T48.4X4	T48.4X5	T48.4X6
stimulant	T48.901	T48.902	T48.903	T48.904	T48.905	T48.906
Retinoic acid	T49.0X1	T49.0X2	T49.0X3	T49.0X4	T49.0X5	T49.0X6
Retinol	T45.2X1	T45.2X2	T45.2X3	T45.2X4	T45.2X5	T45.2X6
Rh (D) immune globulin (human)	T50.Z11	T50.Z12	T50.Z13	T50.Z14	T50.Z15	T50.Z16
Rhodine	T39.011	T39.012	T39.013	T39.014	T39.015	T39.016
RhoGAM	T50.Z11	T50.Z12	T50.Z13	T50.Z14	T50.Z15	T50.Z16
Rhubarb						
dry extract	T47.2X1	T47.2X2	T47.2X3	T47.2X4	T47.2X5	T47.2X6
tincture, compound	T47.2X1	T47.2X2	T47.2X3	T47.2X4	T47.2X5	T47.2X6
Ribavirin	T37.5X1	T37.5X2	T37.5X3	T37.5X4	T37.5X5	T37.5X6
Riboflavin	T45.2X1	T45.2X2	T45.2X3	T45.2X4	T45.2X5	T45.2X6
Ribostamycin	T36.5X1	T36.5X2	T36.5X3	T36.5X4	T36.5X5	T36.5X6
Ricin	T62.2X1	T62.2X2	T62.2X3	T62.2X4	—	—
Ricinus communis	T62.2X1	T62.2X2	T62.2X3	T62.2X4	—	—
Rickettsial vaccine NEC	T50.A91	T50.A92	T50.A93	T50.A94	T50.A95	T50.A96
Rifabutin	T36.6X1	T36.6X2	T36.6X3	T36.6X4	T36.6X5	T36.6X6
Rifamide	T36.6X1	T36.6X2	T36.6X3	T36.6X4	T36.6X5	T36.6X6
Rifampicin	T36.6X1	T36.6X2	T36.6X3	T36.6X4	T36.6X5	T36.6X6
with isoniazid	T37.1X1	T37.1X2	T37.1X3	T37.1X4	T37.1X5	T37.1X6
Rifampin	T36.6X1	T36.6X2	T36.6X3	T36.6X4	T36.6X5	T36.6X6

Substance	Poisoning, Accidental (unintentional)	Poisoning, Intentional Self-harm	Poisoning, Assault	Poisoning, Undetermined	Adverse Effect	Under-dosing
Rifamycin	T36.6X1	T36.6X2	T36.6X3	T36.6X4	T36.6X5	T36.6X6
Rifaximin	T36.6X1	T36.6X2	T36.6X3	T36.6X4	T36.6X5	T36.6X6
Rimantadine	T37.5X1	T37.5X2	T37.5X3	T37.5X4	T37.5X5	T37.5X6
Rimazolium metilsulfate	T39.8X1	T39.8X2	T39.8X3	T39.8X4	T39.8X5	T39.8X6
Rimifon	T37.1X1	T37.1X2	T37.1X3	T37.1X4	T37.1X5	T37.1X6
Rimiterol	T48.6X1	T48.6X2	T48.6X3	T48.6X4	T48.6X5	T48.6X6
Ringer (lactate) solution	T50.3X1	T50.3X2	T50.3X3	T50.3X4	T50.3X5	T50.3X6
Ristocetin	T36.8X1	T36.8X2	T36.8X3	T36.8X4	T36.8X5	T36.8X6
Ritalin	T43.631	T43.632	T43.633	T43.634	T43.635	T43.636
Ritodrine	T44.5X1	T44.5X2	T44.5X3	T44.5X4	T44.5X5	T44.5X6
Roach killer — see Insecticide						
Rociverine	T44.3X1	T44.3X2	T44.3X3	T44.3X4	T44.3X5	T44.3X6
Rocky Mountain spotted fever vaccine	T50.A91	T50.A92	T50.A93	T50.A94	T50.A95	T50.A96
Rodenticide NEC	T60.4X1	T60.4X2	T60.4X3	T60.4X4	—	—
Rohypnol	T42.4X1	T42.4X2	T42.4X3	T42.4X4	T42.4X5	T42.4X6
Rokitamycin	T36.3X1	T36.3X2	T36.3X3	T36.3X4	T36.3X5	T36.3X6
Rolaids	T47.1X1	T47.1X2	T47.1X3	T47.1X4	T47.1X5	T47.1X6
Rolitetracycline	T36.4X1	T36.4X2	T36.4X3	T36.4X4	T36.4X5	T36.4X6
Romilar	T48.3X1	T48.3X2	T48.3X3	T48.3X4	T48.3X5	T48.3X6
Ronifibrate	T46.6X1	T46.6X2	T46.6X3	T46.6X4	T46.6X5	T46.6X6
Rosaprostol	T47.1X1	T47.1X2	T47.1X3	T47.1X4	T47.1X5	T47.1X6
Rose bengal sodium (131I)	T50.8X1	T50.8X2	T50.8X3	T50.8X4	T50.8X5	T50.8X6
Rose water ointment	T49.3X1	T49.3X2	T49.3X3	T49.3X4	T49.3X5	T49.3X6
Rosoxacin	T37.8X1	T37.8X2	T37.8X3	T37.8X4	T37.8X5	T37.8X6
Rotenone	T60.2X1	T60.2X2	T60.2X3	T60.2X4	—	—
Rotoxamine	T45.0X1	T45.0X2	T45.0X3	T45.0X4	T45.0X5	T45.0X6
Rough-on-rats	T60.4X1	T60.4X2	T60.4X3	T60.4X4	—	—
Roxatidine	T47.0X1	T47.0X2	T47.0X3	T47.0X4	T47.0X5	T47.0X6
Roxithromycin	T36.3X1	T36.3X2	T36.3X3	T36.3X4	T36.3X5	T36.3X6
Rt-PA	T45.611	T45.612	T45.613	T45.614	T45.615	T45.616
Rubbing alcohol	T51.2X1	T51.2X2	T51.2X3	T51.2X4	—	—
Rubefacient	T49.4X1	T49.4X2	T49.4X3	T49.4X4	T49.4X5	T49.4X6
Rubella vaccine	T50.B91	T50.B92	T50.B93	T50.B94	T50.B95	T50.B96
Rubeola vaccine	T50.B91	T50.B92	T50.B93	T50.B94	T50.B95	T50.B96
Rubidium chloride Rb82	T50.8X1	T50.8X2	T50.8X3	T50.8X4	T50.8X5	T50.8X6
Rubidomycin	T45.1X1	T45.1X2	T45.1X3	T45.1X4	T45.1X5	T45.1X6
Rue	T62.2X1	T62.2X2	T62.2X3	T62.2X4	—	—
Rufocromomycin	T45.1X1	T45.1X2	T45.1X3	T45.1X4	T45.1X5	T45.1X6
Russel's viper venin	T45.7X1	T45.7X2	T45.7X3	T45.7X4	T45.7X5	T45.7X6
Ruta (graveolens)	T62.2X1	T62.2X2	T62.2X3	T62.2X4	—	—
Rutinum	T46.991	T46.992	T46.993	T46.994	T46.995	T46.996
Rutoside	T46.991	T46.992	T46.993	T46.994	T46.995	T46.996
b-sitosterol(s)	T46.6X1	T46.6X2	T46.6X3	T46.6X4	T46.6X5	T46.6X6
Sabadilla (plant)	T62.2X1	T62.2X2	T62.2X3	T62.2X4	—	—
pesticide	T60.2X1	T60.2X2	T60.2X3	T60.2X4	—	—
Saccharated iron oxide	T45.8X1	T45.8X2	T45.8X3	T45.8X4	T45.8X5	T45.8X6
Saccharin	T50.901	T50.902	T50.903	T50.904	T50.905	T50.906
Saccharomyces boulardii	T47.6X1	T47.6X2	T47.6X3	T47.6X4	T47.6X5	T47.6X6
Safflower oil	T46.6X1	T46.6X2	T46.6X3	T46.6X4	T46.6X5	T46.6X6
Safrazine	T43.1X1	T43.1X2	T43.1X3	T43.1X4	T43.1X5	T43.1X6
Salazosulfapyridine	T37.0X1	T37.0X2	T37.0X3	T37.0X4	T37.0X5	T37.0X6
Salbutamol	T48.6X1	T48.6X2	T48.6X3	T48.6X4	T48.6X5	T48.6X6
Salicylamide	T39.091	T39.092	T39.093	T39.094	T39.095	T39.096
Salicylate NEC	T39.091	T39.092	T39.093	T39.094	T39.095	T39.096
methyl	T49.3X1	T49.3X2	T49.3X3	T49.3X4	T49.3X5	T49.3X6
theobromine calcium	T50.2X1	T50.2X2	T50.2X3	T50.2X4	T50.2X5	T50.2X6
Salicylazosulfapyridine	T37.0X1	T37.0X2	T37.0X3	T37.0X4	T37.0X5	T37.0X6
Salicylhydroxamic acid	T49.0X1	T49.0X2	T49.0X3	T49.0X4	T49.0X5	T49.0X6
Salicylic acid	T49.4X1	T49.4X2	T49.4X3	T49.4X4	T49.4X5	T49.4X6
with benzoic acid	T49.4X1	T49.4X2	T49.4X3	T49.4X4	T49.4X5	T49.4X6
congeners	T39.091	T39.092	T39.093	T39.094	T39.095	T39.096
derivative	T39.091	T39.092	T39.093	T39.094	T39.095	T39.096
salts	T39.091	T39.092	T39.093	T39.094	T39.095	T39.096
Salinazid	T37.1X1	T37.1X2	T37.1X3	T37.1X4	T37.1X5	T37.1X6
Salmeterol	T48.6X1	T48.6X2	T48.6X3	T48.6X4	T48.6X5	T48.6X6
Salol	T49.3X1	T49.3X2	T49.3X3	T49.3X4	T49.3X5	T49.3X6
Salsalate	T39.091	T39.092	T39.093	T39.094	T39.095	T39.096
Salt-replacing drug	T50.901	T50.902	T50.903	T50.904	T50.905	T50.906
Salt-retaining mineralocorticoid	T50.0X1	T50.0X2	T50.0X3	T50.0X4	T50.0X5	T50.0X6
Salt substitute	T50.901	T50.902	T50.903	T50.904	T50.905	T50.906
Saluretic NEC	T50.2X1	T50.2X2	T50.2X3	T50.2X4	T50.2X5	T50.2X6
Saluron	T50.2X1	T50.2X2	T50.2X3	T50.2X4	T50.2X5	T50.2X6
Salvarsan 606 (neosilver) (silver)	T37.8X1	T37.8X2	T37.8X3	T37.8X4	T37.8X5	T37.8X6
Sambucus canadensis	T62.2X1	T62.2X2	T62.2X3	T62.2X4	—	—
berry	T62.1X1	T62.1X2	T62.1X3	T62.1X4	—	—
Sandril	T46.5X1	T46.5X2	T46.5X3	T46.5X4	T46.5X5	T46.5X6
Sanguinaria canadensis	T62.2X1	T62.2X2	T62.2X3	T62.2X4	—	—
Saniflush (cleaner)	T54.2X1	T54.2X2	T54.2X3	T54.2X4	—	—
Santonin	T37.4X1	T37.4X2	T37.4X3	T37.4X4	T37.4X5	T37.4X6
Santyl	T49.8X1	T49.8X2	T49.8X3	T49.8X4	T49.8X5	T49.8X6

Substance	Poisoning, Accidental (unintentional)	Poisoning, Intentional Self-harm	Poisoning, Assault	Poisoning, Undetermined	Adverse Effect	Under-dosing
Saralasin	T46.5X1	T46.5X2	T46.5X3	T46.5X4	T46.5X5	T46.5X6
Sarcolysin	T45.1X1	T45.1X2	T45.1X3	T45.1X4	T45.1X5	T45.1X6
Sarkomycin	T45.1X1	T45.1X2	T45.1X3	T45.1X4	T45.1X5	T45.1X6
Saroten	T43.011	T43.012	T43.013	T43.014	T43.015	T43.016
Saturnine — see Lead						
Savin (oil)	T49.4X1	T49.4X2	T49.4X3	T49.4X4	T49.4X5	T49.4X6
Scammony	T47.2X1	T47.2X2	T47.2X3	T47.2X4	T47.2X5	T47.2X6
Scarlet red	T49.8X1	T49.8X2	T49.8X3	T49.8X4	T49.8X5	T49.8X6
Scheele's green	T57.0X1	T57.0X2	T57.0X3	T57.0X4	—	—
insecticide	T57.0X1	T57.0X2	T57.0X3	T57.0X4	—	—
Schizontozide (blood) (tissue)	T37.2X1	T37.2X2	T37.2X3	T37.2X4	T37.2X5	T37.2X6
Schradan	T60.0X1	T60.0X2	T60.0X3	T60.0X4	—	—
Schweinfurth green	T57.0X1	T57.0X2	T57.0X3	T57.0X4	—	—
insecticide	T57.0X1	T57.0X2	T57.0X3	T57.0X4	—	—
Scilla, rat poison	T60.4X1	T60.4X2	T60.4X3	T60.4X4	—	—
Scillaren	T60.4X1	T60.4X2	T60.4X3	T60.4X4	—	—
Sclerosing agent	T46.8X1	T46.8X2	T46.8X3	T46.8X4	T46.8X5	T46.8X6
Scombrotoxin	T61.11	T61.12	T61.13	T61.14	—	—
Scopolamine	T44.3X1	T44.3X2	T44.3X3	T44.3X4	T44.3X5	T44.3X6
Scopolia extract	T44.3X1	T44.3X2	T44.3X3	T44.3X4	T44.3X5	T44.3X6
Scouring powder	T65.891	T65.892	T65.893	T65.894	—	—
Sea						
anemone (sting)	T63.631	T63.632	T63.633	T63.634	—	—
cucumber (sting)	T63.691	T63.692	T63.693	T63.694	—	—
snake (bite) (venom)	T63.091	T63.092	T63.093	T63.094	—	—
urchin spine (puncture)	T63.691	T63.692	T63.693	T63.694	—	—
Seafood	T61.91	T61.92	T61.93	T61.94	—	—
specified NEC	T61.8X1	T61.8X2	T61.8X3	T61.8X4	—	—
Secbutabarbital	T42.3X1	T42.3X2	T42.3X3	T42.3X4	T42.3X5	T42.3X6
Secbutabarbitone	T42.3X1	T42.3X2	T42.3X3	T42.3X4	T42.3X5	T42.3X6
Secnidazole	T37.3X1	T37.3X2	T37.3X3	T37.3X4	T37.3X5	T37.3X6
Secobarbital	T42.3X1	T42.3X2	T42.3X3	T42.3X4	T42.3X5	T42.3X6
Seconal	T42.3X1	T42.3X2	T42.3X3	T42.3X4	T42.3X5	T42.3X6
Secretin	T50.8X1	T50.8X2	T50.8X3	T50.8X4	T50.8X5	T50.8X6
Sedative NEC	T42.71	T42.72	T42.73	T42.74	T42.75	T42.76
mixed NEC	T42.6X1	T42.6X2	T42.6X3	T42.6X4	T42.6X5	T42.6X6
Sedormid	T42.6X1	T42.6X2	T42.6X3	T42.6X4	T42.6X5	T42.6X6
Seed disinfectant or dressing	T60.8X1	T60.8X2	T60.8X3	T60.8X4	—	—
Seeds (poisonous)	T62.2X1	T62.2X2	T62.2X3	T62.2X4	—	—
Selegiline	T42.8X1	T42.8X2	T42.8X3	T42.8X4	T42.8X5	T42.8X6
Selenium NEC	T56.891	T56.892	T56.893	T56.894	—	—
disulfide or sulfide	T49.4X1	T49.4X2	T49.4X3	T49.4X4	T49.4X5	T49.4X6
fumes	T59.891	T59.892	T59.893	T59.894	—	—
sulfide	T49.4X1	T49.4X2	T49.4X3	T49.4X4	T49.4X5	T49.4X6
Selenomethionine (75Se)	T50.8X1	T50.8X2	T50.8X3	T50.8X4	T50.8X5	T50.8X6
Selsun	T49.4X1	T49.4X2	T49.4X3	T49.4X4	T49.4X5	T49.4X6
Semustine	T45.1X1	T45.1X2	T45.1X3	T45.1X4	T45.1X5	T45.1X6
Senega syrup	T48.4X1	T48.4X2	T48.4X3	T48.4X4	T48.4X5	T48.4X6
Senna	T47.2X1	T47.2X2	T47.2X3	T47.2X4	T47.2X5	T47.2X6
Sennoside A+B	T47.2X1	T47.2X2	T47.2X3	T47.2X4	T47.2X5	T47.2X6
Septisol	T49.2X1	T49.2X2	T49.2X3	T49.2X4	T49.2X5	T49.2X6
Seractide	T38.811	T38.812	T38.813	T38.814	T38.815	T38.816
Serax	T42.4X1	T42.4X2	T42.4X3	T42.4X4	T42.4X5	T42.4X6
Serenesil	T42.6X1	T42.6X2	T42.6X3	T42.6X4	T42.6X5	T42.6X6
Serenium (hydrochloride)	T37.91	T37.92	T37.93	T37.94	T37.95	T37.96
Serepax — see Oxazepam						
Sermorelin	T38.891	T38.892	T38.893	T38.894	T38.895	T38.896
Sernyl	T41.1X1	T41.1X2	T41.1X3	T41.1X4	T41.1X5	T41.1X6
Serotonin	T50.991	T50.992	T50.993	T50.994	T50.995	T50.996
Serpasil	T46.5X1	T46.5X2	T46.5X3	T46.5X4	T46.5X5	T46.5X6
Serrapeptase	T45.3X1	T45.3X2	T45.3X3	T45.3X4	T45.3X5	T45.3X6
Serum						
antibotulinus	T50.Z11	T50.Z12	T50.Z13	T50.Z14	T50.Z15	T50.Z16
anticytotoxic	T50.Z11	T50.Z12	T50.Z13	T50.Z14	T50.Z15	T50.Z16
antidiphtheria	T50.Z11	T50.Z12	T50.Z13	T50.Z14	T50.Z15	T50.Z16
antimeningococcus	T50.Z11	T50.Z12	T50.Z13	T50.Z14	T50.Z15	T50.Z16
anti-Rh	T50.Z11	T50.Z12	T50.Z13	T50.Z14	T50.Z15	T50.Z16
anti-snake-bite	T50.Z11	T50.Z12	T50.Z13	T50.Z14	T50.Z15	T50.Z16
antitetanic	T50.Z11	T50.Z12	T50.Z13	T50.Z14	T50.Z15	T50.Z16
antitoxic	T50.Z11	T50.Z12	T50.Z13	T50.Z14	T50.Z15	T50.Z16
complement (inhibitor)	T45.8X1	T45.8X2	T45.8X3	T45.8X4	T45.8X5	T45.8X6
convalescent	T50.Z11	T50.Z12	T50.Z13	T50.Z14	T50.Z15	T50.Z16
hemolytic complement	T45.8X1	T45.8X2	T45.8X3	T45.8X4	T45.8X5	T45.8X6
immune (human)	T50.Z11	T50.Z12	T50.Z13	T50.Z14	T50.Z15	T50.Z16
protective NEC	T50.Z11	T50.Z12	T50.Z13	T50.Z14	T50.Z15	T50.Z16
Setastine	T45.0X1	T45.0X2	T45.0X3	T45.0X4	T45.0X5	T45.0X6
Setoperone	T43.591	T43.592	T43.593	T43.594	T43.595	T43.596
Sewer gas	T59.91	T59.92	T59.93	T59.94	—	—
Shampoo	T55.0X1	T55.0X2	T55.0X3	T55.0X4	—	—
Shellfish, noxious, nonbacterial	T61.781	T61.782	T61.783	T61.784	—	—

Substance	Poisoning, Accidental (unintentional)	Poisoning, Intentional Self-harm	Poisoning, Assault	Poisoning, Undetermined	Adverse Effect	Under-dosing
Sildenafil	T46.7X1	T46.7X2	T46.7X3	T46.7X4	T46.7X5	T46.7X6
Silibinin	T50.991	T50.992	T50.993	T50.994	T50.995	T50.996
Silicone NEC	T65.891	T65.892	T65.893	T65.894	—	—
medicinal	T49.3X1	T49.3X2	T49.3X3	T49.3X4	T49.3X5	T49.3X6
Silvadene	T49.0X1	T49.0X2	T49.0X3	T49.0X4	T49.0X5	T49.0X6
Silver	T49.0X1	T49.0X2	T49.0X3	T49.0X4	T49.0X5	T49.0X6
anti-infectives	T49.0X1	T49.0X2	T49.0X3	T49.0X4	T49.0X5	T49.0X6
arsphenamine	T37.8X1	T37.8X2	T37.8X3	T37.8X4	T37.8X5	T37.8X6
colloidal	T49.0X1	T49.0X2	T49.0X3	T49.0X4	T49.0X5	T49.0X6
nitrate	T49.0X1	T49.0X2	T49.0X3	T49.0X4	T49.0X5	T49.0X6
ophthalmic preparation	T49.5X1	T49.5X2	T49.5X3	T49.5X4	T49.5X5	T49.5X6
toughened (keratolytic)	T49.4X1	T49.4X2	T49.4X3	T49.4X4	T49.4X5	T49.4X6
nonmedicinal (dust)	T56.891	T56.892	T56.893	T56.894	—	—
protein	T49.5X1	T49.5X2	T49.5X3	T49.5X4	T49.5X5	T49.5X6
salvarsan	T37.8X1	T37.8X2	T37.8X3	T37.8X4	T37.8X5	T37.8X6
sulfadiazine	T49.4X1	T49.4X2	T49.4X3	T49.4X4	T49.4X5	T49.4X6
Silymarin	T50.991	T50.992	T50.993	T50.994	T50.995	T50.996
Simaldrate	T47.1X1	T47.1X2	T47.1X3	T47.1X4	T47.1X5	T47.1X6
Simazine	T60.3X1	T60.3X2	T60.3X3	T60.3X4	—	—
Simethicone	T47.1X1	T47.1X2	T47.1X3	T47.1X4	T47.1X5	T47.1X6
Simfibrate	T46.6X1	T46.6X2	T46.6X3	T46.6X4	T46.6X5	T46.6X6
Simvastatin	T46.6X1	T46.6X2	T46.6X3	T46.6X4	T46.6X5	T46.6X6
Sincalide	T50.8X1	T50.8X2	T50.8X3	T50.8X4	T50.8X5	T50.8X6
Sinequan	T43.011	T43.012	T43.013	T43.014	T43.015	T43.016
Singoserp	T46.5X1	T46.5X2	T46.5X3	T46.5X4	T46.5X5	T46.5X6
Sintrom	T45.511	T45.512	T45.513	T45.514	T45.515	T45.516
Sisomicin	T36.5X1	T36.5X2	T36.5X3	T36.5X4	T36.5X5	T36.5X6
Sitosterols	T46.6X1	T46.6X2	T46.6X3	T46.6X4	T46.6X5	T46.6X6
Skeletal muscle relaxants	T48.1X1	T48.1X2	T48.1X3	T48.1X4	T48.1X5	T48.1X6
Skin						
agents (external)	T49.91	T49.92	T49.93	T49.94	T49.95	T49.96
specified NEC	T49.8X1	T49.8X2	T49.8X3	T49.8X4	T49.8X5	T49.8X6
test antigen	T50.8X1	T50.8X2	T50.8X3	T50.8X4	T50.8X5	T50.8X6
Sleep-eze	T45.0X1	T45.0X2	T45.0X3	T45.0X4	T45.0X5	T45.0X6
Sleeping draught, pill	T42.71	T42.72	T42.73	T42.74	T42.75	T42.76
Smallpox vaccine	T50.B11	T50.B12	T50.B13	T50.B14	T50.B15	T50.B16
Smelter fumes NEC	T56.91	T56.92	T56.93	T56.94	—	—
Smog	T59.1X1	T59.1X2	T59.1X3	T59.1X4	—	—
Smoke NEC	T59.811	T59.812	T59.813	T59.814	—	—
Smooth muscle relaxant	T44.3X1	T44.3X2	T44.3X3	T44.3X4	T44.3X5	T44.3X6
Snail killer NEC	T60.8X1	T60.8X2	T60.8X3	T60.8X4	—	—
Snake venom or bite	T63.001	T63.002	T63.003	T63.004	—	—
hemocoagulase	T45.7X1	T45.7X2	T45.7X3	T45.7X4	T45.7X5	T45.7X6
Snuff	T65.211	T65.212	T65.213	T65.214	—	—
Soap (powder) (product)	T55.0X1	T55.0X2	T55.0X3	T55.0X4	—	—
enema	T47.4X1	T47.4X2	T47.4X3	T47.4X4	T47.4X5	T47.4X6
medicinal, soft	T49.2X1	T49.2X2	T49.2X3	T49.2X4	T49.2X5	T49.2X6
superfatted	T49.2X1	T49.2X2	T49.2X3	T49.2X4	T49.2X5	T49.2X6
Sobrerol	T48.4X1	T48.4X2	T48.4X3	T48.4X4	T48.4X5	T48.4X6
Soda (caustic)	T54.3X1	T54.3X2	T54.3X3	T54.3X4	—	—
bicarb	T47.1X1	T47.1X2	T47.1X3	T47.1X4	T47.1X5	T47.1X6
chlorinated — see Sodium, hypochlorite						
Sodium						
acetosulfone	T37.1X1	T37.1X2	T37.1X3	T37.1X4	T37.1X5	T37.1X6
acetrizoate	T50.8X1	T50.8X2	T50.8X3	T50.8X4	T50.8X5	T50.8X6
acid phosphate	T50.3X1	T50.3X2	T50.3X3	T50.3X4	T50.3X5	T50.3X6
alginate	T47.8X1	T47.8X2	T47.8X3	T47.8X4	T47.8X5	T47.8X6
amidotrizoate	T50.8X1	T50.8X2	T50.8X3	T50.8X4	T50.8X5	T50.8X6
aminopterin	T45.1X1	T45.1X2	T45.1X3	T45.1X4	T45.1X5	T45.1X6
amylosulfate	T47.8X1	T47.8X2	T47.8X3	T47.8X4	T47.8X5	T47.8X6
amytal	T42.3X1	T42.3X2	T42.3X3	T42.3X4	T42.3X5	T42.3X6
antimony gluconate	T37.3X1	T37.3X2	T37.3X3	T37.3X4	T37.3X5	T37.3X6
arsenate	T57.0X1	T57.0X2	T57.0X3	T57.0X4	—	—
aurothiomalate	T39.4X1	T39.4X2	T39.4X3	T39.4X4	T39.4X5	T39.4X6
aurothiosulfate	T39.4X1	T39.4X2	T39.4X3	T39.4X4	T39.4X5	T39.4X6
barbiturate	T42.3X1	T42.3X2	T42.3X3	T42.3X4	T42.3X5	T42.3X6
basic phosphate	T47.4X1	T47.4X2	T47.4X3	T47.4X4	T47.4X5	T47.4X6
bicarbonate	T47.1X1	T47.1X2	T47.1X3	T47.1X4	T47.1X5	T47.1X6
bichromate	T57.8X1	T57.8X2	T57.8X3	T57.8X4	—	—
biphosphate	T50.3X1	T50.3X2	T50.3X3	T50.3X4	T50.3X5	T50.3X6
bisulfate	T65.891	T65.892	T65.893	T65.894	—	—
borate	T57.8X1	T57.8X2	T57.8X3	T57.8X4	—	—
cleanser	T57.8X1	T57.8X2	T57.8X3	T57.8X4	—	—
eye	T49.5X1	T49.5X2	T49.5X3	T49.5X4	T49.5X5	T49.5X6
therapeutic	T49.8X1	T49.8X2	T49.8X3	T49.8X4	T49.8X5	T49.8X6
bromide	T42.6X1	T42.6X2	T42.6X3	T42.6X4	T42.6X5	T42.6X6
cacodylate (nonmedicinal) NEC	T50.8X1	T50.8X2	T50.8X3	T50.8X4	T50.8X5	T50.8X6
anti-infective	T37.8X1	T37.8X2	T37.8X3	T37.8X4	T37.8X5	T37.8X6
herbicide	T60.3X1	T60.3X2	T60.3X3	T60.3X4	—	—
calcium edetate	T45.8X1	T45.8X2	T45.8X3	T45.8X4	T45.8X5	T45.8X6
carbonate NEC	T54.3X1	T54.3X2	T54.3X3	T54.3X4	—	—

Substance	Poisoning, Accidental (unintentional)	Poisoning, Intentional Self-harm	Poisoning, Assault	Poisoning, Undetermined	Adverse Effect	Under-dosing
Sodium — continued						
chlorate NEC	T65.891	T65.892	T65.893	T65.894	—	—
herbicide	T54.91	T54.92	T54.93	T54.94	—	—
chloride	T50.3X1	T50.3X2	T50.3X3	T50.3X4	T50.3X5	T50.3X6
with glucose	T50.3X1	T50.3X2	T50.3X3	T50.3X4	T50.3X5	T50.3X6
chromate	T65.891	T65.892	T65.893	T65.894	—	—
citrate	T50.991	T50.992	T50.993	T50.994	T50.995	T50.996
cromoglicate	T48.6X1	T48.6X2	T48.6X3	T48.6X4	T48.6X5	T48.6X6
cyanide	T65.0X1	T65.0X2	T65.0X3	T65.0X4	—	—
cyclamate	T50.3X1	T50.3X2	T50.3X3	T50.3X4	T50.3X5	T50.3X6
dehydrocholate	T45.8X1	T45.8X2	T45.8X3	T45.8X4	T45.8X5	T45.8X6
diatrizoate	T50.8X1	T50.8X2	T50.8X3	T50.8X4	T50.8X5	T50.8X6
dibunate	T48.4X1	T48.4X2	T48.4X3	T48.4X4	T48.4X5	T48.4X6
dioctyl sulfosuccinate	T47.4X1	T47.4X2	T47.4X3	T47.4X4	T47.4X5	T47.4X6
dipantoyl ferrate	T45.8X1	T45.8X2	T45.8X3	T45.8X4	T45.8X5	T45.8X6
edetate	T45.8X1	T45.8X2	T45.8X3	T45.8X4	T45.8X5	T45.8X6
ethacrynate	T50.1X1	T50.1X2	T50.1X3	T50.1X4	T50.1X5	T50.1X6
feredetate	T45.8X1	T45.8X2	T45.8X3	T45.8X4	T45.8X5	T45.8X6
Fluoride — see Fluoride						
fluoroacetate (dust) (pesticide)	T60.4X1	T60.4X2	T60.4X3	T60.4X4	—	—
free salt	T50.3X1	T50.3X2	T50.3X3	T50.3X4	T50.3X5	T50.3X6
fusidate	T36.8X1	T36.8X2	T36.8X3	T36.8X4	T36.8X5	T36.8X6
glucaldrate	T47.1X1	T47.1X2	T47.1X3	T47.1X4	T47.1X5	T47.1X6
glucosulfone	T37.1X1	T37.1X2	T37.1X3	T37.1X4	T37.1X5	T37.1X6
glutamate	T45.8X1	T45.8X2	T45.8X3	T45.8X4	T45.8X5	T45.8X6
hydrogen carbonate	T50.3X1	T50.3X2	T50.3X3	T50.3X4	T50.3X5	T50.3X6
hydroxide	T54.3X1	T54.3X2	T54.3X3	T54.3X4	—	—
hypochlorite (bleach) NEC	T54.3X1	T54.3X2	T54.3X3	T54.3X4	—	—
disinfectant	T54.3X1	T54.3X2	T54.3X3	T54.3X4	—	—
medicinal (anti-infective) (external)	T49.0X1	T49.0X2	T49.0X3	T49.0X4	T49.0X5	T49.0X6
vapor	T54.3X1	T54.3X2	T54.3X3	T54.3X4	—	—
hyposulfite	T49.0X1	T49.0X2	T49.0X3	T49.0X4	T49.0X5	T49.0X6
indigotin disulfonate	T50.8X1	T50.8X2	T50.8X3	T50.8X4	T50.8X5	T50.8X6
iodide	T50.991	T50.992	T50.993	T50.994	T50.995	T50.996
I-131	T50.8X1	T50.8X2	T50.8X3	T50.8X4	T50.8X5	T50.8X6
therapeutic	T38.2X1	T38.2X2	T38.2X3	T38.2X4	T38.2X5	T38.2X6
iodohippurate (131I)	T50.8X1	T50.8X2	T50.8X3	T50.8X4	T50.8X5	T50.8X6
iopodate	T50.8X1	T50.8X2	T50.8X3	T50.8X4	T50.8X5	T50.8X6
iothalamate	T50.8X1	T50.8X2	T50.8X3	T50.8X4	T50.8X5	T50.8X6
iron edetate	T45.4X1	T45.4X2	T45.4X3	T45.4X4	T45.4X5	T45.4X6
lactate (compound solution)	T45.8X1	T45.8X2	T45.8X3	T45.8X4	T45.8X5	T45.8X6
lauryl (sulfate)	T49.2X1	T49.2X2	T49.2X3	T49.2X4	T49.2X5	T49.2X6
L-triiodothyronine	T38.1X1	T38.1X2	T38.1X3	T38.1X4	T38.1X5	T38.1X6
magnesium citrate	T50.991	T50.992	T50.993	T50.994	T50.995	T50.996
mersalate	T50.2X1	T50.2X2	T50.2X3	T50.2X4	T50.2X5	T50.2X6
metasilicate	T65.891	T65.892	T65.893	T65.894	—	—
metrizoate	T50.8X1	T50.8X2	T50.8X3	T50.8X4	T50.8X5	T50.8X6
monofluoroacetate (pesticide)	T60.1X1	T60.1X2	T60.1X3	T60.1X4	—	—
morrhuate	T46.8X1	T46.8X2	T46.8X3	T46.8X4	T46.8X5	T46.8X6
nafcillin	T36.0X1	T36.0X2	T36.0X3	T36.0X4	T36.0X5	T36.0X6
nitrate (oxidizing agent)	T65.891	T65.892	T65.893	T65.894	—	—
nitrite	T50.6X1	T50.6X2	T50.6X3	T50.6X4	T50.6X5	T50.6X6
nitroferricyanide	T46.5X1	T46.5X2	T46.5X3	T46.5X4	T46.5X5	T46.5X6
nitroprusside	T46.5X1	T46.5X2	T46.5X3	T46.5X4	T46.5X5	T46.5X6
oxalate	T65.891	T65.892	T65.893	T65.894	—	—
oxide/peroxide	T65.891	T65.892	T65.893	T65.894	—	—
oxybate	T41.291	T41.292	T41.293	T41.294	T41.295	T41.296
para-aminohippurate	T50.8X1	T50.8X2	T50.8X3	T50.8X4	T50.8X5	T50.8X6
perborate (nonmedicinal) NEC	T65.891	T65.892	T65.893	T65.894	—	—
medicinal	T49.0X1	T49.0X2	T49.0X3	T49.0X4	T49.0X5	T49.0X6
soap	T55.0X1	T55.0X2	T55.0X3	T55.0X4	—	—
percarbonate — see Sodium, perborate						
pertechnetate Tc99m	T50.8X1	T50.8X2	T50.8X3	T50.8X4	T50.8X5	T50.8X6
phosphate						
cellulose	T45.8X1	T45.8X2	T45.8X3	T45.8X4	T45.8X5	T45.8X6
dibasic	T47.2X1	T47.2X2	T47.2X3	T47.2X4	T47.2X5	T47.2X6
monobasic	T47.2X1	T47.2X2	T47.2X3	T47.2X4	T47.2X5	T47.2X6
phytate	T50.6X1	T50.6X2	T50.6X3	T50.6X4	T50.6X5	T50.6X6
picosulfate	T47.2X1	T47.2X2	T47.2X3	T47.2X4	T47.2X5	T47.2X6
polyhydroxyaluminium monocarbonate	T47.1X1	T47.1X2	T47.1X3	T47.1X4	T47.1X5	T47.1X6
polystyrene sulfonate	T50.3X1	T50.3X2	T50.3X3	T50.3X4	T50.3X5	T50.3X6
propionate	T49.0X1	T49.0X2	T49.0X3	T49.0X4	T49.0X5	T49.0X6
propyl hydroxybenzoate	T50.991	T50.992	T50.993	T50.994	T50.995	T50.996
psylliate	T46.8X1	T46.8X2	T46.8X3	T46.8X4	T46.8X5	T46.8X6
removing resins	T50.3X1	T50.3X2	T50.3X3	T50.3X4	T50.3X5	T50.3X6
salicylate	T39.091	T39.092	T39.093	T39.094	T39.095	T39.096

Substance	Poisoning, Accidental (unintentional)	Poisoning, Intentional Self-harm	Poisoning, Assault	Poisoning, Undetermined	Adverse Effect	Under-dosing
Sodium — continued						
salt NEC	T50.3X1	T50.3X2	T50.3X3	T50.3X4	T50.3X5	T50.3X6
selenate	T60.2X1	T60.2X2	T60.2X3	T60.2X4	—	—
stibogluconate	T37.3X1	T37.3X2	T37.3X3	T37.3X4	T37.3X5	T37.3X6
sulfate	T47.4X1	T47.4X2	T47.4X3	T47.4X4	T47.4X5	T47.4X6
sulfoxone	T37.1X1	T37.1X2	T37.1X3	T37.1X4	T37.1X5	T37.1X6
tetradecyl sulfate	T46.8X1	T46.8X2	T46.8X3	T46.8X4	T46.8X5	T46.8X6
thiopental	T41.1X1	T41.1X2	T41.1X3	T41.1X4	T41.1X5	T41.1X6
thiosalicylate	T39.091	T39.092	T39.093	T39.094	T39.095	T39.096
thiosulfate	T50.6X1	T50.6X2	T50.6X3	T50.6X4	T50.6X5	T50.6X6
tolbutamide	T38.3X1	T38.3X2	T38.3X3	T38.3X4	T38.3X5	T38.3X6
(L)-triiodothyronine	T38.1X1	T38.1X2	T38.1X3	T38.1X4	T38.1X5	T38.1X6
tyropanoate	T50.8X1	T50.8X2	T50.8X3	T50.8X4	T50.8X5	T50.8X6
valproate	T42.6X1	T42.6X2	T42.6X3	T42.6X4	T42.6X5	T42.6X6
versenate	T50.6X1	T50.6X2	T50.6X3	T50.6X4	T50.6X5	T50.6X6
Sodium-free salt	T50.901	T50.902	T50.903	T50.904	T50.905	T50.906
Sodium-removing resin	T50.3X1	T50.3X2	T50.3X3	T50.3X4	T50.3X5	T50.3X6
Soft soap	T55.0X1	T55.0X2	T55.0X3	T55.0X4	—	—
Solanine	T62.2X1	T62.2X2	T62.2X3	T62.2X4	—	—
berries	T62.1X1	T62.1X2	T62.1X3	T62.1X4	—	—
Solanum dulcamara	T62.2X1	T62.2X2	T62.2X3	T62.2X4	—	—
berries	T62.1X1	T62.1X2	T62.1X3	T62.1X4	—	—
Solapsone	T37.1X1	T37.1X2	T37.1X3	T37.1X4	T37.1X5	T37.1X6
Solar lotion	T49.3X1	T49.3X2	T49.3X3	T49.3X4	T49.3X5	T49.3X6
Solasulfone	T37.1X1	T37.1X2	T37.1X3	T37.1X4	T37.1X5	T37.1X6
Soldering fluid	T65.891	T65.892	T65.893	T65.894	—	—
Solid substance	T65.91	T65.92	T65.93	T65.94	—	—
specified NEC	T65.891	T65.892	T65.893	T65.894	—	—
Solvent, industrial NEC	T52.91	T52.92	T52.93	T52.94	—	—
naphtha	T52.0X1	T52.0X2	T52.0X3	T52.0X4	—	—
petroleum	T52.0X1	T52.0X2	T52.0X3	T52.0X4	—	—
specified NEC	T52.8X1	T52.8X2	T52.8X3	T52.8X4	—	—
Soma	T42.8X1	T42.8X2	T42.8X3	T42.8X4	T42.8X5	T42.8X6
Somatorelin	T38.891	T38.892	T38.893	T38.894	T38.895	T38.896
Somatostatin	T38.991	T38.992	T38.993	T38.994	T38.995	T38.996
Somatotropin	T38.811	T38.812	T38.813	T38.814	T38.815	T38.816
Somatrem	T38.811	T38.812	T38.813	T38.814	T38.815	T38.816
Somatropin	T38.811	T38.812	T38.813	T38.814	T38.815	T38.816
Sominex	T45.0X1	T45.0X2	T45.0X3	T45.0X4	T45.0X5	T45.0X6
Somnos	T42.6X1	T42.6X2	T42.6X3	T42.6X4	T42.6X5	T42.6X6
Somonal	T42.3X1	T42.3X2	T42.3X3	T42.3X4	T42.3X5	T42.3X6
Soneryl	T42.3X1	T42.3X2	T42.3X3	T42.3X4	T42.3X5	T42.3X6
Soothing syrup	T50.901	T50.902	T50.903	T50.904	T50.905	T50.906
Sopor	T42.6X1	T42.6X2	T42.6X3	T42.6X4	T42.6X5	T42.6X6
Soporific	T42.71	T42.72	T42.73	T42.74	T42.75	T42.76
Soporific drug	T42.71	T42.72	T42.73	T42.74	T42.75	T42.76
specified type NEC	T42.6X1	T42.6X2	T42.6X3	T42.6X4	T42.6X5	T42.6X6
Sorbide nitrate	T46.3X1	T46.3X2	T46.3X3	T46.3X4	T46.3X5	T46.3X6
Sorbitol	T47.4X1	T47.4X2	T47.4X3	T47.4X4	T47.4X5	T47.4X6
Sotalol	T44.7X1	T44.7X2	T44.7X3	T44.7X4	T44.7X5	T44.7X6
Sotradecol	T46.8X1	T46.8X2	T46.8X3	T46.8X4	T46.8X5	T46.8X6
Soysterol	T46.6X1	T46.6X2	T46.6X3	T46.6X4	T46.6X5	T46.6X6
Spacoline	T44.3X1	T44.3X2	T44.3X3	T44.3X4	T44.3X5	T44.3X6
Spanish fly	T49.8X1	T49.8X2	T49.8X3	T49.8X4	T49.8X5	T49.8X6
Sparine	T43.3X1	T43.3X2	T43.3X3	T43.3X4	T43.3X5	T43.3X6
Sparteine	T48.0X1	T48.0X2	T48.0X3	T48.0X4	T48.0X5	T48.0X6
Spasmolytic						
anticholinergics	T44.3X1	T44.3X2	T44.3X3	T44.3X4	T44.3X5	T44.3X6
autonomic	T44.3X1	T44.3X2	T44.3X3	T44.3X4	T44.3X5	T44.3X6
bronchial NEC	T48.6X1	T48.6X2	T48.6X3	T48.6X4	T48.6X5	T48.6X6
quaternary ammonium	T44.3X1	T44.3X2	T44.3X3	T44.3X4	T44.3X5	T44.3X6
skeletal muscle NEC	T48.1X1	T48.1X2	T48.1X3	T48.1X4	T48.1X5	T48.1X6
Spectinomycin	T36.5X1	T36.5X2	T36.5X3	T36.5X4	T36.5X5	T36.5X6
Speed	T43.621	T43.622	T43.623	T43.624	T43.625	T43.626
Spermicide	T49.8X1	T49.8X2	T49.8X3	T49.8X4	T49.8X5	T49.8X6
Spider (bite) (venom)	T63.391	T63.392	T63.393	T63.394	—	—
antivenin	T50.Z11	T50.Z12	T50.Z13	T50.Z14	T50.Z15	T50.Z16
Spigelia (root)	T37.4X1	T37.4X2	T37.4X3	T37.4X4	T37.4X5	T37.4X6
Spindle inactivator	T50.4X1	T50.4X2	T50.4X3	T50.4X4	T50.4X5	T50.4X6
Spiperone	T43.4X1	T43.4X2	T43.4X3	T43.4X4	T43.4X5	T43.4X6
Spiramycin	T36.3X1	T36.3X2	T36.3X3	T36.3X4	T36.3X5	T36.3X6
Spirapril	T46.4X1	T46.4X2	T46.4X3	T46.4X4	T46.4X5	T46.4X6
Spirilene	T43.591	T43.592	T43.593	T43.594	T43.595	T43.596
Spirit(s) (neutral) **NEC**	T51.0X1	T51.0X2	T51.0X3	T51.0X4	—	—
beverage	T51.0X1	T51.0X2	T51.0X3	T51.0X4	—	—
industrial	T51.0X1	T51.0X2	T51.0X3	T51.0X4	—	—
mineral	T52.0X1	T52.0X2	T52.0X3	T52.0X4	—	—
of salt — see Hydrochloric acid						
surgical	T51.0X1	T51.0X2	T51.0X3	T51.0X4	—	—
Spironolactone	T50.0X1	T50.0X2	T50.0X3	T50.0X4	T50.0X5	T50.0X6
Spiroperidol	T43.4X1	T43.4X2	T43.4X3	T43.4X4	T43.4X5	T43.4X6
Sponge, absorbable (gelatin)	T45.7X1	T45.7X2	T45.7X3	T45.7X4	T45.7X5	T45.7X6
Sporostacin	T49.0X1	T49.0X2	T49.0X3	T49.0X4	T49.0X5	T49.0X6
Spray (aerosol)	T65.91	T65.92	T65.93	T65.94	—	—
cosmetic	T65.891	T65.892	T65.893	T65.894	—	—
medicinal NEC	T50.901	T50.902	T50.903	T50.904	T50.905	T50.906
pesticides — see Pesticides						
specified content — see specific substance						
Spurge flax	T62.2X1	T62.2X2	T62.2X3	T62.2X4	—	—
Spurges	T62.2X1	T62.2X2	T62.2X3	T62.2X4	—	—
Sputum viscosity-lowering drug	T48.4X1	T48.4X2	T48.4X3	T48.4X4	T48.4X5	T48.4X6
Squill	T46.0X1	T46.0X2	T46.0X3	T46.0X4	T46.0X5	T46.0X6
rat poison	T60.4X1	T60.4X2	T60.4X3	T60.4X4	—	—
Squirting cucumber (cathartic)	T47.2X1	T47.2X2	T47.2X3	T47.2X4	T47.2X5	T47.2X6
Stains	T65.6X1	T65.6X2	T65.6X3	T65.6X4	—	—
Stannous fluoride	T49.7X1	T49.7X2	T49.7X3	T49.7X4	T49.7X5	T49.7X6
Stanolone	T38.7X1	T38.7X2	T38.7X3	T38.7X4	T38.7X5	T38.7X6
Stanozolol	T38.7X1	T38.7X2	T38.7X3	T38.7X4	T38.7X5	T38.7X6
Staphisagria or stavesacre (pediculicide)	T49.0X1	T49.0X2	T49.0X3	T49.0X4	T49.0X5	T49.0X6
Starch	T50.901	T50.902	T50.903	T50.904	T50.905	T50.906
Stelazine	T43.3X1	T43.3X2	T43.3X3	T43.3X4	T43.3X5	T43.3X6
Stemetil	T43.3X1	T43.3X2	T43.3X3	T43.3X4	T43.3X5	T43.3X6
Stepronin	T48.4X1	T48.4X2	T48.4X3	T48.4X4	T48.4X5	T48.4X6
Sterculia	T47.4X1	T47.4X2	T47.4X3	T47.4X4	T47.4X5	T47.4X6
Sternutator gas	T59.891	T59.892	T59.893	T59.894	—	—
Steroid	T38.0X1	T38.0X2	T38.0X3	T38.0X4	T38.0X5	T38.0X6
anabolic	T38.7X1	T38.7X2	T38.7X3	T38.7X4	T38.7X5	T38.7X6
androgenic	T38.7X1	T38.7X2	T38.7X3	T38.7X4	T38.7X5	T38.7X6
antineoplastic, hormone	T38.7X1	T38.7X2	T38.7X3	T38.7X4	T38.7X5	T38.7X6
estrogen	T38.5X1	T38.5X2	T38.5X3	T38.5X4	T38.5X5	T38.5X6
ENT agent	T49.6X1	T49.6X2	T49.6X3	T49.6X4	T49.6X5	T49.6X6
ophthalmic preparation	T49.5X1	T49.5X2	T49.5X3	T49.5X4	T49.5X5	T49.5X6
topical NEC	T49.0X1	T49.0X2	T49.0X3	T49.0X4	T49.0X5	T49.0X6
Stibine	T56.891	T56.892	T56.893	T56.894	—	—
Stibogluconate	T37.3X1	T37.3X2	T37.3X3	T37.3X4	T37.3X5	T37.3X6
Stibophen	T37.4X1	T37.4X2	T37.4X3	T37.4X4	T37.4X5	T37.4X6
Stilbamidine (isetionate)	T37.3X1	T37.3X2	T37.3X3	T37.3X4	T37.3X5	T37.3X6
Stilbestrol	T38.5X1	T38.5X2	T38.5X3	T38.5X4	T38.5X5	T38.5X6
Stilboestrol	T38.5X1	T38.5X2	T38.5X3	T38.5X4	T38.5X5	T38.5X6
Stimulant						
central nervous system — see also Psychostimulant	T43.601	T43.602	T43.603	T43.604	T43.605	T43.606
analeptics	T50.7X1	T50.7X2	T50.7X3	T50.7X4	T50.7X5	T50.7X6
opiate antagonist	T50.7X1	T50.7X2	T50.7X3	T50.7X4	T50.7X5	T50.7X6
psychotherapeutic NEC — see also Psychotherapeutic drug	T43.601	T43.602	T43.603	T43.604	T43.605	T43.606
specified NEC	T43.691	T43.692	T43.693	T43.694	T43.695	T43.696
respiratory	T48.901	T48.902	T48.903	T48.904	T48.905	T48.906
Stone-dissolving drug	T50.901	T50.902	T50.903	T50.904	T50.905	T50.906
Storage battery (cells) (acid)	T54.2X1	T54.2X2	T54.2X3	T54.2X4	—	—
Stovaine	T41.3X1	T41.3X2	T41.3X3	T41.3X4	T41.3X5	T41.3X6
infiltration (subcutaneous)	T41.3X1	T41.3X2	T41.3X3	T41.3X4	T41.3X5	T41.3X6
nerve block (peripheral) (plexus)	T41.3X1	T41.3X2	T41.3X3	T41.3X4	T41.3X5	T41.3X6
spinal	T41.3X1	T41.3X2	T41.3X3	T41.3X4	T41.3X5	T41.3X6
topical (surface)	T41.3X1	T41.3X2	T41.3X3	T41.3X4	T41.3X5	T41.3X6
Stovarsal	T37.8X1	T37.8X2	T37.8X3	T37.8X4	T37.8X5	T37.8X6
Stove gas — see Gas, stove						
Stoxil	T49.5X1	T49.5X2	T49.5X3	T49.5X4	T49.5X5	T49.5X6
Stramonium	T48.6X1	T48.6X2	T48.6X3	T48.6X4	T48.6X5	T48.6X6
natural state	T62.2X1	T62.2X2	T62.2X3	T62.2X4	—	—
Streptodornase	T45.3X1	T45.3X2	T45.3X3	T45.3X4	T45.3X5	T45.3X6
Streptoduocin	T36.5X1	T36.5X2	T36.5X3	T36.5X4	T36.5X5	T36.5X6
Streptokinase	T45.611	T45.612	T45.613	T45.614	T45.615	T45.616
Streptomycin (derivative)	T36.5X1	T36.5X2	T36.5X3	T36.5X4	T36.5X5	T36.5X6
Streptonivicin	T36.5X1	T36.5X2	T36.5X3	T36.5X4	T36.5X5	T36.5X6
Streptovarycin	T36.5X1	T36.5X2	T36.5X3	T36.5X4	T36.5X5	T36.5X6
Streptozocin	T45.1X1	T45.1X2	T45.1X3	T45.1X4	T45.1X5	T45.1X6
Streptozotocin	T45.1X1	T45.1X2	T45.1X3	T45.1X4	T45.1X5	T45.1X6
Stripper (paint) (solvent)	T52.8X1	T52.8X2	T52.8X3	T52.8X4	—	—
Strobane	T60.1X1	T60.1X2	T60.1X3	T60.1X4	—	—
Strofantina	T46.0X1	T46.0X2	T46.0X3	T46.0X4	T46.0X5	T46.0X6
Strophanthin (g) (k)	T46.0X1	T46.0X2	T46.0X3	T46.0X4	T46.0X5	T46.0X6
Strophanthus	T46.0X1	T46.0X2	T46.0X3	T46.0X4	T46.0X5	T46.0X6
Strophantin	T46.0X1	T46.0X2	T46.0X3	T46.0X4	T46.0X5	T46.0X6
Strophantin-g	T46.0X1	T46.0X2	T46.0X3	T46.0X4	T46.0X5	T46.0X6
Strychnine (nonmedicinal) (pesticide) (salts)	T65.1X1	T65.1X2	T65.1X3	T65.1X4	—	—
medicinal	T48.291	T48.292	T48.293	T48.294	T48.295	T48.296

Substance	Poisoning, Accidental (unintentional)	Poisoning, Intentional Self-harm	Poisoning, Assault	Poisoning, Undetermined	Adverse Effect	Under-dosing
Strychnos (ignatii) — see Strychnine						
Styramate	T42.8X1	T42.8X2	T42.8X3	T42.8X4	T42.8X5	T42.8X6
Styrene	T65.891	T65.892	T65.893	T65.894	—	—
Succinimide, antiepileptic or anticonvulsant	T42.2X1	T42.2X2	T42.2X3	T42.2X4	T42.2X5	T42.2X6
mercuric — see Mercury						
Succinylcholine	T48.1X1	T48.1X2	T48.1X3	T48.1X4	T48.1X5	T48.1X6
Succinylsulfathiazole	T37.0X1	T37.0X2	T37.0X3	T37.0X4	T37.0X5	T37.0X6
Sucralfate	T47.1X1	T47.1X2	T47.1X3	T47.1X4	T47.1X5	T47.1X6
Sucrose	T50.3X1	T50.3X2	T50.3X3	T50.3X4	T50.3X5	T50.3X6
Sufentanil	T40.4X1	T40.4X2	T40.4X3	T40.4X4	T40.4X5	T40.4X6
Sulbactam	T36.0X1	T36.0X2	T36.0X3	T36.0X4	T36.0X5	T36.0X6
Sulbenicillin	T36.0X1	T36.0X2	T36.0X3	T36.0X4	T36.0X5	T36.0X6
Sulbentine	T49.0X1	T49.0X2	T49.0X3	T49.0X4	T49.0X5	T49.0X6
Sulfacetamide	T49.0X1	T49.0X2	T49.0X3	T49.0X4	T49.0X5	T49.0X6
ophthalmic preparation	T49.5X1	T49.5X2	T49.5X3	T49.5X4	T49.5X5	T49.5X6
Sulfachlorpyridazine	T37.0X1	T37.0X2	T37.0X3	T37.0X4	T37.0X5	T37.0X6
Sulfacitine	T37.0X1	T37.0X2	T37.0X3	T37.0X4	T37.0X5	T37.0X6
Sulfadiasulfone sodium	T37.0X1	T37.0X2	T37.0X3	T37.0X4	T37.0X5	T37.0X6
Sulfadiazine	T37.0X1	T37.0X2	T37.0X3	T37.0X4	T37.0X5	T37.0X6
silver (topical)	T49.0X1	T49.0X2	T49.0X3	T49.0X4	T49.0X5	T49.0X6
Sulfadimethoxine	T37.0X1	T37.0X2	T37.0X3	T37.0X4	T37.0X5	T37.0X6
Sulfadimidine	T37.0X1	T37.0X2	T37.0X3	T37.0X4	T37.0X5	T37.0X6
Sulfadoxine	T37.0X1	T37.0X2	T37.0X3	T37.0X4	T37.0X5	T37.0X6
with pyrimethamine	T37.2X1	T37.2X2	T37.2X3	T37.2X4	T37.2X5	T37.2X6
Sulfaethidole	T37.0X1	T37.0X2	T37.0X3	T37.0X4	T37.0X5	T37.0X6
Sulfafurazole	T37.0X1	T37.0X2	T37.0X3	T37.0X4	T37.0X5	T37.0X6
Sulfaguanidine	T37.0X1	T37.0X2	T37.0X3	T37.0X4	T37.0X5	T37.0X6
Sulfalene	T37.0X1	T37.0X2	T37.0X3	T37.0X4	T37.0X5	T37.0X6
Sulfaloxate	T37.0X1	T37.0X2	T37.0X3	T37.0X4	T37.0X5	T37.0X6
Sulfaloxic acid	T37.0X1	T37.0X2	T37.0X3	T37.0X4	T37.0X5	T37.0X6
Sulfamazone	T39.2X1	T39.2X2	T39.2X3	T39.2X4	T39.2X5	T39.2X6
Sulfamerazine	T37.0X1	T37.0X2	T37.0X3	T37.0X4	T37.0X5	T37.0X6
Sulfameter	T37.0X1	T37.0X2	T37.0X3	T37.0X4	T37.0X5	T37.0X6
Sulfamethazine	T37.0X1	T37.0X2	T37.0X3	T37.0X4	T37.0X5	T37.0X6
Sulfamethizole	T37.0X1	T37.0X2	T37.0X3	T37.0X4	T37.0X5	T37.0X6
Sulfamethoxazole	T37.0X1	T37.0X2	T37.0X3	T37.0X4	T37.0X5	T37.0X6
with trimethoprim	T36.8X1	T36.8X2	T36.8X3	T36.8X4	T36.8X5	T36.8X6
Sulfamethoxydiazine	T37.0X1	T37.0X2	T37.0X3	T37.0X4	T37.0X5	T37.0X6
Sulfamethoxypyridazine	T37.0X1	T37.0X2	T37.0X3	T37.0X4	T37.0X5	T37.0X6
Sulfamethylthiazole	T37.0X1	T37.0X2	T37.0X3	T37.0X4	T37.0X5	T37.0X6
Sulfametoxydiazine	T37.0X1	T37.0X2	T37.0X3	T37.0X4	T37.0X5	T37.0X6
Sulfamidopyrine	T39.2X1	T39.2X2	T39.2X3	T39.2X4	T39.2X5	T39.2X6
Sulfamonomethoxine	T37.0X1	T37.0X2	T37.0X3	T37.0X4	T37.0X5	T37.0X6
Sulfamoxole	T37.0X1	T37.0X2	T37.0X3	T37.0X4	T37.0X5	T37.0X6
Sulfamylon	T49.0X1	T49.0X2	T49.0X3	T49.0X4	T49.0X5	T49.0X6
Sulfan blue (diagnostic dye)	T50.8X1	T50.8X2	T50.8X3	T50.8X4	T50.8X5	T50.8X6
Sulfanilamide	T37.0X1	T37.0X2	T37.0X3	T37.0X4	T37.0X5	T37.0X6
Sulfanilylguanidine	T37.0X1	T37.0X2	T37.0X3	T37.0X4	T37.0X5	T37.0X6
Sulfaperin	T37.0X1	T37.0X2	T37.0X3	T37.0X4	T37.0X5	T37.0X6
Sulfaphenazole	T37.0X1	T37.0X2	T37.0X3	T37.0X4	T37.0X5	T37.0X6
Sulfaphenylthiazole	T37.0X1	T37.0X2	T37.0X3	T37.0X4	T37.0X5	T37.0X6
Sulfaproxyline	T37.0X1	T37.0X2	T37.0X3	T37.0X4	T37.0X5	T37.0X6
Sulfapyridine	T37.0X1	T37.0X2	T37.0X3	T37.0X4	T37.0X5	T37.0X6
Sulfapyrimidine	T37.0X1	T37.0X2	T37.0X3	T37.0X4	T37.0X5	T37.0X6
Sulfarsphenamine	T37.8X1	T37.8X2	T37.8X3	T37.8X4	T37.8X5	T37.8X6
Sulfasalazine	T37.0X1	T37.0X2	T37.0X3	T37.0X4	T37.0X5	T37.0X6
Sulfasuxidine	T37.0X1	T37.0X2	T37.0X3	T37.0X4	T37.0X5	T37.0X6
Sulfasymazine	T37.0X1	T37.0X2	T37.0X3	T37.0X4	T37.0X5	T37.0X6
Sulfated amylopectin	T47.8X1	T47.8X2	T47.8X3	T47.8X4	T47.8X5	T47.8X6
Sulfathiazole	T37.0X1	T37.0X2	T37.0X3	T37.0X4	T37.0X5	T37.0X6
Sulfatostearate	T49.2X1	T49.2X2	T49.2X3	T49.2X4	T49.2X5	T49.2X6
Sulfinpyrazone	T50.4X1	T50.4X2	T50.4X3	T50.4X4	T50.4X5	T50.4X6
Sulfiram	T49.0X1	T49.0X2	T49.0X3	T49.0X4	T49.0X5	T49.0X6
Sulfisomidine	T37.0X1	T37.0X2	T37.0X3	T37.0X4	T37.0X5	T37.0X6
Sulfisoxazole	T37.0X1	T37.0X2	T37.0X3	T37.0X4	T37.0X5	T37.0X6
ophthalmic preparation	T49.5X1	T49.5X2	T49.5X3	T49.5X4	T49.5X5	T49.5X6
Sulfobromophthalein (sodium)	T50.8X1	T50.8X2	T50.8X3	T50.8X4	T50.8X5	T50.8X6
Sulfobromphthalein	T50.8X1	T50.8X2	T50.8X3	T50.8X4	T50.8X5	T50.8X6
Sulfogaiacol	T48.4X1	T48.4X2	T48.4X3	T48.4X4	T48.4X5	T48.4X6
Sulfomyxin	T36.8X1	T36.8X2	T36.8X3	T36.8X4	T36.8X5	T36.8X6
Sulfonal	T42.6X1	T42.6X2	T42.6X3	T42.6X4	T42.6X5	T42.6X6
Sulfonamide NEC	T37.0X1	T37.0X2	T37.0X3	T37.0X4	T37.0X5	T37.0X6
eye	T49.5X1	T49.5X2	T49.5X3	T49.5X4	T49.5X5	T49.5X6
Sulfonazide	T37.1X1	T37.1X2	T37.1X3	T37.1X4	T37.1X5	T37.1X6
Sulfones	T37.1X1	T37.1X2	T37.1X3	T37.1X4	T37.1X5	T37.1X6
Sulfonethylmethane	T42.6X1	T42.6X2	T42.6X3	T42.6X4	T42.6X5	T42.6X6
Sulfonmethane	T42.6X1	T42.6X2	T42.6X3	T42.6X4	T42.6X5	T42.6X6
Sulfonphthal, sulfonphthol	T50.8X1	T50.8X2	T50.8X3	T50.8X4	T50.8X5	T50.8X6

Substance	Poisoning, Accidental (unintentional)	Poisoning, Intentional Self-harm	Poisoning, Assault	Poisoning, Undetermined	Adverse Effect	Under-dosing
Sulfonylurea derivatives, oral	T38.3X1	T38.3X2	T38.3X3	T38.3X4	T38.3X5	T38.3X6
Sulforidazine	T43.3X1	T43.3X2	T43.3X3	T43.3X4	T43.3X5	T43.3X6
Sulfoxone	T37.1X1	T37.1X2	T37.1X3	T37.1X4	T37.1X5	T37.1X6
Sulfuric acid	T54.2X1	T54.2X2	T54.2X3	T54.2X4	—	—
Sulfur, sulfurated, sulfuric, sulfurous, sulfuryl (compounds NEC) (medicinal)	T49.4X1	T49.4X2	T49.4X3	T49.4X4	T49.4X5	T49.4X6
acid	T54.2X1	T54.2X2	T54.2X3	T54.2X4	—	—
dioxide (gas)	T59.1X1	T59.1X2	T59.1X3	T59.1X4	—	—
ether — see Ether(s)						
hydrogen	T59.6X1	T59.6X2	T59.6X3	T59.6X4	—	—
medicinal (keratolytic) (ointment) NEC	T49.4X1	T49.4X2	T49.4X3	T49.4X4	T49.4X5	T49.4X6
ointment	T49.0X1	T49.0X2	T49.0X3	T49.0X4	T49.0X5	T49.0X6
pesticide (vapor)	T60.91	T60.92	T60.93	T60.94	—	—
vapor NEC	T59.891	T59.892	T59.893	T59.894	—	—
Sulglicotide	T47.1X1	T47.1X2	T47.1X3	T47.1X4	T47.1X5	T47.1X6
Sulindac	T39.391	T39.392	T39.393	T39.394	T39.395	T39.396
Sulisatin	T47.2X1	T47.2X2	T47.2X3	T47.2X4	T47.2X5	T47.2X6
Sulisobenzone	T49.3X1	T49.3X2	T49.3X3	T49.3X4	T49.3X5	T49.3X6
Sulkowitch's reagent	T50.8X1	T50.8X2	T50.8X3	T50.8X4	T50.8X5	T50.8X6
Sulmetozine	T44.3X1	T44.3X2	T44.3X3	T44.3X4	T44.3X5	T44.3X6
Suloctidil	T46.7X1	T46.7X2	T46.7X3	T46.7X4	T46.7X5	T46.7X6
Sulph- — see also Sulf-						
Sulphadiazine	T37.0X1	T37.0X2	T37.0X3	T37.0X4	T37.0X5	T37.0X6
Sulphadimethoxine	T37.0X1	T37.0X2	T37.0X3	T37.0X4	T37.0X5	T37.0X6
Sulphadimidine	T37.0X1	T37.0X2	T37.0X3	T37.0X4	T37.0X5	T37.0X6
Sulphadione	T37.1X1	T37.1X2	T37.1X3	T37.1X4	T37.1X5	T37.1X6
Sulphafurazole	T37.0X1	T37.0X2	T37.0X3	T37.0X4	T37.0X5	T37.0X6
Sulphamethizole	T37.0X1	T37.0X2	T37.0X3	T37.0X4	T37.0X5	T37.0X6
Sulphamethoxazole	T37.0X1	T37.0X2	T37.0X3	T37.0X4	T37.0X5	T37.0X6
Sulphan blue	T50.8X1	T50.8X2	T50.8X3	T50.8X4	T50.8X5	T50.8X6
Sulphaphenazole	T37.0X1	T37.0X2	T37.0X3	T37.0X4	T37.0X5	T37.0X6
Sulphapyridine	T37.0X1	T37.0X2	T37.0X3	T37.0X4	T37.0X5	T37.0X6
Sulphasalazine	T37.0X1	T37.0X2	T37.0X3	T37.0X4	T37.0X5	T37.0X6
Sulphinpyrazone	T50.4X1	T50.4X2	T50.4X3	T50.4X4	T50.4X5	T50.4X6
Sulpiride	T43.591	T43.592	T43.593	T43.594	T43.595	T43.596
Sulprostone	T48.0X1	T48.0X2	T48.0X3	T48.0X4	T48.0X5	T48.0X6
Sulpyrine	T39.2X1	T39.2X2	T39.2X3	T39.2X4	T39.2X5	T39.2X6
Sultamicillin	T36.0X1	T36.0X2	T36.0X3	T36.0X4	T36.0X5	T36.0X6
Sulthiame	T42.6X1	T42.6X2	T42.6X3	T42.6X4	T42.6X5	T42.6X6
Sultiame	T42.6X1	T42.6X2	T42.6X3	T42.6X4	T42.6X5	T42.6X6
Sultopride	T43.591	T43.592	T43.593	T43.594	T43.595	T43.596
Sumatriptan	T39.8X1	T39.8X2	T39.8X3	T39.8X4	T39.8X5	T39.8X6
Sunflower seed oil	T46.6X1	T46.6X2	T46.6X3	T46.6X4	T46.6X5	T46.6X6
Superinone	T48.4X1	T48.4X2	T48.4X3	T48.4X4	T48.4X5	T48.4X6
Suprofen	T39.311	T39.312	T39.313	T39.314	T39.315	T39.316
Suramin (sodium)	T37.4X1	T37.4X2	T37.4X3	T37.4X4	T37.4X5	T37.4X6
Surfacaine	T41.3X1	T41.3X2	T41.3X3	T41.3X4	T41.3X5	T41.3X6
Surital	T41.1X1	T41.1X2	T41.1X3	T41.1X4	T41.1X5	T41.1X6
Sutilains	T45.3X1	T45.3X2	T45.3X3	T45.3X4	T45.3X5	T45.3X6
Suxamethonium (chloride)	T48.1X1	T48.1X2	T48.1X3	T48.1X4	T48.1X5	T48.1X6
Suxethonium (chloride)	T48.1X1	T48.1X2	T48.1X3	T48.1X4	T48.1X5	T48.1X6
Suxibuzone	T39.2X1	T39.2X2	T39.2X3	T39.2X4	T39.2X5	T39.2X6
Sweetener	T50.901	T50.902	T50.903	T50.904	T50.905	T50.906
Sweet niter spirit	T46.3X1	T46.3X2	T46.3X3	T46.3X4	T46.3X5	T46.3X6
Sweet oil (birch)	T49.3X1	T49.3X2	T49.3X3	T49.3X4	T49.3X5	T49.3X6
Sym-dichloroethyl ether	T53.6X1	T53.6X2	T53.6X3	T53.6X4	—	—
Sympatholytic NEC	T44.8X1	T44.8X2	T44.8X3	T44.8X4	T44.8X5	T44.8X6
haloalkylamine	T44.8X1	T44.8X2	T44.8X3	T44.8X4	T44.8X5	T44.8X6
Sympathomimetic NEC	T44.901	T44.902	T44.903	T44.904	T44.905	T44.906
anti-common-cold	T48.5X1	T48.5X2	T48.5X3	T48.5X4	T48.5X5	T48.5X6
bronchodilator	T48.6X1	T48.6X2	T48.6X3	T48.6X4	T48.6X5	T48.6X6
specified NEC	T44.991	T44.992	T44.993	T44.994	T44.995	T44.996
Synagis	T50.B91	T50.B92	T50.B93	T50.B94	T50.B95	T50.B96
Synalar	T49.0X1	T49.0X2	T49.0X3	T49.0X4	T49.0X5	T49.0X6
Synthroid	T38.1X1	T38.1X2	T38.1X3	T38.1X4	T38.1X5	T38.1X6
Syntocinon	T48.0X1	T48.0X2	T48.0X3	T48.0X4	T48.0X5	T48.0X6
Syrosingopine	T46.5X1	T46.5X2	T46.5X3	T46.5X4	T46.5X5	T46.5X6
Systemic drug	T45.91	T45.92	T45.93	T45.94	T45.95	T45.96
specified NEC	T45.8X1	T45.8X2	T45.8X3	T45.8X4	T45.8X5	T45.8X6
Tablets — see also specified substance	T50.901	T50.902	T50.903	T50.904	T50.905	T50.906
Tace	T38.5X1	T38.5X2	T38.5X3	T38.5X4	T38.5X5	T38.5X6
Tacrine	T44.0X1	T44.0X2	T44.0X3	T44.0X4	T44.0X5	T44.0X6
Tadalafil	T46.7X1	T46.7X2	T46.7X3	T46.7X4	T46.7X5	T46.7X6
Talampicillin	T36.0X1	T36.0X2	T36.0X3	T36.0X4	T36.0X5	T36.0X6
Talbutal	T42.3X1	T42.3X2	T42.3X3	T42.3X4	T42.3X5	T42.3X6
Talc powder	T49.3X1	T49.3X2	T49.3X3	T49.3X4	T49.3X5	T49.3X6
Talcum	T49.3X1	T49.3X2	T49.3X3	T49.3X4	T49.3X5	T49.3X6
Taleranol	T38.6X1	T38.6X2	T38.6X3	T38.6X4	T38.6X5	T38.6X6

▽ Subterms under main terms may continue to next column or page　　　　　Additional Character May Be Required — Refer to the Tabular List for Character Selection

Substance	Poisoning, Accidental (unintentional)	Poisoning, Intentional Self-harm	Poisoning, Assault	Poisoning, Undetermined	Adverse Effect	Under-dosing
Tamoxifen	T38.6X1	T38.6X2	T38.6X3	T38.6X4	T38.6X5	T38.6X6
Tamsulosin	T44.6X1	T44.6X2	T44.6X3	T44.6X4	T44.6X5	T44.6X6
Tandearil, tanderil	T39.2X1	T39.2X2	T39.2X3	T39.2X4	T39.2X5	T39.2X6
Tannic acid	T49.2X1	T49.2X2	T49.2X3	T49.2X4	T49.2X5	T49.2X6
medicinal (astringent)	T49.2X1	T49.2X2	T49.2X3	T49.2X4	T49.2X5	T49.2X6
Tannin — see Tannic acid						
Tansy	T62.2X1	T62.2X2	T62.2X3	T62.2X4	—	—
TAO	T36.3X1	T36.3X2	T36.3X3	T36.3X4	T36.3X5	T36.3X6
Tapazole	T38.2X1	T38.2X2	T38.2X3	T38.2X4	T38.2X5	T38.2X6
Taractan	T43.591	T43.592	T43.593	T43.594	T43.595	T43.596
Tarantula (venomous)	T63.321	T63.322	T63.323	T63.324	—	—
Tartar emetic	T37.8X1	T37.8X2	T37.8X3	T37.8X4	T37.8X5	T37.8X6
Tartaric acid	T65.891	T65.892	T65.893	T65.894	—	—
Tartrated antimony (anti-infective)	T37.8X1	T37.8X2	T37.8X3	T37.8X4	T37.8X5	T37.8X6
Tartrate, laxative	T47.4X1	T47.4X2	T47.4X3	T47.4X4	T47.4X5	T47.4X6
Tar NEC	T52.0X1	T52.0X2	T52.0X3	T52.0X4	—	—
camphor	T60.1X1	T60.1X2	T60.1X3	T60.1X4	—	—
distillate	T49.1X1	T49.1X2	T49.1X3	T49.1X4	T49.1X5	T49.1X6
fumes	T59.891	T59.892	T59.893	T59.894	—	—
medicinal	T49.1X1	T49.1X2	T49.1X3	T49.1X4	T49.1X5	T49.1X6
ointment	T49.1X1	T49.1X2	T49.1X3	T49.1X4	T49.1X5	T49.1X6
Tauromustine	T45.1X1	T45.1X2	T45.1X3	T45.1X4	T45.1X5	T45.1X6
TCA — see Trichloroacetic acid						
TCDD	T53.7X1	T53.7X2	T53.7X3	T53.7X4	—	—
TDI (vapor)	T65.0X1	T65.0X2	T65.0X3	T65.0X4	—	—
Tear						
gas	T59.3X1	T59.3X2	T59.3X3	T59.3X4	—	—
solution	T49.5X1	T49.5X2	T49.5X3	T49.5X4	T49.5X5	T49.5X6
Teclothiazide	T50.2X1	T50.2X2	T50.2X3	T50.2X4	T50.2X5	T50.2X6
Teclozan	T37.3X1	T37.3X2	T37.3X3	T37.3X4	T37.3X5	T37.3X6
Tegafur	T45.1X1	T45.1X2	T45.1X3	T45.1X4	T45.1X5	T45.1X6
Tegretol	T42.1X1	T42.1X2	T42.1X3	T42.1X4	T42.1X5	T42.1X6
Teicoplanin	T36.8X1	T36.8X2	T36.8X3	T36.8X4	T36.8X5	T36.8X6
Telepaque	T50.8X1	T50.8X2	T50.8X3	T50.8X4	T50.8X5	T50.8X6
Tellurium	T56.891	T56.892	T56.893	T56.894	—	—
fumes	T56.891	T56.892	T56.893	T56.894	—	—
TEM	T45.1X1	T45.1X2	T45.1X3	T45.1X4	T45.1X5	T45.1X6
Temazepam	T42.4X1	T42.4X2	T42.4X3	T42.4X4	T42.4X5	T42.4X6
Temocillin	T36.0X1	T36.0X2	T36.0X3	T36.0X4	T36.0X5	T36.0X6
Tenamfetamine	T43.621	T43.622	T43.623	T43.624	T43.625	T43.626
Teniposide	T45.1X1	T45.1X2	T45.1X3	T45.1X4	T45.1X5	T45.1X6
Tenitramine	T46.3X1	T46.3X2	T46.3X3	T46.3X4	T46.3X5	T46.3X6
Tenoglicin	T48.4X1	T48.4X2	T48.4X3	T48.4X4	T48.4X5	T48.4X6
Tenonitrozole	T37.3X1	T37.3X2	T37.3X3	T37.3X4	T37.3X5	T37.3X6
Tenoxicam	T39.391	T39.392	T39.393	T39.394	T39.395	T39.396
TEPA	T45.1X1	T45.1X2	T45.1X3	T45.1X4	T45.1X5	T45.1X6
TEPP	T60.0X1	T60.0X2	T60.0X3	T60.0X4	—	—
Teprotide	T46.5X1	T46.5X2	T46.5X3	T46.5X4	T46.5X5	T46.5X6
Terazosin	T44.6X1	T44.6X2	T44.6X3	T44.6X4	T44.6X5	T44.6X6
Terbufos	T60.0X1	T60.0X2	T60.0X3	T60.0X4	—	—
Terbutaline	T48.6X1	T48.6X2	T48.6X3	T48.6X4	T48.6X5	T48.6X6
Terconazole	T49.0X1	T49.0X2	T49.0X3	T49.0X4	T49.0X5	T49.0X6
Terfenadine	T45.0X1	T45.0X2	T45.0X3	T45.0X4	T45.0X5	T45.0X6
Teriparatide (acetate)	T50.991	T50.992	T50.993	T50.994	T50.995	T50.996
Terizidone	T37.1X1	T37.1X2	T37.1X3	T37.1X4	T37.1X5	T37.1X6
Terlipressin	T38.891	T38.892	T38.893	T38.894	T38.895	T38.896
Terodiline	T46.3X1	T46.3X2	T46.3X3	T46.3X4	T46.3X5	T46.3X6
Teroxalene	T37.4X1	T37.4X2	T37.4X3	T37.4X4	T37.4X5	T37.4X6
Terpin (cis) hydrate	T48.4X1	T48.4X2	T48.4X3	T48.4X4	T48.4X5	T48.4X6
Terramycin	T36.4X1	T36.4X2	T36.4X3	T36.4X4	T36.4X5	T36.4X6
Tertatolol	T44.7X1	T44.7X2	T44.7X3	T44.7X4	T44.7X5	T44.7X6
Tessalon	T48.3X1	T48.3X2	T48.3X3	T48.3X4	T48.3X5	T48.3X6
Testolactone	T38.7X1	T38.7X2	T38.7X3	T38.7X4	T38.7X5	T38.7X6
Testosterone	T38.7X1	T38.7X2	T38.7X3	T38.7X4	T38.7X5	T38.7X6
Tetanus toxoid or vaccine	T50.A91	T50.A92	T50.A93	T50.A94	T50.A95	T50.A96
antitoxin	T50.Z11	T50.Z12	T50.Z13	T50.Z14	T50.Z15	T50.Z16
immune globulin (human)	T50.Z11	T50.Z12	T50.Z13	T50.Z14	T50.Z15	T50.Z16
toxoid	T50.A91	T50.A92	T50.A93	T50.A94	T50.A95	T50.A96
with diphtheria toxoid	T50.A21	T50.A22	T50.A23	T50.A24	T50.A25	T50.A26
with pertussis	T50.A11	T50.A12	T50.A13	T50.A14	T50.A15	T50.A16
Tetrabenazine	T43.591	T43.592	T43.593	T43.594	T43.595	T43.596
Tetracaine	T41.3X1	T41.3X2	T41.3X3	T41.3X4	T41.3X5	T41.3X6
nerve block (peripheral) (plexus)	T41.3X1	T41.3X2	T41.3X3	T41.3X4	T41.3X5	T41.3X6
regional	T41.3X1	T41.3X2	T41.3X3	T41.3X4	T41.3X5	T41.3X6
spinal	T41.3X1	T41.3X2	T41.3X3	T41.3X4	T41.3X5	T41.3X6
Tetrachlorethylene — see Tetrachloroethylene						
Tetrachlormethiazide	T50.2X1	T50.2X2	T50.2X3	T50.2X4	T50.2X5	T50.2X6
Tetrachloroethane	T53.6X1	T53.6X2	T53.6X3	T53.6X4	—	—
vapor	T53.6X1	T53.6X2	T53.6X3	T53.6X4	—	—
paint or varnish	T53.6X1	T53.6X2	T53.6X3	T53.6X4	—	—

Substance	Poisoning, Accidental (unintentional)	Poisoning, Intentional Self-harm	Poisoning, Assault	Poisoning, Undetermined	Adverse Effect	Under-dosing
Tetrachloroethylene (liquid)	T53.3X1	T53.3X2	T53.3X3	T53.3X4	—	—
medicinal	T37.4X1	T37.4X2	T37.4X3	T37.4X4	T37.4X5	T37.4X6
vapor	T53.3X1	T53.3X2	T53.3X3	T53.3X4	—	—
Tetrachloromethane — see Carbon tetrachloride						
Tetracosactide	T38.811	T38.812	T38.813	T38.814	T38.815	T38.816
Tetracosactrin	T38.811	T38.812	T38.813	T38.814	T38.815	T38.816
Tetracycline	T36.4X1	T36.4X2	T36.4X3	T36.4X4	T36.4X5	T36.4X6
ophthalmic preparation	T49.5X1	T49.5X2	T49.5X3	T49.5X4	T49.5X5	T49.5X6
topical NEC	T49.0X1	T49.0X2	T49.0X3	T49.0X4	T49.0X5	T49.0X6
Tetradifon	T60.8X1	T60.8X2	T60.8X3	T60.8X4	—	—
Tetradotoxin	T61.771	T61.772	T61.773	T61.774	—	—
Tetraethyl						
lead	T56.0X1	T56.0X2	T56.0X3	T56.0X4	—	—
pyrophosphate	T60.0X1	T60.0X2	T60.0X3	T60.0X4	—	—
Tetraethylammonium chloride	T44.2X1	T44.2X2	T44.2X3	T44.2X4	T44.2X5	T44.2X6
Tetraethylthiuram disulfide	T50.6X1	T50.6X2	T50.6X3	T50.6X4	T50.6X5	T50.6X6
Tetrahydroaminoacridine	T44.0X1	T44.0X2	T44.0X3	T44.0X4	T44.0X5	T44.0X6
Tetrahydrocannabinol	T40.7X1	T40.7X2	T40.7X3	T40.7X4	T40.7X5	T40.7X6
Tetrahydrofuran	T52.8X1	T52.8X2	T52.8X3	T52.8X4	—	—
Tetrahydronaphthalene	T52.8X1	T52.8X2	T52.8X3	T52.8X4	—	—
Tetrahydrozoline	T49.5X1	T49.5X2	T49.5X3	T49.5X4	T49.5X5	T49.5X6
Tetralin	T52.8X1	T52.8X2	T52.8X3	T52.8X4	—	—
Tetramethrin	T60.2X1	T60.2X2	T60.2X3	T60.2X4	—	—
Tetramethylthiuram (disulfide) NEC	T60.3X1	T60.3X2	T60.3X3	T60.3X4	—	—
medicinal	T49.0X1	T49.0X2	T49.0X3	T49.0X4	T49.0X5	T49.0X6
Tetramisole	T37.4X1	T37.4X2	T37.4X3	T37.4X4	T37.4X5	T37.4X6
Tetranicotinoyl fructose	T46.7X1	T46.7X2	T46.7X3	T46.7X4	T46.7X5	T46.7X6
Tetrazepam	T42.4X1	T42.4X2	T42.4X3	T42.4X4	T42.4X5	T42.4X6
Tetronal	T42.6X1	T42.6X2	T42.6X3	T42.6X4	T42.6X5	T42.6X6
Tetryl	T65.3X1	T65.3X2	T65.3X3	T65.3X4	—	—
Tetrylammonium chloride	T44.2X1	T44.2X2	T44.2X3	T44.2X4	T44.2X5	T44.2X6
Tetryzoline	T49.5X1	T49.5X2	T49.5X3	T49.5X4	T49.5X5	T49.5X6
Thalidomide	T45.1X1	T45.1X2	T45.1X3	T45.1X4	T45.1X5	T45.1X6
Thallium (compounds) (dust) NEC	T56.811	T56.812	T56.813	T56.814	—	—
pesticide	T60.4X1	T60.4X2	T60.4X3	T60.4X4	—	—
THC	T40.7X1	T40.7X2	T40.7X3	T40.7X4	T40.7X5	T40.7X6
Thebacon	T48.3X1	T48.3X2	T48.3X3	T48.3X4	T48.3X5	T48.3X6
Thebaine	T40.2X1	T40.2X2	T40.2X3	T40.2X4	T40.2X5	T40.2X6
Thenoic acid	T49.6X1	T49.6X2	T49.6X3	T49.6X4	T49.6X5	T49.6X6
Thenyldiamine	T45.0X1	T45.0X2	T45.0X3	T45.0X4	T45.0X5	T45.0X6
Theobromine (calcium salicylate)	T48.6X1	T48.6X2	T48.6X3	T48.6X4	T48.6X5	T48.6X6
sodium salicylate	T48.6X1	T48.6X2	T48.6X3	T48.6X4	T48.6X5	T48.6X6
Theophyllamine	T48.6X1	T48.6X2	T48.6X3	T48.6X4	T48.6X5	T48.6X6
Theophylline	T48.6X1	T48.6X2	T48.6X3	T48.6X4	T48.6X5	T48.6X6
aminobenzoic acid	T48.6X1	T48.6X2	T48.6X3	T48.6X4	T48.6X5	T48.6X6
ethylenediamine	T48.6X1	T48.6X2	T48.6X3	T48.6X4	T48.6X5	T48.6X6
piperazine	T48.6X1	T48.6X2	T48.6X3	T48.6X4	T48.6X5	T48.6X6
p-amino-benzoate						
Thiabendazole	T37.4X1	T37.4X2	T37.4X3	T37.4X4	T37.4X5	T37.4X6
Thialbarbital	T41.1X1	T41.1X2	T41.1X3	T41.1X4	T41.1X5	T41.1X6
Thiamazole	T38.2X1	T38.2X2	T38.2X3	T38.2X4	T38.2X5	T38.2X6
Thiambutosine	T37.1X1	T37.1X2	T37.1X3	T37.1X4	T37.1X5	T37.1X6
Thiamine	T45.2X1	T45.2X2	T45.2X3	T45.2X4	T45.2X5	T45.2X6
Thiamphenicol	T36.2X1	T36.2X2	T36.2X3	T36.2X4	T36.2X5	T36.2X6
Thiamylal	T41.1X1	T41.1X2	T41.1X3	T41.1X4	T41.1X5	T41.1X6
sodium	T41.1X1	T41.1X2	T41.1X3	T41.1X4	T41.1X5	T41.1X6
Thiazesim	T43.291	T43.292	T43.293	T43.294	T43.295	T43.296
Thiazides (diuretics)	T50.2X1	T50.2X2	T50.2X3	T50.2X4	T50.2X5	T50.2X6
Thiazinamium metilsulfate	T43.3X1	T43.3X2	T43.3X3	T43.3X4	T43.3X5	T43.3X6
Thiethylperazine	T43.3X1	T43.3X2	T43.3X3	T43.3X4	T43.3X5	T43.3X6
Thimerosal	T49.0X1	T49.0X2	T49.0X3	T49.0X4	T49.0X5	T49.0X6
ophthalmic preparation	T49.5X1	T49.5X2	T49.5X3	T49.5X4	T49.5X5	T49.5X6
Thioacetazone	T37.1X1	T37.1X2	T37.1X3	T37.1X4	T37.1X5	T37.1X6
with isoniazid	T37.1X1	T37.1X2	T37.1X3	T37.1X4	T37.1X5	T37.1X6
Thiobarbital sodium	T41.1X1	T41.1X2	T41.1X3	T41.1X4	T41.1X5	T41.1X6
Thiobarbiturate anesthetic	T41.1X1	T41.1X2	T41.1X3	T41.1X4	T41.1X5	T41.1X6
Thiobismol	T37.8X1	T37.8X2	T37.8X3	T37.8X4	T37.8X5	T37.8X6
Thiobutabarbital sodium	T41.1X1	T41.1X2	T41.1X3	T41.1X4	T41.1X5	T41.1X6
Thiocarbamate (insecticide)	T60.0X1	T60.0X2	T60.0X3	T60.0X4	—	—
Thiocarbamide	T38.2X1	T38.2X2	T38.2X3	T38.2X4	T38.2X5	T38.2X6
Thiocarbarsone	T37.8X1	T37.8X2	T37.8X3	T37.8X4	T37.8X5	T37.8X6
Thiocarlide	T37.1X1	T37.1X2	T37.1X3	T37.1X4	T37.1X5	T37.1X6
Thioctamide	T50.991	T50.992	T50.993	T50.994	T50.995	T50.996

Substance	Poisoning, Accidental (unintentional)	Poisoning, Intentional Self-harm	Poisoning, Assault	Poisoning, Undetermined	Adverse Effect	Under-dosing
Thioctic acid	T50.991	T50.992	T50.993	T50.994	T50.995	T50.996
Thiofos	T60.0X1	T60.0X2	T60.0X3	T60.0X4	—	—
Thioglycolate	T49.4X1	T49.4X2	T49.4X3	T49.4X4	T49.4X5	T49.4X6
Thioglycolic acid	T65.891	T65.892	T65.893	T65.894		
Thioguanine	T45.1X1	T45.1X2	T45.1X3	T45.1X4	T45.1X5	T45.1X6
Thiomercaptomerin	T50.2X1	T50.2X2	T50.2X3	T50.2X4	T50.2X5	T50.2X6
Thiomerin	T50.2X1	T50.2X2	T50.2X3	T50.2X4	T50.2X5	T50.2X6
Thiomersal	T49.0X1	T49.0X2	T49.0X3	T49.0X4	T49.0X5	T49.0X6
Thionazin	T60.0X1	T60.0X2	T60.0X3	T60.0X4	—	—
Thiopental (sodium)	T41.1X1	T41.1X2	T41.1X3	T41.1X4	T41.1X5	T41.1X6
Thiopentone (sodium)	T41.1X1	T41.1X2	T41.1X3	T41.1X4	T41.1X5	T41.1X6
Thiopropazate	T43.3X1	T43.3X2	T43.3X3	T43.3X4	T43.3X5	T43.3X6
Thioproperazine	T43.3X1	T43.3X2	T43.3X3	T43.3X4	T43.3X5	T43.3X6
Thioridazine	T43.3X1	T43.3X2	T43.3X3	T43.3X4	T43.3X5	T43.3X6
Thiosinamine	T49.3X1	T49.3X2	T49.3X3	T49.3X4	T49.3X5	T49.3X6
Thiotepa	T45.1X1	T45.1X2	T45.1X3	T45.1X4	T45.1X5	T45.1X6
Thiothixene	T43.4X1	T43.4X2	T43.4X3	T43.4X4	T43.4X5	T43.4X6
Thiouracil (benzyl) (methyl) (propyl)	T38.2X1	T38.2X2	T38.2X3	T38.2X4	T38.2X5	T38.2X6
Thiourea	T38.2X1	T38.2X2	T38.2X3	T38.2X4	T38.2X5	T38.2X6
Thiphenamil	T44.3X1	T44.3X2	T44.3X3	T44.3X4	T44.3X5	T44.3X6
Thiram	T60.3X1	T60.3X2	T60.3X3	T60.3X4	—	—
medicinal	T49.2X1	T49.2X2	T49.2X3	T49.2X4	T49.2X5	T49.2X6
Thonzylamine (systemic)	T45.0X1	T45.0X2	T45.0X3	T45.0X4	T45.0X5	T45.0X6
mucosal decongestant	T48.5X1	T48.5X2	T48.5X3	T48.5X4	T48.5X5	T48.5X6
Thorazine	T43.3X1	T43.3X2	T43.3X3	T43.3X4	T43.3X5	T43.3X6
Thorium dioxide suspension	T50.8X1	T50.8X2	T50.8X3	T50.8X4	T50.8X5	T50.8X6
Thornapple	T62.2X1	T62.2X2	T62.2X3	T62.2X4	—	—
Throat drug NEC	T49.6X1	T49.6X2	T49.6X3	T49.6X4	T49.6X5	T49.6X6
Thrombin	T45.7X1	T45.7X2	T45.7X3	T45.7X4	T45.7X5	T45.7X6
Thrombolysin	T45.611	T45.612	T45.613	T45.614	T45.615	T45.616
Thromboplastin	T45.7X1	T45.7X2	T45.7X3	T45.7X4	T45.7X5	T45.7X6
Thurfyl nicotinate	T46.7X1	T46.7X2	T46.7X3	T46.7X4	T46.7X5	T46.7X6
Thymol	T49.0X1	T49.0X2	T49.0X3	T49.0X4	T49.0X5	T49.0X6
Thymopentin	T37.5X1	T37.5X2	T37.5X3	T37.5X4	T37.5X5	T37.5X6
Thymoxamine	T46.7X1	T46.7X2	T46.7X3	T46.7X4	T46.7X5	T46.7X6
Thymus extract	T38.891	T38.892	T38.893	T38.894	T38.895	T38.896
Thyreotrophic hormone	T38.811	T38.812	T38.813	T38.814	T38.815	T38.816
Thyroglobulin	T38.1X1	T38.1X2	T38.1X3	T38.1X4	T38.1X5	T38.1X6
Thyroid (hormone)	T38.1X1	T38.1X2	T38.1X3	T38.1X4	T38.1X5	T38.1X6
Thyrolar	T38.1X1	T38.1X2	T38.1X3	T38.1X4	T38.1X5	T38.1X6
Thyrotrophin	T38.811	T38.812	T38.813	T38.814	T38.815	T38.816
Thyrotropic hormone	T38.811	T38.812	T38.813	T38.814	T38.815	T38.816
Thyroxine	T38.1X1	T38.1X2	T38.1X3	T38.1X4	T38.1X5	T38.1X6
Tiabendazole	T37.4X1	T37.4X2	T37.4X3	T37.4X4	T37.4X5	T37.4X6
Tiamizide	T50.2X1	T50.2X2	T50.2X3	T50.2X4	T50.2X5	T50.2X6
Tianeptine	T43.291	T43.292	T43.293	T43.294	T43.295	T43.296
Tiapamil	T46.1X1	T46.1X2	T46.1X3	T46.1X4	T46.1X5	T46.1X6
Tiapride	T43.591	T43.592	T43.593	T43.594	T43.595	T43.596
Tiaprofenic acid	T39.311	T39.312	T39.313	T39.314	T39.315	T39.316
Tiaramide	T39.8X1	T39.8X2	T39.8X3	T39.8X4	T39.8X5	T39.8X6
Ticarcillin	T36.0X1	T36.0X2	T36.0X3	T36.0X4	T36.0X5	T36.0X6
Ticlatone	T49.0X1	T49.0X2	T49.0X3	T49.0X4	T49.0X5	T49.0X6
Ticlopidine	T45.521	T45.522	T45.523	T45.524	T45.525	T45.526
Ticrynafen	T50.1X1	T50.1X2	T50.1X3	T50.1X4	T50.1X5	T50.1X6
Tidiacic	T50.991	T50.992	T50.993	T50.994	T50.995	T50.996
Tiemonium	T44.3X1	T44.3X2	T44.3X3	T44.3X4	T44.3X5	T44.3X6
iodide	T44.3X1	T44.3X2	T44.3X3	T44.3X4	T44.3X5	T44.3X6
Tienilic acid	T50.1X1	T50.1X2	T50.1X3	T50.1X4	T50.1X5	T50.1X6
Tifenamil	T44.3X1	T44.3X2	T44.3X3	T44.3X4	T44.3X5	T44.3X6
Tigan	T45.0X1	T45.0X2	T45.0X3	T45.0X4	T45.0X5	T45.0X6
Tigloidine	T44.3X1	T44.3X2	T44.3X3	T44.3X4	T44.3X5	T44.3X6
Tilactase	T47.5X1	T47.5X2	T47.5X3	T47.5X4	T47.5X5	T47.5X6
Tiletamine	T41.291	T41.292	T41.293	T41.294	T41.295	T41.296
Tilidine	T40.4X1	T40.4X2	T40.4X3	T40.4X4	—	—
Timepidium bromide	T44.3X1	T44.3X2	T44.3X3	T44.3X4	T44.3X5	T44.3X6
Timiperone	T43.4X1	T43.4X2	T43.4X3	T43.4X4	T43.4X5	T43.4X6
Timolol	T44.7X1	T44.7X2	T44.7X3	T44.7X4	T44.7X5	T44.7X6
Tincture, iodine — see Iodine						
Tindal	T43.3X1	T43.3X2	T43.3X3	T43.3X4	T43.3X5	T43.3X6
Tinidazole	T37.3X1	T37.3X2	T37.3X3	T37.3X4	T37.3X5	T37.3X6
Tin (chloride) (dust) (oxide) NEC	T56.6X1	T56.6X2	T56.6X3	T56.6X4	—	—
anti-infectives	T37.8X1	T37.8X2	T37.8X3	T37.8X4	T37.8X5	T37.8X6
Tinoridine	T39.8X1	T39.8X2	T39.8X3	T39.8X4	T39.8X5	T39.8X6
Tiocarlide	T37.1X1	T37.1X2	T37.1X3	T37.1X4	T37.1X5	T37.1X6
Tioclomarol	T45.511	T45.512	T45.513	T45.514	T45.515	T45.516
Tioconazole	T49.0X1	T49.0X2	T49.0X3	T49.0X4	T49.0X5	T49.0X6
Tioguanine	T45.1X1	T45.1X2	T45.1X3	T45.1X4	T45.1X5	T45.1X6
Tiopronin	T50.991	T50.992	T50.993	T50.994	T50.995	T50.996
Tiotixene	T43.4X1	T43.4X2	T43.4X3	T43.4X4	T43.4X5	T43.4X6
Tioxolone	T49.4X1	T49.4X2	T49.4X3	T49.4X4	T49.4X5	T49.4X6
Tipepidine	T48.3X1	T48.3X2	T48.3X3	T48.3X4	T48.3X5	T48.3X6
Tiquizium bromide	T44.3X1	T44.3X2	T44.3X3	T44.3X4	T44.3X5	T44.3X6
Tiratricol	T38.1X1	T38.1X2	T38.1X3	T38.1X4	T38.1X5	T38.1X6
Tisopurine	T50.4X1	T50.4X2	T50.4X3	T50.4X4	T50.4X5	T50.4X6
Titanium (compounds) (vapor)	T56.891	T56.892	T56.893	T56.894	—	—
dioxide	T49.3X1	T49.3X2	T49.3X3	T49.3X4	T49.3X5	T49.3X6
ointment	T49.3X1	T49.3X2	T49.3X3	T49.3X4	T49.3X5	T49.3X6
oxide	T49.3X1	T49.3X2	T49.3X3	T49.3X4	T49.3X5	T49.3X6
tetrachloride	T56.891	T56.892	T56.893	T56.894		
Titanocene	T56.891	T56.892	T56.893	T56.894		
Titroid	T38.1X1	T38.1X2	T38.1X3	T38.1X4	T38.1X5	T38.1X6
Tizanidine	T42.8X1	T42.8X2	T42.8X3	T42.8X4	T42.8X5	T42.8X6
TMTD	T60.3X1	T60.3X2	T60.3X3	T60.3X4		
TNT (fumes)	T65.3X1	T65.3X2	T65.3X3	T65.3X4		
Toadstool	T62.0X1	T62.0X2	T62.0X3	T62.0X4		
Tobacco NEC	T65.291	T65.292	T65.293	T65.294		
cigarettes	T65.221	T65.222	T65.223	T65.224		
Indian	T62.2X1	T62.2X2	T62.2X3	T62.2X4	—	—
smoke, second-hand	T65.221	T65.222	T65.223	T65.224		
Tobramycin	T36.5X1	T36.5X2	T36.5X3	T36.5X4	T36.5X5	T36.5X6
Tocainide	T46.2X1	T46.2X2	T46.2X3	T46.2X4	T46.2X5	T46.2X6
Tocoferol	T45.2X1	T45.2X2	T45.2X3	T45.2X4	T45.2X5	T45.2X6
Tocopherol	T45.2X1	T45.2X2	T45.2X3	T45.2X4	T45.2X5	T45.2X6
acetate	T45.2X1	T45.2X2	T45.2X3	T45.2X4	T45.2X5	T45.2X6
Tocosamine	T48.0X1	T48.0X2	T48.0X3	T48.0X4	T48.0X5	T48.0X6
Todralazine	T46.5X1	T46.5X2	T46.5X3	T46.5X4	T46.5X5	T46.5X6
Tofisopam	T42.4X1	T42.4X2	T42.4X3	T42.4X4	T42.4X5	T42.4X6
Tofranil	T43.011	T43.012	T43.013	T43.014	T43.015	T43.016
Toilet deodorizer	T65.891	T65.892	T65.893	T65.894		
Tolamolol	T44.7X1	T44.7X2	T44.7X3	T44.7X4	T44.7X5	T44.7X6
Tolazamide	T38.3X1	T38.3X2	T38.3X3	T38.3X4	T38.3X5	T38.3X6
Tolazoline	T46.7X1	T46.7X2	T46.7X3	T46.7X4	T46.7X5	T46.7X6
Tolbutamide (sodium)	T38.3X1	T38.3X2	T38.3X3	T38.3X4	T38.3X5	T38.3X6
Tolciclate	T49.0X1	T49.0X2	T49.0X3	T49.0X4	T49.0X5	T49.0X6
Tolmetin	T39.391	T39.392	T39.393	T39.394	T39.395	T39.396
Tolnaftate	T49.0X1	T49.0X2	T49.0X3	T49.0X4	T49.0X5	T49.0X6
Tolonidine	T46.5X1	T46.5X2	T46.5X3	T46.5X4	T46.5X5	T46.5X6
Toloxatone	T42.6X1	T42.6X2	T42.6X3	T42.6X4	T42.6X5	T42.6X6
Tolperisone	T44.3X1	T44.3X2	T44.3X3	T44.3X4	T44.3X5	T44.3X6
Tolserol	T42.8X1	T42.8X2	T42.8X3	T42.8X4	T42.8X5	T42.8X6
Toluene (liquid)	T52.2X1	T52.2X2	T52.2X3	T52.2X4		
diisocyanate	T65.0X1	T65.0X2	T65.0X3	T65.0X4		
Toluidine	T65.891	T65.892	T65.893	T65.894		
vapor	T59.891	T59.892	T59.893	T59.894		
Toluol (liquid)	T52.2X1	T52.2X2	T52.2X3	T52.2X4		
vapor	T52.2X1	T52.2X2	T52.2X3	T52.2X4		
Toluylenediamine	T65.3X1	T65.3X2	T65.3X3	T65.3X4		
Tolylene-2,4-diisocyanate	T65.0X1	T65.0X2	T65.0X3	T65.0X4		
Tonic NEC	T50.901	T50.902	T50.903	T50.904	T50.905	T50.906
Topical action drug NEC	T49.91	T49.92	T49.93	T49.94	T49.95	T49.96
ear, nose or throat	T49.6X1	T49.6X2	T49.6X3	T49.6X4	T49.6X5	T49.6X6
eye	T49.5X1	T49.5X2	T49.5X3	T49.5X4	T49.5X5	T49.5X6
skin	T49.91	T49.92	T49.93	T49.94	T49.95	T49.96
specified NEC	T49.8X1	T49.8X2	T49.8X3	T49.8X4	T49.8X5	T49.8X6
Toquizine	T44.3X1	T44.3X2	T44.3X3	T44.3X4	T44.3X5	T44.3X6
Toremifene	T38.6X1	T38.6X2	T38.6X3	T38.6X4	T38.6X5	T38.6X6
Tosylchloramide sodium	T49.8X1	T49.8X2	T49.8X3	T49.8X4	T49.8X5	T49.8X6
Toxaphene (dust) (spray)	T60.1X1	T60.1X2	T60.1X3	T60.1X4	—	—
Toxin, diphtheria (Schick Test)	T50.8X1	T50.8X2	T50.8X3	T50.8X4	T50.8X5	T50.8X6
Toxoid						
combined	T50.A21	T50.A22	T50.A23	T50.A24	T50.A25	T50.A26
diphtheria	T50.A91	T50.A92	T50.A93	T50.A94	T50.A95	T50.A96
tetanus	T50.A91	T50.A92	T50.A93	T50.A94	T50.A95	T50.A96
Trace element NEC	T45.8X1	T45.8X2	T45.8X3	T45.8X4	T45.8X5	T45.8X6
Tractor fuel NEC	T52.0X1	T52.0X2	T52.0X3	T52.0X4	—	—
Tragacanth	T50.991	T50.992	T50.993	T50.994	T50.995	T50.996
Tramadol	T40.4X1	T40.4X2	T40.4X3	T40.4X4	T40.4X5	T40.4X6
Tramazoline	T48.5X1	T48.5X2	T48.5X3	T48.5X4	T48.5X5	T48.5X6
Tranexamic acid	T45.621	T45.622	T45.623	T45.624	T45.625	T45.626
Tranilast	T45.0X1	T45.0X2	T45.0X3	T45.0X4	T45.0X5	T45.0X6
Tranquilizer NEC	T43.501	T43.502	T43.503	T43.504	T43.505	T43.506
with hypnotic or sedative	T42.6X1	T42.6X2	T42.6X3	T42.6X4	T42.6X5	T42.6X6
benzodiazepine NEC	T42.4X1	T42.4X2	T42.4X3	T42.4X4	T42.4X5	T42.4X6
butyrophenone NEC	T43.4X1	T43.4X2	T43.4X3	T43.4X4	T43.4X5	T43.4X6
carbamate	T43.591	T43.592	T43.593	T43.594	T43.595	T43.596
dimethylamine	T43.3X1	T43.3X2	T43.3X3	T43.3X4	T43.3X5	T43.3X6
ethylamine	T43.3X1	T43.3X2	T43.3X3	T43.3X4	T43.3X5	T43.3X6
hydroxyzine	T43.591	T43.592	T43.593	T43.594	T43.595	T43.596
major NEC	T43.501	T43.502	T43.503	T43.504	T43.505	T43.506
penothiazine NEC	T43.3X1	T43.3X2	T43.3X3	T43.3X4	T43.3X5	T43.3X6
phenothiazine-based	T43.3X1	T43.3X2	T43.3X3	T43.3X4	T43.3X5	T43.3X6

Substance	Poisoning, Accidental (unintentional)	Poisoning, Intentional Self-harm	Poisoning, Assault	Poisoning, Undetermined	Adverse Effect	Under-dosing
Tranquilizer — *continued*						
piperazine NEC	T43.3X1	T43.3X2	T43.3X3	T43.3X4	T43.3X5	T43.3X6
piperidine	T43.3X1	T43.3X2	T43.3X3	T43.3X4	T43.3X5	T43.3X6
propylamine	T43.3X1	T43.3X2	T43.3X3	T43.3X4	T43.3X5	T43.3X6
specified NEC	T43.591	T43.592	T43.593	T43.594	T43.595	T43.596
thioxanthene NEC	T43.591	T43.592	T43.593	T43.594	T43.595	T43.596
Tranxene	T42.4X1	T42.4X2	T42.4X3	T42.4X4	T42.4X5	T42.4X6
Tranylcypromine	T43.1X1	T43.1X2	T43.1X3	T43.1X4	T43.1X5	T43.1X6
Trapidil	T46.3X1	T46.3X2	T46.3X3	T46.3X4	T46.3X5	T46.3X6
Trasentine	T44.3X1	T44.3X2	T44.3X3	T44.3X4	T44.3X5	T44.3X6
Travert	T50.3X1	T50.3X2	T50.3X3	T50.3X4	T50.3X5	T50.3X6
Trazodone	T43.211	T43.212	T43.213	T43.214	T43.215	T43.216
Trecator	T37.1X1	T37.1X2	T37.1X3	T37.1X4	T37.1X5	T37.1X6
Treosulfan	T45.1X1	T45.1X2	T45.1X3	T45.1X4	T45.1X5	T45.1X6
Tretamine	T45.1X1	T45.1X2	T45.1X3	T45.1X4	T45.1X5	T45.1X6
Tretinoin	T49.0X1	T49.0X2	T49.0X3	T49.0X4	T49.0X5	T49.0X6
Tretoquinol	T48.6X1	T48.6X2	T48.6X3	T48.6X4	T48.6X5	T48.6X6
Triacetin	T49.0X1	T49.0X2	T49.0X3	T49.0X4	T49.0X5	T49.0X6
Triacetoxyanthracene	T49.4X1	T49.4X2	T49.4X3	T49.4X4	T49.4X5	T49.4X6
Triacetyloleandomycin	T36.3X1	T36.3X2	T36.3X3	T36.3X4	T36.3X5	T36.3X6
Triamcinolone	T38.0X1	T38.0X2	T38.0X3	T38.0X4	T38.0X5	T38.0X6
ENT agent	T49.6X1	T49.6X2	T49.6X3	T49.6X4	T49.6X5	T49.6X6
hexacetonide	T49.0X1	T49.0X2	T49.0X3	T49.0X4	T49.0X5	T49.0X6
ophthalmic preparation	T49.5X1	T49.5X2	T49.5X3	T49.5X4	T49.5X5	T49.5X6
topical NEC	T49.0X1	T49.0X2	T49.0X3	T49.0X4	T49.0X5	T49.0X6
Triampyzine	T44.3X1	T44.3X2	T44.3X3	T44.3X4	T44.3X5	T44.3X6
Triamterene	T50.2X1	T50.2X2	T50.2X3	T50.2X4	T50.2X5	T50.2X6
Triazine (herbicide)	T60.3X1	T60.3X2	T60.3X3	T60.3X4	—	—
Triaziquone	T45.1X1	T45.1X2	T45.1X3	T45.1X4	T45.1X5	T45.1X6
Triazolam	T42.4X1	T42.4X2	T42.4X3	T42.4X4	T42.4X5	T42.4X6
Triazole (herbicide)	T60.3X1	T60.3X2	T60.3X3	T60.3X4	—	—
Tribenoside	T46.991	T46.992	T46.993	T46.994	T46.995	T46.996
Tribromacetaldehyde	T42.6X1	T42.6X2	T42.6X3	T42.6X4	T42.6X5	T42.6X6
Tribromoethanol, rectal	T41.291	T41.292	T41.293	T41.294	T41.295	T41.296
Tribromomethane	T42.6X1	T42.6X2	T42.6X3	T42.6X4	T42.6X5	T42.6X6
Trichlorethane	T53.2X1	T53.2X2	T53.2X3	T53.2X4		
Trichlorethylene	T53.2X1	T53.2X2	T53.2X3	T53.2X4		
Trichlorfon	T60.0X1	T60.0X2	T60.0X3	T60.0X4	—	—
Trichlormethiazide	T50.2X1	T50.2X2	T50.2X3	T50.2X4	T50.2X5	T50.2X6
Trichlormethine	T45.1X1	T45.1X2	T45.1X3	T45.1X4	T45.1X5	T45.1X6
Trichloroacetic acid,	T54.2X1	T54.2X2	T54.2X3	T54.2X4		
Trichloracetic acid						
medicinal	T49.4X1	T49.4X2	T49.4X3	T49.4X4	T49.4X5	T49.4X6
Trichloroethane	T53.2X1	T53.2X2	T53.2X3	T53.2X4		
Trichloroethanol	T42.6X1	T42.6X2	T42.6X3	T42.6X4	T42.6X5	T42.6X6
Trichloroethylene (liquid)	T53.2X1	T53.2X2	T53.2X3	T53.2X4		
(vapor)						
anesthetic (gas)	T41.0X1	T41.0X2	T41.0X3	T41.0X4	T41.0X5	T41.0X6
vapor NEC	T53.2X1	T53.2X2	T53.2X3	T53.2X4		
Trichloroethyl phosphate	T42.6X1	T42.6X2	T42.6X3	T42.6X4	T42.6X5	T42.6X6
Trichlorofluoromethane NEC	T53.5X1	T53.5X2	T53.5X3	T53.5X4	—	—
Trichloronate	T60.0X1	T60.0X2	T60.0X3	T60.0X4	—	—
Trichloropropane	T53.6X1	T53.6X2	T53.6X3	T53.6X4	—	—
Trichlorotriethylamine	T45.1X1	T45.1X2	T45.1X3	T45.1X4	T45.1X5	T45.1X6
Trichomonacides NEC	T37.3X1	T37.3X2	T37.3X3	T37.3X4	T37.3X5	T37.3X6
Trichomycin	T36.7X1	T36.7X2	T36.7X3	T36.7X4	T36.7X5	T36.7X6
Triclobisonium chloride	T49.0X1	T49.0X2	T49.0X3	T49.0X4	T49.0X5	T49.0X6
Triclocarban	T49.0X1	T49.0X2	T49.0X3	T49.0X4	T49.0X5	T49.0X6
Triclofos	T42.6X1	T42.6X2	T42.6X3	T42.6X4	T42.6X5	T42.6X6
Triclosan	T49.0X1	T49.0X2	T49.0X3	T49.0X4	T49.0X5	T49.0X6
Tricresyl phosphate	T65.891	T65.892	T65.893	T65.894	—	—
solvent	T52.91	T52.92	T52.93	T52.94	—	—
Tricyclamol chloride	T44.3X1	T44.3X2	T44.3X3	T44.3X4	T44.3X5	T44.3X6
Tridesilon	T49.0X1	T49.0X2	T49.0X3	T49.0X4	T49.0X5	T49.0X6
Tridihexethyl iodide	T44.3X1	T44.3X2	T44.3X3	T44.3X4	T44.3X5	T44.3X6
Tridione	T42.2X1	T42.2X2	T42.2X3	T42.2X4	T42.2X5	T42.2X6
Trientine	T45.8X1	T45.8X2	T45.8X3	T45.8X4	T45.8X5	T45.8X6
Triethanolamine NEC	T54.3X1	T54.3X2	T54.3X3	T54.3X4		
detergent	T54.3X1	T54.3X2	T54.3X3	T54.3X4	—	—
trinitrate (biphosphate)	T46.3X1	T46.3X2	T46.3X3	T46.3X4	T46.3X5	T46.3X6
Triethanomelamine	T45.1X1	T45.1X2	T45.1X3	T45.1X4	T45.1X5	T45.1X6
Triethylenemelamine	T45.1X1	T45.1X2	T45.1X3	T45.1X4	T45.1X5	T45.1X6
Triethylenephosphoramide	T45.1X1	T45.1X2	T45.1X3	T45.1X4	T45.1X5	T45.1X6
Triethylenethiophosphoramide	T45.1X1	T45.1X2	T45.1X3	T45.1X4	T45.1X5	T45.1X6
Trifluoperazine	T43.3X1	T43.3X2	T43.3X3	T43.3X4	T43.3X5	T43.3X6
Trifluoroethyl vinyl ether	T41.0X1	T41.0X2	T41.0X3	T41.0X4	T41.0X5	T41.0X6
Trifluperidol	T43.4X1	T43.4X2	T43.4X3	T43.4X4	T43.4X5	T43.4X6
Triflupromazine	T43.3X1	T43.3X2	T43.3X3	T43.3X4	T43.3X5	T43.3X6
Trifluridine	T37.5X1	T37.5X2	T37.5X3	T37.5X4	T37.5X5	T37.5X6
Triflusal	T45.521	T45.522	T45.523	T45.524	T45.525	T45.526
Trihexyphenidyl	T44.3X1	T44.3X2	T44.3X3	T44.3X4	T44.3X5	T44.3X6
Triiodothyronine	T38.1X1	T38.1X2	T38.1X3	T38.1X4	T38.1X5	T38.1X6

Substance	Poisoning, Accidental (unintentional)	Poisoning, Intentional Self-harm	Poisoning, Assault	Poisoning, Undetermined	Adverse Effect	Under-dosing
Trilene	T41.0X1	T41.0X2	T41.0X3	T41.0X4	T41.0X5	T41.0X6
Trilostane	T38.991	T38.992	T38.993	T38.994	T38.995	T38.996
Trimebutine	T44.3X1	T44.3X2	T44.3X3	T44.3X4	T44.3X5	T44.3X6
Trimecaine	T41.3X1	T41.3X2	T41.3X3	T41.3X4	T41.3X5	T41.3X6
Trimeprazine (tartrate)	T44.3X1	T44.3X2	T44.3X3	T44.3X4	T44.3X5	T44.3X6
Trimetaphan camsilate	T44.2X1	T44.2X2	T44.2X3	T44.2X4	T44.2X5	T44.2X6
Trimetazidine	T46.7X1	T46.7X2	T46.7X3	T46.7X4	T46.7X5	T46.7X6
Trimethadione	T42.2X1	T42.2X2	T42.2X3	T42.2X4	T42.2X5	T42.2X6
Trimethaphan	T44.2X1	T44.2X2	T44.2X3	T44.2X4	T44.2X5	T44.2X6
Trimethidinium	T44.2X1	T44.2X2	T44.2X3	T44.2X4	T44.2X5	T44.2X6
Trimethobenzamide	T45.0X1	T45.0X2	T45.0X3	T45.0X4	T45.0X5	T45.0X6
Trimethoprim	T37.8X1	T37.8X2	T37.8X3	T37.8X4	T37.8X5	T37.8X6
with sulfamethoxazole	T36.8X1	T36.8X2	T36.8X3	T36.8X4	T36.8X5	T36.8X6
Trimethylcarbinol	T51.3X1	T51.3X2	T51.3X3	T51.3X4		
Trimethylpsoralen	T49.3X1	T49.3X2	T49.3X3	T49.3X4	T49.3X5	T49.3X6
Trimeton	T45.0X1	T45.0X2	T45.0X3	T45.0X4	T45.0X5	T45.0X6
Trimetrexate	T45.1X1	T45.1X2	T45.1X3	T45.1X4	T45.1X5	T45.1X6
Trimipramine	T43.011	T43.012	T43.013	T43.014	T43.015	T43.016
Trimustine	T45.1X1	T45.1X2	T45.1X3	T45.1X4	T45.1X5	T45.1X6
Trinitrine	T46.3X1	T46.3X2	T46.3X3	T46.3X4	T46.3X5	T46.3X6
Trinitrobenzol	T65.3X1	T65.3X2	T65.3X3	T65.3X4	—	—
Trinitrophenol	T65.3X1	T65.3X2	T65.3X3	T65.3X4	—	—
Trinitrotoluene (fumes)	T65.3X1	T65.3X2	T65.3X3	T65.3X4	—	—
Trional	T42.6X1	T42.6X2	T42.6X3	T42.6X4	T42.6X5	T42.6X6
Triorthocresyl phosphate	T65.891	T65.892	T65.893	T65.894	—	—
Trioxide of arsenic	T57.0X1	T57.0X2	T57.0X3	T57.0X4	—	—
Trioxysalen	T49.4X1	T49.4X2	T49.4X3	T49.4X4	T49.4X5	T49.4X6
Tripamide	T50.2X1	T50.2X2	T50.2X3	T50.2X4	T50.2X5	T50.2X6
Triparanol	T46.6X1	T46.6X2	T46.6X3	T46.6X4	T46.6X5	T46.6X6
Tripelennamine	T45.0X1	T45.0X2	T45.0X3	T45.0X4	T45.0X5	T45.0X6
Triperiden	T44.3X1	T44.3X2	T44.3X3	T44.3X4	T44.3X5	T44.3X6
Triperidol	T43.4X1	T43.4X2	T43.4X3	T43.4X4	T43.4X5	T43.4X6
Triphenylphosphate	T65.891	T65.892	T65.893	T65.894	—	—
Triple						
bromides	T42.6X1	T42.6X2	T42.6X3	T42.6X4	T42.6X5	T42.6X6
carbonate	T47.1X1	T47.1X2	T47.1X3	T47.1X4	T47.1X5	T47.1X6
vaccine						
DPT	T50.A11	T50.A12	T50.A13	T50.A14	T50.A15	T50.A16
including pertussis	T50.A11	T50.A12	T50.A13	T50.A14	T50.A15	T50.A16
MMR	T50.B91	T50.B92	T50.B93	T50.B94	T50.B95	T50.B96
Triprolidine	T45.0X1	T45.0X2	T45.0X3	T45.0X4	T45.0X5	T45.0X6
Trisodium hydrogen edetate	T50.6X1	T50.6X2	T50.6X3	T50.6X4	T50.6X5	T50.6X6
Trisoralen	T49.3X1	T49.3X2	T49.3X3	T49.3X4	T49.3X5	T49.3X6
Trisulfapyrimidines	T37.0X1	T37.0X2	T37.0X3	T37.0X4	T37.0X5	T37.0X6
Trithiozine	T44.3X1	T44.3X2	T44.3X3	T44.3X4	T44.3X5	T44.3X6
Tritiozine	T44.3X1	T44.3X2	T44.3X3	T44.3X4	T44.3X5	T44.3X6
Tritoqualine	T45.0X1	T45.0X2	T45.0X3	T45.0X4	T45.0X5	T45.0X6
Trofosfamide	T45.1X1	T45.1X2	T45.1X3	T45.1X4	T45.1X5	T45.1X6
Troleandomycin	T36.3X1	T36.3X2	T36.3X3	T36.3X4	T36.3X5	T36.3X6
Trolnitrate (phosphate)	T46.3X1	T46.3X2	T46.3X3	T46.3X4	T46.3X5	T46.3X6
Tromantadine	T37.5X1	T37.5X2	T37.5X3	T37.5X4	T37.5X5	T37.5X6
Trometamol	T50.2X1	T50.2X2	T50.2X3	T50.2X4	T50.2X5	T50.2X6
Tromethamine	T50.2X1	T50.2X2	T50.2X3	T50.2X4	T50.2X5	T50.2X6
Tronothane	T41.3X1	T41.3X2	T41.3X3	T41.3X4	T41.3X5	T41.3X6
Tropacine	T44.3X1	T44.3X2	T44.3X3	T44.3X4	T44.3X5	T44.3X6
Tropatepine	T44.3X1	T44.3X2	T44.3X3	T44.3X4	T44.3X5	T44.3X6
Tropicamide	T44.3X1	T44.3X2	T44.3X3	T44.3X4	T44.3X5	T44.3X6
Trospium chloride	T44.3X1	T44.3X2	T44.3X3	T44.3X4	T44.3X5	T44.3X6
Troxerutin	T46.991	T46.992	T46.993	T46.994	T46.995	T46.996
Troxidone	T42.2X1	T42.2X2	T42.2X3	T42.2X4	T42.2X5	T42.2X6
Tryparsamide	T37.3X1	T37.3X2	T37.3X3	T37.3X4	T37.3X5	T37.3X6
Trypsin	T45.3X1	T45.3X2	T45.3X3	T45.3X4	T45.3X5	T45.3X6
Tryptizol	T43.011	T43.012	T43.013	T43.014	T43.015	T43.016
TSH	T38.811	T38.812	T38.813	T38.814	T38.815	T38.816
Tuaminoheptane	T48.5X1	T48.5X2	T48.5X3	T48.5X4	T48.5X5	T48.5X6
Tuberculin, purified protein derivative (PPD)	T50.8X1	T50.8X2	T50.8X3	T50.8X4	T50.8X5	T50.8X6
Tubocurare	T48.1X1	T48.1X2	T48.1X3	T48.1X4	T48.1X5	T48.1X6
Tubocurarine (chloride)	T48.1X1	T48.1X2	T48.1X3	T48.1X4	T48.1X5	T48.1X6
Tulobuterol	T48.6X1	T48.6X2	T48.6X3	T48.6X4	T48.6X5	T48.6X6
Turpentine (spirits of)	T52.8X1	T52.8X2	T52.8X3	T52.8X4	—	—
vapor	T52.8X1	T52.8X2	T52.8X3	T52.8X4	—	—
Tybamate	T43.591	T43.592	T43.593	T43.594	T43.595	T43.596
Tyloxapol	T48.4X1	T48.4X2	T48.4X3	T48.4X4	T48.4X5	T48.4X6
Tymazoline	T48.5X1	T48.5X2	T48.5X3	T48.5X4	T48.5X5	T48.5X6
Typhoid-paratyphoid vaccine	T50.A91	T50.A92	T50.A93	T50.A94	T50.A95	T50.A96
Typhus vaccine	T50.A91	T50.A92	T50.A93	T50.A94	T50.A95	T50.A96
Tyropanoate	T50.8X1	T50.8X2	T50.8X3	T50.8X4	T50.8X5	T50.8X6
Tyrothricin	T49.6X1	T49.6X2	T49.6X3	T49.6X4	T49.6X5	T49.6X6
ENT agent	T49.6X1	T49.6X2	T49.6X3	T49.6X4	T49.6X5	T49.6X6
ophthalmic preparation	T49.5X1	T49.5X2	T49.5X3	T49.5X4	T49.5X5	T49.5X6

Additional Character May Be Required — Refer to the Tabular List for Character Selection ⬇ Subterms under main terms may continue to next column or page

Substance	Poisoning, Accidental (unintentional)	Poisoning, Intentional Self-harm	Poisoning, Assault	Poisoning, Undetermined	Adverse Effect	Under-dosing
Ufenamate	T39.391	T39.392	T39.393	T39.394	T39.395	T39.396
Ultraviolet light protectant	T49.3X1	T49.3X2	T49.3X3	T49.3X4	T49.3X5	T49.3X6
Undecenoic acid	T49.0X1	T49.0X2	T49.0X3	T49.0X4	T49.0X5	T49.0X6
Undecoylium	T49.0X1	T49.0X2	T49.0X3	T49.0X4	T49.0X5	T49.0X6
Undecylenic acid	T49.0X1	T49.0X2	T49.0X3	T49.0X4	T49.0X5	T49.0X6
(derivatives)	T49.3X1	T49.3X2	T49.3X3	T49.3X4	T49.3X5	T49.3X6
Unna's boot	T49.3X1	T49.3X2	T49.3X3	T49.3X4	T49.3X5	T49.3X6
Unsaturated fatty acid	T46.6X1	T46.6X2	T46.6X3	T46.6X4	T46.6X5	T46.6X6
Uracil mustard	T45.1X1	T45.1X2	T45.1X3	T45.1X4	T45.1X5	T45.1X6
Uramustine	T45.1X1	T45.1X2	T45.1X3	T45.1X4	T45.1X5	T45.1X6
Urapidil	T46.5X1	T46.5X2	T46.5X3	T46.5X4	T46.5X5	T46.5X6
Urari	T48.1X1	T48.1X2	T48.1X3	T48.1X4	T48.1X5	T48.1X6
Urate oxidase	T50.4X1	T50.4X2	T50.4X3	T50.4X4	T50.4X5	T50.4X6
Urea	T47.3X1	T47.3X2	T47.3X3	T47.3X4	T47.3X5	T47.3X6
peroxide	T49.0X1	T49.0X2	T49.0X3	T49.0X4	T49.0X5	T49.0X6
stibamine	T37.4X1	T37.4X2	T37.4X3	T37.4X4	T37.4X5	T37.4X6
topical	T49.8X1	T49.8X2	T49.8X3	T49.8X4	T49.8X5	T49.8X6
Urethane	T45.1X1	T45.1X2	T45.1X3	T45.1X4	T45.1X5	T45.1X6
Urginea (maritima) (scilla) — see Squill						
Uric acid metabolism drug NEC	T50.4X1	T50.4X2	T50.4X3	T50.4X4	T50.4X5	T50.4X6
Uricosuric agent	T50.4X1	T50.4X2	T50.4X3	T50.4X4	T50.4X5	T50.4X6
Urinary anti-infective	T37.8X1	T37.8X2	T37.8X3	T37.8X4	T37.8X5	T37.8X6
Urofollitropin	T38.811	T38.812	T38.813	T38.814	T38.815	T38.816
Urokinase	T45.611	T45.612	T45.613	T45.614	T45.615	T45.616
Urokon	T50.8X1	T50.8X2	T50.8X3	T50.8X4	T50.8X5	T50.8X6
Ursodeoxycholic acid	T50.991	T50.992	T50.993	T50.994	T50.995	T50.996
Ursodiol	T50.991	T50.992	T50.993	T50.994	T50.995	T50.996
Urtica	T62.2X1	T62.2X2	T62.2X3	T62.2X4	—	—
Utility gas — see Gas, utility						
Vaccine NEC	T50.Z91	T50.Z92	T50.Z93	T50.Z94	T50.Z95	T50.Z96
antineoplastic	T50.Z91	T50.Z92	T50.Z93	T50.Z94	T50.Z95	T50.Z96
bacterial NEC	T50.A91	T50.A92	T50.A93	T50.A94	T50.A95	T50.A96
with						
other bacterial component	T50.A21	T50.A22	T50.A23	T50.A24	T50.A25	T50.A26
pertussis component	T50.A11	T50.A12	T50.A13	T50.A14	T50.A15	T50.A16
viral-rickettsial component	T50.A21	T50.A22	T50.A23	T50.A24	T50.A25	T50.A26
mixed NEC	T50.A21	T50.A22	T50.A23	T50.A24	T50.A25	T50.A26
BCG	T50.A91	T50.A92	T50.A93	T50.A94	T50.A95	T50.A96
cholera	T50.A91	T50.A92	T50.A93	T50.A94	T50.A95	T50.A96
diphtheria	T50.A91	T50.A92	T50.A93	T50.A94	T50.A95	T50.A96
with tetanus	T50.A21	T50.A22	T50.A23	T50.A24	T50.A25	T50.A26
and pertussis	T50.A11	T50.A12	T50.A13	T50.A14	T50.A15	T50.A16
influenza	T50.B91	T50.B92	T50.B93	T50.B94	T50.B95	T50.B96
measles	T50.B91	T50.B92	T50.B93	T50.B94	T50.B95	T50.B96
with mumps and rubella	T50.B91	T50.B92	T50.B93	T50.B94	T50.B95	T50.B96
meningococcal	T50.A91	T50.A92	T50.A93	T50.A94	T50.A95	T50.A96
mumps	T50.B91	T50.B92	T50.B93	T50.B94	T50.B95	T50.B96
paratyphoid	T50.A91	T50.A92	T50.A93	T50.A94	T50.A95	T50.A96
pertussis	T50.A11	T50.A12	T50.A13	T50.A14	T50.A15	T50.A16
with diphtheria	T50.A11	T50.A12	T50.A13	T50.A14	T50.A15	T50.A16
and tetanus	T50.A11	T50.A12	T50.A13	T50.A14	T50.A15	T50.A16
with other component	T50.A11	T50.A12	T50.A13	T50.A14	T50.A15	T50.A16
plague	T50.A91	T50.A92	T50.A93	T50.A94	T50.A95	T50.A96
poliomyelitis	T50.B91	T50.B92	T50.B93	T50.B94	T50.B95	T50.B96
poliovirus	T50.B91	T50.B92	T50.B93	T50.B94	T50.B95	T50.B96
rabies	T50.B91	T50.B92	T50.B93	T50.B94	T50.B95	T50.B96
respiratory syncytial virus	T50.B91	T50.B92	T50.B93	T50.B94	T50.B95	T50.B96
rickettsial NEC	T50.A91	T50.A92	T50.A93	T50.A94	T50.A95	T50.A96
with						
bacterial component	T50.A21	T50.A22	T50.A23	T50.A24	T50.A25	T50.A26
Rocky Mountain spotted fever	T50.A91	T50.A92	T50.A93	T50.A94	T50.A95	T50.A96
rubella	T50.B91	T50.B92	T50.B93	T50.B94	T50.B95	T50.B96
sabin oral	T50.B91	T50.B92	T50.B93	T50.B94	T50.B95	T50.B96
smallpox	T50.B11	T50.B12	T50.B13	T50.B14	T50.B15	T50.B16
TAB	T50.A91	T50.A92	T50.A93	T50.A94	T50.A95	T50.A96
tetanus	T50.A91	T50.A92	T50.A93	T50.A94	T50.A95	T50.A96
typhoid	T50.A91	T50.A92	T50.A93	T50.A94	T50.A95	T50.A96
typhus	T50.A91	T50.A92	T50.A93	T50.A94	T50.A95	T50.A96
viral NEC	T50.B91	T50.B92	T50.B93	T50.B94	T50.B95	T50.B96
yellow fever	T50.B91	T50.B92	T50.B93	T50.B94	T50.B95	T50.B96
Vaccinia immune globulin	T50.Z11	T50.Z12	T50.Z13	T50.Z14	T50.Z15	T50.Z16
Vaginal contraceptives	T49.8X1	T49.8X2	T49.8X3	T49.8X4	T49.8X5	T49.8X6
Valerian						
root	T42.6X1	T42.6X2	T42.6X3	T42.6X4	T42.6X5	T42.6X6
tincture	T42.6X1	T42.6X2	T42.6X3	T42.6X4	T42.6X5	T42.6X6
Valethamate bromide	T44.3X1	T44.3X2	T44.3X3	T44.3X4	T44.3X5	T44.3X6
Valisone	T49.0X1	T49.0X2	T49.0X3	T49.0X4	T49.0X5	T49.0X6

Substance	Poisoning, Accidental (unintentional)	Poisoning, Intentional Self-harm	Poisoning, Assault	Poisoning, Undetermined	Adverse Effect	Under-dosing
Valium	T42.4X1	T42.4X2	T42.4X3	T42.4X4	T42.4X5	T42.4X6
Valmid	T42.6X1	T42.6X2	T42.6X3	T42.6X4	T42.6X5	T42.6X6
Valnoctamide	T42.6X1	T42.6X2	T42.6X3	T42.6X4	T42.6X5	T42.6X6
Valproate (sodium)	T42.6X1	T42.6X2	T42.6X3	T42.6X4	T42.6X5	T42.6X6
Valproic acid	T42.6X1	T42.6X2	T42.6X3	T42.6X4	T42.6X5	T42.6X6
Valpromide	T42.6X1	T42.6X2	T42.6X3	T42.6X4	T42.6X5	T42.6X6
Vanadium	T56.891	T56.892	T56.893	T56.894		
Vancomycin	T36.8X1	T36.8X2	T36.8X3	T36.8X4	T36.8X5	T36.8X6
Vapor — see also Gas	T59.91	T59.92	T59.93	T59.94		
kiln (carbon monoxide)	T58.8X1	T58.8X2	T58.8X3	T58.8X4		
lead — see lead						
specified source NEC	T59.891	T59.892	T59.893	T59.894		
Vardenafil	T46.7X1	T46.7X2	T46.7X3	T46.7X4	T46.7X5	T46.7X6
Varicose reduction drug	T46.8X1	T46.8X2	T46.8X3	T46.8X4	T46.8X5	T46.8X6
Varnish	T65.4X1	T65.4X2	T65.4X3	T65.4X4		
cleaner	T52.91	T52.92	T52.93	T52.94	—	—
Vaseline	T49.3X1	T49.3X2	T49.3X3	T49.3X4	T49.3X5	T49.3X6
Vasodilan	T46.7X1	T46.7X2	T46.7X3	T46.7X4	T46.7X5	T46.7X6
Vasodilator						
coronary NEC	T46.3X1	T46.3X2	T46.3X3	T46.3X4	T46.3X5	T46.3X6
peripheral NEC	T46.7X1	T46.7X2	T46.7X3	T46.7X4	T46.7X5	T46.7X6
Vasopressin	T38.891	T38.892	T38.893	T38.894	T38.895	T38.896
Vasopressor drugs	T38.891	T38.892	T38.893	T38.894	T38.895	T38.896
Vecuronium bromide	T48.1X1	T48.1X2	T48.1X3	T48.1X4	T48.1X5	T48.1X6
Vegetable extract, astringent	T49.2X1	T49.2X2	T49.2X3	T49.2X4	T49.2X5	T49.2X6
Venlafaxine	T43.211	T43.212	T43.213	T43.214	T43.215	T43.216
Venom, venomous (bite) (sting)	T63.91	T63.92	T63.93	T63.94	—	—
amphibian NEC	T63.831	T63.832	T63.833	T63.834	—	—
animal NEC	T63.891	T63.892	T63.893	T63.894	—	—
ant	T63.421	T63.422	T63.423	T63.424	—	—
arthropod NEC	T63.481	T63.482	T63.483	T63.484	—	—
bee	T63.441	T63.442	T63.443	T63.444	—	—
centipede	T63.411	T63.412	T63.413	T63.414	—	—
fish	T63.591	T63.592	T63.593	T63.594	—	—
frog	T63.811	T63.812	T63.813	T63.814	—	—
hornet	T63.451	T63.452	T63.453	T63.454	—	—
insect NEC	T63.481	T63.482	T63.483	T63.484	—	—
lizard	T63.121	T63.122	T63.123	T63.124	—	—
marine						
animals	T63.691	T63.692	T63.693	T63.694	—	—
bluebottle	T63.611	T63.612	T63.613	T63.614	—	—
jellyfish NEC	T63.621	T63.622	T63.623	T63.624	—	—
Portugese Man-o-war	T63.611	T63.612	T63.613	T63.614	—	—
sea anemone	T63.631	T63.632	T63.633	T63.634	—	—
specified NEC	T63.691	T63.692	T63.693	T63.694	—	—
fish	T63.591	T63.592	T63.593	T63.594	—	—
plants	T63.711	T63.712	T63.713	T63.714	—	—
sting ray	T63.511	T63.512	T63.513	T63.514	—	—
millipede (tropical)	T63.411	T63.412	T63.413	T63.414	—	—
plant NEC	T63.791	T63.792	T63.793	T63.794	—	—
marine	T63.711	T63.712	T63.713	T63.714	—	—
reptile	T63.191	T63.192	T63.193	T63.194	—	—
gila monster	T63.111	T63.112	T63.113	T63.114	—	—
lizard NEC	T63.121	T63.122	T63.123	T63.124	—	—
scorpion	T63.2X1	T63.2X2	T63.2X3	T63.2X4	—	—
snake	T63.001	T63.002	T63.003	T63.004	—	—
African NEC	T63.081	T63.082	T63.083	T63.084	—	—
American (North) (South) NEC	T63.061	T63.062	T63.063	T63.064	—	—
Asian	T63.081	T63.082	T63.083	T63.084	—	—
Australian	T63.071	T63.072	T63.073	T63.074	—	—
cobra	T63.041	T63.042	T63.043	T63.044	—	—
coral snake	T63.021	T63.022	T63.023	T63.024	—	—
rattlesnake	T63.011	T63.012	T63.013	T63.014	—	—
specified NEC	T63.091	T63.092	T63.093	T63.094	—	—
taipan	T63.031	T63.032	T63.033	T63.034	—	—
specified NEC	T63.891	T63.892	T63.893	T63.894	—	—
spider	T63.301	T63.302	T63.303	T63.304	—	—
black widow	T63.311	T63.312	T63.313	T63.314	—	—
brown recluse	T63.331	T63.332	T63.333	T63.334	—	—
specified NEC	T63.391	T63.392	T63.393	T63.394	—	—
tarantula	T63.321	T63.322	T63.323	T63.324	—	—
sting ray	T63.511	T63.512	T63.513	T63.514	—	—
toad	T63.821	T63.822	T63.823	T63.824	—	—
wasp	T63.461	T63.462	T63.463	T63.464	—	—
Venous sclerosing drug NEC	T46.8X1	T46.8X2	T46.8X3	T46.8X4	T46.8X5	T46.8X6
Ventolin — see Albuterol						
Veramon	T42.3X1	T42.3X2	T42.3X3	T42.3X4	T42.3X5	T42.3X6
Verapamil	T46.1X1	T46.1X2	T46.1X3	T46.1X4	T46.1X5	T46.1X6
Veratrine	T46.5X1	T46.5X2	T46.5X3	T46.5X4	T46.5X5	T46.5X6

Table of Drugs and Chemicals

Ufenamate — Veratrine

Substance	Poisoning, Accidental (unintentional)	Poisoning, Intentional Self-harm	Poisoning, Assault	Poisoning, Undetermined	Adverse Effect	Under-dosing
Veratrum						
album	T62.2X1	T62.2X2	T62.2X3	T62.2X4	—	—
alkaloids	T46.5X1	T46.5X2	T46.5X3	T46.5X4	T46.5X5	T46.5X6
viride	T62.2X1	T62.2X2	T62.2X3	T62.2X4	—	—
Verdigris	T60.3X1	T60.3X2	T60.3X3	T60.3X4	—	—
Veronal	T42.3X1	T42.3X2	T42.3X3	T42.3X4	T42.3X5	T42.3X6
Veroxil	T37.4X1	T37.4X2	T37.4X3	T37.4X4	T37.4X5	T37.4X6
Versenate	T50.6X1	T50.6X2	T50.6X3	T50.6X4	T50.6X5	T50.6X6
Versidyne	T39.8X1	T39.8X2	T39.8X3	T39.8X4	T39.8X5	T39.8X6
Vetrabutine	T48.0X1	T48.0X2	T48.0X3	T48.0X4	T48.0X5	T48.0X6
Vidarabine	T37.5X1	T37.5X2	T37.5X3	T37.5X4	T37.5X5	T37.5X6
Vienna						
green	T57.0X1	T57.0X2	T57.0X3	T57.0X4	—	—
insecticide	T60.2X1	T60.2X2	T60.2X3	T60.2X4	—	—
red	T57.0X1	T57.0X2	T57.0X3	T57.0X4	—	—
pharmaceutical dye	T50.991	T50.992	T50.993	T50.994	T50.995	T50.996
Vigabatrin	T42.6X1	T42.6X2	T42.6X3	T42.6X4	T42.6X5	T42.6X6
Viloxazine	T43.291	T43.292	T43.293	T43.294	T43.295	T43.296
Viminol	T39.8X1	T39.8X2	T39.8X3	T39.8X4	T39.8X5	T39.8X6
Vinbarbital, vinbarbitone	T42.3X1	T42.3X2	T42.3X3	T42.3X4	T42.3X5	T42.3X6
Vinblastine	T45.1X1	T45.1X2	T45.1X3	T45.1X4	T45.1X5	T45.1X6
Vinburnine	T46.7X1	T46.7X2	T46.7X3	T46.7X4	T46.7X5	T46.7X6
Vincamine	T45.1X1	T45.1X2	T45.1X3	T45.1X4	T45.1X5	T45.1X6
Vincristine	T45.1X1	T45.1X2	T45.1X3	T45.1X4	T45.1X5	T45.1X6
Vindesine	T45.1X1	T45.1X2	T45.1X3	T45.1X4	T45.1X5	T45.1X6
Vinesthene, vinethene	T41.0X1	T41.0X2	T41.0X3	T41.0X4	T41.0X5	T41.0X6
Vinorelbine tartrate	T45.1X1	T45.1X2	T45.1X3	T45.1X4	T45.1X5	T45.1X6
Vinpocetine	T46.7X1	T46.7X2	T46.7X3	T46.7X4	T46.7X5	T46.7X6
Vinyl						
acetate	T65.891	T65.892	T65.893	T65.894	—	—
bital	T42.3X1	T42.3X2	T42.3X3	T42.3X4	T42.3X5	T42.3X6
bromide	T65.891	T65.892	T65.893	T65.894	—	—
chloride	T59.891	T59.892	T59.893	T59.894	—	—
ether	T41.0X1	T41.0X2	T41.0X3	T41.0X4	T41.0X5	T41.0X6
Vinylbital	T42.3X1	T42.3X2	T42.3X3	T42.3X4	T42.3X5	T42.3X6
Vinylidene chloride	T65.891	T65.892	T65.893	T65.894	—	—
Vioform	T37.8X1	T37.8X2	T37.8X3	T37.8X4	T37.8X5	T37.8X6
topical	T49.0X1	T49.0X2	T49.0X3	T49.0X4	T49.0X5	T49.0X6
Viomycin	T36.8X1	T36.8X2	T36.8X3	T36.8X4	T36.8X5	T36.8X6
Viosterol	T45.2X1	T45.2X2	T45.2X3	T45.2X4	T45.2X5	T45.2X6
Viper (venom)	T63.091	T63.092	T63.093	T63.094	—	—
Viprynium	T37.4X1	T37.4X2	T37.4X3	T37.4X4	T37.4X5	T37.4X6
Viquidil	T46.7X1	T46.7X2	T46.7X3	T46.7X4	T46.7X5	T46.7X6
Viral vaccine NEC	T50.B91	T50.B92	T50.B93	T50.B94	T50.B95	T50.B96
Virginiamycin	T36.8X1	T36.8X2	T36.8X3	T36.8X4	T36.8X5	T36.8X6
Virugon	T37.5X1	T37.5X2	T37.5X3	T37.5X4	T37.5X5	T37.5X6
Viscous agent	T50.901	T50.902	T50.903	T50.904	T50.905	T50.906
Visine	T49.5X1	T49.5X2	T49.5X3	T49.5X4	T49.5X5	T49.5X6
Visnadine	T46.3X1	T46.3X2	T46.3X3	T46.3X4	T46.3X5	T46.3X6
Vitamin NEC	T45.2X1	T45.2X2	T45.2X3	T45.2X4	T45.2X5	T45.2X6
A	T45.2X1	T45.2X2	T45.2X3	T45.2X4	T45.2X5	T45.2X6
B1	T45.2X1	T45.2X2	T45.2X3	T45.2X4	T45.2X5	T45.2X6
B2	T45.2X1	T45.2X2	T45.2X3	T45.2X4	T45.2X5	T45.2X6
B6	T45.2X1	T45.2X2	T45.2X3	T45.2X4	T45.2X5	T45.2X6
B12	T45.2X1	T45.2X2	T45.2X3	T45.2X4	T45.2X5	T45.2X6
B15	T45.2X1	T45.2X2	T45.2X3	T45.2X4	T45.2X5	T45.2X6
B NEC	T45.2X1	T45.2X2	T45.2X3	T45.2X4	T45.2X5	T45.2X6
nicotinic acid	T46.7X1	T46.7X2	T46.7X3	T46.7X4	T46.7X5	T46.7X6
C	T45.2X1	T45.2X2	T45.2X3	T45.2X4	T45.2X5	T45.2X6
D	T45.2X1	T45.2X2	T45.2X3	T45.2X4	T45.2X5	T45.2X6
D2	T45.2X1	T45.2X2	T45.2X3	T45.2X4	T45.2X5	T45.2X6
D3	T45.2X1	T45.2X2	T45.2X3	T45.2X4	T45.2X5	T45.2X6
E	T45.2X1	T45.2X2	T45.2X3	T45.2X4	T45.2X5	T45.2X6
E acetate	T45.2X1	T45.2X2	T45.2X3	T45.2X4	T45.2X5	T45.2X6
hematopoietic	T45.8X1	T45.8X2	T45.8X3	T45.8X4	T45.8X5	T45.8X6
K1	T45.7X1	T45.7X2	T45.7X3	T45.7X4	T45.7X5	T45.7X6
K2	T45.7X1	T45.7X2	T45.7X3	T45.7X4	T45.7X5	T45.7X6
K NEC	T45.7X1	T45.7X2	T45.7X3	T45.7X4	T45.7X5	T45.7X6
PP	T45.2X1	T45.2X2	T45.2X3	T45.2X4	T45.2X5	T45.2X6
ulceroprotectant	T47.1X1	T47.1X2	T47.1X3	T47.1X4	T47.1X5	T47.1X6
Vleminckx's solution	T49.4X1	T49.4X2	T49.4X3	T49.4X4	T49.4X5	T49.4X6
Voltaren — see Diclofenac						
sodium						
Warfarin	T45.511	T45.512	T45.513	T45.514	T45.515	T45.516
rodenticide	T60.4X1-	T60.4X2-	T60.4X3-	T60.4X4-	—	—
sodium	T45.511	T45.512	T45.513	T45.514	T45.515	T45.516
Wasp (sting)	T63.461	T63.462	T63.463	T63.464	—	—
Water						
balance drug	T50.3X1	T50.3X2	T50.3X3	T50.3X4	T50.3X5	T50.3X6
distilled	T50.3X1	T50.3X2	T50.3X3	T50.3X4	T50.3X5	T50.3X6
gas — see Gas, water						

Substance	Poisoning, Accidental (unintentional)	Poisoning, Intentional Self-harm	Poisoning, Assault	Poisoning, Undetermined	Adverse Effect	Under-dosing
Water — continued						
gas — see Gas, water —						
continued						
incomplete combustion of —						
see Carbon, monoxide,						
fuel, utility						
hemlock	T62.2X1	T62.2X2	T62.2X3	T62.2X4	—	—
moccasin (venom)	T63.061	T63.062	T63.063	T63.064	—	—
purified	T50.3X1	T50.3X2	T50.3X3	T50.3X4	T50.3X5	T50.3X6
Wax (paraffin) (petroleum)	T52.0X1	T52.0X2	T52.0X3	T52.0X4	—	—
automobile	T65.891	T65.892	T65.893	T65.894	—	—
floor	T52.0X1	T52.0X2	T52.0X3	T52.0X4	—	—
Weed killers NEC	T60.3X1	T60.3X2	T60.3X3	T60.3X4	—	—
Welldorm	T42.6X1	T42.6X2	T42.6X3	T42.6X4	T42.6X5	T42.6X6
White						
arsenic	T57.0X1	T57.0X2	T57.0X3	T57.0X4	—	—
hellebore	T62.2X1	T62.2X2	T62.2X3	T62.2X4	—	—
lotion (keratolytic)	T49.4X1	T49.4X2	T49.4X3	T49.4X4	T49.4X5	T49.4X6
spirit	T52.0X1	T52.0X2	T52.0X3	T52.0X4	—	—
Whitewash	T65.891	T65.892	T65.893	T65.894	—	—
Whole blood (human)	T45.8X1	T45.8X2	T45.8X3	T45.8X4	T45.8X5	T45.8X6
Wild						
black cherry	T62.2X1	T62.2X2	T62.2X3	T62.2X4	—	—
poisonous plants NEC	T62.2X1	T62.2X2	T62.2X3	T62.2X4	—	—
Window cleaning fluid	T65.891	T65.892	T65.893	T65.894	—	—
Wintergreen (oil)	T49.3X1	T49.3X2	T49.3X3	T49.3X4	T49.3X5	T49.3X6
Wisterine	T62.2X1	T62.2X2	T62.2X3	T62.2X4	—	—
Witch hazel	T49.2X1	T49.2X2	T49.2X3	T49.2X4	T49.2X5	T49.2X6
Wood alcohol or spirit	T51.1X1	T51.1X2	T51.1X3	T51.1X4	—	—
Wool fat (hydrous)	T49.3X1	T49.3X2	T49.3X3	T49.3X4	T49.3X5	T49.3X6
Woorali	T48.1X1	T48.1X2	T48.1X3	T48.1X4	T48.1X5	T48.1X6
Wormseed, American	T37.4X1	T37.4X2	T37.4X3	T37.4X4	T37.4X5	T37.4X6
Xamoterol	T44.5X1	T44.5X2	T44.5X3	T44.5X4	T44.5X5	T44.5X6
Xanthine diuretics	T50.2X1	T50.2X2	T50.2X3	T50.2X4	T50.2X5	T50.2X6
Xanthinol nicotinate	T46.7X1	T46.7X2	T46.7X3	T46.7X4	T46.7X5	T46.7X6
Xanthotoxin	T49.3X1	T49.3X2	T49.3X3	T49.3X4	T49.3X5	T49.3X6
Xantinol nicotinate	T46.7X1	T46.7X2	T46.7X3	T46.7X4	T46.7X5	T46.7X6
Xantocillin	T36.0X1	T36.0X2	T36.0X3	T36.0X4	T36.0X5	T36.0X6
Xenon (127Xe) (133Xe)	T50.8X1	T50.8X2	T50.8X3	T50.8X4	T50.8X5	T50.8X6
Xenysalate	T49.4X1	T49.4X2	T49.4X3	T49.4X4	T49.4X5	T49.4X6
Xibornol	T37.8X1	T37.8X2	T37.8X3	T37.8X4	T37.8X5	T37.8X6
Xigris	T45.511	T45.512	T45.513	T45.514	T45.515	T45.516
Xipamide	T50.2X1	T50.2X2	T50.2X3	T50.2X4	T50.2X5	T50.2X6
Xylene (vapor)	T52.2X1	T52.2X2	T52.2X3	T52.2X4	—	—
Xylocaine (infiltration) (topical)	T41.3X1	T41.3X2	T41.3X3	T41.3X4	T41.3X5	T41.3X6
nerve block (peripheral) (plexus)	T41.3X1	T41.3X2	T41.3X3	T41.3X4	T41.3X5	T41.3X6
spinal	T41.3X1	T41.3X2	T41.3X3	T41.3X4	T41.3X5	T41.3X6
Xylol (vapor)	T52.2X1	T52.2X2	T52.2X3	T52.2X4	—	—
Xylometazoline	T48.5X1	T48.5X2	T48.5X3	T48.5X4	T48.5X5	T48.5X6
Yeast	T45.2X1	T45.2X2	T45.2X3	T45.2X4	T45.2X5	T45.2X6
dried	T45.2X1	T45.2X2	T45.2X3	T45.2X4	T45.2X5	T45.2X6
Yellow						
fever vaccine	T50.B91	T50.B92	T50.B93	T50.B94	T50.B95	T50.B96
jasmine	T62.2X1	T62.2X2	T62.2X3	T62.2X4	—	—
phenolphthalein	T47.2X1	T47.2X2	T47.2X3	T47.2X4	T47.2X5	T47.2X6
Yew	T62.2X1	T62.2X2	T62.2X3	T62.2X4	—	—
Yohimbic acid	T40.991	T40.992	T40.993	T40.994	T40.995	T40.99●
Zactane	T39.8X1	T39.8X2	T39.8X3	T39.8X4	T39.8X5	T39.8X●
Zalcitabine	T37.5X1	T37.5X2	T37.5X3	T37.5X4	T37.5X5	T37.5X●
Zaroxolyn	T50.2X1	T50.2X2	T50.2X3	T50.2X4	T50.2X5	T50.2X●
Zephiran (topical)	T49.0X1	T49.0X2	T49.0X3	T49.0X4	T49.0X5	T49.0X●
ophthalmic preparation	T49.5X1	T49.5X2	T49.5X3	T49.5X4	T49.5X5	T49.5X●
Zeranol	T38.7X1	T38.7X2	T38.7X3	T38.7X4	T38.7X5	T38.7X
Zerone	T51.1X1	T51.1X2	T51.1X3	T51.1X4	—	—
Zidovudine	T37.5X1	T37.5X2	T37.5X3	T37.5X4	T37.5X5	T37.5X●
Zimeldine	T43.221	T43.222	T43.223	T43.224	T43.225	T43.22●
Zinc (compounds) (fumes) (vapor)	T56.5X1	T56.5X2	T56.5X3	T56.5X4	—	—
NEC						
anti-infectives	T49.0X1	T49.0X2	T49.0X3	T49.0X4	T49.0X5	T49.0X●
antivaricose	T46.8X1	T46.8X2	T46.8X3	T46.8X4	T46.8X5	T46.8X●
bacitracin	T49.0X1	T49.0X2	T49.0X3	T49.0X4	T49.0X5	T49.0X●
chloride (mouthwash)	T49.6X1	T49.6X2	T49.6X3	T49.6X4	T49.6X5	T49.6X●
chromate	T56.5X1	T56.5X2	T56.5X3	T56.5X4	—	—
gelatin	T49.3X1	T49.3X2	T49.3X3	T49.3X4	T49.3X5	T49.3X
oxide	T49.3X1	T49.3X2	T49.3X3	T49.3X4	T49.3X5	T49.3X
plaster	T49.3X1	T49.3X2	T49.3X3	T49.3X4	T49.3X5	T49.3X
peroxide	T49.0X1	T49.0X2	T49.0X3	T49.0X4	T49.0X5	T49.0●
pesticides	T56.5X1	T56.5X2	T56.5X3	T56.5X4	—	—
phosphide	T60.4X1	T60.4X2	T60.4X3	T60.4X4	—	—
pyrithionate	T49.4X1	T49.4X2	T49.4X3	T49.4X4	T49.4X5	T49.4X
stearate	T49.3X1	T49.3X2	T49.3X3	T49.3X4	T49.3X5	T49.3X

Substance	Poisoning, Accidental (unintentional)	Poisoning, Intentional Self-harm	Poisoning, Assault	Poisoning, Undetermined	Adverse Effect	Under-dosing
Zinc (compounds) (fumes) (vapor)						
NEC — *continued*						
sulfate	T49.5X1	T49.5X2	T49.5X3	T49.5X4	T49.5X5	T49.5X6
ENT agent	T49.6X1	T49.6X2	T49.6X3	T49.6X4	T49.6X5	T49.6X6
ophthalmic solution	T49.5X1	T49.5X2	T49.5X3	T49.5X4	T49.5X5	T49.5X6
topical NEC	T49.0X1	T49.0X2	T49.0X3	T49.0X4	T49.0X5	T49.0X6
undecylenate	T49.0X1	T49.0X2	T49.0X3	T49.0X4	T49.0X5	T49.0X6
Zineb	T60.0X1	T60.0X2	T60.0X3	T60.0X4	—	—
Zinostatin	T45.1X1	T45.1X2	T45.1X3	T45.1X4	T45.1X5	T45.1X6
Zipeprol	T48.3X1	T48.3X2	T48.3X3	T48.3X4	T48.3X5	T48.3X6
Zofenopril	T46.4X1	T46.4X2	T46.4X3	T46.4X4	T46.4X5	T46.4X6
Zolpidem	T42.6X1	T42.6X2	T42.6X3	T42.6X4	T42.6X5	T42.6X6
Zomepirac	T39.391	T39.392	T39.393	T39.394	T39.395	T39.396
Zopiclone	T42.6X1	T42.6X2	T42.6X3	T42.6X4	T42.6X5	T42.6X6
Zorubicin	T45.1X1	T45.1X2	T45.1X3	T45.1X4	T45.1X5	T45.1X6
Zotepine	T43.591	T43.592	T43.593	T43.594	T43.595	T43.596
Zovant	T45.511	T45.512	T45.513	T45.514	T45.515	T45.516
Zoxazolamine	T42.8X1	T42.8X2	T42.8X3	T42.8X4	T42.8X5	T42.8X6
Zuclopenthixol	T43.4X1	T43.4X2	T43.4X3	T43.4X4	T43.4X5	T43.4X6
Zygadenus (venenosus)	T62.2X1	T62.2X2	T62.2X3	T62.2X4	—	—
Zyprexa	T43.591	T43.592	T43.593	T43.594	T43.595	T43.596

External Causes Index

A

Abandonment (causing exposure to weather conditions) (with intent to injure or kill) NEC X58 ☑
Abuse (adult) (child) (mental) (physical) (sexual) X58 ☑
Accident (to) X58 ☑
  aircraft (in transit) (powered) — *see also* Accident, transport, aircraft
    due to, caused by cataclysm — *see* Forces of nature, by type
  animal-drawn vehicle — *see* Accident, transport, animal-drawn vehicle occupant
  animal-rider — *see* Accident, transport, animal-rider
  automobile — *see* Accident, transport, car occupant
  bare foot water skier V94.4 ☑
  boat, boating — *see also* Accident, watercraft
    striking swimmer
      powered V94.11 ☑
      unpowered V94.12 ☑
  bus — *see* Accident, transport, bus occupant
  cable car, not on rails V98.0 ☑
    on rails — *see* Accident, transport, streetcar occupant
  car — *see* Accident, transport, car occupant
  caused by, due to
    animal NEC W64 ☑
    chain hoist W24.0 ☑
    cold (excessive) — *see* Exposure, cold
    corrosive liquid, substance — *see* Table of Drugs and Chemicals
    cutting or piercing instrument — *see* Contact, with, by type of instrument
    drive belt W24.0 ☑
    electric
      current — *see* Exposure, electric current
      motor — *see also* Contact, with, by type of machine W31.3 ☑
        current (of) W86.8 ☑
    environmental factor NEC X58 ☑
    explosive material — *see* Explosion
    fire, flames — *see* Exposure, fire
    firearm missile — *see* Discharge, firearm by type
    heat (excessive) — *see* Heat
    hot — *see* Contact, with, hot
    ignition — *see* Ignition
    lifting device W24.0 ☑
    lightning — *see* subcategory T75.0 ☑
      causing fire — *see* Exposure, fire
    machine, machinery — *see* Contact, with, by type of machine
    natural factor NEC X58 ☑
    pulley (block) W24.0 ☑
    radiation — *see* Radiation
    steam X13.1 ☑
      inhalation X13.0 ☑
      pipe X16 ☑
    thunderbolt — *see* subcategory T75.0 ☑
      causing fire — *see* Exposure, fire
    transmission device W24.1 ☑
  coach — *see* Accident, transport, bus occupant
  coal car — *see* Accident, transport, industrial vehicle occupant
  diving — *see also* Fall, into, water
    with
      drowning or submersion — *see* Drowning
  forklift — *see* Accident, transport, industrial vehicle occupant
  heavy transport vehicle NOS — *see* Accident, transport, truck occupant
  ice yacht V98.2 ☑
  in
    medical, surgical procedure
      as, or due to misadventure — *see* Misadventure
      causing an abnormal reaction or later complication without mention of misadventure — *see also* Complication of or following, by type of procedure Y84.9
  land yacht V98.1 ☑
  late effect of — *see* W00-X58 with 7th character S
  logging car — *see* Accident, transport, industrial vehicle occupant
  machine, machinery — *see also* Contact, with, by type of machine
    on board watercraft V93.69 ☑
      explosion — *see* Explosion, in, watercraft

Accident — *continued*
  machine, machinery — *see also* Contact, with, by type of machine — *continued*
    on board watercraft — *continued*
      fire — *see* Burn, on board watercraft
      powered craft V93.63 ☑
        ferry boat V93.61 ☑
        fishing boat V93.62 ☑
        jetskis V93.63 ☑
        liner V93.61 ☑
        merchant ship V93.60 ☑
        passenger ship V93.61 ☑
        sailboat V93.64 ☑
  mine tram — *see* Accident, transport, industrial vehicle occupant
  mobility scooter (motorized) — *see* Accident, transport, pedestrian, conveyance, specified type NEC
  motor scooter — *see* Accident, transport, motorcyclist
  motor vehicle NOS (traffic) — *see also* Accident, transport V89.2 ☑
    nontraffic V89.0 ☑
    three-wheeled NOS — *see* Accident, transport, three-wheeled motor vehicle occupant
  motorcycle NOS — *see* Accident, transport, motorcyclist
  nonmotor vehicle NOS (nontraffic) — *see also* Accident, transport V89.1 ☑
    traffic NOS V89.3 ☑
  nontraffic (victim's mode of transport NOS) V88.9 ☑
    collision (between) V88.7 ☑
      bus and truck V88.5 ☑
      car and:
        bus V88.3 ☑
        pickup V88.2 ☑
        three-wheeled motor vehicle V88.0 ☑
        train V88.6 ☑
        truck V88.4 ☑
        two-wheeled motor vehicle V88.0 ☑
        van V88.2 ☑
      specified vehicle NEC and:
        three-wheeled motor vehicle V88.1 ☑
        two-wheeled motor vehicle V88.1 ☑
      known mode of transport — *see* Accident, transport, by type of vehicle
    noncollision V88.8 ☑
  on board watercraft V93.89 ☑
    powered craft V93.83 ☑
      ferry boat V93.81 ☑
      fishing boat V93.82 ☑
      jetskis V93.83 ☑
      liner V93.81 ☑
      merchant ship V93.80 ☑
      passenger ship V93.81 ☑
    unpowered craft V93.88 ☑
      canoe V93.85 ☑
      inflatable V93.86 ☑
        in tow
          recreational V94.31 ☑
          specified NEC V94.32 ☑
      kayak V93.85 ☑
      sailboat V93.84 ☑
      surf-board V93.88 ☑
      water skis V93.87 ☑
      windsurfer V93.88 ☑
  parachutist V97.29 ☑
    entangled in object V97.21 ☑
    injured on landing V97.22 ☑
  pedal cycle — *see* Accident, transport, pedal cyclist
  pedestrian (on foot)
    with
      another pedestrian W51 ☑
        on pedestrian conveyance NEC V00.09 ☑
        with fall W03 ☑
          due to ice or snow W00.0 ☑
      roller skater (in-line) V00.01 ☑
      skate boarder V00.02 ☑
      transport vehicle — *see* Accident, transport
    on pedestrian conveyance — *see* Accident, transport, pedestrian, conveyance
  pick-up truck or van — *see* Accident, transport, pickup truck occupant
  quarry truck — *see* Accident, transport, industrial vehicle occupant
  railway vehicle (any) (in motion) — *see* Accident, transport, railway vehicle occupant
    due to cataclysm — *see* Forces of nature, by type

Accident — *continued*
  scooter (non-motorized) — *see* Accident, transport, pedestrian, conveyance, scooter
  sequelae of — *see* categories W00-X58 with 7th character S
  skateboard — *see* Accident, transport, pedestrian, conveyance, skateboard
  ski(ing) — *see* Accident, transport, pedestrian, conveyance
    lift V98.3 ☑
  specified cause NEC X58 ☑
  streetcar — *see* Accident, transport, streetcar occupant
  traffic (victim's mode of transport NOS) V87.9 ☑
    collision (between) V87.7 ☑
      bus and truck V87.5 ☑
      car and:
        bus V87.3 ☑
        pickup V87.2 ☑
        three-wheeled motor vehicle V87.0 ☑
        train V87.6 ☑
        truck V87.4 ☑
        two-wheeled motor vehicle V87.0 ☑
        van V87.2 ☑
      specified vehicle NEC V86.39 ☑
        and
          three-wheeled motor vehicle V87.1 ☑
          two-wheeled motor vehicle V87.1 ☑
        driver V86.09 ☑
        passenger V86.19 ☑
        person on outside V86.29 ☑
        while boarding or alighting V86.49 ☑
    known mode of transport — *see* Accident, transport, by type of vehicle
    noncollision V87.8 ☑
  transport (involving injury to) V99 ☑
    18 wheeler — *see* Accident, transport, truck occupant
    agricultural vehicle occupant (nontraffic) V84.9 ☑
      driver V84.5 ☑
      hanger-on V84.7 ☑
      passenger V84.6 ☑
      traffic V84.3 ☑
        driver V84.0 ☑
        hanger-on V84.2 ☑
        passenger V84.1 ☑
      while boarding or alighting V84.4 ☑
    aircraft NEC V97.89 ☑
      military NEC V97.818 ☑
        civilian injured by V97.811 ☑
        with civilian aircraft V97.810 ☑
      occupant injured (in)
        nonpowered craft accident V96.9 ☑
          balloon V96.00 ☑
            collision V96.03 ☑
            crash V96.01 ☑
            explosion V96.05 ☑
            fire V96.04 ☑
            forced landing V96.02 ☑
            specified type NEC V96.09 ☑
          glider V96.20 ☑
            collision V96.23 ☑
            crash V96.21 ☑
            explosion V96.25 ☑
            fire V96.24 ☑
            forced landing V96.22 ☑
            specified type NEC V96.29 ☑
          hang glider V96.10 ☑
            collision V96.13 ☑
            crash V96.11 ☑
            explosion V96.15 ☑
            fire V96.14 ☑
            forced landing V96.12 ☑
            specified type NEC V96.19 ☑
          specified craft NEC V96.8 ☑
        powered craft accident V95.9 ☑
          fixed wing NEC
            commercial V95.30 ☑
              collision V95.33 ☑
              crash V95.31 ☑
              explosion V95.35 ☑
              fire V95.34 ☑
              forced landing V95.32 ☑
              specified type NEC V95.39 ☑
            private V95.20 ☑
              collision V95.23 ☑
              crash V95.21 ☑

Abandonment — Accident

Accident — continued
  transport — continued
    aircraft — continued
      occupant injured — continued
        powered craft accident — continued
          fixed wing — continued
            private — continued
              explosion V95.25 ☑
              fire V95.24 ☑
              forced landing V95.22 ☑
              specified type NEC V95.29 ☑
          glider V95.10 ☑
            collision V95.13 ☑
            crash V95.11 ☑
            explosion V95.15 ☑
            fire V95.14 ☑
            forced landing V95.12 ☑
            specified type NEC V95.19 ☑
          helicopter V95.00 ☑
            collision V95.03 ☑
            crash V95.01 ☑
            explosion V95.05 ☑
            fire V95.04 ☑
            forced landing V95.02 ☑
            specified type NEC V95.09 ☑
          spacecraft V95.40 ☑
            collision V95.43 ☑
            crash V95.41 ☑
            explosion V95.45 ☑
            fire V95.44 ☑
            forced landing V95.42 ☑
            specified type NEC V95.49 ☑
          specified craft NEC V95.8 ☑
          ultralight V95.10 ☑
            collision V95.13 ☑
            crash V95.11 ☑
            explosion V95.15 ☑
            fire V95.14 ☑
            forced landing V95.12 ☑
            specified type NEC V95.19 ☑
         specified accident NEC V97.0 ☑
        while boarding or alighting V97.1 ☑
      person (injured by)
        falling from, in or on aircraft V97.0 ☑
        machinery on aircraft V97.89 ☑
        on ground with aircraft involvement
          V97.39 ☑
        rotating propeller V97.32 ☑
        struck by object falling from aircraft V97.31 ☑
        sucked into aircraft jet V97.33 ☑
        while boarding or alighting aircraft V97.1 ☑
    airport (battery-powered) passenger vehicle — see
      Accident, transport, industrial vehicle occu-
      pant
    all-terrain vehicle occupant (nontraffic) V86.95 ☑
      driver V86.55 ☑
      dune buggy — see Accident, transport, dune
        buggy occupant
      hanger-on V86.75 ☑
      passenger V86.65 ☑
      snowmobile — see Accident, transport, snowmo-
        bile occupant
      specified type NEC V86.99 ☑
        driver V86.59 ☑
        passenger V86.69 ☑
        person on outside V86.79 ☑
      traffic V86.35 ☑
        driver V86.05 ☑
        hanger-on V86.25 ☑
        passenger V86.15 ☑
      while boarding or alighting V86.45 ☑
    ambulance occupant (traffic) V86.31 ☑
      driver V86.01 ☑
      hanger-on V86.21 ☑
      nontraffic V86.91 ☑
        driver V86.51 ☑
        hanger-on V86.71 ☑
        passenger V86.61 ☑
      passenger V86.11 ☑
      while boarding or alighting V86.41 ☑
    animal-drawn vehicle occupant (in) V80.929 ☑
      collision (with)
        animal V80.12 ☑
          being ridden V80.711 ☑
        animal-drawn vehicle V80.721 ☑
        bus V80.42 ☑

Accident — continued
  transport — continued
    animal-drawn vehicle occupant — continued
      collision — continued
        car V80.42 ☑
        fixed or stationary object V80.82 ☑
        military vehicle V80.920 ☑
        nonmotor vehicle V80.791 ☑
        pedal cycle V80.22 ☑
        pedestrian V80.12 ☑
        pickup V80.42 ☑
        railway train or vehicle V80.62 ☑
        specified motor vehicle NEC V80.52 ☑
        streetcar V80.731 ☑
        truck V80.42 ☑
        two- or three-wheeled motor vehicle
          V80.32 ☑
        van V80.42 ☑
      noncollision V80.02 ☑
      specified circumstance NEC V80.928 ☑
    animal-rider V80.919 ☑
      collision (with)
        animal V80.11 ☑
          being ridden V80.710 ☑
        animal-drawn vehicle V80.720 ☑
        bus V80.41 ☑
        car V80.41 ☑
        fixed or stationary object V80.81 ☑
        military vehicle V80.910 ☑
        nonmotor vehicle V80.790 ☑
        pedal cycle V80.21 ☑
        pedestrian V80.11 ☑
        pickup V80.41 ☑
        railway train or vehicle V80.61 ☑
        specified motor vehicle NEC V80.51 ☑
        streetcar V80.730 ☑
        truck V80.41 ☑
        two- or three-wheeled motor vehicle
          V80.31 ☑
        van V80.41 ☑
      noncollision V80.018 ☑
        specified as horse rider V80.010 ☑
      specified circumstance NEC V80.918 ☑
    armored car — see Accident, transport, truck occu-
      pant
    battery-powered truck (baggage) (mail) — see Ac-
      cident, transport, industrial vehicle occupant
    bus occupant V79.9 ☑
      collision (with)
        animal (traffic) V70.9 ☑
          being ridden (traffic) V76.9 ☑
            nontraffic V76.3 ☑
            while boarding or alighting V76.4 ☑
          nontraffic V70.3 ☑
          while boarding or alighting V70.4 ☑
        animal-drawn vehicle (traffic) V76.9 ☑
          nontraffic V76.3 ☑
          while boarding or alighting V76.4 ☑
        bus (traffic) V74.9 ☑
          nontraffic V74.3 ☑
          while boarding or alighting V74.4 ☑
        car (traffic) V73.9 ☑
          nontraffic V73.3 ☑
          while boarding or alighting V73.4 ☑
        motor vehicle NOS (traffic) V79.60 ☑
          nontraffic V79.20 ☑
          specified type NEC (traffic) V79.69 ☑
            nontraffic V79.29 ☑
        pedal cycle (traffic) V71.9 ☑
          nontraffic V71.3 ☑
          while boarding or alighting V71.4 ☑
        pickup truck (traffic) V73.9 ☑
          nontraffic V73.3 ☑
          while boarding or alighting V73.4 ☑
        railway vehicle (traffic) V75.9 ☑
          nontraffic V75.3 ☑
          while boarding or alighting V75.4 ☑
        specified vehicle NEC (traffic) V76.9 ☑
          nontraffic V76.3 ☑
          while boarding or alighting V76.4 ☑
        stationary object (traffic) V77.9 ☑
          nontraffic V77.3 ☑
          while boarding or alighting V77.4 ☑
        streetcar (traffic) V76.9 ☑
          nontraffic V76.3 ☑
          while boarding or alighting V76.4 ☑

Accident — continued
  transport — continued
    bus occupant — continued
      collision — continued
        three wheeled motor vehicle (traffic) V72.9 ☑
          nontraffic V72.3 ☑
          while boarding or alighting V72.4 ☑
        truck (traffic) V74.9 ☑
          nontraffic V74.3 ☑
          while boarding or alighting V74.4 ☑
        two wheeled motor vehicle (traffic) V72.9 ☑
          nontraffic V72.3 ☑
          while boarding or alighting V72.4 ☑
        van (traffic) V73.9 ☑
          nontraffic V73.3 ☑
          while boarding or alighting V73.4 ☑
      driver
        collision (with)
          animal (traffic) V70.5 ☑
            being ridden (traffic) V76.5 ☑
              nontraffic V76.0 ☑
            nontraffic V70.0 ☑
          animal-drawn vehicle (traffic) V76.5 ☑
            nontraffic V76.0 ☑
          bus (traffic) V74.5 ☑
            nontraffic V74.0 ☑
          car (traffic) V73.5 ☑
            nontraffic V73.0 ☑
          motor vehicle NOS (traffic) V79.40 ☑
            nontraffic V79.00 ☑
            specified type NEC (traffic) V79.49 ☑
              nontraffic V79.09 ☑
          pedal cycle (traffic) V71.5 ☑
            nontraffic V71.0 ☑
          pickup truck (traffic) V73.5 ☑
            nontraffic V73.0 ☑
          railway vehicle (traffic) V75.5 ☑
            nontraffic V75.0 ☑
          specified vehicle NEC (traffic) V76.5 ☑
            nontraffic V76.0 ☑
          stationary object (traffic) V77.5 ☑
            nontraffic V77.0 ☑
          streetcar (traffic) V76.5 ☑
            nontraffic V76.0 ☑
          three wheeled motor vehicle (traffic)
            V72.5 ☑
            nontraffic V72.0 ☑
          truck (traffic) V74.5 ☑
            nontraffic V74.0 ☑
          two wheeled motor vehicle (traffic)
            V72.5 ☑
            nontraffic V72.0 ☑
          van (traffic) V73.5 ☑
            nontraffic V73.0 ☑
        noncollision accident (traffic) V78.5 ☑
          nontraffic V78.0 ☑
      hanger-on
        collision (with)
          animal (traffic) V70.7 ☑
            being ridden (traffic) V76.7 ☑
              nontraffic V76.2 ☑
            nontraffic V70.2 ☑
          animal-drawn vehicle (traffic) V76.7 ☑
            nontraffic V76.2 ☑
          bus (traffic) V74.7 ☑
            nontraffic V74.2 ☑
          car (traffic) V73.7 ☑
            nontraffic V73.2 ☑
          pedal cycle (traffic) V71.7 ☑
            nontraffic V71.2 ☑
          pickup truck (traffic) V73.7 ☑
            nontraffic V73.2 ☑
          railway vehicle (traffic) V75.7 ☑
            nontraffic V75.2 ☑
          specified vehicle NEC (traffic) V76.7 ☑
            nontraffic V76.2 ☑
          stationary object (traffic) V77.7 ☑
            nontraffic V77.2 ☑
          streetcar (traffic) V76.7 ☑
            nontraffic V76.2 ☑
          three wheeled motor vehicle (traffic)
            V72.7 ☑
            nontraffic V72.2 ☑
          truck (traffic) V74.7 ☑
            nontraffic V74.2 ☑

External Causes Index

Accident — Accident

Accident — *continued*
  transport — *continued*
    bus occupant — *continued*
      hanger-on — *continued*
        collision — *continued*
          two wheeled motor vehicle (traffic)
            V72.7 ☑
            nontraffic V72.2 ☑
          van (traffic) V73.7 ☑
            nontraffic V73.2 ☑
        noncollision accident (traffic) V78.7 ☑
          nontraffic V78.2 ☑
      noncollision accident (traffic) V78.9 ☑
        nontraffic V78.3 ☑
        while boarding or alighting V78.4 ☑
      nontraffic V79.3 ☑
      passenger
        collision (with)
          animal (traffic) V70.6 ☑
            being ridden (traffic) V76.6 ☑
              nontraffic V76.1 ☑
            nontraffic V70.1 ☑
          animal-drawn vehicle (traffic) V76.6 ☑
            nontraffic V76.1 ☑
          bus (traffic) V74.6 ☑
            nontraffic V74.1 ☑
          car (traffic) V73.6 ☑
            nontraffic V73.1 ☑
          motor vehicle NOS (traffic) V79.50 ☑
            nontraffic V79.10 ☑
            specified type NEC (traffic) V79.59 ☑
              nontraffic V79.19 ☑
          pedal cycle (traffic) V71.6 ☑
            nontraffic V71.1 ☑
          pickup truck (traffic) V73.6 ☑
            nontraffic V73.1 ☑
          railway vehicle (traffic) V75.6 ☑
            nontraffic V75.1 ☑
          specified vehicle NEC (traffic) V76.6 ☑
            nontraffic V76.1 ☑
          stationary object (traffic) V77.6 ☑
            nontraffic V77.1 ☑
          streetcar (traffic) V76.6 ☑
            nontraffic V76.1 ☑
          three wheeled motor vehicle (traffic)
            V72.6 ☑
            nontraffic V72.1 ☑
          truck (traffic) V74.6 ☑
            nontraffic V74.1 ☑
          two wheeled motor vehicle (traffic)
            V72.6 ☑
            nontraffic V72.1 ☑
          van (traffic) V73.6 ☑
            nontraffic V73.1 ☑
        noncollision accident (traffic) V78.6 ☑
          nontraffic V78.1 ☑
      specified type NEC V79.88 ☑
      military vehicle V79.81 ☑
    cable car, not on rails V98.0 ☑
      on rails — *see* Accident, transport, streetcar occupant
    car occupant V49.9 ☑
      ambulance occupant — *see* Accident, transport, ambulance occupant
      collision (with)
        animal (traffic) V40.9 ☑
          being ridden (traffic) V46.9 ☑
            nontraffic V46.3 ☑
            while boarding or alighting V46.4 ☑
          nontraffic V40.3 ☑
          while boarding or alighting V40.4 ☑
        animal-drawn vehicle (traffic) V46.9 ☑
          nontraffic V46.3 ☑
          while boarding or alighting V46.4 ☑
        bus (traffic) V44.9 ☑
          nontraffic V44.3 ☑
          while boarding or alighting V44.4 ☑
        car (traffic) V43.92 ☑
          nontraffic V43.32 ☑
          while boarding or alighting V43.42 ☑
        motor vehicle NOS (traffic) V49.60 ☑
          nontraffic V49.20 ☑
          specified type NEC (traffic) V49.69 ☑
            nontraffic V49.29 ☑
        pedal cycle (traffic) V41.9 ☑
          nontraffic V41.3 ☑

Accident — *continued*
  transport — *continued*
    car occupant — *continued*
      collision — *continued*
        pedal cycle — *continued*
          while boarding or alighting V41.4 ☑
        pickup truck (traffic) V43.93 ☑
          nontraffic V43.33 ☑
          while boarding or alighting V43.43 ☑
        railway vehicle (traffic) V45.9 ☑
          nontraffic V45.3 ☑
          while boarding or alighting V45.4 ☑
        specified vehicle NEC (traffic) V46.9 ☑
          nontraffic V46.3 ☑
          while boarding or alighting V46.4 ☑
        sport utility vehicle (traffic) V43.91 ☑
          nontraffic V43.31 ☑
          while boarding or alighting V43.41 ☑
        stationary object (traffic) V47.9 ☑
          nontraffic V47.3 ☑
          while boarding or alighting V47.4 ☑
        streetcar (traffic) V46.9 ☑
          nontraffic V46.3 ☑
          while boarding or alighting V46.4 ☑
        three wheeled motor vehicle (traffic) V42.9 ☑
          nontraffic V42.3 ☑
          while boarding or alighting V42.4 ☑
        truck (traffic) V44.9 ☑
          nontraffic V44.3 ☑
          while boarding or alighting V44.4 ☑
        two wheeled motor vehicle (traffic) V42.9 ☑
          nontraffic V42.3 ☑
          while boarding or alighting V42.4 ☑
        van (traffic) V43.94 ☑
          nontraffic V43.34 ☑
          while boarding or alighting V43.44 ☑
      driver
        collision (with)
          animal (traffic) V40.5 ☑
            being ridden (traffic) V46.5 ☑
              nontraffic V46.0 ☑
            nontraffic V40.0 ☑
          animal-drawn vehicle (traffic) V46.5 ☑
            nontraffic V46.0 ☑
          bus (traffic) V44.5 ☑
            nontraffic V44.0 ☑
          car (traffic) V43.52 ☑
            nontraffic V43.02 ☑
          motor vehicle NOS (traffic) V49.40 ☑
            nontraffic V49.00 ☑
            specified type NEC (traffic) V49.49 ☑
              nontraffic V49.09 ☑
          pedal cycle (traffic) V41.5 ☑
            nontraffic V41.0 ☑
          pickup truck (traffic) V43.53 ☑
            nontraffic V43.03 ☑
          railway vehicle (traffic) V45.5 ☑
            nontraffic V45.0 ☑
          specified vehicle NEC (traffic) V46.5 ☑
            nontraffic V46.0 ☑
          sport utility vehicle (traffic) V43.51 ☑
            nontraffic V43.01 ☑
          stationary object (traffic) V47.5 ☑
            nontraffic V47.0 ☑
          streetcar (traffic) V46.5 ☑
            nontraffic V46.0 ☑
          three wheeled motor vehicle (traffic)
            V42.5 ☑
            nontraffic V42.0 ☑
          truck (traffic) V44.5 ☑
            nontraffic V44.0 ☑
          two wheeled motor vehicle (traffic)
            V42.5 ☑
            nontraffic V42.0 ☑
          van (traffic) V43.54 ☑
            nontraffic V43.04 ☑
        noncollision accident (traffic) V48.5 ☑
          nontraffic V48.0 ☑
      hanger-on
        collision (with)
          animal (traffic) V40.7 ☑
            being ridden (traffic) V46.7 ☑
              nontraffic V46.2 ☑
            nontraffic V40.2 ☑
          animal-drawn vehicle (traffic) V46.7 ☑
            nontraffic V46.2 ☑

Accident — *continued*
  transport — *continued*
    car occupant — *continued*
      hanger-on — *continued*
        collision — *continued*
          bus (traffic) V44.7 ☑
            nontraffic V44.2 ☑
          car (traffic) V43.72 ☑
            nontraffic V43.22 ☑
          pedal cycle (traffic) V41.7 ☑
            nontraffic V41.2 ☑
          pickup truck (traffic) V43.73 ☑
            nontraffic V43.23 ☑
          railway vehicle (traffic) V45.7 ☑
            nontraffic V45.2 ☑
          specified vehicle NEC (traffic) V46.7 ☑
            nontraffic V46.2 ☑
          sport utility vehicle (traffic) V43.71 ☑
            nontraffic V43.21 ☑
          stationary object (traffic) V47.7 ☑
            nontraffic V47.2 ☑
          streetcar (traffic) V46.7 ☑
            nontraffic V46.2 ☑
          three wheeled motor vehicle (traffic)
            V42.7 ☑
            nontraffic V42.2 ☑
          truck (traffic) V44.7 ☑
            nontraffic V44.2 ☑
          two wheeled motor vehicle (traffic)
            V42.7 ☑
            nontraffic V42.2 ☑
          van (traffic) V43.74 ☑
            nontraffic V43.24 ☑
        noncollision accident (traffic) V48.7 ☑
          nontraffic V48.2 ☑
      noncollision accident (traffic) V48.9 ☑
        nontraffic V48.3 ☑
        while boarding or alighting V48.4 ☑
      nontraffic V49.3 ☑
      passenger
        collision (with)
          animal (traffic) V40.6 ☑
            being ridden (traffic) V46.6 ☑
              nontraffic V46.1 ☑
            nontraffic V40.1 ☑
          animal-drawn vehicle (traffic) V46.6 ☑
            nontraffic V46.1 ☑
          bus (traffic) V44.6 ☑
            nontraffic V44.1 ☑
          car (traffic) V43.62 ☑
            nontraffic V43.12 ☑
          motor vehicle NOS (traffic) V49.50 ☑
            nontraffic V49.10 ☑
            specified type NEC (traffic) V49.59 ☑
              nontraffic V49.19 ☑
          pedal cycle (traffic) V41.6 ☑
            nontraffic V41.1 ☑
          pickup truck (traffic) V43.63 ☑
            nontraffic V43.13 ☑
          railway vehicle (traffic) V45.6 ☑
            nontraffic V45.1 ☑
          specified vehicle NEC (traffic) V46.6 ☑
            nontraffic V46.1 ☑
          sport utility vehicle (traffic) V43.61 ☑
            nontraffic V43.11 ☑
          stationary object (traffic) V47.6 ☑
            nontraffic V47.1 ☑
          streetcar (traffic) V46.6 ☑
            nontraffic V46.1 ☑
          three wheeled motor vehicle (traffic)
            V42.6 ☑
            nontraffic V42.1 ☑
          truck (traffic) V44.6 ☑
            nontraffic V44.1 ☑
          two wheeled motor vehicle (traffic)
            V42.6 ☑
            nontraffic V42.1 ☑
          van (traffic) V43.64 ☑
            nontraffic V43.14 ☑
        noncollision accident (traffic) V48.6 ☑
          nontraffic V48.1 ☑
      specified type NEC V49.88 ☑
      military vehicle V49.81 ☑
    coal car — *see* Accident, transport, industrial vehicle occupant
    construction vehicle occupant (nontraffic) V85.9 ☑

☑ **Additional Character Required — Refer to the Tabular List for Character Selection**   ⬇ **Subterms under main terms may continue to next column or page**

Accident — *continued*
 transport — *continued*
  construction vehicle occupant — *continued*
   driver V85.5 ☑
   hanger-on V85.7 ☑
   passenger V85.6 ☑
   traffic V85.3 ☑
    driver V85.0 ☑
    hanger-on V85.2 ☑
    passenger V85.1 ☑
   while boarding or alighting V85.4 ☑
  dirt bike rider (nontraffic) V86.96 ☑
   driver V86.56 ☑
   hanger-on V86.76 ☑
   passenger V86.66 ☑
   traffic V86.36 ☑
    driver V86.06 ☑
    hanger-on V86.26 ☑
    passenger V86.16 ☑
   while boarding or alighting V86.46 ☑
  due to cataclysm — *see* Forces of nature, by type
  dune buggy occupant (nontraffic) V86.93 ☑
   driver V86.53 ☑
   hanger-on V86.73 ☑
   passenger V86.63 ☑
   traffic V86.33 ☑
    driver V86.03 ☑
    hanger-on V86.23 ☑
    passenger V86.13 ☑
   while boarding or alighting V86.43 ☑
  forklift — *see* Accident, transport, industrial vehicle
    occupant
  go cart — *see* Accident, transport, all-terrain vehicle
    occupant
  golf cart — *see* Accident, transport, all-terrain vehi-
    cle occupant
  heavy transport vehicle occupant — *see* Accident,
    transport, truck occupant
  ice yacht V98.2 ☑
  industrial vehicle occupant (nontraffic) V83.9 ☑
   driver V83.5 ☑
   hanger-on V83.7 ☑
   passenger V83.6 ☑
   traffic V83.3 ☑
    driver V83.0 ☑
    hanger-on V83.2 ☑
    passenger V83.1 ☑
   while boarding or alighting V83.4 ☑
  interurban electric car — *see* Accident, transport,
    streetcar
  land yacht V98.1 ☑
  logging car — *see* Accident, transport, industrial
    vehicle occupant
  military vehicle occupant (traffic) V86.34 ☑
   driver V86.04 ☑
   hanger-on V86.24 ☑
   nontraffic V86.94 ☑
    driver V86.54 ☑
    hanger-on V86.74 ☑
    passenger V86.64 ☑
   passenger V86.14 ☑
   while boarding or alighting V86.44 ☑
  mine tram — *see* Accident, transport, industrial ve-
    hicle occupant
  motor vehicle NEC occupant (traffic) V89.2 ☑
  motorcoach — *see* Accident, transport, bus occu-
    pant
  motor/cross bike rider — *see also* Accident, trans-
    port, dirt bike rider V86.96 ☑
  motorcyclist V29.9 ☑
   collision (with)
    animal (traffic) V20.9 ☑
     being ridden (traffic) V26.9 ☑
      nontraffic V26.2 ☑
      while boarding or alighting V26.3 ☑
     nontraffic V20.2 ☑
     while boarding or alighting V20.3 ☑
    animal-drawn vehicle (traffic) V26.9 ☑
     nontraffic V26.2 ☑
     while boarding or alighting V26.3 ☑
    bus (traffic) V24.9 ☑
     nontraffic V24.2 ☑
     while boarding or alighting V24.3 ☑
    car (traffic) V23.9 ☑
     nontraffic V23.2 ☑
     while boarding or alighting V23.3 ☑

Accident — *continued*
 transport — *continued*
  motorcyclist — *continued*
   collision — *continued*
    motor vehicle NOS (traffic) V29.60 ☑
     nontraffic V29.20 ☑
     specified type NEC (traffic) V29.69 ☑
      nontraffic V29.29 ☑
    pedal cycle (traffic) V21.9 ☑
     nontraffic V21.2 ☑
     while boarding or alighting V21.3 ☑
    pickup truck (traffic) V23.9 ☑
     nontraffic V23.2 ☑
     while boarding or alighting V23.3 ☑
    railway vehicle (traffic) V25.9 ☑
     nontraffic V25.2 ☑
     while boarding or alighting V25.3 ☑
    specified vehicle NEC (traffic) V26.9 ☑
     nontraffic V26.2 ☑
     while boarding or alighting V26.3 ☑
    stationary object (traffic) V27.9 ☑
     nontraffic V27.2 ☑
     while boarding or alighting V27.3 ☑
    streetcar (traffic) V26.9 ☑
     nontraffic V26.2 ☑
     while boarding or alighting V26.3 ☑
    three wheeled motor vehicle (traffic) V22.9 ☑
     nontraffic V22.2 ☑
     while boarding or alighting V22.3 ☑
    truck (traffic) V24.9 ☑
     nontraffic V24.2 ☑
     while boarding or alighting V24.3 ☑
    two wheeled motor vehicle (traffic) V22.9 ☑
     nontraffic V22.2 ☑
     while boarding or alighting V22.3 ☑
    van (traffic) V23.9 ☑
     nontraffic V23.2 ☑
     while boarding or alighting V23.3 ☑
   driver
    collision (with)
     animal (traffic) V20.4 ☑
      being ridden (traffic) V26.4 ☑
       nontraffic V26.0 ☑
      nontraffic V20.0 ☑
     animal-drawn vehicle (traffic) V26.4 ☑
      nontraffic V26.0 ☑
     bus (traffic) V24.4 ☑
      nontraffic V24.0 ☑
     car (traffic) V23.4 ☑
      nontraffic V23.0 ☑
     motor vehicle NOS (traffic) V29.40 ☑
      nontraffic V29.00 ☑
      specified type NEC (traffic) V29.49 ☑
       nontraffic V29.09 ☑
     pedal cycle (traffic) V21.4 ☑
      nontraffic V21.0 ☑
     pickup truck (traffic) V23.4 ☑
      nontraffic V23.0 ☑
     railway vehicle (traffic) V25.4 ☑
      nontraffic V25.0 ☑
     specified vehicle NEC (traffic) V26.4 ☑
      nontraffic V26.0 ☑
     stationary object (traffic) V27.4 ☑
      nontraffic V27.0 ☑
     streetcar (traffic) V26.4 ☑
      nontraffic V26.0 ☑
     three wheeled motor vehicle (traffic)
       V22.4 ☑
      nontraffic V22.0 ☑
     truck (traffic) V24.4 ☑
      nontraffic V24.0 ☑
     two wheeled motor vehicle (traffic)
       V22.4 ☑
      nontraffic V22.0 ☑
     van (traffic) V23.4 ☑
      nontraffic V23.0 ☑
    noncollision accident (traffic) V28.4 ☑
     nontraffic V28.0 ☑
   noncollision accident (traffic) V28.9 ☑
    nontraffic V28.2 ☑
    while boarding or alighting V28.3 ☑
   nontraffic V29.3 ☑
   passenger
    collision (with)
     animal (traffic) V20.5 ☑
      being ridden (traffic) V26.5 ☑

Accident — *continued*
 transport — *continued*
  motorcyclist — *continued*
   passenger — *continued*
    collision — *continued*
     animal — *continued*
      being ridden — *continued*
       nontraffic V26.1 ☑
      nontraffic V20.1 ☑
     animal-drawn vehicle (traffic) V26.5 ☑
      nontraffic V26.1 ☑
     bus (traffic) V24.5 ☑
      nontraffic V24.1 ☑
     car (traffic) V23.5 ☑
      nontraffic V23.1 ☑
     motor vehicle NOS (traffic) V29.50 ☑
      nontraffic V29.10 ☑
      specified type NEC (traffic) V29.59 ☑
       nontraffic V29.19 ☑
     pedal cycle (traffic) V21.5 ☑
      nontraffic V21.1 ☑
     pickup truck (traffic) V23.5 ☑
      nontraffic V23.1 ☑
     railway vehicle (traffic) V25.5 ☑
      nontraffic V25.1 ☑
     specified vehicle NEC (traffic) V26.5 ☑
      nontraffic V26.1 ☑
     stationary object (traffic) V27.5 ☑
      nontraffic V27.1 ☑
     streetcar (traffic) V26.5 ☑
      nontraffic V26.1 ☑
     three wheeled motor vehicle (traffic)
       V22.5 ☑
      nontraffic V22.1 ☑
     truck (traffic) V24.5 ☑
      nontraffic V24.1 ☑
     two wheeled motor vehicle (traffic)
       V22.5 ☑
      nontraffic V22.1 ☑
     van (traffic) V23.5 ☑
      nontraffic V23.1 ☑
    noncollision accident (traffic) V28.5 ☑
     nontraffic V28.1 ☑
   specified type NEC V29.88 ☑
    military vehicle V29.81 ☑
  occupant (of)
   aircraft (powered) V95.9 ☑
    fixed wing
     commercial — *see* Accident, transport,
       aircraft, occupant, powered, fixed
       wing, commercial
     private — *see* Accident, transport, air-
       craft, occupant, powered, fixed
       wing, private
    nonpowered V96.9 ☑
    specified NEC V95.8 ☑
   airport battery-powered vehicle — *see* Accident,
     transport, industrial vehicle occupant
   all-terrain vehicle (ATV) — *see* Accident, trans-
     port, all-terrain vehicle occupant
   animal-drawn vehicle — *see* Accident, transport,
     animal-drawn vehicle occupant
   automobile — *see* Accident, transport, car occu-
     pant
   balloon V96.00 ☑
   battery-powered vehicle — *see* Accident, trans-
     port, industrial vehicle occupant
   bicycle — *see* Accident, transport, pedal cyclist
    motorized — *see* Accident, transport, motor-
      cycle rider
   boat NEC — *see* Accident, watercraft
   bulldozer — *see* Accident, transport, construction
     vehicle occupant
   bus — *see* Accident, transport, bus occupant
   cable car (on rails) — *see also* Accident, transport,
     streetcar occupant
    not on rails V98.0 ☑
   car — *see also* Accident, transport, car occupant
    cable (on rails) — *see also* Accident, transport,
      streetcar occupant
    not on rails V98.0 ☑
   coach — *see* Accident, transport, bus occupant
   coal-car — *see* Accident, transport, industrial
     vehicle occupant
   digger — *see* Accident, transport, construction
     vehicle occupant

Accident — *continued*
  transport — *continued*
    occupant — *continued*
      dump truck — *see* Accident, transport, construction vehicle occupant
      earth-leveler — *see* Accident, transport, construction vehicle occupant
      farm machinery (self-propelled) — *see* Accident, transport, agricultural vehicle occupant
      forklift — *see* Accident, transport, industrial vehicle occupant
      glider (unpowered) V96.20 ☑
        hang V96.10 ☑
        powered (microlight) (ultralight) — *see* Accident, transport, aircraft, occupant, powered, glider
      glider (unpowered) NEC V96.20 ☑
      hang-glider V96.10 ☑
      harvester — *see* Accident, transport, agricultural vehicle occupant
      heavy (transport) vehicle — *see* Accident, transport, truck occupant
      helicopter — *see* Accident, transport, aircraft, occupant, helicopter
      ice-yacht V98.2 ☑
      kite (carrying person) V96.8 ☑
      land-yacht V98.1 ☑
      logging car — *see* Accident, transport, industrial vehicle occupant
      mechanical shovel — *see* Accident, transport, construction vehicle occupant
      microlight — *see* Accident, transport, aircraft, occupant, powered, glider
      minibus — *see* Accident, transport, pickup truck occupant
      minivan — *see* Accident, transport, pickup truck occupant
      moped — *see* Accident, transport, motorcycle
      motor scooter — *see* Accident, transport, motorcycle
      motorcycle (with sidecar) — *see* Accident, transport, motorcycle
      off-road motor-vehicle — *see also* Accident, transport, all-terrain vehicle occupant V86.99 ☑
      pedal cycle — *see also* Accident, transport, pedal cyclist
      pick-up (truck) — *see* Accident, transport, pickup truck occupant
      railway (train) (vehicle) (subterranean) (elevated) — *see* Accident, transport, railway vehicle occupant
      rickshaw — *see* Accident, transport, pedal cycle
        motorized — *see* Accident, transport, three-wheeled motor vehicle
        pedal driven — *see* Accident, transport, pedal cyclist
      road-roller — *see* Accident, transport, construction vehicle occupant
      ship NOS V94.9 ☑
      ski-lift (chair) (gondola) V98.3 ☑
      snowmobile — *see* Accident, transport, snowmobile occupant
      spacecraft, spaceship — *see* Accident, transport, aircraft, occupant, spacecraft
      sport utility vehicle — *see* Accident, transport, pickup truck occupant
      streetcar (interurban) (operating on public street or highway) — *see* Accident, transport, streetcar occupant
      SUV — *see* Accident, transport, pickup truck occupant
      téléférique V98.0 ☑
      three-wheeled vehicle (motorized) — *see also* Accident, transport, three-wheeled motor vehicle occupant
        nonmotorized — *see* Accident, transport, pedal cycle
      tractor (farm) (and trailer) — *see* Accident, transport, agricultural vehicle occupant
      train — *see* Accident, transport, railway vehicle occupant
      tram — *see* Accident, transport, streetcar occupant
        in mine or quarry — *see* Accident, transport, industrial vehicle occupant
      tricycle — *see* Accident, transport, pedal cycle
      tricycle — *see* Accident, transport, pedal cycle
        motorized — *see* Accident, transport, three-wheeled motor vehicle
      trolley — *see* Accident, transport, streetcar occupant
        in mine or quarry — *see* Accident, transport, industrial vehicle occupant
      tub, in mine or quarry — *see* Accident, transport, industrial vehicle occupant
      ultralight — *see* Accident, transport, aircraft, occupant, powered, glider
      van — *see* Accident, transport, van occupant
      vehicle NEC V89.9 ☑
        heavy transport — *see* Accident, transport, truck occupant
        motor (traffic) NEC V89.2 ☑
        nontraffic NEC V89.0 ☑
      watercraft NOS V94.9 ☑
        causing drowning — *see* Drowning, resulting from accident to boat
    off-road motor-vehicle — *see also* Accident, transport, all-terrain vehicle occupant V86.99 ☑
    parachutist V97.29 ☑
      after accident to aircraft — *see* Accident, transport, aircraft
      entangled in object V97.21 ☑
      injured on landing V97.22 ☑
    pedal cyclist V19.9 ☑
      collision (with)
        animal (traffic) V10.9 ☑
          being ridden (traffic) V16.9 ☑
            nontraffic V16.2 ☑
            while boarding or alighting V16.3 ☑
          nontraffic V10.2 ☑
          while boarding or alighting V10.3 ☑
        animal-drawn vehicle (traffic) V16.9 ☑
          nontraffic V16.2 ☑
          while boarding or alighting V16.3 ☑
        bus (traffic) V14.9 ☑
          nontraffic V14.2 ☑
          while boarding or alighting V14.3 ☑
        car (traffic) V13.9 ☑
          nontraffic V13.2 ☑
          while boarding or alighting V13.3 ☑
        motor vehicle NOS (traffic) V19.60 ☑
          nontraffic V19.20 ☑
          specified type NEC (traffic) V19.69 ☑
            nontraffic V19.29 ☑
        pedal cycle (traffic) V11.9 ☑
          nontraffic V11.2 ☑
          while boarding or alighting V11.3 ☑
        pickup truck (traffic) V13.9 ☑
          nontraffic V13.2 ☑
          while boarding or alighting V13.3 ☑
        railway vehicle (traffic) V15.9 ☑
          nontraffic V15.2 ☑
          while boarding or alighting V15.3 ☑
        specified vehicle NEC (traffic) V16.9 ☑
          nontraffic V16.2 ☑
          while boarding or alighting V16.3 ☑
        stationary object (traffic) V17.9 ☑
          nontraffic V17.2 ☑
          while boarding or alighting V17.3 ☑
        streetcar (traffic) V16.9 ☑
          nontraffic V16.2 ☑
          while boarding or alighting V16.3 ☑
        three wheeled motor vehicle (traffic) V12.9 ☑
          nontraffic V12.2 ☑
          while boarding or alighting V12.3 ☑
        truck (traffic) V14.9 ☑
          nontraffic V14.2 ☑
          while boarding or alighting V14.3 ☑
        two wheeled motor vehicle (traffic) V12.9 ☑
          nontraffic V12.2 ☑
          while boarding or alighting V12.3 ☑
        van (traffic) V13.9 ☑
          nontraffic V13.2 ☑
          while boarding or alighting V13.3 ☑
      driver
        collision (with)
          animal (traffic) V10.4 ☑
            being ridden (traffic) V16.4 ☑

Accident — *continued*
  transport — *continued*
    pedal cyclist — *continued*
      driver — *continued*
        collision — *continued*
          animal — *continued*
            being ridden — *continued*
              nontraffic V16.0 ☑
            nontraffic V10.0 ☑
          animal-drawn vehicle (traffic) V16.4 ☑
            nontraffic V16.0 ☑
          bus (traffic) V14.4 ☑
            nontraffic V14.0 ☑
          car (traffic) V13.4 ☑
            nontraffic V13.0 ☑
          motor vehicle NOS (traffic) V19.40 ☑
            nontraffic V19.00 ☑
            specified type NEC (traffic) V19.49 ☑
              nontraffic V19.09 ☑
          pedal cycle (traffic) V11.4 ☑
            nontraffic V11.0 ☑
          pickup truck (traffic) V13.4 ☑
            nontraffic V13.0 ☑
          railway vehicle (traffic) V15.4 ☑
            nontraffic V15.0 ☑
          specified vehicle NEC (traffic) V16.4 ☑
            nontraffic V16.0 ☑
          stationary object (traffic) V17.4 ☑
            nontraffic V17.0 ☑
          streetcar (traffic) V16.4 ☑
            nontraffic V16.0 ☑
          three wheeled motor vehicle (traffic) V12.4 ☑
            nontraffic V12.0 ☑
          truck (traffic) V14.4 ☑
            nontraffic V14.0 ☑
          two wheeled motor vehicle (traffic) V12.4 ☑
            nontraffic V12.0 ☑
          van (traffic) V13.4 ☑
            nontraffic V13.0 ☑
        noncollision accident (traffic) V18.4 ☑
          nontraffic V18.0 ☑
      noncollision accident (traffic) V18.9 ☑
        nontraffic V18.2 ☑
        while boarding or alighting V18.3 ☑
      nontraffic V19.3 ☑
      passenger
        collision (with)
          animal (traffic) V10.5 ☑
            being ridden (traffic) V16.5 ☑
              nontraffic V16.1 ☑
            nontraffic V10.1 ☑
          animal-drawn vehicle (traffic) V16.5 ☑
            nontraffic V16.1 ☑
          bus (traffic) V14.5 ☑
            nontraffic V14.1 ☑
          car (traffic) V13.5 ☑
            nontraffic V13.1 ☑
          motor vehicle NOS (traffic) V19.50 ☑
            nontraffic V19.10 ☑
            specified type NEC (traffic) V19.59 ☑
              nontraffic V19.19 ☑
          pedal cycle (traffic) V11.5 ☑
            nontraffic V11.1 ☑
          pickup truck (traffic) V13.5 ☑
            nontraffic V13.1 ☑
          railway vehicle (traffic) V15.5 ☑
            nontraffic V15.1 ☑
          specified vehicle NEC (traffic) V16.5 ☑
            nontraffic V16.1 ☑
          stationary object (traffic) V17.5 ☑
            nontraffic V17.1 ☑
          streetcar (traffic) V16.5 ☑
            nontraffic V16.1 ☑
          three wheeled motor vehicle (traffic) V12.5 ☑
            nontraffic V12.1 ☑
          truck (traffic) V14.5 ☑
            nontraffic V14.1 ☑
          two wheeled motor vehicle (traffic) V12.5 ☑
            nontraffic V12.1 ☑
          van (traffic) V13.5 ☑
            nontraffic V13.1 ☑
        noncollision accident (traffic) V18.5 ☑

☑ Additional Character Required — Refer to the Tabular List for Character Selection   ▽ Subterms under main terms may continue to next column or page

External Causes Index

Accident — Accident

Accident — *continued*
  transport — *continued*
    pedal cyclist — *continued*
      passenger — *continued*
        noncollision accident — *continued*
          nontraffic V18.1 ☑
      specified type NEC V19.88 ☑
      military vehicle V19.81 ☑
  pedestrian
    conveyance (occupant) V09.9 ☑
      baby stroller V00.828 ☑
        collision (with) V09.9 ☑
          animal being ridden or animal drawn
            vehicle V06.99 ☑
            nontraffic V06.09 ☑
            traffic V06.19 ☑
          bus or heavy transport V04.99 ☑
            nontraffic V04.09 ☑
            traffic V04.19 ☑
          car V03.99 ☑
            nontraffic V03.09 ☑
            traffic V03.19 ☑
          pedal cycle V01.99 ☑
            nontraffic V01.09 ☑
            traffic V01.19 ☑
          pick-up truck or van V03.99 ☑
            nontraffic V03.09 ☑
            traffic V03.19 ☑
          railway (train) (vehicle) V05.99 ☑
            nontraffic V05.09 ☑
            traffic V05.19 ☑
          stationary object V00.822 ☑
          streetcar V06.99 ☑
            nontraffic V06.09 ☑
            traffic V06.19 ☑
          two- or three-wheeled motor vehicle
            V02.99 ☑
            nontraffic V02.09 ☑
            traffic V02.19 ☑
          vehicle V09.9 ☑
            animal-drawn V06.99 ☑
              nontraffic V06.09 ☑
              traffic V06.19 ☑
            motor
              nontraffic V09.00 ☑
              traffic V09.20 ☑
        fall V00.821 ☑
        nontraffic V09.1 ☑
          involving motor vehicle NEC V09.00 ☑
        traffic V09.3 ☑
          involving motor vehicle NEC V09.20 ☑
      flat-bottomed NEC V00.388 ☑
        collision (with) V09.9 ☑
          animal being ridden or animal drawn
            vehicle V06.99 ☑
            nontraffic V06.09 ☑
            traffic V06.19 ☑
          bus or heavy transport V04.99 ☑
            nontraffic V04.09 ☑
            traffic V04.19 ☑
          car V03.99 ☑
            nontraffic V03.09 ☑
            traffic V03.19 ☑
          pedal cycle V01.99 ☑
            nontraffic V01.09 ☑
            traffic V01.19 ☑
          pick-up truck or van V03.99 ☑
            nontraffic V03.09 ☑
            traffic V03.19 ☑
          railway (train) (vehicle) V05.99 ☑
            nontraffic V05.09 ☑
            traffic V05.19 ☑
          stationary object V00.382 ☑
          streetcar V06.99 ☑
            nontraffic V06.09 ☑
            traffic V06.19 ☑
          two- or three-wheeled motor vehicle
            V02.99 ☑
            nontraffic V02.09 ☑
            traffic V02.19 ☑
          vehicle V09.9 ☑
            animal-drawn V06.99 ☑
              nontraffic V06.09 ☑
              traffic V06.19 ☑
            motor
              nontraffic V09.00 ☑

Accident — *continued*
  transport — *continued*
    pedestrian — *continued*
      conveyance — *continued*
        flat-bottomed — *continued*
          collision — *continued*
           vehicle — *continued*
            motor — *continued*
             traffic V09.20 ☑
        fall V00.381 ☑
        nontraffic V09.1 ☑
          involving motor vehicle NEC V09.00 ☑
        snow
          board — *see* Accident, transport,
            pedestrian, conveyance, snow
            board
          ski — *see* Accident, transport, pedes-
            trian, conveyance, skis (snow)
        traffic V09.3 ☑
          involving motor vehicle NEC V09.20 ☑
        gliding type NEC V00.288 ☑
          collision (with) V09.9 ☑
           animal being ridden or animal drawn
             vehicle V06.99 ☑
             nontraffic V06.09 ☑
             traffic V06.19 ☑
           bus or heavy transport V04.99 ☑
             nontraffic V04.09 ☑
             traffic V04.19 ☑
           car V03.99 ☑
             nontraffic V03.09 ☑
             traffic V03.19 ☑
           pedal cycle V01.99 ☑
             nontraffic V01.09 ☑
             traffic V01.19 ☑
           pick-up truck or van V03.99 ☑
             nontraffic V03.09 ☑
             traffic V03.19 ☑
           railway (train) (vehicle) V05.99 ☑
             nontraffic V05.09 ☑
             traffic V05.19 ☑
           stationary object V00.282 ☑
           streetcar V06.99 ☑
             nontraffic V06.09 ☑
             traffic V02.19 ☑
           two- or three-wheeled motor vehicle
             V02.99 ☑
             nontraffic V02.09 ☑
             traffic V02.19 ☑
           vehicle V09.9 ☑
            animal-drawn V06.99 ☑
              nontraffic V06.09 ☑
              traffic V06.19 ☑
            motor
             nontraffic V09.00 ☑
             traffic V09.20 ☑
        fall V00.281 ☑
        heelies — *see* Accident, transport,
          pedestrian, conveyance, heelies
        ice skate — *see* Accident, transport,
          pedestrian, conveyance, ice skate
        nontraffic V09.1 ☑
          involving motor vehicle NEC V09.00 ☑
        sled — *see* Accident, transport, pedestri-
          an, conveyance, sled
        traffic V09.3 ☑
          involving motor vehicle NEC V09.20 ☑
          wheelies — *see* Accident, transport,
           pedestrian, conveyance, heelies
      heelies V00.158 ☑
        colliding with stationary object
          V00.152 ☑
        fall V00.151 ☑
      ice skates V00.218 ☑
        collision (with) V09.9 ☑
          animal being ridden or animal drawn
            vehicle V06.99 ☑
            nontraffic V06.09 ☑
            traffic V06.19 ☑
          bus or heavy transport V04.99 ☑
            nontraffic V04.09 ☑
            traffic V04.19 ☑
          car V03.99 ☑
            nontraffic V03.09 ☑
            traffic V03.19 ☑
          pedal cycle V01.99 ☑

Accident — *continued*
  transport — *continued*
    pedestrian — *continued*
      conveyance — *continued*
        ice skates — *continued*
          collision — *continued*
           pedal cycle — *continued*
            nontraffic V01.09 ☑
            traffic V01.19 ☑
           pick-up truck or van V03.99 ☑
            nontraffic V03.09 ☑
            traffic V03.19 ☑
           railway (train) (vehicle) V05.99 ☑
            nontraffic V05.09 ☑
            traffic V05.19 ☑
           stationary object V00.212 ☑
           streetcar V06.99 ☑
            nontraffic V06.09 ☑
            traffic V06.19 ☑
           two- or three-wheeled motor vehicle
            V02.99 ☑
            nontraffic V02.09 ☑
            traffic V02.19 ☑
           vehicle V09.9 ☑
            animal-drawn V06.99 ☑
             nontraffic V06.09 ☑
             traffic V06.19 ☑
            motor
             nontraffic V09.00 ☑
             traffic V09.20 ☑
        fall V00.211 ☑
        nontraffic V09.1 ☑
          involving motor vehicle NEC V09.00 ☑
        traffic V09.3 ☑
          involving motor vehicle NEC V09.20 ☑
      motorized mobility scooter V00.838 ☑
        collision with stationary object
          V00.832 ☑
        fall from V00.831 ☑
      nontraffic V09.1 ☑
        involving motor vehicle V09.00 ☑
          military V09.01 ☑
          specified type NEC V09.09 ☑
      roller skates (non in-line) V00.128 ☑
        collision (with) V09.9 ☑
          animal being ridden or animal drawn
            vehicle V06.91 ☑
            nontraffic V06.01 ☑
            traffic V06.11 ☑
          bus or heavy transport V04.91 ☑
            nontraffic V04.01 ☑
            traffic V04.11 ☑
          car V03.91 ☑
            nontraffic V03.01 ☑
            traffic V03.11 ☑
          pedal cycle V01.91 ☑
            nontraffic V01.01 ☑
            traffic V01.11 ☑
          pick-up truck or van V03.91 ☑
            nontraffic V03.01 ☑
            traffic V03.11 ☑
          railway (train) (vehicle) V05.91 ☑
            nontraffic V05.01 ☑
            traffic V05.11 ☑
          stationary object V00.122 ☑
          streetcar V06.91 ☑
            nontraffic V06.01 ☑
            traffic V06.11 ☑
          two- or three-wheeled motor vehicle
            V02.91 ☑
            nontraffic V02.01 ☑
            traffic V02.11 ☑
          vehicle V09.9 ☑
           animal-drawn V06.91 ☑
            nontraffic V06.01 ☑
             traffic V06.11 ☑
           motor
            nontraffic V09.00 ☑
            traffic V09.20 ☑
        fall V00.121 ☑
      in-line V00.118 ☑
        collision — *see also* Accident, trans-
          port, pedestrian, conveyance
          occupant, roller skates, collision
          with stationary object V00.112 ☑
        fall V00.111 ☑

Accident — *continued*
  transport — *continued*
    pedestrian — *continued*
      conveyance — *continued*
        roller skates — *continued*
          nontraffic V09.1 ☑
            involving motor vehicle NEC V09.00 ☑
          traffic V09.3 ☑
            involving motor vehicle NEC V09.20 ☑
        rolling shoes V00.158 ☑
          colliding with stationary object V00.152 ☑
          fall V00.151 ☑
        rolling type NEC V00.188 ☑
          collision (with) V09.9 ☑
            animal being ridden or animal drawn vehicle V06.99 ☑
              nontraffic V06.09 ☑
              traffic V06.19 ☑
            bus or heavy transport V04.99 ☑
              nontraffic V04.09 ☑
              traffic V04.19 ☑
            car V03.99 ☑
              nontraffic V03.09 ☑
              traffic V03.19 ☑
            pedal cycle V01.99 ☑
              nontraffic V01.09 ☑
              traffic V01.19 ☑
            pick-up truck or van V03.99 ☑
              nontraffic V03.09 ☑
              traffic V03.19 ☑
            railway (train) (vehicle) V05.99 ☑
              nontraffic V05.09 ☑
              traffic V05.19 ☑
            stationary object V00.182 ☑
            streetcar V06.99 ☑
              nontraffic V06.09 ☑
              traffic V06.19 ☑
            two- or three-wheeled motor vehicle V02.99 ☑
              nontraffic V02.09 ☑
              traffic V02.19 ☑
            vehicle V09.9 ☑
              animal-drawn V06.99 ☑
                nontraffic V06.09 ☑
                traffic V06.19 ☑
              motor
                nontraffic V09.00 ☑
                traffic V09.20 ☑
          fall V00.181 ☑
        in-line roller skate — *see* Accident, transport, pedestrian, conveyance, roller skate, in-line
          nontraffic V09.1 ☑
            involving motor vehicle NEC V09.00 ☑
        roller skate — *see* Accident, transport, pedestrian, conveyance, roller skate
        scooter (non-motorized) — *see* Accident, transport, pedestrian, conveyance, scooter
        skateboard — *see* Accident, transport, pedestrian, conveyance, skateboard
          traffic V09.3 ☑
            involving motor vehicle NEC V09.20 ☑
        scooter (non-motorized) V00.148 ☑
          collision (with) V09.9 ☑
            animal being ridden or animal drawn vehicle V06.99 ☑
              nontraffic V06.09 ☑
              traffic V06.19 ☑
            bus or heavy transport V04.99 ☑
              nontraffic V04.09 ☑
              traffic V04.19 ☑
            car V03.99 ☑
              nontraffic V03.09 ☑
              traffic V03.19 ☑
            pedal cycle V01.99 ☑
              nontraffic V01.09 ☑
              traffic V01.19 ☑
            pick-up truck or van V03.99 ☑
              nontraffic V03.09 ☑
              traffic V03.19 ☑
            railway (train) (vehicle) V05.99 ☑
              nontraffic V05.09 ☑

Accident — *continued*
  transport — *continued*
    pedestrian — *continued*
      conveyance — *continued*
        scooter — *continued*
          collision — *continued*
            railway — *continued*
              traffic V05.19 ☑
            stationary object V00.142 ☑
            streetcar V06.99 ☑
              nontraffic V06.09 ☑
              traffic V06.19 ☑
            two- or three-wheeled motor vehicle V02.99 ☑
              nontraffic V02.09 ☑
              traffic V02.19 ☑
            vehicle V09.9 ☑
              animal-drawn V06.99 ☑
                nontraffic V06.09 ☑
                traffic V06.19 ☑
              motor
                nontraffic V09.00 ☑
                traffic V09.20 ☑
          fall V00.141 ☑
          nontraffic V09.1 ☑
            involving motor vehicle NEC V09.00 ☑
          traffic V09.3 ☑
            involving motor vehicle NEC V09.20 ☑
        skate board V00.138 ☑
          collision (with) V09.9 ☑
            animal being ridden or animal drawn vehicle V06.92 ☑
              nontraffic V06.02 ☑
              traffic V06.12 ☑
            bus or heavy transport V04.92 ☑
              nontraffic V04.02 ☑
              traffic V04.12 ☑
            car V03.92 ☑
              nontraffic V03.02 ☑
              traffic V03.12 ☑
            pedal cycle V01.92 ☑
              nontraffic V01.02 ☑
              traffic V01.12 ☑
            pick-up truck or van V03.92 ☑
              nontraffic V03.02 ☑
              traffic V03.12 ☑
            railway (train) (vehicle) V05.92 ☑
              nontraffic V05.02 ☑
              traffic V05.12 ☑
            stationary object V00.132 ☑
            streetcar V06.92 ☑
              nontraffic V06.02 ☑
              traffic V06.12 ☑
            two- or three-wheeled motor vehicle V02.92 ☑
              nontraffic V02.02 ☑
              traffic V02.12 ☑
            vehicle V09.9 ☑
              animal-drawn V06.92 ☑
                nontraffic V06.02 ☑
                traffic V06.12 ☑
              motor
                nontraffic V09.00 ☑
                traffic V09.20 ☑
          fall V00.131 ☑
          nontraffic V09.1 ☑
            involving motor vehicle NEC V09.00 ☑
          traffic V09.3 ☑
            involving motor vehicle NEC V09.20 ☑
        skis (snow) V00.328 ☑
          collision (with) V09.9 ☑
            animal being ridden or animal drawn vehicle V06.99 ☑
              nontraffic V06.09 ☑
              traffic V06.19 ☑
            bus or heavy transport V04.99 ☑
              nontraffic V04.09 ☑
              traffic V04.19 ☑
            car V03.99 ☑
              nontraffic V03.09 ☑
              traffic V03.19 ☑
            pedal cycle V01.99 ☑
              nontraffic V01.09 ☑
              traffic V01.19 ☑
            pick-up truck or van V03.99 ☑
              nontraffic V03.09 ☑

Accident — *continued*
  transport — *continued*
    pedestrian — *continued*
      conveyance — *continued*
        skis — *continued*
          collision — *continued*
            pick-up truck or van — *continued*
              traffic V03.19 ☑
            railway (train) (vehicle) V05.99 ☑
              nontraffic V05.09 ☑
              traffic V05.19 ☑
            stationary object V00.322 ☑
            streetcar V06.99 ☑
              nontraffic V06.09 ☑
              traffic V06.19 ☑
            two- or three-wheeled motor vehicle V02.99 ☑
              nontraffic V02.09 ☑
              traffic V02.19 ☑
            vehicle V09.9 ☑
              animal-drawn V06.99 ☑
                nontraffic V06.09 ☑
                traffic V06.19 ☑
              motor
                nontraffic V09.00 ☑
                traffic V09.20 ☑
          fall V00.321 ☑
          nontraffic V09.1 ☑
            involving motor vehicle NEC V09.00 ☑
          traffic V09.3 ☑
            involving motor vehicle NEC V09.20 ☑
        sled V00.228 ☑
          collision (with) V09.9 ☑
            animal being ridden or animal drawn vehicle V06.99 ☑
              nontraffic V06.09 ☑
              traffic V06.19 ☑
            bus or heavy transport V04.99 ☑
              nontraffic V04.09 ☑
              traffic V04.19 ☑
            car V03.99 ☑
              nontraffic V03.09 ☑
              traffic V03.19 ☑
            pedal cycle V01.99 ☑
              nontraffic V01.09 ☑
              traffic V01.19 ☑
            pick-up truck or van V03.99 ☑
              nontraffic V03.09 ☑
              traffic V03.19 ☑
            railway (train) (vehicle) V05.99 ☑
              nontraffic V05.09 ☑
              traffic V05.19 ☑
            stationary object V00.222 ☑
            streetcar V06.99 ☑
              nontraffic V06.09 ☑
              traffic V06.19 ☑
            two- or three-wheeled motor vehicle V02.99 ☑
              nontraffic V02.09 ☑
              traffic V02.19 ☑
            vehicle V09.9 ☑
              animal-drawn V06.99 ☑
                nontraffic V06.09 ☑
                traffic V06.19 ☑
              motor
                nontraffic V09.00 ☑
                traffic V09.20 ☑
          fall V00.221 ☑
          nontraffic V09.1 ☑
            involving motor vehicle NEC V09.00 ☑
          traffic V09.3 ☑
            involving motor vehicle NEC V09.20 ☑
        snow board V00.318 ☑
          collision (with) V09.9 ☑
            animal being ridden or animal drawn vehicle V06.99 ☑
              nontraffic V06.09 ☑
              traffic V06.19 ☑
            bus or heavy transport V04.99 ☑
              nontraffic V04.09 ☑
              traffic V04.19 ☑
            car V03.99 ☑
              nontraffic V03.09 ☑
              traffic V03.19 ☑
            pedal cycle V01.99 ☑
              nontraffic V01.09 ☑

☑ **Additional Character Required — Refer to the Tabular List for Character Selection**   ▽ **Subterms under main terms may continue to next column or page**

Accident — *continued*
  transport — *continued*
    pedestrian — *continued*
      conveyance — *continued*
        snow board — *continued*
          collision — *continued*
            pedal cycle — *continued*
              traffic V01.19 ☑
            pick-up truck or van V03.99 ☑
              nontraffic V03.09 ☑
              traffic V03.19 ☑
            railway (train) (vehicle) V05.99 ☑
              nontraffic V05.09 ☑
              traffic V05.19 ☑
            stationary object V00.312 ☑
            streetcar V06.99 ☑
              nontraffic V06.09 ☑
              traffic V06.19 ☑
            two- or three-wheeled motor vehicle V02.99 ☑
              nontraffic V02.09 ☑
              traffic V02.19 ☑
            vehicle V09.9 ☑
              animal-drawn V06.99 ☑
                nontraffic V06.09 ☑
                traffic V06.19 ☑
              motor
                nontraffic V09.00 ☑
                traffic V09.20 ☑
         fall V00.311 ☑
        nontraffic V09.1 ☑
          involving motor vehicle NEC V09.00 ☑
        traffic V09.3 ☑
          involving motor vehicle NEC V09.20 ☑
        specified type NEC V00.898 ☑
          collision (with) V09.9 ☑
            animal being ridden or animal drawn vehicle V06.99 ☑
              nontraffic V06.09 ☑
              traffic V06.19 ☑
            bus or heavy transport V04.99 ☑
              nontraffic V04.09 ☑
              traffic V04.19 ☑
            car V03.99 ☑
              nontraffic V03.09 ☑
              traffic V03.19 ☑
            pedal cycle V01.99 ☑
              nontraffic V01.09 ☑
              traffic V01.19 ☑
            pick-up truck or van V03.99 ☑
              nontraffic V03.09 ☑
              traffic V03.19 ☑
            railway (train) (vehicle) V05.99 ☑
              nontraffic V05.09 ☑
              traffic V05.19 ☑
            stationary object V00.892 ☑
            streetcar V06.99 ☑
              nontraffic V06.09 ☑
              traffic V06.19 ☑
            two- or three-wheeled motor vehicle V02.99 ☑
              nontraffic V02.09 ☑
              traffic V02.19 ☑
            vehicle V09.9 ☑
              animal-drawn V06.99 ☑
                nontraffic V06.09 ☑
                traffic V06.19 ☑
              motor
                nontraffic V09.00 ☑
                traffic V09.20 ☑
         fall V00.891 ☑
        nontraffic V09.1 ☑
          involving motor vehicle NEC V09.00 ☑
        traffic V09.3 ☑
          involving motor vehicle NEC V09.20 ☑
      traffic V09.3 ☑
        involving motor vehicle V09.20 ☑
          military V09.21 ☑
          specified type NEC V09.29 ☑
      wheelchair (powered) V00.818 ☑
        collision (with) V09.9 ☑
          animal being ridden or animal drawn vehicle V06.99 ☑
            nontraffic V06.09 ☑
            traffic V06.19 ☑
          bus or heavy transport V04.99 ☑

Accident — *continued*
  transport — *continued*
    pedestrian — *continued*
      conveyance — *continued*
        wheelchair — *continued*
          collision — *continued*
            bus or heavy transport — *continued*
              nontraffic V04.09 ☑
              traffic V04.19 ☑
            car V03.99 ☑
              nontraffic V03.09 ☑
              traffic V03.19 ☑
            pedal cycle V01.99 ☑
              nontraffic V01.09 ☑
              traffic V01.19 ☑
            pick-up truck or van V03.99 ☑
              nontraffic V03.09 ☑
              traffic V03.19 ☑
            railway (train) (vehicle) V05.99 ☑
              nontraffic V05.09 ☑
              traffic V05.19 ☑
            stationary object V00.812 ☑
            streetcar V06.99 ☑
              nontraffic V06.09 ☑
              traffic V06.19 ☑
            two- or three-wheeled motor vehicle V02.99 ☑
              nontraffic V02.09 ☑
              traffic V02.19 ☑
            vehicle V09.9 ☑
              animal-drawn V06.99 ☑
                nontraffic V06.09 ☑
                traffic V06.19 ☑
              motor
                nontraffic V09.00 ☑
                traffic V09.20 ☑
         fall V00.811 ☑
        nontraffic V09.1 ☑
          involving motor vehicle NEC V09.00 ☑
        traffic V09.3 ☑
          involving motor vehicle NEC V09.20 ☑
      wheeled shoe V00.158 ☑
        colliding with stationary object V00.152 ☑
        fall V00.151 ☑
    on foot — *see also* Accident, pedestrian
      collision (with)
        animal being ridden or animal drawn vehicle V06.90 ☑
          nontraffic V06.00 ☑
          traffic V06.10 ☑
        bus or heavy transport V04.90 ☑
          nontraffic V04.00 ☑
          traffic V04.10 ☑
        car V03.90 ☑
          nontraffic V03.00 ☑
          traffic V03.10 ☑
        pedal cycle V01.90 ☑
          nontraffic V01.00 ☑
          traffic V01.10 ☑
        pick-up truck or van V03.90 ☑
          nontraffic V03.00 ☑
          traffic V03.10 ☑
        railway (train) (vehicle) V05.90 ☑
          nontraffic V05.00 ☑
          traffic V05.10 ☑
        streetcar V06.90 ☑
          nontraffic V06.00 ☑
          traffic V06.10 ☑
        two- or three-wheeled motor vehicle V02.90 ☑
          nontraffic V02.00 ☑
          traffic V02.10 ☑
        vehicle V09.9 ☑
          animal-drawn V06.90 ☑
            nontraffic V06.00 ☑
            traffic V06.10 ☑
          motor
      nontraffic V09.1 ☑
        involving motor vehicle V09.00 ☑
          military V09.01 ☑
          specified type NEC V09.09 ☑
      traffic V09.3 ☑
        involving motor vehicle V09.20 ☑
          military V09.21 ☑

Accident — *continued*
  transport — *continued*
    pedestrian — *continued*
      on foot — *see also* Accident, pedestrian — *continued*
        traffic — *continued*
          involving motor vehicle — *continued*
            specified type NEC V09.29 ☑
      person NEC (unknown way or transportation) V99 ☑
        collision (between)
          bus (with)
            heavy transport vehicle (traffic) V87.5 ☑
              nontraffic V88.5 ☑
          car (with)
            bus (traffic) V87.3 ☑
              nontraffic V88.3 ☑
            heavy transport vehicle (traffic) V87.4 ☑
              nontraffic V88.4 ☑
            nontraffic V88.5 ☑
            pick-up truck or van (traffic) V87.2 ☑
              nontraffic V88.2 ☑
            train or railway vehicle (traffic) V87.6 ☑
              nontraffic V88.6 ☑
            two-or three-wheeled motor vehicle (traffic) V87.0 ☑
              nontraffic V88.0 ☑
          motor vehicle (traffic) NEC V87.7 ☑
            nontraffic V88.7 ☑
          two-or three-wheeled vehicle (with) (traffic)
            motor vehicle NEC V87.1 ☑
              nontraffic V88.1 ☑
          nonmotor vehicle (collision) (noncollision) (traffic) V87.9 ☑
          nontraffic V88.9 ☑
      pickup truck occupant V59.9 ☑
        collision (with)
          animal (traffic) V50.9 ☑
            being ridden (traffic) V56.9 ☑
              nontraffic V56.3 ☑
              while boarding or alighting V56.4 ☑
            nontraffic V50.3 ☑
            while boarding or alighting V50.4 ☑
          animal-drawn vehicle (traffic) V56.9 ☑
            nontraffic V56.3 ☑
            while boarding or alighting V56.4 ☑
          bus (traffic) V54.9 ☑
            nontraffic V54.3 ☑
            while boarding or alighting V54.4 ☑
          car (traffic) V53.9 ☑
            nontraffic V53.3 ☑
            while boarding or alighting V53.4 ☑
          motor vehicle NOS (traffic) V59.60 ☑
            nontraffic V59.20 ☑
            specified type NEC (traffic) V59.69 ☑
              nontraffic V59.29 ☑
          pedal cycle (traffic) V51.9 ☑
            nontraffic V51.3 ☑
            while boarding or alighting V51.4 ☑
          pickup truck (traffic) V53.9 ☑
            nontraffic V53.3 ☑
            while boarding or alighting V53.4 ☑
          railway vehicle (traffic) V55.9 ☑
            nontraffic V55.3 ☑
            while boarding or alighting V55.4 ☑
          specified vehicle NEC (traffic) V56.9 ☑
            nontraffic V56.3 ☑
            while boarding or alighting V56.4 ☑
          stationary object (traffic) V57.9 ☑
            nontraffic V57.3 ☑
            while boarding or alighting V57.4 ☑
          streetcar (traffic) V56.9 ☑
            nontraffic V56.3 ☑
            while boarding or alighting V56.4 ☑
          three wheeled motor vehicle (traffic) V52.9 ☑
            nontraffic V52.3 ☑
            while boarding or alighting V52.4 ☑
          truck (traffic) V54.9 ☑
            nontraffic V54.3 ☑
            while boarding or alighting V54.4 ☑
          two wheeled motor vehicle (traffic) V52.9 ☑
            nontraffic V52.3 ☑
            while boarding or alighting V52.4 ☑
          van (traffic) V53.9 ☑
            nontraffic V53.3 ☑
            while boarding or alighting V53.4 ☑

▽ Subterms under main terms may continue to next column or page   ☑ Additional Character Required — Refer to the Tabular List for Character Selection   **405**

Accident — Accident

External Causes Index

Accident — Accident

Accident — *continued*
  transport — *continued*
    pickup truck occupant — *continued*
      driver
        collision (with)
          animal (traffic) V50.5 ☑
            being ridden (traffic) V56.5 ☑
              nontraffic V56.0 ☑
            nontraffic V50.0 ☑
          animal-drawn vehicle (traffic) V56.5 ☑
            nontraffic V56.0 ☑
          bus (traffic) V54.5 ☑
            nontraffic V54.0 ☑
          car (traffic) V53.5 ☑
            nontraffic V53.0 ☑
          motor vehicle NOS (traffic) V59.40 ☑
            nontraffic V59.00 ☑
            specified type NEC (traffic) V59.49 ☑
              nontraffic V59.09 ☑
          pedal cycle (traffic) V51.5 ☑
            nontraffic V51.0 ☑
          pickup truck (traffic) V53.5 ☑
            nontraffic V53.0 ☑
          railway vehicle (traffic) V55.5 ☑
            nontraffic V55.0 ☑
          specified vehicle NEC (traffic) V56.5 ☑
            nontraffic V56.0 ☑
          stationary object (traffic) V57.5 ☑
            nontraffic V57.0 ☑
          streetcar (traffic) V56.5 ☑
            nontraffic V56.0 ☑
          three wheeled motor vehicle (traffic)
            V52.5 ☑
            nontraffic V52.0 ☑
          truck (traffic) V54.5 ☑
            nontraffic V54.0 ☑
          two wheeled motor vehicle (traffic)
            V52.5 ☑
            nontraffic V52.0 ☑
          van (traffic) V53.5 ☑
            nontraffic V53.0 ☑
        noncollision accident (traffic) V58.5 ☑
          nontraffic V58.0 ☑
      hanger-on
        collision (with)
          animal (traffic) V50.7 ☑
            being ridden (traffic) V56.7 ☑
              nontraffic V56.2 ☑
            nontraffic V50.2 ☑
          animal-drawn vehicle (traffic) V56.7 ☑
            nontraffic V56.2 ☑
          bus (traffic) V54.7 ☑
            nontraffic V54.2 ☑
          car (traffic) V53.7 ☑
            nontraffic V53.2 ☑
          pedal cycle (traffic) V51.7 ☑
            nontraffic V51.2 ☑
          pickup truck (traffic) V53.7 ☑
            nontraffic V53.2 ☑
          railway vehicle (traffic) V55.7 ☑
            nontraffic V55.2 ☑
          specified vehicle NEC (traffic) V56.7 ☑
            nontraffic V56.2 ☑
          stationary object (traffic) V57.7 ☑
            nontraffic V57.2 ☑
          streetcar (traffic) V56.7 ☑
            nontraffic V56.2 ☑
          three wheeled motor vehicle (traffic)
            V52.7 ☑
            nontraffic V52.2 ☑
          truck (traffic) V54.7 ☑
            nontraffic V54.2 ☑
          two wheeled motor vehicle (traffic)
            V52.7 ☑
            nontraffic V52.2 ☑
          van (traffic) V53.7 ☑
            nontraffic V53.2 ☑
        noncollision accident (traffic) V58.7 ☑
          nontraffic V58.2 ☑
      noncollision accident (traffic) V58.9 ☑
        nontraffic V58.3 ☑
        while boarding or alighting V58.4 ☑
      nontraffic V59.3 ☑
      passenger
        collision (with)
          animal (traffic) V50.6 ☑

Accident — *continued*
  transport — *continued*
    pickup truck occupant — *continued*
      passenger — *continued*
        collision — *continued*
          animal — *continued*
            being ridden (traffic) V56.6 ☑
              nontraffic V56.1 ☑
            nontraffic V50.1 ☑
          animal-drawn vehicle (traffic) V56.6 ☑
            nontraffic V56.1 ☑
          bus (traffic) V54.6 ☑
            nontraffic V54.1 ☑
          car (traffic) V53.6 ☑
            nontraffic V53.1 ☑
          motor vehicle NOS (traffic) V59.50 ☑
            nontraffic V59.10 ☑
            specified type NEC (traffic) V59.59 ☑
              nontraffic V59.19 ☑
          pedal cycle (traffic) V51.6 ☑
            nontraffic V51.1 ☑
          pickup truck (traffic) V53.6 ☑
            nontraffic V53.1 ☑
          railway vehicle (traffic) V55.6 ☑
            nontraffic V55.1 ☑
          specified vehicle NEC (traffic) V56.6 ☑
            nontraffic V56.1 ☑
          stationary object (traffic) V57.6 ☑
            nontraffic V57.1 ☑
          streetcar (traffic) V56.6 ☑
            nontraffic V56.1 ☑
          three wheeled motor vehicle (traffic)
            V52.6 ☑
            nontraffic V52.1 ☑
          truck (traffic) V54.6 ☑
            nontraffic V54.1 ☑
          two wheeled motor vehicle (traffic)
            V52.6 ☑
            nontraffic V52.1 ☑
          van (traffic) V53.6 ☑
            nontraffic V53.1 ☑
        noncollision accident (traffic) V58.6 ☑
          nontraffic V58.1 ☑
    specified type NEC V59.88 ☑
    military vehicle V59.81 ☑
  quarry truck — *see* Accident, transport, industrial
      vehicle occupant
  race car — *see* Accident, transport, motor vehicle
      NEC occupant
  railway vehicle occupant V81.9 ☑
    collision (with) V81.3 ☑
      motor vehicle (non-military) (traffic) V81.1 ☑
        military V81.83 ☑
        nontraffic V81.0 ☑
      rolling stock V81.2 ☑
      specified object NEC V81.3 ☑
    during derailment V81.7 ☑
      with antecedent collision — *see* Accident,
          transport, railway vehicle occupant,
          collision
    explosion V81.81 ☑
    fall (in railway vehicle) V81.5 ☑
      during derailment V81.7 ☑
        with antecedent collision — *see* Accident,
            transport, railway vehicle occupant,
            collision
      from railway vehicle V81.6 ☑
        during derailment V81.7 ☑
          with antecedent collision — *see* Acci-
              dent, transport, railway vehicle
              occupant, collision
      while boarding or alighting V81.4 ☑
    fire V81.81 ☑
    object falling onto train V81.82 ☑
    specified type NEC V81.89 ☑
    while boarding or alighting V81.4 ☑
  ski lift V98.3 ☑
  snowmobile occupant (nontraffic) V86.92 ☑
    driver V86.52 ☑
    hanger-on V86.72 ☑
    passenger V86.62 ☑
    traffic V86.32 ☑
      driver V86.02 ☑
      hanger-on V86.22 ☑
      passenger V86.12 ☑
    while boarding or alighting V86.42 ☑

Accident — *continued*
  transport — *continued*
    specified NEC V98.8 ☑
    sport utility vehicle occupant — *see also* Accident,
        transport, pickup truck occupant
    streetcar occupant V82.9 ☑
      collision (with) V82.3 ☑
        motor vehicle (traffic) V82.1 ☑
          nontraffic V82.0 ☑
        rolling stock V82.2 ☑
      during derailment V82.7 ☑
        with antecedent collision — *see* Accident,
            transport, streetcar occupant, collision
      fall (in streetcar) V82.5 ☑
        during derailment V82.7 ☑
          with antecedent collision — *see* Accident,
              transport, streetcar occupant, colli-
              sion
        from streetcar V82.6 ☑
          during derailment V82.7 ☑
            with antecedent collision — *see* Acci-
                dent, transport, streetcar occu-
                pant, collision
          while boarding or alighting V82.4 ☑
        while boarding or alighting V82.4 ☑
      specified type NEC V82.8 ☑
      while boarding or alighting V82.4 ☑
    three-wheeled motor vehicle occupant V39.9 ☑
      collision (with)
        animal (traffic) V30.9 ☑
          being ridden (traffic) V36.9 ☑
            nontraffic V36.3 ☑
            while boarding or alighting V36.4 ☑
          nontraffic V30.3 ☑
          while boarding or alighting V30.4 ☑
        animal-drawn vehicle (traffic) V36.9 ☑
          nontraffic V36.3 ☑
          while boarding or alighting V36.4 ☑
        bus (traffic) V34.9 ☑
          nontraffic V34.3 ☑
          while boarding or alighting V34.4 ☑
        car (traffic) V33.9 ☑
          nontraffic V33.3 ☑
          while boarding or alighting V33.4 ☑
        motor vehicle NOS (traffic) V39.60 ☑
          nontraffic V39.20 ☑
          specified type NEC (traffic) V39.69 ☑
            nontraffic V39.29 ☑
        pedal cycle (traffic) V31.9 ☑
          nontraffic V31.3 ☑
          while boarding or alighting V31.4 ☑
        pickup truck (traffic) V33.9 ☑
          nontraffic V33.3 ☑
          while boarding or alighting V33.4 ☑
        railway vehicle (traffic) V35.9 ☑
          nontraffic V35.3 ☑
          while boarding or alighting V35.4 ☑
        specified vehicle NEC (traffic) V36.9 ☑
          nontraffic V36.3 ☑
          while boarding or alighting V36.4 ☑
        stationary object (traffic) V37.9 ☑
          nontraffic V37.3 ☑
          while boarding or alighting V37.4 ☑
        streetcar (traffic) V36.9 ☑
          nontraffic V36.3 ☑
          while boarding or alighting V36.4 ☑
        three wheeled motor vehicle (traffic) V32.9 ☑
          nontraffic V32.3 ☑
          while boarding or alighting V32.4 ☑
        truck (traffic) V34.9 ☑
          nontraffic V34.3 ☑
          while boarding or alighting V34.4 ☑
        two wheeled motor vehicle (traffic) V32.9 ☑
          nontraffic V32.3 ☑
          while boarding or alighting V32.4 ☑
        van (traffic) V33.9 ☑
          nontraffic V33.3 ☑
          while boarding or alighting V33.4 ☑
      driver
        collision (with)
          animal (traffic) V30.5 ☑
            being ridden (traffic) V36.5 ☑
              nontraffic V36.0 ☑
            nontraffic V30.0 ☑
          animal-drawn vehicle (traffic) V36.5 ☑
            nontraffic V36.0 ☑

☑ **Additional Character Required — Refer to the Tabular List for Character Selection**   ▽ **Subterms under main terms may continue to next column or page**

Accident — *continued*
  transport — *continued*
    three-wheeled motor vehicle occupant — *continued*
      driver — *continued*
        collision — *continued*
          bus (traffic) V34.5 ☑
            nontraffic V34.0 ☑
          car (traffic) V33.5 ☑
            nontraffic V33.0 ☑
          motor vehicle NOS (traffic) V39.40 ☑
            nontraffic V39.00 ☑
            specified type NEC (traffic) V39.49 ☑
              nontraffic V39.09 ☑
          pedal cycle (traffic) V31.5 ☑
            nontraffic V31.0 ☑
          pickup truck (traffic) V33.5 ☑
            nontraffic V33.0 ☑
          railway vehicle (traffic) V35.5 ☑
            nontraffic V35.0 ☑
          specified vehicle NEC (traffic) V36.5 ☑
            nontraffic V36.0 ☑
          stationary object (traffic) V37.5 ☑
            nontraffic V37.0 ☑
          streetcar (traffic) V36.5 ☑
            nontraffic V36.0 ☑
          three wheeled motor vehicle (traffic) V32.5 ☑
            nontraffic V32.0 ☑
          truck (traffic) V34.5 ☑
            nontraffic V34.0 ☑
          two wheeled motor vehicle (traffic) V32.5 ☑
            nontraffic V32.0 ☑
          van (traffic) V33.5 ☑
            nontraffic V33.0 ☑
        noncollision accident (traffic) V38.5 ☑
          nontraffic V38.0 ☑
      hanger-on
        collision (with)
          animal (traffic) V30.7 ☑
            being ridden (traffic) V36.7 ☑
              nontraffic V36.2 ☑
            nontraffic V30.2 ☑
          animal-drawn vehicle (traffic) V36.7 ☑
            nontraffic V36.2 ☑
          bus (traffic) V34.7 ☑
            nontraffic V34.2 ☑
          car (traffic) V33.7 ☑
            nontraffic V33.2 ☑
          pedal cycle (traffic) V31.7 ☑
            nontraffic V31.2 ☑
          pickup truck (traffic) V33.7 ☑
            nontraffic V33.2 ☑
          railway vehicle (traffic) V35.7 ☑
            nontraffic V35.2 ☑
          specified vehicle NEC (traffic) V36.7 ☑
            nontraffic V36.2 ☑
          stationary object (traffic) V37.7 ☑
            nontraffic V37.2 ☑
          streetcar (traffic) V36.7 ☑
            nontraffic V36.2 ☑
          three wheeled motor vehicle (traffic) V32.7 ☑
            nontraffic V32.2 ☑
          truck (traffic) V34.7 ☑
            nontraffic V34.2 ☑
          two wheeled motor vehicle (traffic) V32.7 ☑
            nontraffic V32.2 ☑
          van (traffic) V33.7 ☑
            nontraffic V33.2 ☑
        noncollision accident (traffic) V38.7 ☑
          nontraffic V38.2 ☑
      noncollision accident (traffic) V38.9 ☑
        nontraffic V38.3 ☑
        while boarding or alighting V38.4 ☑
      nontraffic V39.3 ☑
      passenger
        collision (with)
          animal (traffic) V30.6 ☑
            being ridden (traffic) V36.6 ☑
              nontraffic V36.1 ☑
            nontraffic V30.1 ☑
          animal-drawn vehicle (traffic) V36.6 ☑
            nontraffic V36.1 ☑

Accident — *continued*
  transport — *continued*
    three-wheeled motor vehicle occupant — *continued*
      passenger — *continued*
        collision — *continued*
          bus (traffic) V34.6 ☑
            nontraffic V34.1 ☑
          car (traffic) V33.6 ☑
            nontraffic V33.1 ☑
          motor vehicle NOS (traffic) V39.50 ☑
            nontraffic V39.10 ☑
            specified type NEC (traffic) V39.59 ☑
              nontraffic V39.19 ☑
          pedal cycle (traffic) V31.6 ☑
            nontraffic V31.1 ☑
          pickup truck (traffic) V33.6 ☑
            nontraffic V33.1 ☑
          railway vehicle (traffic) V35.6 ☑
            nontraffic V35.1 ☑
          specified vehicle NEC (traffic) V36.6 ☑
            nontraffic V36.1 ☑
          stationary object (traffic) V37.6 ☑
            nontraffic V37.1 ☑
          streetcar (traffic) V36.6 ☑
            nontraffic V36.1 ☑
          three wheeled motor vehicle (traffic) V32.6 ☑
            nontraffic V32.1 ☑
          truck (traffic) V34.6 ☑
            nontraffic V34.1 ☑
          two wheeled motor vehicle (traffic) V32.6 ☑
            nontraffic V32.1 ☑
          van (traffic) V33.6 ☑
            nontraffic V33.1 ☑
        noncollision accident (traffic) V38.6 ☑
          nontraffic V38.1 ☑
      specified type NEC V39.89 ☑
      military vehicle V39.81 ☑
    tractor (farm) (and trailer) — *see* Accident, transport, agricultural vehicle occupant
    tram — *see* Accident, transport, streetcar
      in mine or quarry — *see* Accident, transport, industrial vehicle occupant
    trolley — *see* Accident, transport, streetcar
      in mine or quarry — *see* Accident, transport, industrial vehicle occupant
    truck (heavy) occupant V69.9 ☑
      collision (with)
        animal (traffic) V60.9 ☑
          being ridden (traffic) V66.9 ☑
            nontraffic V66.3 ☑
            while boarding or alighting V66.4 ☑
          nontraffic V60.3 ☑
          while boarding or alighting V60.4 ☑
        animal-drawn vehicle (traffic) V66.9 ☑
          nontraffic V66.3 ☑
          while boarding or alighting V66.4 ☑
        bus (traffic) V64.9 ☑
          nontraffic V64.3 ☑
          while boarding or alighting V64.4 ☑
        car (traffic) V63.9 ☑
          nontraffic V63.3 ☑
          while boarding or alighting V63.4 ☑
        motor vehicle NOS (traffic) V69.60 ☑
          nontraffic V69.20 ☑
          specified type NEC (traffic) V69.69 ☑
            nontraffic V69.29 ☑
        pedal cycle (traffic) V61.9 ☑
          nontraffic V61.3 ☑
          while boarding or alighting V61.4 ☑
        pickup truck (traffic) V63.9 ☑
          nontraffic V63.3 ☑
          while boarding or alighting V63.4 ☑
        railway vehicle (traffic) V65.9 ☑
          nontraffic V65.3 ☑
          while boarding or alighting V65.4 ☑
        specified vehicle NEC (traffic) V66.9 ☑
          nontraffic V66.3 ☑
          while boarding or alighting V66.4 ☑
        stationary object (traffic) V67.9 ☑
          nontraffic V67.3 ☑
          while boarding or alighting V67.4 ☑
        streetcar (traffic) V66.9 ☑
          nontraffic V66.3 ☑

Accident — *continued*
  transport — *continued*
    truck occupant — *continued*
      collision — *continued*
        streetcar (traffic) V66.9 ☑
          while boarding or alighting V66.4 ☑
        three wheeled motor vehicle (traffic) V62.9 ☑
          nontraffic V62.3 ☑
          while boarding or alighting V62.4 ☑
        truck (traffic) V64.9 ☑
          nontraffic V64.3 ☑
          while boarding or alighting V64.4 ☑
        two wheeled motor vehicle (traffic) V62.9 ☑
          nontraffic V62.3 ☑
          while boarding or alighting V62.4 ☑
        van (traffic) V63.9 ☑
          nontraffic V63.3 ☑
          while boarding or alighting V63.4 ☑
      driver
        collision (with)
          animal (traffic) V60.5 ☑
            being ridden (traffic) V66.5 ☑
              nontraffic V66.0 ☑
            nontraffic V60.0 ☑
          animal-drawn vehicle (traffic) V66.5 ☑
            nontraffic V66.0 ☑
          bus (traffic) V64.5 ☑
            nontraffic V64.0 ☑
          car (traffic) V63.5 ☑
            nontraffic V63.0 ☑
          motor vehicle NOS (traffic) V69.40 ☑
            nontraffic V69.00 ☑
            specified type NEC (traffic) V69.49 ☑
              nontraffic V69.09 ☑
          pedal cycle (traffic) V61.5 ☑
            nontraffic V61.0 ☑
          pickup truck (traffic) V63.5 ☑
            nontraffic V63.0 ☑
          railway vehicle (traffic) V65.5 ☑
            nontraffic V65.0 ☑
          specified vehicle NEC (traffic) V66.5 ☑
            nontraffic V66.0 ☑
          stationary object (traffic) V67.5 ☑
            nontraffic V67.0 ☑
          streetcar (traffic) V66.5 ☑
            nontraffic V66.0 ☑
          three wheeled motor vehicle (traffic) V62.5 ☑
            nontraffic V62.0 ☑
          truck (traffic) V64.5 ☑
            nontraffic V64.0 ☑
          two wheeled motor vehicle (traffic) V62.5 ☑
            nontraffic V62.0 ☑
          van (traffic) V63.5 ☑
            nontraffic V63.0 ☑
        noncollision accident (traffic) V68.5 ☑
          nontraffic V68.0 ☑
      dump — *see* Accident, transport, construction vehicle occupant
      hanger-on
        collision (with)
          animal (traffic) V60.7 ☑
            being ridden (traffic) V66.7 ☑
              nontraffic V66.2 ☑
            nontraffic V60.2 ☑
          animal-drawn vehicle (traffic) V66.7 ☑
            nontraffic V66.2 ☑
          bus (traffic) V64.7 ☑
            nontraffic V64.2 ☑
          car (traffic) V63.7 ☑
            nontraffic V63.2 ☑
          pedal cycle (traffic) V61.7 ☑
            nontraffic V61.2 ☑
          pickup truck (traffic) V63.7 ☑
            nontraffic V63.2 ☑
          railway vehicle (traffic) V65.7 ☑
            nontraffic V65.2 ☑
          specified vehicle NEC (traffic) V66.7 ☑
            nontraffic V66.2 ☑
          stationary object (traffic) V67.7 ☑
            nontraffic V67.2 ☑
          streetcar (traffic) V66.7 ☑
            nontraffic V66.2 ☑
          three wheeled motor vehicle (traffic) V62.7 ☑

Accident — *continued*
  transport — *continued*
    truck occupant — *continued*
      hanger-on — *continued*
        collision — *continued*
          three wheeled motor vehicle — *continued*
            nontraffic V62.2 ☑
          truck (traffic) V64.7 ☑
            nontraffic V64.2 ☑
          two wheeled motor vehicle (traffic) V62.7 ☑
            nontraffic V62.2 ☑
          van (traffic) V63.7 ☑
            nontraffic V63.2 ☑
        noncollision accident (traffic) V68.7 ☑
          nontraffic V68.2 ☑
      noncollision accident (traffic) V68.9 ☑
        nontraffic V68.3 ☑
        while boarding or alighting V68.4 ☑
      nontraffic V69.3 ☑
      passenger
        collision (with)
          animal (traffic) V60.6 ☑
            being ridden (traffic) V66.6 ☑
              nontraffic V66.1- ☑
            nontraffic V60.1 ☑
          animal-drawn vehicle (traffic) V66.6 ☑
            nontraffic V66.1 ☑
          bus (traffic) V64.6 ☑
            nontraffic V64.1 ☑
          car (traffic) V63.6 ☑
            nontraffic V63.1 ☑
          motor vehicle NOS (traffic) V69.50 ☑
            nontraffic V69.10 ☑
            specified type NEC (traffic) V69.59 ☑
              nontraffic V69.19 ☑
          pedal cycle (traffic) V61.6 ☑
            nontraffic V61.1 ☑
          pickup truck (traffic) V63.6 ☑
            nontraffic V63.1 ☑
          railway vehicle (traffic) V65.6 ☑
            nontraffic V65.1 ☑
          specified vehicle NEC (traffic) V66.6 ☑
            nontraffic V66.1 ☑
          stationary object (traffic) V67.6 ☑
            nontraffic V67.1 ☑
          streetcar (traffic) V66.6 ☑
            nontraffic V66.1 ☑
          three wheeled motor vehicle (traffic) V62.6 ☑
            nontraffic V62.1 ☑
          truck (traffic) V64.6 ☑
            nontraffic V64.1 ☑
          two wheeled motor vehicle (traffic) V62.6 ☑
            nontraffic V62.1 ☑
          van (traffic) V63.6 ☑
            nontraffic V63.1 ☑
        noncollision accident (traffic) V68.6 ☑
          nontraffic V68.1 ☑
    pickup — *see* Accident, transport, pickup truck occupant
    specified type NEC V69.88 ☑
      military vehicle V69.81 ☑
    van occupant V59.9 ☑
      collision (with)
        animal (traffic) V50.9 ☑
          being ridden (traffic) V56.9 ☑
            nontraffic V56.3 ☑
            while boarding or alighting V56.4 ☑
          nontraffic V50.3 ☑
          while boarding or alighting V50.4 ☑
        animal-drawn vehicle (traffic) V56.9 ☑
          nontraffic V56.3 ☑
          while boarding or alighting V56.4 ☑
        bus (traffic) V54.9 ☑
          nontraffic V54.3 ☑
          while boarding or alighting V54.4 ☑
        car (traffic) V53.9 ☑
          nontraffic V53.3 ☑
          while boarding or alighting V53.4 ☑
        motor vehicle NOS (traffic) V59.60 ☑
          nontraffic V59.20 ☑
          specified type NEC (traffic) V59.69 ☑
            nontraffic V59.29 ☑

Accident — *continued*
  transport — *continued*
    van occupant — *continued*
      collision — *continued*
        pedal cycle (traffic) V51.9 ☑
          nontraffic V51.3 ☑
          while boarding or alighting V51.4 ☑
        pickup truck (traffic) V53.9 ☑
          nontraffic V53.3 ☑
          while boarding or alighting V53.4 ☑
        railway vehicle (traffic) V55.9 ☑
          nontraffic V55.3 ☑
          while boarding or alighting V55.4 ☑
        specified vehicle NEC (traffic) V56.9 ☑
          nontraffic V56.3 ☑
          while boarding or alighting V56.4 ☑
        stationary object (traffic) V57.9 ☑
          nontraffic V57.3 ☑
          while boarding or alighting V57.4 ☑
        streetcar (traffic) V56.9 ☑
          nontraffic V56.3 ☑
          while boarding or alighting V56.4 ☑
        three wheeled motor vehicle (traffic) V52.9 ☑
          nontraffic V52.3 ☑
          while boarding or alighting V52.4 ☑
        truck (traffic) V54.9 ☑
          nontraffic V54.3 ☑
          while boarding or alighting V54.4 ☑
        two wheeled motor vehicle (traffic) V52.9 ☑
          nontraffic V52.3 ☑
          while boarding or alighting V52.4 ☑
        van (traffic) V53.9 ☑
          nontraffic V53.3 ☑
          while boarding or alighting V53.4 ☑
    driver
      collision (with)
        animal (traffic) V50.5 ☑
          being ridden (traffic) V56.5 ☑
            nontraffic V56.0 ☑
          nontraffic V50.0 ☑
        animal-drawn vehicle (traffic) V56.5 ☑
          nontraffic V56.0 ☑
        bus (traffic) V54.5 ☑
          nontraffic V54.0 ☑
        car (traffic) V53.5 ☑
          nontraffic V53.0 ☑
        motor vehicle NOS (traffic) V59.40 ☑
          nontraffic V59.00 ☑
          specified type NEC (traffic) V59.49 ☑
            nontraffic V59.09 ☑
        pedal cycle (traffic) V51.5 ☑
          nontraffic V51.0 ☑
        pickup truck (traffic) V53.5 ☑
          nontraffic V53.0 ☑
        railway vehicle (traffic) V55.5 ☑
          nontraffic V55.0 ☑
        specified vehicle NEC (traffic) V56.5 ☑
          nontraffic V56.0 ☑
        stationary object (traffic) V57.5 ☑
          nontraffic V57.0 ☑
        streetcar (traffic) V56.5 ☑
          nontraffic V56.0 ☑
        three wheeled motor vehicle (traffic) V52.5 ☑
          nontraffic V52.0 ☑
        truck (traffic) V54.5 ☑
          nontraffic V54.0 ☑
        two wheeled motor vehicle (traffic) V52.5 ☑
          nontraffic V52.0 ☑
        van (traffic) V53.5 ☑
          nontraffic V53.0 ☑
      noncollision accident (traffic) V58.5 ☑
        nontraffic V58.0 ☑
    hanger-on
      collision (with)
        animal (traffic) V50.7 ☑
          being ridden (traffic) V56.7 ☑
            nontraffic V56.2 ☑
          nontraffic V50.2 ☑
        animal-drawn vehicle (traffic) V56.7 ☑
          nontraffic V56.2 ☑
        bus (traffic) V54.7 ☑
          nontraffic V54.2 ☑
        car (traffic) V53.7 ☑
          nontraffic V53.2 ☑

Accident — *continued*
  transport — *continued*
    van occupant — *continued*
      hanger-on — *continued*
        collision — *continued*
          pedal cycle (traffic) V51.7 ☑
            nontraffic V51.2 ☑
          pickup truck (traffic) V53.7 ☑
            nontraffic V53.2 ☑
          railway vehicle (traffic) V55.7 ☑
            nontraffic V55.2 ☑
          specified vehicle NEC (traffic) V56.7 ☑
            nontraffic V56.2 ☑
          stationary object (traffic) V57.7 ☑
            nontraffic V57.2 ☑
          streetcar (traffic) V56.7 ☑
            nontraffic V56.2 ☑
          three wheeled motor vehicle (traffic) V52.7 ☑
            nontraffic V52.2 ☑
          truck (traffic) V54.7 ☑
            nontraffic V54.2 ☑
          two wheeled motor vehicle (traffic) V52.7 ☑
            nontraffic V52.2 ☑
          van (traffic) V53.7 ☑
            nontraffic V53.2 ☑
        noncollision accident (traffic) V58.7 ☑
          nontraffic V58.2 ☑
      noncollision accident (traffic) V58.9 ☑
        nontraffic V58.3 ☑
        while boarding or alighting V58.4 ☑
      nontraffic V59.3 ☑
      passenger
        collision (with)
          animal (traffic) V50.6 ☑
            being ridden (traffic) V56.6 ☑
              nontraffic V56.1 ☑
            nontraffic V50.1 ☑
          animal-drawn vehicle (traffic) V56.6 ☑
            nontraffic V56.1 ☑
          bus (traffic) V54.6 ☑
            nontraffic V54.1 ☑
          car (traffic) V53.6 ☑
            nontraffic V53.1 ☑
          motor vehicle NOS (traffic) V59.50 ☑
            nontraffic V59.10 ☑
            specified type NEC (traffic) V59.59 ☑
              nontraffic V59.19 ☑
          pedal cycle (traffic) V51.6 ☑
            nontraffic V51.1 ☑
          pickup truck (traffic) V53.6 ☑
            nontraffic V53.1 ☑
          railway vehicle (traffic) V55.6 ☑
            nontraffic V55.1 ☑
          specified vehicle NEC (traffic) V56.6 ☑
            nontraffic V56.1 ☑
          stationary object (traffic) V57.6 ☑
            nontraffic V57.1 ☑
          streetcar (traffic) V56.6 ☑
            nontraffic V56.1 ☑
          three wheeled motor vehicle (traffic) V52.6 ☑
            nontraffic V52.1 ☑
          truck (traffic) V54.6 ☑
            nontraffic V54.1 ☑
          two wheeled motor vehicle (traffic) V52.6 ☑
            nontraffic V52.1 ☑
          van (traffic) V53.6 ☑
            nontraffic V53.1 ☑
        noncollision accident (traffic) V58.6 ☑
          nontraffic V58.1 ☑
      specified type NEC V59.88 ☑
        military vehicle V59.81 ☑
    watercraft occupant — *see* Accident, watercraft
  vehicle NEC V89.9 ☑
    animal-drawn NEC — *see* Accident, transport, animal-drawn vehicle occupant
    special
      agricultural — *see* Accident, transport, agricultural vehicle occupant
      construction — *see* Accident, transport, construction vehicle occupant
      industrial — *see* Accident, transport, industrial vehicle occupant

☑ **Additional Character Required** — Refer to the Tabular List for Character Selection   ▽ **Subterms under main terms may continue to next column or page**

Accident — *continued*
  vehicle — *continued*
    three-wheeled NEC (motorized) — *see* Accident, transport, three-wheeled motor vehicle occupant
  watercraft V94.9 ☑
    causing
      drowning — *see* Drowning, due to, accident to, watercraft
      injury NEC V91.89 ☑
        crushed between craft and object V91.19 ☑
          powered craft V91.13 ☑
            ferry boat V91.11 ☑
            fishing boat V91.12 ☑
            jetskis V91.13 ☑
            liner V91.11 ☑
            merchant ship V91.10 ☑
            passenger ship V91.11 ☑
          unpowered craft V91.18 ☑
            canoe V91.15 ☑
            inflatable V91.16 ☑
            kayak V91.15 ☑
            sailboat V91.14 ☑
            surf-board V91.18 ☑
            windsurfer V91.18 ☑
        fall on board V91.29 ☑
          powered craft V91.23 ☑
            ferry boat V91.21 ☑
            fishing boat V91.22 ☑
            jetskis V91.23 ☑
            liner V91.21 ☑
            merchant ship V91.20 ☑
            passenger ship V91.21 ☑
          unpowered craft
            canoe V91.25 ☑
            inflatable V91.26 ☑
            kayak V91.25 ☑
            sailboat V91.24 ☑
        fire on board causing burn V91.09 ☑
          powered craft V91.03 ☑
            ferry boat V91.01 ☑
            fishing boat V91.02 ☑
            jetskis V91.03 ☑
            liner V91.01 ☑
            merchant ship V91.00 ☑
            passenger ship V91.01 ☑
          unpowered craft V91.08 ☑
            canoe V91.05 ☑
            inflatable V91.06 ☑
            kayak V91.05 ☑
            sailboat V91.04 ☑
            surf-board V91.08 ☑
            water skis V91.07 ☑
            windsurfer V91.08 ☑
        hit by falling object V91.39 ☑
          powered craft V91.33 ☑
            ferry boat V91.31 ☑
            fishing boat V91.32 ☑
            jetskis V91.33 ☑
            liner V91.31 ☑
            merchant ship V91.30 ☑
            passenger ship V91.31 ☑
          unpowered craft V91.38 ☑
            canoe V91.35 ☑
            inflatable V91.36 ☑
            kayak V91.35 ☑
            sailboat V91.34 ☑
            surf-board V91.38 ☑
            water skis V91.37 ☑
            windsurfer V91.38 ☑
        specified type NEC V91.89 ☑
          powered craft V91.83 ☑
            ferry boat V91.81 ☑
            fishing boat V91.82 ☑
            jetskis V91.83 ☑
            liner V91.81 ☑
            merchant ship V91.80 ☑
            passenger ship V91.81 ☑
          unpowered craft V91.88 ☑
            canoe V91.85 ☑
            inflatable V91.86 ☑
            kayak V91.85 ☑
            sailboat V91.84 ☑
            surf board V91.88 ☑
            water skis V91.87 ☑
            windsurfer V91.88 ☑

Accident — *continued*
  watercraft — *continued*
    due to, caused by cataclysm — *see* Forces of nature, by type
    military NEC V94.818 ☑
      civilian in water injured by V94.811 ☑
      with civilian watercraft V94.810 ☑
    nonpowered, struck by
      nonpowered vessel V94.22 ☑
      powered vessel V94.21 ☑
    specified type NEC V94.89 ☑
    striking swimmer
      powered V94.11 ☑
      unpowered V94.12 ☑
Acid throwing (assault) Y08.89 ☑
Activity (involving) (of victim at time of event) Y93.9
  aerobic and step exercise (class) Y93.A3 (*following* Y93.7)
  alpine skiing Y93.23
  animal care NEC Y93.K9 (*following* Y93.7)
  arts and handcrafts NEC Y93.D9 (*following* Y93.7)
  athletics played as a team or group NEC Y93.69
  athletics played individually NEC Y93.59
  athletics NEC Y93.79
  baking Y93.G3 (*following* Y93.7)
  ballet Y93.41
  barbells Y93.B3 (*following* Y93.7)
  BASE (Building, Antenna, Span, Earth) jumping Y93.33
  baseball Y93.64
  basketball Y93.67
  bathing (personal) Y93.E1 (*following* Y93.7)
  beach volleyball Y93.68
  bike riding Y93.55
  blackout game Y93.85
  boogie boarding Y93.18
  bowling Y93.54
  boxing Y93.71
  brass instrument playing Y93.J4 (*following* Y93.7)
  building construction Y93.H3 (*following* Y93.7)
  bungee jumping Y93.34
  calisthenics Y93.A2 (*following* Y93.7)
  canoeing (in calm and turbulent water) Y93.16
  capture the flag Y93.6A
  cardiorespiratory exercise NEC Y93.A9 (*following* Y93.7)
  caregiving (providing) NEC Y93.F9 (*following* Y93.7)
    bathing Y93.F1 (*following* Y93.7)
    lifting Y93.F2 (*following* Y93.7)
  cellular
    communication device Y93.C2 (*following* Y93.7)
    telephone Y93.C2 (*following* Y93.7)
  challenge course Y93.A5 (*following* Y93.7)
  cheerleading Y93.45
  choking game Y93.85
  circuit training Y93.A4 (*following* Y93.7)
  cleaning
    floor Y93.E5 (*following* Y93.7)
  climbing NEC Y93.39
    mountain Y93.31
    rock Y93.31
    wall Y93.31
  clothing care and maintenance NEC Y93.E9 (*following* Y93.7)
  combatives Y93.75
  computer
    keyboarding Y93.C1 (*following* Y93.7)
    technology NEC Y93.C9 (*following* Y93.7)
  confidence course Y93.A5 (*following* Y93.7)
  construction (building) Y93.H3 (*following* Y93.7)
  cooking and baking Y93.G3 (*following* Y93.7)
  cool down exercises Y93.A2 (*following* Y93.7)
  cricket Y93.69
  crocheting Y93.D1 (*following* Y93.7)
  cross country skiing Y93.24
  dancing (all types) Y93.41
  digging
    dirt Y93.H1 (*following* Y93.7)
  dirt digging Y93.H1 (*following* Y93.7)
  dishwashing Y93.G1 (*following* Y93.7)
  diving (platform) (springboard) Y93.12
    underwater Y93.15
  dodge ball Y93.6A
  downhill skiing Y93.23
  drum playing Y93.J2 (*following* Y93.7)
  dumbbells Y93.B3 (*following* Y93.7)
  electronic
    devices NEC Y93.C9 (*following* Y93.7)
      hand held interactive Y93.C2 (*following* Y93.7)

Activity — *continued*
  electronic — *continued*
    game playing (using) (with)
      interactive device Y93.C2 (*following* Y93.7)
      keyboard or other stationary device Y93.C1 (*following* Y93.7)
  elliptical machine Y93.A1 (*following* Y93.7)
  exercise(s)
    machines ((primarily) for)
      cardiorespiratory conditioning Y93.A1 (*following* Y93.7)
      muscle strengthening Y93.B1 (*following* Y93.7)
    muscle strengthening (non-machine) NEC Y93.B9 (*following* Y93.7)
  external motion NEC Y93.I9 (*following* Y93.7)
    rollercoaster Y93.I1 (*following* Y93.7)
  fainting game Y93.85
  field hockey Y93.65
  figure skating (pairs) (singles) Y93.21
  flag football Y93.62
  floor mopping and cleaning Y93.E5 (*following* Y93.7)
  food preparation and clean up Y93.G1 (*following* Y93.7)
  football (American) NOS Y93.61
    flag Y93.62
    tackle Y93.61
    touch Y93.62
  four square Y93.6A
  free weights Y93.B3 (*following* Y93.7)
  frisbee (ultimate) Y93.74
  furniture
    building Y93.D3 (*following* Y93.7)
    finishing Y93.D3 (*following* Y93.7)
    repair Y93.D3 (*following* Y93.7)
  game playing (electronic)
    using interactive device Y93.C2 (*following* Y93.7)
    using keyboard or other stationary device Y93.C1 (*following* Y93.7)
  gardening Y93.H2 (*following* Y93.7)
  golf Y93.53
  grass drills Y93.A6 (*following* Y93.7)
  grilling and smoking food Y93.G2 (*following* Y93.7)
  grooming and shearing an animal Y93.K3 (*following* Y93.7)
  guerilla drills Y93.A6 (*following* Y93.7)
  gymnastics (rhythmic) Y93.43
  hand held interactive electronic device Y93.C2 (*following* Y93.7)
  handball Y93.73
  handcrafts NEC Y93.D9 (*following* Y93.7)
  hang gliding Y93.35
  hiking (on level or elevated terrain) Y93.01
  hockey (ice) Y93.22
    field Y93.65
  horseback riding Y93.52
  household (interior) maintenance NEC Y93.E9 (*following* Y93.7)
  ice NEC Y93.29
    dancing Y93.21
    hockey Y93.22
    skating Y93.21
  inline roller skating Y93.51
  ironing Y93.E4 (*following* Y93.7)
  judo Y93.75
  jumping jacks Y93.A2 (*following* Y93.7)
  jumping rope Y93.56
  jumping (off) NEC Y93.39
    BASE (Building, Antenna, Span, Earth) Y93.33
    bungee Y93.34
    jacks Y93.A2 (*following* Y93.7)
    rope Y93.56
  karate Y93.75
  kayaking (in calm and turbulent water) Y93.16
  keyboarding (computer) Y93.C1 (*following* Y93.7)
  kickball Y93.6A
  knitting Y93.D1 (*following* Y93.7)
  lacrosse Y93.65
  land maintenance NEC Y93.H9 (*following* Y93.7)
  landscaping Y93.H2 (*following* Y93.7)
  laundry Y93.E2 (*following* Y93.7)
  machines (exercise)
    primarily for cardiorespiratory conditioning Y93.A1 (*following* Y93.7)
    primarily for muscle strengthening Y93.B1 (*following* Y93.7)
  maintenance
    exterior building NEC Y93.H9 (*following* Y93.7)
    household (interior) NEC Y93.E9 (*following* Y93.7)
    land Y93.H9 (*following* Y93.7)
    property Y93.H9 (*following* Y93.7)

Activity — *continued*
- marching (on level or elevated terrain) Y93.Ø1
- martial arts Y93.75
- microwave oven Y93.G3 (*following* Y93.7)
- milking an animal Y93.K2 (*following* Y93.7)
- mopping (floor) Y93.E5 (*following* Y93.7)
- mountain climbing Y93.31
- muscle strengthening
  - exercises (non-machine) NEC Y93.B9 (*following* Y93.7)
  - machines Y93.B1 (*following* Y93.7)
- musical keyboard (electronic) playing Y93.J1 (*following* Y93.7)
- nordic skiing Y93.24
- obstacle course Y93.A5 (*following* Y93.7)
- oven (microwave) Y93.G3 (*following* Y93.7)
- packing up and unpacking in moving to a new residence Y93.E6 (*following* Y93.7)
- parasailing Y93.19
- pass out game Y93.85
- percussion instrument playing NEC Y93.J2 (*following* Y93.7)
- personal
  - bathing and showering Y93.E1 (*following* Y93.7)
  - hygiene NEC Y93.E8 (*following* Y93.7)
  - showering Y93.E1 (*following* Y93.7)
- physical games generally associated with school recess, summer camp and children Y93.6A
- physical training NEC Y93.A9 (*following* Y93.7)
- piano playing Y93.J1 (*following* Y93.7)
- pilates Y93.B4 (*following* Y93.7)
- platform diving Y93.12
- playing musical instrument
  - brass instrument Y93.J4 (*following* Y93.7)
  - drum Y93.J2 (*following* Y93.7)
  - musical keyboard (electronic) Y93.J1 (*following* Y93.7)
  - percussion instrument NEC Y93.J2 (*following* Y93.7)
  - piano Y93.J1 (*following* Y93.7)
  - string instrument Y93.J3 (*following* Y93.7)
  - winds instrument Y93.J4 (*following* Y93.7)
- property maintenance
  - exterior NEC Y93.H9 (*following* Y93.7)
  - interior NEC Y93.E9 (*following* Y93.7)
- pruning (garden and lawn) Y93.H2 (*following* Y93.7)
- pull-ups Y93.B2 (*following* Y93.7)
- push-ups Y93.B2 (*following* Y93.7)
- racquetball Y93.73
- rafting (in calm and turbulent water) Y93.16
- raking (leaves) Y93.H1 (*following* Y93.7)
- rappelling Y93.32
- refereeing a sports activity Y93.81
- residential relocation Y93.E6 (*following* Y93.7)
- rhythmic gymnastics Y93.43
- rhythmic movement NEC Y93.49
- riding
  - horseback Y93.52
  - rollercoaster Y93.I1 (*following* Y93.7)
- rock climbing Y93.31
- roller skating (inline) Y93.51
- rollercoaster riding Y93.I1 (*following* Y93.7)
- rough housing and horseplay Y93.83
- rowing (in calm and turbulent water) Y93.16
- rugby Y93.63
- running Y93.Ø2
- SCUBA diving Y93.15
- sewing Y93.D2 (*following* Y93.7)
- shoveling Y93.H1 (*following* Y93.7)
  - dirt Y93.H1 (*following* Y93.7)
  - snow Y93.H1 (*following* Y93.7)
- showering (personal) Y93.E1 (*following* Y93.7)
- sit-ups Y93.B2 (*following* Y93.7)
- skateboarding Y93.51
- skating (ice) Y93.21
  - roller Y93.51
- skiing (alpine) (downhill) Y93.23
  - cross country Y93.24
  - nordic Y93.24
  - water Y93.17
- sledding (snow) Y93.23
- sleeping (sleep) Y93.84
- smoking and grilling food Y93.G2 (*following* Y93.7)
- snorkeling Y93.15
- snow NEC Y93.29
  - boarding Y93.23
  - shoveling Y93.H1 (*following* Y93.7)
  - sledding Y93.23
  - tubing Y93.23
- soccer Y93.66

Activity — *continued*
- softball Y93.64
- specified NEC Y93.89
- spectator at an event Y93.82
- sports NEC Y93.79
  - sports played as a team or group NEC Y93.69
  - sports played individually NEC Y93.59
- springboard diving Y93.12
- squash Y93.73
- stationary bike Y93.A1 (*following* Y93.7)
- step (stepping) exercise (class) Y93.A3 (*following* Y93.7)
- stepper machine Y93.A1 (*following* Y93.7)
- stove Y93.G3 (*following* Y93.7)
- string instrument playing Y93.J3 (*following* Y93.7)
- surfing Y93.18
  - wind Y93.18
- swimming Y93.11
- tackle football Y93.61
- tap dancing Y93.41
- tennis Y93.73
- tobogganing Y93.23
- touch football Y93.62
- track and field events (non-running) Y93.57
  - running Y93.Ø2
- trampoline Y93.44
- treadmill Y93.A1 (*following* Y93.7)
- trimming shrubs Y93.H2 (*following* Y93.7)
- tubing (in calm and turbulent water) Y93.16
  - snow Y93.23
- ultimate frisbee Y93.74
- underwater diving Y93.15
- unpacking in moving to a new residence Y93.E6 (*following* Y93.7)
- use of stove, oven and microwave oven Y93.G3 (*following* Y93.7)
- vacuuming Y93.E3 (*following* Y93.7)
- volleyball (beach) (court) Y93.68
- wake boarding Y93.17
- walking (on level or elevated terrain) Y93.Ø1
  - an animal Y93.K1 (*following* Y93.7)
- walking an animal Y93.K1 (*following* Y93.7)
- wall climbing Y93.31
- warm up and cool down exercises Y93.A2 (*following* Y93.7)
- water NEC Y93.19
  - aerobics Y93.14
  - craft NEC Y93.19
  - exercise Y93.14
  - polo Y93.13
  - skiing Y93.17
  - sliding Y93.18
  - survival training and testing Y93.19
- weeding (garden and lawn) Y93.H2 (*following* Y93.7)
- wind instrument playing Y93.J4 (*following* Y93.7)
- windsurfing Y93.18
- wrestling Y93.72
- yoga Y93.42

Adverse effect of drugs — *see* Table of Drugs and Chemicals

Aerosinusitis — *see* Air, pressure

After-effect, late — *see* Sequelae

Air
- blast in war operations — *see* War operations, air blast
- pressure
  - change, rapid
    - during
      - ascent W94.29 ☑
        - while (in) (surfacing from)
          - aircraft W94.23 ☑
          - deep water diving W94.21 ☑
          - underground W94.22 ☑
      - descent W94.39 ☑
        - in
          - aircraft W94.31 ☑
          - water W94.32 ☑
    - high, prolonged W94.Ø ☑
    - low, prolonged W94.12 ☑
      - due to residence or long visit at high altitude W94.11 ☑

Alpine sickness W94.11 ☑

Altitude sickness W94.11 ☑

Anaphylactic shock, anaphylaxis — *see* Table of Drugs and Chemicals

Andes disease W94.11 ☑

Arachnidism, arachnoidism X58 ☑

Arson (with intent to injure or kill) X97 ☑

Asphyxia, asphyxiation
- by
  - food (bone) (seed) — *see* categories T17 and T18
  - gas — *see also* Table of Drugs and Chemicals
    - legal
      - execution — *see* Legal, intervention, gas
      - intervention — *see* Legal, intervention, gas
- from
  - fire — *see also* Exposure, fire
    - in war operations — *see* War operations, fire
  - ignition — *see* Ignition
  - vomitus T17.81 ☑
- in war operations — *see* War operations, restriction of airway

Aspiration
- food (any type) (into respiratory tract) (with asphyxia, obstruction respiratory tract, suffocation) — *see* categories T17 and T18 ☑
- foreign body — *see* Foreign body, aspiration
- vomitus (with asphyxia, obstruction respiratory tract, suffocation) T17.81 ☑

Assassination (attempt) — *see* Assault

Assault (homicidal) (by) (in) YØ9
- arson X97 ☑
- bite (of human being) YØ4.1 ☑
- bodily force YØ4.8 ☑
  - bite YØ4.1 ☑
  - bumping into YØ4.2 ☑
  - sexual — *see* subcategories T74.Ø, T76.Ø ☑
  - unarmed fight YØ4.Ø ☑
- bomb X96.9 ☑
  - antipersonnel X96.Ø ☑
  - fertilizer X96.3 ☑
  - gasoline X96.1 ☑
  - letter X96.2 ☑
  - petrol X96.1 ☑
  - pipe X96.3 ☑
  - specified NEC X96.8 ☑
- brawl (hand) (fists) (foot) (unarmed) YØ4.Ø ☑
- burning, burns (by fire) NEC X97 ☑
  - acid YØ8.89 ☑
  - caustic, corrosive substance YØ8.89 ☑
  - chemical from swallowing caustic, corrosive substance — *see* Table of Drugs and Chemicals
  - cigarette(s) X97 ☑
  - hot object X98.9 ☑
    - fluid NEC X98.2 ☑
    - household appliance X98.3 ☑
    - specified NEC X98.8 ☑
    - steam X98.Ø ☑
    - tap water X98.1 ☑
    - vapors X98.Ø ☑
  - scalding — *see* Assault, burning
  - steam X98.Ø ☑
  - vitriol YØ8.89 ☑
- caustic, corrosive substance (gas) YØ8.89 ☑
- crashing of
  - aircraft YØ8.81 ☑
  - motor vehicle YØ3.8 ☑
    - pushed in front of YØ2.Ø ☑
    - run over YØ3.Ø ☑
    - specified NEC YØ3.8 ☑
- cutting or piercing instrument X99.9 ☑
  - dagger X99.2 ☑
  - glass X99.Ø ☑
  - knife X99.1 ☑
  - specified NEC X99.8 ☑
  - sword X99.2 ☑
- dagger X99.2 ☑
- drowning (in) X92.9 ☑
  - bathtub X92.Ø ☑
  - natural water X92.3 ☑
  - specified NEC X92.8 ☑
  - swimming pool X92.1 ☑
    - following fall X92.2 ☑
- dynamite X96.8 ☑
- explosive(s) (material) X96.9 ☑
- fight (hand) (fists) (foot) (unarmed) YØ4.Ø ☑
  - with weapon — *see* Assault, by type of weapon
- fire X97 ☑
- firearm X95.9 ☑
  - airgun X95.Ø1 ☑
  - handgun X93 ☑
  - hunting rifle X94.1 ☑
  - larger X94.9 ☑
    - specified NEC X94.8 ☑

☑ Additional Character Required — Refer to the Tabular List for Character Selection   ▽ Subterms under main terms may continue to next column or page

Assault — *continued*
  firearm — *continued*
    machine gun X94.2 ☑
    shotgun X94.0 ☑
    specified NEC X95.8 ☑
  from high place Y01 ☑
  gunshot (wound) NEC — *see* Assault, firearm, by type
  incendiary device X97 ☑
  injury Y09
    to child due to criminal abortion attempt NEC
      Y08.89 ☑
  knife X99.1 ☑
  late effect of — *see* categories X92-Y08 with 7th character S
  placing before moving object NEC Y02.8 ☑
    motor vehicle Y02.0 ☑
  poisoning — *see* categories T36-T65 with 7th character S
  puncture, any part of body — *see* Assault, cutting or piercing instrument
  pushing
    before moving object NEC Y02.8 ☑
      motor vehicle Y02.0 ☑
      subway train Y02.1 ☑
      train Y02.1 ☑
    from high place Y01 ☑
  rape T74.2-
  scalding — *see* Assault, burning
  sequelae of — *see* categories X92-Y08 with 7th character S
  sexual (by bodily force) T74.2-
  shooting — *see* Assault, firearm
  specified means NEC Y08.89 ☑
  stab, any part of body — *see* Assault, cutting or piercing instrument
  steam X98.0 ☑
  striking against
    other person Y04.2 ☑
    sports equipment Y08.09 ☑
      baseball bat Y08.02 ☑
      hockey stick Y08.01 ☑
  struck by
    sports equipment Y08.09 ☑
      baseball bat Y08.02 ☑
      hockey stick Y08.01 ☑
  submersion — *see* Assault, drowning
  violence Y09
  weapon Y09
    blunt Y00 ☑
    cutting or piercing — *see* Assault, cutting or piercing instrument
    firearm — *see* Assault, firearm
  wound Y09
    cutting — *see* Assault, cutting or piercing instrument
    gunshot — *see* Assault, firearm
    knife X99.1 ☑
    piercing — *see* Assault, cutting or piercing instrument
    puncture — *see* Assault, cutting or piercing instrument
    stab — *see* Assault, cutting or piercing instrument
Attack by mammals NEC W55.89 ☑
Avalanche — *see* Landslide
Aviator's disease — *see* Air, pressure

B

Barotitis, barodontalgia, barosinusitis, barotrauma (otitic) (sinus) — *see* Air, pressure
Battered (baby) (child) (person) (syndrome) X58 ☑
Bayonet wound W26.1 ☑
  in
    legal intervention — *see* Legal, intervention, sharp object, bayonet
    war operations — *see* War operations, combat
  stated as undetermined whether accidental or intentional Y28.8 ☑
  suicide (attempt) X78.2 ☑
Bean in nose — *see* categories T17 and T18 ☑
Bed set on fire NEC — *see* Exposure, fire, uncontrolled, building, bed
Beheading (by guillotine)
  homicide X99.9 ☑
  legal execution — *see* Legal, intervention
Bending, injury in (prolonged) (static) X50.1 ☑

Bends — *see* Air, pressure, change
Bite, bitten by
  alligator W58.01 ☑
  arthropod (nonvenomous) NEC W57 ☑
  bull W55.21 ☑
  cat W55.01 ☑
  cow W55.21 ☑
  crocodile W58.11 ☑
  dog W54.0 ☑
  goat W55.31 ☑
  hoof stock NEC W55.31 ☑
  horse W55.11 ☑
  human being (accidentally) W50.3 ☑
    with intent to injure or kill Y04.1 ☑
    as, or caused by, a crowd or human stampede (with fall) W52
    assault Y04.1 ☑
    homicide (attempt) Y04.1 ☑
    in
      fight Y04.1 ☑
  insect (nonvenomous) W57 ☑
  lizard (nonvenomous) W59.01 ☑
  mammal NEC W55.81 ☑
    marine W56.31 ☑
  marine animal (nonvenomous) W56.81 ☑
  millipede W57 ☑
  moray eel W56.51 ☑
  mouse W53.01 ☑
  person(s) (accidentally) W50.3 ☑
    with intent to injure or kill Y04.1 ☑
    as, or caused by, a crowd or human stampede (with fall) W52
    assault Y04.1 ☑
    homicide (attempt) Y04.1 ☑
    in
      fight Y04.1 ☑
  pig W55.41 ☑
  raccoon W55.51 ☑
  rat W53.11 ☑
  reptile W59.81 ☑
    lizard W59.01 ☑
    snake W59.11 ☑
    turtle W59.21 ☑
      terrestrial W59.81 ☑
  rodent W53.81 ☑
    mouse W53.01 ☑
    rat W53.11 ☑
    specified NEC W53.81 ☑
    squirrel W53.21 ☑
  shark W56.41 ☑
  sheep W55.31 ☑
  snake (nonvenomous) W59.11 ☑
  spider (nonvenomous) W57 ☑
  squirrel W53.21 ☑
Blast (air) in war operations — *see* War operations, blast
Blizzard X37.2 ☑
Blood alcohol level Y90.9
  less than 20mg/100ml Y90.0
  presence in blood, level not specified Y90.9
  20-39mg/100ml Y90.1
  40-59mg/100ml Y90.2
  60-79mg/100ml Y90.3
  80-99mg/100ml Y90.4
  100-119mg/100ml Y90.5
  120-199mg/100ml Y90.6
  200-239mg/100ml Y90.7
Blow X58 ☑
  by law-enforcing agent, police (on duty) — *see* Legal, intervention, manhandling
  blunt object — *see* Legal, intervention, blunt object
Blowing up — *see* Explosion
Brawl (hand) (fists) (foot) Y04.0 ☑
Breakage (accidental) (part of)
  ladder (causing fall) W11 ☑
  scaffolding (causing fall) W12 ☑
Broken
  glass, contact with — *see* Contact, with, glass
  power line (causing electric shock) W85 ☑
Bumping against, into (accidentally)
  object NEC W22.8 ☑
    caused by crowd or human stampede (with fall) W52 ☑
    sports equipment W21.9 ☑
    with fall — *see* Fall, due to, bumping against, object
  person(s) W51 ☑
    with fall W03 ☑

Bumping against, into — *continued*
  person(s) — *continued*
    with fall — *continued*
      due to ice or snow W00.0 ☑
    assault Y04.2 ☑
    caused by, a crowd or human stampede (with fall) W52
    homicide (attempt) Y04.2 ☑
  sports equipment W21.9 ☑
Burn, burned, burning (accidental) (by) (from) (on)
  acid NEC — *see* Table of Drugs and Chemicals
  bed linen — *see* Exposure, fire, uncontrolled, in building, bed
  blowtorch X08.8 ☑
    with ignition of clothing NEC X06.2 ☑
      nightwear X05 ☑
  bonfire, campfire (controlled) — *see also* Exposure, fire, controlled, not in building)
    uncontrolled — *see* Exposure, fire, uncontrolled, not in building
  candle X08.8 ☑
    with ignition of clothing NEC X06.2 ☑
      nightwear X05 ☑
  caustic liquid, substance (external) (internal) NEC — *see* Table of Drugs and Chemicals
  chemical (external) (internal) — *see also* Table of Drugs and Chemicals
    in war operations — *see* War operations. fire
  cigar(s) or cigarette(s) X08.8 ☑
    with ignition of clothing NEC X06.2 ☑
      nightwear X05 ☑
  clothes, clothing NEC (from controlled fire) X06.2 ☑
    with conflagration — *see* Exposure, fire, uncontrolled, building
      not in building or structure — *see* Exposure, fire, uncontrolled, not in building
  cooker (hot) X15.8 ☑
    stated as undetermined whether accidental or intentional Y27.3 ☑
    suicide (attempt) X77.3 ☑
  electric blanket X16 ☑
  engine (hot) X17 ☑
  fire, flames — *see* Exposure, fire
  flare, Very pistol — *see* Discharge, firearm NEC
  heat
    from appliance (electrical) (household) X15.8 ☑
      cooker X15.8 ☑
      hotplate X15.2 ☑
      kettle X15.8 ☑
      light bulb X15.8 ☑
      saucepan X15.3 ☑
      skillet X15.3 ☑
      stated as undetermined whether accidental or intentional Y27.3 ☑
      stove X15.0 ☑
      suicide (attempt) X77.3 ☑
      toaster X15.1 ☑
    in local application or packing during medical or surgical procedure Y63.5
  heating
    appliance, radiator or pipe X16 ☑
  homicide (attempt) — *see* Assault, burning
  hot
    air X14.1 ☑
    cooker X15.8 ☑
    drink X10.0 ☑
    engine X17 ☑
    fat X10.2 ☑
    fluid NEC X12 ☑
    food X10.1 ☑
    gases X14.1 ☑
    heating appliance X16 ☑
    household appliance NEC X15.8 ☑
    kettle X15.8 ☑
    liquid NEC X12 ☑
    machinery X17 ☑
    metal (molten) (liquid) NEC X18 ☑
    object (not producing fire or flames) NEC X19 ☑
    oil (cooking) X10.2 ☑
    pipe(s) X16 ☑
    radiator X16 ☑
    saucepan (glass) (metal) X15.3 ☑
    stove (kitchen) X15.0 ☑
    substance NEC X19 ☑
      caustic or corrosive NEC — *see* Table of Drugs and Chemicals

Burn, burned, burning — *continued*
  hot — *continued*
    toaster X15.1 ☑
    tool X17 ☑
    vapor X13.1 ☑
    water (tap) — *see* Contact, with, hot, tap water
  hotplate X15.2 ☑
    suicide (attempt) X77.3 ☑
  ignition — *see* Ignition
  in war operations — *see* War operations, fire
  inflicted by other person X97 ☑
    by hot objects, hot vapor, and steam — *see* Assault, burning, hot object
  internal, from swallowed caustic, corrosive liquid, substance — *see* Table of Drugs and Chemicals
  iron (hot) X15.8 ☑
    stated as undetermined whether accidental or intentional Y27.3 ☑
    suicide (attempt) X77.3 ☑
  kettle (hot) X15.8 ☑
    stated as undetermined whether accidental or intentional Y27.3 ☑
    suicide (attempt) X77.3 ☑
  lamp (flame) X08.8 ☑
    with ignition of clothing NEC X06.2 ☑
      nightwear X05 ☑
  lighter (cigar) (cigarette) X08.8 ☑
    with ignition of clothing NEC X06.2 ☑
      nightwear X05 ☑
  lightning — *see* subcategory T75.0 ☑
    causing fire — *see* Exposure, fire
  liquid (boiling) (hot) NEC X12 ☑
    stated as undetermined whether accidental or intentional Y27.2 ☑
    suicide (attempt) X77.2 ☑
  local application of externally applied substance in medical or surgical care Y63.5
  machinery (hot) X17 ☑
  matches X08.8 ☑
    with ignition of clothing NEC X06.2 ☑
      nightwear X05 ☑
  mattress — *see* Exposure, fire, uncontrolled, building, bed
  medicament, externally applied Y63.5
  metal (hot) (liquid) (molten) NEC X18 ☑
  nightwear (nightclothes, nightdress, gown, pajamas, robe) X05 ☑
  object (hot) NEC X19 ☑
  on board watercraft
    due to
      accident to watercraft V91.09 ☑
        powered craft V91.03 ☑
          ferry boat V91.01 ☑
          fishing boat V91.02 ☑
          jetskis V91.03 ☑
          liner V91.01 ☑
          merchant ship V91.00 ☑
          passenger ship V91.01 ☑
        unpowered craft V91.08 ☑
          canoe V91.05 ☑
          inflatable V91.06 ☑
          kayak V91.05 ☑
          sailboat V91.04 ☑
          surf-board V91.08 ☑
          water skis V91.07 ☑
          windsurfer V91.08 ☑
      fire on board V93.09 ☑
        ferry boat V93.01 ☑
        fishing boat V93.02 ☑
        jetskis V93.03 ☑
        liner V93.01 ☑
        merchant ship V93.00 ☑
        passenger ship V93.01 ☑
        powered craft NEC V93.03 ☑
        sailboat V93.04 ☑
      specified heat source NEC on board V93.19 ☑
        ferry boat V93.11 ☑
        fishing boat V93.12 ☑
        jetskis V93.13 ☑
        liner V93.11 ☑
        merchant ship V93.10 ☑
        passenger ship V93.11 ☑
        powered craft NEC V93.13 ☑
        sailboat V93.14 ☑
  pipe (hot) X16 ☑
    smoking X08.8 ☑

Burn, burned, burning — *continued*
  pipe — *continued*
    smoking — *continued*
      with ignition of clothing NEC X06.2 ☑
        nightwear X05 ☑
  powder — *see* Powder burn
  radiator (hot) X16 ☑
  saucepan (hot) (glass) (metal) X15.3 ☑
    stated as undetermined whether accidental or intentional Y27.3 ☑
    suicide (attempt) X77.3 ☑
  self-inflicted X76 ☑
    stated as undetermined whether accidental or intentional Y26 ☑
  stated as undetermined whether accidental or intentional Y27.0 ☑
  steam X13.1 ☑
    pipe X16 ☑
      stated as undetermined whether accidental or intentional Y27.8 ☑
    stated as undetermined whether accidental or intentional Y27.0 ☑
    suicide (attempt) X77.0 ☑
  stove (hot) (kitchen) X15.0 ☑
    stated as undetermined whether accidental or intentional Y27.3 ☑
    suicide (attempt) X77.3 ☑
  substance (hot) NEC X19 ☑
    boiling X12 ☑
      stated as undetermined whether accidental or intentional Y27.2 ☑
      suicide (attempt) X77.2 ☑
    molten (metal) X18 ☑
  suicide (attempt) NEC X76 ☑
    hot
      household appliance X77.3 ☑
      object X77.9 ☑
  therapeutic misadventure
    heat in local application or packing during medical or surgical procedure Y63.5
    overdose of radiation Y63.2
  toaster (hot) X15.1 ☑
    stated as undetermined whether accidental or intentional Y27.3 ☑
    suicide (attempt) X77.3 ☑
  tool (hot) X17 ☑
  torch, welding X08.8 ☑
    with ignition of clothing NEC X06.2 ☑
      nightwear X05 ☑
  trash fire (controlled) — *see* Exposure, fire, controlled, not in building
    uncontrolled — *see* Exposure, fire, uncontrolled, not in building
  vapor (hot) X13.1 ☑
    stated as undetermined whether accidental or intentional Y27.0 ☑
    suicide (attempt) X77.0 ☑
  Very pistol — *see* Discharge, firearm NEC
Butted by animal W55.82 ☑
  bull W55.22 ☑
  cow W55.22 ☑
  goat W55.32 ☑
  horse W55.12 ☑
  pig W55.42 ☑
  sheep W55.32 ☑

C

Caisson disease — *see* Air, pressure, change
Campfire (exposure to) (controlled) — *see also* Exposure, fire, controlled, not in building
  uncontrolled — *see* Exposure, fire, uncontrolled, not in building
Capital punishment (any means) — *see* Legal, intervention
Car sickness T75.3 ☑
Casualty (not due to war) NEC X58 ☑
  war — *see* War operations
Cat
  bite W55.01 ☑
  scratch W55.03 ☑
Cataclysm, cataclysmic (any injury) NEC — *see* Forces of nature
Catching fire — *see* Exposure, fire

Caught
  between
    folding object W23.0 ☑
    objects (moving) (stationary and moving) W23.0 ☑
      and machinery — *see* Contact, with, by type of machine
      stationary W23.1 ☑
    sliding door and door frame W23.0 ☑
  by, in
    machinery (moving parts of) — *see* Contact, with, by type of machine
    washing-machine wringer W23.0 ☑
  under packing crate (due to losing grip) W23.1 ☑
Cave-in caused by cataclysmic earth surface movement or eruption — *see* Landslide
Change(s) in air pressure — *see* Air, pressure, change
Choked, choking (on) (any object except food or vomitus)
  food (bone) (seed) — *see* categories T17 and T18 ☑
  vomitus T17.81- ☑
Civil insurrection — *see* War operations
Cloudburst (any injury) X37.8 ☑
Cold, exposure to (accidental) (excessive) (extreme) (natural) (place) NEC — *see* Exposure, cold
Collapse
  building W20.1 ☑
    burning (uncontrolled fire) X00.2 ☑
  dam or man-made structure (causing earth movement) X36.0 ☑
  machinery — *see* Contact, with, by type of machine
  structure W20.1 ☑
    burning (uncontrolled fire) X00.2 ☑
Collision (accidental) NEC — *see also* Accident, transport V89.9 ☑
  pedestrian W51 ☑
    with fall W03 ☑
      due to ice or snow W00.0 ☑
      involving pedestrian conveyance — *see* Accident, transport, pedestrian, conveyance
    and
      crowd or human stampede (with fall) W52 ☑
      object W22.8 ☑
        with fall — *see* Fall, due to, bumping against, object
  person(s) — *see* Collision, pedestrian
  transport vehicle NEC V89.9 ☑
    and
      avalanche, fallen or not moving — *see* Accident, transport
      falling or moving — *see* Landslide
      landslide, fallen or not moving — *see* Accident, transport
      falling or moving — *see* Landslide
    due to cataclysm — *see* Forces of nature, by type
    intentional, purposeful suicide (attempt) — *see* Suicide, collision
Combustion, spontaneous — *see* Ignition
Complication (delayed) **of or following** (medical or surgical procedure) Y84.9
  with misadventure — *see* Misadventure
  amputation of limb(s) Y83.5
  anastomosis (arteriovenous) (blood vessel) (gastrojejunal) (tendon) (natural or artificial material) Y83.2
  aspiration (of fluid) Y84.4
    tissue Y84.8
  biopsy Y84.8
  blood
    sampling Y84.7
    transfusion
      procedure Y84.8
  bypass Y83.2
  catheterization (urinary) Y84.6
    cardiac Y84.0
  colostomy Y83.3
  cystostomy Y83.3
  dialysis (kidney) Y84.1
  drug — *see* Table of Drugs and Chemicals
    due to misadventure — *see* Misadventure
  duodenostomy Y83.3
  electroshock therapy Y84.3
  external stoma, creation of Y83.3
  formation of external stoma Y83.3
  gastrostomy Y83.3
  graft Y83.2
  hypothermia (medically-induced) Y84.8

412

☑ Additional Character Required — Refer to the Tabular List for Character Selection   ▽ Subterms under main terms may continue to next column or page

Complication (delayed) **of or following** —
  continued
  implant, implantation (of)
    artificial
      internal device (cardiac pacemaker) (electrodes in brain) (heart valve prosthesis) (orthopedic) Y83.1
      material or tissue (for anastomosis or bypass) Y83.2
        with creation of external stoma Y83.3
      natural tissues (for anastomosis or bypass) Y83.2
        with creation of external stoma Y83.3
  infusion
    procedure Y84.8
  injection — *see* Table of Drugs and Chemicals
    procedure Y84.8
  insertion of gastric or duodenal sound Y84.5
  insulin-shock therapy Y84.3
  paracentesis (abdominal) (thoracic) (aspirative) Y84.4
  procedures other than surgical operation — *see* Complication of or following, by type of procedure
  radiological procedure or therapy Y84.2
  removal of organ (partial) (total) NEC Y83.6
  sampling
    blood Y84.7
    fluid NEC Y84.4
    tissue Y84.8
  shock therapy Y84.3
  surgical operation NEC — *see also* Complication of or following, by type of operation Y83.9
    reconstructive NEC Y83.4
      with
        anastomosis, bypass or graft Y83.2
        formation of external stoma Y83.3
    specified NEC Y83.8
  transfusion — *see also* Table of Drugs and Chemicals
    procedure Y84.8
  transplant, transplantation (heart) (kidney) (liver) (whole organ, any) Y83.0
    partial organ Y83.4
  ureterostomy Y83.3
  vaccination — *see also* Table of Drugs and Chemicals
    procedure Y84.8
Compression
  divers' squeeze — *see* Air, pressure, change
  trachea by
    food (lodged in esophagus) — *see* categories T17 and T18 ☑
    vomitus (lodged in esophagus) T17.81- ☑
Conflagration — *see* Exposure, fire, uncontrolled
Constriction (external)
  hair W49.01 ☑
  jewelry W49.04 ☑
  ring W49.04 ☑
  rubber band W49.03 ☑
  specified item NEC W49.09 ☑
  string W49.02 ☑
  thread W49.02 ☑
Contact (accidental)
  with
    abrasive wheel (metalworking) W31.1 ☑
    alligator W58.09 ☑
      bite W58.01 ☑
      crushing W58.03 ☑
      strike W58.02 ☑
    amphibian W62.9 ☑
      frog W62.0 ☑
      toad W62.1 ☑
    animal (nonvenomous) NEC W64 ☑
      marine W56.89 ☑
        bite W56.81 ☑
        dolphin — *see* Contact, with, dolphin
        fish NEC — *see* Contact, with, fish
        mammal — *see* Contact, with, mammal, marine
        orca — *see* Contact, with, orca
        sea lion — *see* Contact, with, sea lion
        shark — *see* Contact, with, shark
        strike W56.82 ☑
    animate mechanical force NEC W64 ☑
    arrow W21.89 ☑
      not thrown, projected or falling W45.8 ☑
    arthropods (nonvenomous) W57 ☑
    axe W27.0 ☑
    band-saw (industrial) W31.2 ☑
    bayonet — *see* Bayonet wound
    bee(s) X58 ☑

Contact — *continued*
  with — *continued*
    bench-saw (industrial) W31.2 ☑
    bird W61.99 ☑
      bite W61.91 ☑
      chicken — *see* Contact, with, chicken
      duck — *see* Contact, with, duck
      goose — *see* Contact, with, goose
      macaw — *see* Contact, with, macaw
      parrot — *see* Contact, with, parrot
      psittacine — *see* Contact, with, psittacine
      strike W61.92 ☑
      turkey — *see* Contact, with, turkey
    blender W29.0 ☑
    boiling water X12 ☑
      stated as undetermined whether accidental or intentional Y27.2 ☑
      suicide (attempt) X77.2 ☑
    bore, earth-drilling or mining (land) (seabed) W31.0 ☑
    buffalo — *see* Contact, with, hoof stock NEC
    bull W55.29 ☑
      bite W55.21 ☑
      gored W55.22 ☑
      strike W55.22 ☑
    bumper cars W31.81 ☑
    camel — *see* Contact, with, hoof stock NEC
    can
      lid W26.8 ☑
      opener W27.4 ☑
        powered W29.0 ☑
    cat W55.09 ☑
      bite W55.01 ☑
      scratch W55.03 ☑
    caterpillar (venomous) X58 ☑
    centipede (venomous) X58 ☑
    chain
      hoist W24.0 ☑
        agricultural operations W30.89 ☑
      saw W29.3 ☑
    chicken W61.39 ☑
      peck W61.33 ☑
      strike W61.32 ☑
    chisel W27.0 ☑
    circular saw W31.2 ☑
    cobra X58 ☑
    combine (harvester) W30.0 ☑
    conveyer belt W24.1 ☑
    cooker (hot) X15.8 ☑
      stated as undetermined whether accidental or intentional Y27.3 ☑
      suicide (attempt) X77.3 ☑
    coral X58 ☑
    cotton gin W31.82 ☑
    cow W55.29 ☑
      bite W55.21 ☑
      strike W55.22 ☑
    crane W24.0 ☑
      agricultural operations W30.89 ☑
    crocodile W58.19 ☑
      bite W58.11 ☑
      crushing W58.13 ☑
      strike W58.12 ☑
    dagger W26.1 ☑
      stated as undetermined whether accidental or intentional Y28.2 ☑
      suicide (attempt) X78.2 ☑
    dairy equipment W31.82 ☑
    dart W21.89 ☑
      not thrown, projected or falling W45.8 ☑
    deer — *see* Contact, with, hoof stock NEC
    derrick W24.0 ☑
      agricultural operations W30.89 ☑
        hay W30.2 ☑
    dog W54.8 ☑
      bite W54.0 ☑
      strike W54.1 ☑
    dolphin W56.09 ☑
      bite W56.01 ☑
      strike W56.02 ☑
    donkey — *see* Contact, with, hoof stock NEC
    drill (powered) W29.8 ☑
      earth (land) (seabed) W31.0 ☑
      nonpowered W27.8 ☑
    drive belt W24.0 ☑
      agricultural operations W30.89 ☑

Contact — *continued*
  with — *continued*
    dry ice — *see* Exposure, cold, man-made
    dryer (clothes) (powered) (spin) W29.2 ☑
    duck W61.69 ☑
      bite W61.61 ☑
      strike W61.62 ☑
    earth (-)
      drilling machine (industrial) W31.0 ☑
      scraping machine in stationary use W31.83 ☑
    edge of stiff paper W26.2 ☑
    electric
      beater W29.0 ☑
      blanket X16 ☑
      fan W29.2 ☑
        commercial W31.82 ☑
      knife W29.1 ☑
      mixer W29.0 ☑
    elevator (building) W24.0 ☑
      agricultural operations W30.89 ☑
        grain W30.3 ☑
    engine(s), hot NEC X17 ☑
    excavating machine W31.0 ☑
    farm machine W30.9 ☑
    feces — *see* Contact, with, by type of animal
    fer de lance X58 ☑
    fish W56.59 ☑
      bite W56.51 ☑
      shark — *see* Contact, with, shark
      strike W56.52 ☑
    flying horses W31.81 ☑
    forging (metalworking) machine W31.1 ☑
    fork W27.4 ☑
    forklift (truck) W24.0 ☑
      agricultural operations W30.89 ☑
    frog W62.0 ☑
    garden
      cultivator (powered) W29.3 ☑
        riding W30.89 ☑
      fork W27.1 ☑
    gas turbine W31.3 ☑
    Gila monster X58 ☑
    giraffe — *see* Contact, with, hoof stock NEC
    glass (sharp) (broken) W25 ☑
      assault X99.0 ☑
      due to fall — *see* Fall, by type
      stated as undetermined whether accidental or intentional Y28.0 ☑
      suicide (attempt) X78.0 ☑
      with subsequent fall W18.02 ☑
    goat W55.39 ☑
      bite W55.31 ☑
      strike W55.32 ☑
    goose W61.59 ☑
      bite W61.51 ☑
      strike W61.52 ☑
    hand
      saw W27.0 ☑
      tool (not powered) NEC W27.8 ☑
        powered W29.8 ☑
    harvester W30.0 ☑
    hay-derrick W30.2 ☑
    heating
      appliance (hot) X16 ☑
      pad (electric) X16 ☑
    heat NEC X19 ☑
      from appliance (electrical) (household) — *see* Contact, with, hot, household appliance
      heating appliance X16 ☑
    hedge-trimmer (powered) W29.3 ☑
    hoe W27.1 ☑
    hoist (chain) (shaft) NEC W24.0 ☑
      agricultural W30.89 ☑
    hoof stock NEC W55.39 ☑
      bite W55.31 ☑
      strike W55.32 ☑
    hornet(s) X58 ☑
    horse W55.19 ☑
      bite W55.11 ☑
      strike W55.12 ☑
    hot
      air X14.1 ☑
        inhalation X14.0 ☑
      cooker X15.8 ☑
      drinks X10.0 ☑
      engine X17 ☑

Contact — *continued*
with — *continued*
hot — *continued*
fats X10.2 ☑
fluids NEC X12 ☑
assault X98.2 ☑
suicide (attempt) X77.2 ☑
undetermined whether accidental or intentional Y27.2 ☑
food X10.1 ☑
gases X14.1 ☑
inhalation X14.0 ☑
heating appliance X16 ☑
household appliance X15.8 ☑
assault X98.3 ☑
cooker X15.8 ☑
hotplate X15.2 ☑
kettle X15.8 ☑
light bulb X15.8 ☑
object NEC X19 ☑
assault X98.8 ☑
stated as undetermined whether accidental or intentional Y27.9 ☑
suicide (attempt) X77.8 ☑
saucepan X15.3 ☑
skillet X15.3 ☑
stated as undetermined whether accidental
or intentional Y27.3 ☑
stove X15.0 ☑
suicide (attempt) X77.3 ☑
toaster X15.1 ☑
kettle X15.8 ☑
light bulb X15.8 ☑
liquid NEC — *see also* Burn X12 ☑
drinks X10.0 ☑
stated as undetermined whether accidental
or intentional Y27.2 ☑
suicide (attempt) X77.2 ☑
tap water X11.8 ☑
stated as undetermined whether accidental or intentional Y27.1 ☑
suicide (attempt) X77.1 ☑
machinery X17 ☑
metal (molten) (liquid) NEC X18 ☑
object (not producing fire or flames) NEC X19 ☑
oil (cooking) X10.2 ☑
pipe X16 ☑
plate X15.2 ☑
radiator X16 ☑
saucepan (glass) (metal) X15.3 ☑
skillet X15.3 ☑
stove (kitchen) X15.0 ☑
substance NEC X19 ☑
tap-water X11.8 ☑
assault X98.1 ☑
heated on stove X12 ☑
stated as undetermined whether accidental or intentional Y27.2 ☑
suicide (attempt) X77.2 ☑
in bathtub X11.0 ☑
running X11.1 ☑
stated as undetermined whether accidental
or intentional Y27.1 ☑
suicide (attempt) X77.1 ☑
toaster X15.1 ☑
tool X17 ☑
vapors X13.1 ☑
inhalation X13.0 ☑
water (tap) X11.8 ☑
boiling X12 ☑
stated as undetermined whether accidental or intentional Y27.2 ☑
suicide (attempt) X77.2 ☑
heated on stove X12 ☑
stated as undetermined whether accidental or intentional Y27.2 ☑
suicide (attempt) X77.2 ☑
in bathtub X11.0 ☑
running X11.1 ☑
stated as undetermined whether accidental
or intentional Y27.1 ☑
suicide (attempt) X77.1 ☑
hotplate X15.2 ☑
ice-pick W27.4 ☑
insect (nonvenomous) NEC W57 ☑
kettle (hot) X15.8 ☑

Contact — *continued*
with — *continued*
knife W26.0 ☑
assault X99.1 ☑
electric W29.1 ☑
stated as undetermined whether accidental or
intentional Y28.1 ☑
suicide (attempt) X78.1 ☑
lathe (metalworking) W31.1 ☑
turnings W45.8 ☑
woodworking W31.2 ☑
lawnmower (powered) (ridden) W28 ☑
causing electrocution W86.8 ☑
suicide (attempt) X83.1 ☑
unpowered W27.1 ☑
lift, lifting (devices) W24.0 ☑
agricultural operations W30.89 ☑
shaft W24.0 ☑
liquefied gas — *see* Exposure, cold, man-made
liquid air, hydrogen, nitrogen — *see* Exposure, cold,
man-made
lizard (nonvenomous) W59.09 ☑
bite W59.01 ☑
strike W59.02 ☑
llama — *see* Contact, with, hoof stock NEC
macaw W61.19 ☑
bite W61.11 ☑
strike W61.12 ☑
machine, machinery W31.9 ☑
abrasive wheel W31.1 ☑
agricultural including animal-powered W30.9 ☑
combine harvester W30.0 ☑
grain storage elevator W30.3 ☑
hay derrick W30.2 ☑
power take-off device W30.1 ☑
reaper W30.0 ☑
specified NEC W30.89 ☑
thresher W30.0 ☑
transport vehicle, stationary W30.81 ☑
band saw W31.2 ☑
bench saw W31.2 ☑
circular saw W31.2 ☑
commercial NEC W31.82 ☑
drilling, metal (industrial) W31.1 ☑
earth-drilling W31.0 ☑
earthmoving or scraping W31.89 ☑
excavating W31.89 ☑
forging machine W31.1 ☑
gas turbine W31.3 ☑
hot X17 ☑
internal combustion engine W31.3 ☑
land drill W31.0 ☑
lathe W31.1 ☑
lifting (devices) W24.0 ☑
metal drill W31.1 ☑
metalworking (industrial) W31.1 ☑
milling, metal W31.1 ☑
mining W31.0 ☑
molding W31.2 ☑
overhead plane W31.2 ☑
power press, metal W31.1 ☑
prime mover W31.3 ☑
printing W31.89 ☑
radial saw W31.2 ☑
recreational W31.81 ☑
roller-coaster W31.81 ☑
rolling mill, metal W31.1 ☑
sander W31.2 ☑
seabed drill W31.0 ☑
shaft
hoist W31.0 ☑
lift W31.0 ☑
specified NEC W31.89 ☑
spinning W31.89 ☑
steam engine W31.3 ☑
transmission W24.1 ☑
undercutter W31.0 ☑
water driven turbine W31.3 ☑
weaving W31.89 ☑
woodworking or forming (industrial) W31.2 ☑
mammal (feces) (urine) W55.89 ☑
bull — *see* Contact, with, bull
cat — *see* Contact, with, cat
cow — *see* Contact, with, cow
goat — *see* Contact, with, goat
hoof stock — *see* Contact, with, hoof stock

Contact — *continued*
with — *continued*
mammal — *continued*
horse — *see* Contact, with, horse
marine W56.39 ☑
dolphin — *see* Contact, with, dolphin
orca — *see* Contact, with, orca
sea lion — *see* Contact, with, sea lion
specified NEC W56.39 ☑
bite W56.31 ☑
strike W56.32 ☑
pig — *see* Contact, with, pig
raccoon — *see* Contact, with, raccoon
rodent — *see* Contact, with, rodent
sheep — *see* Contact, with, sheep
specified NEC W55.89 ☑
bite W55.81 ☑
strike W55.82 ☑
marine
animal W56.89 ☑
bite W56.81 ☑
dolphin — *see* Contact, with, dolphin
fish NEC — *see* Contact, with, fish
mammal — *see* Contact, with, mammal, marine
orca — *see* Contact, with, orca
sea lion — *see* Contact, with, sea lion
shark — *see* Contact, with, shark
strike W56.82 ☑
meat
grinder (domestic) W29.0 ☑
industrial W31.82 ☑
nonpowered W27.4 ☑
slicer (domestic) W29.0 ☑
industrial W31.82 ☑
merry go round W31.81 ☑
metal, hot (liquid) (molten) NEC X18 ☑
millipede W57 ☑
nail W45.0 ☑
gun W29.4 ☑
needle (sewing) W27.3 ☑
hypodermic W46.0 ☑
contaminated W46.1 ☑
object (blunt) NEC
hot NEC X19 ☑
legal intervention — *see* Legal, intervention,
blunt object
sharp NEC W45.8 ☑
inflicted by other person NEC W45.8 ☑
stated as
intentional homicide (attempt) — *see*
Assault, cutting or piercing instrument
legal intervention — *see* Legal, intervention,
sharp object
self-inflicted X78.9 ☑
orca W56.29 ☑
bite W56.21 ☑
strike W56.22 ☑
overhead plane W31.2 ☑
paper (as sharp object) W26.2 ☑
paper-cutter W27.5 ☑
parrot W61.09 ☑
bite W61.01 ☑
strike W61.02 ☑
pig W55.49 ☑
bite W55.41 ☑
strike W55.42 ☑
pipe, hot X16 ☑
pitchfork W27.1 ☑
plane (metal) (wood) W27.0 ☑
overhead W31.2 ☑
plant thorns, spines, sharp leaves or other mechanisms W60 ☑
powered
garden cultivator W29.3 ☑
household appliance, implement, or machine
W29.8 ☑
saw (industrial) W31.2 ☑
hand W29.8 ☑
printing machine W31.89 ☑
psittacine bird W61.29 ☑
bite W61.21 ☑
macaw — *see* Contact, with, macaw
parrot — *see* Contact, with, parrot
strike W61.22 ☑

☑ **Additional Character Required** — Refer to the Tabular List for Character Selection   ▽ Subterms under main terms may continue to next column or page

Contact — *continued*
  with — *continued*
    pulley (block) (transmission) W24.0 ☑
      agricultural operations W30.89 ☑
    raccoon W55.59 ☑
      bite W55.51 ☑
      strike W55.52 ☑
    radial-saw (industrial) W31.2 ☑
    radiator (hot) X16 ☑
    rake W27.1 ☑
    rattlesnake X58 ☑
    reaper W30.0 ☑
    reptile W59.89 ☑
      lizard — *see* Contact, with, lizard
      snake — *see* Contact, with, snake
      specified NEC W59.89 ☑
        bite W59.81 ☑
        crushing W59.83 ☑
        strike W59.82 ☑
      turtle — *see* Contact, with, turtle
    rivet gun (powered) W29.4 ☑
    road scraper — *see* Accident, transport, construction
        vehicle
    rodent (feces) (urine) W53.89 ☑
      bite W53.81 ☑
      mouse W53.09 ☑
        bite W53.01 ☑
      rat W53.19 ☑
        bite W53.11 ☑
      specified NEC W53.89 ☑
        bite W53.81 ☑
      squirrel W53.29 ☑
        bite W53.21 ☑
    roller coaster W31.81 ☑
    rope NEC W24.0 ☑
      agricultural operations W30.89 ☑
    saliva — *see* Contact, with, by type of animal
    sander W29.8 ☑
      industrial W31.2 ☑
    saucepan (hot) (glass) (metal) X15.3 ☑
    saw W27.0 ☑
      band (industrial) W31.2 ☑
      bench (industrial) W31.2 ☑
      chain W29.3 ☑
      hand W27.0 ☑
    sawing machine, metal W31.1 ☑
    scissors W27.2 ☑
    scorpion X58 ☑
    screwdriver W27.0 ☑
      powered W29.8 ☑
    sea
      anemone, cucumber or urchin (spine) X58 ☑
      lion W56.19 ☑
        bite W56.11 ☑
        strike W56.12 ☑
    serpent — *see* Contact, with, snake, by type
    sewing-machine (electric) (powered) W29.2 ☑
      not powered W27.8 ☑
    shaft (hoist) (lift) (transmission) NEC W24.0 ☑
      agricultural W30.89 ☑
    shark W56.49 ☑
      bite W56.41 ☑
      strike W56.42 ☑
    sharp object(s) W26.9 ☑
      specified NEC W26.8 ☑
    shears (hand) W27.2 ☑
      powered (industrial) W31.1 ☑
        domestic W29.2 ☑
    sheep W55.39 ☑
      bite W55.31 ☑
      strike W55.32 ☑
    shovel W27.8 ☑
      steam — *see* Accident, transport, construction
          vehicle
    snake (nonvenomous) W59.19 ☑
      bite W59.11 ☑
      crushing W59.13 ☑
      strike W59.12 ☑
    spade W27.1 ☑
    spider (venomous) X58 ☑
    spin-drier W29.2 ☑
    spinning machine W31.89 ☑
    splinter W45.8 ☑
    sports equipment W21.9 ☑
    staple gun (powered) W29.8 ☑
    steam X13.1 ☑

Contact — *continued*
  with — *continued*
    steam — *continued*
      engine W31.3 ☑
      inhalation X13.0 ☑
      pipe X16 ☑
      shovel W31.89 ☑
    stove (hot) (kitchen) X15.0 ☑
    substance, hot NEC X19 ☑
      molten (metal) X18 ☑
    sword W26.1 ☑
      assault X99.2 ☑
      stated as undetermined whether accidental or
          intentional Y28.2 ☑
      suicide (attempt) X78.2 ☑
    tarantula X58 ☑
    thresher W30.0 ☑
    tin can lid W26.8 ☑
    toad W62.1 ☑
    toaster (hot) X15.1 ☑
    tool W27.8 ☑
      hand (not powered) W27.8 ☑
        auger W27.0 ☑
        axe W27.0 ☑
        can opener W27.4 ☑
        chisel W27.0 ☑
        fork W27.4 ☑
        garden W27.1 ☑
        handsaw W27.0 ☑
        hoe W27.1 ☑
        ice-pick W27.4 ☑
        kitchen utensil W27.4 ☑
        manual
          lawn mower W27.1 ☑
          sewing machine W27.8 ☑
        meat grinder W27.4 ☑
        needle (sewing) W27.3 ☑
          hypodermic W46.0 ☑
            contaminated W46.1 ☑
        paper cutter W27.5 ☑
        pitchfork W27.1 ☑
        rake W27.1 ☑
        scissors W27.2 ☑
        screwdriver W27.0 ☑
        specified NEC W27.8 ☑
        workbench W27.0 ☑
      hot X17 ☑
      powered W29.8 ☑
        blender W29.0 ☑
          commercial W31.82 ☑
        can opener W29.0 ☑
          commercial W31.82 ☑
        chainsaw W29.3 ☑
        clothes dryer W29.2 ☑
          commercial W31.82 ☑
        dishwasher W29.2 ☑
          commercial W31.82 ☑
        edger W29.3 ☑
        electric fan W29.2 ☑
          commercial W31.82 ☑
        electric knife W29.1 ☑
        food processor W29.0 ☑
          commercial W31.82 ☑
        garbage disposal W29.0 ☑
          commercial W31.82 ☑
        garden tool W29.3 ☑
        hedge trimmer W29.3 ☑
        ice maker W29.0 ☑
          commercial W31.82 ☑
        kitchen appliance W29.0 ☑
          commercial W31.82 ☑
        lawn mower W28 ☑
        meat grinder W29.0 ☑
          commercial W31.82 ☑
        mixer W29.0 ☑
          commercial W31.82 ☑
        rototiller W29.3 ☑
        sewing machine W29.2 ☑
          commercial W31.82 ☑
        washing machine W29.2 ☑
          commercial W31.82 ☑
    transmission device (belt, cable, chain, gear, pinion,
        shaft) W24.1 ☑
      agricultural operations W30.09 ☑
    turbine (gas) (water-driven) W31.3 ☑
    turkey W61.49 ☑

Contact — *continued*
  with — *continued*
    turkey — *continued*
      peck W61.43 ☑
      strike W61.42 ☑
    turtle (nonvenomous) W59.29 ☑
      bite W59.21 ☑
      strike W59.22 ☑
      terrestrial W59.89 ☑
        bite W59.81 ☑
        crushing W59.83 ☑
        strike W59.82 ☑
    under-cutter W31.0 ☑
    urine — *see* Contact, with, by type of animal
    vehicle
      agricultural use (transport) — *see* Accident,
          transport, agricultural vehicle
        not on public highway W30.81 ☑
      industrial use (transport) — *see* Accident, trans-
          port, industrial vehicle
        not on public highway W31.83 ☑
      off-road use (transport) — *see* Accident, trans-
          port, all-terrain or off-road vehicle
        not on public highway W31.83 ☑
      special construction use (transport) — *see* Acci-
          dent, transport, construction vehicle
        not on public highway W31.83 ☑
    venomous
      animal X58 ☑
      arthropods X58 ☑
      lizard X58 ☑
      marine animal NEC X58 ☑
      marine plant NEC X58 ☑
      millipedes (tropical) X58 ☑
      plant(s) X58 ☑
      snake X58 ☑
      spider X58 ☑
      viper X58 ☑
    washing-machine (powered) W29.2 ☑
    wasp X58 ☑
    weaving-machine W31.89 ☑
    winch W24.0 ☑
      agricultural operations W30.89 ☑
    wire NEC W24.0 ☑
      agricultural operations W30.89 ☑
    wood slivers W45.8 ☑
    yellow jacket X58 ☑
    zebra — *see* Contact, with, hoof stock NEC
  pressure X50.9 ☑
  stress X50.9 ☑
Coup de soleil X32 ☑
Crash
  aircraft (in transit) (powered) V95.9 ☑
    balloon V96.01 ☑
    fixed wing NEC (private) V95.21 ☑
      commercial V95.31 ☑
    glider V96.21 ☑
      hang V96.11 ☑
      powered V95.11 ☑
    helicopter V95.01 ☑
    in war operations — *see* War operations, destruction
        of aircraft
    microlight V95.11 ☑
    nonpowered V96.9 ☑
      specified NEC V96.8 ☑
    powered NEC V95.8 ☑
    stated as
      homicide (attempt) Y08.81 ☑
      suicide (attempt) X83.0 ☑
    ultralight V95.11 ☑
  spacecraft V95.41 ☑
  transport vehicle NEC — *see also* Accident, transport
      V89.9 ☑
    homicide (attempt) Y03.8 ☑
    motor NEC (traffic) V89.2 ☑
      homicide (attempt) Y03.8 ☑
      suicide (attempt) — *see* Suicide, collision
Cruelty (mental) (physical) (sexual) X58 ☑
Crushed (accidentally) X58 ☑
  between objects (moving) (stationary and moving)
      W23.0 ☑
    stationary W23.1 ☑
  by
    alligator W58.03 ☑
    avalanche NEC — *see* Landslide
    cave-in W20.0 ☑

Crushed — *continued*
  by — *continued*
    cave-in — *continued*
      caused by cataclysmic earth surface movement
        — *see* Landslide
    crocodile W58.13 ☑
    crowd or human stampede W52 ☑
    falling
      aircraft V97.39 ☑
        in war operations — *see* War operations, destruction of aircraft
      earth, material W20.0 ☑
        caused by cataclysmic earth surface movement — *see* Landslide
      object NEC W20.8 ☑
    landslide NEC — *see* Landslide
    lizard (nonvenomous) W59.09 ☑
    machinery — *see* Contact, with, by type of machine
    reptile NEC W59.89 ☑
    snake (nonvenomous) W59.13 ☑
  in
    machinery — *see* Contact, with, by type of machine
Cut, cutting (any part of body) (accidental) — *see also* Contact, with, by object or machine
  during medical or surgical treatment as misadventure — *see* Index to Diseases and Injuries, Complications
  homicide (attempt) — *see* Assault, cutting or piercing instrument
  inflicted by other person — *see* Assault, cutting or piercing instrument
  legal
    execution — *see* Legal, intervention
    intervention — *see* Legal, intervention, sharp object
  machine NEC — *see also* Contact, with, by type of machine W31.9 ☑
  self-inflicted — *see* Suicide, cutting or piercing instrument
  suicide (attempt) — *see* Suicide, cutting or piercing instrument
Cyclone (any injury) X37.1 ☑

D

Decapitation (accidental circumstances) NEC X58 ☑
  homicide X99.9 ☑
  legal execution — *see* Legal, intervention
Dehydration from lack of water X58 ☑
Deprivation X58 ☑
Derailment (accidental)
  railway (rolling stock) (train) (vehicle) (without antecedent collision) V81.7 ☑
    with antecedent collision — *see* Accident, transport, railway vehicle occupant
  streetcar (without antecedent collision) V82.7 ☑
    with antecedent collision — *see* Accident, transport, streetcar occupant
Descent
  parachute (voluntary) (without accident to aircraft) V97.29 ☑
    due to accident to aircraft — *see* Accident, transport, aircraft
Desertion X58 ☑
Destitution X58 ☑
Disability, late effect or sequela of injury — *see* Sequelae
Discharge (accidental)
  airgun W34.010 ☑
    assault X95.01 ☑
    homicide (attempt) X95.01 ☑
    stated as undetermined whether accidental or intentional Y24.0 ☑
    suicide (attempt) X74.01 ☑
  BB gun — *see* Discharge, airgun
  firearm (accidental) W34.00 ☑
    assault X95.9 ☑
    handgun (pistol) (revolver) W32.0 ☑
      assault X93 ☑
      homicide (attempt) X93 ☑
      legal intervention — *see* Legal, intervention, firearm, handgun
      stated as undetermined whether accidental or intentional Y22 ☑
      suicide (attempt) X72 ☑
    homicide (attempt) X95.9 ☑
    hunting rifle W33.02 ☑

Discharge — *continued*
  firearm — *continued*
    hunting rifle — *continued*
      assault X94.1 ☑
      homicide (attempt) X94.1 ☑
      legal intervention
        injuring
          bystander Y35.032 ☑
          law enforcement personnel Y35.031 ☑
          suspect Y35.033 ☑
          unspecified person Y35.039 ☑
        stated as undetermined whether accidental or intentional Y23.1 ☑
        suicide (attempt) X73.1 ☑
    larger W33.00 ☑
      assault X94.9 ☑
      homicide (attempt) X94.9 ☑
      hunting rifle — *see* Discharge, firearm, hunting rifle
      legal intervention — *see* Legal, intervention, firearm by type of firearm
      machine gun — *see* Discharge, firearm, machine gun
      shotgun — *see* Discharge, firearm, shotgun
      specified NEC W33.09 ☑
        assault X94.8 ☑
        homicide (attempt) X94.8 ☑
        legal intervention
          injuring
            bystander Y35.092 ☑
            law enforcement personnel Y35.091 ☑
            suspect Y35.093 ☑
            unspecified person Y35.099 ☑
          stated as undetermined whether accidental or intentional Y23.8 ☑
          suicide (attempt) X73.8 ☑
      stated as undetermined whether accidental or intentional Y23.9 ☑
      suicide (attempt) X73.9 ☑
    legal intervention
      injuring
        bystander Y35.002 ☑
        law enforcement personnel Y35.001 ☑
        suspect Y35.03 ☑
        unspecified person Y35.009 ☑
      using rubber bullet
        injuring
          bystander Y35.042 ☑
          law enforcement personnel Y35.041 ☑
          suspect Y35.043 ☑
          unspecified person Y35.049 ☑
    machine gun W33.03 ☑
      assault X94.2 ☑
      homicide (attempt) X94.2 ☑
      legal intervention — *see* Legal, intervention, firearm, machine gun
      stated as undetermined whether accidental or intentional Y23.3 ☑
      suicide (attempt) X73.2 ☑
    pellet gun — *see* Discharge, airgun
    shotgun W33.01 ☑
      assault X94.0 ☑
      homicide (attempt) X94.0 ☑
      legal intervention — *see* Legal, intervention, firearm, specified NEC
      stated as undetermined whether accidental or intentional Y23.0 ☑
      suicide (attempt) X73.0 ☑
    specified NEC W34.09 ☑
      assault X95.8 ☑
      homicide (attempt) X95.8 ☑
      legal intervention — *see* Legal, intervention, firearm, specified NEC
      stated as undetermined whether accidental or intentional Y24.8 ☑
      suicide (attempt) X74.8 ☑
    stated as undetermined whether accidental or intentional Y24.9 ☑
    suicide (attempt) X74.9 ☑
    Very pistol W34.09 ☑
      assault X95.8 ☑
      homicide (attempt) X95.8 ☑
      stated as undetermined whether accidental or intentional Y24.8 ☑
      suicide (attempt) X74.8 ☑

Discharge — *continued*
  firework(s) W39 ☑
    stated as undetermined whether accidental or intentional Y25 ☑
  gas-operated gun NEC W34.018 ☑
    airgun — *see* Discharge, airgun
    assault X95.09 ☑
    homicide (attempt) X95.09 ☑
    paintball gun — *see* Discharge, paintball gun
    stated as undetermined whether accidental or intentional Y24.8 ☑
    suicide (attempt) X74.09 ☑
  gun NEC — *see also* Discharge, firearm NEC
    air — *see* Discharge, airgun
    BB — *see* Discharge, airgun
    for single hand use — *see* Discharge, firearm, handgun
    hand — *see* Discharge, firearm, handgun
    machine — *see* Discharge, firearm, machine gun
    other specified — *see* Discharge, firearm NEC
    paintball — *see* Discharge, paintball gun
    pellet — *see* Discharge, airgun
  handgun — *see* Discharge, firearm, handgun
  machine gun — *see* Discharge, firearm, machine gun
  paintball gun W34.011 ☑
    assault X95.02 ☑
    homicide (attempt) X95.02 ☑
    stated as undetermined whether accidental or intentional Y24.8 ☑
    suicide (attempt) X74.02 ☑
  pistol — *see* Discharge, firearm, handgun
    flare — *see* Discharge, firearm, Very pistol
    pellet — *see* Discharge, airgun
    Very — *see* Discharge, firearm, Very pistol
  revolver — *see* Discharge, firearm, handgun
  rifle (hunting) — *see* Discharge, firearm, hunting rifle
  shotgun — *see* Discharge, firearm, shotgun
  spring-operated gun NEC W34.018 ☑
    assault X95.09 ☑
    homicide (attempt) X95.09 ☑
    stated as undetermined whether accidental or intentional Y24.8 ☑
    suicide (attempt) X74.09 ☑
Disease
  Andes W94.11 ☑
  aviator's — *see* Air, pressure
  range W94.11 ☑
Diver's disease, palsy, paralysis, squeeze — *see* Air, pressure
Diving (into water) — *see* Accident, diving
Dog bite W54.0 ☑
Dragged by transport vehicle NEC — *see also* Accident, transport V09.9 ☑
Drinking poison (accidental) — *see* Table of Drugs and Chemicals
Dropped (accidentally) **while being carried or supported by other person** W04 ☑
Drowning (accidental) W74 ☑
  assault X92.9 ☑
  due to
    accident (to)
      machinery — *see* Contact, with, by type of machine
      watercraft V90.89 ☑
        burning V90.29 ☑
          powered V90.23 ☑
            fishing boat V90.22 ☑
            jetskis V90.23 ☑
            merchant ship V90.20 ☑
            passenger ship V90.21 ☑
          unpowered V90.28 ☑
            canoe V90.25 ☑
            inflatable V90.26 ☑
            kayak V90.25 ☑
            sailboat V90.24 ☑
            water skis V90.27 ☑
        crushed V90.39 ☑
          powered V90.33 ☑
            fishing boat V90.32 ☑
            jetskis V90.33 ☑
            merchant ship V90.30 ☑
            passenger ship V90.31 ☑
          unpowered V90.38 ☑
            canoe V90.35 ☑
            inflatable V90.36 ☑
            kayak V90.35 ☑

☑ **Additional Character Required — Refer to the Tabular List for Character Selection**   ▽ **Subterms under main terms may continue to next column or page**

Drowning — *continued*
  due to — *continued*
    accident — *continued*
      watercraft — *continued*
        crushed — *continued*
          unpowered — *continued*
            sailboat V90.34 ☑
            water skis V90.37 ☑
        overturning V90.09 ☑
          powered V90.03 ☑
            fishing boat V90.02 ☑
            jetskis V90.03 ☑
            merchant ship V90.00 ☑
            passenger ship V90.01 ☑
          unpowered V90.08 ☑
            canoe V90.05 ☑
            inflatable V90.06 ☑
            kayak V90.05 ☑
            sailboat V90.04 ☑
        sinking V90.19 ☑
          powered V90.13 ☑
            fishing boat V90.12 ☑
            jetskis V90.13 ☑
            merchant ship V90.10 ☑
            passenger ship V90.11 ☑
          unpowered V90.18 ☑
            canoe V90.15 ☑
            inflatable V90.16 ☑
            kayak V90.15 ☑
            sailboat V90.14 ☑
        specified type NEC V90.89 ☑
          powered V90.83 ☑
            fishing boat V90.82 ☑
            jetskis V90.83 ☑
            merchant ship V90.80 ☑
            passenger ship V90.81 ☑
          unpowered V90.88 ☑
            canoe V90.85 ☑
            inflatable V90.86 ☑
            kayak V90.85 ☑
            sailboat V90.84 ☑
            water skis V90.87 ☑
    avalanche — *see* Landslide
    cataclysmic
      earth surface movement NEC — *see* Forces of
        nature, earth movement
      storm — *see* Forces of nature, cataclysmic storm
    cloudburst X37.8 ☑
    cyclone X37.1 ☑
    fall overboard (from) V92.09 ☑
      powered craft V92.03 ☑
        ferry boat V92.01 ☑
        fishing boat V92.02 ☑
        jetskis V92.03 ☑
        liner V92.01 ☑
        merchant ship V92.00 ☑
        passenger ship V92.01 ☑
      resulting from
        accident to watercraft — *see* Drowning, due
          to, accident to, watercraft
        being washed overboard (from) V92.29 ☑
          powered craft V92.23 ☑
            ferry boat V92.21 ☑
            fishing boat V92.22 ☑
            jetskis V92.23 ☑
            liner V92.21 ☑
            merchant ship V92.20 ☑
            passenger ship V92.21 ☑
          unpowered craft V92.28 ☑
            canoe V92.25 ☑
            inflatable V92.26 ☑
            kayak V92.25 ☑
            sailboat V92.24 ☑
            surf-board V92.28 ☑
            water skis V92.27 ☑
            windsurfer V92.28 ☑
        motion of watercraft V92.19 ☑
          powered craft V92.13 ☑
            ferry boat V92.11 ☑
            fishing boat V92.12 ☑
            jetskis V92.13 ☑
            liner V92.11 ☑
            merchant ship V92.10 ☑
            passenger ship V92.11 ☑
          unpowered craft
            canoe V92.15 ☑

Drowning — *continued*
  due to — *continued*
    fall overboard — *continued*
      resulting from — *continued*
        motion of watercraft — *continued*
          unpowered craft — *continued*
            inflatable V92.16 ☑
            kayak V92.15 ☑
            sailboat V92.14 ☑
        unpowered craft V92.08 ☑
          canoe V92.05 ☑
          inflatable V92.06 ☑
          kayak V92.05 ☑
          sailboat V92.04 ☑
          surf-board V92.08 ☑
          water skis V92.07 ☑
          windsurfer V92.08 ☑
    hurricane X37.0 ☑
    jumping into water from watercraft (involved in
      accident) — *see also* Drowning, due to, acci-
      dent to, watercraft
      without accident to or on watercraft W16.711 ☑
    tidal wave NEC — *see* Forces of nature, tidal wave
    torrential rain X37.8 ☑
  following
    fall
      into
        bathtub W16.211 ☑
        bucket W16.221 ☑
        fountain — *see* Drowning, following, fall, into,
          water, specified NEC
        quarry — *see* Drowning, following, fall, into,
          water, specified NEC
        reservoir — *see* Drowning, following, fall, into,
          water, specified NEC
        swimming-pool W16.011 ☑
          stated as undetermined whether acciden-
            tal or intentional Y21.3 ☑
          striking
            bottom W16.021 ☑
            wall W16.031 ☑
          suicide (attempt) X71.2 ☑
        water NOS W16.41 ☑
          natural (lake) (open sea) (river) (stream)
            (pond) W16.111 ☑
            striking
              bottom W16.121 ☑
              side W16.131 ☑
          specified NEC W16.311 ☑
            striking
              bottom W16.321 ☑
              wall W16.331 ☑
      overboard NEC — *see* Drowning, due to, fall
        overboard
    jump or dive
      from boat W16.711 ☑
        striking bottom W16.721 ☑
      into
        fountain — *see* Drowning, following, jump
          or dive, into, water, specified NEC
        quarry — *see* Drowning, following, jump or
          dive, into, water, specified NEC
        reservoir — *see* Drowning, following, jump
          or dive, into, water, specified NEC
        swimming-pool W16.511 ☑
          striking
            bottom W16.521 ☑
            wall W16.531 ☑
          suicide (attempt) X71.2 ☑
        water NOS W16.91 ☑
          natural (lake) (open sea) (river) (stream)
            (pond) W16.611 ☑
          specified NEC W16.811 ☑
            bottom W16.821 ☑
            striking
              bottom W16.821 ☑
              wall W16.831 ☑
          striking
            bottom W16.821 ☑
            wall W16.831 ☑
          striking bottom W16.621 ☑
  homicide (attempt) X92.9 ☑
  in
    bathtub (accidental) W65 ☑
      assault X92.0 ☑
      following fall W16.211 ☑

Drowning — *continued*
  in — *continued*
    bathtub — *continued*
      following fall — *continued*
        stated as undetermined whether accidental
          or intentional Y21.1 ☑
      stated as undetermined whether accidental or
        intentional Y21.0 ☑
      suicide (attempt) X71.0 ☑
    lake — *see* Drowning, in, natural water
    natural water (lake) (open sea) (river) (stream)
      (pond) W69 ☑
      assault X92.3 ☑
      following
        dive or jump W16.611 ☑
          striking bottom W16.621 ☑
        fall W16.111 ☑
          striking
            bottom W16.121 ☑
            side W16.131 ☑
      stated as undetermined whether accidental or
        intentional Y21.4 ☑
      suicide (attempt) X71.3 ☑
    quarry — *see* Drowning, in, specified place NEC
    quenching tank — *see* Drowning, in, specified place
      NEC
    reservoir — *see* Drowning, in, specified place NEC
    river — *see* Drowning, in, natural water
    sea — *see* Drowning, in, natural water
    specified place NEC W73 ☑
      assault X92.8 ☑
      following
        dive or jump W16.811 ☑
          striking
            bottom W16.821 ☑
            wall W16.831 ☑
        fall W16.311 ☑
          striking
            bottom W16.321 ☑
            wall W16.331 ☑
      stated as undetermined whether accidental or
        intentional Y21.8 ☑
      suicide (attempt) X71.8 ☑
    stream — *see* Drowning, in, natural water
    swimming-pool W67 ☑
      assault X92.1 ☑
        following fall X92.2 ☑
      following
        dive or jump W16.511 ☑
          striking
            bottom W16.521 ☑
            wall W16.531 ☑
        fall W16.011 ☑
          striking
            bottom W16.021 ☑
            wall W16.031 ☑
      stated as undetermined whether accidental or
        intentional Y21.2 ☑
        following fall Y21.3 ☑
      suicide (attempt) X71.1 ☑
        following fall X71.2 ☑
    war operations — *see* War operations, restriction
      of airway
  resulting from accident to watercraft — *see* Drowning,
    due to, accident to, watercraft
  self-inflicted X71.9 ☑
  stated as undetermined whether accidental or inten-
    tional Y21.9 ☑
  suicide (attempt) X71.9 ☑

E

Earth falling (on) W20.0 ☑
  caused by cataclysmic earth surface movement or
    eruption — *see* Landslide
Earth (surface) **movement NEC** — *see* Forces of nature,
  earth movement
Earthquake (any injury) X34 ☑
Effect(s) (adverse) **of**
  air pressure (any) — *see* Air, pressure
  cold, excessive (exposure to) — *see* Exposure, cold
  heat (excessive) — *see* Heat
  hot place (weather) — *see* Heat
  insolation X30 ☑
  late — *see* Sequelae
  motion — *see* Motion

Effect(s) (adverse) **of** — *continued*
  nuclear explosion or weapon in war operations — *see* War operations, nuclear weapon
  radiation — *see* Radiation
  travel — *see* Travel
Electric shock (accidental) (by) (in) — *see* Exposure, electric current
Electrocution (accidental) — *see* Exposure, electric current
Endotracheal tube wrongly placed during anesthetic procedure
Entanglement
  in
    bed linen, causing suffocation T71 ☑
    wheel of pedal cycle V19.88 ☑
Entry of foreign body or material — *see* Foreign body
Environmental pollution related condition — *see*
  category Z57 ☑
Execution, legal (any method) — *see* Legal, intervention
Exhaustion
  cold — *see* Exposure, cold
  due to excessive exertion — *see also* Overexertion X50.9 ☑
  heat — *see* Heat
Explosion (accidental) (of) (with secondary fire) W40.9 ☑
  acetylene W40.1 ☑
  aerosol can W36.1 ☑
  air tank (compressed) (in machinery) W36.2 ☑
  aircraft (in transit) (powered) NEC V95.9 ☑
    balloon V96.05 ☑
    fixed wing NEC (private) V95.25 ☑
      commercial V95.35 ☑
    glider V96.25 ☑
      hang V96.15 ☑
      powered V95.15 ☑
    helicopter V95.05 ☑
    in war operations — *see* War operations, destruction of aircraft
    microlight V95.15 ☑
    nonpowered V96.9 ☑
      specified NEC V96.8 ☑
    powered NEC V95.8 ☑
    stated as
      homicide (attempt) Y03.8 ☑
      suicide (attempt) X83.0 ☑
    ultralight V95.15 ☑
  anesthetic gas in operating room W40.1 ☑
  antipersonnel bomb W40.8 ☑
    assault X96.0 ☑
    homicide (attempt) X96.0 ☑
    suicide (attempt) X75 ☑
  assault X96.9 ☑
  bicycle tire W37.0 ☑
  blasting (cap) (materials) W40.0 ☑
  boiler (machinery), not on transport vehicle W35 ☑
    on watercraft — *see* Explosion, in, watercraft
  butane W40.1 ☑
  caused by other person X96.9 ☑
  coal gas W40.1 ☑
  detonator W40.0 ☑
  dump (munitions) W40.8 ☑
  dynamite W40.0 ☑
    in
      assault X96.8 ☑
      homicide (attempt) X96.8 ☑
      legal intervention
        injuring
          bystander Y35.112 ☑
          law enforcement personnel Y35.111 ☑
          suspect Y35.113 ☑
          unspecified person Y35.119 ☑
      suicide (attempt) X75 ☑
  explosive (material) W40.9 ☑
    gas W40.1 ☑
    in blasting operation W40.0 ☑
    specified NEC W40.8 ☑
      in
        assault X96.8 ☑
        homicide (attempt) X96.8 ☑
        legal intervention
          injuring
            bystander Y35.192 ☑
            law enforcement personnel Y35.191 ☑
            suspect Y35.193 ☑
            unspecified person Y35.199 ☑

Explosion — *continued*
  explosive — *continued*
    specified — *continued*
      in — *continued*
        suicide (attempt) X75 ☑
  factory (munitions) W40.8 ☑
  fertilizer bomb W40.8 ☑
    assault X96.3 ☑
    homicide (attempt) X96.3 ☑
    suicide (attempt) X75 ☑
  firearm (parts) NEC W34.19 ☑
    airgun W34.110 ☑
    BB gun W34.110 ☑
    gas, air or spring-operated gun NEC W34.118 ☑
    handgun W32.1 ☑
    hunting rifle W33.12 ☑
    larger firearm W33.10 ☑
      specified NEC W33.19 ☑
    machine gun W33.13 ☑
    paintball gun W34.111 ☑
    pellet gun W34.110 ☑
    shotgun W33.11 ☑
    Very pistol [flare] W34.19 ☑
  fire-damp W40.1 ☑
  fireworks W39 ☑
  gas (coal) (explosive) W40.1 ☑
    cylinder W36.9 ☑
      aerosol can W36.1 ☑
      air tank W36.2 ☑
      pressurized W36.3 ☑
      specified NEC W36.8 ☑
  gasoline (fumes) (tank) not in moving motor vehicle W40.1 ☑
    bomb W40.8 ☑
      assault X96.1 ☑
      homicide (attempt) X96.1 ☑
      suicide (attempt) X75 ☑
    in motor vehicle — *see* Accident, transport, by type of vehicle
  grain store W40.8 ☑
  grenade W40.8 ☑
    in
      assault X96.8 ☑
      homicide (attempt) X96.8 ☑
      legal intervention
        injuring
          bystander Y35.192 ☑
          law enforcement personnel Y35.191 ☑
          suspect Y35.193 ☑
          unspecified person Y35.199 ☑
      suicide (attempt) X75 ☑
  handgun (parts) — *see* Explosion, firearm, hangun (parts)
  homicide (attempt) X96.9 ☑
    antipersonnel bomb — *see* Explosion, antipersonnel bomb
    fertilizer bomb — *see* Explosion, fertilizer bomb
    gasoline bomb — *see* Explosion, gasoline bomb
    letter bomb — *see* Explosion, letter bomb
    pipe bomb — *see* Explosion, pipe bomb
    specified NEC X96.8 ☑
  hose, pressurized W37.8 ☑
  hot water heater, tank (in machinery) W35 ☑
    on watercraft — *see* Explosion, in, watercraft
  in, on
    dump W40.8 ☑
    factory W40.8 ☑
    mine (of explosive gases) NEC W40.1 ☑
    watercraft V93.59 ☑
      powered craft V93.53 ☑
        ferry boat V93.51 ☑
        fishing boat V93.52 ☑
        jetskis V93.53 ☑
        liner V93.51 ☑
        merchant ship V93.50 ☑
        passenger ship V93.51 ☑
        sailboat V93.54 ☑
  letter bomb W40.8 ☑
    assault X96.2 ☑
    homicide (attempt) X96.2 ☑
    suicide (attempt) X75 ☑
  machinery — *see also* Contact, with, by type of machine
    on board watercraft — *see* Explosion, in, watercraft
    pressure vessel — *see* Explosion, by type of vessel
  methane W40.1 ☑

Explosion — *continued*
  mine W40.1 ☑
  missile NEC W40.8 ☑
  mortar bomb W40.8 ☑
    in
      assault X96.8 ☑
      homicide (attempt) X96.8 ☑
      legal intervention
        injuring
          bystander Y35.192 ☑
          law enforcement personnel Y35.191 ☑
          suspect Y35.193 ☑
          unspecified person Y35.199 ☑
      suicide (attempt) X75 ☑
  munitions (dump) (factory) W40.8 ☑
  pipe, pressurized W37.8 ☑
    bomb W40.8 ☑
      assault X96.4 ☑
      homicide (attempt) X96.4 ☑
      suicide (attempt) X75 ☑
  pressure, pressurized
    cooker W38 ☑
    gas tank (in machinery) W36.3 ☑
    hose W37.8 ☑
    pipe W37.8 ☑
    specified device NEC W38 ☑
    tire W37.8 ☑
      bicycle W37.0 ☑
    vessel (in machinery) W38 ☑
  propane W40.1 ☑
  self-inflicted X75 ☑
  shell (artillery) NEC W40.8 ☑
    during war operations — *see* War operations, explosion
    in
      legal intervention
        injuring
          bystander Y35.122 ☑
          law enforcement personnel Y35.121 ☑
          suspect Y35.123 ☑
          unspecified person Y35.129 ☑
    war — *see* War operations, explosion
  spacecraft V95.45 ☑
  stated as undetermined whether accidental or intentional Y25 ☑
  steam or water lines (in machinery) W37.8 ☑
  stove W40.9 ☑
  suicide (attempt) X75 ☑
  tire, pressurized W37.8 ☑
    bicycle W37.0 ☑
  undetermined whether accidental or intentional Y25 ☑
  vehicle tire NEC W37.8 ☑
    bicycle W37.0 ☑
  war operations — *see* War operations, explosion
Exposure (to) X58 ☑
  air pressure change — *see* Air, pressure
  cold (accidental) (excessive) (extreme) (natural) (place) X31 ☑
    assault Y08.89 ☑
    due to
      man-made conditions W93.8 ☑
        dry ice (contact) W93.01 ☑
          inhalation W93.02 ☑
        liquid air (contact) (hydrogen) (nitrogen) W93.11 ☑
          inhalation W93.12 ☑
        refrigeration unit (deep freeze) W93.2 ☑
        suicide (attempt) X83.2 ☑
      weather (conditions) X31 ☑
    homicide (attempt) Y08.89 ☑
    self-inflicted X83.2 ☑
  due to abandonment or neglect X58 ☑
  electric current W86.8 ☑
    appliance (faulty) W86.8 ☑
      domestic W86.0 ☑
    caused by other person Y08.89 ☑
    conductor (faulty) W86.1 ☑
    control apparatus (faulty) W86.1 ☑
    electric power generating plant, distribution station W86.1 ☑
    electroshock gun — *see* Exposure, electric current, taser
    high-voltage cable W85 ☑
    homicide (attempt) Y08.89 ☑
    legal execution — *see* Legal, intervention, specified means NEC

Exposure — *continued*
electric current — *continued*
  lightning — *see* subcategory T75.0 ☑
  live rail W86.8 ☑
  misadventure in medical or surgical procedure in electroshock therapy Y63.4
  motor (electric) (faulty) W86.8 ☑
    domestic W86.0 ☑
  self-inflicted X83.1 ☑
  specified NEC W86.8 ☑
    domestic W86.0 ☑
  stun gun — *see* Exposure, electric current, taser
  suicide (attempt) X83.1 ☑
  taser W86.8 ☑
    assault Y08.89 ☑
    legal intervention — *see* category Y35 ☑
    self-harm (intentional) X83.8 ☑
    undetermined intent Y33 ☑
  third rail W86.8 ☑
  transformer (faulty) W86.1 ☑
  transmission lines W85 ☑
environmental tobacco smoke X58 ☑
excessive
  cold — *see* Exposure, cold
  heat (natural) NEC X30 ☑
    man-made W92 ☑
factor(s) NOS X58 ☑
  environmental NEC X58 ☑
  man-made NEC W99 ☑
  natural NEC — *see* Forces of nature
  specified NEC X58 ☑
fire, flames (accidental) X08.8 ☑
  assault X97 ☑
  campfire — *see* Exposure, fire, controlled, not in building
  controlled (in)
    with ignition (of) clothing — *see also* Ignition, clothes X06.2 ☑
      nightwear X05 ☑
    bonfire — *see* Exposure, fire, controlled, not in building
    brazier (in building or structure) — *see also* Exposure, fire, controlled, building
      not in building or structure — *see* Exposure, fire, controlled, not in building
    building or structure X02.0 ☑
      with
        fall from building X02.3 ☑
        from building X02.5 ☑
        injury due to building collapse X02.2 ☑
        smoke inhalation X02.1 ☑
      hit by object from building X02.4 ☑
      specified mode of injury NEC X02.8 ☑
    fireplace, furnace or stove — *see* Exposure, fire, controlled, building
    not in building or structure X03.0 ☑
      with
        fall X03.3 ☑
        smoke inhalation X03.1 ☑
      hit by object X03.4 ☑
      specified mode of injury NEC X03.8 ☑
    trash — *see* Exposure, fire, controlled, not in building
  fireplace — *see* Exposure, fire, controlled, building
  fittings or furniture (in building or structure) (uncontrolled) — *see* Exposure, fire, uncontrolled, building
  forest (uncontrolled) — *see* Exposure, fire, uncontrolled, not in building
  grass (uncontrolled) — *see* Exposure, fire, uncontrolled, not in building
  hay (uncontrolled) — *see* Exposure, fire, uncontrolled, not in building
  homicide (attempt) X97 ☑
  ignition of highly flammable material X04 ☑
  in, of, on, starting in
    machinery — *see* Contact, with, by type of machine
    motor vehicle (in motion) — *see also* Accident, transport, occupant by type of vehicle V87.8 ☑
      with collision — *see* Collision
    railway rolling stock, train, vehicle V81.81 ☑
      with collision — *see* Accident, transport, railway vehicle occupant
    street car (in motion) V82.8 ☑

Exposure — *continued*
fire, flames — *continued*
  in, of, on, starting in — *continued*
    street car — *continued*
      with collision — *see* Accident, transport, streetcar occupant
    transport vehicle NEC — *see also* Accident, transport
      with collision — *see* Collision
    war operations — *see also* War operations, fire
      from nuclear explosion — *see* War operations, nuclear weapons
    watercraft (in transit) (not in transit) V91.09 ☑
      localized — *see* Burn, on board watercraft, due to, fire on board
      powered craft V91.03 ☑
        ferry boat V91.01 ☑
        fishing boat V91.02 ☑
        jet skis V91.03 ☑
        liner V91.01 ☑
        merchant ship V91.00 ☑
        passenger ship V91.01 ☑
      unpowered craft V91.08 ☑
        canoe V91.05 ☑
        inflatable V91.06 ☑
        kayak V91.05 ☑
        sailboat V91.04 ☑
        surf-board V91.08 ☑
        waterskis V91.07 ☑
        windsurfer V91.08 ☑
  lumber (uncontrolled) — *see* Exposure, fire, uncontrolled, not in building
  mine (uncontrolled) — *see* Exposure, fire, uncontrolled, not in building
  prairie (uncontrolled) — *see* Exposure, fire, uncontrolled, not in building
  resulting from
    explosion — *see* Explosion
    lightning X08.8 ☑
  self-inflicted X76 ☑
  specified NEC X08.8 ☑
  started by other person X97 ☑
  stated as undetermined whether accidental or intentional Y26 ☑
  stove — *see* Exposure, fire, controlled, building
  suicide (attempt) X76 ☑
  tunnel (uncontrolled) — *see* Exposure, fire, uncontrolled, not in building
  uncontrolled
    in building or structure X00.0 ☑
      with
        fall from building X00.3 ☑
        injury due to building collapse X00.2 ☑
        jump from building X00.5 ☑
        smoke inhalation X00.1 ☑
      bed X08.00 ☑
        due to
          cigarette X08.01 ☑
          specified material NEC X08.09 ☑
      furniture NEC X08.20 ☑
        due to
          cigarette X08.21 ☑
          specified material NEC X08.29 ☑
      hit by object from building X00.4 ☑
      sofa X08.10 ☑
        due to
          cigarette X08.11 ☑
          specified material NEC X08.19 ☑
      specified mode of injury NEC X08.8 ☑
    not in building or structure (any) X01.0 ☑
      with
        fall X01.3 ☑
        smoke inhalation X01.1 ☑
      hit by object X01.4 ☑
      specified mode of injury NEC X01.8 ☑
  undetermined whether accidental or intentional Y26 ☑
forces of nature NEC — *see* Forces of nature
G-forces (abnormal) W49.9 ☑
gravitational forces (abnormal) W49.9 ☑
heat (natural) NEC — *see* Heat
high-pressure jet (hydraulic) (pneumatic) W49.9 ☑
hydraulic jet W49.9 ☑
inanimate mechanical force W49.9 ☑
jet, high-pressure (hydraulic) (pneumatic) W49.9 ☑
lightning — *see* subcategory T75.0 ☑

Exposure — *continued*
lightning — *see* subcategory — *continued*
  causing fire — *see* Exposure, fire
mechanical forces NEC W49.9 ☑
  animate NEC W64 ☑
  inanimate NEC W49.9 ☑
noise W42.9 ☑
  supersonic W42.0 ☑
noxious substance — *see* Table of Drugs and Chemicals
pneumatic jet W49.9 ☑
prolonged in deep-freeze unit or refrigerator W93.2 ☑
radiation — *see* Radiation
smoke — *see also* Exposure, fire
  tobacco, second hand Z77.22
specified factors NEC X58 ☑
sunlight X32 ☑
  man-made (sun lamp) W89.8 ☑
    tanning bed W89.1 ☑
supersonic waves W42.0 ☑
transmission line(s), electric W85 ☑
vibration W49.9 ☑
waves
  infrasound W49.9 ☑
  sound W42.9 ☑
  supersonic W42.0 ☑
weather NEC — *see* Forces of nature
External cause status Y99.9
  child assisting in compensated work for family Y99.8
  civilian activity done for financial or other compensation Y99.0
  civilian activity done for income or pay Y99.0
  family member assisting in compensated work for other family member Y99.8
  hobby not done for income Y99.8
  leisure activity Y99.8
  military activity Y99.1
  off-duty activity of military personnel Y99.8
  recreation or sport not for income or while a student Y99.8
  specified NEC Y99.8
  student activity Y99.8
  volunteer activity Y99.2

F

Factors, supplemental
alcohol
  blood level
    less than 20mg/100ml Y90.0
    presence in blood, level not specified Y90.9
    20-39mg/100ml Y90.1
    40-59mg/100ml Y90.2
    60-79mg/100ml Y90.3
    80-99mg/100ml Y90.4
    100-119mg/100ml Y90.5
    120-199mg/100ml Y90.6
    200-239mg/100ml Y90.7
    240mg/100ml or more Y90.8
  presence in blood, but level not specified Y90.9
environmental-pollution-related condition- see Z57 ☑
nosocomial condition Y95
work-related condition Y99.0
Failure
in suture or ligature during surgical procedure Y65.2
mechanical, of instrument or apparatus (any) (during any medical or surgical procedure) Y65.8
sterile precautions (during medical and surgical care) — *see* Misadventure, failure, sterile precautions, by type of procedure
to
  introduce tube or instrument Y65.4
    endotracheal tube during anesthesia Y65.3
  make curve (transport vehicle) NEC — *see* Accident, transport
  remove tube or instrument Y65.4
Fall, falling (accidental) W19 ☑
building W20.1 ☑
  burning (uncontrolled fire) X00.3 ☑
down
  embankment W17.81 ☑
  escalator W10.0 ☑
  hill W17.81 ☑
  ladder W11 ☑
  ramp W10.2 ☑
  stairs, steps W10.9 ☑

Fall, falling — *continued*
- due to
  - bumping against
    - object W18.0Ø ☑
      - sharp glass W18.02 ☑
      - specified NEC W18.09 ☑
      - sports equipment W18.01 ☑
    - person W03 ☑
      - due to ice or snow W00.0 ☑
      - on pedestrian conveyance — *see* Accident, transport, pedestrian, conveyance
  - collision with another person W03 ☑
    - due to ice or snow W00.0 ☑
    - involving pedestrian conveyance — *see* Accident, transport, pedestrian, conveyance
  - grocery cart tipping over W17.82 ☑
  - ice or snow W00.9 ☑
    - from one level to another W00.2 ☑
      - on stairs or steps W00.1 ☑
    - involving pedestrian conveyance — *see* Accident, transport, pedestrian, conveyance
    - on same level W00.0 ☑
  - slipping (on moving sidewalk) W01.0 ☑
    - with subsequent striking against object W01.10 ☑
      - furniture W01.190 ☑
      - sharp object W01.119 ☑
        - glass W01.110 ☑
        - power tool or machine W01.111 ☑
        - specified NEC W01.118 ☑
      - specified NEC W01.198 ☑
  - striking against
    - object W18.0Ø ☑
      - sharp glass W18.02 ☑
      - specified NEC W18.09 ☑
      - sports equipment W18.01 ☑
    - person W03 ☑
      - due to ice or snow W00.0 ☑
      - on pedestrian conveyance — *see* Accident, transport, pedestrian, conveyance
  - earth (with asphyxia or suffocation (by pressure)) — *see* Earth, falling
- from, off, out of
  - aircraft NEC (with accident to aircraft NEC) V97.0 ☑
    - while boarding or alighting V97.1 ☑
  - balcony W13.0 ☑
  - bed W06 ☑
  - boat, ship, watercraft NEC (with drowning or submersion) — *see* Drowning, due to, fall overboard
    - with hitting bottom or object V94.0 ☑
  - bridge W13.1 ☑
  - building W13.9 ☑
    - burning (uncontrolled fire) X00.3 ☑
  - cavity W17.2 ☑
  - chair W07 ☑
  - cherry picker W17.89 ☑
  - cliff W15 ☑
  - dock W17.4 ☑
  - embankment W17.81 ☑
  - escalator W10.0 ☑
  - flagpole W13.8 ☑
  - furniture NEC W08 ☑
  - grocery cart W17.82 ☑
  - haystack W17.89 ☑
  - high place NEC W17.89 ☑
    - stated as undetermined whether accidental or intentional Y30 ☑
  - hole W17.2 ☑
  - incline W10.2 ☑
  - ladder W11 ☑
  - lifting device W17.89 ☑
  - machine, machinery — *see also* Contact, with, by type of machine
    - not in operation W17.89 ☑
  - manhole W17.1 ☑
  - mobile elevated work platform [MEWP] W17.89 ☑
  - motorized mobility scooter W05.2 ☑
  - one level to another NEC W17.89 ☑
    - intentional, purposeful, suicide (attempt) X80 ☑
    - stated as undetermined whether accidental or intentional Y30 ☑
  - pit W17.2 ☑
  - playground equipment W09.8 ☑
    - jungle gym W09.2 ☑
    - slide W09.0 ☑

Fall, falling — *continued*
- from, off, out of — *continued*
  - playground equipment — *continued*
    - swing W09.1 ☑
  - quarry W17.89 ☑
  - railing W13.9 ☑
  - ramp W10.2 ☑
  - roof W13.2 ☑
  - scaffolding W12 ☑
  - scooter (nonmotorized) W05.1 ☑
    - motorized mobility W05.2 ☑
  - sky lift W17.89 ☑
  - stairs, steps W10.9 ☑
    - curb W10.1 ☑
    - due to ice or snow W00.1 ☑
    - escalator W10.0 ☑
    - incline W10.2 ☑
    - ramp W10.2 ☑
    - sidewalk curb W10.1 ☑
    - specified NEC W10.8 ☑
  - stepladder W11 ☑
  - storm drain W17.1 ☑
  - streetcar NEC V82.6 ☑
    - while boarding or alighting V82.4 ☑
    - with antecedent collision — *see* Accident, transport, streetcar occupant
  - structure NEC W13.8 ☑
    - burning (uncontrolled fire) X00.3 ☑
  - table W08 ☑
  - toilet W18.11 ☑
    - with subsequent striking against object W18.12 ☑
  - train NEC V81.6 ☑
    - during derailment (without antecedent collision) V81.7 ☑
      - with antecedent collision — *see* Accident, transport, railway vehicle occupant
    - while boarding or alighting V81.4 ☑
  - transport vehicle after collision — *see* Accident, transport, by type of vehicle, collision
  - tree W14 ☑
  - vehicle (in motion) NEC — *see also* Accident, transport V89.9 ☑
    - motor NEC — *see also* Accident, transport, occupant, by type of vehicle V87.8 ☑
    - stationary W17.89 ☑
      - while boarding or alighting — *see* Accident, transport, by type of vehicle, while boarding or alighting
  - viaduct W13.8 ☑
  - wall W13.8 ☑
  - watercraft — *see also* Drowning, due to, fall overboard
    - with hitting bottom or object V94.0 ☑
  - well W17.0 ☑
  - wheelchair, non-moving W05.0 ☑
    - powered — *see* Accident, transport, pedestrian, conveyance occupant, specified type NEC
  - window W13.4 ☑
- in, on
  - aircraft NEC V97.0 ☑
    - while boarding or alighting V97.1 ☑
    - with accident to aircraft V97.0 ☑
  - bathtub (empty) W18.2 ☑
    - filled W16.212 ☑
      - causing drowning W16.211 ☑
  - escalator W10.0 ☑
  - incline W10.2 ☑
  - ladder W11 ☑
  - machine, machinery — *see* Contact, with, by type of machine
  - object, edged, pointed or sharp (with cut) — *see* Fall, by type
  - playground equipment W09.8 ☑
    - jungle gym W09.2 ☑
    - slide W09.0 ☑
    - swing W09.1 ☑
  - ramp W10.2 ☑
  - scaffolding W12 ☑
  - shower W18.2 ☑
    - causing drowning W16.211 ☑
  - staircase, stairs, steps W10.9 ☑
    - curb W10.1 ☑
    - due to ice or snow W00.1 ☑
    - escalator W10.0 ☑
    - incline W10.2 ☑

Fall, falling — *continued*
- in, on — *continued*
  - staircase, stairs, steps — *continued*
    - specified NEC W10.8 ☑
  - streetcar (without antecedent collision) V82.5 ☑
    - with antecedent collision — *see* Accident, transport, streetcar occupant
    - while boarding or alighting V82.4 ☑
  - train (without antecedent collision) V81.5 ☑
    - with antecedent collision — *see* Accident, transport, railway vehicle occupant
    - during derailment (without antecedent collision) V81.7 ☑
      - with antecedent collision — *see* Accident, transport, railway vehicle occupant
    - while boarding or alighting V81.4 ☑
  - transport vehicle after collision — *see* Accident, transport, by type of vehicle, collision
  - watercraft V93.39 ☑
    - due to
      - accident to craft V91.29 ☑
        - powered craft V91.23 ☑
          - ferry boat V91.21 ☑
          - fishing boat V91.22 ☑
          - jetskis V91.23 ☑
          - liner V91.21 ☑
          - merchant ship V91.20 ☑
          - passenger ship V91.21 ☑
        - unpowered craft
          - canoe V91.25 ☑
          - inflatable V91.26 ☑
          - kayak V91.25 ☑
          - sailboat V91.24 ☑
    - powered craft V93.33 ☑
      - ferry boat V93.31 ☑
      - fishing boat V93.32 ☑
      - jetskis V93.33 ☑
      - liner V93.31 ☑
      - merchant ship V93.30 ☑
      - passenger ship V93.31 ☑
    - unpowered craft V93.38 ☑
      - canoe V93.35 ☑
      - inflatable V93.36 ☑
      - kayak V93.35 ☑
      - sailboat V93.34 ☑
      - surf-board V93.38 ☑
      - windsurfer V93.38 ☑
- into
  - cavity W17.2 ☑
  - dock W17.4 ☑
  - fire — *see* Exposure, fire, by type
  - haystack W17.89 ☑
  - hole W17.2 ☑
  - lake — *see* Fall, into, water
  - manhole W17.1 ☑
  - moving part of machinery — *see* Contact, with, by type of machine
  - ocean — *see* Fall, into, water
  - opening in surface NEC W17.89 ☑
  - pit W17.2 ☑
  - pond — *see* Fall, into, water
  - quarry W17.89 ☑
  - river — *see* Fall, into, water
  - shaft W17.89 ☑
  - storm drain W17.1 ☑
  - stream — *see* Fall, into, water
  - swimming pool — *see also* Fall, into, water, in, swimming pool
    - empty W17.3 ☑
  - tank W17.89 ☑
  - water W16.42 ☑
    - causing drowning W16.41 ☑
    - from watercraft — *see* Drowning, due to, fall overboard
    - hitting diving board W21.4 ☑
    - in
      - bathtub W16.212 ☑
        - causing drowning W16.211 ☑
      - bucket W16.222 ☑
        - causing drowning W16.221 ☑
      - natural body of water W16.112 ☑
        - causing drowning W16.111 ☑
        - striking
          - bottom W16.122 ☑
            - causing drowning W16.121 ☑
          - side W16.132 ☑

☑ **Additional Character Required** — Refer to the Tabular List for Character Selection　　🔻 **Subterms under main terms may continue to next column or page**

Fall, falling — *continued*
  into — *continued*
    water — *continued*
      in — *continued*
        natural body of water — *continued*
          striking — *continued*
            side — *continued*
              causing drowning W16.131 ☑
        specified water NEC W16.312 ☑
          causing drowning W16.311 ☑
          striking
            bottom W16.322 ☑
              causing drowning W16.321 ☑
            wall W16.332 ☑
              causing drowning W16.331 ☑
        swimming pool W16.012 ☑
          causing drowning W16.011 ☑
          striking
            bottom W16.022 ☑
              causing drowning W16.031 ☑
            wall W16.032 ☑
              causing drowning W16.021 ☑
        utility bucket W16.222 ☑
          causing drowning W16.221 ☑
    well W17.0 ☑
  involving
    bed W06 ☑
    chair W07 ☑
    furniture NEC W08 ☑
    glass — *see* Fall, by type
    playground equipment W09.8 ☑
      jungle gym W09.2 ☑
      slide W09.0 ☑
      swing W09.1 ☑
    roller blades — *see* Accident, transport, pedestrian, conveyance
    skateboard(s) — *see* Accident, transport, pedestrian, conveyance
    skates (ice) (in line) (roller) — *see* Accident, transport, pedestrian, conveyance
    skis — *see* Accident, transport, pedestrian, conveyance
    table W08 ☑
    wheelchair, non-moving W05.0 ☑
      powered — *see* Accident, transport, pedestrian, conveyance, specified type NEC
  object — *see* Struck by, object, falling
  off
    toilet W18.11 ☑
      with subsequent striking against object W18.12 ☑
  on same level W18.30 ☑
    due to
      specified NEC W18.39 ☑
      stepping on an object W18.31 ☑
  out of
    bed W06 ☑
    building NEC W13.8 ☑
    chair W07 ☑
    furniture NEC W08 ☑
    wheelchair, non-moving W05.0 ☑
      powered — *see* Accident, transport, pedestrian, conveyance, specified type NEC
    window W13.4 ☑
  over
    animal W01.0 ☑
    cliff W15 ☑
    embankment W17.81 ☑
    small object W01.0 ☑
  rock W20.8 ☑
  same level W18.30 ☑
    from
      being crushed, pushed, or stepped on by a crowd or human stampede W52 ☑
      collision, pushing, shoving, by or with other person W03 ☑
      slipping, stumbling, tripping W00.0 ☑
      involving ice or snow W00.0 ☑
        involving skates (ice) (roller), skateboard, skis — *see* Accident, transport, pedestrian, conveyance
  snowslide (avalanche) — *see* Landslide
  stone W20.8 ☑
  structure W20.1 ☑
    burning (uncontrolled fire) X00.3 ☑

Fall, falling — *continued*
  through
    bridge W13.1 ☑
    floor W13.3 ☑
    roof W13.2 ☑
    wall W13.8 ☑
    window W13.4 ☑
  timber W20.8 ☑
  tree (caused by lightning) W20.8 ☑
  while being carried or supported by other person(s) W04 ☑
Fallen on by
  animal (not being ridden) NEC W55.89 ☑
Felo-de-se — *see* Suicide
Fight (hand) (fists) (foot) — *see* Assault, fight
Fire (accidental) — *see* Exposure, fire
Firearm discharge — *see* Discharge, firearm
Fireball effects from nuclear explosion in war operations — *see* War operations, nuclear weapons
Fireworks (explosion) W39 ☑
Flash burns from explosion — *see* Explosion
Flood (any injury) (caused by) X38 ☑
  collapse of man-made structure causing earth movement X36.0 ☑
  tidal wave — *see* Forces of nature, tidal wave
Food (any type) **in**
  air passages (with asphyxia, obstruction, or suffocation) — *see* categories T17 and T18
  alimentary tract causing asphyxia (due to compression of trachea) — *see* categories T17 and T18
Forces of nature X39.8 ☑
  avalanche X36.1 ☑
    causing transport accident — *see* Accident, transport, by type of vehicle
  blizzard X37.2 ☑
  cataclysmic storm X37.9 ☑
    with flood X38 ☑
    blizzard X37.2 ☑
    cloudburst X37.8 ☑
    cyclone X37.1 ☑
    dust storm X37.3 ☑
    hurricane X37.0 ☑
    specified storm NEC X37.8 ☑
    storm surge X37.0 ☑
    tornado X37.1 ☑
    twister X37.1 ☑
    typhoon X37.0 ☑
  cloudburst X37.8 ☑
  cold (natural) X31 ☑
  cyclone X37.1 ☑
  dam collapse causing earth movement X36.0 ☑
  dust storm X37.3 ☑
  earth movement X36.1 ☑
    caused by dam or structure collapse X36.0 ☑
    earthquake X34 ☑
  earthquake X34 ☑
  flood (caused by) X38 ☑
    dam collapse X36.0 ☑
    tidal wave — *see* Forces of nature, tidal wave
  heat (natural) X30 ☑
  hurricane X37.0 ☑
  landslide X36.1 ☑
    causing transport accident — *see* Accident, transport, by type of vehicle
  lightning — *see* subcategory T75.0 ☑
    causing fire — *see* Exposure, fire
  mudslide X36.1 ☑
    causing transport accident — *see* Accident, transport, by type of vehicle
  radiation (natural) X39.08 ☑
    radon X39.01 ☑
  radon X39.01 ☑
  specified force NEC X39.8 ☑
  storm surge X37.0 ☑
  structure collapse causing earth movement X36.0 ☑
  sunlight X32 ☑
  tidal wave X37.41 ☑
    due to
      earthquake X37.41 ☑
      landslide X37.43 ☑
      storm X37.42 ☑
      volcanic eruption X37.41 ☑
  tornado X37.1 ☑
  tsunami X37.41 ☑
  twister X37.1 ☑
  typhoon X37.0 ☑

Forces of nature — *continued*
  volcanic eruption X35 ☑
Foreign body
  aspiration — *see* Index to Diseases and Injuries, Foreign body, respiratory tract
  embedded in skin W45 ☑
  entering through skin W45.8 ☑
    can lid W26.8 ☑
    nail W45.0 ☑
    paper W26.2 ☑
    specified NEC W45.8 ☑
    splinter W45.8 ☑
Forest fire (exposure to) — *see* Exposure, fire, uncontrolled, not in building
Found injured X58 ☑
  from exposure (to) — *see* Exposure
  on
    highway, road(way), street V89.9 ☑
    railway right of way V81.9 ☑
Fracture (circumstances unknown or unspecified) X58 ☑
  due to specified cause NEC X58 ☑
Freezing — *see* Exposure, cold
Frostbite X31 ☑
  due to man-made conditions — *see* Exposure, cold, man-made
Frozen — *see* Exposure, cold

G

Gored by bull W55.22 ☑
Gunshot wound W34.00 ☑

H

Hailstones, injured by X39.8 ☑
Hanged herself or himself — *see* Hanging, self-inflicted
Hanging (accidental) — *see also* category T71 ☑
  legal execution — *see* Legal, intervention, specified means NEC
Heat (effects of) (excessive) X30 ☑
  due to
    man-made conditions W92 ☑
      on board watercraft V93.29 ☑
        fishing boat V93.22 ☑
        merchant ship V93.20 ☑
        passenger ship V93.21 ☑
        sailboat V93.24 ☑
        specified powered craft NEC V93.23 ☑
    weather (conditions) X30 ☑
  from
    electric heating apparatus causing burning X16 ☑
    nuclear explosion in war operations — *see* War operations, nuclear weapons
  inappropriate in local application or packing in medical or surgical procedure Y63.5
Hemorrhage
  delayed following medical or surgical treatment without mention of misadventure — *see* Index to Diseases and Injuries, Complication(s)
  during medical or surgical treatment as misadventure — *see* Index to Diseases and Injuries, Complication(s)
High
  altitude (effects) — *see* Air, pressure, low
  level of radioactivity, effects — *see* Radiation
  pressure (effects) — *see* Air, pressure, high
  temperature, effects — *see* Heat
Hit, hitting (accidental) by — *see* Struck by
Hitting against — *see* Striking against
Homicide (attempt) (justifiable) — *see* Assault
Hot
  place, effects — *see also* Heat
  weather, effects X30 ☑
House fire (uncontrolled) — *see* Exposure, fire, uncontrolled, building
Humidity, causing problem X39.8 ☑
Hunger X58 ☑
Hurricane (any injury) X37.0 ☑
Hypobarism, hypobaropathy — *see* Air, pressure, low

I

Ictus
  caloris — *see also* Heat
  solaris X30 ☑
Ignition (accidental) — *see also* Exposure, fire X08.8 ☑

Ignition — *continued*
  anesthetic gas in operating room W40.1 ☑
  apparel X06.2 ☑
    from highly flammable material X04 ☑
    nightwear X05 ☑
  bed linen (sheets) (spreads) (pillows) (mattress) — *see* Exposure, fire, uncontrolled, building, bed
  benzine X04 ☑
  clothes, clothing NEC (from controlled fire) X06.2 ☑
    from
      highly flammable material X04 ☑
  ether X04 ☑
    in operating room W40.1 ☑
  explosive material — *see* Explosion
  gasoline X04 ☑
  jewelry (plastic) (any) X06.0 ☑
  kerosene X04 ☑
  material
    explosive — *see* Explosion
    highly flammable with secondary explosion X04 ☑
  nightwear X05 ☑
  paraffin X04 ☑
  petrol X04 ☑
Immersion (accidental) — *see also* Drowning
  hand or foot due to cold (excessive) X31 ☑
Implantation of quills of porcupine W55.89 ☑
Inanition (from) (hunger) X58 ☑
  thirst X58 ☑
Inappropriate operation performed
  correct operation on wrong side or body part (wrong side) (wrong site) Y65.53
  operation intended for another patient done on wrong patient Y65.52
  wrong operation performed on correct patient Y65.51
Inattention after, at birth (homicidal intent) (infanticidal intent) X58 ☑
Incident, adverse
  device
    anesthesiology Y70.8
      accessory Y70.2
      diagnostic Y70.0
      miscellaneous Y70.8
      monitoring Y70.0
      prosthetic Y70.2
      rehabilitative Y70.1
      surgical Y70.3
      therapeutic Y70.1
    cardiovascular Y71.8
      accessory Y71.2
      diagnostic Y71.0
      miscellaneous Y71.8
      monitoring Y71.0
      prosthetic Y71.2
      rehabilitative Y71.1
      surgical Y71.3
      therapeutic Y71.1
    gastroenterology Y73.8
      accessory Y73.2
      diagnostic Y73.0
      miscellaneous Y73.8
      monitoring Y73.0
      prosthetic Y73.2
      rehabilitative Y73.1
      surgical Y73.3
      therapeutic Y73.1
    general
      hospital Y74.8
        accessory Y74.2
        diagnostic Y74.0
        miscellaneous Y74.8
        monitoring Y74.0
        prosthetic Y74.2
        rehabilitative Y74.1
        surgical Y74.3
        therapeutic Y74.1
      surgical Y81.8
        accessory Y81.2
        diagnostic Y81.0
        miscellaneous Y81.8
        monitoring Y81.0
        prosthetic Y81.2
        rehabilitative Y81.1
        surgical Y81.3
        therapeutic Y81.1
    gynecological Y76.8
      accessory Y76.2
      diagnostic Y76.0
      miscellaneous Y76.8

Incident, adverse — *continued*
  device — *continued*
    gynecological — *continued*
      monitoring Y76.0
      prosthetic Y76.2
      rehabilitative Y76.1
      surgical Y76.3
      therapeutic Y76.1
    medical Y82.9
      specified type NEC Y82.8
    neurological Y75.8
      accessory Y75.2
      diagnostic Y75.0
      miscellaneous Y75.8
      monitoring Y75.0
      prosthetic Y75.2
      rehabilitative Y75.1
      surgical Y75.3
      therapeutic Y75.1
    obstetrical Y76.8
      accessory Y76.2
      diagnostic Y76.0
      miscellaneous Y76.8
      monitoring Y76.0
      prosthetic Y76.2
      rehabilitative Y76.1
      surgical Y76.3
      therapeutic Y76.1
    ophthalmic Y77.8
      accessory Y77.2
      diagnostic Y77.0
      miscellaneous Y77.8
      monitoring Y77.0
      prosthetic Y77.2
      rehabilitative Y77.1
      surgical Y77.3
      therapeutic Y77.1
    orthopedic Y79.8
      accessory Y79.2
      diagnostic Y79.0
      miscellaneous Y79.8
      monitoring Y79.0
      prosthetic Y79.2
      rehabilitative Y79.1
      surgical Y79.3
      therapeutic Y79.1
    otorhinolaryngological Y72.8
      accessory Y72.2
      diagnostic Y72.0
      miscellaneous Y72.8
      monitoring Y72.0
      prosthetic Y72.2
      rehabilitative Y72.1
      surgical Y72.3
      therapeutic Y72.1
    personal use Y74.8
      accessory Y74.2
      diagnostic Y74.0
      miscellaneous Y74.8
      monitoring Y74.0
      prosthetic Y74.2
      rehabilitative Y74.1
      surgical Y74.3
      therapeutic Y74.1
    physical medicine Y80.8
      accessory Y80.2
      diagnostic Y80.0
      miscellaneous Y80.8
      monitoring Y80.0
      prosthetic Y80.2
      rehabilitative Y80.1
      surgical Y80.3
      therapeutic Y80.1
    plastic surgical Y81.8
      accessory Y81.2
      diagnostic Y81.0
      miscellaneous Y81.8
      monitoring Y81.0
      prosthetic Y81.2
      rehabilitative Y81.1
      surgical Y81.3
      therapeutic Y81.1
    radiological Y78.8
      accessory Y78.2
      diagnostic Y78.0
      miscellaneous Y78.8
      monitoring Y78.0
      prosthetic Y78.2
      rehabilitative Y78.1

Incident, adverse — *continued*
  device — *continued*
    radiological — *continued*
      surgical Y78.3
      therapeutic Y78.1
    urology Y73.8
      accessory Y73.2
      diagnostic Y73.0
      miscellaneous Y73.8
      monitoring Y73.0
      prosthetic Y73.2
      rehabilitative Y73.1
      surgical Y73.3
      therapeutic Y73.1
Incineration (accidental) — *see* Exposure, fire
Infanticide — *see* Assault
Infrasound waves (causing injury) W49.9 ☑
Ingestion
  foreign body (causing injury) (with obstruction) — *see* Foreign body, alimentary canal
  poisonous
    plant(s) X58 ☑
    substance NEC — *see* Table of Drugs and Chemicals
Inhalation
  excessively cold substance, man-made — *see* Exposure, cold, man-made
  food (any type) (into respiratory tract) (with asphyxia, obstruction respiratory tract, suffocation) — *see* categories T17 and T18 ☑
  foreign body — *see* Foreign body, aspiration
  gastric contents (with asphyxia, obstruction respiratory passage, suffocation) T17.81- ☑
  hot air or gases X14.0 ☑
  liquid air, hydrogen, nitrogen W93.12 ☑
    suicide (attempt) X83.2 ☑
  steam X13.0 ☑
    assault X98.0 ☑
    stated as undetermined whether accidental or intentional Y27.0 ☑
    suicide (attempt) X77.0 ☑
  toxic gas — *see* Table of Drugs and Chemicals
  vomitus (with asphyxia, obstruction respiratory passage, suffocation) T17.81- ☑
Injury, injured (accidental(ly)) NOS X58 ☑
  by, caused by, from
    assault — *see* Assault
    law-enforcing agent, police, in course of legal intervention — *see* Legal intervention
    suicide (attempt) X83.8 ☑
  due to, in
    civil insurrection — *see* War operations
    fight — *see also* Assault, fight Y04.0 ☑
    war operations — *see* War operations
  homicide — *see also* Assault Y09
  inflicted (by)
    in course of arrest (attempted), suppression of disturbance, maintenance of order, by law-enforcing agents — *see* Legal intervention
    other person
      stated as
        accidental X58 ☑
        intentional, homicide (attempt) — *see* Assault
        undetermined whether accidental or intentional Y33 ☑
  purposely (inflicted) by other person(s) — *see* Assault
  self-inflicted X83.8 ☑
    stated as accidental X58 ☑
  specified cause NEC X58 ☑
  undetermined whether accidental or intentional Y33 ☑
Insolation, effects X30 ☑
Insufficient nourishment X58 ☑
Interruption of respiration (by)
  food (lodged in esophagus) — *see* categories T17 and T18 ☑
  vomitus (lodged in esophagus) T17.81- ☑
Intervention, legal — *see* Legal intervention
Intoxication
  drug — *see* Table of Drugs and Chemicals
  poison — *see* Table of Drugs and Chemicals

J

Jammed (accidentally)
  between objects (moving) (stationary and moving) W23.0 ☑
    stationary W23.1 ☑

Jumped, jumping

before moving object NEC X81.8 ☑
  motor vehicle X81.0 ☑
  subway train X81.1 ☑
  train X81.1 ☑
  undetermined whether accidental or intentional Y31 ☑
from
  boat (into water) voluntarily, without accident (to or on boat) W16.712 ☑
   striking bottom W16.722 ☑
    causing drowning W16.721 ☑
   with
    accident to or on boat — see Accident, watercraft
    drowning or submersion W16.711 ☑
     suicide (attempt) X71.3 ☑
  building — see also Jumped, from, high place W13.9 ☑
   burning (uncontrolled fire) X00.5 ☑
  high place NEC W17.89 ☑
   suicide (attempt) X80 ☑
   undetermined whether accidental or intentional Y30 ☑
  structure — see also Jumped, from, high place W13.9 ☑
   burning (uncontrolled fire) X00.5 ☑
into water W16.92 ☑
  causing drowning W16.91 ☑
from, off watercraft — see Jumped, from, boat
in
  natural body W16.612 ☑
   causing drowning W16.611 ☑
   striking bottom W16.622 ☑
    causing drowning W16.621 ☑
  specified place NEC W16.812 ☑
   causing drowning W16.811 ☑
   striking
    bottom W16.822 ☑
     causing drowning W16.821 ☑
    wall W16.832 ☑
     causing drowning W16.831 ☑
  swimming pool W16.512 ☑
   causing drowning W16.511 ☑
   striking
    bottom W16.522 ☑
     causing drowning W16.521 ☑
    wall W16.532 ☑
     causing drowning W16.531 ☑
suicide (attempt) X71.3 ☑

K

Kicked by

animal NEC W55.82 ☑
person(s) (accidentally) W50.1 ☑
  with intent to injure or kill Y04.0 ☑
  as, or caused by, a crowd or human stampede (with fall) W52 ☑
  assault Y04.0 ☑
  homicide (attempt) Y04.0 ☑
  in
   fight Y04.0 ☑
   legal intervention
    injuring
     bystander Y35.812 ☑
     law enforcement personnel Y35.811 ☑
     suspect Y35.813 ☑
     unspecified person Y35.819 ☑

Kicking

against
  object W22.8 ☑
   sports equipment W21.9 ☑
   stationary W22.09 ☑
    sports equipment W21.89 ☑
  person — see Striking against, person
  sports equipment W21.9 ☑
carpet stretcher with knee X50.3 ☑

Killed, killing (accidentally) NOS — see also Injury X58 ☑
in
  action — see War operations
  brawl, fight (hand) (fists) (foot) Y04.0 ☑
   by weapon — see also Assault
    cutting, piercing — see Assault, cutting or piercing instrument

Killed, killing — continued

in — continued
  brawl, fight — continued
   by weapon — see also Assault — continued
    firearm — see Discharge, firearm, by type, homicide
self
  stated as
   accident NOS X58 ☑
   suicide — see Suicide
   undetermined whether accidental or intentional Y33 ☑
Kneeling (prolonged (static) X50.1 ☑
Knocked down (accidentally) (by) NOS X58 ☑
animal (not being ridden) NEC — see also Struck by, by type of animal
crowd or human stampede W52 ☑
person W51 ☑
  in brawl, fight Y04.0 ☑
transport vehicle NEC — see also Accident, transport V09.9 ☑

L

Laceration NEC — see Injury
Lack of
care (helpless person) (infant) (newborn) X58 ☑
food except as result of abandonment or neglect X58 ☑
  due to abandonment or neglect X58 ☑
water except as result of transport accident X58 ☑
  due to transport accident — see Accident, transport, by type
  helpless person, infant, newborn X58 ☑
Landslide (falling on transport vehicle) X36.1 ☑
caused by collapse of man-made structure X36.0 ☑
Late effect — see Sequelae
Legal
execution (any method) — see Legal, intervention
intervention (by)
  baton — see Legal, intervention, blunt object, baton
  bayonet — see Legal, intervention, sharp object, bayonet
  blow — see Legal, intervention, manhandling
  blunt object
   baton
    injuring
     bystander Y35.312 ☑
     law enforcement personnel Y35.311 ☑
     suspect Y35.313 ☑
     unspecified person Y35.319 ☑
   injuring
    bystander Y35.302 ☑
    law enforcement personnel Y35.301 ☑
    suspect Y35.303 ☑
    unspecified person Y35.309 ☑
   specified NEC
    injuring
     bystander Y35.392 ☑
     law enforcement personnel Y35.391 ☑
     suspect Y35.393 ☑
     unspecified person Y35.399 ☑
   stave
    injuring
     bystander Y35.392 ☑
     law enforcement personnel Y35.391 ☑
     suspect Y35.393 ☑
     unspecified person Y35.399 ☑
  bomb — see Legal, intervention, explosive
  conducted energy device
   injuring
    bystander Y35.832 ☑
    law enforcement personnel Y35.831 ☑
    suspect Y35.833 ☑
    unspecified person Y35.839 ☑
  cutting or piercing instrument — see Legal, intervention, sharp object
  dynamite — see Legal, intervention, explosive, dynamite
  electroshock device (taser)
   injuring
    bystander Y35.832 ☑
    law enforcement personnel Y35.831 ☑
    suspect Y35.833 ☑
    unspecified person Y35.839 ☑

Legal — continued

intervention — continued
  explosive(s)
   dynamite
    injuring
     bystander Y35.112 ☑
     law enforcement personnel Y35.111 ☑
     suspect Y35.113 ☑
     unspecified person Y35.119 ☑
   grenade
    injuring
     bystander Y35.192 ☑
     law enforcement personnel Y35.191 ☑
     suspect Y35.193 ☑
     unspecified person Y35.199 ☑
   injuring
    bystander Y35.102 ☑
    law enforcement personnel Y35.101 ☑
    suspect Y35.103 ☑
    unspecified person Y35.109 ☑
   mortar bomb
    injuring
     bystander Y35.192 ☑
     law enforcement personnel Y35.191 ☑
     suspect Y35.193 ☑
     unspecified person Y35.199 ☑
   shell
    injuring
     bystander Y35.122 ☑
     law enforcement personnel Y35.121 ☑
     suspect Y35.123 ☑
     unspecified person Y35.129 ☑
   specified NEC
    injuring
     bystander Y35.192 ☑
     law enforcement personnel Y35.191 ☑
     suspect Y35.193 ☑
     unspecified person Y35.199 ☑
  firearm(s) (discharge)
   handgun
    injuring
     bystander Y35.022 ☑
     law enforcement personnel Y35.021 ☑
     suspect Y35.023 ☑
     unspecified person Y35.029 ☑
   injuring
    bystander Y35.002 ☑
    law enforcement personnel Y35.001 ☑
    suspect Y35.003 ☑
    unspecified person Y35.009 ☑
   machine gun
    injuring
     bystander Y35.012 ☑
     law enforcement personnel Y35.011 ☑
     suspect Y35.013 ☑
     unspecified person Y35.019 ☑
   rifle pellet
    injuring
     bystander Y35.032 ☑
     law enforcement personnel Y35.031 ☑
     suspect Y35.033 ☑
     unspecified person Y35.039 ☑
   rubber bullet
    injuring
     bystander Y35.042 ☑
     law enforcement personnel Y35.041 ☑
     suspect Y35.043 ☑
     unspecified person Y35.049 ☑
   shotgun — see Legal, intervention, firearm, specified NEC
   specified NEC
    injuring
     bystander Y35.092 ☑
     law enforcement personnel Y35.091 ☑
     suspect Y35.093 ☑
     unspecified person Y35.099 ☑
  gas (asphyxiation) (poisoning)
   injuring
    bystander Y35.202 ☑
    law enforcement personnel Y35.201 ☑
    suspect Y35.203 ☑
    unspecified person Y35.209 ☑
   specified NEC
    injuring
     bystander Y35.292 ☑
     law enforcement personnel Y35.291 ☑
     suspect Y35.293 ☑

Subterms under main terms may continue to next column or page   ☑ Additional Character Required — Refer to the Tabular List for Character Selection   423

Jumped, jumping — Legal

Legal — *continued*
  intervention — *continued*
    gas — *continued*
      specified — *continued*
        injuring — *continued*
          unspecified person Y35.299 ☑
        tear gas
          injuring
            bystander Y35.212 ☑
            law enforcement personnel Y35.211 ☑
            suspect Y35.213 ☑
            unspecified person Y35.219 ☑
      grenade — *see* Legal, intervention, explosive,
          grenade
      injuring
        bystander Y35.92 ☑
        law enforcement personnel Y35.91 ☑
        suspect Y35.93 ☑
        unspecified person Y35.99 ☑
      late effect (of) — *see* with 7th character S Y35 ☑
      manhandling
        injuring
          bystander Y35.812 ☑
          law enforcement personnel Y35.811 ☑
          suspect Y35.813 ☑
          unspecified person Y35.819 ☑
      sequelae (of) — *see* with 7th character S Y35 ☑
      sharp objects
        bayonet
          injuring
            bystander Y35.412 ☑
            law enforcement personnel Y35.411 ☑
            suspect Y35.413 ☑
            unspecified person Y35.419 ☑
        injuring
          bystander Y35.402 ☑
          law enforcement personnel Y35.401 ☑
          suspect Y35.403 ☑
          unspecified person Y35.409 ☑
        specified NEC
          injuring
            bystander Y35.492 ☑
            law enforcement personnel Y35.491 ☑
            suspect Y35.493 ☑
            unspecified person Y35.499 ☑
      specified means NEC
        injuring
          bystander Y35.892 ☑
          law enforcement personnel Y35.891 ☑
          suspect Y35.893 ☑
      stabbing — *see* Legal, intervention, sharp object
      stave — *see* Legal, intervention, blunt object, stave
      stun gun
        injuring
          bystander Y35.832 ☑
          law enforcement personnel Y35.831 ☑
          suspect Y35.833 ☑
          unspecified person Y35.839 ☑
      taser
        injuring
          bystander Y35.832 ☑
          law enforcement personnel Y35.831 ☑
          suspect Y35.833 ☑
          unspecified person Y35.839 ☑
      tear gas — *see* Legal, intervention, gas, tear gas
      truncheon — *see* Legal, intervention, blunt object,
          stave
Lifting — *see also* Overexertion
  heavy objects X50.0 ☑
  weights X50.0 ☑
Lightning (shock) (stroke) (struck by) — *see* subcategory
      T75.0 ☑
  causing fire — *see* Exposure, fire
Loss of control (transport vehicle) NEC — *see* Accident,
      transport
Lost at sea NOS — *see* Drowning, due to, fall overboard
Low
  pressure (effects) — *see* Air, pressure, low
  temperature (effects) — *see* Exposure, cold
Lying before train, vehicle or other moving object
      X81.8 ☑
  subway train X81.1 ☑
  train X81.1 ☑
  undetermined whether accidental or intentional Y31 ☑
Lynching — *see* Assault

M

Malfunction (mechanism or component) (of)
  firearm W34.10 ☑
    airgun W34.110 ☑
    BB gun W34.110 ☑
    gas, air or spring-operated gun NEC W34.118 ☑
    handgun W32.1 ☑
    hunting rifle W33.12 ☑
    larger firearm W33.10 ☑
      specified NEC W33.19 ☑
    machine gun W33.13 ☑
    paintball gun W34.111 ☑
    pellet gun W34.110 ☑
    shotgun W33.11 ☑
    specified NEC W34.19 ☑
    Very pistol [flare] W34.19 ☑
  handgun — *see* Malfunction, firearm, handgun
Maltreatment — *see* Perpetrator
Mangled (accidentally) NOS X58 ☑
Manhandling (in brawl, fight) Y04.0 ☑
  legal intervention — *see* Legal, intervention, manhan-
      dling
Manslaughter (nonaccidental) — *see* Assault
Mauled by animal NEC W55.89 ☑
Medical procedure, complication of (delayed or as an
      abnormal reaction without mention of misadven-
      ture) — *see* Complication of or following, by speci-
      fied type of procedure
  due to or as a result of misadventure — *see* Misadven-
      ture
Melting (due to fire) — *see also* Exposure, fire
  apparel NEC X06.3 ☑
  clothes, clothing NEC X06.3 ☑
    nightwear X05 ☑
  fittings or furniture (burning building) (uncontrolled
      fire) X00.8 ☑
  nightwear X05 ☑
  plastic jewelry X06.1 ☑
Mental cruelty X58 ☑
Military operations (injuries to military and civilians
      occuring during peacetime on military property and
      during routine military exercises and operations)
      (by) (from) (involving) Y37.90- ☑
  air blast Y37.20- ☑
  aircraft
    destruction — *see* Military operations, destruction
        of aircraft
    airway restriction — *see* Military operations, restriction
        of airways
    asphyxiation — *see* Military operations, restriction of
        airways
  biological weapons Y37.6X- ☑
  blast Y37.20- ☑
  blast fragments Y37.20- ☑
  blast wave Y37.20- ☑
  blast wind Y37.20- ☑
  bomb Y37.20- ☑
    dirty Y37.50- ☑
    gasoline Y37.31- ☑
    incendiary Y37.31- ☑
    petrol Y37.31- ☑
  bullet Y37.43- ☑
    incendiary Y37.32- ☑
    rubber Y37.41- ☑
  chemical weapons Y37.7X- ☑
  combat
    hand to hand (unarmed) combat Y37.44- ☑
    using blunt or piercing object Y37.45- ☑
  conflagration — *see* Military operations, fire
  conventional warfare NEC Y37.49- ☑
  depth-charge Y37.01- ☑
  destruction of aircraft Y37.10- ☑
    due to
      air to air missile Y37.11- ☑
      collision with other aircraft Y37.12- ☑
      detonation (accidental) of onboard munitions
          and explosives Y37.14- ☑
      enemy fire or explosives Y37.11- ☑
      explosive placed on aircraft Y37.11- ☑
      onboard fire Y37.13- ☑
      rocket propelled grenade [RPG] Y37.11- ☑
      small arms fire Y37.11- ☑
      surface to air missile Y37.11- ☑
    specified NEC Y37.19- ☑

Military operations — *continued*
  detonation (accidental) of
    onboard marine weapons Y37.05- ☑
    own munitions or munitions launch device
        Y37.24- ☑
  dirty bomb Y37.50- ☑
  explosion (of) Y37.20- ☑
    aerial bomb Y37.21- ☑
    bomb NOS — *see also* Military operations, bomb(s)
        Y37.20- ☑
    fragments Y37.20- ☑
    grenade Y37.29- ☑
    guided missile Y37.22- ☑
    improvised explosive device [IED] (person-borne)
        (roadside) (vehicle-borne) Y37.23- ☑
    land mine Y37.29- ☑
    marine mine (at sea) (in harbor) Y37.02- ☑
    marine weapon Y37.00- ☑
      specified NEC Y37.09- ☑
    own munitions or munitions launch device (acciden-
        tal) Y37.24- ☑
    sea-based artillery shell Y37.03- ☑
    specified NEC Y37.29- ☑
    torpedo Y37.04- ☑
  fire Y37.30- ☑
    specified NEC Y37.39- ☑
  firearms
    discharge Y37.43- ☑
    pellets Y37.42- ☑
  flamethrower Y37.33- ☑
  fragments (from) (of)
    improvised explosive device [IED] (person-borne)
        (roadside) (vehicle-borne) Y37.26- ☑
    munitions Y37.25- ☑
    specified NEC Y37.29- ☑
    weapons Y37.27- ☑
  friendly fire Y37.92- ☑
  hand to hand (unarmed) combat Y37.44- ☑
  hot substances — *see* Military operations, fire
  incendiary bullet Y37.32- ☑
  nuclear weapon (effects of) Y37.50- ☑
    acute radiation exposure Y37.54- ☑
    blast pressure Y37.51- ☑
    direct blast Y37.51- ☑
    direct heat Y37.53- ☑
    fallout exposure Y37.54- ☑
    fireball Y37.53- ☑
    indirect blast (struck or crushed by blast debris)
        (being thrown by blast) Y37.52- ☑
    ionizing radiation (immediate exposure) Y37.54- ☑
    nuclear radiation Y37.54- ☑
    radiation
      ionizing (immediate exposure) Y37.54- ☑
      nuclear Y37.54- ☑
      thermal Y37.53- ☑
    secondary effects Y37.54- ☑
    specified NEC Y37.59- ☑
    thermal radiation Y37.53- ☑
  restriction of air (airway)
    intentional Y37.46- ☑
    unintentional Y37.47- ☑
  rubber bullets Y37.41- ☑
  shrapnel NOS Y37.29- ☑
  suffocation — *see* Military operations, restriction of
      airways
  unconventional warfare NEC Y37.7X- ☑
  underwater blast NOS Y37.00- ☑
  warfare
    conventional NEC Y37.49- ☑
    unconventional NEC Y37.7X- ☑
  weapon of mass destruction [WMD] Y37.91- ☑
  weapons
    biological weapons Y37.6X- ☑
    chemical Y37.7X- ☑
    nuclear (effects of) Y37.50- ☑
      acute radiation exposure Y37.54- ☑
      blast pressure Y37.51- ☑
      direct blast Y37.51- ☑
      direct heat Y37.53- ☑
      fallout exposure Y37.54- ☑
      fireball Y37.53- ☑
      radiation
        ionizing (immediate exposure) Y37.54- ☑
        nuclear Y37.54- ☑
        thermal Y37.53- ☑
      secondary effects Y37.54- ☑

Military operations — *continued*
  weapons — *continued*
    nuclear — *continued*
      specified NEC Y37.59- ☑
    of mass destruction [WMD] Y37.91- ☑
Misadventure(s) to patient(s) during surgical or
  medical care Y69
  contaminated medical or biological substance (blood,
    drug, fluid) Y64.9
    administered (by) NEC Y64.9
      immunization Y64.1
      infusion Y64.0
      injection Y64.1
      specified means NEC Y64.8
      transfusion Y64.0
      vaccination Y64.1
  excessive amount of blood or other fluid during trans-
    fusion or infusion Y63.0
  failure
    in dosage Y63.9
      electroshock therapy Y63.4
      inappropriate temperature (too hot or too cold)
        in local application and packing Y63.5
      infusion
        excessive amount of fluid Y63.0
        incorrect dilution of fluid Y63.1
      insulin-shock therapy Y63.4
      nonadministration of necessary drug or biologi-
        cal substance Y63.6
      overdose — *see* Table of Drugs and Chemicals
        radiation, in therapy Y63.2
      radiation
        overdose Y63.2
      specified procedure NEC Y63.8
      transfusion
        excessive amount of blood Y63.0
    mechanical, of instrument or apparatus (any) (during
      any procedure) Y65.8
    sterile precautions (during procedure) Y62.9
      aspiration of fluid or tissue (by puncture or
        catheterization, except heart) Y62.6
      biopsy (except needle aspiration) Y62.8
        needle (aspirating) Y62.6
      blood sampling Y62.6
      catheterization Y62.6
        heart Y62.5
      dialysis (kidney) Y62.2
      endoscopic examination Y62.4
      enema Y62.8
      immunization Y62.3
      infusion Y62.1
      injection Y62.3
      needle biopsy Y62.6
      paracentesis (abdominal) (thoracic) Y62.6
      perfusion Y62.2
      puncture (lumbar) Y62.6
      removal of catheter or packing Y62.8
      specified procedure NEC Y62.8
      surgical operation Y62.0
      transfusion Y62.1
      vaccination Y62.3
    suture or ligature during surgical procedure Y65.2
    to introduce or to remove tube or instrument —
      see Failure, to
  hemorrhage — *see* Index to Diseases and Injuries,
    Complication(s)
  inadvertent exposure of patient to radiation Y63.3
  inappropriate
    operation performed — *see* Inappropriate operation
      performed
    temperature (too hot or too cold) in local application
      or packing Y63.5
  infusion — *see also* Misadventure, by type, infusion
    Y69
    excessive amount of fluid Y63.0
    incorrect dilution of fluid Y63.1
    wrong fluid Y65.1
  mismatched blood in transfusion Y65.0
  nonadministration of necessary drug or biological
    substance Y63.6
  overdose — *see* Table of Drugs and Chemicals
    radiation (in therapy) Y63.2
  perforation — *see* Index to Diseases and Injuries,
    Complication(s)
  performance of inappropriate operation — *see* Inap-
    propriate operation performed
  puncture — *see* Index to Diseases and Injuries, Compli-
    cation(s)

Misadventure(s) to patient(s) during surgical or
  medical care — *continued*
  specified type NEC Y65.8
    failure
      suture or ligature during surgical operation Y65.2
      to introduce or to remove tube or instrument —
        see Failure, to
    infusion of wrong fluid Y65.1
    performance of inappropriate operation — *see* In-
      appropriate operation performed
    transfusion of mismatched blood Y65.0
    wrong
      fluid in infusion Y65.1
      placement of endotracheal tube during anesthet-
        ic procedure Y65.3
  transfusion — *see* Misadventure, by type, transfusion
    excessive amount of blood Y63.0
    mismatched blood Y65.0
  wrong
    drug given in error — *see* Table of Drugs and
      Chemicals
    fluid in infusion Y65.1
    placement of endotracheal tube during anesthetic
      procedure Y65.3
Mismatched blood in transfusion Y65.0
Motion sickness T75.3 ☑
Mountain sickness W94.11 ☑
Mudslide (of cataclysmic nature) — *see* Landslide
Murder (attempt) — *see* Assault

N

Nail
  contact with W45.0 ☑
    gun W29.4 ☑
  embedded in skin W45.0 ☑
Neglect (criminal) (homicidal intent) X58 ☑
Noise (causing injury) (pollution) W42.9 ☑
  supersonic W42.0 ☑
Nonadministration (of)
  drug or biological substance (necessary) Y63.6
  surgical and medical care Y66
Nosocomial condition Y95

O

Object
  falling
    from, in, on, hitting
      machinery — *see* Contact, with, by type of ma-
        chine
    set in motion by
      accidental explosion or rupture of pressure vessel
        W38 ☑
      firearm — *see* Discharge, firearm, by type
      machine(ry) — *see* Contact, with, by type of ma-
        chine
Overdose (drug) — *see* Table of Drugs and Chemicals
  radiation Y63.2
Overexertion X50.9 ☑
  from
    prolonged static or awkward postures X50.1 ☑
    repetitive movements X50.3 ☑
    specified strenuous movements or postures NEC
      X50.9 ☑
    strenuous movement or load X50.0 ☑
Overexposure (accidental) (to)
  cold — *see also* Exposure, cold X31 ☑
    due to man-made conditions — *see* Exposure, cold,
      man-made
  heat — *see also* Heat X30 ☑
  radiation — *see* Radiation
  radioactivity W88.0 ☑
  sun (sunburn) X32 ☑
  weather NEC — *see* Forces of nature
  wind NEC — *see* Forces of nature
Overheated — *see* Heat
Overturning (accidental)
  machinery — *see* Contact, with, by type of machine
  transport vehicle NEC — *see also* Accident, transport
    V89.9 ☑
  watercraft (causing drowning, submersion) — *see also*
    Drowning, due to, accident to, watercraft, over-
    turning
    causing injury except drowning or submersion —
      see Accident, watercraft, causing, injury NEC

P

Parachute descent (voluntary) (without accident to aircraft) V97.29 ☑
  due to accident to aircraft — *see* Accident, transport,
    aircraft
Pecked by bird W61.99 ☑
Perforation during medical or surgical treatment as
  misadventure — *see* Index to Diseases and In-
    juries, Complication(s)
Perpetrator, perpetration, of assault, maltreatment
  and neglect (by) Y07.9
  boyfriend Y07.03
  brother Y07.410
    stepbrother Y07.435
  coach Y07.53
  cousin
    female Y07.491
    male Y07.490
  daycare provider Y07.519
    at-home
      adult care Y07.512
      childcare Y07.510
    care center
      adult care Y07.513
      childcare Y07.511
  family member NEC Y07.499
  father Y07.11
    adoptive Y07.13
    foster Y07.420
    stepfather Y07.430
  foster father Y07.420
  foster mother Y07.421
  girl friend Y07.04
  healthcare provider Y07.529
    mental health Y07.521
    specified NEC Y07.528
  husband Y07.01
  instructor Y07.53
  mother Y07.12
    adoptive Y07.14
    foster Y07.421
    stepmother Y07.433
  multiple perpetrators Y07.6
  nonfamily member Y07.50
    specified NEC Y07.59
  nurse Y07.528
  occupational therapist Y07.528
  partner of parent
    female Y07.434
    male Y07.432
  physical therapist Y07.528
  sister Y07.411
  speech therapist Y07.528
  stepbrother Y07.435
  stepfather Y07.430
  stepmother Y07.433
  stepsister Y07.436
  teacher Y07.53
  wife Y07.02
Piercing — *see* Contact, with, by type of object or machine
Pinched
  between objects (moving) (stationary and moving)
    W23.0 ☑
  stationary W23.1 ☑
Pinned under machine(ry) — *see* Contact, with, by type
  of machine
Place of occurrence Y92.9
  abandoned house Y92.89
  airplane Y92.813
  airport Y92.520
  ambulatory health services establishment NEC Y92.538
  ambulatory surgery center Y92.530
  amusement park Y92.831
  apartment (co-op) — *see* Place of occurrence, resi-
    dence, apartment
  assembly hall Y92.29
  bank Y92.510
  barn Y92.71
  baseball field Y92.320
  basketball court Y92.310
  beach Y92.832
  boarding house — *see* Place of occurrence, residence,
    boarding house
  boat Y92.814
  bowling alley Y92.39

Place of occurrence — *continued*
bridge Y92.89
building under construction Y92.61
bus Y92.811
    station Y92.521
cafe Y92.511
campsite Y92.833
campus — *see* Place of occurrence, school
canal Y92.89
car Y92.810
casino Y92.59
children's home — *see* Place of occurrence, residence, institutional, orphanage
church Y92.22
cinema Y92.26
clubhouse Y92.29
coal pit Y92.64
college (community) Y92.214
condominium — *see* Place of occurrence, residence, apartment
construction area — *see* Place of occurrence, industrial and construction area
convalescent home — *see* Place of occurrence, residence, institutional, nursing home
court-house Y92.240
cricket ground Y92.328
cultural building Y92.258
    art gallery Y92.250
    museum Y92.251
    music hall Y92.252
    opera house Y92.253
    specified NEC Y92.258
    theater Y92.254
dancehall Y92.252
day nursery Y92.210
dentist office Y92.531
derelict house Y92.89
desert Y92.820
dockyard Y92.62
dock NOS Y92.89
doctor's office Y92.531
dormitory — *see* Place of occurrence, residence, institutional, school dormitory
dry dock Y92.62
factory (building) (premises) Y92.63
farm (land under cultivation) (outbuildings) Y92.79
    barn Y92.71
    chicken coop Y92.72
    field Y92.73
    hen house Y92.72
    house — *see* Place of occurrence, residence, house
    orchard Y92.74
    specified NEC Y92.79
football field Y92.321
forest Y92.821
freeway Y92.411
gallery Y92.250
garage (commercial) Y92.59
    boarding house Y92.044
    military base Y92.135
    mobile home Y92.025
    nursing home Y92.124
    orphanage Y92.114
    private house Y92.015
    reform school Y92.155
gas station Y92.524
gasworks Y92.69
golf course Y92.39
gravel pit Y92.64
grocery Y92.512
gymnasium Y92.39
handball court Y92.318
harbor Y92.89
harness racing course Y92.39
healthcare provider office Y92.531
highway (interstate) Y92.411
hill Y92.828
hockey rink Y92.330
home — *see* Place of occurrence, residence
hospice — *see* Place of occurrence, residence, institutional, nursing home
hospital Y92.239
    cafeteria Y92.233
    corridor Y92.232
    operating room Y92.234
    patient
        bathroom Y92.231
        room Y92.230

Place of occurrence — *continued*
hospital — *continued*
    specified NEC Y92.238
hotel Y92.59
house — *see also* Place of occurrence, residence
    abandoned Y92.89
    under construction Y92.61
industrial and construction area (yard) Y92.69
    building under construction Y92.61
    dock Y92.62
    dry dock Y92.62
    factory Y92.63
    gasworks Y92.69
    mine Y92.64
    oil rig Y92.65
    pit Y92.64
    power station Y92.69
    shipyard Y92.62
    specified NEC Y92.69
    tunnel under construction Y92.69
    workshop Y92.69
kindergarten Y92.211
lacrosse field Y92.328
lake Y92.828
library Y92.241
mall Y92.59
market Y92.512
marsh Y92.828
military
    base — *see* Place of occurrence, residence, institutional, military base
    training ground Y92.84
mine Y92.64
mosque Y92.22
motel Y92.59
motorway (interstate) Y92.411
mountain Y92.828
movie-house Y92.26
museum Y92.251
music-hall Y92.252
not applicable Y92.9
nuclear power station Y92.69
nursing home — *see* Place of occurrence, residence, institutional, nursing home
office building Y92.59
offshore installation Y92.65
oil rig Y92.65
old people's home — *see* Place of occurrence, residence, institutional, specified NEC
opera-house Y92.253
orphanage — *see* Place of occurrence, residence, institutional, orphanage
outpatient surgery center Y92.530
park (public) Y92.830
    amusement Y92.831
parking garage Y92.89
    lot Y92.481
pavement Y92.480
physician office Y92.531
polo field Y92.328
pond Y92.828
post office Y92.242
power station Y92.69
prairie Y92.828
prison — *see* Place of occurrence, residence, institutional, prison
public
    administration building Y92.248
        city hall Y92.243
        courthouse Y92.240
        library Y92.241
        post office Y92.242
        specified NEC Y92.248
    building NEC Y92.29
    hall Y92.29
    place NOS Y92.89
race course Y92.39
radio station Y92.59
railway line (bridge) Y92.85
ranch (outbuildings) — *see* Place of occurrence, farm
recreation area Y92.838
    amusement park Y92.831
    beach Y92.832
    campsite Y92.833
    park (public) Y92.830
    seashore Y92.832
    specified NEC Y92.838

Place of occurrence — *continued*
reform school - — *see* Place of occurrence, residence, institutional, reform school
religious institution Y92.22
residence (non-institutional) (private) Y92.009
    apartment Y92.039
        bathroom Y92.031
        bedroom Y92.032
        kitchen Y92.030
        specified NEC Y92.038
    bathroom Y92.002
    bedroom Y92.003
    boarding house Y92.049
        bathroom Y92.041
        bedroom Y92.042
        driveway Y92.043
        garage Y92.044
        garden Y92.046
        kitchen Y92.040
        specified NEC Y92.048
        swimming pool Y92.045
        yard Y92.046
    dining room Y92.001
    garden Y92.007
    home Y92.009
    house, single family Y92.019
        bathroom Y92.012
        bedroom Y92.013
        dining room Y92.011
        driveway Y92.014
        garage Y92.015
        garden Y92.017
        kitchen Y92.010
        specified NEC Y92.018
        swimming pool Y92.016
        yard Y92.017
    institutional Y92.10
        children's home — *see* Place of occurrence, residence, institutional, orphanage
        hospice — *see* Place of occurrence, residence, institutional, nursing home
        military base Y92.139
            barracks Y92.133
            garage Y92.135
            garden Y92.137
            kitchen Y92.130
            mess hall Y92.131
            specified NEC Y92.138
            swimming pool Y92.136
            yard Y92.137
        nursing home Y92.129
            bathroom Y92.121
            bedroom Y92.122
            driveway Y92.123
            garage Y92.124
            garden Y92.126
            kitchen Y92.120
            specified NEC Y92.128
            swimming pool Y92.125
            yard Y92.126
        orphanage Y92.119
            bathroom Y92.111
            bedroom Y92.112
            driveway Y92.113
            garage Y92.114
            garden Y92.116
            kitchen Y92.110
            specified NEC Y92.118
            swimming pool Y92.115
            yard Y92.116
        prison Y92.149
            bathroom Y92.142
            cell Y92.143
            courtyard Y92.147
            dining room Y92.141
            kitchen Y92.140
            specified NEC Y92.148
            swimming pool Y92.146
        reform school Y92.159
            bathroom Y92.152
            bedroom Y92.153
            dining room Y92.151
            driveway Y92.154
            garage Y92.155
            garden Y92.157
            kitchen Y92.150
            specified NEC Y92.158
            swimming pool Y92.156
            yard Y92.157

☑ Additional Character Required — Refer to the Tabular List for Character Selection ▽ Subterms under main terms may continue to next column or page

Place of occurrence — *continued*
  residence — *continued*
    institutional — *continued*
      school dormitory Y92.169
        bathroom Y92.162
        bedroom Y92.163
        dining room Y92.161
        kitchen Y92.160
        specified NEC Y92.168
      specified NEC Y92.199
        bathroom Y92.192
        bedroom Y92.193
        dining room Y92.191
        driveway Y92.194
        garage Y92.195
        garden Y92.197
        kitchen Y92.190
        specified NEC Y92.198
        swimming pool Y92.196
        yard Y92.197
    kitchen Y92.000
    mobile home Y92.029
      bathroom Y92.022
      bedroom Y92.023
      dining room Y92.021
      driveway Y92.024
      garage Y92.025
      garden Y92.027
      kitchen Y92.020
      specified NEC Y92.028
      swimming pool Y92.026
      yard Y92.027
    specified place in residence NEC Y92.008
    specified residence type NEC Y92.099
      bathroom Y92.091
      bedroom Y92.092
      driveway Y92.093
      garage Y92.094
      garden Y92.096
      kitchen Y92.090
      specified NEC Y92.098
      swimming pool Y92.095
      yard Y92.096
  restaurant Y92.511
  riding school Y92.39
  river Y92.828
  road Y92.410
  rodeo ring Y92.39
  rugby field Y92.328
  same day surgery center Y92.530
  sand pit Y92.64
  school (private) (public) (state) Y92.219
    college Y92.214
    daycare center Y92.210
    elementary school Y92.211
    high school Y92.213
    kindergarten Y92.211
    middle school Y92.212
    specified NEC Y92.218
    trace school Y92.215
    university Y92.214
    vocational school Y92.215
  sea (shore) Y92.832
  senior citizen center Y92.29
  service area
    airport Y92.520
    bus station Y92.521
    gas station Y92.524
    highway rest stop Y92.523
    railway station Y92.522
  shipyard Y92.62
  shop (commercial) Y92.513
  sidewalk Y92.480
  silo Y92.79
  skating rink (roller) Y92.331
    ice Y92.330
  slaughter house Y92.86
  soccer field Y92.322
  specified place NEC Y92.89
  sports area Y92.39
    athletic
      court Y92.318
        basketball Y92.310
        specified NEC Y92.318
        squash Y92.311
        tennis Y92.312
      field Y92.320
        baseball Y92.320
        cricket ground Y92.328

Place of occurrence — *continued*
  sports area — *continued*
    athletic — *continued*
      field — *continued*
        football Y92.321
        hockey Y92.328
        soccer Y92.322
        specified NEC Y92.328
    golf course Y92.39
    gymnasium Y92.39
    riding school Y92.39
    skating rink (roller) Y92.331
      ice Y92.330
    stadium Y92.39
    swimming pool Y92.34
  squash court Y92.311
  stadium Y92.39
  steeplechasing course Y92.39
  store Y92.512
  stream Y92.828
  street and highway Y92.410
    bike path Y92.482
    freeway Y92.411
    highway ramp Y92.415
    interstate highway Y92.411
    local residential or business street Y92.414
    motorway Y92.411
    parking lot Y92.481
    parkway Y92.412
    sidewalk Y92.480
    specified NEC Y92.488
    state road Y92.413
  subway car Y92.816
  supermarket Y92.512
  swamp Y92.828
  swimming pool (public) Y92.34
    private (at) Y92.095
      boarding house Y92.045
      military base Y92.136
      mobile home Y92.026
      nursing home Y92.125
      orphanage Y92.115
      prison Y92.146
      reform school Y92.156
      single family residence Y92.016
  synagogue Y92.22
  television station Y92.59
  tennis court Y92.312
  theater Y92.254
  trade area Y92.59
    bank Y92.510
    cafe Y92.511
    casino Y92.59
    garage Y92.59
    hotel Y92.59
    market Y92.512
    office building Y92.59
    radio station Y92.59
    restaurant Y92.511
    shop Y92.513
    shopping mall Y92.59
    store Y92.512
    supermarket Y92.512
    television station Y92.59
    warehouse Y92.59
  trailer park, residential — *see* Place of occurrence, residence, mobile home
  trailer site NOS Y92.89
  train Y92.815
    station Y92.522
  truck Y92.812
  tunnel under construction Y92.69
  university Y92.214
  urgent (health) care center Y92.532
  vehicle (transport) Y92.818
    airplane Y92.813
    boat Y92.814
    bus Y92.811
    car Y92.810
    specified NEC Y92.818
    subway car Y92.816
    train Y92.815
    truck Y92.812
  warehouse Y92.59
  water reservoir Y92.89
  wilderness area Y92.828
    desert Y92.020
    forest Y92.821
    marsh Y92.828

Place of occurrence — *continued*
  wilderness area — *continued*
    mountain Y92.828
    prairie Y92.828
    specified NEC Y92.828
    swamp Y92.828
  workshop Y92.69
  yard, private Y92.096
    boarding house Y92.046
    mobile home Y92.027
    single family house Y92.017
  youth center Y92.29
  zoo (zoological garden) Y92.834
Plumbism — *see* Table of Drugs and Chemicals, lead
Poisoning (accidental) (by) — *see also* Table of Drugs and Chemicals
  by plant, thorns, spines, sharp leaves or other mechanisms NEC X58 ☑
  carbon monoxide
    generated by
      motor vehicle — *see* Accident, transport
      watercraft (in transit) (not in transit) V93.89 ☑
        ferry boat V93.81 ☑
        fishing boat V93.82 ☑
        jet skis V93.83 ☑
        liner V93.81 ☑
        merchant ship V93.80 ☑
        passenger ship V93.81 ☑
        powered craft NEC V93.83 ☑
  caused by injection of poisons into skin by plant thorns, spines, sharp leaves X58 ☑
  marine or sea plants (venomous) X58 ☑
  execution — *see* Legal, intervention, gas
    intervention
      by gas — *see* Legal, intervention, gas
      other specified means — *see* Legal, intervention, specified means NEC
  exhaust gas
    generated by
      motor vehicle — *see* Accident, transport
      watercraft (in transit) (not in transit) V93.89 ☑
        ferry boat V93.81 ☑
        fishing boat V93.82 ☑
        jet skis V93.83 ☑
        liner V93.81 ☑
        merchant ship V93.80 ☑
        passenger ship V93.81 ☑
        powered craft NEC V93.83 ☑
  fumes or smoke due to
    explosion — *see also* Explosion W40.9 ☑
    fire — *see* Exposure, fire
    ignition — *see* Ignition
  gas
    in legal intervention — *see* Legal, intervention, gas
    legal execution — *see* Legal, intervention, gas
  in war operations — *see* War operations
  legal
Powder burn (by) (from)
  airgun W34.110 ☑
  BB gun W34.110 ☑
  firearm NEC W34.19 ☑
  gas, air or spring-operated gun NEC W34.118 ☑
  handgun W32.1 ☑
  hunting rifle W33.12 ☑
  larger firearm W33.10 ☑
    specified NEC W33.19 ☑
  machine gun W33.13 ☑
  paintball gun W34.111 ☑
  pellet gun W34.110 ☑
  shotgun W33.11 ☑
  Very pistol [flare] W34.19 ☑
Premature cessation (of) **surgical and medical care** Y66
Privation (food) (water) X58 ☑
Procedure (operation)
  correct, on wrong side or body part (wrong side) (wrong site) Y65.53
  intended for another patient done on wrong patient Y65.52
  performed on patient not scheduled for surgery Y65.52
  performed on wrong patient Y65.52
  wrong, performed on correct patient Y65.51
Prolonged
  sitting in transport vehicle — *see* Travel, by type of vehicle

Prolonged — *continued*
 stay in
  high altitude as cause of anoxia, barodontalgia,
   barotitis or hypoxia W94.11 ☑
  weightless environment X52
Pulling, excessive — *see also* Overexertion X50.9-
Puncture, puncturing — *see also* Contact, with, by type
  of object or machine
 by
  plant thorns, spines, sharp leaves or other mechanisms NEC W60 ☑
 during medical or surgical treatment as misadventure
   — *see* Index to Diseases and Injuries, Complica-
   tion(s)
Pushed, pushing (accidental) (injury in)
 by other person(s) (accidental) W51 ☑
  as, or caused by, a crowd or human stampede (with
   fall) W52 ☑
  before moving object NEC Y02.8 ☑
   motor vehicle Y02.0 ☑
   subway train Y02.1 ☑
   train Y02.1 ☑
  from
   high place NEC
    in accidental circumstances W17.89 ☑
    stated as
     intentional, homicide (attempt) Y01 ☑
     undetermined whether accidental or in-
      tentional Y30 ☑
    transport vehicle NEC — *see also* Accident,
     transport V89.9 ☑
    stated as
     intentional, homicide (attempt) Y08.89 ☑
  with fall W03 ☑
   due to ice or snow W00.0 ☑
 overexertion X50.9 ☑

R

Radiation (exposure to)
 arc lamps W89.0 ☑
 atomic power plant (malfunction) NEC W88.1 ☑
 complication of or abnormal reaction to medical radiotherapy Y84.2
 electromagnetic, ionizing W88.0 ☑
 gamma rays W88.1 ☑
 in
  war operations (from or following nuclear explosion)
   — *see* War operations
 inadvertent exposure of patient (receiving test or
  therapy) Y63.3
 infrared (heaters and lamps) W90.1 ☑
  excessive heat from W92 ☑
 ionized, ionizing (particles, artificially accelerated)
  radioisotopes W88.1 ☑
  specified NEC W88.8 ☑
  x-rays W88.0 ☑
 isotopes, radioactive — *see* Radiation, radioactive isotopes
 laser(s) W90.2 ☑
  in war operations — *see* War operations
  misadventure in medical care Y63.2
 light sources (man-made visible and ultraviolet)
   W89.9 ☑
  natural X32 ☑
  specified NEC W89.8 ☑
  tanning bed W89.1 ☑
  welding light W89.0 ☑
 man-made visible light W89.9 ☑
  specified NEC W89.8 ☑
  tanning bed W89.1 ☑
  welding light W89.0 ☑
 microwave W90.8 ☑
 misadventure in medical or surgical procedure Y63.2
 natural NEC X39.08 ☑
  radon X39.01 ☑
 overdose (in medical or surgical procedure) Y63.2
 radar W90.0 ☑
 radioactive isotopes (any) W88.1 ☑
  atomic power plant malfunction W88.1 ☑
  misadventure in medical or surgical treatment Y63.2
 radiofrequency W90.0 ☑
 radium NEC W88.1 ☑
 sun X32 ☑
 ultraviolet (light) (man-made) W89.9 ☑
  natural X32 ☑

Radiation — *continued*
 ultraviolet — *continued*
  specified NEC W89.8 ☑
  tanning bed W89.1 ☑
  welding light W89.0 ☑
 welding arc, torch, or light W89.0 ☑
  excessive heat from W92 ☑
 x-rays (hard) (soft) W88.0 ☑
Range disease W94.11 ☑
Rape (attempted) T74.2- ☑
Rat bite W53.11 ☑
Reaching (prolonged) (static) X50.1 ☑
Reaction, abnormal to medical procedure — *see also*
  Complication of or following, by type of procedure
  Y84.9
 biologicals — *see* Table of Drugs and Chemicals
 drugs — *see* Table of Drugs and Chemicals
 vaccine — *see* Table of Drugs and Chemicals
 with misadventure — *see* Misadventure
Recoil
 airgun W34.110 ☑
 BB gun W34.110 ☑
 firearm NEC W34.19 ☑
 gas, air or spring-operated gun NEC W34.118 ☑
 handgun W32.1 ☑
 hunting rifle W33.12 ☑
 larger firearm W33.10 ☑
  specified NEC W33.19 ☑
 machine gun W33.13 ☑
 paintball gun W34.111 ☑
 pellet W34.110 ☑
 shotgun W33.11 ☑
 Very pistol [flare] W34.19 ☑
Reduction in
 atmospheric pressure — *see* Air, pressure, change
Rock falling on or hitting (accidentally) (person)
   W20.8 ☑
 in cave-in W20.0 ☑
Run over (accidentally) (by)
 animal (not being ridden) NEC W55.89 ☑
 machinery — *see* Contact, with, by specified type of
  machine
 transport vehicle NEC — *see also* Accident, transport
  V09.9 ☑
  intentional homicide (attempt) Y03.0 ☑
  motor NEC V09.20 ☑
   intentional homicide (attempt) Y03.0 ☑
Running
 before moving object X81.8 ☑
  motor vehicle X81.0 ☑
Running off, away
 animal (being ridden) — *see also* Accident, transport
  V80.918 ☑
  not being ridden W55.89 ☑
 animal-drawn vehicle NEC — *see also* Accident, transport V80.928 ☑
 highway, road(way), street
  transport vehicle NEC — *see also* Accident, transport
   V09.9 ☑
Rupture pressurized devices — *see* Explosion, by type
  of device

S

Saturnism — *see* Table of Drugs and Chemicals, lead
Scald, scalding (accidental) (by) (from) (in) X19 ☑
 air (hot) X14.1 ☑
 gases (hot) X14.1 ☑
 homicide (attempt) — *see* Assault, burning, hot object
 inflicted by other person
  stated as intentional, homicide (attempt) — *see*
   Assault, burning, hot object
 liquid (boiling) (hot) NEC X12 ☑
  stated as undetermined whether accidental or intentional Y27.2 ☑
  suicide (attempt) X77.2 ☑
 local application of externally applied substance in
  medical or surgical care Y63.5
 metal (molten) (liquid) (hot) NEC X18 ☑
 self-inflicted X77.9 ☑
  stated as undetermined whether accidental or intentional Y27.8 ☑
 steam X13.1 ☑
  assault X98.0 ☑
  stated as undetermined whether accidental or intentional Y27.0 ☑

Scald, scalding — *continued*
 steam — *continued*
  suicide (attempt) X77.0 ☑
 suicide (attempt) X77.9 ☑
 vapor (hot) X13.1 ☑
  assault X98.0 ☑
  stated as undetermined whether accidental or intentional Y27.0 ☑
  suicide (attempt) X77.0 ☑
Scratched by
 cat W55.03 ☑
 person(s) (accidentally) W50.4 ☑
  with intent to injure or kill Y04.0 ☑
  as, or caused by, a crowd or human stampede (with
   fall) W52 ☑
  assault Y04.0 ☑
  homicide (attempt) Y04.0 ☑
  in
   fight Y04.0 ☑
   legal intervention
    injuring
     bystander Y35.892 ☑
     law enforcement personnel Y35.891 ☑
     suspect Y35.893 ☑
Seasickness T75.3 ☑
Self-harm NEC — *see also* External cause by type, undetermined whether accidental or intentional
 intentional — *see* Suicide
 poisoning NEC — *see* Table of Drugs and Chemicals,
  poisoning, accidental
Self-inflicted (injury) **NEC** — *see also* External cause by
   type, undetermined whether accidental or intentional
 intentional — *see* Suicide
 poisoning NEC — *see* Table of Drugs and Chemicals,
  poisoning, accidental
Sequelae (of)
 accident NEC — *see* W00-X58 with 7th character S
 assault (homicidal) (any means) — *see* X92-Y08 with
  7th character S
 homicide, attempt (any means) — *see* X92-Y08 with
  7th character S
 injury undetermined whether accidentally or purposely
  inflicted — *see* Y21-Y33 with 7th character S
 intentional self-harm (classifiable to X71-X83) — *see*
  X71-X83 with 7th character S
 legal intervention — *see* with 7th character S Y35
 motor vehicle accident — *see* V00-V99 with 7th character S
 suicide, attempt (any means) — *see* X71-X83 with 7th
  character S
 transport accident — *see* V00-V99 with 7th character
  S
 war operations — *see* War operations
Shock
 electric — *see* Exposure, electric current
 from electric appliance (any) (faulty) W86.8 ☑
  domestic W86.0 ☑
  suicide (attempt) X83.1 ☑
Shooting, shot (accidental(ly)) — *see also* Discharge,
   firearm, by type
 herself or himself — *see* Discharge, firearm by type,
  self-inflicted
 homicide (attempt) — *see* Discharge, firearm by type,
  homicide
 in war operations — *see* War operations
 inflicted by other person — *see* Discharge, firearm by
   type, homicide
  accidental — *see* Discharge, firearm, by type of
   firearm
 legal
  execution — *see* Legal, intervention, firearm
  intervention — *see* Legal, intervention, firearm
 self-inflicted — *see* Discharge, firearm by type, suicide
  accidental — *see* Discharge, firearm, by type of
   firearm
 suicide (attempt) — *see* Discharge, firearm by type,
  suicide
Shoving (accidentally) **by other person** — *see* Pushed,
  by other person
Sickness
 alpine W94.11 ☑
 motion — *see* Motion
 mountain W94.11 ☑
Sinking (accidental)
 watercraft (causing drowning, submersion) — *see also*
  Drowning, due to, accident to, watercraft, sinking

Sinking — *continued*
  watercraft — *see also* Drowning, due to, accident to,
    watercraft, sinking — *continued*
    causing injury except drowning or submersion —
      see Accident, watercraft, causing, injury NEC
Siriasis X32 ☑
Sitting (prolonged) (static) X50.1 ☑
Slashed wrists — *see* Cut, self-inflicted
Slipping (accidental) (on same level) (with fall) W01.0 ☑
  on
    ice W00.0 ☑
      with skates — *see* Accident, transport, pedestri-
        an, conveyance
    mud W01.0 ☑
    oil W01.0 ☑
    snow W00.0 ☑
      with skis — *see* Accident, transport, pedestrian,
        conveyance
    surface (slippery) (wet) NEC W01.0 ☑
  without fall W18.40 ☑
    due to
      specified NEC W18.49 ☑
      stepping from one level to another W18.43 ☑
      stepping into hole or opening W18.42 ☑
      stepping on object W18.41 ☑
Sliver, wood, contact with W45.8 ☑
Smoldering (due to fire) — *see* Exposure, fire
Sodomy (attempted) **by force** T74.2 ☑
Sound waves (causing injury) W42.9 ☑
  supersonic W42.0 ☑
Splinter, contact with W45.8 ☑
Stab, stabbing — *see* Cut
Standing (prolonged) (static) X50.1 ☑
Starvation X58 ☑
Status of external cause Y99.9
  child assisting in compensated work for family Y99.8
  civilian activity done for financial or other compensa-
    tion Y99.0
  civilian activity done for income or pay Y99.0
  family member assisting in compensated work for
    other family member Y99.8
  hobby not done for income Y99.8
  leisure activity Y99.8
  military activity Y99.1
  off-duty activity of military personnel Y99.8
  recreation or sport not for income or while a student
    Y99.8
  specified NEC Y99.8
  student activity Y99.8
  volunteer activity Y99.2
Stepped on
  by
    animal (not being ridden) NEC W55.89 ☑
    crowd or human stampede W52 ☑
    person W50.0 ☑
Stepping on
  object W22.8 ☑
    sports equipment W21.9 ☑
    stationary W22.09 ☑
      sports equipment W21.89 ☑
    with fall W18.31 ☑
  person W51 ☑
    by crowd or human stampede W52 ☑
  sports equipment W21.9 ☑
Sting
  arthropod, nonvenomous W57 ☑
  insect, nonvenomous W57 ☑
Storm (cataclysmic) — *see* Forces of nature, cataclysmic
  storm
Straining, excessive — *see also* Overexertion X50.9 ☑
Strangling — *see* Strangulation
Strangulation (accidental) T71 ☑
Strenuous movements — *see also* Overexertion
  X50.9 ☑
Striking against
  airbag (automobile) W22.10 ☑
    driver side W22.11 ☑
    front passenger side W22.12 ☑
    specified NEC W22.19 ☑
  bottom when
    diving or jumping into water (in) W16.822 ☑
      causing drowning W16.821 ☑
      from boat W16.722 ☑
        causing drowning W16.721 ☑
      natural body W16.622 ☑
        causing drowning W16.821 ☑

Striking against — *continued*
  bottom when — *continued*
    diving or jumping into water — *continued*
      swimming pool W16.522 ☑
        causing drowning W16.521 ☑
    falling into water (in) W16.322 ☑
      causing drowning W16.321 ☑
      fountain — *see* Striking against, bottom when,
        falling into water, specified NEC
      natural body W16.122 ☑
        causing drowning W16.121 ☑
      reservoir — *see* Striking against, bottom when,
        falling into water, specified NEC
      specified NEC W16.322 ☑
        causing drowning W16.321 ☑
      swimming pool W16.022 ☑
        causing drowning W16.021 ☑
  diving board (swimming-pool) W21.4 ☑
  object W22.8 ☑
    caused by crowd or human stampede (with fall)
      W52 ☑
    furniture W22.03 ☑
    lamppost W22.02 ☑
    sports equipment W21.9 ☑
    stationary W22.09 ☑
      sports equipment W21.89 ☑
    wall W22.01 ☑
    with
      drowning or submersion — *see* Drowning
      fall — *see* Fall, due to, bumping against, object
  person(s) W51 ☑
    as, or caused by, a crowd or human stampede (with
      fall) W52 ☑
    assault Y04.2 ☑
    homicide (attempt) Y04.2 ☑
    with fall W03 ☑
      due to ice or snow W00.0 ☑
  sports equipment W21.9 ☑
  wall (when) W22.01 ☑
    diving or jumping into water (in) W16.832 ☑
      causing drowning W16.831 ☑
      swimming pool W16.532 ☑
        causing drowning W16.531 ☑
    falling into water (in) W16.332 ☑
      causing drowning W16.331 ☑
      fountain — *see* Striking against, wall when,
        falling into water, specified NEC
      natural body W16.132 ☑
        causing drowning W16.131 ☑
      reservoir — *see* Striking against, wall when,
        falling into water, specified NEC
      specified NEC W16.332 ☑
        causing drowning W16.331 ☑
      swimming pool W16.032 ☑
        causing drowning W16.031 ☑
    swimming pool (when) W22.042 ☑
      causing drowning W22.041 ☑
      diving or jumping into water W16.532 ☑
        causing drowning W16.531 ☑
      falling into water W16.032 ☑
        causing drowning W16.031 ☑
Struck (accidentally) **by**
  airbag (automobile) W22.10 ☑
    driver side W22.11 ☑
    front passenger side W22.12 ☑
    specified NEC W22.19 ☑
  alligator W58.02 ☑
  animal (not being ridden) NEC W55.89 ☑
  avalanche — *see* Landslide
  ball (hit) (thrown) W21.00 ☑
    assault Y08.09 ☑
    baseball W21.03 ☑
    basketball W21.05 ☑
    football W21.01 ☑
    golf ball W21.04 ☑
    soccer W21.02 ☑
    softball W21.07 ☑
    specified NEC W21.09 ☑
    volleyball W21.06 ☑
  bat or racquet
    baseball bat W21.11 ☑
      assault Y08.02 ☑
    golf club W21.13 ☑
      assault Y08.09 ☑
    specified NEC W21.19 ☑
      assault Y08.09 ☑

Struck (accidentally) **by** — *continued*
  bat or racquet — *continued*
    tennis racquet W21.12 ☑
      assault Y08.09 ☑
  bullet — *see also* Discharge, firearm by type
    in war operations — *see* War operations
  crocodile W58.12 ☑
  dog W54.1 ☑
  flare, Very pistol — *see* Discharge, firearm NEC
  hailstones X39.8 ☑
  hockey (ice)
    field
      puck W21.221 ☑
      stick W21.211 ☑
    puck W21.220 ☑
    stick W21.210 ☑
      assault Y08.01 ☑
  landslide — *see* Landslide
  law-enforcement agent (on duty) — *see* Legal, inter-
    vention, manhandling
    with blunt object — *see* Legal, intervention, blunt
      object
  lightning T75.0 ☑
    causing fire — *see* Exposure, fire
  machine — *see* Contact, with, by type of machine
  mammal NEC W55.89 ☑
    marine W56.32 ☑
  marine animal W56.82 ☑
  missile
    firearm — *see* Discharge, firearm by type
    in war operations — *see* War operations, missile
  object W22.8 ☑
    blunt W22.8 ☑
      assault Y00 ☑
      suicide (attempt) X79 ☑
      undetermined whether accidental or intentional
        Y29 ☑
    falling W20.8 ☑
      from, in, on
        building W20.1 ☑
          burning (uncontrolled fire) X00.4 ☑
        cataclysmic
          earth surface movement NEC — *see*
            Landslide
          storm — *see* Forces of nature, cataclysmic
            storm
        cave-in W20.0 ☑
        earthquake X34 ☑
        machine (in operation) — *see* Contact, with,
          by type of machine
        structure W20.1 ☑
          burning X00.4 ☑
        transport vehicle (in motion) — *see* Accident,
          transport, by type of vehicle
        watercraft V93.49 ☑
          due to
            accident to craft V91.39 ☑
              powered craft V91.33 ☑
                ferry boat V91.31 ☑
                fishing boat V91.32 ☑
                jetskis V91.33 ☑
                liner V91.31 ☑
                merchant ship V91.30 ☑
                passenger ship V91.31 ☑
              unpowered craft V91.38 ☑
                canoe V91.35 ☑
                inflatable V91.36 ☑
                kayak V91.35 ☑
                sailboat V91.34 ☑
                surf-board V91.38 ☑
                windsurfer V91.38 ☑
            powered craft V93.43 ☑
              ferry boat V93.41 ☑
              fishing boat V93.42 ☑
              jetskis V93.43 ☑
              liner V93.41 ☑
              merchant ship V93.40 ☑
              passenger ship V93.41 ☑
            unpowered craft V93.48 ☑
              sailboat V93.44 ☑
              surf-board V93.48 ☑
              windsurfer V93.48 ☑
    moving NEC W20.8 ☑
    projected W20.8 ☑
      assault Y00 ☑
      in sports W21.9 ☑

Struck (accidentally) **by** — *continued*
 object — *continued*
  projected — *continued*
   in sports — *continued*
    assault Y08.09 ☑
    ball W21.00 ☑
     baseball W21.03 ☑
     basketball W21.05 ☑
     football W21.01 ☑
     golf ball W21.04 ☑
     soccer W21.02 ☑
     softball W21.07 ☑
     specified NEC W21.09 ☑
     volleyball W21.06 ☑
    bat or racquet
     baseball bat W21.11 ☑
      assault Y08.02 ☑
     golf club W21.13 ☑
      assault Y08.09 ☑
     specified NEC W21.19 ☑
      assault Y08.09 ☑
     tennis racquet W21.12 ☑
      assault Y08.09 ☑
    hockey (ice)
     field
      puck W21.221 ☑
      stick W21.211 ☑
     puck W21.220 ☑
     stick W21.210 ☑
      assault Y08.01 ☑
    specified NEC W21.89 ☑
 set in motion by explosion — *see* Explosion
 thrown W20.8 ☑
  assault Y00 ☑
  in sports W21.9 ☑
   assault Y08.09 ☑
   ball W21.00 ☑
    baseball W21.03 ☑
    basketball W21.05 ☑
    football W21.01 ☑
    golf ball W21.04 ☑
    soccer W21.02 ☑
    soft ball W21.07 ☑
    specified NEC W21.09 ☑
    volleyball W21.06 ☑
   bat or racquet
    baseball bat W21.11 ☑
     assault Y08.02 ☑
    golf club W21.13 ☑
     assault Y08.09 ☑
    specified NEC W21.19 ☑
     assault Y08.09 ☑
    tennis racquet W21.12 ☑
     assault Y08.09 ☑
   hockey (ice)
    field
     puck W21.221 ☑
     stick W21.211 ☑
    puck W21.220 ☑
    stick W21.210 ☑
     assault Y08.01 ☑
   specified NEC W21.89 ☑
 other person(s) W50.0 ☑
  with
   blunt object W22.8 ☑
    intentional, homicide (attempt) Y00 ☑
   sports equipment W21.9 ☑
    undetermined whether accidental or intentional Y29 ☑
   fall W03 ☑
    due to ice or snow W00.0 ☑
  as, or caused by, a crowd or human stampede (with fall) W52 ☑
  assault Y04.2 ☑
  homicide (attempt) Y04.2 ☑
  in legal intervention
   injuring
    bystander Y35.812 ☑
    law enforcement personnel Y35.811 ☑
    suspect Y35.813 ☑
    unspecified person Y35.819 ☑
  sports equipment W21.9 ☑
  police (on duty) — *see* Legal, intervention, manhandling
   with blunt object — *see* Legal, intervention, blunt object

Struck (accidentally) **by** — *continued*
 sports equipment W21.9 ☑
  assault Y08.09 ☑
  ball W21.00 ☑
   baseball W21.03 ☑
   basketball W21.05 ☑
   football W21.01 ☑
   golf ball W21.04 ☑
   soccer W21.02 ☑
   soft ball W21.07 ☑
   specified NEC W21.09 ☑
   volleyball W21.06 ☑
  bat or racquet
   baseball bat W21.11 ☑
    assault Y08.02 ☑
   golf club W21.13 ☑
    assault Y08.09 ☑
   specified NEC W21.19 ☑
   tennis racquet W21.12 ☑
    assault Y08.09 ☑
  cleats (shoe) W21.31 ☑
  foot wear NEC W21.39 ☑
  football helmet W21.81 ☑
  hockey (ice)
   field
    puck W21.221 ☑
    stick W21.211 ☑
   puck W21.220 ☑
   stick W21.210 ☑
    assault Y08.01 ☑
  skate blades W21.32 ☑
  specified NEC W21.89 ☑
   assault Y08.09 ☑
 thunderbolt — *see* subcategory T75.0 ☑
  causing fire — *see* Exposure, fire
 transport vehicle NEC — *see also* Accident, transport V09.9 ☑
  intentional, homicide (attempt) Y03.0 ☑
 motor NEC — *see also* Accident, transport V09.20 ☑
  homicide Y03.0 ☑
 vehicle (transport) NEC — *see* Accident, transport, by type of vehicle
  stationary (falling from jack, hydraulic lift, ramp) W20.8 ☑

Stumbling
 over
  animal NEC W01.0 ☑
   with fall W18.09 ☑
  carpet, rug or (small) object W22.8 ☑
   with fall W18.09 ☑
  person W51 ☑
   with fall W03 ☑
    due to ice or snow W00.0 ☑
 without fall W18.40 ☑
  due to
   specified NEC W18.49 ☑
   stepping from one level to another W18.43 ☑
   stepping into hole or opening W18.42 ☑
   stepping on object W18.41 ☑
Submersion (accidental) — *see* Drowning
Suffocation (accidental) (by external means) (by pressure) (mechanical) — *see also* category T71 ☑
 due to, by
  avalanche — *see* Landslide
  explosion — *see* Explosion
  fire — *see* Exposure, fire
  food, any type (aspiration) (ingestion) (inhalation) — *see* categories T17 and T18 ☑
  ignition — *see* Ignition
  landslide — *see* Landslide
  machine(ry) — *see* Contact, with, by type of machine
  vomitus (aspiration) (inhalation) T17.81- ☑
 in
  burning building X00.8 ☑
Suicide, suicidal (attempted) (by) X83.8 ☑
 blunt object X79 ☑
 burning, burns X76 ☑
  hot object X77.9 ☑
   fluid NEC X77.2 ☑
   household appliance X77.3 ☑
   specified NEC X77.8 ☑
   steam X77.0 ☑
   tap water X77.1 ☑
   vapors X77.0 ☑
 caustic substance — *see* Table of Drugs and Chemicals

Suicide, suicidal — *continued*
 cold, extreme X83.2 ☑
 collision of motor vehicle with
  motor vehicle X82.0 ☑
  specified NEC X82.8 ☑
  train X82.1 ☑
  tree X82.2 ☑
 crashing of aircraft X83.0 ☑
 cut (any part of body) X78.9 ☑
 cutting or piercing instrument X78.9 ☑
  dagger X78.2 ☑
  glass X78.0 ☑
  knife X78.1 ☑
  specified NEC X78.8 ☑
  sword X78.2 ☑
 drowning (in) X71.9 ☑
  bathtub X71.0 ☑
  natural water X71.3 ☑
  specified NEC X71.8 ☑
  swimming pool X71.1 ☑
   following fall X71.2 ☑
 electrocution X83.1 ☑
 explosive(s) (material) X75 ☑
 fire, flames X76 ☑
 firearm X74.9 ☑
  airgun X74.01 ☑
  handgun X72 ☑
  hunting rifle X73.1 ☑
  larger X73.9 ☑
   specified NEC X73.8 ☑
  machine gun X73.2 ☑
  shotgun X73.0 ☑
  specified NEC X74.8 ☑
 hanging X83.8 ☑
 hot object — *see* Suicide, burning, hot object
 jumping
  before moving object X81.8 ☑
   motor vehicle X81.0 ☑
   subway train X81.1 ☑
   train X81.1 ☑
  from high place X80 ☑
 late effect of attempt — *see* X71-X83 with 7th character S
 lying before moving object, train, vehicle X81.8 ☑
 poisoning — *see* Table of Drugs and Chemicals
 puncture (any part of body) — *see* Suicide, cutting or piercing instrument
 scald — *see* Suicide, burning, hot object
 sequelae of attempt — *see* X71-X83 with 7th character S
 sharp object (any) — *see* Suicide, cutting or piercing instrument
 shooting — *see* Suicide, firearm
 specified means NEC X83.8 ☑
 stab (any part of body) — *see* Suicide, cutting or piercing instrument
 steam, hot vapors X77.0 ☑
 strangulation X83.8 ☑
 submersion — *see* Suicide, drowning
 suffocation X83.8 ☑
 wound NEC X83.8 ☑
Sunstroke X32 ☑
Supersonic waves (causing injury) W42.0 ☑
Surgical procedure, complication of (delayed or as an abnormal reaction without mention of misadventure) — *see also* Complication of or following, by type of procedure
 due to or as a result of misadventure — *see* Misadventure
Swallowed, swallowing
 foreign body — *see* Foreign body, alimentary canal
 poison — *see* Table of Drugs and Chemicals
 substance
  caustic or corrosive — *see* Table of Drugs and Chemicals
  poisonous — *see* Table of Drugs and Chemicals

T

Tackle in sport W03 ☑
Terrorism (involving) Y38.80 ☑
 biological weapons Y38.6X- ☑
 chemical weapons Y38.7X- ☑
 conflagration Y38.3X- ☑
 drowning and submersion Y38.89- ☑
 explosion Y38.2X- ☑

☑ Additional Character Required — Refer to the Tabular List for Character Selection   ▽ Subterms under main terms may continue to next column or page

Terrorism — *continued*
explosion — *continued*
destruction of aircraft Y38.1X- ☑
marine weapons Y38.0X- ☑
fire Y38.3X- ☑
firearms Y38.4X- ☑
hot substances Y38.3X- ☑
lasers Y38.89- ☑
nuclear weapons Y38.5X- ☑
piercing or stabbing instruments Y38.89- ☑
secondary effects Y38.9X- ☑
specified method NEC Y38.89- ☑
suicide bomber Y38.81- ☑
Thirst X58 ☑
Threat to breathing
aspiration — *see* Aspiration
due to cave-in, falling earth or substance NEC T71 ☑
Thrown (accidentally)
against part (any) of or object in transport vehicle (in motion) NEC — *see also* Accident, transport
from
high place, homicide (attempt) Y01 ☑
machinery — *see* Contact, with, by type of machine
transport vehicle NEC — *see also* Accident, transport V89.9 ☑
off — *see* Thrown, from
Thunderbolt — *see* subcategory T75.0 ☑
causing fire — *see* Exposure, fire
Tidal wave (any injury) **NEC** — *see* Forces of nature, tidal wave
Took
overdose (drug) — *see* Table of Drugs and Chemicals
poison — *see* Table of Drugs and Chemicals
Tornado (any injury) X37.1 ☑
Torrential rain (any injury) X37.8 ☑
Torture X58 ☑
Trampled by animal NEC W55.89 ☑
Trapped (accidentally)
between objects (moving) (stationary and moving) — *see* Caught
by part (any) of
motorcycle V29.88 ☑
pedal cycle V19.88 ☑
transport vehicle NEC — *see also* Accident, transport V89.9 ☑
Travel (effects) (sickness) T75.3 ☑
Tree falling on or hitting (accidentally) (person) W20.8 ☑
Tripping
over
animal W01.0 ☑
with fall W01.0 ☑
carpet, rug or (small) object W22.8 ☑
with fall W18.09 ☑
person W51 ☑
with fall W03 ☑
due to ice or snow W00.0 ☑
without fall W18.40 ☑
due to
specified NEC W18.49 ☑
stepping from one level to another W18.43 ☑
stepping into hole or opening W18.42 ☑
stepping on object W18.41 ☑
Twisted by person(s) (accidentally) W50.2 ☑
with intent to injure or kill Y04.0 ☑
as, or caused by, a crowd or human stampede (with fall) W52 ☑
assault Y04.0 ☑
homicide (attempt) Y04.0 ☑
in
fight Y04.0 ☑
legal intervention — *see* Legal, intervention, manhandling
Twisting (prolonged) (static) X50.1- ☑

U

Underdosing of necessary drugs, medicaments or biological substances Y63.6
Undetermined intent (contact) (exposure)
automobile collision Y32 ☑
blunt object Y29 ☑
drowning (submersion) (in) Y21.9 ☑
bathtub Y21.0 ☑
after fall Y21.1 ☑

Undetermined intent — *continued*
drowning — *continued*
natural water (lake) (ocean) (pond) (river) (stream) Y21.4 ☑
specified place NEC Y21.8 ☑
swimming pool Y21.2 ☑
after fall Y21.3 ☑
explosive material Y25 ☑
fall, jump or push from high place Y30 ☑
falling, lying or running before moving object Y31 ☑
fire Y26 ☑
firearm discharge Y24.9 ☑
airgun (BB) (pellet) Y24.0 ☑
handgun (pistol) (revolver) Y22 ☑
hunting rifle Y23.1 ☑
larger Y23.9 ☑
hunting rifle Y23.1 ☑
machine gun Y23.3 ☑
military Y23.2 ☑
shotgun Y23.0 ☑
specified type NEC Y23.8 ☑
machine gun Y23.3 ☑
military Y23.2 ☑
shotgun Y23.0 ☑
specified type NEC Y24.8 ☑
Very pistol Y24.8 ☑
hot object Y27.9 ☑
fluid NEC Y27.2 ☑
household appliance Y27.3 ☑
specified object NEC Y27.8 ☑
steam Y27.0 ☑
tap water Y27.1 ☑
vapor Y27.0 ☑
jump, fall or push from high place Y30 ☑
lying, falling or running before moving object Y31 ☑
motor vehicle crash Y32 ☑
push, fall or jump from high place Y30 ☑
running, falling or lying before moving object Y31 ☑
sharp object Y28.9 ☑
dagger Y28.2 ☑
glass Y28.0 ☑
knife Y28.1 ☑
specified object NEC Y28.8 ☑
sword Y28.2 ☑
smoke Y26 ☑
specified event NEC Y33 ☑
Use of hand as hammer X50.3 ☑

V

Vibration (causing injury) W49.9 ☑
Victim (of)
avalanche — *see* Landslide
earth movements NEC — *see* Forces of nature, earth movement
earthquake X34 ☑
flood — *see* Flood
landslide — *see* Landslide
lightning — *see* subcategory T75.0 ☑
causing fire — *see* Exposure, fire
storm (cataclysmic) NEC — *see* Forces of nature, cataclysmic storm
volcanic eruption X35 ☑
Volcanic eruption (any injury) X35 ☑
Vomitus, gastric contents in air passages (with asphyxia, obstruction or suffocation) T17.81- ☑

W

Walked into stationary object (any) W22.09 ☑
furniture W22.03 ☑
lamppost W22.02 ☑
wall W22.01 ☑
War operations (injuries to military personnel and civilians during war, civil insurrection and peacekeeping missions) (by) (from) (involving) Y36.90 ☑
after cessation of hostilities Y36.89- ☑
explosion (of)
bomb placed during war operations Y36.82- ☑
mine placed during war operations Y36.81- ☑
specified NEC Y36.88- ☑
air blast Y36.20- ☑
aircraft
destruction — *see* War operations, destruction of aircraft

War operations — *continued*
airway restriction — *see* War operations, restriction of airways
asphyxiation — *see* War operations, restriction of airways
biological weapons Y36.6X- ☑
blast Y36.20- ☑
blast fragments Y36.20- ☑
blast wave Y36.20- ☑
blast wind Y36.20- ☑
bomb Y36.20- ☑
dirty Y36.50- ☑
gasoline Y36.31- ☑
incendiary Y36.31- ☑
petrol Y36.31- ☑
bullet Y36.43- ☑
incendiary Y36.32- ☑
rubber Y36.41- ☑
chemical weapons Y36.7X- ☑
combat
hand to hand (unarmed) combat Y36.44- ☑
using blunt or piercing object Y36.45- ☑
conflagration — *see* War operations, fire
conventional warfare NEC Y36.49- ☑
depth-charge Y36.01- ☑
destruction of aircraft Y36.10- ☑
due to
air to air missile Y36.11- ☑
collision with other aircraft Y36.12- ☑
detonation (accidental) of onboard munitions and explosives Y36.14- ☑
enemy fire or explosives Y36.11- ☑
explosive placed on aircraft Y36.11- ☑
onboard fire Y36.13- ☑
rocket propelled grenade [RPG] Y36.11- ☑
small arms fire Y36.11- ☑
surface to air missile Y36.11- ☑
specified NEC Y36.19- ☑
detonation (accidental) of
onboard marine weapons Y36.05- ☑
own munitions or munitions launch device Y36.24- ☑
dirty bomb Y36.50- ☑
explosion (of) Y36.20- ☑
aerial bomb Y36.21- ☑
after cessation of hostilities
bomb placed during war operations Y36.82- ☑
mine placed during war operations Y36.81- ☑
bomb NOS — *see also* War operations, bomb(s) Y36.20- ☑
fragments Y36.20- ☑
grenade Y36.29- ☑
guided missile Y36.22- ☑
improvised explosive device [IED] (person-borne) (roadside) (vehicle-borne) Y36.23- ☑
land mine Y36.29- ☑
marine mine (at sea) (in harbor) Y36.02- ☑
marine weapon Y36.00- ☑
specified NEC Y36.09- ☑
own munitions or munitions launch device (accidental) Y36.24- ☑
sea-based artillery shell Y36.03- ☑
specified NEC Y36.29- ☑
torpedo Y36.04- ☑
fire Y36.30- ☑
specified NEC Y36.39- ☑
firearms
discharge Y36.43- ☑
pellets Y36.42- ☑
flamethrower Y36.33- ☑
fragments (from) (of)
improvised explosive device [IED] (person-borne) (roadside) (vehicle-borne) Y36.26- ☑
munitions Y36.25- ☑
specified NEC Y36.29- ☑
weapons Y36.27- ☑
friendly fire Y36.92- ☑
hand to hand (unarmed) combat Y36.44- ☑
hot substances — *see* War operations, fire
incendiary bullet Y36.32- ☑
nuclear weapon (effects of) Y36.50- ☑
acute radiation exposure Y36.54- ☑
blast pressure Y36.51- ☑
direct blast Y36.51- ☑
direct heat Y36.53- ☑
fallout exposure Y36.54- ☑

War operations — *continued*
nuclear weapon — *continued*
    fireball Y36.53- ☑
    indirect blast (struck or crushed by blast debris)
        (being thrown by blast) Y36.52- ☑
    ionizing radiation (immediate exposure) Y36.54- ☑
    nuclear radiation Y36.54- ☑
    radiation
        ionizing (immediate exposure) Y36.54- ☑
        nuclear Y36.54- ☑
        thermal Y36.53- ☑
    secondary effects Y36.54- ☑
    specified NEC Y36.59- ☑
    thermal radiation Y36.53- ☑
restriction of air (airway)
    intentional Y36.46- ☑
    unintentional Y36.47- ☑
rubber bullets Y36.41- ☑
shrapnel NOS Y36.29- ☑
suffocation — *see* War operations, restriction of airways
unconventional warfare NEC Y36.7X- ☑
underwater blast NOS Y36.00- ☑

War operations — *continued*
warfare
    conventional NEC Y36.49- ☑
    unconventional NEC Y36.7X- ☑
weapon of mass destruction [WMD] Y36.91 ☑
weapons
    biological weapons Y36.6X- ☑
    chemical Y36.7X- ☑
    nuclear (effects of) Y36.50- ☑
        acute radiation exposure Y36.54- ☑
        blast pressure Y36.51- ☑
        direct blast Y36.51- ☑
        direct heat Y36.53- ☑
        fallout exposure Y36.54- ☑
        fireball Y36.53- ☑
        radiation
            ionizing (immediate exposure) Y36.54- ☑
            nuclear Y36.54- ☑
            thermal Y36.53- ☑
        secondary effects Y36.54- ☑
        specified NEC Y36.59- ☑

War operations — *continued*
weapons — *continued*
    of mass destruction [WMD] Y36.91 ☑
Washed
away by flood — *see* Flood
off road by storm (transport vehicle) — *see* Forces of
    nature, cataclysmic storm
Weather exposure NEC — *see* Forces of nature
Weightlessness (causing injury) (effects of) (in spacecraft,
    real or simulated) X52 ☑
Work related condition Y99.0
Wound (accidental) NEC — *see also* Injury X58 ☑
battle — *see also* War operations Y36.90 ☑
gunshot — *see* Discharge, firearm by type
Wreck transport vehicle NEC — *see also* Accident,
    transport V89.9 ☑
Wrong
device implanted into correct surgical site Y65.51
fluid in infusion Y65.1
patient, procedure performed on Y65.52
procedure (operation) on correct patient Y65.51

Chapter 1. Certain Infectious and Parasitic Diseases (A00–B99)

Chapter-specific Guidelines with Coding Examples

The chapter-specific guidelines from the ICD-10-CM Official Guidelines for Coding and Reporting have been provided below. Along with these guidelines are coding examples, contained in the shaded boxes, that have been developed to help illustrate the coding and/or sequencing guidance found in these guidelines.

a. Human immunodeficiency virus (HIV) infections

1) Code only confirmed cases

Code only confirmed cases of HIV infection/illness. This is an exception to the hospital inpatient guideline Section II, H.

In this context, "confirmation" does not require documentation of positive serology or culture for HIV; the provider's diagnostic statement that the patient is HIV positive, or has an HIV-related illness is sufficient.

> Patient admitted with anemia with possible HIV infection
>
> **D64.9 Anemia, unspecified**
>
> *Explanation:* Only the anemia is coded in this scenario because it has not been confirmed that an HIV infection is present.

2) Selection and sequencing of HIV codes

(a) Patient admitted for HIV-related condition

If a patient is admitted for an HIV-related condition, the principal diagnosis should be B20, Human immunodeficiency virus [HIV] disease followed by additional diagnosis codes for all reported HIV-related conditions.

> HIV with PCP
>
> **B20 Human immunodeficiency virus [HIV] disease**
>
> **B59 Pneumocystosis**
>
> *Explanation:* Pneumonia due to *Pneumocystis carinii* is an HIV related condition, so the HIV diagnosis code is reported first, followed by the code for the pneumonia.

(b) Patient with HIV disease admitted for unrelated condition

If a patient with HIV disease is admitted for an unrelated condition (such as a traumatic injury), the code for the unrelated condition (e.g., the nature of injury code) should be the principal diagnosis. Other diagnoses would be B20 followed by additional diagnosis codes for all reported HIV-related conditions.

> Unstable angina, native coronary artery atherosclerosis, HIV
>
> **I25.110 Atherosclerotic heart disease of native coronary artery with unstable angina pectoris**
>
> **B20 Human immunodeficiency virus [HIV] disease**
>
> *Explanation:* The arteriosclerotic coronary artery disease and the unstable angina are not related to HIV, so those conditions are reported first using a combination code, and HIV is reported secondarily.

(c) Whether the patient is newly diagnosed

Whether the patient is newly diagnosed or has had previous admissions/encounters for HIV conditions is irrelevant to the sequencing decision.

> Newly diagnosed multiple cutaneous Kaposi's sarcoma lesions in previously diagnosed HIV disease.
>
> **B20 Human immunodeficiency virus [HIV] disease**
>
> **C46.0 Kaposi's sarcoma of skin**
>
> *Explanation:* Even though the HIV was diagnosed on a previous encounter, it is still sequenced first when coded with an HIV related condition. Kaposi's sarcoma is an HIV-related condition.

(d) Asymptomatic human immunodeficiency virus

Z21, Asymptomatic human immunodeficiency virus [HIV] infection status, is to be applied when the patient without any documentation of symptoms is listed as being "HIV positive," "known HIV," "HIV test positive," or similar terminology. Do not use this code if the term

"AIDS" is used or if the patient is treated for any HIV-related illness or is described as having any condition(s) resulting from his/her HIV positive status; use B20 in these cases.

> Patient admitted for aftercare and rehabilitation post-appendectomy for acute appendicitis; status post-positive HIV test on Atripla, with no prior or current symptoms
>
> **Z48.815 Encounter for surgical aftercare following surgery on the digestive system**
>
> **Z21 Asymptomatic human immunodeficiency virus [HIV] infection status**
>
> *Explanation:* Code Z21 is used to document that the patient has had a positive HIV test but has been asymptomatic. Being on medication for HIV does not indicate that the infection is active and B20 Human immunodeficiency virus [HIV] disease, should not be assigned unless there is documentation that the patient has had *current or prior* symptoms or HIV-related complications. The aftercare being provided post-appendectomy is sequenced first.

(e) Patients with inconclusive HIV serology

Patients with inconclusive HIV serology, but no definitive diagnosis or manifestations of the illness, may be assigned code R75, Inconclusive laboratory evidence of human immunodeficiency virus [HIV].

(f) Previously diagnosed HIV-related illness

Patients with any known prior diagnosis of an HIV-related illness should be coded to B20. Once a patient has developed an HIV-related illness, the patient should always be assigned code B20 on every subsequent admission/encounter. Patients previously diagnosed with any HIV illness (B20) should never be assigned to R75 or Z21, Asymptomatic human immunodeficiency virus [HIV] infection status.

(g) HIV infection in pregnancy, childbirth and the puerperium

During pregnancy, childbirth or the puerperium, a patient admitted (or presenting for a health care encounter) because of an HIV-related illness should receive a principal diagnosis code of O98.7-, Human immunodeficiency [HIV] disease complicating pregnancy, childbirth and the puerperium, followed by B20 and the code(s) for the HIV-related illness(es). Codes from Chapter 15 always take sequencing priority.

Patients with asymptomatic HIV infection status admitted (or presenting for a health care encounter) during pregnancy, childbirth, or the puerperium should receive codes of O98.7- and Z21.

(h) Encounters for testing for HIV

If a patient is being seen to determine his/her HIV status, use code Z11.4, Encounter for screening for human immunodeficiency virus [HIV]. Use additional codes for any associated high risk behavior.

If a patient with signs or symptoms is being seen for HIV testing, code the signs and symptoms. An additional counseling code Z71.7, Human immunodeficiency virus [HIV] counseling, may be used if counseling is provided during the encounter for the test.

When a patient returns to be informed of his/her HIV test results and the test result is negative, use code Z71.7, Human immunodeficiency virus [HIV] counseling.

If the results are positive, see previous guidelines and assign codes as appropriate.

b. Infectious agents as the cause of diseases classified to other chapters

Certain infections are classified in chapters other than Chapter 1 and no organism is identified as part of the infection code. In these instances, it is necessary to use an additional code from Chapter 1 to identify the organism. A code from category B95, Streptococcus, Staphylococcus, and Enterococcus as the cause of diseases classified to other chapters, B96, Other bacterial agents as the cause of diseases classified to other chapters, or B97, Viral agents as the cause of diseases classified to other chapters, is to be used as an additional code to identify the organism. An instructional note will be found at the infection code advising that an additional organism code is required.

E. coli UTI.

N39.Ø	Urinary tract infection, site not specified
B96.2Ø	Unspecified Escherichia coli [E.coli] as the cause of diseases classified elsewhere

Explanation: An instructional note under the code for the urinary tract infection indicates to code also the specific organism.

c. Infections resistant to antibiotics

Many bacterial infections are resistant to current antibiotics. It is necessary to identify all infections documented as antibiotic resistant. Assign a code from category Z16, Resistance to antimicrobial drugs, following the infection code only if the infection code does not identify drug resistance.

Antimycobacterial-resistant primary pulmonary tuberculosis.

A15.Ø	Tuberculosis of lung
Z16.341	Resistance to single antimycobacterial drug

Explanation: Code Z16.341 is assigned as a secondary code to represent the antimycobacterial resistance. This code includes resistance to antimycobacterial drug "NOS"; if multiple drug resistance is not specified, classification defaults to the single drug resistance code.

d. Sepsis, severe sepsis, and septic shock

1) Coding of sepsis and severe sepsis

(a) Sepsis

For a diagnosis of sepsis, assign the appropriate code for the underlying systemic infection. If the type of infection or causal organism is not further specified, assign code A41.9, Sepsis, unspecified organism.

A code from subcategory R65.2, Severe sepsis, should not be assigned unless severe sepsis or an associated acute organ dysfunction is documented.

Gram-negative sepsis.

A41.5Ø	Gram-negative sepsis, unspecified

Staphylococcal sepsis

A41.2	Sepsis due to unspecified staphylococcus

Explanation: In both examples above the organism causing the sepsis is identified, therefore A41.9 Sepsis, unspecified organism, would not be appropriate as this code would not capture the highest degree of specificity found in the documentation. Do not use an additional code for severe sepsis unless an acute organ dysfunction was also documented as "associated with" or "due to" the sepsis or the sepsis was documented as "severe."

(i) Negative or inconclusive blood cultures and sepsis

Negative or inconclusive blood cultures do not preclude a diagnosis of sepsis in patients with clinical evidence of the condition; however, the provider should be queried.

(ii) Urosepsis

The term urosepsis is a nonspecific term. It is not to be considered synonymous with sepsis. It has no default code in the Alphabetic Index. Should a provider use this term, he/she must be queried for clarification.

(iii) Sepsis with organ dysfunction

If a patient has sepsis and associated acute organ dysfunction or multiple organ dysfunction (MOD), follow the instructions for coding severe sepsis.

(iv) Acute organ dysfunction that is not clearly associated with the sepsis

If a patient has sepsis and an acute organ dysfunction, but the medical record documentation indicates that the acute organ dysfunction is related to a medical condition other than the sepsis, do not assign a code from subcategory R65.2, Severe sepsis. An acute organ dysfunction must be associated with the sepsis in order to assign the severe sepsis code. If the documentation is not clear as to whether an acute organ dysfunction is related to the sepsis or another medical condition, query the provider.

Sepsis and acute respiratory failure due to COPD exacerbation.

A41.9	Sepsis, unspecified organism
J44.1	Chronic obstructive pulmonary disease with (acute) exacerbation
J96.ØØ	Acute respiratory failure, unspecified whether with hypoxia or hypercapnia

Explanation: Although acute organ dysfunction is present in the form of acute respiratory failure, severe sepsis (R65.2) is not coded in this example, as the acute respiratory failure is attributed to the COPD exacerbation rather than the sepsis. Sequencing of these codes would be determined by the circumstances of the admission.

(b) Severe sepsis

The coding of severe sepsis requires a minimum of 2 codes: first a code for the underlying systemic infection, followed by a code from subcategory R65.2, Severe sepsis. If the causal organism is not documented, assign code A41.9, Sepsis, unspecified organism, for the infection. Additional code(s) for the associated acute organ dysfunction are also required.

Due to the complex nature of severe sepsis, some cases may require querying the provider prior to assignment of the codes.

2) Septic shock

(a) Septic shock generally refers to circulatory failure associated with severe sepsis, and therefore, it represents a type of acute organ dysfunction.

For cases of septic shock, the code for the systemic infection should be sequenced first, followed by code R65.21, Severe sepsis with septic shock or code T81.12, Postprocedural septic shock. Any additional codes for the other acute organ dysfunctions should also be assigned. As noted in the sequencing instructions in the Tabular List, the code for septic shock cannot be assigned as a principal diagnosis.

Sepsis with septic shock.

A41.9	Sepsis, unspecified organism
R65.21	Severe sepsis with septic shock

Explanation: Documentation of septic shock automatically implies severe sepsis as it is a form of acute organ dysfunction. Septic shock is not coded as the principal diagnosis; it is always preceded by the code for the systemic infection.

3) Sequencing of severe sepsis

If severe sepsis is present on admission, and meets the definition of principal diagnosis, the underlying systemic infection should be assigned as principal diagnosis followed by the appropriate code from subcategory R65.2 as required by the sequencing rules in the Tabular List. A code from subcategory R65.2 can never be assigned as a principal diagnosis.

When severe sepsis develops during an encounter (it was not present on admission), the underlying systemic infection and the appropriate code from subcategory R65.2 should be assigned as secondary diagnoses.

Severe sepsis may be present on admission, but the diagnosis may not be confirmed until sometime after admission. If the documentation is not clear whether severe sepsis was present on admission, the provider should be queried.

4) Sepsis *or* severe sepsis with a localized infection

If the reason for admission is sepsis or severe sepsis and a localized infection, such as pneumonia or cellulitis, a code(s) for the underlying systemic infection should be assigned first and the code for the localized infection should be assigned as a secondary diagnosis. If the patient has severe sepsis, a code from subcategory R65.2 should also be assigned as a secondary diagnosis. If the patient is admitted with a localized infection, such as pneumonia, and sepsis/severe sepsis doesn't develop until after admission, the localized infection should be assigned first, followed by the appropriate sepsis/severe sepsis codes.

Patient presents with acute renal failure due to severe sepsis from *Pseudomonas pneumonia*.

A41.9	Sepsis, unspecified organism
J15.1	Pneumonia due to Pseudomonas
R65.2Ø	Severe sepsis without septic shock
N17.9	Acute kidney failure, unspecified

Explanation: If all conditions are present on admission, the systemic infection (sepsis) is sequenced first followed by the codes for the localized infection (pneumonia), severe sepsis and any organ dysfunction. If only the pneumonia was present on admission with the sepsis and resulting renal failure developing later in the admission, then the pneumonia would be sequenced first.

5) Sepsis due to a postprocedural infection

(a) Documentation of causal relationship

As with all postprocedural complications, code assignment is based on the provider's documentation of the relationship between the infection and the procedure.

(b) Sepsis due to a postprocedural infection

For infections following a procedure, a code from T81.4Ø, to T81.43 Infection following a procedure, or a code from O86.ØØ to O86.Ø3, Infection of obstetric surgical wound, that identifies the site of the infection should be coded first, if known. Assign an additional code for sepsis following a procedure (T81.44) or sepsis following an obstetrical procedure (O86.Ø4). Use an additional code to identify the infectious agent. If the patient has severe sepsis, the appropriate code from subcategory R65.2 should also be assigned with the additional code(s) for any acute organ dysfunction.

For infections following infusion, transfusion, therapeutic injection, or immunization, a code from subcategory T8Ø.2, Infections following infusion, transfusion, and therapeutic injection, or code T88.Ø-, Infection following immunization, should be coded first, followed by the code for the specific infection. If the patient has severe sepsis, the appropriate code from subcategory R65.2 should also be assigned, with the additional codes(s) for any acute organ dysfunction.

(c) Postprocedural infection and postprocedural septic shock

If a postprocedural infection has resulted in postprocedural septic shock, assign the codes indicated above for sepsis due to a postprocedural infection, followed by code T81.12-, Postprocedural septic shock. Do not assign code R65.21, Severe sepsis with septic shock. Additional code(s) should be assigned for any acute organ dysfunction.

6) Sepsis and severe sepsis associated with a noninfectious process (condition)

In some cases a noninfectious process (condition), such as trauma, may lead to an infection which can result in sepsis or severe sepsis. If sepsis or severe sepsis is documented as associated with a noninfectious condition, such as a burn or serious injury, and this condition meets the definition for principal diagnosis, the code for the noninfectious condition should be sequenced first, followed by the code for the resulting infection. If severe sepsis is present, a code from subcategory R65.2 should also be assigned with any associated organ dysfunction(s) codes. It is not necessary to assign a code from subcategory R65.1, Systemic inflammatory response syndrome (SIRS) of non-infectious origin, for these cases.

If the infection meets the definition of principal diagnosis, it should be sequenced before the non-infectious condition. When both the associated non-infectious condition and the infection meet the definition of principal diagnosis, either may be assigned as principal diagnosis.

Only one code from category R65, Symptoms and signs specifically associated with systemic inflammation and infection, should be assigned. Therefore, when a non-infectious condition leads to an infection resulting in severe sepsis, assign the appropriate code from subcategory R65.2, Severe sepsis. Do not additionally assign a code from subcategory R65.1, Systemic inflammatory response syndrome (SIRS) of non-infectious origin.

See Section I.C.18. SIRS due to non-infectious process

7) Sepsis and septic shock complicating abortion, pregnancy, childbirth, and the puerperium

See Section I.C.15. Sepsis and septic shock complicating abortion, pregnancy, childbirth and the puerperium

8) Newborn sepsis

See Section I.C.16. f. Bacterial sepsis of Newborn

e. Methicillin resistant Staphylococcus aureus (MRSA) conditions

1) Selection and sequencing of MRSA codes

(a) Combination codes for MRSA infection

When a patient is diagnosed with an infection that is due to methicillin resistant *Staphylococcus aureus* (MRSA), and that infection has a combination code that includes the causal organism (e.g., sepsis, pneumonia) assign the appropriate combination code for the condition (e.g., code A41.Ø2, Sepsis due to Methicillin resistant Staphylococcus aureus or code J15.212, Pneumonia due to Methicillin resistant Staphylococcus aureus). Do not assign code B95.62, Methicillin resistant Staphylococcus aureus infection as the cause of diseases classified elsewhere, as an additional code, because the combination code includes the type of infection and the MRSA organism. Do not assign a code from subcategory Z16.11, Resistance to penicillins, as an additional diagnosis.

See Section C.1. for instructions on coding and sequencing of sepsis and severe sepsis.

(b) Other codes for MRSA infection

When there is documentation of a current infection (e.g., wound infection, stitch abscess, urinary tract infection) due to MRSA, and that infection does not have a combination code that includes the causal organism, assign the appropriate code to identify the condition along with code B95.62, Methicillin resistant Staphylococcus aureus infection as the cause of diseases classified elsewhere for the MRSA infection. Do not assign a code from subcategory Z16.11, Resistance to penicillins.

(c) Methicillin susceptible Staphylococcus aureus (MSSA) and MRSA colonization

The condition or state of being colonized or carrying MSSA or MRSA is called colonization or carriage, while an individual person is described as being colonized or being a carrier. Colonization means that MSSA or MSRA is present on or in the body without necessarily causing illness. A positive MRSA colonization test might be documented by the provider as "MRSA screen positive" or "MRSA nasal swab positive".

Assign code Z22.322, Carrier or suspected carrier of Methicillin resistant Staphylococcus aureus, for patients documented as having MRSA colonization. Assign code Z22.321, Carrier or suspected carrier of Methicillin susceptible Staphylococcus aureus, for patients documented as having MSSA colonization. Colonization is not necessarily indicative of a disease process or as the cause of a specific condition the patient may have unless documented as such by the provider.

(d) MRSA colonization and infection

If a patient is documented as having both MRSA colonization and infection during a hospital admission, code Z22.322, Carrier or suspected carrier of Methicillin resistant Staphylococcus aureus, and a code for the MRSA infection may both be assigned.

f. Zika virus infections

1) Code only confirmed cases

Code only a confirmed diagnosis of Zika virus (A92.5, Zika virus disease) as documented by the provider. This is an exception to the hospital inpatient guideline Section II, H. In this context, "confirmation" does not require documentation of the type of test performed; the **provider's** diagnostic statement that the condition is confirmed is sufficient. This code should be assigned regardless of the stated mode of transmission.

If the provider documents "suspected", "possible" or "probable" Zika, do not assign code A92.5. Assign a code(s) explaining the reason for encounter (such as fever, rash, or joint pain) or Z20.821, Contact with and (suspected) exposure to Zika virus.

Chapter 1. Certain Infectious and Parasitic Diseases (A00-B99)

INCLUDES diseases generally recognized as communicable or transmissible
Use additional code to identify resistance to antimicrobial drugs (Z16.-)

EXCLUDES 1 certain localized infections — see body system-related chapters

EXCLUDES 2 carrier or suspected carrier of infectious disease (Z22.-)
infectious and parasitic diseases complicating pregnancy, childbirth and the puerperium (O98.-)
infectious and parasitic diseases specific to the perinatal period (P35-P39)
influenza and other acute respiratory infections (J00-J22)

This chapter contains the following blocks:

A00-A09	Intestinal infectious diseases
A15-A19	Tuberculosis
A20-A28	Certain zoonotic bacterial diseases
A30-A49	Other bacterial diseases
A50-A64	Infections with a predominantly sexual mode of transmission
A65-A69	Other spirochetal diseases
A70-A74	Other diseases caused by chlamydiae
A75-A79	Rickettsioses
A80-A89	Viral and prion infections of the central nervous system
A90-A99	Arthropod-borne viral fevers and viral hemorrhagic fevers
B00-B09	Viral infections characterized by skin and mucous membrane lesions
B10	Other human herpesviruses
B15-B19	Viral hepatitis
B20	Human immunodeficiency virus [HIV] disease
B25-B34	Other viral diseases
B35-B49	Mycoses
B50-B64	Protozoal diseases
B65-B83	Helminthiases
B85-B89	Pediculosis, acariasis and other infestations
B90-B94	Sequelae of infectious and parasitic diseases
B95-B97	Bacterial and viral infectious agents
B99	Other infectious diseases

Intestinal infectious diseases (A00-A09)

✓4ᵗʰ A00 Cholera

DEF: Acute infection of the bowel due to vibrio cholerae that presents with profuse diarrhea, cramps, and vomiting, resulting in severe dehydration, electrolyte imbalance, and death. It is spread through ingestion of food or water contaminated with feces of infected persons.

A00.0 Cholera due to Vibrio cholerae 01, biovar cholerae
Classical cholera

A00.1 Cholera due to Vibrio cholerae 01, biovar eltor
Cholera eltor

A00.9 Cholera, unspecified

✓4ᵗʰ A01 Typhoid and paratyphoid fevers

DEF: Typhoid fever: Acute generalized illness caused by Salmonella typhi. Clinical features include fever, headache, abdominal pain, cough, toxemia, leukopenia, abnormal pulse, rose spots on the skin, bacteremia, hyperplasia of intestinal lymph nodes, mesenteric lymphadenopathy, and Peyer's patches in the intestines.
DEF: Paratyphoid fever: Prolonged febrile illness, caused by Salmonella serotypes other than S. typhi, especially S. enterica serotypes paratyphi A, B, and C.

✓5ᵗʰ A01.0 Typhoid fever
Infection due to Salmonella typhi

     A01.00 Typhoid fever, unspecified
     A01.01 Typhoid meningitis
     A01.02 Typhoid fever with heart involvement
         Typhoid endocarditis
         Typhoid myocarditis
     A01.03 Typhoid pneumonia
     A01.04 Typhoid arthritis
     A01.05 Typhoid osteomyelitis
     A01.09 Typhoid fever with other complications

A01.1 Paratyphoid fever A
A01.2 Paratyphoid fever B
A01.3 Paratyphoid fever C
A01.4 Paratyphoid fever, unspecified
     Infection due to Salmonella paratyphi NOS

✓4ᵗʰ A02 Other salmonella infections

INCLUDES infection or foodborne intoxication due to any Salmonella species other than S. typhi and S. paratyphi

A02.0 Salmonella enteritis
Salmonellosis

A02.1 Salmonella sepsis

✓5ᵗʰ A02.2 Localized salmonella infections

     A02.20 Localized salmonella infection, unspecified
     A02.21 Salmonella meningitis
     A02.22 Salmonella pneumonia
     A02.23 Salmonella arthritis
     A02.24 Salmonella osteomyelitis
     A02.25 Salmonella pyelonephritis
         Salmonella tubulo-interstitial nephropathy
     A02.29 Salmonella with other localized infection

A02.8 Other specified salmonella infections
A02.9 Salmonella infection, unspecified

✓4ᵗʰ A03 Shigellosis

DEF: Infection caused by the genus the Shigella, of the family Enterobacteriaceae that is known to cause an acute dysenteric infection of the bowel with fever, drowsiness, anorexia, nausea, vomiting, bloody diarrhea, abdominal cramps, and distention.

A03.0 Shigellosis due to Shigella dysenteriae
Group A shigellosis [Shiga-Kruse dysentery]

A03.1 Shigellosis due to Shigella flexneri
Group B shigellosis

A03.2 Shigellosis due to Shigella boydii
Group C shigellosis

A03.3 Shigellosis due to Shigella sonnei
Group D shigellosis

A03.8 Other shigellosis

A03.9 Shigellosis, unspecified
Bacillary dysentery NOS

✓4ᵗʰ A04 Other bacterial intestinal infections

EXCLUDES 1 bacterial foodborne intoxications, NEC (A05.-)
tuberculous enteritis (A18.32)

DEF: Escherichia coli: Gram negative, anaerobic of the family Enterobacteriaceae found in the large intestine of warm-blooded animals, generally as a nonpathologic entity aiding in digestion. They become pathogenic when an opportunity to grow somewhere outside this relationship presents itself, such as ingestion of fecal contaminated food or water.

A04.0 Enteropathogenic Escherichia coli infection
A04.1 Enterotoxigenic Escherichia coli infection
A04.2 Enteroinvasive Escherichia coli infection
A04.3 Enterohemorrhagic Escherichia coli infection
     DEF: E. coli infection penetrating the intestinal mucosa, producing microscopic ulceration and bleeding.

A04.4 Other intestinal Escherichia coli infections
Escherichia coli enteritis NOS

A04.5 Campylobacter enteritis
A04.6 Enteritis due to Yersinia enterocolitica
     EXCLUDES 1 extraintestinal yersiniosis (A28.2)

✓5ᵗʰ A04.7 Enterocolitis due to Clostridium difficile

Foodborne intoxication by Clostridium difficile
Pseudomembraneous colitis
AHA: 2017,4Q,4

     A04.71 Enterocolitis due to Clostridium difficile, recurrent
     A04.72 Enterocolitis due to Clostridium difficile, not specified as recurrent

A04.8 Other specified bacterial intestinal infections
A04.9 Bacterial intestinal infection, unspecified
Bacterial enteritis NOS

✓4ᵗʰ A05 Other bacterial foodborne intoxications, not elsewhere classified

EXCLUDES 1 Clostridium difficile foodborne intoxication and infection (A04.7-)
Escherichia coli infection (A04.0-A04.4)
listeriosis (A32.-)
salmonella foodborne intoxication and infection (A02.-)
toxic effect of noxious foodstuffs (T61-T62)

A05.0 Foodborne staphylococcal intoxication
A05.1 Botulism food poisoning
Botulism NOS
Classical foodborne intoxication due to Clostridium botulinum
     EXCLUDES 1 infant botulism (A48.51)
         wound botulism (A48.52)
DEF: Muscle-paralyzing neurotoxic disease caused by ingesting pre-formed toxin from the bacterium Clostridium botulinum. It causes vomiting and diarrhea, vision problems, slurred speech, difficulty swallowing, paralysis, and death.

N Newborn: 0   P Pediatric: 0-17   M Maternity: 12-55   A Adult: 15-124   CH Comorbidity High   CL Comorbidity Low   NCDx Noncancer Dx   PDx Primary Dx

436   ICD-10-CM 2020

A05.2   **Foodborne Clostridium perfringens [Clostridium welchii] intoxication**
Enteritis necroticans
Pig-bel

A05.3   **Foodborne Vibrio parahaemolyticus intoxication**

A05.4   **Foodborne Bacillus cereus intoxication**

A05.5   **Foodborne Vibrio vulnificus intoxication**

A05.8   **Other specified bacterial foodborne intoxications**

A05.9   **Bacterial foodborne intoxication, unspecified**

✓4ᵗʰ **A06**   **Amebiasis**
   INCLUDES   infection due to Entamoeba histolytica
   EXCLUDES 1   other protozoal intestinal diseases (A07.-)
   EXCLUDES 2   acanthamebiasis (B60.1-)
              Naegleriasis (B60.2)
   DEF: Infection with a single cell protozoan known as the amoeba. Transmission occurs through ingestion of feces, contaminated food or water, use of human feces as fertilizer, or person-to-person contact.

A06.0   **Acute amebic dysentery**
Acute amebiasis
Intestinal amebiasis NOS

A06.1   **Chronic intestinal amebiasis**

A06.2   **Amebic nondysenteric colitis**

A06.3   **Ameboma of intestine**
Ameboma NOS

A06.4   **Amebic liver abscess**
Hepatic amebiasis

A06.5   **Amebic lung abscess**
Amebic abscess of lung (and liver)

A06.6   **Amebic brain abscess**
Amebic abscess of brain (and liver) (and lung)

A06.7   **Cutaneous amebiasis**

✓5ᵗʰ **A06.8**   **Amebic infection of other sites**

   A06.81   **Amebic cystitis**

   A06.82   **Other amebic genitourinary infections**
       Amebic balanitis
       Amebic vesiculitis
       Amebic vulvovaginitis

   A06.89   **Other amebic infections**
       Amebic appendicitis
       Amebic splenic abscess

A06.9   **Amebiasis, unspecified**

✓4ᵗʰ **A07**   **Other protozoal intestinal diseases**
   DEF: Protozoa: Group comprised of the simplest, single celled organisms, ranging in size from micro to macroscopic. They can live alone or in colonies, and do not show any differentiation in tissues. Most are motile and can live free in nature, but some are parasitic, causing disease in the variety of hosts they inhabit.

A07.0   **Balantidiasis**
Balantidial dysentery

A07.1   **Giardiasis [lambliasis]**
   DEF: Infection caused by the flagellate protozoan *Giardia lamblia* causing gastrointestinal problems such as vomiting, chronic diarrhea, and weight loss. The most common parasite in the US, this is usually transmitted by ingesting contaminated water while in the cyst state and latches onto the wall of the small intestine.

A07.2   **Cryptosporidiosis**
   DEF: Microscopic parasite found in water and one of the most common causes of waterborne gastrointestinal infectious disease in the United States. It is usually transmitted by ingesting contaminated drinking water or recreational water and causes profuse watery diarrhea, flatulence, abdominal pain, and cramping.

A07.3   **Isosporiasis**
Infection due to Isospora belli and Isospora hominis
Intestinal coccidiosis
Isosporosis

A07.4   **Cyclosporiasis**

A07.8   **Other specified protozoal intestinal diseases**
Intestinal microsporidiosis
Intestinal trichomoniasis
Sarcocystosis
Sarcosporidiosis

A07.9   **Protozoal intestinal disease, unspecified**
Flagellate diarrhea
Protozoal colitis
Protozoal diarrhea
Protozoal dysentery

✓4ᵗʰ **A08**   **Viral and other specified intestinal infections**
   EXCLUDES 1   influenza with involvement of gastrointestinal tract (J09.X3, J10.2, J11.2)

A08.0   **Rotaviral enteritis**

✓5ᵗʰ **A08.1**   **Acute gastroenteropathy due to Norwalk agent and other small round viruses**

   A08.11   **Acute gastroenteropathy due to Norwalk agent**
       Acute gastroenteropathy due to Norovirus
       Acute gastroenteropathy due to Norwalk-like agent

   A08.19   **Acute gastroenteropathy due to other small round viruses**
       Acute gastroenteropathy due to small round virus [SRV] NOS

A08.2   **Adenoviral enteritis**

✓5ᵗʰ **A08.3**   **Other viral enteritis**

   A08.31   **Calicivirus enteritis**

   A08.32   **Astrovirus enteritis**

   A08.39   **Other viral enteritis**
       Coxsackie virus enteritis
       Echovirus enteritis
       Enterovirus enteritis NEC
       Torovirus enteritis

A08.4   **Viral intestinal infection, unspecified**
Viral enteritis NOS
Viral gastroenteritis NOS
Viral gastroenteropathy NOS
AHA: 2016,3Q,12

A08.8   **Other specified intestinal infections**

A09   **Infectious gastroenteritis and colitis, unspecified**
Infectious colitis NOS
Infectious enteritis NOS
Infectious gastroenteritis NOS
   EXCLUDES 1   colitis NOS (K52.9)
              diarrhea NOS (R19.7)
              enteritis NOS (K52.9)
              gastroenteritis NOS (K52.9)
              noninfective gastroenteritis and colitis, unspecified (K52.9)
   DEF: Colitis: Inflammation of mucous membranes of the colon.
   DEF: Enteritis: Inflammation of mucous membranes of the small intestine.
   DEF: Gastroenteritis: Inflammation of mucous membranes of the stomach and intestines.

Chapter 1. Certain Infectious and Parasitic Diseases

Tuberculosis (A15-A19)

INCLUDES   infections due to Mycobacterium tuberculosis and Mycobacterium bovis

EXCLUDES 1   congenital tuberculosis (P37.0)
nonspecific reaction to test for tuberculosis without active tuberculosis (R76.1-)
pneumoconiosis associated with tuberculosis, any type in A15 (J65)
positive PPD (R76.11)
positive tuberculin skin test without active tuberculosis (R76.11)
sequelae of tuberculosis (B90.-)
silicotuberculosis (J65)

DEF: Bacterial infection that typically spreads by inhalation of an airborne agent that usually attacks the lungs, but may also affect other organs.

✓4ᵗʰ   A15   Respiratory tuberculosis

     A15.0   Tuberculosis of lung
         Tuberculous bronchiectasis
         Tuberculous fibrosis of lung
         Tuberculous pneumonia
         Tuberculous pneumothorax

Tuberculosis of Lung

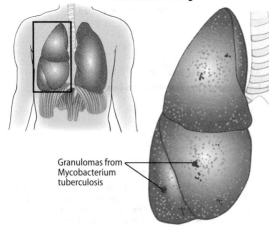

Granulomas from Mycobacterium tuberculosis

     A15.4   Tuberculosis of intrathoracic lymph nodes
         Tuberculosis of hilar lymph nodes
         Tuberculosis of mediastinal lymph nodes
         Tuberculosis of tracheobronchial lymph nodes
         EXCLUDES 1   tuberculosis specified as primary (A15.7)

     A15.5   Tuberculosis of larynx, trachea and bronchus
         Tuberculosis of bronchus
         Tuberculosis of glottis
         Tuberculosis of larynx
         Tuberculosis of trachea

     A15.6   Tuberculous pleurisy
         Tuberculosis of pleura Tuberculous empyema
         EXCLUDES 1   primary respiratory tuberculosis (A15.7)

     A15.7   Primary respiratory tuberculosis

     A15.8   Other respiratory tuberculosis
         Mediastinal tuberculosis
         Nasopharyngeal tuberculosis
         Tuberculosis of nose
         Tuberculosis of sinus [any nasal]

     A15.9   Respiratory tuberculosis unspecified

✓4ᵗʰ   A17   Tuberculosis of nervous system

     A17.0   Tuberculous meningitis
         Tuberculosis of meninges (cerebral)(spinal)
         Tuberculous leptomeningitis
         EXCLUDES 1   tuberculous meningoencephalitis (A17.82)

     A17.1   Meningeal tuberculoma
         Tuberculoma of meninges (cerebral) (spinal)
         EXCLUDES 2   tuberculoma of brain and spinal cord (A17.81)

     ✓5ᵗʰ   **A17.8   Other tuberculosis of nervous system**
         A17.81   Tuberculoma of brain and spinal cord
             Tuberculous abscess of brain and spinal cord
         A17.82   Tuberculous meningoencephalitis
             Tuberculous myelitis

         A17.83   Tuberculous neuritis
             Tuberculous mononeuropathy
         A17.89   Other tuberculosis of nervous system
             Tuberculous polyneuropathy

     A17.9   Tuberculosis of nervous system, unspecified

✓4ᵗʰ   A18   Tuberculosis of other organs

     ✓5ᵗʰ   **A18.0   Tuberculosis of bones and joints**
         A18.01   Tuberculosis of spine
             Pott's disease or curvature of spine
             Tuberculous arthritis
             Tuberculous osteomyelitis of spine
             Tuberculous spondylitis
         A18.02   Tuberculous arthritis of other joints
             Tuberculosis of hip (joint)
             Tuberculosis of knee (joint)
         A18.03   Tuberculosis of other bones
             Tuberculous mastoiditis
             Tuberculous osteomyelitis
         A18.09   Other musculoskeletal tuberculosis
             Tuberculous myositis
             Tuberculous synovitis
             Tuberculous tenosynovitis

     ✓5ᵗʰ   **A18.1   Tuberculosis of genitourinary system**
         A18.10   Tuberculosis of genitourinary system, unspecified
         A18.11   Tuberculosis of kidney and ureter
         A18.12   Tuberculosis of bladder
         A18.13   Tuberculosis of other urinary organs
             Tuberculous urethritis
         A18.14   Tuberculosis of prostate   A ♂
         A18.15   Tuberculosis of other male genital organs   ♂
         A18.16   Tuberculosis of cervix   ♀
         A18.17   Tuberculous female pelvic inflammatory disease   ♀
             Tuberculous endometritis
             Tuberculous oophoritis and salpingitis
         A18.18   Tuberculosis of other female genital organs   ♀
             Tuberculous ulceration of vulva

     A18.2   Tuberculous peripheral lymphadenopathy
         Tuberculous adenitis
         EXCLUDES 2   tuberculosis of bronchial and mediastinal lymph nodes (A15.4)
             tuberculosis of mesenteric and retroperitoneal lymph nodes (A18.39)
             tuberculous tracheobronchial adenopathy (A15.4)

     ✓5ᵗʰ   **A18.3   Tuberculosis of intestines, peritoneum and mesenteric glands**
         A18.31   Tuberculous peritonitis
             Tuberculous ascites
             DEF: Tuberculous inflammation of the membrane lining the abdomen.
         A18.32   Tuberculous enteritis
             Tuberculosis of anus and rectum
             Tuberculosis of intestine (large) (small)
         A18.39   Retroperitoneal tuberculosis
             Tuberculosis of mesenteric glands
             Tuberculosis of retroperitoneal (lymph glands)

     A18.4   Tuberculosis of skin and subcutaneous tissue
         Erythema induratum, tuberculous
         Lupus excedens
         Lupus vulgaris NOS
         Lupus vulgaris of eyelid
         Scrofuloderma
         Tuberculosis of external ear
         EXCLUDES 2   lupus erythematosus (L93.-)
             ~~lupus NOS (M32.9)~~
             ▶systemic lupus erythematosus◀ (M32.-)

     ✓5ᵗʰ   **A18.5   Tuberculosis of eye**
         EXCLUDES 2   lupus vulgaris of eyelid (A18.4)
         A18.50   Tuberculosis of eye, unspecified
         A18.51   Tuberculous episcleritis
         A18.52   Tuberculous keratitis
             Tuberculous interstitial keratitis
             Tuberculous keratoconjunctivitis (interstitial) (phlyctenular)
         A18.53   Tuberculous chorioretinitis

N Newborn: 0   P Pediatric: 0-17   M Maternity: 12-55   A Adult: 15-124   CH Comorbidity High   CL Comorbidity Low   NCDx Noncancer Dx   PDx Primary Dx

438   ICD-10-CM 2020

A18.54 **Tuberculous** iridocyclitis
A18.59 **Other tuberculosis of eye**
    Tuberculous conjunctivitis
A18.6 **Tuberculosis of (inner) (middle) ear**
    Tuberculous otitis media
    EXCLUDES 2   tuberculosis of external ear (A18.4)
             tuberculous mastoiditis (A18.03)
A18.7 **Tuberculosis of** adrenal glands
    Tuberculous Addison's disease
✓5ᵗʰ A18.8 **Tuberculosis of other** specified organs
A18.81 **Tuberculosis of** thyroid gland
A18.82 **Tuberculosis of other** endocrine glands
    Tuberculosis of pituitary gland
    Tuberculosis of thymus gland
A18.83 **Tuberculosis of** digestive tract organs, **not elsewhere classified**
    EXCLUDES 1   tuberculosis of intestine (A18.32)
A18.84 **Tuberculosis of** heart
    Tuberculous cardiomyopathy
    Tuberculous endocarditis
    Tuberculous myocarditis
    Tuberculous pericarditis
A18.85 **Tuberculosis of** spleen
A18.89 **Tuberculosis of other sites**
    Tuberculosis of muscle
    Tuberculous cerebral arteritis

✓4ᵗʰ **A19 Miliary tuberculosis**
INCLUDES   disseminated tuberculosis
         generalized tuberculosis
         tuberculous polyserositis
A19.0 **Acute miliary tuberculosis of a** single specified site
A19.1 **Acute miliary tuberculosis of** multiple sites
A19.2 **Acute miliary tuberculosis, unspecified**
A19.8 **Other miliary tuberculosis**
A19.9 **Miliary tuberculosis, unspecified**

Certain zoonotic bacterial diseases (A20-A28)

✓4ᵗʰ **A20 Plague**
INCLUDES   infection due to Yersinia pestis
A20.0 **Bubonic** plague
A20.1 **Cellulocutaneous** plague
A20.2 **Pneumonic** plague
A20.3 **Plague** meningitis
A20.7 **Septicemic** plague
A20.8 **Other forms of plague**
    Abortive plague
    Asymptomatic plague
    Pestis minor
A20.9 **Plague, unspecified**
✓4ᵗʰ **A21 Tularemia**
INCLUDES   deer-fly fever
         infection due to Francisella tularensis
         rabbit fever
DEF: Febrile disease transmitted to humans by the bites of deer flies, fleas, and ticks, by inhaling aerosolized *F. tularensis*, or by ingesting contaminated food or water. Patients quickly develop fever, chills, weakness, headache, backache, and malaise.
A21.0 **Ulceroglandular** tularemia
A21.1 **Oculoglandular** tularemia
    Ophthalmic tularemia
A21.2 **Pulmonary** tularemia
A21.3 **Gastrointestinal** tularemia
    Abdominal tularemia
A21.7 **Generalized** tularemia
A21.8 **Other forms of tularemia**
A21.9 **Tularemia, unspecified**
✓4ᵗʰ **A22 Anthrax**
INCLUDES   infection due to Bacillus anthracis
A22.0 **Cutaneous** anthrax
    Malignant carbuncle
    Malignant pustule

A22.1 **Pulmonary** anthrax
    Inhalation anthrax
    Ragpicker's disease
    Woolsorter's disease
A22.2 **Gastrointestinal** anthrax
A22.7 **Anthrax** sepsis
A22.8 **Other forms of anthrax**
    Anthrax meningitis
A22.9 **Anthrax, unspecified**
✓4ᵗʰ **A23 Brucellosis**
INCLUDES   Malta fever
         Mediterranean fever
         undulant fever
A23.0 **Brucellosis due to** Brucella melitensis
A23.1 **Brucellosis due to** Brucella abortus
A23.2 **Brucellosis due to** Brucella suis
A23.3 **Brucellosis due to** Brucella canis
A23.8 **Other brucellosis**
A23.9 **Brucellosis, unspecified**
✓4ᵗʰ **A24 Glanders and melioidosis**
A24.0 **Glanders**
    Infection due to Pseudomonas mallei
    Malleus
A24.1 **Acute and fulminating** melioidosis
    Melioidosis pneumonia
    Melioidosis sepsis
A24.2 **Subacute and chronic** melioidosis
A24.3 **Other melioidosis**
A24.9 **Melioidosis, unspecified**
    Infection due to Pseudomonas pseudomallei NOS
    Whitmore's disease
✓4ᵗʰ **A25 Rat-bite fevers**
A25.0 **Spirillosis**
    Sodoku
A25.1 **Streptobacillosis**
    Epidemic arthritic erythema
    Haverhill fever
    Streptobacillary rat-bite fever
A25.9 **Rat-bite fever, unspecified**
✓4ᵗʰ **A26 Erysipeloid**
DEF: Acute cutaneous infection typically caused by trauma to the skin. Presenting as cellulitis, it may become systemic affecting other organs. It is gram positive bacillus and mainly acquired by those who routinely handle meat.
A26.0 **Cutaneous** erysipeloid
    Erythema migrans
A26.7 **Erysipelothrix sepsis**
A26.8 **Other forms of erysipeloid**
A26.9 **Erysipeloid, unspecified**
✓4ᵗʰ **A27 Leptospirosis**
A27.0 **Leptospirosis** icterohemorrhagica
    Leptospiral or spirochetal jaundice (hemorrhagic)
    Weil's disease
✓5ᵗʰ A27.8 **Other forms of leptospirosis**
A27.81 **Aseptic meningitis in leptospirosis**
A27.89 **Other forms of leptospirosis**
A27.9 **Leptospirosis, unspecified**
✓4ᵗʰ **A28 Other zoonotic bacterial diseases, not elsewhere classified**
A28.0 **Pasteurellosis**
A28.1 **Cat-scratch disease**
    Cat-scratch fever
A28.2 **Extraintestinal yersiniosis**
    EXCLUDES 1   enteritis due to Yersinia enterocolitica (A04.6)
             plague (A20.-)
A28.8 **Other specified zoonotic bacterial diseases, not elsewhere classified**
A28.9 **Zoonotic bacterial disease, unspecified**

Other bacterial diseases (A3Ø-A49)

AHA: 2016,3Q,8-14

✓4ᵗʰ A3Ø Leprosy [Hansen's disease]
- **INCLUDES** infection due to Mycobacterium leprae
- **EXCLUDES 1** sequelae of leprosy (B92)

- **A3Ø.Ø Indeterminate leprosy**
  - I leprosy
- **A3Ø.1 Tuberculoid leprosy**
  - TT leprosy
- **A3Ø.2 Borderline tuberculoid leprosy**
  - BT leprosy
- **A3Ø.3 Borderline leprosy**
  - BB leprosy
- **A3Ø.4 Borderline lepromatous leprosy**
  - BL leprosy
- **A3Ø.5 Lepromatous leprosy**
  - LL leprosy
- **A3Ø.8 Other forms of leprosy**
- **A3Ø.9 Leprosy, unspecified**

✓4ᵗʰ A31 Infection due to other mycobacteria
- **EXCLUDES 2** leprosy (A3Ø.-)
  - tuberculosis (A15-A19)

- **A31.Ø Pulmonary mycobacterial infection**
  - Infection due to Mycobacterium avium
  - Infection due to Mycobacterium intracellulare [Battey bacillus]
  - Infection due to Mycobacterium kansasii
- **A31.1 Cutaneous mycobacterial infection**
  - Buruli ulcer
  - Infection due to Mycobacterium marinum
  - Infection due to Mycobacterium ulcerans
- **A31.2 Disseminated mycobacterium avium-intracellulare complex (DMAC)**
  - MAC sepsis
- **A31.8 Other mycobacterial infections**
- **A31.9 Mycobacterial infection, unspecified**
  - Atypical mycobacterial infection NOS
  - Mycobacteriosis NOS

✓4ᵗʰ A32 Listeriosis
- **INCLUDES** listerial foodborne infection
- **EXCLUDES 1** neonatal (disseminated) listeriosis (P37.2)

- **A32.Ø Cutaneous listeriosis**
- **✓5ᵗʰ A32.1 Listerial meningitis and meningoencephalitis**
  - **A32.11 Listerial meningitis**
  - **A32.12 Listerial meningoencephalitis**
- **A32.7 Listerial sepsis**
- **✓5ᵗʰ A32.8 Other forms of listeriosis**
  - **A32.81 Oculoglandular listeriosis**
  - **A32.82 Listerial endocarditis**
  - **A32.89 Other forms of listeriosis**
    - Listerial cerebral arteritis
- **A32.9 Listeriosis, unspecified**

A33 Tetanus neonatorum   N

A34 Obstetrical tetanus   M ♀

A35 Other tetanus
- Tetanus NOS
- **EXCLUDES 1** obstetrical tetanus (A34)
  - tetanus neonatorum (A33)
- **DEF:** Tetanus: Acute, often fatal, infectious disease caused by the anaerobic, spore-forming bacillus Clostridium tetani. The bacillus enters the body through a contaminated wound, burns, surgical wounds, or cutaneous ulcers. Symptoms include lockjaw, spasms, seizures, and paralysis.

✓4ᵗʰ A36 Diphtheria
- **A36.Ø Pharyngeal diphtheria**
  - Diphtheritic membranous angina
  - Tonsillar diphtheria
- **A36.1 Nasopharyngeal diphtheria**
- **A36.2 Laryngeal diphtheria**
  - Diphtheritic laryngotracheitis
- **A36.3 Cutaneous diphtheria**
  - **EXCLUDES 2** erythrasma (LØ8.1)

✓5ᵗʰ A36.8 Other diphtheria
- **A36.81 Diphtheritic cardiomyopathy**
  - Diphtheritic myocarditis
- **A36.82 Diphtheritic radiculomyelitis**
- **A36.83 Diphtheritic polyneuritis**
- **A36.84 Diphtheritic tubulo-interstitial nephropathy**
- **A36.85 Diphtheritic cystitis**
- **A36.86 Diphtheritic conjunctivitis**
- **A36.89 Other diphtheritic complications**
  - Diphtheritic peritonitis

A36.9 Diphtheria, unspecified

✓4ᵗʰ A37 Whooping cough
- **DEF:** Acute, highly contagious respiratory tract infection caused by Bordetella pertussis and B. bronchiseptica. Whooping cough is known by its characteristic paroxysmal cough.

- **✓5ᵗʰ A37.Ø Whooping cough due to Bordetella pertussis**
  - **A37.ØØ Whooping cough due to Bordetella pertussis without pneumonia**
  - **A37.Ø1 Whooping cough due to Bordetella pertussis with pneumonia**
- **✓5ᵗʰ A37.1 Whooping cough due to Bordetella parapertussis**
  - **A37.1Ø Whooping cough due to Bordetella parapertussis without pneumonia**
  - **A37.11 Whooping cough due to Bordetella parapertussis with pneumonia**
- **✓5ᵗʰ A37.8 Whooping cough due to other Bordetella species**
  - **A37.8Ø Whooping cough due to other Bordetella species without pneumonia**
  - **A37.81 Whooping cough due to other Bordetella species with pneumonia**
- **✓5ᵗʰ A37.9 Whooping cough, unspecified species**
  - **A37.9Ø Whooping cough, unspecified species without pneumonia**
  - **A37.91 Whooping cough, unspecified species with pneumonia**

✓4ᵗʰ A38 Scarlet fever
- **INCLUDES** scarlatina
- **EXCLUDES 2** streptococcal sore throat (JØ2.Ø)
- **DEF:** Acute contagious disease caused by Group A bacteria, the same bacterium that causes strep throat. Individuals with strep throat can develop scarlet fever particularly if the infection is not treated with antibiotics. It is characterized by a red blush to the skin of the chest and abdomen and swelling of the nose, throat, and mouth.

- **A38.Ø Scarlet fever with otitis media**
- **A38.1 Scarlet fever with myocarditis**
- **A38.8 Scarlet fever with other complications**
- **A38.9 Scarlet fever, uncomplicated**
  - Scarlet fever, NOS

✓4ᵗʰ A39 Meningococcal infection
- **DEF:** Condition caused by Neisseria meningitidis, a bacteria that may invade the spinal cord, brain, heart, joints, optic nerve, or bloodstream.

- **A39.Ø Meningococcal meningitis**
- **A39.1 Waterhouse-Friderichsen syndrome**
  - Meningococcal hemorrhagic adrenalitis
  - Meningococcic adrenal syndrome
- **A39.2 Acute meningococcemia**
- **A39.3 Chronic meningococcemia**
- **A39.4 Meningococcemia, unspecified**
- **✓5ᵗʰ A39.5 Meningococcal heart disease**
  - **A39.5Ø Meningococcal carditis, unspecified**
  - **A39.51 Meningococcal endocarditis**
  - **A39.52 Meningococcal myocarditis**
  - **A39.53 Meningococcal pericarditis**
- **✓5ᵗʰ A39.8 Other meningococcal infections**
  - **A39.81 Meningococcal encephalitis**
  - **A39.82 Meningococcal retrobulbar neuritis**
  - **A39.83 Meningococcal arthritis**
  - **A39.84 Postmeningococcal arthritis**
  - **A39.89 Other meningococcal infections**
    - Meningococcal conjunctivitis
- **A39.9 Meningococcal infection, unspecified**
  - Meningococcal disease NOS

✓4ᵗʰ A40 Streptococcal sepsis

Code first:

postprocedural streptococcal sepsis (T81.4-)

streptococcal sepsis during labor (O75.3)

streptococcal sepsis following abortion or ectopic or molar pregnancy (O03-O07, O08.0)

streptococcal sepsis following immunization (T88.0)

streptococcal sepsis following infusion, transfusion or therapeutic injection (T80.2-)

EXCLUDES 1   neonatal (P36.0-P36.1)

puerperal sepsis (O85)

sepsis due to Streptococcus, group D (A41.81)

AHA: 2018,4Q,89; 2018,1Q,16; 2016,1Q,32

TIP: Sepsis should not be coded after it has been resolved or documented as resolving; code the underlying infection if still under treatment.

A40.0 Sepsis due to streptococcus, group A

A40.1 Sepsis due to streptococcus, group B

       AHA: 2019,1Q,14

A40.3 Sepsis due to Streptococcus pneumoniae

Pneumococcal sepsis

A40.8 Other streptococcal sepsis

A40.9 Streptococcal sepsis, unspecified

✓4ᵗʰ A41 Other sepsis

Code first:

postprocedural sepsis (T81.4-)

sepsis during labor (O75.3)

sepsis following abortion, ectopic or molar pregnancy (O03-O07, O08.0)

sepsis following immunization (T88.0)

sepsis following infusion, transfusion or therapeutic injection (T80.2-)

EXCLUDES 1   bacteremia NOS (R78.81)

neonatal (P36.-)

puerperal sepsis (O85)

streptococcal sepsis (A40.-)

EXCLUDES 2   sepsis (due to) (in) actinomycotic (A42.7)

sepsis (due to) (in) anthrax (A22.7)

sepsis (due to) (in) candidal (B37.7)

sepsis (due to) (in) Erysipelothrix (A26.7)

sepsis (due to) (in) extraintestinal yersiniosis (A28.2)

sepsis (due to) (in) gonococcal (A54.86)

sepsis (due to) (in) herpesviral (B00.7)

sepsis (due to) (in) listerial (A32.7)

sepsis (due to) (in) melioidosis (A24.1)

sepsis (due to) (in) meningococcal (A39.2-A39.4)

sepsis (due to) (in) plague (A20.7)

sepsis (due to) (in) tularemia (A21.7)

toxic shock syndrome (A48.3)

AHA: 2018,4Q,18; 2018,1Q,16; 2016,1Q,32; 2014,2Q,13

TIP: Sepsis should not be coded after it has been resolved or documented as resolving; code the underlying infection if still under treatment.

✓5ᵗʰ A41.0 Sepsis due to Staphylococcus aureus

   A41.01 Sepsis due to Methicillin susceptible Staphylococcus aureus

MSSA sepsis

Staphylococcus aureus sepsis NOS

   A41.02 Sepsis due to Methicillin resistant Staphylococcus aureus

A41.1 Sepsis due to other specified staphylococcus

Coagulase negative staphylococcus sepsis

A41.2 Sepsis due to unspecified staphylococcus

A41.3 Sepsis due to Hemophilus influenzae

A41.4 Sepsis due to anaerobes

    EXCLUDES 1   gas gangrene (A48.0)

✓5ᵗʰ A41.5 Sepsis due to other Gram-negative organisms

   A41.50 Gram-negative sepsis, unspecified

Gram-negative sepsis NOS

   A41.51 Sepsis due to Escherichia coli [E. coli]

   A41.52 Sepsis due to Pseudomonas

Pseudomonas aeroginosa

   A41.53 Sepsis due to Serratia

   A41.59 Other Gram-negative sepsis

✓5ᵗʰ A41.8 Other specified sepsis

   A41.81 Sepsis due to Enterococcus

   A41.89 Other specified sepsis

      AHA: 2017,1Q,51; 2016,3Q,8-14

A41.9 Sepsis, unspecified organism

Septicemia NOS

✓4ᵗʰ A42 Actinomycosis

   EXCLUDES 1   actinomycetoma (B47.1)

A42.0 Pulmonary actinomycosis

A42.1 Abdominal actinomycosis

A42.2 Cervicofacial actinomycosis

A42.7 Actinomycotic sepsis

✓5ᵗʰ A42.8 Other forms of actinomycosis

   A42.81 Actinomycotic meningitis

   A42.82 Actinomycotic encephalitis

   A42.89 Other forms of actinomycosis

A42.9 Actinomycosis, unspecified

✓4ᵗʰ A43 Nocardiosis

DEF: Rare bacterial infection occurring most often in those with weakened immune systems. Can be acquired in soil, decaying plants, or standing water. It typically begins in the lungs and has a tendency to spread to other body systems.

A43.0 Pulmonary nocardiosis

A43.1 Cutaneous nocardiosis

A43.8 Other forms of nocardiosis

A43.9 Nocardiosis, unspecified

✓4ᵗʰ A44 Bartonellosis

A44.0 Systemic bartonellosis

Oroya fever

A44.1 Cutaneous and mucocutaneous bartonellosis

Verruga peruana

A44.8 Other forms of bartonellosis

A44.9 Bartonellosis, unspecified

A46 Erysipelas

   EXCLUDES 1   postpartum or puerperal erysipelas (O86.89)

DEF: Skin infection affecting the upper dermis and superficial dermal lymphatics. Lesion edges are well-demarcated with distinct raised borders. It is often caused by group A Streptococci.

✓4ᵗʰ A48 Other bacterial diseases, not elsewhere classified

   EXCLUDES 1   actinomycetoma (B47.1)

A48.0 Gas gangrene

Clostridial cellulitis

Clostridial myonecrosis

AHA: 2017,4Q,102

A48.1 Legionnaires' disease

DEF: Severe and often fatal infection by Legionella pneumophila. Symptoms include high fever, gastrointestinal pain, headache, myalgia, dry cough, and pneumonia and it is usually transmitted through airborne water droplets via air conditioning systems or hot tubs.

A48.2 Nonpneumonic Legionnaires' disease [Pontiac fever]

A48.3 Toxic shock syndrome

Use additional code to identify the organism (B95, B96)

   EXCLUDES 1   endotoxic shock NOS (R57.8)

sepsis NOS (A41.9)

DEF: Bacteria producing an endotoxin, such as Staphylococci, flood the body with the toxins producing a high fever, vomiting and diarrhea, decreasing blood pressure, a skin rash, and shock. **Synonym(s):** TSS.

A48.4 Brazilian purpuric fever

Systemic Hemophilus aegyptius infection

✓5ᵗʰ A48.5 Other specified botulism

Non-foodborne intoxication due to toxins of Clostridium botulinum [C. botulinum]

   EXCLUDES 1   food poisoning due to toxins of Clostridium botulinum (A05.1)

   A48.51 Infant botulism   P

   A48.52 Wound botulism

Non-foodborne botulism NOS

Use additional code for associated wound

A48.8 Other specified bacterial diseases

✅ Additional Character Required   ✓x7ᵗʰ Placeholder Alert   Manifestation   Unspecified Dx   ►◄ Revised Text   ● New Code   ▲ Revised Title

✔4ᵗʰ **A49 Bacterial infection of unspecified site**

> EXCLUDES 1   *bacterial agents as the cause of diseases classified elsewhere (B95-B96)*
> *chlamydial infection NOS (A74.9)*
> *meningococcal infection NOS (A39.9)*
> *rickettsial infection NOS (A79.9)*
> *spirochetal infection NOS (A69.9)*

✔5ᵗʰ **A49.0 Staphylococcal infection, unspecified site**

> **A49.01 Methicillin susceptible Staphylococcus aureus infection, unspecified site**
> Methicillin susceptible Staphylococcus aureus (MSSA) infection
> Staphylococcus aureus infection NOS

> **A49.02 Methicillin resistant Staphylococcus aureus infection, unspecified site**
> Methicillin resistant Staphylococcus aureus (MRSA) infection

A49.1 Streptococcal infection, unspecified site

A49.2 Hemophilus influenzae infection, unspecified site

A49.3 Mycoplasma infection, unspecified site

A49.8 Other bacterial infections of unspecified site

A49.9 Bacterial infection, unspecified

> EXCLUDES 1   *bacteremia NOS (R78.81)*

Infections with a predominantly sexual mode of transmission (A50-A64)

> EXCLUDES 1   *human immunodeficiency virus [HIV] disease (B20)*
> *nonspecific and nongonococcal urethritis (N34.1)*
> *Reiter's disease (M02.3-)*

✔4ᵗʰ **A50 Congenital syphilis**

✔5ᵗʰ **A50.0 Early congenital syphilis, symptomatic**

> Any congenital syphilitic condition specified as early or manifest less than two years after birth.

> **A50.01 Early congenital syphilitic oculopathy**
> **A50.02 Early congenital syphilitic osteochondropathy**
> **A50.03 Early congenital syphilitic pharyngitis**
> Early congenital syphilitic laryngitis
> **A50.04 Early congenital syphilitic pneumonia**
> **A50.05 Early congenital syphilitic rhinitis**
> **A50.06 Early cutaneous congenital syphilis**
> **A50.07 Early mucocutaneous congenital syphilis**
> **A50.08 Early visceral congenital syphilis**
> **A50.09 Other early congenital syphilis, symptomatic**

A50.1 Early congenital syphilis, latent

> Congenital syphilis without clinical manifestations, with positive serological reaction and negative spinal fluid test, less than two years after birth.

A50.2 Early congenital syphilis, unspecified

> Congenital syphilis NOS less than two years after birth.

✔5ᵗʰ **A50.3 Late congenital syphilitic oculopathy**

> EXCLUDES 1   *Hutchinson's triad (A50.53)*

> **A50.30 Late congenital syphilitic oculopathy, unspecified**
> **A50.31 Late congenital syphilitic interstitial keratitis**
> **A50.32 Late congenital syphilitic chorioretinitis**
> **A50.39 Other late congenital syphilitic oculopathy**

✔5ᵗʰ **A50.4 Late congenital neurosyphilis [juvenile neurosyphilis]**

> Use additional code to identify any associated mental disorder
> EXCLUDES 1   *Hutchinson's triad (A50.53)*

> **A50.40 Late congenital neurosyphilis, unspecified**
> Juvenile neurosyphilis NOS
> **A50.41 Late congenital syphilitic meningitis**
> **A50.42 Late congenital syphilitic encephalitis**
> **A50.43 Late congenital syphilitic polyneuropathy**
> **A50.44 Late congenital syphilitic optic nerve atrophy**
> **A50.45 Juvenile general paresis**
> Dementia paralytica juvenilis
> Juvenile tabetoparetic neurosyphilis
> **A50.49 Other late congenital neurosyphilis**
> Juvenile tabes dorsalis

✔5ᵗʰ **A50.5 Other late congenital syphilis, symptomatic**

> Any congenital syphilitic condition specified as late or manifest two years or more after birth.

> **A50.51 Clutton's joints**
> **A50.52 Hutchinson's teeth**
> **A50.53 Hutchinson's triad**

A50.54 Late congenital cardiovascular syphilis

A50.55 Late congenital syphilitic arthropathy

A50.56 Late congenital syphilitic osteochondropathy

A50.57 Syphilitic saddle nose

A50.59 Other late congenital syphilis, symptomatic

A50.6 Late congenital syphilis, latent

> Congenital syphilis without clinical manifestations, with positive serological reaction and negative spinal fluid test, two years or more after birth.

A50.7 Late congenital syphilis, unspecified

> Congenital syphilis NOS two years or more after birth.

A50.9 Congenital syphilis, unspecified

✔4ᵗʰ **A51 Early syphilis**

> **DEF:** Syphilis: Sexually transmitted disease caused by the treponema pallidum spirochete. Syphilis usually exhibits cutaneous manifestations and may exist for years without symptoms.

A51.0 Primary genital syphilis

> Syphilitic chancre NOS

A51.1 Primary anal syphilis

A51.2 Primary syphilis of other sites

✔5ᵗʰ **A51.3 Secondary syphilis of skin and mucous membranes**

> **DEF:** Transitory or chronic cutaneous eruptions that present within two to 10 weeks following an initial syphilis infection that may include nontender lymphadenopathy along with alopecia and condylomata lata.

> **A51.31 Condyloma latum**
> **A51.32 Syphilitic alopecia**
> **A51.39 Other secondary syphilis of skin**
> Syphilitic leukoderma
> Syphilitic mucous patch
> EXCLUDES 1   *late syphilitic leukoderma (A52.79)*

✔5ᵗʰ **A51.4 Other secondary syphilis**

> **A51.41 Secondary syphilitic meningitis**
> **A51.42 Secondary syphilitic female pelvic disease** ♀
> **A51.43 Secondary syphilitic oculopathy**
> Secondary syphilitic chorioretinitis
> Secondary syphilitic iridocyclitis, iritis
> Secondary syphilitic uveitis
> **A51.44 Secondary syphilitic nephritis**
> **A51.45 Secondary syphilitic hepatitis**
> **A51.46 Secondary syphilitic osteopathy**
> **A51.49 Other secondary syphilitic conditions**
> Secondary syphilitic lymphadenopathy
> Secondary syphilitic myositis

A51.5 Early syphilis, latent

> Syphilis (acquired) without clinical manifestations, with positive serological reaction and negative spinal fluid test, less than two years after infection.

A51.9 Early syphilis, unspecified

✔4ᵗʰ **A52 Late syphilis**

✔5ᵗʰ **A52.0 Cardiovascular and cerebrovascular syphilis**

> **A52.00 Cardiovascular syphilis, unspecified**
> **A52.01 Syphilitic aneurysm of aorta**
> **A52.02 Syphilitic aortitis**
> **A52.03 Syphilitic endocarditis**
> Syphilitic aortic valve incompetence or stenosis
> Syphilitic mitral valve stenosis
> Syphilitic pulmonary valve regurgitation
> **A52.04 Syphilitic cerebral arteritis**
> **A52.05 Other cerebrovascular syphilis**
> Syphilitic cerebral aneurysm (ruptured) (non-ruptured)
> Syphilitic cerebral thrombosis
> **A52.06 Other syphilitic heart involvement**
> Syphilitic coronary artery disease
> Syphilitic myocarditis
> Syphilitic pericarditis
> **A52.09 Other cardiovascular syphilis**

✔5ᵗʰ **A52.1 Symptomatic neurosyphilis**

> **A52.10 Symptomatic neurosyphilis, unspecified**
> **A52.11 Tabes dorsalis**
> Locomotor ataxia (progressive)
> Tabetic neurosyphilis
> **A52.12 Other cerebrospinal syphilis**
> **A52.13 Late syphilitic meningitis**

| N Newborn: 0 | P Pediatric: 0-17 | M Maternity: 12-55 | A Adult: 15-124 | CH Comorbidity High | CL Comorbidity Low | NCDx Noncancer Dx | PDx Primary Dx |

442   ICD-10-CM 2020

A52.14   **Late syphilitic** encephalitis

A52.15   **Late syphilitic** neuropathy
Late syphilitic acoustic neuritis
Late syphilitic optic (nerve) atrophy
Late syphilitic polyneuropathy
Late syphilitic retrobulbar neuritis

A52.16   **Charcôt's arthropathy (tabetic)**
DEF: Progressive neurologic arthropathy in which chronic degeneration of joints in the weight-bearing areas with peripheral hypertrophy occurs as a complication of a neuropathy disorder. Supporting structures relax from a loss of sensation resulting in chronic joint instability.

A52.17   General paresis
Dementia paralytica

A52.19   **Other symptomatic neurosyphilis**
Syphilitic parkinsonism

A52.2   Asymptomatic **neurosyphilis**

A52.3   **Neurosyphilis, unspecified**
Gumma (syphilitic)
Syphilis (late)
Syphiloma

✓5ᵗʰ A52.7   **Other symptomatic late syphilis**

A52.71   **Late syphilitic** oculopathy
Late syphilitic chorioretinitis
Late syphilitic episcleritis

A52.72   **Syphilis of** lung and bronchus

A52.73   **Symptomatic late syphilis of other respiratory organs**

A52.74   **Syphilis of** liver and other viscera
Late syphilitic peritonitis

A52.75   **Syphilis of** kidney and ureter
Syphilitic glomerular disease

A52.76   **Other genitourinary symptomatic late syphilis**
Late syphilitic female pelvic inflammatory disease

A52.77   **Syphilis of** bone and joint

A52.78   **Syphilis of other musculoskeletal tissue**
Late syphilitic bursitis
Syphilis [stage unspecified] of bursa
Syphilis [stage unspecified] of muscle
Syphilis [stage unspecified] of synovium
Syphilis [stage unspecified] of tendon

A52.79   **Other symptomatic late syphilis**
Late syphilitic leukoderma
Syphilis of adrenal gland
Syphilis of pituitary gland
Syphilis of thyroid gland
Syphilitic splenomegaly
EXCLUDES 1   syphilitic leukoderma (secondary) (A51.39)

A52.8   **Late syphilis,** latent
Syphilis (acquired) without clinical manifestations, with positive serological reaction and negative spinal fluid test, two years or more after infection

A52.9   **Late syphilis, unspecified**

✓4ᵗʰ **A53**   **Other and unspecified syphilis**

A53.0   Latent **syphilis, unspecified as early or late**
Latent syphilis NOS
Positive serological reaction for syphilis

A53.9   **Syphilis, unspecified**
Infection due to Treponema pallidum NOS
Syphilis (acquired) NOS
EXCLUDES 1   syphilis NOS under two years of age (A50.2)

✓4ᵗʰ **A54**   **Gonococcal infection**
DEF: Sexually transmitted bacterial infection caused by Neisseria gonorrhoeae. Women are often asymptomatic, while men tend to develop urinary symptoms quickly.

✓5ᵗʰ A54.0   **Gonococcal infection of** lower genitourinary tract without periurethral or accessory gland abscess
EXCLUDES 1   gonococcal infection with genitourinary gland abscess (A54.1)
gonococcal infection with periurethral abscess (A54.1)

A54.00   **Gonococcal infection of lower genitourinary tract, unspecified**

A54.01   **Gonococcal** cystitis and urethritis, **unspecified**

A54.02   **Gonococcal** vulvovaginitis, **unspecified**   ♀

A54.03   **Gonococcal** cervicitis, **unspecified**   ♀

A54.09   **Other gonococcal infection of lower genitourinary tract**

A54.1   **Gonococcal infection of** lower genitourinary tract with periurethral and accessory gland abscess
Gonococcal Bartholin's gland abscess

✓5ᵗʰ A54.2   **Gonococcal** pelviperitonitis **and other gonococcal genitourinary infection**

A54.21   **Gonococcal infection of** kidney and ureter

A54.22   **Gonococcal** prostatitis   ♂

A54.23   **Gonococcal infection of other** male genital organs   ♂
Gonococcal epididymitis
Gonococcal orchitis

A54.24   **Gonococcal** female pelvic inflammatory **disease**   ♀
Gonococcal pelviperitonitis
EXCLUDES 1   gonococcal peritonitis (A54.85)

A54.29   **Other gonococcal genitourinary infections**

✓5ᵗʰ A54.3   **Gonococcal infection of** eye

A54.30   **Gonococcal infection of eye, unspecified**

A54.31   **Gonococcal** conjunctivitis
Ophthalmia neonatorum due to gonococcus

A54.32   **Gonococcal** iridocyclitis

A54.33   **Gonococcal** keratitis

A54.39   **Other gonococcal eye infection**
Gonococcal endophthalmia

✓5ᵗʰ A54.4   **Gonococcal infection of** musculoskeletal system

A54.40   **Gonococcal infection of musculoskeletal system, unspecified**

A54.41   **Gonococcal** spondylopathy

A54.42   **Gonococcal** arthritis
EXCLUDES 2   gonococcal infection of spine (A54.41)

A54.43   **Gonococcal** osteomyelitis
EXCLUDES 2   gonococcal infection of spine (A54.41)

A54.49   **Gonococcal infection of other musculoskeletal tissue**
Gonococcal bursitis
Gonococcal myositis
Gonococcal synovitis
Gonococcal tenosynovitis

A54.5   **Gonococcal** pharyngitis

A54.6   **Gonococcal infection of** anus and rectum

✓5ᵗʰ A54.8   **Other gonococcal infections**

A54.81   **Gonococcal** meningitis

A54.82   **Gonococcal** brain abscess

A54.83   **Gonococcal** heart infection
Gonococcal endocarditis
Gonococcal myocarditis
Gonococcal pericarditis

A54.84   **Gonococcal** pneumonia

A54.85   **Gonococcal** peritonitis
EXCLUDES 1   gonococcal pelviperitonitis (A54.24)

A54.86   **Gonococcal** sepsis

A54.89   **Other gonococcal infections**
Gonococcal keratoderma
Gonococcal lymphadenitis

A54.9   **Gonococcal infection, unspecified**

A55   **Chlamydial lymphogranuloma (venereum)**
Climatic or tropical bubo
Durand-Nicolas-Favre disease
Esthiomene
Lymphogranuloma inguinale

✓4ᵗʰ A56   Other sexually transmitted chlamydial diseases

> INCLUDES   sexually transmitted diseases due to Chlamydia trachomatis
>
> EXCLUDES 1   neonatal chlamydial conjunctivitis (P39.1)
>   neonatal chlamydial pneumonia (P23.1)
>
> EXCLUDES 2   chlamydial lymphogranuloma (A55)
>   conditions classified to A74.-

DEF: Chlamydia trachomatis: Bacterium that causes a common venereal disease. Symptoms of chlamydia are usually mild or absent, however, serious complications may cause irreversible damage, including cystitis, pelvic inflammatory disease, and infertility in women and discharge from the penis, prostatitis, and infertility in men. Genital chlamydial infection can cause arthritis, skin lesions, and inflammation of the eye and urethra. **Synonym(s):** Reiter's syndrome.

✓5ᵗʰ A56.0   Chlamydial infection of lower genitourinary tract

     A56.00   Chlamydial infection of lower genitourinary tract, unspecified

     A56.01   Chlamydial cystitis and urethritis

     A56.02   Chlamydial vulvovaginitis   ♀

     A56.09   Other chlamydial infection of lower genitourinary tract
              Chlamydial cervicitis

✓5ᵗʰ A56.1   Chlamydial infection of pelviperitoneum and other genitourinary organs

     A56.11   Chlamydial female pelvic inflammatory disease   ♀

     A56.19   Other chlamydial genitourinary infection
              Chlamydial epididymitis
              Chlamydial orchitis

   A56.2   Chlamydial infection of genitourinary tract, unspecified

   A56.3   Chlamydial infection of anus and rectum

   A56.4   Chlamydial infection of pharynx

   A56.8   Sexually transmitted chlamydial infection of other sites

A57   Chancroid
     Ulcus molle
     DEF: Localized infection by *Haemophilus ducreyi,* causing genital ulcers and infecting the inguinal lymph nodes.

A58   Granuloma inguinale
     Donovanosis

✓4ᵗʰ A59   Trichomoniasis

> EXCLUDES 2   intestinal trichomoniasis (A07.8)

DEF: Infection with the parasitic, flagellated protozoa of the genus *Trichomonas*. This protozoon is found in the intestinal and genitourinary tracts of humans and in the mouth around tartar, cavities, and areas of periodontal disease.

✓5ᵗʰ A59.0   Urogenital trichomoniasis

     A59.00   Urogenital trichomoniasis, unspecified
              Fluor (vaginalis) due to Trichomonas
              Leukorrhea (vaginalis) due to Trichomonas

     A59.01   Trichomonal vulvovaginitis   ♀

     A59.02   Trichomonal prostatitis   ♂

     A59.03   Trichomonal cystitis and urethritis

     A59.09   Other urogenital trichomoniasis
              Trichomonas cervicitis

   A59.8   Trichomoniasis of other sites

   A59.9   Trichomoniasis, unspecified

✓4ᵗʰ A60   Anogenital herpesviral [herpes simplex] infections

✓5ᵗʰ A60.0   Herpesviral infection of genitalia and urogenital tract

     A60.00   Herpesviral infection of urogenital system, unspecified

     A60.01   Herpesviral infection of penis   ♂

     A60.02   Herpesviral infection of other male genital organs   ♂

     A60.03   Herpesviral cervicitis   ♀

     A60.04   Herpesviral vulvovaginitis   ♀
              Herpesviral [herpes simplex] ulceration
              Herpesviral [herpes simplex] vaginitis
              Herpesviral [herpes simplex] vulvitis

     A60.09   Herpesviral infection of other urogenital tract

   A60.1   Herpesviral infection of perianal skin and rectum

   A60.9   Anogenital herpesviral infection, unspecified

✓4ᵗʰ A63   Other predominantly sexually transmitted diseases, not elsewhere classified

> EXCLUDES 2   molluscum contagiosum (B08.1)
>   papilloma of cervix (D26.0)

   A63.0   Anogenital (venereal) warts
              Anogenital warts due to (human) papillomavirus [HPV]
              Condyloma acuminatum

   A63.8   Other specified predominantly sexually transmitted diseases

A64   Unspecified sexually transmitted disease

Other spirochetal diseases (A65-A69)

> EXCLUDES 2   leptospirosis (A27.-)
>   syphilis (A50-A53)

A65   Nonvenereal syphilis
     Bejel
     Endemic syphilis
     Njovera

✓4ᵗʰ A66   Yaws

> INCLUDES   bouba
>   frambesia (tropica)
>   pian

   A66.0   Initial lesions of yaws
              Chancre of yaws
              Frambesia, initial or primary
              Initial frambesial ulcer
              Mother yaw

   A66.1   Multiple papillomata and wet crab yaws
              Frambesioma
              Pianoma
              Plantar or palmar papilloma of yaws

   A66.2   Other early skin lesions of yaws
              Cutaneous yaws, less than five years after infection
              Early yaws (cutaneous) (macular) (maculopapular)
                (micropapular) (papular)
              Frambeside of early yaws

   A66.3   Hyperkeratosis of yaws
              Ghoul hand
              Hyperkeratosis, palmar or plantar (early) (late) due to yaws
              Worm-eaten soles

   A66.4   Gummata and ulcers of yaws
              Gummatous frambeside
              Nodular late yaws (ulcerated)

   A66.5   Gangosa
              Rhinopharyngitis mutilans

   A66.6   Bone and joint lesions of yaws
              Yaws ganglion
              Yaws goundou
              Yaws gumma, bone
              Yaws gummatous osteitis or periostitis
              Yaws hydrarthrosis
              Yaws osteitis
              Yaws periostitis (hypertrophic)

   A66.7   Other manifestations of yaws
              Juxta-articular nodules of yaws
              Mucosal yaws

   A66.8   Latent yaws
              Yaws without clinical manifestations, with positive serology

   A66.9   Yaws, unspecified

✓4ᵗʰ A67   Pinta [carate]

   A67.0   Primary lesions of pinta
              Chancre (primary) of pinta
              Papule (primary) of pinta

   A67.1   Intermediate lesions of pinta
              Erythematous plaques of pinta
              Hyperchromic lesions of pinta
              Hyperkeratosis of pinta
              Pintids

   A67.2   Late lesions of pinta
              Achromic skin lesions of pinta
              Cicatricial skin lesions of pinta
              Dyschromic skin lesions of pinta

   A67.3   Mixed lesions of pinta
              Achromic with hyperchromic skin lesions of pinta [carate]

   A67.9   Pinta, unspecified

N Newborn: 0   P Pediatric: 0-17   M Maternity: 12-55   A Adult: 15-124   CH Comorbidity High   CL Comorbidity Low   NCDx Noncancer Dx   PDx Primary Dx

444   ICD-10-CM 2020

✓4ᵗʰ **A68** **Relapsing fevers**

INCLUDES   recurrent fever

EXCLUDES 2   *Lyme disease (A69.2-)*

A68.0 **Louse-borne relapsing fever**
Relapsing fever due to Borrelia recurrentis

A68.1 **Tick-borne relapsing fever**
Relapsing fever due to any Borrelia species other than Borrelia recurrentis

A68.9 **Relapsing fever, unspecified**

✓4ᵗʰ **A69** **Other spirochetal infections**

A69.0 **Necrotizing ulcerative stomatitis**
Cancrum oris
Fusospirochetal gangrene
Noma
Stomatitis gangrenosa

A69.1 **Other Vincent's infections**
Fusospirochetal pharyngitis
Necrotizing ulcerative (acute) gingivitis
Necrotizing ulcerative (acute) gingivostomatitis
Spirochetal stomatitis
Trench mouth
Vincent's angina
Vincent's gingivitis

✓5ᵗʰ **A69.2** **Lyme disease**
Erythema chronicum migrans due to Borrelia burgdorferi
DEF: Recurrent multisystem disorder through tick bites that begins with lesions of erythema chronicum migrans and is followed by arthritis of the large joints, myalgia, malaise, and neurological and cardiac manifestations.

A69.20 **Lyme disease, unspecified**

A69.21 **Meningitis due to Lyme disease**

A69.22 **Other neurologic disorders in Lyme disease**
Cranial neuritis
Meningoencephalitis
Polyneuropathy

A69.23 **Arthritis due to Lyme disease**

A69.29 **Other conditions associated with Lyme disease**
Myopericarditis due to Lyme disease
AHA: 2016,3Q,12

A69.8 **Other specified spirochetal infections**

A69.9 **Spirochetal infection, unspecified**

Other diseases caused by chlamydiae (A70-A74)

EXCLUDES 1   *sexually transmitted chlamydial diseases (A55-A56)*

A70 **Chlamydia psittaci infections**
Ornithosis
Parrot fever
Psittacosis

✓4ᵗʰ **A71** **Trachoma**

EXCLUDES 1   *sequelae of trachoma (B94.0)*

A71.0 **Initial stage of trachoma**
Trachoma dubium

A71.1 **Active stage of trachoma**
Granular conjunctivitis (trachomatous)
Trachomatous follicular conjunctivitis
Trachomatous pannus

A71.9 **Trachoma, unspecified**

✓4ᵗʰ **A74** **Other diseases caused by chlamydiae**

EXCLUDES 1   *neonatal chlamydial conjunctivitis (P39.1)*
neonatal chlamydial pneumonia (P23.1)
Reiter's disease (M02.3-)
sexually transmitted chlamydial diseases (A55-A56)

EXCLUDES 2   *chlamydial pneumonia (J16.0)*

A74.0 **Chlamydial conjunctivitis**
Paratrachoma

✓5ᵗʰ **A74.8** **Other chlamydial diseases**

A74.81 **Chlamydial peritonitis**

A74.89 **Other chlamydial diseases**

A74.9 **Chlamydial infection, unspecified**
Chlamydiosis NOS

Rickettsioses (A75-A79)

DEF: Rickettsia: Condition caused by bacteria that live in lice/ticks transmitted to humans through bites.

✓4ᵗʰ **A75** **Typhus fever**

EXCLUDES 1   *rickettsiosis due to Ehrlichia sennetsu (A79.81)*

A75.0 **Epidemic louse-borne typhus fever due to Rickettsia prowazekii**
Classical typhus (fever)
Epidemic (louse-borne) typhus

A75.1 **Recrudescent typhus [Brill's disease]**
Brill-Zinsser disease

A75.2 **Typhus fever due to Rickettsia typhi**
Murine (flea-borne) typhus

A75.3 **Typhus fever due to Rickettsia tsutsugamushi**
Scrub (mite-borne) typhus
Tsutsugamushi fever

A75.9 **Typhus fever, unspecified**
Typhus (fever) NOS

✓4ᵗʰ **A77** **Spotted fever [tick-borne rickettsioses]**

A77.0 **Spotted fever due to Rickettsia rickettsii**
Rocky Mountain spotted fever
Sao Paulo fever

A77.1 **Spotted fever due to Rickettsia conorii**
African tick typhus
Boutonneuse fever
India tick typhus
Kenya tick typhus
Marseilles fever
Mediterranean tick fever

A77.2 **Spotted fever due to Rickettsia siberica**
North Asian tick fever
Siberian tick typhus

A77.3 **Spotted fever due to Rickettsia australis**
Queensland tick typhus

✓5ᵗʰ **A77.4** **Ehrlichiosis**

EXCLUDES 1   *Rickettsiosis due to Ehrlichia sennetsu (A79.81)*

A77.40 **Ehrlichiosis, unspecified**

A77.41 **Ehrlichiosis chaffeensis [E. chaffeensis]**

A77.49 **Other ehrlichiosis**

A77.8 **Other spotted fevers**

A77.9 **Spotted fever, unspecified**
Tick-borne typhus NOS

A78 **Q fever**
Infection due to Coxiella burnetii
Nine Mile fever
Quadrilateral fever

✓4ᵗʰ **A79** **Other rickettsioses**

A79.0 **Trench fever**
Quintan fever
Wolhynian fever

A79.1 **Rickettsialpox due to Rickettsia akari**
Kew Garden fever
Vesicular rickettsiosis

✓5ᵗʰ **A79.8** **Other specified rickettsioses**

A79.81 **Rickettsiosis due to Ehrlichia sennetsu**

A79.89 **Other specified rickettsioses**

A79.9 **Rickettsiosis, unspecified**
Rickettsial infection NOS

Viral and prion infections of the central nervous system (A80-A89)

EXCLUDES 1   *postpolio syndrome (G14)*
sequelae of poliomyelitis (B91)
sequelae of viral encephalitis (B94.1)

✓4ᵗʰ **A80** **Acute poliomyelitis**

A80.0 **Acute paralytic poliomyelitis, vaccine-associated**

A80.1 **Acute paralytic poliomyelitis, wild virus, imported**

A80.2 **Acute paralytic poliomyelitis, wild virus, indigenous**

✓5ᵗʰ **A80.3** **Acute paralytic poliomyelitis, other and unspecified**

A80.30 **Acute paralytic poliomyelitis, unspecified**

A80.39 **Other acute paralytic poliomyelitis**

A80.4 **Acute nonparalytic poliomyelitis**

A80.9 **Acute poliomyelitis, unspecified**

✓4ᵗʰ **A81 Atypical virus infections of central nervous system**

> INCLUDES   diseases of the central nervous system caused by prions
>
> Use additional code to identify:
> dementia with behavioral disturbance (F02.81)
> dementia without behavioral disturbance (F02.80)

✓5ᵗʰ **A81.0 Creutzfeldt-Jakob disease**

> **DEF:** Communicable, rare spongiform encephalopathy occurring later in life with progressive destruction of the pyramidal and extrapyramidal systems eventually leading to death. Progressive dementia, wasting of muscles, tremor, and other symptoms are present.

     A81.00 Creutzfeldt-Jakob disease, unspecified
         Jakob-Creutzfeldt disease, unspecified

     A81.01 Variant Creutzfeldt-Jakob disease
         vCJD

     A81.09 Other Creutzfeldt-Jakob disease
         CJD
         Familial Creutzfeldt-Jakob disease
         Iatrogenic Creutzfeldt-Jakob disease
         Sporadic Creutzfeldt-Jakob disease
         Subacute spongiform encephalopathy (with dementia)

A81.1 Subacute sclerosing panencephalitis
     Dawson's inclusion body encephalitis
     Van Bogaert's sclerosing leukoencephalopathy

A81.2 Progressive multifocal leukoencephalopathy
     Multifocal leukoencephalopathy NOS

✓5ᵗʰ **A81.8 Other atypical virus infections of central nervous system**

     A81.81 Kuru

     A81.82 Gerstmann-Sträussler-Scheinker syndrome
         GSS syndrome

     A81.83 Fatal familial insomnia
         FFI

     A81.89 Other atypical virus infections of central nervous system

A81.9 Atypical virus infection of central nervous system, unspecified
     Prion diseases of the central nervous system NOS

✓4ᵗʰ **A82 Rabies**

A82.0 Sylvatic rabies

A82.1 Urban rabies

A82.9 Rabies, unspecified

✓4ᵗʰ **A83 Mosquito-borne viral encephalitis**

> INCLUDES   mosquito-borne viral meningoencephalitis
> EXCLUDES 2   Venezuelan equine encephalitis (A92.2)
>   West Nile fever (A92.3-)
>   West Nile virus (A92.3-)

A83.0 Japanese encephalitis

A83.1 Western equine encephalitis

A83.2 Eastern equine encephalitis

A83.3 St Louis encephalitis

A83.4 Australian encephalitis
     Kunjin virus disease

A83.5 California encephalitis
     California meningoencephalitis
     La Crosse encephalitis

A83.6 Rocio virus disease

A83.8 Other mosquito-borne viral encephalitis

A83.9 Mosquito-borne viral encephalitis, unspecified

✓4ᵗʰ **A84 Tick-borne viral encephalitis**

> INCLUDES   tick-borne viral meningoencephalitis

A84.0 Far Eastern tick-borne encephalitis [Russian spring-summer encephalitis]

A84.1 Central European tick-borne encephalitis

A84.8 Other tick-borne viral encephalitis
     Louping ill
     Powassan virus disease

A84.9 Tick-borne viral encephalitis, unspecified

✓4ᵗʰ **A85 Other viral encephalitis, not elsewhere classified**

> INCLUDES   specified viral encephalomyelitis NEC
>   specified viral meningoencephalitis NEC
> EXCLUDES 1   benign myalgic encephalomyelitis (G93.3)
>   encephalitis due to cytomegalovirus (B25.8)
>   encephalitis due to herpesvirus NEC (B10.0-)
>   encephalitis due to herpesvirus [herpes simplex] (B00.4)
>   encephalitis due to measles virus (B05.0)
>   encephalitis due to mumps virus (B26.2)
>   encephalitis due to poliomyelitis virus (A80.-)
>   encephalitis due to zoster (B02.0)
>   lymphocytic choriomeningitis (A87.2)

A85.0 Enteroviral encephalitis
     Enteroviral encephalomyelitis

A85.1 Adenoviral encephalitis
     Adenoviral meningoencephalitis

A85.2 Arthropod-borne viral encephalitis, unspecified
> EXCLUDES 1   West nile virus with encephalitis (A92.31)

A85.8 Other specified viral encephalitis
     Encephalitis lethargica
     Von Economo-Cruchet disease

A86 Unspecified viral encephalitis
     Viral encephalomyelitis NOS
     Viral meningoencephalitis NOS

✓4ᵗʰ **A87 Viral meningitis**

> EXCLUDES 1   meningitis due to herpesvirus [herpes simplex] (B00.3)
>   meningitis due to measles virus (B05.1)
>   meningitis due to mumps virus (B26.1)
>   meningitis due to poliomyelitis virus (A80.-)
>   meningitis due to zoster (B02.1)

> **DEF:** Meningitis: Inflammation of the meningeal layers of the brain and spine.

A87.0 Enteroviral meningitis
     Coxsackievirus meningitis
     Echovirus meningitis

A87.1 Adenoviral meningitis

A87.2 Lymphocytic choriomeningitis
     Lymphocytic meningoencephalitis

A87.8 Other viral meningitis

A87.9 Viral meningitis, unspecified

✓4ᵗʰ **A88 Other viral infections of central nervous system, not elsewhere classified**

> EXCLUDES 1   viral encephalitis NOS (A86)
>   viral meningitis NOS (A87.9)

A88.0 Enteroviral exanthematous fever [Boston exanthem]

A88.1 Epidemic vertigo

A88.8 Other specified viral infections of central nervous system

A89 Unspecified viral infection of central nervous system

Arthropod-borne viral fevers and viral hemorrhagic fevers (A90-A99)

A90 Dengue fever [classical dengue]
> EXCLUDES 1   dengue hemorrhagic fever (A91)
> **AHA:** 2016,3Q,13

A91 Dengue hemorrhagic fever

✓4ᵗʰ **A92 Other mosquito-borne viral fevers**
> EXCLUDES 1   Ross River disease (B33.1)

A92.0 Chikungunya virus disease
     Chikungunya (hemorrhagic) fever

A92.1 O'nyong-nyong fever

A92.2 Venezuelan equine fever
     Venezuelan equine encephalitis
     Venezuelan equine encephalomyelitis virus disease

✓5ᵗʰ **A92.3 West Nile virus infection**
     West Nile fever
     AHA: 2016,3Q,12

     A92.30 West Nile virus infection, unspecified
         West Nile fever NOS
         West Nile fever without complications
         West Nile virus NOS

     A92.31 West Nile virus infection with encephalitis
         West Nile encephalitis
         West Nile encephalomyelitis

A92.32   **West Nile virus infection with other neurologic manifestation**
Use additional code to specify the neurologic manifestation

A92.39   **West Nile virus infection with other complications**
Use additional code to specify the other conditions

A92.4   **Rift Valley fever**

A92.5   **Zika virus disease**
Zika virus fever
Zika virus infection
Zika NOS
EXCLUDES 1   congenital Zika virus disease (P35.4)
AHA: 2016,4Q,4-7
DEF: Virus transmitted via a bite from an infected Aedes species mosquito. Common symptoms of the virus include fever, rash, joint pain, and conjunctivitis; they are usually mild in nature and may last from several days to a week. Most people who have the Zika virus do not require medical attention; however, in pregnant women, the Zika virus can cause a serious birth defect called microcephaly, as well as other severe fetal brain defects.

A92.8   **Other specified mosquito-borne viral fevers**

A92.9   **Mosquito-borne viral fever, unspecified**

✓4ᵗʰ **A93**   **Other arthropod-borne viral fevers, not elsewhere classified**

A93.0   **Oropouche virus disease**
Oropouche fever

A93.1   **Sandfly fever**
Pappataci fever
Phlebotomus fever

A93.2   **Colorado tick fever**

A93.8   **Other specified arthropod-borne viral fevers**
Piry virus disease
Vesicular stomatitis virus disease [Indiana fever]

A94   **Unspecified arthropod-borne viral fever**
Arboviral fever NOS
Arbovirus infection NOS

✓4ᵗʰ **A95**   **Yellow fever**

A95.0   **Sylvatic yellow fever**
Jungle yellow fever

A95.1   **Urban yellow fever**

A95.9   **Yellow fever, unspecified**

✓4ᵗʰ **A96**   **Arenaviral hemorrhagic fever**

A96.0   **Junin hemorrhagic fever**
Argentinian hemorrhagic fever

A96.1   **Machupo hemorrhagic fever**
Bolivian hemorrhagic fever

A96.2   **Lassa fever**

A96.8   **Other arenaviral hemorrhagic fevers**

A96.9   **Arenaviral hemorrhagic fever, unspecified**

✓4ᵗʰ **A98**   **Other viral hemorrhagic fevers, not elsewhere classified**
EXCLUDES 1   chikungunya hemorrhagic fever (A92.0)
dengue hemorrhagic fever (A91)

A98.0   **Crimean-Congo hemorrhagic fever**
Central Asian hemorrhagic fever

A98.1   **Omsk hemorrhagic fever**

A98.2   **Kyasanur Forest disease**

A98.3   **Marburg virus disease**

A98.4   **Ebola virus disease**

A98.5   **Hemorrhagic fever with renal syndrome**
Epidemic hemorrhagic fever
Korean hemorrhagic fever
Russian hemorrhagic fever
Hantaan virus disease
Hantavirus disease with renal manifestations
Nephropathia epidemica
Songo fever
EXCLUDES 1   hantavirus (cardio)-pulmonary syndrome (B33.4)

A98.8   **Other specified viral hemorrhagic fevers**

A99   **Unspecified viral hemorrhagic fever**

Viral infections characterized by skin and mucous membrane lesions (B00-B09)

✓4ᵗʰ **B00**   **Herpesviral [herpes simplex] infections**
EXCLUDES 1   congenital herpesviral infections (P35.2)
EXCLUDES 2   anogenital herpesviral infection (A60.-)
gammaherpesviral mononucleosis (B27.0-)
herpangina (B08.5)

B00.0   **Eczema herpeticum**
Kaposi's varicelliform eruption

B00.1   **Herpesviral vesicular dermatitis**
Herpes simplex facialis
Herpes simplex labialis
Herpes simplex otitis externa
Vesicular dermatitis of ear
Vesicular dermatitis of lip

B00.2   **Herpesviral gingivostomatitis and pharyngotonsillitis**
Herpesviral pharyngitis

B00.3   **Herpesviral meningitis**

B00.4   **Herpesviral encephalitis**
Herpesviral meningoencephalitis
Simian B disease
EXCLUDES 1   herpesviral encephalitis due to herpesvirus 6 and 7 (B10.01, B10.09)
non-simplex herpesviral encephalitis (B10.0-)

✓5ᵗʰ **B00.5**   **Herpesviral ocular disease**

B00.50   **Herpesviral ocular disease, unspecified**

B00.51   **Herpesviral iridocyclitis**
Herpesviral iritis
Herpesviral uveitis, anterior

B00.52   **Herpesviral keratitis**
Herpesviral keratoconjunctivitis

B00.53   **Herpesviral conjunctivitis**

B00.59   **Other herpesviral disease of eye**
Herpesviral dermatitis of eyelid

B00.7   **Disseminated herpesviral disease**
Herpesviral sepsis

✓5ᵗʰ **B00.8**   **Other forms of herpesviral infections**

B00.81   **Herpesviral hepatitis**

B00.82   **Herpes simplex myelitis**

B00.89   **Other herpesviral infection**
Herpesviral whitlow

B00.9   **Herpesviral infection, unspecified**
Herpes simplex infection NOS

✓4ᵗʰ **B01**   **Varicella [chickenpox]**

B01.0   **Varicella meningitis**

✓5ᵗʰ **B01.1**   **Varicella encephalitis, myelitis and encephalomyelitis**
Postchickenpox encephalitis, myelitis and encephalomyelitis

B01.11   **Varicella encephalitis and encephalomyelitis**
Postchickenpox encephalitis and encephalomyelitis

B01.12   **Varicella myelitis**
Postchickenpox myelitis

B01.2   **Varicella pneumonia**

✓5ᵗʰ **B01.8**   **Varicella with other complications**

B01.81   **Varicella keratitis**

B01.89   **Other varicella complications**

B01.9   **Varicella without complication**
Varicella NOS

✓4ᵗʰ **B02**   **Zoster [herpes zoster]**
INCLUDES   shingles
zona

B02.0   **Zoster encephalitis**
Zoster meningoencephalitis

B02.1   **Zoster meningitis**
AHA: 2019,1Q,18

✓5ᵗʰ **B02.2**   **Zoster with other nervous system involvement**

B02.21   **Postherpetic geniculate ganglionitis**

B02.22   **Postherpetic trigeminal neuralgia**

B02.23   **Postherpetic polyneuropathy**

B02.24   **Postherpetic myelitis**
Herpes zoster myelitis

B02.29   **Other postherpetic nervous system involvement**
Postherpetic radiculopathy

☑ Additional Character Required   ✓x7ᵗʰ Placeholder Alert   Manifestation   Unspecified Dx   ►◄ Revised Text   ● New Code   ▲ Revised Title

ICD-10-CM 2020   447

B02.3 Zoster ocular **disease**

     B02.30 Zoster ocular disease, unspecified

     B02.31 Zoster conjunctivitis

     B02.32 Zoster iridocyclitis

     B02.33 Zoster keratitis
         Herpes zoster keratoconjunctivitis

     B02.34 Zoster scleritis

     B02.39 Other herpes zoster eye disease
         Zoster blepharitis

B02.7 Disseminated zoster

B02.8 Zoster with other complications
     Herpes zoster otitis externa

B02.9 Zoster without complications
     Zoster NOS

B03 Smallpox

> **NOTE** In 1980 the 33rd World Health Assembly declared that smallpox had been eradicated.
>
> The classification is maintained for surveillance purposes.

B04 Monkeypox

B05 Measles

> **INCLUDES** morbilli
> **EXCLUDES 1** subacute sclerosing panencephalitis (A81.1)

B05.0 Measles complicated by encephalitis
     Postmeasles encephalitis

B05.1 Measles complicated by meningitis
     Postmeasles meningitis

B05.2 Measles complicated by pneumonia
     Postmeasles pneumonia

B05.3 Measles complicated by otitis media
     Postmeasles otitis media

B05.4 Measles with intestinal **complications**

B05.8 Measles with other complications

     B05.81 Measles keratitis and keratoconjunctivitis

     B05.89 Other measles complications

B05.9 Measles without complication
     Measles NOS

B06 Rubella [German measles]

> **EXCLUDES 1** congenital rubella (P35.0)

DEF: Highly contagious virus in which the symptoms are mild and short-lived in most people. Rubella during pregnancy, however, can result in abortion, stillbirth, or congenital defects.

B06.0 Rubella with neurological complications

     B06.00 Rubella with neurological complication, unspecified

     B06.01 Rubella encephalitis
         Rubella meningoencephalitis

     B06.02 Rubella meningitis

     B06.09 Other neurological complications of rubella

B06.8 Rubella with other complications

     B06.81 Rubella pneumonia

     B06.82 Rubella arthritis

     B06.89 Other rubella complications

B06.9 Rubella without complication
     Rubella NOS

B07 Viral warts

> **INCLUDES** verruca simplex
>   verruca vulgaris
>   viral warts due to human papillomavirus
> **EXCLUDES 2** anogenital (venereal) warts (A63.0)
>   papilloma of bladder (D41.4)
>   papilloma of cervix (D26.0)
>   papilloma larynx (D14.1)

B07.0 Plantar wart
     Verruca plantaris

B07.8 Other viral warts
     Common wart
     Flat wart
     Verruca plana

B07.9 Viral wart, unspecified

B08 Other viral infections characterized by skin and mucous membrane lesions, not elsewhere classified

> **EXCLUDES 1** vesicular stomatitis virus disease (A93.8)

B08.0 Other orthopoxvirus infections

> **EXCLUDES 2** monkeypox (B04)

     B08.01 Cowpox and vaccinia not from vaccine

         B08.010 Cowpox
             DEF: Disease contracted by milking infected cows. The vesicles usually appear on the fingers, hands, and adjacent areas and usually disappear without scarring. Other symptoms include local edema, lymphangitis, and regional lymphadenitis with or without fever.

         B08.011 Vaccinia not from vaccine
             EXCLUDES 1 vaccinia (from vaccination) (generalized) (T88.1)

     B08.02 Orf virus disease
         Contagious pustular dermatitis
         Ecthyma contagiosum

     B08.03 Pseudocowpox [milker's node]

     B08.04 Paravaccinia, unspecified

     B08.09 Other orthopoxvirus infections
         Orthopoxvirus infection NOS

B08.1 Molluscum contagiosum
     DEF: Benign poxvirus infection causing small bumps on the skin or conjunctiva and is transmitted by close contact.

B08.2 Exanthema subitum [sixth disease]

     Roseola infantum

     B08.20 Exanthema subitum [sixth disease], unspecified   P
         Roseola infantum, unspecified

     B08.21 Exanthema subitum [sixth disease] due to human herpesvirus 6   P
         Roseola infantum due to human herpesvirus 6

     B08.22 Exanthema subitum [sixth disease] due to human herpesvirus 7   P
         Roseola infantum due to human herpesvirus 7

B08.3 Erythema infectiosum [fifth disease]
     DEF: Infection with human parvovirus B19, mainly occurring in children. Symptoms include a low-grade fever, malaise, or a "cold" a few days before the appearance of a mild rash illness that presents as a "slapped-cheek" rash on the face and a lacy red rash on the trunk and limbs.

B08.4 Enteroviral vesicular stomatitis with exanthem
     Hand, foot and mouth disease

B08.5 Enteroviral vesicular pharyngitis
     Herpangina
     DEF: Acute infectious Coxsackie virus infection causing throat lesions, fever, and vomiting that generally affects children in the summer.

B08.6 Parapoxvirus infections

     B08.60 Parapoxvirus infection, unspecified

     B08.61 Bovine stomatitis

     B08.62 Sealpox

     B08.69 Other parapoxvirus infections

B08.7 Yatapoxvirus infections

     B08.70 Yatapoxvirus infection, unspecified

     B08.71 Tanapox virus disease

     B08.72 Yaba pox virus disease
         Yaba monkey tumor disease

     B08.79 Other yatapoxvirus infections

B08.8 Other specified viral infections characterized by skin and mucous membrane lesions
     Enteroviral lymphonodular pharyngitis
     Foot-and-mouth disease
     Poxvirus NEC

B09 Unspecified viral infection characterized by skin and mucous membrane lesions
     Viral enanthema NOS
     Viral exanthema NOS

N Newborn: 0   **P** Pediatric: 0-17   **M** Maternity: 12-55   **A** Adult: 15-124   **CH** Comorbidity High   **CL** Comorbidity Low   **NCDx** Noncancer Dx   **PDx** Primary Dx

448   ICD-10-CM 2020

Other human herpesviruses (B10)

☑4ᵗʰ B10 Other human herpesviruses

    EXCLUDES 2   *cytomegalovirus (B25.9)*
               Epstein-Barr virus (B27.0-)
               herpes NOS (B00.9)
               herpes simplex (B00.-)
               herpes zoster (B02.-)
               human herpesvirus NOS (B00.-)
               human herpesvirus 1 and 2 (B00.-)
               human herpesvirus 3 (B01.-, B02.-)
               human herpesvirus 4 (B27.0-)
               human herpesvirus 5 (B25.-)
               varicella (B01.-)
               zoster (B02.-)

  ☑5ᵗʰ B10.0 Other human herpesvirus encephalitis

    EXCLUDES 2   *herpes encephalitis NOS (B00.4)*
               herpes simplex encephalitis (B00.4)
               human herpesvirus encephalitis (B00.4)
               simian B herpes virus encephalitis (B00.4)

    B10.01 Human herpesvirus 6 encephalitis
    B10.09 Other human herpesvirus encephalitis
        Human herpesvirus 7 encephalitis

  ☑5ᵗʰ B10.8 Other human herpesvirus infection

    B10.81 Human herpesvirus 6 infection
    B10.82 Human herpesvirus 7 infection
    B10.89 Other human herpesvirus infection
        Human herpesvirus 8 infection
        Kaposi's sarcoma-associated herpesvirus infection

Viral hepatitis (B15-B19)

  EXCLUDES 1   *sequelae of viral hepatitis (B94.2)*
  EXCLUDES 2   *cytomegaloviral hepatitis (B25.1)*
               herpesviral [herpes simplex] hepatitis (B00.81)

DEF: Hepatitis A: HAV infection that is self-limiting with flulike symptoms. Transmission is fecal-oral.
DEF: Hepatitis B: HBV infection that can be chronic and systemic. Transmission is bodily fluids.
DEF: Hepatitis C: HCV infection that can be chronic and systemic. Transmission is blood transfusion and unidentified agents.
DEF: Hepatitis D (delta): HDV that occurs only in the presence of hepatitis B virus. Transmission is contaminated blood in contact with mucous membranes.
DEF: Hepatitis E: HEV is an epidemic form. Transmission is fecal-oral, most often from contaminated water.

☑4ᵗʰ B15 Acute hepatitis A

  B15.0 Hepatitis A with hepatic coma   NC Dx

  B15.9 Hepatitis A without hepatic coma
      Hepatitis A (acute)(viral) NOS

☑4ᵗʰ B16 Acute hepatitis B

  AHA: 2016,3Q,13

  B16.0 Acute hepatitis B with delta-agent with hepatic coma   NC Dx

  B16.1 Acute hepatitis B with delta-agent without hepatic coma

  B16.2 Acute hepatitis B without delta-agent with hepatic coma   NC Dx

  B16.9 Acute hepatitis B without delta-agent and without hepatic coma
      Hepatitis B (acute) (viral) NOS

☑4ᵗʰ B17 Other acute viral hepatitis

  B17.0 Acute delta-(super) infection of hepatitis B carrier
  ☑5ᵗʰ B17.1 Acute hepatitis C

    B17.10 Acute hepatitis C without hepatic coma
        Acute hepatitis C NOS

    B17.11 Acute hepatitis C with hepatic coma   NC Dx

  B17.2 Acute hepatitis E
  B17.8 Other specified acute viral hepatitis
      Hepatitis non-A non-B (acute) (viral) NEC

  B17.9 Acute viral hepatitis, unspecified
      Acute hepatitis NOS
      Acute infectious hepatitis NOS

☑4ᵗʰ B18 Chronic viral hepatitis

  INCLUDES carrier of viral hepatitis
  AHA: 2017,1Q,41

  B18.0 Chronic viral hepatitis B with delta-agent   NC Dx

  B18.1 Chronic viral hepatitis B without delta-agent   NC Dx
      Carrier of viral hepatitis B
      Chronic (viral) hepatitis B

  B18.2 Chronic viral hepatitis C   NC Dx
      Carrier of viral hepatitis C
      AHA: 2018,1Q,4

  B18.8 Other chronic viral hepatitis   NC Dx
      Carrier of other viral hepatitis

  B18.9 Chronic viral hepatitis, unspecified   NC Dx
      Carrier of unspecified viral hepatitis

☑4ᵗʰ B19 Unspecified viral hepatitis

  B19.0 Unspecified viral hepatitis with hepatic coma   NC Dx

  ☑5ᵗʰ B19.1 Unspecified viral hepatitis B

    B19.10 Unspecified viral hepatitis B without hepatic coma
        Unspecified viral hepatitis B NOS

    B19.11 Unspecified viral hepatitis B with hepatic coma   NC Dx

  ☑5ᵗʰ B19.2 Unspecified viral hepatitis C

    B19.20 Unspecified viral hepatitis C without hepatic coma
        Viral hepatitis C NOS

    B19.21 Unspecified viral hepatitis C with hepatic coma   NC Dx

  B19.9 Unspecified viral hepatitis without hepatic coma
      Viral hepatitis NOS

Human immunodeficiency virus [HIV] disease (B20)

B20 Human immunodeficiency virus [HIV] disease   NC Dx

  INCLUDES acquired immune deficiency syndrome [AIDS]
               AIDS-related complex [ARC]
               HIV infection, symptomatic

Code first Human immunodeficiency virus [HIV] disease complicating pregnancy, childbirth and the puerperium, if applicable (O98.7-)
Use additional code(s) to identify all manifestations of HIV infection

  EXCLUDES 1   *asymptomatic human immunodeficiency virus [HIV] infection status (Z21)*
               exposure to HIV virus (Z20.6)
               inconclusive serologic evidence of HIV (R75)

  AHA: 2019,1Q,8-11

Other viral diseases (B25-B34)

☑4ᵗʰ B25 Cytomegaloviral disease

  EXCLUDES 1   *congenital cytomegalovirus infection (P35.1)*
               cytomegaloviral mononucleosis (B27.1-)

  B25.0 Cytomegaloviral pneumonitis
  B25.1 Cytomegaloviral hepatitis
  B25.2 Cytomegaloviral pancreatitis
  B25.8 Other cytomegaloviral diseases
      Cytomegaloviral encephalitis
  B25.9 Cytomegaloviral disease, unspecified

☑4ᵗʰ B26 Mumps

  INCLUDES epidemic parotitis
               infectious parotitis

  B26.0 Mumps orchitis   ♂

  B26.1 Mumps meningitis
  B26.2 Mumps encephalitis
  B26.3 Mumps pancreatitis
  ☑5ᵗʰ B26.8 Mumps with other complications

    B26.81 Mumps hepatitis
    B26.82 Mumps myocarditis
    B26.83 Mumps nephritis
    B26.84 Mumps polyneuropathy
    B26.85 Mumps arthritis
    B26.89 Other mumps complications

  B26.9 Mumps without complication
      Mumps NOS
      Mumps parotitis NOS

Chapter 1. Certain Infectious and Parasitic Diseases

✓4ᵗʰ **B27 Infectious mononucleosis**

    INCLUDES   glandular fever
                monocytic angina
                Pfeiffer's disease

  ✓5ᵗʰ **B27.0 Gammaherpesviral mononucleosis**

      Mononucleosis due to Epstein-Barr virus

      B27.00 Gammaherpesviral mononucleosis without complication

      B27.01 Gammaherpesviral mononucleosis with polyneuropathy

      B27.02 Gammaherpesviral mononucleosis with meningitis

      B27.09 Gammaherpesviral mononucleosis with other complications
          Hepatomegaly in gammaherpesviral mononucleosis

  ✓5ᵗʰ **B27.1 Cytomegaloviral mononucleosis**

      B27.10 Cytomegaloviral mononucleosis without complications

      B27.11 Cytomegaloviral mononucleosis with polyneuropathy

      B27.12 Cytomegaloviral mononucleosis with meningitis

      B27.19 Cytomegaloviral mononucleosis with other complication
          Hepatomegaly in cytomegaloviral mononucleosis

  ✓5ᵗʰ **B27.8 Other infectious mononucleosis**

      B27.80 Other infectious mononucleosis without complication

      B27.81 Other infectious mononucleosis with polyneuropathy

      B27.82 Other infectious mononucleosis with meningitis

      B27.89 Other infectious mononucleosis with other complication
          Hepatomegaly in other infectious mononucleosis

  ✓5ᵗʰ **B27.9 Infectious mononucleosis, unspecified**

      B27.90 Infectious mononucleosis, unspecified without complication

      B27.91 Infectious mononucleosis, unspecified with polyneuropathy

      B27.92 Infectious mononucleosis, unspecified with meningitis

      B27.99 Infectious mononucleosis, unspecified with other complication
          Hepatomegaly in unspecified infectious mononucleosis

✓4ᵗʰ **B30 Viral conjunctivitis**

    EXCLUDES 1   *herpesviral [herpes simplex] ocular disease (B00.5)*
                ocular zoster (B02.3)

Viral Conjunctivitis

Normal conjunctiva

Inflamed conjunctiva

  B30.0 Keratoconjunctivitis due to adenovirus
      Epidemic keratoconjunctivitis
      Shipyard eye

  B30.1 Conjunctivitis due to adenovirus
      Acute adenoviral follicular conjunctivitis
      Swimming-pool conjunctivitis

  B30.2 Viral pharyngoconjunctivitis

  B30.3 Acute epidemic hemorrhagic conjunctivitis (enteroviral)
      Conjunctivitis due to coxsackievirus 24
      Conjunctivitis due to enterovirus 70
      Hemorrhagic conjunctivitis (acute)(epidemic)

  B30.8 Other viral conjunctivitis
      Newcastle conjunctivitis

  B30.9 Viral conjunctivitis, unspecified

✓4ᵗʰ **B33 Other viral diseases, not elsewhere classified**

  B33.0 Epidemic myalgia
      Bornholm disease

  B33.1 Ross River disease
      Epidemic polyarthritis and exanthema
      Ross River fever

  ✓5ᵗʰ **B33.2 Viral carditis**
      Coxsackie (virus) carditis

      B33.20 Viral carditis, unspecified
      B33.21 Viral endocarditis
      B33.22 Viral myocarditis
      B33.23 Viral pericarditis
      B33.24 Viral cardiomyopathy

  B33.3 Retrovirus infections, not elsewhere classified
      Retrovirus infection NOS

  B33.4 Hantavirus (cardio)-pulmonary syndrome [HPS] [HCPS]
      Hantavirus disease with pulmonary manifestations
      Sin nombre virus disease
      Use additional code to identify any associated acute kidney failure (N17.9)

      EXCLUDES 1   *hantavirus disease with renal manifestations (A98.5)*
                hemorrhagic fever with renal manifestations (A98.5)

  B33.8 Other specified viral diseases
      EXCLUDES 1   *anogenital human papillomavirus infection (A63.0)*
                viral warts due to human papillomavirus infection (B07)

✓4ᵗʰ **B34 Viral infection of unspecified site**

    EXCLUDES 1   *anogenital human papillomavirus infection (A63.0)*
              cytomegaloviral disease NOS (B25.9)
              herpesvirus [herpes simplex] infection NOS (B00.9)
              retrovirus infection NOS (B33.3)
              viral agents as the cause of diseases classified elsewhere (B97.-)
              viral warts due to human papillomavirus infection (B07)

  B34.0 Adenovirus infection, unspecified

  B34.1 Enterovirus infection, unspecified
      Coxsackievirus infection NOS
      Echovirus infection NOS

  B34.2 Coronavirus infection, unspecified
      EXCLUDES 1   *pneumonia due to SARS-associated coronavirus (J12.81)*

  B34.3 Parvovirus infection, unspecified

  B34.4 Papovavirus infection, unspecified

  B34.8 Other viral infections of unspecified site

  B34.9 Viral infection, unspecified
      Viremia NOS
      AHA: 2016,3Q,10

Mycoses (B35-B49)

    EXCLUDES 2   *hypersensitivity pneumonitis due to organic dust (J67.-)*
              mycosis fungoides (C84.0-)

✓4ᵗʰ **B35 Dermatophytosis**

    INCLUDES   favus
                infections due to species of Epidermophyton, Micro-sporum and Trichophyton
                tinea, any type except those in B36.-

  DEF: Contagious superficial fungal infection of the skin that invades and grows in dead keratin.

  B35.0 Tinea barbae and tinea capitis
      Beard ringworm
      Kerion
      Scalp ringworm
      Sycosis, mycotic

B35.1 Tinea unguium
Dermatophytic onychia
Dermatophytosis of nail
Onychomycosis
Ringworm of nails

B35.2 Tinea manuum
Dermatophytosis of hand
Hand ringworm

B35.3 Tinea pedis
Athlete's foot
Dermatophytosis of foot
Foot ringworm

B35.4 Tinea corporis
Ringworm of the body

B35.5 Tinea imbricata
Tokelau

B35.6 Tinea cruris
Dhobi itch
Groin ringworm
Jock itch

B35.8 Other dermatophytoses
Disseminated dermatophytosis
Granulomatous dermatophytosis

B35.9 Dermatophytosis, unspecified
Ringworm NOS

✓4ᵗʰ **B36 Other superficial mycoses**

B36.0 Pityriasis versicolor
Tinea flava
Tinea versicolor

B36.1 Tinea nigra
Keratomycosis nigricans palmaris
Microsporosis nigra
Pityriasis nigra

B36.2 White piedra
Tinea blanca

B36.3 Black piedra

B36.8 Other specified superficial mycoses

B36.9 Superficial mycosis, unspecified

✓4ᵗʰ **B37 Candidiasis**

INCLUDES candidosis
moniliasis

EXCLUDES 1 neonatal candidiasis (P37.5)

DEF: Candida: Genus of yeast-like fungi that are commonly found in the mouth, skin, intestinal tract, and vagina. It may cause a white, cheesy discharge.

B37.0 Candidal stomatitis
Oral thrush

B37.1 Pulmonary candidiasis
Candidal bronchitis
Candidal pneumonia

B37.2 Candidiasis of skin and nail
Candidal onychia
Candidal paronychia

EXCLUDES 2 diaper dermatitis (L22)

B37.3 Candidiasis of vulva and vagina ♀
Candidal vulvovaginitis
Monilial vulvovaginitis
Vaginal thrush

✓5ᵗʰ **B37.4 Candidiasis of other urogenital sites**

     B37.41 Candidal cystitis and urethritis

     B37.42 Candidal balanitis ♂

     B37.49 Other urogenital candidiasis
       Candidal pyelonephritis

B37.5 Candidal meningitis

B37.6 Candidal endocarditis

B37.7 Candidal sepsis
Disseminated candidiasis
Systemic candidiasis
AHA: 2014,4Q,46

✓5ᵗʰ **B37.8 Candidiasis of other sites**

     B37.81 Candidal esophagitis

     B37.82 Candidal enteritis
       Candidal proctitis

     B37.83 Candidal cheilitis

     B37.84 Candidal otitis externa

     B37.89 Other sites of candidiasis
       Candidal osteomyelitis

B37.9 Candidiasis, unspecified
Thrush NOS

✓4ᵗʰ **B38 Coccidioidomycosis**

B38.0 Acute pulmonary coccidioidomycosis

B38.1 Chronic pulmonary coccidioidomycosis

B38.2 Pulmonary coccidioidomycosis, unspecified

B38.3 Cutaneous coccidioidomycosis

B38.4 Coccidioidomycosis meningitis
DEF: Coccidioides immitis infection of the lining of the brain and/or spinal cord.

B38.7 Disseminated coccidioidomycosis
Generalized coccidioidomycosis

✓5ᵗʰ **B38.8 Other forms of coccidioidomycosis**

     B38.81 Prostatic coccidioidomycosis ♂

     B38.89 Other forms of coccidioidomycosis

B38.9 Coccidioidomycosis, unspecified

✓4ᵗʰ **B39 Histoplasmosis**

Code first associated AIDS (B20)
Use additional code for any associated manifestations, such as:
endocarditis (I39)
meningitis (G02)
pericarditis (I32)
retinitis (H32)

DEF: Type of lung infection caused by breathing in fungal spores often found in the droppings of bats and birds or soil contaminated by their droppings.

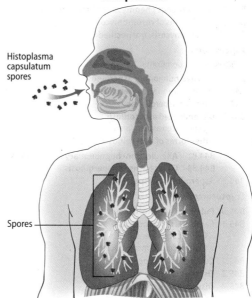

Histoplasmosis

Histoplasma capsulatum spores

Spores

B39.0 Acute pulmonary histoplasmosis capsulati

B39.1 Chronic pulmonary histoplasmosis capsulati

B39.2 Pulmonary histoplasmosis capsulati, unspecified

B39.3 Disseminated histoplasmosis capsulati
Generalized histoplasmosis capsulati

B39.4 Histoplasmosis capsulati, unspecified
American histoplasmosis

B39.5 Histoplasmosis duboisii
African histoplasmosis

B39.9 Histoplasmosis, unspecified

✓4ᵗʰ **B40 Blastomycosis**

EXCLUDES 1 Brazilian blastomycosis (B41.-)
keloidal blastomycosis (B48.0)

B40.0 Acute pulmonary blastomycosis

B40.1 Chronic pulmonary blastomycosis

B40.2 Pulmonary blastomycosis, unspecified

B40.3 Cutaneous blastomycosis

B40.7 Disseminated blastomycosis
Generalized blastomycosis

☑ Additional Character Required   ✓ₓ7ᵗʰ Placeholder Alert   Manifestation   Unspecified Dx   ▶◀ Revised Text   ● New Code   ▲ Revised Title

✓5ᵗʰ **B40.8**   **Other forms of blastomycosis**

     B40.81   **Blastomycotic** meningoencephalitis
                Meningomyelitis due to blastomycosis

     B40.89   **Other forms of blastomycosis**

B40.9   **Blastomycosis, unspecified**

✓4ᵗʰ **B41**   **Paracoccidioidomycosis**

   INCLUDES   Brazilian blastomycosis
               Lutz' disease

   B41.0   **Pulmonary** paracoccidioidomycosis

   B41.7   **Disseminated** paracoccidioidomycosis
             Generalized paracoccidioidomycosis

   B41.8   **Other forms of paracoccidioidomycosis**

   B41.9   **Paracoccidioidomycosis, unspecified**

✓4ᵗʰ **B42**   **Sporotrichosis**

   B42.0   **Pulmonary** sporotrichosis

   B42.1   **Lymphocutaneous** sporotrichosis

   B42.7   **Disseminated** sporotrichosis
             Generalized sporotrichosis

✓5ᵗʰ **B42.8**   **Other forms of sporotrichosis**

     B42.81   **Cerebral** sporotrichosis
               Meningitis due to sporotrichosis

     B42.82   **Sporotrichosis** arthritis

     B42.89   **Other forms of sporotrichosis**

   B42.9   **Sporotrichosis, unspecified**

✓4ᵗʰ **B43**   **Chromomycosis and pheomycotic abscess**

   B43.0   **Cutaneous** chromomycosis
             Dermatitis verrucosa

   B43.1   **Pheomycotic** brain abscess
             Cerebral chromomycosis

   B43.2   **Subcutaneous** pheomycotic abscess and cyst

   B43.8   **Other forms of chromomycosis**

   B43.9   **Chromomycosis, unspecified**

✓4ᵗʰ **B44**   **Aspergillosis**

   INCLUDES   aspergilloma

   B44.0   **Invasive pulmonary** aspergillosis

   B44.1   **Other pulmonary aspergillosis**

   B44.2   **Tonsillar** aspergillosis

   B44.7   **Disseminated** aspergillosis
             Generalized aspergillosis

✓5ᵗʰ **B44.8**   **Other forms of aspergillosis**

     B44.81   **Allergic bronchopulmonary** aspergillosis

     B44.89   **Other forms of aspergillosis**

   B44.9   **Aspergillosis, unspecified**

✓4ᵗʰ **B45**   **Cryptococcosis**

   B45.0   **Pulmonary** cryptococcosis

   B45.1   **Cerebral** cryptococcosis
             Cryptococcal meningitis
             Cryptococcosis meningocerebralis

   B45.2   **Cutaneous** cryptococcosis

   B45.3   **Osseous** cryptococcosis

   B45.7   **Disseminated** cryptococcosis
             Generalized cryptococcosis

   B45.8   **Other forms of cryptococcosis**

   B45.9   **Cryptococcosis, unspecified**

✓4ᵗʰ **B46**   **Zygomycosis**

   B46.0   **Pulmonary** mucormycosis

   B46.1   **Rhinocerebral** mucormycosis

   B46.2   **Gastrointestinal** mucormycosis

   B46.3   **Cutaneous** mucormycosis
             Subcutaneous mucormycosis

   B46.4   **Disseminated** mucormycosis
             Generalized mucormycosis

   B46.5   **Mucormycosis, unspecified**

   B46.8   **Other zygomycoses**
             Entomophthoromycosis

   B46.9   **Zygomycosis, unspecified**
             Phycomycosis NOS

✓4ᵗʰ **B47**   **Mycetoma**

   B47.0   **Eumycetoma**
             Madura foot, mycotic
             Maduromycosis

   B47.1   **Actinomycetoma**

   B47.9   **Mycetoma, unspecified**
             Madura foot NOS

✓4ᵗʰ **B48**   **Other mycoses, not elsewhere classified**

   B48.0   **Lobomycosis**
             Keloidal blastomycosis
             Lobo's disease

   B48.1   **Rhinosporidiosis**

   B48.2   **Allescheriasis**
             Infection due to Pseudallescheria boydii
       EXCLUDES 1   *eumycetoma (B47.0)*

   B48.3   **Geotrichosis**
             Geotrichum stomatitis

   B48.4   **Penicillosis**

   B48.8   **Other specified mycoses**
             Adiaspiromycosis
             Infection of tissue and organs by Alternaria
             Infection of tissue and organs by Drechslera
             Infection of tissue and organs by Fusarium
             Infection of tissue and organs by saprophytic fungi NEC
             AHA: 2014,4Q,46; 2014,2Q,13

B49   **Unspecified mycosis**
         Fungemia NOS

Protozoal diseases (B50-B64)

   EXCLUDES 1   *amebiasis (A06.-)*
               other protozoal intestinal diseases (A07.-)

✓4ᵗʰ **B50**   **Plasmodium** falciparum **malaria**

   INCLUDES   mixed infections of Plasmodium falciparum with any other
               Plasmodium species

   B50.0   **Plasmodium falciparum malaria with** cerebral complications
             Cerebral malaria NOS

   B50.8   **Other severe and complicated Plasmodium falciparum malaria**
             Severe or complicated Plasmodium falciparum malaria NOS

   B50.9   **Plasmodium falciparum malaria, unspecified**

✓4ᵗʰ **B51**   **Plasmodium** vivax **malaria**

   INCLUDES   mixed infections of Plasmodium vivax with other
               Plasmodium species, except Plasmodium falciparum
   EXCLUDES 1   *Plasmodium vivax with Plasmodium falciparum (B50.-)*

   B51.0   **Plasmodium vivax malaria with** rupture of spleen

   B51.8   **Plasmodium vivax malaria with** other complications

   B51.9   **Plasmodium vivax malaria** without complication
             Plasmodium vivax malaria NOS

✓4ᵗʰ **B52**   **Plasmodium** malariae **malaria**

   INCLUDES   mixed infections of Plasmodium malariae with other
               Plasmodium species, except Plasmodium falciparum
               and Plasmodium vivax
   EXCLUDES 1   *Plasmodium falciparum (B50.-)*
               Plasmodium vivax (B51.-)

   B52.0   **Plasmodium malariae malaria with** nephropathy

   B52.8   **Plasmodium malariae malaria with** other complications

   B52.9   **Plasmodium malariae malaria** without complication
             Plasmodium malariae malaria NOS

✓4ᵗʰ **B53**   **Other specified malaria**

   B53.0   **Plasmodium ovale** malaria
       EXCLUDES 1   *Plasmodium ovale with Plasmodium falciparum (B50.-)*
                  Plasmodium ovale with Plasmodium malariae (B52.-)
                  Plasmodium ovale with Plasmodium vivax (B51.-)

   B53.1   **Malaria due to** simian plasmodia
       EXCLUDES 1   *malaria due to simian plasmodia with Plasmodium falciparum (B50.-)*
                  malaria due to simian plasmodia with Plasmodium malariae (B52.-)
                  malaria due to simian plasmodia with Plasmodium ovale (B53.0)
                  malaria due to simian plasmodia with Plasmodium vivax (B51.-)

   B53.8   **Other malaria, not elsewhere classified**

B54   **Unspecified malaria**

N Newborn: 0   P Pediatric: 0-17   M Maternity: 12-55   A Adult: 15-124   CH Comorbidity High   CL Comorbidity Low   NCDx Noncancer Dx   PDx Primary Dx

452   ICD-10-CM 2020

☑4ᵗʰ **B55 Leishmaniasis**

B55.0 Visceral leishmaniasis
Kala-azar
Post-kala-azar dermal leishmaniasis

B55.1 Cutaneous leishmaniasis

B55.2 Mucocutaneous leishmaniasis

B55.9 Leishmaniasis, unspecified

☑4ᵗʰ **B56 African trypanosomiasis**

B56.0 Gambiense trypanosomiasis
Infection due to Trypanosoma brucei gambiense
West African sleeping sickness

B56.1 Rhodesiense trypanosomiasis
East African sleeping sickness
Infection due to Trypanosoma brucei rhodesiense

B56.9 African trypanosomiasis, unspecified
Sleeping sickness NOS

☑4ᵗʰ **B57 Chagas' disease**

INCLUDES   American trypanosomiasis
infection due to Trypanosoma cruzi

B57.0 Acute Chagas' disease with heart involvement
Acute Chagas' disease with myocarditis

B57.1 Acute Chagas' disease without heart involvement
Acute Chagas' disease NOS

B57.2 Chagas' disease (chronic) with heart involvement
American trypanosomiasis NOS
Chagas' disease (chronic) NOS
Chagas' disease (chronic) with myocarditis
Trypanosomiasis NOS

☑5ᵗʰ **B57.3 Chagas' disease (chronic) with digestive system involvement**

B57.30 Chagas' disease with digestive system involvement, unspecified

B57.31 Megaesophagus in Chagas' disease

B57.32 Megacolon in Chagas' disease

B57.39 Other digestive system involvement in Chagas' disease

☑5ᵗʰ **B57.4 Chagas' disease (chronic) with nervous system involvement**

B57.40 Chagas' disease with nervous system involvement, unspecified

B57.41 Meningitis in Chagas' disease

B57.42 Meningoencephalitis in Chagas' disease

B57.49 Other nervous system involvement in Chagas' disease

B57.5 Chagas' disease (chronic) with other organ involvement

☑4ᵗʰ **B58 Toxoplasmosis**

INCLUDES   infection due to Toxoplasma gondii
EXCLUDES 1   congenital toxoplasmosis (P37.1)

☑5ᵗʰ **B58.0 Toxoplasma oculopathy**

B58.00 Toxoplasma oculopathy, unspecified

B58.01 Toxoplasma chorioretinitis

B58.09 Other toxoplasma oculopathy
Toxoplasma uveitis

B58.1 Toxoplasma hepatitis

B58.2 Toxoplasma meningoencephalitis

B58.3 Pulmonary toxoplasmosis

☑5ᵗʰ **B58.8 Toxoplasmosis with other organ involvement**

B58.81 Toxoplasma myocarditis

B58.82 Toxoplasma myositis

B58.83 Toxoplasma tubulo-interstitial nephropathy
Toxoplasma pyelonephritis

B58.89 Toxoplasmosis with other organ involvement

B58.9 Toxoplasmosis, unspecified

B59 Pneumocystosis
Pneumonia due to Pneumocystis carinii
Pneumonia due to Pneumocystis jiroveci

☑4ᵗʰ **B60 Other protozoal diseases, not elsewhere classified**

EXCLUDES 1   cryptosporidiosis (A07.2)
intestinal microsporidiosis (A07.8)
isosporiasis (A07.3)

B60.0 Babesiosis
Piroplasmosis

☑5ᵗʰ **B60.1 Acanthamebiasis**

B60.10 Acanthamebiasis, unspecified

B60.11 Meningoencephalitis due to Acanthamoeba (culbertsoni)

B60.12 Conjunctivitis due to Acanthamoeba

B60.13 Keratoconjunctivitis due to Acanthamoeba

B60.19 Other acanthamebic disease

B60.2 Naegleriasis
Primary amebic meningoencephalitis

B60.8 Other specified protozoal diseases
Microsporidiosis

B64 Unspecified protozoal disease

Helminthiases (B65-B83)

☑4ᵗʰ **B65 Schistosomiasis [bilharziasis]**

INCLUDES   snail fever

B65.0 Schistosomiasis due to Schistosoma haematobium [urinary schistosomiasis]

B65.1 Schistosomiasis due to Schistosoma mansoni [intestinal schistosomiasis]

B65.2 Schistosomiasis due to Schistosoma japonicum
Asiatic schistosomiasis

B65.3 Cercarial dermatitis
Swimmer's itch

B65.8 Other schistosomiasis
Infection due to Schistosoma intercalatum
Infection due to Schistosoma mattheei
Infection due to Schistosoma mekongi

B65.9 Schistosomiasis, unspecified

☑4ᵗʰ **B66 Other fluke infections**

B66.0 Opisthorchiasis
Infection due to cat liver fluke
Infection due to Opisthorchis (felineus)(viverrini)

B66.1 Clonorchiasis
Chinese liver fluke disease
Infection due to Clonorchis sinensis
Oriental liver fluke disease

B66.2 Dicroceliasis
Infection due to Dicrocoelium dendriticum
Lancet fluke infection

B66.3 Fascioliasis
Infection due to Fasciola gigantica
Infection due to Fasciola hepatica
Infection due to Fasciola indica
Sheep liver fluke disease

B66.4 Paragonimiasis
Infection due to Paragonimus species
Lung fluke disease
Pulmonary distomiasis

B66.5 Fasciolopsiasis
Infection due to Fasciolopsis buski
Intestinal distomiasis

B66.8 Other specified fluke infections
Echinostomiasis
Heterophyiasis
Metagonimiasis
Nanophyetiasis
Watsoniasis

B66.9 Fluke infection, unspecified

☑4ᵗʰ **B67 Echinococcosis**

INCLUDES   hydatidosis

B67.0 Echinococcus granulosus infection of liver

B67.1 Echinococcus granulosus infection of lung

B67.2 Echinococcus granulosus infection of bone

☑5ᵗʰ **B67.3 Echinococcus granulosus infection, other and multiple sites**

B67.31 Echinococcus granulosus infection, thyroid gland

B67.32 Echinococcus granulosus infection, multiple sites

B67.39 Echinococcus granulosus infection, other sites

B67.4 Echinococcus granulosus infection, unspecified
Dog tapeworm (infection)

B67.5 Echinococcus multilocularis infection of liver

☑5ᵗʰ **B67.6 Echinococcus multilocularis infection, other and multiple sites**

B67.61 Echinococcus multilocularis infection, multiple sites

B67.69 Echinococcus multilocularis infection, other sites

B67.7 Echinococcus multilocularis infection, unspecified

B67.8 Echinococcosis, unspecified, of liver

☑ Additional Character Required   ✓x7ᵗʰ Placeholder Alert   Manifestation   Unspecified Dx   ▶◀ Revised Text   ● New Code   ▲ Revised Title

ICD-10-CM 2020   **453**

✓5th B67.9 Echinococcosis, other and unspecified

    B67.90 Echinococcosis, unspecified
      Echinococcosis NOS

    B67.99 Other echinococcosis

✓4th B68 Taeniasis

    EXCLUDES 1   cysticercosis (B69.-)

    B68.0 Taenia solium taeniasis
      Pork tapeworm (infection)

    B68.1 Taenia saginata taeniasis
      Beef tapeworm (infection)
      Infection due to adult tapeworm Taenia saginata

    B68.9 Taeniasis, unspecified

✓4th B69 Cysticercosis

    INCLUDES   cysticerciasis infection due to larval form of Taenia solium
    DEF: Condition that is developed when larvae or eggs of the tapeworm *Taenia solium* are ingested, most commonly in fecally contaminated water or undercooked pork.

    B69.0 Cysticercosis of central nervous system

    B69.1 Cysticercosis of eye

    ✓5th B69.8 Cysticercosis of other sites

      B69.81 Myositis in cysticercosis

      B69.89 Cysticercosis of other sites

    B69.9 Cysticercosis, unspecified

✓4th B70 Diphyllobothriasis and sparganosis

    B70.0 Diphyllobothriasis
      Diphyllobothrium (adult) (latum) (pacificum) infection
      Fish tapeworm (infection)
      EXCLUDES 2   larval diphyllobothriasis (B70.1)

    B70.1 Sparganosis
      Infection due to Sparganum (mansoni) (proliferum)
      Infection due to Spirometra larva
      Larval diphyllobothriasis
      Spirometrosis

✓4th B71 Other cestode infections

    B71.0 Hymenolepiasis
      Dwarf tapeworm infection
      Rat tapeworm (infection)

    B71.1 Dipylidiasis

    B71.8 Other specified cestode infections
      Coenurosis

    B71.9 Cestode infection, unspecified
      Tapeworm (infection) NOS

B72 Dracunculiasis

    INCLUDES   guinea worm infection
      infection due to Dracunculus medinensis

✓4th B73 Onchocerciasis

    INCLUDES   onchocerca volvulus infection
      onchocercosis
      river blindness

    ✓5th B73.0 Onchocerciasis with eye disease

      B73.00 Onchocerciasis with eye involvement, unspecified

      B73.01 Onchocerciasis with endophthalmitis

      B73.02 Onchocerciasis with glaucoma

      B73.09 Onchocerciasis with other eye involvement
        Infestation of eyelid due to onchocerciasis

    B73.1 Onchocerciasis without eye disease

✓4th B74 Filariasis

    EXCLUDES 2   onchocerciasis (B73)
      tropical (pulmonary) eosinophilia NOS (J82)

    B74.0 Filariasis due to Wuchereria bancrofti
      Bancroftian elephantiasis
      Bancroftian filariasis

    B74.1 Filariasis due to Brugia malayi

    B74.2 Filariasis due to Brugia timori

    B74.3 Loiasis
      Calabar swelling
      Eyeworm disease of Africa
      Loa loa infection

    B74.4 Mansonelliasis
      Infection due to Mansonella ozzardi
      Infection due to Mansonella perstans
      Infection due to Mansonella streptocerca

B74.8 Other filariases
    Dirofilariasis

B74.9 Filariasis, unspecified

B75 Trichinellosis

    INCLUDES   infection due to Trichinella species
      trichiniasis
    DEF: Infection by *Trichinella spiralis*, the smallest of the parasitic nematodes, that is transmitted by eating undercooked pork or bear meat.
    Synonym(s): Trichinosis.

✓4th B76 Hookworm diseases

    INCLUDES   uncinariasis

    B76.0 Ancylostomiasis
      Infection due to Ancylostoma species

    B76.1 Necatoriasis
      Infection due to Necator americanus

    B76.8 Other hookworm diseases

    B76.9 Hookworm disease, unspecified
      Cutaneous larva migrans NOS

✓4th B77 Ascariasis

    INCLUDES   ascaridiasis
      roundworm infection

    B77.0 Ascariasis with intestinal complications

    ✓5th B77.8 Ascariasis with other complications

      B77.81 Ascariasis pneumonia

      B77.89 Ascariasis with other complications

    B77.9 Ascariasis, unspecified

✓4th B78 Strongyloidiasis

    EXCLUDES 1   trichostrongyliasis (B81.2)

    B78.0 Intestinal strongyloidiasis

    B78.1 Cutaneous strongyloidiasis

    B78.7 Disseminated strongyloidiasis

    B78.9 Strongyloidiasis, unspecified

B79 Trichuriasis

    INCLUDES   trichocephaliasis
      whipworm (disease)(infection)

B80 Enterobiasis

    INCLUDES   oxyuriasis
      pinworm infection
      threadworm infection

✓4th B81 Other intestinal helminthiases, not elsewhere classified

    EXCLUDES 1   angiostrongyliasis due to:
      angiostrongylus cantonensis (B83.2)
      parastrongylus cantonensis (B83.2)

    B81.0 Anisakiasis
      Infection due to Anisakis larva

    B81.1 Intestinal capillariasis
      Capillariasis NOS
      Infection due to Capillaria philippinensis
      EXCLUDES 2   hepatic capillariasis (B83.8)

    B81.2 Trichostrongyliasis

    B81.3 Intestinal angiostrongyliasis
      Angiostrongyliasis due to:
      angiostrongylus costaricensis
      parastrongylus costaricensis

    B81.4 Mixed intestinal helminthiases
      Infection due to intestinal helminths classified to more than one of the categories B65.0-B81.3 and B81.8
      Mixed helminthiasis NOS

    B81.8 Other specified intestinal helminthiases
      Infection due to Oesophagostomum species [esophagostomiasis]
      Infection due to Ternidens diminutus [ternidensiasis]

✓4th B82 Unspecified intestinal parasitism

    B82.0 Intestinal helminthiasis, unspecified

    B82.9 Intestinal parasitism, unspecified

✓4th B83 Other helminthiases

    EXCLUDES 1   capillariasis NOS (B81.1)
    EXCLUDES 2   intestinal capillariasis (B81.1)

    B83.0 Visceral larva migrans
      Toxocariasis

    B83.1 Gnathostomiasis
      Wandering swelling

N Newborn: 0   P Pediatric: 0-17   M Maternity: 12-55   A Adult: 15-124   CH Comorbidity High   CL Comorbidity Low   NCDx Noncancer Dx   PDx Primary Dx

454   ICD-10-CM 2020

B83.2 Angiostrongyliasis due to Parastrongylus cantonensis
Eosinophilic meningoencephalitis due to Parastrongylus cantonensis
EXCLUDES 2   intestinal angiostrongyliasis (B81.3)

B83.3 Syngamiasis
Syngamosis

B83.4 Internal hirudiniasis
EXCLUDES 2   external hirudiniasis (B88.3)

B83.8 Other specified helminthiases
Acanthocephaliasis
Gongylonemiasis
Hepatic capillariasis
Metastrongyliasis
Thelaziasis

B83.9 Helminthiasis, unspecified
Worms NOS
EXCLUDES 1   intestinal helminthiasis NOS (B82.0)

Pediculosis, acariasis and other infestations (B85-B89)

B85 Pediculosis and phthiriasis

B85.0 Pediculosis due to Pediculus humanus capitis
Head-louse infestation

B85.1 Pediculosis due to Pediculus humanus corporis
Body-louse infestation

B85.2 Pediculosis, unspecified

B85.3 Phthiriasis
Infestation by crab-louse
Infestation by Phthirus pubis

B85.4 Mixed pediculosis and phthiriasis
Infestation classifiable to more than one of the categories B85.0-B85.3

B86 Scabies
Sarcoptic itch
DEF: Mite infestation that is caused by Sarcoptes scabiei. Scabies causes intense itching and sometimes secondary infection.

B87 Myiasis
INCLUDES   infestation by larva of flies

B87.0 Cutaneous myiasis
Creeping myiasis

B87.1 Wound myiasis
Traumatic myiasis

B87.2 Ocular myiasis

B87.3 Nasopharyngeal myiasis
Laryngeal myiasis

B87.4 Aural myiasis

B87.8 Myiasis of other sites
B87.81 Genitourinary myiasis
B87.82 Intestinal myiasis
B87.89 Myiasis of other sites

B87.9 Myiasis, unspecified

B88 Other infestations

B88.0 Other acariasis
Acarine dermatitis
Dermatitis due to Demodex species
Dermatitis due to Dermanyssus gallinae
Dermatitis due to Liponyssoides sanguineus
Trombiculosis
EXCLUDES 2   scabies (B86)

B88.1 Tungiasis [sandflea infestation]

B88.2 Other arthropod infestations
Scarabiasis

B88.3 External hirudiniasis
Leech infestation NOS
EXCLUDES 2   internal hirudiniasis (B83.4)

B88.8 Other specified infestations
Ichthyoparasitism due to Vandellia cirrhosa
Linguatulosis
Porocephaliasis

B88.9 Infestation, unspecified
Infestation (skin) NOS
Infestation by mites NOS
Skin parasites NOS

D09 Unspecified parasitic disease

Sequelae of infectious and parasitic diseases (B90-B94)

NOTE   Categories B90-B94 are to be used to indicate conditions in categories A00-B89 as the cause of sequelae, which are themselves classified elsewhere. The "sequelae" include conditions specified as such; they also include residuals of diseases classifiable to the above categories if there is evidence that the disease itself is no longer present. Codes from these categories are not to be used for chronic infections. Code chronic current infections to active infectious disease as appropriate.

Code first condition resulting from (sequela) the infectious or parasitic disease

B90 Sequelae of tuberculosis

B90.0 Sequelae of central nervous system tuberculosis
B90.1 Sequelae of genitourinary tuberculosis
B90.2 Sequelae of tuberculosis of bones and joints
B90.8 Sequelae of tuberculosis of other organs
EXCLUDES 2   sequelae of respiratory tuberculosis (B90.9)

B90.9 Sequelae of respiratory and unspecified tuberculosis
Sequelae of tuberculosis NOS

B91 Sequelae of poliomyelitis
EXCLUDES 1   postpolio syndrome (G14)

B92 Sequelae of leprosy

B94 Sequelae of other and unspecified infectious and parasitic diseases

B94.0 Sequelae of trachoma
B94.1 Sequelae of viral encephalitis
B94.2 Sequelae of viral hepatitis
B94.8 Sequelae of other specified infectious and parasitic diseases
AHA: 2017,4Q,109
B94.9 Sequelae of unspecified infectious and parasitic disease

Bacterial and viral infectious agents (B95-B97)

NOTE   These categories are provided for use as supplementary or additional codes to identify the infectious agent(s) in diseases classified elsewhere.
AHA: 2018,4Q,34; 2018,1Q,16

B95 Streptococcus, Staphylococcus, and Enterococcus as the cause of diseases classified elsewhere

B95.0 Streptococcus, group A, as the cause of diseases classified elsewhere
B95.1 Streptococcus, group B, as the cause of diseases classified elsewhere
AHA: 2019,2Q,8-10
B95.2 Enterococcus as the cause of diseases classified elsewhere
B95.3 Streptococcus pneumoniae as the cause of diseases classified elsewhere
B95.4 Other streptococcus as the cause of diseases classified elsewhere
B95.5 Unspecified streptococcus as the cause of diseases classified elsewhere
B95.6 Staphylococcus aureus as the cause of diseases classified elsewhere
B95.61 Methicillin susceptible Staphylococcus aureus infection as the cause of diseases classified elsewhere
Methicillin susceptible Staphylococcus aureus (MSSA) infection as the cause of diseases classified elsewhere
Staphylococcus aureus infection NOS as the cause of diseases classified elsewhere
B95.62 Methicillin resistant Staphylococcus aureus infection as the cause of diseases classified elsewhere
Methicillin resistant staphylococcus aureus (MRSA) infection as the cause of diseases classified elsewhere
AHA: 2016,1Q,12
B95.7 Other staphylococcus as the cause of diseases classified elsewhere
B95.8 Unspecified staphylococcus as the cause of diseases classified elsewhere

B96 Other bacterial agents as the cause of diseases classified elsewhere

B96.0 Mycoplasma pneumoniae [M. pneumoniae] as the cause of diseases classified elsewhere
Pleuro-pneumonia-like-organism [PPLO]
B96.1 Klebsiella pneumoniae [K. pneumoniae] as the cause of diseases classified elsewhere

Chapter 1. Certain Infectious and Parasitic Diseases

✓5ᵗʰ **B96.2** Escherichia coli [E. coli] as the cause of diseases classified elsewhere

    B96.20 Unspecified Escherichia coli [E. coli] as the cause of diseases classified elsewhere
        Escherichia coli [E. coli] NOS

▲   **B96.21** Shiga toxin-producing Escherichia coli [E. coli] [STEC] O157 as the cause of diseases classified elsewhere
        E. coli O157:H- (nonmotile) with confirmation of Shiga toxin
        E. coli O157 with confirmation of Shiga toxin when H antigen is unknown, or is not H7
        O157:H7 Escherichia coli [E.coli] with or without confirmation of Shiga toxin-production
        Shiga toxin-producing Escherichia coli [E.coli] O157:H7 with or without confirmation of Shiga toxin-production
        STEC O157:H7 with or without confirmation of Shiga toxin-production

▲   **B96.22** Other specified Shiga toxin-producing Escherichia coli [E. coli] [STEC] as the cause of diseases classified elsewhere
        Non-O157 Shiga toxin-producing Escherichia coli [E.coli]
        Non-O157 Shiga toxin-producing Escherichia coli [E.coli] with known O group

▲   **B96.23** Unspecified Shiga toxin-producing Escherichia coli [E. coli] [STEC] as the cause of diseases classified elsewhere
        Shiga toxin-producing Escherichia coli [E. coli] with unspecified O group
        STEC NOS

    B96.29 Other Escherichia coli [E. coli] as the cause of diseases classified elsewhere
        Non-Shiga toxin-producing E. coli

B96.3 Hemophilus influenzae [H. influenzae] as the cause of diseases classified elsewhere

B96.4 Proteus (mirabilis) (morganii) as the cause of diseases classified elsewhere

B96.5 Pseudomonas (aeruginosa) (mallei) (pseudomallei) as the cause of diseases classified elsewhere
    AHA: 2015,1Q,18

B96.6 Bacteroides fragilis [B. fragilis] as the cause of diseases classified elsewhere

B96.7 Clostridium perfringens [C. perfringens] as the cause of diseases classified elsewhere

✓5ᵗʰ **B96.8** Other specified bacterial agents as the cause of diseases classified elsewhere

    B96.81 Helicobacter pylori [H. pylori] as the cause of diseases classified elsewhere

    B96.82 Vibrio vulnificus as the cause of diseases classified elsewhere

    B96.89 Other specified bacterial agents as the cause of diseases classified elsewhere

✓4ᵗʰ **B97** Viral agents as the cause of diseases classified elsewhere
    AHA: 2016,3Q,8-10,14

B97.0 Adenovirus as the cause of diseases classified elsewhere

✓5ᵗʰ **B97.1** Enterovirus as the cause of diseases classified elsewhere

    B97.10 Unspecified enterovirus as the cause of diseases classified elsewhere

    B97.11 Coxsackievirus as the cause of diseases classified elsewhere

    B97.12 Echovirus as the cause of diseases classified elsewhere

    B97.19 Other enterovirus as the cause of diseases classified elsewhere

✓5ᵗʰ **B97.2** Coronavirus as the cause of diseases classified elsewhere

    B97.21 SARS-associated coronavirus as the cause of diseases classified elsewhere
        EXCLUDES 1   pneumonia due to SARS-associated coronavirus (J12.81)

    B97.29 Other coronavirus as the cause of diseases classified elsewhere

✓5ᵗʰ **B97.3** Retrovirus as the cause of diseases classified elsewhere
    EXCLUDES 1   human immunodeficiency virus [HIV] disease (B20)

    B97.30 Unspecified retrovirus as the cause of diseases classified elsewhere

    B97.31 Lentivirus as the cause of diseases classified elsewhere

    B97.32 Oncovirus as the cause of diseases classified elsewhere

    B97.33 Human T-cell lymphotrophic virus, type I [HTLV-I] as the cause of diseases classified elsewhere

    B97.34 Human T-cell lymphotrophic virus, type II [HTLV-II] as the cause of diseases classified elsewhere

    B97.35 Human immunodeficiency virus, type 2 [HIV 2] as the cause of diseases classified elsewhere

    B97.39 Other retrovirus as the cause of diseases classified elsewhere

B97.4 Respiratory syncytial virus as the cause of diseases classified elsewhere
    ►RSV as the cause of diseases classified elsewhere◄
    ►Code first related disorders, such as:◄
        ►otitis media (H65.-)◄
        ►upper respiratory infection (J06.9)◄
        EXCLUDES 2 ►acute bronchiolitis due to respiratory syncytial virus (RSV) (J21.0)◄
            ►acute bronchitis due to respiratory syncytial virus (RSV) (J20.5)◄
            ►respiratory syncytial virus (RSV) pneumonia (J12.1)◄

B97.5 Reovirus as the cause of diseases classified elsewhere

B97.6 Parvovirus as the cause of diseases classified elsewhere

B97.7 Papillomavirus as the cause of diseases classified elsewhere

✓5ᵗʰ **B97.8** Other viral agents as the cause of diseases classified elsewhere

    B97.81 Human metapneumovirus as the cause of diseases classified elsewhere

    B97.89 Other viral agents as the cause of diseases classified elsewhere

Other infectious diseases (B99)

✓4ᵗʰ **B99** Other and unspecified infectious diseases

B99.8 Other infectious disease

B99.9 Unspecified infectious disease

N Newborn: 0   P Pediatric: 0-17   M Maternity: 12-55   A Adult: 15-124   CH Comorbidity High   CL Comorbidity Low   NCDx Noncancer Dx   PDx Primary Dx

456   ICD-10-CM 2020

Chapter 2. Neoplasms (C00–D49)

Chapter-specific Guidelines with Coding Examples

The chapter-specific guidelines from the ICD-10-CM Official Guidelines for Coding and Reporting have been provided below. Along with these guidelines are coding examples, contained in the shaded boxes, that have been developed to help illustrate the coding and/or sequencing guidance found in these guidelines.

General guidelines

Chapter 2 of the ICD-10-CM contains the codes for most benign and all malignant neoplasms. Certain benign neoplasms, such as prostatic adenomas, may be found in the specific body system chapters. To properly code a neoplasm it is necessary to determine from the record if the neoplasm is benign, in-situ, malignant, or of uncertain histologic behavior. If malignant, any secondary (metastatic) sites should also be determined.

Primary malignant neoplasms overlapping site boundaries

A primary malignant neoplasm that overlaps two or more contiguous (next to each other) sites should be classified to the subcategory/code .8 ('overlapping lesion'), unless the combination is specifically indexed elsewhere. For multiple neoplasms of the same site that are not contiguous such as tumors in different quadrants of the same breast, codes for each site should be assigned.

> A 73-year-old white female with a large rapidly growing malignant tumor in the left breast extending from the upper outer quadrant into the axillary tail.
>
> **C50.812**   **Malignant neoplasm of overlapping sites of left female breast**
>
> *Explanation*: Because this is a single large tumor that overlaps two contiguous sites, a single code for overlapping sites is assigned.

> A 52-year old white female with two distinct lesions of the right breast, one (0.5 cm) in the upper outer quadrant and a second (1.5 cm) in the lower outer quadrant; path report indicates both lesions are malignant
>
> **C50.411**   **Malignant neoplasm of upper-outer quadrant of right female breast**
>
> **C50.511**   **Malignant neoplasm of lower-outer quadrant of right female breast**
>
> *Explanation*: This patient has two distinct malignant lesions of right breast in adjacent quadrants. Because the lesions are not contiguous, two codes are reported.

Malignant neoplasm of ectopic tissue

Malignant neoplasms of ectopic tissue are to be coded to the site of origin mentioned, e.g., ectopic pancreatic malignant neoplasms involving the stomach are coded to malignant neoplasm of pancreas, unspecified (C25.9).

The neoplasm table in the Alphabetic Index should be referenced first. However, if the histological term is documented, that term should be referenced first, rather than going immediately to the Neoplasm Table, in order to determine which column in the Neoplasm Table is appropriate. For example, if the documentation indicates "adenoma," refer to the term in the Alphabetic Index to review the entries under this term and the instructional note to "see also neoplasm, by site, benign." The table provides the proper code based on the type of neoplasm and the site. It is important to select the proper column in the table that corresponds to the type of neoplasm. The Tabular List should then be referenced to verify that the correct code has been selected from the table and that a more specific site code does not exist.

See Section I.C.21. Factors influencing health status and contact with health services, Status, for information regarding Z15.0, codes for genetic susceptibility to cancer.

a. Treatment directed at the malignancy

If the treatment is directed at the malignancy, designate the malignancy as the principal diagnosis.

The only exception to this guideline is if a patient admission/encounter is solely for the administration of chemotherapy, immunotherapy or external beam radiation therapy, assign the appropriate Z51.-- code as the first-listed or principal diagnosis, and the diagnosis or problem for which the service is being performed as a secondary diagnosis.

b. Treatment of secondary site

When a patient is admitted because of a primary neoplasm with metastasis and treatment is directed toward the secondary site only, the secondary neoplasm is designated as the principal diagnosis even though the primary malignancy is still present.

> Patient with unresolved primary prostate cancer is admitted for respiratory care and rehabilitation related to new diagnosis of right lung metastasis.
>
> **C78.01**   **Secondary malignant neoplasm of right lung**
>
> **C61**   **Malignant neoplasm of prostate**
>
> *Explanation*: The patient was admitted for treatment of the secondary neoplastic disease of the right lung with respiratory care. The code for the secondary lung metastasis is sequenced before the code for primary prostate cancer.

c. Coding and sequencing of complications

Coding and sequencing of complications associated with the malignancies or with the therapy thereof are subject to the following guidelines:

1) Anemia associated with malignancy

When admission/encounter is for management of an anemia associated with the malignancy, and the treatment is only for anemia, the appropriate code for the malignancy is sequenced as the principal or first-listed diagnosis followed by the appropriate code for the anemia (such as code D63.0, Anemia in neoplastic disease).

> Patient is admitted for treatment of anemia in advanced colon cancer.
>
> **C18.9**   **Malignant neoplasm of colon, unspecified**
>
> **D63.0**   **Anemia in neoplastic disease**
>
> *Explanation*: Even though the admission was solely to treat the anemia, this guideline indicates that the code for the malignancy is sequenced first.

2) Anemia associated with chemotherapy, immunotherapy and radiation therapy

When the admission/encounter is for management of an anemia associated with an adverse effect of the administration of chemotherapy or immunotherapy and the only treatment is for the anemia, the anemia code is sequenced first followed by the appropriate codes for the neoplasm and the adverse effect (T45.1X5, Adverse effect of antineoplastic and immunosuppressive drugs).

> A 52-year-old male with chronic lymphocytic leukemia noted with Richter transformation following acute mononucleosis infection, now resolved, is admitted for assessment and monitoring of labs. The clinical record notes anemia secondary to chemotherapy and weekly lab orders. The patient continues to receive chemotherapy.
>
> **D64.81**   **Anemia due to antineoplastic chemotherapy**
>
> **T45.1X5D**   **Adverse effect of antineoplastic drugs and immunosuppressive drugs, subsequent encounter**
>
> **C91.10**   **Chronic lymphocytic leukemia of B-cell type not having achieved remission**
>
> *Explanation*: The code for anemia is sequenced before the code for the neoplasm and the adverse effect of chemotherapy. The seventh character D is applied to code T45.1X5-, as active treatment of the adverse effect, the anemia, is no longer required.

When the admission/encounter is for management of an anemia associated with an adverse effect of radiotherapy, the anemia code should be sequenced first, followed by the appropriate neoplasm code and code Y84.2, Radiological procedure and radiotherapy as the cause of abnormal reaction of the patient, or of later complication, without mention of misadventure at the time of the procedure.

> A 65-year-old female is admitted following hospitalization for multiple blood transfusions to treat anemia secondary to radiation therapy. She has been receiving radiation treatments for right breast cancer.
>
> **D64.89**   **Other specified anemias**
>
> **C50.911**   **Malignant neoplasm of unspecified site of right female breast**
>
> **Y84.2**   **Radiological procedure and radiotherapy as the cause of abnormal reaction of the patient, or of later complication, without mention of misadventure at the time of the procedure**
>
> *Explanation*: The code for the anemia is sequenced first, followed by the code for the malignancy, and last the code for the abnormal reaction due to radiotherapy.

3) Management of dehydration due to the malignancy

When the admission/encounter is for management of dehydration due to the malignancy and only the dehydration is being treated (intravenous rehydration), the dehydration is sequenced first, followed by the code(s) for the malignancy.

4) Treatment of a complication resulting from a surgical procedure

When the admission/encounter is for treatment of a complication resulting from a surgical procedure, designate the complication as the principal or first-listed diagnosis if treatment is directed at resolving the complication.

d. Primary malignancy previously excised

When a primary malignancy has been previously excised or eradicated from its site and there is no further treatment directed to that site and there is no evidence of any existing primary malignancy at that site, a code from category Z85, Personal history of malignant neoplasm, should be used to indicate the former site of the malignancy. Any mention of extension, invasion, or metastasis to another site is coded as a secondary malignant neoplasm to that site. The secondary site may be the principal or first-listed **diagnosis** with the Z85 code used as a secondary code.

> History of breast cancer, left radical mastectomy 18 months ago with no current treatment; bronchoscopy with lung biopsy shows metastatic disease in the right lung.
>
> **C78.01**   **Secondary malignant neoplasm of right lung**
>
> **Z85.3**   **Personal history of malignant neoplasm of breast**
>
> *Explanation*: The patient has undergone a diagnostic procedure that revealed metastatic breast cancer in the right lung. The code for the secondary (metastatic) site is sequenced first followed by a personal history code to identify the former site of the primary malignancy.

e. Admissions/Encounters involving chemotherapy, immunotherapy and radiation therapy

1) Episode of care involves surgical removal of neoplasm

When an episode of care involves the surgical removal of a neoplasm, primary or secondary site, followed by adjunct chemotherapy or radiation treatment during the same episode of care, the code for the neoplasm should be assigned as principal or first-listed diagnosis.

2) Patient admission/encounter solely for administration of chemotherapy, immunotherapy and radiation therapy

If a patient admission/encounter is solely for the administration of chemotherapy, immunotherapy or external beam radiation therapy assign code Z51.0, Encounter for antineoplastic radiation therapy, or Z51.11, Encounter for antineoplastic chemotherapy, or Z51.12, Encounter for antineoplastic immunotherapy as the first-listed or principal diagnosis. If a patient receives more than one of these therapies during the same admission more than one of these codes may be assigned, in any sequence.

The malignancy for which the therapy is being administered should be assigned as a secondary diagnosis.

If a patient admission/encounter is for the insertion or implantation of radioactive elements (e.g., brachytherapy) the appropriate code for the malignancy is sequenced as the principal or first-listed diagnosis. Code Z51.0 should not be assigned.

3) Patient admitted for radiation therapy, chemotherapy or immunotherapy and develops complications

When a patient is admitted for the purpose of external beam radiotherapy, immunotherapy or chemotherapy and develops complications such as uncontrolled nausea and vomiting or dehydration, the principal or first-listed diagnosis is Z51.0, Encounter for antineoplastic radiation therapy, or Z51.11, Encounter for antineoplastic chemotherapy, or Z51.12, Encounter for antineoplastic immunotherapy followed by any codes for the complications.

When a patient is admitted for the purpose of insertion or implantation of radioactive elements (e.g., brachytherapy)and develops complications such as uncontrolled nausea and vomiting or dehydration, the principal or first-listed diagnosis is the appropriate code for the malignancy followed by any codes for the complications.

f. Admission/encounter to determine extent of malignancy

When the reason for admission/encounter is to determine the extent of the malignancy, or for a procedure such as paracentesis or thoracentesis, the primary malignancy or appropriate metastatic site is designated as the principal or first-listed diagnosis, even though chemotherapy or radiotherapy is administered.

g. Symptoms, signs, and abnormal findings listed in Chapter 18 associated with neoplasms

Symptoms, signs, and ill-defined conditions listed in Chapter 18 characteristic of, or associated with, an existing primary or secondary site malignancy cannot be used to replace the malignancy as principal or first-listed diagnosis, regardless of the number of admissions or encounters for treatment and care of the neoplasm.

See Section I.C.21. Factors influencing health status and contact with health services, Encounter for prophylactic organ removal.

> Patient is admitted for respiratory decline with severe shortness of breath and new onset use of continuous oxygen, related to inoperable neoplasm of the right lung.
>
> **C34.91**   **Malignant neoplasm of unspecified part of right bronchus or lung**
>
> **Z99.81**   **Dependence on supplemental oxygen**
>
> *Explanation*: No code is assigned for shortness of breath, as this symptom is an integral part of the neoplastic lung disease and should not take the place of a code for the neoplasm, regardless of encounter.

h. Admission/encounter for pain control/management

See Section I.C.6. for information on coding admission/encounter for pain control/management.

i. Malignancy in two or more noncontiguous sites

A patient may have more than one malignant tumor in the same organ. These tumors may represent different primaries or metastatic disease, depending on the site. Should the documentation be unclear, the provider should be queried as to the status of each tumor so that the correct codes can be assigned.

j. Disseminated malignant neoplasm, unspecified

Code C80.0, Disseminated malignant neoplasm, unspecified, is for use only in those cases where the patient has advanced metastatic disease and no known primary or secondary sites are specified. It should not be used in place of assigning codes for the primary site and all known secondary sites.

> Patient who has had no regular medical care for over 10 years until recent symptoms developed is admitted post-hospital stay with a new diagnosis of carcinomatosis.
>
> **C80.0**   **Disseminated malignant neoplasm, unspecified**
>
> *Explanation*: Carcinomatosis NOS is an "inclusion term" under code C80.0 Disseminated malignant neoplasm, unspecified. This code should seldom be used but is available for use in cases such as this.

k. Malignant neoplasm without specification of site

Code C80.1, Malignant (primary) neoplasm, unspecified, equates to Cancer, unspecified. This code should only be used when no determination can be made as to the primary site of a malignancy. This code should rarely be used in the inpatient setting.

> Evaluation of painful hip leads to diagnosis of a metastatic bone lesion from an unknown primary neoplasm source.
>
> **C79.51**   **Secondary malignant neoplasm of bone**
>
> **C80.1**   **Malignant (primary) neoplasm, unspecified**
>
> *Explanation*: If only the secondary site is known, use code C80.1 for the unknown primary site.

l. Sequencing of neoplasm codes

1) Encounter for treatment of primary malignancy

If the reason for the encounter is for treatment of a primary malignancy, assign the malignancy as the principal/first-listed diagnosis. The primary site is to be sequenced first, followed by any metastatic sites.

2) Encounter for treatment of secondary malignancy

When an encounter is for a primary malignancy with metastasis and treatment is directed toward the metastatic (secondary) site(s) only, the metastatic site(s) is designated as the principal/first-listed diagnosis. The primary malignancy is coded as an additional code.

> Patient is admitted with primary colon cancer with new onset metastasis to the ribs resulting in shortness of breath and pain.
>
> **C79.51**   **Secondary malignant neoplasm of bone**
>
> **C18.9**   **Malignant neoplasm of colon, unspecified**
>
> **G89.3**   **Neoplasm related pain (acute) (chronic)**
>
> *Explanation*: The focus of care for this admission is on the newly diagnosed metastasis to the ribs (bone) rather than the primary colon cancer, indicating a need to code the metastasis to the bone as primary. Provider documentation supports pain due to neoplastic disease, as well.

3) Malignant neoplasm in a pregnant patient

When a pregnant woman has a malignant neoplasm, a code from subcategory O9A.1-, Malignant neoplasm complicating pregnancy, childbirth, and the puerperium, should be sequenced first, followed by the appropriate code from Chapter 2 to indicate the type of neoplasm.

4) Encounter for complication associated with a neoplasm

When an encounter is for management of a complication associated with a neoplasm, such as dehydration, and the treatment is only for the complication, the complication is coded first, followed by the appropriate code(s) for the neoplasm.

The exception to this guideline is anemia. When the admission/encounter is for management of an anemia associated with the malignancy, and the treatment is only for anemia, the appropriate code for the malignancy is sequenced as the principal or first-listed diagnosis followed by code D63.0, Anemia in neoplastic disease.

> Patient with pancreatic cancer is seen for initiation of TPN for cancer-related moderate protein-calorie malnutrition.
>
> **E44.0**   **Moderate protein-calorie malnutrition**
>
> **C25.9**   **Malignant neoplasm of pancreas, unspecified**
>
> *Explanation*: The encounter is to initiate treatment for malnutrition, a common complication of many types of neoplasms, and is sequenced first.

5) Complication from surgical procedure for treatment of a neoplasm

When an encounter is for treatment of a complication resulting from a surgical procedure performed for the treatment of the neoplasm, designate the complication as the principal/first-listed diagnosis. See **the** guideline regarding the coding of a current malignancy versus personal history to determine if the code for the neoplasm should also be assigned.

6) Pathologic fracture due to a neoplasm

When an encounter is for a pathological fracture due to a neoplasm, and the focus of treatment is the fracture, a code from subcategory M84.5, Pathological fracture in neoplastic disease, should be sequenced first, followed by the code for the neoplasm.

If the focus of treatment is the neoplasm with an associated pathological fracture, the neoplasm code should be sequenced first, followed by a code from M84.5 for the pathological fracture.

m. Current malignancy versus personal history of malignancy

When a primary malignancy has been excised but further treatment, such as an additional surgery for the malignancy, radiation therapy or chemotherapy is directed to that site, the primary malignancy code should be used until treatment is completed.

When a primary malignancy has been previously excised or eradicated from its site, there is no further treatment (of the malignancy) directed to that site, and there is no evidence of any existing primary malignancy at that site, a code from category Z85, Personal history of malignant neoplasm, should be used to indicate the former site of the malignancy.

Subcategories Z85.0 – Z85.7 should only be assigned for the former site of a primary malignancy, not the site of a secondary malignancy. Codes from subcategory Z85.8-, may be assigned for the former site(s) of either a primary or secondary malignancy included in this subcategory.

See Section I.C.21. Factors influencing health status and contact with health services, History (of)

> Female patient with ongoing chemotherapy after right mastectomy for breast cancer.
>
> **C50.911**   **Malignant neoplasm of unspecified site of right female breast**
>
> **Z90.11**   **Acquired absence of right breast and nipple**
>
> *Explanation*: Even though the breast has been removed, the breast cancer is still being treated with chemotherapy and therefore is still coded as a current condition rather than personal history.

n. Leukemia, multiple myeloma, and malignant plasma cell neoplasms in remission versus personal history

The categories for leukemia, and category C90, Multiple myeloma and malignant plasma cell neoplasms, have codes indicating whether or not the leukemia has achieved remission. There are also codes Z85.6, Personal history of leukemia, and Z85.79, Personal history of other malignant neoplasms of lymphoid, hematopoietic and related tissues. If the documentation is unclear as to whether the leukemia has achieved remission, the provider should be queried.

See Section I.C.21. Factors influencing health status and contact with health services, History (of)

o. Aftercare following surgery for neoplasm

See Section I.C.21. Factors influencing health status and contact with health services, Aftercare

p. Follow-up care for completed treatment of a malignancy

See Section I.C.21. Factors influencing health status and contact with health services, Follow-up

q. Prophylactic organ removal for prevention of malignancy

See Section I.C. 21, Factors influencing health status and contact with health services, Prophylactic organ removal

r. Malignant neoplasm associated with transplanted organ

A malignant neoplasm of a transplanted organ should be coded as a transplant complication. Assign first the appropriate code from category T86.-, Complications of transplanted organs and tissue, followed by code C80.2, Malignant neoplasm associated with transplanted organ. Use an additional code for the specific malignancy.

Chapter 2. Neoplasms (C00–D49)

NOTE

Functional activity

All neoplasms are classified in this chapter, whether they are functionally active or not. An additional code from Chapter 4 may be used, to identify functional activity associated with any neoplasm.

Morphology [Histology]

Chapter 2 classifies neoplasms primarily by site (topography), with broad groupings for behavior, malignant, in situ, benign, etc. The Table of Neoplasms should be used to identify the correct topography code. In a few cases, such as for malignant melanoma and certain neuroendocrine tumors, the morphology (histologic type) is included in the category and codes.

Primary malignant neoplasms overlapping site boundaries

A primary malignant neoplasm that overlaps two or more contiguous (next to each other) sites should be classified to the subcategory/code .8 ("overlapping lesion"), unless the combination is specifically indexed elsewhere. For multiple neoplasms of the same site that are not contiguous, such as tumors in different quadrants of the same breast, codes for each site should be assigned.

Malignant neoplasm of ectopic tissue

Malignant neoplasms of ectopic tissue are to be coded to the site mentioned, e.g., ectopic pancreatic malignant neoplasms are coded to pancreas, unspecified (C25.9).

AHA: 2017,4Q,103; 2017,1Q,4,5-6,8

This chapter contains the following blocks:

C00-C14   Malignant neoplasms of lip, oral cavity and pharynx
C15-C26   Malignant neoplasms of digestive organs
C30-C39   Malignant neoplasms of respiratory and intrathoracic organs
C40-C41   Malignant neoplasms of bone and articular cartilage
C43-C44   Melanoma and other malignant neoplasms of skin
C45-C49   Malignant neoplasms of mesothelial and soft tissue
C50   Malignant neoplasms of breast
C51-C58   Malignant neoplasms of female genital organs
C60-C63   Malignant neoplasms of male genital organs
C64-C68   Malignant neoplasms of urinary tract
C69-C72   Malignant neoplasms of eye, brain and other parts of central nervous system
C73-C75   Malignant neoplasms of thyroid and other endocrine glands
C7A   Malignant neuroendocrine tumors
C7B   Secondary neuroendocrine tumors
C76-C80   Malignant neoplasms of ill-defined, other secondary and unspecified sites
C81-C96   Malignant neoplasms of lymphoid, hematopoietic and related tissue
D00-D09   In situ neoplasms
D10-D36   Benign neoplasms, except benign neuroendocrine tumors
D3A   Benign neuroendocrine tumors
D37-D48   Neoplasms of uncertain behavior, polycythemia vera and myelodysplastic syndromes
D49   Neoplasms of unspecified behavior

MALIGNANT NEOPLASMS(C00-C96)

Malignant neoplasms, stated or presumed to be primary (of specified sites), and certain specified histologies, except neuroendocrine, and of lymphoid, hematopoietic and related tissue (C00-C75)

TIP: Codes from this code block can be assigned based on the diagnosis listed in a pathology or cytology report when authenticated by a pathologist and available at the time of code assignment.

Malignant neoplasms of lip, oral cavity and pharynx (C00-C14)

✓4ᵗʰ C00   Malignant neoplasm of lip

Use additional code to identify:
alcohol abuse and dependence (F10.-)
history of tobacco dependence (Z87.891)
tobacco dependence (F17.-)
tobacco use (Z72.0)

     EXCLUDES 1   *malignant melanoma of lip (C43.0)*
                   Merkel cell carcinoma of lip (C4A.0)
                   other and unspecified malignant neoplasm of skin of lip (C44.0-)

    C00.0   Malignant neoplasm of external upper lip   **CL**

       Malignant neoplasm of lipstick area of upper lip
       Malignant neoplasm of upper lip NOS
       Malignant neoplasm of vermilion border of upper lip

    C00.1   Malignant neoplasm of external lower lip   **CL**

       Malignant neoplasm of lower lip NOS
       Malignant neoplasm of lipstick area of lower lip
       Malignant neoplasm of vermilion border of lower lip

    C00.2   Malignant neoplasm of external lip, **unspecified**
       Malignant neoplasm of vermilion border of lip NOS

    C00.3   Malignant neoplasm of upper lip, inner aspect   **CL**

       Malignant neoplasm of buccal aspect of upper lip
       Malignant neoplasm of frenulum of upper lip
       Malignant neoplasm of mucosa of upper lip
       Malignant neoplasm of oral aspect of upper lip

    C00.4   Malignant neoplasm of lower lip, inner aspect   **CL**

       Malignant neoplasm of buccal aspect of lower lip
       Malignant neoplasm of frenulum of lower lip
       Malignant neoplasm of mucosa of lower lip
       Malignant neoplasm of oral aspect of lower lip

    C00.5   Malignant neoplasm of lip, unspecified, inner aspect

       Malignant neoplasm of buccal aspect of lip, unspecified
       Malignant neoplasm of frenulum of lip, unspecified
       Malignant neoplasm of mucosa of lip, unspecified
       Malignant neoplasm of oral aspect of lip, unspecified

    C00.6   Malignant neoplasm of commissure of lip, **unspecified**

    C00.8   Malignant neoplasm of overlapping sites of lip   **CL**

    C00.9   Malignant neoplasm of lip, **unspecified**

C01   Malignant neoplasm of base of tongue   **CL**

       Malignant neoplasm of dorsal surface of base of tongue
       Malignant neoplasm of fixed part of tongue NOS
       Malignant neoplasm of posterior third of tongue
       Use additional code to identify:
          alcohol abuse and dependence (F10.-)
          history of tobacco dependence (Z87.891)
          tobacco dependence (F17.-)
          tobacco use (Z72.0)

Malignant Neoplasm of Tongue

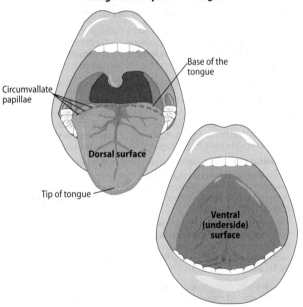

✓4ᵗʰ C02   Malignant neoplasm of other and unspecified parts of tongue

Use additional code to identify:
alcohol abuse and dependence (F10.-)
history of tobacco dependence (Z87.891)
tobacco dependence (F17.-)
tobacco use (Z72.0)

    C02.0   Malignant neoplasm of dorsal surface of tongue   **CL**

       Malignant neoplasm of anterior two-thirds of tongue, dorsal surface

       EXCLUDES 2   *malignant neoplasm of dorsal surface of base of tongue (C01)*

    C02.1   Malignant neoplasm of border of tongue   **CL**

       Malignant neoplasm of tip of tongue

    C02.2   Malignant neoplasm of ventral surface of tongue   **CL**

       Malignant neoplasm of anterior two-thirds of tongue, ventral surface
       Malignant neoplasm of frenulum linguae

N Newborn: 0   **P** Pediatric: 0-17   **M** Maternity: 12-55   **A** Adult: 15-124   **CH** Comorbidity High   **CL** Comorbidity Low   **NCDx** Noncancer Dx   **PDx** Primary Dx

460   ICD-10-CM 2020

C02.3 Malignant neoplasm of anterior two-thirds of tongue, part unspecified `CL`
  Malignant neoplasm of middle third of tongue NOS
  Malignant neoplasm of mobile part of tongue NOS

C02.4 Malignant neoplasm of lingual tonsil `CL`
  EXCLUDES 2   malignant neoplasm of tonsil NOS (C09.9)

C02.8 Malignant neoplasm of overlapping sites of tongue `CL`
  Malignant neoplasm of two or more contiguous sites of tongue

C02.9 Malignant neoplasm of tongue, unspecified `CL`

✓4ᵗʰ **C03 Malignant neoplasm of gum**
  INCLUDES   malignant neoplasm of alveolar (ridge) mucosa
  malignant neoplasm of gingiva
  Use additional code to identify:
    alcohol abuse and dependence (F10.-)
    history of tobacco dependence (Z87.891)
    tobacco dependence (F17.-)
    tobacco use (Z72.0)
  EXCLUDES 2   malignant odontogenic neoplasms (C41.0-C41.1)

C03.0 Malignant neoplasm of upper gum
C03.1 Malignant neoplasm of lower gum `CL`
C03.9 Malignant neoplasm of gum, unspecified

✓4ᵗʰ **C04 Malignant neoplasm of floor of mouth**
  Use additional code to identify:
    alcohol abuse and dependence (F10.-)
    history of tobacco dependence (Z87.891)
    tobacco dependence (F17.-)
    tobacco use (Z72.0)

C04.0 Malignant neoplasm of anterior floor of mouth `CL`
  Malignant neoplasm of anterior to the premolar-canine junction
C04.1 Malignant neoplasm of lateral floor of mouth `CL`
C04.8 Malignant neoplasm of overlapping sites of floor of mouth `CL`
C04.9 Malignant neoplasm of floor of mouth, unspecified `CL`

✓4ᵗʰ **C05 Malignant neoplasm of palate**
  Use additional code to identify:
    alcohol abuse and dependence (F10.-)
    history of tobacco dependence (Z87.891)
    tobacco dependence (F17.-)
    tobacco use (Z72.0)
  EXCLUDES 1   Kaposi's sarcoma of palate (C46.2)

C05.0 Malignant neoplasm of hard palate `CL`
C05.1 Malignant neoplasm of soft palate `CL`
  EXCLUDES 2   malignant neoplasm of nasopharyngeal surface of soft palate (C11.3)
C05.2 Malignant neoplasm of uvula `CL`
C05.8 Malignant neoplasm of overlapping sites of palate `CL`
C05.9 Malignant neoplasm of palate, unspecified `CL`
  Malignant neoplasm of roof of mouth

✓4ᵗʰ **C06 Malignant neoplasm of other and unspecified parts of mouth**
  Use additional code to identify:
    alcohol abuse and dependence (F10.-)
    history of tobacco dependence (Z87.891)
    tobacco dependence (F17.-)
    tobacco use (Z72.0)

C06.0 Malignant neoplasm of cheek mucosa `CL`
  Malignant neoplasm of buccal mucosa NOS
  Malignant neoplasm of internal cheek
C06.1 Malignant neoplasm of vestibule of mouth `CL`
  Malignant neoplasm of buccal sulcus (upper) (lower)
  Malignant neoplasm of labial sulcus (upper) (lower)
C06.2 Malignant neoplasm of retromolar area `CL`
✓5ᵗʰ **C06.8 Malignant neoplasm of overlapping sites of other and unspecified parts of mouth**
  C06.80 Malignant neoplasm of overlapping sites of unspecified parts of mouth `CL`
  C06.89 Malignant neoplasm of overlapping sites of other parts of mouth `CL`
    "book leaf" neoplasm [ventral surface of tongue and floor of mouth]

C06.9 Malignant neoplasm of mouth, unspecified `CL`
  Malignant neoplasm of minor salivary gland, unspecified site
  Malignant neoplasm of oral cavity NOS

C07 Malignant neoplasm of parotid gland `CL`
  Use additional code to identify:
    alcohol abuse and dependence (F10.-)
    exposure to environmental tobacco smoke (Z77.22)
    exposure to tobacco smoke in the perinatal period (P96.81)
    history of tobacco dependence (Z87.891)
    occupational exposure to environmental tobacco smoke (Z57.31)
    tobacco dependence (F17.-)
    tobacco use (Z72.0)

✓4ᵗʰ **C08 Malignant neoplasm of other and unspecified major salivary glands**
  INCLUDES   malignant neoplasm of salivary ducts
  Use additional code to identify:
    alcohol abuse and dependence (F10.-)
    exposure to environmental tobacco smoke (Z77.22)
    exposure to tobacco smoke in the perinatal period (P96.81)
    history of tobacco dependence (Z87.891)
    occupational exposure to environmental tobacco smoke (Z57.31)
    tobacco dependence (F17.-)
    tobacco use (Z72.0)
  EXCLUDES 1   malignant neoplasms of specified minor salivary glands which are classified according to their anatomical location
  EXCLUDES 2   malignant neoplasms of minor salivary glands NOS (C06.9)
    malignant neoplasm of parotid gland (C07)

C08.0 Malignant neoplasm of submandibular gland `CL`
  Malignant neoplasm of submaxillary gland
C08.1 Malignant neoplasm of sublingual gland `CL`
C08.9 Malignant neoplasm of major salivary gland, unspecified `CL`
  Malignant neoplasm of salivary gland (major) NOS

✓4ᵗʰ **C09 Malignant neoplasm of tonsil**
  Use additional code to identify:
    alcohol abuse and dependence (F10.-)
    exposure to environmental tobacco smoke (Z77.22)
    exposure to tobacco smoke in the perinatal period (P96.81)
    history of tobacco dependence (Z87.891)
    occupational exposure to environmental tobacco smoke (Z57.31)
    tobacco dependence (F17.-)
    tobacco use (Z72.0)
  EXCLUDES 2   malignant neoplasm of lingual tonsil (C02.4)
    malignant neoplasm of pharyngeal tonsil (C11.1)

C09.0 Malignant neoplasm of tonsillar fossa `CL`
C09.1 Malignant neoplasm of tonsillar pillar (anterior) (posterior) `CL`
C09.8 Malignant neoplasm of overlapping sites of tonsil `CL`
C09.9 Malignant neoplasm of tonsil, unspecified `CL`
  Malignant neoplasm of tonsil NOS
  Malignant neoplasm of faucial tonsils
  Malignant neoplasm of palatine tonsils

✓4ᵗʰ **C10 Malignant neoplasm of oropharynx**
  Use additional code to identify:
    alcohol abuse and dependence (F10.-)
    exposure to environmental tobacco smoke (Z77.22)
    exposure to tobacco smoke in the perinatal period (P96.81)
    history of tobacco dependence (Z87.891)
    occupational exposure to environmental tobacco smoke (Z57.31)
    tobacco dependence (F17.-)
    tobacco use (Z72.0)
  EXCLUDES 2   malignant neoplasm of tonsil (C09.-)
  DEF: Oropharynx: Middle portion of pharynx (throat); communicates with the oral cavity, nasopharynx and laryngopharynx.

C10.0 Malignant neoplasm of vallecula `CL`
C10.1 Malignant neoplasm of anterior surface of epiglottis `CL`
  Malignant neoplasm of epiglottis, free border [margin]
  Malignant neoplasm of glossoepiglottic fold(s)
  EXCLUDES 2   malignant neoplasm of epiglottis (suprahyoid portion) NOS (C32.1)
C10.2 Malignant neoplasm of lateral wall of oropharynx `CL`
C10.3 Malignant neoplasm of posterior wall of oropharynx `CL`

✓ Additional Character Required   ✓x7ᵗʰ Placeholder Alert   Manifestation   Unspecified Dx   ►◄ Revised Text   ● New Code   ▲ Revised Title
ICD-10-CM 2020   461

C02.3–C10.3

C10.4 **Malignant neoplasm of** branchial cleft `CL`

Malignant neoplasm of branchial cyst [site of neoplasm]

C10.8 **Malignant neoplasm of** overlapping sites **of** `CL`
oropharynx

Malignant neoplasm of junctional region of oropharynx

C10.9 **Malignant neoplasm of oropharynx, unspecified** `CL`

✓4ᵗʰ **C11** **Malignant neoplasm of** nasopharynx

Use additional code to identify:
exposure to environmental tobacco smoke (Z77.22)
exposure to tobacco smoke in the perinatal period (P96.81)
history of tobacco dependence (Z87.891)
occupational exposure to environmental tobacco smoke (Z57.31)
tobacco dependence (F17.-)
tobacco use (Z72.0)

DEF: Nasopharynx: Upper portion of pharynx (throat); communicates with the nasal cavities, oropharynx and tympanic cavities.

C11.0 **Malignant neoplasm of** superior wall **of** `CL`
nasopharynx

Malignant neoplasm of roof of nasopharynx

C11.1 **Malignant neoplasm of** posterior wall **of** `CL`
nasopharynx

Malignant neoplasm of adenoid
Malignant neoplasm of pharyngeal tonsil

C11.2 **Malignant neoplasm of** lateral wall **of** `CL`
nasopharynx

Malignant neoplasm of fossa of Rosenmüller
Malignant neoplasm of opening of auditory tube
Malignant neoplasm of pharyngeal recess

C11.3 **Malignant neoplasm of** anterior wall **of** `CL`
nasopharynx

Malignant neoplasm of floor of nasopharynx
Malignant neoplasm of nasopharyngeal (anterior) (posterior)
surface of soft palate
Malignant neoplasm of posterior margin of nasal choana
Malignant neoplasm of posterior margin of nasal septum

C11.8 **Malignant neoplasm of** overlapping sites **of** `CL`
nasopharynx

C11.9 **Malignant neoplasm of nasopharynx, unspecified**

Malignant neoplasm of nasopharyngeal wall NOS

C12 **Malignant neoplasm of** pyriform sinus `CL`

Malignant neoplasm of pyriform fossa
Use additional code to identify:
exposure to environmental tobacco smoke (Z77.22)
exposure to tobacco smoke in the perinatal period (P96.81)
history of tobacco dependence (Z87.891)
occupational exposure to environmental tobacco smoke (Z57.31)
tobacco dependence (F17.-)
tobacco use (Z72.0)

✓4ᵗʰ **C13** **Malignant neoplasm of** hypopharynx

Use additional code to identify:
exposure to environmental tobacco smoke (Z77.22)
exposure to tobacco smoke in the perinatal period (P96.81)
history of tobacco dependence (Z87.891)
occupational exposure to environmental tobacco smoke (Z57.31)
tobacco dependence (F17.-)
tobacco use (Z72.0)

EXCLUDES 2 *malignant neoplasm of pyriform sinus (C12)*

DEF: Hypopharynx: Lower portion of pharynx (throat); communicates with the oropharynx and the esophagus. ***Synonyms:*** *laryngopharynx.*

C13.0 **Malignant neoplasm of** postcricoid region `CL`

C13.1 **Malignant neoplasm of** aryepiglottic fold, `CL`
hypopharyngeal aspect

Malignant neoplasm of aryepiglottic fold, marginal zone
Malignant neoplasm of aryepiglottic fold NOS
Malignant neoplasm of interarytenoid fold, marginal zone
Malignant neoplasm of interarytenoid fold NOS

EXCLUDES 2 *malignant neoplasm of aryepiglottic fold or*
interarytenoid fold, laryngeal aspect (C32.1)

C13.2 **Malignant neoplasm of** posterior wall **of** `CL`
hypopharynx

C13.8 **Malignant neoplasm of** overlapping sites **of** `CL`
hypopharynx

C13.9 **Malignant neoplasm of hypopharynx, unspecified** `CL`

Malignant neoplasm of hypopharyngeal wall NOS

✓4ᵗʰ **C14** **Malignant neoplasm of** other and ill-defined sites in the lip, oral cavity and pharynx

Use additional code to identify:
alcohol abuse and dependence (F10.-)
exposure to environmental tobacco smoke (Z77.22)
exposure to tobacco smoke in the perinatal period (P96.81)
history of tobacco dependence (Z87.891)
occupational exposure to environmental tobacco smoke (Z57.31)
tobacco dependence (F17.-)
tobacco use (Z72.0)

EXCLUDES 1 *malignant neoplasm of oral cavity NOS (C06.9)*

C14.0 **Malignant neoplasm of pharynx, unspecified** `CL`

C14.2 **Malignant neoplasm of** Waldeyer's ring `CL`

DEF: Waldeyer's ring: Ring of lymphoid tissue that is made up of the two palatine tonsils, the pharyngeal tonsil (adenoid), and the lingual tonsil. It functions as the defense against infection and assists with the development of the immune system.

C14.8 **Malignant neoplasm of** overlapping sites **of lip,** `CL`
oral cavity and pharynx

Primary malignant neoplasm of two or more contiguous sites of lip, oral cavity and pharynx

EXCLUDES 1 *"book leaf" neoplasm [ventral surface of tongue and*
floor of mouth] (C06.89)

Malignant neoplasms of digestive organs (C15-C26)

EXCLUDES 1 *Kaposi's sarcoma of gastrointestinal sites (C46.4)*
EXCLUDES 2 *gastrointestinal stromal tumors (C49.A-)*

✓4ᵗʰ **C15** **Malignant neoplasm of** esophagus

Use additional code to identify:
alcohol abuse and dependence (F10.-)

C15.3 **Malignant neoplasm of** upper third **of esophagus**

C15.4 **Malignant neoplasm of** middle third **of esophagus**

C15.5 **Malignant neoplasm of** lower third **of esophagus**

EXCLUDES 1 *malignant neoplasm of cardio-esophageal junction*
(C16.0)

C15.8 **Malignant neoplasm of** overlapping sites **of esophagus**

C15.9 **Malignant neoplasm of esophagus, unspecified**

✓4ᵗʰ **C16** **Malignant neoplasm of** stomach

Use additional code to identify:
alcohol abuse and dependence (F10.-)

EXCLUDES 2 *malignant carcinoid tumor of the stomach (C7A.092)*

C16.0 **Malignant neoplasm of** cardia

Malignant neoplasm of cardiac orifice
Malignant neoplasm of cardio-esophageal junction
Malignant neoplasm of esophagus and stomach
Malignant neoplasm of gastro-esophageal junction

C16.1 **Malignant neoplasm of** fundus **of stomach**

C16.2 **Malignant neoplasm of** body **of stomach**

C16.3 **Malignant neoplasm of** pyloric antrum

Malignant neoplasm of gastric antrum

C16.4 **Malignant neoplasm of** pylorus

Malignant neoplasm of prepylorus
Malignant neoplasm of pyloric canal

C16.5 **Malignant neoplasm of** lesser curvature **of stomach,**
unspecified

Malignant neoplasm of lesser curvature of stomach, not
classifiable to C16.1-C16.4

C16.6 **Malignant neoplasm of** greater curvature **of stomach,**
unspecified

Malignant neoplasm of greater curvature of stomach, not
classifiable to C16.0-C16.4

C16.8 **Malignant neoplasm of** overlapping sites **of stomach**

C16.9 **Malignant neoplasm of stomach, unspecified**

Gastric cancer NOS

✓4ᵗʰ **C17** **Malignant neoplasm of** small intestine

EXCLUDES 1 *malignant carcinoid tumors of the small intestine (C7A.01)*

AHA: 2016,1Q,19

C17.0 **Malignant neoplasm of** duodenum

C17.1 **Malignant neoplasm of** jejunum

C17.2 **Malignant neoplasm of** ileum

EXCLUDES 1 *malignant neoplasm of ileocecal valve (C18.0)*

N Newborn: 0   P Pediatric: 0-17   M Maternity: 12-55   A Adult: 15-124   CH Comorbidity High   CL Comorbidity Low   NC Dx Noncancer Dx   PDx Primary Dx

462   ICD-10-CM 2020

C17.3   Meckel's diverticulum, **malignant**

> EXCLUDES 1   *Meckel's diverticulum, congenital (Q43.0)*
>
> **DEF:** Congenital, abnormal remnant of embryonic digestive system development that leaves a sacculation or outpouching from the wall of the small intestine near the terminal part of the ileum made of acid-secreting tissue as in the stomach.

C17.8   **Malignant neoplasm of** overlapping sites **of small intestine**

C17.9   **Malignant neoplasm of small intestine, unspecified**

✓4th **C18**   **Malignant neoplasm of** colon

> EXCLUDES 1   *malignant carcinoid tumors of the colon (C7A.02-)*

Colon

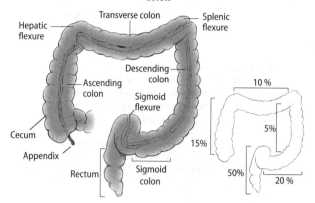

Anatomical distribution of large bowel cancers

C18.0   **Malignant neoplasm of** cecum
Malignant neoplasm of ileocecal valve

C18.1   **Malignant neoplasm of** appendix

C18.2   **Malignant neoplasm of** ascending colon

C18.3   **Malignant neoplasm of** hepatic flexure

C18.4   **Malignant neoplasm of** transverse colon

C18.5   **Malignant neoplasm of** splenic flexure

C18.6   **Malignant neoplasm of** descending colon

C18.7   **Malignant neoplasm of** sigmoid colon
Malignant neoplasm of sigmoid (flexure)

> EXCLUDES 1   *malignant neoplasm of rectosigmoid junction (C19)*

C18.8   **Malignant neoplasm of** overlapping sites **of colon**

C18.9   **Malignant neoplasm of colon, unspecified**
Malignant neoplasm of large intestine NOS

C19   **Malignant neoplasm of** rectosigmoid junction
Malignant neoplasm of colon with rectum
Malignant neoplasm of rectosigmoid (colon)

> EXCLUDES 1   *malignant carcinoid tumors of the colon (C7A.02-)*

C20   **Malignant neoplasm of** rectum
Malignant neoplasm of rectal ampulla

> EXCLUDES 1   *malignant carcinoid tumor of the rectum (C7A.026)*

✓4th **C21**   **Malignant neoplasm of** anus and anal canal

> EXCLUDES 2   *malignant carcinoid tumors of the colon (C7A.02-)*
> *malignant melanoma of anal margin (C43.51)*
> *malignant melanoma of anal skin (C43.51)*
> *malignant melanoma of perianal skin (C43.51)*
> *other and unspecified malignant neoplasm of anal margin (C44.500, C44.510, C44.520, C44.590)*
> *other and unspecified malignant neoplasm of anal skin (C44.500, C44.510, C44.520, C44.590)*
> *other and unspecified malignant neoplasm of perianal skin (C44.500, C44.510, C44.520, C44.590)*

C21.0   **Malignant neoplasm of anus, unspecified**

C21.1   **Malignant neoplasm of** anal canal
Malignant neoplasm of anal sphincter

C21.2   **Malignant neoplasm of** cloacogenic zone

C21.8   **Malignant neoplasm of** overlapping sites **of rectum, anus and anal canal**
Malignant neoplasm of anorectal junction
Malignant neoplasm of anorectum
Primary malignant neoplasm of two or more contiguous sites of rectum, anus and anal canal

✓4th **C22**   **Malignant neoplasm of** liver and intrahepatic bile ducts

> Use additional code to identify:
> alcohol abuse and dependence (F10.-)
> hepatitis B (B16.-, B18.0-B18.1)
> hepatitis C (B17.1-, B18.2)
>
> EXCLUDES 1   *malignant neoplasm of biliary tract NOS (C24.9)*
> *secondary malignant neoplasm of liver and intrahepatic bile duct (C78.7)*

C22.0   Liver cell **carcinoma**
Hepatocellular carcinoma
Hepatoma
AHA: 2016,1Q,18

C22.1   Intrahepatic bile duct **carcinoma**
Cholangiocarcinoma

> EXCLUDES 1   *malignant neoplasm of hepatic duct (C24.0)*

C22.2   **Hepatoblastoma**

C22.3   **Angiosarcoma** of liver
Kupffer cell sarcoma

C22.4   **Other** sarcomas **of liver**

C22.7   **Other specified carcinomas of liver**

C22.8   **Malignant neoplasm of liver,** primary, **unspecified as to type**

C22.9   **Malignant neoplasm of liver, not specified as primary or secondary**

C23   **Malignant neoplasm of** gallbladder

✓4th **C24**   **Malignant neoplasm of** other and unspecified parts of biliary tract

> EXCLUDES 1   *malignant neoplasm of intrahepatic bile duct (C22.1)*

C24.0   **Malignant neoplasm of** extrahepatic bile duct
Malignant neoplasm of biliary duct or passage NOS
Malignant neoplasm of common bile duct
Malignant neoplasm of cystic duct
Malignant neoplasm of hepatic duct

C24.1   **Malignant neoplasm of** ampulla of Vater
DEF: Malignant neoplasm in the area of dilation at the juncture of the common bile and pancreatic ducts near the opening into the lumen of the duodenum.

C24.8   **Malignant neoplasm of** overlapping sites **of biliary tract**
Malignant neoplasm involving both intrahepatic and extrahepatic bile ducts
Primary malignant neoplasm of two or more contiguous sites of biliary tract

C24.9   **Malignant neoplasm of biliary tract, unspecified**

✓4th **C25**   **Malignant neoplasm of** pancreas

> Code also exocrine pancreatic insufficiency (K86.81)
> Use additional code to identify:
> alcohol abuse and dependence (F10.-)

Pancreas

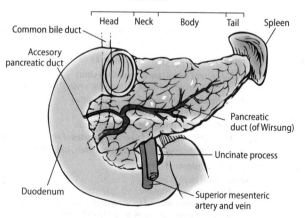

C25.0   **Malignant neoplasm of** head of pancreas

C25.1   **Malignant neoplasm of** body of pancreas

C25.2   **Malignant neoplasm of** tail of pancreas

C25.3   **Malignant neoplasm of** pancreatic duct

C25.4   **Malignant neoplasm of** endocrine pancreas
Malignant neoplasm of islets of Langerhans
Use additional code to identify any functional activity

C25.7   **Malignant neoplasm of other parts of pancreas**
Malignant neoplasm of neck of pancreas

C25.8   **Malignant neoplasm of** overlapping sites **of pancreas**

✓ Additional Character Required   ✓x7th Placeholder Alert   Manifestation   Unspecified Dx   ▶◀ Revised Text   ● New Code   ▲ Revised Title

ICD-10-CM 2020   463

Chapter 2. Neoplasms

C25.9   Malignant neoplasm of pancreas, unspecified

✓4ᵗʰ C26   Malignant neoplasm of other and ill-defined digestive organs

EXCLUDES 1   malignant neoplasm of peritoneum and retroperitoneum (C48.-)

C26.0   Malignant neoplasm of intestinal tract, part unspecified
Malignant neoplasm of intestine NOS

C26.1   Malignant neoplasm of spleen

EXCLUDES 1   Hodgkin lymphoma (C81.-)
non-Hodgkin lymphoma (C82-C85)

C26.9   Malignant neoplasm of ill-defined sites within the digestive system
Malignant neoplasm of alimentary canal or tract NOS
Malignant neoplasm of gastrointestinal tract NOS

EXCLUDES 1   malignant neoplasm of abdominal NOS (C76.2)
malignant neoplasm of intra-abdominal NOS (C76.2)

Malignant neoplasms of respiratory and intrathoracic organs (C30-C39)

INCLUDES   malignant neoplasm of middle ear
EXCLUDES 1   mesothelioma (C45.-)

✓4ᵗʰ C30   Malignant neoplasm of nasal cavity and middle ear

C30.0   Malignant neoplasm of nasal cavity
Malignant neoplasm of cartilage of nose
Malignant neoplasm of nasal concha
Malignant neoplasm of internal nose
Malignant neoplasm of septum of nose
Malignant neoplasm of vestibule of nose

EXCLUDES 1   malignant neoplasm of nasal bone (C41.0)
malignant neoplasm of nose NOS (C76.0)
malignant neoplasm of olfactory bulb (C72.2-)
malignant neoplasm of posterior margin of nasal septum and choana (C11.3)
malignant melanoma of skin of nose (C43.31)
malignant neoplasm of turbinates (C41.0)
other and unspecified malignant neoplasm of skin of nose (C44.301, C44.311, C44.321, C44.391)

C30.1   Malignant neoplasm of middle ear
Malignant neoplasm of antrum tympanicum
Malignant neoplasm of auditory tube
Malignant neoplasm of eustachian tube
Malignant neoplasm of inner ear
Malignant neoplasm of mastoid air cells
Malignant neoplasm of tympanic cavity

EXCLUDES 1   malignant neoplasm of auricular canal (external) (C43.2-,C44.2-)
malignant neoplasm of bone of ear (meatus) (C41.0)
malignant neoplasm of cartilage of ear (C49.0)
malignant melanoma of skin of (external) ear (C43.2-)
other and unspecified malignant neoplasm of skin of (external) ear (C44.2-)

✓4ᵗʰ C31   Malignant neoplasm of accessory sinuses

C31.0   Malignant neoplasm of maxillary sinus
Malignant neoplasm of antrum (Highmore) (maxillary)

C31.1   Malignant neoplasm of ethmoidal sinus

C31.2   Malignant neoplasm of frontal sinus

C31.3   Malignant neoplasm of sphenoid sinus

C31.8   Malignant neoplasm of overlapping sites of accessory sinuses

C31.9   Malignant neoplasm of accessory sinus, unspecified

✓4ᵗʰ C32   Malignant neoplasm of larynx
Use additional code to identify:
alcohol abuse and dependence (F10.-)
exposure to environmental tobacco smoke (Z77.22)
exposure to tobacco smoke in the perinatal period (P96.81)
history of tobacco dependence (Z87.891)
occupational exposure to environmental tobacco smoke (Z57.31)
tobacco dependence (F17.-)
tobacco use (Z72.0)

C32.0   Malignant neoplasm of glottis
Malignant neoplasm of intrinsic larynx
Malignant neoplasm of laryngeal commissure (anterior)(posterior)
Malignant neoplasm of vocal cord (true) NOS

C32.1   Malignant neoplasm of supraglottis
Malignant neoplasm of aryepiglottic fold or interarytenoid fold, laryngeal aspect
Malignant neoplasm of epiglottis (suprahyoid portion) NOS
Malignant neoplasm of extrinsic larynx
Malignant neoplasm of false vocal cord
Malignant neoplasm of posterior (laryngeal) surface of epiglottis
Malignant neoplasm of ventricular bands

EXCLUDES 2   malignant neoplasm of anterior surface of epiglottis (C10.1)
malignant neoplasm of aryepiglottic fold or interarytenoid fold, hypopharyngeal aspect (C13.1)
malignant neoplasm of aryepiglottic fold or interarytenoid fold, marginal zone (C13.1)
malignant neoplasm of aryepiglottic fold or interarytenoid fold NOS (C13.1)

C32.2   Malignant neoplasm of subglottis

C32.3   Malignant neoplasm of laryngeal cartilage

C32.8   Malignant neoplasm of overlapping sites of larynx

C32.9   Malignant neoplasm of larynx, unspecified

C33   Malignant neoplasm of trachea
Use additional code to identify:
exposure to environmental tobacco smoke (Z77.22)
exposure to tobacco smoke in the perinatal period (P96.81)
history of tobacco dependence (Z87.891)
occupational exposure to environmental tobacco smoke (Z57.31)
tobacco dependence (F17.-)
tobacco use (Z72.0)

✓4ᵗʰ C34   Malignant neoplasm of bronchus and lung
Use additional code to identify:
exposure to environmental tobacco smoke (Z77.22)
exposure to tobacco smoke in the perinatal period (P96.81)
history of tobacco dependence (Z87.891)
occupational exposure to environmental tobacco smoke (Z57.31)
tobacco dependence (F17.-)
tobacco use (Z72.0)

EXCLUDES 1   Kaposi's sarcoma of lung (C46.5-)
malignant carcinoid tumor of the bronchus and lung (C7A.090)

AHA: 2019,1Q,16

✓5ᵗʰ C34.0   Malignant neoplasm of main bronchus
Malignant neoplasm of carina
Malignant neoplasm of hilus (of lung)

C34.00   Malignant neoplasm of unspecified main bronchus
C34.01   Malignant neoplasm of right main bronchus
C34.02   Malignant neoplasm of left main bronchus

✓5ᵗʰ C34.1   Malignant neoplasm of upper lobe, bronchus or lung

C34.10   Malignant neoplasm of upper lobe, unspecified bronchus or lung
C34.11   Malignant neoplasm of upper lobe, right bronchus or lung
C34.12   Malignant neoplasm of upper lobe, left bronchus or lung

C34.2   Malignant neoplasm of middle lobe, bronchus or lung

✓5ᵗʰ C34.3   Malignant neoplasm of lower lobe, bronchus or lung

C34.30   Malignant neoplasm of lower lobe, unspecified bronchus or lung
C34.31   Malignant neoplasm of lower lobe, right bronchus or lung
C34.32   Malignant neoplasm of lower lobe, left bronchus or lung

✓5ᵗʰ C34.8   Malignant neoplasm of overlapping sites of bronchus and lung

C34.80   Malignant neoplasm of overlapping sites of unspecified bronchus and lung
C34.81   Malignant neoplasm of overlapping sites of right bronchus and lung
C34.82   Malignant neoplasm of overlapping sites of left bronchus and lung

✓5ᵗʰ C34.9   Malignant neoplasm of unspecified part of bronchus or lung

C34.90   Malignant neoplasm of unspecified part of unspecified bronchus or lung
Lung cancer NOS
C34.91   Malignant neoplasm of unspecified part of right bronchus or lung

N Newborn: 0   P Pediatric: 0-17   M Maternity: 12-55   A Adult: 15-124   CH Comorbidity High   CL Comorbidity Low   NCDx Noncancer Dx   PDx Primary Dx

464   ICD-10-CM 2020

C34.92 Malignant neoplasm of unspecified part of left bronchus or lung

C37 Malignant neoplasm of thymus
> EXCLUDES 1   *malignant carcinoid tumor of the thymus (C7A.091)*

√4th C38 Malignant neoplasm of heart, mediastinum and pleura
> EXCLUDES 1   *mesothelioma (C45.-)*

C38.0 Malignant neoplasm of heart
Malignant neoplasm of pericardium
> EXCLUDES 1   *malignant neoplasm of great vessels (C49.3)*

C38.1 Malignant neoplasm of anterior mediastinum

C38.2 Malignant neoplasm of posterior mediastinum

C38.3 Malignant neoplasm of mediastinum, part unspecified

C38.4 Malignant neoplasm of pleura

C38.8 Malignant neoplasm of overlapping sites of heart, mediastinum and pleura

√4th C39 Malignant neoplasm of other and ill-defined sites in the respiratory system and intrathoracic organs
Use additional code to identify:
exposure to environmental tobacco smoke (Z77.22)
exposure to tobacco smoke in the perinatal period (P96.81)
history of tobacco dependence (Z87.891)
occupational exposure to environmental tobacco smoke (Z57.31)
tobacco dependence (F17.-)
tobacco use (Z72.0)
> EXCLUDES 1   *intrathoracic malignant neoplasm NOS (C76.1)*
> *thoracic malignant neoplasm NOS (C76.1)*

C39.0 Malignant neoplasm of upper respiratory tract, part unspecified

C39.9 Malignant neoplasm of lower respiratory tract, part unspecified
Malignant neoplasm of respiratory tract NOS

Malignant neoplasms of bone and articular cartilage (C40-C41)

> INCLUDES   malignant neoplasm of cartilage (articular) (joint)
> malignant neoplasm of periosteum
> EXCLUDES 1   *malignant neoplasm of bone marrow NOS (C96.9)*
> *malignant neoplasm of synovia (C49.-)*

√4th C40 Malignant neoplasm of bone and articular cartilage of limbs
Use additional code to identify major osseous defect, if applicable (M89.7-)

√5th C40.0 Malignant neoplasm of scapula and long bones of upper limb
> **C40.00 Malignant neoplasm of scapula and long bones of unspecified upper limb**
> **C40.01 Malignant neoplasm of scapula and long bones of right upper limb**
> **C40.02 Malignant neoplasm of scapula and long bones of left upper limb**

√5th C40.1 Malignant neoplasm of short bones of upper limb
> **C40.10 Malignant neoplasm of short bones of unspecified upper limb**
> **C40.11 Malignant neoplasm of short bones of right upper limb**
> **C40.12 Malignant neoplasm of short bones of left upper limb**

√5th C40.2 Malignant neoplasm of long bones of lower limb
> **C40.20 Malignant neoplasm of long bones of unspecified lower limb**
> **C40.21 Malignant neoplasm of long bones of right lower limb**
> **C40.22 Malignant neoplasm of long bones of left lower limb**

√5th C40.3 Malignant neoplasm of short bones of lower limb
> **C40.30 Malignant neoplasm of short bones of unspecified lower limb**
> **C40.31 Malignant neoplasm of short bones of right lower limb**
> **C40.32 Malignant neoplasm of short bones of left lower limb**

√5th C40.8 Malignant neoplasm of overlapping sites of bone and articular cartilage of limb
> **C40.80 Malignant neoplasm of overlapping sites of bone and articular cartilage of unspecified limb**
> **C40.81 Malignant neoplasm of overlapping sites of bone and articular cartilage of right limb**
> **C40.82 Malignant neoplasm of overlapping sites of bone and articular cartilage of left limb**

√5th C40.9 Malignant neoplasm of unspecified bones and articular cartilage of limb
> **C40.90 Malignant neoplasm of unspecified bones and articular cartilage of unspecified limb**
> **C40.91 Malignant neoplasm of unspecified bones and articular cartilage of right limb**
> **C40.92 Malignant neoplasm of unspecified bones and articular cartilage of left limb**

√4th C41 Malignant neoplasm of bone and articular cartilage of other and unspecified sites
> EXCLUDES 1   *malignant neoplasm of bones of limbs (C40.-)*
> *malignant neoplasm of cartilage of ear (C49.0)*
> *malignant neoplasm of cartilage of eyelid (C49.0)*
> *malignant neoplasm of cartilage of larynx (C32.3)*
> *malignant neoplasm of cartilage of limbs (C40.-)*
> *malignant neoplasm of cartilage of nose (C30.0)*

C41.0 Malignant neoplasm of bones of skull and face
Malignant neoplasm of maxilla (superior)
Malignant neoplasm of orbital bone
> EXCLUDES 2   *carcinoma, any type except intraosseous or odontogenic of:*
> *maxillary sinus (C31.0)*
> *upper jaw (C03.0)*
> *malignant neoplasm of jaw bone (lower) (C41.1)*

C41.1 Malignant neoplasm of mandible
Malignant neoplasm of inferior maxilla
Malignant neoplasm of lower jaw bone
> EXCLUDES 2   *carcinoma, any type except intraosseous or odontogenic of:*
> *jaw NOS (C03.9)*
> *lower (C03.1)*
> *malignant neoplasm of upper jaw bone (C41.0)*

C41.2 Malignant neoplasm of vertebral column
> EXCLUDES 1   *malignant neoplasm of sacrum and coccyx (C41.4)*

C41.3 Malignant neoplasm of ribs, sternum and clavicle

C41.4 Malignant neoplasm of pelvic bones, sacrum and coccyx

C41.9 Malignant neoplasm of bone and articular cartilage, unspecified

Melanoma and other malignant neoplasms of skin (C43-C44)

√4th C43 Malignant melanoma of skin
> EXCLUDES 1   *melanoma in situ (D03.-)*
> EXCLUDES 2   *malignant melanoma of skin of genital organs (C51-C52, C60.-, C63.-)*
> *Merkel cell carcinoma (C4A.-)*
> *sites other than skin - code to malignant neoplasm of the site*

C43.0 Malignant melanoma of lip
> EXCLUDES 1   *malignant neoplasm of vermilion border of lip (C00.0-C00.2)*

√5th C43.1 Malignant melanoma of eyelid, including canthus
AHA: 2018,4Q,4
> **C43.10 Malignant melanoma of unspecified eyelid, including canthus**
> **√6th C43.11 Malignant melanoma of right eyelid, including canthus**
> > **C43.111 Malignant melanoma of right upper eyelid, including canthus**
> > **C43.112 Malignant melanoma of right lower eyelid, including canthus**
> **√6th C43.12 Malignant melanoma of left eyelid, including canthus**
> > **C43.121 Malignant melanoma of left upper eyelid, including canthus**
> > **C43.122 Malignant melanoma of left lower eyelid, including canthus**

√5th C43.2 Malignant melanoma of ear and external auricular canal
> **C43.20 Malignant melanoma of unspecified ear and external auricular canal**
> **C43.21 Malignant melanoma of right ear and external auricular canal**
> **C43.22 Malignant melanoma of left ear and external auricular canal**

√5th C43.3 Malignant melanoma of other and unspecified parts of face
> **C43.30 Malignant melanoma of unspecified part of face**
> **C43.31 Malignant melanoma of nose**
> **C43.39 Malignant melanoma of other parts of face**

C43.4 Malignant melanoma of scalp and neck

☑ Additional Character Required   √x7th Placeholder Alert   Manifestation   Unspecified Dx   ►◄ Revised Text   ● New Code   ▲ Revised Title

ICD-10-CM 2020   465

√5ᵗʰ **C43.5** **Malignant melanoma of** trunk
  EXCLUDES 2　*malignant neoplasm of anus NOS (C21.0)*
  　　　　　　malignant neoplasm of scrotum (C63.2)
  C43.51 **Malignant melanoma of** anal skin
  　　　Malignant melanoma of anal margin
  　　　Malignant melanoma of perianal skin
  C43.52 **Malignant melanoma of** skin of breast
  C43.59 **Malignant melanoma of** other part of trunk

√5ᵗʰ **C43.6** **Malignant melanoma of** upper limb, including shoulder
  C43.60 **Malignant melanoma of unspecified upper limb, including shoulder**
  C43.61 **Malignant melanoma of** right upper limb, including shoulder
  C43.62 **Malignant melanoma of** left upper limb, including shoulder

√5ᵗʰ **C43.7** **Malignant melanoma of** lower limb, including hip
  C43.70 **Malignant melanoma of unspecified lower limb, including hip**
  C43.71 **Malignant melanoma of** right lower limb, including hip
  C43.72 **Malignant melanoma of** left lower limb, including hip

  C43.8 **Malignant melanoma of** overlapping sites of skin
  C43.9 **Malignant melanoma of skin, unspecified**
  　　　Malignant melanoma of unspecified site of skin
  　　　Melanoma (malignant) NOS

√4ᵗʰ **C4A** **Merkel cell carcinoma**
  DEF: Malignant cutaneous cancer predominantly found in elderly patients with sun exposure that usually presents as a flesh-colored or bluish-red lump typically seen on the neck, head, and face.
  C4A.0 **Merkel cell carcinoma of** lip
  　　EXCLUDES 1　*malignant neoplasm of vermilion border of lip (C00.0-C00.2)*

√5ᵗʰ **C4A.1** **Merkel cell carcinoma of** eyelid, including canthus
  AHA: 2018,4Q,4
  C4A.10 **Merkel cell carcinoma of unspecified eyelid, including canthus**
  √6ᵗʰ **C4A.11** **Merkel cell carcinoma of** right eyelid, including canthus
  　　C4A.111 **Merkel cell carcinoma of right** upper eyelid, including canthus
  　　C4A.112 **Merkel cell carcinoma of right** lower eyelid, including canthus
  √6ᵗʰ **C4A.12** **Merkel cell carcinoma of** left eyelid, including canthus
  　　C4A.121 **Merkel cell carcinoma of left** upper eyelid, including canthus
  　　C4A.122 **Merkel cell carcinoma of left** lower eyelid, including canthus

√5ᵗʰ **C4A.2** **Merkel cell carcinoma of** ear and external auricular canal
  C4A.20 **Merkel cell carcinoma of unspecified ear and external auricular canal**
  C4A.21 **Merkel cell carcinoma of** right ear and external auricular canal
  C4A.22 **Merkel cell carcinoma of** left ear and external auricular canal

√5ᵗʰ **C4A.3** **Merkel cell carcinoma of other and unspecified** parts of face
  C4A.30 **Merkel cell carcinoma of unspecified part of face**
  C4A.31 **Merkel cell carcinoma of** nose
  C4A.39 **Merkel cell carcinoma of** other parts of face

  C4A.4 **Merkel cell carcinoma of** scalp and neck

√5ᵗʰ **C4A.5** **Merkel cell carcinoma of** trunk
  　　EXCLUDES 2　*malignant neoplasm of anus NOS (C21.0)*
  　　　　　　malignant neoplasm of scrotum (C63.2)
  C4A.51 **Merkel cell carcinoma of** anal skin
  　　　Merkel cell carcinoma of anal margin
  　　　Merkel cell carcinoma of perianal skin
  C4A.52 **Merkel cell carcinoma of** skin of breast
  C4A.59 **Merkel cell carcinoma of** other part of trunk

√5ᵗʰ **C4A.6** **Merkel cell carcinoma of** upper limb, including shoulder
  C4A.60 **Merkel cell carcinoma of unspecified upper limb, including shoulder**
  C4A.61 **Merkel cell carcinoma of** right upper limb, including shoulder
  C4A.62 **Merkel cell carcinoma of** left upper limb, including shoulder

√5ᵗʰ **C4A.7** **Merkel cell carcinoma of** lower limb, including hip
  C4A.70 **Merkel cell carcinoma of unspecified lower limb, including hip**
  C4A.71 **Merkel cell carcinoma of** right lower limb, including hip
  C4A.72 **Merkel cell carcinoma of** left lower limb, including hip

  C4A.8 **Merkel cell carcinoma of** overlapping sites
  C4A.9 **Merkel cell carcinoma, unspecified**
  　　　Merkel cell carcinoma of unspecified site
  　　　Merkel cell carcinoma NOS

√4ᵗʰ **C44** **Other and unspecified malignant neoplasm** of skin
  INCLUDES　malignant neoplasm of sebaceous glands
  　　　　　malignant neoplasm of sweat glands
  EXCLUDES 1　*Kaposi's sarcoma of skin (C46.0)*
  　　　　　malignant melanoma of skin (C43.-)
  　　　　　malignant neoplasm of skin of genital organs (C51-C52, C60.-, C63.2)
  　　　　　Merkel cell carcinoma (C4A.-)
  DEF: Basal cell carcinoma: Abnormal growth of skin cells that arises from the deepest layer of the epidermis and may present as an open sore, red patches, pink growth, or scar. Typically caused by sun exposure, it is one of the most common forms of skin cancer.
  DEF: Squamous cell carcinoma: Uncontrolled growth of abnormal skin cells that arises from the outer layers of the skin (epidermis) and may present as an open sore. It is characterized by a firm, red nodule, elevated growth with a central depression, or a flat sore with a scaly crust.

√5ᵗʰ **C44.0** **Other and unspecified malignant neoplasm of skin of** lip
  　　EXCLUDES 1　*malignant neoplasm of lip (C00.-)*
  C44.00 **Unspecified malignant neoplasm of skin of lip**
  C44.01 Basal cell carcinoma **of skin of lip**
  C44.02 Squamous cell carcinoma **of skin of lip**
  C44.09 **Other specified malignant neoplasm of skin of lip**

√5ᵗʰ **C44.1** **Other and unspecified malignant neoplasm of skin of** eyelid, including canthus
  　　EXCLUDES 1　*connective tissue of eyelid (C49.0)*
  AHA: 2018,4Q,4
  √6ᵗʰ **C44.10** **Unspecified malignant neoplasm of skin of eyelid, including canthus**
  　　C44.101 **Unspecified malignant neoplasm of skin of unspecified eyelid, including canthus**
  　　√7ᵗʰ **C44.102** **Unspecified malignant neoplasm of skin of** right **eyelid, including canthus**
  　　　　C44.1021 **Unspecified malignant neoplasm of skin of right** upper **eyelid, including canthus**
  　　　　C44.1022 **Unspecified malignant neoplasm of skin of right** lower **eyelid, including canthus**
  　　√7ᵗʰ **C44.109** **Unspecified malignant neoplasm of skin of** left **eyelid, including canthus**
  　　　　C44.1091 **Unspecified malignant neoplasm of skin of left** upper **eyelid, including canthus**
  　　　　C44.1092 **Unspecified malignant neoplasm of skin of left** lower **eyelid, including canthus**
  √6ᵗʰ **C44.11** Basal cell carcinoma **of skin of eyelid, including canthus**
  　　C44.111 Basal cell carcinoma of skin of unspecified **eyelid, including canthus**
  　　√7ᵗʰ **C44.112** Basal cell carcinoma of skin of right **eyelid, including canthus**
  　　　　C44.1121 Basal cell carcinoma of skin of right upper **eyelid, including canthus**
  　　　　C44.1122 Basal cell carcinoma of skin of right lower **eyelid, including canthus**
  　　√7ᵗʰ **C44.119** Basal cell carcinoma of skin of left **eyelid, including canthus**
  　　　　C44.1191 Basal cell carcinoma of skin of left upper **eyelid, including canthus**
  　　　　C44.1192 Basal cell carcinoma of skin of left lower **eyelid, including canthus**
  √6ᵗʰ **C44.12** Squamous cell carcinoma **of skin of eyelid, including canthus**
  　　C44.121 Squamous cell carcinoma of skin of unspecified **eyelid, including canthus**

N Newborn: 0　　P Pediatric: 0-17　　M Maternity: 12-55　　A Adult: 15-124　　CH Comorbidity High　　CL Comorbidity Low　　NCDx Noncancer Dx　　PDx Primary Dx

466　　　　　　　　　　　　　　　　　　　　　　　　　　　　ICD-10-CM 2020

√7th **C44.122** Squamous cell carcinoma of skin of right eyelid, including canthus
- **C44.1221** Squamous cell carcinoma of skin of right upper eyelid, including canthus
- **C44.1222** Squamous cell carcinoma of skin of right lower eyelid, including canthus

√7th **C44.129** Squamous cell carcinoma of skin of left eyelid, including canthus
- **C44.1291** Squamous cell carcinoma of skin of left upper eyelid, including canthus
- **C44.1292** Squamous cell carcinoma of skin of left lower eyelid, including canthus

√6th **C44.13** Sebaceous cell carcinoma of skin of eyelid, including canthus
- **C44.131** Sebaceous cell carcinoma of skin of unspecified eyelid, including canthus
- √7th **C44.132** Sebaceous cell carcinoma of skin of right eyelid, including canthus
  - **C44.1321** Sebaceous cell carcinoma of skin of right upper eyelid, including canthus
  - **C44.1322** Sebaceous cell carcinoma of skin of right lower eyelid, including canthus
- √7th **C44.139** Sebaceous cell carcinoma of skin of left eyelid, including canthus
  - **C44.1391** Sebaceous cell carcinoma of skin of left upper eyelid, including canthus
  - **C44.1392** Sebaceous cell carcinoma of skin of left lower eyelid, including canthus

√6th **C44.19** Other specified malignant neoplasm of skin of eyelid, including canthus
- **C44.191** Other specified malignant neoplasm of skin of unspecified eyelid, including canthus
- √7th **C44.192** Other specified malignant neoplasm of skin of right eyelid, including canthus
  - **C44.1921** Other specified malignant neoplasm of skin of right upper eyelid, including canthus
  - **C44.1922** Other specified malignant neoplasm of skin of right lower eyelid, including canthus
- √7th **C44.199** Other specified malignant neoplasm of skin of left eyelid, including canthus
  - **C44.1991** Other specified malignant neoplasm of skin of left upper eyelid, including canthus
  - **C44.1992** Other specified malignant neoplasm of skin of left lower eyelid, including canthus

√5th **C44.2** Other and unspecified malignant neoplasm of skin of ear and external auricular canal
> **EXCLUDES 1**   connective tissue of ear (C49.0)

√6th **C44.20** Unspecified malignant neoplasm of skin of ear and external auricular canal
- **C44.201** Unspecified malignant neoplasm of skin of unspecified ear and external auricular canal
- **C44.202** Unspecified malignant neoplasm of skin of right ear and external auricular canal
- **C44.209** Unspecified malignant neoplasm of skin of left ear and external auricular canal

√6th **C44.21** Basal cell carcinoma of skin of ear and external auricular canal
- **C44.211** Basal cell carcinoma of skin of unspecified ear and external auricular canal
- **C44.212** Basal cell carcinoma of skin of right ear and external auricular canal
- **C44.219** Basal cell carcinoma of skin of left ear and external auricular canal

√6th **C44.22** Squamous cell carcinoma of skin of ear and external auricular canal
- **C44.221** Squamous cell carcinoma of skin of unspecified ear and external auricular canal
- **C44.222** Squamous cell carcinoma of skin of right ear and external auricular canal

C44.229 Squamous cell carcinoma of skin of left ear and external auricular canal

√6th **C44.29** Other specified malignant neoplasm of skin of ear and external auricular canal
- **C44.291** Other specified malignant neoplasm of skin of unspecified ear and external auricular canal
- **C44.292** Other specified malignant neoplasm of skin of right ear and external auricular canal
- **C44.299** Other specified malignant neoplasm of skin of left ear and external auricular canal

√5th **C44.3** Other and unspecified malignant neoplasm of skin of other and unspecified parts of face

√6th **C44.30** Unspecified malignant neoplasm of skin of other and unspecified parts of face
- **C44.300** Unspecified malignant neoplasm of skin of unspecified part of face
- **C44.301** Unspecified malignant neoplasm of skin of nose
- **C44.309** Unspecified malignant neoplasm of skin of other parts of face

√6th **C44.31** Basal cell carcinoma of skin of other and unspecified parts of face
- **C44.310** Basal cell carcinoma of skin of unspecified parts of face
- **C44.311** Basal cell carcinoma of skin of nose
- **C44.319** Basal cell carcinoma of skin of other parts of face

√6th **C44.32** Squamous cell carcinoma of skin of other and unspecified parts of face
- **C44.320** Squamous cell carcinoma of skin of unspecified parts of face
- **C44.321** Squamous cell carcinoma of skin of nose
- **C44.329** Squamous cell carcinoma of skin of other parts of face

√6th **C44.39** Other specified malignant neoplasm of skin of other and unspecified parts of face
- **C44.390** Other specified malignant neoplasm of skin of unspecified parts of face
- **C44.391** Other specified malignant neoplasm of skin of nose
- **C44.399** Other specified malignant neoplasm of skin of other parts of face

√5th **C44.4** Other and unspecified malignant neoplasm of skin of scalp and neck
- **C44.40** Unspecified malignant neoplasm of skin of scalp and neck
- **C44.41** Basal cell carcinoma of skin of scalp and neck
- **C44.42** Squamous cell carcinoma of skin of scalp and neck
- **C44.49** Other specified malignant neoplasm of skin of scalp and neck

√5th **C44.5** Other and unspecified malignant neoplasm of skin of trunk
> **EXCLUDES 1**   anus NOS (C21.0)
> scrotum (C63.2)

√6th **C44.50** Unspecified malignant neoplasm of skin of trunk
- **C44.500** Unspecified malignant neoplasm of anal skin
  - Unspecified malignant neoplasm of anal margin
  - Unspecified malignant neoplasm of perianal skin
- **C44.501** Unspecified malignant neoplasm of skin of breast
- **C44.509** Unspecified malignant neoplasm of skin of other part of trunk

√6th **C44.51** Basal cell carcinoma of skin of trunk
- **C44.510** Basal cell carcinoma of anal skin
  - Basal cell carcinoma of anal margin
  - Basal cell carcinoma of perianal skin
- **C44.511** Basal cell carcinoma of skin of breast
- **C44.519** Basal cell carcinoma of skin of other part of trunk

√6th **C44.52** Squamous cell carcinoma of skin of trunk
- **C44.520** Squamous cell carcinoma of anal skin
  - Squamous cell carcinoma of anal margin
  - Squamous cell carcinoma of perianal skin
- **C44.521** Squamous cell carcinoma of skin of breast
- **C44.529** Squamous cell carcinoma of skin of other part of trunk

☑ Additional Character Required   √x7th Placeholder Alert   Manifestation   Unspecified Dx   ▶◀ Revised Text   ● New Code   ▲ Revised Title

ICD-10-CM 2020   467

Chapter 2. Neoplasms

✓6ᵗʰ **C44.59** Other specified malignant neoplasm of skin of trunk

     C44.590 Other specified malignant neoplasm of anal skin

         Other specified malignant neoplasm of anal margin

         Other specified malignant neoplasm of perianal skin

     C44.591 Other specified malignant neoplasm of skin of breast

     C44.599 Other specified malignant neoplasm of skin of other part of trunk

✓5ᵗʰ **C44.6** Other and unspecified malignant neoplasm of skin of upper limb, including shoulder

     ✓6ᵗʰ **C44.60** Unspecified malignant neoplasm of skin of upper limb, including shoulder

         C44.601 Unspecified malignant neoplasm of skin of unspecified upper limb, including shoulder

         C44.602 Unspecified malignant neoplasm of skin of right upper limb, including shoulder

         C44.609 Unspecified malignant neoplasm of skin of left upper limb, including shoulder

     ✓6ᵗʰ **C44.61** Basal cell carcinoma of skin of upper limb, including shoulder

         C44.611 Basal cell carcinoma of skin of unspecified upper limb, including shoulder

         C44.612 Basal cell carcinoma of skin of right upper limb, including shoulder

         C44.619 Basal cell carcinoma of skin of left upper limb, including shoulder

     ✓6ᵗʰ **C44.62** Squamous cell carcinoma of skin of upper limb, including shoulder

         C44.621 Squamous cell carcinoma of skin of unspecified upper limb, including shoulder

         C44.622 Squamous cell carcinoma of skin of right upper limb, including shoulder

         C44.629 Squamous cell carcinoma of skin of left upper limb, including shoulder

     ✓6ᵗʰ **C44.69** Other specified malignant neoplasm of skin of upper limb, including shoulder

         C44.691 Other specified malignant neoplasm of skin of unspecified upper limb, including shoulder

         C44.692 Other specified malignant neoplasm of skin of right upper limb, including shoulder

         C44.699 Other specified malignant neoplasm of skin of left upper limb, including shoulder

✓5ᵗʰ **C44.7** Other and unspecified malignant neoplasm of skin of lower limb, including hip

     ✓6ᵗʰ **C44.70** Unspecified malignant neoplasm of skin of lower limb, including hip

         C44.701 Unspecified malignant neoplasm of skin of unspecified lower limb, including hip

         C44.702 Unspecified malignant neoplasm of skin of right lower limb, including hip

         C44.709 Unspecified malignant neoplasm of skin of left lower limb, including hip

     ✓6ᵗʰ **C44.71** Basal cell carcinoma of skin of lower limb, including hip

         C44.711 Basal cell carcinoma of skin of unspecified lower limb, including hip

         C44.712 Basal cell carcinoma of skin of right lower limb, including hip

         C44.719 Basal cell carcinoma of skin of left lower limb, including hip

     ✓6ᵗʰ **C44.72** Squamous cell carcinoma of skin of lower limb, including hip

         C44.721 Squamous cell carcinoma of skin of unspecified lower limb, including hip

         C44.722 Squamous cell carcinoma of skin of right lower limb, including hip

         C44.729 Squamous cell carcinoma of skin of left lower limb, including hip

     ✓6ᵗʰ **C44.79** Other specified malignant neoplasm of skin of lower limb, including hip

         C44.791 Other specified malignant neoplasm of skin of unspecified lower limb, including hip

         C44.792 Other specified malignant neoplasm of skin of right lower limb, including hip

     C44.799 Other specified malignant neoplasm of skin of left lower limb, including hip

✓5ᵗʰ **C44.8** Other and unspecified malignant neoplasm of overlapping sites of skin

     C44.80 Unspecified malignant neoplasm of overlapping sites of skin

     C44.81 Basal cell carcinoma of overlapping sites of skin

     C44.82 Squamous cell carcinoma of overlapping sites of skin

     C44.89 Other specified malignant neoplasm of overlapping sites of skin

✓5ᵗʰ **C44.9** Other and unspecified malignant neoplasm of skin, unspecified

     C44.90 Unspecified malignant neoplasm of skin, unspecified

         Malignant neoplasm of unspecified site of skin

     C44.91 Basal cell carcinoma of skin, unspecified

     C44.92 Squamous cell carcinoma of skin, unspecified

     C44.99 Other specified malignant neoplasm of skin, unspecified

Malignant neoplasms of mesothelial and soft tissue (C45-C49)

✓4ᵗʰ **C45 Mesothelioma**

   DEF: Rare type of cancer that forms in the thin layer of protective tissue that covers the majority of internal organs (mesothelium).

   C45.0 Mesothelioma of pleura

     EXCLUDES 1   other malignant neoplasm of pleura (C38.4)

     AHA: 2017,2Q,11

     TIP: For pleural mesothelioma that has metastasized to the chest wall, assign this code for the primary site along with C79.89 for metastatic cancer in the chest wall.

   C45.1 Mesothelioma of peritoneum

     Mesothelioma of cul-de-sac

     Mesothelioma of mesentery

     Mesothelioma of mesocolon

     Mesothelioma of omentum

     Mesothelioma of peritoneum (parietal) (pelvic)

     EXCLUDES 1   other malignant neoplasm of soft tissue of peritoneum (C48.-)

   C45.2 Mesothelioma of pericardium

     EXCLUDES 1   other malignant neoplasm of pericardium (C38.0)

   C45.7 Mesothelioma of other sites

   C45.9 Mesothelioma, unspecified

✓4ᵗʰ **C46 Kaposi's sarcoma**

   Code first any human immunodeficiency virus [HIV] disease (B20)

   DEF: Malignant neoplasm that causes patches of abnormal tissue to grow under the skin, in the lining of the mouth, nose, and throat, in lymph nodes, or in other visceral organs. Kaposi's sarcoma is caused by human herpesvirus8 (HHV8).

   C46.0 Kaposi's sarcoma of skin

   C46.1 Kaposi's sarcoma of soft tissue

     Kaposi's sarcoma of blood vessel

     Kaposi's sarcoma of connective tissue

     Kaposi's sarcoma of fascia

     Kaposi's sarcoma of ligament

     Kaposi's sarcoma of lymphatic(s) NEC

     Kaposi's sarcoma of muscle

     EXCLUDES 2   Kaposi's sarcoma of lymph glands and nodes (C46.3)

   C46.2 Kaposi's sarcoma of palate

   C46.3 Kaposi's sarcoma of lymph nodes

   C46.4 Kaposi's sarcoma of gastrointestinal sites

✓5ᵗʰ **C46.5 Kaposi's sarcoma of lung**

     AHA: 2019,1Q,16

     C46.50 Kaposi's sarcoma of unspecified lung

     C46.51 Kaposi's sarcoma of right lung

     C46.52 Kaposi's sarcoma of left lung

   C46.7 Kaposi's sarcoma of other sites

   C46.9 Kaposi's sarcoma, unspecified

     Kaposi's sarcoma of unspecified site

N Newborn: 0   P Pediatric: 0-17   M Maternity: 12-55   A Adult: 15-124   CH Comorbidity High   CL Comorbidity Low   NCDx Noncancer Dx   PDx Primary Dx

468   ICD-10-CM 2020

☑4ᵗʰ **C47 Malignant neoplasm of peripheral nerves and autonomic nervous system**

     INCLUDES   malignant neoplasm of sympathetic and parasympathetic nerves and ganglia

     EXCLUDES 1   Kaposi's sarcoma of soft tissue (C46.1)

   C47.Ø Malignant neoplasm of peripheral nerves of head, face and neck

       EXCLUDES 1   malignant neoplasm of peripheral nerves of orbit (C69.6-)

   ☑5ᵗʰ **C47.1 Malignant neoplasm of peripheral nerves of** upper limb, including shoulder

     C47.1Ø Malignant neoplasm of peripheral nerves of unspecified upper limb, including shoulder

     C47.11 Malignant neoplasm of peripheral nerves of right **upper limb, including shoulder**

     C47.12 Malignant neoplasm of peripheral nerves of left **upper limb, including shoulder**

   ☑5ᵗʰ **C47.2 Malignant neoplasm of peripheral nerves of** lower limb, including hip

     C47.2Ø Malignant neoplasm of peripheral nerves of unspecified lower limb, including hip

     C47.21 Malignant neoplasm of peripheral nerves of right **lower limb, including hip**

     C47.22 Malignant neoplasm of peripheral nerves of left **lower limb, including hip**

   C47.3 Malignant neoplasm of peripheral nerves of thorax

   C47.4 Malignant neoplasm of peripheral nerves of abdomen

   C47.5 Malignant neoplasm of peripheral nerves of pelvis

   C47.6 Malignant neoplasm of peripheral nerves of trunk, unspecified

     Malignant neoplasm of peripheral nerves of unspecified part of trunk

   C47.8 Malignant neoplasm of overlapping sites **of peripheral nerves and autonomic nervous system**

   C47.9 Malignant neoplasm of peripheral nerves and autonomic nervous system, unspecified

     Malignant neoplasm of unspecified site of peripheral nerves and autonomic nervous system

☑4ᵗʰ **C48 Malignant neoplasm of** retroperitoneum and peritoneum

     EXCLUDES 1   Kaposi's sarcoma of connective tissue (C46.1)

                    mesothelioma (C45.-)

   C48.Ø Malignant neoplasm of retroperitoneum

   C48.1 Malignant neoplasm of specified parts of peritoneum

     Malignant neoplasm of cul-de-sac

     Malignant neoplasm of mesentery

     Malignant neoplasm of mesocolon

     Malignant neoplasm of omentum

     Malignant neoplasm of parietal peritoneum

     Malignant neoplasm of pelvic peritoneum

   C48.2 Malignant neoplasm of peritoneum, unspecified

   C48.8 Malignant neoplasm of overlapping sites **of retroperitoneum and peritoneum**

☑4ᵗʰ **C49 Malignant neoplasm of** other connective and soft tissue

     INCLUDES   malignant neoplasm of blood vessel

                malignant neoplasm of bursa

                malignant neoplasm of cartilage

                malignant neoplasm of fascia

                malignant neoplasm of fat

                malignant neoplasm of ligament, except uterine

                malignant neoplasm of lymphatic vessel

                malignant neoplasm of muscle

                malignant neoplasm of synovia

                malignant neoplasm of tendon (sheath)

     EXCLUDES 1   malignant neoplasm of cartilage (of):

                articular (C40-C41)

                larynx (C32.3)

                nose (C30.Ø)

            malignant neoplasm of connective tissue of breast (C50.-)

     EXCLUDES 2   Kaposi's sarcoma of soft tissue (C46.1)

            malignant neoplasm of heart (C38.Ø)

            malignant neoplasm of peripheral nerves and autonomic nervous system (C47.-)

            malignant neoplasm of peritoneum (C48.2)

            malignant neoplasm of retroperitoneum (C48.Ø)

            malignant neoplasm of uterine ligament (C57.3)

            mesothelioma (C45.-)

   C49.Ø Malignant neoplasm of connective and soft tissue of head, face and neck

     Malignant neoplasm of connective tissue of ear

     Malignant neoplasm of connective tissue of eyelid

     EXCLUDES 1   connective tissue of orbit (C69.6-)

   ☑5ᵗʰ **C49.1 Malignant neoplasm of connective and soft tissue of** upper limb, including shoulder

     C49.1Ø Malignant neoplasm of connective and soft tissue of unspecified upper limb, including shoulder

     C49.11 Malignant neoplasm of connective and soft tissue of right **upper limb, including shoulder**

     C49.12 Malignant neoplasm of connective and soft tissue of left **upper limb, including shoulder**

   ☑5ᵗʰ **C49.2 Malignant neoplasm of connective and soft tissue of** lower limb, including hip

     C49.2Ø Malignant neoplasm of connective and soft tissue of unspecified lower limb, including hip

     C49.21 Malignant neoplasm of connective and soft tissue of right **lower limb, including hip**

     C49.22 Malignant neoplasm of connective and soft tissue of left **lower limb, including hip**

   C49.3 Malignant neoplasm of connective and soft tissue of thorax

     Malignant neoplasm of axilla

     Malignant neoplasm of diaphragm

     Malignant neoplasm of great vessels

     EXCLUDES 1   malignant neoplasm of breast (C50.-)

            malignant neoplasm of heart (C38.Ø)

            malignant neoplasm of mediastinum (C38.1-C38.3)

            malignant neoplasm of thymus (C37)

     AHA: 2015,3Q,19

   C49.4 Malignant neoplasm of connective and soft tissue of abdomen

     Malignant neoplasm of abdominal wall

     Malignant neoplasm of hypochondrium

   C49.5 Malignant neoplasm of connective and soft tissue of pelvis

     Malignant neoplasm of buttock

     Malignant neoplasm of groin

     Malignant neoplasm of perineum

   C49.6 Malignant neoplasm of connective and soft tissue of trunk, unspecified

     Malignant neoplasm of back NOS

   C49.8 Malignant neoplasm of overlapping sites **of connective and soft tissue**

     Primary malignant neoplasm of two or more contiguous sites of connective and soft tissue

   C49.9 Malignant neoplasm of connective and soft tissue, unspecified

   ☑6ᵗʰ **C49.A Gastrointestinal stromal tumor**

     AHA: 2016,4Q,8

     DEF: Uncommon malignant tumor found in the GI tract that originates from interstitial cells of the autonomic nervous system. Most occur in the stomach or small intestine but can originate anywhere in the GI tract.

     C49.AØ Gastrointestinal stromal tumor, unspecified site

☑ Additional Character Required   ☑x7ᵗʰ Placeholder Alert   Manifestation   Unspecified Dx   ▶◀ Revised Text   ● New Code   ▲ Revised Title

ICD-10-CM 2020   469

C49.A1 **Gastrointestinal stromal tumor of** esophagus
C49.A2 **Gastrointestinal stromal tumor of** stomach
C49.A3 **Gastrointestinal stromal tumor of** small intestine
C49.A4 **Gastrointestinal stromal tumor of** large intestine
C49.A5 **Gastrointestinal stromal tumor of** rectum
C49.A9 **Gastrointestinal stromal tumor of other sites**

Malignant neoplasms of breast (C50)

✓4ᵗʰ **C50 Malignant neoplasm of** breast

> INCLUDES   connective tissue of breast
> Paget's disease of breast
> Paget's disease of nipple

Use additional code to identify estrogen receptor status (Z17.0, Z17.1)

> EXCLUDES 1   skin of breast (C44.501, C44.511, C44.521, C44.591)

AHA: 2017,4Q,19

Female Breast

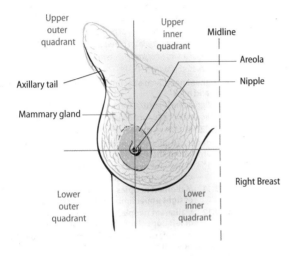

✓5ᵗʰ **C50.0 Malignant neoplasm of** nipple and areola
  ✓6ᵗʰ **C50.01 Malignant neoplasm of nipple and areola,** female
       C50.011 **Malignant neoplasm of nipple and areola,** right **female breast** ♀
       C50.012 **Malignant neoplasm of nipple and areola,** left **female breast** ♀
       C50.019 **Malignant neoplasm of nipple and areola, unspecified female breast** ♀
  ✓6ᵗʰ **C50.02 Malignant neoplasm of nipple and areola,** male
       C50.021 **Malignant neoplasm of nipple and areola,** right **male breast** ♂
       C50.022 **Malignant neoplasm of nipple and areola,** left **male breast** ♂
       C50.029 **Malignant neoplasm of nipple and areola, unspecified male breast** ♂
✓5ᵗʰ **C50.1 Malignant neoplasm of** central portion **of breast**
  ✓6ᵗʰ **C50.11 Malignant neoplasm of central portion of breast,** female
       C50.111 **Malignant neoplasm of central portion of** right **female breast** ♀
       C50.112 **Malignant neoplasm of central portion of** left **female breast** ♀
       C50.119 **Malignant neoplasm of central portion of unspecified female breast** ♀
  ✓6ᵗʰ **C50.12 Malignant neoplasm of central portion of breast,** male
       C50.121 **Malignant neoplasm of central portion of** right **male breast** ♂
       C50.122 **Malignant neoplasm of central portion of** left **male breast** ♂

       C50.129 **Malignant neoplasm of central portion of unspecified male breast** ♂
✓5ᵗʰ **C50.2 Malignant neoplasm of** upper-inner quadrant **of breast**
  ✓6ᵗʰ **C50.21 Malignant neoplasm of upper-inner quadrant of breast,** female
       C50.211 **Malignant neoplasm of upper-inner quadrant of** right **female breast** ♀
       C50.212 **Malignant neoplasm of upper-inner quadrant of** left **female breast** ♀
       C50.219 **Malignant neoplasm of upper-inner quadrant of unspecified female breast** ♀
  ✓6ᵗʰ **C50.22 Malignant neoplasm of upper-inner quadrant of breast,** male
       C50.221 **Malignant neoplasm of upper-inner quadrant of** right **male breast** ♂
       C50.222 **Malignant neoplasm of upper-inner quadrant of** left **male breast** ♂
       C50.229 **Malignant neoplasm of upper-inner quadrant of unspecified male breast** ♂
✓5ᵗʰ **C50.3 Malignant neoplasm of** lower-inner quadrant **of breast**
  ✓6ᵗʰ **C50.31 Malignant neoplasm of lower-inner quadrant of breast,** female
       C50.311 **Malignant neoplasm of lower-inner quadrant of** right **female breast** ♀
       C50.312 **Malignant neoplasm of lower-inner quadrant of** left **female breast** ♀
       C50.319 **Malignant neoplasm of lower-inner quadrant of unspecified female breast** ♀
  ✓6ᵗʰ **C50.32 Malignant neoplasm of lower-inner quadrant of breast,** male
       C50.321 **Malignant neoplasm of lower-inner quadrant of** right **male breast** ♂
       C50.322 **Malignant neoplasm of lower-inner quadrant of** left **male breast** ♂
       C50.329 **Malignant neoplasm of lower-inner quadrant of unspecified male breast** ♂
✓5ᵗʰ **C50.4 Malignant neoplasm of** upper-outer quadrant **of breast**
  ✓6ᵗʰ **C50.41 Malignant neoplasm of upper-outer quadrant of breast,** female
       C50.411 **Malignant neoplasm of upper-outer quadrant of** right **female breast** ♀
       C50.412 **Malignant neoplasm of upper-outer quadrant of** left **female breast** ♀
       C50.419 **Malignant neoplasm of upper-outer quadrant of unspecified female breast** ♀
  ✓6ᵗʰ **C50.42 Malignant neoplasm of upper-outer quadrant of breast,** male
       C50.421 **Malignant neoplasm of upper-outer quadrant of** right **male breast** ♂
       C50.422 **Malignant neoplasm of upper-outer quadrant of** left **male breast** ♂
       C50.429 **Malignant neoplasm of upper-outer quadrant of unspecified male breast** ♂
✓5ᵗʰ **C50.5 Malignant neoplasm of** lower-outer quadrant **of breast**
  ✓6ᵗʰ **C50.51 Malignant neoplasm of lower-outer quadrant of breast,** female
       C50.511 **Malignant neoplasm of lower-outer quadrant of** right **female breast** ♀
       C50.512 **Malignant neoplasm of lower-outer quadrant of** left **female breast** ♀

N Newborn: 0   P Pediatric: 0-17   M Maternity: 12-55   A Adult: 15-124   CH Comorbidity High   CL Comorbidity Low   NCDx Noncancer Dx   PDx Primary Dx

470   ICD-10-CM 2020

C50.519 Malignant neoplasm of lower-outer quadrant of unspecified female breast ♀

✓6ᵗʰ **C50.52** Malignant neoplasm of lower-outer quadrant of breast, male

    C50.521 Malignant neoplasm of lower-outer quadrant of right male breast ♂

    C50.522 Malignant neoplasm of lower-outer quadrant of left male breast ♂

    C50.529 Malignant neoplasm of lower-outer quadrant of unspecified male breast ♂

✓5ᵗʰ **C50.6** Malignant neoplasm of axillary tail of breast

  ✓6ᵗʰ **C50.61** Malignant neoplasm of axillary tail of breast, female

    C50.611 Malignant neoplasm of axillary tail of right female breast ♀

    C50.612 Malignant neoplasm of axillary tail of left female breast ♀

    C50.619 Malignant neoplasm of axillary tail of unspecified female breast ♀

  ✓6ᵗʰ **C50.62** Malignant neoplasm of axillary tail of breast, male

    C50.621 Malignant neoplasm of axillary tail of right male breast ♂

    C50.622 Malignant neoplasm of axillary tail of left male breast ♂

    C50.629 Malignant neoplasm of axillary tail of unspecified male breast ♂

✓5ᵗʰ **C50.8** Malignant neoplasm of overlapping sites of breast

  ✓6ᵗʰ **C50.81** Malignant neoplasm of overlapping sites of breast, female

    C50.811 Malignant neoplasm of overlapping sites of right female breast ♀

    C50.812 Malignant neoplasm of overlapping sites of left female breast ♀

    C50.819 Malignant neoplasm of overlapping sites of unspecified female breast ♀

  ✓6ᵗʰ **C50.82** Malignant neoplasm of overlapping sites of breast, male

    C50.821 Malignant neoplasm of overlapping sites of right male breast ♂

    C50.822 Malignant neoplasm of overlapping sites of left male breast ♂

    C50.829 Malignant neoplasm of overlapping sites of unspecified male breast ♂

✓5ᵗʰ **C50.9** Malignant neoplasm of breast of unspecified site

  ✓6ᵗʰ **C50.91** Malignant neoplasm of breast of unspecified site, female

    C50.911 Malignant neoplasm of unspecified site of right female breast ♀

    C50.912 Malignant neoplasm of unspecified site of left female breast ♀

    C50.919 Malignant neoplasm of unspecified site of unspecified female breast ♀

  ✓6ᵗʰ **C50.92** Malignant neoplasm of breast of unspecified site, male

    C50.921 Malignant neoplasm of unspecified site of right male breast ♂

    C50.922 Malignant neoplasm of unspecified site of left male breast ♂

    C50.929 Malignant neoplasm of unspecified site of unspecified male breast ♂

Malignant neoplasms of female genital organs (C51-C58)

INCLUDES   malignant neoplasm of skin of female genital organs

✓4ᵗʰ **C51** **Malignant neoplasm of vulva**

  EXCLUDES 1   carcinoma in situ of vulva (D07.1)

  C51.0 Malignant neoplasm of labium majus ♀

    Malignant neoplasm of Bartholin's [greater vestibular] gland

  C51.1 Malignant neoplasm of labium minus ♀

  C51.2 Malignant neoplasm of clitoris ♀

  C51.8 Malignant neoplasm of overlapping sites of vulva ♀

  C51.9 Malignant neoplasm of vulva, unspecified ♀

    Malignant neoplasm of external female genitalia NOS

    Malignant neoplasm of pudendum

C52 **Malignant neoplasm of vagina** ♀

  EXCLUDES 1   carcinoma in situ of vagina (D07.2)

✓4ᵗʰ **C53** **Malignant neoplasm of cervix uteri**

  EXCLUDES 1   carcinoma in situ of cervix uteri (D06.-)

  AHA: 2017,4Q,103

  C53.0 Malignant neoplasm of endocervix ♀

  C53.1 Malignant neoplasm of exocervix ♀

  C53.8 Malignant neoplasm of overlapping sites of cervix uteri ♀

  C53.9 Malignant neoplasm of cervix uteri, unspecified ♀

✓4ᵗʰ **C54** **Malignant neoplasm of corpus uteri**

  C54.0 Malignant neoplasm of isthmus uteri ♀

    Malignant neoplasm of lower uterine segment

  C54.1 Malignant neoplasm of endometrium ♀

  C54.2 Malignant neoplasm of myometrium ♀

  C54.3 Malignant neoplasm of fundus uteri ♀

  C54.8 Malignant neoplasm of overlapping sites of corpus uteri ♀

  C54.9 Malignant neoplasm of corpus uteri, unspecified ♀

C55 **Malignant neoplasm of uterus, part unspecified** ♀

✓4ᵗʰ **C56** **Malignant neoplasm of ovary**

  Use additional code to identify any functional activity

  C56.1 Malignant neoplasm of right ovary ♀

  C56.2 Malignant neoplasm of left ovary ♀

  C56.9 Malignant neoplasm of unspecified ovary ♀

✓4ᵗʰ **C57** **Malignant neoplasm of other and unspecified female genital organs**

  ✓5ᵗʰ **C57.0** Malignant neoplasm of fallopian tube

    Malignant neoplasm of oviduct

    Malignant neoplasm of uterine tube

    C57.00 Malignant neoplasm of unspecified fallopian tube ♀

    C57.01 Malignant neoplasm of right fallopian tube ♀

    C57.02 Malignant neoplasm of left fallopian tube ♀

  ✓5ᵗʰ **C57.1** Malignant neoplasm of broad ligament

    C57.10 Malignant neoplasm of unspecified broad ligament ♀

    C57.11 Malignant neoplasm of right broad ligament ♀

    C57.12 Malignant neoplasm of left broad ligament ♀

  ✓5ᵗʰ **C57.2** Malignant neoplasm of round ligament

    C57.20 Malignant neoplasm of unspecified round ligament ♀

    C57.21 Malignant neoplasm of right round ligament ♀

    C57.22 Malignant neoplasm of left round ligament ♀

  C57.3 Malignant neoplasm of parametrium ♀

    Malignant neoplasm of uterine ligament NOS

  C57.4 Malignant neoplasm of uterine adnexa, unspecified ♀

  C57.7 Malignant neoplasm of other specified female genital organs ♀

    Malignant neoplasm of wolffian body or duct

☑ Additional Character Required   ✓x7ᵗʰ Placeholder Alert   Manifestation   Unspecified Dx   ▶◀ Revised Text   ● New Code   ▲ Revised Title

ICD-10-CM 2020   471

Chapter 2. Neoplasms

C57.8   **Malignant neoplasm of** overlapping sites **of** ♀
female genital organs
Primary malignant neoplasm of two or more contiguous sites of the female genital organs whose point of origin cannot be determined
Primary tubo-ovarian malignant neoplasm whose point of origin cannot be determined
Primary utero-ovarian malignant neoplasm whose point of origin cannot be determined

C57.9   **Malignant neoplasm of female genital organ,** ♀
unspecified
Malignant neoplasm of female genitourinary tract NOS

C58   **Malignant neoplasm of** placenta   Ⓜ ♀

INCLUDES   choriocarcinoma NOS
chorionepithelioma NOS

EXCLUDES 1   *chorioadenoma (destruens) (D39.2)*
hydatidiform mole NOS (O01.9)
invasive hydatidiform mole (D39.2)
male choriocarcinoma NOS (C62.9-)
malignant hydatidiform mole (D39.2)

Malignant neoplasms of male genital organs (C60-C63)

INCLUDES   malignant neoplasm of skin of male genital organs

✓4ᵗʰ C60   **Malignant neoplasm of** penis

C60.0   **Malignant neoplasm of** prepuce   ♂
Malignant neoplasm of foreskin

C60.1   **Malignant neoplasm of** glans **penis**   ♂

C60.2   **Malignant neoplasm of** body **of penis**   ♂
Malignant neoplasm of corpus cavernosum

C60.8   **Malignant neoplasm of** overlapping sites **of penis**   ♂

C60.9   **Malignant neoplasm of penis, unspecified**   ♂
Malignant neoplasm of skin of penis NOS

C61   **Malignant neoplasm of** prostate   ♂
Use additional code to identify:
hormone sensitivity status (Z19.1-Z19.2)
rising PSA following treatment for malignant neoplasm of prostate (R97.21)

EXCLUDES 1   *malignant neoplasm of seminal vesicle (C63.7)*
AHA: 2017,1Q,17

✓4ᵗʰ C62   **Malignant neoplasm of** testis
Use additional code to identify any functional activity

✓5ᵗʰ C62.0   **Malignant neoplasm of** undescended **testis**
Malignant neoplasm of ectopic testis
Malignant neoplasm of retained testis

C62.00   **Malignant neoplasm of unspecified** ♂
undescended testis

C62.01   **Malignant neoplasm of undescended** ♂
right testis

C62.02   **Malignant neoplasm of undescended** ♂
left testis

✓5ᵗʰ C62.1   **Malignant neoplasm of** descended **testis**
Malignant neoplasm of scrotal testis

C62.10   **Malignant neoplasm of unspecified** ♂
descended testis

C62.11   **Malignant neoplasm of descended** right ♂
testis

C62.12   **Malignant neoplasm of descended** left ♂
testis

✓5ᵗʰ C62.9   **Malignant neoplasm of testis,** unspecified whether
descended or undescended

C62.90   **Malignant neoplasm of unspecified** ♂
testis, unspecified whether descended or undescended
Malignant neoplasm of testis NOS

C62.91   **Malignant neoplasm of** right **testis,** ♂
unspecified whether descended or undescended

C62.92   **Malignant neoplasm of** left **testis,** ♂
unspecified whether descended or undescended

✓4ᵗʰ C63   **Malignant neoplasm of** other and unspecified male genital organs

✓5ᵗʰ C63.0   **Malignant neoplasm of** epididymis

C63.00   **Malignant neoplasm of unspecified** ♂
epididymis

C63.01   **Malignant neoplasm of** right **epididymis** ♂

C63.02   **Malignant neoplasm of** left **epididymis** ♂

✓5ᵗʰ C63.1   **Malignant neoplasm of** spermatic cord

C63.10   **Malignant neoplasm of unspecified** ♂
spermatic cord

C63.11   **Malignant neoplasm of** right **spermatic** ♂
cord

C63.12   **Malignant neoplasm of** left **spermatic** ♂
cord

C63.2   **Malignant neoplasm of** scrotum ♂
Malignant neoplasm of skin of scrotum

C63.7   **Malignant neoplasm of other specified male** ♂
genital organs
Malignant neoplasm of seminal vesicle
Malignant neoplasm of tunica vaginalis

C63.8   **Malignant neoplasm of** overlapping sites **of male** ♂
genital organs
Primary malignant neoplasm of two or more contiguous sites of male genital organs whose point of origin cannot be determined

C63.9   **Malignant neoplasm of male genital organ,** ♂
unspecified
Malignant neoplasm of male genitourinary tract NOS

Malignant neoplasms of urinary tract (C64-C68)

✓4ᵗʰ C64   **Malignant neoplasm of** kidney, except renal pelvis

EXCLUDES 1   *malignant carcinoid tumor of the kidney (C7A.093)*
malignant neoplasm of renal calyces (C65.-)
malignant neoplasm of renal pelvis (C65.-)

C64.1   **Malignant neoplasm of** right **kidney, except renal pelvis**

C64.2   **Malignant neoplasm of** left **kidney, except renal pelvis**

C64.9   **Malignant neoplasm of unspecified kidney, except renal pelvis**

✓4ᵗʰ C65   **Malignant neoplasm of** renal pelvis

INCLUDES   malignant neoplasm of pelviureteric junction
malignant neoplasm of renal calyces

C65.1   **Malignant neoplasm of** right **renal pelvis**

C65.2   **Malignant neoplasm of** left **renal pelvis**

C65.9   **Malignant neoplasm of unspecified renal pelvis**

✓4ᵗʰ C66   **Malignant neoplasm of** ureter

EXCLUDES 1   *malignant neoplasm of ureteric orifice of bladder (C67.6)*

C66.1   **Malignant neoplasm of** right **ureter**

C66.2   **Malignant neoplasm of** left **ureter**

C66.9   **Malignant neoplasm of unspecified ureter**

✓4ᵗʰ C67   **Malignant neoplasm of** bladder

C67.0   **Malignant neoplasm of** trigone **of bladder**

C67.1   **Malignant neoplasm of** dome **of bladder**

C67.2   **Malignant neoplasm of** lateral wall **of bladder**

C67.3   **Malignant neoplasm of** anterior wall **of bladder**

C67.4   **Malignant neoplasm of** posterior wall **of bladder**

C67.5   **Malignant neoplasm of** bladder neck
Malignant neoplasm of internal urethral orifice

C67.6   **Malignant neoplasm of** ureteric orifice

C67.7   **Malignant neoplasm of** urachus

C67.8   **Malignant neoplasm of** overlapping sites **of bladder**

C67.9   **Malignant neoplasm of bladder, unspecified**
AHA: 2016,1Q,19

✓4ᵗʰ C68   **Malignant neoplasm of other and unspecified** urinary organs

EXCLUDES 1   *malignant neoplasm of female genitourinary tract NOS (C57.9)*
malignant neoplasm of male genitourinary tract NOS (C63.9)

AHA: 2016,1Q,14

C68.0   **Malignant neoplasm of** urethra

EXCLUDES 1   *malignant neoplasm of urethral orifice of bladder (C67.5)*

C68.1   **Malignant neoplasm of** paraurethral glands

C68.8   **Malignant neoplasm of** overlapping sites **of urinary organs**
Primary malignant neoplasm of two or more contiguous sites of urinary organs whose point of origin cannot be determined

C68.9   **Malignant neoplasm of urinary organ, unspecified**
Malignant neoplasm of urinary system NOS

Malignant neoplasms of eye, brain and other parts of central nervous system (C69-C72)

☑4ᵗʰ **C69   Malignant neoplasm of** eye and adnexa

> *EXCLUDES 1*   *malignant neoplasm of connective tissue of eyelid (C49.0)*
> *malignant neoplasm of eyelid (skin) (C43.1-, C44.1-)*
> *malignant neoplasm of optic nerve (C72.3-)*

☑5ᵗʰ **C69.0   Malignant neoplasm of** conjunctiva

C69.00   Malignant neoplasm of unspecified conjunctiva
C69.01   Malignant neoplasm of right conjunctiva
C69.02   Malignant neoplasm of left conjunctiva

☑5ᵗʰ **C69.1   Malignant neoplasm of** cornea

C69.10   Malignant neoplasm of unspecified cornea
C69.11   Malignant neoplasm of right cornea
C69.12   Malignant neoplasm of left cornea

☑5ᵗʰ **C69.2   Malignant neoplasm of** retina

> *EXCLUDES 1*   *dark area on retina (D49.81)*
> *neoplasm of unspecified behavior of retina and choroid (D49.81)*
> *retinal freckle (D49.81)*

C69.20   Malignant neoplasm of unspecified retina
C69.21   Malignant neoplasm of right retina
C69.22   Malignant neoplasm of left retina

☑5ᵗʰ **C69.3   Malignant neoplasm of** choroid

C69.30   Malignant neoplasm of unspecified choroid
C69.31   Malignant neoplasm of right choroid
C69.32   Malignant neoplasm of left choroid

☑5ᵗʰ **C69.4   Malignant neoplasm of** ciliary body

C69.40   Malignant neoplasm of unspecified ciliary body
C69.41   Malignant neoplasm of right ciliary body
C69.42   Malignant neoplasm of left ciliary body

☑5ᵗʰ **C69.5   Malignant neoplasm of** lacrimal gland and duct

   Malignant neoplasm of lacrimal sac
   Malignant neoplasm of nasolacrimal duct

C69.50   Malignant neoplasm of unspecified lacrimal gland and duct
C69.51   Malignant neoplasm of right lacrimal gland and duct
C69.52   Malignant neoplasm of left lacrimal gland and duct

☑5ᵗʰ **C69.6   Malignant neoplasm of** orbit

   Malignant neoplasm of connective tissue of orbit
   Malignant neoplasm of extraocular muscle
   Malignant neoplasm of peripheral nerves of orbit
   Malignant neoplasm of retrobulbar tissue
   Malignant neoplasm of retro-ocular tissue

> *EXCLUDES 1*   *malignant neoplasm of orbital bone (C41.0)*

C69.60   Malignant neoplasm of unspecified orbit
C69.61   Malignant neoplasm of right orbit
C69.62   Malignant neoplasm of left orbit

☑5ᵗʰ **C69.8   Malignant neoplasm of** overlapping sites of eye and adnexa

C69.80   Malignant neoplasm of overlapping sites of unspecified eye and adnexa
C69.81   Malignant neoplasm of overlapping sites of right eye and adnexa
C69.82   Malignant neoplasm of overlapping sites of left eye and adnexa

☑5ᵗʰ **C69.9   Malignant neoplasm of** unspecified site of eye

   Malignant neoplasm of eyeball

C69.90   Malignant neoplasm of unspecified site of unspecified eye
C69.91   Malignant neoplasm of unspecified site of right eye
C69.92   Malignant neoplasm of unspecified site of left eye

☑4ᵗʰ **C70   Malignant neoplasm of** meninges

C70.0   Malignant neoplasm of cerebral meninges
C70.1   Malignant neoplasm of spinal meninges
C70.9   Malignant neoplasm of meninges, unspecified

☑4ᵗʰ **C71   Malignant neoplasm of** brain

> *EXCLUDES 1*   *malignant neoplasm of cranial nerves (C72.2-C72.5)*
> *retrobulbar malignant neoplasm (C69.6-)*

Lobes of the Brain

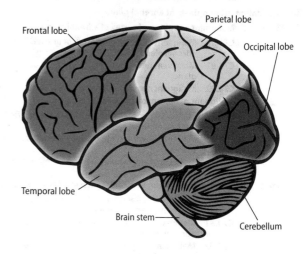

C71.0   Malignant neoplasm of cerebrum, except lobes and ventricles
   Malignant neoplasm of supratentorial NOS
C71.1   Malignant neoplasm of frontal lobe
C71.2   Malignant neoplasm of temporal lobe
C71.3   Malignant neoplasm of parietal lobe
C71.4   Malignant neoplasm of occipital lobe
C71.5   Malignant neoplasm of cerebral ventricle

> *EXCLUDES 1*   *malignant neoplasm of fourth cerebral ventricle (C71.7)*

C71.6   Malignant neoplasm of cerebellum
C71.7   Malignant neoplasm of brain stem
   Malignant neoplasm of fourth cerebral ventricle
   Infratentorial malignant neoplasm NOS
C71.8   Malignant neoplasm of overlapping sites of brain
C71.9   Malignant neoplasm of brain, unspecified
   AHA: 2014,3Q,3

☑4ᵗʰ **C72   Malignant neoplasm of** spinal cord, cranial nerves **and other parts of** central nervous system

> *EXCLUDES 1*   *malignant neoplasm of meninges (C70.-)*
> *malignant neoplasm of peripheral nerves and autonomic nervous system (C47.-)*

C72.0   Malignant neoplasm of spinal cord
C72.1   Malignant neoplasm of cauda equina

☑5ᵗʰ **C72.2   Malignant neoplasm of** olfactory nerve

   Malignant neoplasm of olfactory bulb

C72.20   Malignant neoplasm of unspecified olfactory nerve
C72.21   Malignant neoplasm of right olfactory nerve
C72.22   Malignant neoplasm of left olfactory nerve

☑5ᵗʰ **C72.3   Malignant neoplasm of** optic nerve

C72.30   Malignant neoplasm of unspecified optic nerve
C72.31   Malignant neoplasm of right optic nerve
C72.32   Malignant neoplasm of left optic nerve

☑5ᵗʰ **C72.4   Malignant neoplasm of** acoustic nerve

C72.40   Malignant neoplasm of unspecified acoustic nerve
C72.41   Malignant neoplasm of right acoustic nerve
C72.42   Malignant neoplasm of left acoustic nerve

☑5ᵗʰ **C72.5   Malignant neoplasm of other and unspecified** cranial nerves

C72.50   Malignant neoplasm of unspecified cranial nerve
   Malignant neoplasm of cranial nerve NOS
C72.59   Malignant neoplasm of other cranial nerves
C72.9   Malignant neoplasm of central nervous system, unspecified
   Malignant neoplasm of unspecified site of central nervous system
   Malignant neoplasm of nervous system NOS

☑ Additional Character Required   ☑8/9ᵗʰ Placeholder Alert   Manifestation   Unspecified Dx   ►◄ Revised Text   ● New Code   ▲ Revised Title

ICD-10-CM 2020   **473**

Malignant neoplasms of thyroid and other endocrine glands (C73-C75)

C73 **Malignant neoplasm of** thyroid gland
    Use additional code to identify any functional activity

✓4ᵗʰ **C74** **Malignant neoplasm of** adrenal gland

  ✓5ᵗʰ **C74.0** **Malignant neoplasm of** cortex of adrenal gland

     C74.00 **Malignant neoplasm of cortex of unspecified adrenal gland**

     C74.01 **Malignant neoplasm of cortex of** right **adrenal gland**

     C74.02 **Malignant neoplasm of cortex of** left **adrenal gland**

  ✓5ᵗʰ **C74.1** **Malignant neoplasm of** medulla of adrenal gland

     C74.10 **Malignant neoplasm of medulla of unspecified adrenal gland**

     C74.11 **Malignant neoplasm of medulla of** right **adrenal gland**

     C74.12 **Malignant neoplasm of medulla of** left **adrenal gland**

  ✓5ᵗʰ **C74.9** **Malignant neoplasm of unspecified part of adrenal gland**

     C74.90 **Malignant neoplasm of unspecified part of unspecified adrenal gland**

     C74.91 **Malignant neoplasm of unspecified part of** right **adrenal gland**

     C74.92 **Malignant neoplasm of unspecified part of** left **adrenal gland**

✓4ᵗʰ **C75** **Malignant neoplasm of other** endocrine glands and related structures

    EXCLUDES 1   *malignant carcinoid tumors (C7A.0-)*
                 malignant neoplasm of adrenal gland (C74.-)
                 malignant neoplasm of endocrine pancreas (C25.4)
                 malignant neoplasm of islets of Langerhans (C25.4)
                 malignant neoplasm of ovary (C56.-)
                 malignant neoplasm of testis (C62.-)
                 malignant neoplasm of thymus (C37)
                 malignant neoplasm of thyroid gland (C73)
                 malignant neuroendocrine tumors (C7A.-)

    C75.0 **Malignant neoplasm of** parathyroid **gland**

    C75.1 **Malignant neoplasm of** pituitary **gland**

    C75.2 **Malignant neoplasm of** craniopharyngeal duct

    C75.3 **Malignant neoplasm of** pineal **gland**

    C75.4 **Malignant neoplasm of** carotid body

    C75.5 **Malignant neoplasm of** aortic body **and other** paraganglia

    C75.8 **Malignant neoplasm with** pluriglandular involvement, **unspecified**

    C75.9 **Malignant neoplasm of endocrine gland, unspecified**

Malignant neuroendocrine tumors (C7A)

✓4ᵗʰ **C7A** **Malignant** neuroendocrine tumors

    Code also any associated multiple endocrine neoplasia [MEN] syndromes (E31.2-)
    Use additional code to identify any associated endocrine syndrome, such as:
    carcinoid syndrome (E34.0)
    EXCLUDES 2   *malignant pancreatic islet cell tumors (C25.4)*
                 Merkel cell carcinoma (C4A.-)
    DEF: Tumors comprised of cells that are capable of producing hormonal syndromes in which the normal hormonal balance required to support body system functions is adversely affected.

  ✓5ᵗʰ **C7A.0** **Malignant** carcinoid tumors

     DEF: Specific type of slow-growing benign or malignant neuroendocrine tumors. Carcinoid tumors occur most commonly in the hormone producing cells of the gastrointestinal tracts and can also occur in the pancreas, testes, ovaries, or lungs.

     C7A.00 **Malignant carcinoid tumor of unspecified site**

    ✓6ᵗʰ **C7A.01** **Malignant carcinoid tumors of the** small intestine

      C7A.010 **Malignant carcinoid tumor of the duodenum**

      C7A.011 **Malignant carcinoid tumor of the** jejunum

      C7A.012 **Malignant carcinoid tumor of the** ileum

      C7A.019 **Malignant carcinoid tumor of the small intestine, unspecified portion**

    ✓6ᵗʰ **C7A.02** **Malignant carcinoid tumors of the** appendix, large intestine, and rectum

      C7A.020 **Malignant carcinoid tumor of the appendix**

      C7A.021 **Malignant carcinoid tumor of the** cecum

      C7A.022 **Malignant carcinoid tumor of the ascending colon**

      C7A.023 **Malignant carcinoid tumor of the transverse colon**

      C7A.024 **Malignant carcinoid tumor of the descending colon**

      C7A.025 **Malignant carcinoid tumor of the** sigmoid colon

      C7A.026 **Malignant carcinoid tumor of the** rectum

      C7A.029 **Malignant carcinoid tumor of the large intestine, unspecified portion**
          Malignant carcinoid tumor of the colon NOS

    ✓6ᵗʰ **C7A.09** **Malignant carcinoid tumors of** other sites

      C7A.090 **Malignant carcinoid tumor of the** bronchus and lung
          AHA: 2019,1Q,16

      C7A.091 **Malignant carcinoid tumor of the** thymus

      C7A.092 **Malignant carcinoid tumor of the** stomach

      C7A.093 **Malignant carcinoid tumor of the** kidney

      C7A.094 **Malignant carcinoid tumor of the** foregut, **unspecified**

      C7A.095 **Malignant carcinoid tumor of the** midgut, **unspecified**

      C7A.096 **Malignant carcinoid tumor of the** hindgut, **unspecified**

      C7A.098 **Malignant carcinoid tumors of** other sites

    C7A.1 **Malignant** poorly differentiated **neuroendocrine tumors**
        Malignant poorly differentiated neuroendocrine tumor NOS
        High grade neuroendocrine carcinoma, any site
        Malignant poorly differentiated neuroendocrine carcinoma, any site

    C7A.8 **Other malignant neuroendocrine tumors**

Secondary neuroendocrine tumors (C7B)

✓4ᵗʰ **C7B** Secondary **neuroendocrine tumors**

    Use additional code to identify any functional activity

  ✓5ᵗʰ **C7B.0** **Secondary** carcinoid tumors

     C7B.00 **Secondary carcinoid tumors, unspecified site**

     C7B.01 **Secondary carcinoid tumors of** distant lymph nodes

     C7B.02 **Secondary carcinoid tumors of** liver

     C7B.03 **Secondary carcinoid tumors of** bone

     C7B.04 **Secondary carcinoid tumors of** peritoneum
        Mesentary metastasis of carcinoid tumor

     C7B.09 **Secondary carcinoid tumors of other sites**

    C7B.1 **Secondary** Merkel cell carcinoma
        Merkel cell carcinoma nodal presentation
        Merkel cell carcinoma visceral metastatic presentation

    C7B.8 **Other secondary neuroendocrine tumors**

Malignant neoplasms of ill-defined, other secondary and unspecified sites (C76-C80)

✓4ᵗʰ **C76** **Malignant neoplasm of other and ill-defined sites**

    EXCLUDES 1   *malignant neoplasm of female genitourinary tract NOS (C57.9)*
                 malignant neoplasm of male genitourinary tract NOS (C63.9)
                 malignant neoplasm of lymphoid, hematopoietic and related tissue (C81-C96)
                 malignant neoplasm of skin (C44.-)
                 malignant neoplasm of unspecified site NOS (C80.1)

    C76.0 **Malignant neoplasm of** head, face and neck
        Malignant neoplasm of cheek NOS
        Malignant neoplasm of nose NOS

    C76.1 **Malignant neoplasm of** thorax
        Intrathoracic malignant neoplasm NOS
        Malignant neoplasm of axilla NOS
        Thoracic malignant neoplasm NOS

    C76.2 **Malignant neoplasm of** abdomen

    C76.3 **Malignant neoplasm of** pelvis
        Malignant neoplasm of groin NOS
        Malignant neoplasm of sites overlapping systems within the pelvis
        Rectovaginal (septum) malignant neoplasm
        Rectovesical (septum) malignant neoplasm

Chapter 2. Neoplasms

√5ʰ C76.4 Malignant neoplasm of upper limb

    C76.40 Malignant neoplasm of unspecified upper limb
    C76.41 Malignant neoplasm of right **upper limb**
    C76.42 Malignant neoplasm of left **upper limb**

√5ʰ C76.5 Malignant neoplasm of lower limb

    C76.50 Malignant neoplasm of unspecified lower limb
    C76.51 Malignant neoplasm of right **lower limb**
    C76.52 Malignant neoplasm of left **lower limb**

C76.8 Malignant neoplasm of other specified ill-defined sites
    Malignant neoplasm of overlapping ill-defined sites

√4ʰ C77 Secondary **and unspecified malignant neoplasm of** lymph nodes

    EXCLUDES 1   malignant neoplasm of lymph nodes, specified as primary (C81-C86, C88, C96.-)
           mesentary metastasis of carcinoid tumor (C7B.04)
           secondary carcinoid tumors of distant lymph nodes (C7B.01)

C77.0 Secondary and unspecified malignant neoplasm of lymph nodes of head, face and neck
    Secondary and unspecified malignant neoplasm of supraclavicular lymph nodes

C77.1 Secondary and unspecified malignant neoplasm of intrathoracic **lymph nodes**

C77.2 Secondary and unspecified malignant neoplasm of intra-abdominal **lymph nodes**

C77.3 Secondary and unspecified malignant neoplasm of axilla and upper limb **lymph nodes**
    Secondary and unspecified malignant neoplasm of pectoral lymph nodes

C77.4 Secondary and unspecified malignant neoplasm of inguinal and lower limb **lymph nodes**

C77.5 Secondary and unspecified malignant neoplasm of intrapelvic **lymph nodes**

C77.8 Secondary and unspecified malignant neoplasm of lymph nodes of multiple regions

C77.9 Secondary and unspecified malignant neoplasm of lymph node, unspecified

√4ʰ C78 Secondary **malignant neoplasm of** respiratory and digestive **organs**

    EXCLUDES 1   secondary carcinoid tumors of liver (C7B.02)
           secondary carcinoid tumors of peritoneum (C7B.04)
    EXCLUDES 2   lymph node metastases (C77.0)

√5ʰ C78.0 Secondary malignant neoplasm of lung
    AHA: 2019,1Q,16

    C78.00 Secondary malignant neoplasm of unspecified lung
    C78.01 Secondary malignant neoplasm of right **lung**
    C78.02 Secondary malignant neoplasm of left **lung**

C78.1 Secondary malignant neoplasm of mediastinum

C78.2 Secondary malignant neoplasm of pleura

√5ʰ C78.3 Secondary malignant neoplasm of other and unspecified respiratory organs
    C78.30 Secondary malignant neoplasm of unspecified respiratory organ
    C78.39 Secondary malignant neoplasm of other respiratory organs

C78.4 Secondary malignant neoplasm of small intestine

C78.5 Secondary malignant neoplasm of large intestine and rectum

C78.6 Secondary malignant neoplasm of retroperitoneum and peritoneum
    AHA: 2017,2Q,12

C78.7 Secondary malignant neoplasm of liver and intrahepatic bile duct

√5ʰ C78.8 Secondary malignant neoplasm of other and unspecified digestive organs
    C78.80 Secondary malignant neoplasm of unspecified digestive organ
    C78.89 Secondary malignant neoplasm of other digestive organs
        Code also exocrine pancreatic insufficiency (K86.81)

√4ʰ C79 Secondary **malignant neoplasm of other and unspecified sites**

    EXCLUDES 1   secondary carcinoid tumors (C7B.-)
           secondary neuroendocrine tumors (C7B.-)

√5ʰ C79.0 Secondary malignant neoplasm of kidney and renal pelvis
    C79.00 Secondary malignant neoplasm of unspecified kidney and renal pelvis
    C79.01 Secondary malignant neoplasm of right **kidney and renal pelvis**
    C79.02 Secondary malignant neoplasm of left **kidney and renal pelvis**

√5ʰ C79.1 Secondary malignant neoplasm of bladder **and other and unspecified** urinary organs
    C79.10 Secondary malignant neoplasm of unspecified urinary organs
    C79.11 Secondary malignant neoplasm of bladder
        EXCLUDES 2   lymph node metastases (C77.0)
    C79.19 Secondary malignant neoplasm of other urinary organs

C79.2 Secondary malignant neoplasm of skin
    EXCLUDES 1   secondary Merkel cell carcinoma (C7B.1)

√5ʰ C79.3 Secondary malignant neoplasm of brain and cerebral meninges
    C79.31 Secondary malignant neoplasm of brain
    C79.32 Secondary malignant neoplasm of cerebral meninges

√5ʰ C79.4 Secondary malignant neoplasm of other and unspecified parts of nervous system
    C79.40 Secondary malignant neoplasm of unspecified part of nervous system
    C79.49 Secondary malignant neoplasm of other parts of nervous system

√5ʰ C79.5 Secondary malignant neoplasm of bone and bone marrow
    EXCLUDES 1   secondary carcinoid tumors of bone (C7B.03)
    C79.51 Secondary malignant neoplasm of bone
    C79.52 Secondary malignant neoplasm of bone marrow

√5ʰ C79.6 Secondary malignant neoplasm of ovary
    C79.60 Secondary malignant neoplasm of unspecified ovary ♀
    C79.61 Secondary malignant neoplasm of right **ovary** ♀
    C79.62 Secondary malignant neoplasm of left **ovary** ♀

√5ʰ C79.7 Secondary malignant neoplasm of adrenal gland
    C79.70 Secondary malignant neoplasm of unspecified adrenal gland
    C79.71 Secondary malignant neoplasm of right **adrenal gland**
    C79.72 Secondary malignant neoplasm of left **adrenal gland**

√5ʰ C79.8 Secondary malignant neoplasm of other specified sites
    C79.81 Secondary malignant neoplasm of breast
    C79.82 Secondary malignant neoplasm of genital organs
    C79.89 Secondary malignant neoplasm of other specified sites
        AHA: 2017,2Q,11

C79.9 Secondary malignant neoplasm of unspecified site
    Metastatic cancer NOS
    Metastatic disease NOS
    EXCLUDES 1   carcinomatosis NOS (C80.0)
           generalized cancer NOS (C80.0)
           malignant (primary) neoplasm of unspecified site (C80.1)

√4ʰ C80 Malignant neoplasm without specification of site
    EXCLUDES 1   malignant carcinoid tumor of unspecified site (C7A.00)
           malignant neoplasm of specified multiple sites — code to each site

C80.0 Disseminated **malignant neoplasm, unspecified**
    Carcinomatosis NOS   *Cu all over no*
    Generalized cancer, unspecified site (primary) (secondary)   *effort to*
    Generalized malignancy, unspecified site (primary) (secondary)   *find primary si...*

C80.1 Malignant (primary) **neoplasm, unspecified**
    Cancer NOS   *unknown primary*
    Cancer unspecified site (primary)
    Carcinoma unspecified site (primary)
    Malignancy unspecified site (primary)
    EXCLUDES 1   secondary malignant neoplasm of unspecified site (C79.9)

C80.2 Malignant neoplasm associated with transplanted organ
    Code first complication of transplanted organ (T86.-)
    Use additional code to identify the specific malignancy

Chapter 2. Neoplasms

Malignant neoplasms of lymphoid, hematopoietic and related tissue (C81-C96)

EXCLUDES 2   *Kaposi's sarcoma of lymph nodes (C46.3)*
secondary and unspecified neoplasm of lymph nodes (C77.-)
secondary neoplasm of bone marrow (C79.52)
secondary neoplasm of spleen (C78.89)

✓4ᵗʰ **C81 Hodgkin lymphoma**

EXCLUDES 1   *personal history of Hodgkin lymphoma (Z85.71)*

DEF: Malignant disorder of lymphoid cells characterized by the presence of progressively swollen lymph nodes and spleen that may also involve the liver. A diagnosis of Hodgkin's lymphoma can be confirmed by the presence of Reed-Sternberg cells. *Synonym(s): Hodgkin disease.*

✓5ᵗʰ **C81.0** Nodular lymphocyte predominant **Hodgkin lymphoma**

C81.00 Nodular lymphocyte predominant Hodgkin lymphoma, unspecified site

C81.01 Nodular lymphocyte predominant Hodgkin lymphoma, lymph nodes of head, face, and neck

C81.02 Nodular lymphocyte predominant Hodgkin lymphoma, intrathoracic lymph nodes

C81.03 Nodular lymphocyte predominant Hodgkin lymphoma, intra-abdominal lymph nodes

C81.04 Nodular lymphocyte predominant Hodgkin lymphoma, lymph nodes of axilla and upper limb

C81.05 Nodular lymphocyte predominant Hodgkin lymphoma, lymph nodes of inguinal region and lower limb

C81.06 Nodular lymphocyte predominant Hodgkin lymphoma, intrapelvic lymph nodes

C81.07 Nodular lymphocyte predominant Hodgkin lymphoma, spleen

C81.08 Nodular lymphocyte predominant Hodgkin lymphoma, lymph nodes of multiple sites

C81.09 Nodular lymphocyte predominant Hodgkin lymphoma, extranodal and solid organ sites

✓5ᵗʰ **C81.1** Nodular sclerosis **Hodgkin lymphoma**

Nodular sclerosis classical Hodgkin lymphoma

C81.10 Nodular sclerosis Hodgkin lymphoma, unspecified site

C81.11 Nodular sclerosis Hodgkin lymphoma, lymph nodes of head, face, and neck

C81.12 Nodular sclerosis Hodgkin lymphoma, intrathoracic lymph nodes

C81.13 Nodular sclerosis Hodgkin lymphoma, intra-abdominal lymph nodes

C81.14 Nodular sclerosis Hodgkin lymphoma, lymph nodes of axilla and upper limb

C81.15 Nodular sclerosis Hodgkin lymphoma, lymph nodes of inguinal region and lower limb

C81.16 Nodular sclerosis Hodgkin lymphoma, intrapelvic lymph nodes

C81.17 Nodular sclerosis Hodgkin lymphoma, spleen

C81.18 Nodular sclerosis Hodgkin lymphoma, lymph nodes of multiple sites

C81.19 Nodular sclerosis Hodgkin lymphoma, extranodal and solid organ sites

✓5ᵗʰ **C81.2** Mixed cellularity **Hodgkin lymphoma**

Mixed cellularity classical Hodgkin lymphoma

C81.20 Mixed cellularity Hodgkin lymphoma, unspecified site

C81.21 Mixed cellularity Hodgkin lymphoma, lymph nodes of head, face, and neck

C81.22 Mixed cellularity Hodgkin lymphoma, intrathoracic lymph nodes

C81.23 Mixed cellularity Hodgkin lymphoma, intra-abdominal lymph nodes

C81.24 Mixed cellularity Hodgkin lymphoma, lymph nodes of axilla and upper limb

C81.25 Mixed cellularity Hodgkin lymphoma, lymph nodes of inguinal region and lower limb

C81.26 Mixed cellularity Hodgkin lymphoma, intrapelvic lymph nodes

C81.27 Mixed cellularity Hodgkin lymphoma, spleen

C81.28 Mixed cellularity Hodgkin lymphoma, lymph nodes of multiple sites

C81.29 Mixed cellularity Hodgkin lymphoma, extranodal and solid organ sites

✓5ᵗʰ **C81.3** Lymphocyte depleted **Hodgkin lymphoma**

Lymphocyte depleted classical Hodgkin lymphoma

C81.30 Lymphocyte depleted Hodgkin lymphoma, unspecified site

C81.31 Lymphocyte depleted Hodgkin lymphoma, lymph nodes of head, face, and neck

C81.32 Lymphocyte depleted Hodgkin lymphoma, intrathoracic lymph nodes

C81.33 Lymphocyte depleted Hodgkin lymphoma, intra-abdominal lymph nodes

C81.34 Lymphocyte depleted Hodgkin lymphoma, lymph nodes of axilla and upper limb

C81.35 Lymphocyte depleted Hodgkin lymphoma, lymph nodes of inguinal region and lower limb

C81.36 Lymphocyte depleted Hodgkin lymphoma, intrapelvic lymph nodes

C81.37 Lymphocyte depleted Hodgkin lymphoma, spleen

C81.38 Lymphocyte depleted Hodgkin lymphoma, lymph nodes of multiple sites

C81.39 Lymphocyte depleted Hodgkin lymphoma, extranodal and solid organ sites

✓5ᵗʰ **C81.4** Lymphocyte-rich **Hodgkin lymphoma**

Lymphocyte-rich classical Hodgkin lymphoma

EXCLUDES 1   *nodular lymphocyte predominant Hodgkin lymphoma (C81.0-)*

C81.40 Lymphocyte-rich Hodgkin lymphoma, unspecified site

C81.41 Lymphocyte-rich Hodgkin lymphoma, lymph nodes of head, face, and neck

C81.42 Lymphocyte-rich Hodgkin lymphoma, intrathoracic lymph nodes

C81.43 Lymphocyte-rich Hodgkin lymphoma, intra-abdominal lymph nodes

C81.44 Lymphocyte-rich Hodgkin lymphoma, lymph nodes of axilla and upper limb

C81.45 Lymphocyte-rich Hodgkin lymphoma, lymph nodes of inguinal region and lower limb

C81.46 Lymphocyte-rich Hodgkin lymphoma, intrapelvic lymph nodes

C81.47 Lymphocyte-rich Hodgkin lymphoma, spleen

C81.48 Lymphocyte-rich Hodgkin lymphoma, lymph nodes of multiple sites

C81.49 Lymphocyte-rich Hodgkin lymphoma, extranodal and solid organ sites

✓5ᵗʰ **C81.7** Other Hodgkin lymphoma

Classical Hodgkin lymphoma NOS
Other classical Hodgkin lymphoma

C81.70 Other Hodgkin lymphoma, unspecified site

C81.71 Other Hodgkin lymphoma, lymph nodes of head, face, and neck

C81.72 Other Hodgkin lymphoma, intrathoracic lymph nodes

C81.73 Other Hodgkin lymphoma, intra-abdominal lymph nodes

C81.74 Other Hodgkin lymphoma, lymph nodes of axilla and upper limb

C81.75 Other Hodgkin lymphoma, lymph nodes of inguinal region and lower limb

C81.76 Other Hodgkin lymphoma, intrapelvic lymph nodes

C81.77 Other Hodgkin lymphoma, spleen

C81.78 Other Hodgkin lymphoma, lymph nodes of multiple sites

C81.79 Other Hodgkin lymphoma, extranodal and solid organ sites

✓5ᵗʰ **C81.9** Hodgkin lymphoma, unspecified

C81.90 Hodgkin lymphoma, unspecified, unspecified site

C81.91 Hodgkin lymphoma, unspecified, lymph nodes of head, face, and neck

C81.92 Hodgkin lymphoma, unspecified, intrathoracic lymph nodes

C81.93 Hodgkin lymphoma, unspecified, intra-abdominal lymph nodes

C81.94 Hodgkin lymphoma, unspecified, lymph nodes of axilla and upper limb

C81.95 Hodgkin lymphoma, unspecified, lymph nodes of inguinal region and lower limb

C81.96 Hodgkin lymphoma, unspecified, intrapelvic lymph nodes

C81.97 Hodgkin lymphoma, unspecified, spleen

N Newborn: 0   P Pediatric: 0-17   M Maternity: 12-55   A Adult: 15-124   CH Comorbidity High   CL Comorbidity Low   NCDx Noncancer Dx   PDx Primary Dx

476   ICD-10-CM 2020

C81.98	Hodgkin lymphoma, unspecified, lymph nodes of multiple sites
C81.99	Hodgkin lymphoma, unspecified, extranodal and solid organ sites

✓4ᵗʰ **C82** **Follicular lymphoma**

    INCLUDES   follicular lymphoma with or without diffuse areas

    EXCLUDES 1   *mature T/NK-cell lymphomas (C84.-)*

                personal history of non-Hodgkin lymphoma (Z85.72)

DEF: Most common subgroup of non-Hodgkin lymphomas (NHL), accounting for 20 to 30 percent of all NHLs. NHL is a B-cell lymphoma that is slow growing and characterized by the circular pattern of malignant cell growth with the cells clustered into identifiable nodules or follicles.

✓5ᵗʰ **C82.0** **Follicular lymphoma** grade I

C82.00	Follicular lymphoma grade I, unspecified site
C82.01	Follicular lymphoma grade I, lymph nodes of head, face, and neck
C82.02	Follicular lymphoma grade I, intrathoracic lymph nodes
C82.03	Follicular lymphoma grade I, intra-abdominal lymph nodes
C82.04	Follicular lymphoma grade I, lymph nodes of axilla and upper limb
C82.05	Follicular lymphoma grade I, lymph nodes of inguinal region and lower limb
C82.06	Follicular lymphoma grade I, intrapelvic lymph nodes
C82.07	Follicular lymphoma grade I, spleen
C82.08	Follicular lymphoma grade I, lymph nodes of multiple sites
C82.09	Follicular lymphoma grade I, extranodal and solid organ sites

✓5ᵗʰ **C82.1** **Follicular lymphoma** grade II

C82.10	Follicular lymphoma grade II, unspecified site
C82.11	Follicular lymphoma grade II, lymph nodes of head, face, and neck
C82.12	Follicular lymphoma grade II, intrathoracic lymph nodes
C82.13	Follicular lymphoma grade II, intra-abdominal lymph nodes
C82.14	Follicular lymphoma grade II, lymph nodes of axilla and upper limb
C82.15	Follicular lymphoma grade II, lymph nodes of inguinal region and lower limb
C82.16	Follicular lymphoma grade II, intrapelvic lymph nodes
C82.17	Follicular lymphoma grade II, spleen
C82.18	Follicular lymphoma grade II, lymph nodes of multiple sites
C82.19	Follicular lymphoma grade II, extranodal and solid organ sites

✓5ᵗʰ **C82.2** **Follicular lymphoma** grade III, unspecified

C82.20	Follicular lymphoma grade III, unspecified, unspecified site
C82.21	Follicular lymphoma grade III, unspecified, lymph nodes of head, face, and neck
C82.22	Follicular lymphoma grade III, unspecified, intrathoracic lymph nodes
C82.23	Follicular lymphoma grade III, unspecified, intra-abdominal lymph nodes
C82.24	Follicular lymphoma grade III, unspecified, lymph nodes of axilla and upper limb
C82.25	Follicular lymphoma grade III, unspecified, lymph nodes of inguinal region and lower limb
C82.26	Follicular lymphoma grade III, unspecified, intrapelvic lymph nodes
C82.27	Follicular lymphoma grade III, unspecified, spleen
C82.28	Follicular lymphoma grade III, unspecified, lymph nodes of multiple sites
C82.29	Follicular lymphoma grade III, unspecified, extranodal and solid organ sites

✓5ᵗʰ **C82.3** **Follicular lymphoma** grade IIIa

C82.30	Follicular lymphoma grade IIIa, unspecified site
C82.31	Follicular lymphoma grade IIIa, lymph nodes of head, face, and neck
C82.32	Follicular lymphoma grade IIIa, intrathoracic lymph nodes
C82.33	Follicular lymphoma grade IIIa, intra-abdominal lymph nodes
C82.34	Follicular lymphoma grade IIIa, lymph nodes of axilla and upper limb

C82.35	Follicular lymphoma grade IIIa, lymph nodes of inguinal region and lower limb
C82.36	Follicular lymphoma grade IIIa, intrapelvic lymph nodes
C82.37	Follicular lymphoma grade IIIa, spleen
C82.38	Follicular lymphoma grade IIIa, lymph nodes of multiple sites
C82.39	Follicular lymphoma grade IIIa, extranodal and solid organ sites

✓5ᵗʰ **C82.4** **Follicular lymphoma** grade IIIb

C82.40	Follicular lymphoma grade IIIb, unspecified site
C82.41	Follicular lymphoma grade IIIb, lymph nodes of head, face, and neck
C82.42	Follicular lymphoma grade IIIb, intrathoracic lymph nodes
C82.43	Follicular lymphoma grade IIIb, intra-abdominal lymph nodes
C82.44	Follicular lymphoma grade IIIb, lymph nodes of axilla and upper limb
C82.45	Follicular lymphoma grade IIIb, lymph nodes of inguinal region and lower limb
C82.46	Follicular lymphoma grade IIIb, intrapelvic lymph nodes
C82.47	Follicular lymphoma grade IIIb, spleen
C82.48	Follicular lymphoma grade IIIb, lymph nodes of multiple sites
C82.49	Follicular lymphoma grade IIIb, extranodal and solid organ sites

✓5ᵗʰ **C82.5** **Diffuse follicle center** lymphoma

C82.50	Diffuse follicle center lymphoma, unspecified site
C82.51	Diffuse follicle center lymphoma, lymph nodes of head, face, and neck
C82.52	Diffuse follicle center lymphoma, intrathoracic lymph nodes
C82.53	Diffuse follicle center lymphoma, intra-abdominal lymph nodes
C82.54	Diffuse follicle center lymphoma, lymph nodes of axilla and upper limb
C82.55	Diffuse follicle center lymphoma, lymph nodes of inguinal region and lower limb
C82.56	Diffuse follicle center lymphoma, intrapelvic lymph nodes
C82.57	Diffuse follicle center lymphoma, spleen
C82.58	Diffuse follicle center lymphoma, lymph nodes of multiple sites
C82.59	Diffuse follicle center lymphoma, extranodal and solid organ sites

✓5ᵗʰ **C82.6** **Cutaneous follicle center** lymphoma

C82.60	Cutaneous follicle center lymphoma, unspecified site
C82.61	Cutaneous follicle center lymphoma, lymph nodes of head, face, and neck
C82.62	Cutaneous follicle center lymphoma, intrathoracic lymph nodes
C82.63	Cutaneous follicle center lymphoma, intra-abdominal lymph nodes
C82.64	Cutaneous follicle center lymphoma, lymph nodes of axilla and upper limb
C82.65	Cutaneous follicle center lymphoma, lymph nodes of inguinal region and lower limb
C82.66	Cutaneous follicle center lymphoma, intrapelvic lymph nodes
C82.67	Cutaneous follicle center lymphoma, spleen
C82.68	Cutaneous follicle center lymphoma, lymph nodes of multiple sites
C82.69	Cutaneous follicle center lymphoma, extranodal and solid organ sites

✓5ᵗʰ **C82.8** **Other types of follicular lymphoma**

C82.80	Other types of follicular lymphoma, unspecified site
C82.81	Other types of follicular lymphoma, lymph nodes of head, face, and neck
C82.82	Other types of follicular lymphoma, intrathoracic lymph nodes
C82.83	Other types of follicular lymphoma, intra-abdominal lymph nodes
C82.84	Other types of follicular lymphoma, lymph nodes of axilla and upper limb
C82.85	Other types of follicular lymphoma, lymph nodes of inguinal region and lower limb

☑ Additional Character Required   ✓x7ᵗʰ Placeholder Alert   Manifestation   Unspecified Dx   ►◄ Revised Text   ● New Code   ▲ Revised Title

ICD-10-CM 2020   477

C82.86   **Other types of follicular lymphoma,** intrapelvic lymph nodes

C82.87   **Other types of follicular lymphoma,** spleen

C82.88   **Other types of follicular lymphoma, lymph nodes of** multiple sites

C82.89   **Other types of follicular lymphoma,** extranodal and solid organ sites

√5th **C82.9**   **Follicular lymphoma, unspecified**

C82.90   **Follicular lymphoma, unspecified, unspecified site**

C82.91   **Follicular lymphoma, unspecified, lymph nodes of** head, face, and neck

C82.92   **Follicular lymphoma, unspecified,** intrathoracic lymph nodes

C82.93   **Follicular lymphoma, unspecified,** intra-abdominal lymph nodes

C82.94   **Follicular lymphoma, unspecified, lymph nodes of** axilla and upper limb

C82.95   **Follicular lymphoma, unspecified, lymph nodes of** inguinal region and lower limb

C82.96   **Follicular lymphoma, unspecified,** intrapelvic lymph nodes

C82.97   **Follicular lymphoma, unspecified,** spleen

C82.98   **Follicular lymphoma, unspecified, lymph nodes of** multiple sites

C82.99   **Follicular lymphoma, unspecified,** extranodal and solid organ sites

√4th **C83**   **Non-follicular lymphoma**

EXCLUDES 1   *personal history of non-Hodgkin lymphoma (Z85.72)*

√5th **C83.0**   **Small cell B-cell lymphoma**

Lymphoplasmacytic lymphoma
Nodal marginal zone lymphoma
Non-leukemic variant of B-CLL
Splenic marginal zone lymphoma

EXCLUDES 1   *chronic lymphocytic leukemia (C91.1)*
       mature T/NK-cell lymphomas (C84.-)
       Waldenström macroglobulinemia (C88.0)

DEF: Nonfollicular lymphoma that is rare, slow growing, and usually found in the older population.

C83.00   **Small cell B-cell lymphoma, unspecified site**

C83.01   **Small cell B-cell lymphoma, lymph nodes of** head, face, and neck

C83.02   **Small cell B-cell lymphoma,** intrathoracic lymph nodes

C83.03   **Small cell B-cell lymphoma,** intra-abdominal lymph nodes

C83.04   **Small cell B-cell lymphoma, lymph nodes of** axilla and upper limb

C83.05   **Small cell B-cell lymphoma, lymph nodes of** inguinal region and lower limb

C83.06   **Small cell B-cell lymphoma,** intrapelvic lymph nodes

C83.07   **Small cell B-cell lymphoma,** spleen

C83.08   **Small cell B-cell lymphoma, lymph nodes of** multiple sites

C83.09   **Small cell B-cell lymphoma,** extranodal and solid organ sites

√5th **C83.1**   **Mantle cell lymphoma**

Centrocytic lymphoma
Malignant lymphomatous polyposis

DEF: Rare form of B-cell non-Hodgkin lymphoma named for the location of the tumor cell production, the mantle zone of the lymph nodes.

C83.10   **Mantle cell lymphoma, unspecified site**

C83.11   **Mantle cell lymphoma, lymph nodes of** head, face, and neck

C83.12   **Mantle cell lymphoma,** intrathoracic lymph nodes

C83.13   **Mantle cell lymphoma,** intra-abdominal lymph nodes

C83.14   **Mantle cell lymphoma, lymph nodes of** axilla and upper limb

C83.15   **Mantle cell lymphoma, lymph nodes of** inguinal region and lower limb

C83.16   **Mantle cell lymphoma,** intrapelvic lymph nodes

C83.17   **Mantle cell lymphoma,** spleen

C83.18   **Mantle cell lymphoma, lymph nodes of** multiple sites

C83.19   **Mantle cell lymphoma,** extranodal and solid organ sites

√5th **C83.3**   **Diffuse large B-cell lymphoma**

Anaplastic diffuse large B-cell lymphoma
CD30-positive diffuse large B-cell lymphoma
Centroblastic diffuse large B-cell lymphoma
Diffuse large B-cell lymphoma, subtype not specified
Immunoblastic diffuse large B-cell lymphoma
Plasmablastic diffuse large B-cell lymphoma
T-cell rich diffuse large B-cell lymphoma

EXCLUDES 1   *mediastinal (thymic) large B-cell lymphoma (C85.2-)*
       mature T/NK-cell lymphomas (C84.-)

DEF: Nonfollicular lymphoma that is one of the more common types of lymphoma. This cancer is fast growing and affects any age but is found mostly in the older population.

C83.30   **Diffuse large B-cell lymphoma, unspecified site**

C83.31   **Diffuse large B-cell lymphoma, lymph nodes of** head, face, and neck

C83.32   **Diffuse large B-cell lymphoma,** intrathoracic lymph nodes

C83.33   **Diffuse large B-cell lymphoma,** intra-abdominal lymph nodes

C83.34   **Diffuse large B-cell lymphoma, lymph nodes of** axilla and upper limb

C83.35   **Diffuse large B-cell lymphoma, lymph nodes of** inguinal region and lower limb

C83.36   **Diffuse large B-cell lymphoma,** intrapelvic lymph nodes

C83.37   **Diffuse large B-cell lymphoma,** spleen

C83.38   **Diffuse large B-cell lymphoma, lymph nodes of** multiple sites

C83.39   **Diffuse large B-cell lymphoma,** extranodal and solid organ sites

√5th **C83.5**   **Lymphoblastic (diffuse) lymphoma**

B-precursor lymphoma
Lymphoblastic B-cell lymphoma
Lymphoblastic lymphoma NOS
Lymphoblastic T-cell lymphoma
T-precursor lymphoma

DEF: Type of non-Hodgkin lymphoma considered lymphoma or leukemia—the determination is made based on the amount of bone marrow involvement. The cells are small to medium immature T-cells that often originate in the thymus where many of the T-cells are made.

C83.50   **Lymphoblastic (diffuse) lymphoma, unspecified site**

C83.51   **Lymphoblastic (diffuse) lymphoma, lymph nodes of** head, face, and neck

C83.52   **Lymphoblastic (diffuse) lymphoma,** intrathoracic lymph nodes

C83.53   **Lymphoblastic (diffuse) lymphoma,** intra-abdominal lymph nodes

C83.54   **Lymphoblastic (diffuse) lymphoma, lymph nodes of** axilla and upper limb

C83.55   **Lymphoblastic (diffuse) lymphoma, lymph nodes of** inguinal region and lower limb

C83.56   **Lymphoblastic (diffuse) lymphoma,** intrapelvic lymph nodes

C83.57   **Lymphoblastic (diffuse) lymphoma,** spleen

C83.58   **Lymphoblastic (diffuse) lymphoma, lymph nodes of** multiple sites

C83.59   **Lymphoblastic (diffuse) lymphoma,** extranodal and solid organ sites

√5th **C83.7**   **Burkitt lymphoma**

Atypical Burkitt lymphoma
Burkitt-like lymphoma

EXCLUDES 1   *mature B-cell leukemia Burkitt type (C91.A-)*

DEF: Malignancy of the lymphatic system, most often seen as a large bone-deteriorating lesion within the jaw or as an abdominal mass. It is a form of non-Hodgkin's lymphoma and is recognized as the fastest growing human tumor.

C83.70   **Burkitt lymphoma, unspecified site**

C83.71   **Burkitt lymphoma, lymph nodes of** head, face, and neck

C83.72   **Burkitt lymphoma,** intrathoracic lymph nodes

C83.73   **Burkitt lymphoma,** intra-abdominal lymph nodes

C83.74   **Burkitt lymphoma, lymph nodes of** axilla and upper limb

C83.75   **Burkitt lymphoma, lymph nodes of** inguinal region and lower limb

C83.76   **Burkitt lymphoma,** intrapelvic lymph nodes

C83.77   **Burkitt lymphoma,** spleen

C83.78   **Burkitt lymphoma, lymph nodes of** multiple sites

C83.79   **Burkitt lymphoma,** extranodal and solid organ sites

√5ᵗʰ **C83.8   Other** non-follicular **lymphoma**

     Intravascular large B-cell lymphoma

     Lymphoid granulomatosis

     Primary effusion B-cell lymphoma

     EXCLUDES 1   *mediastinal (thymic) large B-cell lymphoma (C85.2-)*

                T-cell rich B-cell lymphoma (C83.3-)

   C83.80   **Other non-follicular lymphoma, unspecified site**

   C83.81   **Other non-follicular lymphoma, lymph nodes of** head, face, and neck

   C83.82   **Other non-follicular lymphoma,** intrathoracic **lymph nodes**

   C83.83   **Other non-follicular lymphoma,** intra-abdominal **lymph nodes**

   C83.84   **Other non-follicular lymphoma, lymph nodes of** axilla and upper limb

   C83.85   **Other non-follicular lymphoma, lymph nodes of** inguinal region and lower limb

   C83.86   **Other non-follicular lymphoma,** intrapelvic **lymph nodes**

   C83.87   **Other non-follicular lymphoma,** spleen

   C83.88   **Other non-follicular lymphoma, lymph nodes of** multiple sites

   C83.89   **Other non-follicular lymphoma,** extranodal and solid organ sites

√5ᵗʰ **C83.9   Non-follicular (diffuse) lymphoma, unspecified**

   C83.90   **Non-follicular (diffuse) lymphoma, unspecified, unspecified site**

   C83.91   **Non-follicular (diffuse) lymphoma, unspecified, lymph nodes of** head, face, and neck

   C83.92   **Non-follicular (diffuse) lymphoma, unspecified,** intrathoracic **lymph nodes**

   C83.93   **Non-follicular (diffuse) lymphoma, unspecified,** intra-abdominal **lymph nodes**

   C83.94   **Non-follicular (diffuse) lymphoma, unspecified, lymph nodes of** axilla and upper limb

   C83.95   **Non-follicular (diffuse) lymphoma, unspecified, lymph nodes of** inguinal region and lower limb

   C83.96   **Non-follicular (diffuse) lymphoma, unspecified,** intrapelvic **lymph nodes**

   C83.97   **Non-follicular (diffuse) lymphoma, unspecified,** spleen

   C83.98   **Non-follicular (diffuse) lymphoma, unspecified, lymph nodes of** multiple sites

   C83.99   **Non-follicular (diffuse) lymphoma, unspecified,** extranodal and solid organ sites

√4ᵗʰ **C84   Mature T/NK-cell lymphomas**

     EXCLUDES 1   *personal history of non-Hodgkin lymphoma (Z85.72)*

√5ᵗʰ **C84.0   Mycosis fungoides**

     EXCLUDES 1   *peripheral T-cell lymphoma, not classified (C84.4-)*

     DEF: Most common form of cutaneous T-cell lymphoma. A type of non-Hodgkin lymphoma in which white blood cells become cancerous and affect the skin and sometimes internal organs. ***Synonym(s):*** *Alibert-Bazin syndrome.*

   C84.00   **Mycosis fungoides, unspecified site**

   C84.01   **Mycosis fungoides, lymph nodes of** head, face, and neck

   C84.02   **Mycosis fungoides,** intrathoracic **lymph nodes**

   C84.03   **Mycosis fungoides,** intra-abdominal **lymph nodes**

   C84.04   **Mycosis fungoides, lymph nodes of** axilla and upper limb

   C84.05   **Mycosis fungoides, lymph nodes of** inguinal region and lower limb

   C84.06   **Mycosis fungoides,** intrapelvic **lymph nodes**

   C84.07   **Mycosis fungoides,** spleen

   C84.08   **Mycosis fungoides, lymph nodes of** multiple sites

   C84.09   **Mycosis fungoides,** extranodal and solid organ sites

√5ᵗʰ **C84.1   Sézary disease**

     DEF: Extension of mycosis fungoides that affects the blood and all of the skin, appearing as sunburn, rather than patches. It spreads to the lymph nodes and is often linked to a weakened immune system.

   C84.10   **Sézary disease, unspecified site**

   C84.11   **Sézary disease, lymph nodes of** head, face, and neck

   C84.12   **Sézary disease,** intrathoracic **lymph nodes**

   C84.13   **Sézary disease,** intra-abdominal **lymph nodes**

   C84.14   **Sézary disease, lymph nodes of** axilla and upper limb

   C84.15   **Sézary disease, lymph nodes of** inguinal region and lower limb

   C84.16   **Sézary disease,** intrapelvic **lymph nodes**

   C84.17   **Sézary disease,** spleen

   C84.18   **Sézary disease, lymph nodes of** multiple sites

   C84.19   **Sézary disease,** extranodal and solid organ sites

√5ᵗʰ **C84.4   Peripheral T-cell lymphoma, not classified**

     Lennert's lymphoma

     Lymphoepithelioid lymphoma

     Mature T-cell lymphoma, not elsewhere classified

   C84.40   **Peripheral T-cell lymphoma, not classified, unspecified site**

   C84.41   **Peripheral T-cell lymphoma, not classified, lymph nodes of** head, face, and neck

   C84.42   **Peripheral T-cell lymphoma, not classified,** intrathoracic **lymph nodes**

   C84.43   **Peripheral T-cell lymphoma, not classified,** intra-abdominal **lymph nodes**

   C84.44   **Peripheral T-cell lymphoma, not classified, lymph nodes of** axilla and upper limb

   C84.45   **Peripheral T-cell lymphoma, not classified, lymph nodes of** inguinal region and lower limb

   C84.46   **Peripheral T-cell lymphoma, not classified,** intrapelvic **lymph nodes**

   C84.47   **Peripheral T-cell lymphoma, not classified,** spleen

   C84.48   **Peripheral T-cell lymphoma, not classified, lymph nodes of** multiple sites

   C84.49   **Peripheral T-cell lymphoma, not classified,** extranodal and solid organ sites

√5ᵗʰ **C84.6   Anaplastic large cell lymphoma,** ALK-positive

     Anaplastic large cell lymphoma, CD30-positive

   C84.60   **Anaplastic large cell lymphoma, ALK-positive, unspecified site**

   C84.61   **Anaplastic large cell lymphoma, ALK-positive, lymph nodes of** head, face, and neck

   C84.62   **Anaplastic large cell lymphoma, ALK-positive,** intrathoracic **lymph nodes**

   C84.63   **Anaplastic large cell lymphoma, ALK-positive,** intra-abdominal **lymph nodes**

   C84.64   **Anaplastic large cell lymphoma, ALK-positive, lymph nodes of** axilla and upper limb

   C84.65   **Anaplastic large cell lymphoma, ALK-positive, lymph nodes of** inguinal region and lower limb

   C84.66   **Anaplastic large cell lymphoma, ALK-positive,** intrapelvic **lymph nodes**

   C84.67   **Anaplastic large cell lymphoma, ALK-positive,** spleen

   C84.68   **Anaplastic large cell lymphoma, ALK-positive, lymph nodes of** multiple sites

   C84.69   **Anaplastic large cell lymphoma, ALK-positive,** extranodal and solid organ sites

√5ᵗʰ **C84.7   Anaplastic large cell lymphoma,** ALK-negative

     EXCLUDES 1   *primary cutaneous CD30-positive T-cell proliferations (C86.6-)*

   C84.70   **Anaplastic large cell lymphoma, ALK-negative, unspecified site**

   C84.71   **Anaplastic large cell lymphoma, ALK-negative, lymph nodes of** head, face, and neck

   C84.72   **Anaplastic large cell lymphoma, ALK-negative,** intrathoracic **lymph nodes**

   C84.73   **Anaplastic large cell lymphoma, ALK-negative,** intra-abdominal **lymph nodes**

   C84.74   **Anaplastic large cell lymphoma, ALK-negative, lymph nodes of** axilla and upper limb

   C84.75   **Anaplastic large cell lymphoma, ALK-negative, lymph nodes of** inguinal region and lower limb

   C84.76   **Anaplastic large cell lymphoma, ALK-negative,** intrapelvic **lymph nodes**

   C84.77   **Anaplastic large cell lymphoma, ALK-negative,** spleen

   C84.78   **Anaplastic large cell lymphoma, ALK-negative, lymph nodes of** multiple sites

   C84.79   **Anaplastic large cell lymphoma, ALK-negative,** extranodal and solid organ sites

√5ᵗʰ **C84.A   Cutaneous T-cell lymphoma, unspecified**

   C84.A0   **Cutaneous T-cell lymphoma, unspecified, unspecified site**

   C84.A1   **Cutaneous T-cell lymphoma, unspecified lymph** nodes of head, face, and neck

   C84.A2   **Cutaneous T-cell lymphoma, unspecified,** intrathoracic **lymph nodes**

C84.A3   Cutaneous T-cell lymphoma, unspecified, intra-abdominal lymph nodes

C84.A4   Cutaneous T-cell lymphoma, unspecified, lymph nodes of axilla and upper limb

C84.A5   Cutaneous T-cell lymphoma, unspecified, lymph nodes of inguinal region and lower limb

C84.A6   Cutaneous T-cell lymphoma, unspecified, intrapelvic lymph nodes

C84.A7   Cutaneous T-cell lymphoma, unspecified, spleen

C84.A8   Cutaneous T-cell lymphoma, unspecified, lymph nodes of multiple sites

C84.A9   Cutaneous T-cell lymphoma, unspecified, extranodal and solid organ sites

√5th **C84.Z**   Other mature T/NK-cell lymphomas

> **NOTE**   If T-cell lineage or involvement is mentioned in conjunction with a specific lymphoma, code to the more specific description.
>
> **EXCLUDES 1**   angioimmunoblastic T-cell lymphoma (C86.5)
> blastic NK-cell lymphoma (C86.4)
> enteropathy-type T-cell lymphoma (C86.2)
> extranodal NK-cell lymphoma, nasal type (C86.0)
> hepatosplenic T-cell lymphoma (C86.1)
> primary cutaneous CD30-positive T-cell proliferations (C86.6)
> subcutaneous panniculitis-like T-cell lymphoma (C86.3)
> T-cell leukemia (C91.1-)

C84.Z0   Other mature T/NK-cell lymphomas, unspecified site

C84.Z1   Other mature T/NK-cell lymphomas, lymph nodes of head, face, and neck

C84.Z2   Other mature T/NK-cell lymphomas, intrathoracic lymph nodes

C84.Z3   Other mature T/NK-cell lymphomas, intra-abdominal lymph nodes

C84.Z4   Other mature T/NK-cell lymphomas, lymph nodes of axilla and upper limb

C84.Z5   Other mature T/NK-cell lymphomas, lymph nodes of inguinal region and lower limb

C84.Z6   Other mature T/NK-cell lymphomas, intrapelvic lymph nodes

C84.Z7   Other mature T/NK-cell lymphomas, spleen

C84.Z8   Other mature T/NK-cell lymphomas, lymph nodes of multiple sites

C84.Z9   Other mature T/NK-cell lymphomas, extranodal and solid organ sites

√5th **C84.9**   Mature T/NK-cell lymphomas, unspecified

NK/T cell lymphoma NOS

> **EXCLUDES 1**   mature T-cell lymphoma, not elsewhere classified (C84.4-)

C84.90   Mature T/NK-cell lymphomas, unspecified, unspecified site

C84.91   Mature T/NK-cell lymphomas, unspecified, lymph nodes of head, face, and neck

C84.92   Mature T/NK-cell lymphomas, unspecified, intrathoracic lymph nodes

C84.93   Mature T/NK-cell lymphomas, unspecified, intra-abdominal lymph nodes

C84.94   Mature T/NK-cell lymphomas, unspecified, lymph nodes of axilla and upper limb

C84.95   Mature T/NK-cell lymphomas, unspecified, lymph nodes of inguinal region and lower limb

C84.96   Mature T/NK-cell lymphomas, unspecified, intrapelvic lymph nodes

C84.97   Mature T/NK-cell lymphomas, unspecified, spleen

C84.98   Mature T/NK-cell lymphomas, unspecified, lymph nodes of multiple sites

C84.99   Mature T/NK-cell lymphomas, unspecified, extranodal and solid organ sites

√4th **C85**   Other specified and unspecified types of non-Hodgkin lymphoma

> **EXCLUDES 1**   other specified types of T/NK-cell lymphoma (C86.-)
> personal history of non-Hodgkin lymphoma (Z85.72)

√5th **C85.1**   Unspecified B-cell lymphoma

> **NOTE**   If B-cell lineage or involvement is mentioned in conjunction with a specific lymphoma, code to the more specific description.

C85.10   Unspecified B-cell lymphoma, unspecified site

C85.11   Unspecified B-cell lymphoma, lymph nodes of head, face, and neck

C85.12   Unspecified B-cell lymphoma, intrathoracic lymph nodes

C85.13   Unspecified B-cell lymphoma, intra-abdominal lymph nodes

C85.14   Unspecified B-cell lymphoma, lymph nodes of axilla and upper limb

C85.15   Unspecified B-cell lymphoma, lymph nodes of inguinal region and lower limb

C85.16   Unspecified B-cell lymphoma, intrapelvic lymph nodes

C85.17   Unspecified B-cell lymphoma, spleen

C85.18   Unspecified B-cell lymphoma, lymph nodes of multiple sites

C85.19   Unspecified B-cell lymphoma, extranodal and solid organ sites

√5th **C85.2**   Mediastinal (thymic) large B-cell lymphoma

C85.20   Mediastinal (thymic) large B-cell lymphoma, unspecified site

C85.21   Mediastinal (thymic) large B-cell lymphoma, lymph nodes of head, face, and neck

C85.22   Mediastinal (thymic) large B-cell lymphoma, intrathoracic lymph nodes

C85.23   Mediastinal (thymic) large B-cell lymphoma, intra-abdominal lymph nodes

C85.24   Mediastinal (thymic) large B-cell lymphoma, lymph nodes of axilla and upper limb

C85.25   Mediastinal (thymic) large B-cell lymphoma, lymph nodes of inguinal region and lower limb

C85.26   Mediastinal (thymic) large B-cell lymphoma, intrapelvic lymph nodes

C85.27   Mediastinal (thymic) large B-cell lymphoma, spleen

C85.28   Mediastinal (thymic) large B-cell lymphoma, lymph nodes of multiple sites

C85.29   Mediastinal (thymic) large B-cell lymphoma, extranodal and solid organ sites

√5th **C85.8**   Other specified types of non-Hodgkin lymphoma

C85.80   Other specified types of non-Hodgkin lymphoma, unspecified site

C85.81   Other specified types of non-Hodgkin lymphoma, lymph nodes of head, face, and neck

C85.82   Other specified types of non-Hodgkin lymphoma, intrathoracic lymph nodes

C85.83   Other specified types of non-Hodgkin lymphoma, intra-abdominal lymph nodes

C85.84   Other specified types of non-Hodgkin lymphoma, lymph nodes of axilla and upper limb

C85.85   Other specified types of non-Hodgkin lymphoma, lymph nodes of inguinal region and lower limb

C85.86   Other specified types of non-Hodgkin lymphoma, intrapelvic lymph nodes

C85.87   Other specified types of non-Hodgkin lymphoma, spleen

C85.88   Other specified types of non-Hodgkin lymphoma, lymph nodes of multiple sites

C85.89   Other specified types of non-Hodgkin lymphoma, extranodal and solid organ sites

√5th **C85.9**   Non-Hodgkin lymphoma, unspecified

Lymphoma NOS
Malignant lymphoma NOS
Non-Hodgkin lymphoma NOS

C85.90   Non-Hodgkin lymphoma, unspecified, unspecified site

C85.91   Non-Hodgkin lymphoma, unspecified, lymph nodes of head, face, and neck

C85.92   Non-Hodgkin lymphoma, unspecified, intrathoracic lymph nodes

C85.93   Non-Hodgkin lymphoma, unspecified, intra-abdominal lymph nodes

C85.94   Non-Hodgkin lymphoma, unspecified, lymph nodes of axilla and upper limb

C85.95   Non-Hodgkin lymphoma, unspecified, lymph nodes of inguinal region and lower limb

C85.96   Non-Hodgkin lymphoma, unspecified, intrapelvic lymph nodes

C85.97   Non-Hodgkin lymphoma, unspecified, spleen

C85.98   Non-Hodgkin lymphoma, unspecified, lymph nodes of multiple sites

C85.99   Non-Hodgkin lymphoma, unspecified, extranodal and solid organ sites

N Newborn: 0   P Pediatric: 0-17   M Maternity: 12-55   A Adult: 15-124   CH Comorbidity High   CL Comorbidity Low   NCDx Noncancer Dx   PDx Primary Dx

480   ICD-10-CM 2020

☑4ᵗʰ **C86 Other specified types of T/NK-cell lymphoma**

    EXCLUDES 1   *anaplastic large cell lymphoma, ALK negative (C84.7-)*
             anaplastic large cell lymphoma, ALK positive (C84.6-)
             mature T/NK-cell lymphomas (C84.-)
             other specified types of non-Hodgkin lymphoma (C85.8-)

    C86.0 Extranodal NK/T-cell lymphoma, nasal type

    C86.1 Hepatosplenic T-cell lymphoma
        Alpha-beta and gamma delta types

    C86.2 Enteropathy-type (intestinal) T-cell lymphoma
        Enteropathy associated T-cell lymphoma

    C86.3 Subcutaneous panniculitis-like T-cell lymphoma

    C86.4 Blastic NK-cell lymphoma
        Blastic plasmacytoid dendritic cell neoplasm (BPDCN)

    C86.5 Angioimmunoblastic T-cell lymphoma
        Angioimmunoblastic lymphadenopathy with dysproteinemia (AILD)

    C86.6 Primary cutaneous CD30-positive T-cell proliferations
        Lymphomatoid papulosis
        Primary cutaneous anaplastic large cell lymphoma
        Primary cutaneous CD30-positive large T-cell lymphoma

☑4ᵗʰ **C88 Malignant immunoproliferative diseases and certain other B-cell lymphomas**

    EXCLUDES 1   *B-cell lymphoma, unspecified (C85.1-)*
             personal history of other malignant neoplasms of lymphoid, hematopoietic and related tissues (Z85.79)

    C88.0 Waldenström macroglobulinemia
        Lymphoplasmacytic lymphoma with IgM-production
        Macroglobulinemia (idiopathic) (primary)
        EXCLUDES 1   *small cell B-cell lymphoma (C83.0)*

    C88.2 Heavy chain disease
        Franklin disease
        Gamma heavy chain disease
        Mu heavy chain disease

    C88.3 Immunoproliferative small intestinal disease
        Alpha heavy chain disease
        Mediterranean lymphoma

    C88.4 Extranodal marginal zone B-cell lymphoma of mucosa-associated lymphoid tissue [MALT-lymphoma]
        Lymphoma of skin-associated lymphoid tissue [SALT-lymphoma]
        Lymphoma of bronchial-associated lymphoid tissue [BALT-lymphoma]
        EXCLUDES 1   *high malignant (diffuse large B-cell) lymphoma (C83.3-)*

    C88.8 Other malignant immunoproliferative diseases

    C88.9 Malignant immunoproliferative disease, unspecified
        Immunoproliferative disease NOS

☑4ᵗʰ **C90 Multiple myeloma and malignant plasma cell neoplasms**

    EXCLUDES 1   *personal history of other malignant neoplasms of lymphoid, hematopoietic and related tissues (Z85.79)*

    AHA: 2019,2Q,30

☑5ᵗʰ   **C90.0 Multiple myeloma**
        Kahler's disease
        Medullary plasmacytoma
        Myelomatosis
        Plasma cell myeloma
        EXCLUDES 1   *solitary myeloma (C90.3-)*
                   solitary plasmactyoma (C90.3-)

       C90.00 Multiple myeloma not having achieved remission
          Multiple myeloma with failed remission
          Multiple myeloma NOS

       C90.01 Multiple myeloma in remission
       C90.02 Multiple myeloma in relapse

☑5ᵗʰ   **C90.1 Plasma cell leukemia**
        Plasmacytic leukemia
        AHA: 2019,2Q,30

       C90.10 Plasma cell leukemia not having achieved remission
          Plasma cell leukemia with failed remission
          Plasma cell leukemia NOS

       C90.11 Plasma cell leukemia in remission
       C90.12 Plasma cell leukemia in relapse

    C90.2 Extramedullary plasmacytoma

       C90.20 Extramedullary plasmacytoma not having achieved remission
          Extramedullary plasmacytoma with failed remission
          Extramedullary plasmacytoma NOS

       C90.21 Extramedullary plasmacytoma in remission
       C90.22 Extramedullary plasmacytoma in relapse

☑5ᵗʰ   **C90.3 Solitary plasmacytoma**
        Localized malignant plasma cell tumor NOS
        Plasmacytoma NOS
        Solitary myeloma

       C90.30 Solitary plasmacytoma not having achieved remission
          Solitary plasmacytoma with failed remission
          Solitary plasmacytoma NOS

       C90.31 Solitary plasmacytoma in remission
       C90.32 Solitary plasmacytoma in relapse

☑4ᵗʰ **C91 Lymphoid leukemia**

    EXCLUDES 1   *personal history of leukemia (Z85.6)*
    DEF: Malignant proliferation of immature lymphocytes (white blood cells that make up lymphoid tissue), called lymphoblasts, that originate in the bone marrow. Can be acute (ALL) or chronic (CLL).

☑5ᵗʰ   **C91.0 Acute lymphoblastic leukemia [ALL]**

       NOTE   ►Codes in subcategory C91.0- should only be used for T-cell and B-cell precursor leukemia◄

       C91.00 Acute lymphoblastic leukemia not having achieved remission
          Acute lymphoblastic leukemia with failed remission
          Acute lymphoblastic leukemia NOS

       C91.01 Acute lymphoblastic leukemia, in remission
       C91.02 Acute lymphoblastic leukemia, in relapse

☑6ᵗʰ   **C91.1 Chronic lymphocytic leukemia of B-cell type**
        Lymphoplasmacytic leukemia
        Richter syndrome
        EXCLUDES 1   *lymphoplasmacytic lymphoma (C83.0-)*

       C91.10 Chronic lymphocytic leukemia of B-cell type not having achieved remission
          Chronic lymphocytic leukemia of B-cell type with failed remission
          Chronic lymphocytic leukemia of B-cell type NOS

       C91.11 Chronic lymphocytic leukemia of B-cell type in remission

       C91.12 Chronic lymphocytic leukemia of B-cell type in relapse

☑5ᵗʰ   **C91.3 Prolymphocytic leukemia of B-cell type**

       C91.30 Prolymphocytic leukemia of B-cell type not having achieved remission
          Prolymphocytic leukemia of B-cell type with failed remission
          Prolymphocytic leukemia of B-cell type NOS

       C91.31 Prolymphocytic leukemia of B-cell type, in remission

       C91.32 Prolymphocytic leukemia of B-cell type, in relapse

☑5ᵗʰ   **C91.4 Hairy cell leukemia**
        Leukemic reticuloendotheliosis
        DEF: Rare type of leukemia that is slow growing and often also considered a type of lymphoma. The small B-cell lymphocytes appear with "hairy" projections under a microscope and are found mostly in the bone marrow, spleen, and blood.

       C91.40 Hairy cell leukemia not having achieved remission
          Hairy cell leukemia with failed remission
          Hairy cell leukemia NOS

       C91.41 Hairy cell leukemia, in remission
       C91.42 Hairy cell leukemia, in relapse

☑ Additional Character Required   ☑x7ᵗʰ Placeholder Alert   Manifestation   Unspecified Dx   ►◄ Revised Text   ● New Code   ▲ Revised Title

ICD-10-CM 2020   481

Chapter 2. Neoplasms

✓5ᵗʰ **C91.5** Adult T-cell lymphoma/leukemia (HTLV-1-associated)

Acute variant of adult T-cell lymphoma/leukemia (HTLV-1-associated)

Chronic variant of adult T-cell lymphoma/leukemia (HTLV-1-associated)

Lymphomatoid variant of adult T-cell lymphoma/leukemia (HTLV-1-associated)

Smouldering variant of adult T-cell lymphoma/leukemia (HTLV-1-associated)

C91.50 **Adult T-cell lymphoma/leukemia** [A] **(HTLV-1-associated)** not having achieved remission

Adult T-cell lymphoma/leukemia (HTLV-1-associated) with failed remission

Adult T-cell lymphoma/leukemia (HTLV-1-associated) NOS

C91.51 **Adult T-cell lymphoma/leukemia** [A] **(HTLV-1-associated),** in remission

C91.52 **Adult T-cell lymphoma/leukemia** [A] **(HTLV-1-associated),** in relapse

✓5ᵗʰ **C91.6** Prolymphocytic leukemia of T-cell type

C91.60 **Prolymphocytic leukemia of T-cell type** not having achieved remission

Prolymphocytic leukemia of T-cell type with failed remission

Prolymphocytic leukemia of T-cell type NOS

C91.61 **Prolymphocytic leukemia of T-cell type,** in remission

C91.62 **Prolymphocytic leukemia of T-cell type,** in relapse

✓5ᵗʰ **C91.A** Mature B-cell leukemia Burkitt-type

EXCLUDES 1   *Burkitt lymphoma (C83.7-)*

C91.A0 **Mature B-cell leukemia Burkitt-type** not having achieved remission

Mature B-cell leukemia Burkitt-type with failed remission

Mature B-cell leukemia Burkitt-type NOS

C91.A1 **Mature B-cell leukemia Burkitt-type,** in remission

C91.A2 **Mature B-cell leukemia Burkitt-type,** in relapse

✓5ᵗʰ **C91.Z** Other lymphoid leukemia

T-cell large granular lymphocytic leukemia (associated with rheumatoid arthritis)

C91.Z0 **Other lymphoid leukemia** not having achieved remission

Other lymphoid leukemia with failed remission

Other lymphoid leukemia NOS

C91.Z1 **Other lymphoid leukemia,** in remission

C91.Z2 **Other lymphoid leukemia,** in relapse

✓5ᵗʰ **C91.9** Lymphoid leukemia, unspecified

C91.90 **Lymphoid leukemia, unspecified** not having achieved remission

Lymphoid leukemia with failed remission

Lymphoid leukemia NOS

C91.91 **Lymphoid leukemia, unspecified,** in remission

C91.92 **Lymphoid leukemia, unspecified,** in relapse

✓4ᵗʰ **C92** Myeloid leukemia

INCLUDES   granulocytic leukemia
            myelogenous leukemia

EXCLUDES 1   *personal history of leukemia (Z85.6)*

AHA: 2019,1Q,16

DEF: Cancer that develops in immature myelocytes called myeloblasts. These are the cells that become white blood cells (except lymphocytes), red blood cells, or platelet making cells. Can be acute (AML) or chronic (CML).

TIP: Pancytopenia, although common in some types of myeloid leukemias, is not always inherent. When it is documented, code D61.818 can be assigned in addition to a code from this category.

✓5ᵗʰ **C92.0** Acute myeloblastic leukemia

Acute myeloblastic leukemia, minimal differentiation

Acute myeloblastic leukemia (with maturation)

Acute myeloblastic leukemia 1/ETO

Acute myeloblastic leukemia M0

Acute myeloblastic leukemia M1

Acute myeloblastic leukemia M2

Acute myeloblastic leukemia with t(8;21)

Acute myeloblastic leukemia (without a FAB classification) NOS

Refractory anemia with excess blasts in transformation [RAEBT]

EXCLUDES 1   *acute exacerbation of chronic myeloid leukemia (C92.10)*

refractory anemia with excess of blasts not in transformation (D46.2-)

AHA: 2018,4Q,87

C92.00 **Acute myeloblastic leukemia,** not having achieved remission

Acute myeloblastic leukemia with failed remission

Acute myeloblastic leukemia NOS

C92.01 **Acute myeloblastic leukemia,** in remission

C92.02 **Acute myeloblastic leukemia,** in relapse

✓5ᵗʰ **C92.1** Chronic myeloid leukemia, BCR/ABL-positive

Chronic myelogenous leukemia, Philadelphia chromosome (Ph1) positive

Chronic myelogenous leukemia, t(9;22) (q34;q11)

Chronic myelogenous leukemia with crisis of blast cells

EXCLUDES 1   *atypical chronic myeloid leukemia BCR/ABL-negative (C92.2-)*

chronic myelomonocytic leukemia (C93.1-)

chronic myeloproliferative disease (D47.1)

C92.10 **Chronic myeloid leukemia, BCR/ABL-positive,** not having achieved remission

Chronic myeloid leukemia, BCR/ABL-positive with failed remission

Chronic myeloid leukemia, BCR/ABL-positive NOS

C92.11 **Chronic myeloid leukemia, BCR/ABL-positive,** in remission

C92.12 **Chronic myeloid leukemia, BCR/ABL-positive,** in relapse

✓5ᵗʰ **C92.2** Atypical chronic myeloid leukemia, BCR/ABL-negative

C92.20 **Atypical chronic myeloid leukemia, BCR/ABL-negative,** not having achieved remission

Atypical chronic myeloid leukemia, BCR/ABL-negative with failed remission

Atypical chronic myeloid leukemia, BCR/ABL-negative NOS

C92.21 **Atypical chronic myeloid leukemia, BCR/ABL-negative,** in remission

C92.22 **Atypical chronic myeloid leukemia, BCR/ABL-negative,** in relapse

✓5ᵗʰ **C92.3** Myeloid sarcoma

A malignant tumor of immature myeloid cells

Chloroma

Granulocytic sarcoma

C92.30 **Myeloid sarcoma,** not having achieved remission

Myeloid sarcoma with failed remission

Myeloid sarcoma NOS

C92.31 **Myeloid sarcoma,** in remission

C92.32 **Myeloid sarcoma,** in relapse

N Newborn: 0   P Pediatric: 0-17   M Maternity: 12-55   A Adult: 15-124   CH Comorbidity High   CL Comorbidity Low   NCDx Noncancer Dx   PDx Primary Dx

482   ICD-10-CM 2020

√5ᵗʰ **C92.4** Acute promyelocytic **leukemia**

AML M3
AML Me with t(15;17) and variants

C92.40 **Acute promyelocytic leukemia,** not having achieved remission

Acute promyelocytic leukemia with failed remission
Acute promyelocytic leukemia NOS

C92.41 **Acute promyelocytic leukemia,** in remission
C92.42 **Acute promyelocytic leukemia,** in relapse

√5ᵗʰ **C92.5** Acute myelomonocytic **leukemia**

AML M4
AML M4 Eo with inv(16) or t(16;16)

C92.50 **Acute myelomonocytic leukemia,** not having achieved remission

Acute myelomonocytic leukemia with failed remission
Acute myelomonocytic leukemia NOS

C92.51 **Acute myelomonocytic leukemia,** in remission
C92.52 **Acute myelomonocytic leukemia,** in relapse

√5ᵗʰ **C92.6** Acute myeloid **leukemia with** 11q23-abnormality

Acute myeloid leukemia with variation of MLL-gene

C92.60 **Acute myeloid leukemia with 11q23-abnormality** not having achieved remission

Acute myeloid leukemia with 11q23-abnormality with failed remission
Acute myeloid leukemia with 11q23-abnormality NOS

C92.61 **Acute myeloid leukemia with 11q23-abnormality** in remission
C92.62 **Acute myeloid leukemia with 11q23-abnormality** in relapse

√5ᵗʰ **C92.A** Acute myeloid **leukemia with** multilineage dysplasia

Acute myeloid leukemia with dysplasia of remaining hematopoesis and/or myelodysplastic disease in its history

C92.A0 **Acute myeloid leukemia with multilineage dysplasia,** not having achieved remission

Acute myeloid leukemia with multilineage dysplasia with failed remission
Acute myeloid leukemia with multilineage dysplasia NOS

C92.A1 **Acute myeloid leukemia with multilineage dysplasia,** in remission
C92.A2 **Acute myeloid leukemia with multilineage dysplasia,** in relapse

√5ᵗʰ **C92.Z** Other myeloid leukemia

C92.Z0 **Other myeloid leukemia** not having achieved remission

Myeloid leukemia NEC with failed remission
Myeloid leukemia NEC

C92.Z1 **Other myeloid leukemia,** in remission
C92.Z2 **Other myeloid leukemia,** in relapse

√5ᵗʰ **C92.9** Myeloid leukemia, unspecified

C92.90 **Myeloid leukemia, unspecified,** not having achieved remission

Myeloid leukemia, unspecified with failed remission
Myeloid leukemia, unspecified NOS

C92.91 **Myeloid leukemia, unspecified** in remission
C92.92 **Myeloid leukemia, unspecified** in relapse

√4ᵗʰ **C93** Monocytic leukemia

INCLUDES   monocytoid leukemia
EXCLUDES 1   personal history of leukemia (Z85.6)

√5ᵗʰ **C93.0** Acute monoblastic/monocytic **leukemia**

AML M5
AML M5a
AML M5b

C93.00 **Acute monoblastic/monocytic leukemia,** not having achieved remission

Acute monoblastic/monocytic leukemia with failed remission
Acute monoblastic/monocytic leukemia NOS

C93.01 **Acute monoblastic/monocytic leukemia,** in remission
C93.02 **Acute monoblastic/monocytic leukemia,** in relapse

√5ᵗʰ **C93.1** Chronic **myelomonocytic leukemia**

Chronic monocytic leukemia
CMML-1
CMML-2
CMML with eosinophilia

C93.10 **Chronic myelomonocytic leukemia** not having achieved remission

Chronic myelomonocytic leukemia with failed remission
Chronic myelomonocytic leukemia NOS

C93.11 **Chronic myelomonocytic leukemia,** in remission
C93.12 **Chronic myelomonocytic leukemia,** in relapse

√5ᵗʰ **C93.3** Juvenile **myelomonocytic leukemia**

C93.30 **Juvenile myelomonocytic leukemia,** not having achieved remission   P

Juvenile myelomonocytic leukemia with failed remission
Juvenile myelomonocytic leukemia NOS

C93.31 **Juvenile myelomonocytic leukemia,** in remission   P

C93.32 **Juvenile myelomonocytic leukemia,** in relapse   P

√5ᵗʰ **C93.Z** Other monocytic leukemia

C93.Z0 **Other monocytic leukemia,** not having achieved remission

Other monocytic leukemia NOS

C93.Z1 **Other monocytic leukemia,** in remission
C93.Z2 **Other monocytic leukemia,** in relapse

√5ᵗʰ **C93.9** Monocytic leukemia, unspecified

C93.90 **Monocytic leukemia, unspecified,** not having achieved remission

Monocytic leukemia, unspecified with failed remission
Monocytic leukemia, unspecified NOS

C93.91 **Monocytic leukemia, unspecified** in remission
C93.92 **Monocytic leukemia, unspecified** in relapse

√4ᵗʰ **C94** Other leukemias of specified cell type

EXCLUDES 1   leukemic reticuloendotheliosis (C91.4-)
      myelodysplastic syndromes (D46.-)
      personal history of leukemia (Z85.6)
      plasma cell leukemia (C90.1-)

√5ᵗʰ **C94.0** Acute erythroid leukemia

Acute myeloid leukemia M6(a)(b)
Erythroleukemia
DEF: Erythroleukemia: Malignant blood dyscrasia (a myeloproliferative disorder).

C94.00 **Acute erythroid leukemia,** not having achieved remission

Acute erythroid leukemia with failed remission
Acute erythroid leukemia NOS

C94.01 **Acute erythroid leukemia,** in remission
C94.02 **Acute erythroid leukemia,** in relapse

√5ᵗʰ **C94.2** Acute megakaryoblastic leukemia

Acute myeloid leukemia M7
Acute megakaryocytic leukemia

C94.20 **Acute megakaryoblastic leukemia** not having achieved remission

Acute megakaryoblastic leukemia with failed remission
Acute megakaryoblastic leukemia NOS

C94.21 **Acute megakaryoblastic leukemia,** in remission
C94.22 **Acute megakaryoblastic leukemia,** in relapse

√5ᵗʰ **C94.3** Mast cell leukemia

AHA: 2017,4Q,5

C94.30 **Mast cell leukemia** not having achieved remission

Mast cell leukemia with failed remission
Mast cell leukemia NOS

C94.31 **Mast cell leukemia,** in remission
C94.32 **Mast cell leukemia,** in relapse

✓5ᵗʰ **C94.4** **Acute panmyelosis with myelofibrosis**
Acute myelofibrosis
   EXCLUDES 1   *myelofibrosis NOS (D75.81)*
               secondary myelofibrosis NOS (D75.81)

    C94.40 **Acute panmyelosis with myelofibrosis** not having achieved remission
Acute myelofibrosis NOS
Acute panmyelosis with myelofibrosis with failed remission
Acute panmyelosis NOS

    C94.41 **Acute panmyelosis with myelofibrosis,** in remission
    C94.42 **Acute panmyelosis with myelofibrosis,** in relapse

C94.6 **Myelodysplastic disease, not classified**
Myeloproliferative disease, not classified

✓5ᵗʰ **C94.8** **Other specified leukemias**
Aggressive NK-cell leukemia
Acute basophilic leukemia

    C94.80 **Other specified leukemias** not having achieved remission
Other specified leukemia with failed remission
Other specified leukemias NOS

    C94.81 **Other specified leukemias,** in remission
    C94.82 **Other specified leukemias,** in relapse

✓4ᵗʰ **C95** **Leukemia of unspecified** cell type
   EXCLUDES 1   *personal history of leukemia (Z85.6)*

✓5ᵗʰ **C95.0** **Acute** leukemia of unspecified cell type
Acute bilineal leukemia
Acute mixed lineage leukemia
Biphenotypic acute leukemia
Stem cell leukemia of unclear lineage
   EXCLUDES 1   *acute exacerbation of unspecified chronic leukemia (C95.10)*

    C95.00 **Acute leukemia of unspecified cell type** not having achieved remission
Acute leukemia of unspecified cell type with failed remission
Acute leukemia NOS

    C95.01 **Acute leukemia of unspecified cell type,** in remission

    C95.02 **Acute leukemia of unspecified cell type,** in relapse

✓5ᵗʰ **C95.1** **Chronic** leukemia of unspecified cell type

    C95.10 **Chronic leukemia of unspecified cell type** not having achieved remission
Chronic leukemia of unspecified cell type with failed remission
Chronic leukemia NOS

    C95.11 **Chronic leukemia of unspecified cell type,** in remission

    C95.12 **Chronic leukemia of unspecified cell type,** in relapse

✓5ᵗʰ **C95.9** **Leukemia, unspecified**

    C95.90 **Leukemia, unspecified** not having achieved remission
Leukemia, unspecified with failed remission
Leukemia NOS

    C95.91 **Leukemia, unspecified,** in remission
    C95.92 **Leukemia, unspecified,** in relapse

✓4ᵗʰ **C96** **Other and unspecified malignant neoplasms of lymphoid, hematopoietic and related tissue**
   EXCLUDES 1   *personal history of other malignant neoplasms of lymphoid, hematopoietic and related tissues (Z85.79)*

C96.0 **Multifocal and multisystemic (disseminated) Langerhans-cell histiocytosis**
Histiocytosis X, multisystemic
Letterer-Siwe disease
   EXCLUDES 1   *adult pulmonary Langerhans cell histiocytosis (J84.82)*
               multifocal and unisystemic Langerhans-cell histiocytosis (C96.5)
               unifocal Langerhans-cell histiocytosis (C96.6)

✓5ᵗʰ **C96.2** **Malignant mast cell neoplasm**
   EXCLUDES 1   *indolent mastocytosis (D47.02)*
               mast cell leukemia (C94.30)
               mastocytosis (congenital) (cutaneous) (Q82.2)

AHA: 2017,4Q,5
DEF: Mast cell: Type of white blood cell found in the loose connective tissue of blood vessels and bronchioles responsible for acute hypersensitivity reactions, including anaphylactic shock. The IgE receptors on these cells bind with allergens causing cell degranulation and diffuse, widespread histamine release that results in airway constriction and vasodilation with decreased systemic blood pressure.

    C96.20 **Malignant mast cell neoplasm, unspecified**
    C96.21 **Aggressive systemic mastocytosis**
    C96.22 **Mast cell sarcoma**
    C96.29 **Other malignant mast cell neoplasm**

C96.4 **Sarcoma of dendritic cells (accessory cells)**
Follicular dendritic cell sarcoma
Interdigitating dendritic cell sarcoma
Langerhans cell sarcoma

C96.5 **Multifocal and unisystemic Langerhans-cell histiocytosis**
Hand-Schüller-Christian disease
Histiocytosis X, multifocal
   EXCLUDES 1   *multifocal and multisystemic (disseminated) Langerhans-cell histiocytosis (C96.0)*
               unifocal Langerhans-cell histiocytosis (C96.6)

C96.6 **Unifocal Langerhans-cell histiocytosis**
Eosinophilic granuloma
Histiocytosis X, unifocal
Histiocytosis X NOS
Langerhans-cell histiocytosis NOS
   EXCLUDES 1   *multifocal and multisysemic (disseminated) Langerhans-cell histiocytosis (C96.0)*
               multifocal and unisystemic Langerhans-cell histiocytosis (C96.5)

C96.A **Histiocytic sarcoma**
Malignant histiocytosis

C96.Z **Other specified malignant neoplasms of lymphoid, hematopoietic and related tissue**

C96.9 **Malignant neoplasm of lymphoid, hematopoietic and related tissue, unspecified**

In situ neoplasms (D00-D09)

INCLUDES   Bowen's disease
            erythroplasia
            grade III intraepithelial neoplasia
            Queyrat's erythroplasia

✓4ᵗʰ **D00** **Carcinoma in situ of** oral cavity, esophagus and stomach
   EXCLUDES 1   *melanoma in situ (D03.-)*

✓5ᵗʰ **D00.0** **Carcinoma in situ of** lip, oral cavity and pharynx
Use additional code to identify:
exposure to environmental tobacco smoke (Z77.22)
exposure to tobacco smoke in the perinatal period (P96.81)
history of tobacco dependence (Z87.891)
occupational exposure to environmental tobacco smoke (Z57.31)
tobacco dependence (F17.-)
tobacco use (Z72.0)
   EXCLUDES 1   *carcinoma in situ of aryepiglottic fold or interarytenoid fold, laryngeal aspect (D02.0)*
               carcinoma in situ of epiglottis NOS (D02.0)
               carcinoma in situ of epiglottis suprahyoid portion (D02.0)
               carcinoma in situ of skin of lip (D03.0, D04.0)

    D00.00 **Carcinoma in situ of oral cavity, unspecified site**
    D00.01 **Carcinoma in situ of** labial mucosa and vermilion border
    D00.02 **Carcinoma in situ of** buccal mucosa
    D00.03 **Carcinoma in situ of** gingiva and edentulous alveolar ridge
    D00.04 **Carcinoma in situ of** soft palate
    D00.05 **Carcinoma in situ of** hard palate
    D00.06 **Carcinoma in situ of** floor of mouth
    D00.07 **Carcinoma in situ of** tongue

D00.08   **Carcinoma in situ of** pharynx
Carcinoma in situ of aryepiglottic fold NOS
Carcinoma in situ of hypopharyngeal aspect of aryepiglottic fold
Carcinoma in situ of marginal zone of aryepiglottic fold

D00.1   **Carcinoma in situ of** esophagus

D00.2   **Carcinoma in situ of** stomach

√4ᵗʰ **D01**   **Carcinoma in situ of other and unspecified** digestive organs
    EXCLUDES 1   melanoma in situ (D03.-)

D01.0   **Carcinoma in situ of** colon
    EXCLUDES 1   carcinoma in situ of rectosigmoid junction (D01.1)

D01.1   **Carcinoma in situ of** rectosigmoid junction

D01.2   **Carcinoma in situ of** rectum

D01.3   **Carcinoma in situ of** anus and anal canal
Anal intraepithelial neoplasia III [AIN III]
Severe dysplasia of anus
    EXCLUDES 1   anal intraepithelial neoplasia I and II [AIN I and AIN II] (K62.82)
           carcinoma in situ of anal margin (D04.5)
           carcinoma in situ of anal skin (D04.5)
           carcinoma in situ of perianal skin (D04.5)

√5ᵗʰ **D01.4**   **Carcinoma in situ of other and unspecified parts of** intestine
    EXCLUDES 1   carcinoma in situ of ampulla of Vater (D01.5)

    D01.40   **Carcinoma in situ of unspecified part of intestine**
    D01.49   **Carcinoma in situ of other parts of intestine**

D01.5   **Carcinoma in situ of** liver, gallbladder and bile ducts
Carcinoma in situ of ampulla of Vater

D01.7   **Carcinoma in situ of other specified digestive organs**
Carcinoma in situ of pancreas

D01.9   **Carcinoma in situ of digestive organ, unspecified**

√4ᵗʰ **D02**   **Carcinoma in situ of** middle ear and respiratory system
Use additional code to identify:
exposure to environmental tobacco smoke (Z77.22)
exposure to tobacco smoke in the perinatal period (P96.81)
history of tobacco dependence (Z87.891)
occupational exposure to environmental tobacco smoke (Z57.31)
tobacco dependence (F17.-)
tobacco use (Z72.0)
    EXCLUDES 1   melanoma in situ (D03.-)

D02.0   **Carcinoma in situ of** larynx
Carcinoma in situ of aryepiglottic fold or interarytenoid fold, laryngeal aspect
Carcinoma in situ of epiglottis (suprahyoid portion)
    EXCLUDES 1   carcinoma in situ of aryepiglottic fold or interarytenoid fold NOS (D00.08)
           carcinoma in situ of hypopharyngeal aspect (D00.08)
           carcinoma in situ of marginal zone (D00.08)

D02.1   **Carcinoma in situ of** trachea

√5ᵗʰ **D02.2**   **Carcinoma in situ of** bronchus and lung

    D02.20   **Carcinoma in situ of unspecified bronchus and lung**
    D02.21   **Carcinoma in situ of** right **bronchus and lung**
    D02.22   **Carcinoma in situ of** left **bronchus and lung**

D02.3   **Carcinoma in situ of other parts of respiratory system**
Carcinoma in situ of accessory sinuses
Carcinoma in situ of middle ear
Carcinoma in situ of nasal cavities
    EXCLUDES 1   carcinoma in situ of ear (external) (skin) (D04.2-)
           carcinoma in situ of nose NOS (D09.8)
           carcinoma in situ of skin of nose (D04.3)

D02.4   **Carcinoma in situ of respiratory system, unspecified**

√4ᵗʰ **D03**   Melanoma **in situ**

D03.0   **Melanoma in situ of** lip

√5ᵗʰ **D03.1**   **Melanoma in situ of** eyelid, including canthus
    AHA: 2018,4Q,4

    D03.10   **Melanoma in situ of unspecified eyelid, including canthus**

√6ᵗʰ   **D03.11**   **Melanoma in situ of** right **eyelid, including canthus**
       D03.111   **Melanoma in situ of right** upper **eyelid, including canthus**
       D03.112   **Melanoma in situ of right** lower **eyelid, including canthus**

√6ᵗʰ   **D03.12**   **Melanoma in situ of** left **eyelid, including canthus**
       D03.121   **Melanoma in situ of left** upper **eyelid, including canthus**

D03.122   **Melanoma in situ of left** lower **eyelid, including canthus**

√5ᵗʰ **D03.2**   **Melanoma in situ of** ear and external auricular canal

    D03.20   **Melanoma in situ of unspecified ear and external auricular canal**
    D03.21   **Melanoma in situ of** right **ear and external auricular canal**
    D03.22   **Melanoma in situ of** left **ear and external auricular canal**

√5ᵗʰ **D03.3**   **Melanoma in situ of other and unspecified parts of** face

    D03.30   **Melanoma in situ of unspecified part of face**
    D03.39   **Melanoma in situ of other parts of face**

D03.4   **Melanoma in situ of** scalp and neck

√5ᵗʰ **D03.5**   **Melanoma in situ of** trunk

    D03.51   **Melanoma in situ of** anal skin
Melanoma in situ of anal margin
Melanoma in situ of perianal skin
    D03.52   **Melanoma in situ of** breast (skin) (soft tissue)
    D03.59   **Melanoma in situ of other part of trunk**

√5ᵗʰ **D03.6**   **Melanoma in situ of** upper limb, including shoulder

    D03.60   **Melanoma in situ of unspecified upper limb, including shoulder**
    D03.61   **Melanoma in situ of** right **upper limb, including shoulder**
    D03.62   **Melanoma in situ of** left **upper limb, including shoulder**

√5ᵗʰ **D03.7**   **Melanoma in situ of** lower limb, including hip

    D03.70   **Melanoma in situ of unspecified lower limb, including hip**
    D03.71   **Melanoma in situ of** right **lower limb, including hip**
    D03.72   **Melanoma in situ of** left **lower limb, including hip**

D03.8   **Melanoma in situ of other sites**
Melanoma in situ of scrotum
    EXCLUDES 1   carcinoma in situ of scrotum (D07.61)

D03.9   **Melanoma in situ, unspecified**

√4ᵗʰ **D04**   **Carcinoma in situ of** skin
    EXCLUDES 1   erythroplasia of Queyrat (penis) NOS (D07.4)
           melanoma in situ (D03.-)

D04.0   **Carcinoma in situ of skin of** lip
    EXCLUDES 1   carcinoma in situ of vermilion border of lip (D00.01)
    EXCLUDES 2   ▶carcinoma in situ of vermilion border of lip (D00.01)◀

√5ᵗʰ **D04.1**   **Carcinoma in situ of skin of** eyelid, including canthus
    AHA: 2018,4Q,4

    D04.10   **Carcinoma in situ of skin of unspecified eyelid, including canthus**

√6ᵗʰ   **D04.11**   **Carcinoma in situ of skin of** right **eyelid, including canthus**
       D04.111   **Carcinoma in situ of skin of right** upper **eyelid, including canthus**
       D04.112   **Carcinoma in situ of skin of right** lower **eyelid, including canthus**

√6ᵗʰ   **D04.12**   **Carcinoma in situ of skin of** left **eyelid, including canthus**
       D04.121   **Carcinoma in situ of skin of left** upper **eyelid, including canthus**
       D04.122   **Carcinoma in situ of skin of left** lower **eyelid, including canthus**

√5ᵗʰ **D04.2**   **Carcinoma in situ of skin of** ear and external auricular canal

    D04.20   **Carcinoma in situ of skin of unspecified ear and external auricular canal**
    D04.21   **Carcinoma in situ of skin of** right **ear and external auricular canal**
    D04.22   **Carcinoma in situ of skin of** left **ear and external auricular canal**

√5ᵗʰ **D04.3**   **Carcinoma in situ of skin of other and unspecified** parts of face

    D04.30   **Carcinoma in situ of skin of unspecified part of face**
    D04.39   **Carcinoma in situ of skin of other parts of face**

D04.4   **Carcinoma in situ of skin of** scalp and neck

D04.5 **Carcinoma in situ of skin of** trunk
Carcinoma in situ of anal margin
Carcinoma in situ of anal skin
Carcinoma in situ of perianal skin
Carcinoma in situ of skin of breast
EXCLUDES 1 *carcinoma in situ of anus NOS (D01.3)*
carcinoma in situ of scrotum (D07.61)
carcinoma in situ of skin of genital organs (D07.-)

✓5ᵗʰ D04.6 **Carcinoma in situ of skin of** upper limb, including shoulder
D04.60 **Carcinoma in situ of skin of unspecified upper limb, including shoulder**
D04.61 **Carcinoma in situ of skin of** right **upper limb, including shoulder**
D04.62 **Carcinoma in situ of skin of** left **upper limb, including shoulder**

✓5ᵗʰ D04.7 **Carcinoma in situ of skin of** lower limb, including hip
D04.70 **Carcinoma in situ of skin of unspecified lower limb, including hip**
D04.71 **Carcinoma in situ of skin of** right **lower limb, including hip**
D04.72 **Carcinoma in situ of skin of** left **lower limb, including hip**

D04.8 **Carcinoma in situ of skin of other sites**
D04.9 **Carcinoma in situ of skin, unspecified**

✓4ᵗʰ **D05 Carcinoma in situ of** breast
EXCLUDES 1 *carcinoma in situ of skin of breast (D04.5)*
melanoma in situ of breast (skin) (D03.5)
Paget's disease of breast or nipple (C50.-)

✓5ᵗʰ D05.0 Lobular **carcinoma in situ of breast**
D05.00 **Lobular carcinoma in situ of unspecified breast**
D05.01 **Lobular carcinoma in situ of** right **breast**
D05.02 **Lobular carcinoma in situ of** left **breast**

✓5ᵗʰ D05.1 Intraductal **carcinoma in situ of breast**
D05.10 **Intraductal carcinoma in situ of unspecified breast**
D05.11 **Intraductal carcinoma in situ of** right **breast**
D05.12 **Intraductal carcinoma in situ of** left **breast**

✓5ᵗʰ D05.8 **Other specified type of carcinoma in situ of breast**
D05.80 **Other specified type of carcinoma in situ of unspecified breast**
D05.81 **Other specified type of carcinoma in situ of** right **breast**
D05.82 **Other specified type of carcinoma in situ of** left **breast**

✓5ᵗʰ D05.9 **Unspecified type of carcinoma in situ of breast**
D05.90 **Unspecified type of carcinoma in situ of unspecified breast**
D05.91 **Unspecified type of carcinoma in situ of** right **breast**
D05.92 **Unspecified type of carcinoma in situ of** left **breast**

✓4ᵗʰ **D06 Carcinoma in situ of** cervix uteri
INCLUDES cervical adenocarcinoma in situ
cervical intraepithelial glandular neoplasia
cervical intraepithelial neoplasia III [CIN III]
severe dysplasia of cervix uteri
EXCLUDES 1 *cervical intraepithelial neoplasia II [CIN II] (N87.1)*
cytologic evidence of malignancy of cervix without histologic confirmation (R87.614)
high grade squamous intraepithelial lesion (HGSIL) of cervix (R87.613)
melanoma in situ of cervix (D03.5)
moderate cervical dysplasia (N87.1)

D06.0 **Carcinoma in situ of** endocervix ♀
D06.1 **Carcinoma in situ of** exocervix ♀
D06.7 **Carcinoma in situ of other** parts of cervix ♀
D06.9 **Carcinoma in situ of cervix, unspecified** ♀

✓4ᵗʰ **D07 Carcinoma in situ of other and unspecified** genital organs
EXCLUDES 1 *melanoma in situ of trunk (D03.5)*
D07.0 **Carcinoma in situ of** endometrium ♀
D07.1 **Carcinoma in situ of** vulva ♀
Severe dysplasia of vulva
Vulvar intraepithelial neoplasia III [VIN III]
EXCLUDES 1 *moderate dysplasia of vulva (N90.1)*
vulvar intraepithelial neoplasia II [VIN II] (N90.1)

D07.2 **Carcinoma in situ of** vagina ♀
Severe dysplasia of vagina
Vaginal intraepithelial neoplasia III [VAIN III]
EXCLUDES 1 *moderate dysplasia of vagina (N89.1)*
vaginal intraepithelial neoplasia II [VIN II] (N89.1)

✓5ᵗʰ D07.3 **Carcinoma in situ of other and unspecified** female genital organs
D07.30 **Carcinoma in situ of unspecified female genital organs** ♀
D07.39 **Carcinoma in situ of other female genital organs** ♀

D07.4 **Carcinoma in situ of** penis ♂
Erythroplasia of Queyrat NOS
D07.5 **Carcinoma in situ of** prostate ♂
Prostatic intraepithelial neoplasia III (PIN III)
Severe dysplasia of prostate
EXCLUDES 1 *dysplasia (mild) (moderate) of prostate (N42.3-)*
prostatic intraepithelial neoplasia II [PIN II] (N42.3-)

✓5ᵗʰ D07.6 **Carcinoma in situ of other and unspecified** male genital organs
D07.60 **Carcinoma in situ of unspecified male genital organs** ♂
D07.61 **Carcinoma in situ of** scrotum ♂
D07.69 **Carcinoma in situ of other male genital organs** ♂

✓4ᵗʰ **D09 Carcinoma in situ of other and unspecified** sites
EXCLUDES 1 *melanoma in situ (D03.-)*
D09.0 **Carcinoma in situ of** bladder
✓5ᵗʰ D09.1 **Carcinoma in situ of other and unspecified** urinary organs
D09.10 **Carcinoma in situ of unspecified urinary organ**
D09.19 **Carcinoma in situ of other urinary organs**
✓5ᵗʰ D09.2 **Carcinoma in situ of** eye
EXCLUDES 1 *carcinoma in situ of skin of eyelid (D04.1-)*
D09.20 **Carcinoma in situ of unspecified eye**
D09.21 **Carcinoma in situ of** right **eye**
D09.22 **Carcinoma in situ of** left **eye**
D09.3 **Carcinoma in situ of** thyroid **and other** endocrine glands
EXCLUDES 1 *carcinoma in situ of endocrine pancreas (D01.7)*
carcinoma in situ of ovary (D07.39)
carcinoma in situ of testis (D07.69)
D09.8 **Carcinoma in situ of other specified sites**
D09.9 **Carcinoma in situ, unspecified**

Benign neoplasms, except benign neuroendocrine tumors (D10-D36)

✓4ᵗʰ **D10 Benign neoplasm of** mouth and pharynx
D10.0 **Benign neoplasm of** lip
Benign neoplasm of lip (frenulum) (inner aspect) (mucosa) (vermilion border)
EXCLUDES 1 *benign neoplasm of skin of lip (D22.0, D23.0)*
D10.1 **Benign neoplasm of** tongue
Benign neoplasm of lingual tonsil
D10.2 **Benign neoplasm of** floor **of mouth**
✓5ᵗʰ D10.3 **Benign neoplasm of other and unspecified parts of mouth**
D10.30 **Benign neoplasm of unspecified part of mouth**
D10.39 **Benign neoplasm of other parts of mouth**
Benign neoplasm of minor salivary gland NOS
EXCLUDES 1 *benign odontogenic neoplasms (D16.4-D16.5)*
benign neoplasm of mucosa of lip (D10.0)
benign neoplasm of nasopharyngeal surface of soft palate (D10.6)
D10.4 **Benign neoplasm of** tonsil
Benign neoplasm of tonsil (faucial) (palatine)
EXCLUDES 1 *benign neoplasm of lingual tonsil (D10.1)*
benign neoplasm of pharyngeal tonsil (D10.6)
benign neoplasm of tonsillar fossa (D10.5)
benign neoplasm of tonsillar pillars (D10.5)

D10.5   **Benign neoplasm of other parts of** oropharynx
     Benign neoplasm of epiglottis, anterior aspect
     Benign neoplasm of tonsillar fossa
     Benign neoplasm of tonsillar pillars
     Benign neoplasm of vallecula
     EXCLUDES 1   *benign neoplasm of epiglottis NOS (D14.1)*
                 benign neoplasm of epiglottis, suprahyoid portion (D14.1)
     DEF: Oropharynx: Middle portion of pharynx (throat); communicates with the oral cavity, nasopharynx and laryngopharynx.

D10.6   **Benign neoplasm of** nasopharynx
     Benign neoplasm of pharyngeal tonsil
     Benign neoplasm of posterior margin of septum and choanae
     DEF: Nasopharynx: Upper portion of pharynx (throat); communicates with the nasal cavities, oropharynx and tympanic cavities.

D10.7   **Benign neoplasm of** hypopharynx
     DEF: Hypopharynx: Lower portion of pharynx (throat); communicates with the oropharynx and the esophagus.
     Synonyms: laryngopharynx.

D10.9   **Benign neoplasm of pharynx, unspecified**

✓4ᵗʰ D11   **Benign neoplasm of** major salivary glands
     EXCLUDES 1   *benign neoplasms of specified minor salivary glands which are classified according to their anatomical location*
                 benign neoplasms of minor salivary glands NOS (D10.39)

D11.0   **Benign neoplasm of** parotid gland
D11.7   **Benign neoplasm of other major salivary glands**
     Benign neoplasm of sublingual salivary gland
     Benign neoplasm of submandibular salivary gland
D11.9   **Benign neoplasm of major salivary gland, unspecified**

✓4ᵗʰ D12   **Benign neoplasm of** colon, rectum, anus and anal canal
     EXCLUDES 1   *benign carcinoid tumors of the large intestine, and rectum (D3A.02-)*
           ▶*polyp of colon NOS (K63.5)*◀
     AHA: 2018,2Q,14; 2017,1Q,15; 2015,2Q,14

D12.0   **Benign neoplasm of** cecum
     Benign neoplasm of ileocecal valve
D12.1   **Benign neoplasm of** appendix
     EXCLUDES 1   *benign carcinoid tumor of the appendix (D3A.020)*
D12.2   **Benign neoplasm of** ascending colon
D12.3   **Benign neoplasm of** transverse colon
     Benign neoplasm of hepatic flexure
     Benign neoplasm of splenic flexure
     AHA: 2017,1Q,16
D12.4   **Benign neoplasm of** descending colon
D12.5   **Benign neoplasm of** sigmoid colon
D12.6   **Benign neoplasm of colon, unspecified**
     Adenomatosis of colon
     Benign neoplasm of large intestine NOS
     Polyposis (hereditary) of colon
     EXCLUDES 1   *inflammatory polyp of colon (K51.4-)*
                 ~~*polyp of colon NOS (K63.5)*~~
D12.7   **Benign neoplasm of** rectosigmoid junction
D12.8   **Benign neoplasm of** rectum
     EXCLUDES 1   *benign carcinoid tumor of the rectum (D3A.026)*
     AHA: 2018,1Q,6
D12.9   **Benign neoplasm of** anus and anal canal
     Benign neoplasm of anus NOS
     EXCLUDES 1   *benign neoplasm of anal margin (D22.5, D23.5)*
                 benign neoplasm of anal skin (D22.5, D23.5)
                 benign neoplasm of perianal skin (D22.5, D23.5)

✓4ᵗʰ D13   **Benign neoplasm of other and ill-defined parts of** digestive system
     EXCLUDES 1   *benign stromal tumors of digestive system (D21.4)*

D13.0   **Benign neoplasm of** esophagus
D13.1   **Benign neoplasm of** stomach
     EXCLUDES 1   *benign carcinoid tumor of the stomach (D3A.092)*
D13.2   **Benign neoplasm of** duodenum
     EXCLUDES 1   *benign carcinoid tumor of the duodenum (D3A.010)*
✓5ᵗʰ D13.3   **Benign neoplasm of other and unspecified parts of** small intestine
     EXCLUDES 1   *benign carcinoid tumors of the small intestine (D3A.01-)*
                 benign neoplasm of ileocecal valve (D12.0)
     D13.30   **Benign neoplasm of unspecified part of small intestine**

D13.39   **Benign neoplasm of other parts of small intestine**
D13.4   **Benign neoplasm of** liver
     Benign neoplasm of intrahepatic bile ducts
D13.5   **Benign neoplasm of** extrahepatic bile ducts
D13.6   **Benign neoplasm of** pancreas
     EXCLUDES 1   *benign neoplasm of endocrine pancreas (D13.7)*
D13.7   **Benign neoplasm of** endocrine pancreas
     Benign neoplasm of islets of Langerhans
     Islet cell tumor
     Use additional code to identify any functional activity
D13.9   **Benign neoplasm of** ill-defined sites **within the digestive system**
     Benign neoplasm of digestive system NOS
     Benign neoplasm of intestine NOS
     Benign neoplasm of spleen

✓4ᵗʰ D14   **Benign neoplasm of** middle ear and respiratory system
D14.0   **Benign neoplasm of** middle ear, nasal cavity and accessory sinuses
     Benign neoplasm of cartilage of nose
     EXCLUDES 1   *benign neoplasm of auricular canal (external) (D22.2-, D23.2-)*
                 benign neoplasm of bone of ear (D16.4)
                 benign neoplasm of bone of nose (D16.4)
                 benign neoplasm of cartilage of ear (D21.0)
                 benign neoplasm of ear (external)(skin) (D22.2-, D23.2-)
                 benign neoplasm of nose NOS (D36.7)
                 benign neoplasm of skin of nose (D22.39, D23.39)
                 benign neoplasm of olfactory bulb (D33.3)
                 benign neoplasm of posterior margin of septum and choanae (D10.6)
                 polyp of accessory sinus (J33.8)
                 polyp of ear (middle) (H74.4)
                 polyp of nasal (cavity) (J33.-)
D14.1   **Benign neoplasm of** larynx
     Adenomatous polyp of larynx
     Benign neoplasm of epiglottis (suprahyoid portion)
     EXCLUDES 1   *benign neoplasm of epiglottis, anterior aspect (D10.5)*
                 polyp (nonadenomatous) of vocal cord or larynx (J38.1)
D14.2   **Benign neoplasm of** trachea
✓5ᵗʰ D14.3   **Benign neoplasm of** bronchus and lung
     EXCLUDES 1   *benign carcinoid tumor of the bronchus and lung (D3A.090)*
     D14.30   **Benign neoplasm of unspecified bronchus and lung**
     D14.31   **Benign neoplasm of** right **bronchus and lung**
     D14.32   **Benign neoplasm of** left **bronchus and lung**
D14.4   **Benign neoplasm of respiratory system, unspecified**

✓4ᵗʰ D15   **Benign neoplasm of other and unspecified** intrathoracic organs
     EXCLUDES 1   *benign neoplasm of mesothelial tissue (D19.-)*
D15.0   **Benign neoplasm of** thymus
     EXCLUDES 1   *benign carcinoid tumor of the thymus (D3A.091)*
D15.1   **Benign neoplasm of** heart
     EXCLUDES 1   *benign neoplasm of great vessels (D21.3)*
D15.2   **Benign neoplasm of** mediastinum
D15.7   **Benign neoplasm of other specified intrathoracic organs**
D15.9   **Benign neoplasm of intrathoracic organ, unspecified**

✓4ᵗʰ D16   **Benign neoplasm of** bone and articular cartilage
     EXCLUDES 1   *benign neoplasm of connective tissue of ear (D21.0)*
                 benign neoplasm of connective tissue of eyelid (D21.0)
                 benign neoplasm of connective tissue of larynx (D14.1)
                 benign neoplasm of connective tissue of nose (D14.0)
                 benign neoplasm of synovia (D21.-)
✓5ᵗʰ D16.0   **Benign neoplasm of** scapula and long bones of upper limb
     D16.00   **Benign neoplasm of scapula and long bones of unspecified upper limb**
     D16.01   **Benign neoplasm of scapula and long bones of** right **upper limb**
     D16.02   **Benign neoplasm of scapula and long bones of** left **upper limb**
✓5ᵗʰ D16.1   **Benign neoplasm of** short bones of upper limb
     D16.10   **Benign neoplasm of short bones of unspecified upper limb**
     D16.11   **Benign neoplasm of short bones of** right **upper limb**
     D16.12   **Benign neoplasm of short bones of** left **upper limb**

☑ Additional Character Required   ✓x7ᵗʰ Placeholder Alert   Manifestation   Unspecified Dx   ▶◀ Revised Text   ● New Code   ▲ Revised Title

ICD-10-CM 2020   **487**

Chapter 2. Neoplasms *(side tab)*

D16.2–D21.4 *(side tab)*

✓5ᵗʰ **D16.2** **Benign neoplasm of** long bones of lower limb

     D16.20 **Benign neoplasm of long bones of unspecified lower limb**

     D16.21 **Benign neoplasm of long bones of** right **lower limb**

     D16.22 **Benign neoplasm of long bones of** left **lower limb**

✓5ᵗʰ **D16.3** **Benign neoplasm of** short bones of lower limb

     D16.30 **Benign neoplasm of short bones of unspecified lower limb**

     D16.31 **Benign neoplasm of short bones of** right **lower limb**

     D16.32 **Benign neoplasm of short bones of** left **lower limb**

   D16.4 **Benign neoplasm of bones of** skull and face

     Benign neoplasm of maxilla (superior)

     Benign neoplasm of orbital bone

     Keratocyst of maxilla

     Keratocystic odontogenic tumor of maxilla

     EXCLUDES 2   *benign neoplasm of lower jaw bone (D16.5)*

   D16.5 **Benign neoplasm of** lower jaw bone

     Keratocyst of mandible

     Keratocystic odontogenic tumor of mandible

   D16.6 **Benign neoplasm of** vertebral column

     EXCLUDES 1   *benign neoplasm of sacrum and coccyx (D16.8)*

   D16.7 **Benign neoplasm of** ribs, sternum and clavicle

   D16.8 **Benign neoplasm of** pelvic bones, sacrum and coccyx

   D16.9 **Benign neoplasm of bone and articular cartilage, unspecified**

✓4ᵗʰ **D17** **Benign** lipomatous **neoplasm**

   D17.0 **Benign lipomatous neoplasm of** skin and subcutaneous tissue of head, face and neck

   D17.1 **Benign lipomatous neoplasm of** skin and subcutaneous tissue of trunk

✓5ᵗʰ **D17.2** **Benign lipomatous neoplasm of** skin and subcutaneous tissue of limb

     D17.20 **Benign lipomatous neoplasm of skin and subcutaneous tissue of unspecified limb**

     D17.21 **Benign lipomatous neoplasm of skin and subcutaneous tissue of** right arm

     D17.22 **Benign lipomatous neoplasm of skin and subcutaneous tissue of** left arm

     D17.23 **Benign lipomatous neoplasm of skin and subcutaneous tissue of** right leg

     D17.24 **Benign lipomatous neoplasm of skin and subcutaneous tissue of** left leg

✓5ᵗʰ **D17.3** **Benign lipomatous neoplasm of** skin and subcutaneous tissue of other and unspecified sites

     D17.30 **Benign lipomatous neoplasm of skin and subcutaneous tissue of unspecified sites**

     D17.39 **Benign lipomatous neoplasm of skin and subcutaneous tissue of other sites**

   D17.4 **Benign lipomatous neoplasm of** intrathoracic organs

   D17.5 **Benign lipomatous neoplasm of** intra-abdominal organs

     EXCLUDES 1   *benign lipomatous neoplasm of peritoneum and retroperitoneum (D17.79)*

   D17.6 **Benign lipomatous neoplasm of** spermatic cord   ♂

✓5ᵗʰ **D17.7** **Benign lipomatous neoplasm of other sites**

     D17.71 **Benign lipomatous neoplasm of** kidney

     D17.72 **Benign lipomatous neoplasm of other** genitourinary organ

     D17.79 **Benign lipomatous neoplasm of other sites**

        Benign lipomatous neoplasm of peritoneum

        Benign lipomatous neoplasm of retroperitoneum

   D17.9 **Benign lipomatous neoplasm, unspecified**

     Lipoma NOS

✓4ᵗʰ **D18** **Hemangioma and lymphangioma, any site**

     EXCLUDES 1   *benign neoplasm of glomus jugulare (D35.6)*

        blue or pigmented nevus (D22.-)

        nevus NOS (D22.-)

        vascular nevus (Q82.5)

✓5ᵗʰ **D18.0** **Hemangioma**

     Angioma NOS

     Cavernous nevus

     DEF: Common benign tumor usually occurring in infancy that is composed of newly formed blood vessels due to malformation of the angioblastic tissue.

     D18.00 **Hemangioma unspecified site**

     D18.01 **Hemangioma of** skin and subcutaneous tissue

     D18.02 **Hemangioma of** intracranial structures

     D18.03 **Hemangioma of** intra-abdominal structures

     D18.09 **Hemangioma of other sites**

   D18.1 **Lymphangioma, any site**

     AHA: 2018,3Q,31; 2018,2Q,13

✓4ᵗʰ **D19** **Benign neoplasm of** mesothelial tissue

   D19.0 **Benign neoplasm of mesothelial tissue of** pleura

   D19.1 **Benign neoplasm of mesothelial tissue of** peritoneum

   D19.7 **Benign neoplasm of mesothelial tissue of other sites**

   D19.9 **Benign neoplasm of mesothelial tissue, unspecified**

     Benign mesothelioma NOS

✓4ᵗʰ **D20** **Benign neoplasm of soft tissue of** retroperitoneum and peritoneum

     EXCLUDES 1   *benign lipomatous neoplasm of peritoneum and retroperitoneum (D17.79)*

        benign neoplasm of mesothelial tissue (D19.-)

   D20.0 **Benign neoplasm of soft tissue of** retroperitoneum

   D20.1 **Benign neoplasm of soft tissue of** peritoneum

✓4ᵗʰ **D21** **Other benign neoplasms of** connective and other soft tissue

     INCLUDES   benign neoplasm of blood vessel

        benign neoplasm of bursa

        benign neoplasm of cartilage

        benign neoplasm of fascia

        benign neoplasm of fat

        benign neoplasm of ligament, except uterine

        benign neoplasm of lymphatic channel

        benign neoplasm of muscle

        benign neoplasm of synovia

        benign neoplasm of tendon (sheath)

        benign stromal tumors

     EXCLUDES 1   *benign neoplasm of articular cartilage (D16.-)*

        benign neoplasm of cartilage of larynx (D14.1)

        benign neoplasm of cartilage of nose (D14.0)

        benign neoplasm of connective tissue of breast (D24.-)

        benign neoplasm of peripheral nerves and autonomic nervous system (D36.1-)

        benign neoplasm of peritoneum (D20.1)

        benign neoplasm of retroperitoneum (D20.0)

        benign neoplasm of uterine ligament, any (D28.2)

        benign neoplasm of vascular tissue (D18.-)

        hemangioma (D18.0-)

        lipomatous neoplasm (D17.-)

        lymphangioma (D18.1)

        uterine leiomyoma (D25.-)

   D21.0 **Benign neoplasm of connective and other soft tissue of** head, face and neck

     Benign neoplasm of connective tissue of ear

     Benign neoplasm of connective tissue of eyelid

     EXCLUDES 1   *benign neoplasm of connective tissue of orbit (D31.6-)*

✓5ᵗʰ **D21.1** **Benign neoplasm of connective and other soft tissue of** upper limb, including shoulder

     D21.10 **Benign neoplasm of connective and other soft tissue of unspecified upper limb, including shoulder**

     D21.11 **Benign neoplasm of connective and other soft tissue of** right **upper limb, including shoulder**

     D21.12 **Benign neoplasm of connective and other soft tissue of** left **upper limb, including shoulder**

✓5ᵗʰ **D21.2** **Benign neoplasm of connective and other soft tissue of** lower limb, including hip

     D21.20 **Benign neoplasm of connective and other soft tissue of unspecified lower limb, including hip**

     D21.21 **Benign neoplasm of connective and other soft tissue of** right **lower limb, including hip**

     D21.22 **Benign neoplasm of connective and other soft tissue of** left **lower limb, including hip**

   D21.3 **Benign neoplasm of connective and other soft tissue of** thorax

     Benign neoplasm of axilla

     Benign neoplasm of diaphragm

     Benign neoplasm of great vessels

     EXCLUDES 1   *benign neoplasm of heart (D15.1)*

        benign neoplasm of mediastinum (D15.2)

        benign neoplasm of thymus (D15.0)

   D21.4 **Benign neoplasm of connective and other soft tissue of** abdomen

     Benign stromal tumors of abdomen

N Newborn: 0   P Pediatric: 0-17   M Maternity: 12-55   A Adult: 15-124   CH Comorbidity High   CL Comorbidity Low   NCDx Noncancer Dx   PDx Primary Dx

488   ICD-10-CM 2020

D21.5 **Benign neoplasm of connective and other soft tissue of** pelvis
     EXCLUDES 1   *benign neoplasm of any uterine ligament (D28.2)*
                   uterine leiomyoma (D25.-)

D21.6 **Benign neoplasm of connective and other soft tissue of** trunk, **unspecified**
     ▶Benign neoplasm of connective and other soft tissue back NOS◀

D21.9 **Benign neoplasm of connective and other soft tissue, unspecified**

✓4ᵗʰ **D22** **Melanocytic nevi**
     INCLUDES   atypical nevus
              blue hairy pigmented nevus
              nevus NOS

D22.0 **Melanocytic nevi of** lip

✓5ᵗʰ **D22.1** **Melanocytic nevi of** eyelid, including canthus
     AHA: 2018,4Q,4

     D22.10 **Melanocytic nevi of unspecified eyelid, including canthus**

     ✓6ᵗʰ **D22.11** **Melanocytic nevi of** right **eyelid, including canthus**
         D22.111 **Melanocytic nevi of right** upper **eyelid, including canthus**
         D22.112 **Melanocytic nevi of right** lower **eyelid, including canthus**

     ✓6ᵗʰ **D22.12** **Melanocytic nevi of** left **eyelid, including canthus**
         D22.121 **Melanocytic nevi of left** upper **eyelid, including canthus**
         D22.122 **Melanocytic nevi of left** lower **eyelid, including canthus**

✓5ᵗʰ **D22.2** **Melanocytic nevi of** ear and external auricular canal

     D22.20 **Melanocytic nevi of unspecified ear and external auricular canal**

     D22.21 **Melanocytic nevi of** right **ear and external auricular canal**

     D22.22 **Melanocytic nevi of** left **ear and external auricular canal**

✓5ᵗʰ **D22.3** **Melanocytic nevi of other and unspecified** parts of face

     D22.30 **Melanocytic nevi of unspecified part of face**
     D22.39 **Melanocytic nevi of other parts of face**

D22.4 **Melanocytic nevi of** scalp and neck

D22.5 **Melanocytic nevi of** trunk
     Melanocytic nevi of anal margin
     Melanocytic nevi of anal skin
     Melanocytic nevi of perianal skin
     Melanocytic nevi of skin of breast

✓5ᵗʰ **D22.6** **Melanocytic nevi of** upper limb, including shoulder

     D22.60 **Melanocytic nevi of unspecified upper limb, including shoulder**

     D22.61 **Melanocytic nevi of** right **upper limb, including shoulder**

     D22.62 **Melanocytic nevi of** left **upper limb, including shoulder**

✓5ᵗʰ **D22.7** **Melanocytic nevi of** lower limb, including hip

     D22.70 **Melanocytic nevi of unspecified lower limb, including hip**

     D22.71 **Melanocytic nevi of** right **lower limb, including hip**
     D22.72 **Melanocytic nevi of** left **lower limb, including hip**

D22.9 **Melanocytic nevi, unspecified**

✓4ᵗʰ **D23** **Other benign neoplasms of** skin
     INCLUDES   benign neoplasm of hair follicles
              benign neoplasm of sebaceous glands
              benign neoplasm of sweat glands
     EXCLUDES 1   *benign lipomatous neoplasms of skin (D17.0-D17.3)*
               ~~*melanocytic nevi (D22.-)*~~
     EXCLUDES 2   ▶*melanocytic nevi (D22.-)*◀

D23.0 **Other benign neoplasm of skin of** lip
     EXCLUDES 1   *benign neoplasm of vermilion border of lip (D10.0)*

✓5ᵗʰ **D23.1** **Other benign neoplasm of skin of** eyelid, including canthus
     AHA: 2018,4Q,4

     D23.10 **Other benign neoplasm of skin of unspecified eyelid, including canthus**

     ✓6ᵗʰ **D23.11** **Other benign neoplasm of skin of** right **eyelid, including canthus**
         D23.111 **Other benign neoplasm of skin of right** upper **eyelid, including canthus**
         D23.112 **Other benign neoplasm of skin of right** lower **eyelid, including canthus**

     ✓6ᵗʰ **D23.12** **Other benign neoplasm of skin of** left **eyelid, including canthus**
         D23.121 **Other benign neoplasm of skin of left** upper **eyelid, including canthus**
         D23.122 **Other benign neoplasm of skin of left** lower **eyelid, including canthus**

✓5ᵗʰ **D23.2** **Other benign neoplasm of skin of** ear and external auricular canal

     D23.20 **Other benign neoplasm of skin of unspecified ear and external auricular canal**

     D23.21 **Other benign neoplasm of skin of** right **ear and external auricular canal**

     D23.22 **Other benign neoplasm of skin of** left **ear and external auricular canal**

✓5ᵗʰ **D23.3** **Other benign neoplasm of skin of other and unspecified parts of** face

     D23.30 **Other benign neoplasm of skin of unspecified part of face**

     D23.39 **Other benign neoplasm of skin of other parts of face**

D23.4 **Other benign neoplasm of skin of** scalp and neck

D23.5 **Other benign neoplasm of skin of** trunk
     Other benign neoplasm of anal margin
     Other benign neoplasm of anal skin
     Other benign neoplasm of perianal skin
     Other benign neoplasm of skin of breast
     EXCLUDES 1   *benign neoplasm of anus NOS (D12.9)*

✓5ᵗʰ **D23.6** **Other benign neoplasm of skin of** upper limb, including shoulder

     D23.60 **Other benign neoplasm of skin of unspecified upper limb, including shoulder**

     D23.61 **Other benign neoplasm of skin of** right **upper limb, including shoulder**

     D23.62 **Other benign neoplasm of skin of** left **upper limb, including shoulder**

✓5ᵗʰ **D23.7** **Other benign neoplasm of skin of** lower limb, including hip

     D23.70 **Other benign neoplasm of skin of unspecified lower limb, including hip**

     D23.71 **Other benign neoplasm of skin of** right **lower limb, including hip**

     D23.72 **Other benign neoplasm of skin of** left **lower limb, including hip**

D23.9 **Other benign neoplasm of skin, unspecified**

✓4ᵗʰ **D24** **Benign neoplasm of** breast
     INCLUDES   benign neoplasm of connective tissue of breast
              benign neoplasm of soft parts of breast
              fibroadenoma of breast
     EXCLUDES 2   *adenofibrosis of breast (N60.2)*
               benign cyst of breast (N60.-)
               benign mammary dysplasia (N60.-)
               benign neoplasm of skin of breast (D22.5, D23.5)
               fibrocystic disease of breast (N60.-)

D24.1 **Benign neoplasm of** right **breast**

D24.2 **Benign neoplasm of** left **breast**

D24.9 **Benign neoplasm of unspecified breast**

☑ Additional Character Required   ✓x 7ᵗʰ Placeholder Alert   Manifestation   Unspecified Dx   ▶◀ Revised Text   ● New Code   ▲ Revised Title

Chapter 2. Neoplasms

✓4th D25 Leiomyoma of uterus

> INCLUDES   uterine fibroid
> uterine fibromyoma
> uterine myoma

Uterine Leiomyomas (Fibroids)

- Cornual
- Pedunculated
- Uterine cavity
- Intramural
- Subserosal
- Submucosal
- Cervical

D25.0	Submucous **leiomyoma of uterus**	♀
D25.1	Intramural **leiomyoma of uterus**	♀
	Interstitial leiomyoma of uterus	
D25.2	Subserosal **leiomyoma of uterus**	♀
	Subperitoneal leiomyoma of uterus	
D25.9	**Leiomyoma of uterus, unspecified**	♀

✓4th D26 Other benign neoplasms of uterus

D26.0	**Other benign neoplasm of** cervix uteri	♀
D26.1	**Other benign neoplasm of** corpus uteri	♀
D26.7	**Other benign neoplasm of other** parts **of uterus**	♀
D26.9	**Other benign neoplasm of uterus, unspecified**	♀

✓4th D27 Benign neoplasm of ovary

> Use additional code to identify any functional activity
> EXCLUDES 2   corpus albicans cyst (N83.2-)
> corpus luteum cyst (N83.1-)
> endometrial cyst (N80.1)
> follicular (atretic) cyst (N83.0-)
> graafian follicle cyst (N83.0-)
> ovarian cyst NEC (N83.2-)
> ovarian retention cyst (N83.2-)

D27.0	**Benign neoplasm of** right **ovary**	♀
D27.1	**Benign neoplasm of** left **ovary**	♀
D27.9	**Benign neoplasm of unspecified ovary**	♀

✓4th D28 Benign neoplasm of other and unspecified female genital organs

> INCLUDES   adenomatous polyp
> benign neoplasm of skin of female genital organs
> benign teratoma
> EXCLUDES 1   epoophoron cyst (Q50.5)
> fimbrial cyst (Q50.4)
> Gartner's duct cyst (Q52.4)
> parovarian cyst (Q50.5)

D28.0	**Benign neoplasm of** vulva	♀
D28.1	**Benign neoplasm of** vagina	♀
D28.2	**Benign neoplasm of** uterine tubes and ligaments	♀
	Benign neoplasm of fallopian tube	
	Benign neoplasm of uterine ligament (broad) (round)	
D28.7	**Benign neoplasm of other specified female genital organs**	♀
D28.9	**Benign neoplasm of female genital organ, unspecified**	♀

✓4th D29 Benign neoplasm of male genital organs

> INCLUDES   benign neoplasm of skin of male genital organs

D29.0	**Benign neoplasm of** penis	♂

D29.1	**Benign neoplasm of** prostate	♂
	EXCLUDES 1 enlarged prostate (N40.-)	

✓5th D29.2 Benign neoplasm of testis

> Use additional code to identify any functional activity

D29.20	**Benign neoplasm of unspecified testis**	♂
D29.21	**Benign neoplasm of** right **testis**	♂
D29.22	**Benign neoplasm of** left **testis**	♂

✓5th D29.3 Benign neoplasm of epididymis

D29.30	**Benign neoplasm of unspecified epididymis**	♂
D29.31	**Benign neoplasm of** right **epididymis**	♂
D29.32	**Benign neoplasm of** left **epididymis**	♂

D29.4	**Benign neoplasm of** scrotum	♂
	Benign neoplasm of skin of scrotum	
D29.8	**Benign neoplasm of other specified male genital organs**	♂
	Benign neoplasm of seminal vesicle	
	Benign neoplasm of spermatic cord	
	Benign neoplasm of tunica vaginalis	
D29.9	**Benign neoplasm of male genital organ, unspecified**	♂

✓4th D30 Benign neoplasm of urinary organs

✓5th D30.0 Benign neoplasm of kidney

> EXCLUDES 1   benign carcinoid tumor of the kidney (D3A.093)
> benign neoplasm of renal calyces (D30.1-)
> benign neoplasm of renal pelvis (D30.1-)

D30.00	**Benign neoplasm of unspecified kidney**
D30.01	**Benign neoplasm of** right **kidney**
D30.02	**Benign neoplasm of** left **kidney**

✓5th D30.1 Benign neoplasm of renal pelvis

D30.10	**Benign neoplasm of unspecified renal pelvis**
D30.11	**Benign neoplasm of** right **renal pelvis**
D30.12	**Benign neoplasm of** left **renal pelvis**

✓5th D30.2 Benign neoplasm of ureter

> EXCLUDES 1   benign neoplasm of ureteric orifice of bladder (D30.3)

D30.20	**Benign neoplasm of unspecified ureter**
D30.21	**Benign neoplasm of** right **ureter**
D30.22	**Benign neoplasm of** left **ureter**

D30.3	**Benign neoplasm of** bladder
	Benign neoplasm of ureteric orifice of bladder
	Benign neoplasm of urethral orifice of bladder
D30.4	**Benign neoplasm of** urethra
	EXCLUDES 1 benign neoplasm of urethral orifice of bladder (D30.3)
D30.8	**Benign neoplasm of other specified urinary organs**
	Benign neoplasm of paraurethral glands
D30.9	**Benign neoplasm of urinary organ, unspecified**
	Benign neoplasm of urinary system NOS

✓4th D31 Benign neoplasm of eye and adnexa

> EXCLUDES 1   benign neoplasm of connective tissue of eyelid (D21.0)
> benign neoplasm of optic nerve (D33.3)
> benign neoplasm of skin of eyelid (D22.1-, D23.1-)

✓5th D31.0 Benign neoplasm of conjunctiva

D31.00	**Benign neoplasm of unspecified conjunctiva**
D31.01	**Benign neoplasm of** right **conjunctiva**
D31.02	**Benign neoplasm of** left **conjunctiva**

✓5th D31.1 Benign neoplasm of cornea

D31.10	**Benign neoplasm of unspecified cornea**
D31.11	**Benign neoplasm of** right **cornea**
D31.12	**Benign neoplasm of** left **cornea**

✓5th D31.2 Benign neoplasm of retina

> EXCLUDES 1   dark area on retina (D49.81)
> hemangioma of retina (D49.81)
> neoplasm of unspecified behavior of retina and choroid (D49.81)
> retinal freckle (D49.81)

D31.20	**Benign neoplasm of unspecified retina**
D31.21	**Benign neoplasm of** right **retina**
D31.22	**Benign neoplasm of** left **retina**

✓5th D31.3 Benign neoplasm of choroid

D31.30	**Benign neoplasm of unspecified choroid**
D31.31	**Benign neoplasm of** right **choroid**
D31.32	**Benign neoplasm of** left **choroid**

N Newborn: 0   P Pediatric: 0-17   M Maternity: 12-55   A Adult: 15-124   CH Comorbidity High   CL Comorbidity Low   NC-Dx Noncancer Dx   PDx Primary Dx

490   ICD-10-CM 2020

Chapter 2. Neoplasms

√5ᵗʰ **D31.4** **Benign neoplasm of** ciliary body

    D31.40 **Benign neoplasm of unspecified ciliary body**

    D31.41 **Benign neoplasm of** right **ciliary body**

    D31.42 **Benign neoplasm of** left **ciliary body**

√5ᵗʰ **D31.5** **Benign neoplasm of** lacrimal gland and duct

    Benign neoplasm of lacrimal sac

    Benign neoplasm of nasolacrimal duct

    D31.50 **Benign neoplasm of unspecified lacrimal gland and duct**

    D31.51 **Benign neoplasm of** right **lacrimal gland and duct**

    D31.52 **Benign neoplasm of** left **lacrimal gland and duct**

√5ᵗʰ **D31.6** **Benign neoplasm of unspecified site of** orbit

    Benign neoplasm of connective tissue of orbit

    Benign neoplasm of extraocular muscle

    Benign neoplasm of peripheral nerves of orbit

    Benign neoplasm of retrobulbar tissue

    Benign neoplasm of retro-ocular tissue

    EXCLUDES 1   benign neoplasm of orbital bone (D16.4)

    D31.60 **Benign neoplasm of unspecified site of unspecified orbit**

    D31.61 **Benign neoplasm of unspecified site of** right **orbit**

    D31.62 **Benign neoplasm of unspecified site of** left **orbit**

√5ᵗʰ **D31.9** **Benign neoplasm of unspecified** part of eye

    Benign neoplasm of eyeball

    D31.90 **Benign neoplasm of unspecified part of unspecified eye**

    D31.91 **Benign neoplasm of unspecified part of** right **eye**

    D31.92 **Benign neoplasm of unspecified part of** left **eye**

√4ᵗʰ **D32** **Benign neoplasm of** meninges

    D32.0 **Benign neoplasm of** cerebral **meninges**

    D32.1 **Benign neoplasm of** spinal **meninges**

    D32.9 **Benign neoplasm of meninges, unspecified**

        Meningioma NOS

√4ᵗʰ **D33** **Benign neoplasm of** brain and other parts of central nervous system

    EXCLUDES 1   angioma (D18.0-)

        benign neoplasm of meninges (D32.-)

        benign neoplasm of peripheral nerves and autonomic nervous system (D36.1-)

        hemangioma (D18.0-)

        neurofibromatosis (Q85.0-)

        retro-ocular benign neoplasm (D31.6-)

    D33.0 **Benign neoplasm of** brain, supratentorial

    Benign neoplasm of cerebral ventricle

    Benign neoplasm of cerebrum

    Benign neoplasm of frontal lobe

    Benign neoplasm of occipital lobe

    Benign neoplasm of parietal lobe

    Benign neoplasm of temporal lobe

    EXCLUDES 1   benign neoplasm of fourth ventricle (D33.1)

    D33.1 **Benign neoplasm of** brain, infratentorial

    Benign neoplasm of brain stem

    Benign neoplasm of cerebellum

    Benign neoplasm of fourth ventricle

    D33.2 **Benign neoplasm of brain, unspecified**

    D33.3 **Benign neoplasm of** cranial nerves

    Benign neoplasm of olfactory bulb

    D33.4 **Benign neoplasm of** spinal cord

    D33.7 **Benign neoplasm of other specified parts of central nervous system**

    D33.9 **Benign neoplasm of central nervous system, unspecified**

        Benign neoplasm of nervous system (central) NOS

D34 **Benign neoplasm of** thyroid gland

    Use additional code to identify any functional activity

√4ᵗʰ **D35** **Benign neoplasm of other and unspecified** endocrine glands

    Use additional code to identify any functional activity

    EXCLUDES 1   benign neoplasm of endocrine pancreas (D13.7)

        benign neoplasm of ovary (D27.-)

        benign neoplasm of testis (D29.2.-)

        benign neoplasm of thymus (D15.0)

√5ᵗʰ **D35.0** **Benign neoplasm of** adrenal gland

    D35.00 **Benign neoplasm of unspecified adrenal gland**

    D35.01 **Benign neoplasm of** right **adrenal gland**

    D35.02 **Benign neoplasm of** left **adrenal gland**

    D35.1 **Benign neoplasm of** parathyroid gland

D35.2 **Benign neoplasm of** pituitary gland

    AHA: 2014,3Q,22

D35.3 **Benign neoplasm of** craniopharyngeal duct

D35.4 **Benign neoplasm of** pineal gland

D35.5 **Benign neoplasm of** carotid body

D35.6 **Benign neoplasm of** aortic body and other paraganglia

    Benign tumor of glomus jugulare

D35.7 **Benign neoplasm of other specified endocrine glands**

D35.9 **Benign neoplasm of endocrine gland, unspecified**

    Benign neoplasm of unspecified endocrine gland

√4ᵗʰ **D36** **Benign neoplasm of other and unspecified sites**

    D36.0 **Benign neoplasm of** lymph nodes

        EXCLUDES 1   lymphangioma (D18.1)

√5ᵗʰ   **D36.1** **Benign neoplasm of** peripheral nerves and autonomic nervous system

        EXCLUDES 1   benign neoplasm of peripheral nerves of orbit (D31.6-)

            neurofibromatosis (Q85.0-)

    D36.10 **Benign neoplasm of peripheral nerves and autonomic nervous system, unspecified**

    D36.11 **Benign neoplasm of peripheral nerves and autonomic nervous system of** face, head, and neck

    D36.12 **Benign neoplasm of peripheral nerves and autonomic nervous system,** upper limb, including shoulder

    D36.13 **Benign neoplasm of peripheral nerves and autonomic nervous system of** lower limb, including hip

    D36.14 **Benign neoplasm of peripheral nerves and autonomic nervous system of** thorax

    D36.15 **Benign neoplasm of peripheral nerves and autonomic nervous system of** abdomen

    D36.16 **Benign neoplasm of peripheral nerves and autonomic nervous system of** pelvis

    D36.17 **Benign neoplasm of peripheral nerves and autonomic nervous system of** trunk, **unspecified**

D36.7 **Benign neoplasm of other specified sites**

    ▶Benign neoplasm of back NOS◀

    Benign neoplasm of nose NOS

D36.9 **Benign neoplasm, unspecified site**

Benign neuroendocrine tumors (D3A)

√4ᵗʰ **D3A** **Benign neuroendocrine tumors**

    Code also any associated multiple endocrine neoplasia [MEN] syndromes (E31.2-)

    Use additional code to identify any associated endocrine syndrome, such as:

    carcinoid syndrome (E34.0)

    EXCLUDES 2   benign pancreatic islet cell tumors (D13.7)

√5ᵗʰ   **D3A.0** **Benign** carcinoid tumors

    D3A.00 **Benign carcinoid tumor of unspecified site**

        Carcinoid tumor NOS

√6ᵗʰ   **D3A.01** **Benign carcinoid tumors of the** small intestine

        D3A.010 **Benign carcinoid tumor of the** duodenum

        D3A.011 **Benign carcinoid tumor of the** jejunum

        D3A.012 **Benign carcinoid tumor of the** ileum

        D3A.019 **Benign carcinoid tumor of the small intestine, unspecified portion**

√6ᵗʰ   **D3A.02** **Benign carcinoid tumors of the** appendix, large intestine, and rectum

        D3A.020 **Benign carcinoid tumor of the** appendix

        D3A.021 **Benign carcinoid tumor of the** cecum

        D3A.022 **Benign carcinoid tumor of the** ascending colon

        D3A.023 **Benign carcinoid tumor of the** transverse colon

        D3A.024 **Benign carcinoid tumor of the** descending colon

        D3A.025 **Benign carcinoid tumor of the** sigmoid colon

        D3A.026 **Benign carcinoid tumor of the** rectum

        D3A.029 **Benign carcinoid tumor of the large intestine, unspecified portion**

            Benign carcinoid tumor of the colon NOS

√6ᵗʰ   **D3A.09** **Benign carcinoid tumors of other sites**

        D3A.090 **Benign carcinoid tumor of the** bronchus and lung

        D3A.091 **Benign carcinoid tumor of the** thymus

☑ Additional Character Required   √ˣ7ᵗʰ Placeholder Alert   Manifestation   Unspecified Dx   ▶◀ Revised Text   ● New Code   ▲ Revised Title

D3A.092   Benign carcinoid tumor of the stomach
D3A.093   Benign carcinoid tumor of the kidney
D3A.094   Benign carcinoid tumor of the foregut, unspecified
D3A.095   Benign carcinoid tumor of the midgut, unspecified
D3A.096   Benign carcinoid tumor of the hindgut, unspecified
D3A.098   Benign carcinoid tumors of other sites
D3A.8   Other benign neuroendocrine tumors
   Neuroendocrine tumor NOS

Neoplasms of uncertain behavior, polycythemia vera and myelodysplastic syndromes (D37-D48)

NOTE   Categories D37-D44, and D48 classify by site neoplasms of uncertain behavior, i.e., histologic confirmation whether the neoplasm is malignant or benign cannot be made.

EXCLUDES 1   neoplasms of unspecified behavior (D49.-)

✓4ᵗʰ D37   Neoplasm of uncertain behavior of oral cavity and digestive organs
   EXCLUDES 1   stromal tumors of uncertain behavior of digestive system (D48.1)

✓5ᵗʰ D37.0   Neoplasm of uncertain behavior of lip, oral cavity and pharynx
   EXCLUDES 1   neoplasm of uncertain behavior of aryepiglottic fold or interarytenoid fold, laryngeal aspect (D38.0)
   neoplasm of uncertain behavior of epiglottis NOS (D38.0)
   neoplasm of uncertain behavior of skin of lip (D48.5)
   neoplasm of uncertain behavior of suprahyoid portion of epiglottis (D38.0)

D37.01   Neoplasm of uncertain behavior of lip
   Neoplasm of uncertain behavior of vermilion border of lip

D37.02   Neoplasm of uncertain behavior of tongue

✓6ᵗʰ D37.03   Neoplasm of uncertain behavior of the major salivary glands
   D37.030   Neoplasm of uncertain behavior of the parotid salivary glands
   D37.031   Neoplasm of uncertain behavior of the sublingual salivary glands
   D37.032   Neoplasm of uncertain behavior of the submandibular salivary glands
   D37.039   Neoplasm of uncertain behavior of the major salivary glands, unspecified

D37.04   Neoplasm of uncertain behavior of the minor salivary glands
   Neoplasm of uncertain behavior of submucosal salivary glands of lip
   Neoplasm of uncertain behavior of submucosal salivary glands of cheek
   Neoplasm of uncertain behavior of submucosal salivary glands of hard palate
   Neoplasm of uncertain behavior of submucosal salivary glands of soft palate

D37.05   Neoplasm of uncertain behavior of pharynx
   Neoplasm of uncertain behavior of aryepiglottic fold of pharynx NOS
   Neoplasm of uncertain behavior of hypopharyngeal aspect of aryepiglottic fold of pharynx
   Neoplasm of uncertain behavior of marginal zone of aryepiglottic fold of pharynx

D37.09   Neoplasm of uncertain behavior of other specified sites of the oral cavity

D37.1   Neoplasm of uncertain behavior of stomach
D37.2   Neoplasm of uncertain behavior of small intestine
D37.3   Neoplasm of uncertain behavior of appendix
D37.4   Neoplasm of uncertain behavior of colon
D37.5   Neoplasm of uncertain behavior of rectum
   Neoplasm of uncertain behavior of rectosigmoid junction
D37.6   Neoplasm of uncertain behavior of liver, gallbladder and bile ducts
   Neoplasm of uncertain behavior of ampulla of Vater

D37.8   Neoplasm of uncertain behavior of other specified digestive organs
   Neoplasm of uncertain behavior of anal canal
   Neoplasm of uncertain behavior of anal sphincter
   Neoplasm of uncertain behavior of anus NOS
   Neoplasm of uncertain behavior of esophagus
   Neoplasm of uncertain behavior of intestine NOS
   Neoplasm of uncertain behavior of pancreas
   EXCLUDES 1   neoplasm of uncertain behavior of anal margin (D48.5)
   neoplasm of uncertain behavior of anal skin (D48.5)
   neoplasm of uncertain behavior of perianal skin (D48.5)

D37.9   Neoplasm of uncertain behavior of digestive organ, unspecified

✓4ᵗʰ D38   Neoplasm of uncertain behavior of middle ear and respiratory and intrathoracic organs
   EXCLUDES 1   neoplasm of uncertain behavior of heart (D48.7)

D38.0   Neoplasm of uncertain behavior of larynx
   Neoplasm of uncertain behavior of aryepiglottic fold or interarytenoid fold, laryngeal aspect
   Neoplasm of uncertain behavior of epiglottis (suprahyoid portion)
   EXCLUDES 1   neoplasm of uncertain behavior of aryepiglottic fold or interarytenoid fold NOS (D37.05)
   neoplasm of uncertain behavior of hypopharyngeal aspect of aryepiglottic fold (D37.05)
   neoplasm of uncertain behavior of marginal zone of aryepiglottic fold (D37.05)

D38.1   Neoplasm of uncertain behavior of trachea, bronchus and lung
D38.2   Neoplasm of uncertain behavior of pleura
D38.3   Neoplasm of uncertain behavior of mediastinum
D38.4   Neoplasm of uncertain behavior of thymus
D38.5   Neoplasm of uncertain behavior of other respiratory organs
   Neoplasm of uncertain behavior of accessory sinuses
   Neoplasm of uncertain behavior of cartilage of nose
   Neoplasm of uncertain behavior of middle ear
   Neoplasm of uncertain behavior of nasal cavities
   EXCLUDES 1   neoplasm of uncertain behavior of ear (external) (skin) (D48.5)
   neoplasm of uncertain behavior of nose NOS (D48.7)
   neoplasm of uncertain behavior of skin of nose (D48.5)

D38.6   Neoplasm of uncertain behavior of respiratory organ, unspecified

✓4ᵗʰ D39   Neoplasm of uncertain behavior of female genital organs

D39.0   Neoplasm of uncertain behavior of uterus   ♀

✓5ᵗʰ D39.1   Neoplasm of uncertain behavior of ovary
   Use additional code to identify any functional activity
   D39.10   Neoplasm of uncertain behavior of unspecified ovary   ♀
   D39.11   Neoplasm of uncertain behavior of right ovary   ♀
   D39.12   Neoplasm of uncertain behavior of left ovary   ♀

D39.2   Neoplasm of uncertain behavior of placenta   Ⓜ ♀
   Chorioadenoma destruens
   Invasive hydatidiform mole
   Malignant hydatidiform mole
   EXCLUDES 1   hydatidiform mole NOS (O01.9)

D39.8   Neoplasm of uncertain behavior of other specified female genital organs   ♀
   Neoplasm of uncertain behavior of skin of female genital organs

D39.9   Neoplasm of uncertain behavior of female genital organ, unspecified   ♀

✓4ᵗʰ D40   Neoplasm of uncertain behavior of male genital organs

D40.0   Neoplasm of uncertain behavior of prostate   ♂

✓5ᵗʰ D40.1   Neoplasm of uncertain behavior of testis
   D40.10   Neoplasm of uncertain behavior of unspecified testis   ♂
   D40.11   Neoplasm of uncertain behavior of right testis   ♂
   D40.12   Neoplasm of uncertain behavior of left testis   ♂

D40.8　**Neoplasm of uncertain behavior of other**　　　♂
　　　　　specified male genital organs
　　　　　Neoplasm of uncertain behavior of skin of male genital organs

D40.9　**Neoplasm of uncertain behavior of male genital**　　　♂
　　　　　organ, unspecified

✓4ᵗʰ **D41**　**Neoplasm of uncertain behavior of** urinary organs

　✓5ᵗʰ **D41.0**　**Neoplasm of uncertain behavior of** kidney

　　　　EXCLUDES 1　neoplasm of uncertain behavior of renal pelvis
　　　　　　　　　(D41.1-)

　　　D41.00　**Neoplasm of uncertain behavior of unspecified**
　　　　　　　　kidney

　　　D41.01　**Neoplasm of uncertain behavior of** right **kidney**

　　　D41.02　**Neoplasm of uncertain behavior of** left **kidney**

　✓5ᵗʰ **D41.1**　**Neoplasm of uncertain behavior of** renal pelvis

　　　D41.10　**Neoplasm of uncertain behavior of unspecified**
　　　　　　　　renal pelvis

　　　D41.11　**Neoplasm of uncertain behavior of** right **renal pelvis**

　　　D41.12　**Neoplasm of uncertain behavior of** left **renal pelvis**

　✓5ᵗʰ **D41.2**　**Neoplasm of uncertain behavior of** ureter

　　　D41.20　**Neoplasm of uncertain behavior of unspecified**
　　　　　　　　ureter

　　　D41.21　**Neoplasm of uncertain behavior of** right **ureter**

　　　D41.22　**Neoplasm of uncertain behavior of** left **ureter**

　　D41.3　**Neoplasm of uncertain behavior of** urethra

　　D41.4　**Neoplasm of uncertain behavior of** bladder

　　D41.8　**Neoplasm of uncertain behavior of other specified urinary**
　　　　　　organs

　　D41.9　**Neoplasm of uncertain behavior of unspecified urinary organ**

✓4ᵗʰ **D42**　**Neoplasm of uncertain behavior of** meninges

　　D42.0　**Neoplasm of uncertain behavior of** cerebral **meninges**

　　D42.1　**Neoplasm of uncertain behavior of** spinal **meninges**

　　D42.9　**Neoplasm of uncertain behavior of meninges, unspecified**

✓4ᵗʰ **D43**　**Neoplasm of uncertain behavior of** brain and central nervous
　　　　system

　　　EXCLUDES 1　neoplasm of uncertain behavior of peripheral nerves and
　　　　　　　　autonomic nervous system (D48.2)

　　D43.0　**Neoplasm of uncertain behavior of** brain, supratentorial
　　　　　　Neoplasm of uncertain behavior of cerebral ventricle
　　　　　　Neoplasm of uncertain behavior of cerebrum
　　　　　　Neoplasm of uncertain behavior of frontal lobe
　　　　　　Neoplasm of uncertain behavior of occipital lobe
　　　　　　Neoplasm of uncertain behavior of parietal lobe
　　　　　　Neoplasm of uncertain behavior of temporal lobe

　　　EXCLUDES 1　neoplasm of uncertain behavior of fourth ventricle
　　　　　　　　(D43.1)

　　D43.1　**Neoplasm of uncertain behavior of** brain, infratentorial
　　　　　　Neoplasm of uncertain behavior of brain stem
　　　　　　Neoplasm of uncertain behavior of cerebellum
　　　　　　Neoplasm of uncertain behavior of fourth ventricle

　　D43.2　**Neoplasm of uncertain behavior of** brain, **unspecified**

　　D43.3　**Neoplasm of uncertain behavior of** cranial nerves

　　D43.4　**Neoplasm of uncertain behavior of** spinal cord

　　D43.8　**Neoplasm of uncertain behavior of other** specified parts of
　　　　　　central nervous system

　　D43.9　**Neoplasm of uncertain behavior of central nervous system,**
　　　　　　unspecified
　　　　　　Neoplasm of uncertain behavior of nervous system (central)
　　　　　　　NOS

✓4ᵗʰ **D44**　**Neoplasm of uncertain behavior of** endocrine glands

　　　EXCLUDES 1　multiple endocrine adenomatosis (E31.2-)
　　　　　　　　multiple endocrine neoplasia (E31.2-)
　　　　　　　　neoplasm of uncertain behavior of endocrine pancreas (D37.8)
　　　　　　　　neoplasm of uncertain behavior of ovary (D39.1-)
　　　　　　　　neoplasm of uncertain behavior of testis (D40.1-)
　　　　　　　　neoplasm of uncertain behavior of thymus (D38.4)

　　D44.0　**Neoplasm of uncertain behavior of** thyroid gland

　✓5ᵗʰ **D44.1**　**Neoplasm of uncertain behavior of** adrenal gland
　　　　　　Use additional code to identify any functional activity

　　　D44.10　**Neoplasm of uncertain behavior of unspecified**
　　　　　　　　adrenal gland

　　　D44.11　**Neoplasm of uncertain behavior of** right **adrenal**
　　　　　　　　gland

　　　D44.12　**Neoplasm of uncertain behavior of** left **adrenal**
　　　　　　　　gland

　　D44.2　**Neoplasm of uncertain behavior of** parathyroid gland

D44.3　**Neoplasm of uncertain behavior of** pituitary gland
　　　　Use additional code to identify any functional activity

D44.4　**Neoplasm of uncertain behavior of** craniopharyngeal duct

D44.5　**Neoplasm of uncertain behavior of** pineal gland

D44.6　**Neoplasm of uncertain behavior of** carotid body

D44.7　**Neoplasm of uncertain behavior of** aortic body and other
　　　　paraganglia
　　　　AHA: 2016,4Q,26

D44.9　**Neoplasm of uncertain behavior of unspecified endocrine**
　　　　gland

D45　**Polycythemia vera**

　　EXCLUDES 1　familial polycythemia (D75.0)
　　　　　　　secondary polycythemia (D75.1)

　　DEF: Abnormal proliferation of all bone marrow elements, increased red
　　cell mass, and total blood volume. The etiology is unknown, but it is
　　frequently associated with splenomegaly, leukocytosis, and
　　thrombocythemia.

✓4ᵗʰ **D46**　**Myelodysplastic syndromes**

　　Use additional code for adverse effect, if applicable, to identify drug
　　(T36-T50 with fifth or sixth character 5)

　　EXCLUDES 2　drug-induced aplastic anemia (D61.1)

　　D46.0　**Refractory anemia** without ring sideroblasts, **so stated**
　　　　　　Refractory anemia without sideroblasts, without excess of blasts

　　D46.1　**Refractory anemia** with ring sideroblasts
　　　　　　RARS

　✓5ᵗʰ **D46.2**　**Refractory anemia** with excess of blasts [RAEB]

　　　D46.20　**Refractory anemia with excess of blasts, unspecified**
　　　　　　　　RAEB NOS

　　　D46.21　**Refractory anemia with excess of** blasts 1
　　　　　　　　RAEB 1

　　　D46.22　**Refractory anemia with excess of** blasts 2
　　　　　　　　RAEB 2

　　D46.A　**Refractory** cytopenia with multilineage dysplasia

　　D46.B　**Refractory** cytopenia with multilineage dysplasia and ring
　　　　　　sideroblasts
　　　　　　RCMD RS

　　D46.C　**Myelodysplastic syndrome** with isolated del(5q)
　　　　　　chromosomal abnormality
　　　　　　Myelodysplastic syndrome with 5q deletion
　　　　　　5q minus syndrome NOS

　　D46.4　**Refractory anemia, unspecified**

　　D46.Z　**Other myelodysplastic syndromes**
　　　　　　EXCLUDES 1　chronic myelomonocytic leukemia (C93.1-)

　　D46.9　**Myelodysplastic syndrome, unspecified**
　　　　　　Myelodysplasia NOS

✓4ᵗʰ **D47**　**Other neoplasms of uncertain behavior of** lymphoid,
　　　　hematopoietic and related tissue

　✓5ᵗʰ **D47.0**　**Mast cell neoplasms of uncertain behavior**

　　　　EXCLUDES 1　congenital cutaneous mastocytosis (Q82.2)
　　　　　　　　　histiocytic neoplasms of uncertain behavior (D47.Z9)
　　　　　　　　　malignant mast cell neoplasm (C96.2-)

　　　　AHA: 2017,4Q,5

　　　D47.01　Cutaneous **mastocytosis**
　　　　　　　　Diffuse cutaneous mastocytosis
　　　　　　　　Maculopapular cutaneous mastocytosis
　　　　　　　　Solitary mastocytoma
　　　　　　　　Telangiectasia macularis eruptiva perstans
　　　　　　　　Urticaria pigmentosa
　　　　　　　　EXCLUDES 1　congenital (diffuse) (maculopapular)
　　　　　　　　　　　　　cutaneous mastocytosis (Q82.2)
　　　　　　　　　　　　congenital urticaria pigmentosa (Q82.2)
　　　　　　　　　　　　extracutaneous mastocytoma (D47.09)

☑ Additional Character Required　　✓x7ᵗʰ Placeholder Alert　　Manifestation　　Unspecified Dx　　▶◀ Revised Text　　● New Code　　▲ Revised Title

ICD-10-CM 2020　　　　　　　　　　　　　　　　　　　　　　　　　　　　　　　　　　　　　**493**

D47.02 Systemic mastocytosis
Indolent systemic mastocytosis
Isolated bone marrow mastocytosis
Smoldering systemic mastocytosis
Systemic mastocytosis, with an associated hematological non-mast cell lineage disease (SM-AHNMD)
Code also, if applicable, any associated hematological non-mast cell lineage disease, such as:
acute myeloid leukemia (C92.6-, C92.A-)
chronic myelomonocytic leukemia (C93.1-)
essential thrombocytosis (D47.3)
hypereosinophilic syndrome (D72.1)
myelodysplastic syndrome (D46.9)
myeloproliferative syndrome (D47.1)
non-Hodgkin lymphoma (C82-C85)
plasma cell myeloma (C90.0-)
polycythemia vera (D45)
EXCLUDES 1   *aggressive systemic mastocytosis (C96.21)*
mast cell leukemia (C94.3-)

D47.09 Other mast cell neoplasms of uncertain behavior
Extracutaneous mastocytoma
Mast cell tumor NOS
Mastocytoma NOS
Mastocytosis NOS

D47.1 Chronic myeloproliferative disease
Chronic neutrophilic leukemia
Myeloproliferative disease, unspecified
EXCLUDES 1   *atypical chronic myeloid leukemia BCR/ABL-negative (C92.2-)*
chronic myeloid leukemia BCR/ABL-positive (C92.1-)
myelofibrosis NOS (D75.81)
myelophthisic anemia (D61.82)
myelophthisis (D61.82)
secondary myelofibrosis NOS (D75.81)

D47.2 Monoclonal gammopathy
Monoclonal gammopathy of undetermined significance [MGUS]

D47.3 Essential (hemorrhagic) thrombocythemia
Essential thrombocytosis
Idiopathic hemorrhagic thrombocythemia
DEF: Chronic myeloproliferative neoplasm involving production of excess blood platelets that may result in abnormal clotting or hemorrhaging.

D47.4 Osteomyelofibrosis
Chronic idiopathic myelofibrosis
Myelofibrosis (idiopathic) (with myeloid metaplasia)
Myelosclerosis (megakaryocytic) with myeloid metaplasia
Secondary myelofibrosis in myeloproliferative disease
EXCLUDES 1   *acute myelofibrosis (C94.4-)*

✓5ᵗʰ D47.Z Other specified neoplasms of uncertain behavior of lymphoid, hematopoietic and related tissue
AHA: 2016,4Q,8

D47.Z1 Post-transplant lymphoproliferative disorder (PTLD)
Code first complications of transplanted organs and tissue (T86.-)
DEF: Excessive proliferation of B-cell lymphocytes following Epstein-Barr virus infection in organ transplant patients. It may progress to non-Hodgkin lymphoma.

D47.Z2 Castleman disease
Code also if applicable human herpesvirus 8 infection (B10.89)
EXCLUDES 2   *Kaposi's sarcoma (C46-)*
DEF: Rare disease of the lymph nodes and lymphoid tissues that closely mimics lymphoma.

D47.Z9 Other specified neoplasms of uncertain behavior of lymphoid, hematopoietic and related tissue
Histiocytic tumors of uncertain behavior

D47.9 Neoplasm of uncertain behavior of lymphoid, hematopoietic and related tissue, unspecified
Lymphoproliferative disease NOS

✓4ᵗʰ D48 Neoplasm of uncertain behavior of other and unspecified sites
EXCLUDES 1   *neurofibromatosis (nonmalignant) (Q85.0-)*

D48.0 Neoplasm of uncertain behavior of bone and articular cartilage
EXCLUDES 1   *neoplasm of uncertain behavior of cartilage of ear (D48.1)*
neoplasm of uncertain behavior of cartilage of larynx (D38.0)
neoplasm of uncertain behavior of cartilage of nose (D38.5)
neoplasm of uncertain behavior of connective tissue of eyelid (D48.1)
neoplasm of uncertain behavior of synovia (D48.1)

D48.1 Neoplasm of uncertain behavior of connective and other soft tissue
Neoplasm of uncertain behavior of connective tissue of ear
Neoplasm of uncertain behavior of connective tissue of eyelid
Stromal tumors of uncertain behavior of digestive system
EXCLUDES 1   *neoplasm of uncertain behavior of articular cartilage (D48.0)*
neoplasm of uncertain behavior of cartilage of larynx (D38.0)
neoplasm of uncertain behavior of cartilage of nose (D38.5)
neoplasm of uncertain behavior of connective tissue of breast (D48.6-)

D48.2 Neoplasm of uncertain behavior of peripheral nerves and autonomic nervous system
EXCLUDES 1   *neoplasm of uncertain behavior of peripheral nerves of orbit (D48.7)*

D48.3 Neoplasm of uncertain behavior of retroperitoneum

D48.4 Neoplasm of uncertain behavior of peritoneum

D48.5 Neoplasm of uncertain behavior of skin
Neoplasm of uncertain behavior of anal margin
Neoplasm of uncertain behavior of anal skin
Neoplasm of uncertain behavior of perianal skin
Neoplasm of uncertain behavior of skin of breast
EXCLUDES 1   *neoplasm of uncertain behavior of anus NOS (D37.8)*
neoplasm of uncertain behavior of skin of genital organs (D39.8, D40.8)
neoplasm of uncertain behavior of vermilion border of lip (D37.0)

✓5ᵗʰ D48.6 Neoplasm of uncertain behavior of breast
Neoplasm of uncertain behavior of connective tissue of breast
Cystosarcoma phyllodes
EXCLUDES 1   *neoplasm of uncertain behavior of skin of breast (D48.5)*

D48.60 Neoplasm of uncertain behavior of unspecified breast

D48.61 Neoplasm of uncertain behavior of right breast

D48.62 Neoplasm of uncertain behavior of left breast

D48.7 Neoplasm of uncertain behavior of other specified sites
Neoplasm of uncertain behavior of eye
Neoplasm of uncertain behavior of heart
Neoplasm of uncertain behavior of peripheral nerves of orbit
EXCLUDES 1   *neoplasm of uncertain behavior of connective tissue (D48.1)*
neoplasm of uncertain behavior of skin of eyelid (D48.5)

D48.9 Neoplasm of uncertain behavior, unspecified

Neoplasms of unspecified behavior (D49)

✓4ᵗʰ D49 Neoplasms of unspecified behavior

> **NOTE** Category D49 classifies by site neoplasms of unspecified morphology and behavior. The term "mass", unless otherwise stated, is not to be regarded as a neoplastic growth.
>
> **INCLUDES** "growth" NOS
> neoplasm NOS
> new growth NOS
> tumor NOS
>
> **EXCLUDES 1** neoplasms of uncertain behavior (D37-D44, D48)

D49.Ø Neoplasm of unspecified behavior of digestive system
> **EXCLUDES 1** neoplasm of unspecified behavior of margin of anus (D49.2)
> neoplasm of unspecified behavior of perianal skin (D49.2)
> neoplasm of unspecified behavior of skin of anus (D49.2)

D49.1 Neoplasm of unspecified behavior of respiratory system

D49.2 Neoplasm of unspecified behavior of bone, soft tissue, and skin
> **EXCLUDES 1** neoplasm of unspecified behavior of anal canal (D49.Ø)
> neoplasm of unspecified behavior of anus NOS (D49.Ø)
> neoplasm of unspecified behavior of bone marrow (D49.89)
> neoplasm of unspecified behavior of cartilage of larynx (D49.1)
> neoplasm of unspecified behavior of cartilage of nose (D49.1)
> neoplasm of unspecified behavior of connective tissue of breast (D49.3)
> neoplasm of unspecified behavior of skin of genital organs (D49.59)
> neoplasm of unspecified behavior of vermilion border of lip (D49.Ø)

D49.3 Neoplasm of unspecified behavior of breast
> **EXCLUDES 1** neoplasm of unspecified behavior of skin of breast (D49.2)

D49.4 Neoplasm of unspecified behavior of bladder

✓5ᵗʰ D49.5 Neoplasm of unspecified behavior of other genitourinary organs
> **AHA:** 2016,4Q,9

> **✓6ᵗʰ D49.51 Neoplasm of unspecified behavior of kidney**
> > **D49.511 Neoplasm of unspecified behavior of right kidney**
> > **D49.512 Neoplasm of unspecified behavior of left kidney**
> > **D49.519 Neoplasm of unspecified behavior of unspecified kidney**
>
> **D49.59 Neoplasm of unspecified behavior of other genitourinary organ**

D49.6 Neoplasm of unspecified behavior of brain
> **EXCLUDES 1** neoplasm of unspecified behavior of cerebral meninges (D49.7)
> neoplasm of unspecified behavior of cranial nerves (D49.7)

D49.7 Neoplasm of unspecified behavior of endocrine glands and other parts of nervous system
> **EXCLUDES 1** neoplasm of unspecified behavior of peripheral, sympathetic, and parasympathetic nerves and ganglia (D49.2)

✓5ᵗʰ D49.8 Neoplasm of unspecified behavior of other specified sites
> **EXCLUDES 1** neoplasm of unspecified behavior of eyelid (skin) (D49.2)
> neoplasm of unspecified behavior of eyelid cartilage (D49.2)
> neoplasm of unspecified behavior of great vessels (D49.2)
> neoplasm of unspecified behavior of optic nerve (D49.7)

> **D49.81 Neoplasm of unspecified behavior of retina and choroid**
> > Dark area on retina
> > Retinal freckle
>
> **D49.89 Neoplasm of unspecified behavior of other specified sites**

D49.9 Neoplasm of unspecified behavior of unspecified site

☑ Additional Character Required   ✓ˣ7ᵗʰ Placeholder Alert   Manifestation   Unspecified Dx   ▶◀ Revised Text   ● New Code   ▲ Revised Title

ICD-10-CM 2020   495

Chapter 3. Diseases of the Blood and Blood-forming Organs and Certain Disorders Involving the Immune Mechanism (D50–D89)

Chapter-specific Coding Guidelines and Examples
Reserved for future guideline expansion

Chapter 3. Diseases of the Blood and Blood-forming Organs and Certain Disorders Involving the Immune Mechanism (D5Ø-D89)

EXCLUDES 2   autoimmune disease (systemic) NOS (M35.9)
certain conditions originating in the perinatal period (PØØ-P96)
complications of pregnancy, childbirth and the puerperium (OØØ-O9A)
congenital malformations, deformations and chromosomal abnormalities (QØØ-Q99)
endocrine, nutritional and metabolic diseases (EØØ-E88)
human immunodeficiency virus [HIV] disease (B2Ø)
injury, poisoning and certain other consequences of external causes (SØØ-T88)
neoplasms (CØØ-D49)
symptoms, signs and abnormal clinical and laboratory findings, not elsewhere classified (RØØ-R94)

This chapter contains the following blocks:

D5Ø-D53   Nutritional anemias
D55-D59   Hemolytic anemias
D6Ø-D64   Aplastic and other anemias and other bone marrow failure syndromes
D65-D69   Coagulation defects, purpura and other hemorrhagic conditions
D7Ø-D77   Other disorders of blood and blood-forming organs
D78   Intraoperative and postprocedural complications of the spleen
D8Ø-D89   Certain disorders involving the immune mechanism

Nutritional anemias (D5Ø-D53)

DEF: Nutritional anemia: The result of inadequate intake or absorption of a vitamin or mineral that impacts the production of red blood cells or causes them to develop abnormally affecting the size and shape.

✓4ᵗʰ D5Ø   Iron deficiency anemia

   INCLUDES   asiderotic anemia
               hypochromic anemia

   D5Ø.Ø   Iron deficiency anemia secondary to blood loss (chronic)
       Posthemorrhagic anemia (chronic)
       EXCLUDES 1   acute posthemorrhagic anemia (D62)
                     congenital anemia from fetal blood loss (P61.3)

   D5Ø.1   Sideropenic dysphagia
       Kelly-Paterson syndrome
       Plummer-Vinson syndrome

   D5Ø.8   Other iron deficiency anemias
       Iron deficiency anemia due to inadequate dietary iron intake

   D5Ø.9   Iron deficiency anemia, unspecified

✓4ᵗʰ D51   Vitamin B12 deficiency anemia

   EXCLUDES 1   vitamin B12 deficiency (E53.8)

   D51.Ø   Vitamin B12 deficiency anemia due to intrinsic factor deficiency
       Addison anemia
       Biermer anemia
       Pernicious (congenital) anemia
       Congenital intrinsic factor deficiency
       DEF: Chronic progressive anemia due to vitamin B12 malabsorption, caused by lack of secretion of intrinsic factor, which is produced by the gastric mucosa of the stomach.

   D51.1   Vitamin B12 deficiency anemia due to selective vitamin B12 malabsorption with proteinuria
       Imerslund (Gräsbeck) syndrome
       Megaloblastic hereditary anemia

   D51.2   Transcobalamin II deficiency

   D51.3   Other dietary vitamin B12 deficiency anemia
       Vegan anemia

   D51.8   Other vitamin B12 deficiency anemias
   D51.9   Vitamin B12 deficiency anemia, unspecified

✓4ᵗʰ D52   Folate deficiency anemia

   EXCLUDES 1   folate deficiency without anemia (E53.8)
   DEF: Deficiency in a B complex vitamin needed for the production of healthy red blood cells. Lack of folate, or folic acid, and other absorption conditions can cause anemia resulting in large, misshapen red blood cells called megaloblasts.

   D52.Ø   Dietary folate deficiency anemia
       Nutritional megaloblastic anemia
       DEF: Result of a poor diet with inadequate intake of folate, which is needed to produce healthy red blood cells.

   D52.1   Drug-induced folate deficiency anemia
       Use additional code for adverse effect, if applicable, to identify drug (T36-T5Ø with fifth or sixth character 5)

   D52.8   Other folate deficiency anemias

   D52.9   Folate deficiency anemia, unspecified
       Folic acid deficiency anemia NOS

✓4ᵗʰ D53   Other nutritional anemias

   INCLUDES   megaloblastic anemia unresponsive to vitamin B12 or folate therapy

   D53.Ø   Protein deficiency anemia
       Amino-acid deficiency anemia
       Orotaciduric anemia
       EXCLUDES 1   Lesch-Nyhan syndrome (E79.1)

   D53.1   Other megaloblastic anemias, not elsewhere classified
       Megaloblastic anemia NOS
       EXCLUDES 1   Di Guglielmo's disease (C94.Ø)

   D53.2   Scorbutic anemia
       EXCLUDES 1   scurvy (E54)

   D53.8   Other specified nutritional anemias
       Anemia associated with deficiency of copper
       Anemia associated with deficiency of molybdenum
       Anemia associated with deficiency of zinc
       EXCLUDES 1   nutritional deficiencies without anemia, such as:
                   copper deficiency NOS (E61.Ø)
                   molybdenum deficiency NOS (E61.5)
                   zinc deficiency NOS (E6Ø)

   D53.9   Nutritional anemia, unspecified
       Simple chronic anemia
       EXCLUDES 1   anemia NOS (D64.9)
       AHA: 2018,4Q,88

Hemolytic anemias (D55-D59)

✓4ᵗʰ D55   Anemia due to enzyme disorders

   EXCLUDES 1   drug-induced enzyme deficiency anemia (D59.2)

   D55.Ø   Anemia due to glucose-6-phosphate dehydrogenase [G6PD] deficiency
       Favism
       G6PD deficiency anemia
       EXCLUDES 1   ▶glucose-6-phosphate dehydrogenase (G6PD) deficiency without anemia (D75.A)◀

   D55.1   Anemia due to other disorders of glutathione metabolism
       Anemia (due to) enzyme deficiencies, except G6PD, related to the hexose monophosphate [HMP] shunt pathway
       Anemia (due to) hemolytic nonspherocytic (hereditary), type I

   D55.2   Anemia due to disorders of glycolytic enzymes
       Hemolytic nonspherocytic (hereditary) anemia, type II
       Hexokinase deficiency anemia
       Pyruvate kinase [PK] deficiency anemia
       Triose-phosphate isomerase deficiency anemia
       EXCLUDES 1   disorders of glycolysis not associated with anemia (E74.8)

   D55.3   Anemia due to disorders of nucleotide metabolism
   D55.8   Other anemias due to enzyme disorders
   D55.9   Anemia due to enzyme disorder, unspecified

Ⓝ Newborn: 0   Ⓟ Pediatric: 0-17   Ⓜ Maternity: 12-55   Ⓐ Adult: 15-124   **CH** Comorbidity High   **CL** Comorbidity Low   **NCDx** Noncancer Dx   **PDx** Primary Dx

498   ICD-10-CM 2020

☑️4ᵗʰ **D56   Thalassemia**

> *EXCLUDES 1*   *sickle-cell thalassemia (D57.4-)*
>
> **DEF:** Group of inherited disorders of hemoglobin metabolism causing mild to severe anemia. It is usually found in people of Mediterranean, African, Chinese, or Asian descent.

Thalassemia

Misshapen RBC

Misshapen RBC

Healthy RBC

D56.Ø   Alpha thalassemia
> Alpha thalassemia major
> Hemoglobin H Constant Spring
> Hemoglobin H disease
> Hydrops fetalis due to alpha thalassemia
> Severe alpha thalassemia
> Triple gene defect alpha thalassemia
> Use additional code, if applicable, for hydrops fetalis due to alpha thalassemia (P56.99)
>
> > *EXCLUDES 1*   *alpha thalassemia trait or minor (D56.3)*
> > *asymptomatic alpha thalassemia (D56.3)*
> > *hydrops fetalis due to isoimmunization (P56.Ø)*
> > *hydrops fetalis not due to immune hemolysis (P83.2)*
>
> **DEF:** HBA1 and HBA2 genetic variant of chromosome 16 prevalent among those of African and Southeast Asian descent. Alpha thalassemia is associated with a wide spectrum of anemic presentation and includes hemoglobin H disease subtypes.

D56.1   Beta thalassemia
> Beta thalassemia major
> Cooley's anemia
> Homozygous beta thalassemia
> Severe beta thalassemia
> Thalassemia intermedia
> Thalassemia major
>
> > *EXCLUDES 1*   *beta thalassemia minor (D56.3)*
> > *beta thalassemia trait (D56.3)*
> > *delta-beta thalassemia (D56.2)*
> > *hemoglobin E-beta thalassemia (D56.5)*
> > *sickle-cell beta thalassemia (D57.4-)*

D56.2   Delta-beta thalassemia
> Homozygous delta-beta thalassemia
>
> > *EXCLUDES 1*   *delta-beta thalassemia minor (D56.3)*
> > *delta-beta thalassemia trait (D56.3)*

D56.3   Thalassemia minor
> Alpha thalassemia minor
> Alpha thalassemia silent carrier
> Alpha thalassemia trait
> Beta thalassemia minor
> Beta thalassemia trait
> Delta-beta thalassemia minor
> Delta-beta thalassemia trait
> Thalassemia trait NOS
>
> > *EXCLUDES 1*   *alpha thalassemia (D56.Ø)*
> > *beta thalassemia (D56.1)*
> > *delta-beta thalassemia (D56.2)*
> > *hemoglobin E-beta thalassemia (D56.5)*
> > *sickle-cell trait (D57.3)*
>
> **DEF:** Solitary abnormal gene that identifies a carrier of the disease, yet with an absence of symptoms or a clinically mild anemic presentation.

D56.4   Hereditary persistence of fetal hemoglobin [HPFH]

D56.5   Hemoglobin E-beta thalassemia
> > *EXCLUDES 1*   *beta thalassemia (D56.1)*
> > *beta thalassemia minor (D56.3)*
> > *beta thalassemia trait (D56.3)*
> > *delta-beta thalassemia (D56.2)*
> > *delta-beta thalassemia trait (D56.3)*
> > *hemoglobin E disease (D58.2)*
> > *other hemoglobinopathies (D58.2)*
> > *sickle-cell beta thalassemia (D57.4-)*

D56.8   Other thalassemias
> Dominant thalassemia
> Hemoglobin C thalassemia
> Mixed thalassemia
> Thalassemia with other hemoglobinopathy
>
> > *EXCLUDES 1*   *hemoglobin C disease (D58.2)*
> > *hemoglobin E disease (D58.2)*
> > *other hemoglobinopathies (D58.2)*
> > *sickle-cell anemia (D57.-)*
> > *sickle-cell thalassemia (D57.4)*

D56.9   Thalassemia, unspecified
> Mediterranean anemia (with other hemoglobinopathy)

☑️4ᵗʰ **D57   Sickle-cell disorders**

> Use additional code for any associated fever (R5Ø.81)
>
> *EXCLUDES 1*   *other hemoglobinopathies (D58.-)*
>
> **DEF:** Severe, chronic inherited diseases caused by a genetic variation in hemoglobin protein of the red blood cell. The gene mutation causes the red blood cell to become hard, sticky, and crescent or sickle shaped making it harder for red blood cells to travel through the bloodstream disrupting blood flow and decreasing oxygen transport to tissues.

Sickle cell

Sickle cells

Normal RBCs

☑️5ᵗʰ **D57.Ø   Hb-SS disease with crisis**
> Sickle-cell disease NOS with crisis
> Hb-SS disease with vasoocclusive pain
>
> **D57.ØØ   Hb-SS disease with crisis, unspecified**
> **D57.Ø1   Hb-SS disease with acute chest syndrome**
> **D57.Ø2   Hb-SS disease with splenic sequestration**

☑️ Additional Character Required   √x7ᵗʰ Placeholder Alert   Manifestation   Unspecified Dx   ►◄ Revised Text   ● New Code   ▲ Revised Title

ICD-10-CM 2020   499

Chapter 3. Diseases of the Blood and Blood-forming Organs

D57.1 Sickle-cell disease without crisis
Hb-SS disease without crisis
Sickle-cell anemia NOS
Sickle-cell disease NOS
Sickle-cell disorder NOS

√5ᵗʰ **D57.2 Sickle-cell/Hb-C disease**
Hb-SC disease
Hb-S/Hb-C disease

    D57.20 Sickle-cell/Hb-C disease without crisis
√6ᵗʰ **D57.21 Sickle-cell/Hb-C disease** with crisis
      D57.211 Sickle-cell/Hb-C disease with acute chest syndrome
      D57.212 Sickle-cell/Hb-C disease with splenic sequestration
      D57.219 Sickle-cell/Hb-C disease with crisis, unspecified
        Sickle-cell/Hb-C disease with crisis NOS

D57.3 Sickle-cell trait
Hb-S trait
Heterozygous hemoglobin S
DEF: Heterozygous genetic makeup characterized by one gene for normal hemoglobin and one for sickle-cell hemoglobin. The clinical disease is rarely present.

√5ᵗʰ **D57.4 Sickle-cell** thalassemia
Sickle-cell beta thalassemia
Thalassemia Hb-S disease

    D57.40 Sickle-cell thalassemia without crisis
      Microdrepanocytosis
      Sickle-cell thalassemia NOS
√6ᵗʰ **D57.41 Sickle-cell thalassemia** with crisis
      Sickle-cell thalassemia with vasoocclusive pain
      D57.411 Sickle-cell thalassemia with acute chest syndrome
      D57.412 Sickle-cell thalassemia with splenic sequestration
      D57.419 Sickle-cell thalassemia with crisis, unspecified
        Sickle-cell thalassemia with crisis NOS

√5ᵗʰ **D57.8 Other sickle-cell disorders**
Hb-SD disease
Hb-SE disease

    D57.80 Other sickle-cell disorders without crisis
√6ᵗʰ **D57.81 Other sickle-cell disorders** with crisis
      D57.811 Other sickle-cell disorders with acute chest syndrome
      D57.812 Other sickle-cell disorders with splenic sequestration
      D57.819 Other sickle-cell disorders with crisis, unspecified
        Other sickle-cell disorders with crisis NOS

√4ᵗʰ **D58 Other** hereditary **hemolytic anemias**
EXCLUDES 1   hemolytic anemia of the newborn (P55.-)

D58.0 Hereditary spherocytosis
Acholuric (familial) jaundice
Congenital (spherocytic) hemolytic icterus
Minkowski-Chauffard syndrome
DEF: Inherited condition caused by mutations to genes responsible for the production of proteins that form the membranes of red blood cells. The shape and flexibility of the red blood cell membrane is altered diminishing the cells ability to traverse the spleen, therefore becoming trapped and destroyed before the red blood cell has reached maturity.

D58.1 Hereditary elliptocytosis
Elliptocytosis (congenital)
Ovalocytosis (congenital) (hereditary)

D58.2 Other hemoglobinopathies
Abnormal hemoglobin NOS
Congenital Heinz body anemia
Hb-C disease
Hb-D disease
Hb-E disease
Hemoglobinopathy NOS
Unstable hemoglobin hemolytic disease
EXCLUDES 1   familial polycythemia (D75.0)
       Hb-M disease (D74.0)
       hemoglobin E-beta thalassemia (D56.5)
       hereditary persistence of fetal hemoglobin [HPFH] (D56.4)
       high-altitude polycythemia (D75.1)
       methemoglobinemia (D74.-)
       other hemoglobinopathies with thalassemia (D56.8)

D58.8 Other specified hereditary hemolytic anemias
Stomatocytosis

D58.9 Hereditary hemolytic anemia, unspecified

√4ᵗʰ **D59** Acquired **hemolytic anemia**
DEF: Non-hereditary anemia characterized by premature destruction of red blood cells caused by infectious organisms, poisons, and physical agents.

D59.0 Drug-induced autoimmune hemolytic anemia
Use additional code for adverse effect, if applicable, to identify drug (T36-T50 with fifth or sixth character 5)

D59.1 Other autoimmune hemolytic anemias
Autoimmune hemolytic disease (cold type) (warm type)
Chronic cold hemagglutinin disease
Cold agglutinin disease
Cold agglutinin hemoglobinuria
Cold type (secondary) (symptomatic) hemolytic anemia
Warm type (secondary) (symptomatic) hemolytic anemia
EXCLUDES 1   Evans syndrome (D69.41)
       hemolytic disease of newborn (P55.-)
       paroxysmal cold hemoglobinuria (D59.6)

D59.2 Drug-induced nonautoimmune hemolytic anemia
Drug-induced enzyme deficiency anemia
Use additional code for adverse effect, if applicable, to identify drug (T36-T50 with fifth or sixth character 5)

D59.3 Hemolytic-uremic syndrome
Use additional code to identify associated:
    E. coli infection (B96.2-)
    Pneumococcal pneumonia (J13)
    Shigella dysenteriae (A03.9)
DEF: Condition typically precipitated by infection causing low platelets and destruction of red blood cells resulting in hemolytic anemia. This cell damage and blockage of renal capillaries lead to kidney failure. Mainly affects children.

D59.4 Other nonautoimmune hemolytic anemias
Mechanical hemolytic anemia
Microangiopathic hemolytic anemia
Toxic hemolytic anemia

D59.5 Paroxysmal nocturnal hemoglobinuria [Marchiafava-Micheli]
EXCLUDES 1   hemoglobinuria NOS (R82.3)

D59.6 Hemoglobinuria due to hemolysis from other external causes
Hemoglobinuria from exertion
March hemoglobinuria
Paroxysmal cold hemoglobinuria
Use additional code (Chapter 20) to identify external cause
EXCLUDES 1   hemoglobinuria NOS (R82.3)

D59.8 Other acquired hemolytic anemias

D59.9 Acquired hemolytic anemia, unspecified
Idiopathic hemolytic anemia, chronic

Aplastic and other anemias and other bone marrow failure syndromes (D60-D64)

√4ᵗʰ **D60 Acquired pure red cell aplasia [erythroblastopenia]**
INCLUDES   red cell aplasia (acquired) (adult) (with thymoma)
EXCLUDES 1   congenital red cell aplasia (D61.01)
DEF: Bone marrow failure characterized by underproduction of red blood cells while white blood cell and platelet production remains normal.

D60.0 Chronic acquired pure red cell aplasia
D60.1 Transient acquired pure red cell aplasia
D60.8 Other acquired pure red cell aplasias
D60.9 Acquired pure red cell aplasia, unspecified

✓4ᵗʰ D61 Other aplastic anemias and other bone marrow failure syndromes

    EXCLUDES 1   *neutropenia (D70.-)*

    AHA: 2014,4Q,22

    DEF: Aplastic anemia: Bone marrow failure characterized by underproduction of red bloods cells, white blood cells and platelets.

    ✓5ᵗʰ D61.0 Constitutional aplastic anemia

        D61.01 Constitutional (pure) red blood cell aplasia

            Blackfan-Diamond syndrome

            Congenital (pure) red cell aplasia

            Familial hypoplastic anemia

            Primary (pure) red cell aplasia

            Red cell (pure) aplasia of infants

            EXCLUDES 1   *acquired red cell aplasia (D60.9)*

        D61.09 Other constitutional aplastic anemia

            Fanconi's anemia

            Pancytopenia with malformations

    D61.1 Drug-induced aplastic anemia

        Use additional code for adverse effect, if applicable, to identify drug (T36-T50 with fifth or sixth character 5)

    D61.2 Aplastic anemia due to other external agents

        Code first, if applicable, toxic effects of substances chiefly nonmedicinal as to source (T51-T65)

    D61.3 Idiopathic aplastic anemia

    ✓5ᵗʰ D61.8 Other specified aplastic anemias and other bone marrow failure syndromes

        ✓6ᵗʰ D61.81 Pancytopenia

            EXCLUDES 1   *pancytopenia (due to) (with) aplastic anemia (D61.9)*

                      pancytopenia (due to) (with) bone marrow infiltration (D61.82)

                      pancytopenia (due to) (with) congenital (pure) red cell aplasia (D61.01)

                      pancytopenia (due to) (with) hairy cell leukemia (C91.4-)

                      pancytopenia (due to) (with) human immunodeficiency virus disease (B20)

                      pancytopenia (due to) (with) leukoerythroblastic anemia (D61.82)

                      pancytopenia (due to) (with) myeloproliferative disease (D47.1)

            EXCLUDES 2   *pancytopenia (due to) (with) myelodysplastic syndromes (D46.-)*

            DEF: Shortage of all three blood cells: white, red, and platelets.

            D61.810 Antineoplastic chemotherapy induced pancytopenia

                EXCLUDES 2   *aplastic anemia due to antineoplastic chemotherapy (D61.1)*

            D61.811 Other drug-induced pancytopenia

                EXCLUDES 2   *aplastic anemia due to drugs (D61.1)*

            D61.818 Other pancytopenia

                AHA: 2019,1Q,16

                TIP: Assign this code in addition to myeloid leukemia codes (C92.-) when pancytopenia is documented. Although common in some types of myeloid leukemia, pancytopenia is not always inherent.

        D61.82 Myelophthisis

            Leukoerythroblastic anemia

            Myelophthisic anemia

            Panmyelophthisis

            Code also the underlying disorder, such as:

                malignant neoplasm of breast (C50.-)

                tuberculosis (A15.-)

            EXCLUDES 1   *idiopathic myelofibrosis (D47.1)*

                      myelofibrosis NOS (D75.81)

                      myelofibrosis with myeloid metaplasia (D47.4)

                      primary myelofibrosis (D47.1)

                      secondary myelofibrosis (D75.81)

            DEF: Condition that occurs when normal hematopoietic tissue in the bone marrow is replaced with abnormal tissue, such as fibrous tissue or tumors. Most commonly seen during the advanced stages of cancer.

        D61.89 Other specified aplastic anemias and other bone marrow failure syndromes

D61.9 Aplastic anemia, unspecified

    Hypoplastic anemia NOS

    Medullary hypoplasia

D62 Acute posthemorrhagic anemia

    EXCLUDES 1   *anemia due to chronic blood loss (D50.0)*

                  blood loss anemia NOS (D50.0)

                  congenital anemia from fetal blood loss (P61.3)

✓4ᵗʰ D63 Anemia in chronic diseases classified elsewhere

    D63.0 Anemia in neoplastic disease

        Code first neoplasm (C00-D49)

        EXCLUDES 1   *aplastic anemia due to antineoplastic chemotherapy (D61.1)*

        EXCLUDES 2   *anemia due to antineoplastic chemotherapy (D64.81)*

    D63.1 Anemia in chronic kidney disease

        Erythropoietin resistant anemia (EPO resistant anemia)

        Code first underlying chronic kidney disease (CKD) (N18.-)

    D63.8 Anemia in other chronic diseases classified elsewhere

        Code first underlying disease, such as:

            diphyllobothriasis (B70.0)

            hookworm disease (B76.0-B76.9)

            hypothyroidism (E00.0-E03.9)

            malaria (B50.0-B54)

            symptomatic late syphilis (A52.79)

            tuberculosis (A18.89)

✓4ᵗʰ D64 Other anemias

    EXCLUDES 1   *refractory anemia (D46.-)*

                  refractory anemia with excess blasts in transformation [RAEB T] (C92.0-)

    DEF: Sideroblastic anemia: Hereditary or secondary disorder in which the red blood cells cannot effectively use iron, a nutrient needed to make hemoglobin. Although the iron can enter the red blood cell it is not assimilated into the hemoglobin molecule and builds up ringed sideroblasts around the cell nucleus.

    D64.0 Hereditary sideroblastic anemia

        Sex-linked hypochromic sideroblastic anemia

    D64.1 Secondary sideroblastic anemia due to disease

        Code first underlying disease

    D64.2 Secondary sideroblastic anemia due to drugs and toxins

        Code first poisoning due to drug or toxin, if applicable (T36-T65 with fifth or sixth character 1-4 or 6)

        Use additional code for adverse effect, if applicable, to identify drug (T36-T50 with fifth or sixth character 5)

    D64.3 Other sideroblastic anemias

        Sideroblastic anemia NOS

        Pyridoxine-responsive sideroblastic anemia NEC

    D64.4 Congenital dyserythropoietic anemia

        Dyshematopoietic anemia (congenital)

        EXCLUDES 1   *Blackfan-Diamond syndrome (D61.01)*

                    Di Guglielmo's disease (C94.0)

    ✓5ᵗʰ D64.8 Other specified anemias

        D64.81 Anemia due to antineoplastic chemotherapy

            Antineoplastic chemotherapy induced anemia

            EXCLUDES 1   *aplastic anemia due to antineoplastic chemotherapy (D61.1)*

            EXCLUDES 2   *anemia in neoplastic disease (D63.0)*

            AHA: 2014,4Q,22

            DEF: Reversible adverse effect of chemotherapy, causing inhibition of bone marrow production. A decrease in red blood cell production prevents adequate oxygenation of the tissues and organs causing fatigue, shortness of breath (SOB), and exacerbation of other medical conditions.

        D64.89 Other specified anemias

            Infantile pseudoleukemia

    D64.9 Anemia, unspecified

        AHA: 2018,4Q,88; 2017,1Q,7

☑ Additional Character Required   ✓x7ᵗʰ Placeholder Alert   Manifestation   Unspecified Dx   ►◄ Revised Text   ● New Code   ▲ Revised Title

Chapter 3. Diseases of the Blood and Blood-forming Organs

Coagulation defects, purpura and other hemorrhagic conditions (D65-D69)

D65 Disseminated intravascular coagulation [defibrination syndrome]
Afibrinogenemia, acquired
Consumption coagulopathy
Diffuse or disseminated intravascular coagulation [DIC]
Fibrinolytic hemorrhage, acquired
Fibrinolytic purpura
Purpura fulminans

> **EXCLUDES 1** disseminated intravascular coagulation (complicating): abortion or ectopic or molar pregnancy (O00-O07, O08.1)
> in newborn (P60)
> pregnancy, childbirth and the puerperium (O45.0, O46.0, O67.0, O72.3)

Coagulation

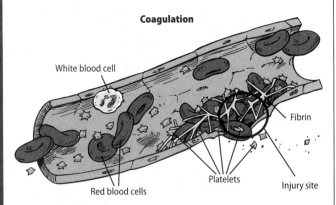

White blood cell
Fibrin
Red blood cells
Platelets
Injury site

D66 Hereditary factor VIII deficiency
Classical hemophilia
Deficiency factor VIII (with functional defect)
Hemophilia A
Hemophilia NOS

> **EXCLUDES 1** factor VIII deficiency with vascular defect (D68.0)

DEF: Hereditary, sex-linked lack of antihemophilic globulin (AHG) (factor VIII) that causes abnormal coagulation characterized by increased bleeding; large bruises of skin; bleeding in the mouth, nose, and gastrointestinal tract; and hemorrhages into joints, resulting in swelling and impaired function.

D67 Hereditary factor IX deficiency
Christmas disease
Factor IX deficiency (with functional defect)
Hemophilia B
Plasma thromboplastin component [PTC] deficiency

D68 Other coagulation defects

> **EXCLUDES 1** abnormal coagulation profile (R79.1)
> coagulation defects complicating abortion or ectopic or molar pregnancy (O00-O07, O08.1)
> coagulation defects complicating pregnancy, childbirth and the puerperium (O45.0, O46.0, O67.0, O72.3)

AHA: 2016,1Q,14

D68.0 Von Willebrand's disease
Angiohemophilia
Factor VIII deficiency with vascular defect
Vascular hemophilia

> **EXCLUDES 1** capillary fragility (hereditary) (D69.8)
> factor VIII deficiency NOS (D66)
> factor VIII deficiency with functional defect (D66)

DEF: Congenital, abnormal blood coagulation caused by deficient blood factor VII. Symptoms include excess or prolonged bleeding.

D68.1 Hereditary factor XI deficiency
Hemophilia C
Plasma thromboplastin antecedent [PTA] deficiency
Rosenthal's disease

D68.2 Hereditary deficiency of other clotting factors
AC globulin deficiency
Congenital afibrinogenemia
Deficiency of factor I [fibrinogen]
Deficiency of factor II [prothrombin]
Deficiency of factor V [labile]
Deficiency of factor VII [stable]
Deficiency of factor X [Stuart-Prower]
Deficiency of factor XII [Hageman]
Deficiency of factor XIII [fibrin stabilizing]
Dysfibrinogenemia (congenital)
Hypoproconvertinemia
Owren's disease
Proaccelerin deficiency

D68.3 Hemorrhagic disorder due to circulating anticoagulants

D68.31 Hemorrhagic disorder due to intrinsic circulating anticoagulants, antibodies, or inhibitors

D68.311 Acquired hemophilia
Autoimmune hemophilia
Autoimmune inhibitors to clotting factors
Secondary hemophilia

D68.312 Antiphospholipid antibody with hemorrhagic disorder
Lupus anticoagulant (LAC) with hemorrhagic disorder
Systemic lupus erythematosus [SLE] inhibitor with hemorrhagic disorder

> **EXCLUDES 1** antiphospholipid antibody, finding without diagnosis (R76.0)
> antiphospholipid antibody syndrome (D68.61)
> antiphospholipid antibody with hypercoagulable state (D68.61)
> lupus anticoagulant (LAC) finding without diagnosis (R76.0)
> lupus anticoagulant (LAC) with hypercoagulable state (D68.62)
> systemic lupus erythematosus [SLE] inhibitor finding without diagnosis (R76.0)
> systemic lupus erythematosus [SLE] inhibitor with hypercoagulable state (D68.62)

D68.318 Other hemorrhagic disorder due to intrinsic circulating anticoagulants, antibodies, or inhibitors
Antithromboplastinemia
Antithromboplastinogenemia
Hemorrhagic disorder due to intrinsic increase in antithrombin
Hemorrhagic disorder due to intrinsic increase in anti-VIIIa
Hemorrhagic disorder due to intrinsic increase in anti-IXa
Hemorrhagic disorder due to intrinsic increase in anti-XIa

D68.32 Hemorrhagic disorder due to extrinsic circulating anticoagulants
Drug-induced hemorrhagic disorder
Hemorrhagic disorder due to increase in anti-IIa
Hemorrhagic disorder due to increase in anti-Xa
Hyperheparinemia
Use additional code for adverse effect, if applicable, to identify drug (T45.515, T45.525)

AHA: 2016,1Q,14-15

TIP: Do not assign to identify routine therapeutic anticoagulation effects; assign only for documented adverse effects. An adverse effect code (T36–T50) identifying the specific therapeutic agent should also be assigned.

N Newborn: 0   P Pediatric: 0-17   M Maternity: 12-55   A Adult: 15-124   CH Comorbidity High   CL Comorbidity Low   NC Dx Noncancer Dx   PDx Primary Dx

502   ICD-10-CM 2020

Chapter 3. Diseases of the Blood and Blood-forming Organs

D68.4 Acquired coagulation factor deficiency
Deficiency of coagulation factor due to liver disease
Deficiency of coagulation factor due to vitamin K deficiency
  EXCLUDES 1 *vitamin K deficiency of newborn (P53)*

✓5ᵗʰ **D68.5 Primary thrombophilia**
Primary hypercoagulable states
  EXCLUDES 1 *antiphospholipid syndrome (D68.61)*
  lupus anticoagulant (D68.62)
  secondary activated protein C resistance (D68.69)
  secondary antiphospholipid antibody syndrome (D68.69)
  secondary lupus anticoagulant with hypercoagulable state (D68.69)
  secondary systemic lupus erythematosus [SLE] inhibitor with hypercoagulable state (D68.69)
  systemic lupus erythematosus [SLE] inhibitor finding without diagnosis (R76.0)
  systemic lupus erythematosus [SLE] inhibitor with hemorrhagic disorder (D68.312)
  thrombotic thrombocytopenic purpura (M31.1)
DEF: Thrombophilia: Increased tendency of the blood to clot, which can lead to thrombus or embolus formation.

D68.51 Activated protein C resistance
Factor V Leiden mutation

D68.52 Prothrombin gene mutation

D68.59 Other primary thrombophilia
Antithrombin III deficiency
Hypercoagulable state NOS
Primary hypercoagulable state NEC
Primary thrombophilia NEC
Protein C deficiency
Protein S deficiency
Thrombophilia NOS

✓5ᵗʰ **D68.6 Other thrombophilia**
Other hypercoagulable states
  EXCLUDES 1 *diffuse or disseminated intravascular coagulation [DIC] (D65)*
  heparin induced thrombocytopenia (HIT) (D75.82)
  hyperhomocysteinemia (E72.11)

D68.61 Antiphospholipid syndrome
Anticardiolipin syndrome
Antiphospholipid antibody syndrome
  EXCLUDES 1 *anti-phospholipid antibody, finding without diagnosis (R76.0)*
  anti-phospholipid antibody with hemorrhagic disorder (D68.312)
  lupus anticoagulant syndrome (D68.62)

D68.62 Lupus anticoagulant syndrome
Lupus anticoagulant
Presence of systemic lupus erythematosus [SLE] inhibitor
  EXCLUDES 1 *anticardiolipin syndrome (D68.61)*
  antiphospholipid syndrome (D68.61)
  lupus anticoagulant (LAC) finding without diagnosis (R76.0)
  lupus anticoagulant (LAC) with hemorrhagic disorder (D68.312)

D68.69 Other thrombophilia
Hypercoagulable states NEC
Secondary hypercoagulable state NOS

D68.8 Other specified coagulation defects
  EXCLUDES 1 *hemorrhagic disease of newborn (P53)*

D68.9 Coagulation defect, unspecified

✓4ᵗʰ **D69 Purpura and other hemorrhagic conditions**
  EXCLUDES 1 *benign hypergammaglobulinemic purpura (D89.0)*
  cryoglobulinemic purpura (D89.1)
  essential (hemorrhagic) thrombocythemia (D47.3)
  hemorrhagic thrombocythemia (D47.3)
  purpura fulminans (D65)
  thrombotic thrombocytopenic purpura (M31.1)
  Waldenström hypergammaglobulinemic purpura (D89.0)

D69.0 Allergic purpura
Allergic vasculitis
Nonthrombocytopenic hemorrhagic purpura
Nonthrombocytopenic idiopathic purpura
Purpura anaphylactoid
Purpura Henoch(-Schönlein)
Purpura rheumatica
Vascular purpura
  EXCLUDES 1 *thrombocytopenic hemorrhagic purpura (D69.3)*
DEF: Any hemorrhagic condition, thrombocytic or nonthrombocytopenic in origin, caused by a presumed allergic reaction.

D69.1 Qualitative platelet defects
Bernard-Soulier [giant platelet] syndrome
Glanzmann's disease
Grey platelet syndrome
Thromboasthenia (hemorrhagic) (hereditary)
Thrombocytopathy
  EXCLUDES 1 *von Willebrand's disease (D68.0)*

D69.2 Other nonthrombocytopenic purpura
Purpura NOS
Purpura simplex
Senile purpura

D69.3 Immune thrombocytopenic purpura
Hemorrhagic (thrombocytopenic) purpura
Idiopathic thrombocytopenic purpura
Tidal platelet dysgenesis
DEF: Tidal platelet dysgenesis: Fluctuation of platelet counts from normal to very low within periods of 20 to 40 days and may involve autoimmune platelet destruction.

✓5ᵗʰ **D69.4 Other primary thrombocytopenia**
  EXCLUDES 1 *transient neonatal thrombocytopenia (P61.0)*
  Wiskott-Aldrich syndrome (D82.0)

D69.41 Evans syndrome

D69.42 Congenital and hereditary thrombocytopenia purpura
Congenital thrombocytopenia
Hereditary thrombocytopenia
Code first congenital or hereditary disorder, such as:
  thrombocytopenia with absent radius (TAR syndrome) (Q87.2)

D69.49 Other primary thrombocytopenia
Megakaryocytic hypoplasia
Primary thrombocytopenia NOS

✓5ᵗʰ **D69.5 Secondary thrombocytopenia**
  EXCLUDES 1 *heparin induced thrombocytopenia (HIT) (D75.82)*
  transient thrombocytopenia of newborn (P61.0)

D69.51 Posttransfusion purpura
Posttransfusion purpura from whole blood (fresh) or blood products
PTP

D69.59 Other secondary thrombocytopenia
AHA: 2014,4Q,22

D69.6 Thrombocytopenia, unspecified

D69.8 Other specified hemorrhagic conditions
Capillary fragility (hereditary)
Vascular pseudohemophilia

D69.9 Hemorrhagic condition, unspecified

✓ Additional Character Required   ✓x7ᵗʰ Placeholder Alert   Manifestation   Unspecified Dx   ►◄ Revised Text   ● New Code   ▲ Revised Title

Other disorders of blood and blood-forming organs (D70-D77)

✓4ᵗʰ D70 Neutropenia

INCLUDES   agranulocytosis
decreased absolute neurophile count (ANC)

Use additional code for any associated:
fever (R50.81)
mucositis (J34.81, K12.3-, K92.81, N76.81)

EXCLUDES 1   neutropenic splenomegaly (D73.81)
transient neonatal neutropenia (P61.5)

DEF: Abnormally low number of neutrophils. Neutrophils are phagocytic, meaning they surround and consume harmful pathogens, primarily bacteria. When neutrophil counts decrease the risk of infection increases.

D70.0 Congenital agranulocytosis
Congenital neutropenia
Infantile genetic agranulocytosis
Kostmann's disease

D70.1 Agranulocytosis secondary to cancer chemotherapy
Code also underlying neoplasm
Use additional code for adverse effect, if applicable, to identify drug (T45.1X5)
AHA: 2014,4Q,22

D70.2 Other drug-induced agranulocytosis
Use additional code for adverse effect, if applicable, to identify drug (T36-T50 with fifth or sixth character 5)

D70.3 Neutropenia due to infection

D70.4 Cyclic neutropenia
Cyclic hematopoiesis
Periodic neutropenia

D70.8 Other neutropenia

D70.9 Neutropenia, unspecified

D71 Functional disorders of polymorphonuclear neutrophils
Cell membrane receptor complex [CR3] defect
Chronic (childhood) granulomatous disease
Congenital dysphagocytosis
Progressive septic granulomatosis

✓4ᵗʰ D72 Other disorders of white blood cells

EXCLUDES 1   basophilia (D72.824)
immunity disorders (D80-D89)
neutropenia (D70)
preleukemia (syndrome) (D46.9)

D72.0 Genetic anomalies of leukocytes
Alder (granulation) (granulocyte) anomaly
Alder syndrome
Hereditary leukocytic hypersegmentation
Hereditary leukocytic hyposegmentation
Hereditary leukomelanopathy
May-Hegglin (granulation) (granulocyte) anomaly
May-Hegglin syndrome
Pelger-Huët (granulation) (granulocyte) anomaly
Pelger-Huët syndrome
EXCLUDES 1   Chédiak (-Steinbrinck)-Higashi syndrome (E70.330)

D72.1 Eosinophilia
Allergic eosinophilia
Hereditary eosinophilia
EXCLUDES 1   Löffler's syndrome (J82)
pulmonary eosinophilia (J82)

✓5ᵗʰ D72.8 Other specified disorders of white blood cells
EXCLUDES 1   leukemia (C91-C95)

✓6ᵗʰ D72.81 Decreased white blood cell count
EXCLUDES 1   neutropenia (D70.-)

D72.810 Lymphocytopenia
Decreased lymphocytes

D72.818 Other decreased white blood cell count
Basophilic leukopenia
Eosinophilic leukopenia
Monocytopenia
Other decreased leukocytes
Plasmacytopenia

D72.819 Decreased white blood cell count, unspecified
Decreased leukocytes, unspecified
Leukocytopenia, unspecified
Leukopenia
EXCLUDES 1   malignant leukopenia (D70.9)

✓6ᵗʰ D72.82 Elevated white blood cell count
EXCLUDES 1   eosinophilia (D72.1)

D72.820 Lymphocytosis (symptomatic)
Elevated lymphocytes

D72.821 Monocytosis (symptomatic)
EXCLUDES 1   infectious mononucleosis (B27.-)

D72.822 Plasmacytosis

D72.823 Leukemoid reaction
Basophilic leukemoid reaction
Leukemoid reaction NOS
Lymphocytic leukemoid reaction
Monocytic leukemoid reaction
Myelocytic leukemoid reaction
Neutrophilic leukemoid reaction

D72.824 Basophilia
DEF: Increase in the basophils of the blood, a type of white blood cell, often seen in conjunction with neoplastic disorders.

D72.825 Bandemia
Bandemia without diagnosis of specific infection
EXCLUDES 1   confirmed infection — code to infection
leukemia (C91.-, C92.-, C93.-, C94.-, C95.-)
DEF: Increase in early neutrophil cells, called band cells that may indicate infection.

D72.828 Other elevated white blood cell count

D72.829 Elevated white blood cell count, unspecified
Elevated leukocytes, unspecified
Leukocytosis, unspecified

D72.89 Other specified disorders of white blood cells
Abnormality of white blood cells NEC

D72.9 Disorder of white blood cells, unspecified
Abnormal leukocyte differential NOS

✓4ᵗʰ D73 Diseases of spleen

D73.0 Hyposplenism
Atrophy of spleen
EXCLUDES 1   asplenia (congenital) (Q89.01)
postsurgical absence of spleen (Z90.81)

D73.1 Hypersplenism
EXCLUDES 1   neutropenic splenomegaly (D73.81)
primary splenic neutropenia (D73.81)
splenitis, splenomegaly in late syphilis (A52.79)
splenitis, splenomegaly in tuberculosis (A18.85)
splenomegaly NOS (R16.1)
splenomegaly congenital (Q89.0)

D73.2 Chronic congestive splenomegaly

D73.3 Abscess of spleen

D73.4 Cyst of spleen

D73.5 Infarction of spleen
Splenic rupture, nontraumatic
Torsion of spleen
EXCLUDES 1   rupture of spleen due to Plasmodium vivax malaria (B51.0)
traumatic rupture of spleen (S36.03-)

✓5ᵗʰ D73.8 Other diseases of spleen

D73.81 Neutropenic splenomegaly
Werner-Schultz disease

D73.89 Other diseases of spleen
Fibrosis of spleen NOS
Perisplenitis
Splenitis NOS

D73.9 Disease of spleen, unspecified

✓4ᵗʰ **D74 Methemoglobinemia**

D74.0 Congenital methemoglobinemia
Congenital NADH-methemoglobin reductase deficiency
Hemoglobin-M [Hb-M] disease
Methemoglobinemia, hereditary

D74.8 Other methemoglobinemias
Acquired methemoglobinemia (with sulfhemoglobinemia)
Toxic methemoglobinemia

D74.9 Methemoglobinemia, unspecified

✓4ᵗʰ **D75 Other and unspecified diseases of blood and blood-forming organs**
EXCLUDES 2　acute lymphadenitis (L04.-)
chronic lymphadenitis (I88.1)
enlarged lymph nodes (R59.-)
hypergammaglobulinemia NOS (D89.2)
lymphadenitis NOS (I88.9)
mesenteric lymphadenitis (acute) (chronic) (I88.0)

D75.0 Familial erythrocytosis
Benign polycythemia
Familial polycythemia
EXCLUDES 1　hereditary ovalocytosis (D58.1)

D75.1 Secondary polycythemia
Acquired polycythemia
Emotional polycythemia
Erythrocytosis NOS
Hypoxemic polycythemia
Nephrogenous polycythemia
Polycythemia due to erythropoietin
Polycythemia due to fall in plasma volume
Polycythemia due to high altitude
Polycythemia due to stress
Polycythemia NOS
Relative polycythemia
EXCLUDES 1　polycythemia neonatorum (P61.1)
polycythemia vera (D45)
DEF: Elevated number of red blood cells in circulating blood as a result of reduced oxygen supply to the tissues.

✓5ᵗʰ **D75.8 Other specified diseases of blood and blood-forming organs**

D75.81 Myelofibrosis
Myelofibrosis NOS
Secondary myelofibrosis NOS
Code first the underlying disorder, such as:
malignant neoplasm of breast (C50.-)
Use additional code, if applicable, for associated therapy-related myelodysplastic syndrome (D46.-)
Use additional code for adverse effect, if applicable, to identify drug (T45.1X5)
EXCLUDES 1　acute myelofibrosis (C94.4-)
idiopathic myelofibrosis (D47.1)
leukoerythroblastic anemia (D61.82)
myelofibrosis with myeloid metaplasia (D47.4)
myelophthisic anemia (D61.82)
myelophthisis (D61.82)
primary myelofibrosis (D47.1)

D75.82 Heparin induced thrombocytopenia (HIT)
DEF: Immune-mediated reaction to heparin therapy causing an abrupt fall in platelet count and serious complications such as pulmonary embolism, stroke, AMI, or DVT.

D75.89 Other specified diseases of blood and blood-forming organs

D75.9 Disease of blood and blood-forming organs, unspecified

● **D75.A Glucose-6-phosphate dehydrogenase (G6PD) deficiency without anemia**
EXCLUDES 1　glucose-6-phosphate dehydrogenase (G6PD) deficiency with anemia (D55.0)

✓4ᵗʰ **D76 Other specified diseases with participation of lymphoreticular and reticulohistiocytic tissue**
EXCLUDES 1　(Abt-) Letterer-Siwe disease (C96.0)
eosinophilic granuloma (C96.6)
Hand-Schüller-Christian disease (C96.5)
histiocytic medullary reticulosis (C96.9)
histiocytic sarcoma (C96.A)
histiocytosis X, multifocal (C96.5)
histiocytosis X, unifocal (C96.6)
Langerhans-cell histiocytosis, multifocal (C96.5)
Langerhans-cell histiocytosis NOS (C96.6)
Langerhans-cell histiocytosis, unifocal (C96.6)
leukemic reticuloendotheliosis (C91.4-)
lipomelanotic reticulosis (I89.8)
malignant histiocytosis (C96.A)
malignant reticulosis (C86.0)
nonlipid reticuloendotheliosis (C96.0)

D76.1 Hemophagocytic lymphohistiocytosis
Familial hemophagocytic reticulosis
Histiocytoses of mononuclear phagocytes

D76.2 Hemophagocytic syndrome, infection-associated
Use additional code to identify infectious agent or disease

D76.3 Other histiocytosis syndromes
Reticulohistiocytoma (giant-cell)
Sinus histiocytosis with massive lymphadenopathy
Xanthogranuloma

D77 Other disorders of blood and blood-forming organs in diseases classified elsewhere
Code first underlying disease, such as:
amyloidosis (E85.-)
congenital early syphilis (A50.0)
echinococcosis (B67.0-B67.9)
malaria (B50.0-B54)
schistosomiasis [bilharziasis] (B65.0-B65.9)
vitamin C deficiency (E54)
EXCLUDES 1　rupture of spleen due to Plasmodium vivax malaria (B51.0)
splenitis, splenomegaly in late syphilis (A52.79)
splenitis, splenomegaly in tuberculosis (A18.85)

Intraoperative and postprocedural complications of the spleen (D78)

✓4ᵗʰ **D78 Intraoperative and postprocedural complications of the spleen**
AHA: 2016,4Q,9-10

✓5ᵗʰ **D78.0 Intraoperative hemorrhage and hematoma of the spleen complicating a procedure**
EXCLUDES 1　intraoperative hemorrhage and hematoma of the spleen due to accidental puncture or laceration during a procedure (D78.1-)

D78.01 Intraoperative hemorrhage and hematoma of the spleen complicating a procedure on the spleen

D78.02 Intraoperative hemorrhage and hematoma of the spleen complicating other procedure

✓5ᵗʰ **D78.1 Accidental puncture and laceration of the spleen during a procedure**

D78.11 Accidental puncture and laceration of the spleen during a procedure on the spleen

D78.12 Accidental puncture and laceration of the spleen during other procedure

✓5ᵗʰ **D78.2 Postprocedural hemorrhage of the spleen following a procedure**

D78.21 Postprocedural hemorrhage of the spleen following a procedure on the spleen

D78.22 Postprocedural hemorrhage of the spleen following other procedure

✓5ᵗʰ **D78.3 Postprocedural hematoma and seroma of the spleen following a procedure**

D78.31 Postprocedural hematoma of the spleen following a procedure on the spleen

D78.32 Postprocedural hematoma of the spleen following other procedure

D78.33 Postprocedural seroma of the spleen following a procedure on the spleen

D78.34 Postprocedural seroma of the spleen following other procedure

✓5ᵗʰ **D78.8 Other intraoperative and postprocedural complications of the spleen**
Use additional code, if applicable, to further specify disorder

D78.81 Other intraoperative complications of the spleen

☑ Additional Character Required　　✓x7ᵗʰ Placeholder Alert　　Manifestation　　Unspecified Dx　　►◄ Revised Text　　● New Code　　▲ Revised Title

Chapter 3. Diseases of the Blood and Blood-forming Organs

D78.89   **Other** postprocedural **complications of the spleen**

Certain disorders involving the immune mechanism (D80-D89)

INCLUDES   defects in the complement system
immunodeficiency disorders, except human immunodeficiency virus [HIV] disease
sarcoidosis

EXCLUDES 1   *autoimmune disease (systemic) NOS (M35.9)*
functional disorders of polymorphonuclear neutrophils (D71)
human immunodeficiency virus [HIV] disease (B20)

✓4ᵗʰ **D80**   **Immunodeficiency with predominantly antibody defects**

D80.0   **Hereditary** hypogammaglobulinemia
Autosomal recessive agammaglobulinemia (Swiss type)
X-linked agammaglobulinemia [Bruton] (with growth hormone deficiency)

D80.1   **Nonfamilial** hypogammaglobulinemia
Agammaglobulinemia with immunoglobulin-bearing B-lymphocytes
Common variable agammaglobulinemia [CVAgamma]
Hypogammaglobulinemia NOS

D80.2   **Selective deficiency of** immunoglobulin A [IgA]

D80.3   **Selective deficiency of** immunoglobulin G [IgG] subclasses

D80.4   **Selective deficiency of** immunoglobulin M [IgM]

D80.5   **Immunodeficiency with** increased immunoglobulin M [IgM]

D80.6   **Antibody deficiency with** near-normal immunoglobulins or with hyperimmunoglobulinemia

D80.7   **Transient hypogammaglobulinemia** of infancy

D80.8   **Other immunodeficiencies with predominantly antibody defects**
Kappa light chain deficiency

D80.9   **Immunodeficiency with predominantly antibody defects, unspecified**

✓4ᵗʰ **D81**   **Combined immunodeficiencies**

EXCLUDES 1   *autosomal recessive agammaglobulinemia (Swiss type) (D80.0)*

D81.0   **Severe** combined immunodeficiency [SCID] with reticular dysgenesis

D81.1   **Severe** combined immunodeficiency [SCID] with low T- and B-cell numbers

D81.2   **Severe** combined immunodeficiency [SCID] with low or normal B-cell numbers

▲   ✓5ᵗʰ **D81.3**   **Adenosine deaminase [ADA] deficiency**

●   **D81.30**   **Adenosine deaminase deficiency, unspecified**
ADA deficiency NOS

●   **D81.31**   **Severe combined immunodeficiency** due to **adenosine deaminase deficiency**
ADA deficiency with SCID
Adenosine deaminase [ADA] deficiency with severe combined immunodeficiency

●   **D81.32**   **Adenosine deaminase 2 deficiency**
ADA2 deficiency
Adenosine deaminase deficiency type 2
Code also, if applicable, any associated manifestations, such as:
polyarteritis nodosa (M30.0)
stroke (I63.-)

●   **D81.39**   **Other adenosine deaminase deficiency**
Adenosine deaminase [ADA] deficiency type 1, NOS
Adenosine deaminase [ADA] deficiency type 1, without SCID
Adenosine deaminase [ADA] deficiency type 1, without severe combined immunodeficiency
Partial ADA deficiency (type 1)
Partial adenosine deaminase deficiency (type 1)

D81.4   **Nezelof's syndrome**

D81.5   **Purine nucleoside phosphorylase [PNP] deficiency**

D81.6   **Major histocompatibility complex class I deficiency**
Bare lymphocyte syndrome

D81.7   **Major histocompatibility complex class II deficiency**

✓5ᵗʰ **D81.8**   **Other combined immunodeficiencies**

✓6ᵗʰ **D81.81**   **Biotin-dependent carboxylase deficiency**
Multiple carboxylase deficiency
EXCLUDES 1   *biotin-dependent carboxylase deficiency due to dietary deficiency of biotin (E53.8)*

D81.810   **Biotinidase deficiency**

D81.818   **Other biotin-dependent carboxylase deficiency**
Holocarboxylase synthetase deficiency
Other multiple carboxylase deficiency

D81.819   **Biotin-dependent carboxylase deficiency, unspecified**
Multiple carboxylase deficiency, unspecified

D81.89   **Other combined immunodeficiencies**

D81.9   **Combined immunodeficiency, unspecified**
Severe combined immunodeficiency disorder [SCID] NOS

✓4ᵗʰ **D82**   **Immunodeficiency associated with other major defects**

EXCLUDES 1   *ataxia telangiectasia [Louis-Bar] (G11.3)*

D82.0   **Wiskott-Aldrich syndrome**
Immunodeficiency with thrombocytopenia and eczema

D82.1   **Di George's syndrome**
Pharyngeal pouch syndrome
Thymic alymphoplasia
Thymic aplasia or hypoplasia with immunodeficiency

D82.2   **Immunodeficiency with short-limbed stature**

D82.3   **Immunodeficiency following hereditary defective response to Epstein-Barr virus**
X-linked lymphoproliferative disease

D82.4   **Hyperimmunoglobulin E [IgE] syndrome**

D82.8   **Immunodeficiency associated with other specified major defects**

D82.9   **Immunodeficiency associated with major defect, unspecified**

✓4ᵗʰ **D83**   **Common variable immunodeficiency**

D83.0   **Common variable immunodeficiency** with predominant abnormalities of B-cell numbers and function

D83.1   **Common variable immunodeficiency** with predominant immunoregulatory T-cell disorders

D83.2   **Common variable immunodeficiency** with autoantibodies to B- or T-cells

D83.8   **Other common variable immunodeficiencies**

D83.9   **Common variable immunodeficiency, unspecified**

✓4ᵗʰ **D84**   **Other immunodeficiencies**

D84.0   **Lymphocyte function antigen-1 [LFA-1] defect**

D84.1   **Defects in the** complement system
C1 esterase inhibitor [C1-INH] deficiency

D84.8   **Other specified immunodeficiencies**

D84.9   **Immunodeficiency, unspecified**

✓4ᵗʰ **D86**   **Sarcoidosis**

DEF: Clustering of immune cells resulting in granuloma formation. Often affects the lungs and lymphatic system but can occur in other body sites.

D86.0   **Sarcoidosis of lung**

D86.1   **Sarcoidosis of lymph nodes**

D86.2   **Sarcoidosis of lung with sarcoidosis of lymph nodes**

D86.3   **Sarcoidosis of skin**

✓5ᵗʰ **D86.8**   **Sarcoidosis of other sites**

D86.81   **Sarcoid meningitis**

D86.82   **Multiple cranial nerve palsies in sarcoidosis**

D86.83   **Sarcoid iridocyclitis**

D86.84   **Sarcoid pyelonephritis**
Tubulo-interstitial nephropathy in sarcoidosis

D86.85   **Sarcoid myocarditis**

D86.86   **Sarcoid arthropathy**
Polyarthritis in sarcoidosis

D86.87   **Sarcoid myositis**

D86.89   **Sarcoidosis of other sites**
Hepatic granuloma
Uveoparotid fever [Heerfordt]

D86.9   **Sarcoidosis, unspecified**

✓4ᵗʰ **D89**   **Other disorders involving the immune mechanism, not elsewhere classified**

EXCLUDES 1   *hyperglobulinemia NOS (R77.1)*
monoclonal gammopathy (of undetermined significance) (D47.2)

EXCLUDES 2   *transplant failure and rejection (T86.-)*

D89.0   **Polyclonal hypergammaglobulinemia**
Benign hypergammaglobulinemic purpura
Polyclonal gammopathy NOS

N Newborn: 0   P Pediatric: 0-17   M Maternity: 12-55   A Adult: 15-124   CH Comorbidity High   CL Comorbidity Low   NCDx Noncancer Dx   PDx Primary Dx

506   ICD-10-CM 2020

D89.1 Cryoglobulinemia
   Cryoglobulinemic purpura
   Cryoglobulinemic vasculitis
   Essential cryoglobulinemia
   Idiopathic cryoglobulinemia
   Mixed cryoglobulinemia
   Primary cryoglobulinemia
   Secondary cryoglobulinemia

D89.2 Hypergammaglobulinemia, unspecified

D89.3 Immune reconstitution syndrome
   Immune reconstitution inflammatory syndrome [IRIS]
   Use additional code for adverse effect, if applicable, to identify
      drug (T36-T50 with fifth or sixth character 5)

✓5ᵗʰ **D89.4 Mast cell activation syndrome and related disorders**
   EXCLUDES 1   aggressive systemic mastocytosis (C96.21)
               congenital cutaneous mastocytosis (Q82.2)
               (non-congenital) cutaneous mastocytosis (D47.01)
               (indolent) systemic mastocytosis (D47.02)
               malignant mast cell neoplasm (C96.2-)
               malignant mastocytoma (C96.29)
               mast cell leukemia (C94.3-)
               mast cell sarcoma (C96.22)
               mastocytoma NOS (D47.09)
               other mast cell neoplasms of uncertain behavior
                  (D47.09)
               systemic mastocytosis associated with a clonal
                  hematologic non-mast cell lineage disease
                  (SM-AHNMD) (D47.02)
   AHA: 2016,4Q,11

   D89.40 Mast cell activation, unspecified
      Mast cell activation disorder, unspecified
      Mast cell activation syndrome, NOS

   D89.41 Monoclonal mast cell activation syndrome
   D89.42 Idiopathic mast cell activation syndrome
   D89.43 Secondary mast cell activation
      Secondary mast cell activation syndrome
      Code also underlying etiology, if known

   D89.49 Other mast cell activation disorder
      Other mast cell activation syndrome

✓5ᵗʰ **D89.8 Other specified disorders involving the immune mechanism,
         not elsewhere classified**

   ✓6ᵗʰ **D89.81 Graft-versus-host disease**
      Code first underlying cause, such as:
         complications of transplanted organs and tissue
            (T86.-)
         complications of blood transfusion (T80.89)
      Use additional code to identify associated
            manifestations, such as:
         desquamative dermatitis (L30.8)
         diarrhea (R19.7)
         elevated bilirubin (R17)
         hair loss (L65.9)

      D89.810 Acute graft-versus-host disease
      D89.811 Chronic graft-versus-host disease
      **D89.812 Acute on chronic graft-versus-host
                 disease**
      D89.813 Graft-versus-host disease, unspecified

   D89.82 Autoimmune lymphoproliferative syndrome [ALPS]
      DEF: Rare genetic alteration of the Fas protein that
      impairs normal cellular apoptosis (normal cell death),
      causing abnormal accumulation of lymphocytes in the
      lymph glands, liver, and spleen. Symptoms include
      neutropenia, anemia, and thrombocytopenia.

   **D89.89 Other specified disorders involving the immune
            mechanism, not elsewhere classified**
      EXCLUDES 1   human immunodeficiency virus disease
                       (B20)
      AHA: 2017,4Q,109

D89.9 Disorder involving the immune mechanism, unspecified
   Immune disease NOS
   AHA: 2015,3Q,22

☑ Additional Character Required   ✓x7ᵗʰ Placeholder Alert   Manifestation   Unspecified Dx   ▶◀ Revised Text   ● New Code   ▲ Revised Title

Chapter 4. Endocrine, Nutritional and Metabolic Diseases (E00–E89)

Chapter-specific Guidelines with Coding Examples

The chapter-specific guidelines from the ICD-10-CM Official Guidelines for Coding and Reporting have been provided below. Along with these guidelines are coding examples, contained in the shaded boxes, that have been developed to help illustrate the coding and/or sequencing guidance found in these guidelines.

a. Diabetes mellitus

The diabetes mellitus codes are combination codes that include the type of diabetes mellitus, the body system affected, and the complications affecting that body system. As many codes within a particular category as are necessary to describe all of the complications of the disease may be used. They should be sequenced based on the reason for a particular encounter. Assign as many codes from categories E08–E13 as needed to identify all of the associated conditions that the patient has.

> Patient is admitted with reported diagnoses of uncontrolled diabetes, type 2, with diabetic polyneuropathy and diabetic retinopathy with macular edema. Endocrinology clinical notes indicate a current HgA1c of 12.4 and "persistent blood glucose elevations over 300."
>
> **E11.65**   **Type 2 diabetes mellitus with hyperglycemia**
>
> **E11.311**   **Type 2 diabetes mellitus with unspecified diabetic retinopathy with macular edema**
>
> **E11.42**   **Type 2 diabetes mellitus with diabetic polyneuropathy**
>
> *Explanation*: Use as many codes to describe the diabetic complications as needed. Many are combination codes that describe more than one condition. "Uncontrolled" may reference hypo- or hyperglycemia, based upon available provider documentation.

1) Type of diabetes

The age of a patient is not the sole determining factor, though most type 1 diabetics develop the condition before reaching puberty. For this reason type 1 diabetes mellitus is also referred to as juvenile diabetes.

> A 45-year-old patient is diagnosed with Type 1 diabetes.
>
> **E10.9**   **Type 1 diabetes mellitus without complications**
>
> *Explanation*: Although most type 1 diabetics are diagnosed in childhood or adolescence, it can also begin in adults.

2) Type of diabetes mellitus not documented

If the type of diabetes mellitus is not documented in the medical record the default is E11.-, Type 2 diabetes mellitus.

> Patient is referred with new diagnoses reported in provider clinical notes as diabetes and hypertension.
>
> **E11.9**   **Type 2 diabetes mellitus without complications**
>
> **I10**   **Essential (primary) hypertension**
>
> *Explanation*: Since the type of diabetes was not documented and no complications were noted, the default code is E11.9.

3) Diabetes mellitus and the use of insulin and oral hypoglycemics

If the documentation in a medical record does not indicate the type of diabetes but does indicate that the patient uses insulin, code E11-, Type 2 diabetes mellitus, should be assigned. An additional code should be assigned from category Z79 to identify the long-term (current) use of insulin or oral hypoglycemic drugs. If the patient is treated with both oral medications and insulin, only the code for long-term (current) use of insulin should be assigned. Code Z79.4 should not be assigned if insulin is given temporarily to bring a type 2 patient's blood sugar under control during an encounter.

> Patient is referred with documented provider notes reporting 10-year history of diabetes requiring daily insulin use.
>
> **E11.9**   **Type 2 diabetes mellitus without complication**
>
> **Z79.4**   **Long term (current) use of insulin**
>
> *Explanation*: Do not assume that a patient requiring insulin use must have type 1 diabetes. The default for diabetes without further specification defaults to type 2. Add the code for long-term use of insulin.

4) Diabetes mellitus in pregnancy and gestational diabetes

See Section I.C.15. Diabetes mellitus in pregnancy.

See Section I.C.15. Gestational (pregnancy induced) diabetes

5) Complications due to insulin pump malfunction

(a) Underdose of insulin due to insulin pump failure

An underdose of insulin due to an insulin pump failure should be assigned to a code from subcategory T85.6, Mechanical complication of other specified internal and external prosthetic devices, implants and grafts, that specifies the type of pump malfunction, as the principal or first-listed code, followed by code T38.3X6-, Underdosing of insulin and oral hypoglycemic [antidiabetic] drugs. Additional codes for the type of diabetes mellitus and any associated complications due to the underdosing should also be assigned.

> A 76-year-old male with diabetic ESRD is admitted for rehabilitation and develops hyperglycemia. He has had an implanted insulin pump for 14 years and after returning from the ER, is noted to have experienced hyperglycemia due to a pump malfunction resulting in too little insulin being administered. On return, the blood sugars are resolving.
>
> **T85.614D**   **Breakdown (mechanical) of insulin pump, subsequent encounter**
>
> **T38.3X6D**   **Underdosing of insulin and oral hypoglycemic [antidiabetic] drugs, subsequent encounter**
>
> **E11.65**   **Type 2 diabetes mellitus with hyperglycemia**
>
> **E11.22**   **Type 2 diabetes mellitus with diabetic chronic kidney disease**
>
> **N18.6**   **End stage renal disease**
>
> *Explanation*: The complication code for the mechanical breakdown of the pump is sequenced first, followed by the underdosing code and type of diabetes with complication. If two or more diabetic complications are present, assign all codes needed to capture each complication. The seventh character D is used for a subsequent encounter.

(b) Overdose of insulin due to insulin pump failure

The principal or first-listed code for an encounter due to an insulin pump malfunction resulting in an overdose of insulin, should also be T85.6-, Mechanical complication of other specified internal and external prosthetic devices, implants and grafts, followed by code T38.3X1-, Poisoning by insulin and oral hypoglycemic [antidiabetic] drugs, accidental (unintentional).

> A 70-year-old female with type 2 diabetes is found on the floor and sent to the ER. On her return from the hospital, it is noted that a failure of her insulin pump, resulting in excess insulin administration, caused the hypoglycemia, resulting in her condition.
>
> **T85.614D**   **Breakdown (mechanical) of insulin pump, subsequent encounter**
>
> **T38.3X1D**   **Poisoning by insulin and oral hypoglycemic [antidiabetic] drugs, accidental (unintentional), subsequent encounter**
>
> **E11.649**   **Type 2 diabetes mellitus with hypoglycemia without coma**
>
> *Explanation*: The complication code for the mechanical breakdown of the pump is sequenced first, followed by the code for poisoning and type of diabetes with any associated complications. The seventh character D is used for subsequent encounter.

6) Secondary diabetes mellitus

Codes under categories E08, Diabetes mellitus due to underlying condition, E09, Drug or chemical induced diabetes mellitus, and E13, Other specified diabetes mellitus, identify complications/manifestations associated with secondary diabetes mellitus. Secondary diabetes is always caused by another condition or event (e.g., cystic fibrosis, malignant neoplasm of pancreas, pancreatectomy, adverse effect of drug, or poisoning).

(a) Secondary diabetes mellitus and the use of insulin or oral hypoglycemic drugs

For patients with secondary diabetes mellitus who routinely use insulin or oral hypoglycemic drugs, an additional code from category Z79 should be assigned to identify the long-term (current) use of insulin or oral hypoglycemic drugs. If the patient is treated with both oral medications and insulin, only the code for long-term (current) use of insulin should be assigned. Code Z79.4 should not be assigned if insulin is given temporarily to bring a secondary diabetic patient's blood sugar under control during an encounter.

Type 2 diabetic with diabetic polyneuropathy on insulin.

E11.42 **Type 2 diabetes mellitus with diabetic polyneuropathy**

Z79.4 **Long-term (current) use of insulin**

Explanation: Add the Z code for the long-term use of insulin because the insulin is taken chronically.

(b) Assigning and sequencing secondary diabetes codes and its causes

The sequencing of the secondary diabetes codes in relationship to codes for the cause of the diabetes is based on the Tabular List instructions for categories E08, E09 and E13.

(i) Secondary diabetes mellitus due to pancreatectomy

For postpancreatectomy diabetes mellitus (lack of insulin due to the surgical removal of all or part of the pancreas), assign code E89.1, Postprocedural hypoinsulinemia. Assign a code from category E13 and a code from subcategory Z90.41, Acquired absence of pancreas, as additional codes.

Patient with newly diagnosed diabetes after surgical removal of part of pancreas. Patient is now insulin-dependent following the procedure.

E89.1 **Postprocedural hypoinsulinemia**

E13.9 **Other specified diabetes mellitus without complications**

Z90.411 **Acquired partial absence of pancreas**

Z79.4 **Long term (current) use of insulin**

Explanation: Sequence the postprocedural complication of the hypoinsulinemia due to the partial removal of the pancreas as the first-listed code, followed by the other specified diabetes (NEC) with or without complications and the partial or total acquired absence of the pancreas. Instructional notes at E89.1 specify to "use additional code" for insulin use.

(ii) Secondary diabetes due to drugs

Secondary diabetes may be caused by an adverse effect of correctly administered medications, poisoning or sequela of poisoning.

See section I.C.19.e for coding of adverse effects and poisoning, and section I.C.20 for external cause code reporting.

Subsequent encounter for corticosteroid-induced diabetes mellitus.

E09.9 **Drug or chemical induced diabetes mellitus without complications**

T38.0X5D **Adverse effect of glucocorticoids and synthetic analogues, subsequent encounter**

Explanation: If the diabetes is caused by an adverse effect of a drug, the diabetic condition is coded first. If it occurs from a poisoning or overdose, the poisoning code causing the diabetes is sequenced first.

Chapter 4. Endocrine, Nutritional and Metabolic Diseases (E00-E89)

NOTE All neoplasms, whether functionally active or not, are classified in Chapter 2. Appropriate codes in this chapter (i.e. E05.8, E07.0, E16-E31, E34.-) may be used as additional codes to indicate either functional activity by neoplasms and ectopic endocrine tissue or hyperfunction and hypofunction of endocrine glands associated with neoplasms and other conditions classified elsewhere.

EXCLUDES 1 *transitory endocrine and metabolic disorders specific to newborn (P70-P74)*

AHA: 2018,2Q,6

This chapter contains the following blocks:

E00-E07	Disorders of thyroid gland
E08-E13	Diabetes mellitus
E15-E16	Other disorders of glucose regulation and pancreatic internal secretion
E20-E35	Disorders of other endocrine glands
E36	Intraoperative complications of endocrine system
E40-E46	Malnutrition
E50-E64	Other nutritional deficiencies
E65-E68	Overweight, obesity and other hyperalimentation
E70-E88	Metabolic disorders
E89	Postprocedural endocrine and metabolic complications and disorders, not elsewhere classified

Disorders of thyroid gland (E00-E07)

✓4ᵗʰ E00 Congenital iodine-deficiency syndrome

Use additional code (F70-F79) to identify associated intellectual disabilities

EXCLUDES 1 *subclinical iodine-deficiency hypothyroidism (E02)*

E00.0 Congenital iodine-deficiency syndrome, neurological type
Endemic cretinism, neurological type

E00.1 Congenital iodine-deficiency syndrome, myxedematous type
Endemic hypothyroid cretinism
Endemic cretinism, myxedematous type

E00.2 Congenital iodine-deficiency syndrome, mixed type
Endemic cretinism, mixed type

E00.9 Congenital iodine-deficiency syndrome, unspecified
Congenital iodine-deficiency hypothyroidism NOS
Endemic cretinism NOS

✓4ᵗʰ E01 Iodine-deficiency related thyroid disorders and allied conditions

EXCLUDES 1 *congenital iodine-deficiency syndrome (E00.-)*
subclinical iodine-deficiency hypothyroidism (E02)

E01.0 Iodine-deficiency related diffuse (endemic) goiter

E01.1 Iodine-deficiency related multinodular (endemic) goiter
Iodine-deficiency related nodular goiter

E01.2 Iodine-deficiency related (endemic) goiter, unspecified
Endemic goiter NOS

E01.8 Other iodine-deficiency related thyroid disorders and allied conditions
Acquired iodine-deficiency hypothyroidism NOS

E02 Subclinical iodine-deficiency hypothyroidism

✓4ᵗʰ E03 Other hypothyroidism

EXCLUDES 1 *iodine-deficiency related hypothyroidism (E00-E02)*
postprocedural hypothyroidism (E89.0)

DEF: Hypothyroidism: Underproduction of thyroid hormone.

E03.0 Congenital hypothyroidism with diffuse goiter
Congenital parenchymatous goiter (nontoxic)
Congenital goiter (nontoxic) NOS
EXCLUDES 1 *transitory congenital goiter with normal function (P72.0)*

E03.1 Congenital hypothyroidism without goiter
Aplasia of thyroid (with myxedema)
Congenital atrophy of thyroid
Congenital hypothyroidism NOS

E03.2 Hypothyroidism due to medicaments and other exogenous substances
Code first poisoning due to drug or toxin, if applicable (T36-T65 with fifth or sixth character 1-4 or 6)
Use additional code for adverse effect, if applicable, to identify drug (T36-T50 with fifth or sixth character 5)

E03.3 Postinfectious hypothyroidism

E03.4 Atrophy of thyroid (acquired)
EXCLUDES 1 *congenital atrophy of thyroid (E03.1)*

E03.5 Myxedema coma   **HCC**

E03.8 Other specified hypothyroidism

E03.9 Hypothyroidism, unspecified
Myxedema NOS

✓4ᵗʰ E04 Other nontoxic goiter

EXCLUDES 1 *congenital goiter (NOS) (diffuse) (parenchymatous) (E03.0)*
iodine-deficiency related goiter (E00-E02)

E04.0 Nontoxic diffuse goiter
Diffuse (colloid) nontoxic goiter
Simple nontoxic goiter

E04.1 Nontoxic single thyroid nodule
Colloid nodule (cystic) (thyroid)
Nontoxic uninodular goiter
Thyroid (cystic) nodule NOS
DEF: Enlarged thyroid, commonly due to decreased thyroid production, with a single nodule. No clinical hypothyroidism.

E04.2 Nontoxic multinodular goiter
Cystic goiter NOS
Multinodular (cystic) goiter NOS
DEF: Enlarged thyroid, commonly due to decreased thyroid production with multiple nodules. No clinical hypothyroidism.

E04.8 Other specified nontoxic goiter

E04.9 Nontoxic goiter, unspecified
Goiter NOS
Nodular goiter (nontoxic) NOS

✓4ᵗʰ E05 Thyrotoxicosis [hyperthyroidism]

EXCLUDES 1 *chronic thyroiditis with transient thyrotoxicosis (E06.2)*
neonatal thyrotoxicosis (P72.1)

DEF: Excessive quantities of hormones from the thyroid gland caused by overproduction or loss of storage ability.

✓5ᵗʰ E05.0 Thyrotoxicosis with diffuse goiter
Exophthalmic or toxic goiter NOS
Graves' disease
Toxic diffuse goiter
DEF: Diffuse thyroid enlargement accompanied by hyperthyroidism, bulging eyes, and dermopathy.

E05.00 Thyrotoxicosis with diffuse goiter without thyrotoxic crisis or storm

E05.01 Thyrotoxicosis with diffuse goiter with thyrotoxic crisis or storm

Goiter

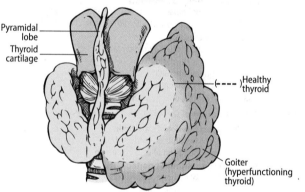

Labels: Pyramidal lobe; Thyroid cartilage; Healthy thyroid; Goiter (hyperfunctioning thyroid)

✓5ᵗʰ E05.1 Thyrotoxicosis with toxic single thyroid nodule
Thyrotoxicosis with toxic uninodular goiter
DEF: Symptomatic hyperthyroidism with a single nodule on the enlarged thyroid gland. Onset of symptoms can be abrupt and include extreme nervousness, insomnia, weight loss, tremors, and psychosis or coma.

E05.10 Thyrotoxicosis with toxic single thyroid nodule without thyrotoxic crisis or storm

E05.11 Thyrotoxicosis with toxic single thyroid nodule with thyrotoxic crisis or storm

✓5ᵗʰ E05.2 Thyrotoxicosis with toxic multinodular goiter
Toxic nodular goiter NOS

E05.20 Thyrotoxicosis with toxic multinodular goiter without thyrotoxic crisis or storm

E05.21 Thyrotoxicosis with toxic multinodular goiter with thyrotoxic crisis or storm

✓5ᵗʰ E05.3 Thyrotoxicosis from ectopic thyroid tissue

E05.30 Thyrotoxicosis from ectopic thyroid tissue without thyrotoxic crisis or storm

E05.31 Thyrotoxicosis from ectopic thyroid tissue with thyrotoxic crisis or storm

☑ Additional Character Required   ✓x7ᵗʰ Placeholder Alert   Manifestation   Unspecified Dx   ▶◀ Revised Text   ● New Code   ▲ Revised Title

ICD-10-CM 2020   511

Chapter 4. Endocrine, Nutritional and Metabolic Diseases

E05.4–E08.29

✓5ᵗʰ **E05.4 Thyrotoxicosis factitia**

     E05.40 Thyrotoxicosis factitia without thyrotoxic crisis or storm

     E05.41 Thyrotoxicosis factitia with thyrotoxic crisis or storm

✓5ᵗʰ **E05.8 Other thyrotoxicosis**

     Overproduction of thyroid-stimulating hormone

     E05.80 Other thyrotoxicosis without thyrotoxic crisis or storm

     E05.81 Other thyrotoxicosis with thyrotoxic crisis or storm

✓5ᵗʰ **E05.9 Thyrotoxicosis, unspecified**

     Hyperthyroidism NOS

     E05.90 Thyrotoxicosis, unspecified without thyrotoxic crisis or storm

     E05.91 Thyrotoxicosis, unspecified with thyrotoxic crisis or storm

✓4ᵗʰ **E06 Thyroiditis**

     EXCLUDES 1   postpartum thyroiditis (O90.5)

     DEF: Inflammation of the thyroid gland.

     E06.0 Acute thyroiditis

         Abscess of thyroid

         Pyogenic thyroiditis

         Suppurative thyroiditis

         Use additional code (B95-B97) to identify infectious agent

     E06.1 Subacute thyroiditis

         de Quervain thyroiditis

         Giant-cell thyroiditis

         Granulomatous thyroiditis

         Nonsuppurative thyroiditis

         Viral thyroiditis

         EXCLUDES 1   autoimmune thyroiditis (E06.3)

     E06.2 Chronic thyroiditis with transient thyrotoxicosis

         EXCLUDES 1   autoimmune thyroiditis (E06.3)

     E06.3 Autoimmune thyroiditis

         Hashimoto's thyroiditis

         Hashitoxicosis (transient)

         Lymphadenoid goiter

         Lymphocytic thyroiditis

         Struma lymphomatosa

     E06.4 Drug-induced thyroiditis

         Use additional code for adverse effect, if applicable, to identify drug (T36-T50 with fifth or sixth character 5)

     E06.5 Other chronic thyroiditis

         Chronic fibrous thyroiditis

         Chronic thyroiditis NOS

         Ligneous thyroiditis

         Riedel thyroiditis

     E06.9 Thyroiditis, unspecified

✓4ᵗʰ **E07 Other disorders of thyroid**

     E07.0 Hypersecretion of calcitonin

         C-cell hyperplasia of thyroid

         Hypersecretion of thyrocalcitonin

     E07.1 Dyshormogenetic goiter

         Familial dyshormogenetic goiter

         Pendred's syndrome

         EXCLUDES 1   transitory congenital goiter with normal function (P72.0)

✓5ᵗʰ **E07.8 Other specified disorders of thyroid**

     E07.81 Sick-euthyroid syndrome

         Euthyroid sick-syndrome

         DEF: Thyroid dysfunction caused by abnormal levels of thyroid hormones T3 and/or T4. This syndrome is often associated with starvation or critical illness.

     E07.89 Other specified disorders of thyroid

         Abnormality of thyroid-binding globulin

         Hemorrhage of thyroid

         Infarction of thyroid

     E07.9 Disorder of thyroid, unspecified

Diabetes mellitus (E08-E13)

AHA: 2018,4Q,88; 2018,3Q,3-4; 2018,2Q,6; 2017,4Q,6; 2017,1Q,42; 2016,4Q,11-13; 2016,2Q,36; 2016,1Q,11-13

TIP: There is no default code for diabetes mellitus documented only as uncontrolled. The provider must indicate whether the diabetic patient is hypoglycemic or hyperglycemic to determine the appropriate code.

✓4ᵗʰ **E08 Diabetes mellitus** due to underlying condition

     Code first the underlying condition, such as:

         congenital rubella (P35.0)

         Cushing's syndrome (E24.-)

         cystic fibrosis (E84.-)

         malignant neoplasm (C00-C96)

         malnutrition (E40-E46)

         pancreatitis and other diseases of the pancreas (K85-K86.-)

     Use additional code to identify control using:

         insulin (Z79.4)

         oral antidiabetic drugs (Z79.84)

         oral hypoglycemic drugs (Z79.84)

     EXCLUDES 1   *drug or chemical induced diabetes mellitus (E09.-)*

         gestational diabetes (O24.4-)

         neonatal diabetes mellitus (P70.2)

         postpancreatectomy diabetes mellitus (E13.-)

         postprocedural diabetes mellitus (E13.-)

         secondary diabetes mellitus NEC (E13.-)

         type 1 diabetes mellitus (E10.-)

         type 2 diabetes mellitus (E11.-)

     AHA: 2013,4Q,114; 2013,3Q,20

✓5ᵗʰ **E08.0 Diabetes mellitus due to underlying condition with** hyperosmolarity

     DEF: Diabetic hyperosmolarity: Extremely high levels of glucose in the blood without ketones.

     E08.00 *Diabetes mellitus due to underlying condition with hyperosmolarity* without nonketotic hyperglycemic-hyperosmolar coma (NKHHC)

     E08.01 *Diabetes mellitus due to underlying condition with hyperosmolarity* with coma

✓5ᵗʰ **E08.1 Diabetes mellitus due to underlying condition with** ketoacidosis

     DEF: Diabetic ketoacidosis: Potentially life-threatening complication due to a shortage of insulin in which the body switches to burning fatty acids and producing acidic ketone bodies.

     E08.10 *Diabetes mellitus due to underlying condition with ketoacidosis* without coma

     E08.11 *Diabetes mellitus due to underlying condition with ketoacidosis* with coma

✓5ᵗʰ **E08.2 Diabetes mellitus due to underlying condition with** kidney complications

     E08.21 *Diabetes mellitus due to underlying condition with diabetic* nephropathy

         Diabetes mellitus due to underlying condition with intercapillary glomerulosclerosis

         Diabetes mellitus due to underlying condition with intracapillary glomerulonephrosis

         Diabetes mellitus due to underlying condition with Kimmelstiel-Wilson disease

     E08.22 *Diabetes mellitus due to underlying condition with diabetic chronic kidney disease*

         Use additional code to identify stage of chronic kidney disease (N18.1-N18.6)

     E08.29 *Diabetes mellitus due to underlying condition with other diabetic kidney complication*

         Renal tubular degeneration in diabetes mellitus due to underlying condition

Ⓝ Newborn: 0   Ⓟ Pediatric: 0-17   Ⓜ Maternity: 12-55   Ⓐ Adult: 15-124   CH Comorbidity High   CL Comorbidity Low   NC DX Noncancer Dx   PD X Primary Dx

512

ICD-10-CM 2020

√5ᵗʰ **E08.3 Diabetes mellitus due to underlying condition with ophthalmic complications**

One of the following 7th characters is to be assigned to codes in subcategories E08.32, E08.33, E08.34, E08.35, and E08.37 to designate laterality of the disease:
1 right eye
2 left eye
3 bilateral
9 unspecified eye

√6ᵗʰ **E08.31 Diabetes mellitus due to underlying condition with unspecified diabetic retinopathy**
DEF: Diabetic retinopathy: Diabetic complication from damage to the retinal vessels resulting in vision problems that can progress to blindness.

E08.311 *Diabetes mellitus due to underlying condition with unspecified diabetic retinopathy with macular edema* CL

E08.319 *Diabetes mellitus due to underlying condition with unspecified diabetic retinopathy without macular edema*

√6ᵗʰ **E08.32 Diabetes mellitus due to underlying condition with mild nonproliferative diabetic retinopathy**
Diabetes mellitus due to underlying condition with nonproliferative diabetic retinopathy NOS

√7ᵗʰ E08.321 *Diabetes mellitus due to underlying condition with mild nonproliferative diabetic retinopathy with macular edema* CL

√7ᵗʰ E08.329 *Diabetes mellitus due to underlying condition with mild nonproliferative diabetic retinopathy without macular edema*

√6ᵗʰ **E08.33 Diabetes mellitus due to underlying condition with moderate nonproliferative diabetic retinopathy**

√7ᵗʰ E08.331 *Diabetes mellitus due to underlying condition with moderate nonproliferative diabetic retinopathy with macular edema* CL

√7ᵗʰ E08.339 *Diabetes mellitus due to underlying condition with moderate nonproliferative diabetic retinopathy without macular edema*

√6ᵗʰ **E08.34 Diabetes mellitus due to underlying condition with severe nonproliferative diabetic retinopathy**

√7ᵗʰ E08.341 *Diabetes mellitus due to underlying condition with severe nonproliferative diabetic retinopathy with macular edema* CL

√7ᵗʰ E08.349 *Diabetes mellitus due to underlying condition with severe nonproliferative diabetic retinopathy without macular edema*

√6ᵗʰ **E08.35 Diabetes mellitus due to underlying condition with proliferative diabetic retinopathy**

√7ᵗʰ E08.351 *Diabetes mellitus due to underlying condition with proliferative diabetic retinopathy with macular edema* CL

√7ᵗʰ E08.352 *Diabetes mellitus due to underlying condition with proliferative diabetic retinopathy with traction retinal detachment involving the macula*

√7ᵗʰ E08.353 *Diabetes mellitus due to underlying condition with proliferative diabetic retinopathy with traction retinal detachment not involving the macula*

√7ᵗʰ E08.354 *Diabetes mellitus due to underlying condition with proliferative diabetic retinopathy with combined traction retinal detachment and rhegmatogenous retinal detachment*

√7ᵗʰ E08.355 *Diabetes mellitus due to underlying condition with stable proliferative diabetic retinopathy*

√7ᵗʰ E08.359 *Diabetes mellitus due to underlying condition with proliferative diabetic retinopathy without macular edema*

E08.36 *Diabetes mellitus due to underlying condition with diabetic cataract*
AHA: 2019,2Q,30-31; 2016,4Q,142

√x7ᵗʰ E08.37 *Diabetes mellitus due to underlying condition with diabetic macular edema, resolved following treatment*

E08.39 *Diabetes mellitus due to underlying condition with other diabetic ophthalmic complication*
Use additional code to identify manifestation, such as:
diabetic glaucoma (H40-H42)

√5ᵗʰ **E08.4 Diabetes mellitus due to underlying condition with neurological complications**

E08.40 *Diabetes mellitus due to underlying condition with diabetic neuropathy, unspecified* CH CL

E08.41 **Diabetes mellitus due to underlying condition with diabetic mononeuropathy**

E08.42 **Diabetes mellitus due to underlying condition with diabetic polyneuropathy** CH CL
Diabetes mellitus due to underlying condition with diabetic neuralgia

E08.43 **Diabetes mellitus due to underlying condition with diabetic autonomic (poly)neuropathy**
Diabetes mellitus due to underlying condition with diabetic gastroparesis
AHA: 2013,4Q,114

E08.44 **Diabetes mellitus due to underlying condition with diabetic amyotrophy**

E08.49 **Diabetes mellitus due to underlying condition with other diabetic neurological complication**

√5ᵗʰ **E08.5 Diabetes mellitus due to underlying condition with circulatory complications**

E08.51 **Diabetes mellitus due to underlying condition with diabetic peripheral angiopathy without gangrene**
AHA: 2018,2Q,7

E08.52 **Diabetes mellitus due to underlying condition with diabetic peripheral angiopathy with gangrene**
Diabetes mellitus due to underlying condition with diabetic gangrene
AHA: 2018,2Q,7; 2017,4Q,102

E08.59 **Diabetes mellitus due to underlying condition with other circulatory complications**

√5ᵗʰ **E08.6 Diabetes mellitus due to underlying condition with other specified complications**

√6ᵗʰ **E08.61 Diabetes mellitus due to underlying condition with diabetic arthropathy**

E08.610 *Diabetes mellitus due to underlying condition with diabetic neuropathic arthropathy*
Diabetes mellitus due to underlying condition with Charcôt's joints
DEF: Charcot's joint: Progressive neurologic arthropathy in which chronic degeneration of joints in the weight-bearing areas with peripheral hypertrophy occurs as a complication of a neuropathy disorder. Supporting structures relax from a loss of sensation resulting in chronic joint instability.

E08.618 *Diabetes mellitus due to underlying condition with other diabetic arthropathy*
AHA: 2018,2Q,6

√6ᵗʰ **E08.62 Diabetes mellitus due to underlying condition with skin complications**

E08.620 *Diabetes mellitus due to underlying condition with diabetic dermatitis*
Diabetes mellitus due to underlying condition with diabetic necrobiosis lipoidica

E08.621 *Diabetes mellitus due to underlying condition with foot ulcer*
Use additional code to identify site of ulcer (L97.4-, L97.5-)
TIP: Do not assign a code for diabetic ulcer when the ulcer is closed/resolved or to report history of diabetic ulcers; Z86.31 Personal history of diabetic foot ulcer, may be assigned.

E08.622 Diabetes mellitus due to underlying condition with other skin ulcer
Use additional code to identify site of ulcer (L97.1-L97.9, L98.41-L98.49)
AHA: 2017,4Q,17

E08.628 Diabetes mellitus due to underlying condition with other skin complications
AHA: 2017,4Q,100-101

√6ᵗʰ **E08.63 Diabetes mellitus due to underlying condition with oral complications**

E08.630 Diabetes mellitus due to underlying condition with periodontal disease

E08.638 Diabetes mellitus due to underlying condition with other oral complications

√6ᵗʰ **E08.64 Diabetes mellitus due to underlying condition with hypoglycemia**

E08.641 Diabetes mellitus due to underlying condition with hypoglycemia with coma

E08.649 Diabetes mellitus due to underlying condition with hypoglycemia without coma
AHA: 2016,3Q,42; 2015,3Q,21

E08.65 Diabetes mellitus due to underlying condition with hyperglycemia

E08.69 Diabetes mellitus due to underlying condition with other specified complication
Use additional code to identify complication
AHA: 2016,4Q,141; 2016,1Q,13

E08.8 Diabetes mellitus due to underlying condition with unspecified complications

E08.9 Diabetes mellitus due to underlying condition without complications

√4ᵗʰ **E09 Drug or chemical induced diabetes mellitus**
Code first poisoning due to drug or toxin, if applicable (T36-T65 with fifth or sixth character 1-4 or 6)
Use additional code for adverse effect, if applicable, to identify drug (T36-T50 with fifth or sixth character 5)
Use additional code to identify control using:
insulin (Z79.4)
oral antidiabetic drugs (Z79.84)
oral hypoglycemic drugs (Z79.84)
EXCLUDES 1   diabetes mellitus due to underlying condition (E08.-)
gestational diabetes (O24.4-)
neonatal diabetes mellitus (P70.2)
postpancreatectomy diabetes mellitus (E13.-)
postprocedural diabetes mellitus (E13.-)
secondary diabetes mellitus NEC (E13.-)
type 1 diabetes mellitus (E10.-)
type 2 diabetes mellitus (E11.-)
AHA: 2013,4Q,114; 2013,3Q,20

√5ᵗʰ **E09.0 Drug or chemical induced diabetes mellitus with hyperosmolarity**
DEF: Diabetic hyperosmolarity: Extremely high levels of glucose in the blood without ketones.

E09.00 Drug or chemical induced diabetes mellitus with hyperosmolarity without nonketotic hyperglycemic-hyperosmolar coma (NKHHC)

E09.01 Drug or chemical induced diabetes mellitus with hyperosmolarity with coma

√5ᵗʰ **E09.1 Drug or chemical induced diabetes mellitus with ketoacidosis**
DEF: Diabetic ketoacidosis: Potentially life-threatening complication due to a shortage of insulin in which the body switches to burning fatty acids and producing acidic ketone bodies.

E09.10 Drug or chemical induced diabetes mellitus with ketoacidosis without coma

E09.11 Drug or chemical induced diabetes mellitus with ketoacidosis with coma

√5ᵗʰ **E09.2 Drug or chemical induced diabetes mellitus with kidney complications**

E09.21 Drug or chemical induced diabetes mellitus with diabetic nephropathy
Drug or chemical induced diabetes mellitus with intercapillary glomerulosclerosis
Drug or chemical induced diabetes mellitus with intracapillary glomerulonephrosis
Drug or chemical induced diabetes mellitus with Kimmelstiel-Wilson disease

E09.22 Drug or chemical induced diabetes mellitus with diabetic chronic kidney disease
Use additional code to identify stage of chronic kidney disease (N18.1-N18.6)

E09.29 Drug or chemical induced diabetes mellitus with other diabetic kidney complication
Drug or chemical induced diabetes mellitus with renal tubular degeneration

√5ᵗʰ **E09.3 Drug or chemical induced diabetes mellitus with ophthalmic complications**

One of the following 7th characters is to be assigned to codes in subcategories E09.32, E09.33, E09.34, E09.35, and E09.37 to designate laterality of the disease:
1   right eye
2   left eye
3   bilateral
9   unspecified eye

√6ᵗʰ **E09.31 Drug or chemical induced diabetes mellitus with unspecified diabetic retinopathy**
DEF: Diabetic retinopathy: Diabetic complication from damage to the retinal vessels resulting in vision problems that can progress to blindness.

E09.311 Drug or chemical induced diabetes mellitus with unspecified diabetic retinopathy with macular edema CL

E09.319 Drug or chemical induced diabetes mellitus with unspecified diabetic retinopathy without macular edema

√6ᵗʰ **E09.32 Drug or chemical induced diabetes mellitus with mild nonproliferative diabetic retinopathy**
Drug or chemical induced diabetes mellitus with nonproliferative diabetic retinopathy NOS

√7ᵗʰ **E09.321 Drug or chemical induced diabetes mellitus with mild nonproliferative diabetic retinopathy with macular edema** CL

√7ᵗʰ **E09.329 Drug or chemical induced diabetes mellitus with mild nonproliferative diabetic retinopathy without macular edema**

√6ᵗʰ **E09.33 Drug or chemical induced diabetes mellitus with moderate nonproliferative diabetic retinopathy**

√7ᵗʰ **E09.331 Drug or chemical induced diabetes mellitus with moderate nonproliferative diabetic retinopathy with macular edema** CL

√7ᵗʰ **E09.339 Drug or chemical induced diabetes mellitus with moderate nonproliferative diabetic retinopathy without macular edema**

√6ᵗʰ **E09.34 Drug or chemical induced diabetes mellitus with severe nonproliferative diabetic retinopathy**

√7ᵗʰ **E09.341 Drug or chemical induced diabetes mellitus with severe nonproliferative diabetic retinopathy with macular edema** CL

√7ᵗʰ **E09.349 Drug or chemical induced diabetes mellitus with severe nonproliferative diabetic retinopathy without macular edema**

√6ᵗʰ **E09.35 Drug or chemical induced diabetes mellitus with proliferative diabetic retinopathy**

√7ᵗʰ **E09.351 Drug or chemical induced diabetes mellitus with proliferative diabetic retinopathy with macular edema** CL

√7ᵗʰ **E09.352 Drug or chemical induced diabetes mellitus with proliferative diabetic retinopathy with traction retinal detachment involving the macula**

√7ᵗʰ **E09.353 Drug or chemical induced diabetes mellitus with proliferative diabetic retinopathy with traction retinal detachment not involving the macula**

√7ᵗʰ **E09.354 Drug or chemical induced diabetes mellitus with proliferative diabetic retinopathy** with combined traction retinal detachment and rhegmatogenous retinal detachment

√7ᵗʰ **E09.355 Drug or chemical induced diabetes mellitus** with stable proliferative diabetic retinopathy

√7ᵗʰ **E09.359 Drug or chemical induced diabetes mellitus with proliferative diabetic retinopathy** without macular edema

E09.36 Drug or chemical induced diabetes mellitus with diabetic cataract
    AHA: 2019,2Q,30-31; 2016,4Q,142

√x7ᵗʰ **E09.37 Drug or chemical induced diabetes mellitus with diabetic** macular edema, resolved following treatment

E09.39 Drug or chemical induced diabetes mellitus with other diabetic ophthalmic complication
    Use additional code to identify manifestation, such as:
      diabetic glaucoma (H40-H42)

√5ᵗʰ **E09.4 Drug or chemical induced diabetes mellitus with** neurological complications

E09.40 Drug or chemical induced diabetes mellitus with neurological complications with diabetic neuropathy, unspecified   CM CL

E09.41 Drug or chemical induced diabetes mellitus with neurological complications with diabetic mononeuropathy

E09.42 Drug or chemical induced diabetes mellitus with neurological complications with diabetic polyneuropathy   CM CL
    Drug or chemical induced diabetes mellitus with diabetic neuralgia

E09.43 Drug or chemical induced diabetes mellitus with neurological complications with diabetic autonomic (poly)neuropathy
    Drug or chemical induced diabetes mellitus with diabetic gastroparesis
    AHA: 2013,4Q,114

E09.44 Drug or chemical induced diabetes mellitus with neurological complications with diabetic amyotrophy

E09.49 Drug or chemical induced diabetes mellitus with neurological complications with other diabetic neurological complication

√5ᵗʰ **E09.5 Drug or chemical induced diabetes mellitus with** circulatory complications

E09.51 Drug or chemical induced diabetes mellitus with diabetic peripheral angiopathy without gangrene
    AHA: 2018,2Q,7

E09.52 Drug or chemical induced diabetes mellitus with diabetic peripheral angiopathy with gangrene
    Drug or chemical induced diabetes mellitus with diabetic gangrene
    AHA: 2018,2Q,7; 2017,4Q,102

E09.59 Drug or chemical induced diabetes mellitus with other circulatory complications

√5ᵗʰ **E09.6 Drug or chemical induced diabetes mellitus with other specified complications**

√6ᵗʰ **E09.61 Drug or chemical induced diabetes mellitus with diabetic** arthropathy

E09.610 Drug or chemical induced diabetes mellitus with diabetic neuropathic arthropathy
    Drug or chemical induced diabetes mellitus with Charcôt's joints
    DEF: Charcot's joint: Progressive neurologic arthropathy in which chronic degeneration of joints in the weight-bearing areas with peripheral hypertrophy occurs as a complication of a neuropathy disorder. Supporting structures relax from a loss of sensation resulting in chronic joint instability.

E09.618 Drug or chemical induced diabetes mellitus with other diabetic arthropathy
    AHA: 2018,2Q,6

√6ᵗʰ **E09.62 Drug or chemical induced diabetes mellitus with** skin complications

E09.620 Drug or chemical induced diabetes mellitus with diabetic dermatitis
    Drug or chemical induced diabetes mellitus with diabetic necrobiosis lipoidica

E09.621 Drug or chemical induced diabetes mellitus with foot ulcer
    Use additional code to identify site of ulcer (L97.4-, L97.5-)
    TIP: Do not assign a code for diabetic ulcer when the ulcer is closed/resolved or to report history of diabetic ulcers; Z86.31 Personal history of diabetic foot ulcer, may be assigned.

E09.622 Drug or chemical induced diabetes mellitus with other skin ulcer
    Use additional code to identify site of ulcer (L97.1-L97.9, L98.41-L98.49)
    AHA: 2017,4Q,17

E09.628 Drug or chemical induced diabetes mellitus with other skin complications
    AHA: 2017,4Q,100-101

√6ᵗʰ **E09.63 Drug or chemical induced diabetes mellitus with** oral complications

E09.630 Drug or chemical induced diabetes mellitus with periodontal disease

E09.638 Drug or chemical induced diabetes mellitus with other oral complications

√6ᵗʰ **E09.64 Drug or chemical induced diabetes mellitus with** hypoglycemia

E09.641 Drug or chemical induced diabetes mellitus with hypoglycemia with coma

E09.649 Drug or chemical induced diabetes mellitus with hypoglycemia without coma
    AHA: 2016,3Q,42; 2015,3Q,21

E09.65 Drug or chemical induced diabetes mellitus with hyperglycemia

E09.69 Drug or chemical induced diabetes mellitus with other specified complication
    Use additional code to identify complication
    AHA: 2016,4Q,141; 2016,1Q,13

E09.8 Drug or chemical induced diabetes mellitus with unspecified complications

E09.9 Drug or chemical induced diabetes mellitus without complications

√4ᵗʰ **E10 Type 1 diabetes mellitus**

    INCLUDES   brittle diabetes (mellitus)
        diabetes (mellitus) due to autoimmune process
        diabetes (mellitus) due to immune mediated pancreatic islet beta-cell destruction
        idiopathic diabetes (mellitus)
        juvenile onset diabetes (mellitus)
        ketosis-prone diabetes (mellitus)

    EXCLUDES 1   *diabetes mellitus due to underlying condition (E08.-)*
        drug or chemical induced diabetes mellitus (E09.-)
        gestational diabetes (O24.4-)
        hyperglycemia NOS (R73.9)
        neonatal diabetes mellitus (P70.2)
        postpancreatectomy diabetes mellitus (E13.-)
        postprocedural diabetes mellitus (E13.-)
        secondary diabetes mellitus NEC (E13.-)
        type 2 diabetes mellitus (E11.-)
    AHA: 2013,4Q,114; 2013,3Q,20

√5ᵗʰ **E10.1 Type 1 diabetes mellitus with** ketoacidosis
    AHA: 2013,3Q,20
    DEF: Diabetic ketoacidosis: Potentially life-threatening complication due to a shortage of insulin in which the body switches to burning fatty acids and producing acidic ketone bodies.

E10.10 Type 1 diabetes mellitus with ketoacidosis without coma   CM

E10.11 Type 1 diabetes mellitus with ketoacidosis with coma   CM

☑ Additional Character Required   √7ᵗʰ Placeholder Alert   Manifestation   Unspecified Dx   ▶◀ Revised Text   ● New Code   ▲ Revised Title

ICD-10-CM 2020   515

Chapter 4. Endocrine, Nutritional and Metabolic Diseases

E10.2–E10.620

√5ᵗʰ **E10.2 Type 1 diabetes mellitus with kidney complications**

E10.21 Type 1 diabetes mellitus with diabetic nephropathy `CH`

Type 1 diabetes mellitus with intercapillary glomerulosclerosis

Type 1 diabetes mellitus with intracapillary glomerulonephrosis

Type 1 diabetes mellitus with Kimmelstiel-Wilson disease

E10.22 Type 1 diabetes mellitus with diabetic chronic kidney disease `CH`

Use additional code to identify stage of chronic kidney disease (N18.1-N18.6)

E10.29 Type 1 diabetes mellitus with other diabetic kidney complication `CH`

Type 1 diabetes mellitus with renal tubular degeneration

AHA: 2016,1Q,13

√5ᵗʰ **E10.3 Type 1 diabetes mellitus with ophthalmic complications**

One of the following 7th characters is to be assigned to codes in subcategories E10.32, E10.33, E10.34, E10.35, and E10.37 to designate laterality of the disease:
1 right eye
2 left eye
3 bilateral
9 unspecified eye

√6ᵗʰ **E10.31 Type 1 diabetes mellitus with unspecified diabetic retinopathy**

DEF: Diabetic retinopathy: Diabetic complication from damage to the retinal vessels resulting in vision problems that can progress to blindness.

E10.311 Type 1 diabetes mellitus with unspecified diabetic retinopathy with macular edema `CL`

E10.319 Type 1 diabetes mellitus with unspecified diabetic retinopathy without macular edema `CH`

√6ᵗʰ **E10.32 Type 1 diabetes mellitus with mild nonproliferative diabetic retinopathy**

Type 1 diabetes mellitus with nonproliferative diabetic retinopathy NOS

√7ᵗʰ **E10.321 Type 1 diabetes mellitus with mild nonproliferative diabetic retinopathy with macular edema** `CL`

√7ᵗʰ **E10.329 Type 1 diabetes mellitus with mild nonproliferative diabetic retinopathy without macular edema** `CH`

√6ᵗʰ **E10.33 Type 1 diabetes mellitus with moderate nonproliferative diabetic retinopathy**

√7ᵗʰ **E10.331 Type 1 diabetes mellitus with moderate nonproliferative diabetic retinopathy with macular edema** `CL`

√7ᵗʰ **E10.339 Type 1 diabetes mellitus with moderate nonproliferative diabetic retinopathy without macular edema** `CH`

√6ᵗʰ **E10.34 Type 1 diabetes mellitus with severe nonproliferative diabetic retinopathy**

√7ᵗʰ **E10.341 Type 1 diabetes mellitus with severe nonproliferative diabetic retinopathy with macular edema** `CL`

√7ᵗʰ **E10.349 Type 1 diabetes mellitus with severe nonproliferative diabetic retinopathy without macular edema** `CH`

√6ᵗʰ **E10.35 Type 1 diabetes mellitus with proliferative diabetic retinopathy**

√7ᵗʰ **E10.351 Type 1 diabetes mellitus with proliferative diabetic retinopathy with macular edema** `CL`

√7ᵗʰ **E10.352 Type 1 diabetes mellitus with proliferative diabetic retinopathy with traction retinal detachment involving the macula** `CH`

√7ᵗʰ **E10.353 Type 1 diabetes mellitus with proliferative diabetic retinopathy with traction retinal detachment not involving the macula** `CH`

√7ᵗʰ **E10.354 Type 1 diabetes mellitus with proliferative diabetic retinopathy with combined traction retinal detachment and rhegmatogenous retinal detachment** `CH`

√7ᵗʰ **E10.355 Type 1 diabetes mellitus with stable proliferative diabetic retinopathy** `CH`

√7ᵗʰ **E10.359 Type 1 diabetes mellitus with proliferative diabetic retinopathy without macular edema** `CH`

E10.36 Type 1 diabetes mellitus with diabetic cataract `CH`

AHA: 2019,2Q,30-31; 2016,4Q,142

√×7ᵗʰ **E10.37 Type 1 diabetes mellitus with diabetic macular edema, resolved following treatment** `CH`

E10.39 Type 1 diabetes mellitus with other diabetic ophthalmic complication `CH`

Use additional code to identify manifestation, such as:
diabetic glaucoma (H40-H42)

√5ᵗʰ **E10.4 Type 1 diabetes mellitus with neurological complications**

E10.40 Type 1 diabetes mellitus with diabetic neuropathy, unspecified `CH` `CL`

E10.41 Type 1 diabetes mellitus with diabetic mononeuropathy `CH`

E10.42 Type 1 diabetes mellitus with diabetic polyneuropathy `CH` `CL`

Type 1 diabetes mellitus with diabetic neuralgia

E10.43 Type 1 diabetes mellitus with diabetic autonomic (poly)neuropathy `CH`

Type 1 diabetes mellitus with diabetic gastroparesis

AHA: 2013,4Q,114

E10.44 Type 1 diabetes mellitus with diabetic amyotrophy `CH`

E10.49 Type 1 diabetes mellitus with other diabetic neurological complication `CH`

√5ᵗʰ **E10.5 Type 1 diabetes mellitus with circulatory complications**

E10.51 Type 1 diabetes mellitus with diabetic peripheral angiopathy without gangrene `CH`

AHA: 2018,2Q,7

E10.52 Type 1 diabetes mellitus with diabetic peripheral angiopathy with gangrene `CH`

Type 1 diabetes mellitus with diabetic gangrene

AHA: 2018,2Q,7; 2017,4Q,102

E10.59 Type 1 diabetes mellitus with other circulatory complications `CH`

√5ᵗʰ **E10.6 Type 1 diabetes mellitus with other specified complications**

√6ᵗʰ **E10.61 Type 1 diabetes mellitus with diabetic arthropathy**

E10.610 Type 1 diabetes mellitus with diabetic neuropathic arthropathy `CH`

Type 1 diabetes mellitus with Charcôt's joints

DEF: Charcot's joint: Progressive neurologic arthropathy in which chronic degeneration of joints in the weight-bearing areas with peripheral hypertrophy occurs as a complication of a neuropathy disorder. Supporting structures relax from a loss of sensation resulting in chronic joint instability.

E10.618 Type 1 diabetes mellitus with other diabetic arthropathy `CH`

AHA: 2018,2Q,6

√6ᵗʰ **E10.62 Type 1 diabetes mellitus with skin complications**

E10.620 Type 1 diabetes mellitus with diabetic dermatitis `CH`

Type 1 diabetes mellitus with diabetic necrobiosis lipoidica

`N` Newborn: 0   `P` Pediatric: 0-17   `M` Maternity: 12-55   `A` Adult: 15-124   `CH` Comorbidity High   `CL` Comorbidity Low   `NCDx` Noncancer Dx   `PDx` Primary Dx

516   ICD-10-CM 2020

E10.621 **Type 1 diabetes mellitus with** `CH`
foot ulcer
Use additional code to identify site of ulcer (L97.4-, L97.5-)
TIP: Do not assign a code for diabetic ulcer when the ulcer is closed/resolved or to report history of diabetic ulcers; Z86.31 Personal history of diabetic foot ulcer, may be assigned.

E10.622 **Type 1 diabetes mellitus with** `CH`
other skin ulcer
Use additional code to identify site of ulcer (L97.1-L97.9, L98.41-L98.49)
AHA: 2017,4Q,17

E10.628 **Type 1 diabetes mellitus with** `CH`
other skin complications
AHA: 2017,4Q,100-101

√6ᵗʰ E10.63 **Type 1 diabetes mellitus with** oral complications

E10.630 **Type 1 diabetes mellitus with** `CH`
periodontal disease

E10.638 **Type 1 diabetes mellitus with** `CH`
other oral complications

√6ᵗʰ E10.64 **Type 1 diabetes mellitus with** hypoglycemia

E10.641 **Type 1 diabetes mellitus with** `CH`
hypoglycemia with coma

E10.649 **Type 1 diabetes mellitus with** `CH`
hypoglycemia without coma
AHA: 2016,3Q,42; 2016,1Q,13; 2015,3Q,21

E10.65 **Type 1 diabetes mellitus with** `CH`
hyperglycemia
AHA: 2013,3Q,20

E10.69 **Type 1 diabetes mellitus with other** `CH`
specified complication
Use additional code to identify complication
AHA: 2016,4Q,141; 2016,1Q,13

E10.8 **Type 1 diabetes mellitus with unspecified complications**

E10.9 **Type 1 diabetes mellitus** without complications `CH`

√4ᵗʰ **E11** Type 2 diabetes mellitus

`INCLUDES` diabetes (mellitus) due to insulin secretory defect
diabetes NOS
insulin resistant diabetes (mellitus)
Use additional code to identify control using:
insulin (Z79.4)
oral antidiabetic drugs (Z79.84)
oral hypoglycemic drugs (Z79.84)

`EXCLUDES 1` diabetes mellitus due to underlying condition (E08.-)
drug or chemical induced diabetes mellitus (E09.-)
gestational diabetes (O24.4-)
neonatal diabetes mellitus (P70.2)
postpancreatectomy diabetes mellitus (E13.-)
postprocedural diabetes mellitus (E13.-)
secondary diabetes mellitus NEC (E13.-)
type 1 diabetes mellitus (E10.-)

AHA: 2016,2Q,10; 2013,4Q,114; 2013,3Q,20; 2013,1Q,26

√5ᵗʰ **E11.0** Type 2 diabetes mellitus with hyperosmolarity
DEF: Diabetic hyperosmolarity: Extremely high levels of glucose in the blood without ketones.

E11.00 **Type 2 diabetes mellitus with** `CH`
hyperosmolarity without nonketotic hyperglycemic-hyperosmolar coma (NKHHC)

E11.01 **Type 2 diabetes mellitus with** `CH`
hyperosmolarity with coma

√5ᵗʰ **E11.1** Type 2 diabetes mellitus with ketoacidosis
DEF: Diabetic ketoacidosis: Potentially life-threatening complication due to a shortage of insulin in which the body switches to burning fatty acids and producing acidic ketone bodies.

E11.10 **Type 2 diabetes mellitus with** `CH`
ketoacidosis without coma

E11.11 **Type 2 diabetes mellitus with** `CH`
ketoacidosis with coma

√5ᵗʰ **E11.2** Type 2 diabetes mellitus with kidney complications

E11.21 **Type 2 diabetes mellitus with diabetic** `CH`
nephropathy
Type 2 diabetes mellitus with intercapillary glomerulosclerosis
Type 2 diabetes mellitus with intracapillary glomerulonephrosis
Type 2 diabetes mellitus with Kimmelstiel-Wilson disease

E11.22 **Type 2 diabetes mellitus with diabetic** `CH`
chronic kidney disease
Use additional code to identify stage of chronic kidney disease (N18.1-N18.6)
AHA: 2016,1Q,12

E11.29 **Type 2 diabetes mellitus with other** `CH`
diabetic kidney complication
Type 2 diabetes mellitus with renal tubular degeneration

√5ᵗʰ **E11.3** Type 2 diabetes mellitus with ophthalmic complications

One of the following 7th characters is to be assigned to codes in subcategories E11.32, E11.33, E11.34, E11.35, and E11.37 to designate laterality of the disease:
1   right eye
2   left eye
3   bilateral
9   unspecified eye

√6ᵗʰ E11.31 **Type 2 diabetes mellitus with unspecified diabetic**
retinopathy
DEF: Diabetic retinopathy: Diabetic complication from damage to the retinal vessels resulting in vision problems that can progress to blindness.

E11.311 **Type 2 diabetes mellitus with** `CL`
unspecified diabetic retinopathy with macular edema

E11.319 **Type 2 diabetes mellitus with** `CH`
unspecified diabetic retinopathy without macular edema

√6ᵗʰ E11.32 **Type 2 diabetes mellitus with** mild nonproliferative diabetic retinopathy
Type 2 diabetes mellitus with nonproliferative diabetic retinopathy NOS

√7ᵗʰ E11.321 **Type 2 diabetes mellitus with** `CL`
mild nonproliferative diabetic retinopathy with macular edema

√7ᵗʰ E11.329 **Type 2 diabetes mellitus with** `CH`
mild nonproliferative diabetic retinopathy without macular edema

√6ᵗʰ E11.33 **Type 2 diabetes mellitus with** moderate nonproliferative diabetic retinopathy

√7ᵗʰ E11.331 **Type 2 diabetes mellitus with** `CL`
moderate nonproliferative diabetic retinopathy with macular edema

√7ᵗʰ E11.339 **Type 2 diabetes mellitus with** `CH`
moderate nonproliferative diabetic retinopathy without macular edema

√6ᵗʰ E11.34 **Type 2 diabetes mellitus with** severe nonproliferative diabetic retinopathy

√7ᵗʰ E11.341 **Type 2 diabetes mellitus with** `CL`
severe nonproliferative diabetic retinopathy with macular edema

√7ᵗʰ E11.349 **Type 2 diabetes mellitus with** `CH`
severe nonproliferative diabetic retinopathy without macular edema

√6ᵗʰ E11.35 **Type 2 diabetes mellitus with** proliferative diabetic retinopathy

√7ᵗʰ E11.351 **Type 2 diabetes mellitus with** `CL`
proliferative diabetic retinopathy with macular edema

√7ᵗʰ E11.352 **Type 2 diabetes mellitus with** `CH`
proliferative diabetic retinopathy with traction retinal detachment involving the macula

Chapter 4. Endocrine, Nutritional and Metabolic Diseases

✓7ᵗʰ **E11.353** **Type 2 diabetes mellitus with proliferative diabetic retinopathy** with traction retinal detachment not involving the macula   CH

✓7ᵗʰ **E11.354** **Type 2 diabetes mellitus with proliferative diabetic retinopathy** with combined traction retinal detachment and rhegmatogenous retinal detachment   CH

✓7ᵗʰ **E11.355** **Type 2 diabetes mellitus** with **stable proliferative diabetic retinopathy**   CH

✓7ᵗʰ **E11.359** **Type 2 diabetes mellitus with proliferative diabetic retinopathy** without macular edema   CH

E11.36 **Type 2 diabetes mellitus with diabetic cataract**   CH
     AHA: 2019,2Q,30-31; 2016,4Q,142

✓x7ᵗʰ **E11.37** **Type 2 diabetes mellitus with diabetic macular edema, resolved following treatment**   CH

E11.39 **Type 2 diabetes mellitus with other diabetic ophthalmic complication**   CH
     Use additional code to identify manifestation, such as:
         diabetic glaucoma (H40-H42)

✓5ᵗʰ **E11.4** **Type 2 diabetes mellitus with** neurological complications

E11.40 **Type 2 diabetes mellitus with diabetic neuropathy, unspecified**   CH CL
     AHA: 2013,4Q,129

E11.41 **Type 2 diabetes mellitus with diabetic mononeuropathy**   CH

E11.42 **Type 2 diabetes mellitus with diabetic polyneuropathy**   CH CL
     Type 2 diabetes mellitus with diabetic neuralgia
     AHA: 2016,1Q,12

E11.43 **Type 2 diabetes mellitus with diabetic autonomic (poly)neuropathy**   CH
     Type 2 diabetes mellitus with diabetic gastroparesis
     AHA: 2013,4Q,114

E11.44 **Type 2 diabetes mellitus with diabetic amyotrophy**   CH

E11.49 **Type 2 diabetes mellitus with other diabetic neurological complication**   CH

✓5ᵗʰ **E11.5** **Type 2 diabetes mellitus with** circulatory complications

E11.51 **Type 2 diabetes mellitus with diabetic peripheral angiopathy without gangrene**   CH
     AHA: 2018,2Q,7

E11.52 **Type 2 diabetes mellitus with diabetic peripheral angiopathy with gangrene**   CH
     Type 2 diabetes mellitus with diabetic gangrene
     AHA: 2018,2Q,7; 2017,4Q,102

E11.59 **Type 2 diabetes mellitus with other circulatory complications**   CH

✓5ᵗʰ **E11.6** **Type 2 diabetes mellitus with other specified complications**

✓6ᵗʰ **E11.61** **Type 2 diabetes mellitus with diabetic** arthropathy

E11.610 **Type 2 diabetes mellitus with diabetic** neuropathic **arthropathy**   CH
     Type 2 diabetes mellitus with Charcôt's joints
     DEF: Charcot's joint: Progressive neurologic arthropathy in which chronic degeneration of joints in the weight-bearing areas with peripheral hypertrophy occurs as a complication of a neuropathy disorder. Supporting structures relax from a loss of sensation resulting in chronic joint instability.

E11.618 **Type 2 diabetes mellitus with other diabetic arthropathy**   CH
     AHA: 2018,2Q,6

✓6ᵗʰ **E11.62** **Type 2 diabetes mellitus with** skin complications

E11.620 **Type 2 diabetes mellitus with** diabetic dermatitis   CH
     Type 2 diabetes mellitus with diabetic necrobiosis lipoidica

E11.621 **Type 2 diabetes mellitus with foot ulcer**   CH
     Use additional code to identify site of ulcer (L97.4-, L97.5-)
     AHA: 2016,1Q,12
     TIP: Do not assign a code for diabetic ulcer when the ulcer is closed/resolved or to report history of diabetic ulcers; Z86.31 Personal history of diabetic foot ulcer may be assigned.

E11.622 **Type 2 diabetes mellitus with other skin ulcer**   CH
     Use additional code to identify site of ulcer (L97.1-L97.9, L98.41-L98.49)
     AHA: 2017,4Q,17

E11.628 **Type 2 diabetes mellitus with other skin complications**   CH
     AHA: 2017,4Q,100-101

✓6ᵗʰ **E11.63** **Type 2 diabetes mellitus with** oral complications

E11.630 **Type 2 diabetes mellitus with** periodontal disease   CH

E11.638 **Type 2 diabetes mellitus with other oral complications**   CH

✓6ᵗʰ **E11.64** **Type 2 diabetes mellitus with** hypoglycemia

E11.641 **Type 2 diabetes mellitus with hypoglycemia** with coma   CH

E11.649 **Type 2 diabetes mellitus with hypoglycemia** without coma   CH
     AHA: 2016,3Q,42; 2015,3Q,21

E11.65 **Type 2 diabetes mellitus with** hyperglycemia   CH
     AHA: 2013,3Q,20

E11.69 **Type 2 diabetes mellitus with other specified complication**   CH
     Use additional code to identify complication
     AHA: 2016,4Q,141; 2016,1Q,13

E11.8 **Type 2 diabetes mellitus with unspecified complications**

E11.9 **Type 2 diabetes mellitus** without complications   CH

✓4ᵗʰ **E13** **Other specified diabetes mellitus**
     INCLUDES   diabetes mellitus due to genetic defects of beta-cell function
         diabetes mellitus due to genetic defects in insulin action
         postpancreatectomy diabetes mellitus
         postprocedural diabetes mellitus
         secondary diabetes mellitus NEC
     Use additional code to identify control using:
     insulin (Z79.4)
     oral antidiabetic drugs (Z79.84)
     oral hypoglycemic drugs (Z79.84)
     EXCLUDES 1   diabetes (mellitus) due to autoimmune process (E10.-)
         diabetes (mellitus) due to immune mediated pancreatic islet beta-cell destruction (E10.-)
         diabetes mellitus due to underlying condition (E08.-)
         drug or chemical induced diabetes mellitus (E09.-)
         gestational diabetes (O24.4-)
         neonatal diabetes mellitus (P70.2)
         type 1 diabetes mellitus (E10.-)
     AHA: 2018,3Q,4; 2016,1Q,11-13; 2013,4Q,114; 2013,3Q,20
     TIP: When postprocedural or postpancreatectomy hypoinsulinemia (E89.1) is documented with postprocedural or postpancreatectomy diabetes mellitus (E13.-), code E89.1 should be sequenced first.
     TIP: Use this category when the diabetes is documented as diabetes type 1.5. Synonymous terms used in the documentation may also include combined diabetes type 1 and type 2, latent autoimmune diabetes of adults (LADA), slow-progressing type 1 diabetes, or double diabetes.

✓5ᵗʰ **E13.0** **Other specified diabetes mellitus with** hyperosmolarity
     DEF: Diabetic hyperosmolarity: Extremely high levels of glucose in the blood without ketones.

E13.00 **Other specified diabetes mellitus with hyperosmolarity** without nonketotic hyperglycemic-hyperosmolar coma (NKHHC)   CH
     EXCLUDES 2   type 2 diabetes mellitus (E11.-)

E13.01   Other specified diabetes mellitus with hyperosmolarity with coma `CH`

√5ᵗʰ **E13.1   Other specified diabetes mellitus with** ketoacidosis

> **AHA:** 2016,2Q,10; 2013,1Q,26
> **DEF:** Diabetic ketoacidosis: Potentially life-threatening complication due to a shortage of insulin in which the body switches to burning fatty acids and producing acidic ketone bodies.

E13.10   Other specified diabetes mellitus with ketoacidosis without coma `CH`

E13.11   Other specified diabetes mellitus with ketoacidosis with coma `CH`

√5ᵗʰ **E13.2   Other specified diabetes mellitus with** kidney complications

E13.21   Other specified diabetes mellitus with diabetic nephropathy `CH`
> Other specified diabetes mellitus with intercapillary glomerulosclerosis
> Other specified diabetes mellitus with intracapillary glomerulonephrosis
> Other specified diabetes mellitus with Kimmelstiel-Wilson disease

E13.22   Other specified diabetes mellitus with diabetic chronic kidney disease `CH`
> Use additional code to identify stage of chronic kidney disease (N18.1-N18.6)

E13.29   Other specified diabetes mellitus with other diabetic kidney complication `CH`
> Other specified diabetes mellitus with renal tubular degeneration

√5ᵗʰ **E13.3   Other specified diabetes mellitus with** ophthalmic complications

> One of the following 7th characters is to be assigned to codes in subcategories E13.32, E13.33, E13.34, E13.35, and E13.37 to designate laterality of the disease:
> 1   right eye
> 2   left eye
> 3   bilateral
> 9   unspecified eye

√6ᵗʰ **E13.31   Other specified diabetes mellitus with unspecified diabetic** retinopathy
> **DEF:** Diabetic retinopathy: Diabetic complication from damage to the retinal vessels resulting in vision problems that can progress to blindness.

E13.311   Other specified diabetes mellitus with unspecified diabetic retinopathy with macular edema `CL`

E13.319   Other specified diabetes mellitus with unspecified diabetic retinopathy without macular edema `CH`

√6ᵗʰ **E13.32   Other specified diabetes mellitus with** mild nonproliferative **diabetic** retinopathy
> Other specified diabetes mellitus with nonproliferative diabetic retinopathy NOS

√7ᵗʰ **E13.321   Other specified diabetes mellitus with mild nonproliferative diabetic retinopathy with** macular edema `CL`

√7ᵗʰ **E13.329   Other specified diabetes mellitus with mild nonproliferative diabetic retinopathy without** macular edema `CH`

√6ᵗʰ **E13.33   Other specified diabetes mellitus with** moderate nonproliferative **diabetic** retinopathy

√7ᵗʰ **E13.331   Other specified diabetes mellitus with moderate nonproliferative diabetic retinopathy with** macular edema `CL`

√7ᵗʰ **E13.339   Other specified diabetes mellitus with moderate nonproliferative diabetic retinopathy without** macular edema `CH`

√6ᵗʰ **E13.34   Other specified diabetes mellitus with** severe nonproliferative **diabetic** retinopathy

√7ᵗʰ **E13.341   Other specified diabetes mellitus with severe nonproliferative diabetic retinopathy with** macular edema `CL`

√7ᵗʰ **E13.349   Other specified diabetes mellitus with severe nonproliferative diabetic retinopathy without** macular edema `CH`

√6ᵗʰ **E13.35   Other specified diabetes mellitus with** proliferative **diabetic** retinopathy

√7ᵗʰ **E13.351   Other specified diabetes mellitus with proliferative diabetic retinopathy with** macular edema `CL`

√7ᵗʰ **E13.352   Other specified diabetes mellitus with proliferative diabetic retinopathy with** traction retinal detachment involving the macula `CH`

√7ᵗʰ **E13.353   Other specified diabetes mellitus with proliferative diabetic retinopathy with** traction retinal detachment not involving the macula `CH`

√7ᵗʰ **E13.354   Other specified diabetes mellitus with proliferative diabetic retinopathy with** combined traction retinal detachment and rhegmatogenous retinal detachment `CH`

√7ᵗʰ **E13.355   Other specified diabetes mellitus with** stable proliferative diabetic retinopathy `CH`

√7ᵗʰ **E13.359   Other specified diabetes mellitus with proliferative diabetic retinopathy without** macular edema `CH`

E13.36   Other specified diabetes mellitus with diabetic cataract `CH`
> **AHA:** 2019,2Q,30-31; 2016,4Q,142

√x7ᵗʰ **E13.37   Other specified diabetes mellitus with diabetic** macular edema, resolved following treatment `CH`

E13.39   Other specified diabetes mellitus with other diabetic ophthalmic complication `CH`
> Use additional code to identify manifestation, such as:
> diabetic glaucoma (H40-H42)

√5ᵗʰ **E13.4   Other specified diabetes mellitus with** neurological complications

E13.40   Other specified diabetes mellitus with diabetic neuropathy, unspecified `CH` `CL`

E13.41   Other specified diabetes mellitus with diabetic mononeuropathy `CH`

E13.42   Other specified diabetes mellitus with diabetic polyneuropathy `CH` `CL`
> Other specified diabetes mellitus with diabetic neuralgia

E13.43   Other specified diabetes mellitus with diabetic autonomic (poly)neuropathy `CH`
> Other specified diabetes mellitus with diabetic gastroparesis
> **AHA:** 2013,4Q,114

E13.44   Other specified diabetes mellitus with diabetic amyotrophy `CH`

E13.49   Other specified diabetes mellitus with other diabetic neurological complication `CH`

√5ᵗʰ **E13.5   Other specified diabetes mellitus with** circulatory complications

E13.51   Other specified diabetes mellitus with diabetic peripheral angiopathy without gangrene `CH`
> **AHA:** 2018,2Q,7

Chapter 4. Endocrine, Nutritional and Metabolic Diseases

E13.01–E13.51

Chapter 4. Endocrine, Nutritional and Metabolic Diseases

E13.52   **Other specified diabetes mellitus with diabetic** peripheral angiopathy with gangrene   `CH`
Other specified diabetes mellitus with diabetic gangrene
AHA: 2018,2Q,7; 2017,4Q,102

E13.59   **Other specified diabetes mellitus with other circulatory complications**   `CH`

✓5ᵗʰ **E13.6**   **Other specified diabetes mellitus with other specified complications**

✓6ᵗʰ **E13.61**   **Other specified diabetes mellitus with diabetic arthropathy**

E13.610   **Other specified diabetes mellitus with diabetic neuropathic arthropathy**   `CH`
Other specified diabetes mellitus with Charcôt's joints
DEF: Charcôt's joint: Progressive neurologic arthropathy in which chronic degeneration of joints in the weight-bearing areas with peripheral hypertrophy occurs as a complication of a neuropathy disorder. Supporting structures relax from a loss of sensation resulting in chronic joint instability.

E13.618   **Other specified diabetes mellitus with other diabetic arthropathy**   `CH`
AHA: 2018,2Q,6

✓6ᵗʰ **E13.62**   **Other specified diabetes mellitus with skin complications**

E13.620   **Other specified diabetes mellitus with diabetic dermatitis**   `CH`
Other specified diabetes mellitus with diabetic necrobiosis lipoidica

E13.621   **Other specified diabetes mellitus with foot ulcer**   `CH`
Use additional code to identify site of ulcer (L97.4-, L97.5-)
TIP: Do not assign a code for diabetic ulcer when the ulcer is closed/resolved or to report history of diabetic ulcers; Z86.31 Personal history of diabetic foot ulcer, may be assigned.

E13.622   **Other specified diabetes mellitus with other skin ulcer**   `CH`
Use additional code to identify site of ulcer (L97.1-L97.9, L98.41-L98.49)
AHA: 2017,4Q,17

E13.628   **Other specified diabetes mellitus with other skin complications**   `CH`
AHA: 2017,4Q,100-101

✓6ᵗʰ **E13.63**   **Other specified diabetes mellitus with oral complications**

E13.630   **Other specified diabetes mellitus with periodontal disease**   `CH`

E13.638   **Other specified diabetes mellitus with other oral complications**   `CH`

✓6ᵗʰ **E13.64**   **Other specified diabetes mellitus with hypoglycemia**

E13.641   **Other specified diabetes mellitus with hypoglycemia with coma**   `CH`

E13.649   **Other specified diabetes mellitus with hypoglycemia without coma**   `CH`
AHA: 2016,3Q,42; 2015,3Q,21

E13.65   **Other specified diabetes mellitus with hyperglycemia**   `CH`

E13.69   **Other specified diabetes mellitus with other specified complication**   `CH`
Use additional code to identify complication
AHA: 2016,4Q,141; 2016,1Q,13

E13.8   **Other specified diabetes mellitus with unspecified complications**

E13.9   **Other specified diabetes mellitus without complications**   `CH`

Other disorders of glucose regulation and pancreatic internal secretion (E15-E16)

E15   **Nondiabetic hypoglycemic coma**
`INCLUDES` drug-induced insulin coma in nondiabetic
hyperinsulinism with hypoglycemic coma
hypoglycemic coma NOS

✓4ᵗʰ **E16**   **Other disorders of pancreatic internal secretion**

E16.0   **Drug-induced hypoglycemia without coma**
Use additional code for adverse effect, if applicable, to identify drug (T36-T50 with fifth or sixth character 5)
`EXCLUDES 1` diabetes with hypoglycemia without coma (E09.649)

E16.1   **Other hypoglycemia**
Functional hyperinsulinism
Functional nonhyperinsulinemic hypoglycemia
Hyperinsulinism NOS
Hyperplasia of pancreatic islet beta cells NOS
`EXCLUDES 1` diabetes with hypoglycemia (E08.649, E10.649, E11.649, E13.649)
hypoglycemia in infant of diabetic mother (P70.1)
neonatal hypoglycemia (P70.4)

E16.2   **Hypoglycemia, unspecified**
`EXCLUDES 1` diabetes with hypoglycemia (E08.649, E10.649, E11.649, E13.649)
AHA: 2016,3Q,42

E16.3   **Increased secretion of glucagon**
Hyperplasia of pancreatic endocrine cells with glucagon excess

E16.4   **Increased secretion of gastrin**
Hypergastrinemia
Hyperplasia of pancreatic endocrine cells with gastrin excess
Zollinger-Ellison syndrome

E16.8   **Other specified disorders of pancreatic internal secretion**
Increased secretion from endocrine pancreas of growth hormone-releasing hormone
Increased secretion from endocrine pancreas of pancreatic polypeptide
Increased secretion from endocrine pancreas of somatostatin
Increased secretion from endocrine pancreas of vasoactive-intestinal polypeptide

E16.9   **Disorder of pancreatic internal secretion, unspecified**
Islet-cell hyperplasia NOS
Pancreatic endocrine cell hyperplasia NOS

Disorders of other endocrine glands (E20-E35)

`EXCLUDES 1` galactorrhea (N64.3)
gynecomastia (N62)

✓4ᵗʰ **E20**   **Hypoparathyroidism**
`EXCLUDES 1` Di George's syndrome (D82.1)
postprocedural hypoparathyroidism (E89.2)
tetany NOS (R29.0)
transitory neonatal hypoparathyroidism (P71.4)

E20.0   **Idiopathic hypoparathyroidism**
DEF: Abnormally low secretion of parathyroid hormones, with unknown cause, which causes decreased calcium and increased phosphorus in the blood, resulting in muscle cramps, tetany, tingling, or burning in the lips, fingers, and toes, and cataracts.

E20.1   **Pseudohypoparathyroidism**

E20.8   **Other hypoparathyroidism**

E20.9   **Hypoparathyroidism, unspecified**
Parathyroid tetany

✓4ᵗʰ **E21**   **Hyperparathyroidism and other disorders of parathyroid gland**
`EXCLUDES 1` adult osteomalacia (M83.-)
ectopic hyperparathyroidism (E34.2)
familial hypocalciuric hypercalcemia (E83.52)
hungry bone syndrome (E83.81)
infantile and juvenile osteomalacia (E55.0)

E21.0   **Primary hyperparathyroidism**
Hyperplasia of parathyroid
Osteitis fibrosa cystica generalisata [von Recklinghausen's disease of bone]
DEF: Parathyroid dysfunction commonly caused by hyperplasia of two or more glands. Symptoms include hypercalcemia and increased parathyroid hormone levels.

Chapter 4. Endocrine, Nutritional and Metabolic Diseases

E21.1 Secondary **hyperparathyroidism, not elsewhere classified**
> EXCLUDES 1   secondary hyperparathyroidism of renal origin (N25.81)

E21.2 **Other hyperparathyroidism**
Tertiary hyperparathyroidism
> EXCLUDES 1   familial hypocalciuric hypercalcemia (E83.52)

E21.3 **Hyperparathyroidism, unspecified**
E21.4 **Other specified disorders of parathyroid gland**
E21.5 **Disorder of parathyroid gland, unspecified**

✓4ᵗʰ **E22** **Hyperfunction of pituitary gland**
> EXCLUDES 1   Cushing's syndrome (E24.-)
> Nelson's syndrome (E24.1)
> overproduction of ACTH not associated with Cushing's disease (E27.0)
> overproduction of pituitary ACTH (E24.0)
> overproduction of thyroid-stimulating hormone (E05.8-)

E22.0 **Acromegaly and pituitary gigantism**
Overproduction of growth hormone
> EXCLUDES 1   constitutional gigantism (E34.4)
> constitutional tall stature (E34.4)
> increased secretion from endocrine pancreas of growth hormone-releasing hormone (E16.8)

DEF: Acromegaly: Chronic condition caused by overproduction of the pituitary growth hormone resulting in enlarged skeletal parts and facial features.

E22.1 **Hyperprolactinemia**
Use additional code for adverse effect, if applicable, to identify drug (T36-T50 with fifth or sixth character 5)

E22.2 **Syndrome of inappropriate secretion of antidiuretic hormone**
E22.8 **Other hyperfunction of pituitary gland**
Central precocious puberty
E22.9 **Hyperfunction of pituitary gland, unspecified**

✓4ᵗʰ **E23** **Hypofunction and other disorders of the pituitary gland**
> INCLUDES   the listed conditions whether the disorder is in the pituitary or the hypothalamus
> EXCLUDES 1   postprocedural hypopituitarism (E89.3)

E23.0 **Hypopituitarism**
Fertile eunuch syndrome
Hypogonadotropic hypogonadism
Idiopathic growth hormone deficiency
Isolated deficiency of gonadotropin
Isolated deficiency of growth hormone
Isolated deficiency of pituitary hormone
Kallmann's syndrome
Lorain-Levi short stature
Necrosis of pituitary gland (postpartum)
Panhypopituitarism
Pituitary cachexia
Pituitary insufficiency NOS
Pituitary short stature
Sheehan's syndrome
Simmonds' disease

E23.1 **Drug-induced hypopituitarism**
Use additional code for adverse effect, if applicable, to identify drug (T36-T50 with fifth or sixth character 5)

E23.2 **Diabetes insipidus**
> EXCLUDES 1   nephrogenic diabetes insipidus (N25.1)

E23.3 **Hypothalamic dysfunction, not elsewhere classified**
> EXCLUDES 1   Prader-Willi syndrome ▶(Q87.11)◀
> Russell-Silver syndrome ▶(Q87.19)◀

E23.6 **Other disorders of pituitary gland**
Abscess of pituitary
Adiposogenital dystrophy
E23.7 **Disorder of pituitary gland, unspecified**

✓4ᵗʰ **E24** **Cushing's syndrome**
> EXCLUDES 1   congenital adrenal hyperplasia (E25.0)

DEF: Abdominal striae, acne, hypertension, decreased carbohydrate tolerance, moon face, obesity, protein catabolism, and psychiatric disturbances resulting from increased adrenocortical secretion of cortisol caused by ACTH-dependent adrenocortical hyperplasia or tumor, or by steroid effects.

E24.0 Pituitary-dependent **Cushing's disease**
Overproduction of pituitary ACTH
Pituitary-dependent hypercorticalism

E24.1 **Nelson's syndrome**

E24.2 **Drug-induced Cushing's syndrome**
Use additional code for adverse effect, if applicable, to identify drug (T36-T50 with fifth or sixth character 5)

E24.3 **Ectopic ACTH syndrome**
E24.4 **Alcohol-induced pseudo-Cushing's syndrome**
E24.8 **Other Cushing's syndrome**
E24.9 **Cushing's syndrome, unspecified**

✓4ᵗʰ **E25** **Adrenogenital disorders**
> INCLUDES   adrenogenital syndromes, virilizing or feminizing, whether acquired or due to adrenal hyperplasia
> consequent on inborn enzyme defects in hormone synthesis
> female adrenal pseudohermaphroditism
> female heterosexual precocious pseudopuberty
> male isosexual precocious pseudopuberty
> male macrogenitosomia praecox
> male sexual precocity with adrenal hyperplasia
> male virilization (female)
> EXCLUDES 1   indeterminate sex and pseudohermaphroditism (Q56)
> chromosomal abnormalities (Q90-Q99)

E25.0 Congenital **adrenogenital disorders** associated with enzyme deficiency
Congenital adrenal hyperplasia
21-Hydroxylase deficiency
Salt-losing congenital adrenal hyperplasia

E25.8 **Other adrenogenital disorders**
Idiopathic adrenogenital disorder
Use additional code for adverse effect, if applicable, to identify drug (T36-T50 with fifth or sixth character 5)

E25.9 **Adrenogenital disorder, unspecified**
Adrenogenital syndrome NOS

✓4ᵗʰ **E26** **Hyperaldosteronism**
✓5ᵗʰ **E26.0** Primary **hyperaldosteronism**

E26.01 **Conn's syndrome**
Code also adrenal adenoma (D35.0-)

E26.02 **Glucocorticoid-remediable aldosteronism**
Familial aldosteronism type I
DEF: Rare autosomal dominant familial form of primary aldosteronism in which the secretion of aldosterone is under the influence of adrenocorticotrophic hormone (ACTH) rather than the renin-angiotensin mechanism. Moderate hypersecretion of aldosterone and suppressed plasma renin activity that are rapidly reversed by administration of glucosteroids. Symptoms include hypertension and mild hypokalemia.

E26.09 **Other primary hyperaldosteronism**
Primary aldosteronism due to adrenal hyperplasia (bilateral)

E26.1 Secondary **hyperaldosteronism**
✓5ᵗʰ **E26.8** **Other hyperaldosteronism**
E26.81 **Bartter's syndrome**
E26.89 **Other hyperaldosteronism**
E26.9 **Hyperaldosteronism, unspecified**
Aldosteronism NOS
Hyperaldosteronism NOS

✓4ᵗʰ **E27** **Other disorders of adrenal gland**

E27.0 **Other adrenocortical overactivity**
Overproduction of ACTH, not associated with Cushing's disease
Premature adrenarche
> EXCLUDES 1   Cushing's syndrome (E24.-)

E27.1 **Primary adrenocortical insufficiency**
Addison's disease
Autoimmune adrenalitis
> EXCLUDES 1   Addison only phenotype adrenoleukodystrophy (E71.528)
> amyloidosis (E85.-)
> tuberculous Addison's disease (A18.7)
> Waterhouse-Friderichsen syndrome (A39.1)

E27.2 **Addisonian crisis**
Adrenal crisis
Adrenocortical crisis
DEF: Life-threatening condition that occurs when there is not enough cortisol excreted from the adrenal glands. This condition may be due to injury to the adrenal glands or to the pituitary gland, which controls adrenal hormone secretion, or when a patient stops hydrocortisone treatment too quickly or too early.

E27.3   **Drug-induced adrenocortical insufficiency**
Use additional code for adverse effect, if applicable, to identify drug (T36-T50 with fifth or sixth character 5)

✓5ᵗʰ **E27.4**   **Other and unspecified adrenocortical insufficiency**
> EXCLUDES 1   adrenoleukodystrophy [Addison-Schilder] (E71.528)
> Waterhouse-Friderichsen syndrome (A39.1)

     E27.40   **Unspecified adrenocortical insufficiency**
Adrenocortical insufficiency NOS
Hypoaldosteronism

     E27.49   **Other adrenocortical insufficiency**
Adrenal hemorrhage
Adrenal infarction

E27.5   **Adrenomedullary hyperfunction**
Adrenomedullary hyperplasia
Catecholamine hypersecretion

E27.8   **Other specified disorders of adrenal gland**
Abnormality of cortisol-binding globulin

E27.9   **Disorder of adrenal gland, unspecified**

✓4ᵗʰ **E28**   **Ovarian dysfunction**
> EXCLUDES 1   isolated gonadotropin deficiency (E23.0)
> postprocedural ovarian failure (E89.4-)

E28.0   **Estrogen excess**   ♀
Use additional code for adverse effect, if applicable, to identify drug (T36-T50 with fifth or sixth character 5)

E28.1   **Androgen excess**   ♀
Hypersecretion of ovarian androgens
Use additional code for adverse effect, if applicable, to identify drug (T36-T50 with fifth or sixth character 5)

E28.2   **Polycystic ovarian syndrome**   ♀
Sclerocystic ovary syndrome
Stein-Leventhal syndrome
DEF: Common hormonal disorder among women of reproductive age that involves enlarged ovaries with numerous small cysts located along the outer ovarian edge.

✓5ᵗʰ **E28.3**   **Primary ovarian failure**
> EXCLUDES 1   pure gonadal dysgenesis (Q99.1)
> Turner's syndrome (Q96.-)

     ✓6ᵗʰ **E28.31**   **Premature menopause**

         E28.310   **Symptomatic premature menopause**   A ♀
Symptoms such as flushing, sleeplessness, headache, lack of concentration, associated with premature menopause

         E28.319   **Asymptomatic premature menopause**   A ♀
Premature menopause NOS

     E28.39   **Other primary ovarian failure**   ♀
Decreased estrogen
Resistant ovary syndrome

E28.8   **Other ovarian dysfunction**   ♀
Ovarian hyperfunction NOS
> EXCLUDES 1   postprocedural ovarian failure (E89.4-)

E28.9   **Ovarian dysfunction, unspecified**   ♀

✓4ᵗʰ **E29**   **Testicular dysfunction**
> EXCLUDES 1   androgen insensitivity syndrome (E34.5-)
> azoospermia or oligospermia NOS (N46.0-N46.1)
> isolated gonadotropin deficiency (E23.0)
> Klinefelter's syndrome (Q98.0-Q98.1, Q98.4)

E29.0   **Testicular hyperfunction**   ♂
Hypersecretion of testicular hormones

E29.1   **Testicular hypofunction**   ♂
Defective biosynthesis of testicular androgen NOS
5-delta-Reductase deficiency (with male pseudohermaphroditism)
Testicular hypogonadism NOS
Use additional code for adverse effect, if applicable, to identify drug (T36-T50 with fifth or sixth character 5)
> EXCLUDES 1   postprocedural testicular hypofunction (E89.5)

E29.8   **Other testicular dysfunction**   ♂

E29.9   **Testicular dysfunction, unspecified**   ♂

✓4ᵗʰ **E30**   **Disorders of puberty, not elsewhere classified**

E30.0   **Delayed puberty**
Constitutional delay of puberty
Delayed sexual development

E30.1   **Precocious puberty**   P
Precocious menstruation
> EXCLUDES 1   Albright (-McCune) (-Sternberg) syndrome (Q78.1)
> central precocious puberty (E22.8)
> congenital adrenal hyperplasia (E25.0)
> female heterosexual precocious pseudopuberty (E25.-)
> male isosexual precocious pseudopuberty (E25.-)

E30.8   **Other disorders of puberty**   P
Premature thelarche

E30.9   **Disorder of puberty, unspecified**

✓4ᵗʰ **E31**   **Polyglandular dysfunction**
> EXCLUDES 1   ataxia telangiectasia [Louis-Bar] (G11.3)
> dystrophia myotonica [Steinert] (G71.11)
> pseudohypoparathyroidism (E20.1)

E31.0   **Autoimmune polyglandular failure**
Schmidt's syndrome

E31.1   **Polyglandular hyperfunction**
> EXCLUDES 1   multiple endocrine adenomatosis (E31.2-)
> multiple endocrine neoplasia (E31.2-)

✓5ᵗʰ **E31.2**   **Multiple endocrine neoplasia [MEN] syndromes**
Multiple endocrine adenomatosis
Code also any associated malignancies and other conditions associated with the syndromes
DEF: Group of conditions in which several endocrine glands grow excessively (such as in adenomatous hyperplasia) and/or develop benign or malignant tumors. Tumors and hyperplasia associated with MEN often produce excess hormones, which impede normal physiology. There is no comprehensive cure known for MEN syndrome. Treatment is directed at the hyperplasia or tumors in each individual gland. Tumors are usually surgically removed and oral medications or hormonal injections are used to correct hormone imbalances.

     E31.20   **Multiple endocrine neoplasia [MEN] syndrome, unspecified**
Multiple endocrine adenomatosis NOS
Multiple endocrine neoplasia [MEN] syndrome NOS

     E31.21   **Multiple endocrine neoplasia [MEN] type I**
Wermer's syndrome

     E31.22   **Multiple endocrine neoplasia [MEN] type IIA**
Sipple's syndrome

     E31.23   **Multiple endocrine neoplasia [MEN] type IIB**

E31.8   **Other polyglandular dysfunction**

E31.9   **Polyglandular dysfunction, unspecified**

✓4ᵗʰ **E32**   **Diseases of thymus**
> EXCLUDES 1   aplasia or hypoplasia of thymus with immunodeficiency (D82.1)
> myasthenia gravis (G70.0)

E32.0   **Persistent hyperplasia of thymus**
Hypertrophy of thymus

E32.1   **Abscess of thymus**

E32.8   **Other diseases of thymus**
> EXCLUDES 1   aplasia or hypoplasia with immunodeficiency (D82.1)
> thymoma (D15.0)

E32.9   **Disease of thymus, unspecified**

✓4ᵗʰ **E34**   **Other endocrine disorders**
> EXCLUDES 1   pseudohypoparathyroidism (E20.1)

E34.0   **Carcinoid syndrome**
> NOTE   May be used as an additional code to identify functional activity associated with a carcinoid tumor.

E34.1   **Other hypersecretion of intestinal hormones**

E34.2   **Ectopic hormone secretion, not elsewhere classified**
> EXCLUDES 1   ectopic ACTH syndrome (E24.3)

N Newborn: 0   P Pediatric: 0-17   M Maternity: 12-55   A Adult: 15-124   CH Comorbidity High   CL Comorbidity Low   NC Dx Noncancer Dx   PDx Primary Dx

522   ICD-10-CM 2020

E34.3 **Short stature due to endocrine disorder**
Constitutional short stature
Laron-type short stature
EXCLUDES 1   *achondroplastic short stature (Q77.4)*
hypochondroplastic short stature (Q77.4)
nutritional short stature (E45)
pituitary short stature (E23.0)
progeria (E34.8)
renal short stature (N25.0)
Russell-Silver syndrome ▶(Q87.19)◀
short-limbed stature with immunodeficiency (D82.2)
short stature in specific dysmorphic syndromes —
code to syndrome — see Alphabetical Index
short stature NOS (R62.52)

E34.4 **Constitutional tall stature**
Constitutional gigantism

✓5ᵗʰ **E34.5** **Androgen insensitivity syndrome**
DEF: X-linked recessive condition in which individuals that are chromosomally male fail to develop normal male external genitalia due to an abnormality on the X chromosome that prohibits the body, completely or in part, from recognizing the androgens produced. *Synonym(s): AIS*

E34.50 **Androgen insensitivity syndrome, unspecified**
Androgen insensitivity NOS

E34.51 **Complete androgen insensitivity syndrome**
Complete androgen insensitivity
de Quervain syndrome
Goldberg-Maxwell syndrome

E34.52 **Partial androgen insensitivity syndrome**
Partial androgen insensitivity
Reifenstein syndrome

E34.8 **Other specified endocrine disorders**
Pineal gland dysfunction
Progeria
EXCLUDES 2   *pseudohypoparathyroidism (E20.1)*

E34.9 **Endocrine disorder, unspecified**
Endocrine disturbance NOS
Hormone disturbance NOS

E35 *Disorders of endocrine glands in diseases classified elsewhere*
Code first underlying disease, such as:
late congenital syphilis of thymus gland [Dubois disease] (A50.5)
Use additional code, if applicable, to identify:
sequelae of tuberculosis of other organs (B90.8)
EXCLUDES 1   *Echinococcus granulosus infection of thyroid gland (B67.3)*
meningococcal hemorrhagic adrenalitis (A39.1)
syphilis of endocrine gland (A52.79)
tuberculosis of adrenal gland, except calcification (A18.7)
tuberculosis of endocrine gland NEC (A18.82)
tuberculosis of thyroid gland (A18.81)
Waterhouse-Friderichsen syndrome (A39.1)

Intraoperative complications of endocrine system (E36)

✓4ᵗʰ **E36** **Intraoperative complications of endocrine system**
EXCLUDES 2   *postprocedural endocrine and metabolic complications and disorders, not elsewhere classified (E89.-)*

✓5ᵗʰ **E36.0** **Intraoperative hemorrhage and hematoma of an endocrine system organ or structure complicating a procedure**
EXCLUDES 1   *intraoperative hemorrhage and hematoma of an endocrine system organ or structure due to accidental puncture or laceration during a procedure (E36.1-)*

E36.01 **Intraoperative hemorrhage and hematoma of an endocrine system organ or structure complicating an endocrine system procedure**

E36.02 **Intraoperative hemorrhage and hematoma of an endocrine system organ or structure complicating other procedure**

✓5ᵗʰ **E36.1** **Accidental puncture and laceration of an endocrine system organ or structure during a procedure**

E36.11 **Accidental puncture and laceration of an endocrine system organ or structure during an endocrine system procedure**

E36.12 **Accidental puncture and laceration of an endocrine system organ or structure during other procedure**

E36.8 **Other intraoperative complications of endocrine system**
Use additional code, if applicable, to further specify disorder

Malnutrition (E40-E46)

EXCLUDES 1   *intestinal malabsorption (K90.-)*
sequelae of protein-calorie malnutrition (E64.0)
EXCLUDES 2   *nutritional anemias (D50-D53)*
starvation (T73.0)
AHA: 2017,4Q,108; 2017,3Q,25

E40 **Kwashiorkor**
Severe malnutrition with nutritional edema with dyspigmentation of skin and hair
EXCLUDES 1   *marasmic kwashiorkor (E42)*

E41 **Nutritional marasmus**
Severe malnutrition with marasmus
EXCLUDES 1   *marasmic kwashiorkor (E42)*
AHA: 2017,3Q,24
DEF: Protein-calorie malabsorption or malnutrition in children characterized by tissue wasting, dehydration, and subcutaneous fat depletion. It may occur with infectious disease.
TIP: Assign code R64 when emaciated or emaciation is documented without documentation of malnutrition.

E42 **Marasmic kwashiorkor**
Intermediate form severe protein-calorie malnutrition
Severe protein-calorie malnutrition with signs of both kwashiorkor and marasmus

E43 **Unspecified severe protein-calorie malnutrition**
Starvation edema
AHA: 2017,4Q,108
TIP: If a patient is diagnosed with both severe malnutrition and severe malabsorption, regardless of the Excludes 1 note, it is appropriate to assign this code as well as K90.9 for malabsorption since these are separate conditions that can exist independently.

✓4ᵗʰ **E44** **Protein-calorie malnutrition of moderate and mild degree**

E44.0 **Moderate protein-calorie malnutrition**

E44.1 **Mild protein-calorie malnutrition**

E45 **Retarded development following protein-calorie malnutrition**
Nutritional short stature
Nutritional stunting
Physical retardation due to malnutrition

E46 **Unspecified protein-calorie malnutrition**
Malnutrition NOS
Protein-calorie imbalance NOS
EXCLUDES 1   *nutritional deficiency NOS (E63.9)*
AHA: 2018,4Q,82

Other nutritional deficiencies (E50-E64)

EXCLUDES 2   *nutritional anemias (D50-D53)*

✓4ᵗʰ **E50** **Vitamin A deficiency**
EXCLUDES 1   *sequelae of vitamin A deficiency (E64.1)*

E50.0 **Vitamin A deficiency with conjunctival xerosis**

E50.1 **Vitamin A deficiency with Bitot's spot and conjunctival xerosis**
Bitot's spot in the young child
DEF: Vitamin A deficiency with conjunctival dryness and superficial spots of keratinized epithelium.

E50.2 **Vitamin A deficiency with corneal xerosis**

E50.3 **Vitamin A deficiency with corneal ulceration and xerosis**

E50.4 **Vitamin A deficiency with keratomalacia**
DEF: Vitamin A deficiency creating corneal dryness that progresses to corneal insensitivity, softness, and necrosis. It is usually bilateral.

E50.5 **Vitamin A deficiency with night blindness**

E50.6 **Vitamin A deficiency with xerophthalmic scars of cornea**

E50.7 **Other ocular manifestations of vitamin A deficiency**
Xerophthalmia NOS

E50.8 **Other manifestations of vitamin A deficiency**
Follicular keratosis
Xeroderma

E50.9 **Vitamin A deficiency, unspecified**
Hypovitaminosis A NOS

✓4ᵗʰ **E51** **Thiamine deficiency**
EXCLUDES 1   *sequelae of thiamine deficiency (E64.8)*

✓5ᵗʰ **E51.1** **Beriberi**

E51.11 **Dry beriberi**
Beriberi NOS
Beriberi with polyneuropathy

☑ Additional Character Required   ✓x7ᵗʰ Placeholder Alert   Manifestation   Unspecified Dx   ▶◀ Revised Text   ● New Code   ▲ Revised Title

Chapter 4. Endocrine, Nutritional and Metabolic Diseases *(left margin)*

E51.12–E66.2 *(left margin)*

    E51.12   **Wet beriberi**
           Beriberi with cardiovascular manifestations
           Cardiovascular beriberi
           Shoshin disease

    E51.2   **Wernicke's encephalopathy**
        DEF: Deficiency of vitamin B1 resulting in a triad of acute mental confusion, ataxia, and ophthalmoplegia. The vast majority of affected patients are alcoholics.

    E51.8   **Other manifestations of thiamine deficiency**

    E51.9   **Thiamine deficiency, unspecified**

E52   **Niacin deficiency [pellagra]**
      Niacin (-tryptophan) deficiency
      Nicotinamide deficiency
      Pellagra (alcoholic)
      EXCLUDES 1   *sequelae of niacin deficiency (E64.8)*

✓4ᵗʰ **E53**   **Deficiency of other B group vitamins**
      EXCLUDES 1   *sequelae of vitamin B deficiency (E64.8)*

    E53.0   **Riboflavin deficiency**
        Ariboflavinosis
        Vitamin B2 deficiency

    E53.1   **Pyridoxine deficiency**
        Vitamin B6 deficiency
        EXCLUDES 1   *pyridoxine-responsive sideroblastic anemia (D64.3)*

    E53.8   **Deficiency of other specified B group vitamins**
        Biotin deficiency
        Cyanocobalamin deficiency
        Folate deficiency
        Folic acid deficiency
        Pantothenic acid deficiency
        Vitamin B12 deficiency
        EXCLUDES 1   *folate deficiency anemia (D52.-)*
                  vitamin B12 deficiency anemia (D51.-)

    E53.9   **Vitamin B deficiency, unspecified**

E54   **Ascorbic acid deficiency**
      Deficiency of vitamin C
      Scurvy
      EXCLUDES 1   *scorbutic anemia (D53.2)*
                  sequelae of vitamin C deficiency (E64.2)
      DEF: Vitamin C deficiency causing swollen gums, myalgia, weight loss, and weakness.

✓4ᵗʰ **E55**   **Vitamin D deficiency**
      EXCLUDES 1   *adult osteomalacia (M83.-)*
                  osteoporosis (M80.-)
                  sequelae of rickets (E64.3)

    E55.0   **Rickets, active**
        Infantile osteomalacia
        Juvenile osteomalacia
        EXCLUDES 1   *celiac rickets (K90.0)*
                Crohn's rickets (K50.-)
                hereditary vitamin D-dependent rickets (E83.32)
                inactive rickets (E64.3)
                renal rickets (N25.0)
                sequelae of rickets (E64.3)
                vitamin D-resistant rickets (E83.31)
        DEF: Rickets: Softening or weakening of the bones due to a lack of vitamin D, calcium, and phosphate.

    E55.9   **Vitamin D deficiency, unspecified**
        Avitaminosis D

✓4ᵗʰ **E56**   **Other vitamin deficiencies**
      EXCLUDES 1   *sequelae of other vitamin deficiencies (E64.8)*

    E56.0   **Deficiency of vitamin E**

    E56.1   **Deficiency of vitamin K**
        EXCLUDES 1   *deficiency of coagulation factor due to vitamin K deficiency (D68.4)*
                  vitamin K deficiency of newborn (P53)

    E56.8   **Deficiency of other vitamins**

    E56.9   **Vitamin deficiency, unspecified**

E58   **Dietary calcium deficiency**
      EXCLUDES 1   *disorders of calcium metabolism (E83.5-)*
                  sequelae of calcium deficiency (E64.8)

E59   **Dietary selenium deficiency**
      Keshan disease
      EXCLUDES 1   *sequelae of selenium deficiency (E64.8)*

E60   **Dietary zinc deficiency**

✓4ᵗʰ **E61**   **Deficiency of other nutrient elements**
      Use additional code for adverse effect, if applicable, to identify drug (T36-T50 with fifth or sixth character 5)
      EXCLUDES 1   *disorders of mineral metabolism (E83.-)*
                  iodine deficiency related thyroid disorders (E00-E02)
                  sequelae of malnutrition and other nutritional deficiencies (E64.-)

    E61.0   **Copper deficiency**

    E61.1   **Iron deficiency**
        EXCLUDES 1   *iron deficiency anemia (D50.-)*

    E61.2   **Magnesium deficiency**

    E61.3   **Manganese deficiency**

    E61.4   **Chromium deficiency**

    E61.5   **Molybdenum deficiency**

    E61.6   **Vanadium deficiency**

    E61.7   **Deficiency of multiple nutrient elements**

    E61.8   **Deficiency of other specified nutrient elements**

    E61.9   **Deficiency of nutrient element, unspecified**

✓4ᵗʰ **E63**   **Other nutritional deficiencies**
      EXCLUDES 1   *dehydration (E86.0)*
                  failure to thrive, adult (R62.7)
                  failure to thrive, child (R62.51)
                  feeding problems in newborn (P92.-)
                  sequelae of malnutrition and other nutritional deficiencies (E64.-)

    E63.0   **Essential fatty acid [EFA] deficiency**

    E63.1   **Imbalance of constituents of food intake**

    E63.8   **Other specified nutritional deficiencies**

    E63.9   **Nutritional deficiency, unspecified**

✓4ᵗʰ **E64**   **Sequelae of malnutrition and other nutritional deficiencies**
      NOTE   This category is to be used to indicate conditions in categories E43, E44, E46, E50-E63 as the cause of sequelae, which are themselves classified elsewhere. The 'sequelae' include conditions specified as such; they also include the late effects of diseases classifiable to the above categories if the disease itself is no longer present
      Code first condition resulting from (sequela) of malnutrition and other nutritional deficiencies

    E64.0   **Sequelae of protein-calorie malnutrition**
        EXCLUDES 2   *retarded development following protein-calorie malnutrition (E45)*

    E64.1   **Sequelae of vitamin A deficiency**

    E64.2   **Sequelae of vitamin C deficiency**

    E64.3   **Sequelae of rickets**

    E64.8   **Sequelae of other nutritional deficiencies**

    E64.9   **Sequelae of unspecified nutritional deficiency**

Overweight, obesity and other hyperalimentation (E65-E68)

E65   **Localized adiposity**
      Fat pad

✓4ᵗʰ **E66**   **Overweight and obesity**
      Code first obesity complicating pregnancy, childbirth and the puerperium, if applicable (O99.21-)
      Use additional code to identify body mass index (BMI), if known (Z68.-)
      EXCLUDES 1   *adiposogenital dystrophy (E23.6)*
                  lipomatosis NOS (E88.2)
                  lipomatosis dolorosa [Dercum] (E88.2)
                  Prader-Willi syndrome ▶(Q87.11)◀
      AHA: 2018,4Q,77,79-80
      TIP: BMI may be calculated and assigned as a secondary diagnosis based on documentation of clinicians other than the diagnosing provider.

    ✓5ᵗʰ **E66.0**   **Obesity due to excess calories**
        E66.01   **Morbid (severe) obesity due to excess calories**
            EXCLUDES 1   *morbid (severe) obesity with alveolar hypoventilation (E66.2)*
        E66.09   **Other obesity due to excess calories**

    E66.1   **Drug-induced obesity**
        Use additional code for adverse effect, if applicable, to identify drug (T36-T50 with fifth or sixth character 5)

    E66.2   **Morbid (severe) obesity with alveolar hypoventilation**
        Obesity hypoventilation syndrome (OHS)
        Pickwickian syndrome

N Newborn: 0   P Pediatric: 0-17   M Maternity: 12-55   A Adult: 15-124   CH Comorbidity High   CL Comorbidity Low   NCDx Noncancer Dx   PDx Primary Dx

524   ICD-10-CM 2020

E66.3   Overweight
> **AHA:** 2018,4Q,78

E66.8   **Other obesity**

E66.9   **Obesity, unspecified**
> Obesity NOS

☑4ᵗʰ   **E67   Other hyperalimentation**
> **EXCLUDES 1**   hyperalimentation NOS (R63.2)
>   sequelae of hyperalimentation (E68)

E67.0   **Hypervitaminosis A**

E67.1   **Hypercarotenemia**
> **DEF:** Elevated blood carotene level as a result of excessive carotenoid ingestion or an inability to convert carotenoids to vitamin A. Characteristics often include yellow discoloration of the skin, which may follow overeating of carotenoid-rich foods such as carrots, sweet potatoes, or squash.

E67.2   **Megavitamin-B6 syndrome**

E67.3   **Hypervitaminosis D**

E67.8   **Other specified hyperalimentation**

E68   Sequelae of hyperalimentation
> Code first condition resulting from (sequela) of hyperalimentation

Metabolic disorders (E70-E88)

EXCLUDES 1   androgen insensitivity syndrome (E34.5-)
           congenital adrenal hyperplasia (E25.0)
           Ehlers-Danlos syndrome ▶(Q79.6-)◀
           hemolytic anemias attributable to enzyme disorders (D55.-)
           Marfan's syndrome (Q87.4)
           5-alpha-reductase deficiency (E29.1)

AHA: 2018,2Q,6

☑4ᵗʰ   **E70   Disorders of aromatic amino-acid metabolism**

E70.0   **Classical phenylketonuria**

E70.1   **Other hyperphenylalaninemias**

☑5ᵗʰ   E70.2   **Disorders of tyrosine metabolism**
> **EXCLUDES 1**   transitory tyrosinemia of newborn (P74.5)

E70.20   **Disorder of tyrosine metabolism, unspecified**

E70.21   **Tyrosinemia**
> Hypertyrosinemia

E70.29   **Other disorders of tyrosine metabolism**
> Alkaptonuria
> Ochronosis

☑5ᵗʰ   E70.3   Albinism
> **DEF:** Absence of pigment in skin, hair, and eyes. This genetic condition is often accompanied by astigmatism, photophobia, and nystagmus.

E70.30   **Albinism, unspecified**

☑6ᵗʰ   E70.31   Ocular albinism
> E70.310   X-linked ocular albinism
> E70.311   Autosomal recessive ocular albinism
> E70.318   **Other ocular albinism**
> E70.319   **Ocular albinism, unspecified**

☑6ᵗʰ   E70.32   Oculocutaneous albinism
> **EXCLUDES 1**   Chediak-Higashi syndrome (E70.330)
>   Hermansky-Pudlak syndrome (E70.331)
>
> E70.320   Tyrosinase negative oculocutaneous albinism
> > Albinism I
> > Oculocutaneous albinism ty-neg
>
> E70.321   Tyrosinase positive oculocutaneous albinism
> > Albinism II
> > Oculocutaneous albinism ty-pos
>
> E70.328   **Other oculocutaneous albinism**
> > Cross syndrome
>
> E70.329   **Oculocutaneous albinism, unspecified**

☑6ᵗʰ   E70.33   **Albinism with hematologic abnormality**
> E70.330   Chediak-Higashi syndrome
> E70.331   Hermansky-Pudlak syndrome
> E70.338   **Other albinism with hematologic abnormality**
> E70.339   **Albinism with hematologic abnormality, unspecified**

E70.39   **Other specified albinism**
> Piebaldism

☑5ᵗʰ   E70.4   **Disorders of histidine metabolism**

E70.40   **Disorders of histidine metabolism, unspecified**

E70.41   Histidinemia

E70.49   **Other disorders of histidine metabolism**

E70.5   **Disorders of tryptophan metabolism**

E70.8   **Other disorders of aromatic amino-acid metabolism**

E70.9   **Disorder of aromatic amino-acid metabolism, unspecified**

☑4ᵗʰ   **E71   Disorders of branched-chain amino-acid metabolism and fatty-acid metabolism**

E71.0   **Maple-syrup-urine disease**

☑5ᵗʰ   E71.1   **Other disorders of branched-chain amino-acid metabolism**

☑6ᵗʰ   E71.11   **Branched-chain organic acidurias**
> E71.110   Isovaleric acidemia
> E71.111   3-methylglutaconic aciduria
> E71.118   **Other branched-chain organic acidurias**

☑6ᵗʰ   E71.12   **Disorders of propionate metabolism**
> E71.120   Methylmalonic acidemia
> E71.121   Propionic acidemia
> E71.128   **Other disorders of propionate metabolism**

E71.19   **Other disorders of branched-chain amino-acid metabolism**
> Hyperleucine-isoleucinemia
> Hypervalinemia

E71.2   **Disorder of branched-chain amino-acid metabolism, unspecified**

☑5ᵗʰ   E71.3   **Disorders of fatty-acid metabolism**
> **EXCLUDES 1**   peroxisomal disorders (E71.5)
>   Refsum's disease (G60.1)
>   Schilder's disease (G37.0)
>
> **EXCLUDES 2**   carnitine deficiency due to inborn error of metabolism (E71.42)

E71.30   **Disorder of fatty-acid metabolism, unspecified**

☑6ᵗʰ   E71.31   **Disorders of fatty-acid oxidation**
> E71.310   Long chain/very long chain acyl CoA dehydrogenase deficiency
> > LCAD
> > VLCAD
>
> E71.311   Medium chain acyl CoA dehydrogenase deficiency
> > MCAD
>
> E71.312   Short chain acyl CoA dehydrogenase deficiency
> > SCAD
>
> E71.313   Glutaric aciduria type II
> > Glutaric aciduria type II A
> > Glutaric aciduria type II B
> > Glutaric aciduria type II C
> > **EXCLUDES 1**   glutaric aciduria (type 1) NOS (E72.3)
>
> E71.314   Muscle carnitine palmitoyltransferase deficiency
>
> E71.318   **Other disorders of fatty-acid oxidation**

E71.32   **Disorders of ketone metabolism**

E71.39   **Other disorders of fatty-acid metabolism**

☑5ᵗʰ   E71.4   **Disorders of carnitine metabolism**
> **EXCLUDES 1**   muscle carnitine palmitoyltransferase deficiency (E71.314)

E71.40   **Disorder of carnitine metabolism, unspecified**

E71.41   Primary carnitine deficiency

E71.42   **Carnitine deficiency due to inborn errors of metabolism**
> Code also associated inborn error or metabolism

E71.43   Iatrogenic carnitine deficiency
> Carnitine deficiency due to hemodialysis
> Carnitine deficiency due to Valproic acid therapy

☑6ᵗʰ   E71.44   **Other secondary carnitine deficiency**
> E71.440   Ruvalcaba-Myhre-Smith syndrome
> E71.448   **Other secondary carnitine deficiency**

☑5ᵗʰ   E71.5   Peroxisomal disorders
> **EXCLUDES 1**   Schilder's disease (G37.0)

E71.50   **Peroxisomal disorder, unspecified**

☑6ᵗʰ   E71.51   **Disorders of peroxisome biogenesis**
> Group 1 peroxisomal disorders
> **EXCLUDES 1**   Refsum's disease (G60.1)
>
> E71.510   Zellweger syndrome

    E71.511 Neonatal adrenoleukodystrophy
        EXCLUDES 1   *X-linked adrenoleukodystrophy (E71.42-)*

    E71.518 Other disorders of peroxisome biogenesis

✓6ᵗʰ **E71.52 X-linked adrenoleukodystrophy**

    E71.520 Childhood cerebral X-linked adrenoleukodystrophy

    E71.521 Adolescent X-linked adrenoleukodystrophy

    E71.522 Adrenomyeloneuropathy

    E71.528 Other X-linked adrenoleukodystrophy
        Addison only phenotype adrenoleukodystrophy
        Addison-Schilder adrenoleukodystrophy

    E71.529 X-linked adrenoleukodystrophy, unspecified type

E71.53 Other group 2 peroxisomal disorders

✓6ᵗʰ **E71.54 Other peroxisomal disorders**

    E71.540 Rhizomelic chondrodysplasia punctata
        EXCLUDES 1   *chondrodysplasia punctata NOS (Q77.3)*

    E71.541 Zellweger-like syndrome

    E71.542 Other group 3 peroxisomal disorders

    E71.548 Other peroxisomal disorders

✓4ᵗʰ **E72 Other disorders of amino-acid metabolism**
    EXCLUDES 1   disorders of:
        aromatic amino-acid metabolism (E70.-)
        branched-chain amino-acid metabolism (E71.0-E71.2)
        fatty-acid metabolism (E71.3)
        purine and pyrimidine metabolism (E79.-)
        gout (M1A.-, M10.-)

✓5ᵗʰ **E72.0 Disorders of amino-acid transport**
    EXCLUDES 1   *disorders of tryptophan metabolism (E70.5)*

    E72.00 Disorders of amino-acid transport, unspecified

    E72.01 Cystinuria

    E72.02 Hartnup's disease

    E72.03 Lowe's syndrome
        Use additional code for associated glaucoma (H42)

    E72.04 Cystinosis
        Fanconi (-de Toni) (-Debré) syndrome with cystinosis
        EXCLUDES 1   *Fanconi (-de Toni) (-Debré) syndrome without cystinosis (E72.09)*

    E72.09 Other disorders of amino-acid transport
        Fanconi (-de Toni) (-Debré) syndrome, unspecified

✓5ᵗʰ **E72.1 Disorders of sulfur-bearing amino-acid metabolism**
    EXCLUDES 1   *cystinosis (E72.04)*
        cystinuria (E72.01)
        transcobalamin II deficiency (D51.2)

    E72.10 Disorders of sulfur-bearing amino-acid metabolism, unspecified

    E72.11 Homocystinuria
        Cystathionine synthase deficiency

    E72.12 Methylenetetrahydrofolate reductase deficiency

    E72.19 Other disorders of sulfur-bearing amino-acid metabolism
        Cystathioninuria
        Methioninemia
        Sulfite oxidase deficiency

✓5ᵗʰ **E72.2 Disorders of urea cycle metabolism**
    EXCLUDES 1   *disorders of ornithine metabolism (E72.4)*

    E72.20 Disorder of urea cycle metabolism, unspecified
        Hyperammonemia
        EXCLUDES 1   *hyperammonemia- hyperornithinemia-homocitrullinemia syndrome E72.4*
        transient hyperammonemia of newborn (P74.6)

    E72.21 Argininemia

    E72.22 Arginosuccinic aciduria

    E72.23 Citrullinemia

    E72.29 Other disorders of urea cycle metabolism

E72.3 Disorders of lysine and hydroxylysine metabolism
    Glutaric aciduria NOS
    Glutaric aciduria (type I)
    Hydroxylysinemia
    Hyperlysinemia
    EXCLUDES 1   *glutaric aciduria type II (E71.313)*
        Refsum's disease (G60.1)
        Zellweger syndrome (E71.510)

E72.4 Disorders of ornithine metabolism
    Hyperammonemia-Hyperornithinemia-Homocitrullinemia syndrome
    Ornithinemia (types I, II)
    Ornithine transcarbamylase deficiency
    EXCLUDES 1   *hereditary choroidal dystrophy (H31.2-)*

✓5ᵗʰ **E72.5 Disorders of glycine metabolism**

    E72.50 Disorder of glycine metabolism, unspecified

    E72.51 Non-ketotic hyperglycinemia

    E72.52 Trimethylaminuria

    E72.53 Primary hyperoxaluria
        Oxalosis
        Oxaluria
        AHA: 2018,4Q,29

    E72.59 Other disorders of glycine metabolism
        D-glycericacidemia
        Hyperhydroxyprolinemia
        Hyperprolinemia (types I, II)
        Sarcosinemia

✓5ᵗʰ **E72.8 Other specified disorders of amino-acid metabolism**
    AHA: 2018,4Q,5

    E72.81 Disorders of gamma aminobutyric acid metabolism
        4-hydroxybutyric aciduria
        Disorders of GABA metabolism
        GABA metabolic defect
        GABA transaminase deficiency
        GABA-T deficiency
        Gamma-hydroxybutyric aciduria
        SSADHD
        Succinic semialdehyde dehydrogenase deficiency

    E72.89 Other specified disorders of amino-acid metabolism
        Disorders of beta-amino-acid metabolism
        Disorders of gamma-glutamyl cycle

E72.9 Disorder of amino-acid metabolism, unspecified

✓4ᵗʰ **E73 Lactose intolerance**
    DEF: Inability to break down sugar in dairy products due to a deficiency in the enzyme lactase.

E73.0 Congenital lactase deficiency

E73.1 Secondary lactase deficiency

E73.8 Other lactose intolerance

E73.9 Lactose intolerance, unspecified

✓4ᵗʰ **E74 Other disorders of carbohydrate metabolism**
    EXCLUDES 1   *diabetes mellitus (E08-E13)*
        hypoglycemia NOS (E16.2)
        increased secretion of glucagon (E16.3)
        mucopolysaccharidosis (E76.0-E76.3)

✓5ᵗʰ **E74.0 Glycogen storage disease**

    E74.00 Glycogen storage disease, unspecified

    E74.01 von Gierke disease
        Type I glycogen storage disease

    E74.02 Pompe disease
        Cardiac glycogenosis
        Type II glycogen storage disease

    E74.03 Cori disease
        Forbes disease
        Type III glycogen storage disease

    E74.04 McArdle disease
        Type V glycogen storage disease

    E74.09 Other glycogen storage disease
        Andersen disease
        Hers disease
        Tauri disease
        Glycogen storage disease, types 0, IV, VI-XI
        Liver phosphorylase deficiency
        Muscle phosphofructokinase deficiency

N Newborn: 0   P Pediatric: 0-17   M Maternity: 12-55   A Adult: 15-124   CH Comorbidity High   CL Comorbidity Low   NCDx Noncancer Dx   PDx Primary Dx

526   ICD-10-CM 2020

√5ᵗʰ **E74.1** **Disorders of fructose metabolism**

     EXCLUDES 1   *muscle phosphofructokinase deficiency (E74.09)*

     E74.10 **Disorder of fructose metabolism, unspecified**

     E74.11 **Essential fructosuria**

       Fructokinase deficiency

     E74.12 **Hereditary fructose intolerance**

       Fructosemia

     E74.19 **Other disorders of fructose metabolism**

       Fructose-1, 6-diphosphatase deficiency

√5ᵗʰ **E74.2** **Disorders of galactose metabolism**

     E74.20 **Disorders of galactose metabolism, unspecified**

     E74.21 **Galactosemia**

       DEF: Any of three genetic disorders caused by a defective galactose metabolism. Symptoms include failure to thrive in infancy, jaundice, liver and spleen damage, cataracts, and mental retardation.

     E74.29 **Other disorders of galactose metabolism**

       Galactokinase deficiency

√5ᵗʰ **E74.3** **Other disorders of intestinal carbohydrate absorption**

     EXCLUDES 2   *lactose intolerance (E73.-)*

     E74.31 **Sucrase-isomaltase deficiency**

     E74.39 **Other disorders of intestinal carbohydrate absorption**

       Disorder of intestinal carbohydrate absorption NOS

       Glucose-galactose malabsorption

       Sucrase deficiency

E74.4 **Disorders of pyruvate metabolism and gluconeogenesis**

     Deficiency of phosphoenolpyruvate carboxykinase

     Deficiency of pyruvate carboxylase

     Deficiency of pyruvate dehydrogenase

     EXCLUDES 1   *disorders of pyruvate metabolism and gluconeogenesis with anemia (D55.-)*

             Leigh's syndrome (G31.82)

E74.8 **Other specified disorders of carbohydrate metabolism**

     Essential pentosuria

     Renal glycosuria

E74.9 **Disorder of carbohydrate metabolism, unspecified**

√4ᵗʰ **E75** **Disorders of sphingolipid metabolism and other lipid storage disorders**

     EXCLUDES 1   *mucolipidosis, types I-III (E77.0-E77.1)*

             Refsum's disease (G60.1)

√5ᵗʰ **E75.0** **GM2 gangliosidosis**

     E75.00 **GM2 gangliosidosis, unspecified**

     E75.01 **Sandhoff disease**

     E75.02 **Tay-Sachs disease**

       DEF: Genetic mutation of the HEXA gene that inhibits the breakdown of a toxic substance called ganglioside. The accumulation of ganglioside results in destruction of the neurons in the brain and spinal cord.

Tay-Sachs Disease

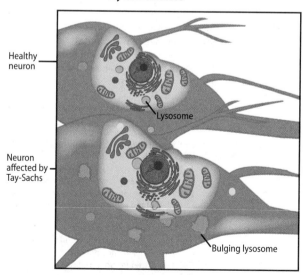

Healthy neuron

Lysosome

Neuron affected by Tay-Sachs

Bulging lysosome

E75.09 **Other GM2 gangliosidosis**

     Adult GM2 gangliosidosis

     Juvenile GM2 gangliosidosis

√5ᵗʰ **E75.1** **Other and unspecified gangliosidosis**

     E75.10 **Unspecified gangliosidosis**

       Gangliosidosis NOS

     E75.11 **Mucolipidosis IV**

     E75.19 **Other gangliosidosis**

       GM1 gangliosidosis

       GM3 gangliosidosis

√5ᵗʰ **E75.2** **Other sphingolipidosis**

     EXCLUDES 1   *adrenoleukodystrophy [Addison-Schilder] (E71.528)*

     E75.21 **Fabry (-Anderson) disease**

     E75.22 **Gaucher disease**

     E75.23 **Krabbe disease**

√6ᵗʰ   **E75.24** **Niemann-Pick disease**

       E75.240 **Niemann-Pick disease type A**

       E75.241 **Niemann-Pick disease type B**

       E75.242 **Niemann-Pick disease type C**

       E75.243 **Niemann-Pick disease type D**

       E75.248 **Other Niemann-Pick disease**

       E75.249 **Niemann-Pick disease, unspecified**

     E75.25 **Metachromatic leukodystrophy**

     E75.26 **Sulfatase deficiency**

       Multiple sulfatase deficiency (MSD)

       AHA: 2018,4Q,5-6

     E75.29 **Other sphingolipidosis**

       Farber's syndrome

       Sulfatide lipidosis

E75.3 **Sphingolipidosis, unspecified**

E75.4 **Neuronal ceroid lipofuscinosis**

     Batten disease

     Bielschowsky-Jansky disease

     Kufs disease

     Spielmeyer-Vogt disease

E75.5 **Other lipid storage disorders**

     Cerebrotendinous cholesterosis [van Bogaert-Scherer-Epstein]

     Wolman's disease

E75.6 **Lipid storage disorder, unspecified**

√4ᵗʰ **E76** **Disorders of glycosaminoglycan metabolism**

√5ᵗʰ **E76.0** **Mucopolysaccharidosis, type I**

     E76.01 **Hurler's syndrome**

     E76.02 **Hurler-Scheie syndrome**

     E76.03 **Scheie's syndrome**

E76.1 **Mucopolysaccharidosis, type II**

     Hunter's syndrome

√5ᵗʰ **E76.2** **Other mucopolysaccharidoses**

√6ᵗʰ   **E76.21** **Morquio mucopolysaccharidoses**

       E76.210 **Morquio A mucopolysaccharidoses**

         Classic Morquio syndrome

         Morquio syndrome A

         Mucopolysaccharidosis, type IVA

       E76.211 **Morquio B mucopolysaccharidoses**

         Morquio-like mucopolysaccharidoses

         Morquio-like syndrome

         Morquio syndrome B

         Mucopolysaccharidosis, type IVB

       E76.219 **Morquio mucopolysaccharidoses, unspecified**

         Morquio syndrome

         Mucopolysaccharidosis, type IV

     E76.22 **Sanfilippo mucopolysaccharidoses**

       Mucopolysaccharidosis, type III (A) (B) (C) (D)

       Sanfilippo A syndrome

       Sanfilippo B syndrome

       Sanfilippo C syndrome

       Sanfilippo D syndrome

     E76.29 **Other mucopolysaccharidoses**

       beta-Glucuronidase deficiency

       Maroteaux-Lamy (mild) (severe) syndrome

       Mucopolysaccharidosis, types VI, VII

E76.3 **Mucopolysaccharidosis, unspecified**

E76.8 **Other disorders of glucosaminoglycan metabolism**

E76.9 **Glucosaminoglycan metabolism disorder, unspecified**

✔ Additional Character Required   √ᵗ Tᵗ Placeholder Alert   Manifestation   Unspecified Dx   ►◄ Revised Text   ● New Code   ▲ Revised Title

ICD-10-CM 2020   527

Chapter 4. Endocrine, Nutritional and Metabolic Diseases

E77–E83.119

✓4ᵗʰ E77 Disorders of glycoprotein metabolism

E77.Ø Defects in post-translational modification of lysosomal enzymes
Mucolipidosis II [I-cell disease]
Mucolipidosis III [pseudo-Hurler polydystrophy]

E77.1 Defects in glycoprotein degradation
Aspartylglucosaminuria
Fucosidosis
Mannosidosis
Sialidosis [mucolipidosis I]

E77.8 Other disorders of glycoprotein metabolism

E77.9 Disorder of glycoprotein metabolism, unspecified

✓4ᵗʰ E78 Disorders of lipoprotein metabolism and other lipidemias
EXCLUDES 1   *sphingolipidosis (E75.Ø-E75.3)*

✓5ᵗʰ E78.Ø Pure hypercholesterolemia
AHA: 2016,4Q,13-14

E78.ØØ Pure hypercholesterolemia, unspecified
Fredrickson's hyperlipoproteinemia, type IIa
Hyperbetalipoproteinemia
Low-density-lipoprotein-type [LDL] hyperlipoproteinemia
(Pure) hypercholesterolemia NOS

E78.Ø1 Familial hypercholesterolemia

E78.1 Pure hyperglyceridemia
Elevated fasting triglycerides
Endogenous hyperglyceridemia
Fredrickson's hyperlipoproteinemia, type IV
Hyperlipidemia, group B
Hyperprebetalipoproteinemia
Very-low-density-lipoprotein-type [VLDL] hyperlipoproteinemia

E78.2 Mixed hyperlipidemia
Broad- or floating-betalipoproteinemia
Combined hyperlipidemia NOS
Elevated cholesterol with elevated triglycerides NEC
Fredrickson's hyperlipoproteinemia, type IIb or III
Hyperbetalipoproteinemia with prebetalipoproteinemia
Hypercholesteremia with endogenous hyperglyceridemia
Hyperlipidemia, group C
Tubo-eruptive xanthoma
Xanthoma tuberosum
EXCLUDES 1   *cerebrotendinous cholesterosis [van Bogaert-Scherer-Epstein] (E75.5)*
familial combined hyperlipidemia (E78.49)

E78.3 Hyperchylomicronemia
Chylomicron retention disease
Fredrickson's hyperlipoproteinemia, type I or V
Hyperlipidemia, group D
Mixed hyperglyceridemia

✓5ᵗʰ E78.4 Other hyperlipidemia
AHA: 2018,4Q,6

E78.41 Elevated Lipoprotein(a)
Elevated Lp(a)

E78.49 Other hyperlipidemia
Familial combined hyperlipidemia

E78.5 Hyperlipidemia, unspecified

E78.6 Lipoprotein deficiency
Abetalipoproteinemia
Depressed HDL cholesterol
High-density lipoprotein deficiency
Hypoalphalipoproteinemia
Hypobetalipoproteinemia (familial)
Lecithin cholesterol acyltransferase deficiency
Tangier disease

✓6ᵗʰ E78.7 Disorders of bile acid and cholesterol metabolism
EXCLUDES 1   *Niemann-Pick disease type C (E75.242)*

E78.7Ø Disorder of bile acid and cholesterol metabolism, unspecified

E78.71 Barth syndrome

E78.72 Smith-Lemli-Opitz syndrome

E78.79 Other disorders of bile acid and cholesterol metabolism

✓5ᵗʰ E78.8 Other disorders of lipoprotein metabolism

E78.81 Lipoid dermatoarthritis

E78.89 Other lipoprotein metabolism disorders

E78.9 Disorder of lipoprotein metabolism, unspecified

✓4ᵗʰ E79 Disorders of purine and pyrimidine metabolism
EXCLUDES 1   *Ataxia-telangiectasia ▶(Q87.19)◀*
Bloom's syndrome (Q82.8)
Cockayne's syndrome ▶(Q87.19)◀
calculus of kidney (N2Ø.Ø)
combined immunodeficiency disorders (D81.-)
Fanconi's anemia (D61.Ø9)
gout (M1A.-, M1Ø.-)
orotaciduric anemia (D53.Ø)
progeria (E34.8)
Werner's syndrome (E34.8)
xeroderma pigmentosum (Q82.1)

E79.Ø Hyperuricemia without signs of inflammatory arthritis and tophaceous disease
Asymptomatic hyperuricemia

E79.1 Lesch-Nyhan syndrome
HGPRT deficiency

E79.2 Myoadenylate deaminase deficiency

E79.8 Other disorders of purine and pyrimidine metabolism
Hereditary xanthinuria

E79.9 Disorder of purine and pyrimidine metabolism, unspecified

✓4ᵗʰ E8Ø Disorders of porphyrin and bilirubin metabolism
INCLUDES   defects of catalase and peroxidase

E8Ø.Ø Hereditary erythropoietic porphyria
Congenital erythropoietic porphyria
Erythropoietic protoporphyria

E8Ø.1 Porphyria cutanea tarda

✓5ᵗʰ E8Ø.2 Other and unspecified porphyria

E8Ø.2Ø Unspecified porphyria
Porphyria NOS

E8Ø.21 Acute intermittent (hepatic) porphyria

E8Ø.29 Other porphyria
Hereditary coproporphyria

E8Ø.3 Defects of catalase and peroxidase
Acatalasia [Takahara]

E8Ø.4 Gilbert syndrome

E8Ø.5 Crigler-Najjar syndrome

E8Ø.6 Other disorders of bilirubin metabolism
Dubin-Johnson syndrome
Rotor's syndrome

E8Ø.7 Disorder of bilirubin metabolism, unspecified

✓4ᵗʰ E83 Disorders of mineral metabolism
EXCLUDES 1   *dietary mineral deficiency (E58-E61)*
parathyroid disorders (E2Ø-E21)
vitamin D deficiency (E55.-)

✓5ᵗʰ E83.Ø Disorders of copper metabolism

E83.ØØ Disorder of copper metabolism, unspecified

E83.Ø1 Wilson's disease
Code also associated Kayser Fleischer ring (H18.Ø4-)

E83.Ø9 Other disorders of copper metabolism
Menkes' (kinky hair) (steely hair) disease

✓5ᵗʰ E83.1 Disorders of iron metabolism
EXCLUDES 1   *iron deficiency anemia (D5Ø.-)*
sideroblastic anemia (D64.Ø-D64.3)

E83.1Ø Disorder of iron metabolism, unspecified

✓6ᵗʰ E83.11 Hemochromatosis
EXCLUDES 1   *GALD (P78.84)*
gestational alloimmune liver disease (P78.84)
neonatal hemochromatosis (P78.84)

E83.11Ø Hereditary hemochromatosis
Bronzed diabetes
Pigmentary cirrhosis (of liver)
Primary (hereditary) hemochromatosis

E83.111 Hemochromatosis due to repeated red blood cell transfusions
Iron overload due to repeated red blood cell transfusions
Transfusion (red blood cell) associated hemochromatosis

E83.118 Other hemochromatosis

E83.119 Hemochromatosis, unspecified

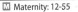

E83.19 **Other disorders of iron metabolism**
Use additional code, if applicable, for idiopathic
pulmonary hemosiderosis (J84.03)

E83.2 **Disorders of zinc metabolism**
Acrodermatitis enteropathica

✓5ᵗʰ **E83.3** **Disorders of phosphorus metabolism and phosphatases**
EXCLUDES 1   adult osteomalacia (M83.-)
osteoporosis (M80.-)

E83.30 **Disorder of phosphorus metabolism, unspecified**
E83.31 **Familial hypophosphatemia**
Vitamin D-resistant osteomalacia
Vitamin D-resistant rickets
EXCLUDES 1   vitamin D-deficiency rickets (E55.0)

E83.32 **Hereditary vitamin D-dependent rickets (type 1) (type 2)**
25-hydroxyvitamin D 1-alpha-hydroxylase deficiency
Pseudovitamin D deficiency
Vitamin D receptor defect

E83.39 **Other disorders of phosphorus metabolism**
Acid phosphatase deficiency
Hypophosphatasia

✓5ᵗʰ **E83.4** **Disorders of magnesium metabolism**
E83.40 **Disorders of magnesium metabolism, unspecified**
E83.41 **Hypermagnesemia**
AHA: 2016,4Q,54
E83.42 **Hypomagnesemia**
E83.49 **Other disorders of magnesium metabolism**

✓5ᵗʰ **E83.5** **Disorders of calcium metabolism**
EXCLUDES 1   chondrocalcinosis (M11.1-M11.2)
hungry bone syndrome (E83.81)
hyperparathyroidism (E21.0-E21.3)

E83.50 **Unspecified disorder of calcium metabolism**
E83.51 **Hypocalcemia**
E83.52 **Hypercalcemia**
Familial hypocalciuric hypercalcemia
E83.59 **Other disorders of calcium metabolism**

✓5ᵗʰ **E83.8** **Other disorders of mineral metabolism**
E83.81 **Hungry bone syndrome**
E83.89 **Other disorders of mineral metabolism**
E83.9 **Disorder of mineral metabolism, unspecified**

✓4ᵗʰ **E84** **Cystic fibrosis**
INCLUDES   mucoviscidosis
Code also exocrine pancreatic insufficiency (K86.81)
DEF: Genetic disorder affecting the respiratory, digestive, and reproductive systems in infants to young adults by disturbing exocrine gland function and causing chronic pulmonary disease with excess mucus production and pancreatic deficiency.

E84.0 **Cystic fibrosis with pulmonary manifestations**
Use additional code to identify any infectious organism present, such as:
Pseudomonas (B96.5)

✓5ᵗʰ **E84.1** **Cystic fibrosis with intestinal manifestations**
E84.11 **Meconium ileus in cystic fibrosis**   N
EXCLUDES 1   meconium ileus not due to cystic fibrosis (P76.0)

E84.19 **Cystic fibrosis with other intestinal manifestations**
Distal intestinal obstruction syndrome

E84.8 **Cystic fibrosis with other manifestations**
E84.9 **Cystic fibrosis, unspecified**

✓4ᵗʰ **E85** **Amyloidosis**
EXCLUDES 2   Alzheimer's disease (G30.0-)
DEF: Conditions of diverse etiologies characterized by the accumulation of insoluble fibrillar proteins (amyloid) in various organs and tissues of the body, compromising vital functions.

E85.0 **Non-neuropathic heredofamilial amyloidosis**
Hereditary amyloid nephropathy
Code also associated disorders, such as:
autoinflammatory syndromes (M04.-)
EXCLUDES 2   transthyretin-related (ATTR) familial amyloid cardiomyopathy (E85.4)

E85.1 **Neuropathic heredofamilial amyloidosis**
Amyloid polyneuropathy (Portuguese)
Transthyretin-related (ATTR) familial amyloid polyneuropathy
AHA: 2012,4Q,99

E85.2 **Heredofamilial amyloidosis, unspecified**

E85.3 **Secondary systemic amyloidosis**
Hemodialysis-associated amyloidosis

E85.4 **Organ-limited amyloidosis**
Localized amyloidosis
Transthyretin-related (ATTR) familial amyloid cardiomyopathy

✓5ᵗʰ **E85.8** **Other amyloidosis**
AHA: 2017,4Q,7
E85.81 **Light chain (AL) amyloidosis**
E85.82 **Wild-type transthyretin-related (ATTR) amyloidosis**
Senile systemic amyloidosis (SSA)
E85.89 **Other amyloidosis**
E85.9 **Amyloidosis, unspecified**

✓4ᵗʰ **E86** **Volume depletion**
Use additional code(s) for any associated disorders of electrolyte and acid-base balance (E87.-)
EXCLUDES 1   dehydration of newborn (P74.1)
hypovolemic shock NOS (R57.1)
postprocedural hypovolemic shock (T81.19)
traumatic hypovolemic shock (T79.4)
AHA: 2019,2Q,7; 2018,2Q,6

E86.0 **Dehydration**
AHA: 2019,2Q,7; 2019,1Q,12; 2014,1Q,7

E86.1 **Hypovolemia**
Depletion of volume of plasma

E86.9 **Volume depletion, unspecified**
DEF: Depletion of total body water (dehydration) and/or contraction of total intravascular plasma (hypovolemia).

✓4ᵗʰ **E87** **Other disorders of fluid, electrolyte and acid-base balance**
EXCLUDES 1   diabetes insipidus (E23.2)
electrolyte imbalance associated with hyperemesis gravidarum (O21.1)
electrolyte imbalance following ectopic or molar pregnancy (O08.5)
familial periodic paralysis (G72.3)
AHA: 2018,2Q,6

E87.0 **Hyperosmolality and hypernatremia**
Sodium [Na] excess
Sodium [Na] overload
AHA: 2014,1Q,7

E87.1 **Hypo-osmolality and hyponatremia**
Sodium [Na] deficiency
EXCLUDES 1   syndrome of inappropriate secretion of antidiuretic hormone (E22.2)
AHA: 2014,1Q,7

E87.2 **Acidosis**
Acidosis NOS
Lactic acidosis
Metabolic acidosis
Respiratory acidosis
EXCLUDES 1   diabetic acidosis — see categories E08-E10, E13 with ketoacidosis
DEF: Reduction of alkaline in the blood and tissues caused by an increase in acid and decrease in bicarbonate.

E87.3 **Alkalosis**
Alkalosis NOS
Metabolic alkalosis
Respiratory alkalosis

E87.4 **Mixed disorder of acid-base balance**

E87.5 **Hyperkalemia**
Potassium [K] excess
Potassium [K] overload

E87.6 **Hypokalemia**
Potassium [K] deficiency

✓5ᵗʰ **E87.7** **Fluid overload**
EXCLUDES 1   edema NOS (R60.9)
fluid retention (R60.9)

E87.70 **Fluid overload, unspecified**
E87.71 **Transfusion associated circulatory overload**
Fluid overload due to transfusion (blood) (blood components)
TACO
E87.79 **Other fluid overload**

✓ Additional Character Required   ✓x7ᵗʰ Placeholder Alert   Manifestation   Unspecified Dx   ►◄ Revised Text   ● New Code   ▲ Revised Title

E87.8   **Other disorders of electrolyte and fluid balance, not elsewhere classified**
Electrolyte imbalance NOS
Hyperchloremia
Hypochloremia

✓4ᵗʰ **E88**   **Other and unspecified metabolic disorders**
Use additional codes for associated conditions
EXCLUDES 1   *histiocytosis X (chronic) (C96.6)*

✓5ᵗʰ **E88.0**   **Disorders of plasma-protein metabolism, not elsewhere classified**
EXCLUDES 1   *disorder of lipoprotein metabolism (E78.-)*
monoclonal gammopathy (of undetermined significance) (D47.2)
polyclonal hypergammaglobulinemia (D89.0)
Waldenström macroglobulinemia (C88.0)

E88.01   **Alpha-1-antitrypsin deficiency**
AAT deficiency

E88.02   **Plasminogen deficiency**
Dysplasminogenemia
Hypoplasminogenemia
Type 1 plasminogen deficiency
Type 2 plasminogen deficiency
Code also, if applicable, ligneous conjunctivitis (H10.51)
Use additional code for associated findings, such as:
hydrocephalus (G91.4)
~~ligneous conjunctivitis (H10.51)~~
otitis media (H67.-)
respiratory disorder related to plasminogen deficiency (J99)
AHA: 2018,4Q,6-7

E88.09   **Other disorders of plasma-protein metabolism, not elsewhere classified**
Bisalbuminemia

E88.1   **Lipodystrophy, not elsewhere classified**
Lipodystrophy NOS
EXCLUDES 1   *Whipple's disease (K90.81)*

E88.2   **Lipomatosis, not elsewhere classified**
Lipomatosis NOS
Lipomatosis (Check) dolorosa [Dercum]

E88.3   **Tumor lysis syndrome**
Tumor lysis syndrome (spontaneous)
Tumor lysis syndrome following antineoplastic drug chemotherapy
Use additional code for adverse effect, if applicable, to identify drug (T45.1X5)
AHA: 2019,2Q,24
DEF: Potentially fatal metabolic complication of tumor necrosis caused by spontaneous or treatment-related accumulation of byproducts from dying cancer cells. Symptoms include hyperkalemia, hyperphosphatemia, hypocalcemia, hyperuricemia, and hyperuricosuria.

✓5ᵗʰ **E88.4**   **Mitochondrial metabolism disorders**
EXCLUDES 1   *disorders of pyruvate metabolism (E74.4)*
Kearns-Sayre syndrome (H49.81)
Leber's disease (H47.22)
Leigh's encephalopathy (G31.82)
mitochondrial myopathy, NEC (G71.3)
Reye's syndrome (G93.7)

E88.40   **Mitochondrial metabolism disorder, unspecified**

E88.41   **MELAS syndrome**
Mitochondrial myopathy, encephalopathy, lactic acidosis and stroke-like episodes

E88.42   **MERRF syndrome**
Myoclonic epilepsy associated with ragged-red fibers
Code also progressive myoclonic epilepsy (G40.3-)

E88.49   **Other mitochondrial metabolism disorders**

✓5ᵗʰ **E88.8**   **Other specified metabolic disorders**

E88.81   **Metabolic syndrome**
Dysmetabolic syndrome X
Use additional codes for associated manifestations, such as:
obesity (E66.-)
DEF: Group of health risks that increase the likelihood of developing heart disease, stroke, and diabetes. These risks include certain parameters for blood pressure, cholesterol, and glucose levels.

E88.89   **Other specified metabolic disorders**
Launois-Bensaude adenolipomatosis
EXCLUDES 1   *adult pulmonary Langerhans cell histiocytosis (J84.82)*

E88.9   **Metabolic disorder, unspecified**

Postprocedural endocrine and metabolic complications and disorders, not elsewhere classified (E89)

✓4ᵗʰ **E89**   **Postprocedural endocrine and metabolic complications and disorders, not elsewhere classified**
EXCLUDES 2   *intraoperative complications of endocrine system organ or structure (E36.0-, E36.1-, E36.8)*

E89.0   **Postprocedural hypothyroidism**
Postirradiation hypothyroidism
Postsurgical hypothyroidism

E89.1   **Postprocedural hypoinsulinemia**
Postpancreatectomy hyperglycemia
Postsurgical hypoinsulinemia
Use additional code, if applicable, to identify:
acquired absence of pancreas (Z90.41-)
diabetes mellitus (postpancreatectomy) (postprocedural) (E13.-)
insulin use (Z79.4)
EXCLUDES 1   *transient postprocedural hyperglycemia (R73.9)*
transient postprocedural hypoglycemia (E16.2)

E89.2   **Postprocedural hypoparathyroidism**
Parathyroprival tetany

E89.3   **Postprocedural hypopituitarism**
Postirradiation hypopituitarism

✓5ᵗʰ **E89.4**   **Postprocedural ovarian failure**

E89.40   **Asymptomatic postprocedural ovarian failure**   ♀
Postprocedural ovarian failure NOS

E89.41   **Symptomatic postprocedural ovarian failure**   ♀
Symptoms such as flushing, sleeplessness, headache, lack of concentration, associated with postprocedural menopause

E89.5   **Postprocedural testicular hypofunction**   ♂

E89.6   **Postprocedural adrenocortical (-medullary) hypofunction**

✓5ᵗʰ **E89.8**   **Other postprocedural endocrine and metabolic complications and disorders**
AHA: 2016,4Q,9-10

✓6ᵗʰ **E89.81**   **Postprocedural hemorrhage of an endocrine system organ or structure following a procedure**

E89.810   **Postprocedural hemorrhage of an endocrine system organ or structure following an endocrine system procedure**

E89.811   **Postprocedural hemorrhage of an endocrine system organ or structure following other procedure**

✓6ᵗʰ **E89.82**   **Postprocedural hematoma and seroma of an endocrine system organ or structure**

E89.820   **Postprocedural hematoma of an endocrine system organ or structure following an endocrine system procedure**

E89.821   **Postprocedural hematoma of an endocrine system organ or structure following other procedure**

E89.822   **Postprocedural seroma of an endocrine system organ or structure following an endocrine system procedure**

E89.823   **Postprocedural seroma of an endocrine system organ or structure following other procedure**

E89.89 Other postprocedural endocrine and metabolic complications and disorders

Use additional code, if applicable, to further specify disorder

☑ Additional Character Required   √x7ᵗʰ Placeholder Alert   Manifestation   Unspecified Dx   ►◄ Revised Text   ● New Code   ▲ Revised Title

ICD-10-CM 2020   531

Chapter 5. Mental, Behavioral and Neurodevelopmental Disorders (FØ1–F99)

Chapter-specific Guidelines with Coding Examples

The chapter-specific guidelines from the ICD-10-CM Official Guidelines for Coding and Reporting have been provided below. Along with these guidelines are coding examples, contained in the shaded boxes, that have been developed to help illustrate the coding and/or sequencing guidance found in these guidelines.

a. Pain disorders related to psychological factors

Assign code F45.41, for pain that is exclusively related to psychological disorders. As indicated by the Excludes 1 note under category G89, a code from category G89 should not be assigned with code F45.41.

> Perceived abdominal pain determined to be persistent somatoform pain disorder.
>
> **F45.41   Pain disorder exclusively related to psychological factors**
>
> *Explanation*: This pain was diagnosed as being exclusively psychological; therefore, no code from category G89 is added.

Code F45.42, Pain disorders with related psychological factors, should be used with a code from category G89, Pain, not elsewhere classified, if there is documentation of a psychological component for a patient with acute or chronic pain.

See Section I.C.6. Pain

b. Mental and behavioral disorders due to psychoactive substance use

1) In remission

Selection of codes for "in remission" for categories F1Ø-F19, Mental and behavioral disorders due to psychoactive substance use (categories F1Ø-F19 with -11, -.21) requires the provider's clinical judgment. The appropriate codes for "in remission" are assigned only on the basis of provider documentation (as defined in the Official Guidelines for Coding and Reporting), unless otherwise instructed by the classification.

Mild substance use disorders in early or sustained remission are classified to the appropriate codes for substance abuse in remission, and moderate or severe substance use disorders in early or sustained remission are classified to the appropriate codes for substance dependence in remission.

2) Psychoactive substance use, abuse and dependence

When the provider documentation refers to use, abuse and dependence of the same substance (e.g. alcohol, opioid, cannabis, etc.), only one code should be assigned to identify the pattern of use based on the following hierarchy:

- If both use and abuse are documented, assign only the code for abuse
- If both abuse and dependence are documented, assign only the code for dependence
- If use, abuse and dependence are all documented, assign only the code for dependence
- If both use and dependence are documented, assign only the code for dependence.

> History and physical notes cannabis dependence; progress note says cannabis abuse.
>
> **F12.2Ø   Cannabis dependence, uncomplicated**
>
> *Explanation*: In the hierarchy, the dependence code is used if both abuse and dependence are documented.

> Discharge summary says cocaine abuse; progress notes list cocaine use.
>
> **F14.1Ø   Cocaine abuse, uncomplicated**
>
> *Explanation*: In the hierarchy, the abuse code is used if both abuse and use are documented.

3) Psychoactive substance use, unspecified

As with all other unspecified diagnoses, the codes for unspecified psychoactive substance use disorders (F1Ø.9-, F11.9-, F12.9-, F13.9-, F14.9-, F15.9-, F16.9-, F18.9-, F19.9-) should only be assigned based on provider documentation and when they meet the definition of a reportable diagnosis (see Section III, Reporting Additional Diagnoses). These codes are to be used only when the psychoactive substance use is associated with a physical, mental or behavioral disorder, and such a relationship is documented by the provider.

c. Factitious disorder

Factitious disorder imposed on self or Munchausen's syndrome is a disorder in which a person falsely reports or causes his or her own physical or psychological signs or symptoms. For patients with documented factitious disorder on self or Munchausen's syndrome, assign the appropriate code from subcategory F68.1-, Factitious disorder imposed on self.

Munchausen's syndrome by proxy (MSBP) is a disorder in which a caregiver (perpetrator) falsely reports or causes an illness or injury in another person (victim) under his or her care, such as a child, an elderly adult, or a person who has a disability. The condition is also referred to as "factitious disorder imposed on another" or "factitious disorder by proxy." The perpetrator, not the victim, receives this diagnosis. Assign code F68.A, Factitious disorder imposed on another, to the perpetrator's record. For the victim of a patient suffering from MSBP, assign the appropriate code from categories T74, Adult and child abuse, neglect and other maltreatment, confirmed, or T76, Adult and child abuse, neglect and other maltreatment, suspected.

See Section I.C.19.f. Adult and child abuse, neglect and other maltreatment

Chapter 5. Mental, Behavioral and Neurodevelopmental Disorders (F01-F99)

INCLUDES   disorders of psychological development

EXCLUDES 2   symptoms, signs and abnormal clinical laboratory findings, not elsewhere classified (R00-R99)

This chapter contains the following blocks:

F01-F09	Mental disorders due to known physiological conditions
F10-F19	Mental and behavioral disorders due to psychoactive substance use
F20-F29	Schizophrenia, schizotypal, delusional, and other non-mood psychotic disorders
F30-F39	Mood [affective] disorders
F40-F48	Anxiety, dissociative, stress-related, somatoform and other nonpsychotic mental disorders
F50-F59	Behavioral syndromes associated with physiological disturbances and physical factors
F60-F69	Disorders of adult personality and behavior
F70-F79	Intellectual disabilities
F80-F89	Pervasive and specific developmental disorders
F90-F98	Behavioral and emotional disorders with onset usually occurring in childhood and adolescence
F99	Unspecified mental disorder

Mental disorders due to known physiological conditions (F01-F09)

NOTE   This block comprises a range of mental disorders grouped together on the basis of their having in common a demonstrable etiology in cerebral disease, brain injury, or other insult leading to cerebral dysfunction. The dysfunction may be primary, as in diseases, injuries, and insults that affect the brain directly and selectively; or secondary, as in systemic diseases and disorders that attack the brain only as one of the multiple organs or systems of the body that are involved.

✓4ᵗʰ F01 Vascular dementia   *Rejected HH/Hospice as primary*

Vascular dementia as a result of infarction of the brain due to vascular disease, including hypertensive cerebrovascular disease.

INCLUDES   arteriosclerotic dementia

→ Code first the underlying physiological condition or sequelae of cerebrovascular disease.

✓5ᵗʰ F01.5 Vascular dementia

F01.50 Vascular dementia without behavioral disturbance   Ⓐ

Major neurocognitive disorder without behavioral disturbance

F01.51 Vascular dementia with behavioral disturbance   Ⓐ

Major neurocognitive disorder due to vascular disease, with behavioral disturbance

Major neurocognitive disorder with aggressive behavior

Major neurocognitive disorder with combative behavior

Major neurocognitive disorder with violent behavior

Vascular dementia with aggressive behavior

Vascular dementia with combative behavior

Vascular dementia with violent behavior

Use additional code, if applicable, to identify wandering in vascular dementia (Z91.83)

✓4ᵗʰ F02 Dementia in other diseases classified elsewhere

INCLUDES   major neurocognitive disorder in other diseases classified elsewhere

Code first the underlying physiological condition, such as:

Alzheimer's (G30.-)

cerebral lipidosis (E75.4)

Creutzfeldt-Jakob disease (A81.0-)

dementia with Lewy bodies (G31.83)

dementia with Parkinsonism (G31.83)

epilepsy and recurrent seizures (G40.-)

frontotemporal dementia (G31.09)

hepatolenticular degeneration (E83.0)

human immunodeficiency virus [HIV] disease (B20)

Huntington's disease (G10)

hypercalcemia (E83.52)

hypothyroidism, acquired (E00-E03.-)

intoxications (T36-T65)

Jakob-Creutzfeldt disease (A81.0-)

multiple sclerosis (G35)

neurosyphilis (A52.17)

niacin deficiency [pellagra] (E52)

Parkinson's disease (G20)

Pick's disease (G31.01)

polyarteritis nodosa (M30.0)

prion disease (A81.9)

systemic lupus erythematosus (M32.-)

traumatic brain injury (S06.-)

trypanosomiasis (B56.-, B57.-)

vitamin B deficiency (E53.8)

EXCLUDES 2   dementia in alcohol and psychoactive substance disorders (F10-F19, with .17, .27, .97)

vascular dementia (F01.5-)

✓5ᵗʰ F02.8 Dementia in other diseases classified elsewhere

AHA: 2017,2Q,7; 2016,4Q,141; 2016,2Q,6

F02.80 Dementia in other diseases classified elsewhere without behavioral disturbance   CH

Dementia in other diseases classified elsewhere NOS

Major neurocognitive disorder in other diseases classified elsewhere

F02.81 Dementia in other diseases classified elsewhere with behavioral disturbance   CH

Dementia in other diseases classified elsewhere with aggressive behavior

Dementia in other diseases classified elsewhere with combative behavior

Dementia in other diseases classified elsewhere with violent behavior

Major neurocognitive disorder in other diseases classified elsewhere with aggressive behavior

Major neurocognitive disorder in other diseases classified elsewhere with combative behavior

Major neurocognitive disorder in other diseases classified elsewhere with violent behavior

Use additional code, if applicable, to identify wandering in dementia in conditions classified elsewhere (Z91.83)

✓4ᵗʰ F03 Unspecified dementia

Presenile dementia NOS

Presenile psychosis NOS

Primary degenerative dementia NOS

Senile dementia NOS

Senile dementia depressed or paranoid type

Senile psychosis NOS

EXCLUDES 1   senility NOS (R41.81)

EXCLUDES 2   mild memory disturbance due to known physiological condition (F06.8)

senile dementia with delirium or acute confusional state (F05)

✓5ᵗʰ F03.9 Unspecified dementia

F03.90 Unspecified dementia without behavioral disturbance   CH NCDx Ⓐ

Dementia NOS

AHA: 2012,4Q,92

TIP: This code would be viewed by Medicare as a questionable admission if used as the admitting diagnosis for a hospice encounter.

Ⓝ Newborn: 0   Ⓟ Pediatric: 0-17   Ⓜ Maternity: 12-55   Ⓐ Adult: 15-124   CH Comorbidity High   CL Comorbidity Low   NCDx Noncancer Dx   PDx Primary Dx

F03.91 Unspecified dementia with behavioral `CH` `NCDx` `A`
disturbance
     Unspecified dementia with aggressive behavior
     Unspecified dementia with combative behavior
     Unspecified dementia with violent behavior
     Use additional code, if applicable, to identify
       wandering in unspecified dementia (Z91.83)
     TIP: This code would be viewed by Medicare as a
     questionable admission if used as the admitting
     diagnosis for a hospice encounter.

F04 Amnestic disorder due to known physiological   `CH`
condition
     Korsakov's psychosis or syndrome, nonalcoholic
     Code first the underlying physiological condition
     EXCLUDES 1   *amnesia NOS (R41.3)*
                anterograde amnesia (R41.1)
                dissociative amnesia (F44.0)
                retrograde amnesia (R41.2)
     EXCLUDES 2   *alcohol-induced or unspecified Korsakov's syndrome (F10.26, F10.96)*
                Korsakov's syndrome induced by other psychoactive substances (F13.26, F13.96, F19.16, F19.26, F19.96)

F05 Delirium due to known physiological condition   `CH`
     Acute or subacute brain syndrome
     Acute or subacute confusional state (nonalcoholic)
     Acute or subacute infective psychosis
     Acute or subacute organic reaction
     Acute or subacute psycho-organic syndrome
     Delirium of mixed etiology
     Delirium superimposed on dementia
     Sundowning
     Code first the underlying physiological condition
     EXCLUDES 1   *delirium NOS (R41.0)*
     EXCLUDES 2   *delirium tremens alcohol-induced or unspecified (F10.231, F10.921)*
     AHA: 2019,2Q,34

`√4th` **F06 Other mental disorders due to known physiological condition**
     `INCLUDES`   mental disorders due to endocrine disorder
                mental disorders due to exogenous hormone
                mental disorders due to exogenous toxic substance
                mental disorders due to primary cerebral disease
                mental disorders due to somatic illness
                mental disorders due to systemic disease affecting the brain
     Code first the underlying physiological condition
     EXCLUDES 1   *unspecified dementia (F03)*
     EXCLUDES 2   *delirium due to known physiological condition (F05)*
                dementia as classified in F01-F02
                other mental disorders associated with alcohol and other psychoactive substances (F10-F19)

F06.0 Psychotic disorder with hallucinations **due to known**
physiological condition
     Organic hallucinatory state (nonalcoholic)
     EXCLUDES 2   *hallucinations and perceptual disturbance induced by alcohol and other psychoactive substances (F10-F19 with .151, .251, .951)*
                schizophrenia (F20.-)

F06.1 Catatonic disorder due to known physiological   `CH`
condition
     Catatonia associated with another mental disorder
     Catatonia NOS
     EXCLUDES 1   *catatonic stupor (R40.1)*
                stupor NOS (R40.1)
     EXCLUDES 2   *catatonic schizophrenia (F20.2)*
                dissociative stupor (F44.2)
     DEF: Catatonic: Abnormal neuropsychiatric state characterized
     by stupor, immobility or purposeless movements, or
     unresponsiveness in a person who otherwise appears awake.

F06.2 Psychotic disorder with delusions **due to known physiological**
condition
     Paranoid and paranoid-hallucinatory organic states
     Schizophrenia-like psychosis in epilepsy
     EXCLUDES 2   *alcohol and drug-induced psychotic disorder (F10-F19 with .150, .250, .950)*
                brief psychotic disorder (F23)
                delusional disorder (F22)
                schizophrenia (F20.-)

`√5th` **F06.3 Mood disorder due to known physiological condition**
     EXCLUDES 2   *mood disorders due to alcohol and other psychoactive substances (F10-F19 with .14, .24, .94)*
                mood disorders, not due to known physiological condition or unspecified (F30-F39)

     F06.30 Mood disorder due to known physiological
              condition, unspecified
     F06.31 Mood disorder due to known physiological
              condition with depressive features
              Depressive disorder due to known physiological
              condition, with depressive features
     F06.32 Mood disorder due to known physiological
              condition with major depressive-like episode
              Depressive disorder due to known physiological
              condition, with major depressive-like episode
     F06.33 Mood disorder due to known physiological
              condition with manic features
              Bipolar and related disorder due to a known
              physiological condition, with manic features
              Bipolar and related disorder due to known
              physiological condition, with manic- or
              hypomanic-like episodes
     F06.34 Mood disorder due to known physiological
              condition with mixed features
              Bipolar and related disorder due to known
              physiological condition, with mixed features
              Depressive disorder due to known physiological
              condition, with mixed features

F06.4 Anxiety disorder due to known physiological condition
     EXCLUDES 2   *anxiety disorders due to alcohol and other psychoactive substances (F10-F19 with .180, .280, .980)*
                anxiety disorders, not due to known physiological condition or unspecified (F40.-, F41.-)

F06.8 Other specified mental disorders due to known   `CH`
physiological condition
     Epileptic psychosis NOS
     Obsessive-compulsive and related disorder due to a known
       physiological condition
     Organic dissociative disorder
     Organic emotionally labile [asthenic] disorder

`√4th` **F07 Personality and behavioral disorders due to known physiological**
condition
     Code first the underlying physiological condition
     F07.0 Personality change due to known physiological condition
              Frontal lobe syndrome
              Limbic epilepsy personality syndrome
              Lobotomy syndrome
              Organic personality disorder
              Organic pseudopsychopathic personality
              Organic pseudoretarded personality
              Postleucotomy syndrome
              Code first underlying physiological condition
              EXCLUDES 1   *mild cognitive impairment (G31.84)*
                        postconcussional syndrome (F07.81)
                        postencephalitic syndrome (F07.89)
                        signs and symptoms involving emotional state (R45.-)
              EXCLUDES 2   *specific personality disorder (F60.-)*

☑ Additional Character Required   `√x7th` Placeholder Alert   <u>Manifestation</u>   <u>Unspecified Dx</u>   ►◄ Revised Text   ● New Code   ▲ Revised Title

ICD-10-CM 2020   **535**

Chapter 5. Mental, Behavioral and Neurodevelopmental Disorders

F07.8–F10.280

✓5ᵗʰ **F07.8 Other personality and behavioral disorders due to known physiological condition**

    F07.81 Postconcussional syndrome
        Postcontusional syndrome (encephalopathy)
        Post-traumatic brain syndrome, nonpsychotic
        Use additional code to identify associated
            post-traumatic headache, if applicable (G44.3-)
        EXCLUDES 1   *current concussion (brain) (S06.0-)*
                       postencephalitic syndrome (F07.89)
        DEF: Concussion symptoms that persist for weeks or months after a head injury. These symptoms may include headache, giddiness, fatigue, insomnia, mood fluctuation, and a subjective feeling of impaired intellectual function with extreme reaction to normal stressors.

    F07.89 Other personality and behavioral disorders due to known physiological condition
        Postencephalitic syndrome
        Right hemispheric organic affective disorder

F07.9 Unspecified personality and behavioral disorder due to known physiological condition
    Organic psychosyndrome

F09 Unspecified mental disorder due to known physiological condition
    Mental disorder NOS due to known physiological condition
    Organic brain syndrome NOS
    Organic mental disorder NOS
    Organic psychosis NOS
    Symptomatic psychosis NOS
    Code first the underlying physiological condition
    EXCLUDES 1   *psychosis NOS (F29)*

Mental and behavioral disorders due to psychoactive substance use (F10-F19)

AHA: 2018,4Q,69-70; 2017,4Q,8; 2017,2Q,27

✓4ᵗʰ **F10 Alcohol related disorders**

    Use additional code for blood alcohol level, if applicable (Y90.-)

✓5ᵗʰ **F10.1 Alcohol abuse**
      EXCLUDES 1   *alcohol dependence (F10.2-)*
                    alcohol use, unspecified (F10.9-)
      AHA: 2018,1Q,16; 2015,2Q,15

    F10.10 Alcohol abuse, uncomplicated
        Alcohol use disorder, mild

    F10.11 Alcohol abuse, in remission
        Alcohol use disorder, mild, in early remission
        Alcohol use disorder, mild, in sustained remission

    ✓6ᵗʰ **F10.12 Alcohol abuse with intoxication**
        F10.120 Alcohol abuse with intoxication, uncomplicated
        F10.121 Alcohol abuse with intoxication delirium
        F10.129 Alcohol abuse with intoxication, unspecified

    F10.14 Alcohol abuse with alcohol-induced mood disorder
        Alcohol use disorder, mild, with alcohol-induced bipolar or related disorder
        Alcohol use disorder, mild, with alcohol-induced depressive disorder

    ✓6ᵗʰ **F10.15 Alcohol abuse with alcohol-induced psychotic disorder**
        F10.150 Alcohol abuse with alcohol-induced psychotic disorder with delusions
        F10.151 Alcohol abuse with alcohol-induced psychotic disorder with hallucinations
            DEF: Psychosis lasting less than six months with slight or no clouding of consciousness in which auditory hallucinations predominate.
        F10.159 Alcohol abuse with alcohol-induced psychotic disorder, unspecified

    ✓6ᵗʰ **F10.18 Alcohol abuse with other alcohol-induced disorders**
        F10.180 Alcohol abuse with alcohol-induced anxiety disorder
        F10.181 Alcohol abuse with alcohol-induced sexual dysfunction
        F10.182 Alcohol abuse with alcohol-induced sleep disorder
        F10.188 Alcohol abuse with other alcohol-induced disorder

    F10.19 Alcohol abuse with unspecified alcohol-induced disorder

✓5ᵗʰ **F10.2 Alcohol dependence**
      EXCLUDES 1   *alcohol abuse (F10.1-)*
                    alcohol use, unspecified (F10.9-)
      EXCLUDES 2   *toxic effect of alcohol (T51.0-)*

    F10.20 Alcohol dependence, uncomplicated
        Alcohol use disorder, moderate
        Alcohol use disorder, severe

    F10.21 Alcohol dependence, in remission
        Alcohol use disorder, moderate, in early remission
        Alcohol use disorder, moderate, in sustained remission
        Alcohol use disorder, severe, in early remission
        Alcohol use disorder, severe, in sustained remission

    ✓6ᵗʰ **F10.22 Alcohol dependence with intoxication**
        Acute drunkenness (in alcoholism)
        EXCLUDES 2   *alcohol dependence with withdrawal (F10.23-)*
        F10.220 Alcohol dependence with intoxication, uncomplicated
        F10.221 Alcohol dependence with intoxication delirium
        F10.229 Alcohol dependence with intoxication, unspecified

    ✓6ᵗʰ **F10.23 Alcohol dependence with withdrawal**
        EXCLUDES 2   *alcohol dependence with intoxication (F10.22-)*
        AHA: 2018,1Q,16; 2015,2Q,15
        F10.230 Alcohol dependence with withdrawal, uncomplicated
        F10.231 Alcohol dependence with withdrawal delirium
        F10.232 Alcohol dependence with withdrawal with perceptual disturbance
        F10.239 Alcohol dependence with withdrawal, unspecified

    F10.24 Alcohol dependence with alcohol-induced mood disorder
        Alcohol use disorder, moderate, with alcohol-induced bipolar or related disorder
        Alcohol use disorder, moderate, with alcohol-induced depressive disorder
        Alcohol use disorder, severe, with alcohol-induced bipolar or related disorder
        Alcohol use disorder, severe, with alcohol-induced depressive disorder

    ✓6ᵗʰ **F10.25 Alcohol dependence with alcohol-induced psychotic disorder**
        F10.250 Alcohol dependence with alcohol-induced psychotic disorder with delusions
        F10.251 Alcohol dependence with alcohol-induced psychotic disorder with hallucinations
        F10.259 Alcohol dependence with alcohol-induced psychotic disorder, unspecified

    F10.26 Alcohol dependence with alcohol-induced persisting amnestic disorder
        Alcohol use disorder, moderate, with alcohol-induced major neurocognitive disorder, amnestic-confabulatory type
        Alcohol use disorder, severe, with alcohol-induced major neurocognitive disorder, amnestic-confabulatory type
        DEF: Prominent and lasting reduced memory span and disordered time appreciation and confabulation that occurs in alcoholics as sequel to acute alcoholic psychosis.

    F10.27 Alcohol dependence with alcohol-induced persisting dementia
        Alcohol use disorder, moderate, with alcohol-induced major neurocognitive disorder, nonamnestic-confabulatory type
        Alcohol use disorder, severe, with alcohol-induced major neurocognitive disorder, nonamnestic-confabulatory type

    ✓6ᵗʰ **F10.28 Alcohol dependence with other alcohol-induced disorders**
        F10.280 Alcohol dependence with alcohol-induced anxiety disorder

[handwritten margin notes: F10.13 - Withdrawal codes; 0 - uncomp; 1 - delirm; 2 w perceptul disturbnc; 9 - unsp]

N Newborn: 0   P Pediatric: 0-17   M Maternity: 12-55   A Adult: 15-124   CH Comorbidity High   CL Comorbidity Low   NCDx Noncancer Dx   PDx Primary Dx

536   ICD-10-CM 2020

F10.281 Alcohol dependence with alcohol-induced sexual dysfunction
F10.282 Alcohol dependence with alcohol-induced sleep disorder
F10.288 Alcohol dependence with other alcohol-induced disorder
Alcohol use disorder, moderate, with alcohol-induced mild neurocognitive disorder
Alcohol use disorder, severe, with alcohol-induced mild neurocognitive disorder

F10.29 Alcohol dependence with unspecified alcohol-induced disorder

√5ᵗʰ **F10.9 Alcohol** use, **unspecified**
    EXCLUDES 1   alcohol abuse (F10.1-)
                   alcohol dependence (F10.2-)
AHA: 2018,2Q,10-11
TIP: Assign a substance use code only when the provider documents a relationship between the use and an associated physical, mental, or behavioral disorder. As with all diagnoses, substance use codes must meet the definition of a reportable diagnosis.

√6ᵗʰ **F10.92 Alcohol use, unspecified with** intoxication
    F10.920 Alcohol use, unspecified with intoxication, uncomplicated
        AHA: 2018,2Q,10-11
    F10.921 Alcohol use, unspecified with intoxication delirium
    F10.929 Alcohol use, unspecified with intoxication, unspecified

F10.94 Alcohol use, unspecified with alcohol-induced mood disorder
Alcohol induced bipolar or related disorder, without use disorder
Alcohol induced depressive disorder, without use disorder

√6ᵗʰ **F10.95 Alcohol use, unspecified with alcohol-induced** psychotic disorder
    F10.950 Alcohol use, unspecified with alcohol-induced psychotic disorder with delusions
    F10.951 Alcohol use, unspecified with alcohol-induced psychotic disorder with hallucinations
    F10.959 Alcohol use, unspecified with alcohol-induced psychotic disorder, unspecified
        Alcohol-induced psychotic disorder without use disorder

F10.96 Alcohol use, unspecified with alcohol-induced persisting amnestic disorder
Alcohol-induced major neurocognitive disorder, amnestic-confabulatory type, without use disorder

F10.97 Alcohol use, unspecified with alcohol-induced persisting dementia
Alcohol-induced major neurocognitive disorder, nonamnestic-confabulatory type, without use disorder

√6ᵗʰ **F10.98 Alcohol use, unspecified with other alcohol-induced disorders**
    F10.980 Alcohol use, unspecified with alcohol-induced anxiety disorder
        Alcohol induced anxiety disorder, without use disorder
    F10.981 Alcohol use, unspecified with alcohol-induced sexual dysfunction
        Alcohol induced sexual dysfunction, without use disorder
    F10.982 Alcohol use, unspecified with alcohol-induced sleep disorder
        Alcohol induced sleep disorder, without use disorder
    F10.988 Alcohol use, unspecified with other alcohol-induced disorder
        Alcohol induced mild neurocognitive disorder, without use disorder

F10.99 Alcohol use, unspecified with unspecified alcohol-induced disorder

√4ᵗʰ **F11 Opioid related disorders**
√5ᵗʰ **F11.1 Opioid** abuse
    EXCLUDES 1   opioid dependence (F11.2-)
                   opioid use, unspecified (F11.9-)
    F11.10 Opioid abuse, uncomplicated
        Opioid use disorder, mild
    F11.11 Opioid abuse, in remission
        Opioid use disorder, mild, in early remission
        Opioid use disorder, mild, in sustained remission
√6ᵗʰ **F11.12 Opioid abuse with** intoxication
    F11.120 Opioid abuse with intoxication, uncomplicated
    F11.121 Opioid abuse with intoxication delirium
    F11.122 Opioid abuse with intoxication with perceptual disturbance
    F11.129 Opioid abuse with intoxication, unspecified
    F11.14 Opioid abuse with opioid-induced mood disorder
        Opioid use disorder, mild, with opioid-induced depressive disorder
√6ᵗʰ **F11.15 Opioid abuse with opioid-induced** psychotic disorder
    F11.150 Opioid abuse with opioid-induced psychotic disorder with delusions
    F11.151 Opioid abuse with opioid-induced psychotic disorder with hallucinations
    F11.159 Opioid abuse with opioid-induced psychotic disorder, unspecified
√6ᵗʰ **F11.18 Opioid abuse with other opioid-induced disorder**
    F11.181 Opioid abuse with opioid-induced sexual dysfunction
    F11.182 Opioid abuse with opioid-induced sleep disorder
    F11.188 Opioid abuse with other opioid-induced disorder
F11.19 Opioid abuse with unspecified opioid-induced disorder
√5ᵗʰ **F11.2 Opioid** dependence
    EXCLUDES 1   opioid abuse (F11.1-)
                   opioid use, unspecified (F11.9-)
    EXCLUDES 2   opioid poisoning (T40.0-T40.2-)
    F11.20 Opioid dependence, uncomplicated
        Opioid use disorder, moderate
        Opioid use disorder, severe
    F11.21 Opioid dependence, in remission
        Opioid use disorder, moderate, in early remission
        Opioid use disorder, moderate, in sustained remission
        Opioid use disorder, severe, in early remission
        Opioid use disorder, severe, in sustained remission
√6ᵗʰ **F11.22 Opioid dependence with** intoxication
    EXCLUDES 1   opioid dependence with withdrawal (F11.23)
    F11.220 Opioid dependence with intoxication, uncomplicated
    F11.221 Opioid dependence with intoxication delirium
    F11.222 Opioid dependence with intoxication with perceptual disturbance
    F11.229 Opioid dependence with intoxication, unspecified
    F11.23 Opioid dependence with withdrawal
        EXCLUDES 1   opioid dependence with intoxication (F11.22-)
    F11.24 Opioid dependence with opioid-induced mood disorder
        Opioid use disorder, moderate, with opioid induced depressive disorder
√6ᵗʰ **F11.25 Opioid dependence with opioid-induced** psychotic disorder
    F11.250 Opioid dependence with opioid-induced psychotic disorder with delusions
    F11.251 Opioid dependence with opioid-induced psychotic disorder with hallucinations
    F11.259 Opioid dependence with opioid-induced psychotic disorder, unspecified
√6ᵗʰ **F11.28 Opioid dependence with other opioid-induced disorder**
    F11.281 Opioid dependence with opioid induced sexual dysfunction

Chapter 5. Mental, Behavioral and Neurodevelopmental Disorders

F11.282–F12.922

     F11.282   Opioid dependence with opioid-induced sleep disorder

     F11.288   Opioid dependence with other opioid-induced disorder

   F11.29   Opioid dependence with unspecified opioid-induced disorder

✓5th **F11.9**   Opioid use, unspecified

    EXCLUDES 1   opioid abuse (F11.1-)

           opioid dependence (F11.2-)

    TIP: Assign a substance use code only when the provider documents a relationship between the use and an associated physical, mental, or behavioral disorder. As with all diagnoses, substance use codes must meet the definition of a reportable diagnosis.

   F11.90   Opioid use, unspecified, uncomplicated
        AHA: 2018,2Q,10-11

   ✓6th **F11.92**   Opioid use, unspecified with intoxication

    EXCLUDES 1   opioid use, unspecified with withdrawal (F11.93)

     F11.920   Opioid use, unspecified with intoxication, uncomplicated

     F11.921   Opioid use, unspecified with intoxication delirium
         Opioid-induced delirium

     F11.922   Opioid use, unspecified with intoxication with perceptual disturbance

     F11.929   Opioid use, unspecified with intoxication, unspecified

   F11.93   Opioid use, unspecified with withdrawal
    EXCLUDES 1   opioid use, unspecified with intoxication (F11.92-)

   F11.94   Opioid use, unspecified with opioid-induced mood disorder
     Opioid induced depressive disorder, without use disorder

   ✓6th **F11.95**   Opioid use, unspecified with opioid-induced psychotic disorder

     F11.950   Opioid use, unspecified with opioid-induced psychotic disorder with delusions

     F11.951   Opioid use, unspecified with opioid-induced psychotic disorder with hallucinations

     F11.959   Opioid use, unspecified with opioid-induced psychotic disorder, unspecified

   ✓6th **F11.98**   Opioid use, unspecified with other specified opioid-induced disorder

     F11.981   Opioid use, unspecified with opioid-induced sexual dysfunction
         Opioid induced sexual dysfunction, without use disorder

     F11.982   Opioid use, unspecified with opioid-induced sleep disorder
         Opioid induced sleep disorder, without use disorder

     F11.988   Opioid use, unspecified with other opioid-induced disorder
         Opioid induced anxiety disorder, without use disorder

   F11.99   Opioid use, unspecified with unspecified opioid-induced disorder

✓4th **F12**   Cannabis related disorders
    INCLUDES   marijuana

✓5th **F12.1**   Cannabis abuse
    EXCLUDES 1   cannabis dependence (F12.2-)
          cannabis use, unspecified (F12.9-)

   F12.10   Cannabis abuse, uncomplicated
     Cannabis use disorder, mild

   F12.11   Cannabis abuse, in remission
     Cannabis use disorder, mild, in early remission
     Cannabis use disorder, mild, in sustained remission

   ✓6th **F12.12**   Cannabis abuse with intoxication

     F12.120   Cannabis abuse with intoxication, uncomplicated

     F12.121   Cannabis abuse with intoxication delirium

     F12.122   Cannabis abuse with intoxication with perceptual disturbance

     F12.129   Cannabis abuse with intoxication, unspecified

   ✓6th **F12.15**   Cannabis abuse with psychotic disorder

     F12.150   Cannabis abuse with psychotic disorder with delusions

     F12.151   Cannabis abuse with psychotic disorder with hallucinations

     F12.159   Cannabis abuse with psychotic disorder, unspecified

   ✓6th **F12.18**   Cannabis abuse with other cannabis-induced disorder

     F12.180   Cannabis abuse with cannabis-induced anxiety disorder

     F12.188   Cannabis abuse with other cannabis-induced disorder
         Cannabis use disorder, mild, with cannabis-induced sleep disorder

   F12.19   Cannabis abuse with unspecified cannabis-induced disorder

✓5th **F12.2**   Cannabis dependence
    EXCLUDES 1   cannabis abuse (F12.1-)
          cannabis use, unspecified (F12.9-)
    EXCLUDES 2   cannabis poisoning (T40.7-)

   F12.20   Cannabis dependence, uncomplicated
     Cannabis use disorder, moderate
     Cannabis use disorder, severe

   F12.21   Cannabis dependence, in remission
     Cannabis use disorder, moderate, in early remission
     Cannabis use disorder, moderate, in sustained remission
     Cannabis use disorder, severe, in early remission
     Cannabis use disorder, severe, in sustained remission

   ✓6th **F12.22**   Cannabis dependence with intoxication

     F12.220   Cannabis dependence with intoxication, uncomplicated

     F12.221   Cannabis dependence with intoxication delirium

     F12.222   Cannabis dependence with intoxication with perceptual disturbance

     F12.229   Cannabis dependence with intoxication, unspecified

   F12.23   Cannabis dependence with withdrawal
     AHA: 2018,4Q,7

   ✓6th **F12.25**   Cannabis dependence with psychotic disorder

     F12.250   Cannabis dependence with psychotic disorder with delusions

     F12.251   Cannabis dependence with psychotic disorder with hallucinations

     F12.259   Cannabis dependence with psychotic disorder, unspecified

   ✓6th **F12.28**   Cannabis dependence with other cannabis-induced disorder

     F12.280   Cannabis dependence with cannabis-induced anxiety disorder

     F12.288   Cannabis dependence with other cannabis-induced disorder
         Cannabis use disorder, moderate, with cannabis-induced sleep disorder
         Cannabis use disorder, severe, with cannabis-induced sleep disorder

   F12.29   Cannabis dependence with unspecified cannabis-induced disorder

✓5th **F12.9**   Cannabis use, unspecified
    EXCLUDES 1   cannabis abuse (F12.1-)
          cannabis dependence (F12.2-)

    TIP: Assign a substance use code only when the provider documents a relationship between the use and an associated physical, mental, or behavioral disorder. As with all diagnoses, substance use codes must meet the definition of a reportable diagnosis.

   F12.90   Cannabis use, unspecified, uncomplicated
     AHA: 2018,2Q,10-11

   ✓6th **F12.92**   Cannabis use, unspecified with intoxication

     F12.920   Cannabis use, unspecified with intoxication, uncomplicated

     F12.921   Cannabis use, unspecified with intoxication delirium

     F12.922   Cannabis use, unspecified with intoxication with perceptual disturbance

N Newborn: 0   P Pediatric: 0-17   M Maternity: 12-55   A Adult: 15-124   CH Comorbidity High   CL Comorbidity Low   NCDx Noncancer Dx   PDx Primary Dx

538   ICD-10-CM 2020

F12.929 **Cannabis use, unspecified with intoxication, unspecified**

F12.93 **Cannabis use, unspecified with** withdrawal
AHA: 2018,4Q,7

√6ᵗʰ F12.95 **Cannabis use, unspecified with** psychotic disorder

F12.950 **Cannabis use, unspecified with psychotic disorder with** delusions

F12.951 **Cannabis use, unspecified with psychotic disorder with** hallucinations

F12.959 **Cannabis use, unspecified with psychotic disorder, unspecified**
Cannabis induced psychotic disorder, without use disorder

√6ᵗʰ F12.98 **Cannabis use, unspecified with other cannabis-induced disorder**

F12.980 **Cannabis use, unspecified with** anxiety disorder
Cannabis induced anxiety disorder, without use disorder

F12.988 **Cannabis use, unspecified with other cannabis-induced disorder**
Cannabis induced sleep disorder, without use disorder

F12.99 **Cannabis use, unspecified with unspecified cannabis-induced disorder**

√4ᵗʰ **F13** Sedative, hypnotic, or anxiolytic **related disorders**

√5ᵗʰ **F13.1 Sedative, hypnotic or anxiolytic-related** abuse

EXCLUDES 1   *sedative, hypnotic or anxiolytic-related dependence (F13.2-)*
sedative, hypnotic, or anxiolytic use, unspecified (F13.9-)

F13.10 **Sedative, hypnotic or anxiolytic abuse,** uncomplicated
Sedative, hypnotic, or anxiolytic use disorder, mild

F13.11 **Sedative, hypnotic or anxiolytic abuse, in remission**
Sedative, hypnotic or anxiolytic use disorder, mild, in early remission
Sedative, hypnotic or anxiolytic use disorder, mild, in sustained remission

√6ᵗʰ F13.12 **Sedative, hypnotic or anxiolytic abuse with** intoxication

F13.120 **Sedative, hypnotic or anxiolytic abuse with intoxication,** uncomplicated

F13.121 **Sedative, hypnotic or anxiolytic abuse with intoxication** delirium

F13.129 **Sedative, hypnotic or anxiolytic abuse with intoxication, unspecified**

F13.14 **Sedative, hypnotic or anxiolytic abuse with sedative, hypnotic or anxiolytic-induced** mood disorder
Sedative, hypnotic, or anxiolytic use disorder, mild, with sedative, hypnotic, or anxiolytic-induced bipolar or related disorder
Sedative, hypnotic, or anxiolytic use disorder, mild, with sedative, hypnotic, or anxiolytic-induced depressive disorder

√6ᵗʰ F13.15 **Sedative, hypnotic or anxiolytic abuse with sedative, hypnotic or anxiolytic-induced** psychotic disorder

F13.150 **Sedative, hypnotic or anxiolytic abuse with sedative, hypnotic or anxiolytic-induced psychotic disorder with** delusions

F13.151 **Sedative, hypnotic or anxiolytic abuse with sedative, hypnotic or anxiolytic-induced psychotic disorder with** hallucinations

F13.159 **Sedative, hypnotic or anxiolytic abuse with sedative, hypnotic or anxiolytic-induced psychotic disorder, unspecified**

√6ᵗʰ F13.18 **Sedative, hypnotic or anxiolytic abuse with other sedative, hypnotic or anxiolytic-induced disorders**

F13.180 **Sedative, hypnotic or anxiolytic abuse with sedative, hypnotic or anxiolytic-induced** anxiety disorder

F13.181 **Sedative, hypnotic or anxiolytic abuse with sedative, hypnotic or anxiolytic-induced** sexual dysfunction

F13.182 **Sedative, hypnotic or anxiolytic abuse with sedative, hypnotic or anxiolytic-induced** sleep disorder

F13.188 **Sedative, hypnotic or anxiolytic abuse with other sedative, hypnotic or anxiolytic-induced disorder**

F13.19 **Sedative, hypnotic or anxiolytic abuse with unspecified sedative, hypnotic or anxiolytic-induced disorder**

√5ᵗʰ **F13.2 Sedative, hypnotic or anxiolytic-related** dependence

EXCLUDES 1   *sedative, hypnotic or anxiolytic-related abuse (F13.1-)*
sedative, hypnotic, or anxiolytic use, unspecified (F13.9-)

EXCLUDES 2   *sedative, hypnotic, or anxiolytic poisoning (T42.-)*

F13.20 **Sedative, hypnotic or anxiolytic dependence,** uncomplicated

F13.21 **Sedative, hypnotic or anxiolytic dependence, in** remission
Sedative, hypnotic or anxiolytic use disorder, moderate, in early remission
Sedative, hypnotic or anxiolytic use disorder, moderate, in sustained remission
Sedative, hypnotic or anxiolytic use disorder, severe, in early remission
Sedative, hypnotic or anxiolytic use disorder, severe, in sustained remission

√6ᵗʰ F13.22 **Sedative, hypnotic or anxiolytic dependence with** intoxication

EXCLUDES 1   *sedative, hypnotic or anxiolytic dependence with withdrawal (F13.23-)*

F13.220 **Sedative, hypnotic or anxiolytic dependence with intoxication,** uncomplicated

F13.221 **Sedative, hypnotic or anxiolytic dependence with intoxication** delirium

F13.229 **Sedative, hypnotic or anxiolytic dependence with intoxication, unspecified**

√6ᵗʰ F13.23 **Sedative, hypnotic or anxiolytic dependence with** withdrawal
Sedative, hypnotic, or anxiolytic use disorder, moderate
Sedative, hypnotic, or anxiolytic use disorder, severe

EXCLUDES 1   *sedative, hypnotic or anxiolytic dependence with intoxication (F13.22-)*

F13.230 **Sedative, hypnotic or anxiolytic dependence with withdrawal,** uncomplicated

F13.231 **Sedative, hypnotic or anxiolytic dependence with withdrawal** delirium

F13.232 **Sedative, hypnotic or anxiolytic dependence with withdrawal with** perceptual disturbance
Sedative, hypnotic, or anxiolytic withdrawal with perceptual disturbances

F13.239 **Sedative, hypnotic or anxiolytic dependence with withdrawal, unspecified**
Sedative, hypnotic, or anxiolytic withdrawal without perceptual disturbances

F13.24 **Sedative, hypnotic or anxiolytic dependence with sedative, hypnotic or anxiolytic-induced** mood disorder
Sedative, hypnotic, or anxiolytic use disorder, moderate, with sedative, hypnotic, or anxiolytic-induced bipolar or related disorder
Sedative, hypnotic, or anxiolytic use disorder, moderate, with sedative, hypnotic, or anxiolytic-induced depressive disorder
Sedative, hypnotic, or anxiolytic use disorder, severe, with sedative, hypnotic, or anxiolytic-induced bipolar or related disorder
Sedative, hypnotic, or anxiolytic use disorder, severe, with sedative, hypnotic, or anxiolytic-induced depressive disorder

Chapter 5. Mental, Behavioral and Neurodevelopmental Disorders

√6ᵗʰ **F13.25** Sedative, hypnotic or anxiolytic dependence with sedative, hypnotic or anxiolytic-induced psychotic disorder

     F13.250 Sedative, hypnotic or anxiolytic dependence with sedative, hypnotic or anxiolytic-induced psychotic disorder with delusions

     F13.251 Sedative, hypnotic or anxiolytic dependence with sedative, hypnotic or anxiolytic-induced psychotic disorder with hallucinations

     F13.259 Sedative, hypnotic or anxiolytic dependence with sedative, hypnotic or anxiolytic-induced psychotic disorder, unspecified

F13.26 Sedative, hypnotic or anxiolytic dependence with sedative, hypnotic or anxiolytic-induced persisting amnestic disorder

F13.27 Sedative, hypnotic or anxiolytic dependence with sedative, hypnotic or anxiolytic-induced persisting dementia

     Sedative, hypnotic, or anxiolytic use disorder, moderate, with sedative, hypnotic, or anxiolytic induced major neurocognitive disorder

     Sedative, hypnotic, or anxiolytic use disorder, severe, with sedative, hypnotic, or anxiolytic-induced major neurocognitive disorder

√6ᵗʰ **F13.28** Sedative, hypnotic or anxiolytic dependence with other sedative, hypnotic or anxiolytic-induced disorders

     F13.280 Sedative, hypnotic or anxiolytic dependence with sedative, hypnotic or anxiolytic-induced anxiety disorder

     F13.281 Sedative, hypnotic or anxiolytic dependence with sedative, hypnotic or anxiolytic-induced sexual dysfunction

     F13.282 Sedative, hypnotic or anxiolytic dependence with sedative, hypnotic or anxiolytic-induced sleep disorder

     F13.288 Sedative, hypnotic or anxiolytic dependence with other sedative, hypnotic or anxiolytic-induced disorder

         Sedative, hypnotic, or anxiolytic use disorder, moderate, with sedative, hypnotic, or anxiolytic-induced mild neurocognitive disorder

         Sedative, hypnotic, or anxiolytic use disorder, severe, with sedative, hypnotic, or anxiolytic-induced mild neurocognitive disorder

     F13.29 Sedative, hypnotic or anxiolytic dependence with unspecified sedative, hypnotic or anxiolytic-induced disorder

√5ᵗʰ **F13.9** Sedative, hypnotic or anxiolytic-related use, unspecified

     EXCLUDES 1   sedative, hypnotic or anxiolytic-related abuse (F13.1-)

                sedative, hypnotic or anxiolytic-related dependence (F13.2-)

     TIP: Assign a substance use code only when the provider documents a relationship between the use and an associated physical, mental, or behavioral disorder. As with all diagnoses, substance use codes must meet the definition of a reportable diagnosis.

     F13.90 Sedative, hypnotic, or anxiolytic use, unspecified, uncomplicated

         AHA: 2018,2Q,10-11

√6ᵗʰ **F13.92** Sedative, hypnotic or anxiolytic use, unspecified with intoxication

     EXCLUDES 1   sedative, hypnotic or anxiolytic use, unspecified with withdrawal (F13.93-)

     F13.920 Sedative, hypnotic or anxiolytic use, unspecified with intoxication, uncomplicated

     F13.921 Sedative, hypnotic or anxiolytic use, unspecified with intoxication delirium

         Sedative, hypnotic, or anxiolytic-induced delirium

     F13.929 Sedative, hypnotic or anxiolytic use, unspecified with intoxication, unspecified

√6ᵗʰ **F13.93** Sedative, hypnotic or anxiolytic use, unspecified with withdrawal

     EXCLUDES 1   sedative, hypnotic or anxiolytic use, unspecified with intoxication (F13.92-)

     F13.930 Sedative, hypnotic or anxiolytic use, unspecified with withdrawal, uncomplicated

     F13.931 Sedative, hypnotic or anxiolytic use, unspecified with withdrawal delirium

     F13.932 Sedative, hypnotic or anxiolytic use, unspecified with withdrawal with perceptual disturbances

     F13.939 Sedative, hypnotic or anxiolytic use, unspecified with withdrawal, unspecified

F13.94 Sedative, hypnotic or anxiolytic use, unspecified with sedative, hypnotic or anxiolytic-induced mood disorder

     Sedative, hypnotic, or anxiolytic-induced bipolar or related disorder, without use disorder

     Sedative, hypnotic, or anxiolytic-induced depressive disorder, without use disorder

√6ᵗʰ **F13.95** Sedative, hypnotic or anxiolytic use, unspecified with sedative, hypnotic or anxiolytic-induced psychotic disorder

     F13.950 Sedative, hypnotic or anxiolytic use, unspecified with sedative, hypnotic or anxiolytic-induced psychotic disorder with delusions

     F13.951 Sedative, hypnotic or anxiolytic use, unspecified with sedative, hypnotic or anxiolytic-induced psychotic disorder with hallucinations

     F13.959 Sedative, hypnotic or anxiolytic use, unspecified with sedative, hypnotic or anxiolytic-induced psychotic disorder, unspecified

         Sedative, hypnotic, or anxiolytic-induced psychotic disorder, without use disorder

F13.96 Sedative, hypnotic or anxiolytic use, unspecified with sedative, hypnotic or anxiolytic-induced persisting amnestic disorder

F13.97 Sedative, hypnotic or anxiolytic use, unspecified with sedative, hypnotic or anxiolytic-induced persisting dementia

     Sedative, hypnotic, or anxiolytic-induced major neurocognitive disorder, without use disorder

√6ᵗʰ **F13.98** Sedative, hypnotic or anxiolytic use, unspecified with other sedative, hypnotic or anxiolytic-induced disorders

     F13.980 Sedative, hypnotic or anxiolytic use, unspecified with sedative, hypnotic or anxiolytic-induced anxiety disorder

         Sedative, hypnotic, or anxiolytic-induced anxiety disorder, without use disorder

     F13.981 Sedative, hypnotic or anxiolytic use, unspecified with sedative, hypnotic or anxiolytic-induced sexual dysfunction

         Sedative, hypnotic, or anxiolytic-induced sexual dysfunction disorder, without use disorder

     F13.982 Sedative, hypnotic or anxiolytic use, unspecified with sedative, hypnotic or anxiolytic-induced sleep disorder

         Sedative, hypnotic, or anxiolytic-induced sleep disorder, without use disorder

     F13.988 Sedative, hypnotic or anxiolytic use, unspecified with other sedative, hypnotic or anxiolytic-induced disorder

         Sedative, hypnotic, or anxiolytic-induced mild neurocognitive disorder

     F13.99 Sedative, hypnotic or anxiolytic use, unspecified with unspecified sedative, hypnotic or anxiolytic-induced disorder

---

N Newborn: 0   P Pediatric: 0-17   M Maternity: 12-55   A Adult: 15-124   CH Comorbidity High   CL Comorbidity Low   NCDx Noncancer Dx   PDx Primary Dx

✓4ᵗʰ **F14** Cocaine related disorders

    EXCLUDES 2   *other stimulant-related disorders (F15.-)*

✓5ᵗʰ **F14.1** Cocaine abuse

    EXCLUDES 1   *cocaine dependence (F14.2-)*

              cocaine use, unspecified (F14.9-)

    F14.10 Cocaine abuse, uncomplicated

        Cocaine use disorder, mild

    F14.11 Cocaine abuse, in remission

        Cocaine use disorder, mild, in early remission

        Cocaine use disorder, mild, in sustained remission

   ✓6ᵗʰ **F14.12** Cocaine abuse with intoxication

        F14.120 Cocaine abuse with intoxication, uncomplicated

        F14.121 Cocaine abuse with intoxication with delirium

        F14.122 Cocaine abuse with intoxication with perceptual disturbance

        F14.129 Cocaine abuse with intoxication, unspecified

    F14.14 Cocaine abuse with cocaine-induced mood disorder

        Cocaine use disorder, mild, with cocaine-induced bipolar or related disorder

        Cocaine use disorder, mild, with cocaine-induced depressive disorder

   ✓6ᵗʰ **F14.15** Cocaine abuse with cocaine-induced psychotic disorder

        F14.150 Cocaine abuse with cocaine-induced psychotic disorder with delusions

        F14.151 Cocaine abuse with cocaine-induced psychotic disorder with hallucinations

        F14.159 Cocaine abuse with cocaine-induced psychotic disorder, unspecified

   ✓6ᵗʰ **F14.18** Cocaine abuse with other cocaine-induced disorder

        F14.180 Cocaine abuse with cocaine-induced anxiety disorder

        F14.181 Cocaine abuse with cocaine-induced sexual dysfunction

        F14.182 Cocaine abuse with cocaine-induced sleep disorder

        F14.188 Cocaine abuse with other cocaine-induced disorder

            Cocaine use disorder, mild, with cocaine-induced obsessive compulsive or related disorder

    F14.19 Cocaine abuse with unspecified cocaine-induced disorder

✓5ᵗʰ **F14.2** Cocaine dependence

    EXCLUDES 1   *cocaine abuse (F14.1-)*

              cocaine use, unspecified (F14.9-)

    EXCLUDES 2   *cocaine poisoning (T40.5-)*

    F14.20 Cocaine dependence, uncomplicated

        Cocaine use disorder, moderate

        Cocaine use disorder, severe

    F14.21 Cocaine dependence, in remission

        Cocaine use disorder, moderate, in early remission

        Cocaine use disorder, moderate, in sustained remission

        Cocaine use disorder, severe, in early remission

        Cocaine use disorder, severe, in sustained remission

   ✓6ᵗʰ **F14.22** Cocaine dependence with intoxication

        EXCLUDES 1   *cocaine dependence with withdrawal (F14.23)*

        F14.220 Cocaine dependence with intoxication, uncomplicated

        F14.221 Cocaine dependence with intoxication delirium

        F14.222 Cocaine dependence with intoxication with perceptual disturbance

        F14.229 Cocaine dependence with intoxication, unspecified

    F14.23 Cocaine dependence with withdrawal

        EXCLUDES 1   *cocaine dependence with intoxication (F14.22-)*

F14.24 Cocaine dependence with cocaine-induced mood disorder

    Cocaine use disorder, moderate, with cocaine-induced bipolar or related disorder

    Cocaine use disorder, moderate, with cocaine-induced depressive disorder

    Cocaine use disorder, severe, with cocaine-induced bipolar or related disorder

    Cocaine use disorder, severe, with cocaine-induced depressive disorder

✓6ᵗʰ **F14.25** Cocaine dependence with cocaine-induced psychotic disorder

    F14.250 Cocaine dependence with cocaine-induced psychotic disorder with delusions

    F14.251 Cocaine dependence with cocaine-induced psychotic disorder with hallucinations

    F14.259 Cocaine dependence with cocaine-induced psychotic disorder, unspecified

✓6ᵗʰ **F14.28** Cocaine dependence with other cocaine-induced disorder

    F14.280 Cocaine dependence with cocaine-induced anxiety disorder

    F14.281 Cocaine dependence with cocaine-induced sexual dysfunction

    F14.282 Cocaine dependence with cocaine-induced sleep disorder

    F14.288 Cocaine dependence with other cocaine-induced disorder

        Cocaine use disorder, moderate, with cocaine-induced obsessive compulsive or related disorder

        Cocaine use disorder, severe, with cocaine-induced obsessive compulsive or related disorder

F14.29 Cocaine dependence with unspecified cocaine-induced disorder

✓5ᵗʰ **F14.9** Cocaine use, unspecified

    EXCLUDES 1   *cocaine abuse (F14.1-)*

              cocaine dependence (F14.2-)

    TIP: Assign a substance use code only when the provider documents a relationship between the use and an associated physical, mental, or behavioral disorder. As with all diagnoses, substance use codes must meet the definition of a reportable diagnosis.

    F14.90 Cocaine use, unspecified, uncomplicated

        AHA: 2018,2Q,10-11

   ✓6ᵗʰ **F14.92** Cocaine use, unspecified with intoxication

        F14.920 Cocaine use, unspecified with intoxication, uncomplicated

        F14.921 Cocaine use, unspecified with intoxication delirium

        F14.922 Cocaine use, unspecified with intoxication with perceptual disturbance

        F14.929 Cocaine use, unspecified with intoxication, unspecified

    F14.94 Cocaine use, unspecified with cocaine-induced mood disorder

        Cocaine induced bipolar or related disorder, without use disorder

        Cocaine induced depressive disorder, without use disorder

   ✓6ᵗʰ **F14.95** Cocaine use, unspecified with cocaine-induced psychotic disorder

        F14.950 Cocaine use, unspecified with cocaine-induced psychotic disorder with delusions

        F14.951 Cocaine use, unspecified with cocaine-induced psychotic disorder with hallucinations

        F14.959 Cocaine use, unspecified with cocaine-induced psychotic disorder, unspecified

            Cocaine induced psychotic disorder, without use disorder

☑ Additional Character Required   ✓x7ᵗʰ Placeholder Alert   Manifestation   Unspecified Dx   ►◄ Revised Text   ● New Code   ▲ Revised Title

ICD-10-CM 2020   **541**

✓6ᵗʰ **F14.98 Cocaine use, unspecified with other specified cocaine-induced disorder**

F14.980 Cocaine use, unspecified with cocaine-induced anxiety disorder

Cocaine induced anxiety disorder, without use disorder

F14.981 Cocaine use, unspecified with cocaine-induced sexual dysfunction

Cocaine induced sexual dysfunction, without use disorder

F14.982 Cocaine use, unspecified with cocaine-induced sleep disorder

Cocaine induced sleep disorder, without use disorder

F14.988 Cocaine use, unspecified with other cocaine-induced disorder

Cocaine induced obsessive compulsive or related disorder

F14.99 Cocaine use, unspecified with unspecified cocaine-induced disorder

✓4ᵗʰ **F15 Other** stimulant **related disorders**

INCLUDES   amphetamine-related disorders
                       caffeine
EXCLUDES 2   cocaine-related disorders (F14.-)

✓5ᵗʰ **F15.1 Other stimulant** abuse

EXCLUDES 1   other stimulant dependence (F15.2-)
                       other stimulant use, unspecified (F15.9-)

F15.10 Other stimulant abuse, uncomplicated

Amphetamine type substance use disorder, mild
Other or unspecified stimulant use disorder, mild

F15.11 Other stimulant abuse, in remission

Amphetamine type substance use disorder, mild, in early remission
Amphetamine type substance use disorder, mild, in sustained remission
Other or unspecified stimulant use disorder, mild, in early remission
Other or unspecified stimulant use disorder, mild, in sustained remission

✓6ᵗʰ **F15.12 Other stimulant abuse with** intoxication

F15.120 Other stimulant abuse with intoxication, uncomplicated

F15.121 Other stimulant abuse with intoxication delirium

F15.122 Other stimulant abuse with intoxication with perceptual disturbance

Amphetamine or other stimulant use disorder, mild, with amphetamine or other stimulant intoxication, with perceptual disturbances

F15.129 Other stimulant abuse with intoxication, unspecified

Amphetamine or other stimulant use disorder, mild, with amphetamine or other stimulant intoxication, without perceptual disturbances

F15.14 Other stimulant abuse with stimulant-induced mood disorder

Amphetamine or other stimulant use disorder, mild, with amphetamine or other stimulant induced bipolar or related disorder
Amphetamine or other stimulant use disorder, mild, with amphetamine or other stimulant induced depressive disorder

✓6ᵗʰ **F15.15 Other stimulant abuse with stimulant-induced** psychotic disorder

F15.150 Other stimulant abuse with stimulant-induced psychotic disorder with delusions

F15.151 Other stimulant abuse with stimulant-induced psychotic disorder with hallucinations

F15.159 Other stimulant abuse with stimulant-induced psychotic disorder, unspecified

✓6ᵗʰ **F15.18 Other stimulant abuse with other stimulant-induced disorder**

F15.180 Other stimulant abuse with stimulant-induced anxiety disorder

F15.181 Other stimulant abuse with stimulant-induced sexual dysfunction

F15.182 Other stimulant abuse with stimulant-induced sleep disorder

F15.188 Other stimulant abuse with other stimulant-induced disorder

Amphetamine or other stimulant use disorder, mild, with amphetamine or other stimulant induced obsessive-compulsive or related disorder

F15.19 Other stimulant abuse with unspecified stimulant-induced disorder

✓5ᵗʰ **F15.2 Other stimulant** dependence

EXCLUDES 1   other stimulant abuse (F15.1-)
                       other stimulant use, unspecified (F15.9-)

F15.20 Other stimulant dependence, uncomplicated

Amphetamine type substance use disorder, moderate
Amphetamine type substance use disorder, severe
Other or unspecified stimulant use disorder, moderate
Other or unspecified stimulant use disorder, severe

F15.21 Other stimulant dependence, in remission

Amphetamine type substance use disorder, moderate, in early remission
Amphetamine type substance use disorder, moderate, in sustained remission
Amphetamine type substance use disorder, severe, in early remission
Amphetamine type substance use disorder, severe, in sustained remission
Other or unspecified stimulant use disorder, moderate, in early remission
Other or unspecified stimulant use disorder, moderate, in sustained remission
Other or unspecified stimulant use disorder, severe, in early remission
Other or unspecified stimulant use disorder, severe, in sustained remission

✓6ᵗʰ **F15.22 Other stimulant dependence with** intoxication

EXCLUDES 1   other stimulant dependence with withdrawal (F15.23)

F15.220 Other stimulant dependence with intoxication, uncomplicated

F15.221 Other stimulant dependence with intoxication delirium

F15.222 Other stimulant dependence with intoxication with perceptual disturbance

Amphetamine or other stimulant use disorder, moderate, with amphetamine or other stimulant intoxication, with perceptual disturbances
Amphetamine or other stimulant use disorder, severe, with amphetamine or other stimulant intoxication, with perceptual disturbances

F15.229 Other stimulant dependence with intoxication, unspecified

Amphetamine or other stimulant use disorder, moderate, with amphetamine or other stimulant intoxication, without perceptual disturbances
Amphetamine or other stimulant use disorder, severe, with amphetamine or other stimulant intoxication, without perceptual disturbances

F15.23 Other stimulant dependence with withdrawal

Amphetamine or other stimulant withdrawal
EXCLUDES 1   other stimulant dependence with intoxication (F15.22-)

F15.24   **Other stimulant dependence with stimulant-induced** mood disorder

Amphetamine or other stimulant use disorder, moderate, with amphetamine or other stimulant-induced bipolar or related disorder

Amphetamine or other stimulant use disorder, moderate, with amphetamine or other stimulant induced depressive disorder

Amphetamine or other stimulant use disorder, severe, with amphetamine or other stimulant-induced bipolar or related disorder

Amphetamine or other stimulant use disorder, severe, with amphetamine or other stimulant-induced depressive disorder

✓6ᵗʰ **F15.25**   **Other stimulant dependence with stimulant-induced** psychotic disorder

   F15.250   **Other stimulant dependence with stimulant-induced psychotic disorder with** delusions

   F15.251   **Other stimulant dependence with stimulant-induced psychotic disorder with** hallucinations

   F15.259   **Other stimulant dependence with stimulant-induced psychotic disorder, unspecified**

✓6ᵗʰ **F15.28**   **Other stimulant dependence with other stimulant-induced disorder**

   F15.280   **Other stimulant dependence with stimulant-induced** anxiety disorder

   F15.281   **Other stimulant dependence with stimulant-induced** sexual dysfunction

   F15.282   **Other stimulant dependence with stimulant-induced** sleep disorder

   F15.288   **Other stimulant dependence with other stimulant-induced disorder**

Amphetamine or other stimulant use disorder, moderate, with amphetamine orother stimulant induced obsessive compulsive or related disorder

Amphetamine or other stimulant use disorder, severe, with amphetamine or otherstimulant induced obsessive compulsive or related disorder

F15.29   **Other stimulant dependence with unspecified stimulant-induced disorder**

✓5ᵗʰ **F15.9**   **Other stimulant** use, unspecified

> EXCLUDES 1   other stimulant abuse (F15.1-)
> other stimulant dependence (F15.2-)

TIP: Assign a substance use code only when the provider documents a relationship between the use and an associated physical, mental, or behavioral disorder. As with all diagnoses, substance use codes must meet the definition of a reportable diagnosis.

F15.90   **Other stimulant use, unspecified,** uncomplicated
   AHA: 2018,2Q,10-11

✓6ᵗʰ **F15.92**   **Other stimulant use, unspecified with** intoxication

> EXCLUDES 1   other stimulant use, unspecified with withdrawal (F15.93)

   F15.920   **Other stimulant use, unspecified with intoxication,** uncomplicated

   F15.921   **Other stimulant use, unspecified with intoxication** delirium
     Amphetamine or other stimulant-induced delirium

   F15.922   **Other stimulant use, unspecified with intoxication with** perceptual disturbance

   F15.929   **Other stimulant use, unspecified with intoxication, unspecified**
     Caffeine intoxication

F15.93   **Other stimulant use, unspecified with** withdrawal
   Caffeine withdrawal
> EXCLUDES 1   other stimulant use, unspecified with intoxication (F15.92-)

F15.94   **Other stimulant use, unspecified with stimulant-induced** mood disorder

Amphetamine or other stimulant-induced bipolar or related disorder, without use disorder

Amphetamine or other stimulant-induced depressive disorder, without use disorder

✓6ᵗʰ **F15.95**   **Other stimulant use, unspecified with stimulant-induced** psychotic disorder

   F15.950   **Other stimulant use, unspecified with stimulant-induced psychotic disorder with** delusions

   F15.951   **Other stimulant use, unspecified with stimulant-induced psychotic disorder with** hallucinations

   F15.959   **Other stimulant use, unspecified with stimulant-induced psychotic disorder, unspecified**
     Amphetamine or other stimulant-induced psychotic disorder, without use disorder

✓6ᵗʰ **F15.98**   **Other stimulant use, unspecified with other stimulant-induced disorder**

   F15.980   **Other stimulant use, unspecified with stimulant-induced** anxiety disorder
     Amphetamine or other stimulant-induced anxiety disorder, without use disorder
     Caffeine induced anxiety disorder, without use disorder

   F15.981   **Other stimulant use, unspecified with stimulant-induced** sexual dysfunction
     Amphetamine or other stimulant-induced sexual dysfunction, without use disorder

   F15.982   **Other stimulant use, unspecified with stimulant-induced** sleep disorder
     Amphetamine or other stimulant-induced sleep disorder, without use disorder
     Caffeine induced sleep disorder, without use disorder

   F15.988   **Other stimulant use, unspecified with other stimulant-induced disorder**
     Amphetamine or other stimulant-induced obsessive compulsive or related disorder, without use disorder

F15.99   **Other stimulant use, unspecified with unspecified stimulant-induced disorder**

✓4ᵗʰ **F16**   Hallucinogen related disorders

> INCLUDES   ecstasy
> PCP
> phencyclidine

AHA: 2018,4Q,31

✓5ᵗʰ **F16.1**   **Hallucinogen** abuse

> EXCLUDES 1   hallucinogen dependence (F16.2-)
> hallucinogen use, unspecified (F16.9-)

F16.10   **Hallucinogen abuse,** uncomplicated
   Other hallucinogen use disorder, mild
   Phencyclidine use disorder, mild

F16.11   **Hallucinogen abuse,** in remission
   Other hallucinogen use disorder, mild, in early remission
   Other hallucinogen use disorder, mild, in sustained remission
   Phencyclidine use disorder, mild, in early remission
   Phencyclidine use disorder, mild, in sustained remission

✓6ᵗʰ **F16.12**   **Hallucinogen abuse with** intoxication

   F16.120   **Hallucinogen abuse with intoxication,** uncomplicated

   F16.121   **Hallucinogen abuse with intoxication with** delirium

   F16.122   **Hallucinogen abuse with intoxication with** perceptual disturbance

   F16.129   **Hallucinogen abuse with intoxication, unspecified**

✔ Additional Character Required   ✓x7ᵗʰ Placeholder Alert   Manifestation   Unspecified Dx   ▶◀ Revised Text   ● New Code   ▲ Revised Title

ICD-10-CM 2020   **543**

F16.14 **Hallucinogen abuse with hallucinogen-induced mood disorder**
Other hallucinogen use disorder, mild, with other hallucinogen induced bipolar or related disorder
Other hallucinogen use disorder, mild, with other hallucinogen induced depressive disorder
Phencyclidine use disorder, mild, with phencyclidine induced bipolar or related disorder
Phencyclidine use disorder, mild, with phencyclidine induced depressive disorder

√6ᵗʰ F16.15 **Hallucinogen abuse with hallucinogen-induced psychotic disorder**
F16.150 **Hallucinogen abuse with hallucinogen-induced psychotic disorder with delusions**
F16.151 **Hallucinogen abuse with hallucinogen-induced psychotic disorder with hallucinations**
F16.159 **Hallucinogen abuse with hallucinogen-induced psychotic disorder, unspecified**

√6ᵗʰ F16.18 **Hallucinogen abuse with other hallucinogen-induced disorder**
F16.180 **Hallucinogen abuse with hallucinogen-induced anxiety disorder**
F16.183 **Hallucinogen abuse with hallucinogen persisting perception disorder (flashbacks)**
F16.188 **Hallucinogen abuse with other hallucinogen-induced disorder**

F16.19 **Hallucinogen abuse with unspecified hallucinogen-induced disorder**

√5ᵗʰ F16.2 **Hallucinogen dependence**
EXCLUDES 1 *hallucinogen abuse (F16.1-)*
hallucinogen use, unspecified (F16.9-)

F16.20 **Hallucinogen dependence, uncomplicated**
Other hallucinogen use disorder, moderate
Other hallucinogen use disorder, severe
Phencyclidine use disorder, moderate
Phencyclidine use disorder, severe

F16.21 **Hallucinogen dependence, in remission**
Other hallucinogen use disorder, moderate, in early remission
Other hallucinogen use disorder, moderate, in sustained remission
Other hallucinogen use disorder, severe, in early remission
Other hallucinogen use disorder, severe, in sustained remission
Phencyclidine use disorder, moderate, in early remission
Phencyclidine use disorder, moderate, in sustained remission
Phencyclidine use disorder, severe, in early remission
Phencyclidine use disorder, severe, in sustained remission

√6ᵗʰ F16.22 **Hallucinogen dependence with intoxication**
F16.220 **Hallucinogen dependence with intoxication, uncomplicated**
F16.221 **Hallucinogen dependence with intoxication with delirium**
F16.229 **Hallucinogen dependence with intoxication, unspecified**

F16.24 **Hallucinogen dependence with hallucinogen-induced mood disorder**
Other hallucinogen use disorder, moderate, with other hallucinogen induced bipolar or related disorder
Other hallucinogen use disorder, moderate, with other hallucinogen induced depressive disorder
Other hallucinogen use disorder, severe, with other hallucinogen-induced bipolar or related disorder
Other hallucinogen use disorder, severe, with other hallucinogen-induced depressive disorder
Phencyclidine use disorder, moderate, with phencyclidine induced bipolar or related disorder
Phencyclidine use disorder, moderate, with phencyclidine induced depressive disorder
Phencyclidine use disorder, severe, with phencyclidine induced bipolar or related disorder
Phencyclidine use disorder, severe, with phencyclidine-induced depressive disorder

√6ᵗʰ F16.25 **Hallucinogen dependence with hallucinogen-induced psychotic disorder**
F16.250 **Hallucinogen dependence with hallucinogen-induced psychotic disorder with delusions**
F16.251 **Hallucinogen dependence with hallucinogen-induced psychotic disorder with hallucinations**
F16.259 **Hallucinogen dependence with hallucinogen-induced psychotic disorder, unspecified**

√6ᵗʰ F16.28 **Hallucinogen dependence with other hallucinogen-induced disorder**
F16.280 **Hallucinogen dependence with hallucinogen-induced anxiety disorder**
F16.283 **Hallucinogen dependence with hallucinogen persisting perception disorder (flashbacks)**
F16.288 **Hallucinogen dependence with other hallucinogen-induced disorder**

F16.29 **Hallucinogen dependence with unspecified hallucinogen-induced disorder**

√5ᵗʰ F16.9 **Hallucinogen use, unspecified**
EXCLUDES 1 *hallucinogen abuse (F16.1-)*
hallucinogen dependence (F16.2-)
TIP: Assign a substance use code only when the provider documents a relationship between the use and an associated physical, mental, or behavioral disorder. As with all diagnoses, substance use codes must meet the definition of a reportable diagnosis.

F16.90 **Hallucinogen use, unspecified, uncomplicated**
AHA: 2018,2Q,10-11

√6ᵗʰ F16.92 **Hallucinogen use, unspecified with intoxication**
F16.920 **Hallucinogen use, unspecified with intoxication, uncomplicated**
F16.921 **Hallucinogen use, unspecified with intoxication with delirium**
Other hallucinogen intoxication delirium
F16.929 **Hallucinogen use, unspecified with intoxication, unspecified**

F16.94 **Hallucinogen use, unspecified with hallucinogen-induced mood disorder**
Other hallucinogen induced bipolar or related disorder, without use disorder
Other hallucinogen induced depressive disorder, without use disorder
Phencyclidine induced bipolar or related disorder, without use disorder
Phencyclidine induced depressive disorder, without use disorder

√6ᵗʰ F16.95 **Hallucinogen use, unspecified with hallucinogen-induced psychotic disorder**
F16.950 **Hallucinogen use, unspecified with hallucinogen-induced psychotic disorder with delusions**
F16.951 **Hallucinogen use, unspecified with hallucinogen-induced psychotic disorder with hallucinations**

F16.959   **Hallucinogen use, unspecified with hallucinogen-induced psychotic disorder, unspecified**
Other hallucinogen induced psychotic disorder, without use disorder
Phencyclidine induced psychotic disorder, without use disorder

√6ᵗʰ   **F16.98**   **Hallucinogen use, unspecified with other specified hallucinogen-induced disorder**

F16.980   **Hallucinogen use, unspecified with hallucinogen-induced** anxiety disorder
Other hallucinogen-induced anxiety disorder, without use disorder
Phencyclidine induced anxiety disorder, without use disorder

F16.983   **Hallucinogen use, unspecified with hallucinogen** persisting perception disorder (flashbacks)

F16.988   **Hallucinogen use, unspecified with other hallucinogen-induced disorder**

F16.99   **Hallucinogen use, unspecified with unspecified hallucinogen-induced disorder**

√4ᵗʰ   **F17**   Nicotine **dependence**

> **EXCLUDES 1**   history of tobacco dependence (Z87.891) ●
> tobacco use NOS (Z72.0) ●
> **EXCLUDES 2**   tobacco use (smoking) during pregnancy, childbirth and the puerperium (O99.33-)
> toxic effect of nicotine (T65.2-)

AHA: 2013,4Q,108-109
TIP: Provider documentation indicating "smoker" without further specification should be coded to F17.200 Nicotine dependence, unspecified, uncomplicated.

√5ᵗʰ   **F17.2**   Nicotine dependence

√6ᵗʰ   **F17.20**   **Nicotine dependence, unspecified**

F17.200   **Nicotine dependence, unspecified, uncomplicated**
Tobacco use disorder, mild
Tobacco use disorder, moderate
Tobacco use disorder, severe
AHA: 2016,1Q,36

F17.201   **Nicotine dependence, unspecified, in** remission
Tobacco use disorder, mild, in early remission
Tobacco use disorder, mild, in sustained remission
Tobacco use disorder, moderate, in early remission
Tobacco use disorder, moderate, in sustained remission
Tobacco use disorder, severe, in early remission
Tobacco use disorder, severe, in sustained remission

F17.203   **Nicotine dependence unspecified, with** withdrawal
Tobacco withdrawal

F17.208   **Nicotine dependence, unspecified, with other nicotine-induced disorders**

F17.209   **Nicotine dependence, unspecified, with unspecified nicotine-induced disorders**

√6ᵗʰ   **F17.21**   Nicotine dependence, cigarettes

F17.210   **Nicotine dependence, cigarettes, uncomplicated**
AHA: 2017,2Q,28-29

F17.211   **Nicotine dependence, cigarettes, in** remission
Tobacco use disorder, cigarettes, mild, in early remission
Tobacco use disorder, cigarettes, mild, in sustained remission
Tobacco use disorder, cigarettes, moderate, in early remission
Tobacco use disorder, cigarettes, moderate, in sustained remission
Tobacco use disorder, cigarettes, severe, in early remission
Tobacco use disorder, cigarettes, severe, in sustained remission

F17.213   **Nicotine dependence, cigarettes, with** withdrawal

F17.218   **Nicotine dependence, cigarettes, with other nicotine-induced disorders**

F17.219   **Nicotine dependence, cigarettes, with unspecified nicotine-induced disorders**

√6ᵗʰ   **F17.22**   Nicotine dependence, chewing tobacco

F17.220   **Nicotine dependence, chewing tobacco, uncomplicated**

F17.221   **Nicotine dependence, chewing tobacco, in remission**
Tobacco use disorder, chewing tobacco, mild, in early remission
Tobacco use disorder, chewing tobacco, mild, in sustained remission
Tobacco use disorder, chewing tobacco, moderate, in early remission
Tobacco use disorder, chewing tobacco, moderate, in sustained remission
Tobacco use disorder, chewing tobacco, severe, in early remission
Tobacco use disorder, chewing tobacco, severe, in sustained remission

F17.223   **Nicotine dependence, chewing tobacco, with** withdrawal

F17.228   **Nicotine dependence, chewing tobacco, with other nicotine-induced disorders**

F17.229   **Nicotine dependence, chewing tobacco, with unspecified nicotine-induced disorders**

√6ᵗʰ   **F17.29**   Nicotine dependence, other tobacco product

F17.290   **Nicotine dependence, other tobacco product, uncomplicated**
AHA: 2017,2Q,28-29

F17.291   **Nicotine dependence, other tobacco product, in remission**
Tobacco use disorder, other tobacco product, mild, in early remission
Tobacco use disorder, other tobacco product, mild, in sustained remission
Tobacco use disorder, other tobacco product, moderate, in early remission
Tobacco use disorder, other tobacco product, moderate, in sustained remission
Tobacco use disorder, other tobacco product, severe, in early remission
Tobacco use disorder, other tobacco product, severe, in sustained remission

F17.293   **Nicotine dependence, other tobacco product, with** withdrawal

F17.298   **Nicotine dependence, other tobacco product, with other nicotine-induced disorders**

F17.299   **Nicotine dependence, other tobacco product, with unspecified nicotine-induced disorders**

Chapter 5. Mental, Behavioral and Neurodevelopmental Disorders

✓4th **F18** Inhalant related disorders
INCLUDES volatile solvents

✓5th **F18.1** Inhalant abuse
EXCLUDES 1 inhalant dependence (F18.2-)
inhalant use, unspecified (F18.9-)

F18.10 Inhalant abuse, uncomplicated
Inhalant use disorder, mild

F18.11 Inhalant abuse, in remission
Inhalant use disorder, mild, in early remission
Inhalant use disorder, mild, in sustained remission

✓6th **F18.12** Inhalant abuse with intoxication
F18.120 Inhalant abuse with intoxication, uncomplicated
F18.121 Inhalant abuse with intoxication delirium
F18.129 Inhalant abuse with intoxication, unspecified

F18.14 Inhalant abuse with inhalant-induced mood disorder
Inhalant use disorder, mild, with inhalant induced depressive disorder

✓6th **F18.15** Inhalant abuse with inhalant-induced psychotic disorder
F18.150 Inhalant abuse with inhalant-induced psychotic disorder with delusions
F18.151 Inhalant abuse with inhalant-induced psychotic disorder with hallucinations
F18.159 Inhalant abuse with inhalant-induced psychotic disorder, unspecified

F18.17 Inhalant abuse with inhalant-induced dementia
Inhalant use disorder, mild, with inhalant induced major neurocognitive disorder

✓6th **F18.18** Inhalant abuse with other inhalant-induced disorders
F18.180 Inhalant abuse with inhalant-induced anxiety disorder
F18.188 Inhalant abuse with other inhalant-induced disorder
Inhalant use disorder, mild, with inhalant induced mild neurocognitive disorder

F18.19 Inhalant abuse with unspecified inhalant-induced disorder

✓5th **F18.2** Inhalant dependence
EXCLUDES 1 inhalant abuse (F18.1-)
inhalant use, unspecified (F18.9-)

F18.20 Inhalant dependence, uncomplicated
Inhalant use disorder, moderate
Inhalant use disorder, severe

F18.21 Inhalant dependence, in remission
Inhalant use disorder, moderate, in early remission
Inhalant use disorder, moderate, in sustained remission
Inhalant use disorder, severe, in early remission
Inhalant use disorder, severe, in sustained remission

✓6th **F18.22** Inhalant dependence with intoxication
F18.220 Inhalant dependence with intoxication, uncomplicated
F18.221 Inhalant dependence with intoxication delirium
F18.229 Inhalant dependence with intoxication, unspecified

F18.24 Inhalant dependence with inhalant-induced mood disorder
Inhalant use disorder, moderate, with inhalant induced depressive disorder
Inhalant use disorder, severe, with inhalant induced depressive disorder

✓6th **F18.25** Inhalant dependence with inhalant-induced psychotic disorder
F18.250 Inhalant dependence with inhalant-induced psychotic disorder with delusions
F18.251 Inhalant dependence with inhalant-induced psychotic disorder with hallucinations
F18.259 Inhalant dependence with inhalant-induced psychotic disorder, unspecified

F18.27 Inhalant dependence with inhalant-induced dementia
Inhalant use disorder, moderate, with inhalant induced major neurocognitive disorder
Inhalant use disorder, severe, with inhalant induced major neurocognitive disorder

✓6th **F18.28** Inhalant dependence with other inhalant-induced disorders
F18.280 Inhalant dependence with inhalant-induced anxiety disorder
F18.288 Inhalant dependence with other inhalant-induced disorder
Inhalant use disorder, moderate, with inhalant-induced mild neurocognitive disorder
Inhalant use disorder, severe, with inhalant-induced mild neurocognitive disorder

F18.29 Inhalant dependence with unspecified inhalant-induced disorder

✓5th **F18.9** Inhalant use, unspecified
EXCLUDES 1 inhalant abuse (F18.1-)
inhalant dependence (F18.2-)

F18.90 Inhalant use, unspecified, uncomplicated
AHA: 2018,2Q,10-11

✓6th **F18.92** Inhalant use, unspecified with intoxication
F18.920 Inhalant use, unspecified with intoxication, uncomplicated
F18.921 Inhalant use, unspecified with intoxication with delirium
F18.929 Inhalant use, unspecified with intoxication, unspecified

F18.94 Inhalant use, unspecified with inhalant-induced mood disorder
Inhalant induced depressive disorder

✓6th **F18.95** Inhalant use, unspecified with inhalant-induced psychotic disorder
F18.950 Inhalant use, unspecified with inhalant-induced psychotic disorder with delusions
F18.951 Inhalant use, unspecified with inhalant-induced psychotic disorder with hallucinations
F18.959 Inhalant use, unspecified with inhalant-induced psychotic disorder, unspecified

F18.97 Inhalant use, unspecified with inhalant-induced persisting dementia
Inhalant-induced major neurocognitive disorder

✓6th **F18.98** Inhalant use, unspecified with other inhalant-induced disorders
F18.980 Inhalant use, unspecified with inhalant-induced anxiety disorder
F18.988 Inhalant use, unspecified with other inhalant-induced disorder
Inhalant-induced mild neurocognitive disorder

F18.99 Inhalant use, unspecified with unspecified inhalant-induced disorder

✓4th **F19** Other psychoactive substance related disorders
INCLUDES polysubstance drug use (indiscriminate drug use)

✓5th **F19.1** Other psychoactive substance abuse
EXCLUDES 1 other psychoactive substance dependence (F19.2-)
other psychoactive substance use, unspecified (F19.9-)

F19.10 Other psychoactive substance abuse, uncomplicated
Other (or unknown) substance use disorder, mild

F19.11 Other psychoactive substance abuse, in remission
Other (or unknown) substance use disorder, mild, in early remission
Other (or unknown) substance use disorder, mild, in sustained remission

✓6th **F19.12** Other psychoactive substance abuse with intoxication
F19.120 Other psychoactive substance abuse with intoxication, uncomplicated
F19.121 Other psychoactive substance abuse with intoxication delirium

          F19.122 Other psychoactive substance abuse with intoxication with perceptual disturbances

          F19.129 Other psychoactive substance abuse with intoxication, unspecified

    F19.14 Other psychoactive substance abuse with psychoactive substance-induced mood disorder

        Other (or unknown) substance use disorder, mild, with other (or unknown) substance-induced bipolar or related disorder

        Other (or unknown) substance use disorder, mild, with other (or unknown) substance-induced depressive disorder

✓6ᵗʰ **F19.15** Other psychoactive substance abuse with psychoactive substance-induced psychotic disorder

          F19.150 Other psychoactive substance abuse with psychoactive substance-induced psychotic disorder with delusions

          F19.151 Other psychoactive substance abuse with psychoactive substance-induced psychotic disorder with hallucinations

          F19.159 Other psychoactive substance abuse with psychoactive substance-induced psychotic disorder, unspecified

    F19.16 Other psychoactive substance abuse with psychoactive substance-induced persisting amnestic disorder

    F19.17 Other psychoactive substance abuse with psychoactive substance-induced persisting dementia

        Other (or unknown) substance use disorder, mild, with other (or unknown) substance-induced major neurocognitive disorder

✓6ᵗʰ **F19.18** Other psychoactive substance abuse with other psychoactive substance-induced disorders

          F19.180 Other psychoactive substance abuse with psychoactive substance-induced anxiety disorder

          F19.181 Other psychoactive substance abuse with psychoactive substance-induced sexual dysfunction

          F19.182 Other psychoactive substance abuse with psychoactive substance-induced sleep disorder

          F19.188 Other psychoactive substance abuse with other psychoactive substance-induced disorder

            Other (or unknown) substance use disorder, mild, with other (or unknown) substance induced mild neurocognitive disorder

            Other (or unknown) substance use disorder, mild, with other (or unknown) substance induced obsessive-compulsive or related disorder

    F19.19 Other psychoactive substance abuse with unspecified psychoactive substance-induced disorder

✓5ᵗʰ **F19.2** Other psychoactive substance dependence

      EXCLUDES 1   other psychoactive substance abuse (F19.1-)

                other psychoactive substance use, unspecified (F19.9-)

    F19.20 Other psychoactive substance dependence, uncomplicated

        Other (or unknown) substance use disorder, moderate

        Other (or unknown) substance use disorder, severe

    F19.21 Other psychoactive substance dependence, in remission

        Other (or unknown) substance use disorder, moderate, in early remission

        Other (or unknown) substance use disorder, moderate, in sustained remission

        Other (or unknown) substance use disorder, severe, in early remission

        Other (or unknown) substance use disorder, severe, in sustained remission

✓6ᵗʰ **F19.22** Other psychoactive substance dependence with intoxication

      EXCLUDES 1   other psychoactive substance dependence with withdrawal (F19.23-)

          F19.220 Other psychoactive substance dependence with intoxication, uncomplicated

          F19.221 Other psychoactive substance dependence with intoxication delirium

          F19.222 Other psychoactive substance dependence with intoxication with perceptual disturbance

          F19.229 Other psychoactive substance dependence with intoxication, unspecified

✓6ᵗʰ **F19.23** Other psychoactive substance dependence with withdrawal

      EXCLUDES 1   other psychoactive substance dependence with intoxication (F19.22-)

          F19.230 Other psychoactive substance dependence with withdrawal, uncomplicated

          F19.231 Other psychoactive substance dependence with withdrawal delirium

          F19.232 Other psychoactive substance dependence with withdrawal with perceptual disturbance

          F19.239 Other psychoactive substance dependence with withdrawal, unspecified

    F19.24 Other psychoactive substance dependence with psychoactive substance-induced mood disorder

        Other (or unknown) substance use disorder, moderate, with other (or unknown) substance induced bipolar or related disorder

        Other (or unknown) substance use disorder, moderate, with other (or unknown) substance induced depressive disorder

        Other (or unknown) substance use disorder, severe, with other (or unknown) substance induced bipolar or related disorder

        Other (or unknown) substance use disorder, severe, with other (or unknown) substance induced depressive disorder

✓6ᵗʰ **F19.25** Other psychoactive substance dependence with psychoactive substance-induced psychotic disorder

          F19.250 Other psychoactive substance dependence with psychoactive substance-induced psychotic disorder with delusions

          F19.251 Other psychoactive substance dependence with psychoactive substance-induced psychotic disorder with hallucinations

          F19.259 Other psychoactive substance dependence with psychoactive substance-induced psychotic disorder, unspecified

    F19.26 Other psychoactive substance dependence with psychoactive substance-induced persisting amnestic disorder

    F19.27 Other psychoactive substance dependence with psychoactive substance-induced persisting dementia

        Other (or unknown) substance use disorder, moderate, with other (or unknown) substance induced major neurocognitive disorder

        Other (or unknown) substance use disorder, severe, with other (or unknown) substance induced major neurocognitive disorder

✓6ᵗʰ **F19.28** Other psychoactive substance dependence with other psychoactive substance-induced disorders

          F19.280 Other psychoactive substance dependence with psychoactive substance-induced anxiety disorder

          F19.281 Other psychoactive substance dependence with psychoactive substance-induced sexual dysfunction

          F19.282 Other psychoactive substance dependence with psychoactive substance-induced sleep disorder

✓ Additional Character Required   ✓x7ᵗʰ Placeholder Alert   Manifestation   Unspecified Dx   ►◄ Revised Text   ● New Code   ▲ Revised Title

ICD-10-CM 2020   547

F19.288 **Other psychoactive substance dependence with other psychoactive substance-induced disorder**
Other (or unknown) substance use disorder, moderate, with other (or unknown) substance induced mild neurocognitive disorder
Other (or unknown) substance use disorder, severe, with other (or unknown) substance induced mild neurocognitive disorder
Other (or unknown) substance use disorder, moderate, with other (or unknown) substance induced obsessive compulsive or related disorder
Other (or unknown) substance use disorder, severe, with other (or unknown) substance induced obsessive-compulsive or related disorder

F19.29 **Other psychoactive substance dependence with unspecified psychoactive substance-induced disorder**

√5ᵗʰ **F19.9** **Other psychoactive substance use, unspecified**
> EXCLUDES 1   *other psychoactive substance abuse (F19.1-)*
> *other psychoactive substance dependence (F19.2-)*

F19.90 **Other psychoactive substance use, unspecified, uncomplicated**
AHA: 2018,2Q,10-11

√6ᵗʰ **F19.92** **Other psychoactive substance use, unspecified with intoxication**
> EXCLUDES 1   *other psychoactive substance use, unspecified with withdrawal (F19.93)*

F19.920 **Other psychoactive substance use, unspecified with intoxication, uncomplicated**

F19.921 **Other psychoactive substance use, unspecified with intoxication with delirium**
Other (or unknown) substance-induced delirium

F19.922 **Other psychoactive substance use, unspecified with intoxication with perceptual disturbance**

F19.929 **Other psychoactive substance use, unspecified with intoxication, unspecified**

√6ᵗʰ **F19.93** **Other psychoactive substance use, unspecified with withdrawal**
> EXCLUDES 1   *other psychoactive substance use, unspecified with intoxication (F19.92-)*

F19.930 **Other psychoactive substance use, unspecified with withdrawal, uncomplicated**

F19.931 **Other psychoactive substance use, unspecified with withdrawal delirium**

F19.932 **Other psychoactive substance use, unspecified with withdrawal with perceptual disturbance**

F19.939 **Other psychoactive substance use, unspecified with withdrawal, unspecified**

F19.94 **Other psychoactive substance use, unspecified with psychoactive substance-induced mood disorder**
Other (or unknown) substance-induced bipolar or related disorder, without use disorder
Other (or unknown) substance-induced depressive disorder, without use disorder

√6ᵗʰ **F19.95** **Other psychoactive substance use, unspecified with psychoactive substance-induced psychotic disorder**

F19.950 **Other psychoactive substance use, unspecified with psychoactive substance-induced psychotic disorder with delusions**

F19.951 **Other psychoactive substance use, unspecified with psychoactive substance-induced psychotic disorder with hallucinations**

F19.959 **Other psychoactive substance use, unspecified with psychoactive substance-induced psychotic disorder, unspecified**
Other or unknown substance-induced psychotic disorder, without use disorder

F19.96 **Other psychoactive substance use, unspecified with psychoactive substance-induced persisting amnestic disorder**

F19.97 **Other psychoactive substance use, unspecified with psychoactive substance-induced persisting dementia**
Other (or unknown) substance-induced major neurocognitive disorder, without use disorder

√6ᵗʰ **F19.98** **Other psychoactive substance use, unspecified with other psychoactive substance-induced disorders**

F19.980 **Other psychoactive substance use, unspecified with psychoactive substance-induced anxiety disorder**
Other (or unknown) substance-induced anxiety disorder, without use disorder

F19.981 **Other psychoactive substance use, unspecified with psychoactive substance-induced sexual dysfunction**
Other (or unknown) substance-induced sexual dysfunction, without use disorder

F19.982 **Other psychoactive substance use, unspecified with psychoactive substance-induced sleep disorder**
Other (or unknown) substance-induced sleep disorder, without use disorder

F19.988 **Other psychoactive substance use, unspecified with other psychoactive substance-induced disorder**
Other (or unknown) substance-induced mild neurocognitive disorder, without use disorder
Other (or unknown) substance-induced obsessive-compulsive or related disorder, without use disorder

F19.99 **Other psychoactive substance use, unspecified with unspecified psychoactive substance-induced disorder**

Schizophrenia, schizotypal, delusional, and other non-mood psychotic disorders (F20-F29)

√4ᵗʰ **F20** **Schizophrenia**
> EXCLUDES 1   *brief psychotic disorder (F23)*
> *cyclic schizophrenia (F25.0)*
> *mood [affective] disorders with psychotic symptoms (F30.2, F31.2, F31.5, F31.64, F32.3, F33.3)*
> *schizoaffective disorder (F25.-)*
> *schizophrenic reaction NOS (F23)*
> EXCLUDES 2   *schizophrenic reaction in:*
> *alcoholism (F10.15-, F10.25-, F10.95-)*
> *brain disease (F06.2)*
> *epilepsy (F06.2)*
> *psychoactive drug use (F11-F19 with .15, .25, .95)*
> *schizotypal disorder (F21)*

DEF: Group of disorders with disturbances in thought (delusions, hallucinations), mood (blunted, flattened, inappropriate affect), and sense of self. Schizophrenia also includes bizarre, purposeless behavior, repetitious activity, or inactivity.

F20.0 **Paranoid schizophrenia**
Paraphrenic schizophrenia
> EXCLUDES 1   *involutional paranoid state (F22)*
> *paranoia (F22)*

DEF: Preoccupied with delusional suspicions and auditory hallucinations related to a single theme. This type of schizophrenia is usually hostile, grandiose, threatening, persecutory, and occasionally hypochondriacal.

F20.1 **Disorganized schizophrenia**
Hebephrenic schizophrenia
Hebephrenia

F20.2 Catatonic schizophrenia
Schizophrenic catalepsy
Schizophrenic catatonia
Schizophrenic flexibilitas cerea
EXCLUDES 1 *catatonic stupor (R40.1)*
DEF: Extreme changes in motor activity. One extreme is a decreased response or reaction to the environment and the other is spontaneous activity.

F20.3 Undifferentiated schizophrenia
Atypical schizophrenia
EXCLUDES 1 *acute schizophrenia-like psychotic disorder (F23)*
EXCLUDES 2 *post-schizophrenic depression (F32.89)*

F20.5 Residual schizophrenia
Restzustand (schizophrenic)
Schizophrenic residual state

✓6ᵗʰ F20.8 Other schizophrenia
F20.81 Schizophreniform disorder
Schizophreniform psychosis NOS
F20.89 Other schizophrenia
Cenesthopathic schizophrenia
Simple schizophrenia

F20.9 Schizophrenia, unspecified
AHA: 2019,2Q,32

F21 Schizotypal disorder
Borderline schizophrenia
Latent schizophrenia
Latent schizophrenic reaction
Prepsychotic schizophrenia
Prodromal schizophrenia
Pseudoneurotic schizophrenia
Pseudopsychopathic schizophrenia
Schizotypal personality disorder
EXCLUDES 2 *Asperger's syndrome (F84.5)*
schizoid personality disorder (F60.1)
DEF: Disorder characterized by various oddities of thinking, perception, communication, and behavior that may be manifested as magical thinking, ideas of reference, paranoid ideation, recurrent illusions and derealization (depersonalization), or social isolation.

F22 Delusional disorders
Delusional dysmorphophobia
Involutional paranoid state
Paranoia
Paranoia querulans
Paranoid psychosis
Paranoid state
Paraphrenia (late)
Sensitiver Beziehungswahn
EXCLUDES 1 *mood [affective] disorders with psychotic symptoms (F30.2, F31.2, F31.5, F31.64, F32.3, F33.3)*
paranoid schizophrenia (F20.0)
EXCLUDES 2 *paranoid personality disorder (F60.0)*
paranoid psychosis, psychogenic (F23)
paranoid reaction (F23)

F23 Brief psychotic disorder
Paranoid reaction
Psychogenic paranoid psychosis
EXCLUDES 2 *mood [affective] disorders with psychotic symptoms (F30.2, F31.2, F31.5, F31.64, F32.3, F33.3)*
AHA: 2019,2Q,32

F24 Shared psychotic disorder
Folie à deux
Induced paranoid disorder
Induced psychotic disorder

✓4ᵗʰ F25 Schizoaffective disorders
EXCLUDES 1 *mood [affective] disorders with psychotic symptoms (F30.2, F31.2, F31.5, F31.64, F32.3, F33.3)*
schizophrenia (F20.-)
F25.0 Schizoaffective disorder, bipolar type
Cyclic schizophrenia
Schizoaffective disorder, manic type
Schizoaffective disorder, mixed type
Schizoaffective psychosis, bipolar type
F25.1 Schizoaffective disorder, depressive type
Schizoaffective psychosis, depressive type
F25.8 Other schizoaffective disorders

F25.9 Schizoaffective disorder, unspecified
Schizoaffective psychosis NOS

F28 Other psychotic disorder not due to a substance or known physiological condition
Chronic hallucinatory psychosis
Other specified schizophrenia spectrum and other psychotic disorder

F29 Unspecified psychosis not due to a substance or known physiological condition
Psychosis NOS
Unspecified schizophrenia spectrum and other psychotic disorder
EXCLUDES 1 *mental disorder NOS (F99)*
unspecified mental disorder due to known physiological condition (F09)

Mood [affective] disorders (F30-F39)

✓4ᵗʰ F30 Manic episode
INCLUDES bipolar disorder, single manic episode
mixed affective episode
EXCLUDES 1 *bipolar disorder (F31.-)*
major depressive disorder, recurrent (F33.-)
major depressive disorder, single episode (F32.-)
DEF: Mania: Characterized by abnormal states of elation or excitement out of keeping with the individual's circumstances and varying from enhanced liveliness (hypomania) to violent, almost uncontrollable, excitement. Aggression and anger, flight of ideas, distractibility, impaired judgment, and grandiose ideas are common.

✓5ᵗʰ F30.1 Manic episode without psychotic symptoms
F30.10 Manic episode without psychotic symptoms, unspecified CH
F30.11 Manic episode without psychotic symptoms, mild CH
F30.12 Manic episode without psychotic symptoms, moderate CH
F30.13 Manic episode, severe, without psychotic symptoms CH
F30.2 Manic episode, severe with psychotic symptoms CH
Manic stupor
Mania with mood-congruent psychotic symptoms
Mania with mood-incongruent psychotic symptoms
F30.3 Manic episode in partial remission CH
F30.4 Manic episode in full remission CH
F30.8 Other manic episodes CH
Hypomania
F30.9 Manic episode, unspecified CH
Mania NOS

✓4ᵗʰ F31 Bipolar disorder
INCLUDES bipolar I disorder
bipolar type I disorder
manic-depressive illness
manic-depressive psychosis
manic-depressive reaction
EXCLUDES 1 *bipolar disorder, single manic episode (F30.-)*
major depressive disorder, recurrent (F33.-)
major depressive disorder, single episode (F32.-)
EXCLUDES 2 *cyclothymia (F34.0)*
F31.0 Bipolar disorder, current episode hypomanic CH
✓5ᵗʰ F31.1 Bipolar disorder, current episode manic without psychotic features
F31.10 Bipolar disorder, current episode manic without psychotic features, unspecified CH
F31.11 Bipolar disorder, current episode manic without psychotic features, mild CH
F31.12 Bipolar disorder, current episode manic without psychotic features, moderate CH
F31.13 Bipolar disorder, current episode manic without psychotic features, severe CH
F31.2 Bipolar disorder, current episode manic severe with psychotic features CH
Bipolar disorder, current episode manic with mood-congruent psychotic symptoms
Bipolar disorder, current episode manic with mood-incongruent psychotic symptoms
Bipolar I disorder, current or most recent episode manic with psychotic features

Chapter 5. Mental, Behavioral and Neurodevelopmental Disorders

√5ᵗʰ **F31.3** **Bipolar disorder, current episode** depressed, mild or moderate severity

    F31.30 **Bipolar disorder, current episode depressed, mild or moderate severity, unspecified** `CH`

    F31.31 **Bipolar disorder, current episode depressed,** mild `CH`

    F31.32 **Bipolar disorder, current episode depressed,** moderate `CH`

F31.4 **Bipolar disorder, current episode** depressed, severe, without psychotic features `CH`

F31.5 **Bipolar disorder, current episode** depressed, severe, with psychotic features `CH`

    Bipolar disorder, current episode depressed with mood-congruent psychotic symptoms

    Bipolar disorder, current episode depressed with mood-incongruent psychotic symptoms

    Bipolar I disorder, current or most recent episode depressed, with psychotic features

√5ᵗʰ **F31.6** **Bipolar disorder, current episode** mixed

    F31.60 **Bipolar disorder, current episode mixed, unspecified** `CH`

    F31.61 **Bipolar disorder, current episode mixed,** mild `CH`

    F31.62 **Bipolar disorder, current episode mixed,** moderate `CH`

    F31.63 **Bipolar disorder, current episode mixed,** severe, without psychotic features `CH`

    F31.64 **Bipolar disorder, current episode mixed,** severe, with psychotic features `CH`

        Bipolar disorder, current episode mixed with mood-congruent psychotic symptoms

        Bipolar disorder, current episode mixed with mood-incongruent psychotic symptoms

√5ᵗʰ **F31.7** **Bipolar disorder, currently** in remission

    F31.70 **Bipolar disorder, currently in remission, most recent episode unspecified** `CH`

    F31.71 **Bipolar disorder,** in partial remission, **most recent episode** hypomanic `CH`

    F31.72 **Bipolar disorder,** in full remission, **most recent episode** hypomanic `CH`

    F31.73 **Bipolar disorder,** in partial remission, **most recent episode** manic `CH`

    F31.74 **Bipolar disorder,** in full remission, **most recent episode** manic

    F31.75 **Bipolar disorder,** in partial remission, **most recent episode** depressed

    F31.76 **Bipolar disorder,** in full remission, **most recent episode** depressed

    F31.77 **Bipolar disorder,** in partial remission, **most recent episode** mixed `CH`

    F31.78 **Bipolar disorder,** in full remission, **most recent episode** mixed `CH`

√5ᵗʰ **F31.8** **Other bipolar disorders**

    F31.81 **Bipolar II disorder** `CH`

        Bipolar disorder, type 2

    F31.89 **Other bipolar disorder** `CH`

        Recurrent manic episodes NOS

F31.9 **Bipolar disorder, unspecified** `CH`

    Manic depression

√4ᵗʰ **F32** **Major depressive disorder,** single episode

    `INCLUDES` single episode of agitated depression
              single episode of depressive reaction
              single episode of major depression
              single episode of psychogenic depression
              single episode of reactive depression
              single episode of vital depression

    `EXCLUDES 1` bipolar disorder (F31.-)
              manic episode (F30.-)
              recurrent depressive disorder (F33.-)

    `EXCLUDES 2` adjustment disorder (F43.2)

    DEF: Mood disorder that produces depression that may exhibit as sadness, low self-esteem, or guilt feelings. Other manifestations may be withdrawal from friends and family and interrupted sleep.

F32.0 **Major depressive disorder, single episode,** mild `CH`

F32.1 **Major depressive disorder, single episode,** moderate `CH`

F32.2 **Major depressive disorder, single episode,** severe without psychotic features `CH`

F32.3 **Major depressive disorder, single episode,** severe with psychotic features

    Single episode of major depression with mood-congruent psychotic symptoms

    Single episode of major depression with mood-incongruent psychotic symptoms

    Single episode of major depression with psychotic symptoms

    Single episode of psychogenic depressive psychosis

    Single episode of psychotic depression

    Single episode of reactive depressive psychosis

F32.4 **Major depressive disorder, single episode, in partial remission** `CH`

F32.5 **Major depressive disorder, single episode, in full remission** `CH`

√5ᵗʰ **F32.8** **Other depressive episodes**

    AHA: 2016,4Q,14

    F32.81 **Premenstrual dysphoric disorder** ♀

        `EXCLUDES 1` premenstrual tension syndrome (N94.3)

        DEF: Severe manifestation of premenstrual syndrome (PMS) that can be disabling and destructive to day-to-day activities. It can exacerbate pre-existing emotional disorders, like depression and anxiety, and cause feelings of loss of control, fatigue, and irritability.

    F32.89 **Other specified depressive episodes** `CH`

        Atypical depression

        Post-schizophrenic depression

        Single episode of 'masked' depression NOS

F32.9 **Major depressive disorder, single episode, unspecified** `CH`

    Depression NOS

    Depressive disorder NOS

    Major depression NOS

    AHA: 2013,4Q,107

    TIP: Use for chronic depression, not further specified.

√4ᵗʰ **F33** **Major depressive disorder,** recurrent

    `INCLUDES` recurrent episodes of depressive reaction
              recurrent episodes of endogenous depression
              recurrent episodes of major depression
              recurrent episodes of psychogenic depression
              recurrent episodes of reactive depression
              recurrent episodes of seasonal depressive disorder
              recurrent episodes of vital depression

    `EXCLUDES 1` bipolar disorder (F31.-)
              manic episode (F30.-)

    DEF: Mood disorder that produces depression that may exhibit as sadness, low self-esteem, or guilt feelings. Other manifestations may be withdrawal from friends and family and interrupted sleep.

F33.0 **Major depressive disorder, recurrent,** mild `CH`

F33.1 **Major depressive disorder, recurrent,** moderate `CH`

F33.2 **Major depressive disorder, recurrent,** severe without psychotic features `CH`

F33.3 **Major depressive disorder, recurrent,** severe with psychotic symptoms

    Endogenous depression with psychotic symptoms

    Major depressive disorder, recurrent, with psychotic features

    Recurrent severe episodes of major depression with mood-congruent psychotic symptoms

    Recurrent severe episodes of major depression with mood-incongruent psychotic symptoms

    Recurrent severe episodes of major depression with psychotic symptoms

    Recurrent severe episodes of psychogenic depressive psychosis

    Recurrent severe episodes of psychotic depression

    Recurrent severe episodes of reactive depressive psychosis

√5ᵗʰ **F33.4** **Major depressive disorder, recurrent,** in remission

    F33.40 **Major depressive disorder, recurrent, in remission, unspecified** `CH`

    F33.41 **Major depressive disorder, recurrent, in** partial **remission** `CH`

    F33.42 **Major depressive disorder, recurrent, in** full **remission**

F33.8 **Other recurrent depressive disorders** `CH`

    Recurrent brief depressive episodes

F33.9 **Major depressive disorder, recurrent, unspecified** `CH`

    Monopolar depression NOS

`N` Newborn: 0   `P` Pediatric: 0-17   `M` Maternity: 12-55   `A` Adult: 15-124   `CH` Comorbidity High   `CL` Comorbidity Low   `NCDx` Noncancer Dx   `PDx` Primary Dx

550   ICD-10-CM 2020

F34 Persistent mood [affective] disorders

F34.0 Cyclothymic disorder
Affective personality disorder
Cycloid personality
Cyclothymia
Cyclothymic personality
DEF: Mood disorder characterized by fast and repeated alterations between hypomanic and depressed moods.

F34.1 Dysthymic disorder
Depressive neurosis
Depressive personality disorder
Dysthymia
Neurotic depression
Persistent anxiety depression
Persistent depressive disorder
EXCLUDES 2 anxiety depression (mild or not persistent) (F41.8)
DEF: Depression without psychosis. It is a less severe but persistent depression and is considered a mild to moderate chronic form of depression.

F34.8 Other persistent mood [affective] disorders
AHA: 2016,4Q,14

F34.81 Disruptive mood dysregulation disorder
F34.89 Other specified persistent mood disorders
F34.9 Persistent mood [affective] disorder, unspecified

F39 Unspecified mood [affective] disorder
Affective psychosis NOS

Anxiety, dissociative, stress-related, somatoform and other nonpsychotic mental disorders (F40-F48)

F40 Phobic anxiety disorders
DEF: Phobia: Broad-range anxiety with abnormally intense dread of certain objects or specific situations that would not normally have that effect.

F40.0 Agoraphobia
DEF: Profound anxiety or fear of leaving familiar settings like home, or being in unfamiliar locations or with strangers or crowds. Agoraphobia may or may not be preceded by recurrent panic attacks.
F40.00 Agoraphobia, unspecified
F40.01 Agoraphobia with panic disorder
Panic disorder with agoraphobia
EXCLUDES 1 panic disorder without agoraphobia (F41.0)
F40.02 Agoraphobia without panic disorder

F40.1 Social phobias
Anthropophobia
Social anxiety disorder
Social anxiety disorder of childhood
Social neurosis
F40.10 Social phobia, unspecified
F40.11 Social phobia, generalized

F40.2 Specific (isolated) phobias
EXCLUDES 2 dysmorphophobia (nondelusional) (F45.22)
nosophobia (F45.22)
F40.21 Animal type phobia
F40.210 Arachnophobia
Fear of spiders
F40.218 Other animal type phobia
F40.22 Natural environment type phobia
F40.220 Fear of thunderstorms
F40.228 Other natural environment type phobia
F40.23 Blood, injection, injury type phobia
F40.230 Fear of blood
F40.231 Fear of injections and transfusions
F40.232 Fear of other medical care
F40.233 Fear of injury
F40.24 Situational type phobia
F40.240 Claustrophobia
F40.241 Acrophobia
F40.242 Fear of bridges
F40.243 Fear of flying
F40.248 Other situational type phobia

F40.29 Other specified phobia
F40.290 Androphobia
Fear of men
F40.291 Gynephobia
Fear of women
F40.298 Other specified phobia
F40.8 Other phobic anxiety disorders
Phobic anxiety disorder of childhood
F40.9 Phobic anxiety disorder, unspecified
Phobia NOS
Phobic state NOS

F41 Other anxiety disorders
EXCLUDES 2 anxiety in:
acute stress reaction (F43.0)
neurasthenia (F48.8)
psychophysiologic disorders (F45.-)
transient adjustment reaction (F43.2)
separation anxiety (F93.0)

F41.0 Panic disorder [episodic paroxysmal anxiety]
Panic attack
Panic state
EXCLUDES 1 panic disorder with agoraphobia (F40.01)
DEF: Neurotic disorder characterized by recurrent panic or anxiety, apprehension, fear, or terror. Symptoms include shortness of breath, palpitations, dizziness, and shakiness; fear of dying may persist.

F41.1 Generalized anxiety disorder
Anxiety neurosis
Anxiety reaction
Anxiety state
Overanxious disorder
EXCLUDES 2 neurasthenia (F48.8)
F41.3 Other mixed anxiety disorders
F41.8 Other specified anxiety disorders
Anxiety depression (mild or not persistent)
Anxiety hysteria
Mixed anxiety and depressive disorder
F41.9 Anxiety disorder, unspecified
Anxiety NOS

F42 Obsessive-compulsive disorder
EXCLUDES 2 obsessive-compulsive personality (disorder) (F60.5)
obsessive-compulsive symptoms occurring in depression (F32-F33)
obsessive-compulsive symptoms occurring in schizophrenia (F20.-)
AHA: 2016,4Q,14-15
F42.2 Mixed obsessional thoughts and acts
F42.3 Hoarding disorder
F42.4 Excoriation (skin-picking) disorder
EXCLUDES 1 factitial dermatitis (L98.1)
other specified behavioral and emotional disorders with onset usually occurring in early childhood and adolescence (F98.8)
F42.8 Other obsessive-compulsive disorder
Anancastic neurosis
Obsessive-compulsive neurosis
F42.9 Obsessive-compulsive disorder, unspecified

F43 Reaction to severe stress, and adjustment disorders
F43.0 Acute stress reaction
Acute crisis reaction
Acute reaction to stress
Combat and operational stress reaction
Combat fatigue
Crisis state
Psychic shock
F43.1 Post-traumatic stress disorder (PTSD)
Traumatic neurosis
DEF: Preoccupation with traumatic events beyond normal experience (i.e., rape, personal assault, etc.) that may also include recurring flashbacks of the trauma. Symptoms include difficulty remembering, sleeping, or concentrating, and guilt feelings for surviving.
F43.10 Post-traumatic stress disorder, unspecified
F43.11 Post-traumatic stress disorder, acute
F43.12 Post-traumatic stress disorder, chronic

Chapter 5. Mental, Behavioral and Neurodevelopmental Disorders

✓5ᵗʰ **F43.2 Adjustment disorders**
Culture shock
Grief reaction
Hospitalism in children
EXCLUDES 2 *separation anxiety disorder of childhood (F93.0)*

F43.20 Adjustment disorder, unspecified
F43.21 Adjustment disorder with depressed mood
AHA: 2014,1Q,25
F43.22 Adjustment disorder with anxiety
F43.23 Adjustment disorder with mixed anxiety and depressed mood
F43.24 Adjustment disorder with disturbance of conduct
F43.25 Adjustment disorder with mixed disturbance of emotions and conduct
F43.29 Adjustment disorder with other symptoms
F43.8 Other reactions to severe stress
Other specified trauma and stressor-related disorder
F43.9 Reaction to severe stress, unspecified
Trauma and stressor-related disorder, NOS

✓4ᵗʰ **F44 Dissociative and conversion disorders**
INCLUDES conversion hysteria
conversion reaction
hysteria
hysterical psychosis
EXCLUDES 2 *malingering [conscious simulation] (Z76.5)*

F44.0 Dissociative amnesia
EXCLUDES 1 *amnesia NOS (R41.3)*
anterograde amnesia (R41.1)
dissociative amnesia with dissociative fugue (F44.1)
retrograde amnesia (R41.2)
EXCLUDES 2 *alcohol-or other psychoactive substance-induced amnestic disorder (F10, F13, F19 with .26, .96)*
amnestic disorder due to known physiological condition (F04)
postictal amnesia in epilepsy (G40.-)

F44.1 Dissociative fugue
Dissociative amnesia with dissociative fugue
EXCLUDES 2 *postictal fugue in epilepsy (G40.-)*
DEF: Dissociative hysteria identified by memory loss and flight from familiar surroundings to a completely separate environment. Episodes may last hours or days. Conscious activity is not associated with perception of surroundings and there is no later memory of the episode.

F44.2 Dissociative stupor
EXCLUDES 1 *catatonic stupor (R40.1)*
stupor NOS (R40.1)
EXCLUDES 2 *catatonic disorder due to known physiological condition (F06.1)*
depressive stupor (F32, F33)
manic stupor (F30, F31)

F44.4 Conversion disorder with motor symptom or deficit
Conversion disorder with abnormal movement
Conversion disorder with speech symptoms
Conversion disorder with swallowing symptoms
Conversion disorder with weakness/paralysis
Dissociative motor disorders
Psychogenic aphonia
Psychogenic dysphonia

F44.5 Conversion disorder with seizures or convulsions
Conversion disorder with attacks or seizures
Dissociative convulsions
AHA: 2019,1Q,19

F44.6 Conversion disorder with sensory symptom or deficit
Conversion disorder with anesthesia or sensory loss
Conversion disorder with special sensory symptoms
Dissociative anesthesia and sensory loss
Psychogenic deafness

F44.7 Conversion disorder with mixed symptom presentation
✓5ᵗʰ **F44.8 Other dissociative and conversion disorders**

F44.81 Dissociative identity disorder
Multiple personality disorder
F44.89 Other dissociative and conversion disorders
Ganser's syndrome
Psychogenic confusion
Psychogenic twilight state
Trance and possession disorders

F44.9 Dissociative and conversion disorder, unspecified
Dissociative disorder NOS

✓4ᵗʰ **F45 Somatoform disorders**
EXCLUDES 2 *dissociative and conversion disorders (F44.-)*
factitious disorders (F68.1-, F68.A)
hair-plucking (F63.3)
lalling (F80.0)
lisping (F80.0)
malingering [conscious simulation] (Z76.5)
nail-biting (F98.8)
psychological or behavioral factors associated with disorders or diseases classified elsewhere (F54)
sexual dysfunction, not due to a substance or known physiological condition (F52.-)
thumb-sucking (F98.8)
tic disorders (in childhood and adolescence) (F95.-)
Tourette's syndrome (F95.2)
trichotillomania (F63.3)
DEF: Types of disorders causing inconsistent physical symptoms that cannot be explained.

F45.0 Somatization disorder
Briquet's disorder
Multiple psychosomatic disorder
F45.1 Undifferentiated somatoform disorder
Somatic symptom disorder
Undifferentiated psychosomatic disorder
✓5ᵗʰ **F45.2 Hypochondriacal disorders**
EXCLUDES 2 *delusional dysmorphophobia (F22)*
fixed delusions about bodily functions or shape (F22)

F45.20 Hypochondriacal disorder, unspecified
F45.21 Hypochondriasis
Hypochondriacal neurosis
Illness anxiety disorder
F45.22 Body dysmorphic disorder
Dysmorphophobia (nondelusional)
Nosophobia
F45.29 Other hypochondriacal disorders
✓5ᵗʰ **F45.4 Pain disorders related to psychological factors**
EXCLUDES 1 *pain NOS (R52)*

F45.41 Pain disorder exclusively related to psychological factors
Somatoform pain disorder (persistent)
F45.42 Pain disorder with related psychological factors
Code also associated acute or chronic pain (G89.-)
F45.8 Other somatoform disorders
Psychogenic dysmenorrhea
Psychogenic dysphagia, including 'globus hystericus'
Psychogenic pruritus
Psychogenic torticollis
Somatoform autonomic dysfunction
Teeth grinding
EXCLUDES 1 *sleep related teeth grinding (G47.63)*
F45.9 Somatoform disorder, unspecified
Psychosomatic disorder NOS

✓4ᵗʰ **F48 Other nonpsychotic mental disorders**
F48.1 Depersonalization-derealization syndrome
F48.2 Pseudobulbar affect
Involuntary emotional expression disorder
Code first underlying cause, if known, such as:
amyotrophic lateral sclerosis (G12.21)
multiple sclerosis (G35)
sequelae of cerebrovascular disease (I69.-)
sequelae of traumatic intracranial injury (S06.-)
F48.8 Other specified nonpsychotic mental disorders
Dhat syndrome
Neurasthenia
Occupational neurosis, including writer's cramp
Psychasthenia
Psychasthenic neurosis
Psychogenic syncope
F48.9 Nonpsychotic mental disorder, unspecified
Neurosis NOS

Behavioral syndromes associated with physiological disturbances and physical factors (F50-F59)

✓4ᵗʰ F50 Eating disorders

   EXCLUDES 1   anorexia NOS (R63.0)
         feeding difficulties (R63.3)
         feeding problems of newborn (P92.-)
         polyphagia (R63.2)
   EXCLUDES 2   feeding disorder in infancy or childhood (F98.2-)
   AHA: 2018,4Q,82

✓5ᵗʰ F50.0 Anorexia nervosa

   EXCLUDES 1   loss of appetite (R63.0)
         psychogenic loss of appetite (F50.89)
   DEF: Psychological eating disorder characterized by an intense fear of gaining weight and an unrealistic perception of body image that perpetuates the feeling of being fat or having too much fat. Avoidance of food and restrictive or unhealthy eating are common.

   F50.00 Anorexia nervosa, unspecified
   F50.01 Anorexia nervosa, restricting type
   F50.02 Anorexia nervosa, binge eating/purging type
      EXCLUDES 1   bulimia nervosa (F50.2)

F50.2 Bulimia nervosa
   Bulimia NOS
   Hyperorexia nervosa
   EXCLUDES 1   anorexia nervosa, binge eating/purging type (F50.02)
   DEF: Episodic pattern of overeating (binge eating) followed by purging or extreme exercise accompanied by an awareness of the abnormal eating pattern with a fear of not being able to stop eating.

✓5ᵗʰ F50.8 Other eating disorders
   EXCLUDES 2   pica of infancy and childhood (F98.3)
   AHA: 2017,4Q,9; 2016,4Q,15-16

   F50.81 Binge eating disorder
   F50.82 Avoidant/restrictive food intake disorder
   F50.89 Other specified eating disorder
      Pica in adults
      Psychogenic loss of appetite

F50.9 Eating disorder, unspecified
   Atypical anorexia nervosa
   Atypical bulimia nervosa
   Feeding or eating disorder, unspecified
   Other specified feeding disorder

✓4ᵗʰ F51 Sleep disorders not due to a substance or known physiological condition
   EXCLUDES 2   organic sleep disorders (G47.-)

✓5ᵗʰ F51.0 Insomnia not due to a substance or known physiological condition
   EXCLUDES 2   alcohol related insomnia (F10.182, F10.282, F10.982)
         drug-related insomnia (F11.182, F11.282, F11.982, F13.182, F13.282, F13.982, F14.182, F14.282, F15.182, F15.282, F15.982, F19.182, F19.282, F19.982)
         insomnia NOS (G47.0-)
         insomnia due to known physiological condition (G47.0-)
         organic insomnia (G47.0-)
         sleep deprivation (Z72.820)

   F51.01 Primary insomnia
      Idiopathic insomnia
   F51.02 Adjustment insomnia
   F51.03 Paradoxical insomnia
   F51.04 Psychophysiologic insomnia
   F51.05 Insomnia due to other mental disorder
      Code also associated mental disorder
   F51.09 Other insomnia not due to a substance or known physiological condition

✓5ᵗʰ F51.1 Hypersomnia not due to a substance or known physiological condition
   EXCLUDES 2   alcohol related hypersomnia (F10.182, F10.282, F10.982)
         drug-related hypersomnia (F11.182, F11.282, F11.982, F13.182, F13.282, F13.982, F14.182, F14.282, F14.982, F15.182, F15.282, F15.982, F19.182, F19.282, F19.982)
         hypersomnia NOS (G47.10)
         hypersomnia due to known physiological condition (G47.10)
         idiopathic hypersomnia (G47.11, G47.12)
         narcolepsy (G47.4-)

   F51.11 Primary hypersomnia
   F51.12 Insufficient sleep syndrome
      EXCLUDES 1   sleep deprivation (Z72.820)
   F51.13 Hypersomnia due to other mental disorder
      Code also associated mental disorder
   F51.19 Other hypersomnia not due to a substance or known physiological condition

F51.3 Sleepwalking [somnambulism]
   Non-rapid eye movement sleep arousal disorders, sleepwalking type

F51.4 Sleep terrors [night terrors]
   Non-rapid eye movement sleep arousal disorders, sleep terror type

F51.5 Nightmare disorder
   Dream anxiety disorder

F51.8 Other sleep disorders not due to a substance or known physiological condition

F51.9 Sleep disorder not due to a substance or known physiological condition, unspecified
   Emotional sleep disorder NOS

✓4ᵗʰ F52 Sexual dysfunction not due to a substance or known physiological condition
   EXCLUDES 2   Dhat syndrome (F48.8)

F52.0 Hypoactive sexual desire disorder
   Lack or loss of sexual desire
   Male hypoactive sexual desire disorder
   Sexual anhedonia
   EXCLUDES 1   decreased libido (R68.82)

F52.1 Sexual aversion disorder
   Sexual aversion and lack of sexual enjoyment

✓5ᵗʰ F52.2 Sexual arousal disorders
   Failure of genital response

   F52.21 Male erectile disorder ♂
      Erectile disorder
      Psychogenic impotence
      EXCLUDES 1   impotence of organic origin (N52.-)
           impotence NOS (N52.-)
   F52.22 Female sexual arousal disorder ♀
      Female sexual interest/arousal disorder

✓5ᵗʰ F52.3 Orgasmic disorder
   Inhibited orgasm
   Psychogenic anorgasmy

   F52.31 Female orgasmic disorder ♀
   F52.32 Male orgasmic disorder ♂
      Delayed ejaculation

F52.4 Premature ejaculation ♂

F52.5 Vaginismus not due to a substance or known physiological condition ♀
   Psychogenic vaginismus
   EXCLUDES 2   vaginismus (due to a known physiological condition) (N94.2)
   DEF: Psychogenic response resulting in painful contractions of the vaginal canal muscles. This condition can be severe enough to prevent sexual intercourse.

F52.6 Dyspareunia not due to a substance or known physiological condition
   Genito-pelvic pain penetration disorder
   Psychogenic dyspareunia
   EXCLUDES 2   dyspareunia (due to a known physiological condition) (N94.1-)

☑ Additional Character Required   ✓x7ᵗʰ Placeholder Alert   Manifestation   Unspecified Dx   ▶◀ Revised Text   ● New Code   ▲ Revised Title

ICD-10-CM 2020   553

Chapter 5. Mental, Behavioral and Neurodevelopmental Disorders

F52.8 Other sexual dysfunction not due to a substance or known physiological condition
Excessive sexual drive
Nymphomania
Satyriasis

F52.9 Unspecified sexual dysfunction not due to a substance or known physiological condition
Sexual dysfunction NOS

☑4ᵗʰ **F53 Mental and behavioral disorders associated with the puerperium, not elsewhere classified**
EXCLUDES 1   *mood disorders with psychotic features (F30.2, F31.2, F31.5, F31.64, F32.3, F33.3)*
postpartum dysphoria (O90.6)
psychosis in schizophrenia, schizotypal, delusional, and other psychotic disorders (F20-F29)

AHA: 2018,4Q,8

F53.0 Postpartum depression   Ⓜ ♀
Postnatal depression, NOS
Postpartum depression, NOS

F53.1 Puerperal psychosis   Ⓜ ♀
Postpartum psychosis
Puerperal psychosis, NOS

F54 *Psychological and behavioral factors associated with disorders or diseases classified elsewhere*
Psychological factors affecting physical conditions
Code first the associated physical disorder, such as:
asthma (J45.-)
dermatitis (L23-L25)
gastric ulcer (K25.-)
mucous colitis (K58.-)
ulcerative colitis (K51.-)
urticaria (L50.-)
EXCLUDES 2   *tension-type headache (G44.2)*

☑4ᵗʰ **F55 Abuse of non-psychoactive substances**
EXCLUDES 2   *abuse of psychoactive substances (F10-F19)*

F55.0 Abuse of antacids
F55.1 Abuse of herbal or folk remedies
F55.2 Abuse of laxatives
F55.3 Abuse of steroids or hormones
F55.4 Abuse of vitamins
F55.8 Abuse of other non-psychoactive substances

F59 Unspecified behavioral syndromes associated with physiological disturbances and physical factors
Psychogenic physiological dysfunction NOS

Disorders of adult personality and behavior (F60-F69)

☑4ᵗʰ **F60 Specific personality disorders**

F60.0 Paranoid personality disorder
Expansive paranoid personality (disorder)
Fanatic personality (disorder)
Paranoid personality (disorder)
Querulant personality (disorder)
Sensitive paranoid personality (disorder)
EXCLUDES 2   *paranoia (F22)*
paranoia querulans (F22)
paranoid psychosis (F22)
paranoid schizophrenia (F20.0)
paranoid state (F22)

F60.1 Schizoid personality disorder
EXCLUDES 2   *Asperger's syndrome (F84.5)*
delusional disorder (F22)
schizoid disorder of childhood (F84.5)
schizophrenia (F20.-)
schizotypal disorder (F21)

F60.2 Antisocial personality disorder
Amoral personality (disorder)
Asocial personality (disorder)
Dissocial personality disorder
Psychopathic personality (disorder)
Sociopathic personality (disorder)
EXCLUDES 1   *conduct disorders (F91.-)*
EXCLUDES 2   *borderline personality disorder (F60.3)*

F60.3 Borderline personality disorder
Aggressive personality (disorder)
Emotionally unstable personality disorder
Explosive personality (disorder)
EXCLUDES 2   *antisocial personality disorder (F60.2)*

F60.4 Histrionic personality disorder
Hysterical personality (disorder)
Psychoinfantile personality (disorder)

F60.5 Obsessive-compulsive personality disorder
Anankastic personality (disorder)
Compulsive personality (disorder)
Obsessional personality (disorder)
EXCLUDES 2   *obsessive-compulsive disorder (F42-)*

F60.6 Avoidant personality disorder
Anxious personality disorder

F60.7 Dependent personality disorder
Asthenic personality (disorder)
Inadequate personality (disorder)
Passive personality (disorder)
DEF: Lack of self-confidence, fear of abandonment, and an obsessive need to be taken care of.

☑5ᵗʰ **F60.8 Other specific personality disorders**

F60.81 Narcissistic personality disorder
F60.89 Other specific personality disorders
Eccentric personality disorder
"Haltlose" type personality disorder
Immature personality disorder
Passive-aggressive personality disorder
Psychoneurotic personality disorder
Self-defeating personality disorder

F60.9 Personality disorder, unspecified
Character disorder NOS
Character neurosis NOS
Pathological personality NOS

☑4ᵗʰ **F63 Impulse disorders**
EXCLUDES 2   *habitual excessive use of alcohol or psychoactive substances (F10-F19)*
impulse disorders involving sexual behavior (F65.-)

F63.0 Pathological gambling
Compulsive gambling
Gambling disorder
EXCLUDES 1   *gambling and betting NOS (Z72.6)*
EXCLUDES 2   *excessive gambling by manic patients (F30, F31)*
gambling in antisocial personality disorder (F60.2)

F63.1 Pyromania
Pathological fire-setting
EXCLUDES 2   *fire-setting (by) (in):*
adult with antisocial personality disorder (F60.2)
alcohol or psychoactive substance intoxication (F10-F19)
conduct disorders (F91.-)
mental disorders due to known physiological condition (F01-F09)
schizophrenia (F20.-)

F63.2 Kleptomania
Pathological stealing
EXCLUDES 1   *shoplifting as the reason for observation for suspected mental disorder (Z03.8)*
EXCLUDES 2   *depressive disorder with stealing (F31-F33)*
stealing due to underlying mental condition - code to mental condition
stealing in mental disorders due to known physiological condition (F01-F09)

F63.3 Trichotillomania
Hair plucking
EXCLUDES 2   *other stereotyped movement disorder (F98.4)*

☑5ᵗʰ **F63.8 Other impulse disorders**

F63.81 Intermittent explosive disorder
F63.89 Other impulse disorders
F63.9 Impulse disorder, unspecified
Impulse control disorder NOS

Ⓝ Newborn: 0   Ⓟ Pediatric: 0-17   Ⓜ Maternity: 12-55   Ⓐ Adult: 15-124   **CH** Comorbidity High   **CL** Comorbidity Low   **NCDx** Noncancer Dx   **PDx** Primary Dx

554   ICD-10-CM 2020

✓4ᵗʰ **F64 Gender identity disorders**

AHA: 2016,4Q,16

F64.0 Transsexualism
Gender identity disorder in adolescence and adulthood
Gender dysphoria in adolescents and adults

F64.1 Dual role transvestism
Use additional code to identify sex reassignment status (Z87.890)
EXCLUDES 1   *gender identity disorder in childhood (F64.2)*
EXCLUDES 2   *fetishistic transvestism (F65.1)*

F64.2 Gender identity disorder of childhood   P
Gender dysphoria in children
EXCLUDES 1   *gender identity disorder in adolescence and adulthood (F64.0)*
EXCLUDES 2   *sexual maturation disorder (F66)*

F64.8 Other gender identity disorders
Other specified gender dysphoria

F64.9 Gender identity disorder, unspecified
Gender dysphoria, unspecified
Gender-role disorder NOS

✓4ᵗʰ **F65 Paraphilias**

F65.0 Fetishism
Fetishistic disorder

F65.1 Transvestic fetishism
Fetishistic transvestism
Transvestic disorder

F65.2 Exhibitionism
Exhibitionistic disorder

F65.3 Voyeurism
Voyeuristic disorder

F65.4 Pedophilia
Pedophilic disorder

✓5ᵗʰ **F65.5 Sadomasochism**

F65.50 Sadomasochism, unspecified
F65.51 Sexual masochism
Sexual masochism disorder
F65.52 Sexual sadism
Sexual sadism disorder

✓5ᵗʰ **F65.8 Other paraphilias**

F65.81 Frotteurism
Frotteuristic disorder
F65.89 Other paraphilias
Necrophilia
Other specified paraphilic disorder

F65.9 Paraphilia, unspecified
Paraphilic disorder, unspecified
Sexual deviation NOS

F66 Other sexual disorders
Sexual maturation disorder
Sexual relationship disorder

✓4ᵗʰ **F68 Other disorders of adult personality and behavior**

AHA: 2018,4Q,9,65

✓5ᵗʰ **F68.1 Factitious disorder** imposed on self
Compensation neurosis
Elaboration of physical symptoms for psychological reasons
Hospital hopper syndrome
Münchausen's syndrome
Peregrinating patient
EXCLUDES 2   *factitial dermatitis (L98.1)*
person feigning illness (with obvious motivation) (Z76.5)

F68.10 Factitious disorder imposed on self, unspecified
F68.11 Factitious disorder imposed on self, with predominantly psychological signs and symptoms
F68.12 Factitious disorder imposed on self, with predominantly physical signs and symptoms
F68.13 Factitious disorder imposed on self, with combined psychological and physical signs and symptoms

F68.A Factitious disorder imposed on another
Factitious disorder by proxy
Münchausen's by proxy

F68.8 Other specified disorders of adult personality and behavior

F69 Unspecified disorder of adult personality and behavior   A

Intellectual disabilities (F70-F79)

Code first any associated physical or developmental disorders
EXCLUDES 1   *borderline intellectual functioning, IQ above 70 to 84 (R41.83)*

F70 Mild intellectual disabilities
IQ level 50-55 to approximately 70
Mild mental subnormality

F71 Moderate intellectual disabilities
IQ level 35-40 to 50-55
Moderate mental subnormality

F72 Severe intellectual disabilities
IQ 20-25 to 35-40
Severe mental subnormality

F73 Profound intellectual disabilities
IQ level below 20-25
Profound mental subnormality

F78 Other intellectual disabilities

F79 Unspecified intellectual disabilities
Mental deficiency NOS
Mental subnormality NOS

Pervasive and specific developmental disorders (F80-F89)

✓4ᵗʰ **F80 Specific developmental disorders of speech and language**

F80.0 Phonological disorder
Dyslalia
Functional speech articulation disorder
Lalling
Lisping
Phonological developmental disorder
Speech articulation developmental disorder
Speech-sound disorder
EXCLUDES 1   *speech articulation impairment due to aphasia NOS (R47.01)*
speech articulation impairment due to apraxia (R48.2)
EXCLUDES 2   *speech articulation impairment due to hearing loss (F80.4)*
speech articulation impairment due to intellectual disabilities (F70-F79)
speech articulation impairment with expressive language developmental disorder (F80.1)
speech articulation impairment with mixed receptive expressive language developmental disorder (F80.2)

F80.1 Expressive language disorder
Developmental dysphasia or aphasia, expressive type
EXCLUDES 1   *mixed receptive-expressive language disorder (F80.2)*
dysphasia and aphasia NOS (R47.-)
EXCLUDES 2   *acquired aphasia with epilepsy [Landau-Kleffner] (G40.80-)*
selective mutism (F94.0)
intellectual disabilities (F70-F79)
pervasive developmental disorders (F84.-)

F80.2 Mixed receptive-expressive language disorder
Developmental dysphasia or aphasia, receptive type
Developmental Wernicke's aphasia
EXCLUDES 1   *central auditory processing disorder (H93.25)*
dysphasia or aphasia NOS (R47.-)
expressive language disorder (F80.1)
expressive type dysphasia or aphasia (F80.1)
word deafness (H93.25)
EXCLUDES 2   *acquired aphasia with epilepsy [Landau-Kleffner] (G40.80-)*
pervasive developmental disorders (F84.-)
selective mutism (F94.0)
intellectual disabilities (F70-F79)

F80.4 Speech and language development delay due to hearing loss
Code also type of hearing loss (H90.-, H91.-)

✓5ᵗʰ **F80.8　Other developmental disorders of speech and language**
　　AHA: 2017,1Q,27
　F80.81　Childhood onset fluency disorder
　　　Cluttering NOS
　　　Stuttering NOS
　　　EXCLUDES 1　*adult onset fluency disorder (F98.5)*
　　　　　　fluency disorder in conditions classified elsewhere (R47.82)
　　　　　　fluency disorder (stuttering) following cerebrovascular disease (I69. with final characters -23)
　F80.82　Social pragmatic communication disorder
　　　EXCLUDES 1　*Asperger's syndrome (F84.5)*
　　　　　　autistic disorder (F84.0)
　　　AHA: 2016,4Q,16
　F80.89　Other developmental disorders of speech and language
F80.9　Developmental disorder of speech and language, unspecified
　　Communication disorder NOS
　　Language disorder NOS

✓4ᵗʰ **F81　Specific developmental disorders of scholastic skills**
F81.0　Specific reading disorder
　　"Backward reading"
　　Developmental dyslexia
　　Specific learning disorder, with impairment in reading
　　Specific reading retardation
　　EXCLUDES 1　*alexia NOS (R48.0)*
　　　　　　dyslexia NOS (R48.0)
　　DEF: Serious impairment of reading skills unexplained in relation to general intelligence and teaching processes.
F81.2　Mathematics disorder
　　Developmental acalculia
　　Developmental arithmetical disorder
　　Developmental Gerstmann's syndrome
　　Specific learning disorder, with impairment in mathematics
　　EXCLUDES 1　*acalculia NOS (R48.8)*
　　EXCLUDES 2　*arithmetical difficulties associated with a reading disorder (F81.0)*
　　　　　　arithmetical difficulties associated with a spelling disorder (F81.81)
　　　　　　arithmetical difficulties due to inadequate teaching (Z55.8)
✓5ᵗʰ **F81.8　Other developmental disorders of scholastic skills**
　F81.81　Disorder of written expression
　　　Specific learning disorder, with impairment in written expression
　　　Specific spelling disorder
　F81.89　Other developmental disorders of scholastic skills
F81.9　Developmental disorder of scholastic skills, unspecified
　　Knowledge acquisition disability NOS
　　Learning disability NOS
　　Learning disorder NOS

F82　Specific developmental disorder of motor function
　　Clumsy child syndrome
　　Developmental coordination disorder
　　Developmental dyspraxia
　　EXCLUDES 1　*abnormalities of gait and mobility (R26.-)*
　　　　　　lack of coordination (R27.-)
　　EXCLUDES 2　*lack of coordination secondary to intellectual disabilities (F70-F79)*

✓4ᵗʰ **F84　Pervasive developmental disorders**
　　Use additional code to identify any associated medical condition and intellectual disabilities.
F84.0　Autistic disorder
　　Autism spectrum disorder
　　Infantile autism
　　Infantile psychosis
　　Kanner's syndrome
　　EXCLUDES 1　*Asperger's syndrome (F84.5)*
　　AHA: 2017,1Q,27
　　TIP: When the encounter is focused on treatment of conditions related to autism spectrum disorder, first assign codes to identify the problem or manifestation of autism receiving therapeutic services.

F84.2　Rett's syndrome
　　EXCLUDES 1　*Asperger's syndrome (F84.5)*
　　　　　　autistic disorder (F84.0)
　　　　　　other childhood disintegrative disorder (F84.3)
F84.3　Other childhood disintegrative disorder　P
　　Dementia infantilis
　　Disintegrative psychosis
　　Heller's syndrome
　　Symbiotic psychosis
　　Use additional code to identify any associated neurological condition
　　EXCLUDES 1　*Asperger's syndrome (F84.5)*
　　　　　　autistic disorder (F84.0)
　　　　　　Rett's syndrome (F84.2)
F84.5　Asperger's syndrome
　　Asperger's disorder
　　Autistic psychopathy
　　Schizoid disorder of childhood
　　DEF: High-functioning form of autism. Children with this syndrome usually develop speech on schedule, are generally very intelligent, and communicate well, but have considerable social shortcomings. Synonym(s): AS.
F84.8　Other pervasive developmental disorders
　　Overactive disorder associated with intellectual disabilities and stereotyped movements
F84.9　Pervasive developmental disorder, unspecified
　　Atypical autism

F88　Other disorders of psychological development
　　Developmental agnosia
　　Global developmental delay
　　Other specified neurodevelopmental disorder

F89　Unspecified disorder of psychological development
　　Developmental disorder NOS
　　Neurodevelopmental disorder NOS

Behavioral and emotional disorders with onset usually occurring in childhood and adolescence (F90-F98)

NOTE　Codes within categories F90-F98 may be used regardless of the age of a patient. These disorders generally have onset within the childhood or adolescent years, but may continue throughout life or not be diagnosed until adulthood

✓4ᵗʰ **F90　Attention-deficit hyperactivity disorders**
　　INCLUDES　attention deficit disorder with hyperactivity
　　　　attention deficit syndrome with hyperactivity
　　EXCLUDES 2　*anxiety disorders (F40.-, F41.-)*
　　　　　　mood [affective] disorders (F30-F39)
　　　　　　pervasive developmental disorders (F84.-)
　　　　　　schizophrenia (F20.-)
F90.0　Attention-deficit hyperactivity disorder, predominantly inattentive type
　　Attention-deficit/hyperactivity disorder, predominantly inattentive presentation
F90.1　Attention-deficit hyperactivity disorder, predominantly hyperactive type
　　Attention-deficit/hyperactivity disorder, predominantly hyperactive impulsive presentation
F90.2　Attention-deficit hyperactivity disorder, combined type
　　Attention-deficit/hyperactivity disorder, combined presentation
F90.8　Attention-deficit hyperactivity disorder, other type
F90.9　Attention-deficit hyperactivity disorder, unspecified type
　　Attention-deficit hyperactivity disorder of childhood or adolescence NOS
　　Attention-deficit hyperactivity disorder NOS

✓4ᵗʰ **F91　Conduct disorders**
　　EXCLUDES 1　*antisocial behavior (Z72.81-)*
　　　　　　antisocial personality disorder (F60.2)
　　EXCLUDES 2　*conduct problems associated with attention-deficit hyperactivity disorder (F90.-)*
　　　　　　mood [affective] disorders (F30-F39)
　　　　　　pervasive developmental disorders (F84.-)
　　　　　　schizophrenia (F20.-)
F91.0　Conduct disorder confined to family context

F91.1 Conduct disorder, childhood-onset type
    Unsocialized conduct disorder
    Conduct disorder, solitary aggressive type
    Unsocialized aggressive disorder

F91.2 Conduct disorder, adolescent-onset type
    Socialized conduct disorder
    Conduct disorder, group type

F91.3 Oppositional defiant disorder

F91.8 Other conduct disorders
    Other specified conduct disorder
    Other specified disruptive disorder

F91.9 Conduct disorder, unspecified
    Behavioral disorder NOS
    Conduct disorder NOS
    Disruptive behavior disorder NOS
    Disruptive disorder NOS

✓4ᵗʰ **F93 Emotional disorders with onset specific to childhood**

F93.0 Separation anxiety disorder of childhood
    EXCLUDES 2   *mood [affective] disorders (F30-F39)*
               nonpsychotic mental disorders (F40-F48)
               phobic anxiety disorder of childhood (F40.8)
               social phobia (F40.1)

F93.8 Other childhood emotional disorders
    Identity disorder
    EXCLUDES 2   *gender identity disorder of childhood (F64.2)*

F93.9 Childhood emotional disorder, unspecified

✓4ᵗʰ **F94 Disorders of social functioning with onset specific to childhood and adolescence**

F94.0 Selective mutism
    Elective mutism
    EXCLUDES 2   *pervasive developmental disorders (F84.-)*
               schizophrenia (F20.-)
               specific developmental disorders of speech and language (F80.-)
               transient mutism as part of separation anxiety in young children (F93.0)

F94.1 Reactive attachment disorder of childhood
    Use additional code to identify any associated failure to thrive or growth retardation
    EXCLUDES 1   *disinhibited attachment disorder of childhood (F94.2)*
               normal variation in pattern of selective attachment
    EXCLUDES 2   *Asperger's syndrome (F84.5)*
               maltreatment syndromes (T74.-)
               sexual or physical abuse in childhood, resulting in psychosocial problems (Z62.81-)

F94.2 Disinhibited attachment disorder of childhood
    Affectionless psychopathy
    Institutional syndrome
    EXCLUDES 1   *reactive attachment disorder of childhood (F94.1)*
    EXCLUDES 2   *Asperger's syndrome (F84.5)*
               attention-deficit hyperactivity disorders (F90.-)
               hospitalism in children (F43.2-)

F94.8 Other childhood disorders of social functioning

F94.9 Childhood disorder of social functioning, unspecified

✓4ᵗʰ **F95 Tic disorder**

F95.0 Transient tic disorder
    Provisional tic disorder

F95.1 Chronic motor or vocal tic disorder

F95.2 Tourette's disorder
    Combined vocal and multiple motor tic disorder [de la Tourette]
    Tourette's syndrome

F95.8 Other tic disorders

F95.9 Tic disorder, unspecified
    Tic NOS

✓4ᵗʰ **F98 Other behavioral and emotional disorders with onset usually occurring in childhood and adolescence**
    EXCLUDES 2   *breath-holding spells (R06.89)*
               gender identity disorder of childhood (F64.2)
               Kleine-Levin syndrome (G47.13)
               obsessive-compulsive disorder (F42-)
               sleep disorders not due to a substance or known physiological condition (F51.-)

F98.0 Enuresis not due to a substance or known physiological condition
    Enuresis (primary) (secondary) of nonorganic origin
    Functional enuresis
    Psychogenic enuresis
    Urinary incontinence of nonorganic origin
    EXCLUDES 1   *enuresis NOS (R32)*

F98.1 Encopresis not due to a substance or known physiological condition
    Functional encopresis
    Incontinence of feces of nonorganic origin
    Psychogenic encopresis
    Use additional code to identify the cause of any coexisting constipation
    EXCLUDES 1   *encopresis NOS (R15.-)*

✓5ᵗʰ **F98.2 Other feeding disorders of infancy and childhood**
    EXCLUDES 1   *feeding difficulties (R63.3)*
    EXCLUDES 2   *anorexia nervosa and other eating disorders (F50.-)*
               feeding problems of newborn (P92.-)
               pica of infancy or childhood (F98.3)

    F98.21 Rumination disorder of infancy
    F98.29 Other feeding disorders of infancy and early childhood

F98.3 Pica of infancy and childhood

F98.4 Stereotyped movement disorders
    Stereotype/habit disorder
    EXCLUDES 1   *abnormal involuntary movements (R25.-)*
    EXCLUDES 2   *compulsions in obsessive-compulsive disorder (F42-)*
               hair plucking (F63.3)
               movement disorders of organic origin (G20-G25)
               nail-biting (F98.8)
               nose-picking (F98.8)
               stereotypies that are part of a broader psychiatric condition (F01-F95)
               thumb-sucking (F98.8)
               tic disorders (F95.-)
               trichotillomania (F63.3)

F98.5 Adult onset fluency disorder
    EXCLUDES 1   *childhood onset fluency disorder (F80.81)*
               dysphasia (R47.02)
               fluency disorder in conditions classified elsewhere (R47.82)
               fluency disorder (stuttering) following cerebrovascular disease (I69. with final characters -23)
               tic disorders (F95.-)

F98.8 Other specified behavioral and emotional disorders with onset usually occurring in childhood and adolescence
    Excessive masturbation
    Nail-biting
    Nose-picking
    Thumb-sucking

F98.9 Unspecified behavioral and emotional disorders with onset usually occurring in childhood and adolescence

Unspecified mental disorder (F99)

F99 Mental disorder, not otherwise specified
    Mental illness NOS
    EXCLUDES 1   *unspecified mental disorder due to known physiological condition (F09)*

Chapter 6. Diseases of the Nervous System (GØØ-G99)

Chapter-specific Guidelines with Coding Examples

The chapter-specific guidelines from the ICD-10-CM Official Guidelines for Coding and Reporting have been provided below. Along with these guidelines are coding examples, contained in the shaded boxes, that have been developed to help illustrate the coding and/or sequencing guidance found in these guidelines.

a. Dominant/nondominant side

Codes from category G81, Hemiplegia and hemiparesis, and subcategories G83.1, Monoplegia of lower limb, G83.2, Monoplegia of upper limb, and G83.3, Monoplegia, unspecified, identify whether the dominant or nondominant side is affected. Should the affected side be documented, but not specified as dominant or nondominant, and the classification system does not indicate a default, code selection is as follows:

- For ambidextrous patients, the default should be dominant.
- If the left side is affected, the default is non-dominant.
- If the right side is affected, the default is dominant.

> Hemiplegia affecting left side of ambidextrous patient.
>
> **G81.92   Hemiplegia, unspecified affecting left dominant side**
>
> *Explanation*: Documentation states that the left side is affected and dominant is used for ambidextrous persons.

> Right spastic hemiplegia, unknown whether patient is right- or left-handed.
>
> **G81.11   Spastic hemiplegia affecting right dominant side**
>
> *Explanation*: Since it is unknown whether the patient is right- or left-handed, if the right side is affected, the default is dominant.

b. Pain—Category G89

1) General coding information

Codes in category G89, Pain, not elsewhere classified, may be used in conjunction with codes from other categories and chapters to provide more detail about acute or chronic pain and neoplasm-related pain, unless otherwise indicated below.

If the pain is not specified as acute or chronic, post-thoracotomy, postprocedural, or neoplasm-related, do not assign codes from category G89.

A code from category G89 should not be assigned if the underlying (definitive) diagnosis is known, unless the reason for the encounter is pain control/ management and not management of the underlying condition.

When an admission or encounter is for a procedure aimed at treating the underlying condition (e.g., spinal fusion, kyphoplasty), a code for the underlying condition (e.g., vertebral fracture, spinal stenosis) should be assigned as the principal diagnosis. No code from category G89 should be assigned.

(a) Category G89 codes as principal or first-listed diagnosis

Category G89 codes are acceptable as principal diagnosis or the first-listed code:

- When pain control or pain management is the reason for the admission/encounter (e.g., a patient with displaced intervertebral disc, nerve impingement and severe back pain presents for injection of steroid into the spinal canal). The underlying cause of the pain should be reported as an additional diagnosis, if known.

> A patient is admitted for rehabilitation focused on pain management. Provider notes indicate malignant neoplasm of the bone, with associated pain and debility.
>
> **G89.3   Neoplasm related pain (acute) (chronic)**
>
> **C41.9   Malignant neoplasm of bone and articular cartilage, unspecified**
>
> *Explanation*: Since the care focuses on controlling neoplasm-related pain, rather than treating the bone cancer, the pain code is sequenced first followed by the code for the underlying condition.

- When a patient is admitted for the insertion of a neurostimulator for pain control, assign the appropriate pain code as the principal or first-listed diagnosis. When an admission or encounter is for a procedure aimed at treating the underlying condition and a neurostimulator is inserted for pain control during the same admission/encounter, a code for the underlying condition should be assigned as the principal diagnosis and the appropriate pain code should be assigned as a secondary diagnosis.

(b) Use of category G89 codes in conjunction with site specific pain codes

(i) Assigning category G89 and site-specific pain codes

Codes from category G89 may be used in conjunction with codes that identify the site of pain (including codes from chapter 18) if the category G89 code provides additional information. For example, if the code describes the site of the pain, but does not fully describe whether the pain is acute or chronic, then both codes should be assigned.

(ii) Sequencing of category G89 codes with site-specific pain codes

The sequencing of category G89 codes with site-specific pain codes (including chapter 18 codes), is dependent on the circumstances of the encounter/admission as follows:

- If the encounter is for pain control or pain management, assign the code from category G89 followed by the code identifying the specific site of pain (e.g., encounter for pain management for acute neck pain from trauma is assigned code G89.11, Acute pain due to trauma, followed by code M54.2, Cervicalgia, to identify the site of pain).

> Patient is admitted for rehabilitation following hospitalization for a fall. Provider orders specify rehabilitative therapy services due to acute post-fall right knee pain. Nursing will medically manage pain control.
>
> **G89.11   Acute pain due to trauma**
>
> **M25.561   Pain in right knee**
>
> *Explanation*: The focus of the skilled care is rehabilitation for pain management, so code G89.11 is sequenced first. Since this does not fully describe the condition, an additional code to indicate the site of the pain is added.

- If the encounter is for any other reason except pain control or pain management, and a related definitive diagnosis has not been established (confirmed) by the provider, assign the code for the specific site of pain first, followed by the appropriate code from category G89.

2) Pain due to devices, implants and grafts

See Section I.C.19. Pain due to medical devices

3) Postoperative pain

The provider's documentation should be used to guide the coding of postoperative pain, as well as *Section III. Reporting Additional Diagnoses* and *Section IV. Diagnostic Coding and Reporting in the Outpatient Setting*.

The default for post-thoracotomy and other postoperative pain not specified as acute or chronic is the code for the acute form.

Routine or expected postoperative pain immediately after surgery should not be coded.

> Patient is admitted for skilled care following surgery for repair of a large abdominal hernia. He requires skilled nursing for postoperative pain management and observation and home health aide due to unexpected and severe pain that is impacting self-care.
>
> **G89.18   Other acute postprocedural pain**
>
> **Z48.815   Encounter for surgical aftercare following surgery on the digestive system**
>
> *Explanation*: When acute or chronic is not documented, default to acute. Some postoperative pain is expected, but the above documentation indicates this patient had pain that was unexpected and severe, limiting the patient's ability to return home and necessitating a skilled stay.

(a) Postoperative pain not associated with specific postoperative complication

Postoperative pain not associated with a specific postoperative complication is assigned to the appropriate postoperative pain code in category G89.

(b) Postoperative pain associated with specific postoperative complication

Postoperative pain associated with a specific postoperative complication (such as painful wire sutures) is assigned to the appropriate code(s) found in Chapter 19, Injury, poisoning, and certain other consequences of external causes. If appropriate, use additional code(s) from category G89 to identify acute or chronic pain (G89.18 or G89.28).

4) Chronic pain

Chronic pain is classified to subcategory G89.2. There is no time frame defining when pain becomes chronic pain. The provider's documentation should be used to guide use of these codes.

5) Neoplasm related pain

Code G89.3 is assigned to pain documented as being related, associated or due to cancer, primary or secondary malignancy, or tumor. This code is assigned regardless of whether the pain is acute or chronic.

This code may be assigned as the principal or first-listed code when the stated reason for the admission/encounter is documented as pain control/pain management. The underlying neoplasm should be reported as an additional diagnosis.

Patient with history of primary cancer of the prostate and pain due to bone metastasis is admitted to skilled care for continued pain control post-hospitalization.

G89.3   **Neoplasm related pain (acute)(chronic)**

C79.51   **Secondary malignant neoplasm of bone**

Z85.46   **Personal history of malignant neoplasm of prostate**

Explanation: After hospitalization, the patient was admitted to skilled home health care for continued management of pain secondary to bone metastasis. The neoplasm was not the reason for the skilled care and is sequenced after the code for the neoplasm-related pain. Code G89.3 is used for both acute and chronic cancer-related pain.

When the reason for the admission/encounter is management of the neoplasm and the pain associated with the neoplasm is also documented, code G89.3 may be assigned as an additional diagnosis. It is not necessary to assign an additional code for the site of the pain.

See Section I.C.2 for instructions on the sequencing of neoplasms for all other stated reasons for the admission/encounter (except for pain control/pain management).

Provider notes bone neoplasm with current neoplastic fracture of right femur. The fracture is healing normally, but diffuse pain due to extensive neoplastic bone disease in that lower extremity is documented.

M84.551D   **Pathological fracture in neoplastic disease, right femur, subsequent encounter for fracture with routine healing**

C40.21   **Malignant neoplasm of long bones of right lower limb**

G89.3   **Neoplasm related pain (acute) (chronic)**

Explanation: The reason for the encounter is the treatment of the pathological femur fracture due to bone cancer. Additional codes to identify the neoplasm and neoplastic pain should also be assigned.

6) Chronic pain syndrome

Central pain syndrome (G89.0) and chronic pain syndrome (G89.4) are different than the term "chronic pain," and therefore codes should only be used when the provider has specifically documented this condition.

See Section I.C.5. Pain disorders related to psychological factors

Chapter 6. Diseases of the Nervous System (G00-G99)

EXCLUDES 2   certain conditions originating in the perinatal period (P04-P96)
       certain infectious and parasitic diseases (A00-B99)
       complications of pregnancy, childbirth and the puerperium (O00-O9A)
       congenital malformations, deformations, and chromosomal abnormalities (Q00-Q99)
       endocrine, nutritional and metabolic diseases (E00-E88)
       injury, poisoning and certain other consequences of external causes (S00-T88)
       neoplasms (C00-D49)
       symptoms, signs and abnormal clinical and laboratory findings, not elsewhere classified (R00-R94)

This chapter contains the following blocks:

G00-G09   Inflammatory diseases of the central nervous system
G10-G14   Systemic atrophies primarily affecting the central nervous system
G20-G26   Extrapyramidal and movement disorders
G30-G32   Other degenerative diseases of the nervous system
G35-G37   Demyelinating diseases of the central nervous system
G40-G47   Episodic and paroxysmal disorders
G50-G59   Nerve, nerve root and plexus disorders
G60-G65   Polyneuropathies and other disorders of the peripheral nervous system
G70-G73   Diseases of myoneural junction and muscle
G80-G83   Cerebral palsy and other paralytic syndromes
G89-G99   Other disorders of the nervous system

Inflammatory diseases of the central nervous system (G00-G09)

✓4th G00   Bacterial meningitis, not elsewhere classified

INCLUDES   bacterial arachnoiditis
       bacterial leptomeningitis
       bacterial meningitis
       bacterial pachymeningitis
EXCLUDES 1   bacterial meningoencephalitis (G04.2)
       bacterial meningomyelitis (G04.2)

DEF: Inflammation of meningeal layers of the brain and spinal cord due to a bacterial infection.

G00.0   Hemophilus meningitis
Meningitis due to Hemophilus influenzae

G00.1   Pneumococcal meningitis
Meningtitis due to Streptococcal pneumoniae

G00.2   Streptococcal meningitis
Use additional code to further identify organism (B95.0-B95.5)

G00.3   Staphylococcal meningitis
Use additional code to further identify organism (B95.61-B95.8)

G00.8   Other bacterial meningitis
Meningitis due to Escherichia coli
Meningitis due to Friedländer's bacillus
Meningitis due to Klebsiella
Use additional code to further identify organism (B96.-)

G00.9   Bacterial meningitis, unspecified
Meningitis due to gram-negative bacteria, unspecified
Purulent meningitis NOS
Pyogenic meningitis NOS
Suppurative meningitis NOS

G01   Meningitis in bacterial diseases classified elsewhere

Code first underlying disease
EXCLUDES 1   meningitis (in):
       gonococcal (A54.81)
       leptospirosis (A27.81)
       listeriosis (A32.11)
       Lyme disease (A69.21)
       meningococcal (A39.0)
       neurosyphilis (A52.13)
       tuberculosis (A17.0)
       meningoencephalitis and meningomyelitis in bacterial diseases classified elsewhere (G05)

G02   Meningitis in other infectious and parasitic diseases classified elsewhere

Code first underlying disease, such as:
       African trypanosomiasis (B56.-)
       poliovirus infection (A80.-)
EXCLUDES 1   candidal meningitis (B37.5)
       coccidioidomycosis meningitis (B38.4)
       cryptococcal meningitis (B45.1)
       herpesviral [herpes simplex] meningitis (B00.3)
       infectious mononucleosis complicated by meningitis (B27.- with fourth character 2)
       measles complicated by meningitis (B05.1)
       meningoencephalitis and meningomyelitis in other infectious and parasitic diseases classified elsewhere (G05)
       mumps meningitis (B26.1)
       rubella meningitis (B06.02)
       varicella [chickenpox] meningitis (B01.0)
       zoster meningitis (B02.1)

✓4th G03   Meningitis due to other and unspecified causes

INCLUDES   arachnoiditis NOS
       leptomeningitis NOS
       meningitis NOS
       pachymeningitis NOS
EXCLUDES 1   meningoencephalitis (G04.-)
       meningomyelitis (G04.-)

G03.0   Nonpyogenic meningitis
Aseptic meningitis
Nonbacterial meningitis
DEF: Type of meningitis where no bacterial, viral, or other infectious source exists that explains the meningitis symptomology.

G03.1   Chronic meningitis

G03.2   Benign recurrent meningitis [Mollaret]
DEF: Aseptic or noninfectious inflammation of the meninges with the presence of Mollaret cells in the spinal fluid. The patient experiences recurrent bouts of inflammation, lasting anywhere from two to five days.

G03.8   Meningitis due to other specified causes

G03.9   Meningitis, unspecified
Arachnoiditis (spinal) NOS

✓4th G04   Encephalitis, myelitis and encephalomyelitis

INCLUDES   acute ascending myelitis
       meningoencephalitis
       meningomyelitis
EXCLUDES 1   encephalopathy NOS (G93.40)
EXCLUDES 2   acute transverse myelitis (G37.3-)
       alcoholic encephalopathy (G31.2)
       benign myalgic encephalomyelitis (G93.3)
       multiple sclerosis (G35)
       subacute necrotizing myelitis (G37.4)
       toxic encephalitis (G92)
       toxic encephalopathy (G92)

DEF: Encephalitis: Inflammation of the brain, often caused by viral or bacterial infection.
DEF: Encephalomyelitis: Inflammatory disease, often viral in nature, that affects the brain and spinal cord.
DEF: Myelitis: Inflammation of the spinal cord.

✓5th G04.0   Acute disseminated encephalitis and encephalomyelitis (ADEM)
EXCLUDES 1   acute necrotizing hemorrhagic encephalopathy (G04.3-)
       other noninfectious acute disseminated encephalomyelitis (noninfectious ADEM) (G04.81)

G04.00   Acute disseminated encephalitis and encephalomyelitis, unspecified

G04.01   Postinfectious acute disseminated encephalitis and encephalomyelitis (postinfectious ADEM)
EXCLUDES 1   post chickenpox encephalitis (B01.1)
       post measles encephalitis (B05.0)
       post measles myelitis (B05.1)

Chapter 6. Diseases of the Nervous System

G04.02   *Postimmunization* **acute disseminated encephalitis, myelitis and encephalomyelitis**
Encephalitis, post immunization
Encephalomyelitis, post immunization
Use additional code to identify the vaccine (T50.A-, T50.B-, T50.Z-)

G04.1 Tropical spastic paraplegia   **CH** **CL**

G04.2 Bacterial meningoencephalitis and meningomyelitis, not elsewhere classified

✓5ᵗʰ G04.3 Acute necrotizing hemorrhagic encephalopathy
   EXCLUDES 1   *acute disseminated encephalitis and encephalomyelitis (G04.0-)*

   G04.30   **Acute necrotizing hemorrhagic encephalopathy, unspecified**

   G04.31   *Postinfectious* **acute necrotizing hemorrhagic encephalopathy**

   G04.32   *Postimmunization* **acute necrotizing hemorrhagic encephalopathy**
     Use additional code to identify the vaccine (T50.A-, T50.B-, T50.Z-)

   G04.39   **Other acute necrotizing hemorrhagic encephalopathy**
     Code also underlying etiology, if applicable

✓5ᵗʰ G04.8 Other encephalitis, myelitis and encephalomyelitis
   Code also any associated seizure (G40.-, R56.9)

   G04.81   **Other encephalitis and encephalomyelitis**   **NC Dx**
     Noninfectious acute disseminated encephalomyelitis (noninfectious ADEM)

   G04.89   **Other myelitis**   **NC Dx**

✓5ᵗʰ G04.9 Encephalitis, myelitis and encephalomyelitis, unspecified

   G04.90   **Encephalitis and encephalomyelitis, unspecified**
     Ventriculitis (cerebral) NOS

   G04.91   **Myelitis, unspecified**

✓4ᵗʰ G05 Encephalitis, myelitis and encephalomyelitis in diseases classified elsewhere
   Code first underlying disease, such as:
     human immunodeficiency virus [HIV] disease (B20)
     poliovirus (A80.-)
     suppurative otitis media (H66.01-H66.4)
     trichinellosis (B75)
   EXCLUDES 1   *adenoviral encephalitis, myelitis and encephalomyelitis (A85.1)*
     congenital toxoplasmosis encephalitis, myelitis and encephalomyelitis (P37.1)
     cytomegaloviral encephalitis, myelitis and encephalomyelitis (B25.8)
     encephalitis, myelitis and encephalomyelitis (in) measles (B05.0)
     encephalitis, myelitis and encephalomyelitis (in) systemic lupus erythematosus (M32.19)
     enteroviral encephalitis, myelitis and encephalomyelitis (A85.0)
     eosinophilic meningoencephalitis (B83.2)
     herpesviral [herpes simplex] encephalitis, myelitis and encephalomyelitis (B00.4)
     listerial encephalitis, myelitis and encephalomyelitis (A32.12)
     meningococcal encephalitis, myelitis and encephalomyelitis (A39.81)
     mumps encephalitis, myelitis and encephalomyelitis (B26.2)
     postchickenpox encephalitis, myelitis and encephalomyelitis (B01.1-)
     rubella encephalitis, myelitis and encephalomyelitis (B06.01)
     toxoplasmosis encephalitis, myelitis and encephalomyelitis (B58.2)
     zoster encephalitis, myelitis and encephalomyelitis (B02.0)

   G05.3   *Encephalitis and encephalomyelitis in diseases classified elsewhere*
     Meningoencephalitis in diseases classified elsewhere

   G05.4   *Myelitis in diseases classified elsewhere*
     Meningomyelitis in diseases classified elsewhere

✓4ᵗʰ G06 Intracranial and intraspinal abscess and granuloma
   Use additional code (B95-B97) to identify infectious agent
   DEF: Abscess: Circumscribed collection of pus resulting from bacteria, frequently associated with swelling and other signs of inflammation.
   DEF: Granuloma: Abnormal, dense collections or cells forming a mass or nodule of chronically inflamed tissue with granulations that is usually associated with an infective process.

   G06.0   *Intracranial* **abscess and granuloma**
     Brain [any part] abscess (embolic)
     Cerebellar abscess (embolic)
     Cerebral abscess (embolic)
     Intracranial epidural abscess or granuloma
     Intracranial extradural abscess or granuloma
     Intracranial subdural abscess or granuloma
     Otogenic abscess (embolic)
     EXCLUDES 1   *tuberculous intracranial abscess and granuloma (A17.81)*

   G06.1   *Intraspinal* **abscess and granuloma**
     Abscess (embolic) of spinal cord [any part]
     Intraspinal epidural abscess or granuloma
     Intraspinal extradural abscess or granuloma
     Intraspinal subdural abscess or granuloma
     EXCLUDES 1   *tuberculous intraspinal abscess and granuloma (A17.81)*

   G06.2   **Extradural and subdural abscess, unspecified**

G07 Intracranial and intraspinal abscess and granuloma in diseases classified elsewhere
   Code first underlying disease, such as:
     schistosomiasis granuloma of brain (B65.-)
   EXCLUDES 1   *abscess of brain:*
     amebic (A06.6)
     chromomycotic (B43.1)
     gonococcal (A54.82)
     tuberculous (A17.81)
     tuberculoma of meninges (A17.1)

G08 Intracranial and intraspinal phlebitis and thrombophlebitis
   Septic embolism of intracranial or intraspinal venous sinuses and veins
   Septic endophlebitis of intracranial or intraspinal venous sinuses and veins
   Septic phlebitis of intracranial or intraspinal venous sinuses and veins
   Septic thrombophlebitis of intracranial or intraspinal venous sinuses and veins
   Septic thrombosis of intracranial or intraspinal venous sinuses and veins
   EXCLUDES 1   *intracranial phlebitis and thrombophlebitis complicating:*
     abortion, ectopic or molar pregnancy (O00-O07, O08.7)
     pregnancy, childbirth and the puerperium (O22.5, O87.3)
     nonpyogenic intracranial phlebitis and thrombophlebitis (I67.6)
   EXCLUDES 2   *intracranial phlebitis and thrombophlebitis complicating nonpyogenic intraspinal phlebitis and thrombophlebitis (G95.1)*
   DEF: Inflammation and formation of a blood clot in a vein within the brain or spine, or their linings.

G09 Sequelae of inflammatory diseases of central nervous system
   NOTE   Category G09 is to be used to indicate conditions whose primary classification is to G00-G08 as the cause of sequelae, themselves classifiable elsewhere. The "sequelae" include conditions specified as residuals.
   Code first condition resulting from (sequela) of inflammatory diseases of central nervous system

Systemic atrophies primarily affecting the central nervous system (G10-G14)

G10 Huntington's disease
   Huntington's chorea
   Huntington's dementia
   Code also dementia in other diseases classified elsewhere without behavioral disturbance (F02.80)
   DEF: Genetic disease caused by degeneration of nerve cells in the brain, characterized by chronic progressive mental deterioration. Dementia and death occur within 15 to 20 years of onset.

N Newborn: 0   **P** Pediatric: 0-17   **M** Maternity: 12-55   **A** Adult: 15-124   **CH** Comorbidity High   **CL** Comorbidity Low   **NC Dx** Noncancer Dx   **PDx** Primary Dx

562   ICD-10-CM 2020

√4ᵗʰ **G11 Hereditary ataxia**

     EXCLUDES 2   cerebral palsy (G80.-)

                hereditary and idiopathic neuropathy (G60.-)

                metabolic disorders (E70-E88)

     DEF: Ataxia: Defect in muscular control or coordination due to a central nervous system disorder, particularly when voluntary muscular movements are attempted.

     G11.0   Congenital nonprogressive **ataxia**

     G11.1   **Early-onset cerebellar** ataxia

           Early-onset cerebellar ataxia with essential tremor

           Early-onset cerebellar ataxia with myoclonus [Hunt's ataxia]

           Early-onset cerebellar ataxia with retained tendon reflexes

           Friedreich's ataxia (autosomal recessive)

           X-linked recessive spinocerebellar ataxia

     G11.2   Late-onset cerebellar **ataxia**   A

     G11.3   Cerebellar **ataxia** with defective DNA repair

           Ataxia telangiectasia [Louis-Bar]

           EXCLUDES 2   Cockayne's syndrome ▶(Q87.19)◀

                other disorders of purine and pyrimidine metabolism (E79.-)

                xeroderma pigmentosum (Q82.1)

     G11.4   **Hereditary spastic paraplegia**

     G11.8   **Other hereditary ataxias**

     G11.9   **Hereditary ataxia, unspecified**

           Hereditary cerebellar ataxia NOS

           Hereditary cerebellar degeneration

           Hereditary cerebellar disease

           Hereditary cerebellar syndrome

√4ᵗʰ **G12 Spinal muscular atrophy and related syndromes**

     G12.0   **Infantile** spinal muscular atrophy, type I [Werdnig-Hoffman]

     G12.1   **Other inherited spinal muscular atrophy**

           Adult form spinal muscular atrophy

           Childhood form, type II spinal muscular atrophy

           Distal spinal muscular atrophy

           Juvenile form, type III spinal muscular atrophy [Kugelberg-Welander]

           Progressive bulbar palsy of childhood [Fazio-Londe]

           Scapuloperoneal form spinal muscular atrophy

   √5ᵗʰ **G12.2**   **Motor neuron disease**

           AHA: 2017,4Q,9-10

       G12.20   **Motor neuron disease, unspecified**

       G12.21   **Amyotrophic lateral sclerosis**   NC Dx   A

       G12.22   **Progressive bulbar palsy**

       G12.23   **Primary lateral sclerosis**

       G12.24   **Familial motor neuron disease**

       G12.25   **Progressive spinal muscle atrophy**

       G12.29   **Other motor neuron disease**

     G12.8   **Other spinal muscular atrophies and related syndromes**

     G12.9   **Spinal muscular atrophy, unspecified**

√4ᵗʰ **G13 Systemic atrophies primarily affecting central nervous system in diseases classified elsewhere**

     G13.0   *Paraneoplastic neuromyopathy and neuropathy*

           Carcinomatous neuromyopathy

           Sensorial paraneoplastic neuropathy [Denny Brown]

           Code first underlying neoplasm (C00-D49)

     G13.1   *Other systemic atrophy primarily affecting central nervous system in neoplastic disease*

           Paraneoplastic limbic encephalopathy

           Code first underlying neoplasm (C00-D49)

     G13.2   *Systemic atrophy primarily affecting the central nervous system in myxedema*

           Code first underlying disease, such as:

                hypothyroidism (E03.-)

                myxedematous congenital iodine deficiency (E00.1)

     G13.8   *Systemic atrophy primarily affecting central nervous system in other diseases classified elsewhere*

           Code first underlying disease

G14 Postpolio syndrome

     INCLUDES   postpolio myelitic syndrome

     EXCLUDES 1   sequelae of poliomyelitis (B91)

Extrapyramidal and movement disorders (G20-G26)

   G20 Parkinson's disease   CH   CL   NC Dx

           Hemiparkinsonism

           Idiopathic Parkinsonism or Parkinson's disease

           Paralysis agitans

           Parkinsonism or Parkinson's disease NOS

           Primary Parkinsonism or Parkinson's disease

       EXCLUDES 1   dementia with Parkinsonism (G31.83)

       AHA: 2017,2Q,7; 2016,2Q,6

       TIP: Repeated falls (R29.6) are not integral to Parkinson's disease and can be separately coded.

√4ᵗʰ **G21 Secondary parkinsonism**

     EXCLUDES 1   dementia with Parkinsonism (G31.83)

               Huntington's disease (G10)

               Shy-Drager syndrome (G90.3)

               syphilitic Parkinsonism (A52.19)

     G21.0   **Malignant neuroleptic** syndrome

           Use additional code for adverse effect, if applicable, to identify drug (T43.3X5, T43.4X5, T43.505, T43.595)

           EXCLUDES 1   neuroleptic induced parkinsonism (G21.11)

   √5ᵗʰ **G21.1**   **Other drug-induced secondary parkinsonism**

       G21.11   **Neuroleptic** induced parkinsonism   CH   CL

              Use additional code for adverse effect, if applicable, to identify drug (T43.3X5, T43.4X5, T43.505, T43.595)

              EXCLUDES 1   malignant neuroleptic syndrome (G21.0)

       G21.19   **Other drug induced secondary parkinsonism**   CH   CL

              Other medication-induced parkinsonism

              Use additional code for adverse effect, if applicable, to identify drug (T36-T50 with fifth or sixth character 5)

     G21.2   **Secondary parkinsonism due to other external agents**   CH   CL

           Code first (T51-T65) to identify external agent

     G21.3   **Postencephalitic** parkinsonism   CH   CL

     G21.4   **Vascular** parkinsonism   CH   CL

     G21.8   **Other secondary parkinsonism**   CH   CL

     G21.9   **Secondary parkinsonism, unspecified**   CH   CL

√4ᵗʰ **G23 Other degenerative diseases of basal ganglia**

     EXCLUDES 2   multi-system degeneration of the autonomic nervous system (G90.3)

     G23.0   **Hallervorden-Spatz disease**

           Pigmentary pallidal degeneration

     G23.1   **Progressive supranuclear ophthalmoplegia [Steele-Richardson-Olszewski]**

           Progressive supranuclear palsy

     G23.2   **Striatonigral degeneration**

     G23.8   **Other specified degenerative diseases of basal ganglia**

           Calcification of basal ganglia

     G23.9   **Degenerative disease of basal ganglia, unspecified**

√4ᵗʰ **G24 Dystonia**

     INCLUDES   dyskinesia

     EXCLUDES 2   athetoid cerebral palsy (G80.3)

     DEF: Disorder of abnormal muscle tone, excessive or inadequate. Involuntary movements and prolonged muscle contractions result in tremors, abnormalities in posture, and twisting body motions that affect an isolated area or the whole body.

   √5ᵗʰ **G24.0**   **Drug induced dystonia**

           Use additional code for adverse effect, if applicable, to identify drug (T36-T50 with fifth or sixth character 5)

       G24.01   **Drug induced subacute dyskinesia**

              Drug induced blepharospasm

              Drug induced orofacial dyskinesia

              Neuroleptic induced tardive dyskinesia

              Tardive dyskinesia

       G24.02   **Drug induced acute dystonia**

              Acute dystonic reaction to drugs

              Neuroleptic induced acute dystonia

       G24.09   **Other drug induced dystonia**

☑ Additional Character Required   √x7ᵗʰ Placeholder Alert   Manifestation   Unspecified Dx   ▶◀ Revised Text   ● New Code   ▲ Revised Title

ICD-10-CM 2020   563

G24.1 Genetic torsion dystonia
Dystonia deformans progressiva
Dystonia musculorum deformans
Familial torsion dystonia
Idiopathic familial dystonia
Idiopathic (torsion) dystonia NOS
(Schwalbe-) Ziehen-Oppenheim disease

G24.2 Idiopathic nonfamilial dystonia

G24.3 Spasmodic torticollis
> EXCLUDES 1   congenital torticollis (Q68.0)
> hysterical torticollis (F44.4)
> ocular torticollis (R29.891)
> psychogenic torticollis (F45.8)
> torticollis NOS (M43.6)
> traumatic recurrent torticollis (S13.4)

DEF: Twisted, unnatural position of the neck due to contracted cervical muscles that pull the head to one side or cause involuntary shaking of the head.

G24.4 Idiopathic orofacial dystonia
Orofacial dyskinesia
> EXCLUDES 1   drug induced orofacial dyskinesia (G24.01)

G24.5 Blepharospasm
> EXCLUDES 1   drug induced blepharospasm (G24.01)

DEF: Involuntary contraction of the orbicularis oculi muscle, resulting in the eyelids being completely closed.

G24.8 Other dystonia
Acquired torsion dystonia NOS

G24.9 Dystonia, unspecified
Dyskinesia NOS

☑4ᵗʰ G25 Other extrapyramidal and movement disorders
> EXCLUDES 2   sleep related movement disorders (G47.6-)

G25.0 Essential tremor
Familial tremor
> EXCLUDES 1   tremor NOS (R25.1)

G25.1 Drug-induced tremor
Use additional code for adverse effect, if applicable, to identify drug (T36-T50 with fifth or sixth character 5)

G25.2 Other specified forms of tremor
Intention tremor

G25.3 Myoclonus
Drug-induced myoclonus
Palatal myoclonus
Use additional code for adverse effect, if applicable, to identify drug (T36-T50 with fifth or sixth character 5)
> EXCLUDES 1   facial myokymia (G51.4)
> myoclonic epilepsy (G40.-)

DEF: Spasmodic, brief, involuntary muscle contractions that can be due to an undetermined etiology, drug-induced, or caused by a disease process.

G25.4 Drug-induced chorea
Use additional code for adverse effect, if applicable, to identify drug (T36-T50 with fifth or sixth character 5)

G25.5 Other chorea
Chorea NOS
> EXCLUDES 1   chorea NOS with heart involvement (I02.0)
> Huntington's chorea (G10)
> rheumatic chorea (I02.-)
> Sydenham's chorea (I02.-)

☑5ᵗʰ G25.6 Drug induced tics and other tics of organic origin

G25.61 Drug induced tics
Use additional code for adverse effect, if applicable, to identify drug (T36-T50 with fifth or sixth character 5)

G25.69 Other tics of organic origin
> EXCLUDES 1   habit spasm (F95.9)
> tic NOS (F95.9)
> Tourette's syndrome (F95.2)

☑5ᵗʰ G25.7 Other and unspecified drug induced movement disorders
Use additional code for adverse effect, if applicable, to identify drug (T36-T50 with fifth or sixth character 5)

G25.70 Drug induced movement disorder, unspecified
G25.71 Drug induced akathisia
Drug induced acathisia
Neuroleptic induced acute akathisia
Tardive akathisia

G25.79 Other drug induced movement disorders

☑5ᵗʰ G25.8 Other specified extrapyramidal and movement disorders

G25.81 Restless legs syndrome
DEF: Neurological disorder of unknown etiology creating an irresistible urge to move the legs, which may temporarily relieve the symptoms. This syndrome is accompanied by motor restlessness and sensations of pain, burning, prickling, or tingling.

G25.82 Stiff-man syndrome
G25.83 Benign shuddering attacks
G25.89 Other specified extrapyramidal and movement disorders

G25.9 Extrapyramidal and movement disorder, unspecified

G26 Extrapyramidal and movement disorders in diseases classified elsewhere
Code first underlying disease

Other degenerative diseases of the nervous system (G30-G32)

☑4ᵗʰ G30 Alzheimer's disease
> INCLUDES   Alzheimer's dementia senile and presenile forms

Use additional code to identify:
delirium, if applicable (F05)
dementia with behavioral disturbance (F02.81)
dementia without behavioral disturbance (F02.80)
> EXCLUDES 1   senile degeneration of brain NEC (G31.1)
> senile dementia NOS (F03)
> senility NOS (R41.81)

AHA: 2017,1Q,43
TIP: Sundowning (F05) is not integral to Alzheimer's disease and can be coded separately.
TIP: Functional quadriplegia (R53.2) is not integral to Alzheimer's disease and can be coded in addition to codes from category G30.

G30.0 Alzheimer's disease with early onset   NC Dx

G30.1 Alzheimer's disease with late onset   NC Dx A

G30.8 Other Alzheimer's disease   NC Dx

G30.9 Alzheimer's disease, unspecified   NC Dx
AHA: 2016,2Q,6; 2012,4Q,95

☑4ᵗʰ G31 Other degenerative diseases of nervous system, not elsewhere classified
▶For codes G31.0–G31.83, G31.85–G31.9, use additional code to identify:◀
dementia with behavioral disturbance (F02.81)
dementia without behavioral disturbance (F02.80)
> EXCLUDES 2   Reye's syndrome (G93.7)

☑5ᵗʰ G31.0 Frontotemporal dementia

G31.01 Pick's disease   NC Dx
Primary progressive aphasia
Progressive isolated aphasia
DEF: Progressive frontotemporal dementia with asymmetrical atrophy of the frontal and temporal regions of the cerebral cortex and abnormal rounded brain cells called Pick cells with the presence of abnormal staining of protein (called tau). Symptoms include prominent apathy, behavioral changes such as disinhibition and restlessness, echolalia, impairment of language, memory, and intellect, increased carelessness, poor personal hygiene, and decreased attention span.

G31.09 Other frontotemporal dementia   NC Dx
Frontal dementia

G31.1 Senile degeneration of brain, not elsewhere classified   NC Dx
> EXCLUDES 1   Alzheimer's disease (G30.-)
> senility NOS (R41.81)

G31.2 Degeneration of nervous system due to alcohol
Alcoholic cerebellar ataxia
Alcoholic cerebellar degeneration
Alcoholic cerebral degeneration
Alcoholic encephalopathy
Dysfunction of the autonomic nervous system due to alcohol
Code also associated alcoholism (F10.-)

☑5ᵗʰ G31.8 Other specified degenerative diseases of nervous system

G31.81 Alpers disease
Grey-matter degeneration

N Newborn: 0   P Pediatric: 0-17   M Maternity: 12-55   A Adult: 15-124   CH Comorbidity High   CL Comorbidity Low   NC Dx Noncancer Dx   PDx Primary Dx

564   ICD-10-CM 2020

G31.82　Leigh's disease
　　　Subacute necrotizing encephalopathy

G31.83　Dementia with Lewy bodies `NC Dx`

　　　Dementia with Parkinsonism
　　　Lewy body dementia
　　　Lewy body disease
　　　AHA: 2017,2Q,7; 2016,4Q,141
　　　DEF: Cerebral dementia with neurophysiologic changes, increased hippocampal volume, hypoperfusion in the occipital lobes, beta amyloid deposits with neurofibrillary tangles, and atrophy of the cortex and brainstem. Hallmark neuropsychological characteristics include fluctuating cognition with pronounced variation in attention and alertness, recurrent hallucinations, and Parkinsonism.

G31.84　Mild cognitive impairment, so stated
　　　Mild neurocognitive disorder
　　　　EXCLUDES 1　　*age related cognitive decline (R41.81)*
　　　　　　altered mental status (R41.82)
　　　　　　cerebral degeneration (G31.9)
　　　　　　change in mental status (R41.82)
　　　　　　cognitive deficits following (sequelae of) cerebral hemorrhage or infarction (I69.01-, I69.11-, I69.21-, I69.31-, I69.81-, I69.91-)
　　　　　　cognitive impairment due to intracranial or head injury (S06.-)
　　　　　　dementia (F01.-, F02.-, F03)
　　　　　　mild memory disturbance (F06.8)
　　　　　　neurologic neglect syndrome (R41.4)
　　　　　　personality change, nonpsychotic (F68.8)

G31.85　Corticobasal degeneration `NC Dx`

G31.89　Other specified degenerative diseases of nervous system

G31.9　Degenerative disease of nervous system, unspecified

`√4th` **G32　Other degenerative disorders of nervous system in diseases classified elsewhere**

　　G32.0　*Subacute combined degeneration of spinal cord in diseases classified elsewhere*
　　　　Dana-Putnam syndrome
　　　　Sclerosis of spinal cord (combined) (dorsolateral) (posterolateral)
　　　　Code first underlying disease, such as:
　　　　　anemia (D51.9)
　　　　　dietary (D51.3)
　　　　　pernicious (D51.0)
　　　　　vitamin B12 deficiency (E53.8)
　　　　　EXCLUDES 1　*syphilitic combined degeneration of spinal cord (A52.11)*

　`√5th` **G32.8　Other specified degenerative disorders of nervous system in diseases classified elsewhere**
　　　　Code first underlying disease, such as:
　　　　　amyloidosis cerebral degeneration (E85.-)
　　　　　cerebral degeneration (due to) hypothyroidism (E00.0-E03.9)
　　　　　cerebral degeneration (due to) neoplasm (C00-D49)
　　　　　cerebral degeneration (due to) vitamin B deficiency, except thiamine (E52-E53.-)
　　　　　EXCLUDES 1　*superior hemorrhagic polioencephalitis [Wernicke's encephalopathy] (E51.2)*

　　G32.81　*Cerebellar ataxia in diseases classified elsewhere*
　　　　Code first underlying disease, such as:
　　　　　celiac disease (with gluten ataxia) (K90.0)
　　　　　cerebellar ataxia (in) neoplastic disease (paraneoplastic cerebellar degeneration) (C00-D49)
　　　　　non-celiac gluten ataxia (M35.9)
　　　　　EXCLUDES 1　*systemic atrophy primarily affecting the central nervous system in alcoholic cerebellar ataxia (G31.2)*
　　　　　　systemic atrophy primarily affecting the central nervous system in myxedema (G13.2)

　　G32.89　*Other specified degenerative disorders of nervous system in diseases classified elsewhere*
　　　　Degenerative encephalopathy in diseases classified elsewhere

Demyelinating diseases of the central nervous system (G35-G37)

G35　Multiple sclerosis `CH` `CL` `NC Dx`
　　　Disseminated multiple sclerosis
　　　Generalized multiple sclerosis
　　　Multiple sclerosis NOS
　　　Multiple sclerosis of brain stem
　　　Multiple sclerosis of cord

`√4th` **G36　Other acute disseminated demyelination**
　　　　EXCLUDES 1　*postinfectious encephalitis and encephalomyelitis NOS (G04.01)*
　　　DEF: Demyelination: Abnormal loss of myelin, the protective white matter that insulates nerve endings and facilitates neuroreception and neurotransmission. When this substance is damaged, the nerve is short-circuited, resulting in impaired or loss of function.

　　G36.0　Neuromyelitis optica [Devic]
　　　　Demyelination in optic neuritis
　　　　EXCLUDES 1　*optic neuritis NOS (H46)*

　　G36.1　Acute and subacute hemorrhagic leukoencephalitis [Hurst]
　　G36.8　Other specified acute disseminated demyelination
　　G36.9　Acute disseminated demyelination, unspecified

`√4th` **G37　Other demyelinating diseases of central nervous system**

　　G37.0　Diffuse sclerosis of central nervous system
　　　　Periaxial encephalitis
　　　　Schilder's disease
　　　　EXCLUDES 1　*X linked adrenoleukodystrophy (E71.52-)*

　　G37.1　Central demyelination of corpus callosum
　　G37.2　Central pontine myelinolysis
　　G37.3　Acute transverse myelitis in demyelinating disease of central nervous system
　　　　Acute transverse myelitis NOS
　　　　Acute transverse myelopathy
　　　　EXCLUDES 1　*multiple sclerosis (G35)*
　　　　　　neuromyelitis optica [Devic] (G36.0)

　　G37.4　Subacute necrotizing myelitis of central nervous system
　　G37.5　Concentric sclerosis [Balo] of central nervous system
　　G37.8　Other specified demyelinating diseases of central nervous system
　　G37.9　Demyelinating disease of central nervous system, unspecified

Episodic and paroxysmal disorders (G40-G47)

`√4th` **G40　Epilepsy and recurrent seizures**

　　　`NOTE`　The following terms are to be considered equivalent to intractable: pharmacoresistant (pharmacologically resistant), treatment resistant, refractory (medically) and poorly controlled

　　　EXCLUDES 1　*conversion disorder with seizures (F44.5)*
　　　　convulsions NOS (R56.9)
　　　　post traumatic seizures (R56.1)
　　　　seizure (convulsive) NOS (R56.9)
　　　　seizure of newborn (P90)
　　　EXCLUDES 2　*hippocampal sclerosis (G93.81)*
　　　　mesial temporal sclerosis (G93.81)
　　　　temporal sclerosis (G93.81)
　　　　Todd's paralysis (G83.84)

　`√5th` **G40.0　Localization-related (focal) (partial) idiopathic epilepsy and epileptic syndromes with seizures of localized onset**
　　　　Benign childhood epilepsy with centrotemporal EEG spikes
　　　　Childhood epilepsy with occipital EEG paroxysms
　　　　EXCLUDES 1　*adult onset localization-related epilepsy (G40.1-, G40.2-)*

　　`√6th` **G40.00　Localization-related (focal) (partial) idiopathic epilepsy and epileptic syndromes with seizures of localized onset, not intractable**
　　　　Localization-related (focal) (partial) idiopathic epilepsy and epileptic syndromes with seizures of localized onset without intractability

　　　　G40.001　Localization-related (focal) (partial) idiopathic epilepsy and epileptic syndromes with seizures of localized onset, not intractable, with status epilepticus

Chapter 6. Diseases of the Nervous System

G31.82–G40.001

Chapter 6. Diseases of the Nervous System

G40.009–G40.401

G40.009 Localization-related (focal) (partial) idiopathic epilepsy and epileptic syndromes with seizures of localized onset, not intractable, without status epilepticus

Localization-related (focal) (partial) idiopathic epilepsy and epileptic syndromes with seizures of localized onset NOS

√6th **G40.01** Localization-related (focal) (partial) idiopathic epilepsy and epileptic syndromes with seizures of localized onset, intractable

G40.011 Localization-related (focal) (partial) idiopathic epilepsy and epileptic syndromes with seizures of localized onset, intractable, with status epilepticus

G40.019 Localization-related (focal) (partial) idiopathic epilepsy and epileptic syndromes with seizures of localized onset, intractable, without status epilepticus

√5th **G40.1** Localization-related (focal) (partial) symptomatic epilepsy and epileptic syndromes with simple partial seizures

Attacks without alteration of consciousness
Epilepsia partialis continua [Kozhevnikof]
Simple partial seizures developing into secondarily generalized seizures

√6th **G40.10** Localization-related (focal) (partial) symptomatic epilepsy and epileptic syndromes with simple partial seizures, not intractable

Localization-related (focal) (partial) symptomatic epilepsy and epileptic syndromes with simple partial seizures without intractability

G40.101 Localization-related (focal) (partial) symptomatic epilepsy and epileptic syndromes with simple partial seizures, not intractable, with status epilepticus

G40.109 Localization-related (focal) (partial) symptomatic epilepsy and epileptic syndromes with simple partial seizures, not intractable, without status epilepticus

Localization-related (focal) (partial) symptomatic epilepsy and epileptic syndromes with simple partial seizures NOS

√6th **G40.11** Localization-related (focal) (partial) symptomatic epilepsy and epileptic syndromes with simple partial seizures, intractable

G40.111 Localization-related (focal) (partial) symptomatic epilepsy and epileptic syndromes with simple partial seizures, intractable, with status epilepticus

G40.119 Localization-related (focal) (partial) symptomatic epilepsy and epileptic syndromes with simple partial seizures, intractable, without status epilepticus

√5th **G40.2** Localization-related (focal) (partial) symptomatic epilepsy and epileptic syndromes with complex partial seizures

Attacks with alteration of consciousness, often with automatisms
Complex partial seizures developing into secondarily generalized seizures

√6th **G40.20** Localization-related (focal) (partial) symptomatic epilepsy and epileptic syndromes with complex partial seizures, not intractable

Localization-related (focal) (partial) symptomatic epilepsy and epileptic syndromes with complex partial seizures without intractability

G40.201 Localization-related (focal) (partial) symptomatic epilepsy and epileptic syndromes with complex partial seizures, not intractable, with status epilepticus

G40.209 Localization-related (focal) (partial) symptomatic epilepsy and epileptic syndromes with complex partial seizures, not intractable, without status epilepticus

Localization-related (focal) (partial) symptomatic epilepsy and epileptic syndromes with complex partial seizures NOS

√6th **G40.21** Localization-related (focal) (partial) symptomatic epilepsy and epileptic syndromes with complex partial seizures, intractable

G40.211 Localization-related (focal) (partial) symptomatic epilepsy and epileptic syndromes with complex partial seizures, intractable, with status epilepticus

G40.219 Localization-related (focal) (partial) symptomatic epilepsy and epileptic syndromes with complex partial seizures, intractable, without status epilepticus

√5th **G40.3** Generalized idiopathic epilepsy and epileptic syndromes

Code also MERRF syndrome, if applicable (E88.42)

√6th **G40.30** Generalized idiopathic epilepsy and epileptic syndromes, not intractable

Generalized idiopathic epilepsy and epileptic syndromes without intractability

G40.301 Generalized idiopathic epilepsy and epileptic syndromes, not intractable, with status epilepticus

G40.309 Generalized idiopathic epilepsy and epileptic syndromes, not intractable, without status epilepticus

Generalized idiopathic epilepsy and epileptic syndromes NOS

√6th **G40.31** Generalized idiopathic epilepsy and epileptic syndromes, intractable

G40.311 Generalized idiopathic epilepsy and epileptic syndromes, intractable, with status epilepticus

G40.319 Generalized idiopathic epilepsy and epileptic syndromes, intractable, without status epilepticus

√5th **G40.A** Absence epileptic syndrome

Childhood absence epilepsy [pyknolepsy]
Juvenile absence epilepsy
Absence epileptic syndrome, NOS

√6th **G40.A0** Absence epileptic syndrome, not intractable

G40.A01 Absence epileptic syndrome, not intractable, with status epilepticus

G40.A09 Absence epileptic syndrome, not intractable, without status epilepticus

√6th **G40.A1** Absence epileptic syndrome, intractable

G40.A11 Absence epileptic syndrome, intractable, with status epilepticus

G40.A19 Absence epileptic syndrome, intractable, without status epilepticus

√5th **G40.B** Juvenile myoclonic epilepsy [impulsive petit mal]

√6th **G40.B0** Juvenile myoclonic epilepsy, not intractable

G40.B01 Juvenile myoclonic epilepsy, not intractable, with status epilepticus

G40.B09 Juvenile myoclonic epilepsy, not intractable, without status epilepticus

√6th **G40.B1** Juvenile myoclonic epilepsy, intractable

G40.B11 Juvenile myoclonic epilepsy, intractable, with status epilepticus

G40.B19 Juvenile myoclonic epilepsy, intractable, without status epilepticus

√5th **G40.4** Other generalized epilepsy and epileptic syndromes

Epilepsy with grand mal seizures on awakening
Epilepsy with myoclonic absences
Epilepsy with myoclonic-astatic seizures
Grand mal seizure NOS
Nonspecific atonic epileptic seizures
Nonspecific clonic epileptic seizures
Nonspecific myoclonic epileptic seizures
Nonspecific tonic epileptic seizures
Nonspecific tonic-clonic epileptic seizures
Symptomatic early myoclonic encephalopathy

√6th **G40.40** Other generalized epilepsy and epileptic syndromes, not intractable

Other generalized epilepsy and epileptic syndromes without intractability
Other generalized epilepsy and epileptic syndromes NOS

G40.401 Other generalized epilepsy and epileptic syndromes, not intractable, with status epilepticus

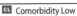
N Newborn: 0   **P** Pediatric: 0-17   **M** Maternity: 12-55   **A** Adult: 15-124   **CH** Comorbidity High   **CL** Comorbidity Low   **NCDx** Noncancer Dx   **PDx** Primary Dx

566   ICD-10-CM 2020

G40.409 Other generalized epilepsy and epileptic syndromes, not intractable, **without status epilepticus**

✓6ᵗʰ **G40.41** Other generalized epilepsy and epileptic syndromes, **intractable**

G40.411 Other generalized epilepsy and epileptic syndromes, intractable, **with status epilepticus**

G40.419 Other generalized epilepsy and epileptic syndromes, intractable, **without status epilepticus**

✓5ᵗʰ **G40.5** Epileptic seizures related to **external causes**

Epileptic seizures related to alcohol
Epileptic seizures related to drugs
Epileptic seizures related to hormonal changes
Epileptic seizures related to sleep deprivation
Epileptic seizures related to stress
Code also, if applicable, associated epilepsy and recurrent seizures (G40.-)
Use additional code for adverse effect, if applicable, to identify drug (T36-T50 with fifth or sixth character 5)

✓6ᵗʰ **G40.50** Epileptic seizures related to external causes, **not intractable**

G40.501 Epileptic seizures related to external causes, not intractable, **with status epilepticus**

G40.509 Epileptic seizures related to external causes, not intractable, **without status epilepticus**

Epileptic seizures related to external causes, NOS

✓5ᵗʰ **G40.8** Other epilepsy and recurrent seizures

Epilepsies and epileptic syndromes undetermined as to whether they are focal or generalized
Landau-Kleffner syndrome

✓6ᵗʰ **G40.80** Other epilepsy

G40.801 Other epilepsy, not intractable, **with status epilepticus**

Other epilepsy without intractability with status epilepticus

G40.802 Other epilepsy, not intractable, **without status epilepticus**

Other epilepsy NOS
Other epilepsy without intractability without status epilepticus

G40.803 Other epilepsy, intractable, **with status epilepticus**

G40.804 Other epilepsy, intractable, **without status epilepticus**

✓6ᵗʰ **G40.81** Lennox-Gastaut syndrome

DEF: Severe form of epilepsy with usual onset in early childhood. Seizures are frequent and difficult to treat, causing falls and intellectual impairment.

G40.811 Lennox-Gastaut syndrome, **not intractable, with status epilepticus**

G40.812 Lennox-Gastaut syndrome, **not intractable, without status epilepticus**

G40.813 Lennox-Gastaut syndrome, **intractable, with status epilepticus**

G40.814 Lennox-Gastaut syndrome, **intractable, without status epilepticus**

✓6ᵗʰ **G40.82** Epileptic spasms

Infantile spasms
Salaam attacks
West's syndrome

G40.821 Epileptic spasms, **not intractable, with status epilepticus**

G40.822 Epileptic spasms, **not intractable, without status epilepticus**

G40.823 Epileptic spasms, **intractable, with status epilepticus**

G40.824 Epileptic spasms, **intractable, without status epilepticus**

G40.89 Other seizures

EXCLUDES 1   post traumatic seizures (R56.1)
     recurrent seizures NOS (G40.909)
     seizure NOS (R56.9)

✓5ᵗʰ **G40.9** Epilepsy, unspecified

AHA: 2019, 1Q, 19

✓6ᵗʰ **G40.90** Epilepsy, unspecified, **not intractable**

Epilepsy, unspecified, without intractability

G40.901 Epilepsy, unspecified, not intractable, **with status epilepticus**

G40.909 Epilepsy, unspecified, not intractable, **without status epilepticus**

Epilepsy NOS
Epileptic convulsions NOS
Epileptic fits NOS
Epileptic seizures NOS
Recurrent seizures NOS
Seizure disorder NOS

✓6ᵗʰ **G40.91** Epilepsy, unspecified, **intractable**

Intractable seizure disorder NOS

G40.911 Epilepsy, unspecified, intractable, **with status epilepticus**

G40.919 Epilepsy, unspecified, intractable, **without status epilepticus**

✓4ᵗʰ **G43** Migraine

NOTE The following terms are to be considered equivalent to intractable: pharmacoresistant (pharmacologically resistant), treatment resistant, refractory (medically) and poorly controlled

Use additional code for adverse effect, if applicable, to identify drug (T36-T50 with fifth or sixth character 5)

EXCLUDES 1   headache NOS (R51)
     lower half migraine (G44.00)
EXCLUDES 2   headache syndromes (G44.-)

DEF: Headaches that occur periodically on one or both sides of the head that may be associated with nausea and vomiting, sensitivity to light and sound, dizziness, distorted vision, and cognitive disturbances.

✓5ᵗʰ **G43.0** Migraine **without aura**

Common migraine
EXCLUDES 1   chronic migraine without aura (G43.7-)

✓6ᵗʰ **G43.00** Migraine without aura, **not intractable**

Migraine without aura without mention of refractory migraine

G43.001 Migraine without aura, not intractable, **with status migrainosus**

G43.009 Migraine without aura, not intractable, **without status migrainosus**

Migraine without aura NOS

✓6ᵗʰ **G43.01** Migraine without aura, **intractable**

Migraine without aura with refractory migraine

G43.011 Migraine without aura, intractable, **with status migrainosus**

G43.019 Migraine without aura, intractable, **without status migrainosus**

✓5ᵗʰ **G43.1** Migraine **with aura**

Basilar migraine
Classical migraine
Migraine equivalents
Migraine preceded or accompanied by transient focal neurological phenomena
Migraine triggered seizures
Migraine with acute-onset aura
Migraine with aura without headache (migraine equivalents)
Migraine with prolonged aura
Migraine with typical aura
Retinal migraine
Code also any associated seizure (G40.-, R56.9)
EXCLUDES 1   persistent migraine aura (G43.5-, G43.6-)

✓6ᵗʰ **G43.10** Migraine with aura, **not intractable**

Migraine with aura without mention of refractory migraine

G43.101 Migraine with aura, not intractable, **with status migrainosus**

G43.109 Migraine with aura, not intractable, **without status migrainosus**

Migraine with aura NOS

✓6ᵗʰ **G43.11** Migraine with aura, **intractable**

Migraine with aura with refractory migraine

G43.111 Migraine with aura, intractable, **with status migrainosus**

☑ Additional Character Required   √x7ᵗʰ Placeholder Alert   Manifestation   Unspecified Dx   ►◄ Revised Text   ● New Code   ▲ Revised Title

ICD-10-CM 2020   567

G43.119 Migraine with aura, intractable, without status migrainosus

✓5ᵗʰ **G43.4 Hemiplegic migraine**

Familial migraine
Sporadic migraine

✓6ᵗʰ **G43.40 Hemiplegic migraine,** not intractable

Hemiplegic migraine without refractory migraine

G43.401 Hemiplegic migraine, not intractable, with status migrainosus

G43.409 Hemiplegic migraine, not intractable, without status migrainosus

Hemiplegic migraine NOS

✓6ᵗʰ **G43.41 Hemiplegic migraine,** intractable

Hemiplegic migraine with refractory migraine

G43.411 Hemiplegic migraine, intractable, with status migrainosus

G43.419 Hemiplegic migraine, intractable, without status migrainosus

✓5ᵗʰ **G43.5 Persistent migraine** aura without cerebral infarction

✓6ᵗʰ **G43.50 Persistent migraine aura without cerebral infarction,** not intractable

Persistent migraine aura without cerebral infarction, without refractory migraine

G43.501 Persistent migraine aura without cerebral infarction, not intractable, with status migrainosus

G43.509 Persistent migraine aura without cerebral infarction, not intractable, without status migrainosus

Persistent migraine aura NOS

✓6ᵗʰ **G43.51 Persistent migraine aura without cerebral infarction,** intractable

Persistent migraine aura without cerebral infarction, with refractory migraine

G43.511 Persistent migraine aura without cerebral infarction, intractable, with status migrainosus

G43.519 Persistent migraine aura without cerebral infarction, intractable, without status migrainosus

✓5ᵗʰ **G43.6 Persistent migraine** aura with cerebral infarction

Code also the type of cerebral infarction (I63.-)

✓6ᵗʰ **G43.60 Persistent migraine aura with cerebral infarction,** not intractable

Persistent migraine aura with cerebral infarction, without refractory migraine

G43.601 Persistent migraine aura with cerebral infarction, not intractable, with status migrainosus

G43.609 Persistent migraine aura with cerebral infarction, not intractable, without status migrainosus

✓6ᵗʰ **G43.61 Persistent migraine aura with cerebral infarction,** intractable

Persistent migraine aura with cerebral infarction, with refractory migraine

G43.611 Persistent migraine aura with cerebral infarction, intractable, with status migrainosus

G43.619 Persistent migraine aura with cerebral infarction, intractable, without status migrainosus

✓5ᵗʰ **G43.7 Chronic migraine** without aura

Transformed migraine

EXCLUDES 1   migraine without aura (G43.0-)

✓6ᵗʰ **G43.70 Chronic migraine without aura,** not intractable

Chronic migraine without aura, without refractory migraine

G43.701 Chronic migraine without aura, not intractable, with status migrainosus

G43.709 Chronic migraine without aura, not intractable, without status migrainosus

Chronic migraine without aura NOS

✓6ᵗʰ **G43.71 Chronic migraine without aura,** intractable

Chronic migraine without aura, with refractory migraine

G43.711 Chronic migraine without aura, intractable, with status migrainosus

G43.719 Chronic migraine without aura, intractable, without status migrainosus

✓5ᵗʰ **G43.A Cyclical vomiting**

EXCLUDES 1   ▶cyclical vomiting syndrome unrelated to migraine (R11.15)◀

▲ **G43.A0 Cyclical vomiting, in migraine,** not intractable

Cyclical vomiting, without refractory migraine

▲ **G43.A1 Cyclical vomiting, in migraine,** intractable

Cyclical vomiting, with refractory migraine

✓5ᵗʰ **G43.B Ophthalmoplegic migraine**

G43.B0 Ophthalmoplegic migraine, not intractable

Ophthalmoplegic migraine, without refractory migraine

G43.B1 Ophthalmoplegic migraine, intractable

Ophthalmoplegic migraine, with refractory migraine

✓5ᵗʰ **G43.C Periodic headache syndromes in child or adult**

G43.C0 Periodic headache syndromes in child or adult, not intractable

Periodic headache syndromes in child or adult, without refractory migraine

G43.C1 Periodic headache syndromes in child or adult, intractable

Periodic headache syndromes in child or adult, with refractory migraine

✓5ᵗʰ **G43.D Abdominal migraine**

G43.D0 Abdominal migraine, not intractable

Abdominal migraine, without refractory migraine

G43.D1 Abdominal migraine, intractable

Abdominal migraine, with refractory migraine

✓5ᵗʰ **G43.8 Other migraine**

✓6ᵗʰ **G43.80 Other migraine,** not intractable

Other migraine, without refractory migraine

G43.801 Other migraine, not intractable, with status migrainosus

G43.809 Other migraine, not intractable, without status migrainosus

✓6ᵗʰ **G43.81 Other migraine,** intractable

Other migraine, with refractory migraine

G43.811 Other migraine, intractable, with status migrainosus

G43.819 Other migraine, intractable, without status migrainosus

✓6ᵗʰ **G43.82 Menstrual migraine,** not intractable

Menstrual headache, not intractable
Menstrual migraine, without refractory migraine
Menstrually related migraine, not intractable
Pre-menstrual headache, not intractable
Pre-menstrual migraine, not intractable
Pure menstrual migraine, not intractable
Code also associated premenstrual tension syndrome (N94.3)

G43.821 Menstrual migraine, not intractable, with status migrainosus   ♀

G43.829 Menstrual migraine, not intractable, without status migrainosus   ♀

Menstrual migraine NOS

✓6ᵗʰ **G43.83 Menstrual migraine,** intractable

Menstrual headache, intractable
Menstrual migraine, with refractory migraine
Menstrually related migraine, intractable
Pre-menstrual headache, intractable
Pre-menstrual migraine, intractable
Pure menstrual migraine, intractable
Code also associated premenstrual tension syndrome (N94.3)

G43.831 Menstrual migraine, intractable, with status migrainosus   ♀

G43.839 Menstrual migraine, intractable, without status migrainosus   ♀

N Newborn: 0   P Pediatric: 0-17   M Maternity: 12-55   A Adult: 15-124   CH Comorbidity High   CL Comorbidity Low   NCDx Noncancer Dx   PDx Primary Dx

568

ICD-10-CM 2020

√5ᵗʰ **G43.9** **Migraine, unspecified**

√6ᵗʰ **G43.90** **Migraine, unspecified,** not intractable

Migraine, unspecified, without refractory migraine

G43.901 **Migraine, unspecified, not intractable, with status migrainosus**
Status migrainosus NOS

G43.909 **Migraine, unspecified, not intractable, without status migrainosus**
Migraine NOS

√6ᵗʰ **G43.91** **Migraine, unspecified,** intractable

Migraine, unspecified, with refractory migraine

G43.911 **Migraine, unspecified, intractable, with status migrainosus**

G43.919 **Migraine, unspecified, intractable, without status migrainosus**

√4ᵗʰ **G44** **Other** headache **syndromes**

EXCLUDES 1   headache NOS (R51)

EXCLUDES 2   atypical facial pain (G50.1)
headache due to lumbar puncture (G97.1)
migraines (G43.-)
trigeminal neuralgia (G50.0)

√5ᵗʰ **G44.0** **Cluster headaches and other trigeminal autonomic cephalgias (TAC)**
DEF: Cluster headache: Characteristic grouping or clustering of headaches that can last for a number of weeks or months and then completely disappear for months or years. They are typically not associated with gastrointestinal upset or light sensitivity as experienced in migraines.

√6ᵗʰ **G44.00** **Cluster headache syndrome, unspecified**

Ciliary neuralgia
Cluster headache NOS
Histamine cephalgia
Lower half migraine
Migrainous neuralgia

G44.001 **Cluster headache syndrome, unspecified, intractable**

G44.009 **Cluster headache syndrome, unspecified, not intractable**
Cluster headache syndrome NOS

√6ᵗʰ **G44.01** **Episodic** cluster headache

G44.011 **Episodic cluster headache,** intractable

G44.019 **Episodic cluster headache,** not intractable
Episodic cluster headache NOS

√6ᵗʰ **G44.02** **Chronic** cluster headache

G44.021 **Chronic cluster headache,** intractable

G44.029 **Chronic cluster headache,** not intractable
Chronic cluster headache NOS

√6ᵗʰ **G44.03** **Episodic** paroxysmal hemicrania

Paroxysmal hemicrania NOS

G44.031 **Episodic paroxysmal hemicrania, intractable**

G44.039 **Episodic paroxysmal hemicrania,** not intractable
Episodic paroxysmal hemicrania NOS

√6ᵗʰ **G44.04** **Chronic** paroxysmal hemicrania

G44.041 **Chronic paroxysmal hemicrania, intractable**

G44.049 **Chronic paroxysmal hemicrania,** not intractable
Chronic paroxysmal hemicrania NOS

√6ᵗʰ **G44.05** **Short lasting unilateral** neuralgiform headache **with conjunctival injection and tearing (SUNCT)**

G44.051 **Short lasting unilateral neuralgiform headache with conjunctival injection and tearing (SUNCT),** intractable

G44.059 **Short lasting unilateral neuralgiform headache with conjunctival injection and tearing (SUNCT),** not intractable
Short lasting unilateral neuralgiform headache with conjunctival injection and tearing (SUNCT) NOS

√6ᵗʰ **G44.09** **Other** trigeminal autonomic cephalgias **(TAC)**

G44.091 **Other trigeminal autonomic cephalgias (TAC),** intractable

G44.099 **Other trigeminal autonomic cephalgias (TAC),** not intractable

G44.1 **Vascular** headache, not elsewhere classified

EXCLUDES 2   cluster headache (G44.0)
complicated headache syndromes (G44.5-)
drug-induced headache (G44.4-)
migraine (G43.-)
other specified headache syndromes (G44.8-)
post-traumatic headache (G44.3-)
tension-type headache (G44.2-)

√5ᵗʰ **G44.2** **Tension-type** headache

√6ᵗʰ **G44.20** **Tension-type headache, unspecified**

G44.201 **Tension-type headache, unspecified, intractable**

G44.209 **Tension-type headache, unspecified,** not intractable
Tension headache NOS

√6ᵗʰ **G44.21** **Episodic** tension-type headache

G44.211 **Episodic tension-type headache, intractable**

G44.219 **Episodic tension-type headache,** not intractable
Episodic tension-type headache NOS

√6ᵗʰ **G44.22** **Chronic** tension-type headache

G44.221 **Chronic tension-type headache, intractable**

G44.229 **Chronic tension-type headache,** not intractable
Chronic tension-type headache NOS

√5ᵗʰ **G44.3** **Post-traumatic** headache

√6ᵗʰ **G44.30** **Post-traumatic headache, unspecified**

G44.301 **Post-traumatic headache, unspecified, intractable**

G44.309 **Post-traumatic headache, unspecified, not intractable**
Post-traumatic headache NOS

√6ᵗʰ **G44.31** **Acute** post-traumatic headache

G44.311 **Acute post-traumatic headache, intractable**

G44.319 **Acute post-traumatic headache,** not intractable
Acute post-traumatic headache NOS

√6ᵗʰ **G44.32** **Chronic** post-traumatic headache

G44.321 **Chronic post-traumatic headache, intractable**

G44.329 **Chronic post-traumatic headache,** not intractable
Chronic post-traumatic headache NOS

√5ᵗʰ **G44.4** **Drug-induced** headache, not elsewhere classified

Medication overuse headache
Use additional code for adverse effect, if applicable, to identify drug (T36-T50 with fifth or sixth character 5)

G44.40 **Drug-induced headache, not elsewhere classified,** not intractable

G44.41 **Drug-induced headache, not elsewhere classified, intractable**

√5ᵗʰ **G44.5** **Complicated** headache syndromes

G44.51 **Hemicrania** continua
DEF: Persistent primary headache of unknown causation occurring on one side of the face and head. May last for more than three months, with daily and continuous pain of moderate intensity with severe exacerbations.

G44.52 **New daily persistent headache (NDPH)**

G44.53 **Primary thunderclap** headache

G44.59 **Other complicated headache syndrome**

√5ᵗʰ **G44.8** **Other specified headache syndromes**

G44.81 **Hypnic** headache

G44.82 **Headache associated with** sexual activity
Orgasmic headache
Preorgasmic headache

G44.83 **Primary cough** headache

G44.84 **Primary exertional** headache

G44.85 **Primary stabbing** headache

G44.89 **Other headache syndrome**

Chapter 6. Diseases of the Nervous System

✓4ᵗʰ G45 Transient cerebral ischemic attacks and related syndromes

> *EXCLUDES 1*   neonatal cerebral ischemia (P91.0)
> transient retinal artery occlusion (H34.0-)

AHA: 2018,2Q,9

DEF: Transient cerebral ischemic attack: Intermittent or brief cerebral dysfunction from lack of oxygenation with no persistent neurological deficits associated with occlusive vascular disease. TIA may denote an impending cerebrovascular accident.

G45.0 Vertebro-basilar artery syndrome

G45.1 Carotid artery syndrome (hemispheric)

G45.2 Multiple and bilateral precerebral artery syndromes

G45.3 Amaurosis fugax

G45.4 Transient global amnesia

> *EXCLUDES 1*   amnesia NOS (R41.3)

G45.8 Other transient cerebral ischemic attacks and related syndromes

G45.9 Transient cerebral ischemic attack, unspecified
Spasm of cerebral artery
TIA
Transient cerebral ischemia NOS

✓4ᵗʰ G46 Vascular syndromes of brain in cerebrovascular diseases
Code first underlying cerebrovascular disease (I60-I69)

G46.0 Middle cerebral artery syndrome

G46.1 Anterior cerebral artery syndrome

G46.2 Posterior cerebral artery syndrome

G46.3 Brain stem stroke syndrome
Benedikt syndrome
Claude syndrome
Foville syndrome
Millard-Gubler syndrome
Wallenberg syndrome
Weber syndrome

G46.4 Cerebellar stroke syndrome

G46.5 Pure motor lacunar syndrome

G46.6 Pure sensory lacunar syndrome

G46.7 Other lacunar syndromes

G46.8 Other vascular syndromes of brain in cerebrovascular diseases

✓4ᵗʰ G47 Sleep disorders

> *EXCLUDES 2*   nightmares (F51.5)
> nonorganic sleep disorders (F51.-)
> sleep terrors (F51.4)
> sleepwalking (F51.3)

✓5ᵗʰ G47.0 Insomnia

> *EXCLUDES 2*   alcohol related insomnia (F10.182, F10.282, F10.982)
> drug-related insomnia (F11.182, F11.282, F11.982, F13.182, F13.282, F13.982, F14.182, F14.282, F14.982, F15.182, F15.282, F15.982, F19.182, F19.282, F19.982)
> idiopathic insomnia (F51.01)
> insomnia due to a mental disorder (F51.05)
> insomnia not due to a substance or known physiological condition (F51.0-)
> nonorganic insomnia (F51.0-)
> primary insomnia (F51.01)
> sleep apnea (G47.3-)

G47.00 Insomnia, unspecified
Insomnia NOS

G47.01 Insomnia due to medical condition
Code also associated medical condition

G47.09 Other insomnia

✓5ᵗʰ G47.1 Hypersomnia

> *EXCLUDES 2*   alcohol-related hypersomnia (F10.182, F10.282, F10.982)
> drug-related hypersomnia (F11.182, F11.282, F11.982, F13.182, F13.282, F13.982, F14.182, F14.282, F14.982, F15.182, F15.282, F15.982, F19.182, F19.282, F19.982)
> hypersomnia due to a mental disorder (F51.13)
> hypersomnia not due to a substance or known physiological condition (F51.1-)
> primary hypersomnia (F51.11)
> sleep apnea (G47.3-)

G47.10 Hypersomnia, unspecified
Hypersomnia NOS

G47.11 Idiopathic hypersomnia with long sleep time
Idiopathic hypersomnia NOS

G47.12 Idiopathic hypersomnia without long sleep time

G47.13 Recurrent hypersomnia
Kleine-Levin syndrome
Menstrual related hypersomnia

G47.14 Hypersomnia due to medical condition
Code also associated medical condition

G47.19 Other hypersomnia

✓5ᵗʰ G47.2 Circadian rhythm sleep disorders
Disorders of the sleep wake schedule
Inversion of nyctohemeral rhythm
Inversion of sleep rhythm

DEF: Circadian rhythm: Daily cycle (24-hour period) of physical, mental and behavioral changes. It is largely influenced by environmental ques, such as changes in light or temperature.
Synonyms: sleep/wake cycle.

G47.20 Circadian rhythm sleep disorder, unspecified type
Sleep wake schedule disorder NOS

G47.21 Circadian rhythm sleep disorder, delayed sleep phase type
Delayed sleep phase syndrome

G47.22 Circadian rhythm sleep disorder, advanced sleep phase type

G47.23 Circadian rhythm sleep disorder, irregular sleep wake type
Irregular sleep-wake pattern

G47.24 Circadian rhythm sleep disorder, free running type
Circadian rhythm sleep disorder, non-24-hour sleep-wake type

G47.25 Circadian rhythm sleep disorder, jet lag type

G47.26 Circadian rhythm sleep disorder, shift work type

G47.27 Circadian rhythm sleep disorder in conditions classified elsewhere
Code first underlying condition

G47.29 Other circadian rhythm sleep disorder

✓5ᵗʰ G47.3 Sleep apnea
Code also any associated underlying condition

> *EXCLUDES 1*   apnea NOS (R06.81)
> Cheyne-Stokes breathing (R06.3)
> pickwickian syndrome (E66.2)
> sleep apnea of newborn (P28.3)

G47.30 Sleep apnea, unspecified
Sleep apnea NOS

G47.31 Primary central sleep apnea
Idiopathic central sleep apnea

G47.32 High altitude periodic breathing

G47.33 Obstructive sleep apnea (adult) (pediatric)
Obstructive sleep apnea hypopnea

> *EXCLUDES 1*   obstructive sleep apnea of newborn (P28.3)

G47.34 Idiopathic sleep related nonobstructive alveolar hypoventilation
Sleep related hypoxia

G47.35 Congenital central alveolar hypoventilation syndrome

G47.36 Sleep related hypoventilation in conditions classified elsewhere
Sleep related hypoxemia in conditions classified elsewhere
Code first underlying condition

G47.37 Central sleep apnea in conditions classified elsewhere
Code first underlying condition

G47.39 Other sleep apnea

Ⓝ Newborn: 0   Ⓟ Pediatric: 0-17   Ⓜ Maternity: 12-55   Ⓐ Adult: 15-124   CH Comorbidity High   CL Comorbidity Low   NCDx Noncancer Dx   PDx Primary Dx

570   ICD-10-CM 2020

√5ᵗʰ **G47.4 Narcolepsy and cataplexy**

√6ᵗʰ   **G47.41 Narcolepsy**

     G47.411 Narcolepsy with cataplexy

     G47.419 Narcolepsy without cataplexy
               Narcolepsy NOS

√6ᵗʰ   **G47.42 Narcolepsy in conditions classified elsewhere**
         Code first underlying condition

     G47.421 Narcolepsy in conditions classified elsewhere with cataplexy

     G47.429 Narcolepsy in conditions classified elsewhere without cataplexy

√5ᵗʰ **G47.5 Parasomnia**

   EXCLUDES 1   *alcohol induced parasomnia (F10.182, F10.282, F10.982)*

            drug induced parasomnia (F11.182, F11.282, F11.982, F13.182, F13.282, F13.982, F14.182, F14.282, F14.982, F15.182, F15.282, F15.982, F19.182, F19.282, F19.982)

            parasomnia not due to a substance or known physiological condition (F51.8)

   G47.50 Parasomnia, unspecified
       Parasomnia NOS

   G47.51 Confusional arousals

   G47.52 REM sleep behavior disorder

   G47.53 Recurrent isolated sleep paralysis

   G47.54 Parasomnia in conditions classified elsewhere
       Code first underlying condition

   G47.59 Other parasomnia

√5ᵗʰ **G47.6 Sleep related movement disorders**

   EXCLUDES 2   *restless legs syndrome (G25.81)*

   G47.61 Periodic limb movement disorder

   G47.62 Sleep related leg cramps

   G47.63 Sleep related bruxism
     EXCLUDES 1   *psychogenic bruxism (F45.8)*

   G47.69 Other sleep related movement disorders

G47.8 Other sleep disorders
   Other specified sleep-wake disorder

G47.9 Sleep disorder, unspecified
   Sleep disorder NOS
   Unspecified sleep-wake disorder

Nerve, nerve root and plexus disorders (G50-G59)

   EXCLUDES 1   *current traumatic nerve, nerve root and plexus disorders — see Injury, nerve by body region*
            neuralgia NOS (M79.2)
            neuritis NOS (M79.2)
            peripheral neuritis in pregnancy (O26.82-)
            radiculitis NOS (M54.1-)

√4ᵗʰ **G50 Disorders of trigeminal nerve**
   INCLUDES   disorders of 5th cranial nerve

Trigeminal and Facial Nerve Branches

Supratrochlear nerve

Supraorbital nerve

V2 branch

Infraorbital nerve

V1 branch

Trigeminal nerve (CN V) branches in infratemporal fossa

V3 branch

Mental nerve

Mental foramen

   G50.0 Trigeminal neuralgia
       Syndrome of paroxysmal facial pain
       Tic douloureux

   G50.1 Atypical facial pain

   G50.8 Other disorders of trigeminal nerve

   G50.9 Disorder of trigeminal nerve, unspecified

√4ᵗʰ **G51 Facial nerve disorders**
   INCLUDES   disorders of 7th cranial nerve

   G51.0 Bell's palsy
       Facial palsy

   G51.1 Geniculate ganglionitis
     EXCLUDES 1   *postherpetic geniculate ganglionitis (B02.21)*

   G51.2 Melkersson's syndrome
       Melkersson-Rosenthal syndrome

√5ᵗʰ   **G51.3 Clonic hemifacial spasm**
     AHA: 2018,4Q,10

     G51.31 Clonic hemifacial spasm, right

     G51.32 Clonic hemifacial spasm, left

     G51.33 Clonic hemifacial spasm, bilateral

     G51.39 Clonic hemifacial spasm, unspecified

   G51.4 Facial myokymia

   G51.8 Other disorders of facial nerve

   G51.9 Disorder of facial nerve, unspecified

√4ᵗʰ **G52 Disorders of other cranial nerves**
   EXCLUDES 2   *disorders of acoustic [8th] nerve (H93.3)*
            disorders of optic [2nd] nerve (H46, H47.0)
            paralytic strabismus due to nerve palsy (H49.0-H49.2)

   G52.0 Disorders of olfactory nerve
       Disorders of 1st cranial nerve

   G52.1 Disorders of glossopharyngeal nerve
       Disorder of 9th cranial nerve
       Glossopharyngeal neuralgia

   G52.2 Disorders of vagus nerve
       Disorders of pneumogastric [10th] nerve

   G52.3 Disorders of hypoglossal nerve
       Disorders of 12th cranial nerve

   G52.7 Disorders of multiple cranial nerves
       Polyneuritis cranialis

   G52.8 Disorders of other specified cranial nerves

   G52.9 Cranial nerve disorder, unspecified

Chapter 6. Diseases of the Nervous System

G53 **Cranial nerve disorders in diseases classified elsewhere**
Code first underlying disease, such as:
neoplasm (C00-D49)
> **EXCLUDES 1**   multiple cranial nerve palsy in sarcoidosis (D86.82)
> multiple cranial nerve palsy in syphilis (A52.15)
> postherpetic geniculate ganglionitis (B02.21)
> postherpetic trigeminal neuralgia (B02.22)

✓4th **G54**   Nerve root and plexus **disorders**
> **EXCLUDES 1**   current traumatic nerve root and plexus disorders — see nerve injury by body region
> intervertebral disc disorders (M50-M51)
> neuralgia or neuritis NOS (M79.2)
> neuritis or radiculitis brachial NOS (M54.13)
> neuritis or radiculitis lumbar NOS (M54.16)
> neuritis or radiculitis lumbosacral NOS (M54.17)
> neuritis or radiculitis thoracic NOS (M54.14)
> radiculitis NOS (M54.10)
> radiculopathy NOS (M54.10)
> spondylosis (M47.-)

G54.0   Brachial plexus **disorders**
Thoracic outlet syndrome
DEF: Acquired disorder affecting the spinal nerves that send signals to the shoulder, arm, and hand, causing corresponding motor and sensory dysfunction. This disorder is characterized by regional paresthesia, pain, muscle weakness, and in severe cases paralysis.

G54.1   Lumbosacral plexus **disorders**
G54.2   Cervical root **disorders, not elsewhere classified**
G54.3   Thoracic root **disorders, not elsewhere classified**
G54.4   Lumbosacral root **disorders, not elsewhere classified**
G54.5   Neuralgic amyotrophy
Parsonage-Aldren-Turner syndrome
Shoulder-girdle neuritis
> **EXCLUDES 1**   neuralgic amyotrophy in diabetes mellitus (E08-E13 with .44)

G54.6   Phantom limb **syndrome with pain**
G54.7   Phantom limb **syndrome without pain**
Phantom limb syndrome NOS
G54.8   **Other nerve root and plexus disorders**
G54.9   **Nerve root and plexus disorder, unspecified**

G55 **Nerve root and plexus compressions in diseases classified elsewhere**
Code first underlying disease, such as:
neoplasm (C00-D49)
> **EXCLUDES 1**   nerve root compression (due to) (in) ankylosing spondylitis (M45.-)
> nerve root compression (due to) (in) dorsopathies (M53.-, M54.-)
> nerve root compression (due to) (in) intervertebral disc disorders (M50.1-, M51.1.-)
> nerve root compression (due to) (in) spondylopathies (M46.-, M48.-)
> nerve root compression (due to) (in) spondylosis (M47.0-M47.2-)

✓4th **G56**   Mononeuropathies of upper limb
> **EXCLUDES 1**   current traumatic nerve disorder — see nerve injury by body region
> **AHA:** 2016,4Q,17-18

Nerves of Upper Limb

Radial
Deep branch of radial
Ulnar
Superficial branch of radial
Median

✓5th **G56.0**   Carpal tunnel **syndrome**
DEF: Swelling and inflammation in the tendons or bursa surrounding the median nerve caused by repetitive activity. The resulting compression on the nerve causes pain, numbness, and tingling especially to the palm, index, middle finger, and thumb.
G56.00   Carpal tunnel syndrome, unspecified upper limb
G56.01   Carpal tunnel syndrome, right upper limb
G56.02   Carpal tunnel syndrome, left upper limb
G56.03   Carpal tunnel syndrome, bilateral upper limbs

✓5th **G56.1**   Other lesions of median nerve
G56.10   Other lesions of median nerve, unspecified upper limb
G56.11   Other lesions of median nerve, right upper limb
G56.12   Other lesions of median nerve, left upper limb
G56.13   Other lesions of median nerve, bilateral upper limbs

✓5th **G56.2**   Lesion of ulnar nerve
Tardy ulnar nerve palsy
G56.20   Lesion of ulnar nerve, unspecified upper limb
G56.21   Lesion of ulnar nerve, right upper limb
G56.22   Lesion of ulnar nerve, left upper limb
G56.23   Lesion of ulnar nerve, bilateral upper limbs

✓5th **G56.3**   Lesion of radial nerve
G56.30   Lesion of radial nerve, unspecified upper limb
G56.31   Lesion of radial nerve, right upper limb
G56.32   Lesion of radial nerve, left upper limb
G56.33   Lesion of radial nerve, bilateral upper limbs

✓5th **G56.4**   Causalgia of upper limb
Complex regional pain syndrome II of upper limb
> **EXCLUDES 1**   complex regional pain syndrome I of lower limb (G90.52-)
> complex regional pain syndrome I of upper limb (G90.51-)
> complex regional pain syndrome II of lower limb (G57.7-)
> reflex sympathetic dystrophy of lower limb (G90.52-)
> reflex sympathetic dystrophy of upper limb (G90.51-)

G56.40   Causalgia of unspecified upper limb
G56.41   Causalgia of right upper limb
G56.42   Causalgia of left upper limb
G56.43   Causalgia of bilateral upper limbs

✓5th **G56.8**   Other specified mononeuropathies of upper limb
Interdigital neuroma of upper limb
G56.80   **Other specified mononeuropathies of unspecified upper limb**

N Newborn: 0   P Pediatric: 0-17   M Maternity: 12-55   A Adult: 15-124   CH Comorbidity High   CL Comorbidity Low   NC Dx Noncancer Dx   PDx Primary Dx

572

ICD-10-CM 2020

G56.81   Other specified mononeuropathies of right upper limb

G56.82   Other specified mononeuropathies of left upper limb

G56.83   Other specified mononeuropathies of bilateral upper limbs

✓5ᵗʰ **G56.9 Unspecified mononeuropathy of upper limb**

G56.90   Unspecified mononeuropathy of unspecified upper limb

G56.91   Unspecified mononeuropathy of right upper limb

G56.92   Unspecified mononeuropathy of left upper limb

G56.93   Unspecified mononeuropathy of bilateral upper limbs

✓4ᵗʰ **G57 Mononeuropathies of lower limb**

> EXCLUDES 1   current traumatic nerve disorder — see nerve injury by body region
>
> AHA: 2016,4Q,17-18

Nerves of Lower Limb

Obturator nerve
Sciatic nerve
Femoral nerve
Saphenous nerve
Common fibular (peroneal) nerve
Deep fibular (peroneal) nerve
Tibial nerve
Superficial fibular (peroneal) nerve

Mononeuropathy

✓5ᵗʰ **G57.0 Lesion of sciatic nerve**

> EXCLUDES 1   sciatica NOS (M54.3-)
>
> EXCLUDES 2   sciatica attributed to intervertebral disc disorder (M51.1.-)

G57.00   Lesion of sciatic nerve, unspecified lower limb

G57.01   Lesion of sciatic nerve, right lower limb

G57.02   Lesion of sciatic nerve, left lower limb

G57.03   Lesion of sciatic nerve, bilateral lower limbs

✓5ᵗʰ **G57.1 Meralgia paresthetica**

Lateral cutaneous nerve of thigh syndrome

G57.10   Meralgia paresthetica, unspecified lower limb

G57.11   Meralgia paresthetica, right lower limb

G57.12   Meralgia paresthetica, left lower limb

G57.13   Meralgia paresthetica, bilateral lower limbs

✓5ᵗʰ **G57.2 Lesion of femoral nerve**

G57.20   Lesion of femoral nerve, unspecified lower limb

G57.21   Lesion of femoral nerve, right lower limb

G57.22   Lesion of femoral nerve, left lower limb

G57.23   Lesion of femoral nerve, bilateral lower limbs

✓5ᵗʰ **G57.3 Lesion of lateral popliteal nerve**

Peroneal nerve palsy

G57.30   Lesion of lateral popliteal nerve, unspecified lower limb

G57.31   Lesion of lateral popliteal nerve, right lower limb

G57.32   Lesion of lateral popliteal nerve, left lower limb

G57.33   Lesion of lateral popliteal nerve, bilateral lower limbs

✓5ᵗʰ **G57.4 Lesion of medial popliteal nerve**

G57.40   Lesion of medial popliteal nerve, unspecified lower limb

G57.41   Lesion of medial popliteal nerve, right lower limb

G57.42   Lesion of medial popliteal nerve, left lower limb

G57.43   Lesion of medial popliteal nerve, bilateral lower limbs

✓5ᵗʰ **G57.5 Tarsal tunnel syndrome**

G57.50   Tarsal tunnel syndrome, unspecified lower limb

G57.51   Tarsal tunnel syndrome, right lower limb

G57.52   Tarsal tunnel syndrome, left lower limb

G57.53   Tarsal tunnel syndrome, bilateral lower limbs

✓5ᵗʰ **G57.6 Lesion of plantar nerve**

Morton's metatarsalgia

G57.60   Lesion of plantar nerve, unspecified lower limb

G57.61   Lesion of plantar nerve, right lower limb

G57.62   Lesion of plantar nerve, left lower limb

G57.63   Lesion of plantar nerve, bilateral lower limbs

✓5ᵗʰ **G57.7 Causalgia of lower limb**

Complex regional pain syndrome II of lower limb

> EXCLUDES 1   complex regional pain syndrome I of lower limb (G90.52-)
>
> complex regional pain syndrome I of upper limb (G90.51-)
>
> complex regional pain syndrome II of upper limb (G56.4-)
>
> reflex sympathetic dystrophy of lower limb (G90.52-)
>
> reflex sympathetic dystrophy of upper limb (G90.51-)

G57.70   Causalgia of unspecified lower limb

G57.71   Causalgia of right lower limb

G57.72   Causalgia of left lower limb

G57.73   Causalgia of bilateral lower limbs

✓5ᵗʰ **G57.8 Other specified mononeuropathies of lower limb**

Interdigital neuroma of lower limb

G57.80   Other specified mononeuropathies of unspecified lower limb

G57.81   Other specified mononeuropathies of right lower limb

G57.82   Other specified mononeuropathies of left lower limb

G57.83   Other specified mononeuropathies of bilateral lower limbs

✓5ᵗʰ **G57.9 Unspecified mononeuropathy of lower limb**

G57.90   Unspecified mononeuropathy of unspecified lower limb

G57.91   Unspecified mononeuropathy of right lower limb

G57.92   Unspecified mononeuropathy of left lower limb

G57.93   Unspecified mononeuropathy of bilateral lower limbs

✓4ᵗʰ **G58 Other mononeuropathies**

G58.0   Intercostal neuropathy

G58.7   Mononeuritis multiplex

G58.8   Other specified mononeuropathies

G58.9   Mononeuropathy, unspecified

G59 *Mononeuropathy in diseases classified elsewhere*

Code first underlying disease

> EXCLUDES 1   diabetic mononeuropathy (E08-E13 with .41)
>
> syphilitic nerve paralysis (A52.19)
>
> syphilitic neuritis (A52.15)
>
> tuberculous mononeuropathy (A17.83)

☑ Additional Character Required   ✓ₓ7ᵗʰ Placeholder Alert   Manifestation   Unspecified Dx   ▶◀ Revised Text   ● New Code   ▲ Revised Title

ICD-10-CM 2020

573

G56.81–G59

Polyneuropathies and other disorders of the peripheral nervous system (G60-G65)

EXCLUDES 1   neuralgia NOS (M79.2)
neuritis NOS (M79.2)
peripheral neuritis in pregnancy (O26.82-)
radiculitis NOS (M54.10)

✓4ᵗʰ **G60**   **Hereditary and idiopathic neuropathy**

G60.0   **Hereditary motor and sensory neuropathy**
Charcôt-Marie-Tooth disease
Déjérine-Sottas disease
Hereditary motor and sensory neuropathy, types I-IV
Hypertrophic neuropathy of infancy
Peroneal muscular atrophy (axonal type) (hypertrophic type)
Roussy-Levy syndrome

G60.1   **Refsum's disease**
Infantile Refsum disease
DEF: Genetic disorder of the lipid metabolism characterized by retinitis pigmentosa, degenerative nerve disease, ataxia, and dry, rough, scaly skin.

G60.2   **Neuropathy in association with hereditary ataxia**

G60.3   **Idiopathic progressive neuropathy**

G60.8   **Other hereditary and idiopathic neuropathies**
Dominantly inherited sensory neuropathy
Morvan's disease
Nelaton's syndrome
Recessively inherited sensory neuropathy

G60.9   **Hereditary and idiopathic neuropathy, unspecified**

✓4ᵗʰ **G61**   **Inflammatory polyneuropathy**

G61.0   **Guillain-Barre syndrome**
Acute (post-)infective polyneuritis
Miller Fisher syndrome
AHA: 2014,2Q,4
DEF: Autoimmune disorder due to an immune response to foreign antigens with paraplegia of limbs, flaccid paralysis, ophthalmoplegia, ataxia, and areflexia. In most cases, this disorder is triggered by a mild viral infection, surgery, or following an immunization.

G61.1   **Serum neuropathy**
Use additional code for adverse effect, if applicable, to identify serum (T50.-)

✓5ᵗʰ **G61.8**   **Other inflammatory polyneuropathies**

G61.81   **Chronic inflammatory demyelinating polyneuritis**

G61.82   **Multifocal motor neuropathy**
MMN
AHA: 2016,4Q,18

G61.89   **Other inflammatory polyneuropathies**

G61.9   **Inflammatory polyneuropathy, unspecified**

✓4ᵗʰ **G62**   **Other and unspecified polyneuropathies**

G62.0   **Drug-induced polyneuropathy**   CL
Use additional code for adverse effect, if applicable, to identify drug (T36-T50 with fifth or sixth character 5)

G62.1   **Alcoholic polyneuropathy**   CL

G62.2   **Polyneuropathy due to other toxic agents**   CL
Code first (T51-T65) to identify toxic agent

✓5ᵗʰ **G62.8**   **Other specified polyneuropathies**

G62.81   **Critical illness polyneuropathy**   CL
Acute motor neuropathy

G62.82   **Radiation-induced polyneuropathy**   CL
Use additional external cause code (W88-W90, X39.0-) to identify cause

G62.89   **Other specified polyneuropathies**   CL
AHA: 2016,2Q,11

G62.9   **Polyneuropathy, unspecified**   CL
Neuropathy NOS

G63   **Polyneuropathy in diseases classified elsewhere**
Code first underlying disease, such as:
amyloidosis (E85.-)
endocrine disease, except diabetes (E00-E07, E15-E16, E20-E34)
metabolic diseases (E70-E88)
neoplasm (C00-D49)
nutritional deficiency (E40-E64)
EXCLUDES 1   polyneuropathy (in):
diabetes mellitus (E08-E13 with .42)
diphtheria (A36.83)
infectious mononucleosis (B27.0-B27.9 with 1)
Lyme disease (A69.22)
mumps (B26.84)
postherpetic (B02.23)
rheumatoid arthritis ▶(M05.5-)◀
scleroderma (M34.83)
systemic lupus erythematosus (M32.19)
AHA: 2012,4Q,99

G64   **Other disorders of peripheral nervous system**
Disorder of peripheral nervous system NOS

✓4ᵗʰ **G65**   **Sequelae of inflammatory and toxic polyneuropathies**
Code first condition resulting from (sequela) of inflammatory and toxic polyneuropathies

G65.0   **Sequelae of Guillain-Barré syndrome**

G65.1   **Sequelae of other inflammatory polyneuropathy**

G65.2   **Sequelae of toxic polyneuropathy**

Diseases of myoneural junction and muscle (G70-G73)

✓4ᵗʰ **G70**   **Myasthenia gravis and other myoneural disorders**
EXCLUDES 1   botulism (A05.1, A48.51-A48.52)
transient neonatal myasthenia gravis (P94.0)

✓5ᵗʰ **G70.0**   **Myasthenia gravis**
DEF: Autoimmune neuromuscular disorder caused by antibodies to the acetylcholine receptors at the neuromuscular junction, interfering with proper binding of the neurotransmitter from the neuron to the target muscle, causing muscle weakness, fatigue, and exhaustion, without pain or atrophy.

G70.00   **Myasthenia gravis without (acute) exacerbation**
Myasthenia gravis NOS

G70.01   **Myasthenia gravis with (acute) exacerbation**   NC Dx
Myasthenia gravis in crisis

G70.1   **Toxic myoneural disorders**
Code first (T51-T65) to identify toxic agent

G70.2   **Congenital and developmental myasthenia**

✓5ᵗʰ **G70.8**   **Other specified myoneural disorders**

G70.80   **Lambert-Eaton syndrome, unspecified**
Lambert-Eaton syndrome NOS

G70.81   **Lambert-Eaton syndrome in disease classified elsewhere**
Code first underlying disease
EXCLUDES 1   Lambert-Eaton syndrome in neoplastic disease (G73.1)

G70.89   **Other specified myoneural disorders**

G70.9   **Myoneural disorder, unspecified**

✓4ᵗʰ **G71**   **Primary disorders of muscles**
EXCLUDES 2   arthrogryposis multiplex congenita (Q74.3)
metabolic disorders (E70-E88)
myositis (M60.-)

✓5ᵗʰ **G71.0**   **Muscular dystrophy**
AHA: 2018,4Q,11-12

G71.00   **Muscular dystrophy, unspecified**

G71.01   **Duchenne or Becker muscular dystrophy**
Autosomal recessive, childhood type, muscular dystrophy resembling Duchenne or Becker muscular dystrophy
Benign [Becker] muscular dystrophy
Severe [Duchenne] muscular dystrophy

G71.02   **Facioscapulohumeral muscular dystrophy**
Scapulohumeral muscular dystrophy

G71.09   **Other specified muscular dystrophies**
Benign scapuloperoneal muscular dystrophy with early contractures [Emery-Dreifuss]
Congenital muscular dystrophy NOS
Congenital muscular dystrophy with specific morphological abnormalities of the muscle fiber
Distal muscular dystrophy
Limb-girdle muscular dystrophy
Ocular muscular dystrophy
Oculopharyngeal muscular dystrophy
Scapuloperoneal muscular dystrophy

√5ᵗʰ **G71.1**   **Myotonic disorders**

G71.11   **Myotonic muscular dystrophy**   NC Dx
Dystrophia myotonica [Steinert]
Myotonia atrophica
Myotonic dystrophy
Proximal myotonic myopathy (PROMM)
Steinert disease

G71.12   **Myotonia congenita**
Acetazolamide responsive myotonia congenita
Dominant myotonia congenita [Thomsen disease]
Myotonia levior
Recessive myotonia congenita [Becker disease]

G71.13   **Myotonic chondrodystrophy**
Chondrodystrophic myotonia
Congenital myotonic chondrodystrophy
Schwartz-Jampel disease

G71.14   **Drug induced myotonia**
Use additional code for adverse effect, if applicable, to identify drug (T36-T50 with fifth or sixth character 5)

G71.19   **Other specified myotonic disorders**
Myotonia fluctuans
Myotonia permanens
Neuromyotonia [Isaacs]
Paramyotonia congenita (of von Eulenburg)
Pseudomyotonia
Symptomatic myotonia

G71.2   **Congenital myopathies**
Central core disease
Fiber-type disproportion
Minicore disease
Multicore disease
Myotubular (centronuclear) myopathy
Nemaline myopathy
EXCLUDES 1   *arthrogryposis multiplex congenita (Q74.3)*

G71.3   **Mitochondrial myopathy, not elsewhere classified**
EXCLUDES 1   *Kearns-Sayre syndrome (H49.81)*
Leber's disease (H47.21)
Leigh's encephalopathy (G31.82)
mitochondrial metabolism disorders (E88.4.-)
Reye's syndrome (G93.7)

G71.8   **Other primary disorders of muscles**

G71.9   **Primary disorder of muscle, unspecified**
Hereditary myopathy NOS

√4ᵗʰ **G72**   **Other and unspecified myopathies**
EXCLUDES 1   *arthrogryposis multiplex congenita (Q74.3)*
dermatopolymyositis (M33.-)
ischemic infarction of muscle (M62.2-)
myositis (M60.-)
polymyositis (M33.2.-)

G72.0   **Drug-induced myopathy**
Use additional code for adverse effect, if applicable, to identify drug (T36-T50 with fifth or sixth character 5)

G72.1   **Alcoholic myopathy**
Use additional code to identify alcoholism (F10.-)

G72.2   **Myopathy due to other toxic agents**
Code first (T51-T65) to identify toxic agent

G72.3   **Periodic paralysis**
Familial periodic paralysis
Hyperkalemic periodic paralysis (familial)
Hypokalemic periodic paralysis (familial)
Myotonic periodic paralysis (familial)
Normokalemic paralysis (familial)
Potassium sensitive periodic paralysis
EXCLUDES 1   *paramyotonia congenita (of von Eulenburg) (G71.19)*

√5ᵗʰ **G72.4**   **Inflammatory and immune myopathies, not elsewhere classified**

G72.41   **Inclusion body myositis [IBM]**

G72.49   **Other inflammatory and immune myopathies, not elsewhere classified**
Inflammatory myopathy NOS

√5ᵗʰ **G72.8**   **Other specified myopathies**

G72.81   **Critical illness myopathy**
Acute necrotizing myopathy
Acute quadriplegic myopathy
Intensive care (ICU) myopathy
Myopathy of critical illness

G72.89   **Other specified myopathies**

G72.9   **Myopathy, unspecified**

√4ᵗʰ **G73**   **Disorders of myoneural junction and muscle in diseases classified elsewhere**

G73.1   *Lambert-Eaton syndrome in neoplastic disease*
Code first underlying neoplasm (C00-D49)
EXCLUDES 1   *Lambert-Eaton syndrome not associated with neoplasm (G70.80-G70.81)*

G73.3   *Myasthenic syndromes in other diseases classified elsewhere*
Code first underlying disease, such as:
neoplasm (C00-D49)
thyrotoxicosis (E05.-)

G73.7   *Myopathy in diseases classified elsewhere*
Code first underlying disease, such as:
hyperparathyroidism (E21.0, E21.3)
hypoparathyroidism (E20.-)
glycogen storage disease (E74.0)
lipid storage disorders (E75.-)
EXCLUDES 1   *myopathy in:*
rheumatoid arthritis (M05.32)
sarcoidosis (D86.87)
scleroderma (M34.82)
sicca syndrome [Sjögren] (M35.03)
systemic lupus erythematosus (M32.19)

Cerebral palsy and other paralytic syndromes (G80-G83)

√4ᵗʰ **G80**   **Cerebral palsy**
EXCLUDES 1   *hereditary spastic paraplegia (G11.4)*

G80.0   **Spastic quadriplegic cerebral palsy**
Congenital spastic paralysis (cerebral)

G80.1   **Spastic diplegic cerebral palsy**
Spastic cerebral palsy NOS

G80.2   **Spastic hemiplegic cerebral palsy**

G80.3   **Athetoid cerebral palsy**
Double athetosis (syndrome)
Dyskinetic cerebral palsy
Dystonic cerebral palsy
Vogt disease

G80.4   **Ataxic cerebral palsy**

G80.8   **Other cerebral palsy**
Mixed cerebral palsy syndromes

G80.9   **Cerebral palsy, unspecified**
Cerebral palsy NOS

✔ Additional Character Required   √x7ᵗʰ Placeholder Alert   Manifestation   Unspecified Dx   ►◄ Revised Text   ● New Code   ▲ Revised Title

Chapter 6. Diseases of the Nervous System

G81–G83.9

✓4ᵗʰ **G81   Hemiplegia and hemiparesis**

> **NOTE**   This category is to be used only when hemiplegia (complete)(incomplete) is reported without further specification, or is stated to be old or longstanding but of unspecified cause. The category is also for use in multiple coding to identify these types of hemiplegia resulting from any cause.

> **EXCLUDES 1**   congenital cerebral palsy (G80.-)
> hemiplegia and hemiparesis due to sequela of cerebrovascular disease (I69.05-, I69.15-, I69.25-, I69.35-, I69.85-, I69.95-)

> **AHA:** 2015,1Q,25

✓5ᵗʰ **G81.0   Flaccid hemiplegia**

> **G81.00**   Flaccid hemiplegia affecting unspecified side
> **G81.01**   Flaccid hemiplegia affecting right dominant side   CH CL
> **G81.02**   Flaccid hemiplegia affecting left dominant side   CH CL
> **G81.03**   Flaccid hemiplegia affecting right nondominant side   CH CL
> **G81.04**   Flaccid hemiplegia affecting left nondominant side   CH CL

✓5ᵗʰ **G81.1   Spastic hemiplegia**

> **G81.10**   Spastic hemiplegia affecting unspecified side
> **G81.11**   Spastic hemiplegia affecting right dominant side   CH CL
> **G81.12**   Spastic hemiplegia affecting left dominant side   CH CL
> **G81.13**   Spastic hemiplegia affecting right nondominant side   CH CL
> **G81.14**   Spastic hemiplegia affecting left nondominant side   CH CL

✓5ᵗʰ **G81.9   Hemiplegia, unspecified**

> **AHA:** 2014,1Q,23

> **G81.90**   Hemiplegia, unspecified affecting unspecified side
> **G81.91**   Hemiplegia, unspecified affecting right dominant side   CH CL
> **G81.92**   Hemiplegia, unspecified affecting left dominant side   CH CL
> **G81.93**   Hemiplegia, unspecified affecting right nondominant side   CH CL
> **G81.94**   Hemiplegia, unspecified affecting left nondominant side   CH CL

✓4ᵗʰ **G82   Paraplegia (paraparesis) and quadriplegia (quadriparesis)**

> **NOTE**   This category is to be used only when the listed conditions are reported without further specification, or are stated to be old or longstanding but of unspecified cause. The category is also for use in multiple coding to identify these conditions resulting from any cause

> **EXCLUDES 1**   congenital cerebral palsy (G80.-)
> functional quadriplegia (R53.2)
> hysterical paralysis (F44.4)

✓5ᵗʰ **G82.2   Paraplegia**

> Paralysis of both lower limbs NOS
> Paraparesis (lower) NOS
> Paraplegia (lower) NOS
> **AHA:** 2017,3Q,3

> **G82.20**   Paraplegia, unspecified   CH CL
> **G82.21**   Paraplegia, complete   CH CL
> **G82.22**   Paraplegia, incomplete   CH CL

✓5ᵗʰ **G82.5   Quadriplegia**

> **G82.50**   Quadriplegia, unspecified   CH CL
> **G82.51**   Quadriplegia, C1-C4 complete   CH CL
> **G82.52**   Quadriplegia, C1-C4 incomplete   CH CL
> **G82.53**   Quadriplegia, C5-C7 complete   CH CL
> **G82.54**   Quadriplegia, C5-C7 incomplete   CH CL

✓4ᵗʰ **G83   Other paralytic syndromes**

> **NOTE**   This category is to be used only when the listed conditions are reported without further specification, or are stated to be old or longstanding but of unspecified cause. The category is also for use in multiple coding to identify these conditions resulting from any cause.

> **INCLUDES**   paralysis (complete) (incomplete), except as in G80-G82

G83.0   Diplegia of upper limbs

> Diplegia (upper)
> Paralysis of both upper limbs

✓5ᵗʰ **G83.1   Monoplegia of lower limb**

> Paralysis of lower limb
> **EXCLUDES 1**   monoplegia of lower limbs due to sequela of cerebrovascular disease (I69.04-, I69.14-, I69.24-, I69.34-, I69.84-, I69.94-)

> **G83.10**   Monoplegia of lower limb affecting unspecified side
> **G83.11**   Monoplegia of lower limb affecting right dominant side
> **G83.12**   Monoplegia of lower limb affecting left dominant side
> **G83.13**   Monoplegia of lower limb affecting right nondominant side
> **G83.14**   Monoplegia of lower limb affecting left nondominant side

✓5ᵗʰ **G83.2   Monoplegia of upper limb**

> Paralysis of upper limb
> **EXCLUDES 1**   monoplegia of upper limbs due to sequela of cerebrovascular disease (I69.03-, I69.13-, I69.23-, I69.33-, I69.83-, I69.93-)

> **G83.20**   Monoplegia of upper limb affecting unspecified side
> **G83.21**   Monoplegia of upper limb affecting right dominant side
> **G83.22**   Monoplegia of upper limb affecting left dominant side
> **G83.23**   Monoplegia of upper limb affecting right nondominant side
> **G83.24**   Monoplegia of upper limb affecting left nondominant side

✓5ᵗʰ **G83.3   Monoplegia, unspecified**

> **G83.30**   Monoplegia, unspecified affecting unspecified side
> **G83.31**   Monoplegia, unspecified affecting right dominant side
> **G83.32**   Monoplegia, unspecified affecting left dominant side
> **G83.33**   Monoplegia, unspecified affecting right nondominant side
> **G83.34**   Monoplegia, unspecified affecting left nondominant side

G83.4   Cauda equina syndrome

> Neurogenic bladder due to cauda equina syndrome
> **EXCLUDES 1**   cord bladder NOS (G95.89)
> neurogenic bladder NOS (N31.9)

> **DEF:** Compression of the spinal nerve roots presenting with pain and tingling radiating down the buttocks, back of the thigh and calf, and into the foot in a sciatic manner with aching in the bladder, perineum, and sacrum. Loss of bowel and bladder control may also occur.

G83.5   Locked-in state

✓5ᵗʰ **G83.8   Other specified paralytic syndromes**

> **EXCLUDES 1**   paralytic syndromes due to current spinal cord injury — code to spinal cord injury (S14, S24, S34)

> **G83.81**   Brown-Séquard syndrome
> **G83.82**   Anterior cord syndrome
> **G83.83**   Posterior cord syndrome
> **G83.84**   Todd's paralysis (postepileptic)
> **G83.89**   Other specified paralytic syndromes

G83.9   Paralytic syndrome, unspecified

N Newborn: 0   P Pediatric: 0-17   M Maternity: 12-55   A Adult: 15-124   CH Comorbidity High   CL Comorbidity Low   NCDx Noncancer Dx   PDx Primary Dx

576   ICD-10-CM 2020

Other disorders of the nervous system (G89-G99)

✓4ᵗʰ **G89   Pain, not elsewhere classified**
　　　　Code also related psychological factors associated with pain (F45.42)
　　　EXCLUDES 1　*generalized pain NOS (R52)*
　　　　　　pain disorders exclusively related to psychological factors
　　　　　　　(F45.41)
　　　　　　pain NOS (R52)
　　　EXCLUDES 2　*atypical face pain (G50.1)*
　　　　　　headache syndromes (G44.-)
　　　　　　localized pain, unspecified type — code to pain by site, such
　　　　　　　as:
　　　　　　　abdomen pain (R10.-)
　　　　　　　back pain (M54.9)
　　　　　　　breast pain (N64.4)
　　　　　　　chest pain (R07.1-R07.9)
　　　　　　　ear pain (H92.0-)
　　　　　　　eye pain (H57.1)
　　　　　　　headache (R51)
　　　　　　　joint pain (M25.5-)
　　　　　　　limb pain (M79.6-)
　　　　　　　lumbar region pain (M54.5)
　　　　　　　painful urination (R30.9)
　　　　　　　pelvic and perineal pain (R10.2)
　　　　　　　renal colic (N23)
　　　　　　　shoulder pain (M25.51-)
　　　　　　　spine pain (M54.-)
　　　　　　　throat pain (R07.0)
　　　　　　　tongue pain (K14.6)
　　　　　　　tooth pain (K08.8)
　　　　　　migraines (G43.-)
　　　　　　myalgia (M79.1-)
　　　　　　pain from prosthetic devices, implants, and grafts (T82.84,
　　　　　　　T83.84, T84.84, T85.84-)
　　　　　　phantom limb syndrome with pain (G54.6)
　　　　　　vulvar vestibulitis (N94.810)
　　　　　　vulvodynia (N94.81-)

　　G89.0   Central pain syndrome
　　　　　Déjérine-Roussy syndrome
　　　　　Myelopathic pain syndrome
　　　　　Thalamic pain syndrome (hyperesthetic)

✓5ᵗʰ **G89.1   Acute pain, not elsewhere classified**
　　　　G89.11   Acute pain due to trauma
　　　　G89.12   Acute post-thoracotomy pain
　　　　　　Post-thoracotomy pain NOS
　　　　G89.18   Other acute postprocedural pain
　　　　　　Postoperative pain NOS
　　　　　　Postprocedural pain NOS

✓5ᵗʰ **G89.2   Chronic pain, not elsewhere classified**
　　　　EXCLUDES 1　*causalgia, lower limb (G57.7-)*
　　　　　　causalgia, upper limb (G56.4-)
　　　　　　central pain syndrome (G89.0)
　　　　　　chronic pain syndrome (G89.4)
　　　　　　complex regional pain syndrome II, lower limb
　　　　　　　(G57.7-)
　　　　　　complex regional pain syndrome II, upper limb
　　　　　　　(G56.4-)
　　　　　　neoplasm related chronic pain (G89.3)
　　　　　　reflex sympathetic dystrophy (G90.5-)
　　　　G89.21   Chronic pain due to trauma
　　　　G89.22   Chronic post-thoracotomy pain
　　　　G89.28   Other chronic postprocedural pain
　　　　　　Other chronic postoperative pain
　　　　G89.29   Other chronic pain
　　G89.3   Neoplasm related pain (acute) (chronic)
　　　　　Cancer associated pain
　　　　　Pain due to malignancy (primary) (secondary)
　　　　　Tumor associated pain
　　G89.4   Chronic pain syndrome
　　　　　Chronic pain associated with significant psychosocial
　　　　　　dysfunction

✓4ᵗʰ **G90   Disorders of autonomic nervous system**
　　　EXCLUDES 1　*dysfunction of the autonomic nervous system due to alcohol*
　　　　　　(G31.2)

✓6ᵗʰ **G90.0   Idiopathic peripheral autonomic neuropathy**
　　　　G90.01   Carotid sinus syncope
　　　　　　Carotid sinus syndrome
　　　　　　DEF: Vagal activation caused by pressure on the carotid
　　　　　　sinus baroreceptors. Sympathetic nerve impulses may
　　　　　　cause sinus arrest or AV block.
　　　　G90.09   Other idiopathic peripheral autonomic neuropathy
　　　　　　Idiopathic peripheral autonomic neuropathy NOS

　　G90.1   Familial dysautonomia [Riley-Day]
　　G90.2   Horner's syndrome
　　　　　Bernard(-Horner) syndrome
　　　　　Cervical sympathetic dystrophy or paralysis
　　G90.3   Multi-system degeneration of the autonomic nervous system
　　　　　Neurogenic orthostatic hypotension [Shy-Drager]
　　　　EXCLUDES 1　*orthostatic hypotension NOS (I95.1)*
　　G90.4   Autonomic dysreflexia
　　　　　Use additional code to identify the cause, such as:
　　　　　　fecal impaction (K56.41)
　　　　　　pressure ulcer (pressure area) (L89.-)
　　　　　　urinary tract infection (N39.0)

✓5ᵗʰ **G90.5   Complex regional pain syndrome I (CRPS I)**
　　　　　Reflex sympathetic dystrophy
　　　　EXCLUDES 1　*causalgia of lower limb (G57.7-)*
　　　　　　causalgia of upper limb (G56.4-)
　　　　　　complex regional pain syndrome II of lower limb
　　　　　　　(G57.7-)
　　　　　　complex regional pain syndrome II of upper limb
　　　　　　　(G56.4-)
　　　　G90.50   Complex regional pain syndrome I, unspecified
　　✓6ᵗʰ **G90.51   Complex regional pain syndrome I of upper limb**
　　　　　　G90.511   Complex regional pain syndrome I of
　　　　　　　right upper limb
　　　　　　G90.512   Complex regional pain syndrome I of left
　　　　　　　upper limb
　　　　　　G90.513   Complex regional pain syndrome I of
　　　　　　　upper limb, bilateral
　　　　　　G90.519   Complex regional pain syndrome I of
　　　　　　　unspecified upper limb
　　✓6ᵗʰ **G90.52   Complex regional pain syndrome I of lower limb**
　　　　　　G90.521   Complex regional pain syndrome I of
　　　　　　　right lower limb
　　　　　　G90.522   Complex regional pain syndrome I of left
　　　　　　　lower limb
　　　　　　G90.523   Complex regional pain syndrome I of
　　　　　　　lower limb, bilateral
　　　　　　G90.529   Complex regional pain syndrome I of
　　　　　　　unspecified lower limb
　　　　G90.59   Complex regional pain syndrome I of other
　　　　　　specified site
　　G90.8   Other disorders of autonomic nervous system
　　G90.9   Disorder of the autonomic nervous system, unspecified

✓4ᵗʰ G91 Hutdrocephalus

INCLUDES   acquired hydrocephalus
EXCLUDES 1   *Arnold-Chiari syndrome with hydrocephalus (Q07.-)*
           congenital hydrocephalus (Q03.-)
           spina bifida with hydrocephalus (Q05.-)
DEF: Abnormal buildup of cerebrospinal fluid in the brain causing dilation of the ventricles.

Hydrocephalus (Acquired)

Normal ventricles   Hydrocephalic ventricles

G91.0   **Communicating hydrocephalus**
      Secondary normal pressure hydrocephalus
G91.1   **Obstructive hydrocephalus**
      DEF: Obstruction of the cerebrospinal fluid passage from the brain into the spinal canal characterized by headaches, drowsiness, poor coordination, urinary incontinence, nausea, vomiting, and papilledema.
G91.2   **(Idiopathic) normal pressure hydrocephalus**
      Normal pressure hydrocephalus NOS
G91.3   **Post-traumatic hydrocephalus, unspecified**
G91.4   *Hydrocephalus in diseases classified elsewhere*
      Code first underlying condition, such as:
           congenital syphilis (A50.4-)
           neoplasm (C00-D49)
           plasminogen deficiency (E88.02)
      EXCLUDES 1   *hydrocephalus due to congenital toxoplasmosis (P37.1)*
      AHA: 2014,3Q,3
G91.8   **Other hydrocephalus**
G91.9   **Hydrocephalus, unspecified**

G92 Toxic encephalopathy

Toxic encephalitis
Toxic metabolic encephalopathy
Code first, if applicable, drug induced (T36-T50)
Code first (T51-T65) to identify toxic agent
AHA: 2017,1Q,39-40
DEF: Brain tissue degeneration due to a toxic substance.

✓4ᵗʰ G93 Other disorders of brain

G93.0   **Cerebral cysts**
      Arachnoid cyst
      Porencephalic cyst, acquired
      EXCLUDES 1   *acquired periventricular cysts of newborn (P91.1)*
                congenital cerebral cysts (Q04.6)
G93.1   **Anoxic brain damage, not elsewhere classified**
      EXCLUDES 1   *cerebral anoxia due to anesthesia during labor and delivery (O74.3)*
                cerebral anoxia due to anesthesia during the puerperium (O89.2)
                neonatal anoxia (P84)
      DEF: Brain injury not resulting from birth trauma that is due to lack of oxygen. Brain cells, when deprived of oxygen; begin to expire after 4 minutes.
G93.2   **Benign intracranial hypertension**
      EXCLUDES 1   *hypertensive encephalopathy (I67.4)*

G93.3   **Postviral fatigue syndrome**
      Benign myalgic encephalomyelitis
      EXCLUDES 1   *chronic fatigue syndrome NOS (R53.82)*
✓5ᵗʰ G93.4   **Other and unspecified encephalopathy**
      EXCLUDES 1   *alcoholic encephalopathy (G31.2)*
                encephalopathy in diseases classified elsewhere (G94)
                hypertensive encephalopathy (I67.4)
                toxic (metabolic) encephalopathy (G92)
      G93.40   **Encephalopathy, unspecified**
           AHA: 2017,2Q,8
      G93.41   **Metabolic encephalopathy**
           Septic encephalopathy
           AHA: 2017,2Q,8; 2016,3Q,42; 2015,3Q,21
      G93.49   **Other encephalopathy**
           Encephalopathy NEC
           AHA: 2018,4Q,16; 2018,2Q,22,24; 2017,2Q,9
G93.5   **Compression of brain**
      Arnold-Chiari type 1 compression of brain
      Compression of brain (stem)
      Herniation of brain (stem)
      EXCLUDES 1   *diffuse traumatic compression of brain (S06.2-)*
                focal traumatic compression of brain (S06.3-)
G93.6   **Cerebral edema**
      EXCLUDES 1   *cerebral edema due to birth injury (P11.0)*
                traumatic cerebral edema (S06.1-)
G93.7   **Reye's syndrome**   🄿
      Code first poisoning due to salicylates, if applicable (T39.0-, with sixth character 1-4)
      Use additional code for adverse effect due to salicylates, if applicable (T39.0-, with sixth character 5)
      DEF: Rare childhood illness often developed after a viral upper respiratory infection. Symptoms include vomiting, elevated serum transaminase, brain swelling, disturbances of consciousness, seizures, and changes in liver and other viscera and it can be fatal.
✓5ᵗʰ G93.8   **Other specified disorders of brain**
      G93.81   **Temporal sclerosis**
           Hippocampal sclerosis
           Mesial temporal sclerosis
      G93.82   **Brain death**
      G93.89   **Other specified disorders of brain**
           Postradiation encephalopathy
G93.9   **Disorder of brain, unspecified**

G94 *Other disorders of brain in diseases classified elsewhere*

Code first underlying disease
EXCLUDES 1   *encephalopathy in congenital syphilis (A50.49)*
            encephalopathy in influenza (J09.X9, J10.81, J11.81)
            encephalopathy in syphilis (A52.19)
            hydrocephalus in diseases classified elsewhere (G91.4)
AHA: 2018,2Q,22; 2017,2Q,8-9

✓4ᵗʰ G95 Other and unspecified diseases of spinal cord

EXCLUDES 2   *myelitis (G04.-)*
G95.0   **Syringomyelia and syringobulbia**
✓5ᵗʰ G95.1   **Vascular myelopathies**
      EXCLUDES 2   *intraspinal phlebitis and thrombophlebitis, except non-pyogenic (G08)*
      G95.11   **Acute infarction of spinal cord (embolic) (nonembolic)**
           Anoxia of spinal cord
           Arterial thrombosis of spinal cord
      G95.19   **Other vascular myelopathies**
           Edema of spinal cord
           Hematomyelia
           Nonpyogenic intraspinal phlebitis and thrombophlebitis
           Subacute necrotic myelopathy
✓5ᵗʰ G95.2   **Other and unspecified cord compression**
      G95.20   **Unspecified cord compression**
      G95.29   **Other cord compression**
✓5ᵗʰ G95.8   **Other specified diseases of spinal cord**
      EXCLUDES 1   *neurogenic bladder NOS (N31.9)*
                neurogenic bladder due to cauda equina syndrome (G83.4)
                neuromuscular dysfunction of bladder without spinal cord lesion (N31.-)
      G95.81   **Conus medullaris syndrome**

N Newborn: 0   **P** Pediatric: 0-17   **M** Maternity: 12-55   **A** Adult: 15-124   **CH** Comorbidity High   **CL** Comorbidity Low   **NCDx** Noncancer Dx   **PDx** Primary Dx

578   ICD-10-CM 2020

G95.89 Other specified diseases of spinal cord
Cord bladder NOS
Drug-induced myelopathy
Radiation-induced myelopathy
EXCLUDES 1   *myelopathy NOS (G95.9)*

G95.9 Disease of spinal cord, unspecified
Myelopathy NOS

☑4ᵗʰ **G96 Other disorders of central nervous system**

G96.0 Cerebrospinal fluid leak
EXCLUDES 1   *cerebrospinal fluid leak from spinal puncture (G97.0)*
AHA: 2018,2Q,13
DEF: Cerebrospinal fluid discharging from the nose or the ear caused by a fracture of the frontal bone with tearing of dura mater and arachnoid. It is characterized by watery drainage usually from only one side of the nose or one ear, headache, vision changes, and hearing loss.

☑5ᵗʰ **G96.1 Disorders of meninges, not elsewhere classified**

G96.11 Dural tear
EXCLUDES 1   *accidental puncture or laceration of dura during a procedure (G97.41)*
AHA: 2014,4Q,24

G96.12 Meningeal adhesions (cerebral) (spinal)

G96.19 Other disorders of meninges, not elsewhere classified

G96.8 Other specified disorders of central nervous system

G96.9 Disorder of central nervous system, unspecified

☑4ᵗʰ **G97 Intraoperative and postprocedural complications and disorders of nervous system, not elsewhere classified**
EXCLUDES 2   *intraoperative and postprocedural cerebrovascular infarction (I97.81-, I97.82-)*
AHA: 2016,4Q,9-10

G97.0 Cerebrospinal fluid leak from spinal puncture

Spinal Puncture

Spinal cord
Epidural space
Subarachnoid space
Vertebra
Spinal needle

Lumbar area

G97.1 Other reaction to spinal and lumbar puncture
Headache due to lumbar puncture

G97.2 Intracranial hypotension following ventricular shunting

☑5ᵗʰ **G97.3 Intraoperative hemorrhage and hematoma of a nervous system organ or structure complicating a procedure**
EXCLUDES 1   *intraoperative hemorrhage and hematoma of a nervous system organ or structure due to accidental puncture and laceration during a procedure (G97.4-)*

G97.31 Intraoperative hemorrhage and hematoma of a nervous system organ or structure complicating a nervous system procedure

G97.32 Intraoperative hemorrhage and hematoma of a nervous system organ or structure complicating other procedure

☑5ᵗʰ **G97.4 Accidental puncture and laceration of a nervous system organ or structure during a procedure**

G97.41 Accidental puncture or laceration of dura during a procedure
Incidental (inadvertent) durotomy
AHA: 2014,4Q,24

G97.48 Accidental puncture and laceration of other nervous system organ or structure during a nervous system procedure

G97.49 Accidental puncture and laceration of other nervous system organ or structure during other procedure

☑5ᵗʰ **G97.5 Postprocedural hemorrhage of a nervous system organ or structure following a procedure**

G97.51 Postprocedural hemorrhage of a nervous system organ or structure following a nervous system procedure

G97.52 Postprocedural hemorrhage of a nervous system organ or structure following other procedure

☑5ᵗʰ **G97.6 Postprocedural hematoma and seroma of a nervous system organ or structure following a procedure**

G97.61 Postprocedural hematoma of a nervous system organ or structure following a nervous system procedure

G97.62 Postprocedural hematoma of a nervous system organ or structure following other procedure

G97.63 Postprocedural seroma of a nervous system organ or structure following a nervous system procedure

G97.64 Postprocedural seroma of a nervous system organ or structure following other procedure

☑5ᵗʰ **G97.8 Other intraoperative and postprocedural complications and disorders of nervous system**
Use additional code to further specify disorder

G97.81 Other intraoperative complications of nervous system

G97.82 Other postprocedural complications and disorders of nervous system

☑4ᵗʰ **G98 Other disorders of nervous system not elsewhere classified**
INCLUDES   nervous system disorder NOS

G98.0 Neurogenic arthritis, not elsewhere classified
Nonsyphilitic neurogenic arthropathy NEC
Nonsyphilitic neurogenic spondylopathy NEC
EXCLUDES 1   *spondylopathy (in):*
     syringomyelia and syringobulbia (G95.0)
     tabes dorsalis (A52.11)

G98.8 Other disorders of nervous system
Nervous system disorder NOS

☑4ᵗʰ **G99 Other disorders of nervous system in diseases classified elsewhere**

G99.0 *Autonomic neuropathy in diseases classified elsewhere*
Code first underlying disease, such as:
     amyloidosis (E85.-)
     gout (M1A.-, M10.-)
     hyperthyroidism (E05.-)
EXCLUDES 1   *diabetic autonomic neuropathy (E08-E13 with .43)*

G99.2 *Myelopathy in diseases classified elsewhere*
Code first underlying disease, such as:
     neoplasm (C00-D49)
EXCLUDES 1   *myelopathy in:*
     intervertebral disease (M50.0-, M51.0-)
     spondylosis (M47.0-, M47.1-)
AHA: 2018,3Q,18-19
TIP: Use this code in addition to a spondylolisthesis code (M43.1-) or a spinal stenosis code (M48.0-) when either of these disorders is documented as the cause of the myelopathy.

G99.8 *Other specified disorders of nervous system in diseases classified elsewhere*
Code first underlying disorder, such as:
     amyloidosis (E85.-)
     avitaminosis (E56.9)
EXCLUDES 1   *nervous system involvement in:*
     cysticercosis (B69.0)
     rubella (B06.0-)
     syphilis (A52.1-)

Chapter 7. Diseases of the Eye and Adnexa (H00–H59)

Chapter-specific Guidelines with Coding Examples

The chapter-specific guidelines from the ICD-10-CM Official Guidelines for Coding and Reporting have been provided below. Along with these guidelines are coding examples, contained in the shaded boxes, that have been developed to help illustrate the coding and/or sequencing guidance found in these guidelines.

a. Glaucoma

1) Assigning glaucoma codes

Assign as many codes from category H40, Glaucoma, as needed to identify the type of glaucoma, the affected eye, and the glaucoma stage.

2) Bilateral glaucoma with same type and stage

When a patient has bilateral glaucoma and both eyes are documented as being the same type and stage, and there is a code for bilateral glaucoma, report only the code for the type of glaucoma, bilateral, with the seventh character for the stage.

> Bilateral severe stage pigmentary glaucoma.
>
> **H40.1333　　Pigmentary glaucoma, bilateral, severe stage**
>
> *Explanation*: In this scenario, the patient has the same type and stage of glaucoma in both eyes. As this type of glaucoma has a code for bilateral, assign only the code for the bilateral glaucoma with the seventh character for the stage.

When a patient has bilateral glaucoma and both eyes are documented as being the same type and stage, and the classification does not provide a code for bilateral glaucoma (i.e. subcategories H40.10 and H40.20) report only one code for the type of glaucoma with the appropriate seventh character for the stage.

> Bilateral open-angle glaucoma; not specified as to type and stage indeterminate in both eyes.
>
> **H40.10X4　　Unspecified open-angle glaucoma, indeterminate stage**
>
> *Explanation*: In this scenario, the patient has glaucoma of the same type and stage of both eyes, but there is no code specifically for bilateral glaucoma. Only one code is assigned with the appropriate seventh character for the stage.

3) Bilateral glaucoma stage with different types or stages

When a patient has bilateral glaucoma and each eye is documented as having a different type or stage, and the classification distinguishes laterality, assign the appropriate code for each eye rather than the code for bilateral glaucoma.

> Bilateral chronic angle-closure glaucoma; right eye is documented as mild stage and left eye as moderate stage.
>
> **H40.2211　　Chronic angle-closure glaucoma, right eye, mild stage**
>
> **H40.2222　　Chronic angle-closure glaucoma, left eye, moderate stage**
>
> *Explanation*: In this scenario the patient has the same type of glaucoma in both eyes, but each eye is at a different stage. Because the subcategory for this condition identifies laterality, one code is assigned for the right eye and one code is assigned for the left eye, each with the appropriate seventh character for the stage appended.

When a patient has bilateral glaucoma and each eye is documented as having a different type, and the classification does not distinguish laterality (i.e. subcategories H40.10 and H40.20), assign one code for each type of glaucoma with the appropriate seventh character for the stage.

> Documentation relates mild, unspecified primary angle-closure glaucoma of the left eye with mild unspecified open-angle glaucoma of the right eye.
>
> **H40.20X1　　Unspecified primary angle-closure glaucoma, mild stage**
>
> **H40.10X1　　Unspecified open-angle glaucoma, mild stage**
>
> *Explanation*: In this scenario the patient has a different type of glaucoma in each eye and the classification does not distinguish laterality. A code for each type of glaucoma is assigned, each with the appropriate seventh character for the stage.

When a patient has bilateral glaucoma and each eye is documented as having the same type, but different stage, and the classification does not distinguish laterality (i.e. subcategories H40.10 and H40.20), assign a code for the type of glaucoma for each eye with the seventh character for the specific glaucoma stage documented for each eye.

> Bilateral open-angle glaucoma, not specified as to type; the right eye is documented to be in mild stage and the left eye as being in moderate stage.
>
> **H40.10X2　　Unspecified open-angle glaucoma, moderate stage**
>
> **H40.10X1　　Unspecified open-angle glaucoma, mild stage**
>
> *Explanation*: In this scenario the patient has the same type of glaucoma in each eye but each eye is at a different stage, and the classification does not distinguish laterality at this subcategory level. Two codes are assigned; both codes represent the same type of glaucoma but each has a different seventh character identifying the appropriate stage for each eye.

4) Patient admitted with glaucoma and stage evolves during the admission

If a patient is admitted with glaucoma and the stage progresses during the admission, assign the code for highest stage documented.

5) Indeterminate stage glaucoma

Assignment of the seventh character "4" for "indeterminate stage" should be based on the clinical documentation. The seventh character "4" is used for glaucomas whose stage cannot be clinically determined. This seventh character should not be confused with the seventh character "0", unspecified, which should be assigned when there is no documentation regarding the stage of the glaucoma.

b. Blindness

If "blindness" or "low vision" of both eyes is documented but the visual impairment category is not documented, assign code H54.3, Unqualified visual loss, both eyes. If "blindness" or "low vision" in one eye is documented but the visual impairment category is not documented, assign a code from H54.6-, Unqualified visual loss, one eye. If "blindness" or "visual loss" is documented without any information about whether one or both eyes are affected, assign code H54.7, Unspecified visual loss.

Chapter 7. Diseases of the Eye and Adnexa (H00-H59)

NOTE Use an external cause code following the code for the eye condition, if applicable, to identify the cause of the eye condition

EXCLUDES 2
certain conditions originating in the perinatal period (P04-P96)
certain infectious and parasitic diseases (A00-B99)
complications of pregnancy, childbirth and the puerperium (O00-O9A)
congenital malformations, deformations, and chromosomal abnormalities (Q00-Q99)
diabetes mellitus related eye conditions (E09.3-, E10.3-, E11.3-, E13.3-)
endocrine, nutritional and metabolic diseases (E00-E88)
injury (trauma) of eye and orbit (S05.-)
injury, poisoning and certain other consequences of external causes (S00-T88)
neoplasms (C00-D49)
symptoms, signs and abnormal clinical and laboratory findings, not elsewhere classified (R00-R94)
syphilis related eye disorders (A50.01, A50.3-, A51.43, A52.71)

This chapter contains the following blocks:
H00-H05 Disorders of eyelid, lacrimal system and orbit
H10-H11 Disorders of conjunctiva
H15-H22 Disorders of sclera, cornea, iris and ciliary body
H25-H28 Disorders of lens
H30-H36 Disorders of choroid and retina
H40-H42 Glaucoma
H43-H44 Disorders of vitreous body and globe
H46-H47 Disorders of optic nerve and visual pathways
H49-H52 Disorders of ocular muscles, binocular movement, accommodation and refraction
H53-H54 Visual disturbances and blindness
H55-H57 Other disorders of eye and adnexa
H59 Intraoperative and postprocedural complications and disorders of eye and adnexa, not elsewhere classified

Disorders of eyelid, lacrimal system and orbit (H00-H05)

EXCLUDES 2 open wound of eyelid (S01.1-)
superficial injury of eyelid (S00.1-, S00.2-)

✓4ᵗʰ **H00 Hordeolum and chalazion**

✓5ᵗʰ **H00.0 Hordeolum (externum) (internum) of eyelid**
DEF: Acute localized infection of the gland of Zeis (external hordeolum) or Molt or of the meibomian glands (internal hordeolum) of the orbit.

✓6ᵗʰ **H00.01 Hordeolum externum**
Hordeolum NOS
Stye
H00.011 Hordeolum externum right upper eyelid
H00.012 Hordeolum externum right lower eyelid
H00.013 Hordeolum externum right eye, unspecified eyelid
H00.014 Hordeolum externum left upper eyelid
H00.015 Hordeolum externum left lower eyelid
H00.016 Hordeolum externum left eye, unspecified eyelid
H00.019 Hordeolum externum unspecified eye, unspecified eyelid

✓6ᵗʰ **H00.02 Hordeolum internum**
Infection of meibomian gland
H00.021 Hordeolum internum right upper eyelid
H00.022 Hordeolum internum right lower eyelid
H00.023 Hordeolum internum right eye, unspecified eyelid
H00.024 Hordeolum internum left upper eyelid
H00.025 Hordeolum internum left lower eyelid
H00.026 Hordeolum internum left eye, unspecified eyelid
H00.029 Hordeolum internum unspecified eye, unspecified eyelid

✓6ᵗʰ **H00.03 Abscess of eyelid**
Furuncle of eyelid
H00.031 Abscess of right upper eyelid
H00.032 Abscess of right lower eyelid
H00.033 Abscess of eyelid right eye, unspecified eyelid
H00.034 Abscess of left upper eyelid
H00.035 Abscess of left lower eyelid
H00.036 Abscess of eyelid left eye, unspecified eyelid
H00.039 Abscess of eyelid unspecified eye, unspecified eyelid

✓5ᵗʰ **H00.1 Chalazion**
Meibomian (gland) cyst
EXCLUDES 2 infected meibomian gland (H00.02-)
DEF: Noninfectious, obstructive mass in the oil gland of the eyelid that results in a small chronic lump or inflammation.
H00.11 Chalazion right upper eyelid
H00.12 Chalazion right lower eyelid
H00.13 Chalazion right eye, unspecified eyelid
H00.14 Chalazion left upper eyelid
H00.15 Chalazion left lower eyelid
H00.16 Chalazion left eye, unspecified eyelid
H00.19 Chalazion unspecified eye, unspecified eyelid

✓4ᵗʰ **H01 Other inflammation of eyelid**

✓5ᵗʰ **H01.0 Blepharitis**
EXCLUDES 1 blepharoconjunctivitis (H10.5-)

✓6ᵗʰ **H01.00 Unspecified blepharitis**
AHA: 2018,4Q,13
H01.001 Unspecified blepharitis right upper eyelid
H01.002 Unspecified blepharitis right lower eyelid
H01.003 Unspecified blepharitis right eye, unspecified eyelid
H01.004 Unspecified blepharitis left upper eyelid
H01.005 Unspecified blepharitis left lower eyelid
H01.006 Unspecified blepharitis left eye, unspecified eyelid
H01.009 Unspecified blepharitis unspecified eye, unspecified eyelid
H01.00A Unspecified blepharitis right eye, upper and lower eyelids
H01.00B Unspecified blepharitis left eye, upper and lower eyelids

✓6ᵗʰ **H01.01 Ulcerative blepharitis**
AHA: 2018,4Q,13
H01.011 Ulcerative blepharitis right upper eyelid
H01.012 Ulcerative blepharitis right lower eyelid
H01.013 Ulcerative blepharitis right eye, unspecified eyelid
H01.014 Ulcerative blepharitis left upper eyelid
H01.015 Ulcerative blepharitis left lower eyelid
H01.016 Ulcerative blepharitis left eye, unspecified eyelid
H01.019 Ulcerative blepharitis unspecified eye, unspecified eyelid
H01.01A Ulcerative blepharitis right eye, upper and lower eyelids
H01.01B Ulcerative blepharitis left eye, upper and lower eyelids

✓6ᵗʰ **H01.02 Squamous blepharitis**
AHA: 2018,4Q,13
H01.021 Squamous blepharitis right upper eyelid
H01.022 Squamous blepharitis right lower eyelid
H01.023 Squamous blepharitis right eye, unspecified eyelid
H01.024 Squamous blepharitis left upper eyelid
H01.025 Squamous blepharitis left lower eyelid
H01.026 Squamous blepharitis left eye, unspecified eyelid
H01.029 Squamous blepharitis unspecified eye, unspecified eyelid
H01.02A Squamous blepharitis right eye, upper and lower eyelids
H01.02B Squamous blepharitis left eye, upper and lower eyelids

✓5ᵗʰ **H01.1 Noninfectious dermatoses of eyelid**

✓6ᵗʰ **H01.11 Allergic dermatitis of eyelid**
Contact dermatitis of eyelid
H01.111 Allergic dermatitis of right upper eyelid
H01.112 Allergic dermatitis of right lower eyelid
H01.113 Allergic dermatitis of right eye, unspecified eyelid
H01.114 Allergic dermatitis of left upper eyelid
H01.115 Allergic dermatitis of left lower eyelid
H01.116 Allergic dermatitis of left eye, unspecified eyelid
H01.119 Allergic dermatitis of unspecified eye, unspecified eyelid

√6ᵗʰ **H01.12** Discoid lupus erythematosus of eyelid

     H01.121 Discoid lupus erythematosus of right upper eyelid

     H01.122 Discoid lupus erythematosus of right lower eyelid

     H01.123 Discoid lupus erythematosus of right eye, unspecified eyelid

     H01.124 Discoid lupus erythematosus of left upper eyelid

     H01.125 Discoid lupus erythematosus of left lower eyelid

     H01.126 Discoid lupus erythematosus of left eye, unspecified eyelid

     H01.129 Discoid lupus erythematosus of unspecified eye, unspecified eyelid

√6ᵗʰ **H01.13** Eczematous dermatitis of eyelid

     H01.131 Eczematous dermatitis of right upper eyelid

     H01.132 Eczematous dermatitis of right lower eyelid

     H01.133 Eczematous dermatitis of right eye, unspecified eyelid

     H01.134 Eczematous dermatitis of left upper eyelid

     H01.135 Eczematous dermatitis of left lower eyelid

     H01.136 Eczematous dermatitis of left eye, unspecified eyelid

     H01.139 Eczematous dermatitis of unspecified eye, unspecified eyelid

√6ᵗʰ **H01.14** Xeroderma of eyelid

     H01.141 Xeroderma of right upper eyelid

     H01.142 Xeroderma of right lower eyelid

     H01.143 Xeroderma of right eye, unspecified eyelid

     H01.144 Xeroderma of left upper eyelid

     H01.145 Xeroderma of left lower eyelid

     H01.146 Xeroderma of left eye, unspecified eyelid

     H01.149 Xeroderma of unspecified eye, unspecified eyelid

H01.8 Other specified inflammations of eyelid

H01.9 Unspecified inflammation of eyelid

     Inflammation of eyelid NOS

√4ᵗʰ **H02** Other disorders of eyelid

     EXCLUDES 1   *congenital malformations of eyelid (Q10.0-Q10.3)*

Entropion and Ectropion

Normal eyelid   Entropion   Ectropion

√5ᵗʰ **H02.0** Entropion and trichiasis of eyelid

     DEF: Entropion: Inversion of the eyelid, turning the edge in toward the eyeball and causing irritation from contact of the lashes with the surface of the eye.

     DEF: Trichiasis: Condition wherein the eyelid is in a normal position but lashes are ingrown or misdirected in their growth so that they irritate the tissues of the eye.

√6ᵗʰ **H02.00** Unspecified entropion of eyelid

     H02.001 Unspecified entropion of right upper eyelid

     H02.002 Unspecified entropion of right lower eyelid

     H02.003 Unspecified entropion of right eye, unspecified eyelid

     H02.004 Unspecified entropion of left upper eyelid

     H02.005 Unspecified entropion of left lower eyelid

     H02.006 Unspecified entropion of left eye, unspecified eyelid

     H02.009 Unspecified entropion of unspecified eye, unspecified eyelid

√6ᵗʰ **H02.01** Cicatricial entropion of eyelid

     H02.011 Cicatricial entropion of right upper eyelid

     H02.012 Cicatricial entropion of right lower eyelid

     H02.013 Cicatricial entropion of right eye, unspecified eyelid

     H02.014 Cicatricial entropion of left upper eyelid

     H02.015 Cicatricial entropion of left lower eyelid

     H02.016 Cicatricial entropion of left eye, unspecified eyelid

     H02.019 Cicatricial entropion of unspecified eye, unspecified eyelid

√6ᵗʰ **H02.02** Mechanical entropion of eyelid

     H02.021 Mechanical entropion of right upper eyelid

     H02.022 Mechanical entropion of right lower eyelid

     H02.023 Mechanical entropion of right eye, unspecified eyelid

     H02.024 Mechanical entropion of left upper eyelid

     H02.025 Mechanical entropion of left lower eyelid

     H02.026 Mechanical entropion of left eye, unspecified eyelid

     H02.029 Mechanical entropion of unspecified eye, unspecified eyelid

√6ᵗʰ **H02.03** Senile entropion of eyelid

     H02.031 Senile entropion of right upper eyelid   A

     H02.032 Senile entropion of right lower eyelid   A

     H02.033 Senile entropion of right eye, unspecified eyelid   A

     H02.034 Senile entropion of left upper eyelid   A

     H02.035 Senile entropion of left lower eyelid   A

     H02.036 Senile entropion of left eye, unspecified eyelid   A

     H02.039 Senile entropion of unspecified eye, unspecified eyelid   A

√6ᵗʰ **H02.04** Spastic entropion of eyelid

     H02.041 Spastic entropion of right upper eyelid

     H02.042 Spastic entropion of right lower eyelid

     H02.043 Spastic entropion of right eye, unspecified eyelid

     H02.044 Spastic entropion of left upper eyelid

     H02.045 Spastic entropion of left lower eyelid

     H02.046 Spastic entropion of left eye, unspecified eyelid

     H02.049 Spastic entropion of unspecified eye, unspecified eyelid

√6ᵗʰ **H02.05** Trichiasis without entropion

     H02.051 Trichiasis without entropion right upper eyelid

     H02.052 Trichiasis without entropion right lower eyelid

     H02.053 Trichiasis without entropion right eye, unspecified eyelid

     H02.054 Trichiasis without entropion left upper eyelid

     H02.055 Trichiasis without entropion left lower eyelid

     H02.056 Trichiasis without entropion left eye, unspecified eyelid

     H02.059 Trichiasis without entropion unspecified eye, unspecified eyelid

√5ᵗʰ **H02.1** Ectropion of eyelid

     DEF: Drooping of the lower eyelid away from the eye or outward turning or eversion of the edge of the eyelid, exposing the palpebral conjunctiva and causing irritation.

√6ᵗʰ **H02.10** Unspecified ectropion of eyelid

     H02.101 Unspecified ectropion of right upper eyelid

     H02.102 Unspecified ectropion of right lower eyelid

     H02.103 Unspecified ectropion of right eye, unspecified eyelid

     H02.104 Unspecified ectropion of left upper eyelid

     H02.105 Unspecified ectropion of left lower eyelid

H02.106 Unspecified ectropion of left eye, unspecified eyelid

H02.109 Unspecified ectropion of unspecified eye, unspecified eyelid

√6ᵗʰ **H02.11** Cicatricial ectropion of eyelid

H02.111 Cicatricial ectropion of right upper eyelid

H02.112 Cicatricial ectropion of right lower eyelid

H02.113 Cicatricial ectropion of right eye, unspecified eyelid

H02.114 Cicatricial ectropion of left upper eyelid

H02.115 Cicatricial ectropion of left lower eyelid

H02.116 Cicatricial ectropion of left eye, unspecified eyelid

H02.119 Cicatricial ectropion of unspecified eye, unspecified eyelid

√6ᵗʰ **H02.12** Mechanical ectropion of eyelid

H02.121 Mechanical ectropion of right upper eyelid

H02.122 Mechanical ectropion of right lower eyelid

H02.123 Mechanical ectropion of right eye, unspecified eyelid

H02.124 Mechanical ectropion of left upper eyelid

H02.125 Mechanical ectropion of left lower eyelid

H02.126 Mechanical ectropion of left eye, unspecified eyelid

H02.129 Mechanical ectropion of unspecified eye, unspecified eyelid

√6ᵗʰ **H02.13** Senile ectropion of eyelid

H02.131 Senile ectropion of right upper eyelid   🅐

H02.132 Senile ectropion of right lower eyelid   🅐

H02.133 Senile ectropion of right eye, unspecified eyelid   🅐

H02.134 Senile ectropion of left upper eyelid   🅐

H02.135 Senile ectropion of left lower eyelid   🅐

H02.136 Senile ectropion of left eye, unspecified eyelid   🅐

H02.139 Senile ectropion of unspecified eye, unspecified eyelid   🅐

√6ᵗʰ **H02.14** Spastic ectropion of eyelid

H02.141 Spastic ectropion of right upper eyelid

H02.142 Spastic ectropion of right lower eyelid

H02.143 Spastic ectropion of right eye, unspecified eyelid

H02.144 Spastic ectropion of left upper eyelid

H02.145 Spastic ectropion of left lower eyelid

H02.146 Spastic ectropion of left eye, unspecified eyelid

H02.149 Spastic ectropion of unspecified eye, unspecified eyelid

√6ᵗʰ **H02.15** Paralytic ectropion of eyelid

AHA: 2018,4Q,13

H02.151 Paralytic ectropion of right upper eyelid

H02.152 Paralytic ectropion of right lower eyelid

H02.153 Paralytic ectropion of right eye, unspecified eyelid

H02.154 Paralytic ectropion of left upper eyelid

H02.155 Paralytic ectropion of left lower eyelid

H02.156 Paralytic ectropion of left eye, unspecified eyelid

H02.159 Paralytic ectropion of unspecified eye, unspecified eyelid

√5ᵗʰ **H02.2** Lagophthalmos

AHA: 2018,4Q,14

DEF: Condition of the eye that prevents it from closing completely.

√6ᵗʰ **H02.20** Unspecified lagophthalmos

H02.201 Unspecified lagophthalmos right upper eyelid

H02.202 Unspecified lagophthalmos right lower eyelid

H02.203 Unspecified lagophthalmos right eye, unspecified eyelid

H02.204 Unspecified lagophthalmos left upper eyelid

H02.205 Unspecified lagophthalmos left lower eyelid

H02.206 Unspecified lagophthalmos left eye, unspecified eyelid

H02.209 Unspecified lagophthalmos unspecified eye, unspecified eyelid

H02.20A Unspecified lagophthalmos right eye, upper and lower eyelids

H02.20B Unspecified lagophthalmos left eye, upper and lower eyelids

H02.20C Unspecified lagophthalmos, bilateral, upper and lower eyelids

√6ᵗʰ **H02.21** Cicatricial lagophthalmos

H02.211 Cicatricial lagophthalmos right upper eyelid

H02.212 Cicatricial lagophthalmos right lower eyelid

H02.213 Cicatricial lagophthalmos right eye, unspecified eyelid

H02.214 Cicatricial lagophthalmos left upper eyelid

H02.215 Cicatricial lagophthalmos left lower eyelid

H02.216 Cicatricial lagophthalmos left eye, unspecified eyelid

H02.219 Cicatricial lagophthalmos unspecified eye, unspecified eyelid

H02.21A Cicatricial lagophthalmos right eye, upper and lower eyelids

H02.21B Cicatricial lagophthalmos left eye, upper and lower eyelids

H02.21C Cicatricial lagophthalmos, bilateral, upper and lower eyelids

√6ᵗʰ **H02.22** Mechanical lagophthalmos

H02.221 Mechanical lagophthalmos right upper eyelid

H02.222 Mechanical lagophthalmos right lower eyelid

H02.223 Mechanical lagophthalmos right eye, unspecified eyelid

H02.224 Mechanical lagophthalmos left upper eyelid

H02.225 Mechanical lagophthalmos left lower eyelid

H02.226 Mechanical lagophthalmos left eye, unspecified eyelid

H02.229 Mechanical lagophthalmos unspecified eye, unspecified eyelid

H02.22A Mechanical lagophthalmos right eye, upper and lower eyelids

H02.22B Mechanical lagophthalmos left eye, upper and lower eyelids

H02.22C Mechanical lagophthalmos, bilateral, upper and lower eyelids

√6ᵗʰ **H02.23** Paralytic lagophthalmos

H02.231 Paralytic lagophthalmos right upper eyelid

H02.232 Paralytic lagophthalmos right lower eyelid

H02.233 Paralytic lagophthalmos right eye, unspecified eyelid

H02.234 Paralytic lagophthalmos left upper eyelid

H02.235 Paralytic lagophthalmos left lower eyelid

H02.236 Paralytic lagophthalmos left eye, unspecified eyelid

H02.239 Paralytic lagophthalmos unspecified eye, unspecified eyelid

H02.23A Paralytic lagophthalmos right eye, upper and lower eyelids

H02.23B Paralytic lagophthalmos left eye, upper and lower eyelids

H02.23C Paralytic lagophthalmos, bilateral, upper and lower eyelids

√5ᵗʰ **H02.3** Blepharochalasis

Pseudoptosis

DEF: Loss of elasticity and relaxation of skin of the eyelid, thickened or indurated skin on the eyelid associated with recurrent episodes of edema, and intracellular atrophy.

H02.30 Blepharochalasis unspecified eye, unspecified eyelid

H02.31 Blepharochalasis right upper eyelid

H02.32 Blepharochalasis right lower eyelid

H02.33 Blepharochalasis right eye, unspecified eyelid

H02.34 Blepharochalasis left upper eyelid

🅝 Newborn: 0   🅟 Pediatric: 0-17   🅜 Maternity: 12-55   🅐 Adult: 15-124   CH Comorbidity High   CL Comorbidity Low   NCDx Noncancer Dx   PDx Primary Dx

584   ICD-10-CM 2020

H02.35   Blepharochalasis left lower eyelid
H02.36   Blepharochalasis left eye, unspecified eyelid

✓5ᵗʰ **H02.4   Ptosis of eyelid**

✓6ᵗʰ   H02.40   Unspecified ptosis of eyelid
    H02.401   Unspecified ptosis of right eyelid
    H02.402   Unspecified ptosis of left eyelid
    H02.403   Unspecified ptosis of bilateral eyelids
    H02.409   Unspecified ptosis of unspecified eyelid

✓6ᵗʰ   H02.41   Mechanical ptosis of eyelid
    H02.411   Mechanical ptosis of right eyelid
    H02.412   Mechanical ptosis of left eyelid
    H02.413   Mechanical ptosis of bilateral eyelids
    H02.419   Mechanical ptosis of unspecified eyelid

✓6ᵗʰ   H02.42   Myogenic ptosis of eyelid
    H02.421   Myogenic ptosis of right eyelid
    H02.422   Myogenic ptosis of left eyelid
    H02.423   Myogenic ptosis of bilateral eyelids
    H02.429   Myogenic ptosis of unspecified eyelid

✓6ᵗʰ   H02.43   Paralytic ptosis of eyelid
    Neurogenic ptosis of eyelid
    H02.431   Paralytic ptosis of right eyelid
    H02.432   Paralytic ptosis of left eyelid
    H02.433   Paralytic ptosis of bilateral eyelids
    H02.439   Paralytic ptosis unspecified eyelid

✓5ᵗʰ **H02.5   Other disorders affecting eyelid function**
   EXCLUDES 2   blepharospasm (G24.5)
     organic tic (G25.69)
     psychogenic tic (F95.-)

✓6ᵗʰ   H02.51   Abnormal innervation syndrome
    H02.511   Abnormal innervation syndrome right upper eyelid
    H02.512   Abnormal innervation syndrome right lower eyelid
    H02.513   Abnormal innervation syndrome right eye, unspecified eyelid
    H02.514   Abnormal innervation syndrome left upper eyelid
    H02.515   Abnormal innervation syndrome left lower eyelid
    H02.516   Abnormal innervation syndrome left eye, unspecified eyelid
    H02.519   Abnormal innervation syndrome unspecified eye, unspecified eyelid

✓6ᵗʰ   H02.52   Blepharophimosis
    Ankyloblepharon
    H02.521   Blepharophimosis right upper eyelid
    H02.522   Blepharophimosis right lower eyelid
    H02.523   Blepharophimosis right eye, unspecified eyelid
    H02.524   Blepharophimosis left upper eyelid
    H02.525   Blepharophimosis left lower eyelid
    H02.526   Blepharophimosis left eye, unspecified eyelid
    H02.529   Blepharophimosis unspecified eye, unspecified lid

✓6ᵗʰ   H02.53   Eyelid retraction
    Eyelid lag
    H02.531   Eyelid retraction right upper eyelid
    H02.532   Eyelid retraction right lower eyelid
    H02.533   Eyelid retraction right eye, unspecified eyelid
    H02.534   Eyelid retraction left upper eyelid
    H02.535   Eyelid retraction left lower eyelid
    H02.536   Eyelid retraction left eye, unspecified eyelid
    H02.539   Eyelid retraction unspecified eye, unspecified lid

  H02.59   Other disorders affecting eyelid function
    Deficient blink reflex
    Sensory disorders

✓5ᵗʰ **H02.6   Xanthelasma of eyelid**
   DEF: Condition in which there are small yellow tumors that occur on the eyelid, usually appearing near the nose.
   H02.60   Xanthelasma of unspecified eye, unspecified eyelid
   H02.61   Xanthelasma of right upper eyelid
   H02.62   Xanthelasma of right lower eyelid
   H02.63   Xanthelasma of right eye, unspecified eyelid
   H02.64   Xanthelasma of left upper eyelid
   H02.65   Xanthelasma of left lower eyelid
   H02.66   Xanthelasma of left eye, unspecified eyelid

✓5ᵗʰ **H02.7   Other and unspecified degenerative disorders of eyelid and periocular area**
   H02.70   Unspecified degenerative disorders of eyelid and periocular area

✓6ᵗʰ   H02.71   Chloasma of eyelid and periocular area
    Dyspigmentation of eyelid
    Hyperpigmentation of eyelid
    H02.711   Chloasma of right upper eyelid and periocular area
    H02.712   Chloasma of right lower eyelid and periocular area
    H02.713   Chloasma of right eye, unspecified eyelid and periocular area
    H02.714   Chloasma of left upper eyelid and periocular area
    H02.715   Chloasma of left lower eyelid and periocular area
    H02.716   Chloasma of left eye, unspecified eyelid and periocular area
    H02.719   Chloasma of unspecified eye, unspecified eyelid and periocular area

✓6ᵗʰ   H02.72   Madarosis of eyelid and periocular area
    Hypotrichosis of eyelid
    H02.721   Madarosis of right upper eyelid and periocular area
    H02.722   Madarosis of right lower eyelid and periocular area
    H02.723   Madarosis of right eye, unspecified eyelid and periocular area
    H02.724   Madarosis of left upper eyelid and periocular area
    H02.725   Madarosis of left lower eyelid and periocular area
    H02.726   Madarosis of left eye, unspecified eyelid and periocular area
    H02.729   Madarosis of unspecified eye, unspecified eyelid and periocular area

✓6ᵗʰ   H02.73   Vitiligo of eyelid and periocular area
    Hypopigmentation of eyelid
    H02.731   Vitiligo of right upper eyelid and periocular area
    H02.732   Vitiligo of right lower eyelid and periocular area
    H02.733   Vitiligo of right eye, unspecified eyelid and periocular area
    H02.734   Vitiligo of left upper eyelid and periocular area
    H02.735   Vitiligo of left lower eyelid and periocular area
    H02.736   Vitiligo of left eye, unspecified eyelid and periocular area
    H02.739   Vitiligo of unspecified eye, unspecified eyelid and periocular area

  H02.79   Other degenerative disorders of eyelid and periocular area

✓5ᵗʰ **H02.8   Other specified disorders of eyelid**

✓6ᵗʰ   H02.81   Retained foreign body in eyelid
    Use additional code to identify the type of retained foreign body (Z18.-)
    EXCLUDES 1   laceration of eyelid with foreign body (S01.12-)
     retained intraocular foreign body (H44.6-, H44.7-)
     superficial foreign body of eyelid and periocular area (S00.25-)
    H02.811   Retained foreign body in right upper eyelid
    H02.812   Retained foreign body in right lower eyelid
    H02.813   Retained foreign body in right eye, unspecified eyelid
    H02.814   Retained foreign body in left upper eyelid
    H02.815   Retained foreign body in left lower eyelid
    H02.816   Retained foreign body in left eye, unspecified eyelid
    H02.819   Retained foreign body in unspecified eye, unspecified eyelid

☑ Additional Character Required   ✓x7ᵗʰ Placeholder Alert   Manifestation   Unspecified Dx   ►◄ Revised Text   ● New Code   ▲ Revised Title
ICD-10-CM 2020   585
H02.35–H02.819

✓6ᵗʰ **H02.82** Cysts of eyelid
  Sebaceous cyst of eyelid
     H02.821 Cysts of right upper eyelid
     H02.822 Cysts of right lower eyelid
     H02.823 Cysts of right eye, unspecified eyelid
     H02.824 Cysts of left upper eyelid
     H02.825 Cysts of left lower eyelid
     H02.826 Cysts of left eye, unspecified eyelid
     H02.829 Cysts of unspecified eye, unspecified eyelid

✓6ᵗʰ **H02.83** Dermatochalasis of eyelid
  DEF: Acquired form of connective tissue disorder associated with decreased elastic tissue and abnormal elastin formation, resulting in loss of elasticity of the skin of the eyelid. It is generally associated with aging.
     H02.831 Dermatochalasis of right upper eyelid
     H02.832 Dermatochalasis of right lower eyelid
     H02.833 Dermatochalasis of right eye, unspecified eyelid
     H02.834 Dermatochalasis of left upper eyelid
     H02.835 Dermatochalasis of left lower eyelid
     H02.836 Dermatochalasis of left eye, unspecified eyelid
     H02.839 Dermatochalasis of unspecified eye, unspecified eyelid

✓6ᵗʰ **H02.84** Edema of eyelid
  Hyperemia of eyelid
     H02.841 Edema of right upper eyelid
     H02.842 Edema of right lower eyelid
     H02.843 Edema of right eye, unspecified eyelid
     H02.844 Edema of left upper eyelid
     H02.845 Edema of left lower eyelid
     H02.846 Edema of left eye, unspecified eyelid
     H02.849 Edema of unspecified eye, unspecified eyelid

✓6ᵗʰ **H02.85** Elephantiasis of eyelid
     H02.851 Elephantiasis of right upper eyelid
     H02.852 Elephantiasis of right lower eyelid
     H02.853 Elephantiasis of right eye, unspecified eyelid
     H02.854 Elephantiasis of left upper eyelid
     H02.855 Elephantiasis of left lower eyelid
     H02.856 Elephantiasis of left eye, unspecified eyelid
     H02.859 Elephantiasis of unspecified eye, unspecified eyelid

✓6ᵗʰ **H02.86** Hypertrichosis of eyelid
     H02.861 Hypertrichosis of right upper eyelid
     H02.862 Hypertrichosis of right lower eyelid
     H02.863 Hypertrichosis of right eye, unspecified eyelid
     H02.864 Hypertrichosis of left upper eyelid
     H02.865 Hypertrichosis of left lower eyelid
     H02.866 Hypertrichosis of left eye, unspecified eyelid
     H02.869 Hypertrichosis of unspecified eye, unspecified eyelid

✓6ᵗʰ **H02.87** Vascular anomalies of eyelid
     H02.871 Vascular anomalies of right upper eyelid
     H02.872 Vascular anomalies of right lower eyelid
     H02.873 Vascular anomalies of right eye, unspecified eyelid
     H02.874 Vascular anomalies of left upper eyelid
     H02.875 Vascular anomalies of left lower eyelid
     H02.876 Vascular anomalies of left eye, unspecified eyelid
     H02.879 Vascular anomalies of unspecified eye, unspecified eyelid

✓6ᵗʰ **H02.88** Meibomian gland dysfunction of eyelid
  AHA: 2018,4Q,14-15
     H02.881 Meibomian gland dysfunction right upper eyelid
     H02.882 Meibomian gland dysfunction right lower eyelid
     H02.883 Meibomian gland dysfunction of right eye, unspecified eyelid
     H02.884 Meibomian gland dysfunction left upper eyelid
     H02.885 Meibomian gland dysfunction left lower eyelid

     H02.886 Meibomian gland dysfunction of left eye, unspecified eyelid
     H02.889 Meibomian gland dysfunction of unspecified eye, unspecified eyelid
     H02.88A Meibomian gland dysfunction right eye, upper and lower eyelids
     H02.88B Meibomian gland dysfunction left eye, upper and lower eyelids

H02.89 Other specified disorders of eyelid
  Hemorrhage of eyelid

H02.9 Unspecified disorder of eyelid
  Disorder of eyelid NOS

✓4ᵗʰ **H04** Disorders of lacrimal system
  EXCLUDES 1   congenital malformations of lacrimal system (Q10.4-Q10.6)

✓5ᵗʰ **H04.0** Dacryoadenitis
  DEF: Inflammation of the lacrimal gland.

     ✓6ᵗʰ **H04.00** Unspecified dacryoadenitis
         H04.001 Unspecified dacryoadenitis, right lacrimal gland
         H04.002 Unspecified dacryoadenitis, left lacrimal gland
         H04.003 Unspecified dacryoadenitis, bilateral lacrimal glands
         H04.009 Unspecified dacryoadenitis, unspecified lacrimal gland

     ✓6ᵗʰ **H04.01** Acute dacryoadenitis
         H04.011 Acute dacryoadenitis, right lacrimal gland
         H04.012 Acute dacryoadenitis, left lacrimal gland
         H04.013 Acute dacryoadenitis, bilateral lacrimal glands
         H04.019 Acute dacryoadenitis, unspecified lacrimal gland

     ✓6ᵗʰ **H04.02** Chronic dacryoadenitis
         H04.021 Chronic dacryoadenitis, right lacrimal gland
         H04.022 Chronic dacryoadenitis, left lacrimal gland
         H04.023 Chronic dacryoadenitis, bilateral lacrimal gland
         H04.029 Chronic dacryoadenitis, unspecified lacrimal gland

     ✓6ᵗʰ **H04.03** Chronic enlargement of lacrimal gland
         H04.031 Chronic enlargement of right lacrimal gland
         H04.032 Chronic enlargement of left lacrimal gland
         H04.033 Chronic enlargement of bilateral lacrimal glands
         H04.039 Chronic enlargement of unspecified lacrimal gland

✓5ᵗʰ **H04.1** Other disorders of lacrimal gland

     ✓6ᵗʰ **H04.11** Dacryops
         H04.111 Dacryops of right lacrimal gland
         H04.112 Dacryops of left lacrimal gland
         H04.113 Dacryops of bilateral lacrimal glands
         H04.119 Dacryops of unspecified lacrimal gland

     ✓6ᵗʰ **H04.12** Dry eye syndrome
       Tear film insufficiency, NOS
         H04.121 Dry eye syndrome of right lacrimal gland
         H04.122 Dry eye syndrome of left lacrimal gland
         H04.123 Dry eye syndrome of bilateral lacrimal glands
         H04.129 Dry eye syndrome of unspecified lacrimal gland

     ✓6ᵗʰ **H04.13** Lacrimal cyst
       Lacrimal cystic degeneration
         H04.131 Lacrimal cyst, right lacrimal gland
         H04.132 Lacrimal cyst, left lacrimal gland
         H04.133 Lacrimal cyst, bilateral lacrimal glands
         H04.139 Lacrimal cyst, unspecified lacrimal gland

     ✓6ᵗʰ **H04.14** Primary lacrimal gland atrophy
         H04.141 Primary lacrimal gland atrophy, right lacrimal gland
         H04.142 Primary lacrimal gland atrophy, left lacrimal gland
         H04.143 Primary lacrimal gland atrophy, bilateral lacrimal glands
         H04.149 Primary lacrimal gland atrophy, unspecified lacrimal gland

N Newborn: 0   P Pediatric: 0-17   M Maternity: 12-55   A Adult: 15-124   CH Comorbidity High   CL Comorbidity Low   NCDx Noncancer Dx   PDx Primary Dx

586   ICD-10-CM 2020

✓6ᵗʰ **H04.15** Secondary lacrimal gland atrophy

   H04.151 **Secondary lacrimal gland atrophy,** right **lacrimal gland**

   H04.152 **Secondary lacrimal gland atrophy,** left **lacrimal gland**

   H04.153 **Secondary lacrimal gland atrophy,** bilateral **lacrimal glands**

   H04.159 **Secondary lacrimal gland atrophy, unspecified lacrimal gland**

✓6ᵗʰ **H04.16** **Lacrimal gland dislocation**

   H04.161 **Lacrimal gland dislocation,** right **lacrimal gland**

   H04.162 **Lacrimal gland dislocation,** left **lacrimal gland**

   H04.163 **Lacrimal gland dislocation,** bilateral **lacrimal glands**

   H04.169 **Lacrimal gland dislocation, unspecified lacrimal gland**

  H04.19 **Other specified disorders of lacrimal gland**

✓5ᵗʰ **H04.2** **Epiphora**

  DEF: Excessive tearing or overflow of tears down the cheeks often due to a stricture in the lacrimal passages but can be caused by other conditions.

  ✓6ᵗʰ **H04.20** **Unspecified epiphora**

   H04.201 **Unspecified epiphora,** right **side**

   H04.202 **Unspecified epiphora,** left **side**

   H04.203 **Unspecified epiphora,** bilateral

   H04.209 **Unspecified epiphora, unspecified side**

  ✓6ᵗʰ **H04.21** **Epiphora** due to excess lacrimation

   H04.211 **Epiphora due to excess lacrimation,** right **lacrimal gland**

   H04.212 **Epiphora due to excess lacrimation,** left **lacrimal gland**

   H04.213 **Epiphora due to excess lacrimation,** bilateral **lacrimal glands**

   H04.219 **Epiphora due to excess lacrimation, unspecified lacrimal gland**

  ✓6ᵗʰ **H04.22** **Epiphora** due to insufficient drainage

   H04.221 **Epiphora due to insufficient drainage,** right **side**

   H04.222 **Epiphora due to insufficient drainage,** left **side**

   H04.223 **Epiphora due to insufficient drainage,** bilateral

   H04.229 **Epiphora due to insufficient drainage, unspecified side**

✓5ᵗʰ **H04.3** **Acute and unspecified inflammation of lacrimal passages**

  EXCLUDES 1 *neonatal dacryocystitis (P39.1)*

  ✓6ᵗʰ **H04.30** **Unspecified dacryocystitis**

   H04.301 **Unspecified dacryocystitis of** right **lacrimal passage**

   H04.302 **Unspecified dacryocystitis of** left **lacrimal passage**

   H04.303 **Unspecified dacryocystitis of** bilateral **lacrimal passages**

   H04.309 **Unspecified dacryocystitis of unspecified lacrimal passage**

  ✓6ᵗʰ **H04.31** Phlegmonous **dacryocystitis**

   H04.311 **Phlegmonous dacryocystitis of** right **lacrimal passage**

   H04.312 **Phlegmonous dacryocystitis of** left **lacrimal passage**

   H04.313 **Phlegmonous dacryocystitis of** bilateral **lacrimal passages**

   H04.319 **Phlegmonous dacryocystitis of unspecified lacrimal passage**

  ✓6ᵗʰ **H04.32** Acute **dacryocystitis**

   Acute dacryopericystitis

   H04.321 **Acute dacryocystitis of** right **lacrimal passage**

   H04.322 **Acute dacryocystitis of** left **lacrimal passage**

   H04.323 **Acute dacryocystitis of** bilateral **lacrimal passages**

   H04.329 **Acute dacryocystitis of unspecified lacrimal passage**

  ✓6ᵗʰ **H04.33** Acute lacrimal canaliculitis

   H04.331 **Acute lacrimal canaliculitis of** right **lacrimal passage**

   H04.332 **Acute lacrimal canaliculitis of** left **lacrimal passage**

   H04.333 **Acute lacrimal canaliculitis of** bilateral **lacrimal passages**

   H04.339 **Acute lacrimal canaliculitis of unspecified lacrimal passage**

✓5ᵗʰ **H04.4** **Chronic inflammation of lacrimal passages**

  ✓6ᵗʰ **H04.41** Chronic dacryocystitis

   H04.411 **Chronic dacryocystitis of** right **lacrimal passage**

   H04.412 **Chronic dacryocystitis of** left **lacrimal passage**

   H04.413 **Chronic dacryocystitis of** bilateral **lacrimal passages**

   H04.419 **Chronic dacryocystitis of unspecified lacrimal passage**

  ✓6ᵗʰ **H04.42** Chronic **lacrimal** canaliculitis

   H04.421 **Chronic lacrimal canaliculitis of** right **lacrimal passage**

   H04.422 **Chronic lacrimal canaliculitis of** left **lacrimal passage**

   H04.423 **Chronic lacrimal canaliculitis of** bilateral **lacrimal passages**

   H04.429 **Chronic lacrimal canaliculitis of unspecified lacrimal passage**

  ✓6ᵗʰ **H04.43** Chronic **lacrimal** mucocele

   H04.431 **Chronic lacrimal mucocele of** right **lacrimal passage**

   H04.432 **Chronic lacrimal mucocele of** left **lacrimal passage**

   H04.433 **Chronic lacrimal mucocele of** bilateral **lacrimal passages**

   H04.439 **Chronic lacrimal mucocele of unspecified lacrimal passage**

✓5ᵗʰ **H04.5** **Stenosis and insufficiency of lacrimal passages**

  ✓6ᵗʰ **H04.51** Dacryolith

   H04.511 **Dacryolith of** right **lacrimal passage**

   H04.512 **Dacryolith of** left **lacrimal passage**

   H04.513 **Dacryolith of** bilateral **lacrimal passages**

   H04.519 **Dacryolith of unspecified lacrimal passage**

  ✓6ᵗʰ **H04.52** Eversion **of lacrimal** punctum

   H04.521 **Eversion of** right **lacrimal punctum**

   H04.522 **Eversion of** left **lacrimal punctum**

   H04.523 **Eversion of** bilateral **lacrimal punctum**

   H04.529 **Eversion of unspecified lacrimal punctum**

  ✓6ᵗʰ **H04.53** Neonatal obstruction **of nasolacrimal duct**

   EXCLUDES 1 *congenital stenosis and stricture of lacrimal duct (Q10.5)*

   H04.531 **Neonatal obstruction of** right **nasolacrimal duct** Ⓝ

   H04.532 **Neonatal obstruction of** left **nasolacrimal duct** Ⓝ

   H04.533 **Neonatal obstruction of** bilateral **nasolacrimal duct** Ⓝ

   H04.539 **Neonatal obstruction of unspecified nasolacrimal duct** Ⓝ

  ✓6ᵗʰ **H04.54** **Stenosis of lacrimal** canaliculi

   H04.541 **Stenosis of** right **lacrimal canaliculi**

   H04.542 **Stenosis of** left **lacrimal canaliculi**

   H04.543 **Stenosis of** bilateral **lacrimal canaliculi**

   H04.549 **Stenosis of unspecified lacrimal canaliculi**

  ✓6ᵗʰ **H04.55** **Acquired stenosis of nasolacrimal** duct

   H04.551 **Acquired stenosis of** right **nasolacrimal duct**

   H04.552 **Acquired stenosis of** left **nasolacrimal duct**

   H04.553 **Acquired stenosis of** bilateral **nasolacrimal duct**

   H04.559 **Acquired stenosis of unspecified nasolacrimal duct**

  ✓6ᵗʰ **H04.56** **Stenosis of lacrimal** punctum

   H04.561 **Stenosis of** right **lacrimal punctum**

   H04.562 **Stenosis of** left **lacrimal punctum**

   H04.563 **Stenosis of** bilateral **lacrimal punctum**

   H04.569 **Stenosis of unspecified lacrimal punctum**

  ✓6ᵗʰ **H04.57** **Stenosis of lacrimal** sac

   H04.571 **Stenosis of** right **lacrimal sac**

   H04.572 **Stenosis of** left **lacrimal sac**

✔ Additional Character Required   ✓x7ᵗʰ Placeholder Alert   Manifestation   Unspecified Dx   ▶◀ Revised Text   ● New Code   ▲ Revised Title

Chapter 7. Diseases of the Eye and Adnexa

H04.573 Stenosis of bilateral lacrimal sac
H04.579 Stenosis of unspecified lacrimal sac

☑5ᵗʰ **H04.6 Other changes of lacrimal passages**

☑6ᵗʰ H04.61 Lacrimal fistula
H04.611 Lacrimal fistula right lacrimal passage
H04.612 Lacrimal fistula left lacrimal passage
H04.613 Lacrimal fistula bilateral lacrimal passages
H04.619 Lacrimal fistula unspecified lacrimal passage

H04.69 Other changes of lacrimal passages

☑5ᵗʰ **H04.8 Other disorders of lacrimal system**

☑6ᵗʰ H04.81 Granuloma of lacrimal passages
H04.811 Granuloma of right lacrimal passage
H04.812 Granuloma of left lacrimal passage
H04.813 Granuloma of bilateral lacrimal passages
H04.819 Granuloma of unspecified lacrimal passage

H04.89 Other disorders of lacrimal system

H04.9 Disorder of lacrimal system, unspecified

☑4ᵗʰ **H05 Disorders of orbit**

EXCLUDES 1   congenital malformation of orbit (Q10.7)

☑5ᵗʰ **H05.0 Acute inflammation of orbit**

H05.00 Unspecified acute inflammation of orbit

☑6ᵗʰ H05.01 Cellulitis of orbit
Abscess of orbit
H05.011 Cellulitis of right orbit
H05.012 Cellulitis of left orbit
H05.013 Cellulitis of bilateral orbits
H05.019 Cellulitis of unspecified orbit

☑6ᵗʰ H05.02 Osteomyelitis of orbit
H05.021 Osteomyelitis of right orbit
H05.022 Osteomyelitis of left orbit
H05.023 Osteomyelitis of bilateral orbits
H05.029 Osteomyelitis of unspecified orbit

☑6ᵗʰ H05.03 Periostitis of orbit
H05.031 Periostitis of right orbit
H05.032 Periostitis of left orbit
H05.033 Periostitis of bilateral orbits
H05.039 Periostitis of unspecified orbit

☑6ᵗʰ H05.04 Tenonitis of orbit
H05.041 Tenonitis of right orbit
H05.042 Tenonitis of left orbit
H05.043 Tenonitis of bilateral orbits
H05.049 Tenonitis of unspecified orbit

☑5ᵗʰ **H05.1 Chronic inflammatory disorders of orbit**

H05.10 Unspecified chronic inflammatory disorders of orbit

☑6ᵗʰ H05.11 Granuloma of orbit
Pseudotumor (inflammatory) of orbit
H05.111 Granuloma of right orbit
H05.112 Granuloma of left orbit
H05.113 Granuloma of bilateral orbits
H05.119 Granuloma of unspecified orbit

☑6ᵗʰ H05.12 Orbital myositis
H05.121 Orbital myositis, right orbit
H05.122 Orbital myositis, left orbit
H05.123 Orbital myositis, bilateral
H05.129 Orbital myositis, unspecified orbit

☑5ᵗʰ **H05.2 Exophthalmic conditions**

H05.20 Unspecified exophthalmos

☑6ᵗʰ H05.21 Displacement (lateral) of globe
H05.211 Displacement (lateral) of globe, right eye
H05.212 Displacement (lateral) of globe, left eye
H05.213 Displacement (lateral) of globe, bilateral
H05.219 Displacement (lateral) of globe, unspecified eye

☑6ᵗʰ H05.22 Edema of orbit
Orbital congestion
H05.221 Edema of right orbit
H05.222 Edema of left orbit
H05.223 Edema of bilateral orbit
H05.229 Edema of unspecified orbit

☑6ᵗʰ H05.23 Hemorrhage of orbit
H05.231 Hemorrhage of right orbit
H05.232 Hemorrhage of left orbit

H05.233 Hemorrhage of bilateral orbit
H05.239 Hemorrhage of unspecified orbit

☑6ᵗʰ H05.24 Constant exophthalmos
H05.241 Constant exophthalmos, right eye
H05.242 Constant exophthalmos, left eye
H05.243 Constant exophthalmos, bilateral
H05.249 Constant exophthalmos, unspecified eye

☑6ᵗʰ H05.25 Intermittent exophthalmos
H05.251 Intermittent exophthalmos, right eye
H05.252 Intermittent exophthalmos, left eye
H05.253 Intermittent exophthalmos, bilateral
H05.259 Intermittent exophthalmos, unspecified eye

☑6ᵗʰ H05.26 Pulsating exophthalmos
H05.261 Pulsating exophthalmos, right eye
H05.262 Pulsating exophthalmos, left eye
H05.263 Pulsating exophthalmos, bilateral
H05.269 Pulsating exophthalmos, unspecified eye

☑5ᵗʰ **H05.3 Deformity of orbit**

EXCLUDES 1   congenital deformity of orbit (Q10.7)
hypertelorism (Q75.2)

H05.30 Unspecified deformity of orbit

☑6ᵗʰ H05.31 Atrophy of orbit
H05.311 Atrophy of right orbit
H05.312 Atrophy of left orbit
H05.313 Atrophy of bilateral orbit
H05.319 Atrophy of unspecified orbit

☑6ᵗʰ H05.32 Deformity of orbit due to bone disease
Code also associated bone disease
H05.321 Deformity of right orbit due to bone disease
H05.322 Deformity of left orbit due to bone disease
H05.323 Deformity of bilateral orbits due to bone disease
H05.329 Deformity of unspecified orbit due to bone disease

☑6ᵗʰ H05.33 Deformity of orbit due to trauma or surgery
H05.331 Deformity of right orbit due to trauma or surgery
H05.332 Deformity of left orbit due to trauma or surgery
H05.333 Deformity of bilateral orbits due to trauma or surgery
H05.339 Deformity of unspecified orbit due to trauma or surgery

☑6ᵗʰ H05.34 Enlargement of orbit
H05.341 Enlargement of right orbit
H05.342 Enlargement of left orbit
H05.343 Enlargement of bilateral orbits
H05.349 Enlargement of unspecified orbit

☑6ᵗʰ H05.35 Exostosis of orbit
H05.351 Exostosis of right orbit
H05.352 Exostosis of left orbit
H05.353 Exostosis of bilateral orbits
H05.359 Exostosis of unspecified orbit

☑5ᵗʰ **H05.4 Enophthalmos**

☑6ᵗʰ H05.40 Unspecified enophthalmos
H05.401 Unspecified enophthalmos, right eye
H05.402 Unspecified enophthalmos, left eye
H05.403 Unspecified enophthalmos, bilateral
H05.409 Unspecified enophthalmos, unspecified eye

☑6ᵗʰ H05.41 Enophthalmos due to atrophy of orbital tissue
H05.411 Enophthalmos due to atrophy of orbital tissue, right eye
H05.412 Enophthalmos due to atrophy of orbital tissue, left eye
H05.413 Enophthalmos due to atrophy of orbital tissue, bilateral
H05.419 Enophthalmos due to atrophy of orbital tissue, unspecified eye

☑6ᵗʰ H05.42 Enophthalmos due to trauma or surgery
H05.421 Enophthalmos due to trauma or surgery, right eye
H05.422 Enophthalmos due to trauma or surgery, left eye

N Newborn: 0   P Pediatric: 0-17   M Maternity: 12-55   A Adult: 15-124   CH Comorbidity High   CL Comorbidity Low   NCDx Noncancer Dx   PDx Primary Dx

588

ICD-10-CM 2020

H05.423   Enophthalmos due to trauma or surgery, bilateral

H05.429   Enophthalmos due to trauma or surgery, unspecified eye

✓5ᵗʰ **H05.5   Retained (old) foreign body following penetrating wound of orbit**

Retrobulbar foreign body

Use additional code to identify the type of retained foreign body (Z18.-)

EXCLUDES 1   current penetrating wound of orbit (S05.4-)

EXCLUDES 2   retained foreign body of eyelid (H02.81-)

retained intraocular foreign body (H44.6-, H44.7-)

H05.50   Retained (old) foreign body following penetrating wound of unspecified orbit

H05.51   Retained (old) foreign body following penetrating wound of right orbit

H05.52   Retained (old) foreign body following penetrating wound of left orbit

H05.53   Retained (old) foreign body following penetrating wound of bilateral orbits

✓5ᵗʰ **H05.8   Other disorders of orbit**

✓6ᵗʰ **H05.81   Cyst of orbit**

Encephalocele of orbit

H05.811   Cyst of right orbit

H05.812   Cyst of left orbit

H05.813   Cyst of bilateral orbits

H05.819   Cyst of unspecified orbit

✓6ᵗʰ **H05.82   Myopathy of extraocular muscles**

H05.821   Myopathy of extraocular muscles, right orbit

H05.822   Myopathy of extraocular muscles, left orbit

H05.823   Myopathy of extraocular muscles, bilateral

H05.829   Myopathy of extraocular muscles, unspecified orbit

H05.89   Other disorders of orbit

H05.9   Unspecified disorder of orbit

Disorders of conjunctiva (H10-H11)

✓4ᵗʰ **H10   Conjunctivitis**

EXCLUDES 1   keratoconjunctivitis (H16.2-)

✓5ᵗʰ **H10.0   Mucopurulent conjunctivitis**

✓6ᵗʰ **H10.01   Acute follicular conjunctivitis**

H10.011   Acute follicular conjunctivitis, right eye

H10.012   Acute follicular conjunctivitis, left eye

H10.013   Acute follicular conjunctivitis, bilateral

H10.019   Acute follicular conjunctivitis, unspecified eye

✓6ᵗʰ **H10.02   Other mucopurulent conjunctivitis**

H10.021   Other mucopurulent conjunctivitis, right eye

H10.022   Other mucopurulent conjunctivitis, left eye

H10.023   Other mucopurulent conjunctivitis, bilateral

H10.029   Other mucopurulent conjunctivitis, unspecified eye

✓5ᵗʰ **H10.1   Acute atopic conjunctivitis**

Acute papillary conjunctivitis

H10.10   Acute atopic conjunctivitis, unspecified eye

H10.11   Acute atopic conjunctivitis, right eye

H10.12   Acute atopic conjunctivitis, left eye

H10.13   Acute atopic conjunctivitis, bilateral

✓5ᵗʰ **H10.2   Other acute conjunctivitis**

✓6ᵗʰ **H10.21   Acute toxic conjunctivitis**

Acute chemical conjunctivitis

Code first (T51-T65) to identify chemical and intent

EXCLUDES 1   burn and corrosion of eye and adnexa (T26.-)

H10.211   Acute toxic conjunctivitis, right eye

H10.212   Acute toxic conjunctivitis, left eye

H10.213   Acute toxic conjunctivitis, bilateral

H10.219   Acute toxic conjunctivitis, unspecified eye

✓6ᵗʰ **H10.22   Pseudomembranous conjunctivitis**

H10.221   Pseudomembranous conjunctivitis, right eye

H10.222   Pseudomembranous conjunctivitis, left eye

H10.223   Pseudomembranous conjunctivitis, bilateral

H10.229   Pseudomembranous conjunctivitis, unspecified eye

✓6ᵗʰ **H10.23   Serous conjunctivitis, except viral**

EXCLUDES 1   viral conjunctivitis (B30.-)

H10.231   Serous conjunctivitis, except viral, right eye

H10.232   Serous conjunctivitis, except viral, left eye

H10.233   Serous conjunctivitis, except viral, bilateral

H10.239   Serous conjunctivitis, except viral, unspecified eye

✓5ᵗʰ **H10.3   Unspecified acute conjunctivitis**

EXCLUDES 1   ophthalmia neonatorum NOS (P39.1)

H10.30   Unspecified acute conjunctivitis, unspecified eye

H10.31   Unspecified acute conjunctivitis, right eye

H10.32   Unspecified acute conjunctivitis, left eye

H10.33   Unspecified acute conjunctivitis, bilateral

✓5ᵗʰ **H10.4   Chronic conjunctivitis**

✓6ᵗʰ **H10.40   Unspecified chronic conjunctivitis**

H10.401   Unspecified chronic conjunctivitis, right eye

H10.402   Unspecified chronic conjunctivitis, left eye

H10.403   Unspecified chronic conjunctivitis, bilateral

H10.409   Unspecified chronic conjunctivitis, unspecified eye

✓6ᵗʰ **H10.41   Chronic giant papillary conjunctivitis**

H10.411   Chronic giant papillary conjunctivitis, right eye

H10.412   Chronic giant papillary conjunctivitis, left eye

H10.413   Chronic giant papillary conjunctivitis, bilateral

H10.419   Chronic giant papillary conjunctivitis, unspecified eye

✓6ᵗʰ **H10.42   Simple chronic conjunctivitis**

H10.421   Simple chronic conjunctivitis, right eye

H10.422   Simple chronic conjunctivitis, left eye

H10.423   Simple chronic conjunctivitis, bilateral

H10.429   Simple chronic conjunctivitis, unspecified eye

✓6ᵗʰ **H10.43   Chronic follicular conjunctivitis**

H10.431   Chronic follicular conjunctivitis, right eye

H10.432   Chronic follicular conjunctivitis, left eye

H10.433   Chronic follicular conjunctivitis, bilateral

H10.439   Chronic follicular conjunctivitis, unspecified eye

H10.44   Vernal conjunctivitis

EXCLUDES 1   vernal keratoconjunctivitis with limbar and corneal involvement (H16.26-)

H10.45   Other chronic allergic conjunctivitis

✓5ᵗʰ **H10.5   Blepharoconjunctivitis**

✓6ᵗʰ **H10.50   Unspecified blepharoconjunctivitis**

H10.501   Unspecified blepharoconjunctivitis, right eye

H10.502   Unspecified blepharoconjunctivitis, left eye

H10.503   Unspecified blepharoconjunctivitis, bilateral

H10.509   Unspecified blepharoconjunctivitis, unspecified eye

✓6ᵗʰ **H10.51   Ligneous conjunctivitis**

Code also underlying condition if known, such as: plasminogen deficiency (E88.02)

H10.511   Ligneous conjunctivitis, right eye

H10.512   Ligneous conjunctivitis, left eye

H10.513   Ligneous conjunctivitis, bilateral

H10.519   Ligneous conjunctivitis, unspecified eye

☑ Additional Character Required   ✓ₓ7ᵗʰ Placeholder Alert   Manifestation   Unspecified Dx   ►◄ Revised Text   ● New Code   ▲ Revised Title

ICD-10-CM 2020   589

Chapter 7. Diseases of the Eye and Adnexa

H10.52–H11.149

✓6ᵗʰ **H10.52** **Angular** blepharoconjunctivitis
     H10.521 Angular blepharoconjunctivitis, **right eye**
     H10.522 Angular blepharoconjunctivitis, **left eye**
     H10.523 Angular blepharoconjunctivitis, **bilateral**
     H10.529 Angular blepharoconjunctivitis, **unspecified eye**

✓6ᵗʰ **H10.53** **Contact** blepharoconjunctivitis
     H10.531 Contact blepharoconjunctivitis, **right eye**
     H10.532 Contact blepharoconjunctivitis, **left eye**
     H10.533 Contact blepharoconjunctivitis, **bilateral**
     H10.539 Contact blepharoconjunctivitis, **unspecified eye**

✓5ᵗʰ **H10.8** **Other conjunctivitis**

✓6ᵗʰ **H10.81** **Pingueculitis**
     EXCLUDES 1   *pinguecula (H11.15-)*
     H10.811 Pingueculitis, **right eye**
     H10.812 Pingueculitis, **left eye**
     H10.813 Pingueculitis, **bilateral**
     H10.819 Pingueculitis, unspecified eye

✓6ᵗʰ **H10.82** **Rosacea** conjunctivitis
     Code first underlying rosacea dermatitis (L71.-)
     AHA: 2018,4Q,15
     H10.821 Rosacea conjunctivitis, **right eye**
     H10.822 Rosacea conjunctivitis, **left eye**
     H10.823 Rosacea conjunctivitis, **bilateral**
     H10.829 Rosacea conjunctivitis, unspecified eye

     H10.89 **Other conjunctivitis**

H10.9 **Unspecified conjunctivitis**

✓4ᵗʰ **H11** **Other disorders of conjunctiva**
     EXCLUDES 1   *keratoconjunctivitis (H16.2-)*

✓5ᵗʰ **H11.0** **Pterygium of eye**
     EXCLUDES 1   *pseudopterygium (H11.81-)*
     DEF: Benign, wedge-shaped, conjunctival thickening that advances from the inner corner of the eye toward the cornea.

Pterygium

Pterygium

✓6ᵗʰ **H11.00** **Unspecified pterygium of eye**
     H11.001 Unspecified pterygium of **right eye**
     H11.002 Unspecified pterygium of **left eye**
     H11.003 Unspecified pterygium of eye, **bilateral**
     H11.009 Unspecified pterygium of unspecified eye

✓6ᵗʰ **H11.01** **Amyloid** pterygium
     H11.011 Amyloid pterygium of **right eye**
     H11.012 Amyloid pterygium of **left eye**
     H11.013 Amyloid pterygium of eye, **bilateral**
     H11.019 Amyloid pterygium of unspecified eye

✓6ᵗʰ **H11.02** **Central** pterygium of eye
     H11.021 Central pterygium of **right eye**
     H11.022 Central pterygium of **left eye**
     H11.023 Central pterygium of eye, **bilateral**
     H11.029 Central pterygium of unspecified eye

✓6ᵗʰ **H11.03** **Double** pterygium of eye
     H11.031 Double pterygium of **right eye**
     H11.032 Double pterygium of **left eye**
     H11.033 Double pterygium of eye, **bilateral**
     H11.039 Double pterygium of unspecified eye

✓6ᵗʰ **H11.04** **Peripheral** pterygium of eye, **stationary**
     H11.041 Peripheral pterygium, stationary, **right eye**
     H11.042 Peripheral pterygium, stationary, **left eye**
     H11.043 Peripheral pterygium, stationary, **bilateral**
     H11.049 Peripheral pterygium, stationary, unspecified eye

✓6ᵗʰ **H11.05** **Peripheral** pterygium of eye, **progressive**
     H11.051 Peripheral pterygium, progressive, **right eye**
     H11.052 Peripheral pterygium, progressive, **left eye**
     H11.053 Peripheral pterygium, progressive, **bilateral**
     H11.059 Peripheral pterygium, progressive, unspecified eye

✓6ᵗʰ **H11.06** **Recurrent** pterygium of eye
     H11.061 Recurrent pterygium of **right eye**
     H11.062 Recurrent pterygium of **left eye**
     H11.063 Recurrent pterygium of eye, **bilateral**
     H11.069 Recurrent pterygium of unspecified eye

✓5ᵗʰ **H11.1** **Conjunctival degenerations and deposits**
     EXCLUDES 2   *pseudopterygium (H11.81)*

     H11.10 **Unspecified conjunctival degenerations**

✓6ᵗʰ **H11.11** **Conjunctival** deposits
     H11.111 Conjunctival deposits, **right eye**
     H11.112 Conjunctival deposits, **left eye**
     H11.113 Conjunctival deposits, **bilateral**
     H11.119 Conjunctival deposits, unspecified eye

✓6ᵗʰ **H11.12** **Conjunctival** concretions
     H11.121 Conjunctival concretions, **right eye**
     H11.122 Conjunctival concretions, **left eye**
     H11.123 Conjunctival concretions, **bilateral**
     H11.129 Conjunctival concretions, unspecified eye

✓6ᵗʰ **H11.13** **Conjunctival** pigmentations
     Conjunctival argyrosis [argyria]
     H11.131 Conjunctival pigmentations, **right eye**
     H11.132 Conjunctival pigmentations, **left eye**
     H11.133 Conjunctival pigmentations, **bilateral**
     H11.139 Conjunctival pigmentations, unspecified eye

✓6ᵗʰ **H11.14** **Conjunctival xerosis, unspecified**
     EXCLUDES 1   *xerosis of conjunctiva due to vitamin A deficiency (E50.0, E50.1)*
     DEF: Abnormal dryness of the conjunctiva due to lack of insufficient tears or conjunctival secretions.
     H11.141 Conjunctival xerosis, unspecified, **right eye**
     H11.142 Conjunctival xerosis, unspecified, **left eye**
     H11.143 Conjunctival xerosis, unspecified, **bilateral**
     H11.149 Conjunctival xerosis, unspecified, unspecified eye

√6ᵗʰ **H11.15** Pinguecula

> **EXCLUDES 1**   *pingueculitis (H10.81-)*
>
> **DEF:** Proliferation on the conjunctiva near the sclerocorneal junction, usually of the side of the nose and usually in older patients.

Pinguecula

Pinguecula

     H11.151 Pinguecula, right eye
     H11.152 Pinguecula, left eye
     H11.153 Pinguecula, bilateral
     H11.159 Pinguecula, unspecified eye

√5ᵗʰ **H11.2** Conjunctival scars

   √6ᵗʰ **H11.21** Conjunctival adhesions and strands (localized)

     H11.211 Conjunctival adhesions and strands (localized), right eye
     H11.212 Conjunctival adhesions and strands (localized), left eye
     H11.213 Conjunctival adhesions and strands (localized), bilateral
     H11.219 Conjunctival adhesions and strands (localized), unspecified eye

   √6ᵗʰ **H11.22** Conjunctival granuloma

     H11.221 Conjunctival granuloma, right eye
     H11.222 Conjunctival granuloma, left eye
     H11.223 Conjunctival granuloma, bilateral
     H11.229 Conjunctival granuloma, unspecified

   √6ᵗʰ **H11.23** Symblepharon

     H11.231 Symblepharon, right eye
     H11.232 Symblepharon, left eye
     H11.233 Symblepharon, bilateral
     H11.239 Symblepharon, unspecified eye

   √6ᵗʰ **H11.24** Scarring of conjunctiva

     H11.241 Scarring of conjunctiva, right eye
     H11.242 Scarring of conjunctiva, left eye
     H11.243 Scarring of conjunctiva, bilateral
     H11.249 Scarring of conjunctiva, unspecified eye

√5ᵗʰ **H11.3** Conjunctival hemorrhage

   Subconjunctival hemorrhage

     H11.30 Conjunctival hemorrhage, unspecified eye
     H11.31 Conjunctival hemorrhage, right eye
     H11.32 Conjunctival hemorrhage, left eye
     H11.33 Conjunctival hemorrhage, bilateral

√5ᵗʰ **H11.4** Other conjunctival vascular disorders and cysts

   √6ᵗʰ **H11.41** Vascular abnormalities of conjunctiva

     Conjunctival aneurysm
     H11.411 Vascular abnormalities of conjunctiva, right eye
     H11.412 Vascular abnormalities of conjunctiva, left eye
     H11.413 Vascular abnormalities of conjunctiva, bilateral
     H11.419 Vascular abnormalities of conjunctiva, unspecified eye

   √6ᵗʰ **H11.42** Conjunctival edema

     H11.421 Conjunctival edema, right eye
     H11.422 Conjunctival edema, left eye
     H11.423 Conjunctival edema, bilateral
     H11.429 Conjunctival edema, unspecified eye

   √6ᵗʰ **H11.43** Conjunctival hyperemia

     H11.431 Conjunctival hyperemia, right eye
     H11.432 Conjunctival hyperemia, left eye
     H11.433 Conjunctival hyperemia, bilateral
     H11.439 Conjunctival hyperemia, unspecified eye

   √6ᵗʰ **H11.44** Conjunctival cysts

     H11.441 Conjunctival cysts, right eye
     H11.442 Conjunctival cysts, left eye
     H11.443 Conjunctival cysts, bilateral
     H11.449 Conjunctival cysts, unspecified eye

√5ᵗʰ **H11.8** Other specified disorders of conjunctiva

   √6ᵗʰ **H11.81** Pseudopterygium of conjunctiva

     H11.811 Pseudopterygium of conjunctiva, right eye
     H11.812 Pseudopterygium of conjunctiva, left eye
     H11.813 Pseudopterygium of conjunctiva, bilateral
     H11.819 Pseudopterygium of conjunctiva, unspecified eye

   √6ᵗʰ **H11.82** Conjunctivochalasis

     H11.821 Conjunctivochalasis, right eye
     H11.822 Conjunctivochalasis, left eye
     H11.823 Conjunctivochalasis, bilateral
     H11.829 Conjunctivochalasis, unspecified eye

     H11.89 Other specified disorders of conjunctiva

H11.9 Unspecified disorder of conjunctiva

Disorders of sclera, cornea, iris and ciliary body (H15-H22)

√4ᵗʰ **H15** Disorders of sclera

   √5ᵗʰ **H15.0** Scleritis

   √6ᵗʰ **H15.00** Unspecified scleritis

     H15.001 Unspecified scleritis, right eye
     H15.002 Unspecified scleritis, left eye
     H15.003 Unspecified scleritis, bilateral
     H15.009 Unspecified scleritis, unspecified eye

   √6ᵗʰ **H15.01** Anterior scleritis

     H15.011 Anterior scleritis, right eye
     H15.012 Anterior scleritis, left eye
     H15.013 Anterior scleritis, bilateral
     H15.019 Anterior scleritis, unspecified eye

   √6ᵗʰ **H15.02** Brawny scleritis

     H15.021 Brawny scleritis, right eye
     H15.022 Brawny scleritis, left eye
     H15.023 Brawny scleritis, bilateral
     H15.029 Brawny scleritis, unspecified eye

   √6ᵗʰ **H15.03** Posterior scleritis

     Sclerotenonitis
     H15.031 Posterior scleritis, right eye
     H15.032 Posterior scleritis, left eye
     H15.033 Posterior scleritis, bilateral
     H15.039 Posterior scleritis, unspecified eye

   √6ᵗʰ **H15.04** Scleritis with corneal involvement

     H15.041 Scleritis with corneal involvement, right eye
     H15.042 Scleritis with corneal involvement, left eye
     H15.043 Scleritis with corneal involvement, bilateral
     H15.049 Scleritis with corneal involvement, unspecified eye

   √6ᵗʰ **H15.05** Scleromalacia perforans

     H15.051 Scleromalacia perforans, right eye
     H15.052 Scleromalacia perforans, left eye
     H15.053 Scleromalacia perforans, bilateral
     H15.059 Scleromalacia perforans, unspecified eye

   √6ᵗʰ **H15.09** Other scleritis

     Scleral abscess
     H15.091 Other scleritis, right eye
     H15.092 Other scleritis, left eye
     H15.093 Other scleritis, bilateral
     H15.099 Other scleritis, unspecified eye

   √5ᵗʰ **H15.1** Episcleritis

   √6ᵗʰ **H15.10** Unspecified episcleritis

     H15.101 Unspecified episcleritis, right eye
     H15.102 Unspecified episcleritis, left eye
     H15.103 Unspecified episcleritis, bilateral
     H15.109 Unspecified episcleritis, unspecified eye

☑ Additional Character Required   √x7ᵗʰ Placeholder Alert   Manifestation   Unspecified Dx   ►◄ Revised Text   ● New Code   ▲ Revised Title

ICD-10-CM 2020   **591**

✓6ᵗʰ **H15.11** **Episcleritis** periodica fugax

    H15.111 **Episcleritis periodica fugax,** right eye

    H15.112 **Episcleritis periodica fugax,** left eye

    H15.113 **Episcleritis periodica fugax,** bilateral

    H15.119 **Episcleritis periodica fugax, unspecified eye**

✓6ᵗʰ **H15.12** **Nodular** episcleritis

    H15.121 **Nodular episcleritis,** right eye

    H15.122 **Nodular episcleritis,** left eye

    H15.123 **Nodular episcleritis,** bilateral

    H15.129 **Nodular episcleritis, unspecified eye**

✓5ᵗʰ **H15.8** **Other disorders of sclera**

    EXCLUDES 2   blue sclera (Q13.5)

                   degenerative myopia (H44.2-)

✓6ᵗʰ **H15.81** **Equatorial** staphyloma

    H15.811 **Equatorial staphyloma,** right eye

    H15.812 **Equatorial staphyloma,** left eye

    H15.813 **Equatorial staphyloma,** bilateral

    H15.819 **Equatorial staphyloma, unspecified eye**

✓6ᵗʰ **H15.82** **Localized anterior** staphyloma

    H15.821 **Localized anterior staphyloma,** right eye

    H15.822 **Localized anterior staphyloma,** left eye

    H15.823 **Localized anterior staphyloma,** bilateral

    H15.829 **Localized anterior staphyloma, unspecified eye**

✓6ᵗʰ **H15.83** **Staphyloma posticum**

    H15.831 **Staphyloma posticum,** right eye

    H15.832 **Staphyloma posticum,** left eye

    H15.833 **Staphyloma posticum,** bilateral

    H15.839 **Staphyloma posticum, unspecified eye**

✓6ᵗʰ **H15.84** **Scleral** ectasia

    H15.841 **Scleral ectasia,** right eye

    H15.842 **Scleral ectasia,** left eye

    H15.843 **Scleral ectasia,** bilateral

    H15.849 **Scleral ectasia, unspecified eye**

✓6ᵗʰ **H15.85** **Ring** staphyloma

    H15.851 **Ring staphyloma,** right eye

    H15.852 **Ring staphyloma,** left eye

    H15.853 **Ring staphyloma,** bilateral

    H15.859 **Ring staphyloma, unspecified eye**

    H15.89 **Other disorders of sclera**

H15.9 **Unspecified disorder of sclera**

✓4ᵗʰ **H16** **Keratitis**

    DEF: Condition in which the cornea becomes inflamed and irritated.

✓5ᵗʰ **H16.0** **Corneal ulcer**

✓6ᵗʰ **H16.00** **Unspecified corneal ulcer**

    H16.001 **Unspecified corneal ulcer,** right eye

    H16.002 **Unspecified corneal ulcer,** left eye

    H16.003 **Unspecified corneal ulcer,** bilateral

    H16.009 **Unspecified corneal ulcer, unspecified eye**

✓6ᵗʰ **H16.01** **Central** corneal ulcer

    H16.011 **Central corneal ulcer,** right eye

    H16.012 **Central corneal ulcer,** left eye

    H16.013 **Central corneal ulcer,** bilateral

    H16.019 **Central corneal ulcer, unspecified eye**

✓6ᵗʰ **H16.02** **Ring** corneal ulcer

    H16.021 **Ring corneal ulcer,** right eye

    H16.022 **Ring corneal ulcer,** left eye

    H16.023 **Ring corneal ulcer,** bilateral

    H16.029 **Ring corneal ulcer, unspecified eye**

✓6ᵗʰ **H16.03** **Corneal ulcer** with hypopyon

    H16.031 **Corneal ulcer with hypopyon,** right eye

    H16.032 **Corneal ulcer with hypopyon,** left eye

    H16.033 **Corneal ulcer with hypopyon,** bilateral

    H16.039 **Corneal ulcer with hypopyon, unspecified eye**

✓6ᵗʰ **H16.04** **Marginal** corneal ulcer

    H16.041 **Marginal corneal ulcer,** right eye

    H16.042 **Marginal corneal ulcer,** left eye

    H16.043 **Marginal corneal ulcer,** bilateral

    H16.049 **Marginal corneal ulcer, unspecified eye**

✓6ᵗʰ **H16.05** **Mooren's** corneal ulcer

    H16.051 **Mooren's corneal ulcer,** right eye

    H16.052 **Mooren's corneal ulcer,** left eye

    H16.053 **Mooren's corneal ulcer,** bilateral

    H16.059 **Mooren's corneal ulcer, unspecified eye**

✓6ᵗʰ **H16.06** **Mycotic** corneal ulcer

    H16.061 **Mycotic corneal ulcer,** right eye

    H16.062 **Mycotic corneal ulcer,** left eye

    H16.063 **Mycotic corneal ulcer,** bilateral

    H16.069 **Mycotic corneal ulcer, unspecified eye**

✓6ᵗʰ **H16.07** **Perforated** corneal ulcer

    H16.071 **Perforated corneal ulcer,** right eye

    H16.072 **Perforated corneal ulcer,** left eye

    H16.073 **Perforated corneal ulcer,** bilateral

    H16.079 **Perforated corneal ulcer, unspecified eye**

✓5ᵗʰ **H16.1** **Other and unspecified superficial keratitis without conjunctivitis**

✓6ᵗʰ **H16.10** **Unspecified** superficial **keratitis**

    H16.101 **Unspecified superficial keratitis,** right eye

    H16.102 **Unspecified superficial keratitis,** left eye

    H16.103 **Unspecified superficial keratitis,** bilateral

    H16.109 **Unspecified superficial keratitis, unspecified eye**

✓6ᵗʰ **H16.11** **Macular keratitis**

    Areolar keratitis

    Nummular keratitis

    Stellate keratitis

    Striate keratitis

    H16.111 **Macular keratitis,** right eye

    H16.112 **Macular keratitis,** left eye

    H16.113 **Macular keratitis,** bilateral

    H16.119 **Macular keratitis, unspecified eye**

✓6ᵗʰ **H16.12** **Filamentary keratitis**

    H16.121 **Filamentary keratitis,** right eye

    H16.122 **Filamentary keratitis,** left eye

    H16.123 **Filamentary keratitis,** bilateral

    H16.129 **Filamentary keratitis, unspecified eye**

✓6ᵗʰ **H16.13** **Photokeratitis**

    Snow blindness

    Welders keratitis

    H16.131 **Photokeratitis,** right eye

    H16.132 **Photokeratitis,** left eye

    H16.133 **Photokeratitis,** bilateral

    H16.139 **Photokeratitis, unspecified eye**

✓6ᵗʰ **H16.14** **Punctate keratitis**

    H16.141 **Punctate keratitis,** right eye

    H16.142 **Punctate keratitis,** left eye

    H16.143 **Punctate keratitis,** bilateral

    H16.149 **Punctate keratitis, unspecified eye**

✓5ᵗʰ **H16.2** **Keratoconjunctivitis**

✓6ᵗʰ **H16.20** **Unspecified keratoconjunctivitis**

    Superficial keratitis with conjunctivitis NOS

    H16.201 **Unspecified keratoconjunctivitis,** right eye

    H16.202 **Unspecified keratoconjunctivitis,** left eye

    H16.203 **Unspecified keratoconjunctivitis, bilateral**

    H16.209 **Unspecified keratoconjunctivitis, unspecified eye**

✓6ᵗʰ **H16.21** **Exposure keratoconjunctivitis**

    H16.211 **Exposure keratoconjunctivitis,** right eye

    H16.212 **Exposure keratoconjunctivitis,** left eye

    H16.213 **Exposure keratoconjunctivitis,** bilateral

    H16.219 **Exposure keratoconjunctivitis, unspecified eye**

✓6ᵗʰ **H16.22** **Keratoconjunctivitis sicca, not specified as Sjögren's**

    EXCLUDES 1   Sjögren's syndrome (M35.01)

    H16.221 **Keratoconjunctivitis sicca, not specified as Sjögren's,** right eye

    H16.222 **Keratoconjunctivitis sicca, not specified as Sjögren's,** left eye

    H16.223 **Keratoconjunctivitis sicca, not specified as Sjögren's,** bilateral

    H16.229 **Keratoconjunctivitis sicca, not specified as Sjögren's, unspecified eye**

✓6ᵗʰ **H16.23** **Neurotrophic keratoconjunctivitis**

    H16.231 **Neurotrophic keratoconjunctivitis,** right eye

    H16.232 **Neurotrophic keratoconjunctivitis,** left eye

N Newborn: 0   P Pediatric: 0-17   M Maternity: 12-55   A Adult: 15-124   CH Comorbidity High   CL Comorbidity Low   NC Dx Noncancer Dx   PD x Primary Dx

592   ICD-10-CM 2020

         H16.233   **Neurotrophic keratoconjunctivitis, bilateral**

         H16.239   **Neurotrophic keratoconjunctivitis, unspecified eye**

√6ᵗʰ **H16.24**   Ophthalmia nodosa

         H16.241   **Ophthalmia nodosa,** right **eye**

         H16.242   **Ophthalmia nodosa,** left **eye**

         H16.243   **Ophthalmia nodosa,** bilateral

         H16.249   **Ophthalmia nodosa, unspecified eye**

√6ᵗʰ **H16.25**   Phlyctenular **keratoconjunctivitis**

         H16.251   **Phlyctenular keratoconjunctivitis,** right **eye**

         H16.252   **Phlyctenular keratoconjunctivitis,** left **eye**

         H16.253   **Phlyctenular keratoconjunctivitis,** bilateral

         H16.259   **Phlyctenular keratoconjunctivitis, unspecified eye**

√6ᵗʰ **H16.26**   Vernal **keratoconjunctivitis, with** limbar and corneal involvement

         EXCLUDES 1   *vernal conjunctivitis without limbar and corneal involvement (H10.44)*

         H16.261   **Vernal keratoconjunctivitis, with limbar and corneal involvement,** right **eye**

         H16.262   **Vernal keratoconjunctivitis, with limbar and corneal involvement,** left **eye**

         H16.263   **Vernal keratoconjunctivitis, with limbar and corneal involvement,** bilateral

         H16.269   **Vernal keratoconjunctivitis, with limbar and corneal involvement, unspecified eye**

√6ᵗʰ **H16.29**   Other keratoconjunctivitis

         H16.291   **Other keratoconjunctivitis,** right **eye**

         H16.292   **Other keratoconjunctivitis,** left **eye**

         H16.293   **Other keratoconjunctivitis,** bilateral

         H16.299   **Other keratoconjunctivitis, unspecified eye**

√5ᵗʰ **H16.3**   Interstitial and deep keratitis

√6ᵗʰ **H16.30**   Unspecified interstitial keratitis

         H16.301   **Unspecified interstitial keratitis,** right **eye**

         H16.302   **Unspecified interstitial keratitis,** left **eye**

         H16.303   **Unspecified interstitial keratitis,** bilateral

         H16.309   **Unspecified interstitial keratitis, unspecified eye**

√6ᵗʰ **H16.31**   Corneal **abscess**

         H16.311   **Corneal abscess,** right **eye**

         H16.312   **Corneal abscess,** left **eye**

         H16.313   **Corneal abscess,** bilateral

         H16.319   **Corneal abscess, unspecified eye**

√6ᵗʰ **H16.32**   Diffuse **interstitial keratitis**

         Cogan's syndrome

         H16.321   **Diffuse interstitial keratitis,** right **eye**

         H16.322   **Diffuse interstitial keratitis,** left **eye**

         H16.323   **Diffuse interstitial keratitis,** bilateral

         H16.329   **Diffuse interstitial keratitis, unspecified eye**

√6ᵗʰ **H16.33**   Sclerosing **keratitis**

         H16.331   **Sclerosing keratitis,** right **eye**

         H16.332   **Sclerosing keratitis,** left **eye**

         H16.333   **Sclerosing keratitis,** bilateral

         H16.339   **Sclerosing keratitis, unspecified eye**

√6ᵗʰ **H16.39**   Other interstitial and deep keratitis

         H16.391   **Other interstitial and deep keratitis,** right **eye**

         H16.392   **Other interstitial and deep keratitis,** left **eye**

         H16.393   **Other interstitial and deep keratitis,** bilateral

         H16.399   **Other interstitial and deep keratitis, unspecified eye**

√5ᵗʰ **H16.4**   Corneal neovascularization

√6ᵗʰ **H16.40**   Unspecified corneal neovascularization

         H16.401   **Unspecified corneal neovascularization,** right **eye**

         H16.402   **Unspecified corneal neovascularization,** left **eye**

         H16.403   **Unspecified corneal neovascularization,** bilateral

         H16.409   **Unspecified corneal neovascularization, unspecified eye**

√6ᵗʰ **H16.41**   Ghost vessels (corneal)

         H16.411   **Ghost vessels (corneal),** right **eye**

         H16.412   **Ghost vessels (corneal),** left **eye**

         H16.413   **Ghost vessels (corneal),** bilateral

         H16.419   **Ghost vessels (corneal), unspecified eye**

√6ᵗʰ **H16.42**   Pannus (corneal)

         H16.421   **Pannus (corneal),** right **eye**

         H16.422   **Pannus (corneal),** left **eye**

         H16.423   **Pannus (corneal),** bilateral

         H16.429   **Pannus (corneal), unspecified eye**

√6ᵗʰ **H16.43**   Localized vascularization of cornea

         H16.431   **Localized vascularization of cornea,** right **eye**

         H16.432   **Localized vascularization of cornea,** left **eye**

         H16.433   **Localized vascularization of cornea,** bilateral

         H16.439   **Localized vascularization of cornea, unspecified eye**

√6ᵗʰ **H16.44**   Deep vascularization of cornea

         H16.441   **Deep vascularization of cornea,** right **eye**

         H16.442   **Deep vascularization of cornea,** left **eye**

         H16.443   **Deep vascularization of cornea,** bilateral

         H16.449   **Deep vascularization of cornea, unspecified eye**

H16.8   Other keratitis

H16.9   Unspecified keratitis

√4ᵗʰ **H17**   **Corneal scars and opacities**

√5ᵗʰ **H17.0**   Adherent leukoma

         H17.00   **Adherent leukoma, unspecified eye**

         H17.01   **Adherent leukoma,** right **eye**

         H17.02   **Adherent leukoma,** left **eye**

         H17.03   **Adherent leukoma,** bilateral

√5ᵗʰ **H17.1**   Central corneal opacity

         H17.10   **Central corneal opacity, unspecified eye**

         H17.11   **Central corneal opacity,** right **eye**

         H17.12   **Central corneal opacity,** left **eye**

         H17.13   **Central corneal opacity,** bilateral

√5ᵗʰ **H17.8**   Other corneal scars and opacities

√6ᵗʰ **H17.81**   Minor **opacity of cornea**

         Corneal nebula

         H17.811   **Minor opacity of cornea,** right **eye**

         H17.812   **Minor opacity of cornea,** left **eye**

         H17.813   **Minor opacity of cornea,** bilateral

         H17.819   **Minor opacity of cornea, unspecified eye**

√6ᵗʰ **H17.82**   Peripheral **opacity of cornea**

         H17.821   **Peripheral opacity of cornea,** right **eye**

         H17.822   **Peripheral opacity of cornea,** left **eye**

         H17.823   **Peripheral opacity of cornea,** bilateral

         H17.829   **Peripheral opacity of cornea, unspecified eye**

         H17.89   **Other corneal scars and opacities**

H17.9   Unspecified corneal scar and opacity

√4ᵗʰ **H18**   **Other disorders of cornea**

√5ᵗʰ **H18.0**   Corneal pigmentations and deposits

√6ᵗʰ **H18.00**   Unspecified corneal deposit

         H18.001   **Unspecified corneal deposit,** right **eye**

         H18.002   **Unspecified corneal deposit,** left **eye**

         H18.003   **Unspecified corneal deposit,** bilateral

         H18.009   **Unspecified corneal deposit, unspecified eye**

√6ᵗʰ **H18.01**   Anterior **corneal pigmentations**

         Staehli's line

         H18.011   **Anterior corneal pigmentations,** right **eye**

         H18.012   **Anterior corneal pigmentations,** left **eye**

         H18.013   **Anterior corneal pigmentations,** bilateral

         H18.019   **Anterior corneal pigmentations, unspecified eye**

√6ᵗʰ **H18.02**   Argentous **corneal deposits**

         H18.021   **Argentous corneal deposits,** right **eye**

         H18.022   **Argentous corneal deposits,** left **eye**

         H18.023   **Argentous corneal deposits,** bilateral

         H18.029   **Argentous corneal deposits, unspecified eye**

☑ Additional Character Required   √x7ᵗʰ Placeholder Alert   Manifestation   Unspecified Dx   ►◄ Revised Text   ● New Code   ▲ Revised Title

ICD-10-CM 2020   593

Chapter 7. Diseases of the Eye and Adnexa

✓6ᵗʰ **H18.Ø3 Corneal deposits in** metabolic disorders
  Code also associated metabolic disorder
  H18.Ø31 Corneal deposits in metabolic disorders, right eye
  H18.Ø32 Corneal deposits in metabolic disorders, left eye
  H18.Ø33 Corneal deposits in metabolic disorders, bilateral
  H18.Ø39 Corneal deposits in metabolic disorders, unspecified eye

✓6ᵗʰ **H18.Ø4** Kayser-Fleischer ring
  Code also associated Wilson's disease (E83.Ø1)
  H18.Ø41 Kayser-Fleischer ring, right eye
  H18.Ø42 Kayser-Fleischer ring, left eye
  H18.Ø43 Kayser-Fleischer ring, bilateral
  H18.Ø49 Kayser-Fleischer ring, unspecified eye

✓6ᵗʰ **H18.Ø5** Posterior **corneal pigmentations**
  Krukenberg's spindle
  H18.Ø51 Posterior corneal pigmentations, right eye
  H18.Ø52 Posterior corneal pigmentations, left eye
  H18.Ø53 Posterior corneal pigmentations, bilateral
  H18.Ø59 Posterior corneal pigmentations, unspecified eye

✓6ᵗʰ **H18.Ø6** Stromal **corneal pigmentations**
  Hematocornea
  H18.Ø61 Stromal corneal pigmentations, right eye
  H18.Ø62 Stromal corneal pigmentations, left eye
  H18.Ø63 Stromal corneal pigmentations, bilateral
  H18.Ø69 Stromal corneal pigmentations, unspecified eye

✓5ᵗʰ **H18.1 Bullous keratopathy**
  DEF: Corneal swelling due to a damaged corneal endothelium. Bullous keratopathy is characterized by recurring, rupturing epithelial blisters causing glaucoma, iridocyclitis, and Fuchs dystrophy.
  H18.1Ø Bullous keratopathy, unspecified eye
  H18.11 Bullous keratopathy, right eye
  H18.12 Bullous keratopathy, left eye
  H18.13 Bullous keratopathy, bilateral

✓5ᵗʰ **H18.2 Other and unspecified corneal edema**
  H18.2Ø Unspecified corneal edema
✓6ᵗʰ **H18.21 Corneal edema** secondary to contact lens
  EXCLUDES 2 other corneal disorders due to contact lens (H18.82-)
  H18.211 Corneal edema secondary to contact lens, right eye
  H18.212 Corneal edema secondary to contact lens, left eye
  H18.213 Corneal edema secondary to contact lens, bilateral
  H18.219 Corneal edema secondary to contact lens, unspecified eye
✓6ᵗʰ **H18.22** Idiopathic **corneal edema**
  H18.221 Idiopathic corneal edema, right eye
  H18.222 Idiopathic corneal edema, left eye
  H18.223 Idiopathic corneal edema, bilateral
  H18.229 Idiopathic corneal edema, unspecified eye
✓6ᵗʰ **H18.23** Secondary **corneal edema**
  H18.231 Secondary corneal edema, right eye
  H18.232 Secondary corneal edema, left eye
  H18.233 Secondary corneal edema, bilateral
  H18.239 Secondary corneal edema, unspecified eye

✓5ᵗʰ **H18.3 Changes of corneal membranes**
  H18.3Ø Unspecified corneal membrane change
✓6ᵗʰ **H18.31 Folds and rupture in** Bowman's membrane
  H18.311 Folds and rupture in Bowman's membrane, right eye
  H18.312 Folds and rupture in Bowman's membrane, left eye
  H18.313 Folds and rupture in Bowman's membrane, bilateral
  H18.319 Folds and rupture in Bowman's membrane, unspecified eye
✓6ᵗʰ **H18.32** Folds in Descemet's membrane
  H18.321 Folds in Descemet's membrane, right eye

H18.322 Folds in Descemet's membrane, left eye
H18.323 Folds in Descemet's membrane, bilateral
H18.329 Folds in Descemet's membrane, unspecified eye
✓6ᵗʰ **H18.33** Rupture in Descemet's membrane
  H18.331 Rupture in Descemet's membrane, right eye
  H18.332 Rupture in Descemet's membrane, left eye
  H18.333 Rupture in Descemet's membrane, bilateral
  H18.339 Rupture in Descemet's membrane, unspecified eye

✓5ᵗʰ **H18.4 Corneal degeneration**
  EXCLUDES 1 Mooren's ulcer (H16.Ø-)
        recurrent erosion of cornea (H18.83-)
  H18.4Ø Unspecified corneal degeneration
✓6ᵗʰ **H18.41** Arcus senilis
  Senile corneal changes
  H18.411 Arcus senilis, right eye
  H18.412 Arcus senilis, left eye
  H18.413 Arcus senilis, bilateral
  H18.419 Arcus senilis, unspecified eye
✓6ᵗʰ **H18.42** Band **keratopathy**
  H18.421 Band keratopathy, right eye
  H18.422 Band keratopathy, left eye
  H18.423 Band keratopathy, bilateral
  H18.429 Band keratopathy, unspecified eye
  H18.43 Other calcerous corneal degeneration
✓6ᵗʰ **H18.44 Keratomalacia**
  EXCLUDES 1 keratomalacia due to vitamin A deficiency (E5Ø.4)
  H18.441 Keratomalacia, right eye
  H18.442 Keratomalacia, left eye
  H18.443 Keratomalacia, bilateral
  H18.449 Keratomalacia, unspecified eye
✓6ᵗʰ **H18.45** Nodular **corneal degeneration**
  H18.451 Nodular corneal degeneration, right eye
  H18.452 Nodular corneal degeneration, left eye
  H18.453 Nodular corneal degeneration, bilateral
  H18.459 Nodular corneal degeneration, unspecified eye
✓6ᵗʰ **H18.46** Peripheral **corneal degeneration**
  H18.461 Peripheral corneal degeneration, right eye
  H18.462 Peripheral corneal degeneration, left eye
  H18.463 Peripheral corneal degeneration, bilateral
  H18.469 Peripheral corneal degeneration, unspecified eye
  H18.49 Other corneal degeneration

✓5ᵗʰ **H18.5 Hereditary corneal dystrophies**
  H18.5Ø Unspecified hereditary corneal dystrophies
  H18.51 Endothelial **corneal dystrophy**
    Fuchs' dystrophy
  H18.52 Epithelial (juvenile) **corneal dystrophy**
  H18.53 Granular **corneal dystrophy**
  H18.54 Lattice **corneal dystrophy**
  H18.55 Macular **corneal dystrophy**
  H18.59 Other **hereditary corneal dystrophies**

✓5ᵗʰ **H18.6 Keratoconus**
✓6ᵗʰ **H18.6Ø Keratoconus, unspecified**
  H18.6Ø1 Keratoconus, unspecified, right eye
  H18.6Ø2 Keratoconus, unspecified, left eye
  H18.6Ø3 Keratoconus, unspecified, bilateral
  H18.6Ø9 Keratoconus, unspecified, unspecified eye
✓6ᵗʰ **H18.61 Keratoconus,** stable
  H18.611 Keratoconus, stable, right eye
  H18.612 Keratoconus, stable, left eye
  H18.613 Keratoconus, stable, bilateral
  H18.619 Keratoconus, stable, unspecified eye
✓6ᵗʰ **H18.62 Keratoconus,** unstable
  Acute hydrops
  H18.621 Keratoconus, unstable, right eye
  H18.622 Keratoconus, unstable, left eye
  H18.623 Keratoconus, unstable, bilateral

H18.629 **Keratoconus, unstable, unspecified eye**

√5ᵗʰ **H18.7 Other and unspecified corneal deformities**

    EXCLUDES 1   *congenital malformations of cornea (Q13.3-Q13.4)*

    H18.70 Unspecified corneal deformity

    √6ᵗʰ **H18.71 Corneal** ectasia

        H18.711 **Corneal ectasia,** right **eye**

        H18.712 **Corneal ectasia,** left **eye**

        H18.713 **Corneal ectasia,** bilateral

        H18.719 **Corneal ectasia, unspecified eye**

    √6ᵗʰ **H18.72 Corneal** staphyloma

        H18.721 **Corneal staphyloma,** right **eye**

        H18.722 **Corneal staphyloma,** left **eye**

        H18.723 **Corneal staphyloma,** bilateral

        H18.729 **Corneal staphyloma, unspecified eye**

    √6ᵗʰ **H18.73** Descemetocele

        H18.731 **Descemetocele,** right **eye**

        H18.732 **Descemetocele,** left **eye**

        H18.733 **Descemetocele,** bilateral

        H18.739 **Descemetocele, unspecified eye**

    √6ᵗʰ **H18.79 Other corneal deformities**

        H18.791 **Other corneal deformities,** right **eye**

        H18.792 **Other corneal deformities,** left **eye**

        H18.793 **Other corneal deformities,** bilateral

        H18.799 **Other corneal deformities, unspecified eye**

√5ᵗʰ **H18.8 Other specified disorders of cornea**

    √6ᵗʰ **H18.81 Anesthesia and hypoesthesia of cornea**

        H18.811 **Anesthesia and hypoesthesia of cornea,** right **eye**

        H18.812 **Anesthesia and hypoesthesia of cornea,** left **eye**

        H18.813 **Anesthesia and hypoesthesia of cornea,** bilateral

        H18.819 **Anesthesia and hypoesthesia of cornea, unspecified eye**

    √6ᵗʰ **H18.82 Corneal disorder due to contact lens**

        EXCLUDES 2   *corneal edema due to contact lens (H18.21-)*

        H18.821 **Corneal disorder due to contact lens,** right **eye**

        H18.822 **Corneal disorder due to contact lens,** left **eye**

        H18.823 **Corneal disorder due to contact lens,** bilateral

        H18.829 **Corneal disorder due to contact lens, unspecified eye**

    √6ᵗʰ **H18.83 Recurrent erosion of cornea**

        H18.831 **Recurrent erosion of cornea,** right **eye**

        H18.832 **Recurrent erosion of cornea,** left **eye**

        H18.833 **Recurrent erosion of cornea,** bilateral

        H18.839 **Recurrent erosion of cornea, unspecified eye**

    √6ᵗʰ **H18.89 Other specified disorders of cornea**

        H18.891 **Other specified disorders of cornea,** right **eye**

        H18.892 **Other specified disorders of cornea,** left **eye**

        H18.893 **Other specified disorders of cornea,** bilateral

        H18.899 **Other specified disorders of cornea, unspecified eye**

H18.9 Unspecified disorder of cornea

√4ᵗʰ **H20 Iridocyclitis**

    √5ᵗʰ **H20.0 Acute and subacute iridocyclitis**

        Acute anterior uveitis

        Acute cyclitis

        Acute iritis

        Subacute anterior uveitis

        Subacute cyclitis

        Subacute iritis

        EXCLUDES 1   *iridocyclitis, iritis, uveitis (due to) (in) diabetes mellitus (E08-E13 with .39)*

                iridocyclitis, iritis, uveitis (due to) (in) diphtheria (A36.89)

                iridocyclitis, iritis, uveitis (due to) (in) gonococcal (A54.32)

                iridocyclitis, iritis, uveitis (due to) (in) herpes (simplex) (B00.51)

                iridocyclitis, iritis, uveitis (due to) (in) herpes zoster (B02.32)

                iridocyclitis, iritis, uveitis (due to) (in) late congenital syphilis (A50.39)

                iridocyclitis, iritis, uveitis (due to) (in) late syphilis (A52.71)

                iridocyclitis, iritis, uveitis (due to) (in) sarcoidosis (D86.83)

                iridocyclitis, iritis, uveitis (due to) (in) syphilis (A51.43)

                iridocyclitis, iritis, uveitis (due to) (in) toxoplasmosis (B58.09)

                iridocyclitis, iritis, uveitis (due to) (in) tuberculosis (A18.54)

        H20.00 Unspecified acute and subacute iridocyclitis

    √6ᵗʰ **H20.01 Primary iridocyclitis**

        H20.011 **Primary iridocyclitis,** right **eye**

        H20.012 **Primary iridocyclitis,** left **eye**

        H20.013 **Primary iridocyclitis,** bilateral

        H20.019 **Primary iridocyclitis, unspecified eye**

    √6ᵗʰ **H20.02 Recurrent acute iridocyclitis**

        H20.021 **Recurrent acute iridocyclitis,** right **eye**

        H20.022 **Recurrent acute iridocyclitis,** left **eye**

        H20.023 **Recurrent acute iridocyclitis,** bilateral

        H20.029 **Recurrent acute iridocyclitis, unspecified eye**

    √6ᵗʰ **H20.03 Secondary infectious iridocyclitis**

        H20.031 **Secondary infectious iridocyclitis,** right **eye**

        H20.032 **Secondary infectious iridocyclitis,** left **eye**

        H20.033 **Secondary infectious iridocyclitis,** bilateral

        H20.039 **Secondary infectious iridocyclitis, unspecified eye**

    √6ᵗʰ **H20.04 Secondary noninfectious iridocyclitis**

        H20.041 **Secondary noninfectious iridocyclitis,** right **eye**

        H20.042 **Secondary noninfectious iridocyclitis,** left **eye**

        H20.043 **Secondary noninfectious iridocyclitis,** bilateral

        H20.049 **Secondary noninfectious iridocyclitis, unspecified eye**

    √6ᵗʰ **H20.05 Hypopyon**

        H20.051 **Hypopyon,** right **eye**

        H20.052 **Hypopyon,** left **eye**

        H20.053 **Hypopyon,** bilateral

        H20.059 **Hypopyon, unspecified eye**

    √5ᵗʰ **H20.1 Chronic iridocyclitis**

        Use additional code for any associated cataract (H26.21-)

        EXCLUDES 2   *posterior cyclitis (H30.2-)*

        H20.10 Chronic iridocyclitis, unspecified eye

        H20.11 **Chronic iridocyclitis,** right **eye**

        H20.12 **Chronic iridocyclitis,** left **eye**

        H20.13 **Chronic iridocyclitis,** bilateral

    √5ᵗʰ **H20.2 Lens-induced iridocyclitis**

        H20.20 Lens-induced iridocyclitis, unspecified eye

        H20.21 **Lens-induced iridocyclitis,** right **eye**

        H20.22 **Lens-induced iridocyclitis,** left **eye**

        H20.23 **Lens-induced iridocyclitis,** bilateral

☑ Additional Character Required   √x7ᵗʰ Placeholder Alert   Manifestation   Unspecified Dx   ▶◀ Revised Text   ● New Code   ▲ Revised Title

ICD-10-CM 2020   595

Chapter 7. Diseases of the Eye and Adnexa

✓5ᵗʰ **H20.8 Other iridocyclitis**

EXCLUDES 2   *glaucomatocyclitis crises (H40.4-)*
posterior cyclitis (H30.2-)
sympathetic uveitis (H44.13-)

✓6ᵗʰ **H20.81 Fuchs' heterochromic cyclitis**

H20.811 Fuchs' heterochromic cyclitis, right eye
H20.812 Fuchs' heterochromic cyclitis, left eye
H20.813 Fuchs' heterochromic cyclitis, bilateral
H20.819 Fuchs' heterochromic cyclitis, unspecified eye

✓6ᵗʰ **H20.82 Vogt-Koyanagi syndrome**

H20.821 Vogt-Koyanagi syndrome, right eye
H20.822 Vogt-Koyanagi syndrome, left eye
H20.823 Vogt-Koyanagi syndrome, bilateral
H20.829 Vogt-Koyanagi syndrome, unspecified eye

H20.9 Unspecified iridocyclitis
Uveitis NOS

✓4ᵗʰ **H21 Other disorders of iris and ciliary body**

EXCLUDES 2   *sympathetic uveitis (H44.1-)*

✓5ᵗʰ **H21.0 Hyphema**

EXCLUDES 1   *traumatic hyphema (S05.1-)*

Hyphema

- Iris
- Cornea
- Hyphema

H21.00 Hyphema, unspecified eye
H21.01 Hyphema, right eye
H21.02 Hyphema, left eye
H21.03 Hyphema, bilateral

✓5ᵗʰ **H21.1 Other vascular disorders of iris and ciliary body**
Neovascularization of iris or ciliary body
Rubeosis iridis
Rubeosis of iris

✓6ᵗʰ **H21.1X Other vascular disorders of iris and ciliary body**

H21.1X1 Other vascular disorders of iris and ciliary body, right eye
H21.1X2 Other vascular disorders of iris and ciliary body, left eye
H21.1X3 Other vascular disorders of iris and ciliary body, bilateral
H21.1X9 Other vascular disorders of iris and ciliary body, unspecified eye

✓5ᵗʰ **H21.2 Degeneration of iris and ciliary body**

✓6ᵗʰ **H21.21 Degeneration of chamber angle**

H21.211 Degeneration of chamber angle, right eye
H21.212 Degeneration of chamber angle, left eye
H21.213 Degeneration of chamber angle, bilateral
H21.219 Degeneration of chamber angle, unspecified eye

✓6ᵗʰ **H21.22 Degeneration of ciliary body**

H21.221 Degeneration of ciliary body, right eye
H21.222 Degeneration of ciliary body, left eye
H21.223 Degeneration of ciliary body, bilateral
H21.229 Degeneration of ciliary body, unspecified eye

✓6ᵗʰ **H21.23 Degeneration of iris (pigmentary)**
Translucency of iris

H21.231 Degeneration of iris (pigmentary), right eye
H21.232 Degeneration of iris (pigmentary), left eye

H21.233 Degeneration of iris (pigmentary), bilateral
H21.239 Degeneration of iris (pigmentary), unspecified eye

✓6ᵗʰ **H21.24 Degeneration of pupillary margin**

H21.241 Degeneration of pupillary margin, right eye
H21.242 Degeneration of pupillary margin, left eye
H21.243 Degeneration of pupillary margin, bilateral
H21.249 Degeneration of pupillary margin, unspecified eye

✓6ᵗʰ **H21.25 Iridoschisis**

H21.251 Iridoschisis, right eye
H21.252 Iridoschisis, left eye
H21.253 Iridoschisis, bilateral
H21.259 Iridoschisis, unspecified eye

✓6ᵗʰ **H21.26 Iris atrophy (essential) (progressive)**

H21.261 Iris atrophy (essential) (progressive), right eye
H21.262 Iris atrophy (essential) (progressive), left eye
H21.263 Iris atrophy (essential) (progressive), bilateral
H21.269 Iris atrophy (essential) (progressive), unspecified eye

✓6ᵗʰ **H21.27 Miotic pupillary cyst**

H21.271 Miotic pupillary cyst, right eye
H21.272 Miotic pupillary cyst, left eye
H21.273 Miotic pupillary cyst, bilateral
H21.279 Miotic pupillary cyst, unspecified eye

H21.29 Other iris atrophy

✓5ᵗʰ **H21.3 Cyst of iris, ciliary body and anterior chamber**

EXCLUDES 2   *miotic pupillary cyst (H21.27-)*

✓6ᵗʰ **H21.30 Idiopathic cysts of iris, ciliary body or anterior chamber**
Cyst of iris, ciliary body or anterior chamber NOS

H21.301 Idiopathic cysts of iris, ciliary body or anterior chamber, right eye
H21.302 Idiopathic cysts of iris, ciliary body or anterior chamber, left eye
H21.303 Idiopathic cysts of iris, ciliary body or anterior chamber, bilateral
H21.309 Idiopathic cysts of iris, ciliary body or anterior chamber, unspecified eye

✓6ᵗʰ **H21.31 Exudative cysts of iris or anterior chamber**

H21.311 Exudative cysts of iris or anterior chamber, right eye
H21.312 Exudative cysts of iris or anterior chamber, left eye
H21.313 Exudative cysts of iris or anterior chamber, bilateral
H21.319 Exudative cysts of iris or anterior chamber, unspecified eye

✓6ᵗʰ **H21.32 Implantation cysts of iris, ciliary body or anterior chamber**

H21.321 Implantation cysts of iris, ciliary body or anterior chamber, right eye
H21.322 Implantation cysts of iris, ciliary body or anterior chamber, left eye
H21.323 Implantation cysts of iris, ciliary body or anterior chamber, bilateral
H21.329 Implantation cysts of iris, ciliary body or anterior chamber, unspecified eye

✓6ᵗʰ **H21.33 Parasitic cyst of iris, ciliary body or anterior chamber**

H21.331 Parasitic cyst of iris, ciliary body or anterior chamber, right eye
H21.332 Parasitic cyst of iris, ciliary body or anterior chamber, left eye
H21.333 Parasitic cyst of iris, ciliary body or anterior chamber, bilateral
H21.339 Parasitic cyst of iris, ciliary body or anterior chamber, unspecified eye

✓6ᵗʰ **H21.34 Primary cyst of pars plana**

H21.341 Primary cyst of pars plana, right eye
H21.342 Primary cyst of pars plana, left eye
H21.343 Primary cyst of pars plana, bilateral

    H21.349   Primary cyst of pars plana, unspecified eye

✓6ᵗʰ **H21.35**   Exudative cyst of pars plana

    DEF: Protein, fatty-filled bullous elevation of the nonpigmented outermost ciliary epithelium of pars plana, due to fluid leak from blood vessels.

    H21.351   Exudative cyst of pars plana, right eye
    H21.352   Exudative cyst of pars plana, left eye
    H21.353   Exudative cyst of pars plana, bilateral
    H21.359   Exudative cyst of pars plana, unspecified eye

✓5ᵗʰ **H21.4**   **Pupillary membranes**

    Iris bombé
    Pupillary occlusion
    Pupillary seclusion
    EXCLUDES 1   congenital pupillary membranes (Q13.8)

    H21.40   Pupillary membranes, unspecified eye
    H21.41   Pupillary membranes, right eye
    H21.42   Pupillary membranes, left eye
    H21.43   Pupillary membranes, bilateral

✓5ᵗʰ **H21.5**   **Other and unspecified adhesions and disruptions of iris and ciliary body**

    EXCLUDES 1   corectopia (Q13.2)

    ✓6ᵗʰ **H21.50**   Unspecified adhesions of iris

        Synechia (iris) NOS

        H21.501   Unspecified adhesions of iris, right eye
        H21.502   Unspecified adhesions of iris, left eye
        H21.503   Unspecified adhesions of iris, bilateral
        H21.509   Unspecified adhesions of iris and ciliary body, unspecified eye

    ✓6ᵗʰ **H21.51**   Anterior synechiae (iris)

        H21.511   Anterior synechiae (iris), right eye
        H21.512   Anterior synechiae (iris), left eye
        H21.513   Anterior synechiae (iris), bilateral
        H21.519   Anterior synechiae (iris), unspecified eye

    ✓6ᵗʰ **H21.52**   Goniosynechiae

        H21.521   Goniosynechiae, right eye
        H21.522   Goniosynechiae, left eye
        H21.523   Goniosynechiae, bilateral
        H21.529   Goniosynechiae, unspecified eye

    ✓6ᵗʰ **H21.53**   Iridodialysis

        H21.531   Iridodialysis, right eye
        H21.532   Iridodialysis, left eye
        H21.533   Iridodialysis, bilateral
        H21.539   Iridodialysis, unspecified eye

    ✓6ᵗʰ **H21.54**   Posterior synechiae (iris)

        H21.541   Posterior synechiae (iris), right eye
        H21.542   Posterior synechiae (iris), left eye
        H21.543   Posterior synechiae (iris), bilateral
        H21.549   Posterior synechiae (iris), unspecified eye

    ✓6ᵗʰ **H21.55**   Recession of chamber angle

        H21.551   Recession of chamber angle, right eye
        H21.552   Recession of chamber angle, left eye
        H21.553   Recession of chamber angle, bilateral
        H21.559   Recession of chamber angle, unspecified eye

    ✓6ᵗʰ **H21.56**   Pupillary abnormalities

        Deformed pupil
        Ectopic pupil
        Rupture of sphincter, pupil
        EXCLUDES 1   congenital deformity of pupil (Q13.2-)

        H21.561   Pupillary abnormality, right eye
        H21.562   Pupillary abnormality, left eye
        H21.563   Pupillary abnormality, bilateral
        H21.569   Pupillary abnormality, unspecified eye

✓5ᵗʰ **H21.8**   **Other specified disorders of iris and ciliary body**

    H21.81   Floppy iris syndrome

        Intraoperative floppy iris syndrome (IFIS)
        Use additional code for adverse effect, if applicable, to identify drug (T36-T50 with fifth or sixth character 5)

    H21.82   Plateau iris syndrome (post-iridectomy) (postprocedural)

    H21.89   Other specified disorders of iris and ciliary body

H21.9   Unspecified disorder of iris and ciliary body

H22   *Disorders of iris and ciliary body in diseases classified elsewhere*

    Code first underlying disease, such as:
    gout (M1A.-, M10.-)
    leprosy (A30.-)
    parasitic disease (B89)

Disorders of lens (H25-H28)

✓4ᵗʰ **H25**   **Age-related cataract**

    Senile cataract
    EXCLUDES 2   capsular glaucoma with pseudoexfoliation of lens (H40.1-)

Cataracts

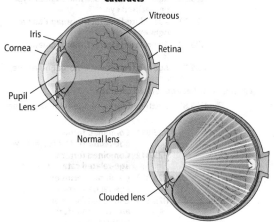

Normal lens

Clouded lens

Lens affected by cataracts

    ✓5ᵗʰ **H25.0**   Age-related incipient cataract

        ✓6ᵗʰ **H25.01**   Cortical age-related cataract

            H25.011   Cortical age-related cataract, right eye   A
            H25.012   Cortical age-related cataract, left eye   A
            H25.013   Cortical age-related cataract, bilateral   A
            H25.019   Cortical age-related cataract, unspecified eye   A

        ✓6ᵗʰ **H25.03**   Anterior subcapsular polar age-related cataract

            H25.031   Anterior subcapsular polar age-related cataract, right eye   A
            H25.032   Anterior subcapsular polar age-related cataract, left eye   A
            H25.033   Anterior subcapsular polar age-related cataract, bilateral   A
            H25.039   Anterior subcapsular polar age-related cataract, unspecified eye   A

        ✓6ᵗʰ **H25.04**   Posterior subcapsular polar age-related cataract

            H25.041   Posterior subcapsular polar age-related cataract, right eye   A
            H25.042   Posterior subcapsular polar age-related cataract, left eye   A
            H25.043   Posterior subcapsular polar age-related cataract, bilateral   A
            H25.049   Posterior subcapsular polar age-related cataract, unspecified eye   A

        ✓6ᵗʰ **H25.09**   Other age-related incipient cataract

            Coronary age-related cataract
            Punctate age-related cataract
            Water clefts

            H25.091   Other age-related incipient cataract, right eye   A
            H25.092   Other age-related incipient cataract, left eye   A
            H25.093   Other age-related incipient cataract, bilateral   A
            H25.099   Other age-related incipient cataract, unspecified eye   A

✓ Additional Character Required   ✓x7ᵗʰ Placeholder Alert   Manifestation   Unspecified Dx   ►◄ Revised Text   ● New Code   ▲ Revised Title

ICD-10-CM 2020   597

√5ᵗʰ **H25.1** Age-related nuclear cataract

    Cataracta brunescens

    Nuclear sclerosis cataract

    AHA: 2019,2Q,31; 2016,1Q,32

    H25.10 Age-related nuclear cataract, unspecified eye   [A]

    H25.11 Age-related nuclear cataract, right eye   [A]

    H25.12 Age-related nuclear cataract, left eye   [A]

    H25.13 Age-related nuclear cataract, bilateral   [A]

√5ᵗʰ **H25.2** Age-related cataract, morgagnian type

    Age-related hypermature cataract

    H25.20 Age-related cataract, morgagnian type, unspecified eye   [A]

    H25.21 Age-related cataract, morgagnian type, right eye   [A]

    H25.22 Age-related cataract, morgagnian type, left eye   [A]

    H25.23 Age-related cataract, morgagnian type, bilateral   [A]

√5ᵗʰ **H25.8** Other age-related cataract

    √6ᵗʰ **H25.81** Combined forms of age-related cataract

        AHA: 2019,2Q,30

        H25.811 Combined forms of age-related cataract, right eye   [A]

        H25.812 Combined forms of age-related cataract, left eye   [A]

        H25.813 Combined forms of age-related cataract, bilateral   [A]

        H25.819 Combined forms of age-related cataract, unspecified eye   [A]

    H25.89 Other age-related cataract   [A]

    H25.9 Unspecified age-related cataract   [A]

√4ᵗʰ **H26** Other cataract

    EXCLUDES 1   congenital cataract (Q12.0)

    √5ᵗʰ **H26.0** Infantile and juvenile cataract

        √6ᵗʰ **H26.00** Unspecified infantile and juvenile cataract

            H26.001 Unspecified infantile and juvenile cataract, right eye   [P]

            H26.002 Unspecified infantile and juvenile cataract, left eye   [P]

            H26.003 Unspecified infantile and juvenile cataract, bilateral   [P]

            H26.009 Unspecified infantile and juvenile cataract, unspecified eye   [P]

        √6ᵗʰ **H26.01** Infantile and juvenile cortical, lamellar, or zonular cataract

            H26.011 Infantile and juvenile cortical, lamellar, or zonular cataract, right eye   [P]

            H26.012 Infantile and juvenile cortical, lamellar, or zonular cataract, left eye   [P]

            H26.013 Infantile and juvenile cortical, lamellar, or zonular cataract, bilateral   [P]

            H26.019 Infantile and juvenile cortical, lamellar, or zonular cataract, unspecified eye   [P]

        √6ᵗʰ **H26.03** Infantile and juvenile nuclear cataract

            H26.031 Infantile and juvenile nuclear cataract, right eye   [P]

            H26.032 Infantile and juvenile nuclear cataract, left eye   [P]

            H26.033 Infantile and juvenile nuclear cataract, bilateral   [P]

            H26.039 Infantile and juvenile nuclear cataract, unspecified eye   [P]

        √6ᵗʰ **H26.04** Anterior subcapsular polar infantile and juvenile cataract

            H26.041 Anterior subcapsular polar infantile and juvenile cataract, right eye   [P]

            H26.042 Anterior subcapsular polar infantile and juvenile cataract, left eye   [P]

            H26.043 Anterior subcapsular polar infantile and juvenile cataract, bilateral   [P]

            H26.049 Anterior subcapsular polar infantile and juvenile cataract, unspecified eye   [P]

        √6ᵗʰ **H26.05** Posterior subcapsular polar infantile and juvenile cataract

            H26.051 Posterior subcapsular polar infantile and juvenile cataract, right eye   [P]

            H26.052 Posterior subcapsular polar infantile and juvenile cataract, left eye   [P]

            H26.053 Posterior subcapsular polar infantile and juvenile cataract, bilateral   [P]

            H26.059 Posterior subcapsular polar infantile and juvenile cataract, unspecified eye   [P]

        √6ᵗʰ **H26.06** Combined forms of infantile and juvenile cataract

            H26.061 Combined forms of infantile and juvenile cataract, right eye   [P]

            H26.062 Combined forms of infantile and juvenile cataract, left eye   [P]

            H26.063 Combined forms of infantile and juvenile cataract, bilateral   [P]

            H26.069 Combined forms of infantile and juvenile cataract, unspecified eye   [P]

        H26.09 Other infantile and juvenile cataract   [P]

    √5ᵗʰ **H26.1** Traumatic cataract

        Use additional code (Chapter 20) to identify external cause

        √6ᵗʰ **H26.10** Unspecified traumatic cataract

            H26.101 Unspecified traumatic cataract, right eye

            H26.102 Unspecified traumatic cataract, left eye

            H26.103 Unspecified traumatic cataract, bilateral

            H26.109 Unspecified traumatic cataract, unspecified eye

        √6ᵗʰ **H26.11** Localized traumatic opacities

            H26.111 Localized traumatic opacities, right eye

            H26.112 Localized traumatic opacities, left eye

            H26.113 Localized traumatic opacities, bilateral

            H26.119 Localized traumatic opacities, unspecified eye

        √6ᵗʰ **H26.12** Partially resolved traumatic cataract

            H26.121 Partially resolved traumatic cataract, right eye

            H26.122 Partially resolved traumatic cataract, left eye

            H26.123 Partially resolved traumatic cataract, bilateral

            H26.129 Partially resolved traumatic cataract, unspecified eye

        √6ᵗʰ **H26.13** Total traumatic cataract

            H26.131 Total traumatic cataract, right eye

            H26.132 Total traumatic cataract, left eye

            H26.133 Total traumatic cataract, bilateral

            H26.139 Total traumatic cataract, unspecified eye

    √5ᵗʰ **H26.2** Complicated cataract

        H26.20 Unspecified complicated cataract

            Cataracta complicata NOS

        √6ᵗʰ **H26.21** Cataract with neovascularization

            Code also associated condition, such as:

                chronic iridocyclitis (H20.1-)

            H26.211 Cataract with neovascularization, right eye

            H26.212 Cataract with neovascularization, left eye

            H26.213 Cataract with neovascularization, bilateral

            H26.219 Cataract with neovascularization, unspecified eye

        √6ᵗʰ **H26.22** Cataract secondary to ocular disorders (degenerative) (inflammatory)

            Code also associated ocular disorder

            H26.221 Cataract secondary to ocular disorders (degenerative) (inflammatory), right eye

[N] Newborn: 0   [P] Pediatric: 0-17   [M] Maternity: 12-55   [A] Adult: 15-124   [CH] Comorbidity High   [CL] Comorbidity Low   [NCDx] Noncancer Dx   [PDx] Primary Dx

598   ICD-10-CM 2020

           H26.222 **Cataract secondary to ocular disorders (degenerative) (inflammatory),** left **eye**

           H26.223 **Cataract secondary to ocular disorders (degenerative) (inflammatory),** bilateral

           H26.229 **Cataract secondary to ocular disorders (degenerative) (inflammatory), unspecified eye**

    ✓6ᵗʰ **H26.23** Glaucomatous flecks (subcapsular)

         Code first underlying glaucoma (H40-H42)

           H26.231 **Glaucomatous flecks (subcapsular),** right **eye**

           H26.232 **Glaucomatous flecks (subcapsular),** left **eye**

           H26.233 **Glaucomatous flecks (subcapsular),** bilateral

           H26.239 **Glaucomatous flecks (subcapsular), unspecified eye**

   ✓5ᵗʰ **H26.3** Drug-induced **cataract**

         Toxic cataract

         Use additional code for adverse effect, if applicable, to identify drug (T36-T50 with fifth or sixth character 5)

         H26.30 **Drug-induced cataract, unspecified eye**

         H26.31 **Drug-induced cataract,** right **eye**

         H26.32 **Drug-induced cataract,** left **eye**

         H26.33 **Drug-induced cataract,** bilateral

   ✓5ᵗʰ **H26.4** Secondary **cataract**

         H26.40 **Unspecified secondary cataract**

    ✓6ᵗʰ **H26.41** Soemmering's ring

           H26.411 **Soemmering's ring,** right **eye**

           H26.412 **Soemmering's ring,** left **eye**

           H26.413 **Soemmering's ring,** bilateral

           H26.419 **Soemmering's ring, unspecified eye**

    ✓6ᵗʰ **H26.49** Other secondary cataract

           AHA: 2018,2Q,14

           H26.491 **Other secondary cataract,** right **eye**

           H26.492 **Other secondary cataract,** left **eye**

           H26.493 **Other secondary cataract,** bilateral

           H26.499 **Other secondary cataract, unspecified eye**

   H26.8 Other specified cataract

   H26.9 Unspecified cataract

✓4ᵗʰ **H27** Other disorders of lens

    EXCLUDES 1   *congenital lens malformations (Q12.-)*

                   mechanical complications of intraocular lens implant (T85.2)

                   pseudophakia (Z96.1)

   ✓5ᵗʰ **H27.0** Aphakia

         Acquired absence of lens

         Acquired aphakia

         Aphakia due to trauma

       EXCLUDES 1   *cataract extraction status (Z98.4-)*

                     congenital absence of lens (Q12.3)

                     congenital aphakia (Q12.3)

         H27.00 **Aphakia, unspecified eye**

         H27.01 **Aphakia,** right **eye**

         H27.02 **Aphakia,** left **eye**

         H27.03 **Aphakia,** bilateral

   ✓5ᵗʰ **H27.1** Dislocation of lens

         H27.10 **Unspecified dislocation of lens**

    ✓6ᵗʰ **H27.11** Subluxation of lens

           H27.111 **Subluxation of lens,** right **eye**

           H27.112 **Subluxation of lens,** left **eye**

           H27.113 **Subluxation of lens,** bilateral

           H27.119 **Subluxation of lens, unspecified eye**

    ✓6ᵗʰ **H27.12** Anterior dislocation of lens

           H27.121 **Anterior dislocation of lens,** right **eye**

           H27.122 **Anterior dislocation of lens,** left **eye**

           H27.123 **Anterior dislocation of lens,** bilateral

           H27.129 **Anterior dislocation of lens, unspecified eye**

    ✓6ᵗʰ **H27.13** Posterior dislocation of lens

           H27.131 **Posterior dislocation of lens,** right **eye**

           H27.132 **Posterior dislocation of lens,** left **eye**

           H27.133 **Posterior dislocation of lens,** bilateral

           H27.139 **Posterior dislocation of lens, unspecified eye**

   H27.8 Other specified disorders of lens

   H27.9 Unspecified disorder of lens

H28 *Cataract in diseases classified elsewhere*

         Code first underlying disease, such as:

           hypoparathyroidism (E20.-)

           myotonia (G71.1-)

           myxedema (E03.-)

           protein-calorie malnutrition (E40-E46)

       EXCLUDES 1   *cataract in diabetes mellitus (E08.36, E09.36, E10.36, E11.36, E13.36)*

Disorders of choroid and retina (H30-H36)

✓4ᵗʰ **H30** Chorioretinal inflammation

   ✓5ᵗʰ **H30.0** Focal chorioretinal inflammation

         Focal chorioretinitis

         Focal choroiditis

         Focal retinitis

         Focal retinochoroiditis

    ✓6ᵗʰ **H30.00** Unspecified focal chorioretinal inflammation

           Focal chorioretinitis NOS

           Focal choroiditis NOS

           Focal retinitis NOS

           Focal retinochoroiditis NOS

           H30.001 **Unspecified focal chorioretinal inflammation,** right **eye**

           H30.002 **Unspecified focal chorioretinal inflammation,** left **eye**

           H30.003 **Unspecified focal chorioretinal inflammation,** bilateral

           H30.009 **Unspecified focal chorioretinal inflammation, unspecified eye**

    ✓6ᵗʰ **H30.01** Focal chorioretinal inflammation, juxtapapillary

           H30.011 **Focal chorioretinal inflammation, juxtapapillary,** right **eye**

           H30.012 **Focal chorioretinal inflammation, juxtapapillary,** left **eye**

           H30.013 **Focal chorioretinal inflammation, juxtapapillary,** bilateral

           H30.019 **Focal chorioretinal inflammation, juxtapapillary, unspecified eye**

    ✓6ᵗʰ **H30.02** Focal chorioretinal inflammation of posterior pole

           H30.021 **Focal chorioretinal inflammation of posterior pole,** right **eye**

           H30.022 **Focal chorioretinal inflammation of posterior pole,** left **eye**

           H30.023 **Focal chorioretinal inflammation of posterior pole,** bilateral

           H30.029 **Focal chorioretinal inflammation of posterior pole, unspecified eye**

    ✓6ᵗʰ **H30.03** Focal chorioretinal inflammation, peripheral

           H30.031 **Focal chorioretinal inflammation, peripheral,** right **eye**

           H30.032 **Focal chorioretinal inflammation, peripheral,** left **eye**

           H30.033 **Focal chorioretinal inflammation, peripheral,** bilateral

           H30.039 **Focal chorioretinal inflammation, peripheral, unspecified eye**

    ✓6ᵗʰ **H30.04** Focal chorioretinal inflammation, macular or paramacular

           H30.041 **Focal chorioretinal inflammation, macular or paramacular,** right **eye**

           H30.042 **Focal chorioretinal inflammation, macular or paramacular,** left **eye**

           H30.043 **Focal chorioretinal inflammation, macular or paramacular,** bilateral

           H30.049 **Focal chorioretinal inflammation, macular or paramacular, unspecified eye**

✓ Additional Character Required   ✓x7ᵗʰ Placeholder Alert   Manifestation   Unspecified Dx   ▶◀ Revised Text   ● New Code   ▲ Revised Title

ICD-10-CM 2020   **599**

✓5th **H30.1** Disseminated **chorioretinal inflammation**
    Disseminated chorioretinitis
    Disseminated choroiditis
    Disseminated retinitis
    Disseminated retinochoroiditis
    EXCLUDES 2   exudative retinopathy (H35.02-)

✓6th **H30.10** **Unspecified disseminated chorioretinal inflammation**
    Disseminated chorioretinitis NOS
    Disseminated choroiditis NOS
    Disseminated retinitis NOS
    Disseminated retinochoroiditis NOS

    H30.101 Unspecified disseminated chorioretinal inflammation, right eye
    H30.102 Unspecified disseminated chorioretinal inflammation, left eye
    H30.103 Unspecified disseminated chorioretinal inflammation, bilateral
    H30.109 Unspecified disseminated chorioretinal inflammation, unspecified eye

✓6th **H30.11** **Disseminated chorioretinal inflammation of posterior pole**
    H30.111 Disseminated chorioretinal inflammation of posterior pole, right eye
    H30.112 Disseminated chorioretinal inflammation of posterior pole, left eye
    H30.113 Disseminated chorioretinal inflammation of posterior pole, bilateral
    H30.119 Disseminated chorioretinal inflammation of posterior pole, unspecified eye

✓6th **H30.12** **Disseminated chorioretinal inflammation, peripheral**
    H30.121 Disseminated chorioretinal inflammation, peripheral right eye
    H30.122 Disseminated chorioretinal inflammation, peripheral, left eye
    H30.123 Disseminated chorioretinal inflammation, peripheral, bilateral
    H30.129 Disseminated chorioretinal inflammation, peripheral, unspecified eye

✓6th **H30.13** **Disseminated chorioretinal inflammation, generalized**
    H30.131 Disseminated chorioretinal inflammation, generalized, right eye
    H30.132 Disseminated chorioretinal inflammation, generalized, left eye
    H30.133 Disseminated chorioretinal inflammation, generalized, bilateral
    H30.139 Disseminated chorioretinal inflammation, generalized, unspecified eye

✓6th **H30.14** **Acute posterior multifocal placoid pigment epitheliopathy**
    H30.141 Acute posterior multifocal placoid pigment epitheliopathy, right eye
    H30.142 Acute posterior multifocal placoid pigment epitheliopathy, left eye
    H30.143 Acute posterior multifocal placoid pigment epitheliopathy, bilateral
    H30.149 Acute posterior multifocal placoid pigment epitheliopathy, unspecified eye

✓5th **H30.2** Posterior cyclitis
    Pars planitis
    H30.20 Posterior cyclitis, unspecified eye
    H30.21 Posterior cyclitis, right eye
    H30.22 Posterior cyclitis, left eye
    H30.23 Posterior cyclitis, bilateral

✓5th **H30.8** Other chorioretinal inflammations
✓6th **H30.81** Harada's disease
    H30.811 Harada's disease, right eye
    H30.812 Harada's disease, left eye
    H30.813 Harada's disease, bilateral
    H30.819 Harada's disease, unspecified eye
✓6th **H30.89** Other chorioretinal inflammations
    H30.891 Other chorioretinal inflammations, right eye
    H30.892 Other chorioretinal inflammations, left eye
    H30.893 Other chorioretinal inflammations, bilateral
    H30.899 Other chorioretinal inflammations, unspecified eye

✓5th **H30.9** **Unspecified chorioretinal inflammation**
    Chorioretinitis NOS
    Choroiditis NOS
    Neuroretinitis NOS
    Retinitis NOS
    Retinochoroiditis NOS
    H30.90 Unspecified chorioretinal inflammation, unspecified eye
    H30.91 Unspecified chorioretinal inflammation, right eye
    H30.92 Unspecified chorioretinal inflammation, left eye
    H30.93 Unspecified chorioretinal inflammation, bilateral

✓4th **H31** **Other disorders of choroid**
✓5th **H31.0** Chorioretinal scars
    EXCLUDES 2   postsurgical chorioretinal scars (H59.81-)
✓6th **H31.00** **Unspecified chorioretinal scars**
    H31.001 Unspecified chorioretinal scars, right eye
    H31.002 Unspecified chorioretinal scars, left eye
    H31.003 Unspecified chorioretinal scars, bilateral
    H31.009 Unspecified chorioretinal scars, unspecified eye

✓6th **H31.01** **Macula scars of posterior pole (postinflammatory) (post-traumatic)**
    EXCLUDES 1   postprocedural choriorentinal scar (H59.81-)
    H31.011 Macula scars of posterior pole (postinflammatory) (post-traumatic), right eye
    H31.012 Macula scars of posterior pole (postinflammatory) (post-traumatic), left eye
    H31.013 Macula scars of posterior pole (postinflammatory) (post-traumatic), bilateral
    H31.019 Macula scars of posterior pole (postinflammatory) (post-traumatic), unspecified eye

✓6th **H31.02** **Solar retinopathy**
    H31.021 Solar retinopathy, right eye
    H31.022 Solar retinopathy, left eye
    H31.023 Solar retinopathy, bilateral
    H31.029 Solar retinopathy, unspecified eye

✓6th **H31.09** **Other chorioretinal scars**
    H31.091 Other chorioretinal scars, right eye
    H31.092 Other chorioretinal scars, left eye
    H31.093 Other chorioretinal scars, bilateral
    H31.099 Other chorioretinal scars, unspecified eye

✓5th **H31.1** Choroidal degeneration
    EXCLUDES 2   angioid streaks of macula (H35.33)
✓6th **H31.10** **Unspecified choroidal degeneration**
    Choroidal sclerosis NOS
    H31.101 Choroidal degeneration, unspecified, right eye
    H31.102 Choroidal degeneration, unspecified, left eye
    H31.103 Choroidal degeneration, unspecified, bilateral
    H31.109 Choroidal degeneration, unspecified, unspecified eye

✓6th **H31.11** Age-related choroidal atrophy
    H31.111 Age-related choroidal atrophy, right eye   A
    H31.112 Age-related choroidal atrophy, left eye   A
    H31.113 Age-related choroidal atrophy, bilateral   A
    H31.119 Age-related choroidal atrophy, unspecified eye   A

✓6th **H31.12** Diffuse secondary atrophy of choroid
    H31.121 Diffuse secondary atrophy of choroid, right eye
    H31.122 Diffuse secondary atrophy of choroid, left eye
    H31.123 Diffuse secondary atrophy of choroid, bilateral
    H31.129 Diffuse secondary atrophy of choroid, unspecified eye

√5ᵗʰ **H31.2 Hereditary choroidal dystrophy**

     EXCLUDES 2   *hyperornithinemia (E72.4)*
                   ornithinemia (E72.4)

    H31.20 Hereditary choroidal dystrophy, unspecified
    H31.21 Choroideremia
    H31.22 Choroidal dystrophy (central areolar) (generalized) (peripapillary)
    H31.23 Gyrate atrophy, choroid
    H31.29 Other hereditary choroidal dystrophy

√5ᵗʰ **H31.3 Choroidal hemorrhage and rupture**

    √6ᵗʰ **H31.30 Unspecified choroidal hemorrhage**
        H31.301 Unspecified choroidal hemorrhage, right eye
        H31.302 Unspecified choroidal hemorrhage, left eye
        H31.303 Unspecified choroidal hemorrhage, bilateral
        H31.309 Unspecified choroidal hemorrhage, unspecified eye

    √6ᵗʰ **H31.31 Expulsive choroidal hemorrhage**
        H31.311 Expulsive choroidal hemorrhage, right eye
        H31.312 Expulsive choroidal hemorrhage, left eye
        H31.313 Expulsive choroidal hemorrhage, bilateral
        H31.319 Expulsive choroidal hemorrhage, unspecified eye

    √6ᵗʰ **H31.32 Choroidal rupture**
        H31.321 Choroidal rupture, right eye
        H31.322 Choroidal rupture, left eye
        H31.323 Choroidal rupture, bilateral
        H31.329 Choroidal rupture, unspecified eye

√5ᵗʰ **H31.4 Choroidal detachment**

    √6ᵗʰ **H31.40 Unspecified choroidal detachment**
        H31.401 Unspecified choroidal detachment, right eye
        H31.402 Unspecified choroidal detachment, left eye
        H31.403 Unspecified choroidal detachment, bilateral
        H31.409 Unspecified choroidal detachment, unspecified eye

    √6ᵗʰ **H31.41 Hemorrhagic choroidal detachment**
        H31.411 Hemorrhagic choroidal detachment, right eye
        H31.412 Hemorrhagic choroidal detachment, left eye
        H31.413 Hemorrhagic choroidal detachment, bilateral
        H31.419 Hemorrhagic choroidal detachment, unspecified eye

    √6ᵗʰ **H31.42 Serous choroidal detachment**
        H31.421 Serous choroidal detachment, right eye
        H31.422 Serous choroidal detachment, left eye
        H31.423 Serous choroidal detachment, bilateral
        H31.429 Serous choroidal detachment, unspecified eye

    H31.8 Other specified disorders of choroid
    H31.9 Unspecified disorder of choroid

H32 **Chorioretinal disorders in diseases classified elsewhere**

    Code first underlying disease, such as:
      congenital toxoplasmosis (P37.1)
      histoplasmosis (B39.-)
      leprosy (A30.-)
     EXCLUDES 1 *chorioretinitis (in):*
               toxoplasmosis (acquired) (B58.01)
               tuberculosis (A18.53)

√4ᵗʰ **H33 Retinal detachments and breaks**

    EXCLUDES 1 *detachment of retinal pigment epithelium (H35.72-, H35.73-)*

Retinal Detachment

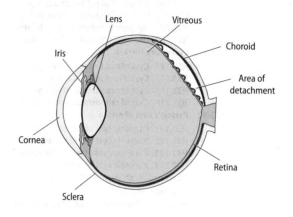

Lens — Vitreous — Choroid — Area of detachment — Iris — Cornea — Sclera — Retina

√5ᵗʰ **H33.0 Retinal detachment with retinal break**

    Rhegmatogenous retinal detachment
     EXCLUDES 1 *serous retinal detachment (without retinal break) (H33.2-)*

    √6ᵗʰ **H33.00 Unspecified retinal detachment with retinal break**
        H33.001 Unspecified retinal detachment with retinal break, right eye
        H33.002 Unspecified retinal detachment with retinal break, left eye
        H33.003 Unspecified retinal detachment with retinal break, bilateral
        H33.009 Unspecified retinal detachment with retinal break, unspecified eye

    √6ᵗʰ **H33.01 Retinal detachment with single break**
        H33.011 Retinal detachment with single break, right eye
        H33.012 Retinal detachment with single break, left eye
        H33.013 Retinal detachment with single break, bilateral
        H33.019 Retinal detachment with single break, unspecified eye

    √6ᵗʰ **H33.02 Retinal detachment with multiple breaks**
        H33.021 Retinal detachment with multiple breaks, right eye
        H33.022 Retinal detachment with multiple breaks, left eye
        H33.023 Retinal detachment with multiple breaks, bilateral
        H33.029 Retinal detachment with multiple breaks, unspecified eye

    √6ᵗʰ **H33.03 Retinal detachment with giant retinal tear**
        H33.031 Retinal detachment with giant retinal tear, right eye
        H33.032 Retinal detachment with giant retinal tear, left eye
        H33.033 Retinal detachment with giant retinal tear, bilateral
        H33.039 Retinal detachment with giant retinal tear, unspecified eye

    √6ᵗʰ **H33.04 Retinal detachment with retinal dialysis**
        H33.041 Retinal detachment with retinal dialysis, right eye
        H33.042 Retinal detachment with retinal dialysis, left eye
        H33.043 Retinal detachment with retinal dialysis, bilateral
        H33.049 Retinal detachment with retinal dialysis, unspecified eye

    √6ᵗʰ **H33.05 Total retinal detachment**
        H33.051 Total retinal detachment, right eye
        H33.052 Total retinal detachment, left eye
        H33.053 Total retinal detachment, bilateral
        H33.059 Total retinal detachment, unspecified eye

√5ᵗʰ H33.1 Retinoschisis and retinal cysts

> **EXCLUDES 1**   congenital retinoschisis (Q14.1)
> microcystoid degeneration of retina (H35.42-)

    √6ᵗʰ H33.10 Unspecified retinoschisis

        H33.101 Unspecified retinoschisis, right eye
        H33.102 Unspecified retinoschisis, left eye
        H33.103 Unspecified retinoschisis, bilateral
        H33.109 Unspecified retinoschisis, unspecified eye

    √6ᵗʰ H33.11 Cyst of ora serrata

        H33.111 Cyst of ora serrata, right eye
        H33.112 Cyst of ora serrata, left eye
        H33.113 Cyst of ora serrata, bilateral
        H33.119 Cyst of ora serrata, unspecified eye

    √6ᵗʰ H33.12 Parasitic cyst of retina

        H33.121 Parasitic cyst of retina, right eye
        H33.122 Parasitic cyst of retina, left eye
        H33.123 Parasitic cyst of retina, bilateral
        H33.129 Parasitic cyst of retina, unspecified eye

    √6ᵗʰ H33.19 Other retinoschisis and retinal cysts

      Pseudocyst of retina

        H33.191 Other retinoschisis and retinal cysts, right eye
        H33.192 Other retinoschisis and retinal cysts, left eye
        H33.193 Other retinoschisis and retinal cysts, bilateral
        H33.199 Other retinoschisis and retinal cysts, unspecified eye

√5ᵗʰ H33.2 Serous retinal detachment

    Retinal detachment NOS
    Retinal detachment without retinal break

> **EXCLUDES 1**   central serous chorioretinopathy (H35.71-)

    H33.20 Serous retinal detachment, unspecified eye
    H33.21 Serous retinal detachment, right eye
    H33.22 Serous retinal detachment, left eye
    H33.23 Serous retinal detachment, bilateral

√5ᵗʰ H33.3 Retinal breaks without detachment

> **EXCLUDES 1**   chorioretinal scars after surgery for detachment (H59.81-)
> peripheral retinal degeneration without break (H35.4-)

    √6ᵗʰ H33.30 Unspecified retinal break

        H33.301 Unspecified retinal break, right eye
        H33.302 Unspecified retinal break, left eye
        H33.303 Unspecified retinal break, bilateral
        H33.309 Unspecified retinal break, unspecified eye

    √6ᵗʰ H33.31 Horseshoe tear of retina without detachment

      Operculum of retina without detachment

        H33.311 Horseshoe tear of retina without detachment, right eye
        H33.312 Horseshoe tear of retina without detachment, left eye
        H33.313 Horseshoe tear of retina without detachment, bilateral
        H33.319 Horseshoe tear of retina without detachment, unspecified eye

    √6ᵗʰ H33.32 Round hole of retina without detachment

        H33.321 Round hole, right eye
        H33.322 Round hole, left eye
        H33.323 Round hole, bilateral
        H33.329 Round hole, unspecified eye

    √6ᵗʰ H33.33 Multiple defects of retina without detachment

        H33.331 Multiple defects of retina without detachment, right eye
        H33.332 Multiple defects of retina without detachment, left eye
        H33.333 Multiple defects of retina without detachment, bilateral
        H33.339 Multiple defects of retina without detachment, unspecified eye

√5ᵗʰ H33.4 Traction detachment of retina

    Proliferative vitreo-retinopathy with retinal detachment

    H33.40 Traction detachment of retina, unspecified eye
    H33.41 Traction detachment of retina, right eye
    H33.42 Traction detachment of retina, left eye
    H33.43 Traction detachment of retina, bilateral

H33.8 Other retinal detachments

√4ᵗʰ H34 Retinal vascular occlusions

> **EXCLUDES 1**   amaurosis fugax (G45.3)

    √5ᵗʰ H34.0 Transient retinal artery occlusion

        H34.00 Transient retinal artery occlusion, unspecified eye
        H34.01 Transient retinal artery occlusion, right eye
        H34.02 Transient retinal artery occlusion, left eye
        H34.03 Transient retinal artery occlusion, bilateral

    √5ᵗʰ H34.1 Central retinal artery occlusion

        H34.10 Central retinal artery occlusion, unspecified eye
        H34.11 Central retinal artery occlusion, right eye
        H34.12 Central retinal artery occlusion, left eye
        H34.13 Central retinal artery occlusion, bilateral

    √5ᵗʰ H34.2 Other retinal artery occlusions

    √6ᵗʰ H34.21 Partial retinal artery occlusion

      Hollenhorst's plaque
      Retinal microembolism

        H34.211 Partial retinal artery occlusion, right eye
        H34.212 Partial retinal artery occlusion, left eye
        H34.213 Partial retinal artery occlusion, bilateral
        H34.219 Partial retinal artery occlusion, unspecified eye

    √6ᵗʰ H34.23 Retinal artery branch occlusion

        H34.231 Retinal artery branch occlusion, right eye
        H34.232 Retinal artery branch occlusion, left eye
        H34.233 Retinal artery branch occlusion, bilateral
        H34.239 Retinal artery branch occlusion, unspecified eye

    √5ᵗʰ H34.8 Other retinal vascular occlusions

      AHA: 2016,4Q,19

    √6ᵗʰ H34.81 Central retinal vein occlusion

> One of the following 7th characters is to be assigned to codes in subcategory H34.81 to designate the severity of the occlusion:
> 0   with macular edema
> 1   with retinal neovascularization
> 2   stable
>   old central retinal vein occlusion

        √7ᵗʰ H34.811 Central retinal vein occlusion, right eye
        √7ᵗʰ H34.812 Central retinal vein occlusion, left eye
        √7ᵗʰ H34.813 Central retinal vein occlusion, bilateral
        √7ᵗʰ H34.819 Central retinal vein occlusion, unspecified eye

    √6ᵗʰ H34.82 Venous engorgement

      Incipient retinal vein occlusion
      Partial retinal vein occlusion

        H34.821 Venous engorgement, right eye
        H34.822 Venous engorgement, left eye
        H34.823 Venous engorgement, bilateral
        H34.829 Venous engorgement, unspecified eye

    √6ᵗʰ H34.83 Tributary (branch) retinal vein occlusion

> One of the following 7th characters is to be assigned to codes in subcategory H34.83 to designate the severity of the occlusion:
> 0   with macular edema
> 1   with retinal neovascularization
> 2   stable
>   old tributary (branch) retinal vein occlusion

        √7ᵗʰ H34.831 Tributary (branch) retinal vein occlusion, right eye
        √7ᵗʰ H34.832 Tributary (branch) retinal vein occlusion, left eye
        √7ᵗʰ H34.833 Tributary (branch) retinal vein occlusion, bilateral
        √7ᵗʰ H34.839 Tributary (branch) retinal vein occlusion, unspecified eye

    H34.9 Unspecified retinal vascular occlusion

√4ᵗʰ H35 Other retinal disorders

> **EXCLUDES 2**   diabetic retinal disorders (E08.311-E08.359, E09.311-E09.359, E10.311-E10.359, E11.311-E11.359, E13.311-E13.359)

    √5ᵗʰ H35.0 Background retinopathy and retinal vascular changes

      Code also any associated hypertension (I10.-)

        H35.00 Unspecified background retinopathy

N Newborn: 0   **P** Pediatric: 0-17   **M** Maternity: 12-55   **A** Adult: 15-124   **CH** Comorbidity High   **CL** Comorbidity Low   **NC Dx** Noncancer Dx   **PDx** Primary Dx

602   ICD-10-CM 2020

√6ᵗʰ **H35.01 Changes in retinal vascular appearance**
Retinal vascular sheathing
H35.011 Changes in retinal vascular appearance, right eye
H35.012 Changes in retinal vascular appearance, left eye
H35.013 Changes in retinal vascular appearance, bilateral
H35.019 Changes in retinal vascular appearance, unspecified eye

√6ᵗʰ **H35.02 Exudative retinopathy**
Coats retinopathy
H35.021 Exudative retinopathy, right eye
H35.022 Exudative retinopathy, left eye
H35.023 Exudative retinopathy, bilateral
H35.029 Exudative retinopathy, unspecified eye

√6ᵗʰ **H35.03 Hypertensive retinopathy**
H35.031 Hypertensive retinopathy, right eye
H35.032 Hypertensive retinopathy, left eye
H35.033 Hypertensive retinopathy, bilateral
H35.039 Hypertensive retinopathy, unspecified eye

√6ᵗʰ **H35.04 Retinal micro-aneurysms, unspecified**
H35.041 Retinal micro-aneurysms, unspecified, right eye
H35.042 Retinal micro-aneurysms, unspecified, left eye
H35.043 Retinal micro-aneurysms, unspecified, bilateral
H35.049 Retinal micro-aneurysms, unspecified, unspecified eye

√6ᵗʰ **H35.05 Retinal neovascularization, unspecified**
H35.051 Retinal neovascularization, unspecified, right eye
H35.052 Retinal neovascularization, unspecified, left eye
H35.053 Retinal neovascularization, unspecified, bilateral
H35.059 Retinal neovascularization, unspecified, unspecified eye

√6ᵗʰ **H35.06 Retinal vasculitis**
Eales disease
Retinal perivasculitis
DEF: Sight-threatening intraocular inflammation of the retinal blood vessels that causes minimal, partial, or even complete blindness.
H35.061 Retinal vasculitis, right eye
H35.062 Retinal vasculitis, left eye
H35.063 Retinal vasculitis, bilateral
H35.069 Retinal vasculitis, unspecified eye

√6ᵗʰ **H35.07 Retinal telangiectasis**
H35.071 Retinal telangiectasis, right eye
H35.072 Retinal telangiectasis, left eye
H35.073 Retinal telangiectasis, bilateral
H35.079 Retinal telangiectasis, unspecified eye

H35.09 Other intraretinal microvascular abnormalities
Retinal varices

√5ᵗʰ **H35.1 Retinopathy of prematurity**
√6ᵗʰ **H35.10 Retinopathy of prematurity, unspecified**
Retinopathy of prematurity NOS
H35.101 Retinopathy of prematurity, unspecified, right eye
H35.102 Retinopathy of prematurity, unspecified, left eye
H35.103 Retinopathy of prematurity, unspecified, bilateral
H35.109 Retinopathy of prematurity, unspecified, unspecified eye

√6ᵗʰ **H35.11 Retinopathy of prematurity, stage 0**
H35.111 Retinopathy of prematurity, stage 0, right eye
H35.112 Retinopathy of prematurity, stage 0, left eye
H35.113 Retinopathy of prematurity, stage 0, bilateral
H35.119 Retinopathy of prematurity, stage 0, unspecified eye

√6ᵗʰ **H35.12 Retinopathy of prematurity, stage 1**
H35.121 Retinopathy of prematurity, stage 1, right eye
H35.122 Retinopathy of prematurity, stage 1, left eye
H35.123 Retinopathy of prematurity, stage 1, bilateral
H35.129 Retinopathy of prematurity, stage 1, unspecified eye

√6ᵗʰ **H35.13 Retinopathy of prematurity, stage 2**
H35.131 Retinopathy of prematurity, stage 2, right eye
H35.132 Retinopathy of prematurity, stage 2, left eye
H35.133 Retinopathy of prematurity, stage 2, bilateral
H35.139 Retinopathy of prematurity, stage 2, unspecified eye

√6ᵗʰ **H35.14 Retinopathy of prematurity, stage 3**
H35.141 Retinopathy of prematurity, stage 3, right eye
H35.142 Retinopathy of prematurity, stage 3, left eye
H35.143 Retinopathy of prematurity, stage 3, bilateral
H35.149 Retinopathy of prematurity, stage 3, unspecified eye

√6ᵗʰ **H35.15 Retinopathy of prematurity, stage 4**
H35.151 Retinopathy of prematurity, stage 4, right eye
H35.152 Retinopathy of prematurity, stage 4, left eye
H35.153 Retinopathy of prematurity, stage 4, bilateral
H35.159 Retinopathy of prematurity, stage 4, unspecified eye

√6ᵗʰ **H35.16 Retinopathy of prematurity, stage 5**
H35.161 Retinopathy of prematurity, stage 5, right eye
H35.162 Retinopathy of prematurity, stage 5, left eye
H35.163 Retinopathy of prematurity, stage 5, bilateral
H35.169 Retinopathy of prematurity, stage 5, unspecified eye

√6ᵗʰ **H35.17 Retrolental fibroplasia**
H35.171 Retrolental fibroplasia, right eye
H35.172 Retrolental fibroplasia, left eye
H35.173 Retrolental fibroplasia, bilateral
H35.179 Retrolental fibroplasia, unspecified eye

√5ᵗʰ **H35.2 Other non-diabetic proliferative retinopathy**
Proliferative vitreo-retinopathy
EXCLUDES 1   *proliferative vitreo-retinopathy with retinal detachment (H33.4-)*
H35.20 Other non-diabetic proliferative retinopathy, unspecified eye
H35.21 Other non-diabetic proliferative retinopathy, right eye
H35.22 Other non-diabetic proliferative retinopathy, left eye
H35.23 Other non-diabetic proliferative retinopathy, bilateral

√5ᵗʰ **H35.3 Degeneration of macula and posterior pole**
H35.30 Unspecified macular degeneration   CL A
Age-related macular degeneration

✓6ᵗʰ H35.31 Nonexudative age-related macular degeneration

Atrophic age-related macular degeneration
Dry age-related macular degeneration
AHA: 2016,4Q,20-21

One of the following 7th characters is to be assigned to each code in subcategory H35.31 to designate the stage of the disease:
Ø stage unspecified
1 early dry stage
2 intermediate dry stage
3 advanced atrophic without subfoveal involvement
　advanced dry stage
4 advanced atrophic with subfoveal involvement

✓7ᵗʰ H35.311 Nonexudative age-related macular degeneration, right eye CL A

✓7ᵗʰ H35.312 Nonexudative age-related macular degeneration, left eye CL A

✓7ᵗʰ H35.313 Nonexudative age-related macular degeneration, bilateral CL A

✓7ᵗʰ H35.319 Nonexudative age-related macular degeneration, unspecified eye A

✓6ᵗʰ H35.32 Exudative age-related macular degeneration

Wet age-related macular degeneration
AHA: 2016,4Q,20-21

One of the following 7th characters is to be assigned to each code in subcategory H35.32 to designate the stage of the disease:
Ø stage unspecified
1 with active choroidal neovascularization
2 with inactive choroidal neovascularization
　with involuted or regressed neovascularization
3 with inactive scar

✓7ᵗʰ H35.321 Exudative age-related macular degeneration, right eye CL A

✓7ᵗʰ H35.322 Exudative age-related macular degeneration, left eye CL A

✓7ᵗʰ H35.323 Exudative age-related macular degeneration, bilateral CL A

✓7ᵗʰ H35.329 Exudative age-related macular degeneration, unspecified eye A

H35.33 Angioid streaks of macula
DEF: Degeneration of the choroid; characterized by broad, irregular, dark brown streaks radiating from optic disc; occurs with pseudoxanthoma elasticum or Paget's disease.

✓6ᵗʰ H35.34 Macular cyst, hole, or pseudohole

H35.341 Macular cyst, hole, or pseudohole, right eye CL

H35.342 Macular cyst, hole, or pseudohole, left eye CL

H35.343 Macular cyst, hole, or pseudohole, bilateral CL

H35.349 Macular cyst, hole, or pseudohole, unspecified eye

✓6ᵗʰ H35.35 Cystoid macular degeneration

EXCLUDES 1 cystoid macular edema following cataract surgery (H59.Ø3-)

H35.351 Cystoid macular degeneration, right eye CL

H35.352 Cystoid macular degeneration, left eye CL

H35.353 Cystoid macular degeneration, bilateral CL

H35.359 Cystoid macular degeneration, unspecified eye

✓6ᵗʰ H35.36 Drusen (degenerative) of macula

AHA: 2017,1Q,51; 2016,4Q,21

H35.361 Drusen (degenerative) of macula, right eye CL

H35.362 Drusen (degenerative) of macula, left eye CL

H35.363 Drusen (degenerative) of macula, bilateral CL

H35.369 Drusen (degenerative) of macula, unspecified eye

✓6ᵗʰ H35.37 Puckering of macula

H35.371 Puckering of macula, right eye CL

H35.372 Puckering of macula, left eye CL

H35.373 Puckering of macula, bilateral CL

H35.379 Puckering of macula, unspecified eye

✓6ᵗʰ H35.38 Toxic maculopathy

Code first poisoning due to drug or toxin, if applicable (T36-T65 with fifth or sixth character 1-4 or 6)
Use additional code for adverse effect, if applicable, to identify drug (T36-T5Ø with fifth or sixth character 5)

H35.381 Toxic maculopathy, right eye CL

H35.382 Toxic maculopathy, left eye CL

H35.383 Toxic maculopathy, bilateral CL

H35.389 Toxic maculopathy, unspecified eye

✓5ᵗʰ H35.4 Peripheral retinal degeneration

EXCLUDES 1 hereditary retinal degeneration (dystrophy) (H35.5-)
peripheral retinal degeneration with retinal break (H33.3-)

H35.4Ø Unspecified peripheral retinal degeneration

✓6ᵗʰ H35.41 Lattice degeneration of retina

Palisade degeneration of retina
DEF: Degeneration of the retina, often bilateral, that is usually benign. It is characterized by lines intersecting at irregular intervals in the peripheral retina. Retinal thinning and retinal holes may occur.

H35.411 Lattice degeneration of retina, right eye

H35.412 Lattice degeneration of retina, left eye

H35.413 Lattice degeneration of retina, bilateral

H35.419 Lattice degeneration of retina, unspecified eye

✓6ᵗʰ H35.42 Microcystoid degeneration of retina

H35.421 Microcystoid degeneration of retina, right eye

H35.422 Microcystoid degeneration of retina, left eye

H35.423 Microcystoid degeneration of retina, bilateral

H35.429 Microcystoid degeneration of retina, unspecified eye

✓6ᵗʰ H35.43 Paving stone degeneration of retina

H35.431 Paving stone degeneration of retina, right eye

H35.432 Paving stone degeneration of retina, left eye

H35.433 Paving stone degeneration of retina, bilateral

H35.439 Paving stone degeneration of retina, unspecified eye

✓6ᵗʰ H35.44 Age-related reticular degeneration of retina

H35.441 Age-related reticular degeneration of retina, right eye A

H35.442 Age-related reticular degeneration of retina, left eye A

H35.443 Age-related reticular degeneration of retina, bilateral A

H35.449 Age-related reticular degeneration of retina, unspecified eye A

✓6ᵗʰ H35.45 Secondary pigmentary degeneration

H35.451 Secondary pigmentary degeneration, right eye

H35.452 Secondary pigmentary degeneration, left eye

H35.453 Secondary pigmentary degeneration, bilateral

H35.459 Secondary pigmentary degeneration, unspecified eye

✓6ᵗʰ H35.46 Secondary vitreoretinal degeneration

H35.461 Secondary vitreoretinal degeneration, right eye

    H35.462 Secondary vitreoretinal degeneration, left eye

    H35.463 Secondary vitreoretinal degeneration, bilateral

    H35.469 Secondary vitreoretinal degeneration, unspecified eye

√5ᵗʰ **H35.5** **Hereditary retinal dystrophy**

    EXCLUDES 1 dystrophies primarily involving Bruch's membrane (H31.1-)

  H35.50 **Unspecified hereditary retinal dystrophy**

  H35.51 **Vitreoretinal dystrophy**

  H35.52 **Pigmentary retinal dystrophy**
    Albipunctate retinal dystrophy
    Retinitis pigmentosa
    Tapetoretinal dystrophy

  H35.53 **Other dystrophies primarily involving the sensory retina**
    Stargardt's disease

  H35.54 **Dystrophies primarily involving the retinal pigment epithelium**
    Vitelliform retinal dystrophy

√5ᵗʰ **H35.6** **Retinal hemorrhage**

  H35.60 **Retinal hemorrhage, unspecified eye**

  H35.61 **Retinal hemorrhage, right eye**

  H35.62 **Retinal hemorrhage, left eye**

  H35.63 **Retinal hemorrhage, bilateral**

√5ᵗʰ **H35.7** **Separation of retinal layers**

    EXCLUDES 1 retinal detachment (serous) (H33.2-)
      rhegmatogenous retinal detachment (H33.0-)

  H35.70 **Unspecified separation of retinal layers**

√6ᵗʰ H35.71 **Central serous chorioretinopathy**

    H35.711 **Central serous chorioretinopathy, right eye**

    H35.712 **Central serous chorioretinopathy, left eye**

    H35.713 **Central serous chorioretinopathy, bilateral**

    H35.719 **Central serous chorioretinopathy, unspecified eye**

√6ᵗʰ H35.72 **Serous detachment of retinal pigment epithelium**

    H35.721 **Serous detachment of retinal pigment epithelium, right eye**

    H35.722 **Serous detachment of retinal pigment epithelium, left eye**

    H35.723 **Serous detachment of retinal pigment epithelium, bilateral**

    H35.729 **Serous detachment of retinal pigment epithelium, unspecified eye**

√6ᵗʰ H35.73 **Hemorrhagic detachment of retinal pigment epithelium**

    H35.731 **Hemorrhagic detachment of retinal pigment epithelium, right eye**

    H35.732 **Hemorrhagic detachment of retinal pigment epithelium, left eye**

    H35.733 **Hemorrhagic detachment of retinal pigment epithelium, bilateral**

    H35.739 **Hemorrhagic detachment of retinal pigment epithelium, unspecified eye**

√5ᵗʰ **H35.8** **Other specified retinal disorders**

    EXCLUDES 2 retinal hemorrhage (H35.6-)

  H35.81 **Retinal edema**
    Retinal cotton wool spots

  H35.82 **Retinal ischemia**

  H35.89 **Other specified retinal disorders**

  H35.9 **Unspecified retinal disorder**

H36 *Retinal disorders in diseases classified elsewhere*
    Code first underlying disease, such as:
      lipid storage disorders (E75.-)
      sickle-cell disorders (D57.-)
    EXCLUDES 1 arteriosclerotic retinopathy (H35.0-)
      diabetic retinopathy (E08.3-, E09.3-, E10.3-, E11.3-, E13.3-)

Glaucoma (H40-H42)

√4ᵗʰ **H40** **Glaucoma**

    EXCLUDES 1 absolute glaucoma (H44.51-)
      congenital glaucoma (Q15.0)
      traumatic glaucoma due to birth injury (P15.3)

Open Angle/Angle Closure Glaucoma

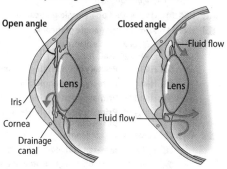

√5ᵗʰ **H40.0** **Glaucoma suspect**

  √6ᵗʰ H40.00 **Preglaucoma, unspecified**

    H40.001 **Preglaucoma, unspecified, right eye**

    H40.002 **Preglaucoma, unspecified, left eye**

    H40.003 **Preglaucoma, unspecified, bilateral**

    H40.009 **Preglaucoma, unspecified, unspecified eye**

  √6ᵗʰ H40.01 **Open angle with borderline findings, low risk**
    Open angle, low risk

    H40.011 **Open angle with borderline findings, low risk, right eye**

    H40.012 **Open angle with borderline findings, low risk, left eye**

    H40.013 **Open angle with borderline findings, low risk, bilateral**

    H40.019 **Open angle with borderline findings, low risk, unspecified eye**

  √6ᵗʰ H40.02 **Open angle with borderline findings, high risk**
    Open angle, high risk

    H40.021 **Open angle with borderline findings, high risk, right eye**

    H40.022 **Open angle with borderline findings, high risk, left eye**

    H40.023 **Open angle with borderline findings, high risk, bilateral**

    H40.029 **Open angle with borderline findings, high risk, unspecified eye**

  √6ᵗʰ H40.03 **Anatomical narrow angle**
    Primary angle closure suspect

    H40.031 **Anatomical narrow angle, right eye**

    H40.032 **Anatomical narrow angle, left eye**

    H40.033 **Anatomical narrow angle, bilateral**

    H40.039 **Anatomical narrow angle, unspecified eye**

  √6ᵗʰ H40.04 **Steroid responder**

    H40.041 **Steroid responder, right eye**

    H40.042 **Steroid responder, left eye**

    H40.043 **Steroid responder, bilateral**

    H40.049 **Steroid responder, unspecified eye**

  √6ᵗʰ H40.05 **Ocular hypertension**

    H40.051 **Ocular hypertension, right eye**

    H40.052 **Ocular hypertension, left eye**

    H40.053 **Ocular hypertension, bilateral**

    H40.059 **Ocular hypertension, unspecified eye**

  √6ᵗʰ H40.06 **Primary angle closure without glaucoma damage**

    H40.061 **Primary angle closure without glaucoma damage, right eye**

    H40.062 **Primary angle closure without glaucoma damage, left eye**

    H40.063 **Primary angle closure without glaucoma damage, bilateral**

    H40.069 **Primary angle closure without glaucoma damage, unspecified eye**

✔ Additional Character Required   ✔×7ᵗʰ Placeholder Alert   Manifestation   Unspecified Dx   ▶◀ Revised Text   ● New Code   ▲ Revised Title

ICD-10-CM 2020   **605**

✓5ᵗʰ **H40.1 Open-angle glaucoma**

One of the following 7th characters is to be assigned to each code in subcategories H40.10, H40.11, H40.12, H40.13, and H40.14 to designate the stage of glaucoma.
- Ø stage unspecified
- 1 mild stage
- 2 moderate stage
- 3 severe stage
- 4 indeterminate stage

✓x7ᵗʰ **H40.10 Unspecified open-angle glaucoma**

✓6ᵗʰ **H40.11 Primary open-angle glaucoma**

Chronic simple glaucoma
AHA: 2016,4Q,22

     ✓7ᵗʰ **H40.111 Primary open-angle glaucoma, right eye**

     ✓7ᵗʰ **H40.112 Primary open-angle glaucoma, left eye**

     ✓7ᵗʰ **H40.113 Primary open-angle glaucoma, bilateral**

     ✓7ᵗʰ **H40.119 Primary open-angle glaucoma, unspecified eye**

✓6ᵗʰ **H40.12 Low-tension glaucoma**

     ✓7ᵗʰ **H40.121 Low-tension glaucoma, right eye**

     ✓7ᵗʰ **H40.122 Low-tension glaucoma, left eye**

     ✓7ᵗʰ **H40.123 Low-tension glaucoma, bilateral**

     ✓7ᵗʰ **H40.129 Low-tension glaucoma, unspecified eye**

✓6ᵗʰ **H40.13 Pigmentary glaucoma**

     ✓7ᵗʰ **H40.131 Pigmentary glaucoma, right eye**

     ✓7ᵗʰ **H40.132 Pigmentary glaucoma, left eye**

     ✓7ᵗʰ **H40.133 Pigmentary glaucoma, bilateral**

     ✓7ᵗʰ **H40.139 Pigmentary glaucoma, unspecified eye**

✓6ᵗʰ **H40.14 Capsular glaucoma with pseudoexfoliation of lens**

     ✓7ᵗʰ **H40.141 Capsular glaucoma with pseudoexfoliation of lens, right eye**

     ✓7ᵗʰ **H40.142 Capsular glaucoma with pseudoexfoliation of lens, left eye**

     ✓7ᵗʰ **H40.143 Capsular glaucoma with pseudoexfoliation of lens, bilateral**

     ✓7ᵗʰ **H40.149 Capsular glaucoma with pseudoexfoliation of lens, unspecified eye**

✓6ᵗʰ **H40.15 Residual stage of open-angle glaucoma**

     H40.151 Residual stage of open-angle glaucoma, right eye

     H40.152 Residual stage of open-angle glaucoma, left eye

     H40.153 Residual stage of open-angle glaucoma, bilateral

     H40.159 Residual stage of open-angle glaucoma, unspecified eye

✓5ᵗʰ **H40.2 Primary angle-closure glaucoma**

EXCLUDES 1   aqueous misdirection (H40.83-)
           malignant glaucoma (H40.83-)

One of the following 7th characters is to be assigned to code H40.20 and H40.22- to designate the stage of glaucoma.
- Ø stage unspecified
- 1 mild stage
- 2 moderate stage
- 3 severe stage
- 4 indeterminate stage

✓x7ᵗʰ **H40.20 Unspecified primary angle-closure glaucoma**

✓6ᵗʰ **H40.21 Acute angle-closure glaucoma**

Acute angle-closure glaucoma attack
Acute angle-closure glaucoma crisis

     H40.211 Acute angle-closure glaucoma, right eye

     H40.212 Acute angle-closure glaucoma, left eye

     H40.213 Acute angle-closure glaucoma, bilateral

     H40.219 Acute angle-closure glaucoma, unspecified eye

✓6ᵗʰ **H40.22 Chronic angle-closure glaucoma**

Chronic primary angle closure glaucoma

     ✓7ᵗʰ **H40.221 Chronic angle-closure glaucoma, right eye**

     ✓7ᵗʰ **H40.222 Chronic angle-closure glaucoma, left eye**

     ✓7ᵗʰ **H40.223 Chronic angle-closure glaucoma, bilateral**

     ✓7ᵗʰ **H40.229 Chronic angle-closure glaucoma, unspecified eye**

✓6ᵗʰ **H40.23 Intermittent angle-closure glaucoma**

     H40.231 Intermittent angle-closure glaucoma, right eye

     H40.232 Intermittent angle-closure glaucoma, left eye

     H40.233 Intermittent angle-closure glaucoma, bilateral

     H40.239 Intermittent angle-closure glaucoma, unspecified eye

✓6ᵗʰ **H40.24 Residual stage of angle-closure glaucoma**

     H40.241 Residual stage of angle-closure glaucoma, right eye

     H40.242 Residual stage of angle-closure glaucoma, left eye

     H40.243 Residual stage of angle-closure glaucoma, bilateral

     H40.249 Residual stage of angle-closure glaucoma, unspecified eye

✓5ᵗʰ **H40.3 Glaucoma secondary to eye trauma**

Code also underlying condition

One of the following 7th characters is to be assigned to each code in subcategory H40.3- to designate the stage of glaucoma.
- Ø stage unspecified
- 1 mild stage
- 2 moderate stage
- 3 severe stage
- 4 indeterminate stage

✓x7ᵗʰ **H40.30 Glaucoma secondary to eye trauma, unspecified eye**

✓x7ᵗʰ **H40.31 Glaucoma secondary to eye trauma, right eye**

✓x7ᵗʰ **H40.32 Glaucoma secondary to eye trauma, left eye**

✓x7ᵗʰ **H40.33 Glaucoma secondary to eye trauma, bilateral**

✓5ᵗʰ **H40.4 Glaucoma secondary to eye inflammation**

Code also underlying condition

One of the following 7th characters is to be assigned to each code in subcategory H40.4- to designate the stage of glaucoma.
- Ø stage unspecified
- 1 mild stage
- 2 moderate stage
- 3 severe stage
- 4 indeterminate stage

✓x7ᵗʰ **H40.40 Glaucoma secondary to eye inflammation, unspecified eye**

✓x7ᵗʰ **H40.41 Glaucoma secondary to eye inflammation, right eye**

✓x7ᵗʰ **H40.42 Glaucoma secondary to eye inflammation, left eye**

✓x7ᵗʰ **H40.43 Glaucoma secondary to eye inflammation, bilateral**

✓5ᵗʰ **H40.5 Glaucoma secondary to other eye disorders**

Code also underlying eye disorder

One of the following 7th characters is to be assigned to each code in subcategory H40.5- to designate the stage of glaucoma.
- Ø stage unspecified
- 1 mild stage
- 2 moderate stage
- 3 severe stage
- 4 indeterminate stage

✓x7ᵗʰ **H40.50 Glaucoma secondary to other eye disorders, unspecified eye**

✓x7ᵗʰ **H40.51 Glaucoma secondary to other eye disorders, right eye**

✓x7ᵗʰ **H40.52 Glaucoma secondary to other eye disorders, left eye**

✓x7ᵗʰ **H40.53 Glaucoma secondary to other eye disorders, bilateral**

Ⓝ Newborn: 0   Ⓟ Pediatric: 0-17   Ⓜ Maternity: 12-55   Ⓐ Adult: 15-124   CH Comorbidity High   CL Comorbidity Low   NCDx Noncancer Dx   PDx Primary Dx

606   ICD-10-CM 2020

√5ᵗʰ **H40.6** **Glaucoma** secondary to **drugs**

> Use additional code for adverse effect, if applicable, to identify drug (T36-T50 with fifth or sixth character 5)
>
> One of the following 7th characters is to be assigned to each code in subcategory H40.6- to designate the stage of glaucoma
> 0   stage unspecified
> 1   mild stage
> 2   moderate stage
> 3   severe stage
> 4   indeterminate stage

√x7ᵗʰ **H40.60**   Glaucoma secondary to drugs, unspecified eye
√x7ᵗʰ **H40.61**   Glaucoma secondary to drugs, right eye
√x7ᵗʰ **H40.62**   Glaucoma secondary to drugs, left eye
√x7ᵗʰ **H40.63**   Glaucoma secondary to drugs, bilateral

√5ᵗʰ **H40.8** **Other glaucoma**

   √6ᵗʰ **H40.81**   **Glaucoma with** increased episcleral venous pressure

     H40.811   Glaucoma with increased episcleral venous pressure, right eye
     H40.812   Glaucoma with increased episcleral venous pressure, left eye
     H40.813   Glaucoma with increased episcleral venous pressure, bilateral
     H40.819   Glaucoma with increased episcleral venous pressure, unspecified eye

   √6ᵗʰ **H40.82**   **Hypersecretion glaucoma**

     H40.821   Hypersecretion glaucoma, right eye
     H40.822   Hypersecretion glaucoma, left eye
     H40.823   Hypersecretion glaucoma, bilateral
     H40.829   Hypersecretion glaucoma, unspecified eye

   √6ᵗʰ **H40.83**   **Aqueous misdirection**

     Malignant glaucoma
     H40.831   Aqueous misdirection, right eye
     H40.832   Aqueous misdirection, left eye
     H40.833   Aqueous misdirection, bilateral
     H40.839   Aqueous misdirection, unspecified eye

   H40.89   Other specified glaucoma

H40.9   **Unspecified glaucoma**

H42   *Glaucoma in diseases classified elsewhere*

> Code first underlying condition, such as:
> amyloidosis (E85.-)
> aniridia (Q13.1)
> glaucoma (in) diabetes mellitus (E08.39, E09.39, E10.39, E11.39, E13.39)
> Lowe's syndrome (E72.03)
> Reiger's anomaly (Q13.81)
> specified metabolic disorder (E70-E88)
>
> EXCLUDES 1   glaucoma (in) onchocerciasis (B73.02)
>   glaucoma (in) syphilis (A52.71)
>   glaucoma (in) tuberculous (A18.59)

Disorders of vitreous body and globe (H43-H44)

√4ᵗʰ **H43** **Disorders of vitreous body**

   √5ᵗʰ **H43.0**   **Vitreous** prolapse

> EXCLUDES 1   traumatic vitreous prolapse (S05.2-)
>   vitreous syndrome following cataract surgery (H59.0-)

     H43.00   Vitreous prolapse, unspecified eye
     H43.01   Vitreous prolapse, right eye
     H43.02   Vitreous prolapse, left eye
     H43.03   Vitreous prolapse, bilateral

   √5ᵗʰ **H43.1**   **Vitreous** hemorrhage

     H43.10   Vitreous hemorrhage, unspecified eye
     H43.11   Vitreous hemorrhage, right eye
     H43.12   Vitreous hemorrhage, left eye
     H43.13   Vitreous hemorrhage, bilateral

   √5ᵗʰ **H43.2**   **Crystalline deposits** in vitreous body

     H43.20   Crystalline deposits in vitreous body, unspecified eye
     H43.21   Crystalline deposits in vitreous body, right eye
     H43.22   Crystalline deposits in vitreous body, left eye
     H43.23   Crystalline deposits in vitreous body, bilateral

---

   √5ᵗʰ **H43.3**   **Other vitreous opacities**

   √6ᵗʰ **H43.31**   **Vitreous** membranes and strands

     H43.311   Vitreous membranes and strands, right eye
     H43.312   Vitreous membranes and strands, left eye
     H43.313   Vitreous membranes and strands, bilateral
     H43.319   Vitreous membranes and strands, unspecified eye

   √6ᵗʰ **H43.39**   **Other vitreous opacities**

     Vitreous floaters
     H43.391   Other vitreous opacities, right eye
     H43.392   Other vitreous opacities, left eye
     H43.393   Other vitreous opacities, bilateral
     H43.399   Other vitreous opacities, unspecified eye

   √5ᵗʰ **H43.8**   **Other disorders of vitreous body**

> EXCLUDES 1   proliferative vitreo-retinopathy with retinal detachment (H33.4-)
> EXCLUDES 2   vitreous abscess (H44.02-)

   √6ᵗʰ **H43.81**   **Vitreous** degeneration

     Vitreous detachment
     H43.811   Vitreous degeneration, right eye
     H43.812   Vitreous degeneration, left eye
     H43.813   Vitreous degeneration, bilateral
     H43.819   Vitreous degeneration, unspecified eye

   √6ᵗʰ **H43.82**   **Vitreomacular** adhesion

     Vitreomacular traction
     H43.821   Vitreomacular adhesion, right eye   Ⓐ
     H43.822   Vitreomacular adhesion, left eye   Ⓐ
     H43.823   Vitreomacular adhesion, bilateral   Ⓐ
     H43.829   Vitreomacular adhesion, unspecified eye   Ⓐ

     H43.89   Other disorders of vitreous body

   H43.9   **Unspecified disorder of vitreous body**

√4ᵗʰ **H44** **Disorders of globe**

> INCLUDES   disorders affecting multiple structures of eye

   √5ᵗʰ **H44.0**   **Purulent endophthalmitis**

> Use additional code to identify organism
> EXCLUDES 1   bleb associated endophthalmitis (H59.4-)

   √6ᵗʰ **H44.00**   **Unspecified purulent endophthalmitis**

     H44.001   Unspecified purulent endophthalmitis, right eye
     H44.002   Unspecified purulent endophthalmitis, left eye
     H44.003   Unspecified purulent endophthalmitis, bilateral
     H44.009   Unspecified purulent endophthalmitis, unspecified eye

   √6ᵗʰ **H44.01**   **Panophthalmitis (acute)**

     H44.011   Panophthalmitis (acute), right eye
     H44.012   Panophthalmitis (acute), left eye
     H44.013   Panophthalmitis (acute), bilateral
     H44.019   Panophthalmitis (acute), unspecified eye

   √6ᵗʰ **H44.02**   **Vitreous abscess (chronic)**

     H44.021   Vitreous abscess (chronic), right eye
     H44.022   Vitreous abscess (chronic), left eye
     H44.023   Vitreous abscess (chronic), bilateral
     H44.029   Vitreous abscess (chronic), unspecified eye

   √5ᵗʰ **H44.1**   **Other endophthalmitis**

> EXCLUDES 1   bleb associated endophthalmitis (H59.4-)
> EXCLUDES 2   ophthalmia nodosa (H16.2-)

   √6ᵗʰ **H44.11**   **Panuveitis**

     DEF: Inflammation of all layers of the uvea of the eye, including the choroid, iris, and ciliary body. It also typically involves the lens, retina, optic nerve, and vitreous and causes reduced vision or blindness.
     H44.111   Panuveitis, right eye
     H44.112   Panuveitis, left eye
     H44.113   Panuveitis, bilateral
     H44.119   Panuveitis, unspecified eye

   √6ᵗʰ **H44.12**   **Parasitic endophthalmitis, unspecified**

     H44.121   Parasitic endophthalmitis, unspecified, right eye

---

☑ Additional Character Required   √x7ᵗʰ Placeholder Alert   Manifestation   Unspecified Dx   ▶◀ Revised Text   ● New Code   ▲ Revised Title

ICD-10-CM 2020   **607**

Chapter 7. Diseases of the Eye and Adnexa

        H44.122 Parasitic endophthalmitis, unspecified, left eye

        H44.123 Parasitic endophthalmitis, unspecified, bilateral

        H44.129 Parasitic endophthalmitis, unspecified, unspecified eye

   ✓6ᵗʰ **H44.13** **Sympathetic uveitis**

        H44.131 Sympathetic uveitis, right eye

        H44.132 Sympathetic uveitis, left eye

        H44.133 Sympathetic uveitis, bilateral

        H44.139 Sympathetic uveitis, unspecified eye

     H44.19 **Other endophthalmitis**

  ✓5ᵗʰ **H44.2** **Degenerative myopia**

     Malignant myopia

     AHA: 2017,4Q,10-11

     H44.20 **Degenerative myopia, unspecified eye**

     H44.21 Degenerative myopia, right eye

     H44.22 Degenerative myopia, left eye

     H44.23 Degenerative myopia, bilateral

   ✓6ᵗʰ **H44.2A** **Degenerative myopia with choroidal neovascularization**

       Use additional code for any associated choroid disorders (H31.-)

        H44.2A1 Degenerative myopia with choroidal neovascularization, right eye

        H44.2A2 Degenerative myopia with choroidal neovascularization, left eye

        H44.2A3 Degenerative myopia with choroidal neovascularization, bilateral eye

        H44.2A9 Degenerative myopia with choroidal neovascularization, unspecified eye

   ✓6ᵗʰ **H44.2B** **Degenerative myopia with macular hole**

        H44.2B1 Degenerative myopia with macular hole, right eye

        H44.2B2 Degenerative myopia with macular hole, left eye

        H44.2B3 Degenerative myopia with macular hole, bilateral eye

        H44.2B9 Degenerative myopia with macular hole, unspecified eye

   ✓6ᵗʰ **H44.2C** **Degenerative myopia with retinal detachment**

       Use additional code to identify the retinal detachment (H33.-)

        H44.2C1 Degenerative myopia with retinal detachment, right eye

        H44.2C2 Degenerative myopia with retinal detachment, left eye

        H44.2C3 Degenerative myopia with retinal detachment, bilateral eye

        H44.2C9 Degenerative myopia with retinal detachment, unspecified eye

   ✓6ᵗʰ **H44.2D** **Degenerative myopia with foveoschisis**

        H44.2D1 Degenerative myopia with foveoschisis, right eye

        H44.2D2 Degenerative myopia with foveoschisis, left eye

        H44.2D3 Degenerative myopia with foveoschisis, bilateral eye

        H44.2D9 Degenerative myopia with foveoschisis, unspecified eye

   ✓6ᵗʰ **H44.2E** **Degenerative myopia with other maculopathy**

        H44.2E1 Degenerative myopia with other maculopathy, right eye

        H44.2E2 Degenerative myopia with other maculopathy, left eye

        H44.2E3 Degenerative myopia with other maculopathy, bilateral eye

        H44.2E9 Degenerative myopia with other maculopathy, unspecified eye

  ✓5ᵗʰ **H44.3** **Other and unspecified degenerative disorders of globe**

     H44.30 **Unspecified degenerative disorder of globe**

   ✓6ᵗʰ **H44.31** **Chalcosis**

        H44.311 Chalcosis, right eye

        H44.312 Chalcosis, left eye

        H44.313 Chalcosis, bilateral

        H44.319 Chalcosis, unspecified eye

   ✓6ᵗʰ **H44.32** **Siderosis of eye**

      DEF: Iron pigment deposits within tissue of the eyeball caused by high iron content of the blood. Symptoms include cataracts, rust-colored anterior subcapsular deposits, iris heterochromia, pupillary mydriasis, and depressed electroretinogram amplitudes.

        H44.321 Siderosis of eye, right eye

        H44.322 Siderosis of eye, left eye

        H44.323 Siderosis of eye, bilateral

        H44.329 Siderosis of eye, unspecified eye

   ✓6ᵗʰ **H44.39** **Other degenerative disorders of globe**

        H44.391 Other degenerative disorders of globe, right eye

        H44.392 Other degenerative disorders of globe, left eye

        H44.393 Other degenerative disorders of globe, bilateral

        H44.399 Other degenerative disorders of globe, unspecified eye

  ✓5ᵗʰ **H44.4** **Hypotony of eye**

     H44.40 **Unspecified hypotony of eye**

   ✓6ᵗʰ **H44.41** **Flat anterior chamber hypotony of eye**

        H44.411 Flat anterior chamber hypotony of right eye

        H44.412 Flat anterior chamber hypotony of left eye

        H44.413 Flat anterior chamber hypotony of eye, bilateral

        H44.419 Flat anterior chamber hypotony of unspecified eye

   ✓6ᵗʰ **H44.42** **Hypotony of eye due to ocular fistula**

        H44.421 Hypotony of right eye due to ocular fistula

        H44.422 Hypotony of left eye due to ocular fistula

        H44.423 Hypotony of eye due to ocular fistula, bilateral

        H44.429 Hypotony of unspecified eye due to ocular fistula

   ✓6ᵗʰ **H44.43** **Hypotony of eye due to other ocular disorders**

        H44.431 Hypotony of eye due to other ocular disorders, right eye

        H44.432 Hypotony of eye due to other ocular disorders, left eye

        H44.433 Hypotony of eye due to other ocular disorders, bilateral

        H44.439 Hypotony of eye due to other ocular disorders, unspecified eye

   ✓6ᵗʰ **H44.44** **Primary hypotony of eye**

        H44.441 Primary hypotony of right eye

        H44.442 Primary hypotony of left eye

        H44.443 Primary hypotony of eye, bilateral

        H44.449 Primary hypotony of unspecified eye

  ✓5ᵗʰ **H44.5** **Degenerated conditions of globe**

     H44.50 **Unspecified degenerated conditions of globe**

   ✓6ᵗʰ **H44.51** **Absolute glaucoma**

        H44.511 Absolute glaucoma, right eye

        H44.512 Absolute glaucoma, left eye

        H44.513 Absolute glaucoma, bilateral

        H44.519 Absolute glaucoma, unspecified eye

   ✓6ᵗʰ **H44.52** **Atrophy of globe**

      Phthisis bulbi

        H44.521 Atrophy of globe, right eye

        H44.522 Atrophy of globe, left eye

        H44.523 Atrophy of globe, bilateral

        H44.529 Atrophy of globe, unspecified eye

   ✓6ᵗʰ **H44.53** **Leucocoria**

        H44.531 Leucocoria, right eye

        H44.532 Leucocoria, left eye

        H44.533 Leucocoria, bilateral

        H44.539 Leucocoria, unspecified eye

Ⓝ Newborn: 0   Ⓟ Pediatric: 0-17   Ⓜ Maternity: 12-55   Ⓐ Adult: 15-124   **CH** Comorbidity High   **CL** Comorbidity Low   **NCDx** Noncancer Dx   **PDx** Primary Dx

608

ICD-10-CM 2020

✓5ᵗʰ **H44.6** **Retained (old) intraocular foreign body, magnetic**
Use additional code to identify magnetic foreign body (Z18.11)
> **EXCLUDES 1**   current intraocular foreign body (S05.-)
> **EXCLUDES 2**   retained foreign body in eyelid (H02.81-)
> retained (old) foreign body following penetrating wound of orbit (H05.5-)
> retained (old) intraocular foreign body, nonmagnetic (H44.7-)

✓6ᵗʰ **H44.60** **Unspecified retained (old) intraocular foreign body, magnetic**
- **H44.601** Unspecified retained (old) intraocular foreign body, magnetic, **right** eye
- **H44.602** Unspecified retained (old) intraocular foreign body, magnetic, **left** eye
- **H44.603** Unspecified retained (old) intraocular foreign body, magnetic, **bilateral**
- **H44.609** Unspecified retained (old) intraocular foreign body, magnetic, unspecified eye

✓6ᵗʰ **H44.61** **Retained (old) magnetic foreign body in anterior chamber**
- **H44.611** Retained (old) magnetic foreign body in anterior chamber, **right** eye
- **H44.612** Retained (old) magnetic foreign body in anterior chamber, **left** eye
- **H44.613** Retained (old) magnetic foreign body in anterior chamber, **bilateral**
- **H44.619** Retained (old) magnetic foreign body in anterior chamber, unspecified eye

✓6ᵗʰ **H44.62** **Retained (old) magnetic foreign body in iris or ciliary body**
- **H44.621** Retained (old) magnetic foreign body in iris or ciliary body, **right** eye
- **H44.622** Retained (old) magnetic foreign body in iris or ciliary body, **left** eye
- **H44.623** Retained (old) magnetic foreign body in iris or ciliary body, **bilateral**
- **H44.629** Retained (old) magnetic foreign body in iris or ciliary body, unspecified eye

✓6ᵗʰ **H44.63** **Retained (old) magnetic foreign body in lens**
- **H44.631** Retained (old) magnetic foreign body in lens, **right** eye
- **H44.632** Retained (old) magnetic foreign body in lens, **left** eye
- **H44.633** Retained (old) magnetic foreign body in lens, **bilateral**
- **H44.639** Retained (old) magnetic foreign body in lens, unspecified eye

✓6ᵗʰ **H44.64** **Retained (old) magnetic foreign body in posterior wall of globe**
- **H44.641** Retained (old) magnetic foreign body in posterior wall of globe, **right** eye
- **H44.642** Retained (old) magnetic foreign body in posterior wall of globe, **left** eye
- **H44.643** Retained (old) magnetic foreign body in posterior wall of globe, **bilateral**
- **H44.649** Retained (old) magnetic foreign body in posterior wall of globe, unspecified eye

✓6ᵗʰ **H44.65** **Retained (old) magnetic foreign body in vitreous body**
- **H44.651** Retained (old) magnetic foreign body in vitreous body, **right** eye
- **H44.652** Retained (old) magnetic foreign body in vitreous body, **left** eye
- **H44.653** Retained (old) magnetic foreign body in vitreous body, **bilateral**
- **H44.659** Retained (old) magnetic foreign body in vitreous body, unspecified eye

✓6ᵗʰ **H44.69** **Retained (old) intraocular foreign body, magnetic, in other or multiple sites**
- **H44.691** Retained (old) intraocular foreign body, magnetic, in other or multiple sites, **right** eye
- **H44.692** Retained (old) intraocular foreign body, magnetic, in other or multiple sites, **left** eye
- **H44.693** Retained (old) intraocular foreign body, magnetic, in other or multiple sites, **bilateral**
- **H44.699** Retained (old) intraocular foreign body, magnetic, in other or multiple sites, unspecified eye

✓5ᵗʰ **H44.7** **Retained (old) intraocular foreign body, nonmagnetic**
Use additional code to identify nonmagnetic foreign body (Z18.01-Z18.10, Z18.12, Z18.2-Z18.9)
> **EXCLUDES 1**   current intraocular foreign body (S05.-)
> **EXCLUDES 2**   retained foreign body in eyelid (H02.81-)
> retained (old) foreign body following penetrating wound of orbit (H05.5-)
> retained (old) intraocular foreign body, magnetic (H44.6-)

✓6ᵗʰ **H44.70** **Unspecified retained (old) intraocular foreign body, nonmagnetic**
- **H44.701** Unspecified retained (old) intraocular foreign body, nonmagnetic, **right** eye
- **H44.702** Unspecified retained (old) intraocular foreign body, nonmagnetic, **left** eye
- **H44.703** Unspecified retained (old) intraocular foreign body, nonmagnetic, **bilateral**
- **H44.709** Unspecified retained (old) intraocular foreign body, nonmagnetic, unspecified eye
    Retained (old) intraocular foreign body NOS

✓6ᵗʰ **H44.71** **Retained (nonmagnetic) (old) foreign body in anterior chamber**
- **H44.711** Retained (nonmagnetic) (old) foreign body in anterior chamber, **right** eye
- **H44.712** Retained (nonmagnetic) (old) foreign body in anterior chamber, **left** eye
- **H44.713** Retained (nonmagnetic) (old) foreign body in anterior chamber, **bilateral**
- **H44.719** Retained (nonmagnetic) (old) foreign body in anterior chamber, unspecified eye

✓6ᵗʰ **H44.72** **Retained (nonmagnetic) (old) foreign body in iris or ciliary body**
- **H44.721** Retained (nonmagnetic) (old) foreign body in iris or ciliary body, **right** eye
- **H44.722** Retained (nonmagnetic) (old) foreign body in iris or ciliary body, **left** eye
- **H44.723** Retained (nonmagnetic) (old) foreign body in iris or ciliary body, **bilateral**
- **H44.729** Retained (nonmagnetic) (old) foreign body in iris or ciliary body, unspecified eye

✓6ᵗʰ **H44.73** **Retained (nonmagnetic) (old) foreign body in lens**
- **H44.731** Retained (nonmagnetic) (old) foreign body in lens, **right** eye
- **H44.732** Retained (nonmagnetic) (old) foreign body in lens, **left** eye
- **H44.733** Retained (nonmagnetic) (old) foreign body in lens, **bilateral**
- **H44.739** Retained (nonmagnetic) (old) foreign body in lens, unspecified eye

✓6ᵗʰ **H44.74** **Retained (nonmagnetic) (old) foreign body in posterior wall of globe**
- **H44.741** Retained (nonmagnetic) (old) foreign body in posterior wall of globe, **right** eye
- **H44.742** Retained (nonmagnetic) (old) foreign body in posterior wall of globe, **left** eye
- **H44.743** Retained (nonmagnetic) (old) foreign body in posterior wall of globe, **bilateral**
- **H44.749** Retained (nonmagnetic) (old) foreign body in posterior wall of globe, unspecified eye

✓6ᵗʰ **H44.75** **Retained (nonmagnetic) (old) foreign body in vitreous body**
- **H44.751** Retained (nonmagnetic) (old) foreign body in vitreous body, **right** eye
- **H44.752** Retained (nonmagnetic) (old) foreign body in vitreous body, **left** eye
- **H44.753** Retained (nonmagnetic) (old) foreign body in vitreous body, **bilateral**
- **H44.759** Retained (nonmagnetic) (old) foreign body in vitreous body, unspecified eye

✓6ᵗʰ **H44.79** **Retained (old) intraocular foreign body, nonmagnetic, in other or multiple sites**
- **H44.791** Retained (old) intraocular foreign body, nonmagnetic, in other or multiple sites, **right** eye
- **H44.792** Retained (old) intraocular foreign body, nonmagnetic, in other or multiple sites, **left** eye

---

✔ Additional Character Required   ✓x7ᵗʰ Placeholder Alert   Manifestation   Unspecified Dx   ▶◀ Revised Text   ● New Code   ▲ Revised Title

H44.793 Retained (old) intraocular foreign body, nonmagnetic, in other or multiple sites, bilateral

H44.799 Retained (old) intraocular foreign body, nonmagnetic, in other or multiple sites, unspecified eye

✓5ᵗʰ **H44.8 Other disorders of globe**

✓6ᵗʰ **H44.81 Hemophthalmos**

DEF: Pool of blood within the eyeball, not from a current injury.

H44.811 Hemophthalmos, right eye
H44.812 Hemophthalmos, left eye
H44.813 Hemophthalmos, bilateral
H44.819 Hemophthalmos, unspecified eye

✓6ᵗʰ **H44.82 Luxation of globe**

H44.821 Luxation of globe, right eye
H44.822 Luxation of globe, left eye
H44.823 Luxation of globe, bilateral
H44.829 Luxation of globe, unspecified eye

H44.89 Other disorders of globe

H44.9 Unspecified disorder of globe

Disorders of optic nerve and visual pathways (H46-H47)

✓4ᵗʰ **H46 Optic neuritis**

EXCLUDES 2   ischemic optic neuropathy (H47.01-)
neuromyelitis optica [Devic] (G36.0)

✓5ᵗʰ **H46.0 Optic papillitis**

H46.00 Optic papillitis, unspecified eye
H46.01 Optic papillitis, right eye
H46.02 Optic papillitis, left eye
H46.03 Optic papillitis, bilateral

✓5ᵗʰ **H46.1 Retrobulbar neuritis**

Retrobulbar neuritis NOS
EXCLUDES 1   syphilitic retrobulbar neuritis (A52.15)

H46.10 Retrobulbar neuritis, unspecified eye
H46.11 Retrobulbar neuritis, right eye
H46.12 Retrobulbar neuritis, left eye
H46.13 Retrobulbar neuritis, bilateral

H46.2 Nutritional optic neuropathy

H46.3 Toxic optic neuropathy
Code first (T51-T65) to identify cause

H46.8 Other optic neuritis

H46.9 Unspecified optic neuritis

✓4ᵗʰ **H47 Other disorders of optic [2nd] nerve and visual pathways**

✓5ᵗʰ **H47.0 Disorders of optic nerve, not elsewhere classified**

✓6ᵗʰ **H47.01 Ischemic optic neuropathy**

H47.011 Ischemic optic neuropathy, right eye
H47.012 Ischemic optic neuropathy, left eye
H47.013 Ischemic optic neuropathy, bilateral
H47.019 Ischemic optic neuropathy, unspecified eye

✓6ᵗʰ **H47.02 Hemorrhage in optic nerve sheath**

H47.021 Hemorrhage in optic nerve sheath, right eye
H47.022 Hemorrhage in optic nerve sheath, left eye
H47.023 Hemorrhage in optic nerve sheath, bilateral
H47.029 Hemorrhage in optic nerve sheath, unspecified eye

✓6ᵗʰ **H47.03 Optic nerve hypoplasia**

H47.031 Optic nerve hypoplasia, right eye
H47.032 Optic nerve hypoplasia, left eye
H47.033 Optic nerve hypoplasia, bilateral
H47.039 Optic nerve hypoplasia, unspecified eye

✓6ᵗʰ **H47.09 Other disorders of optic nerve, not elsewhere classified**

Compression of optic nerve
H47.091 Other disorders of optic nerve, not elsewhere classified, right eye
H47.092 Other disorders of optic nerve, not elsewhere classified, left eye
H47.093 Other disorders of optic nerve, not elsewhere classified, bilateral
H47.099 Other disorders of optic nerve, not elsewhere classified, unspecified eye

✓5ᵗʰ **H47.1 Papilledema**

DEF: Swelling of the optic papilla, the raised area connected to the optic disk made up of nerves that enter the eyeball. It may be caused by increased intracranial pressure, decreased ocular pressure, or a retinal disorder.

H47.10 Unspecified papilledema
H47.11 Papilledema associated with increased intracranial pressure
H47.12 Papilledema associated with decreased ocular pressure
H47.13 Papilledema associated with retinal disorder

✓6ᵗʰ **H47.14 Foster-Kennedy syndrome**

H47.141 Foster-Kennedy syndrome, right eye
H47.142 Foster-Kennedy syndrome, left eye
H47.143 Foster-Kennedy syndrome, bilateral
H47.149 Foster-Kennedy syndrome, unspecified eye

✓5ᵗʰ **H47.2 Optic atrophy**

H47.20 Unspecified optic atrophy

✓6ᵗʰ **H47.21 Primary optic atrophy**

H47.211 Primary optic atrophy, right eye
H47.212 Primary optic atrophy, left eye
H47.213 Primary optic atrophy, bilateral
H47.219 Primary optic atrophy, unspecified eye

H47.22 Hereditary optic atrophy
Leber's optic atrophy

✓6ᵗʰ **H47.23 Glaucomatous optic atrophy**

H47.231 Glaucomatous optic atrophy, right eye
H47.232 Glaucomatous optic atrophy, left eye
H47.233 Glaucomatous optic atrophy, bilateral
H47.239 Glaucomatous optic atrophy, unspecified eye

✓6ᵗʰ **H47.29 Other optic atrophy**

Temporal pallor of optic disc
H47.291 Other optic atrophy, right eye
H47.292 Other optic atrophy, left eye
H47.293 Other optic atrophy, bilateral
H47.299 Other optic atrophy, unspecified eye

✓5ᵗʰ **H47.3 Other disorders of optic disc**

✓6ᵗʰ **H47.31 Coloboma of optic disc**

H47.311 Coloboma of optic disc, right eye
H47.312 Coloboma of optic disc, left eye
H47.313 Coloboma of optic disc, bilateral
H47.319 Coloboma of optic disc, unspecified eye

✓6ᵗʰ **H47.32 Drusen of optic disc**

H47.321 Drusen of optic disc, right eye
H47.322 Drusen of optic disc, left eye
H47.323 Drusen of optic disc, bilateral
H47.329 Drusen of optic disc, unspecified eye

✓6ᵗʰ **H47.33 Pseudopapilledema of optic disc**

H47.331 Pseudopapilledema of optic disc, right eye
H47.332 Pseudopapilledema of optic disc, left eye
H47.333 Pseudopapilledema of optic disc, bilateral
H47.339 Pseudopapilledema of optic disc, unspecified eye

✓6ᵗʰ **H47.39 Other disorders of optic disc**

H47.391 Other disorders of optic disc, right eye
H47.392 Other disorders of optic disc, left eye
H47.393 Other disorders of optic disc, bilateral
H47.399 Other disorders of optic disc, unspecified eye

✓5ᵗʰ **H47.4 Disorders of optic chiasm**

Code also underlying condition
H47.41 Disorders of optic chiasm in (due to) inflammatory disorders
H47.42 Disorders of optic chiasm in (due to) neoplasm
H47.43 Disorders of optic chiasm in (due to) vascular disorders
H47.49 Disorders of optic chiasm in (due to) other disorders

✓5ᵗʰ **H47.5 Disorders of other visual pathways**

Disorders of optic tracts, geniculate nuclei and optic radiations
Code also underlying condition

✓6ᵗʰ **H47.51 Disorders of visual pathways in (due to) inflammatory disorders**

H47.511 Disorders of visual pathways in (due to) inflammatory disorders, right side

---

Ⓝ Newborn: 0   Ⓟ Pediatric: 0-17   Ⓜ Maternity: 12-55   Ⓐ Adult: 15-124   CH Comorbidity High   CL Comorbidity Low   NCDx Noncancer Dx   PDx Primary Dx

610   ICD-10-CM 2020

H47.512 Disorders of visual pathways in (due to) inflammatory disorders, left side

H47.519 Disorders of visual pathways in (due to) inflammatory disorders, unspecified side

☑6ᵗʰ H47.52 Disorders of visual pathways in (due to) neoplasm

H47.521 Disorders of visual pathways in (due to) neoplasm, right side

H47.522 Disorders of visual pathways in (due to) neoplasm, left side

H47.529 Disorders of visual pathways in (due to) neoplasm, unspecified side

☑6ᵗʰ H47.53 Disorders of visual pathways in (due to) vascular disorders

H47.531 Disorders of visual pathways in (due to) vascular disorders, right side

H47.532 Disorders of visual pathways in (due to) vascular disorders, left side

H47.539 Disorders of visual pathways in (due to) vascular disorders, unspecified side

☑5ᵗʰ H47.6 Disorders of visual cortex

Code also underlying condition

EXCLUDES 1   injury to visual cortex ▶S04.04-◀

☑6ᵗʰ H47.61 Cortical blindness

H47.611 Cortical blindness, right side of brain

H47.612 Cortical blindness, left side of brain

H47.619 Cortical blindness, unspecified side of brain

☑6ᵗʰ H47.62 Disorders of visual cortex in (due to) inflammatory disorders

H47.621 Disorders of visual cortex in (due to) inflammatory disorders, right side of brain

H47.622 Disorders of visual cortex in (due to) inflammatory disorders, left side of brain

H47.629 Disorders of visual cortex in (due to) inflammatory disorders, unspecified side of brain

☑6ᵗʰ H47.63 Disorders of visual cortex in (due to) neoplasm

H47.631 Disorders of visual cortex in (due to) neoplasm, right side of brain

H47.632 Disorders of visual cortex in (due to) neoplasm, left side of brain

H47.639 Disorders of visual cortex in (due to) neoplasm, unspecified side of brain

☑6ᵗʰ H47.64 Disorders of visual cortex in (due to) vascular disorders

H47.641 Disorders of visual cortex in (due to) vascular disorders, right side of brain

H47.642 Disorders of visual cortex in (due to) vascular disorders, left side of brain

H47.649 Disorders of visual cortex in (due to) vascular disorders, unspecified side of brain

H47.9 Unspecified disorder of visual pathways

Disorders of ocular muscles, binocular movement, accommodation and refraction (H49-H52)

EXCLUDES 2   nystagmus and other irregular eye movements (H55)

☑4ᵗʰ H49 Paralytic strabismus

EXCLUDES 2   internal ophthalmoplegia (H52.51-)

internuclear ophthalmoplegia (H51.2-)

progressive supranuclear ophthalmoplegia (G23.1)

DEF: Strabismus: Misalignment of the eyes with the inability to move and focus in the same direction due to conditions affecting the muscles controlling them.

☑5ᵗʰ H49.0 Third [oculomotor] nerve palsy

H49.00 Third [oculomotor] nerve palsy, unspecified eye

H49.01 Third [oculomotor] nerve palsy, right eye

H49.02 Third [oculomotor] nerve palsy, left eye

H49.03 Third [oculomotor] nerve palsy, bilateral

☑5ᵗʰ H49.1 Fourth [trochlear] nerve palsy

H49.10 Fourth [trochlear] nerve palsy, unspecified eye

H49.11 Fourth [trochlear] nerve palsy, right eye

H49.12 Fourth [trochlear] nerve palsy, left eye

H49.13 Fourth [trochlear] nerve palsy, bilateral

☑5ᵗʰ H49.2 Sixth [abducent] nerve palsy

H49.20 Sixth [abducent] nerve palsy, unspecified eye

H49.21 Sixth [abducent] nerve palsy, right eye

H49.22 Sixth [abducent] nerve palsy, left eye

H49.23 Sixth [abducent] nerve palsy, bilateral

☑5ᵗʰ H49.3 Total (external) ophthalmoplegia

H49.30 Total (external) ophthalmoplegia, unspecified eye

H49.31 Total (external) ophthalmoplegia, right eye

H49.32 Total (external) ophthalmoplegia, left eye

H49.33 Total (external) ophthalmoplegia, bilateral

☑5ᵗʰ H49.4 Progressive external ophthalmoplegia

EXCLUDES 1   Kearns-Sayre syndrome (H49.81-)

H49.40 Progressive external ophthalmoplegia, unspecified eye

H49.41 Progressive external ophthalmoplegia, right eye

H49.42 Progressive external ophthalmoplegia, left eye

H49.43 Progressive external ophthalmoplegia, bilateral

☑5ᵗʰ H49.8 Other paralytic strabismus

☑6ᵗʰ H49.81 Kearns-Sayre syndrome

Progressive external ophthalmoplegia with pigmentary retinopathy

Use additional code for other manifestation, such as: heart block (I45.9)

H49.811 Kearns-Sayre syndrome, right eye

H49.812 Kearns-Sayre syndrome, left eye

H49.813 Kearns-Sayre syndrome, bilateral

H49.819 Kearns-Sayre syndrome, unspecified eye

☑6ᵗʰ H49.88 Other paralytic strabismus

External ophthalmoplegia NOS

H49.881 Other paralytic strabismus, right eye

H49.882 Other paralytic strabismus, left eye

H49.883 Other paralytic strabismus, bilateral

H49.889 Other paralytic strabismus, unspecified eye

H49.9 Unspecified paralytic strabismus

☑4ᵗʰ H50 Other strabismus

DEF: Strabismus: Misalignment of the eyes with the inability to move and focus in the same direction due to conditions affecting the muscles controlling them.

☑5ᵗʰ H50.0 Esotropia

Convergent concomitant strabismus

EXCLUDES 1   intermittent esotropia (H50.31-, H50.32)

H50.00 Unspecified esotropia

☑6ᵗʰ H50.01 Monocular esotropia

H50.011 Monocular esotropia, right eye

H50.012 Monocular esotropia, left eye

☑6ᵗʰ H50.02 Monocular esotropia with A pattern

H50.021 Monocular esotropia with A pattern, right eye

H50.022 Monocular esotropia with A pattern, left eye

☑6ᵗʰ H50.03 Monocular esotropia with V pattern

H50.031 Monocular esotropia with V pattern, right eye

H50.032 Monocular esotropia with V pattern, left eye

☑6ᵗʰ H50.04 Monocular esotropia with other noncomitancies

H50.041 Monocular esotropia with other noncomitancies, right eye

H50.042 Monocular esotropia with other noncomitancies, left eye

H50.05 Alternating esotropia

H50.06 Alternating esotropia with A pattern

H50.07 Alternating esotropia with V pattern

☑ Additional Character Required   ☑x7ᵗʰ Placeholder Alert   Manifestation   Unspecified Dx   ▶◀ Revised Text   ● New Code   ▲ Revised Title

ICD-10-CM 2020   611

H50.08　Alternating esotropia with other noncomitancies

Eye Muscle Diseases

R.　　　L.
Monocular (one eye only) esotropia (inward)

Monocular exotropia (outward)

Monocular hypertropia (upward)

✓5ᵗʰ **H50.1**　**Exotropia**
　　　Divergent concomitant strabismus
　　　EXCLUDES 1　intermittent exotropia (H50.33-, H50.34)
　　H50.10　Unspecified exotropia
　✓6ᵗʰ **H50.11**　Monocular exotropia
　　　　H50.111 Monocular exotropia, right eye
　　　　H50.112 Monocular exotropia, left eye
　✓6ᵗʰ **H50.12**　Monocular exotropia with A pattern
　　　　H50.121 Monocular exotropia with A pattern, right eye
　　　　H50.122 Monocular exotropia with A pattern, left eye
　✓6ᵗʰ **H50.13**　Monocular exotropia with V pattern
　　　　H50.131 Monocular exotropia with V pattern, right eye
　　　　H50.132 Monocular exotropia with V pattern, left eye
　✓6ᵗʰ **H50.14**　Monocular exotropia with other noncomitancies
　　　　H50.141 Monocular exotropia with other noncomitancies, right eye
　　　　H50.142 Monocular exotropia with other noncomitancies, left eye
　　H50.15　Alternating exotropia
　　H50.16　Alternating exotropia with A pattern
　　H50.17　Alternating exotropia with V pattern
　　H50.18　Alternating exotropia with other noncomitancies
✓5ᵗʰ **H50.2**　**Vertical strabismus**
　　　Hypertropia
　　H50.21　Vertical strabismus, right eye
　　H50.22　Vertical strabismus, left eye
✓5ᵗʰ **H50.3**　**Intermittent heterotropia**
　　H50.30　Unspecified intermittent heterotropia
　✓6ᵗʰ **H50.31**　Intermittent monocular esotropia
　　　　H50.311 Intermittent monocular esotropia, right eye
　　　　H50.312 Intermittent monocular esotropia, left eye
　　H50.32　Intermittent alternating esotropia
　✓6ᵗʰ **H50.33**　Intermittent monocular exotropia
　　　　H50.331 Intermittent monocular exotropia, right eye
　　　　H50.332 Intermittent monocular exotropia, left eye
　　H50.34　Intermittent alternating exotropia
✓5ᵗʰ **H50.4**　**Other and unspecified heterotropia**
　　H50.40　Unspecified heterotropia
　✓6ᵗʰ **H50.41**　Cyclotropia
　　　　H50.411 Cyclotropia, right eye
　　　　H50.412 Cyclotropia, left eye
　　H50.42　Monofixation syndrome

H50.43　Accommodative component in esotropia
✓5ᵗʰ **H50.5**　**Heterophoria**
　　H50.50　Unspecified heterophoria
　　H50.51　Esophoria
　　H50.52　Exophoria
　　H50.53　Vertical heterophoria
　　H50.54　Cyclophoria
　　H50.55　Alternating heterophoria
✓5ᵗʰ **H50.6**　**Mechanical strabismus**
　　H50.60　Mechanical strabismus, unspecified
　✓6ᵗʰ **H50.61**　Brown's sheath syndrome
　　　　H50.611 Brown's sheath syndrome, right eye
　　　　H50.612 Brown's sheath syndrome, left eye
　　H50.69　Other mechanical strabismus
　　　　Strabismus due to adhesions
　　　　Traumatic limitation of duction of eye muscle
✓5ᵗʰ **H50.8**　**Other specified strabismus**
　✓6ᵗʰ **H50.81**　Duane's syndrome
　　　　H50.811 Duane's syndrome, right eye
　　　　H50.812 Duane's syndrome, left eye
　　H50.89　Other specified strabismus
　　H50.9　Unspecified strabismus
✓4ᵗʰ **H51**　**Other disorders of binocular movement**
　　H51.0　Palsy (spasm) of conjugate gaze
✓5ᵗʰ **H51.1**　Convergence insufficiency and excess
　　H51.11　Convergence insufficiency
　　H51.12　Convergence excess
✓5ᵗʰ **H51.2**　Internuclear ophthalmoplegia
　　H51.20　Internuclear ophthalmoplegia, unspecified eye
　　H51.21　Internuclear ophthalmoplegia, right eye
　　H51.22　Internuclear ophthalmoplegia, left eye
　　H51.23　Internuclear ophthalmoplegia, bilateral
　　H51.8　Other specified disorders of binocular movement
　　H51.9　Unspecified disorder of binocular movement
✓4ᵗʰ **H52**　**Disorders of refraction and accommodation**
✓5ᵗʰ **H52.0**　Hypermetropia
　　H52.00　Hypermetropia, unspecified eye
　　H52.01　Hypermetropia, right eye
　　H52.02　Hypermetropia, left eye
　　H52.03　Hypermetropia, bilateral
✓5ᵗʰ **H52.1**　Myopia
　　　EXCLUDES 1　degenerative myopia (H44.2-)
　　H52.10　Myopia, unspecified eye
　　H52.11　Myopia, right eye
　　H52.12　Myopia, left eye
　　H52.13　Myopia, bilateral
✓5ᵗʰ **H52.2**　Astigmatism
　✓6ᵗʰ **H52.20**　Unspecified astigmatism
　　　　H52.201 Unspecified astigmatism, right eye
　　　　H52.202 Unspecified astigmatism, left eye
　　　　H52.203 Unspecified astigmatism, bilateral
　　　　H52.209 Unspecified astigmatism, unspecified eye
　✓6ᵗʰ **H52.21**　Irregular astigmatism
　　　　H52.211 Irregular astigmatism, right eye
　　　　H52.212 Irregular astigmatism, left eye
　　　　H52.213 Irregular astigmatism, bilateral
　　　　H52.219 Irregular astigmatism, unspecified eye
　✓6ᵗʰ **H52.22**　Regular astigmatism
　　　　H52.221 Regular astigmatism, right eye
　　　　H52.222 Regular astigmatism, left eye
　　　　H52.223 Regular astigmatism, bilateral
　　　　H52.229 Regular astigmatism, unspecified eye
✓5ᵗʰ **H52.3**　Anisometropia and aniseikonia
　　H52.31　Anisometropia
　　H52.32　Aniseikonia
　　H52.4　Presbyopia
✓5ᵗʰ **H52.5**　Disorders of accommodation
　✓6ᵗʰ **H52.51**　Internal ophthalmoplegia (complete) (total)
　　　　H52.511 Internal ophthalmoplegia (complete) (total), right eye
　　　　H52.512 Internal ophthalmoplegia (complete) (total), left eye

N Newborn: 0　**P** Pediatric: 0-17　**M** Maternity: 12-55　**A** Adult: 15-124　**CH** Comorbidity High　**CL** Comorbidity Low　**NC Dx** Noncancer Dx　**PDx** Primary Dx

612　　　　　　　　　　　　　　　　　　　　　　　　　　　　　　ICD-10-CM 2020

H52.513 Internal ophthalmoplegia (complete) (total), **bilateral**

H52.519 Internal ophthalmoplegia (complete) (total), unspecified eye

√6ᵗʰ **H52.52** **Paresis** of accommodation

H52.521 Paresis of accommodation, **right** eye

H52.522 Paresis of accommodation, **left** eye

H52.523 Paresis of accommodation, **bilateral**

H52.529 Paresis of accommodation, unspecified eye

√6ᵗʰ **H52.53** **Spasm** of accommodation

H52.531 Spasm of accommodation, **right** eye

H52.532 Spasm of accommodation, **left** eye

H52.533 Spasm of accommodation, **bilateral**

H52.539 Spasm of accommodation, unspecified eye

H52.6 **Other disorders of refraction**

H52.7 **Unspecified disorder of refraction**

Visual disturbances and blindness (H53-H54)

√4ᵗʰ **H53** **Visual disturbances**

√5ᵗʰ **H53.0** **Amblyopia ex anopsia**

EXCLUDES 1 *amblyopia due to vitamin A deficiency (E50.5)*

√6ᵗʰ **H53.00** **Unspecified amblyopia**

H53.001 Unspecified amblyopia, **right** eye

H53.002 Unspecified amblyopia, **left** eye

H53.003 Unspecified amblyopia, **bilateral**

H53.009 Unspecified amblyopia, unspecified eye

√6ᵗʰ **H53.01** **Deprivation amblyopia**

H53.011 Deprivation amblyopia, **right** eye

H53.012 Deprivation amblyopia, **left** eye

H53.013 Deprivation amblyopia, **bilateral**

H53.019 Deprivation amblyopia, unspecified eye

√6ᵗʰ **H53.02** **Refractive amblyopia**

H53.021 Refractive amblyopia, **right** eye

H53.022 Refractive amblyopia, **left** eye

H53.023 Refractive amblyopia, **bilateral**

H53.029 Refractive amblyopia, unspecified eye

√6ᵗʰ **H53.03** **Strabismic amblyopia**

EXCLUDES 1 *strabismus (H50.-)*

H53.031 Strabismic amblyopia, **right** eye

H53.032 Strabismic amblyopia, **left** eye

H53.033 Strabismic amblyopia, **bilateral**

H53.039 Strabismic amblyopia, unspecified eye

√6ᵗʰ **H53.04** **Amblyopia suspect**

AHA: 2016,4Q,22-23

H53.041 Amblyopia suspect, **right** eye

H53.042 Amblyopia suspect, **left** eye

H53.043 Amblyopia suspect, **bilateral**

H53.049 Amblyopia suspect, unspecified eye

√5ᵗʰ **H53.1** **Subjective visual disturbances**

EXCLUDES 1 *subjective visual disturbances due to vitamin A deficiency (E50.5)*

visual hallucinations (R44.1)

H53.10 **Unspecified subjective visual disturbances**

H53.11 **Day blindness**

Hemeralopia

√6ᵗʰ **H53.12** **Transient visual loss**

Scintillating scotoma

EXCLUDES 1 *amaurosis fugax (G45.3-)*

transient retinal artery occlusion (H34.0-)

H53.121 Transient visual loss, **right** eye

H53.122 Transient visual loss, **left** eye

H53.123 Transient visual loss, **bilateral**

H53.129 Transient visual loss, unspecified eye

√6ᵗʰ **H53.13** **Sudden visual loss**

H53.131 Sudden visual loss, **right** eye

H53.132 Sudden visual loss, **left** eye

H53.133 Sudden visual loss, **bilateral**

H53.139 Sudden visual loss, unspecified eye

√6ᵗʰ **H53.14** **Visual discomfort**

Asthenopia

Photophobia

H53.141 Visual discomfort, **right** eye

H53.142 Visual discomfort, **left** eye

H53.143 Visual discomfort, **bilateral**

H53.149 Visual discomfort, unspecified

H53.15 **Visual distortions of shape and size**

Metamorphopsia

H53.16 **Psychophysical visual disturbances**

H53.19 **Other subjective visual disturbances**

Visual halos

H53.2 **Diplopia**

Double vision

√5ᵗʰ **H53.3** **Other and unspecified disorders of binocular vision**

H53.30 **Unspecified disorder of binocular vision**

H53.31 **Abnormal retinal correspondence**

H53.32 **Fusion with defective stereopsis**

H53.33 **Simultaneous visual perception without fusion**

H53.34 **Suppression of binocular vision**

√5ᵗʰ **H53.4** **Visual field defects**

H53.40 **Unspecified visual field defects**

√6ᵗʰ **H53.41** **Scotoma involving central area**

Central scotoma

H53.411 Scotoma involving central area, **right** eye

H53.412 Scotoma involving central area, **left** eye

H53.413 Scotoma involving central area, **bilateral**

H53.419 Scotoma involving central area, unspecified eye

√6ᵗʰ **H53.42** **Scotoma of blind spot area**

Enlarged blind spot

H53.421 Scotoma of blind spot area, **right** eye

H53.422 Scotoma of blind spot area, **left** eye

H53.423 Scotoma of blind spot area, **bilateral**

H53.429 Scotoma of blind spot area, unspecified eye

√6ᵗʰ **H53.43** **Sector or arcuate defects**

Arcuate scotoma

Bjerrum scotoma

H53.431 Sector or arcuate defects, **right** eye

H53.432 Sector or arcuate defects, **left** eye

H53.433 Sector or arcuate defects, **bilateral**

H53.439 Sector or arcuate defects, unspecified eye

√6ᵗʰ **H53.45** **Other localized visual field defect**

Peripheral visual field defect

Ring scotoma NOS

Scotoma NOS

H53.451 Other localized visual field defect, **right** eye

H53.452 Other localized visual field defect, **left** eye

H53.453 Other localized visual field defect, **bilateral**

H53.459 Other localized visual field defect, unspecified eye

√6ᵗʰ **H53.46** **Homonymous bilateral field defects**

Homonymous hemianopia

Homonymous hemianopsia

Quadrant anopia

Quadrant anopsia

H53.461 Homonymous bilateral field defects, **right** side

H53.462 Homonymous bilateral field defects, **left** side

H53.469 Homonymous bilateral field defects, unspecified side

Homonymous bilateral field defects NOS

H53.47 **Heteronymous bilateral field defects**

Heteronymous hemianop(s)ia

√6ᵗʰ **H53.48** **Generalized contraction of visual field**

H53.481 Generalized contraction of visual field, **right** eye

H53.482 Generalized contraction of visual field, **left** eye

H53.483 Generalized contraction of visual field, **bilateral**

H53.489 Generalized contraction of visual field, unspecified eye

✔ Additional Character Required   √x7ᵗʰ Placeholder Alert   Manifestation   Unspecified Dx   ▶◀ Revised Text   ● New Code   ▲ Revised Title

CD-10-CM 2020   613

H52.513-H53.489

Chapter 7. Diseases of the Eye and Adnexa

H53.5–H54.415

✓5ᵗʰ **H53.5 Color vision deficiencies**
Color blindness
EXCLUDES 2   day blindness (H53.11)

H53.50 Unspecified color vision deficiencies
Color blindness NOS

H53.51 Achromatopsia
DEF: Nonprogressive genetic visual disorder characterized by complete color blindness, decreased vision, and light sensitivity.

H53.52 Acquired color vision deficiency

H53.53 Deuteranomaly
Deuteranopia
DEF: Male-only genetic disorder causing difficulty in distinguishing green and red; no shortened spectrum.

H53.54 Protanomaly
Protanopia

H53.55 Tritanomaly
Tritanopia

H53.59 Other color vision deficiencies

✓5ᵗʰ **H53.6 Night blindness**
EXCLUDES 1   night blindness due to vitamin A deficiency (E50.5)

H53.60 Unspecified night blindness

H53.61 Abnormal dark adaptation curve

H53.62 Acquired night blindness

H53.63 Congenital night blindness

H53.69 Other night blindness

✓5ᵗʰ **H53.7 Vision sensitivity deficiencies**

H53.71 Glare sensitivity

H53.72 Impaired contrast sensitivity

H53.8 Other visual disturbances

H53.9 Unspecified visual disturbance

✓4ᵗʰ **H54 Blindness and low vision**

NOTE   For definition of visual impairment categories see table below

Code first any associated underlying cause of the blindness
EXCLUDES 1   amaurosis fugax (G45.3)
AHA: 2017,4Q,11-12

✓5ᵗʰ **H54.0 Blindness, both eyes**
Visual impairment categories 3, 4, 5 in both eyes.

✓6ᵗʰ **H54.0X Blindness, both eyes, different category levels**

✓7ᵗʰ **H54.0X3 Blindness right eye, category 3**

H54.0X33 Blindness right eye category 3, blindness left eye category 3 CL

H54.0X34 Blindness right eye category 3, blindness left eye category 4 CL

H54.0X35 Blindness right eye category 3, blindness left eye category 5 CL

✓7ᵗʰ **H54.0X4 Blindness right eye, category 4**

H54.0X43 Blindness right eye category 4, blindness left eye category 3 CL

H54.0X44 Blindness right eye category 4, blindness left eye category 4 CL

H54.0X45 Blindness right eye category 4, blindness left eye category 5 CL

✓7ᵗʰ **H54.0X5 Blindness right eye, category 5**

H54.0X53 Blindness right eye category 5, blindness left eye category 3 CL

H54.0X54 Blindness right eye category 5, blindness left eye category 4 CL

H54.0X55 Blindness right eye category 5, blindness left eye category 5 CL

✓5ᵗʰ **H54.1 Blindness, one eye, low vision other eye**
Visual impairment categories 3, 4, 5 in one eye, with categories 1 or 2 in the other eye.

H54.10 Blindness, one eye, low vision other eye, unspecified eyes CL

✓6ᵗʰ **H54.11 Blindness, right eye, low vision left eye**

✓7ᵗʰ **H54.113 Blindness right eye category 3, low vision left eye**

H54.1131 Blindness right eye category 3, low vision left eye category 1 CL

H54.1132 Blindness right eye category 3, low vision left eye category 2 CL

✓7ᵗʰ **H54.114 Blindness right eye category 4, low vision left eye**

H54.1141 Blindness right eye category 4, low vision left eye category 1 CL

H54.1142 Blindness right eye category 4, low vision left eye category 2 CL

✓7ᵗʰ **H54.115 Blindness right eye category 5, low vision left eye**

H54.1151 Blindness right eye category 5, low vision left eye category 1 CL

H54.1152 Blindness right eye category 5, low vision left eye category 2 CL

✓6ᵗʰ **H54.12 Blindness, left eye, low vision right eye**

✓7ᵗʰ **H54.121 Low vision right eye category 1, blindness left eye**

H54.1213 Low vision right eye category 1, blindness left eye category 3 CL

H54.1214 Low vision right eye category 1, blindness left eye category 4 CL

H54.1215 Low vision right eye category 1, blindness left eye category 5 CL

✓7ᵗʰ **H54.122 Low vision right eye category 2, blindness left eye**

H54.1223 Low vision right eye category 2, blindness left eye category 3 CL

H54.1224 Low vision right eye category 2, blindness left eye category 4 CL

H54.1225 Low vision right eye category 2, blindness left eye category 5 CL

✓5ᵗʰ **H54.2 Low vision, both eyes**
Visual impairment categories 1 or 2 in both eyes.

✓6ᵗʰ **H54.2X Low vision, both eyes, different category levels**

✓7ᵗʰ **H54.2X1 Low vision, right eye, category 1**

H54.2X11 Low vision right eye category 1, low vision left eye category 1 CL

H54.2X12 Low vision right eye category 1, low vision left eye category 2 CL

✓7ᵗʰ **H54.2X2 Low vision, right eye, category 2**

H54.2X21 Low vision right eye category 2, low vision left eye category 1 CL

H54.2X22 Low vision right eye category 2, low vision left eye category 2 CL

H54.3 Unqualified visual loss, both eyes CL
Visual impairment category 9 in both eyes.

✓5ᵗʰ **H54.4 Blindness, one eye**
Visual impairment categories 3, 4, 5 in one eye [normal vision in other eye]

H54.40 Blindness, one eye, unspecified eye

✓6ᵗʰ **H54.41 Blindness, right eye, normal vision left eye**

✓7ᵗʰ **H54.413 Blindness, right eye, category 3**

H54.413A Blindness right eye category 3, normal vision left eye CL

✓7ᵗʰ **H54.414 Blindness, right eye, category 4**

H54.414A Blindness right eye category 4, normal vision left eye CL

✓7ᵗʰ **H54.415 Blindness, right eye, category 5**

N Newborn: 0   P Pediatric: 0-17   M Maternity: 12-55   A Adult: 15-124   CH Comorbidity High   CL Comorbidity Low   NCDx Noncancer Dx   PDx Primary Dx

614   ICD-10-CM 2020

H54.415A   Blindness right eye category 5, normal vision left eye   `CL`

√6ᵗʰ   **H54.42**   Blindness, left eye, normal vision right eye

√7ᵗʰ   **H54.42A**   Blindness, left eye, category 3-5

H54.42A3   Blindness left eye category 3, normal vision right eye   `CL`

H54.42A4   Blindness left eye category 4, normal vision right eye   `CL`

H54.42A5   Blindness left eye category 5, normal vision right eye   `CL`

√5ᵗʰ   **H54.5**   Low vision, one eye

Visual impairment categories 1 or 2 in one eye [normal vision in other eye].

H54.50   Low vision, one eye, unspecified eye

√6ᵗʰ   **H54.51**   Low vision, right eye, normal vision left eye

√7ᵗʰ   **H54.511**   Low vision, right eye, category 1-2

H54.511A   Low vision right eye category 1, normal vision left eye   `CL`

H54.512A   Low vision right eye category 2, normal vision left eye   `CL`

√7ᵗʰ   **H54.52**   Low vision, left eye, normal vision right eye

√7ᵗʰ   **H54.52A**   Low vision, left eye, category 1-2

H54.52A1   Low vision left eye category 1, normal vision right eye   `CL`

H54.52A2   Low vision left eye category 2, normal vision right eye   `CL`

√5ᵗʰ   **H54.6**   Unqualified visual loss, one eye

Visual impairment category 9 in one eye [normal vision in other eye].

H54.60   Unqualified visual loss, one eye, unspecified

H54.61   Unqualified visual loss, right eye, normal vision left eye

H54.62   Unqualified visual loss, left eye, normal vision right eye

H54.7   Unspecified visual loss

Visual impairment category 9 NOS

H54.8   Legal blindness, as defined in USA   `CL`

Blindness NOS according to USA definition

EXCLUDES 1   legal blindness with specification of impairment level (H54.0-H54.7)

NOTE   The table below gives a classification of severity of visual impairment recommended by a WHO Study Group on the Prevention of Blindness, Geneva, 6-10 November 1972.

The term "low vision" in category H54 comprises categories 1 and 2 of the table, the term "blindness" categories 3, 4 and 5, and the term "unqualified visual loss" category 9.

If the extent of the visual field is taken into account, patients with a field no greater than 10 but greater than 5 around central fixation should be placed in category 3 and patients with a field no greater than 5 around central fixation should be placed in category 4, even if the central acuity is not impaired.

Category of visual impairment	Visual acuity with best possible correction	
	Maximum less than:	**Minimum equal to or better than:**
1	6/18 3/10 (0.3) 20/70	6/60 1/10 (0.1) 20/200
2	6/60 1/10 (0.1) 20/200	3/60 1/20 (0.05) 20/400
3	3/60 1/200 (0.05) 20/400	1/60 (finger counting at one meter) 1/50 (0.02) 5/300 (20/1200)
4	1/60 (finger counting at one meter) 1/50 (0.02) 5/300	Light perception
5	No light perception	
9	Undetermined or unspecified	

Other disorders of eye and adnexa (H55-H57)

√4ᵗʰ   **H55**   Nystagmus and other irregular eye movements

√5ᵗʰ   **H55.0**   Nystagmus

DEF: Rapid, rhythmic, involuntary movements of the eyeball in vertical, horizontal, rotational, or mixed directions.

H55.00   Unspecified nystagmus

H55.01   Congenital nystagmus

H55.02   Latent nystagmus

H55.03   Visual deprivation nystagmus

H55.04   Dissociated nystagmus

H55.09   Other forms of nystagmus

√5ᵗʰ   **H55.8**   Other irregular eye movements

H55.81   Saccadic eye movements

H55.89   Other irregular eye movements

√4ᵗʰ   **H57**   Other disorders of eye and adnexa

√5ᵗʰ   **H57.0**   Anomalies of pupillary function

H57.00   Unspecified anomaly of pupillary function

H57.01   Argyll Robertson pupil, atypical

EXCLUDES 1   syphilitic Argyll Robertson pupil (A52.19)

H57.02   Anisocoria

H57.03   Miosis

H57.04   Mydriasis

√6ᵗʰ   **H57.05**   Tonic pupil

H57.051   Tonic pupil, right eye

H57.052   Tonic pupil, left eye

H57.053   Tonic pupil, bilateral

H57.059   Tonic pupil, unspecified eye

H57.09   Other anomalies of pupillary function

√5ᵗʰ   **H57.1**   Ocular pain

H57.10   Ocular pain, unspecified eye

H57.11   Ocular pain, right eye

☑ Additional Character Required   √x7ᵗʰ Placeholder Alert   Manifestation   Unspecified Dx   ▶◀ Revised Text   ● New Code   ▲ Revised Title

ICD-10-CM 2020   615

H57.12   Ocular pain, left eye

H57.13   Ocular pain, bilateral

√5ᵗʰ   **H57.8**   **Other specified disorders of eye and adnexa**

      AHA: 2018,4Q,15-16

   √6ᵗʰ   **H57.81**   **Brow ptosis**

      H57.811   Brow ptosis, right

      H57.812   Brow ptosis, left

      H57.813   Brow ptosis, bilateral

      H57.819   Brow ptosis, unspecified

   H57.89   Other specified disorders of eye and adnexa

H57.9   **Unspecified disorder of eye and adnexa**

Intraoperative and postprocedural complications and disorders of eye and adnexa, not elsewhere classified (H59)

√4ᵗʰ   **H59**   **Intraoperative and postprocedural complications and disorders of eye and adnexa, not elsewhere classified**

     EXCLUDES 1   mechanical complication of intraocular lens (T85.2)

          mechanical complication of other ocular prosthetic devices, implants and grafts (T85.3)

          pseudophakia (Z96.1)

          secondary cataracts (H26.4-)

  √5ᵗʰ   **H59.0**   **Disorders of the eye following cataract surgery**

   √6ᵗʰ   **H59.01**   **Keratopathy (bullous aphakic) following cataract surgery**

      Vitreal corneal syndrome

      Vitreous (touch) syndrome

      H59.011   Keratopathy (bullous aphakic) following cataract surgery, right eye

      H59.012   Keratopathy (bullous aphakic) following cataract surgery, left eye

      H59.013   Keratopathy (bullous aphakic) following cataract surgery, bilateral

      H59.019   Keratopathy (bullous aphakic) following cataract surgery, unspecified eye

   √6ᵗʰ   **H59.02**   **Cataract (lens) fragments in eye following cataract surgery**

      H59.021   Cataract (lens) fragments in eye following cataract surgery, right eye

      H59.022   Cataract (lens) fragments in eye following cataract surgery, left eye

      H59.023   Cataract (lens) fragments in eye following cataract surgery, bilateral

      H59.029   Cataract (lens) fragments in eye following cataract surgery, unspecified eye

   √6ᵗʰ   **H59.03**   **Cystoid macular edema following cataract surgery**

      H59.031   Cystoid macular edema following cataract surgery, right eye

      H59.032   Cystoid macular edema following cataract surgery, left eye

      H59.033   Cystoid macular edema following cataract surgery, bilateral

      H59.039   Cystoid macular edema following cataract surgery, unspecified eye

   √6ᵗʰ   **H59.09**   **Other disorders of the eye following cataract surgery**

      H59.091   Other disorders of the right eye following cataract surgery

      H59.092   Other disorders of the left eye following cataract surgery

      H59.093   Other disorders of the eye following cataract surgery, bilateral

      H59.099   Other disorders of unspecified eye following cataract surgery

  √5ᵗʰ   **H59.1**   **Intraoperative hemorrhage and hematoma of eye and adnexa complicating a procedure**

     EXCLUDES 1   intraoperative hemorrhage and hematoma of eye and adnexa due to accidental puncture or laceration during a procedure (H59.2-)

   √6ᵗʰ   **H59.11**   **Intraoperative hemorrhage and hematoma of eye and adnexa complicating an ophthalmic procedure**

      H59.111   Intraoperative hemorrhage and hematoma of right eye and adnexa complicating an ophthalmic procedure

      H59.112   Intraoperative hemorrhage and hematoma of left eye and adnexa complicating an ophthalmic procedure

      H59.113   Intraoperative hemorrhage and hematoma of eye and adnexa complicating an ophthalmic procedure, bilateral

      H59.119   Intraoperative hemorrhage and hematoma of unspecified eye and adnexa complicating an ophthalmic procedure

   √6ᵗʰ   **H59.12**   **Intraoperative hemorrhage and hematoma of eye and adnexa complicating other procedure**

      H59.121   Intraoperative hemorrhage and hematoma of right eye and adnexa complicating other procedure

      H59.122   Intraoperative hemorrhage and hematoma of left eye and adnexa complicating other procedure

      H59.123   Intraoperative hemorrhage and hematoma of eye and adnexa complicating other procedure, bilateral

      H59.129   Intraoperative hemorrhage and hematoma of unspecified eye and adnexa complicating other procedure

  √5ᵗʰ   **H59.2**   **Accidental puncture and laceration of eye and adnexa during a procedure**

   √6ᵗʰ   **H59.21**   **Accidental puncture and laceration of eye and adnexa during an ophthalmic procedure**

      H59.211   Accidental puncture and laceration of right eye and adnexa during an ophthalmic procedure

      H59.212   Accidental puncture and laceration of left eye and adnexa during an ophthalmic procedure

      H59.213   Accidental puncture and laceration of eye and adnexa during an ophthalmic procedure, bilateral

      H59.219   Accidental puncture and laceration of unspecified eye and adnexa during an ophthalmic procedure

   √6ᵗʰ   **H59.22**   **Accidental puncture and laceration of eye and adnexa during other procedure**

      H59.221   Accidental puncture and laceration of right eye and adnexa during other procedure

      H59.222   Accidental puncture and laceration of left eye and adnexa during other procedure

      H59.223   Accidental puncture and laceration of eye and adnexa during other procedure, bilateral

      H59.229   Accidental puncture and laceration of unspecified eye and adnexa during other procedure

  √5ᵗʰ   **H59.3**   **Postprocedural hemorrhage, hematoma, and seroma of eye and adnexa following a procedure**

      AHA: 2016,4Q,9-10

   √6ᵗʰ   **H59.31**   **Postprocedural hemorrhage of eye and adnexa following an ophthalmic procedure**

      H59.311   Postprocedural hemorrhage of right eye and adnexa following an ophthalmic procedure

      H59.312   Postprocedural hemorrhage of left eye and adnexa following an ophthalmic procedure

      H59.313   Postprocedural hemorrhage of eye and adnexa following an ophthalmic procedure, bilateral

      H59.319   Postprocedural hemorrhage of unspecified eye and adnexa following an ophthalmic procedure

   √6ᵗʰ   **H59.32**   **Postprocedural hemorrhage of eye and adnexa following other procedure**

      H59.321   Postprocedural hemorrhage of right eye and adnexa following other procedure

      H59.322   Postprocedural hemorrhage of left eye and adnexa following other procedure

      H59.323   Postprocedural hemorrhage of eye and adnexa following other procedure, bilateral

      H59.329   Postprocedural hemorrhage of unspecified eye and adnexa following other procedure

   √6ᵗʰ   **H59.33**   **Postprocedural hematoma of eye and adnexa following an ophthalmic procedure**

      H59.331   Postprocedural hematoma of right eye and adnexa following an ophthalmic procedure

      H59.332   Postprocedural hematoma of left eye and adnexa following an ophthalmic procedure

H59.333   Postprocedural hematoma of eye and adnexa following an ophthalmic procedure, bilateral

H59.339   Postprocedural hematoma of unspecified eye and adnexa following an ophthalmic procedure

√6ᵗʰ   **H59.34**   Postprocedural hematoma of eye and adnexa following other procedure

H59.341   Postprocedural hematoma of right eye and adnexa following other procedure

H59.342   Postprocedural hematoma of left eye and adnexa following other procedure

H59.343   Postprocedural hematoma of eye and adnexa following other procedure, bilateral

H59.349   Postprocedural hematoma of unspecified eye and adnexa following other procedure

√6ᵗʰ   **H59.35**   Postprocedural seroma of eye and adnexa following an ophthalmic procedure

H59.351   Postprocedural seroma of right eye and adnexa following an ophthalmic procedure

H59.352   Postprocedural seroma of left eye and adnexa following an ophthalmic procedure

H59.353   Postprocedural seroma of eye and adnexa following an ophthalmic procedure, bilateral

H59.359   Postprocedural seroma of unspecified eye and adnexa following an ophthalmic procedure

√6ᵗʰ   **H59.36**   Postprocedural seroma of eye and adnexa following other procedure

H59.361   Postprocedural seroma of right eye and adnexa following other procedure

H59.362   Postprocedural seroma of left eye and adnexa following other procedure

H59.363   Postprocedural seroma of eye and adnexa following other procedure, bilateral

H59.369   Postprocedural seroma of unspecified eye and adnexa following other procedure

√5ᵗʰ   **H59.4**   Inflammation (infection) of postprocedural bleb

Postprocedural blebitis

EXCLUDES 1   filtering (vitreous) bleb after glaucoma surgery status (Z98.83)

H59.40   Inflammation (infection) of postprocedural bleb, unspecified

H59.41   Inflammation (infection) of postprocedural bleb, stage 1

H59.42   Inflammation (infection) of postprocedural bleb, stage 2

H59.43   Inflammation (infection) of postprocedural bleb, stage 3

Bleb endophthalmitis

√5ᵗʰ   **H59.8**   Other intraoperative and postprocedural complications and disorders of eye and adnexa, not elsewhere classified

√6ᵗʰ   **H59.81**   Chorioretinal scars after surgery for detachment

H59.811   Chorioretinal scars after surgery for detachment, right eye

H59.812   Chorioretinal scars after surgery for detachment, left eye

H59.813   Chorioretinal scars after surgery for detachment, bilateral

H59.819   Chorioretinal scars after surgery for detachment, unspecified eye

H59.88   Other intraoperative complications of eye and adnexa, not elsewhere classified

H59.89   Other postprocedural complications and disorders of eye and adnexa, not elsewhere classified

☑ Additional Character Required   √x7ᵗʰ Placeholder Alert   Manifestation   Unspecified Dx   ►◄ Revised Text   ● New Code   ▲ Revised Title

ICD-10-CM 2020   **617**

H59.333–H59.89

Chapter 8. Diseases of the Ear and Mastoid Process (H6Ø–H95)

Chapter-specific Coding Guidelines and Examples
Reserved for future guideline expansion.

Chapter 8. Diseases of the Ear and Mastoid Process (H60–H95)

NOTE Use an external cause code following the code for the ear condition, if applicable, to identify the cause of the ear condition

EXCLUDES 2
certain conditions originating in the perinatal period (P04-P96)
certain infectious and parasitic diseases (A00-B99)
complications of pregnancy, childbirth and the puerperium (O00-O9A)
congenital malformations, deformations and chromosomal abnormalities (Q00-Q99)
endocrine, nutritional and metabolic diseases (E00-E88)
injury, poisoning and certain other consequences of external causes (S00-T88)
neoplasms (C00-D49)
symptoms, signs and abnormal clinical and laboratory findings, not elsewhere classified (R00-R94)

This chapter contains the following blocks:
H60-H62 Diseases of external ear
H65-H75 Diseases of middle ear and mastoid
H80-H83 Diseases of inner ear
H90-H94 Other disorders of ear
H95 Intraoperative and postprocedural complications and disorders of ear and mastoid process, not elsewhere classified

Diseases of external ear (H60-H62)

H60 Otitis externa

H60.0 Abscess of external ear
Boil of external ear
Carbuncle of auricle or external auditory canal
Furuncle of external ear
H60.00 Abscess of external ear, unspecified ear
H60.01 Abscess of right external ear
H60.02 Abscess of left external ear
H60.03 Abscess of external ear, bilateral

H60.1 Cellulitis of external ear
Cellulitis of auricle
Cellulitis of external auditory canal
H60.10 Cellulitis of external ear, unspecified ear
H60.11 Cellulitis of right external ear
H60.12 Cellulitis of left external ear
H60.13 Cellulitis of external ear, bilateral

H60.2 Malignant otitis externa
H60.20 Malignant otitis externa, unspecified ear
H60.21 Malignant otitis externa, right ear
H60.22 Malignant otitis externa, left ear
H60.23 Malignant otitis externa, bilateral

H60.3 Other infective otitis externa
H60.31 Diffuse otitis externa
H60.311 Diffuse otitis externa, right ear
H60.312 Diffuse otitis externa, left ear
H60.313 Diffuse otitis externa, bilateral
H60.319 Diffuse otitis externa, unspecified ear
H60.32 Hemorrhagic otitis externa
H60.321 Hemorrhagic otitis externa, right ear
H60.322 Hemorrhagic otitis externa, left ear
H60.323 Hemorrhagic otitis externa, bilateral
H60.329 Hemorrhagic otitis externa, unspecified ear
H60.33 Swimmer's ear
DEF: Commonly occurs when water gets trapped in the ear after swimming.
H60.331 Swimmer's ear, right ear
H60.332 Swimmer's ear, left ear
H60.333 Swimmer's ear, bilateral
H60.339 Swimmer's ear, unspecified ear
H60.39 Other infective otitis externa
H60.391 Other infective otitis externa, right ear
H60.392 Other infective otitis externa, left ear
H60.393 Other infective otitis externa, bilateral
H60.399 Other infective otitis externa, unspecified ear

H60.4 Cholesteatoma of external ear
Keratosis obturans of external ear (canal)
EXCLUDES 2 *cholesteatoma of middle ear (H71.-)*
recurrent cholesteatoma of postmastoidectomy cavity (H95.0-)
DEF: Cholesteatoma: Noncancerous cyst-like mass of cell debris, including cholesterol and epithelial cells resulting from trauma, repeated or improperly healed infections, and congenital enclosure of epidermal cells.
H60.40 Cholesteatoma of external ear, unspecified ear
H60.41 Cholesteatoma of right external ear
H60.42 Cholesteatoma of left external ear
H60.43 Cholesteatoma of external ear, bilateral

H60.5 Acute noninfective otitis externa
H60.50 Unspecified acute noninfective otitis externa
Acute otitis externa NOS
H60.501 Unspecified acute noninfective otitis externa, right ear
H60.502 Unspecified acute noninfective otitis externa, left ear
H60.503 Unspecified acute noninfective otitis externa, bilateral
H60.509 Unspecified acute noninfective otitis externa, unspecified ear
H60.51 Acute actinic otitis externa
H60.511 Acute actinic otitis externa, right ear
H60.512 Acute actinic otitis externa, left ear
H60.513 Acute actinic otitis externa, bilateral
H60.519 Acute actinic otitis externa, unspecified ear
H60.52 Acute chemical otitis externa
H60.521 Acute chemical otitis externa, right ear
H60.522 Acute chemical otitis externa, left ear
H60.523 Acute chemical otitis externa, bilateral
H60.529 Acute chemical otitis externa, unspecified ear
H60.53 Acute contact otitis externa
H60.531 Acute contact otitis externa, right ear
H60.532 Acute contact otitis externa, left ear
H60.533 Acute contact otitis externa, bilateral
H60.539 Acute contact otitis externa, unspecified ear
H60.54 Acute eczematoid otitis externa
H60.541 Acute eczematoid otitis externa, right ear
H60.542 Acute eczematoid otitis externa, left ear
H60.543 Acute eczematoid otitis externa, bilateral
H60.549 Acute eczematoid otitis externa, unspecified ear
H60.55 Acute reactive otitis externa
H60.551 Acute reactive otitis externa, right ear
H60.552 Acute reactive otitis externa, left ear
H60.553 Acute reactive otitis externa, bilateral
H60.559 Acute reactive otitis externa, unspecified ear
H60.59 Other noninfective acute otitis externa
H60.591 Other noninfective acute otitis externa, right ear
H60.592 Other noninfective acute otitis externa, left ear
H60.593 Other noninfective acute otitis externa, bilateral
H60.599 Other noninfective acute otitis externa, unspecified ear

H60.6 Unspecified chronic otitis externa
H60.60 Unspecified chronic otitis externa, unspecified ear
H60.61 Unspecified chronic otitis externa, right ear
H60.62 Unspecified chronic otitis externa, left ear
H60.63 Unspecified chronic otitis externa, bilateral

H60.8 Other otitis externa
H60.8X Other otitis externa
H60.8X1 Other otitis externa, right ear
H60.8X2 Other otitis externa, left ear
H60.8X3 Other otitis externa, bilateral
H60.8X9 Other otitis externa, unspecified ear

H60.9 Unspecified otitis externa
H60.90 Unspecified otitis externa, unspecified ear
H60.91 Unspecified otitis externa, right ear

H60.92   Unspecified otitis externa, left ear

H60.93   Unspecified otitis externa, bilateral

✓4ᵗʰ **H61**   **Other disorders of external ear**

   ✓5ᵗʰ **H61.0**   **Chondritis and perichondritis of external ear**

        Chondrodermatitis nodularis chronica helicis

        Perichondritis of auricle

        Perichondritis of pinna

    ✓6ᵗʰ **H61.00**   **Unspecified perichondritis of external ear**

        H61.001   Unspecified perichondritis of right external ear

        H61.002   Unspecified perichondritis of left external ear

        H61.003   Unspecified perichondritis of external ear, bilateral

        H61.009   Unspecified perichondritis of external ear, unspecified ear

    ✓6ᵗʰ **H61.01**   **Acute perichondritis of external ear**

        H61.011   Acute perichondritis of right external ear

        H61.012   Acute perichondritis of left external ear

        H61.013   Acute perichondritis of external ear, bilateral

        H61.019   Acute perichondritis of external ear, unspecified ear

    ✓6ᵗʰ **H61.02**   **Chronic perichondritis of external ear**

        H61.021   Chronic perichondritis of right external ear

        H61.022   Chronic perichondritis of left external ear

        H61.023   Chronic perichondritis of external ear, bilateral

        H61.029   Chronic perichondritis of external ear, unspecified ear

    ✓6ᵗʰ **H61.03**   **Chondritis of external ear**

        Chondritis of auricle

        Chondritis of pinna

        AHA: 2015,1Q,18

        DEF: Infection that has progressed into the cartilage and presents as indurated and edematous skin over the pinna. Vascular compromise occurs with tissue necrosis and deformity.

        H61.031   Chondritis of right external ear

        H61.032   Chondritis of left external ear

        H61.033   Chondritis of external ear, bilateral

        H61.039   Chondritis of external ear, unspecified ear

   ✓5ᵗʰ **H61.1**   **Noninfective disorders of pinna**

        EXCLUDES 2   cauliflower ear (M95.1-)

                    gouty tophi of ear (M1A.-)

    ✓6ᵗʰ **H61.10**   **Unspecified noninfective disorders of pinna**

        Disorder of pinna NOS

        H61.101   Unspecified noninfective disorders of pinna, right ear

        H61.102   Unspecified noninfective disorders of pinna, left ear

        H61.103   Unspecified noninfective disorders of pinna, bilateral

        H61.109   Unspecified noninfective disorders of pinna, unspecified ear

    ✓6ᵗʰ **H61.11**   **Acquired deformity of pinna**

        Acquired deformity of auricle

        EXCLUDES 2   cauliflower ear (M95.1-)

        H61.111   Acquired deformity of pinna, right ear

        H61.112   Acquired deformity of pinna, left ear

        H61.113   Acquired deformity of pinna, bilateral

        H61.119   Acquired deformity of pinna, unspecified ear

    ✓6ᵗʰ **H61.12**   **Hematoma of pinna**

        Hematoma of auricle

        H61.121   Hematoma of pinna, right ear

        H61.122   Hematoma of pinna, left ear

        H61.123   Hematoma of pinna, bilateral

        H61.129   Hematoma of pinna, unspecified ear

    ✓6ᵗʰ **H61.19**   **Other noninfective disorders of pinna**

        H61.191   Noninfective disorders of pinna, right ear

        H61.192   Noninfective disorders of pinna, left ear

        H61.193   Noninfective disorders of pinna, bilateral

        H61.199   Noninfective disorders of pinna, unspecified ear

   ✓5ᵗʰ **H61.2**   **Impacted cerumen**

        Wax in ear

        H61.20   Impacted cerumen, unspecified ear

        H61.21   Impacted cerumen, right ear

        H61.22   Impacted cerumen, left ear

        H61.23   Impacted cerumen, bilateral

   ✓5ᵗʰ **H61.3**   **Acquired stenosis of external ear canal**

        Collapse of external ear canal

        EXCLUDES 1   postprocedural stenosis of external ear canal (H95.81-)

    ✓6ᵗʰ **H61.30**   **Acquired stenosis of external ear canal, unspecified**

        H61.301   Acquired stenosis of right external ear canal, unspecified

        H61.302   Acquired stenosis of left external ear canal, unspecified

        H61.303   Acquired stenosis of external ear canal, unspecified, bilateral

        H61.309   Acquired stenosis of external ear canal, unspecified, unspecified ear

    ✓6ᵗʰ **H61.31**   **Acquired stenosis of external ear canal secondary to trauma**

        H61.311   Acquired stenosis of right external ear canal secondary to trauma

        H61.312   Acquired stenosis of left external ear canal secondary to trauma

        H61.313   Acquired stenosis of external ear canal secondary to trauma, bilateral

        H61.319   Acquired stenosis of external ear canal secondary to trauma, unspecified ear

    ✓6ᵗʰ **H61.32**   **Acquired stenosis of external ear canal secondary to inflammation and infection**

        DEF: Narrowing of the external ear canal due to chronic inflammation or infection.

        H61.321   Acquired stenosis of right external ear canal secondary to inflammation and infection

        H61.322   Acquired stenosis of left external ear canal secondary to inflammation and infection

        H61.323   Acquired stenosis of external ear canal secondary to inflammation and infection, bilateral

        H61.329   Acquired stenosis of external ear canal secondary to inflammation and infection, unspecified ear

    ✓6ᵗʰ **H61.39**   **Other acquired stenosis of external ear canal**

        H61.391   Other acquired stenosis of right external ear canal

        H61.392   Other acquired stenosis of left external ear canal

        H61.393   Other acquired stenosis of external ear canal, bilateral

        H61.399   Other acquired stenosis of external ear canal, unspecified ear

   ✓5ᵗʰ **H61.8**   **Other specified disorders of external ear**

    ✓6ᵗʰ **H61.81**   **Exostosis of external canal**

        H61.811   Exostosis of right external canal

        H61.812   Exostosis of left external canal

        H61.813   Exostosis of external canal, bilateral

        H61.819   Exostosis of external canal, unspecified ear

    ✓6ᵗʰ **H61.89**   **Other specified disorders of external ear**

        H61.891   Other specified disorders of right external ear

        H61.892   Other specified disorders of left external ear

        H61.893   Other specified disorders of external ear, bilateral

        H61.899   Other specified disorders of external ear, unspecified ear

   ✓5ᵗʰ **H61.9**   **Disorder of external ear, unspecified**

        H61.90   Disorder of external ear, unspecified, unspecified ear

        H61.91   Disorder of right external ear, unspecified

        H61.92   Disorder of left external ear, unspecified

        H61.93   Disorder of external ear, unspecified, bilateral

☑ Additional Character Required   ✓x7ᵗʰ Placeholder Alert   Manifestation   Unspecified Dx   ▶◀ Revised Text   ● New Code   ▲ Revised Title

ICD-10-CM 2020   621

Chapter 8. Diseases of the Ear and Mastoid Process

✓4ᵗʰ **H62** **Disorders of external ear in diseases classified elsewhere**

  ✓5ᵗʰ **H62.4** **Otitis externa in other diseases classified elsewhere**

    Code first underlying disease, such as:
      erysipelas (A46)
      impetigo (L01.0)

     EXCLUDES 1   *otitis externa (in):*
          candidiasis (B37.84)
          herpes viral [herpes simplex] (B00.1)
          herpes zoster (B02.8)

    H62.40 *Otitis externa in other diseases classified elsewhere, unspecified ear*

    H62.41 *Otitis externa in other diseases classified elsewhere, right ear*

    H62.42 *Otitis externa in other diseases classified elsewhere, left ear*

    H62.43 *Otitis externa in other diseases classified elsewhere, bilateral*

  ✓5ᵗʰ **H62.8** **Other disorders of external ear in diseases classified elsewhere**

    Code first underlying disease, such as:
      gout (M1A.-, M10.-)

    ✓6ᵗʰ **H62.8X** **Other disorders of external ear in diseases classified elsewhere**

      H62.8X1 *Other disorders of right external ear in diseases classified elsewhere*

      H62.8X2 *Other disorders of left external ear in diseases classified elsewhere*

      H62.8X3 *Other disorders of external ear in diseases classified elsewhere, bilateral*

      H62.8X9 *Other disorders of external ear in diseases classified elsewhere, unspecified ear*

Diseases of middle ear and mastoid (H65-H75)

✓4ᵗʰ **H65** **Nonsuppurative otitis media**

  INCLUDES   nonsuppurative otitis media with myringitis

  Use additional code for any associated perforated tympanic membrane (H72.-)

  ▶Use additional code, if applicable, to identify:◀
    exposure to environmental tobacco smoke (Z77.22)
    exposure to tobacco smoke in the perinatal period (P96.81)
    history of tobacco dependence (Z87.891)
  ▶infectious agent (B95-B97)◀
    occupational exposure to environmental tobacco smoke (Z57.31)
    tobacco dependence (F17.-)
    tobacco use (Z72.0)

  ✓5ᵗʰ **H65.0** **Acute serous otitis media**

    Acute and subacute secretory otitis

    H65.00 **Acute serous otitis media, unspecified ear**
    H65.01 **Acute serous otitis media, right ear**
    H65.02 **Acute serous otitis media, left ear**
    H65.03 **Acute serous otitis media, bilateral**
    H65.04 **Acute serous otitis media, recurrent, right ear**
    H65.05 **Acute serous otitis media, recurrent, left ear**
    H65.06 **Acute serous otitis media, recurrent, bilateral**
    H65.07 **Acute serous otitis media, recurrent, unspecified ear**

  ✓5ᵗʰ **H65.1** **Other acute nonsuppurative otitis media**

    EXCLUDES 1 *otitic barotrauma (T70.0)*
               otitis media (acute) NOS (H66.9)

    ✓6ᵗʰ **H65.11** **Acute and subacute allergic otitis media (mucoid) (sanguinous) (serous)**

      H65.111 **Acute and subacute allergic otitis media (mucoid) (sanguinous) (serous), right ear**

      H65.112 **Acute and subacute allergic otitis media (mucoid) (sanguinous) (serous), left ear**

      H65.113 **Acute and subacute allergic otitis media (mucoid) (sanguinous) (serous), bilateral**

      H65.114 **Acute and subacute allergic otitis media (mucoid) (sanguinous) (serous), recurrent, right ear**

      H65.115 **Acute and subacute allergic otitis media (mucoid) (sanguinous) (serous), recurrent, left ear**

      H65.116 **Acute and subacute allergic otitis media (mucoid) (sanguinous) (serous), recurrent, bilateral**

      H65.117 **Acute and subacute allergic otitis media (mucoid) (sanguinous) (serous), recurrent, unspecified ear**

      H65.119 **Acute and subacute allergic otitis media (mucoid) (sanguinous) (serous), unspecified ear**

    ✓6ᵗʰ **H65.19** **Other acute nonsuppurative otitis media**

      Acute and subacute mucoid otitis media
      Acute and subacute nonsuppurative otitis media NOS
      Acute and subacute sanguinous otitis media
      Acute and subacute seromucinous otitis media

      H65.191 **Other acute nonsuppurative otitis media, right ear**
      H65.192 **Other acute nonsuppurative otitis media, left ear**
      H65.193 **Other acute nonsuppurative otitis media, bilateral**
      H65.194 **Other acute nonsuppurative otitis media, recurrent, right ear**
      H65.195 **Other acute nonsuppurative otitis media, recurrent, left ear**
      H65.196 **Other acute nonsuppurative otitis media, recurrent, bilateral**
      H65.197 **Other acute nonsuppurative otitis media, recurrent, unspecified ear**
      H65.199 **Other acute nonsuppurative otitis media, unspecified ear**

  ✓5ᵗʰ **H65.2** **Chronic serous otitis media**

    Chronic tubotympanal catarrh

    H65.20 **Chronic serous otitis media, unspecified ear**
    H65.21 **Chronic serous otitis media, right ear**
    H65.22 **Chronic serous otitis media, left ear**
    H65.23 **Chronic serous otitis media, bilateral**

  ✓5ᵗʰ **H65.3** **Chronic mucoid otitis media**

    Chronic mucinous otitis media
    Chronic secretory otitis media
    Chronic transudative otitis media
    Glue ear

    EXCLUDES 1 *adhesive middle ear disease (H74.1)*

    H65.30 **Chronic mucoid otitis media, unspecified ear**
    H65.31 **Chronic mucoid otitis media, right ear**
    H65.32 **Chronic mucoid otitis media, left ear**
    H65.33 **Chronic mucoid otitis media, bilateral**

  ✓5ᵗʰ **H65.4** **Other chronic nonsuppurative otitis media**

    ✓6ᵗʰ **H65.41** **Chronic allergic otitis media**

      H65.411 **Chronic allergic otitis media, right ear**
      H65.412 **Chronic allergic otitis media, left ear**
      H65.413 **Chronic allergic otitis media, bilateral**
      H65.419 **Chronic allergic otitis media, unspecified ear**

    ✓6ᵗʰ **H65.49** **Other chronic nonsuppurative otitis media**

      Chronic exudative otitis media
      Chronic nonsuppurative otitis media NOS
      Chronic otitis media with effusion (nonpurulent)
      Chronic seromucinous otitis media

      H65.491 **Other chronic nonsuppurative otitis media, right ear**
      H65.492 **Other chronic nonsuppurative otitis media, left ear**
      H65.493 **Other chronic nonsuppurative otitis media, bilateral**
      H65.499 **Other chronic nonsuppurative otitis media, unspecified ear**

  ✓5ᵗʰ **H65.9** **Unspecified nonsuppurative otitis media**

    Allergic otitis media NOS
    Catarrhal otitis media NOS
    Exudative otitis media NOS
    Mucoid otitis media NOS
    Otitis media with effusion (nonpurulent) NOS
    Secretory otitis media NOS
    Seromucinous otitis media NOS
    Serous otitis media NOS
    Transudative otitis media NOS

    H65.90 **Unspecified nonsuppurative otitis media, unspecified ear**
    H65.91 **Unspecified nonsuppurative otitis media, right ear**
    H65.92 **Unspecified nonsuppurative otitis media, left ear**
    H65.93 **Unspecified nonsuppurative otitis media, bilateral**

Ⓝ Newborn: 0   Ⓟ Pediatric: 0-17   Ⓜ Maternity: 12-55   Ⓐ Adult: 15-124   **CH** Comorbidity High   **CL** Comorbidity Low   **NCDx** Noncancer Dx   **PDx** Primary Dx

622   ICD-10-CM 2020

☑4ᵗʰ **H66** **Suppurative and unspecified otitis media**

    INCLUDES   suppurative and unspecified otitis media with myringitis
    Use additional code to identify:
      exposure to environmental tobacco smoke (Z77.22)
      exposure to tobacco smoke in the perinatal period (P96.81)
      history of tobacco dependence (Z87.891)
      occupational exposure to environmental tobacco smoke (Z57.31)
      tobacco dependence (F17.-)
      tobacco use (Z72.0)
    AHA: 2016,1Q,34

  ☑5ᵗʰ **H66.0** **Acute suppurative** otitis media

    ☑6ᵗʰ **H66.00** **Acute suppurative otitis media** without spontaneous rupture of ear drum

      H66.001 Acute suppurative otitis media without spontaneous rupture of ear drum, right ear

      H66.002 Acute suppurative otitis media without spontaneous rupture of ear drum, left ear

      H66.003 Acute suppurative otitis media without spontaneous rupture of ear drum, bilateral

      H66.004 Acute suppurative otitis media without spontaneous rupture of ear drum, recurrent, right ear

      H66.005 Acute suppurative otitis media without spontaneous rupture of ear drum, recurrent, left ear

      H66.006 Acute suppurative otitis media without spontaneous rupture of ear drum, recurrent, bilateral

      H66.007 Acute suppurative otitis media without spontaneous rupture of ear drum, recurrent, unspecified ear

      H66.009 Acute suppurative otitis media without spontaneous rupture of ear drum, unspecified ear

    ☑6ᵗʰ **H66.01** **Acute suppurative otitis media** with spontaneous rupture of ear drum

      DEF: Sudden, severe inflammation of the middle ear, causing pressure that perforates the ear drum tissue.

      H66.011 Acute suppurative otitis media with spontaneous rupture of ear drum, right ear

      H66.012 Acute suppurative otitis media with spontaneous rupture of ear drum, left ear

      H66.013 Acute suppurative otitis media with spontaneous rupture of ear drum, bilateral

      H66.014 Acute suppurative otitis media with spontaneous rupture of ear drum, recurrent, right ear

      H66.015 Acute suppurative otitis media with spontaneous rupture of ear drum, recurrent, left ear

      H66.016 Acute suppurative otitis media with spontaneous rupture of ear drum, recurrent, bilateral

      H66.017 Acute suppurative otitis media with spontaneous rupture of ear drum, recurrent, unspecified ear

      H66.019 Acute suppurative otitis media with spontaneous rupture of ear drum, unspecified ear

  ☑5ᵗʰ **H66.1** **Chronic tubotympanic** suppurative otitis media

    Benign chronic suppurative otitis media
    Chronic tubotympanic disease
    Use additional code for any associated perforated tympanic membrane (H72.-)

    H66.10 Chronic tubotympanic suppurative otitis media, unspecified

    H66.11 Chronic tubotympanic suppurative otitis media, right ear

    H66.12 Chronic tubotympanic suppurative otitis media, left ear

    H66.13 Chronic tubotympanic suppurative otitis media, bilateral

  ☑5ᵗʰ **H66.2** **Chronic atticoantral** suppurative otitis media

    Chronic atticoantral disease
    Use additional code for any associated perforated tympanic membrane (H72.-)

    H66.20 Chronic atticoantral suppurative otitis media, unspecified ear

    H66.21 Chronic atticoantral suppurative otitis media, right ear

    H66.22 Chronic atticoantral suppurative otitis media, left ear

    H66.23 Chronic atticoantral suppurative otitis media, bilateral

  ☑5ᵗʰ **H66.3** **Other chronic suppurative otitis media**

    Chronic suppurative otitis media NOS
    Use additional code for any associated perforated tympanic membrane (H72.-)

    EXCLUDES 1   tuberculous otitis media (A18.6)

    ☑6ᵗʰ **H66.3X** **Other chronic suppurative otitis media**

      H66.3X1 Other chronic suppurative otitis media, right ear

      H66.3X2 Other chronic suppurative otitis media, left ear

      H66.3X3 Other chronic suppurative otitis media, bilateral

      H66.3X9 Other chronic suppurative otitis media, unspecified ear

  ☑5ᵗʰ **H66.4** **Suppurative otitis media, unspecified**

    Purulent otitis media NOS
    Use additional code for any associated perforated tympanic membrane (H72.-)

    H66.40 Suppurative otitis media, unspecified, unspecified ear

    H66.41 Suppurative otitis media, unspecified, right ear

    H66.42 Suppurative otitis media, unspecified, left ear

    H66.43 Suppurative otitis media, unspecified, bilateral

  ☑5ᵗʰ **H66.9** **Otitis media, unspecified**

    Otitis media NOS
    Acute otitis media NOS
    Chronic otitis media NOS
    Use additional code for any associated perforated tympanic membrane (H72.-)

    H66.90 Otitis media, unspecified, unspecified ear

    H66.91 Otitis media, unspecified, right ear

    H66.92 Otitis media, unspecified, left ear

    H66.93 Otitis media, unspecified, bilateral

☑4ᵗʰ **H67** **Otitis media in diseases classified elsewhere**

    Code first underlying disease, such as:
      plasminogen deficiency (E88.02)
      viral disease NEC (B00-B34)
    Use additional code for any associated perforated tympanic membrane (H72.-)

    EXCLUDES 1   otitis media in:
      influenza (J09.X9, J10.83, J11.83)
      measles (B05.3)
      scarlet fever (A38.0)
      tuberculosis (A18.6)

  H67.1 *Otitis media in diseases classified elsewhere, right ear*

  H67.2 *Otitis media in diseases classified elsewhere, left ear*

  H67.3 *Otitis media in diseases classified elsewhere, bilateral*

  H67.9 *Otitis media in diseases classified elsewhere, unspecified ear*

☑4ᵗʰ **H68** **Eustachian salpingitis and obstruction**

    DEF: Eustachian tube: Internal channel between the tympanic cavity and the nasopharynx that equalizes internal pressure to the outside pressure and drains mucous production from the middle ear.

  ☑5ᵗʰ **H68.0** **Eustachian** salpingitis

    ☑6ᵗʰ **H68.00** **Unspecified Eustachian salpingitis**

      H68.001 Unspecified Eustachian salpingitis, right ear

      H68.002 Unspecified Eustachian salpingitis, left ear

      H68.003 Unspecified Eustachian salpingitis, bilateral

      H68.009 Unspecified Eustachian salpingitis, unspecified ear

    ☑6ᵗʰ **H68.01** **Acute Eustachian salpingitis**

      H68.011 Acute Eustachian salpingitis, right ear

      H68.012 Acute Eustachian salpingitis, left ear

      H68.013 Acute Eustachian salpingitis, bilateral

      H68.019 Acute Eustachian salpingitis, unspecified ear

    ☑6ᵗʰ **H68.02** **Chronic Eustachian salpingitis**

      H68.021 Chronic Eustachian salpingitis, right ear

      H68.022 Chronic Eustachian salpingitis, left ear

H68.Ø23   **Chronic Eustachian salpingitis,** bilateral

H68.Ø29   **Chronic Eustachian salpingitis, unspecified ear**

√5ᵗʰ **H68.1**   **Obstruction** of Eustachian tube

    Stenosis of Eustachian tube

    Stricture of Eustachian tube

√6ᵗʰ **H68.10**   **Unspecified obstruction of Eustachian tube**

H68.1Ø1   **Unspecified obstruction of Eustachian tube,** right ear

H68.1Ø2   **Unspecified obstruction of Eustachian tube,** left ear

H68.1Ø3   **Unspecified obstruction of Eustachian tube,** bilateral

H68.1Ø9   **Unspecified obstruction of Eustachian tube, unspecified ear**

√6ᵗʰ **H68.11**   **Osseous obstruction of Eustachian tube**

H68.111   **Osseous obstruction of Eustachian tube,** right ear

H68.112   **Osseous obstruction of Eustachian tube,** left ear

H68.113   **Osseous obstruction of Eustachian tube,** bilateral

H68.119   **Osseous obstruction of Eustachian tube, unspecified ear**

√6ᵗʰ **H68.12**   **Intrinsic cartilagenous obstruction of Eustachian tube**

H68.121   **Intrinsic cartilagenous obstruction of Eustachian tube,** right ear

H68.122   **Intrinsic cartilagenous obstruction of Eustachian tube,** left ear

H68.123   **Intrinsic cartilagenous obstruction of Eustachian tube,** bilateral

H68.129   **Intrinsic cartilagenous obstruction of Eustachian tube, unspecified ear**

√6ᵗʰ **H68.13**   **Extrinsic cartilagenous obstruction of Eustachian tube**

    Compression of Eustachian tube

H68.131   **Extrinsic cartilagenous obstruction of Eustachian tube,** right ear

H68.132   **Extrinsic cartilagenous obstruction of Eustachian tube,** left ear

H68.133   **Extrinsic cartilagenous obstruction of Eustachian tube,** bilateral

H68.139   **Extrinsic cartilagenous obstruction of Eustachian tube, unspecified ear**

√4ᵗʰ **H69**   **Other and unspecified disorders of Eustachian tube**

    DEF: Eustachian tube: Internal channel between the tympanic cavity and the nasopharynx that equalizes internal pressure to the outside pressure and drains mucous production from the middle ear.

√5ᵗʰ **H69.Ø**   **Patulous Eustachian tube**

H69.ØØ   **Patulous Eustachian tube, unspecified ear**

H69.Ø1   **Patulous Eustachian tube,** right ear

H69.Ø2   **Patulous Eustachian tube,** left ear

H69.Ø3   **Patulous Eustachian tube,** bilateral

√5ᵗʰ **H69.8**   **Other specified disorders of Eustachian tube**

H69.8Ø   **Other specified disorders of Eustachian tube, unspecified ear**

H69.81   **Other specified disorders of Eustachian tube,** right ear

H69.82   **Other specified disorders of Eustachian tube,** left ear

H69.83   **Other specified disorders of Eustachian tube,** bilateral

√5ᵗʰ **H69.9**   **Unspecified Eustachian tube disorder**

H69.9Ø   **Unspecified Eustachian tube disorder, unspecified ear**

H69.91   **Unspecified Eustachian tube disorder,** right ear

H69.92   **Unspecified Eustachian tube disorder,** left ear

H69.93   **Unspecified Eustachian tube disorder,** bilateral

√4ᵗʰ **H7Ø**   **Mastoiditis and related conditions**

√5ᵗʰ **H7Ø.Ø**   **Acute mastoiditis**

    Abscess of mastoid

    Empyema of mastoid

√6ᵗʰ **H7Ø.ØØ**   **Acute mastoiditis** without complications

H7Ø.ØØ1   **Acute mastoiditis without complications,** right ear

H7Ø.ØØ2   **Acute mastoiditis without complications,** left ear

H7Ø.ØØ3   **Acute mastoiditis without complications,** bilateral

H7Ø.ØØ9   **Acute mastoiditis without complications, unspecified ear**

√6ᵗʰ **H7Ø.Ø1**   **Subperiosteal abscess** of mastoid

H7Ø.Ø11   **Subperiosteal abscess of mastoid,** right ear

H7Ø.Ø12   **Subperiosteal abscess of mastoid,** left ear

H7Ø.Ø13   **Subperiosteal abscess of mastoid,** bilateral

H7Ø.Ø19   **Subperiosteal abscess of mastoid, unspecified ear**

√6ᵗʰ **H7Ø.Ø9**   **Acute mastoiditis with other complications**

H7Ø.Ø91   **Acute mastoiditis with other complications,** right ear

H7Ø.Ø92   **Acute mastoiditis with other complications,** left ear

H7Ø.Ø93   **Acute mastoiditis with other complications,** bilateral

H7Ø.Ø99   **Acute mastoiditis with other complications, unspecified ear**

√5ᵗʰ **H7Ø.1**   Chronic **mastoiditis**

    Caries of mastoid

    Fistula of mastoid

    EXCLUDES 1   *tuberculous mastoiditis (A18.Ø3)*

H7Ø.1Ø   **Chronic mastoiditis, unspecified ear**

H7Ø.11   **Chronic mastoiditis,** right ear

H7Ø.12   **Chronic mastoiditis,** left ear

H7Ø.13   **Chronic mastoiditis,** bilateral

√5ᵗʰ **H7Ø.2**   **Petrositis**

    Inflammation of petrous bone

√6ᵗʰ **H7Ø.2Ø**   **Unspecified petrositis**

H7Ø.2Ø1   **Unspecified petrositis,** right ear

H7Ø.2Ø2   **Unspecified petrositis,** left ear

H7Ø.2Ø3   **Unspecified petrositis,** bilateral

H7Ø.2Ø9   **Unspecified petrositis, unspecified ear**

√6ᵗʰ **H7Ø.21**   **Acute petrositis**

    DEF: Sudden, severe inflammation of the petrous temporal bone behind the ear, associated with a middle ear infection.

H7Ø.211   **Acute petrositis,** right ear

H7Ø.212   **Acute petrositis,** left ear

H7Ø.213   **Acute petrositis,** bilateral

H7Ø.219   **Acute petrositis, unspecified ear**

√6ᵗʰ **H7Ø.22**   Chronic **petrositis**

H7Ø.221   **Chronic petrositis,** right ear

H7Ø.222   **Chronic petrositis,** left ear

H7Ø.223   **Chronic petrositis,** bilateral

H7Ø.229   **Chronic petrositis, unspecified ear**

√5ᵗʰ **H7Ø.8**   **Other mastoiditis and related conditions**

    EXCLUDES 1   *preauricular sinus and cyst (Q18.1)*

                      sinus, fistula, and cyst of branchial cleft (Q18.Ø)

√6ᵗʰ **H7Ø.81**   Postauricular fistula

H7Ø.811   **Postauricular fistula,** right ear

H7Ø.812   **Postauricular fistula,** left ear

H7Ø.813   **Postauricular fistula,** bilateral

H7Ø.819   **Postauricular fistula, unspecified ear**

√6ᵗʰ **H7Ø.89**   **Other mastoiditis and related conditions**

H7Ø.891   Other mastoiditis and related conditions, right ear

H7Ø.892   **Other mastoiditis and related conditions,** left ear

H7Ø.893   **Other mastoiditis and related conditions,** bilateral

H7Ø.899   **Other mastoiditis and related conditions, unspecified ear**

√5ᵗʰ **H7Ø.9**   **Unspecified mastoiditis**

H7Ø.9Ø   **Unspecified mastoiditis, unspecified ear**

H7Ø.91   **Unspecified mastoiditis,** right ear

H7Ø.92   **Unspecified mastoiditis,** left ear

H7Ø.93   **Unspecified mastoiditis,** bilateral

✓4th **H71 Cholesteatoma of middle ear**

> EXCLUDES 2   cholesteatoma of external ear (H60.4-)
> recurrent cholesteatoma of postmastoidectomy cavity (H95.0-)

DEF: Cholesteatoma: Noncancerous cyst-like mass of cell debris, including cholesterol and epithelial cells resulting from trauma, repeated or improperly healed infections, and congenital enclosure of epidermal cells.

Cholesteatoma of Middle Ear

- Middle ear chamber
- Ear drum
- Cholesteatoma sac

✓5th **H71.0 Cholesteatoma of attic**
- **H71.00 Cholesteatoma of attic, unspecified ear**
- **H71.01 Cholesteatoma of attic, right ear**
- **H71.02 Cholesteatoma of attic, left ear**
- **H71.03 Cholesteatoma of attic, bilateral**

✓5th **H71.1 Cholesteatoma of tympanum**
- **H71.10 Cholesteatoma of tympanum, unspecified ear**
- **H71.11 Cholesteatoma of tympanum, right ear**
- **H71.12 Cholesteatoma of tympanum, left ear**
- **H71.13 Cholesteatoma of tympanum, bilateral**

✓5th **H71.2 Cholesteatoma of mastoid**
- **H71.20 Cholesteatoma of mastoid, unspecified ear**
- **H71.21 Cholesteatoma of mastoid, right ear**
- **H71.22 Cholesteatoma of mastoid, left ear**
- **H71.23 Cholesteatoma of mastoid, bilateral**

✓5th **H71.3 Diffuse cholesteatosis**
- **H71.30 Diffuse cholesteatosis, unspecified ear**
- **H71.31 Diffuse cholesteatosis, right ear**
- **H71.32 Diffuse cholesteatosis, left ear**
- **H71.33 Diffuse cholesteatosis, bilateral**

✓5th **H71.9 Unspecified cholesteatoma**
- **H71.90 Unspecified cholesteatoma, unspecified ear**
- **H71.91 Unspecified cholesteatoma, right ear**
- **H71.92 Unspecified cholesteatoma, left ear**
- **H71.93 Unspecified cholesteatoma, bilateral**

✓4th **H72 Perforation of tympanic membrane**

> INCLUDES   persistent post-traumatic perforation of ear drum
> postinflammatory perforation of ear drum

Code first any associated otitis media (H65.-, H66.1-, H66.2-, H66.3-, H66.4-, H66.9-, H67.-)

> EXCLUDES 1   acute suppurative otitis media with rupture of the tympanic membrane (H66.01-)
> traumatic rupture of ear drum (S09.2-)

✓5th **H72.0 Central perforation of tympanic membrane**
- **H72.00 Central perforation of tympanic membrane, unspecified ear**
- **H72.01 Central perforation of tympanic membrane, right ear**
- **H72.02 Central perforation of tympanic membrane, left ear**
- **H72.03 Central perforation of tympanic membrane, bilateral**

✓5th **H72.1 Attic perforation of tympanic membrane**

Perforation of pars flaccida
- **H72.10 Attic perforation of tympanic membrane, unspecified ear**
- **H72.11 Attic perforation of tympanic membrane, right ear**
- **H72.12 Attic perforation of tympanic membrane, left ear**

- **H72.13 Attic perforation of tympanic membrane, bilateral**

✓5th **H72.2 Other marginal perforations of tympanic membrane**

✓6th **H72.2X Other marginal perforations of tympanic membrane**
- **H72.2X1 Other marginal perforations of tympanic membrane, right ear**
- **H72.2X2 Other marginal perforations of tympanic membrane, left ear**
- **H72.2X3 Other marginal perforations of tympanic membrane, bilateral**
- **H72.2X9 Other marginal perforations of tympanic membrane, unspecified ear**

✓5th **H72.8 Other perforations of tympanic membrane**

✓6th **H72.81 Multiple perforations of tympanic membrane**
- **H72.811 Multiple perforations of tympanic membrane, right ear**
- **H72.812 Multiple perforations of tympanic membrane, left ear**
- **H72.813 Multiple perforations of tympanic membrane, bilateral**
- **H72.819 Multiple perforations of tympanic membrane, unspecified ear**

✓6th **H72.82 Total perforations of tympanic membrane**
- **H72.821 Total perforations of tympanic membrane, right ear**
- **H72.822 Total perforations of tympanic membrane, left ear**
- **H72.823 Total perforations of tympanic membrane, bilateral**
- **H72.829 Total perforations of tympanic membrane, unspecified ear**

✓5th **H72.9 Unspecified perforation of tympanic membrane**
- **H72.90 Unspecified perforation of tympanic membrane, unspecified ear**
- **H72.91 Unspecified perforation of tympanic membrane, right ear**
- **H72.92 Unspecified perforation of tympanic membrane, left ear**
- **H72.93 Unspecified perforation of tympanic membrane, bilateral**

✓4th **H73 Other disorders of tympanic membrane**

✓5th **H73.0 Acute myringitis**

> EXCLUDES 1   acute myringitis with otitis media (H65, H66)

✓6th **H73.00 Unspecified acute myringitis**

Acute tympanitis NOS
- **H73.001 Acute myringitis, right ear**
- **H73.002 Acute myringitis, left ear**
- **H73.003 Acute myringitis, bilateral**
- **H73.009 Acute myringitis, unspecified ear**

✓6th **H73.01 Bullous myringitis**

DEF: Bacterial or viral otitis media that is characterized by the appearance of serous or hemorrhagic blebs on the ear drum and sudden onset of severe pain in ear.
- **H73.011 Bullous myringitis, right ear**
- **H73.012 Bullous myringitis, left ear**
- **H73.013 Bullous myringitis, bilateral**
- **H73.019 Bullous myringitis, unspecified ear**

✓6th **H73.09 Other acute myringitis**
- **H73.091 Other acute myringitis, right ear**
- **H73.092 Other acute myringitis, left ear**
- **H73.093 Other acute myringitis, bilateral**
- **H73.099 Other acute myringitis, unspecified ear**

✓5th **H73.1 Chronic myringitis**

Chronic tympanitis

> EXCLUDES 1   chronic myringitis with otitis media (H65, H66)
- **H73.10 Chronic myringitis, unspecified ear**
- **H73.11 Chronic myringitis, right ear**
- **H73.12 Chronic myringitis, left ear**
- **H73.13 Chronic myringitis, bilateral**

✓5th **H73.2 Unspecified myringitis**
- **H73.20 Unspecified myringitis, unspecified ear**
- **H73.21 Unspecified myringitis, right ear**
- **H73.22 Unspecified myringitis, left ear**
- **H73.23 Unspecified myringitis, bilateral**

✓5th **H73.8 Other specified disorders of tympanic membrane**

✓6th **H73.81 Atrophic flaccid tympanic membrane**
- **H73.811 Atrophic flaccid tympanic membrane, right ear**

✓ Additional Character Required   ✓x7th Placeholder Alert   Manifestation   Unspecified Dx   ▶◀ Revised Text   ● New Code   ▲ Revised Title

Chapter 8. Diseases of the Ear and Mastoid Process

H73.812–H80.23

H73.812   **Atrophic flaccid tympanic membrane,** left **ear**

H73.813   **Atrophic flaccid tympanic membrane,** bilateral

H73.819   **Atrophic flaccid tympanic membrane,** unspecified ear

✓6ᵗʰ **H73.82**   Atrophic nonflaccid **tympanic membrane**

H73.821   **Atrophic nonflaccid tympanic membrane,** right **ear**

H73.822   **Atrophic nonflaccid tympanic membrane,** left **ear**

H73.823   **Atrophic nonflaccid tympanic membrane,** bilateral

H73.829   **Atrophic nonflaccid tympanic membrane,** unspecified ear

✓6ᵗʰ **H73.89**   **Other specified disorders of tympanic membrane**

H73.891   **Other specified disorders of tympanic membrane,** right **ear**

H73.892   **Other specified disorders of tympanic membrane,** left **ear**

H73.893   **Other specified disorders of tympanic membrane,** bilateral

H73.899   **Other specified disorders of tympanic membrane,** unspecified ear

✓5ᵗʰ **H73.9**   **Unspecified disorder of tympanic membrane**

H73.90   **Unspecified disorder of tympanic membrane, unspecified ear**

H73.91   **Unspecified disorder of tympanic membrane,** right **ear**

H73.92   **Unspecified disorder of tympanic membrane,** left **ear**

H73.93   **Unspecified disorder of tympanic membrane,** bilateral

✓4ᵗʰ **H74**   **Other disorders of middle ear mastoid**

EXCLUDES 2   mastoiditis (H70.-)

✓5ᵗʰ **H74.0**   **Tympanosclerosis**

DEF: Calcification of tissue in the ear drum, middle ear bones, and middle ear canal.

H74.01   **Tympanosclerosis,** right **ear**

H74.02   **Tympanosclerosis,** left **ear**

H74.03   **Tympanosclerosis,** bilateral

H74.09   **Tympanosclerosis, unspecified ear**

✓5ᵗʰ **H74.1**   **Adhesive middle ear disease**

Adhesive otitis

EXCLUDES 1   glue ear (H65.3-)

H74.11   **Adhesive** right **middle ear disease**

H74.12   **Adhesive** left **middle ear disease**

H74.13   **Adhesive middle ear disease,** bilateral

H74.19   **Adhesive middle ear disease, unspecified ear**

✓5ᵗʰ **H74.2**   **Discontinuity and dislocation of ear ossicles**

H74.20   **Discontinuity and dislocation of ear ossicles, unspecified ear**

H74.21   **Discontinuity and dislocation of** right **ear ossicles**

H74.22   **Discontinuity and dislocation of** left **ear ossicles**

H74.23   **Discontinuity and dislocation of ear ossicles,** bilateral

✓5ᵗʰ **H74.3**   **Other acquired abnormalities of ear ossicles**

✓6ᵗʰ **H74.31**   Ankylosis **of ear ossicles**

H74.311   **Ankylosis of ear ossicles,** right **ear**

H74.312   **Ankylosis of ear ossicles,** left **ear**

H74.313   **Ankylosis of ear ossicles,** bilateral

H74.319   **Ankylosis of ear ossicles, unspecified ear**

✓6ᵗʰ **H74.32**   Partial loss **of ear ossicles**

H74.321   **Partial loss of ear ossicles,** right **ear**

H74.322   **Partial loss of ear ossicles,** left **ear**

H74.323   **Partial loss of ear ossicles,** bilateral

H74.329   **Partial loss of ear ossicles, unspecified ear**

✓6ᵗʰ **H74.39**   **Other acquired abnormalities of ear ossicles**

H74.391   **Other acquired abnormalities of** right **ear ossicles**

H74.392   **Other acquired abnormalities of** left **ear ossicles**

H74.393   **Other acquired abnormalities of ear ossicles,** bilateral

H74.399   **Other acquired abnormalities of ear ossicles, unspecified ear**

✓5ᵗʰ **H74.4**   **Polyp of middle ear**

H74.40   **Polyp of middle ear, unspecified ear**

H74.41   **Polyp of** right **middle ear**

H74.42   **Polyp of** left **middle ear**

H74.43   **Polyp of middle ear,** bilateral

✓5ᵗʰ **H74.8**   **Other specified disorders of middle ear and mastoid**

✓6ᵗʰ **H74.8X**   **Other specified disorders of middle ear and mastoid**

H74.8X1   **Other specified disorders of** right **middle ear and mastoid**

H74.8X2   **Other specified disorders of** left **middle ear and mastoid**

H74.8X3   **Other specified disorders of middle ear and mastoid,** bilateral

H74.8X9   **Other specified disorders of middle ear and mastoid, unspecified ear**

✓5ᵗʰ **H74.9**   **Unspecified disorder of middle ear and mastoid**

H74.90   **Unspecified disorder of middle ear and mastoid, unspecified ear**

H74.91   **Unspecified disorder of** right **middle ear and mastoid**

H74.92   **Unspecified disorder of** left **middle ear and mastoid**

H74.93   **Unspecified disorder of middle ear and mastoid,** bilateral

✓4ᵗʰ **H75**   **Other disorders of middle ear and mastoid in diseases classified elsewhere**

Code first underlying disease

✓5ᵗʰ **H75.0**   **Mastoiditis in infectious and parasitic diseases classified elsewhere**

EXCLUDES 1   mastoiditis (in):
syphilis (A52.77)
tuberculosis (A18.03)

H75.00   *Mastoiditis in infectious and parasitic diseases classified elsewhere, unspecified ear*

H75.01   *Mastoiditis in infectious and parasitic diseases classified elsewhere, right ear*

H75.02   *Mastoiditis in infectious and parasitic diseases classified elsewhere, left ear*

H75.03   *Mastoiditis in infectious and parasitic diseases classified elsewhere, bilateral*

✓5ᵗʰ **H75.8**   **Other specified disorders of middle ear and mastoid in diseases classified elsewhere**

H75.80   *Other specified disorders of middle ear and mastoid in diseases classified elsewhere, unspecified ear*

H75.81   *Other specified disorders of right middle ear and mastoid in diseases classified elsewhere*

H75.82   *Other specified disorders of left middle ear and mastoid in diseases classified elsewhere*

H75.83   *Other specified disorders of middle ear and mastoid in diseases classified elsewhere, bilateral*

Diseases of inner ear (H80-H83)

✓4ᵗʰ **H80**   **Otosclerosis**

INCLUDES   otospongiosis

✓5ᵗʰ **H80.0**   **Otosclerosis involving oval window,** nonobliterative

H80.00   **Otosclerosis involving oval window, nonobliterative, unspecified ear**

H80.01   **Otosclerosis involving oval window, nonobliterative,** right **ear**

H80.02   **Otosclerosis involving oval window, nonobliterative,** left **ear**

H80.03   **Otosclerosis involving oval window, nonobliterative,** bilateral

✓5ᵗʰ **H80.1**   **Otosclerosis involving oval window,** obliterative

H80.10   **Otosclerosis involving oval window, obliterative, unspecified ear**

H80.11   **Otosclerosis involving oval window, obliterative,** right **ear**

H80.12   **Otosclerosis involving oval window, obliterative,** left **ear**

H80.13   **Otosclerosis involving oval window, obliterative,** bilateral

✓5ᵗʰ **H80.2**   Cochlear **otosclerosis**

Otosclerosis involving otic capsule
Otosclerosis involving round window

H80.20   **Cochlear otosclerosis, unspecified ear**

H80.21   **Cochlear otosclerosis,** right **ear**

H80.22   **Cochlear otosclerosis,** left **ear**

H80.23   **Cochlear otosclerosis,** bilateral

N Newborn: 0   P Pediatric: 0-17   M Maternity: 12-55   A Adult: 15-124   CH Comorbidity High   CL Comorbidity Low   NCDx Noncancer Dx   PDx Primary Dx

626   ICD-10-CM 2020

Chapter 8. Diseases of the Ear and Mastoid Process

✓5ᵗʰ **H80.8 Other otosclerosis**

    H80.80 Other otosclerosis, unspecified ear

    H80.81 Other otosclerosis, right ear

    H80.82 Other otosclerosis, left ear

    H80.83 Other otosclerosis, bilateral

✓5ᵗʰ **H80.9 Unspecified otosclerosis**

    H80.90 Unspecified otosclerosis, unspecified ear

    H80.91 Unspecified otosclerosis, right ear

    H80.92 Unspecified otosclerosis, left ear

    H80.93 Unspecified otosclerosis, bilateral

✓4ᵗʰ **H81 Disorders of vestibular function**

    EXCLUDES 1   epidemic vertigo (A88.1)

                vertigo NOS (R42)

✓5ᵗʰ **H81.0 Ménière's disease**

    Labyrinthine hydrops

    Ménière's syndrome or vertigo

    DEF: Distended membranous labyrinth of the middle ear from fluctuating pressure of fluid (hydrops) that causes vertigo, tinnitus, pressure, and hearing loss that may last on and off for several hours. Episodes may occur in clusters or may subside for weeks, months, or even years.

    H81.01 Ménière's disease, right ear

    H81.02 Ménière's disease, left ear

    H81.03 Ménière's disease, bilateral

    H81.09 Ménière's disease, unspecified ear

✓5ᵗʰ **H81.1 Benign paroxysmal vertigo**

    H81.10 Benign paroxysmal vertigo, unspecified ear

    H81.11 Benign paroxysmal vertigo, right ear

    H81.12 Benign paroxysmal vertigo, left ear

    H81.13 Benign paroxysmal vertigo, bilateral

✓5ᵗʰ **H81.2 Vestibular neuronitis**

    DEF: Transient benign vertigo caused by inflammation of the vestibular nerve. It is characterized by response to caloric stimulation on one side and nystagmus with rhythmic movement of the eyes. Normal auditory function is present.

    H81.20 Vestibular neuronitis, unspecified ear

    H81.21 Vestibular neuronitis, right ear

    H81.22 Vestibular neuronitis, left ear

    H81.23 Vestibular neuronitis, bilateral

✓5ᵗʰ **H81.3 Other peripheral vertigo**

    ✓6ᵗʰ **H81.31 Aural vertigo**

        H81.311 Aural vertigo, right ear

        H81.312 Aural vertigo, left ear

        H81.313 Aural vertigo, bilateral

        H81.319 Aural vertigo, unspecified ear

    ✓6ᵗʰ **H81.39 Other peripheral vertigo**

        Lermoyez' syndrome

        Otogenic vertigo

        Peripheral vertigo NOS

        H81.391 Other peripheral vertigo, right ear

        H81.392 Other peripheral vertigo, left ear

        H81.393 Other peripheral vertigo, bilateral

        H81.399 Other peripheral vertigo, unspecified ear

▲ **H81.4 Vertigo of central origin**

    Central positional nystagmus

    ~~H81.41 Vertigo of central origin, right ear~~

    ~~H81.42 Vertigo of central origin, left ear~~

    ~~H81.43 Vertigo of central origin, bilateral~~

    ~~H81.49 Vertigo of central origin, unspecified ear~~

✓5ᵗʰ **H81.8 Other disorders of vestibular function**

    ✓6ᵗʰ **H81.8X Other disorders of vestibular function**

        H81.8X1 Other disorders of vestibular function, right ear

        H81.8X2 Other disorders of vestibular function, left ear

        H81.8X3 Other disorders of vestibular function, bilateral

        H81.8X9 Other disorders of vestibular function, unspecified ear

✓5ᵗʰ **H81.9 Unspecified disorder of vestibular function**

    Vertiginous syndrome NOS

    H81.90 Unspecified disorder of vestibular function, unspecified ear

    H81.91 Unspecified disorder of vestibular function, right ear

    H81.92 Unspecified disorder of vestibular function, left ear

    H81.93 Unspecified disorder of vestibular function, bilateral

✓4ᵗʰ **H82 Vertiginous syndromes in diseases classified elsewhere**

    Code first underlying disease

    EXCLUDES 1   epidemic vertigo (A88.1)

    H82.1 Vertiginous syndromes in diseases classified elsewhere, right ear

    H82.2 Vertiginous syndromes in diseases classified elsewhere, left ear

    H82.3 Vertiginous syndromes in diseases classified elsewhere, bilateral

    H82.9 Vertiginous syndromes in diseases classified elsewhere, unspecified ear

✓4ᵗʰ **H83 Other diseases of inner ear**

    ✓5ᵗʰ **H83.0 Labyrinthitis**

        DEF: Inflammation of the inner ear, or labyrinth, characterized by pus, vertigo, dizziness, nausea, and hearing loss.

        H83.01 Labyrinthitis, right ear

        H83.02 Labyrinthitis, left ear

        H83.03 Labyrinthitis, bilateral

        H83.09 Labyrinthitis, unspecified ear

    ✓5ᵗʰ **H83.1 Labyrinthine fistula**

        H83.11 Labyrinthine fistula, right ear

        H83.12 Labyrinthine fistula, left ear

        H83.13 Labyrinthine fistula, bilateral

        H83.19 Labyrinthine fistula, unspecified ear

    ✓5ᵗʰ **H83.2 Labyrinthine dysfunction**

        Labyrinthine hypersensitivity

        Labyrinthine hypofunction

        Labyrinthine loss of function

        DEF: Decreased function of the labyrinth sensors.

        ✓6ᵗʰ **H83.2X Labyrinthine dysfunction**

            H83.2X1 Labyrinthine dysfunction, right ear

            H83.2X2 Labyrinthine dysfunction, left ear

            H83.2X3 Labyrinthine dysfunction, bilateral

            H83.2X9 Labyrinthine dysfunction, unspecified ear

    ✓5ᵗʰ **H83.3 Noise effects on inner ear**

        Acoustic trauma of inner ear

        Noise-induced hearing loss of inner ear

        ✓6ᵗʰ **H83.3X Noise effects on inner ear**

            H83.3X1 Noise effects on right inner ear

            H83.3X2 Noise effects on left inner ear

            H83.3X3 Noise effects on inner ear, bilateral

            H83.3X9 Noise effects on inner ear, unspecified ear

    ✓5ᵗʰ **H83.8 Other specified diseases of inner ear**

        ✓6ᵗʰ **H83.8X Other specified diseases of inner ear**

            H83.8X1 Other specified diseases of right inner ear

            H83.8X2 Other specified diseases of left inner ear

            H83.8X3 Other specified diseases of inner ear, bilateral

            H83.8X9 Other specified diseases of inner ear, unspecified ear

    ✓5ᵗʰ **H83.9 Unspecified disease of inner ear**

        H83.90 Unspecified disease of inner ear, unspecified ear

        H83.91 Unspecified disease of right inner ear

        H83.92 Unspecified disease of left inner ear

        H83.93 Unspecified disease of inner ear, bilateral

Other disorders of ear (H90-H94)

✓4ᵗʰ **H90 Conductive and sensorineural hearing loss**

    EXCLUDES 1   deaf nonspeaking NEC (H91.3)

                deafness NOS (H91.9-)

                hearing loss NOS (H91.9-)

                noise-induced hearing loss (H83.3-)

                ototoxic hearing loss (H91.0-)

                sudden (idiopathic) hearing loss (H91.2-)

    AHA: 2015,2Q,7

    DEF: Conductive hearing loss: Hearing Loss due to the inability of sound waves to move from the outer (external ear) to the inner ear.

    DEF: Sensorineural hearing loss: Hearing loss that occurs from damage to the hair cells of the inner ear or problems with the nerve pathways from the inner ear to the brain.

    H90.0 Conductive hearing loss, bilateral

☑ Additional Character Required   ✓x7ᵗʰ Placeholder Alert   Manifestation   Unspecified Dx   ▶◀ Revised Text   ● New Code   ▲ Revised Title

✓5ᵗʰ **H90.1** Conductive hearing loss, unilateral with unrestricted hearing on the contralateral side

    H90.11 Conductive hearing loss, unilateral, right ear, with unrestricted hearing on the contralateral side

    H90.12 Conductive hearing loss, unilateral, left ear, with unrestricted hearing on the contralateral side

H90.2 Conductive hearing loss, unspecified
    Conductive deafness NOS

H90.3 Sensorineural hearing loss, bilateral

✓5ᵗʰ **H90.4** Sensorineural hearing loss, unilateral with unrestricted hearing on the contralateral side

    H90.41 Sensorineural hearing loss, unilateral, right ear, with unrestricted hearing on the contralateral side

    H90.42 Sensorineural hearing loss, unilateral, left ear, with unrestricted hearing on the contralateral side

H90.5 Unspecified sensorineural hearing loss
    Central hearing loss NOS
    Congenital deafness NOS
    Neural hearing loss NOS
    Perceptive hearing loss NOS
    Sensorineural deafness NOS
    Sensory hearing loss NOS

    EXCLUDES 1 *abnormal auditory perception (H93.2-)*
                  psychogenic deafness (F44.6)

H90.6 Mixed conductive and sensorineural hearing loss, bilateral
    AHA: 2015,2Q,7

✓5ᵗʰ **H90.7** Mixed conductive and sensorineural hearing loss, unilateral with unrestricted hearing on the contralateral side

    H90.71 Mixed conductive and sensorineural hearing loss, unilateral, right ear, with unrestricted hearing on the contralateral side

    H90.72 Mixed conductive and sensorineural hearing loss, unilateral, left ear, with unrestricted hearing on the contralateral side

H90.8 Mixed conductive and sensorineural hearing loss, unspecified

✓5ᵗʰ **H90.A** Conductive and sensorineural hearing loss with restricted hearing on the contralateral side
    AHA: 2016,4Q,23-25

  ✓6ᵗʰ **H90.A1** Conductive hearing loss, unilateral, with restricted hearing on the contralateral side

    H90.A11 Conductive hearing loss, unilateral, right ear with restricted hearing on the contralateral side

    H90.A12 Conductive hearing loss, unilateral, left ear with restricted hearing on the contralateral side

  ✓6ᵗʰ **H90.A2** Sensorineural hearing loss, unilateral, with restricted hearing on the contralateral side

    H90.A21 Sensorineural hearing loss, unilateral, right ear, with restricted hearing on the contralateral side

    H90.A22 Sensorineural hearing loss, unilateral, left ear, with restricted hearing on the contralateral side

  ✓6ᵗʰ **H90.A3** Mixed conductive and sensorineural hearing loss, unilateral with restricted hearing on the contralateral side

    H90.A31 Mixed conductive and sensorineural hearing loss, unilateral, right ear with restricted hearing on the contralateral side

    H90.A32 Mixed conductive and sensorineural hearing, unilateral, left ear with restricted hearing on the contralateral side

✓4ᵗʰ **H91** Other and unspecified hearing loss

    EXCLUDES 1 *abnormal auditory perception (H93.2-)*
                  hearing loss as classified in H90.-
                  impacted cerumen (H61.2-)
                  noise-induced hearing loss (H83.3-)
                  psychogenic deafness (F44.6)
                  transient ischemic deafness (H93.01-)

✓5ᵗʰ **H91.0** Ototoxic hearing loss
    Code first poisoning due to drug or toxin, if applicable (T36-T65 with fifth or sixth character 1-4 or 6)
    Use additional code for adverse effect, if applicable, to identify drug (T36-T50 with fifth or sixth character 5)

    H91.01 Ototoxic hearing loss, right ear
    H91.02 Ototoxic hearing loss, left ear
    H91.03 Ototoxic hearing loss, bilateral
    H91.09 Ototoxic hearing loss, unspecified ear

✓5ᵗʰ **H91.1** Presbycusis
    Presbyacusia

    H91.10 Presbycusis, unspecified ear
    H91.11 Presbycusis, right ear
    H91.12 Presbycusis, left ear
    H91.13 Presbycusis, bilateral

✓5ᵗʰ **H91.2** Sudden idiopathic hearing loss
    Sudden hearing loss NOS

    H91.20 Sudden idiopathic hearing loss, unspecified ear
    H91.21 Sudden idiopathic hearing loss, right ear
    H91.22 Sudden idiopathic hearing loss, left ear
    H91.23 Sudden idiopathic hearing loss, bilateral

H91.3 Deaf nonspeaking, not elsewhere classified

✓5ᵗʰ **H91.8** Other specified hearing loss

  ✓6ᵗʰ **H91.8X** Other specified hearing loss

    H91.8X1 Other specified hearing loss, right ear
    H91.8X2 Other specified hearing loss, left ear
    H91.8X3 Other specified hearing loss, bilateral
    H91.8X9 Other specified hearing loss, unspecified ear

✓5ᵗʰ **H91.9** Unspecified hearing loss
    Deafness NOS
    High frequency deafness
    Low frequency deafness

    H91.90 Unspecified hearing loss, unspecified ear
    H91.91 Unspecified hearing loss, right ear
    H91.92 Unspecified hearing loss, left ear
    H91.93 Unspecified hearing loss, bilateral

✓4ᵗʰ **H92** Otalgia and effusion of ear

✓5ᵗʰ **H92.0** Otalgia
    H92.01 Otalgia, right ear
    H92.02 Otalgia, left ear
    H92.03 Otalgia, bilateral
    H92.09 Otalgia, unspecified ear

✓5ᵗʰ **H92.1** Otorrhea
    EXCLUDES 1 *leakage of cerebrospinal fluid through ear (G96.0)*

    H92.10 Otorrhea, unspecified ear
    H92.11 Otorrhea, right ear
    H92.12 Otorrhea, left ear
    H92.13 Otorrhea, bilateral

✓5ᵗʰ **H92.2** Otorrhagia
    EXCLUDES 1 *traumatic otorrhagia — code to injury*

    H92.20 Otorrhagia, unspecified ear
    H92.21 Otorrhagia, right ear
    H92.22 Otorrhagia, left ear
    H92.23 Otorrhagia, bilateral

✓4ᵗʰ **H93** Other disorders of ear, not elsewhere classified

✓5ᵗʰ **H93.0** Degenerative and vascular disorders of ear
    EXCLUDES 1 *presbycusis (H91.1)*

  ✓6ᵗʰ **H93.01** Transient ischemic deafness
    H93.011 Transient ischemic deafness, right ear
    H93.012 Transient ischemic deafness, left ear
    H93.013 Transient ischemic deafness, bilateral
    H93.019 Transient ischemic deafness, unspecified ear

  ✓6ᵗʰ **H93.09** Unspecified degenerative and vascular disorders of ear
    H93.091 Unspecified degenerative and vascular disorders of right ear
    H93.092 Unspecified degenerative and vascular disorders of left ear
    H93.093 Unspecified degenerative and vascular disorders of ear, bilateral
    H93.099 Unspecified degenerative and vascular disorders of unspecified ear

✓5ᵗʰ **H93.1** Tinnitus
    H93.11 Tinnitus, right ear
    H93.12 Tinnitus, left ear
    H93.13 Tinnitus, bilateral
    H93.19 Tinnitus, unspecified ear

✓5ᵗʰ **H93.A** Pulsatile tinnitus
    AHA: 2016,4Q,25-26

    H93.A1 Pulsatile tinnitus, right ear
    H93.A2 Pulsatile tinnitus, left ear
    H93.A3 Pulsatile tinnitus, bilateral

N Newborn: 0   P Pediatric: 0-17   M Maternity: 12-55   A Adult: 15-124   CH Comorbidity High   CL Comorbidity Low   NCDx Noncancer Dx   PDx Primary Dx

H93.A9 Pulsatile tinnitus, unspecified ear

✓5th **H93.2 Other abnormal auditory perceptions**
   EXCLUDES 2   auditory hallucinations (R44.0)

  ✓6th **H93.21 Auditory recruitment**
    H93.211 Auditory recruitment, right ear
    H93.212 Auditory recruitment, left ear
    H93.213 Auditory recruitment, bilateral
    H93.219 Auditory recruitment, unspecified ear

  ✓6th **H93.22 Diplacusis**
    H93.221 Diplacusis, right ear
    H93.222 Diplacusis, left ear
    H93.223 Diplacusis, bilateral
    H93.229 Diplacusis, unspecified ear

  ✓6th **H93.23 Hyperacusis**
    DEF: Exceptionally acute sense of hearing caused by such conditions as Bell's palsy. This term may also refer to painful sensitivity to sounds.
    H93.231 Hyperacusis, right ear
    H93.232 Hyperacusis, left ear
    H93.233 Hyperacusis, bilateral
    H93.239 Hyperacusis, unspecified ear

  ✓6th **H93.24 Temporary auditory threshold shift**
    H93.241 Temporary auditory threshold shift, right ear
    H93.242 Temporary auditory threshold shift, left ear
    H93.243 Temporary auditory threshold shift, bilateral
    H93.249 Temporary auditory threshold shift, unspecified ear

  H93.25 Central auditory processing disorder
    Congenital auditory imperception
    Word deafness
    EXCLUDES 1   mixed receptive-expressive language disorder (F80.2)

  ✓6th **H93.29 Other abnormal auditory perceptions**
    H93.291 Other abnormal auditory perceptions, right ear
    H93.292 Other abnormal auditory perceptions, left ear
    H93.293 Other abnormal auditory perceptions, bilateral
    H93.299 Other abnormal auditory perceptions, unspecified ear

✓5th **H93.3 Disorders of acoustic nerve**
   Disorder of 8th cranial nerve
   EXCLUDES 1   acoustic neuroma (D33.3)
    syphilitic acoustic neuritis (A52.15)

  ✓6th **H93.3X Disorders of acoustic nerve**
    H93.3X1 Disorders of right acoustic nerve
    H93.3X2 Disorders of left acoustic nerve
    H93.3X3 Disorders of bilateral acoustic nerves
    H93.3X9 Disorders of unspecified acoustic nerve

✓5th **H93.8 Other specified disorders of ear**
  ✓6th **H93.8X Other specified disorders of ear**
    H93.8X1 Other specified disorders of right ear
    H93.8X2 Other specified disorders of left ear
    H93.8X3 Other specified disorders of ear, bilateral
    H93.8X9 Other specified disorders of ear, unspecified ear

✓5th **H93.9 Unspecified disorder of ear**
  H93.90 Unspecified disorder of ear, unspecified ear
  H93.91 Unspecified disorder of right ear
  H93.92 Unspecified disorder of left ear
  H93.93 Unspecified disorder of ear, bilateral

✓4th **H94 Other disorders of ear in diseases classified elsewhere**
  ✓5th **H94.0 Acoustic neuritis in infectious and parasitic diseases classified elsewhere**
    Code first underlying disease, such as:
    parasitic disease (B65-B89)
    EXCLUDES 1   acoustic neuritis (in):
     herpes zoster (B02.29)
     syphilis (A52.15)
    H94.00 Acoustic neuritis in infectious and parasitic diseases classified elsewhere, unspecified ear
    H94.01 Acoustic neuritis in infectious and parasitic diseases classified elsewhere, right ear

H94.02 Acoustic neuritis in infectious and parasitic diseases classified elsewhere, left ear
H94.03 Acoustic neuritis in infectious and parasitic diseases classified elsewhere, bilateral

✓5th **H94.8 Other specified disorders of ear in diseases classified elsewhere**
  Code first underlying disease, such as:
  congenital syphilis (A50.0)
  EXCLUDES 1   aural myiasis (B87.4)
    syphilitic labyrinthitis (A52.79)
  H94.80 Other specified disorders of ear in diseases classified elsewhere, unspecified ear
  H94.81 Other specified disorders of right ear in diseases classified elsewhere
  H94.82 Other specified disorders of left ear in diseases classified elsewhere
  H94.83 Other specified disorders of ear in diseases classified elsewhere, bilateral

Intraoperative and postprocedural complications and disorders of ear and mastoid process, not elsewhere classified (H95)

✓4th **H95 Intraoperative and postprocedural complications and disorders of ear and mastoid process, not elsewhere classified**
  AHA: 2016,4Q,9-10

  ✓5th **H95.0 Recurrent cholesteatoma of postmastoidectomy cavity**
    H95.00 Recurrent cholesteatoma of postmastoidectomy cavity, unspecified ear
    H95.01 Recurrent cholesteatoma of postmastoidectomy cavity, right ear
    H95.02 Recurrent cholesteatoma of postmastoidectomy cavity, left ear
    H95.03 Recurrent cholesteatoma of postmastoidectomy cavity, bilateral ears

  ✓5th **H95.1 Other disorders of ear and mastoid process following mastoidectomy**
   ✓6th **H95.11 Chronic inflammation of postmastoidectomy cavity**
    H95.111 Chronic inflammation of postmastoidectomy cavity, right ear
    H95.112 Chronic inflammation of postmastoidectomy cavity, left ear
    H95.113 Chronic inflammation of postmastoidectomy cavity, bilateral ears
    H95.119 Chronic inflammation of postmastoidectomy cavity, unspecified ear

   ✓6th **H95.12 Granulation of postmastoidectomy cavity**
    H95.121 Granulation of postmastoidectomy cavity, right ear
    H95.122 Granulation of postmastoidectomy cavity, left ear
    H95.123 Granulation of postmastoidectomy cavity, bilateral ears
    H95.129 Granulation of postmastoidectomy cavity, unspecified ear

   ✓6th **H95.13 Mucosal cyst of postmastoidectomy cavity**
    H95.131 Mucosal cyst of postmastoidectomy cavity, right ear
    H95.132 Mucosal cyst of postmastoidectomy cavity, left ear
    H95.133 Mucosal cyst of postmastoidectomy cavity, bilateral ears
    H95.139 Mucosal cyst of postmastoidectomy cavity, unspecified ear

   ✓6th **H95.19 Other disorders following mastoidectomy**
    H95.191 Other disorders following mastoidectomy, right ear
    H95.192 Other disorders following mastoidectomy, left ear
    H95.193 Other disorders following mastoidectomy, bilateral ears
    H95.199 Other disorders following mastoidectomy, unspecified ear

✓5ᵗʰ **H95.2** Intraoperative hemorrhage and hematoma **of ear and mastoid process complicating a procedure**

> EXCLUDES 1   *intraoperative hemorrhage and hematoma of ear and mastoid process due to accidental puncture or laceration during a procedure (H95.3-)*

H95.21 **Intraoperative hemorrhage and hematoma of ear and mastoid process complicating a** procedure on the ear and mastoid process

H95.22 **Intraoperative hemorrhage and hematoma of ear and mastoid process complicating** other procedure

✓5ᵗʰ **H95.3** Accidental puncture and laceration **of ear and mastoid process during a procedure**

H95.31 **Accidental puncture and laceration of the ear and mastoid process during a** procedure on the ear and mastoid process

H95.32 **Accidental puncture and laceration of the ear and mastoid process during** other procedure

✓5ᵗʰ **H95.4** Postprocedural hemorrhage **of ear and mastoid process following a procedure**

H95.41 **Postprocedural hemorrhage of ear and mastoid process following a** procedure on the ear and mastoid process

H95.42 **Postprocedural hemorrhage of ear and mastoid process following** other procedure

✓5ᵗʰ **H95.5** Postprocedural hematoma and seroma **of ear and mastoid process following a procedure**

H95.51 **Postprocedural** hematoma **of ear and mastoid process following a** procedure on the ear and mastoid process

H95.52 **Postprocedural** hematoma **of ear and mastoid process following** other procedure

H95.53 **Postprocedural** seroma **of ear and mastoid process following a** procedure on the ear and mastoid process

H95.54 **Postprocedural** seroma **of ear and mastoid process following** other procedure

✓5ᵗʰ **H95.8** **Other intraoperative and postprocedural complications and disorders of the ear and mastoid process, not elsewhere classified**

> EXCLUDES 2   *postprocedural complications and disorders following mastoidectomy (H95.0-, H95.1-)*

✓6ᵗʰ **H95.81** Postprocedural stenosis **of external ear canal**

H95.811 **Postprocedural stenosis of** right **external ear canal**

H95.812 **Postprocedural stenosis of** left **external ear canal**

H95.813 **Postprocedural stenosis of external ear canal,** bilateral

H95.819 **Postprocedural stenosis of unspecified external ear canal**

H95.88 **Other intraoperative complications and disorders of the ear and mastoid process, not elsewhere classified**

> Use additional code, if applicable, to further specify disorder

H95.89 **Other postprocedural complications and disorders of the ear and mastoid process, not elsewhere classified**

> Use additional code, if applicable, to further specify disorder

✓5ᵗʰ **H95.2** Intraoperative hemorrhage and hematoma **of ear and mastoid process complicating a procedure**

Ⓝ Newborn: 0   Ⓟ Pediatric: 0-17   Ⓜ Maternity: 12-55   Ⓐ Adult: 15-124   CH Comorbidity High   CL Comorbidity Low   NCDx Noncancer Dx   PDx Primary Dx

630

ICD-10-CM 2020

H95.2–H95.89

Chapter 9. Diseases of the Circulatory System (I00–I99)

Chapter-specific Guidelines with Coding Examples

The chapter-specific guidelines from the ICD-10-CM Official Guidelines for Coding and Reporting have been provided below. Along with these guidelines are coding examples, contained in the shaded boxes, that have been developed to help illustrate the coding and/or sequencing guidance found in these guidelines.

a. Hypertension

The classification presumes a causal relationship between hypertension and heart involvement and between hypertension and kidney involvement, as the two conditions are linked by the term "with" in the Alphabetic Index. These conditions should be coded as related even in the absence of provider documentation explicitly linking them, unless the documentation clearly states the conditions are unrelated.

For hypertension and conditions not specifically linked by relational terms such as "with," "associated with" or "due to" in the classification, provider documentation must link the conditions in order to code them as related.

1) Hypertension with heart disease

Hypertension with heart conditions classified to I50.- or I51.4-I51.7, I51.89, I51.9, are assigned to a code from category I11, Hypertensive heart disease. Use additional code(s) from category I50, Heart failure, to identify the type(s) of heart failure in those patients with heart failure.

The same heart conditions (I50.-, I51.4-I51.7, I51.89, I51.9) with hypertension are coded separately if the provider has documented they are unrelated to the hypertension. Sequence according to the circumstances of the admission/encounter.

> Hypertensive heart disease with left heart failure
>
> **I11.0**   **Hypertensive heart disease with heart failure**
>
> **I50.1**   **Left ventricular failure, unspecified**
>
> *Explanation*: A causal relationship between hypertension and heart disease must be stated or implied to report codes from category I11 Hypertensive heart disease. Use an additional code to identify type of heart failure (I50.-).

2) Hypertensive chronic kidney disease

Assign codes from category I12, Hypertensive chronic kidney disease, when both hypertension and a condition classifiable to category N18, Chronic kidney disease (CKD), are present. CKD should not be coded as hypertension if the provider indicates the CKD is not related to the hypertension.

The appropriate code from category N18 should be used as a secondary code with a code from category I12 to identify the stage of chronic kidney disease.

See Section I.C.14. Chronic kidney disease.

If a patient has hypertensive chronic kidney disease and acute renal failure, an additional code for the acute renal failure is required.

> Patient is admitted with stage IV chronic kidney disease (CKD). The physician has also documented hypertension for this patient.
>
> **I12.9**   **Hypertensive chronic kidney disease with stage 1 through stage 4 chronic kidney disease, or unspecified chronic kidney disease**
>
> **N18.4**   **Chronic kidney disease, stage 4 (severe)**
>
> *Explanation*: A causal relationship between hypertension and chronic kidney disease (CKD) is assumed unless otherwise documented. Use an additional code to identify the stage of chronic kidney disease.

3) Hypertensive heart and chronic kidney disease

Assign codes from combination category I13, Hypertensive heart and chronic kidney disease, when there is hypertension with both heart and kidney involvement. If heart failure is present, assign an additional code from category I50 to identify the type of heart failure.

The appropriate code from category N18, Chronic kidney disease, should be used as a secondary code with a code from category I13 to identify the stage of chronic kidney disease.

See Section I.C.14. Chronic kidney disease.

The codes in category I13, Hypertensive heart and chronic kidney disease, are combination codes that include hypertension, heart disease and chronic kidney disease. The Includes note at I13 specifies that the conditions included at I11 and I12 are included together in I13. If a patient has hypertension, heart disease and chronic kidney disease then a code from I13 should be used, not individual codes for hypertension, heart disease and chronic kidney disease, or codes from I11 or I12.

For patients with both acute renal failure and chronic kidney disease an additional code for acute renal failure is required.

> Hypertensive heart and kidney disease with congestive heart failure and stage 2 chronic kidney disease.
>
> **I13.0**   **Hypertensive heart and chronic kidney disease with heart failure and stage 1 through stage 4 chronic kidney disease, or unspecified chronic kidney disease**
>
> **I50.9**   **Heart failure, unspecified**
>
> **N18.2**   **Chronic kidney disease, stage 2 (mild)**
>
> *Explanation*: Combination codes in category I13 are used to report conditions classifiable to *both* categories I11 and I12. Do not report conditions classifiable to I11 and I12 separately. Use additional codes to report type of heart failure and stage of CKD.

4) Hypertensive cerebrovascular disease

For hypertensive cerebrovascular disease, first assign the appropriate code from categories I60-I69, followed by the appropriate hypertension code.

5) Hypertensive retinopathy

Subcategory H35.0, Background retinopathy and retinal vascular changes, should be used with a code from category I10 – I15, Hypertensive disease to include the systemic hypertension. The sequencing is based on the reason for the encounter.

> Hypertensive retinopathy of the right eye.
>
> **H35.031**   **Hypertensive retinopathy, right eye**
>
> **I10**   **Essential (primary) hypertension**
>
> *Explanation*: Hypertensive retinopathy requires two codes: the appropriate subcategory H35.0 code and a code for the hypertension.

6) Hypertension, secondary

Secondary hypertension is due to an underlying condition. Two codes are required: one to identify the underlying etiology and one from category I15 to identify the hypertension. Sequencing of codes is determined by the reason for admission/encounter.

7) Hypertension, transient

Assign code R03.0, Elevated blood pressure reading without diagnosis of hypertension, unless patient has an established diagnosis of hypertension. Assign code O13.-, Gestational [pregnancy-induced] hypertension without significant proteinuria, or O14.-, Pre-eclampsia, for transient hypertension of pregnancy.

8) Hypertension, controlled

This diagnostic statement usually refers to an existing state of hypertension under control by therapy. Assign the appropriate code from categories I10-I15, Hypertensive diseases.

9) Hypertension, uncontrolled

Uncontrolled hypertension may refer to untreated hypertension or hypertension not responding to current therapeutic regimen. In either case, assign the appropriate code from categories I10-I15, Hypertensive diseases.

10) Hypertensive crisis

Assign a code from category I16, Hypertensive crisis, for documented hypertensive urgency, hypertensive emergency or unspecified hypertensive crisis. Code also any identified hypertensive disease (I10-I15). The sequencing is based on the reason for the encounter.

11) Pulmonary hypertension

Pulmonary hypertension is classified to category I27, Other pulmonary heart diseases. For secondary pulmonary hypertension (I27.1, I27.2-), code also any associated conditions or adverse effects of drugs or toxins. The sequencing is based on the reason for the encounter, except for adverse effects of drugs (See Section I.C.19.e.).

b. Atherosclerotic coronary artery disease and angina

ICD-10-CM has combination codes for atherosclerotic heart disease with angina pectoris. The subcategories for these codes are I25.11, Atherosclerotic heart disease of native coronary artery with angina pectoris and I25.7, Atherosclerosis of coronary artery bypass graft(s) and coronary artery of transplanted heart with angina pectoris.

When using one of these combination codes it is not necessary to use an additional code for angina pectoris. A causal relationship can be assumed in a patient with both atherosclerosis and angina pectoris, unless the documentation indicates the angina is due to something other than the atherosclerosis.

If a patient with coronary artery disease is admitted due to an acute myocardial infarction (AMI), the AMI should be sequenced before the coronary artery disease.

See Section I.C.9. Acute myocardial infarction (AMI)

c. Intraoperative and postprocedural cerebrovascular accident

Medical record documentation should clearly specify the cause- and- effect relationship between the medical intervention and the cerebrovascular accident in order to assign a code for intraoperative or postprocedural cerebrovascular accident.

Proper code assignment depends on whether it was an infarction or hemorrhage and whether it occurred intraoperatively or postoperatively. If it was a cerebral hemorrhage, code assignment depends on the type of procedure performed.

d. Sequelae of cerebrovascular disease

1) Category I69, Sequelae of cerebrovascular disease

Category I69 is used to indicate conditions classifiable to categories I60-I67 as the causes of sequela (neurologic deficits), themselves classified elsewhere. These "late effects" include neurologic deficits that persist after initial onset of conditions classifiable to categories I60-I67. The neurologic deficits caused by cerebrovascular disease may be present from the onset or may arise at any time after the onset of the condition classifiable to categories I60-I67.

Patient admitted for skilled services following hospital stay for stroke due to thrombosis of posterior cerebral artery. Provider documentation indicates residual memory deficit.

I69.311 **Memory deficit following cerebral infarction**

I69.392 **Facial weakness following cerebral infarction**

Explanation: In the post-acute care setting, the residual sequelae of an acute cerebral vascular accident are the focus of care for the encounter. The residual deficits may not be present from the onset and may occur at any time following the initial stroke. All deficits should be coded when documented as related to the cerebrovascular disease, regardless of when they develop. If it is unclear if a condition may be sequelae of cerebrovascular disease, the provider should be queried as to the relationship between the conditions.

Codes from category I69, Sequelae of cerebrovascular disease, that specify hemiplegia, hemiparesis and monoplegia identify whether the dominant or nondominant side is affected. Should the affected side be documented, but not specified as dominant or nondominant, and the classification system does not indicate a default, code selection is as follows:

- For ambidextrous patients, the default should be dominant.
- If the left side is affected, the default is non-dominant.
- If the right side is affected, the default is dominant.

2) Codes from category I69 with codes from I60-I67

Codes from category I69 may be assigned on a health care record with codes from I60-I67, if the patient has a current cerebrovascular disease and deficits from an old cerebrovascular disease.

3) Codes from category I69 and personal history of transient ischemic attack (TIA) and cerebral infarction (Z86.73)

Codes from category I69 should not be assigned if the patient does not have neurologic deficits.

See Section I.C.21. 4. History (of) for use of personal history codes

An 86-year-old female patient was hospitalized due to transient ischemic attack. The patient is now being discharged with orders for home health for skilled nursing and physical therapy. Provider notes also report hypertension and stage III CKD.

I12.9 **Hypertensive chronic kidney disease with stage 1 through stage 4 chronic kidney disease, or unspecified chronic kidney disease**

N18.3 **Chronic kidney disease, stage 3 (moderate)**

Z86.73 **Personal history of transient ischemic attack (TIA), and cerebral infarction without residual deficits**

Explanation: A transient ischemic attack is an event in which blood flow to the brain is blocked temporarily and then restored. Acute symptoms may mimic those of a stroke but, by definition, are transient and therefore resolve quickly and completely. Because no residual deficits are present, code Z86.73 should be assigned to indicate a history of TIA.

e. Acute myocardial infarction (AMI)

1) Type 1 ST elevation myocardial infarction (STEMI) and non-ST elevation myocardial infarction (NSTEMI)

The ICD-10-CM codes for type 1 acute myocardial infarction (AMI) identify the site, such as anterolateral wall or true posterior wall. Subcategories I21.0-I21.2 and I21.3 are used for type 1 ST elevation myocardial infarction (STEMI). Code I21.4, Non-ST elevation (NSTEMI) myocardial infarction, is used for type 1 non ST elevation myocardial infarction (NSTEMI) and nontransmural MIs.

If a type 1 NSTEMI evolves to STEMI, assign the STEMI code. If a type 1 STEMI converts to NSTEMI due to thrombolytic therapy, it is still coded as STEMI.

For encounters occurring while the myocardial infarction is equal to, or less than, four weeks old, including transfers to another acute setting or a postacute setting, and the myocardial infarction meets the definition for "other diagnoses" (see Section III, Reporting Additional Diagnoses), codes from category I21 may continue to be reported. For encounters after the 4 week time frame and the patient is still receiving care related to the myocardial infarction, the appropriate aftercare code should be assigned, rather than a code from category I21. For old or healed myocardial infarctions not requiring further care, code I25.2, Old myocardial infarction, may be assigned.

2) Acute myocardial infarction, unspecified

Code I21.9, Acute myocardial infarction, unspecified, is the default for unspecified acute myocardial infarction or unspecified type. If only type 1 STEMI or transmural MI without the site is documented, assign code I21.3, ST elevation (STEMI) myocardial infarction of unspecified site.

3) AMI documented as nontransmural or subendocardial but site provided

If an AMI is documented as nontransmural or subendocardial, but the site is provided, it is still coded as a subendocardial AMI.

See Section I.C.21.3 for information on coding status post administration of tPA in a different facility within the last 24 hours.

4) Subsequent acute myocardial infarction

A code from category I22, Subsequent ST elevation (STEMI) and non-ST elevation (NSTEMI) myocardial infarction, is to be used when a patient who has suffered a type 1 or unspecified AMI has a new AMI within the 4 week time frame of the initial AMI. A code from category I22 must be used in conjunction with a code from category I21. The sequencing of the I22 and I21 codes depends on the circumstances of the encounter.

Do not assign code I22 for subsequent myocardial infarctions other than type 1 or unspecified. For subsequent type 2 AMI assign only code I21.A1. For subsequent type 4 or type 5 AMI, assign only code I21.A9.

If a subsequent myocardial infarction of one type occurs within 4 weeks of a myocardial infarction of a different type, assign the appropriate codes from category I21 to identify each type. Do not assign a code from I22. Codes from category I22 should only be assigned if both the initial and subsequent myocardial infarctions are type 1 or unspecified.

5) Other Types of Myocardial Infarction

The ICD-10-CM provides codes for different types of myocardial infarction. Type 1 myocardial infarctions are assigned to codes I21.0-I21.4.

Type 2 myocardial infarction (myocardial infarction due to demand ischemia or secondary to ischemic **im**balance) is assigned to code I21.A1, Myocardial infarction type 2 with the underlying cause **coded first**. Do not assign code I24.8, Other forms of acute ischemic heart disease, for the demand ischemia. **If** a type 2 AMI is described as NSTEMI or STEMI, only assign code I21.A1. Codes I21.01-I21.4 should only be assigned for type 1 AMIs.

Acute myocardial infarctions type 3, 4a, 4b, 4c and 5 are assigned to code I21.A9, Other myocardial infarction type.

The "Code also" and "Code first" notes should be followed related to complications, and for coding of postprocedural myocardial infarctions during or following cardiac surgery.

Chapter 9. Diseases of the Circulatory System (I00-I99)

EXCLUDES 2   *certain conditions originating in the perinatal period (P04-P96)*
certain infectious and parasitic diseases (A00-B99)
complications of pregnancy, childbirth and the puerperium (O00-O9A)
congenital malformations, deformations, and chromosomal abnormalities (Q00-Q99)
endocrine, nutritional and metabolic diseases (E00-E88)
injury, poisoning and certain other consequences of external causes (S00-T88)
neoplasms (C00-D49)
symptoms, signs and abnormal clinical and laboratory findings, not elsewhere classified (R00-R94)
systemic connective tissue disorders (M30-M36)
transient cerebral ischemic attacks and related syndromes (G45.-)

This chapter contains the following blocks:

I00-I02	Acute rheumatic fever
I05-I09	Chronic rheumatic heart diseases
I10-I16	Hypertensive diseases
I20-I25	Ischemic heart diseases
I26-I28	Pulmonary heart disease and diseases of pulmonary circulation
I30-I52	Other forms of heart disease
I60-I69	Cerebrovascular diseases
I70-I79	Diseases of arteries, arterioles and capillaries
I80-I89	Diseases of veins, lymphatic vessels and lymph nodes, not elsewhere classified
I95-I99	Other and unspecified disorders of the circulatory system

Acute rheumatic fever (I00-I02)

DEF: Inflammatory disease that can follow a throat infection by group A streptococci. Complications can involve the joints (arthritis), subcutaneous tissue (nodules), skin (erythema marginatum), heart (carditis), or brain (chorea).

I00   **Rheumatic fever without heart involvement**
    INCLUDES   arthritis, rheumatic, acute or subacute
    EXCLUDES 1   *rheumatic fever with heart involvement (I01.0-I01.9)*

✓4ᵗʰ **I01**   **Rheumatic fever with heart involvement**
    EXCLUDES 1   *chronic diseases of rheumatic origin (I05-I09) unless rheumatic fever is also present or there is evidence of reactivation or activity of the rheumatic process*

   I01.0   **Acute rheumatic pericarditis**
      Any condition in I00 with pericarditis
      Rheumatic pericarditis (acute)
      EXCLUDES 1   *acute pericarditis not specified as rheumatic (I30.-)*

   I01.1   **Acute rheumatic endocarditis**
      Any condition in I00 with endocarditis or valvulitis
      Acute rheumatic valvulitis

   I01.2   **Acute rheumatic myocarditis**
      Any condition in I00 with myocarditis

   I01.8   **Other acute rheumatic heart disease**
      Any condition in I00 with other or multiple types of heart involvement
      Acute rheumatic pancarditis

   I01.9   **Acute rheumatic heart disease, unspecified**
      Any condition in I00 with unspecified type of heart involvement
      Rheumatic carditis, acute
      Rheumatic heart disease, active or acute

✓4ᵗʰ **I02**   **Rheumatic chorea**
    INCLUDES   Sydenham's chorea
    EXCLUDES 1   *chorea NOS (G25.5)*
                  Huntington's chorea (G10)

   I02.0   **Rheumatic chorea with heart involvement**
      Chorea NOS with heart involvement
      Rheumatic chorea with heart involvement of any type classifiable under I01.-

   I02.9   **Rheumatic chorea without heart involvement**
      Rheumatic chorea NOS

Chronic rheumatic heart diseases (I05-I09)

✓4ᵗʰ **I05**   **Rheumatic mitral valve diseases**
    INCLUDES   conditions classifiable to both I05.0 and I05.2-I05.9, whether specified as rheumatic or not
    EXCLUDES 1   *mitral valve disease specified as nonrheumatic (I34.-)*
                  mitral valve disease with aortic and/or tricuspid valve involvement (I08.-)

   I05.0   **Rheumatic mitral stenosis**
      Mitral (valve) obstruction (rheumatic)
      DEF: Narrowing of the mitral valve between the left atrium and left ventricle due to rheumatic fever. Symptoms include shortness of breath during or after exercise, fatigue, palpitations, chest discomfort, and swelling of feet or legs.

   I05.1   **Rheumatic mitral insufficiency**
      Rheumatic mitral incompetence
      Rheumatic mitral regurgitation
      EXCLUDES 1   *mitral insufficiency not specified as rheumatic (I34.0)*

   I05.2   **Rheumatic mitral stenosis with insufficiency**
      Rheumatic mitral stenosis with incompetence or regurgitation

   I05.8   **Other rheumatic mitral valve disease**
      Rheumatic mitral (valve) failure

   I05.9   **Rheumatic mitral valve disease, unspecified**
      Rheumatic mitral (valve) disorder (chronic) NOS

✓4ᵗʰ **I06**   **Rheumatic aortic valve diseases**
    EXCLUDES 1   *aortic valve disease not specified as rheumatic (I35.-)*
                  aortic valve disease with mitral and/or tricuspid valve involvement (I08.-)

   I06.0   **Rheumatic aortic stenosis**
      Rheumatic aortic (valve) obstruction

   I06.1   **Rheumatic aortic insufficiency**
      Rheumatic aortic incompetence
      Rheumatic aortic regurgitation

   I06.2   **Rheumatic aortic stenosis with insufficiency**
      Rheumatic aortic stenosis with incompetence or regurgitation

   I06.8   **Other rheumatic aortic valve diseases**

   I06.9   **Rheumatic aortic valve disease, unspecified**
      Rheumatic aortic (valve) disease NOS

✓4ᵗʰ **I07**   **Rheumatic tricuspid valve diseases**
    INCLUDES   rheumatic tricuspid valve diseases specified as rheumatic or unspecified
    EXCLUDES 1   *tricuspid valve disease specified as nonrheumatic (I36.-)*
                  tricuspid valve disease with aortic and/or mitral valve involvement (I08.-)

   I07.0   **Rheumatic tricuspid stenosis**
      Tricuspid (valve) stenosis (rheumatic)

   I07.1   **Rheumatic tricuspid insufficiency**
      Tricuspid (valve) insufficiency (rheumatic)

   I07.2   **Rheumatic tricuspid stenosis and insufficiency**

   I07.8   **Other rheumatic tricuspid valve diseases**

   I07.9   **Rheumatic tricuspid valve disease, unspecified**
      Rheumatic tricuspid valve disorder NOS

✓4ᵗʰ **I08**   **Multiple valve diseases**
    INCLUDES   multiple valve diseases specified as rheumatic or unspecified
    EXCLUDES 1   *endocarditis, valve unspecified (I38)*
                  multiple valve disease specified a nonrheumatic (I34.-, I35.-, I36.-, I37.-, I38.-, Q22.-, Q23.-, Q24.8-)
                  rheumatic valve disease NOS (I09.1)

   I08.0   **Rheumatic disorders of both mitral and aortic valves**
      Involvement of both mitral and aortic valves specified as rheumatic or unspecified
      AHA: 2019,2Q,5

   I08.1   **Rheumatic disorders of both mitral and tricuspid valves**

   I08.2   **Rheumatic disorders of both aortic and tricuspid valves**

   I08.3   **Combined rheumatic disorders of mitral, aortic and tricuspid valves**

   I08.8   **Other rheumatic multiple valve diseases**

   I08.9   **Rheumatic multiple valve disease, unspecified**

✓4ᵗʰ **I09**   **Other rheumatic heart diseases**

   I09.0   **Rheumatic myocarditis**
      EXCLUDES 1   *myocarditis not specified as rheumatic (I51.4)*

☑ Additional Character Required   ✓x7ᵗʰ Placeholder Alert   Manifestation   Unspecified Dx   ▶◀ Revised Text   ● New Code   ▲ Revised Title

ICD-10-CM 2020   **633**

Chapter 9. Diseases of the Circulatory System

I09.1   **Rheumatic diseases of endocardium, valve unspecified**
Rheumatic endocarditis (chronic)
Rheumatic valvulitis (chronic)
EXCLUDES 1   endocarditis, valve unspecified (I38)

I09.2   **Chronic rheumatic pericarditis**
Adherent pericardium, rheumatic
Chronic rheumatic mediastinopericarditis
Chronic rheumatic myopericarditis
EXCLUDES 1   chronic pericarditis not specified as rheumatic (I31.-)

☑5ᵗʰ **I09.8**   **Other specified rheumatic heart diseases**

I09.81   **Rheumatic heart failure**   CH CL NC Dx
Use additional code to identify type of heart failure (I50.-)
DEF: Decreased cardiac output, edema, and hypertension due to rheumatic heart disease.

I09.89   **Other specified rheumatic heart diseases**
Rheumatic disease of pulmonary valve

I09.9   **Rheumatic heart disease, unspecified**
Rheumatic carditis
EXCLUDES 1   rheumatoid carditis (M05.31)

Hypertensive diseases (I10-I16)

Use additional code to identify:
exposure to environmental tobacco smoke (Z77.22)
history of tobacco dependence (Z87.891)
occupational exposure to environmental tobacco smoke (Z57.31)
tobacco dependence (F17.-)
tobacco use (Z72.0)
EXCLUDES 1   neonatal hypertension (P29.2)
   primary pulmonary hypertension (I27.0)
EXCLUDES 2   hypertensive disease complicating pregnancy, childbirth and the puerperium (O10-O11, O13-O16)

I10   **Essential (primary) hypertension**
INCLUDES   high blood pressure
hypertension (arterial) (benign) (essential) (malignant) (primary) (systemic)
EXCLUDES 1   hypertensive disease complicating pregnancy, childbirth and the puerperium (O10-O11, O13-O16)
EXCLUDES 2   essential (primary) hypertension involving vessels of brain (I60-I69)
   essential (primary) hypertension involving vessels of eye (H35.0-)
AHA: 2018,2Q,9; 2016,4Q,27

☑4ᵗʰ **I11**   **Hypertensive heart disease**
INCLUDES   any condition in I50.-, I51.4-I51.9 due to hypertension
AHA: 2018,2Q,9
TIP: Do not assign a code from this category when provider documentation indicates the heart disease is attributable to another cause.

I11.0   **Hypertensive heart disease with heart failure**   CH CL NC Dx
Hypertensive heart failure
Use additional code to identify type of heart failure (I50.-)
AHA: 2017,1Q,47

I11.9   **Hypertensive heart disease without heart failure**
Hypertensive heart disease NOS

☑4ᵗʰ **I12**   **Hypertensive chronic kidney disease**
INCLUDES   any condition in N18 and N26 — due to hypertension
arteriosclerosis of kidney
arteriosclerotic nephritis (chronic) (interstitial)
hypertensive nephropathy
nephrosclerosis
EXCLUDES 1   hypertension due to kidney disease (I15.0, I15.1)
   renovascular hypertension (I15.0)
   secondary hypertension (I15.-)
EXCLUDES 2   acute kidney failure (N17.-)
AHA: 2018,4Q,88; 2016,3Q,22
TIP: Do not assign a code from this category when provider documentation indicates the chronic kidney disease (CKD) is attributable to another cause.

I12.0   **Hypertensive chronic kidney disease with stage 5 chronic kidney disease or end stage renal disease**   CH NC Dx
Use additional code to identify the stage of chronic kidney disease (N18.5, N18.6)

I12.9   **Hypertensive chronic kidney disease with stage 1 through stage 4 chronic kidney disease, or unspecified chronic kidney disease**   CH
Hypertensive chronic kidney disease NOS
Hypertensive renal disease NOS
Use additional code to identify the stage of chronic kidney disease (N18.1-N18.4, N18.9)

☑4ᵗʰ **I13**   **Hypertensive heart and chronic kidney disease**
INCLUDES   any condition in I11.- with any condition in I12.-
cardiorenal disease
cardiovascular renal disease
TIP: Do not assign a code from this category when provider documentation indicates the heart and/or chronic kidney disease is attributable to another cause.

I13.0   **Hypertensive heart and chronic kidney disease with heart failure and stage 1 through stage 4 chronic kidney disease, or unspecified chronic kidney disease**   CH NC Dx
Use additional code to identify type of heart failure (I50.-)
Use additional code to identify stage of chronic kidney disease (N18.1-N18.4, N18.9)

☑5ᵗʰ **I13.1**   **Hypertensive heart and chronic kidney disease without heart failure**

I13.10   **Hypertensive heart and chronic kidney disease without heart failure, with stage 1 through stage 4 chronic kidney disease, or unspecified chronic kidney disease**   CH
Hypertensive heart disease and hypertensive chronic kidney disease NOS
Use additional code to identify the stage of chronic kidney disease (N18.1-N18.4, N18.9)

I13.11   **Hypertensive heart and chronic kidney disease without heart failure, with stage 5 chronic kidney disease, or end stage renal disease**   CH NC Dx
Use additional code to identify the stage of chronic kidney disease (N18.5, N18.6)

I13.2   **Hypertensive heart and chronic kidney disease with heart failure and with stage 5 chronic kidney disease, or end stage renal disease**   CH NC Dx
Use additional code to identify type of heart failure (I50.-)
Use additional code to identify the stage of chronic kidney disease (N18.5, N18.6)

☑4ᵗʰ **I15**   **Secondary hypertension**
Code also underlying condition
EXCLUDES 1   postprocedural hypertension (I97.3)
EXCLUDES 2   secondary hypertension involving vessels of brain (I60-I69)
   secondary hypertension involving vessels of eye (H35.0-)

I15.0   **Renovascular hypertension**

I15.1   **Hypertension secondary to other renal disorders**
AHA: 2016,3Q,22

I15.2   **Hypertension secondary to endocrine disorders**

I15.8   **Other secondary hypertension**

I15.9   **Secondary hypertension, unspecified**

☑4ᵗʰ **I16**   **Hypertensive crisis**
Code also any identified hypertensive disease (I10-I15)
AHA: 2016,4Q,26-28

I16.0   **Hypertensive urgency**

I16.1   **Hypertensive emergency**

I16.9   **Hypertensive crisis, unspecified**

Ischemic heart diseases (I20-I25)

Use additional code to identify presence of hypertension (I10-I16)

✓4th I20 Angina pectoris

Use additional code to identify:
exposure to environmental tobacco smoke (Z77.22)
history of tobacco dependence (Z87.891)
occupational exposure to environmental tobacco smoke (Z57.31)
tobacco dependence (F17.-)
tobacco use (Z72.0)

EXCLUDES1   angina pectoris with atherosclerotic heart disease of native
coronary arteries (I25.1-)
atherosclerosis of coronary artery bypass graft(s) and
coronary artery of transplanted heart with angina
pectoris (I25.7-)
postinfarction angina (I23.7)

DEF: Chest pain due to reduced blood flow resulting in a lack of oxygen
to the heart muscles.

I20.0 Unstable angina   `CH`

Accelerated angina
Crescendo angina
De novo effort angina
Intermediate coronary syndrome
Preinfarction syndrome
Worsening effort angina
DEF: Condition representing an intermediate stage between
angina of effort and acute myocardial infarction.

I20.1 Angina pectoris with documented spasm   `CH`

Angiospastic angina
Prinzmetal angina
Spasm-induced angina
Variant angina

I20.8 Other forms of angina pectoris   `CH`

Angina equivalent
Angina of effort
Coronary slow flow syndrome
Stable angina
Stenocardia
Use additional code(s) for symptoms associated with angina
equivalent

I20.9 Angina pectoris, unspecified   `CH`

Angina NOS / w/o ASHD
Anginal syndrome
Cardiac angina
Ischemic chest pain

✓4th I21 Acute myocardial infarction

INCLUDES   cardiac infarction
coronary (artery) embolism
coronary (artery) occlusion
coronary (artery) rupture
coronary (artery) thrombosis
infarction of heart, myocardium, or ventricle
4 wk/less Acute → myocardial infarction specified as acute or with a stated
duration of 4 weeks (28 days) or less from onset

Use additional code, if applicable, to identify:
exposure to environmental tobacco smoke (Z77.22)
history of tobacco dependence (Z87.891)
occupational exposure to environmental tobacco smoke (Z57.31)
status post administration of tPA (rtPA) in a different facility within
the last 24 hours prior to admission to current facility (Z92.82)
tobacco dependence (F17.-)
tobacco use (Z72.0)

EXCLUDES2   old myocardial infarction (I25.2)
postmyocardial infarction syndrome (I24.1)
subsequent type 1 myocardial infarction (I22.-)

AHA: 2019,2Q,5; 2018,4Q,68; 2018,3Q,5; 2017,4Q,12-14; 2017,1Q,44-45;
2016,4Q,140; 2015,2Q,16; 2013,1Q,25; 2012,4Q,96,102-103

✓5th I21.0 ST elevation (STEMI) myocardial infarction of anterior wall

Type 1 ST elevation myocardial infarction of anterior wall
DEF: ST elevation myocardial infarction: Complete obstruction
of one or more coronary arteries causing decreased blood flow
(ischemia) and necrosis of myocardial muscle cells.

I21.01 ST elevation (STEMI) myocardial infarction involving left main coronary artery

I21.02 ST elevation (STEMI) myocardial infarction involving left anterior descending coronary artery

ST elevation (STEMI) myocardial infarction involving
diagonal coronary artery
AHA: 2013,1Q,25

I21.09 ST elevation (STEMI) myocardial infarction involving other coronary artery of anterior wall

Acute transmural myocardial infarction of anterior
wall
Anteroapical transmural (Q wave) infarction (acute)
Anterolateral transmural (Q wave) infarction (acute)
Anteroseptal transmural (Q wave) infarction (acute)
Transmural (Q wave) infarction (acute) (of) anterior
(wall) NOS
AHA: 2012,4Q,102-103

✓5th I21.1 ST elevation (STEMI) myocardial infarction of inferior wall

Type 1 ST elevation myocardial infarction of inferior wall
DEF: ST elevation myocardial infarction: Complete obstruction
of one or more coronary arteries causing decreased blood flow
(ischemia) and necrosis of myocardial muscle cells.

I21.11 ST elevation (STEMI) myocardial infarction involving right coronary artery

Inferoposterior transmural (Q wave) infarction (acute)

I21.19 ST elevation (STEMI) myocardial infarction involving other coronary artery of inferior wall

Acute transmural myocardial infarction of inferior
wall
Inferolateral transmural (Q wave) infarction (acute)
Transmural (Q wave) infarction (acute) (of)
diaphragmatic wall
Transmural (Q wave) infarction (acute) (of) inferior
(wall) NOS

EXCLUDES2   ST elevation (STEMI) myocardial infarction
involving left circumflex coronary
artery (I21.21)

AHA: 2012,4Q,96

✓5th I21.2 ST elevation (STEMI) myocardial infarction of other sites

Type 1 ST elevation myocardial infarction of other sites
DEF: ST elevation myocardial infarction: Complete obstruction
of one or more coronary arteries causing decreased blood flow
(ischemia) and necrosis of myocardial muscle cells.

I21.21 ST elevation (STEMI) myocardial infarction involving left circumflex coronary artery

ST elevation (STEMI) myocardial infarction involving
oblique marginal coronary artery

I21.29 ST elevation (STEMI) myocardial infarction involving other sites

Acute transmural myocardial infarction of other sites
Apical-lateral transmural (Q wave) infarction (acute)
Basal-lateral transmural (Q wave) infarction (acute)
High lateral transmural (Q wave) infarction (acute)
Lateral (wall) NOS transmural (Q wave) infarction
(acute)
Posterior (true) transmural (Q wave) infarction (acute)
Posterobasal transmural (Q wave) infarction (acute)
Posterolateral transmural (Q wave) infarction (acute)
Posteroseptal transmural (Q wave) infarction (acute)
Septal transmural (Q wave) infarction (acute) NOS

I21.3 ST elevation (STEMI) myocardial infarction of unspecified site

Acute transmural myocardial infarction of unspecified site
Transmural (Q wave) myocardial infarction NOS
Type 1 ST elevation myocardial infarction of unspecified site
DEF: ST elevation myocardial infarction: Complete obstruction
of one or more coronary arteries causing decreased blood flow
(ischemia) and necrosis of myocardial muscle cells.

I21.4 Non-ST elevation (NSTEMI) myocardial infarction

Acute subendocardial myocardial infarction
Non-Q wave myocardial infarction NOS
Nontransmural myocardial infarction NOS
Type 1 non-ST elevation myocardial infarction
AHA: 2019,2Q,33; 2017,1Q,44-45
DEF: Partial obstruction of one or more coronary arteries that
causes decreased blood flow (ischemia) and may cause partial
thickness necrosis of myocardial muscle cells.

I21.9 Acute myocardial infarction, unspecified

Myocardial infarction (acute) NOS

✓ Additional Character Required   ✓x7th Placeholder Alert   Manifestation   Unspecified Dx   ►◄ Revised Text   ● New Code   ▲ Revised Title

ICD-10-CM 2020   635

Chapter 9. Diseases of the Circulatory System

✓5th I21.A   Other type of myocardial infarction

AHA: 2019,2Q,5

I21.A1   Myocardial infarction type 2

Handwritten note: See Notes Block I20–125 P 635 Excludes 1 124.8

Myocardial infarction due to demand ischemia

Myocardial infarction secondary to ischemic imbalance

▸Code first the underlying cause, such as:◂
  - ▸anemia (D50.0-D64.9)◂
  - ▸chronic obstructive pulmonary disease (J44.-)◂
  - ▸paroxysmal tachycardia (I47.0-I47.9)◂
  - ▸shock (R57.0-R57.9)◂

~~Code also the underlying cause, if known and applicable, such as:~~
  - ~~anemia (D50.0-D64.9)~~
  - ~~chronic obstructive pulmonary disease (J44.-)~~
  - ~~heart failure (I50.-)~~
  - ~~paroxysmal tachycardia (I47.0-I47.9)~~
  - ~~renal failure (N17.0-N19)~~
  - ~~shock (R57.0-R57.9)~~

AHA: 2017,4Q,13-14

DEF: Often referred to as due to demand ischemia, myocardial infarction (MI) type 2 refers to an MI due to ischemia and necrosis resulting from an oxygen imbalance to the heart. This mismatch between oxygen decreased supply and increased demand is caused by conditions other than coronary artery disease such as vasospasm, embolism, anemia, hypertension, hypotension, or arrhythmias.

I21.A9   Other myocardial infarction type

Myocardial infarction associated with revascularization procedure

Myocardial infarction type 3

Myocardial infarction type 4a

Myocardial infarction type 4b

Myocardial infarction type 4c

Myocardial infarction type 5

Code first, if applicable, postprocedural myocardial infarction following cardiac surgery (I97.190), or postprocedural myocardial infarction during cardiac surgery (I97.790)

Code also complication, if known and applicable, such as:
  - (acute) stent occlusion (T82.897-)
  - (acute) stent stenosis ▸(T82.855-)◂
  - (acute) stent thrombosis (T82.867-)
  - cardiac arrest due to underlying cardiac condition (I46.2)
  - complication of percutaneous coronary intervention (PCI) (I97.89)
  - occlusion of coronary artery bypass graft (T82.218-)

AHA: 2019,2Q,33

✓4th I22   Subsequent ST elevation (STEMI) and non-ST elevation (NSTEMI) myocardial infarction

INCLUDES   acute myocardial infarction occurring within four weeks (28 days) of a previous acute myocardial infarction, regardless of site

Handwritten note: use for Type I or NOS Re-MI in the 200 day window only use with I21.-

cardiac infarction

coronary (artery) embolism

coronary (artery) occlusion

coronary (artery) rupture

coronary (artery) thrombosis

infarction of heart, myocardium, or ventricle

recurrent myocardial infarction

reinfarction of myocardium

rupture of heart, myocardium, or ventricle

subsequent type 1 myocardial infarction

Use additional code, if applicable, to identify:

exposure to environmental tobacco smoke (Z77.22)

history of tobacco dependence (Z87.891)

occupational exposure to environmental tobacco smoke (Z57.31)

status post administration of tPA (rtPA) in a different facility within the last 24 hours prior to admission to current facility (Z92.82)

tobacco dependence (F17.-)

tobacco use (Z72.0)

EXCLUDES 1   *subsequent myocardial infarction, type 2 (I21.A1)*

subsequent myocardial infarction of other type (type 3) (type 4) (type 5) (I21.A9)

AHA: 2018,4Q,68; 2018,3Q,5; 2017,4Q,12-13; 2017,2Q,11; 2013,1Q,25; 2012,4Q,97,102-103

DEF: Non-ST elevation myocardial infarction: Partial obstruction of one or more coronary arteries that causes decreased blood flow (ischemia) and may cause partial thickness necrosis of myocardial muscle cells.

DEF: ST elevation myocardial infarction: Complete obstruction of one or more coronary arteries causing decreased blood flow (ischemia) and necrosis of myocardial muscle cells.

I22.0   Subsequent ST elevation (STEMI) myocardial infarction of anterior wall

Subsequent acute transmural myocardial infarction of anterior wall

Subsequent transmural (Q wave) infarction (acute)(of) anterior (wall) NOS

Subsequent anteroapical transmural (Q wave) infarction (acute)

Subsequent anterolateral transmural (Q wave) infarction (acute)

Subsequent anteroseptal transmural (Q wave) infarction (acute)

I22.1   Subsequent ST elevation (STEMI) myocardial infarction of inferior wall

Subsequent acute transmural myocardial infarction of inferior wall

Subsequent transmural (Q wave) infarction (acute)(of) diaphragmatic wall

Subsequent transmural (Q wave) infarction (acute)(of) inferior (wall) NOS

Subsequent inferolateral transmural (Q wave) infarction (acute)

Subsequent inferoposterior transmural (Q wave) infarction (acute)

AHA: 2012,4Q,102

I22.2   Subsequent non-ST elevation (NSTEMI) myocardial infarction

Subsequent acute subendocardial myocardial infarction

Subsequent non-Q wave myocardial infarction NOS

Subsequent nontransmural myocardial infarction NOS

N Newborn: 0   P Pediatric: 0-17   M Maternity: 12-55   A Adult: 15-124   CH Comorbidity High   CL Comorbidity Low   NCDx Noncancer Dx   PDx Primary Dx

636   ICD-10-CM 2020

I22.8   **Subsequent ST elevation (STEMI) myocardial infarction of other sites**

Subsequent acute transmural myocardial infarction of other sites

Subsequent apical-lateral transmural (Q wave) myocardial infarction (acute)

Subsequent basal-lateral transmural (Q wave) myocardial infarction (acute)

Subsequent high lateral transmural (Q wave) myocardial infarction (acute)

Subsequent transmural (Q wave) myocardial infarction (acute)(of) lateral (wall) NOS

Subsequent posterior (true) transmural (Q wave) myocardial infarction (acute)

Subsequent posterobasal transmural (Q wave) myocardial infarction (acute)

Subsequent posterolateral transmural (Q wave) myocardial infarction (acute)

Subsequent posteroseptal transmural (Q wave) myocardial infarction (acute)

Subsequent septal NOS transmural (Q wave) myocardial infarction (acute)

I22.9   **Subsequent ST elevation (STEMI) myocardial infarction of unspecified site**

Subsequent acute myocardial infarction of unspecified site

Subsequent myocardial infarction (acute) NOS

☑4ᵗʰ I23   Certain current complications following ST elevation (STEMI) and non-ST elevation (NSTEMI) myocardial infarction (within the 28 day period)

AHA: 2017,2Q,11

DEF: ST elevation myocardial infarction: Complete obstruction of one or more coronary arteries causing decreased blood flow (ischemia) and necrosis of myocardial muscle cells.

DEF: Non-ST elevation myocardial infarction: Partial obstruction of one or more coronary arteries that causes decreased blood flow (ischemia) and may cause partial thickness necrosis of myocardial muscle cells.

I23.0   **Hemopericardium as current complication following acute myocardial infarction**   🅰

EXCLUDES 1   *hemopericardium not specified as current complication following acute myocardial infarction (I31.2)*

I23.1   **Atrial septal defect as current complication following acute myocardial infarction**   🅰

EXCLUDES 1   *acquired atrial septal defect not specified as current complication following acute myocardial infarction (I51.0)*

I23.2   **Ventricular septal defect as current complication following acute myocardial infarction**   🅰

EXCLUDES 1   *acquired ventricular septal defect not specified as current complication following acute myocardial infarction (I51.0)*

I23.3   **Rupture of cardiac wall without hemopericardium as current complication following acute myocardial infarction**   🅰

I23.4   **Rupture of chordae tendineae as current complication following acute myocardial infarction**   🅰

EXCLUDES 1   *rupture of chordae tendineae not specified as current complication following acute myocardial infarction (I51.1)*

I23.5   **Rupture of papillary muscle as current complication following acute myocardial infarction**   🅰

EXCLUDES 1   *rupture of papillary muscle not specified as current complication following acute myocardial infarction (I51.2)*

I23.6   **Thrombosis of atrium, auricular appendage, and ventricle as current complications following acute myocardial infarction**   🅰

EXCLUDES 1   *thrombosis of atrium, auricular appendage, and ventricle not specified as current complication following acute myocardial infarction (I51.3)*

I23.7   **Postinfarction angina**   *P 4 wks from initial*   🅰

AHA: 2015,2Q,16   *MI use → I25.118*

I23.8   **Other current complications following acute myocardial infarction**   🅰

☑4ᵗʰ I24   Other acute ischemic heart diseases

EXCLUDES 1   *angina pectoris (I20.-)*

     transient myocardial ischemia in newborn (P29.4)

I24.0   **Acute coronary thrombosis not resulting in myocardial infarction**   CH

Acute coronary (artery) (vein) embolism not resulting in myocardial infarction

Acute coronary (artery) (vein) occlusion not resulting in myocardial infarction

Acute coronary (artery) (vein) thromboembolism not resulting in myocardial infarction

EXCLUDES 1   *atherosclerotic heart disease (I25.1-)*

AHA: 2013,1Q,24

I24.1   **Dressler's syndrome**   CH

Postmyocardial infarction syndrome

EXCLUDES 1   *postinfarction angina (I23.7)*

DEF: Fever, leukocytosis, chest pain, evidence of pericarditis, pleurisy, and pneumonia occurring days or weeks after a myocardial infarction.

I24.8   **Other forms of acute ischemic heart disease**   CH

EXCLUDES 1   *myocardial infarction due to demand ischemia (I21.A1)*

AHA: 2017,4Q,13

I24.9   **Acute ischemic heart disease, unspecified**   CH

EXCLUDES 1   *ischemic heart disease (chronic) NOS (I25.9)*

☑4ᵗʰ I25   Chronic ischemic heart disease   *code HTN also*

Use additional code to identify:

chronic total occlusion of coronary artery (I25.82)

exposure to environmental tobacco smoke (Z77.22)

history of tobacco dependence (Z87.891)

occupational exposure to environmental tobacco smoke (Z57.31)

tobacco dependence (F17.-)

tobacco use (Z72.0)

☑5ᵗʰ I25.1   **Atherosclerotic heart disease of native coronary artery**

Atherosclerotic cardiovascular disease

Coronary (artery) atheroma

Coronary (artery) atherosclerosis

Coronary (artery) disease

Coronary (artery) sclerosis

Use additional code, if applicable, to identify:

coronary atherosclerosis due to calcified coronary lesion (I25.84)

coronary atherosclerosis due to lipid rich plaque (I25.83)

EXCLUDES 2   *atheroembolism (I75.-)*

     atherosclerosis of coronary artery bypass graft(s) and transplanted heart (I25.7-)

Atheromas

Atheromas (fatty tissue and/or plaque)   Lumen

I25.10   **Atherosclerotic heart disease of native coronary artery without angina pectoris**   CH 🅰

Atherosclerotic heart disease NOS

AHA: 2015,2Q,16; 2012,4Q,92

☑6ᵗʰ I25.11   **Atherosclerotic heart disease of native coronary artery with angina pectoris**

I25.110   **Atherosclerotic heart disease of native coronary artery with unstable angina pectoris**   🅰

EXCLUDES 1   *unstable angina without atherosclerotic heart disease (I20.0)*

☑ Additional Character Required   ☑x7ᵗʰ Placeholder Alert   Manifestation   Unspecified Dx   ▶◀ Revised Text   ● New Code   ▲ Revised Title

ICD-10-CM 2020   637

I25.111 Atherosclerotic heart disease of native coronary artery with angina pectoris with documented spasm [A]
> EXCLUDES 1   angina pectoris with documented spasm without atherosclerotic heart disease (I20.1)

I25.118 Atherosclerotic heart disease of native coronary artery with other forms of angina pectoris [A]
> EXCLUDES 1   other forms of angina pectoris without atherosclerotic heart disease (I20.8)

AHA: 2015,2Q,16

I25.119 Atherosclerotic heart disease of native coronary artery with unspecified angina pectoris [A]
Atherosclerotic heart disease with angina NOS
Atherosclerotic heart disease with ischemic chest pain
> EXCLUDES 1   unspecified angina pectoris without atherosclerotic heart disease (I20.9)

old MI

I25.2 Old myocardial infarction
Healed myocardial infarction
Past myocardial infarction diagnosed by ECG or other investigation, but currently presenting no symptoms

I25.3 Aneurysm of heart NC Dx
Mural aneurysm
Ventricular aneurysm

✓5ᵗʰ I25.4 Coronary artery aneurysm and dissection

I25.41 Coronary artery aneurysm NC Dx
Coronary arteriovenous fistula, acquired
> EXCLUDES 1   congenital coronary (artery) aneurysm (Q24.5)

I25.42 Coronary artery dissection NC Dx
> DEF: Tear in the intimal arterial wall of a coronary artery resulting in the sudden intrusion of blood within the layers of the wall.

I25.5 Ischemic cardiomyopathy NC Dx
> EXCLUDES 2   coronary atherosclerosis (I25.1-, I25.7-)

I25.6 Silent myocardial ischemia NC Dx

✓5ᵗʰ I25.7 Atherosclerosis of coronary artery bypass graft(s) and coronary artery of transplanted heart with angina pectoris
Use additional code, if applicable, to identify:
coronary atherosclerosis due to calcified coronary lesion (I25.84)
coronary atherosclerosis due to lipid rich plaque (I25.83)
> EXCLUDES 1   atherosclerosis of bypass graft(s) of transplanted heart without angina pectoris (I25.812)
> atherosclerosis of coronary artery bypass graft(s) without angina pectoris (I25.810)
> atherosclerosis of native coronary artery of transplanted heart without angina pectoris (I25.811)

✓6ᵗʰ I25.70 Atherosclerosis of coronary artery bypass graft(s), unspecified, with angina pectoris

I25.700 Atherosclerosis of coronary artery bypass graft(s), unspecified, with unstable angina pectoris [A]
> EXCLUDES 1   unstable angina pectoris without atherosclerosis of coronary artery bypass graft (I20.0)

I25.701 Atherosclerosis of coronary artery bypass graft(s), unspecified, with angina pectoris with documented spasm [A]
> EXCLUDES 1   angina pectoris with documented spasm without atherosclerosis of coronary artery bypass graft (I20.1)

I25.708 Atherosclerosis of coronary artery bypass graft(s), unspecified, with other forms of angina pectoris [A]
> EXCLUDES 1   other forms of angina pectoris without atherosclerosis of coronary artery bypass graft (I20.8)

I25.709 Atherosclerosis of coronary artery bypass graft(s), unspecified, with unspecified angina pectoris [A]
> EXCLUDES 1   unspecified angina pectoris without atherosclerosis of coronary artery bypass graft (I20.9)

✓6ᵗʰ I25.71 Atherosclerosis of autologous vein coronary artery bypass graft(s) with angina pectoris

I25.710 Atherosclerosis of autologous vein coronary artery bypass graft(s) with unstable angina pectoris [A]
> EXCLUDES 1   unstable angina without atherosclerosis of autologous vein coronary artery bypass graft(s) (I20.0)
> EXCLUDES 2   embolism or thrombus of coronary artery bypass graft(s) (T82.8-)

I25.711 Atherosclerosis of autologous vein coronary artery bypass graft(s) with angina pectoris with documented spasm [A]
> EXCLUDES 1   angina pectoris with documented spasm without atherosclerosis of autologous vein coronary artery bypass graft(s) (I20.1)

I25.718 Atherosclerosis of autologous vein coronary artery bypass graft(s) with other forms of angina pectoris [A]
> EXCLUDES 1   other forms of angina pectoris without atherosclerosis of autologous vein coronary artery bypass graft(s) (I20.8)

I25.719 Atherosclerosis of autologous vein coronary artery bypass graft(s) with unspecified angina pectoris [A]
> EXCLUDES 1   unspecified angina pectoris without atherosclerosis of autologous vein coronary artery bypass graft(s) (I20.9)

✓6ᵗʰ I25.72 Atherosclerosis of autologous artery coronary artery bypass graft(s) with angina pectoris
Atherosclerosis of internal mammary artery graft with angina pectoris

I25.720 Atherosclerosis of autologous artery coronary artery bypass graft(s) with unstable angina pectoris [A]
> EXCLUDES 1   unstable angina without atherosclerosis of autologous artery coronary artery bypass graft(s) (I20.0)

[N] Newborn: 0   [P] Pediatric: 0-17   [M] Maternity: 12-55   [A] Adult: 15-124   [CH] Comorbidity High   [CL] Comorbidity Low   [NC Dx] Noncancer Dx   [PDx] Primary Dx

638   ICD-10-CM 2020

I25.721 Atherosclerosis of autologous artery coronary artery bypass graft(s) with angina pectoris with documented spasm [A]

> EXCLUDES 1   *angina pectoris with documented spasm without atherosclerosis of autologous artery coronary artery bypass graft(s) (I20.1)*

I25.728 Atherosclerosis of autologous artery coronary artery bypass graft(s) with other forms of angina pectoris [A]

> EXCLUDES 1   *other forms of angina pectoris without atherosclerosis of autologous artery coronary artery bypass graft(s) (I20.8)*

I25.729 Atherosclerosis of autologous artery coronary artery bypass graft(s) with unspecified angina pectoris [A]

> EXCLUDES 1   *unspecified angina pectoris without atherosclerosis of autologous artery coronary artery bypass graft(s) (I20.9)*

√6th **I25.73 Atherosclerosis of nonautologous biological coronary artery bypass graft(s) with angina pectoris**

I25.730 Atherosclerosis of nonautologous biological coronary artery bypass graft(s) with unstable angina pectoris [A]

> EXCLUDES 1   *unstable angina without atherosclerosis of nonautologous biological coronary artery bypass graft(s) (I20.0)*

I25.731 Atherosclerosis of nonautologous biological coronary artery bypass graft(s) with angina pectoris with documented spasm [A]

> EXCLUDES 1   *angina pectoris with documented spasm without atherosclerosis of nonautologous biological coronary artery bypass graft(s) (I20.1)*

I25.738 Atherosclerosis of nonautologous biological coronary artery bypass graft(s) with other forms of angina pectoris [A]

> EXCLUDES 1   *other forms of angina pectoris without atherosclerosis of nonautologous biological coronary artery bypass graft(s) (I20.8)*

I25.739 Atherosclerosis of nonautologous biological coronary artery bypass graft(s) with unspecified angina pectoris [A]

> EXCLUDES 1   *unspecified angina pectoris without atherosclerosis of nonautologous biological coronary artery bypass graft(s) (I20.9)*

√6th **I25.75 Atherosclerosis of native coronary artery of transplanted heart with angina pectoris**

> EXCLUDES 1   *atherosclerosis of native coronary artery of transplanted heart without angina pectoris (I25.811)*

I25.750 Atherosclerosis of native coronary artery of transplanted heart with unstable angina

I25.751 Atherosclerosis of native coronary artery of transplanted heart with angina pectoris with documented spasm

I25.758 Atherosclerosis of native coronary artery of transplanted heart with other forms of angina pectoris

I25.759 Atherosclerosis of native coronary artery of transplanted heart with unspecified angina pectoris

√6th **I25.76 Atherosclerosis of bypass graft of coronary artery of transplanted heart with angina pectoris**

> EXCLUDES 1   *atherosclerosis of bypass graft of coronary artery of transplanted heart without angina pectoris (I25.812)*

I25.760 Atherosclerosis of bypass graft of coronary artery of transplanted heart with unstable angina [A]

I25.761 Atherosclerosis of bypass graft of coronary artery of transplanted heart with angina pectoris with documented spasm [A]

I25.768 Atherosclerosis of bypass graft of coronary artery of transplanted heart with other forms of angina pectoris [A]

I25.769 Atherosclerosis of bypass graft of coronary artery of transplanted heart with unspecified angina pectoris [A]

√6th **I25.79 Atherosclerosis of other coronary artery bypass graft(s) with angina pectoris**

I25.790 Atherosclerosis of other coronary artery bypass graft(s) with unstable angina pectoris [A]

> EXCLUDES 1   *unstable angina without atherosclerosis of other coronary artery bypass graft(s) (I20.0)*

I25.791 Atherosclerosis of other coronary artery bypass graft(s) with angina pectoris with documented spasm [A]

> EXCLUDES 1   *angina pectoris with documented spasm without atherosclerosis of other coronary artery bypass graft(s) (I20.1)*

I25.798 Atherosclerosis of other coronary artery bypass graft(s) with other forms of angina pectoris [A]

> EXCLUDES 1   *other forms of angina pectoris without atherosclerosis of other coronary artery bypass graft(s) (I20.8)*

I25.799 Atherosclerosis of other coronary artery bypass graft(s) with unspecified angina pectoris [A]

> EXCLUDES 1   *unspecified angina pectoris without atherosclerosis of other coronary artery bypass graft(s) (I20.9)*

✓ Additional Character Required   ✓x7th Placeholder Alert   Manifestation   Unspecified Dx   ►◄ Revised Text   ● New Code   ▲ Revised Title

ICD-10-CM 2020   639

Chapter 9. Diseases of the Circulatory System

✓5ᵗʰ **I25.8 Other forms of chronic ischemic heart disease**

✓6ᵗʰ **I25.81 Atherosclerosis of other coronary vessels without angina pectoris**

Use additional code, if applicable, to identify:
coronary atherosclerosis due to calcified coronary lesion (I25.84)
coronary atherosclerosis due to lipid rich plaque (I25.83)

EXCLUDES 1   ~~atherosclerotic heart disease of native coronary artery without angina pectoris (I25.10)~~

EXCLUDES 2   ▶atherosclerotic heart disease of native coronary artery without angina pectoris (I25.10)◀

I25.810 Atherosclerosis of coronary artery bypass graft(s) without angina pectoris 🅰

Atherosclerosis of coronary artery bypass graft NOS

EXCLUDES 1   atherosclerosis of coronary bypass graft(s) with angina pectoris (I25.70-I25.73-, I25.79-)

I25.811 Atherosclerosis of native coronary artery of transplanted heart without angina pectoris

Atherosclerosis of native coronary artery of transplanted heart NOS

EXCLUDES 1   atherosclerosis of native coronary artery of transplanted heart with angina pectoris (I25.75-)

I25.812 Atherosclerosis of bypass graft of coronary artery of transplanted heart without angina pectoris 🅰

Atherosclerosis of bypass graft of transplanted heart NOS

EXCLUDES 1   atherosclerosis of bypass graft of transplanted heart with angina pectoris (I25.76)

I25.82 Chronic total occlusion of coronary artery

Complete occlusion of coronary artery
Total occlusion of coronary artery
Code first coronary atherosclerosis (I25.1-, I25.7-, I25.81-)

EXCLUDES 1   acute coronary occlusion with myocardial infarction (I21.0-I21.9, I22.-)
acute coronary occlusion without myocardial infarction (I24.0)

AHA: 2018,3Q,5
DEF: Complete blockage of the coronary artery due to plaque accumulation over an extended period of time, resulting in substantial reduction of blood flow. Symptoms include angina or chest pain.

I25.83 Coronary atherosclerosis due to lipid rich plaque 🅰

Code first coronary atherosclerosis (I25.1-, I25.7-, I25.81-)

I25.84 Coronary atherosclerosis due to calcified coronary lesion

Coronary atherosclerosis due to severely calcified coronary lesion
Code first coronary atherosclerosis (I25.1-, I25.7-, I25.81-)

I25.89 Other forms of chronic ischemic heart disease ᴺᶜ ᴰˣ

I25.9 Chronic ischemic heart disease, unspecified ᴺᶜ ᴰˣ

Ischemic heart disease (chronic) NOS

Pulmonary heart disease and diseases of pulmonary circulation (I26-I28)

✓4ᵗʰ **I26 Pulmonary embolism**

INCLUDES   pulmonary (acute)(artery)(vein) infarction
pulmonary (acute) (artery)(vein) thromboembolism
pulmonary (acute)(artery)(vein) thrombosis

EXCLUDES 2   chronic pulmonary embolism (I27.82)
personal history of pulmonary embolism (Z86.711)
pulmonary embolism complicating abortion, ectopic or molar pregnancy (O00-O07, O08.2)
pulmonary embolism complicating pregnancy, childbirth and the puerperium (O88.-)
pulmonary embolism due to trauma (T79.0, T79.1)
pulmonary embolism due to complications of surgical and medical care (T80.0, T81.7-, T82.8-)
septic (non-pulmonary) arterial embolism (I76)

✓5ᵗʰ **I26.0 Pulmonary embolism with acute cor pulmonale**

DEF: Cor pulmonale: Heart-lung disease appearing in identifiable forms as chronic or acute. The chronic form of this heart-lung disease is marked by dilation, hypertrophy and failure of the right ventricle due to a disease that has affected the function of the lungs, excluding congenital or left heart diseases and is also called chronic cardiopulmonary disease. The acute form is an overload of the right ventricle from a rapid onset of pulmonary hypertension, usually arising from a pulmonary embolism.

I26.01 Septic pulmonary embolism with acute cor pulmonale

Code first underlying infection

I26.02 Saddle embolus of pulmonary artery with acute cor pulmonale ᴺᶜ ᴰˣ

I26.09 Other pulmonary embolism with acute cor pulmonale ᶜᴸ ᴺᶜ ᴰˣ

Acute cor pulmonale NOS
AHA: 2014,4Q,21

✓5ᵗʰ **I26.9 Pulmonary embolism without acute cor pulmonale**

I26.90 Septic pulmonary embolism without acute cor pulmonale

Code first underlying infection

I26.92 Saddle embolus of pulmonary artery without acute cor pulmonale ᴺᶜ ᴰˣ

I26.93 Single subsegmental pulmonary embolism without acute cor pulmonale

Subsegmental pulmonary embolism NOS

I26.94 Multiple subsegmental pulmonary emboli without acute cor pulmonale

I26.99 Other pulmonary embolism without acute cor pulmonale ᶜᴸ ᴺᶜ ᴰˣ

Acute pulmonary embolism NOS
Pulmonary embolism NOS
AHA: 2019,2Q,22

✓4ᵗʰ **I27 Other pulmonary heart diseases**

I27.0 Primary pulmonary hypertension ᴺᶜ ᴰˣ

Heritable pulmonary arterial hypertension
Idiopathic pulmonary arterial hypertension
Primary group 1 pulmonary hypertension
Primary pulmonary arterial hypertension

EXCLUDES 1   persistent pulmonary hypertension of newborn (P29.30)
pulmonary hypertension NOS (I27.20)
secondary pulmonary arterial hypertension (I27.21)
secondary pulmonary hypertension (I27.29)

DEF: Condition that occurs when pressure within the pulmonary artery is elevated and vascular resistance is observed in the lungs.

I27.1 Kyphoscoliotic heart disease ᴺᶜ ᴰˣ

✓5ᵗʰ **I27.2 Other secondary pulmonary hypertension**

Code also associated underlying condition

EXCLUDES 1   Eisenmenger's syndrome (I27.83)
AHA: 2017,4Q,14-15; 2014,4Q,21
DEF: Condition that occurs when pressure within the pulmonary artery is elevated and vascular resistance is observed in the lungs.

I27.20 Pulmonary hypertension, unspecified

Pulmonary hypertension NOS

Ⓝ Newborn: 0   Ⓟ Pediatric: 0-17   Ⓜ Maternity: 12-55   🅰 Adult: 15-124   ᶜᴴ Comorbidity High   ᶜᴸ Comorbidity Low   ᴺᶜ ᴰˣ Noncancer Dx   ᴾᴰˣ Primary Dx

640   ICD-10-CM 2020

I25.8–I27.20

I27.21 Secondary pulmonary arterial hypertension
(Associated) (drug-induced) (toxin-induced)
  pulmonary arterial hypertension NOS
(Associated) (drug-induced) (toxin-induced)
  (secondary) group 1 pulmonary hypertension
Code also associated conditions if applicable, or
  adverse effects of drugs or toxins, such as:
  adverse effect of appetite depressants (T50.5X5)
  congenital heart disease (Q20-Q28)
  human immunodeficiency virus [HIV] disease (B20)
  polymyositis (M33.2-)
  portal hypertension (K76.6)
  rheumatoid arthritis (M05.-)
  schistosomiasis (B65.-)
  Sjögren syndrome (M35.0-)
  systemic sclerosis (M34.-)

I27.22 Pulmonary hypertension due to left heart disease
Group 2 pulmonary hypertension
Code also associated left heart disease, if known, such
  as:
  multiple valve disease (I08.-)
  rheumatic aortic valve diseases (I06.-)
  rheumatic mitral valve diseases (I05.-)

I27.23 Pulmonary hypertension due to lung diseases and hypoxia
Group 3 pulmonary hypertension
Code also associated lung disease, if known, such as:
  bronchiectasis (J47.-)
  cystic fibrosis with pulmonary manifestations
    (E84.0)
  interstitial lung disease (J84.-)
  pleural effusion (J90)
  sleep apnea (G47.3-)

I27.24 Chronic thromboembolic pulmonary hypertension
Group 4 pulmonary hypertension
Code also associated pulmonary embolism, if
  applicable (I26.-, I27.82)

I27.29 Other secondary pulmonary hypertension
Group 5 pulmonary hypertension
Pulmonary hypertension with unclear multifactorial
  mechanisms
Pulmonary hypertension due to hematologic
  disorders
Pulmonary hypertension due to metabolic disorders
Pulmonary hypertension due to other systemic
  disorders
Code also other associated disorders, if known, such
  as:
  chronic myeloid leukemia (C92.10- C92.22)
  essential thrombocythemia (D47.3)
  Gaucher disease (E75.22)
  hypertensive chronic kidney disease with end stage
    renal disease (I12.0, I13.11, I13.2)
  hyperthyroidism (E05.-)
  hypothyroidism (E00-E03)
  polycythemia vera (D45)
  sarcoidosis (D86.-)
AHA: 2016,2Q,8

✓5ᵗʰ I27.8 Other specified pulmonary heart diseases

I27.81 Cor pulmonale (chronic)   `NC Dx`
Cor pulmonale NOS
EXCLUDES 1   *acute cor pulmonale (I26.0-)*
AHA: 2014,4Q,21
DEF: Heart-lung disease appearing in identifiable forms
as chronic or acute. The chronic form of this heart-lung
disease is marked by dilation, hypertrophy and failure
of the right ventricle due to a disease that has affected
the function of the lungs, excluding congenital or left
heart diseases and is also called chronic
cardiopulmonary disease. The acute form is an overload
of the right ventricle from a rapid onset of pulmonary
hypertension, usually arising from a pulmonary
embolism.

I27.82 Chronic pulmonary embolism   `NC Dx`
Use additional code, if applicable, for associated
  long-term (current) use of anticoagulants
  (Z79.01)
EXCLUDES 1   *personal history of pulmonary embolism*
    (Z86.711)
DEF: Long-standing condition commonly associated
with pulmonary hypertension in which small blood
clots travel to the lungs repeatedly over many weeks,
months, or years, requiring continuation of established
anticoagulant or thrombolytic therapy.

I27.83 Eisenmenger's syndrome
Eisenmenger's complex
(Irreversible) Eisenmenger's disease
Pulmonary hypertension with right to left shunt
  related to congenital heart disease
Code also underlying heart defect, if known, such as:
  atrial septal defect (Q21.1)
  Eisenmenger's defect (Q21.8)
  patent ductus arteriosus (Q25.0)
  ventricular septal defect (Q21.0)
DEF: Pulmonary hypertension with congenital
communication between two circulations resulting in
a right to left shunt. This causes reduced oxygen
saturation in the arterial blood, leading to cyanosis and
organ damage. Once it develops, this life-threating
condition is irreversible.

I27.89 Other specified pulmonary heart diseases   `NC Dx`

I27.9 Pulmonary heart disease, unspecified   `NC Dx`
Chronic cardiopulmonary disease

✓4ᵗʰ I28 Other diseases of pulmonary vessels

I28.0 Arteriovenous fistula of pulmonary vessels   `NC Dx`
EXCLUDES 1   *congenital arteriovenous fistula (Q25.72)*

I28.1 Aneurysm of pulmonary artery   `NC Dx`
EXCLUDES 1   *congenital aneurysm (Q25.79)*
    congenital arteriovenous aneurysm (Q25.72)

I28.8 Other diseases of pulmonary vessels
Pulmonary arteritis
Pulmonary endarteritis
Rupture of pulmonary vessels
Stenosis of pulmonary vessels
Stricture of pulmonary vessels

I28.9 Disease of pulmonary vessels, unspecified

Other forms of heart disease (I30-I52)

✓4ᵗʰ I30 Acute pericarditis
INCLUDES   acute mediastinopericarditis
  acute myopericarditis
  acute pericardial effusion
  acute pleuropericarditis
  acute pneumopericarditis
EXCLUDES 1   *Dressler's syndrome (I24.1)*
  rheumatic pericarditis (acute) (I01.0)
  viral pericarditis due to Coxsakie virus (B33.23)
DEF: Pericarditis: Inflammation affecting the pericardium, the fibroserous
membrane that surrounds the heart.

I30.0 Acute nonspecific idiopathic pericarditis

I30.1 Infective pericarditis
Pneumococcal pericarditis
Pneumopyopericardium
Purulent pericarditis
Pyopericarditis
Pyopericardium
Pyopneumopericardium
Staphylococcal pericarditis
Streptococcal pericarditis
Suppurative pericarditis
Viral pericarditis
Use additional code (B95-B97) to identify infectious agent

I30.8 Other forms of acute pericarditis

I30.9 Acute pericarditis, unspecified

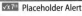
☑ Additional Character Required   ✓x7ᵗʰ Placeholder Alert   Manifestation   Unspecified Dx   ►◄ Revised Text   ● New Code   ▲ Revised Title

ICD-10-CM 2020   641

Chapter 9. Diseases of the Circulatory System

I31–I37.0

✓4ᵗʰ **I31 Other diseases of pericardium**

> *EXCLUDES 1*   diseases of pericardium specified as rheumatic (I09.2)
> postcardiotomy syndrome (I97.0)
> traumatic injury to pericardium (S26.-)

I31.0 Chronic adhesive pericarditis
Accretio cordis
Adherent pericardium
Adhesive mediastinopericarditis

I31.1 Chronic constrictive pericarditis
Concretio cordis
Pericardial calcification

I31.2 Hemopericardium, not elsewhere classified

> *EXCLUDES 1*   hemopericardium as current complication following
> acute myocardial infarction (I23.0)

DEF: Presence of blood in the pericardial sac (pericardium). It can lead to potentially fatal cardiac tamponade if enough blood enters the pericardial cavity.

I31.3 Pericardial effusion (noninflammatory)
Chylopericardium

> *EXCLUDES 1*   acute pericardial effusion (I30.9)

AHA: 2019,1Q,16

I31.4 Cardiac tamponade
Code first underlying cause
DEF: Life-threatening condition in which fluid or blood accumulates in the space between the muscle of the heart (myocardium) and the outer sac that covers the heart (pericardium), resulting in compression of the heart.

Cardiac Tamponade

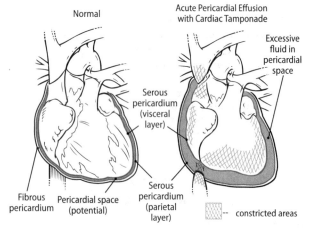

Normal

Acute Pericardial Effusion with Cardiac Tamponade

Excessive fluid in pericardial space

Serous pericardium (visceral layer)

Serous pericardium (parietal layer)

Fibrous pericardium   Pericardial space (potential)

▨ -- constricted areas

I31.8 Other specified diseases of pericardium
Epicardial plaques
Focal pericardial adhesions

I31.9 Disease of pericardium, unspecified
Pericarditis (chronic) NOS

I32 Pericarditis in diseases classified elsewhere
Code first underlying disease

> *EXCLUDES 1*   pericarditis (in):
> coxsackie (virus) (B33.23)
> gonococcal (A54.83)
> meningococcal (A39.53)
> rheumatoid (arthritis) (M05.31)
> syphilitic (A52.06)
> systemic lupus erythematosus (M32.12)
> tuberculosis (A18.84)

DEF: Pericarditis: Inflammation affecting the pericardium, the fibroserous membrane that surrounds the heart.

✓4ᵗʰ **I33 Acute and subacute endocarditis**

> *EXCLUDES 1*   acute rheumatic endocarditis (I01.1)
> endocarditis NOS (I38)

DEF: Endocarditis: Inflammatory disease of the interior lining of the heart chamber and heart valves.

I33.0 Acute and subacute infective endocarditis
Bacterial endocarditis (acute) (subacute)
Infective endocarditis (acute) (subacute) NOS
Endocarditis lenta (acute) (subacute)
Malignant endocarditis (acute) (subacute)
Purulent endocarditis (acute) (subacute)
Septic endocarditis (acute) (subacute)
Ulcerative endocarditis (acute) (subacute)
Vegetative endocarditis (acute) (subacute)
Use additional code (B95-B97) to identify infectious agent

I33.9 Acute and subacute endocarditis, unspecified
Acute endocarditis NOS
Acute myoendocarditis NOS
Acute periendocarditis NOS
Subacute endocarditis NOS
Subacute myoendocarditis NOS
Subacute periendocarditis NOS

✓4ᵗʰ **I34 Nonrheumatic mitral valve disorders**

> *EXCLUDES 1*   mitral valve disease (I05.9)
> mitral valve failure (I05.8)
> mitral valve stenosis (I05.0)
> mitral valve disorder of unspecified cause with diseases of aortic and/or tricuspid valve(s) (I08.-)
> mitral valve disorder of unspecified cause with mitral stenosis or obstruction (I05.0)
> mitral valve disorder specified as congenital (Q23.2, Q23.9)
> mitral valve disorder specified as rheumatic (I05.-)

I34.0 Nonrheumatic mitral (valve) insufficiency
Nonrheumatic mitral (valve) incompetence NOS
Nonrheumatic mitral (valve) regurgitation NOS

I34.1 Nonrheumatic mitral (valve) prolapse
Floppy nonrheumatic mitral valve syndrome

> *EXCLUDES 1*   Marfan's syndrome (Q87.4-)

I34.2 Nonrheumatic mitral (valve) stenosis
I34.8 Other nonrheumatic mitral valve disorders
I34.9 Nonrheumatic mitral valve disorder, unspecified

✓4ᵗʰ **I35 Nonrheumatic aortic valve disorders**

> *EXCLUDES 1*   aortic valve disorder of unspecified cause but with diseases of mitral and/or tricuspid valve(s) (I08.-)
> aortic valve disorder specified as congenital (Q23.0, Q23.1)
> aortic valve disorder specified as rheumatic (I06.-)
> hypertrophic subaortic stenosis (I42.1)

I35.0 Nonrheumatic aortic (valve) stenosis
I35.1 Nonrheumatic aortic (valve) insufficiency
Nonrheumatic aortic (valve) incompetence NOS
Nonrheumatic aortic (valve) regurgitation NOS

I35.2 Nonrheumatic aortic (valve) stenosis with insufficiency
I35.8 Other nonrheumatic aortic valve disorders
I35.9 Nonrheumatic aortic valve disorder, unspecified

✓4ᵗʰ **I36 Nonrheumatic tricuspid valve disorders**

> *EXCLUDES 1*   tricuspid valve disorders of unspecified cause (I07.-)
> tricuspid valve disorders specified as congenital (Q22.4, Q22.8, Q22.9)
> tricuspid valve disorders specified as rheumatic (I07.-)
> tricuspid valve disorders with aortic and/or mitral valve involvement (I08.-)

I36.0 Nonrheumatic tricuspid (valve) stenosis
I36.1 Nonrheumatic tricuspid (valve) insufficiency
Nonrheumatic tricuspid (valve) incompetence
Nonrheumatic tricuspid (valve) regurgitation

I36.2 Nonrheumatic tricuspid (valve) stenosis with insufficiency
I36.8 Other nonrheumatic tricuspid valve disorders
I36.9 Nonrheumatic tricuspid valve disorder, unspecified

✓4ᵗʰ **I37 Nonrheumatic pulmonary valve disorders**

> *EXCLUDES 1*   pulmonary valve disorder specified as congenital (Q22.1, Q22.2, Q22.3)
> pulmonary valve disorder specified as rheumatic (I09.89)

I37.0 Nonrheumatic pulmonary valve stenosis

Ⓝ Newborn: 0   Ⓟ Pediatric: 0-17   Ⓜ Maternity: 12-55   Ⓐ Adult: 15-124   CH Comorbidity High   CL Comorbidity Low   NCDx Noncancer Dx   PDx Primary Dx

642   ICD-10-CM 2020

I37.1   **Nonrheumatic pulmonary valve** insufficiency
> Nonrheumatic pulmonary valve incompetence
> Nonrheumatic pulmonary valve regurgitation

I37.2   **Nonrheumatic pulmonary valve** stenosis with insufficiency

I37.8   **Other nonrheumatic pulmonary valve disorders**

I37.9   **Nonrheumatic pulmonary valve disorder, unspecified**

I38   Endocarditis, valve unspecified

> INCLUDES   endocarditis (chronic) NOS
> valvular incompetence NOS
> valvular insufficiency NOS
> valvular regurgitation NOS
> valvular stenosis NOS
> valvulitis (chronic) NOS

> EXCLUDES 1   *congenital insufficiency of cardiac valve NOS (Q24.8)*
> *congenital stenosis of cardiac valve NOS (Q24.8)*
> *endocardial fibroelastosis (I42.4)*
> *endocarditis specified as rheumatic (I09.1)*

DEF: Endocarditis: Inflammatory disease of the interior lining of the heart chamber and heart valves.

I39   *Endocarditis and heart valve disorders in diseases classified elsewhere*

> Code first underlying disease, such as:
> Q fever (A78)

> EXCLUDES 1   *endocardial involvement in:*
> *candidiasis (B37.6)*
> *gonococcal infection (A54.83)*
> *Libman-Sacks disease (M32.11)*
> *listerosis (A32.82)*
> *meningococcal infection (A39.51)*
> *rheumatoid arthritis (M05.31)*
> *syphilis (A52.03)*
> *tuberculosis (A18.84)*
> *typhoid fever (A01.02)*

DEF: Endocarditis: Inflammatory disease of the interior lining of the heart chamber and heart valves.

✓4th I40   Acute myocarditis

> INCLUDES   subacute myocarditis
> EXCLUDES 1   *acute rheumatic myocarditis (I01.2)*

DEF: Myocarditis: Inflammation of the middle layer of the heart, which is composed of muscle tissue.

I40.0   **Infective myocarditis**
> Septic myocarditis
> Use additional code (B95-B97) to identify infectious agent

I40.1   **Isolated myocarditis**
> Fiedler's myocarditis
> Giant cell myocarditis
> Idiopathic myocarditis

I40.8   **Other acute myocarditis**

I40.9   **Acute myocarditis, unspecified**

I41   *Myocarditis in diseases classified elsewhere*

> Code first underlying disease, such as:
> typhus (A75.0-A75.9)

> EXCLUDES 1   *myocarditis (in):*
> *Chagas' disease (chronic) (B57.2)*
> *acute (B57.0)*
> *coxsackie (virus) infection (B33.22)*
> *diphtheritic (A36.81)*
> *gonococcal (A54.83)*
> *influenzal (J09.X9, J10.82, J11.82)*
> *meningococcal (A39.52)*
> *mumps (B26.82)*
> *rheumatoid arthritis (M05.31)*
> *sarcoid (D86.85)*
> *syphilis (A52.06)*
> *toxoplasmosis (B58.81)*
> *tuberculous (A18.84)*

DEF: Myocarditis: Inflammation of the middle layer of the heart, which is composed of muscle tissue.

✓4th I42   Cardiomyopathy

> INCLUDES   myocardiopathy
> Code first pre-existing cardiomyopathy complicating pregnancy and puerperium (O99.4)

> EXCLUDES 2   *ischemic cardiomyopathy (I25.5)*
> *peripartum cardiomyopathy (O90.3)*
> *ventricular hypertrophy (I51.7)*

I42.0   **Dilated cardiomyopathy**
> Congestive cardiomyopathy

I42.1   **Obstructive hypertrophic cardiomyopathy**
> Hypertrophic subaortic stenosis (idiopathic)
> **DEF:** Cardiomyopathy marked by left ventricle hypertrophy and an enlarged septum that result in obstructed blood flow, arrhythmias, mitral regurgitation, and sudden cardiac death.

I42.2   **Other hypertrophic cardiomyopathy**
> Nonobstructive hypertrophic cardiomyopathy

I42.3   **Endomyocardial (eosinophilic) disease**
> Endomyocardial (tropical) fibrosis
> Löffler's endocarditis

I42.4   **Endocardial fibroelastosis**
> Congenital cardiomyopathy
> Elastomyofibrosis

I42.5   **Other restrictive cardiomyopathy**
> Constrictive cardiomyopathy NOS

I42.6   **Alcoholic cardiomyopathy**
> Code also presence of alcoholism (F10.-)

I42.7   **Cardiomyopathy due to drug and external agent**
> Code first poisoning due to drug or toxin, if applicable (T36-T65 with fifth or sixth character 1-4 or 6)
> Use additional code for adverse effect, if applicable, to identify drug (T36-T50 with fifth or sixth character 5)

I42.8   **Other cardiomyopathies**

I42.9   **Cardiomyopathy, unspecified**
> Cardiomyopathy (primary) (secondary) NOS

I43   *Cardiomyopathy in diseases classified elsewhere*

> Code first underlying disease, such as:
> amyloidosis (E85.-)
> glycogen storage disease (E74.0)
> gout (M10.0-)
> thyrotoxicosis (E05.0-E05.9-)

> EXCLUDES 1   *cardiomyopathy (in):*
> *coxsackie (virus) (B33.24)*
> *diphtheria (A36.81)*
> *sarcoidosis (D86.85)*
> *tuberculosis (A18.84)*

✓4th I44   Atrioventricular and left bundle-branch block

[handwritten: Z95.0 pacer]

I44.0   **Atrioventricular block, first degree**

I44.1   **Atrioventricular block, second degree**
> Atrioventricular block, type I and II
> Möbitz block, type I and II
> Second degree block, type I and II
> Wenckebach's block

I44.2   **Atrioventricular block, complete**
> Complete heart block NOS
> Third degree block
> **AHA:** 2019,2Q,4

✓5th I44.3   **Other and unspecified atrioventricular block**
> Atrioventricular block NOS

I44.30   **Unspecified atrioventricular block**

I44.39   **Other atrioventricular block**

I44.4   **Left anterior fascicular block**

I44.5   **Left posterior fascicular block**

✓5th I44.6   **Other and unspecified fascicular block**

I44.60   **Unspecified fascicular block**
> Left bundle-branch hemiblock NOS

I44.69   **Other fascicular block**

☑ Additional Character Required   ✓×7th Placeholder Alert   Manifestation   Unspecified Dx   ►◄ Revised Text   ● New Code   ▲ Revised Title

ICD-10-CM 2020   643

Chapter 9. Diseases of the Circulatory System

I44.7 Left bundle-branch block, unspecified

Conduction Disorders

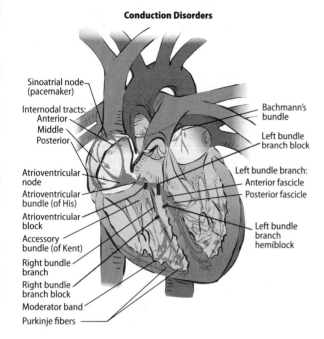

Sinoatrial node (pacemaker)
Internodal tracts:
Anterior
Middle
Posterior
Atrioventricular node
Atrioventricular bundle (of His)
Atrioventricular block
Accessory bundle (of Kent)
Right bundle branch
Right bundle branch block
Moderator band
Purkinje fibers

Bachmann's bundle
Left bundle branch block
Left bundle branch:
Anterior fascicle
Posterior fascicle
Left bundle branch hemiblock

I45 Other conduction disorders

I45.0 Right fascicular block

I45.1 Other and unspecified right bundle-branch block

I45.10 Unspecified right bundle-branch block
Right bundle-branch block NOS

I45.19 Other right bundle-branch block

I45.2 Bifascicular block

I45.3 Trifascicular block

I45.4 Nonspecific intraventricular block
Bundle-branch block NOS

I45.5 Other specified heart block
Sinoatrial block
Sinoauricular block
EXCLUDES 1　heart block NOS (I45.9)

I45.6 Pre-excitation syndrome
Accelerated atrioventricular conduction
Accessory atrioventricular conduction
Anomalous atrioventricular excitation
Lown-Ganong-Levine syndrome
Pre-excitation atrioventricular conduction
Wolff-Parkinson-White syndrome

I45.8 Other specified conduction disorders

I45.81 Long QT syndrome
DEF: Condition characterized by recurrent syncope, malignant arrhythmias, and sudden death. This syndrome has a characteristic prolonged Q-T interval on an electrocardiogram.

I45.89 Other specified conduction disorders
Atrioventricular [AV] dissociation
Interference dissociation
Isorhythmic dissociation
Nonparoxysmal AV nodal tachycardia
AHA: 2013,2Q,31

I45.9 Conduction disorder, unspecified
Heart block NOS
Stokes-Adams syndrome

I46 Cardiac arrest
EXCLUDES 1　cardiogenic shock (R57.0)
AHA: 2019,2Q,4-5

I46.2 Cardiac arrest due to underlying cardiac condition
Code first underlying cardiac condition

I46.8 Cardiac arrest due to other underlying condition
Code first underlying condition

I46.9 Cardiac arrest, cause unspecified

I47 Paroxysmal tachycardia
Code first tachycardia complicating:
abortion or ectopic or molar pregnancy (O00-O07, O08.8)
obstetric surgery and procedures (O75.4)
EXCLUDES 1　tachycardia NOS (R00.0)
sinoauricular tachycardia NOS (R00.0)
sinus [sinusal] tachycardia NOS (R00.0)

I47.0 Re-entry ventricular arrhythmia

I47.1 Supraventricular tachycardia
Atrial (paroxysmal) tachycardia
Atrioventricular [AV] (paroxysmal) tachycardia
Atrioventricular re-entrant (nodal) tachycardia [AVNRT] [AVRT]
Junctional (paroxysmal) tachycardia
Nodal (paroxysmal) tachycardia

I47.2 Ventricular tachycardia
AHA: 2013,3Q,23

I47.9 Paroxysmal tachycardia, unspecified
Bouveret (-Hoffman) syndrome

I48 Atrial fibrillation and flutter

I48.0 Paroxysmal atrial fibrillation　　CH CL
AHA: 2018,3Q,6

▲ **I48.1** Persistent atrial fibrillation
EXCLUDES 1　►permanent atrial fibrillation (I48.21)◄
AHA: 2019,2Q,3; 2018,3Q,6

● **I48.11** Longstanding persistent atrial fibrillation

● **I48.19** Other persistent atrial fibrillation
Chronic persistent atrial fibrillation
Persistent atrial fibrillation, NOS

▲ **I48.2** Chronic atrial fibrillation
~~Permanent atrial fibrillation~~
AHA: 2019,2Q,3; 2018,3Q,6

● **I48.20** Chronic atrial fibrillation, unspecified
EXCLUDES 1　chronic persistent atrial fibrillation (I48.19)

● **I48.21** Permanent atrial fibrillation

I48.3 Typical atrial flutter　　CH CL
Type I atrial flutter

I48.4 Atypical atrial flutter　　CH CL
Type II atrial flutter

I48.9 Unspecified atrial fibrillation and atrial flutter

I48.91 Unspecified atrial fibrillation　　CH CL

I48.92 Unspecified atrial flutter　　CH CL

I49 Other cardiac arrhythmias
Code first cardiac arrhythmia complicating:
abortion or ectopic or molar pregnancy (O00-O07, O08.8)
obstetric surgery and procedures (O75.4)
EXCLUDES 1　neonatal dysrhythmia (P29.1-)
sinoatrial bradycardia (R00.1)
sinus bradycardia (R00.1)
vagal bradycardia (R00.1)
EXCLUDES 2　bradycardia NOS (R00.1)

I49.0 Ventricular fibrillation and flutter

I49.01 Ventricular fibrillation

I49.02 Ventricular flutter

I49.1 Atrial premature depolarization
Atrial premature beats

I49.2 Junctional premature depolarization

I49.3 Ventricular premature depolarization

I49.4 Other and unspecified premature depolarization

I49.40 Unspecified premature depolarization
Premature beats NOS

I49.49 Other premature depolarization
Ectopic beats
Extrasystoles
Extrasystolic arrhythmias
Premature contractions

I49.5 Sick sinus syndrome　　CH CL
Tachycardia-bradycardia syndrome
AHA: 2019,1Q,33

N Newborn: 0　P Pediatric: 0-17　M Maternity: 12-55　A Adult: 15-124　CH Comorbidity High　CL Comorbidity Low　NC Dx Noncancer Dx　PDx Primary Dx

644

ICD-10-CM 2020

I49.8   **Other specified cardiac arrhythmias**   `CH` `CL`

Brugada syndrome
Coronary sinus rhythm disorder
Ectopic rhythm disorder
Nodal rhythm disorder

I49.9   **Cardiac arrhythmia, unspecified**   `CH` `CL`

Arrhythmia (cardiac) NOS

✓4ᵗʰ I50   **Heart failure**

Code first:

heart failure complicating abortion or ectopic or molar pregnancy (O00-O07, O08.8)
heart failure due to hypertension (I11.0)
heart failure due to hypertension with chronic kidney disease (I13.-)
heart failure following surgery (I97.13-)
obstetric surgery and procedures (O75.4)
rheumatic heart failure (I09.81)

EXCLUDES 1   *neonatal cardiac failure (P29.0)*
EXCLUDES 2   *cardiac arrest (I46.-)*

AHA: 2018,4Q,67; 2018,2Q,9; 2017,1Q,47; 2014,1Q,25; 2013,2Q,33

I50.1   **Left ventricular failure, unspecified**   `CH` `CL` `NC Dx`

Cardiac asthma
Edema of lung with heart disease NOS
Edema of lung with heart failure
Left heart failure
Pulmonary edema with heart disease NOS
Pulmonary edema with heart failure

EXCLUDES 1   *edema of lung without heart disease or heart failure (J81.-)*
         pulmonary edema without heart disease or failure (J81.-)

✓5ᵗʰ I50.2   **Systolic (congestive) heart failure**

Heart failure with reduced ejection fraction [HFrEF]
Systolic left ventricular heart failure
Code also end stage heart failure, if applicable (I50.84)

EXCLUDES 1   *combined systolic (congestive) and diastolic (congestive) heart failure (I50.4-)*

AHA: 2017,1Q,46; 2016,1Q,10

I50.20   **Unspecified systolic (congestive) heart failure**   `CH` `CL` `NC Dx`

TIP: This code would be viewed by Medicare as a questionable admission if used as the admitting diagnosis for a hospice encounter.

I50.21   **Acute systolic (congestive) heart failure**   `CH` `CL` `NC Dx`

I50.22   **Chronic systolic (congestive) heart failure**   `CH` `CL` `NC Dx`

I50.23   **Acute on chronic systolic (congestive) heart failure**   `CH` `CL` `NC Dx`

✓5ᵗʰ I50.3   **Diastolic (congestive) heart failure**

Diastolic left ventricular heart failure
Heart failure with normal ejection fraction
Heart failure with preserved ejection fraction [HFpEF]
Code also end stage heart failure, if applicable (I50.84)

EXCLUDES 1   *combined systolic (congestive) and diastolic (congestive) heart failure (I50.4-)*

AHA: 2017,1Q,46; 2016,1Q,10

I50.30   **Unspecified diastolic (congestive) heart failure**   `CH` `CL` `NC Dx`

TIP: This code would be viewed by Medicare as a questionable admission if used as the admitting diagnosis for a hospice encounter.

I50.31   **Acute diastolic (congestive) heart failure**   `CH` `CL` `NC Dx`

I50.32   **Chronic diastolic (congestive) heart failure**   `CH` `CL` `NC Dx`

I50.33   **Acute on chronic diastolic (congestive) heart failure**   `CH` `CL` `NC Dx`

✓5ᵗʰ I50.4   **Combined systolic (congestive) and diastolic (congestive) heart failure**

Combined systolic and diastolic left ventricular heart failure
Heart failure with reduced ejection fraction and diastolic dysfunction
Code also end stage heart failure, if applicable (I50.84)

AHA: 2017,1Q,46; 2016,1Q,10

I50.40   **Unspecified combined systolic (congestive) and diastolic (congestive) heart failure**   `CH` `CL` `NC Dx`

TIP: This code would be viewed by Medicare as a questionable admission if used as the admitting diagnosis for a hospice encounter.

I50.41   **Acute combined systolic (congestive) and diastolic (congestive) heart failure**   `CH` `CL` `NC Dx`

I50.42   **Chronic combined systolic (congestive) and diastolic (congestive) heart failure**   `CH` `CL` `NC Dx`

I50.43   **Acute on chronic combined systolic (congestive) and diastolic (congestive) heart failure**   `CH` `CL` `NC Dx`

✓5ᵗʰ I50.8   **Other heart failure**

AHA: 2017,4Q,15-16

✓6ᵗʰ I50.81   **Right heart failure**

Right ventricular failure

I50.810   **Right heart failure, unspecified**   `CH` `CL` `NC Dx`

Right heart failure without mention of left heart failure
Right ventricular failure NOS

I50.811   **Acute right heart failure**   `CH` `CL` `NC Dx`

Acute isolated right heart failure
Acute (isolated) right ventricular failure

I50.812   **Chronic right heart failure**   `CH` `CL` `NC Dx`

Chronic isolated right heart failure
Chronic (isolated) right ventricular failure

I50.813   **Acute on chronic right heart failure**   `CH` `CL` `NC Dx`

Acute on chronic isolated right heart failure
Acute on chronic (isolated) right ventricular failure
Acute decompensation of chronic (isolated) right ventricular failure
Acute exacerbation of chronic (isolated) right ventricular failure

I50.814   **Right heart failure due to left heart failure**   `CH` `CL` `NC Dx`

Right ventricular failure secondary to left ventricular failure
Code also the type of left ventricular failure, if known (I50.2-I50.43)

EXCLUDES 1   *right heart failure with but not due to left heart failure (I50.82)*

I50.82   **Biventricular heart failure**   `CH` `CL` `NC Dx`

Code also the type of left ventricular failure as systolic, diastolic, or combined, if known (I50.2-I50.43)

I50.83   **High output heart failure**   `CH` `CL` `NC Dx`

DEF: Occurs when the high demand for blood exceeds the capacity of a normally functioning heart to meet the demand.

I50.84   **End stage heart failure**   `CH` `CL` `NC Dx`

Stage D heart failure
Code also the type of heart failure as systolic, diastolic, or combined, if known (I50.2-I50.43)

I50.89   **Other heart failure**   `CH` `CL` `NC Dx`

I50.9   **Heart failure, unspecified**   `CH` `CL` `NC Dx`

Cardiac, heart or myocardial failure NOS
Congestive heart disease
Congestive heart failure NOS

EXCLUDES 2   ▶*fluid overload unrelated to congestive heart failure*◀ *(E87.70)*

AHA: 2017,4Q,15-16; 2017,1Q,45-46; 2014,4Q,21; 2012,4Q,92
TIP: This code would be viewed by Medicare as a questionable admission if used as the admitting diagnosis for a hospice encounter.

✓ Additional Character Required   ✓x7ᵗʰ Placeholder Alert   Manifestation   Unspecified Dx   ▶◀ Revised Text   ● New Code   ▲ Revised Title

ICD-10-CM 2020   645

I49.8–I50.9

Chapter 9. Diseases of the Circulatory System

☑4ᵗʰ **I51   Complications and ill-defined descriptions of heart disease**

> EXCLUDES 1   any condition in I51.4-I51.9 due to hypertension (I11.-)
> any condition in I51.4-I51.9 due to hypertension and chronic kidney disease (I13.-)
> heart disease specified as rheumatic (I00-I09)

I51.0   Cardiac septal defect, acquired   Ⓐ

Acquired septal atrial defect (old)
Acquired septal auricular defect (old)
Acquired septal ventricular defect (old)

> EXCLUDES 1   cardiac septal defect as current complication following acute myocardial infarction (I23.1, I23.2)

DEF: Abnormal communication between opposite heart chambers due to a defect of the septum. It is not present at birth.

I51.1   Rupture of chordae tendineae, not elsewhere classified   NC Dx

> EXCLUDES 1   rupture of chordae tendineae as current complication following acute myocardial infarction (I23.4)

I51.2   Rupture of papillary muscle, not elsewhere classified   NC Dx

> EXCLUDES 1   rupture of papillary muscle as current complication following acute myocardial infarction (I23.5)

I51.3   Intracardiac thrombosis, not elsewhere classified   CH NC Dx

Apical thrombosis (old)
Atrial thrombosis (old)
Auricular thrombosis (old)
Mural thrombosis (old)
Ventricular thrombosis (old)

> EXCLUDES 1   intracardiac thrombosis as current complication following acute myocardial infarction (I23.6)

AHA: 2013,1Q,24

I51.4   Myocarditis, unspecified   NC Dx

Chronic (interstitial) myocarditis
Myocardial fibrosis
Myocarditis NOS

> EXCLUDES 1   acute or subacute myocarditis (I40.-)

AHA: 2018,4Q,67; 2018,2Q,9

I51.5   Myocardial degeneration   NC Dx

Fatty degeneration of heart or myocardium
Myocardial disease
Senile degeneration of heart or myocardium

AHA: 2018,4Q,67; 2018,2Q,9

I51.7   Cardiomegaly

Cardiac dilatation
Cardiac hypertrophy
Ventricular dilatation

AHA: 2018,4Q,67; 2018,2Q,9

☑5ᵗʰ **I51.8   Other ill-defined heart diseases**

AHA: 2018,2Q,9

I51.81   Takotsubo syndrome

Reversible left ventricular dysfunction following sudden emotional stress
Stress induced cardiomyopathy
Takotsubo cardiomyopathy
Transient left ventricular apical ballooning syndrome

DEF: Complex of symptoms mimicking myocardial infarct in absence of heart disease, with the majority of cases occurring in postmenopausal women. Heart muscles are temporarily weakened, and a sudden, massive surge of adrenalin stuns the heart, greatly reducing the ability to pump blood.

I51.89   Other ill-defined heart diseases   CH

Carditis (acute)(chronic)
Pancarditis (acute)(chronic)

AHA: 2019,2Q,5; 2018,4Q,67

I51.9   Heart disease, unspecified

AHA: 2018,4Q,67; 2018,2Q,9

I52   Other heart disorders in diseases classified elsewhere

Code first underlying disease, such as:
congenital syphilis (A50.5)
mucopolysaccharidosis (E76.3)
schistosomiasis (B65.0-B65.9)

> EXCLUDES 1   heart disease (in):
> gonococcal infection (A54.83)
> meningococcal infection (A39.50)
> rheumatoid arthritis (M05.31)
> syphilis (A52.06)

Cerebrovascular diseases (I60-I69)

Use additional code to identify presence of:
alcohol abuse and dependence (F10.-)
exposure to environmental tobacco smoke (Z77.22)
history of tobacco dependence (Z87.891)
hypertension (I10-I16)
occupational exposure to environmental tobacco smoke (Z57.31)
tobacco dependence (F17.-)
tobacco use (Z72.0)

> EXCLUDES 1   traumatic intracranial hemorrhage (S06.-)

AHA: 2014,3Q,5; 2012,4Q,91-92

☑4ᵗʰ **I60   Nontraumatic subarachnoid hemorrhage**

> EXCLUDES 1   syphilitic ruptured cerebral aneurysm (A52.05)
> EXCLUDES 2   sequelae of subarachnoid hemorrhage (I69.0-)

☑5ᵗʰ **I60.0   Nontraumatic subarachnoid hemorrhage from carotid siphon and bifurcation**

I60.00   Nontraumatic subarachnoid hemorrhage from unspecified carotid siphon and bifurcation   NC Dx

I60.01   Nontraumatic subarachnoid hemorrhage from right carotid siphon and bifurcation   NC Dx

I60.02   Nontraumatic subarachnoid hemorrhage from left carotid siphon and bifurcation   NC Dx

☑5ᵗʰ **I60.1   Nontraumatic subarachnoid hemorrhage from middle cerebral artery**

I60.10   Nontraumatic subarachnoid hemorrhage from unspecified middle cerebral artery   NC Dx

I60.11   Nontraumatic subarachnoid hemorrhage from right middle cerebral artery   NC Dx

I60.12   Nontraumatic subarachnoid hemorrhage from left middle cerebral artery   NC Dx

I60.2   Nontraumatic subarachnoid hemorrhage from anterior communicating artery   NC Dx

☑5ᵗʰ **I60.3   Nontraumatic subarachnoid hemorrhage from posterior communicating artery**

I60.30   Nontraumatic subarachnoid hemorrhage from unspecified posterior communicating artery   NC Dx

I60.31   Nontraumatic subarachnoid hemorrhage from right posterior communicating artery   NC Dx

I60.32   Nontraumatic subarachnoid hemorrhage from left posterior communicating artery   NC Dx

I60.4   Nontraumatic subarachnoid hemorrhage from basilar artery   NC Dx

☑5ᵗʰ **I60.5   Nontraumatic subarachnoid hemorrhage from vertebral artery**

I60.50   Nontraumatic subarachnoid hemorrhage from unspecified vertebral artery   NC Dx

I60.51   Nontraumatic subarachnoid hemorrhage from right vertebral artery   NC Dx

I60.52   Nontraumatic subarachnoid hemorrhage from left vertebral artery   NC Dx

I60.6   Nontraumatic subarachnoid hemorrhage from other intracranial arteries   NC Dx

Ⓝ Newborn: 0   Ⓟ Pediatric: 0-17   Ⓜ Maternity: 12-55   Ⓐ Adult: 15-124   CH Comorbidity High   CL Comorbidity Low   NC Dx Noncancer Dx   PDx Primary Dx

646   ICD-10-CM 2020

I60.7 Nontraumatic subarachnoid hemorrhage from unspecified intracranial artery `NC Dx`
Ruptured (congenital) berry aneurysm
Ruptured (congenital) cerebral aneurysm
Subarachnoid hemorrhage (nontraumatic) from cerebral artery NOS
Subarachnoid hemorrhage (nontraumatic) from communicating artery NOS
> EXCLUDES 1   berry aneurysm, nonruptured (I67.1)

I60.8 Other nontraumatic subarachnoid hemorrhage `NC Dx`
Meningeal hemorrhage
Rupture of cerebral arteriovenous malformation

I60.9 Nontraumatic subarachnoid hemorrhage, unspecified `NC Dx`

√4th I61 Nontraumatic intracerebral hemorrhage
> EXCLUDES 2   sequelae of intracerebral hemorrhage (I69.1-)
AHA: 2017,2Q,9-10

Acute Care

I61.0 Nontraumatic intracerebral hemorrhage in hemisphere, subcortical `NC Dx`
Deep intracerebral hemorrhage (nontraumatic)
AHA: 2016,4Q,27

I61.1 Nontraumatic intracerebral hemorrhage in hemisphere, cortical `NC Dx`
Cerebral lobe hemorrhage (nontraumatic)
Superficial intracerebral hemorrhage (nontraumatic)

I61.2 Nontraumatic intracerebral hemorrhage in hemisphere, unspecified `NC Dx`

I61.3 Nontraumatic intracerebral hemorrhage in brain stem `NC Dx`

I61.4 Nontraumatic intracerebral hemorrhage in cerebellum `NC Dx`

I61.5 Nontraumatic intracerebral hemorrhage, intraventricular `NC Dx`

I61.6 Nontraumatic intracerebral hemorrhage, multiple localized `NC Dx`

I61.8 Other nontraumatic intracerebral hemorrhage `NC Dx`

I61.9 Nontraumatic intracerebral hemorrhage, unspecified `NC Dx`

√4th I62 Other and unspecified nontraumatic intracranial hemorrhage
> EXCLUDES 2   sequelae of intracranial hemorrhage (I69.2)

Acute Care

√5th I62.0 Nontraumatic subdural hemorrhage
  I62.00 Nontraumatic subdural hemorrhage, unspecified `NC Dx`
  I62.01 Nontraumatic acute subdural hemorrhage `NC Dx`
  I62.02 Nontraumatic subacute subdural hemorrhage `NC Dx`
  I62.03 Nontraumatic chronic subdural hemorrhage `NC Dx`

I62.1 Nontraumatic extradural hemorrhage `NC Dx`
Nontraumatic epidural hemorrhage

I62.9 Nontraumatic intracranial hemorrhage, unspecified `NC Dx`

√4th I63 Cerebral infarction
> INCLUDES   occlusion and stenosis of cerebral and precerebral arteries, resulting in cerebral infarction
Use additional code, if applicable, to identify status post administration of tPA (rtPA) in a different facility within the last 24 hours prior to admission to current facility (Z92.82)
Use additional code, if known, to indicate National Institutes of Health Stroke Scale (NIHSS) score (R29.7-)
> EXCLUDES 2   sequelae of cerebral infarction (I69.3-)
AHA: 2017,2Q,9-10; 2016,4Q,28,61-62; 2014,1Q,23

Acute Care

√5th I63.0 Cerebral infarction due to thrombosis of precerebral arteries
  I63.00 Cerebral infarction due to thrombosis of unspecified precerebral artery `NC Dx`
  √6th I63.01 Cerebral infarction due to thrombosis of vertebral artery
    I63.011 Cerebral infarction due to thrombosis of right vertebral artery `NC Dx`
    I63.012 Cerebral infarction due to thrombosis of left vertebral artery `NC Dx`
    I63.013 Cerebral infarction due to thrombosis of bilateral vertebral arteries `NC Dx`

Acute care

    I63.019 Cerebral infarction due to thrombosis of unspecified vertebral artery `NC Dx`
  I63.02 Cerebral infarction due to thrombosis of basilar artery `NC Dx`
  √6th I63.03 Cerebral infarction due to thrombosis of carotid artery
    I63.031 Cerebral infarction due to thrombosis of right carotid artery `NC Dx`
    I63.032 Cerebral infarction due to thrombosis of left carotid artery `NC Dx`
    I63.033 Cerebral infarction due to thrombosis of bilateral carotid arteries `NC Dx`
    I63.039 Cerebral infarction due to thrombosis of unspecified carotid artery `NC Dx`
  I63.09 Cerebral infarction due to thrombosis of other precerebral artery `NC Dx`

√5th I63.1 Cerebral infarction due to embolism of precerebral arteries
  I63.10 Cerebral infarction due to embolism of unspecified precerebral artery `NC Dx`
  √6th I63.11 Cerebral infarction due to embolism of vertebral artery
    I63.111 Cerebral infarction due to embolism of right vertebral artery `NC Dx`
    I63.112 Cerebral infarction due to embolism of left vertebral artery `NC Dx`
    I63.113 Cerebral infarction due to embolism of bilateral vertebral arteries
    I63.119 Cerebral infarction due to embolism of unspecified vertebral artery `NC Dx`
  I63.12 Cerebral infarction due to embolism of basilar artery `NC Dx`
  √6th I63.13 Cerebral infarction due to embolism of carotid artery
    I63.131 Cerebral infarction due to embolism of right carotid artery `NC Dx`
    I63.132 Cerebral infarction due to embolism of left carotid artery `NC Dx`
    I63.133 Cerebral infarction due to embolism of bilateral carotid arteries `NC Dx`
    I63.139 Cerebral infarction due to embolism of unspecified carotid artery `NC Dx`
  I63.19 Cerebral infarction due to embolism of other precerebral artery `NC Dx`

√5th I63.2 Cerebral infarction due to unspecified occlusion or stenosis of precerebral arteries
  I63.20 Cerebral infarction due to unspecified occlusion or stenosis of unspecified precerebral arteries `NC Dx`
  √6th I63.21 Cerebral infarction due to unspecified occlusion or stenosis of vertebral arteries
    I63.211 Cerebral infarction due to unspecified occlusion or stenosis of right vertebral artery `NC Dx`
    I63.212 Cerebral infarction due to unspecified occlusion or stenosis of left vertebral artery `NC Dx`
    I63.213 Cerebral infarction due to unspecified occlusion or stenosis of bilateral vertebral arteries `NC Dx`
    I63.219 Cerebral infarction due to unspecified occlusion or stenosis of unspecified vertebral artery `NC Dx`
  I63.22 Cerebral infarction due to unspecified occlusion or stenosis of basilar artery `NC Dx`

✓6ᵗʰ **I63.23** **Cerebral infarction due to unspecified occlusion or stenosis of carotid arteries**

   I63.231 Cerebral infarction due to unspecified occlusion or stenosis of right carotid arteries   NC Dx

   I63.232 Cerebral infarction due to unspecified occlusion or stenosis of left carotid arteries   NC Dx

   I63.233 Cerebral infarction due to unspecified occlusion or stenosis of bilateral carotid arteries   NC Dx

   I63.239 Cerebral infarction due to unspecified occlusion or stenosis of unspecified carotid artery   NC Dx

  I63.29 Cerebral infarction due to unspecified occlusion or stenosis of other precerebral arteries   NC Dx

✓5ᵗʰ **I63.3** **Cerebral infarction due to thrombosis of cerebral arteries**

  I63.30 Cerebral infarction due to thrombosis of unspecified cerebral artery   NC Dx

✓6ᵗʰ **I63.31** Cerebral infarction due to thrombosis of middle cerebral artery

   I63.311 Cerebral infarction due to thrombosis of right middle cerebral artery   NC Dx

   I63.312 Cerebral infarction due to thrombosis of left middle cerebral artery   NC Dx

   I63.313 Cerebral infarction due to thrombosis of bilateral middle cerebral arteries   NC Dx

   I63.319 Cerebral infarction due to thrombosis of unspecified middle cerebral artery   NC Dx

✓6ᵗʰ **I63.32** Cerebral infarction due to thrombosis of anterior cerebral artery

   I63.321 Cerebral infarction due to thrombosis of right anterior cerebral artery   NC Dx

   I63.322 Cerebral infarction due to thrombosis of left anterior cerebral artery   NC Dx

   I63.323 Cerebral infarction due to thrombosis of bilateral anterior cerebral arteries   NC Dx

   I63.329 Cerebral infarction due to thrombosis of unspecified anterior cerebral artery   NC Dx

✓6ᵗʰ **I63.33** Cerebral infarction due to thrombosis of posterior cerebral artery

   I63.331 Cerebral infarction due to thrombosis of right posterior cerebral artery   NC Dx

   I63.332 Cerebral infarction due to thrombosis of left posterior cerebral artery   NC Dx

   I63.333 Cerebral infarction due to thrombosis of bilateral posterior cerebral arteries   NC Dx

   I63.339 Cerebral infarction due to thrombosis of unspecified posterior cerebral artery   NC Dx

✓6ᵗʰ **I63.34** Cerebral infarction due to thrombosis of cerebellar artery

   I63.341 Cerebral infarction due to thrombosis of right cerebellar artery   NC Dx

   I63.342 Cerebral infarction due to thrombosis of left cerebellar artery   NC Dx

   I63.343 Cerebral infarction due to thrombosis of bilateral cerebellar arteries   NC Dx

   I63.349 Cerebral infarction due to thrombosis of unspecified cerebellar artery   NC Dx

  I63.39 Cerebral infarction due to thrombosis of other cerebral artery   NC Dx

✓5ᵗʰ **I63.4** **Cerebral infarction due to embolism of cerebral arteries**

  I63.40 Cerebral infarction due to embolism of unspecified cerebral artery   NC Dx

✓6ᵗʰ **I63.41** **Cerebral infarction due to embolism of middle cerebral artery**

   I63.411 Cerebral infarction due to embolism of right middle cerebral artery   NC Dx

   I63.412 Cerebral infarction due to embolism of left middle cerebral artery   NC Dx

   I63.413 Cerebral infarction due to embolism of bilateral middle cerebral arteries   NC Dx

   I63.419 Cerebral infarction due to embolism of unspecified middle cerebral artery   NC Dx

✓6ᵗʰ **I63.42** Cerebral infarction due to embolism of anterior cerebral artery

   I63.421 Cerebral infarction due to embolism of right anterior cerebral artery   NC Dx

   I63.422 Cerebral infarction due to embolism of left anterior cerebral artery   NC Dx

   I63.423 Cerebral infarction due to embolism of bilateral anterior cerebral arteries   NC Dx

   I63.429 Cerebral infarction due to embolism of unspecified anterior cerebral artery   NC Dx

✓6ᵗʰ **I63.43** Cerebral infarction due to embolism of posterior cerebral artery

   I63.431 Cerebral infarction due to embolism of right posterior cerebral artery   NC Dx

   I63.432 Cerebral infarction due to embolism of left posterior cerebral artery   NC Dx

   I63.433 Cerebral infarction due to embolism of bilateral posterior cerebral arteries   NC Dx

   I63.439 Cerebral infarction due to embolism of unspecified posterior cerebral artery   NC Dx

✓6ᵗʰ **I63.44** Cerebral infarction due to embolism of cerebellar artery

   I63.441 Cerebral infarction due to embolism of right cerebellar artery   NC Dx

   I63.442 Cerebral infarction due to embolism of left cerebellar artery   NC Dx

   I63.443 Cerebral infarction due to embolism of bilateral cerebellar arteries   NC Dx

   I63.449 Cerebral infarction due to embolism of unspecified cerebellar artery   NC Dx

  I63.49 Cerebral infarction due to embolism of other cerebral artery   NC Dx

✓5ᵗʰ **I63.5** **Cerebral infarction due to unspecified occlusion or stenosis of cerebral arteries**

  I63.50 Cerebral infarction due to unspecified occlusion or stenosis of unspecified cerebral artery   NC Dx

✓6ᵗʰ **I63.51** Cerebral infarction due to unspecified occlusion or stenosis of middle cerebral artery

   I63.511 Cerebral infarction due to unspecified occlusion or stenosis of right middle cerebral artery   NC Dx

   I63.512 Cerebral infarction due to unspecified occlusion or stenosis of left middle cerebral artery   NC Dx

   I63.513 Cerebral infarction due to unspecified occlusion or stenosis of bilateral middle cerebral arteries   NC Dx

   I63.519 Cerebral infarction due to unspecified occlusion or stenosis of unspecified middle cerebral artery   NC Dx

---

N Newborn: 0   P Pediatric: 0-17   M Maternity: 12-55   A Adult: 15-124   CH Comorbidity High   CL Comorbidity Low   NC Dx Noncancer Dx   PDx Primary Dx

648

ICD-10-CM 2020

√6ᵗʰ **I63.52** **Cerebral infarction due to unspecified occlusion or stenosis of** anterior **cerebral artery**

I63.521 **Cerebral infarction due to unspecified occlusion or stenosis of** right **anterior cerebral artery** `NC Dx`

I63.522 **Cerebral infarction due to unspecified occlusion or stenosis of** left **anterior cerebral artery** `NC Dx`

I63.523 **Cerebral infarction due to unspecified occlusion or stenosis of** bilateral **anterior cerebral arteries** `NC Dx`

I63.529 **Cerebral infarction due to unspecified occlusion or stenosis of unspecified anterior cerebral artery** `NC Dx`

√6ᵗʰ **I63.53** **Cerebral infarction due to unspecified occlusion or stenosis of** posterior **cerebral artery**

I63.531 **Cerebral infarction due to unspecified occlusion or stenosis of** right **posterior cerebral artery** `NC Dx`

I63.532 **Cerebral infarction due to unspecified occlusion or stenosis of** left **posterior cerebral artery** `NC Dx`

I63.533 **Cerebral infarction due to unspecified occlusion or stenosis of** bilateral **posterior cerebral arteries** `NC Dx`

I63.539 **Cerebral infarction due to unspecified occlusion or stenosis of unspecified posterior cerebral artery** `NC Dx`

√6ᵗʰ **I63.54** **Cerebral infarction due to unspecified occlusion or stenosis of** cerebellar **artery**

I63.541 **Cerebral infarction due to unspecified occlusion or stenosis of** right **cerebellar artery** `NC Dx`

I63.542 **Cerebral infarction due to unspecified occlusion or stenosis of** left **cerebellar artery** `NC Dx`

I63.543 **Cerebral infarction due to unspecified occlusion or stenosis of** bilateral **cerebellar arteries** `NC Dx`

I63.549 **Cerebral infarction due to unspecified occlusion or stenosis of unspecified cerebellar artery** `NC Dx`

I63.59 **Cerebral infarction due to unspecified occlusion or stenosis of other cerebral artery** `NC Dx`

I63.6 **Cerebral infarction due to** cerebral venous thrombosis, nonpyogenic `NC Dx`

√5ᵗʰ **I63.8** **Other cerebral infarction**

AHA: 2018,4Q,16

I63.81 **Other cerebral infarction due to** occlusion or stenosis **of small artery**
Lacunar infarction

I63.89 **Other cerebral infarction**

I63.9 **Cerebral infarction, unspecified** `NC Dx`
Stroke NOS
EXCLUDES 2   *transient cerebral ischemic attacks and related syndromes (G45.-)*

AHA: 2015,1Q,25

√4ᵗʰ **I65** **Occlusion and stenosis of** precerebral **arteries,** not resulting in cerebral infarction
INCLUDES   embolism of precerebral artery
narrowing of precerebral artery
obstruction (complete) (partial) of precerebral artery
thrombosis of precerebral artery
EXCLUDES 1   *insufficiency, NOS, of precerebral artery (G45.-)*
insufficiency of precerebral arteries causing cerebral infarction (I63.0-I63.2)

AHA: 2018,2Q,9

√6ᵗʰ **I65.0** **Occlusion and stenosis of** vertebral **artery**

I65.01 **Occlusion and stenosis of** right **vertebral artery**

I65.02 **Occlusion and stenosis of** left **vertebral artery**

I65.03 **Occlusion and stenosis of** bilateral **vertebral arteries**

I65.09 **Occlusion and stenosis of unspecified vertebral artery**

I65.1 **Occlusion and stenosis of** basilar **artery**

√5ᵗʰ **I65.2** **Occlusion and stenosis of** carotid **artery**

I65.21 **Occlusion and stenosis of** right **carotid artery**

I65.22 **Occlusion and stenosis of** left **carotid artery**

I65.23 **Occlusion and stenosis of** bilateral **carotid arteries**

I65.29 **Occlusion and stenosis of unspecified carotid artery**

I65.8 **Occlusion and stenosis of other precerebral arteries**

I65.9 **Occlusion and stenosis of unspecified precerebral artery**
Occlusion and stenosis of precerebral artery NOS

√4ᵗʰ **I66** **Occlusion and stenosis of** cerebral **arteries,** not resulting in cerebral infarction
INCLUDES   embolism of cerebral artery
narrowing of cerebral artery
obstruction (complete) (partial) of cerebral artery
thrombosis of cerebral artery
EXCLUDES 1   *occlusion and stenosis of cerebral artery causing cerebral infarction (I63.3-I63.5)*

√5ᵗʰ **I66.0** **Occlusion and stenosis of** middle **cerebral artery**

I66.01 **Occlusion and stenosis of** right **middle cerebral artery**

I66.02 **Occlusion and stenosis of** left **middle cerebral artery**

I66.03 **Occlusion and stenosis of** bilateral **middle cerebral arteries**

I66.09 **Occlusion and stenosis of unspecified middle cerebral artery**

√5ᵗʰ **I66.1** **Occlusion and stenosis of** anterior **cerebral artery**

I66.11 **Occlusion and stenosis of** right **anterior cerebral artery**

I66.12 **Occlusion and stenosis of** left **anterior cerebral artery**

I66.13 **Occlusion and stenosis of** bilateral **anterior cerebral arteries**

I66.19 **Occlusion and stenosis of unspecified anterior cerebral artery**

√5ᵗʰ **I66.2** **Occlusion and stenosis of** posterior **cerebral artery**

I66.21 **Occlusion and stenosis of** right **posterior cerebral artery**

I66.22 **Occlusion and stenosis of** left **posterior cerebral artery**

I66.23 **Occlusion and stenosis of** bilateral **posterior cerebral arteries**

I66.29 **Occlusion and stenosis of unspecified posterior cerebral artery**

I66.3 **Occlusion and stenosis of** cerebellar **arteries**

I66.8 **Occlusion and stenosis of other cerebral arteries**
Occlusion and stenosis of perforating arteries

I66.9 **Occlusion and stenosis of unspecified cerebral artery**

√4ᵗʰ **I67** **Other cerebrovascular diseases**
EXCLUDES 2   *sequelae of the listed conditions (I69.8)*

I67.0 **Dissection of cerebral arteries, nonruptured**
EXCLUDES 1   *ruptured cerebral arteries (I60.7)*

I67.1   Cerebral aneurysm, nonruptured
Cerebral aneurysm NOS
Cerebral arteriovenous fistula, acquired
Internal carotid artery aneurysm, intracranial portion
Internal carotid artery aneurysm, NOS
> **EXCLUDES 1**   congenital cerebral aneurysm, nonruptured (Q28.-)
> ruptured cerebral aneurysm (I60.7)

Berry Aneurysm

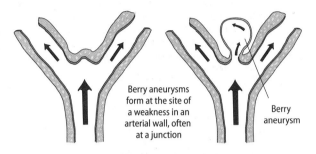

Berry aneurysms form at the site of a weakness in an arterial wall, often at a junction

Berry aneurysm

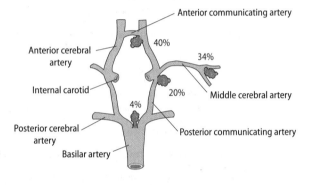

Anterior communicating artery
40%
Anterior cerebral artery
34%
Internal carotid
20%
Middle cerebral artery
4%
Posterior cerebral artery
Posterior communicating artery
Basilar artery

Common sites of berry aneurysms in the circle of Willis arteries

I67.2   Cerebral atherosclerosis   `CH` `CL` `NC Dx` `A`
Atheroma of cerebral and precerebral arteries

I67.3   Progressive vascular leukoencephalopathy
Binswanger's disease

I67.4   Hypertensive encephalopathy   `NC Dx`
> **EXCLUDES 2**   insufficiency, NOS, of precerebral arteries (G45.2)

I67.5   Moyamoya disease   `NC Dx`
DEF: Cerebrovascular ischemia. Vessels occlude and rupture, causing tiny hemorrhages at the base of brain. It affects predominantly Japanese people.

I67.6   Nonpyogenic thrombosis of intracranial venous system   `NC Dx`
Nonpyogenic thrombosis of cerebral vein
Nonpyogenic thrombosis of intracranial venous sinus
> **EXCLUDES 1**   nonpyogenic thrombosis of intracranial venous system causing infarction (I63.6)

I67.7   Cerebral arteritis, not elsewhere classified   `NC Dx`
Granulomatous angiitis of the nervous system
> **EXCLUDES 1**   allergic granulomatous angiitis (M30.1)

`√5ᵗʰ` **I67.8   Other specified cerebrovascular diseases**

   I67.81   Acute cerebrovascular insufficiency   `CH` `CL` `NC Dx`
     Acute cerebrovascular insufficiency unspecified as to location or reversibility

   I67.82   Cerebral ischemia   `CH` `CL` `NC Dx`
     Chronic cerebral ischemia

   I67.83   Posterior reversible encephalopathy syndrome
     PRES

   `√6ᵗʰ` **I67.84   Cerebral vasospasm and vasoconstriction**

     I67.841   Reversible cerebrovascular vasoconstriction syndrome
       Call-Fleming syndrome
       Code first underlying condition, if applicable, such as eclampsia (O15.00-O15.9)

     I67.848   Other cerebrovascular vasospasm and vasoconstriction

`√6ᵗʰ` **I67.85   Hereditary cerebrovascular diseases**
   AHA: 2018,4Q,17

   I67.850   Cerebral autosomal dominant arteriopathy with subcortical infarcts and leukoencephalopathy
     CADASIL
     Code also any associated diagnoses, such as:
       epilepsy (G40.-)
       stroke (I63.-)
       vascular dementia (F01.-)

   I67.858   Other hereditary cerebrovascular disease

I67.89   Other cerebrovascular disease   `CH` `CL` `NC Dx`

I67.9   Cerebrovascular disease, unspecified   `NC Dx`
> **TIP:** This code would be viewed by Medicare as a questionable admission if used as the admitting diagnosis for a hospice encounter.

`√4ᵗʰ` **I68   Cerebrovascular disorders in diseases classified elsewhere**

I68.0   Cerebral amyloid angiopathy
Code first underlying amyloidosis (E85.-)

I68.2   Cerebral arteritis in other diseases classified elsewhere
Code first underlying disease
> **EXCLUDES 1**   cerebral arteritis (in):
> listerosis (A32.89)
> syphilis (A52.04)
> systemic lupus erythematosus (M32.19)
> tuberculosis (A18.89)

I68.8   Other cerebrovascular disorders in diseases classified elsewhere
Code first underlying disease
> **EXCLUDES 1**   syphilitic cerebral aneurysm (A52.05)

`√4ᵗʰ` **I69   Sequelae of cerebrovascular disease**

> **NOTE**   Category I69 is to be used to indicate conditions in I60-I67 as the cause of sequelae. The "sequelae" include conditions specified as such or as residuals which may occur at any time after the onset of the causal condition
>
> **EXCLUDES 1**   personal history of cerebral infarction without residual deficit (Z86.73)
> personal history of prolonged reversible ischemic neurologic deficit (PRIND) (Z86.73)
> personal history of reversible ischemic neurologcial deficit (RIND) (Z86.73)
> sequelae of traumatic intracranial injury (S06.-)

AHA: 2017,1Q,47; 2016,4Q,28; 2015,1Q,25; 2012,4Q,106
TIP: Weakness on one side of the body (unilateral weakness) documented as secondary to old cerebrovascular disease is synonymous with hemiparesis/hemiplegia. Weakness of one limb documented as secondary to old cerebrovascular disease is synonymous with monoplegia.

`√5ᵗʰ` **I69.0   Sequelae of nontraumatic subarachnoid hemorrhage**

   I69.00   Unspecified sequelae of nontraumatic subarachnoid hemorrhage

   `√6ᵗʰ` **I69.01   Cognitive deficits following nontraumatic subarachnoid hemorrhage**

[handwritten: STROKE CAUSED BY Hemorrhage]

     I69.010   Attention and concentration deficit following nontraumatic subarachnoid hemorrhage   `CH` `CL`

     I69.011   Memory deficit following nontraumatic subarachnoid hemorrhage   `CH` `CL`

     I69.012   Visuospatial deficit and spatial neglect following nontraumatic subarachnoid hemorrhage   `CH` `CL`

     I69.013   Psychomotor deficit following nontraumatic subarachnoid hemorrhage   `CH` `CL`

     I69.014   Frontal lobe and executive function deficit following nontraumatic subarachnoid hemorrhage   `CH` `CL`

     I69.015   Cognitive social or emotional deficit following nontraumatic subarachnoid hemorrhage   `CH` `CL`

     I69.018   Other symptoms and signs involving cognitive functions following nontraumatic subarachnoid hemorrhage   `CH` `CL`

`N` Newborn: 0   `P` Pediatric: 0-17   `M` Maternity: 12-55   `A` Adult: 15-124   `CH` Comorbidity High   `CL` Comorbidity Low   `NC Dx` Noncancer Dx   `PDx` Primary Dx

650   ICD-10-CM 2020

I69.019   Unspecified symptoms and signs involving cognitive functions following nontraumatic subarachnoid hemorrhage

✓6ᵗʰ **I69.02**   **Speech and language deficits** following nontraumatic subarachnoid hemorrhage

I69.020   Aphasia following nontraumatic subarachnoid hemorrhage   `CH` `CL`

I69.021   Dysphasia following nontraumatic subarachnoid hemorrhage   `CH` `CL`

I69.022   Dysarthria following nontraumatic subarachnoid hemorrhage   `CH` `CL`

I69.023   Fluency disorder following nontraumatic subarachnoid hemorrhage   `CH` `CL`
> Stuttering following nontraumatic subarachnoid hemorrhage

I69.028   Other speech and language deficits following nontraumatic subarachnoid hemorrhage   `CH` `CL`

✓6ᵗʰ **I69.03**   **Monoplegia of upper limb** following nontraumatic subarachnoid hemorrhage
> **AHA:** 2017,1Q,47

I69.031   Monoplegia of upper limb following nontraumatic subarachnoid hemorrhage affecting right dominant side   `CH` `CL`

I69.032   Monoplegia of upper limb following nontraumatic subarachnoid hemorrhage affecting left dominant side   `CH` `CL`

I69.033   Monoplegia of upper limb following nontraumatic subarachnoid hemorrhage affecting right non-dominant side   `CH` `CL`

I69.034   Monoplegia of upper limb following nontraumatic subarachnoid hemorrhage affecting left non-dominant side   `CH` `CL`

I69.039   Monoplegia of upper limb following nontraumatic subarachnoid hemorrhage affecting unspecified side

✓6ᵗʰ **I69.04**   **Monoplegia of lower limb** following nontraumatic subarachnoid hemorrhage
> **AHA:** 2017,1Q,47

I69.041   Monoplegia of lower limb following nontraumatic subarachnoid hemorrhage affecting right dominant side   `CH` `CL`

I69.042   Monoplegia of lower limb following nontraumatic subarachnoid hemorrhage affecting left dominant side   `CH` `CL`

I69.043   Monoplegia of lower limb following nontraumatic subarachnoid hemorrhage affecting right non-dominant side   `CH` `CL`

I69.044   Monoplegia of lower limb following nontraumatic subarachnoid hemorrhage affecting left non-dominant side   `CH` `CL`

I69.049   Monoplegia of lower limb following nontraumatic subarachnoid hemorrhage affecting unspecified side

✓6ᵗʰ **I69.05**   **Hemiplegia and hemiparesis** following nontraumatic subarachnoid hemorrhage
> **AHA:** 2015,1Q,25

I69.051   Hemiplegia and hemiparesis following nontraumatic subarachnoid hemorrhage affecting right dominant side   `CH` `CL`

I69.052   Hemiplegia and hemiparesis following nontraumatic subarachnoid hemorrhage affecting left dominant side   `CH` `CL`

I69.053   Hemiplegia and hemiparesis following nontraumatic subarachnoid hemorrhage affecting right non-dominant side   `CH` `CL`

I69.054   Hemiplegia and hemiparesis following nontraumatic subarachnoid hemorrhage affecting left non-dominant side   `CH` `CL`

I69.059   Hemiplegia and hemiparesis following nontraumatic subarachnoid hemorrhage affecting unspecified side

✓6ᵗʰ **I69.06**   Other paralytic syndrome following nontraumatic subarachnoid hemorrhage
> Use additional code to identify type of paralytic syndrome, such as:
> locked-in state (G83.5)
> quadriplegia (G82.5-)

> **EXCLUDES 1**   hemiplegia/hemiparesis following nontraumatic subarachnoid hemorrhage (I69.05-)
> monoplegia of lower limb following nontraumatic subarachnoid hemorrhage (I69.04-)
> monoplegia of upper limb following nontraumatic subarachnoid hemorrhage (I69.03-)

I69.061   Other paralytic syndrome following nontraumatic subarachnoid hemorrhage affecting right dominant side   `CH` `CL`

I69.062   Other paralytic syndrome following nontraumatic subarachnoid hemorrhage affecting left dominant side   `CH` `CL`

I69.063   Other paralytic syndrome following nontraumatic subarachnoid hemorrhage affecting right non-dominant side   `CH` `CL`

I69.064   Other paralytic syndrome following nontraumatic subarachnoid hemorrhage affecting left non-dominant side   `CH` `CL`

I69.065   Other paralytic syndrome following nontraumatic subarachnoid hemorrhage, bilateral   `CH` `CL`

I69.069   Other paralytic syndrome following nontraumatic subarachnoid hemorrhage affecting unspecified side

✓6ᵗʰ **I69.09**   Other sequelae of nontraumatic subarachnoid hemorrhage

I69.090   Apraxia following nontraumatic subarachnoid hemorrhage   `CH` `CL`

I69.091   Dysphagia following nontraumatic subarachnoid hemorrhage   `CH` `CL`
> Use additional code to identify the type of dysphagia, if known (R13.1-)

I69.092   Facial weakness following nontraumatic subarachnoid hemorrhage
> Facial droop following nontraumatic subarachnoid hemorrhage

I69.093   Ataxia following nontraumatic subarachnoid hemorrhage   `CH` `CL`

I69.098   Other sequelae following nontraumatic subarachnoid hemorrhage   `CH` `CL`
> Alterations of sensation following nontraumatic subarachnoid hemorrhage
> Disturbance of vision following nontraumatic subarachnoid hemorrhage
> Use additional code to identify the sequelae

☑ Additional Character Required   ✓x7ᵗʰ Placeholder Alert   Manifestation   Unspecified Dx   ►◄ Revised Text   ● New Code   ▲ Revised Title

ICD-10-CM 2020   651

Chapter 9. Diseases of the Circulatory System

✓5th **I69.1** **Sequelae of nontraumatic** intracerebral **hemorrhage**

    I69.10 **Unspecified sequelae of nontraumatic intracerebral hemorrhage**

✓6th **I69.11** Cognitive deficits **following nontraumatic intracerebral hemorrhage**

    I69.110 Attention and concentration deficit following nontraumatic intracerebral hemorrhage `CH` `CL`

    I69.111 Memory deficit following nontraumatic intracerebral hemorrhage `CH` `CL`

    I69.112 Visuospatial deficit and spatial neglect following nontraumatic intracerebral hemorrhage `CH` `CL`

    I69.113 Psychomotor deficit following nontraumatic intracerebral hemorrhage `CH` `CL`

    I69.114 Frontal lobe and executive function deficit following nontraumatic intracerebral hemorrhage `CH` `CL`

    I69.115 Cognitive social or emotional deficit following nontraumatic intracerebral hemorrhage `CH` `CL`

    I69.118 **Other symptoms and signs involving cognitive functions following nontraumatic intracerebral hemorrhage** `CH` `CL`

    I69.119 **Unspecified symptoms and signs involving cognitive functions following nontraumatic intracerebral hemorrhage**

✓6th **I69.12** Speech and language deficits **following nontraumatic intracerebral hemorrhage**

    I69.120 Aphasia following nontraumatic intracerebral hemorrhage `CH` `CL`

    I69.121 Dysphasia following nontraumatic intracerebral hemorrhage `CH` `CL`

    I69.122 Dysarthria following nontraumatic intracerebral hemorrhage `CH` `CL`

    I69.123 Fluency disorder **following nontraumatic intracerebral hemorrhage** `CH` `CL`

        Stuttering following nontraumatic intracerebral hemorrhage

    I69.128 **Other speech and language deficits following nontraumatic intracerebral hemorrhage** `CH` `CL`

✓6th **I69.13** Monoplegia of upper limb **following nontraumatic intracerebral hemorrhage**

    AHA: 2017,1Q,47

    I69.131 **Monoplegia of upper limb following nontraumatic intracerebral hemorrhage affecting** right dominant **side** `CH` `CL`

    I69.132 **Monoplegia of upper limb following nontraumatic intracerebral hemorrhage affecting** left dominant **side** `CH` `CL`

    I69.133 **Monoplegia of upper limb following nontraumatic intracerebral hemorrhage affecting** right non-dominant side `CH` `CL`

    I69.134 **Monoplegia of upper limb following nontraumatic intracerebral hemorrhage affecting** left non-dominant side `CH` `CL`

    I69.139 **Monoplegia of upper limb following nontraumatic intracerebral hemorrhage affecting unspecified side**

✓6th **I69.14** Monoplegia of lower limb **following nontraumatic intracerebral hemorrhage**

    AHA: 2017,1Q,47

    I69.141 **Monoplegia of lower limb following nontraumatic intracerebral hemorrhage affecting** right dominant **side** `CH` `CL`

    I69.142 **Monoplegia of lower limb following nontraumatic intracerebral hemorrhage affecting** left dominant **side** `CH` `CL`

    I69.143 **Monoplegia of lower limb following nontraumatic intracerebral hemorrhage affecting** right non-dominant side `CH` `CL`

    I69.144 **Monoplegia of lower limb following nontraumatic intracerebral hemorrhage affecting** left non-dominant side `CH` `CL`

    I69.149 **Monoplegia of lower limb following nontraumatic intracerebral hemorrhage affecting unspecified side**

✓6th **I69.15** Hemiplegia and hemiparesis **following nontraumatic intracerebral hemorrhage**

    AHA: 2015,1Q,25

    I69.151 **Hemiplegia and hemiparesis following nontraumatic intracerebral hemorrhage affecting** right dominant **side** `CH` `CL`

    I69.152 **Hemiplegia and hemiparesis following nontraumatic intracerebral hemorrhage affecting** left dominant **side** `CH` `CL`

    I69.153 **Hemiplegia and hemiparesis following nontraumatic intracerebral hemorrhage affecting** right non-dominant side `CH` `CL`

    I69.154 **Hemiplegia and hemiparesis following nontraumatic intracerebral hemorrhage affecting** left non-dominant side `CH` `CL`

    I69.159 **Hemiplegia and hemiparesis following nontraumatic intracerebral hemorrhage affecting unspecified side**

✓6th **I69.16** **Other** paralytic syndrome **following nontraumatic intracerebral hemorrhage**

    Use additional code to identify type of paralytic syndrome, such as:

    locked-in state (G83.5)

    quadriplegia (G82.5-)

    EXCLUDES 1 hemiplegia/hemiparesis following nontraumatic intracerebral hemorrhage (I69.15-)

        monoplegia of lower limb following nontraumatic intracerebral hemorrhage (I69.14-)

        monoplegia of upper limb following nontraumatic intracerebral hemorrhage (I69.13-)

    I69.161 **Other paralytic syndrome following nontraumatic intracerebral hemorrhage affecting** right dominant **side** `CH` `CL`

    I69.162 **Other paralytic syndrome following nontraumatic intracerebral hemorrhage affecting** left dominant **side** `CH` `CL`

    I69.163 **Other paralytic syndrome following nontraumatic intracerebral hemorrhage affecting** right non-dominant side `CH` `CL`

    I69.164 **Other paralytic syndrome following nontraumatic intracerebral hemorrhage affecting** left non-dominant side `CH` `CL`

    I69.165 **Other paralytic syndrome following nontraumatic intracerebral hemorrhage,** bilateral `CH` `CL`

    I69.169 **Other paralytic syndrome following nontraumatic intracerebral hemorrhage affecting unspecified side**

`N` Newborn: 0   `P` Pediatric: 0-17   `M` Maternity: 12-55   `A` Adult: 15-124   `CH` Comorbidity High   `CL` Comorbidity Low   `NCDx` Noncancer Dx   `PDx` Primary Dx

652   ICD-10-CM 2020

☑6ᵗʰ **I69.19 Other sequelae of nontraumatic intracerebral hemorrhage**

     I69.190 Apraxia following nontraumatic intracerebral hemorrhage `CH` `CL`

     I69.191 Dysphagia following nontraumatic intracerebral hemorrhage `CH` `CL`

       Use additional code to identify the type of dysphagia, if known (R13.1-)

     I69.192 Facial weakness following nontraumatic intracerebral hemorrhage

       Facial droop following nontraumatic intracerebral hemorrhage

     I69.193 Ataxia following nontraumatic intracerebral hemorrhage `CH` `CL`

     I69.198 Other sequelae of nontraumatic intracerebral hemorrhage `CH` `CL`

       Alteration of sensations following nontraumatic intracerebral hemorrhage

       Disturbance of vision following nontraumatic intracerebral hemorrhage

       Use additional code to identify the sequelae

☑5ᵗʰ **I69.2 Sequelae of other nontraumatic intracranial hemorrhage**

   I69.20 Unspecified sequelae of other nontraumatic intracranial hemorrhage

☑6ᵗʰ **I69.21 Cognitive deficits following other nontraumatic intracranial hemorrhage**

     I69.210 Attention and concentration deficit following other nontraumatic intracranial hemorrhage `CH` `CL`

     I69.211 Memory deficit following other nontraumatic intracranial hemorrhage `CH` `CL`

     I69.212 Visuospatial deficit and spatial neglect following other nontraumatic intracranial hemorrhage `CH` `CL`

     I69.213 Psychomotor deficit following other nontraumatic intracranial hemorrhage `CH` `CL`

     I69.214 Frontal lobe and executive function deficit following other nontraumatic intracranial hemorrhage `CH` `CL`

     I69.215 Cognitive social or emotional deficit following other nontraumatic intracranial hemorrhage `CH` `CL`

     I69.218 Other symptoms and signs involving cognitive functions following other nontraumatic intracranial hemorrhage `CH` `CL`

     I69.219 Unspecified symptoms and signs involving cognitive functions following other nontraumatic intracranial hemorrhage

☑6ᵗʰ **I69.22 Speech and language deficits following other nontraumatic intracranial hemorrhage**

     I69.220 Aphasia following other nontraumatic intracranial hemorrhage `CH` `CL`

     I69.221 Dysphasia following other nontraumatic intracranial hemorrhage `CH` `CL`

     I69.222 Dysarthria following other nontraumatic intracranial hemorrhage `CH` `CL`

     I69.223 Fluency disorder following other nontraumatic intracranial hemorrhage `CH` `CL`

       Stuttering following other nontraumatic intracranial hemorrhage

     I69.228 Other speech and language deficits following other nontraumatic intracranial hemorrhage `CH` `CL`

☑6ᵗʰ **I69.23 Monoplegia of upper limb following other nontraumatic intracranial hemorrhage**

   AHA: 2017,1Q,47

     I69.231 Monoplegia of upper limb following other nontraumatic intracranial hemorrhage affecting right dominant side `CH` `CL`

     I69.232 Monoplegia of upper limb following other nontraumatic intracranial hemorrhage affecting left dominant side `CH` `CL`

     I69.233 Monoplegia of upper limb following other nontraumatic intracranial hemorrhage affecting right non-dominant side `CH` `CL`

     I69.234 Monoplegia of upper limb following other nontraumatic intracranial hemorrhage affecting left non-dominant side `CH` `CL`

     I69.239 Monoplegia of upper limb following other nontraumatic intracranial hemorrhage affecting unspecified side

☑6ᵗʰ **I69.24 Monoplegia of lower limb following other nontraumatic intracranial hemorrhage**

   AHA: 2017,1Q,47

     I69.241 Monoplegia of lower limb following other nontraumatic intracranial hemorrhage affecting right dominant side `CH` `CL`

     I69.242 Monoplegia of lower limb following other nontraumatic intracranial hemorrhage affecting left dominant side `CH` `CL`

     I69.243 Monoplegia of lower limb following other nontraumatic intracranial hemorrhage affecting right non-dominant side `CH` `CL`

     I69.244 Monoplegia of lower limb following other nontraumatic intracranial hemorrhage affecting left non-dominant side `CH` `CL`

     I69.249 Monoplegia of lower limb following other nontraumatic intracranial hemorrhage affecting unspecified side

☑6ᵗʰ **I69.25 Hemiplegia and hemiparesis following other nontraumatic intracranial hemorrhage**

   AHA: 2015,1Q,25

     I69.251 Hemiplegia and hemiparesis following other nontraumatic intracranial hemorrhage affecting right dominant side `CH` `CL`

     I69.252 Hemiplegia and hemiparesis following other nontraumatic intracranial hemorrhage affecting left dominant side `CH` `CL`

     I69.253 Hemiplegia and hemiparesis following other nontraumatic intracranial hemorrhage affecting right non-dominant side `CH` `CL`

     I69.254 Hemiplegia and hemiparesis following other nontraumatic intracranial hemorrhage affecting left non-dominant side `CH` `CL`

     I69.259 Hemiplegia and hemiparesis following other nontraumatic intracranial hemorrhage affecting unspecified side

---

☑ Additional Character Required   √x7ᵗʰ Placeholder Alert   Manifestation   Unspecified Dx   ▶◀ Revised Text   ● New Code   ▲ Revised Title

√6ᵗʰ I69.26 Other paralytic syndrome following other nontraumatic intracranial hemorrhage

Use additional code to identify type of paralytic syndrome, such as:

locked-in state (G83.5)
quadriplegia (G82.5-)

EXCLUDES 1   hemiplegia/hemiparesis following other nontraumatic intracranial hemorrhage (I69.25-)
monoplegia of lower limb following other nontraumatic intracranial hemorrhage (I69.24-)
monoplegia of upper limb following other nontraumatic intracranial hemorrhage (I69.23-)

I69.261 Other paralytic syndrome following other nontraumatic intracranial hemorrhage affecting right dominant side CH CL

I69.262 Other paralytic syndrome following other nontraumatic intracranial hemorrhage affecting left dominant side CH CL

I69.263 Other paralytic syndrome following other nontraumatic intracranial hemorrhage affecting right non-dominant side CH CL

I69.264 Other paralytic syndrome following other nontraumatic intracranial hemorrhage affecting left non-dominant side CH CL

I69.265 Other paralytic syndrome following other nontraumatic intracranial hemorrhage, bilateral CH CL

I69.269 Other paralytic syndrome following other nontraumatic intracranial hemorrhage affecting unspecified side

√6ᵗʰ I69.29 Other sequelae of other nontraumatic intracranial hemorrhage

I69.290 Apraxia following other nontraumatic intracranial hemorrhage CH CL

I69.291 Dysphagia following other nontraumatic intracranial hemorrhage CH CL

Use additional code to identify the type of dysphagia, if known (R13.1-)

I69.292 Facial weakness following other nontraumatic intracranial hemorrhage

Facial droop following other nontraumatic intracranial hemorrhage

I69.293 Ataxia following other nontraumatic intracranial hemorrhage CH CL

I69.298 Other sequelae of other nontraumatic intracranial hemorrhage CH CL

Alteration of sensation following other nontraumatic intracranial hemorrhage
Disturbance of vision following other nontraumatic intracranial hemorrhage
Use additional code to identify the sequelae

√5ᵗʰ I69.3 Sequelae of cerebral infarction

Should not be used I69.30

Sequelae of stroke NOS
AHA: 2013,4Q,127-128; 2012,4Q,92,94

I69.30 Unspecified sequelae of cerebral infarction

√6ᵗʰ I69.31 Cognitive deficits following cerebral infarction

I69.310 Attention and concentration deficit following cerebral infarction CH CL

I69.311 Memory deficit following cerebral infarction CH CL

I69.312 Visuospatial deficit and spatial neglect following cerebral infarction CH CL

I69.313 Psychomotor deficit following cerebral infarction CH CL

I69.314 Frontal lobe and executive function deficit following cerebral infarction CH CL

I69.315 Cognitive social or emotional deficit following cerebral infarction CH CL

I69.318 Other symptoms and signs involving cognitive functions following cerebral infarction CH CL

I69.319 Unspecified symptoms and signs involving cognitive functions following cerebral infarction

√6ᵗʰ I69.32 Speech and language deficits following cerebral infarction

I69.320 Aphasia following cerebral infarction CH CL

I69.321 Dysphasia following cerebral infarction CH CL

AHA: 2012,4Q,91

I69.322 Dysarthria following cerebral infarction CH CL

EXCLUDES 2   transient ischemic attack (TIA) (G45.9)

I69.323 Fluency disorder following cerebral infarction CH CL

Stuttering following cerebral infarction

I69.328 Other speech and language deficits following cerebral infarction CH CL

√6ᵗʰ I69.33 Monoplegia of upper limb following cerebral infarction

AHA: 2017,1Q,47

I69.331 Monoplegia of upper limb following cerebral infarction affecting right dominant side CH CL

I69.332 Monoplegia of upper limb following cerebral infarction affecting left dominant side CH CL

I69.333 Monoplegia of upper limb following cerebral infarction affecting right non-dominant side CH CL

I69.334 Monoplegia of upper limb following cerebral infarction affecting left non-dominant side CH CL

I69.339 Monoplegia of upper limb following cerebral infarction affecting unspecified side

√6ᵗʰ I69.34 Monoplegia of lower limb following cerebral infarction

AHA: 2017,1Q,47

I69.341 Monoplegia of lower limb following cerebral infarction affecting right dominant side CH CL

I69.342 Monoplegia of lower limb following cerebral infarction affecting left dominant side CH CL

I69.343 Monoplegia of lower limb following cerebral infarction affecting right non-dominant side CH CL

I69.344 Monoplegia of lower limb following cerebral infarction affecting left non-dominant side CH CL

I69.349 Monoplegia of lower limb following cerebral infarction affecting unspecified side

√6ᵗʰ I69.35 Hemiplegia and hemiparesis following cerebral infarction

AHA: 2015,1Q,25

I69.351 Hemiplegia and hemiparesis following cerebral infarction affecting right dominant side CH CL

EXCLUDES 2   transient ischemic attack (TIA) (G45.9)

I69.352 Hemiplegia and hemiparesis following cerebral infarction affecting left dominant side CH CL

N Newborn: 0   P Pediatric: 0-17   M Maternity: 12-55   A Adult: 15-124   CH Comorbidity High   CL Comorbidity Low   NCDx Noncancer Dx   PDx Primary Dx

654   ICD-10-CM 2020

I69.353 Hemiplegia and hemiparesis following cerebral infarction affecting right non-dominant side `CH` `CL`

I69.354 Hemiplegia and hemiparesis following cerebral infarction affecting left non-dominant side `CH` `CL`
    AHA: 2012,4Q,91

I69.359 Hemiplegia and hemiparesis following cerebral infarction affecting unspecified side

√6th **I69.36** Other paralytic syndrome following cerebral infarction
  Use additional code to identify type of paralytic syndrome, such as:
  locked-in state (G83.5)
  quadriplegia (G82.5-)
  EXCLUDES 1   hemiplegia/hemiparesis following cerebral infarction (I69.35-)
    monoplegia of lower limb following cerebral infarction (I69.34-)
    monoplegia of upper limb following cerebral infarction (I69.33-)

I69.361 Other paralytic syndrome following cerebral infarction affecting right dominant side `CH` `CL`

I69.362 Other paralytic syndrome following cerebral infarction affecting left dominant side `CH` `CL`

I69.363 Other paralytic syndrome following cerebral infarction affecting right non-dominant side `CH` `CL`

I69.364 Other paralytic syndrome following cerebral infarction affecting left non-dominant side `CH` `CL`

I69.365 Other paralytic syndrome following cerebral infarction, bilateral `CH` `CL`

I69.369 Other paralytic syndrome following cerebral infarction affecting unspecified side

√6th **I69.39** Other sequelae of cerebral infarction

I69.390 Apraxia following cerebral infarction `CH` `CL`

I69.391 Dysphagia following cerebral infarction `CH` `CL`
  Use additional code to identify the type of dysphagia, if known (R13.1-)

I69.392 Facial weakness following cerebral infarction `CH` `CL`
  Facial droop following cerebral infarction

I69.393 Ataxia following cerebral infarction `CH` `CL`

I69.398 Other sequelae of cerebral infarction `CH` `CL`
  Alteration of sensation following cerebral infarction
  Disturbance of vision following cerebral infarction
  Use additional code to identify the sequelae

√5th **I69.8** Sequelae of other cerebrovascular diseases
  EXCLUDES 1   sequelae of traumatic intracranial injury (S06.-)

I69.80 Unspecified sequelae of other cerebrovascular disease

√6th **I69.81** Cognitive deficits following other cerebrovascular disease

I69.810 Attention and concentration deficit following other cerebrovascular disease `CH` `CL`

I69.811 Memory deficit following other cerebrovascular disease `CH` `CL`

I69.812 Visuospatial deficit and spatial neglect following other cerebrovascular disease `CH` `CL`

I69.813 Psychomotor deficit following other cerebrovascular disease `CH` `CL`

I69.814 Frontal lobe and executive function deficit following other cerebrovascular disease `CH` `CL`

I69.815 Cognitive social or emotional deficit following other cerebrovascular disease `CH` `CL`

I69.818 Other symptoms and signs involving cognitive functions following other cerebrovascular disease `CH` `CL`

I69.819 Unspecified symptoms and signs involving cognitive functions following other cerebrovascular disease

√6th **I69.82** Speech and language deficits following other cerebrovascular disease

I69.820 Aphasia following other cerebrovascular disease `CH` `CL`

I69.821 Dysphasia following other cerebrovascular disease `CH` `CL`

I69.822 Dysarthria following other cerebrovascular disease `CH` `CL`

I69.823 Fluency disorder following other cerebrovascular disease `CH` `CL`
  Stuttering following other cerebrovascular disease

I69.828 Other speech and language deficits following other cerebrovascular disease `CH` `CL`

√6th **I69.83** Monoplegia of upper limb following other cerebrovascular disease
  AHA: 2017,1Q,47

I69.831 Monoplegia of upper limb following other cerebrovascular disease affecting right dominant side `CH` `CL`

I69.832 Monoplegia of upper limb following other cerebrovascular disease affecting left dominant side `CH` `CL`

I69.833 Monoplegia of upper limb following other cerebrovascular disease affecting right non-dominant side `CH` `CL`

I69.834 Monoplegia of upper limb following other cerebrovascular disease affecting left non-dominant side `CH` `CL`

I69.839 Monoplegia of upper limb following other cerebrovascular disease affecting unspecified side

√6th **I69.84** Monoplegia of lower limb following other cerebrovascular disease
  AHA: 2017,1Q,47

I69.841 Monoplegia of lower limb following other cerebrovascular disease affecting right dominant side `CH` `CL`

I69.842 Monoplegia of lower limb following other cerebrovascular disease affecting left dominant side `CH` `CL`

I69.843 Monoplegia of lower limb following other cerebrovascular disease affecting right non-dominant side `CH` `CL`

I69.844 Monoplegia of lower limb following other cerebrovascular disease affecting left non-dominant side `CH` `CL`

I69.849 Monoplegia of lower limb following other cerebrovascular disease affecting unspecified side

√6th **I69.85** Hemiplegia and hemiparesis following other cerebrovascular disease
  AHA: 2015,1Q,25

I69.851 Hemiplegia and hemiparesis following other cerebrovascular disease affecting right dominant side `CH` `CL`

I69.852 Hemiplegia and hemiparesis following other cerebrovascular disease affecting left dominant side `CH` `CL`

I69.853 Hemiplegia and hemiparesis following other cerebrovascular disease affecting right non-dominant side `CH` `CL`

I69.854 Hemiplegia and hemiparesis following other cerebrovascular disease affecting left non-dominant side `CH` `CL`

I69.859 Hemiplegia and hemiparesis following other cerebrovascular disease affecting unspecified side

√6th **I69.86** Other paralytic syndrome following other cerebrovascular disease

Use additional code to identify type of paralytic syndrome, such as:
locked-in state (G83.5)
quadriplegia (G82.5-)

EXCLUDES 1   hemiplegia/hemiparesis following other cerebrovascular disease (I69.85-)
monoplegia of lower limb following other cerebrovascular disease (I69.84-)
monoplegia of upper limb following other cerebrovascular disease (I69.83-)

I69.861 Other paralytic syndrome following other cerebrovascular disease affecting right dominant side `CH` `CL`

I69.862 Other paralytic syndrome following other cerebrovascular disease affecting left dominant side `CH` `CL`

I69.863 Other paralytic syndrome following other cerebrovascular disease affecting right non-dominant side `CH` `CL`

I69.864 Other paralytic syndrome following other cerebrovascular disease affecting left non-dominant side `CH` `CL`

I69.865 Other paralytic syndrome following other cerebrovascular disease, bilateral `CH` `CL`

I69.869 Other paralytic syndrome following other cerebrovascular disease affecting unspecified side

√6th **I69.89** Other sequelae of other cerebrovascular disease

I69.890 Apraxia following other cerebrovascular disease `CH` `CL`

I69.891 Dysphagia following other cerebrovascular disease `CH` `CL`
Use additional code to identify the type of dysphagia, if known (R13.1-)

I69.892 Facial weakness following other cerebrovascular disease
Facial droop following other cerebrovascular disease

I69.893 Ataxia following other cerebrovascular disease `CH` `CL`

I69.898 Other sequelae of other cerebrovascular disease `CH` `CL`
Alteration of sensation following other cerebrovascular disease
Disturbance of vision following other cerebrovascular disease
Use additional code to identify the sequelae

√5th **I69.9** Sequelae of unspecified cerebrovascular diseases

EXCLUDES 1   sequelae of stroke (I69.3)
sequelae of traumatic intracranial injury (S06.-)

I69.90 Unspecified sequelae of unspecified cerebrovascular disease `NC Dx`
TIP: This code would be viewed by Medicare as a questionable admission if used as the admitting diagnosis for a hospice encounter.

√6th **I69.91** Cognitive deficits following unspecified cerebrovascular disease

I69.910 Attention and concentration deficit following unspecified cerebrovascular disease `CH` `CL`

I69.911 Memory deficit following unspecified cerebrovascular disease `CH` `CL`

I69.912 Visuospatial deficit and spatial neglect following unspecified cerebrovascular disease `CH` `CL`

I69.913 Psychomotor deficit following unspecified cerebrovascular disease `CH` `CL`

I69.914 Frontal lobe and executive function deficit following unspecified cerebrovascular disease `CH` `CL`

I69.915 Cognitive social or emotional deficit following unspecified cerebrovascular disease `CH` `CL`

I69.918 Other symptoms and signs involving cognitive functions following unspecified cerebrovascular disease `CH` `CL`

I69.919 Unspecified symptoms and signs involving cognitive functions following unspecified cerebrovascular disease

√6th **I69.92** Speech and language deficits following unspecified cerebrovascular disease

I69.920 Aphasia following unspecified cerebrovascular disease `CH` `CL`

I69.921 Dysphasia following unspecified cerebrovascular disease `CH` `CL`

I69.922 Dysarthria following unspecified cerebrovascular disease `CH` `CL`

I69.923 Fluency disorder following unspecified cerebrovascular disease `CH` `CL`
Stuttering following unspecified cerebrovascular disease

I69.928 Other speech and language deficits following unspecified cerebrovascular disease `CH` `CL`

√6th **I69.93** Monoplegia of upper limb following unspecified cerebrovascular disease
AHA: 2017,1Q,47

I69.931 Monoplegia of upper limb following unspecified cerebrovascular disease affecting right dominant side `CH` `CL`

I69.932 Monoplegia of upper limb following unspecified cerebrovascular disease affecting left dominant side `CH` `CL`

I69.933 Monoplegia of upper limb following unspecified cerebrovascular disease affecting right non-dominant side `CH` `CL`

I69.934 Monoplegia of upper limb following unspecified cerebrovascular disease affecting left non-dominant side `CH` `CL`

I69.939 Monoplegia of upper limb following unspecified cerebrovascular disease affecting unspecified side

√6ᵗʰ **I69.94** Monoplegia of lower limb following unspecified cerebrovascular disease
AHA: 2017,1Q,47

     I69.941 Monoplegia of lower limb following unspecified cerebrovascular disease affecting right dominant side   CH CL

     I69.942 Monoplegia of lower limb following unspecified cerebrovascular disease affecting left dominant side   CH CL

     I69.943 Monoplegia of lower limb following unspecified cerebrovascular disease affecting right non-dominant side   CH CL

     I69.944 Monoplegia of lower limb following unspecified cerebrovascular disease affecting left non-dominant side   CH CL

     I69.949 Monoplegia of lower limb following unspecified cerebrovascular disease affecting unspecified side

√6ᵗʰ **I69.95** Hemiplegia and hemiparesis following unspecified cerebrovascular disease
AHA: 2015,1Q,25

     I69.951 Hemiplegia and hemiparesis following unspecified cerebrovascular disease affecting right dominant side   CH CL

     I69.952 Hemiplegia and hemiparesis following unspecified cerebrovascular disease affecting left dominant side   CH CL

     I69.953 Hemiplegia and hemiparesis following unspecified cerebrovascular disease affecting right non-dominant side   CH CL

     I69.954 Hemiplegia and hemiparesis following unspecified cerebrovascular disease affecting left non-dominant side   CH CL

     I69.959 Hemiplegia and hemiparesis following unspecified cerebrovascular disease affecting unspecified side

√6ᵗʰ **I69.96** Other paralytic syndrome following unspecified cerebrovascular disease
Use additional code to identify type of paralytic syndrome, such as:
locked-in state (G83.5)
quadriplegia (G82.5-)

     EXCLUDES 1   *hemiplegia/hemiparesis following unspecified cerebrovascular disease (I69.95-)*
monoplegia of lower limb following unspecified cerebrovascular disease (I69.94-)
monoplegia of upper limb following unspecified cerebrovascular disease (I69.93-)

     I69.961 Other paralytic syndrome following unspecified cerebrovascular disease affecting right dominant side   CH CL

     I69.962 Other paralytic syndrome following unspecified cerebrovascular disease affecting left dominant side   CH CL

     I69.963 Other paralytic syndrome following unspecified cerebrovascular disease affecting right non-dominant side   CH CL

     I69.964 Other paralytic syndrome following unspecified cerebrovascular disease affecting left non-dominant side   CH CL

     I69.965 Other paralytic syndrome following unspecified cerebrovascular disease, bilateral   CH CL

     I69.969 Other paralytic syndrome following unspecified cerebrovascular disease affecting unspecified side

√6ᵗʰ **I69.99** Other sequelae of unspecified cerebrovascular disease

     I69.990 Apraxia following unspecified cerebrovascular disease   CH CL

     I69.991 Dysphagia following unspecified cerebrovascular disease   CH CL
Use additional code to identify the type of dysphagia, if known (R13.1-)

     I69.992 Facial weakness following unspecified cerebrovascular disease
Facial droop following unspecified cerebrovascular disease

     I69.993 Ataxia following unspecified cerebrovascular disease   CH CL

     I69.998 Other sequelae following unspecified cerebrovascular disease   CH CL
Alteration in sensation following unspecified cerebrovascular disease
Disturbance of vision following unspecified cerebrovascular disease
Use additional code to identify the sequelae

Diseases of arteries, arterioles and capillaries (I70-I79)

√4ᵗʰ **I70** Atherosclerosis

   INCLUDES   arterial degeneration
arteriolosclerosis
arteriosclerosis
arteriosclerotic vascular disease
arteriovascular degeneration
atheroma
endarteritis deformans or obliterans
senile arteritis
senile endarteritis
vascular degeneration

Use additional code to identify:
exposure to environmental tobacco smoke (Z77.22)
history of tobacco dependence (Z87.891)
occupational exposure to environmental tobacco smoke (Z57.31)
tobacco dependence (F17.-)
tobacco use (Z72.0)

   EXCLUDES 2   *arteriosclerotic cardiovascular disease (I25.1-)*
arteriosclerotic heart disease (I25.1-)
atheroembolism (I75.-)
cerebral atherosclerosis (I67.2)
coronary atherosclerosis (I25.1-)
mesenteric atherosclerosis (K55.1)
precerebral atherosclerosis (I67.2)
primary pulmonary atherosclerosis (I27.0)

I70.0 Atherosclerosis of aorta   CH A

I70.1 Atherosclerosis of renal artery   CH A
Goldblatt's kidney
   EXCLUDES 2   *atherosclerosis of renal arterioles (I12.-)*

√5ᵗʰ **I70.2** Atherosclerosis of native arteries of the extremities
Mönckeberg's (medial) sclerosis
Use additional code, if applicable, to identify chronic total occlusion of artery of extremity (I70.92)
   EXCLUDES 2   *atherosclerosis of bypass graft of extremities (I70.30-I70.79)*
AHA: 2018,3Q,4; 2018,2Q,7

√6ᵗʰ **I70.20** Unspecified atherosclerosis of native arteries of extremities

     I70.201 Unspecified atherosclerosis of native arteries of extremities, right leg   CH A

     I70.202 Unspecified atherosclerosis of native arteries of extremities, left leg   CH A

I70.203 Unspecified atherosclerosis of native arteries of extremities, bilateral legs   CH A

I70.208 Unspecified atherosclerosis of native arteries of extremities, other extremity   CH A

I70.209 Unspecified atherosclerosis of native arteries of extremities, unspecified extremity   A

√6th **I70.21** Atherosclerosis of native arteries of extremities with intermittent claudication

I70.211 Atherosclerosis of native arteries of extremities with intermittent claudication, right leg   CH A

I70.212 Atherosclerosis of native arteries of extremities with intermittent claudication, left leg   CH A

I70.213 Atherosclerosis of native arteries of extremities with intermittent claudication, bilateral legs   CH A

I70.218 Atherosclerosis of native arteries of extremities with intermittent claudication, other extremity   CH A

I70.219 Atherosclerosis of native arteries of extremities with intermittent claudication, unspecified extremity   A

√6th **I70.22** Atherosclerosis of native arteries of extremities with rest pain

INCLUDES   any condition classifiable to I70.21-

I70.221 Atherosclerosis of native arteries of extremities with rest pain, right leg   CH A

I70.222 Atherosclerosis of native arteries of extremities with rest pain, left leg   CH A

I70.223 Atherosclerosis of native arteries of extremities with rest pain, bilateral legs   CH A

I70.228 Atherosclerosis of native arteries of extremities with rest pain, other extremity   CH A

I70.229 Atherosclerosis of native arteries of extremities with rest pain, unspecified extremity   A

√6th **I70.23** Atherosclerosis of native arteries of right leg with ulceration

INCLUDES   any condition classifiable to I70.211 and I70.221

Use additional code to identify severity of ulcer (L97.-)

I70.231 Atherosclerosis of native arteries of right leg with ulceration of thigh   CH CL A

I70.232 Atherosclerosis of native arteries of right leg with ulceration of calf   CH CL A

I70.233 Atherosclerosis of native arteries of right leg with ulceration of ankle   CH CL A

I70.234 Atherosclerosis of native arteries of right leg with ulceration of heel and midfoot   CH CL A

Atherosclerosis of native arteries of right leg with ulceration of plantar surface of midfoot

I70.235 Atherosclerosis of native arteries of right leg with ulceration of other part of foot   CH CL A

Atherosclerosis of native arteries of right leg extremities with ulceration of toe

I70.238 Atherosclerosis of native arteries of right leg with ulceration of other part of lower leg   CH CL A

I70.239 Atherosclerosis of native arteries of right leg with ulceration of unspecified site   A

√6th **I70.24** Atherosclerosis of native arteries of left leg with ulceration

INCLUDES   any condition classifiable to I70.212 and I70.222

Use additional code to identify severity of ulcer (L97.-)

I70.241 Atherosclerosis of native arteries of left leg with ulceration of thigh   CH CL A

I70.242 Atherosclerosis of native arteries of left leg with ulceration of calf   CH CL A

I70.243 Atherosclerosis of native arteries of left leg with ulceration of ankle   CH CL A

I70.244 Atherosclerosis of native arteries of left leg with ulceration of heel and midfoot   CH CL A

Atherosclerosis of native arteries of left leg with ulceration of plantar surface of midfoot

I70.245 Atherosclerosis of native arteries of left leg with ulceration of other part of foot   CH CL A

Atherosclerosis of native arteries of left leg extremities with ulceration of toe

I70.248 Atherosclerosis of native arteries of left leg with ulceration of other part of lower leg   CH CL A

I70.249 Atherosclerosis of native arteries of left leg with ulceration of unspecified site   A

I70.25 Atherosclerosis of native arteries of other extremities with ulceration   A

INCLUDES   any condition classifiable to I70.218 and I70.228

Use additional code to identify the severity of the ulcer (L98.49-)

√6th **I70.26** Atherosclerosis of native arteries of extremities with gangrene

INCLUDES   any condition classifiable to I70.21-, I70.22-, I70.23-, I70.24-, and I70.25-

Use additional code to identify the severity of any ulcer (L97.-, L98.49-), if applicable

I70.261 Atherosclerosis of native arteries of extremities with gangrene, right leg   CH A

I70.262 Atherosclerosis of native arteries of extremities with gangrene, left leg   CH A

I70.263 Atherosclerosis of native arteries of extremities with gangrene, bilateral legs   CH A

I70.268 Atherosclerosis of native arteries of extremities with gangrene, other extremity   CH A

I70.269 Atherosclerosis of native arteries of extremities with gangrene, unspecified extremity   A

√6th **I70.29** Other atherosclerosis of native arteries of extremities

I70.291 Other atherosclerosis of native arteries of extremities, right leg   A

I70.292 Other atherosclerosis of native arteries of extremities, left leg   A

I70.293 Other atherosclerosis of native arteries of extremities, bilateral legs   A

I70.298 Other atherosclerosis of native arteries of extremities, other extremity   A

I70.299 Other atherosclerosis of native arteries of extremities, unspecified extremity   A

N Newborn: 0   P Pediatric: 0-17   M Maternity: 12-55   A Adult: 15-124   CH Comorbidity High   CL Comorbidity Low   NCDx Noncancer Dx   PDx Primary Dx

658   ICD-10-CM 2020

Chapter 9. Diseases of the Circulatory System

I70.203-I70.299

✓5ᵗʰ I70.3 **Atherosclerosis of** unspecified type of bypass graft(s) **of the** extremities

Use additional code, if applicable, to identify chronic total occlusion of artery of extremity (I70.92)

> **EXCLUDES 1** embolism or thrombus of bypass graft(s) of extremities (T82.8-)

✓6ᵗʰ I70.30 **Unspecified atherosclerosis of unspecified type of bypass graft(s) of the extremities**

I70.301 Unspecified atherosclerosis of unspecified type of bypass graft(s) of the extremities, right leg   A

I70.302 Unspecified atherosclerosis of unspecified type of bypass graft(s) of the extremities, left leg   A

I70.303 Unspecified atherosclerosis of unspecified type of bypass graft(s) of the extremities, bilateral legs   A

I70.308 Unspecified atherosclerosis of unspecified type of bypass graft(s) of the extremities, other extremity   A

I70.309 Unspecified atherosclerosis of unspecified type of bypass graft(s) of the extremities, unspecified extremity   A

✓6ᵗʰ I70.31 **Atherosclerosis of unspecified type of bypass graft(s) of the extremities with** intermittent claudication

I70.311 Atherosclerosis of unspecified type of bypass graft(s) of the extremities with intermittent claudication, right leg   A

I70.312 Atherosclerosis of unspecified type of bypass graft(s) of the extremities with intermittent claudication, left leg   A

I70.313 Atherosclerosis of unspecified type of bypass graft(s) of the extremities with intermittent claudication, bilateral legs   A

I70.318 Atherosclerosis of unspecified type of bypass graft(s) of the extremities with intermittent claudication, other extremity   A

I70.319 Atherosclerosis of unspecified type of bypass graft(s) of the extremities with intermittent claudication, unspecified extremity   A

✓6ᵗʰ I70.32 **Atherosclerosis of unspecified type of bypass graft(s) of the extremities with** rest pain

> **INCLUDES** any condition classifiable to I70.31-

I70.321 Atherosclerosis of unspecified type of bypass graft(s) of the extremities with rest pain, right leg   A

I70.322 Atherosclerosis of unspecified type of bypass graft(s) of the extremities with rest pain, left leg   A

I70.323 Atherosclerosis of unspecified type of bypass graft(s) of the extremities with rest pain, bilateral legs   A

I70.328 Atherosclerosis of unspecified type of bypass graft(s) of the extremities with rest pain, other extremity   A

I70.329 Atherosclerosis of unspecified type of bypass graft(s) of the extremities with rest pain, unspecified extremity   A

✓6ᵗʰ I70.33 **Atherosclerosis of unspecified type of bypass graft(s) of the** right leg with ulceration

> **INCLUDES** any condition classifiable to I70.311 and I70.321

Use additional code to identify severity of ulcer (L97.-)

I70.331 Atherosclerosis of unspecified type of bypass graft(s) of the right leg with ulceration of thigh   CH CL A

I70.332 Atherosclerosis of unspecified type of bypass graft(s) of the right leg with ulceration of calf   CH CL A

I70.333 Atherosclerosis of unspecified type of bypass graft(s) of the right leg with ulceration of ankle   CH CL A

I70.334 Atherosclerosis of unspecified type of bypass graft(s) of the right leg with ulceration of heel and midfoot   CH CL A

Atherosclerosis of unspecified type of bypass graft(s) of right leg with ulceration of plantar surface of midfoot

I70.335 Atherosclerosis of unspecified type of bypass graft(s) of the right leg with ulceration of other part of foot   CH CL A

Atherosclerosis of unspecified type of bypass graft(s) of the right leg with ulceration of toe

I70.338 Atherosclerosis of unspecified type of bypass graft(s) of the right leg with ulceration of other part of lower leg   CH CL A

I70.339 Atherosclerosis of unspecified type of bypass graft(s) of the right leg with ulceration of unspecified site   CH CL A

✓6ᵗʰ I70.34 **Atherosclerosis of unspecified type of bypass graft(s) of the** left leg with ulceration

> **INCLUDES** any condition classifiable to I70.312 and I70.322

Use additional code to identify severity of ulcer (L97.-)

I70.341 Atherosclerosis of unspecified type of bypass graft(s) of the left leg with ulceration of thigh   CH CL A

I70.342 Atherosclerosis of unspecified type of bypass graft(s) of the left leg with ulceration of calf   CH CL A

I70.343 Atherosclerosis of unspecified type of bypass graft(s) of the left leg with ulceration of ankle   CH CL A

I70.344 Atherosclerosis of unspecified type of bypass graft(s) of the left leg with ulceration of heel and midfoot   CH CL A

Atherosclerosis of unspecified type of bypass graft(s) of left leg with ulceration of plantar surface of midfoot

I70.345 Atherosclerosis of unspecified type of bypass graft(s) of the left leg with ulceration of other part of foot   CH CL A

Atherosclerosis of unspecified type of bypass graft(s) of the left leg with ulceration of toe

I70.348 Atherosclerosis of unspecified type of bypass graft(s) of the left leg with ulceration of other part of lower leg   CH CL A

I70.349 Atherosclerosis of unspecified type of bypass graft(s) of the left leg with ulceration of unspecified site   CH CL A

I70.35 **Atherosclerosis of unspecified type of bypass graft(s) of other extremity with** ulceration   A

> **INCLUDES** any condition classifiable to I70.318 and I70.328

Use additional code to identify severity of ulcer (L98.49-)

✅ Additional Character Required   ✓x7ᵗʰ Placeholder Alert   Manifestation   Unspecified Dx   ▶◀ Revised Text   ● New Code   ▲ Revised Title

ICD-10-CM 2020   659

Chapter 9. Diseases of the Circulatory System

I70.36–I70.441

√6ᵗʰ **I70.36 Atherosclerosis of unspecified type of bypass graft(s) of the extremities with** gangrene

INCLUDES   any condition classifiable to I70.31-, I70.32-, I70.33-, I70.34-, I70.35

Use additional code to identify the severity of any ulcer (L97.-, L98.49-), if applicable

I70.361 Atherosclerosis of unspecified type of bypass graft(s) of the extremities with gangrene, right leg A

I70.362 Atherosclerosis of unspecified type of bypass graft(s) of the extremities with gangrene, left leg A

I70.363 Atherosclerosis of unspecified type of bypass graft(s) of the extremities with gangrene, bilateral legs A

I70.368 Atherosclerosis of unspecified type of bypass graft(s) of the extremities with gangrene, other extremity A

I70.369 Atherosclerosis of unspecified type of bypass graft(s) of the extremities with gangrene, unspecified extremity A

√6ᵗʰ **I70.39 Other atherosclerosis of unspecified type of bypass graft(s) of the extremities**

I70.391 Other atherosclerosis of unspecified type of bypass graft(s) of the extremities, right leg A

I70.392 Other atherosclerosis of unspecified type of bypass graft(s) of the extremities, left leg A

I70.393 Other atherosclerosis of unspecified type of bypass graft(s) of the extremities, bilateral legs A

I70.398 Other atherosclerosis of unspecified type of bypass graft(s) of the extremities, other extremity A

I70.399 Other atherosclerosis of unspecified type of bypass graft(s) of the extremities, unspecified extremity A

√5ᵗʰ **I70.4 Atherosclerosis of** autologous vein bypass graft(s) **of the extremities**

Use additional code, if applicable, to identify chronic total occlusion of artery of extremity (I70.92)

√6ᵗʰ **I70.40 Unspecified atherosclerosis of autologous vein bypass graft(s) of the extremities**

I70.401 Unspecified atherosclerosis of autologous vein bypass graft(s) of the extremities, right leg A

I70.402 Unspecified atherosclerosis of autologous vein bypass graft(s) of the extremities, left leg A

I70.403 Unspecified atherosclerosis of autologous vein bypass graft(s) of the extremities, bilateral legs A

I70.408 Unspecified atherosclerosis of autologous vein bypass graft(s) of the extremities, other extremity A

I70.409 Unspecified atherosclerosis of autologous vein bypass graft(s) of the extremities, unspecified extremity A

√6ᵗʰ **I70.41 Atherosclerosis of autologous vein bypass graft(s) of the extremities with** intermittent claudication

I70.411 Atherosclerosis of autologous vein bypass graft(s) of the extremities with intermittent claudication, right leg A

I70.412 Atherosclerosis of autologous vein bypass graft(s) of the extremities with intermittent claudication, left leg A

I70.413 Atherosclerosis of autologous vein bypass graft(s) of the extremities with intermittent claudication, bilateral legs A

I70.418 Atherosclerosis of autologous vein bypass graft(s) of the extremities with intermittent claudication, other extremity A

I70.419 Atherosclerosis of autologous vein bypass graft(s) of the extremities with intermittent claudication, unspecified extremity A

√6ᵗʰ **I70.42 Atherosclerosis of autologous vein bypass graft(s) of the extremities with** rest pain

INCLUDES   any condition classifiable to I70.41-

I70.421 Atherosclerosis of autologous vein bypass graft(s) of the extremities with rest pain, right leg A

I70.422 Atherosclerosis of autologous vein bypass graft(s) of the extremities with rest pain, left leg A

I70.423 Atherosclerosis of autologous vein bypass graft(s) of the extremities with rest pain, bilateral legs A

I70.428 Atherosclerosis of autologous vein bypass graft(s) of the extremities with rest pain, other extremity A

I70.429 Atherosclerosis of autologous vein bypass graft(s) of the extremities with rest pain, unspecified extremity A

√6ᵗʰ **I70.43 Atherosclerosis of autologous vein bypass graft(s) of the** right leg **with** ulceration

INCLUDES   any condition classifiable to I70.411 and I70.421

Use additional code to identify severity of ulcer (L97.-)

I70.431 Atherosclerosis of autologous vein bypass graft(s) of the right leg with ulceration of thigh CH CL A

I70.432 Atherosclerosis of autologous vein bypass graft(s) of the right leg with ulceration of calf CH CL A

I70.433 Atherosclerosis of autologous vein bypass graft(s) of the right leg with ulceration of ankle CH CL A

I70.434 Atherosclerosis of autologous vein bypass graft(s) of the right leg with ulceration of heel and midfoot CH CL A

Atherosclerosis of autologous vein bypass graft(s) of right leg with ulceration of plantar surface of midfoot

I70.435 Atherosclerosis of autologous vein bypass graft(s) of the right leg with ulceration of other part of foot CH CL A

Atherosclerosis of autologous vein bypass graft(s) of right leg with ulceration of toe

I70.438 Atherosclerosis of autologous vein bypass graft(s) of the right leg with ulceration of other part of lower leg CH CL A

I70.439 Atherosclerosis of autologous vein bypass graft(s) of the right leg with ulceration of unspecified site CH CL A

√6ᵗʰ **I70.44 Atherosclerosis of autologous vein bypass graft(s) of the** left leg **with** ulceration

INCLUDES   any condition classifiable to I70.412 and I70.422

Use additional code to identify severity of ulcer (L97.-)

I70.441 Atherosclerosis of autologous vein bypass graft(s) of the left leg with ulceration of thigh CH CL A

N Newborn: 0   P Pediatric: 0-17   M Maternity: 12-55   A Adult: 15-124   CH Comorbidity High   CL Comorbidity Low   NCDx Noncancer Dx   PDx Primary Dx

660   ICD-10-CM 2020

I70.442   **Atherosclerosis of autologous vein bypass graft(s) of the left leg with ulceration of** calf   CH CL A

I70.443   **Atherosclerosis of autologous vein bypass graft(s) of the left leg with ulceration of** ankle   CH CL A

I70.444   **Atherosclerosis of autologous vein bypass graft(s) of the left leg with ulceration of** heel and midfoot   CH CL A

     Atherosclerosis of autologous vein bypass graft(s) of left leg with ulceration of plantar surface of midfoot

I70.445   **Atherosclerosis of autologous vein bypass graft(s) of the left leg with ulceration of other part of foot**   CH CL A

     Atherosclerosis of autologous vein bypass graft(s) of left leg with ulceration of toe

I70.448   **Atherosclerosis of autologous vein bypass graft(s) of the left leg with ulceration of other part of lower leg**   CH CL A

I70.449   **Atherosclerosis of autologous vein bypass graft(s) of the left leg with ulceration of unspecified site**   CH CL A

I70.45   **Atherosclerosis of autologous vein bypass graft(s) of other extremity with** ulceration   A

     INCLUDES   any condition classifiable to I70.418, I70.428, and I70.438

     Use additional code to identify severity of ulcer (L98.49)

√6ᵗʰ   I70.46   **Atherosclerosis of autologous vein bypass graft(s) of the extremities with** gangrene

     INCLUDES   any condition classifiable to I70.41-, I70.42-, and I70.43-, I70.44-, I70.45

     Use additional code to identify the severity of any ulcer (L97.-, L98.49-), if applicable

I70.461   **Atherosclerosis of autologous vein bypass graft(s) of the extremities with gangrene, right leg**   A

I70.462   **Atherosclerosis of autologous vein bypass graft(s) of the extremities with gangrene, left leg**   A

I70.463   **Atherosclerosis of autologous vein bypass graft(s) of the extremities with gangrene, bilateral legs**   A

I70.468   **Atherosclerosis of autologous vein bypass graft(s) of the extremities with gangrene, other extremity**   A

I70.469   **Atherosclerosis of autologous vein bypass graft(s) of the extremities with gangrene, unspecified extremity**   A

√6ᵗʰ   I70.49   **Other atherosclerosis of autologous vein bypass graft(s) of the extremities**

I70.491   **Other atherosclerosis of autologous vein bypass graft(s) of the extremities, right leg**   A

I70.492   **Other atherosclerosis of autologous vein bypass graft(s) of the extremities,** left leg   A

I70.493   **Other atherosclerosis of autologous vein bypass graft(s) of the extremities,** bilateral legs   A

I70.498   **Other atherosclerosis of autologous vein bypass graft(s) of the extremities, other extremity**   A

I70.499   **Other atherosclerosis of autologous vein bypass graft(s) of the extremities, unspecified extremity**   A

√6ᵗʰ   I70.5   **Atherosclerosis of** nonautologous biological bypass graft(s) **of the** extremities

     Use additional code, if applicable, to identify chronic total occlusion of artery of extremity (I70.92)

√6ᵗʰ   I70.50   **Unspecified atherosclerosis of nonautologous biological bypass graft(s) of the extremities**

I70.501   **Unspecified atherosclerosis of nonautologous biological bypass graft(s) of the extremities,** right leg   A

I70.502   **Unspecified atherosclerosis of nonautologous biological bypass graft(s) of the extremities,** left leg   A

I70.503   **Unspecified atherosclerosis of nonautologous biological bypass graft(s) of the extremities,** bilateral legs   A

I70.508   **Unspecified atherosclerosis of nonautologous biological bypass graft(s) of the extremities, other extremity**   A

I70.509   **Unspecified atherosclerosis of nonautologous biological bypass graft(s) of the extremities, unspecified extremity**   A

√6ᵗʰ   I70.51   **Atherosclerosis of nonautologous biological bypass graft(s) of the extremities** intermittent claudication

I70.511   **Atherosclerosis of nonautologous biological bypass graft(s) of the extremities with intermittent claudication,** right leg   A

I70.512   **Atherosclerosis of nonautologous biological bypass graft(s) of the extremities with intermittent claudication,** left leg   A

I70.513   **Atherosclerosis of nonautologous biological bypass graft(s) of the extremities with intermittent claudication,** bilateral legs   A

I70.518   **Atherosclerosis of nonautologous biological bypass graft(s) of the extremities with intermittent claudication, other extremity**   A

I70.519   **Atherosclerosis of nonautologous biological bypass graft(s) of the extremities with intermittent claudication, unspecified extremity**   A

√6ᵗʰ   I70.52   **Atherosclerosis of nonautologous biological bypass graft(s) of the extremities with** rest pain

     INCLUDES   any condition classifiable to I70.51-

I70.521   **Atherosclerosis of nonautologous biological bypass graft(s) of the extremities with rest pain,** right leg   A

I70.522   **Atherosclerosis of nonautologous biological bypass graft(s) of the extremities with rest pain,** left leg   A

I70.523   **Atherosclerosis of nonautologous biological bypass graft(s) of the extremities with rest pain,** bilateral legs   A

I70.528   **Atherosclerosis of nonautologous biological bypass graft(s) of the extremities with rest pain, other extremity**   A

I70.529   **Atherosclerosis of nonautologous biological bypass graft(s) of the extremities with rest pain, unspecified extremity**   A

✓ Additional Character Required   √x7ᵗʰ Placeholder Alert   Manifestation   Unspecified Dx   ►◄ Revised Text   ● New Code   ▲ Revised Title

ICD-10-CM 2020   661

√6ᵗʰ **I70.53** **Atherosclerosis of nonautologous biological bypass graft(s) of the right leg with ulceration**

INCLUDES   any condition classifiable to I70.511 and I70.521

Use additional code to identify severity of ulcer (L97.-)

I70.531 Atherosclerosis of nonautologous biological bypass graft(s) of the right leg with ulceration of thigh   CH CL A

I70.532 Atherosclerosis of nonautologous biological bypass graft(s) of the right leg with ulceration of calf   CH CL A

I70.533 Atherosclerosis of nonautologous biological bypass graft(s) of the right leg with ulceration of ankle   CH CL A

I70.534 Atherosclerosis of nonautologous biological bypass graft(s) of the right leg with ulceration of heel and midfoot   CH CL A

Atherosclerosis of nonautologous biological bypass graft(s) of right leg with ulceration of plantar surface of midfoot

I70.535 Atherosclerosis of nonautologous biological bypass graft(s) of the right leg with ulceration of other part of foot   CH CL A

Atherosclerosis of nonautologous biological bypass graft(s) of the right leg with ulceration of toe

I70.538 Atherosclerosis of nonautologous biological bypass graft(s) of the right leg with ulceration of other part of lower leg   CH CL A

I70.539 Atherosclerosis of nonautologous biological bypass graft(s) of the right leg with ulceration of unspecified site   CH CL A

√6ᵗʰ **I70.54** **Atherosclerosis of nonautologous biological bypass graft(s) of the left leg with ulceration**

INCLUDES   any condition classifiable to I70.512 and I70.522

Use additional code to identify severity of ulcer (L97.-)

I70.541 Atherosclerosis of nonautologous biological bypass graft(s) of the left leg with ulceration of thigh   CH CL A

I70.542 Atherosclerosis of nonautologous biological bypass graft(s) of the left leg with ulceration of calf   CH CL A

I70.543 Atherosclerosis of nonautologous biological bypass graft(s) of the left leg with ulceration of ankle   CH CL A

I70.544 Atherosclerosis of nonautologous biological bypass graft(s) of the left leg with ulceration of heel and midfoot   CH CL A

Atherosclerosis of nonautologous biological bypass graft(s) of left leg with ulceration of plantar surface of midfoot

I70.545 Atherosclerosis of nonautologous biological bypass graft(s) of the left leg with ulceration of other part of foot   CH CL A

Atherosclerosis of nonautologous biological bypass graft(s) of the left leg with ulceration of toe

I70.548 Atherosclerosis of nonautologous biological bypass graft(s) of the left leg with ulceration of other part of lower leg   CH CL A

I70.549 Atherosclerosis of nonautologous biological bypass graft(s) of the left leg with ulceration of unspecified site   CH CL A

I70.55 **Atherosclerosis of nonautologous biological bypass graft(s) of other extremity with ulceration**   A

INCLUDES   any condition classifiable to I70.518, I70.528, and I70.538

Use additional code to identify severity of ulcer (L98.49)

√6ᵗʰ **I70.56** **Atherosclerosis of nonautologous biological bypass graft(s) of the extremities with gangrene**

INCLUDES   any condition classifiable to I70.51-, I70.53-, I70.54-, I70.55

Use additional code to identify the severity of any ulcer (L97.-, L98.49-), if applicable

I70.561 Atherosclerosis of nonautologous biological bypass graft(s) of the extremities with gangrene, right leg   A

I70.562 Atherosclerosis of nonautologous biological bypass graft(s) of the extremities with gangrene, left leg   A

I70.563 Atherosclerosis of nonautologous biological bypass graft(s) of the extremities with gangrene, bilateral legs   A

I70.568 Atherosclerosis of nonautologous biological bypass graft(s) of the extremities with gangrene, other extremity   A

I70.569 Atherosclerosis of nonautologous biological bypass graft(s) of the extremities with gangrene, unspecified extremity   A

√6ᵗʰ **I70.59** **Other atherosclerosis of nonautologous biological bypass graft(s) of the extremities**

I70.591 Other atherosclerosis of nonautologous biological bypass graft(s) of the extremities, right leg   A

I70.592 Other atherosclerosis of nonautologous biological bypass graft(s) of the extremities, left leg   A

I70.593 Other atherosclerosis of nonautologous biological bypass graft(s) of the extremities, bilateral legs   A

I70.598 Other atherosclerosis of nonautologous biological bypass graft(s) of the extremities, other extremity   A

I70.599 Other atherosclerosis of nonautologous biological bypass graft(s) of the extremities, unspecified extremity   A

√5ᵗʰ **I70.6** **Atherosclerosis of nonbiological bypass graft(s) of the extremities**

Use additional code, if applicable, to identify chronic total occlusion of artery of extremity (I70.92)

√6ᵗʰ **I70.60** **Unspecified atherosclerosis of nonbiological bypass graft(s) of the extremities**

I70.601 Unspecified atherosclerosis of nonbiological bypass graft(s) of the extremities, right leg   A

I70.602 Unspecified atherosclerosis of nonbiological bypass graft(s) of the extremities, left leg   A

I70.603 Unspecified atherosclerosis of nonbiological bypass graft(s) of the extremities, bilateral legs   A

N Newborn: 0   P Pediatric: 0-17   M Maternity: 12-55   A Adult: 15-124   CH Comorbidity High   CL Comorbidity Low   NCDx Noncancer Dx   PDx Primary Dx

662   ICD-10-CM 2020

I70.608   **Unspecified atherosclerosis of nonbiological bypass graft(s) of the extremities, other extremity**   A

I70.609   **Unspecified atherosclerosis of nonbiological bypass graft(s) of the extremities, unspecified extremity**   A

√6ᵗʰ   I70.61   **Atherosclerosis of nonbiological bypass graft(s) of the extremities with** intermittent claudication

I70.611   **Atherosclerosis of nonbiological bypass graft(s) of the extremities with intermittent claudication,** right leg   A

I70.612   **Atherosclerosis of nonbiological bypass graft(s) of the extremities with intermittent claudication,** left leg   A

I70.613   **Atherosclerosis of nonbiological bypass graft(s) of the extremities with intermittent claudication,** bilateral legs   A

I70.618   **Atherosclerosis of nonbiological bypass graft(s) of the extremities with intermittent claudication, other extremity**   A

I70.619   **Atherosclerosis of nonbiological bypass graft(s) of the extremities with intermittent claudication, unspecified extremity**   A

√6ᵗʰ   I70.62   **Atherosclerosis of nonbiological bypass graft(s) of the extremities with** rest pain
> INCLUDES   any condition classifiable to I70.61-

I70.621   **Atherosclerosis of nonbiological bypass graft(s) of the extremities with rest pain,** right leg   A

I70.622   **Atherosclerosis of nonbiological bypass graft(s) of the extremities with rest pain,** left leg   A

I70.623   **Atherosclerosis of nonbiological bypass graft(s) of the extremities with rest pain,** bilateral legs   A

I70.628   **Atherosclerosis of nonbiological bypass graft(s) of the extremities with rest pain, other extremity**   A

I70.629   **Atherosclerosis of nonbiological bypass graft(s) of the extremities with rest pain, unspecified extremity**   A

√6ᵗʰ   I70.63   **Atherosclerosis of nonbiological bypass graft(s) of the** right leg **with** ulceration
> INCLUDES   any condition classifiable to I70.611 and I70.621

Use additional code to identify severity of ulcer (L97.-)

I70.631   **Atherosclerosis of nonbiological bypass graft(s) of the right leg with ulceration of** thigh   CH CL A

I70.632   **Atherosclerosis of nonbiological bypass graft(s) of the right leg with ulceration of** calf   CH CL A

I70.633   **Atherosclerosis of nonbiological bypass graft(s) of the right leg with ulceration of** ankle   CH CL A

I70.634   **Atherosclerosis of nonbiological bypass graft(s) of the right leg with ulceration of** heel and midfoot   CH CL A
> Atherosclerosis of nonbiological bypass graft(s) of right leg with ulceration of plantar surface of midfoot

I70.635   **Atherosclerosis of nonbiological bypass graft(s) of the right leg with ulceration of other part of foot**   CH CL A
> Atherosclerosis of nonbiological bypass graft(s) of the right leg with ulceration of toe

I70.638   **Atherosclerosis of nonbiological bypass graft(s) of the right leg with ulceration of other part of lower leg**   CH CL A

I70.639   **Atherosclerosis of nonbiological bypass graft(s) of the right leg with ulceration of unspecified site**   CH CL A

√6ᵗʰ   I70.64   **Atherosclerosis of nonbiological bypass graft(s) of the** left leg **with** ulceration
> INCLUDES   any condition classifiable to I70.612 and I70.622

Use additional code to identify severity of ulcer (L97.-)

I70.641   **Atherosclerosis of nonbiological bypass graft(s) of the left leg with ulceration of** thigh   CH CL A

I70.642   **Atherosclerosis of nonbiological bypass graft(s) of the left leg with ulceration of** calf   CH CL A

I70.643   **Atherosclerosis of nonbiological bypass graft(s) of the left leg with ulceration of** ankle   CH CL A

I70.644   **Atherosclerosis of nonbiological bypass graft(s) of the left leg with ulceration of** heel and midfoot   CH CL A
> Atherosclerosis of nonbiological bypass graft(s) of left leg with ulceration of plantar surface of midfoot

I70.645   **Atherosclerosis of nonbiological bypass graft(s) of the left leg with ulceration of other part of foot**   CH CL A
> Atherosclerosis of nonbiological bypass graft(s) of the left leg with ulceration of toe

I70.648   **Atherosclerosis of nonbiological bypass graft(s) of the left leg with ulceration of other part of lower leg**   CH CL A

I70.649   **Atherosclerosis of nonbiological bypass graft(s) of the left leg with ulceration of unspecified site**   CH CL A

I70.65   **Atherosclerosis of nonbiological bypass graft(s) of other extremity with** ulceration   A
> INCLUDES   any condition classifiable to I70.618 and I70.628

Use additional code to identify severity of ulcer (L98.49)

√6ᵗʰ   I70.66   **Atherosclerosis of nonbiological bypass graft(s) of the extremities with** gangrene
> INCLUDES   any condition classifiable to I70.61-, I70.62-, I70.63-, I70.64-, I70.65

Use additional code to identify the severity of any ulcer (L97.-, L98.49-), if applicable

I70.661   **Atherosclerosis of nonbiological bypass graft(s) of the extremities with gangrene,** right leg   A

I70.662   **Atherosclerosis of nonbiological bypass graft(s) of the extremities with gangrene,** left leg   A

I70.663   **Atherosclerosis of nonbiological bypass graft(s) of the extremities with gangrene,** bilateral legs   A

☑ Additional Character Required   √x7ᵗʰ Placeholder Alert   Manifestation   Unspecified Dx   ▶◀ Revised Text   ● New Code   ▲ Revised Title

ICD-10-CM 2020   **663**

Chapter 9. Diseases of the Circulatory System

I70.668 Atherosclerosis of nonbiological bypass graft(s) of the extremities with gangrene, other extremity A

I70.669 Atherosclerosis of nonbiological bypass graft(s) of the extremities with gangrene, unspecified extremity A

✓6th **I70.69 Other atherosclerosis of nonbiological bypass graft(s) of the extremities**

I70.691 Other atherosclerosis of nonbiological bypass graft(s) of the extremities, right leg A

I70.692 Other atherosclerosis of nonbiological bypass graft(s) of the extremities, left leg A

I70.693 Other atherosclerosis of nonbiological bypass graft(s) of the extremities, bilateral legs A

I70.698 Other atherosclerosis of nonbiological bypass graft(s) of the extremities, other extremity A

I70.699 Other atherosclerosis of nonbiological bypass graft(s) of the extremities, unspecified extremity A

✓5th **I70.7 Atherosclerosis of other type of bypass graft(s) of the extremities**
Use additional code, if applicable, to identify chronic total occlusion of artery of extremity (I70.92)

✓6th **I70.70 Unspecified atherosclerosis of other type of bypass graft(s) of the extremities**

I70.701 Unspecified atherosclerosis of other type of bypass graft(s) of the extremities, right leg A

I70.702 Unspecified atherosclerosis of other type of bypass graft(s) of the extremities, left leg A

I70.703 Unspecified atherosclerosis of other type of bypass graft(s) of the extremities, bilateral legs A

I70.708 Unspecified atherosclerosis of other type of bypass graft(s) of the extremities, other extremity A

I70.709 Unspecified atherosclerosis of other type of bypass graft(s) of the extremities, unspecified extremity A

✓6th **I70.71 Atherosclerosis of other type of bypass graft(s) of the extremities with intermittent claudication**

I70.711 Atherosclerosis of other type of bypass graft(s) of the extremities with intermittent claudication, right leg A

I70.712 Atherosclerosis of other type of bypass graft(s) of the extremities with intermittent claudication, left leg A

I70.713 Atherosclerosis of other type of bypass graft(s) of the extremities with intermittent claudication, bilateral legs A

I70.718 Atherosclerosis of other type of bypass graft(s) of the extremities with intermittent claudication, other extremity A

I70.719 Atherosclerosis of other type of bypass graft(s) of the extremities with intermittent claudication, unspecified extremity A

✓6th **I70.72 Atherosclerosis of other type of bypass graft(s) of the extremities with rest pain**
INCLUDES any condition classifiable to I70.71-

I70.721 Atherosclerosis of other type of bypass graft(s) of the extremities with rest pain, right leg A

I70.722 Atherosclerosis of other type of bypass graft(s) of the extremities with rest pain, left leg A

I70.723 Atherosclerosis of other type of bypass graft(s) of the extremities with rest pain, bilateral legs A

I70.728 Atherosclerosis of other type of bypass graft(s) of the extremities with rest pain, other extremity A

I70.729 Atherosclerosis of other type of bypass graft(s) of the extremities with rest pain, unspecified extremity A

✓6th **I70.73 Atherosclerosis of other type of bypass graft(s) of the right leg with ulceration**
INCLUDES any condition classifiable to I70.711 and I70.721
Use additional code to identify severity of ulcer (L97.-)

I70.731 Atherosclerosis of other type of bypass graft(s) of the right leg with ulceration of thigh CH CL A

I70.732 Atherosclerosis of other type of bypass graft(s) of the right leg with ulceration of calf CH CL A

I70.733 Atherosclerosis of other type of bypass graft(s) of the right leg with ulceration of ankle CH CL A

I70.734 Atherosclerosis of other type of bypass graft(s) of the right leg with ulceration of heel and midfoot CH CL A
Atherosclerosis of other type of bypass graft(s) of right leg with ulceration of plantar surface of midfoot

I70.735 Atherosclerosis of other type of bypass graft(s) of the right leg with ulceration of other part of foot CH CL A
Atherosclerosis of other type of bypass graft(s) of right leg with ulceration of toe

I70.738 Atherosclerosis of other type of bypass graft(s) of the right leg with ulceration of other part of lower leg CH CL A

I70.739 Atherosclerosis of other type of bypass graft(s) of the right leg with ulceration of unspecified site CH CL A

✓6th **I70.74 Atherosclerosis of other type of bypass graft(s) of the left leg with ulceration**
INCLUDES any condition classifiable to I70.712 and I70.722
Use additional code to identify severity of ulcer (L97.-)

I70.741 Atherosclerosis of other type of bypass graft(s) of the left leg with ulceration of thigh CH CL A

I70.742 Atherosclerosis of other type of bypass graft(s) of the left leg with ulceration of calf CH CL A

I70.743 Atherosclerosis of other type of bypass graft(s) of the left leg with ulceration of ankle CH CL A

I70.744 Atherosclerosis of other type of bypass graft(s) of the left leg with ulceration of heel and midfoot CH CL A
Atherosclerosis of other type of bypass graft(s) of left leg with ulceration of plantar surface of midfoot

I70.745 Atherosclerosis of other type of bypass graft(s) of the left leg with ulceration of other part of foot CH CL A
Atherosclerosis of other type of bypass graft(s) of left leg with ulceration of toe

I70.748 Atherosclerosis of other type of bypass graft(s) of the left leg with ulceration of other part of lower leg CH CL A

I70.749 Atherosclerosis of other type of bypass graft(s) of the left leg with ulceration of unspecified site   `CH` `CL` `A`

I70.75 Atherosclerosis of other type of bypass graft(s) of other extremity with ulceration   `A`

> `INCLUDES` any condition classifiable to I70.718 and I70.728
>
> Use additional code to identify severity of ulcer (L98.49)

√6ᵗʰ **I70.76** Atherosclerosis of other type of bypass graft(s) of the extremities with gangrene

> `INCLUDES` any condition classifiable to I70.71-, I70.72-, I70.73-, I70.74-, I70.75
>
> Use additional code to identify the severity of any ulcer (L97.-, L98.49-), if applicable

I70.761 Atherosclerosis of other type of bypass graft(s) of the extremities with gangrene, right leg   `A`

I70.762 Atherosclerosis of other type of bypass graft(s) of the extremities with gangrene, left leg   `A`

I70.763 Atherosclerosis of other type of bypass graft(s) of the extremities with gangrene, bilateral legs   `A`

I70.768 Atherosclerosis of other type of bypass graft(s) of the extremities with gangrene, other extremity   `A`

I70.769 Atherosclerosis of other type of bypass graft(s) of the extremities with gangrene, unspecified extremity   `A`

√6ᵗʰ **I70.79** Other atherosclerosis of other type of bypass graft(s) of the extremities

I70.791 Other atherosclerosis of other type of bypass graft(s) of the extremities, right leg   `A`

I70.792 Other atherosclerosis of other type of bypass graft(s) of the extremities, left leg   `A`

I70.793 Other atherosclerosis of other type of bypass graft(s) of the extremities, bilateral legs   `A`

I70.798 Other atherosclerosis of other type of bypass graft(s) of the extremities, other extremity   `A`

I70.799 Other atherosclerosis of other type of bypass graft(s) of the extremities, unspecified extremity   `A`

I70.8 Atherosclerosis of other arteries   `A`

> **TIP:** Arteriosclerosis of the iliac arteries is coded here.

√5ᵗʰ **I70.9** Other and unspecified atherosclerosis

I70.90 Unspecified atherosclerosis   `CH` `A`

I70.91 Generalized atherosclerosis   `CH` `A`

I70.92 Chronic total occlusion of artery of the extremities   `A`

> Complete occlusion of artery of the extremities
> Total occlusion of artery of the extremities
> Code first atherosclerosis of arteries of the extremities (I70.2-, I70.3-, I70.4-, I70.5-, I70.6-, I70.7-)

√4ᵗʰ **I71 Aortic aneurysm and dissection**

> `EXCLUDES 1` aortic ectasia (I77.81-)
> syphilitic aortic aneurysm (A52.01)
> traumatic aortic aneurysm (S25.09, S35.09)

√5ᵗʰ **I71.0** Dissection of aorta

I71.00 Dissection of unspecified site of aorta

I71.01 Dissection of thoracic aorta

I71.02 Dissection of abdominal aorta

I71.03 Dissection of thoracoabdominal aorta

I71.1 Thoracic aortic aneurysm, ruptured

I71.2 Thoracic aortic aneurysm, without rupture   `CH`

I71.3 Abdominal aortic aneurysm, ruptured

I71.4 Abdominal aortic aneurysm, without rupture   `CH`

I71.5 Thoracoabdominal aortic aneurysm, ruptured

I71.6 Thoracoabdominal aortic aneurysm, without rupture   `CH`

I71.8 Aortic aneurysm of unspecified site, ruptured
> Rupture of aorta NOS

I71.9 Aortic aneurysm of unspecified site, without rupture
> Aneurysm of aorta
> Dilatation of aorta
> Hyaline necrosis of aorta

√4ᵗʰ **I72 Other aneurysm**

> `INCLUDES` aneurysm (cirsoid) (false) (ruptured)
>
> `EXCLUDES 2` acquired aneurysm (I77.0)
> aneurysm (of) aorta (I71.-)
> aneurysm (of) arteriovenous NOS (Q27.3-)
> carotid artery dissection (I77.71)
> cerebral (nonruptured) aneurysm (I67.1)
> coronary aneurysm (I25.4)
> coronary artery dissection (I25.42)
> dissection of artery NEC (I77.79)
> dissection of precerebral artery, congenital (nonruptured) (Q28.1)
> heart aneurysm (I25.3)
> iliac artery dissection (I77.72)
> precerebral artery, congenital (nonruptured) (Q28.1)
> pulmonary artery aneurysm (I28.1)
> renal artery dissection (I77.73)
> retinal aneurysm (H35.0)
> ruptured cerebral aneurysm (I60.7)
> varicose aneurysm (I77.0)
> vertebral artery dissection (I77.74)

AHA: 2016,4Q,28-29

I72.0 Aneurysm of carotid artery
> Aneurysm of common carotid artery
> Aneurysm of external carotid artery
> Aneurysm of internal carotid artery, extracranial portion
>> `EXCLUDES 1` aneurysm of internal carotid artery, intracranial portion (I67.1)
>> aneurysm of internal carotid artery NOS (I67.1)

I72.1 Aneurysm of artery of upper extremity

I72.2 Aneurysm of renal artery

I72.3 Aneurysm of iliac artery

I72.4 Aneurysm of artery of lower extremity
> **AHA:** 2019,2Q,21

I72.5 Aneurysm of other precerebral arteries
> Aneurysm of basilar artery (trunk)
>> `EXCLUDES 2` aneurysm of carotid artery (I72.0)
>> aneurysm of vertebral artery (I72.6)
>> dissection of carotid artery (I77.71)
>> dissection of other precerebral arteries (I77.75)
>> dissection of vertebral artery (I77.74)

I72.6 Aneurysm of vertebral artery
>> `EXCLUDES 2` dissection of vertebral artery (I77.74)

I72.8 Aneurysm of other specified arteries

I72.9 Aneurysm of unspecified site

Aneurysm

- Layers of muscular and elastic tissue
- Outer layer
- Inner layer
- Aneurysm

☑ Additional Character Required   √x7ᵗʰ Placeholder Alert   Manifestation   Unspecified Dx   ▶◀ Revised Text   ● New Code   ▲ Revised Title

Chapter 9. Diseases of the Circulatory System

✓4ᵗʰ **I73 Other peripheral vascular diseases**

EXCLUDES 2   *chilblains (T69.1)*
            frostbite (T33-T34)
            immersion hand or foot (T69.0-)
            spasm of cerebral artery (G45.9)

AHA: 2018,4Q,87

✓5ᵗʰ **I73.0 Raynaud's syndrome**

Raynaud's disease
Raynaud's phenomenon (secondary)
DEF: Constriction of the arteries of the digits caused by cold or by nerve or arterial damage and can be prompted by stress or emotion. Blood cannot reach the skin and soft tissues and the skin turns white with blue mottling.

I73.00 Raynaud's syndrome without gangrene
I73.01 Raynaud's syndrome with gangrene

I73.1 Thromboangiitis obliterans [Buerger's disease]
DEF: Inflammatory disease of the extremity blood vessels, mainly the lower blood vessels. This disease is associated with heavy tobacco use. The arteries are more affected than veins. It occurs primarily in young men and leads to tissue ischemia and gangrene.

✓5ᵗʰ **I73.8 Other specified peripheral vascular diseases**

EXCLUDES 1   *diabetic (peripheral) angiopathy (E08-E13 with .51-.52)*

I73.81 Erythromelalgia
I73.89 Other specified peripheral vascular diseases
Acrocyanosis
Erythrocyanosis
Simple acroparesthesia [Schultze's type]
Vasomotor acroparesthesia [Nothnagel's type]

I73.9 Peripheral vascular disease, unspecified CH

Intermittent claudication
Peripheral angiopathy NOS
Spasm of artery
EXCLUDES 1   *atherosclerosis of the extremities (I70.2-I70.7-)*
AHA: 2018,2Q,7

✓4ᵗʰ **I74 Arterial embolism and thrombosis**

INCLUDES   embolic infarction
            embolic occlusion
            thrombotic infarction
            thrombotic occlusion

Code first:
embolism and thrombosis complicating abortion or ectopic or molar pregnancy (O00-O07, O08.2)
embolism and thrombosis complicating pregnancy, childbirth and the puerperium (O88.-)

EXCLUDES 2   *atheroembolism (I75.-)*
            basilar embolism and thrombosis (I63.0-I63.2, I65.1)
            carotid embolism and thrombosis (I63.0-I63.2, I65.2)
            cerebral embolism and thrombosis (I63.3-I63.5, I66.-)
            coronary embolism and thrombosis (I21-I25)
            mesenteric embolism and thrombosis (K55.0-)
            ophthalmic embolism and thrombosis (H34.-)
            precerebral embolism and thrombosis NOS (I63.0-I63.2, I65.9)
            pulmonary embolism and thrombosis (I26.-)
            renal embolism and thrombosis (N28.0)
            retinal embolism and thrombosis (H34.-)
            septic embolism and thrombosis (I76)
            vertebral embolism and thrombosis (I63.0-I63.2, I65.0)

✓5ᵗʰ **I74.0 Embolism and thrombosis of** abdominal aorta

I74.01 Saddle embolus of abdominal aorta
I74.09 Other arterial embolism and thrombosis of abdominal aorta
Aortic bifurcation syndrome
Aortoiliac obstruction
Leriche's syndrome

✓5ᵗʰ **I74.1 Embolism and thrombosis of other and unspecified parts of aorta**

I74.10 Embolism and thrombosis of unspecified parts of aorta
I74.11 Embolism and thrombosis of thoracic **aorta**
I74.19 Embolism and thrombosis of other parts of aorta
I74.2 Embolism and thrombosis of arteries of the upper extremities
I74.3 Embolism and thrombosis of arteries of the lower extremities

I74.4 Embolism and thrombosis of arteries of extremities, unspecified
Peripheral arterial embolism NOS
I74.5 Embolism and thrombosis of iliac **artery**
I74.8 Embolism and thrombosis of other arteries
I74.9 Embolism and thrombosis of unspecified artery

✓4ᵗʰ **I75 Atheroembolism**

INCLUDES   atherothrombotic microembolism
            cholesterol embolism

✓5ᵗʰ **I75.0 Atheroembolism of** extremities

✓6ᵗʰ **I75.01 Atheroembolism of** upper **extremity**

I75.011 Atheroembolism of right **upper extremity**
I75.012 Atheroembolism of left **upper extremity**
I75.013 Atheroembolism of bilateral **upper extremities**
I75.019 Atheroembolism of unspecified upper extremity

✓6ᵗʰ **I75.02 Atheroembolism of** lower **extremity**

I75.021 Atheroembolism of right **lower extremity**
I75.022 Atheroembolism of left **lower extremity**
I75.023 Atheroembolism of bilateral **lower extremities**
I75.029 Atheroembolism of unspecified lower extremity

✓5ᵗʰ **I75.8 Atheroembolism of other sites**

I75.81 Atheroembolism of kidney
Use additional code for any associated acute kidney failure and chronic kidney disease (N17.-, N18.-)
I75.89 Atheroembolism of other site

I76 Septic arterial embolism
Code first underlying infection, such as:
infective endocarditis (I33.0)
lung abscess (J85.-)
Use additional code to identify the site of the embolism (I74.-)
EXCLUDES 2   *septic pulmonary embolism (I26.01, I26.90)*

✓4ᵗʰ **I77 Other disorders of arteries and arterioles**

EXCLUDES 2   *collagen (vascular) diseases (M30-M36)*
            hypersensitivity angiitis (M31.0)
            pulmonary artery (I28.-)

I77.0 Arteriovenous fistula, acquired
Aneurysmal varix
Arteriovenous aneurysm, acquired
EXCLUDES 1   *arteriovenous aneurysm NOS (Q27.3-)*
            presence of arteriovenous shunt (fistula) for dialysis (Z99.2)
            traumatic — see injury of blood vessel by body region
EXCLUDES 2   *cerebral (I67.1)*
            coronary (I25.4)
DEF: Communication between an artery and vein caused by trauma or invasive procedures.

I77.1 Stricture of artery
Narrowing of artery

I77.2 Rupture of artery
Erosion of artery
Fistula of artery
Ulcer of artery
EXCLUDES 1   *traumatic rupture of artery — see injury of blood vessel by body region*

I77.3 Arterial fibromuscular dysplasia
Fibromuscular hyperplasia (of) carotid artery
Fibromuscular hyperplasia (of) renal artery

I77.4 Celiac artery compression syndrome
I77.5 Necrosis of artery
I77.6 Arteritis, unspecified
Aortitis NOS
Endarteritis NOS
EXCLUDES 1   *arteritis or endarteritis:*
            aortic arch (M31.4)
            cerebral NEC (I67.7)
            coronary (I25.89)
            deformans (I70.-)
            giant cell (M31.5, M31.6)
            obliterans (I70.-)
            senile (I70.-)

N Newborn: 0   P Pediatric: 0-17   M Maternity: 12-55   A Adult: 15-124   CH Comorbidity High   CL Comorbidity Low   NCDx Noncancer Dx   PDx Primary Dx

666   ICD-10-CM 2020

✓5ᵗʰ **I77.7 Other arterial dissection**
- EXCLUDES 2   *dissection of aorta (I71.0-)*
- *dissection of coronary artery (I25.42)*
- **AHA:** 2016,4Q,28-29

  I77.70 Dissection of unspecified artery
  I77.71 Dissection of carotid artery
  I77.72 Dissection of iliac artery
  I77.73 Dissection of renal artery
  I77.74 Dissection of vertebral artery
  - EXCLUDES 2   *aneurysm of vertebral artery (I72.6)*

  I77.75 Dissection of other precerebral arteries
  Dissection of basilar artery (trunk)
  - EXCLUDES 2   *aneurysm of carotid artery (I72.0)*
  - *aneurysm of other precerebral arteries (I72.5)*
  - *aneurysm of vertebral artery (I72.6)*
  - *dissection of carotid artery (I77.71)*
  - *dissection of vertebral artery (I77.74)*

  I77.76 Dissection of artery of upper extremity
  I77.77 Dissection of artery of lower extremity
  I77.79 Dissection of other specified artery

✓5ᵗʰ **I77.8 Other specified disorders of arteries and arterioles**

  ✓6ᵗʰ **I77.81 Aortic ectasia**
  Ectasis aorta
  - EXCLUDES 1   *aortic aneurysm and dissection (I71.0-)*

    I77.810 Thoracic aortic ectasia
    I77.811 Abdominal aortic ectasia
    I77.812 Thoracoabdominal aortic ectasia
    I77.819 Aortic ectasia, unspecified site
  I77.89 Other specified disorders of arteries and arterioles
I77.9 Disorder of arteries and arterioles, unspecified
  AHA: 2018,2Q,7

✓4ᵗʰ **I78 Diseases of capillaries**

I78.0 Hereditary hemorrhagic telangiectasia
  Rendu-Osler-Weber disease

I78.1 Nevus, non-neoplastic
  Araneus nevus
  Senile nevus
  Spider nevus
  Stellar nevus
  - EXCLUDES 1   *nevus NOS (D22.-)*
  - *vascular NOS (Q82.5)*
  - EXCLUDES 2   *blue nevus (D22.-)*
  - *flammeus nevus (Q82.5)*
  - *hairy nevus (D22.-)*
  - *melanocytic nevus (D22.-)*
  - *pigmented nevus (D22.-)*
  - *portwine nevus (Q82.5)*
  - *sanguineous nevus (Q82.5)*
  - *strawberry nevus (Q82.5)*
  - *verrucous nevus (Q82.5)*
  - **AHA:** 2019,1Q,21

I78.8 Other diseases of capillaries
I78.9 Disease of capillaries, unspecified

✓4ᵗʰ **I79 Disorders of arteries, arterioles and capillaries in diseases classified elsewhere**

I79.0 Aneurysm of aorta in diseases classified elsewhere   CM
  Code first underlying disease
  - EXCLUDES 1   *syphilitic aneurysm (A52.01)*

I79.1 Aortitis in diseases classified elsewhere
  Code first underlying disease
  - EXCLUDES 1   *syphilitic aortitis (A52.02)*

I79.8 Other disorders of arteries, arterioles and capillaries in diseases classified elsewhere
  Code first underlying disease, such as:
  amyloidosis (E85.-)
  - EXCLUDES 1   *diabetic (peripheral) angiopathy (E08-E13 with .51-.52)*
  - *syphilitic endarteritis (A52.09)*
  - *tuberculous endarteritis (A18.89)*

Diseases of veins, lymphatic vessels and lymph nodes, not elsewhere classified (I80-I89)

✓4ᵗʰ **I80 Phlebitis and thrombophlebitis**
- INCLUDES   endophlebitis
  inflammation, vein
  periphlebitis
  suppurative phlebitis
- Code first:
  phlebitis and thrombophlebitis complicating abortion, ectopic or molar pregnancy (O00-O07, O08.7)
  phlebitis and thrombophlebitis complicating pregnancy, childbirth and the puerperium (O22.-, O87.-)
- EXCLUDES 1   *venous embolism and thrombosis of lower extremities (I82.4-, I82.5-, I82.81-)*

✓5ᵗʰ **I80.0 Phlebitis and thrombophlebitis of superficial vessels of lower extremities**
  Phlebitis and thrombophlebitis of femoropopliteal vein

  I80.00 Phlebitis and thrombophlebitis of superficial vessels of unspecified lower extremity
  I80.01 Phlebitis and thrombophlebitis of superficial vessels of right lower extremity
  I80.02 Phlebitis and thrombophlebitis of superficial vessels of left lower extremity
  I80.03 Phlebitis and thrombophlebitis of superficial vessels of lower extremities, bilateral

✓5ᵗʰ **I80.1 Phlebitis and thrombophlebitis of femoral vein**
  ▶Phlebitis and thrombophlebitis of common femoral vein◀
  ▶Phlebitis and thrombophlebitis of deep femoral vein◀

  I80.10 Phlebitis and thrombophlebitis of unspecified femoral vein
  I80.11 Phlebitis and thrombophlebitis of right femoral vein
  I80.12 Phlebitis and thrombophlebitis of left femoral vein
  I80.13 Phlebitis and thrombophlebitis of femoral vein, bilateral

✓5ᵗʰ **I80.2 Phlebitis and thrombophlebitis of other and unspecified deep vessels of lower extremities**

  ✓6ᵗʰ **I80.20 Phlebitis and thrombophlebitis of unspecified deep vessels of lower extremities**
    I80.201 Phlebitis and thrombophlebitis of unspecified deep vessels of right lower extremity
    I80.202 Phlebitis and thrombophlebitis of unspecified deep vessels of left lower extremity
    I80.203 Phlebitis and thrombophlebitis of unspecified deep vessels of lower extremities, bilateral
    I80.209 Phlebitis and thrombophlebitis of unspecified deep vessels of unspecified lower extremity

  ✓6ᵗʰ **I80.21 Phlebitis and thrombophlebitis of iliac vein**
    ▶Phlebitis and thrombophlebitis of common iliac vein◀
    ▶Phlebitis and thrombophlebitis of external iliac vein◀
    ▶Phlebitis and thrombophlebitis of internal iliac vein◀
    I80.211 Phlebitis and thrombophlebitis of right iliac vein
    I80.212 Phlebitis and thrombophlebitis of left iliac vein
    I80.213 Phlebitis and thrombophlebitis of iliac vein, bilateral
    I80.219 Phlebitis and thrombophlebitis of unspecified iliac vein

  ✓6ᵗʰ **I80.22 Phlebitis and thrombophlebitis of popliteal vein**
    I80.221 Phlebitis and thrombophlebitis of right popliteal vein
    I80.222 Phlebitis and thrombophlebitis of left popliteal vein
    I80.223 Phlebitis and thrombophlebitis of popliteal vein, bilateral
    I80.229 Phlebitis and thrombophlebitis of unspecified popliteal vein

  ✓6ᵗʰ **I80.23 Phlebitis and thrombophlebitis of tibial vein**
    ▶Phlebitis and thrombophlebitis of anterior tibial vein◀
    ▶Phlebitis and thrombophlebitis of posterior tibial vein◀
    I80.231 Phlebitis and thrombophlebitis of right tibial vein

✅ Additional Character Required   ✓x7ᵗʰ Placeholder Alert   Manifestation   Unspecified Dx   ▶◀ Revised Text   ● New Code   ▲ Revised Title

ICD-10-CM 2020   **667**

I80.232 Phlebitis and thrombophlebitis of left tibial vein

I80.233 Phlebitis and thrombophlebitis of tibial vein, bilateral

I80.239 Phlebitis and thrombophlebitis of unspecified tibial vein

√6ᵗʰ **I80.24 Phlebitis and thrombophlebitis of peroneal vein**

I80.241 Phlebitis and thrombophlebitis of right peroneal vein

I80.242 Phlebitis and thrombophlebitis of left peroneal vein

I80.243 Phlebitis and thrombophlebitis of peroneal vein, bilateral

I80.249 Phlebitis and thrombophlebitis of unspecified peroneal vein

√6ᵗʰ **I80.25 Phlebitis and thrombophlebitis of calf muscular vein**

Phlebitis and thrombophlebitis of calf muscular vein, NOS
Phlebitis and thrombophlebitis of gastrocnemial vein
Phlebitis and thrombophlebitis of soleal vein

I80.251 Phlebitis and thrombophlebitis of right calf muscular vein

I80.252 Phlebitis and thrombophlebitis of left calf muscular vein

I80.253 Phlebitis and thrombophlebitis of calf muscular vein, bilateral

I80.259 Phlebitis and thrombophlebitis of unspecified calf muscular vein

√6ᵗʰ **I80.29 Phlebitis and thrombophlebitis of other deep vessels of lower extremities**

I80.291 Phlebitis and thrombophlebitis of other deep vessels of right lower extremity

I80.292 Phlebitis and thrombophlebitis of other deep vessels of left lower extremity

I80.293 Phlebitis and thrombophlebitis of other deep vessels of lower extremity, bilateral

I80.299 Phlebitis and thrombophlebitis of other deep vessels of unspecified lower extremity

I80.3 Phlebitis and thrombophlebitis of lower extremities, unspecified

I80.8 Phlebitis and thrombophlebitis of other sites

I80.9 Phlebitis and thrombophlebitis of unspecified site

I81 Portal vein thrombosis

Portal (vein) obstruction

EXCLUDES 2   hepatic vein thrombosis (I82.0)
phlebitis of portal vein (K75.1)

√4ᵗʰ **I82 Other venous embolism and thrombosis**

Code first venous embolism and thrombosis complicating:
abortion, ectopic or molar pregnancy (O00-O07, O08.7)
pregnancy, childbirth and the puerperium (O22.-, O87.-)

EXCLUDES 2   venous embolism and thrombosis (of):
cerebral (I63.6, I67.6)
coronary (I21-I25)
intracranial and intraspinal, septic or NOS (G08)
intracranial, nonpyogenic (I67.6)
intraspinal, nonpyogenic (G95.1)
mesenteric (K55.0-)
portal (I81)
pulmonary (I26.-)

I82.0 Budd-Chiari syndrome   CL

Hepatic vein thrombosis
DEF: Thrombosis or other obstruction of the hepatic veins. Symptoms include an enlarged liver, extensive collateral vessels, intractable ascites, and severe portal hypertension.

I82.1 Thrombophlebitis migrans   CL

√5ᵗʰ **I82.2 Embolism and thrombosis of vena cava and other thoracic veins**

√6ᵗʰ **I82.21 Embolism and thrombosis of superior vena cava**

I82.210 Acute embolism and thrombosis of superior vena cava   CL

Embolism and thrombosis of superior vena cava NOS

I82.211 Chronic embolism and thrombosis of superior vena cava   CL

√6ᵗʰ **I82.22 Embolism and thrombosis of inferior vena cava**

I82.220 Acute embolism and thrombosis of inferior vena cava   CL

Embolism and thrombosis of inferior vena cava NOS

I82.221 Chronic embolism and thrombosis of inferior vena cava   CL

√6ᵗʰ **I82.29 Embolism and thrombosis of other thoracic veins**

Embolism and thrombosis of brachiocephalic (innominate) vein

I82.290 Acute embolism and thrombosis of other thoracic veins   CL

I82.291 Chronic embolism and thrombosis of other thoracic veins   CL

I82.3 Embolism and thrombosis of renal vein   CL

√5ᵗʰ **I82.4 Acute embolism and thrombosis of deep veins of lower extremity**

√6ᵗʰ **I82.40 Acute embolism and thrombosis of unspecified deep veins of lower extremity**

Deep vein thrombosis NOS
DVT NOS

EXCLUDES 1   acute embolism and thrombosis of unspecified deep veins of distal lower extremity (I82.4Z-)
acute embolism and thrombosis of unspecified deep veins of proximal lower extremity (I82.4Y-)

I82.401 Acute embolism and thrombosis of unspecified deep veins of right lower extremity   CL

I82.402 Acute embolism and thrombosis of unspecified deep veins of left lower extremity   CL

I82.403 Acute embolism and thrombosis of unspecified deep veins of lower extremity, bilateral   CL

I82.409 Acute embolism and thrombosis of unspecified deep veins of unspecified lower extremity

√6ᵗʰ **I82.41 Acute embolism and thrombosis of femoral vein**

▶Acute embolism and thrombosis of common femoral vein◀
▶Acute embolism and thrombosis of deep femoral vein◀

I82.411 Acute embolism and thrombosis of right femoral vein   CL

I82.412 Acute embolism and thrombosis of left femoral vein   CL

I82.413 Acute embolism and thrombosis of femoral vein, bilateral   CL

I82.419 Acute embolism and thrombosis of unspecified femoral vein

√6ᵗʰ **I82.42 Acute embolism and thrombosis of iliac vein**

▶Acute embolism and thrombosis of common iliac vein◀
▶Acute embolism and thrombosis of external iliac vein◀
▶Acute embolism and thrombosis of internal iliac vein◀

I82.421 Acute embolism and thrombosis of right iliac vein   CL

I82.422 Acute embolism and thrombosis of left iliac vein   CL

I82.423 Acute embolism and thrombosis of iliac vein, bilateral   CL

I82.429 Acute embolism and thrombosis of unspecified iliac vein

N Newborn: 0   P Pediatric: 0-17   M Maternity: 12-55   A Adult: 15-124   CH Comorbidity High   CL Comorbidity Low   NCDx Noncancer Dx   PDx Primary Dx

668   ICD-10-CM 2020

√6ᵗʰ **I82.43** **Acute embolism and thrombosis of popliteal vein**

I82.431 **Acute embolism and thrombosis of right popliteal vein** `CL`

I82.432 **Acute embolism and thrombosis of left popliteal vein** `CL`

I82.433 **Acute embolism and thrombosis of popliteal vein, bilateral** `CL`

I82.439 **Acute embolism and thrombosis of unspecified popliteal vein**

√6ᵗʰ **I82.44** **Acute embolism and thrombosis of tibial vein**

►Acute embolism and thrombosis of anterior tibial vein◄

►Acute embolism and thrombosis of posterior tibial vein◄

I82.441 **Acute embolism and thrombosis of right tibial vein** `CL`

I82.442 **Acute embolism and thrombosis of left tibial vein** `CL`

I82.443 **Acute embolism and thrombosis of tibial vein, bilateral** `CL`

I82.449 **Acute embolism and thrombosis of unspecified tibial vein**

• √6ᵗʰ **I82.45** **Acute embolism and thrombosis of peroneal vein**

• **I82.451** **Acute embolism and thrombosis of right peroneal vein**

• **I82.452** **Acute embolism and thrombosis of left peroneal vein**

• **I82.453** **Acute embolism and thrombosis of peroneal vein, bilateral**

• **I82.459** **Acute embolism and thrombosis of unspecified peroneal vein**

• √6ᵗʰ **I82.46** **Acute embolism and thrombosis of calf muscular vein**

Acute embolism and thrombosis of calf muscular vein, NOS

Acute embolism and thrombosis of gastrocnemial vein

Acute embolism and thrombosis of soleal vein

• **I82.461** **Acute embolism and thrombosis of right calf muscular vein**

• **I82.462** **Acute embolism and thrombosis of left calf muscular vein**

• **I82.463** **Acute embolism and thrombosis of calf muscular vein, bilateral**

• **I82.469** **Acute embolism and thrombosis of unspecified calf muscular vein**

√6ᵗʰ **I82.49** **Acute embolism and thrombosis of other specified deep vein of lower extremity**

I82.491 **Acute embolism and thrombosis of other specified deep vein of right lower extremity** `CL`

I82.492 **Acute embolism and thrombosis of other specified deep vein of left lower extremity** `CL`

I82.493 **Acute embolism and thrombosis of other specified deep vein of lower extremity, bilateral** `CL`

I82.499 **Acute embolism and thrombosis of other specified deep vein of unspecified lower extremity**

√6ᵗʰ **I82.4Y** **Acute embolism and thrombosis of unspecified deep veins of proximal lower extremity**

Acute embolism and thrombosis of deep vein of thigh NOS

Acute embolism and thrombosis of deep vein of upper leg NOS

I82.4Y1 **Acute embolism and thrombosis of unspecified deep veins of right proximal lower extremity** `CL`

I82.4Y2 **Acute embolism and thrombosis of unspecified deep veins of left proximal lower extremity** `CL`

I82.4Y3 **Acute embolism and thrombosis of unspecified deep veins of proximal lower extremity, bilateral** `CL`

I82.4Y9 **Acute embolism and thrombosis of unspecified deep veins of unspecified proximal lower extremity**

√6ᵗʰ **I82.4Z** **Acute embolism and thrombosis of unspecified deep veins of distal lower extremity**

Acute embolism and thrombosis of deep vein of calf NOS

Acute embolism and thrombosis of deep vein of lower leg NOS

I82.4Z1 **Acute embolism and thrombosis of unspecified deep veins of right distal lower extremity** `CL`

I82.4Z2 **Acute embolism and thrombosis of unspecified deep veins of left distal lower extremity** `CL`

I82.4Z3 **Acute embolism and thrombosis of unspecified deep veins of distal lower extremity, bilateral** `CL`

I82.4Z9 **Acute embolism and thrombosis of unspecified deep veins of unspecified distal lower extremity**

√5ᵗʰ **I82.5** **Chronic embolism and thrombosis of deep veins of lower extremity**

Use additional code, if applicable, for associated long-term (current) use of anticoagulants (Z79.01)

EXCLUDES 1   personal history of venous embolism and thrombosis (Z86.718)

√6ᵗʰ **I82.50** **Chronic embolism and thrombosis of unspecified deep veins of lower extremity**

EXCLUDES 1   chronic embolism and thrombosis of unspecified deep veins of distal lower extremity (I82.5Z-)

chronic embolism and thrombosis of unspecified deep veins of proximal lower extremity (I82.5Y-)

I82.501 **Chronic embolism and thrombosis of unspecified deep veins of right lower extremity** `CL`

I82.502 **Chronic embolism and thrombosis of unspecified deep veins of left lower extremity** `CL`

I82.503 **Chronic embolism and thrombosis of unspecified deep veins of lower extremity, bilateral** `CL`

I82.509 **Chronic embolism and thrombosis of unspecified deep veins of unspecified lower extremity**

√6ᵗʰ **I82.51** **Chronic embolism and thrombosis of femoral vein**

►Chronic embolism and thrombosis of common femoral vein◄

►Chronic embolism and thrombosis of deep femoral vein◄

I82.511 **Chronic embolism and thrombosis of right femoral vein** `CL`

I82.512 **Chronic embolism and thrombosis of left femoral vein** `CL`

I82.513 **Chronic embolism and thrombosis of femoral vein, bilateral** `CL`

I82.519 **Chronic embolism and thrombosis of unspecified femoral vein**

√6ᵗʰ **I82.52** **Chronic embolism and thrombosis of iliac vein**

►Chronic embolism and thrombosis of common iliac vein◄

►Chronic embolism and thrombosis of external iliac vein◄

►Chronic embolism and thrombosis of internal iliac vein◄

I82.521 **Chronic embolism and thrombosis of right iliac vein** `CL`

☑ Additional Character Required   √x7ᵗʰ Placeholder Alert   Manifestation   Unspecified Dx   ►◄ Revised Text   ● New Code   ▲ Revised Title

I82.522   **Chronic embolism and thrombosis of** left **iliac vein** `CL`

I82.523   **Chronic embolism and thrombosis of iliac vein,** bilateral `CL`

I82.529   **Chronic embolism and thrombosis of unspecified iliac vein**

✓6ᵗʰ **I82.53**   **Chronic embolism and thrombosis of** popliteal vein

    I82.531   **Chronic embolism and thrombosis of** right **popliteal vein** `CL`

    I82.532   **Chronic embolism and thrombosis of** left **popliteal vein** `CL`

    I82.533   **Chronic embolism and thrombosis of popliteal vein,** bilateral `CL`

    I82.539   **Chronic embolism and thrombosis of unspecified popliteal vein**

✓6ᵗʰ **I82.54**   **Chronic embolism and thrombosis of** tibial vein

    ▶Chronic embolism and thrombosis of anterior tibial vein◀

    ▶Chronic embolism and thrombosis of posterior tibial vein◀

    I82.541   **Chronic embolism and thrombosis of** right **tibial vein** `CL`

    I82.542   **Chronic embolism and thrombosis of** left **tibial vein** `CL`

    I82.543   **Chronic embolism and thrombosis of tibial vein,** bilateral `CL`

    I82.549   **Chronic embolism and thrombosis of unspecified tibial vein**

● ✓6ᵗʰ **I82.55**   **Chronic embolism and thrombosis of** peroneal vein

●   **I82.551**   **Chronic embolism and thrombosis of** right peroneal vein

●   **I82.552**   **Chronic embolism and thrombosis of** left peroneal vein

●   **I82.553**   **Chronic embolism and thrombosis of** peroneal vein, bilateral

●   **I82.559**   **Chronic embolism and thrombosis of unspecified peroneal vein**

● ✓6ᵗʰ **I82.56**   **Chronic embolism and thrombosis of** calf muscular vein

    Chronic embolism and thrombosis of calf muscular vein NOS

    Chronic embolism and thrombosis of gastrocnemial vein

    Chronic embolism and thrombosis of soleal vein

●   **I82.561**   **Chronic embolism and thrombosis of** right calf muscular vein

●   **I82.562**   **Chronic embolism and thrombosis of** left calf muscular vein

●   **I82.563**   **Chronic embolism and thrombosis of calf muscular vein,** bilateral

●   **I82.569**   **Chronic embolism and thrombosis of unspecified calf muscular vein**

✓6ᵗʰ **I82.59**   **Chronic embolism and thrombosis of other specified deep vein of lower extremity**

    I82.591   **Chronic embolism and thrombosis of other specified deep vein of** right **lower extremity** `CL`

    I82.592   **Chronic embolism and thrombosis of other specified deep vein of** left **lower extremity** `CL`

    I82.593   **Chronic embolism and thrombosis of other specified deep vein of lower extremity,** bilateral `CL`

    I82.599   **Chronic embolism and thrombosis of other specified deep vein of unspecified lower extremity**

✓6ᵗʰ **I82.5Y**   **Chronic embolism and thrombosis of unspecified deep veins of** proximal **lower extremity**

    Chronic embolism and thrombosis of deep veins of thigh NOS

    Chronic embolism and thrombosis of deep veins of upper leg NOS

    I82.5Y1   **Chronic embolism and thrombosis of unspecified deep veins of** right **proximal lower extremity** `CL`

    I82.5Y2   **Chronic embolism and thrombosis of unspecified deep veins of** left **proximal lower extremity** `CL`

    I82.5Y3   **Chronic embolism and thrombosis of unspecified deep veins of proximal lower extremity,** bilateral `CL`

    I82.5Y9   **Chronic embolism and thrombosis of unspecified deep veins of unspecified proximal lower extremity**

✓6ᵗʰ **I82.5Z**   **Chronic embolism and thrombosis of unspecified deep veins of** distal **lower extremity**

    Chronic embolism and thrombosis of deep veins of calf NOS

    Chronic embolism and thrombosis of deep veins of lower leg NOS

    I82.5Z1   **Chronic embolism and thrombosis of unspecified deep veins of** right **distal lower extremity** `CL`

    I82.5Z2   **Chronic embolism and thrombosis of unspecified deep veins of** left **distal lower extremity** `CL`

    I82.5Z3   **Chronic embolism and thrombosis of unspecified deep veins of distal lower extremity,** bilateral `CL`

    I82.5Z9   **Chronic embolism and thrombosis of unspecified deep veins of unspecified distal lower extremity**

✓5ᵗʰ **I82.6**   Acute **embolism and thrombosis of veins of** upper extremity

✓6ᵗʰ **I82.60**   **Acute embolism and thrombosis of unspecified veins of upper extremity**

    I82.601   **Acute embolism and thrombosis of unspecified veins of** right **upper extremity** `CL`

    I82.602   **Acute embolism and thrombosis of unspecified veins of** left **upper extremity** `CL`

    I82.603   **Acute embolism and thrombosis of unspecified veins of upper extremity,** bilateral `CL`

    I82.609   **Acute embolism and thrombosis of unspecified veins of unspecified upper extremity**

✓6ᵗʰ **I82.61**   **Acute embolism and thrombosis of** superficial veins **of upper extremity**

    Acute embolism and thrombosis of antecubital vein

    Acute embolism and thrombosis of basilic vein

    Acute embolism and thrombosis of cephalic vein

    I82.611   **Acute embolism and thrombosis of superficial veins of** right **upper extremity** `CL`

    I82.612   **Acute embolism and thrombosis of superficial veins of** left **upper extremity** `CL`

    I82.613   **Acute embolism and thrombosis of superficial veins of upper extremity,** bilateral `CL`

    I82.619   **Acute embolism and thrombosis of superficial veins of unspecified upper extremity**

✓6ᵗʰ **I82.62**   **Acute embolism and thrombosis of** deep veins **of upper extremity**

    Acute embolism and thrombosis of brachial vein

    Acute embolism and thrombosis of radial vein

    Acute embolism and thrombosis of ulnar vein

    I82.621   **Acute embolism and thrombosis of deep veins of** right **upper extremity** `CL`

N Newborn: 0   P Pediatric: 0-17   M Maternity: 12-55   A Adult: 15-124   `CH` Comorbidity High   `CL` Comorbidity Low   `NCDx` Noncancer Dx   `PDx` Primary Dx

670   ICD-10-CM 2020

I82.622   **Acute embolism and thrombosis of deep veins of left upper extremity** `CL`

I82.623   **Acute embolism and thrombosis of deep veins of upper extremity, bilateral** `CL`

I82.629   **Acute embolism and thrombosis of deep veins of unspecified upper extremity**

√5ᵗʰ **I82.7** Chronic embolism and thrombosis of veins of upper extremity

Use additional code, if applicable, for associated long-term (current) use of anticoagulants (Z79.01)

EXCLUDES 1   personal history of venous embolism and thrombosis (Z86.718)

√6ᵗʰ **I82.70** **Chronic embolism and thrombosis of unspecified veins of upper extremity**

I82.701   **Chronic embolism and thrombosis of unspecified veins of right upper extremity** `CL`

I82.702   **Chronic embolism and thrombosis of unspecified veins of left upper extremity** `CL`

I82.703   **Chronic embolism and thrombosis of unspecified veins of upper extremity, bilateral** `CL`

I82.709   **Chronic embolism and thrombosis of unspecified veins of unspecified upper extremity**

√6ᵗʰ **I82.71** **Chronic embolism and thrombosis of superficial veins of upper extremity**

Chronic embolism and thrombosis of antecubital vein
Chronic embolism and thrombosis of basilic vein
Chronic embolism and thrombosis of cephalic vein

I82.711   **Chronic embolism and thrombosis of superficial veins of right upper extremity** `CL`

I82.712   **Chronic embolism and thrombosis of superficial veins of left upper extremity** `CL`

I82.713   **Chronic embolism and thrombosis of superficial veins of upper extremity, bilateral** `CL`

I82.719   **Chronic embolism and thrombosis of superficial veins of unspecified upper extremity**

√6ᵗʰ **I82.72** **Chronic embolism and thrombosis of deep veins of upper extremity**

Chronic embolism and thrombosis of brachial vein
Chronic embolism and thrombosis of radial vein
Chronic embolism and thrombosis of ulnar vein

I82.721   **Chronic embolism and thrombosis of deep veins of right upper extremity** `CL`

I82.722   **Chronic embolism and thrombosis of deep veins of left upper extremity** `CL`

I82.723   **Chronic embolism and thrombosis of deep veins of upper extremity, bilateral** `CL`

I82.729   **Chronic embolism and thrombosis of deep veins of unspecified upper extremity**

√5ᵗʰ **I82.A** Embolism and thrombosis of axillary vein

√6ᵗʰ **I82.A1** Acute embolism and thrombosis of axillary vein

I82.A11   **Acute embolism and thrombosis of right axillary vein** `CL`

I82.A12   **Acute embolism and thrombosis of left axillary vein** `CL`

I82.A13   **Acute embolism and thrombosis of axillary vein, bilateral** `CL`

I82.A19   **Acute embolism and thrombosis of unspecified axillary vein**

√6ᵗʰ **I82.A2** Chronic embolism and thrombosis of axillary vein

I82.A21   **Chronic embolism and thrombosis of right axillary vein** `CL`

I82.A22   **Chronic embolism and thrombosis of left axillary vein** `CL`

I82.A23   **Chronic embolism and thrombosis of axillary vein, bilateral** `CL`

I82.A29   **Chronic embolism and thrombosis of unspecified axillary vein**

√5ᵗʰ **I82.B** Embolism and thrombosis of subclavian vein

√6ᵗʰ **I82.B1** Acute embolism and thrombosis of subclavian vein

I82.B11   **Acute embolism and thrombosis of right subclavian vein** `CL`

I82.B12   **Acute embolism and thrombosis of left subclavian vein** `CL`

I82.B13   **Acute embolism and thrombosis of subclavian vein, bilateral** `CL`

I82.B19   **Acute embolism and thrombosis of unspecified subclavian vein**

√6ᵗʰ **I82.B2** Chronic embolism and thrombosis of subclavian vein

I82.B21   **Chronic embolism and thrombosis of right subclavian vein** `CL`

I82.B22   **Chronic embolism and thrombosis of left subclavian vein** `CL`

I82.B23   **Chronic embolism and thrombosis of subclavian vein, bilateral** `CL`

I82.B29   **Chronic embolism and thrombosis of unspecified subclavian vein**

√5ᵗʰ **I82.C** Embolism and thrombosis of internal jugular vein

√6ᵗʰ **I82.C1** Acute embolism and thrombosis of internal jugular vein

I82.C11   **Acute embolism and thrombosis of right internal jugular vein** `CL`

I82.C12   **Acute embolism and thrombosis of left internal jugular vein** `CL`

I82.C13   **Acute embolism and thrombosis of internal jugular vein, bilateral** `CL`

I82.C19   **Acute embolism and thrombosis of unspecified internal jugular vein**

√6ᵗʰ **I82.C2** Chronic embolism and thrombosis of internal jugular vein

I82.C21   **Chronic embolism and thrombosis of right internal jugular vein** `CL`

I82.C22   **Chronic embolism and thrombosis of left internal jugular vein** `CL`

I82.C23   **Chronic embolism and thrombosis of internal jugular vein, bilateral** `CL`

I82.C29   **Chronic embolism and thrombosis of unspecified internal jugular vein**

√5ᵗʰ **I82.8** Embolism and thrombosis of other specified veins

Use additional code, if applicable, for associated long-term (current) use of anticoagulants (Z79.01)

√6ᵗʰ **I82.81** **Embolism and thrombosis of superficial veins of lower extremities**

Embolism and thrombosis of saphenous vein (greater) (lesser)

I82.811   **Embolism and thrombosis of superficial veins of right lower extremity** `CL`

I82.812   **Embolism and thrombosis of superficial veins of left lower extremity** `CL`

I82.813   **Embolism and thrombosis of superficial veins of lower extremities, bilateral** `CL`

I82.819   **Embolism and thrombosis of superficial veins of unspecified lower extremity**

√6ᵗʰ **I82.89** **Embolism and thrombosis of other specified veins**

I82.890   **Acute embolism and thrombosis of other specified veins** `CL`

☑ Additional Character Required   √x7ᵗʰ Placeholder Alert   Manifestation   Unspecified Dx   ►◄ Revised Text   ● New Code   ▲ Revised Title

ICD-10-CM 2020   671

I82.891 Chronic embolism and thrombosis of other specified veins   `CL`

√5ᵗʰ **I82.9 Embolism and thrombosis of unspecified vein**

I82.90 Acute embolism and thrombosis of unspecified vein
Embolism of vein NOS
Thrombosis (vein) NOS

I82.91 Chronic embolism and thrombosis of unspecified vein

√4ᵗʰ **I83 Varicose veins of lower extremities**

EXCLUDES 1   *varicose veins complicating pregnancy (O22.0-)*
varicose veins complicating the puerperium (O87.4)

√5ᵗʰ **I83.0 Varicose veins of lower extremities with ulcer**
Use additional code to identify severity of ulcer (L97.-)

√6ᵗʰ **I83.00 Varicose veins of unspecified lower extremity with ulcer**

I83.001 Varicose veins of unspecified lower extremity with ulcer of thigh   `A`

I83.002 Varicose veins of unspecified lower extremity with ulcer of calf   `A`

I83.003 Varicose veins of unspecified lower extremity with ulcer of ankle   `A`

I83.004 Varicose veins of unspecified lower extremity with ulcer of heel and midfoot   `A`
Varicose veins of unspecified lower extremity with ulcer of plantar surface of midfoot

I83.005 Varicose veins of unspecified lower extremity with ulcer other part of foot   `A`
Varicose veins of unspecified lower extremity with ulcer of toe

I83.008 Varicose veins of unspecified lower extremity with ulcer other part of lower leg   `A`

I83.009 Varicose veins of unspecified lower extremity with ulcer of unspecified site   `A`

√6ᵗʰ **I83.01 Varicose veins of right lower extremity with ulcer**

I83.011 Varicose veins of right lower extremity with ulcer of thigh   `CH` `CL` `A`

I83.012 Varicose veins of right lower extremity with ulcer of calf   `CH` `CL` `A`

I83.013 Varicose veins of right lower extremity with ulcer of ankle   `CH` `CL` `A`

I83.014 Varicose veins of right lower extremity with ulcer of heel and midfoot   `CH` `CL` `A`
Varicose veins of right lower extremity with ulcer of plantar surface of midfoot

I83.015 Varicose veins of right lower extremity with ulcer other part of foot   `CH` `CL` `A`
Varicose veins of right lower extremity with ulcer of toe

I83.018 Varicose veins of right lower extremity with ulcer other part of lower leg   `CH` `CL` `A`

I83.019 Varicose veins of right lower extremity with ulcer of unspecified site   `A`

√6ᵗʰ **I83.02 Varicose veins of left lower extremity with ulcer**

I83.021 Varicose veins of left lower extremity with ulcer of thigh   `CH` `CL` `A`

I83.022 Varicose veins of left lower extremity with ulcer of calf   `CH` `CL` `A`

I83.023 Varicose veins of left lower extremity with ulcer of ankle   `CH` `CL` `A`

I83.024 Varicose veins of left lower extremity with ulcer of heel and midfoot   `CH` `CL` `A`
Varicose veins of left lower extremity with ulcer of plantar surface of midfoot

I83.025 Varicose veins of left lower extremity with ulcer other part of foot   `CH` `CL` `A`
Varicose veins of left lower extremity with ulcer of toe

I83.028 Varicose veins of left lower extremity with ulcer other part of lower leg   `CH` `CL` `A`

I83.029 Varicose veins of left lower extremity with ulcer of unspecified site   `A`

√5ᵗʰ **I83.1 Varicose veins of lower extremities with inflammation**

I83.10 Varicose veins of unspecified lower extremity with inflammation   `A`

I83.11 Varicose veins of right lower extremity with inflammation   `CH` `CL` `A`

I83.12 Varicose veins of left lower extremity with inflammation   `CH` `CL` `A`

√5ᵗʰ **I83.2 Varicose veins of lower extremities with both ulcer and inflammation**
Use additional code to identify severity of ulcer (L97.-)

√6ᵗʰ **I83.20 Varicose veins of unspecified lower extremity with both ulcer and inflammation**

I83.201 Varicose veins of unspecified lower extremity with both ulcer of thigh and inflammation   `A`

I83.202 Varicose veins of unspecified lower extremity with both ulcer of calf and inflammation   `A`

I83.203 Varicose veins of unspecified lower extremity with both ulcer of ankle and inflammation   `A`

I83.204 Varicose veins of unspecified lower extremity with both ulcer of heel and midfoot and inflammation   `A`
Varicose veins of unspecified lower extremity with both ulcer of plantar surface of midfoot and inflammation

I83.205 Varicose veins of unspecified lower extremity with both ulcer of other part of foot and inflammation   `A`
Varicose veins of unspecified lower extremity with both ulcer of toe and inflammation

I83.208 Varicose veins of unspecified lower extremity with both ulcer of other part of lower extremity and inflammation   `A`

I83.209 Varicose veins of unspecified lower extremity with both ulcer of unspecified site and inflammation   `A`

√6ᵗʰ **I83.21 Varicose veins of right lower extremity with both ulcer and inflammation**

I83.211 Varicose veins of right lower extremity with both ulcer of thigh and inflammation   `CH` `CL` `A`

I83.212 Varicose veins of right lower extremity with both ulcer of calf and inflammation   `CH` `CL` `A`

I83.213 Varicose veins of right lower extremity with both ulcer of ankle and inflammation   `CH` `CL` `A`

I83.214 Varicose veins of right lower extremity with both ulcer of heel and midfoot and inflammation   `CH` `CL` `A`
Varicose veins of right lower extremity with both ulcer of plantar surface of midfoot and inflammation

I83.215 Varicose veins of right lower extremity with both ulcer other part of foot and inflammation   `CH` `CL` `A`
Varicose veins of right lower extremity with both ulcer of toe and inflammation

I83.218 Varicose veins of right lower extremity with both ulcer of other part of lower extremity and inflammation   `CH` `CL` `A`

I83.219　Varicose veins of right lower extremity with both ulcer of unspecified site and inflammation　[A]

✓6ᵗʰ I83.22　Varicose veins of left lower extremity with both ulcer and inflammation

I83.221　Varicose veins of left lower extremity with both ulcer of thigh and inflammation　[CH] [CL] [A]

I83.222　Varicose veins of left lower extremity with both ulcer of calf and inflammation　[CH] [CL] [A]

I83.223　Varicose veins of left lower extremity with both ulcer of ankle and inflammation　[CH] [CL] [A]

I83.224　Varicose veins of left lower extremity with both ulcer of heel and midfoot and inflammation　[CH] [CL] [A]
　　Varicose veins of left lower extremity with both ulcer of plantar surface of midfoot and inflammation

I83.225　Varicose veins of left lower extremity with both ulcer other part of foot and inflammation　[CH] [CL] [A]
　　Varicose veins of left lower extremity with both ulcer of toe and inflammation

I83.228　Varicose veins of left lower extremity with both ulcer of other part of lower extremity and inflammation　[CH] [CL] [A]

I83.229　Varicose veins of left lower extremity with both ulcer of unspecified site and inflammation　[A]

✓5ᵗʰ I83.8　Varicose veins of lower extremities with other complications

✓6ᵗʰ I83.81　Varicose veins of lower extremities with pain

I83.811　Varicose veins of right lower extremity with pain　[A]

I83.812　Varicose veins of left lower extremity with pain　[A]

I83.813　Varicose veins of bilateral lower extremities with pain　[A]

I83.819　Varicose veins of unspecified lower extremity with pain　[A]

✓6ᵗʰ I83.89　Varicose veins of lower extremities with other complications
　　Varicose veins of lower extremities with edema
　　Varicose veins of lower extremities with swelling

I83.891　Varicose veins of right lower extremity with other complications　[A]

I83.892　Varicose veins of left lower extremity with other complications　[A]

I83.893　Varicose veins of bilateral lower extremities with other complications　[A]

I83.899　Varicose veins of unspecified lower extremity with other complications　[A]

✓5ᵗʰ I83.9　Asymptomatic varicose veins of lower extremities
　　Phlebectasia of lower extremities
　　Varicose veins of lower extremities
　　Varix of lower extremities

I83.90　Asymptomatic varicose veins of unspecified lower extremity　[A]
　　Varicose veins NOS

I83.91　Asymptomatic varicose veins of right lower extremity　[A]

I83.92　Asymptomatic varicose veins of left lower extremity　[A]

I83.93　Asymptomatic varicose veins of bilateral lower extremities　[A]

✓4ᵗʰ I85　Esophageal varices
　　Use additional code to identify:
　　alcohol abuse and dependence (F10.-)

✓5ᵗʰ I85.0　Esophageal varices
　　Idiopathic esophageal varices
　　Primary esophageal varices

I85.00　Esophageal varices without bleeding　[CH] [CL]
　　Esophageal varices NOS

I85.01　Esophageal varices with bleeding

✓5ᵗʰ I85.1　Secondary esophageal varices
　　Esophageal varices secondary to alcoholic liver disease
　　Esophageal varices secondary to cirrhosis of liver
　　Esophageal varices secondary to schistosomiasis
　　Esophageal varices secondary to toxic liver disease
　　Code first underlying disease

I85.10　Secondary esophageal varices without bleeding

I85.11　Secondary esophageal varices with bleeding

✓4ᵗʰ I86　Varicose veins of other sites
　　EXCLUDES 1　varicose veins of unspecified site (I83.9-)
　　EXCLUDES 2　retinal varices (H35.0-)

I86.0　Sublingual varices
　　DEF: Distended, tortuous veins beneath the tongue.

I86.1　Scrotal varices　♂
　　Varicocele

I86.2　Pelvic varices

I86.3　Vulval varices　♀
　　EXCLUDES 1　vulval varices complicating childbirth and the puerperium (O87.8)
　　vulval varices complicating pregnancy (O22.1-)

I86.4　Gastric varices

I86.8　Varicose veins of other specified sites　[A]
　　Varicose ulcer of nasal septum

✓4ᵗʰ I87　Other disorders of veins

✓5ᵗʰ I87.0　Postthrombotic syndrome
　　Chronic venous hypertension due to deep vein thrombosis
　　Postphlebitic syndrome
　　EXCLUDES 1　chronic venous hypertension without deep vein thrombosis (I87.3-)

✓6ᵗʰ I87.00　Postthrombotic syndrome without complications
　　Asymptomatic postthrombotic syndrome

I87.001　Postthrombotic syndrome without complications of right lower extremity

I87.002　Postthrombotic syndrome without complications of left lower extremity

I87.003　Postthrombotic syndrome without complications of bilateral lower extremity

I87.009　Postthrombotic syndrome without complications of unspecified extremity
　　Postthrombotic syndrome NOS

✓6ᵗʰ I87.01　Postthrombotic syndrome with ulcer
　　Use additional code to specify site and severity of ulcer (L97.-)

I87.011　Postthrombotic syndrome with ulcer of right lower extremity

I87.012　Postthrombotic syndrome with ulcer of left lower extremity

I87.013　Postthrombotic syndrome with ulcer of bilateral lower extremity

I87.019　Postthrombotic syndrome with ulcer of unspecified lower extremity

✓6ᵗʰ I87.02　Postthrombotic syndrome with inflammation

I87.021　Postthrombotic syndrome with inflammation of right lower extremity

I87.022　Postthrombotic syndrome with inflammation of left lower extremity

I87.023　Postthrombotic syndrome with inflammation of bilateral lower extremity

I87.029　Postthrombotic syndrome with inflammation of unspecified lower extremity

✓6ᵗʰ I87.03　Postthrombotic syndrome with ulcer and inflammation
　　Use additional code to specify site and severity of ulcer (L97.-)

I87.031　Postthrombotic syndrome with ulcer and inflammation of right lower extremity

☑ Additional Character Required　　✓x7ᵗʰ Placeholder Alert　　Manifestation　　Unspecified Dx　　►◄ Revised Text　　● New Code　　▲ Revised Title

I87.Ø32   **Postthrombotic syndrome with ulcer and inflammation of** left lower **extremity**

I87.Ø33   **Postthrombotic syndrome with ulcer and inflammation of** bilateral lower **extremity**

I87.Ø39   **Postthrombotic syndrome with ulcer and inflammation of unspecified lower extremity**

✓6ᵗʰ   **I87.Ø9**   **Postthrombotic syndrome with other complications**

I87.Ø91   **Postthrombotic syndrome with other complications of** right lower **extremity**

I87.Ø92   **Postthrombotic syndrome with other complications of** left lower **extremity**

I87.Ø93   **Postthrombotic syndrome with other complications of** bilateral lower **extremity**

I87.Ø99   **Postthrombotic syndrome with other complications of unspecified lower extremity**

I87.1   **Compression of vein**
Stricture of vein
Vena cava syndrome (inferior) (superior)
> EXCLUDES 2   *compression of pulmonary vein (I28.8)*

I87.2   **Venous insufficiency (chronic) (peripheral)**

[handwritten margin note: Also code site + severity of ulcer]

Stasis dermatitis
> EXCLUDES 1   *stasis dermatitis with varicose veins of lower extremities (I83.1-, I83.2-)*

DEF: Insufficient drainage of venous blood in any part of the body that results in edema or dermatosis.

✓5ᵗʰ   **I87.3**   **Chronic venous hypertension (idiopathic)**
Stasis edema
> EXCLUDES 1   *chronic venous hypertension due to deep vein thrombosis (I87.Ø-)*
> *varicose veins of lower extremities (I83.-)*

✓6ᵗʰ   **I87.3Ø**   **Chronic venous hypertension (idiopathic) without complications**
Asymptomatic chronic venous hypertension (idiopathic)

I87.3Ø1   **Chronic venous hypertension (idiopathic) without complications of** right lower **extremity**

I87.3Ø2   **Chronic venous hypertension (idiopathic) without complications of** left lower **extremity**

I87.3Ø3   **Chronic venous hypertension (idiopathic) without complications of** bilateral lower **extremity**

I87.3Ø9   **Chronic venous hypertension (idiopathic) without complications of unspecified lower extremity**
Chronic venous hypertension NOS

✓6ᵗʰ   **I87.31**   **Chronic venous hypertension (idiopathic) with** ulcer
Use additional code to specify site and severity of ulcer (L97.-)

I87.311   **Chronic venous hypertension (idiopathic) with ulcer of** right lower **extremity**

I87.312   **Chronic venous hypertension (idiopathic) with ulcer of** left lower **extremity**

I87.313   **Chronic venous hypertension (idiopathic) with ulcer of** bilateral lower **extremity**

I87.319   **Chronic venous hypertension (idiopathic) with ulcer of unspecified lower extremity**

✓6ᵗʰ   **I87.32**   **Chronic venous hypertension (idiopathic) with inflammation**

I87.321   **Chronic venous hypertension (idiopathic) with inflammation of** right lower **extremity**

I87.322   **Chronic venous hypertension (idiopathic) with inflammation of** left lower **extremity**

I87.323   **Chronic venous hypertension (idiopathic) with inflammation of** bilateral lower **extremity**

I87.329   **Chronic venous hypertension (idiopathic) with inflammation of unspecified lower extremity**

✓6ᵗʰ   **I87.33**   **Chronic venous hypertension (idiopathic) with** ulcer and inflammation
Use additional code to specify site and severity of ulcer (L97.-)

I87.331   **Chronic venous hypertension (idiopathic) with ulcer and inflammation of** right lower **extremity**

I87.332   **Chronic venous hypertension (idiopathic) with ulcer and inflammation of** left lower **extremity**

I87.333   **Chronic venous hypertension (idiopathic) with ulcer and inflammation of** bilateral lower **extremity**

I87.339   **Chronic venous hypertension (idiopathic) with ulcer and inflammation of unspecified lower extremity**

✓6ᵗʰ   **I87.39**   **Chronic venous hypertension (idiopathic) with other complications**

I87.391   **Chronic venous hypertension (idiopathic) with other complications of** right lower **extremity**

I87.392   **Chronic venous hypertension (idiopathic) with other complications of** left lower **extremity**

I87.393   **Chronic venous hypertension (idiopathic) with other complications of** bilateral lower **extremity**

I87.399   **Chronic venous hypertension (idiopathic) with other complications of unspecified lower extremity**

I87.8   **Other specified disorders of veins**
Phlebosclerosis
Venofibrosis

I87.9   **Disorder of vein, unspecified**

✓4ᵗʰ   **I88**   **Nonspecific lymphadenitis**
> EXCLUDES 1   *acute lymphadenitis, except mesenteric (LØ4.-)*
> *enlarged lymph nodes NOS (R59.-)*
> *human immunodeficiency virus [HIV] disease resulting in generalized lymphadenopathy (B2Ø)*

I88.Ø   **Nonspecific mesenteric lymphadenitis**
Mesenteric lymphadenitis (acute)(chronic)

I88.1   **Chronic lymphadenitis, except mesenteric**
Adenitis
Lymphadenitis

I88.8   **Other nonspecific lymphadenitis**

I88.9   **Nonspecific lymphadenitis, unspecified**
Lymphadenitis NOS

✓4ᵗʰ   **I89**   **Other noninfective disorders of lymphatic vessels and lymph nodes**
> EXCLUDES 1   *chylocele, tunica vaginalis (nonfilarial) NOS (N5Ø.89)*
> *enlarged lymph nodes NOS (R59.-)*
> *filarial chylocele (B74.-)*
> *hereditary lymphedema (Q82.Ø)*

I89.Ø   **Lymphedema, not elsewhere classified**   CH   CL
Elephantiasis (nonfilarial) NOS
Lymphangiectasis
Obliteration, lymphatic vessel
Praecox lymphedema
Secondary lymphedema
> EXCLUDES 1   *postmastectomy lymphedema (I97.2)*

I89.1   **Lymphangitis**
Chronic lymphangitis
Lymphangitis NOS
Subacute lymphangitis
> EXCLUDES 1   *acute lymphangitis (LØ3.-)*

I89.8   **Other specified noninfective disorders of lymphatic vessels and lymph nodes**
Chylocele (nonfilarial)
Chylous ascites
Chylous cyst
Lipomelanotic reticulosis
Lymph node or vessel fistula
Lymph node or vessel infarction
Lymph node or vessel rupture

I89.9   **Noninfective disorder of lymphatic vessels and lymph nodes, unspecified**
Disease of lymphatic vessels NOS

N Newborn: 0   P Pediatric: 0-17   M Maternity: 12-55   A Adult: 15-124   CH Comorbidity High   CL Comorbidity Low   NCDx Noncancer Dx   PDx Primary Dx

674   ICD-10-CM 2020

Other and unspecified disorders of the circulatory system (I95-I99)

✓4ᵗʰ I95 Hypotension

> **EXCLUDES 1** cardiovascular collapse (R57.9) (~R57.9)
> maternal hypotension syndrome (O26.5-)
> nonspecific low blood pressure reading NOS (R03.1)

I95.0 Idiopathic **hypotension**

I95.1 Orthostatic **hypotension**   CH

Hypotension, postural

> **EXCLUDES 1** neurogenic orthostatic hypotension [Shy-Drager]
> (G90.3)
> orthostatic hypotension due to drugs (I95.2)

I95.2 **Hypotension** due to drugs

Orthostatic hypotension due to drugs
Use additional code for adverse effect, if applicable, to identify drug (T36-T50 with fifth or sixth character 5)

I95.3 **Hypotension of** hemodialysis

Intra-dialytic hypotension

✓5ᵗʰ I95.8 **Other hypotension**

I95.81 Postprocedural **hypotension**

I95.89 **Other hypotension**   CH

Chronic hypotension

I95.9 **Hypotension, unspecified**   CH

I96 Gangrene, not elsewhere classified

Gangrenous cellulitis

> **EXCLUDES 1** gangrene in atherosclerosis of native arteries of the extremities
> (I70.26)
> gangrene in hernia (K40.1, K40.4, K41.1, K41.4, K42.1, K43.1-,
> K44.1, K45.1, K46.1)
> gangrene in other peripheral vascular diseases (I73.-)
> gangrene of certain specified sites — see Alphabetical Index
> gas gangrene (A48.0)
> pyoderma gangrenosum (L88)
> **EXCLUDES 2** gangrene in diabetes mellitus (E08-E13 with .52)

AHA: 2018,4Q,87; 2018,3Q,3; 2017,3Q,6; 2013,2Q,34

✓4ᵗʰ I97 Intraoperative and postprocedural complications and disorders of circulatory system, not elsewhere classified

> **EXCLUDES 2** postprocedural shock (T81.1-)

AHA: 2019,2Q,21

I97.0 **Postcardiotomy syndrome**

✓5ᵗʰ I97.1 **Other postprocedural cardiac** functional disturbances

> **EXCLUDES 2** acute pulmonary insufficiency following thoracic
> surgery (J95.1)
> intraoperative cardiac functional disturbances
> (I97.7-)

✓6ᵗʰ I97.11 **Postprocedural** cardiac insufficiency

I97.110 **Postprocedural cardiac insufficiency following** cardiac surgery

I97.111 **Postprocedural cardiac insufficiency following** other surgery

✓6ᵗʰ I97.12 **Postprocedural** cardiac arrest

I97.120 **Postprocedural cardiac arrest following** cardiac surgery

I97.121 **Postprocedural cardiac arrest following** other surgery

✓6ᵗʰ I97.13 **Postprocedural** heart failure

Use additional code to identify the heart failure (I50.-)

I97.130 **Postprocedural heart failure following** cardiac surgery

I97.131 **Postprocedural heart failure following** other surgery

✓6ᵗʰ I97.19 **Other postprocedural cardiac functional disturbances**

Use additional code, if applicable, to further specify disorder

I97.190 **Other postprocedural cardiac functional disturbances following** cardiac surgery

Use additional code, if applicable, for type 4 or type 5 myocardial infarction, to further specify disorder

AHA: 2019,2Q,33

I97.191 **Other postprocedural cardiac functional disturbances following** other surgery

I97.2 **Postmastectomy lymphedema syndrome**   CH CL A

Elephantiasis due to mastectomy
Obliteration of lymphatic vessels

I97.3 **Postprocedural hypertension**

✓5ᵗʰ I97.4 Intraoperative hemorrhage and hematoma **of a circulatory system organ or structure complicating a procedure**

> **EXCLUDES 1** intraoperative hemorrhage and hematoma of a
> circulatory system organ or structure due to
> accidental puncture and laceration during a
> procedure (I97.5-)
> **EXCLUDES 2** intraoperative cerebrovascular hemorrhage
> complicating a procedure (G97.3-)

✓6ᵗʰ I97.41 **Intraoperative hemorrhage and hematoma of a circulatory system organ or structure complicating a** circulatory system procedure

I97.410 **Intraoperative hemorrhage and hematoma of a circulatory system organ or structure complicating a** cardiac catheterization

I97.411 **Intraoperative hemorrhage and hematoma of a circulatory system organ or structure complicating a** cardiac bypass

I97.418 **Intraoperative hemorrhage and hematoma of a circulatory system organ or structure complicating** other circulatory system procedure

I97.42 **Intraoperative hemorrhage and hematoma of a circulatory system organ or structure complicating** other procedure

✓5ᵗʰ I97.5 Accidental puncture and laceration **of a circulatory system organ or structure during a procedure**

> **EXCLUDES 2** accidental puncture and laceration of brain during
> a procedure (G97.4-)

I97.51 **Accidental puncture and laceration of a circulatory system organ or structure during a** circulatory system procedure

AHA: 2019,2Q,24

I97.52 **Accidental puncture and laceration of a circulatory system organ or structure during** other procedure

✓5ᵗʰ I97.6 Postprocedural hemorrhage, hematoma and seroma **of a circulatory system organ or structure following a procedure**

> **EXCLUDES 2** postprocedural cerebrovascular hemorrhage
> complicating a procedure (G97.5-)

AHA: 2016,4Q,9-10

✓6ᵗʰ I97.61 Postprocedural hemorrhage **of a circulatory system organ or structure following a** circulatory system procedure

I97.610 **Postprocedural hemorrhage of a circulatory system organ or structure following a** cardiac catheterization

I97.611 **Postprocedural hemorrhage of a circulatory system organ or structure following** cardiac bypass

I97.618 **Postprocedural hemorrhage of a circulatory system organ or structure following** other circulatory system procedure

✓6ᵗʰ I97.62 Postprocedural hemorrhage, hematoma and seroma **of a circulatory system organ or structure following** other procedure

I97.620 **Postprocedural** hemorrhage **of a circulatory system organ or structure following other procedure**

I97.621 **Postprocedural** hematoma **of a circulatory system organ or structure following other procedure**

I97.622 **Postprocedural** seroma **of a circulatory system organ or structure following other procedure**

✓6ᵗʰ I97.63 Postprocedural hematoma **of a circulatory system organ or structure following a** circulatory system procedure

I97.630 **Postprocedural hematoma of a circulatory system organ or structure following a** cardiac catheterization

I97.631 **Postprocedural hematoma of a circulatory system organ or structure following** cardiac bypass

I97.638 **Postprocedural hematoma of a circulatory system organ or structure following** other circulatory system procedure

☑ Additional Character Required   ✓x7ᵗʰ Placeholder Alert   Manifestation   Unspecified Dx   ►◄ Revised Text   ● New Code   ▲ Revised Title

ICD-10-CM 2020   675

Chapter 9. Diseases of the Circulatory System

✓6ᵗʰ   **I97.64**   Postprocedural seroma **of a circulatory system organ or structure following a circulatory system procedure**

     I97.640   **Postprocedural seroma of a circulatory system organ or structure following a** cardiac catheterization

     I97.641   **Postprocedural seroma of a circulatory system organ or structure following** cardiac bypass

     I97.648   **Postprocedural seroma of a circulatory system organ or structure following other** circulatory system procedure

✓5ᵗʰ   **I97.7**   Intraoperative **cardiac** functional disturbances

     EXCLUDES 2   *acute pulmonary insufficiency following thoracic surgery (J95.1)*

         postprocedural cardiac functional disturbances (I97.1-)

✓6ᵗʰ   **I97.71**   **Intraoperative** cardiac arrest

     I97.710   **Intraoperative cardiac arrest during** cardiac surgery

     I97.711   **Intraoperative cardiac arrest during** other surgery

✓6ᵗʰ   **I97.79**   **Other intraoperative cardiac functional disturbances**

     Use additional code, if applicable, to further specify disorder

     I97.790   **Other intraoperative cardiac functional disturbances during** cardiac surgery

     I97.791   **Other intraoperative cardiac functional disturbances during** other surgery

✓5ᵗʰ   **I97.8**   **Other intraoperative and postprocedural complications and disorders of the circulatory system, not elsewhere classified**

     Use additional code, if applicable, to further specify disorder

✓6ᵗʰ   **I97.81**   Intraoperative **cerebrovascular infarction**

     I97.810   **Intraoperative cerebrovascular infarction during** cardiac surgery

     I97.811   **Intraoperative cerebrovascular infarction during** other surgery

✓6ᵗʰ   **I97.82**   Postprocedural **cerebrovascular infarction**

     I97.820   **Postprocedural cerebrovascular infarction following** cardiac surgery

     I97.821   **Postprocedural cerebrovascular infarction following** other surgery

     I97.88   **Other intraoperative complications of the circulatory system, not elsewhere classified**

     I97.89   **Other postprocedural complications and disorders of the circulatory system, not elsewhere classified**

         AHA: 2019,2Q,33

✓4ᵗʰ   **I99**   **Other and unspecified disorders of circulatory system**

     I99.8   **Other disorder of circulatory system**

     I99.9   **Unspecified disorder of circulatory system**

N Newborn: 0   P Pediatric: 0-17   M Maternity: 12-55   A Adult: 15-124   CH Comorbidity High   CL Comorbidity Low   NC Dx Noncancer Dx   PDx Primary Dx

676   ICD-10-CM 2020

Chapter 10. Diseases of the Respiratory System (JØØ–J99)

Chapter-specific Guidelines with Coding Examples

The chapter-specific guidelines from the ICD-10-CM Official Guidelines for Coding and Reporting have been provided below. Along with these guidelines are coding examples, contained in the shaded boxes, that have been developed to help illustrate the coding and/or sequencing guidance found in these guidelines.

a. Chronic obstructive pulmonary disease [COPD] and asthma

1) Acute exacerbation of chronic obstructive bronchitis and asthma

The codes in categories J44 and J45 distinguish between uncomplicated cases and those in acute exacerbation. An acute exacerbation is a worsening or a decompensation of a chronic condition. An acute exacerbation is not equivalent to an infection superimposed on a chronic condition, though an exacerbation may be triggered by an infection.

Patient is admitted for continued IV antibiotic administration and physical therapy with diagnoses of MRSA pneumonia with acute exacerbation of COPD. Provider documentation indicates comorbid moderate persistent asthma.

J15.212	Pneumonia due to methicillin resistant Staphylococcus aureus
J44.Ø	Chronic obstructive pulmonary disease with (acute) lower respiratory infection
J44.1	Chronic obstructive pulmonary disease with (acute) exacerbation
J45.4Ø	Moderate persistent asthma, uncomplicated

Explanation: ICD-1Ø-CM uses combination codes to create organism-specific classifications for many types of pneumonia. Category J44 distinguishes between COPD that is exacerbated, COPD with acute lower respiratory infection, and COPD without mention of a complication (unspecified). When a lower respiratory infection is present and COPD is diagnosed, two codes would be required, J44.Ø and the code for the infection. Sequencing will be dependent on the condition that is the focus of treatment upon admission to the post-acute setting, which in this case is the MRSA pneumonia.

An acute exacerbation is a worsening or decompensation of a chronic condition and must be specified by the provider as such. When both COPD and asthma are diagnosed and the provider reports an acute exacerbation of COPD, an acute exacerbation of asthma cannot be assumed unless specifically stated by the provider.

Exacerbation of moderate persistent asthma with status asthmaticus.

J45.42	Moderate persistent asthma with status asthmaticus

Explanation: Category J45 Asthma includes severity-specific subcategories and fifth-character codes to distinguish between uncomplicated cases, those in acute exacerbation, and those with status asthmaticus.

---

b. Acute respiratory failure

1) Acute respiratory failure as principal diagnosis

A code from subcategory J96.Ø, Acute respiratory failure, or subcategory J96.2, Acute and chronic respiratory failure, may be assigned as a principal diagnosis when it is the condition established after study to be chiefly responsible for occasioning the admission to the hospital, and the selection is supported by the Alphabetic Index and Tabular List. However, chapter-specific coding guidelines (such as obstetrics, poisoning, HIV, newborn) that provide sequencing direction take precedence.

2) Acute respiratory failure as secondary diagnosis

Respiratory failure may be listed as a secondary diagnosis if it occurs after admission, or if it is present on admission, but does not meet the definition of principal diagnosis.

Acute pneumococcal pneumonia with subsequent development of acute respiratory failure.

J13	Pneumonia due to Streptococcus pneumoniae
J96.ØØ	Acute respiratory failure, unspecified whether with hypoxia or hypercapnia

Explanation: Acute respiratory failure may be listed as a secondary diagnosis if it occurs after admission, or if it is present on admission but does not meet the definition of principal diagnosis.

---

3) Sequencing of acute respiratory failure and another acute condition

When a patient is admitted with respiratory failure and another acute condition, (e.g., myocardial infarction, cerebrovascular accident, aspiration pneumonia), the principal diagnosis will not be the same in every situation. This applies whether the other acute condition is a respiratory or nonrespiratory condition. Selection of the principal diagnosis will be dependent on the circumstances of admission. If both the respiratory failure and the other acute condition are equally responsible for occasioning the admission to the hospital, and there are no chapter-specific sequencing rules, the guideline regarding two or more diagnoses that equally meet the definition for principal diagnosis (Section II, C.) may be applied in these situations.

If the documentation is not clear as to whether acute respiratory failure and another condition are equally responsible for occasioning the admission, query the provider for clarification.

c. Influenza due to certain identified influenza viruses

Code only confirmed cases of influenza due to certain identified influenza viruses (category JØ9), and due to other identified influenza virus (category J10). This is an exception to the hospital inpatient guideline Section II, H. (Uncertain Diagnosis).

In this context, "confirmation" does not require documentation of positive laboratory testing specific for avian or other novel influenza A or other identified influenza virus. However, coding should be based on the provider's diagnostic statement that the patient has avian influenza, or other novel influenza A, for category JØ9, or has another particular identified strain of influenza, such as H1N1 or H3N2, but not identified as novel or variant, for category J10.

If the provider records "suspected" or "possible" or "probable" avian influenza, or novel influenza, or other identified influenza, then the appropriate influenza code from category J11, Influenza due to unidentified influenza virus, should be assigned. A code from category JØ9, Influenza due to certain identified influenza viruses, should not be assigned nor should a code from category J10, Influenza due to other identified influenza virus.

Influenza due to avian influenza virus with pneumonia.

JØ9.X1	Influenza due to identified novel influenza A virus with pneumonia

Explanation: Codes in category JØ9 Influenza due to certain identified influenza viruses should be assigned only for confirmed cases. "Confirmation" does not require positive laboratory testing of a specific influenza virus but does need to be based on the provider's diagnostic statement, which should not include terms such as "possible," "probable," or "suspected."

---

d. Ventilator associated pneumonia

1) Documentation of ventilator associated pneumonia

As with all procedural or postprocedural complications, code assignment is based on the provider's documentation of the relationship between the condition and the procedure.

Code J95.851, Ventilator associated pneumonia, should be assigned only when the provider has documented ventilator associated pneumonia (VAP). An additional code to identify the organism (e.g., Pseudomonas aeruginosa, code B96.5) should also be assigned. Do not assign an additional code from categories J12-J18 to identify the type of pneumonia.

Code J95.851 should not be assigned for cases where the patient has pneumonia and is on a mechanical ventilator and the provider has not specifically stated that the pneumonia is ventilator-associated pneumonia. If the documentation is unclear as to whether the patient has a pneumonia that is a complication attributable to the mechanical ventilator, query the provider.

2) Ventilator associated pneumonia develops after admission

A patient may be admitted with one type of pneumonia (e.g., code J13, Pneumonia due to Streptococcus pneumonia) and subsequently develop VAP. In this instance, the principal diagnosis would be the appropriate code from categories J12-J18 for the pneumonia diagnosed at the time of admission. Code J95.851, Ventilator associated pneumonia, would be assigned as an additional diagnosis when the provider has also documented the presence of ventilator associated pneumonia.

Patient with pneumonia due to *Klebsiella pneumoniae* develops superimposed MRSA ventilator-associated pneumonia.

J15.Ø	**Pneumonia due to Klebsiella pneumoniae**
J95.851	**Ventilator associated pneumonia**
B95.62	**Methicillin resistant Staphylococcus aureus infection as the cause of diseases classified elsewhere**

Explanation: Code assignment for ventilator-associated pneumonia is based on the provider's documentation of the relationship between the condition and the procedure and is reported only when the provider has documented ventilator-associated pneumonia (VAP).

A patient may be admitted with one type of pneumonia and subsequently develop VAP. In this example, the principal diagnosis code describes the pneumonia diagnosed at the time of admission, with code J95.851 Ventilator associated pneumonia, assigned as secondary.

Chapter 10. Diseases of the Respiratory System (J00-J99)

NOTE When a respiratory condition is described as occurring in more than one site and is not specifically indexed, it should be classified to the lower anatomic site (e.g., tracheobronchitis to bronchitis in J40).

Use additional code, where applicable, to identify:
exposure to environmental tobacco smoke (Z77.22)
exposure to tobacco smoke in the perinatal period (P96.81)
history of tobacco dependence (Z87.891)
occupational exposure to environmental tobacco smoke (Z57.31)
tobacco dependence (F17.-)
tobacco use (Z72.0)

EXCLUDES 2   certain conditions originating in the perinatal period (P04-P96)
certain infectious and parasitic diseases (A00-B99)
complications of pregnancy, childbirth and the puerperium (O00-O9A)
congenital malformations, deformations and chromosomal abnormalities (Q00-Q99)
endocrine, nutritional and metabolic diseases (E00-E88)
injury, poisoning and certain other consequences of external causes (S00-T88)
neoplasms (C00-D49)
smoke inhalation (T59.81-)
symptoms, signs and abnormal clinical and laboratory findings, not elsewhere classified (R00-R94)

This chapter contains the following blocks:
J00-J06 Acute upper respiratory infections
J09-J18 Influenza and pneumonia
J20-J22 Other acute lower respiratory infections
J30-J39 Other diseases of upper respiratory tract
J40-J47 Chronic lower respiratory diseases
J60-J70 Lung diseases due to external agents
J80-J84 Other respiratory diseases principally affecting the interstitium
J85-J86 Suppurative and necrotic conditions of the lower respiratory tract
J90-J94 Other diseases of the pleura
J95   Intraoperative and postprocedural complications and disorders of respiratory system, not elsewhere classified
J96-J99 Other diseases of the respiratory system

Acute upper respiratory infections (J00-J06)

EXCLUDES 1   chronic obstructive pulmonary disease with acute lower respiratory infection (J44.0)
influenza virus with other respiratory manifestations (J09.X2, J10.1, J11.1)

J00 Acute nasopharyngitis [common cold]
Acute rhinitis
Coryza (acute)
Infective nasopharyngitis NOS
Infective rhinitis
Nasal catarrh, acute
Nasopharyngitis NOS
EXCLUDES 1   acute pharyngitis (J02.-)
acute sore throat NOS (J02.9)
pharyngitis NOS (J02.9)
rhinitis NOS (J31.0)
sore throat NOS (J02.9)
EXCLUDES 2   allergic rhinitis (J30.1-J30.9)
chronic pharyngitis (J31.2)
chronic rhinitis (J31.0)
chronic sore throat (J31.2)
nasopharyngitis, chronic (J31.1)
vasomotor rhinitis (J30.0)

DEF: Acute inflammation of the mucous membranes that extends from the nares to the pharynx. It is characterized by nasal obstruction, sneezing, runny nose, and sore throat.

✓4th J01 Acute sinusitis
INCLUDES acute abscess of sinus
acute empyema of sinus
acute infection of sinus
acute inflammation of sinus
acute suppuration of sinus
Use additional code (B95-B97) to identify infectious agent
EXCLUDES 1   sinusitis NOS (J32.9)
EXCLUDES 2   chronic sinusitis (J32.0-J32.8)

✓5th J01.0 Acute maxillary sinusitis
Acute antritis
J01.00 Acute maxillary sinusitis, unspecified
J01.01 Acute recurrent maxillary sinusitis

✓5th J01.1 Acute frontal sinusitis
J01.10 Acute frontal sinusitis, unspecified
J01.11 Acute recurrent frontal sinusitis

✓5th J01.2 Acute ethmoidal sinusitis
J01.20 Acute ethmoidal sinusitis, unspecified
J01.21 Acute recurrent ethmoidal sinusitis

✓5th J01.3 Acute sphenoidal sinusitis
J01.30 Acute sphenoidal sinusitis, unspecified
J01.31 Acute recurrent sphenoidal sinusitis

✓5th J01.4 Acute pansinusitis
J01.40 Acute pansinusitis, unspecified
J01.41 Acute recurrent pansinusitis

✓5th J01.8 Other acute sinusitis
J01.80 Other acute sinusitis
Acute sinusitis involving more than one sinus but not pansinusitis
J01.81 Other acute recurrent sinusitis
Acute recurrent sinusitis involving more than one sinus but not pansinusitis

✓5th J01.9 Acute sinusitis, unspecified
J01.90 Acute sinusitis, unspecified
J01.91 Acute recurrent sinusitis, unspecified

✓4th J02 Acute pharyngitis
INCLUDES acute sore throat
EXCLUDES 1   acute laryngopharyngitis (J06.0)
peritonsillar abscess (J36)
pharyngeal abscess (J39.1)
retropharyngeal abscess (J39.0)
EXCLUDES 2   chronic pharyngitis (J31.2)

J02.0 Streptococcal pharyngitis
Septic pharyngitis
Streptococcal sore throat
EXCLUDES 2   scarlet fever (A38.-)

J02.8 Acute pharyngitis due to other specified organisms
Use additional code (B95-B97) to identify infectious agent
EXCLUDES 1   acute pharyngitis due to coxsackie virus (B08.5)
acute pharyngitis due to gonococcus (A54.5)
acute pharyngitis due to herpes [simplex] virus (B00.2)
acute pharyngitis due to infectious mononucleosis (B27.-)
enteroviral vesicular pharyngitis (B08.5)

J02.9 Acute pharyngitis, unspecified
Gangrenous pharyngitis (acute)
Infective pharyngitis (acute) NOS
Pharyngitis (acute) NOS
Sore throat (acute) NOS
Suppurative pharyngitis (acute)
Ulcerative pharyngitis (acute)

✓4th J03 Acute tonsillitis
EXCLUDES 1   acute sore throat (J02.-)
hypertrophy of tonsils (J35.1)
peritonsillar abscess (J36)
sore throat NOS (J02.9)
streptococcal sore throat (J02.0)
EXCLUDES 2   chronic tonsillitis (J35.0)

✓5th J03.0 Streptococcal tonsillitis
J03.00 Acute streptococcal tonsillitis, unspecified
J03.01 Acute recurrent streptococcal tonsillitis

✓5th J03.8 Acute tonsillitis due to other specified organisms
Use additional code (B95-B97) to identify infectious agent
EXCLUDES 1   diphtheritic tonsillitis (A36.0)
herpesviral pharyngotonsillitis (B00.2)
streptococcal tonsillitis (J03.0)
tuberculous tonsillitis (A15.8)
Vincent's tonsillitis (A69.1)

J03.80 Acute tonsillitis due to other specified organisms
J03.81 Acute recurrent tonsillitis due to other specified organisms

---

☑ Additional Character Required   ✓x7th Placeholder Alert   Manifestation   Unspecified Dx   ►◄ Revised Text   ● New Code   ▲ Revised Title

√5ᵗʰ **J03.9 Acute tonsillitis, unspecified**
Follicular tonsillitis (acute)
Gangrenous tonsillitis (acute)
Infective tonsillitis (acute)
Tonsillitis (acute) NOS
Ulcerative tonsillitis (acute)
- **J03.90 Acute tonsillitis, unspecified**
- **J03.91 Acute recurrent tonsillitis, unspecified**

√4ᵗʰ **J04 Acute laryngitis and tracheitis**
Use additional code (B95-B97) to identify infectious agent
EXCLUDES 1 acute obstructive laryngitis [croup] and epiglottitis (J05.-)
EXCLUDES 2 laryngismus (stridulus) (J38.5)

J04.0 Acute laryngitis
Edematous laryngitis (acute)
Laryngitis (acute) NOS
Subglottic laryngitis (acute)
Suppurative laryngitis (acute)
Ulcerative laryngitis (acute)
EXCLUDES 1 acute obstructive laryngitis (J05.0)
EXCLUDES 2 chronic laryngitis (J37.0)

√5ᵗʰ **J04.1 Acute tracheitis**
Acute viral tracheitis
Catarrhal tracheitis (acute)
Tracheitis (acute) NOS
EXCLUDES 2 chronic tracheitis (J42)
- **J04.10 Acute tracheitis without obstruction**
- **J04.11 Acute tracheitis with obstruction**

J04.2 Acute laryngotracheitis
Laryngotracheitis NOS
Tracheitis (acute) with laryngitis (acute)
EXCLUDES 1 acute obstructive laryngotracheitis (J05.0)
EXCLUDES 2 chronic laryngotracheitis (J37.1)

√5ᵗʰ **J04.3 Supraglottitis, unspecified**
- **J04.30 Supraglottitis, unspecified, without obstruction**
- **J04.31 Supraglottitis, unspecified, with obstruction**

√4ᵗʰ **J05 Acute obstructive laryngitis [croup] and epiglottitis**
Use additional code (B95-B97) to identify infectious agent

J05.0 Acute obstructive laryngitis [croup]
Obstructive laryngitis (acute) NOS
Obstructive laryngotracheitis NOS
DEF: Acute laryngeal obstruction due to allergies, foreign bodies, or in the majority of cases a viral infection. Symptoms include a harsh, barking cough, hoarseness, and a persistent, high-pitched respiratory sound (stridor).

√5ᵗʰ **J05.1 Acute epiglottitis**
EXCLUDES 2 epiglottitis, chronic (J37.0)
- **J05.10 Acute epiglottitis without obstruction**
Epiglottitis NOS
- **J05.11 Acute epiglottitis with obstruction**

√4ᵗʰ **J06 Acute upper respiratory infections of multiple and unspecified sites**
EXCLUDES 1 acute respiratory infection NOS (J22)
streptococcal pharyngitis (J02.0)

J06.0 Acute laryngopharyngitis
J06.9 Acute upper respiratory infection, unspecified
Upper respiratory disease, acute
Upper respiratory infection NOS
►Use additional code (B95-B97) to identify infectious agent, if known, such as:◄
►respiratory syncytial virus (RSV) (B97.4)◄

Influenza and pneumonia (J09-J18)

EXCLUDES 2 allergic or eosinophilic pneumonia (J82)
aspiration pneumonia NOS (J69.0)
meconium pneumonia (P24.01)
neonatal aspiration pneumonia (P24.-)
pneumonia due to solids and liquids (J69.-)
congenital pneumonia (P23.9)
lipid pneumonia (J69.1)
rheumatic pneumonia (I00)
ventilator associated pneumonia (J95.851)

AHA: 2017,4Q,96
TIP: Documentation of lobar pneumonia or multilobar pneumonia should be coded to J18.1 when the specific organism causing the pneumonia is not identified. When the organism is documented, lobar pneumonia or multilobar pneumonia should be coded using categories J12-J16, depending on the organism that is present.

√4ᵗʰ **J09 Influenza due to certain identified influenza viruses**
EXCLUDES 1 influenza A/H1N1 (J10.-)
influenza due to other identified influenza virus (J10.-)
influenza due to unidentified influenza virus (J11.-)
seasonal influenza due to other identified influenza virus (J10.-)
seasonal influenza due to unidentified influenza virus (J11.-)

√5ᵗʰ **J09.X Influenza due to identified novel influenza A virus**
Avian influenza
Bird influenza
Influenza A/H5N1
Influenza of other animal origin, not bird or swine
Swine influenza virus (viruses that normally cause infections in pigs)
AHA: 2016,3Q,10
J09.X1 Influenza due to identified novel influenza A virus with pneumonia
Code also, if applicable, associated:
lung abscess (J85.1)
other specified type of pneumonia
J09.X2 Influenza due to identified novel influenza A virus with other respiratory manifestations
Influenza due to identified novel influenza A virus NOS
Influenza due to identified novel influenza A virus with laryngitis
Influenza due to identified novel influenza A virus with pharyngitis
Influenza due to identified novel influenza A virus with upper respiratory symptoms
Use additional code, if applicable, for associated:
pleural effusion (J91.8)
sinusitis (J01.-)
J09.X3 Influenza due to identified novel influenza A virus with gastrointestinal manifestations
Influenza due to identified novel influenza A virus gastroenteritis
EXCLUDES 1 'intestinal flu' [viral gastroenteritis] (A08.-)
J09.X9 Influenza due to identified novel influenza A virus with other manifestations
Influenza due to identified novel influenza A virus with encephalopathy
Influenza due to identified novel influenza A virus with myocarditis
Influenza due to identified novel influenza A virus with otitis media
Use additional code to identify manifestation

√4ᵗʰ **J10 Influenza due to other identified influenza virus**
EXCLUDES 1 influenza due to avian influenza virus (J09.X-)
influenza due to swine flu (J09.X-)
influenza due to unidentifed influenza virus (J11.-)

√5ᵗʰ **J10.0 Influenza due to other identified influenza virus with pneumonia**
Code also associated lung abscess, if applicable (J85.1)
- **J10.00 Influenza due to other identified influenza virus with unspecified type of pneumonia**
- **J10.01 Influenza due to other identified influenza virus with the same other identified influenza virus pneumonia**

J10.08   **Influenza due to other identified influenza virus with other specified pneumonia**
       Code also other specified type of pneumonia

J10.1   **Influenza due to other identified influenza virus with other respiratory manifestations**
     Influenza due to other identified influenza virus NOS
     Influenza due to other identified influenza virus with laryngitis
     Influenza due to other identified influenza virus with pharyngitis
     Influenza due to other identified influenza virus with upper respiratory symptoms
     Use additional code for associated pleural effusion, if applicable (J91.8)
     Use additional code for associated sinusitis, if applicable (J01.-)
     AHA: 2016,3Q,10-11

J10.2   **Influenza due to other identified influenza virus with gastrointestinal manifestations**
     Influenza due to other identified influenza virus gastroenteritis
     EXCLUDES 1   "intestinal flu" [viral gastroenteritis] (A08.-)

✓5ᵗʰ **J10.8**   **Influenza due to other identified influenza virus with other manifestations**

     J10.81   **Influenza due to other identified influenza virus with encephalopathy**

     J10.82   **Influenza due to other identified influenza virus with myocarditis**

     J10.83   **Influenza due to other identified influenza virus with otitis media**
         Use additional code for any associated perforated tympanic membrane (H72.-)

     J10.89   **Influenza due to other identified influenza virus with other manifestations**
         Use additional codes to identify the manifestations

✓4ᵗʰ **J11**   **Influenza due to unidentified influenza virus**

✓5ᵗʰ **J11.0**   **Influenza due to unidentified influenza virus with pneumonia**
     Code also associated lung abscess, if applicable (J85.1)
     AHA: 2016,3Q,11

     J11.00   **Influenza due to unidentified influenza virus with unspecified type of pneumonia**
         Influenza with pneumonia NOS

     J11.08   **Influenza due to unidentified influenza virus with specified pneumonia**
         Code also other specified type of pneumonia

J11.1   **Influenza due to unidentified influenza virus with other respiratory manifestations**
     Influenza NOS
     Influenzal laryngitis NOS
     Influenzal pharyngitis NOS
     Influenza with upper respiratory symptoms NOS
     Use additional code for associated pleural effusion, if applicable (J91.8)
     Use additional code for associated sinusitis, if applicable (J01.-)

J11.2   **Influenza due to unidentified influenza virus with gastrointestinal manifestations**
     Influenza gastroenteritis NOS
     EXCLUDES 1   "intestinal flu" [viral gastroenteritis] (A08.-)

✓5ᵗʰ **J11.8**   **Influenza due to unidentified influenza virus with other manifestations**

     J11.81   **Influenza due to unidentified influenza virus with encephalopathy**
         Influenzal encephalopathy NOS

     J11.82   **Influenza due to unidentified influenza virus with myocarditis**
         Influenzal myocarditis NOS

     J11.83   **Influenza due to unidentified influenza virus with otitis media**
         Influenzal otitis media NOS
         Use additional code for any associated perforated tympanic membrane (H72.-)

     J11.89   **Influenza due to unidentified influenza virus with other manifestations**
         Use additional codes to identify the manifestations

✓4ᵗʰ **J12**   **Viral pneumonia, not elsewhere classified**
     INCLUDES   bronchopneumonia due to viruses other than influenza viruses
     Code first associated influenza, if applicable (J09.X1, J10.-, J11.0-)
     Code also associated abscess, if applicable (J85.1)
     EXCLUDES 1   aspiration pneumonia due to anesthesia during labor and delivery (O74.0)
         aspiration pneumonia due to anesthesia during pregnancy (O29)
         aspiration pneumonia due to anesthesia during puerperium (O89.0)
         aspiration pneumonia due to solids and liquids (J69.-)
         aspiration pneumonia NOS (J69.0)
         congenital pneumonia (P23.0)
         congenital rubella pneumonitis (P35.0)
         interstitial pneumonia NOS (J84.9)
         lipid pneumonia (J69.1)
         neonatal aspiration pneumonia (P24.-)
     AHA: 2019,1Q,35; 2018,3Q,24; 2016,3Q,15; 2013,4Q,118

     J12.0   **Adenoviral pneumonia**

     J12.1   **Respiratory syncytial virus pneumonia**
         ▶RSV pneumonia◀

     J12.2   **Parainfluenza virus pneumonia**

     J12.3   **Human metapneumovirus pneumonia**

✓5ᵗʰ   **J12.8**   **Other viral pneumonia**

       J12.81   **Pneumonia due to SARS-associated coronavirus**
           Severe acute respiratory syndrome NOS
           DEF: Severe adult respiratory syndrome caused by the coronavirus, specified as inflammation of the lungs with consolidation.

       J12.89   **Other viral pneumonia**

     J12.9   **Viral pneumonia, unspecified**

J13   **Pneumonia due to Streptococcus pneumoniae**
     Bronchopneumonia due to S. pneumoniae
     Code first associated influenza, if applicable (J09.X1, J10.0-, J11.0-)
     Code also associated abscess, if applicable (J85.1)
     EXCLUDES 1   congenital pneumonia due to S. pneumoniae (P23.6)
         lobar pneumonia, unspecified organism (J18.1)
         pneumonia due to other streptococci (J15.3-J15.4)
     AHA: 2019,1Q,35; 2018,3Q,24; 2016,3Q,15; 2013,4Q,118

J14   **Pneumonia due to Hemophilus influenzae**
     Bronchopneumonia due to H. influenzae
     Code first associated influenza, if applicable (J09.X1, J10.0-, J11.0-)
     Code also associated abscess, if applicable (J85.1)
     EXCLUDES 1   congenital pneumonia due to H. influenzae (P23.6)
     AHA: 2019,1Q,35; 2018,3Q,24; 2016,3Q,15; 2013,4Q,118

✓4ᵗʰ **J15**   **Bacterial pneumonia, not elsewhere classified**
     INCLUDES   Bronchopneumonia due to bacteria other than S. pneumoniae and H. influenzae
     Code first associated influenza, if applicable (J09.X1, J10.0-, -J11.0-)
     Code also associated abscess, if applicable (J85.1)
     EXCLUDES 1   chlamydial pneumonia (J16.0)
         congenital pneumonia (P23.-)
         Legionnaires' disease (A48.1)
         spirochetal pneumonia (A69.8)
     AHA: 2019,1Q,35; 2018,3Q,24; 2016,3Q,15; 2013,4Q,118

     J15.0   **Pneumonia due to Klebsiella pneumoniae**

     J15.1   **Pneumonia due to Pseudomonas**

✓5ᵗʰ   **J15.2**   **Pneumonia due to staphylococcus**

       J15.20   **Pneumonia due to staphylococcus, unspecified**

✓6ᵗʰ   **J15.21**   **Pneumonia due to Staphylococcus aureus**

         J15.211   **Pneumonia due to methicillin susceptible Staphylococcus aureus**
            MSSA pneumonia
            Pneumonia due to Staphylococcus aureus NOS

         J15.212   **Pneumonia due to methicillin resistant Staphylococcus aureus**

       J15.29   **Pneumonia due to other staphylococcus**

     J15.3   **Pneumonia due to streptococcus, group B**

     J15.4   **Pneumonia due to other streptococci**
       EXCLUDES 1   pneumonia due to streptococcus, group B (J15.3)
         pneumonia due to Streptococcus pneumoniae (J13)

     J15.5   **Pneumonia due to Escherichia coli**

Handwritten margin notes: Code also J44.0 if + COPD   Z87.01 Hx pneumonia

Chapter 10. Diseases of the Respiratory System

J15.6   **Pneumonia due to** other Gram-negative bacteria
Pneumonia due to other aerobic Gram-negative bacteria
Pneumonia due to Serratia marcescens

J15.7   **Pneumonia due to** Mycoplasma pneumoniae

J15.8   **Pneumonia due to other specified bacteria**

J15.9   **Unspecified bacterial pneumonia**
Pneumonia due to gram-positive bacteria

✓4ᵗʰ **J16**   **Pneumonia due to other infectious organisms, not elsewhere classified**
Code first associated influenza, if applicable (J09.X1, J10.0-, J11.0-)
Code also associated abscess, if applicable (J85.1)
EXCLUDES 1   congenital pneumonia (P23.-)
ornithosis (A70)
pneumocystosis (B59)
pneumonia NOS (J18.9)
AHA: 2019,1Q,35; 2018,3Q,24; 2016,3Q,15; 2013,4Q,118

J16.0   Chlamydial **pneumonia**

J16.8   **Pneumonia due to other specified infectious organisms**

J17   *Pneumonia in diseases classified elsewhere*
Code first underlying disease, such as:
Q fever (A78)
rheumatic fever (I00)
schistosomiasis (B65.0-B65.9)
EXCLUDES 1   candidial pneumonia (B37.1)
chlamydial pneumonia (J16.0)
gonorrheal pneumonia (A54.84)
histoplasmosis pneumonia (B39.0-B39.2)
measles pneumonia (B05.2)
nocardiosis pneumonia (A43.0)
pneumocystosis (B59)
pneumonia due to Pneumocystis carinii (B59)
pneumonia due to Pneumocystis jiroveci (B59)
pneumonia in actinomycosis (A42.0)
pneumonia in anthrax (A22.1)
pneumonia in ascariasis (B77.81)
pneumonia in aspergillosis (B44.0-B44.1)
pneumonia in coccidioidomycosis (B38.0-B38.2)
pneumonia in cytomegalovirus disease (B25.0)
pneumonia in toxoplasmosis (B58.3)
rubella pneumonia (B06.81)
salmonella pneumonia (A02.22)
spirochetal infection NEC with pneumonia (A69.8)
tularemia pneumonia (A21.2)
typhoid fever with pneumonia (A01.03)
varicella pneumonia (B01.2)
whooping cough with pneumonia (A37 with fifth character 1)
AHA: 2019,1Q,35; 2016,3Q,15; 2013,4Q,118

✓4ᵗʰ **J18**   **Pneumonia, unspecified organism**
Code first associated influenza, if applicable (J09.X1, J10.0-, J11.0-)
EXCLUDES 1   abscess of lung with pneumonia (J85.1)
aspiration pneumonia due to anesthesia during labor and delivery (O74.0)
aspiration pneumonia due to anesthesia during pregnancy (O29)
aspiration pneumonia due to anesthesia during puerperium (O89.0)
aspiration pneumonia due to solids and liquids (J69.-)
aspiration pneumonia NOS (J69.0)
congenital pneumonia (P23.0)
drug-induced interstitial lung disorder (J70.2-J70.4)
interstitial pneumonia NOS (J84.9)
lipid pneumonia (J69.1)
neonatal aspiration pneumonia (P24.-)
pneumonitis due to external agents (J67-J70)
pneumonitis due to fumes and vapors (J68.0)
usual interstitial pneumonia (J84.17)
AHA: 2019,1Q,35; 2016,3Q,15; 2013,4Q,118
TIP: Hemoptysis (R04.2) is not integral to pneumonia and can be coded separately.

J18.0   Bronchopneumonia**, unspecified organism**
EXCLUDES 1   hypostatic bronchopneumonia (J18.2)
lipid pneumonia (J69.1)
EXCLUDES 2   acute bronchiolitis (J21.-)
chronic bronchiolitis (J44.9)

J18.1   Lobar **pneumonia, unspecified organism**
AHA: 2018,3Q,24

J18.2   Hypostatic **pneumonia, unspecified organism**
Hypostatic bronchopneumonia
Passive pneumonia

J18.8   **Other pneumonia, unspecified organism**

J18.9   **Pneumonia, unspecified organism**
AHA: 2019,2Q,28; 2014,3Q,4; 2013,4Q,119; 2012,4Q,94

Other acute lower respiratory infections (J20-J22)

EXCLUDES 2   *chronic obstructive pulmonary disease with acute lower respiratory infection (J44.0)*

✓4ᵗʰ **J20**   **Acute bronchitis**
INCLUDES   acute and subacute bronchitis (with) bronchospasm
acute and subacute bronchitis (with) tracheitis
acute and subacute bronchitis (with) tracheobronchitis, acute
acute and subacute fibrinous bronchitis
acute and subacute membranous bronchitis
acute and subacute purulent bronchitis
acute and subacute septic bronchitis
EXCLUDES 1   *bronchitis NOS (J40)*
tracheobronchitis NOS (J40)
EXCLUDES 2   *acute bronchitis with bronchiectasis (J47.0)*
acute bronchitis with chronic obstructive asthma (J44.0)
acute bronchitis with chronic obstructive pulmonary disease (J44.0)
allergic bronchitis NOS (J45.909-)
bronchitis due to chemicals, fumes and vapors (J68.0)
chronic bronchitis NOS (J42)
chronic mucopurulent bronchitis (J41.1)
chronic obstructive bronchitis (J44.-)
chronic obstructive tracheobronchitis (J44.-)
chronic simple bronchitis (J41.0)
chronic tracheobronchitis (J42)
AHA: 2019,1Q,35; 2016,3Q,10,16
DEF: Acute inflammation of the main branches of the bronchial tree due to infectious or irritant agents. Symptoms include cough with a varied production of sputum, fever, substernal soreness, and lung rales. Bronchitis usually lasts three to 10 days.

J20.0   **Acute bronchitis due to** Mycoplasma pneumoniae

J20.1   **Acute bronchitis due to** Hemophilus influenzae

J20.2   **Acute bronchitis due to** streptococcus

J20.3   **Acute bronchitis due to** coxsackievirus

J20.4   **Acute bronchitis due to** parainfluenza virus

J20.5   **Acute bronchitis due to** respiratory syncytial virus
▶Acute bronchitis due to RSV◀

J20.6   **Acute bronchitis due to** rhinovirus

J20.7   **Acute bronchitis due to** echovirus

J20.8   **Acute bronchitis due to other specified organisms**

J20.9   **Acute bronchitis, unspecified**

✓4ᵗʰ **J21**   **Acute bronchiolitis**
INCLUDES   acute bronchiolitis with bronchospasm
EXCLUDES 2   *respiratory bronchiolitis interstitial lung disease (J84.115)*

J21.0   **Acute bronchiolitis due to** respiratory syncytial virus
▶Acute bronchiolitis due to RSV◀

J21.1   **Acute bronchiolitis due to** human metapneumovirus

J21.8   **Acute bronchiolitis due to other specified organisms**

J21.9   **Acute bronchiolitis, unspecified**
Bronchiolitis (acute)
EXCLUDES 1   *chronic bronchiolitis (J44.-)*

J22   **Unspecified acute lower respiratory infection**
Acute (lower) respiratory (tract) infection NOS
EXCLUDES 1   *upper respiratory infection (acute) (J06.9)*

N Newborn: 0   P Pediatric: 0-17   M Maternity: 12-55   A Adult: 15-124   CH Comorbidity High   CL Comorbidity Low   NC Dx Noncancer Dx   PDx Primary Dx

682   ICD-10-CM 2020

Other diseases of upper respiratory tract (J30-J39)

✓4ᵗʰ **J30 Vasomotor and allergic rhinitis**
  INCLUDES spasmodic rhinorrhea
  EXCLUDES 1 *allergic rhinitis with asthma (bronchial) (J45.909)*
      rhinitis NOS (J31.0)

J30.0 Vasomotor rhinitis
  DEF: Noninfectious and nonallergic type of rhinitis for which the cause is often unknown. Symptoms often mimic those of allergic rhinitis with a diagnosis of vasomotor rhinitis typically made after ruling out allergens as the cause.

J30.1 Allergic rhinitis due to pollen
  Allergy NOS due to pollen
  Hay fever
  Pollinosis

J30.2 Other seasonal allergic rhinitis

J30.5 Allergic rhinitis due to food

✓5ᵗʰ **J30.8 Other allergic rhinitis**
  J30.81 Allergic rhinitis due to animal (cat) (dog) hair and dander
  J30.89 Other allergic rhinitis
    Perennial allergic rhinitis

J30.9 Allergic rhinitis, unspecified

✓4ᵗʰ **J31 Chronic rhinitis, nasopharyngitis and pharyngitis**
  Use additional code to identify:
  exposure to environmental tobacco smoke (Z77.22)
  exposure to tobacco smoke in the perinatal period (P96.81)
  history of tobacco dependence (Z87.891)
  occupational exposure to environmental tobacco smoke (Z57.31)
  tobacco dependence (F17.-)
  tobacco use (Z72.0)

J31.0 Chronic rhinitis
  Atrophic rhinitis (chronic)
  Granulomatous rhinitis (chronic)
  Hypertrophic rhinitis (chronic)
  Obstructive rhinitis (chronic)
  Ozena
  Purulent rhinitis (chronic)
  Rhinitis (chronic) NOS
  Ulcerative rhinitis (chronic)
  EXCLUDES 1 *allergic rhinitis (J30.1-J30.9)*
    vasomotor rhinitis (J30.0)
  DEF: Persistent inflammation of the mucous membranes of the nose, characterized by a postnasal drip.

J31.1 Chronic nasopharyngitis
  EXCLUDES 2 *acute nasopharyngitis (J00)*
  DEF: Persistent inflammation of the mucous membranes extending from the nares to the pharynx. It is characterized by constant irritation in the nasopharynx and postnasal drip.

J31.2 Chronic pharyngitis
  Atrophic pharyngitis (chronic)
  Chronic sore throat
  Granular pharyngitis (chronic)
  Hypertrophic pharyngitis (chronic)
  EXCLUDES 2 *acute pharyngitis (J02.9)*

✓4ᵗʰ **J32 Chronic sinusitis**
  INCLUDES sinus abscess
    sinus empyema
    sinus infection
    sinus suppuration
  Use additional code to identify:
  exposure to environmental tobacco smoke (Z77.22)
  exposure to tobacco smoke in the perinatal period (P96.81)
  history of tobacco dependence (Z87.891)
  infectious agent (B95-B97)
  occupational exposure to environmental tobacco smoke (Z57.31)
  tobacco dependence (F17.-)
  tobacco use (Z72.0)
  EXCLUDES 2 *acute sinusitis (J01.-)*

J32.0 Chronic maxillary sinusitis
  Antritis (chronic)
  Maxillary sinusitis NOS

J32.1 Chronic frontal sinusitis
  Frontal sinusitis NOS

J32.2 Chronic ethmoidal sinusitis
  Ethmoidal sinusitis NOS
  EXCLUDES 1 *Woakes' ethmoiditis (J33.1)*

J32.3 Chronic sphenoidal sinusitis
  Sphenoidal sinusitis NOS

J32.4 Chronic pansinusitis
  Pansinusitis NOS

J32.8 Other chronic sinusitis
  Sinusitis (chronic) involving more than one sinus but not pansinusitis

J32.9 Chronic sinusitis, unspecified
  Sinusitis (chronic) NOS

✓4ᵗʰ **J33 Nasal polyp**
  Use additional code to identify:
  exposure to environmental tobacco smoke (Z77.22)
  exposure to tobacco smoke in the perinatal period (P96.81)
  history of tobacco dependence (Z87.891)
  occupational exposure to environmental tobacco smoke (Z57.31)
  tobacco dependence (F17.-)
  tobacco use (Z72.0)
  EXCLUDES 1 *adenomatous polyps (D14.0)*

J33.0 Polyp of nasal cavity
  Choanal polyp
  Nasopharyngeal polyp

J33.1 Polypoid sinus degeneration
  Woakes' syndrome or ethmoiditis

J33.8 Other polyp of sinus
  Accessory polyp of sinus
  Ethmoidal polyp of sinus
  Maxillary polyp of sinus
  Sphenoidal polyp of sinus

J33.9 Nasal polyp, unspecified

✓4ᵗʰ **J34 Other and unspecified disorders of nose and nasal sinuses**
  EXCLUDES 2 *varicose ulcer of nasal septum (I86.8)*

J34.0 Abscess, furuncle and carbuncle of nose
  Cellulitis of nose
  Necrosis of nose
  Ulceration of nose

[handwritten: Y82.8 Y82.9 mucous membrane pressure ulcer]

J34.1 Cyst and mucocele of nose and nasal sinus

J34.2 Deviated nasal septum
  Deflection or deviation of septum (nasal) (acquired)
  EXCLUDES 1 *congenital deviated nasal septum (Q67.4)*
  DEF: Condition in which the nasal septum, a thin wall composed of cartilage and bone that separates the two nostrils, is crooked or displaced from the midline.

J34.3 Hypertrophy of nasal turbinates
  DEF: Overgrowth of bones within the nasal turbinate, which are ridges of bone and soft tissue that project from the sidewalls of the nasal passages. Hypertrophy can cause obstruction of the nasal passages.

✓5ᵗʰ **J34.8 Other specified disorders of nose and nasal sinuses**
  J34.81 Nasal mucositis (ulcerative)
    Code also type of associated therapy, such as:
    antineoplastic and immunosuppressive drugs (T45.1X-)
    radiological procedure and radiotherapy (Y84.2)
    EXCLUDES 2 *gastrointestinal mucositis (ulcerative) (K92.81)*
      mucositis (ulcerative) of vagina and vulva (N76.81)
      oral mucositis (ulcerative) (K12.3-)
  J34.89 Other specified disorders of nose and nasal sinuses
    Perforation of nasal septum NOS
    Rhinolith

J34.9 Unspecified disorder of nose and nasal sinuses

✓4ᵗʰ **J35 Chronic diseases of tonsils and adenoids**
  Use additional code to identify:
  exposure to environmental tobacco smoke (Z77.22)
  exposure to tobacco smoke in the perinatal period (P96.81)
  history of tobacco dependence (Z87.891)
  occupational exposure to environmental tobacco smoke (Z57.31)
  tobacco dependence (F17.-)
  tobacco use (Z72.0)

✓5ᵗʰ **J35.0 Chronic tonsillitis and adenoiditis**
  EXCLUDES 2 *acute tonsillitis (J03.-)*
  J35.01 Chronic tonsillitis

Chapter 10. Diseases of the Respiratory System

J35.Ø2   **Chronic** adenoiditis

J35.Ø3   **Chronic** tonsillitis and adenoiditis

J35.1   **Hypertrophy of** tonsils
Enlargement of tonsils
> EXCLUDES 1   *hypertrophy of tonsils with tonsillitis (J35.Ø-)*

J35.2   **Hypertrophy of** adenoids
Enlargement of adenoids
> EXCLUDES 1   *hypertrophy of adenoids with adenoiditis (J35.Ø-)*

J35.3   **Hypertrophy of** tonsils with hypertrophy of adenoids
> EXCLUDES 1   *hypertrophy of tonsils and adenoids with tonsillitis and adenoiditis (J35.Ø3)*

J35.8   **Other chronic diseases of tonsils and adenoids**
Adenoid vegetations
Amygdalolith ·
Calculus, tonsil
Cicatrix of tonsil (and adenoid)
Tonsillar tag
Ulcer of tonsil

J35.9   **Chronic disease of tonsils and adenoids, unspecified**
Disease (chronic) of tonsils and adenoids NOS

J36 Peritonsillar abscess
> INCLUDES   abscess of tonsil
> peritonsillar cellulitis
> quinsy

Use additional code (B95-B97) to identify infectious agent
> EXCLUDES 1   *acute tonsillitis (JØ3.-)*
> *chronic tonsillitis (J35.Ø)*
> *retropharyngeal abscess (J39.Ø)*
> *tonsillitis NOS (JØ3.9-)*

✓4ᵗʰ J37 Chronic laryngitis and laryngotracheitis
Use additional code to identify:
exposure to environmental tobacco smoke (Z77.22)
exposure to tobacco smoke in the perinatal period (P96.81)
history of tobacco dependence (Z87.891)
infectious agent (B95-B97)
occupational exposure to environmental tobacco smoke (Z57.31)
tobacco dependence (F17.-)
tobacco use (Z72.Ø)

J37.Ø   **Chronic** laryngitis
Catarrhal laryngitis
Hypertrophic laryngitis
Sicca laryngitis
> EXCLUDES 2   *acute laryngitis (JØ4.Ø)*
> *obstructive (acute) laryngitis (JØ5.Ø)*

J37.1   **Chronic** laryngotracheitis
Laryngitis, chronic, with tracheitis (chronic)
Tracheitis, chronic, with laryngitis
> EXCLUDES 1   *chronic tracheitis (J42)*
> EXCLUDES 2   *acute laryngotracheitis (JØ4.2)*
> *acute tracheitis (JØ4.1)*

✓4ᵗʰ J38 Diseases of vocal cords and larynx, not elsewhere classified
Use additional code to identify:
exposure to environmental tobacco smoke (Z77.22)
exposure to tobacco smoke in the perinatal period (P96.81)
history of tobacco dependence (Z87.891)
occupational exposure to environmental tobacco smoke (Z57.31)
tobacco dependence (F17.-)
tobacco use (Z72.Ø)
> EXCLUDES 1   *congenital laryngeal stridor (P28.89)*
> *obstructive laryngitis (acute) (JØ5.Ø)*
> *postprocedural subglottic stenosis (J95.5)*
> *stridor (RØ6.1)*
> *ulcerative laryngitis (JØ4.Ø)*

✓5ᵗʰ J38.Ø   **Paralysis of vocal cords and larynx**
Laryngoplegia
Paralysis of glottis

J38.ØØ   **Paralysis of vocal cords and larynx, unspecified**

J38.Ø1   **Paralysis of vocal cords and larynx,** unilateral

J38.Ø2   **Paralysis of vocal cords and larynx,** bilateral

J38.1   **Polyp of vocal cord and larynx**
> EXCLUDES 1   *adenomatous polyps (D14.1)*

J38.2   **Nodules of vocal cords**
Chorditis (fibrinous)(nodosa)(tuberosa)
Singer's nodes
Teacher's nodes

J38.3   **Other diseases of vocal cords**
Abscess of vocal cords
Cellulitis of vocal cords
Granuloma of vocal cords
Leukokeratosis of vocal cords
Leukoplakia of vocal cords

J38.4   **Edema of larynx**
Edema (of) glottis
Subglottic edema
Supraglottic edema
> EXCLUDES 1   *acute obstructive laryngitis [croup] (JØ5.Ø)*
> *edematous laryngitis (JØ4.Ø)*

J38.5   **Laryngeal spasm**
Laryngismus (stridulus)

J38.6   **Stenosis of larynx**

J38.7   **Other diseases of larynx**
Abscess of larynx
Cellulitis of larynx
Disease of larynx NOS
Necrosis of larynx
Pachyderma of larynx
Perichondritis of larynx
Ulcer of larynx

✓4ᵗʰ J39 Other diseases of upper respiratory tract
> EXCLUDES 1   *acute respiratory infection NOS (J22)*
> *acute upper respiratory infection (JØ6.9)*
> *upper respiratory inflammation due to chemicals, gases, fumes or vapors (J68.2)*

J39.Ø   **Retropharyngeal and parapharyngeal abscess**
Peripharyngeal abscess
> EXCLUDES 1   *peritonsillar abscess (J36)*

DEF: Purulent infection behind the pharynx and the front of the precerebral fascia, characterized by neck stiffness, cervical lymphadenopathy, sore throat, fever, and stridor.

J39.1   **Other abscess of pharynx**
Cellulitis of pharynx
Nasopharyngeal abscess

J39.2   **Other diseases of pharynx**
Cyst of pharynx
Edema of pharynx
> EXCLUDES 2   *chronic pharyngitis (J31.2)*
> *ulcerative pharyngitis (JØ2.9)*

J39.3   **Upper respiratory tract hypersensitivity reaction, site unspecified**
> EXCLUDES 1   *hypersensitivity reaction of upper respiratory tract, such as:*
> *extrinsic allergic alveolitis (J67.9)*
> *pneumoconiosis (J6Ø-J67.9)*

J39.8   **Other specified diseases of upper respiratory tract**

J39.9   **Disease of upper respiratory tract, unspecified**

Chronic lower respiratory diseases (J4Ø-J47)

> EXCLUDES 1   *bronchitis due to chemicals, gases, fumes and vapors (J68.Ø)*
> EXCLUDES 2   *cystic fibrosis (E84.-)*

J4Ø Bronchitis, not specified as acute or chronic
Bronchitis NOS
Bronchitis with tracheitis NOS
Catarrhal bronchitis
Tracheobronchitis NOS
Use additional code to identify:
exposure to environmental tobacco smoke (Z77.22)
exposure to tobacco smoke in the perinatal period (P96.81)
history of tobacco dependence (Z87.891)
occupational exposure to environmental tobacco smoke (Z57.31)
tobacco dependence (F17.-)
tobacco use (Z72.Ø)
> EXCLUDES 1   *acute bronchitis (J2Ø.-)*
> *allergic bronchitis NOS (J45.9Ø9-)*
> *asthmatic bronchitis NOS (J45.9-)*
> *bronchitis due to chemicals, gases, fumes and vapors (J68.Ø)*

N Newborn: 0   P Pediatric: 0-17   M Maternity: 12-55   A Adult: 15-124   CH Comorbidity High   CL Comorbidity Low   NCDx Noncancer Dx   PDx Primary Dx

684   ICD-10-CM 2020

✓4ᵗʰ **J41 Simple and mucopurulent chronic bronchitis**

Use additional code to identify:

exposure to environmental tobacco smoke (Z77.22)
exposure to tobacco smoke in the perinatal period (P96.81)
history of tobacco dependence (Z87.891)
occupational exposure to environmental tobacco smoke (Z57.31)
tobacco dependence (F17.-)
tobacco use (Z72.0)

EXCLUDES 1   *chronic bronchitis NOS (J42)*
                chronic obstructive bronchitis (J44.-)

J41.0 Simple chronic bronchitis

J41.1 Mucopurulent chronic bronchitis

J41.8 Mixed simple and mucopurulent chronic bronchitis

J42 Unspecified chronic bronchitis

Chronic bronchitis NOS
Chronic tracheitis
Chronic tracheobronchitis

Use additional code to identify:

exposure to environmental tobacco smoke (Z77.22)
exposure to tobacco smoke in the perinatal period (P96.81)
history of tobacco dependence (Z87.891)
occupational exposure to environmental tobacco smoke (Z57.31)
tobacco dependence (F17.-)
tobacco use (Z72.0)

EXCLUDES 1   *chronic asthmatic bronchitis (J44.-)*
                chronic bronchitis with airways obstruction (J44.-)
                chronic emphysematous bronchitis (J44.-)
                chronic obstructive pulmonary disease NOS (J44.9)
                simple and mucopurulent chronic bronchitis (J41.-)

✓4ᵗʰ **J43 Emphysema**

Use additional code to identify:

exposure to environmental tobacco smoke (Z77.22)
history of tobacco dependence (Z87.891)
occupational exposure to environmental tobacco smoke (Z57.31)
tobacco dependence (F17.-)
tobacco use (Z72.0)

EXCLUDES 1   *compensatory emphysema (J98.3)*
                emphysema due to inhalation of chemicals, gases, fumes or vapors (J68.4)
                emphysema with chronic (obstructive) bronchitis (J44.-)
                emphysematous (obstructive) bronchitis (J44.-)
                interstitial emphysema (J98.2)
                mediastinal emphysema (J98.2)
                neonatal interstitial emphysema (P25.0)
                surgical (subcutaneous) emphysema (T81.82)
                traumatic subcutaneous emphysema (T79.7)

DEF: Pathological condition in which there is destructive enlargement of the air sacs in the lungs resulting in damage and lack of elasticity to the alveolar walls, commonly seen in long-term smokers.

Emphysema

Healthy alveoli | Alveoli w/ Emphysema
Patent bronchiole
Collapsed bronchiole
Well-vascularized
Enlarged alveoli | Broken/ fewer capillaries
Dilated alveoli | Alveolar membranes break down
Excess mucus

J43.0 Unilateral pulmonary emphysema [MacLeod's syndrome]

Swyer-James syndrome
Unilateral emphysema
Unilateral hyperlucent lung
Unilateral pulmonary artery functional hypoplasia
Unilateral transparency of lung

J43.1 Panlobular emphysema

Panacinar emphysema

J43.2 Centrilobular emphysema

J43.8 Other emphysema

J43.9 Emphysema, unspecified

Bullous emphysema (lung)(pulmonary)
Emphysema (lung)(pulmonary) NOS
Emphysematous bleb
Vesicular emphysema (lung)(pulmonary)
AHA: 2019,1Q,34-36; 2017,4Q,97-98

✓4ᵗʰ **J44 Other chronic obstructive pulmonary disease**

INCLUDES   asthma with chronic obstructive pulmonary disease
              chronic asthmatic (obstructive) bronchitis
              chronic bronchitis with airways obstruction
              chronic bronchitis with emphysema
              chronic emphysematous bronchitis
              chronic obstructive asthma
              chronic obstructive bronchitis
              chronic obstructive tracheobronchitis

Code also type of asthma, if applicable (J45.-)

Use additional code to identify:

exposure to environmental tobacco smoke (Z77.22)
history of tobacco dependence (Z87.891)
occupational exposure to environmental tobacco smoke (Z57.31)
tobacco dependence (F17.-)
tobacco use (Z72.0)

EXCLUDES 1   *bronchiectasis (J47.-)*
                chronic bronchitis NOS (J42)
                chronic simple and mucopurulent bronchitis (J41.-)
                chronic tracheitis (J42)
                chronic tracheobronchitis (J42)
                emphysema without chronic bronchitis (J43.-)

AHA: 2019,1Q,34-36; 2017,4Q,97-98; 2017,1Q,25-26; 2016,3Q,15-16; 2013,4Q,109

J44.0 Chronic obstructive pulmonary disease with   CH NC Dx
(acute) lower respiratory infection

Code also to identify the infection
AHA: 2019,1Q,35; 2017,4Q,96; 2017,1Q,24-25

J44.1 Chronic obstructive pulmonary disease with   CH NC Dx
(acute) exacerbation

Decompensated COPD
Decompensated COPD with (acute) exacerbation

EXCLUDES 2   *chronic obstructive pulmonary disease [COPD] with acute bronchitis (J44.0)*
                lung diseases due to external agents (J60-J70)

AHA: 2019,1Q,34; 2017,4Q,96; 2017,1Q,26; 2016,1Q,36
TIP: Exacerbation of COPD should not be assumed based upon worsening of a concomitant respiratory disease or when COPD is described as end-stage.
TIP: Assign J43.9 when COPD exacerbation with emphysema is documented.

J44.9 Chronic obstructive pulmonary disease,   CH NC Dx
unspecified

Chronic obstructive airway disease NOS
Chronic obstructive lung disease NOS

EXCLUDES 2   *lung diseases due to external agents (J60-J70)*

AHA: 2019,1Q,36; 2017,4Q,96-97; 2016,1Q,36; 2014,4Q,21; 2013,4Q,109

Chapter 10. Diseases of the Respiratory System

☑️4ᵗʰ **J45 Asthma**

INCLUDES   allergic (predominantly) asthma
    allergic bronchitis NOS
    allergic rhinitis with asthma
    atopic asthma
    extrinsic allergic asthma
    hay fever with asthma
    idiosyncratic asthma
    intrinsic nonallergic asthma
    nonallergic asthma

Use additional code to identify:
    exposure to environmental tobacco smoke (Z77.22)
    exposure to tobacco smoke in the perinatal period (P96.81)
    history of tobacco dependence (Z87.891)
    occupational exposure to environmental tobacco smoke (Z57.31)
    tobacco dependence (F17.-)
    tobacco use (Z72.0)

EXCLUDES 1   *detergent asthma (J69.8)*
    eosinophilic asthma (J82)
    miner's asthma (J60)
    wheezing NOS (R06.2)
    wood asthma (J67.8)

EXCLUDES 2   *asthma with chronic obstructive pulmonary disease (J44.9)*
    chronic asthmatic (obstructive) bronchitis (J44.9)
    chronic obstructive asthma (J44.9)

AHA: 2019,1Q,36; 2017,1Q,25-26; 2012,4Q,99
DEF: Status asthmaticus: Severe, intractable episode of asthma that is unresponsive to normal therapeutic measures.
TIP: When asthma is present concurrent to COPD but not specified as to type or current exacerbation, assign only a code from J44.

Asthma

Respiratory bronchiole
Smooth muscle fibers
Contraction of smooth muscle fibers
Mucus lining bronchial tubes
Extra mucus secretion in inflamed bronchial tubes
Air trapped within alveoli
Alveoli

Normal alveoli   Asthmatic alveoli

☑️5ᵗʰ **J45.2 Mild intermittent asthma**

   J45.20 Mild intermittent asthma, uncomplicated   CH
     Mild intermittent asthma NOS

   J45.21 Mild intermittent asthma with (acute) exacerbation   CH

   J45.22 Mild intermittent asthma with status asthmaticus   CH

☑️5ᵗʰ **J45.3 Mild persistent asthma**

   J45.30 Mild persistent asthma, uncomplicated   CH
     Mild persistent asthma NOS

   J45.31 Mild persistent asthma with (acute) exacerbation   CH
     AHA: 2016,1Q,35

   J45.32 Mild persistent asthma with status asthmaticus   CH

☑️5ᵗʰ **J45.4 Moderate persistent asthma**

   J45.40 Moderate persistent asthma, uncomplicated   CH
     Moderate persistent asthma NOS

   J45.41 Moderate persistent asthma with (acute) exacerbation   CH
     AHA: 2017,1Q,26

   J45.42 Moderate persistent asthma with status asthmaticus   CH

☑️5ᵗʰ **J45.5 Severe persistent asthma**

   J45.50 Severe persistent asthma, uncomplicated   CH
     Severe persistent asthma NOS

   J45.51 Severe persistent asthma with (acute) exacerbation   CH

   J45.52 Severe persistent asthma with status asthmaticus   CH

☑️5ᵗʰ **J45.9 Other and unspecified asthma**

   ☑️6ᵗʰ **J45.90 Unspecified asthma**
     Asthmatic bronchitis NOS
     Childhood asthma NOS
     Late onset asthma
     AHA: 2017,4Q,96; 2017,1Q,25

     J45.901 Unspecified asthma with (acute) exacerbation   CH

     J45.902 Unspecified asthma with status asthmaticus   CH

     J45.909 Unspecified asthma, uncomplicated   CH
       Asthma NOS
       EXCLUDES 2   *lung diseases due to external agents (J60-J70)*
       AHA: 2017,1Q,25

   ☑️6ᵗʰ **J45.99 Other asthma**

     J45.990 Exercise induced bronchospasm   CH

     J45.991 Cough variant asthma   CH

     J45.998 Other asthma   CH

☑️4ᵗʰ **J47 Bronchiectasis**

INCLUDES   bronchiolectasis

Use additional code to identify:
    exposure to environmental tobacco smoke (Z77.22)
    exposure to tobacco smoke in the perinatal period (P96.81)
    history of tobacco dependence (Z87.891)
    occupational exposure to environmental tobacco smoke (Z57.31)
    tobacco dependence (F17.-)
    tobacco use (Z72.0)

EXCLUDES 1   *congenital bronchiectasis (Q33.4)*
    tuberculous bronchiectasis (current disease) (A15.0)

DEF: Dilation of the bronchi with mucus production and persistent cough due to infection or chronic conditions that causes diminished lung capacity and frequent infections of the lung.

   J47.0 Bronchiectasis with acute lower respiratory infection   CH
     Bronchiectasis with acute bronchitis
     Use additional code to identify the infection

   J47.1 Bronchiectasis with (acute) exacerbation   CH

   J47.9 Bronchiectasis, uncomplicated   CH
     Bronchiectasis NOS

Lung diseases due to external agents (J60-J70)

EXCLUDES 2   *asthma (J45.-)*
    malignant neoplasm of bronchus and lung (C34.-)

DEF: Pneumoconiosis: Condition caused by inhaling inorganic dust particles, typically associated with occupations that require regular exposure to mineral dusts. A form of interstitial lung disease that contributes to the inflammation of the air sacs, causing the lung tissue to harden.

J60 Coalworker's pneumoconiosis   A
   Anthracosilicosis
   Anthracosis
   Black lung disease
   Coalworker's lung
   EXCLUDES 1   *coalworker pneumoconiosis with tuberculosis, any type in A15 (J65)*

J61 Pneumoconiosis due to asbestos and other mineral fibers   A
   Asbestosis
   EXCLUDES 1   *pleural plaque with asbestosis (J92.0)*
    pneumoconiosis with tuberculosis, any type in A15 (J65)

☑️4ᵗʰ **J62 Pneumoconiosis due to dust containing silica**
   INCLUDES   silicotic fibrosis (massive) of lung
   EXCLUDES 1   *pneumoconiosis with tuberculosis, any type in A15 (J65)*

   J62.0 Pneumoconiosis due to talc dust

J62.8   **Pneumoconiosis due to** other dust containing silica
     Silicosis NOS

✓4ᵗʰ   **J63**   **Pneumoconiosis due to other** inorganic dusts
     EXCLUDES 1   *pneumoconiosis with tuberculosis, any type in A15 (J65)*

     J63.0   **Aluminosis (of lung)**

     J63.1   **Bauxite fibrosis (of lung)**

     J63.2   **Berylliosis**

     J63.3   **Graphite fibrosis (of lung)**

     J63.4   **Siderosis**

     J63.5   **Stannosis**

     J63.6   **Pneumoconiosis due to other specified inorganic dusts**

J64   **Unspecified pneumoconiosis**
     EXCLUDES 1   *pneumonoconiosis with tuberculosis, any type in A15 (J65)*

J65   **Pneumoconiosis** associated with tuberculosis
     Any condition in J60-J64 with tuberculosis, any type in A15
     Silicotuberculosis

✓4ᵗʰ   **J66**   **Airway disease due to specific** organic dust
     EXCLUDES 2   *allergic alveolitis (J67.-)*
         asbestosis (J61)
         bagassosis (J67.1)
         farmer's lung (J67.0)
         hypersensitivity pneumonitis due to organic dust (J67.-)
         reactive airways dysfunction syndrome (J68.3)

     J66.0   **Byssinosis**
         Airway disease due to cotton dust

     J66.1   **Flax-dressers' disease**

     J66.2   **Cannabinosis**

     J66.8   **Airway disease due to other specific organic dusts**

✓4ᵗʰ   **J67**   **Hypersensitivity pneumonitis due to organic dust**
     INCLUDES   allergic alveolitis and pneumonitis due to inhaled organic
         dust and particles of fungal, actinomycetic or other
         origin
     EXCLUDES 1   *pneumonitis due to inhalation of chemicals, gases, fumes or*
         vapors (J68.0)

     J67.0   **Farmer's lung**
         Harvester's lung
         Haymaker's lung
         Moldy hay disease

     J67.1   **Bagassosis**
         Bagasse disease
         Bagasse pneumonitis

     J67.2   **Bird fancier's lung**
         Budgerigar fancier's disease or lung
         Pigeon fancier's disease or lung

     J67.3   **Suberosis**
         Corkhandler's disease or lung
         Corkworker's disease or lung

     J67.4   **Maltworker's lung**
         Alveolitis due to Aspergillus clavatus

     J67.5   **Mushroom-worker's lung**

     J67.6   **Maple-bark-stripper's lung**
         Alveolitis due to Cryptostroma corticale
         Cryptostromosis

     J67.7   **Air conditioner and humidifier lung**
         Allergic alveolitis due to fungal, thermophilic actinomycetes
         and other organisms growing in ventilation [air
         conditioning] systems

     J67.8   **Hypersensitivity pneumonitis due to other organic dusts**
         Cheese-washer's lung
         Coffee-worker's lung
         Fish-meal worker's lung
         Furrier's lung
         Sequoiosis

     J67.9   **Hypersensitivity pneumonitis due to unspecified organic dust**
         Allergic alveolitis (extrinsic) NOS
         Hypersensitivity pneumonitis NOS

✓4ᵗʰ   **J68**   **Respiratory conditions due to inhalation of chemicals, gases, fumes and vapors**
     Code first (T51-T65) to identify cause
     Use additional code to identify associated respiratory conditions, such as:
     acute respiratory failure (J96.0-)

     J68.0   **Bronchitis and pneumonitis due to chemicals, gases, fumes and vapors**
         Chemical bronchitis (acute)
         AHA: 2019,2Q,31

     J68.1   **Pulmonary edema due to chemicals, gases, fumes and vapors**
         Chemical pulmonary edema (acute) (chronic)
         EXCLUDES 1   *pulmonary edema (acute) (chronic) NOS (J81.-)*

     J68.2   **Upper respiratory inflammation due to chemicals, gases, fumes and vapors, not elsewhere classified**

     J68.3   **Other** acute and subacute respiratory conditions **due to chemicals, gases, fumes and vapors**
         Reactive airways dysfunction syndrome

     J68.4   **Chronic respiratory conditions due to chemicals, gases, fumes and vapors**
         Emphysema (diffuse) (chronic) due to inhalation of chemicals,
         gases, fumes and vapors
         Obliterative bronchiolitis (chronic) (subacute) due to inhalation
         of chemicals, gases, fumes and vapors
         Pulmonary fibrosis (chronic) due to inhalation of chemicals,
         gases, fumes and vapors
         EXCLUDES 1   *chronic pulmonary edema due to chemicals, gases,*
           fumes and vapors (J68.1)

     J68.8   **Other respiratory conditions due to chemicals, gases, fumes and vapors**

     J68.9   **Unspecified respiratory condition due to chemicals, gases, fumes and vapors**

✓4ᵗʰ   **J69**   **Pneumonitis due to solids and liquids**
     EXCLUDES 1   *neonatal aspiration syndromes (P24.-)*
         postprocedural pneumonitis (J95.4)

     AHA: 2017,1Q,24
     DEF: Pneumonitis: Noninfectious inflammation of the walls of the alveoli
     in the lung tissue due to inhalation of food, vomit, oils, essences, or other
     solids or liquids.

     J69.0   **Pneumonitis due to** inhalation of food and vomit
         Aspiration pneumonia NOS
         Aspiration pneumonia (due to) food (regurgitated)
         Aspiration pneumonia (due to) gastric secretions
         Aspiration pneumonia (due to) milk
         Aspiration pneumonia (due to) vomit
         Code also any associated foreign body in respiratory tract (T17.-)
         EXCLUDES 1   *chemical pneumonitis due to anesthesia (J95.4)*
           obstetric aspiration pneumonitis (O74.0)

         AHA: 2019,2Q,6,31
         TIP: Aspiration pneumonia is not classified to respiratory infection
         codes and does not warrant the assignment of J44.0 Chronic
         obstructive pulmonary disease with acute lower respiratory
         infection, when present concurrently with COPD.

     J69.1   **Pneumonitis due to** inhalation of oils and essences
         Exogenous lipoid pneumonia
         Lipid pneumonia NOS
         Code first (T51-T65) to identify substance
         EXCLUDES 1   *endogenous lipoid pneumonia (J84.89)*

     J69.8   **Pneumonitis due to inhalation of other solids and liquids**
         Pneumonitis due to aspiration of blood
         Pneumonitis due to aspiration of detergent
         Code first (T51-T65) to identify substance

✓4ᵗʰ   **J70**   **Respiratory conditions due to other external agents**

     J70.0   **Acute pulmonary manifestations due to** radiation
         Radiation pneumonitis
         Use additional code (W88-W90, X39.0-) to identify the external
         cause

     J70.1   **Chronic and other pulmonary manifestations due to** radiation
         Fibrosis of lung following radiation
         Use additional code (W88-W90, X39.0-) to identify the external
         cause

     J70.2   **Acute drug-induced interstitial lung disorders**
         Use additional code for adverse effect, if applicable, to identify
         drug (T36-T50 with fifth or sixth character 5)
         EXCLUDES 1   *interstitial pneumonia NOS (J84.9)*
           lymphoid interstitial pneumonia (J84.2)

         AHA: 2019,2Q,28

✓ Additional Character Required   ✓x7ᵗʰ Placeholder Alert   Manifestation   Unspecified Dx   ▶◀ Revised Text   ● New Code   ▲ Revised Title

ICD-10-CM 2020   687

J70.3 Chronic drug-induced interstitial **lung disorders**
> Use additional code for adverse effect, if applicable, to identify drug (T36-T50 with fifth or sixth character 5)
> **EXCLUDES 1** *interstitial pneumonia NOS (J84.9)*
> *lymphoid interstitial pneumonia (J84.2)*

J70.4 **Drug-induced interstitial lung disorders, unspecified**
> Use additional code for adverse effect, if applicable, to identify drug (T36-T50 with fifth or sixth character 5)
> **EXCLUDES 1** *interstitial pneumonia NOS (J84.9)*
> *lymphoid interstitial pneumonia (J84.2)*
> **AHA:** 2019,2Q,28

J70.5 **Respiratory conditions due to** smoke inhalation
> Smoke inhalation NOS
> **EXCLUDES 1** *smoke inhalation due to chemicals, gases, fumes and vapors (J68.9)*
> **AHA:** 2013,4Q,121

J70.8 **Respiratory conditions due to other specified external agents**
> Code first (T51-T65) to identify the external agent

J70.9 **Respiratory conditions due to unspecified external agent**
> Code first (T51-T65) to identify the external agent

Other respiratory diseases principally affecting the interstitium (J80-J84)

J80 Acute respiratory distress syndrome
> Acute respiratory distress syndrome in adult or child
> Adult hyaline membrane disease
> **EXCLUDES 1** *respiratory distress syndrome in newborn (perinatal) (P22.0)*
> **AHA:** 2017,1Q,26
> **DEF:** Lung inflammation or injury resulting in a build-up of fluid in the air sacs, preventing the passage of oxygen from the air into the bloodstream.
> **TIP:** Assign only when acute respiratory distress *syndrome* (ARDS) is specified. When provider documentation indicates only "respiratory distress" or "acute respiratory distress," assign R06.03.

✓4ᵗʰ J81 Pulmonary edema
> Use additional code to identify:
> exposure to environmental tobacco smoke (Z77.22)
> history of tobacco dependence (Z87.891)
> occupational exposure to environmental tobacco smoke (Z57.31)
> tobacco dependence (F17.-)
> tobacco use (Z72.0)
> **EXCLUDES 1** *chemical (acute) pulmonary edema (J68.1)*
> *hypostatic pneumonia (J18.2)*
> *passive pneumonia (J18.2)*
> *pulmonary edema due to external agents (J60-J70)*
> *pulmonary edema with heart disease NOS (I50.1)*
> *pulmonary edema with heart failure (I50.1)*
> **DEF:** Accumulation of fluid in the air sacs of the lungs, making it difficult to breath.

> **J81.0** Acute **pulmonary edema**
> > Acute edema of lung

> **J81.1** Chronic **pulmonary edema**
> > Pulmonary congestion (chronic) (passive)
> > Pulmonary edema NOS

J82 Pulmonary eosinophilia, not elsewhere classified
> Allergic pneumonia
> Eosinophilic asthma
> Eosinophilic pneumonia
> Löffler's pneumonia
> Tropical (pulmonary) eosinophilia NOS
> **EXCLUDES 1** *pulmonary eosinophilia due to aspergillosis (B44.-)*
> *pulmonary eosinophilia due to drugs (J70.2-J70.4)*
> *pulmonary eosinophilia due to specified parasitic infection (B50-B83)*
> *pulmonary eosinophilia due to systemic connective tissue disorders (M30-M36)*
> *pulmonary infiltrate NOS (R91.8)*
> **DEF:** Infiltration of eosinophils (white blood cells of the immune system) into the parenchyma of the lungs, resulting in cough, fever, and dyspnea.

✓4ᵗʰ J84 Other interstitial **pulmonary diseases**
> **EXCLUDES 1** *drug-induced interstitial lung disorders (J70.2-J70.4)*
> *interstitial emphysema (J98.2)*
> **EXCLUDES 2** *lung diseases due to external agents (J60-J70)*
> **DEF:** Interstitial: Within the small spaces or gaps occurring in tissue or organs.

✓5ᵗʰ J84.0 Alveolar and parieto-alveolar conditions

> **J84.01** **Alveolar** proteinosis
> > **DEF:** Reduced ventilation due to proteinaceous deposits on alveoli. Symptoms include dyspnea, cough, chest pain, weakness, weight loss, and hemoptysis.

> **J84.02** **Pulmonary alveolar** microlithiasis

> **J84.03** *Idiopathic pulmonary* hemosiderosis
> > Essential brown induration of lung
> > Code first underlying disease, such as:
> > disorders of iron metabolism (E83.1-)
> > **EXCLUDES 1** *acute idiopathic pulmonary hemorrhage in infants [AIPHI] (R04.81)*
> > **DEF:** Fibrosis of the alveolar walls marked by abnormal accumulation of iron as hemosiderin in the lungs. It primarily affects children and symptoms include anemia, fluid in the lungs, and blood in the sputum. Etiology is unknown.

> **J84.09** **Other alveolar and parieto-alveolar conditions**

✓5ᵗʰ J84.1 Other interstitial pulmonary diseases with fibrosis
> **EXCLUDES 1** *pulmonary fibrosis (chronic) due to inhalation of chemicals, gases, fumes or vapors (J68.4)*
> *pulmonary fibrosis (chronic) following radiation (J70.1)*

> **J84.10** **Pulmonary fibrosis, unspecified**
> > Capillary fibrosis of lung
> > Cirrhosis of lung (chronic) NOS
> > Fibrosis of lung (atrophic) (chronic) (confluent) (massive) (perialveolar) (peribronchial) NOS
> > Induration of lung (chronic) NOS
> > Postinflammatory pulmonary fibrosis

> **✓6ᵗʰ J84.11** **Idiopathic interstitial pneumonia**
> > **EXCLUDES 1** *lymphoid interstitial pneumonia (J84.2)*
> > *pneumocystis pneumonia (B59)*

> > **J84.111** **Idiopathic interstitial** pneumonia, **not otherwise specified**

> > **J84.112** **Idiopathic** pulmonary fibrosis
> > > Cryptogenic fibrosing alveolitis
> > > Idiopathic fibrosing alveolitis

> > **J84.113** **Idiopathic** non-specific **interstitial pneumonitis**
> > > **EXCLUDES 1** *non-specific interstitial pneumonia NOS, or due to known underlying cause (J84.89)*

> > **J84.114** Acute **interstitial pneumonitis**
> > > Hamman-Rich syndrome
> > > **EXCLUDES 1** *pneumocystis pneumonia (B59)*

> > **J84.115** Respiratory bronchiolitis **interstitial lung disease**

> > **J84.116** Cryptogenic organizing **pneumonia**
> > > **EXCLUDES 1** *organizing pneumonia NOS, or due to known underlying cause (J84.89)*

> > **J84.117** Desquamative **interstitial pneumonia**

> **J84.17** *Other interstitial pulmonary diseases with fibrosis in diseases classified elsewhere*
> > Interstitial pneumonia (nonspecific) (usual) due to collagen vascular disease
> > Interstitial pneumonia (nonspecific) (usual) in diseases classified elsewhere
> > Organizing pneumonia due to collagen vascular disease
> > Organizing pneumonia in diseases classified elsewhere
> > Code first underlying disease, such as:
> > progressive systemic sclerosis (M34.0)
> > rheumatoid arthritis (M05.00-M06.9)
> > systemic lupus erythematosis (M32.0-M32.9)

> **J84.2** Lymphoid **interstitial pneumonia**
> > Lymphoid interstitial pneumonitis

Ⓝ Newborn: 0   Ⓟ Pediatric: 0-17   Ⓜ Maternity: 12-55   Ⓐ Adult: 15-124   CH Comorbidity High   CL Comorbidity Low   NC Dx Noncancer Dx   PDx Primary Dx

688

ICD-10-CM 2020

✓5ᵗʰ **J84.8 Other specified interstitial pulmonary diseases**

     EXCLUDES 1   *exogenous lipoid pneumonia (J69.1)*
               unspecified lipoid pneumonia (J69.1)

   J84.81 Lymphangioleiomyomatosis
         Lymphangiomyomatosis

   J84.82 Adult pulmonary Langerhans cell   🅰
         histiocytosis
         Adult PLCH

   J84.83 Surfactant mutations of the lung
         DEF: Genetic disorder resulting in insufficient secretion of a complex mixture of phospholipids and proteins that reduce surface tension in the alveoli following the onset of breathing to facilitate lung expansion in the newborn. It is the leading indication for pediatric lung transplantation.

✓6ᵗʰ   **J84.84 Other interstitial lung diseases of** childhood

     J84.841 Neuroendocrine cell hyperplasia of infancy

     J84.842 Pulmonary interstitial glycogenosis

     J84.843 Alveolar capillary dysplasia with vein misalignment

     J84.848 Other interstitial lung diseases of childhood

   J84.89 Other specified interstitial pulmonary diseases
         Endogenous lipoid pneumonia
         Interstitial pneumonitis
         Non-specific interstitial pneumonitis NOS
         Organizing pneumonia NOS
         Code first, if applicable:
            poisoning due to drug or toxin (T51-T65 with fifth or sixth character to indicate intent), for toxic pneumonopathy
            underlying cause of pneumonopathy, if known
         Use additional code, for adverse effect, to identify drug (T36-T50 with fifth or sixth character 5), if drug-induced

         EXCLUDES 1   *cryptogenic organizing pneumonia (J84.116)*
                   idiopathic non-specific interstitial pneumonitis (J84.113)
                   lymphoid interstitial pneumonia (J84.2)
                   lipoid pneumonia, exogenous or unspecified (J69.1)

         AHA: 2019,2Q,28

J84.9 Interstitial pulmonary disease, unspecified
     Interstitial pneumonia NOS

Suppurative and necrotic conditions of the lower respiratory tract (J85-J86)

✓4ᵗʰ **J85 Abscess of lung and mediastinum**
     Use additional code (B95-B97) to identify infectious agent

   J85.0 Gangrene and necrosis of lung

   J85.1 Abscess of lung with pneumonia
         Code also the type of pneumonia

   J85.2 Abscess of lung without pneumonia
         Abscess of lung NOS

   J85.3 Abscess of mediastinum

✓4ᵗʰ **J86 Pyothorax**
     Use additional code (B95-B97) to identify infectious agent
     EXCLUDES 1   *abscess of lung (J85.-)*
                pyothorax due to tuberculosis (A15.6)
     DEF: Collection of pus in the pleural space that is commonly caused by an infection that spreads from the lung, such as bacterial pneumonia or a lung abscess.

   J86.0 Pyothorax with fistula
         Bronchocutaneous fistula
         Bronchopleural fistula
         Hepatopleural fistula
         Mediastinal fistula
         Pleural fistula
         Thoracic fistula
         Any condition classifiable to J86.9 with fistula
         DEF: Purulent infection of the respiratory cavity, with communication from a cavity to another structure.

   J86.9 Pyothorax without fistula
         Abscess of pleura
         Abscess of thorax
         Empyema (chest) (lung) (pleura)
         Fibrinopurulent pleurisy
         Purulent pleurisy
         Pyopneumothorax
         Septic pleurisy
         Seropurulent pleurisy
         Suppurative pleurisy

Other diseases of the pleura (J90-J94)

J90 Pleural effusion, not elsewhere classified
     Encysted pleurisy
     Pleural effusion NOS
     Pleurisy with effusion (exudative) (serous)
     EXCLUDES 1   *chylous (pleural) effusion (J94.0)*
                malignant pleural effusion (J91.0))
                pleurisy NOS (R09.1)
                tuberculous pleural effusion (A15.6)
     DEF: Collection of lymph and other fluid within the pleural space.

✓4ᵗʰ **J91 Pleural effusion in conditions classified elsewhere**
     EXCLUDES 2   *pleural effusion in heart failure (I50.-)*
                pleural effusion in systemic lupus erythematosus (M32.13)
     DEF: Collection of lymph and other fluid within the pleural space.

   J91.0 Malignant pleural effusion
         Code first underlying neoplasm

   J91.8 Pleural effusion in other conditions classified elsewhere
         Code first underlying disease, such as:
            filariasis (B74.0-B74.9)
            influenza (J09.X2, J10.1, J11.1)
         AHA: 2015,2Q,15

Pleural Effusion

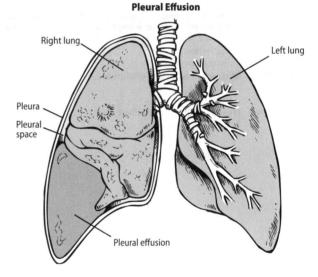

Right lung / Left lung / Pleura / Pleural space / Pleural effusion

✓4ᵗʰ **J92 Pleural plaque**
     INCLUDES   pleural thickening
     DEF: Areas of fibrous thickening that form on the parietal or visceral pleura, the membranes that line the ribs and lungs.

   J92.0 Pleural plaque with presence of asbestos

   J92.9 Pleural plaque without asbestos
         Pleural plaque NOS

✓4ᵗʰ **J93 Pneumothorax and air leak**
     EXCLUDES 1   *congenital or perinatal pneumothorax (P25.1)*
                postprocedural air leak (J95.812)
                postprocedural pneumothorax (J95.811)
                pyopneumothorax (J86.-)
                traumatic pneumothorax (S27.0)
                tuberculous (current disease) pneumothorax (A15.-)
     DEF: Pneumothorax: Lung displacement due to abnormal leakage of air or gas that is trapped in the pleural space formed by the membrane that encloses the lungs and lines the thoracic cavity.

   J93.0 Spontaneous tension pneumothorax
         DEF: Leaking air from the lung into the lining, causing collapse.

✓ Additional Character Required   ✓x7ᵗʰ Placeholder Alert   Manifestation   Unspecified Dx   ▶◀ Revised Text   ● New Code   ▲ Revised Title

ICD-10-CM 2020   689

✓5ᵗʰ **J93.1 Other** spontaneous **pneumothorax**

    J93.11 Primary **spontaneous pneumothorax**

    J93.12 Secondary **spontaneous pneumothorax**
        Code first underlying condition, such as:
            catamenial pneumothorax due to endometriosis
              (N80.8)
            cystic fibrosis (E84.-)
            eosinophilic pneumonia (J82)
            lymphangioleiomyomatosis (J84.81)
            malignant neoplasm of bronchus and lung (C34.-)
            Marfan's syndrome (Q87.4)
            pneumonia due to Pneumocystis carinii (B59)
            secondary malignant neoplasm of lung (C78.0-)
            spontaneous rupture of the esophagus (K22.3)

✓5ᵗʰ **J93.8 Other** pneumothorax and air leak

    J93.81 Chronic **pneumothorax**

    J93.82 Other air leak
        Persistent air leak

    J93.83 Other pneumothorax
        Acute pneumothorax
        Spontaneous pneumothorax NOS

J93.9 Pneumothorax, unspecified
    Pneumothorax NOS

✓4ᵗʰ **J94 Other pleural conditions**

    EXCLUDES 1   pleurisy NOS (R09.1)
               traumatic hemopneumothorax (S27.2)
               traumatic hemothorax (S27.1)
               tuberculous pleural conditions (current disease) (A15.-)

    J94.0 Chylous effusion
        Chyliform effusion
        DEF: Fluid within the pleural space due to the leaking of lymph
        contents into the space, usually as a result of thoracic duct
        damage or injury or mediastinal lymphoma.

    J94.1 Fibrothorax
        DEF: Fibrosis within the pleural lining of the lungs commonly
        seen as a stiff layer surrounding the lung typically attributed to
        traumatic hemothorax or pleural effusion.

    J94.2 Hemothorax
        Hemopneumothorax

    J94.8 Other specified pleural conditions
        Hydropneumothorax
        Hydrothorax

    J94.9 Pleural condition, unspecified

Intraoperative and postprocedural complications and disorders of respiratory system, not elsewhere classified (J95)

✓4ᵗʰ **J95 Intraoperative and postprocedural complications and disorders of respiratory system, not elsewhere classified**

    EXCLUDES 2   aspiration pneumonia (J69.-)
               emphysema (subcutaneous) resulting from a procedure
                 (T81.82)
               hypostatic pneumonia (J18.2)
               pulmonary manifestations due to radiation (J70.0-J70.1)

✓5ᵗʰ **J95.0 Tracheostomy complications**
        DEF: Tracheostomy: Formation of a tracheal opening on the neck
        surface with tube insertion to allow for respiration in cases of
        obstruction or decreased patency. A tracheostomy may be
        planned or performed on an emergency basis for temporary or
        long-term use.

Tracheostomy

Tracheostomy
in place

Incision
in trachea

Trachea

Tracheostomy
tube

    J95.00 Unspecified tracheostomy complication

    J95.01 Hemorrhage **from tracheostomy stoma**

    J95.02 Infection of tracheostomy stoma
        Use additional code to identify type of infection, such
          as:
        cellulitis of neck (L03.221)
        sepsis (A40, A41.-)

    J95.03 Malfunction **of tracheostomy stoma**
        Mechanical complication of tracheostomy stoma
        Obstruction of tracheostomy airway
        Tracheal stenosis due to tracheostomy

    J95.04 Tracheo-esophageal fistula **following tracheostomy**

    J95.09 Other tracheostomy complication

J95.1 Acute pulmonary insufficiency **following** thoracic surgery
    EXCLUDES 2   functional disturbances following cardiac surgery
               (I97.0, I97.1-)

J95.2 Acute pulmonary insufficiency **following** nonthoracic surgery
    EXCLUDES 2   functional disturbances following cardiac surgery
               (I97.0, I97.1-)

J95.3 Chronic pulmonary insufficiency **following surgery**
    EXCLUDES 2   functional disturbances following cardiac surgery
               (I97.0, I97.1-)

N Newborn: 0   P Pediatric: 0-17   M Maternity: 12-55   A Adult: 15-124   CH Comorbidity High   CL Comorbidity Low   NCDx Noncancer Dx   PDx Primary Dx

690   ICD-10-CM 2020

J95.4   Chemical pneumonitis **due to** anesthesia
     Mendelson's syndrome
     Postprocedural aspiration pneumonia
     Use additional code for adverse effect, if applicable, to identify drug (T41.- with fifth or sixth character 5)

     EXCLUDES 1   aspiration pneumonitis due to anesthesia complicating labor and delivery (O74.0)
         aspiration pneumonitis due to anesthesia complicating pregnancy (O29)
         aspiration pneumonitis due to anesthesia complicating the puerperium (O89.01)

J95.5   Postprocedural subglottic stenosis

✓5ᵗʰ **J95.6**   Intraoperative hemorrhage and hematoma **of a respiratory system organ or structure complicating a procedure**

     EXCLUDES 1   intraoperative hemorrhage and hematoma of a respiratory system organ or structure due to accidental puncture and laceration during procedure (J95.7-)

   J95.61   Intraoperative hemorrhage and hematoma of a respiratory system organ or structure complicating **a** respiratory system procedure

   J95.62   Intraoperative hemorrhage and hematoma of a respiratory system organ or structure complicating other procedure

✓5ᵗʰ **J95.7**   Accidental puncture and laceration **of a respiratory system organ or structure during a procedure**

     EXCLUDES 2   postprocedural pneumothorax (J95.811)

   J95.71   Accidental puncture and laceration of a respiratory system organ or structure during a respiratory system procedure

   J95.72   Accidental puncture and laceration of a respiratory system organ or structure during other procedure

✓5ᵗʰ **J95.8**   Other intraoperative and postprocedural complications and disorders of respiratory system, not elsewhere classified
     AHA: 2016,4Q,9-10

  ✓6ᵗʰ **J95.81**   Postprocedural pneumothorax and air leak

     J95.811   Postprocedural pneumothorax
     J95.812   Postprocedural air leak

  ✓6ᵗʰ **J95.82**   Postprocedural respiratory failure

     EXCLUDES 1   respiratory failure in other conditions (J96.-)

     J95.821   Acute postprocedural respiratory failure
         Postprocedural respiratory failure NOS

     J95.822   Acute and chronic postprocedural respiratory failure

  ✓6ᵗʰ **J95.83**   Postprocedural hemorrhage of a respiratory system organ or structure following a procedure

     J95.830   Postprocedural hemorrhage of a respiratory system organ or structure following a respiratory system procedure

     J95.831   Postprocedural hemorrhage of a respiratory system organ or structure following other procedure

   J95.84   Transfusion-related acute lung injury **(TRALI)**
     DEF: Relatively rare, but serious, pulmonary complication of blood transfusion, with acute respiratory distress, noncardiogenic pulmonary edema, cyanosis, hypoxemia, hypotension, fever, and chills.

  ✓6ᵗʰ **J95.85**   **Complication of** respirator **[ventilator]**

     J95.850   Mechanical **complication of** respirator

         EXCLUDES 1   encounter for respirator [ventilator] dependence during power failure (Z99.12)

     J95.851   **Ventilator** associated pneumonia
         Ventilator associated pneumonitis
         Use additional code to identify the organism, if known (B95.-, B96.-, B97.-)

         EXCLUDES 1   ventilator lung in newborn (P27.8)

         AHA: 2017,1Q,25

     J95.859   **Other complication of** respirator **[ventilator]**

  ✓6ᵗʰ **J95.86**   Postprocedural hematoma and seroma **of a respiratory system organ or structure following a procedure**

     J95.860   **Postprocedural** hematoma **of a respiratory system organ or structure following a** respiratory system procedure

     J95.861   **Postprocedural** hematoma **of a respiratory system organ or structure following** other procedure

     J95.862   **Postprocedural** seroma **of a respiratory system organ or structure following a** respiratory system **procedure**

     J95.863   **Postprocedural** seroma **of a respiratory system organ or structure following** other procedure

   J95.88   **Other intraoperative complications of respiratory system, not elsewhere classified**

   J95.89   **Other postprocedural complications and disorders of respiratory system, not elsewhere classified**
     Use additional code to identify disorder, such as:
       aspiration pneumonia (J69.-)
       bacterial or viral pneumonia (J12-J18)

     EXCLUDES 2   acute pulmonary insufficiency following thoracic surgery (J95.1)
         postprocedural subglottic stenosis (J95.5)

Other diseases of the respiratory system (J96-J99)

✓4ᵗʰ **J96**   **Respiratory failure, not elsewhere classified**

     EXCLUDES 1   acute respiratory distress syndrome (J80)
         cardiorespiratory failure (R09.2)
         newborn respiratory distress syndrome (P22.0)
         postprocedural respiratory failure (J95.82-)
         respiratory arrest (R09.2)
         respiratory arrest of newborn (P28.81)
         respiratory failure of newborn (P28.5)

  ✓5ᵗʰ **J96.0**   Acute **respiratory failure**

     J96.00   **Acute respiratory failure, unspecified whether with hypoxia or hypercapnia**
       AHA: 2016,3Q,14; 2013,4Q,121

     J96.01   **Acute respiratory failure with** hypoxia
     J96.02   **Acute respiratory failure with** hypercapnia

  ✓5ᵗʰ **J96.1**   Chronic **respiratory failure**

     J96.10   **Chronic respiratory failure, unspecified whether with hypoxia or hypercapnia**
       AHA: 2016,1Q,38; 2015,1Q,21

     J96.11   **Chronic respiratory failure with** hypoxia
       AHA: 2013,4Q,129

     J96.12   **Chronic respiratory failure with** hypercapnia

  ✓5ᵗʰ **J96.2**   Acute and chronic **respiratory failure**
     Acute on chronic respiratory failure

     J96.20   **Acute and chronic respiratory failure, unspecified whether with hypoxia or hypercapnia**

     J96.21   **Acute and chronic respiratory failure with** hypoxia

     J96.22   **Acute and chronic respiratory failure with** hypercapnia

  ✓5ᵗʰ **J96.9**   **Respiratory failure, unspecified**

     J96.90   **Respiratory failure, unspecified, unspecified whether with hypoxia or hypercapnia**

     J96.91   **Respiratory failure, unspecified with** hypoxia

     J96.92   **Respiratory failure, unspecified with** hypercapnia

✓4ᵗʰ **J98**   **Other respiratory disorders**
     Use additional code to identify:
       exposure to environmental tobacco smoke (Z77.22)
       exposure to tobacco smoke in the perinatal period (P96.81)
       history of tobacco dependence (Z87.891)
       occupational exposure to environmental tobacco smoke (Z57.31)
       tobacco dependence (F17.-)
       tobacco use (Z72.0)

     EXCLUDES 1   newborn apnea (P28.4)
         newborn sleep apnea (P28.3)

     EXCLUDES 2   apnea NOS (R06.81)
         sleep apnea (G47.3-)

  ✓5ᵗʰ **J98.0**   **Diseases of bronchus, not elsewhere classified**

     J98.01   **Acute bronchospasm**

       EXCLUDES 1   acute bronchiolitis with bronchospasm (J21.-)
         acute bronchitis with bronchospasm (J20.-)
         asthma (J45.-)
         exercise induced bronchospasm (J45.990)

J98.09   Other diseases of bronchus, not elsewhere classified
> Broncholithiasis
> Calcification of bronchus
> Stenosis of bronchus
> Tracheobronchial collapse
> Tracheobronchial dyskinesia
> Ulcer of bronchus

√5ᵗʰ **J98.1   Pulmonary collapse**
> EXCLUDES 1   *therapeutic collapse of lung status (Z98.3)*

J98.11   Atelectasis
> EXCLUDES 1   *newborn atelectasis*
> *tuberculous atelectasis (current disease) (A15)*
>
> **DEF:** Collapse of lung tissue affecting part or all of one lung, preventing normal oxygen absorption to healthy tissues.

J98.19   Other pulmonary collapse

J98.2   Interstitial emphysema
> Mediastinal emphysema
> EXCLUDES 1   *emphysema NOS (J43.9)*
> *emphysema in newborn (P25.0)*
> *surgical emphysema (subcutaneous) (T81.82)*
> *traumatic subcutaneous emphysema (T79.7)*

J98.3   Compensatory emphysema
> **DEF:** Distention of all or part of the lung caused by disease processes or surgical intervention that decreased volume in another part of the lung, causing an overcompensation reaction. Compensatory emphysema occurs in association with pneumonias, pleural effusions, atelectasis, empyema, and pneumothorax.

J98.4   Other disorders of lung
> Calcification of lung
> Cystic lung disease (acquired)
> Lung disease NOS
> Pulmolithiasis
> EXCLUDES 1   *acute interstitial pneumonitis (J84.114)*
> *pulmonary insufficiency following surgery (J95.1-J95.2)*

√5ᵗʰ **J98.5   Diseases of mediastinum, not elsewhere classified**
> EXCLUDES 2   *abscess of mediastinum (J85.3)*
> **AHA:** 2016,4Q,29

J98.51   Mediastinitis
> Code first underlying condition, if applicable, such as postoperative mediastinitis (T81.-)

J98.59   Other diseases of mediastinum, not elsewhere classified
> Fibrosis of mediastinum
> Hernia of mediastinum
> Retraction of mediastinum

J98.6   Disorders of diaphragm
> Diaphragmatitis
> Paralysis of diaphragm
> Relaxation of diaphragm
> EXCLUDES 1   *congenital malformation of diaphragm NEC (Q79.1)*
> *congenital diaphragmatic hernia (Q79.0)*
> EXCLUDES 2   *diaphragmatic hernia (K44.-)*

J98.8   Other specified respiratory disorders

J98.9   Respiratory disorder, unspecified
> Respiratory disease (chronic) NOS

J99   Respiratory disorders in diseases classified elsewhere
> Code first underlying disease, such as:
> amyloidosis (E85.-)
> ankylosing spondylitis (M45)
> congenital syphilis (A50.5)
> cryoglobulinemia (D89.1)
> early congenital syphilis (A50.0)
> plasminogen deficiency (E88.02)
> schistosomiasis (B65.0-B65.9)
> EXCLUDES 1   *respiratory disorders in:*
> *amebiasis (A06.5)*
> *blastomycosis (B40.0-B40.2)*
> *candidiasis (B37.1)*
> *coccidioidomycosis (B38.0-B38.2)*
> *cystic fibrosis with pulmonary manifestations (E84.0)*
> *dermatomyositis (M33.01, M33.11)*
> *histoplasmosis (B39.0-B39.2)*
> *late syphilis (A52.72, A52.73)*
> *polymyositis (M33.21)*
> *sicca syndrome (M35.02)*
> *systemic lupus erythematosus (M32.13)*
> *systemic sclerosis (M34.81)*
> *Wegener's granulomatosis (M31.30-M31.31)*

Chapter 11. Diseases of the Digestive System (K00–K95)

Chapter-specific Coding Guidelines and Examples
Reserved for future guideline expansion.

Chapter 11. Diseases of the Digestive System (K00-K95)

EXCLUDES 2   *certain conditions originating in the perinatal period (P04-P96)*
certain infectious and parasitic diseases (A00-B99)
complications of pregnancy, childbirth and the puerperium (O00-O9A)
congenital malformations, deformations and chromosomal abnormalities (Q00-Q99)
endocrine, nutritional and metabolic diseases (E00-E88)
injury, poisoning and certain other consequences of external causes (S00-T88)
neoplasms (C00-D49)
symptoms, signs and abnormal clinical and laboratory findings, not elsewhere classified (R00-R94)

This chapter contains the following blocks:

K00-K14 Diseases of oral cavity and salivary glands
K20-K31 Diseases of esophagus, stomach and duodenum
K35-K38 Diseases of appendix
K40-K46 Hernia
K50-K52 Noninfective enteritis and colitis
K55-K64 Other diseases of intestines
K65-K68 Diseases of peritoneum and retroperitoneum
K70-K77 Diseases of liver
K80-K87 Disorders of gallbladder, biliary tract and pancreas
K90-K95 Other diseases of the digestive system

Diseases of oral cavity and salivary glands (K00-K14)

✓4ᵗʰ **K00 Disorders of tooth development and eruption**
  EXCLUDES 2   *embedded and impacted teeth (K01.-)*

K00.0 Anodontia
Hypodontia
Oligodontia
EXCLUDES 1   *acquired absence of teeth (K08.1-)*
DEF: Partial or complete absence of teeth due to a congenital defect involving the tooth bud.

K00.1 Supernumerary teeth
Distomolar
Fourth molar
Mesiodens
Paramolar
Supplementary teeth
EXCLUDES 2   *supernumerary roots (K00.2)*

K00.2 Abnormalities of size and form of teeth
Concrescence of teeth
Dens evaginatus
Dens in dente
Dens invaginatus
Enamel pearls
Fusion of teeth
Gemination of teeth
Macrodontia
Microdontia
Peg-shaped [conical] teeth
Supernumerary roots
Taurodontism
Tuberculum paramolare
EXCLUDES 1   *abnormalities of teeth due to congenital syphilis (A50.5)*
          tuberculum Carabelli, which is regarded as a normal variation and should not be coded

K00.3 Mottled teeth
Dental fluorosis
Mottling of enamel
Nonfluoride enamel opacities
EXCLUDES 2   *deposits [accretions] on teeth (K03.6)*

K00.4 Disturbances in tooth formation
Aplasia and hypoplasia of cementum
Dilaceration of tooth
Enamel hypoplasia (neonatal) (postnatal) (prenatal)
Regional odontodysplasia
Turner's tooth
EXCLUDES 1   *Hutchinson's teeth and mulberry molars in congenital syphilis (A50.5)*
EXCLUDES 2   *mottled teeth (K00.3)*

K00.5 Hereditary disturbances in tooth structure, not elsewhere classified
Amelogenesis imperfecta
Dentinogenesis imperfecta
Odontogenesis imperfecta
Dentinal dysplasia
Shell teeth

K00.6 Disturbances in tooth eruption
Dentia praecox
Natal tooth
Neonatal tooth
Premature eruption of tooth
Premature shedding of primary [deciduous] tooth
Prenatal teeth
Retained [persistent] primary tooth
EXCLUDES 2   *embedded and impacted teeth (K01.-)*

K00.7 Teething syndrome

K00.8 Other disorders of tooth development
Color changes during tooth formation
Intrinsic staining of teeth NOS
EXCLUDES 2   *posteruptive color changes (K03.7)*

K00.9 Disorder of tooth development, unspecified
Disorder of odontogenesis NOS

✓4ᵗʰ **K01 Embedded and impacted teeth**
  EXCLUDES 1   *abnormal position of fully erupted teeth (M26.3-)*

K01.0 Embedded teeth

K01.1 Impacted teeth

✓4ᵗʰ **K02 Dental caries**
  INCLUDES   caries of dentine
           dental cavities
           early childhood caries
           pre-eruptive caries
           recurrent caries (dentino enamel junction) (enamel) (to the pulp)
           tooth decay
DEF: Localized section of tooth decay that begins on the tooth surface with destruction of the calcified enamel, allowing bacterial destruction to continue and form cavities and may extend to the dentin and pulp.

Tooth Anatomy

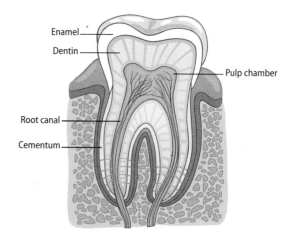

Enamel
Dentin
Pulp chamber
Root canal
Cementum

K02.3 Arrested dental caries
Arrested coronal and root caries

✓5ᵗʰ **K02.5 Dental caries on pit and fissure surface**
Dental caries on chewing surface of tooth

K02.51 Dental caries on pit and fissure surface limited to enamel
White spot lesions [initial caries] on pit and fissure surface of tooth

K02.52 Dental caries on pit and fissure surface penetrating into dentin
Primary dental caries, cervical origin

K02.53 Dental caries on pit and fissure surface penetrating into pulp

N Newborn: 0   P Pediatric: 0-17   M Maternity: 12-55   A Adult: 15-124   CH Comorbidity High   CL Comorbidity Low   NC Dx Noncancer Dx   P Dx Primary Dx

694
ICD-10-CM 2020

Chapter 11. Diseases of the Digestive System

✓5ᵗʰ **K02.6** **Dental caries on** smooth surface

    K02.61 **Dental caries on smooth surface** limited to enamel
        White spot lesions [initial caries] on smooth surface of tooth

    K02.62 **Dental caries on smooth surface** penetrating into dentin

    K02.63 **Dental caries on smooth surface** penetrating into pulp

K02.7 **Dental** root **caries**

K02.9 **Dental caries, unspecified**

✓4ᵗʰ **K03** **Other diseases of hard tissues of teeth**

    EXCLUDES 2   bruxism (F45.8)
                dental caries (K02.-)
                teeth-grinding NOS (F45.8)

K03.0 **Excessive attrition of teeth**
    Approximal wear of teeth
    Occlusal wear of teeth
    DEF: Attrition: In dentistry, wearing away or erosion of tooth surface from abrasive food or grinding teeth.

K03.1 **Abrasion of teeth**
    Dentifrice abrasion of teeth
    Habitual abrasion of teeth
    Occupational abrasion of teeth
    Ritual abrasion of teeth
    Traditional abrasion of teeth
    Wedge defect NOS

K03.2 **Erosion of teeth**
    Erosion of teeth due to diet
    Erosion of teeth due to drugs and medicaments
    Erosion of teeth due to persistent vomiting
    Erosion of teeth NOS
    Idiopathic erosion of teeth
    Occupational erosion of teeth

K03.3 **Pathological resorption of teeth**
    Internal granuloma of pulp
    Resorption of teeth (external)

K03.4 **Hypercementosis**
    Cementation hyperplasia

K03.5 **Ankylosis of teeth**

K03.6 **Deposits [accretions] on teeth**
    Betel deposits [accretions] on teeth
    Black deposits [accretions] on teeth
    Extrinsic staining of teeth NOS
    Green deposits [accretions] on teeth
    Materia alba deposits [accretions] on teeth
    Orange deposits [accretions] on teeth
    Staining of teeth NOS
    Subgingival dental calculus
    Supragingival dental calculus
    Tobacco deposits [accretions] on teeth

K03.7 **Posteruptive color changes of dental hard tissues**
    EXCLUDES 2   deposits [accretions] on teeth (K03.6)

✓5ᵗʰ **K03.8** **Other specified diseases of hard tissues of teeth**

    K03.81 **Cracked tooth**
        EXCLUDES 1   asymptomatic craze lines in enamel - omit code
              broken or fractured tooth due to trauma (S02.5)

    K03.89 **Other specified diseases of hard tissues of teeth**

K03.9 **Disease of hard tissues of teeth, unspecified**

✓4ᵗʰ **K04** **Diseases of pulp and periapical tissues**
    AHA: 2016,4Q,29-30

✓5ᵗʰ **K04.0** **Pulpitis**
    Acute pulpitis
    Chronic (hyperplastic) (ulcerative) pulpitis
    K04.01 **Reversible pulpitis**
    K04.02 **Irreversible pulpitis**

K04.1 **Necrosis of pulp**
    Pulpal gangrene

K04.2 **Pulp degeneration**
    Denticles
    Pulpal calcifications
    Pulpal stones

K04.3 **Abnormal hard tissue formation in pulp**
    Secondary or irregular dentine

K04.4 **Acute apical periodontitis of pulpal origin**
    Acute apical periodontitis NOS
    EXCLUDES 1   acute periodontitis (K05.2-)
    DEF: Severe inflammation of the area surrounding the tip of a tooth's root that is often secondary to infection or trauma.

K04.5 **Chronic apical periodontitis**
    Apical or periapical granuloma
    Apical periodontitis NOS
    EXCLUDES 1   chronic periodontitis (K05.3-)

K04.6 **Periapical abscess with sinus**
    Dental abscess with sinus
    Dentoalveolar abscess with sinus

K04.7 **Periapical abscess without sinus**
    Dental abscess without sinus
    Dentoalveolar abscess without sinus

K04.8 **Radicular cyst**
    Apical (periodontal) cyst
    Periapical cyst
    Residual radicular cyst
    EXCLUDES 2   lateral periodontal cyst (K09.0)
    DEF: Most common odontogenic cyst in tissue around the tooth apex due to chronic inflammation of dental pulp.

✓5ᵗʰ **K04.9** **Other and unspecified diseases of pulp and periapical tissues**
    K04.90 **Unspecified diseases of pulp and periapical tissues**
    K04.99 **Other diseases of pulp and periapical tissues**

✓4ᵗʰ **K05** **Gingivitis and periodontal diseases**
    Use additional code to identify:
    alcohol abuse and dependence (F10.-)
    exposure to environmental tobacco smoke (Z77.22)
    exposure to tobacco smoke in the perinatal period (P96.81)
    history of tobacco dependence (Z87.891)
    occupational exposure to environmental tobacco smoke (Z57.31)
    tobacco dependence (F17.-)
    tobacco use (Z72.0)
    AHA: 2016,4Q,29-30

✓5ᵗʰ **K05.0** **Acute gingivitis**
    EXCLUDES 1   acute necrotizing ulcerative gingivitis (A69.1)
              herpesviral [herpes simplex] gingivostomatitis (B00.2)
    K05.00 **Acute gingivitis,** plaque induced
        Acute gingivitis NOS
        Plaque induced gingival disease
    K05.01 **Acute gingivitis,** non-plaque induced

✓5ᵗʰ **K05.1** **Chronic gingivitis**
    Desquamative gingivitis (chronic)
    Gingivitis (chronic) NOS
    Hyperplastic gingivitis (chronic)
    Pregnancy associated gingivitis
    Simple marginal gingivitis (chronic)
    Ulcerative gingivitis (chronic)
    Code first, if applicable, diseases of the digestive system complicating pregnacy (O99.61-)
    K05.10 **Chronic gingivitis,** plaque induced
        Chronic gingivitis NOS
        Gingivitis NOS
    K05.11 **Chronic gingivitis,** non-plaque induced

✓5ᵗʰ **K05.2** **Aggressive periodontitis**
    Acute pericoronitis
    EXCLUDES 1   acute apical periodontitis (K04.4)
              periapical abscess (K04.7)
              periapical abscess with sinus (K04.6)
    K05.20 **Aggressive periodontitis, unspecified**
    ✓6ᵗʰ **K05.21** **Aggressive periodontitis,** localized
        Periodontal abscess
        K05.211 **Aggressive periodontitis, localized,** slight
        K05.212 **Aggressive periodontitis, localized, moderate**
        K05.213 **Aggressive periodontitis, localized, severe**
        K05.219 **Aggressive periodontitis, localized, unspecified severity**
    ✓6ᵗʰ **K05.22** **Aggressive periodontitis,** generalized
        K05.221 **Aggressive periodontitis, generalized, slight**
        K05.222 **Aggressive periodontitis, generalized, moderate**
        K05.223 **Aggressive periodontitis, generalized, severe**

Chapter 11. Diseases of the Digestive System

K05.229 Aggressive periodontitis, generalized, unspecified severity

√5ᵗʰ **K05.3 Chronic periodontitis**
Chronic pericoronitis
Complex periodontitis
Periodontitis NOS
Simplex periodontitis
EXCLUDES 1   chronic apical periodontitis (K04.5)

K05.30 Chronic periodontitis, unspecified
√6ᵗʰ **K05.31** Chronic periodontitis, localized
K05.311 Chronic periodontitis, localized, slight
K05.312 Chronic periodontitis, localized, moderate
K05.313 Chronic periodontitis, localized, severe
K05.319 Chronic periodontitis, localized, unspecified severity
√6ᵗʰ **K05.32** Chronic periodontitis, generalized
K05.321 Chronic periodontitis, generalized, slight
K05.322 Chronic periodontitis, generalized, moderate
K05.323 Chronic periodontitis, generalized, severe
K05.329 Chronic periodontitis, generalized, unspecified

K05.4 Periodontosis
Juvenile periodontosis
K05.5 Other periodontal diseases
Combined periodontic-endodontic lesion
Narrow gingival width (of periodontal soft tissue)
EXCLUDES 2   leukoplakia of gingiva (K13.21)
K05.6 Periodontal disease, unspecified

√4ᵗʰ **K06 Other disorders of gingiva and edentulous alveolar ridge**
EXCLUDES 2   acute gingivitis (K05.0)
atrophy of edentulous alveolar ridge (K08.2)
chronic gingivitis (K05.1)
gingivitis NOS (K05.1)
AHA: 2016,4Q,29-30

√5ᵗʰ **K06.0 Gingival recession**
Gingival recession (postinfective) (postprocedural)
AHA: 2017,4Q,16
√6ᵗʰ **K06.01** Gingival recession, localized
K06.010 Localized gingival recession, unspecified
Localized gingival recession, NOS
K06.011 Localized gingival recession, minimal
K06.012 Localized gingival recession, moderate
K06.013 Localized gingival recession, severe
√6ᵗʰ **K06.02** Gingival recession, generalized
K06.020 Generalized gingival recession, unspecified
Generalized gingival recession, NOS
K06.021 Generalized gingival recession, minimal
K06.022 Generalized gingival recession, moderate
K06.023 Generalized gingival recession, severe

K06.1 Gingival enlargement
Gingival fibromatosis
K06.2 Gingival and edentulous alveolar ridge lesions associated with trauma
Irritative hyperplasia of edentulous ridge [denture hyperplasia]
Use additional code (Chapter 20) to identify external cause or denture status (Z97.2)
K06.3 Horizontal alveolar bone loss
K06.8 Other specified disorders of gingiva and edentulous alveolar ridge
Fibrous epulis
Flabby alveolar ridge
Giant cell epulis
Peripheral giant cell granuloma of gingiva
Pyogenic granuloma of gingiva
Vertical ridge deficiency
EXCLUDES 2   gingival cyst (K09.0)
K06.9 Disorder of gingiva and edentulous alveolar ridge, unspecified

√4ᵗʰ **K08 Other disorders of teeth and supporting structures**
EXCLUDES 2   dentofacial anomalies [including malocclusion] (M26.-)
disorders of jaw (M27.-)
AHA: 2016,4Q,29-30

K08.0 Exfoliation of teeth due to systemic causes
Code also underlying systemic condition
√5ᵗʰ **K08.1 Complete loss of teeth**
Acquired loss of teeth, complete
EXCLUDES 1   congenital absence of teeth (K00.0)
exfoliation of teeth due to systemic causes (K08.0)
partial loss of teeth (K08.4-)
DEF: Loss of all teeth as a result of caries, trauma, extraction, periodontal disease, or other specified or unspecified causes.
Synonym(s): complete edentulism
√6ᵗʰ **K08.10** Complete loss of teeth, unspecified cause
K08.101 Complete loss of teeth, unspecified cause, class I
K08.102 Complete loss of teeth, unspecified cause, class II
K08.103 Complete loss of teeth, unspecified cause, class III
K08.104 Complete loss of teeth, unspecified cause, class IV
K08.109 Complete loss of teeth, unspecified cause, unspecified class
Edentulism NOS
√6ᵗʰ **K08.11** Complete loss of teeth due to trauma
K08.111 Complete loss of teeth due to trauma, class I
K08.112 Complete loss of teeth due to trauma, class II
K08.113 Complete loss of teeth due to trauma, class III
K08.114 Complete loss of teeth due to trauma, class IV
K08.119 Complete loss of teeth due to trauma, unspecified class
√6ᵗʰ **K08.12** Complete loss of teeth due to periodontal diseases
K08.121 Complete loss of teeth due to periodontal diseases, class I
K08.122 Complete loss of teeth due to periodontal diseases, class II
K08.123 Complete loss of teeth due to periodontal diseases, class III
K08.124 Complete loss of teeth due to periodontal diseases, class IV
K08.129 Complete loss of teeth due to periodontal diseases, unspecified class
√6ᵗʰ **K08.13** Complete loss of teeth due to caries
K08.131 Complete loss of teeth due to caries, class I
K08.132 Complete loss of teeth due to caries, class II
K08.133 Complete loss of teeth due to caries, class III
K08.134 Complete loss of teeth due to caries, class IV
K08.139 Complete loss of teeth due to caries, unspecified class
√6ᵗʰ **K08.19** Complete loss of teeth due to other specified cause
K08.191 Complete loss of teeth due to other specified cause, class I
K08.192 Complete loss of teeth due to other specified cause, class II
K08.193 Complete loss of teeth due to other specified cause, class III
K08.194 Complete loss of teeth due to other specified cause, class IV
K08.199 Complete loss of teeth due to other specified cause, unspecified class
√5ᵗʰ **K08.2 Atrophy of edentulous alveolar ridge**
K08.20 Unspecified atrophy of edentulous alveolar ridge
Atrophy of the mandible NOS
Atrophy of the maxilla NOS
K08.21 Minimal atrophy of the mandible
Minimal atrophy of the edentulous mandible
K08.22 Moderate atrophy of the mandible
Moderate atrophy of the edentulous mandible

K08.23 **Severe atrophy of the** mandible
Severe atrophy of the edentulous mandible

K08.24 **Minimal atrophy of** maxilla
Minimal atrophy of the edentulous maxilla

K08.25 **Moderate atrophy of the** maxilla
Moderate atrophy of the edentulous maxilla

K08.26 **Severe atrophy of the** maxilla
Severe atrophy of the edentulous maxilla

K08.3 **Retained dental root**

√5ᵗʰ K08.4 **Partial loss of teeth**
Acquired loss of teeth, partial
EXCLUDES 1   *complete loss of teeth (K08.1-)*
congenital absence of teeth (K00.0)
EXCLUDES 2   *exfoliation of teeth due to systemic causes (K08.0)*

√6ᵗʰ K08.40 **Partial loss of teeth, unspecified cause**

K08.401 **Partial loss of teeth, unspecified cause,** class I

K08.402 **Partial loss of teeth, unspecified cause,** class II

K08.403 **Partial loss of teeth, unspecified cause,** class III

K08.404 **Partial loss of teeth, unspecified cause,** class IV

K08.409 **Partial loss of teeth, unspecified cause, unspecified class**
Tooth extraction status NOS

√6ᵗʰ K08.41 **Partial loss of teeth due to** trauma

K08.411 **Partial loss of teeth due to trauma,** class I

K08.412 **Partial loss of teeth due to trauma,** class II

K08.413 **Partial loss of teeth due to trauma,** class III

K08.414 **Partial loss of teeth due to trauma,** class IV

K08.419 **Partial loss of teeth due to trauma, unspecified class**

√6ᵗʰ K08.42 **Partial loss of teeth due to** periodontal diseases

K08.421 **Partial loss of teeth due to periodontal diseases,** class I

K08.422 **Partial loss of teeth due to periodontal diseases,** class II

K08.423 **Partial loss of teeth due to periodontal diseases,** class III

K08.424 **Partial loss of teeth due to periodontal diseases,** class IV

K08.429 **Partial loss of teeth due to periodontal diseases, unspecified class**

√6ᵗʰ K08.43 **Partial loss of teeth due to** caries

K08.431 **Partial loss of teeth due to caries,** class I
K08.432 **Partial loss of teeth due to caries,** class II
K08.433 **Partial loss of teeth due to caries,** class III
K08.434 **Partial loss of teeth due to caries,** class IV
K08.439 **Partial loss of teeth due to caries, unspecified class**

√6ᵗʰ K08.49 **Partial loss of teeth due to other specified cause**

K08.491 **Partial loss of teeth due to other specified cause,** class I

K08.492 **Partial loss of teeth due to other specified cause,** class II

K08.493 **Partial loss of teeth due to other specified cause,** class III

K08.494 **Partial loss of teeth due to other specified cause,** class IV

K08.499 **Partial loss of teeth due to other specified cause, unspecified class**

√5ᵗʰ K08.5 **Unsatisfactory restoration of tooth**
Defective bridge, crown, filling
Defective dental restoration
EXCLUDES 1   *dental restoration status (Z98.811)*
EXCLUDES 2   *endosseous dental implant failure (M27.6-)*
unsatisfactory endodontic treatment (M27.5-)

K08.50 **Unsatisfactory restoration of tooth, unspecified**
Defective dental restoration NOS

K08.51 **Open restoration margins of tooth**
Dental restoration failure of marginal integrity
Open margin on tooth restoration
Poor gingival margin to tooth restoration

K08.52 **Unrepairable overhanging of dental restorative materials**
Overhanging of tooth restoration

√6ᵗʰ K08.53 **Fractured dental restorative material**
EXCLUDES 1   *cracked tooth (K03.81)*
traumatic fracture of tooth (S02.5)

K08.530 **Fractured dental restorative material without loss of material**

K08.531 **Fractured dental restorative material with loss of material**

K08.539 **Fractured dental restorative material, unspecified**

K08.54 **Contour of existing restoration of tooth biologically incompatible with oral health**
Dental restoration failure of periodontal anatomical integrity
Unacceptable contours of existing restoration of tooth
Unacceptable morphology of existing restoration of tooth

K08.55 **Allergy to existing dental restorative material**
Use additional code to identify the specific type of allergy

K08.56 **Poor aesthetic of existing restoration of tooth**
Dental restoration aesthetically inadequate or displeasing

K08.59 **Other unsatisfactory restoration of tooth**
Other defective dental restoration

√5ᵗʰ K08.8 **Other specified disorders of teeth and supporting structures**

K08.81 **Primary occlusal trauma**
K08.82 **Secondary occlusal trauma**
K08.89 **Other specified disorders of teeth and supporting structures**
Enlargement of alveolar ridge NOS
Insufficient anatomic crown height
Insufficient clinical crown length
Irregular alveolar process
Toothache NOS

K08.9 **Disorder of teeth and supporting structures, unspecified**

√4ᵗʰ **K09 Cysts of oral region, not elsewhere classified**
INCLUDES   lesions showing histological features both of aneurysmal cyst and of another fibro-osseous lesion
EXCLUDES 2   *cysts of jaw (M27.0-, M27.4-)*
radicular cyst (K04.8)

K09.0 **Developmental odontogenic cysts**
Dentigerous cyst
Eruption cyst
Follicular cyst
Gingival cyst
Lateral periodontal cyst
Primordial cyst
EXCLUDES 2   *keratocysts (D16.4, D16.5)*
odontogenic keratocystic tumors (D16.4, D16.5)

K09.1 **Developmental (nonodontogenic) cysts of oral region**
Cyst (of) incisive canal
Cyst (of) palatine of papilla
Globulomaxillary cyst
Median palatal cyst
Nasoalveolar cyst
Nasolabial cyst
Nasopalatine duct cyst

K09.8 **Other cysts of oral region, not elsewhere classified**
Dermoid cyst
Epidermoid cyst
Lymphoepithelial cyst
Epstein's pearl

K09.9 **Cyst of oral region, unspecified**

√4ᵗʰ **K11 Diseases of salivary glands**
Use additional code to identify:
alcohol abuse and dependence (F10.-)
exposure to environmental tobacco smoke (Z77.22)
exposure to tobacco smoke in the perinatal period (P96.81)
history of tobacco dependence (Z87.891)
occupational exposure to environmental tobacco smoke (Z57.31)
tobacco dependence (F17.-)
tobacco use (Z72.0)

K11.0 **Atrophy of salivary gland**

☑ Additional Character Required   √x7ᵗʰ Placeholder Alert   Manifestation   <u>Unspecified Dx</u>   ▶◀ Revised Text   ● New Code   ▲ Revised Title

Chapter 11. Diseases of the Digestive System

K11.1   **Hypertrophy of salivary gland**
> **DEF:** Overgrowth of or enlarged salivary gland tissue caused by infection, salivary duct blockage, autoimmune diseases, and benign and malignant tumors.

✓5ᵗʰ **K11.2**   **Sialoadenitis**
> Parotitis
> *EXCLUDES 1*   *epidemic parotitis (B26.-)*
>   *mumps (B26.-)*
>   *uveoparotid fever [Heerfordt] (D86.89)*
> **DEF:** Inflammation of the salivary gland.

     K11.20   **Sialoadenitis, unspecified**
     K11.21   **Acute sialoadenitis**
>   *EXCLUDES 1*   *acute recurrent sialoadenitis (K11.22)*

     K11.22   **Acute recurrent sialoadenitis**
     K11.23   **Chronic sialoadenitis**

K11.3   **Abscess of salivary gland**

K11.4   **Fistula of salivary gland**
> *EXCLUDES 1*   *congenital fistula of salivary gland (Q38.4)*

K11.5   **Sialolithiasis**
> Calculus of salivary gland or duct
> Stone of salivary gland or duct

K11.6   **Mucocele of salivary gland**
> Mucous extravasation cyst of salivary gland
> Mucous retention cyst of salivary gland
> Ranula

K11.7   **Disturbances of salivary secretion**
> Hypoptyalism
> Ptyalism
> Xerostomia
> *EXCLUDES 2*   *dry mouth NOS (R68.2)*

K11.8   **Other diseases of salivary glands**
> Benign lymphoepithelial lesion of salivary gland
> Mikulicz' disease
> Necrotizing sialometaplasia
> Sialectasia
> Stenosis of salivary duct
> Stricture of salivary duct
> *EXCLUDES 1*   *sicca syndrome [Sjögren] (M35.0-)*

K11.9   **Disease of salivary gland, unspecified**
> Sialoadenopathy NOS

✓4ᵗʰ **K12**   **Stomatitis and related lesions**
> Use additional code to identify:
>   alcohol abuse and dependence (F10.-)
>   exposure to environmental tobacco smoke (Z77.22)
>   exposure to tobacco smoke in the perinatal period (P96.81)
>   history of tobacco dependence (Z87.891)
>   occupational exposure to environmental tobacco smoke (Z57.31)
>   tobacco dependence (F17.-)
>   tobacco use (Z72.0)
> *EXCLUDES 1*   *cancrum oris (A69.0)*
>   *cheilitis (K13.0)*
>   *gangrenous stomatitis (A69.0)*
>   *herpesviral [herpes simplex] gingivostomatitis (B00.2)*
>   *noma (A69.0)*

K12.0   **Recurrent oral aphthae**
> Aphthous stomatitis (major) (minor)
> Bednar's aphthae
> Periadenitis mucosa necrotica recurrens
> Recurrent aphthous ulcer
> Stomatitis herpetiformis
> **DEF:** Disorder of unknown etiology with small oval or round painful ulcers of the mouth marked by a grayish exudate and a red halo effect.

K12.1   **Other forms of stomatitis**
> Stomatitis NOS
> Denture stomatitis
> Ulcerative stomatitis
> Vesicular stomatitis
> *EXCLUDES 1*   *acute necrotizing ulcerative stomatitis (A69.1)*
>   *Vincent's stomatitis (A69.1)*

[handwritten: P ll oral mucosa]

K12.2   **Cellulitis and abscess of mouth**
> Cellulitis of mouth (floor)
> Submandibular abscess
> *EXCLUDES 2*   *abscess of salivary gland (K11.3)*
>   *abscess of tongue (K14.0)*
>   *periapical abscess (K04.6-K04.7)*
>   *periodontal abscess (K05.21)*
>   *peritonsillar abscess (J36)*

✓5ᵗʰ **K12.3**   **Oral mucositis (ulcerative)**
> Mucositis (oral) (oropharyneal)
> *EXCLUDES 2*   *gastrointestinal mucositis (ulcerative) (K92.81)*
>   *mucositis (ulcerative) of vagina and vulva (N76.81)*
>   *nasal mucositis (ulcerative) (J34.81)*

     K12.30   **Oral mucositis (ulcerative), unspecified**
     K12.31   **Oral mucositis (ulcerative) due to antineoplastic therapy**
>   Use additional code for adverse effect, if applicable, to identify antineoplastic and immunosuppressive drugs (T45.1X5)
>   Use additional code for other antineoplastic therapy, such as:
>   radiological procedure and radiotherapy (Y84.2)

     K12.32   **Oral mucositis (ulcerative) due to other drugs**
>   Use additional code for adverse effect, if applicable, to identify drug (T36-T50 with fifth or sixth character 5)

     K12.33   **Oral mucositis (ulcerative) due to radiation**
>   Use additional external cause code (W88-W90, X39.0-) to identify cause

     K12.39   **Other oral mucositis (ulcerative)**
>   Viral oral mucositis (ulcerative)

✓4ᵗʰ **K13**   **Other diseases of lip and oral mucosa**
> *INCLUDES*   epithelial disturbances of tongue
> Use additional code to identify:
>   alcohol abuse and dependence (F10.-)
>   exposure to environmental tobacco smoke (Z77.22)
>   exposure to tobacco smoke in the perinatal period (P96.81)
>   history of tobacco dependence (Z87.891)
>   occupational exposure to environmental tobacco smoke (Z57.31)
>   tobacco dependence (F17.-)
>   tobacco use (Z72.0)
> *EXCLUDES 2*   *certain disorders of gingiva and edentulous alveolar ridge (K05-K06)*
>   *cysts of oral region (K09.-)*
>   *diseases of tongue (K14.-)*
>   *stomatitis and related lesions (K12.-)*

K13.0   **Diseases of lips**
> Abscess of lips
> Angular cheilitis
> Cellulitis of lips
> Cheilitis NOS
> Cheilodynia
> Cheilosis
> Exfoliative cheilitis
> Fistula of lips
> Glandular cheilitis
> Hypertrophy of lips
> Perlèche NEC
> *EXCLUDES 1*   *ariboflavinosis (E53.0)*
>   *cheilitis due to radiation-related disorders (L55-L59)*
>   *congenital fistula of lips (Q38.0)*
>   *congenital hypertrophy of lips (Q18.6)*
>   *perlèche due to candidiasis (B37.83)*
>   *perlèche due to riboflavin deficiency (E53.0)*

K13.1   **Cheek and lip biting**

N Newborn: 0   P Pediatric: 0-17   M Maternity: 12-55   A Adult: 15-124   CH Comorbidity High   CL Comorbidity Low   NCDx Noncancer Dx   PDx Primary Dx

698   ICD-10-CM 2020

☑5ᵗʰ **K13.2 Leukoplakia and other disturbances of oral epithelium, including tongue**

     EXCLUDES 1   *carcinoma in situ of oral epithelium (D00.0-)*

                hairy leukoplakia (K13.3)

     DEF: Leukoplakia: Thickened white patches or lesions appearing on a mucous membrane, such as oral mucosa or tongue.

     K13.21 Leukoplakia of oral mucosa, including tongue

         Leukokeratosis of oral mucosa

         Leukoplakia of gingiva, lips, tongue

         EXCLUDES 1   *hairy leukoplakia (K13.3)*

                   leukokeratosis nicotina palati (K13.24)

     K13.22 Minimal keratinized residual ridge mucosa

         Minimal keratinization of alveolar ridge mucosa

     K13.23 Excessive keratinized residual ridge mucosa

         Excessive keratinization of alveolar ridge mucosa

     K13.24 Leukokeratosis nicotina palati

         Smoker's palate

     K13.29 Other disturbances of oral epithelium, including tongue

         Erythroplakia of mouth or tongue

         Focal epithelial hyperplasia of mouth or tongue

         Leukoedema of mouth or tongue

         Other oral epithelium disturbances

K13.3 Hairy leukoplakia

K13.4 Granuloma and granuloma-like lesions of oral mucosa

     Eosinophilic granuloma

     Granuloma pyogenicum

     Verrucous xanthoma

K13.5 Oral submucous fibrosis

     Submucous fibrosis of tongue

K13.6 Irritative hyperplasia of oral mucosa

     EXCLUDES 2   *irritative hyperplasia of edentulous ridge [denture hyperplasia] (K06.2)*

☑5ᵗʰ **K13.7 Other and unspecified lesions of oral mucosa**

     K13.70 Unspecified lesions of oral mucosa

     K13.79 Other lesions of oral mucosa

         Focal oral mucinosis

☑4ᵗʰ **K14 Diseases of tongue**

     Use additional code to identify:

         alcohol abuse and dependence (F10.-)

         exposure to environmental tobacco smoke (Z77.22)

         history of tobacco dependence (Z87.891)

         occupational exposure to environmental tobacco smoke (Z57.31)

         tobacco dependence (F17.-)

         tobacco use (Z72.0)

     EXCLUDES 2   *erythroplakia (K13.29)*

                   focal epithelial hyperplasia (K13.29)

                   leukedema of tongue (K13.29)

                   leukoplakia of tongue (K13.21)

                   hairy leukoplakia (K13.3)

                   macroglossia (congenital) (Q38.2)

                   submucous fibrosis of tongue (K13.5)

     K14.0 Glossitis

         Abscess of tongue

         Ulceration (traumatic) of tongue

         EXCLUDES 1   *atrophic glossitis (K14.4)*

         DEF: Inflammation and swelling of the tongue that may be associated with infection, adverse drug reactions, smoking, or injury.

     K14.1 Geographic tongue

         Benign migratory glossitis

         Glossitis areata exfoliativa

     K14.2 Median rhomboid glossitis

     K14.3 Hypertrophy of tongue papillae

         Black hairy tongue

         Coated tongue

         Hypertrophy of foliate papillae

         Lingua villosa nigra

     K14.4 Atrophy of tongue papillae

         Atrophic glossitis

     K14.5 Plicated tongue

         Fissured tongue

         Furrowed tongue

         Scrotal tongue

         EXCLUDES 1   *fissured tongue, congenital (Q38.3)*

     K14.6 Glossodynia

         Glossopyrosis

         Painful tongue

     K14.8 Other diseases of tongue

         Atrophy of tongue

         Crenated tongue

         Enlargement of tongue

         Glossocele

         Glossoptosis

         Hypertrophy of tongue

     K14.9 Disease of tongue, unspecified

         Glossopathy NOS

Diseases of esophagus, stomach and duodenum (K20-K31)

     EXCLUDES 2   *hiatus hernia (K44.-)*

☑4ᵗʰ **K20 Esophagitis**

     Use additional code to identify:

         alcohol abuse and dependence (F10.-)

     EXCLUDES 1   *erosion of esophagus (K22.1-)*

                   esophagitis with gastro-esophageal reflux disease (K21.0)

                   reflux esophagitis (K21.0)

                   ulcerative esophagitis (K22.1-)

     EXCLUDES 2   *eosinophilic gastritis or gastroenteritis (K52.81)*

     K20.0 Eosinophilic esophagitis

     K20.8 Other esophagitis

         Abscess of esophagus

     K20.9 Esophagitis, unspecified

         Esophagitis NOS

☑4ᵗʰ **K21 Gastro-esophageal reflux disease**

     EXCLUDES 1   *newborn esophageal reflux (P78.83)*

     K21.0 Gastro-esophageal reflux disease with esophagitis

         Reflux esophagitis

     K21.9 Gastro-esophageal reflux disease without esophagitis

         Esophageal reflux NOS

         AHA: 2016,1Q,18

☑4ᵗʰ **K22 Other diseases of esophagus**

     EXCLUDES 2   *esophageal varices (I85.-)*

     K22.0 Achalasia of cardia

         Achalasia NOS

         Cardiospasm

         EXCLUDES 1   *congenital cardiospasm (Q39.5)*

         DEF: Esophageal motility disorder that is caused by absence of the esophageal peristalsis and impaired relaxation of the lower esophageal sphincter. It is characterized by dysphagia, regurgitation, and heartburn.

☑5ᵗʰ   **K22.1 Ulcer of esophagus**

         Barrett's ulcer

         Erosion of esophagus

         Fungal ulcer of esophagus

         Peptic ulcer of esophagus

         Ulcer of esophagus due to ingestion of chemicals

         Ulcer of esophagus due to ingestion of drugs and medicaments

         Ulcerative esophagitis

         Code first poisoning due to drug or toxin, if applicable (T36-T65 with fifth or sixth character 1-4 or 6)

         Use additional code for adverse effect, if applicable, to identify drug (T36-T50 with fifth or sixth character 5)

         EXCLUDES 1   *Barrett's esophagus (K22.7-)*

         AHA: 2018,3Q,22; 2017,3Q,27

     K22.10 Ulcer of esophagus without bleeding

         Ulcer of esophagus NOS

     K22.11 Ulcer of esophagus with bleeding

         EXCLUDES 2   *bleeding esophageal varices (I85.01, I85.11)*

     K22.2 Esophageal obstruction

         Compression of esophagus

         Constriction of esophagus

         Stenosis of esophagus

         Stricture of esophagus

         EXCLUDES 1   *congenital stenosis or stricture of esophagus (Q39.3)*

     K22.3 Perforation of esophagus

         Rupture of esophagus

         EXCLUDES 1   *traumatic perforation of (thoracic) esophagus (S27.0-)*

☑ Additional Character Required   ☑x7ᵗʰ Placeholder Alert   Manifestation   Unspecified Dx   ▶◀ Revised Text   ● New Code   ▲ Revised Title

K22.4 Dyskinesia of esophagus
Corkscrew esophagus
Diffuse esophageal spasm
Spasm of esophagus
EXCLUDES 1   cardiospasm (K22.0)

K22.5 Diverticulum of esophagus, acquired
Esophageal pouch, acquired
EXCLUDES 1   diverticulum of esophagus (congenital) (Q39.6)

K22.6 Gastro-esophageal laceration-hemorrhage syndrome
Mallory-Weiss syndrome

√5ᵗʰ **K22.7 Barrett's esophagus**
Barrett's disease
Barrett's syndrome
EXCLUDES 1   Barrett's ulcer (K22.1)
            malignant neoplasm of esophagus (C15.-)
DEF: Metaplastic disorder in which specialized columnar epithelial cells replace the normal squamous epithelial cells. Secondary to chronic gastroesophageal reflux damage to the mucosa, this disorder increases the risk of developing adenocarcinoma.

     K22.70 Barrett's esophagus without dysplasia
          Barrett's esophagus NOS

√6ᵗʰ   **K22.71 Barrett's esophagus with dysplasia**

         K22.710 Barrett's esophagus with low grade dysplasia

         K22.711 Barrett's esophagus with high grade dysplasia

         K22.719 Barrett's esophagus with dysplasia, unspecified

K22.8 Other specified diseases of esophagus
Hemorrhage of esophagus NOS
EXCLUDES 2   esophageal varices (I85.-)
            Paterson-Kelly syndrome (D50.1)

K22.9 Disease of esophagus, unspecified

K23 Disorders of esophagus in diseases classified elsewhere
Code first underlying disease, such as:
congenital syphilis (A50.5)
EXCLUDES 1   late syphilis (A52.79)
            megaesophagus due to Chagas' disease (B57.31)
            tuberculosis (A18.83)

√4ᵗʰ **K25 Gastric ulcer**
INCLUDES   erosion (acute) of stomach
          pylorus ulcer (peptic)
          stomach ulcer (peptic)
Use additional code to identify:
alcohol abuse and dependence (F10.-)
EXCLUDES 1   acute gastritis (K29.0-)
            peptic ulcer NOS (K27.-)
AHA: 2017,3Q,27

K25.0 Acute gastric ulcer with hemorrhage
K25.1 Acute gastric ulcer with perforation
K25.2 Acute gastric ulcer with both hemorrhage and perforation
K25.3 Acute gastric ulcer without hemorrhage or perforation
K25.4 Chronic or unspecified gastric ulcer with hemorrhage
K25.5 Chronic or unspecified gastric ulcer with perforation
K25.6 Chronic or unspecified gastric ulcer with both hemorrhage and perforation
K25.7 Chronic gastric ulcer without hemorrhage or perforation

K25.9 Gastric ulcer, unspecified as acute or chronic, without hemorrhage or perforation

Gastrointestinal Ulcers

Esophagus
Esophageal ulcer
Stomach
Duodenal ulcer
Gastric ulcer
Small intestine

√4ᵗʰ **K26 Duodenal ulcer**
INCLUDES   erosion (acute) of duodenum
          duodenum ulcer (peptic)
          postpyloric ulcer (peptic)
Use additional code to identify:
alcohol abuse and dependence (F10.-)
EXCLUDES 1   peptic ulcer NOS (K27.-)
AHA: 2017,3Q,27

K26.0 Acute duodenal ulcer with hemorrhage
K26.1 Acute duodenal ulcer with perforation
K26.2 Acute duodenal ulcer with both hemorrhage and perforation
K26.3 Acute duodenal ulcer without hemorrhage or perforation
K26.4 Chronic or unspecified duodenal ulcer with hemorrhage
     AHA: 2016,1Q,14
     TIP: Use for bleeding duodenal ulcer resulting from anticoagulant therapy. When the adverse effect of an anticoagulant is the cause of such bleeding, additional codes D68.32 Hemorrhagic disorder due to extrinsic circulating anticoagulant, and T45.515- Adverse effect of anticoagulants, should be assigned.
K26.5 Chronic or unspecified duodenal ulcer with perforation
K26.6 Chronic or unspecified duodenal ulcer with both hemorrhage and perforation
K26.7 Chronic duodenal ulcer without hemorrhage or perforation
K26.9 Duodenal ulcer, unspecified as acute or chronic, without hemorrhage or perforation

√4ᵗʰ **K27 Peptic ulcer, site unspecified**
INCLUDES   gastroduodenal ulcer NOS
          peptic ulcer NOS
Use additional code to identify:
alcohol abuse and dependence (F10.-)
EXCLUDES 1   peptic ulcer of newborn (P78.82)
AHA: 2017,3Q,27

K27.0 Acute peptic ulcer, site unspecified, with hemorrhage
K27.1 Acute peptic ulcer, site unspecified, with perforation
K27.2 Acute peptic ulcer, site unspecified, with both hemorrhage and perforation
K27.3 Acute peptic ulcer, site unspecified, without hemorrhage or perforation
K27.4 Chronic or unspecified peptic ulcer, site unspecified, with hemorrhage
K27.5 Chronic or unspecified peptic ulcer, site unspecified, with perforation
K27.6 Chronic or unspecified peptic ulcer, site unspecified, with both hemorrhage and perforation
K27.7 Chronic peptic ulcer, site unspecified, without hemorrhage or perforation
K27.9 Peptic ulcer, site unspecified, unspecified as acute or chronic, without hemorrhage or perforation

√4ᵗʰ K28 Gastrojejunal ulcer

INCLUDES   anastomotic ulcer (peptic) or erosion
gastrocolic ulcer (peptic) or erosion
gastrointestinal ulcer (peptic) or erosion
gastrojejunal ulcer (peptic) or erosion
jejunal ulcer (peptic) or erosion
marginal ulcer (peptic) or erosion
stomal ulcer (peptic) or erosion

Use additional code to identify:
alcohol abuse and dependence (F10.-)

EXCLUDES 1   *primary ulcer of small intestine (K63.3)*

AHA: 2017,3Q,27

K28.0   Acute gastrojejunal ulcer with hemorrhage

K28.1   Acute gastrojejunal ulcer with perforation

K28.2   Acute gastrojejunal ulcer with both hemorrhage and perforation

K28.3   Acute gastrojejunal ulcer without hemorrhage or perforation

K28.4   Chronic or unspecified gastrojejunal ulcer with hemorrhage

K28.5   Chronic or unspecified gastrojejunal ulcer with perforation

K28.6   Chronic or unspecified gastrojejunal ulcer with both hemorrhage and perforation

K28.7   Chronic gastrojejunal ulcer without hemorrhage or perforation

K28.9   Gastrojejunal ulcer, unspecified as acute or chronic, without hemorrhage or perforation

√4ᵗʰ K29 Gastritis and duodenitis

EXCLUDES 1   *eosinophilic gastritis or gastroenteritis (K52.81)*
Zollinger-Ellison syndrome (E16.4)

AHA: 2018,3Q,22

√5ᵗʰ K29.0   Acute gastritis

Use additional code to identify:
alcohol abuse and dependence (F10.-)

EXCLUDES 1   *erosion (acute) of stomach (K25.-)*

K29.00   Acute gastritis without bleeding

K29.01   Acute gastritis with bleeding

√5ᵗʰ K29.2   Alcoholic gastritis

Use additional code to identify:
alcohol abuse and dependence (F10.-)

K29.20   Alcoholic gastritis without bleeding

K29.21   Alcoholic gastritis with bleeding

√5ᵗʰ K29.3   Chronic superficial gastritis

K29.30   Chronic superficial gastritis without bleeding

K29.31   Chronic superficial gastritis with bleeding

√5ᵗʰ K29.4   Chronic atrophic gastritis

Gastric atrophy

K29.40   Chronic atrophic gastritis without bleeding

K29.41   Chronic atrophic gastritis with bleeding

√5ᵗʰ K29.5   Unspecified chronic gastritis

Chronic antral gastritis
Chronic fundal gastritis

K29.50   Unspecified chronic gastritis without bleeding

K29.51   Unspecified chronic gastritis with bleeding

√5ᵗʰ K29.6   Other gastritis

Giant hypertrophic gastritis
Granulomatous gastritis
Ménétrier's disease

K29.60   Other gastritis without bleeding

K29.61   Other gastritis with bleeding

√5ᵗʰ K29.7   Gastritis, unspecified

K29.70   Gastritis, unspecified, without bleeding

K29.71   Gastritis, unspecified, with bleeding

√5ᵗʰ K29.8   Duodenitis

K29.80   Duodenitis without bleeding

K29.81   Duodenitis with bleeding

√5ᵗʰ K29.9   Gastroduodenitis, unspecified

K29.90   Gastroduodenitis, unspecified, without bleeding

K29.91   Gastroduodenitis, unspecified, with bleeding

K30 Functional dyspepsia

Indigestion

EXCLUDES 1   *dyspepsia NOS (R10.13)*
heartburn (R12)
nervous dyspepsia (F45.8)
neurotic dyspepsia (F45.8)
psychogenic dyspepsia (F45.8)

√4ᵗʰ K31 Other diseases of stomach and duodenum

INCLUDES   functional disorders of stomach

EXCLUDES 2   *diabetic gastroparesis (E08.43, E09.43, E10.43, E11.43, E13.43)*
diverticulum of duodenum (K57.00-K57.13)

K31.0   Acute dilatation of stomach

Acute distention of stomach

K31.1   Adult hypertrophic pyloric stenosis   A

Pyloric stenosis NOS

EXCLUDES 1   *congenital or infantile pyloric stenosis (Q40.0)*

K31.2   Hourglass stricture and stenosis of stomach

EXCLUDES 1   *congenital hourglass stomach (Q40.2)*
hourglass contraction of stomach (K31.89)

K31.3   Pylorospasm, not elsewhere classified

EXCLUDES 1   *congenital or infantile pylorospasm (Q40.0)*
neurotic pylorospasm (F45.8)
psychogenic pylorospasm (F45.8)

K31.4   Gastric diverticulum

EXCLUDES 1   *congenital diverticulum of stomach (Q40.2)*

K31.5   Obstruction of duodenum

Constriction of duodenum
Duodenal ileus (chronic)
Stenosis of duodenum
Stricture of duodenum
Volvulus of duodenum

EXCLUDES 1   *congenital stenosis of duodenum (Q41.0)*

K31.6   Fistula of stomach and duodenum

Gastrocolic fistula
Gastrojejunocolic fistula

K31.7   Polyp of stomach and duodenum

EXCLUDES 1   *adenomatous polyp of stomach (D13.1)*

√5ᵗʰ K31.8   Other specified diseases of stomach and duodenum

√6ᵗʰ K31.81   Angiodysplasia of stomach and duodenum

K31.811   Angiodysplasia of stomach and duodenum with bleeding

K31.819   Angiodysplasia of stomach and duodenum without bleeding
Angiodysplasia of stomach and duodenum NOS

K31.82   Dieulafoy lesion (hemorrhagic) of stomach and duodenum

EXCLUDES 2   *Dieulafoy lesion of intestine (K63.81)*

DEF: Abnormally large submucosal artery protruding through a defect in the stomach mucosa or intestines that can cause massive and life-threatening hemorrhaging.

K31.83   Achlorhydria

DEF: Absence of hydrochloric acid in gastric secretions due to gastric mucosa atrophy. Achlorhydria is unresponsive to histamines.

K31.84   Gastroparesis
Gastroparalysis

Code first underlying disease, if known, such as:
anorexia nervosa (F50.0-)
diabetes mellitus (E08.43, E09.43, E10.43, E11.43, E13.43)
scleroderma (M34.-)

AHA: 2013,4Q,114

K31.89   Other diseases of stomach and duodenum

AHA: 2017,1Q,28

K31.9   Disease of stomach and duodenum, unspecified

☑ Additional Character Required   √x7ᵗʰ Placeholder Alert   Manifestation   Unspecified Dx   ►◄ Revised Text   ● New Code   ▲ Revised Title

ICD-10-CM 2020   701

Chapter 11. Diseases of the Digestive System

Diseases of appendix (K35-K38)

☑4ᵗʰ K35 Acute appendicitis

> AHA: 2018,4Q,17-18

☑5ᵗʰ K35.2 Acute appendicitis with generalized peritonitis

> Appendicitis (acute) with generalized (diffuse) peritonitis following rupture or perforation of appendix

>> **K35.20 Acute appendicitis with generalized peritonitis, without abscess**
>> (Acute) appendicitis with generalized peritonitis NOS

>> **K35.21 Acute appendicitis with generalized peritonitis, with abscess**

☑5ᵗʰ K35.3 Acute appendicitis with localized peritonitis

>> **K35.30 Acute appendicitis with localized peritonitis, without perforation or gangrene**
>> Acute appendicitis with localized peritonitis NOS

>> **K35.31 Acute appendicitis with localized peritonitis and gangrene, without perforation**

>> **K35.32 Acute appendicitis with perforation and localized peritonitis, without abscess**
>> (Acute) appendicitis with perforation NOS
>> Perforated appendix NOS
>> Ruptured appendix (with localized peritonitis) NOS

>> **K35.33 Acute appendicitis with perforation and localized peritonitis, with abscess**
>> (Acute) appendicitis with (peritoneal) abscess NOS
>> Ruptured appendix with localized peritonitis and abscess

☑5ᵗʰ K35.8 Other and unspecified acute appendicitis

>> **K35.80 Unspecified acute appendicitis**
>> Acute appendicitis NOS
>> Acute appendicitis without (localized) (generalized) peritonitis

>> **☑6ᵗʰ K35.89 Other acute appendicitis**

>>> **K35.890 Other acute appendicitis without perforation or gangrene**

>>> **K35.891 Other acute appendicitis without perforation, with gangrene**
>>> (Acute) appendicitis with gangrene NOS

K36 Other appendicitis
> Chronic appendicitis
> Recurrent appendicitis

K37 Unspecified appendicitis
> EXCLUDES 1   unspecified appendicitis with peritonitis (K35.2-, K35.3-)

☑4ᵗʰ K38 Other diseases of appendix

> **K38.0 Hyperplasia of appendix**

> **K38.1 Appendicular concretions**
>> Fecalith of appendix
>> Stercolith of appendix

> **K38.2 Diverticulum of appendix**

> **K38.3 Fistula of appendix**

> **K38.8 Other specified diseases of appendix**
>> Intussusception of appendix

> **K38.9 Disease of appendix, unspecified**

Hernia (K40-K46)

> **NOTE**   Hernia with both gangrene and obstruction is classified to hernia with gangrene.

> **INCLUDES**   acquired hernia
> congenital [except diaphragmatic or hiatus] hernia
> recurrent hernia

☑4ᵗʰ K40 Inguinal hernia

> **INCLUDES**   bubonocele
> direct inguinal hernia
> double inguinal hernia
> indirect inguinal hernia
> inguinal hernia NOS
> oblique inguinal hernia
> scrotal hernia

> **DEF:** Within the groin region.

☑5ᵗʰ K40.0 Bilateral inguinal hernia, with obstruction, without gangrene

> Inguinal hernia (bilateral) causing obstruction without gangrene
> Incarcerated inguinal hernia (bilateral) without gangrene
> Irreducible inguinal hernia (bilateral) without gangrene
> Strangulated inguinal hernia (bilateral) without gangrene

>> **K40.00 Bilateral inguinal hernia, with obstruction, without gangrene, not specified as recurrent**
>> Bilateral inguinal hernia, with obstruction, without gangrene NOS

>> **K40.01 Bilateral inguinal hernia, with obstruction, without gangrene, recurrent**

☑5ᵗʰ K40.1 Bilateral inguinal hernia, with gangrene

>> **K40.10 Bilateral inguinal hernia, with gangrene, not specified as recurrent**
>> Bilateral inguinal hernia, with gangrene NOS

>> **K40.11 Bilateral inguinal hernia, with gangrene, recurrent**

☑5ᵗʰ K40.2 Bilateral inguinal hernia, without obstruction or gangrene

>> **K40.20 Bilateral inguinal hernia, without obstruction or gangrene, not specified as recurrent**
>> Bilateral inguinal hernia NOS

>> **K40.21 Bilateral inguinal hernia, without obstruction or gangrene, recurrent**

☑5ᵗʰ K40.3 Unilateral inguinal hernia, with obstruction, without gangrene

> Inguinal hernia (unilateral) causing obstruction without gangrene
> Incarcerated inguinal hernia (unilateral) without gangrene
> Irreducible inguinal hernia (unilateral) without gangrene
> Strangulated inguinal hernia (unilateral) without gangrene

>> **K40.30 Unilateral inguinal hernia, with obstruction, without gangrene, not specified as recurrent**
>> Inguinal hernia, with obstruction NOS
>> Unilateral inguinal hernia, with obstruction, without gangrene NOS

>> **K40.31 Unilateral inguinal hernia, with obstruction, without gangrene, recurrent**

☑5ᵗʰ K40.4 Unilateral inguinal hernia, with gangrene

>> **K40.40 Unilateral inguinal hernia, with gangrene, not specified as recurrent**
>> Inguinal hernia with gangrene NOS
>> Unilateral inguinal hernia with gangrene NOS

>> **K40.41 Unilateral inguinal hernia, with gangrene, recurrent**

☑6ᵗʰ K40.9 Unilateral inguinal hernia, without obstruction or gangrene

>> **K40.90 Unilateral inguinal hernia, without obstruction or gangrene, not specified as recurrent**
>> Inguinal hernia NOS
>> Unilateral inguinal hernia NOS

Ⓝ Newborn: 0   Ⓟ Pediatric: 0-17   Ⓜ Maternity: 12-55   Ⓐ Adult: 15-124   CH Comorbidity High   CL Comorbidity Low   NCDx Noncancer Dx   PDx Primary Dx

702   ICD-10-CM 2020

K35–K40.90

K40.91   **Unilateral inguinal hernia, without obstruction or gangrene,** recurrent

Hernia Sites

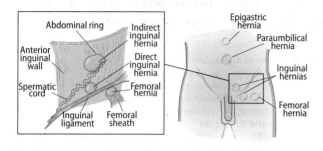

Abdominal ring | Indirect inguinal hernia | Epigastric hernia | Paraumbilical hernia | Anterior inguinal wall | Direct inguinal hernia | Inguinal hernias | Spermatic cord | Femoral hernia | Inguinal ligament | Femoral sheath | Femoral hernia

☑4ᵗʰ **K41**   **Femoral hernia**

   ☑5ᵗʰ **K41.0**   **Bilateral femoral hernia, with obstruction, without gangrene**
Femoral hernia (bilateral) causing obstruction, without gangrene
Incarcerated femoral hernia (bilateral), without gangrene
Irreducible femoral hernia (bilateral), without gangrene
Strangulated femoral hernia (bilateral), without gangrene

     K41.00   **Bilateral femoral hernia, with obstruction, without gangrene,** not specified as recurrent
Bilateral femoral hernia, with obstruction, without gangrene NOS

     K41.01   **Bilateral femoral hernia, with obstruction, without gangrene,** recurrent

   ☑5ᵗʰ **K41.1**   **Bilateral femoral hernia, with gangrene**

     K41.10   **Bilateral femoral hernia, with gangrene,** not specified as recurrent
Bilateral femoral hernia, with gangrene NOS

     K41.11   **Bilateral femoral hernia, with gangrene,** recurrent

   ☑5ᵗʰ **K41.2**   **Bilateral femoral hernia, without obstruction or gangrene**

     K41.20   **Bilateral femoral hernia, without obstruction or gangrene,** not specified as recurrent
Bilateral femoral hernia NOS

     K41.21   **Bilateral femoral hernia, without obstruction or gangrene,** recurrent

   ☑5ᵗʰ **K41.3**   **Unilateral femoral hernia, with obstruction, without gangrene**
Femoral hernia (unilateral) causing obstruction, without gangrene
Incarcerated femoral hernia (unilateral), without gangrene
Irreducible femoral hernia (unilateral), without gangrene
Strangulated femoral hernia (unilateral), without gangrene

     K41.30   **Unilateral femoral hernia, with obstruction, without gangrene,** not specified as recurrent
Femoral hernia, with obstruction NOS
Unilateral femoral hernia, with obstruction NOS

     K41.31   **Unilateral femoral hernia, with obstruction, without gangrene,** recurrent

   ☑5ᵗʰ **K41.4**   **Unilateral femoral hernia, with gangrene**

     K41.40   **Unilateral femoral hernia, with gangrene,** not specified as recurrent
Femoral hernia, with gangrene NOS
Unilateral femoral hernia, with gangrene NOS

     K41.41   **Unilateral femoral hernia, with gangrene,** recurrent

   ☑5ᵗʰ **K41.9**   **Unilateral femoral hernia, without obstruction or gangrene**

     K41.90   **Unilateral femoral hernia, without obstruction or gangrene,** not specified as recurrent
Femoral hernia NOS
Unilateral femoral hernia NOS

     K41.91   **Unilateral femoral hernia, without obstruction or gangrene,** recurrent

☑4ᵗʰ **K42**   **Umbilical hernia**

   INCLUDES   paraumbilical hernia
   EXCLUDES 1   *omphalocele (Q79.2)*

   K42.0   **Umbilical hernia with obstruction, without gangrene**
Umbilical hernia causing obstruction, without gangrene
Incarcerated umbilical hernia, without gangrene
Irreducible umbilical hernia, without gangrene
Strangulated umbilical hernia, without gangrene

K42.1   **Umbilical hernia with gangrene**
Gangrenous umbilical hernia

K42.9   **Umbilical hernia without obstruction or gangrene**
Umbilical hernia NOS

☑4ᵗʰ **K43**   **Ventral hernia**
DEF: Condition in which a loop of bowel protrudes through a weakness in the abdominal wall muscles that may occur as a birth defect, past surgical site (incisional), or form at a stomal site (parastomal).

   K43.0   **Incisional hernia with obstruction, without gangrene**
Incisional hernia causing obstruction, without gangrene
Incarcerated incisional hernia, without gangrene
Irreducible incisional hernia, without gangrene
Strangulated incisional hernia, without gangrene

   K43.1   **Incisional hernia with gangrene**
Gangrenous incisional herniá

   K43.2   **Incisional hernia without obstruction or gangrene**
Incisional hernia NOS

   K43.3   **Parastomal hernia with obstruction, without gangrene**
Incarcerated parastomal hernia, without gangrene
Irreducible parastomal hernia, without gangrene
Parastomal hernia causing obstruction, without gangrene
Strangulated parastomal hernia, without gangrene

   K43.4   **Parastomal hernia with gangrene**
Gangrenous parastomal hernia

   K43.5   **Parastomal hernia without obstruction or gangrene**
Parastomal hernia NOS

   K43.6   **Other and unspecified ventral hernia with obstruction, without gangrene**
Epigastric hernia causing obstruction, without gangrene
Hypogastric hernia causing obstruction, without gangrene
Incarcerated epigastric hernia without gangrene
Incarcerated hypogastric hernia without gangrene
Incarcerated midline hernia without gangrene
Incarcerated spigelian hernia without gangrene
Incarcerated subxiphoid hernia without gangrene
Irreducible epigastric hernia without gangrene
Irreducible hypogastric hernia without gangrene
Irreducible midline hernia without gangrene
Irreducible spigelian hernia without gangrene
Irreducible subxiphoid hernia without gangrene
Midline hernia causing obstruction, without gangrene
Spigelian hernia causing obstruction, without gangrene
Strangulated epigastric hernia without gangrene
Strangulated hypogastric hernia without gangrene
Strangulated midline hernia without gangrene
Strangulated spigelian hernia without gangrene
Strangulated subxiphoid hernia without gangrene
Subxiphoid hernia causing obstruction, without gangrene

   K43.7   **Other and unspecified ventral hernia with gangrene**
Any condition listed under K43.6 specified as gangrenous

   K43.9   **Ventral hernia without obstruction or gangrene**
Epigastric hernia
Ventral hernia NOS

✅4ᵗʰ **K44** Diaphragmatic **hernia**

INCLUDES   hiatus hernia (esophageal) (sliding)
paraesophageal hernia

EXCLUDES 1   *congenital diaphragmatic hernia (Q79.0)*
congenital hiatus hernia (Q40.1)

DEF: Protrusion of an abdominal organ, usually the stomach, through the esophageal opening within the diaphragm and occurring in two types: the sliding hiatal hernia and the paraesophageal hernia.

Hiatal Hernia

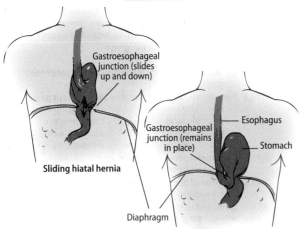

Sliding hiatal hernia

Paraesophageal hiatal hernia

K44.0 Diaphragmatic hernia with obstruction, without gangrene
Diaphragmatic hernia causing obstruction
Incarcerated diaphragmatic hernia
Irreducible diaphragmatic hernia
Strangulated diaphragmatic hernia

K44.1 Diaphragmatic hernia with gangrene
Gangrenous diaphragmatic hernia

K44.9 Diaphragmatic hernia without obstruction or gangrene
Diaphragmatic hernia NOS

✅4ᵗʰ **K45** Other abdominal hernia

INCLUDES   abdominal hernia, specified site NEC
lumbar hernia
obturator hernia
pudendal hernia
retroperitoneal hernia
sciatic hernia

K45.0 Other specified abdominal hernia with obstruction, without gangrene
Other specified abdominal hernia causing obstruction
Other specified incarcerated abdominal hernia
Other specified irreducible abdominal hernia
Other specified strangulated abdominal hernia

K45.1 Other specified abdominal hernia with gangrene
Any condition listed under K45 specified as gangrenous

K45.8 Other specified abdominal hernia without obstruction or gangrene

✅4ᵗʰ **K46** Unspecified abdominal hernia

INCLUDES   enterocele
epiplocele
hernia NOS
interstitial hernia
intestinal hernia
intra-abdominal hernia

EXCLUDES 1   *vaginal enterocele (N81.5)*

K46.0 Unspecified abdominal hernia with obstruction, without gangrene
Unspecified abdominal hernia causing obstruction
Unspecified incarcerated abdominal hernia
Unspecified irreducible abdominal hernia
Unspecified strangulated abdominal hernia

K46.1 Unspecified abdominal hernia with gangrene
Any condition listed under K46 specified as gangrenous

K46.9 Unspecified abdominal hernia without obstruction or gangrene
Abdominal hernia NOS

Noninfective enteritis and colitis (K50-K52)

INCLUDES   noninfective inflammatory bowel disease

EXCLUDES 1   *irritable bowel syndrome (K58.-)*
megacolon (K59.3-)

✅4ᵗʰ **K50** Crohn's disease [regional enteritis]

INCLUDES   granulomatous enteritis
Use additional code to identify manifestations, such as:
pyoderma gangrenosum (L88)

EXCLUDES 1   *ulcerative colitis (K51.-)*

AHA: 2012,4Q,104

DEF: Chronic inflammation of the gastrointestinal tract characterized by chronic granulomatous disease, most commonly affecting the intestines and the terminal ileum.

✅5ᵗʰ **K50.0** Crohn's disease of small intestine
Crohn's disease [regional enteritis] of duodenum
Crohn's disease [regional enteritis] of ileum
Crohn's disease [regional enteritis] of jejunum
Regional ileitis
Terminal ileitis

EXCLUDES 1   *Crohn's disease of both small and large intestine (K50.8-)*

K50.00 Crohn's disease of small intestine without complications

✅6ᵗʰ **K50.01** Crohn's disease of small intestine with complications

K50.011 Crohn's disease of small intestine with rectal bleeding

K50.012 Crohn's disease of small intestine with intestinal obstruction

K50.013 Crohn's disease of small intestine with fistula

K50.014 Crohn's disease of small intestine with abscess
AHA: 2012,4Q,104

K50.018 Crohn's disease of small intestine with other complication

K50.019 Crohn's disease of small intestine with unspecified complications

✅5ᵗʰ **K50.1** Crohn's disease of large intestine
Crohn's disease [regional enteritis] of colon
Crohn's disease [regional enteritis] of large bowel
Crohn's disease [regional enteritis] of rectum
Granulomatous colitis
Regional colitis

EXCLUDES 1   *Crohn's disease of both small and large intestine (K50.8)*

K50.10 Crohn's disease of large intestine without complications

✅6ᵗʰ **K50.11** Crohn's disease of large intestine with complications

K50.111 Crohn's disease of large intestine with rectal bleeding

K50.112 Crohn's disease of large intestine with intestinal obstruction

K50.113 Crohn's disease of large intestine with fistula

K50.114 Crohn's disease of large intestine with abscess

K50.118 Crohn's disease of large intestine with other complication

K50.119 Crohn's disease of large intestine with unspecified complications

✅5ᵗʰ **K50.8** Crohn's disease of both small and large intestine

K50.80 Crohn's disease of both small and large intestine without complications

✅6ᵗʰ **K50.81** Crohn's disease of both small and large intestine with complications

K50.811 Crohn's disease of both small and large intestine with rectal bleeding

K50.812 Crohn's disease of both small and large intestine with intestinal obstruction

K50.813 Crohn's disease of both small and large intestine with fistula

K50.814 Crohn's disease of both small and large intestine with abscess

N Newborn: 0   P Pediatric: 0-17   M Maternity: 12-55   A Adult: 15-124   CH Comorbidity High   CL Comorbidity Low   NCDx Noncancer Dx   PDx Primary Dx

704   ICD-10-CM 2020

K50.818   **Crohn's disease of both small and large intestine with other complication**

K50.819   **Crohn's disease of both small and large intestine with unspecified complications**

√5ᵗʰ   **K50.9**   **Crohn's disease, unspecified**

    K50.90   **Crohn's disease, unspecified,** without complications

       Crohn's disease NOS

       Regional enteritis NOS

   √6ᵗʰ   **K50.91**   **Crohn's disease, unspecified,** with complications

       K50.911   **Crohn's disease, unspecified, with** rectal bleeding

       K50.912   **Crohn's disease, unspecified, with intestinal obstruction**

       K50.913   **Crohn's disease, unspecified, with** fistula

       K50.914   **Crohn's disease, unspecified, with** abscess

       K50.918   **Crohn's disease, unspecified, with other complication**

       K50.919   **Crohn's disease, unspecified, with unspecified complications**

√4ᵗʰ   **K51**   **Ulcerative colitis**

    Use additional code to identify manifestations, such as: pyoderma gangrenosum (L88)

    EXCLUDES 1   *Crohn's disease [regional enteritis] (K50.-)*

   √5ᵗʰ   **K51.0**   **Ulcerative (chronic)** pancolitis

       Backwash ileitis

    K51.00   **Ulcerative (chronic) pancolitis** without complications

       Ulcerative (chronic) pancolitis NOS

   √6ᵗʰ   **K51.01**   **Ulcerative (chronic) pancolitis** with complications

       K51.011   **Ulcerative (chronic) pancolitis with** rectal bleeding

       K51.012   **Ulcerative (chronic) pancolitis with intestinal obstruction**

       K51.013   **Ulcerative (chronic) pancolitis with** fistula

       K51.014   **Ulcerative (chronic) pancolitis with** abscess

       K51.018   **Ulcerative (chronic) pancolitis with other complication**

       K51.019   **Ulcerative (chronic) pancolitis with unspecified complications**

   √5ᵗʰ   **K51.2**   **Ulcerative (chronic)** proctitis

    K51.20   **Ulcerative (chronic) proctitis** without complications

       Ulcerative (chronic) proctitis NOS

   √6ᵗʰ   **K51.21**   **Ulcerative (chronic) proctitis** with complications

       K51.211   **Ulcerative (chronic) proctitis with** rectal bleeding

       K51.212   **Ulcerative (chronic) proctitis with intestinal obstruction**

       K51.213   **Ulcerative (chronic) proctitis with** fistula

       K51.214   **Ulcerative (chronic) proctitis with** abscess

       K51.218   **Ulcerative (chronic) proctitis with other complication**

       K51.219   **Ulcerative (chronic) proctitis with unspecified complications**

   √5ᵗʰ   **K51.3**   **Ulcerative (chronic)** rectosigmoiditis

    K51.30   **Ulcerative (chronic) rectosigmoiditis** without complications

       Ulcerative (chronic) rectosigmoiditis NOS

   √6ᵗʰ   **K51.31**   **Ulcerative (chronic) rectosigmoiditis** with complications

       K51.311   **Ulcerative (chronic) rectosigmoiditis with** rectal bleeding

       K51.312   **Ulcerative (chronic) rectosigmoiditis with intestinal obstruction**

       K51.313   **Ulcerative (chronic) rectosigmoiditis with** fistula

       K51.314   **Ulcerative (chronic) rectosigmoiditis with** abscess

       K51.318   **Ulcerative (chronic) rectosigmoiditis with other complication**

       K51.319   **Ulcerative (chronic) rectosigmoiditis with unspecified complications**

√5ᵗʰ   **K51.4**   **Inflammatory polyps of colon**

    EXCLUDES 1   *adenomatous polyp of colon (D12.6)*

              polyposis of colon (D12.6)

              polyps of colon NOS (K63.5)

    K51.40   **Inflammatory polyps of colon** without complications

       Inflammatory polyps of colon NOS

   √6ᵗʰ   **K51.41**   **Inflammatory polyps of colon** with complications

       K51.411   **Inflammatory polyps of colon with** rectal bleeding

       K51.412   **Inflammatory polyps of colon with intestinal obstruction**

       K51.413   **Inflammatory polyps of colon with** fistula

       K51.414   **Inflammatory polyps of colon with** abscess

       K51.418   **Inflammatory polyps of colon with other complication**

       K51.419   **Inflammatory polyps of colon with unspecified complications**

√5ᵗʰ   **K51.5**   **Left sided colitis**

    Left hemicolitis

    K51.50   **Left sided colitis** without complications

       Left sided colitis NOS

   √6ᵗʰ   **K51.51**   **Left sided colitis** with complications

       K51.511   **Left sided colitis with** rectal bleeding

       K51.512   **Left sided colitis with** intestinal obstruction

       K51.513   **Left sided colitis with** fistula

       K51.514   **Left sided colitis with** abscess

       K51.518   **Left sided colitis with other complication**

       K51.519   **Left sided colitis with unspecified complications**

√5ᵗʰ   **K51.8**   **Other ulcerative colitis**

    K51.80   **Other ulcerative colitis** without complications

   √6ᵗʰ   **K51.81**   **Other ulcerative colitis** with complications

       K51.811   **Other ulcerative colitis with** rectal bleeding

       K51.812   **Other ulcerative colitis with** intestinal obstruction

       K51.813   **Other ulcerative colitis with** fistula

       K51.814   **Other ulcerative colitis with** abscess

       K51.818   **Other ulcerative colitis with other complication**

       K51.819   **Other ulcerative colitis with unspecified complications**

√5ᵗʰ   **K51.9**   **Ulcerative colitis, unspecified**

    K51.90   **Ulcerative colitis, unspecified,** without complications

   √6ᵗʰ   **K51.91**   **Ulcerative colitis, unspecified,** with complications

       K51.911   **Ulcerative colitis, unspecified with** rectal bleeding

       K51.912   **Ulcerative colitis, unspecified with intestinal obstruction**

       K51.913   **Ulcerative colitis, unspecified with** fistula

       K51.914   **Ulcerative colitis, unspecified with abscess**

       K51.918   **Ulcerative colitis, unspecified with other complication**

       K51.919   **Ulcerative colitis, unspecified with unspecified complications**

√4ᵗʰ   **K52**   **Other and unspecified noninfective gastroenteritis and colitis**

    AHA: 2016,4Q,30-31

    K52.0   **Gastroenteritis and colitis due to** radiation

    K52.1   **Toxic gastroenteritis and colitis**

       Drug-induced gastroenteritis and colitis

       Code first (T51-T65) to identify toxic agent

       Use additional code for adverse effect, if applicable, to identify drug (T36-T50 with fifth or sixth character 5)

       AHA: 2019,1Q,17

       TIP: This code is assigned for diarrhea due to drug use such as antibiotics or chemotherapy and is sequenced before a code for the adverse effect of the specific drug from category T36-T50.

☑ Additional Character Required   √x7ᵗʰ Placeholder Alert   Manifestation   Unspecified Dx   ►◄ Revised Text   ● New Code   ▲ Revised Title

ICD-10-CM 2020   705

√5ᵗʰ K52.2 Allergic and dietetic gastroenteritis and colitis
Food hypersensitivity gastroenteritis or colitis
Use additional code to identify type of food allergy (Z91.01-, Z91.02-)
> EXCLUDES 2   allergic eosinophilic colitis (K52.82)
> allergic eosinophilic esophagitis (K20.0)
> allergic eosinophilic gastritis (K52.81)
> allergic eosinophilic gastroenteritis (K52.81)
> food protein-induced proctocolitis (K52.82)

DEF: True immunoglobulin E (IgE)-mediated allergic reaction of the lining of the stomach, intestines, or colon to food proteins. It causes nausea, vomiting, diarrhea, and abdominal cramping.

K52.21 Food protein-induced enterocolitis syndrome
FPIES
Use additional code for hypovolemic shock, if present (R57.1)

K52.22 Food protein-induced enteropathy

K52.29 Other allergic and dietetic gastroenteritis and colitis
Food hypersensitivity gastroenteritis or colitis
Immediate gastrointestinal hypersensitivity

K52.3 Indeterminate colitis
Colonic inflammatory bowel disease unclassified (IBDU)
> EXCLUDES 1   unspecified colitis (K52.9)

√5ᵗʰ K52.8 Other specified noninfective gastroenteritis and colitis

K52.81 Eosinophilic gastritis or gastroenteritis
Eosinophilic enteritis
> EXCLUDES 2   eosinophilic esophagitis (K20.0)

DEF: Disorder involving the accumulation of eosinophil in the lining of the stomach or multiple levels of the gastrointestinal tract, but without a known cause such as connective tissue disease, drug reaction, malignancy, or parasitic infection.

K52.82 Eosinophilic colitis
Allergic proctocolitis
Food-induced eosinophilic proctocolitis
Food protein-induced proctocolitis
Milk protein-induced proctocolitis
DEF: Disorder involving the accumulation of eosinophil in the tissues lining the colon, but without a known cause such as connective tissue disease, drug reaction, malignancy, or parasitic infection. The resultant inflammation may cause extreme abdominal pain, diarrhea, or bloody stool.

√6ᵗʰ K52.83 Microscopic colitis
K52.831 Collagenous colitis
K52.832 Lymphocytic colitis
K52.838 Other microscopic colitis
K52.839 Microscopic colitis, unspecified

K52.89 Other specified noninfective gastroenteritis and colitis
AHA: 2019,1Q,20
TIP: This code is assigned for neutropenic colitis due to chemotherapy and is sequenced before T45.1X5- Adverse effect of antineoplastic and immunosuppressive drugs.

K52.9 Noninfective gastroenteritis and colitis, unspecified
Colitis NOS
Enteritis NOS
Gastroenteritis NOS
Ileitis NOS
Jejunitis NOS
Sigmoiditis NOS
> EXCLUDES 1   diarrhea NOS (R19.7)
> functional diarrhea (K59.1)
> infectious gastroenteritis and colitis NOS (A09)
> neonatal diarrhea (noninfective) (P78.3)
> psychogenic diarrhea (F45.8)

Other diseases of intestines (K55-K64)

√4ᵗʰ K55 Vascular disorders of intestine
> EXCLUDES 1   necrotizing enterocolitis of newborn (P77.-)
AHA: 2016,4Q,32

√5ᵗʰ K55.0 Acute vascular disorders of intestine
Infarction of appendices epiploicae
Mesenteric (artery) (vein) embolism
Mesenteric (artery) (vein) infarction
Mesenteric (artery) (vein) thrombosis

√6ᵗʰ K55.01 Acute (reversible) ischemia of small intestine
K55.011 Focal (segmental) acute (reversible) ischemia of small intestine
K55.012 Diffuse acute (reversible) ischemia of small intestine
K55.019 Acute (reversible) ischemia of small intestine, extent unspecified

√6ᵗʰ K55.02 Acute infarction of small intestine
Gangrene of small intestine
Necrosis of small intestine
K55.021 Focal (segmental) acute infarction of small intestine
K55.022 Diffuse acute infarction of small intestine
K55.029 Acute infarction of small intestine, extent unspecified

√6ᵗʰ K55.03 Acute (reversible) ischemia of large intestine
Acute fulminant ischemic colitis
Subacute ischemic colitis
K55.031 Focal (segmental) acute (reversible) ischemia of large intestine
K55.032 Diffuse acute (reversible) ischemia of large intestine
K55.039 Acute (reversible) ischemia of large intestine, extent unspecified

√6ᵗʰ K55.04 Acute infarction of large intestine
Gangrene of large intestine
Necrosis of large intestine
K55.041 Focal (segmental) acute infarction of large intestine
K55.042 Diffuse acute infarction of large intestine
K55.049 Acute infarction of large intestine, extent unspecified

√6ᵗʰ K55.05 Acute (reversible) ischemia of intestine, part unspecified
K55.051 Focal (segmental) acute (reversible) ischemia of intestine, part unspecified
K55.052 Diffuse acute (reversible) ischemia of intestine, part unspecified
K55.059 Acute (reversible) ischemia of intestine, part and extent unspecified

√6ᵗʰ K55.06 Acute infarction of intestine, part unspecified
Acute intestinal infarction
Gangrene of intestine
Necrosis of intestine
K55.061 Focal (segmental) acute infarction of intestine, part unspecified
K55.062 Diffuse acute infarction of intestine, part unspecified
K55.069 Acute infarction of intestine, part and extent unspecified

K55.1 Chronic vascular disorders of intestine
Chronic ischemic colitis
Chronic ischemic enteritis
Chronic ischemic enterocolitis
Ischemic stricture of intestine
Mesenteric atherosclerosis
Mesenteric vascular insufficiency

√5ᵗʰ K55.2 Angiodysplasia of colon
AHA: 2018,3Q,21
K55.20 Angiodysplasia of colon without hemorrhage
K55.21 Angiodysplasia of colon with hemorrhage
DEF: Small vascular abnormalities due to fragile blood vessels in the colon, resulting in blood loss from the gastrointestinal (GI) tract.

✓5ᵗʰ **K55.3 Necrotizing enterocolitis**

     EXCLUDES 1   *necrotizing enterocolitis of newborn (P77.-)*
     EXCLUDES 2   *necrotizing enterocolitis due to Clostridium difficile (A04.7-)*

     K55.30 Necrotizing enterocolitis, unspecified
       Necrotizing enterocolitis, NOS

     K55.31 Stage 1 necrotizing enterocolitis
       Necrotizing enterocolitis without pneumatosis, without perforation

     K55.32 Stage 2 necrotizing enterocolitis
       Necrotizing enterocolitis with pneumatosis, without perforation

     K55.33 Stage 3 necrotizing enterocolitis
       Necrotizing enterocolitis with perforation
       Necrotizing enterocolitis with pneumatosis and perforation

K55.8 Other vascular disorders of intestine

K55.9 Vascular disorder of intestine, unspecified
     Ischemic colitis
     Ischemic enteritis
     Ischemic enterocolitis

✓4ᵗʰ **K56 Paralytic ileus and intestinal obstruction without hernia**

     EXCLUDES 1   *congenital stricture or stenosis of intestine (Q41-Q42)*
       cystic fibrosis with meconium ileus (E84.11)
       ischemic stricture of intestine (K55.1)
       meconium ileus NOS (P76.0)
       neonatal intestinal obstructions classifiable to P76.-
       obstruction of duodenum (K31.5)
       postprocedural intestinal obstruction (K91.3-)
       stenosis of anus or rectum (K62.4)

K56.0 Paralytic ileus
     Paralysis of bowel
     Paralysis of colon
     Paralysis of intestine
     EXCLUDES 1   *gallstone ileus (K56.3)*
       ileus NOS (K56.7)
       obstructive ileus NOS (K56.69-)
     DEF: Intestinal obstruction due to paralysis of bowel motility or peristalsis.

K56.1 Intussusception
     Intussusception or invagination of bowel
     Intussusception or invagination of colon
     Intussusception or invagination of intestine
     Intussusception or invagination of rectum
     EXCLUDES 2   *intussusception of appendix (K38.8)*
     DEF: Intestinal obstruction due to prolapse of a bowel section into an adjacent section. It occurs primarily in children and symptoms include acute abdominal pain, vomiting, and passage of blood and mucus from the rectum.

K56.2 Volvulus
     Strangulation of colon or intestine
     Torsion of colon or intestine
     Twist of colon or intestine
     EXCLUDES 2   *volvulus of duodenum (K31.5)*
     DEF: Twisting, knotting, or entanglement of the bowel on itself that may quickly compromise oxygen supply to the intestinal tissues. A volvulus usually occurs at the sigmoid and ileocecal areas of the intestines.

Volvulus

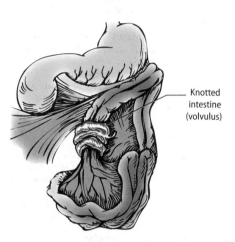

Knotted intestine (volvulus)

K56.3 Gallstone ileus
     Obstruction of intestine by gallstone

✓5ᵗʰ **K56.4 Other impaction of intestine**

     K56.41 Fecal impaction
       EXCLUDES 1   *constipation (K59.0-)*
         incomplete defecation (R15.0)

     K56.49 Other impaction of intestine

✓5ᵗʰ **K56.5 Intestinal adhesions [bands] with obstruction (postinfection)**
     Abdominal hernia due to adhesions with obstruction
     Peritoneal adhesions [bands] with intestinal obstruction (postinfection)
     AHA: 2017,4Q,16-17

     K56.50 Intestinal adhesions [bands], unspecified as to partial versus complete obstruction
       Intestinal adhesions with obstruction NOS

     K56.51 Intestinal adhesions [bands], with partial obstruction
       Intestinal adhesions with incomplete obstruction

     K56.52 Intestinal adhesions [bands] with complete obstruction

✓5ᵗʰ **K56.6 Other and unspecified intestinal obstruction**
     AHA: 2017,4Q,16-17; 2017,2Q,12

     ✓6ᵗʰ **K56.60 Unspecified intestinal obstruction**
       EXCLUDES 1   *intestinal obstruction due to specified condition - code to condition*

       K56.600 Partial intestinal obstruction, unspecified as to cause
         Incomplete intestinal obstruction, NOS

       K56.601 Complete intestinal obstruction, unspecified as to cause

       K56.609 Unspecified intestinal obstruction, unspecified as to partial versus complete obstruction
         Intestinal obstruction NOS

     ✓6ᵗʰ **K56.69 Other intestinal obstruction**
       Enterostenosis NOS
       Obstructive ileus NOS
       Occlusion of colon or intestine NOS
       Stenosis of colon or intestine NOS
       Stricture of colon or intestine NOS
       EXCLUDES 1   *intestinal obstruction due to specified condition - code to condition*

       K56.690 Other partial intestinal obstruction
         Other incomplete intestinal obstruction

       K56.691 Other complete intestinal obstruction

☑ Additional Character Required   ✓x7ᵗʰ Placeholder Alert   Manifestation   Unspecified Dx   ►◄ Revised Text   ● New Code   ▲ Revised Title

ICD-10-CM 2020   707

Chapter 11. Diseases of the Digestive System

K56.699   **Other intestinal obstruction unspecified as to partial versus complete obstruction**
Other intestinal obstruction, NEC

K56.7   **Ileus, unspecified**
EXCLUDES 1   *obstructive ileus (K56.69-)*
EXCLUDES 2   *intestinal obstruction with hernia (K40-K46)*
AHA: 2017,1Q,40

✓4ᵗʰ **K57**   **Diverticular disease of intestine**
Code also if applicable peritonitis K65.-
EXCLUDES 1   *congenital diverticulum of intestine (Q43.8)*
Meckel's diverticulum (Q43.0)
EXCLUDES 2   *diverticulum of appendix (K38.2)*
AHA: 2018,3Q,21

✓5ᵗʰ **K57.0**   **Diverticulitis of small intestine with perforation and abscess**
Diverticulitis of small intestine with peritonitis
EXCLUDES 1   *diverticulitis of both small and large intestine with perforation and abscess (K57.4-)*

K57.00   **Diverticulitis of small intestine with perforation and abscess without bleeding**

K57.01   **Diverticulitis of small intestine with perforation and abscess with bleeding**

✓5ᵗʰ **K57.1**   **Diverticular disease of small intestine without perforation or abscess**
EXCLUDES 1   *diverticular disease of both small and large intestine without perforation or abscess (K57.5-)*

K57.10   **Diverticulosis of small intestine without perforation or abscess without bleeding**
Diverticular disease of small intestine NOS

K57.11   **Diverticulosis of small intestine without perforation or abscess with bleeding**

K57.12   **Diverticulitis of small intestine without perforation or abscess without bleeding**

K57.13   **Diverticulitis of small intestine without perforation or abscess with bleeding**

✓5ᵗʰ **K57.2**   **Diverticulitis of large intestine with perforation and abscess**
Diverticulitis of colon with peritonitis
EXCLUDES 1   *diverticulitis of both small and large intestine with perforation and abscess (K57.4-)*

K57.20   **Diverticulitis of large intestine with perforation and abscess without bleeding**

K57.21   **Diverticulitis of large intestine with perforation and abscess with bleeding**

✓5ᵗʰ **K57.3**   **Diverticular disease of large intestine without perforation or abscess**
EXCLUDES 1   *diverticular disease of both small and large intestine without perforation or abscess (K57.5-)*

K57.30   **Diverticulosis of large intestine without perforation or abscess without bleeding**
Diverticular disease of colon NOS

K57.31   **Diverticulosis of large intestine without perforation or abscess with bleeding**

K57.32   **Diverticulitis of large intestine without perforation or abscess without bleeding**

K57.33   **Diverticulitis of large intestine without perforation or abscess with bleeding**

✓5ᵗʰ **K57.4**   **Diverticulitis of both small and large intestine with perforation and abscess**
Diverticulitis of both small and large intestine with peritonitis

K57.40   **Diverticulitis of both small and large intestine with perforation and abscess without bleeding**

K57.41   **Diverticulitis of both small and large intestine with perforation and abscess with bleeding**

✓5ᵗʰ **K57.5**   **Diverticular disease of both small and large intestine without perforation or abscess**

K57.50   **Diverticulosis of both small and large intestine without perforation or abscess without bleeding**
Diverticular disease of both small and large intestine NOS

K57.51   **Diverticulosis of both small and large intestine without perforation or abscess with bleeding**

K57.52   **Diverticulitis of both small and large intestine without perforation or abscess without bleeding**

K57.53   **Diverticulitis of both small and large intestine without perforation or abscess with bleeding**

✓5ᵗʰ **K57.8**   **Diverticulitis of intestine, part unspecified, with perforation and abscess**
Diverticulitis of intestine NOS with peritonitis

K57.80   **Diverticulitis of intestine, part unspecified, with perforation and abscess without bleeding**

K57.81   **Diverticulitis of intestine, part unspecified, with perforation and abscess with bleeding**

✓5ᵗʰ **K57.9**   **Diverticular disease of intestine, part unspecified, without perforation or abscess**

K57.90   **Diverticulosis of intestine, part unspecified, without perforation or abscess without bleeding**
Diverticular disease of intestine NOS

K57.91   **Diverticulosis of intestine, part unspecified, without perforation or abscess with bleeding**

K57.92   **Diverticulitis of intestine, part unspecified, without perforation or abscess without bleeding**

K57.93   **Diverticulitis of intestine, part unspecified, without perforation or abscess with bleeding**

✓4ᵗʰ **K58**   **Irritable bowel syndrome**
INCLUDES   irritable colon
spastic colon
AHA: 2016,4Q,32-33

K58.0   **Irritable bowel syndrome with diarrhea**

K58.1   **Irritable bowel syndrome with constipation**

K58.2   **Mixed irritable bowel syndrome**

K58.8   **Other irritable bowel syndrome**

K58.9   **Irritable bowel syndrome without diarrhea**
Irritable bowel syndrome NOS

✓4ᵗʰ **K59**   **Other functional intestinal disorders**
EXCLUDES 1   *change in bowel habit NOS (R19.4)*
intestinal malabsorption (K90.-)
psychogenic intestinal disorders (F45.8)
EXCLUDES 2   *functional disorders of stomach (K31.-)*

✓5ᵗʰ **K59.0**   **Constipation**
Use additional code for adverse effect, if applicable, to identify drug (T36-T50 with fifth or sixth character 5)
EXCLUDES 1   *fecal impaction (K56.41)*
incomplete defecation (R15.0)
AHA: 2016,4Q,33

K59.00   **Constipation, unspecified**

K59.01   **Slow transit constipation**
DEF: Delay in the transit of fecal material through the colon secondary to smooth muscle dysfunction or decreased peristaltic contractions along the colon.

K59.02   **Outlet dysfunction constipation**

K59.03   **Drug induced constipation**
Use additional code for adverse effect, if applicable, to identify drug (T36-T50 with fifth or sixth character 5)

K59.04   **Chronic idiopathic constipation**
Functional constipation

K59.09   **Other constipation**
Chronic constipation

K59.1   **Functional diarrhea**
EXCLUDES 1   *diarrhea NOS (R19.7)*
irritable bowel syndrome with diarrhea (K58.0)

K59.2   **Neurogenic bowel, not elsewhere classified**
DEF: Disorder of bowel due to a spinal cord lesion due to injury or as a complication of conditions such as multiple sclerosis (MS) or spina bifida. Loss of bowel control is the primary symptom, manifested as constipation or bowel incontinence.

✓5ᵗʰ **K59.3**   **Megacolon, not elsewhere classified**
Dilatation of colon
Code first, if applicable (T51-T65) to identify toxic agent
EXCLUDES 1   *congenital megacolon (aganglionic) (Q43.1)*
megacolon (due to) (in) Chagas' disease (B57.32)
megacolon (due to) (in) Clostridium difficile (A04.7-)
megacolon (due to) (in) Hirschsprung's disease (Q43.1)
AHA: 2016,4Q,33-34

K59.31   **Toxic megacolon**

K59.39   **Other megacolon**
Megacolon NOS

K59.4   **Anal spasm**
Proctalgia fugax

K59.8   **Other specified functional intestinal disorders**
Atony of colon
Pseudo-obstruction (acute) (chronic) of intestine

K59.9   **Functional intestinal disorder, unspecified**

☑4ᵗʰ **K60 Fissure and fistula of anal and rectal regions**

> *EXCLUDES 1*   fissure and fistula of anal and rectal regions with abscess or cellulitis (K61.-)
>
> *EXCLUDES 2*   anal sphincter tear (healed) (nontraumatic) (old) (K62.81)

K60.0   Acute **anal fissure**

K60.1   Chronic **anal fissure**

K60.2   **Anal fissure, unspecified**

K60.3   Anal **fistula**

K60.4   Rectal **fistula**

> Fistula of rectum to skin
>
> *EXCLUDES 1*   rectovaginal fistula (N82.3)
>
>   vesicorectal fistual (N32.1)

K60.5   Anorectal **fistula**

☑4ᵗʰ **K61 Abscess of anal and rectal regions**

> **INCLUDES**   abscess of anal and rectal regions
>
>   cellulitis of anal and rectal regions

K61.0   Anal **abscess**

> Perianal abscess
>
> *EXCLUDES 2*   intrasphincteric abscess (K61.4)

K61.1   Rectal **abscess**

> Perirectal abscess
>
> *EXCLUDES 1*   ischiorectal abscess (K61.39)
>
> **AHA:** 2012,4Q,104

K61.2   Anorectal **abscess**

☑5ᵗʰ **K61.3**   Ischiorectal **abscess**

> **AHA:** 2018,4Q,19

     K61.31   Horseshoe **abscess**

     K61.39   **Other ischiorectal abscess**

>   Abscess of ischiorectal fossa
>
>   Ischiorectal abscess, NOS

K61.4   Intrasphincteric **abscess**

> Intersphincteric abscess

K61.5   Supralevator **abscess**

> **AHA:** 2018,4Q,19

☑4ᵗʰ **K62 Other diseases of anus and rectum**

> **INCLUDES**   anal canal
>
> *EXCLUDES 2*   colostomy and enterostomy malfunction (K94.0-, K94.1-)
>
>   fecal incontinence (R15.-)
>
>   hemorrhoids (K64.-)

K62.0   **Anal polyp**

K62.1   **Rectal polyp**

> *EXCLUDES 1*   adenomatous polyp (D12.8)
>
> **AHA:** 2018,1Q,6

K62.2   **Anal prolapse**

> Prolapse of anal canal

K62.3   **Rectal prolapse**

> Prolapse of rectal mucosa

K62.4   **Stenosis of anus and rectum**

> Stricture of anus (sphincter)
>
> **AHA:** 2019,2Q,13

K62.5   **Hemorrhage of anus and rectum**

> *EXCLUDES 1*   gastrointestinal bleeding NOS (K92.2)
>
>   melena (K92.1)
>
>   neonatal rectal hemorrhage (P54.2)
>
> **AHA:** 2019,1Q,21

K62.6   **Ulcer of anus and rectum**

> Solitary ulcer of anus and rectum
>
> Stercoral ulcer of anus and rectum
>
> *EXCLUDES 1*   fissure and fistula of anus and rectum (K60.-)
>
>   ulcerative colitis (K51.-)

K62.7   **Radiation proctitis**

> Use additional code to identify the type of radiation (W90.-)
>
> **AHA:** 2019,1Q,21

☑5ᵗʰ **K62.8**   **Other specified diseases of anus and rectum**

> *EXCLUDES 2*   ulcerative proctitis (K51.2)

     K62.81   **Anal sphincter tear (healed) (nontraumatic) (old)**

>   Tear of anus, nontraumatic
>
>   Use additional code for any associated fecal incontinence (R15.-)
>
>   *EXCLUDES 2*   anal fissure (K60.-)
>
>   anal sphincter tear (healed) (old) complicating delivery (O34.7-)
>
>   traumatic tear of anal sphincter (S31.831)

K62.82   **Dysplasia of anus**

> Anal intraepithelial neoplasia I and II (AIN I and II) (histologically confirmed)
>
> Dysplasia of anus NOS
>
> Mild and moderate dysplasia of anus (histologically confirmed)
>
> *EXCLUDES 1*   abnormal results from anal cytologic examination without histologic confirmation (R85.61-)
>
>   anal intraepithelial neoplasia III (D01.3)
>
>   carcinoma in situ of anus (D01.3)
>
>   HGSIL of anus (R85.613)
>
>   severe dysplasia of anus (D01.3)

K62.89   **Other specified diseases of anus and rectum**

> Proctitis NOS
>
> Use additional code for any associated fecal incontinence (R15.-)

K62.9   **Disease of anus and rectum, unspecified**

☑4ᵗʰ **K63 Other diseases of intestine**

K63.0   Abscess **of intestine**

> *EXCLUDES 1*   abscess of intestine with Crohn's disease (K50.014, K50.114, K50.814, K50.914)
>
>   abscess of intestine with diverticular disease (K57.0, K57.2, K57.4, K57.8)
>
>   abscess of intestine with ulcerative colitis (K51.014, K51.214, K51.314, K51.414, K51.514, K51.814, K51.914)
>
> *EXCLUDES 2*   abscess of anal and rectal regions (K61.-)
>
>   abscess of appendix (K35.3-)

K63.1   Perforation **of intestine (nontraumatic)**

> Perforation (nontraumatic) of rectum
>
> *EXCLUDES 1*   perforation (nontraumatic) of duodenum (K26.-)
>
>   perforation (nontraumatic) of intestine with diverticular disease (K57.0, K57.2, K57.4, K57.8)
>
> *EXCLUDES 2*   perforation (nontraumatic) of appendix (K35.2-, K35.3-)

K63.2   Fistula **of intestine**

> *EXCLUDES 1*   fistula of duodenum (K31.6)
>
>   fistula of intestine with Crohn's disease (K50.013, K50.113, K50.813, K50.913)
>
>   fistula of intestine with ulcerative colitis (K51.013, K51.213, K51.313, K51.413, K51.513, K51.813, K51.913)
>
> *EXCLUDES 2*   fistula of anal and rectal regions (K60.-)
>
>   fistula of appendix (K38.3)
>
>   intestinal-genital fistula, female (N82.2-N82.4)
>
>   vesicointestinal fistula (N32.1)
>
> **AHA:** 2017,3Q,4

K63.3   Ulcer **of intestine**

> Primary ulcer of small intestine
>
> *EXCLUDES 1*   duodenal ulcer (K26.-)
>
>   gastrointestinal ulcer (K28.-)
>
>   gastrojejunal ulcer (K28.-)
>
>   jejunal ulcer (K28.-)
>
>   peptic ulcer, site unspecified (K27.-)
>
>   ulcer of intestine with perforation (K63.1)
>
>   ulcer of anus or rectum (K62.6)
>
>   ulcerative colitis (K51.-)

K63.4   Enteroptosis

K63.5   Polyp **of colon**

> *EXCLUDES 1*   adenomatous polyp of colon ▶(D12.-)◀
>
>   inflammatory polyp of colon (K51.4-)
>
>   polyposis of colon (D12.6)
>
> **AHA:** 2019,1Q,33; 2018,2Q,14; 2017,1Q,15; 2015,2Q,14

☑5ᵗʰ **K63.8**   **Other specified diseases of intestine**

     K63.81   **Dieulafoy lesion of intestine**

>   *EXCLUDES 2*   Dieulafoy lesion of stomach and duodenum (K31.82)
>
>   **DEF:** Abnormally large submucosal artery protruding through a defect in the stomach mucosa or intestines that can cause massive and life-threatening hemorrhage.

     K63.89   **Other specified diseases of intestine**

>   **AHA:** 2013,2Q,31

K63.9   **Disease of intestine, unspecified**

☑ Additional Character Required   ✓x7ᵗʰ Placeholder Alert   Manifestation   Unspecified Dx   ▶◀ Revised Text   ● New Code   ▲ Revised Title

Chapter 11. Diseases of the Digestive System

✓4ᵗʰ K64 Hemorrhoids and perianal venous thrombosis

INCLUDES   piles

EXCLUDES 1   *hemorrhoids complicating childbirth and the puerperium (O87.2)*
             hemorrhoids complicating pregnancy (O22.4)

Hemorrhoids

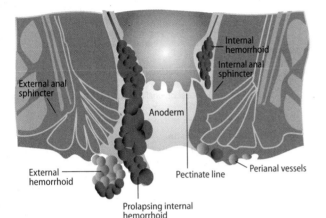

K64.0 First degree hemorrhoids
     Grade/stage I hemorrhoids
     Hemorrhoids (bleeding) without prolapse outside of anal canal

K64.1 Second degree hemorrhoids
     Grade/stage II hemorrhoids
     Hemorrhoids (bleeding) that prolapse with straining, but retract spontaneously

K64.2 Third degree hemorrhoids
     Grade/stage III hemorrhoids
     Hemorrhoids (bleeding) that prolapse with straining and require manual replacement back inside anal canal

K64.3 Fourth degree hemorrhoids
     Grade/stage IV hemorrhoids
     Hemorrhoids (bleeding) with prolapsed tissue that cannot be manually replaced

K64.4 Residual hemorrhoidal skin tags
     External hemorrhoids, NOS
     Skin tags of anus

K64.5 Perianal venous thrombosis
     External hemorrhoids with thrombosis
     Perianal hematoma
     Thrombosed hemorrhoids NOS

K64.8 Other hemorrhoids
     Internal hemorrhoids, without mention of degree
     Prolapsed hemorrhoids, degree not specified

K64.9 Unspecified hemorrhoids
     Hemorrhoids (bleeding) NOS
     Hemorrhoids (bleeding) without mention of degree

Diseases of peritoneum and retroperitoneum (K65-K68)

✓4ᵗʰ K65 Peritonitis

Use additional code (B95-B97), to identify infectious agent, if known
Code also if applicable diverticular disease of intestine (K57.-)

EXCLUDES 1   *acute appendicitis with generalized peritonitis (K35.2-)*
             aseptic peritonitis (T81.6)
             benign paroxysmal peritonitis (E85.0)
             chemical peritonitis (T81.6)
             gonococcal peritonitis (A54.85)
             neonatal peritonitis (P78.0-P78.1)
             pelvic peritonitis, female (N73.3-N73.5)
             periodic familial peritonitis (E85.0)
             peritonitis due to talc or other foreign substance (T81.6)
             peritonitis in chlamydia (A74.81)
             peritonitis in diphtheria (A36.89)
             peritonitis in syphilis (late) (A52.74)
             peritonitis in tuberculosis (A18.31)
             peritonitis with or following abortion or ectopic or molar pregnancy (O00-O07, O08.0)
             peritonitis with or following appendicitis (K35.-)
             puerperal peritonitis (O85)
             retroperitoneal infections (K68.-)

K65.0 Generalized (acute) peritonitis
     Pelvic peritonitis (acute), male
     Subphrenic peritonitis (acute)
     Suppurative peritonitis (acute)

K65.1 Peritoneal abscess
     Abdominopelvic abscess
     Abscess (of) omentum
     Abscess (of) peritoneum
     Mesenteric abscess
     Retrocecal abscess
     Subdiaphragmatic abscess
     Subhepatic abscess
     Subphrenic abscess
     AHA: 2019,1Q,15

K65.2 Spontaneous bacterial peritonitis
     EXCLUDES 1   *bacterial peritonitis NOS (K65.9)*

K65.3 Choleperitonitis
     Peritonitis due to bile
     DEF: Inflammation of the peritoneum due to leakage of bile into the peritoneal cavity resulting from rupture of the bile passages or gallbladder.

K65.4 Sclerosing mesenteritis
     Fat necrosis of peritoneum
     (Idiopathic) sclerosing mesenteric fibrosis
     Mesenteric lipodystrophy
     Mesenteric panniculitis
     Retractile mesenteritis

K65.8 Other peritonitis
     Chronic proliferative peritonitis
     Peritonitis due to urine

K65.9 Peritonitis, unspecified
     Bacterial peritonitis NOS
     AHA: 2013,2Q,31

✓4ᵗʰ K66 Other disorders of peritoneum

EXCLUDES 2   *ascites (R18.-)*
             peritoneal effusion (chronic) (R18.8)

K66.0 Peritoneal adhesions (postprocedural) (postinfection)
     Adhesions (of) abdominal (wall)
     Adhesions (of) diaphragm
     Adhesions (of) intestine
     Adhesions (of) male pelvis
     Adhesions (of) omentum
     Adhesions (of) stomach
     Adhesive bands
     Mesenteric adhesions
     EXCLUDES 1   *female pelvic adhesions [bands] (N73.6)*
                   peritoneal adhesions with intestinal obstruction (K56.5-)

K66.1 Hemoperitoneum
     EXCLUDES 1   *traumatic hemoperitoneum (S36.8-)*

K66.8 Other specified disorders of peritoneum

K66.9 Disorder of peritoneum, unspecified

N Newborn: 0   P Pediatric: 0-17   M Maternity: 12-55   A Adult: 15-124   CH Comorbidity High   CL Comorbidity Low   NCDx Noncancer Dx   PDx Primary Dx

710   ICD-10-CM 2020

K64–K66.9

K67   *Disorders of peritoneum in infectious diseases classified elsewhere*
> Code first underlying disease, such as:
> congenital syphilis (A50.0)
> helminthiasis (B65.0-B83.9)
>> EXCLUDES 1   *peritonitis in chlamydia (A74.81)*
>> *peritonitis in diphtheria (A36.89)*
>> *peritonitis in gonococcal (A54.85)*
>> *peritonitis in syphilis (late) (A52.74)*
>> *peritonitis in tuberculosis (A18.31)*

✓4th **K68**   **Disorders of retroperitoneum**

   ✓5th **K68.1**   **Retroperitoneal abscess**

     K68.11   **Postprocedural** retroperitoneal **abscess**
       EXCLUDES 2   *infection following procedure (T81.4-)*

     K68.12   **Psoas muscle abscess**

     K68.19   **Other retroperitoneal abscess**
       AHA: 2019,1Q,15
       TIP: This code should be used for a diagnosis of internal presacral abscess. If an intra-abdominal abscess is also present, code K65.1 can also be assigned; sequencing depends on the circumstances of admission.

   K68.9   **Other disorders of retroperitoneum**

Diseases of liver (K70-K77)

EXCLUDES 1   *jaundice NOS (R17)*
EXCLUDES 2   *hemochromatosis (E83.11-)*
     Reye's syndrome (G93.7)
     viral hepatitis (B15-B19)
     Wilson's disease (E83.0)

✓4th **K70**   **Alcoholic liver disease**
> Use additional code to identify:
> alcohol abuse and dependence (F10.-)

   K70.0   **Alcoholic** fatty liver   A

   ✓5th **K70.1**   **Alcoholic** hepatitis

     K70.10   **Alcoholic hepatitis** without ascites   A

     K70.11   **Alcoholic hepatitis** with ascites   A

   K70.2   **Alcoholic fibrosis and sclerosis of liver**   NC Dx A

   ✓5th **K70.3**   **Alcoholic** cirrhosis **of liver**
     Alcoholic cirrhosis NOS

     K70.30   **Alcoholic cirrhosis of liver** without ascites   NC Dx A

     K70.31   **Alcoholic cirrhosis of liver** with ascites   NC Dx A
       AHA: 2018,1Q,4

   ✓5th **K70.4**   **Alcoholic** hepatic failure
     Acute alcoholic hepatic failure
     Alcoholic hepatic failure NOS
     Chronic alcoholic hepatic failure
     Subacute alcoholic hepatic failure

     K70.40   **Alcoholic hepatic failure** without coma   A

     K70.41   **Alcoholic hepatic failure** with coma   NC Dx A

   K70.9   **Alcoholic liver disease, unspecified**   A

✓4th **K71**   **Toxic liver disease**
   INCLUDES   drug-induced idiosyncratic (unpredictable) liver disease
       drug-induced toxic (predictable) liver disease
> Code first poisoning due to drug or toxin, if applicable (T36-T65 with fifth or sixth character 1-4 or 6)
> Use additional code for adverse effect, if applicable, to identify drug (T36-T50 with fifth or sixth character 5)
>> EXCLUDES 2   *alcoholic liver disease (K70.-)*
>> *Budd-Chiari syndrome (I82.0)*

   K71.0   **Toxic liver disease with** cholestasis   NC Dx
     Cholestasis with hepatocyte injury
     "Pure" cholestasis

   ✓5th **K71.1**   **Toxic liver disease with** hepatic necrosis
     Hepatic failure (acute) (chronic) due to drugs

     K71.10   **Toxic liver disease with hepatic necrosis, without coma**   NC Dx

     K71.11   **Toxic liver disease with hepatic necrosis, with coma**   NC Dx

   K71.2   **Toxic liver disease with** acute hepatitis   NC Dx

   K71.3   **Toxic liver disease with** chronic persistent hepatitis   NC Dx

   K71.4   **Toxic liver disease with** chronic lobular hepatitis   NC Dx

   ✓5th **K71.5**   **Toxic liver disease with** chronic active hepatitis
     Toxic liver disease with lupoid hepatitis

     K71.50   **Toxic liver disease with chronic active hepatitis** without ascites   NC Dx

     K71.51   **Toxic liver disease with chronic active hepatitis** with ascites   NC Dx
       AHA: 2018,1Q,4

   K71.6   **Toxic liver disease with** hepatitis, not elsewhere classified   NC Dx

   K71.7   **Toxic liver disease with** fibrosis and cirrhosis **of liver**   NC Dx

   K71.8   **Toxic liver disease with other disorders of liver**   NC Dx
     Toxic liver disease with focal nodular hyperplasia
     Toxic liver disease with hepatic granulomas
     Toxic liver disease with peliosis hepatis
     Toxic liver disease with veno-occlusive disease of liver

   K71.9   **Toxic liver disease, unspecified**   NC Dx

✓4th **K72**   **Hepatic failure, not elsewhere classified**
   INCLUDES   fulminant hepatitis NEC, with hepatic failure
       hepatic encephalopathy NOS
       liver (cell) necrosis with hepatic failure
       malignant hepatitis NEC, with hepatic failure
       yellow liver atrophy or dystrophy
   EXCLUDES 1   *alcoholic hepatic failure (K70.4)*
       hepatic failure with toxic liver disease (K71.1-)
       icterus of newborn (P55-P59)
       postprocedural hepatic failure (K91.82)
   EXCLUDES 2   *hepatic failure complicating abortion or ectopic or molar pregnancy (O00-O07, O08.8)*
       hepatic failure complicating pregnancy, childbirth and the puerperium (O26.6-)
       viral hepatitis with hepatic coma (B15-B19)
   AHA: 2017,1Q,41

   ✓5th **K72.0**   **Acute and subacute** hepatic failure
     Acute non-viral hepatitis NOS
     AHA: 2015,2Q,17; 2014,2Q,13

     K72.00   **Acute and subacute hepatic failure without coma**   NC Dx

     K72.01   **Acute and subacute hepatic failure** with coma   NC Dx

   ✓5th **K72.1**   **Chronic** hepatic failure

     K72.10   **Chronic hepatic failure** without coma

     K72.11   **Chronic hepatic failure** with coma   NC Dx

   ✓5th **K72.9**   **Hepatic failure, unspecified**

     K72.90   **Hepatic failure, unspecified** without coma
       AHA: 2018,4Q,20; 2016,2Q,35

     K72.91   **Hepatic failure, unspecified** with coma   NC Dx
       Hepatic coma NOS

✓4th **K73**   **Chronic hepatitis, not elsewhere classified**
   EXCLUDES 1   *alcoholic hepatitis (chronic) (K70.1-)*
       drug-induced hepatitis (chronic) (K71.-)
       granulomatous hepatitis (chronic) NEC (K75.3)
       reactive, nonspecific hepatitis (chronic) (K75.2)
       viral hepatitis (chronic) (B15-B19)

   K73.0   **Chronic** persistent **hepatitis, not elsewhere classified**   NC Dx

   K73.1   **Chronic** lobular **hepatitis, not elsewhere classified**   NC Dx

   K73.2   **Chronic** active **hepatitis, not elsewhere classified**   NC Dx

   K73.8   **Other chronic hepatitis, not elsewhere classified**   NC Dx

   K73.9   **Chronic hepatitis, unspecified**   NC Dx

✓4th **K74**   **Fibrosis and cirrhosis of liver**
> Code also, if applicable, viral hepatitis (acute) (chronic) (B15-B19)
>> EXCLUDES 1   *alcoholic cirrhosis (of liver) (K70.3)*
>> *alcoholic fibrosis of liver (K70.2)*
>> *cardiac sclerosis of liver (K76.1)*
>> *cirrhosis (of liver) with toxic liver disease (K71.7)*
>> *congenital cirrhosis (of liver) (P78.81)*
>> *pigmentary cirrhosis (of liver) (E83.110)*

   K74.0   **Hepatic** fibrosis   NC Dx

   K74.1   **Hepatic** sclerosis

   K74.2   **Hepatic** fibrosis with hepatic sclerosis

☑ Additional Character Required   ✓x7th Placeholder Alert   Manifestation   Unspecified Dx   ▶◀ Revised Text   ● New Code   ▲ Revised Title

ICD-10-CM 2020   711

K74.3   Primary **biliary cirrhosis**   `NC Dx`

     Chronic nonsuppurative destructive cholangitis
     Primary biliary cholangitis
     EXCLUDES 2   ▶*primary sclerosing cholangitis*◀ *(K83.01)*

K74.4   Secondary **biliary cirrhosis**   `NC Dx`

K74.5   **Biliary cirrhosis, unspecified**   `NC Dx`

✓5ᵗʰ **K74.6**   **Other and unspecified cirrhosis of liver**

     K74.60   **Unspecified cirrhosis of liver**   `NC Dx`

         Cirrhosis (of liver) NOS
         AHA: 2018,1Q,4

     K74.69   **Other cirrhosis of liver**   `NC Dx`

         Cryptogenic cirrhosis (of liver)
         Macronodular cirrhosis (of liver)
         Micronodular cirrhosis (of liver)
         Mixed type cirrhosis (of liver)
         Portal cirrhosis (of liver)
         Postnecrotic cirrhosis (of liver)

✓4ᵗʰ **K75**   **Other inflammatory liver diseases**

     EXCLUDES 2   *toxic liver disease (K71.-)*

K75.0   **Abscess of liver**

     Cholangitic hepatic abscess
     Hematogenic hepatic abscess
     Hepatic abscess NOS
     Lymphogenic hepatic abscess
     Pylephlebitic hepatic abscess
     EXCLUDES 1   *amebic liver abscess (A06.4)*
              cholangitis without liver abscess (K83.09)
              pylephlebitis without liver abscess (K75.1)
     EXCLUDES 2   *acute or subacute hepatitis NOS (B17.9)*
              acute or subacute non-viral hepatitis (K72.0)
              chronic hepatitis NEC (K73.8)

K75.1   **Phlebitis of portal vein**
     Pylephlebitis
     EXCLUDES 1   *pylephlebitic liver abscess (K75.0)*
     DEF: Inflammation of the portal vein or branches due to diverticulitis, perforated appendicitis, or peritonitis. Symptoms include fever, chills, jaundice, sweating, and abscess in various body parts.

K75.2   **Nonspecific reactive hepatitis**   `NC Dx`

     EXCLUDES 1   *acute or subacute hepatitis (K72.0-)*
              chronic hepatitis NEC (K73.-)
              viral hepatitis (B15-B19)

K75.3   **Granulomatous hepatitis, not elsewhere classified**   `NC Dx`

     EXCLUDES 1   *acute or subacute hepatitis (K72.0-)*
              chronic hepatitis NEC (K73.-)
              viral hepatitis (B15-B19)

K75.4   **Autoimmune hepatitis**   `NC Dx`

     Lupoid hepatitis NEC

✓5ᵗʰ **K75.8**   **Other specified inflammatory liver diseases**

     K75.81   **Nonalcoholic steatohepatitis (NASH)**   `NC Dx`

     K75.89   **Other specified inflammatory liver diseases**

K75.9   **Inflammatory liver disease, unspecified**
     Hepatitis NOS
     EXCLUDES 1   *acute or subacute hepatitis (K72.0-)*
              chronic hepatitis NEC (K73.-)
              viral hepatitis (B15-B19)
     AHA: 2015,2Q,17

✓4ᵗʰ **K76**   **Other diseases of liver**

     EXCLUDES 2   *alcoholic liver disease (K70.-)*
              amyloid degeneration of liver (E85.-)
              cystic disease of liver (congenital) (Q44.6)
              hepatic vein thrombosis (I82.0)
              hepatomegaly NOS (R16.0)
              pigmentary cirrhosis (of liver) (E83.110)
              portal vein thrombosis (I81)
              toxic liver disease (K71.-)

K76.0   **Fatty (change of) liver, not elsewhere classified**
     Nonalcoholic fatty liver disease (NAFLD)
     EXCLUDES 1   *nonalcoholic steatohepatitis (NASH) (K75.81)*

K76.1   **Chronic passive congestion of liver**
     Cardiac cirrhosis
     Cardiac sclerosis

K76.2   **Central hemorrhagic necrosis of liver**
     EXCLUDES 1   *liver necrosis with hepatic failure (K72.-)*

K76.3   **Infarction of liver**

K76.4   **Peliosis hepatis**   `NC Dx`

     Hepatic angiomatosis

K76.5   **Hepatic veno-occlusive disease**
     EXCLUDES 1   *Budd-Chiari syndrome (I82.0)*

K76.6   **Portal hypertension**
     Use additional code for any associated complications, such as:
       portal hypertensive gastropathy (K31.89)

K76.7   **Hepatorenal syndrome**   `NC Dx`

     EXCLUDES 1   *hepatorenal syndrome following labor and delivery (O90.4)*
              postprocedural hepatorenal syndrome (K91.83)

✓5ᵗʰ **K76.8**   **Other specified diseases of liver**

     K76.81   **Hepatopulmonary syndrome**   `NC Dx`

         Code first underlying liver disease, such as:
           alcoholic cirrhosis of liver (K70.3-)
           cirrhosis of liver without mention of alcohol (K74.6-)

     K76.89   **Other specified diseases of liver**
         Cyst (simple) of liver
         Focal nodular hyperplasia of liver
         Hepatoptosis

K76.9   **Liver disease, unspecified**

K77   *Liver disorders in diseases classified elsewhere*
     Code first underlying disease, such as:
       amyloidosis (E85.-)
       congenital syphilis (A50.0, A50.5)
       congenital toxoplasmosis (P37.1)
       schistosomiasis (B65.0-B65.9)
     EXCLUDES 1   *alcoholic hepatitis (K70.1-)*
              alcoholic liver disease (K70.-)
              cytomegaloviral hepatitis (B25.1)
              herpesviral [herpes simplex] hepatitis (B00.81)
              infectious mononucleosis with liver disease (B27.0-B27.9 with .9)
              mumps hepatitis (B26.81)
              sarcoidosis with liver disease (D86.89)
              secondary syphilis with liver disease (A51.45)
              syphilis (late) with liver disease (A52.74)
              toxoplasmosis (acquired) hepatitis (B58.1)
              tuberculosis with liver disease (A18.83)

Ⓝ Newborn: 0   Ⓟ Pediatric: 0-17   Ⓜ Maternity: 12-55   Ⓐ Adult: 15-124   `CH` Comorbidity High   `CL` Comorbidity Low   `NC Dx` Noncancer Dx   `PDx` Primary Dx

712   ICD-10-CM 2020

Disorders of gallbladder, biliary tract and pancreas (K80-K87)

✓4ᵗʰ **K80 Cholelithiasis**

> **EXCLUDES 1** *retained cholelithiasis following cholecystectomy (K91.86)*
>
> **AHA:** 2018,4Q,20
>
> **DEF:** Presence or formation of concretions (calculi or "gallstones") in the gallbladder. The stones contain cholesterol, calcium carbonate, or calcium bilirubinate in pure forms or in various combinations.

Cholelithiasis

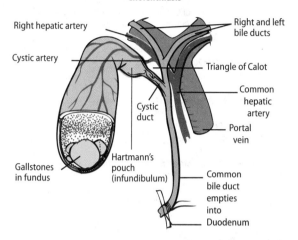

Right hepatic artery

Cystic artery

Cystic duct

Gallstones in fundus

Hartmann's pouch (infundibulum)

Right and left bile ducts

Triangle of Calot

Common hepatic artery

Portal vein

Common bile duct empties into Duodenum

✓5ᵗʰ **K80.0 Calculus of** gallbladder with acute cholecystitis

> Any condition listed in K80.2 with acute cholecystitis
> Use additional code if applicable for associated gangrene of gallbladder (K82.A1), or perforation of gallbladder (K82.A2)

K80.00 Calculus of gallbladder with acute cholecystitis without obstruction

K80.01 Calculus of gallbladder with acute cholecystitis with obstruction

✓5ᵗʰ **K80.1 Calculus of** gallbladder with other cholecystitis

> Use additional code if applicable for associated gangrene of gallbladder (K82.A1), or perforation of gallbladder (K82.A2)

K80.10 Calculus of gallbladder with chronic **cholecystitis** without obstruction

> Cholelithiasis with cholecystitis NOS

K80.11 Calculus of gallbladder with chronic **cholecystitis** with obstruction

K80.12 Calculus of gallbladder with acute and chronic **cholecystitis** without obstruction

K80.13 Calculus of gallbladder with acute and chronic **cholecystitis** with obstruction

K80.18 Calculus of gallbladder with other cholecystitis without obstruction

K80.19 Calculus of gallbladder with other cholecystitis with obstruction

✓5ᵗʰ **K80.2 Calculus of** gallbladder without cholecystitis

> Cholecystolithiasis without cholecystitis
> Cholelithiasis (without cholecystitis)
> Colic (recurrent) of gallbladder (without cholecystitis)
> Gallstone (impacted) of cystic duct (without cholecystitis)
> Gallstone (impacted) of gallbladder (without cholecystitis)

K80.20 Calculus of gallbladder without cholecystitis without obstruction

K80.21 Calculus of gallbladder without cholecystitis with obstruction

✓5ᵗʰ **K80.3 Calculus of** bile duct with cholangitis

> Any condition listed in K80.5 with cholangitis
> **DEF:** Cholangitis: Inflammation of the bile ducts.

K80.30 Calculus of bile duct with cholangitis, unspecified, without obstruction

K80.31 Calculus of bile duct with cholangitis, unspecified, with obstruction

K80.32 Calculus of bile duct with acute **cholangitis** without obstruction

K80.33 Calculus of bile duct with acute **cholangitis** with obstruction

K80.34 Calculus of bile duct with chronic **cholangitis** without obstruction

K80.35 Calculus of bile duct with chronic **cholangitis with** obstruction

K80.36 Calculus of bile duct with acute and chronic **cholangitis** without obstruction

K80.37 Calculus of bile duct with acute and chronic **cholangitis** with obstruction

✓5ᵗʰ **K80.4 Calculus of** bile duct with cholecystitis

> Any condition listed in K80.5 with cholecystitis (with cholangitis)
> Use additional code if applicable for associated gangrene of gallbladder (K82.A1), or perforation of gallbladder (K82.A2)
> **AHA:** 2019,1Q,17

K80.40 Calculus of bile duct with cholecystitis, unspecified, without obstruction

K80.41 Calculus of bile duct with cholecystitis, unspecified, with obstruction

> **AHA:** 2019,1Q,17

K80.42 Calculus of bile duct with acute **cholecystitis** without obstruction

K80.43 Calculus of bile duct with acute **cholecystitis with** obstruction

K80.44 Calculus of bile duct with chronic **cholecystitis** without obstruction

K80.45 Calculus of bile duct with chronic **cholecystitis with** obstruction

K80.46 Calculus of bile duct with acute and chronic **cholecystitis** without obstruction

K80.47 Calculus of bile duct with acute and chronic **cholecystitis** with obstruction

✓5ᵗʰ **K80.5 Calculus of** bile duct without cholangitis or cholecystitis

> Choledocholithiasis (without cholangitis or cholecystitis)
> Gallstone (impacted) of bile duct NOS (without cholangitis or cholecystitis)
> Gallstone (impacted) of common duct (without cholangitis or cholecystitis)
> Gallstone (impacted) of hepatic duct (without cholangitis or cholecystitis)
> Hepatic cholelithiasis (without cholangitis or cholecystitis)
> Hepatic colic (recurrent) (without cholangitis or cholecystitis)
> **DEF:** Cholangitis: Inflammation of the bile ducts.

K80.50 Calculus of bile duct without cholangitis or cholecystitis without obstruction

K80.51 Calculus of bile duct without cholangitis or cholecystitis with obstruction

✓5ᵗʰ **K80.6 Calculus of** gallbladder and bile duct with cholecystitis

> Use additional code if applicable for associated gangrene of gallbladder (K82.A1), or perforation of gallbladder (K82.A2)

K80.60 Calculus of gallbladder and bile duct with cholecystitis, unspecified, without obstruction

K80.61 Calculus of gallbladder and bile duct with cholecystitis, unspecified, with obstruction

K80.62 Calculus of gallbladder and bile duct with acute **cholecystitis** without obstruction

K80.63 Calculus of gallbladder and bile duct with acute **cholecystitis** with obstruction

K80.64 Calculus of gallbladder and bile duct with chronic **cholecystitis** without obstruction

K80.65 Calculus of gallbladder and bile duct with chronic **cholecystitis** with obstruction

K80.66 Calculus of gallbladder and bile duct with acute and chronic **cholecystitis** without obstruction

K80.67 Calculus of gallbladder and bile duct with acute and chronic **cholecystitis** with obstruction

✓5ᵗʰ **K80.7 Calculus of** gallbladder and bile duct without cholecystitis

K80.70 Calculus of gallbladder and bile duct without cholecystitis without obstruction

K80.71 Calculus of gallbladder and bile duct without cholecystitis with obstruction

✓5ᵗʰ **K80.8 Other cholelithiasis**

K80.80 Other cholelithiasis without obstruction

K80.81 Other cholelithiasis with obstruction

☑ Additional Character Required   ✓x7ᵗʰ Placeholder Alert   Manifestation   Unspecified Dx   ►◄ Revised Text   ● New Code   ▲ Revised Title

ICD-10-CM 2020   713

K80–K80.81

☑4ᵗʰ K81　Cholecystitis

Use additional code if applicable for associated gangrene of gallbladder (K82.A1), or perforation of gallbladder (K82.A2)

EXCLUDES 1　*cholecystitis with cholelithiasis (K80.-)*

AHA: 2018,4Q,20

K81.0　Acute cholecystitis
Abscess of gallbladder
Angiocholecystitis
Emphysematous (acute) cholecystitis
Empyema of gallbladder
Gangrene of gallbladder
Gangrenous cholecystitis
Suppurative cholecystitis

K81.1　Chronic cholecystitis

K81.2　Acute cholecystitis with chronic cholecystitis

K81.9　Cholecystitis, unspecified

☑4ᵗʰ K82　Other diseases of gallbladder

EXCLUDES 1　*nonvisualization of gallbladder (R93.2)*
postcholecystectomy syndrome (K91.5)

K82.0　Obstruction of gallbladder
Occlusion of cystic duct or gallbladder without cholelithiasis
Stenosis of cystic duct or gallbladder without cholelithiasis
Stricture of cystic duct or gallbladder without cholelithiasis

EXCLUDES 1　*obstruction of gallbladder with cholelithiasis (K80.-)*

K82.1　Hydrops of gallbladder
Mucocele of gallbladder

K82.2　Perforation of gallbladder
Rupture of cystic duct or gallbladder

EXCLUDES 1　*perforation of gallbladder in cholecystitis (K82.A2)*

K82.3　Fistula of gallbladder
Cholecystocolic fistula
Cholecystoduodenal fistula

K82.4　Cholesterolosis of gallbladder
Strawberry gallbladder

EXCLUDES 1　*cholesterolosis of gallbladder with cholecystitis (K81.-)*
cholesterolosis of gallbladder with cholelithiasis (K80.-)

K82.8　Other specified diseases of gallbladder
Adhesions of cystic duct or gallbladder
Atrophy of cystic duct or gallbladder
Cyst of cystic duct or gallbladder
Dyskinesia of cystic duct or gallbladder
Hypertrophy of cystic duct or gallbladder
Nonfunctioning of cystic duct or gallbladder
Ulcer of cystic duct or gallbladder

K82.9　Disease of gallbladder, unspecified

☑5ᵗʰ K82.A　Disorders of gallbladder in diseases classified elsewhere
Code first the type of cholecystitis (K81.-), or cholelithiasis with cholecystitis (K80.00-K80.19, K80.40-K80.47, K80.60-K80.67)

AHA: 2018,4Q,19-20

K82.A1　Gangrene of gallbladder in cholecystitis

K82.A2　Perforation of gallbladder in cholecystitis

☑4ᵗʰ K83　Other diseases of biliary tract

EXCLUDES 1　*postcholecystectomy syndrome (K91.5)*
EXCLUDES 2　*conditions involving the gallbladder (K81-K82)*
conditions involving the cystic duct (K81-K82)

☑5ᵗʰ K83.0　Cholangitis

EXCLUDES 1　*cholangitic liver abscess (K75.0)*
cholangitis with choledocholithiasis (K80.3-, K80.4-)
EXCLUDES 2　*chronic nonsuppurative destructive cholangitis (K74.3)*
primary biliary cholangitis (K74.3)
primary biliary cirrhosis (K74.3)

AHA: 2018,4Q,20

K83.01　Primary sclerosing cholangitis　　　NC Dx

K83.09　Other cholangitis
Ascending cholangitis
Cholangitis NOS
Primary cholangitis
Recurrent cholangitis
Sclerosing cholangitis
Secondary cholangitis
Stenosing cholangitis
Suppurative cholangitis

K83.1　Obstruction of bile duct
Occlusion of bile duct without cholelithiasis
Stenosis of bile duct without cholelithiasis
Stricture of bile duct without cholelithiasis

EXCLUDES 1　*congenital obstruction of bile duct (Q44.3)*
obstruction of bile duct with cholelithiasis (K80.-)

AHA: 2016,1Q,18

K83.2　Perforation of bile duct
Rupture of bile duct

K83.3　Fistula of bile duct
Choledochoduodenal fistula

AHA: 2019,1Q,17

K83.4　Spasm of sphincter of Oddi

K83.5　Biliary cyst

K83.8　Other specified diseases of biliary tract
Adhesions of biliary tract
Atrophy of biliary tract
Hypertrophy of biliary tract
Ulcer of biliary tract

K83.9　Disease of biliary tract, unspecified

☑4ᵗʰ K85　Acute pancreatitis

INCLUDES　acute (recurrent) pancreatitis
subacute pancreatitis

AHA: 2016,4Q,34

☑5ᵗʰ K85.0　Idiopathic acute pancreatitis

K85.00　Idiopathic acute pancreatitis without necrosis or infection

K85.01　Idiopathic acute pancreatitis with uninfected necrosis

K85.02　Idiopathic acute pancreatitis with infected necrosis

☑5ᵗʰ K85.1　Biliary acute pancreatitis
Gallstone pancreatitis

K85.10　Biliary acute pancreatitis without necrosis or infection

K85.11　Biliary acute pancreatitis with uninfected necrosis

K85.12　Biliary acute pancreatitis with infected necrosis

☑5ᵗʰ K85.2　Alcohol induced acute pancreatitis

EXCLUDES 2　*alcohol induced chronic pancreatitis (K86.0)*

K85.20　Alcohol induced acute pancreatitis without necrosis or infection

K85.21　Alcohol induced acute pancreatitis with uninfected necrosis

K85.22　Alcohol induced acute pancreatitis with infected necrosis

☑5ᵗʰ K85.3　Drug induced acute pancreatitis
Use additional code for adverse effect, if applicable, to identify drug (T36-T50 with fifth or sixth character 5)
Use additional code to identify drug abuse and dependence (F11.- F17.-)

K85.30　Drug induced acute pancreatitis without necrosis or infection

K85.31　Drug induced acute pancreatitis with uninfected necrosis

K85.32　Drug induced acute pancreatitis with infected necrosis

☑5ᵗʰ K85.8　Other acute pancreatitis

K85.80　Other acute pancreatitis without necrosis or infection

K85.81　Other acute pancreatitis with uninfected necrosis

K85.82　Other acute pancreatitis with infected necrosis

☑5ᵗʰ K85.9　Acute pancreatitis, unspecified
Pancreatitis NOS

K85.90　Acute pancreatitis without necrosis or infection, unspecified

K85.91　Acute pancreatitis with uninfected necrosis, unspecified

K85.92　Acute pancreatitis with infected necrosis, unspecified

Ⓝ Newborn: 0　　Ⓟ Pediatric: 0-17　　Ⓜ Maternity: 12-55　　Ⓐ Adult: 15-124　　CH Comorbidity High　　CL Comorbidity Low　　NC Dx Noncancer Dx　　PDx Primary Dx

714　　　ICD-10-CM 2020

Chapter 11. Diseases of the Digestive System

✓4ᵗʰ K86 Other diseases of pancreas

     EXCLUDES 2   *fibrocystic disease of pancreas (E84.-)*
                    islet cell tumor (of pancreas) (D13.7)
                    pancreatic steatorrhea (K90.3)

   K86.0 Alcohol-induced chronic pancreatitis
       Use additional code to identify:
         alcohol abuse and dependence (F10.-)
       Code also exocrine pancreatic insufficiency (K86.81)
       EXCLUDES 2   *alcohol induced acute pancreatitis (K85.2-)*

   K86.1 Other chronic pancreatitis
       Chronic pancreatitis NOS
       Infectious chronic pancreatitis
       Recurrent chronic pancreatitis
       Relapsing chronic pancreatitis
       Code also exocrine pancreatic insufficiency (K86.81)

   K86.2 Cyst of pancreas
   K86.3 Pseudocyst of pancreas
   ✓5ᵗʰ K86.8 Other specified diseases of pancreas
       AHA: 2016,4Q,34-35

     K86.81 Exocrine pancreatic insufficiency
     K86.89 Other specified diseases of pancreas
         Aseptic pancreatic necrosis, unrelated to acute
            pancreatitis
         Atrophy of pancreas
         Calculus of pancreas
         Cirrhosis of pancreas
         Fibrosis of pancreas
         Pancreatic fat necrosis, unrelated to acute pancreatitis
         Pancreatic infantilism
         Pancreatic necrosis NOS, unrelated to acute
            pancreatitis

   K86.9 Disease of pancreas, unspecified

K87 Disorders of gallbladder, biliary tract and pancreas in diseases classified elsewhere
     Code first underlying disease
     EXCLUDES 1   *cytomegaloviral pancreatitis (B25.2)*
                 mumps pancreatitis (B26.3)
                 syphilitic gallbladder (A52.74)
                 syphilitic pancreas (A52.74)
                 tuberculosis of gallbladder (A18.83)
                 tuberculosis of pancreas (A18.83)

Other diseases of the digestive system (K90-K95)

✓4ᵗʰ K90 Intestinal malabsorption

     EXCLUDES 1   *intestinal malabsorption following gastrointestinal surgery*
                 (K91.2)

   AHA: 2017,4Q,108

   K90.0 Celiac disease
       Celiac disease with steatorrhea
       Celiac gluten-sensitive enteropathy
       Nontropical sprue
       Use additional code for associated disorders including:
         dermatitis herpetiformis (L13.0)
         gluten ataxia (G32.81)
       Code also exocrine pancreatic insufficiency (K86.81)
       DEF: Malabsorption syndrome due to gluten consumption. Symptoms include fetid, bulky, frothy, oily stools; a distended abdomen; gas; asthenia; electrolyte depletion; and vitamin B, D, and K deficiency.

   K90.1 Tropical sprue
       Sprue NOS
       Tropical steatorrhea

   K90.2 Blind loop syndrome, not elsewhere classified
       Blind loop syndrome NOS
       EXCLUDES 1   *congenital blind loop syndrome (Q43.8)*
                  postsurgical blind loop syndrome (K91.2)

   K90.3 Pancreatic steatorrhea
   ✓5ᵗʰ K90.4 Other malabsorption due to intolerance
       EXCLUDES 2   *celiac gluten-sensitive enteropathy (K90.0)*
                  lactose intolerance (E73.-)
       AHA: 2016,4Q,35-36

     K90.41 Non-celiac gluten sensitivity
         Gluten sensitivity NOS
         Non-celiac gluten sensitive enteropathy

     K90.49 Malabsorption due to intolerance, not elsewhere classified
         Malabsorption due to intolerance to carbohydrate
         Malabsorption due to intolerance to fat
         Malabsorption due to intolerance to protein
         Malabsorption due to intolerance to starch

   ✓5ᵗʰ K90.8 Other intestinal malabsorption

     K90.81 Whipple's disease
     K90.89 Other intestinal malabsorption
   K90.9 Intestinal malabsorption, unspecified
       TIP: If a patient is diagnosed with both severe malnutrition and severe malabsorption, it is appropriate to assign this code as well as code E43 Unspecified severe protein-calorie malnutrition, regardless of the Excludes 1 note at code E43. This is allowable since these are separate conditions that can exist independently.

✓4ᵗʰ K91 Intraoperative and postprocedural complications and disorders of digestive system, not elsewhere classified
     EXCLUDES 2   *complications of artificial opening of digestive system (K94.-)*
                 complications of bariatric procedures (K95.-)
                 gastrojejunal ulcer (K28.-)
                 postprocedural (radiation) retroperitoneal abscess (K68.11)
                 radiation colitis (K52.0)
                 radiation gastroenteritis (K52.0)
                 radiation proctitis (K62.7)

   AHA: 2016,4Q,9-10

   K91.0 Vomiting following gastrointestinal surgery
   K91.1 Postgastric surgery syndromes
       Dumping syndrome
       Postgastrectomy syndrome
       Postvagotomy syndrome

   K91.2 Postsurgical malabsorption, not elsewhere classified
       Postsurgical blind loop syndrome
       EXCLUDES 1   *malabsorption osteomalacia in adults (M83.2)*
                 malabsorption osteoporosis, postsurgical (M80.8-, M81.8)

   ✓5ᵗʰ K91.3 Postprocedural intestinal obstruction
       AHA: 2017,4Q,16-17; 2017,1Q,40

     K91.30 Postprocedural intestinal obstruction, unspecified as to partial versus complete
         Postprocedural intestinal obstruction NOS
     K91.31 Postprocedural partial intestinal obstruction
         Postprocedural incomplete intestinal obstruction
     K91.32 Postprocedural complete intestinal obstruction
   K91.5 Postcholecystectomy syndrome
   ✓5ᵗʰ K91.6 Intraoperative hemorrhage and hematoma of a digestive system organ or structure complicating a procedure
       EXCLUDES 1   *intraoperative hemorrhage and hematoma of a digestive system organ or structure due to accidental puncture and laceration during a procedure (K91.7-)*

     K91.61 Intraoperative hemorrhage and hematoma of a digestive system organ or structure complicating a digestive system procedure
     K91.62 Intraoperative hemorrhage and hematoma of a digestive system organ or structure complicating other procedure
   ✓5ᵗʰ K91.7 Accidental puncture and laceration of a digestive system organ or structure during a procedure
     K91.71 Accidental puncture and laceration of a digestive system organ or structure during a digestive system procedure
     K91.72 Accidental puncture and laceration of a digestive system organ or structure during other procedure
         AHA: 2019,2Q,23
   ✓5ᵗʰ K91.8 Other intraoperative and postprocedural complications and disorders of digestive system
     K91.81 Other intraoperative complications of digestive system
     K91.82 Postprocedural hepatic failure
     K91.83 Postprocedural hepatorenal syndrome
     ✓6ᵗʰ K91.84 Postprocedural hemorrhage of a digestive system organ or structure following a procedure
       K91.840 Postprocedural hemorrhage of a digestive system organ or structure following a digestive system procedure
         AHA: 2016,1Q,15
       K91.841 Postprocedural hemorrhage of a digestive system organ or structure following other procedure

✓ Additional Character Required   ✓x7ᵗʰ Placeholder Alert   Manifestation   Unspecified Dx   ▶◀ Revised Text   ● New Code   ▲ Revised Title

ICD-10-CM 2020   715

✓6ᵗʰ **K91.85** **Complications of** intestinal pouch

    K91.850 **Pouchitis**

        Inflammation of internal ileoanal pouch

        DEF: Inflammatory complication of an existing surgically created ileoanal pouch, resulting in multiple GI complaints, including diarrhea, abdominal pain, rectal bleeding, fecal urgency, or incontinence.

    K91.858 **Other complications of intestinal pouch**

        AHA: 2019,2Q,13

K91.86 Retained cholelithiasis following cholecystectomy

✓6ᵗʰ **K91.87** Postprocedural hematoma and seroma of a digestive system organ or structure following a procedure

    K91.870 **Postprocedural** hematoma **of a digestive system organ or structure following a** digestive system procedure

    K91.871 **Postprocedural** hematoma **of a digestive system organ or structure following** other procedure

    K91.872 **Postprocedural** seroma **of a digestive system organ or structure following a** digestive system procedure

    K91.873 **Postprocedural** seroma **of a digestive system organ or structure following** other procedure

K91.89 **Other postprocedural complications and disorders of digestive system**

    Use additional code, if applicable, to further specify disorder

    EXCLUDES 2   postprocedural retroperitoneal abscess (K68.11)

    AHA: 2017,1Q,40

✓4ᵗʰ **K92** **Other diseases of digestive system**

    EXCLUDES 1   neonatal gastrointestinal hemorrhage (P54.0-P54.3)

K92.0 **Hematemesis**

K92.1 **Melena**

    EXCLUDES 1   occult blood in feces (R19.5)

K92.2 **Gastrointestinal hemorrhage, unspecified**

    Gastric hemorrhage NOS

    Intestinal hemorrhage NOS

    EXCLUDES 1   acute hemorrhagic gastritis (K29.01)

        hemorrhage of anus and rectum (K62.5)

        angiodysplasia of stomach with hemorrhage (K31.811)

        diverticular disease with hemorrhage (K57.-)

        gastritis and duodenitis with hemorrhage (K29.-)

        peptic ulcer with hemorrhage (K25-K28)

✓5ᵗʰ **K92.8** **Other specified diseases of the digestive system**

    K92.81 **Gastrointestinal mucositis (ulcerative)**

        Code also type of associated therapy, such as: antineoplastic and immunosuppressive drugs (T45.1X-)

        radiological procedure and radiotherapy (Y84.2)

        EXCLUDES 2   mucositis (ulcerative) of vagina and vulva (N76.81)

            nasal mucositis (ulcerative) (J34.81)

            oral mucositis (ulcerative) (K12.3-)

    K92.89 **Other specified diseases of the digestive system**

K92.9 **Disease of digestive system, unspecified**

✓4ᵗʰ **K94** **Complications of artificial openings of the digestive system**

✓5ᵗʰ **K94.0** Colostomy complications

    K94.00 **Colostomy complication, unspecified**

    K94.01 **Colostomy** hemorrhage

    K94.02 **Colostomy** infection

        Use additional code to specify type of infection, such as:

        cellulitis of abdominal wall (L03.311)

        sepsis (A40.-, A41.-)

    K94.03 **Colostomy** malfunction

        Mechanical complication of colostomy

    K94.09 **Other complications of colostomy**

✓5ᵗʰ **K94.1** Enterostomy complications

    K94.10 **Enterostomy complication, unspecified**

    K94.11 **Enterostomy** hemorrhage

K94.12 **Enterostomy** infection

    Use additional code to specify type of infection, such as:

    cellulitis of abdominal wall (L03.311)

    sepsis (A40.-, A41.-)

K94.13 **Enterostomy** malfunction

    Mechanical complication of enterostomy

K94.19 **Other complications of enterostomy**

✓5ᵗʰ **K94.2** Gastrostomy complications

    K94.20 **Gastrostomy complication, unspecified**

    K94.21 **Gastrostomy** hemorrhage

    K94.22 **Gastrostomy** infection

        Use additional code to specify type of infection, such as:

        cellulitis of abdominal wall (L03.311)

        sepsis (A40.-, A41.-)

    K94.23 **Gastrostomy** malfunction

        Mechanical complication of gastrostomy

        AHA: 2019,1Q,26

        TIP: Assign this code for a gastrostomy tube that has become clogged.

    K94.29 **Other complications of gastrostomy**

✓5ᵗʰ **K94.3** Esophagostomy complications

    K94.30 **Esophagostomy complications, unspecified**

    K94.31 **Esophagostomy** hemorrhage

    K94.32 **Esophagostomy** infection

        Use additional code to identify the infection

    K94.33 **Esophagostomy** malfunction

        Mechanical complication of esophagostomy

    K94.39 **Other complications of esophagostomy**

✓4ᵗʰ **K95** **Complications of bariatric procedures**

✓5ᵗʰ **K95.0** **Complications of** gastric band procedure

    K95.01 **Infection due to gastric band procedure**

        Use additional code to specify type of infection or organism, such as:

        bacterial and viral infectious agents (B95.-, B96.-)

        cellulitis of abdominal wall (L03.311)

        sepsis (A40.-, A41.-)

[handwritten: B95.61 (S) / B95.62 (R)]

    K95.09 **Other complications of gastric band procedure**

        Use additional code, if applicable, to further specify complication

✓5ᵗʰ **K95.8** **Complications of other bariatric procedure**

    EXCLUDES 1   complications of gastric band surgery (K95.0-)

    K95.81 **Infection due to other bariatric procedure**

        Use additional code to specify type of infection or organism, such as:

        bacterial and viral infectious agents (B95.-, B96.-)

        cellulitis of abdominal wall (L03.311)

        sepsis (A40.-, A41.-)

    K95.89 **Other complications of other bariatric procedure**

        Use additional code, if applicable, to further specify complication

N Newborn: 0   P Pediatric: 0-17   M Maternity: 12-55   A Adult: 15-124   CH Comorbidity High   CL Comorbidity Low   NCDx Noncancer Dx   PDx Primary Dx

716   ICD-10-CM 2020

Chapter 12. Diseases of the Skin and Subcutaneous Tissue (LØØ–L99)

Chapter-specific Guidelines with Coding Examples

The chapter-specific guidelines from the ICD-10-CM Official Guidelines for Coding and Reporting have been provided below. Along with these guidelines are coding examples, contained in the shaded boxes, that have been developed to help illustrate the coding and/or sequencing guidance found in these guidelines.

a. Pressure ulcer stage codes

1) Pressure ulcer stages

Codes **in** category L89, Pressure ulcer, identify the site **and stage** of the pressure ulcer.

The ICD-10-CM classifies pressure ulcer stages based on severity, which is designated by stages 1-4, **deep tissue pressure injury,** unspecified stage, and unstageable.

Assign as many codes from category L89 as needed to identify all the pressure ulcers the patient has, if applicable.

See Section I.B.14 for pressure ulcer stage documentation by clinicians other than patient's provider

> Stage 4 pressure ulcer right heel, 9 x 10 cm that invades the muscle and fascia; stage 2 pressure ulcer of left elbow.
>
> **L89.614   Pressure ulcer of right heel, stage 4**
>
> **L89.Ø22   Pressure ulcer of left elbow, stage 2**
>
> *Explanation:* Patient has a right heel pressure ulcer documented as stage 4 and a left elbow pressure ulcer documented as stage 2. Combination codes from category L89 Pressure ulcer, identify the site of the pressure ulcer as well as the stage. Assign as many codes from category L89 as needed to identify all the pressure ulcers the patient has.

2) Unstageable pressure ulcers

Assignment of the code for unstageable pressure ulcer (L89.--Ø) should be based on the clinical documentation. These codes are used for pressure ulcers whose stage cannot be clinically determined (e.g., the ulcer is covered by eschar or has been treated with a skin or muscle graft). This code should not be confused with the codes for unspecified stage (L89.--9). When there is no documentation regarding the stage of the pressure ulcer, assign the appropriate code for unspecified stage (L89.--9).

> Pressure ulcer of the right lower back documented as unstageable due to the presence of thick eschar covering the ulcer.
>
> **L89.13Ø   Pressure ulcer of right lower back, unstageable**
>
> *Explanation:* Codes for unstageable pressure ulcers are assigned when the stage cannot be clinically determined (e.g., the ulcer is covered by eschar or has been treated with a skin or muscle graft).

3) Documented pressure ulcer stage

Assignment of the pressure ulcer stage code should be guided by clinical documentation of the stage or documentation of the terms found in the Alphabetic Index. For clinical terms describing the stage that are not found in the Alphabetic Index, and there is no documentation of the stage, the provider should be queried.

> Left heel pressure ulcer with partial thickness skin loss involving the dermis.
>
> **L89.622   Pressure ulcer of left heel, stage 2**
>
> *Explanation:* Code assignment for the pressure ulcer stage should be guided by either the clinical documentation of the stage or the documentation of terms found in the Alphabetic Index. The clinical documentation describing the left heel pressure ulcer "partial thickness skin loss involving the dermis" matches the ICD-10-CM index parenthetical description for stage 2 "(abrasion, blister, partial thickness skin loss involving epidermis and/or dermis)."

4) Patients admitted with pressure ulcers documented as healed

No code is assigned if the documentation states that the pressure ulcer is completely healed **at the time of admission.**

5) Pressure ulcers documented as healing

Pressure ulcers described as healing should be assigned the appropriate pressure ulcer stage code based on the documentation in the medical record. If the documentation does not provide information about the stage of the healing pressure ulcer, assign the appropriate code for unspecified stage.

If the documentation is unclear as to whether the patient has a current (new) pressure ulcer or if the patient is being treated for a healing pressure ulcer, query the provider.

For ulcers that were present on admission but healed at the time of discharge, assign the code for the site and stage of the pressure ulcer at the time of admission.

6) Patient admitted with pressure ulcer evolving into another stage during the admission

If a patient is admitted to an inpatient hospital with a pressure ulcer at one stage and it progresses to a higher stage, two separate codes should be assigned: one code for the site and stage of the ulcer on admission and a second code for the same ulcer site and the highest stage reported during the stay.

7) Pressure-induced deep tissue damage

For pressure-induced deep tissue damage or deep tissue pressure injury, assign only the appropriate code for pressure-induced deep tissue damage (L89.--6).

b. Non-pressure chronic ulcers

1) Patients admitted with non-pressure ulcers documented as healed

No code is assigned if the documentation states that the non-pressure ulcer is completely healed **at the time of admission**.

2) Non-pressure ulcers documented as healing

Non-pressure ulcers described as healing should be assigned the appropriate non-pressure ulcer code based on the documentation in the medical record. If the documentation does not provide information about the severity of the healing non-pressure ulcer, assign the appropriate code for unspecified severity.

If the documentation is unclear as to whether the patient has a current (new) non-pressure ulcer or if the patient is being treated for a healing non-pressure ulcer, query the provider.

For ulcers that were present on admission but healed at the time of discharge, assign the code for the site and severity of the non-pressure ulcer at the time of admission.

3) Patient admitted with non-pressure ulcer that progresses to another severity level during the admission

If a patient is admitted to an inpatient hospital with a non-pressure ulcer at one severity level and it progresses to a higher severity level, two separate codes should be assigned: one code for the site and severity level of the ulcer on admission and a second code for the same ulcer site and the highest severity level reported during the stay.

See Section I.B.14 for pressure ulcer stage documentation by clinicians other than patient's provider

Chapter 12. Diseases of the Skin and Subcutaneous Tissue (L00-L99)

EXCLUDES 2   *certain conditions originating in the perinatal period (P04-P96)*
certain infectious and parasitic diseases (A00-B99)
complications of pregnancy, childbirth and the puerperium (O00-O9A)
congenital malformations, deformations, and chromosomal abnormalities (Q00-Q99)
endocrine, nutritional and metabolic diseases (E00-E88)
lipomelanotic reticulosis (I89.8)
neoplasms (C00-D49)
symptoms, signs and abnormal clinical and laboratory findings, not elsewhere classified (R00-R94)
systemic connective tissue disorders (M30-M36)
viral warts (B07.-)

This chapter contains the following blocks:
L00-L08   Infections of the skin and subcutaneous tissue
L10-L14   Bullous disorders
L20-L30   Dermatitis and eczema
L40-L45   Papulosquamous disorders
L49-L54   Urticaria and erythema
L55-L59   Radiation-related disorders of the skin and subcutaneous tissue
L60-L75   Disorders of skin appendages
L76   Intraoperative and postprocedural complications of skin and subcutaneous tissue
L80-L99   Other disorders of the skin and subcutaneous tissue

Infections of the skin and subcutaneous tissue (L00-L08)

Use additional code (B95-B97) to identify infectious agent
EXCLUDES 2   *hordeolum (H00.0)*
infective dermatitis (L30.3)
local infections of skin classified in Chapter 1
lupus panniculitis (L93.2)
panniculitis NOS (M79.3)
panniculitis of neck and back (M54.0-)
perlèche NOS (K13.0)
perlèche due to candidiasis (B37.0)
perlèche due to riboflavin deficiency (E53.0)
pyogenic granuloma (L98.0)
relapsing panniculitis [Weber-Christian] (M35.6)
viral warts (B07.-)
zoster (B02.-)

L00   Staphylococcal scalded skin syndrome
Ritter's disease
Use additional code to identify percentage of skin exfoliation (L49.-)
EXCLUDES 1   *bullous impetigo (L01.03)*
pemphigus neonatorum (L01.03)
toxic epidermal necrolysis [Lyell] (L51.2)
DEF: Infectious skin disease of children younger than 5 years marked by eruptions ranging from a few localized blisters to widespread, easily ruptured, fine vesicles and bullae affecting almost the entire body. It results in exfoliation of large planes of skin and leaves raw areas.

✓4ᵗʰ L01   Impetigo
EXCLUDES 1   *impetigo herpetiformis (L40.1)*
DEF: Acute, superficial, highly contagious skin infection commonly occurring in children. Skin lesions usually appear on the face and consist of vesicles and bullae that burst and form yellow crusts.

✓5ᵗʰ L01.0   Impetigo
Impetigo contagiosa
Impetigo vulgaris

    L01.00   Impetigo, unspecified
      Impetigo NOS

    L01.01   Non-bullous impetigo

    L01.02   Bockhart's impetigo
      Impetigo follicularis
      Perifolliculitis NOS
      Superficial pustular perifolliculitis
      DEF: Superficial inflammation of the hair follicles most commonly caused by staph aureus that manifests as rounded, sphere-shaped, pustular eruptions in the areas of the scalp, beard, underarms, extremities, and buttocks.

    L01.03   Bullous impetigo
      Impetigo neonatorum
      Pemphigus neonatorum

    L01.09   Other impetigo
      Ulcerative impetigo

L01.1   Impetiginization of other dermatoses

✓4ᵗʰ L02   Cutaneous abscess, furuncle and carbuncle
Use additional code to identify organism (B95-B96)
EXCLUDES 2   *abscess of anus and rectal regions (K61.-)*
abscess of female genital organs (external) (N76.4)
abscess of male genital organs (external) (N48.2, N49.-)
DEF: Carbuncle: Infection of the skin that arises from a collection of interconnected infected boils or furuncles, usually from hair follicles infected by *Staphylococcus*. This condition can produce pus and form drainage cavities.
DEF: Furuncle: Inflamed, painful abscess, cyst, or nodule on the skin caused by bacteria, often *Staphylococcus*, entering along the hair follicle.

✓5ᵗʰ L02.0   Cutaneous abscess, furuncle and carbuncle of face
EXCLUDES 2   *abscess of ear, external (H60.0)*
abscess of eyelid (H00.0)
abscess of head [any part, except face] (L02.8)
abscess of lacrimal gland (H04.0)
abscess of lacrimal passages (H04.3)
abscess of mouth (K12.2)
abscess of nose (J34.0)
abscess of orbit (H05.0)
submandibular abscess (K12.2)

    L02.01   Cutaneous abscess of face
    L02.02   Furuncle of face
      Boil of face
      Folliculitis of face
    L02.03   Carbuncle of face

✓5ᵗʰ L02.1   Cutaneous abscess, furuncle and carbuncle of neck
    L02.11   Cutaneous abscess of neck   CH CL
    L02.12   Furuncle of neck
      Boil of neck
      Folliculitis of neck
    L02.13   Carbuncle of neck

✓5ᵗʰ L02.2   Cutaneous abscess, furuncle and carbuncle of trunk
EXCLUDES 1   *non-newborn omphalitis (L08.82)*
omphalitis of newborn (P38.-)
EXCLUDES 2   *abscess of breast (N61.1)*
abscess of buttocks (L02.3)
abscess of female external genital organs (N76.4)
abscess of hip (L02.4)
abscess of male external genital organs (N48.2, N49.-)

    ✓6ᵗʰ **L02.21   Cutaneous abscess of trunk**
      L02.211   Cutaneous abscess of abdominal wall   CH CL
      L02.212   Cutaneous abscess of back [any part, except buttock]   CH CL
      L02.213   Cutaneous abscess of chest wall   CH CL
      L02.214   Cutaneous abscess of groin   CH CL
      L02.215   Cutaneous abscess of perineum   CH CL
      L02.216   Cutaneous abscess of umbilicus   CH CL
      L02.219   Cutaneous abscess of trunk, unspecified   CH CL

    ✓6ᵗʰ **L02.22   Furuncle of trunk**
      Boil of trunk
      Folliculitis of trunk
      L02.221   Furuncle of abdominal wall
      L02.222   Furuncle of back [any part, except buttock]
      L02.223   Furuncle of chest wall
      L02.224   Furuncle of groin
      L02.225   Furuncle of perineum
      L02.226   Furuncle of umbilicus
      L02.229   Furuncle of trunk, unspecified

    ✓6ᵗʰ **L02.23   Carbuncle of trunk**
      L02.231   Carbuncle of abdominal wall
      L02.232   Carbuncle of back [any part, except buttock]
      L02.233   Carbuncle of chest wall
      L02.234   Carbuncle of groin
      L02.235   Carbuncle of perineum
      L02.236   Carbuncle of umbilicus
      L02.239   Carbuncle of trunk, unspecified

✓5ᵗʰ **L02.3** **Cutaneous abscess, furuncle and carbuncle of buttock**
  EXCLUDES 1 pilonidal cyst with abscess (L05.01)
  L02.31 Cutaneous abscess of buttock CH CL
    Cutaneous abscess of gluteal region
  L02.32 Furuncle of buttock
    Boil of buttock
    Folliculitis of buttock
    Furuncle of gluteal region
  L02.33 Carbuncle of buttock
    Carbuncle of gluteal region

✓5ᵗʰ **L02.4** **Cutaneous abscess, furuncle and carbuncle of limb**
  EXCLUDES 2 cutaneous abscess, furuncle and carbuncle of groin
    (L02.214, L02.224, L02.234)
    cutaneous abscess, furuncle and carbuncle of hand
    (L02.5-)
    cutaneous abscess, furuncle and carbuncle of foot
    (L02.6-)
  ✓6ᵗʰ **L02.41** Cutaneous abscess of limb
    L02.411 Cutaneous abscess of right axilla CH CL
    L02.412 Cutaneous abscess of left axilla CH CL
    L02.413 Cutaneous abscess of right upper limb CH CL
    L02.414 Cutaneous abscess of left upper limb CH CL
    L02.415 Cutaneous abscess of right lower limb CH CL
    L02.416 Cutaneous abscess of left lower limb CH CL
    L02.419 Cutaneous abscess of limb, unspecified
  ✓6ᵗʰ **L02.42** Furuncle of limb
    Boil of limb
    Folliculitis of limb
    L02.421 Furuncle of right axilla
    L02.422 Furuncle of left axilla
    L02.423 Furuncle of right upper limb
    L02.424 Furuncle of left upper limb
    L02.425 Furuncle of right lower limb
    L02.426 Furuncle of left lower limb
    L02.429 Furuncle of limb, unspecified
  ✓6ᵗʰ **L02.43** Carbuncle of limb
    L02.431 Carbuncle of right axilla
    L02.432 Carbuncle of left axilla
    L02.433 Carbuncle of right upper limb
    L02.434 Carbuncle of left upper limb
    L02.435 Carbuncle of right lower limb
    L02.436 Carbuncle of left lower limb
    L02.439 Carbuncle of limb, unspecified

✓5ᵗʰ **L02.5** **Cutaneous abscess, furuncle and carbuncle of hand**
  ✓6ᵗʰ **L02.51** Cutaneous abscess of hand
    L02.511 Cutaneous abscess of right hand CH CL
    L02.512 Cutaneous abscess of left hand CH CL
    L02.519 Cutaneous abscess of unspecified hand
  ✓6ᵗʰ **L02.52** Furuncle hand
    Boil of hand
    Folliculitis of hand
    L02.521 Furuncle right hand
    L02.522 Furuncle left hand
    L02.529 Furuncle unspecified hand
  ✓6ᵗʰ **L02.53** Carbuncle of hand
    L02.531 Carbuncle of right hand
    L02.532 Carbuncle of left hand
    L02.539 Carbuncle of unspecified hand

✓5ᵗʰ **L02.6** **Cutaneous abscess, furuncle and carbuncle of foot**
  ✓6ᵗʰ **L02.61** Cutaneous abscess of foot
    L02.611 Cutaneous abscess of right foot CH CL
    L02.612 Cutaneous abscess of left foot CH CL
    L02.619 Cutaneous abscess of unspecified foot
  ✓6ᵗʰ **L02.62** Furuncle of foot
    Boil of foot
    Folliculitis of foot
    L02.621 Furuncle of right foot

    L02.622 Furuncle of left foot
    L02.629 Furuncle of unspecified foot
  ✓6ᵗʰ **L02.63** Carbuncle of foot
    L02.631 Carbuncle of right foot
    L02.632 Carbuncle of left foot
    L02.639 Carbuncle of unspecified foot

✓5ᵗʰ **L02.8** **Cutaneous abscess, furuncle and carbuncle of other sites**
  ✓6ᵗʰ **L02.81** Cutaneous abscess of other sites
    L02.811 Cutaneous abscess of head [any part, except face] CH CL
    L02.818 Cutaneous abscess of other sites CH CL
  ✓6ᵗʰ **L02.82** Furuncle of other sites
    Boil of other sites
    Folliculitis of other sites
    L02.821 Furuncle of head [any part, except face]
    L02.828 Furuncle of other sites
  ✓6ᵗʰ **L02.83** Carbuncle of other sites
    L02.831 Carbuncle of head [any part, except face]
    L02.838 Carbuncle of other sites

✓5ᵗʰ **L02.9** **Cutaneous abscess, furuncle and carbuncle, unspecified**
    L02.91 Cutaneous abscess, unspecified
    L02.92 Furuncle, unspecified
      Boil NOS
      Furunculosis NOS
    L02.93 Carbuncle, unspecified

✓4ᵗʰ **L03** **Cellulitis and acute lymphangitis**
  EXCLUDES 2 cellulitis of anal and rectal region (K61.-)
    cellulitis of external auditory canal (H60.1)
    cellulitis of eyelid (H00.0)
    cellulitis of female external genital organs (N76.4)
    cellulitis of lacrimal apparatus (H04.3)
    cellulitis of male external genital organs (N48.2, N49.-)
    cellulitis of mouth (K12.2)
    cellulitis of nose (J34.0)
    eosinophilic cellulitis [Wells] (L98.3)
    febrile neutrophilic dermatosis [Sweet] (L98.2)
    lymphangitis (chronic) (subacute) (I89.1)
  AHA: 2017,4Q,100
  DEF: Cellulitis: Infection of the skin and subcutaneous tissues, most often caused by *Staphylococcus* or *Streptococcus* bacteria secondary to a cutaneous lesion. Progression of the inflammation may lead to abscess and tissue death, or even systemic infection-like bacteremia.
  DEF: Lymphangitis: Inflammation of the lymph channels most often caused by *Streptococcus*.
  ✓5ᵗʰ **L03.0** **Cellulitis and acute lymphangitis of finger and toe**
    Infection of nail
    Onychia
    Paronychia
    Perionychia
    ✓6ᵗʰ **L03.01** Cellulitis of finger
      Felon
      Whitlow
      EXCLUDES 1 herpetic whitlow (B00.89)
      DEF: Felon: Superficial bacterial skin infection at the tip of the finger.
      L03.011 Cellulitis of right finger
      L03.012 Cellulitis of left finger
      L03.019 Cellulitis of unspecified finger
    ✓6ᵗʰ **L03.02** Acute lymphangitis of finger
      Hangnail with lymphangitis of finger
      L03.021 Acute lymphangitis of right finger
      L03.022 Acute lymphangitis of left finger
      L03.029 Acute lymphangitis of unspecified finger
    ✓6ᵗʰ **L03.03** Cellulitis of toe
      L03.031 Cellulitis of right toe
      L03.032 Cellulitis of left toe
      L03.039 Cellulitis of unspecified toe
    ✓6ᵗʰ **L03.04** Acute lymphangitis of toe
      Hangnail with lymphangitis of toe
      L03.041 Acute lymphangitis of right toe
      L03.042 Acute lymphangitis of left toe
      L03.049 Acute lymphangitis of unspecified toe

✓5ᵗʰ **L03.1** **Cellulitis and acute lymphangitis of other parts of limb**

    ✓6ᵗʰ **L03.11** Cellulitis of other parts of limb

        EXCLUDES 2   *cellulitis of fingers (L03.01-)*
                     cellulitis of toes (L03.03-)
                     groin (L03.314)

        L03.111 Cellulitis of right axilla   CH CL
        L03.112 Cellulitis of left axilla   CH CL
        L03.113 Cellulitis of right upper limb   CH CL
        L03.114 Cellulitis of left upper limb   CH CL
        L03.115 Cellulitis of right lower limb   CH CL
        L03.116 Cellulitis of left lower limb   CH CL
        L03.119 Cellulitis of unspecified part of limb

    ✓6ᵗʰ **L03.12** Acute lymphangitis of other parts of limb

        EXCLUDES 2   *acute lymphangitis of fingers (L03.2-)*
                     acute lymphangitis of groin (L03.324)
                     acute lymphangitis of toes (L03.04-)

        L03.121 Acute lymphangitis of right axilla   CH CL
        L03.122 Acute lymphangitis of left axilla   CH CL
        L03.123 Acute lymphangitis of right upper limb   CH CL
        L03.124 Acute lymphangitis of left upper limb   CH CL
        L03.125 Acute lymphangitis of right lower limb   CH CL
        L03.126 Acute lymphangitis of left lower limb   CH CL
        L03.129 Acute lymphangitis of unspecified part of limb

✓5ᵗʰ **L03.2** **Cellulitis and acute lymphangitis of face and neck**

    ✓6ᵗʰ **L03.21** Cellulitis and acute lymphangitis of face

        L03.211 Cellulitis of face

            EXCLUDES 2   *abscess of orbit (H05.01-)*
                        cellulitis of ear (H60.1-)
                        cellulitis of eyelid (H00.0-)
                        cellulitis of head (L03.81)
                        cellulitis of lacrimal apparatus (H04.3)
                        cellulitis of lip (K13.0)
                        cellulitis of mouth (K12.2)
                        cellulitis of nose (internal) (J34.0)
                        cellulitis of orbit (H05.01-)
                        cellulitis of scalp (L03.81)

            AHA: 2013,4Q,123

        L03.212 Acute lymphangitis of face
        L03.213 Periorbital cellulitis
            Preseptal cellulitis
            AHA: 2016,4Q,36

    ✓6ᵗʰ **L03.22** Cellulitis and acute lymphangitis of neck

        L03.221 Cellulitis of neck   CH CL
        L03.222 Acute lymphangitis of neck   CH CL

✓5ᵗʰ **L03.3** **Cellulitis and acute lymphangitis of trunk**

    ✓6ᵗʰ **L03.31** Cellulitis of trunk

        EXCLUDES 2   *cellulitis of anal and rectal regions (K61.-)*
                     cellulitis of breast NOS (N61.0)
                     cellulitis of female external genital organs (N76.4)
                     cellulitis of male external genital organs (N48.2, N49.-)
                     omphalitis of newborn (P38.-)
                     puerperal cellulitis of breast (O91.2)

        L03.311 Cellulitis of abdominal wall   CH CL

            EXCLUDES 2   *cellulitis of umbilicus (L03.316)*
                          cellulitis of groin (L03.314)

        L03.312 Cellulitis of back [any part except buttock]   CH CL
        L03.313 Cellulitis of chest wall   CH CL
        L03.314 Cellulitis of groin   CH CL
        L03.315 Cellulitis of perineum   CH CL
        L03.316 Cellulitis of umbilicus   CH CL
        L03.317 Cellulitis of buttock   CH CL

        L03.319 Cellulitis of trunk, unspecified   CH CL

    ✓6ᵗʰ **L03.32** Acute lymphangitis of trunk

        L03.321 Acute lymphangitis of abdominal wall   CH CL
        L03.322 Acute lymphangitis of back [any part except buttock]   CH CL
        L03.323 Acute lymphangitis of chest wall   CH CL
        L03.324 Acute lymphangitis of groin   CH CL
        L03.325 Acute lymphangitis of perineum   CH CL
        L03.326 Acute lymphangitis of umbilicus   CH CL
        L03.327 Acute lymphangitis of buttock   CH CL
        L03.329 Acute lymphangitis of trunk, unspecified   CH CL

✓5ᵗʰ **L03.8** **Cellulitis and acute lymphangitis of other sites**

    ✓6ᵗʰ **L03.81** Cellulitis of other sites

        L03.811 Cellulitis of head [any part, except face]   CH CL
            Cellulitis of scalp

            EXCLUDES 2   *cellulitis of face (L03.211)*

        L03.818 Cellulitis of other sites   CH CL

    ✓6ᵗʰ **L03.89** Acute lymphangitis of other sites

        L03.891 Acute lymphangitis of head [any part, except face]   CH CL
        L03.898 Acute lymphangitis of other sites   CH CL

✓5ᵗʰ **L03.9** **Cellulitis and acute lymphangitis, unspecified**

    L03.90 Cellulitis, unspecified
    L03.91 Acute lymphangitis, unspecified

        EXCLUDES 1   *lymphangitis NOS (I89.1)*

✓4ᵗʰ **L04** **Acute lymphadenitis**

    INCLUDES   abscess (acute) of lymph nodes, except mesenteric
                   acute lymphadenitis, except mesenteric

    EXCLUDES 1   *chronic or subacute lymphadenitis, except mesenteric (I88.1)*
                   enlarged lymph nodes (R59.-)
                   human immunodeficiency virus [HIV] disease resulting in generalized lymphadenopathy (B20)
                   lymphadenitis NOS (I88.9)
                   nonspecific mesenteric lymphadenitis (I88.0)

    DEF: Inflammation or enlargement of the lymph nodes.

    L04.0 Acute lymphadenitis of face, head and neck
    L04.1 Acute lymphadenitis of trunk
    L04.2 Acute lymphadenitis of upper limb
        Acute lymphadenitis of axilla
        Acute lymphadenitis of shoulder
    L04.3 Acute lymphadenitis of lower limb
        Acute lymphadenitis of hip

        EXCLUDES 2   *acute lymphadenitis of groin (L04.1)*

    L04.8 Acute lymphadenitis of other sites
    L04.9 Acute lymphadenitis, unspecified

N Newborn: 0   P Pediatric: 0-17   M Maternity: 12-55   A Adult: 15-124   CH Comorbidity High   CL Comorbidity Low   NCDx Noncancer Dx   PDx Primary Dx

720   **ICD-10-CM 2020**

✓4ᵗʰ L05 Pilonidal cyst and sinus

DEF: Pilonidal cyst: Sac or sinus cavity of trapped epithelial tissues in the sacrococcygeal region, usually associated with ingrown hair.
DEF: Pilonidal sinus: Fistula, tract, or channel that extends from an infected area of ingrown hair to another site within the skin or out to the skin surface.

Pilonidal Cyst

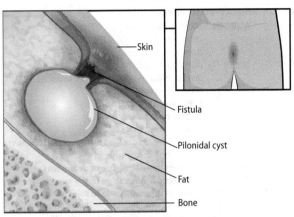

- Skin
- Fistula
- Pilonidal cyst
- Fat
- Bone

✓5ᵗʰ L05.0 Pilonidal cyst and sinus with abscess

L05.01 Pilonidal cyst with abscess
Pilonidal abscess
Pilonidal dimple with abscess
Postanal dimple with abscess
EXCLUDES 2   congenital sacral dimple (Q82.6)
             parasacral dimple (Q82.6)

L05.02 Pilonidal sinus with abscess
Coccygeal fistula with abscess
Coccygeal sinus with abscess
Pilonidal fistula with abscess

✓5ᵗʰ L05.9 Pilonidal cyst and sinus without abscess

L05.91 Pilonidal cyst without abscess
Pilonidal dimple
Postanal dimple
Pilonidal cyst NOS
EXCLUDES 2   congenital sacral dimple (Q82.6)
             parasacral dimple (Q82.6)

L05.92 Pilonidal sinus without abscess
Coccygeal fistula
Coccygeal sinus without abscess
Pilonidal fistula

✓4ᵗʰ L08 Other local infections of skin and subcutaneous tissue

L08.0 Pyoderma
Dermatitis gangrenosa
Purulent dermatitis
Septic dermatitis
Suppurative dermatitis
EXCLUDES 1   pyoderma gangrenosum (L88)
             pyoderma vegetans (L08.81)
DEF: Any superficial skin disease commonly characterized by the discharging of pus not attributed to another condition.

L08.1 Erythrasma
DEF: Chronic, superficial skin infection of brown scaly patches, commonly found in skin folds most prevalent in the overweight or diabetic population.

✓5ᵗʰ L08.8 Other specified local infections of the skin and subcutaneous tissue

L08.81 Pyoderma vegetans
EXCLUDES 1   pyoderma gangrenosum (L88)
             pyoderma NOS (L08.0)

L08.82 Omphalitis not of newborn
EXCLUDES 1   omphalitis of newborn (P38.-)

L08.89 Other specified local infections of the skin and subcutaneous tissue

L08.9 Local infection of the skin and subcutaneous tissue, unspecified

Bullous disorders (L10-L14)

EXCLUDES 1   benign familial pemphigus [Hailey-Hailey] (Q82.8)
             staphylococcal scalded skin syndrome (L00)
             toxic epidermal necrolysis [Lyell] (L51.2)

✓4ᵗʰ L10 Pemphigus

EXCLUDES 1   pemphigus neonatorum (L01.03)

L10.0 Pemphigus vulgaris
L10.1 Pemphigus vegetans
L10.2 Pemphigus foliaceous
L10.3 Brazilian pemphigus [fogo selvagem]
L10.4 Pemphigus erythematosus
     Senear-Usher syndrome
L10.5 Drug-induced pemphigus
     Use additional code for adverse effect, if applicable, to identify drug (T36-T50 with fifth or sixth character 5)

✓5ᵗʰ L10.8 Other pemphigus
L10.81 Paraneoplastic pemphigus
L10.89 Other pemphigus
L10.9 Pemphigus, unspecified

✓4ᵗʰ L11 Other acantholytic disorders

L11.0 Acquired keratosis follicularis
EXCLUDES 1   keratosis follicularis (congenital) [Darier-White] (Q82.8)
L11.1 Transient acantholytic dermatosis [Grover]
L11.8 Other specified acantholytic disorders
L11.9 Acantholytic disorder, unspecified

✓4ᵗʰ L12 Pemphigoid

EXCLUDES 1   herpes gestationis (O26.4-)
             impetigo herpetiformis (L40.1)

L12.0 Bullous pemphigoid
L12.1 Cicatricial pemphigoid
     Benign mucous membrane pemphigoid
     DEF: Chronic autoimmune disease characterized by subepidermal blistering lesions of the mucosa, including the conjunctiva. It is seen predominantly in the elderly and produces adhesions and scarring.
L12.2 Chronic bullous disease of childhood   P
     Juvenile dermatitis herpetiformis

✓5ᵗʰ L12.3 Acquired epidermolysis bullosa
EXCLUDES 1   epidermolysis bullosa (congenital) (Q81.-)
L12.30 Acquired epidermolysis bullosa, unspecified
L12.31 Epidermolysis bullosa due to drug
     Use additional code for adverse effect, if applicable, to identify drug (T36-T50 with fifth or sixth character 5)
L12.35 Other acquired epidermolysis bullosa
L12.8 Other pemphigoid
L12.9 Pemphigoid, unspecified

✓4ᵗʰ L13 Other bullous disorders

L13.0 Dermatitis herpetiformis
     Duhring's disease
     Hydroa herpetiformis
EXCLUDES 1   juvenile dermatitis herpetiformis (L12.2)
             senile dermatitis herpetiformis (L12.0)
     DEF: Skin disease to which people are genetically predisposed resulting from an immunological response to gluten. Dermatitis herpetiformis is an extremely pruritic eruption of various lesions that frequently heal, leaving hyperpigmentation or hypopigmentation and occasionally scarring. It is usually associated with asymptomatic gluten-sensitive enteropathy.

L13.1 Subcorneal pustular dermatitis
     Sneddon-Wilkinson disease
L13.8 Other specified bullous disorders
L13.9 Bullous disorder, unspecified

L14 Bullous disorders in diseases classified elsewhere
     Code first underlying disease

✓ Additional Character Required   ✓x7ᵗʰ Placeholder Alert   Manifestation   Unspecified Dx   ►◄ Revised Text   ● New Code   ▲ Revised Title

Chapter 12. Diseases of the Skin and Subcutaneous Tissue

Dermatitis and eczema (L20-L30)

NOTE   In this block the terms dermatitis and eczema are used synonymously and interchangeably.

EXCLUDES 2   chronic (childhood) granulomatous disease (D71)
dermatitis gangrenosa (L08.0)
dermatitis herpetiformis (L13.0)
dry skin dermatitis (L85.3)
factitial dermatitis (L98.1)
perioral dermatitis (L71.0)
radiation-related disorders of the skin and subcutaneous tissue (L55-L59)
stasis dermatitis (I87.2)

√4th **L20** Atopic **dermatitis**

L20.0 Besnier's prurigo

√5th **L20.8** **Other atopic dermatitis**

EXCLUDES 2   circumscribed neurodermatitis (L28.0)

L20.81 Atopic neurodermatitis
Diffuse neurodermatitis

L20.82 Flexural eczema

L20.83 Infantile (acute) (chronic) eczema   P

L20.84 Intrinsic (allergic) eczema

L20.89 Other atopic dermatitis

L20.9 Atopic dermatitis, unspecified

√4th **L21** Seborrheic **dermatitis**

EXCLUDES 2   infective dermatitis (L30.3)
seborrheic keratosis (L82.-)

L21.0 Seborrhea capitis
Cradle cap
AHA: 2018,1Q,6

L21.1 Seborrheic infantile dermatitis   P

L21.8 Other seborrheic dermatitis

L21.9 Seborrheic dermatitis, unspecified
Seborrhea NOS

L22 Diaper **dermatitis**
Diaper erythema
Diaper rash
Psoriasiform diaper rash

√4th **L23** Allergic contact **dermatitis**

EXCLUDES 1   allergy NOS (T78.40)
contact dermatitis NOS (L25.9)
dermatitis NOS (L30.9)

EXCLUDES 2   dermatitis due to substances taken internally (L27.-)
dermatitis of eyelid (H01.1-)
diaper dermatitis (L22)
eczema of external ear (H60.5-)
irritant contact dermatitis (L24.-)
perioral dermatitis (L71.0)
radiation-related disorders of the skin and subcutaneous tissue (L55-L59)

L23.0 Allergic contact dermatitis due to metals
Allergic contact dermatitis due to chromium
Allergic contact dermatitis due to nickel

L23.1 Allergic contact dermatitis due to adhesives

L23.2 Allergic contact dermatitis due to cosmetics

L23.3 Allergic contact dermatitis due to drugs in contact with skin
Use additional code for adverse effect, if applicable, to identify drug (T36-T50 with fifth or sixth character 5)
EXCLUDES 2   dermatitis due to ingested drugs and medicaments (L27.0-L27.1)

L23.4 Allergic contact dermatitis due to dyes

L23.5 Allergic contact dermatitis due to other chemical products
Allergic contact dermatitis due to cement
Allergic contact dermatitis due to insecticide
Allergic contact dermatitis due to plastic
Allergic contact dermatitis due to rubber

L23.6 Allergic contact dermatitis due to food in contact with the skin
EXCLUDES 2   dermatitis due to ingested food (L27.2)

L23.7 Allergic contact dermatitis due to plants, except food
EXCLUDES 2   allergy NOS due to pollen (J30.1)

√5th **L23.8** **Allergic contact dermatitis due to other agents**

L23.81 Allergic contact dermatitis due to animal (cat) (dog) dander
Allergic contact dermatitis due to animal (cat) (dog) hair

L23.89 Allergic contact dermatitis due to other agents

L23.9 Allergic contact dermatitis, unspecified cause
Allergic contact eczema NOS

√4th **L24** Irritant contact **dermatitis**

EXCLUDES 1   allergy NOS (T78.40)
contact dermatitis NOS (L25.9)
dermatitis NOS (L30.9)

EXCLUDES 2   allergic contact dermatitis (L23.-)
dermatitis due to substances taken internally (L27.-)
dermatitis of eyelid (H01.1-)
diaper dermatitis (L22)
eczema of external ear (H60.5-)
perioral dermatitis (L71.0)
radiation-related disorders of the skin and subcutaneous tissue (L55-L59)

L24.0 Irritant contact dermatitis due to detergents

L24.1 Irritant contact dermatitis due to oils and greases

L24.2 Irritant contact dermatitis due to solvents
Irritant contact dermatitis due to chlorocompound
Irritant contact dermatitis due to cyclohexane
Irritant contact dermatitis due to ester
Irritant contact dermatitis due to glycol
Irritant contact dermatitis due to hydrocarbon
Irritant contact dermatitis due to ketone

L24.3 Irritant contact dermatitis due to cosmetics

L24.4 Irritant contact dermatitis due to drugs in contact with skin
Use additional code for adverse effect, if applicable, to identify drug (T36-T50 with fifth or sixth character 5)

L24.5 Irritant contact dermatitis due to other chemical products
Irritant contact dermatitis due to cement
Irritant contact dermatitis due to insecticide
Irritant contact dermatitis due to plastic
Irritant contact dermatitis due to rubber

L24.6 Irritant contact dermatitis due to food in contact with skin
EXCLUDES 2   dermatitis due to ingested food (L27.2)

L24.7 Irritant contact dermatitis due to plants, except food
EXCLUDES 2   allergy NOS to pollen (J30.1)

√5th **L24.8** **Irritant contact dermatitis due to other agents**

L24.81 Irritant contact dermatitis due to metals
Irritant contact dermatitis due to chromium
Irritant contact dermatitis due to nickel

L24.89 Irritant contact dermatitis due to other agents
Irritant contact dermatitis due to dyes

L24.9 Irritant contact dermatitis, unspecified cause
Irritant contact eczema NOS

√4th **L25** Unspecified contact **dermatitis**

EXCLUDES 1   allergic contact dermatitis (L23.-)
allergy NOS (T78.40)
dermatitis NOS (L30.9)
irritant contact dermatitis (L24.-)

EXCLUDES 2   dermatitis due to ingested substances (L27.-)
dermatitis of eyelid (H01.1-)
eczema of external ear (H60.5-)
perioral dermatitis (L71.0)
radiation-related disorders of the skin and subcutaneous tissue (L55-L59)

L25.0 Unspecified contact dermatitis due to cosmetics

L25.1 Unspecified contact dermatitis due to drugs in contact with skin
Use additional code for adverse effect, if applicable, to identify drug (T36-T50 with fifth or sixth character 5)
EXCLUDES 2   dermatitis due to ingested drugs and medicaments (L27.0-L27.1)

L25.2 Unspecified contact dermatitis due to dyes

L25.3 Unspecified contact dermatitis due to other chemical products
Unspecified contact dermatitis due to cement
Unspecified contact dermatitis due to insecticide

N Newborn: 0   P Pediatric: 0-17   M Maternity: 12-55   A Adult: 15-124   CH Comorbidity High   CL Comorbidity Low   NCDx Noncancer Dx   PDx Primary Dx

722   ICD-10-CM 2020

L25.4   Unspecified contact dermatitis due to food in contact with skin
> EXCLUDES 2   dermatitis due to ingested food (L27.2)

L25.5   Unspecified contact dermatitis due to plants, except food
> EXCLUDES 1   nettle rash (L50.9)
> EXCLUDES 2   allergy NOS due to pollen (J30.1)

L25.8   Unspecified contact dermatitis due to other agents

L25.9   Unspecified contact dermatitis, unspecified cause
> Contact dermatitis (occupational) NOS
> Contact eczema (occupational) NOS

L26   Exfoliative dermatitis
> Hebra's pityriasis
> EXCLUDES 1   Ritter's disease (L00)

✓4ᵗʰ **L27**   Dermatitis due to substances taken internally
> EXCLUDES 1   allergy NOS (T78.40)
> EXCLUDES 2   adverse food reaction, except dermatitis (T78.0-T78.1)
>   contact dermatitis (L23-L25)
>   drug photoallergic response (L56.1)
>   drug phototoxic response (L56.0)
>   urticaria (L50.-)

L27.0   Generalized skin eruption due to drugs and medicaments taken internally
> Use additional code for adverse effect, if applicable, to identify drug (T36-T50 with fifth or sixth character 5)

L27.1   Localized skin eruption due to drugs and medicaments taken internally
> Use additional code for adverse effect, if applicable, to identify drug (T36-T50 with fifth or sixth character 5)

L27.2   Dermatitis due to ingested food
> EXCLUDES 2   dermatitis due to food in contact with skin (L23.6, L24.6, L25.4)

L27.8   Dermatitis due to other substances taken internally

L27.9   Dermatitis due to unspecified substance taken internally

✓4ᵗʰ **L28**   Lichen simplex chronicus and prurigo

L28.0   Lichen simplex chronicus
> Circumscribed neurodermatitis
> Lichen NOS

L28.1   Prurigo nodularis

L28.2   Other prurigo
> Prurigo NOS
> Prurigo Hebra
> Prurigo mitis
> Urticaria papulosa

✓4ᵗʰ **L29**   Pruritus
> EXCLUDES 1   neurotic excoriation (L98.1)
>   psychogenic pruritus (F45.8)

L29.0   Pruritus ani

L29.1   Pruritus scroti   ♂

L29.2   Pruritus vulvae   ♀

L29.3   Anogenital pruritus, unspecified

L29.8   Other pruritus

L29.9   Pruritus, unspecified
> Itch NOS

✓4ᵗʰ **L30**   Other and unspecified dermatitis
> EXCLUDES 2   contact dermatitis (L23-L25)
>   dry skin dermatitis (L85.3)
>   small plaque parapsoriasis (L41.3)
>   stasis dermatitis (I87.2)

L30.0   Nummular dermatitis

L30.1   Dyshidrosis [pompholyx]

L30.2   Cutaneous autosensitization
> Candidid [levurid]
> Dermatophytid
> Eczematid

L30.3   Infective dermatitis
> Infectious eczematoid dermatitis

L30.4   Erythema intertrigo

L30.5   Pityriasis alba
> AHA: 2018,1Q,6

L30.8   Other specified dermatitis

L30.9   Dermatitis, unspecified
> Eczema NOS

Papulosquamous disorders (L40-L45)

✓4ᵗʰ **L40**   Psoriasis
> DEF: Chronic autoimmune condition that speeds up skin cell growth, causing excessive immature skin cells to form raised, rounded erythematous lesions covered by dry, silvery scaling patches. Most commonly found on the scalp, elbows, knees, hands, feet, and genitals, it can also affect the joints with stiffness and swelling.

L40.0   Psoriasis vulgaris
> Nummular psoriasis
> Plaque psoriasis

L40.1   Generalized pustular psoriasis
> Impetigo herpetiformis
> Von Zumbusch's disease

L40.2   Acrodermatitis continua

L40.3   Pustulosis palmaris et plantaris

L40.4   Guttate psoriasis

✓5ᵗʰ **L40.5**   Arthropathic psoriasis

     L40.50   Arthropathic psoriasis, unspecified

     L40.51   Distal interphalangeal psoriatic arthropathy

     L40.52   Psoriatic arthritis mutilans

     L40.53   Psoriatic spondylitis

     L40.54   Psoriatic juvenile arthropathy

     L40.59   Other psoriatic arthropathy

L40.8   Other psoriasis
> Flexural psoriasis

L40.9   Psoriasis, unspecified

✓4ᵗʰ **L41**   Parapsoriasis
> EXCLUDES 1   poikiloderma vasculare atrophicans (L94.5)

L41.0   Pityriasis lichenoides et varioliformis acuta
> Mucha-Habermann disease

L41.1   Pityriasis lichenoides chronica

L41.3   Small plaque parapsoriasis

L41.4   Large plaque parapsoriasis

L41.5   Retiform parapsoriasis

L41.8   Other parapsoriasis

L41.9   Parapsoriasis, unspecified

L42   Pityriasis rosea

✓4ᵗʰ **L43**   Lichen planus
> EXCLUDES 1   lichen planopilaris (L66.1)

L43.0   Hypertrophic lichen planus

L43.1   Bullous lichen planus

L43.2   Lichenoid drug reaction
> Use additional code for adverse effect, if applicable, to identify drug (T36-T50 with fifth or sixth character 5)

L43.3   Subacute (active) lichen planus
> Lichen planus tropicus

L43.8   Other lichen planus

L43.9   Lichen planus, unspecified

✓4ᵗʰ **L44**   Other papulosquamous disorders

L44.0   Pityriasis rubra pilaris

L44.1   Lichen nitidus
> DEF: Chronic, inflammatory, asymptomatic skin disorder, characterized by numerous glistening, flat-topped, discrete, skin-colored micropapules, most often on the penis, lower abdomen, inner thighs, wrists, forearms, breasts, and buttocks.

L44.2   Lichen striatus

L44.3   Lichen ruber moniliformis

L44.4   Infantile papular acrodermatitis [Gianotti-Crosti]   P

L44.8   Other specified papulosquamous disorders

L44.9   Papulosquamous disorder, unspecified

L45   *Papulosquamous disorders in diseases classified elsewhere*
> Code first underlying disease

| ✓ Additional Character Required | ✓x7ᵗʰ Placeholder Alert | Manifestation | Unspecified Dx | ►◄ Revised Text | ● New Code | ▲ Revised Title |

ICD-10-CM 2020   723

Urticaria and erythema (L49-L54)

EXCLUDES 1   *Lyme disease (A69.2-)*
       rosacea (L71.-)

✓4ᵗʰ **L49 Exfoliation due to erythematous conditions according to extent of body surface involved**
     Code first erythematous condition causing exfoliation, such as:
       Ritter's disease (L00)
       ▶(Staphylococcal) scalded skin syndrome◄ (L00)
       Stevens-Johnson syndrome (L51.1)
       Stevens-Johnson syndrome-toxic epidermal necrolysis overlap syndrome (L51.3)
       toxic epidermal necrolysis (L51.2)
     DEF: Exfoliation: Falling or sloughing off skin in layers.

     L49.0 Exfoliation due to erythematous condition involving less than 10 percent of body surface
       Exfoliation due to erythematous condition NOS

     L49.1 Exfoliation due to erythematous condition involving 10-19 percent of body surface

     L49.2 Exfoliation due to erythematous condition involving 20-29 percent of body surface

     L49.3 Exfoliation due to erythematous condition involving 30-39 percent of body surface

     L49.4 Exfoliation due to erythematous condition involving 40-49 percent of body surface

     L49.5 Exfoliation due to erythematous condition involving 50-59 percent of body surface

     L49.6 Exfoliation due to erythematous condition involving 60-69 percent of body surface

     L49.7 Exfoliation due to erythematous condition involving 70-79 percent of body surface

     L49.8 Exfoliation due to erythematous condition involving 80-89 percent of body surface

     L49.9 Exfoliation due to erythematous condition involving 90 or more percent of body surface

✓4ᵗʰ **L50 Urticaria**
     EXCLUDES 1   *allergic contact dermatitis (L23.-)*
           angioneurotic edema (T78.3)
           giant urticaria (T78.3)
           hereditary angio-edema (D84.1)
           Quincke's edema (T78.3)
           serum urticaria (T80.6-)
           solar urticaria (L56.3)
           urticaria neonatorum (P83.8)
           urticaria papulosa (L28.2)
           urticaria pigmentosa ▶(D47.01)◄
     DEF: Eruption of itching edema of the skin. **Synonym(s):** *hives.*

     L50.0 Allergic urticaria

     L50.1 Idiopathic urticaria

     L50.2 Urticaria due to cold and heat
       EXCLUDES 2   *familial cold urticaria (M04.2)*

     L50.3 Dermatographic urticaria

     L50.4 Vibratory urticaria

     L50.5 Cholinergic urticaria

     L50.6 Contact urticaria

     L50.8 Other urticaria
       Chronic urticaria
       Recurrent periodic urticaria

     L50.9 Urticaria, unspecified

✓4ᵗʰ **L51 Erythema multiforme**
     Use additional code for adverse effect, if applicable, to identify drug (T36-T50 with fifth or sixth character 5)
     Use additional code to identify associated manifestations, such as:
       arthropathy associated with dermatological disorders (M14.8-)
       conjunctival edema (H11.42)
       conjunctivitis (H10.22-)
       corneal scars and opacities (H17.-)
       corneal ulcer (H16.0-)
       edema of eyelid (H02.84-)
       inflammation of eyelid (H01.8)
       keratoconjunctivitis sicca (H16.22-)
       mechanical lagophthalmos (H02.22-)
       stomatitis (K12.-)
       symblepharon (H11.23-)
     Use additional code to identify percentage of skin exfoliation (L49.-)
     EXCLUDES 1   *staphylococcal scalded skin syndrome (L00)*
           Ritter's disease (L00)
     DEF: Acute complex of symptoms with a varied pattern of skin eruptions, such as macular, bullous, popular, nodose, or vesicular lesions on the neck, face, and legs. Erythema (redness of skin and mucous membranes) multiforme (multiple forms) is a hypersensitivity (allergic) reaction that can occur at any age but primarily affects children or young adults.

     L51.0 Nonbullous erythema multiforme

     L51.1 Stevens-Johnson syndrome

     L51.2 Toxic epidermal necrolysis [Lyell]

     L51.3 Stevens-Johnson syndrome-toxic epidermal necrolysis overlap syndrome
       SJS-TEN overlap syndrome

     L51.8 Other erythema multiforme

     L51.9 Erythema multiforme, unspecified
       Erythema iris
       Erythema multiforme major NOS
       Erythema multiforme minor NOS
       Herpes iris

L52 Erythema nodosum
     EXCLUDES 1   *tuberculous erythema nodosum (A18.4)*
     DEF: Form of panniculitis (inflammation of the fat layer beneath the skin) most often occurring in women. Commonly seen as a hypersensitivity reaction to infections, drugs, sarcoidosis, and specific enteropathies. The acute stage is associated with fever, malaise, and arthralgia. The lesions are pink to blue in color as tender nodules and are found on the front of the legs below the knees.

✓4ᵗʰ **L53 Other erythematous conditions**
     EXCLUDES 1   *erythema ab igne (L59.0)*
           erythema due to external agents in contact with skin (L23-L25)
           erythema intertrigo (L30.4)

     L53.0 Toxic erythema
       Code first poisoning due to drug or toxin, if applicable (T36-T65 with fifth or sixth character 1-4 or 6)
       Use additional code for adverse effect, if applicable, to identify drug (T36-T50 with fifth or sixth character 5)
       EXCLUDES 1   *neonatal erythema toxicum (P83.1)*

     L53.1 Erythema annulare centrifugum

     L53.2 Erythema marginatum

     L53.3 Other chronic figurate erythema

     L53.8 Other specified erythematous conditions

     L53.9 Erythematous condition, unspecified
       Erythema NOS
       Erythroderma NOS

L54 Erythema in diseases classified elsewhere
     Code first underlying disease

Radiation-related disorders of the skin and subcutaneous tissue (L55-L59)

✓4ᵗʰ **L55 Sunburn**
     L55.0 Sunburn of first degree
     L55.1 Sunburn of second degree
     L55.2 Sunburn of third degree
     L55.9 Sunburn, unspecified

N Newborn: 0   P Pediatric: 0-17   M Maternity: 12-55   A Adult: 15-124   CH Comorbidity High   CL Comorbidity Low   NCDx Noncancer Dx   PDx Primary Dx

724   ICD-10-CM 2020

✓4ᵗʰ **L56 Other acute skin changes due to ultraviolet radiation**

Use additional code to identify the source of the ultraviolet radiation (W89, X32)

L56.0 Drug phototoxic response

Use additional code for adverse effect, if applicable, to identify drug (T36-T50 with fifth or sixth character 5)

L56.1 Drug photoallergic response

Use additional code for adverse effect, if applicable, to identify drug (T36-T50 with fifth or sixth character 5)

L56.2 Photocontact dermatitis [berloque dermatitis]

L56.3 Solar urticaria

L56.4 Polymorphous light eruption

L56.5 Disseminated superficial actinic porokeratosis (DSAP)

DEF: Autosomal dominant skin condition occurring in sun-exposed areas of the skin (particularly the arms and legs), characterized by superficial annular, keratotic, brownish-red spots or thickenings with depressed centers and sharp, ridged borders. It may evolve into squamous cell carcinoma.

L56.8 Other specified acute skin changes due to ultraviolet radiation

L56.9 Acute skin change due to ultraviolet radiation, unspecified

✓4ᵗʰ **L57 Skin changes due to chronic exposure to nonionizing radiation**

Use additional code to identify the source of the ultraviolet radiation (W89)

L57.0 Actinic keratosis

Keratosis NOS
Senile keratosis
Solar keratosis

L57.1 Actinic reticuloid

L57.2 Cutis rhomboidalis nuchae

L57.3 Poikiloderma of Civatte

L57.4 Cutis laxa senilis

Elastosis senilis

L57.5 Actinic granuloma

L57.8 Other skin changes due to chronic exposure to nonionizing radiation

Farmer's skin
Sailor's skin
Solar dermatitis

L57.9 Skin changes due to chronic exposure to nonionizing radiation, unspecified

✓4ᵗʰ **L58 Radiodermatitis**

Use additional code to identify the source of the radiation (W88, W90)

L58.0 Acute radiodermatitis

L58.1 Chronic radiodermatitis

L58.9 Radiodermatitis, unspecified

✓4ᵗʰ **L59 Other disorders of skin and subcutaneous tissue related to radiation**

L59.0 Erythema ab igne [dermatitis ab igne]

L59.8 Other specified disorders of the skin and subcutaneous tissue related to radiation

AHA: 2017,1Q,33

L59.9 Disorder of the skin and subcutaneous tissue related to radiation, unspecified

Disorders of skin appendages (L60-L75)

EXCLUDES 1   *congenital malformations of integument (Q84.-)*

✓4ᵗʰ **L60 Nail disorders**

EXCLUDES 2   *clubbing of nails (R68.3)*
                onychia and paronychia (L03.0-)

Nail Disorders

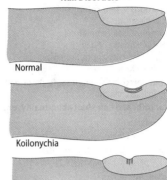

Normal

Koilonychia

Beau's Lines

L60.0 Ingrowing nail

L60.1 Onycholysis

L60.2 Onychogryphosis

L60.3 Nail dystrophy

L60.4 Beau's lines

L60.5 Yellow nail syndrome

L60.8 Other nail disorders

L60.9 Nail disorder, unspecified

L62 Nail disorders in diseases classified elsewhere

Code first underlying disease, such as:
pachydermoperiostosis (M89.4-)

✓4ᵗʰ **L63 Alopecia areata**

L63.0 Alopecia (capitis) totalis

L63.1 Alopecia universalis

L63.2 Ophiasis

L63.8 Other alopecia areata

L63.9 Alopecia areata, unspecified

✓4ᵗʰ **L64 Androgenic alopecia**

INCLUDES   male-pattern baldness

L64.0 Drug-induced androgenic alopecia

Use additional code for adverse effect, if applicable, to identify drug (T36-T50 with fifth or sixth character 5)

L64.8 Other androgenic alopecia

L64.9 Androgenic alopecia, unspecified

✓4ᵗʰ **L65 Other nonscarring hair loss**

Use additional code for adverse effect, if applicable, to identify drug (T36-T50 with fifth or sixth character 5)

EXCLUDES 1   *trichotillomania (F63.3)*

L65.0 Telogen effluvium

DEF: Form of nonscarring alopecia characterized by shedding of hair from premature telogen development in follicles due to stress, including shock, childbirth, surgery, drugs, or weight loss.

L65.1 Anagen effluvium

L65.2 Alopecia mucinosa

L65.8 Other specified nonscarring hair loss

L65.9 Nonscarring hair loss, unspecified

Alopecia NOS

✓4ᵗʰ **L66 Cicatricial alopecia [scarring hair loss]**

L66.0 Pseudopelade

L66.1 Lichen planopilaris

Follicular lichen planus

L66.2 Folliculitis decalvans

L66.3 Perifolliculitis capitis abscedens

L66.4 Folliculitis ulerythematosa reticulata

✔ Additional Character Required   ✓x7ᵗʰ Placeholder Alert   Manifestation   Unspecified Dx   ▶◀ Revised Text   ● New Code   ▲ Revised Title

ICD-10-CM 2020   725

L66.8   **Other cicatricial alopecia**
    AHA: 2015,1Q,19

L66.9   **Cicatricial alopecia, unspecified**

✓4ᵗʰ **L67**   **Hair color and hair shaft abnormalities**
    EXCLUDES 1   *monilethrix (Q84.1)*
       pili annulati (Q84.1)
       telogen effluvium (L65.0)

L67.0   **Trichorrhexis nodosa**

L67.1   **Variations in hair color**
    Canities
    Greyness, hair (premature)
    Heterochromia of hair
    Poliosis circumscripta, acquired
    Poliosis NOS

L67.8   **Other hair color and hair shaft abnormalities**
    Fragilitas crinium

L67.9   **Hair color and hair shaft abnormality, unspecified**

✓4ᵗʰ **L68**   **Hypertrichosis**
    INCLUDES   excess hair
    EXCLUDES 1   *congenital hypertrichosis (Q84.2)*
       persistent lanugo (Q84.2)

L68.0   **Hirsutism**

L68.1   **Acquired hypertrichosis lanuginosa**

L68.2   **Localized hypertrichosis**

L68.3   **Polytrichia**

L68.8   **Other hypertrichosis**

L68.9   **Hypertrichosis, unspecified**

✓4ᵗʰ **L70**   **Acne**
    EXCLUDES 2   *acne keloid (L73.0)*

L70.0   **Acne** vulgaris

L70.1   **Acne** conglobata

L70.2   **Acne** varioliformis
    Acne necrotica miliaris
    DEF: Rare form of acne characterized by development of persistent brown papulopustules followed by scar formation. This type of acne usually presents on the brow and temporoparietal part of the scalp.

L70.3   **Acne** tropica

L70.4   Infantile **acne**   P

L70.5   Acné excoriée
    Acné excoriée des jeunes filles
    Picker's acne

L70.8   **Other acne**

L70.9   **Acne, unspecified**

✓4ᵗʰ **L71**   **Rosacea**
    Use additional code for adverse effect, if applicable, to identify drug (T36-T50 with fifth or sixth character 5)

L71.0   **Perioral dermatitis**

L71.1   **Rhinophyma**

L71.8   **Other rosacea**
    AHA: 2018,4Q,15

L71.9   **Rosacea, unspecified**

✓4ᵗʰ **L72**   **Follicular cysts of skin and subcutaneous tissue**

L72.0   **Epidermal cyst**

✓5ᵗʰ **L72.1**   **Pilar and trichodermal cyst**

    L72.11   **Pilar cyst**

    L72.12   **Trichodermal cyst**
       Trichilemmal (proliferating) cyst

L72.2   **Steatocystoma multiplex**

L72.3   **Sebaceous cyst**
    EXCLUDES 2   *pilar cyst (L72.11)*
       trichilemmal (proliferating) cyst (L72.12)

L72.8   **Other follicular cysts of the skin and subcutaneous tissue**

L72.9   **Follicular cyst of the skin and subcutaneous tissue, unspecified**

✓4ᵗʰ **L73**   **Other follicular disorders**

L73.0   **Acne keloid**

L73.1   **Pseudofolliculitis barbae**

L73.2   **Hidradenitis suppurativa**

L73.8   **Other specified follicular disorders**
    Sycosis barbae

L73.9   **Follicular disorder, unspecified**

✓4ᵗʰ **L74**   **Eccrine sweat disorders**
    EXCLUDES 2   *generalized hyperhidrosis (R61)*
    DEF: Eccrine sweat glands: Glands found in the dermal and hypodermal layer of the skin throughout the body, particularly on the forehead, scalp, axillae, palms, and soles. These glands produce watery and neutral or slightly acidic sweat.

L74.0   **Miliaria** rubra

L74.1   **Miliaria** crystallina

L74.2   **Miliaria** profunda
    Miliaria tropicalis

L74.3   **Miliaria, unspecified**

L74.4   **Anhidrosis**
    Hypohidrosis
    DEF: Inability to sweat normally. When the body can't cool itself through perspiration it can lead to heatstroke, a life-threatening condition.

✓5ᵗʰ **L74.5**   **Focal hyperhidrosis**

✓6ᵗʰ **L74.51**   Primary **focal hyperhidrosis**

      L74.510   **Primary focal hyperhidrosis,** axilla
      L74.511   **Primary focal hyperhidrosis,** face
      L74.512   **Primary focal hyperhidrosis,** palms
      L74.513   **Primary focal hyperhidrosis,** soles
      L74.519   **Primary focal hyperhidrosis, unspecified**

    L74.52   Secondary **focal hyperhidrosis**
       Frey's syndrome

L74.8   **Other eccrine sweat disorders**

L74.9   **Eccrine sweat disorder, unspecified**
    Sweat gland disorder NOS

✓4ᵗʰ **L75**   **Apocrine sweat disorders**
    EXCLUDES 1   *dyshidrosis (L30.1)*
       hidradenitis suppurativa (L73.2)
    DEF: Apocrine sweat glands: Found in the axilla, areola, and circumanal region, these glands begin to function in puberty and produce viscid milky secretions in response to external stimuli.

L75.0   **Bromhidrosis**

L75.1   **Chromhidrosis**

L75.2   **Apocrine miliaria**
    Fox-Fordyce disease
    DEF: Chronic, usually pruritic disease evidenced by small follicular papular eruptions, especially in the axillary and pubic areas. Apocrine miliaria develops from the closure and rupture of the affected apocrine glands' intraepidermal portion of the ducts.

L75.8   **Other apocrine sweat disorders**

L75.9   **Apocrine sweat disorder, unspecified**

Intraoperative and postprocedural complications of skin and subcutaneous tissue (L76)

✓4ᵗʰ **L76**   **Intraoperative and postprocedural complications of skin and subcutaneous tissue**
    AHA: 2016,4Q,9-10

✓5ᵗʰ **L76.0**   Intraoperative hemorrhage and hematoma of skin and subcutaneous tissue complicating a procedure
    EXCLUDES 1   *intraoperative hemorrhage and hematoma of skin and subcutaneous tissue due to accidental puncture and laceration during a procedure (L76.1-)*

    L76.01   **Intraoperative hemorrhage and hematoma of skin and subcutaneous tissue complicating a** dermatologic procedure

    L76.02   **Intraoperative hemorrhage and hematoma of skin and subcutaneous tissue complicating** other procedure

✓5ᵗʰ **L76.1**   Accidental puncture and laceration of skin and subcutaneous tissue during a procedure

    L76.11   **Accidental puncture and laceration of skin and subcutaneous tissue during a** dermatologic procedure

    L76.12   **Accidental puncture and laceration of skin and subcutaneous tissue during** other procedure

✓5ᵗʰ **L76.2**   Postprocedural hemorrhage of skin and subcutaneous tissue following a procedure

    L76.21   **Postprocedural hemorrhage of skin and subcutaneous tissue following a** dermatologic procedure

    L76.22   **Postprocedural hemorrhage of skin and subcutaneous tissue following** other procedure

√5ᵗʰ **L76.3** Postprocedural hematoma and seroma of skin and subcutaneous tissue following a procedure

     L76.31 Postprocedural hematoma of skin and subcutaneous tissue following a dermatologic procedure

     L76.32 Postprocedural hematoma of skin and subcutaneous tissue following other procedure

     L76.33 Postprocedural seroma of skin and subcutaneous tissue following a dermatologic procedure

     L76.34 Postprocedural seroma of skin and subcutaneous tissue following other procedure

√5ᵗʰ **L76.8** Other intraoperative and postprocedural complications of skin and subcutaneous tissue

     Use additional code, if applicable, to further specify disorder

     L76.81 Other intraoperative complications of skin and subcutaneous tissue

     L76.82 Other postprocedural complications of skin and subcutaneous tissue

         AHA: 2017,3Q,6

Other disorders of the skin and subcutaneous tissue (L80-L99)

L80 Vitiligo

     EXCLUDES 2   vitiligo of eyelids (H02.73-)

                     vitiligo of vulva (N90.89)

     DEF: Persistent, progressive development of nonpigmented white patches on otherwise normal skin.

√4ᵗʰ **L81 Other disorders of pigmentation**

     EXCLUDES 1   birthmark NOS (Q82.5)

                     Peutz-Jeghers syndrome (Q85.8)

     EXCLUDES 2   nevus — see Alphabetical Index

     L81.0 Postinflammatory hyperpigmentation

     L81.1 Chloasma

     L81.2 Freckles

     L81.3 Café au lait spots

     L81.4 Other melanin hyperpigmentation

         Lentigo

     L81.5 Leukoderma, not elsewhere classified

     L81.6 Other disorders of diminished melanin formation

     L81.7 Pigmented purpuric dermatosis

         Angioma serpiginosum

     L81.8 Other specified disorders of pigmentation

         Iron pigmentation

         Tattoo pigmentation

     L81.9 Disorder of pigmentation, unspecified

√4ᵗʰ **L82 Seborrheic keratosis**

     INCLUDES   basal cell papilloma

                 dermatosis papulosa nigra

                 Leser-Trélat disease

     EXCLUDES 2   seborrheic dermatitis (L21.-)

     DEF: Common, benign, noninvasive, lightly pigmented, warty growth composed of basaloid cells that usually appear at middle age as soft, easily crumbling plaques on the face, trunk, and extremities.

     L82.0 Inflamed seborrheic keratosis

     L82.1 Other seborrheic keratosis

         Seborrheic keratosis NOS

L83 Acanthosis nigricans

     Confluent and reticulated papillomatosis

     DEF: Diffuse, velvety hyperplasia of the spinous skin layer of the axilla and other body folds marked by gray, brown, or black pigmentation. In adult form, it is often associated with malignant acanthosis nigricans in a benign, nevoid form relatively generalized.

L84 Corns and callosities

     Callus

     Clavus

√4ᵗʰ **L85 Other epidermal thickening**

     EXCLUDES 2   hypertrophic disorders of the skin (L91.-)

     L85.0 Acquired ichthyosis

         EXCLUDES 1   congenital ichthyosis (Q80.-)

     L85.1 Acquired keratosis [keratoderma] palmaris et plantaris

         EXCLUDES 1   inherited keratosis palmaris et plantaris (Q82.8)

     L85.2 Keratosis punctata (palmaris et plantaris)

     L85.3 Xerosis cutis

         Dry skin dermatitis

     L85.8 Other specified epidermal thickening

         Cutaneous horn

     L85.9 Epidermal thickening, unspecified

L86 Keratoderma in diseases classified elsewhere

     Code first underlying disease, such as:

     Reiter's disease (M02.3-)

     EXCLUDES 1   gonococcal keratoderma (A54.89)

                     gonococcal keratosis (A54.89)

                     keratoderma due to vitamin A deficiency (E50.8)

                     keratosis due to vitamin A deficiency (E50.8)

                     xeroderma due to vitamin A deficiency (E50.8)

√4ᵗʰ **L87 Transepidermal elimination disorders**

     EXCLUDES 1   granuloma annulare (perforating) (L92.0)

     L87.0 Keratosis follicularis et parafollicularis in cutem penetrans

         Hyperkeratosis follicularis penetrans

         Kyrle disease

     L87.1 Reactive perforating collagenosis

     L87.2 Elastosis perforans serpiginosa

     L87.8 Other transepidermal elimination disorders

     L87.9 Transepidermal elimination disorder, unspecified

L88 Pyoderma gangrenosum

     Phagedenic pyoderma

     EXCLUDES 1   dermatitis gangrenosa (L08.0)

     DEF: Persistent debilitating skin disease characterized by irregular, boggy, blue-red ulcerations, with central healing and undermined edges.

√4ᵗʰ **L89 Pressure ulcer**

     INCLUDES   bed sore

                 decubitus ulcer

                 plaster ulcer

                 pressure area

                 pressure sore

     Code first any associated gangrene (I96)

     EXCLUDES 2   decubitus (trophic) ulcer of cervix (uteri) (N86)

                     diabetic ulcers (E08.621, E08.622, E09.621, E09.622, E10.621, E10.622, E11.621, E11.622, E13.621, E13.622)

                     non-pressure chronic ulcer of skin (L97.-)

                     skin infections (L00-L08)

                     varicose ulcer (I83.0, I83.2)

     AHA: 2018,4Q,69; 2018,3Q,3; 2018,2Q,21; 2017,4Q,109; 2017,1Q,49; 2016,4Q,143

     TIP: Ulcers documented as Kennedy ulcers are coded in this category with the appropriate code for site and stage specificity. Kennedy ulcer is a rapidly developing ulcer occurring in terminally ill patients due to multi-organ failure and not typically responsive to treatment.

     TIP: ICD-10-CM guideline I.C.12.a.6 regarding evolving pressure ulcer stages applies to inpatient encounters and is not applicable to home health services.

Four Stages of Pressure Ulcer

Stage 1
Persistent focal edema

Stage 2
Abrasion, blister, partial thickness skin loss involving epidermis and/or dermis

Stage 3
Full thickness skin loss involving damage or necrosis of subcutaneous tissue

Stage 4
Necrosis of soft tissues through to underlying muscle, tendon, or bone

√5ᵗʰ **L89.0** Pressure ulcer of elbow

     √6ᵗʰ **L89.00** Pressure ulcer of unspecified elbow

         L89.000 Pressure ulcer of unspecified elbow, unstageable

☑ Additional Character Required   √x7ᵗʰ Placeholder Alert   Manifestation   Unspecified Dx   ▶◀ Revised Text   ● New Code   ▲ Revised Title

ICD-10-CM 2020   **727**

Chapter 12. Diseases of the Skin and Subcutaneous Tissue

L89.001 Pressure ulcer of unspecified elbow, stage 1

Healing pressure ulcer of unspecified elbow, stage 1

Pressure pre-ulcer skin changes limited to persistent focal edema, unspecified elbow

L89.002 Pressure ulcer of unspecified elbow, stage 2

Healing pressure ulcer of unspecified elbow, stage 2

Pressure ulcer with abrasion, blister, partial thickness skin loss involving epidermis and/or dermis, unspecified elbow

L89.003 Pressure ulcer of unspecified elbow, stage 3

Healing pressure ulcer of unspecified elbow, stage 3

Pressure ulcer with full thickness skin loss involving damage or necrosis of subcutaneous tissue, unspecified elbow

L89.004 Pressure ulcer of unspecified elbow, stage 4

Healing pressure ulcer of unspecified elbow, stage 4

Pressure ulcer with necrosis of soft tissues through to underlying muscle, tendon, or bone, unspecified elbow

L89.006 Pressure-induced deep tissue damage of unspecified elbow

L89.009 Pressure ulcer of unspecified elbow, unspecified stage

Healing pressure ulcer of elbow NOS

Healing pressure ulcer of unspecified elbow, unspecified stage

√6ᵗʰ **L89.01 Pressure ulcer of right elbow**

L89.010 Pressure ulcer of right elbow, unstageable `CH` `CL`

L89.011 Pressure ulcer of right elbow, stage 1

Healing pressure ulcer of right elbow, stage 1

Pressure pre-ulcer skin changes limited to persistent focal edema, right elbow

L89.012 Pressure ulcer of right elbow, stage 2 `CH` `CL`

Healing pressure ulcer of right elbow, stage 2

Pressure ulcer with abrasion, blister, partial thickness skin loss involving epidermis and/or dermis, right elbow

L89.013 Pressure ulcer of right elbow, stage 3 `CH` `CL`

Healing pressure ulcer of right elbow, stage 3

Pressure ulcer with full thickness skin loss involving damage or necrosis of subcutaneous tissue, right elbow

L89.014 Pressure ulcer of right elbow, stage 4 `CH` `CL`

Healing pressure ulcer of right elbow, stage 4

Pressure ulcer with necrosis of soft tissues through to underlying muscle, tendon, or bone, right elbow

L89.016 Pressure-induced deep tissue damage of right elbow

L89.019 Pressure ulcer of right elbow, unspecified stage

Healing pressure right of elbow NOS

Healing pressure ulcer of right elbow, unspecified stage

√6ᵗʰ **L89.02 Pressure ulcer of left elbow**

L89.020 Pressure ulcer of left elbow, unstageable

L89.021 Pressure ulcer of left elbow, stage 1

Healing pressure ulcer of left elbow, stage 1

Pressure pre-ulcer skin changes limited to persistent focal edema, left elbow

L89.022 Pressure ulcer of left elbow, stage 2 `CH` `CL`

Healing pressure ulcer of left elbow, stage 2

Pressure ulcer with abrasion, blister, partial thickness skin loss involving epidermis and/or dermis, left elbow

L89.023 Pressure ulcer of left elbow, stage 3 `CH` `CL`

Healing pressure ulcer of left elbow, stage 3

Pressure ulcer with full thickness skin loss involving damage or necrosis of subcutaneous tissue, left elbow

L89.024 Pressure ulcer of left elbow, stage 4 `CH` `CL`

Healing pressure ulcer of left elbow, stage 4

Pressure ulcer with necrosis of soft tissues through to underlying muscle, tendon, or bone, left elbow

L89.026 Pressure-induced deep tissue damage of left elbow

L89.029 Pressure ulcer of left elbow, unspecified stage

Healing pressure ulcer of left of elbow NOS

Healing pressure ulcer of left elbow, unspecified stage

√5ᵗʰ **L89.1 Pressure ulcer of back**

√6ᵗʰ **L89.10 Pressure ulcer of unspecified part of back**

L89.100 Pressure ulcer of unspecified part of back, unstageable

L89.101 Pressure ulcer of unspecified part of back, stage 1

Healing pressure ulcer of unspecified part of back, stage 1

Pressure pre-ulcer skin changes limited to persistent focal edema, unspecified part of back

L89.102 Pressure ulcer of unspecified part of back, stage 2 `CH` `CL`

Healing pressure ulcer of unspecified part of back, stage 2

Pressure ulcer with abrasion, blister, partial thickness skin loss involving epidermis and/or dermis, unspecified part of back

L89.103 Pressure ulcer of unspecified part of back, stage 3 `CH` `CL`

Healing pressure ulcer of unspecified part of back, stage 3

Pressure ulcer with full thickness skin loss involving damage or necrosis of subcutaneous tissue, unspecified part of back

L89.104 Pressure ulcer of unspecified part of back, stage 4 `CH` `CL`

Healing pressure ulcer of unspecified part of back, stage 4

Pressure ulcer with necrosis of soft tissues through to underlying muscle, tendon, or bone, unspecified part of back

L89.106 Pressure-induced deep tissue damage of unspecified part of back

L89.109 Pressure ulcer of unspecified part of back, unspecified stage

Healing pressure ulcer of unspecified part of back NOS

Healing pressure ulcer of unspecified part of back, unspecified stage

---

N Newborn: 0   P Pediatric: 0-17   M Maternity: 12-55   A Adult: 15-124   CH Comorbidity High   CL Comorbidity Low   NCDx Noncancer Dx   PDx Primary Dx

728   ICD-10-CM 2020

✓6ᵗʰ **L89.11** **Pressure ulcer of** right upper **back**
- Pressure ulcer of right shoulder blade

L89.11Ø **Pressure ulcer of right upper** `CH` `CL`
back, unstageable

L89.111 **Pressure ulcer of right upper back,** stage 1
- Healing pressure ulcer of right upper back, stage 1
- Pressure pre-ulcer skin changes limited to persistent focal edema, right upper back

L89.112 **Pressure ulcer of right upper** `CH` `CL`
back, stage 2
- Healing pressure ulcer of right upper back, stage 2
- Pressure ulcer with abrasion, blister, partial thickness skin loss involving epidermis and/or dermis, right upper back

L89.113 **Pressure ulcer of right upper** `CH` `CL`
back, stage 3
- Healing pressure ulcer of right upper back, stage 3
- Pressure ulcer with full thickness skin loss involving damage or necrosis of subcutaneous tissue, right upper back

L89.114 **Pressure ulcer of right upper** `CH` `CL`
back, stage 4
- Healing pressure ulcer of right upper back, stage 4
- Pressure ulcer with necrosis of soft tissues through to underlying muscle, tendon, or bone, right upper back

● **L89.116** **Pressure-induced** deep tissue damage **of right upper back**

L89.119 **Pressure ulcer of right upper back, unspecified stage**
- Healing pressure ulcer of right upper back NOS
- Healing pressure ulcer of right upper back, unspecified stage

✓6ᵗʰ **L89.12** **Pressure ulcer of** left upper **back**
- Pressure ulcer of left shoulder blade

L89.12Ø **Pressure ulcer of left upper** `CH` `CL`
back, unstageable

L89.121 **Pressure ulcer of left upper back,** stage 1
- Healing pressure ulcer of left upper back, stage 1
- Pressure pre-ulcer skin changes limited to persistent focal edema, left upper back

L89.122 **Pressure ulcer of left upper** `CH` `CL`
back, stage 2
- Healing pressure ulcer of left upper back, stage 2
- Pressure ulcer with abrasion, blister, partial thickness skin loss involving epidermis and/or dermis, left upper back

L89.123 **Pressure ulcer of left upper** `CH` `CL`
back, stage 3
- Healing pressure ulcer of left upper back, stage 3
- Pressure ulcer with full thickness skin loss involving damage or necrosis of subcutaneous tissue, left upper back

L89.124 **Pressure ulcer of left upper** `CH` `CL`
back, stage 4
- Healing pressure ulcer of left upper back, stage 4
- Pressure ulcer with necrosis of soft tissues through to underlying muscle, tendon, or bone, left upper back

● **L89.126** **Pressure-induced** deep tissue damage **of left upper back**

L89.129 **Pressure ulcer of left upper back, unspecified stage**
- Healing pressure ulcer of left upper back NOS
- Healing pressure ulcer of left upper back, unspecified stage

✓6ᵗʰ **L89.13** **Pressure ulcer of** right lower **back**

L89.13Ø **Pressure ulcer of right lower** `CH` `CL`
back, unstageable

L89.131 **Pressure ulcer of right lower back,** stage 1
- Healing pressure ulcer of right lower back, stage 1
- Pressure pre-ulcer skin changes limited to persistent focal edema, right lower back

L89.132 **Pressure ulcer of right lower** `CH` `CL`
back, stage 2
- Healing pressure ulcer of right lower back, stage 2
- Pressure ulcer with abrasion, blister, partial thickness skin loss involving epidermis and/or dermis, right lower back

L89.133 **Pressure ulcer of right lower** `CH` `CL`
back, stage 3
- Healing pressure ulcer of right lower back, stage 3
- Pressure ulcer with full thickness skin loss involving damage or necrosis of subcutaneous tissue, right lower back

L89.134 **Pressure ulcer of right lower** `CH` `CL`
back, stage 4
- Healing pressure ulcer of right lower back, stage 4
- Pressure ulcer with necrosis of soft tissues through to underlying muscle, tendon, or bone, right lower back

● **L89.136** **Pressure-induced** deep tissue damage **of right lower back**

L89.139 **Pressure ulcer of right lower back, unspecified stage**
- Healing pressure ulcer of right lower back NOS
- Healing pressure ulcer of right lower back, unspecified stage

✓6ᵗʰ **L89.14** **Pressure ulcer of** left lower **back**

L89.14Ø **Pressure ulcer of left lower** `CH` `CL`
back, unstageable

L89.141 **Pressure ulcer of left lower back,** stage 1
- Healing pressure ulcer of left lower back, stage 1
- Pressure pre-ulcer skin changes limited to persistent focal edema, left lower back

L89.142 **Pressure ulcer of left lower** `CH` `CL`
back, stage 2
- Healing pressure ulcer of left lower back, stage 2
- Pressure ulcer with abrasion, blister, partial thickness skin loss involving epidermis and/or dermis, left lower back

L89.143 **Pressure ulcer of left lower** `CH` `CL`
back, stage 3
- Healing pressure ulcer of left lower back, stage 3
- Pressure ulcer with full thickness skin loss involving damage or necrosis of subcutaneous tissue, left lower back

L89.144 **Pressure ulcer of left lower** `CH` `CL`
back, stage 4
- Healing pressure ulcer of left lower back, stage 4
- Pressure ulcer with necrosis of soft tissues through to underlying muscle, tendon, or bone, left lower back

● **L89.146** **Pressure-induced** deep tissue damage **of left lower back**

☑ Additional Character Required   ✓ₓ7ᵗʰ Placeholder Alert   Manifestation   Unspecified Dx   ►◄ Revised Text   ● New Code   ▲ Revised Title

ICD-10-CM 2020   729

L89.149 Pressure ulcer of left lower back, unspecified stage
Healing pressure ulcer of left lower back NOS
Healing pressure ulcer of left lower back, unspecified stage

✓6ᵗʰ **L89.15 Pressure ulcer of sacral region**
Pressure ulcer of coccyx
Pressure ulcer of tailbone

L89.150 Pressure ulcer of sacral CH CL **region, unstageable**

L89.151 Pressure ulcer of sacral region, stage 1
Healing pressure ulcer of sacral region, stage 1
Pressure pre-ulcer skin changes limited to persistent focal edema, sacral region

L89.152 Pressure ulcer of sacral CH CL **region, stage 2**
Healing pressure ulcer of sacral region, stage 2
Pressure ulcer with abrasion, blister, partial thickness skin loss involving epidermis and/or dermis, sacral region

L89.153 Pressure ulcer of sacral CH CL **region, stage 3**
Healing pressure ulcer of sacral region, stage 3
Pressure ulcer with full thickness skin loss involving damage or necrosis of subcutaneous tissue, sacral region

L89.154 Pressure ulcer of sacral CH CL **region, stage 4**
Healing pressure ulcer of sacral region, stage 4
Pressure ulcer with necrosis of soft tissues through to underlying muscle, tendon, or bone, sacral region

● **L89.156 Pressure-induced deep tissue damage of sacral region**

L89.159 Pressure ulcer of sacral region, unspecified stage
Healing pressure ulcer of sacral region NOS
Healing pressure ulcer of sacral region, unspecified stage

✓5ᵗʰ **L89.2 Pressure ulcer of hip**

✓6ᵗʰ **L89.20 Pressure ulcer of unspecified hip**

L89.200 Pressure ulcer of unspecified hip, unstageable

L89.201 Pressure ulcer of unspecified hip, stage 1
Healing pressure ulcer of unspecified hip back, stage 1
Pressure pre-ulcer skin changes limited to persistent focal edema, unspecified hip

L89.202 Pressure ulcer of unspecified hip, stage 2
Healing pressure ulcer of unspecified hip, stage 2
Pressure ulcer with abrasion, blister, partial thickness skin loss involving epidermis and/or dermis, unspecified hip

L89.203 Pressure ulcer of unspecified hip, stage 3
Healing pressure ulcer of unspecified hip, stage 3
Pressure ulcer with full thickness skin loss involving damage or necrosis of subcutaneous tissue, unspecified hip

L89.204 Pressure ulcer of unspecified hip, stage 4
Healing pressure ulcer of unspecified hip, stage 4
Pressure ulcer with necrosis of soft tissues through to underlying muscle, tendon, or bone, unspecified hip

● **L89.206 Pressure-induced deep tissue damage of unspecified hip**

L89.209 Pressure ulcer of unspecified hip, unspecified stage
Healing pressure ulcer of unspecified hip NOS
Healing pressure ulcer of unspecified hip, unspecified stage

✓6ᵗʰ **L89.21 Pressure ulcer of right hip**

L89.210 Pressure ulcer of right hip, CH CL **unstageable**

L89.211 Pressure ulcer of right hip, stage 1
Healing pressure ulcer of right hip back, stage 1
Pressure pre-ulcer skin changes limited to persistent focal edema, right hip

L89.212 Pressure ulcer of right hip, CH CL **stage 2**
Healing pressure ulcer of right hip, stage 2
Pressure ulcer with abrasion, blister, partial thickness skin loss involving epidermis and/or dermis, right hip

L89.213 Pressure ulcer of right hip, CH CL **stage 3**
Healing pressure ulcer of right hip, stage 3
Pressure ulcer with full thickness skin loss involving damage or necrosis of subcutaneous tissue, right hip

L89.214 Pressure ulcer of right hip, CH CL **stage 4**
Healing pressure ulcer of right hip, stage 4
Pressure ulcer with necrosis of soft tissues through to underlying muscle, tendon, or bone, right hip

● **L89.216 Pressure-induced deep tissue damage of right hip**

L89.219 Pressure ulcer of right hip, unspecified stage
Healing pressure ulcer of right hip NOS
Healing pressure ulcer of right hip, unspecified stage

✓6ᵗʰ **L89.22 Pressure ulcer of left hip**

L89.220 Pressure ulcer of left hip, CH CL **unstageable**

L89.221 Pressure ulcer of left hip, stage 1
Healing pressure ulcer of left hip back, stage 1
Pressure pre-ulcer skin changes limited to persistent focal edema, left hip

L89.222 Pressure ulcer of left hip, CH CL **stage 2**
Healing pressure ulcer of left hip, stage 2
Pressure ulcer with abrasion, blister, partial thickness skin loss involving epidermis and/or dermis, left hip

L89.223 Pressure ulcer of left hip, CH CL **stage 3**
Healing pressure ulcer of left hip, stage 3
Pressure ulcer with full thickness skin loss involving damage or necrosis of subcutaneous tissue, left hip

L89.224 Pressure ulcer of left hip, CH CL **stage 4**
Healing pressure ulcer of left hip, stage 4
Pressure ulcer with necrosis of soft tissues through to underlying muscle, tendon, or bone, left hip

● **L89.226 Pressure-induced deep tissue damage of left hip**

L89.229 Pressure ulcer of left hip, unspecified stage
Healing pressure ulcer of left hip NOS
Healing pressure ulcer of left hip, unspecified stage

✓5ᵗʰ **L89.3 Pressure ulcer of buttock**

✓6ᵗʰ **L89.30 Pressure ulcer of unspecified buttock**

L89.300 Pressure ulcer of unspecified buttock, unstageable

L89.301 Pressure ulcer of unspecified buttock, stage 1
Healing pressure ulcer of unspecified buttock, stage 1
Pressure pre-ulcer skin changes limited to persistent focal edema, unspecified buttock

L89.302 Pressure ulcer of unspecified buttock, stage 2
Healing pressure ulcer of unspecified buttock, stage 2
Pressure ulcer with abrasion, blister, partial thickness skin loss involving epidermis and/or dermis, unspecified buttock

L89.303 Pressure ulcer of unspecified buttock, stage 3
Healing pressure ulcer of unspecified buttock, stage 3
Pressure ulcer with full thickness skin loss involving damage or necrosis of subcutaneous tissue, unspecified buttock

L89.304 Pressure ulcer of unspecified buttock, stage 4
Healing pressure ulcer of unspecified buttock, stage 4
Pressure ulcer with necrosis of soft tissues through to underlying muscle, tendon, or bone, unspecified buttock

L89.306 Pressure-induced deep tissue damage of unspecified buttock

L89.309 Pressure ulcer of unspecified buttock, unspecified stage
Healing pressure ulcer of unspecified buttock NOS
Healing pressure ulcer of unspecified buttock, unspecified stage

√6ᵗʰ **L89.31 Pressure ulcer of right buttock**

L89.310 Pressure ulcer of right buttock, unstageable CH CL

L89.311 Pressure ulcer of right buttock, stage 1
Healing pressure ulcer of right buttock, stage 1
Pressure pre-ulcer skin changes limited to persistent focal edema, right buttock

L89.312 Pressure ulcer of right buttock, stage 2 CH CL
Healing pressure ulcer of right buttock, stage 2
Pressure ulcer with abrasion, blister, partial thickness skin loss involving epidermis and/or dermis, right buttock

L89.313 Pressure ulcer of right buttock, stage 3 CH CL
Healing pressure ulcer of right buttock, stage 3
Pressure ulcer with full thickness skin loss involving damage or necrosis of subcutaneous tissue, right buttock

L89.314 Pressure ulcer of right buttock, stage 4 CH CL
Healing pressure ulcer of right buttock, stage 4
Pressure ulcer with necrosis of soft tissues through to underlying muscle, tendon, or bone, right buttock

L89.316 Pressure-induced deep tissue damage of right buttock

L89.319 Pressure ulcer of right buttock, unspecified stage
Healing pressure ulcer of right buttock NOS
Healing pressure ulcer of right buttock, unspecified stage

√6ᵗʰ **L89.32 Pressure ulcer of left buttock**

L89.320 Pressure ulcer of left buttock, unstageable CH CL

L89.321 Pressure ulcer of left buttock, stage 1
Healing pressure ulcer of left buttock, stage 1
Pressure pre-ulcer skin changes limited to persistent focal edema, left buttock

L89.322 Pressure ulcer of left buttock, stage 2 CH CL
Healing pressure ulcer of left buttock, stage 2
Pressure ulcer with abrasion, blister, partial thickness skin loss involving epidermis and/or dermis, left buttock

L89.323 Pressure ulcer of left buttock, stage 3 CH CL
Healing pressure ulcer of left buttock, stage 3
Pressure ulcer with full thickness skin loss involving damage or necrosis of subcutaneous tissue, left buttock

L89.324 Pressure ulcer of left buttock, stage 4 CH CL
Healing pressure ulcer of left buttock, stage 4
Pressure ulcer with necrosis of soft tissues through to underlying muscle, tendon, or bone, left buttock

L89.326 Pressure-induced deep tissue damage of left buttock

L89.329 Pressure ulcer of left buttock, unspecified stage
Healing pressure ulcer of left buttock NOS
Healing pressure ulcer of left buttock, unspecified stage

√5ᵗʰ **L89.4 Pressure ulcer of contiguous site of back, buttock and hip**

L89.40 Pressure ulcer of contiguous site of back, buttock and hip, unspecified stage
Healing pressure ulcer of contiguous site of back, buttock and hip NOS
Healing pressure ulcer of contiguous site of back, buttock and hip, unspecified stage

L89.41 Pressure ulcer of contiguous site of back, buttock and hip, stage 1
Healing pressure ulcer of contiguous site of back, buttock and hip, stage 1
Pressure pre-ulcer skin changes limited to persistent focal edema, contiguous site of back, buttock and hip

L89.42 Pressure ulcer of contiguous site of back, buttock and hip, stage 2 CH CL
Healing pressure ulcer of contiguous site of back, buttock and hip, stage 2
Pressure ulcer with abrasion, blister, partial thickness skin loss involving epidermis and/or dermis, contiguous site of back, buttock and hip

L89.43 Pressure ulcer of contiguous site of back, buttock and hip, stage 3 CH CL
Healing pressure ulcer of contiguous site of back, buttock and hip, stage 3
Pressure ulcer with full thickness skin loss involving damage or necrosis of subcutaneous tissue, contiguous site of back, buttock and hip

L89.44 Pressure ulcer of contiguous site of back, buttock and hip, stage 4 CH CL
Healing pressure ulcer of contiguous site of back, buttock and hip, stage 4
Pressure ulcer with necrosis of soft tissues through to underlying muscle, tendon, or bone, contiguous site of back, buttock and hip

L89.45 Pressure ulcer of contiguous site of back, buttock and hip, unstageable CH CL

L89.46 Pressure-induced deep tissue damage of contiguous site of back, buttock and hip

√5ᵗʰ **L89.5 Pressure ulcer of ankle**

√6ᵗʰ **L89.50 Pressure ulcer of unspecified ankle**

L89.500 Pressure ulcer of unspecified ankle, unstageable

Chapter 12. Diseases of the Skin and Subcutaneous Tissue *(left margin)*

L89.501 **Pressure ulcer of unspecified ankle,** stage 1
> Healing pressure ulcer of unspecified ankle, stage 1
> Pressure pre-ulcer skin changes limited to persistent focal edema, unspecified ankle

L89.502 **Pressure ulcer of unspecified ankle,** stage 2
> Healing pressure ulcer of unspecified ankle, stage 2
> Pressure ulcer with abrasion, blister, partial thickness skin loss involving epidermis and/or dermis, unspecified ankle

L89.503 **Pressure ulcer of unspecified ankle,** stage 3
> Healing pressure ulcer of unspecified ankle, stage 3
> Pressure ulcer with full thickness skin loss involving damage or necrosis of subcutaneous tissue, unspecified ankle

L89.504 **Pressure ulcer of unspecified ankle,** stage 4
> Healing pressure ulcer of unspecified ankle, stage 4
> Pressure ulcer with necrosis of soft tissues through to underlying muscle, tendon, or bone, unspecified ankle

L89.506 **Pressure-induced** deep tissue damage **of unspecified ankle**

L89.509 **Pressure ulcer of unspecified ankle, unspecified stage**
> Healing pressure ulcer of unspecified ankle NOS
> Healing pressure ulcer of unspecified ankle, unspecified stage

✓6ᵗʰ **L89.51** **Pressure ulcer of** right **ankle**

L89.510 **Pressure ulcer of right ankle, unstageable** [CH] [CL]

L89.511 **Pressure ulcer of right ankle,** stage 1
> Healing pressure ulcer of right ankle, stage 1
> Pressure pre-ulcer skin changes limited to persistent focal edema, right ankle

L89.512 **Pressure ulcer of right ankle, stage 2** [CH] [CL]
> Healing pressure ulcer of right ankle, stage 2
> Pressure ulcer with abrasion, blister, partial thickness skin loss involving epidermis and/or dermis, right ankle

L89.513 **Pressure ulcer of right ankle, stage 3** [CH] [CL]
> Healing pressure ulcer of right ankle, stage 3
> Pressure ulcer with full thickness skin loss involving damage or necrosis of subcutaneous tissue, right ankle

L89.514 **Pressure ulcer of right ankle, stage 4** [CH] [CL]
> Healing pressure ulcer of right ankle, stage 4
> Pressure ulcer with necrosis of soft tissues through to underlying muscle, tendon, or bone, right ankle

L89.516 **Pressure-induced** deep tissue damage **of right ankle**

L89.519 **Pressure ulcer of right ankle, unspecified stage**
> Healing pressure ulcer of right ankle NOS
> Healing pressure ulcer of right ankle, unspecified stage

✓6ᵗʰ **L89.52** **Pressure ulcer of** left **ankle**

L89.520 **Pressure ulcer of left ankle, unstageable** [CH] [CL]

L89.521 **Pressure ulcer of left ankle,** stage 1
> Healing pressure ulcer of left ankle, stage 1
> Pressure pre-ulcer skin changes limited to persistent focal edema, left ankle

L89.522 **Pressure ulcer of left ankle, stage 2** [CH] [CL]
> Healing pressure ulcer of left ankle, stage 2
> Pressure ulcer with abrasion, blister, partial thickness skin loss involving epidermis and/or dermis, left ankle

L89.523 **Pressure ulcer of left ankle, stage 3** [CH] [CL]
> Healing pressure ulcer of left ankle, stage 3
> Pressure ulcer with full thickness skin loss involving damage or necrosis of subcutaneous tissue, left ankle

L89.524 **Pressure ulcer of left ankle, stage 4** [CH] [CL]
> Healing pressure ulcer of left ankle, stage 4
> Pressure ulcer with necrosis of soft tissues through to underlying muscle, tendon, or bone, left ankle

L89.526 **Pressure-induced** deep tissue damage **of left ankle**

L89.529 **Pressure ulcer of left ankle, unspecified stage**
> Healing pressure ulcer of left ankle NOS
> Healing pressure ulcer of left ankle, unspecified stage

✓5ᵗʰ **L89.6** **Pressure ulcer of** heel

✓6ᵗʰ **L89.60** **Pressure ulcer of unspecified heel**

L89.600 **Pressure ulcer of unspecified heel, unstageable**

L89.601 **Pressure ulcer of unspecified heel,** stage 1
> Healing pressure ulcer of unspecified heel, stage 1
> Pressure pre-ulcer skin changes limited to persistent focal edema, unspecified heel

L89.602 **Pressure ulcer of unspecified heel,** stage 2
> Healing pressure ulcer of unspecified heel, stage 2
> Pressure ulcer with abrasion, blister, partial thickness skin loss involving epidermis and/or dermis, unspecified heel

L89.603 **Pressure ulcer of unspecified heel,** stage 3
> Healing pressure ulcer of unspecified heel, stage 3
> Pressure ulcer with full thickness skin loss involving damage or necrosis of subcutaneous tissue, unspecified heel

L89.604 **Pressure ulcer of unspecified heel,** stage 4
> Healing pressure ulcer of unspecified heel, stage 4
> Pressure ulcer with necrosis of soft tissues through to underlying muscle, tendon, or bone, unspecified heel

L89.606 **Pressure-induced** deep tissue damage **of unspecified heel**

L89.609 **Pressure ulcer of unspecified heel, unspecified stage**
> Healing pressure ulcer of unspecified heel NOS
> Healing pressure ulcer of unspecified heel, unspecified stage

✓6ᵗʰ **L89.61** **Pressure ulcer of** right **heel**

L89.610 **Pressure ulcer of right heel, unstageable** [CH] [CL]

L89.611 **Pressure ulcer of right heel,** stage 1
> Healing pressure ulcer of right heel, stage 1
> Pressure pre-ulcer skin changes limited to persistent focal edema, right heel

N Newborn: 0   P Pediatric: 0-17   M Maternity: 12-55   A Adult: 15-124   CH Comorbidity High   CL Comorbidity Low   NCDx Noncancer Dx   PDx Primary Dx

732   ICD-10-CM 2020

L89.612 Pressure ulcer of right heel, stage 2 `CH` `CL`
    Healing pressure ulcer of right heel, stage 2
    Pressure ulcer with abrasion, blister, partial thickness skin loss involving epidermis and/or dermis, right heel

L89.613 Pressure ulcer of right heel, stage 3 `CH` `CL`
    Healing pressure ulcer of right heel, stage 3
    Pressure ulcer with full thickness skin loss involving damage or necrosis of subcutaneous tissue, right heel

L89.614 Pressure ulcer of right heel, stage 4 `CH` `CL`
    Healing pressure ulcer of right heel, stage 4
    Pressure ulcer with necrosis of soft tissues through to underlying muscle, tendon, or bone, right heel

L89.616 Pressure-induced deep tissue damage of right heel

L89.619 Pressure ulcer of right heel, unspecified stage
    Healing pressure ulcer of right heel NOS
    Healing pressure ulcer of right heel, unspecified stage

√6ᵗʰ **L89.62 Pressure ulcer of left heel**

L89.620 Pressure ulcer of left heel, unstageable `CH` `CL`

L89.621 Pressure ulcer of left heel, stage 1
    Healing pressure ulcer of left heel, stage 1
    Pressure pre-ulcer skin changes limited to persistent focal edema, left heel

L89.622 Pressure ulcer of left heel, stage 2 `CH` `CL`
    Healing pressure ulcer of left heel, stage 2
    Pressure ulcer with abrasion, blister, partial thickness skin loss involving epidermis and/or dermis, left heel

L89.623 Pressure ulcer of left heel, stage 3 `CH` `CL`
    Healing pressure ulcer of left heel, stage 3
    Pressure ulcer with full thickness skin loss involving damage or necrosis of subcutaneous tissue, left heel

L89.624 Pressure ulcer of left heel, stage 4 `CH` `CL`
    Healing pressure ulcer of left heel, stage 4
    Pressure ulcer with necrosis of soft tissues through to underlying muscle, tendon, or bone, left heel

L89.626 Pressure-induced deep tissue damage of left heel

L89.629 Pressure ulcer of left heel, unspecified stage
    Healing pressure ulcer of left heel NOS
    Healing pressure ulcer of left heel, unspecified stage

√5ᵗʰ **L89.8 Pressure ulcer of other site**

√6ᵗʰ **L89.81 Pressure ulcer of head**
    Pressure ulcer of face

L89.810 Pressure ulcer of head, unstageable `CH` `CL`

L89.811 Pressure ulcer of head, stage 1
    Healing pressure ulcer of head, stage 1
    Pressure pre-ulcer skin changes limited to persistent focal edema, head

L89.812 Pressure ulcer of head, stage 2 `CH` `CL`
    Healing pressure ulcer of head, stage 2
    Pressure ulcer with abrasion, blister, partial thickness skin loss involving epidermis and/or dermis, head

L89.813 Pressure ulcer of head, stage 3 `CH` `CL`
    Healing pressure ulcer of head, stage 3
    Pressure ulcer with full thickness skin loss involving damage or necrosis of subcutaneous tissue, head

L89.814 Pressure ulcer of head, stage 4 `CH` `CL`
    Healing pressure ulcer of head, stage 4
    Pressure ulcer with necrosis of soft tissues through to underlying muscle, tendon, or bone, head

L89.816 Pressure-induced deep tissue damage of head

L89.819 Pressure ulcer of head, unspecified stage
    Healing pressure ulcer of head NOS
    Healing pressure ulcer of head, unspecified stage

√6ᵗʰ **L89.89 Pressure ulcer of other site**

L89.890 Pressure ulcer of other site, unstageable `CH` `CL`

L89.891 Pressure ulcer of other site, stage 1
    Healing pressure ulcer of other site, stage 1
    Pressure pre-ulcer skin changes limited to persistent focal edema, other site

L89.892 Pressure ulcer of other site, stage 2 `CH` `CL`
    Healing pressure ulcer of other site, stage 2
    Pressure ulcer with abrasion, blister, partial thickness skin loss involving epidermis and/or dermis, other site

L89.893 Pressure ulcer of other site, stage 3 `CH` `CL`
    Healing pressure ulcer of other site, stage 3
    Pressure ulcer with full thickness skin loss involving damage or necrosis of subcutaneous tissue, other site

L89.894 Pressure ulcer of other site, stage 4 `CH` `CL`
    Healing pressure ulcer of other site, stage 4
    Pressure ulcer with necrosis of soft tissues through to underlying muscle, tendon, or bone, other site

L89.896 Pressure-induced deep tissue damage of other site

L89.899 Pressure ulcer of other site, unspecified stage
    Healing pressure ulcer of other site NOS
    Healing pressure ulcer of other site, unspecified stage

√5ᵗʰ **L89.9 Pressure ulcer of unspecified site**

L89.90 Pressure ulcer of unspecified site, unspecified stage
    Healing pressure ulcer of unspecified site NOS
    Healing pressure ulcer of unspecified site, unspecified stage

L89.91 Pressure ulcer of unspecified site, stage 1
    Healing pressure ulcer of unspecified site, stage 1
    Pressure pre-ulcer skin changes limited to persistent focal edema, unspecified site

L89.92 Pressure ulcer of unspecified site, stage 2
    Healing pressure ulcer of unspecified site, stage 2
    Pressure ulcer with abrasion, blister, partial thickness skin loss involving epidermis and/or dermis, unspecified site

L89.93 Pressure ulcer of unspecified site, stage 3
    Healing pressure ulcer of unspecified site, stage 3
    Pressure ulcer with full thickness skin loss involving damage or necrosis of subcutaneous tissue, unspecified site

L89.94 Pressure ulcer of unspecified site, stage 4
    Healing pressure ulcer of unspecified site, stage 4
    Pressure ulcer with necrosis of soft tissues through to underlying muscle, tendon, or bone, unspecified site

L89.95 Pressure ulcer of unspecified site, unstageable

L89.96 Pressure-induced deep tissue damage of unspecified site

√4ᵗʰ **L90 Atrophic disorders of skin**

L90.0 Lichen sclerosus et atrophicus
    EXCLUDES 2   *lichen sclerosus of external female genital organs (N90.4)*
                    lichen sclerosus of external male genital organs (N48.0)

L90.1 Anetoderma of Schweninger-Buzzi

☑ Additional Character Required   √x7ᵗʰ Placeholder Alert   Manifestation   Unspecified Dx   ►◄ Revised Text   ● New Code   ▲ Revised Title

ICD-10-CM 2020   733

L90.2 Anetoderma of Jadassohn-Pellizzari
L90.3 Atrophoderma of Pasini and Pierini
L90.4 Acrodermatitis chronica atrophicans
L90.5 Scar conditions and fibrosis of skin
Adherent scar (skin)
Cicatrix
Disfigurement of skin due to scar
Fibrosis of skin NOS
Scar NOS
EXCLUDES 2 hypertrophic scar (L91.0)
keloid scar (L91.0)
AHA: 2016,2Q,5; 2015,1Q,19
L90.6 Striae atrophicae
L90.8 Other atrophic disorders of skin
L90.9 Atrophic disorder of skin, unspecified

L91 Hypertrophic disorders of skin
L91.0 Hypertrophic scar
Keloid
Keloid scar
EXCLUDES 2 acne keloid (L73.0)
scar NOS (L90.5)
DEF: Overgrowth of scar tissue due to excess amounts of collagen during connective tissue repair, occurring mainly on the upper trunk and face.
L91.8 Other hypertrophic disorders of the skin
L91.9 Hypertrophic disorder of the skin, unspecified

L92 Granulomatous disorders of skin and subcutaneous tissue
EXCLUDES 2 actinic granuloma (L57.5)
L92.0 Granuloma annulare
Perforating granuloma annulare
L92.1 Necrobiosis lipoidica, not elsewhere classified
EXCLUDES 1 necrobiosis lipoidica associated with diabetes mellitus (E08-E13 with .620)
L92.2 Granuloma faciale [eosinophilic granuloma of skin]
L92.3 Foreign body granuloma of the skin and subcutaneous tissue
Use additional code to identify the type of retained foreign body (Z18.-)
L92.8 Other granulomatous disorders of the skin and subcutaneous tissue
L92.9 Granulomatous disorder of the skin and subcutaneous tissue, unspecified
EXCLUDES 2 umbilical granuloma (P83.81)
AHA: 2017,4Q,21-22

L93 Lupus erythematosus
Use additional code for adverse effect, if applicable, to identify drug (T36-T50 with fifth or sixth character 5)
EXCLUDES 1 lupus exedens (A18.4)
lupus vulgaris (A18.4)
scleroderma (M34.-)
systemic lupus erythematosus (M32.-)
DEF: Inflammatory, autoimmune skin condition in which the body's autoimmune system attacks healthy tissue of the integumentary system.
L93.0 Discoid lupus erythematosus
Lupus erythematosus NOS
L93.1 Subacute cutaneous lupus erythematosus
L93.2 Other local lupus erythematosus
Lupus erythematosus profundus
Lupus panniculitis

L94 Other localized connective tissue disorders
EXCLUDES 1 systemic connective tissue disorders (M30-M36)
L94.0 Localized scleroderma [morphea]
Circumscribed scleroderma
L94.1 Linear scleroderma
En coup de sabre lesion
L94.2 Calcinosis cutis
L94.3 Sclerodactyly
L94.4 Gottron's papules
L94.5 Poikiloderma vasculare atrophicans
L94.6 Ainhum
L94.8 Other specified localized connective tissue disorders
L94.9 Localized connective tissue disorder, unspecified

L95 Vasculitis limited to skin, not elsewhere classified
EXCLUDES 1 angioma serpiginosum (L81.7)
Henoch(-Schönlein) purpura (D69.0)
hypersensitivity angiitis (M31.0)
lupus panniculitis (L93.2)
panniculitis NOS (M79.3)
panniculitis of neck and back (M54.0-)
polyarteritis nodosa (M30.0)
relapsing panniculitis (M35.6)
rheumatoid vasculitis (M05.2)
serum sickness (T80.6-)
urticaria (L50.-)
Wegener's granulomatosis (M31.3-)
L95.0 Livedoid vasculitis
Atrophie blanche (en plaque)
L95.1 Erythema elevatum diutinum
L95.8 Other vasculitis limited to the skin
L95.9 Vasculitis limited to the skin, unspecified

L97 Non-pressure chronic ulcer of lower limb, not elsewhere classified
INCLUDES chronic ulcer of skin of lower limb NOS
non-healing ulcer of skin
non-infected sinus of skin
trophic ulcer NOS
tropical ulcer NOS
ulcer of skin of lower limb NOS
Code first any associated underlying condition, such as:
any associated gangrene (I96)
atherosclerosis of the lower extremities (I70.23-, I70.24-, I70.33-, I70.34-, I70.43-, I70.44-, I70.53-, I70.54-, I70.63-, I70.64-, I70.73-, I70.74-)
chronic venous hypertension (I87.31-, I87.33-)
diabetic ulcers (E08.621, E08.622, E09.621, E09.622, E10.621, E10.622, E11.621, E11.622, E13.621, E13.622)
postphlebitic syndrome (I87.01-, I87.03-)
postthrombotic syndrome (I87.01-, I87.03-)
varicose ulcer (I83.0-, I83.2-)
EXCLUDES 2 pressure ulcer (pressure area) (L89.-)
skin infections (L00-L08)
specific infections classified to A00-B99
AHA: 2018,4Q,69; 2017,4Q,17
TIP: The depth and/or severity of a diagnosed nonpressure ulcer can be determined based on medical record documentation from clinicians who are not the patient's provider.

L97.1 Non-pressure chronic ulcer of thigh
L97.10 Non-pressure chronic ulcer of unspecified thigh
L97.101 Non-pressure chronic ulcer of unspecified thigh limited to breakdown of skin
L97.102 Non-pressure chronic ulcer of unspecified thigh with fat layer exposed
L97.103 Non-pressure chronic ulcer of unspecified thigh with necrosis of muscle
L97.104 Non-pressure chronic ulcer of unspecified thigh with necrosis of bone
L97.105 Non-pressure chronic ulcer of unspecified thigh with muscle involvement without evidence of necrosis
L97.106 Non-pressure chronic ulcer of unspecified thigh with bone involvement without evidence of necrosis
L97.108 Non-pressure chronic ulcer of unspecified thigh with other specified severity
L97.109 Non-pressure chronic ulcer of unspecified thigh with unspecified severity
L97.11 Non-pressure chronic ulcer of right thigh
L97.111 Non-pressure chronic ulcer of right thigh limited to breakdown of skin CH CL
L97.112 Non-pressure chronic ulcer of right thigh with fat layer exposed CH CL
L97.113 Non-pressure chronic ulcer of right thigh with necrosis of muscle CH CL
L97.114 Non-pressure chronic ulcer of right thigh with necrosis of bone CH CL

     L97.115 **Non-pressure chronic ulcer of right thigh** with muscle involvement without evidence of necrosis `CH` `CL`

     L97.116 **Non-pressure chronic ulcer of right thigh** with bone involvement without evidence of necrosis `CH` `CL`

     L97.118 **Non-pressure chronic ulcer of right thigh with other specified severity** `CH` `CL`

     L97.119 **Non-pressure chronic ulcer of right thigh with unspecified severity** `CH` `CL`

√6th **L97.12** **Non-pressure chronic ulcer of** left **thigh**

     L97.121 **Non-pressure chronic ulcer of left thigh** limited to breakdown of skin

     L97.122 **Non-pressure chronic ulcer of left thigh** with fat layer exposed

     L97.123 **Non-pressure chronic ulcer of left thigh** with necrosis of muscle

     L97.124 **Non-pressure chronic ulcer of left thigh** with necrosis of bone

     L97.125 **Non-pressure chronic ulcer of left thigh** with muscle involvement without evidence of necrosis

     L97.126 **Non-pressure chronic ulcer of left thigh** with bone involvement without evidence of necrosis

     L97.128 **Non-pressure chronic ulcer of left thigh with other specified severity**

     L97.129 **Non-pressure chronic ulcer of left thigh with unspecified severity**

√5th **L97.2** **Non-pressure chronic ulcer of** calf

  √6th **L97.20** **Non-pressure chronic ulcer of unspecified calf**

     L97.201 **Non-pressure chronic ulcer of unspecified calf** limited to breakdown of skin

     L97.202 **Non-pressure chronic ulcer of unspecified calf** with fat layer exposed

     L97.203 **Non-pressure chronic ulcer of unspecified calf** with necrosis of muscle

     L97.204 **Non-pressure chronic ulcer of unspecified calf** with necrosis of bone

     L97.205 **Non-pressure chronic ulcer of unspecified calf** with muscle involvement without evidence of necrosis

     L97.206 **Non-pressure chronic ulcer of unspecified calf** with bone involvement without evidence of necrosis

     L97.208 **Non-pressure chronic ulcer of unspecified calf with other specified severity**

     L97.209 **Non-pressure chronic ulcer of unspecified calf with unspecified severity**

  √6th **L97.21** **Non-pressure chronic ulcer of** right **calf**

     L97.211 **Non-pressure chronic ulcer of right calf** limited to breakdown of skin

     L97.212 **Non-pressure chronic ulcer of right calf** with fat layer exposed `CH` `CL`

     L97.213 **Non-pressure chronic ulcer of right calf** with necrosis of muscle `CH` `CL`

     L97.214 **Non-pressure chronic ulcer of right calf** with necrosis of bone `CH` `CL`

     L97.215 **Non-pressure chronic ulcer of right calf** with muscle involvement without evidence of necrosis `CH` `CL`

     L97.216 **Non-pressure chronic ulcer of right calf** with bone involvement without evidence of necrosis

     L97.218 **Non-pressure chronic ulcer of right calf with other specified severity** `CH` `CL`

     L97.219 **Non-pressure chronic ulcer of right calf with unspecified severity** `CH` `CL`

  √6th **L97.22** **Non-pressure chronic ulcer of** left **calf**

     L97.221 **Non-pressure chronic ulcer of left calf** limited to breakdown of skin `CH` `CL`

     L97.222 **Non-pressure chronic ulcer of left calf** with fat layer exposed `CH` `CL`

     L97.223 **Non-pressure chronic ulcer of left calf** with necrosis of muscle `CH` `CL`

     L97.224 **Non-pressure chronic ulcer of left calf** with necrosis of bone `CH` `CL`

     L97.225 **Non-pressure chronic ulcer of left calf** with muscle involvement without evidence of necrosis `CH` `CL`

     L97.226 **Non-pressure chronic ulcer of left calf** with bone involvement without evidence of necrosis `CH` `CL`

     L97.228 **Non-pressure chronic ulcer of left calf with other specified severity** `CH` `CL`

     L97.229 **Non-pressure chronic ulcer of left calf with unspecified severity** `CH` `CL`

√5th **L97.3** **Non-pressure chronic ulcer of** ankle

  √6th **L97.30** **Non-pressure chronic ulcer of unspecified ankle**

     L97.301 **Non-pressure chronic ulcer of unspecified ankle** limited to breakdown of skin

     L97.302 **Non-pressure chronic ulcer of unspecified ankle** with fat layer exposed

     L97.303 **Non-pressure chronic ulcer of unspecified ankle** with necrosis of muscle

     L97.304 **Non-pressure chronic ulcer of unspecified ankle** with necrosis of bone

     L97.305 **Non-pressure chronic ulcer of unspecified ankle** with muscle involvement without evidence of necrosis

     L97.306 **Non-pressure chronic ulcer of unspecified ankle** with bone involvement without evidence of necrosis

     L97.308 **Non-pressure chronic ulcer of unspecified ankle with other specified severity**

     L97.309 **Non-pressure chronic ulcer of unspecified ankle with unspecified severity**

  √6th **L97.31** **Non-pressure chronic ulcer of** right **ankle**

     L97.311 **Non-pressure chronic ulcer of right ankle** limited to breakdown of skin `CH` `CL`

     L97.312 **Non-pressure chronic ulcer of right ankle** with fat layer exposed `CH` `CL`

     L97.313 **Non-pressure chronic ulcer of right ankle** with necrosis of muscle `CH` `CL`

     L97.314 **Non-pressure chronic ulcer of right ankle** with necrosis of bone `CH` `CL`

     L97.315 **Non-pressure chronic ulcer of right ankle** with muscle involvement without evidence of necrosis `CH` `CL`

     L97.316 **Non-pressure chronic ulcer of right ankle** with bone involvement without evidence of necrosis `CH` `CL`

     L97.318 **Non-pressure chronic ulcer of right ankle with other specified severity** `CH` `CL`

     L97.319 **Non-pressure chronic ulcer of right ankle with unspecified severity** `CH` `CL`

  √6th **L97.32** **Non-pressure chronic ulcer of** left **ankle**

     L97.321 **Non-pressure chronic ulcer of left ankle** limited to breakdown of skin `CH` `CL`

☑ Additional Character Required   √x7th Placeholder Alert   Manifestation   Unspecified Dx   ►◄ Revised Text   ● New Code   ▲ Revised Title

ICD-10-CM 2020   735

L97.322 Non-pressure chronic ulcer of left ankle with fat layer exposed `CH` `CL`

L97.323 Non-pressure chronic ulcer of left ankle with necrosis of muscle `CH` `CL`

L97.324 Non-pressure chronic ulcer of left ankle with necrosis of bone `CH` `CL`

L97.325 Non-pressure chronic ulcer of left ankle with muscle involvement without evidence of necrosis `CH` `CL`

L97.326 Non-pressure chronic ulcer of left ankle with bone involvement without evidence of necrosis `CH` `CL`

L97.328 Non-pressure chronic ulcer of left ankle with other specified severity `CH` `CL`

L97.329 Non-pressure chronic ulcer of left ankle with unspecified severity `CH` `CL`

✓5ᵗʰ **L97.4** Non-pressure chronic ulcer of heel and midfoot

Non-pressure chronic ulcer of plantar surface of midfoot

  ✓6ᵗʰ **L97.40** Non-pressure chronic ulcer of unspecified heel and midfoot

L97.401 Non-pressure chronic ulcer of unspecified heel and midfoot limited to breakdown of skin

L97.402 Non-pressure chronic ulcer of unspecified heel and midfoot with fat layer exposed

L97.403 Non-pressure chronic ulcer of unspecified heel and midfoot with necrosis of muscle

L97.404 Non-pressure chronic ulcer of unspecified heel and midfoot with necrosis of bone

L97.405 Non-pressure chronic ulcer of unspecified heel and midfoot with muscle involvement without evidence of necrosis

L97.406 Non-pressure chronic ulcer of unspecified heel and midfoot with bone involvement without evidence of necrosis

L97.408 Non-pressure chronic ulcer of unspecified heel and midfoot with other specified severity

L97.409 Non-pressure chronic ulcer of unspecified heel and midfoot with unspecified severity

  ✓6ᵗʰ **L97.41** Non-pressure chronic ulcer of right heel and midfoot

L97.411 Non-pressure chronic ulcer of right heel and midfoot limited to breakdown of skin `CH` `CL`

L97.412 Non-pressure chronic ulcer of right heel and midfoot with fat layer exposed `CH` `CL`

L97.413 Non-pressure chronic ulcer of right heel and midfoot with necrosis of muscle `CH` `CL`

L97.414 Non-pressure chronic ulcer of right heel and midfoot with necrosis of bone `CH` `CL`

L97.415 Non-pressure chronic ulcer of right heel and midfoot with muscle involvement without evidence of necrosis `CH` `CL`

L97.416 Non-pressure chronic ulcer of right heel and midfoot with bone involvement without evidence of necrosis `CH` `CL`

L97.418 Non-pressure chronic ulcer of right heel and midfoot with other specified severity `CH` `CL`

L97.419 Non-pressure chronic ulcer of right heel and midfoot with unspecified severity `CH` `CL`

  ✓6ᵗʰ **L97.42** Non-pressure chronic ulcer of left heel and midfoot

L97.421 Non-pressure chronic ulcer of left heel and midfoot limited to breakdown of skin `CH` `CL`

AHA: 2016,1Q,12

L97.422 Non-pressure chronic ulcer of left heel and midfoot with fat layer exposed `CH` `CL`

L97.423 Non-pressure chronic ulcer of left heel and midfoot with necrosis of muscle `CH` `CL`

L97.424 Non-pressure chronic ulcer of left heel and midfoot with necrosis of bone `CH` `CL`

L97.425 Non-pressure chronic ulcer of left heel and midfoot with muscle involvement without evidence of necrosis `CH` `CL`

L97.426 Non-pressure chronic ulcer of left heel and midfoot with bone involvement without evidence of necrosis `CH` `CL`

L97.428 Non-pressure chronic ulcer of left heel and midfoot with other specified severity `CH` `CL`

L97.429 Non-pressure chronic ulcer of left heel and midfoot with unspecified severity `CH` `CL`

✓5ᵗʰ **L97.5** Non-pressure chronic ulcer of other part of foot

Non-pressure chronic ulcer of toe

  ✓6ᵗʰ **L97.50** Non-pressure chronic ulcer of other part of unspecified foot

L97.501 Non-pressure chronic ulcer of other part of unspecified foot limited to breakdown of skin

L97.502 Non-pressure chronic ulcer of other part of unspecified foot with fat layer exposed

L97.503 Non-pressure chronic ulcer of other part of unspecified foot with necrosis of muscle

L97.504 Non-pressure chronic ulcer of other part of unspecified foot with necrosis of bone

L97.505 Non-pressure chronic ulcer of other part of unspecified foot with muscle involvement without evidence of necrosis

L97.506 Non-pressure chronic ulcer of other part of unspecified foot with bone involvement without evidence of necrosis

L97.508 Non-pressure chronic ulcer of other part of unspecified foot with other specified severity

L97.509 Non-pressure chronic ulcer of other part of unspecified foot with unspecified severity

  ✓6ᵗʰ **L97.51** Non-pressure chronic ulcer of other part of right foot

L97.511 Non-pressure chronic ulcer of other part of right foot limited to breakdown of skin `CH` `CL`

L97.512 Non-pressure chronic ulcer of other part of right foot with fat layer exposed `CH` `CL`

L97.513 Non-pressure chronic ulcer of other part of right foot with necrosis of muscle `CH` `CL`

L97.514 Non-pressure chronic ulcer of other part of right foot with necrosis of bone `CH` `CL`

L97.515 Non-pressure chronic ulcer of other part of right foot with muscle involvement without evidence of necrosis `CH` `CL`

L97.516 Non-pressure chronic ulcer of other part of right foot with bone involvement without evidence of necrosis `CH` `CL`

L97.518 Non-pressure chronic ulcer of other part of right foot with other specified severity `CH` `CL`

L97.519 Non-pressure chronic ulcer of other part of right foot with unspecified severity `CH` `CL`

  ✓6ᵗʰ **L97.52** Non-pressure chronic ulcer of other part of left foot

L97.521 Non-pressure chronic ulcer of other part of left foot limited to breakdown of skin `CH` `CL`

L97.522 Non-pressure chronic ulcer of other part of left foot with fat layer exposed `CH` `CL`

L97.523 Non-pressure chronic ulcer of other part of left foot with necrosis of muscle `CH` `CL`

Ⓝ Newborn: 0   Ⓟ Pediatric: 0-17   Ⓜ Maternity: 12-55   Ⓐ Adult: 15-124   `CH` Comorbidity High   `CL` Comorbidity Low   `NCDx` Noncancer Dx   `PDx` Primary Dx

736

ICD-10-CM 2020

L97.524 Non-pressure chronic ulcer of other part of left foot with necrosis of bone `CM` `CL`

L97.525 Non-pressure chronic ulcer of other part of left foot with muscle involvement without evidence of necrosis `CM` `CL`

L97.526 Non-pressure chronic ulcer of other part of left foot with bone involvement without evidence of necrosis `CM` `CL`

L97.528 Non-pressure chronic ulcer of other part of left foot with other specified severity `CM` `CL`

L97.529 Non-pressure chronic ulcer of other part of left foot with unspecified severity `CM` `CL`

√5ᵗʰ **L97.8** Non-pressure chronic ulcer of other part of lower leg

    √6ᵗʰ **L97.80** Non-pressure chronic ulcer of other part of unspecified lower leg

        L97.801 Non-pressure chronic ulcer of other part of unspecified lower leg limited to breakdown of skin

        L97.802 Non-pressure chronic ulcer of other part of unspecified lower leg with fat layer exposed

        L97.803 Non-pressure chronic ulcer of other part of unspecified lower leg with necrosis of muscle

        L97.804 Non-pressure chronic ulcer of other part of unspecified lower leg with necrosis of bone

        L97.805 Non-pressure chronic ulcer of other part of unspecified lower leg with muscle involvement without evidence of necrosis

        L97.806 Non-pressure chronic ulcer of other part of unspecified lower leg with bone involvement without evidence of necrosis

        L97.808 Non-pressure chronic ulcer of other part of unspecified lower leg with other specified severity

        L97.809 Non-pressure chronic ulcer of other part of unspecified lower leg with unspecified severity

    √6ᵗʰ **L97.81** Non-pressure chronic ulcer of other part of right lower leg

        L97.811 Non-pressure chronic ulcer of other part of right lower leg limited to breakdown of skin `CM` `CL`

        L97.812 Non-pressure chronic ulcer of other part of right lower leg with fat layer exposed `CM` `CL`

        L97.813 Non-pressure chronic ulcer of other part of right lower leg with necrosis of muscle `CM` `CL`

        L97.814 Non-pressure chronic ulcer of other part of right lower leg with necrosis of bone `CM` `CL`

        L97.815 Non-pressure chronic ulcer of other part of right lower leg with muscle involvement without evidence of necrosis `CM` `CL`

        L97.816 Non-pressure chronic ulcer of other part of right lower leg with bone involvement without evidence of necrosis `CM` `CL`

        L97.818 Non-pressure chronic ulcer of other part of right lower leg with other specified severity `CM` `CL`

        L97.819 Non-pressure chronic ulcer of other part of right lower leg with unspecified severity `CM` `CL`

    √6ᵗʰ **L97.82** Non-pressure chronic ulcer of other part of left lower leg

        L97.821 Non-pressure chronic ulcer of other part of left lower leg limited to breakdown of skin `CM` `CL`

        L97.822 Non-pressure chronic ulcer of other part of left lower leg with fat layer exposed `CM` `CL`

        L97.823 Non-pressure chronic ulcer of other part of left lower leg with necrosis of muscle `CM` `CL`

L97.824 Non-pressure chronic ulcer of other part of left lower leg with necrosis of bone `CM` `CL`

L97.825 Non-pressure chronic ulcer of other part of left lower leg with muscle involvement without evidence of necrosis `CM` `CL`

L97.826 Non-pressure chronic ulcer of other part of left lower leg with bone involvement without evidence of necrosis `CM` `CL`

L97.828 Non-pressure chronic ulcer of other part of left lower leg with other specified severity `CM` `CL`

L97.829 Non-pressure chronic ulcer of other part of left lower leg with unspecified severity `CM` `CL`

√5ᵗʰ **L97.9** Non-pressure chronic ulcer of unspecified part of lower leg

    √6ᵗʰ **L97.90** Non-pressure chronic ulcer of unspecified part of unspecified lower leg

        L97.901 Non-pressure chronic ulcer of unspecified part of unspecified lower leg limited to breakdown of skin

        L97.902 Non-pressure chronic ulcer of unspecified part of unspecified lower leg with fat layer exposed

        L97.903 Non-pressure chronic ulcer of unspecified part of unspecified lower leg with necrosis of muscle

        L97.904 Non-pressure chronic ulcer of unspecified part of unspecified lower leg with necrosis of bone

        L97.905 Non-pressure chronic ulcer of unspecified part of unspecified lower leg with muscle involvement without evidence of necrosis

        L97.906 Non-pressure chronic ulcer of unspecified part of unspecified lower leg with bone involvement without evidence of necrosis

        L97.908 Non-pressure chronic ulcer of unspecified part of unspecified lower leg with other specified severity

        L97.909 Non-pressure chronic ulcer of unspecified part of unspecified lower leg with unspecified severity

    √6ᵗʰ **L97.91** Non-pressure chronic ulcer of unspecified part of right lower leg

        L97.911 Non-pressure chronic ulcer of unspecified part of right lower leg limited to breakdown of skin `CM` `CL`

        L97.912 Non-pressure chronic ulcer of unspecified part of right lower leg with fat layer exposed `CM` `CL`

        L97.913 Non-pressure chronic ulcer of unspecified part of right lower leg with necrosis of muscle `CM` `CL`

        L97.914 Non-pressure chronic ulcer of unspecified part of right lower leg with necrosis of bone `CM` `CL`

        L97.915 Non-pressure chronic ulcer of unspecified part of right lower leg with muscle involvement without evidence of necrosis `CM` `CL`

        L97.916 Non-pressure chronic ulcer of unspecified part of right lower leg with bone involvement without evidence of necrosis `CM` `CL`

        L97.918 Non-pressure chronic ulcer of unspecified part of right lower leg with other specified severity `CM` `CL`

        L97.919 Non-pressure chronic ulcer of unspecified part of right lower leg with unspecified severity `CM` `CL`

    √6ᵗʰ **L97.92** Non-pressure chronic ulcer of unspecified part of left lower leg

        L97.921 Non-pressure chronic ulcer of unspecified part of left lower leg limited to breakdown of skin `CM` `CL`

        L97.922 Non-pressure chronic ulcer of unspecified part of left lower leg with fat layer exposed `CM` `CL`

☑ Additional Character Required   √x7ᵗʰ Placeholder Alert   Manifestation   Unspecified Dx   ►◄ Revised Text   ● New Code   ▲ Revised Title

L97.923 Non-pressure chronic ulcer of unspecified part of left lower leg with necrosis of muscle `CH` `CL`

L97.924 Non-pressure chronic ulcer of unspecified part of left lower leg with necrosis of bone `CH` `CL`

L97.925 Non-pressure chronic ulcer of unspecified part of left lower leg with muscle involvement without evidence of necrosis `CH` `CL`

L97.926 Non-pressure chronic ulcer of unspecified part of left lower leg with bone involvement without evidence of necrosis `CH` `CL`

L97.928 Non-pressure chronic ulcer of unspecified part of left lower leg with other specified severity `CH` `CL`

L97.929 Non-pressure chronic ulcer of unspecified part of left lower leg with unspecified severity `CH` `CL`

✓4ᵗʰ **L98 Other disorders of skin and subcutaneous tissue, not elsewhere classified**

L98.0 Pyogenic granuloma

> EXCLUDES 2 *pyogenic granuloma of gingiva (K06.8)*
> *pyogenic granuloma of maxillary alveolar ridge (K04.5)*
> *pyogenic granuloma of oral mucosa (K13.4)*

DEF: Solitary polypoid capillary hemangioma often associated with local irritation, trauma, and superimposed inflammation. Located on the skin and gingival or oral mucosa, they bleed easily and may ulcerate and form crusted sores.

L98.1 Factitial dermatitis

Neurotic excoriation

> EXCLUDES 1 *excoriation (skin-picking) disorder (F42.4)*

AHA: 2016,4Q,15

DEF: Self-inflicted skin lesions to satisfy an unconscious psychological or emotional need. Methods used to injure the skin include deep excoriations with a sharp instrument, scarification with a knife, or the application of caustic chemicals and burning, sometimes with a cigarette.

L98.2 Febrile neutrophilic dermatosis [Sweet]

L98.3 Eosinophilic cellulitis [Wells] `CH` `CL`

✓5ᵗʰ **L98.4 Non-pressure chronic ulcer of skin, not elsewhere classified**

Chronic ulcer of skin NOS
Tropical ulcer NOS
Ulcer of skin NOS

> EXCLUDES 2 *gangrene (I96)*
> *pressure ulcer (pressure area) (L89.-)*
> *skin infections (L00-L08)*
> *specific infections classified to A00-B99*
> *ulcer of lower limb NEC (L97.-)*
> *varicose ulcer (I83.0-I82.2)*

AHA: 2017,4Q,17

TIP: The depth and/or severity of a diagnosed nonpressure ulcer can be determined based on medical record documentation from clinicians who are not the patient's provider.

✓6ᵗʰ **L98.41 Non-pressure chronic ulcer of buttock**

L98.411 Non-pressure chronic ulcer of buttock limited to breakdown of skin

L98.412 Non-pressure chronic ulcer of buttock with fat layer exposed

L98.413 Non-pressure chronic ulcer of buttock with necrosis of muscle

L98.414 Non-pressure chronic ulcer of buttock with necrosis of bone

L98.415 Non-pressure chronic ulcer of buttock with muscle involvement without evidence of necrosis

L98.416 Non-pressure chronic ulcer of buttock with bone involvement without evidence of necrosis

L98.418 Non-pressure chronic ulcer of buttock with other specified severity

L98.419 Non-pressure chronic ulcer of buttock with unspecified severity

✓6ᵗʰ **L98.42 Non-pressure chronic ulcer of back**

L98.421 Non-pressure chronic ulcer of back limited to breakdown of skin

L98.422 Non-pressure chronic ulcer of back with fat layer exposed

L98.423 Non-pressure chronic ulcer of back with necrosis of muscle

L98.424 Non-pressure chronic ulcer of back with necrosis of bone

L98.425 Non-pressure chronic ulcer of back with muscle involvement without evidence of necrosis

L98.426 Non-pressure chronic ulcer of back with bone involvement without evidence of necrosis

L98.428 Non-pressure chronic ulcer of back with other specified severity

L98.429 Non-pressure chronic ulcer of back with unspecified severity

✓6ᵗʰ **L98.49 Non-pressure chronic ulcer of skin of other sites**

Non-pressure chronic ulcer of skin NOS

L98.491 Non-pressure chronic ulcer of skin of other sites limited to breakdown of skin

L98.492 Non-pressure chronic ulcer of skin of other sites with fat layer exposed

L98.493 Non-pressure chronic ulcer of skin of other sites with necrosis of muscle

L98.494 Non-pressure chronic ulcer of skin of other sites with necrosis of bone

L98.495 Non-pressure chronic ulcer of skin of other sites with muscle involvement without evidence of necrosis

L98.496 Non-pressure chronic ulcer of skin of other sites with bone involvement without evidence of necrosis

L98.498 Non-pressure chronic ulcer of skin of other sites with other specified severity

L98.499 Non-pressure chronic ulcer of skin of other sites with unspecified severity

L98.5 Mucinosis of the skin

Focal mucinosis
Lichen myxedematosus
Reticular erythematous mucinosis

> EXCLUDES 1 *focal oral mucinosis (K13.79)*
> *myxedema (E03.9)*

L98.6 Other infiltrative disorders of the skin and subcutaneous tissue

> EXCLUDES 1 *hyalinosis cutis et mucosae (E78.89)*

L98.7 Excessive and redundant skin and subcutaneous tissue

Loose or sagging skin, following bariatric surgery weight loss
Loose or sagging skin following dietary weight loss
Loose or sagging skin, NOS

> EXCLUDES 2 *acquired excess or redundant skin of eyelid (H02.3-)*
> *congenital excess or redundant skin of eyelid (Q10.3)*
> *skin changes due to chronic exposure to nonionizing radiation (L57.-)*

AHA: 2016,4Q,36

L98.8 Other specified disorders of the skin and subcutaneous tissue

AHA: 2013,2Q,32

L98.9 Disorder of the skin and subcutaneous tissue, unspecified

L99 Other disorders of skin and subcutaneous tissue in diseases classified elsewhere

Code first underlying disease, such as:
amyloidosis (E85.-)

> EXCLUDES 1 *skin disorders in diabetes (E08-E13 with .62)*
> *skin disorders in gonorrhea (A54.89)*
> *skin disorders in syphilis (A51.31, A52.79)*

Chapter 13. Diseases of the Musculoskeletal System and Connective Tissue (M00–M99)

Chapter-specific Guidelines with Coding Examples

The chapter-specific guidelines from the ICD-10-CM Official Guidelines for Coding and Reporting have been provided below. Along with these guidelines are coding examples, contained in the shaded boxes, that have been developed to help illustrate the coding and/or sequencing guidance found in these guidelines.

a. Site and laterality

Most of the codes within Chapter 13 have site and laterality designations. The site represents the bone, joint or the muscle involved. For some conditions where more than one bone, joint or muscle is usually involved, such as osteoarthritis, there is a "multiple sites" code available. For categories where no multiple site code is provided and more than one bone, joint or muscle is involved, multiple codes should be used to indicate the different sites involved.

> Right elbow infective bursitis
>
> **M71.121   Other infective bursitis, right elbow**
>
> *Explanation:* Most of the codes within chapter 13 have site and laterality designations. The site represents the bone, joint, or the muscle involved.

> Rheumatoid arthritis of multiple sites without rheumatoid factor
>
> **M06.09   Rheumatoid arthritis without rheumatoid factor, multiple sites**
>
> *Explanation:* For some conditions where more than one bone, joint or muscle is usually involved, such as osteoarthritis, there is a "multiple sites" code available.

> Osteomyelitis of the fourth thoracic and second lumbar vertebrae
>
> **M46.24   Osteomyelitis of vertebra, thoracic region**
>
> **M46.26   Osteomyelitis of vertebra, lumbar region**
>
> *Explanation:* For categories without a multiple site code and more than one bone, joint, or muscle is involved, multiple codes should be used to indicate the different sites involved.

1) Bone versus joint

For certain conditions, the bone may be affected at the upper or lower end, (e.g., avascular necrosis of bone, M87, Osteoporosis, M80, M81). Though the portion of the bone affected may be at the joint, the site designation will be the bone, not the joint.

> Idiopathic avascular necrosis of the femoral head of the left hip joint
>
> **M87.052   Idiopathic aseptic necrosis of left femur**
>
> *Explanation:* For certain conditions such as avascular necrosis, the bone may be affected at the joint, but the site designation is the bone, not the joint.

b. Acute traumatic versus chronic or recurrent musculoskeletal conditions

Many musculoskeletal conditions are a result of previous injury or trauma to a site, or are recurrent conditions. Bone, joint or muscle conditions that are the result of a healed injury are usually found in chapter 13. Recurrent bone, joint or muscle conditions are also usually found in chapter 13. Any current, acute injury should be coded to the appropriate injury code from chapter 19. Chronic or recurrent conditions should generally be coded with a code from chapter 13. If it is difficult to determine from the documentation in the record which code is best to describe a condition, query the provider.

> Old bucket-handle tear of right medial meniscus
>
> **M23.203   Derangement of unspecified medial meniscus due to old tear or injury, right knee**
>
> *Explanation:* Chronic or recurrent conditions should generally be coded with a code from chapter 13.

c. Coding of pathologic fractures

7th character A is for use as long as the patient is receiving active treatment for the fracture. Examples of active treatment are: surgical treatment, emergency department encounter, evaluation and continuing treatment by the same or a different physician. While the patient may be seen by a new or different provider over the course of treatment for a pathological fracture, assignment of the 7th character is based on whether the patient is undergoing active treatment and not whether the provider is seeing the patient for the first time.

7th character D is to be used for encounters after the patient has completed active treatment for the fracture and is receiving routine care for the fracture during the healing or recovery phase. The other 7th characters, listed under each subcategory in the Tabular List, are to be used for subsequent encounters for treatment of problems associated with the healing, such as malunions, nonunions, and sequelae.

> Following a hospital and inpatient rehabilitation stay for treatment of a pathological fracture of the right femur, a 72-year-old woman is admitted to home health for continued physical therapy and pain management.
>
> **M84.451D   Pathological fracture, right femur, subsequent encounter for fracture with routine healing**
>
> *Explanation:* The use of seventh character D is appropriate when the patient is receiving routine care for the fracture during the healing and recovery phase. Depending on the category/subcategory, other seventh characters are available to designate subsequent care related to complications associated with the healing phase. For subcategory M84.4- these include delayed healing (seventh character G), nonunion (seventh character K), malunion (seventh character P), and sequela (seventh character S).

Care for complications of surgical treatment for fracture repairs during the healing or recovery phase should be coded with the appropriate complication codes.

See Section I.C.19. Coding of traumatic fractures.

d. Osteoporosis

Osteoporosis is a systemic condition, meaning that all bones of the musculoskeletal system are affected. Therefore, site is not a component of the codes under category M81, Osteoporosis without current pathological fracture. The site codes under category M80, Osteoporosis with current pathological fracture, identify the site of the fracture, not the osteoporosis.

1) Osteoporosis without pathological fracture

Category M81, Osteoporosis without current pathological fracture, is for use for patients with osteoporosis who do not currently have a pathologic fracture due to the osteoporosis, even if they have had a fracture in the past. For patients with a history of osteoporosis fractures, status code Z87.310, Personal history of (healed) osteoporosis fracture, should follow the code from M81.

> Age-related osteoporosis with healed osteoporotic fracture of the lumbar vertebra
>
> **M81.0   Age-related osteoporosis without current pathological fracture**
>
> **Z87.310   Personal history of (healed) osteoporosis fracture**
>
> *Explanation:* Category M81 is used for patients with osteoporosis who do not currently have a pathologic fracture due to the osteoporosis. To report a previous (healed) fracture, status code Z87.310 Personal history of (healed) osteoporosis fracture, should follow the code from M81.

2) Osteoporosis with current pathological fracture

Category M80, Osteoporosis with current pathological fracture, is for patients who have a current pathologic fracture at the time of an encounter. The codes under M80 identify the site of the fracture. A code from category M80, not a traumatic fracture code, should be used for any patient with known osteoporosis who suffers a fracture, even if the patient had a minor fall or trauma, if that fall or trauma would not usually break a normal, healthy bone.

> Disuse osteoporosis with current fracture of right shoulder sustained lifting a grocery bag, subsequent encounter
>
> **M80.811D   Other osteoporosis with current pathological fracture, right shoulder, subsequent encounter for fracture with routine healing**
>
> *Explanation:* A code from category M80, not a traumatic fracture code, should be used for any patient with known osteoporosis who suffers a fracture, even if the patient had a minor fall or trauma, if that fall or trauma would not usually break a normal, healthy bone.

Muscle/Tendon Table

ICD-10-CM categorizes certain muscles and tendons in the upper and lower extremities by their action (e.g., extension, flexion), their anatomical location (e.g., posterior, anterior), and/or whether they are intrinsic or extrinsic to a certain anatomical area. The Muscle/Tendon Table is provided at the beginning of chapters 13 and 19 as a resource to help users when code selection depends on one or more of these characteristics. Please note that this table is not all-inclusive, and proper code assignment should be based on the provider's documentation.

Body Region	Muscle	Extensor Tendon	Flexor Tendon	Other Tendon
Shoulder				
	Deltoid	Posterior deltoid	Anterior deltoid	
	Rotator cuff			
	Infraspinatus			Infraspinatus
	Subscapularis			Subscapularis
	Supraspinatus			Supraspinatus
	Teres minor			Teres minor
	Teres major	Teres major		
Upper arm				
	Anterior muscles			
	Biceps brachii — long head		Biceps brachii — long head	
	Biceps brachii — short head		Biceps brachii — short head	
	Brachialis		Brachialis	
	Coracobrachialis		Coracobrachialis	
	Posterior muscles			
	Triceps brachii	Triceps brachii		
Forearm				
	Anterior muscles			
	Flexors			
	Deep			
	Flexor digitorum profundus		Flexor digitorum profundus	
	Flexor pollicis longus		Flexor pollicis longus	
	Intermediate			
	Flexor digitorum superficialis		Flexor digitorum superficialis	
	Superficial			
	Flexor carpi radialis		Flexor carpi radialis	
	Flexor carpi ulnaris		Flexor carpi ulnaris	
	Palmaris longus		Palmaris longus	
	Pronators			
	Pronator quadratus			Pronator quadratus
	Pronator teres			Pronator teres
	Posterior muscles			
	Extensors			
	Deep			
	Abductor pollicis longus			Abductor pollicis longus
	Extensor indicis	Extensor indicis		
	Extensor pollicis brevis	Extensor pollicis brevis		
	Extensor pollicis longus	Extensor pollicis longus		
	Superficial			
	Brachioradialis			Brachioradialis
	Extensor carpi radialis brevis	Extensor carpi radialis brevis		
	Extensor carpi radialis longus	Extensor carpi radialis longus		
	Extensor carpi ulnaris	Extensor carpi ulnaris		
	Extensor digiti minimi	Extensor digiti minimi		
	Extensor digitorum	Extensor digitorum		
	Anconeus	Anconeus		
	Supinator			Supinator

Body Region	Muscle	Extensor Tendon	Flexor Tendon	Other Tendon
Hand				
Extrinsic — attach to a site in the forearm as well as a site in the hand with action related to hand movement at the wrist				
	Extensor carpi radialis brevis	Extensor carpi radialis brevis		
	Extensor carpi radialis longus	Extensor carpie radialis longus		
	Extensor carpi ulnaris	Extensor carpi ulnaris		
	Flexor carpi radialis		Flexor carpi radialis	
	Flexor carpi ulnaris		Flexor carpi ulnaris	
	Flexor digitorum superficialis		Flexor digitorum superficialis	
	Palmaris longus		Palmaris longus	
Extrinsic — attach to a site in the forearm as well as a site in the hand with action in the hand related to finger movement				
	Adductor pollicis longus			Adductor pollicis longus
	Extensor digiti minimi	Extensor digiti minimi		
	Extensor digitorum	Extensor digitorum		
	Extensor indicis	Extensor indicis		
	Flexor digitorum profundus		Flexor digitorum profundus	
	Flexor digitorum superficialis		Flexor digitorum superficialis	
Extrinsic — attach to a site in the forearm as well as a site in the hand with action in the hand related to thumb movement				
	Extensor pollicis brevis	Extensor pollicis brevis		
	Extensor pollicis longus	Extensor pollicis longus		
	Flexor pollicis longus		Flexor pollicis longus	
Intrinsic — found within the hand only				
	Adductor pollicis			Adductor pollicis
	Dorsal interossei	Dorsal interossei	Dorsal interossei	
	Lumbricals	Lumbricals	Lumbricals	
	Palmaris brevis			Palmaris brevis
	Palmar interossei	Palmar interossei	Palmar interossei	
	Hypothenar muscles			
	Abductor digiti minimi			Abductor digiti minimi
	Flexor digiti minimi brevis		Flexor digiti minimi brevis	
	Oppenens digiti minimi		Oppenens digiti minimi	
	Thenar muscles			
	Abductor pollicis brevis			Abductor pollicis brevis
	Flexor pollicis brevis		Flexor pollicis brevis	
	Oppenens pollicis		Oppenens pollicis	
Thigh				
	Anterior muscles			
	Iliopsoas		Iliopsoas	
	Pectineus		Pectineus	
	Quadriceps	Quadriceps		
	Rectus femoris	Rectus femoris — Extends knee	Rectus femoris — Flexes hip	
	Vastus intermedius	Vastus intermedius		
	Vastus lateralis	Vastus lateralis		
	Vastus medialis	Vastus medialis		
	Sartorius		Sartorius	
	Medial muscles			
	Adductor brevis			Adductor brevis
	Adductor longus			Adductor longus
	Adductor magnus			Adductor magnus
	Gracilis			Gracilis
	Obturator externus			Obturator externus
	Posterior muscles			
	Hamstring	Hamstring — Extends hip	Hamstring — Flexes knee	
	Biceps femoris	Biceps femoris	Biceps femoris	
	Semimembranosus	Semimembranosus	Semimembranosus	
	Semitendinosus	Semitendinosus	Semitendinosus	

Body Region	Muscle	Extensor Tendon	Flexor Tendon	Other Tendon
Lower leg				
	Anterior muscles			
	Extensor digitorum longus	Extensor digitorum longus		
	Extensor hallucis longus	Extensor hallucis longus		
	Fibularis (peroneus) tertius	Fibularis (peroneus) tertius		
	Tibialis anterior	Tibialis anterior		Tibialis anterior
	Lateral muscles			
	Fibularis (peroneus) brevis		Fibularis (peroneus) brevis	
	Fibularis (peroneus) longus		Fibularis (peroneus) longus	
	Posterior muscles			
	Deep			
	Flexor digitorum longus		Flexor digitorum longus	
	Flexor hallucis longus		Flexor hallucis longus	
	Popliteus		Popliteus	
	Tibialis posterior		Tibialis posterior	
	Superficial			
	Gastrocnemius		Gastrocnemius	
	Plantaris		Plantaris	
	Soleus		Soleus	
				Calcaneal (Achilles)
Ankle/Foot				
Extrinsic — attach to a site in the lower leg as well as a site in the foot with action related to foot movement at the ankle				
	Plantaris		Plantaris	
	Soleus		Soleus	
	Tibialis anterior	Tibialis anterior		
	Tibialis posterior		Tibialis posterior	
Extrinsic — attach to a site in the lower leg as well as a site in the foot with action in the foot related to toe movement				
	Extensor digitorum longus	Extensor digitorum longus		
	Extensor hallucis longus	Extensor hallucis longus		
	Flexor digitorum longus		Flexor digitorum longus	
	Flexor hallucis longus		Flexor hallucis longus	
Intrinsic — found within the ankle/foot only				
	Dorsal muscles			
	Extensor digitorum brevis	Extensor digitorum brevis		
	Extensor hallucis brevis	Extensor hallucis brevis		
	Plantar muscles			
	Abductor digiti minimi		Abductor digiti minimi	
	Abductor hallucis		Abductor hallucis	
	Dorsal interossei	Dorsal interossei	Dorsal interossei	
	Flexor digiti minimi brevis		Flexor digiti minimi brevis	
	Flexor digitorum brevis		Flexor digitorum brevis	
	Flexor hallucis brevis		Flexor hallucis brevis	
	Lumbricals	Lumbricals	Lumbricals	
	Quadratus plantae		Quadratus plantae	
	Plantar interossei	Plantar interossei	Plantar interossei	

Chapter 13. Diseases of the Musculoskeletal System and Connective Tissue (M00–M99)

NOTE   Use an external cause code following the code for the musculoskeletal condition, if applicable, to identify the cause of the musculoskeletal condition

EXCLUDES 2   *arthropathic psoriasis (L40.5-)*
certain conditions originating in the perinatal period (P04-P96)
certain infectious and parasitic diseases (A00-B99)
compartment syndrome (traumatic) (T79.A-)
complications of pregnancy, childbirth and the puerperium (O00-O9A)
congenital malformations, deformations, and chromosomal abnormalities (Q00-Q99)
endocrine, nutritional and metabolic diseases (E00-E88)
injury, poisoning and certain other consequences of external causes (S00-T88)
neoplasms (C00-D49)
symptoms, signs and abnormal clinical and laboratory findings, not elsewhere classified (R00-R94)

This chapter contains the following blocks:

M00-M02   Infectious arthropathies
M04   Autoinflammatory syndromes
M05-M14   Inflammatory polyarthropathies
M15-M19   Osteoarthritis
M20-M25   Other joint disorders
M26-M27   Dentofacial anomalies [including malocclusion] and other disorders of jaw
M30-M36   Systemic connective tissue disorders
M40-M43   Deforming dorsopathies
M45-M49   Spondylopathies
M50-M54   Other dorsopathies
M60-M63   Disorders of muscles
M65-M67   Disorders of synovium and tendon
M70-M79   Other soft tissue disorders
M80-M85   Disorders of bone density and structure
M86-M90   Other osteopathies
M91-M94   Chondropathies
M95   Other disorders of the musculoskeletal system and connective tissue
M96   Intraoperative and postprocedural complications and disorders of musculoskeletal system, not elsewhere classified
M97   Periprosthetic fracture around internal prosthetic joint
M99   Biomechanical lesions, not elsewhere classified

ARTHROPATHIES (M00-M25)

INCLUDES   disorders affecting predominantly peripheral (limb) joints

Infectious arthropathies (M00-M02)

NOTE   This block comprises arthropathies due to microbiological agents. Distinction is made between the following types of etiological relationship:

a) direct infection of joint, where organisms invade synovial tissue and microbial antigen is present in the joint;

b) indirect infection, which may be of two types: a reactive arthropathy, where microbial infection of the body is established but neither organisms nor antigens can be identified in the joint, and a postinfective arthropathy, where microbial antigen is present but recovery of an organism is inconstant and evidence of local multiplication is lacking.

✓4th **M00 Pyogenic arthritis**

DEF: Pyogenic: Relating to or involving pus production, often referred to as suppurative or purulent.

✓5th **M00.0 Staphylococcal arthritis and polyarthritis**

Use additional code (B95.61-B95.8) to identify bacterial agent

EXCLUDES 2   *infection and inflammatory reaction due to internal joint prosthesis (T84.5-)*

M00.00   Staphylococcal arthritis, unspecified joint
✓6th M00.01   Staphylococcal arthritis, shoulder

M00.011   Staphylococcal arthritis, right shoulder
M00.012   Staphylococcal arthritis, left shoulder
M00.019   Staphylococcal arthritis, unspecified shoulder

✓6th M00.02   Staphylococcal arthritis, elbow

M00.021   Staphylococcal arthritis, right elbow
M00.022   Staphylococcal arthritis, left elbow
M00.029   Staphylococcal arthritis, unspecified elbow

✓6th M00.03   Staphylococcal arthritis, wrist

Staphylococcal arthritis of carpal bones
M00.031   Staphylococcal arthritis, right wrist
M00.032   Staphylococcal arthritis, left wrist

M00.039   Staphylococcal arthritis, unspecified wrist
✓6th M00.04   Staphylococcal arthritis, hand

Staphylococcal arthritis of metacarpus and phalanges
M00.041   Staphylococcal arthritis, right hand
M00.042   Staphylococcal arthritis, left hand
M00.049   Staphylococcal arthritis, unspecified hand

✓6th M00.05   Staphylococcal arthritis, hip

M00.051   Staphylococcal arthritis, right hip
M00.052   Staphylococcal arthritis, left hip
M00.059   Staphylococcal arthritis, unspecified hip

✓6th M00.06   Staphylococcal arthritis, knee

M00.061   Staphylococcal arthritis, right knee
M00.062   Staphylococcal arthritis, left knee
M00.069   Staphylococcal arthritis, unspecified knee

✓6th M00.07   Staphylococcal arthritis, ankle and foot

Staphylococcal arthritis, tarsus, metatarsus and phalanges
M00.071   Staphylococcal arthritis, right ankle and foot
M00.072   Staphylococcal arthritis, left ankle and foot
M00.079   Staphylococcal arthritis, unspecified ankle and foot

M00.08   Staphylococcal arthritis, vertebrae
M00.09   Staphylococcal polyarthritis

✓5th **M00.1 Pneumococcal arthritis and polyarthritis**

M00.10   Pneumococcal arthritis, unspecified joint
✓6th M00.11   Pneumococcal arthritis, shoulder

M00.111   Pneumococcal arthritis, right shoulder
M00.112   Pneumococcal arthritis, left shoulder
M00.119   Pneumococcal arthritis, unspecified shoulder

✓6th M00.12   Pneumococcal arthritis, elbow

M00.121   Pneumococcal arthritis, right elbow
M00.122   Pneumococcal arthritis, left elbow
M00.129   Pneumococcal arthritis, unspecified elbow

✓6th M00.13   Pneumococcal arthritis, wrist

Pneumococcal arthritis of carpal bones
M00.131   Pneumococcal arthritis, right wrist
M00.132   Pneumococcal arthritis, left wrist
M00.139   Pneumococcal arthritis, unspecified wrist

✓6th M00.14   Pneumococcal arthritis, hand

Pneumococcal arthritis of metacarpus and phalanges
M00.141   Pneumococcal arthritis, right hand
M00.142   Pneumococcal arthritis, left hand
M00.149   Pneumococcal arthritis, unspecified hand

✓6th M00.15   Pneumococcal arthritis, hip

M00.151   Pneumococcal arthritis, right hip
M00.152   Pneumococcal arthritis, left hip
M00.159   Pneumococcal arthritis, unspecified hip

✓6th M00.16   Pneumococcal arthritis, knee

M00.161   Pneumococcal arthritis, right knee
M00.162   Pneumococcal arthritis, left knee
M00.169   Pneumococcal arthritis, unspecified knee

✓6th M00.17   Pneumococcal arthritis, ankle and foot

Pneumococcal arthritis, tarsus, metatarsus and phalanges
M00.171   Pneumococcal arthritis, right ankle and foot
M00.172   Pneumococcal arthritis, left ankle and foot
M00.179   Pneumococcal arthritis, unspecified ankle and foot

M00.18   Pneumococcal arthritis, vertebrae
M00.19   Pneumococcal polyarthritis

✓5th **M00.2 Other streptococcal arthritis and polyarthritis**

Use additional code (B95.0-B95.2, B95.4-B95.5) to identify bacterial agent

M00.20   Other streptococcal arthritis, unspecified joint
✓6th M00.21   Other streptococcal arthritis, shoulder

M00.211   Other streptococcal arthritis, right shoulder
M00.212   Other streptococcal arthritis, left shoulder
M00.219   Other streptococcal arthritis, unspecified shoulder

---

☑ Additional Character Required   ✓x7th Placeholder Alert   Manifestation   Unspecified Dx   ▶◀ Revised Text   ● New Code   ▲ Revised Title

Chapter 13. Diseases of the Musculoskeletal System and Connective Tissue

√6ᵗʰ **M00.22 Other streptococcal arthritis,** elbow

     M00.221 Other streptococcal arthritis, right elbow
     M00.222 Other streptococcal arthritis, left elbow
     M00.229 Other streptococcal arthritis, unspecified elbow

√6ᵗʰ **M00.23 Other streptococcal arthritis,** wrist

     Other streptococcal arthritis of carpal bones
     M00.231 Other streptococcal arthritis, right wrist
     M00.232 Other streptococcal arthritis, left wrist
     M00.239 Other streptococcal arthritis, unspecified wrist

√6ᵗʰ **M00.24 Other streptococcal arthritis,** hand

     Other streptococcal arthritis metacarpus and phalanges
     M00.241 Other streptococcal arthritis, right hand
     M00.242 Other streptococcal arthritis, left hand
     M00.249 Other streptococcal arthritis, unspecified hand

√6ᵗʰ **M00.25 Other streptococcal arthritis,** hip

     M00.251 Other streptococcal arthritis, right hip
     M00.252 Other streptococcal arthritis, left hip
     M00.259 Other streptococcal arthritis, unspecified hip

√6ᵗʰ **M00.26 Other streptococcal arthritis,** knee

     M00.261 Other streptococcal arthritis, right knee
     M00.262 Other streptococcal arthritis, left knee
     M00.269 Other streptococcal arthritis, unspecified knee

√6ᵗʰ **M00.27 Other streptococcal arthritis,** ankle and foot

     Other streptococcal arthritis, tarsus, metatarsus and phalanges
     M00.271 Other streptococcal arthritis, right ankle and foot
     M00.272 Other streptococcal arthritis, left ankle and foot
     M00.279 Other streptococcal arthritis, unspecified ankle and foot

     M00.28 Other streptococcal arthritis, vertebrae
     M00.29 Other streptococcal polyarthritis

√5ᵗʰ **M00.8 Arthritis and polyarthritis due to other bacteria**

     Use additional code (B96) to identify bacteria

     M00.80 Arthritis due to other bacteria, unspecified joint

√6ᵗʰ **M00.81 Arthritis due to other bacteria,** shoulder

     M00.811 Arthritis due to other bacteria, right shoulder
     M00.812 Arthritis due to other bacteria, left shoulder
     M00.819 Arthritis due to other bacteria, unspecified shoulder

√6ᵗʰ **M00.82 Arthritis due to other bacteria,** elbow

     M00.821 Arthritis due to other bacteria, right elbow
     M00.822 Arthritis due to other bacteria, left elbow
     M00.829 Arthritis due to other bacteria, unspecified elbow

√6ᵗʰ **M00.83 Arthritis due to other bacteria,** wrist

     Arthritis due to other bacteria, carpal bones
     M00.831 Arthritis due to other bacteria, right wrist
     M00.832 Arthritis due to other bacteria, left wrist
     M00.839 Arthritis due to other bacteria, unspecified wrist

√6ᵗʰ **M00.84 Arthritis due to other bacteria,** hand

     Arthritis due to other bacteria, metacarpus and phalanges
     M00.841 Arthritis due to other bacteria, right hand
     M00.842 Arthritis due to other bacteria, left hand
     M00.849 Arthritis due to other bacteria, unspecified hand

√6ᵗʰ **M00.85 Arthritis due to other bacteria,** hip

     M00.851 Arthritis due to other bacteria, right hip
     M00.852 Arthritis due to other bacteria, left hip
     M00.859 Arthritis due to other bacteria, unspecified hip

√6ᵗʰ **M00.86 Arthritis due to other bacteria,** knee

     M00.861 Arthritis due to other bacteria, right knee
     M00.862 Arthritis due to other bacteria, left knee
     M00.869 Arthritis due to other bacteria, unspecified knee

√6ᵗʰ **M00.87 Arthritis due to other bacteria,** ankle and foot

     Arthritis due to other bacteria, tarsus, metatarsus, and phalanges
     M00.871 Arthritis due to other bacteria, right ankle and foot
     M00.872 Arthritis due to other bacteria, left ankle and foot
     M00.879 Arthritis due to other bacteria, unspecified ankle and foot

     M00.88 Arthritis due to other bacteria, vertebrae
     M00.89 Polyarthritis due to other bacteria

M00.9 Pyogenic arthritis, unspecified

     Infective arthritis NOS

√4ᵗʰ **M01 Direct infections of joint in infectious and parasitic diseases classified elsewhere**

     Code first underlying disease, such as:
     leprosy [Hansen's disease] (A30.-)
     mycoses (B35-B49)
     O'nyong-nyong fever (A92.1)
     paratyphoid fever (A01.1-A01.4)

     EXCLUDES 1   *arthropathy in Lyme disease (A69.23)*
         gonococcal arthritis (A54.42)
         meningococcal arthritis (A39.83)
         mumps arthritis (B26.85)
         postinfective arthropathy (M02.-)
         postmeningococcal arthritis (A39.84)
         reactive arthritis (M02.3)
         rubella arthritis (B06.82)
         sarcoidosis arthritis (D86.86)
         typhoid fever arthritis (A01.04)
         tuberculosis arthritis (A18.01-A18.02)

√5ᵗʰ **M01.X Direct infection of joint in infectious and parasitic diseases classified elsewhere**

     M01.X0 Direct infection of unspecified joint in infectious and parasitic diseases classified elsewhere

√6ᵗʰ **M01.X1 Direct infection of** shoulder **joint in infectious and parasitic diseases classified elsewhere**

     M01.X11 Direct infection of right shoulder in infectious and parasitic diseases classified elsewhere
     M01.X12 Direct infection of left shoulder in infectious and parasitic diseases classified elsewhere
     M01.X19 Direct infection of unspecified shoulder in infectious and parasitic diseases classified elsewhere

√6ᵗʰ **M01.X2 Direct infection of** elbow **in infectious and parasitic diseases classified elsewhere**

     M01.X21 Direct infection of right elbow in infectious and parasitic diseases classified elsewhere
     M01.X22 Direct infection of left elbow in infectious and parasitic diseases classified elsewhere
     M01.X29 Direct infection of unspecified elbow in infectious and parasitic diseases classified elsewhere

√6ᵗʰ **M01.X3 Direct infection of** wrist **in infectious and parasitic diseases classified elsewhere**

     Direct infection of carpal bones in infectious and parasitic diseases classified elsewhere
     M01.X31 Direct infection of right wrist in infectious and parasitic diseases classified elsewhere
     M01.X32 Direct infection of left wrist in infectious and parasitic diseases classified elsewhere
     M01.X39 Direct infection of unspecified wrist in infectious and parasitic diseases classified elsewhere

√6ᵗʰ **M01.X4 Direct infection of** hand **in infectious and parasitic diseases classified elsewhere**

     Direct infection of metacarpus and phalanges in infectious and parasitic diseases classified elsewhere
     M01.X41 Direct infection of right hand in infectious and parasitic diseases classified elsewhere
     M01.X42 Direct infection of left hand in infectious and parasitic diseases classified elsewhere
     M01.X49 Direct infection of unspecified hand in infectious and parasitic diseases classified elsewhere

N Newborn: 0   P Pediatric: 0-17   M Maternity: 12-55   A Adult: 15-124   CH Comorbidity High   CL Comorbidity Low   NCDx Noncancer Dx   PDx Primary Dx

744   ICD-10-CM 2020

✓6ᵗʰ **M01.X5** **Direct infection of hip in infectious and parasitic diseases classified elsewhere**

    M01.X51 *Direct infection of right hip in infectious and parasitic diseases classified elsewhere*

    M01.X52 *Direct infection of left hip in infectious and parasitic diseases classified elsewhere*

    M01.X59 *Direct infection of unspecified hip in infectious and parasitic diseases classified elsewhere*

✓6ᵗʰ **M01.X6** **Direct infection of knee in infectious and parasitic diseases classified elsewhere**

    M01.X61 *Direct infection of right knee in infectious and parasitic diseases classified elsewhere*

    M01.X62 *Direct infection of left knee in infectious and parasitic diseases classified elsewhere*

    M01.X69 *Direct infection of unspecified knee in infectious and parasitic diseases classified elsewhere*

✓6ᵗʰ **M01.X7** **Direct infection of ankle and foot in infectious and parasitic diseases classified elsewhere**

    Direct infection of tarsus, metatarsus and phalanges in infectious and parasitic diseases classified elsewhere

    M01.X71 *Direct infection of right ankle and foot in infectious and parasitic diseases classified elsewhere*

    M01.X72 *Direct infection of left ankle and foot in infectious and parasitic diseases classified elsewhere*

    M01.X79 *Direct infection of unspecified ankle and foot in infectious and parasitic diseases classified elsewhere*

    M01.X8 *Direct infection of vertebrae in infectious and parasitic diseases classified elsewhere*

    M01.X9 *Direct infection of multiple joints in infectious and parasitic diseases classified elsewhere*

✓4ᵗʰ **M02** **Postinfective and reactive arthropathies**

    Code first underlying disease, such as:

        congenital syphilis [Clutton's joints] (A50.5)

        enteritis due to Yersinia enterocolitica (A04.6)

        infective endocarditis (I33.0)

        viral hepatitis (B15-B19)

    EXCLUDES 1 *Behçet's disease (M35.2)*

        direct infections of joint in infectious and parasitic diseases classified elsewhere (M01.-)

        mumps arthritis (B26.85)

        postmeningococcal arthritis (A39.84)

        rheumatic fever (I00)

        rubella arthritis (B06.82)

        syphilis arthritis (late) (A52.77)

        tabetic arthropathy [Charcôt's] (A52.16)

✓5ᵗʰ **M02.0** **Arthropathy following intestinal bypass**

    M02.00 **Arthropathy following intestinal bypass, unspecified site**

    ✓6ᵗʰ **M02.01** **Arthropathy following intestinal bypass, shoulder**

        M02.011 **Arthropathy following intestinal bypass, right shoulder**

        M02.012 **Arthropathy following intestinal bypass, left shoulder**

        M02.019 **Arthropathy following intestinal bypass, unspecified shoulder**

    ✓6ᵗʰ **M02.02** **Arthropathy following intestinal bypass, elbow**

        M02.021 **Arthropathy following intestinal bypass, right elbow**

        M02.022 **Arthropathy following intestinal bypass, left elbow**

        M02.029 **Arthropathy following intestinal bypass, unspecified elbow**

    ✓6ᵗʰ **M02.03** **Arthropathy following intestinal bypass, wrist**

        Arthropathy following intestinal bypass, carpal bones

        M02.031 **Arthropathy following intestinal bypass, right wrist**

        M02.032 **Arthropathy following intestinal bypass, left wrist**

        M02.039 **Arthropathy following intestinal bypass, unspecified wrist**

✓6ᵗʰ **M02.04** **Arthropathy following intestinal bypass, hand**

    Arthropathy following intestinal bypass, metacarpals and phalanges

    M02.041 **Arthropathy following intestinal bypass, right hand**

    M02.042 **Arthropathy following intestinal bypass, left hand**

    M02.049 **Arthropathy following intestinal bypass, unspecified hand**

✓6ᵗʰ **M02.05** **Arthropathy following intestinal bypass, hip**

    M02.051 **Arthropathy following intestinal bypass, right hip**

    M02.052 **Arthropathy following intestinal bypass, left hip**

    M02.059 **Arthropathy following intestinal bypass, unspecified hip**

✓6ᵗʰ **M02.06** **Arthropathy following intestinal bypass, knee**

    M02.061 **Arthropathy following intestinal bypass, right knee**

    M02.062 **Arthropathy following intestinal bypass, left knee**

    M02.069 **Arthropathy following intestinal bypass, unspecified knee**

✓6ᵗʰ **M02.07** **Arthropathy following intestinal bypass, ankle and foot**

    Arthropathy following intestinal bypass, tarsus, metatarsus and phalanges

    M02.071 **Arthropathy following intestinal bypass, right ankle and foot**

    M02.072 **Arthropathy following intestinal bypass, left ankle and foot**

    M02.079 **Arthropathy following intestinal bypass, unspecified ankle and foot**

    M02.08 **Arthropathy following intestinal bypass, vertebrae**

    M02.09 **Arthropathy following intestinal bypass, multiple sites**

✓5ᵗʰ **M02.1** **Postdysenteric arthropathy**

    M02.10 **Postdysenteric arthropathy, unspecified site**

    ✓6ᵗʰ **M02.11** **Postdysenteric arthropathy, shoulder**

        M02.111 **Postdysenteric arthropathy, right shoulder**

        M02.112 **Postdysenteric arthropathy, left shoulder**

        M02.119 **Postdysenteric arthropathy, unspecified shoulder**

    ✓6ᵗʰ **M02.12** **Postdysenteric arthropathy, elbow**

        M02.121 **Postdysenteric arthropathy, right elbow**

        M02.122 **Postdysenteric arthropathy, left elbow**

        M02.129 **Postdysenteric arthropathy, unspecified elbow**

    ✓6ᵗʰ **M02.13** **Postdysenteric arthropathy, wrist**

        Postdysenteric arthropathy, carpal bones

        M02.131 **Postdysenteric arthropathy, right wrist**

        M02.132 **Postdysenteric arthropathy, left wrist**

        M02.139 **Postdysenteric arthropathy, unspecified wrist**

    ✓6ᵗʰ **M02.14** **Postdysenteric arthropathy, hand**

        Postdysenteric arthropathy, metacarpus and phalanges

        M02.141 **Postdysenteric arthropathy, right hand**

        M02.142 **Postdysenteric arthropathy, left hand**

        M02.149 **Postdysenteric arthropathy, unspecified hand**

    ✓6ᵗʰ **M02.15** **Postdysenteric arthropathy, hip**

        M02.151 **Postdysenteric arthropathy, right hip**

        M02.152 **Postdysenteric arthropathy, left hip**

        M02.159 **Postdysenteric arthropathy, unspecified hip**

    ✓6ᵗʰ **M02.16** **Postdysenteric arthropathy, knee**

        M02.161 **Postdysenteric arthropathy, right knee**

        M02.162 **Postdysenteric arthropathy, left knee**

        M02.169 **Postdysenteric arthropathy, unspecified knee**

    ✓6ᵗʰ **M02.17** **Postdysenteric arthropathy, ankle and foot**

        Postdysenteric arthropathy, tarsus, metatarsus and phalanges

        M02.171 **Postdysenteric arthropathy, right ankle and foot**

        M02.172 **Postdysenteric arthropathy, left ankle and foot**

☑ Additional Character Required   ✓x7ᵗʰ Placeholder Alert   Manifestation   Unspecified Dx   ▶◀ Revised Text   ● New Code   ▲ Revised Title

ICD-10-CM 2020   745

M02.179   Postdysenteric arthropathy, unspecified ankle and foot
M02.18   Postdysenteric arthropathy, vertebrae
M02.19   Postdysenteric arthropathy, multiple sites
✓5ᵗʰ M02.2   Postimmunization arthropathy

M02.20   Postimmunization arthropathy, unspecified site
✓6ᵗʰ M02.21   Postimmunization arthropathy, shoulder
   M02.211   Postimmunization arthropathy, right shoulder
   M02.212   Postimmunization arthropathy, left shoulder
   M02.219   Postimmunization arthropathy, unspecified shoulder
✓6ᵗʰ M02.22   Postimmunization arthropathy, elbow
   M02.221   Postimmunization arthropathy, right elbow
   M02.222   Postimmunization arthropathy, left elbow
   M02.229   Postimmunization arthropathy, unspecified elbow
✓6ᵗʰ M02.23   Postimmunization arthropathy, wrist
   Postimmunization arthropathy, carpal bones
   M02.231   Postimmunization arthropathy, right wrist
   M02.232   Postimmunization arthropathy, left wrist
   M02.239   Postimmunization arthropathy, unspecified wrist
✓6ᵗʰ M02.24   Postimmunization arthropathy, hand
   Postimmunization arthropathy, metacarpus and phalanges
   M02.241   Postimmunization arthropathy, right hand
   M02.242   Postimmunization arthropathy, left hand
   M02.249   Postimmunization arthropathy, unspecified hand
✓6ᵗʰ M02.25   Postimmunization arthropathy, hip
   M02.251   Postimmunization arthropathy, right hip
   M02.252   Postimmunization arthropathy, left hip
   M02.259   Postimmunization arthropathy, unspecified hip
✓6ᵗʰ M02.26   Postimmunization arthropathy, knee
   M02.261   Postimmunization arthropathy, right knee
   M02.262   Postimmunization arthropathy, left knee
   M02.269   Postimmunization arthropathy, unspecified knee
✓6ᵗʰ M02.27   Postimmunization arthropathy, ankle and foot
   Postimmunization arthropathy, tarsus, metatarsus and phalanges
   M02.271   Postimmunization arthropathy, right ankle and foot
   M02.272   Postimmunization arthropathy, left ankle and foot
   M02.279   Postimmunization arthropathy, unspecified ankle and foot
M02.28   Postimmunization arthropathy, vertebrae
M02.29   Postimmunization arthropathy, multiple sites
✓5ᵗʰ M02.3   Reiter's disease
   Reactive arthritis
   DEF: Arthritis, iridocyclitis, and urethritis, sometimes with diarrhea. While symptoms may recur, arthritis is constant.
M02.30   Reiter's disease, unspecified site
✓6ᵗʰ M02.31   Reiter's disease, shoulder
   M02.311   Reiter's disease, right shoulder
   M02.312   Reiter's disease, left shoulder
   M02.319   Reiter's disease, unspecified shoulder
✓6ᵗʰ M02.32   Reiter's disease, elbow
   M02.321   Reiter's disease, right elbow
   M02.322   Reiter's disease, left elbow
   M02.329   Reiter's disease, unspecified elbow
✓6ᵗʰ M02.33   Reiter's disease, wrist
   Reiter's disease, carpal bones
   M02.331   Reiter's disease, right wrist
   M02.332   Reiter's disease, left wrist
   M02.339   Reiter's disease, unspecified wrist
✓6ᵗʰ M02.34   Reiter's disease, hand
   Reiter's disease, metacarpus and phalanges
   M02.341   Reiter's disease, right hand

M02.342   Reiter's disease, left hand
M02.349   Reiter's disease, unspecified hand
✓6ᵗʰ M02.35   Reiter's disease, hip
   M02.351   Reiter's disease, right hip
   M02.352   Reiter's disease, left hip
   M02.359   Reiter's disease, unspecified hip
✓6ᵗʰ M02.36   Reiter's disease, knee
   M02.361   Reiter's disease, right knee
   M02.362   Reiter's disease, left knee
   M02.369   Reiter's disease, unspecified knee
✓6ᵗʰ M02.37   Reiter's disease, ankle and foot
   Reiter's disease, tarsus, metatarsus and phalanges
   M02.371   Reiter's disease, right ankle and foot
   M02.372   Reiter's disease, left ankle and foot
   M02.379   Reiter's disease, unspecified ankle and foot
M02.38   Reiter's disease, vertebrae
M02.39   Reiter's disease, multiple sites
✓5ᵗʰ M02.8   Other reactive arthropathies

M02.80   Other reactive arthropathies, unspecified site
✓6ᵗʰ M02.81   Other reactive arthropathies, shoulder
   M02.811   Other reactive arthropathies, right shoulder
   M02.812   Other reactive arthropathies, left shoulder
   M02.819   Other reactive arthropathies, unspecified shoulder
✓6ᵗʰ M02.82   Other reactive arthropathies, elbow
   M02.821   Other reactive arthropathies, right elbow
   M02.822   Other reactive arthropathies, left elbow
   M02.829   Other reactive arthropathies, unspecified elbow
✓6ᵗʰ M02.83   Other reactive arthropathies, wrist
   Other reactive arthropathies, carpal bones
   M02.831   Other reactive arthropathies, right wrist
   M02.832   Other reactive arthropathies, left wrist
   M02.839   Other reactive arthropathies, unspecified wrist
✓6ᵗʰ M02.84   Other reactive arthropathies, hand
   Other reactive arthropathies, metacarpus and phalanges
   M02.841   Other reactive arthropathies, right hand
   M02.842   Other reactive arthropathies, left hand
   M02.849   Other reactive arthropathies, unspecified hand
✓6ᵗʰ M02.85   Other reactive arthropathies, hip
   M02.851   Other reactive arthropathies, right hip
   M02.852   Other reactive arthropathies, left hip
   M02.859   Other reactive arthropathies, unspecified hip
✓6ᵗʰ M02.86   Other reactive arthropathies, knee
   M02.861   Other reactive arthropathies, right knee
   M02.862   Other reactive arthropathies, left knee
   M02.869   Other reactive arthropathies, unspecified knee
✓6ᵗʰ M02.87   Other reactive arthropathies, ankle and foot
   Other reactive arthropathies, tarsus, metatarsus and phalanges
   M02.871   Other reactive arthropathies, right ankle and foot
   M02.872   Other reactive arthropathies, left ankle and foot
   M02.879   Other reactive arthropathies, unspecified ankle and foot
M02.88   Other reactive arthropathies, vertebrae
M02.89   Other reactive arthropathies, multiple sites
M02.9   Reactive arthropathy, unspecified

Autoinflammatory syndromes (M04)

✓4ᵗʰ M04 Autoinflammatory syndromes
   EXCLUDES 2   *Crohn's disease (K50.-)*
   AHA: 2016,4Q,37

M04.1 Periodic fever syndromes
Familial Mediterranean fever
Hyperimmunoglobin D syndrome
Mevalonate kinase deficiency
Tumor necrosis factor receptor associated periodic syndrome [TRAPS]

M04.2 Cryopyrin-associated periodic syndromes
Chronic infantile neurological, cutaneous and articular syndrome [CINCA]
Familial cold autoinflammatory syndrome
Familial cold urticaria
Muckle-Wells syndrome
Neonatal onset multisystemic inflammatory disorder [NOMID]

M04.8 Other autoinflammatory syndromes
Blau syndrome
Deficiency of interleukin 1 receptor antagonist [DIRA]
Majeed syndrome
Periodic fever, aphthous stomatitis, pharyngitis, and adenopathy syndrome [PFAPA]
Pyogenic arthritis, pyoderma gangrenosum, and acne syndrome [PAPA]

M04.9 Autoinflammatory syndrome, unspecified

Inflammatory polyarthropathies (M05-M14)

✓4ᵗʰ M05 Rheumatoid arthritis with rheumatoid factor
   EXCLUDES 1   *rheumatic fever (I00)*
      juvenile rheumatoid arthritis (M08.-)
      rheumatoid arthritis of spine (M45.-)
DEF: Rheumatoid arthritis: Autoimmune systemic disease that causes chronic inflammation of the joints and other areas of the body, manifested by inflammatory changes in articular structures and synovial membranes, atrophy, and loss in bone density.

✓5ᵗʰ M05.0 Felty's syndrome
Rheumatoid arthritis with splenoadenomegaly and leukopenia
  M05.00 Felty's syndrome, unspecified site
  ✓6ᵗʰ M05.01 Felty's syndrome, shoulder
    M05.011 Felty's syndrome, right shoulder
    M05.012 Felty's syndrome, left shoulder
    M05.019 Felty's syndrome, unspecified shoulder
  ✓6ᵗʰ M05.02 Felty's syndrome, elbow
    M05.021 Felty's syndrome, right elbow
    M05.022 Felty's syndrome, left elbow
    M05.029 Felty's syndrome, unspecified elbow
  ✓6ᵗʰ M05.03 Felty's syndrome, wrist
    Felty's syndrome, carpal bones
    M05.031 Felty's syndrome, right wrist
    M05.032 Felty's syndrome, left wrist
    M05.039 Felty's syndrome, unspecified wrist
  ✓6ᵗʰ M05.04 Felty's syndrome, hand
    Felty's syndrome, metacarpus and phalanges
    M05.041 Felty's syndrome, right hand
    M05.042 Felty's syndrome, left hand
    M05.049 Felty's syndrome, unspecified hand
  ✓6ᵗʰ M05.05 Felty's syndrome, hip
    M05.051 Felty's syndrome, right hip
    M05.052 Felty's syndrome, left hip
    M05.059 Felty's syndrome, unspecified hip
  ✓6ᵗʰ M05.06 Felty's syndrome, knee
    M05.061 Felty's syndrome, right knee
    M05.062 Felty's syndrome, left knee
    M05.069 Felty's syndrome, unspecified knee
  ✓6ᵗʰ M05.07 Felty's syndrome, ankle and foot
    Felty's syndrome, tarsus, metatarsus and phalanges
    M05.071 Felty's syndrome, right ankle and foot
    M05.072 Felty's syndrome, left ankle and foot
    M05.079 Felty's syndrome, unspecified ankle and foot
  M05.09 Felty's syndrome, multiple sites

✓5ᵗʰ M05.1 Rheumatoid lung disease with rheumatoid arthritis
   DEF: Lung disorders associated with rheumatoid arthritis.
  M05.10 Rheumatoid lung disease with rheumatoid arthritis of unspecified site
  ✓6ᵗʰ M05.11 Rheumatoid lung disease with rheumatoid arthritis of shoulder
    M05.111 Rheumatoid lung disease with rheumatoid arthritis of right shoulder
    M05.112 Rheumatoid lung disease with rheumatoid arthritis of left shoulder
    M05.119 Rheumatoid lung disease with rheumatoid arthritis of unspecified shoulder
  ✓6ᵗʰ M05.12 Rheumatoid lung disease with rheumatoid arthritis of elbow
    M05.121 Rheumatoid lung disease with rheumatoid arthritis of right elbow
    M05.122 Rheumatoid lung disease with rheumatoid arthritis of left elbow
    M05.129 Rheumatoid lung disease with rheumatoid arthritis of unspecified elbow
  ✓6ᵗʰ M05.13 Rheumatoid lung disease with rheumatoid arthritis of wrist
    Rheumatoid lung disease with rheumatoid arthritis, carpal bones
    M05.131 Rheumatoid lung disease with rheumatoid arthritis of right wrist
    M05.132 Rheumatoid lung disease with rheumatoid arthritis of left wrist
    M05.139 Rheumatoid lung disease with rheumatoid arthritis of unspecified wrist
  ✓6ᵗʰ M05.14 Rheumatoid lung disease with rheumatoid arthritis of hand
    Rheumatoid lung disease with rheumatoid arthritis, metacarpus and phalanges
    M05.141 Rheumatoid lung disease with rheumatoid arthritis of right hand
    M05.142 Rheumatoid lung disease with rheumatoid arthritis of left hand
    M05.149 Rheumatoid lung disease with rheumatoid arthritis of unspecified hand
  ✓6ᵗʰ M05.15 Rheumatoid lung disease with rheumatoid arthritis of hip
    M05.151 Rheumatoid lung disease with rheumatoid arthritis of right hip
    M05.152 Rheumatoid lung disease with rheumatoid arthritis of left hip
    M05.159 Rheumatoid lung disease with rheumatoid arthritis of unspecified hip
  ✓6ᵗʰ M05.16 Rheumatoid lung disease with rheumatoid arthritis of knee
    M05.161 Rheumatoid lung disease with rheumatoid arthritis of right knee
    M05.162 Rheumatoid lung disease with rheumatoid arthritis of left knee
    M05.169 Rheumatoid lung disease with rheumatoid arthritis of unspecified knee
  ✓6ᵗʰ M05.17 Rheumatoid lung disease with rheumatoid arthritis of ankle and foot
    Rheumatoid lung disease with rheumatoid arthritis, tarsus, metatarsus and phalanges
    M05.171 Rheumatoid lung disease with rheumatoid arthritis of right ankle and foot
    M05.172 Rheumatoid lung disease with rheumatoid arthritis of left ankle and foot
    M05.179 Rheumatoid lung disease with rheumatoid arthritis of unspecified ankle and foot
  M05.19 Rheumatoid lung disease with rheumatoid arthritis of multiple sites

✓5ᵗʰ M05.2 Rheumatoid vasculitis with rheumatoid arthritis
  M05.20 Rheumatoid vasculitis with rheumatoid arthritis of unspecified site
  ✓6ᵗʰ M05.21 Rheumatoid vasculitis with rheumatoid arthritis of shoulder
    M05.211 Rheumatoid vasculitis with rheumatoid arthritis of right shoulder
    M05.212 Rheumatoid vasculitis with rheumatoid arthritis of left shoulder
    M05.219 Rheumatoid vasculitis with rheumatoid arthritis of unspecified shoulder

√6ᵗʰ **M05.22 Rheumatoid vasculitis with rheumatoid arthritis of elbow**
- **M05.221 Rheumatoid vasculitis with rheumatoid arthritis of right elbow**
- **M05.222 Rheumatoid vasculitis with rheumatoid arthritis of left elbow**
- **M05.229 Rheumatoid vasculitis with rheumatoid arthritis of unspecified elbow**

√6ᵗʰ **M05.23 Rheumatoid vasculitis with rheumatoid arthritis of wrist**
Rheumatoid vasculitis with rheumatoid arthritis, carpal bones
- **M05.231 Rheumatoid vasculitis with rheumatoid arthritis of right wrist**
- **M05.232 Rheumatoid vasculitis with rheumatoid arthritis of left wrist**
- **M05.239 Rheumatoid vasculitis with rheumatoid arthritis of unspecified wrist**

√6ᵗʰ **M05.24 Rheumatoid vasculitis with rheumatoid arthritis of hand**
Rheumatoid vasculitis with rheumatoid arthritis, metacarpus and phalanges
- **M05.241 Rheumatoid vasculitis with rheumatoid arthritis of right hand**
- **M05.242 Rheumatoid vasculitis with rheumatoid arthritis of left hand**
- **M05.249 Rheumatoid vasculitis with rheumatoid arthritis of unspecified hand**

√6ᵗʰ **M05.25 Rheumatoid vasculitis with rheumatoid arthritis of hip**
- **M05.251 Rheumatoid vasculitis with rheumatoid arthritis of right hip**
- **M05.252 Rheumatoid vasculitis with rheumatoid arthritis of left hip**
- **M05.259 Rheumatoid vasculitis with rheumatoid arthritis of unspecified hip**

√6ᵗʰ **M05.26 Rheumatoid vasculitis with rheumatoid arthritis of knee**
- **M05.261 Rheumatoid vasculitis with rheumatoid arthritis of right knee**
- **M05.262 Rheumatoid vasculitis with rheumatoid arthritis of left knee**
- **M05.269 Rheumatoid vasculitis with rheumatoid arthritis of unspecified knee**

√6ᵗʰ **M05.27 Rheumatoid vasculitis with rheumatoid arthritis of ankle and foot**
Rheumatoid vasculitis with rheumatoid arthritis, tarsus, metatarsus and phalanges
- **M05.271 Rheumatoid vasculitis with rheumatoid arthritis of right ankle and foot**
- **M05.272 Rheumatoid vasculitis with rheumatoid arthritis of left ankle and foot**
- **M05.279 Rheumatoid vasculitis with rheumatoid arthritis of unspecified ankle and foot**

M05.29 Rheumatoid vasculitis with rheumatoid arthritis of multiple sites

√5ᵗʰ **M05.3 Rheumatoid heart disease with rheumatoid arthritis**
Rheumatoid carditis
Rheumatoid endocarditis
Rheumatoid myocarditis
Rheumatoid pericarditis

M05.30 Rheumatoid heart disease with rheumatoid arthritis of unspecified site

√6ᵗʰ **M05.31 Rheumatoid heart disease with rheumatoid arthritis of shoulder**
- **M05.311 Rheumatoid heart disease with rheumatoid arthritis of right shoulder**
- **M05.312 Rheumatoid heart disease with rheumatoid arthritis of left shoulder**
- **M05.319 Rheumatoid heart disease with rheumatoid arthritis of unspecified shoulder**

√6ᵗʰ **M05.32 Rheumatoid heart disease with rheumatoid arthritis of elbow**
- **M05.321 Rheumatoid heart disease with rheumatoid arthritis of right elbow**
- **M05.322 Rheumatoid heart disease with rheumatoid arthritis of left elbow**
- **M05.329 Rheumatoid heart disease with rheumatoid arthritis of unspecified elbow**

√6ᵗʰ **M05.33 Rheumatoid heart disease with rheumatoid arthritis of wrist**
Rheumatoid heart disease with rheumatoid arthritis, carpal bones
- **M05.331 Rheumatoid heart disease with rheumatoid arthritis of right wrist**
- **M05.332 Rheumatoid heart disease with rheumatoid arthritis of left wrist**
- **M05.339 Rheumatoid heart disease with rheumatoid arthritis of unspecified wrist**

√6ᵗʰ **M05.34 Rheumatoid heart disease with rheumatoid arthritis of hand**
Rheumatoid heart disease with rheumatoid arthritis, metacarpus and phalanges
- **M05.341 Rheumatoid heart disease with rheumatoid arthritis of right hand**
- **M05.342 Rheumatoid heart disease with rheumatoid arthritis of left hand**
- **M05.349 Rheumatoid heart disease with rheumatoid arthritis of unspecified hand**

√6ᵗʰ **M05.35 Rheumatoid heart disease with rheumatoid arthritis of hip**
- **M05.351 Rheumatoid heart disease with rheumatoid arthritis of right hip**
- **M05.352 Rheumatoid heart disease with rheumatoid arthritis of left hip**
- **M05.359 Rheumatoid heart disease with rheumatoid arthritis of unspecified hip**

√6ᵗʰ **M05.36 Rheumatoid heart disease with rheumatoid arthritis of knee**
- **M05.361 Rheumatoid heart disease with rheumatoid arthritis of right knee**
- **M05.362 Rheumatoid heart disease with rheumatoid arthritis of left knee**
- **M05.369 Rheumatoid heart disease with rheumatoid arthritis of unspecified knee**

√6ᵗʰ **M05.37 Rheumatoid heart disease with rheumatoid arthritis of ankle and foot**
Rheumatoid heart disease with rheumatoid arthritis, tarsus, metatarsus and phalanges
- **M05.371 Rheumatoid heart disease with rheumatoid arthritis of right ankle and foot**
- **M05.372 Rheumatoid heart disease with rheumatoid arthritis of left ankle and foot**
- **M05.379 Rheumatoid heart disease with rheumatoid arthritis of unspecified ankle and foot**

M05.39 Rheumatoid heart disease with rheumatoid arthritis of multiple sites

√5ᵗʰ **M05.4 Rheumatoid myopathy with rheumatoid arthritis**

M05.40 Rheumatoid myopathy with rheumatoid arthritis of unspecified site

√6ᵗʰ **M05.41 Rheumatoid myopathy with rheumatoid arthritis of shoulder**
- **M05.411 Rheumatoid myopathy with rheumatoid arthritis of right shoulder**
- **M05.412 Rheumatoid myopathy with rheumatoid arthritis of left shoulder**
- **M05.419 Rheumatoid myopathy with rheumatoid arthritis of unspecified shoulder**

√6ᵗʰ **M05.42 Rheumatoid myopathy with rheumatoid arthritis of elbow**
- **M05.421 Rheumatoid myopathy with rheumatoid arthritis of right elbow**
- **M05.422 Rheumatoid myopathy with rheumatoid arthritis of left elbow**
- **M05.429 Rheumatoid myopathy with rheumatoid arthritis of unspecified elbow**

√6ᵗʰ **M05.43 Rheumatoid myopathy with rheumatoid arthritis of wrist**
Rheumatoid myopathy with rheumatoid arthritis, carpal bones
- **M05.431 Rheumatoid myopathy with rheumatoid arthritis of right wrist**
- **M05.432 Rheumatoid myopathy with rheumatoid arthritis of left wrist**
- **M05.439 Rheumatoid myopathy with rheumatoid arthritis of unspecified wrist**

√6ᵗʰ **M05.44 Rheumatoid myopathy with rheumatoid arthritis of** hand
> Rheumatoid myopathy with rheumatoid arthritis, metacarpus and phalanges

    M05.441 Rheumatoid myopathy with rheumatoid arthritis of right **hand**
    M05.442 Rheumatoid myopathy with rheumatoid arthritis of left **hand**
    M05.449 Rheumatoid myopathy with rheumatoid arthritis of unspecified hand

√6ᵗʰ **M05.45 Rheumatoid myopathy with rheumatoid arthritis of** hip

    M05.451 Rheumatoid myopathy with rheumatoid arthritis of right **hip**
    M05.452 Rheumatoid myopathy with rheumatoid arthritis of left **hip**
    M05.459 Rheumatoid myopathy with rheumatoid arthritis of unspecified hip

√6ᵗʰ **M05.46 Rheumatoid myopathy with rheumatoid arthritis of** knee

    M05.461 Rheumatoid myopathy with rheumatoid arthritis of right **knee**
    M05.462 Rheumatoid myopathy with rheumatoid arthritis of left **knee**
    M05.469 Rheumatoid myopathy with rheumatoid arthritis of unspecified knee

√6ᵗʰ **M05.47 Rheumatoid myopathy with rheumatoid arthritis of** ankle and foot
> Rheumatoid myopathy with rheumatoid arthritis, tarsus, metatarsus and phalanges

    M05.471 Rheumatoid myopathy with rheumatoid arthritis of right **ankle and foot**
    M05.472 Rheumatoid myopathy with rheumatoid arthritis of left **ankle and foot**
    M05.479 Rheumatoid myopathy with rheumatoid arthritis of unspecified ankle and foot

M05.49 Rheumatoid myopathy with rheumatoid arthritis of multiple sites

√5ᵗʰ **M05.5 Rheumatoid** polyneuropathy with rheumatoid arthritis

    M05.50 Rheumatoid polyneuropathy with rheumatoid arthritis of unspecified site

√6ᵗʰ **M05.51 Rheumatoid polyneuropathy with rheumatoid arthritis of** shoulder

    M05.511 Rheumatoid polyneuropathy with rheumatoid arthritis of right **shoulder**
    M05.512 Rheumatoid polyneuropathy with rheumatoid arthritis of left **shoulder**
    M05.519 Rheumatoid polyneuropathy with rheumatoid arthritis of unspecified shoulder

√6ᵗʰ **M05.52 Rheumatoid polyneuropathy with rheumatoid arthritis of** elbow

    M05.521 Rheumatoid polyneuropathy with rheumatoid arthritis of right **elbow**
    M05.522 Rheumatoid polyneuropathy with rheumatoid arthritis of left **elbow**
    M05.529 Rheumatoid polyneuropathy with rheumatoid arthritis of unspecified elbow

√6ᵗʰ **M05.53 Rheumatoid polyneuropathy with rheumatoid arthritis of** wrist
> Rheumatoid polyneuropathy with rheumatoid arthritis, carpal bones

    M05.531 Rheumatoid polyneuropathy with rheumatoid arthritis of right **wrist**
    M05.532 Rheumatoid polyneuropathy with rheumatoid arthritis of left **wrist**
    M05.539 Rheumatoid polyneuropathy with rheumatoid arthritis of unspecified wrist

√6ᵗʰ **M05.54 Rheumatoid polyneuropathy with rheumatoid arthritis of** hand
> Rheumatoid polyneuropathy with rheumatoid arthritis, metacarpus and phalanges

    M05.541 Rheumatoid polyneuropathy with rheumatoid arthritis of right **hand**
    M05.542 Rheumatoid polyneuropathy with rheumatoid arthritis of left **hand**
    M05.549 Rheumatoid polyneuropathy with rheumatoid arthritis of unspecified hand

√6ᵗʰ **M05.55 Rheumatoid polyneuropathy with rheumatoid arthritis of** hip

    M05.551 Rheumatoid polyneuropathy with rheumatoid arthritis of right **hip**
    M05.552 Rheumatoid polyneuropathy with rheumatoid arthritis of left **hip**
    M05.559 Rheumatoid polyneuropathy with rheumatoid arthritis of unspecified hip

√6ᵗʰ **M05.56 Rheumatoid polyneuropathy with rheumatoid arthritis of** knee

    M05.561 Rheumatoid polyneuropathy with rheumatoid arthritis of right **knee**
    M05.562 Rheumatoid polyneuropathy with rheumatoid arthritis of left **knee**
    M05.569 Rheumatoid polyneuropathy with rheumatoid arthritis of unspecified knee

√6ᵗʰ **M05.57 Rheumatoid polyneuropathy with rheumatoid arthritis of** ankle and foot
> Rheumatoid polyneuropathy with rheumatoid arthritis, tarsus, metatarsus and phalanges

    M05.571 Rheumatoid polyneuropathy with rheumatoid arthritis of right **ankle and foot**
    M05.572 Rheumatoid polyneuropathy with rheumatoid arthritis of left **ankle and foot**
    M05.579 Rheumatoid polyneuropathy with rheumatoid arthritis of unspecified ankle and foot

M05.59 Rheumatoid polyneuropathy with rheumatoid arthritis of multiple sites

√5ᵗʰ **M05.6 Rheumatoid arthritis** with involvement of other organs and systems

    M05.60 Rheumatoid arthritis of unspecified site with involvement of other organs and systems

√6ᵗʰ **M05.61 Rheumatoid arthritis of** shoulder **with involvement of other organs and systems**

    M05.611 Rheumatoid arthritis of right **shoulder with involvement of other organs and systems**
    M05.612 Rheumatoid arthritis of left **shoulder with involvement of other organs and systems**
    M05.619 Rheumatoid arthritis of unspecified shoulder with involvement of other organs and systems

√6ᵗʰ **M05.62 Rheumatoid arthritis of** elbow **with involvement of other organs and systems**

    M05.621 Rheumatoid arthritis of right **elbow with involvement of other organs and systems**
    M05.622 Rheumatoid arthritis of left **elbow with involvement of other organs and systems**
    M05.629 Rheumatoid arthritis of unspecified elbow with involvement of other organs and systems

√6ᵗʰ **M05.63 Rheumatoid arthritis of** wrist **with involvement of other organs and systems**
> Rheumatoid arthritis of carpal bones with involvement of other organs and systems

    M05.631 Rheumatoid arthritis of right **wrist with involvement of other organs and systems**
    M05.632 Rheumatoid arthritis of left **wrist with involvement of other organs and systems**
    M05.639 Rheumatoid arthritis of unspecified wrist with involvement of other organs and systems

√6ᵗʰ **M05.64 Rheumatoid arthritis of** hand **with involvement of other organs and systems**
> Rheumatoid arthritis of metacarpus and phalanges with involvement of other organs and systems

    M05.641 Rheumatoid arthritis of right **hand with involvement of other organs and systems**
    M05.642 Rheumatoid arthritis of left **hand with involvement of other organs and systems**
    M05.649 Rheumatoid arthritis of unspecified hand with involvement of other organs and systems

√6ᵗʰ **M05.65 Rheumatoid arthritis of** hip **with involvement of other organs and systems**

    M05.651 Rheumatoid arthritis of right **hip with involvement of other organs and systems**
    M05.652 Rheumatoid arthritis of left **hip with involvement of other organs and systems**
    M05.659 Rheumatoid arthritis of unspecified hip with involvement of other organs and systems

✔ Additional Character Required   √x7ᵗʰ Placeholder Alert   Manifestation   Unspecified Dx   ►◄ Revised Text   ● New Code   ▲ Revised Title

ICD-10-CM 2020   749

√6ᵗʰ M05.66 Rheumatoid arthritis of knee with involvement of other organs and systems

- M05.661 Rheumatoid arthritis of right knee with involvement of other organs and systems
- M05.662 Rheumatoid arthritis of left knee with involvement of other organs and systems
- M05.669 Rheumatoid arthritis of unspecified knee with involvement of other organs and systems

√6ᵗʰ M05.67 Rheumatoid arthritis of ankle and foot with involvement of other organs and systems

Rheumatoid arthritis of tarsus, metatarsus and phalanges with involvement of other organs and systems

- M05.671 Rheumatoid arthritis of right ankle and foot with involvement of other organs and systems
- M05.672 Rheumatoid arthritis of left ankle and foot with involvement of other organs and systems
- M05.679 Rheumatoid arthritis of unspecified ankle and foot with involvement of other organs and systems

M05.69 Rheumatoid arthritis of multiple sites with involvement of other organs and systems

√5ᵗʰ M05.7 Rheumatoid arthritis with rheumatoid factor without organ or systems involvement

M05.70 Rheumatoid arthritis with rheumatoid factor of unspecified site without organ or systems involvement

√6ᵗʰ M05.71 Rheumatoid arthritis with rheumatoid factor of shoulder without organ or systems involvement

- M05.711 Rheumatoid arthritis with rheumatoid factor of right shoulder without organ or systems involvement
- M05.712 Rheumatoid arthritis with rheumatoid factor of left shoulder without organ or systems involvement
- M05.719 Rheumatoid arthritis with rheumatoid factor of unspecified shoulder without organ or systems involvement

√6ᵗʰ M05.72 Rheumatoid arthritis with rheumatoid factor of elbow without organ or systems involvement

- M05.721 Rheumatoid arthritis with rheumatoid factor of right elbow without organ or systems involvement
- M05.722 Rheumatoid arthritis with rheumatoid factor of left elbow without organ or systems involvement
- M05.729 Rheumatoid arthritis with rheumatoid factor of unspecified elbow without organ or systems involvement

√6ᵗʰ M05.73 Rheumatoid arthritis with rheumatoid factor of wrist without organ or systems involvement

- M05.731 Rheumatoid arthritis with rheumatoid factor of right wrist without organ or systems involvement
- M05.732 Rheumatoid arthritis with rheumatoid factor of left wrist without organ or systems involvement
- M05.739 Rheumatoid arthritis with rheumatoid factor of unspecified wrist without organ or systems involvement

√6ᵗʰ M05.74 Rheumatoid arthritis with rheumatoid factor of hand without organ or systems involvement

- M05.741 Rheumatoid arthritis with rheumatoid factor of right hand without organ or systems involvement
- M05.742 Rheumatoid arthritis with rheumatoid factor of left hand without organ or systems involvement
- M05.749 Rheumatoid arthritis with rheumatoid factor of unspecified hand without organ or systems involvement

√6ᵗʰ M05.75 Rheumatoid arthritis with rheumatoid factor of hip without organ or systems involvement

- M05.751 Rheumatoid arthritis with rheumatoid factor of right hip without organ or systems involvement
- M05.752 Rheumatoid arthritis with rheumatoid factor of left hip without organ or systems involvement

- M05.759 Rheumatoid arthritis with rheumatoid factor of unspecified hip without organ or systems involvement

√6ᵗʰ M05.76 Rheumatoid arthritis with rheumatoid factor of knee without organ or systems involvement

- M05.761 Rheumatoid arthritis with rheumatoid factor of right knee without organ or systems involvement
- M05.762 Rheumatoid arthritis with rheumatoid factor of left knee without organ or systems involvement
- M05.769 Rheumatoid arthritis with rheumatoid factor of unspecified knee without organ or systems involvement

√6ᵗʰ M05.77 Rheumatoid arthritis with rheumatoid factor of ankle and foot without organ or systems involvement

- M05.771 Rheumatoid arthritis with rheumatoid factor of right ankle and foot without organ or systems involvement
- M05.772 Rheumatoid arthritis with rheumatoid factor of left ankle and foot without organ or systems involvement
- M05.779 Rheumatoid arthritis with rheumatoid factor of unspecified ankle and foot without organ or systems involvement

M05.79 Rheumatoid arthritis with rheumatoid factor of multiple sites without organ or systems involvement

√5ᵗʰ M05.8 Other rheumatoid arthritis with rheumatoid factor

M05.80 Other rheumatoid arthritis with rheumatoid factor of unspecified site

√6ᵗʰ M05.81 Other rheumatoid arthritis with rheumatoid factor of shoulder

- M05.811 Other rheumatoid arthritis with rheumatoid factor of right shoulder
- M05.812 Other rheumatoid arthritis with rheumatoid factor of left shoulder
- M05.819 Other rheumatoid arthritis with rheumatoid factor of unspecified shoulder

√6ᵗʰ M05.82 Other rheumatoid arthritis with rheumatoid factor of elbow

- M05.821 Other rheumatoid arthritis with rheumatoid factor of right elbow
- M05.822 Other rheumatoid arthritis with rheumatoid factor of left elbow
- M05.829 Other rheumatoid arthritis with rheumatoid factor of unspecified elbow

√6ᵗʰ M05.83 Other rheumatoid arthritis with rheumatoid factor of wrist

- M05.831 Other rheumatoid arthritis with rheumatoid factor of right wrist
- M05.832 Other rheumatoid arthritis with rheumatoid factor of left wrist
- M05.839 Other rheumatoid arthritis with rheumatoid factor of unspecified wrist

√6ᵗʰ M05.84 Other rheumatoid arthritis with rheumatoid factor of hand

- M05.841 Other rheumatoid arthritis with rheumatoid factor of right hand
- M05.842 Other rheumatoid arthritis with rheumatoid factor of left hand
- M05.849 Other rheumatoid arthritis with rheumatoid factor of unspecified hand

√6ᵗʰ M05.85 Other rheumatoid arthritis with rheumatoid factor of hip

- M05.851 Other rheumatoid arthritis with rheumatoid factor of right hip
- M05.852 Other rheumatoid arthritis with rheumatoid factor of left hip
- M05.859 Other rheumatoid arthritis with rheumatoid factor of unspecified hip

√6ᵗʰ M05.86 Other rheumatoid arthritis with rheumatoid factor of knee

- M05.861 Other rheumatoid arthritis with rheumatoid factor of right knee
- M05.862 Other rheumatoid arthritis with rheumatoid factor of left knee
- M05.869 Other rheumatoid arthritis with rheumatoid factor of unspecified knee

√6ᵗʰ **M05.87** **Other rheumatoid arthritis with rheumatoid factor of** ankle and foot

     M05.871 **Other rheumatoid arthritis with rheumatoid factor of** right **ankle and foot**

     M05.872 **Other rheumatoid arthritis with rheumatoid factor of** left **ankle and foot**

     M05.879 **Other rheumatoid arthritis with rheumatoid factor of unspecified ankle and foot**

     M05.89 **Other rheumatoid arthritis with rheumatoid factor of** multiple sites

     M05.9 **Rheumatoid arthritis with rheumatoid factor, unspecified**

√4ᵗʰ **M06** **Other rheumatoid arthritis**

     DEF: Rheumatoid arthritis: Autoimmune systemic disease that causes chronic inflammation of the joints and other areas of the body, manifested by inflammatory changes in articular structures and synovial membranes, atrophy, and loss in bone density.

√5ᵗʰ **M06.0** **Rheumatoid arthritis** without rheumatoid factor

     M06.00 **Rheumatoid arthritis without rheumatoid factor, unspecified site**

     √6ᵗʰ **M06.01** **Rheumatoid arthritis without rheumatoid factor,** shoulder

         M06.011 **Rheumatoid arthritis without rheumatoid factor,** right **shoulder**

         M06.012 **Rheumatoid arthritis without rheumatoid factor,** left **shoulder**

         M06.019 **Rheumatoid arthritis without rheumatoid factor, unspecified shoulder**

     √6ᵗʰ **M06.02** **Rheumatoid arthritis without rheumatoid factor,** elbow

         M06.021 **Rheumatoid arthritis without rheumatoid factor,** right **elbow**

         M06.022 **Rheumatoid arthritis without rheumatoid factor,** left **elbow**

         M06.029 **Rheumatoid arthritis without rheumatoid factor, unspecified elbow**

     √6ᵗʰ **M06.03** **Rheumatoid arthritis without rheumatoid factor,** wrist

         M06.031 **Rheumatoid arthritis without rheumatoid factor,** right **wrist**

         M06.032 **Rheumatoid arthritis without rheumatoid factor,** left **wrist**

         M06.039 **Rheumatoid arthritis without rheumatoid factor, unspecified wrist**

     √6ᵗʰ **M06.04** **Rheumatoid arthritis without rheumatoid factor,** hand

         M06.041 **Rheumatoid arthritis without rheumatoid factor,** right **hand**

         M06.042 **Rheumatoid arthritis without rheumatoid factor,** left **hand**

         M06.049 **Rheumatoid arthritis without rheumatoid factor, unspecified hand**

     √6ᵗʰ **M06.05** **Rheumatoid arthritis without rheumatoid factor,** hip

         M06.051 **Rheumatoid arthritis without rheumatoid factor,** right **hip**

         M06.052 **Rheumatoid arthritis without rheumatoid factor,** left **hip**

         M06.059 **Rheumatoid arthritis without rheumatoid factor, unspecified hip**

     √6ᵗʰ **M06.06** **Rheumatoid arthritis without rheumatoid factor,** knee

         M06.061 **Rheumatoid arthritis without rheumatoid factor,** right **knee**

         M06.062 **Rheumatoid arthritis without rheumatoid factor,** left **knee**

         M06.069 **Rheumatoid arthritis without rheumatoid factor, unspecified knee**

     √6ᵗʰ **M06.07** **Rheumatoid arthritis without rheumatoid factor,** ankle and foot

         M06.071 **Rheumatoid arthritis without rheumatoid factor,** right **ankle and foot**

         M06.072 **Rheumatoid arthritis without rheumatoid factor,** left **ankle and foot**

         M06.079 **Rheumatoid arthritis without rheumatoid factor, unspecified ankle and foot**

     M06.08 **Rheumatoid arthritis without rheumatoid factor,** vertebrae

     M06.09 **Rheumatoid arthritis without rheumatoid factor,** multiple sites

M06.1 **Adult-onset Still's disease**   A

     EXCLUDES 1   *Still's disease NOS (M08.2-)*

     DEF: Type of systemic arthritis characterized by a transient rash and spiking fevers. This condition may resolve or develop into a chronic condition and may affect internal organs, as well as joints.

     Synonym(s): AOSD

√5ᵗʰ **M06.2** **Rheumatoid bursitis**

     M06.20 **Rheumatoid bursitis, unspecified site**

     √6ᵗʰ **M06.21** **Rheumatoid bursitis,** shoulder

         M06.211 **Rheumatoid bursitis,** right **shoulder**

         M06.212 **Rheumatoid bursitis,** left **shoulder**

         M06.219 **Rheumatoid bursitis, unspecified shoulder**

     √6ᵗʰ **M06.22** **Rheumatoid bursitis,** elbow

         M06.221 **Rheumatoid bursitis,** right **elbow**

         M06.222 **Rheumatoid bursitis,** left **elbow**

         M06.229 **Rheumatoid bursitis, unspecified elbow**

     √6ᵗʰ **M06.23** **Rheumatoid bursitis,** wrist

         M06.231 **Rheumatoid bursitis,** right **wrist**

         M06.232 **Rheumatoid bursitis,** left **wrist**

         M06.239 **Rheumatoid bursitis, unspecified wrist**

     √6ᵗʰ **M06.24** **Rheumatoid bursitis,** hand

         M06.241 **Rheumatoid bursitis,** right **hand**

         M06.242 **Rheumatoid bursitis,** left **hand**

         M06.249 **Rheumatoid bursitis, unspecified hand**

     √6ᵗʰ **M06.25** **Rheumatoid bursitis,** hip

         M06.251 **Rheumatoid bursitis,** right **hip**

         M06.252 **Rheumatoid bursitis,** left **hip**

         M06.259 **Rheumatoid bursitis, unspecified hip**

     √6ᵗʰ **M06.26** **Rheumatoid bursitis,** knee

         M06.261 **Rheumatoid bursitis,** right **knee**

         M06.262 **Rheumatoid bursitis,** left **knee**

         M06.269 **Rheumatoid bursitis, unspecified knee**

     √6ᵗʰ **M06.27** **Rheumatoid bursitis,** ankle and foot

         M06.271 **Rheumatoid bursitis,** right **ankle and foot**

         M06.272 **Rheumatoid bursitis,** left **ankle and foot**

         M06.279 **Rheumatoid bursitis, unspecified ankle and foot**

     M06.28 **Rheumatoid bursitis,** vertebrae

     M06.29 **Rheumatoid bursitis,** multiple sites

√5ᵗʰ **M06.3** **Rheumatoid nodule**

     M06.30 **Rheumatoid nodule, unspecified site**

     √6ᵗʰ **M06.31** **Rheumatoid nodule,** shoulder

         M06.311 **Rheumatoid nodule,** right **shoulder**

         M06.312 **Rheumatoid nodule,** left **shoulder**

         M06.319 **Rheumatoid nodule, unspecified shoulder**

     √6ᵗʰ **M06.32** **Rheumatoid nodule,** elbow

         M06.321 **Rheumatoid nodule,** right **elbow**

         M06.322 **Rheumatoid nodule,** left **elbow**

         M06.329 **Rheumatoid nodule, unspecified elbow**

     √6ᵗʰ **M06.33** **Rheumatoid nodule,** wrist

         M06.331 **Rheumatoid nodule,** right **wrist**

         M06.332 **Rheumatoid nodule,** left **wrist**

         M06.339 **Rheumatoid nodule, unspecified wrist**

     √6ᵗʰ **M06.34** **Rheumatoid nodule,** hand

         M06.341 **Rheumatoid nodule,** right **hand**

         M06.342 **Rheumatoid nodule,** left **hand**

         M06.349 **Rheumatoid nodule, unspecified hand**

     √6ᵗʰ **M06.35** **Rheumatoid nodule,** hip

         M06.351 **Rheumatoid nodule,** right **hip**

         M06.352 **Rheumatoid nodule,** left **hip**

         M06.359 **Rheumatoid nodule, unspecified hip**

     √6ᵗʰ **M06.36** **Rheumatoid nodule,** knee

         M06.361 **Rheumatoid nodule,** right **knee**

         M06.362 **Rheumatoid nodule,** left **knee**

         M06.369 **Rheumatoid nodule, unspecified knee**

     √6ᵗʰ **M06.37** **Rheumatoid nodule,** ankle and foot

         M06.371 **Rheumatoid nodule,** right **ankle and foot**

         M06.372 **Rheumatoid nodule,** left **ankle and foot**

         M06.379 **Rheumatoid nodule, unspecified ankle and foot**

     M06.38 **Rheumatoid nodule,** vertebrae

     M06.39 **Rheumatoid nodule,** multiple sites

☑ Additional Character Required   ✓x7ᵗʰ Placeholder Alert   Manifestation   Unspecified Dx   ►◄ Revised Text   ● New Code   ▲ Revised Title

ICD-10-CM 2020   751

M06.4 Inflammatory polyarthropathy
> EXCLUDES 1 polyarthritis NOS (M13.0)

✓5ᵗʰ **M06.8 Other specified rheumatoid arthritis**

M06.80 Other specified rheumatoid arthritis, unspecified site

✓6ᵗʰ **M06.81 Other specified rheumatoid arthritis, shoulder**
- M06.811 Other specified rheumatoid arthritis, right shoulder
- M06.812 Other specified rheumatoid arthritis, left shoulder
- M06.819 Other specified rheumatoid arthritis, unspecified shoulder

✓6ᵗʰ **M06.82 Other specified rheumatoid arthritis, elbow**
- M06.821 Other specified rheumatoid arthritis, right elbow
- M06.822 Other specified rheumatoid arthritis, left elbow
- M06.829 Other specified rheumatoid arthritis, unspecified elbow

✓6ᵗʰ **M06.83 Other specified rheumatoid arthritis, wrist**
- M06.831 Other specified rheumatoid arthritis, right wrist
- M06.832 Other specified rheumatoid arthritis, left wrist
- M06.839 Other specified rheumatoid arthritis, unspecified wrist

✓6ᵗʰ **M06.84 Other specified rheumatoid arthritis, hand**
- M06.841 Other specified rheumatoid arthritis, right hand
- M06.842 Other specified rheumatoid arthritis, left hand
- M06.849 Other specified rheumatoid arthritis, unspecified hand

✓6ᵗʰ **M06.85 Other specified rheumatoid arthritis, hip**
- M06.851 Other specified rheumatoid arthritis, right hip
- M06.852 Other specified rheumatoid arthritis, left hip
- M06.859 Other specified rheumatoid arthritis, unspecified hip

✓6ᵗʰ **M06.86 Other specified rheumatoid arthritis, knee**
- M06.861 Other specified rheumatoid arthritis, right knee
- M06.862 Other specified rheumatoid arthritis, left knee
- M06.869 Other specified rheumatoid arthritis, unspecified knee

✓6ᵗʰ **M06.87 Other specified rheumatoid arthritis, ankle and foot**
- M06.871 Other specified rheumatoid arthritis, right ankle and foot
- M06.872 Other specified rheumatoid arthritis, left ankle and foot
- M06.879 Other specified rheumatoid arthritis, unspecified ankle and foot

M06.88 Other specified rheumatoid arthritis, vertebrae

M06.89 Other specified rheumatoid arthritis, multiple sites

M06.9 Rheumatoid arthritis, unspecified

✓4ᵗʰ **M07 Enteropathic arthropathies**
> Code also associated enteropathy, such as:
> regional enteritis [Crohn's disease] (K50.-)
> ulcerative colitis (K51.-)
> EXCLUDES 1 psoriatic arthropathies (L40.5-)

✓5ᵗʰ **M07.6 Enteropathic arthropathies**

M07.60 Enteropathic arthropathies, unspecified site

✓6ᵗʰ **M07.61 Enteropathic arthropathies, shoulder**
- M07.611 Enteropathic arthropathies, right shoulder
- M07.612 Enteropathic arthropathies, left shoulder
- M07.619 Enteropathic arthropathies, unspecified shoulder

✓6ᵗʰ **M07.62 Enteropathic arthropathies, elbow**
- M07.621 Enteropathic arthropathies, right elbow
- M07.622 Enteropathic arthropathies, left elbow
- M07.629 Enteropathic arthropathies, unspecified elbow

✓6ᵗʰ **M07.63 Enteropathic arthropathies, wrist**
- M07.631 Enteropathic arthropathies, right wrist
- M07.632 Enteropathic arthropathies, left wrist

M07.639 Enteropathic arthropathies, unspecified wrist

✓6ᵗʰ **M07.64 Enteropathic arthropathies, hand**
- M07.641 Enteropathic arthropathies, right hand
- M07.642 Enteropathic arthropathies, left hand
- M07.649 Enteropathic arthropathies, unspecified hand

✓6ᵗʰ **M07.65 Enteropathic arthropathies, hip**
- M07.651 Enteropathic arthropathies, right hip
- M07.652 Enteropathic arthropathies, left hip
- M07.659 Enteropathic arthropathies, unspecified hip

✓6ᵗʰ **M07.66 Enteropathic arthropathies, knee**
- M07.661 Enteropathic arthropathies, right knee
- M07.662 Enteropathic arthropathies, left knee
- M07.669 Enteropathic arthropathies, unspecified knee

✓6ᵗʰ **M07.67 Enteropathic arthropathies, ankle and foot**
- M07.671 Enteropathic arthropathies, right ankle and foot
- M07.672 Enteropathic arthropathies, left ankle and foot
- M07.679 Enteropathic arthropathies, unspecified ankle and foot

M07.68 Enteropathic arthropathies, vertebrae

M07.69 Enteropathic arthropathies, multiple sites

✓4ᵗʰ **M08 Juvenile arthritis**
> Code also any associated underlying condition, such as:
> regional enteritis [Crohn's disease] (K50.-)
> ulcerative colitis (K51.-)
> EXCLUDES 1 arthropathy in Whipple's disease (M14.8)
> Felty's syndrome (M05.0)
> juvenile dermatomyositis (M33.0-)
> psoriatic juvenile arthropathy (L40.54)

✓5ᵗʰ **M08.0 Unspecified juvenile rheumatoid arthritis**
> Juvenile rheumatoid arthritis with or without rheumatoid factor

M08.00 Unspecified juvenile rheumatoid arthritis of unspecified site

✓6ᵗʰ **M08.01 Unspecified juvenile rheumatoid arthritis, shoulder**
- M08.011 Unspecified juvenile rheumatoid arthritis, right shoulder
- M08.012 Unspecified juvenile rheumatoid arthritis, left shoulder
- M08.019 Unspecified juvenile rheumatoid arthritis, unspecified shoulder

✓6ᵗʰ **M08.02 Unspecified juvenile rheumatoid arthritis of elbow**
- M08.021 Unspecified juvenile rheumatoid arthritis, right elbow
- M08.022 Unspecified juvenile rheumatoid arthritis, left elbow
- M08.029 Unspecified juvenile rheumatoid arthritis, unspecified elbow

✓6ᵗʰ **M08.03 Unspecified juvenile rheumatoid arthritis, wrist**
- M08.031 Unspecified juvenile rheumatoid arthritis, right wrist
- M08.032 Unspecified juvenile rheumatoid arthritis, left wrist
- M08.039 Unspecified juvenile rheumatoid arthritis, unspecified wrist

✓6ᵗʰ **M08.04 Unspecified juvenile rheumatoid arthritis, hand**
- M08.041 Unspecified juvenile rheumatoid arthritis, right hand
- M08.042 Unspecified juvenile rheumatoid arthritis, left hand
- M08.049 Unspecified juvenile rheumatoid arthritis, unspecified hand

✓6ᵗʰ **M08.05 Unspecified juvenile rheumatoid arthritis, hip**
- M08.051 Unspecified juvenile rheumatoid arthritis, right hip
- M08.052 Unspecified juvenile rheumatoid arthritis, left hip
- M08.059 Unspecified juvenile rheumatoid arthritis, unspecified hip

✓6ᵗʰ **M08.06 Unspecified juvenile rheumatoid arthritis, knee**
- M08.061 Unspecified juvenile rheumatoid arthritis, right knee
- M08.062 Unspecified juvenile rheumatoid arthritis, left knee

Ⓝ Newborn: 0 Ⓟ Pediatric: 0-17 Ⓜ Maternity: 12-55 Ⓐ Adult: 15-124   CH Comorbidity High   CL Comorbidity Low   NCDx Noncancer Dx   PDx Primary Dx

752

ICD-10-CM 2020

M08.069 Unspecified juvenile rheumatoid arthritis, unspecified knee

✓6ᵗʰ **M08.07** Unspecified juvenile rheumatoid arthritis, ankle and foot

    M08.071 Unspecified juvenile rheumatoid arthritis, right ankle and foot

    M08.072 Unspecified juvenile rheumatoid arthritis, left ankle and foot

    M08.079 Unspecified juvenile rheumatoid arthritis, unspecified ankle and foot

M08.08 Unspecified juvenile rheumatoid arthritis, vertebrae

M08.09 Unspecified juvenile rheumatoid arthritis, multiple sites

M08.1 Juvenile ankylosing spondylitis

   EXCLUDES 1   ankylosing spondylitis in adults (M45.0-)

✓5ᵗʰ **M08.2** Juvenile rheumatoid arthritis with systemic onset

Still's disease NOS

   EXCLUDES 1   adult-onset Still's disease (M06.1-)

DEF: Systemic juvenile rheumatoid arthritis characterized by a transient rash and spiking fevers that may affect internal organs, as well as joints.

M08.20 Juvenile rheumatoid arthritis with systemic onset, unspecified site

✓6ᵗʰ **M08.21** Juvenile rheumatoid arthritis with systemic onset, shoulder

    M08.211 Juvenile rheumatoid arthritis with systemic onset, right shoulder

    M08.212 Juvenile rheumatoid arthritis with systemic onset, left shoulder

    M08.219 Juvenile rheumatoid arthritis with systemic onset, unspecified shoulder

✓6ᵗʰ **M08.22** Juvenile rheumatoid arthritis with systemic onset, elbow

    M08.221 Juvenile rheumatoid arthritis with systemic onset, right elbow

    M08.222 Juvenile rheumatoid arthritis with systemic onset, left elbow

    M08.229 Juvenile rheumatoid arthritis with systemic onset, unspecified elbow

✓6ᵗʰ **M08.23** Juvenile rheumatoid arthritis with systemic onset, wrist

    M08.231 Juvenile rheumatoid arthritis with systemic onset, right wrist

    M08.232 Juvenile rheumatoid arthritis with systemic onset, left wrist

    M08.239 Juvenile rheumatoid arthritis with systemic onset, unspecified wrist

✓6ᵗʰ **M08.24** Juvenile rheumatoid arthritis with systemic onset, hand

    M08.241 Juvenile rheumatoid arthritis with systemic onset, right hand

    M08.242 Juvenile rheumatoid arthritis with systemic onset, left hand

    M08.249 Juvenile rheumatoid arthritis with systemic onset, unspecified hand

✓6ᵗʰ **M08.25** Juvenile rheumatoid arthritis with systemic onset, hip

    M08.251 Juvenile rheumatoid arthritis with systemic onset, right hip

    M08.252 Juvenile rheumatoid arthritis with systemic onset, left hip

    M08.259 Juvenile rheumatoid arthritis with systemic onset, unspecified hip

✓6ᵗʰ **M08.26** Juvenile rheumatoid arthritis with systemic onset, knee

    M08.261 Juvenile rheumatoid arthritis with systemic onset, right knee

    M08.262 Juvenile rheumatoid arthritis with systemic onset, left knee

    M08.269 Juvenile rheumatoid arthritis with systemic onset, unspecified knee

✓6ᵗʰ **M08.27** Juvenile rheumatoid arthritis with systemic onset, ankle and foot

    M08.271 Juvenile rheumatoid arthritis with systemic onset, right ankle and foot

    M08.272 Juvenile rheumatoid arthritis with systemic onset, left ankle and foot

    M08.279 Juvenile rheumatoid arthritis with systemic onset, unspecified ankle and foot

M08.28 Juvenile rheumatoid arthritis with systemic onset, vertebrae

M08.29 Juvenile rheumatoid arthritis with systemic onset, multiple sites

M08.3 Juvenile rheumatoid polyarthritis (seronegative)

✓5ᵗʰ **M08.4** Pauciarticular juvenile rheumatoid arthritis

M08.40 Pauciarticular juvenile rheumatoid arthritis, unspecified site

✓6ᵗʰ **M08.41** Pauciarticular juvenile rheumatoid arthritis, shoulder

    M08.411 Pauciarticular juvenile rheumatoid arthritis, right shoulder

    M08.412 Pauciarticular juvenile rheumatoid arthritis, left shoulder

    M08.419 Pauciarticular juvenile rheumatoid arthritis, unspecified shoulder

✓6ᵗʰ **M08.42** Pauciarticular juvenile rheumatoid arthritis, elbow

    M08.421 Pauciarticular juvenile rheumatoid arthritis, right elbow

    M08.422 Pauciarticular juvenile rheumatoid arthritis, left elbow

    M08.429 Pauciarticular juvenile rheumatoid arthritis, unspecified elbow

✓6ᵗʰ **M08.43** Pauciarticular juvenile rheumatoid arthritis, wrist

    M08.431 Pauciarticular juvenile rheumatoid arthritis, right wrist

    M08.432 Pauciarticular juvenile rheumatoid arthritis, left wrist

    M08.439 Pauciarticular juvenile rheumatoid arthritis, unspecified wrist

✓6ᵗʰ **M08.44** Pauciarticular juvenile rheumatoid arthritis, hand

    M08.441 Pauciarticular juvenile rheumatoid arthritis, right hand

    M08.442 Pauciarticular juvenile rheumatoid arthritis, left hand

    M08.449 Pauciarticular juvenile rheumatoid arthritis, unspecified hand

✓6ᵗʰ **M08.45** Pauciarticular juvenile rheumatoid arthritis, hip

    M08.451 Pauciarticular juvenile rheumatoid arthritis, right hip

    M08.452 Pauciarticular juvenile rheumatoid arthritis, left hip

    M08.459 Pauciarticular juvenile rheumatoid arthritis, unspecified hip

✓6ᵗʰ **M08.46** Pauciarticular juvenile rheumatoid arthritis, knee

    M08.461 Pauciarticular juvenile rheumatoid arthritis, right knee

    M08.462 Pauciarticular juvenile rheumatoid arthritis, left knee

    M08.469 Pauciarticular juvenile rheumatoid arthritis, unspecified knee

✓6ᵗʰ **M08.47** Pauciarticular juvenile rheumatoid arthritis, ankle and foot

    M08.471 Pauciarticular juvenile rheumatoid arthritis, right ankle and foot

    M08.472 Pauciarticular juvenile rheumatoid arthritis, left ankle and foot

    M08.479 Pauciarticular juvenile rheumatoid arthritis, unspecified ankle and foot

M08.48 Pauciarticular juvenile rheumatoid arthritis, vertebrae

✓5ᵗʰ **M08.8** Other juvenile arthritis

M08.80 Other juvenile arthritis, unspecified site

✓6ᵗʰ **M08.81** Other juvenile arthritis, shoulder

    M08.811 Other juvenile arthritis, right shoulder

    M08.812 Other juvenile arthritis, left shoulder

    M08.819 Other juvenile arthritis, unspecified shoulder

✓6ᵗʰ **M08.82** Other juvenile arthritis, elbow

    M08.821 Other juvenile arthritis, right elbow

    M08.822 Other juvenile arthritis, left elbow

    M08.829 Other juvenile arthritis, unspecified elbow

✓6ᵗʰ **M08.83** Other juvenile arthritis, wrist

    M08.831 Other juvenile arthritis, right wrist

    M08.832 Other juvenile arthritis, left wrist

    M08.839 Other juvenile arthritis, unspecified wrist

✓6ᵗʰ **M08.84** Other juvenile arthritis, hand

    M08.841 Other juvenile arthritis, right hand

    M08.842 Other juvenile arthritis, left hand

    M08.849 Other juvenile arthritis, unspecified hand

☑ Additional Character Required   ✓x7ᵗʰ Placeholder Alert   Manifestation   Unspecified Dx   ►◄ Revised Text   ● New Code   ▲ Revised Title

ICD-10-CM 2020   753

√6ᵗʰ **M08.85** **Other juvenile arthritis,** hip

  M08.851 **Other juvenile arthritis,** right **hip**
  M08.852 **Other juvenile arthritis,** left **hip**
  M08.859 **Other juvenile arthritis,** unspecified **hip**

√6ᵗʰ **M08.86** **Other juvenile arthritis,** knee

  M08.861 **Other juvenile arthritis,** right **knee**
  M08.862 **Other juvenile arthritis,** left **knee**
  M08.869 **Other juvenile arthritis,** unspecified **knee**

√6ᵗʰ **M08.87** **Other juvenile arthritis,** ankle and foot

  M08.871 **Other juvenile arthritis,** right **ankle and foot**
  M08.872 **Other juvenile arthritis,** left **ankle and foot**
  M08.879 **Other juvenile arthritis,** unspecified **ankle and foot**

M08.88 **Other juvenile arthritis, other specified site**
  Other juvenile arthritis, vertebrae

M08.89 **Other juvenile arthritis,** multiple sites

√5ᵗʰ **M08.9** **Juvenile arthritis, unspecified**

  EXCLUDES 1   *juvenile rheumatoid arthritis, unspecified (M08.0-)*

  M08.90 **Juvenile arthritis, unspecified, unspecified site**

√6ᵗʰ **M08.91** **Juvenile arthritis, unspecified,** shoulder

  M08.911 **Juvenile arthritis, unspecified,** right **shoulder**
  M08.912 **Juvenile arthritis, unspecified,** left **shoulder**
  M08.919 **Juvenile arthritis, unspecified, unspecified shoulder**

√6ᵗʰ **M08.92** **Juvenile arthritis, unspecified,** elbow

  M08.921 **Juvenile arthritis, unspecified,** right **elbow**
  M08.922 **Juvenile arthritis, unspecified,** left **elbow**
  M08.929 **Juvenile arthritis, unspecified, unspecified elbow**

√6ᵗʰ **M08.93** **Juvenile arthritis, unspecified,** wrist

  M08.931 **Juvenile arthritis, unspecified,** right **wrist**
  M08.932 **Juvenile arthritis, unspecified,** left **wrist**
  M08.939 **Juvenile arthritis, unspecified, unspecified wrist**

√6ᵗʰ **M08.94** **Juvenile arthritis, unspecified,** hand

  M08.941 **Juvenile arthritis, unspecified,** right **hand**
  M08.942 **Juvenile arthritis, unspecified,** left **hand**
  M08.949 **Juvenile arthritis, unspecified, unspecified hand**

√6ᵗʰ **M08.95** **Juvenile arthritis, unspecified,** hip

  M08.951 **Juvenile arthritis, unspecified,** right **hip**
  M08.952 **Juvenile arthritis, unspecified,** left **hip**
  M08.959 **Juvenile arthritis, unspecified, unspecified hip**

√6ᵗʰ **M08.96** **Juvenile arthritis, unspecified,** knee

  M08.961 **Juvenile arthritis, unspecified,** right **knee**
  M08.962 **Juvenile arthritis, unspecified,** left **knee**
  M08.969 **Juvenile arthritis, unspecified, unspecified knee**

√6ᵗʰ **M08.97** **Juvenile arthritis, unspecified,** ankle and foot

  M08.971 **Juvenile arthritis, unspecified,** right **ankle and foot**
  M08.972 **Juvenile arthritis, unspecified,** left **ankle and foot**
  M08.979 **Juvenile arthritis, unspecified, unspecified ankle and foot**

M08.98 **Juvenile arthritis, unspecified,** vertebrae
M08.99 **Juvenile arthritis, unspecified,** multiple sites

√4ᵗʰ **M1A** **Chronic gout**

  Use additional code to identify:
    autonomic neuropathy in diseases classified elsewhere (G99.0)
    calculus of urinary tract in diseases classified elsewhere (N22)
    cardiomyopathy in diseases classified elsewhere (I43)
    disorders of external ear in diseases classified elsewhere (H61.1-, H62.8-)
    disorders of iris and ciliary body in diseases classified elsewhere (H22)
    glomerular disorders in diseases classified elsewhere (N08)

  EXCLUDES 1   gout NOS (M10.-)
  EXCLUDES 2   acute gout (M10.-)

  The appropriate 7th character is to be added to each code from category M1A.
  0   without tophus (tophi)
  1   with tophus (tophi)

√5ᵗʰ **M1A.0** **Idiopathic** chronic gout

  Chronic gouty bursitis
  Primary chronic gout

  √x7ᵗʰ **M1A.00** **Idiopathic chronic gout, unspecified site**

  √6ᵗʰ **M1A.01** **Idiopathic chronic gout,** shoulder

    √7ᵗʰ **M1A.011** **Idiopathic chronic gout,** right **shoulder**
    √7ᵗʰ **M1A.012** **Idiopathic chronic gout,** left **shoulder**
    √7ᵗʰ **M1A.019** **Idiopathic chronic gout, unspecified shoulder**

  √6ᵗʰ **M1A.02** **Idiopathic chronic gout,** elbow

    √7ᵗʰ **M1A.021** **Idiopathic chronic gout,** right **elbow**
    √7ᵗʰ **M1A.022** **Idiopathic chronic gout,** left **elbow**
    √7ᵗʰ **M1A.029** **Idiopathic chronic gout, unspecified elbow**

  √6ᵗʰ **M1A.03** **Idiopathic chronic gout,** wrist

    √7ᵗʰ **M1A.031** **Idiopathic chronic gout,** right **wrist**
    √7ᵗʰ **M1A.032** **Idiopathic chronic gout,** left **wrist**
    √7ᵗʰ **M1A.039** **Idiopathic chronic gout, unspecified wrist**

  √6ᵗʰ **M1A.04** **Idiopathic chronic gout,** hand

    √7ᵗʰ **M1A.041** **Idiopathic chronic gout,** right **hand**
    √7ᵗʰ **M1A.042** **Idiopathic chronic gout,** left **hand**
    √7ᵗʰ **M1A.049** **Idiopathic chronic gout, unspecified hand**

  √6ᵗʰ **M1A.05** **Idiopathic chronic gout,** hip

    √7ᵗʰ **M1A.051** **Idiopathic chronic gout,** right **hip**
    √7ᵗʰ **M1A.052** **Idiopathic chronic gout,** left **hip**
    √7ᵗʰ **M1A.059** **Idiopathic chronic gout, unspecified hip**

  √6ᵗʰ **M1A.06** **Idiopathic chronic gout,** knee

    √7ᵗʰ **M1A.061** **Idiopathic chronic gout,** right **knee**
    √7ᵗʰ **M1A.062** **Idiopathic chronic gout,** left **knee**
    √7ᵗʰ **M1A.069** **Idiopathic chronic gout, unspecified knee**

  √6ᵗʰ **M1A.07** **Idiopathic chronic gout,** ankle and foot

    √7ᵗʰ **M1A.071** **Idiopathic chronic gout,** right **ankle and foot**
    √7ᵗʰ **M1A.072** **Idiopathic chronic gout,** left **ankle and foot**
    √7ᵗʰ **M1A.079** **Idiopathic chronic gout, unspecified ankle and foot**

  √x7ᵗʰ **M1A.08** **Idiopathic chronic gout,** vertebrae
  √x7ᵗʰ **M1A.09** **Idiopathic chronic gout,** multiple sites

√5ᵗʰ **M1A.1** **Lead-induced** chronic gout

  Code first toxic effects of lead and its compounds (T56.0-)

  √x7ᵗʰ **M1A.10** **Lead-induced chronic gout, unspecified site**

  √6ᵗʰ **M1A.11** **Lead-induced chronic gout,** shoulder

    √7ᵗʰ **M1A.111** **Lead-induced chronic gout,** right **shoulder**
    √7ᵗʰ **M1A.112** **Lead-induced chronic gout,** left **shoulder**
    √7ᵗʰ **M1A.119** **Lead-induced chronic gout, unspecified shoulder**

  √6ᵗʰ **M1A.12** **Lead-induced chronic gout,** elbow

    √7ᵗʰ **M1A.121** **Lead-induced chronic gout,** right **elbow**
    √7ᵗʰ **M1A.122** **Lead-induced chronic gout,** left **elbow**
    √7ᵗʰ **M1A.129** **Lead-induced chronic gout, unspecified elbow**

  √6ᵗʰ **M1A.13** **Lead-induced chronic gout,** wrist

    √7ᵗʰ **M1A.131** **Lead-induced chronic gout,** right **wrist**
    √7ᵗʰ **M1A.132** **Lead-induced chronic gout,** left **wrist**

N Newborn: 0   P Pediatric: 0-17   M Maternity: 12-55   A Adult: 15-124   CH Comorbidity High   CL Comorbidity Low   NCDx Noncancer Dx   PDx Primary Dx

754   ICD-10-CM 2020

√7ᵗʰ **M1A.139** Lead-induced chronic gout, unspecified wrist

√6ᵗʰ **M1A.14** Lead-induced chronic gout, hand

√7ᵗʰ **M1A.141** Lead-induced chronic gout, right hand

√7ᵗʰ **M1A.142** Lead-induced chronic gout, left hand

√7ᵗʰ **M1A.149** Lead-induced chronic gout, unspecified hand

√6ᵗʰ **M1A.15** Lead-induced chronic gout, hip

√7ᵗʰ **M1A.151** Lead-induced chronic gout, right hip

√7ᵗʰ **M1A.152** Lead-induced chronic gout, left hip

√7ᵗʰ **M1A.159** Lead-induced chronic gout, unspecified hip

√6ᵗʰ **M1A.16** Lead-induced chronic gout, knee

√7ᵗʰ **M1A.161** Lead-induced chronic gout, right knee

√7ᵗʰ **M1A.162** Lead-induced chronic gout, left knee

√7ᵗʰ **M1A.169** Lead-induced chronic gout, unspecified knee

√6ᵗʰ **M1A.17** Lead-induced chronic gout, ankle and foot

√7ᵗʰ **M1A.171** Lead-induced chronic gout, right ankle and foot

√7ᵗʰ **M1A.172** Lead-induced chronic gout, left ankle and foot

√7ᵗʰ **M1A.179** Lead-induced chronic gout, unspecified ankle and foot

√x7ᵗʰ **M1A.18** Lead-induced chronic gout, vertebrae

√x7ᵗʰ **M1A.19** Lead-induced chronic gout, multiple sites

√5ᵗʰ **M1A.2** Drug-induced chronic gout

Use additional code for adverse effect, if applicable, to identify drug (T36-T50 with fifth or sixth character 5)

√x7ᵗʰ **M1A.20** Drug-induced chronic gout, unspecified site

√6ᵗʰ **M1A.21** Drug-induced chronic gout, shoulder

√7ᵗʰ **M1A.211** Drug-induced chronic gout, right shoulder

√7ᵗʰ **M1A.212** Drug-induced chronic gout, left shoulder

√7ᵗʰ **M1A.219** Drug-induced chronic gout, unspecified shoulder

√6ᵗʰ **M1A.22** Drug-induced chronic gout, elbow

√7ᵗʰ **M1A.221** Drug-induced chronic gout, right elbow

√7ᵗʰ **M1A.222** Drug-induced chronic gout, left elbow

√7ᵗʰ **M1A.229** Drug-induced chronic gout, unspecified elbow

√6ᵗʰ **M1A.23** Drug-induced chronic gout, wrist

√7ᵗʰ **M1A.231** Drug-induced chronic gout, right wrist

√7ᵗʰ **M1A.232** Drug-induced chronic gout, left wrist

√7ᵗʰ **M1A.239** Drug-induced chronic gout, unspecified wrist

√6ᵗʰ **M1A.24** Drug-induced chronic gout, hand

√7ᵗʰ **M1A.241** Drug-induced chronic gout, right hand

√7ᵗʰ **M1A.242** Drug-induced chronic gout, left hand

√7ᵗʰ **M1A.249** Drug-induced chronic gout, unspecified hand

√6ᵗʰ **M1A.25** Drug-induced chronic gout, hip

√7ᵗʰ **M1A.251** Drug-induced chronic gout, right hip

√7ᵗʰ **M1A.252** Drug-induced chronic gout, left hip

√7ᵗʰ **M1A.259** Drug-induced chronic gout, unspecified hip

√6ᵗʰ **M1A.26** Drug-induced chronic gout, knee

√7ᵗʰ **M1A.261** Drug-induced chronic gout, right knee

√7ᵗʰ **M1A.262** Drug-induced chronic gout, left knee

√7ᵗʰ **M1A.269** Drug-induced chronic gout, unspecified knee

√6ᵗʰ **M1A.27** Drug-induced chronic gout, ankle and foot

√7ᵗʰ **M1A.271** Drug-induced chronic gout, right ankle and foot

√7ᵗʰ **M1A.272** Drug-induced chronic gout, left ankle and foot

√7ᵗʰ **M1A.279** Drug-induced chronic gout, unspecified ankle and foot

√x7ᵗʰ **M1A.28** Drug-induced chronic gout, vertebrae

√x7ᵗʰ **M1A.29** Drug-induced chronic gout, multiple sites

√5ᵗʰ **M1A.3** Chronic gout due to renal impairment

Code first associated renal disease

√x7ᵗʰ **M1A.30** Chronic gout due to renal impairment, unspecified site

√6ᵗʰ **M1A.31** Chronic gout due to renal impairment, shoulder

√7ᵗʰ **M1A.311** Chronic gout due to renal impairment, right shoulder

√7ᵗʰ **M1A.312** Chronic gout due to renal impairment, left shoulder

√7ᵗʰ **M1A.319** Chronic gout due to renal impairment, unspecified shoulder

√6ᵗʰ **M1A.32** Chronic gout due to renal impairment, elbow

√7ᵗʰ **M1A.321** Chronic gout due to renal impairment, right elbow

√7ᵗʰ **M1A.322** Chronic gout due to renal impairment, left elbow

√7ᵗʰ **M1A.329** Chronic gout due to renal impairment, unspecified elbow

√6ᵗʰ **M1A.33** Chronic gout due to renal impairment, wrist

√7ᵗʰ **M1A.331** Chronic gout due to renal impairment, right wrist

√7ᵗʰ **M1A.332** Chronic gout due to renal impairment, left wrist

√7ᵗʰ **M1A.339** Chronic gout due to renal impairment, unspecified wrist

√6ᵗʰ **M1A.34** Chronic gout due to renal impairment, hand

√7ᵗʰ **M1A.341** Chronic gout due to renal impairment, right hand

√7ᵗʰ **M1A.342** Chronic gout due to renal impairment, left hand

√7ᵗʰ **M1A.349** Chronic gout due to renal impairment, unspecified hand

√6ᵗʰ **M1A.35** Chronic gout due to renal impairment, hip

√7ᵗʰ **M1A.351** Chronic gout due to renal impairment, right hip

√7ᵗʰ **M1A.352** Chronic gout due to renal impairment, left hip

√7ᵗʰ **M1A.359** Chronic gout due to renal impairment, unspecified hip

√6ᵗʰ **M1A.36** Chronic gout due to renal impairment, knee

√7ᵗʰ **M1A.361** Chronic gout due to renal impairment, right knee

√7ᵗʰ **M1A.362** Chronic gout due to renal impairment, left knee

√7ᵗʰ **M1A.369** Chronic gout due to renal impairment, unspecified knee

√6ᵗʰ **M1A.37** Chronic gout due to renal impairment, ankle and foot

√7ᵗʰ **M1A.371** Chronic gout due to renal impairment, right ankle and foot

√7ᵗʰ **M1A.372** Chronic gout due to renal impairment, left ankle and foot

√7ᵗʰ **M1A.379** Chronic gout due to renal impairment, unspecified ankle and foot

√x7ᵗʰ **M1A.38** Chronic gout due to renal impairment, vertebrae

√x7ᵗʰ **M1A.39** Chronic gout due to renal impairment, multiple sites

√5ᵗʰ **M1A.4** Other secondary chronic gout

Code first associated condition

√x7ᵗʰ **M1A.40** Other secondary chronic gout, unspecified site

√6ᵗʰ **M1A.41** Other secondary chronic gout, shoulder

√7ᵗʰ **M1A.411** Other secondary chronic gout, right shoulder

√7ᵗʰ **M1A.412** Other secondary chronic gout, left shoulder

√7ᵗʰ **M1A.419** Other secondary chronic gout, unspecified shoulder

√6ᵗʰ **M1A.42** Other secondary chronic gout, elbow

√7ᵗʰ **M1A.421** Other secondary chronic gout, right elbow

√7ᵗʰ **M1A.422** Other secondary chronic gout, left elbow

√7ᵗʰ **M1A.429** Other secondary chronic gout, unspecified elbow

√6ᵗʰ **M1A.43** Other secondary chronic gout, wrist

√7ᵗʰ **M1A.431** Other secondary chronic gout, right wrist

√7ᵗʰ **M1A.432** Other secondary chronic gout, left wrist

√7ᵗʰ **M1A.439** Other secondary chronic gout, unspecified wrist

Chapter 13. Diseases of the Musculoskeletal System and Connective Tissue

√6ᵗʰ **M1A.44 Other secondary chronic gout,** hand

    √7ᵗʰ **M1A.441 Other secondary chronic gout,** right hand

    √7ᵗʰ **M1A.442 Other secondary chronic gout,** left hand

    √7ᵗʰ **M1A.449 Other secondary chronic gout, unspecified hand**

√6ᵗʰ **M1A.45 Other secondary chronic gout,** hip

    √7ᵗʰ **M1A.451 Other secondary chronic gout,** right hip

    √7ᵗʰ **M1A.452 Other secondary chronic gout,** left hip

    √7ᵗʰ **M1A.459 Other secondary chronic gout, unspecified hip**

√6ᵗʰ **M1A.46 Other secondary chronic gout,** knee

    √7ᵗʰ **M1A.461 Other secondary chronic gout,** right knee

    √7ᵗʰ **M1A.462 Other secondary chronic gout,** left knee

    √7ᵗʰ **M1A.469 Other secondary chronic gout, unspecified knee**

√6ᵗʰ **M1A.47 Other secondary chronic gout,** ankle and foot

    √7ᵗʰ **M1A.471 Other secondary chronic gout,** right ankle and foot

    √7ᵗʰ **M1A.472 Other secondary chronic gout,** left ankle and foot

    √7ᵗʰ **M1A.479 Other secondary chronic gout, unspecified ankle and foot**

√×7ᵗʰ **M1A.48 Other secondary chronic gout,** vertebrae

√×7ᵗʰ **M1A.49 Other secondary chronic gout,** multiple sites

√×7ᵗʰ **M1A.9 Chronic gout, unspecified**

√4ᵗʰ **M10 Gout**

Acute gout
Gout attack
Gout flare
Podagra
Use additional code to identify:
    autonomic neuropathy in diseases classified elsewhere (G99.0)
    calculus of urinary tract in diseases classified elsewhere (N22)
    cardiomyopathy in diseases classified elsewhere (I43)
    disorders of external ear in diseases classified elsewhere (H61.1-, H62.8-)
    disorders of iris and ciliary body in diseases classified elsewhere (H22)
    glomerular disorders in diseases classified elsewhere (N08)

EXCLUDES 2   chronic gout (M1A.-)

DEF: Purine and pyrimidine metabolic disorders, manifested by hyperuricemia and recurrent acute inflammatory arthritis. Monosodium urate or monohydrate crystals may be deposited in and around the joints, leading to joint destruction and severe crippling.

√5ᵗʰ **M10.0** Idiopathic gout

Gouty bursitis
Primary gout

M10.00 Idiopathic gout, unspecified site

√6ᵗʰ **M10.01 Idiopathic gout,** shoulder

    M10.011 Idiopathic gout, right shoulder
    M10.012 Idiopathic gout, left shoulder
    M10.019 Idiopathic gout, unspecified shoulder

√6ᵗʰ **M10.02 Idiopathic gout,** elbow

    M10.021 Idiopathic gout, right elbow
    M10.022 Idiopathic gout, left elbow
    M10.029 Idiopathic gout, unspecified elbow

√6ᵗʰ **M10.03 Idiopathic gout,** wrist

    M10.031 Idiopathic gout, right wrist
    M10.032 Idiopathic gout, left wrist
    M10.039 Idiopathic gout, unspecified wrist

√6ᵗʰ **M10.04 Idiopathic gout,** hand

    M10.041 Idiopathic gout, right hand
    M10.042 Idiopathic gout, left hand
    M10.049 Idiopathic gout, unspecified hand

√6ᵗʰ **M10.05 Idiopathic gout,** hip

    M10.051 Idiopathic gout, right hip
    M10.052 Idiopathic gout, left hip
    M10.059 Idiopathic gout, unspecified hip

√6ᵗʰ **M10.06 Idiopathic gout,** knee

    M10.061 Idiopathic gout, right knee
    M10.062 Idiopathic gout, left knee
    M10.069 Idiopathic gout, unspecified knee

√6ᵗʰ **M10.07 Idiopathic gout,** ankle and foot

    M10.071 Idiopathic gout, right ankle and foot
    M10.072 Idiopathic gout, left ankle and foot

    M10.079 Idiopathic gout, unspecified ankle and foot

M10.08 Idiopathic gout, vertebrae

M10.09 Idiopathic gout, multiple sites

√5ᵗʰ **M10.1** Lead-induced gout

Code first toxic effects of lead and its compounds (T56.0-)

M10.10 Lead-induced gout, unspecified site

√6ᵗʰ **M10.11 Lead-induced gout,** shoulder

    M10.111 Lead-induced gout, right shoulder
    M10.112 Lead-induced gout, left shoulder
    M10.119 Lead-induced gout, unspecified shoulder

√6ᵗʰ **M10.12 Lead-induced gout,** elbow

    M10.121 Lead-induced gout, right elbow
    M10.122 Lead-induced gout, left elbow
    M10.129 Lead-induced gout, unspecified elbow

√6ᵗʰ **M10.13 Lead-induced gout,** wrist

    M10.131 Lead-induced gout, right wrist
    M10.132 Lead-induced gout, left wrist
    M10.139 Lead-induced gout, unspecified wrist

√6ᵗʰ **M10.14 Lead-induced gout,** hand

    M10.141 Lead-induced gout, right hand
    M10.142 Lead-induced gout, left hand
    M10.149 Lead-induced gout, unspecified hand

√6ᵗʰ **M10.15 Lead-induced gout,** hip

    M10.151 Lead-induced gout, right hip
    M10.152 Lead-induced gout, left hip
    M10.159 Lead-induced gout, unspecified hip

√6ᵗʰ **M10.16 Lead-induced gout,** knee

    M10.161 Lead-induced gout, right knee
    M10.162 Lead-induced gout, left knee
    M10.169 Lead-induced gout, unspecified knee

√6ᵗʰ **M10.17 Lead-induced gout,** ankle and foot

    M10.171 Lead-induced gout, right ankle and foot
    M10.172 Lead-induced gout, left ankle and foot
    M10.179 Lead-induced gout, unspecified ankle and foot

M10.18 Lead-induced gout, vertebrae

M10.19 Lead-induced gout, multiple sites

√5ᵗʰ **M10.2** Drug-induced gout

Use additional code for adverse effect, if applicable, to identify drug (T36-T50 with fifth or sixth character 5)

M10.20 Drug-induced gout, unspecified site

√6ᵗʰ **M10.21 Drug-induced gout,** shoulder

    M10.211 Drug-induced gout, right shoulder
    M10.212 Drug-induced gout, left shoulder
    M10.219 Drug-induced gout, unspecified shoulder

√6ᵗʰ **M10.22 Drug-induced gout,** elbow

    M10.221 Drug-induced gout, right elbow
    M10.222 Drug-induced gout, left elbow
    M10.229 Drug-induced gout, unspecified elbow

√6ᵗʰ **M10.23 Drug-induced gout,** wrist

    M10.231 Drug-induced gout, right wrist
    M10.232 Drug-induced gout, left wrist
    M10.239 Drug-induced gout, unspecified wrist

√6ᵗʰ **M10.24 Drug-induced gout,** hand

    M10.241 Drug-induced gout, right hand
    M10.242 Drug-induced gout, left hand
    M10.249 Drug-induced gout, unspecified hand

√6ᵗʰ **M10.25 Drug-induced gout,** hip

    M10.251 Drug-induced gout, right hip
    M10.252 Drug-induced gout, left hip
    M10.259 Drug-induced gout, unspecified hip

√6ᵗʰ **M10.26 Drug-induced gout,** knee

    M10.261 Drug-induced gout, right knee
    M10.262 Drug-induced gout, left knee
    M10.269 Drug-induced gout, unspecified knee

√6ᵗʰ **M10.27 Drug-induced gout,** ankle and foot

    M10.271 Drug-induced gout, right ankle and foot
    M10.272 Drug-induced gout, left ankle and foot
    M10.279 Drug-induced gout, unspecified ankle and foot

M10.28 Drug-induced gout, vertebrae

M10.29 Drug-induced gout, multiple sites

N Newborn: 0   P Pediatric: 0-17   M Maternity: 12-55   A Adult: 15-124   CH Comorbidity High   CL Comorbidity Low   NCDx Noncancer Dx   PDx Primary Dx

756   ICD-10-CM 2020

√5ᵗʰ **M10.3** **Gout due to** renal impairment

Code first associated renal disease

M10.30 **Gout due to renal impairment, unspecified site**

√6ᵗʰ **M10.31** **Gout due to renal impairment,** shoulder

M10.311 Gout due to renal impairment, right shoulder

M10.312 Gout due to renal impairment, left shoulder

M10.319 Gout due to renal impairment, unspecified shoulder

√6ᵗʰ **M10.32** **Gout due to renal impairment,** elbow

M10.321 Gout due to renal impairment, right elbow

M10.322 Gout due to renal impairment, left elbow

M10.329 Gout due to renal impairment, unspecified elbow

√6ᵗʰ **M10.33** **Gout due to renal impairment,** wrist

M10.331 Gout due to renal impairment, right wrist

M10.332 Gout due to renal impairment, left wrist

M10.339 Gout due to renal impairment, unspecified wrist

√6ᵗʰ **M10.34** **Gout due to renal impairment,** hand

M10.341 Gout due to renal impairment, right hand

M10.342 Gout due to renal impairment, left hand

M10.349 Gout due to renal impairment, unspecified hand

√6ᵗʰ **M10.35** **Gout due to renal impairment,** hip

M10.351 Gout due to renal impairment, right hip

M10.352 Gout due to renal impairment, left hip

M10.359 Gout due to renal impairment, unspecified hip

√6ᵗʰ **M10.36** **Gout due to renal impairment,** knee

M10.361 Gout due to renal impairment, right knee

M10.362 Gout due to renal impairment, left knee

M10.369 Gout due to renal impairment, unspecified knee

√6ᵗʰ **M10.37** **Gout due to renal impairment,** ankle and foot

M10.371 Gout due to renal impairment, right ankle and foot

M10.372 Gout due to renal impairment, left ankle and foot

M10.379 Gout due to renal impairment, unspecified ankle and foot

M10.38 **Gout due to renal impairment,** vertebrae

M10.39 **Gout due to renal impairment,** multiple sites

√5ᵗʰ **M10.4** **Other** secondary gout

Code first associated condition

M10.40 **Other secondary gout, unspecified site**

√6ᵗʰ **M10.41** **Other secondary gout,** shoulder

M10.411 Other secondary gout, right shoulder

M10.412 Other secondary gout, left shoulder

M10.419 Other secondary gout, unspecified shoulder

√6ᵗʰ **M10.42** **Other secondary gout,** elbow

M10.421 Other secondary gout, right elbow

M10.422 Other secondary gout, left elbow

M10.429 Other secondary gout, unspecified elbow

√6ᵗʰ **M10.43** **Other secondary gout,** wrist

M10.431 Other secondary gout, right wrist

M10.432 Other secondary gout, left wrist

M10.439 Other secondary gout, unspecified wrist

√6ᵗʰ **M10.44** **Other secondary gout,** hand

M10.441 Other secondary gout, right hand

M10.442 Other secondary gout, left hand

M10.449 Other secondary gout, unspecified hand

√6ᵗʰ **M10.45** **Other secondary gout,** hip

M10.451 Other secondary gout, right hip

M10.452 Other secondary gout, left hip

M10.459 Other secondary gout, unspecified hip

√6ᵗʰ **M10.46** **Other secondary gout,** knee

M10.461 Other secondary gout, right knee

M10.462 Other secondary gout, left knee

M10.469 Other secondary gout, unspecified knee

√6ᵗʰ **M10.47** **Other secondary gout,** ankle and foot

M10.471 Other secondary gout, right ankle and foot

M10.472 Other secondary gout, left ankle and foot

M10.479 Other secondary gout, unspecified ankle and foot

M10.48 **Other secondary gout,** vertebrae

M10.49 **Other secondary gout,** multiple sites

M10.9 **Gout, unspecified**

Gout NOS

√4ᵗʰ **M11** **Other crystal arthropathies**

√5ᵗʰ **M11.0** **Hydroxyapatite deposition disease**

DEF: Disease caused by deposits of calcium phosphate crystals in the soft tissues close to the joint (especially tendons) or in the joints. These calcifications can be mono or polyarticular and can cause destruction of the joint involved.

M11.00 **Hydroxyapatite deposition disease, unspecified site**

√6ᵗʰ **M11.01** **Hydroxyapatite deposition disease,** shoulder

M11.011 Hydroxyapatite deposition disease, right shoulder

M11.012 Hydroxyapatite deposition disease, left shoulder

M11.019 Hydroxyapatite deposition disease, unspecified shoulder

√6ᵗʰ **M11.02** **Hydroxyapatite deposition disease,** elbow

M11.021 Hydroxyapatite deposition disease, right elbow

M11.022 Hydroxyapatite deposition disease, left elbow

M11.029 Hydroxyapatite deposition disease, unspecified elbow

√6ᵗʰ **M11.03** **Hydroxyapatite deposition disease,** wrist

M11.031 Hydroxyapatite deposition disease, right wrist

M11.032 Hydroxyapatite deposition disease, left wrist

M11.039 Hydroxyapatite deposition disease, unspecified wrist

√6ᵗʰ **M11.04** **Hydroxyapatite deposition disease,** hand

M11.041 Hydroxyapatite deposition disease, right hand

M11.042 Hydroxyapatite deposition disease, left hand

M11.049 Hydroxyapatite deposition disease, unspecified hand

√6ᵗʰ **M11.05** **Hydroxyapatite deposition disease,** hip

M11.051 Hydroxyapatite deposition disease, right hip

M11.052 Hydroxyapatite deposition disease, left hip

M11.059 Hydroxyapatite deposition disease, unspecified hip

√6ᵗʰ **M11.06** **Hydroxyapatite deposition disease,** knee

M11.061 Hydroxyapatite deposition disease, right knee

M11.062 Hydroxyapatite deposition disease, left knee

M11.069 Hydroxyapatite deposition disease, unspecified knee

√6ᵗʰ **M11.07** **Hydroxyapatite deposition disease,** ankle and foot

M11.071 Hydroxyapatite deposition disease, right ankle and foot

M11.072 Hydroxyapatite deposition disease, left ankle and foot

M11.079 Hydroxyapatite deposition disease, unspecified ankle and foot

M11.08 **Hydroxyapatite deposition disease,** vertebrae

M11.09 **Hydroxyapatite deposition disease,** multiple sites

√5ᵗʰ **M11.1** **Familial chondrocalcinosis**

M11.10 **Familial chondrocalcinosis, unspecified site**

√6ᵗʰ **M11.11** **Familial chondrocalcinosis,** shoulder

M11.111 Familial chondrocalcinosis, right shoulder

M11.112 Familial chondrocalcinosis, left shoulder

M11.119 Familial chondrocalcinosis, unspecified shoulder

√6ᵗʰ **M11.12** **Familial chondrocalcinosis,** elbow

M11.121 Familial chondrocalcinosis, right elbow

M11.122 Familial chondrocalcinosis, left elbow

M11.129 Familial chondrocalcinosis, unspecified elbow

√6ᵗʰ **M11.13** **Familial chondrocalcinosis,** wrist

M11.131 Familial chondrocalcinosis, right wrist

☑ Additional Character Required   √x7ᵗʰ Placeholder Alert   Manifestation   Unspecified Dx   ▶◀ Revised Text   ● New Code   ▲ Revised Title

Chapter 13. Diseases of the Musculoskeletal System and Connective Tissue

M10.3–M11.131

M11.132 Familial chondrocalcinosis, left wrist
M11.139 Familial chondrocalcinosis, unspecified wrist

√6ᵗʰ **M11.14** Familial chondrocalcinosis, hand

M11.141 Familial chondrocalcinosis, right hand
M11.142 Familial chondrocalcinosis, left hand
M11.149 Familial chondrocalcinosis, unspecified hand

√6ᵗʰ **M11.15** Familial chondrocalcinosis, hip

M11.151 Familial chondrocalcinosis, right hip
M11.152 Familial chondrocalcinosis, left hip
M11.159 Familial chondrocalcinosis, unspecified hip

√6ᵗʰ **M11.16** Familial chondrocalcinosis, knee

M11.161 Familial chondrocalcinosis, right knee
M11.162 Familial chondrocalcinosis, left knee
M11.169 Familial chondrocalcinosis, unspecified knee

√6ᵗʰ **M11.17** Familial chondrocalcinosis, ankle and foot

M11.171 Familial chondrocalcinosis, right ankle and foot
M11.172 Familial chondrocalcinosis, left ankle and foot
M11.179 Familial chondrocalcinosis, unspecified ankle and foot

M11.18 Familial chondrocalcinosis, vertebrae
M11.19 Familial chondrocalcinosis, multiple sites

√5ᵗʰ **M11.2** Other chondrocalcinosis

Chondrocalcinosis NOS
AHA: 2018,3Q,20
TIP: Pseudogout is captured with codes in this subcategory.

M11.20 Other chondrocalcinosis, unspecified site

√6ᵗʰ **M11.21** Other chondrocalcinosis, shoulder

M11.211 Other chondrocalcinosis, right shoulder
M11.212 Other chondrocalcinosis, left shoulder
M11.219 Other chondrocalcinosis, unspecified shoulder

√6ᵗʰ **M11.22** Other chondrocalcinosis, elbow

M11.221 Other chondrocalcinosis, right elbow
M11.222 Other chondrocalcinosis, left elbow
M11.229 Other chondrocalcinosis, unspecified elbow

√6ᵗʰ **M11.23** Other chondrocalcinosis, wrist

M11.231 Other chondrocalcinosis, right wrist
M11.232 Other chondrocalcinosis, left wrist
M11.239 Other chondrocalcinosis, unspecified wrist

√6ᵗʰ **M11.24** Other chondrocalcinosis, hand

M11.241 Other chondrocalcinosis, right hand
M11.242 Other chondrocalcinosis, left hand
M11.249 Other chondrocalcinosis, unspecified hand

√6ᵗʰ **M11.25** Other chondrocalcinosis, hip

M11.251 Other chondrocalcinosis, right hip
M11.252 Other chondrocalcinosis, left hip
M11.259 Other chondrocalcinosis, unspecified hip

√6ᵗʰ **M11.26** Other chondrocalcinosis, knee

M11.261 Other chondrocalcinosis, right knee
M11.262 Other chondrocalcinosis, left knee
M11.269 Other chondrocalcinosis, unspecified knee

√6ᵗʰ **M11.27** Other chondrocalcinosis, ankle and foot

M11.271 Other chondrocalcinosis, right ankle and foot
M11.272 Other chondrocalcinosis, left ankle and foot
M11.279 Other chondrocalcinosis, unspecified ankle and foot

M11.28 Other chondrocalcinosis, vertebrae
M11.29 Other chondrocalcinosis, multiple sites

√5ᵗʰ **M11.8** Other specified crystal arthropathies

M11.80 Other specified crystal arthropathies, unspecified site

√6ᵗʰ **M11.81** Other specified crystal arthropathies, shoulder

M11.811 Other specified crystal arthropathies, right shoulder
M11.812 Other specified crystal arthropathies, left shoulder

M11.819 Other specified crystal arthropathies, unspecified shoulder

√6ᵗʰ **M11.82** Other specified crystal arthropathies, elbow

M11.821 Other specified crystal arthropathies, right elbow
M11.822 Other specified crystal arthropathies, left elbow
M11.829 Other specified crystal arthropathies, unspecified elbow

√6ᵗʰ **M11.83** Other specified crystal arthropathies, wrist

M11.831 Other specified crystal arthropathies, right wrist
M11.832 Other specified crystal arthropathies, left wrist
M11.839 Other specified crystal arthropathies, unspecified wrist

√6ᵗʰ **M11.84** Other specified crystal arthropathies, hand

M11.841 Other specified crystal arthropathies, right hand
M11.842 Other specified crystal arthropathies, left hand
M11.849 Other specified crystal arthropathies, unspecified hand

√6ᵗʰ **M11.85** Other specified crystal arthropathies, hip

M11.851 Other specified crystal arthropathies, right hip
M11.852 Other specified crystal arthropathies, left hip
M11.859 Other specified crystal arthropathies, unspecified hip

√6ᵗʰ **M11.86** Other specified crystal arthropathies, knee

M11.861 Other specified crystal arthropathies, right knee
M11.862 Other specified crystal arthropathies, left knee
M11.869 Other specified crystal arthropathies, unspecified knee

√6ᵗʰ **M11.87** Other specified crystal arthropathies, ankle and foot

M11.871 Other specified crystal arthropathies, right ankle and foot
M11.872 Other specified crystal arthropathies, left ankle and foot
M11.879 Other specified crystal arthropathies, unspecified ankle and foot

M11.88 Other specified crystal arthropathies, vertebrae
M11.89 Other specified crystal arthropathies, multiple sites

M11.9 Crystal arthropathy, unspecified

√4ᵗʰ **M12** Other and unspecified arthropathy

EXCLUDES 1   arthrosis (M15-M19)
         cricoarytenoid arthropathy (J38.7)

√5ᵗʰ **M12.0** Chronic postrheumatic arthropathy [Jaccoud]

M12.00 Chronic postrheumatic arthropathy [Jaccoud], unspecified site

√6ᵗʰ **M12.01** Chronic postrheumatic arthropathy [Jaccoud], shoulder

M12.011 Chronic postrheumatic arthropathy [Jaccoud], right shoulder
M12.012 Chronic postrheumatic arthropathy [Jaccoud], left shoulder
M12.019 Chronic postrheumatic arthropathy [Jaccoud], unspecified shoulder

√6ᵗʰ **M12.02** Chronic postrheumatic arthropathy [Jaccoud], elbow

M12.021 Chronic postrheumatic arthropathy [Jaccoud], right elbow
M12.022 Chronic postrheumatic arthropathy [Jaccoud], left elbow
M12.029 Chronic postrheumatic arthropathy [Jaccoud], unspecified elbow

√6ᵗʰ **M12.03** Chronic postrheumatic arthropathy [Jaccoud], wrist

M12.031 Chronic postrheumatic arthropathy [Jaccoud], right wrist
M12.032 Chronic postrheumatic arthropathy [Jaccoud], left wrist
M12.039 Chronic postrheumatic arthropathy [Jaccoud], unspecified wrist

√6ᵗʰ **M12.04** Chronic postrheumatic arthropathy [Jaccoud], hand

M12.041 Chronic postrheumatic arthropathy [Jaccoud], right hand

N Newborn: 0   P Pediatric: 0-17   M Maternity: 12-55   A Adult: 15-124   CH Comorbidity High   CL Comorbidity Low   NCDx Noncancer Dx   PDx Primary Dx

758   ICD-10-CM 2020

M12.042 Chronic postrheumatic arthropathy [Jaccoud], left hand
M12.049 Chronic postrheumatic arthropathy [Jaccoud], unspecified hand
✓6ᵗʰ **M12.05** Chronic postrheumatic arthropathy [Jaccoud], hip
  M12.051 Chronic postrheumatic arthropathy [Jaccoud], right hip
  M12.052 Chronic postrheumatic arthropathy [Jaccoud], left hip
  M12.059 Chronic postrheumatic arthropathy [Jaccoud], unspecified hip
✓6ᵗʰ **M12.06** Chronic postrheumatic arthropathy [Jaccoud], knee
  M12.061 Chronic postrheumatic arthropathy [Jaccoud], right knee
  M12.062 Chronic postrheumatic arthropathy [Jaccoud], left knee
  M12.069 Chronic postrheumatic arthropathy [Jaccoud], unspecified knee
✓6ᵗʰ **M12.07** Chronic postrheumatic arthropathy [Jaccoud], ankle and foot
  M12.071 Chronic postrheumatic arthropathy [Jaccoud], right ankle and foot
  M12.072 Chronic postrheumatic arthropathy [Jaccoud], left ankle and foot
  M12.079 Chronic postrheumatic arthropathy [Jaccoud], unspecified ankle and foot
M12.08 Chronic postrheumatic arthropathy [Jaccoud], other specified site
  Chronic postrheumatic arthropathy [Jaccoud], vertebrae
M12.09 Chronic postrheumatic arthropathy [Jaccoud], multiple sites
✓5ᵗʰ **M12.1** Kaschin-Beck disease
  Osteochondroarthrosis deformans endemica
  M12.10 Kaschin-Beck disease, unspecified site
✓6ᵗʰ **M12.11** Kaschin-Beck disease, shoulder
  M12.111 Kaschin-Beck disease, right shoulder
  M12.112 Kaschin-Beck disease, left shoulder
  M12.119 Kaschin-Beck disease, unspecified shoulder
✓6ᵗʰ **M12.12** Kaschin-Beck disease, elbow
  M12.121 Kaschin-Beck disease, right elbow
  M12.122 Kaschin-Beck disease, left elbow
  M12.129 Kaschin-Beck disease, unspecified elbow
✓6ᵗʰ **M12.13** Kaschin-Beck disease, wrist
  M12.131 Kaschin-Beck disease, right wrist
  M12.132 Kaschin-Beck disease, left wrist
  M12.139 Kaschin-Beck disease, unspecified wrist
✓6ᵗʰ **M12.14** Kaschin-Beck disease, hand
  M12.141 Kaschin-Beck disease, right hand
  M12.142 Kaschin-Beck disease, left hand
  M12.149 Kaschin-Beck disease, unspecified hand
✓6ᵗʰ **M12.15** Kaschin-Beck disease, hip
  M12.151 Kaschin-Beck disease, right hip
  M12.152 Kaschin-Beck disease, left hip
  M12.159 Kaschin-Beck disease, unspecified hip
✓6ᵗʰ **M12.16** Kaschin-Beck disease, knee
  M12.161 Kaschin-Beck disease, right knee
  M12.162 Kaschin-Beck disease, left knee
  M12.169 Kaschin-Beck disease, unspecified knee
✓6ᵗʰ **M12.17** Kaschin-Beck disease, ankle and foot
  M12.171 Kaschin-Beck disease, right ankle and foot
  M12.172 Kaschin-Beck disease, left ankle and foot
  M12.179 Kaschin-Beck disease, unspecified ankle and foot
M12.18 Kaschin-Beck disease, vertebrae
M12.19 Kaschin-Beck disease, multiple sites
✓5ᵗʰ **M12.2** Villonodular synovitis (pigmented)
  M12.20 Villonodular synovitis (pigmented), unspecified site
✓6ᵗʰ **M12.21** Villonodular synovitis (pigmented), shoulder
  M12.211 Villonodular synovitis (pigmented), right shoulder
  M12.212 Villonodular synovitis (pigmented), left shoulder
  M12.219 Villonodular synovitis (pigmented), unspecified shoulder

✓6ᵗʰ **M12.22** Villonodular synovitis (pigmented), elbow
  M12.221 Villonodular synovitis (pigmented), right elbow
  M12.222 Villonodular synovitis (pigmented), left elbow
  M12.229 Villonodular synovitis (pigmented), unspecified elbow
✓6ᵗʰ **M12.23** Villonodular synovitis (pigmented), wrist
  M12.231 Villonodular synovitis (pigmented), right wrist
  M12.232 Villonodular synovitis (pigmented), left wrist
  M12.239 Villonodular synovitis (pigmented), unspecified wrist
✓6ᵗʰ **M12.24** Villonodular synovitis (pigmented), hand
  M12.241 Villonodular synovitis (pigmented), right hand
  M12.242 Villonodular synovitis (pigmented), left hand
  M12.249 Villonodular synovitis (pigmented), unspecified hand
✓6ᵗʰ **M12.25** Villonodular synovitis (pigmented), hip
  M12.251 Villonodular synovitis (pigmented), right hip
  M12.252 Villonodular synovitis (pigmented), left hip
  M12.259 Villonodular synovitis (pigmented), unspecified hip
✓6ᵗʰ **M12.26** Villonodular synovitis (pigmented), knee
  M12.261 Villonodular synovitis (pigmented), right knee
  M12.262 Villonodular synovitis (pigmented), left knee
  M12.269 Villonodular synovitis (pigmented), unspecified knee
✓6ᵗʰ **M12.27** Villonodular synovitis (pigmented), ankle and foot
  M12.271 Villonodular synovitis (pigmented), right ankle and foot
  M12.272 Villonodular synovitis (pigmented), left ankle and foot
  M12.279 Villonodular synovitis (pigmented), unspecified ankle and foot
M12.28 Villonodular synovitis (pigmented), other specified site
  Villonodular synovitis (pigmented), vertebrae
M12.29 Villonodular synovitis (pigmented), multiple sites
✓5ᵗʰ **M12.3** Palindromic rheumatism
  DEF: Sudden and recurring attacks of moderate to severe joint pain and swelling generally occurring in the hands or feet of unknown etiology. After the attack subsides, the joints appear normal again.
  M12.30 Palindromic rheumatism, unspecified site
✓6ᵗʰ **M12.31** Palindromic rheumatism, shoulder
  M12.311 Palindromic rheumatism, right shoulder
  M12.312 Palindromic rheumatism, left shoulder
  M12.319 Palindromic rheumatism, unspecified shoulder
✓6ᵗʰ **M12.32** Palindromic rheumatism, elbow
  M12.321 Palindromic rheumatism, right elbow
  M12.322 Palindromic rheumatism, left elbow
  M12.329 Palindromic rheumatism, unspecified elbow
✓6ᵗʰ **M12.33** Palindromic rheumatism, wrist
  M12.331 Palindromic rheumatism, right wrist
  M12.332 Palindromic rheumatism, left wrist
  M12.339 Palindromic rheumatism, unspecified wrist
✓6ᵗʰ **M12.34** Palindromic rheumatism, hand
  M12.341 Palindromic rheumatism, right hand
  M12.342 Palindromic rheumatism, left hand
  M12.349 Palindromic rheumatism, unspecified hand
✓6ᵗʰ **M12.35** Palindromic rheumatism, hip
  M12.351 Palindromic rheumatism, right hip
  M12.352 Palindromic rheumatism, left hip
  M12.359 Palindromic rheumatism, unspecified hip
✓6ᵗʰ **M12.36** Palindromic rheumatism, knee
  M12.361 Palindromic rheumatism, right knee
  M12.362 Palindromic rheumatism, left knee

Chapter 13. Diseases of the Musculoskeletal System and Connective Tissue

M12.369   Palindromic rheumatism, unspecified knee

√6th   M12.37   **Palindromic rheumatism,** ankle and foot

    M12.371   Palindromic rheumatism, right ankle and foot

    M12.372   Palindromic rheumatism, left ankle and foot

    M12.379   Palindromic rheumatism, unspecified ankle and foot

M12.38   **Palindromic rheumatism, other specified site**
    Palindromic rheumatism, vertebrae

M12.39   **Palindromic rheumatism,** multiple sites

√5th   M12.4   **Intermittent hydrarthrosis**

M12.40   **Intermittent hydrarthrosis, unspecified site**

√6th   M12.41   **Intermittent hydrarthrosis,** shoulder

    M12.411   Intermittent hydrarthrosis, right shoulder
    M12.412   Intermittent hydrarthrosis, left shoulder
    M12.419   Intermittent hydrarthrosis, unspecified shoulder

√6th   M12.42   **Intermittent hydrarthrosis,** elbow

    M12.421   Intermittent hydrarthrosis, right elbow
    M12.422   Intermittent hydrarthrosis, left elbow
    M12.429   Intermittent hydrarthrosis, unspecified elbow

√6th   M12.43   **Intermittent hydrarthrosis,** wrist

    M12.431   Intermittent hydrarthrosis, right wrist
    M12.432   Intermittent hydrarthrosis, left wrist
    M12.439   Intermittent hydrarthrosis, unspecified wrist

√6th   M12.44   **Intermittent hydrarthrosis,** hand

    M12.441   Intermittent hydrarthrosis, right hand
    M12.442   Intermittent hydrarthrosis, left hand
    M12.449   Intermittent hydrarthrosis, unspecified hand

√6th   M12.45   **Intermittent hydrarthrosis,** hip

    M12.451   Intermittent hydrarthrosis, right hip
    M12.452   Intermittent hydrarthrosis, left hip
    M12.459   Intermittent hydrarthrosis, unspecified hip

√6th   M12.46   **Intermittent hydrarthrosis,** knee

    M12.461   Intermittent hydrarthrosis, right knee
    M12.462   Intermittent hydrarthrosis, left knee
    M12.469   Intermittent hydrarthrosis, unspecified knee

√6th   M12.47   **Intermittent hydrarthrosis,** ankle and foot

    M12.471   Intermittent hydrarthrosis, right ankle and foot
    M12.472   Intermittent hydrarthrosis, left ankle and foot
    M12.479   Intermittent hydrarthrosis, unspecified ankle and foot

M12.48   **Intermittent hydrarthrosis, other site**

M12.49   **Intermittent hydrarthrosis,** multiple sites

√5th   M12.5   **Traumatic arthropathy**

    EXCLUDES 1   current injury–see Alphabetic Index
       post-traumatic osteoarthritis of first carpometacarpal joint (M18.2-M18.3)
       post-traumatic osteoarthritis of hip (M16.4-M16.5)
       post-traumatic osteoarthritis of knee (M17.2-M17.3)
       post-traumatic osteoarthritis NOS (M19.1-)
       post-traumatic osteoarthritis of other single joints (M19.1-)

    AHA: 2015,1Q,17

M12.50   **Traumatic arthropathy, unspecified site**

√6th   M12.51   **Traumatic arthropathy,** shoulder

    M12.511   Traumatic arthropathy, right shoulder
    M12.512   Traumatic arthropathy, left shoulder
    M12.519   Traumatic arthropathy, unspecified shoulder

√6th   M12.52   **Traumatic arthropathy,** elbow

    M12.521   Traumatic arthropathy, right elbow
    M12.522   Traumatic arthropathy, left elbow
    M12.529   Traumatic arthropathy, unspecified elbow

√6th   M12.53   **Traumatic arthropathy,** wrist

    M12.531   Traumatic arthropathy, right wrist
    M12.532   Traumatic arthropathy, left wrist

    M12.539   Traumatic arthropathy, unspecified wrist

√6th   M12.54   **Traumatic arthropathy,** hand

    M12.541   Traumatic arthropathy, right hand
    M12.542   Traumatic arthropathy, left hand
    M12.549   Traumatic arthropathy, unspecified hand

√6th   M12.55   **Traumatic arthropathy,** hip

    M12.551   Traumatic arthropathy, right hip
    M12.552   Traumatic arthropathy, left hip
    M12.559   Traumatic arthropathy, unspecified hip

√6th   M12.56   **Traumatic arthropathy,** knee

    M12.561   Traumatic arthropathy, right knee
    M12.562   Traumatic arthropathy, left knee
    M12.569   Traumatic arthropathy, unspecified knee

√6th   M12.57   **Traumatic arthropathy,** ankle and foot

    M12.571   Traumatic arthropathy, right ankle and foot
    M12.572   Traumatic arthropathy, left ankle and foot
    M12.579   Traumatic arthropathy, unspecified ankle and foot

M12.58   **Traumatic arthropathy, other specified site**
    Traumatic arthropathy, vertebrae

M12.59   **Traumatic arthropathy,** multiple sites

√5th   M12.8   **Other specific arthropathies, not elsewhere classified**
    Transient arthropathy

M12.80   **Other specific arthropathies, not elsewhere classified, unspecified site**

√6th   M12.81   **Other specific arthropathies, not elsewhere classified,** shoulder

    M12.811   Other specific arthropathies, not elsewhere classified, right shoulder
    M12.812   Other specific arthropathies, not elsewhere classified, left shoulder
    M12.819   Other specific arthropathies, not elsewhere classified, unspecified shoulder

√6th   M12.82   **Other specific arthropathies, not elsewhere classified,** elbow

    M12.821   Other specific arthropathies, not elsewhere classified, right elbow
    M12.822   Other specific arthropathies, not elsewhere classified, left elbow
    M12.829   Other specific arthropathies, not elsewhere classified, unspecified elbow

√6th   M12.83   **Other specific arthropathies, not elsewhere classified,** wrist

    M12.831   Other specific arthropathies, not elsewhere classified, right wrist
    M12.832   Other specific arthropathies, not elsewhere classified, left wrist
    M12.839   Other specific arthropathies, not elsewhere classified, unspecified wrist

√6th   M12.84   **Other specific arthropathies, not elsewhere classified,** hand

    M12.841   Other specific arthropathies, not elsewhere classified, right hand
    M12.842   Other specific arthropathies, not elsewhere classified, left hand
    M12.849   Other specific arthropathies, not elsewhere classified, unspecified hand

√6th   M12.85   **Other specific arthropathies, not elsewhere classified,** hip

    M12.851   Other specific arthropathies, not elsewhere classified, right hip
    M12.852   Other specific arthropathies, not elsewhere classified, left hip
    M12.859   Other specific arthropathies, not elsewhere classified, unspecified hip

√6th   M12.86   **Other specific arthropathies, not elsewhere classified,** knee

    M12.861   Other specific arthropathies, not elsewhere classified, right knee
    M12.862   Other specific arthropathies, not elsewhere classified, left knee
    M12.869   Other specific arthropathies, not elsewhere classified, unspecified knee

√6th   M12.87   **Other specific arthropathies, not elsewhere classified,** ankle and foot

    M12.871   Other specific arthropathies, not elsewhere classified, right ankle and foot

N Newborn: 0   P Pediatric: 0-17   M Maternity: 12-55   A Adult: 15-124   CH Comorbidity High   CL Comorbidity Low   NCDx Noncancer Dx   PDx Primary Dx

760   ICD-10-CM 2020

M12.872 Other specific arthropathies, not elsewhere classified, left ankle and foot

M12.879 Other specific arthropathies, not elsewhere classified, unspecified ankle and foot

M12.88 Other specific arthropathies, not elsewhere classified, other specified site
Other specific arthropathies, not elsewhere classified, vertebrae

M12.89 Other specific arthropathies, not elsewhere classified, multiple sites

M12.9 Arthropathy, unspecified

✓4ᵗʰ **M13 Other arthritis**
EXCLUDES 1 arthrosis (M15-M19)
osteoarthritis (M15-M19)

M13.0 Polyarthritis, unspecified

✓5ᵗʰ M13.1 Monoarthritis, not elsewhere classified
M13.10 Monoarthritis, not elsewhere classified, unspecified site

✓6ᵗʰ M13.11 Monoarthritis, not elsewhere classified, shoulder
M13.111 Monoarthritis, not elsewhere classified, right shoulder
M13.112 Monoarthritis, not elsewhere classified, left shoulder
M13.119 Monoarthritis, not elsewhere classified, unspecified shoulder

✓6ᵗʰ M13.12 Monoarthritis, not elsewhere classified, elbow
M13.121 Monoarthritis, not elsewhere classified, right elbow
M13.122 Monoarthritis, not elsewhere classified, left elbow
M13.129 Monoarthritis, not elsewhere classified, unspecified elbow

✓6ᵗʰ M13.13 Monoarthritis, not elsewhere classified, wrist
M13.131 Monoarthritis, not elsewhere classified, right wrist
M13.132 Monoarthritis, not elsewhere classified, left wrist
M13.139 Monoarthritis, not elsewhere classified, unspecified wrist

✓6ᵗʰ M13.14 Monoarthritis, not elsewhere classified, hand
M13.141 Monoarthritis, not elsewhere classified, right hand
M13.142 Monoarthritis, not elsewhere classified, left hand
M13.149 Monoarthritis, not elsewhere classified, unspecified hand

✓6ᵗʰ M13.15 Monoarthritis, not elsewhere classified, hip
M13.151 Monoarthritis, not elsewhere classified, right hip
M13.152 Monoarthritis, not elsewhere classified, left hip
M13.159 Monoarthritis, not elsewhere classified, unspecified hip

✓6ᵗʰ M13.16 Monoarthritis, not elsewhere classified, knee
M13.161 Monoarthritis, not elsewhere classified, right knee
M13.162 Monoarthritis, not elsewhere classified, left knee
M13.169 Monoarthritis, not elsewhere classified, unspecified knee

✓6ᵗʰ M13.17 Monoarthritis, not elsewhere classified, ankle and foot
M13.171 Monoarthritis, not elsewhere classified, right ankle and foot
M13.172 Monoarthritis, not elsewhere classified, left ankle and foot
M13.179 Monoarthritis, not elsewhere classified, unspecified ankle and foot

✓5ᵗʰ M13.8 Other specified arthritis
Allergic arthritis
EXCLUDES 1 osteoarthritis (M15-M19)
M13.80 Other specified arthritis, unspecified site

✓6ᵗʰ M13.81 Other specified arthritis, shoulder
M13.811 Other specified arthritis, right shoulder
M13.812 Other specified arthritis, left shoulder
M13.819 Other specified arthritis, unspecified shoulder

✓6ᵗʰ M13.82 Other specified arthritis, elbow
M13.821 Other specified arthritis, right elbow
M13.822 Other specified arthritis, left elbow
M13.829 Other specified arthritis, unspecified elbow

✓6ᵗʰ M13.83 Other specified arthritis, wrist
M13.831 Other specified arthritis, right wrist
M13.832 Other specified arthritis, left wrist
M13.839 Other specified arthritis, unspecified wrist

✓6ᵗʰ M13.84 Other specified arthritis, hand
M13.841 Other specified arthritis, right hand
M13.842 Other specified arthritis, left hand
M13.849 Other specified arthritis, unspecified hand

✓6ᵗʰ M13.85 Other specified arthritis, hip
M13.851 Other specified arthritis, right hip
M13.852 Other specified arthritis, left hip
M13.859 Other specified arthritis, unspecified hip

✓6ᵗʰ M13.86 Other specified arthritis, knee
M13.861 Other specified arthritis, right knee
M13.862 Other specified arthritis, left knee
M13.869 Other specified arthritis, unspecified knee

✓6ᵗʰ M13.87 Other specified arthritis, ankle and foot
M13.871 Other specified arthritis, right ankle and foot
M13.872 Other specified arthritis, left ankle and foot
M13.879 Other specified arthritis, unspecified ankle and foot

M13.88 Other specified arthritis, other site
M13.89 Other specified arthritis, multiple sites

✓4ᵗʰ **M14 Arthropathies in other diseases classified elsewhere**
EXCLUDES 1 arthropathy in:
diabetes mellitus (E08-E13 with .61-)
hematological disorders (M36.2-M36.3)
hypersensitivity reactions (M36.4)
neoplastic disease (M36.1)
neurosyphilis (A52.16)
sarcoidosis (D86.86)
enteropathic arthropathies (M07.-)
juvenile psoriatic arthropathy (L40.54)
lipoid dermatoarthritis (E78.81)

✓5ᵗʰ M14.6 Charcôt's joint
Neuropathic arthropathy
EXCLUDES 1 Charcôt's joint in diabetes mellitus (E08-E13 with .610)
Charcôt's joint in tabes dorsalis (A52.16)
DEF: Progressive neurologic arthropathy in which chronic degeneration of joints in the weight-bearing areas with peripheral hypertrophy occurs as a complication of a neuropathy disorder. Supporting structures relax from a loss of sensation resulting in chronic joint instability.

M14.60 Charcôt's joint, unspecified site

✓6ᵗʰ M14.61 Charcôt's joint, shoulder
M14.611 Charcôt's joint, right shoulder
M14.612 Charcôt's joint, left shoulder
M14.619 Charcôt's joint, unspecified shoulder

✓6ᵗʰ M14.62 Charcôt's joint, elbow
M14.621 Charcôt's joint, right elbow
M14.622 Charcôt's joint, left elbow
M14.629 Charcôt's joint, unspecified elbow

✓6ᵗʰ M14.63 Charcôt's joint, wrist
M14.631 Charcôt's joint, right wrist
M14.632 Charcôt's joint, left wrist
M14.639 Charcôt's joint, unspecified wrist

✓6ᵗʰ M14.64 Charcôt's joint, hand
M14.641 Charcôt's joint, right hand
M14.642 Charcôt's joint, left hand
M14.649 Charcôt's joint, unspecified hand

✓6ᵗʰ M14.65 Charcôt's joint, hip
M14.651 Charcôt's joint, right hip
M14.652 Charcôt's joint, left hip
M14.659 Charcôt's joint, unspecified hip

✓6ᵗʰ M14.66 Charcôt's joint, knee
M14.661 Charcôt's joint, right knee

M14.662 Charcôt's joint, left knee
M14.669 Charcôt's joint, unspecified knee
✓6ᵗʰ M14.67 Charcôt's joint, ankle and foot
M14.671 Charcôt's joint, right ankle and foot
M14.672 Charcôt's joint, left ankle and foot
M14.679 Charcôt's joint, unspecified ankle and foot
M14.68 Charcôt's joint, vertebrae
M14.69 Charcôt's joint, multiple sites
✓5ᵗʰ M14.8 Arthropathies in other specified diseases classified elsewhere
Code first underlying disease, such as:
amyloidosis (E85.-)
erythema multiforme (L51.-)
erythema nodosum (L52)
hemochromatosis (E83.11-)
hyperparathyroidism (E21.-)
hypothyroidism (E00-E03)
sickle-cell disorders (D57.-)
thyrotoxicosis [hyperthyroidism] (E05.-)
Whipple's disease (K90.81)
M14.80 *Arthropathies in other specified diseases classified elsewhere, unspecified site*
✓6ᵗʰ M14.81 Arthropathies in other specified diseases classified elsewhere, shoulder
M14.811 *Arthropathies in other specified diseases classified elsewhere, right shoulder*
M14.812 *Arthropathies in other specified diseases classified elsewhere, left shoulder*
M14.819 *Arthropathies in other specified diseases classified elsewhere, unspecified shoulder*
✓6ᵗʰ M14.82 Arthropathies in other specified diseases classified elsewhere, elbow
M14.821 *Arthropathies in other specified diseases classified elsewhere, right elbow*
M14.822 *Arthropathies in other specified diseases classified elsewhere, left elbow*
M14.829 *Arthropathies in other specified diseases classified elsewhere, unspecified elbow*
✓6ᵗʰ M14.83 Arthropathies in other specified diseases classified elsewhere, wrist
M14.831 *Arthropathies in other specified diseases classified elsewhere, right wrist*
M14.832 *Arthropathies in other specified diseases classified elsewhere, left wrist*
M14.839 *Arthropathies in other specified diseases classified elsewhere, unspecified wrist*
✓6ᵗʰ M14.84 Arthropathies in other specified diseases classified elsewhere, hand
M14.841 *Arthropathies in other specified diseases classified elsewhere, right hand*
M14.842 *Arthropathies in other specified diseases classified elsewhere, left hand*
M14.849 *Arthropathies in other specified diseases classified elsewhere, unspecified hand*
✓6ᵗʰ M14.85 Arthropathies in other specified diseases classified elsewhere, hip
M14.851 *Arthropathies in other specified diseases classified elsewhere, right hip*
M14.852 *Arthropathies in other specified diseases classified elsewhere, left hip*
M14.859 *Arthropathies in other specified diseases classified elsewhere, unspecified hip*
✓6ᵗʰ M14.86 Arthropathies in other specified diseases classified elsewhere, knee
M14.861 *Arthropathies in other specified diseases classified elsewhere, right knee*
M14.862 *Arthropathies in other specified diseases classified elsewhere, left knee*
M14.869 *Arthropathies in other specified diseases classified elsewhere, unspecified knee*
✓6ᵗʰ M14.87 Arthropathies in other specified diseases classified elsewhere, ankle and foot
M14.871 *Arthropathies in other specified diseases classified elsewhere, right ankle and foot*
M14.872 *Arthropathies in other specified diseases classified elsewhere, left ankle and foot*
M14.879 *Arthropathies in other specified diseases classified elsewhere, unspecified ankle and foot*
M14.88 *Arthropathies in other specified diseases classified elsewhere, vertebrae*

M14.89 *Arthropathies in other specified diseases classified elsewhere, multiple sites*

Osteoarthritis (M15-M19)

EXCLUDES 2   osteoarthritis of spine (M47.-)

✓4ᵗʰ M15 Polyosteoarthritis
INCLUDES   arthritis of multiple sites
EXCLUDES 1   bilateral involvement of single joint (M16-M19)
M15.0 Primary generalized (osteo)arthritis
M15.1 Heberden's nodes (with arthropathy)
Interphalangeal distal osteoarthritis
M15.2 Bouchard's nodes (with arthropathy)
Juxtaphalangeal distal osteoarthritis
M15.3 Secondary multiple arthritis
Post-traumatic polyosteoarthritis
M15.4 Erosive (osteo)arthritis
M15.8 Other polyosteoarthritis
M15.9 Polyosteoarthritis, unspecified
Generalized osteoarthritis NOS

✓4ᵗʰ M16 Osteoarthritis of hip
AHA: 2016,4Q,146
M16.0 Bilateral primary osteoarthritis of hip
AHA: 2018,2Q,15
✓5ᵗʰ M16.1 Unilateral primary osteoarthritis of hip
Primary osteoarthritis of hip NOS
AHA: 2018,2Q,15
M16.10 Unilateral primary osteoarthritis, unspecified hip
M16.11 Unilateral primary osteoarthritis, right hip
M16.12 Unilateral primary osteoarthritis, left hip
M16.2 Bilateral osteoarthritis resulting from hip dysplasia
✓5ᵗʰ M16.3 Unilateral osteoarthritis resulting from hip dysplasia
Dysplastic osteoarthritis of hip NOS
M16.30 Unilateral osteoarthritis resulting from hip dysplasia, unspecified hip
M16.31 Unilateral osteoarthritis resulting from hip dysplasia, right hip
M16.32 Unilateral osteoarthritis resulting from hip dysplasia, left hip
M16.4 Bilateral post-traumatic osteoarthritis of hip
✓5ᵗʰ M16.5 Unilateral post-traumatic osteoarthritis of hip
Post-traumatic osteoarthritis of hip NOS
M16.50 Unilateral post-traumatic osteoarthritis, unspecified hip
M16.51 Unilateral post-traumatic osteoarthritis, right hip
M16.52 Unilateral post-traumatic osteoarthritis, left hip
M16.6 Other bilateral secondary osteoarthritis of hip
M16.7 Other unilateral secondary osteoarthritis of hip
Secondary osteoarthritis of hip NOS
M16.9 Osteoarthritis of hip, unspecified

✓4ᵗʰ M17 Osteoarthritis of knee
AHA: 2016,4Q,146-147
M17.0 Bilateral primary osteoarthritis of knee
AHA: 2018,2Q,15
✓5ᵗʰ M17.1 Unilateral primary osteoarthritis of knee
Primary osteoarthritis of knee NOS
AHA: 2018,2Q,15
M17.10 Unilateral primary osteoarthritis, unspecified knee
M17.11 Unilateral primary osteoarthritis, right knee
M17.12 Unilateral primary osteoarthritis, left knee
M17.2 Bilateral post-traumatic osteoarthritis of knee
✓5ᵗʰ M17.3 Unilateral post-traumatic osteoarthritis of knee
Post-traumatic osteoarthritis of knee NOS
M17.30 Unilateral post-traumatic osteoarthritis, unspecified knee
M17.31 Unilateral post-traumatic osteoarthritis, right knee
M17.32 Unilateral post-traumatic osteoarthritis, left knee
M17.4 Other bilateral secondary osteoarthritis of knee
M17.5 Other unilateral secondary osteoarthritis of knee
Secondary osteoarthritis of knee NOS
M17.9 Osteoarthritis of knee, unspecified

✓4ᵗʰ M18 Osteoarthritis of first carpometacarpal joint
M18.0 Bilateral primary osteoarthritis of first carpometacarpal joints

√6ᵗʰ **M18.1** Unilateral primary osteoarthritis of first carpometacarpal joint
Primary osteoarthritis of first carpometacarpal joint NOS
    M18.10 Unilateral primary osteoarthritis of first carpometacarpal joint, unspecified hand
    M18.11 Unilateral primary osteoarthritis of first carpometacarpal joint, right hand
    M18.12 Unilateral primary osteoarthritis of first carpometacarpal joint, left hand
M18.2 Bilateral post-traumatic osteoarthritis of first carpometacarpal joints
√5ᵗʰ **M18.3** Unilateral post-traumatic osteoarthritis of first carpometacarpal joint
Post-traumatic osteoarthritis of first carpometacarpal joint NOS
    M18.30 Unilateral post-traumatic osteoarthritis of first carpometacarpal joint, unspecified hand
    M18.31 Unilateral post-traumatic osteoarthritis of first carpometacarpal joint, right hand
    M18.32 Unilateral post-traumatic osteoarthritis of first carpometacarpal joint, left hand
M18.4 Other bilateral secondary osteoarthritis of first carpometacarpal joints
√5ᵗʰ **M18.5** Other unilateral secondary osteoarthritis of first carpometacarpal joint
Secondary osteoarthritis of first carpometacarpal joint NOS
    M18.50 Other unilateral secondary osteoarthritis of first carpometacarpal joint, unspecified hand
    M18.51 Other unilateral secondary osteoarthritis of first carpometacarpal joint, right hand
    M18.52 Other unilateral secondary osteoarthritis of first carpometacarpal joint, left hand
M18.9 Osteoarthritis of first carpometacarpal joint, unspecified

√4ᵗʰ **M19** Other and unspecified osteoarthritis
EXCLUDES 1   polyarthritis (M15.-)
EXCLUDES 2   arthrosis of spine (M47.-)
          hallux rigidus (M20.2)
          osteoarthritis of spine (M47.-)

√5ᵗʰ **M19.0** Primary osteoarthritis of other joints
AHA: 2018,2Q,15; 2016,4Q,145
    √6ᵗʰ **M19.01** Primary osteoarthritis, shoulder
       M19.011 Primary osteoarthritis, right shoulder
       M19.012 Primary osteoarthritis, left shoulder
       M19.019 Primary osteoarthritis, unspecified shoulder
    √6ᵗʰ **M19.02** Primary osteoarthritis, elbow
       M19.021 Primary osteoarthritis, right elbow
       M19.022 Primary osteoarthritis, left elbow
       M19.029 Primary osteoarthritis, unspecified elbow
    √6ᵗʰ **M19.03** Primary osteoarthritis, wrist
       M19.031 Primary osteoarthritis, right wrist
       M19.032 Primary osteoarthritis, left wrist
       M19.039 Primary osteoarthritis, unspecified wrist
    √6ᵗʰ **M19.04** Primary osteoarthritis, hand
       EXCLUDES 2   primary osteoarthritis of first carpometacarpal joint (M18.0-, M18.1-)
       M19.041 Primary osteoarthritis, right hand
       M19.042 Primary osteoarthritis, left hand
       M19.049 Primary osteoarthritis, unspecified hand
    √6ᵗʰ **M19.07** Primary osteoarthritis ankle and foot
       M19.071 Primary osteoarthritis, right ankle and foot
       M19.072 Primary osteoarthritis, left ankle and foot
       M19.079 Primary osteoarthritis, unspecified ankle and foot

√5ᵗʰ **M19.1** Post-traumatic osteoarthritis of other joints
    √6ᵗʰ **M19.11** Post-traumatic osteoarthritis, shoulder
       M19.111 Post-traumatic osteoarthritis, right shoulder
       M19.112 Post-traumatic osteoarthritis, left shoulder
       M19.119 Post-traumatic osteoarthritis, unspecified shoulder
    √6ᵗʰ **M19.12** Post-traumatic osteoarthritis, elbow
       M19.121 Post-traumatic osteoarthritis, right elbow
       M19.122 Post-traumatic osteoarthritis, left elbow
       M19.129 Post-traumatic osteoarthritis, unspecified elbow

√6ᵗʰ **M19.13** Post-traumatic osteoarthritis, wrist
    M19.131 Post-traumatic osteoarthritis, right wrist
    M19.132 Post-traumatic osteoarthritis, left wrist
    M19.139 Post-traumatic osteoarthritis, unspecified wrist
√6ᵗʰ **M19.14** Post-traumatic osteoarthritis, hand
    EXCLUDES 2   post-traumatic osteoarthritis of first carpometacarpal joint (M18.2-, M18.3-)
    M19.141 Post-traumatic osteoarthritis, right hand
    M19.142 Post-traumatic osteoarthritis, left hand
    M19.149 Post-traumatic osteoarthritis, unspecified hand
√6ᵗʰ **M19.17** Post-traumatic osteoarthritis, ankle and foot
    M19.171 Post-traumatic osteoarthritis, right ankle and foot
    M19.172 Post-traumatic osteoarthritis, left ankle and foot
    M19.179 Post-traumatic osteoarthritis, unspecified ankle and foot

√5ᵗʰ **M19.2** Secondary osteoarthritis of other joints
    √6ᵗʰ **M19.21** Secondary osteoarthritis, shoulder
       M19.211 Secondary osteoarthritis, right shoulder
       M19.212 Secondary osteoarthritis, left shoulder
       M19.219 Secondary osteoarthritis, unspecified shoulder
    √6ᵗʰ **M19.22** Secondary osteoarthritis, elbow
       M19.221 Secondary osteoarthritis, right elbow
       M19.222 Secondary osteoarthritis, left elbow
       M19.229 Secondary osteoarthritis, unspecified elbow
    √6ᵗʰ **M19.23** Secondary osteoarthritis, wrist
       M19.231 Secondary osteoarthritis, right wrist
       M19.232 Secondary osteoarthritis, left wrist
       M19.239 Secondary osteoarthritis, unspecified wrist
    √6ᵗʰ **M19.24** Secondary osteoarthritis, hand
       M19.241 Secondary osteoarthritis, right hand
       M19.242 Secondary osteoarthritis, left hand
       M19.249 Secondary osteoarthritis, unspecified hand
    √6ᵗʰ **M19.27** Secondary osteoarthritis, ankle and foot
       M19.271 Secondary osteoarthritis, right ankle and foot
       M19.272 Secondary osteoarthritis, left ankle and foot
       M19.279 Secondary osteoarthritis, unspecified ankle and foot

√5ᵗʰ **M19.9** Osteoarthritis, unspecified site
    M19.90 Unspecified osteoarthritis, unspecified site
       Arthrosis NOS
       Arthritis NOS
       Osteoarthritis NOS
       AHA: 2016,4Q,147
    M19.91 Primary osteoarthritis, unspecified site
       Primary osteoarthritis NOS
    M19.92 Post-traumatic osteoarthritis, unspecified site
       Post-traumatic osteoarthritis NOS
    M19.93 Secondary osteoarthritis, unspecified site
       Secondary osteoarthritis NOS

Other joint disorders (M20-M25)

EXCLUDES 2   joints of the spine (M40-M54)

√4ᵗʰ **M20** Acquired deformities of fingers and toes
EXCLUDES 1   acquired absence of fingers and toes (Z89.-)
          congenital absence of fingers and toes (Q71.3-, Q72.3-)
          congenital deformities and malformations of fingers and toes (Q66.-, Q68-Q70, Q74.-)
    √5ᵗʰ **M20.0** Deformity of finger(s)
       EXCLUDES 1   clubbing of fingers (R68.3)
            palmar fascial fibromatosis [Dupuytren] (M72.0)
            trigger finger (M65.3)
    √6ᵗʰ **M20.00** Unspecified deformity of finger(s)
       M20.001 Unspecified deformity of right finger(s)
       M20.002 Unspecified deformity of left finger(s)

✔ Additional Character Required   √x7ᵗʰ Placeholder Alert   Manifestation   Unspecified Dx   ▶◀ Revised Text   ● New Code   ▲ Revised Title

M20.009   Unspecified deformity of unspecified finger(s)

✓6ᵗʰ M20.01   **Mallet finger**

    M20.011   Mallet finger of right finger(s)
    M20.012   Mallet finger of left finger(s)
    M20.019   Mallet finger of unspecified finger(s)

✓6ᵗʰ M20.02   **Boutonnière deformity**

    DEF: Deformity of the finger caused by flexion of the proximal interphalangeal joint and hyperextension of the distal joint. The deformity results from rheumatoid arthritis, osteoarthritis, or injury.

    M20.021   Boutonnière deformity of right finger(s)
    M20.022   Boutonnière deformity of left finger(s)
    M20.029   Boutonnière deformity of unspecified finger(s)

✓6ᵗʰ M20.03   **Swan-neck deformity**

    DEF: Flexed distal and hyperextended proximal interphalangeal joint most commonly caused by rheumatoid arthritis.

    M20.031   Swan-neck deformity of right finger(s)
    M20.032   Swan-neck deformity of left finger(s)
    M20.039   Swan-neck deformity of unspecified finger(s)

✓6ᵗʰ M20.09   **Other deformity of finger(s)**

    M20.091   Other deformity of right finger(s)
    M20.092   Other deformity of left finger(s)
    M20.099   Other deformity of finger(s), unspecified finger(s)

✓5ᵗʰ M20.1   **Hallux valgus (acquired)**

    EXCLUDES 2   bunion (M21.6-)
    AHA: 2016,4Q,38
    DEF: Deformity in which the great toe deviates toward the other toes and may even be positioned over or under the second toe.

Hallux Valgus

Hallux valgus

Medial eminence of metatarsal bone

Right foot

    M20.10   Hallux valgus (acquired), unspecified foot
    M20.11   Hallux valgus (acquired), right foot
    M20.12   Hallux valgus (acquired), left foot

✓5ᵗʰ M20.2   **Hallux rigidus**

    M20.20   Hallux rigidus, unspecified foot
    M20.21   Hallux rigidus, right foot
    M20.22   Hallux rigidus, left foot

✓5ᵗʰ M20.3   **Hallux varus (acquired)**

    DEF: Deformity in which the great toe deviates away from the other toes.

    M20.30   Hallux varus (acquired), unspecified foot
    M20.31   Hallux varus (acquired), right foot
    M20.32   Hallux varus (acquired), left foot

✓5ᵗʰ M20.4   **Other hammer toe(s) (acquired)**

    M20.40   Other hammer toe(s) (acquired), unspecified foot
    M20.41   Other hammer toe(s) (acquired), right foot
    M20.42   Other hammer toe(s) (acquired), left foot

✓5ᵗʰ M20.5   **Other deformities of toe(s) (acquired)**

    ✓6ᵗʰ M20.5X   Other deformities of toe(s) (acquired)

      M20.5X1   Other deformities of toe(s) (acquired), right foot
      M20.5X2   Other deformities of toe(s) (acquired), left foot
      M20.5X9   Other deformities of toe(s) (acquired), unspecified foot

✓5ᵗʰ M20.6   **Acquired deformities of toe(s), unspecified**

    M20.60   Acquired deformities of toe(s), unspecified, unspecified foot
    M20.61   Acquired deformities of toe(s), unspecified, right foot
    M20.62   Acquired deformities of toe(s), unspecified, left foot

✓4ᵗʰ **M21   Other acquired deformities of limbs**

    EXCLUDES 1   acquired absence of limb (Z89.-)
             congenital absence of limbs (Q71-Q73)
             congenital deformities and malformations of limbs (Q65-Q66, Q68-Q74)
    EXCLUDES 2   acquired deformities of fingers or toes (M20.-)
             coxa plana (M91.2)

✓5ᵗʰ M21.0   **Valgus deformity, not elsewhere classified**

    EXCLUDES 1   metatarsus valgus (Q66.6)
             talipes calcaneovalgus ▶(Q66.4-)◀

    M21.00   Valgus deformity, not elsewhere classified, unspecified site

    ✓6ᵗʰ M21.02   Valgus deformity, not elsewhere classified, elbow
      Cubitus valgus
      M21.021   Valgus deformity, not elsewhere classified, right elbow
      M21.022   Valgus deformity, not elsewhere classified, left elbow
      M21.029   Valgus deformity, not elsewhere classified, unspecified elbow

    ✓6ᵗʰ M21.05   Valgus deformity, not elsewhere classified, hip
      M21.051   Valgus deformity, not elsewhere classified, right hip
      M21.052   Valgus deformity, not elsewhere classified, left hip
      M21.059   Valgus deformity, not elsewhere classified, unspecified hip

    ✓6ᵗʰ M21.06   Valgus deformity, not elsewhere classified, knee
      Genu valgum
      Knock knee
      DEF: Genu valga/valgum: Condition in which the thighs slant inward, causing the knees to be angled abnormally close together, leaving the space between the ankles wider than normal.

Genu Valga (knock-knee)

      M21.061   Valgus deformity, not elsewhere classified, right knee
      M21.062   Valgus deformity, not elsewhere classified, left knee

    M21.069 Valgus deformity, not elsewhere classified, unspecified knee

✓6ᵗʰ M21.07 Valgus deformity, not elsewhere classified, ankle

    M21.071 Valgus deformity, not elsewhere classified, right ankle

    M21.072 Valgus deformity, not elsewhere classified, left ankle

    M21.079 Valgus deformity, not elsewhere classified, unspecified ankle

✓5ᵗʰ M21.1 Varus deformity, not elsewhere classified

    EXCLUDES 1   *metatarsus varus* ▶*(Q66.22-)*◀
                 tibia vara (M92.5)

    M21.10 Varus deformity, not elsewhere classified, unspecified site

✓6ᵗʰ M21.12 Varus deformity, not elsewhere classified, elbow
      Cubitus varus, elbow

    M21.121 Varus deformity, not elsewhere classified, right elbow

    M21.122 Varus deformity, not elsewhere classified, left elbow

    M21.129 Varus deformity, not elsewhere classified, unspecified elbow

✓6ᵗʰ M21.15 Varus deformity, not elsewhere classified, hip

    M21.151 Varus deformity, not elsewhere classified, right hip

    M21.152 Varus deformity, not elsewhere classified, left hip

    M21.159 Varus deformity, not elsewhere classified, unspecified

✓6ᵗʰ M21.16 Varus deformity, not elsewhere classified, knee
      Bow leg
      Genu varum
      DEF: Genu varus/varum: Condition in which the thighs and/or legs are bowed in an outward curve with an abnormally increased space between the knees.

Genu Varus (bowleg)

    M21.161 Varus deformity, not elsewhere classified, right knee

    M21.162 Varus deformity, not elsewhere classified, left knee

    M21.169 Varus deformity, not elsewhere classified, unspecified knee

✓6ᵗʰ M21.17 Varus deformity, not elsewhere classified, ankle

    M21.171 Varus deformity, not elsewhere classified, right ankle

    M21.172 Varus deformity, not elsewhere classified, left ankle

    M21.179 Varus deformity, not elsewhere classified, unspecified ankle

✓5ᵗʰ M21.2 Flexion deformity

    M21.20 Flexion deformity, unspecified site

✓6ᵗʰ M21.21 Flexion deformity, shoulder

    M21.211 Flexion deformity, right shoulder

    M21.212 Flexion deformity, left shoulder

    M21.219 Flexion deformity, unspecified shoulder

✓6ᵗʰ M21.22 Flexion deformity, elbow

    M21.221 Flexion deformity, right elbow

    M21.222 Flexion deformity, left elbow

    M21.229 Flexion deformity, unspecified elbow

✓6ᵗʰ M21.23 Flexion deformity, wrist

    M21.231 Flexion deformity, right wrist

    M21.232 Flexion deformity, left wrist

    M21.239 Flexion deformity, unspecified wrist

✓6ᵗʰ M21.24 Flexion deformity, finger joints

    M21.241 Flexion deformity, right finger joints

    M21.242 Flexion deformity, left finger joints

    M21.249 Flexion deformity, unspecified finger joints

✓6ᵗʰ M21.25 Flexion deformity, hip

    M21.251 Flexion deformity, right hip

    M21.252 Flexion deformity, left hip

    M21.259 Flexion deformity, unspecified hip

✓6ᵗʰ M21.26 Flexion deformity, knee

    M21.261 Flexion deformity, right knee

    M21.262 Flexion deformity, left knee

    M21.269 Flexion deformity, unspecified knee

✓6ᵗʰ M21.27 Flexion deformity, ankle and toes

    M21.271 Flexion deformity, right ankle and toes

    M21.272 Flexion deformity, left ankle and toes

    M21.279 Flexion deformity, unspecified ankle and toes

✓5ᵗʰ M21.3 Wrist or foot drop (acquired)

✓6ᵗʰ M21.33 Wrist drop (acquired)

    M21.331 Wrist drop, right wrist

    M21.332 Wrist drop, left wrist

    M21.339 Wrist drop, unspecified wrist

✓6ᵗʰ M21.37 Foot drop (acquired)

    M21.371 Foot drop, right foot

    M21.372 Foot drop, left foot

    M21.379 Foot drop, unspecified foot

✓5ᵗʰ M21.4 Flat foot [pes planus] (acquired)

    EXCLUDES 1   *congenital pes planus (Q66.5-)*

    M21.40 Flat foot [pes planus] (acquired), unspecified foot

    M21.41 Flat foot [pes planus] (acquired), right foot

    M21.42 Flat foot [pes planus] (acquired), left foot

✓5ᵗʰ M21.5 Acquired clawhand, clubhand, clawfoot and clubfoot

    EXCLUDES 1   *clubfoot, not specified as acquired (Q66.89)*

✓6ᵗʰ M21.51 Acquired clawhand

    M21.511 Acquired clawhand, right hand

    M21.512 Acquired clawhand, left hand

    M21.519 Acquired clawhand, unspecified hand

✓6ᵗʰ M21.52 Acquired clubhand

    M21.521 Acquired clubhand, right hand

    M21.522 Acquired clubhand, left hand

    M21.529 Acquired clubhand, unspecified hand

✓6ᵗʰ M21.53 Acquired clawfoot
      DEF: High foot arch with hyperextended toes at the metatarsophalangeal joint and flexed toes at the distal joints.

    M21.531 Acquired clawfoot, right foot

    M21.532 Acquired clawfoot, left foot

    M21.539 Acquired clawfoot, unspecified foot

✓6ᵗʰ M21.54 Acquired clubfoot
      DEF: Acquired anomaly of the foot with the heel elevated and rotated outward and the toes pointing inward.

    M21.541 Acquired clubfoot, right foot

    M21.542 Acquired clubfoot, left foot

    M21.549 Acquired clubfoot, unspecified foot

✓5ᵗʰ M21.6 Other acquired deformities of foot

    EXCLUDES 2   *deformities of toe (acquired) (M20.1-M20.6-)*
    AHA: 2016,4Q,38

✓6ᵗʰ M21.61 Bunion

    M21.611 Bunion of right foot

    M21.612 Bunion of left foot

    M21.619 Bunion of unspecified foot

✓6ᵗʰ M21.62 Bunionette

    M21.621 Bunionette of right foot

    M21.622 Bunionette of left foot

M21.629 Bunionette of unspecified foot
✓6ᵗʰ M21.6X Other acquired deformities of foot
M21.6X1 Other acquired deformities of right foot
M21.6X2 Other acquired deformities of left foot
M21.6X9 Other acquired deformities of unspecified foot
✓5ᵗʰ M21.7 Unequal limb length (acquired)
NOTE The site used should correspond to the shorter limb
M21.70 Unequal limb length (acquired), unspecified site
✓6ᵗʰ M21.72 Unequal limb length (acquired), humerus
M21.721 Unequal limb length (acquired), right humerus
M21.722 Unequal limb length (acquired), left humerus
M21.729 Unequal limb length (acquired), unspecified humerus
✓6ᵗʰ M21.73 Unequal limb length (acquired), ulna and radius
M21.731 Unequal limb length (acquired), right ulna
M21.732 Unequal limb length (acquired), left ulna
M21.733 Unequal limb length (acquired), right radius
M21.734 Unequal limb length (acquired), left radius
M21.739 Unequal limb length (acquired), unspecified ulna and radius
✓6ᵗʰ M21.75 Unequal limb length (acquired), femur
M21.751 Unequal limb length (acquired), right femur
M21.752 Unequal limb length (acquired), left femur
M21.759 Unequal limb length (acquired), unspecified femur
✓6ᵗʰ M21.76 Unequal limb length (acquired), tibia and fibula
M21.761 Unequal limb length (acquired), right tibia
M21.762 Unequal limb length (acquired), left tibia
M21.763 Unequal limb length (acquired), right fibula
M21.764 Unequal limb length (acquired), left fibula
M21.769 Unequal limb length (acquired), unspecified tibia and fibula
✓5ᵗʰ M21.8 Other specified acquired deformities of limbs
EXCLUDES2 coxa plana (M91.2)
M21.80 Other specified acquired deformities of unspecified limb
✓6ᵗʰ M21.82 Other specified acquired deformities of upper arm
M21.821 Other specified acquired deformities of right upper arm
M21.822 Other specified acquired deformities of left upper arm
M21.829 Other specified acquired deformities of unspecified upper arm
✓6ᵗʰ M21.83 Other specified acquired deformities of forearm
M21.831 Other specified acquired deformities of right forearm
M21.832 Other specified acquired deformities of left forearm
M21.839 Other specified acquired deformities of unspecified forearm
✓6ᵗʰ M21.85 Other specified acquired deformities of thigh
M21.851 Other specified acquired deformities of right thigh
M21.852 Other specified acquired deformities of left thigh
M21.859 Other specified acquired deformities of unspecified thigh
✓6ᵗʰ M21.86 Other specified acquired deformities of lower leg
M21.861 Other specified acquired deformities of right lower leg
M21.862 Other specified acquired deformities of left lower leg
M21.869 Other specified acquired deformities of unspecified lower leg
✓5ᵗʰ M21.9 Unspecified acquired deformity of limb and hand
M21.90 Unspecified acquired deformity of unspecified limb

✓6ᵗʰ M21.92 Unspecified acquired deformity of upper arm
M21.921 Unspecified acquired deformity of right upper arm
M21.922 Unspecified acquired deformity of left upper arm
M21.929 Unspecified acquired deformity of unspecified upper arm
✓6ᵗʰ M21.93 Unspecified acquired deformity of forearm
M21.931 Unspecified acquired deformity of right forearm
M21.932 Unspecified acquired deformity of left forearm
M21.939 Unspecified acquired deformity of unspecified forearm
✓6ᵗʰ M21.94 Unspecified acquired deformity of hand
M21.941 Unspecified acquired deformity of hand, right hand
M21.942 Unspecified acquired deformity of hand, left hand
M21.949 Unspecified acquired deformity of hand, unspecified hand
✓6ᵗʰ M21.95 Unspecified acquired deformity of thigh
M21.951 Unspecified acquired deformity of right thigh
M21.952 Unspecified acquired deformity of left thigh
M21.959 Unspecified acquired deformity of unspecified thigh
✓6ᵗʰ M21.96 Unspecified acquired deformity of lower leg
M21.961 Unspecified acquired deformity of right lower leg
M21.962 Unspecified acquired deformity of left lower leg
M21.969 Unspecified acquired deformity of unspecified lower leg

✓4ᵗʰ M22 Disorder of patella
EXCLUDES1 traumatic dislocation of patella (S83.0-)
✓5ᵗʰ M22.0 Recurrent dislocation of patella
M22.00 Recurrent dislocation of patella, unspecified knee
M22.01 Recurrent dislocation of patella, right knee
M22.02 Recurrent dislocation of patella, left knee
✓5ᵗʰ M22.1 Recurrent subluxation of patella
Incomplete dislocation of patella
M22.10 Recurrent subluxation of patella, unspecified knee
M22.11 Recurrent subluxation of patella, right knee
M22.12 Recurrent subluxation of patella, left knee
✓5ᵗʰ M22.2 Patellofemoral disorders
✓6ᵗʰ M22.2X Patellofemoral disorders
M22.2X1 Patellofemoral disorders, right knee
M22.2X2 Patellofemoral disorders, left knee
M22.2X9 Patellofemoral disorders, unspecified knee
✓5ᵗʰ M22.3 Other derangements of patella
✓6ᵗʰ M22.3X Other derangements of patella
M22.3X1 Other derangements of patella, right knee
M22.3X2 Other derangements of patella, left knee
M22.3X9 Other derangements of patella, unspecified knee
✓5ᵗʰ M22.4 Chondromalacia patellae
M22.40 Chondromalacia patellae, unspecified knee
M22.41 Chondromalacia patellae, right knee
M22.42 Chondromalacia patellae, left knee
✓5ᵗʰ M22.8 Other disorders of patella
✓6ᵗʰ M22.8X Other disorders of patella
M22.8X1 Other disorders of patella, right knee
M22.8X2 Other disorders of patella, left knee
M22.8X9 Other disorders of patella, unspecified knee
✓5ᵗʰ M22.9 Unspecified disorder of patella
M22.90 Unspecified disorder of patella, unspecified knee
M22.91 Unspecified disorder of patella, right knee
M22.92 Unspecified disorder of patella, left knee

✔4ᵗʰ **M23 Internal derangement of knee**

     EXCLUDES 1   ankylosis (M24.66)
                    current injury — see injury of knee and lower leg (S80-S89)
                    deformity of knee (M21.-)
                    osteochondritis dissecans (M93.2)
                    recurrent dislocation or subluxation of joints (M24.4)
                    recurrent dislocation or subluxation of patella (M22.0-M22.1)

✔5ᵗʰ **M23.0 Cystic meniscus**

    ✔6ᵗʰ **M23.00 Cystic meniscus, unspecified meniscus**

        Cystic meniscus, unspecified lateral meniscus
        Cystic meniscus, unspecified medial meniscus

        M23.000 Cystic meniscus, unspecified lateral meniscus, **right** knee
        M23.001 Cystic meniscus, unspecified lateral meniscus, **left** knee
        M23.002 Cystic meniscus, unspecified lateral meniscus, unspecified knee
        M23.003 Cystic meniscus, unspecified medial meniscus, **right** knee
        M23.004 Cystic meniscus, unspecified medial meniscus, **left** knee
        M23.005 Cystic meniscus, unspecified medial meniscus, unspecified knee
        M23.006 Cystic meniscus, unspecified meniscus, **right** knee
        M23.007 Cystic meniscus, unspecified meniscus, **left** knee
        M23.009 Cystic meniscus, unspecified meniscus, unspecified knee

    ✔6ᵗʰ **M23.01 Cystic meniscus, anterior horn of medial meniscus**

        M23.011 Cystic meniscus, anterior horn of medial meniscus, **right** knee
        M23.012 Cystic meniscus, anterior horn of medial meniscus, **left** knee
        M23.019 Cystic meniscus, anterior horn of medial meniscus, unspecified knee

    ✔6ᵗʰ **M23.02 Cystic meniscus, posterior horn of medial meniscus**

        M23.021 Cystic meniscus, posterior horn of medial meniscus, **right** knee
        M23.022 Cystic meniscus, posterior horn of medial meniscus, **left** knee
        M23.029 Cystic meniscus, posterior horn of medial meniscus, unspecified knee

    ✔6ᵗʰ **M23.03 Cystic meniscus, other medial meniscus**

        M23.031 Cystic meniscus, other medial meniscus, **right** knee
        M23.032 Cystic meniscus, other medial meniscus, **left** knee
        M23.039 Cystic meniscus, other medial meniscus, unspecified knee

    ✔6ᵗʰ **M23.04 Cystic meniscus, anterior horn of lateral meniscus**

        M23.041 Cystic meniscus, anterior horn of lateral meniscus, **right** knee
        M23.042 Cystic meniscus, anterior horn of lateral meniscus, **left** knee
        M23.049 Cystic meniscus, anterior horn of lateral meniscus, unspecified knee

    ✔6ᵗʰ **M23.05 Cystic meniscus, posterior horn of lateral meniscus**

        M23.051 Cystic meniscus, posterior horn of lateral meniscus, **right** knee
        M23.052 Cystic meniscus, posterior horn of lateral meniscus, **left** knee
        M23.059 Cystic meniscus, posterior horn of lateral meniscus, unspecified knee

    ✔6ᵗʰ **M23.06 Cystic meniscus, other lateral meniscus**

        M23.061 Cystic meniscus, other lateral meniscus, **right** knee
        M23.062 Cystic meniscus, other lateral meniscus, **left** knee
        M23.069 Cystic meniscus, other lateral meniscus, unspecified knee

✔5ᵗʰ **M23.2 Derangement of meniscus due to old tear or injury**

     Old bucket-handle tear
     AHA: 2019,2Q,26

Derangement of Meniscus

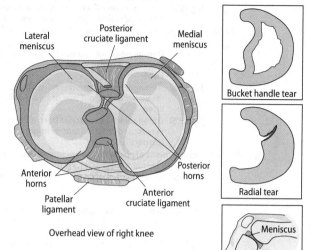

Lateral meniscus — Posterior cruciate ligament — Medial meniscus — Anterior horns — Posterior horns — Patellar ligament — Anterior cruciate ligament — Bucket handle tear — Radial tear — Meniscus

Overhead view of right knee

    ✔6ᵗʰ **M23.20 Derangement of unspecified meniscus due to old tear or injury**

        Derangement of unspecified lateral meniscus due to old tear or injury
        Derangement of unspecified medial meniscus due to old tear or injury

        M23.200 Derangement of unspecified lateral meniscus due to old tear or injury, **right** knee
        M23.201 Derangement of unspecified lateral meniscus due to old tear or injury, **left** knee
        M23.202 Derangement of unspecified lateral meniscus due to old tear or injury, unspecified knee
        M23.203 Derangement of unspecified medial meniscus due to old tear or injury, **right** knee
        M23.204 Derangement of unspecified medial meniscus due to old tear or injury, **left** knee
        M23.205 Derangement of unspecified medial meniscus due to old tear or injury, unspecified knee
        M23.206 Derangement of unspecified meniscus due to old tear or injury, **right** knee
        M23.207 Derangement of unspecified meniscus due to old tear or injury, **left** knee
        M23.209 Derangement of unspecified meniscus due to old tear or injury, unspecified knee

    ✔6ᵗʰ **M23.21 Derangement of anterior horn of medial meniscus due to old tear or injury**

        M23.211 Derangement of anterior horn of medial meniscus due to old tear or injury, **right** knee
        M23.212 Derangement of anterior horn of medial meniscus due to old tear or injury, **left** knee
        M23.219 Derangement of anterior horn of medial meniscus due to old tear or injury, unspecified knee

    ✔6ᵗʰ **M23.22 Derangement of posterior horn of medial meniscus due to old tear or injury**

        M23.221 Derangement of posterior horn of medial meniscus due to old tear or injury, **right** knee
        M23.222 Derangement of posterior horn of medial meniscus due to old tear or injury, **left** knee
        M23.229 Derangement of posterior horn of medial meniscus due to old tear or injury, unspecified knee

✔ Additional Character Required   ✔x7ᵗʰ Placeholder Alert   Manifestation   Unspecified Dx   ▶◀ Revised Text   ● New Code   ▲ Revised Title

ICD-10-CM 2020   767

✓6ᵗʰ **M23.23** Derangement of other medial meniscus due to old tear or injury

    M23.231 Derangement of other medial meniscus due to old tear or injury, **right** knee

    M23.232 Derangement of other medial meniscus due to old tear or injury, **left** knee

    M23.239 Derangement of other medial meniscus due to old tear or injury, unspecified knee

✓6ᵗʰ **M23.24** Derangement of anterior horn of lateral meniscus due to old tear or injury

    M23.241 Derangement of anterior horn of lateral meniscus due to old tear or injury, **right** knee

    M23.242 Derangement of anterior horn of lateral meniscus due to old tear or injury, **left** knee

    M23.249 Derangement of anterior horn of lateral meniscus due to old tear or injury, unspecified knee

✓6ᵗʰ **M23.25** Derangement of posterior horn of lateral meniscus due to old tear or injury

    M23.251 Derangement of posterior horn of lateral meniscus due to old tear or injury, **right** knee

    M23.252 Derangement of posterior horn of lateral meniscus due to old tear or injury, **left** knee

    M23.259 Derangement of posterior horn of lateral meniscus due to old tear or injury, unspecified knee

✓6ᵗʰ **M23.26** Derangement of other lateral meniscus due to old tear or injury

    M23.261 Derangement of other lateral meniscus due to old tear or injury, **right** knee

    M23.262 Derangement of other lateral meniscus due to old tear or injury, **left** knee

    M23.269 Derangement of other lateral meniscus due to old tear or injury, unspecified knee

✓5ᵗʰ **M23.3** Other meniscus derangements

    Degenerate meniscus

    Detached meniscus

    Retained meniscus

✓6ᵗʰ **M23.30** Other meniscus derangements, unspecified meniscus

    Other meniscus derangements, unspecified lateral meniscus

    Other meniscus derangements, unspecified medial meniscus

    M23.300 Other meniscus derangements, unspecified lateral meniscus, **right** knee

    M23.301 Other meniscus derangements, unspecified lateral meniscus, **left** knee

    M23.302 Other meniscus derangements, unspecified lateral meniscus, unspecified knee

    M23.303 Other meniscus derangements, unspecified medial meniscus, **right** knee

    M23.304 Other meniscus derangements, unspecified medial meniscus, **left** knee

    M23.305 Other meniscus derangements, unspecified medial meniscus, unspecified knee

    M23.306 Other meniscus derangements, unspecified meniscus, **right** knee

    M23.307 Other meniscus derangements, unspecified meniscus, **left** knee

    M23.309 Other meniscus derangements, unspecified meniscus, unspecified knee

✓6ᵗʰ **M23.31** Other meniscus derangements, anterior horn of medial meniscus

    M23.311 Other meniscus derangements, anterior horn of medial meniscus, **right** knee

    M23.312 Other meniscus derangements, anterior horn of medial meniscus, **left** knee

    M23.319 Other meniscus derangements, anterior horn of medial meniscus, unspecified knee

✓6ᵗʰ **M23.32** Other meniscus derangements, posterior horn of medial meniscus

    M23.321 Other meniscus derangements, posterior horn of medial meniscus, **right** knee

    M23.322 Other meniscus derangements, posterior horn of medial meniscus, **left** knee

    M23.329 Other meniscus derangements, posterior horn of medial meniscus, unspecified knee

✓6ᵗʰ **M23.33** Other meniscus derangements, other medial meniscus

    M23.331 Other meniscus derangements, other medial meniscus, **right** knee

    M23.332 Other meniscus derangements, other medial meniscus, **left** knee

    M23.339 Other meniscus derangements, other medial meniscus, unspecified knee

✓6ᵗʰ **M23.34** Other meniscus derangements, anterior horn of lateral meniscus

    M23.341 Other meniscus derangements, anterior horn of lateral meniscus, **right** knee

    M23.342 Other meniscus derangements, anterior horn of lateral meniscus, **left** knee

    M23.349 Other meniscus derangements, anterior horn of lateral meniscus, unspecified knee

✓6ᵗʰ **M23.35** Other meniscus derangements, posterior horn of lateral meniscus

    M23.351 Other meniscus derangements, posterior horn of lateral meniscus, **right** knee

    M23.352 Other meniscus derangements, posterior horn of lateral meniscus, **left** knee

    M23.359 Other meniscus derangements, posterior horn of lateral meniscus, unspecified knee

✓6ᵗʰ **M23.36** Other meniscus derangements, other lateral meniscus

    M23.361 Other meniscus derangements, other lateral meniscus, **right** knee

    M23.362 Other meniscus derangements, other lateral meniscus, **left** knee

    M23.369 Other meniscus derangements, other lateral meniscus, unspecified knee

✓5ᵗʰ **M23.4** Loose body in knee

    M23.40 Loose body in knee, unspecified knee

    M23.41 Loose body in knee, **right** knee

    M23.42 Loose body in knee, **left** knee

✓5ᵗʰ **M23.5** Chronic instability of knee

    M23.50 Chronic instability of knee, unspecified knee

    M23.51 Chronic instability of knee, **right** knee

    M23.52 Chronic instability of knee, **left** knee

✓5ᵗʰ **M23.6** Other spontaneous disruption of ligament(s) of knee

    ✓6ᵗʰ **M23.60** Other spontaneous disruption of unspecified ligament of knee

      M23.601 Other spontaneous disruption of unspecified ligament of **right** knee

      M23.602 Other spontaneous disruption of unspecified ligament of **left** knee

      M23.609 Other spontaneous disruption of unspecified ligament of unspecified knee

    ✓6ᵗʰ **M23.61** Other spontaneous disruption of anterior cruciate ligament of knee

      M23.611 Other spontaneous disruption of anterior cruciate ligament of **right** knee

      M23.612 Other spontaneous disruption of anterior cruciate ligament of **left** knee

      M23.619 Other spontaneous disruption of anterior cruciate ligament of unspecified knee

    ✓6ᵗʰ **M23.62** Other spontaneous disruption of posterior cruciate ligament of knee

      M23.621 Other spontaneous disruption of posterior cruciate ligament of **right** knee

      M23.622 Other spontaneous disruption of posterior cruciate ligament of **left** knee

      M23.629 Other spontaneous disruption of posterior cruciate ligament of unspecified knee

    ✓6ᵗʰ **M23.63** Other spontaneous disruption of medial collateral ligament of knee

      M23.631 Other spontaneous disruption of medial collateral ligament of **right** knee

      M23.632 Other spontaneous disruption of medial collateral ligament of **left** knee

      M23.639 Other spontaneous disruption of medial collateral ligament of unspecified knee

Ⓝ Newborn: 0   Ⓟ Pediatric: 0-17   Ⓜ Maternity: 12-55   Ⓐ Adult: 15-124   **CH** Comorbidity High   **CL** Comorbidity Low   **NCDx** Noncancer Dx   **PDx** Primary Dx

768

ICD-10-CM 2020

✓6ᵗʰ **M23.64** Other spontaneous disruption of lateral collateral ligament of knee

M23.641 Other spontaneous disruption of lateral collateral ligament of right knee

M23.642 Other spontaneous disruption of lateral collateral ligament of left knee

M23.649 Other spontaneous disruption of lateral collateral ligament of unspecified knee

✓6ᵗʰ **M23.67** Other spontaneous disruption of capsular ligament of knee

M23.671 Other spontaneous disruption of capsular ligament of right knee

M23.672 Other spontaneous disruption of capsular ligament of left knee

M23.679 Other spontaneous disruption of capsular ligament of unspecified knee

✓5ᵗʰ **M23.8** Other internal derangements of knee

Laxity of ligament of knee
Snapping knee

✓6ᵗʰ **M23.8X** Other internal derangements of knee

M23.8X1 Other internal derangements of right knee

M23.8X2 Other internal derangements of left knee

M23.8X9 Other internal derangements of unspecified knee

✓5ᵗʰ **M23.9** Unspecified internal derangement of knee

M23.90 Unspecified internal derangement of unspecified knee

M23.91 Unspecified internal derangement of right knee

M23.92 Unspecified internal derangement of left knee

✓4ᵗʰ **M24** Other specific joint derangements

EXCLUDES 1 current injury — see injury of joint by body region

EXCLUDES 2 ganglion (M67.4)
snapping knee (M23.8-)
temporomandibular joint disorders (M26.6-)

✓5ᵗʰ **M24.0** Loose body in joint

EXCLUDES 2 loose body in knee (M23.4)

M24.00 Loose body in unspecified joint

✓6ᵗʰ **M24.01** Loose body in shoulder

M24.011 Loose body in right shoulder
M24.012 Loose body in left shoulder
M24.019 Loose body in unspecified shoulder

✓6ᵗʰ **M24.02** Loose body in elbow

M24.021 Loose body in right elbow
M24.022 Loose body in left elbow
M24.029 Loose body in unspecified elbow

✓6ᵗʰ **M24.03** Loose body in wrist

M24.031 Loose body in right wrist
M24.032 Loose body in left wrist
M24.039 Loose body in unspecified wrist

✓6ᵗʰ **M24.04** Loose body in finger joints

M24.041 Loose body in right finger joint(s)
M24.042 Loose body in left finger joint(s)
M24.049 Loose body in unspecified finger joint(s)

✓6ᵗʰ **M24.05** Loose body in hip

M24.051 Loose body in right hip
M24.052 Loose body in left hip
M24.059 Loose body in unspecified hip

✓6ᵗʰ **M24.07** Loose body in ankle and toe joints

M24.071 Loose body in right ankle
M24.072 Loose body in left ankle
M24.073 Loose body in unspecified ankle
M24.074 Loose body in right toe joint(s)
M24.075 Loose body in left toe joint(s)
M24.076 Loose body in unspecified toe joints

M24.08 Loose body, other site

✓5ᵗʰ **M24.1** Other articular cartilage disorders

EXCLUDES 2 chondrocalcinosis (M11.1, M11.2-)
internal derangement of knee (M23.-)
metastatic calcification (E83.5)
ochronosis (E70.2)

M24.10 Other articular cartilage disorders, unspecified site

✓6ᵗʰ **M24.11** Other articular cartilage disorders, shoulder

M24.111 Other articular cartilage disorders, right shoulder

M24.112 Other articular cartilage disorders, left shoulder

M24.119 Other articular cartilage disorders, unspecified shoulder

✓6ᵗʰ **M24.12** Other articular cartilage disorders, elbow

M24.121 Other articular cartilage disorders, right elbow

M24.122 Other articular cartilage disorders, left elbow

M24.129 Other articular cartilage disorders, unspecified elbow

✓6ᵗʰ **M24.13** Other articular cartilage disorders, wrist

M24.131 Other articular cartilage disorders, right wrist

M24.132 Other articular cartilage disorders, left wrist

M24.139 Other articular cartilage disorders, unspecified wrist

✓6ᵗʰ **M24.14** Other articular cartilage disorders, hand

M24.141 Other articular cartilage disorders, right hand

M24.142 Other articular cartilage disorders, left hand

M24.149 Other articular cartilage disorders, unspecified hand

✓6ᵗʰ **M24.15** Other articular cartilage disorders, hip

M24.151 Other articular cartilage disorders, right hip

M24.152 Other articular cartilage disorders, left hip

M24.159 Other articular cartilage disorders, unspecified hip

✓6ᵗʰ **M24.17** Other articular cartilage disorders, ankle and foot

M24.171 Other articular cartilage disorders, right ankle

M24.172 Other articular cartilage disorders, left ankle

M24.173 Other articular cartilage disorders, unspecified ankle

M24.174 Other articular cartilage disorders, right foot

M24.175 Other articular cartilage disorders, left foot

M24.176 Other articular cartilage disorders, unspecified foot

✓5ᵗʰ **M24.2** Disorder of ligament

Instability secondary to old ligament injury
Ligamentous laxity NOS

EXCLUDES 1 familial ligamentous laxity (M35.7)

EXCLUDES 2 internal derangement of knee ▶(M23.5-M23.8X9)◀

M24.20 Disorder of ligament, unspecified site

✓6ᵗʰ **M24.21** Disorder of ligament, shoulder

M24.211 Disorder of ligament, right shoulder
M24.212 Disorder of ligament, left shoulder
M24.219 Disorder of ligament, unspecified shoulder

✓6ᵗʰ **M24.22** Disorder of ligament, elbow

M24.221 Disorder of ligament, right elbow
M24.222 Disorder of ligament, left elbow
M24.229 Disorder of ligament, unspecified elbow

✓6ᵗʰ **M24.23** Disorder of ligament, wrist

M24.231 Disorder of ligament, right wrist
M24.232 Disorder of ligament, left wrist
M24.239 Disorder of ligament, unspecified wrist

✓6ᵗʰ **M24.24** Disorder of ligament, hand

M24.241 Disorder of ligament, right hand
M24.242 Disorder of ligament, left hand
M24.249 Disorder of ligament, unspecified hand

✓6ᵗʰ **M24.25** Disorder of ligament, hip

M24.251 Disorder of ligament, right hip
M24.252 Disorder of ligament, left hip
M24.259 Disorder of ligament, unspecified hip

✓6ᵗʰ **M24.27** Disorder of ligament, ankle and foot

M24.271 Disorder of ligament, right ankle
M24.272 Disorder of ligament, left ankle
M24.273 Disorder of ligament, unspecified ankle
M24.274 Disorder of ligament, right foot
M24.275 Disorder of ligament, left foot

☑ Additional Character Required   ✓x7ᵗʰ Placeholder Alert   Manifestation   Unspecified Dx   ▶◀ Revised Text   ● New Code   ▲ Revised Title

ICD-10-CM 2020   769

M24.276   **Disorder of ligament, unspecified foot**
M24.28   **Disorder of ligament,** vertebrae
✓5ᵗʰ M24.3   **Pathological dislocation of joint, not elsewhere classified**

> EXCLUDES 1   *congenital dislocation or displacement of joint —*
> *see congenital malformations and deformations*
> *of the musculoskeletal system (Q65-Q79)*
> *current injury — see injury of joints and ligaments*
> *by body region*
> *recurrent dislocation of joint (M24.4-)*

M24.30   **Pathological dislocation of unspecified joint, not elsewhere classified**
✓6ᵗʰ M24.31   **Pathological dislocation of** shoulder, **not elsewhere classified**
  M24.311   **Pathological dislocation of** right **shoulder, not elsewhere classified**
  M24.312   **Pathological dislocation of** left **shoulder, not elsewhere classified**
  M24.319   **Pathological dislocation of unspecified shoulder, not elsewhere classified**
✓6ᵗʰ M24.32   **Pathological dislocation of** elbow, **not elsewhere classified**
  M24.321   **Pathological dislocation of** right **elbow, not elsewhere classified**
  M24.322   **Pathological dislocation of** left **elbow, not elsewhere classified**
  M24.329   **Pathological dislocation of unspecified elbow, not elsewhere classified**
✓6ᵗʰ M24.33   **Pathological dislocation of** wrist, **not elsewhere classified**
  M24.331   **Pathological dislocation of** right **wrist, not elsewhere classified**
  M24.332   **Pathological dislocation of** left **wrist, not elsewhere classified**
  M24.339   **Pathological dislocation of unspecified wrist, not elsewhere classified**
✓6ᵗʰ M24.34   **Pathological dislocation of** hand, **not elsewhere classified**
  M24.341   **Pathological dislocation of** right **hand, not elsewhere classified**
  M24.342   **Pathological dislocation of** left **hand, not elsewhere classified**
  M24.349   **Pathological dislocation of unspecified hand, not elsewhere classified**
✓6ᵗʰ M24.35   **Pathological dislocation of** hip, **not elsewhere classified**
  M24.351   **Pathological dislocation of** right **hip, not elsewhere classified**
  M24.352   **Pathological dislocation of** left **hip, not elsewhere classified**
  M24.359   **Pathological dislocation of unspecified hip, not elsewhere classified**
✓6ᵗʰ M24.36   **Pathological dislocation of** knee, **not elsewhere classified**
  M24.361   **Pathological dislocation of** right **knee, not elsewhere classified**
  M24.362   **Pathological dislocation of** left **knee, not elsewhere classified**
  M24.369   **Pathological dislocation of unspecified knee, not elsewhere classified**
✓6ᵗʰ M24.37   **Pathological dislocation of** ankle and foot, **not elsewhere classified**
  M24.371   **Pathological dislocation of** right **ankle, not elsewhere classified**
  M24.372   **Pathological dislocation of** left **ankle, not elsewhere classified**
  M24.373   **Pathological dislocation of unspecified ankle, not elsewhere classified**
  M24.374   **Pathological dislocation of** right **foot, not elsewhere classified**
  M24.375   **Pathological dislocation of** left **foot, not elsewhere classified**
  M24.376   **Pathological dislocation of unspecified foot, not elsewhere classified**
✓5ᵗʰ M24.4   **Recurrent dislocation of joint**
  Recurrent subluxation of joint

> EXCLUDES 2   *recurrent dislocation of patella (M22.0-M22.1)*
> *recurrent vertebral dislocation (M43.3-, M43.4,*
> *M43.5-)*

M24.40   **Recurrent dislocation, unspecified joint**
✓6ᵗʰ M24.41   **Recurrent dislocation,** shoulder
  M24.411   **Recurrent dislocation,** right **shoulder**

M24.412   **Recurrent dislocation,** left **shoulder**
M24.419   **Recurrent dislocation, unspecified shoulder**
✓6ᵗʰ M24.42   **Recurrent dislocation,** elbow
  M24.421   **Recurrent dislocation,** right **elbow**
  M24.422   **Recurrent dislocation,** left **elbow**
  M24.429   **Recurrent dislocation, unspecified elbow**
✓6ᵗʰ M24.43   **Recurrent dislocation,** wrist
  M24.431   **Recurrent dislocation,** right **wrist**
  M24.432   **Recurrent dislocation,** left **wrist**
  M24.439   **Recurrent dislocation, unspecified wrist**
✓6ᵗʰ M24.44   **Recurrent dislocation,** hand and finger(s)
  M24.441   **Recurrent dislocation,** right **hand**
  M24.442   **Recurrent dislocation,** left **hand**
  M24.443   **Recurrent dislocation, unspecified hand**
  M24.444   **Recurrent dislocation,** right **finger**
  M24.445   **Recurrent dislocation,** left **finger**
  M24.446   **Recurrent dislocation, unspecified finger**
✓6ᵗʰ M24.45   **Recurrent dislocation,** hip
  M24.451   **Recurrent dislocation,** right **hip**
  M24.452   **Recurrent dislocation,** left **hip**
  M24.459   **Recurrent dislocation, unspecified hip**
✓6ᵗʰ M24.46   **Recurrent dislocation,** knee
  M24.461   **Recurrent dislocation,** right **knee**
  M24.462   **Recurrent dislocation,** left **knee**
  M24.469   **Recurrent dislocation, unspecified knee**
✓6ᵗʰ M24.47   **Recurrent dislocation,** ankle, foot and toes
  M24.471   **Recurrent dislocation,** right **ankle**
  M24.472   **Recurrent dislocation,** left **ankle**
  M24.473   **Recurrent dislocation, unspecified ankle**
  M24.474   **Recurrent dislocation,** right **foot**
  M24.475   **Recurrent dislocation,** left **foot**
  M24.476   **Recurrent dislocation, unspecified foot**
  M24.477   **Recurrent dislocation,** right **toe(s)**
  M24.478   **Recurrent dislocation,** left **toe(s)**
  M24.479   **Recurrent dislocation, unspecified toe(s)**
✓5ᵗʰ M24.5   **Contracture of joint**

> EXCLUDES 1   *contracture of muscle without contracture of joint*
> *(M62.4-)*
> *contracture of tendon (sheath) without contracture*
> *of joint (M62.4-)*
> *Dupuytren's contracture (M72.0)*
> EXCLUDES 2   *acquired deformities of limbs (M20-M21)*
> AHA: 2016,2Q,6

M24.50   **Contracture, unspecified joint**
✓6ᵗʰ M24.51   **Contracture,** shoulder
  M24.511   **Contracture,** right **shoulder**
  M24.512   **Contracture,** left **shoulder**
  M24.519   **Contracture, unspecified shoulder**
✓6ᵗʰ M24.52   **Contracture,** elbow
  M24.521   **Contracture,** right **elbow**
  M24.522   **Contracture,** left **elbow**
  M24.529   **Contracture, unspecified elbow**
✓6ᵗʰ M24.53   **Contracture,** wrist
  M24.531   **Contracture,** right **wrist**
  M24.532   **Contracture,** left **wrist**
  M24.539   **Contracture, unspecified wrist**
✓6ᵗʰ M24.54   **Contracture,** hand
  M24.541   **Contracture,** right **hand**
  M24.542   **Contracture,** left **hand**
  M24.549   **Contracture, unspecified hand**
✓6ᵗʰ M24.55   **Contracture,** hip
  M24.551   **Contracture,** right **hip**
  M24.552   **Contracture,** left **hip**
  M24.559   **Contracture, unspecified hip**
✓6ᵗʰ M24.56   **Contracture,** knee
  M24.561   **Contracture,** right **knee**
  M24.562   **Contracture,** left **knee**
  M24.569   **Contracture, unspecified knee**
✓6ᵗʰ M24.57   **Contracture,** ankle and foot
  M24.571   **Contracture,** right **ankle**
  M24.572   **Contracture,** left **ankle**
  M24.573   **Contracture, unspecified ankle**
  M24.574   **Contracture,** right **foot**
  M24.575   **Contracture,** left **foot**
  M24.576   **Contracture, unspecified foot**

M23.64 Other spontaneous disruption of lateral collateral ligament of knee

    M23.641 Other spontaneous disruption of lateral collateral ligament of right knee

    M23.642 Other spontaneous disruption of lateral collateral ligament of left knee

    M23.649 Other spontaneous disruption of lateral collateral ligament of unspecified knee

M23.67 Other spontaneous disruption of capsular ligament of knee

    M23.671 Other spontaneous disruption of capsular ligament of right knee

    M23.672 Other spontaneous disruption of capsular ligament of left knee

    M23.679 Other spontaneous disruption of capsular ligament of unspecified knee

M23.8 Other internal derangements of knee

    Laxity of ligament of knee
    Snapping knee

  M23.8X Other internal derangements of knee

    M23.8X1 Other internal derangements of right knee

    M23.8X2 Other internal derangements of left knee

    M23.8X9 Other internal derangements of unspecified knee

M23.9 Unspecified internal derangement of knee

  M23.90 Unspecified internal derangement of unspecified knee

  M23.91 Unspecified internal derangement of right knee

  M23.92 Unspecified internal derangement of left knee

M24 Other specific joint derangements

  EXCLUDES 1   current injury — see injury of joint by body region

  EXCLUDES 2   ganglion (M67.4)

               snapping knee (M23.8-)

               temporomandibular joint disorders (M26.6-)

M24.0 Loose body in joint

  EXCLUDES 2   loose body in knee (M23.4)

  M24.00 Loose body in unspecified joint

  M24.01 Loose body in shoulder

    M24.011 Loose body in right shoulder
    M24.012 Loose body in left shoulder
    M24.019 Loose body in unspecified shoulder

  M24.02 Loose body in elbow

    M24.021 Loose body in right elbow
    M24.022 Loose body in left elbow
    M24.029 Loose body in unspecified elbow

  M24.03 Loose body in wrist

    M24.031 Loose body in right wrist
    M24.032 Loose body in left wrist
    M24.039 Loose body in unspecified wrist

  M24.04 Loose body in finger joints

    M24.041 Loose body in right finger joint(s)
    M24.042 Loose body in left finger joint(s)
    M24.049 Loose body in unspecified finger joint(s)

  M24.05 Loose body in hip

    M24.051 Loose body in right hip
    M24.052 Loose body in left hip
    M24.059 Loose body in unspecified hip

  M24.07 Loose body in ankle and toe joints

    M24.071 Loose body in right ankle
    M24.072 Loose body in left ankle
    M24.073 Loose body in unspecified ankle
    M24.074 Loose body in right toe joint(s)
    M24.075 Loose body in left toe joint(s)
    M24.076 Loose body in unspecified toe joints

  M24.08 Loose body, other site

M24.1 Other articular cartilage disorders

  EXCLUDES 2   chondrocalcinosis (M11.1, M11.2-)

               internal derangement of knee (M23.-)

               metastatic calcification (E83.5)

               ochronosis (E70.2)

  M24.10 Other articular cartilage disorders, unspecified site

  M24.11 Other articular cartilage disorders, shoulder

    M24.111 Other articular cartilage disorders, right shoulder

    M24.112 Other articular cartilage disorders, left shoulder

    M24.119 Other articular cartilage disorders, unspecified shoulder

  M24.12 Other articular cartilage disorders, elbow

    M24.121 Other articular cartilage disorders, right elbow

    M24.122 Other articular cartilage disorders, left elbow

    M24.129 Other articular cartilage disorders, unspecified elbow

  M24.13 Other articular cartilage disorders, wrist

    M24.131 Other articular cartilage disorders, right wrist

    M24.132 Other articular cartilage disorders, left wrist

    M24.139 Other articular cartilage disorders, unspecified wrist

  M24.14 Other articular cartilage disorders, hand

    M24.141 Other articular cartilage disorders, right hand

    M24.142 Other articular cartilage disorders, left hand

    M24.149 Other articular cartilage disorders, unspecified hand

  M24.15 Other articular cartilage disorders, hip

    M24.151 Other articular cartilage disorders, right hip

    M24.152 Other articular cartilage disorders, left hip

    M24.159 Other articular cartilage disorders, unspecified hip

  M24.17 Other articular cartilage disorders, ankle and foot

    M24.171 Other articular cartilage disorders, right ankle

    M24.172 Other articular cartilage disorders, left ankle

    M24.173 Other articular cartilage disorders, unspecified ankle

    M24.174 Other articular cartilage disorders, right foot

    M24.175 Other articular cartilage disorders, left foot

    M24.176 Other articular cartilage disorders, unspecified foot

M24.2 Disorder of ligament

  Instability secondary to old ligament injury
  Ligamentous laxity NOS

  EXCLUDES 1   familial ligamentous laxity (M35.7)

  EXCLUDES 2   internal derangement of knee ▶(M23.5-M23.8X9)◀

  M24.20 Disorder of ligament, unspecified site

  M24.21 Disorder of ligament, shoulder

    M24.211 Disorder of ligament, right shoulder
    M24.212 Disorder of ligament, left shoulder
    M24.219 Disorder of ligament, unspecified shoulder

  M24.22 Disorder of ligament, elbow

    M24.221 Disorder of ligament, right elbow
    M24.222 Disorder of ligament, left elbow
    M24.229 Disorder of ligament, unspecified elbow

  M24.23 Disorder of ligament, wrist

    M24.231 Disorder of ligament, right wrist
    M24.232 Disorder of ligament, left wrist
    M24.239 Disorder of ligament, unspecified wrist

  M24.24 Disorder of ligament, hand

    M24.241 Disorder of ligament, right hand
    M24.242 Disorder of ligament, left hand
    M24.249 Disorder of ligament, unspecified hand

  M24.25 Disorder of ligament, hip

    M24.251 Disorder of ligament, right hip
    M24.252 Disorder of ligament, left hip
    M24.259 Disorder of ligament, unspecified hip

  M24.27 Disorder of ligament, ankle and foot

    M24.271 Disorder of ligament, right ankle
    M24.272 Disorder of ligament, left ankle
    M24.273 Disorder of ligament, unspecified ankle
    M24.274 Disorder of ligament, right foot
    M24.275 Disorder of ligament, left foot

✓ Additional Character Required   ✓x7th Placeholder Alert   Manifestation   Unspecified Dx   ▶◀ Revised Text   ● New Code   ▲ Revised Title

ICD-10-CM 2020   769

M24.276 Disorder of ligament, unspecified foot

M24.28 Disorder of ligament, vertebrae

√5ᵗʰ **M24.3** Pathological dislocation of joint, not elsewhere classified

> EXCLUDES 1   congenital dislocation or displacement of joint — see congenital malformations and deformations of the musculoskeletal system (Q65-Q79)
> current injury — see injury of joints and ligaments by body region
> recurrent dislocation of joint (M24.4-)

M24.30 Pathological dislocation of unspecified joint, not elsewhere classified

√6ᵗʰ **M24.31** Pathological dislocation of shoulder, not elsewhere classified

M24.311 Pathological dislocation of right shoulder, not elsewhere classified

M24.312 Pathological dislocation of left shoulder, not elsewhere classified

M24.319 Pathological dislocation of unspecified shoulder, not elsewhere classified

√6ᵗʰ **M24.32** Pathological dislocation of elbow, not elsewhere classified

M24.321 Pathological dislocation of right elbow, not elsewhere classified

M24.322 Pathological dislocation of left elbow, not elsewhere classified

M24.329 Pathological dislocation of unspecified elbow, not elsewhere classified

√6ᵗʰ **M24.33** Pathological dislocation of wrist, not elsewhere classified

M24.331 Pathological dislocation of right wrist, not elsewhere classified

M24.332 Pathological dislocation of left wrist, not elsewhere classified

M24.339 Pathological dislocation of unspecified wrist, not elsewhere classified

√6ᵗʰ **M24.34** Pathological dislocation of hand, not elsewhere classified

M24.341 Pathological dislocation of right hand, not elsewhere classified

M24.342 Pathological dislocation of left hand, not elsewhere classified

M24.349 Pathological dislocation of unspecified hand, not elsewhere classified

√6ᵗʰ **M24.35** Pathological dislocation of hip, not elsewhere classified

M24.351 Pathological dislocation of right hip, not elsewhere classified

M24.352 Pathological dislocation of left hip, not elsewhere classified

M24.359 Pathological dislocation of unspecified hip, not elsewhere classified

√6ᵗʰ **M24.36** Pathological dislocation of knee, not elsewhere classified

M24.361 Pathological dislocation of right knee, not elsewhere classified

M24.362 Pathological dislocation of left knee, not elsewhere classified

M24.369 Pathological dislocation of unspecified knee, not elsewhere classified

√6ᵗʰ **M24.37** Pathological dislocation of ankle and foot, not elsewhere classified

M24.371 Pathological dislocation of right ankle, not elsewhere classified

M24.372 Pathological dislocation of left ankle, not elsewhere classified

M24.373 Pathological dislocation of unspecified ankle, not elsewhere classified

M24.374 Pathological dislocation of right foot, not elsewhere classified

M24.375 Pathological dislocation of left foot, not elsewhere classified

M24.376 Pathological dislocation of unspecified foot, not elsewhere classified

√5ᵗʰ **M24.4** Recurrent dislocation of joint

Recurrent subluxation of joint

> EXCLUDES 2   recurrent dislocation of patella (M22.0-M22.1)
> recurrent vertebral dislocation (M43.3-, M43.4, M43.5-)

M24.40 Recurrent dislocation, unspecified joint

√6ᵗʰ **M24.41** Recurrent dislocation, shoulder

M24.411 Recurrent dislocation, right shoulder

M24.412 Recurrent dislocation, left shoulder

M24.419 Recurrent dislocation, unspecified shoulder

√6ᵗʰ **M24.42** Recurrent dislocation, elbow

M24.421 Recurrent dislocation, right elbow

M24.422 Recurrent dislocation, left elbow

M24.429 Recurrent dislocation, unspecified elbow

√6ᵗʰ **M24.43** Recurrent dislocation, wrist

M24.431 Recurrent dislocation, right wrist

M24.432 Recurrent dislocation, left wrist

M24.439 Recurrent dislocation, unspecified wrist

√6ᵗʰ **M24.44** Recurrent dislocation, hand and finger(s)

M24.441 Recurrent dislocation, right hand

M24.442 Recurrent dislocation, left hand

M24.443 Recurrent dislocation, unspecified hand

M24.444 Recurrent dislocation, right finger

M24.445 Recurrent dislocation, left finger

M24.446 Recurrent dislocation, unspecified finger

√6ᵗʰ **M24.45** Recurrent dislocation, hip

M24.451 Recurrent dislocation, right hip

M24.452 Recurrent dislocation, left hip

M24.459 Recurrent dislocation, unspecified hip

√6ᵗʰ **M24.46** Recurrent dislocation, knee

M24.461 Recurrent dislocation, right knee

M24.462 Recurrent dislocation, left knee

M24.469 Recurrent dislocation, unspecified knee

√6ᵗʰ **M24.47** Recurrent dislocation, ankle, foot and toes

M24.471 Recurrent dislocation, right ankle

M24.472 Recurrent dislocation, left ankle

M24.473 Recurrent dislocation, unspecified ankle

M24.474 Recurrent dislocation, right foot

M24.475 Recurrent dislocation, left foot

M24.476 Recurrent dislocation, unspecified foot

M24.477 Recurrent dislocation, right toe(s)

M24.478 Recurrent dislocation, left toe(s)

M24.479 Recurrent dislocation, unspecified toe(s)

√5ᵗʰ **M24.5** Contracture of joint

> EXCLUDES 1   contracture of muscle without contracture of joint (M62.4-)
> contracture of tendon (sheath) without contracture of joint (M62.4-)
> Dupuytren's contracture (M72.0)
> EXCLUDES 2   acquired deformities of limbs (M20-M21)

AHA: 2016,2Q,6

M24.50 Contracture, unspecified joint

√6ᵗʰ **M24.51** Contracture, shoulder

M24.511 Contracture, right shoulder

M24.512 Contracture, left shoulder

M24.519 Contracture, unspecified shoulder

√6ᵗʰ **M24.52** Contracture, elbow

M24.521 Contracture, right elbow

M24.522 Contracture, left elbow

M24.529 Contracture, unspecified elbow

√6ᵗʰ **M24.53** Contracture, wrist

M24.531 Contracture, right wrist

M24.532 Contracture, left wrist

M24.539 Contracture, unspecified wrist

√6ᵗʰ **M24.54** Contracture, hand

M24.541 Contracture, right hand

M24.542 Contracture, left hand

M24.549 Contracture, unspecified hand

√6ᵗʰ **M24.55** Contracture, hip

M24.551 Contracture, right hip

M24.552 Contracture, left hip

M24.559 Contracture, unspecified hip

√6ᵗʰ **M24.56** Contracture, knee

M24.561 Contracture, right knee

M24.562 Contracture, left knee

M24.569 Contracture, unspecified knee

√6ᵗʰ **M24.57** Contracture, ankle and foot

M24.571 Contracture, right ankle

M24.572 Contracture, left ankle

M24.573 Contracture, unspecified ankle

M24.574 Contracture, right foot

M24.575 Contracture, left foot

M24.576 Contracture, unspecified foot

✓6ᵗʰ **M25.52 Pain in** elbow

    M25.521 Pain in right **elbow**
    M25.522 Pain in left **elbow**
    M25.529 Pain in unspecified elbow

✓6ᵗʰ **M25.53 Pain in** wrist

    M25.531 Pain in right **wrist**
    M25.532 Pain in left **wrist**
    M25.539 Pain in unspecified wrist

✓6ᵗʰ **M25.54 Pain in** joints of hand

    AHA: 2016,4Q,38

    M25.541 Pain in joints of right **hand**
    M25.542 Pain in joints of left **hand**
    M25.549 Pain in joints of unspecified hand
        Pain in joints of hand NOS

✓6ᵗʰ **M25.55 Pain in** hip

    M25.551 Pain in right **hip**
    M25.552 Pain in left **hip**
    M25.559 Pain in unspecified hip

✓6ᵗʰ **M25.56 Pain in** knee

    M25.561 Pain in right **knee**
    M25.562 Pain in left **knee**
    M25.569 Pain in unspecified knee

✓6ᵗʰ **M25.57 Pain in** ankle and joints of foot

    M25.571 Pain in right **ankle and joints of right foot**
    M25.572 Pain in left **ankle and joints of left foot**
    M25.579 Pain in unspecified ankle and joints of unspecified foot

✓5ᵗʰ **M25.6 Stiffness of joint, not elsewhere classified**

    EXCLUDES 1 ankylosis of joint (M24.6-)
        contracture of joint (M24.5-)

    M25.60 Stiffness of unspecified joint, not elsewhere classified

✓6ᵗʰ **M25.61 Stiffness of** shoulder, **not elsewhere classified**

    M25.611 Stiffness of right **shoulder, not elsewhere classified**
    M25.612 Stiffness of left **shoulder, not elsewhere classified**
    M25.619 Stiffness of unspecified shoulder, not elsewhere classified

✓6ᵗʰ **M25.62 Stiffness of** elbow, **not elsewhere classified**

    M25.621 Stiffness of right **elbow, not elsewhere classified**
    M25.622 Stiffness of left **elbow, not elsewhere classified**
    M25.629 Stiffness of unspecified elbow, not elsewhere classified

✓6ᵗʰ **M25.63 Stiffness of** wrist, **not elsewhere classified**

    M25.631 Stiffness of right **wrist, not elsewhere classified**
    M25.632 Stiffness of left **wrist, not elsewhere classified**
    M25.639 Stiffness of unspecified wrist, not elsewhere classified

✓6ᵗʰ **M25.64 Stiffness of** hand, **not elsewhere classified**

    M25.641 Stiffness of right **hand, not elsewhere classified**
    M25.642 Stiffness of left **hand, not elsewhere classified**
    M25.649 Stiffness of unspecified hand, not elsewhere classified

✓6ᵗʰ **M25.65 Stiffness of** hip, **not elsewhere classified**

    M25.651 Stiffness of right **hip, not elsewhere classified**
    M25.652 Stiffness of left **hip, not elsewhere classified**
    M25.659 Stiffness of unspecified hip, not elsewhere classified

✓6ᵗʰ **M25.66 Stiffness of** knee, **not elsewhere classified**

    M25.661 Stiffness of right **knee, not elsewhere classified**
    M25.662 Stiffness of left **knee, not elsewhere classified**
    M25.669 Stiffness of unspecified knee, not elsewhere classified

✓6ᵗʰ **M25.67 Stiffness of** ankle and foot, **not elsewhere classified**

    M25.671 Stiffness of right **ankle, not elsewhere classified**

    M25.672 Stiffness of left **ankle, not elsewhere classified**
    M25.673 Stiffness of unspecified ankle, not elsewhere classified
    M25.674 Stiffness of right **foot, not elsewhere classified**
    M25.675 Stiffness of left **foot, not elsewhere classified**
    M25.676 Stiffness of unspecified foot, not elsewhere classified

✓5ᵗʰ **M25.7 Osteophyte**

    M25.70 Osteophyte, unspecified joint

✓6ᵗʰ **M25.71 Osteophyte,** shoulder

    M25.711 Osteophyte, right **shoulder**
    M25.712 Osteophyte, left **shoulder**
    M25.719 Osteophyte, unspecified shoulder

✓6ᵗʰ **M25.72 Osteophyte,** elbow

    M25.721 Osteophyte, right **elbow**
    M25.722 Osteophyte, left **elbow**
    M25.729 Osteophyte, unspecified elbow

✓6ᵗʰ **M25.73 Osteophyte,** wrist

    M25.731 Osteophyte, right **wrist**
    M25.732 Osteophyte, left **wrist**
    M25.739 Osteophyte, unspecified wrist

✓6ᵗʰ **M25.74 Osteophyte,** hand

    M25.741 Osteophyte, right **hand**
    M25.742 Osteophyte, left **hand**
    M25.749 Osteophyte, unspecified hand

✓6ᵗʰ **M25.75 Osteophyte,** hip

    M25.751 Osteophyte, right **hip**
    M25.752 Osteophyte, left **hip**
    M25.759 Osteophyte, unspecified hip

✓6ᵗʰ **M25.76 Osteophyte,** knee

    M25.761 Osteophyte, right **knee**
    M25.762 Osteophyte, left **knee**
    M25.769 Osteophyte, unspecified knee

✓6ᵗʰ **M25.77 Osteophyte,** ankle and foot

    M25.771 Osteophyte, right **ankle**
    M25.772 Osteophyte, left **ankle**
    M25.773 Osteophyte, unspecified ankle
    M25.774 Osteophyte, right **foot**
    M25.775 Osteophyte, left **foot**
    M25.776 Osteophyte, unspecified foot

    M25.78 Osteophyte, vertebrae

✓5ᵗʰ **M25.8 Other specified joint disorders**

    M25.80 Other specified joint disorders, unspecified joint

✓6ᵗʰ **M25.81 Other specified joint disorders,** shoulder

    M25.811 Other specified joint disorders, right **shoulder**
    M25.812 Other specified joint disorders, left **shoulder**
    M25.819 Other specified joint disorders, unspecified shoulder

✓6ᵗʰ **M25.82 Other specified joint disorders,** elbow

    M25.821 Other specified joint disorders, right **elbow**
    M25.822 Other specified joint disorders, left **elbow**
    M25.829 Other specified joint disorders, unspecified elbow

✓6ᵗʰ **M25.83 Other specified joint disorders,** wrist

    M25.831 Other specified joint disorders, right **wrist**
    M25.832 Other specified joint disorders, left **wrist**
    M25.839 Other specified joint disorders, unspecified wrist

✓6ᵗʰ **M25.84 Other specified joint disorders,** hand

    M25.841 Other specified joint disorders, right **hand**
    M25.842 Other specified joint disorders, left **hand**
    M25.849 Other specified joint disorders, unspecified hand

✓6ᵗʰ **M25.85 Other specified joint disorders,** hip

    AHA: 2014,4Q,25

    M25.851 Other specified joint disorders, right **hip**
    M25.852 Other specified joint disorders, left **hip**
    M25.859 Other specified joint disorders, unspecified hip

✓6ᵗʰ **M25.86 Other specified joint disorders,** knee

    M25.861 Other specified joint disorders, right **knee**

☑ Additional Character Required   ✓x7ᵗʰ Placeholder Alert   Manifestation   Unspecified Dx   ►◄ Revised Text   ● New Code   ▲ Revised Title

ICD-10-CM 2020   **773**

        M25.862   **Other specified joint disorders,** left knee
        M25.869   **Other specified joint disorders, unspecified knee**
  ✓6ᵗʰ **M25.87**   **Other specified joint disorders,** ankle and foot
        M25.871   **Other specified joint disorders,** right ankle and foot
        M25.872   **Other specified joint disorders,** left ankle and foot
        M25.879   **Other specified joint disorders, unspecified ankle and foot**
M25.9   **Joint disorder, unspecified**

Dentofacial anomalies [including malocclusion] and other disorders of jaw (M26-M27)

EXCLUDES 1   *hemifacial atrophy or hypertrophy (Q67.4)*
         unilateral condylar hyperplasia or hypoplasia (M27.8)

✓4ᵗʰ **M26**   **Dentofacial anomalies [including malocclusion]**

  ✓5ᵗʰ **M26.0**   **Major anomalies of jaw size**
      EXCLUDES 1   *acromegaly (E22.0)*
             Robin's syndrome (Q87.0)
      M26.00   **Unspecified anomaly of jaw size**
      M26.01   **Maxillary hyperplasia**
      M26.02   **Maxillary hypoplasia**
          AHA: 2014,3Q,23
      M26.03   **Mandibular hyperplasia**
      M26.04   **Mandibular hypoplasia**
      M26.05   **Macrogenia**
      M26.06   **Microgenia**
      M26.07   **Excessive tuberosity of jaw**
          Entire maxillary tuberosity
      M26.09   **Other specified anomalies of jaw size**
  ✓5ᵗʰ **M26.1**   **Anomalies of jaw-cranial base relationship**
      M26.10   **Unspecified anomaly of jaw-cranial base relationship**
      M26.11   **Maxillary asymmetry**
      M26.12   **Other jaw asymmetry**
      M26.19   **Other specified anomalies of jaw-cranial base relationship**
  ✓5ᵗʰ **M26.2**   **Anomalies of dental arch relationship**
      M26.20   **Unspecified anomaly of dental arch relationship**
    ✓6ᵗʰ **M26.21**   **Malocclusion, Angle's class**
        M26.211   **Malocclusion, Angle's** class I
          Neutro-occlusion
        M26.212   **Malocclusion, Angle's** class II
          Disto-occlusion Division I
          Disto-occlusion Division II
        M26.213   **Malocclusion, Angle's** class III
          Mesio-occlusion
        M26.219   **Malocclusion, Angle's class, unspecified**
    ✓6ᵗʰ **M26.22**   **Open occlusal relationship**
        M26.220   **Open** anterior **occlusal relationship**
          Anterior open bite
        M26.221   **Open** posterior **occlusal relationship**
          Posterior open bite
      M26.23   **Excessive horizontal overlap**
          Excessive horizontal overjet
      M26.24   **Reverse articulation**
          Crossbite (anterior) (posterior)
      M26.25   **Anomalies of interarch distance**
      M26.29   **Other anomalies of dental arch relationship**
          Midline deviation of dental arch
          Overbite (excessive) deep
          Overbite (excessive) horizontal
          Overbite (excessive) vertical
          Posterior lingual occlusion of mandibular teeth
  ✓5ᵗʰ **M26.3**   **Anomalies of tooth position of fully erupted tooth or teeth**
      EXCLUDES 2   *embedded and impacted teeth (K01.-)*
      M26.30   **Unspecified anomaly of tooth position of fully erupted tooth or teeth**
          Abnormal spacing of fully erupted tooth or teeth NOS
          Displacement of fully erupted tooth or teeth NOS
          Transposition of fully erupted tooth or teeth NOS
      M26.31   **Crowding of fully erupted teeth**
      M26.32   **Excessive spacing of fully erupted teeth**
          Diastema of fully erupted tooth or teeth NOS

      M26.33   **Horizontal displacement of fully erupted tooth or teeth**
          Tipped tooth or teeth
          Tipping of fully erupted tooth
      M26.34   **Vertical displacement of fully erupted tooth or teeth**
          Extruded tooth
          Infraeruption of tooth or teeth
          Supraeruption of tooth or teeth
      M26.35   **Rotation of fully erupted tooth or teeth**
      M26.36   **Insufficient interocclusal distance of fully erupted teeth (ridge)**
          Lack of adequate intermaxillary vertical dimension of fully erupted teeth
      M26.37   **Excessive interocclusal distance of fully erupted teeth**
          Excessive intermaxillary vertical dimension of fully erupted teeth
          Loss of occlusal vertical dimension of fully erupted teeth
      M26.39   **Other anomalies of tooth position of fully erupted tooth or teeth**
M26.4   **Malocclusion, unspecified**
✓5ᵗʰ **M26.5**   **Dentofacial functional abnormalities**
      EXCLUDES 1   *bruxism (F45.8)*
             teeth-grinding NOS (F45.8)
      M26.50   **Dentofacial functional abnormalities, unspecified**
      M26.51   **Abnormal jaw closure**
      M26.52   **Limited mandibular range of motion**
      M26.53   **Deviation in opening and closing of the mandible**
      M26.54   **Insufficient anterior guidance**
          Insufficient anterior occlusal guidance
      M26.55   **Centric occlusion maximum intercuspation discrepancy**
          EXCLUDES 1   *centric occlusion NOS (M26.59)*
      M26.56   **Non-working side interference**
          Balancing side interference
      M26.57   **Lack of posterior occlusal support**
      M26.59   **Other dentofacial functional abnormalities**
          Centric occlusion (of teeth) NOS
          Malocclusion due to abnormal swallowing
          Malocclusion due to mouth breathing
          Malocclusion due to tongue, lip or finger habits
✓5ᵗʰ **M26.6**   **Temporomandibular joint disorders**
      EXCLUDES 2   *current temporomandibular joint dislocation (S03.0)*
           current temporomandibular joint sprain (S03.4)
      AHA: 2016,4Q,38-39

Temporomandibular Joint

Cutaway view of temporomandibular joint (TMJ)

    ✓6ᵗʰ **M26.60**   **Temporomandibular joint disorder, unspecified**
        M26.601   Right **temporomandibular joint disorder, unspecified**
        M26.602   Left **temporomandibular joint disorder, unspecified**
        M26.603   Bilateral **temporomandibular joint disorder, unspecified**
        M26.609   **Unspecified temporomandibular joint disorder, unspecified side**
          Temporomandibular joint disorder NOS
    ✓6ᵗʰ **M26.61**   Adhesions and ankylosis **of temporomandibular joint**
        M26.611   **Adhesions and ankylosis of** right **temporomandibular joint**
        M26.612   **Adhesions and ankylosis of** left **temporomandibular joint**

M26.613 **Adhesions and ankylosis of** bilateral **temporomandibular joint**

M26.619 **Adhesions and ankylosis of temporomandibular joint, unspecified side**

√6ᵗʰ **M26.62** Arthralgia **of temporomandibular joint**

  M26.621 **Arthralgia of** right **temporomandibular joint**

  M26.622 **Arthralgia of** left **temporomandibular joint**

  M26.623 **Arthralgia of** bilateral **temporomandibular joint**

  M26.629 **Arthralgia of temporomandibular joint, unspecified side**

√6ᵗʰ **M26.63** Articular disc disorder **of temporomandibular joint**

  M26.631 **Articular disc disorder of** right **temporomandibular joint**

  M26.632 **Articular disc disorder of** left **temporomandibular joint**

  M26.633 **Articular disc disorder of** bilateral **temporomandibular joint**

  M26.639 **Articular disc disorder of temporomandibular joint, unspecified side**

M26.69 **Other specified disorders of temporomandibular joint**

√5ᵗʰ **M26.7 Dental alveolar anomalies**

  M26.70 **Unspecified alveolar anomaly**

  M26.71 **Alveolar** maxillary hyperplasia

  M26.72 **Alveolar** mandibular hyperplasia

  M26.73 **Alveolar** maxillary hypoplasia

  M26.74 **Alveolar** mandibular hypoplasia

  M26.79 **Other specified alveolar anomalies**

√5ᵗʰ **M26.8 Other dentofacial anomalies**

  M26.81 Anterior **soft tissue impingement**
    Anterior soft tissue impingement on teeth

  M26.82 Posterior **soft tissue impingement**
    Posterior soft tissue impingement on teeth

  M26.89 **Other dentofacial anomalies**

M26.9 Dentofacial anomaly, unspecified

√4ᵗʰ **M27 Other diseases of jaws**

M27.0 Developmental disorders of jaws
  Latent bone cyst of jaw
  Stafne's cyst
  Torus mandibularis
  Torus palatinus

M27.1 Giant cell granuloma, central
  Giant cell granuloma NOS
  EXCLUDES 1   *peripheral giant cell granuloma (K06.8)*

M27.2 Inflammatory conditions of jaws
  Osteitis of jaw(s)
  Osteomyelitis (neonatal) jaw(s)
  Osteoradionecrosis jaw(s)
  Periostitis jaw(s)
  Sequestrum of jaw bone
  Use additional code (W88-W90, X39.0) to identify radiation, if radiation-induced
  EXCLUDES 2   *osteonecrosis of jaw due to drug (M87.180)*

M27.3 Alveolitis of jaws
  Alveolar osteitis
  Dry socket

√5ᵗʰ **M27.4 Other and unspecified cysts of jaw**
  EXCLUDES 1   *cysts of oral region (K09.-)*
          latent bone cyst of jaw (M27.0)
          Stafne's cyst (M27.0)

  M27.40 **Unspecified cyst of jaw**
    Cyst of jaw NOS

  M27.49 **Other cysts of jaw**
    Aneurysmal cyst of jaw
    Hemorrhagic cyst of jaw
    Traumatic cyst of jaw

√5ᵗʰ **M27.5 Periradicular pathology associated with previous endodontic treatment**
  M27.51 **Perforation of root canal space due to endodontic treatment**
  M27.52 **Endodontic overfill**
  M27.53 **Endodontic underfill**

M27.59 **Other periradicular pathology associated with previous endodontic treatment**

√5ᵗʰ **M27.6 Endosseous dental implant failure**

M27.61 Osseointegration **failure of dental implant**
  Hemorrhagic complications of dental implant placement
  Iatrogenic osseointegration failure of dental implant
  Osseointegration failure of dental implant due to complications of systemic disease
  Osseointegration failure of dental implant due to poor bone quality
  Pre-integration failure of dental implant NOS
  Pre-osseointegration failure of dental implant

M27.62 Post-osseointegration biological **failure of dental implant**
  Failure of dental implant due to lack of attached gingiva
  Failure of dental implant due to occlusal trauma (caused by poor prosthetic design)
  Failure of dental implant due to parafunctional habits
  Failure of dental implant due to periodontal infection (peri-implantitis)
  Failure of dental implant due to poor oral hygiene
  Iatrogenic post-osseointegration failure of dental implant
  Post-osseointegration failure of dental implant due to complications of systemic disease

M27.63 Post-osseointegration mechanical **failure of dental implant**
  Failure of dental prosthesis causing loss of dental implant
  Fracture of dental implant
    EXCLUDES 2   *cracked tooth (K03.81)*
           fractured dental restorative material with loss of material (K08.531)
           fractured dental restorative material without loss of material (K08.530)
           fractured tooth (S02.5)

M27.69 **Other endosseous dental implant failure**
  Dental implant failure NOS

M27.8 Other specified diseases of jaws
  Cherubism
  Exostosis
  Fibrous dysplasia
  Unilateral condylar hyperplasia
  Unilateral condylar hypoplasia
  EXCLUDES 1   *jaw pain (R68.84)*

M27.9 Disease of jaws, unspecified

Systemic connective tissue disorders (M30-M36)

INCLUDES   autoimmune disease NOS
          collagen (vascular) disease NOS
          systemic autoimmune disease
          systemic collagen (vascular) disease

EXCLUDES 1   *autoimmune disease, single organ or single cell-type-code to relevant condition category*

√4ᵗʰ **M30 Polyarteritis nodosa and related conditions**
  EXCLUDES 1   *microscopic polyarteritis (M31.7)*

M30.0 Polyarteritis nodosa

M30.1 Polyarteritis with lung involvement [Churg-Strauss]
  Allergic granulomatous angiitis

M30.2 Juvenile polyarteritis

M30.3 Mucocutaneous lymph node syndrome [Kawasaki]

M30.8 Other conditions related to polyarteritis nodosa
  Polyangiitis overlap syndrome

√4ᵗʰ **M31 Other necrotizing vasculopathies**

M31.0 Hypersensitivity angiitis
  Goodpasture's syndrome

M31.1 Thrombotic microangiopathy
  Thrombotic thrombocytopenic purpura

M31.2 Lethal midline granuloma

√5ᵗʰ **M31.3 Wegener's granulomatosis**
  Necrotizing respiratory granulomatosis

  M31.30 **Wegener's granulomatosis** without renal involvement
    Wegener's granulomatosis NOS

  M31.31 **Wegener's granulomatosis** with renal involvement

☑ Additional Character Required   √x7ᵗʰ Placeholder Alert   Manifestation   Unspecified Dx   ►◄ Revised Text   ● New Code   ▲ Revised Title

ICD-10-CM 2020   775

M31.4   **Aortic arch syndrome [Takayasu]**

M31.5   **Giant cell arteritis with polymyalgia rheumatica**

M31.6   **Other giant cell arteritis**

M31.7   **Microscopic polyangiitis**
     Microscopic polyarteritis
     EXCLUDES 1   polyarteritis nodosa (M30.0)

M31.8   **Other specified necrotizing vasculopathies**
     Hypocomplementemic vasculitis
     Septic vasculitis

M31.9   **Necrotizing vasculopathy, unspecified**

✓4ᵗʰ **M32**   **Systemic lupus erythematosus (SLE)**
     EXCLUDES 1   lupus erythematosus (discoid) (NOS) (L93.0)
     AHA: 2018,3Q,14

M32.0   **Drug-induced systemic lupus erythematosus**
     Use additional code for adverse effect, if applicable, to identify drug (T36-T50 with fifth or sixth character 5)

✓5ᵗʰ **M32.1**   **Systemic lupus erythematosus with organ or system involvement**

     M32.10   **Systemic lupus erythematosus, organ or system involvement unspecified**

     M32.11   **Endocarditis in systemic lupus erythematosus**
         Libman-Sacks disease

     M32.12   **Pericarditis in systemic lupus erythematosus**
         Lupus pericarditis

     M32.13   **Lung involvement in systemic lupus erythematosus**
         Pleural effusion due to systemic lupus erythematosus

     M32.14   **Glomerular disease in systemic lupus erythematosus**
         Lupus renal disease NOS
         AHA: 2013,4Q,125

     M32.15   **Tubulo-interstitial nephropathy in systemic lupus erythematosus**

     M32.19   **Other organ or system involvement in systemic lupus erythematosus**

M32.8   **Other forms of systemic lupus erythematosus**

M32.9   **Systemic lupus erythematosus, unspecified**
     SLE NOS
     Systemic lupus erythematosus NOS
     Systemic lupus erythematosus without organ involvement

✓4ᵗʰ **M33**   **Dermatopolymyositis**
     AHA: 2017,4Q,18

✓5ᵗʰ **M33.0**   **Juvenile dermatomyositis**

     M33.00   **Juvenile dermatomyositis, organ involvement unspecified**

     M33.01   **Juvenile dermatomyositis with respiratory involvement**

     M33.02   **Juvenile dermatomyositis with myopathy**

     M33.03   **Juvenile dermatomyositis without myopathy**

     M33.09   **Juvenile dermatomyositis with other organ involvement**

✓5ᵗʰ **M33.1**   **Other dermatomyositis**
     Adult dermatomyositis

     M33.10   **Other dermatomyositis, organ involvement unspecified**

     M33.11   **Other dermatomyositis with respiratory involvement**

     M33.12   **Other dermatomyositis with myopathy**

     M33.13   **Other dermatomyositis without myopathy**
         Dermatomyositis NOS

     M33.19   **Other dermatomyositis with other organ involvement**

✓5ᵗʰ **M33.2**   **Polymyositis**

     M33.20   **Polymyositis, organ involvement unspecified**

     M33.21   **Polymyositis with respiratory involvement**

     M33.22   **Polymyositis with myopathy**

     M33.29   **Polymyositis with other organ involvement**

✓5ᵗʰ **M33.9**   **Dermatopolymyositis, unspecified**

     M33.90   **Dermatopolymyositis, unspecified, organ involvement unspecified**

     M33.91   **Dermatopolymyositis, unspecified with respiratory involvement**

     M33.92   **Dermatopolymyositis, unspecified with myopathy**

     M33.93   **Dermatopolymyositis, unspecified without myopathy**

     M33.99   **Dermatopolymyositis, unspecified with other organ involvement**

✓4ᵗʰ **M34**   **Systemic sclerosis [scleroderma]**
     EXCLUDES 1   circumscribed scleroderma (L94.0)
         neonatal scleroderma ▶(P83.88)◄

M34.0   **Progressive systemic sclerosis**

M34.1   **CR(E)ST syndrome**
     Combination of calcinosis, Raynaud's phenomenon, esophageal dysfunction, sclerodactyly, telangiectasia

M34.2   **Systemic sclerosis induced by drug and chemical**
     Code first poisoning due to drug or toxin, if applicable (T36-T65 with fifth or sixth character 1-4 or 6)
     Use additional code for adverse effect, if applicable, to identify drug (T36-T50 with fifth or sixth character 5)

✓5ᵗʰ **M34.8**   **Other forms of systemic sclerosis**

     M34.81   **Systemic sclerosis with lung involvement**

     M34.82   **Systemic sclerosis with myopathy**

     M34.83   **Systemic sclerosis with polyneuropathy**

     M34.89   **Other systemic sclerosis**

M34.9   **Systemic sclerosis, unspecified**

✓4ᵗʰ **M35**   **Other systemic involvement of connective tissue**
     EXCLUDES 1   reactive perforating collagenosis (L87.1)

✓5ᵗʰ **M35.0**   **Sicca syndrome [Sjögren]**
     DEF: Autoimmune disease associated with keratoconjunctivitis, laryngopharyngitis, rhinitis, dry mouth, enlarged parotid gland, and chronic polyarthritis.

     M35.00   **Sicca syndrome, unspecified**

     M35.01   **Sicca syndrome with keratoconjunctivitis**

     M35.02   **Sicca syndrome with lung involvement**

     M35.03   **Sicca syndrome with myopathy**

     M35.04   **Sicca syndrome with tubulo-interstitial nephropathy**
         Renal tubular acidosis in sicca syndrome

     M35.09   **Sicca syndrome with other organ involvement**

M35.1   **Other overlap syndromes**
     Mixed connective tissue disease
     EXCLUDES 1   polyangiitis overlap syndrome (M30.8)

M35.2   **Behçet's disease**

M35.3   **Polymyalgia rheumatica**
     EXCLUDES 1   polymyalgia rheumatica with giant cell arteritis (M31.5)

M35.4   **Diffuse (eosinophilic) fasciitis**

M35.5   **Multifocal fibrosclerosis**

M35.6   **Relapsing panniculitis [Weber-Christian]**
     EXCLUDES 1   lupus panniculitis (L93.2)
         panniculitis NOS (M79.3-)

M35.7   **Hypermobility syndrome**
     Familial ligamentous laxity
     EXCLUDES 1   Ehlers-Danlos syndrome ▶(Q79.6-)◄
         ligamentous laxity, NOS (M24.2-)

M35.8   **Other specified systemic involvement of connective tissue**

M35.9   **Systemic involvement of connective tissue, unspecified**
     Autoimmune disease (systemic) NOS
     Collagen (vascular) disease NOS

✓4ᵗʰ **M36**   **Systemic disorders of connective tissue in diseases classified elsewhere**
     EXCLUDES 2   arthropathies in diseases classified elsewhere (M14.-)

M36.0   **Dermato(poly)myositis in neoplastic disease**
     Code first underlying neoplasm (C00-D49)

M36.1   **Arthropathy in neoplastic disease**
     Code first underlying neoplasm, such as:
         leukemia (C91-C95)
         malignant histiocytosis (C96.A)
         multiple myeloma (C90.0)

M36.2   **Hemophilic arthropathy**
     Hemarthrosis in hemophilic arthropathy
     Code first underlying disease, such as:
         factor VIII deficiency (D66)
           with vascular defect (D68.0)
         factor IX deficiency (D67)
         hemophilia (classical) (D66)
         hemophilia B (D67)
         hemophilia C (D68.1)

M36.3   **Arthropathy in other blood disorders**

N Newborn: 0   P Pediatric: 0-17   M Maternity: 12-55   A Adult: 15-124   CH Comorbidity High   CL Comorbidity Low   NCDx Noncancer Dx   PDx Primary Dx

776   ICD-10-CM 2020

M36.4 *Arthropathy in hypersensitivity reactions classified elsewhere*
    Code first underlying disease, such as:
        Henoch (-Schönlein) purpura (D69.0)
        serum sickness (T80.6-)

M36.8 *Systemic disorders of connective tissue in other diseases classified elsewhere*
    Code first underlying disease, such as:
        alkaptonuria (E70.2)
        hypogammaglobulinemia (D80.-)
        ochronosis (E70.2)

DORSOPATHIES (M40-M54)

Deforming dorsopathies (M40-M43)

✓4ᵗʰ M40 Kyphosis and lordosis
    EXCLUDES 1   congenital kyphosis and lordosis (Q76.4)
                kyphoscoliosis (M41.-)
                postprocedural kyphosis and lordosis (M96.-)

Kyphosis and Lordosis

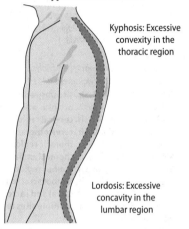

Kyphosis: Excessive convexity in the thoracic region

Lordosis: Excessive concavity in the lumbar region

✓5ᵗʰ M40.0 Postural kyphosis
    EXCLUDES 1   osteochondrosis of spine (M42.-)
    M40.00 Postural kyphosis, site unspecified
    M40.03 Postural kyphosis, cervicothoracic region
    M40.04 Postural kyphosis, thoracic region
    M40.05 Postural kyphosis, thoracolumbar region

✓5ᵗʰ M40.1 Other secondary kyphosis
    M40.10 Other secondary kyphosis, site unspecified
    M40.12 Other secondary kyphosis, cervical region
    M40.13 Other secondary kyphosis, cervicothoracic region
    M40.14 Other secondary kyphosis, thoracic region
    M40.15 Other secondary kyphosis, thoracolumbar region

✓5ᵗʰ M40.2 Other and unspecified kyphosis
    ✓6ᵗʰ M40.20   Unspecified kyphosis
        M40.202 Unspecified kyphosis, cervical region
        M40.203 Unspecified kyphosis, cervicothoracic region
        M40.204 Unspecified kyphosis, thoracic region
        M40.205 Unspecified kyphosis, thoracolumbar region
        M40.209 Unspecified kyphosis, site unspecified
    ✓6ᵗʰ M40.29   Other kyphosis
        M40.292 Other kyphosis, cervical region
        M40.293 Other kyphosis, cervicothoracic region
        M40.294 Other kyphosis, thoracic region
        M40.295 Other kyphosis, thoracolumbar region
        M40.299 Other kyphosis, site unspecified

✓5ᵗʰ M40.3 Flatback syndrome
    M40.30 Flatback syndrome, site unspecified
    M40.35 Flatback syndrome, thoracolumbar region
    M40.36 Flatback syndrome, lumbar region
    M40.37 Flatback syndrome, lumbosacral region

✓5ᵗʰ M40.4 Postural lordosis
    Acquired lordosis
    M40.40 Postural lordosis, site unspecified

M40.45 Postural lordosis, thoracolumbar region
M40.46 Postural lordosis, lumbar region
M40.47 Postural lordosis, lumbosacral region
✓5ᵗʰ M40.5 Lordosis, unspecified
    M40.50 Lordosis, unspecified, site unspecified
    M40.55 Lordosis, unspecified, thoracolumbar region
    M40.56 Lordosis, unspecified, lumbar region
    M40.57 Lordosis, unspecified, lumbosacral region

✓4ᵗʰ M41 Scoliosis
    INCLUDES   kyphoscoliosis
    EXCLUDES 1   congenital scoliosis due to bony malformation (Q76.3)
                congenital scoliosis NOS (Q67.5)
                kyphoscoliotic heart disease (I27.1)
                postprocedural scoliosis (M96.-)
                postural congenital scoliosis (Q67.5)

Scoliosis

Lateral curvature of spine

✓5ᵗʰ M41.0 Infantile idiopathic scoliosis
    AHA: 2014,4Q,26
    M41.00 Infantile idiopathic scoliosis, site unspecified
    M41.02 Infantile idiopathic scoliosis, cervical region
    M41.03 Infantile idiopathic scoliosis, cervicothoracic region
    M41.04 Infantile idiopathic scoliosis, thoracic region
    M41.05 Infantile idiopathic scoliosis, thoracolumbar region
    M41.06 Infantile idiopathic scoliosis, lumbar region
    M41.07 Infantile idiopathic scoliosis, lumbosacral region
    M41.08 Infantile idiopathic scoliosis, sacral and sacrococcygeal region

✓5ᵗʰ M41.1 Juvenile and adolescent idiopathic scoliosis
    ✓6ᵗʰ M41.11   Juvenile idiopathic scoliosis
        AHA: 2014,4Q,28
        M41.112 Juvenile idiopathic scoliosis, cervical region
        M41.113 Juvenile idiopathic scoliosis, cervicothoracic region
        M41.114 Juvenile idiopathic scoliosis, thoracic region
        M41.115 Juvenile idiopathic scoliosis, thoracolumbar region
        M41.116 Juvenile idiopathic scoliosis, lumbar region
        M41.117 Juvenile idiopathic scoliosis, lumbosacral region
        M41.119 Juvenile idiopathic scoliosis, site unspecified
    ✓6ᵗʰ M41.12   Adolescent scoliosis
        M41.122 Adolescent idiopathic scoliosis, cervical region
        M41.123 Adolescent idiopathic scoliosis, cervicothoracic region
        M41.124 Adolescent idiopathic scoliosis, thoracic region
        M41.125 Adolescent idiopathic scoliosis, thoracolumbar region
        M41.126 Adolescent idiopathic scoliosis, lumbar region

M41.127 **Adolescent idiopathic scoliosis, lumbosacral region**
M41.129 **Adolescent idiopathic scoliosis, site unspecified**

√5ᵗʰ **M41.2 Other idiopathic scoliosis**
M41.20 **Other idiopathic scoliosis, site unspecified**
M41.22 **Other idiopathic scoliosis, cervical region**
M41.23 **Other idiopathic scoliosis, cervicothoracic region**
M41.24 **Other idiopathic scoliosis, thoracic region**
M41.25 **Other idiopathic scoliosis, thoracolumbar region**
M41.26 **Other idiopathic scoliosis, lumbar region**
M41.27 **Other idiopathic scoliosis, lumbosacral region**

√5ᵗʰ **M41.3 Thoracogenic scoliosis**
M41.30 **Thoracogenic scoliosis, site unspecified**
M41.34 **Thoracogenic scoliosis, thoracic region**
M41.35 **Thoracogenic scoliosis, thoracolumbar region**

√5ᵗʰ **M41.4 Neuromuscular scoliosis**
Scoliosis secondary to cerebral palsy, Friedreich's ataxia, poliomyelitis and other neuromuscular disorders
Code also underlying condition
AHA: 2014,4Q,27
M41.40 **Neuromuscular scoliosis, site unspecified**
M41.41 **Neuromuscular scoliosis, occipito-atlanto-axial region**
M41.42 **Neuromuscular scoliosis, cervical region**
M41.43 **Neuromuscular scoliosis, cervicothoracic region**
M41.44 **Neuromuscular scoliosis, thoracic region**
M41.45 **Neuromuscular scoliosis, thoracolumbar region**
M41.46 **Neuromuscular scoliosis, lumbar region**
M41.47 **Neuromuscular scoliosis, lumbosacral region**

√5ᵗʰ **M41.5 Other secondary scoliosis**
AHA: 2019,1Q,19
M41.50 **Other secondary scoliosis, site unspecified**
M41.52 **Other secondary scoliosis, cervical region**
M41.53 **Other secondary scoliosis, cervicothoracic region**
M41.54 **Other secondary scoliosis, thoracic region**
M41.55 **Other secondary scoliosis, thoracolumbar region**
M41.56 **Other secondary scoliosis, lumbar region**
M41.57 **Other secondary scoliosis, lumbosacral region**

√5ᵗʰ **M41.8 Other forms of scoliosis**
M41.80 **Other forms of scoliosis, site unspecified**
M41.82 **Other forms of scoliosis, cervical region**
M41.83 **Other forms of scoliosis, cervicothoracic region**
M41.84 **Other forms of scoliosis, thoracic region**
M41.85 **Other forms of scoliosis, thoracolumbar region**
M41.86 **Other forms of scoliosis, lumbar region**
M41.87 **Other forms of scoliosis, lumbosacral region**

M41.9 **Scoliosis, unspecified**

√4ᵗʰ **M42 Spinal osteochondrosis**

√5ᵗʰ **M42.0 Juvenile osteochondrosis of spine**
Calvé's disease
Scheuermann's disease
EXCLUDES 1 postural kyphosis (M40.0)
M42.00 **Juvenile osteochondrosis of spine, site unspecified**
M42.01 **Juvenile osteochondrosis of spine, occipito-atlanto-axial region**
M42.02 **Juvenile osteochondrosis of spine, cervical region**
M42.03 **Juvenile osteochondrosis of spine, cervicothoracic region**
M42.04 **Juvenile osteochondrosis of spine, thoracic region**
M42.05 **Juvenile osteochondrosis of spine, thoracolumbar region**
M42.06 **Juvenile osteochondrosis of spine, lumbar region**
M42.07 **Juvenile osteochondrosis of spine, lumbosacral region**
M42.08 **Juvenile osteochondrosis of spine, sacral and sacrococcygeal region**
M42.09 **Juvenile osteochondrosis of spine, multiple sites in spine**

√5ᵗʰ **M42.1 Adult osteochondrosis of spine**
M42.10 **Adult osteochondrosis of spine, site unspecified** Ⓐ
M42.11 **Adult osteochondrosis of spine, occipito-atlanto-axial region** Ⓐ
M42.12 **Adult osteochondrosis of spine, cervical region** Ⓐ
M42.13 **Adult osteochondrosis of spine, cervicothoracic region** Ⓐ
M42.14 **Adult osteochondrosis of spine, thoracic region** Ⓐ
M42.15 **Adult osteochondrosis of spine, thoracolumbar region** Ⓐ
M42.16 **Adult osteochondrosis of spine, lumbar region** Ⓐ
M42.17 **Adult osteochondrosis of spine, lumbosacral region** Ⓐ
M42.18 **Adult osteochondrosis of spine, sacral and sacrococcygeal region** Ⓐ
M42.19 **Adult osteochondrosis of spine, multiple sites in spine** Ⓐ

M42.9 **Spinal osteochondrosis, unspecified**

√4ᵗʰ **M43 Other deforming dorsopathies**
EXCLUDES 1 congenital spondylolysis and spondylolisthesis (Q76.2)
hemivertebra (Q76.3-Q76.4)
Klippel-Feil syndrome (Q76.1)
lumbarization and sacralization (Q76.4)
platyspondylisis (Q76.4)
spina bifida occulta (Q76.0)
spinal curvature in osteoporosis (M80.-)
spinal curvature in Paget's disease of bone [osteitis deformans] (M88.-)

√5ᵗʰ **M43.0 Spondylolysis**
EXCLUDES 1 congenital spondylolysis (Q76.2)
spondylolisthesis (M43.1)
M43.00 **Spondylolysis, site unspecified**
M43.01 **Spondylolysis, occipito-atlanto-axial region**
M43.02 **Spondylolysis, cervical region**
M43.03 **Spondylolysis, cervicothoracic region**
M43.04 **Spondylolysis, thoracic region**
M43.05 **Spondylolysis, thoracolumbar region**
M43.06 **Spondylolysis, lumbar region**
M43.07 **Spondylolysis, lumbosacral region**
M43.08 **Spondylolysis, sacral and sacrococcygeal region**
M43.09 **Spondylolysis, multiple sites in spine**

√5ᵗʰ **M43.1 Spondylolisthesis**
EXCLUDES 1 acute traumatic of lumbosacral region (S33.1)
acute traumatic of sites other than lumbosacral — code to Fracture, vertebra, by region
congenital spondylolisthesis (Q76.2)
AHA: 2018,3Q,18
TIP: Code also any associated radiculopathy (M54.1-) and/or myelopathy (G99.2).
M43.10 **Spondylolisthesis, site unspecified**
M43.11 **Spondylolisthesis, occipito-atlanto-axial region**
M43.12 **Spondylolisthesis, cervical region**
M43.13 **Spondylolisthesis, cervicothoracic region**
M43.14 **Spondylolisthesis, thoracic region**
M43.15 **Spondylolisthesis, thoracolumbar region**
M43.16 **Spondylolisthesis, lumbar region**
M43.17 **Spondylolisthesis, lumbosacral region**
M43.18 **Spondylolisthesis, sacral and sacrococcygeal region**
M43.19 **Spondylolisthesis, multiple sites in spine**

√5ᵗʰ **M43.2 Fusion of spine**
Ankylosis of spinal joint
EXCLUDES 1 ankylosing spondylitis (M45.0-)
congenital fusion of spine (Q76.4)
EXCLUDES 2 arthrodesis status (Z98.1)
pseudoarthrosis after fusion or arthrodesis (M96.0)
M43.20 **Fusion of spine, site unspecified**
M43.21 **Fusion of spine, occipito-atlanto-axial region**
M43.22 **Fusion of spine, cervical region**
M43.23 **Fusion of spine, cervicothoracic region**
M43.24 **Fusion of spine, thoracic region**
M43.25 **Fusion of spine, thoracolumbar region**
M43.26 **Fusion of spine, lumbar region**
M43.27 **Fusion of spine, lumbosacral region**
M43.28 **Fusion of spine, sacral and sacrococcygeal region**

M43.3 **Recurrent atlantoaxial dislocation with myelopathy**
M43.4 **Other recurrent atlantoaxial dislocation**

✓5ᵗʰ **M43.5 Other recurrent vertebral dislocation**

　　EXCLUDES 1　biomechanical lesions NEC (M99.-)

　✓6ᵗʰ **M43.5X Other recurrent vertebral dislocation**

　　　M43.5X2 Other recurrent vertebral dislocation, cervical region

　　　M43.5X3 Other recurrent vertebral dislocation, cervicothoracic region

　　　M43.5X4 Other recurrent vertebral dislocation, thoracic region

　　　M43.5X5 Other recurrent vertebral dislocation, thoracolumbar region

　　　M43.5X6 Other recurrent vertebral dislocation, lumbar region

　　　M43.5X7 Other recurrent vertebral dislocation, lumbosacral region

　　　M43.5X8 Other recurrent vertebral dislocation, sacral and sacrococcygeal region

　　　M43.5X9 Other recurrent vertebral dislocation, site unspecified

M43.6 Torticollis

　　EXCLUDES 1　congenital (sternomastoid) torticollis (Q68.Ø)
　　　　current injury — see Injury, of spine, by body region
　　　　ocular torticollis (R29.891)
　　　　psychogenic torticollis (F45.8)
　　　　spasmodic torticollis (G24.3)
　　　　torticollis due to birth injury (P15.2)

　　DEF: Twisted, unnatural position of the neck due to contracted cervical muscles that pull the head to one side.

✓5ᵗʰ **M43.8 Other specified deforming dorsopathies**

　　EXCLUDES 2　kyphosis and lordosis (M4Ø.-)
　　　　scoliosis (M41.-)

　✓6ᵗʰ **M43.8X Other specified deforming dorsopathies**

　　　M43.8X1 Other specified deforming dorsopathies, occipito-atlanto-axial region

　　　M43.8X2 Other specified deforming dorsopathies, cervical region

　　　M43.8X3 Other specified deforming dorsopathies, cervicothoracic region

　　　M43.8X4 Other specified deforming dorsopathies, thoracic region

　　　M43.8X5 Other specified deforming dorsopathies, thoracolumbar region

　　　M43.8X6 Other specified deforming dorsopathies, lumbar region

　　　M43.8X7 Other specified deforming dorsopathies, lumbosacral region

　　　M43.8X8 Other specified deforming dorsopathies, sacral and sacrococcygeal region

　　　M43.8X9 Other specified deforming dorsopathies, site unspecified

M43.9 Deforming dorsopathy, unspecified

　　Curvature of spine NOS

Spondylopathies (M45-M49)

✓4ᵗʰ **M45 Ankylosing spondylitis**

　　Rheumatoid arthritis of spine

　　EXCLUDES 1　arthropathy in Reiter's disease (MØ2.3-)
　　　　juvenile (ankylosing) spondylitis (MØ8.1)

　　EXCLUDES 2　Behçet's disease (M35.2)

M45.Ø Ankylosing spondylitis of multiple sites in spine

M45.1 Ankylosing spondylitis of occipito-atlanto-axial region

M45.2 Ankylosing spondylitis of cervical region

M45.3 Ankylosing spondylitis of cervicothoracic region

M45.4 Ankylosing spondylitis of thoracic region

M45.5 Ankylosing spondylitis of thoracolumbar region

M45.6 Ankylosing spondylitis lumbar region

M45.7 Ankylosing spondylitis of lumbosacral region

M45.8 Ankylosing spondylitis sacral and sacrococcygeal region

M45.9 Ankylosing spondylitis of unspecified sites in spine

✓4ᵗʰ **M46 Other inflammatory spondylopathies**

　✓5ᵗʰ **M46.Ø Spinal enthesopathy**

　　　Disorder of ligamentous or muscular attachments of spine

　　　M46.ØØ Spinal enthesopathy, site unspecified

　　　M46.Ø1 Spinal enthesopathy, occipito-atlanto-axial region

　　　M46.Ø2 Spinal enthesopathy, cervical region

　　　M46.Ø3 Spinal enthesopathy, cervicothoracic region

　　　M46.Ø4 Spinal enthesopathy, thoracic region

　　　M46.Ø5 Spinal enthesopathy, thoracolumbar region

　　　M46.Ø6 Spinal enthesopathy, lumbar region

　　　M46.Ø7 Spinal enthesopathy, lumbosacral region

　　　M46.Ø8 Spinal enthesopathy, sacral and sacrococcygeal region

　　　M46.Ø9 Spinal enthesopathy, multiple sites in spine

M46.1 Sacroiliitis, not elsewhere classified

　　DEF: Inflammation of the sacroiliac joint (situated at the juncture of the sacrum and hip). Symptoms include pain in the buttocks or lower back that can extend down one or both legs.

✓5ᵗʰ **M46.2 Osteomyelitis of vertebra**

　　M46.2Ø Osteomyelitis of vertebra, site unspecified

　　M46.21 Osteomyelitis of vertebra, occipito-atlanto-axial region

　　M46.22 Osteomyelitis of vertebra, cervical region

　　M46.23 Osteomyelitis of vertebra, cervicothoracic region

　　M46.24 Osteomyelitis of vertebra, thoracic region

　　M46.25 Osteomyelitis of vertebra, thoracolumbar region

　　M46.26 Osteomyelitis of vertebra, lumbar region

　　M46.27 Osteomyelitis of vertebra, lumbosacral region

　　M46.28 Osteomyelitis of vertebra, sacral and sacrococcygeal region

✓5ᵗʰ **M46.3 Infection of intervertebral disc (pyogenic)**

　　Use additional code (B95-B97) to identify infectious agent

　　M46.3Ø Infection of intervertebral disc (pyogenic), site unspecified

　　M46.31 Infection of intervertebral disc (pyogenic), occipito-atlanto-axial region

　　M46.32 Infection of intervertebral disc (pyogenic), cervical region

　　M46.33 Infection of intervertebral disc (pyogenic), cervicothoracic region

　　M46.34 Infection of intervertebral disc (pyogenic), thoracic region

　　M46.35 Infection of intervertebral disc (pyogenic), thoracolumbar region

　　M46.36 Infection of intervertebral disc (pyogenic), lumbar region

　　M46.37 Infection of intervertebral disc (pyogenic), lumbosacral region

　　M46.38 Infection of intervertebral disc (pyogenic), sacral and sacrococcygeal region

　　M46.39 Infection of intervertebral disc (pyogenic), multiple sites in spine

✓5ᵗʰ **M46.4 Discitis, unspecified**

　　M46.4Ø Discitis, unspecified, site unspecified

　　M46.41 Discitis, unspecified, occipito-atlanto-axial region

　　M46.42 Discitis, unspecified, cervical region

　　M46.43 Discitis, unspecified, cervicothoracic region

　　M46.44 Discitis, unspecified, thoracic region

　　M46.45 Discitis, unspecified, thoracolumbar region

　　M46.46 Discitis, unspecified, lumbar region

　　M46.47 Discitis, unspecified, lumbosacral region

　　M46.48 Discitis, unspecified, sacral and sacrococcygeal region

　　M46.49 Discitis, unspecified, multiple sites in spine

✓5ᵗʰ **M46.5 Other infective spondylopathies**

　　M46.5Ø Other infective spondylopathies, site unspecified

　　M46.51 Other infective spondylopathies, occipito-atlanto-axial region

　　M46.52 Other infective spondylopathies, cervical region

　　M46.53 Other infective spondylopathies, cervicothoracic region

　　M46.54 Other infective spondylopathies, thoracic region

　　M46.55 Other infective spondylopathies, thoracolumbar region

　　M46.56 Other infective spondylopathies, lumbar region

　　M46.57 Other infective spondylopathies, lumbosacral region

　　M46.58 Other infective spondylopathies, sacral and sacrococcygeal region

　　M46.59 Other infective spondylopathies, multiple sites in spine

✓5ᵗʰ **M46.8 Other specified inflammatory spondylopathies**

　　M46.8Ø Other specified inflammatory spondylopathies, site unspecified

　　M46.81 Other specified inflammatory spondylopathies, occipito-atlanto-axial region

☑ Additional Character Required　✓ₓ7ᵗʰ Placeholder Alert　Manifestation　Unspecified Dx　▶◀ Revised Text　● New Code　▲ Revised Title

ICD-10-CM 2020

779

M46.82 **Other specified inflammatory spondylopathies,** cervical **region**

M46.83 **Other specified inflammatory spondylopathies,** cervicothoracic **region**

M46.84 **Other specified inflammatory spondylopathies,** thoracic **region**

M46.85 **Other specified inflammatory spondylopathies,** thoracolumbar **region**

M46.86 **Other specified inflammatory spondylopathies,** lumbar **region**

M46.87 **Other specified inflammatory spondylopathies,** lumbosacral **region**

M46.88 **Other specified inflammatory spondylopathies,** sacral and sacrococcygeal **region**

M46.89 **Other specified inflammatory spondylopathies,** multiple sites **in spine**

✓5ᵗʰ M46.9 **Unspecified inflammatory spondylopathy**

M46.90 **Unspecified inflammatory spondylopathy, site unspecified**

M46.91 **Unspecified inflammatory spondylopathy,** occipito-atlanto-axial **region**

M46.92 **Unspecified inflammatory spondylopathy,** cervical **region**

M46.93 **Unspecified inflammatory spondylopathy,** cervicothoracic **region**

M46.94 **Unspecified inflammatory spondylopathy,** thoracic **region**

M46.95 **Unspecified inflammatory spondylopathy,** thoracolumbar **region**

M46.96 **Unspecified inflammatory spondylopathy,** lumbar **region**

M46.97 **Unspecified inflammatory spondylopathy,** lumbosacral **region**

M46.98 **Unspecified inflammatory spondylopathy, sacral** and sacrococcygeal **region**

M46.99 **Unspecified inflammatory spondylopathy,** multiple sites **in spine**

✓4ᵗʰ M47 **Spondylosis**

INCLUDES   arthrosis or osteoarthritis of spine
degeneration of facet joints

✓5ᵗʰ M47.0 **Anterior spinal and vertebral artery** compression syndromes

✓6ᵗʰ M47.01 Anterior spinal artery **compression syndromes**

M47.011 **Anterior spinal artery compression syndromes,** occipito-atlanto-axial **region**

M47.012 **Anterior spinal artery compression syndromes,** cervical **region**

M47.013 **Anterior spinal artery compression syndromes,** cervicothoracic **region**

M47.014 **Anterior spinal artery compression syndromes,** thoracic **region**

M47.015 **Anterior spinal artery compression syndromes,** thoracolumbar **region**

M47.016 **Anterior spinal artery compression syndromes,** lumbar **region**

M47.019 **Anterior spinal artery compression syndromes, site unspecified**

✓6ᵗʰ M47.02 Vertebral artery **compression syndromes**

M47.021 **Vertebral artery compression syndromes,** occipito-atlanto-axial **region**

M47.022 **Vertebral artery compression syndromes,** cervical **region**

M47.029 **Vertebral artery compression syndromes, site unspecified**

✓5ᵗʰ M47.1 **Other spondylosis** with myelopathy

Spondylogenic compression of spinal cord
EXCLUDES 1   vertebral subluxation ▶(M43.3-M43.5X9)◀

M47.10 **Other spondylosis with myelopathy, site unspecified**

M47.11 **Other spondylosis with myelopathy,** occipito-atlanto-axial **region**

M47.12 **Other spondylosis with myelopathy,** cervical **region**

M47.13 **Other spondylosis with myelopathy,** cervicothoracic **region**

M47.14 **Other spondylosis with myelopathy,** thoracic **region**

M47.15 **Other spondylosis with myelopathy,** thoracolumbar **region**

M47.16 **Other spondylosis with myelopathy,** lumbar **region**

✓5ᵗʰ M47.2 **Other spondylosis** with radiculopathy

M47.20 **Other spondylosis with radiculopathy, site unspecified**

M47.21 **Other spondylosis with radiculopathy,** occipito-atlanto-axial **region**

M47.22 **Other spondylosis with radiculopathy,** cervical **region**

M47.23 **Other spondylosis with radiculopathy,** cervicothoracic **region**

M47.24 **Other spondylosis with radiculopathy,** thoracic **region**

M47.25 **Other spondylosis with radiculopathy,** thoracolumbar **region**

M47.26 **Other spondylosis with radiculopathy,** lumbar **region**

M47.27 **Other spondylosis with radiculopathy,** lumbosacral **region**

M47.28 **Other spondylosis with radiculopathy,** sacral and sacrococcygeal **region**

✓5ᵗʰ M47.8 **Other spondylosis**

✓6ᵗʰ M47.81 **Spondylosis** without myelopathy or radiculopathy
AHA: 2018,2Q,14

M47.811 **Spondylosis without myelopathy or radiculopathy,** occipito-atlanto-axial **region**

M47.812 **Spondylosis without myelopathy or radiculopathy,** cervical **region**

M47.813 **Spondylosis without myelopathy or radiculopathy,** cervicothoracic **region**

M47.814 **Spondylosis without myelopathy or radiculopathy,** thoracic **region**

M47.815 **Spondylosis without myelopathy or radiculopathy,** thoracolumbar **region**

M47.816 **Spondylosis without myelopathy or radiculopathy,** lumbar **region**

M47.817 **Spondylosis without myelopathy or radiculopathy,** lumbosacral **region**

M47.818 **Spondylosis without myelopathy or radiculopathy,** sacral and sacrococcygeal **region**

M47.819 **Spondylosis without myelopathy or radiculopathy, site unspecified**

✓6ᵗʰ M47.89 **Other spondylosis**

M47.891 **Other spondylosis,** occipito-atlanto-axial **region**

M47.892 **Other spondylosis,** cervical **region**

M47.893 **Other spondylosis,** cervicothoracic **region**

M47.894 **Other spondylosis,** thoracic **region**

M47.895 **Other spondylosis,** thoracolumbar **region**

M47.896 **Other spondylosis,** lumbar **region**

M47.897 **Other spondylosis,** lumbosacral **region**

M47.898 **Other spondylosis,** sacral and sacrococcygeal **region**

M47.899 **Other spondylosis, site unspecified**

M47.9 **Spondylosis, unspecified**

✓4ᵗʰ M48 **Other spondylopathies**

✓5ᵗʰ M48.0 **Spinal stenosis**

Caudal stenosis
AHA: 2018,3Q,18-19
TIP: Code also any associated radiculopathy (M54.1-) and/or myelopathy (G99.2).

M48.00 **Spinal stenosis, site unspecified**

M48.01 **Spinal stenosis,** occipito-atlanto-axial **region**

M48.02 **Spinal stenosis,** cervical **region**

M48.03 **Spinal stenosis,** cervicothoracic **region**

M48.04 **Spinal stenosis,** thoracic **region**

M48.05 **Spinal stenosis,** thoracolumbar **region**

✓6ᵗʰ M48.06 **Spinal stenosis, lumbar region**

AHA: 2018,3Q,19; 2017,4Q,18-19
DEF: Spinal canal narrowing in the lumbar area with nerve root compression, causing muscle pain, fatigue, and weakness during extension of the lumbar spine. Pain is relieved by sitting or bending.

M48.061 **Spinal stenosis, lumbar region** without neurogenic claudication
Spinal stenosis, lumbar region NOS

M48.062 **Spinal stenosis, lumbar region** with neurogenic claudication

M48.07 **Spinal stenosis,** lumbosacral **region**

M48.08 **Spinal stenosis,** sacral and sacrococcygeal **region**

√5ᵗʰ **M48.1 Ankylosing hyperostosis [Forestier]**

Diffuse idiopathic skeletal hyperostosis [DISH]

M48.10 Ankylosing hyperostosis [Forestier], site unspecified

M48.11 Ankylosing hyperostosis [Forestier], occipito-atlanto-axial region

M48.12 Ankylosing hyperostosis [Forestier], cervical region

M48.13 Ankylosing hyperostosis [Forestier], cervicothoracic region

M48.14 Ankylosing hyperostosis [Forestier], thoracic region

M48.15 Ankylosing hyperostosis [Forestier], thoracolumbar region

M48.16 Ankylosing hyperostosis [Forestier], lumbar region

M48.17 Ankylosing hyperostosis [Forestier], lumbosacral region

M48.18 Ankylosing hyperostosis [Forestier], sacral and sacrococcygeal region

M48.19 Ankylosing hyperostosis [Forestier], multiple sites in spine

√5ᵗʰ **M48.2 Kissing spine**

M48.20 Kissing spine, site unspecified

M48.21 Kissing spine, occipito-atlanto-axial region

M48.22 Kissing spine, cervical region

M48.23 Kissing spine, cervicothoracic region

M48.24 Kissing spine, thoracic region

M48.25 Kissing spine, thoracolumbar region

M48.26 Kissing spine, lumbar region

M48.27 Kissing spine, lumbosacral region

√5ᵗʰ **M48.3 Traumatic spondylopathy**

M48.30 Traumatic spondylopathy, site unspecified

M48.31 Traumatic spondylopathy, occipito-atlanto-axial region

M48.32 Traumatic spondylopathy, cervical region

M48.33 Traumatic spondylopathy, cervicothoracic region

M48.34 Traumatic spondylopathy, thoracic region

M48.35 Traumatic spondylopathy, thoracolumbar region

M48.36 Traumatic spondylopathy, lumbar region

M48.37 Traumatic spondylopathy, lumbosacral region

M48.38 Traumatic spondylopathy, sacral and sacrococcygeal region

√5ᵗʰ **M48.4 Fatigue fracture of vertebra**

Stress fracture of vertebra

EXCLUDES 1   pathological fracture NOS (M84.4-)
pathological fracture of vertebra due to neoplasm (M84.58)
pathological fracture of vertebra due to osteoporosis (M80.-)
pathological fracture of vertebra due to other diagnosis (M84.68)
traumatic fracture of vertebrae (S12.0-S12.3-, S22.0-, S32.0-)

The appropriate 7th character is to be added to each code from subcategory M48.4.
A   initial encounter for fracture
D   subsequent encounter for fracture with routine healing
G   subsequent encounter for fracture with delayed healing
S   sequela of fracture

√x7ᵗʰ **M48.40 Fatigue fracture of vertebra, site unspecified**

√x7ᵗʰ **M48.41 Fatigue fracture of vertebra, occipito-atlanto-axial region**

√x7ᵗʰ **M48.42 Fatigue fracture of vertebra, cervical region**

√x7ᵗʰ **M48.43 Fatigue fracture of vertebra, cervicothoracic region**

√x7ᵗʰ **M48.44 Fatigue fracture of vertebra, thoracic region**

√x7ᵗʰ **M48.45 Fatigue fracture of vertebra, thoracolumbar region**

√x7ᵗʰ **M48.46 Fatigue fracture of vertebra, lumbar region**

√x7ᵗʰ **M48.47 Fatigue fracture of vertebra, lumbosacral region**

√x7ᵗʰ **M48.48 Fatigue fracture of vertebra, sacral and sacrococcygeal region**

√5ᵗʰ **M48.5 Collapsed vertebra, not elsewhere classified**

Collapsed vertebra NOS
Compression fracture of vertebra NOS
Wedging of vertebra NOS

EXCLUDES 1   current injury — see Injury of spine, by body region
fatigue fracture of vertebra (M48.4)
pathological fracture NOS (M84.4-)
pathological fracture of vertebra due to neoplasm (M84.58)
pathological fracture of vertebra due to osteoporosis (M80.-)
pathological fracture of vertebra due to other diagnosis (M84.68)
stress fracture of vertebra (M48.4-)
traumatic fracture of vertebra (S12.-, S22.-, S32.-)

The appropriate 7th character is to be added to each code from subcategory M48.5.
A   initial encounter for fracture
D   subsequent encounter for fracture with routine healing
G   subsequent encounter for fracture with delayed healing
S   sequela of fracture

√x7ᵗʰ **M48.50 Collapsed vertebra, not elsewhere classified, site unspecified**

√x7ᵗʰ **M48.51 Collapsed vertebra, not elsewhere classified, occipito-atlanto-axial region**

√x7ᵗʰ **M48.52 Collapsed vertebra, not elsewhere classified, cervical region**

√x7ᵗʰ **M48.53 Collapsed vertebra, not elsewhere classified, cervicothoracic region**

√x7ᵗʰ **M48.54 Collapsed vertebra, not elsewhere classified, thoracic region**

√x7ᵗʰ **M48.55 Collapsed vertebra, not elsewhere classified, thoracolumbar region**

√x7ᵗʰ **M48.56 Collapsed vertebra, not elsewhere classified, lumbar region**

√x7ᵗʰ **M48.57 Collapsed vertebra, not elsewhere classified, lumbosacral region**

√x7ᵗʰ **M48.58 Collapsed vertebra, not elsewhere classified, sacral and sacrococcygeal region**

√5ᵗʰ **M48.8 Other specified spondylopathies**

Ossification of posterior longitudinal ligament

√6ᵗʰ **M48.8X Other specified spondylopathies**

M48.8X1 Other specified spondylopathies, occipito-atlanto-axial region

M48.8X2 Other specified spondylopathies, cervical region

M48.8X3 Other specified spondylopathies, cervicothoracic region

M48.8X4 Other specified spondylopathies, thoracic region

M48.8X5 Other specified spondylopathies, thoracolumbar region

M48.8X6 Other specified spondylopathies, lumbar region

M48.8X7 Other specified spondylopathies, lumbosacral region

M48.8X8 Other specified spondylopathies, sacral and sacrococcygeal region

M48.8X9 Other specified spondylopathies, site unspecified

M48.9 Spondylopathy, unspecified

☑ Additional Character Required   √x7ᵗʰ Placeholder Alert   Manifestation   Unspecified Dx   ▶◀ Revised Text   ● New Code   ▲ Revised Title

☑4ᵗʰ **M49 Spondylopathies in diseases classified elsewhere**

> **INCLUDES** curvature of spine in diseases classified elsewhere
> deformity of spine in diseases classified elsewhere
> kyphosis in diseases classified elsewhere
> scoliosis in diseases classified elsewhere
> spondylopathy in diseases classified elsewhere

> Code first underlying disease, such as:
> brucellosis (A23.-)
> Charcôt-Marie-Tooth disease (G60.0)
> enterobacterial infections (A01-A04)
> osteitis fibrosa cystica (E21.0)

> **EXCLUDES 1** curvature of spine in tuberculosis [Pott's] (A18.01)
> enteropathic arthropathies (M07.-)
> gonococcal spondylitis (A54.41)
> neuropathic spondylopathy in syringomyelia (G95.0)
> neuropathic spondylopathy in tabes dorsalis (A52.11)
> neuropathic [tabes dorsalis] spondylitis (A52.11)
> nonsyphilitic neuropathic spondylopathy NEC (G98.0)
> spondylitis in syphilis (acquired) (A52.77)
> tuberculous spondylitis (A18.01)
> typhoid fever spondylitis (A01.05)

☑5ᵗʰ **M49.8 Spondylopathy in diseases classified elsewhere**

> **M49.80** *Spondylopathy in diseases classified elsewhere, site unspecified*
>
> **M49.81** *Spondylopathy in diseases classified elsewhere, occipito-atlanto-axial region*
>
> **M49.82** *Spondylopathy in diseases classified elsewhere, cervical region*
>
> **M49.83** *Spondylopathy in diseases classified elsewhere, cervicothoracic region*
>
> **M49.84** *Spondylopathy in diseases classified elsewhere, thoracic region*
>
> **M49.85** *Spondylopathy in diseases classified elsewhere, thoracolumbar region*
>
> **M49.86** *Spondylopathy in diseases classified elsewhere, lumbar region*
>
> **M49.87** *Spondylopathy in diseases classified elsewhere, lumbosacral region*
>
> **M49.88** *Spondylopathy in diseases classified elsewhere, sacral and sacrococcygeal region*
>
> **M49.89** *Spondylopathy in diseases classified elsewhere, multiple sites in spine*

Other dorsopathies (M50-M54)

> **EXCLUDES 1** current injury — see injury of spine by body region
> discitis NOS (M46.4-)

☑4ᵗʰ **M50 Cervical disc disorders**

> **NOTE** Code to the most superior level of disorder
>
> **INCLUDES** cervicothoracic disc disorders
> cervicothoracic disc disorders with cervicalgia
>
> **AHA:** 2016,4Q,39-40; 2016,1Q,17

☑5ᵗʰ **M50.0 Cervical disc disorder with myelopathy**

> **AHA:** 2018,3Q,19
>
> **M50.00** **Cervical disc disorder with myelopathy, unspecified cervical region**
>
> **M50.01** **Cervical disc disorder with myelopathy, high cervical region**
> C2-C3 disc disorder with myelopathy
> C3-C4 disc disorder with myelopathy
>
> ☑6ᵗʰ **M50.02** **Cervical disc disorder with myelopathy, mid-cervical region**
>> **M50.020** **Cervical disc disorder with myelopathy, mid-cervical region, unspecified level**
>> **M50.021** **Cervical disc disorder at C4-C5 level with myelopathy**
>> C4-C5 disc disorder with myelopathy
>> **M50.022** **Cervical disc disorder at C5-C6 level with myelopathy**
>> C5-C6 disc disorder with myelopathy
>> **M50.023** **Cervical disc disorder at C6-C7 level with myelopathy**
>> C6-C7 disc disorder with myelopathy
>
> **M50.03** **Cervical disc disorder with myelopathy, cervicothoracic region**
> C7-T1 disc disorder with myelopathy

☑5ᵗʰ **M50.1 Cervical disc disorder with radiculopathy**

> **EXCLUDES 2** brachial radiculitis NOS (M54.13)
>
> **AHA:** 2018,3Q,19
>
> **M50.10** **Cervical disc disorder with radiculopathy, unspecified cervical region**
>
> **M50.11** **Cervical disc disorder with radiculopathy, high cervical region**
> C2-C3 disc disorder with radiculopathy
> C3 radiculopathy due to disc disorder
> C3-C4 disc disorder with radiculopathy
> C4 radiculopathy due to disc disorder
>
> ☑6ᵗʰ **M50.12** **Cervical disc disorder with radiculopathy, mid-cervical region**
>> **M50.120** **Mid-cervical disc disorder, unspecified level**
>> **M50.121** **Cervical disc disorder at C4-C5 level with radiculopathy**
>> C4-C5 disc disorder with radiculopathy
>> C5 radiculopathy due to disc disorder
>> **M50.122** **Cervical disc disorder at C5-C6 level with radiculopathy**
>> C5-C6 disc disorder with radiculopathy
>> C6 radiculopathy due to disc disorder
>> **M50.123** **Cervical disc disorder at C6-C7 level with radiculopathy**
>> C6-C7 disc disorder with radiculopathy
>> C7 radiculopathy due to disc disorder
>
> **M50.13** **Cervical disc disorder with radiculopathy, cervicothoracic region**
> C7-T1 disc disorder with radiculopathy
> C8 radiculopathy due to disc disorder

☑5ᵗʰ **M50.2 Other cervical disc displacement**

> **M50.20** **Other cervical disc displacement, unspecified cervical region**
>
> **M50.21** **Other cervical disc displacement, high cervical region**
> Other C2-C3 cervical disc displacement
> Other C3-C4 cervical disc displacement
>
> ☑6ᵗʰ **M50.22** **Other cervical disc displacement, mid-cervical region**
>> **M50.220** **Other cervical disc displacement, mid-cervical region, unspecified level**
>> **M50.221** **Other cervical disc displacement at C4-C5 level**
>> Other C4-C5 cervical disc displacement
>> **M50.222** **Other cervical disc displacement at C5-C6 level**
>> Other C5-C6 cervical disc displacement
>> **M50.223** **Other cervical disc displacement at C6-C7 level**
>> Other C6-C7 cervical disc displacement
>
> **M50.23** **Other cervical disc displacement, cervicothoracic region**
> Other C7-T1 cervical disc displacement

☑5ᵗʰ **M50.3 Other cervical disc degeneration**

> **M50.30** **Other cervical disc degeneration, unspecified cervical region**
>
> **M50.31** **Other cervical disc degeneration, high cervical region**
> Other C2-C3 cervical disc degeneration
> Other C3-C4 cervical disc degeneration
>
> ☑6ᵗʰ **M50.32** **Other cervical disc degeneration, mid-cervical region**
>> **M50.320** **Other cervical disc degeneration, mid-cervical region, unspecified level**
>> **M50.321** **Other cervical disc degeneration at C4-C5 level**
>> Other C4-C5 cervical disc degeneration
>> **M50.322** **Other cervical disc degeneration at C5-C6 level**
>> Other C5-C6 cervical disc degeneration
>> **M50.323** **Other cervical disc degeneration at C6-C7 level**
>> Other C6-C7 cervical disc degeneration
>
> **M50.33** **Other cervical disc degeneration, cervicothoracic region**
> Other C7-T1 cervical disc degeneration

☑5ᵗʰ **M50.8 Other cervical disc disorders**

> **M50.80** **Other cervical disc disorders, unspecified cervical region**

M50.81 **Other cervical disc disorders, high cervical region**
Other C2-C3 cervical disc disorders
Other C3-C4 cervical disc disorders

✓6th M50.82 **Other cervical disc disorders, mid-cervical region**

     M50.820 **Other cervical disc disorders, mid-cervical region, unspecified level**

     M50.821 **Other cervical disc disorders at C4-C5 level**
Other C4-C5 cervical disc disorders

     M50.822 **Other cervical disc disorders at C5-C6 level**
Other C5-C6 cervical disc disorders

     M50.823 **Other cervical disc disorders at C6-C7 level**
Other C6-C7 cervical disc disorders

M50.83 **Other cervical disc disorders, cervicothoracic region**
Other C7-T1 cervical disc disorders

✓5th M50.9 **Cervical disc disorder, unspecified**

     M50.90 **Cervical disc disorder, unspecified, unspecified cervical region**

     M50.91 **Cervical disc disorder, unspecified, high cervical region**
C2-C3 cervical disc disorder, unspecified
C3-C4 cervical disc disorder, unspecified

✓6th M50.92 **Cervical disc disorder, unspecified, mid-cervical region**

     M50.920 **Unspecified cervical disc disorder, mid-cervical region, unspecified level**

     M50.921 **Unspecified cervical disc disorder at C4-C5 level**
Unspecified C4-C5 cervical disc disorder

     M50.922 **Unspecified cervical disc disorder at C5-C6 level**
Unspecified C5-C6 cervical disc disorder

     M50.923 **Unspecified cervical disc disorder at C6-C7 level**
Unspecified C6-C7 cervical disc disorder

     M50.93 **Cervical disc disorder, unspecified, cervicothoracic region**
C7-T1 cervical disc disorder, unspecified

✓4th **M51 Thoracic, thoracolumbar, and lumbosacral intervertebral disc disorders**

     EXCLUDES 2   cervical and cervicothoracic disc disorders (M50.-)
                sacral and sacrococcygeal disorders (M53.3)

✓5th M51.0 **Thoracic, thoracolumbar and lumbosacral intervertebral disc disorders with myelopathy**

     M51.04 **Intervertebral disc disorders with myelopathy, thoracic region**

     M51.05 **Intervertebral disc disorders with myelopathy, thoracolumbar region**

     M51.06 **Intervertebral disc disorders with myelopathy, lumbar region**

✓5th M51.1 **Thoracic, thoracolumbar and lumbosacral intervertebral disc disorders with radiculopathy**
Sciatica due to intervertebral disc disorder
     EXCLUDES 1   lumbar radiculitis NOS (M54.16)
                sciatica NOS (M54.3)
     AHA: 2018,3Q,18

     M51.14 **Intervertebral disc disorders with radiculopathy, thoracic region**

     M51.15 **Intervertebral disc disorders with radiculopathy, thoracolumbar region**

     M51.16 **Intervertebral disc disorders with radiculopathy, lumbar region**

     M51.17 **Intervertebral disc disorders with radiculopathy, lumbosacral region**

✓5th M51.2 **Other thoracic, thoracolumbar and lumbosacral intervertebral disc displacement**
Lumbago due to displacement of intervertebral disc

Displacement Intervertebral Disc

Normal Top View   Herniated Top View

Lamina   Nucleus pulposus   Ligamentum flavum   Spinal cord   Spinal nerve   Disc annulus   Nucleus pulposus   Herniates through annulus

M51.24 **Other intervertebral disc displacement, thoracic region**

M51.25 **Other intervertebral disc displacement, thoracolumbar region**

M51.26 **Other intervertebral disc displacement, lumbar region**

M51.27 **Other intervertebral disc displacement, lumbosacral region**

✓5th M51.3 **Other thoracic, thoracolumbar and lumbosacral intervertebral disc degeneration**
     AHA: 2018,2Q,15; 2013,3Q,22

M51.34 **Other intervertebral disc degeneration, thoracic region**

M51.35 **Other intervertebral disc degeneration, thoracolumbar region**

M51.36 **Other intervertebral disc degeneration, lumbar region**

M51.37 **Other intervertebral disc degeneration, lumbosacral region**

✓5th M51.4 **Schmorl's nodes**
     DEF: Irregular bone defect in the margin of the vertebral body that causes herniation into the end plate of the vertebral body.

M51.44 **Schmorl's nodes, thoracic region**

M51.45 **Schmorl's nodes, thoracolumbar region**

M51.46 **Schmorl's nodes, lumbar region**

M51.47 **Schmorl's nodes, lumbosacral region**

✓5th M51.8 **Other thoracic, thoracolumbar and lumbosacral intervertebral disc disorders**

M51.84 **Other intervertebral disc disorders, thoracic region**

M51.85 **Other intervertebral disc disorders, thoracolumbar region**

M51.86 **Other intervertebral disc disorders, lumbar region**

M51.87 **Other intervertebral disc disorders, lumbosacral region**

M51.9 **Unspecified thoracic, thoracolumbar and lumbosacral intervertebral disc disorder**

✓4th **M53 Other and unspecified dorsopathies, not elsewhere classified**

M53.0 **Cervicocranial syndrome**
Posterior cervical sympathetic syndrome

M53.1 **Cervicobrachial syndrome**
     EXCLUDES 2   cervical disc disorder (M50.-)
                thoracic outlet syndrome (G54.0)

✓5th M53.2 **Spinal instabilities**

     ✓6th M53.2X **Spinal instabilities**

         M53.2X1 **Spinal instabilities, occipito-atlanto-axial region**

         M53.2X2 **Spinal instabilities, cervical region**

         M53.2X3 **Spinal instabilities, cervicothoracic region**

         M53.2X4 **Spinal instabilities, thoracic region**

         M53.2X5 **Spinal instabilities, thoracolumbar region**

         M53.2X6 **Spinal instabilities, lumbar region**

         M53.2X7 **Spinal instabilities, lumbosacral region**

         M53.2X8 **Spinal instabilities, sacral and sacrococcygeal region**

         M53.2X9 **Spinal instabilities, site unspecified**

✔ Additional Character Required   ✔x7th Placeholder Alert   Manifestation   Unspecified Dx   ▶◀ Revised Text   ● New Code   ▲ Revised Title

ICD-10-CM 2020   783

M53.3 Sacrococcygeal disorders, not elsewhere classified
Coccygodynia

✓5ᵗʰ **M53.8 Other specified dorsopathies**

M53.80 Other specified dorsopathies, site unspecified

M53.81 Other specified dorsopathies, occipito-atlanto-axial region

M53.82 Other specified dorsopathies, cervical region

M53.83 Other specified dorsopathies, cervicothoracic region

M53.84 Other specified dorsopathies, thoracic region

M53.85 Other specified dorsopathies, thoracolumbar region

M53.86 Other specified dorsopathies, lumbar region

M53.87 Other specified dorsopathies, lumbosacral region

M53.88 Other specified dorsopathies, sacral and sacrococcygeal region

M53.9 Dorsopathy, unspecified

✓4ᵗʰ **M54 Dorsalgia**

EXCLUDES 1   psychogenic dorsalgia (F45.41)

✓5ᵗʰ **M54.0 Panniculitis affecting regions of neck and back**

EXCLUDES 1   lupus panniculitis (L93.2)
panniculitis NOS (M79.3)
relapsing [Weber-Christian] panniculitis (M35.6)

M54.00 Panniculitis affecting regions of neck and back, site unspecified

M54.01 Panniculitis affecting regions of neck and back, occipito-atlanto-axial region

M54.02 Panniculitis affecting regions of neck and back, cervical region

M54.03 Panniculitis affecting regions of neck and back, cervicothoracic region

M54.04 Panniculitis affecting regions of neck and back, thoracic region

M54.05 Panniculitis affecting regions of neck and back, thoracolumbar region

M54.06 Panniculitis affecting regions of neck and back, lumbar region

M54.07 Panniculitis affecting regions of neck and back, lumbosacral region

M54.08 Panniculitis affecting regions of neck and back, sacral and sacrococcygeal region

M54.09 Panniculitis affecting regions, neck and back, multiple sites in spine

✓5ᵗʰ **M54.1 Radiculopathy**

Brachial neuritis or radiculitis NOS
Lumbar neuritis or radiculitis NOS
Lumbosacral neuritis or radiculitis NOS
Thoracic neuritis or radiculitis NOS
Radiculitis NOS

EXCLUDES 1   neuralgia and neuritis NOS (M79.2)
radiculopathy with cervical disc disorder (M50.1)
radiculopathy with lumbar and other intervertebral disc disorder (M51.1-)
radiculopathy with spondylosis (M47.2-)

AHA: 2018,3Q,18

TIP: A code from this subcategory can be used in addition to a spondylolisthesis code (M43.1-) or a spinal stenosis code (M48.0-) when either condition is documented as the cause of the radiculopathy.

M54.10 Radiculopathy, site unspecified

M54.11 Radiculopathy, occipito-atlanto-axial region

M54.12 Radiculopathy, cervical region

M54.13 Radiculopathy, cervicothoracic region

M54.14 Radiculopathy, thoracic region

M54.15 Radiculopathy, thoracolumbar region

M54.16 Radiculopathy, lumbar region

M54.17 Radiculopathy, lumbosacral region

M54.18 Radiculopathy, sacral and sacrococcygeal region

M54.2 Cervicalgia

EXCLUDES 1   cervicalgia due to intervertebral cervical disc disorder (M50.-)

✓5ᵗʰ **M54.3 Sciatica**

EXCLUDES 1   lesion of sciatic nerve (G57.0)
sciatica due to intervertebral disc disorder (M51.1-)
sciatica with lumbago (M54.4-)

M54.30 Sciatica, unspecified side

M54.31 Sciatica, right side

M54.32 Sciatica, left side

✓5ᵗʰ **M54.4 Lumbago with sciatica**

EXCLUDES 1   lumbago with sciatica due to intervertebral disc disorder (M51.1-)

AHA: 2016,2Q,7

M54.40 Lumbago with sciatica, unspecified side

M54.41 Lumbago with sciatica, right side

M54.42 Lumbago with sciatica, left side

M54.5 Low back pain
Loin pain
Lumbago NOS

EXCLUDES 1   low back strain (S39.012)
lumbago due to intervertebral disc displacement (M51.2-)
lumbago with sciatica (M54.4-)

M54.6 Pain in thoracic spine

EXCLUDES 1   pain in thoracic spine due to intervertebral disc disorder (M51.-)

✓5ᵗʰ **M54.8 Other dorsalgia**

EXCLUDES 1   dorsalgia in thoracic region (M54.6)
low back pain (M54.5)

M54.81 Occipital neuralgia

M54.89 Other dorsalgia

M54.9 Dorsalgia, unspecified
Backache NOS
Back pain NOS

SOFT TISSUE DISORDERS (M60-M79)

Disorders of muscles (M60-M63)

EXCLUDES 1   dermatopolymyositis (M33.-)
muscular dystrophies and myopathies (G71-G72)
myopathy in amyloidosis (E85.-)
myopathy in polyarteritis nodosa (M30.0)
myopathy in rheumatoid arthritis (M05.32)
myopathy in scleroderma (M34.-)
myopathy in Sjögren's syndrome (M35.03)
myopathy in systemic lupus erythematosus (M32.-)

✓4ᵗʰ **M60 Myositis**

EXCLUDES 2   inclusion body myositis [IBM] (G72.41)

✓5ᵗʰ **M60.0 Infective myositis**

Tropical pyomyositis
Use additional code (B95-B97) to identify infectious agent

✓6ᵗʰ **M60.00 Infective myositis, unspecified site**

M60.000 Infective myositis, unspecified right arm
Infective myositis, right upper limb NOS

M60.001 Infective myositis, unspecified left arm
Infective myositis, left upper limb NOS

M60.002 Infective myositis, unspecified arm
Infective myositis, upper limb NOS

M60.003 Infective myositis, unspecified right leg
Infective myositis, right lower limb NOS

M60.004 Infective myositis, unspecified left leg
Infective myositis, left lower limb NOS

M60.005 Infective myositis, unspecified leg
Infective myositis, lower limb NOS

M60.009 Infective myositis, unspecified site

✓6ᵗʰ **M60.01 Infective myositis, shoulder**

M60.011 Infective myositis, right shoulder

M60.012 Infective myositis, left shoulder

M60.019 Infective myositis, unspecified shoulder

✓6ᵗʰ **M60.02 Infective myositis, upper arm**

M60.021 Infective myositis, right upper arm

M60.022 Infective myositis, left upper arm

M60.029 Infective myositis, unspecified upper arm

✓6ᵗʰ **M60.03 Infective myositis, forearm**

M60.031 Infective myositis, right forearm

M60.032 Infective myositis, left forearm

M60.039 Infective myositis, unspecified forearm

✓6ᵗʰ **M60.04 Infective myositis, hand and fingers**

M60.041 Infective myositis, right hand

M60.042 Infective myositis, left hand

M60.043 Infective myositis, unspecified hand

M60.044 Infective myositis, right finger(s)

M60.045 Infective myositis, left finger(s)

M60.046 Infective myositis, unspecified finger(s)

√6ᵗʰ **M60.05** Infective myositis, thigh

    M60.051 Infective myositis, right thigh
    M60.052 Infective myositis, left thigh
    M60.059 Infective myositis, unspecified thigh

√6ᵗʰ **M60.06** Infective myositis, lower leg

    M60.061 Infective myositis, right lower leg
    M60.062 Infective myositis, left lower leg
    M60.069 Infective myositis, unspecified lower leg

√6ᵗʰ **M60.07** Infective myositis, ankle, foot and toes

    M60.070 Infective myositis, right ankle
    M60.071 Infective myositis, left ankle
    M60.072 Infective myositis, unspecified ankle
    M60.073 Infective myositis, right foot
    M60.074 Infective myositis, left foot
    M60.075 Infective myositis, unspecified foot
    M60.076 Infective myositis, right toe(s)
    M60.077 Infective myositis, left toe(s)
    M60.078 Infective myositis, unspecified toe(s)

M60.08 Infective myositis, other site
M60.09 Infective myositis, multiple sites

√5ᵗʰ **M60.1** Interstitial myositis

    M60.10 Interstitial myositis of unspecified site

√6ᵗʰ **M60.11** Interstitial myositis, shoulder

    M60.111 Interstitial myositis, right shoulder
    M60.112 Interstitial myositis, left shoulder
    M60.119 Interstitial myositis, unspecified shoulder

√6ᵗʰ **M60.12** Interstitial myositis, upper arm

    M60.121 Interstitial myositis, right upper arm
    M60.122 Interstitial myositis, left upper arm
    M60.129 Interstitial myositis, unspecified upper arm

√6ᵗʰ **M60.13** Interstitial myositis, forearm

    M60.131 Interstitial myositis, right forearm
    M60.132 Interstitial myositis, left forearm
    M60.139 Interstitial myositis, unspecified forearm

√6ᵗʰ **M60.14** Interstitial myositis, hand

    M60.141 Interstitial myositis, right hand
    M60.142 Interstitial myositis, left hand
    M60.149 Interstitial myositis, unspecified hand

√6ᵗʰ **M60.15** Interstitial myositis, thigh

    M60.151 Interstitial myositis, right thigh
    M60.152 Interstitial myositis, left thigh
    M60.159 Interstitial myositis, unspecified thigh

√6ᵗʰ **M60.16** Interstitial myositis, lower leg

    M60.161 Interstitial myositis, right lower leg
    M60.162 Interstitial myositis, left lower leg
    M60.169 Interstitial myositis, unspecified lower leg

√6ᵗʰ **M60.17** Interstitial myositis, ankle and foot

    M60.171 Interstitial myositis, right ankle and foot
    M60.172 Interstitial myositis, left ankle and foot
    M60.179 Interstitial myositis, unspecified ankle and foot

M60.18 Interstitial myositis, other site
M60.19 Interstitial myositis, multiple sites

√5ᵗʰ **M60.2** Foreign body granuloma of soft tissue, not elsewhere classified

    Use additional code to identify the type of retained foreign body (Z18.-)

    EXCLUDES 1   *foreign body granuloma of skin and subcutaneous tissue (L92.3)*

    M60.20 Foreign body granuloma of soft tissue, not elsewhere classified, unspecified site

√6ᵗʰ **M60.21** Foreign body granuloma of soft tissue, not elsewhere classified, shoulder

    M60.211 Foreign body granuloma of soft tissue, not elsewhere classified, right shoulder
    M60.212 Foreign body granuloma of soft tissue, not elsewhere classified, left shoulder
    M60.219 Foreign body granuloma of soft tissue, not elsewhere classified, unspecified shoulder

√6ᵗʰ **M60.22** Foreign body granuloma of soft tissue, not elsewhere classified, upper arm

    M60.221 Foreign body granuloma of soft tissue, not elsewhere classified, right upper arm
    M60.222 Foreign body granuloma of soft tissue, not elsewhere classified, left upper arm

    M60.229 Foreign body granuloma of soft tissue, not elsewhere classified, unspecified upper arm

√6ᵗʰ **M60.23** Foreign body granuloma of soft tissue, not elsewhere classified, forearm

    M60.231 Foreign body granuloma of soft tissue, not elsewhere classified, right forearm
    M60.232 Foreign body granuloma of soft tissue, not elsewhere classified, left forearm
    M60.239 Foreign body granuloma of soft tissue, not elsewhere classified, unspecified forearm

√6ᵗʰ **M60.24** Foreign body granuloma of soft tissue, not elsewhere classified, hand

    M60.241 Foreign body granuloma of soft tissue, not elsewhere classified, right hand
    M60.242 Foreign body granuloma of soft tissue, not elsewhere classified, left hand
    M60.249 Foreign body granuloma of soft tissue, not elsewhere classified, unspecified hand

√6ᵗʰ **M60.25** Foreign body granuloma of soft tissue, not elsewhere classified, thigh

    M60.251 Foreign body granuloma of soft tissue, not elsewhere classified, right thigh
    M60.252 Foreign body granuloma of soft tissue, not elsewhere classified, left thigh
    M60.259 Foreign body granuloma of soft tissue, not elsewhere classified, unspecified thigh

√6ᵗʰ **M60.26** Foreign body granuloma of soft tissue, not elsewhere classified, lower leg

    M60.261 Foreign body granuloma of soft tissue, not elsewhere classified, right lower leg
    M60.262 Foreign body granuloma of soft tissue, not elsewhere classified, left lower leg
    M60.269 Foreign body granuloma of soft tissue, not elsewhere classified, unspecified lower leg

√6ᵗʰ **M60.27** Foreign body granuloma of soft tissue, not elsewhere classified, ankle and foot

    M60.271 Foreign body granuloma of soft tissue, not elsewhere classified, right ankle and foot
    M60.272 Foreign body granuloma of soft tissue, not elsewhere classified, left ankle and foot
    M60.279 Foreign body granuloma of soft tissue, not elsewhere classified, unspecified ankle and foot

M60.28 Foreign body granuloma of soft tissue, not elsewhere classified, other site

√5ᵗʰ **M60.8** Other myositis

    M60.80 Other myositis, unspecified site

√6ᵗʰ **M60.81** Other myositis shoulder

    M60.811 Other myositis, right shoulder
    M60.812 Other myositis, left shoulder
    M60.819 Other myositis, unspecified shoulder

√6ᵗʰ **M60.82** Other myositis, upper arm

    M60.821 Other myositis, right upper arm
    M60.822 Other myositis, left upper arm
    M60.829 Other myositis, unspecified upper arm

√6ᵗʰ **M60.83** Other myositis, forearm

    M60.831 Other myositis, right forearm
    M60.832 Other myositis, left forearm
    M60.839 Other myositis, unspecified forearm

√6ᵗʰ **M60.84** Other myositis, hand

    M60.841 Other myositis, right hand
    M60.842 Other myositis, left hand
    M60.849 Other myositis, unspecified hand

√6ᵗʰ **M60.85** Other myositis, thigh

    M60.851 Other myositis, right thigh
    M60.852 Other myositis, left thigh
    M60.859 Other myositis, unspecified thigh

√6ᵗʰ **M60.86** Other myositis, lower leg

    M60.861 Other myositis, right lower leg
    M60.862 Other myositis, left lower leg
    M60.869 Other myositis, unspecified lower leg

√6ᵗʰ **M60.87** Other myositis, ankle and foot

    M60.871 Other myositis, right ankle and foot

✔ Additional Character Required   √×7ᵗʰ Placeholder Alert   Manifestation   Unspecified Dx   ▶◀ Revised Text   ● New Code   ▲ Revised Title

ICD-10-CM 2020   785

M60.872 Other myositis, left ankle and foot
M60.879 Other myositis, unspecified ankle and foot
M60.88 Other myositis, other site
M60.89 Other myositis, multiple sites
M60.9 Myositis, unspecified

M61 Calcification and ossification of muscle
  M61.0 Myositis ossificans traumatica
    M61.00 Myositis ossificans traumatica, unspecified site
    M61.01 Myositis ossificans traumatica, shoulder
      M61.011 Myositis ossificans traumatica, right shoulder
      M61.012 Myositis ossificans traumatica, left shoulder
      M61.019 Myositis ossificans traumatica, unspecified shoulder
    M61.02 Myositis ossificans traumatica, upper arm
      M61.021 Myositis ossificans traumatica, right upper arm
      M61.022 Myositis ossificans traumatica, left upper arm
      M61.029 Myositis ossificans traumatica, unspecified upper arm
    M61.03 Myositis ossificans traumatica, forearm
      M61.031 Myositis ossificans traumatica, right forearm
      M61.032 Myositis ossificans traumatica, left forearm
      M61.039 Myositis ossificans traumatica, unspecified forearm
    M61.04 Myositis ossificans traumatica, hand
      M61.041 Myositis ossificans traumatica, right hand
      M61.042 Myositis ossificans traumatica, left hand
      M61.049 Myositis ossificans traumatica, unspecified hand
    M61.05 Myositis ossificans traumatica, thigh
      M61.051 Myositis ossificans traumatica, right thigh
      M61.052 Myositis ossificans traumatica, left thigh
      M61.059 Myositis ossificans traumatica, unspecified thigh
    M61.06 Myositis ossificans traumatica, lower leg
      M61.061 Myositis ossificans traumatica, right lower leg
      M61.062 Myositis ossificans traumatica, left lower leg
      M61.069 Myositis ossificans traumatica, unspecified lower leg
    M61.07 Myositis ossificans traumatica, ankle and foot
      M61.071 Myositis ossificans traumatica, right ankle and foot
      M61.072 Myositis ossificans traumatica, left ankle and foot
      M61.079 Myositis ossificans traumatica, unspecified ankle and foot
    M61.08 Myositis ossificans traumatica, other site
    M61.09 Myositis ossificans traumatica, multiple sites
  M61.1 Myositis ossificans progressiva
      Fibrodysplasia ossificans progressiva
    M61.10 Myositis ossificans progressiva, unspecified site
    M61.11 Myositis ossificans progressiva, shoulder
      M61.111 Myositis ossificans progressiva, right shoulder
      M61.112 Myositis ossificans progressiva, left shoulder
      M61.119 Myositis ossificans progressiva, unspecified shoulder
    M61.12 Myositis ossificans progressiva, upper arm
      M61.121 Myositis ossificans progressiva, right upper arm
      M61.122 Myositis ossificans progressiva, left upper arm
      M61.129 Myositis ossificans progressiva, unspecified arm
    M61.13 Myositis ossificans progressiva, forearm
      M61.131 Myositis ossificans progressiva, right forearm
      M61.132 Myositis ossificans progressiva, left forearm

M61.139 Myositis ossificans progressiva, unspecified forearm
M61.14 Myositis ossificans progressiva, hand and finger(s)
  M61.141 Myositis ossificans progressiva, right hand
  M61.142 Myositis ossificans progressiva, left hand
  M61.143 Myositis ossificans progressiva, unspecified hand
  M61.144 Myositis ossificans progressiva, right finger(s)
  M61.145 Myositis ossificans progressiva, left finger(s)
  M61.146 Myositis ossificans progressiva, unspecified finger(s)
M61.15 Myositis ossificans progressiva, thigh
  M61.151 Myositis ossificans progressiva, right thigh
  M61.152 Myositis ossificans progressiva, left thigh
  M61.159 Myositis ossificans progressiva, unspecified thigh
M61.16 Myositis ossificans progressiva, lower leg
  M61.161 Myositis ossificans progressiva, right lower leg
  M61.162 Myositis ossificans progressiva, left lower leg
  M61.169 Myositis ossificans progressiva, unspecified lower leg
M61.17 Myositis ossificans progressiva, ankle, foot and toe(s)
  M61.171 Myositis ossificans progressiva, right ankle
  M61.172 Myositis ossificans progressiva, left ankle
  M61.173 Myositis ossificans progressiva, unspecified ankle
  M61.174 Myositis ossificans progressiva, right foot
  M61.175 Myositis ossificans progressiva, left foot
  M61.176 Myositis ossificans progressiva, unspecified foot
  M61.177 Myositis ossificans progressiva, right toe(s)
  M61.178 Myositis ossificans progressiva, left toe(s)
  M61.179 Myositis ossificans progressiva, unspecified toe(s)
M61.18 Myositis ossificans progressiva, other site
M61.19 Myositis ossificans progressiva, multiple sites
M61.2 Paralytic calcification and ossification of muscle
    Myositis ossificans associated with quadriplegia or paraplegia
  M61.20 Paralytic calcification and ossification of muscle, unspecified site
  M61.21 Paralytic calcification and ossification of muscle, shoulder
    M61.211 Paralytic calcification and ossification of muscle, right shoulder
    M61.212 Paralytic calcification and ossification of muscle, left shoulder
    M61.219 Paralytic calcification and ossification of muscle, unspecified shoulder
  M61.22 Paralytic calcification and ossification of muscle, upper arm
    M61.221 Paralytic calcification and ossification of muscle, right upper arm
    M61.222 Paralytic calcification and ossification of muscle, left upper arm
    M61.229 Paralytic calcification and ossification of muscle, unspecified upper arm
  M61.23 Paralytic calcification and ossification of muscle, forearm
    M61.231 Paralytic calcification and ossification of muscle, right forearm
    M61.232 Paralytic calcification and ossification of muscle, left forearm
    M61.239 Paralytic calcification and ossification of muscle, unspecified forearm
  M61.24 Paralytic calcification and ossification of muscle, hand
    M61.241 Paralytic calcification and ossification of muscle, right hand
    M61.242 Paralytic calcification and ossification of muscle, left hand
    M61.249 Paralytic calcification and ossification of muscle, unspecified hand

✓6ᵗʰ **M61.25** Paralytic calcification and ossification of muscle, thigh
- **M61.251** Paralytic calcification and ossification of muscle, right thigh
- **M61.252** Paralytic calcification and ossification of muscle, left thigh
- **M61.259** Paralytic calcification and ossification of muscle, unspecified thigh

✓6ᵗʰ **M61.26** Paralytic calcification and ossification of muscle, lower leg
- **M61.261** Paralytic calcification and ossification of muscle, right lower leg
- **M61.262** Paralytic calcification and ossification of muscle, left lower leg
- **M61.269** Paralytic calcification and ossification of muscle, unspecified lower leg

✓6ᵗʰ **M61.27** Paralytic calcification and ossification of muscle, ankle and foot
- **M61.271** Paralytic calcification and ossification of muscle, right ankle and foot
- **M61.272** Paralytic calcification and ossification of muscle, left ankle and foot
- **M61.279** Paralytic calcification and ossification of muscle, unspecified ankle and foot

M61.28 Paralytic calcification and ossification of muscle, other site

M61.29 Paralytic calcification and ossification of muscle, multiple sites

✓5ᵗʰ **M61.3** Calcification and ossification of muscles associated with burns
  Myositis ossificans associated with burns

M61.30 Calcification and ossification of muscles associated with burns, unspecified site

✓6ᵗʰ **M61.31** Calcification and ossification of muscles associated with burns, shoulder
- **M61.311** Calcification and ossification of muscles associated with burns, right shoulder
- **M61.312** Calcification and ossification of muscles associated with burns, left shoulder
- **M61.319** Calcification and ossification of muscles associated with burns, unspecified shoulder

✓6ᵗʰ **M61.32** Calcification and ossification of muscles associated with burns, upper arm
- **M61.321** Calcification and ossification of muscles associated with burns, right upper arm
- **M61.322** Calcification and ossification of muscles associated with burns, left upper arm
- **M61.329** Calcification and ossification of muscles associated with burns, unspecified upper arm

✓6ᵗʰ **M61.33** Calcification and ossification of muscles associated with burns, forearm
- **M61.331** Calcification and ossification of muscles associated with burns, right forearm
- **M61.332** Calcification and ossification of muscles associated with burns, left forearm
- **M61.339** Calcification and ossification of muscles associated with burns, unspecified forearm

✓6ᵗʰ **M61.34** Calcification and ossification of muscles associated with burns, hand
- **M61.341** Calcification and ossification of muscles associated with burns, right hand
- **M61.342** Calcification and ossification of muscles associated with burns, left hand
- **M61.349** Calcification and ossification of muscles associated with burns, unspecified hand

✓6ᵗʰ **M61.35** Calcification and ossification of muscles associated with burns, thigh
- **M61.351** Calcification and ossification of muscles associated with burns, right thigh
- **M61.352** Calcification and ossification of muscles associated with burns, left thigh
- **M61.359** Calcification and ossification of muscles associated with burns, unspecified thigh

✓6ᵗʰ **M61.36** Calcification and ossification of muscles associated with burns, lower leg
- **M61.361** Calcification and ossification of muscles associated with burns, right lower leg
- **M61.362** Calcification and ossification of muscles associated with burns, left lower leg

M61.369 Calcification and ossification of muscles associated with burns, unspecified lower leg

✓6ᵗʰ **M61.37** Calcification and ossification of muscles associated with burns, ankle and foot
- **M61.371** Calcification and ossification of muscles associated with burns, right ankle and foot
- **M61.372** Calcification and ossification of muscles associated with burns, left ankle and foot
- **M61.379** Calcification and ossification of muscles associated with burns, unspecified ankle and foot

M61.38 Calcification and ossification of muscles associated with burns, other site

M61.39 Calcification and ossification of muscles associated with burns, multiple sites

✓5ᵗʰ **M61.4** Other calcification of muscle
  EXCLUDES 1 calcific tendinitis NOS (M65.2-)
    calcific tendinitis of shoulder (M75.3)

M61.40 Other calcification of muscle, unspecified site

✓6ᵗʰ **M61.41** Other calcification of muscle, shoulder
- **M61.411** Other calcification of muscle, right shoulder
- **M61.412** Other calcification of muscle, left shoulder
- **M61.419** Other calcification of muscle, unspecified shoulder

✓6ᵗʰ **M61.42** Other calcification of muscle, upper arm
- **M61.421** Other calcification of muscle, right upper arm
- **M61.422** Other calcification of muscle, left upper arm
- **M61.429** Other calcification of muscle, unspecified upper arm

✓6ᵗʰ **M61.43** Other calcification of muscle, forearm
- **M61.431** Other calcification of muscle, right forearm
- **M61.432** Other calcification of muscle, left forearm
- **M61.439** Other calcification of muscle, unspecified forearm

✓6ᵗʰ **M61.44** Other calcification of muscle, hand
- **M61.441** Other calcification of muscle, right hand
- **M61.442** Other calcification of muscle, left hand
- **M61.449** Other calcification of muscle, unspecified hand

✓6ᵗʰ **M61.45** Other calcification of muscle, thigh
- **M61.451** Other calcification of muscle, right thigh
- **M61.452** Other calcification of muscle, left thigh
- **M61.459** Other calcification of muscle, unspecified thigh

✓6ᵗʰ **M61.46** Other calcification of muscle, lower leg
- **M61.461** Other calcification of muscle, right lower leg
- **M61.462** Other calcification of muscle, left lower leg
- **M61.469** Other calcification of muscle, unspecified lower leg

✓6ᵗʰ **M61.47** Other calcification of muscle, ankle and foot
- **M61.471** Other calcification of muscle, right ankle and foot
- **M61.472** Other calcification of muscle, left ankle and foot
- **M61.479** Other calcification of muscle, unspecified ankle and foot

M61.48 Other calcification of muscle, other site

M61.49 Other calcification of muscle, multiple sites

✓5ᵗʰ **M61.5** Other ossification of muscle

M61.50 Other ossification of muscle, unspecified site

✓6ᵗʰ **M61.51** Other ossification of muscle, shoulder
- **M61.511** Other ossification of muscle, right shoulder
- **M61.512** Other ossification of muscle, left shoulder
- **M61.519** Other ossification of muscle, unspecified shoulder

✓6ᵗʰ **M61.52** Other ossification of muscle, upper arm
- **M61.521** Other ossification of muscle, right upper arm

✓ Additional Character Required ✓x7ᵗʰ Placeholder Alert Manifestation Unspecified Dx ▶◀ Revised Text ● New Code ▲ Revised Title

M61.522 Other ossification of muscle, left upper arm

M61.529 Other ossification of muscle, unspecified upper arm

√6th **M61.53** Other ossification of muscle, forearm

M61.531 Other ossification of muscle, right forearm

M61.532 Other ossification of muscle, left forearm

M61.539 Other ossification of muscle, unspecified forearm

√6th **M61.54** Other ossification of muscle, hand

M61.541 Other ossification of muscle, right hand

M61.542 Other ossification of muscle, left hand

M61.549 Other ossification of muscle, unspecified hand

√6th **M61.55** Other ossification of muscle, thigh

M61.551 Other ossification of muscle, right thigh

M61.552 Other ossification of muscle, left thigh

M61.559 Other ossification of muscle, unspecified thigh

√6th **M61.56** Other ossification of muscle, lower leg

M61.561 Other ossification of muscle, right lower leg

M61.562 Other ossification of muscle, left lower leg

M61.569 Other ossification of muscle, unspecified lower leg

√6th **M61.57** Other ossification of muscle, ankle and foot

M61.571 Other ossification of muscle, right ankle and foot

M61.572 Other ossification of muscle, left ankle and foot

M61.579 Other ossification of muscle, unspecified ankle and foot

M61.58 Other ossification of muscle, other site

M61.59 Other ossification of muscle, multiple sites

M61.9 Calcification and ossification of muscle, unspecified

√4th **M62** Other disorders of muscle

EXCLUDES 1   alcoholic myopathy (G72.1)

       cramp and spasm (R25.2)

       drug-induced myopathy (G72.0)

       myalgia (M79.1-)

       stiff-man syndrome (G25.82)

EXCLUDES 2   nontraumatic hematoma of muscle (M79.81)

√5th **M62.0** Separation of muscle (nontraumatic)

Diastasis of muscle

EXCLUDES 1   diastasis recti complicating pregnancy, labor and delivery (O71.8)

       traumatic separation of muscle — see strain of muscle by body region

M62.00 Separation of muscle (nontraumatic), unspecified site

√6th **M62.01** Separation of muscle (nontraumatic), shoulder

M62.011 Separation of muscle (nontraumatic), right shoulder

M62.012 Separation of muscle (nontraumatic), left shoulder

M62.019 Separation of muscle (nontraumatic), unspecified shoulder

√6th **M62.02** Separation of muscle (nontraumatic), upper arm

M62.021 Separation of muscle (nontraumatic), right upper arm

M62.022 Separation of muscle (nontraumatic), left upper arm

M62.029 Separation of muscle (nontraumatic), unspecified upper arm

√6th **M62.03** Separation of muscle (nontraumatic), forearm

M62.031 Separation of muscle (nontraumatic), right forearm

M62.032 Separation of muscle (nontraumatic), left forearm

M62.039 Separation of muscle (nontraumatic), unspecified forearm

√6th **M62.04** Separation of muscle (nontraumatic), hand

M62.041 Separation of muscle (nontraumatic), right hand

M62.042 Separation of muscle (nontraumatic), left hand

M62.049 Separation of muscle (nontraumatic), unspecified hand

√6th **M62.05** Separation of muscle (nontraumatic), thigh

M62.051 Separation of muscle (nontraumatic), right thigh

M62.052 Separation of muscle (nontraumatic), left thigh

M62.059 Separation of muscle (nontraumatic), unspecified thigh

√6th **M62.06** Separation of muscle (nontraumatic), lower leg

M62.061 Separation of muscle (nontraumatic), right lower leg

M62.062 Separation of muscle (nontraumatic), left lower leg

M62.069 Separation of muscle (nontraumatic), unspecified lower leg

√6th **M62.07** Separation of muscle (nontraumatic), ankle and foot

M62.071 Separation of muscle (nontraumatic), right ankle and foot

M62.072 Separation of muscle (nontraumatic), left ankle and foot

M62.079 Separation of muscle (nontraumatic), unspecified ankle and foot

M62.08 Separation of muscle (nontraumatic), other site

√5th **M62.1** Other rupture of muscle (nontraumatic)

EXCLUDES 1   traumatic rupture of muscle — see strain of muscle by body region

EXCLUDES 2   rupture of tendon (M66.-)

M62.10 Other rupture of muscle (nontraumatic), unspecified site

√6th **M62.11** Other rupture of muscle (nontraumatic), shoulder

M62.111 Other rupture of muscle (nontraumatic), right shoulder

M62.112 Other rupture of muscle (nontraumatic), left shoulder

M62.119 Other rupture of muscle (nontraumatic), unspecified shoulder

√6th **M62.12** Other rupture of muscle (nontraumatic), upper arm

M62.121 Other rupture of muscle (nontraumatic), right upper arm

M62.122 Other rupture of muscle (nontraumatic), left upper arm

M62.129 Other rupture of muscle (nontraumatic), unspecified upper arm

√6th **M62.13** Other rupture of muscle (nontraumatic), forearm

M62.131 Other rupture of muscle (nontraumatic), right forearm

M62.132 Other rupture of muscle (nontraumatic), left forearm

M62.139 Other rupture of muscle (nontraumatic), unspecified forearm

√6th **M62.14** Other rupture of muscle (nontraumatic), hand

M62.141 Other rupture of muscle (nontraumatic), right hand

M62.142 Other rupture of muscle (nontraumatic), left hand

M62.149 Other rupture of muscle (nontraumatic), unspecified hand

√6th **M62.15** Other rupture of muscle (nontraumatic), thigh

M62.151 Other rupture of muscle (nontraumatic), right thigh

M62.152 Other rupture of muscle (nontraumatic), left thigh

M62.159 Other rupture of muscle (nontraumatic), unspecified thigh

√6th **M62.16** Other rupture of muscle (nontraumatic), lower leg

M62.161 Other rupture of muscle (nontraumatic), right lower leg

M62.162 Other rupture of muscle (nontraumatic), left lower leg

M62.169 Other rupture of muscle (nontraumatic), unspecified lower leg

√6th **M62.17** Other rupture of muscle (nontraumatic), ankle and foot

M62.171 Other rupture of muscle (nontraumatic), right ankle and foot

M62.172 Other rupture of muscle (nontraumatic), left ankle and foot

N Newborn: 0   P Pediatric: 0-17   M Maternity: 12-55   A Adult: 15-124   CH Comorbidity High   CL Comorbidity Low   NCDx Noncancer Dx   PDx Primary Dx

788   ICD-10-CM 2020

M62.179   Other rupture of muscle (nontraumatic), unspecified ankle and foot

M62.18   Other rupture of muscle (nontraumatic), other site

☑5ᵗʰ **M62.2**   **Nontraumatic ischemic infarction of muscle**

> EXCLUDES 1   *compartment syndrome (traumatic) (T79.A-)*
> *nontraumatic compartment syndrome (M79.A-)*
> *rhabdomyolysis (M62.82)*
> *traumatic ischemia of muscle (T79.6)*
> *Volkmann's ischemic contracture (T79.6)*

M62.20   Nontraumatic ischemic infarction of muscle, unspecified site

☑6ᵗʰ M62.21   Nontraumatic ischemic infarction of muscle, shoulder

> M62.211   Nontraumatic ischemic infarction of muscle, right shoulder
> M62.212   Nontraumatic ischemic infarction of muscle, left shoulder
> M62.219   Nontraumatic ischemic infarction of muscle, unspecified shoulder

☑6ᵗʰ M62.22   Nontraumatic ischemic infarction of muscle, upper arm

> M62.221   Nontraumatic ischemic infarction of muscle, right upper arm
> M62.222   Nontraumatic ischemic infarction of muscle, left upper arm
> M62.229   Nontraumatic ischemic infarction of muscle, unspecified upper arm

☑6ᵗʰ M62.23   Nontraumatic ischemic infarction of muscle, forearm

> M62.231   Nontraumatic ischemic infarction of muscle, right forearm
> M62.232   Nontraumatic ischemic infarction of muscle, left forearm
> M62.239   Nontraumatic ischemic infarction of muscle, unspecified forearm

☑6ᵗʰ M62.24   Nontraumatic ischemic infarction of muscle, hand

> M62.241   Nontraumatic ischemic infarction of muscle, right hand
> M62.242   Nontraumatic ischemic infarction of muscle, left hand
> M62.249   Nontraumatic ischemic infarction of muscle, unspecified hand

☑6ᵗʰ M62.25   Nontraumatic ischemic infarction of muscle, thigh

> M62.251   Nontraumatic ischemic infarction of muscle, right thigh
> M62.252   Nontraumatic ischemic infarction of muscle, left thigh
> M62.259   Nontraumatic ischemic infarction of muscle, unspecified thigh

☑6ᵗʰ M62.26   Nontraumatic ischemic infarction of muscle, lower leg

> M62.261   Nontraumatic ischemic infarction of muscle, right lower leg
> M62.262   Nontraumatic ischemic infarction of muscle, left lower leg
> M62.269   Nontraumatic ischemic infarction of muscle, unspecified lower leg

☑6ᵗʰ M62.27   Nontraumatic ischemic infarction of muscle, ankle and foot

> M62.271   Nontraumatic ischemic infarction of muscle, right ankle and foot
> M62.272   Nontraumatic ischemic infarction of muscle, left ankle and foot
> M62.279   Nontraumatic ischemic infarction of muscle, unspecified ankle and foot

M62.28   Nontraumatic ischemic infarction of muscle, other site

M62.3   **Immobility syndrome (paraplegic)**

☑5ᵗʰ **M62.4**   **Contracture of muscle**

> Contracture of tendon (sheath)
> EXCLUDES 1   *contracture of joint (M24.5-)*

M62.40   Contracture of muscle, unspecified site

☑6ᵗʰ M62.41   Contracture of muscle, shoulder

> M62.411   Contracture of muscle, right shoulder
> M62.412   Contracture of muscle, left shoulder
> M62.419   Contracture of muscle, unspecified shoulder

☑6ᵗʰ M62.42   Contracture of muscle, upper arm

> M62.421   Contracture of muscle, right upper arm
> M62.422   Contracture of muscle, left upper arm

M62.429   Contracture of muscle, unspecified upper arm

☑6ᵗʰ M62.43   Contracture of muscle, forearm

> M62.431   Contracture of muscle, right forearm
> M62.432   Contracture of muscle, left forearm
> M62.439   Contracture of muscle, unspecified forearm

☑6ᵗʰ M62.44   Contracture of muscle, hand

> M62.441   Contracture of muscle, right hand
> M62.442   Contracture of muscle, left hand
> M62.449   Contracture of muscle, unspecified hand

☑6ᵗʰ M62.45   Contracture of muscle, thigh

> M62.451   Contracture of muscle, right thigh
> M62.452   Contracture of muscle, left thigh
> M62.459   Contracture of muscle, unspecified thigh

☑6ᵗʰ M62.46   Contracture of muscle, lower leg

> M62.461   Contracture of muscle, right lower leg
> M62.462   Contracture of muscle, left lower leg
> M62.469   Contracture of muscle, unspecified lower leg

☑6ᵗʰ M62.47   Contracture of muscle, ankle and foot

> M62.471   Contracture of muscle, right ankle and foot
> M62.472   Contracture of muscle, left ankle and foot
> M62.479   Contracture of muscle, unspecified ankle and foot

M62.48   Contracture of muscle, other site

M62.49   Contracture of muscle, multiple sites

☑5ᵗʰ **M62.5**   **Muscle wasting and atrophy, not elsewhere classified**

> Disuse atrophy NEC
> EXCLUDES 1   *neuralgic amyotrophy (G54.5)*
> *progressive muscular atrophy (G12.21)*
> *sarcopenia (M62.84)*
> EXCLUDES 2   *pelvic muscle wasting (N81.84)*

M62.50   Muscle wasting and atrophy, not elsewhere classified, unspecified site

☑6ᵗʰ M62.51   Muscle wasting and atrophy, not elsewhere classified, shoulder

> M62.511   Muscle wasting and atrophy, not elsewhere classified, right shoulder
> M62.512   Muscle wasting and atrophy, not elsewhere classified, left shoulder
> M62.519   Muscle wasting and atrophy, not elsewhere classified, unspecified shoulder

☑6ᵗʰ M62.52   Muscle wasting and atrophy, not elsewhere classified, upper arm

> M62.521   Muscle wasting and atrophy, not elsewhere classified, right upper arm
> M62.522   Muscle wasting and atrophy, not elsewhere classified, left upper arm
> M62.529   Muscle wasting and atrophy, not elsewhere classified, unspecified upper arm

☑6ᵗʰ M62.53   Muscle wasting and atrophy, not elsewhere classified, forearm

> M62.531   Muscle wasting and atrophy, not elsewhere classified, right forearm
> M62.532   Muscle wasting and atrophy, not elsewhere classified, left forearm
> M62.539   Muscle wasting and atrophy, not elsewhere classified, unspecified forearm

☑6ᵗʰ M62.54   Muscle wasting and atrophy, not elsewhere classified, hand

> M62.541   Muscle wasting and atrophy, not elsewhere classified, right hand
> M62.542   Muscle wasting and atrophy, not elsewhere classified, left hand
> M62.549   Muscle wasting and atrophy, not elsewhere classified, unspecified hand

☑6ᵗʰ M62.55   Muscle wasting and atrophy, not elsewhere classified, thigh

> M62.551   Muscle wasting and atrophy, not elsewhere classified, right thigh
> M62.552   Muscle wasting and atrophy, not elsewhere classified, left thigh
> M62.559   Muscle wasting and atrophy, not elsewhere classified, unspecified thigh

---

☑ Additional Character Required   ✓x7ᵗʰ Placeholder Alert   Manifestation   Unspecified Dx   ▶◀ Revised Text   ● New Code   ▲ Revised Title

√6ᵗʰ **M62.56** **Muscle wasting and atrophy, not elsewhere classified, lower leg**
    M62.561 Muscle wasting and atrophy, not elsewhere classified, right lower leg
    M62.562 Muscle wasting and atrophy, not elsewhere classified, left lower leg
    M62.569 Muscle wasting and atrophy, not elsewhere classified, unspecified lower leg

√6ᵗʰ **M62.57** **Muscle wasting and atrophy, not elsewhere classified, ankle and foot**
    M62.571 Muscle wasting and atrophy, not elsewhere classified, right ankle and foot
    M62.572 Muscle wasting and atrophy, not elsewhere classified, left ankle and foot
    M62.579 Muscle wasting and atrophy, not elsewhere classified, unspecified ankle and foot

M62.58 **Muscle wasting and atrophy, not elsewhere classified, other site**

M62.59 **Muscle wasting and atrophy, not elsewhere classified, multiple sites**

√5ᵗʰ **M62.8** **Other specified disorders of muscle**
    EXCLUDES 2   nontraumatic hematoma of muscle (M79.81)

M62.81 **Muscle weakness (generalized)**
    EXCLUDES 1   muscle weakness in sarcopenia (M62.84)

M62.82 **Rhabdomyolysis**
    EXCLUDES 1   traumatic rhabdomyolysis (T79.6)
    AHA: 2019,2Q,12
    DEF: Rapid disintegration or destruction of skeletal muscle caused by direct or indirect injury, resulting in the excretion of muscle protein myoglobin into the urine.

√6ᵗʰ **M62.83** **Muscle spasm**
    M62.830 Muscle spasm of back
    M62.831 Muscle spasm of calf
        Charley-horse
    M62.838 Other muscle spasm

M62.84 **Sarcopenia**
    Age-related sarcopenia
    Code first underlying disease, if applicable, such as:
        disorders of myoneural junction and muscle disease in diseases classified elsewhere (G73.-)
        other and unspecified myopathies (G72.-)
        primary disorders of muscles (G71.-)
    AHA: 2016,4Q,41

M62.89 **Other specified disorders of muscle**
    Muscle (sheath) hernia

M62.9 **Disorder of muscle, unspecified**

√4ᵗʰ **M63** **Disorders of muscle in diseases classified elsewhere**
    Code first underlying disease, such as:
    leprosy (A30.-)
    neoplasm (C49.-, C79.89, D21.-, D48.1)
    schistosomiasis (B65.-)
    trichinellosis (B75)
    EXCLUDES 1   myopathy in cysticercosis (B69.81)
        myopathy in endocrine diseases (G73.7)
        myopathy in metabolic diseases (G73.7)
        myopathy in sarcoidosis (D86.87)
        myopathy in secondary syphilis (A51.49)
        myopathy in syphilis (late) (A52.78)
        myopathy in toxoplasmosis (B58.82)
        myopathy in tuberculosis (A18.09)

√5ᵗʰ **M63.8** **Disorders of muscle in diseases classified elsewhere**
    M63.80 *Disorders of muscle in diseases classified elsewhere, unspecified site*

√6ᵗʰ *M63.81* *Disorders of muscle in diseases classified elsewhere, shoulder*
    M63.811 *Disorders of muscle in diseases classified elsewhere, right shoulder*
    M63.812 *Disorders of muscle in diseases classified elsewhere, left shoulder*
    M63.819 *Disorders of muscle in diseases classified elsewhere, unspecified shoulder*

√6ᵗʰ *M63.82* *Disorders of muscle in diseases classified elsewhere, upper arm*
    M63.821 *Disorders of muscle in diseases classified elsewhere, right upper arm*

M63.822 *Disorders of muscle in diseases classified elsewhere, left upper arm*
M63.829 *Disorders of muscle in diseases classified elsewhere, unspecified upper arm*

√6ᵗʰ *M63.83* *Disorders of muscle in diseases classified elsewhere, forearm*
    M63.831 *Disorders of muscle in diseases classified elsewhere, right forearm*
    M63.832 *Disorders of muscle in diseases classified elsewhere, left forearm*
    M63.839 *Disorders of muscle in diseases classified elsewhere, unspecified forearm*

√6ᵗʰ *M63.84* *Disorders of muscle in diseases classified elsewhere, hand*
    M63.841 *Disorders of muscle in diseases classified elsewhere, right hand*
    M63.842 *Disorders of muscle in diseases classified elsewhere, left hand*
    M63.849 *Disorders of muscle in diseases classified elsewhere, unspecified hand*

√6ᵗʰ *M63.85* *Disorders of muscle in diseases classified elsewhere, thigh*
    M63.851 *Disorders of muscle in diseases classified elsewhere, right thigh*
    M63.852 *Disorders of muscle in diseases classified elsewhere, left thigh*
    M63.859 *Disorders of muscle in diseases classified elsewhere, unspecified thigh*

√6ᵗʰ *M63.86* *Disorders of muscle in diseases classified elsewhere, lower leg*
    M63.861 *Disorders of muscle in diseases classified elsewhere, right lower leg*
    M63.862 *Disorders of muscle in diseases classified elsewhere, left lower leg*
    M63.869 *Disorders of muscle in diseases classified elsewhere, unspecified lower leg*

√6ᵗʰ *M63.87* *Disorders of muscle in diseases classified elsewhere, ankle and foot*
    M63.871 *Disorders of muscle in diseases classified elsewhere, right ankle and foot*
    M63.872 *Disorders of muscle in diseases classified elsewhere, left ankle and foot*
    M63.879 *Disorders of muscle in diseases classified elsewhere, unspecified ankle and foot*

M63.88 *Disorders of muscle in diseases classified elsewhere, other site*

M63.89 *Disorders of muscle in diseases classified elsewhere, multiple sites*

Disorders of synovium and tendon (M65-M67)

√4ᵗʰ **M65** **Synovitis and tenosynovitis**
    EXCLUDES 1   chronic crepitant synovitis of hand and wrist (M70.0-)
        current injury — see injury of ligament or tendon by body region
        soft tissue disorders related to use, overuse and pressure (M70.-)

√5ᵗʰ **M65.0** **Abscess of tendon sheath**
    Use additional code (B95-B96) to identify bacterial agent.
    M65.00 Abscess of tendon sheath, unspecified site

√6ᵗʰ **M65.01** Abscess of tendon sheath, shoulder
    M65.011 Abscess of tendon sheath, right shoulder
    M65.012 Abscess of tendon sheath, left shoulder
    M65.019 Abscess of tendon sheath, unspecified shoulder

√6ᵗʰ **M65.02** Abscess of tendon sheath, upper arm
    M65.021 Abscess of tendon sheath, right upper arm
    M65.022 Abscess of tendon sheath, left upper arm
    M65.029 Abscess of tendon sheath, unspecified upper arm

√6ᵗʰ **M65.03** Abscess of tendon sheath, forearm
    M65.031 Abscess of tendon sheath, right forearm
    M65.032 Abscess of tendon sheath, left forearm
    M65.039 Abscess of tendon sheath, unspecified forearm

√6ᵗʰ **M65.04** Abscess of tendon sheath, hand
    M65.041 Abscess of tendon sheath, right hand
    M65.042 Abscess of tendon sheath, left hand
    M65.049 Abscess of tendon sheath, unspecified hand

√6ᵗʰ **M65.05** Abscess of tendon sheath, thigh
 M65.051 Abscess of tendon sheath, right thigh
 M65.052 Abscess of tendon sheath, left thigh
 M65.059 Abscess of tendon sheath, unspecified thigh
√6ᵗʰ **M65.06** Abscess of tendon sheath, lower leg
 M65.061 Abscess of tendon sheath, right lower leg
 M65.062 Abscess of tendon sheath, left lower leg
 M65.069 Abscess of tendon sheath, unspecified lower leg
√6ᵗʰ **M65.07** Abscess of tendon sheath, ankle and foot
 M65.071 Abscess of tendon sheath, right ankle and foot
 M65.072 Abscess of tendon sheath, left ankle and foot
 M65.079 Abscess of tendon sheath, unspecified ankle and foot
 M65.08 Abscess of tendon sheath, other site
√5ᵗʰ **M65.1** Other infective (teno)synovitis
 M65.10 Other infective (teno)synovitis, unspecified site
√6ᵗʰ **M65.11** Other infective (teno)synovitis, shoulder
 M65.111 Other infective (teno)synovitis, right shoulder
 M65.112 Other infective (teno)synovitis, left shoulder
 M65.119 Other infective (teno)synovitis, unspecified shoulder
√6ᵗʰ **M65.12** Other infective (teno)synovitis, elbow
 M65.121 Other infective (teno)synovitis, right elbow
 M65.122 Other infective (teno)synovitis, left elbow
 M65.129 Other infective (teno)synovitis, unspecified elbow
√6ᵗʰ **M65.13** Other infective (teno)synovitis, wrist
 M65.131 Other infective (teno)synovitis, right wrist
 M65.132 Other infective (teno)synovitis, left wrist
 M65.139 Other infective (teno)synovitis, unspecified wrist
√6ᵗʰ **M65.14** Other infective (teno)synovitis, hand
 M65.141 Other infective (teno)synovitis, right hand
 M65.142 Other infective (teno)synovitis, left hand
 M65.149 Other infective (teno)synovitis, unspecified hand
√6ᵗʰ **M65.15** Other infective (teno)synovitis, hip
 M65.151 Other infective (teno)synovitis, right hip
 M65.152 Other infective (teno)synovitis, left hip
 M65.159 Other infective (teno)synovitis, unspecified hip
√6ᵗʰ **M65.16** Other infective (teno)synovitis, knee
 M65.161 Other infective (teno)synovitis, right knee
 M65.162 Other infective (teno)synovitis, left knee
 M65.169 Other infective (teno)synovitis, unspecified knee
√6ᵗʰ **M65.17** Other infective (teno)synovitis, ankle and foot
 M65.171 Other infective (teno)synovitis, right ankle and foot
 M65.172 Other infective (teno)synovitis, left ankle and foot
 M65.179 Other infective (teno)synovitis, unspecified ankle and foot
 M65.18 Other infective (teno)synovitis, other site
 M65.19 Other infective (teno)synovitis, multiple sites
√5ᵗʰ **M65.2** Calcific tendinitis
 EXCLUDES 1 tendinitis as classified in M75-M77
 calcified tendinitis of shoulder (M75.3)
 M65.20 Calcific tendinitis, unspecified site
√6ᵗʰ **M65.22** Calcific tendinitis, upper arm
 M65.221 Calcific tendinitis, right upper arm
 M65.222 Calcific tendinitis, left upper arm
 M65.229 Calcific tendinitis, unspecified upper arm
√6ᵗʰ **M65.23** Calcific tendinitis, forearm
 M65.231 Calcific tendinitis, right forearm
 M65.232 Calcific tendinitis, left forearm
 M65.239 Calcific tendinitis, unspecified forearm
√6ᵗʰ **M65.24** Calcific tendinitis, hand
 M65.241 Calcific tendinitis, right hand

 M65.242 Calcific tendinitis, left hand
 M65.249 Calcific tendinitis, unspecified hand
√6ᵗʰ **M65.25** Calcific tendinitis, thigh
 M65.251 Calcific tendinitis, right thigh
 M65.252 Calcific tendinitis, left thigh
 M65.259 Calcific tendinitis, unspecified thigh
√6ᵗʰ **M65.26** Calcific tendinitis, lower leg
 M65.261 Calcific tendinitis, right lower leg
 M65.262 Calcific tendinitis, left lower leg
 M65.269 Calcific tendinitis, unspecified lower leg
√6ᵗʰ **M65.27** Calcific tendinitis, ankle and foot
 M65.271 Calcific tendinitis, right ankle and foot
 M65.272 Calcific tendinitis, left ankle and foot
 M65.279 Calcific tendinitis, unspecified ankle and foot
 M65.28 Calcific tendinitis, other site
 M65.29 Calcific tendinitis, multiple sites
√5ᵗʰ **M65.3** Trigger finger
 Nodular tendinous disease
 M65.30 Trigger finger, unspecified finger
√6ᵗʰ **M65.31** Trigger thumb
 M65.311 Trigger thumb, right thumb
 M65.312 Trigger thumb, left thumb
 M65.319 Trigger thumb, unspecified thumb
√6ᵗʰ **M65.32** Trigger finger, index finger
 M65.321 Trigger finger, right index finger
 M65.322 Trigger finger, left index finger
 M65.329 Trigger finger, unspecified index finger
√6ᵗʰ **M65.33** Trigger finger, middle finger
 M65.331 Trigger finger, right middle finger
 M65.332 Trigger finger, left middle finger
 M65.339 Trigger finger, unspecified middle finger
√6ᵗʰ **M65.34** Trigger finger, ring finger
 M65.341 Trigger finger, right ring finger
 M65.342 Trigger finger, left ring finger
 M65.349 Trigger finger, unspecified ring finger
√6ᵗʰ **M65.35** Trigger finger, little finger
 M65.351 Trigger finger, right little finger
 M65.352 Trigger finger, left little finger
 M65.359 Trigger finger, unspecified little finger
 M65.4 Radial styloid tenosynovitis [de Quervain]
√5ᵗʰ **M65.8** Other synovitis and tenosynovitis
 M65.80 Other synovitis and tenosynovitis, unspecified site
√6ᵗʰ **M65.81** Other synovitis and tenosynovitis, shoulder
 M65.811 Other synovitis and tenosynovitis, right shoulder
 M65.812 Other synovitis and tenosynovitis, left shoulder
 M65.819 Other synovitis and tenosynovitis, unspecified shoulder
√6ᵗʰ **M65.82** Other synovitis and tenosynovitis, upper arm
 M65.821 Other synovitis and tenosynovitis, right upper arm
 M65.822 Other synovitis and tenosynovitis, left upper arm
 M65.829 Other synovitis and tenosynovitis, unspecified upper arm
√6ᵗʰ **M65.83** Other synovitis and tenosynovitis, forearm
 M65.831 Other synovitis and tenosynovitis, right forearm
 M65.832 Other synovitis and tenosynovitis, left forearm
 M65.839 Other synovitis and tenosynovitis, unspecified forearm
√6ᵗʰ **M65.84** Other synovitis and tenosynovitis, hand
 M65.841 Other synovitis and tenosynovitis, right hand
 M65.842 Other synovitis and tenosynovitis, left hand
 M65.849 Other synovitis and tenosynovitis, unspecified hand
√6ᵗʰ **M65.85** Other synovitis and tenosynovitis, thigh
 M65.851 Other synovitis and tenosynovitis, right thigh
 M65.852 Other synovitis and tenosynovitis, left thigh

M65.859   Other synovitis and tenosynovitis, unspecified thigh

✓6ᵗʰ   M65.86   Other synovitis and tenosynovitis, lower leg

    M65.861   Other synovitis and tenosynovitis, right lower leg

    M65.862   Other synovitis and tenosynovitis, left lower leg

    M65.869   Other synovitis and tenosynovitis, unspecified lower leg

✓6ᵗʰ   M65.87   Other synovitis and tenosynovitis, ankle and foot

    M65.871   Other synovitis and tenosynovitis, right ankle and foot

    M65.872   Other synovitis and tenosynovitis, left ankle and foot

    M65.879   Other synovitis and tenosynovitis, unspecified ankle and foot

    M65.88   Other synovitis and tenosynovitis, other site

    M65.89   Other synovitis and tenosynovitis, multiple sites

M65.9   Synovitis and tenosynovitis, unspecified

✓4ᵗʰ   **M66**   **Spontaneous rupture of synovium and tendon**

    INCLUDES   rupture that occurs when a normal force is applied to tissues that are inferred to have less than normal strength

    EXCLUDES 2   rotator cuff syndrome (M75.1-)

    rupture where an abnormal force is applied to normal tissue — see injury of tendon by body region

    M66.0   Rupture of popliteal cyst

✓5ᵗʰ   M66.1   Rupture of synovium

    Rupture of synovial cyst

    EXCLUDES 2   rupture of popliteal cyst (M66.0)

    M66.10   Rupture of synovium, unspecified joint

✓6ᵗʰ   M66.11   Rupture of synovium, shoulder

    M66.111   Rupture of synovium, right shoulder

    M66.112   Rupture of synovium, left shoulder

    M66.119   Rupture of synovium, unspecified shoulder

✓6ᵗʰ   M66.12   Rupture of synovium, elbow

    M66.121   Rupture of synovium, right elbow

    M66.122   Rupture of synovium, left elbow

    M66.129   Rupture of synovium, unspecified elbow

✓6ᵗʰ   M66.13   Rupture of synovium, wrist

    M66.131   Rupture of synovium, right wrist

    M66.132   Rupture of synovium, left wrist

    M66.139   Rupture of synovium, unspecified wrist

✓6ᵗʰ   M66.14   Rupture of synovium, hand and fingers

    M66.141   Rupture of synovium, right hand

    M66.142   Rupture of synovium, left hand

    M66.143   Rupture of synovium, unspecified hand

    M66.144   Rupture of synovium, right finger(s)

    M66.145   Rupture of synovium, left finger(s)

    M66.146   Rupture of synovium, unspecified finger(s)

✓6ᵗʰ   M66.15   Rupture of synovium, hip

    M66.151   Rupture of synovium, right hip

    M66.152   Rupture of synovium, left hip

    M66.159   Rupture of synovium, unspecified hip

✓6ᵗʰ   M66.17   Rupture of synovium, ankle, foot and toes

    M66.171   Rupture of synovium, right ankle

    M66.172   Rupture of synovium, left ankle

    M66.173   Rupture of synovium, unspecified ankle

    M66.174   Rupture of synovium, right foot

    M66.175   Rupture of synovium, left foot

    M66.176   Rupture of synovium, unspecified foot

    M66.177   Rupture of synovium, right toe(s)

    M66.178   Rupture of synovium, left toe(s)

    M66.179   Rupture of synovium, unspecified toe(s)

    M66.18   Rupture of synovium, other site

✓5ᵗʰ   M66.2   Spontaneous rupture of extensor tendons

    TIP: Refer to the Muscle/Tendon table at the beginning of this chapter.

    M66.20   Spontaneous rupture of extensor tendons, unspecified site

✓6ᵗʰ   M66.21   Spontaneous rupture of extensor tendons, shoulder

    M66.211   Spontaneous rupture of extensor tendons, right shoulder

    M66.212   Spontaneous rupture of extensor tendons, left shoulder

    M66.219   Spontaneous rupture of extensor tendons, unspecified shoulder

✓6ᵗʰ   M66.22   Spontaneous rupture of extensor tendons, upper arm

    M66.221   Spontaneous rupture of extensor tendons, right upper arm

    M66.222   Spontaneous rupture of extensor tendons, left upper arm

    M66.229   Spontaneous rupture of extensor tendons, unspecified upper arm

✓6ᵗʰ   M66.23   Spontaneous rupture of extensor tendons, forearm

    M66.231   Spontaneous rupture of extensor tendons, right forearm

    M66.232   Spontaneous rupture of extensor tendons, left forearm

    M66.239   Spontaneous rupture of extensor tendons, unspecified forearm

✓6ᵗʰ   M66.24   Spontaneous rupture of extensor tendons, hand

    M66.241   Spontaneous rupture of extensor tendons, right hand

    M66.242   Spontaneous rupture of extensor tendons, left hand

    M66.249   Spontaneous rupture of extensor tendons, unspecified hand

✓6ᵗʰ   M66.25   Spontaneous rupture of extensor tendons, thigh

    M66.251   Spontaneous rupture of extensor tendons, right thigh

    M66.252   Spontaneous rupture of extensor tendons, left thigh

    M66.259   Spontaneous rupture of extensor tendons, unspecified thigh

✓6ᵗʰ   M66.26   Spontaneous rupture of extensor tendons, lower leg

    M66.261   Spontaneous rupture of extensor tendons, right lower leg

    M66.262   Spontaneous rupture of extensor tendons, left lower leg

    M66.269   Spontaneous rupture of extensor tendons, unspecified lower leg

✓6ᵗʰ   M66.27   Spontaneous rupture of extensor tendons, ankle and foot

    M66.271   Spontaneous rupture of extensor tendons, right ankle and foot

    M66.272   Spontaneous rupture of extensor tendons, left ankle and foot

    M66.279   Spontaneous rupture of extensor tendons, unspecified ankle and foot

    M66.28   Spontaneous rupture of extensor tendons, other site

    M66.29   Spontaneous rupture of extensor tendons, multiple sites

✓5ᵗʰ   M66.3   Spontaneous rupture of flexor tendons

    TIP: Refer to the Muscle/Tendon table at the beginning of this chapter.

    M66.30   Spontaneous rupture of flexor tendons, unspecified site

✓6ᵗʰ   M66.31   Spontaneous rupture of flexor tendons, shoulder

    M66.311   Spontaneous rupture of flexor tendons, right shoulder

    M66.312   Spontaneous rupture of flexor tendons, left shoulder

    M66.319   Spontaneous rupture of flexor tendons, unspecified shoulder

✓6ᵗʰ   M66.32   Spontaneous rupture of flexor tendons, upper arm

    M66.321   Spontaneous rupture of flexor tendons, right upper arm

    M66.322   Spontaneous rupture of flexor tendons, left upper arm

    M66.329   Spontaneous rupture of flexor tendons, unspecified upper arm

✓6ᵗʰ   M66.33   Spontaneous rupture of flexor tendons, forearm

    M66.331   Spontaneous rupture of flexor tendons, right forearm

    M66.332   Spontaneous rupture of flexor tendons, left forearm

    M66.339   Spontaneous rupture of flexor tendons, unspecified forearm

✓6ᵗʰ   M66.34   Spontaneous rupture of flexor tendons, hand

    M66.341   Spontaneous rupture of flexor tendons, right hand

N Newborn: 0   P Pediatric: 0-17   M Maternity: 12-55   A Adult: 15-124   CH Comorbidity High   CL Comorbidity Low   NCDx Noncancer Dx   PDx Primary Dx

792   ICD-10-CM 2020

    M66.342 Spontaneous rupture of flexor tendons, left hand

    M66.349 Spontaneous rupture of flexor tendons, unspecified hand

√6ᵗʰ M66.35 Spontaneous rupture of flexor tendons, thigh

    M66.351 Spontaneous rupture of flexor tendons, right thigh

    M66.352 Spontaneous rupture of flexor tendons, left thigh

    M66.359 Spontaneous rupture of flexor tendons, unspecified thigh

√6ᵗʰ M66.36 Spontaneous rupture of flexor tendons, lower leg

    M66.361 Spontaneous rupture of flexor tendons, right lower leg

    M66.362 Spontaneous rupture of flexor tendons, left lower leg

    M66.369 Spontaneous rupture of flexor tendons, unspecified lower leg

√6ᵗʰ M66.37 Spontaneous rupture of flexor tendons, ankle and foot

    M66.371 Spontaneous rupture of flexor tendons, right ankle and foot

    M66.372 Spontaneous rupture of flexor tendons, left ankle and foot

    M66.379 Spontaneous rupture of flexor tendons, unspecified ankle and foot

M66.38 Spontaneous rupture of flexor tendons, other site

M66.39 Spontaneous rupture of flexor tendons, multiple sites

√5ᵗʰ M66.8 Spontaneous rupture of other tendons

    TIP: Refer to the Muscle/Tendon table at the beginning of this chapter.

    M66.80 Spontaneous rupture of other tendons, unspecified site

√6ᵗʰ M66.81 Spontaneous rupture of other tendons, shoulder

    M66.811 Spontaneous rupture of other tendons, right shoulder

    M66.812 Spontaneous rupture of other tendons, left shoulder

    M66.819 Spontaneous rupture of other tendons, unspecified shoulder

√6ᵗʰ M66.82 Spontaneous rupture of other tendons, upper arm

    M66.821 Spontaneous rupture of other tendons, right upper arm

    M66.822 Spontaneous rupture of other tendons, left upper arm

    M66.829 Spontaneous rupture of other tendons, unspecified upper arm

√6ᵗʰ M66.83 Spontaneous rupture of other tendons, forearm

    M66.831 Spontaneous rupture of other tendons, right forearm

    M66.832 Spontaneous rupture of other tendons, left forearm

    M66.839 Spontaneous rupture of other tendons, unspecified forearm

√6ᵗʰ M66.84 Spontaneous rupture of other tendons, hand

    M66.841 Spontaneous rupture of other tendons, right hand

    M66.842 Spontaneous rupture of other tendons, left hand

    M66.849 Spontaneous rupture of other tendons, unspecified hand

√6ᵗʰ M66.85 Spontaneous rupture of other tendons, thigh

    M66.851 Spontaneous rupture of other tendons, right thigh

    M66.852 Spontaneous rupture of other tendons, left thigh

    M66.859 Spontaneous rupture of other tendons, unspecified thigh

√6ᵗʰ M66.86 Spontaneous rupture of other tendons, lower leg

    M66.861 Spontaneous rupture of other tendons, right lower leg

    M66.862 Spontaneous rupture of other tendons, left lower leg

    M66.869 Spontaneous rupture of other tendons, unspecified lower leg

√6ᵗʰ M66.87 Spontaneous rupture of other tendons, ankle and foot

    M66.871 Spontaneous rupture of other tendons, right ankle and foot

    M66.872 Spontaneous rupture of other tendons, left ankle and foot

    M66.879 Spontaneous rupture of other tendons, unspecified ankle and foot

▲   M66.88 Spontaneous rupture of other tendons, other sites

    M66.89 Spontaneous rupture of other tendons, multiple sites

M66.9 Spontaneous rupture of unspecified tendon

    Rupture at musculotendinous junction, nontraumatic

√4ᵗʰ **M67 Other disorders of synovium and tendon**

    EXCLUDES 1   palmar fascial fibromatosis [Dupuytren] (M72.0)
               tendinitis NOS (M77.9-)
               xanthomatosis localized to tendons (E78.2)

√5ᵗʰ M67.0 Short Achilles tendon (acquired)

    M67.00 Short Achilles tendon (acquired), unspecified ankle

    M67.01 Short Achilles tendon (acquired), right ankle

    M67.02 Short Achilles tendon (acquired), left ankle

√5ᵗʰ M67.2 Synovial hypertrophy, not elsewhere classified

    EXCLUDES 1   villonodular synovitis (pigmented) (M12.2-)

    M67.20 Synovial hypertrophy, not elsewhere classified, unspecified site

√6ᵗʰ M67.21 Synovial hypertrophy, not elsewhere classified, shoulder

    M67.211 Synovial hypertrophy, not elsewhere classified, right shoulder

    M67.212 Synovial hypertrophy, not elsewhere classified, left shoulder

    M67.219 Synovial hypertrophy, not elsewhere classified, unspecified shoulder

√6ᵗʰ M67.22 Synovial hypertrophy, not elsewhere classified, upper arm

    M67.221 Synovial hypertrophy, not elsewhere classified, right upper arm

    M67.222 Synovial hypertrophy, not elsewhere classified, left upper arm

    M67.229 Synovial hypertrophy, not elsewhere classified, unspecified upper arm

√6ᵗʰ M67.23 Synovial hypertrophy, not elsewhere classified, forearm

    M67.231 Synovial hypertrophy, not elsewhere classified, right forearm

    M67.232 Synovial hypertrophy, not elsewhere classified, left forearm

    M67.239 Synovial hypertrophy, not elsewhere classified, unspecified forearm

√6ᵗʰ M67.24 Synovial hypertrophy, not elsewhere classified, hand

    M67.241 Synovial hypertrophy, not elsewhere classified, right hand

    M67.242 Synovial hypertrophy, not elsewhere classified, left hand

    M67.249 Synovial hypertrophy, not elsewhere classified, unspecified hand

√6ᵗʰ M67.25 Synovial hypertrophy, not elsewhere classified, thigh

    M67.251 Synovial hypertrophy, not elsewhere classified, right thigh

    M67.252 Synovial hypertrophy, not elsewhere classified, left thigh

    M67.259 Synovial hypertrophy, not elsewhere classified, unspecified thigh

√6ᵗʰ M67.26 Synovial hypertrophy, not elsewhere classified, lower leg

    M67.261 Synovial hypertrophy, not elsewhere classified, right lower leg

    M67.262 Synovial hypertrophy, not elsewhere classified, left lower leg

    M67.269 Synovial hypertrophy, not elsewhere classified, unspecified lower leg

√6ᵗʰ M67.27 Synovial hypertrophy, not elsewhere classified, ankle and foot

    M67.271 Synovial hypertrophy, not elsewhere classified, right ankle and foot

    M67.272 Synovial hypertrophy, not elsewhere classified, left ankle and foot

    M67.279 Synovial hypertrophy, not elsewhere classified, unspecified ankle and foot

M67.28 Synovial hypertrophy, not elsewhere classified, other site

M67.29 Synovial hypertrophy, not elsewhere classified, multiple sites

☑ Additional Character Required   √x7ᵗʰ Placeholder Alert   Manifestation   Unspecified Dx   ►◄ Revised Text   ● New Code   ▲ Revised Title

ICD-10-CM 2020   793

√5ᵗʰ **M67.3 Transient synovitis**

     Toxic synovitis

     EXCLUDES 1   *palindromic rheumatism (M12.3-)*

     M67.30 Transient synovitis, unspecified site

√6ᵗʰ **M67.31 Transient synovitis, shoulder**

     M67.311 Transient synovitis, right shoulder

     M67.312 Transient synovitis, left shoulder

     M67.319 Transient synovitis, unspecified shoulder

√6ᵗʰ **M67.32 Transient synovitis, elbow**

     M67.321 Transient synovitis, right elbow

     M67.322 Transient synovitis, left elbow

     M67.329 Transient synovitis, unspecified elbow

√6ᵗʰ **M67.33 Transient synovitis, wrist**

     M67.331 Transient synovitis, right wrist

     M67.332 Transient synovitis, left wrist

     M67.339 Transient synovitis, unspecified wrist

√6ᵗʰ **M67.34 Transient synovitis, hand**

     M67.341 Transient synovitis, right hand

     M67.342 Transient synovitis, left hand

     M67.349 Transient synovitis, unspecified hand

√6ᵗʰ **M67.35 Transient synovitis, hip**

     M67.351 Transient synovitis, right hip

     M67.352 Transient synovitis, left hip

     M67.359 Transient synovitis, unspecified hip

√6ᵗʰ **M67.36 Transient synovitis, knee**

     M67.361 Transient synovitis, right knee

     M67.362 Transient synovitis, left knee

     M67.369 Transient synovitis, unspecified knee

√6ᵗʰ **M67.37 Transient synovitis, ankle and foot**

     M67.371 Transient synovitis, right ankle and foot

     M67.372 Transient synovitis, left ankle and foot

     M67.379 Transient synovitis, unspecified ankle and foot

     M67.38 Transient synovitis, other site

     M67.39 Transient synovitis, multiple sites

√5ᵗʰ **M67.4 Ganglion**

     Ganglion of joint or tendon (sheath)

     EXCLUDES 1   *ganglion in yaws (A66.6)*

     EXCLUDES 2   *cyst of bursa (M71.2-M71.3)*

                 cyst of synovium (M71.2-M71.3)

     DEF: Fluid-filled, benign cyst appearing on a tendon sheath or aponeurosis, frequently connecting to an underlying joint.

     M67.40 Ganglion, unspecified site

√6ᵗʰ **M67.41 Ganglion, shoulder**

     M67.411 Ganglion, right shoulder

     M67.412 Ganglion, left shoulder

     M67.419 Ganglion, unspecified shoulder

√6ᵗʰ **M67.42 Ganglion, elbow**

     M67.421 Ganglion, right elbow

     M67.422 Ganglion, left elbow

     M67.429 Ganglion, unspecified elbow

√6ᵗʰ **M67.43 Ganglion, wrist**

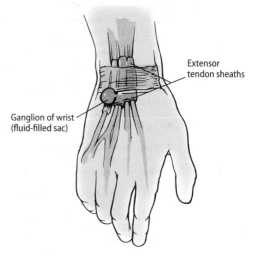

Ganglion of Wrist

Extensor tendon sheaths

Ganglion of wrist (fluid-filled sac)

     M67.431 Ganglion, right wrist

     M67.432 Ganglion, left wrist

     M67.439 Ganglion, unspecified wrist

√6ᵗʰ **M67.44 Ganglion, hand**

     M67.441 Ganglion, right hand

     M67.442 Ganglion, left hand

     M67.449 Ganglion, unspecified hand

√6ᵗʰ **M67.45 Ganglion, hip**

     M67.451 Ganglion, right hip

     M67.452 Ganglion, left hip

     M67.459 Ganglion, unspecified hip

√6ᵗʰ **M67.46 Ganglion, knee**

     M67.461 Ganglion, right knee

     M67.462 Ganglion, left knee

     M67.469 Ganglion, unspecified knee

√6ᵗʰ **M67.47 Ganglion, ankle and foot**

     M67.471 Ganglion, right ankle and foot

     M67.472 Ganglion, left ankle and foot

     M67.479 Ganglion, unspecified ankle and foot

     M67.48 Ganglion, other site

     M67.49 Ganglion, multiple sites

√5ᵗʰ **M67.5 Plica syndrome**

     Plica knee

     M67.50 Plica syndrome, unspecified knee

     M67.51 Plica syndrome, right knee

     M67.52 Plica syndrome, left knee

√5ᵗʰ **M67.8 Other specified disorders of synovium and tendon**

     M67.80 Other specified disorders of synovium and tendon, unspecified site

√6ᵗʰ **M67.81 Other specified disorders of synovium and tendon, shoulder**

     M67.811 Other specified disorders of synovium, right shoulder

     M67.812 Other specified disorders of synovium, left shoulder

     M67.813 Other specified disorders of tendon, right shoulder

     M67.814 Other specified disorders of tendon, left shoulder

     M67.819 Other specified disorders of synovium and tendon, unspecified shoulder

√6ᵗʰ **M67.82 Other specified disorders of synovium and tendon, elbow**

     M67.821 Other specified disorders of synovium, right elbow

     M67.822 Other specified disorders of synovium, left elbow

     M67.823 Other specified disorders of tendon, right elbow

     M67.824 Other specified disorders of tendon, left elbow

N Newborn: 0   P Pediatric: 0-17   M Maternity: 12-55   A Adult: 15-124   CH Comorbidity High   CL Comorbidity Low   NC Dx Noncancer Dx   PDx Primary Dx

794   ICD-10-CM 2020

M67.829 Other specified disorders of synovium and tendon, unspecified elbow

✓6ᵗʰ M67.83 Other specified disorders of synovium and tendon, wrist
  M67.831 Other specified disorders of synovium, right wrist
  M67.832 Other specified disorders of synovium, left wrist
  M67.833 Other specified disorders of tendon, right wrist
  M67.834 Other specified disorders of tendon, left wrist
  M67.839 Other specified disorders of synovium and tendon, unspecified wrist

✓6ᵗʰ M67.84 Other specified disorders of synovium and tendon, hand
  M67.841 Other specified disorders of synovium, right hand
  M67.842 Other specified disorders of synovium, left hand
  M67.843 Other specified disorders of tendon, right hand
  M67.844 Other specified disorders of tendon, left hand
  M67.849 Other specified disorders of synovium and tendon, unspecified hand

✓6ᵗʰ M67.85 Other specified disorders of synovium and tendon, hip
  M67.851 Other specified disorders of synovium, right hip
  M67.852 Other specified disorders of synovium, left hip
  M67.853 Other specified disorders of tendon, right hip
  M67.854 Other specified disorders of tendon, left hip
  M67.859 Other specified disorders of synovium and tendon, unspecified hip

✓6ᵗʰ M67.86 Other specified disorders of synovium and tendon, knee
  M67.861 Other specified disorders of synovium, right knee
  M67.862 Other specified disorders of synovium, left knee
  M67.863 Other specified disorders of tendon, right knee
  M67.864 Other specified disorders of tendon, left knee
  M67.869 Other specified disorders of synovium and tendon, unspecified knee

✓6ᵗʰ M67.87 Other specified disorders of synovium and tendon, ankle and foot
  M67.871 Other specified disorders of synovium, right ankle and foot
  M67.872 Other specified disorders of synovium, left ankle and foot
  M67.873 Other specified disorders of tendon, right ankle and foot
  M67.874 Other specified disorders of tendon, left ankle and foot
  M67.879 Other specified disorders of synovium and tendon, unspecified ankle and foot
M67.88 Other specified disorders of synovium and tendon, other site
M67.89 Other specified disorders of synovium and tendon, multiple sites

✓5ᵗʰ M67.9 Unspecified disorder of synovium and tendon
  M67.90 Unspecified disorder of synovium and tendon, unspecified site
✓6ᵗʰ M67.91 Unspecified disorder of synovium and tendon, shoulder
  M67.911 Unspecified disorder of synovium and tendon, right shoulder
  M67.912 Unspecified disorder of synovium and tendon, left shoulder
  M67.919 Unspecified disorder of synovium and tendon, unspecified shoulder
✓6ᵗʰ M67.92 Unspecified disorder of synovium and tendon, upper arm
  M67.921 Unspecified disorder of synovium and tendon, right upper arm
  M67.922 Unspecified disorder of synovium and tendon, left upper arm

M67.929 Unspecified disorder of synovium and tendon, unspecified upper arm
✓6ᵗʰ M67.93 Unspecified disorder of synovium and tendon, forearm
  M67.931 Unspecified disorder of synovium and tendon, right forearm
  M67.932 Unspecified disorder of synovium and tendon, left forearm
  M67.939 Unspecified disorder of synovium and tendon, unspecified forearm
✓6ᵗʰ M67.94 Unspecified disorder of synovium and tendon, hand
  M67.941 Unspecified disorder of synovium and tendon, right hand
  M67.942 Unspecified disorder of synovium and tendon, left hand
  M67.949 Unspecified disorder of synovium and tendon, unspecified hand
✓6ᵗʰ M67.95 Unspecified disorder of synovium and tendon, thigh
  M67.951 Unspecified disorder of synovium and tendon, right thigh
  M67.952 Unspecified disorder of synovium and tendon, left thigh
  M67.959 Unspecified disorder of synovium and tendon, unspecified thigh
✓6ᵗʰ M67.96 Unspecified disorder of synovium and tendon, lower leg
  M67.961 Unspecified disorder of synovium and tendon, right lower leg
  M67.962 Unspecified disorder of synovium and tendon, left lower leg
  M67.969 Unspecified disorder of synovium and tendon, unspecified lower leg
✓6ᵗʰ M67.97 Unspecified disorder of synovium and tendon, ankle and foot
  M67.971 Unspecified disorder of synovium and tendon, right ankle and foot
  M67.972 Unspecified disorder of synovium and tendon, left ankle and foot
  M67.979 Unspecified disorder of synovium and tendon, unspecified ankle and foot
M67.98 Unspecified disorder of synovium and tendon, other site
M67.99 Unspecified disorder of synovium and tendon, multiple sites

Other soft tissue disorders (M70-M79)

✓4ᵗʰ M70 Soft tissue disorders related to use, overuse and pressure
  INCLUDES soft tissue disorders of occupational origin
  Use additional external cause code to identify activity causing disorder (Y93.-)
  EXCLUDES 1 bursitis NOS (M71.9-)
  EXCLUDES 2 bursitis of shoulder (M75.5)
    enthesopathies (M76-M77)
    pressure ulcer (pressure area) (L89.-)
✓5ᵗʰ M70.0 Crepitant synovitis (acute) (chronic) of hand and wrist
  ✓6ᵗʰ M70.03 Crepitant synovitis (acute) (chronic), wrist
    M70.031 Crepitant synovitis (acute) (chronic), right wrist
    M70.032 Crepitant synovitis (acute) (chronic), left wrist
    M70.039 Crepitant synovitis (acute) (chronic), unspecified wrist
  ✓6ᵗʰ M70.04 Crepitant synovitis (acute) (chronic), hand
    M70.041 Crepitant synovitis (acute) (chronic), right hand
    M70.042 Crepitant synovitis (acute) (chronic), left hand
    M70.049 Crepitant synovitis (acute) (chronic), unspecified hand
✓5ᵗʰ M70.1 Bursitis of hand
  M70.10 Bursitis, unspecified hand
  M70.11 Bursitis, right hand
  M70.12 Bursitis, left hand
✓5ᵗʰ M70.2 Olecranon bursitis
  M70.20 Olecranon bursitis, unspecified elbow
  M70.21 Olecranon bursitis, right elbow
  M70.22 Olecranon bursitis, left elbow

Chapter 13. Diseases of the Musculoskeletal System and Connective Tissue

✓5ᵗʰ **M70.3** **Other bursitis of** elbow

    M70.30 Other bursitis of elbow, unspecified elbow

    M70.31 Other bursitis of elbow, right elbow

    M70.32 Other bursitis of elbow, left elbow

✓5ᵗʰ **M70.4** **Prepatellar** bursitis

    M70.40 Prepatellar bursitis, unspecified knee

    M70.41 Prepatellar bursitis, right knee

    M70.42 Prepatellar bursitis, left knee

Knee Bursae

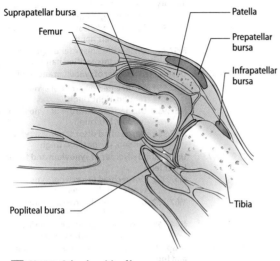

Suprapatellar bursa — Patella — Femur — Prepatellar bursa — Infrapatellar bursa — Popliteal bursa — Tibia

✓5ᵗʰ **M70.5** **Other bursitis of** knee

    M70.50 Other bursitis of knee, unspecified knee

    M70.51 Other bursitis of knee, right knee

    M70.52 Other bursitis of knee, left knee

✓6ᵗʰ **M70.6** **Trochanteric** bursitis

    Trochanteric tendinitis

    M70.60 Trochanteric bursitis, unspecified hip

    M70.61 Trochanteric bursitis, right hip

    M70.62 Trochanteric bursitis, left hip

✓5ᵗʰ **M70.7** **Other bursitis of** hip

    Ischial bursitis

    M70.70 Other bursitis of hip, unspecified hip

    M70.71 Other bursitis of hip, right hip

    M70.72 Other bursitis of hip, left hip

✓5ᵗʰ **M70.8** Other soft tissue disorders related to use, overuse and pressure

    M70.80 Other soft tissue disorders related to use, overuse and pressure of unspecified site

✓6ᵗʰ   **M70.81** Other soft tissue disorders related to use, overuse and pressure of shoulder

        M70.811 Other soft tissue disorders related to use, overuse and pressure, right shoulder

        M70.812 Other soft tissue disorders related to use, overuse and pressure, left shoulder

        M70.819 Other soft tissue disorders related to use, overuse and pressure, unspecified shoulder

✓6ᵗʰ   **M70.82** Other soft tissue disorders related to use, overuse and pressure of upper arm

        M70.821 Other soft tissue disorders related to use, overuse and pressure, right upper arm

        M70.822 Other soft tissue disorders related to use, overuse and pressure, left upper arm

        M70.829 Other soft tissue disorders related to use, overuse and pressure, unspecified upper arms

✓6ᵗʰ   **M70.83** Other soft tissue disorders related to use, overuse and pressure of forearm

        M70.831 Other soft tissue disorders related to use, overuse and pressure, right forearm

        M70.832 Other soft tissue disorders related to use, overuse and pressure, left forearm

        M70.839 Other soft tissue disorders related to use, overuse and pressure, unspecified forearm

✓6ᵗʰ **M70.84** Other soft tissue disorders related to use, overuse and pressure of hand

    M70.841 Other soft tissue disorders related to use, overuse and pressure, right hand

    M70.842 Other soft tissue disorders related to use, overuse and pressure, left hand

    M70.849 Other soft tissue disorders related to use, overuse and pressure, unspecified hand

✓6ᵗʰ **M70.85** Other soft tissue disorders related to use, overuse and pressure of thigh

    M70.851 Other soft tissue disorders related to use, overuse and pressure, right thigh

    M70.852 Other soft tissue disorders related to use, overuse and pressure, left thigh

    M70.859 Other soft tissue disorders related to use, overuse and pressure, unspecified thigh

✓6ᵗʰ **M70.86** Other soft tissue disorders related to use, overuse and pressure lower leg

    M70.861 Other soft tissue disorders related to use, overuse and pressure, right lower leg

    M70.862 Other soft tissue disorders related to use, overuse and pressure, left lower leg

    M70.869 Other soft tissue disorders related to use, overuse and pressure, unspecified leg

✓6ᵗʰ **M70.87** Other soft tissue disorders related to use, overuse and pressure of ankle and foot

    M70.871 Other soft tissue disorders related to use, overuse and pressure, right ankle and foot

    M70.872 Other soft tissue disorders related to use, overuse and pressure, left ankle and foot

    M70.879 Other soft tissue disorders related to use, overuse and pressure, unspecified ankle and foot

    M70.88 Other soft tissue disorders related to use, overuse and pressure other site

    M70.89 Other soft tissue disorders related to use, overuse and pressure multiple sites

✓5ᵗʰ **M70.9** Unspecified soft tissue disorder related to use, overuse and pressure

    M70.90 Unspecified soft tissue disorder related to use, overuse and pressure of unspecified site

✓6ᵗʰ   **M70.91** Unspecified soft tissue disorder related to use, overuse and pressure of shoulder

        M70.911 Unspecified soft tissue disorder related to use, overuse and pressure, right shoulder

        M70.912 Unspecified soft tissue disorder related to use, overuse and pressure, left shoulder

        M70.919 Unspecified soft tissue disorder related to use, overuse and pressure, unspecified shoulder

✓6ᵗʰ   **M70.92** Unspecified soft tissue disorder related to use, overuse and pressure of upper arm

        M70.921 Unspecified soft tissue disorder related to use, overuse and pressure, right upper arm

        M70.922 Unspecified soft tissue disorder related to use, overuse and pressure, left upper arm

        M70.929 Unspecified soft tissue disorder related to use, overuse and pressure, unspecified upper arm

✓6ᵗʰ   **M70.93** Unspecified soft tissue disorder related to use, overuse and pressure of forearm

        M70.931 Unspecified soft tissue disorder related to use, overuse and pressure, right forearm

        M70.932 Unspecified soft tissue disorder related to use, overuse and pressure, left forearm

        M70.939 Unspecified soft tissue disorder related to use, overuse and pressure, unspecified forearm

✓6ᵗʰ   **M70.94** Unspecified soft tissue disorder related to use, overuse and pressure of hand

        M70.941 Unspecified soft tissue disorder related to use, overuse and pressure, right hand

        M70.942 Unspecified soft tissue disorder related to use, overuse and pressure, left hand

        M70.949 Unspecified soft tissue disorder related to use, overuse and pressure, unspecified hand

N Newborn: 0   P Pediatric: 0-17   M Maternity: 12-55   A Adult: 15-124   CH Comorbidity High   CL Comorbidity Low   NCDx Noncancer Dx   PDx Primary Dx

796   ICD-10-CM 2020

✓6ᵗʰ **M70.95 Unspecified soft tissue disorder related to use, overuse and pressure of** thigh

    M70.951 Unspecified soft tissue disorder related to use, overuse and pressure, right **thigh**

    M70.952 Unspecified soft tissue disorder related to use, overuse and pressure, left **thigh**

    M70.959 Unspecified soft tissue disorder related to use, overuse and pressure, unspecified thigh

✓6ᵗʰ **M70.96 Unspecified soft tissue disorder related to use, overuse and pressure** lower leg

    M70.961 Unspecified soft tissue disorder related to use, overuse and pressure, right **lower leg**

    M70.962 Unspecified soft tissue disorder related to use, overuse and pressure, left **lower leg**

    M70.969 Unspecified soft tissue disorder related to use, overuse and pressure, unspecified lower leg

✓6ᵗʰ **M70.97 Unspecified soft tissue disorder related to use, overuse and pressure of** ankle and foot

    M70.971 Unspecified soft tissue disorder related to use, overuse and pressure, right **ankle and foot**

    M70.972 Unspecified soft tissue disorder related to use, overuse and pressure, left **ankle and foot**

    M70.979 Unspecified soft tissue disorder related to use, overuse and pressure, unspecified ankle and foot

M70.98 Unspecified soft tissue disorder related to use, overuse and pressure other

M70.99 Unspecified soft tissue disorder related to use, overuse and pressure multiple sites

✓4ᵗʰ **M71 Other bursopathies**

    EXCLUDES 1   bunion (M20.1)

                bursitis related to use, overuse or pressure (M70.-)

                enthesopathies (M76-M77)

✓5ᵗʰ **M71.0 Abscess of bursa**

    Use additional code (B95.-, B96.-) to identify causative organism

    M71.00 Abscess of bursa, unspecified site

    ✓6ᵗʰ **M71.01 Abscess of bursa,** shoulder

        M71.011 Abscess of bursa, right **shoulder**

        M71.012 Abscess of bursa, left **shoulder**

        M71.019 Abscess of bursa, unspecified shoulder

    ✓6ᵗʰ **M71.02 Abscess of bursa,** elbow

        M71.021 Abscess of bursa, right **elbow**

        M71.022 Abscess of bursa, left **elbow**

        M71.029 Abscess of bursa, unspecified elbow

    ✓6ᵗʰ **M71.03 Abscess of bursa,** wrist

        M71.031 Abscess of bursa, right **wrist**

        M71.032 Abscess of bursa, left **wrist**

        M71.039 Abscess of bursa, unspecified wrist

    ✓6ᵗʰ **M71.04 Abscess of bursa,** hand

        M71.041 Abscess of bursa, right **hand**

        M71.042 Abscess of bursa, left **hand**

        M71.049 Abscess of bursa, unspecified hand

    ✓6ᵗʰ **M71.05 Abscess of bursa,** hip

        M71.051 Abscess of bursa, right **hip**

        M71.052 Abscess of bursa, left **hip**

        M71.059 Abscess of bursa, unspecified hip

    ✓6ᵗʰ **M71.06 Abscess of bursa,** knee

        M71.061 Abscess of bursa, right **knee**

        M71.062 Abscess of bursa, left **knee**

        M71.069 Abscess of bursa, unspecified knee

    ✓6ᵗʰ **M71.07 Abscess of bursa,** ankle and foot

        M71.071 Abscess of bursa, right **ankle and foot**

        M71.072 Abscess of bursa, left **ankle and foot**

        M71.079 Abscess of bursa, unspecified ankle and foot

    M71.08 Abscess of bursa, other site

    M71.09 Abscess of bursa, multiple sites

✓5ᵗʰ **M71.1 Other infective bursitis**

    Use additional code (B95.-, B96.-) to identify causative organism

    M71.10 Other infective bursitis, unspecified site

    ✓6ᵗʰ **M71.11 Other infective bursitis,** shoulder

        M71.111 Other infective bursitis, right **shoulder**

        M71.112 Other infective bursitis, left **shoulder**

        M71.119 Other infective bursitis, unspecified shoulder

    ✓6ᵗʰ **M71.12 Other infective bursitis,** elbow

        M71.121 Other infective bursitis, right **elbow**

        M71.122 Other infective bursitis, left **elbow**

        M71.129 Other infective bursitis, unspecified elbow

    ✓6ᵗʰ **M71.13 Other infective bursitis,** wrist

        M71.131 Other infective bursitis, right **wrist**

        M71.132 Other infective bursitis, left **wrist**

        M71.139 Other infective bursitis, unspecified wrist

    ✓6ᵗʰ **M71.14 Other infective bursitis,** hand

        M71.141 Other infective bursitis, right **hand**

        M71.142 Other infective bursitis, left **hand**

        M71.149 Other infective bursitis, unspecified hand

    ✓6ᵗʰ **M71.15 Other infective bursitis,** hip

        M71.151 Other infective bursitis, right **hip**

        M71.152 Other infective bursitis, left **hip**

        M71.159 Other infective bursitis, unspecified hip

    ✓6ᵗʰ **M71.16 Other infective bursitis,** knee

        M71.161 Other infective bursitis, right **knee**

        M71.162 Other infective bursitis, left **knee**

        M71.169 Other infective bursitis, unspecified knee

    ✓6ᵗʰ **M71.17 Other infective bursitis,** ankle and foot

        M71.171 Other infective bursitis, right **ankle and foot**

        M71.172 Other infective bursitis, left **ankle and foot**

        M71.179 Other infective bursitis, unspecified ankle and foot

    M71.18 Other infective bursitis, other site

    M71.19 Other infective bursitis, multiple sites

✓5ᵗʰ **M71.2 Synovial cyst of popliteal space [Baker]**

    EXCLUDES 1   synovial cyst of popliteal space with rupture (M66.0)

    DEF: Sac filled with clear synovial fluid in adults, usually secondary to disease inside the joint, located on the back of the knee in the popliteal fossa area. In children, the cyst usually represents a ganglion of one of the tendons in the knee.

Baker's Cyst

Baker's cyst connected to knee joint synovial cavity

    M71.20 Synovial cyst of popliteal space [Baker], unspecified knee

    M71.21 Synovial cyst of popliteal space [Baker], right **knee**

    M71.22 Synovial cyst of popliteal space [Baker], left **knee**

✓5ᵗʰ **M71.3 Other bursal cyst**

    Synovial cyst NOS

    EXCLUDES 1   synovial cyst with rupture (M66.1-)

    M71.30 Other bursal cyst, unspecified site

    ✓6ᵗʰ **M71.31 Other bursal cyst,** shoulder

        M71.311 Other bursal cyst, right **shoulder**

        M71.312 Other bursal cyst, left **shoulder**

        M71.319 Other bursal cyst, unspecified shoulder

    ✓6ᵗʰ **M71.32 Other bursal cyst,** elbow

        M71.321 Other bursal cyst, right **elbow**

✓ Additional Character Required   ✓x7ᵗʰ Placeholder Alert   Manifestation   Unspecified Dx   ▶◀ Revised Text   ● New Code   ▲ Revised Title

ICD-10-CM 2020   797

      M71.322 Other bursal cyst, left elbow
      M71.329 Other bursal cyst, unspecified elbow

√6ᵗʰ **M71.33** Other bursal cyst, wrist
      M71.331 Other bursal cyst, right wrist
      M71.332 Other bursal cyst, left wrist
      M71.339 Other bursal cyst, unspecified wrist

√6ᵗʰ **M71.34** Other bursal cyst, hand
      M71.341 Other bursal cyst, right hand
      M71.342 Other bursal cyst, left hand
      M71.349 Other bursal cyst, unspecified hand

√6ᵗʰ **M71.35** Other bursal cyst, hip
      M71.351 Other bursal cyst, right hip
      M71.352 Other bursal cyst, left hip
      M71.359 Other bursal cyst, unspecified hip

√6ᵗʰ **M71.37** Other bursal cyst, ankle and foot
      M71.371 Other bursal cyst, right ankle and foot
      M71.372 Other bursal cyst, left ankle and foot
      M71.379 Other bursal cyst, unspecified ankle and foot

   M71.38 Other bursal cyst, other site
   M71.39 Other bursal cyst, multiple sites

√5ᵗʰ **M71.4** Calcium deposit in bursa
      EXCLUDES 2   calcium deposit in bursa of shoulder (M75.3)

   M71.40 Calcium deposit in bursa, unspecified site

√6ᵗʰ **M71.42** Calcium deposit in bursa, elbow
      M71.421 Calcium deposit in bursa, right elbow
      M71.422 Calcium deposit in bursa, left elbow
      M71.429 Calcium deposit in bursa, unspecified elbow

√6ᵗʰ **M71.43** Calcium deposit in bursa, wrist
      M71.431 Calcium deposit in bursa, right wrist
      M71.432 Calcium deposit in bursa, left wrist
      M71.439 Calcium deposit in bursa, unspecified wrist

√6ᵗʰ **M71.44** Calcium deposit in bursa, hand
      M71.441 Calcium deposit in bursa, right hand
      M71.442 Calcium deposit in bursa, left hand
      M71.449 Calcium deposit in bursa, unspecified hand

√6ᵗʰ **M71.45** Calcium deposit in bursa, hip
      M71.451 Calcium deposit in bursa, right hip
      M71.452 Calcium deposit in bursa, left hip
      M71.459 Calcium deposit in bursa, unspecified hip

√6ᵗʰ **M71.46** Calcium deposit in bursa, knee
      M71.461 Calcium deposit in bursa, right knee
      M71.462 Calcium deposit in bursa, left knee
      M71.469 Calcium deposit in bursa, unspecified knee

√6ᵗʰ **M71.47** Calcium deposit in bursa, ankle and foot
      M71.471 Calcium deposit in bursa, right ankle and foot
      M71.472 Calcium deposit in bursa, left ankle and foot
      M71.479 Calcium deposit in bursa, unspecified ankle and foot

   M71.48 Calcium deposit in bursa, other site
   M71.49 Calcium deposit in bursa, multiple sites

√5ᵗʰ **M71.5** Other bursitis, not elsewhere classified
      EXCLUDES 1   bursitis NOS (M71.9-)
      EXCLUDES 2   bursitis of shoulder (M75.5)
             bursitis of tibial collateral [Pellegrini-Stieda] (M76.4-)

   M71.50 Other bursitis, not elsewhere classified, unspecified site

√6ᵗʰ **M71.52** Other bursitis, not elsewhere classified, elbow
      M71.521 Other bursitis, not elsewhere classified, right elbow
      M71.522 Other bursitis, not elsewhere classified, left elbow
      M71.529 Other bursitis, not elsewhere classified, unspecified elbow

√6ᵗʰ **M71.53** Other bursitis, not elsewhere classified, wrist
      M71.531 Other bursitis, not elsewhere classified, right wrist
      M71.532 Other bursitis, not elsewhere classified, left wrist
      M71.539 Other bursitis, not elsewhere classified, unspecified wrist

√6ᵗʰ **M71.54** Other bursitis, not elsewhere classified, hand
      M71.541 Other bursitis, not elsewhere classified, right hand
      M71.542 Other bursitis, not elsewhere classified, left hand
      M71.549 Other bursitis, not elsewhere classified, unspecified hand

√6ᵗʰ **M71.55** Other bursitis, not elsewhere classified, hip
      M71.551 Other bursitis, not elsewhere classified, right hip
      M71.552 Other bursitis, not elsewhere classified, left hip
      M71.559 Other bursitis, not elsewhere classified, unspecified hip

√6ᵗʰ **M71.56** Other bursitis, not elsewhere classified, knee
      M71.561 Other bursitis, not elsewhere classified, right knee
      M71.562 Other bursitis, not elsewhere classified, left knee
      M71.569 Other bursitis, not elsewhere classified, unspecified knee

√6ᵗʰ **M71.57** Other bursitis, not elsewhere classified, ankle and foot
      M71.571 Other bursitis, not elsewhere classified, right ankle and foot
      M71.572 Other bursitis, not elsewhere classified, left ankle and foot
      M71.579 Other bursitis, not elsewhere classified, unspecified ankle and foot

   M71.58 Other bursitis, not elsewhere classified, other site

√5ᵗʰ **M71.8** Other specified bursopathies
   M71.80 Other specified bursopathies, unspecified site

√6ᵗʰ **M71.81** Other specified bursopathies, shoulder
      M71.811 Other specified bursopathies, right shoulder
      M71.812 Other specified bursopathies, left shoulder
      M71.819 Other specified bursopathies, unspecified shoulder

√6ᵗʰ **M71.82** Other specified bursopathies, elbow
      M71.821 Other specified bursopathies, right elbow
      M71.822 Other specified bursopathies, left elbow
      M71.829 Other specified bursopathies, unspecified elbow

√6ᵗʰ **M71.83** Other specified bursopathies, wrist
      M71.831 Other specified bursopathies, right wrist
      M71.832 Other specified bursopathies, left wrist
      M71.839 Other specified bursopathies, unspecified wrist

√6ᵗʰ **M71.84** Other specified bursopathies, hand
      M71.841 Other specified bursopathies, right hand
      M71.842 Other specified bursopathies, left hand
      M71.849 Other specified bursopathies, unspecified hand

√6ᵗʰ **M71.85** Other specified bursopathies, hip
      M71.851 Other specified bursopathies, right hip
      M71.852 Other specified bursopathies, left hip
      M71.859 Other specified bursopathies, unspecified hip

√6ᵗʰ **M71.86** Other specified bursopathies, knee
      M71.861 Other specified bursopathies, right knee
      M71.862 Other specified bursopathies, left knee
      M71.869 Other specified bursopathies, unspecified knee

√6ᵗʰ **M71.87** Other specified bursopathies, ankle and foot
      M71.871 Other specified bursopathies, right ankle and foot
      M71.872 Other specified bursopathies, left ankle and foot
      M71.879 Other specified bursopathies, unspecified ankle and foot

   M71.88 Other specified bursopathies, other site
   M71.89 Other specified bursopathies, multiple sites

M71.9 Bursopathy, unspecified
   Bursitis NOS

Ⓝ Newborn: 0   Ⓟ Pediatric: 0-17   Ⓜ Maternity: 12-55   Ⓐ Adult: 15-124   **CH** Comorbidity High   **CL** Comorbidity Low   **NCDx** Noncancer Dx   **PDx** Primary Dx

798   ICD-10-CM 2020

✓4th **M72 Fibroblastic disorders**
> EXCLUDES 2   retroperitoneal fibromatosis (D48.3)

M72.0 Palmar fascial fibromatosis [Dupuytren]   A
> **DEF:** Dupuytren's contracture: Flexion deformity of a finger, due to shortened, thickened fibrosing of palmar fascia. The cause is unknown, but it is associated with long-standing epilepsy.

M72.1 Knuckle pads

M72.2 Plantar fascial fibromatosis
> Plantar fasciitis
> **DEF:** Rapid-growing and multiplanar nodular swellings and pain in the foot that is not associated with contractures.

M72.4 Pseudosarcomatous fibromatosis
> Nodular fasciitis

M72.6 Necrotizing fasciitis
> Use additional code (B95.-, B96.-) to identify causative organism

M72.8 Other fibroblastic disorders
> Abscess of fascia
> Fasciitis NEC
> Other infective fasciitis
> Use additional code to (B95.-, B96.-) identify causative organism
> EXCLUDES 1   diffuse (eosinophilic) fasciitis (M35.4)
>   necrotizing fasciitis (M72.6)
>   nodular fasciitis (M72.4)
>   perirenal fasciitis NOS (N13.5)
>   perirenal fasciitis with infection (N13.6)
>   plantar fasciitis (M72.2)

M72.9 Fibroblastic disorder, unspecified
> Fasciitis NOS
> Fibromatosis NOS

✓4th **M75 Shoulder lesions**
> EXCLUDES 2   shoulder-hand syndrome (M89.0-)

✓5th **M75.0 Adhesive capsulitis of shoulder**
> Frozen shoulder
> Periarthritis of shoulder
> **AHA:** 2015,2Q,23

   M75.00 Adhesive capsulitis of unspecified shoulder
   M75.01 Adhesive capsulitis of right shoulder
   M75.02 Adhesive capsulitis of left shoulder

✓5th **M75.1 Rotator cuff tear or rupture, not specified as traumatic**
> Rotator cuff syndrome
> Supraspinatus syndrome
> Supraspinatus tear or rupture, not specified as traumatic
> EXCLUDES 1   tear of rotator cuff, traumatic (S46.01-)

   ✓6th **M75.10 Unspecified rotator cuff tear or rupture, not specified as traumatic**
     M75.100 Unspecified rotator cuff tear or rupture of unspecified shoulder, not specified as traumatic
     M75.101 Unspecified rotator cuff tear or rupture of right shoulder, not specified as traumatic
     M75.102 Unspecified rotator cuff tear or rupture of left shoulder, not specified as traumatic

   ✓6th **M75.11 Incomplete rotator cuff tear or rupture not specified as traumatic**
     M75.110 Incomplete rotator cuff tear or rupture of unspecified shoulder, not specified as traumatic
     M75.111 Incomplete rotator cuff tear or rupture of right shoulder, not specified as traumatic
     M75.112 Incomplete rotator cuff tear or rupture of left shoulder, not specified as traumatic

   ✓6th **M75.12 Complete rotator cuff tear or rupture not specified as traumatic**
     M75.120 Complete rotator cuff tear or rupture of unspecified shoulder, not specified as traumatic
     M75.121 Complete rotator cuff tear or rupture of right shoulder, not specified as traumatic
     M75.122 Complete rotator cuff tear or rupture of left shoulder, not specified as traumatic

✓5th **M75.2 Bicipital tendinitis**
   M75.20 Bicipital tendinitis, unspecified shoulder
   M75.21 Bicipital tendinitis, right shoulder
   M75.22 Bicipital tendinitis, left shoulder

✓5th **M75.3 Calcific tendinitis of shoulder**
> Calcified bursa of shoulder
   M75.30 Calcific tendinitis of unspecified shoulder
   M75.31 Calcific tendinitis of right shoulder
   M75.32 Calcific tendinitis of left shoulder

✓5th **M75.4 Impingement syndrome of shoulder**
   M75.40 Impingement syndrome of unspecified shoulder
   M75.41 Impingement syndrome of right shoulder
   M75.42 Impingement syndrome of left shoulder

✓5th **M75.5 Bursitis of shoulder**
   M75.50 Bursitis of unspecified shoulder
   M75.51 Bursitis of right shoulder
   M75.52 Bursitis of left shoulder

✓5th **M75.8 Other shoulder lesions**
   M75.80 Other shoulder lesions, unspecified shoulder
   M75.81 Other shoulder lesions, right shoulder
   M75.82 Other shoulder lesions, left shoulder

✓5th **M75.9 Shoulder lesion, unspecified**
   M75.90 Shoulder lesion, unspecified, unspecified shoulder
   M75.91 Shoulder lesion, unspecified, right shoulder
   M75.92 Shoulder lesion, unspecified, left shoulder

✓4th **M76 Enthesopathies, lower limb, excluding foot**
> EXCLUDES 2   bursitis due to use, overuse and pressure (M70.-)
>   enthesopathies of ankle and foot (M77.5-)

✓5th **M76.0 Gluteal tendinitis**
   M76.00 Gluteal tendinitis, unspecified hip
   M76.01 Gluteal tendinitis, right hip
   M76.02 Gluteal tendinitis, left hip

✓5th **M76.1 Psoas tendinitis**
   M76.10 Psoas tendinitis, unspecified hip
   M76.11 Psoas tendinitis, right hip
   M76.12 Psoas tendinitis, left hip

✓5th **M76.2 Iliac crest spur**
   M76.20 Iliac crest spur, unspecified hip
   M76.21 Iliac crest spur, right hip
   M76.22 Iliac crest spur, left hip

✓5th **M76.3 Iliotibial band syndrome**
   M76.30 Iliotibial band syndrome, unspecified leg
   M76.31 Iliotibial band syndrome, right leg
   M76.32 Iliotibial band syndrome, left leg

✓5th **M76.4 Tibial collateral bursitis [Pellegrini-Stieda]**
   M76.40 Tibial collateral bursitis [Pellegrini-Stieda], unspecified leg
   M76.41 Tibial collateral bursitis [Pellegrini-Stieda], right leg
   M76.42 Tibial collateral bursitis [Pellegrini-Stieda], left leg

✓5th **M76.5 Patellar tendinitis**
   M76.50 Patellar tendinitis, unspecified knee
   M76.51 Patellar tendinitis, right knee
   M76.52 Patellar tendinitis, left knee

✓5th **M76.6 Achilles tendinitis**
> Achilles bursitis
   M76.60 Achilles tendinitis, unspecified leg
   M76.61 Achilles tendinitis, right leg
   M76.62 Achilles tendinitis, left leg

✓5th **M76.7 Peroneal tendinitis**
   M76.70 Peroneal tendinitis, unspecified leg
   M76.71 Peroneal tendinitis, right leg
   M76.72 Peroneal tendinitis, left leg

✓5th **M76.8 Other specified enthesopathies of lower limb, excluding foot**
   ✓6th **M76.81 Anterior tibial syndrome**
     M76.811 Anterior tibial syndrome, right leg
     M76.812 Anterior tibial syndrome, left leg
     M76.819 Anterior tibial syndrome, unspecified leg
   ✓6th **M76.82 Posterior tibial tendinitis**
     M76.821 Posterior tibial tendinitis, right leg
     M76.822 Posterior tibial tendinitis, left leg
     M76.829 Posterior tibial tendinitis, unspecified leg
   ✓6th **M76.89 Other specified enthesopathies of lower limb, excluding foot**
     M76.891 Other specified enthesopathies of right lower limb, excluding foot
     M76.892 Other specified enthesopathies of left lower limb, excluding foot

M76.899 Other specified enthesopathies of unspecified lower limb, excluding foot

M76.9 Unspecified enthesopathy, lower limb, excluding foot

✓4ᵗʰ **M77** Other enthesopathies

> *EXCLUDES 1*   bursitis NOS (M71.9-)
>
> *EXCLUDES 2*   bursitis due to use, overuse and pressure (M70.-)
> osteophyte (M25.7)
> spinal enthesopathy (M46.0-)

✓5ᵗʰ **M77.0** Medial epicondylitis

M77.00 Medial epicondylitis, unspecified elbow
M77.01 Medial epicondylitis, right elbow
M77.02 Medial epicondylitis, left elbow

✓5ᵗʰ **M77.1** Lateral epicondylitis

Tennis elbow

M77.10 Lateral epicondylitis, unspecified elbow
M77.11 Lateral epicondylitis, right elbow
M77.12 Lateral epicondylitis, left elbow

✓5ᵗʰ **M77.2** Periarthritis of wrist

M77.20 Periarthritis, unspecified wrist
M77.21 Periarthritis, right wrist
M77.22 Periarthritis, left wrist

✓5ᵗʰ **M77.3** Calcaneal spur

> **DEF:** Overgrowth of calcaneus bone on the underside of the heel that causes pain on walking. Calcaneal spur is due to a chronic avulsion injury of the plantar fascia from the calcaneus.

M77.30 Calcaneal spur, unspecified foot
M77.31 Calcaneal spur, right foot
M77.32 Calcaneal spur, left foot

✓5ᵗʰ **M77.4** Metatarsalgia

> *EXCLUDES 1*   Morton's metatarsalgia (G57.6)

M77.40 Metatarsalgia, unspecified foot
M77.41 Metatarsalgia, right foot
M77.42 Metatarsalgia, left foot

▲ ✓5ᵗʰ **M77.5** Other enthesopathy of foot and ankle

▲   **M77.50** Other enthesopathy of unspecified foot and ankle
▲   **M77.51** Other enthesopathy of right foot and ankle
▲   **M77.52** Other enthesopathy of left foot and ankle

M77.8 Other enthesopathies, not elsewhere classified
M77.9 Enthesopathy, unspecified

Bone spur NOS
Capsulitis NOS
Periarthritis NOS
Tendinitis NOS

✓4ᵗʰ **M79** Other and unspecified soft tissue disorders, not elsewhere classified

> *EXCLUDES 1*   psychogenic rheumatism (F45.8)
> soft tissue pain, psychogenic (F45.41)

M79.0 Rheumatism, unspecified

> *EXCLUDES 1*   fibromyalgia (M79.7)
> palindromic rheumatism (M12.3-)

✓5ᵗʰ **M79.1** Myalgia

Myofascial pain syndrome

> *EXCLUDES 1*   fibromyalgia (M79.7)
> myositis (M60.-)

AHA: 2018,4Q,21

M79.10 Myalgia, unspecified site
M79.11 Myalgia of mastication muscle
M79.12 Myalgia of auxiliary muscles, head and neck
M79.18 Myalgia, other site

M79.2 Neuralgia and neuritis, unspecified

> *EXCLUDES 1*   brachial radiculitis NOS (M54.1)
> lumbosacral radiculitis NOS (M54.1)
> mononeuropathies (G56-G58)
> radiculitis NOS (M54.1)
> sciatica (M54.3-M54.4)

M79.3 Panniculitis, unspecified

> *EXCLUDES 1*   lupus panniculitis (L93.2)
> neck and back panniculitis (M54.0-)
> relapsing [Weber-Christian] panniculitis (M35.6)

M79.4 Hypertrophy of (infrapatellar) fat pad

M79.5 Residual foreign body in soft tissue

> *EXCLUDES 1*   foreign body granuloma of skin and subcutaneous tissue (L92.3)
> foreign body granuloma of soft tissue (M60.2-)

✓5ᵗʰ **M79.6** Pain in limb, hand, foot, fingers and toes

> *EXCLUDES 2*   pain in joint (M25.5-)

✓6ᵗʰ **M79.60** Pain in limb, unspecified

M79.601 Pain in right arm
Pain in right upper limb NOS
M79.602 Pain in left arm
Pain in left upper limb NOS
M79.603 Pain in arm, unspecified
Pain in upper limb NOS
M79.604 Pain in right leg
Pain in right lower limb NOS
M79.605 Pain in left leg
Pain in left lower limb NOS
M79.606 Pain in leg, unspecified
Pain in lower limb NOS
M79.609 Pain in unspecified limb
Pain in limb NOS

✓6ᵗʰ **M79.62** Pain in upper arm

Pain in axillary region

M79.621 Pain in right upper arm
M79.622 Pain in left upper arm
M79.629 Pain in unspecified upper arm

✓6ᵗʰ **M79.63** Pain in forearm

M79.631 Pain in right forearm
M79.632 Pain in left forearm
M79.639 Pain in unspecified forearm

✓6ᵗʰ **M79.64** Pain in hand and fingers

M79.641 Pain in right hand
M79.642 Pain in left hand
M79.643 Pain in unspecified hand
M79.644 Pain in right finger(s)
M79.645 Pain in left finger(s)
M79.646 Pain in unspecified finger(s)

✓6ᵗʰ **M79.65** Pain in thigh

M79.651 Pain in right thigh
M79.652 Pain in left thigh
M79.659 Pain in unspecified thigh

✓6ᵗʰ **M79.66** Pain in lower leg

M79.661 Pain in right lower leg
M79.662 Pain in left lower leg
M79.669 Pain in unspecified lower leg

✓6ᵗʰ **M79.67** Pain in foot and toes

M79.671 Pain in right foot
M79.672 Pain in left foot
M79.673 Pain in unspecified foot
M79.674 Pain in right toe(s)
M79.675 Pain in left toe(s)
M79.676 Pain in unspecified toe(s)

M79.7 Fibromyalgia

Fibromyositis
Fibrositis
Myofibrositis

✓5ᵗʰ **M79.A** Nontraumatic compartment syndrome

Code first, if applicable, associated postprocedural complication

> *EXCLUDES 1*   compartment syndrome NOS (T79.A-)
> fibromyalgia (M79.7)
> nontraumatic ischemic infarction of muscle (M62.2-)
> traumatic compartment syndrome (T79.A-)

✓6ᵗʰ **M79.A1** Nontraumatic compartment syndrome of upper extremity

Nontraumatic compartment syndrome of shoulder, arm, forearm, wrist, hand, and fingers

M79.A11 Nontraumatic compartment syndrome of right upper extremity
M79.A12 Nontraumatic compartment syndrome of left upper extremity
M79.A19 Nontraumatic compartment syndrome of unspecified upper extremity

N Newborn: 0   P Pediatric: 0-17   M Maternity: 12-55   A Adult: 15-124   CH Comorbidity High   CL Comorbidity Low   NCDx Noncancer Dx   PDx Primary Dx

800

ICD-10-CM 2020

√6ᵗʰ **M79.A2 Nontraumatic compartment syndrome of** lower extremity
Nontraumatic compartment syndrome of hip, buttock, thigh, leg, foot, and toes

    M79.A21 Nontraumatic compartment syndrome of right **lower extremity**

    M79.A22 Nontraumatic compartment syndrome of left **lower extremity**

    M79.A29 Nontraumatic compartment syndrome of unspecified lower extremity

    M79.A3 Nontraumatic compartment syndrome of abdomen

    M79.A9 Nontraumatic compartment syndrome of other sites

√5ᵗʰ **M79.8 Other specified soft tissue disorders**

    M79.81 Nontraumatic hematoma of soft tissue
Nontraumatic hematoma of muscle
Nontraumatic seroma of muscle and soft tissue

    M79.89 Other specified soft tissue disorders
Polyalgia

M79.9 Soft tissue disorder, unspecified

OSTEOPATHIES AND CHONDROPATHIES (M80-M94)

Disorders of bone density and structure (M80-M85)

√4ᵗʰ **M80 Osteoporosis** with current pathological fracture

INCLUDES osteoporosis with current fragility fracture
Use additional code to identify major osseous defect, if applicable (M89.7-)

EXCLUDES 1 collapsed vertebra NOS (M48.5)
pathological fracture NOS (M84.4)
wedging of vertebra NOS (M48.5)

EXCLUDES 2 personal history of (healed) osteoporosis fracture (Z87.310)

AHA: 2018,2Q,12

TIP: The term "improper alignment" is not synonymous with malunion or nonunion of a fracture when noted in provider documentation.

The appropriate 7th character is to be added to each code from category M80:
A initial encounter for fracture
D subsequent encounter for fracture with routine healing
G subsequent encounter for fracture with delayed healing
K subsequent encounter for fracture with nonunion
P subsequent encounter for fracture with malunion
S sequela

√5ᵗʰ **M80.0 Age-related osteoporosis with current pathological fracture**
Involutional osteoporosis with current pathological fracture
Osteoporosis NOS with current pathological fracture
Postmenopausal osteoporosis with current pathological fracture
Senile osteoporosis with current pathological fracture

√x7ᵗʰ **M80.00 Age-related osteoporosis with current pathological fracture, unspecified site** Ⓐ

√6ᵗʰ **M80.01 Age-related osteoporosis with current pathological fracture,** shoulder

    √7ᵗʰ **M80.011 Age-related osteoporosis with current pathological fracture,** right **shoulder** Ⓐ

    √7ᵗʰ **M80.012 Age-related osteoporosis with current pathological fracture,** left **shoulder** Ⓐ

    √7ᵗʰ **M80.019 Age-related osteoporosis with current pathological fracture, unspecified shoulder** Ⓐ

√6ᵗʰ **M80.02 Age-related osteoporosis with current pathological fracture,** humerus

    √7ᵗʰ **M80.021 Age-related osteoporosis with current pathological fracture,** right **humerus** Ⓐ

    √7ᵗʰ **M80.022 Age-related osteoporosis with current pathological fracture,** left **humerus** Ⓐ

    √7ᵗʰ **M80.029 Age-related osteoporosis with current pathological fracture, unspecified humerus** Ⓐ

√6ᵗʰ **M80.03 Age-related osteoporosis with current pathological fracture,** forearm
Age-related osteoporosis with current pathological fracture of wrist

    √7ᵗʰ **M80.031 Age-related osteoporosis with current pathological fracture,** right **forearm** Ⓐ

    √7ᵗʰ **M80.032 Age-related osteoporosis with current pathological fracture,** left **forearm** Ⓐ

    √7ᵗʰ **M80.039 Age-related osteoporosis with current pathological fracture, unspecified forearm** Ⓐ

√6ᵗʰ **M80.04 Age-related osteoporosis with current pathological fracture,** hand

    √7ᵗʰ **M80.041 Age-related osteoporosis with current pathological fracture,** right **hand** Ⓐ

    √7ᵗʰ **M80.042 Age-related osteoporosis with current pathological fracture,** left **hand** Ⓐ

    √7ᵗʰ **M80.049 Age-related osteoporosis with current pathological fracture, unspecified hand** Ⓐ

√6ᵗʰ **M80.05 Age-related osteoporosis with current pathological fracture,** femur
Age-related osteoporosis with current pathological fracture of hip

    √7ᵗʰ **M80.051 Age-related osteoporosis with current pathological fracture,** right **femur** Ⓐ

    √7ᵗʰ **M80.052 Age-related osteoporosis with current pathological fracture,** left **femur** Ⓐ

    √7ᵗʰ **M80.059 Age-related osteoporosis with current pathological fracture, unspecified femur** Ⓐ

√6ᵗʰ **M80.06 Age-related osteoporosis with current pathological fracture,** lower leg

    √7ᵗʰ **M80.061 Age-related osteoporosis with current pathological fracture,** right **lower leg** Ⓐ

    √7ᵗʰ **M80.062 Age-related osteoporosis with current pathological fracture,** left **lower leg** Ⓐ

    √7ᵗʰ **M80.069 Age-related osteoporosis with current pathological fracture, unspecified lower leg** Ⓐ

√6ᵗʰ **M80.07 Age-related osteoporosis with current pathological fracture,** ankle and foot

    √7ᵗʰ **M80.071 Age-related osteoporosis with current pathological fracture,** right **ankle and foot** Ⓐ

    √7ᵗʰ **M80.072 Age-related osteoporosis with current pathological fracture,** left **ankle and foot** Ⓐ

    √7ᵗʰ **M80.079 Age-related osteoporosis with current pathological fracture, unspecified ankle and foot** Ⓐ

√x7ᵗʰ **M80.08 Age-related osteoporosis with current pathological fracture,** vertebra(e) Ⓐ

√5ᵗʰ **M80.8 Other osteoporosis with current pathological fracture**
Drug-induced osteoporosis with current pathological fracture
Idiopathic osteoporosis with current pathological fracture
Osteoporosis of disuse with current pathological fracture
Postoophorectomy osteoporosis with current pathological fracture
Postsurgical malabsorption osteoporosis with current pathological fracture
Post-traumatic osteoporosis with current pathological fracture
Use additional code for adverse effect, if applicable, to identify drug (T36-T50 with fifth or sixth character 5)

√x7ᵗʰ **M80.80 Other osteoporosis with current pathological fracture, unspecified site**

√6ᵗʰ **M80.81 Other osteoporosis with pathological fracture,** shoulder

    √7ᵗʰ **M80.811 Other osteoporosis with current pathological fracture,** right **shoulder**

    √7ᵗʰ **M80.812 Other osteoporosis with current pathological fracture,** left **shoulder**

    √7ᵗʰ **M80.819 Other osteoporosis with current pathological fracture, unspecified shoulder**

√6ᵗʰ **M80.82 Other osteoporosis with current pathological fracture,** humerus

    √7ᵗʰ **M80.821 Other osteoporosis with current pathological fracture,** right **humerus**

    √7ᵗʰ **M80.022 Other osteoporosis with current pathological fracture,** left **humerus**

☑ Additional Character Required   √x7ᵗʰ Placeholder Alert   Manifestation   Unspecified Dx   ►◄ Revised Text   ● New Code   ▲ Revised Title

ICD-10-CM 2020   **801**

M79.A2–M80.822

Chapter 13. Diseases of the Musculoskeletal System and Connective Tissue

    √7ᵗʰ **M80.829** Other osteoporosis with current pathological fracture, unspecified humerus

  √6ᵗʰ **M80.83** Other osteoporosis with current pathological fracture, forearm

       Other osteoporosis with current pathological fracture of wrist

    √7ᵗʰ **M80.831** Other osteoporosis with current pathological fracture, right forearm

    √7ᵗʰ **M80.832** Other osteoporosis with current pathological fracture, left forearm

    √7ᵗʰ **M80.839** Other osteoporosis with current pathological fracture, unspecified forearm

  √6ᵗʰ **M80.84** Other osteoporosis with current pathological fracture, hand

    √7ᵗʰ **M80.841** Other osteoporosis with current pathological fracture, right hand

    √7ᵗʰ **M80.842** Other osteoporosis with current pathological fracture, left hand

    √7ᵗʰ **M80.849** Other osteoporosis with current pathological fracture, unspecified hand

  √6ᵗʰ **M80.85** Other osteoporosis with current pathological fracture, femur

       Other osteoporosis with current pathological fracture of hip

    √7ᵗʰ **M80.851** Other osteoporosis with current pathological fracture, right femur

    √7ᵗʰ **M80.852** Other osteoporosis with current pathological fracture, left femur

    √7ᵗʰ **M80.859** Other osteoporosis with current pathological fracture, unspecified femur

  √6ᵗʰ **M80.86** Other osteoporosis with current pathological fracture, lower leg

    √7ᵗʰ **M80.861** Other osteoporosis with current pathological fracture, right lower leg

    √7ᵗʰ **M80.862** Other osteoporosis with current pathological fracture, left lower leg

    √7ᵗʰ **M80.869** Other osteoporosis with current pathological fracture, unspecified lower leg

  √6ᵗʰ **M80.87** Other osteoporosis with current pathological fracture, ankle and foot

    √7ᵗʰ **M80.871** Other osteoporosis with current pathological fracture, right ankle and foot

    √7ᵗʰ **M80.872** Other osteoporosis with current pathological fracture, left ankle and foot

    √7ᵗʰ **M80.879** Other osteoporosis with current pathological fracture, unspecified ankle and foot

  √x7ᵗʰ **M80.88** Other osteoporosis with current pathological fracture, vertebra(e)

√4ᵗʰ **M81 Osteoporosis without current pathological fracture**

   Use additional code to identify:

   major osseous defect, if applicable (M89.7-)

   personal history of (healed) osteoporosis fracture, if applicable (Z87.310)

     EXCLUDES 1   osteoporosis with current pathological fracture (M80.-)

           Sudeck's atrophy (M89.0)

M81.0 Age-related osteoporosis without current pathological fracture   Ⓐ

     Involutional osteoporosis without current pathological fracture

     Osteoporosis NOS

     Postmenopausal osteoporosis without current pathological fracture

     Senile osteoporosis without current pathological fracture

M81.6 Localized osteoporosis [Lequesne]

     EXCLUDES 1   Sudeck's atrophy (M89.0)

M81.8 Other osteoporosis without current pathological fracture

   Drug-induced osteoporosis without current pathological fracture

   Idiopathic osteoporosis without current pathological fracture

   Osteoporosis of disuse without current pathological fracture

   Postoophorectomy osteoporosis without current pathological fracture

   Postsurgical malabsorption osteoporosis without current pathological fracture

   Post-traumatic osteoporosis without current pathological fracture

   Use additional code for adverse effect, if applicable, to identify drug (T36-T50 with fifth or sixth character 5)

√4ᵗʰ **M83 Adult osteomalacia**

     EXCLUDES 1   *infantile and juvenile osteomalacia (E55.0)*

           renal osteodystrophy (N25.0)

           rickets (active) (E55.0)

           rickets (active) sequelae (E64.3)

           vitamin D-resistant osteomalacia (E83.3)

           vitamin D-resistant rickets (active) (E83.3)

  M83.0 Puerperal osteomalacia   Ⓜ ♀

  M83.1 Senile osteomalacia   Ⓐ

  M83.2 Adult osteomalacia due to malabsorption   Ⓐ

     Postsurgical malabsorption osteomalacia in adults

  M83.3 Adult osteomalacia due to malnutrition   Ⓐ

  M83.4 Aluminum bone disease

  M83.5 Other drug-induced osteomalacia in adults   Ⓐ

     Use additional code for adverse effect, if applicable, to identify drug (T36-T50 with fifth or sixth character 5)

  M83.8 Other adult osteomalacia   Ⓐ

  M83.9 Adult osteomalacia, unspecified   Ⓐ

√4ᵗʰ **M84 Disorder of continuity of bone**

     EXCLUDES 2   *traumatic fracture of bone-see fracture, by site*

     TIP: The term "improper alignment" is not synonymous with malunion or nonunion of a fracture when noted in provider documentation.

  √5ᵗʰ **M84.3 Stress fracture**

     Fatigue fracture

     March fracture

     Stress fracture NOS

     Stress reaction

     Use additional external cause code(s) to identify the cause of the stress fracture

     EXCLUDES 1   *pathological fracture due to osteoporosis (M80.-)*

           pathological fracture NOS (M84.4.-)

           traumatic fracture (S12.-, S22.-, S32.-, S42.-, S52.-, S62.-, S72.-, S82.-, S92.-)

     EXCLUDES 2   *personal history of (healed) stress (fatigue) fracture (Z87.312)*

           stress fracture of vertebra (M48.4-)

> The appropriate 7th character is to be added to each code from subcategory M84.3.
> A   initial encounter for fracture
> D   subsequent encounter for fracture with routine healing
> G   subsequent encounter for fracture with delayed healing
> K   subsequent encounter for fracture with nonunion
> P   subsequent encounter for fracture with malunion
> S   sequela

  √x7ᵗʰ **M84.30** Stress fracture, unspecified site

  √6ᵗʰ **M84.31** Stress fracture, shoulder

    √7ᵗʰ **M84.311** Stress fracture, right shoulder

    √7ᵗʰ **M84.312** Stress fracture, left shoulder

    √7ᵗʰ **M84.319** Stress fracture, unspecified shoulder

  √6ᵗʰ **M84.32** Stress fracture, humerus

    √7ᵗʰ **M84.321** Stress fracture, right humerus

    √7ᵗʰ **M84.322** Stress fracture, left humerus

    √7ᵗʰ **M84.329** Stress fracture, unspecified humerus

  √6ᵗʰ **M84.33** Stress fracture, ulna and radius

    √7ᵗʰ **M84.331** Stress fracture, right ulna

    √7ᵗʰ **M84.332** Stress fracture, left ulna

    √7ᵗʰ **M84.333** Stress fracture, right radius

    √7ᵗʰ **M84.334** Stress fracture, left radius

Ⓝ Newborn: 0   Ⓟ Pediatric: 0-17   Ⓜ Maternity: 12-55   Ⓐ Adult: 15-124   CH Comorbidity High   CL Comorbidity Low   NCDx Noncancer Dx   PDx Primary Dx

802   ICD-10-CM 2020

√7ᵗʰ **M84.339** Stress fracture, unspecified ulna and radius

✓6ᵗʰ **M84.34** Stress fracture, **hand and fingers**

  √7ᵗʰ **M84.341** Stress fracture, **right hand**

  √7ᵗʰ **M84.342** Stress fracture, **left hand**

  √7ᵗʰ **M84.343** Stress fracture, **unspecified hand**

  √7ᵗʰ **M84.344** Stress fracture, **right finger(s)**

  √7ᵗʰ **M84.345** Stress fracture, **left finger(s)**

  √7ᵗʰ **M84.346** Stress fracture, **unspecified finger(s)**

✓6ᵗʰ **M84.35** Stress fracture, **pelvis and femur**

  Stress fracture, hip

  √7ᵗʰ **M84.350** Stress fracture, **pelvis**

  √7ᵗʰ **M84.351** Stress fracture, **right femur**

  √7ᵗʰ **M84.352** Stress fracture, **left femur**

  √7ᵗʰ **M84.353** Stress fracture, **unspecified femur**

  √7ᵗʰ **M84.359** Stress fracture, **hip, unspecified**

✓6ᵗʰ **M84.36** Stress fracture, **tibia and fibula**

  √7ᵗʰ **M84.361** Stress fracture, **right tibia**

  √7ᵗʰ **M84.362** Stress fracture, **left tibia**

  √7ᵗʰ **M84.363** Stress fracture, **right fibula**

  √7ᵗʰ **M84.364** Stress fracture, **left fibula**

  √7ᵗʰ **M84.369** Stress fracture, **unspecified tibia and fibula**

✓6ᵗʰ **M84.37** Stress fracture, **ankle, foot and toes**

  √7ᵗʰ **M84.371** Stress fracture, **right ankle**

  √7ᵗʰ **M84.372** Stress fracture, **left ankle**

  √7ᵗʰ **M84.373** Stress fracture, **unspecified ankle**

  √7ᵗʰ **M84.374** Stress fracture, **right foot**

  √7ᵗʰ **M84.375** Stress fracture, **left foot**

  √7ᵗʰ **M84.376** Stress fracture, **unspecified foot**

  √7ᵗʰ **M84.377** Stress fracture, **right toe(s)**

  √7ᵗʰ **M84.378** Stress fracture, **left toe(s)**

  √7ᵗʰ **M84.379** Stress fracture, **unspecified toe(s)**

√x7ᵗʰ **M84.38** Stress fracture, **other site**

  EXCLUDES 2   stress fracture of vertebra (M48.4-)

✓5ᵗʰ **M84.4** Pathological fracture, **not elsewhere classified**

  Chronic fracture

  Pathological fracture NOS

  EXCLUDES 1   collapsed vertebra NEC (M48.5)

     pathological fracture in neoplastic disease (M84.5-)

     pathological fracture in osteoporosis (M80.-)

     pathological fracture in other disease (M84.6-)

     stress fracture (M84.3-)

     traumatic fracture (S12.-, S22.-, S32.-, S42.-, S52.-, S62.-, S72.-, S82.-, S92.-)

  EXCLUDES 2   personal history of (healed) pathological fracture (Z87.311)

  The appropriate 7th character is to be added to each code from subcategory M84.4.

  A   initial encounter for fracture

  D   subsequent encounter for fracture with routine healing

  G   subsequent encounter for fracture with delayed healing

  K   subsequent encounter for fracture with nonunion

  P   subsequent encounter for fracture with malunion

  S   sequela

√x7ᵗʰ **M84.40** Pathological fracture, **unspecified site**

✓6ᵗʰ **M84.41** Pathological fracture, **shoulder**

  √7ᵗʰ **M84.411** Pathological fracture, **right shoulder**

  √7ᵗʰ **M84.412** Pathological fracture, **left shoulder**

  √7ᵗʰ **M84.419** Pathological fracture, **unspecified shoulder**

✓6ᵗʰ **M84.42** Pathological fracture, **humerus**

  √7ᵗʰ **M84.421** Pathological fracture, **right humerus**

  √7ᵗʰ **M84.422** Pathological fracture, **left humerus**

  √7ᵗʰ **M84.429** Pathological fracture, **unspecified humerus**

✓6ᵗʰ **M84.43** Pathological fracture, **ulna and radius**

  √7ᵗʰ **M84.431** Pathological fracture, **right ulna**

  √7ᵗʰ **M84.432** Pathological fracture, **left ulna**

  √7ᵗʰ **M84.433** Pathological fracture, **right radius**

  √7ᵗʰ **M84.434** Pathological fracture, **left radius**

  √7ᵗʰ **M84.439** Pathological fracture, **unspecified ulna and radius**

✓6ᵗʰ **M84.44** Pathological fracture, **hand and fingers**

  √7ᵗʰ **M84.441** Pathological fracture, **right hand**

  √7ᵗʰ **M84.442** Pathological fracture, **left hand**

  √7ᵗʰ **M84.443** Pathological fracture, **unspecified hand**

  √7ᵗʰ **M84.444** Pathological fracture, **right finger(s)**

  √7ᵗʰ **M84.445** Pathological fracture, **left finger(s)**

  √7ᵗʰ **M84.446** Pathological fracture, **unspecified finger(s)**

✓6ᵗʰ **M84.45** Pathological fracture, **femur and pelvis**

  AHA: 2016,4Q,43

  √7ᵗʰ **M84.451** Pathological fracture, **right femur**

  √7ᵗʰ **M84.452** Pathological fracture, **left femur**

  √7ᵗʰ **M84.453** Pathological fracture, **unspecified femur**

  √7ᵗʰ **M84.454** Pathological fracture, **pelvis**

  √7ᵗʰ **M84.459** Pathological fracture, **hip, unspecified**

✓6ᵗʰ **M84.46** Pathological fracture, **tibia and fibula**

  √7ᵗʰ **M84.461** Pathological fracture, **right tibia**

  √7ᵗʰ **M84.462** Pathological fracture, **left tibia**

  √7ᵗʰ **M84.463** Pathological fracture, **right fibula**

  √7ᵗʰ **M84.464** Pathological fracture, **left fibula**

  √7ᵗʰ **M84.469** Pathological fracture, **unspecified tibia and fibula**

✓6ᵗʰ **M84.47** Pathological fracture, **ankle, foot and toes**

  √7ᵗʰ **M84.471** Pathological fracture, **right ankle**

  √7ᵗʰ **M84.472** Pathological fracture, **left ankle**

  √7ᵗʰ **M84.473** Pathological fracture, **unspecified ankle**

  √7ᵗʰ **M84.474** Pathological fracture, **right foot**

  √7ᵗʰ **M84.475** Pathological fracture, **left foot**

  √7ᵗʰ **M84.476** Pathological fracture, **unspecified foot**

  √7ᵗʰ **M84.477** Pathological fracture, **right toe(s)**

  √7ᵗʰ **M84.478** Pathological fracture, **left toe(s)**

  √7ᵗʰ **M84.479** Pathological fracture, **unspecified toe(s)**

√x7ᵗʰ **M84.48** Pathological fracture, **other site**

✓5ᵗʰ **M84.5** Pathological fracture in **neoplastic disease**

  Code also underlying neoplasm

  The appropriate 7th character is to be added to each code from subcategory M84.5.

  A   initial encounter for fracture

  D   subsequent encounter for fracture with routine healing

  G   subsequent encounter for fracture with delayed healing

  K   subsequent encounter for fracture with nonunion

  P   subsequent encounter for fracture with malunion

  S   sequela

√x7ᵗʰ **M84.50** Pathological fracture in neoplastic disease, **unspecified site**

✓6ᵗʰ **M84.51** Pathological fracture in neoplastic disease, **shoulder**

  √7ᵗʰ **M84.511** Pathological fracture in neoplastic disease, **right shoulder**

  √7ᵗʰ **M84.512** Pathological fracture in neoplastic disease, **left shoulder**

  √7ᵗʰ **M84.519** Pathological fracture in neoplastic disease, **unspecified shoulder**

✓6ᵗʰ **M84.52** Pathological fracture in neoplastic disease, **humerus**

  √7ᵗʰ **M84.521** Pathological fracture in neoplastic disease, **right humerus**

  √7ᵗʰ **M84.522** Pathological fracture in neoplastic disease, **left humerus**

  √7ᵗʰ **M84.529** Pathological fracture in neoplastic disease, **unspecified humerus**

✓6ᵗʰ **M84.53** Pathological fracture in neoplastic disease, **ulna and radius**

  √7ᵗʰ **M84.531** Pathological fracture in neoplastic disease, **right ulna**

  √7ᵗʰ **M84.532** Pathological fracture in neoplastic disease, **left ulna**

  √7ᵗʰ **M84.533** Pathological fracture in neoplastic disease, **right radius**

  √7ᵗʰ **M84.534** Pathological fracture in neoplastic disease, **left radius**

☑ Additional Character Required   √x7ᵗʰ Placeholder Alert   Manifestation   Unspecified Dx   ►◄ Revised Text   ● New Code   ▲ Revised Title

ICD-10-CM 2020   803

M84.339–M84.534

Chapter 13. Diseases of the Musculoskeletal System and Connective Tissue

✓7ᵗʰ **M84.539** Pathological fracture in neoplastic disease, unspecified ulna and radius

✓6ᵗʰ **M84.54** Pathological fracture in neoplastic disease, hand

  ✓7ᵗʰ **M84.541** Pathological fracture in neoplastic disease, right hand

  ✓7ᵗʰ **M84.542** Pathological fracture in neoplastic disease, left hand

  ✓7ᵗʰ **M84.549** Pathological fracture in neoplastic disease, unspecified hand

✓6ᵗʰ **M84.55** Pathological fracture in neoplastic disease, pelvis and femur

  ✓7ᵗʰ **M84.550** Pathological fracture in neoplastic disease, pelvis

  ✓7ᵗʰ **M84.551** Pathological fracture in neoplastic disease, right femur

  ✓7ᵗʰ **M84.552** Pathological fracture in neoplastic disease, left femur

  ✓7ᵗʰ **M84.553** Pathological fracture in neoplastic disease, unspecified femur

  ✓7ᵗʰ **M84.559** Pathological fracture in neoplastic disease, hip, unspecified

✓6ᵗʰ **M84.56** Pathological fracture in neoplastic disease, tibia and fibula

  ✓7ᵗʰ **M84.561** Pathological fracture in neoplastic disease, right tibia

  ✓7ᵗʰ **M84.562** Pathological fracture in neoplastic disease, left tibia

  ✓7ᵗʰ **M84.563** Pathological fracture in neoplastic disease, right fibula

  ✓7ᵗʰ **M84.564** Pathological fracture in neoplastic disease, left fibula

  ✓7ᵗʰ **M84.569** Pathological fracture in neoplastic disease, unspecified tibia and fibula

✓6ᵗʰ **M84.57** Pathological fracture in neoplastic disease, ankle and foot

  ✓7ᵗʰ **M84.571** Pathological fracture in neoplastic disease, right ankle

  ✓7ᵗʰ **M84.572** Pathological fracture in neoplastic disease, left ankle

  ✓7ᵗʰ **M84.573** Pathological fracture in neoplastic disease, unspecified ankle

  ✓7ᵗʰ **M84.574** Pathological fracture in neoplastic disease, right foot

  ✓7ᵗʰ **M84.575** Pathological fracture in neoplastic disease, left foot

  ✓7ᵗʰ **M84.576** Pathological fracture in neoplastic disease, unspecified foot

✓x7ᵗʰ **M84.58** Pathological fracture in neoplastic disease, other specified site

     Pathological fracture in neoplastic disease, vertebrae

✓5ᵗʰ **M84.6** Pathological fracture in other disease

   Code also underlying condition

   EXCLUDES 1 *pathological fracture in osteoporosis (M80.-)*

   The appropriate 7th character is to be added to each code from subcategory M84.6.
   A   initial encounter for fracture
   D   subsequent encounter for fracture with routine healing
   G   subsequent encounter for fracture with delayed healing
   K   subsequent encounter for fracture with nonunion
   P   subsequent encounter for fracture with malunion
   S   sequela

✓x7ᵗʰ **M84.60** Pathological fracture in other disease, unspecified site

✓6ᵗʰ **M84.61** Pathological fracture in other disease, shoulder

  ✓7ᵗʰ **M84.611** Pathological fracture in other disease, right shoulder

  ✓7ᵗʰ **M84.612** Pathological fracture in other disease, left shoulder

  ✓7ᵗʰ **M84.619** Pathological fracture in other disease, unspecified shoulder

✓6ᵗʰ **M84.62** Pathological fracture in other disease, humerus

  ✓7ᵗʰ **M84.621** Pathological fracture in other disease, right humerus

  ✓7ᵗʰ **M84.622** Pathological fracture in other disease, left humerus

  ✓7ᵗʰ **M84.629** Pathological fracture in other disease, unspecified humerus

✓6ᵗʰ **M84.63** Pathological fracture in other disease, ulna and radius

  ✓7ᵗʰ **M84.631** Pathological fracture in other disease, right ulna

✓7ᵗʰ **M84.632** Pathological fracture in other disease, left ulna

✓7ᵗʰ **M84.633** Pathological fracture in other disease, right radius

✓7ᵗʰ **M84.634** Pathological fracture in other disease, left radius

✓7ᵗʰ **M84.639** Pathological fracture in other disease, unspecified ulna and radius

✓6ᵗʰ **M84.64** Pathological fracture in other disease, hand

  ✓7ᵗʰ **M84.641** Pathological fracture in other disease, right hand

  ✓7ᵗʰ **M84.642** Pathological fracture in other disease, left hand

  ✓7ᵗʰ **M84.649** Pathological fracture in other disease, unspecified hand

✓6ᵗʰ **M84.65** Pathological fracture in other disease, pelvis and femur

  ✓7ᵗʰ **M84.650** Pathological fracture in other disease, pelvis

  ✓7ᵗʰ **M84.651** Pathological fracture in other disease, right femur

  ✓7ᵗʰ **M84.652** Pathological fracture in other disease, left femur

  ✓7ᵗʰ **M84.653** Pathological fracture in other disease, unspecified femur

  ✓7ᵗʰ **M84.659** Pathological fracture in other disease, hip, unspecified

✓6ᵗʰ **M84.66** Pathological fracture in other disease, tibia and fibula

  ✓7ᵗʰ **M84.661** Pathological fracture in other disease, right tibia

  ✓7ᵗʰ **M84.662** Pathological fracture in other disease, left tibia

  ✓7ᵗʰ **M84.663** Pathological fracture in other disease, right fibula

  ✓7ᵗʰ **M84.664** Pathological fracture in other disease, left fibula

  ✓7ᵗʰ **M84.669** Pathological fracture in other disease, unspecified tibia and fibula

✓6ᵗʰ **M84.67** Pathological fracture in other disease, ankle and foot

  ✓7ᵗʰ **M84.671** Pathological fracture in other disease, right ankle

  ✓7ᵗʰ **M84.672** Pathological fracture in other disease, left ankle

  ✓7ᵗʰ **M84.673** Pathological fracture in other disease, unspecified ankle

  ✓7ᵗʰ **M84.674** Pathological fracture in other disease, right foot

  ✓7ᵗʰ **M84.675** Pathological fracture in other disease, left foot

  ✓7ᵗʰ **M84.676** Pathological fracture in other disease, unspecified foot

✓x7ᵗʰ **M84.68** Pathological fracture in other disease, other site

✓5ᵗʰ **M84.7** Nontraumatic fracture, not elsewhere classified

✓6ᵗʰ **M84.75** Atypical femoral fracture

     AHA: 2016,4Q,41-42

   The appropriate 7th character is to be added to each code from M84.75.
   A   initial encounter for fracture
   D   subsequent encounter for fracture with routine healing
   G   subsequent encounter for fracture with delayed healing
   K   subsequent encounter for fracture with nonunion
   P   subsequent encounter for fracture with malunion
   S   sequela

  ✓7ᵗʰ **M84.750** Atypical femoral fracture, unspecified

  ✓7ᵗʰ **M84.751** Incomplete atypical femoral fracture, right leg

  ✓7ᵗʰ **M84.752** Incomplete atypical femoral fracture, left leg

  ✓7ᵗʰ **M84.753** Incomplete atypical femoral fracture, unspecified leg

  ✓7ᵗʰ **M84.754** Complete transverse atypical femoral fracture, right leg

  ✓7ᵗʰ **M84.755** Complete transverse atypical femoral fracture, left leg

N Newborn: 0   **P** Pediatric: 0-17   **M** Maternity: 12-55   **A** Adult: 15-124   **CH** Comorbidity High   **CL** Comorbidity Low   **NCDx** Noncancer Dx   **PDx** Primary Dx

804   ICD-10-CM 2020

✓7ᵗʰ **M84.756** Complete transverse atypical femoral fracture, unspecified leg

✓7ᵗʰ **M84.757** Complete oblique atypical femoral fracture, right leg

✓7ᵗʰ **M84.758** Complete oblique atypical femoral fracture, left leg

✓7ᵗʰ **M84.759** Complete oblique atypical femoral fracture, unspecified leg

✓5ᵗʰ **M84.8 Other disorders of continuity of bone**

M84.80 Other disorders of continuity of bone, unspecified site

✓6ᵗʰ **M84.81** Other disorders of continuity of bone, shoulder

    M84.811 Other disorders of continuity of bone, right shoulder

    M84.812 Other disorders of continuity of bone, left shoulder

    M84.819 Other disorders of continuity of bone, unspecified shoulder

✓6ᵗʰ **M84.82** Other disorders of continuity of bone, humerus

    M84.821 Other disorders of continuity of bone, right humerus

    M84.822 Other disorders of continuity of bone, left humerus

    M84.829 Other disorders of continuity of bone, unspecified humerus

✓6ᵗʰ **M84.83** Other disorders of continuity of bone, ulna and radius

    M84.831 Other disorders of continuity of bone, right ulna

    M84.832 Other disorders of continuity of bone, left ulna

    M84.833 Other disorders of continuity of bone, right radius

    M84.834 Other disorders of continuity of bone, left radius

    M84.839 Other disorders of continuity of bone, unspecified ulna and radius

✓6ᵗʰ **M84.84** Other disorders of continuity of bone, hand

    M84.841 Other disorders of continuity of bone, right hand

    M84.842 Other disorders of continuity of bone, left hand

    M84.849 Other disorders of continuity of bone, unspecified hand

✓6ᵗʰ **M84.85** Other disorders of continuity of bone, pelvic region and thigh

    M84.851 Other disorders of continuity of bone, right pelvic region and thigh

    M84.852 Other disorders of continuity of bone, left pelvic region and thigh

    M84.859 Other disorders of continuity of bone, unspecified pelvic region and thigh

✓6ᵗʰ **M84.86** Other disorders of continuity of bone, tibia and fibula

    M84.861 Other disorders of continuity of bone, right tibia

    M84.862 Other disorders of continuity of bone, left tibia

    M84.863 Other disorders of continuity of bone, right fibula

    M84.864 Other disorders of continuity of bone, left fibula

    M84.869 Other disorders of continuity of bone, unspecified tibia and fibula

✓6ᵗʰ **M84.87** Other disorders of continuity of bone, ankle and foot

    M84.871 Other disorders of continuity of bone, right ankle and foot

    M84.872 Other disorders of continuity of bone, left ankle and foot

    M84.879 Other disorders of continuity of bone, unspecified ankle and foot

M84.88 Other disorders of continuity of bone, other site

M84.9 Disorder of continuity of bone, unspecified

✓4ᵗʰ **M85 Other disorders of bone density and structure**

EXCLUDES 1   osteogenesis imperfecta (Q78.0)
        osteopetrosis (Q78.2)
        osteopoikilosis (Q78.8)
        polyostotic fibrous dysplasia (Q78.1)

✓6ᵗʰ **M85.0 Fibrous dysplasia (monostotic)**

EXCLUDES 2   fibrous dysplasia of jaw (M27.8)

M85.00 Fibrous dysplasia (monostotic), unspecified site

✓6ᵗʰ **M85.01** Fibrous dysplasia (monostotic), shoulder

    M85.011 Fibrous dysplasia (monostotic), right shoulder

    M85.012 Fibrous dysplasia (monostotic), left shoulder

    M85.019 Fibrous dysplasia (monostotic), unspecified shoulder

✓6ᵗʰ **M85.02** Fibrous dysplasia (monostotic), upper arm

    M85.021 Fibrous dysplasia (monostotic), right upper arm

    M85.022 Fibrous dysplasia (monostotic), left upper arm

    M85.029 Fibrous dysplasia (monostotic), unspecified upper arm

✓6ᵗʰ **M85.03** Fibrous dysplasia (monostotic), forearm

    M85.031 Fibrous dysplasia (monostotic), right forearm

    M85.032 Fibrous dysplasia (monostotic), left forearm

    M85.039 Fibrous dysplasia (monostotic), unspecified forearm

✓6ᵗʰ **M85.04** Fibrous dysplasia (monostotic), hand

    M85.041 Fibrous dysplasia (monostotic), right hand

    M85.042 Fibrous dysplasia (monostotic), left hand

    M85.049 Fibrous dysplasia (monostotic), unspecified hand

✓6ᵗʰ **M85.05** Fibrous dysplasia (monostotic), thigh

    M85.051 Fibrous dysplasia (monostotic), right thigh

    M85.052 Fibrous dysplasia (monostotic), left thigh

    M85.059 Fibrous dysplasia (monostotic), unspecified thigh

✓6ᵗʰ **M85.06** Fibrous dysplasia (monostotic), lower leg

    M85.061 Fibrous dysplasia (monostotic), right lower leg

    M85.062 Fibrous dysplasia (monostotic), left lower leg

    M85.069 Fibrous dysplasia (monostotic), unspecified lower leg

✓6ᵗʰ **M85.07** Fibrous dysplasia (monostotic), ankle and foot

    M85.071 Fibrous dysplasia (monostotic), right ankle and foot

    M85.072 Fibrous dysplasia (monostotic), left ankle and foot

    M85.079 Fibrous dysplasia (monostotic), unspecified ankle and foot

M85.08 Fibrous dysplasia (monostotic), other site

M85.09 Fibrous dysplasia (monostotic), multiple sites

✓5ᵗʰ **M85.1 Skeletal fluorosis**

M85.10 Skeletal fluorosis, unspecified site

✓6ᵗʰ **M85.11** Skeletal fluorosis, shoulder

    M85.111 Skeletal fluorosis, right shoulder

    M85.112 Skeletal fluorosis, left shoulder

    M85.119 Skeletal fluorosis, unspecified shoulder

✓6ᵗʰ **M85.12** Skeletal fluorosis, upper arm

    M85.121 Skeletal fluorosis, right upper arm

    M85.122 Skeletal fluorosis, left upper arm

    M85.129 Skeletal fluorosis, unspecified upper arm

✓6ᵗʰ **M85.13** Skeletal fluorosis, forearm

    M85.131 Skeletal fluorosis, right forearm

    M85.132 Skeletal fluorosis, left forearm

    M85.139 Skeletal fluorosis, unspecified forearm

✓6ᵗʰ **M85.14** Skeletal fluorosis, hand

    M85.141 Skeletal fluorosis, right hand

    M85.142 Skeletal fluorosis, left hand

    M85.149 Skeletal fluorosis, unspecified hand

✓6ᵗʰ **M85.15** Skeletal fluorosis, thigh

    M85.151 Skeletal fluorosis, right thigh

☑ Additional Character Required   ✓x7ᵗʰ Placeholder Alert   Manifestation   Unspecified Dx   ▶◀ Revised Text   ● New Code   ▲ Revised Title

ICD-10-CM 2020

805

Chapter 13. Diseases of the Musculoskeletal System and Connective Tissue

        M85.152   Skeletal fluorosis, left thigh
        M85.159   Skeletal fluorosis, unspecified thigh

√6ᵗʰ M85.16   Skeletal fluorosis, lower leg
        M85.161   Skeletal fluorosis, right lower leg
        M85.162   Skeletal fluorosis, left lower leg
        M85.169   Skeletal fluorosis, unspecified lower leg

√6ᵗʰ M85.17   Skeletal fluorosis, ankle and foot
        M85.171   Skeletal fluorosis, right ankle and foot
        M85.172   Skeletal fluorosis, left ankle and foot
        M85.179   Skeletal fluorosis, unspecified ankle and foot

   M85.18   Skeletal fluorosis, other site
   M85.19   Skeletal fluorosis, multiple sites

M85.2   **Hyperostosis of skull**
    DEF: Abnormal bone growth on the inner aspect of the cranial bones.

√5ᵗʰ M85.3   **Osteitis condensans**

   M85.30   Osteitis condensans, unspecified site
√6ᵗʰ M85.31   Osteitis condensans, shoulder
        M85.311   Osteitis condensans, right shoulder
        M85.312   Osteitis condensans, left shoulder
        M85.319   Osteitis condensans, unspecified shoulder

√6ᵗʰ M85.32   Osteitis condensans, upper arm
        M85.321   Osteitis condensans, right upper arm
        M85.322   Osteitis condensans, left upper arm
        M85.329   Osteitis condensans, unspecified upper arm

√6ᵗʰ M85.33   Osteitis condensans, forearm
        M85.331   Osteitis condensans, right forearm
        M85.332   Osteitis condensans, left forearm
        M85.339   Osteitis condensans, unspecified forearm

√6ᵗʰ M85.34   Osteitis condensans, hand
        M85.341   Osteitis condensans, right hand
        M85.342   Osteitis condensans, left hand
        M85.349   Osteitis condensans, unspecified hand

√6ᵗʰ M85.35   Osteitis condensans, thigh
        M85.351   Osteitis condensans, right thigh
        M85.352   Osteitis condensans, left thigh
        M85.359   Osteitis condensans, unspecified thigh

√6ᵗʰ M85.36   Osteitis condensans, lower leg
        M85.361   Osteitis condensans, right lower leg
        M85.362   Osteitis condensans, left lower leg
        M85.369   Osteitis condensans, unspecified lower leg

√6ᵗʰ M85.37   Osteitis condensans, ankle and foot
        M85.371   Osteitis condensans, right ankle and foot
        M85.372   Osteitis condensans, left ankle and foot
        M85.379   Osteitis condensans, unspecified ankle and foot

   M85.38   Osteitis condensans, other site
   M85.39   Osteitis condensans, multiple sites

√5ᵗʰ M85.4   **Solitary bone cyst**
    EXCLUDES 2   solitary cyst of jaw (M27.4)

   M85.40   Solitary bone cyst, unspecified site
√6ᵗʰ M85.41   Solitary bone cyst, shoulder
        M85.411   Solitary bone cyst, right shoulder
        M85.412   Solitary bone cyst, left shoulder
        M85.419   Solitary bone cyst, unspecified shoulder

√6ᵗʰ M85.42   Solitary bone cyst, humerus
        M85.421   Solitary bone cyst, right humerus
        M85.422   Solitary bone cyst, left humerus
        M85.429   Solitary bone cyst, unspecified humerus

√6ᵗʰ M85.43   Solitary bone cyst, ulna and radius
        M85.431   Solitary bone cyst, right ulna and radius
        M85.432   Solitary bone cyst, left ulna and radius
        M85.439   Solitary bone cyst, unspecified ulna and radius

√6ᵗʰ M85.44   Solitary bone cyst, hand
        M85.441   Solitary bone cyst, right hand
        M85.442   Solitary bone cyst, left hand
        M85.449   Solitary bone cyst, unspecified hand

√6ᵗʰ M85.45   Solitary bone cyst, pelvis
        M85.451   Solitary bone cyst, right pelvis
        M85.452   Solitary bone cyst, left pelvis
        M85.459   Solitary bone cyst, unspecified pelvis

√6ᵗʰ M85.46   Solitary bone cyst, tibia and fibula
        M85.461   Solitary bone cyst, right tibia and fibula
        M85.462   Solitary bone cyst, left tibia and fibula
        M85.469   Solitary bone cyst, unspecified tibia and fibula

√6ᵗʰ M85.47   Solitary bone cyst, ankle and foot
        M85.471   Solitary bone cyst, right ankle and foot
        M85.472   Solitary bone cyst, left ankle and foot
        M85.479   Solitary bone cyst, unspecified ankle and foot

   M85.48   Solitary bone cyst, other site

√5ᵗʰ M85.5   **Aneurysmal bone cyst**
    EXCLUDES 2   aneurysmal cyst of jaw (M27.4)
    DEF: Solitary bone lesion that bulges into the periosteum and is marked by a calcified rim.

   M85.50   Aneurysmal bone cyst, unspecified site
√6ᵗʰ M85.51   Aneurysmal bone cyst, shoulder
        M85.511   Aneurysmal bone cyst, right shoulder
        M85.512   Aneurysmal bone cyst, left shoulder
        M85.519   Aneurysmal bone cyst, unspecified shoulder

√6ᵗʰ M85.52   Aneurysmal bone cyst, upper arm
        M85.521   Aneurysmal bone cyst, right upper arm
        M85.522   Aneurysmal bone cyst, left upper arm
        M85.529   Aneurysmal bone cyst, unspecified upper arm

√6ᵗʰ M85.53   Aneurysmal bone cyst, forearm
        M85.531   Aneurysmal bone cyst, right forearm
        M85.532   Aneurysmal bone cyst, left forearm
        M85.539   Aneurysmal bone cyst, unspecified forearm

√6ᵗʰ M85.54   Aneurysmal bone cyst, hand
        M85.541   Aneurysmal bone cyst, right hand
        M85.542   Aneurysmal bone cyst, left hand
        M85.549   Aneurysmal bone cyst, unspecified hand

√6ᵗʰ M85.55   Aneurysmal bone cyst, thigh
        M85.551   Aneurysmal bone cyst, right thigh
        M85.552   Aneurysmal bone cyst, left thigh
        M85.559   Aneurysmal bone cyst, unspecified thigh

√6ᵗʰ M85.56   Aneurysmal bone cyst, lower leg
        M85.561   Aneurysmal bone cyst, right lower leg
        M85.562   Aneurysmal bone cyst, left lower leg
        M85.569   Aneurysmal bone cyst, unspecified lower leg

√6ᵗʰ M85.57   Aneurysmal bone cyst, ankle and foot
        M85.571   Aneurysmal bone cyst, right ankle and foot
        M85.572   Aneurysmal bone cyst, left ankle and foot
        M85.579   Aneurysmal bone cyst, unspecified ankle and foot

   M85.58   Aneurysmal bone cyst, other site
   M85.59   Aneurysmal bone cyst, multiple sites

√5ᵗʰ M85.6   **Other cyst of bone**
    EXCLUDES 1   cyst of jaw NEC (M27.4)
         osteitis fibrosa cystica generalisata [von Recklinghausen's disease of bone] (E21.0)

   M85.60   Other cyst of bone, unspecified site
√6ᵗʰ M85.61   Other cyst of bone, shoulder
        M85.611   Other cyst of bone, right shoulder
        M85.612   Other cyst of bone, left shoulder
        M85.619   Other cyst of bone, unspecified shoulder

√6ᵗʰ M85.62   Other cyst of bone, upper arm
        M85.621   Other cyst of bone, right upper arm
        M85.622   Other cyst of bone, left upper arm
        M85.629   Other cyst of bone, unspecified upper arm

√6ᵗʰ M85.63   Other cyst of bone, forearm
        M85.631   Other cyst of bone, right forearm
        M85.632   Other cyst of bone, left forearm
        M85.639   Other cyst of bone, unspecified forearm

√6ᵗʰ M85.64   Other cyst of bone, hand
        M85.641   Other cyst of bone, right hand
        M85.642   Other cyst of bone, left hand
        M85.649   Other cyst of bone, unspecified hand

√6ᵗʰ M85.65   Other cyst of bone, thigh
        M85.651   Other cyst of bone, right thigh
        M85.652   Other cyst of bone, left thigh

Ⓝ Newborn: 0   Ⓟ Pediatric: 0-17   Ⓜ Maternity: 12-55   Ⓐ Adult: 15-124   CH Comorbidity High   CL Comorbidity Low   NCDx Noncancer Dx   PDx Primary Dx

M85.659 Other cyst of bone, unspecified thigh

✓6ᵗʰ **M85.66** Other cyst of bone, lower leg

    M85.661 Other cyst of bone, right lower leg

    M85.662 Other cyst of bone, left lower leg

    M85.669 Other cyst of bone, unspecified lower leg

✓6ᵗʰ **M85.67** Other cyst of bone, ankle and foot

    M85.671 Other cyst of bone, right ankle and foot

    M85.672 Other cyst of bone, left ankle and foot

    M85.679 Other cyst of bone, unspecified ankle and foot

    M85.68 Other cyst of bone, other site

    M85.69 Other cyst of bone, multiple sites

✓5ᵗʰ **M85.8** Other specified disorders of bone density and structure

    Hyperostosis of bones, except skull

    Osteosclerosis, acquired

    EXCLUDES 1 *diffuse idiopathic skeletal hyperostosis [DISH] (M48.1)*
        osteosclerosis congenita (Q77.4)
        osteosclerosis fragilitas (generalista) (Q78.2)
        osteosclerosis myelofibrosis (D75.81)

    M85.80 Other specified disorders of bone density and structure, unspecified site

✓6ᵗʰ **M85.81** Other specified disorders of bone density and structure, shoulder

    M85.811 Other specified disorders of bone density and structure, right shoulder

    M85.812 Other specified disorders of bone density and structure, left shoulder

    M85.819 Other specified disorders of bone density and structure, unspecified shoulder

✓6ᵗʰ **M85.82** Other specified disorders of bone density and structure, upper arm

    M85.821 Other specified disorders of bone density and structure, right upper arm

    M85.822 Other specified disorders of bone density and structure, left upper arm

    M85.829 Other specified disorders of bone density and structure, unspecified upper arm

✓6ᵗʰ **M85.83** Other specified disorders of bone density and structure, forearm

    M85.831 Other specified disorders of bone density and structure, right forearm

    M85.832 Other specified disorders of bone density and structure, left forearm

    M85.839 Other specified disorders of bone density and structure, unspecified forearm

✓6ᵗʰ **M85.84** Other specified disorders of bone density and structure, hand

    M85.841 Other specified disorders of bone density and structure, right hand

    M85.842 Other specified disorders of bone density and structure, left hand

    M85.849 Other specified disorders of bone density and structure, unspecified hand

✓6ᵗʰ **M85.85** Other specified disorders of bone density and structure, thigh

    M85.851 Other specified disorders of bone density and structure, right thigh

    M85.852 Other specified disorders of bone density and structure, left thigh

    M85.859 Other specified disorders of bone density and structure, unspecified thigh

✓6ᵗʰ **M85.86** Other specified disorders of bone density and structure, lower leg

    M85.861 Other specified disorders of bone density and structure, right lower leg

    M85.862 Other specified disorders of bone density and structure, left lower leg

    M85.869 Other specified disorders of bone density and structure, unspecified lower leg

✓6ᵗʰ **M85.87** Other specified disorders of bone density and structure, ankle and foot

    M85.871 Other specified disorders of bone density and structure, right ankle and foot

    M85.872 Other specified disorders of bone density and structure, left ankle and foot

    M85.879 Other specified disorders of bone density and structure, unspecified ankle and foot

    M85.88 Other specified disorders of bone density and structure, other site

    M85.89 Other specified disorders of bone density and structure, multiple sites

M85.9 Disorder of bone density and structure, unspecified

Other osteopathies (M86-M90)

EXCLUDES 1 *postprocedural osteopathies (M96.-)*

✓4ᵗʰ **M86 Osteomyelitis**

    Use additional code (B95-B97) to identify infectious agent

    Use additional code to identify major osseous defect, if applicable (M89.7-)

    EXCLUDES 1 *osteomyelitis due to:*
        echinococcus (B67.2)
        gonococcus (A54.43)
        salmonella (A02.24)

    EXCLUDES 2 *ostemyelitis of:*
        orbit (H05.0-)
        petrous bone (H70.2-)
        vertebra (M46.2-)

✓5ᵗʰ **M86.0** Acute hematogenous osteomyelitis

    M86.00 Acute hematogenous osteomyelitis, unspecified site

✓6ᵗʰ **M86.01** Acute hematogenous osteomyelitis, shoulder

    M86.011 Acute hematogenous osteomyelitis, right shoulder

    M86.012 Acute hematogenous osteomyelitis, left shoulder

    M86.019 Acute hematogenous osteomyelitis, unspecified shoulder

✓6ᵗʰ **M86.02** Acute hematogenous osteomyelitis, humerus

    M86.021 Acute hematogenous osteomyelitis, right humerus

    M86.022 Acute hematogenous osteomyelitis, left humerus

    M86.029 Acute hematogenous osteomyelitis, unspecified humerus

✓6ᵗʰ **M86.03** Acute hematogenous osteomyelitis, radius and ulna

    M86.031 Acute hematogenous osteomyelitis, right radius and ulna

    M86.032 Acute hematogenous osteomyelitis, left radius and ulna

    M86.039 Acute hematogenous osteomyelitis, unspecified radius and ulna

✓6ᵗʰ **M86.04** Acute hematogenous osteomyelitis, hand

    M86.041 Acute hematogenous osteomyelitis, right hand

    M86.042 Acute hematogenous osteomyelitis, left hand

    M86.049 Acute hematogenous osteomyelitis, unspecified hand

✓6ᵗʰ **M86.05** Acute hematogenous osteomyelitis, femur

    M86.051 Acute hematogenous osteomyelitis, right femur

    M86.052 Acute hematogenous osteomyelitis, left femur

    M86.059 Acute hematogenous osteomyelitis, unspecified femur

✓6ᵗʰ **M86.06** Acute hematogenous osteomyelitis, tibia and fibula

    M86.061 Acute hematogenous osteomyelitis, right tibia and fibula

    M86.062 Acute hematogenous osteomyelitis, left tibia and fibula

    M86.069 Acute hematogenous osteomyelitis, unspecified tibia and fibula

✓6ᵗʰ **M86.07** Acute hematogenous osteomyelitis, ankle and foot

    M86.071 Acute hematogenous osteomyelitis, right ankle and foot

    M86.072 Acute hematogenous osteomyelitis, left ankle and foot

    M86.079 Acute hematogenous osteomyelitis, unspecified ankle and foot

    M86.08 Acute hematogenous osteomyelitis, other sites

    M86.09 Acute hematogenous osteomyelitis, multiple sites

✓5ᵗʰ **M86.1** Other acute osteomyelitis

    M86.10 Other acute osteomyelitis, unspecified site

✓6ᵗʰ **M86.11** Other acute osteomyelitis, shoulder

    M86.111 Other acute osteomyelitis, right shoulder

    M86.112 Other acute osteomyelitis, left shoulder

    M86.119 Other acute osteomyelitis, unspecified shoulder

☑ Additional Character Required   ✓x7ᵗʰ Placeholder Alert   Manifestation   Unspecified Dx   ►◄ Revised Text   ● New Code   ▲ Revised Title

ICD-10-CM 2020   807

✓6ᵗʰ **M86.12 Other acute osteomyelitis, humerus**
    M86.121 Other acute osteomyelitis, right humerus
    M86.122 Other acute osteomyelitis, left humerus
    M86.129 Other acute osteomyelitis, unspecified humerus

✓6ᵗʰ **M86.13 Other acute osteomyelitis, radius and ulna**
    M86.131 Other acute osteomyelitis, right radius and ulna
    M86.132 Other acute osteomyelitis, left radius and ulna
    M86.139 Other acute osteomyelitis, unspecified radius and ulna

✓6ᵗʰ **M86.14 Other acute osteomyelitis, hand**
    M86.141 Other acute osteomyelitis, right hand
    M86.142 Other acute osteomyelitis, left hand
    M86.149 Other acute osteomyelitis, unspecified hand

✓6ᵗʰ **M86.15 Other acute osteomyelitis, femur**
    M86.151 Other acute osteomyelitis, right femur
    M86.152 Other acute osteomyelitis, left femur
    M86.159 Other acute osteomyelitis, unspecified femur

✓6ᵗʰ **M86.16 Other acute osteomyelitis, tibia and fibula**
    M86.161 Other acute osteomyelitis, right tibia and fibula
    M86.162 Other acute osteomyelitis, left tibia and fibula
    M86.169 Other acute osteomyelitis, unspecified tibia and fibula

✓6ᵗʰ **M86.17 Other acute osteomyelitis, ankle and foot**
    M86.171 Other acute osteomyelitis, right ankle and foot
    M86.172 Other acute osteomyelitis, left ankle and foot
    M86.179 Other acute osteomyelitis, unspecified ankle and foot

M86.18 Other acute osteomyelitis, other site
M86.19 Other acute osteomyelitis, multiple sites

✓5ᵗʰ **M86.2 Subacute osteomyelitis**
    M86.20 Subacute osteomyelitis, unspecified site

✓6ᵗʰ **M86.21 Subacute osteomyelitis, shoulder**
    M86.211 Subacute osteomyelitis, right shoulder
    M86.212 Subacute osteomyelitis, left shoulder
    M86.219 Subacute osteomyelitis, unspecified shoulder

✓6ᵗʰ **M86.22 Subacute osteomyelitis, humerus**
    M86.221 Subacute osteomyelitis, right humerus
    M86.222 Subacute osteomyelitis, left humerus
    M86.229 Subacute osteomyelitis, unspecified humerus

✓6ᵗʰ **M86.23 Subacute osteomyelitis, radius and ulna**
    M86.231 Subacute osteomyelitis, right radius and ulna
    M86.232 Subacute osteomyelitis, left radius and ulna
    M86.239 Subacute osteomyelitis, unspecified radius and ulna

✓6ᵗʰ **M86.24 Subacute osteomyelitis, hand**
    M86.241 Subacute osteomyelitis, right hand
    M86.242 Subacute osteomyelitis, left hand
    M86.249 Subacute osteomyelitis, unspecified hand

✓6ᵗʰ **M86.25 Subacute osteomyelitis, femur**
    M86.251 Subacute osteomyelitis, right femur
    M86.252 Subacute osteomyelitis, left femur
    M86.259 Subacute osteomyelitis, unspecified femur

✓6ᵗʰ **M86.26 Subacute osteomyelitis, tibia and fibula**
    M86.261 Subacute osteomyelitis, right tibia and fibula
    M86.262 Subacute osteomyelitis, left tibia and fibula
    M86.269 Subacute osteomyelitis, unspecified tibia and fibula

✓6ᵗʰ **M86.27 Subacute osteomyelitis, ankle and foot**
    M86.271 Subacute osteomyelitis, right ankle and foot
    M86.272 Subacute osteomyelitis, left ankle and foot
    M86.279 Subacute osteomyelitis, unspecified ankle and foot

M86.28 Subacute osteomyelitis, other site
M86.29 Subacute osteomyelitis, multiple sites

✓5ᵗʰ **M86.3 Chronic multifocal osteomyelitis**
    M86.30 Chronic multifocal osteomyelitis, unspecified site

✓6ᵗʰ **M86.31 Chronic multifocal osteomyelitis, shoulder**
    M86.311 Chronic multifocal osteomyelitis, right shoulder
    M86.312 Chronic multifocal osteomyelitis, left shoulder
    M86.319 Chronic multifocal osteomyelitis, unspecified shoulder

✓6ᵗʰ **M86.32 Chronic multifocal osteomyelitis, humerus**
    M86.321 Chronic multifocal osteomyelitis, right humerus
    M86.322 Chronic multifocal osteomyelitis, left humerus
    M86.329 Chronic multifocal osteomyelitis, unspecified humerus

✓6ᵗʰ **M86.33 Chronic multifocal osteomyelitis, radius and ulna**
    M86.331 Chronic multifocal osteomyelitis, right radius and ulna
    M86.332 Chronic multifocal osteomyelitis, left radius and ulna
    M86.339 Chronic multifocal osteomyelitis, unspecified radius and ulna

✓6ᵗʰ **M86.34 Chronic multifocal osteomyelitis, hand**
    M86.341 Chronic multifocal osteomyelitis, right hand
    M86.342 Chronic multifocal osteomyelitis, left hand
    M86.349 Chronic multifocal osteomyelitis, unspecified hand

✓6ᵗʰ **M86.35 Chronic multifocal osteomyelitis, femur**
    M86.351 Chronic multifocal osteomyelitis, right femur
    M86.352 Chronic multifocal osteomyelitis, left femur
    M86.359 Chronic multifocal osteomyelitis, unspecified femur

✓6ᵗʰ **M86.36 Chronic multifocal osteomyelitis, tibia and fibula**
    M86.361 Chronic multifocal osteomyelitis, right tibia and fibula
    M86.362 Chronic multifocal osteomyelitis, left tibia and fibula
    M86.369 Chronic multifocal osteomyelitis, unspecified tibia and fibula

✓6ᵗʰ **M86.37 Chronic multifocal osteomyelitis, ankle and foot**
    M86.371 Chronic multifocal osteomyelitis, right ankle and foot
    M86.372 Chronic multifocal osteomyelitis, left ankle and foot
    M86.379 Chronic multifocal osteomyelitis, unspecified ankle and foot

M86.38 Chronic multifocal osteomyelitis, other site
M86.39 Chronic multifocal osteomyelitis, multiple sites

✓5ᵗʰ **M86.4 Chronic osteomyelitis with draining sinus**
    M86.40 Chronic osteomyelitis with draining sinus, unspecified site

✓6ᵗʰ **M86.41 Chronic osteomyelitis with draining sinus, shoulder**
    M86.411 Chronic osteomyelitis with draining sinus, right shoulder
    M86.412 Chronic osteomyelitis with draining sinus, left shoulder
    M86.419 Chronic osteomyelitis with draining sinus, unspecified shoulder

✓6ᵗʰ **M86.42 Chronic osteomyelitis with draining sinus, humerus**
    M86.421 Chronic osteomyelitis with draining sinus, right humerus
    M86.422 Chronic osteomyelitis with draining sinus, left humerus
    M86.429 Chronic osteomyelitis with draining sinus, unspecified humerus

✓6ᵗʰ **M86.43 Chronic osteomyelitis with draining sinus, radius and ulna**
    M86.431 Chronic osteomyelitis with draining sinus, right radius and ulna
    M86.432 Chronic osteomyelitis with draining sinus, left radius and ulna

M86.439 Chronic osteomyelitis with draining sinus, unspecified radius and ulna

✓6ᵗʰ **M86.44** Chronic osteomyelitis with draining sinus, hand
- **M86.441** Chronic osteomyelitis with draining sinus, right hand
- **M86.442** Chronic osteomyelitis with draining sinus, left hand
- **M86.449** Chronic osteomyelitis with draining sinus, unspecified hand

✓6ᵗʰ **M86.45** Chronic osteomyelitis with draining sinus, femur
- **M86.451** Chronic osteomyelitis with draining sinus, right femur
- **M86.452** Chronic osteomyelitis with draining sinus, left femur
- **M86.459** Chronic osteomyelitis with draining sinus, unspecified femur

✓6ᵗʰ **M86.46** Chronic osteomyelitis with draining sinus, tibia and fibula
- **M86.461** Chronic osteomyelitis with draining sinus, right tibia and fibula
- **M86.462** Chronic osteomyelitis with draining sinus, left tibia and fibula
- **M86.469** Chronic osteomyelitis with draining sinus, unspecified tibia and fibula

✓6ᵗʰ **M86.47** Chronic osteomyelitis with draining sinus, ankle and foot
- **M86.471** Chronic osteomyelitis with draining sinus, right ankle and foot
- **M86.472** Chronic osteomyelitis with draining sinus, left ankle and foot
- **M86.479** Chronic osteomyelitis with draining sinus, unspecified ankle and foot

M86.48 Chronic osteomyelitis with draining sinus, other site

M86.49 Chronic osteomyelitis with draining sinus, multiple sites

✓5ᵗʰ **M86.5** Other chronic hematogenous osteomyelitis
- **M86.50** Other chronic hematogenous osteomyelitis, unspecified site
- ✓6ᵗʰ **M86.51** Other chronic hematogenous osteomyelitis, shoulder
  - **M86.511** Other chronic hematogenous osteomyelitis, right shoulder
  - **M86.512** Other chronic hematogenous osteomyelitis, left shoulder
  - **M86.519** Other chronic hematogenous osteomyelitis, unspecified shoulder
- ✓6ᵗʰ **M86.52** Other chronic hematogenous osteomyelitis, humerus
  - **M86.521** Other chronic hematogenous osteomyelitis, right humerus
  - **M86.522** Other chronic hematogenous osteomyelitis, left humerus
  - **M86.529** Other chronic hematogenous osteomyelitis, unspecified humerus
- ✓6ᵗʰ **M86.53** Other chronic hematogenous osteomyelitis, radius and ulna
  - **M86.531** Other chronic hematogenous osteomyelitis, right radius and ulna
  - **M86.532** Other chronic hematogenous osteomyelitis, left radius and ulna
  - **M86.539** Other chronic hematogenous osteomyelitis, unspecified radius and ulna
- ✓6ᵗʰ **M86.54** Other chronic hematogenous osteomyelitis, hand
  - **M86.541** Other chronic hematogenous osteomyelitis, right hand
  - **M86.542** Other chronic hematogenous osteomyelitis, left hand
  - **M86.549** Other chronic hematogenous osteomyelitis, unspecified hand
- ✓6ᵗʰ **M86.55** Other chronic hematogenous osteomyelitis, femur
  - **M86.551** Other chronic hematogenous osteomyelitis, right femur
  - **M86.552** Other chronic hematogenous osteomyelitis, left femur
  - **M86.559** Other chronic hematogenous osteomyelitis, unspecified femur
- ✓6ᵗʰ **M86.56** Other chronic hematogenous osteomyelitis, tibia and fibula
  - **M86.561** Other chronic hematogenous osteomyelitis, right tibia and fibula
  - **M86.562** Other chronic hematogenous osteomyelitis, left tibia and fibula
  - **M86.569** Other chronic hematogenous osteomyelitis, unspecified tibia and fibula
- ✓6ᵗʰ **M86.57** Other chronic hematogenous osteomyelitis, ankle and foot
  - **M86.571** Other chronic hematogenous osteomyelitis, right ankle and foot
  - **M86.572** Other chronic hematogenous osteomyelitis, left ankle and foot
  - **M86.579** Other chronic hematogenous osteomyelitis, unspecified ankle and foot
- **M86.58** Other chronic hematogenous osteomyelitis, other site
- **M86.59** Other chronic hematogenous osteomyelitis, multiple sites

✓5ᵗʰ **M86.6** Other chronic osteomyelitis
- **M86.60** Other chronic osteomyelitis, unspecified site
- ✓6ᵗʰ **M86.61** Other chronic osteomyelitis, shoulder
  - **M86.611** Other chronic osteomyelitis, right shoulder
  - **M86.612** Other chronic osteomyelitis, left shoulder
  - **M86.619** Other chronic osteomyelitis, unspecified shoulder
- ✓6ᵗʰ **M86.62** Other chronic osteomyelitis, humerus
  - **M86.621** Other chronic osteomyelitis, right humerus
  - **M86.622** Other chronic osteomyelitis, left humerus
  - **M86.629** Other chronic osteomyelitis, unspecified humerus
- ✓6ᵗʰ **M86.63** Other chronic osteomyelitis, radius and ulna
  - **M86.631** Other chronic osteomyelitis, right radius and ulna
  - **M86.632** Other chronic osteomyelitis, left radius and ulna
  - **M86.639** Other chronic osteomyelitis, unspecified radius and ulna
- ✓6ᵗʰ **M86.64** Other chronic osteomyelitis, hand
  - **M86.641** Other chronic osteomyelitis, right hand
  - **M86.642** Other chronic osteomyelitis, left hand
  - **M86.649** Other chronic osteomyelitis, unspecified hand
- ✓6ᵗʰ **M86.65** Other chronic osteomyelitis, thigh
  - **M86.651** Other chronic osteomyelitis, right thigh
  - **M86.652** Other chronic osteomyelitis, left thigh
  - **M86.659** Other chronic osteomyelitis, unspecified thigh
- ✓6ᵗʰ **M86.66** Other chronic osteomyelitis, tibia and fibula
  - **M86.661** Other chronic osteomyelitis, right tibia and fibula
  - **M86.662** Other chronic osteomyelitis, left tibia and fibula
  - **M86.669** Other chronic osteomyelitis, unspecified tibia and fibula
- ✓6ᵗʰ **M86.67** Other chronic osteomyelitis, ankle and foot
  - **M86.671** Other chronic osteomyelitis, right ankle and foot
    - AHA: 2016,1Q,13
  - **M86.672** Other chronic osteomyelitis, left ankle and foot
  - **M86.679** Other chronic osteomyelitis, unspecified ankle and foot
- **M86.68** Other chronic osteomyelitis, other site
- **M86.69** Other chronic osteomyelitis, multiple sites

✓5ᵗʰ **M86.8** Other osteomyelitis
- Brodie's abscess
- ✓6ᵗʰ **M86.8X** Other osteomyelitis
  - **M86.8X0** Other osteomyelitis, multiple sites
  - **M86.8X1** Other osteomyelitis, shoulder
  - **M86.8X2** Other osteomyelitis, upper arm
  - **M86.8X3** Other osteomyelitis, forearm
  - **M86.8X4** Other osteomyelitis, hand
  - **M86.8X5** Other osteomyelitis, thigh
  - **M86.8X6** Other osteomyelitis, lower leg
  - **M86.8X7** Other osteomyelitis, ankle and foot
  - **M86.8X8** Other osteomyelitis, other site
  - **M86.8X9** Other osteomyelitis, unspecified sites

☑ Additional Character Required   ✓✗7ᵗʰ Placeholder Alert   Manifestation   Unspecified Dx   ▶◀ Revised Text   ● New Code   ▲ Revised Title

ICD-10-CM 2020   **809**

M86.9 **Osteomyelitis, unspecified**
Infection of bone NOS
Periostitis without osteomyelitis

✓4ᵗʰ M87 **Osteonecrosis**

    INCLUDES   avascular necrosis of bone
    Use additional code to identify major osseous defect, if applicable (M89.7-)
    EXCLUDES 1   juvenile osteonecrosis (M91-M92)
             osteochondropathies (M90-M93)

✓5ᵗʰ M87.0 **Idiopathic aseptic necrosis of bone**

    M87.00 **Idiopathic aseptic necrosis of unspecified bone**

    ✓6ᵗʰ M87.01 **Idiopathic aseptic necrosis of shoulder**
        Idiopathic aseptic necrosis of clavicle and scapula
        M87.011 **Idiopathic aseptic necrosis of right shoulder**
        M87.012 **Idiopathic aseptic necrosis of left shoulder**
        M87.019 **Idiopathic aseptic necrosis of unspecified shoulder**

    ✓6ᵗʰ M87.02 **Idiopathic aseptic necrosis of humerus**
        M87.021 **Idiopathic aseptic necrosis of right humerus**
        M87.022 **Idiopathic aseptic necrosis of left humerus**
        M87.029 **Idiopathic aseptic necrosis of unspecified humerus**

    ✓6ᵗʰ M87.03 **Idiopathic aseptic necrosis of radius, ulna and carpus**
        M87.031 **Idiopathic aseptic necrosis of right radius**
        M87.032 **Idiopathic aseptic necrosis of left radius**
        M87.033 **Idiopathic aseptic necrosis of unspecified radius**
        M87.034 **Idiopathic aseptic necrosis of right ulna**
        M87.035 **Idiopathic aseptic necrosis of left ulna**
        M87.036 **Idiopathic aseptic necrosis of unspecified ulna**
        M87.037 **Idiopathic aseptic necrosis of right carpus**
        M87.038 **Idiopathic aseptic necrosis of left carpus**
        M87.039 **Idiopathic aseptic necrosis of unspecified carpus**

    ✓6ᵗʰ M87.04 **Idiopathic aseptic necrosis of hand and fingers**
        Idiopathic aseptic necrosis of metacarpals and phalanges of hands
        M87.041 **Idiopathic aseptic necrosis of right hand**
        M87.042 **Idiopathic aseptic necrosis of left hand**
        M87.043 **Idiopathic aseptic necrosis of unspecified hand**
        M87.044 **Idiopathic aseptic necrosis of right finger(s)**
        M87.045 **Idiopathic aseptic necrosis of left finger(s)**
        M87.046 **Idiopathic aseptic necrosis of unspecified finger(s)**

    ✓6ᵗʰ M87.05 **Idiopathic aseptic necrosis of pelvis and femur**
        M87.050 **Idiopathic aseptic necrosis of pelvis**
        M87.051 **Idiopathic aseptic necrosis of right femur**
        M87.052 **Idiopathic aseptic necrosis of left femur**
        M87.059 **Idiopathic aseptic necrosis of unspecified femur**

    ✓6ᵗʰ M87.06 **Idiopathic aseptic necrosis of tibia and fibula**
        M87.061 **Idiopathic aseptic necrosis of right tibia**
        M87.062 **Idiopathic aseptic necrosis of left tibia**
        M87.063 **Idiopathic aseptic necrosis of unspecified tibia**
        M87.064 **Idiopathic aseptic necrosis of right fibula**
        M87.065 **Idiopathic aseptic necrosis of left fibula**
        M87.066 **Idiopathic aseptic necrosis of unspecified fibula**

    ✓6ᵗʰ M87.07 **Idiopathic aseptic necrosis of ankle, foot and toes**
        Idiopathic aseptic necrosis of metatarsus, tarsus, and phalanges of toes
        M87.071 **Idiopathic aseptic necrosis of right ankle**
        M87.072 **Idiopathic aseptic necrosis of left ankle**
        M87.073 **Idiopathic aseptic necrosis of unspecified ankle**
        M87.074 **Idiopathic aseptic necrosis of right foot**
        M87.075 **Idiopathic aseptic necrosis of left foot**
        M87.076 **Idiopathic aseptic necrosis of unspecified foot**
        M87.077 **Idiopathic aseptic necrosis of right toe(s)**
        M87.078 **Idiopathic aseptic necrosis of left toe(s)**
        M87.079 **Idiopathic aseptic necrosis of unspecified toe(s)**

    M87.08 **Idiopathic aseptic necrosis of bone, other site**
    M87.09 **Idiopathic aseptic necrosis of bone, multiple sites**

✓5ᵗʰ M87.1 **Osteonecrosis due to drugs**
    Use additional code for adverse effect, if applicable, to identify drug (T36-T50 with fifth or sixth character 5)

    M87.10 **Osteonecrosis due to drugs, unspecified bone**

    ✓6ᵗʰ M87.11 **Osteonecrosis due to drugs, shoulder**
        M87.111 **Osteonecrosis due to drugs, right shoulder**
        M87.112 **Osteonecrosis due to drugs, left shoulder**
        M87.119 **Osteonecrosis due to drugs, unspecified shoulder**

    ✓6ᵗʰ M87.12 **Osteonecrosis due to drugs, humerus**
        M87.121 **Osteonecrosis due to drugs, right humerus**
        M87.122 **Osteonecrosis due to drugs, left humerus**
        M87.129 **Osteonecrosis due to drugs, unspecified humerus**

    ✓6ᵗʰ M87.13 **Osteonecrosis due to drugs of radius, ulna and carpus**
        M87.131 **Osteonecrosis due to drugs of right radius**
        M87.132 **Osteonecrosis due to drugs of left radius**
        M87.133 **Osteonecrosis due to drugs of unspecified radius**
        M87.134 **Osteonecrosis due to drugs of right ulna**
        M87.135 **Osteonecrosis due to drugs of left ulna**
        M87.136 **Osteonecrosis due to drugs of unspecified ulna**
        M87.137 **Osteonecrosis due to drugs of right carpus**
        M87.138 **Osteonecrosis due to drugs of left carpus**
        M87.139 **Osteonecrosis due to drugs of unspecified carpus**

    ✓6ᵗʰ M87.14 **Osteonecrosis due to drugs, hand and fingers**
        M87.141 **Osteonecrosis due to drugs, right hand**
        M87.142 **Osteonecrosis due to drugs, left hand**
        M87.143 **Osteonecrosis due to drugs, unspecified hand**
        M87.144 **Osteonecrosis due to drugs, right finger(s)**
        M87.145 **Osteonecrosis due to drugs, left finger(s)**
        M87.146 **Osteonecrosis due to drugs, unspecified finger(s)**

    ✓6ᵗʰ M87.15 **Osteonecrosis due to drugs, pelvis and femur**
        M87.150 **Osteonecrosis due to drugs, pelvis**
        M87.151 **Osteonecrosis due to drugs, right femur**
        M87.152 **Osteonecrosis due to drugs, left femur**
        M87.159 **Osteonecrosis due to drugs, unspecified femur**

    ✓6ᵗʰ M87.16 **Osteonecrosis due to drugs, tibia and fibula**
        M87.161 **Osteonecrosis due to drugs, right tibia**
        M87.162 **Osteonecrosis due to drugs, left tibia**
        M87.163 **Osteonecrosis due to drugs, unspecified tibia**
        M87.164 **Osteonecrosis due to drugs, right fibula**
        M87.165 **Osteonecrosis due to drugs, left fibula**
        M87.166 **Osteonecrosis due to drugs, unspecified fibula**

    ✓6ᵗʰ M87.17 **Osteonecrosis due to drugs, ankle, foot and toes**
        M87.171 **Osteonecrosis due to drugs, right ankle**
        M87.172 **Osteonecrosis due to drugs, left ankle**
        M87.173 **Osteonecrosis due to drugs, unspecified ankle**
        M87.174 **Osteonecrosis due to drugs, right foot**
        M87.175 **Osteonecrosis due to drugs, left foot**
        M87.176 **Osteonecrosis due to drugs, unspecified foot**
        M87.177 **Osteonecrosis due to drugs, right toe(s)**
        M87.178 **Osteonecrosis due to drugs, left toe(s)**
        M87.179 **Osteonecrosis due to drugs, unspecified toe(s)**

    ✓6ᵗʰ M87.18 **Osteonecrosis due to drugs, other site**
        M87.180 **Osteonecrosis due to drugs, jaw**
        M87.188 **Osteonecrosis due to drugs, other site**
    M87.19 **Osteonecrosis due to drugs, multiple sites**

N Newborn: 0   **P** Pediatric: 0-17   **M** Maternity: 12-55   **A** Adult: 15-124   **CH** Comorbidity High   **CL** Comorbidity Low   **NCDx** Noncancer Dx   **PDx** Primary Dx

810   ICD-10-CM 2020

✓5ᵗʰ M87.2 Osteonecrosis due to previous trauma

    M87.20 Osteonecrosis due to previous trauma, unspecified bone

    ✓6ᵗʰ M87.21 Osteonecrosis due to previous trauma, shoulder

        M87.211 Osteonecrosis due to previous trauma, right shoulder

        M87.212 Osteonecrosis due to previous trauma, left shoulder

        M87.219 Osteonecrosis due to previous trauma, unspecified shoulder

    ✓6ᵗʰ M87.22 Osteonecrosis due to previous trauma, humerus

        M87.221 Osteonecrosis due to previous trauma, right humerus

        M87.222 Osteonecrosis due to previous trauma, left humerus

        M87.229 Osteonecrosis due to previous trauma, unspecified humerus

    ✓6ᵗʰ M87.23 Osteonecrosis due to previous trauma of radius, ulna and carpus

        M87.231 Osteonecrosis due to previous trauma of right radius

        M87.232 Osteonecrosis due to previous trauma of left radius

        M87.233 Osteonecrosis due to previous trauma of unspecified radius

        M87.234 Osteonecrosis due to previous trauma of right ulna

        M87.235 Osteonecrosis due to previous trauma of left ulna

        M87.236 Osteonecrosis due to previous trauma of unspecified ulna

        M87.237 Osteonecrosis due to previous trauma of right carpus

        M87.238 Osteonecrosis due to previous trauma of left carpus

        M87.239 Osteonecrosis due to previous trauma of unspecified carpus

    ✓6ᵗʰ M87.24 Osteonecrosis due to previous trauma, hand and fingers

        M87.241 Osteonecrosis due to previous trauma, right hand

        M87.242 Osteonecrosis due to previous trauma, left hand

        M87.243 Osteonecrosis due to previous trauma, unspecified hand

        M87.244 Osteonecrosis due to previous trauma, right finger(s)

        M87.245 Osteonecrosis due to previous trauma, left finger(s)

        M87.246 Osteonecrosis due to previous trauma, unspecified finger(s)

    ✓6ᵗʰ M87.25 Osteonecrosis due to previous trauma, pelvis and femur

        M87.250 Osteonecrosis due to previous trauma, pelvis

        M87.251 Osteonecrosis due to previous trauma, right femur

        M87.252 Osteonecrosis due to previous trauma, left femur

        M87.256 Osteonecrosis due to previous trauma, unspecified femur

    ✓6ᵗʰ M87.26 Osteonecrosis due to previous trauma, tibia and fibula

        M87.261 Osteonecrosis due to previous trauma, right tibia

        M87.262 Osteonecrosis due to previous trauma, left tibia

        M87.263 Osteonecrosis due to previous trauma, unspecified tibia

        M87.264 Osteonecrosis due to previous trauma, right fibula

        M87.265 Osteonecrosis due to previous trauma, left fibula

        M87.266 Osteonecrosis due to previous trauma, unspecified fibula

    ✓6ᵗʰ M87.27 Osteonecrosis due to previous trauma, ankle, foot and toes

        M87.271 Osteonecrosis due to previous trauma, right ankle

        M87.272 Osteonecrosis due to previous trauma, left ankle

        M87.273 Osteonecrosis due to previous trauma, unspecified ankle

        M87.274 Osteonecrosis due to previous trauma, right foot

        M87.275 Osteonecrosis due to previous trauma, left foot

        M87.276 Osteonecrosis due to previous trauma, unspecified foot

        M87.277 Osteonecrosis due to previous trauma, right toe(s)

        M87.278 Osteonecrosis due to previous trauma, left toe(s)

        M87.279 Osteonecrosis due to previous trauma, unspecified toe(s)

    M87.28 Osteonecrosis due to previous trauma, other site

    M87.29 Osteonecrosis due to previous trauma, multiple sites

✓5ᵗʰ M87.3 Other secondary osteonecrosis

    M87.30 Other secondary osteonecrosis, unspecified bone

    ✓6ᵗʰ M87.31 Other secondary osteonecrosis, shoulder

        M87.311 Other secondary osteonecrosis, right shoulder

        M87.312 Other secondary osteonecrosis, left shoulder

        M87.319 Other secondary osteonecrosis, unspecified shoulder

    ✓6ᵗʰ M87.32 Other secondary osteonecrosis, humerus

        M87.321 Other secondary osteonecrosis, right humerus

        M87.322 Other secondary osteonecrosis, left humerus

        M87.329 Other secondary osteonecrosis, unspecified humerus

    ✓6ᵗʰ M87.33 Other secondary osteonecrosis of radius, ulna and carpus

        M87.331 Other secondary osteonecrosis of right radius

        M87.332 Other secondary osteonecrosis of left radius

        M87.333 Other secondary osteonecrosis of unspecified radius

        M87.334 Other secondary osteonecrosis of right ulna

        M87.335 Other secondary osteonecrosis of left ulna

        M87.336 Other secondary osteonecrosis of unspecified ulna

        M87.337 Other secondary osteonecrosis of right carpus

        M87.338 Other secondary osteonecrosis of left carpus

        M87.339 Other secondary osteonecrosis of unspecified carpus

    ✓6ᵗʰ M87.34 Other secondary osteonecrosis, hand and fingers

        M87.341 Other secondary osteonecrosis, right hand

        M87.342 Other secondary osteonecrosis, left hand

        M87.343 Other secondary osteonecrosis, unspecified hand

        M87.344 Other secondary osteonecrosis, right finger(s)

        M87.345 Other secondary osteonecrosis, left finger(s)

        M87.346 Other secondary osteonecrosis, unspecified finger(s)

    ✓6ᵗʰ M87.35 Other secondary osteonecrosis, pelvis and femur

        M87.350 Other secondary osteonecrosis, pelvis

        M87.351 Other secondary osteonecrosis, right femur

        M87.352 Other secondary osteonecrosis, left femur

        M87.353 Other secondary osteonecrosis, unspecified femur

    ✓6ᵗʰ M87.36 Other secondary osteonecrosis, tibia and fibula

        M87.361 Other secondary osteonecrosis, right tibia

        M87.362 Other secondary osteonecrosis, left tibia

        M87.363 Other secondary osteonecrosis, unspecified tibia

        M87.364 Other secondary osteonecrosis, right fibula

        M87.365 Other secondary osteonecrosis, left fibula

        M87.366 Other secondary osteonecrosis, unspecified fibula

---

✓ Additional Character Required   ✓x7ᵗʰ Placeholder Alert   Manifestation   Unspecified Dx   ►◄ Revised Text   ● New Code   ▲ Revised Title

Chapter 13. Diseases of the Musculoskeletal System and Connective Tissue

√6ᵗʰ **M87.37** **Other secondary osteonecrosis**, ankle and foot

     M87.371 **Other secondary osteonecrosis**, right ankle

     M87.372 **Other secondary osteonecrosis**, left ankle

     M87.373 **Other secondary osteonecrosis, unspecified ankle**

     M87.374 **Other secondary osteonecrosis**, right foot

     M87.375 **Other secondary osteonecrosis**, left foot

     M87.376 **Other secondary osteonecrosis, unspecified foot**

     M87.377 **Other secondary osteonecrosis**, right toe(s)

     M87.378 **Other secondary osteonecrosis**, left toe(s)

     M87.379 **Other secondary osteonecrosis, unspecified toe(s)**

  M87.38 **Other secondary osteonecrosis, other site**

  M87.39 **Other secondary osteonecrosis**, multiple sites

√5ᵗʰ **M87.8** **Other osteonecrosis**

   M87.80 **Other osteonecrosis, unspecified bone**

√6ᵗʰ **M87.81** **Other osteonecrosis**, shoulder

     M87.811 **Other osteonecrosis**, right shoulder

     M87.812 **Other osteonecrosis**, left shoulder

     M87.819 **Other osteonecrosis, unspecified shoulder**

√6ᵗʰ **M87.82** **Other osteonecrosis**, humerus

     M87.821 **Other osteonecrosis**, right humerus

     M87.822 **Other osteonecrosis**, left humerus

     M87.829 **Other osteonecrosis, unspecified humerus**

√6ᵗʰ **M87.83** **Other osteonecrosis of** radius, ulna and carpus

     M87.831 **Other osteonecrosis of** right radius

     M87.832 **Other osteonecrosis of** left radius

     M87.833 **Other osteonecrosis of unspecified radius**

     M87.834 **Other osteonecrosis of** right ulna

     M87.835 **Other osteonecrosis of** left ulna

     M87.836 **Other osteonecrosis of unspecified ulna**

     M87.837 **Other osteonecrosis of** right carpus

     M87.838 **Other osteonecrosis of** left carpus

     M87.839 **Other osteonecrosis of unspecified carpus**

√6ᵗʰ **M87.84** **Other osteonecrosis**, hand and fingers

     M87.841 **Other osteonecrosis**, right hand

     M87.842 **Other osteonecrosis**, left hand

     M87.843 **Other osteonecrosis, unspecified hand**

     M87.844 **Other osteonecrosis**, right finger(s)

     M87.845 **Other osteonecrosis**, left finger(s)

     M87.849 **Other osteonecrosis, unspecified finger(s)**

√6ᵗʰ **M87.85** **Other osteonecrosis**, pelvis and femur

     M87.850 **Other osteonecrosis**, pelvis

     M87.851 **Other osteonecrosis**, right femur

     M87.852 **Other osteonecrosis**, left femur

     M87.859 **Other osteonecrosis, unspecified femur**

√6ᵗʰ **M87.86** **Other osteonecrosis**, tibia and fibula

     M87.861 **Other osteonecrosis**, right tibia

     M87.862 **Other osteonecrosis**, left tibia

     M87.863 **Other osteonecrosis, unspecified tibia**

     M87.864 **Other osteonecrosis**, right fibula

     M87.865 **Other osteonecrosis**, left fibula

     M87.869 **Other osteonecrosis, unspecified fibula**

√6ᵗʰ **M87.87** **Other osteonecrosis**, ankle, foot and toes

     M87.871 **Other osteonecrosis**, right ankle

     M87.872 **Other osteonecrosis**, left ankle

     M87.873 **Other osteonecrosis, unspecified ankle**

     M87.874 **Other osteonecrosis**, right foot

     M87.875 **Other osteonecrosis**, left foot

     M87.876 **Other osteonecrosis, unspecified foot**

     M87.877 **Other osteonecrosis**, right toe(s)

     M87.878 **Other osteonecrosis**, left toe(s)

     M87.879 **Other osteonecrosis, unspecified toe(s)**

  M87.88 **Other osteonecrosis, other site**

  M87.89 **Other osteonecrosis**, multiple sites

M87.9 **Osteonecrosis, unspecified**

     Necrosis of bone NOS

√4ᵗʰ **M88** **Osteitis deformans [Paget's disease of bone]**

     EXCLUDES 1   *osteitis deformans in neoplastic disease (M90.6)*

     DEF: Bone disease characterized by numerous cycles of bone resorption by the body. Resorption is followed by accelerated repair attempts, causing bone deformities and bowing, with associated fractures and pain.

  M88.0 **Osteitis deformans of** skull

  M88.1 **Osteitis deformans of** vertebrae

√5ᵗʰ **M88.8** **Osteitis deformans of other bones**

√6ᵗʰ **M88.81** **Osteitis deformans of** shoulder

     M88.811 **Osteitis deformans of** right shoulder

     M88.812 **Osteitis deformans of** left shoulder

     M88.819 **Osteitis deformans of unspecified shoulder**

√6ᵗʰ **M88.82** **Osteitis deformans of** upper arm

     M88.821 **Osteitis deformans of** right upper arm

     M88.822 **Osteitis deformans of** left upper arm

     M88.829 **Osteitis deformans of unspecified upper arm**

√6ᵗʰ **M88.83** **Osteitis deformans of** forearm

     M88.831 **Osteitis deformans of** right forearm

     M88.832 **Osteitis deformans of** left forearm

     M88.839 **Osteitis deformans of unspecified forearm**

√6ᵗʰ **M88.84** **Osteitis deformans of** hand

     M88.841 **Osteitis deformans of** right hand

     M88.842 **Osteitis deformans of** left hand

     M88.849 **Osteitis deformans of unspecified hand**

√6ᵗʰ **M88.85** **Osteitis deformans of** thigh

     M88.851 **Osteitis deformans of** right thigh

     M88.852 **Osteitis deformans of** left thigh

     M88.859 **Osteitis deformans of unspecified thigh**

√6ᵗʰ **M88.86** **Osteitis deformans of** lower leg

     M88.861 **Osteitis deformans of** right lower leg

     M88.862 **Osteitis deformans of** left lower leg

     M88.869 **Osteitis deformans of unspecified lower leg**

√6ᵗʰ **M88.87** **Osteitis deformans of** ankle and foot

     M88.871 **Osteitis deformans of** right ankle and foot

     M88.872 **Osteitis deformans of** left ankle and foot

     M88.879 **Osteitis deformans of unspecified ankle and foot**

  M88.88 **Osteitis deformans of other bones**

     EXCLUDES 2   *osteitis deformans of skull (M88.0)*

             osteitis deformans of vertebrae (M88.1)

  M88.89 **Osteitis deformans of** multiple sites

M88.9 **Osteitis deformans of unspecified bone**

√4ᵗʰ **M89** **Other disorders of bone**

√5ᵗʰ **M89.0** **Algoneurodystrophy**

     Shoulder-hand syndrome

     Sudeck's atrophy

     EXCLUDES 1   *causalgia, lower limb (G57.7-)*

             causalgia, upper limb (G56.4-)

             complex regional pain syndrome II, lower limb (G57.7-)

             complex regional pain syndrome II, upper limb (G56.4-)

             reflex sympathetic dystrophy (G90.5-)

   M89.00 **Algoneurodystrophy, unspecified site**

√6ᵗʰ **M89.01** **Algoneurodystrophy**, shoulder

     M89.011 **Algoneurodystrophy**, right shoulder

     M89.012 **Algoneurodystrophy**, left shoulder

     M89.019 **Algoneurodystrophy, unspecified shoulder**

√6ᵗʰ **M89.02** **Algoneurodystrophy**, upper arm

     M89.021 **Algoneurodystrophy**, right upper arm

     M89.022 **Algoneurodystrophy**, left upper arm

     M89.029 **Algoneurodystrophy, unspecified upper arm**

√6ᵗʰ **M89.03** **Algoneurodystrophy**, forearm

     M89.031 **Algoneurodystrophy**, right forearm

     M89.032 **Algoneurodystrophy**, left forearm

     M89.039 **Algoneurodystrophy, unspecified forearm**

√6ᵗʰ **M89.04** **Algoneurodystrophy**, hand

     M89.041 **Algoneurodystrophy**, right hand

     M89.042 **Algoneurodystrophy**, left hand

N Newborn: 0   P Pediatric: 0-17   M Maternity: 12-55   A Adult: 15-124   CH Comorbidity High   CL Comorbidity Low   NCDx Noncancer Dx   PDx Primary Dx

812   ICD-10-CM 2020

M89.049   Algoneurodystrophy, unspecified hand

☑6ᵗʰ   **M89.05**   Algoneurodystrophy, thigh

    M89.051   Algoneurodystrophy, right thigh
    M89.052   Algoneurodystrophy, left thigh
    M89.059   Algoneurodystrophy, unspecified thigh

☑6ᵗʰ   **M89.06**   Algoneurodystrophy, lower leg

    M89.061   Algoneurodystrophy, right lower leg
    M89.062   Algoneurodystrophy, left lower leg
    M89.069   Algoneurodystrophy, unspecified lower leg

☑6ᵗʰ   **M89.07**   Algoneurodystrophy, ankle and foot

    M89.071   Algoneurodystrophy, right ankle and foot
    M89.072   Algoneurodystrophy, left ankle and foot
    M89.079   Algoneurodystrophy, unspecified ankle and foot

    M89.08   Algoneurodystrophy, other site
    M89.09   Algoneurodystrophy, multiple sites

☑5ᵗʰ   **M89.1**   Physeal arrest

    Arrest of growth plate
    Epiphyseal arrest
    Growth plate arrest

☑6ᵗʰ   **M89.12**   Physeal arrest, humerus

    M89.121   Complete physeal arrest, right proximal humerus
    M89.122   Complete physeal arrest, left proximal humerus
    M89.123   Partial physeal arrest, right proximal humerus
    M89.124   Partial physeal arrest, left proximal humerus
    M89.125   Complete physeal arrest, right distal humerus
    M89.126   Complete physeal arrest, left distal humerus
    M89.127   Partial physeal arrest, right distal humerus
    M89.128   Partial physeal arrest, left distal humerus
    M89.129   Physeal arrest, humerus, unspecified

☑6ᵗʰ   **M89.13**   Physeal arrest, forearm

    M89.131   Complete physeal arrest, right distal radius
    M89.132   Complete physeal arrest, left distal radius
    M89.133   Partial physeal arrest, right distal radius
    M89.134   Partial physeal arrest, left distal radius
    M89.138   Other physeal arrest of forearm
    M89.139   Physeal arrest, forearm, unspecified

☑6ᵗʰ   **M89.15**   Physeal arrest, femur

    M89.151   Complete physeal arrest, right proximal femur
    M89.152   Complete physeal arrest, left proximal femur
    M89.153   Partial physeal arrest, right proximal femur
    M89.154   Partial physeal arrest, left proximal femur
    M89.155   Complete physeal arrest, right distal femur
    M89.156   Complete physeal arrest, left distal femur
    M89.157   Partial physeal arrest, right distal femur
    M89.158   Partial physeal arrest, left distal femur
    M89.159   Physeal arrest, femur, unspecified

☑6ᵗʰ   **M89.16**   Physeal arrest, lower leg

    M89.160   Complete physeal arrest, right proximal tibia
    M89.161   Complete physeal arrest, left proximal tibia
    M89.162   Partial physeal arrest, right proximal tibia
    M89.163   Partial physeal arrest, left proximal tibia
    M89.164   Complete physeal arrest, right distal tibia
    M89.165   Complete physeal arrest, left distal tibia
    M89.166   Partial physeal arrest, right distal tibia
    M89.167   Partial physeal arrest, left distal tibia
    M89.168   Other physeal arrest of lower leg
    M89.169   Physeal arrest, lower leg, unspecified

    M89.18   Physeal arrest, other site

☑5ᵗʰ   **M89.2**   Other disorders of bone development and growth

    M89.20   Other disorders of bone development and growth, unspecified site

☑6ᵗʰ   **M89.21**   Other disorders of bone development and growth, shoulder

    M89.211   Other disorders of bone development and growth, right shoulder
    M89.212   Other disorders of bone development and growth, left shoulder
    M89.219   Other disorders of bone development and growth, unspecified shoulder

☑6ᵗʰ   **M89.22**   Other disorders of bone development and growth, humerus

    M89.221   Other disorders of bone development and growth, right humerus
    M89.222   Other disorders of bone development and growth, left humerus
    M89.229   Other disorders of bone development and growth, unspecified humerus

☑6ᵗʰ   **M89.23**   Other disorders of bone development and growth, ulna and radius

    M89.231   Other disorders of bone development and growth, right ulna
    M89.232   Other disorders of bone development and growth, left ulna
    M89.233   Other disorders of bone development and growth, right radius
    M89.234   Other disorders of bone development and growth, left radius
    M89.239   Other disorders of bone development and growth, unspecified ulna and radius

☑6ᵗʰ   **M89.24**   Other disorders of bone development and growth, hand

    M89.241   Other disorders of bone development and growth, right hand
    M89.242   Other disorders of bone development and growth, left hand
    M89.249   Other disorders of bone development and growth, unspecified hand

☑6ᵗʰ   **M89.25**   Other disorders of bone development and growth, femur

    M89.251   Other disorders of bone development and growth, right femur
    M89.252   Other disorders of bone development and growth, left femur
    M89.259   Other disorders of bone development and growth, unspecified femur

☑6ᵗʰ   **M89.26**   Other disorders of bone development and growth, tibia and fibula

    M89.261   Other disorders of bone development and growth, right tibia
    M89.262   Other disorders of bone development and growth, left tibia
    M89.263   Other disorders of bone development and growth, right fibula
    M89.264   Other disorders of bone development and growth, left fibula
    M89.269   Other disorders of bone development and growth, unspecified lower leg

☑6ᵗʰ   **M89.27**   Other disorders of bone development and growth, ankle and foot

    M89.271   Other disorders of bone development and growth, right ankle and foot
    M89.272   Other disorders of bone development and growth, left ankle and foot
    M89.279   Other disorders of bone development and growth, unspecified ankle and foot

    M89.28   Other disorders of bone development and growth, other site
    M89.29   Other disorders of bone development and growth, multiple sites

☑5ᵗʰ   **M89.3**   Hypertrophy of bone

    M89.30   Hypertrophy of bone, unspecified site

☑6ᵗʰ   **M89.31**   Hypertrophy of bone, shoulder

    M89.311   Hypertrophy of bone, right shoulder
    M89.312   Hypertrophy of bone, left shoulder
    M89.319   Hypertrophy of bone, unspecified shoulder

☑6ᵗʰ   **M89.32**   Hypertrophy of bone, humerus

    M89.321   Hypertrophy of bone, right humerus
    M89.322   Hypertrophy of bone, left humerus
    M89.329   Hypertrophy of bone, unspecified humerus

☑5ᵗʰ   **M89.33**   Hypertrophy of bone, ulna and radius

    M89.331   Hypertrophy of bone, right ulna

M89.332   Hypertrophy of bone, left ulna
M89.333   Hypertrophy of bone, right radius
M89.334   Hypertrophy of bone, left radius
M89.339   Hypertrophy of bone, unspecified ulna and radius
✓6ᵗʰ M89.34   Hypertrophy of bone, hand
M89.341   Hypertrophy of bone, right hand
M89.342   Hypertrophy of bone, left hand
M89.349   Hypertrophy of bone, unspecified hand
✓6ᵗʰ M89.35   Hypertrophy of bone, femur
M89.351   Hypertrophy of bone, right femur
M89.352   Hypertrophy of bone, left femur
M89.359   Hypertrophy of bone, unspecified femur
✓6ᵗʰ M89.36   Hypertrophy of bone, tibia and fibula
M89.361   Hypertrophy of bone, right tibia
M89.362   Hypertrophy of bone, left tibia
M89.363   Hypertrophy of bone, right fibula
M89.364   Hypertrophy of bone, left fibula
M89.369   Hypertrophy of bone, unspecified tibia and fibula
✓6ᵗʰ M89.37   Hypertrophy of bone, ankle and foot
M89.371   Hypertrophy of bone, right ankle and foot
M89.372   Hypertrophy of bone, left ankle and foot
M89.379   Hypertrophy of bone, unspecified ankle and foot
M89.38   Hypertrophy of bone, other site
M89.39   Hypertrophy of bone, multiple sites
✓5ᵗʰ M89.4   Other hypertrophic osteoarthropathy
Marie-Bamberger disease
Pachydermoperiostosis
M89.40   Other hypertrophic osteoarthropathy, unspecified site
✓6ᵗʰ M89.41   Other hypertrophic osteoarthropathy, shoulder
M89.411   Other hypertrophic osteoarthropathy, right shoulder
M89.412   Other hypertrophic osteoarthropathy, left shoulder
M89.419   Other hypertrophic osteoarthropathy, unspecified shoulder
✓6ᵗʰ M89.42   Other hypertrophic osteoarthropathy, upper arm
M89.421   Other hypertrophic osteoarthropathy, right upper arm
M89.422   Other hypertrophic osteoarthropathy, left upper arm
M89.429   Other hypertrophic osteoarthropathy, unspecified upper arm
✓6ᵗʰ M89.43   Other hypertrophic osteoarthropathy, forearm
M89.431   Other hypertrophic osteoarthropathy, right forearm
M89.432   Other hypertrophic osteoarthropathy, left forearm
M89.439   Other hypertrophic osteoarthropathy, unspecified forearm
✓6ᵗʰ M89.44   Other hypertrophic osteoarthropathy, hand
M89.441   Other hypertrophic osteoarthropathy, right hand
M89.442   Other hypertrophic osteoarthropathy, left hand
M89.449   Other hypertrophic osteoarthropathy, unspecified hand
✓6ᵗʰ M89.45   Other hypertrophic osteoarthropathy, thigh
M89.451   Other hypertrophic osteoarthropathy, right thigh
M89.452   Other hypertrophic osteoarthropathy, left thigh
M89.459   Other hypertrophic osteoarthropathy, unspecified thigh
✓6ᵗʰ M89.46   Other hypertrophic osteoarthropathy, lower leg
M89.461   Other hypertrophic osteoarthropathy, right lower leg
M89.462   Other hypertrophic osteoarthropathy, left lower leg
M89.469   Other hypertrophic osteoarthropathy, unspecified lower leg
✓6ᵗʰ M89.47   Other hypertrophic osteoarthropathy, ankle and foot
M89.471   Other hypertrophic osteoarthropathy, right ankle and foot

M89.472   Other hypertrophic osteoarthropathy, left ankle and foot
M89.479   Other hypertrophic osteoarthropathy, unspecified ankle and foot
M89.48   Other hypertrophic osteoarthropathy, other site
M89.49   Other hypertrophic osteoarthropathy, multiple sites
✓5ᵗʰ M89.5   Osteolysis
Use additional code to identify major osseous defect, if applicable (M89.7-)
EXCLUDES 2   periprosthetic osteolysis of internal prosthetic joint (T84.05-)
M89.50   Osteolysis, unspecified site
✓6ᵗʰ M89.51   Osteolysis, shoulder
M89.511   Osteolysis, right shoulder
M89.512   Osteolysis, left shoulder
M89.519   Osteolysis, unspecified shoulder
✓6ᵗʰ M89.52   Osteolysis, upper arm
M89.521   Osteolysis, right upper arm
M89.522   Osteolysis, left upper arm
M89.529   Osteolysis, unspecified upper arm
✓6ᵗʰ M89.53   Osteolysis, forearm
M89.531   Osteolysis, right forearm
M89.532   Osteolysis, left forearm
M89.539   Osteolysis, unspecified forearm
✓6ᵗʰ M89.54   Osteolysis, hand
M89.541   Osteolysis, right hand
M89.542   Osteolysis, left hand
M89.549   Osteolysis, unspecified hand
✓6ᵗʰ M89.55   Osteolysis, thigh
M89.551   Osteolysis, right thigh
M89.552   Osteolysis, left thigh
M89.559   Osteolysis, unspecified thigh
✓6ᵗʰ M89.56   Osteolysis, lower leg
M89.561   Osteolysis, right lower leg
M89.562   Osteolysis, left lower leg
M89.569   Osteolysis, unspecified lower leg
✓6ᵗʰ M89.57   Osteolysis, ankle and foot
M89.571   Osteolysis, right ankle and foot
M89.572   Osteolysis, left ankle and foot
M89.579   Osteolysis, unspecified ankle and foot
M89.58   Osteolysis, other site
M89.59   Osteolysis, multiple sites
✓6ᵗʰ M89.6   Osteopathy after poliomyelitis
Use additional code (B91) to identify previous poliomyelitis
EXCLUDES 1   postpolio syndrome (G14)
M89.60   Osteopathy after poliomyelitis, unspecified site
✓6ᵗʰ M89.61   Osteopathy after poliomyelitis, shoulder
M89.611   Osteopathy after poliomyelitis, right shoulder
M89.612   Osteopathy after poliomyelitis, left shoulder
M89.619   Osteopathy after poliomyelitis, unspecified shoulder
✓6ᵗʰ M89.62   Osteopathy after poliomyelitis, upper arm
M89.621   Osteopathy after poliomyelitis, right upper arm
M89.622   Osteopathy after poliomyelitis, left upper arm
M89.629   Osteopathy after poliomyelitis, unspecified upper arm
✓6ᵗʰ M89.63   Osteopathy after poliomyelitis, forearm
M89.631   Osteopathy after poliomyelitis, right forearm
M89.632   Osteopathy after poliomyelitis, left forearm
M89.639   Osteopathy after poliomyelitis, unspecified forearm
✓6ᵗʰ M89.64   Osteopathy after poliomyelitis, hand
M89.641   Osteopathy after poliomyelitis, right hand
M89.642   Osteopathy after poliomyelitis, left hand
M89.649   Osteopathy after poliomyelitis, unspecified hand
✓6ᵗʰ M89.65   Osteopathy after poliomyelitis, thigh
M89.651   Osteopathy after poliomyelitis, right thigh

M89.652 **Osteopathy after poliomyelitis,** left **thigh**

M89.659 **Osteopathy after poliomyelitis, unspecified thigh**

✓6ᵗʰ M89.66 **Osteopathy after poliomyelitis,** lower leg

     M89.661 **Osteopathy after poliomyelitis,** right **lower leg**

     M89.662 **Osteopathy after poliomyelitis,** left **lower leg**

     M89.669 **Osteopathy after poliomyelitis, unspecified lower leg**

✓6ᵗʰ M89.67 **Osteopathy after poliomyelitis,** ankle and foot

     M89.671 **Osteopathy after poliomyelitis,** right **ankle and foot**

     M89.672 **Osteopathy after poliomyelitis,** left **ankle and foot**

     M89.679 **Osteopathy after poliomyelitis, unspecified ankle and foot**

M89.68 **Osteopathy after poliomyelitis, other site**

M89.69 **Osteopathy after poliomyelitis,** multiple sites

✓5ᵗʰ **M89.7 Major osseous defect**

     Code first underlying disease, if known, such as:
     aseptic necrosis of bone (M87.-)
     malignant neoplasm of bone (C40.-)
     osteolysis (M89.5)
     osteomyelitis (M86.-)
     osteonecrosis (M87.-)
     osteoporosis (M80.-, M81.-)
     periprosthetic osteolysis (T84.05-)

M89.70 **Major osseous defect, unspecified site**

✓6ᵗʰ M89.71 **Major osseous defect,** shoulder **region**

     Major osseous defect clavicle or scapula

     M89.711 **Major osseous defect,** right **shoulder region**

     M89.712 **Major osseous defect,** left **shoulder region**

     M89.719 **Major osseous defect, unspecified shoulder region**

✓6ᵗʰ M89.72 **Major osseous defect,** humerus

     M89.721 **Major osseous defect,** right **humerus**

     M89.722 **Major osseous defect,** left **humerus**

     M89.729 **Major osseous defect, unspecified humerus**

✓6ᵗʰ M89.73 **Major osseous defect,** forearm

     Major osseous defect of radius and ulna

     M89.731 **Major osseous defect,** right **forearm**

     M89.732 **Major osseous defect,** left **forearm**

     M89.739 **Major osseous defect, unspecified forearm**

✓6ᵗʰ M89.74 **Major osseous defect,** hand

     Major osseous defect of carpus, fingers, metacarpus

     M89.741 **Major osseous defect,** right **hand**

     M89.742 **Major osseous defect,** left **hand**

     M89.749 **Major osseous defect, unspecified hand**

✓6ᵗʰ M89.75 **Major osseous defect,** pelvic region and thigh

     Major osseous defect of femur and pelvis

     M89.751 **Major osseous defect,** right **pelvic region and thigh**

     M89.752 **Major osseous defect,** left **pelvic region and thigh**

     M89.759 **Major osseous defect, unspecified pelvic region and thigh**

✓6ᵗʰ M89.76 **Major osseous defect,** lower leg

     Major osseous defect of fibula and tibia

     M89.761 **Major osseous defect,** right **lower leg**

     M89.762 **Major osseous defect,** left **lower leg**

     M89.769 **Major osseous defect, unspecified lower leg**

✓6ᵗʰ M89.77 **Major osseous defect,** ankle and foot

     Major osseous defect of metatarsus, tarsus, toes

     M89.771 **Major osseous defect,** right **ankle and foot**

     M89.772 **Major osseous defect,** left **ankle and foot**

     M89.779 **Major osseous defect, unspecified ankle and foot**

M89.78 **Major osseous defect, other site**

M89.79 **Major osseous defect,** multiple sites

✓5ᵗʰ M89.8 **Other specified disorders of bone**

     Infantile cortical hyperostoses
     Post-traumatic subperiosteal ossification

✓6ᵗʰ M89.8X **Other specified disorders of bone**

     M89.8X0 **Other specified disorders of bone,** multiple sites

     M89.8X1 **Other specified disorders of bone,** shoulder

     M89.8X2 **Other specified disorders of bone,** upper arm

     M89.8X3 **Other specified disorders of bone,** forearm

     M89.8X4 **Other specified disorders of bone,** hand

     M89.8X5 **Other specified disorders of bone,** thigh

     M89.8X6 **Other specified disorders of bone,** lower leg

     M89.8X7 **Other specified disorders of bone,** ankle and foot

     M89.8X8 **Other specified disorders of bone, other site**

     M89.8X9 **Other specified disorders of bone, unspecified site**

M89.9 **Disorder of bone, unspecified**

✓4ᵗʰ M90 **Osteopathies in diseases classified elsewhere**

     EXCLUDES 1   *osteochondritis, osteomyelitis, and osteopathy (in):*
         cryptococcosis (B45.3)
         diabetes mellitus (E08-E13 with .69-)
         gonococcal (A54.43)
         neurogenic syphilis (A52.11)
         renal osteodystrophy (N25.0)
         salmonellosis (A02.24)
         secondary syphilis (A51.46)
         syphilis (late) (A52.77)

✓5ᵗʰ M90.5 **Osteonecrosis in diseases classified elsewhere**

     Code first underlying disease, such as:
     caisson disease (T70.3)
     hemoglobinopathy (D50-D64)

     M90.50 *Osteonecrosis in diseases classified elsewhere, unspecified site*

✓6ᵗʰ M90.51 **Osteonecrosis in diseases classified elsewhere,** shoulder

     M90.511 *Osteonecrosis in diseases classified elsewhere,* right *shoulder*

     M90.512 *Osteonecrosis in diseases classified elsewhere,* left *shoulder*

     M90.519 *Osteonecrosis in diseases classified elsewhere, unspecified shoulder*

✓6ᵗʰ M90.52 **Osteonecrosis in diseases classified elsewhere,** upper arm

     M90.521 *Osteonecrosis in diseases classified elsewhere,* right *upper arm*

     M90.522 *Osteonecrosis in diseases classified elsewhere,* left *upper arm*

     M90.529 *Osteonecrosis in diseases classified elsewhere, unspecified upper arm*

✓6ᵗʰ M90.53 **Osteonecrosis in diseases classified elsewhere,** forearm

     M90.531 *Osteonecrosis in diseases classified elsewhere,* right *forearm*

     M90.532 *Osteonecrosis in diseases classified elsewhere,* left *forearm*

     M90.539 *Osteonecrosis in diseases classified elsewhere, unspecified forearm*

✓6ᵗʰ M90.54 **Osteonecrosis in diseases classified elsewhere,** hand

     M90.541 *Osteonecrosis in diseases classified elsewhere,* right *hand*

     M90.542 *Osteonecrosis in diseases classified elsewhere,* left *hand*

     M90.549 *Osteonecrosis in diseases classified elsewhere, unspecified hand*

✓6ᵗʰ M90.55 **Osteonecrosis in diseases classified elsewhere,** thigh

     M90.551 *Osteonecrosis in diseases classified elsewhere,* right *thigh*

     M90.552 *Osteonecrosis in diseases classified elsewhere,* left *thigh*

     M90.559 *Osteonecrosis in diseases classified elsewhere, unspecified thigh*

☑ Additional Character Required   ✓x7ᵗʰ Placeholder Alert   Manifestation   Unspecified Dx   ►◄ Revised Text   ● New Code   ▲ Revised Title

ICD-10-CM 2020   815

✓6ᵗʰ M90.56 Osteonecrosis in diseases classified elsewhere, lower leg

     M90.561 Osteonecrosis in diseases classified elsewhere, right lower leg

     M90.562 Osteonecrosis in diseases classified elsewhere, left lower leg

     M90.569 Osteonecrosis in diseases classified elsewhere, unspecified lower leg

✓6ᵗʰ M90.57 Osteonecrosis in diseases classified elsewhere, ankle and foot

     M90.571 Osteonecrosis in diseases classified elsewhere, right ankle and foot

     M90.572 Osteonecrosis in diseases classified elsewhere, left ankle and foot

     M90.579 Osteonecrosis in diseases classified elsewhere, unspecified ankle and foot

     M90.58 *Osteonecrosis in diseases classified elsewhere, other site*

     M90.59 *Osteonecrosis in diseases classified elsewhere, multiple sites*

✓5ᵗʰ M90.6 Osteitis deformans in neoplastic diseases

     Osteitis deformans in malignant neoplasm of bone

     Code first the neoplasm (C40.-, C41.-)

     EXCLUDES 1   osteitis deformans [Paget's disease of bone] (M88.-)

     M90.60 *Osteitis deformans in neoplastic diseases, unspecified site*

✓6ᵗʰ M90.61 Osteitis deformans in neoplastic diseases, shoulder

     M90.611 Osteitis deformans in neoplastic diseases, right shoulder

     M90.612 Osteitis deformans in neoplastic diseases, left shoulder

     M90.619 Osteitis deformans in neoplastic diseases, unspecified shoulder

✓6ᵗʰ M90.62 Osteitis deformans in neoplastic diseases, upper arm

     M90.621 Osteitis deformans in neoplastic diseases, right upper arm

     M90.622 Osteitis deformans in neoplastic diseases, left upper arm

     M90.629 Osteitis deformans in neoplastic diseases, unspecified upper arm

✓6ᵗʰ M90.63 Osteitis deformans in neoplastic diseases, forearm

     M90.631 Osteitis deformans in neoplastic diseases, right forearm

     M90.632 Osteitis deformans in neoplastic diseases, left forearm

     M90.639 Osteitis deformans in neoplastic diseases, unspecified forearm

✓6ᵗʰ M90.64 Osteitis deformans in neoplastic diseases, hand

     M90.641 Osteitis deformans in neoplastic diseases, right hand

     M90.642 Osteitis deformans in neoplastic diseases, left hand

     M90.649 Osteitis deformans in neoplastic diseases, unspecified hand

✓6ᵗʰ M90.65 Osteitis deformans in neoplastic diseases, thigh

     M90.651 Osteitis deformans in neoplastic diseases, right thigh

     M90.652 Osteitis deformans in neoplastic diseases, left thigh

     M90.659 Osteitis deformans in neoplastic diseases, unspecified thigh

✓6ᵗʰ M90.66 Osteitis deformans in neoplastic diseases, lower leg

     M90.661 Osteitis deformans in neoplastic diseases, right lower leg

     M90.662 Osteitis deformans in neoplastic diseases, left lower leg

     M90.669 Osteitis deformans in neoplastic diseases, unspecified lower leg

✓6ᵗʰ M90.67 Osteitis deformans in neoplastic diseases, ankle and foot

     M90.671 Osteitis deformans in neoplastic diseases, right ankle and foot

     M90.672 Osteitis deformans in neoplastic diseases, left ankle and foot

     M90.679 Osteitis deformans in neoplastic diseases, unspecified ankle and foot

     M90.68 *Osteitis deformans in neoplastic diseases, other site*

     M90.69 *Osteitis deformans in neoplastic diseases, multiple sites*

✓5ᵗʰ M90.8 Osteopathy in diseases classified elsewhere

     Code first underlying disease, such as:

     rickets (E55.0)

     vitamin-D-resistant rickets (E83.3)

     M90.80 *Osteopathy in diseases classified elsewhere, unspecified site*

✓6ᵗʰ M90.81 Osteopathy in diseases classified elsewhere, shoulder

     M90.811 Osteopathy in diseases classified elsewhere, right shoulder

     M90.812 Osteopathy in diseases classified elsewhere, left shoulder

     M90.819 Osteopathy in diseases classified elsewhere, unspecified shoulder

✓6ᵗʰ M90.82 Osteopathy in diseases classified elsewhere, upper arm

     M90.821 Osteopathy in diseases classified elsewhere, right upper arm

     M90.822 Osteopathy in diseases classified elsewhere, left upper arm

     M90.829 Osteopathy in diseases classified elsewhere, unspecified upper arm

✓6ᵗʰ M90.83 Osteopathy in diseases classified elsewhere, forearm

     M90.831 Osteopathy in diseases classified elsewhere, right forearm

     M90.832 Osteopathy in diseases classified elsewhere, left forearm

     M90.839 Osteopathy in diseases classified elsewhere, unspecified forearm

✓6ᵗʰ M90.84 Osteopathy in diseases classified elsewhere, hand

     M90.841 Osteopathy in diseases classified elsewhere, right hand

     M90.842 Osteopathy in diseases classified elsewhere, left hand

     M90.849 Osteopathy in diseases classified elsewhere, unspecified hand

✓6ᵗʰ M90.85 Osteopathy in diseases classified elsewhere, thigh

     M90.851 Osteopathy in diseases classified elsewhere, right thigh

     M90.852 Osteopathy in diseases classified elsewhere, left thigh

     M90.859 Osteopathy in diseases classified elsewhere, unspecified thigh

✓6ᵗʰ M90.86 Osteopathy in diseases classified elsewhere, lower leg

     M90.861 Osteopathy in diseases classified elsewhere, right lower leg

     M90.862 Osteopathy in diseases classified elsewhere, left lower leg

     M90.869 Osteopathy in diseases classified elsewhere, unspecified lower leg

✓6ᵗʰ M90.87 Osteopathy in diseases classified elsewhere, ankle and foot

     M90.871 Osteopathy in diseases classified elsewhere, right ankle and foot

     M90.872 Osteopathy in diseases classified elsewhere, left ankle and foot

     M90.879 Osteopathy in diseases classified elsewhere, unspecified ankle and foot

     M90.88 *Osteopathy in diseases classified elsewhere, other site*

     M90.89 *Osteopathy in diseases classified elsewhere, multiple sites*

Chondropathies (M91-M94)

     EXCLUDES 1   postprocedural chondropathies (M96.-)

✓4ᵗʰ M91 Juvenile osteochondrosis of hip and pelvis

     EXCLUDES 1   slipped upper femoral epiphysis (nontraumatic) (M93.0)

     M91.0 Juvenile osteochondrosis of pelvis

        Osteochondrosis (juvenile) of acetabulum

        Osteochondrosis (juvenile) of iliac crest [Buchanan]

        Osteochondrosis (juvenile) of ischiopubic synchondrosis [van Neck]

        Osteochondrosis (juvenile) of symphysis pubis [Pierson]

     ✓5ᵗʰ M91.1 Juvenile osteochondrosis of head of femur [Legg-Calvé-Perthes]

        M91.10 Juvenile osteochondrosis of head of femur [Legg-Calvé-Perthes], unspecified leg

        M91.11 Juvenile osteochondrosis of head of femur [Legg-Calvé-Perthes], right leg

N Newborn: 0   **P** Pediatric: 0-17   **M** Maternity: 12-55   **A** Adult: 15-124   **CH** Comorbidity High   **CL** Comorbidity Low   **NCDx** Noncancer Dx   **PDx** Primary Dx

816   ICD-10-CM 2020

Chapter 13. Diseases of the Musculoskeletal System and Connective Tissue

M90.56–M91.11

M91.12   **Juvenile osteochondrosis of head of femur [Legg-Calvé-Perthes], left leg**

✓5ᵗʰ **M91.2**   Coxa plana

    Hip deformity due to previous juvenile osteochondrosis

    M91.20   Coxa plana, unspecified hip
    M91.21   Coxa plana, right hip
    M91.22   Coxa plana, left hip

✓5ᵗʰ **M91.3**   Pseudocoxalgia

    M91.30   Pseudocoxalgia, unspecified hip
    M91.31   Pseudocoxalgia, right hip
    M91.32   Pseudocoxalgia, left hip

✓5ᵗʰ **M91.4**   Coxa magna

    M91.40   Coxa magna, unspecified hip
    M91.41   Coxa magna, right hip
    M91.42   Coxa magna, left hip

✓5ᵗʰ **M91.8**   Other juvenile osteochondrosis of hip and pelvis

    Juvenile osteochondrosis after reduction of congenital dislocation of hip

    M91.80   Other juvenile osteochondrosis of hip and pelvis, unspecified leg
    M91.81   Other juvenile osteochondrosis of hip and pelvis, right leg
    M91.82   Other juvenile osteochondrosis of hip and pelvis, left leg

✓5ᵗʰ **M91.9**   Juvenile osteochondrosis of hip and pelvis, unspecified

    M91.90   Juvenile osteochondrosis of hip and pelvis, unspecified, unspecified leg
    M91.91   Juvenile osteochondrosis of hip and pelvis, unspecified, right leg
    M91.92   Juvenile osteochondrosis of hip and pelvis, unspecified, left leg

✓4ᵗʰ **M92**   **Other juvenile osteochondrosis**

✓5ᵗʰ **M92.0**   Juvenile osteochondrosis of humerus

    Osteochondrosis (juvenile) of capitulum of humerus [Panner]
    Osteochondrosis (juvenile) of head of humerus [Haas]

    M92.00   Juvenile osteochondrosis of humerus, unspecified arm
    M92.01   Juvenile osteochondrosis of humerus, right arm
    M92.02   Juvenile osteochondrosis of humerus, left arm

✓5ᵗʰ **M92.1**   Juvenile osteochondrosis of radius and ulna

    Osteochondrosis (juvenile) of lower ulna [Burns]
    Osteochondrosis (juvenile) of radial head [Brailsford]

    M92.10   Juvenile osteochondrosis of radius and ulna, unspecified arm
    M92.11   Juvenile osteochondrosis of radius and ulna, right arm
    M92.12   Juvenile osteochondrosis of radius and ulna, left arm

✓5ᵗʰ **M92.2**   Juvenile osteochondrosis, hand

    ✓6ᵗʰ **M92.20**   Unspecified juvenile osteochondrosis, hand
       M92.201   Unspecified juvenile osteochondrosis, right hand
       M92.202   Unspecified juvenile osteochondrosis, left hand
       M92.209   Unspecified juvenile osteochondrosis, unspecified hand

    ✓6ᵗʰ **M92.21**   Osteochondrosis (juvenile) of carpal lunate [Kienböck]
       M92.211   Osteochondrosis (juvenile) of carpal lunate [Kienböck], right hand
       M92.212   Osteochondrosis (juvenile) of carpal lunate [Kienböck], left hand
       M92.219   Osteochondrosis (juvenile) of carpal lunate [Kienböck], unspecified hand

    ✓6ᵗʰ **M92.22**   Osteochondrosis (juvenile) of metacarpal heads [Mauclaire]
       M92.221   Osteochondrosis (juvenile) of metacarpal heads [Mauclaire], right hand
       M92.222   Osteochondrosis (juvenile) of metacarpal heads [Mauclaire], left hand
       M92.229   Osteochondrosis (juvenile) of metacarpal heads [Mauclaire], unspecified hand

    ✓6ᵗʰ **M92.29**   Other juvenile osteochondrosis, hand
       M92.291   Other juvenile osteochondrosis, right hand
       M92.292   Other juvenile osteochondrosis, left hand
       M92.299   Other juvenile osteochondrosis, unspecified hand

✓5ᵗʰ **M92.3**   Other juvenile osteochondrosis, upper limb

    M92.30   Other juvenile osteochondrosis, unspecified upper limb
    M92.31   Other juvenile osteochondrosis, right upper limb
    M92.32   Other juvenile osteochondrosis, left upper limb

✓5ᵗʰ **M92.4**   Juvenile osteochondrosis of patella

    Osteochondrosis (juvenile) of primary patellar center [Köhler]
    Osteochondrosis (juvenile) of secondary patellar centre [Sinding Larsen]

    M92.40   Juvenile osteochondrosis of patella, unspecified knee
    M92.41   Juvenile osteochondrosis of patella, right knee
    M92.42   Juvenile osteochondrosis of patella, left knee

✓5ᵗʰ **M92.5**   Juvenile osteochondrosis of tibia and fibula

    Osteochondrosis (juvenile) of proximal tibia [Blount]
    Osteochondrosis (juvenile) of tibial tubercle [Osgood-Schlatter]
    Tibia vara

    M92.50   Juvenile osteochondrosis of tibia and fibula, unspecified leg
    M92.51   Juvenile osteochondrosis of tibia and fibula, right leg
    M92.52   Juvenile osteochondrosis of tibia and fibula, left leg

✓5ᵗʰ **M92.6**   Juvenile osteochondrosis of tarsus

    Osteochondrosis (juvenile) of calcaneum [Sever]
    Osteochondrosis (juvenile) of os tibiale externum [Haglund]
    Osteochondrosis (juvenile) of talus [Diaz]
    Osteochondrosis (juvenile) of tarsal navicular [Köhler]

    M92.60   Juvenile osteochondrosis of tarsus, unspecified ankle
    M92.61   Juvenile osteochondrosis of tarsus, right ankle
    M92.62   Juvenile osteochondrosis of tarsus, left ankle

✓5ᵗʰ **M92.7**   Juvenile osteochondrosis of metatarsus

    Osteochondrosis (juvenile) of fifth metatarsus [Iselin]
    Osteochondrosis (juvenile) of second metatarsus [Freiberg]

    M92.70   Juvenile osteochondrosis of metatarsus, unspecified foot
    M92.71   Juvenile osteochondrosis of metatarsus, right foot
    M92.72   Juvenile osteochondrosis of metatarsus, left foot

   M92.8   Other specified juvenile osteochondrosis

    Calcaneal apophysitis
    DEF: Calcaneal apophysitis: Inflammation of the calcaneus at the point of Achilles tendon insertion usually occurring in boys ages 8 to 14. Pain, tenderness, and localized swelling are present.

   M92.9   Juvenile osteochondrosis, unspecified

    Juvenile apophysitis NOS
    Juvenile epiphysitis NOS
    Juvenile osteochondritis NOS
    Juvenile osteochondrosis NOS

✓4ᵗʰ **M93**   **Other osteochondropathies**

    EXCLUDES 2   osteochondrosis of spine (M42.-)

✓5ᵗʰ **M93.0**   Slipped upper femoral epiphysis (nontraumatic)

    Use additional code for associated chondrolysis (M94.3)

    ✓6ᵗʰ **M93.00**   Unspecified slipped upper femoral epiphysis (nontraumatic)
       M93.001   Unspecified slipped upper femoral epiphysis (nontraumatic), right hip
       M93.002   Unspecified slipped upper femoral epiphysis (nontraumatic), left hip
       M93.003   Unspecified slipped upper femoral epiphysis (nontraumatic), unspecified hip

    ✓6ᵗʰ **M93.01**   Acute slipped upper femoral epiphysis (nontraumatic)
       M93.011   Acute slipped upper femoral epiphysis (nontraumatic), right hip
       M93.012   Acute slipped upper femoral epiphysis (nontraumatic), left hip
       M93.013   Acute slipped upper femoral epiphysis (nontraumatic), unspecified hip

    ✓6ᵗʰ **M93.02**   Chronic slipped upper femoral epiphysis (nontraumatic)
       M93.021   Chronic slipped upper femoral epiphysis (nontraumatic), right hip
       M93.022   Chronic slipped upper femoral epiphysis (nontraumatic), left hip
       M93.023   Chronic slipped upper femoral epiphysis (nontraumatic), unspecified hip

---

✓ Additional Character Required   ✓x7ᵗʰ Placeholder Alert   Manifestation   Unspecified Dx   ▶◀ Revised Text   ● New Code   ▲ Revised Title

☑6ᵗʰ **M93.Ø3** Acute on chronic slipped upper femoral epiphysis (nontraumatic)

  M93.Ø31 Acute on chronic slipped upper femoral epiphysis (nontraumatic), right hip

  M93.Ø32 Acute on chronic slipped upper femoral epiphysis (nontraumatic), left hip

  M93.Ø33 Acute on chronic slipped upper femoral epiphysis (nontraumatic), unspecified hip

M93.1 Kienböck's disease of adults   Ⓐ

  Adult osteochondrosis of carpal lunates

☑5ᵗʰ **M93.2** Osteochondritis dissecans

  DEF: Avascular necrosis caused by lack of blood flow to the bone and cartilage of a joint causing the bone to die. This can result in splinters or pieces of cartilage breaking off in the joint.

  M93.2Ø Osteochondritis dissecans of unspecified site

☑6ᵗʰ **M93.21** Osteochondritis dissecans of shoulder

  M93.211 Osteochondritis dissecans, right shoulder
  M93.212 Osteochondritis dissecans, left shoulder
  M93.219 Osteochondritis dissecans, unspecified shoulder

☑6ᵗʰ **M93.22** Osteochondritis dissecans of elbow

  M93.221 Osteochondritis dissecans, right elbow
  M93.222 Osteochondritis dissecans, left elbow
  M93.229 Osteochondritis dissecans, unspecified elbow

☑6ᵗʰ **M93.23** Osteochondritis dissecans of wrist

  M93.231 Osteochondritis dissecans, right wrist
  M93.232 Osteochondritis dissecans, left wrist
  M93.239 Osteochondritis dissecans, unspecified wrist

☑6ᵗʰ **M93.24** Osteochondritis dissecans of joints of hand

  M93.241 Osteochondritis dissecans, joints of right hand
  M93.242 Osteochondritis dissecans, joints of left hand
  M93.249 Osteochondritis dissecans, joints of unspecified hand

☑6ᵗʰ **M93.25** Osteochondritis dissecans of hip

  M93.251 Osteochondritis dissecans, right hip
  M93.252 Osteochondritis dissecans, left hip
  M93.259 Osteochondritis dissecans, unspecified hip

☑6ᵗʰ **M93.26** Osteochondritis dissecans knee

  M93.261 Osteochondritis dissecans, right knee
  M93.262 Osteochondritis dissecans, left knee
  M93.269 Osteochondritis dissecans, unspecified knee

☑6ᵗʰ **M93.27** Osteochondritis dissecans of ankle and joints of foot

  M93.271 Osteochondritis dissecans, right ankle and joints of right foot
  M93.272 Osteochondritis dissecans, left ankle and joints of left foot
  M93.279 Osteochondritis dissecans, unspecified ankle and joints of foot

  M93.28 Osteochondritis dissecans other site

  M93.29 Osteochondritis dissecans multiple sites

☑5ᵗʰ **M93.8** Other specified osteochondropathies

  M93.8Ø Other specified osteochondropathies of unspecified site

☑6ᵗʰ **M93.81** Other specified osteochondropathies of shoulder

  M93.811 Other specified osteochondropathies, right shoulder
  M93.812 Other specified osteochondropathies, left shoulder
  M93.819 Other specified osteochondropathies, unspecified shoulder

☑6ᵗʰ **M93.82** Other specified osteochondropathies of upper arm

  M93.821 Other specified osteochondropathies, right upper arm
  M93.822 Other specified osteochondropathies, left upper arm
  M93.829 Other specified osteochondropathies, unspecified upper arm

☑6ᵗʰ **M93.83** Other specified osteochondropathies of forearm

  M93.831 Other specified osteochondropathies, right forearm
  M93.832 Other specified osteochondropathies, left forearm

  M93.839 Other specified osteochondropathies, unspecified forearm

☑6ᵗʰ **M93.84** Other specified osteochondropathies of hand

  M93.841 Other specified osteochondropathies, right hand
  M93.842 Other specified osteochondropathies, left hand
  M93.849 Other specified osteochondropathies, unspecified hand

☑6ᵗʰ **M93.85** Other specified osteochondropathies of thigh

  M93.851 Other specified osteochondropathies, right thigh
  M93.852 Other specified osteochondropathies, left thigh
  M93.859 Other specified osteochondropathies, unspecified thigh

☑6ᵗʰ **M93.86** Other specified osteochondropathies lower leg

  M93.861 Other specified osteochondropathies, right lower leg
  M93.862 Other specified osteochondropathies, left lower leg
  M93.869 Other specified osteochondropathies, unspecified lower leg

☑6ᵗʰ **M93.87** Other specified osteochondropathies of ankle and foot

  M93.871 Other specified osteochondropathies, right ankle and foot
  M93.872 Other specified osteochondropathies, left ankle and foot
  M93.879 Other specified osteochondropathies, unspecified ankle and foot

  M93.88 Other specified osteochondropathies other site

  M93.89 Other specified osteochondropathies multiple sites

☑5ᵗʰ **M93.9** Osteochondropathy, unspecified

  Apophysitis NOS
  Epiphysitis NOS
  Osteochondritis NOS
  Osteochondrosis NOS

  M93.9Ø Osteochondropathy, unspecified of unspecified site

☑6ᵗʰ **M93.91** Osteochondropathy, unspecified of shoulder

  M93.911 Osteochondropathy, unspecified, right shoulder
  M93.912 Osteochondropathy, unspecified, left shoulder
  M93.919 Osteochondropathy, unspecified, unspecified shoulder

☑6ᵗʰ **M93.92** Osteochondropathy, unspecified of upper arm

  M93.921 Osteochondropathy, unspecified, right upper arm
  M93.922 Osteochondropathy, unspecified, left upper arm
  M93.929 Osteochondropathy, unspecified, unspecified upper arm

☑6ᵗʰ **M93.93** Osteochondropathy, unspecified of forearm

  M93.931 Osteochondropathy, unspecified, right forearm
  M93.932 Osteochondropathy, unspecified, left forearm
  M93.939 Osteochondropathy, unspecified, unspecified forearm

☑6ᵗʰ **M93.94** Osteochondropathy, unspecified of hand

  M93.941 Osteochondropathy, unspecified, right hand
  M93.942 Osteochondropathy, unspecified, left hand
  M93.949 Osteochondropathy, unspecified, unspecified hand

☑6ᵗʰ **M93.95** Osteochondropathy, unspecified of thigh

  M93.951 Osteochondropathy, unspecified, right thigh
  M93.952 Osteochondropathy, unspecified, left thigh
  M93.959 Osteochondropathy, unspecified, unspecified thigh

☑6ᵗʰ **M93.96** Osteochondropathy, unspecified lower leg

  M93.961 Osteochondropathy, unspecified, right lower leg
  M93.962 Osteochondropathy, unspecified, left lower leg

Ⓝ Newborn: 0   Ⓟ Pediatric: 0-17   Ⓜ Maternity: 12-55   Ⓐ Adult: 15-124   CH Comorbidity High   CL Comorbidity Low   NCDx Noncancer Dx   PDx Primary Dx

818   ICD-10-CM 2020

M93.969 Osteochondropathy, unspecified, unspecified lower leg

√6ᵗʰ **M93.97** Osteochondropathy, unspecified of ankle and foot

M93.971 Osteochondropathy, unspecified, right ankle and foot

M93.972 Osteochondropathy, unspecified, left ankle and foot

M93.979 Osteochondropathy, unspecified, unspecified ankle and foot

M93.98 Osteochondropathy, unspecified other site

M93.99 Osteochondropathy, unspecified multiple sites

√4ᵗʰ **M94** Other disorders of cartilage

M94.0 Chondrocostal junction syndrome [Tietze]
Costochondritis

M94.1 Relapsing polychondritis

√5ᵗʰ **M94.2** Chondromalacia

EXCLUDES 1 chondromalacia patellae (M22.4)

M94.20 Chondromalacia, unspecified site

√6ᵗʰ **M94.21** Chondromalacia, shoulder

M94.211 Chondromalacia, right shoulder
M94.212 Chondromalacia, left shoulder
M94.219 Chondromalacia, unspecified shoulder

√6ᵗʰ **M94.22** Chondromalacia, elbow

M94.221 Chondromalacia, right elbow
M94.222 Chondromalacia, left elbow
M94.229 Chondromalacia, unspecified elbow

√6ᵗʰ **M94.23** Chondromalacia, wrist

M94.231 Chondromalacia, right wrist
M94.232 Chondromalacia, left wrist
M94.239 Chondromalacia, unspecified wrist

√6ᵗʰ **M94.24** Chondromalacia, joints of hand

M94.241 Chondromalacia, joints of right hand
M94.242 Chondromalacia, joints of left hand
M94.249 Chondromalacia, joints of unspecified hand

√6ᵗʰ **M94.25** Chondromalacia, hip

M94.251 Chondromalacia, right hip
M94.252 Chondromalacia, left hip
M94.259 Chondromalacia, unspecified hip

√6ᵗʰ **M94.26** Chondromalacia, knee

M94.261 Chondromalacia, right knee
M94.262 Chondromalacia, left knee
M94.269 Chondromalacia, unspecified knee

√6ᵗʰ **M94.27** Chondromalacia, ankle and joints of foot

M94.271 Chondromalacia, right ankle and joints of right foot
M94.272 Chondromalacia, left ankle and joints of left foot
M94.279 Chondromalacia, unspecified ankle and joints of foot

M94.28 Chondromalacia, other site
M94.29 Chondromalacia, multiple sites

√5ᵗʰ **M94.3** Chondrolysis

Code first any associated slipped upper femoral epiphysis (nontraumatic) (M93.0-)

√6ᵗʰ **M94.35** Chondrolysis, hip

M94.351 Chondrolysis, right hip
M94.352 Chondrolysis, left hip
M94.359 Chondrolysis, unspecified hip

√5ᵗʰ **M94.8** Other specified disorders of cartilage

√6ᵗʰ **M94.8X** Other specified disorders of cartilage

M94.8X0 Other specified disorders of cartilage, multiple sites
M94.8X1 Other specified disorders of cartilage, shoulder
M94.8X2 Other specified disorders of cartilage, upper arm
M94.8X3 Other specified disorders of cartilage, forearm
M94.8X4 Other specified disorders of cartilage, hand
M94.8X5 Other specified disorders of cartilage, thigh
M94.8X6 Other specified disorders of cartilage, lower leg
M94.8X7 Other specified disorders of cartilage, ankle and foot

M94.8X8 Other specified disorders of cartilage, other site
M94.8X9 Other specified disorders of cartilage, unspecified sites

M94.9 Disorder of cartilage, unspecified

Other disorders of the musculoskeletal system and connective tissue (M95)

√4ᵗʰ **M95** Other acquired deformities of musculoskeletal system and connective tissue

EXCLUDES 2 acquired absence of limbs and organs (Z89-Z90)
acquired deformities of limbs (M20-M21)
congenital malformations and deformations of the musculoskeletal system (Q65-Q79)
deforming dorsopathies (M40-M43)
dentofacial anomalies [including malocclusion] (M26.-)
postprocedural musculoskeletal disorders (M96.-)

M95.0 Acquired deformity of nose
EXCLUDES 2 deviated nasal septum (J34.2)

√5ᵗʰ **M95.1** Cauliflower ear
EXCLUDES 2 other acquired deformities of ear (H61.1)
DEF: Acquired deformity of the external ear due to injury or subsequent perichondritis.

M95.10 Cauliflower ear, unspecified ear
M95.11 Cauliflower ear, right ear
M95.12 Cauliflower ear, left ear

M95.2 Other acquired deformity of head
M95.3 Acquired deformity of neck
M95.4 Acquired deformity of chest and rib
AHA: 2014,4Q,26-27
M95.5 Acquired deformity of pelvis
EXCLUDES 1 maternal care for known or suspected disproportion (O33.-)
M95.8 Other specified acquired deformities of musculoskeletal system
M95.9 Acquired deformity of musculoskeletal system, unspecified

Intraoperative and postprocedural complications and disorders of musculoskeletal system, not elsewhere classified (M96)

√4ᵗʰ **M96** Intraoperative and postprocedural complications and disorders of musculoskeletal system, not elsewhere classified

EXCLUDES 2 arthropathy following intestinal bypass (M02.0-)
complications of internal orthopedic prosthetic devices, implants and grafts (T84.-)
disorders associated with osteoporosis (M80)
periprosthetic fracture around internal prosthetic joint (M97.-)
presence of functional implants and other devices (Z96-Z97)

M96.0 Pseudarthrosis after fusion or arthrodesis
M96.1 Postlaminectomy syndrome, not elsewhere classified
M96.2 Postradiation kyphosis
M96.3 Postlaminectomy kyphosis
M96.4 Postsurgical lordosis
M96.5 Postradiation scoliosis

√5ᵗʰ **M96.6** Fracture of bone following insertion of orthopedic implant, joint prosthesis, or bone plate
Intraoperative fracture of bone during insertion of orthopedic implant, joint prosthesis, or bone plate
EXCLUDES 2 complication of internal orthopedic devices, implants or grafts (T84.-)

√6ᵗʰ **M96.62** Fracture of humerus following insertion of orthopedic implant, joint prosthesis, or bone plate
M96.621 Fracture of humerus following insertion of orthopedic implant, joint prosthesis, or bone plate, right arm
M96.622 Fracture of humerus following insertion of orthopedic implant, joint prosthesis, or bone plate, left arm
M96.629 Fracture of humerus following insertion of orthopedic implant, joint prosthesis, or bone plate, unspecified arm

√6ᵗʰ **M96.63** Fracture of radius or ulna following insertion of orthopedic implant, joint prosthesis, or bone plate
M96.631 Fracture of radius or ulna following insertion of orthopedic implant, joint prosthesis, or bone plate, right arm

M96.632   Fracture of radius or ulna following insertion of orthopedic implant, joint prosthesis, or bone plate, left arm

M96.639   Fracture of radius or ulna following insertion of orthopedic implant, joint prosthesis, or bone plate, unspecified arm

M96.65   Fracture of pelvis following insertion of orthopedic implant, joint prosthesis, or bone plate

✓6th M96.66   Fracture of femur following insertion of orthopedic implant, joint prosthesis, or bone plate

M96.661   Fracture of femur following insertion of orthopedic implant, joint prosthesis, or bone plate, right leg

M96.662   Fracture of femur following insertion of orthopedic implant, joint prosthesis, or bone plate, left leg

M96.669   Fracture of femur following insertion of orthopedic implant, joint prosthesis, or bone plate, unspecified leg

✓6th M96.67   Fracture of tibia or fibula following insertion of orthopedic implant, joint prosthesis, or bone plate

M96.671   Fracture of tibia or fibula following insertion of orthopedic implant, joint prosthesis, or bone plate, right leg

M96.672   Fracture of tibia or fibula following insertion of orthopedic implant, joint prosthesis, or bone plate, left leg

M96.679   Fracture of tibia or fibula following insertion of orthopedic implant, joint prosthesis, or bone plate, unspecified leg

M96.69   Fracture of other bone following insertion of orthopedic implant, joint prosthesis, or bone plate

✓5th M96.8   Other intraoperative and postprocedural complications and disorders of musculoskeletal system, not elsewhere classified

AHA: 2016,4Q,9-10

✓6th M96.81   Intraoperative hemorrhage and hematoma of a musculoskeletal structure complicating a procedure

EXCLUDES 1   intraoperative hemorrhage and hematoma of a musculoskeletal structure due to accidental puncture and laceration during a procedure (M96.82-)

M96.810   Intraoperative hemorrhage and hematoma of a musculoskeletal structure complicating a musculoskeletal system procedure

M96.811   Intraoperative hemorrhage and hematoma of a musculoskeletal structure complicating other procedure

✓6th M96.82   Accidental puncture and laceration of a musculoskeletal structure during a procedure

M96.820   Accidental puncture and laceration of a musculoskeletal structure during a musculoskeletal system procedure

M96.821   Accidental puncture and laceration of a musculoskeletal structure during other procedure

✓6th M96.83   Postprocedural hemorrhage of a musculoskeletal structure following a procedure

M96.830   Postprocedural hemorrhage of a musculoskeletal structure following a musculoskeletal system procedure

M96.831   Postprocedural hemorrhage of a musculoskeletal structure following other procedure

✓6th M96.84   Postprocedural hematoma and seroma of a musculoskeletal structure following a procedure

M96.840   Postprocedural hematoma of a musculoskeletal structure following a musculoskeletal system procedure

M96.841   Postprocedural hematoma of a musculoskeletal structure following other procedure

AHA: 2016,4Q,10

M96.842   Postprocedural seroma of a musculoskeletal structure following a musculoskeletal system procedure

M96.843   Postprocedural seroma of a musculoskeletal structure following other procedure

AHA: 2018,3Q,6

M96.89   Other intraoperative and postprocedural complications and disorders of the musculoskeletal system

Instability of joint secondary to removal of joint prosthesis

Use additional code, if applicable, to further specify disorder

Periprosthetic fractures around internal prosthetic joint (M97)

✓4th M97   Periprosthetic fracture around internal prosthetic joint

EXCLUDES 2   breakage (fracture) of prosthetic joint (T84.01-)
fracture of bone following insertion of orthopedic implant, joint prosthesis or bone plate (M96.6-)

AHA: 2016,4Q,42-43

The appropriate 7th character is to be added to each code from category M97.
A   initial encounter
D   subsequent encounter
S   sequela

✓5th M97.0   Periprosthetic fracture around internal prosthetic hip joint

AHA: 2018,1Q,21; 2016,4Q,42

✓x7th M97.01   Periprosthetic fracture around internal prosthetic right hip joint

✓x7th M97.02   Periprosthetic fracture around internal prosthetic left hip joint

✓5th M97.1   Periprosthetic fracture around internal prosthetic knee joint

✓x7th M97.11   Periprosthetic fracture around internal prosthetic right knee joint

✓x7th M97.12   Periprosthetic fracture around internal prosthetic left knee joint

✓5th M97.2   Periprosthetic fracture around internal prosthetic ankle joint

✓x7th M97.21   Periprosthetic fracture around internal prosthetic right ankle joint

✓x7th M97.22   Periprosthetic fracture around internal prosthetic left ankle joint

✓5th M97.3   Periprosthetic fracture around internal prosthetic shoulder joint

✓x7th M97.31   Periprosthetic fracture around internal prosthetic right shoulder joint

✓x7th M97.32   Periprosthetic fracture around internal prosthetic left shoulder joint

✓5th M97.4   Periprosthetic fracture around internal prosthetic elbow joint

✓x7th M97.41   Periprosthetic fracture around internal prosthetic right elbow joint

✓x7th M97.42   Periprosthetic fracture around internal prosthetic left elbow joint

✓x7th M97.8   Periprosthetic fracture around other internal prosthetic joint

Periprosthetic fracture around internal prosthetic finger joint
Periprosthetic fracture around internal prosthetic spinal joint
Periprosthetic fracture around internal prosthetic toe joint
Periprosthetic fracture around internal prosthetic wrist joint
Use additional code to identify the joint (Z96.6-)

✓x7th M97.9   Periprosthetic fracture around unspecified internal prosthetic joint

Biomechanical lesions, not elsewhere classified (M99)

✓4th M99   Biomechanical lesions, not elsewhere classified

NOTE   This category should not be used if the condition can be classified elsewhere.

DEF: Biomechanical lesion: Term used by osteopathic and chiropractic physicians to describe musculoskeletal conditions treated that are not more appropriately classified elsewhere.

✓5th M99.0   Segmental and somatic dysfunction

M99.00   Segmental and somatic dysfunction of head region

M99.01   Segmental and somatic dysfunction of cervical region

M99.02   Segmental and somatic dysfunction of thoracic region

M99.03   Segmental and somatic dysfunction of lumbar region

M99.04   Segmental and somatic dysfunction of sacral region

M99.05   Segmental and somatic dysfunction of pelvic region

M99.06   Segmental and somatic dysfunction of lower extremity

M99.07   Segmental and somatic dysfunction of upper extremity

N Newborn: 0   P Pediatric: 0-17   M Maternity: 12-55   A Adult: 15-124   CH Comorbidity High   CL Comorbidity Low   NCDx Noncancer Dx   PDx Primary Dx

820   ICD-10-CM 2020

M99.Ø8 **Segmental and somatic dysfunction of** rib cage
M99.Ø9 **Segmental and somatic dysfunction of** abdomen and other **regions**

√5ᵗʰ **M99.1 Subluxation complex (vertebral)**

M99.1Ø **Subluxation complex (vertebral) of** head **region**
M99.11 **Subluxation complex (vertebral) of** cervical **region**
M99.12 **Subluxation complex (vertebral) of** thoracic **region**
M99.13 **Subluxation complex (vertebral) of** lumbar **region**
M99.14 **Subluxation complex (vertebral) of** sacral **region**
M99.15 **Subluxation complex (vertebral) of** pelvic **region**
M99.16 **Subluxation complex (vertebral) of** lower extremity
M99.17 **Subluxation complex (vertebral) of** upper extremity
M99.18 **Subluxation complex (vertebral) of** rib cage
M99.19 **Subluxation complex (vertebral) of** abdomen and other **regions**

√5ᵗʰ **M99.2 Subluxation stenosis of neural canal**

M99.2Ø **Subluxation stenosis of neural canal of** head **region**
M99.21 **Subluxation stenosis of neural canal of** cervical **region**
M99.22 **Subluxation stenosis of neural canal of** thoracic **region**
M99.23 **Subluxation stenosis of neural canal of** lumbar **region**
M99.24 **Subluxation stenosis of neural canal of** sacral **region**
M99.25 **Subluxation stenosis of neural canal of** pelvic **region**
M99.26 **Subluxation stenosis of neural canal of** lower extremity
M99.27 **Subluxation stenosis of neural canal of** upper extremity
M99.28 **Subluxation stenosis of neural canal of** rib cage
M99.29 **Subluxation stenosis of neural canal of** abdomen and other **regions**

√5ᵗʰ **M99.3 Osseous stenosis of neural canal**

M99.3Ø **Osseous stenosis of neural canal of** head **region**
M99.31 **Osseous stenosis of neural canal of** cervical **region**
M99.32 **Osseous stenosis of neural canal of** thoracic **region**
M99.33 **Osseous stenosis of neural canal of** lumbar **region**
M99.34 **Osseous stenosis of neural canal of** sacral **region**
M99.35 **Osseous stenosis of neural canal of** pelvic **region**
M99.36 **Osseous stenosis of neural canal of** lower extremity
M99.37 **Osseous stenosis of neural canal of** upper extremity
M99.38 **Osseous stenosis of neural canal of** rib cage
M99.39 **Osseous stenosis of neural canal of** abdomen and other **regions**

√5ᵗʰ **M99.4 Connective tissue stenosis of neural canal**

M99.4Ø **Connective tissue stenosis of neural canal of** head **region**
M99.41 **Connective tissue stenosis of neural canal of** cervical **region**
M99.42 **Connective tissue stenosis of neural canal of** thoracic **region**
M99.43 **Connective tissue stenosis of neural canal of** lumbar **region**
M99.44 **Connective tissue stenosis of neural canal of** sacral **region**
M99.45 **Connective tissue stenosis of neural canal of** pelvic **region**
M99.46 **Connective tissue stenosis of neural canal of** lower extremity
M99.47 **Connective tissue stenosis of neural canal of** upper extremity
M99.48 **Connective tissue stenosis of neural canal of** rib cage
M99.49 **Connective tissue stenosis of neural canal of** abdomen and other **regions**

√5ᵗʰ **M99.5 Intervertebral disc stenosis of neural canal**

M99.5Ø **Intervertebral disc stenosis of neural canal of** head **region**
M99.51 **Intervertebral disc stenosis of neural canal of** cervical **region**
M99.52 **Intervertebral disc stenosis of neural canal of** thoracic **region**
M99.53 **Intervertebral disc stenosis of neural canal of** lumbar **region**
M99.54 **Intervertebral disc stenosis of neural canal of** sacral **region**
M99.55 **Intervertebral disc stenosis of neural canal of** pelvic **region**

M99.56 **Intervertebral disc stenosis of neural canal of** lower extremity
M99.57 **Intervertebral disc stenosis of neural canal of** upper extremity
M99.58 **Intervertebral disc stenosis of neural canal of** rib cage
M99.59 **Intervertebral disc stenosis of neural canal of** abdomen and other **regions**

√5ᵗʰ **M99.6 Osseous and subluxation stenosis of intervertebral foramina**

M99.6Ø **Osseous and subluxation stenosis of intervertebral foramina of** head **region**
M99.61 **Osseous and subluxation stenosis of intervertebral foramina of** cervical **region**
M99.62 **Osseous and subluxation stenosis of intervertebral foramina of** thoracic **region**
M99.63 **Osseous and subluxation stenosis of intervertebral foramina of** lumbar **region**
M99.64 **Osseous and subluxation stenosis of intervertebral foramina of** sacral **region**
M99.65 **Osseous and subluxation stenosis of intervertebral foramina of** pelvic **region**
M99.66 **Osseous and subluxation stenosis of intervertebral foramina of** lower extremity
M99.67 **Osseous and subluxation stenosis of intervertebral foramina of** upper extremity
M99.68 **Osseous and subluxation stenosis of intervertebral foramina of** rib cage
M99.69 **Osseous and subluxation stenosis of intervertebral foramina of** abdomen and other **regions**

√5ᵗʰ **M99.7 Connective tissue and disc stenosis of intervertebral foramina**

M99.7Ø **Connective tissue and disc stenosis of intervertebral foramina of** head **region**
M99.71 **Connective tissue and disc stenosis of intervertebral foramina of** cervical **region**
M99.72 **Connective tissue and disc stenosis of intervertebral foramina of** thoracic **region**
M99.73 **Connective tissue and disc stenosis of intervertebral foramina of** lumbar **region**
M99.74 **Connective tissue and disc stenosis of intervertebral foramina of** sacral **region**
M99.75 **Connective tissue and disc stenosis of intervertebral foramina of** pelvic **region**
M99.76 **Connective tissue and disc stenosis of intervertebral foramina of** lower extremity
M99.77 **Connective tissue and disc stenosis of intervertebral foramina of** upper extremity
M99.78 **Connective tissue and disc stenosis of intervertebral foramina of** rib cage
M99.79 **Connective tissue and disc stenosis of intervertebral foramina of** abdomen and other **regions**

√5ᵗʰ **M99.8 Other biomechanical lesions**

M99.8Ø **Other biomechanical lesions of** head **region**
M99.81 **Other biomechanical lesions of** cervical **region**
M99.82 **Other biomechanical lesions of** thoracic **region**
M99.83 **Other biomechanical lesions of** lumbar **region**
M99.84 **Other biomechanical lesions of** sacral **region**
M99.85 **Other biomechanical lesions of** pelvic **region**
M99.86 **Other biomechanical lesions of** lower extremity
M99.87 **Other biomechanical lesions of** upper extremity
M99.88 **Other biomechanical lesions of** rib cage
M99.89 **Other biomechanical lesions of** abdomen and other regions

M99.9 **Biomechanical lesion, unspecified**

☑ Additional Character Required   √x7ᵗʰ Placeholder Alert   Manifestation   Unspecified Dx   ►◄ Revised Text   ● New Code   ▲ Revised Title

Chapter 14. Diseases of Genitourinary System (NØØ–N99)

Chapter-specific Guidelines with Coding Examples

The chapter-specific guidelines from the ICD-10-CM Official Guidelines for Coding and Reporting have been provided below. Along with these guidelines are coding examples, contained in the shaded boxes, that have been developed to help illustrate the coding and/or sequencing guidance found in these guidelines.

a. Chronic kidney disease

1) Stages of chronic kidney disease (CKD)

The ICD-10-CM classifies CKD based on severity. The severity of CKD is designated by stages 1-5. Stage 2, code N18.2, equates to mild CKD; stage 3, code N18.3, equates to moderate CKD; and stage 4, code N18.4, equates to severe CKD. Code N18.6, End stage renal disease (ESRD), is assigned when the provider has documented end-stage renal disease (ESRD).

If both a stage of CKD and ESRD are documented, assign code N18.6 only.

Stage 5 chronic kidney disease with ESRD requiring chronic dialysis

N18.6	End stage renal disease
Z99.2	Dependence on renal dialysis

Explanation: The diagnostic statement indicates the patient has chronic kidney disease, documented both as stage 5 and as ESRD requiring chronic dialysis. Code N18.6 End stage renal disease (ESRD), is assigned when the provider has documented end-stage-renal disease (ESRD). If both a stage of CKD and ESRD are documented, assign code N18.6 only.

---

2) Chronic kidney disease and kidney transplant status

Patients who have undergone kidney transplant may still have some form of chronic kidney disease (CKD) because the kidney transplant may not fully restore kidney function. Therefore, the presence of CKD alone does not constitute a transplant complication. Assign the appropriate N18 code for the patient's stage of CKD and code Z94.0, Kidney transplant status. If a transplant complication such as failure or rejection or other transplant complication is documented, see section I.C.19.g for information on coding complications of a kidney transplant. If the documentation is unclear as to whether the patient has a complication of the transplant, query the provider.

Patient with residual chronic kidney disease stage 1 after kidney transplant

N18.1	Chronic kidney disease, stage 1
Z94.0	Kidney transplant status

Explanation: Patients who have undergone kidney transplant may still have some form of chronic kidney disease (CKD) because the kidney transplant may not fully restore kidney function. The presence of CKD alone does not constitute a transplant complication. Assign the appropriate N18 code for the patient's stage of CKD and code Z94.0 Kidney transplant status.

---

3) Chronic kidney disease with other conditions

Patients with CKD may also suffer from other serious conditions, most commonly diabetes mellitus and hypertension. The sequencing of the CKD code in relationship to codes for other contributing conditions is based on the conventions in the Tabular List.

See I.C.9. Hypertensive chronic kidney disease.

See I.C.19. Chronic kidney disease and kidney transplant complications.

Type 1 diabetic chronic kidney disease, stage 2

E10.22	Type 1 diabetes mellitus with diabetic chronic kidney disease
N18.2	Chronic kidney disease, stage 2 (mild)

Explanation: Patients with CKD may also suffer from other serious conditions such as diabetes mellitus. The sequencing of the CKD code in relationship to codes for other contributing conditions is based on the conventions in the Tabular List. Diabetic CKD code E10.22 includes an instructional note to "Use additional code to identify stage of chronic kidney disease (N18.1–N18.6)," thus providing sequencing direction.

Chapter 14. Diseases of the Genitourinary System (N00-N99)

EXCLUDES 2   certain conditions originating in the perinatal period (P04-P96)
certain infectious and parasitic diseases (A00-B99)
complications of pregnancy, childbirth and the puerperium (O00-O9A)
congenital malformations, deformations and chromosomal abnormalities (Q00-Q99)
endocrine, nutritional and metabolic diseases (E00-E88)
injury, poisoning and certain other consequences of external causes (S00-T88)
neoplasms (C00-D49)
symptoms, signs and abnormal clinical and laboratory findings, not elsewhere classified (R00-R94)

This chapter contains the following blocks:

N00-N08   Glomerular diseases
N10-N16   Renal tubulo-interstitial diseases
N17-N19   Acute kidney failure and chronic kidney disease
N20-N23   Urolithiasis
N25-N29   Other disorders of kidney and ureter
N30-N39   Other diseases of the urinary system
N40-N53   Diseases of male genital organs
N60-N65   Disorders of breast
N70-N77   Inflammatory diseases of female pelvic organs
N80-N98   Noninflammatory disorders of female genital tract
N99   Intraoperative and postprocedural complications and disorders of genitourinary system, not elsewhere classified

Glomerular diseases (N00-N08)

Code also any associated kidney failure (N17-N19).

EXCLUDES 1   hypertensive chronic kidney disease (I12.-)

DEF: Glomeruli: Clusters of microscopic blood vessels located within the kidneys containing small pores through which waste products are filtered from the blood and urine is formed.

DEF: Glomerulonephritis: Disease of the kidney with diffuse inflammation of the capillary loops of the glomeruli.

√4ᵗʰ **N00**   **Acute nephritic syndrome**

INCLUDES   acute glomerular disease
acute glomerulonephritis
acute nephritis

EXCLUDES 1   acute tubulo-interstitial nephritis (N10)
nephritic syndrome NOS (N05.-)

N00.0   **Acute nephritic syndrome with minor glomerular abnormality**
Acute nephritic syndrome with minimal change lesion

N00.1   **Acute nephritic syndrome with focal and segmental glomerular lesions**
Acute nephritic syndrome with focal and segmental hyalinosis
Acute nephritic syndrome with focal and segmental sclerosis
Acute nephritic syndrome with focal glomerulonephritis

N00.2   **Acute nephritic syndrome with diffuse membranous glomerulonephritis**

N00.3   **Acute nephritic syndrome with diffuse mesangial proliferative glomerulonephritis**

N00.4   **Acute nephritic syndrome with diffuse endocapillary proliferative glomerulonephritis**

N00.5   **Acute nephritic syndrome with diffuse mesangiocapillary glomerulonephritis**
Acute nephritic syndrome with membranoproliferative glomerulonephritis, types 1 and 3, or NOS

N00.6   **Acute nephritic syndrome with dense deposit disease**
Acute nephritic syndrome with membranoproliferative glomerulonephritis, type 2

N00.7   **Acute nephritic syndrome with diffuse crescentic glomerulonephritis**
Acute nephritic syndrome with extracapillary glomerulonephritis

N00.8   **Acute nephritic syndrome with other morphologic changes**
Acute nephritic syndrome with proliferative glomerulonephritis NOS

N00.9   **Acute nephritic syndrome with unspecified morphologic changes**

√4ᵗʰ **N01**   **Rapidly progressive nephritic syndrome**

INCLUDES   rapidly progressive glomerular disease
rapidly progressive glomerulonephritis
rapidly progressive nephritis

EXCLUDES 1   nephritic syndrome NOS (N05.-)

N01.0   **Rapidly progressive nephritic syndrome with minor glomerular abnormality**
Rapidly progressive nephritic syndrome with minimal change lesion

N01.1   **Rapidly progressive nephritic syndrome with focal and segmental glomerular lesions**
Rapidly progressive nephritic syndrome with focal and segmental hyalinosis
Rapidly progressive nephritic syndrome with focal and segmental sclerosis
Rapidly progressive nephritic syndrome with focal glomerulonephritis

N01.2   **Rapidly progressive nephritic syndrome with diffuse membranous glomerulonephritis**

N01.3   **Rapidly progressive nephritic syndrome with diffuse mesangial proliferative glomerulonephritis**

N01.4   **Rapidly progressive nephritic syndrome with diffuse endocapillary proliferative glomerulonephritis**

N01.5   **Rapidly progressive nephritic syndrome with diffuse mesangiocapillary glomerulonephritis**
Rapidly progressive nephritic syndrome with membranoproliferative glomerulonephritis, types 1 and 3, or NOS

N01.6   **Rapidly progressive nephritic syndrome with dense deposit disease**
Rapidly progressive nephritic syndrome with membranoproliferative glomerulonephritis, type 2

N01.7   **Rapidly progressive nephritic syndrome with diffuse crescentic glomerulonephritis**
Rapidly progressive nephritic syndrome with extracapillary glomerulonephritis

N01.8   **Rapidly progressive nephritic syndrome with other morphologic changes**
Rapidly progressive nephritic syndrome with proliferative glomerulonephritis NOS

N01.9   **Rapidly progressive nephritic syndrome with unspecified morphologic changes**

√4ᵗʰ **N02**   **Recurrent and persistent hematuria**

EXCLUDES 1   acute cystitis with hematuria (N30.01)
hematuria NOS (R31.9)
hematuria not associated with specified morphologic lesions (R31.-)

N02.0   **Recurrent and persistent hematuria with minor glomerular abnormality**
Recurrent and persistent hematuria with minimal change lesion

N02.1   **Recurrent and persistent hematuria with focal and segmental glomerular lesions**
Recurrent and persistent hematuria with focal and segmental hyalinosis
Recurrent and persistent hematuria with focal and segmental sclerosis
Recurrent and persistent hematuria with focal glomerulonephritis

N02.2   **Recurrent and persistent hematuria with diffuse membranous glomerulonephritis**

N02.3   **Recurrent and persistent hematuria with diffuse mesangial proliferative glomerulonephritis**

N02.4   **Recurrent and persistent hematuria with diffuse endocapillary proliferative glomerulonephritis**

N02.5   **Recurrent and persistent hematuria with diffuse mesangiocapillary glomerulonephritis**
Recurrent and persistent hematuria with membranoproliferative glomerulonephritis, types 1 and 3, or NOS

N02.6   **Recurrent and persistent hematuria with dense deposit disease**
Recurrent and persistent hematuria with membranoproliferative glomerulonephritis, type 2

N02.7   **Recurrent and persistent hematuria with diffuse crescentic glomerulonephritis**
Recurrent and persistent hematuria with extracapillary glomerulonephritis

N   Newborn: 0   P   Pediatric: 0-17   M   Maternity: 12-55   A   Adult: 15-124   CH   Comorbidity High   CL   Comorbidity Low   NCDx   Noncancer Dx   PDx   Primary Dx

824   ICD-10-CM 2020

N02.8 **Recurrent and persistent hematuria with other morphologic changes**
Recurrent and persistent hematuria with proliferative glomerulonephritis NOS

N02.9 **Recurrent and persistent hematuria with unspecified morphologic changes**
AHA: 2017,2Q,5

☑4ᵗʰ **N03** Chronic **nephritic syndrome**

INCLUDES   chronic glomerular disease
chronic glomerulonephritis
chronic nephritis

EXCLUDES 1   chronic tubulo-interstitial nephritis (N11.-)
diffuse sclerosing glomerulonephritis (N05.8-)
nephritic syndrome NOS (N05.-)

DEF: Slow, progressive type of nephritis characterized by inflammation of the capillary loops in the glomeruli of the kidney, which leads to renal failure.

N03.0 **Chronic nephritic syndrome with** minor glomerular abnormality
Chronic nephritic syndrome with minimal change lesion

N03.1 **Chronic nephritic syndrome with** focal and segmental glomerular lesions
Chronic nephritic syndrome with focal and segmental hyalinosis
Chronic nephritic syndrome with focal and segmental sclerosis
Chronic nephritic syndrome with focal glomerulonephritis

N03.2 **Chronic nephritic syndrome with** diffuse membranous glomerulonephritis

N03.3 **Chronic nephritic syndrome with** diffuse mesangial proliferative glomerulonephritis

N03.4 **Chronic nephritic syndrome with** diffuse endocapillary proliferative glomerulonephritis

N03.5 **Chronic nephritic syndrome with diffuse** mesangiocapillary glomerulonephritis
Chronic nephritic syndrome with membranoproliferative glomerulonephritis, types 1 and 3, or NOS

N03.6 **Chronic nephritic syndrome with** dense deposit disease
Chronic nephritic syndrome with membranoproliferative glomerulonephritis, type 2

N03.7 **Chronic nephritic syndrome with** diffuse crescentic glomerulonephritis
Chronic nephritic syndrome with extracapillary glomerulonephritis

N03.8 **Chronic nephritic syndrome with other morphologic changes**
Chronic nephritic syndrome with proliferative glomerulonephritis NOS

N03.9 **Chronic nephritic syndrome with unspecified morphologic changes**

☑4ᵗʰ **N04** **Nephrotic syndrome**

INCLUDES   congenital nephrotic syndrome
lipoid nephrosis

N04.0 **Nephrotic syndrome with** minor glomerular abnormality
Nephrotic syndrome with minimal change lesion

N04.1 **Nephrotic syndrome with** focal and segmental glomerular lesions
Nephrotic syndrome with focal and segmental hyalinosis
Nephrotic syndrome with focal and segmental sclerosis
Nephrotic syndrome with focal glomerulonephritis

N04.2 **Nephrotic syndrome with** diffuse membranous glomerulonephritis

N04.3 **Nephrotic syndrome with** diffuse mesangial proliferative glomerulonephritis

N04.4 **Nephrotic syndrome with** diffuse endocapillary proliferative glomerulonephritis

N04.5 **Nephrotic syndrome with** diffuse mesangiocapillary glomerulonephritis
Nephrotic syndrome with membranoproliferative glomerulonephritis, types 1 and 3, or NOS

N04.6 **Nephrotic syndrome with** dense deposit disease
Nephrotic syndrome with membranoproliferative glomerulonephritis, type 2

N04.7 **Nephrotic syndrome with** diffuse crescentic glomerulonephritis
Nephrotic syndrome with extracapillary glomerulonephritis

N04.8 **Nephrotic syndrome with other morphologic changes**
Nephrotic syndrome with proliferative glomerulonephritis NOS

N04.9 **Nephrotic syndrome with unspecified morphologic changes**

☑4ᵗʰ **N05** **Unspecified nephritic syndrome**

INCLUDES   glomerular disease NOS
glomerulonephritis NOS
nephritis NOS
nephropathy NOS and renal disease NOS with morphological lesion specified in .0-.8

EXCLUDES 1   nephropathy NOS with no stated morphological lesion (N28.9)
renal disease NOS with no stated morphological lesion (N28.9)
tubulo-interstitial nephritis NOS (N12)

N05.0 **Unspecified nephritic syndrome with** minor glomerular abnormality
Unspecified nephritic syndrome with minimal change lesion

N05.1 **Unspecified nephritic syndrome with** focal and segmental glomerular lesions
Unspecified nephritic syndrome with focal and segmental hyalinosis
Unspecified nephritic syndrome with focal and segmental sclerosis
Unspecified nephritic syndrome with focal glomerulonephritis

N05.2 **Unspecified nephritic syndrome with** diffuse membranous glomerulonephritis

N05.3 **Unspecified nephritic syndrome with** diffuse mesangial proliferative glomerulonephritis

N05.4 **Unspecified nephritic syndrome with** diffuse endocapillary proliferative glomerulonephritis

N05.5 **Unspecified nephritic syndrome with** diffuse mesangiocapillary glomerulonephritis
Unspecified nephritic syndrome with membranoproliferative glomerulonephritis, types 1 and 3, or NOS

N05.6 **Unspecified nephritic syndrome with** dense deposit disease
Unspecified nephritic syndrome with membranoproliferative glomerulonephritis, type 2

N05.7 **Unspecified nephritic syndrome with** diffuse crescentic glomerulonephritis
Unspecified nephritic syndrome with extracapillary glomerulonephritis

N05.8 **Unspecified nephritic syndrome with other morphologic changes**
Unspecified nephritic syndrome with proliferative glomerulonephritis NOS

N05.9 **Unspecified nephritic syndrome with unspecified morphologic changes**

☑4ᵗʰ **N06** **Isolated proteinuria with specified morphological lesion**

EXCLUDES 1   proteinuria not associated with specific morphologic lesions (R80.0)

N06.0 **Isolated proteinuria with** minor glomerular abnormality
Isolated proteinuria with minimal change lesion

N06.1 **Isolated proteinuria with** focal and segmental glomerular lesions
Isolated proteinuria with focal and segmental hyalinosis
Isolated proteinuria with focal and segmental sclerosis
Isolated proteinuria with focal glomerulonephritis

N06.2 **Isolated proteinuria with** diffuse membranous glomerulonephritis

N06.3 **Isolated proteinuria with** diffuse mesangial proliferative glomerulonephritis

N06.4 **Isolated proteinuria with** diffuse endocapillary proliferative glomerulonephritis

N06.5 **Isolated proteinuria with** diffuse mesangiocapillary glomerulonephritis
Isolated proteinuria with membranoproliferative glomerulonephritis, types 1 and 3, or NOS

N06.6 **Isolated proteinuria with** dense deposit disease
Isolated proteinuria with membranoproliferative glomerulonephritis, type 2

N06.7 **Isolated proteinuria with** diffuse crescentic glomerulonephritis
Isolated proteinuria with extracapillary glomerulonephritis

N06.8 **Isolated proteinuria with other morphologic lesion**
Isolated proteinuria with proliferative glomerulonephritis NOS

N06.9 **Isolated proteinuria with unspecified morphologic lesion**

☑ Additional Character Required   ✓x7ᵗʰ Placeholder Alert   Manifestation   Unspecified Dx   ▶◀ Revised Text   ● New Code   ▲ Revised Title

✓4ᵗʰ N07 Hereditary nephropathy, not elsewhere classified

EXCLUDES 2   Alport's syndrome (Q87.81-)
hereditary amyloid nephropathy (E85.-)
nail patella syndrome (Q87.2)
non-neuropathic heredofamilial amyloidosis (E85.-)

N07.0 Hereditary nephropathy, not elsewhere classified with minor glomerular abnormality
Hereditary nephropathy, not elsewhere classified with minimal change lesion

N07.1 Hereditary nephropathy, not elsewhere classified with focal and segmental glomerular lesions
Hereditary nephropathy, not elsewhere classified with focal and segmental hyalinosis
Hereditary nephropathy, not elsewhere classified with focal and segmental sclerosis
Hereditary nephropathy, not elsewhere classified with focal glomerulonephritis

N07.2 Hereditary nephropathy, not elsewhere classified with diffuse membranous glomerulonephritis

N07.3 Hereditary nephropathy, not elsewhere classified with diffuse mesangial proliferative glomerulonephritis

N07.4 Hereditary nephropathy, not elsewhere classified with diffuse endocapillary proliferative glomerulonephritis

N07.5 Hereditary nephropathy, not elsewhere classified with diffuse mesangiocapillary glomerulonephritis
Hereditary nephropathy, not elsewhere classified with membranoproliferative glomerulonephritis, types 1 and 3, or NOS

N07.6 Hereditary nephropathy, not elsewhere classified with dense deposit disease
Hereditary nephropathy, not elsewhere classified with membranoproliferative glomerulonephritis, type 2

N07.7 Hereditary nephropathy, not elsewhere classified with diffuse crescentic glomerulonephritis
Hereditary nephropathy, not elsewhere classified with extracapillary glomerulonephritis

N07.8 Hereditary nephropathy, not elsewhere classified with other morphologic lesions
Hereditary nephropathy, not elsewhere classified with proliferative glomerulonephritis NOS

N07.9 Hereditary nephropathy, not elsewhere classified with unspecified morphologic lesions

N08 Glomerular disorders in diseases classified elsewhere
Glomerulonephritis
Nephritis
Nephropathy
Code first underlying disease, such as:
amyloidosis (E85.-)
congenital syphilis (A50.5)
cryoglobulinemia (D89.1)
disseminated intravascular coagulation (D65)
gout (M1A.-, M10.-)
microscopic polyangiitis (M31.7)
multiple myeloma (C90.0-)
sepsis (A40.0-A41.9)
sickle-cell disease (D57.0-D57.8)

EXCLUDES 1   glomerulonephritis, nephritis and nephropathy (in):
antiglomerular basement membrane disease (M31.0)
diabetes (E08-E13 with .21)
gonococcal (A54.21)
Goodpasture's syndrome (M31.0)
hemolytic-uremic syndrome (D59.3)
lupus (M32.14)
mumps (B26.83)
syphilis (A52.75)
systemic lupus erythematosus (M32.14)
Wegener's granulomatosis (M31.31)
pyelonephritis in diseases classified elsewhere (N16)
renal tubulo-interstitial disorders classified elsewhere (N16)

Renal tubulo-interstitial diseases (N10-N16)

INCLUDES   pyelonephritis
EXCLUDES 1   pyeloureteritis cystica (N28.85)

N10 Acute pyelonephritis
Acute infectious interstitial nephritis
Acute pyelitis
Acute tubulo-interstitial nephritis
Hemoglobin nephrosis
Myoglobin nephrosis
Use additional code (B95-B97), to identify infectious agent

✓4ᵗʰ N11 Chronic tubulo-interstitial nephritis
INCLUDES   chronic infectious interstitial nephritis
chronic pyelitis
chronic pyelonephritis
Use additional code (B95-B97), to identify infectious agent

N11.0 Nonobstructive reflux-associated chronic pyelonephritis `CH`
Pyelonephritis (chronic) associated with (vesicoureteral) reflux
EXCLUDES 1   vesicoureteral reflux NOS (N13.70)

N11.1 Chronic obstructive pyelonephritis `CH`
Pyelonephritis (chronic) associated with anomaly of pelviureteric junction
Pyelonephritis (chronic) associated with anomaly of pyeloureteric junction
Pyelonephritis (chronic) associated with crossing of vessel
Pyelonephritis (chronic) associated with kinking of ureter
Pyelonephritis (chronic) associated with obstruction of ureter
Pyelonephritis (chronic) associated with stricture of pelviureteric junction
Pyelonephritis (chronic) associated with stricture of ureter
EXCLUDES 1   calculous pyelonephritis (N20.9)
obstructive uropathy (N13.-)

N11.8 Other chronic tubulo-interstitial nephritis `CH`
Nonobstructive chronic pyelonephritis NOS

N11.9 Chronic tubulo-interstitial nephritis, unspecified
Chronic interstitial nephritis NOS
Chronic pyelitis NOS
Chronic pyelonephritis NOS

N12 Tubulo-interstitial nephritis, not specified as acute or chronic
Interstitial nephritis NOS
Pyelitis NOS
Pyelonephritis NOS
EXCLUDES 1   calculous pyelonephritis (N20.9)

✓4th N13 Obstructive and reflux uropathy

> EXCLUDES 2   calculus of kidney and ureter without hydronephrosis (N20.-)
> congenital obstructive defects of renal pelvis and ureter (Q62.0-Q62.3)
> hydronephrosis with ureteropelvic junction obstruction (Q62.11)
> obstructive pyelonephritis (N11.1)

DEF: Hydronephrosis: Distension of the kidney caused by an accumulation of urine that cannot flow out due to an obstruction that may be caused by conditions such as kidney stones or vesicoureteral reflux.

N13.0 Hydronephrosis with ureteropelvic junction obstruction
Hydronephrosis due to acquired occlusion of ureteropelvic junction

> EXCLUDES 2   hydronephrosis with ureteropelvic junction obstruction due to calculus (N13.2)

AHA: 2016,4Q,43

Hydronephrosis/UPJ Obstruction

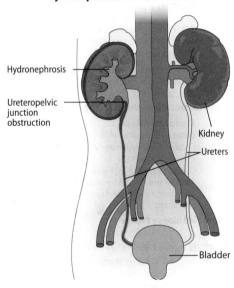

Hydronephrosis

Ureteropelvic junction obstruction

Kidney

Ureters

Bladder

N13.1 Hydronephrosis with ureteral stricture, not elsewhere classified

> EXCLUDES 1   hydronephrosis with ureteral stricture with infection (N13.6)

N13.2 Hydronephrosis with renal and ureteral calculous obstruction   `CH`

> EXCLUDES 1   hydronephrosis with renal and ureteral calculous obstruction with infection (N13.6)

✓5th N13.3 Other and unspecified hydronephrosis

> EXCLUDES 1   hydronephrosis with infection (N13.6)

    N13.30 Unspecified hydronephrosis
    N13.39 Other hydronephrosis

N13.4 Hydroureter

> EXCLUDES 1   congenital hydroureter (Q62.3-)
> hydroureter with infection (N13.6)
> vesicoureteral-reflux with hydroureter (N13.73-)

DEF: Abnormal enlargement or distension of the ureter with water or urine caused by an obstruction.

N13.5 Crossing vessel and stricture of ureter without hydronephrosis
Kinking and stricture of ureter without hydronephrosis

> EXCLUDES 1   crossing vessel and stricture of ureter without hydronephrosis with infection (N13.6)

N13.6 Pyonephrosis
Conditions in N13.0-N13.5 with infection
Obstructive uropathy with infection
Use additional code (B95-B97), to identify infectious agent
AHA: 2018,2Q,21

✓5th N13.7 Vesicoureteral-reflux

> EXCLUDES 1   reflux-associated pyelonephritis (N11.0)

DEF: Urine passage from the bladder flows backward up into the ureter and kidneys that can lead to bacterial infection and an increase in hydrostatic pressure, causing kidney damage.

Vesicoureteral Reflux

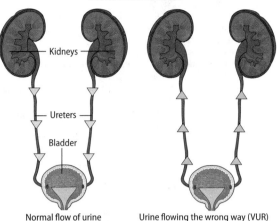

Kidneys

Ureters

Bladder

Normal flow of urine   Urine flowing the wrong way (VUR)

    N13.70 Vesicoureteral-reflux, unspecified
       Vesicoureteral-reflux NOS
    N13.71 Vesicoureteral-reflux without reflux nephropathy
    ✓6th N13.72 Vesicoureteral-reflux with reflux nephropathy without hydroureter
       N13.721 Vesicoureteral-reflux with reflux nephropathy without hydroureter, unilateral
       N13.722 Vesicoureteral-reflux with reflux nephropathy without hydroureter, bilateral
       N13.729 Vesicoureteral-reflux with reflux nephropathy without hydroureter, unspecified
    ✓6th N13.73 Vesicoureteral-reflux with reflux nephropathy with hydroureter
       N13.731 Vesicoureteral-reflux with reflux nephropathy with hydroureter, unilateral
       N13.732 Vesicoureteral-reflux with reflux nephropathy with hydroureter, bilateral
       N13.739 Vesicoureteral-reflux with reflux nephropathy with hydroureter, unspecified

N13.8 Other obstructive and reflux uropathy
Urinary tract obstruction due to specified cause
Code first, if applicable, any causal condition, such as:
    enlarged prostate (N40.1)

N13.9 Obstructive and reflux uropathy, unspecified
Urinary tract obstruction NOS

✓4th N14 Drug- and heavy-metal-induced tubulo-interstitial and tubular conditions
Code first poisoning due to drug or toxin, if applicable (T36-T65 with fifth or sixth character 1-4 or 6)
Use additional code for adverse effect, if applicable, to identify drug (T36-T50 with fifth or sixth character 5)

N14.0 Analgesic nephropathy
N14.1 Nephropathy induced by other drugs, medicaments and biological substances
N14.2 Nephropathy induced by unspecified drug, medicament or biological substance
N14.3 Nephropathy induced by heavy metals
N14.4 Toxic nephropathy, not elsewhere classified

✓4th N15 Other renal tubulo-interstitial diseases

N15.0 Balkan nephropathy
Balkan endemic nephropathy
N15.1 Renal and perinephric abscess
N15.8 Other specified renal tubulo-interstitial diseases
N15.9 Renal tubulo-interstitial disease, unspecified
Infection of kidney NOS

> EXCLUDES 1   urinary tract infection NOS (N39.0)

☑ Additional Character Required   ✓x7th Placeholder Alert   Manifestation   Unspecified Dx   ►◄ Revised Text   ● New Code   ▲ Revised Title

ICD-10-CM 2020   **827**

N13–N15.9

N16 Renal tubulo-interstitial disorders in diseases classified elsewhere

Pyelonephritis
Tubulo-interstitial nephritis
Code first underlying disease, such as:
brucellosis (A23.0-A23.9)
cryoglobulinemia (D89.1)
glycogen storage disease (E74.0)
leukemia (C91-C95)
lymphoma (C81.0-C85.9, C96.0-C96.9)
multiple myeloma (C90.0-)
sepsis (A40.0-A41.9)
Wilson's disease (E83.0)

EXCLUDES 1 diphtheritic pyelonephritis and tubulo-interstitial nephritis (A36.84)
pyelonephritis and tubulo-interstitial nephritis in candidiasis (B37.49)
pyelonephritis and tubulo-interstitial nephritis in cystinosis (E72.04)
pyelonephritis and tubulo-interstitial nephritis in salmonella infection (A02.25)
pyelonephritis and tubulo-interstitial nephritis in sarcoidosis (D86.84)
pyelonephritis and tubulo-interstitial nephritis in sicca syndrome [Sjogren's] (M35.04)
pyelonephritis and tubulo-interstitial nephritis in systemic lupus erythematosus (M32.15)
pyelonephritis and tubulo-interstitial nephritis in toxoplasmosis (B58.83)
renal tubular degeneration in diabetes (E08-E13 with .29)
syphilitic pyelonephritis and tubulo-interstitial nephritis (A52.75)

Acute kidney failure and chronic kidney disease (N17-N19)

EXCLUDES 2 congenital renal failure (P96.0)
drug- and heavy-metal-induced tubulo-interstitial and tubular conditions (N14.-)
extrarenal uremia (R39.2)
hemolytic-uremic syndrome (D59.3)
hepatorenal syndrome (K76.7)
postpartum hepatorenal syndrome (O90.4)
posttraumatic renal failure (T79.5)
prerenal uremia (R39.2)
renal failure complicating abortion or ectopic or molar pregnancy (O00-O07, O08.4)
renal failure following labor and delivery (O90.4)
renal failure postprocedural (N99.0)

✓4ᵗʰ **N17 Acute kidney failure**

Code also associated underlying condition
EXCLUDES 1 posttraumatic renal failure (T79.5)
AHA: 2019,2Q,7; 2019,1Q,12; 2013,4Q,124

N17.0 Acute kidney failure with tubular necrosis `NC Dx`

Acute tubular necrosis
Renal tubular necrosis
Tubular necrosis NOS

N17.1 Acute kidney failure with acute cortical necrosis `NC Dx`

Acute cortical necrosis
Cortical necrosis NOS
Renal cortical necrosis

N17.2 Acute kidney failure with medullary necrosis `NC Dx`

Medullary [papillary] necrosis NOS
Acute medullary [papillary] necrosis
Renal medullary [papillary] necrosis

N17.8 Other acute kidney failure `NC Dx`

N17.9 Acute kidney failure, unspecified `NC Dx`

Acute kidney injury (nontraumatic)
EXCLUDES 2 traumatic kidney injury (S37.0-)

✓4ᵗʰ **N18 Chronic kidney disease (CKD)**

Code first any associated:
diabetic chronic kidney disease (E08.22, E09.22, E10.22, E11.22, E13.22)
hypertensive chronic kidney disease (I12.-, I13.-)
Use additional code to identify kidney transplant status, if applicable, (Z94.0)
AHA: 2013,1Q,24
TIP: CKD/ESRD occurring in an individual with a history of kidney transplant should not be assumed to be a transplant complication unless specifically indicated as such by provider documentation.
TIP: The term "chronic renal impairment" should not be interpreted as CKD or chronic renal insufficiency and should be coded as N28.9.

N18.1 Chronic kidney disease, stage 1 `CH`

N18.2 Chronic kidney disease, stage 2 (mild) `CH`

N18.3 Chronic kidney disease, stage 3 (moderate) `CH`

N18.4 Chronic kidney disease, stage 4 (severe) `CH`

N18.5 Chronic kidney disease, stage 5 `CH`

EXCLUDES 1 chronic kidney disease, stage 5 requiring chronic dialysis (N18.6)
DEF: End-stage renal disease (ESRD) with a GFR value of 15 ml/min or less not yet requiring chronic dialysis.

N18.6 End stage renal disease `CH` `NC Dx`

Chronic kidney disease requiring chronic dialysis
Use additional code to identify dialysis status (Z99.2)
AHA: 2016,3Q,22; 2016,1Q,12; 2013,4Q,124-125

N18.9 Chronic kidney disease, unspecified `NC Dx`

Chronic renal disease
Chronic renal failure NOS
Chronic renal insufficiency
Chronic uremia NOS
Diffuse sclerosing glomerulonephritis NOS
TIP: This code would be viewed by Medicare as a questionable admission if used as the admitting diagnosis for a hospice encounter.

N19 Unspecified kidney failure `NC Dx`

Uremia NOS
EXCLUDES 1 acute kidney failure (N17.-)
chronic kidney disease (N18.-)
chronic uremia (N18.9)
extrarenal uremia (R39.2)
prerenal uremia (R39.2)
renal insufficiency (acute) (N28.9)
uremia of newborn (P96.0)
TIP: This code would be viewed by Medicare as a questionable admission if used as the admitting diagnosis for a hospice encounter.

Urolithiasis (N20-N23)

AHA: 2017,1Q,5; 2015,2Q,8
TIP: Codes from this code block can be assigned based on the diagnosis listed in a radiology report when authenticated by a radiologist and available at the time of code assignment.

✓4ᵗʰ **N20 Calculus of kidney and ureter**

Calculous pyelonephritis
EXCLUDES 1 nephrocalcinosis (E83.5)
that with hydronephrosis (N13.2)

N20.0 Calculus of kidney `CH`

Nephrolithiasis NOS
Renal calculus
Renal stone
Staghorn calculus
Stone in kidney

N20.1 Calculus of ureter

Ureteric stone
AHA: 2016,3Q,22

N20.2 Calculus of kidney with calculus of ureter `CH`

N20.9 Urinary calculus, unspecified

✓4ᵗʰ **N21 Calculus of lower urinary tract**

INCLUDES calculus of lower urinary tract with cystitis and urethritis

N21.0 Calculus in bladder

Calculus in diverticulum of bladder
Urinary bladder stone
EXCLUDES 2 staghorn calculus (N20.0)

(handwritten annotations in margin:)
Oct 1 2021
N18.30 - N18.39
N18.31 - 3A
N18.32 - 3B

N Newborn: 0   P Pediatric: 0-17   M Maternity: 12-55   A Adult: 15-124   CH Comorbidity High   CL Comorbidity Low   NC Dx Noncancer Dx   PDx Primary Dx

N21.1   **Calculus in** urethra
> EXCLUDES 2   calculus of prostate (N42.0)

N21.8   **Other lower urinary tract calculus**

N21.9   **Calculus of lower urinary tract, unspecified**
> EXCLUDES 1   calculus of urinary tract NOS (N20.9)

N22   *Calculus of urinary tract in diseases classified elsewhere*
> Code first underlying disease, such as:
> gout (M1A.-, M10.-)
> schistosomiasis (B65.0-B65.9)

N23   **Unspecified renal colic**

Other disorders of kidney and ureter (N25-N29)

> EXCLUDES 2   disorders of kidney and ureter with urolithiasis (N20-N23)

✓4th N25   **Disorders resulting from impaired renal tubular function**

N25.0   **Renal osteodystrophy**
> Azotemic osteodystrophy
> Phosphate-losing tubular disorders
> Renal rickets
> Renal short stature
> EXCLUDES 2   metabolic disorders classifiable to E70-E88
> **DEF:** Various bone diseases occurring when kidney function is impaired or fails. Abnormal levels of phosphorous and calcium can lead to osteomalacia, osteoporosis, or osteosclerosis.

N25.1   **Nephrogenic diabetes insipidus**   CH
> EXCLUDES 1   diabetes insipidus NOS (E23.2)
> **DEF:** Type of diabetes due to the inability of renal tubules to reabsorb water back into the body. It is not responsive to vasopressin (antidiuretic hormone) and it is characterized by excessive thirst and excessive urine production. It may develop into chronic renal insufficiency.

✓6th N25.8   **Other disorders resulting from impaired renal tubular function**

N25.81   **Secondary hyperparathyroidism of renal origin**
> EXCLUDES 1   secondary hyperparathyroidism, non-renal (E21.1)
> EXCLUDES 2   metabolic disorders classifiable to E70-E88
> **DEF:** Parathyroid dysfunction caused by chronic renal failure. Phosphate clearance and vitamin D production is impaired resulting in lowered calcium blood levels and an excessive production of parathyroid hormone.

N25.89   **Other disorders resulting from impaired renal tubular function**
> Hypokalemic nephropathy
> Lightwood-Albright syndrome
> Renal tubular acidosis NOS

N25.9   **Disorder resulting from impaired renal tubular function, unspecified**

✓4th N26   **Unspecified contracted kidney**
> EXCLUDES 1   contracted kidney due to hypertension (I12.-)
> diffuse sclerosing glomerulonephritis (N05.8-)
> hypertensive nephrosclerosis (arteriolar) (arteriosclerotic) (I12.-)
> small kidney of unknown cause (N27.-)

N26.1   **Atrophy of kidney (terminal)**

N26.2   **Page kidney**

N26.9   **Renal sclerosis, unspecified**

✓4th N27   **Small kidney of unknown cause**
> INCLUDES   oligonephronia

N27.0   **Small kidney, unilateral**

N27.1   **Small kidney, bilateral**

N27.9   **Small kidney, unspecified**

✓4th N28   **Other disorders of kidney and ureter, not elsewhere classified**

N28.0   **Ischemia and infarction of kidney**
> Renal artery embolism
> Renal artery obstruction
> Renal artery occlusion
> Renal artery thrombosis
> Renal infarct
> EXCLUDES 1   atherosclerosis of renal artery (extrarenal part) (I70.1)
> congenital stenosis of renal artery (Q27.1)
> Goldblatt's kidney (I70.1)

N28.1   **Cyst of kidney, acquired**
> Cyst (multiple) (solitary) of kidney (acquired)
> EXCLUDES 1   cystic kidney disease (congenital) (Q61.-)

✓5th N28.8   **Other specified disorders of kidney and ureter**
> EXCLUDES 1   hydroureter (N13.4)
> ureteric stricture with hydronephrosis (N13.1)
> ureteric stricture without hydronephrosis (N13.5)

N28.81   **Hypertrophy of kidney**

N28.82   **Megaloureter**

N28.83   **Nephroptosis**

N28.84   **Pyelitis cystica**

N28.85   **Pyeloureteritis cystica**

N28.86   **Ureteritis cystica**

N28.89   **Other specified disorders of kidney and ureter**

N28.9   **Disorder of kidney and ureter, unspecified**
> Nephropathy NOS
> Renal disease (acute) NOS
> Renal insufficiency (acute)
> EXCLUDES 1   chronic renal insufficiency (N18.9)
> unspecified nephritic syndrome (N05.-)
> **AHA:** 2016,1Q,13
> **TIP:** The term "chronic renal impairment" should not be interpreted as CKD or chronic renal insufficiency and should be coded as N28.9.

N29   *Other disorders of kidney and ureter in diseases classified*   CH *elsewhere*
> Code first underlying disease, such as:
> amyloidosis (E85.-)
> nephrocalcinosis (E83.5)
> schistosomiasis (B65.0-B65.9)
> EXCLUDES 1   disorders of kidney and ureter in:
> cystinosis (E72.0)
> gonorrhea (A54.21)
> syphilis (A52.75)
> tuberculosis (A18.11)

Other diseases of the urinary system (N30-N39)

> EXCLUDES 1   urinary infection (complicating):
> abortion or ectopic or molar pregnancy (O00-O07, O08.8)
> pregnancy, childbirth and the puerperium (O23.-, O75.3, O86.2-)

✓4th N30   **Cystitis**
> Use additional code to identify infectious agent (B95-B97)
> EXCLUDES 1   prostatocystitis (N41.3)
> **AHA:** 2017,1Q,6
> **DEF:** Inflammation of the urinary bladder. Symptoms include dysuria, frequency of urination, urgency, and hematuria.

✓5th N30.0   **Acute** cystitis
> EXCLUDES 1   irradiation cystitis (N30.4-)
> trigonitis (N30.3-)

N30.00   **Acute cystitis** without hematuria

N30.01   **Acute cystitis** with hematuria

✓5th N30.1   **Interstitial** cystitis (chronic)

N30.10   **Interstitial cystitis (chronic)** without hematuria

N30.11   **Interstitial cystitis (chronic)** with hematuria

✓5th N30.2   **Other** chronic cystitis

N30.20   **Other chronic cystitis** without hematuria

N30.21   **Other chronic cystitis** with hematuria

✓5th N30.3   **Trigonitis**
> Urethrotrigonitis

N30.30   **Trigonitis** without hematuria

N30.31   **Trigonitis** with hematuria

✓5th N30.4   **Irradiation** cystitis

N30.40   **Irradiation cystitis** without hematuria

N30.41   **Irradiation cystitis** with hematuria

✓5th N30.8   **Other cystitis**
> Abscess of bladder

N30.80   **Other cystitis** without hematuria

N30.81   **Other cystitis** with hematuria

✓5th N30.9   **Cystitis, unspecified**

N30.90   **Cystitis, unspecified** without hematuria

N30.91   **Cystitis, unspecified** with hematuria

☑ Additional Character Required   ✓x7th Placeholder Alert   Manifestation   Unspecified Dx   ►◄ Revised Text   ● New Code   ▲ Revised Title

ICD-10-CM 2020   829

Chapter 14. Diseases of the Genitourinary System

✔4ᵗʰ **N31** **Neuromuscular dysfunction of bladder, not elsewhere classified**
Use additional code to identify any associated urinary incontinence (N39.3-N39.4-)
EXCLUDES 1　cord bladder NOS (G95.89)
neurogenic bladder due to cauda equina syndrome (G83.4)
neuromuscular dysfunction due to spinal cord lesion (G95.89)

N31.0 **Uninhibited** neuropathic bladder, not elsewhere classified　CH

N31.1 **Reflex** neuropathic bladder, not elsewhere classified　CH

N31.2 **Flaccid** neuropathic bladder, not elsewhere classified
Atonic (motor) (sensory) neuropathic bladder
Autonomous neuropathic bladder
Nonreflex neuropathic bladder

N31.8 **Other neuromuscular dysfunction of bladder**

N31.9 **Neuromuscular dysfunction of bladder, unspecified**　CH
Neurogenic bladder dysfunction NOS

✔4ᵗʰ **N32** **Other disorders of bladder**
EXCLUDES 2　calculus of bladder (N21.0)
cystocele (N81.1-)
hernia or prolapse of bladder, female (N81.1-)

N32.0 **Bladder-neck obstruction**
Bladder-neck stenosis (acquired)
EXCLUDES 1　congenital bladder-neck obstruction (Q64.3-)
DEF: Bladder outlet and vesicourethral obstruction that occurs as a consequence of benign prostatic hypertrophy or prostatic cancer. It may also occur in either sex due to strictures, radiation, cystoscopy, catheterization, injury, infection, blood clots, bladder cancer, impaction, or other disease that compresses the bladder neck.

N32.1 **Vesicointestinal fistula**
Vesicorectal fistula

N32.2 **Vesical fistula, not elsewhere classified**
EXCLUDES 1　fistula between bladder and female genital tract (N82.0-N82.1)

N32.3 **Diverticulum of bladder**
EXCLUDES 1　congenital diverticulum of bladder (Q64.6)
diverticulitis of bladder (N30.8-)

✔5ᵗʰ **N32.8** **Other specified disorders of bladder**

N32.81 **Overactive bladder**
Detrusor muscle hyperactivity
EXCLUDES 1　frequent urination due to specified bladder condition — code to condition
DEF: Sudden involuntary contractions of the muscular wall of the bladder that results in a sudden, strong urge to urinate.

N32.89 **Other specified disorders of bladder**
Bladder hemorrhage
Bladder hypertrophy
Calcified bladder
Contracted bladder

N32.9 **Bladder disorder, unspecified**

N33 *Bladder disorders in diseases classified elsewhere*
Code first underlying disease, such as:
schistosomiasis (B65.0-B65.9)
EXCLUDES 1　bladder disorder in syphilis (A52.76)
bladder disorder in tuberculosis (A18.12)
candidal cystitis (B37.41)
chlamydial cystitis (A56.01)
cystitis in gonorrhea (A54.01)
cystitis in neurogenic bladder (N31.-)
diphtheritic cystitis (A36.85)
neurogenic bladder (N31.-)
syphilitic cystitis (A52.76)
trichomonal cystitis (A59.03)

✔4ᵗʰ **N34** **Urethritis and urethral syndrome**
Use additional code (B95-B97), to identify infectious agent
EXCLUDES 2　Reiter's disease (M02.3-)
urethritis in diseases with a predominantly sexual mode of transmission (A50-A64)
urethrotrigonitis (N30.3-)
AHA: 2017,1Q,6

N34.0 **Urethral abscess**
Abscess (of) Cowper's gland
Abscess (of) Littré's gland
Abscess (of) urethral (gland)
Periurethral abscess
EXCLUDES 1　urethral caruncle (N36.2)

N34.1 **Nonspecific urethritis**
Nongonococcal urethritis
Nonvenereal urethritis

N34.2 **Other urethritis**
Meatitis, urethral
Postmenopausal urethritis
Ulcer of urethra (meatus) — P. u. ?
Urethritis NOS

N34.3 **Urethral syndrome, unspecified**

✔4ᵗʰ **N35** **Urethral stricture**
EXCLUDES 1　congenital urethral stricture (Q64.3-)
postprocedural urethral stricture (N99.1-)
AHA: 2018,4Q,21-22

✔5ᵗʰ **N35.0** **Post-traumatic** urethral stricture
Urethral stricture due to injury
EXCLUDES 1　postprocedural urethral stricture (N99.1-)

✔6ᵗʰ **N35.01** **Post-traumatic urethral stricture, male**

N35.010 **Post-traumatic urethral stricture, male, meatal**　♂

N35.011 **Post-traumatic bulbous urethral stricture**　♂

N35.012 **Post-traumatic membranous urethral stricture**　♂

N35.013 **Post-traumatic anterior urethral stricture**　♂

N35.014 **Post-traumatic urethral stricture, male, unspecified**　♂

N35.016 **Post-traumatic urethral stricture, male, overlapping sites**　♂

✔6ᵗʰ **N35.02** **Post-traumatic urethral stricture, female**

N35.021 **Urethral stricture due to childbirth**　♀

N35.028 **Other post-traumatic urethral stricture, female**　♀

✔5ᵗʰ **N35.1** **Postinfective** urethral stricture, not elsewhere classified
EXCLUDES 1　gonococcal urethral stricture (A54.01)
syphilitic urethral stricture (A52.76)
urethral stricture associated with schistosomiasis (B65.-, N29)

✔6ᵗʰ **N35.11** **Postinfective urethral stricture, not elsewhere classified, male**

N35.111 **Postinfective urethral stricture, not elsewhere classified, male, meatal**　♂

N35.112 **Postinfective bulbous urethral stricture, not elsewhere classified, male**　♂

N35.113 **Postinfective membranous urethral stricture, not elsewhere classified, male**　♂

N35.114 **Postinfective anterior urethral stricture, not elsewhere classified, male**　♂

N35.116 **Postinfective urethral stricture, not elsewhere classified, male, overlapping sites**　♂

N35.119 **Postinfective urethral stricture, not elsewhere classified, male, unspecified**　♂

N35.12 **Postinfective urethral stricture, not elsewhere classified, female**　♀

N35.8 Other urethral stricture
   EXCLUDES 1   postprocedural urethral stricture (N99.1-)
- **N35.81 Other urethral stricture, male**
  - **N35.811 Other urethral stricture, male, meatal** ♂
  - **N35.812 Other urethral bulbous stricture, male** ♂
  - **N35.813 Other membranous urethral stricture, male** ♂
  - **N35.814 Other anterior urethral stricture, male** ♂
  - **N35.816 Other urethral stricture, male, overlapping sites** ♂
  - **N35.819 Other urethral stricture, male, unspecified site** ♂
- **N35.82 Other urethral stricture, female** ♀
- **N35.9 Urethral stricture, unspecified**
  - **N35.91 Urethral stricture, unspecified, male**
    - **N35.911 Unspecified urethral stricture, male, meatal** ♂
    - **N35.912 Unspecified bulbous urethral stricture, male** ♂
    - **N35.913 Unspecified membranous urethral stricture, male** ♂
    - **N35.914 Unspecified anterior urethral stricture, male** ♂
    - **N35.916 Unspecified urethral stricture, male, overlapping sites** ♂
    - **N35.919 Unspecified urethral stricture, male, unspecified site** ♂
      - Pinhole meatus NOS
      - Urethral stricture NOS
  - **N35.92 Unspecified urethral stricture, female** ♀

N36 Other disorders of urethra
- **N36.0 Urethral fistula**
  - Urethroperineal fistula
  - Urethrorectal fistula
  - Urinary fistula NOS
  - EXCLUDES 1   urethroscrotal fistula (N50.89)
  - urethrovaginal fistula (N82.1)
  - urethrovesicovaginal fistula (N82.1)
- **N36.1 Urethral diverticulum**
- **N36.2 Urethral caruncle**
- **N36.4 Urethral functional and muscular disorders**
  - Use additional code to identify associated urinary stress incontinence (N39.3)
  - **N36.41 Hypermobility of urethra**
  - **N36.42 Intrinsic sphincter deficiency (ISD)**
  - **N36.43 Combined hypermobility of urethra and intrinsic sphincter deficiency**
  - **N36.44 Muscular disorders of urethra**
    - Bladder sphincter dyssynergy
- **N36.5 Urethral false passage**
- **N36.8 Other specified disorders of urethra**
  - EXCLUDES 1   congenital urethrocele (Q64.7)
  - female urethrocele (N81.0)
- **N36.9 Urethral disorder, unspecified**

N37 Urethral disorders in diseases classified elsewhere
- Code first underlying disease
- EXCLUDES 1   urethritis (in):
  - candidal infection (B37.41)
  - chlamydial (A56.01)
  - gonorrhea (A54.01)
  - syphilis (A52.76)
  - trichomonal infection (A59.03)
  - tuberculosis (A18.13)

N39 Other disorders of urinary system
   EXCLUDES 2   hematuria NOS (R31.-)
    recurrent or persistent hematuria (N02.-)
    recurrent or persistent hematuria with specified morphological lesion (N02.-)
    proteinuria NOS (R80.-)
- **N39.0 Urinary tract infection, site not specified** CH
  - Use additional code (B95-B97), to identify infectious agent
  - EXCLUDES 1   candidiasis of urinary tract (B37.4-)
  - neonatal urinary tract infection (P39.3)
  - ▶pyuria (R82.81)◀
  - urinary tract infection of specified site, such as:
    - cystitis (N30.-)
    - urethritis (N34.-)
  - **AHA:** 2018,2Q,21,22; 2018,1Q,16; 2017,1Q,6; 2012,4Q,94
  - **TIP:** Do not assign code based solely on laboratory results indicating positive bacterial growth unless such results have been interpreted by the provider, who confirmed a UTI diagnosis.
- **N39.3 Stress incontinence (female) (male)**
  - Code also any associated overactive bladder (N32.81)
  - EXCLUDES 1   mixed incontinence (N39.46)
- **N39.4 Other specified urinary incontinence**
  - Code also any associated overactive bladder (N32.81)
  - EXCLUDES 1   enuresis NOS (R32)
  - functional urinary incontinence (R39.81)
  - urinary incontinence associated with cognitive impairment (R39.81)
  - urinary incontinence NOS (R32)
  - urinary incontinence of nonorganic origin (F98.0)
  - **N39.41 Urge incontinence**
    - EXCLUDES 1   mixed incontinence (N39.46)
  - **N39.42 Incontinence without sensory awareness**
    - Insensible (urinary) incontinence
  - **N39.43 Post-void dribbling**
  - **N39.44 Nocturnal enuresis**
  - **N39.45 Continuous leakage**
  - **N39.46 Mixed incontinence**
    - Urge and stress incontinence
  - **N39.49 Other specified urinary incontinence**
    - **AHA:** 2016,4Q,44
    - **N39.490 Overflow incontinence**
    - **N39.491 Coital incontinence**
    - **N39.492 Postural (urinary) incontinence**
    - **N39.498 Other specified urinary incontinence**
      - Reflex incontinence
      - Total incontinence
- **N39.8 Other specified disorders of urinary system**
- **N39.9 Disorder of urinary system, unspecified**

Diseases of male genital organs (N40-N53)

N40 Benign prostatic hyperplasia
- INCLUDES   adenofibromatous hypertrophy of prostate
  - benign hypertrophy of the prostate
  - benign prostatic hypertrophy
  - BPH
  - enlarged prostate
  - nodular prostate
  - polyp of prostate
- EXCLUDES 1   benign neoplasms of prostate (adenoma, benign) (fibroadenoma) (fibroma) (myoma) (D29.1)
- EXCLUDES 2   malignant neoplasm of prostate (C61)
- **DEF:** Enlargement of the prostate gland due to an abnormal proliferation of fibrostromal tissue in the paraurethral glands. This condition causes impingement of the urethra resulting in obstructed urinary flow.
- **N40.0 Benign prostatic hyperplasia without lower urinary tract symptoms** A ♂
  - Enlarged prostate NOS
  - Enlarged prostate without LUTS

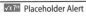

N40.1 Benign prostatic hyperplasia with lower urinary tract symptoms CH A ♂
Enlarged prostate with LUTS
Use additional code for associated symptoms, when specified:
incomplete bladder emptying (R39.14)
nocturia (R35.1)
straining on urination (R39.16)
urinary frequency (R35.0)
urinary hesitancy (R39.11)
urinary incontinence (N39.4-)
urinary obstruction (N13.8)
urinary retention (R33.8)
urinary urgency (R39.15)
weak urinary stream (R39.12)
AHA: 2018,4Q,55

N40.2 Nodular prostate without lower urinary tract symptoms A ♂
Nodular prostate without LUTS

N40.3 Nodular prostate with lower urinary tract symptoms A ♂
Use additional code for associated symptoms, when specified:
incomplete bladder emptying (R39.14)
nocturia (R35.1)
straining on urination (R39.16)
urinary frequency (R35.0)
urinary hesitancy (R39.11)
urinary incontinence (N39.4-)
urinary obstruction (N13.8)
urinary retention (R33.8)
urinary urgency (R39.15)
weak urinary stream (R39.12)

√4th N41 Inflammatory diseases of prostate
Use additional code (B95-B97), to identify infectious agent
N41.0 Acute prostatitis A ♂
N41.1 Chronic prostatitis A ♂
N41.2 Abscess of prostate A ♂
N41.3 Prostatocystitis A ♂
N41.4 Granulomatous prostatitis A ♂
N41.8 Other inflammatory diseases of prostate A ♂
N41.9 Inflammatory disease of prostate, unspecified A ♂
Prostatitis NOS

√4th N42 Other and unspecified disorders of prostate
N42.0 Calculus of prostate A ♂
Prostatic stone
DEF: Formation of a small, solid stone often composed of calcium carbonate or calcium phosphate in the prostate gland.
N42.1 Congestion and hemorrhage of prostate A ♂
EXCLUDES 1 enlarged prostate (N40.-)
hematuria (R31.-)
hyperplasia of prostate (N40.-)
inflammatory diseases of prostate (N41.-)
√5th N42.3 Dysplasia of prostate
AHA: 2016,4Q,44
N42.30 Unspecified dysplasia of prostate ♂
N42.31 Prostatic intraepithelial neoplasia ♂
PIN
Prostatic intraepithelial neoplasia I (PIN I)
Prostatic intraepithelial neoplasia II (PIN II)
EXCLUDES 1 prostatic intraepithelial neoplasia III (PIN III) (D07.5)
DEF: Abnormality of shape and size of the intraepithelial tissues of the prostate. It is a premalignant condition characterized by stalks and absence of a basilar cell layer.
N42.32 Atypical small acinar proliferation of prostate ♂
N42.39 Other dysplasia of prostate ♂
√5th N42.8 Other specified disorders of prostate
N42.81 Prostatodynia syndrome A ♂
Painful prostate syndrome
N42.82 Prostatosis syndrome A ♂
N42.83 Cyst of prostate A ♂
N42.89 Other specified disorders of prostate A ♂

N42.9 Disorder of prostate, unspecified A ♂

√4th N43 Hydrocele and spermatocele
INCLUDES hydrocele of spermatic cord, testis or tunica vaginalis
EXCLUDES 1 congenital hydrocele (P83.5)
DEF: Hydrocele: Serous fluid that collects in the tunica vaginalis of the scrotum along the spermatic cord in males.
N43.0 Encysted hydrocele ♂
N43.1 Infected hydrocele ♂
Use additional code (B95-B97), to identify infectious agent
N43.2 Other hydrocele ♂

Hydrocele

Normal | Noncommunicating hydrocele | Communicating hydrocele | Hydrocele of the cord

N43.3 Hydrocele, unspecified ♂
√6th N43.4 Spermatocele of epididymis
Spermatic cyst
DEF: Spermatocele: Noncancerous accumulation of fluid and dead sperm cells normally located at the head of the epididymis that exhibits itself as a hard, smooth scrotal mass and do not normally require treatment unless they become enlarged or cause pain.
N43.40 Spermatocele of epididymis, unspecified ♂
N43.41 Spermatocele of epididymis, single ♂
N43.42 Spermatocele of epididymis, multiple ♂

√4th N44 Noninflammatory disorders of testis
√5th N44.0 Torsion of testis
N44.00 Torsion of testis, unspecified ♂
N44.01 Extravaginal torsion of spermatic cord ♂
DEF: Torsion of the spermatic cord just below the tunica vaginalis attachments.
N44.02 Intravaginal torsion of spermatic cord ♂
Torsion of spermatic cord NOS
N44.03 Torsion of appendix testis ♂
N44.04 Torsion of appendix epididymis ♂
N44.1 Cyst of tunica albuginea testis ♂
N44.2 Benign cyst of testis ♂
N44.8 Other noninflammatory disorders of the testis ♂

√4th N45 Orchitis and epididymitis
Use additional code (B95-B97), to identify infectious agent
N45.1 Epididymitis ♂
N45.2 Orchitis ♂
N45.3 Epididymo-orchitis ♂
N45.4 Abscess of epididymis or testis ♂

√4th N46 Male infertility
EXCLUDES 1 vasectomy status (Z98.52)
√5th N46.0 Azoospermia
Absolute male infertility
Male infertility due to germinal (cell) aplasia
Male infertility due to spermatogenic arrest (complete)
DEF: Failure of the development of sperm or the absence of sperm in semen.
N46.01 Organic azoospermia A ♂
Azoospermia NOS

√6ᵗʰ N46.Ø2 Azoospermia due to extratesticular causes
    Code also associated cause

    N46.Ø21 Azoospermia due to drug therapy   A ♂
    N46.Ø22 Azoospermia due to infection   A ♂
    N46.Ø23 Azoospermia due to obstruction of efferent ducts   A ♂
    N46.Ø24 Azoospermia due to radiation   A ♂
    N46.Ø25 Azoospermia due to systemic disease   A ♂
    N46.Ø29 Azoospermia due to other extratesticular causes   A ♂

√5ᵗʰ N46.1 Oligospermia
    Male infertility due to germinal cell desquamation
    Male infertility due to hypospermatogenesis
    Male infertility due to incomplete spermatogenic arrest
    DEF: Insufficient production of sperm in semen.

    N46.11 Organic oligospermia   A ♂
      Oligospermia NOS

    √6ᵗʰ N46.12 Oligospermia due to extratesticular causes
      Code also associated cause

      N46.121 Oligospermia due to drug therapy   A ♂
      N46.122 Oligospermia due to infection   A ♂
      N46.123 Oligospermia due to obstruction of efferent ducts   A ♂
      N46.124 Oligospermia due to radiation   A ♂
      N46.125 Oligospermia due to systemic disease   A ♂
      N46.129 Oligospermia due to other extratesticular causes

N46.8 Other male infertility   A ♂
N46.9 Male infertility, unspecified   A ♂

√4ᵗʰ N47 Disorders of prepuce

N47.Ø Adherent prepuce, newborn   N ♂
N47.1 Phimosis   ♂
    DEF: Condition in which the foreskin is contracted and cannot be drawn back behind the glans penis.
N47.2 Paraphimosis   ♂
N47.3 Deficient foreskin   ♂
N47.4 Benign cyst of prepuce   ♂
N47.5 Adhesions of prepuce and glans penis   ♂
N47.6 Balanoposthitis   ♂
    Use additional code (B95-B97), to identify infectious agent
    EXCLUDES 1   balanitis (N48.1)
N47.7 Other inflammatory diseases of prepuce   ♂
    Use additional code (B95-B97), to identify infectious agent
N47.8 Other disorders of prepuce   ♂

√4ᵗʰ N48 Other disorders of penis

N48.Ø Leukoplakia of penis   ♂
    Balanitis xerotica obliterans
    Kraurosis of penis
    Lichen sclerosus of external male genital organs
    EXCLUDES 1   carcinoma in situ of penis (DØ7.4)
N48.1 Balanitis   ♂
    Use additional code (B95-B97), to identify infectious agent
    EXCLUDES 1   amebic balanitis (AØ6.8)
      balanitis xerotica obliterans (N48.Ø)
      candidal balanitis (B37.42)
      gonococcal balanitis (A54.23)
      herpesviral [herpes simplex] balanitis (A6Ø.Ø1)
    DEF: Inflammation of the glans penis, most often affecting uncircumcised males.
√5ᵗʰ N48.2 Other inflammatory disorders of penis
    Use additional code (B95-B97), to identify infectious agent
    EXCLUDES 1   balanitis (N48.1)
      balanitis xerotica obliterans (N48.Ø)
      balanoposthitis (N47.6)
    N48.21 Abscess of corpus cavernosum and penis   ♂
    N48.22 Cellulitis of corpus cavernosum and penis   ♂
    N48.29 Other inflammatory disorders of penis   ♂

√5ᵗʰ N48.3 Priapism
    Painful erection
    Code first underlying cause

    N48.3Ø Priapism, unspecified   ♂
    N48.31 Priapism due to trauma   ♂
    N48.32 Priapism due to disease classified elsewhere   ♂
    N48.33 Priapism, drug-induced   ♂
    N48.39 Other priapism   ♂

N48.5 Ulcer of penis   ♂
N48.6 Induration penis plastica   ♂
    Peyronie's disease
    Plastic induration of penis
√5ᵗʰ N48.8 Other specified disorders of penis
    N48.81 Thrombosis of superficial vein of penis   ♂
    N48.82 Acquired torsion of penis   ♂
      Acquired torsion of penis NOS
      EXCLUDES 1   congenital torsion of penis (Q55.63)
    N48.83 Acquired buried penis   ♂
      EXCLUDES 1   congenital hidden penis (Q55.64)
    N48.89 Other specified disorders of penis   ♂
N48.9 Disorder of penis, unspecified   ♂

√4ᵗʰ N49 Inflammatory disorders of male genital organs, not elsewhere classified
    Use additional code (B95-B97), to identify infectious agent
    EXCLUDES 1   inflammation of penis (N48.1, N48.2-)
      orchitis and epididymitis (N45.-)

N49.Ø Inflammatory disorders of seminal vesicle   ♂
    Vesiculitis NOS
N49.1 Inflammatory disorders of spermatic cord, tunica vaginalis and vas deferens   ♂
    Vasitis
N49.2 Inflammatory disorders of scrotum   ♂
N49.3 Fournier gangrene   ♂
N49.8 Inflammatory disorders of other specified male genital organs   ♂
    Inflammation of multiple sites in male genital organs
N49.9 Inflammatory disorder of unspecified male genital organ   ♂
    Abscess of unspecified male genital organ
    Boil of unspecified male genital organ
    Carbuncle of unspecified male genital organ
    Cellulitis of unspecified male genital organ

√4ᵗʰ N5Ø Other and unspecified disorders of male genital organs
    EXCLUDES 2   torsion of testis (N44.Ø-)
N5Ø.Ø Atrophy of testis   ♂
N5Ø.1 Vascular disorders of male genital organs   ♂
    Hematocele, NOS, of male genital organs
    Hemorrhage of male genital organs
    Thrombosis of male genital organs
N5Ø.3 Cyst of epididymis   ♂
√5ᵗʰ N5Ø.8 Other specified disorders of male genital organs
    AHA: 2016,4Q,45
    √6ᵗʰ N5Ø.81 Testicular pain
      N5Ø.811 Right testicular pain   ♂
      N5Ø.812 Left testicular pain   ♂
      N5Ø.819 Testicular pain, unspecified   ♂
    N5Ø.82 Scrotal pain   ♂

N50.89 **Other specified disorders of the male genital organs** ♂

Atrophy of scrotum, seminal vesicle, spermatic cord, tunica vaginalis and vas deferens

Chylocele, tunica vaginalis (nonfilarial) NOS

Edema of scrotum, seminal vesicle, spermatic cord, tunica vaginalis and vas deferens

Hypertrophy of scrotum, seminal vesicle, spermatic cord, tunica vaginalis and vas deferens

Stricture of spermatic cord, tunica vaginalis, and vas deferens

Ulcer of scrotum, seminal vesicle, spermatic cord, testis, tunica vaginalis and vas deferens

Urethroscrotal fistula

N50.9 **Disorder of male genital organs, unspecified** ♂

N51 *Disorders of male genital organs in diseases classified elsewhere* ♂

Code first underlying disease, such as:
filariasis (B74.0-B74.9)

EXCLUDES 1 *amebic balanitis (A06.8)*
candidal balanitis (B37.42)
gonococcal balanitis (A54.23)
gonococcal prostatitis (A54.22)
herpesviral [herpes simplex] balanitis (A60.01)
trichomonal prostatitis (A59.02)
tuberculous prostatitis (A18.14)

√4ᵗʰ **N52** **Male erectile dysfunction**

EXCLUDES 1 *psychogenic impotence (F52.21)*

√5ᵗʰ **N52.0** **Vasculogenic erectile dysfunction**

N52.01 **Erectile dysfunction due to arterial insufficiency** Ⓐ♂

N52.02 **Corporo-venous occlusive erectile dysfunction** Ⓐ♂

N52.03 **Combined arterial insufficiency and corporo-venous occlusive erectile dysfunction** Ⓐ♂

N52.1 *Erectile dysfunction due to diseases classified elsewhere* Ⓐ♂

Code first underlying disease

N52.2 **Drug-induced erectile dysfunction** Ⓐ♂

√5ᵗʰ **N52.3** **Postprocedural erectile dysfunction**

AHA: 2016,4Q,45

N52.31 **Erectile dysfunction following radical prostatectomy** Ⓐ♂

N52.32 **Erectile dysfunction following radical cystectomy** Ⓐ♂

N52.33 **Erectile dysfunction following urethral surgery** Ⓐ♂

N52.34 **Erectile dysfunction following simple prostatectomy** Ⓐ♂

N52.35 **Erectile dysfunction following radiation therapy** Ⓐ♂

N52.36 **Erectile dysfunction following interstitial seed therapy** Ⓐ♂

N52.37 **Erectile dysfunction following prostate ablative therapy** Ⓐ♂

Erectile dysfunction following cryotherapy

Erectile dysfunction following other prostate ablative therapies

Erectile dysfunction following ultrasound ablative therapies

N52.39 **Other and unspecified postprocedural erectile dysfunction** Ⓐ♂

N52.8 **Other male erectile dysfunction** Ⓐ♂

N52.9 **Male erectile dysfunction, unspecified** Ⓐ♂

Impotence NOS

√4ᵗʰ **N53** **Other male sexual dysfunction**

EXCLUDES 1 *psychogenic sexual dysfunction (F52.-)*

√5ᵗʰ **N53.1** **Ejaculatory dysfunction**

EXCLUDES 1 *premature ejaculation (F52.4)*

N53.11 **Retarded ejaculation** ♂

N53.12 **Painful ejaculation** ♂

N53.13 **Anejaculatory orgasm** ♂

N53.14 **Retrograde ejaculation** ♂

DEF: Form of male sexual dysfunction in which the semen enters the bladder instead of going out through the urethra during ejaculation.

N53.19 **Other ejaculatory dysfunction** ♂

Ejaculatory dysfunction NOS

N53.8 **Other male sexual dysfunction** ♂

N53.9 **Unspecified male sexual dysfunction** ♂

Disorders of breast (N60-N65)

EXCLUDES 1 *disorders of breast associated with childbirth (O91-O92)*

√4ᵗʰ **N60** **Benign mammary dysplasia**

INCLUDES fibrocystic mastopathy

√5ᵗʰ **N60.0** **Solitary cyst of breast**

Cyst of breast

N60.01 **Solitary cyst of right breast**

N60.02 **Solitary cyst of left breast**

N60.09 **Solitary cyst of unspecified breast**

√5ᵗʰ **N60.1** **Diffuse cystic mastopathy**

Cystic breast

Fibrocystic disease of breast

EXCLUDES 1 *diffuse cystic mastopathy with epithelial proliferation (N60.3-)*

N60.11 **Diffuse cystic mastopathy of right breast** Ⓐ

N60.12 **Diffuse cystic mastopathy of left breast** Ⓐ

N60.19 **Diffuse cystic mastopathy of unspecified breast** Ⓐ

√5ᵗʰ **N60.2** **Fibroadenosis of breast**

Adenofibrosis of breast

EXCLUDES 2 *fibroadenoma of breast (D24.-)*

N60.21 **Fibroadenosis of right breast**

N60.22 **Fibroadenosis of left breast**

N60.29 **Fibroadenosis of unspecified breast**

√5ᵗʰ **N60.3** **Fibrosclerosis of breast**

Cystic mastopathy with epithelial proliferation

N60.31 **Fibrosclerosis of right breast**

N60.32 **Fibrosclerosis of left breast**

N60.39 **Fibrosclerosis of unspecified breast**

√5ᵗʰ **N60.4** **Mammary duct ectasia**

N60.41 **Mammary duct ectasia of right breast**

N60.42 **Mammary duct ectasia of left breast**

N60.49 **Mammary duct ectasia of unspecified breast**

√5ᵗʰ **N60.8** **Other benign mammary dysplasias**

N60.81 **Other benign mammary dysplasias of right breast**

N60.82 **Other benign mammary dysplasias of left breast**

N60.89 **Other benign mammary dysplasias of unspecified breast**

√5ᵗʰ **N60.9** **Unspecified benign mammary dysplasia**

N60.91 **Unspecified benign mammary dysplasia of right breast**

N60.92 **Unspecified benign mammary dysplasia of left breast**

N60.99 **Unspecified benign mammary dysplasia of unspecified breast**

√4ᵗʰ **N61** **Inflammatory disorders of breast**

EXCLUDES 1 *inflammatory carcinoma of breast (C50.9)*
inflammatory disorder of breast associated with childbirth (O91.-)
neonatal infective mastitis (P39.0)
thrombophlebitis of breast [Mondor's disease] (I80.8)

N61.0 **Mastitis without abscess**

Infective mastitis (acute) (nonpuerperal) (subacute)

Mastitis (acute) (nonpuerperal) (subacute) NOS

Cellulitis (acute) (nonpuerperal) (subacute) of breast NOS

Cellulitis (acute) (nonpuerperal) (subacute) of nipple NOS

N61.1 **Abscess of the breast and nipple**

Abscess (acute) (chronic) (nonpuerperal) of areola

Abscess (acute) (chronic) (nonpuerperal) of breast

Carbuncle of breast

Mastitis with abscess

Ⓝ Newborn: 0 Ⓟ Pediatric: 0-17 Ⓜ Maternity: 12-55 Ⓐ Adult: 15-124 CH Comorbidity High CL Comorbidity Low NCDx Noncancer Dx PDx Primary Dx

834

ICD-10-CM 2020

N62   Hypertrophy of breast
Gynecomastia
Hypertrophy of breast NOS
Massive pubertal hypertrophy of breast
EXCLUDES 1   breast engorgement of newborn (P83.4)
          disproportion of reconstructed breast (N65.1)

✓4ᵗʰ N63   Unspecified lump in breast
Nodule(s) NOS in breast
AHA: 2017,4Q,19

N63.0   Unspecified lump in unspecified breast

✓5ᵗʰ N63.1   Unspecified lump in right breast

   N63.10   Unspecified lump in the right breast, unspecified quadrant

   N63.11   Unspecified lump in the right breast, upper outer quadrant

   N63.12   Unspecified lump in the right breast, upper inner quadrant

   N63.13   Unspecified lump in the right breast, lower outer quadrant

   N63.14   Unspecified lump in the right breast, lower inner quadrant

●   **N63.15   Unspecified lump in the right breast, overlapping quadrants**

✓5ᵗʰ N63.2   Unspecified lump in left breast

   N63.20   Unspecified lump in the left breast, unspecified quadrant

   N63.21   Unspecified lump in the left breast, upper outer quadrant

   N63.22   Unspecified lump in the left breast, upper inner quadrant

   N63.23   Unspecified lump in the left breast, lower outer quadrant

   N63.24   Unspecified lump in the left breast, lower inner quadrant

●   **N63.25   Unspecified lump in the left breast, overlapping quadrants**

✓5ᵗʰ N63.3   Unspecified lump in axillary tail

   N63.31   Unspecified lump in axillary tail of the right breast
   N63.32   Unspecified lump in axillary tail of the left breast

✓5ᵗʰ N63.4   Unspecified lump in breast, subareolar

   N63.41   Unspecified lump in right breast, subareolar
   N63.42   Unspecified lump in left breast, subareolar

✓4ᵗʰ N64   Other disorders of breast
EXCLUDES 2   mechanical complication of breast prosthesis and implant (T85.4-)

N64.0   Fissure and fistula of nipple

N64.1   Fat necrosis of breast
Fat necrosis (segmental) of breast
Code first breast necrosis due to breast graft (T85.898)

N64.2   Atrophy of breast

N64.3   Galactorrhea not associated with childbirth

N64.4   Mastodynia

✓5ᵗʰ N64.5   Other signs and symptoms in breast
EXCLUDES 2   abnormal findings on diagnostic imaging of breast (R92.-)

   N64.51   Induration of breast

   N64.52   Nipple discharge
     EXCLUDES 1   abnormal findings in nipple discharge (R89.-)

   N64.53   Retraction of nipple

   N64.59   Other signs and symptoms in breast

✓5ᵗʰ N64.8   Other specified disorders of breast

   N64.81   Ptosis of breast   🅰
     EXCLUDES 1   ptosis of native breast in relation to reconstructed breast (N65.1)

   N64.82   Hypoplasia of breast   🅰
     Micromastia
     EXCLUDES 1   congenital absence of breast (Q83.0)
          hypoplasia of native breast in relation to reconstructed breast (N65.1)

   N64.89   Other specified disorders of breast
     Galactocele
     Subinvolution of breast (postlactational)
     AHA: 2019,1Q,32; 2018,1Q,3

N64.9   Disorder of breast, unspecified

✓4ᵗʰ N65   Deformity and disproportion of reconstructed breast

N65.0   Deformity of reconstructed breast   🅰
Contour irregularity in reconstructed breast
Excess tissue in reconstructed breast
Misshapen reconstructed breast

N65.1   Disproportion of reconstructed breast   🅰
Breast asymmetry between native breast and reconstructed breast
Disproportion between native breast and reconstructed breast

Inflammatory diseases of female pelvic organs (N70-N77)

EXCLUDES 1   inflammatory diseases of female pelvic organs complicating:
     abortion or ectopic or molar pregnancy (O00-O07, O08.0)
     pregnancy, childbirth and the puerperium (O23.-, O75.3, O85, O86.-)

✓4ᵗʰ N70   Salpingitis and oophoritis
INCLUDES   abscess (of) fallopian tube
          abscess (of) ovary
          pyosalpinx
          salpingo-oophoritis
          tubo-ovarian abscess
          tubo-ovarian inflammatory disease
Use additional code (B95-B97), to identify infectious agent
EXCLUDES 1   gonococcal infection (A54.24)
          tuberculous infection (A18.17)

✓5ᵗʰ N70.0   Acute salpingitis and oophoritis

   N70.01   Acute salpingitis   ♀
   N70.02   Acute oophoritis   ♀
   N70.03   Acute salpingitis and oophoritis   ♀

✓5ᵗʰ N70.1   Chronic salpingitis and oophoritis
Hydrosalpinx
   N70.11   Chronic salpingitis   ♀
   N70.12   Chronic oophoritis   ♀
   N70.13   Chronic salpingitis and oophoritis   ♀

✓5ᵗʰ N70.9   Salpingitis and oophoritis, unspecified

   N70.91   Salpingitis, unspecified   ♀
   N70.92   Oophoritis, unspecified   ♀
   N70.93   Salpingitis and oophoritis, unspecified   ♀

✓4ᵗʰ N71   Inflammatory disease of uterus, except cervix
INCLUDES   endo (myo) metritis
          metritis
          myometritis
          pyometra
          uterine abscess
Use additional code (B95-B97), to identify infectious agent
EXCLUDES 1   hyperplastic endometritis (N85.0-)
          infection of uterus following delivery (O85, O86.-)

N71.0   Acute inflammatory disease of uterus   ♀

N71.1   Chronic inflammatory disease of uterus   ♀

N71.9   Inflammatory disease of uterus, unspecified   ♀

N72   Inflammatory disease of cervix uteri   ♀
INCLUDES   cervicitis (with or without erosion or ectropion)
          endocervicitis (with or without erosion or ectropion)
          exocervicitis (with or without erosion or ectropion)
Use additional code (B95-B97), to identify infectious agent
EXCLUDES 1   erosion and ectropion of cervix without cervicitis (N86)

✓4ᵗʰ N73   Other female pelvic inflammatory diseases
Use additional code (B95-B97), to identify infectious agent

N73.0   Acute parametritis and pelvic cellulitis   ♀
Abscess of broad ligament
Abscess of parametrium
Pelvic cellulitis, female
DEF: Parametritis: Inflammation of the parametrium.

N73.1   Chronic parametritis and pelvic cellulitis   ♀
Any condition in N73.0 specified as chronic
EXCLUDES 1   tuberculous parametritis and pelvic cellultis (A18.17)

N73.2   Unspecified parametritis and pelvic cellulitis   ♀
Any condition in N73.0 unspecified whether acute or chronic

N73.3   Female acute pelvic peritonitis   ♀

✅ Additional Character Required   ✓x7ᵗʰ Placeholder Alert   Manifestation   Unspecified Dx   ►◄ Revised Text   ● New Code   ▲ Revised Title

ICD-10-CM 2020   835

N73.4 Female chronic **pelvic peritonitis** ♀
> EXCLUDES 1   *tuberculous pelvic (female) peritonitis (A18.17)*

N73.5 Female pelvic peritonitis, unspecified ♀

N73.6 Female pelvic peritoneal adhesions **(postinfective)** ♀
> EXCLUDES 2   postprocedural pelvic peritoneal adhesions (N99.4)

> AHA: 2014,1Q,6

N73.8 Other specified female pelvic inflammatory diseases ♀

N73.9 Female pelvic inflammatory disease, unspecified ♀
> Female pelvic infection or inflammation NOS

N74 Female pelvic inflammatory disorders in diseases classified elsewhere ♀
> Code first underlying disease
> EXCLUDES 1   *chlamydial cervicitis (A56.02)*
> *chlamydial pelvic inflammatory disease (A56.11)*
> *gonococcal cervicitis (A54.03)*
> *gonococcal pelvic inflammatory disease (A54.24)*
> *herpesviral [herpes simplex] cervicitis (A60.03)*
> *herpesviral [herpes simplex] pelvic inflammatory disease (A60.09)*
> *syphilitic cervicitis (A52.76)*
> *syphilitic pelvic inflammatory disease (A52.76)*
> *trichomonal cervicitis (A59.09)*
> *tuberculous cervicitis (A18.16)*
> *tuberculous pelvic inflammatory disease (A18.17)*

✓4ᵗʰ **N75 Diseases of Bartholin's gland**
> **DEF:** Bartholin's gland: Mucous-producing gland found in the vestibular bulbs on either side of the vaginal orifice and connected to the mucosal membrane at the opening by a duct.

N75.0 Cyst **of Bartholin's gland** ♀

N75.1 Abscess **of Bartholin's gland** ♀

N75.8 Other diseases of Bartholin's gland ♀
> Bartholinitis

N75.9 Disease of Bartholin's gland, unspecified ♀

✓4ᵗʰ **N76 Other inflammation of vagina and vulva**
> Use additional code (B95-B97), to identify infectious agent
> EXCLUDES 2   senile (atrophic) vaginitis (N95.2)
> vulvar vestibulitis (N94.810)

N76.0 Acute vaginitis ♀
> Acute vulvovaginitis
> Vaginitis NOS
> Vulvovaginitis NOS

N76.1 Subacute and chronic vaginitis ♀
> Chronic vulvovaginitis
> Subacute vulvovaginitis

N76.2 Acute vulvitis ♀
> Vulvitis NOS

N76.3 Subacute and chronic vulvitis ♀

N76.4 Abscess of vulva ♀
> Furuncle of vulva

N76.5 Ulceration of vagina ♀

N76.6 Ulceration of vulva ♀

✓5ᵗʰ **N76.8 Other specified inflammation of vagina and vulva**

N76.81 Mucositis (ulcerative) of vagina and vulva ♀
> Code also type of associated therapy, such as:
> antineoplastic and immunosuppressive drugs (T45.1X-)
> radiological procedure and radiotherapy (Y84.2)
> EXCLUDES 2   gastrointestinal mucositis (ulcerative) (K92.81)
> nasal mucositis (ulcerative) (J34.81)
> oral mucositis (ulcerative) (K12.3-)

N76.89 Other specified inflammation of vagina and vulva ♀

✓4ᵗʰ **N77 Vulvovaginal ulceration and inflammation in diseases classified elsewhere**

N77.0 Ulceration of vulva in diseases classified elsewhere ♀
> Code first underlying disease, such as:
> Behçet's disease (M35.2)
> EXCLUDES 1   *ulceration of vulva in gonococcal infection (A54.02)*
> *ulceration of vulva in herpesviral [herpes simplex] infection (A60.04)*
> *ulceration of vulva in syphilis (A51.0)*
> *ulceration of vulva in tuberculosis (A18.18)*

N77.1 Vaginitis, vulvitis and vulvovaginitis in diseases classified elsewhere ♀
> Code first underlying disease, such as:
> pinworm (B80)
> EXCLUDES 1   *candidal vulvovaginitis (B37.3)*
> *chlamydial vulvovaginitis (A56.02)*
> *gonococcal vulvovaginitis (A54.02)*
> *herpesviral [herpes simplex] vulvovaginitis (A60.04)*
> *trichomonal vulvovaginitis (A59.01)*
> *tuberculous vulvovaginitis (A18.18)*
> *vulvovaginitis in early syphilis (A51.0)*
> *vulvovaginitis in late syphilis (A52.76)*

Noninflammatory disorders of female genital tract (N80-N98)

✓4ᵗʰ **N80 Endometriosis**
> **DEF:** Aberrant uterine mucosal tissue appearing in areas of the pelvic cavity outside of its normal location, lining the uterus, and inflaming surrounding tissues often resulting in infertility or spontaneous abortion.

N80.0 Endometriosis of uterus ♀
> Adenomyosis
> EXCLUDES 1   *stromal endometriosis (D39.0)*

N80.1 Endometriosis of ovary ♀

N80.2 Endometriosis of fallopian tube ♀

N80.3 Endometriosis of pelvic peritoneum ♀

N80.4 Endometriosis of rectovaginal septum and vagina ♀

N80.5 Endometriosis of intestine ♀

N80.6 Endometriosis in cutaneous scar ♀

N80.8 Other endometriosis ♀
> Endometriosis of thorax

N80.9 Endometriosis, unspecified ♀

Ⓝ Newborn: 0   Ⓟ Pediatric: 0-17   Ⓜ Maternity: 12-55   Ⓐ Adult: 15-124   CH Comorbidity High   CL Comorbidity Low   NCDx Noncancer Dx   PDx Primary Dx

836   ICD-10-CM 2020

☑4ᵗʰ **N81 Female genital prolapse**

    EXCLUDES 1   genital prolapse complicating pregnancy, labor or delivery (O34.5-)
           prolapse and hernia of ovary and fallopian tube (N83.4-)
           prolapse of vaginal vault after hysterectomy (N99.3)

Types of Pelvic Organ Prolapse

Urethrocele   Cystocele

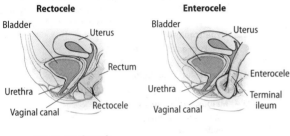

Rectocele   Enterocele

N81.0 Urethrocele ♀

    EXCLUDES 1   urethrocele with cystocele (N81.1-)
           urethrocele with prolapse of uterus (N81.2-N81.4)

☑5ᵗʰ **N81.1 Cystocele**

    Cystocele with urethrocele
    Cystourethrocele
    EXCLUDES 1   cystocele with prolapse of uterus (N81.2-N81.4)

    N81.10 Cystocele, unspecified ♀
        Prolapse of (anterior) vaginal wall NOS

    N81.11 Cystocele, midline ♀

    N81.12 Cystocele, lateral ♀
        Paravaginal cystocele
        DEF: Detachment of the lateral support connections of the vagina at the arcus tendineus fasciae pelvis (ATFP) that results in bladder drop. The bladder herniates into the vagina laterally.

N81.2 Incomplete uterovaginal prolapse ♀
    First degree uterine prolapse
    Prolapse of cervix NOS
    Second degree uterine prolapse
    EXCLUDES 1   cervical stump prolapse (N81.85)

N81.3 Complete uterovaginal prolapse ♀
    Procidentia (uteri) NOS
    Third degree uterine prolapse

N81.4 Uterovaginal prolapse, unspecified ♀
    Prolapse of uterus NOS

N81.5 Vaginal enterocele ♀
    EXCLUDES 1   enterocele with prolapse of uterus (N81.2-N81.4)

N81.6 Rectocele ♀
    Prolapse of posterior vaginal wall
    Use additional code for any associated fecal incontinence, if applicable (R15.-)
    EXCLUDES 2   perineocele (N81.81)
           rectal prolapse (K62.3)
           rectocele with prolapse of uterus (N81.2-N81.4)

☑5ᵗʰ **N81.8 Other female genital prolapse**

    N81.81 Perineocele ♀

    N81.82 Incompetence or weakening of pubocervical tissue ♀

    N81.83 Incompetence or weakening of rectovaginal tissue ♀

    N81.84 Pelvic muscle wasting ♀
        Disuse atrophy of pelvic muscles and anal sphincter

    N81.85 Cervical stump prolapse ♀

    N81.89 Other female genital prolapse ♀
        Deficient perineum
        Old laceration of muscles of pelvic floor

N81.9 Female genital prolapse, unspecified ♀

☑4ᵗʰ **N82 Fistulae involving female genital tract**

    EXCLUDES 1   vesicointestinal fistulae (N32.1)

N82.0 Vesicovaginal fistula ♀

N82.1 Other female urinary-genital tract fistulae ♀
    Cervicovesical fistula
    Ureterovaginal fistula
    Urethrovaginal fistula
    Uteroureteric fistula
    Uterovesical fistula
    AHA: 2017,3Q,3

N82.2 Fistula of vagina to small intestine ♀

N82.3 Fistula of vagina to large intestine ♀
    Rectovaginal fistula

N82.4 Other female intestinal-genital tract fistulae ♀
    Intestinouterine fistula

N82.5 Female genital tract-skin fistulae ♀
    Uterus to abdominal wall fistula
    Vaginoperineal fistula

N82.8 Other female genital tract fistulae ♀

N82.9 Female genital tract fistula, unspecified ♀

☑4ᵗʰ **N83 Noninflammatory disorders of ovary, fallopian tube and broad ligament**

    EXCLUDES 2   hydrosalpinx (N70.1-)
    AHA: 2016,4Q,46

☑5ᵗʰ **N83.0 Follicular cyst of ovary**
    Cyst of graafian follicle
    Hemorrhagic follicular cyst (of ovary)

    N83.00 Follicular cyst of ovary, unspecified side ♀

    N83.01 Follicular cyst of right ovary ♀

    N83.02 Follicular cyst of left ovary ♀

☑5ᵗʰ **N83.1 Corpus luteum cyst**
    Hemorrhagic corpus luteum cyst

    N83.10 Corpus luteum cyst of ovary, unspecified side ♀

    N83.11 Corpus luteum cyst of right ovary ♀

    N83.12 Corpus luteum cyst of left ovary ♀

☑5ᵗʰ **N83.2 Other and unspecified ovarian cysts**
    EXCLUDES 1   developmental ovarian cyst (Q50.1)
           neoplastic ovarian cyst (D27.-)
           polycystic ovarian syndrome (E28.2)
           Stein-Leventhal syndrome (E28.2)

    ☑6ᵗʰ **N83.20 Unspecified ovarian cysts**

        N83.201 Unspecified ovarian cyst, right side ♀

        N83.202 Unspecified ovarian cyst, left side ♀

        N83.209 Unspecified ovarian cyst, unspecified side ♀
           Ovarian cyst, NOS

    ☑6ᵗʰ **N83.29 Other ovarian cysts**
        Retention cyst of ovary
        Simple cyst of ovary

        N83.291 Other ovarian cyst, right side ♀

        N83.292 Other ovarian cyst, left side ♀

        N83.299 Other ovarian cyst, unspecified side ♀

☑5ᵗʰ **N83.3 Acquired atrophy of ovary and fallopian tube**

    ☑6ᵗʰ **N83.31 Acquired atrophy of ovary**

        N83.311 Acquired atrophy of right ovary ♀

        N83.312 Acquired atrophy of left ovary ♀

        N83.319 Acquired atrophy of ovary, unspecified side ♀
           Acquired atrophy of ovary, NOS

    ☑6ᵗʰ **N83.32 Acquired atrophy of fallopian tube**

        N83.321 Acquired atrophy of right fallopian tube ♀

Chapter 14. Diseases of the Genitourinary System

   N83.322   **Acquired atrophy of** left **fallopian tube** ♀

   N83.329   **Acquired atrophy of fallopian tube, unspecified side** ♀
     Acquired atrophy of fallopian tube, NOS

  ✓6ᵗʰ N83.33   **Acquired atrophy of** ovary and fallopian tube

   N83.331   **Acquired atrophy of** right **ovary and fallopian tube** ♀

   N83.332   **Acquired atrophy of** left **ovary and fallopian tube** ♀

   N83.339   **Acquired atrophy of ovary and fallopian tube, unspecified side** ♀
     Acquired atrophy of ovary and fallopian tube, NOS

 ✓5ᵗʰ N83.4   **Prolapse and hernia of ovary and fallopian tube**

  N83.40   **Prolapse and hernia of ovary and fallopian tube, unspecified side** ♀
   Prolapse and hernia of ovary and fallopian tube, NOS

  N83.41   **Prolapse and hernia of** right **ovary and fallopian tube** ♀

  N83.42   **Prolapse and hernia of** left **ovary and fallopian tube** ♀

 ✓5ᵗʰ N83.5   **Torsion of ovary, ovarian pedicle and fallopian tube**
  Torsion of accessory tube

  ✓6ᵗʰ N83.51   **Torsion of** ovary and ovarian pedicle

   N83.511   **Torsion of** right **ovary and ovarian pedicle** ♀

   N83.512   **Torsion of** left **ovary and ovarian pedicle** ♀

   N83.519   **Torsion of ovary and ovarian pedicle, unspecified side** ♀
    Torsion of ovary and ovarian pedicle, NOS

  ✓6ᵗʰ N83.52   **Torsion of** fallopian tube
   Torsion of hydatid of Morgagni

   N83.521   **Torsion of** right **fallopian tube** ♀

   N83.522   **Torsion of** left **fallopian tube** ♀

   N83.529   **Torsion of fallopian tube, unspecified side** ♀
    Torsion of fallopian tube, NOS

  N83.53   **Torsion of** ovary, ovarian pedicle and fallopian tube ♀

 N83.6   **Hematosalpinx** ♀
   EXCLUDES 1   *hematosalpinx (with) (in):*
    hematocolpos (N89.7)
    hematometra (N85.7)
    tubal pregnancy (O00.1-)

 N83.7   **Hematoma of broad ligament** ♀

 N83.8   **Other noninflammatory disorders of ovary, fallopian tube and broad ligament** ♀
  Broad ligament laceration syndrome [Allen-Masters]

 N83.9   **Noninflammatory disorder of ovary, fallopian tube and broad ligament, unspecified** ♀

✓4ᵗʰ **N84   Polyp of female genital tract**
  EXCLUDES 1   *adenomatous polyp (D28.-)*
   placental polyp (O90.89)

 N84.0   **Polyp of** corpus uteri ♀
  Polyp of endometrium
  Polyp of uterus NOS
  EXCLUDES 1   *polypoid endometrial hyperplasia (N85.0-)*

 N84.1   **Polyp of** cervix uteri ♀
  Mucous polyp of cervix

 N84.2   **Polyp of** vagina ♀

 N84.3   **Polyp of** vulva ♀
  Polyp of labia

 N84.8   **Polyp of other parts of female genital tract** ♀

 N84.9   **Polyp of female genital tract, unspecified** ♀

✓4ᵗʰ **N85   Other noninflammatory disorders of uterus, except cervix**
  EXCLUDES 1   *endometriosis (N80.-)*
   inflammatory diseases of uterus (N71.-)
   noninflammatory disorders of cervix, except malposition (N86-N88)
   polyp of corpus uteri (N84.0)
   uterine prolapse (N81.-)

 ✓5ᵗʰ N85.0   **Endometrial hyperplasia**

  N85.00   **Endometrial hyperplasia, unspecified** ♀
   Hyperplasia (adenomatous) (cystic) (glandular) of endometrium
   Hyperplastic endometritis

  N85.01   Benign **endometrial hyperplasia** ♀
   Endometrial hyperplasia (complex) (simple) without atypia

  N85.02   Endometrial intraepithelial neoplasia [EIN] ♀
   Endometrial hyperplasia with atypia
   EXCLUDES 1   *malignant neoplasm of endometrium (with endometrial intraepithelial neoplasia [EIN]) (C54.1)*

 N85.2   **Hypertrophy of uterus** ♀
  Bulky or enlarged uterus
  EXCLUDES 1   *puerperal hypertrophy of uterus (O90.89)*

 N85.3   **Subinvolution of uterus** ♀
  EXCLUDES 1   *puerperal subinvolution of uterus (O90.89)*

 N85.4   **Malposition of uterus** ♀
  Anteversion of uterus
  Retroflexion of uterus
  Retroversion of uterus
  EXCLUDES 1   *malposition of uterus complicating pregnancy, labor or delivery (O34.5-, O65.5)*

 N85.5   **Inversion of uterus** ♀
  EXCLUDES 1   *current obstetric trauma (O71.2)*
   postpartum inversion of uterus (O71.2)
  DEF: Abnormality in which the uterus turns inside out.

Inversion of Uterus

Uterus

 N85.6   **Intrauterine synechiae** ♀

 N85.7   **Hematometra** ♀
  Hematosalpinx with hematometra
  EXCLUDES 1   *hematometra with hematocolpos (N89.7)*
  DEF: Accumulation of blood within the uterus.

 N85.8   **Other specified noninflammatory disorders of uterus** ♀
  Atrophy of uterus, acquired
  Fibrosis of uterus NOS

 N85.9   **Noninflammatory disorder of uterus, unspecified** ♀
  Disorder of uterus NOS

N86   Erosion and ectropion of cervix uteri ♀
  Decubitus (trophic) ulcer of cervix
  Eversion of cervix
  EXCLUDES 1   *erosion and ectropion of cervix with cervicitis (N72)*

N Newborn: 0   P Pediatric: 0-17   M Maternity: 12-55   A Adult: 15-124   CH Comorbidity High   CL Comorbidity Low   NC Dx Noncancer Dx   P Dx Primary Dx

838   ICD-10-CM 2020

N83.322–N86

x uteri

rmal results from cervical cytologic examination without
histologic confirmation (R87.61-)
noma in situ of cervix uteri (D06.-)
ical intraepithelial neoplasia III [CIN III] (D06.-)
L of cervix (R87.613)
re dysplasia of cervix uteri (D06.-)

cal dysplasia   ♀

intraepithelial neoplasia I [CIN I]

e cervical dysplasia   ♀

intraepithelial neoplasia II [CIN II]

a of cervix uteri, unspecified   ♀

sia of cervix
l atypism
al dysplasia NOS

mmatory disorders of cervix uteri

flammatory disease of cervix (N72)
lyp of cervix (N84.1)

akia of cervix uteri   ♀

eration of cervix uteri   ♀

sions of cervix
DES 1   current obstetric trauma (O71.3)

re and stenosis of cervix uteri   ♀

DES 1   stricture and stenosis of cervix uteri complicating
labor (O65.5)

petence of cervix uteri   ♀

stigation and management of (suspected) cervical
incompetence in a nonpregnant woman
UDES 1   cervical incompetence complicating pregnancy
(O34.3-)
: Inadequate functioning of the cervix marked by abnormal
ening during pregnancy and causing premature birth or
carriage.

rtrophic elongation of cervix uteri   ♀

**r specified noninflammatory disorders of
x uteri**   ♀
LUDES 1   current obstetric trauma (O71.3)

**inflammatory disorder of cervix uteri,
ecified**   ♀

nflammatory disorders of vagina

abnormal results from vaginal cytologic examination without
histologic confirmation (R87.62-)
carcinoma in situ of vagina (D07.2)
HGSIL of vagina (R87.623)
inflammation of vagina (N76.-)
senile (atrophic) vaginitis (N95.2)
severe dysplasia of vagina (D07.2)
trichomonal leukorrhea (A59.00)
vaginal intraepithelial neoplasia [VAIN], grade III (D07.2)

d vaginal dysplasia   ♀

Vaginal intraepithelial neoplasia [VAIN], grade I

oderate vaginal dysplasia   ♀

Vaginal intraepithelial neoplasia [VAIN], grade II

ysplasia of vagina, unspecified   ♀

eukoplakia of vagina   ♀

tricture and atresia of vagina   ♀

Vaginal adhesions
Vaginal stenosis
EXCLUDES 1   congenital atresia or stricture (Q52.4)
postprocedural adhesions of vagina (N99.2)

Tight hymenal ring   ♀

Rigid hymen
Tight introitus
EXCLUDES 1   imperforate hymen (Q52.3)

Hematocolpos   ♀

Hematocolpos with hematometra or hematosalpinx
AHA: 2016,4Q,58

N89.8 **Other specified noninflammatory disorders of vagina**   ♀

Leukorrhea NOS
Old vaginal laceration
Pessary ulcer of vagina
EXCLUDES 1   current obstetric trauma (O70.-, O71.4, O71.7-O71.8)
old laceration involving muscles of pelvic floor
(N81.8)

N89.9 **Noninflammatory disorder of vagina, unspecified**   ♀

√4ᵗʰ **N90** **Other noninflammatory disorders of vulva and perineum**

EXCLUDES 1   anogenital (venereal) warts (A63.0)
carcinoma in situ of vulva (D07.1)
condyloma acuminatum (A63.0)
current obstetric trauma (O70.-, O71.7-O71.8)
inflammation of vulva (N76.-)
severe dysplasia of vulva (D07.1)
vulvar intraepithelial neoplasm III [VIN III] (D07.1)

N90.0 Mild **vulvar dysplasia**   ♀

Vulvar intraepithelial neoplasia [VIN], grade I

N90.1 Moderate **vulvar dysplasia**   ♀

Vulvar intraepithelial neoplasia [VIN], grade II

N90.3 **Dysplasia of vulva, unspecified**   ♀

N90.4 **Leukoplakia of vulva**   ♀

Dystrophy of vulva
Kraurosis of vulva
Lichen sclerosus of external female genital organs

N90.5 **Atrophy of vulva**   ♀

Stenosis of vulva

√5ᵗʰ **N90.6** **Hypertrophy of vulva**

AHA: 2016,4Q,46

N90.60 **Unspecified hypertrophy of vulva**   ♀

Unspecified hypertrophy of labia

N90.61 **Childhood asymmetric labium majus
enlargement**   ♀

CALME

N90.69 **Other specified hypertrophy of vulva**   ♀

Other specified hypertrophy of labia

N90.7 **Vulvar cyst**   ♀

√5ᵗʰ **N90.8** **Other specified noninflammatory disorders of vulva and
perineum**

√6ᵗʰ **N90.81** **Female genital mutilation status**

Female genital cutting status

N90.810 **Female genital mutilation
status, unspecified**   ♀

Female genital cutting status, unspecified
Female genital mutilation status NOS

N90.811 **Female genital mutilation
Type I status**   ♀

Clitorectomy status
Female genital cutting Type I status

N90.812 **Female genital mutilation
Type II status**   ♀

Clitorectomy with excision of labia minora
status
Female genital cutting Type II status

N90.813 **Female genital mutilation
Type III status**   ♀

Female genital cutting Type III status
Infibulation status

N90.818 **Other female genital
mutilation status**   ♀

Female genital cutting Type IV status
Female genital mutilation Type IV status
Other female genital cutting status

N90.89 **Other specified noninflammatory
disorders of vulva and perineum**   ♀

Adhesions of vulva
Hypertrophy of clitoris

N90.9 **Noninflammatory disorder of vulva and
perineum, unspecified**   ♀

√4ᵗʰ **N91** **Absent, scanty and rare menstruation**

EXCLUDES 1   ovarian dysfunction (E28.-)

N91.0 **Primary amenorrhea**   ♀

N91.1 **Secondary amenorrhea**   ♀

N91.2 **Amenorrhea, unspecified** ♀

N91.3 **Primary oligomenorrhea** ♀

N91.4 **Secondary oligomenorrhea** ♀

N91.5 **Oligomenorrhea, unspecified** ♀
     Hypomenorrhea NOS

✓4ᵗʰ **N92** **Excessive, frequent and irregular menstruation**
     EXCLUDES 1   postmenopausal bleeding (N95.0)
          precocious puberty (menstruation) (E30.1)

N92.0 **Excessive and frequent menstruation** with regular cycle ♀
     Heavy periods NOS
     Menorrhagia NOS
     Polymenorrhea

N92.1 **Excessive and frequent menstruation** with irregular cycle ♀
     Irregular intermenstrual bleeding
     Irregular, shortened intervals between menstrual bleeding
     Menometrorrhagia
     Metrorrhagia

N92.2 **Excessive menstruation at puberty** P♀
     Excessive bleeding associated with onset of menstrual periods
     Pubertal menorrhagia
     Puberty bleeding

N92.3 **Ovulation bleeding** ♀
     Regular intermenstrual bleeding

N92.4 **Excessive bleeding in the premenopausal period** ♀
     Climacteric menorrhagia or metrorrhagia
     Menopausal menorrhagia or metrorrhagia
     ▶Perimenopausal bleeding◀
     ▶Perimenopausal menorrhagia or metrorrhagia◀
     Preclimacteric menorrhagia or metrorrhagia
     Premenopausal menorrhagia or metrorrhagia

N92.5 **Other specified irregular menstruation** ♀

N92.6 **Irregular menstruation, unspecified** ♀
     Irregular bleeding NOS
     Irregular periods NOS
     EXCLUDES 1   irregular menstruation with:
          lengthened intervals or scanty bleeding (N91.3-N91.5)
          shortened intervals or excessive bleeding (N92.1)

✓4ᵗʰ **N93** **Other abnormal uterine and vaginal bleeding**
     EXCLUDES 1   neonatal vaginal hemorrhage (P54.6)
          precocious puberty (menstruation) (E30.1)
          pseudomenses (P54.6)

N93.0 **Postcoital and contact bleeding** ♀

N93.1 **Pre-pubertal vaginal bleeding** ♀
     AHA: 2016,4Q,47

N93.8 **Other specified abnormal uterine and vaginal bleeding** ♀
     Dysfunctional or functional uterine or vaginal bleeding NOS

N93.9 **Abnormal uterine and vaginal bleeding, unspecified** ♀

✓4ᵗʰ **N94** **Pain and other conditions associated with female genital organs and menstrual cycle**

N94.0 **Mittelschmerz** ♀
     DEF: One-sided, lower abdominal pain occurring between menstrual periods that is associated with ovulation.

✓5ᵗʰ **N94.1** **Dyspareunia**
     EXCLUDES 1   psychogenic dyspareunia (F52.6)
     AHA: 2016,4Q,47

N94.10 **Unspecified dyspareunia** ♀

N94.11 **Superficial** (introital) **dyspareunia** ♀

N94.12 **Deep** dyspareunia ♀

N94.19 **Other specified dyspareunia** ♀

N94.2 **Vaginismus** ♀
     EXCLUDES 1   psychogenic vaginismus (F52.5)
     DEF: Spontaneous contractions of the muscles surrounding the vagina, causing it to constrict or close.

N94.3 **Premenstrual tension syndrome** ♀
     Code also associated menstrual migraine (G43.82-, G43.83-)
     EXCLUDES 1   premenstrual dysphoric disorder (F32.81)

N94.4 **Primary dysmenorrhea** ♀

N94.5 **Secondary dysmenorrhea**

N94.6 **Dysmenorrhea, unspecified**
     EXCLUDES 1   psychogenic dysm

✓5ᵗʰ **N94.8** **Other specified conditions ass** organs and menstrual cycle

✓6ᵗʰ **N94.81** **Vulvodynia**

N94.810 **Vulvar vest**

N94.818 **Other vulvo**

N94.819 **Vulvodynia,**
     Vulvodynia

N94.89 **Other specified condit** with female genital or menstrual cycle
     DEF: Hydrocele: Serous of Nuck in females.

N94.9 **Unspecified condition associate** genital organs and menstrual cy

✓4ᵗʰ **N95** **Menopausal and other perimenopausa**
     Menopausal and other perimenopausal c occurring (age-related) menopause
     EXCLUDES 1   excessive bleeding in the prem menopausal and perimenopa or premature menopause premature menopause (E28.3
     EXCLUDES 2   postmenopausal osteoporosis postmenopausal osteoporosis fracture (M80.0-) postmenopausal urethritis (N3

N95.0 **Postmenopausal bleeding**

N95.1 **Menopausal and female climacter**
     Symptoms such as flushing, sleeple concentration, associated with menopause
     Use additional code for associated s
     EXCLUDES 1   asymptomatic menopa symptoms associated w (E89.41) symptoms associated w (E28.310)

N95.2 **Postmenopausal atrophic vaginitis**
     Senile (atrophic) vaginitis

N95.8 **Other specified menopausal and peri** disorders

N95.9 **Unspecified menopausal and perime** disorder

N96 **Recurrent pregnancy loss**
     Investigation or care in a nonpregnant woman pregnancy loss
     EXCLUDES 1   recurrent pregnancy loss with curre

✓4ᵗʰ **N97** **Female infertility**
     INCLUDES   inability to achieve a pregnancy sterility, female NOS
     EXCLUDES 1   female infertility associated with: hypopituitarism (E23.0) Stein-Leventhal syndrome (E28.2)
     EXCLUDES 2   incompetence of cervix uteri (N88.3)
     DEF: Infertility: Inability to conceive for at least or intercourse.
     DEF: Primary infertility: Infertility occurring in pati conceived.
     DEF: Secondary infertility: Infertility occurring in p previously conceived.

N97.0 **Female infertility** associated with anov

N97.1 **Female infertility of** tubal origin
     Female infertility associated with congen
     Female infertility due to tubal block
     Female infertility due to tubal occlusion
     Female infertility due to tubal stenosis

N97.2 **Female infertility of** uterine origin
     Female infertility associated with congenit
     Female infertility due to nonimplantation

N97.8 **Female infertility of other origin**

N97.9 **Female infertility, unspecified**

N Newborn: 0   P Pediatric: 0-17   M Maternity: 12-55   A Adult: 15-124   CH Comorbidity High   CL Comorbidity Low   NCDx Noncancer Dx

840

☑4ᵗʰ **N98 Complications associated with artificial fertilization**

N98.0 Infection associated with artificial insemination ♀

N98.1 Hyperstimulation of ovaries ♀
Hyperstimulation of ovaries NOS
Hyperstimulation of ovaries associated with induced ovulation

N98.2 Complications of attempted introduction of fertilized ovum following in vitro fertilization ♀

N98.3 Complications of attempted introduction of embryo in embryo transfer ♀

N98.8 Other complications associated with artificial fertilization ♀

N98.9 Complication associated with artificial fertilization, unspecified ♀

Intraoperative and postprocedural complications and disorders of genitourinary system, not elsewhere classified (N99)

☑4ᵗʰ **N99 Intraoperative and postprocedural complications and disorders of genitourinary system, not elsewhere classified**
EXCLUDES 2   irradiation cystitis (N30.4-)
postoophorectomy osteoporosis with current pathological fracture (M80.8-)
postoophorectomy osteoporosis without current pathological fracture (M81.8)

N99.0 Postprocedural (acute) (chronic) kidney failure
Use additional code to type of kidney disease

☑5ᵗʰ **N99.1** Postprocedural urethral stricture
Postcatheterization urethral stricture

☑6ᵗʰ **N99.11 Postprocedural urethral stricture, male**
AHA: 2016,4Q,47-48

N99.110 Postprocedural urethral stricture, male, meatal ♂

N99.111 Postprocedural bulbous urethral stricture, male ♂

N99.112 Postprocedural membranous urethral stricture, male ♂

N99.113 Postprocedural anterior bulbous urethral stricture, male ♂

N99.114 Postprocedural urethral stricture, male, unspecified ♂

N99.115 Postprocedural fossa navicularis urethral stricture ♂

N99.116 Postprocedural urethral stricture, male, overlapping sites ♂

N99.12 Postprocedural urethral stricture, female ♀

N99.2 Postprocedural adhesions of vagina ♀

N99.3 Prolapse of vaginal vault after hysterectomy ♀

N99.4 Postprocedural pelvic peritoneal adhesions
EXCLUDES 2   pelvic peritoneal adhesions NOS (N73.6)
postinfective pelvic peritoneal adhesions (N73.6)

☑5ᵗʰ **N99.5** Complications of stoma of urinary tract
EXCLUDES 2   mechanical complication of urinary catheter (T83.0-)
AHA: 2016,4Q,48

☑6ᵗʰ **N99.51 Complication of cystostomy**
N99.510 Cystostomy hemorrhage
N99.511 Cystostomy infection
N99.512 Cystostomy malfunction
N99.518 Other cystostomy complication

☑6ᵗʰ **N99.52 Complication of incontinent external stoma of urinary tract**
N99.520 Hemorrhage of incontinent external stoma of urinary tract
N99.521 Infection of incontinent external stoma of urinary tract
N99.522 Malfunction of incontinent external stoma of urinary tract
N99.523 Herniation of incontinent stoma of urinary tract
N99.524 Stenosis of incontinent stoma of urinary tract
N99.528 Other complication of incontinent external stoma of urinary tract

☑6ᵗʰ **N99.53 Complication of continent stoma of urinary tract**
N99.530 Hemorrhage of continent stoma of urinary tract
N99.531 Infection of continent stoma of urinary tract
N99.532 Malfunction of continent stoma of urinary tract
N99.533 Herniation of continent stoma of urinary tract
N99.534 Stenosis of continent stoma of urinary tract
N99.538 Other complication of continent stoma of urinary tract

☑5ᵗʰ **N99.6** Intraoperative hemorrhage and hematoma of a genitourinary system organ or structure complicating a procedure
EXCLUDES 1   intraoperative hemorrhage and hematoma of a genitourinary system organ or structure due to accidental puncture or laceration during a procedure (N99.7-)

N99.61 Intraoperative hemorrhage and hematoma of a genitourinary system organ or structure complicating a genitourinary system procedure

N99.62 Intraoperative hemorrhage and hematoma of a genitourinary system organ or structure complicating other procedure

☑5ᵗʰ **N99.7** Accidental puncture and laceration of a genitourinary system organ or structure during a procedure

N99.71 Accidental puncture and laceration of a genitourinary system organ or structure during a genitourinary system procedure

N99.72 Accidental puncture and laceration of a genitourinary system organ or structure during other procedure

☑5ᵗʰ **N99.8** Other intraoperative and postprocedural complications and disorders of genitourinary system
AHA: 2016,4Q,9-10

N99.81 Other intraoperative complications of genitourinary system

☑6ᵗʰ **N99.82** Postprocedural hemorrhage of a genitourinary system organ or structure following a procedure
N99.820 Postprocedural hemorrhage of a genitourinary system organ or structure following a genitourinary system procedure
N99.821 Postprocedural hemorrhage of a genitourinary system organ or structure following other procedure

N99.83 Residual ovary syndrome ♀

☑6ᵗʰ **N99.84** Postprocedural hematoma and seroma of a genitourinary system organ or structure following a procedure
N99.840 Postprocedural hematoma of a genitourinary system organ or structure following a genitourinary system procedure
N99.841 Postprocedural hematoma of a genitourinary system organ or structure following other procedure
N99.842 Postprocedural seroma of a genitourinary system organ or structure following a genitourinary system procedure
N99.843 Postprocedural seroma of a genitourinary system organ or structure following other procedure

● **N99.85** Post endometrial ablation syndrome

N99.89 Other postprocedural complications and disorders of genitourinary system

Chapter 15. Pregnancy, Childbirth and the Puerperium (O00–O9A)

Chapter-specific Guidelines with Coding Examples

The chapter-specific guidelines from the ICD-10-CM Official Guidelines for Coding and Reporting have been provided below. Along with these guidelines are coding examples, contained in the shaded boxes, that have been developed to help illustrate the coding and/or sequencing guidance found in these guidelines.

a. General rules for obstetric cases

1) Codes from chapter 15 and sequencing priority

Obstetric cases require codes from chapter 15, codes in the range O00-O9A, Pregnancy, Childbirth, and the Puerperium. Chapter 15 codes have sequencing priority over codes from other chapters. Additional codes from other chapters may be used in conjunction with chapter 15 codes to further specify conditions. Should the provider document that the pregnancy is incidental to the encounter, then code Z33.1, Pregnant state, incidental, should be used in place of any chapter 15 codes. It is the provider's responsibility to state that the condition being treated is not affecting the pregnancy.

Bladder abscess in pregnant patient at 25 weeks' gestation	
O23.12	Infections of bladder in pregnancy, second trimester
N30.80	Other cystitis without hematuria
Z3A.25	25 weeks gestation of pregnancy

Explanation: The documentation does not indicate that the pregnancy is incidental or in any way unaffected by the bladder abscess; therefore, an obstetrics code should be sequenced first. An additional code was provided to identify the specific bladder condition as this information is not called out specifically in the obstetrics code.

2) Chapter 15 codes used only on the maternal record

Chapter 15 codes are to be used only on the maternal record, never on the record of the newborn.

3) Final character for trimester

The majority of codes in Chapter 15 have a final character indicating the trimester of pregnancy. The timeframes for the trimesters are indicated at the beginning of the chapter. If trimester is not a component of a code, it is because the condition always occurs in a specific trimester, or the concept of trimester of pregnancy is not applicable. Certain codes have characters for only certain trimesters because the condition does not occur in all trimesters, but it may occur in more than just one.

Assignment of the final character for trimester should be based on the provider's documentation of the trimester (or number of weeks) for the current admission/encounter. This applies to the assignment of trimester for pre-existing conditions as well as those that develop during or are due to the pregnancy. The provider's documentation of the number of weeks may be used to assign the appropriate code identifying the trimester.

Whenever delivery occurs during the current admission, and there is an "in childbirth" option for the obstetric complication being coded, the "in childbirth" code should be assigned.

Pregnant patient at 21 weeks' gestation admitted with excessive vomiting	
O21.2	Late vomiting of pregnancy
Z3A.21	21 weeks gestation of pregnancy

Explanation: Category O21 classifies vomiting in pregnancy. Although code selection is based on whether the vomiting is before or after 20 completed weeks, these codes are not further classified by trimester. If vomiting only in the second trimester was documented, the provider should be queried for the specific week of gestation, as this will affect code selection.

4) Selection of trimester for inpatient admissions that encompass more than one trimester

In instances when a patient is admitted to a hospital for complications of pregnancy during one trimester and remains in the hospital into a subsequent trimester, the trimester character for the antepartum complication code should be assigned on the basis of the trimester when the complication developed, not the trimester of the discharge. If the condition developed prior to the current admission/encounter or represents a pre-existing condition, the trimester character for the trimester at the time of the admission/encounter should be assigned.

5) Unspecified trimester

Each category that includes codes for trimester has a code for "unspecified trimester." The "unspecified trimester" code should rarely be used, such as when the documentation in the record is insufficient to determine the trimester and it is not possible to obtain clarification.

6) 7th character for fetus identification

Where applicable, a 7th character is to be assigned for certain categories (O31, O32, O33.3 - O33.6, O35, O36, O40, O41, O60.1, O60.2, O64, and O69) to identify the fetus for which the complication code applies.

Assign 7th character "0":

- For single gestations
- When the documentation in the record is insufficient to determine the fetus affected and it is not possible to obtain clarification.
- When it is not possible to clinically determine which fetus is affected.

b. Selection of OB principal or first-listed diagnosis

1) Routine outpatient prenatal visits

For routine outpatient prenatal visits when no complications are present, a code from category Z34, Encounter for supervision of normal pregnancy, should be used as the first-listed diagnosis. These codes should not be used in conjunction with chapter 15 codes.

2) Supervision of high-risk pregnancy

Codes from category O09, Supervision of high-risk pregnancy, are intended for use only during the prenatal period. For complications during the labor or delivery episode as a result of a high-risk pregnancy, assign the applicable complication codes from Chapter 15. If there are no complications during the labor or delivery episode, assign code O80, Encounter for full-term uncomplicated delivery.

For routine prenatal outpatient visits for patients with high-risk pregnancies, a code from category O09, Supervision of high-risk pregnancy, should be used as the first-listed diagnosis. Secondary chapter 15 codes may be used in conjunction with these codes if appropriate.

3) Episodes when no delivery occurs

In episodes when no delivery occurs, the principal diagnosis should correspond to the principal complication of the pregnancy which necessitated the encounter. Should more than one complication exist, all of which are treated or monitored, any of the complication codes may be sequenced first.

4) When a delivery occurs

When an obstetric patient is admitted and delivers during that admission, the condition that prompted the admission should be sequenced as the principal diagnosis. If multiple conditions prompted the admission, sequence the one most related to the delivery as the principal diagnosis. A code for any complication of the delivery should be assigned as an additional diagnosis. In cases of cesarean delivery, if the patient was admitted with a condition that resulted in the performance of a cesarean procedure, that condition should be selected as the principal diagnosis. If the reason for the admission was unrelated to the condition resulting in the cesarean delivery, the condition related to the reason for the admission should be selected as the principal diagnosis.

5) Outcome of delivery

A code from category Z37, Outcome of delivery, should be included on every maternal record when a delivery has occurred. These codes are not to be used on subsequent records or on the newborn record.

c. Pre-existing conditions versus conditions due to the pregnancy

Certain categories in Chapter 15 distinguish between conditions of the mother that existed prior to pregnancy (pre-existing) and those that are a direct result of pregnancy. When assigning codes from Chapter 15, it is important to assess if a condition was pre-existing prior to pregnancy or developed during or due to the pregnancy in order to assign the correct code.

Categories that do not distinguish between pre-existing and pregnancy-related conditions may be used for either. It is acceptable to use codes specifically for the puerperium with codes complicating pregnancy and childbirth if a condition arises postpartum during the delivery encounter.

Chapter 15. Pregnancy, Childbirth and the Puerperium

d. Pre-existing hypertension in pregnancy

Category O1Ø, Pre-existing hypertension complicating pregnancy, childbirth and the puerperium, includes codes for hypertensive heart and hypertensive chronic kidney disease. When assigning one of the O1Ø codes that includes hypertensive heart disease or hypertensive chronic kidney disease, it is necessary to add a secondary code from the appropriate hypertension category to specify the type of heart failure or chronic kidney disease.

See Section I.C.9. Hypertension.

e. Fetal conditions affecting the management of the mother

1) Codes from categories O35 and O36

Codes from categories O35, Maternal care for known or suspected fetal abnormality and damage, and O36, Maternal care for other fetal problems, are assigned only when the fetal condition is actually responsible for modifying the management of the mother, i.e., by requiring diagnostic studies, additional observation, special care, or termination of pregnancy. The fact that the fetal condition exists does not justify assigning a code from this series to the mother's record.

2) In utero surgery

In cases when surgery is performed on the fetus, a diagnosis code from category O35, Maternal care for known or suspected fetal abnormality and damage, should be assigned identifying the fetal condition. Assign the appropriate procedure code for the procedure performed.

No code from Chapter 16, the perinatal codes, should be used on the mother's record to identify fetal conditions. Surgery performed in utero on a fetus is still to be coded as an obstetric encounter.

f. HIV infection in pregnancy, childbirth and the puerperium

During pregnancy, childbirth or the puerperium, a patient admitted because of an HIV-related illness should receive a principal diagnosis from subcategory O98.7-, Human immunodeficiency [HIV] disease complicating pregnancy, childbirth and the puerperium, followed by the code(s) for the HIV-related illness(es).

Patients with asymptomatic HIV infection status admitted during pregnancy, childbirth, or the puerperium should receive codes of O98.7- and Z21, Asymptomatic human immunodeficiency virus [HIV] infection status.

An HIV-positive female, age 42, with a history of Down syndrome is admitted for skilled nursing care, medication management, and observation due to worsening HIV-associated nephritis during her pregnancy. Current provider reports indicate she is 13 weeks pregnant.

O98.711	Human immunodeficiency virus [HIV] disease complicating pregnancy, first trimester
B2Ø	Human immunodeficiency virus [HIV] disease
NØ8	Glomerular disorders in diseases classified elsewhere
O99.89	Other specified diseases and conditions complicating pregnancy, childbirth and the puerperium
Q9Ø.9	Down syndrome, unspecified
Z3A.13	13 weeks gestation of pregnancy

Explanation: When HIV and associated complications require treatment during the course of a pregnancy, a code from subcategory O98.7- must be assigned, followed by the codes for the HIV infection and any manifestation(s) related to the HIV. Code Z3A.13 should also be used in this scenario to report the current gestation.

g. Diabetes mellitus in pregnancy

Diabetes mellitus is a significant complicating factor in pregnancy. Pregnant women who are diabetic should be assigned a code from category O24, Diabetes mellitus in pregnancy, childbirth, and the puerperium, first, followed by the appropriate diabetes code(s) (E08-E13) from Chapter 4.

h. Long term use of insulin and oral hypoglycemics

See section I.C.4.a.3 for information on the long term use of insulin and oral hypoglycemic.

i. Gestational (pregnancy induced) diabetes

Gestational (pregnancy induced) diabetes can occur during the second and third trimester of pregnancy in women who were not diabetic prior to pregnancy. Gestational diabetes can cause complications in the pregnancy similar to those of pre-existing diabetes mellitus. It also puts the woman at greater risk of developing diabetes after the pregnancy. Codes for gestational diabetes are in subcategory O24.4, Gestational diabetes mellitus. No other code from category O24, Diabetes mellitus in pregnancy, childbirth, and the puerperium, should be used with a code from O24.4.

The codes under subcategory O24.4 include diet controlled, insulin controlled, and controlled by oral hypoglycemic drugs. If a patient with gestational diabetes is treated with both diet and insulin, only the code for insulin-controlled is required. If a patient with gestational diabetes is treated with both diet and oral hypoglycemic medications, only the code for "controlled by oral hypoglycemic drugs" is required. Code Z79.4, Long-term (current) use of insulin or code Z79.84, Long-term (current) use of oral hypoglycemic drugs, should not be assigned with codes from subcategory O24.4.

An abnormal glucose tolerance in pregnancy is assigned a code from subcategory O99.81, Abnormal glucose complicating pregnancy, childbirth, and the puerperium.

j. Sepsis and septic shock complicating abortion, pregnancy, childbirth and the puerperium

When assigning a chapter 15 code for sepsis complicating abortion, pregnancy, childbirth, and the puerperium, a code for the specific type of infection should be assigned as an additional diagnosis. If severe sepsis is present, a code from subcategory R65.2, Severe sepsis, and code(s) for associated organ dysfunction(s) should also be assigned as additional diagnoses.

Patient is admitted to the skilled home health nursing for an extended course of intravenous antibiotic administration due to MSSA sepsis that resulted from a miscarriage 1 week ago.

OØ3.87	Sepsis following complete or unspecified spontaneous abortion
B95.61	Methicillin susceptible Staphylococcus aureus infection as the cause of diseases classified elsewhere

Explanation: The type of infection that caused this patient to become septic was methicillin susceptible *Staphylococcus aureus* (MSSA), which as a secondary code helps capture all aspects related to this patient's septic condition.

k. Puerperal sepsis

Code O85, Puerperal sepsis, should be assigned with a secondary code to identify the causal organism (e.g., for a bacterial infection, assign a code from category B95-B96, Bacterial infections in conditions classified elsewhere). A code from category A40, Streptococcal sepsis, or A41, Other sepsis, should not be used for puerperal sepsis. If applicable, use additional codes to identify severe sepsis (R65.2-) and any associated acute organ dysfunction.

l. Alcohol, tobacco and drug use during pregnancy, childbirth and the puerperium

1) Alcohol use during pregnancy, childbirth and the puerperium

Codes under subcategory O99.31, Alcohol use complicating pregnancy, childbirth, and the puerperium, should be assigned for any pregnancy case when a mother uses alcohol during the pregnancy or postpartum. A secondary code from category F10, Alcohol related disorders, should also be assigned to identify manifestations of the alcohol use.

2) Tobacco use during pregnancy, childbirth and the puerperium

Codes under subcategory O99.33, Smoking (tobacco) complicating pregnancy, childbirth, and the puerperium, should be assigned for any pregnancy case when a mother uses any type of tobacco product during the pregnancy or postpartum. A secondary code from category F17, Nicotine dependence, should also be assigned to identify the type of nicotine dependence.

3) Drug use during pregnancy, childbirth and the puerperium

Codes under subcategory O99.32, Drug use complicating pregnancy, childbirth, and the puerperium, should be assigned for any pregnancy case when a mother uses drugs during the pregnancy or postpartum. This can involve illegal drugs, or inappropriate use or abuse of prescription drugs. Secondary code(s) from categories F11-F16 and F18-F19 should also be assigned to identify manifestations of the drug use.

m. Poisoning, toxic effects, adverse effects and underdosing in a pregnant patient

A code from subcategory O9A.2, Injury, poisoning and certain other consequences of external causes complicating pregnancy, childbirth, and the puerperium, should be sequenced first, followed by the appropriate injury, poisoning, toxic effect, adverse effect or underdosing code, and then the additional code(s) that specifies the condition caused by the poisoning, toxic effect, adverse effect or underdosing.

See Section I.C.19. Adverse effects, poisoning, underdosing and toxic effects.

An 18-week pregnant female, who is wheelchair-bound due to paraplegia, is admitted for skilled nursing care with medication instruction after developing severe hypotension due to taking an incorrect dose of nifedipine. The drug was ordered to control her transient hypertension during the pregnancy, and she remains on the drug now with the correct dose administered.

O9A.212	Injury, poisoning and certain other consequences of external causes complicating pregnancy, second trimester
T46.1X1D	Poisoning by calcium-channel blockers, accidental (unintentional), subsequent encounter
I95.2	Hypotension due to drugs
O13.2	Gestational [pregnancy-induced] hypertension without significant proteinuria, second trimester
O99.352	Diseases of the nervous system complicating pregnancy, second trimester
G82.20	Paraplegia, unspecified
Z3A.18	18 weeks gestation of pregnancy

Explanation: Although the poisoning with resulting hypotension is the reason for admission, a code from the obstetrics chapter must first be assigned. Codes from chapter 15 have sequencing priority over codes from other chapters.

n. Normal delivery, code O80

1) Encounter for full term uncomplicated delivery

Code O80 should be assigned when a woman is admitted for a full-term normal delivery and delivers a single, healthy infant without any complications antepartum, during the delivery, or postpartum during the delivery episode. Code O80 is always a principal diagnosis. It is not to be used if any other code from chapter 15 is needed to describe a current complication of the antenatal, delivery, or **postnatal** period. Additional codes from other chapters may be used with code O80 if they are not related to or are in any way complicating the pregnancy.

2) Uncomplicated delivery with resolved antepartum complication

Code O80 may be used if the patient had a complication at some point during the pregnancy, but the complication is not present at the time of the admission for delivery.

3) Outcome of delivery for O80

Z37.0, Single live birth, is the only outcome of delivery code appropriate for use with O80.

o. The peripartum and postpartum periods

1) Peripartum and postpartum periods

The postpartum period begins immediately after delivery and continues for six weeks following delivery. The peripartum period is defined as the last month of pregnancy to five months postpartum.

2) Peripartum and postpartum complication

A postpartum complication is any complication occurring within the six-week period.

3) Pregnancy-related complications after 6 week period

Chapter 15 codes may also be used to describe pregnancy-related complications after the peripartum or postpartum period if the provider documents that a condition is pregnancy related.

A 46-year-old woman had a baby boy 7 weeks ago. Following delivery, she quickly developed severe pseudomonas pyelonephritis, necessitating IV antibiotic therapy. She is referred to home health where she will be continued on antibiotics via PICC line. The physician reports "puerperal pseudomonas pyelonephritis."

Code	Description
O86.21	Infection of kidney following delivery
B96.5	Pseudomonas (aeruginosa) (mallei) (pseudomallei) as the cause of diseases classified elsewhere
Z45.2	Encounter for adjustment and management of vascular access device
Z79.2	Long term (current) use of antibiotics

Explanation: While not all infections of the urinary tract occurring after delivery are related directly to the delivery, in this case the physician reports "puerperal" in reference to the pyelonephritis. This indicates a need to assign a code from chapter 15 for the infection.

4) Admission for routine postpartum care following delivery outside hospital

When the mother delivers outside the hospital prior to admission and is admitted for routine postpartum care and no complications are noted, code Z39.0, Encounter for care and examination of mother immediately after delivery, should be assigned as the principal diagnosis.

5) Pregnancy associated cardiomyopathy

Pregnancy associated cardiomyopathy, code O90.3, is unique in that it may be diagnosed in the third trimester of pregnancy but may continue to progress months after delivery. For this reason, it is referred to as peripartum cardiomyopathy. Code O90.3 is only for use when the cardiomyopathy develops as a result of pregnancy in a woman who did not have pre-existing heart disease.

A 36-year-old woman with no pre-existing conditions started experiencing heart failure symptoms late in the 3rd trimester of her second pregnancy. After an extensive workup she was diagnosed with nonobstructive hypertrophic cardiomyopathy. She made it through the delivery without any further complications but was referred to home health for observation of her condition and physical therapy to address reduced endurance. The cardiologist reports that the cardiomyopathy was directly related to the pregnancy and remains unresolved.

Code	Description
O90.3	Peripartum cardiomyopathy
I42.2	Other hypertrophic cardiomyopathy

Explanation: Because this patient has no cardiac history and no other conditions were found to be the cause of her cardiomyopathy, code O90.3 is most appropriate. An additional code for the specific type of cardiomyopathy may also be assigned, according to the inclusion term at code O90.3 as well as the Excludes 2 note at category I42.

Since this patient has no cardiac history, continues to experience cardiomyopathy in the postpartum period, and was diagnosed during the pregnancy, code O90.3 must be used. Also assign a code sequenced after O90.3 to specify the specific type of cardiomyopathy, as peripartum cardiomyopathy and codes from category I42 are listed as Excludes 2 conditions.

p. Code O94, Sequelae of complication of pregnancy, childbirth, and the puerperium

1) Code O94

Code O94, Sequelae of complication of pregnancy, childbirth, and the puerperium, is for use in those cases when an initial complication of a pregnancy develops a sequelae requiring care or treatment at a future date.

2) After the initial postpartum period

This code may be used at any time after the initial postpartum period.

3) Sequencing of code O94

This code, like all sequela codes, is to be sequenced following the code describing the sequelae of the complication.

q. Termination of pregnancy and spontaneous abortions

1) Abortion with liveborn fetus

When an attempted termination of pregnancy results in a liveborn fetus, assign code Z33.2, Encounter for elective termination of pregnancy and a code from category Z37, Outcome of Delivery.

2) Retained products of conception following an abortion

Subsequent encounters for retained products of conception following a spontaneous abortion or elective termination of pregnancy, without complications are assigned O03.4, Incomplete spontaneous abortion without complication, or code O07.4, Failed attempted termination of pregnancy without complication. This advice is appropriate even when the patient was discharged previously with a discharge diagnosis of complete abortion. If the patient has a specific complication associated with the spontaneous abortion or elective termination of pregnancy in addition to retained products of conception, assign the appropriate complication **code (e.g., O03.-, O04.-, O07.-)** instead of code O03.4 or O07.4.

3) Complications leading to abortion

Codes from Chapter 15 may be used as additional codes to identify any documented complications of the pregnancy in conjunction with codes in categories in O04, O07 and O08.

r. **Abuse in a pregnant patient**

For suspected or confirmed cases of abuse of a pregnant patient, a code(s) from subcategories O9A.3, Physical abuse complicating pregnancy, childbirth, and the puerperium, O9A.4, Sexual abuse complicating pregnancy, childbirth, and the puerperium, and O9A.5, Psychological abuse complicating pregnancy, childbirth, and the puerperium, should be sequenced first, followed by the appropriate codes (if applicable) to identify any associated current injury due to physical abuse, sexual abuse, and the perpetrator of abuse.

See Section I.C.19. Adult and child abuse, neglect and other maltreatment.

Chapter 15. Pregnancy, Childbirth and the Puerperium (O00-O9A)

NOTE   CODES FROM THIS CHAPTER ARE FOR USE ONLY ON MATERNAL RECORDS, NEVER ON NEWBORN RECORDS

Codes from this chapter are for use for conditions related to or aggravated by the pregnancy, childbirth, or by the puerperium (maternal causes or obstetric causes)

NOTE   Trimesters are counted from the first day of the last menstrual period. They are defined as follows:

1st trimester- less than 14 weeks 0 days

2nd trimester- 14 weeks 0 days to less than 28 weeks 0 days

3rd trimester- 28 weeks 0 days until delivery

Use additional code from category Z3A, Weeks of gestation, to identify the specific week of the pregnancy, if known.

EXCLUDES 1   supervision of normal pregnancy (Z34.-)

EXCLUDES 2   mental and behavioral disorders associated with the puerperium (F53.-)
obstetrical tetanus (A34)
postpartum necrosis of pituitary gland (E23.0)
puerperal osteomalacia (M83.0)

AHA: 2016,1Q,3-5; 2014,3Q,17

This chapter contains the following blocks:

O00-O08   Pregnancy with abortive outcome
O09   Supervision of high risk pregnancy
O10-O16   Edema, proteinuria and hypertensive disorders in pregnancy, childbirth and the puerperium
O20-O29   Other maternal disorders predominantly related to pregnancy
O30-O48   Maternal care related to the fetus and amniotic cavity and possible delivery problems
O60-O77   Complications of labor and delivery
O80-O82   Encounter for delivery
O85-O92   Complications predominantly related to the puerperium
O94-O9A   Other obstetric conditions, not elsewhere classified

Pregnancy with abortive outcome (O00-O08)

EXCLUDES 1   continuing pregnancy in multiple gestation after abortion of one fetus or more (O31.1-, O31.3-)

✓4ᵗʰ O00 Ectopic pregnancy

INCLUDES   ruptured ectopic pregnancy

Use additional code from category O08 to identify any associated complication

AHA: 2016,4Q,48-50; 2014,3Q,17

DEF: Implantation of a fertilized egg outside the uterus, usually in the fallopian tube or abdomen that requires emergency treatment.

Ectopic Pregnancy

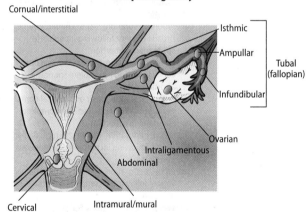

Cornual/interstitial
Isthmic
Ampullar
Tubal (fallopian)
Infundibular
Ovarian
Intraligamentous
Abdominal
Cervical
Intramural/mural

✓5ᵗʰ O00.0 Abdominal pregnancy

EXCLUDES 1   maternal care for viable fetus in abdominal pregnancy (O36.7-)

O00.00 Abdominal pregnancy without intrauterine pregnancy   ⓜ♀
Abdominal pregnancy NOS

O00.01 Abdominal pregnancy with intrauterine pregnancy   ⓜ♀

✓5ᵗʰ O00.1 Tubal pregnancy
Fallopian pregnancy
Rupture of (fallopian) tube due to pregnancy
Tubal abortion
AHA: 2017,4Q,20

✓6ᵗʰ O00.10 Tubal pregnancy without intrauterine pregnancy
Tubal pregnancy NOS

O00.101 Right tubal pregnancy without intrauterine pregnancy   ⓜ♀

O00.102 Left tubal pregnancy without intrauterine pregnancy   ⓜ♀

O00.109 Unspecified tubal pregnancy without intrauterine pregnancy   ⓜ♀

✓6ᵗʰ O00.11 Tubal pregnancy with intrauterine pregnancy

O00.111 Right tubal pregnancy with intrauterine pregnancy   ⓜ♀

O00.112 Left tubal pregnancy with intrauterine pregnancy   ⓜ♀

O00.119 Unspecified tubal pregnancy with intrauterine pregnancy   ⓜ♀

✓5ᵗʰ O00.2 Ovarian pregnancy

AHA: 2017,4Q,20

✓6ᵗʰ O00.20 Ovarian pregnancy without intrauterine pregnancy
Ovarian pregnancy NOS

O00.201 Right ovarian pregnancy without intrauterine pregnancy   ⓜ♀

O00.202 Left ovarian pregnancy without intrauterine pregnancy   ⓜ♀

O00.209 Unspecified ovarian pregnancy without intrauterine pregnancy   ⓜ♀

✓6ᵗʰ O00.21 Ovarian pregnancy with intrauterine pregnancy

O00.211 Right ovarian pregnancy with intrauterine pregnancy   ⓜ♀

O00.212 Left ovarian pregnancy with intrauterine pregnancy   ⓜ♀

O00.219 Unspecified ovarian pregnancy with intrauterine pregnancy   ⓜ♀

✓5ᵗʰ O00.8 Other ectopic pregnancy
Cervical pregnancy
Cornual pregnancy
Intraligamentous pregnancy
Mural pregnancy

O00.80 Other ectopic pregnancy without intrauterine pregnancy   ⓜ♀
Other ectopic pregnancy NOS

O00.81 Other ectopic pregnancy with intrauterine pregnancy   ⓜ♀

✓5ᵗʰ O00.9 Ectopic pregnancy, unspecified

O00.90 Unspecified ectopic pregnancy without intrauterine pregnancy   ⓜ♀
Ectopic pregnancy NOS

O00.91 Unspecified ectopic pregnancy with intrauterine pregnancy   ⓜ♀

✓4ᵗʰ O01 Hydatidiform mole

Use additional code from category O08 to identify any associated complication

EXCLUDES 1   chorioadenoma (destruens) (D39.2)
malignant hydatidiform mole (D39.2)

AHA: 2014,3Q,17

DEF: Abnormal product of pregnancy, marked by a mass of cysts resembling a bunch of grapes due to chorionic villi proliferation and dissolution. It must be surgically removed.

O01.0 Classical hydatidiform mole   ⓜ♀
Complete hydatidiform mole

O01.1 Incomplete and partial hydatidiform mole   ⓜ♀

O01.9 Hydatidiform mole, unspecified   ⓜ♀
Trophoblastic disease NOS
Vesicular mole NOS

✓ Additional Character Required   ✓x7ᵗʰ Placeholder Alert   Manifestation   Unspecified Dx   ▶◀ Revised Text   ● New Code   ▲ Revised Title

ICD-10-CM 2020   847

O02 Other abnormal products of conception
Use additional code from category O08 to identify any associated complication

EXCLUDES 1　papyraceous fetus (O31.0-)

AHA: 2014,3Q,17

O02.0 Blighted ovum and nonhydatidiform mole Ⓜ♀
Carneous mole
Fleshy mole
Intrauterine mole NOS
Molar pregnancy NEC
Pathological ovum

O02.1 Missed abortion Ⓜ♀
Early fetal death, before completion of 20 weeks of gestation, with retention of dead fetus

EXCLUDES 1　failed induced abortion (O07.-)
fetal death (intrauterine) (late) (O36.4)
missed abortion with blighted ovum (O02.0)
missed abortion with hydatidiform mole (O01.-)
missed abortion with nonhydatidiform (O02.0)
missed abortion with other abnormal products of conception (O02.8-)
missed delivery (O36.4)
stillbirth (P95)

O02.8 Other specified abnormal products of conception

EXCLUDES 1　abnormal products of conception with blighted ovum (O02.0)
abnormal products of conception with hydatidiform mole (O01.-)
abnormal products of conception with nonhydatidiform mole (O02.0)

O02.81 Inappropriate change in quantitative human chorionic gonadotropin (hCG) in early pregnancy Ⓜ♀
Biochemical pregnancy
Chemical pregnancy
Inappropriate level of quantitative human chorionic gonadotropin (hCG) for gestational age in early pregnancy

O02.89 Other abnormal products of conception Ⓜ♀

O02.9 Abnormal product of conception, unspecified Ⓜ♀

O03 Spontaneous abortion
NOTE　Incomplete abortion includes retained products of conception following spontaneous abortion

INCLUDES　miscarriage

O03.0 Genital tract and pelvic infection following incomplete spontaneous abortion Ⓜ♀
Endometritis following incomplete spontaneous abortion
Oophoritis following incomplete spontaneous abortion
Parametritis following incomplete spontaneous abortion
Pelvic peritonitis following incomplete spontaneous abortion
Salpingitis following incomplete spontaneous abortion
Salpingo-oophoritis following incomplete spontaneous abortion

EXCLUDES 1　sepsis following incomplete spontaneous abortion (O03.37)
urinary tract infection following incomplete spontaneous abortion (O03.38)

O03.1 Delayed or excessive hemorrhage following incomplete spontaneous abortion Ⓜ♀
Afibrinogenemia following incomplete spontaneous abortion
Defibrination syndrome following incomplete spontaneous abortion
Hemolysis following incomplete spontaneous abortion
Intravascular coagulation following incomplete spontaneous abortion

O03.2 Embolism following incomplete spontaneous abortion Ⓜ♀
Air embolism following incomplete spontaneous abortion
Amniotic fluid embolism following incomplete spontaneous abortion
Blood-clot embolism following incomplete spontaneous abortion
Embolism NOS following incomplete spontaneous abortion
Fat embolism following incomplete spontaneous abortion
Pulmonary embolism following incomplete spontaneous abortion
Pyemic embolism following incomplete spontaneous abortion
Septic or septicopyemic embolism following incomplete spontaneous abortion
Soap embolism following incomplete spontaneous abortion

O03.3 Other and unspecified complications following incomplete spontaneous abortion

O03.30 Unspecified complication following incomplete spontaneous abortion Ⓜ♀

O03.31 Shock following incomplete spontaneous abortion Ⓜ♀
Circulatory collapse following incomplete spontaneous abortion
Shock (postprocedural) following incomplete spontaneous abortion

EXCLUDES 1　shock due to infection following incomplete spontaneous abortion (O03.37)

O03.32 Renal failure following incomplete spontaneous abortion Ⓜ♀
Kidney failure (acute) following incomplete spontaneous abortion
Oliguria following incomplete spontaneous abortion
Renal shutdown following incomplete spontaneous abortion
Renal tubular necrosis following incomplete spontaneous abortion
Uremia following incomplete spontaneous abortion

O03.33 Metabolic disorder following incomplete spontaneous abortion Ⓜ♀

O03.34 Damage to pelvic organs following incomplete spontaneous abortion Ⓜ♀
Laceration, perforation, tear or chemical damage of bladder following incomplete spontaneous abortion
Laceration, perforation, tear or chemical damage of bowel following incomplete spontaneous abortion
Laceration, perforation, tear or chemical damage of broad ligament following incomplete spontaneous abortion
Laceration, perforation, tear or chemical damage of cervix following incomplete spontaneous abortion
Laceration, perforation, tear or chemical damage of periurethral tissue following incomplete spontaneous abortion
Laceration, perforation, tear or chemical damage of uterus following incomplete spontaneous abortion
Laceration, perforation, tear or chemical damage of vagina following incomplete spontaneous abortion

O03.35 Other venous complications following incomplete spontaneous abortion Ⓜ♀

O03.36 Cardiac arrest following incomplete spontaneous abortion Ⓜ♀

O03.37 Sepsis following incomplete spontaneous abortion Ⓜ♀
Use additional code to identify infectious agent (B95-B97)
Use additional code to identify severe sepsis, if applicable (R65.2-)

EXCLUDES 1　septic or septicopyemic embolism following incomplete spontaneous abortion (O03.2)

O03.38 Urinary tract infection following incomplete spontaneous abortion ▫ ♀
   Cystitis following incomplete spontaneous abortion

O03.39 Incomplete spontaneous abortion with other complications ▫ ♀

O03.4 Incomplete spontaneous abortion without complication ▫ ♀

O03.5 Genital tract and pelvic infection following complete or unspecified spontaneous abortion ▫ ♀
   Endometritis following complete or unspecified spontaneous abortion
   Oophoritis following complete or unspecified spontaneous abortion
   Parametritis following complete or unspecified spontaneous abortion
   Pelvic peritonitis following complete or unspecified spontaneous abortion
   Salpingitis following complete or unspecified spontaneous abortion
   Salpingo-oophoritis following complete or unspecified spontaneous abortion
   EXCLUDES 1   sepsis following complete or unspecified spontaneous abortion (O03.87)
    urinary tract infection following complete or unspecified spontaneous abortion (O03.88)

O03.6 Delayed or excessive hemorrhage following complete or unspecified spontaneous abortion ▫ ♀
   Afibrinogenemia following complete or unspecified spontaneous abortion
   Defibrination syndrome following complete or unspecified spontaneous abortion
   Hemolysis following complete or unspecified spontaneous abortion
   Intravascular coagulation following complete or unspecified spontaneous abortion

O03.7 Embolism following complete or unspecified spontaneous abortion ▫ ♀
   Air embolism following complete or unspecified spontaneous abortion
   Amniotic fluid embolism following complete or unspecified spontaneous abortion
   Blood-clot embolism following complete or unspecified spontaneous abortion
   Embolism NOS following complete or unspecified spontaneous abortion
   Fat embolism following complete or unspecified spontaneous abortion
   Pulmonary embolism following complete or unspecified spontaneous abortion
   Pyemic embolism following complete or unspecified spontaneous abortion
   Septic or septicopyemic embolism following complete or unspecified spontaneous abortion
   Soap embolism following complete or unspecified spontaneous abortion

✓5ᵗʰ **O03.8** Other and unspecified complications following complete or unspecified spontaneous abortion

O03.80 Unspecified complication following complete or unspecified spontaneous abortion ▫ ♀

O03.81 Shock following complete or unspecified spontaneous abortion ▫ ♀
   Circulatory collapse following complete or unspecified spontaneous abortion
   Shock (postprocedural) following complete or unspecified spontaneous abortion
   EXCLUDES 1   shock due to infection following complete or unspecified spontaneous abortion (O03.87)

O03.82 Renal failure following complete or unspecified spontaneous abortion ▫ ♀
   Kidney failure (acute) following complete or unspecified spontaneous abortion
   Oliguria following complete or unspecified spontaneous abortion
   Renal shutdown following complete or unspecified spontaneous abortion
   Renal tubular necrosis following complete or unspecified spontaneous abortion
   Uremia following complete or unspecified spontaneous abortion

O03.83 Metabolic disorder following complete or unspecified spontaneous abortion ▫ ♀

O03.84 Damage to pelvic organs following complete or unspecified spontaneous abortion ▫ ♀
   Laceration, perforation, tear or chemical damage of bladder following complete or unspecified spontaneous abortion
   Laceration, perforation, tear or chemical damage of bowel following complete or unspecified spontaneous abortion
   Laceration, perforation, tear or chemical damage of broad ligament following complete or unspecified spontaneous abortion
   Laceration, perforation, tear or chemical damage of cervix following complete or unspecified spontaneous abortion
   Laceration, perforation, tear or chemical damage of periurethral tissue following complete or unspecified spontaneous abortion
   Laceration, perforation, tear or chemical damage of uterus following complete or unspecified spontaneous abortion
   Laceration, perforation, tear or chemical damage of vagina following complete or unspecified spontaneous abortion

O03.85 Other venous complications following complete or unspecified spontaneous abortion ▫ ♀

O03.86 Cardiac arrest following complete or unspecified spontaneous abortion ▫ ♀

O03.87 Sepsis following complete or unspecified spontaneous abortion ▫ ♀
   Use additional code to identify infectious agent (B95-B97)
   Use additional code to identify severe sepsis, if applicable (R65.2-)
   EXCLUDES 1   septic or septicopyemic embolism following complete or unspecified spontaneous abortion (O03.7)

O03.88 Urinary tract infection following complete or unspecified spontaneous abortion ▫ ♀
   Cystitis following complete or unspecified spontaneous abortion

O03.89 Complete or unspecified spontaneous abortion with other complications ▫ ♀

O03.9 Complete or unspecified spontaneous abortion without complication ▫ ♀
   Miscarriage NOS
   Spontaneous abortion NOS

Chapter 15. Pregnancy, Childbirth and the Puerperium

✓4ᵗʰ **O04 Complications following (induced) termination of pregnancy**

INCLUDES   complications following (induced) termination of pregnancy

EXCLUDES 1   *encounter for elective termination of pregnancy, uncomplicated (Z33.2)*
failed attempted termination of pregnancy (O07.-)

O04.5 Genital tract and pelvic infection following Ⓜ♀ **(induced) termination of pregnancy**

Endometritis following (induced) termination of pregnancy
Oophoritis following (induced) termination of pregnancy
Parametritis following (induced) termination of pregnancy
Pelvic peritonitis following (induced) termination of pregnancy
Salpingitis following (induced) termination of pregnancy
Salpingo-oophoritis following (induced) termination of pregnancy

EXCLUDES 1   *sepsis following (induced) termination of pregnancy (O04.87)*
urinary tract infection following (induced) termination of pregnancy (O04.88)

O04.6 Delayed or excessive hemorrhage following Ⓜ♀ **(induced) termination of pregnancy**

Afibrinogenemia following (induced) termination of pregnancy
Defibrination syndrome following (induced) termination of pregnancy
Hemolysis following (induced) termination of pregnancy
Intravascular coagulation following (induced) termination of pregnancy

O04.7 Embolism following (induced) termination of Ⓜ♀ **pregnancy**

Air embolism following (induced) termination of pregnancy
Amniotic fluid embolism following (induced) termination of pregnancy
Blood-clot embolism following (induced) termination of pregnancy
Embolism NOS following (induced) termination of pregnancy
Fat embolism following (induced) termination of pregnancy
Pulmonary embolism following (induced) termination of pregnancy
Pyemic embolism following (induced) termination of pregnancy
Septic or septicopyemic embolism following (induced) termination of pregnancy
Soap embolism following (induced) termination of pregnancy

✓5ᵗʰ **O04.8 (Induced) termination of pregnancy with other and unspecified complications**

O04.80 (Induced) termination of pregnancy Ⓜ♀ **with unspecified complications**

O04.81 Shock following (induced) termination Ⓜ♀ **of pregnancy**

Circulatory collapse following (induced) termination of pregnancy
Shock (postprocedural) following (induced) termination of pregnancy

EXCLUDES 1   *shock due to infection following (induced) termination of pregnancy (O04.87)*

O04.82 Renal failure following (induced) Ⓜ♀ **termination of pregnancy**

Kidney failure (acute) following (induced) termination of pregnancy
Oliguria following (induced) termination of pregnancy
Renal shutdown following (induced) termination of pregnancy
Renal tubular necrosis following (induced) termination of pregnancy
Uremia following (induced) termination of pregnancy

O04.83 Metabolic disorder following (induced) Ⓜ♀ **termination of pregnancy**

O04.84 Damage to pelvic organs following Ⓜ♀ **(induced) termination of pregnancy**

Laceration, perforation, tear or chemical damage of bladder following (induced) termination of pregnancy
Laceration, perforation, tear or chemical damage of bowel following (induced) termination of pregnancy
Laceration, perforation, tear or chemical damage of broad ligament following (induced) termination of pregnancy
Laceration, perforation, tear or chemical damage of cervix following (induced) termination of pregnancy
Laceration, perforation, tear or chemical damage of periurethral tissue following (induced) termination of pregnancy
Laceration, perforation, tear or chemical damage of uterus following (induced) termination of pregnancy
Laceration, perforation, tear or chemical damage of vagina following (induced) termination of pregnancy

O04.85 Other venous complications following Ⓜ♀ **(induced) termination of pregnancy**

O04.86 Cardiac arrest following (induced) Ⓜ♀ **termination of pregnancy**

O04.87 Sepsis following (induced) termination Ⓜ♀ **of pregnancy**

Use additional code to identify infectious agent (B95-B97)
Use additional code to identify severe sepsis, if applicable (R65.2-)

EXCLUDES 1   *septic or septicopyemic embolism following (induced) termination of pregnancy (O04.7)*

O04.88 Urinary tract infection following Ⓜ♀ **(induced) termination of pregnancy**

Cystitis following (induced) termination of pregnancy

O04.89 (Induced) termination of pregnancy Ⓜ♀ **with other complications**

✓4ᵗʰ **O07 Failed attempted termination of pregnancy**

INCLUDES   failure of attempted induction of termination of pregnancy
incomplete elective abortion

EXCLUDES 1   *incomplete spontaneous abortion (O03.0-)*

O07.0 Genital tract and pelvic infection following failed Ⓜ♀ **attempted termination of pregnancy**

Endometritis following failed attempted termination of pregnancy
Oophoritis following failed attempted termination of pregnancy
Parametritis following failed attempted termination of pregnancy
Pelvic peritonitis following failed attempted termination of pregnancy
Salpingitis following failed attempted termination of pregnancy
Salpingo-oophoritis following failed attempted termination of pregnancy

EXCLUDES 1   *sepsis following failed attempted termination of pregnancy (O07.37)*
urinary tract infection following failed attempted termination of pregnancy (O07.38)

O07.1 Delayed or excessive hemorrhage following failed Ⓜ♀ **attempted termination of pregnancy**

Afibrinogenemia following failed attempted termination of pregnancy
Defibrination syndrome following failed attempted termination of pregnancy
Hemolysis following failed attempted termination of pregnancy
Intravascular coagulation following failed attempted termination of pregnancy

O07.2 Embolism **following failed attempted termination of pregnancy**   Ⓜ ♀

Air embolism following failed attempted termination of pregnancy

Amniotic fluid embolism following failed attempted termination of pregnancy

Blood-clot embolism following failed attempted termination of pregnancy

Embolism NOS following failed attempted termination of pregnancy

Fat embolism following failed attempted termination of pregnancy

Pulmonary embolism following failed attempted termination of pregnancy

Pyemic embolism following failed attempted termination of pregnancy

Septic or septicopyemic embolism following failed attempted termination of pregnancy

Soap embolism following failed attempted termination of pregnancy

✓5ᵗʰ **O07.3** **Failed attempted termination of pregnancy with other and unspecified complications**

O07.30 **Failed attempted termination of pregnancy with unspecified complications**   Ⓜ ♀

O07.31 Shock **following failed attempted termination of pregnancy**   Ⓜ ♀

Circulatory collapse following failed attempted termination of pregnancy

Shock (postprocedural) following failed attempted termination of pregnancy

EXCLUDES 1   *shock due to infection following failed attempted termination of pregnancy (O07.37)*

O07.32 Renal failure **following failed attempted termination of pregnancy**   Ⓜ ♀

Kidney failure (acute) following failed attempted termination of pregnancy

Oliguria following failed attempted termination of pregnancy

Renal shutdown following failed attempted termination of pregnancy

Renal tubular necrosis following failed attempted termination of pregnancy

Uremia following failed attempted termination of pregnancy

O07.33 Metabolic disorder **following failed attempted termination of pregnancy**   Ⓜ ♀

O07.34 Damage to pelvic organs **following failed attempted termination of pregnancy**   Ⓜ ♀

Laceration, perforation, tear or chemical damage of bladder following failed attempted termination of pregnancy

Laceration, perforation, tear or chemical damage of bowel following failed attempted termination of pregnancy

Laceration, perforation, tear or chemical damage of broad ligament following failed attempted termination of pregnancy

Laceration, perforation, tear or chemical damage of cervix following failed attempted termination of pregnancy

Laceration, perforation, tear or chemical damage of periurethral tissue following failed attempted termination of pregnancy

Laceration, perforation, tear or chemical damage of uterus following failed attempted termination of pregnancy

Laceration, perforation, tear or chemical damage of vagina following failed attempted termination of pregnancy

O07.35 **Other venous complications following failed attempted termination of pregnancy**   Ⓜ ♀

O07.36 Cardiac arrest **following failed attempted termination of pregnancy**   Ⓜ ♀

O07.37 Sepsis **following failed attempted termination of pregnancy**   Ⓜ ♀

Use additional code (B95-B97), to identify infectious agent

Use additional code (R65.2-) to identify severe sepsis, if applicable

EXCLUDES 1   *septic or septicopyemic embolism following failed attempted termination of pregnancy (O07.2)*

O07.38 Urinary tract infection **following failed attempted termination of pregnancy**   Ⓜ ♀

Cystitis following failed attempted termination of pregnancy

O07.39 **Failed attempted termination of pregnancy with other complications**   Ⓜ ♀

O07.4 **Failed attempted termination of pregnancy without complication**   Ⓜ ♀

✓4ᵗʰ **O08** Complications following ectopic and molar **pregnancy**

This category is for use with categories O00-O02 to identify any associated complications

O08.0 Genital tract and pelvic infection **following ectopic and molar pregnancy**   Ⓜ ♀

Endometritis following ectopic and molar pregnancy

Oophoritis following ectopic and molar pregnancy

Parametritis following ectopic and molar pregnancy

Pelvic peritonitis following ectopic and molar pregnancy

Salpingitis following ectopic and molar pregnancy

Salpingo-oophoritis following ectopic and molar pregnancy

EXCLUDES 1   *sepsis following ectopic and molar pregnancy (O08.82)*

urinary tract infection (O08.83)

O08.1 Delayed or excessive hemorrhage **following ectopic and molar pregnancy**   Ⓜ ♀

Afibrinogenemia following ectopic and molar pregnancy

Defibrination syndrome following ectopic and molar pregnancy

Hemolysis following ectopic and molar pregnancy

Intravascular coagulation following ectopic and molar pregnancy

EXCLUDES 1   *delayed or excessive hemorrhage due to incomplete abortion (O03.1)*

O08.2 Embolism **following ectopic and molar pregnancy**   Ⓜ ♀

Air embolism following ectopic and molar pregnancy

Amniotic fluid embolism following ectopic and molar pregnancy

Blood-clot embolism following ectopic and molar pregnancy

Embolism NOS following ectopic and molar pregnancy

Fat embolism following ectopic and molar pregnancy

Pulmonary embolism following ectopic and molar pregnancy

Pyemic embolism following ectopic and molar pregnancy

Septic or septicopyemic embolism following ectopic and molar pregnancy

Soap embolism following ectopic and molar pregnancy

O08.3 Shock **following ectopic and molar pregnancy**   Ⓜ ♀

Circulatory collapse following ectopic and molar pregnancy

Shock (postprocedural) following ectopic and molar pregnancy

EXCLUDES 1   *shock due to infection following ectopic and molar pregnancy (O08.82)*

O08.4 Renal failure **following ectopic and molar pregnancy**   Ⓜ ♀

Kidney failure (acute) following ectopic and molar pregnancy

Oliguria following ectopic and molar pregnancy

Renal shutdown following ectopic and molar pregnancy

Renal tubular necrosis following ectopic and molar pregnancy

Uremia following ectopic and molar pregnancy

O08.5 Metabolic disorders **following an ectopic and molar pregnancy**   Ⓜ ♀

✅ Additional Character Required   ✓x7ᵗʰ Placeholder Alert   Manifestation   Unspecified Dx   ►◄ Revised Text   ● New Code   ▲ Revised Title

Chapter 15. Pregnancy, Childbirth and the Puerperium

O08.6 Damage to pelvic organs and tissues following an ectopic and molar pregnancy Ⓜ♀
Laceration, perforation, tear or chemical damage of bladder following an ectopic and molar pregnancy
Laceration, perforation, tear or chemical damage of bowel following an ectopic and molar pregnancy
Laceration, perforation, tear or chemical damage of broad ligament following an ectopic and molar pregnancy
Laceration, perforation, tear or chemical damage of cervix following an ectopic and molar pregnancy
Laceration, perforation, tear or chemical damage of periurethral tissue following an ectopic and molar pregnancy
Laceration, perforation, tear or chemical damage of uterus following an ectopic and molar pregnancy
Laceration, perforation, tear or chemical damage of vagina following an ectopic and molar pregnancy

O08.7 Other venous complications following an ectopic and molar pregnancy Ⓜ♀

✓5ᵗʰ **O08.8 Other complications following an ectopic and molar pregnancy**

O08.81 Cardiac arrest following an ectopic and molar pregnancy Ⓜ♀

O08.82 Sepsis following ectopic and molar pregnancy Ⓜ♀
Use additional code (B95-B97), to identify infectious agent
Use additional code (R65.2-) to identify severe sepsis, if applicable
EXCLUDES 1   septic or septicopyemic embolism following ectopic and molar pregnancy (O08.2)

O08.83 Urinary tract infection following an ectopic and molar pregnancy Ⓜ♀
Cystitis following an ectopic and molar pregnancy

O08.89 Other complications following an ectopic and molar pregnancy Ⓜ♀

O08.9 Unspecified complication following an ectopic and molar pregnancy Ⓜ♀

Supervision of high risk pregnancy (O09)

✓4ᵗʰ **O09 Supervision of high risk pregnancy**
AHA: 2016,4Q,48-50,150

✓5ᵗʰ **O09.0 Supervision of pregnancy with history of infertility**
DEF: Infertility: Inability to conceive for at least one year with regular intercourse.

O09.00 Supervision of pregnancy with history of infertility, unspecified trimester Ⓜ♀

O09.01 Supervision of pregnancy with history of infertility, first trimester Ⓜ♀

O09.02 Supervision of pregnancy with history of infertility, second trimester Ⓜ♀

O09.03 Supervision of pregnancy with history of infertility, third trimester Ⓜ♀

✓5ᵗʰ **O09.1 Supervision of pregnancy with history of ectopic pregnancy**
DEF: Ectopic pregnancy: Implantation of a fertilized egg outside the uterus, usually in the fallopian tube or abdomen that requires emergency treatment.

O09.10 Supervision of pregnancy with history of ectopic pregnancy, unspecified trimester Ⓜ♀

O09.11 Supervision of pregnancy with history of ectopic pregnancy, first trimester Ⓜ♀

O09.12 Supervision of pregnancy with history of ectopic pregnancy, second trimester Ⓜ♀

O09.13 Supervision of pregnancy with history of ectopic pregnancy, third trimester Ⓜ♀

✓5ᵗʰ **O09.A Supervision of pregnancy with history of molar pregnancy**
DEF: Molar pregnancy: Trophoblastic neoplasm that mimics pregnancy by proliferating from a pathologic ovum and resulting only in a mass of cysts resembling grapes, 80 percent of which are benign, but require surgical removal.

O09.A0 Supervision of pregnancy with history of molar pregnancy, unspecified trimester Ⓜ♀

O09.A1 Supervision of pregnancy with history of molar pregnancy, first trimester Ⓜ♀

O09.A2 Supervision of pregnancy with history of molar pregnancy, second trimester Ⓜ♀

O09.A3 Supervision of pregnancy with history of molar pregnancy, third trimester Ⓜ♀

✓5ᵗʰ **O09.2 Supervision of pregnancy with other poor reproductive or obstetric history**
EXCLUDES 2   pregnancy care for patient with history of recurrent pregnancy loss (O26.2-)

✓6ᵗʰ **O09.21 Supervision of pregnancy with history of pre-term labor**

O09.211 Supervision of pregnancy with history of pre-term labor, first trimester Ⓜ♀

O09.212 Supervision of pregnancy with history of pre-term labor, second trimester Ⓜ♀

O09.213 Supervision of pregnancy with history of pre-term labor, third trimester Ⓜ♀

O09.219 Supervision of pregnancy with history of pre-term labor, unspecified trimester Ⓜ♀

✓6ᵗʰ **O09.29 Supervision of pregnancy with other poor reproductive or obstetric history**
Supervision of pregnancy with history of neonatal death
Supervision of pregnancy with history of stillbirth

O09.291 Supervision of pregnancy with other poor reproductive or obstetric history, first trimester Ⓜ♀

O09.292 Supervision of pregnancy with other poor reproductive or obstetric history, second trimester Ⓜ♀

O09.293 Supervision of pregnancy with other poor reproductive or obstetric history, third trimester Ⓜ♀

O09.299 Supervision of pregnancy with other poor reproductive or obstetric history, unspecified trimester Ⓜ♀

✓5ᵗʰ **O09.3 Supervision of pregnancy with insufficient antenatal care**
Supervision of concealed pregnancy
Supervision of hidden pregnancy

O09.30 Supervision of pregnancy with insufficient antenatal care, unspecified trimester Ⓜ♀

O09.31 Supervision of pregnancy with insufficient antenatal care, first trimester Ⓜ♀

O09.32 Supervision of pregnancy with insufficient antenatal care, second trimester Ⓜ♀

O09.33 Supervision of pregnancy with insufficient antenatal care, third trimester Ⓜ♀

✓5ᵗʰ **O09.4 Supervision of pregnancy with grand multiparity**

O09.40 Supervision of pregnancy with grand multiparity, unspecified trimester Ⓜ♀

O09.41 Supervision of pregnancy with grand multiparity, first trimester Ⓜ♀

O09.42 Supervision of pregnancy with grand multiparity, second trimester Ⓜ♀

O09.43 Supervision of pregnancy with grand multiparity, third trimester Ⓜ♀

✓5ᵗʰ **O09.5 Supervision of elderly primigravida and multigravida**
Pregnancy for a female 35 years and older at expected date of delivery

✓6ᵗʰ **O09.51 Supervision of elderly primigravida**

O09.511 Supervision of elderly primigravida, first trimester Ⓜ♀

O09.512 Supervision of elderly primigravida, second trimester Ⓜ♀

O09.513 Supervision of elderly primigravida, third trimester Ⓜ♀

O09.519 Supervision of elderly primigravida, unspecified trimester Ⓜ♀

✓6ᵗʰ **O09.52 Supervision of elderly multigravida**

O09.521 Supervision of elderly multigravida, first trimester Ⓜ♀

O09.522 **Supervision of elderly multigravida, second trimester** Ⓜ ♀

O09.523 **Supervision of elderly multigravida, third trimester** Ⓜ ♀

O09.529 **Supervision of elderly multigravida, unspecified trimester** Ⓜ ♀

✓5ᵗʰ O09.6 **Supervision of** young primigravida and multigravida

Supervision of pregnancy for a female less than 16 years old at expected date of delivery

✓6ᵗʰ O09.61 **Supervision of** young primigravida

O09.611 **Supervision of young primigravida, first trimester** Ⓜ ♀

O09.612 **Supervision of young primigravida, second trimester** Ⓜ ♀

O09.613 **Supervision of young primigravida, third trimester** Ⓜ ♀

O09.619 **Supervision of young primigravida, unspecified trimester** Ⓜ ♀

✓6ᵗʰ O09.62 **Supervision of** young multigravida

O09.621 **Supervision of young multigravida, first trimester** Ⓜ ♀

O09.622 **Supervision of young multigravida, second trimester** Ⓜ ♀

O09.623 **Supervision of young multigravida, third trimester** Ⓜ ♀

O09.629 **Supervision of young multigravida, unspecified trimester** Ⓜ ♀

✓5ᵗʰ O09.7 **Supervision of high risk pregnancy due to** social problems

O09.70 **Supervision of high risk pregnancy due to social problems, unspecified trimester** Ⓜ ♀

O09.71 **Supervision of high risk pregnancy due to social problems, first trimester** Ⓜ ♀

O09.72 **Supervision of high risk pregnancy due to social problems, second trimester** Ⓜ ♀

O09.73 **Supervision of high risk pregnancy due to social problems, third trimester** Ⓜ ♀

✓5ᵗʰ O09.8 **Supervision of other high risk pregnancies**

✓6ᵗʰ O09.81 **Supervision of pregnancy** resulting from assisted reproductive technology

Supervision of pregnancy resulting from in-vitro fertilization

EXCLUDES 2   gestational carrier status (Z33.3)

O09.811 **Supervision of pregnancy resulting from assisted reproductive technology, first trimester** Ⓜ ♀

O09.812 **Supervision of pregnancy resulting from assisted reproductive technology, second trimester** Ⓜ ♀

O09.813 **Supervision of pregnancy resulting from assisted reproductive technology, third trimester** Ⓜ ♀

O09.819 **Supervision of pregnancy resulting from assisted reproductive technology, unspecified trimester** Ⓜ ♀

✓6ᵗʰ O09.82 **Supervision of pregnancy with** history of in utero procedure during previous pregnancy

O09.821 **Supervision of pregnancy with history of in utero procedure during previous pregnancy, first trimester** Ⓜ ♀

O09.822 **Supervision of pregnancy with history of in utero procedure during previous pregnancy, second trimester** Ⓜ ♀

O09.823 **Supervision of pregnancy with history of in utero procedure during previous pregnancy, third trimester** Ⓜ ♀

O09.829 **Supervision of pregnancy with history of in utero procedure during previous pregnancy, unspecified trimester** Ⓜ ♀

EXCLUDES 1   supervision of pregnancy affected by in utero procedure during current pregnancy (O35.7)

✓6ᵗʰ O09.89 **Supervision of other high risk pregnancies**

O09.891 **Supervision of other high risk pregnancies, first trimester** Ⓜ ♀

O09.892 **Supervision of other high risk pregnancies, second trimester** Ⓜ ♀

O09.893 **Supervision of other high risk pregnancies, third trimester** Ⓜ ♀

O09.899 **Supervision of other high risk pregnancies, unspecified trimester** Ⓜ ♀

✓5ᵗʰ O09.9 **Supervision of high risk pregnancy, unspecified**

O09.90 **Supervision of high risk pregnancy, unspecified, unspecified trimester** Ⓜ ♀

O09.91 **Supervision of high risk pregnancy, unspecified, first trimester** Ⓜ ♀

O09.92 **Supervision of high risk pregnancy, unspecified, second trimester** Ⓜ ♀

O09.93 **Supervision of high risk pregnancy, unspecified, third trimester** Ⓜ ♀

Edema, proteinuria and hypertensive disorders in pregnancy, childbirth and the puerperium (O10-O16)

AHA: 2016,4Q,50

✓4ᵗʰ O10 Pre-existing hypertension complicating pregnancy, childbirth and the puerperium

INCLUDES   pre-existing hypertension with pre-existing proteinuria complicating pregnancy, childbirth and the puerperium

EXCLUDES 2   pre-existing hypertension with superimposed pre-eclampsia complicating pregnancy, childbirth and the puerperium (O11.-)

✓5ᵗʰ O10.0 **Pre-existing** essential **hypertension complicating pregnancy, childbirth and the puerperium**

Any condition in I10 specified as a reason for obstetric care during pregnancy, childbirth or the puerperium

✓6ᵗʰ O10.01 **Pre-existing essential hypertension complicating** pregnancy

O10.011 **Pre-existing essential hypertension complicating pregnancy, first trimester** Ⓜ ♀

O10.012 **Pre-existing essential hypertension complicating pregnancy, second trimester** Ⓜ ♀

O10.013 **Pre-existing essential hypertension complicating pregnancy, third trimester** Ⓜ ♀

O10.019 **Pre-existing essential hypertension complicating pregnancy, unspecified trimester** Ⓜ ♀

O10.02 **Pre-existing essential hypertension complicating** childbirth Ⓜ ♀

O10.03 **Pre-existing essential hypertension complicating the** puerperium Ⓜ ♀

✓5ᵗʰ O10.1 **Pre-existing** hypertensive heart disease **complicating pregnancy, childbirth and the puerperium**

Any condition in I11 specified as a reason for obstetric care during pregnancy, childbirth or the puerperium

Use additional code from I11 to identify the type of hypertensive heart disease

✓6ᵗʰ O10.11 **Pre-existing hypertensive heart disease complicating** pregnancy

O10.111 **Pre-existing hypertensive heart disease complicating pregnancy, first trimester** Ⓜ ♀

O10.112 **Pre-existing hypertensive heart disease complicating pregnancy, second trimester** Ⓜ ♀

O10.113 **Pre-existing hypertensive heart disease complicating pregnancy, third trimester** Ⓜ ♀

☑ Additional Character Required   ✓x7ᵗʰ Placeholder Alert   Manifestation   Unspecified Dx   ►◄ Revised Text   ● New Code   ▲ Revised Title

ICD-10-CM 2020   853

          O10.119 Pre-existing hypertensive heart disease complicating pregnancy, unspecified trimester   Ⓜ♀

    O10.12 Pre-existing hypertensive heart disease complicating childbirth   Ⓜ♀

    O10.13 Pre-existing hypertensive heart disease complicating the puerperium   Ⓜ♀

√5ᵗʰ **O10.2** Pre-existing hypertensive chronic kidney disease complicating pregnancy, childbirth and the puerperium

      Any condition in I12 specified as a reason for obstetric care during pregnancy, childbirth or the puerperium

      Use additional code from I12 to identify the type of hypertensive chronic kidney disease

  √6ᵗʰ **O10.21** Pre-existing hypertensive chronic kidney disease complicating pregnancy

          O10.211 Pre-existing hypertensive chronic kidney disease complicating pregnancy, first trimester   Ⓜ♀

          O10.212 Pre-existing hypertensive chronic kidney disease complicating pregnancy, second trimester   Ⓜ♀

          O10.213 Pre-existing hypertensive chronic kidney disease complicating pregnancy, third trimester   Ⓜ♀

          O10.219 Pre-existing hypertensive chronic kidney disease complicating pregnancy, unspecified trimester   Ⓜ♀

    O10.22 Pre-existing hypertensive chronic kidney disease complicating childbirth   Ⓜ♀

    O10.23 Pre-existing hypertensive chronic kidney disease complicating the puerperium   Ⓜ♀

√5ᵗʰ **O10.3** Pre-existing hypertensive heart and chronic kidney disease complicating pregnancy, childbirth and the puerperium

      Any condition in I13 specified as a reason for obstetric care during pregnancy, childbirth or the puerperium

      Use additional code from I13 to identify the type of hypertensive heart and chronic kidney disease

  √6ᵗʰ **O10.31** Pre-existing hypertensive heart and chronic kidney disease complicating pregnancy

          O10.311 Pre-existing hypertensive heart and chronic kidney disease complicating pregnancy, first trimester   Ⓜ♀

          O10.312 Pre-existing hypertensive heart and chronic kidney disease complicating pregnancy, second trimester   Ⓜ♀

          O10.313 Pre-existing hypertensive heart and chronic kidney disease complicating pregnancy, third trimester   Ⓜ♀

          O10.319 Pre-existing hypertensive heart and chronic kidney disease complicating pregnancy, unspecified trimester   Ⓜ♀

    O10.32 Pre-existing hypertensive heart and chronic kidney disease complicating childbirth   Ⓜ♀

    O10.33 Pre-existing hypertensive heart and chronic kidney disease complicating the puerperium   Ⓜ♀

√5ᵗʰ **O10.4** Pre-existing secondary hypertension complicating pregnancy, childbirth and the puerperium

      Any condition in I15 specified as a reason for obstetric care during pregnancy, childbirth or the puerperium

      Use additional code from I15 to identify the type of secondary hypertension

  √6ᵗʰ **O10.41** Pre-existing secondary hypertension complicating pregnancy

          O10.411 Pre-existing secondary hypertension complicating pregnancy, first trimester   Ⓜ♀

          O10.412 Pre-existing secondary hypertension complicating pregnancy, second trimester   Ⓜ♀

          O10.413 Pre-existing secondary hypertension complicating pregnancy, third trimester   Ⓜ♀

          O10.419 Pre-existing secondary hypertension complicating pregnancy, unspecified trimester   Ⓜ♀

    O10.42 Pre-existing secondary hypertension complicating childbirth   Ⓜ♀

    O10.43 Pre-existing secondary hypertension complicating the puerperium   Ⓜ♀

√5ᵗʰ **O10.9** Unspecified pre-existing hypertension complicating pregnancy, childbirth and the puerperium

  √6ᵗʰ **O10.91** Unspecified pre-existing hypertension complicating pregnancy

          O10.911 Unspecified pre-existing hypertension complicating pregnancy, first trimester   Ⓜ♀

          O10.912 Unspecified pre-existing hypertension complicating pregnancy, second trimester   Ⓜ♀

          O10.913 Unspecified pre-existing hypertension complicating pregnancy, third trimester   Ⓜ♀

          O10.919 Unspecified pre-existing hypertension complicating pregnancy, unspecified trimester   Ⓜ♀

    O10.92 Unspecified pre-existing hypertension complicating childbirth   Ⓜ♀

    O10.93 Unspecified pre-existing hypertension complicating the puerperium   Ⓜ♀

√4ᵗʰ **O11** Pre-existing hypertension with pre-eclampsia

   INCLUDES   conditions in O10 complicated by pre-eclampsia

          pre-eclampsia superimposed pre-existing in hypertension

  Use additional code from O10 to identify the type of hypertension

  DEF: Complication of pregnancy manifesting in the development of borderline hypertension, protein in the urine, and unresponsive swelling between the 20th week of pregnancy and the end of the first week following birth in mild to moderate cases. Severe preeclampsia presents with hypertension, associated with marked swelling, proteinuria, abdominal pain, and/or visual changes.

    O11.1 Pre-existing hypertension with pre-eclampsia, first trimester   Ⓜ♀

    O11.2 Pre-existing hypertension with pre-eclampsia, second trimester   Ⓜ♀

    O11.3 Pre-existing hypertension with pre-eclampsia, third trimester   Ⓜ♀

    O11.4 Pre-existing hypertension with pre-eclampsia, complicating childbirth   Ⓜ♀

    O11.5 Pre-existing hypertension with pre-eclampsia, complicating the puerperium   Ⓜ♀

    O11.9 Pre-existing hypertension with pre-eclampsia, unspecified trimester   Ⓜ♀

√4ᵗʰ **O12** Gestational [pregnancy-induced] edema and proteinuria without hypertension

  √5ᵗʰ **O12.0** Gestational edema

    O12.00 Gestational edema, unspecified trimester   Ⓜ♀

    O12.01 Gestational edema, first trimester   Ⓜ♀

    O12.02 Gestational edema, second trimester   Ⓜ♀

    O12.03 Gestational edema, third trimester   Ⓜ♀

    O12.04 Gestational edema, complicating childbirth   Ⓜ♀

    O12.05 Gestational edema, complicating the puerperium   Ⓜ♀

  √5ᵗʰ **O12.1** Gestational proteinuria

    O12.10 Gestational proteinuria, unspecified trimester   Ⓜ♀

    O12.11 Gestational proteinuria, first trimester   Ⓜ♀

    O12.12 Gestational proteinuria, second trimester   Ⓜ♀

    O12.13 Gestational proteinuria, third trimester   Ⓜ♀

    O12.14 Gestational proteinuria, complicating childbirth   Ⓜ♀

    O12.15 Gestational proteinuria, complicating the puerperium   Ⓜ♀

  √5ᵗʰ **O12.2** Gestational edema with proteinuria

    O12.20 Gestational edema with proteinuria, unspecified trimester   Ⓜ♀

Ⓝ Newborn: 0   Ⓟ Pediatric: 0-17   Ⓜ Maternity: 12-55   Ⓐ Adult: 15-124   ᴄʜ Comorbidity High   ᴄʟ Comorbidity Low   ɴᴄᴅx Noncancer Dx   ᴘᴅx Primary Dx

854   ICD-10-CM 2020

O12.21   **Gestational edema with proteinuria, first trimester**   M ♀

O12.22   **Gestational edema with proteinuria, second trimester**   M ♀

O12.23   **Gestational edema with proteinuria, third trimester**   M ♀

O12.24   **Gestational edema with proteinuria, complicating** childbirth   M ♀

O12.25   **Gestational edema with proteinuria, complicating the** puerperium   M ♀

✓4th **O13** Gestational [**pregnancy-induced**] hypertension without significant proteinuria

    INCLUDES   gestational hypertension NOS

           transient hypertension of pregnancy

    AHA: 2016,1Q,5

O13.1   **Gestational [pregnancy-induced] hypertension without significant proteinuria, first trimester**   M ♀

O13.2   **Gestational [pregnancy-induced] hypertension without significant proteinuria, second trimester**   M ♀

O13.3   **Gestational [pregnancy-induced] hypertension without significant proteinuria, third trimester**   M ♀

O13.4   **Gestational [pregnancy-induced] hypertension without significant proteinuria, complicating childbirth**   M ♀

O13.5   **Gestational [pregnancy-induced] hypertension without significant proteinuria, complicating the puerperium**   M ♀

O13.9   **Gestational [pregnancy-induced] hypertension without significant proteinuria, unspecified trimester**   M ♀

✓4th **O14** Pre-eclampsia

    EXCLUDES 1   pre-existing hypertension with pre-eclampsia (O11)

    DEF: Complication of pregnancy manifesting in the development of borderline hypertension, protein in the urine, and unresponsive swelling between the 20th week of pregnancy and the end of the first week following birth in mild to moderate cases. Severe preeclampsia presents with hypertension, associated with marked swelling, proteinuria, abdominal pain, and/or visual changes.

    ✓5th **O14.0**   Mild to moderate **pre-eclampsia**

        AHA: 2019,2Q,8

O14.00   **Mild to moderate pre-eclampsia, unspecified trimester**   M ♀

O14.02   **Mild to moderate pre-eclampsia, second trimester**   M ♀

O14.03   **Mild to moderate pre-eclampsia, third trimester**   M ♀

O14.04   **Mild to moderate pre-eclampsia, complicating** childbirth   M ♀

        AHA: 2019,2Q,8

O14.05   **Mild to moderate pre-eclampsia, complicating the** puerperium   M ♀

    ✓5th **O14.1**   Severe **pre-eclampsia**

        EXCLUDES 1   HELLP syndrome (O14.2-)

O14.10   **Severe pre-eclampsia, unspecified trimester**   M ♀

O14.12   **Severe pre-eclampsia,** second trimester   M ♀

O14.13   **Severe pre-eclampsia,** third trimester   M ♀

O14.14   **Severe pre-eclampsia complicating** childbirth   M ♀

O14.15   **Severe pre-eclampsia, complicating the** puerperium   M ♀

    ✓5th **O14.2**   HELLP syndrome

        Severe pre-eclampsia with hemolysis, elevated liver enzymes and low platelet count (HELLP)

O14.20   **HELLP syndrome (HELLP), unspecified trimester**   M ♀

O14.22   **HELLP syndrome (HELLP),** second trimester   M ♀

O14.23   **HELLP syndrome (HELLP),** third trimester   M ♀

O14.24   **HELLP syndrome, complicating** childbirth   M ♀

O14.25   **HELLP syndrome, complicating the** puerperium   M ♀

    ✓5th **O14.9**   Unspecified pre-eclampsia

O14.90   **Unspecified pre-eclampsia, unspecified trimester**   M ♀

O14.92   **Unspecified pre-eclampsia,** second trimester   M ♀

O14.93   **Unspecified pre-eclampsia,** third trimester   M ♀

O14.94   **Unspecified pre-eclampsia, complicating** childbirth   M ♀

O14.95   **Unspecified pre-eclampsia, complicating the** puerperium   M ♀

✓4th **O15** Eclampsia

    INCLUDES   convulsions following conditions in O10-O14 and O16

    DEF: Tetany and toxemia producing seizure activity or coma in a pregnant patient who most often has presented with prior preeclampsia (i.e., hypertension, albuminuria, and edema).

    ✓5th **O15.0**   Eclampsia complicating pregnancy

O15.00   **Eclampsia complicating pregnancy, unspecified trimester**   M ♀

O15.02   **Eclampsia complicating pregnancy,** second trimester   M ♀

O15.03   **Eclampsia complicating pregnancy,** third trimester   M ♀

O15.1   **Eclampsia complicating** labor   M ♀

O15.2   **Eclampsia complicating the** puerperium   M ♀

O15.9   **Eclampsia, unspecified as to time period**   M ♀

        Eclampsia NOS

✓4th **O16** Unspecified maternal hypertension

O16.1   **Unspecified maternal hypertension,** first trimester   M ♀

O16.2   **Unspecified maternal hypertension,** second trimester   M ♀

O16.3   **Unspecified maternal hypertension,** third trimester   M ♀

O16.4   **Unspecified maternal hypertension, complicating** childbirth   M ♀

O16.5   **Unspecified maternal hypertension, complicating the** puerperium   M ♀

O16.9   **Unspecified maternal hypertension, unspecified** trimester   M ♀

Other maternal disorders predominantly related to pregnancy (O20-O29)

    EXCLUDES 2   maternal care related to the fetus and amniotic cavity and possible delivery problems (O30-O48)

           maternal diseases classifiable elsewhere but complicating pregnancy, labor and delivery, and the puerperium (O98-O99)

✓4th **O20** Hemorrhage in early pregnancy

    INCLUDES   hemorrhage before completion of 20 weeks gestation

    EXCLUDES 1   pregnancy with abortive outcome (O00-O08)

O20.0   **Threatened abortion**   M ♀

        Hemorrhage specified as due to threatened abortion

        DEF: Bloody discharge during pregnancy. The cervix may be dilated and pregnancy threatened, but the pregnancy is not terminated.

O20.8   **Other hemorrhage in early pregnancy**   M ♀

O20.9   **Hemorrhage in early pregnancy, unspecified**   M ♀

✓4th **O21** Excessive vomiting in pregnancy

O21.0   Mild hyperemesis gravidarum   M ♀

        Hyperemesis gravidarum, mild or unspecified, starting before the end of the 20th week of gestation

O21.1   **Hyperemesis gravidarum with** metabolic disturbance   M ♀

        Hyperemesis gravidarum, starting before the end of the 20th week of gestation, with metabolic disturbance such as carbohydrate depletion

        Hyperemesis gravidarum, starting before the end of the 20th week of gestation, with metabolic disturbance such as dehydration

        Hyperemesis gravidarum, starting before the end of the 20th week of gestation, with metabolic disturbance such as electrolyte imbalance

O21.2   Late **vomiting of pregnancy**   M ♀

        Excessive vomiting starting after 20 completed weeks of gestation

O21.8   **Other vomiting complicating pregnancy**   M ♀

        Vomiting due to diseases classified elsewhere, complicating pregnancy

        Use additional code, to identify cause

O21.9   **Vomiting of pregnancy, unspecified**   M ♀

✓ Additional Character Required   ✓x7th Placeholder Alert   Manifestation   Unspecified Dx   ►◄ Revised Text   ● New Code   ▲ Revised Title

ICD-10-CM 2020   855

√4ᵗʰ **O22 Venous complications and hemorrhoids in pregnancy**

EXCLUDES 1   venous complications of:
- abortion NOS (O03.9)
- ectopic or molar pregnancy (O08.7)
- failed attempted abortion (O07.35)
- induced abortion (O04.85)
- spontaneous abortion (O03.89)

EXCLUDES 2   obstetric pulmonary embolism (O88.-)
- venous complications and hemorrhoids of childbirth and the puerperium (O87.-)

√5ᵗʰ **O22.0 Varicose veins of lower extremity in pregnancy**

Varicose veins NOS in pregnancy
DEF: Distended, tortuous veins of the lower extremities associated with pregnancy.

- **O22.00 Varicose veins of lower extremity in pregnancy, unspecified trimester** Ⓜ♀
- **O22.01 Varicose veins of lower extremity in pregnancy, first trimester** Ⓜ♀
- **O22.02 Varicose veins of lower extremity in pregnancy, second trimester** Ⓜ♀
- **O22.03 Varicose veins of lower extremity in pregnancy, third trimester** Ⓜ♀

√5ᵗʰ **O22.1 Genital varices in pregnancy**

Perineal varices in pregnancy
Vaginal varices in pregnancy
Vulval varices in pregnancy

- **O22.10 Genital varices in pregnancy, unspecified trimester** Ⓜ♀
- **O22.11 Genital varices in pregnancy, first trimester** Ⓜ♀
- **O22.12 Genital varices in pregnancy, second trimester** Ⓜ♀
- **O22.13 Genital varices in pregnancy, third trimester** Ⓜ♀

√5ᵗʰ **O22.2 Superficial thrombophlebitis in pregnancy**

Phlebitis in pregnancy NOS
Thrombophlebitis of legs in pregnancy
Thrombosis in pregnancy NOS
Use additional code to identify the superficial thrombophlebitis (I80.0-)

- **O22.20 Superficial thrombophlebitis in pregnancy, unspecified trimester** Ⓜ♀
- **O22.21 Superficial thrombophlebitis in pregnancy, first trimester** Ⓜ♀
- **O22.22 Superficial thrombophlebitis in pregnancy, second trimester** Ⓜ♀
- **O22.23 Superficial thrombophlebitis in pregnancy, third trimester** Ⓜ♀

√5ᵗʰ **O22.3 Deep phlebothrombosis in pregnancy**

Deep vein thrombosis, antepartum
Use additional code to identify the deep vein thrombosis (I82.4-, I82.5-, I82.62-, I82.72-)
Use additional code, if applicable, for associated long-term (current) use of anticoagulants (Z79.01)

- **O22.30 Deep phlebothrombosis in pregnancy, unspecified trimester** Ⓜ♀
- **O22.31 Deep phlebothrombosis in pregnancy, first trimester** Ⓜ♀
- **O22.32 Deep phlebothrombosis in pregnancy, second trimester** Ⓜ♀
- **O22.33 Deep phlebothrombosis in pregnancy, third trimester** Ⓜ♀

√5ᵗʰ **O22.4 Hemorrhoids in pregnancy**

- **O22.40 Hemorrhoids in pregnancy, unspecified trimester** Ⓜ♀
- **O22.41 Hemorrhoids in pregnancy, first trimester** Ⓜ♀
- **O22.42 Hemorrhoids in pregnancy, second trimester** Ⓜ♀
- **O22.43 Hemorrhoids in pregnancy, third trimester** Ⓜ♀

√5ᵗʰ **O22.5 Cerebral venous thrombosis in pregnancy**

Cerebrovenous sinus thrombosis in pregnancy

- **O22.50 Cerebral venous thrombosis in pregnancy, unspecified trimester** Ⓜ♀
- **O22.51 Cerebral venous thrombosis in pregnancy, first trimester** Ⓜ♀
- **O22.52 Cerebral venous thrombosis in pregnancy, second trimester** Ⓜ♀

- **O22.53 Cerebral venous thrombosis in pregnancy, third trimester** Ⓜ♀

√5ᵗʰ **O22.8 Other venous complications in pregnancy**

√6ᵗʰ **O22.8X Other venous complications in pregnancy**

- **O22.8X1 Other venous complications in pregnancy, first trimester** Ⓜ♀
- **O22.8X2 Other venous complications in pregnancy, second trimester** Ⓜ♀
- **O22.8X3 Other venous complications in pregnancy, third trimester** Ⓜ♀
- **O22.8X9 Other venous complications in pregnancy, unspecified trimester** Ⓜ♀

√5ᵗʰ **O22.9 Venous complication in pregnancy, unspecified**

Gestational phlebitis NOS
Gestational phlebopathy NOS
Gestational thrombosis NOS

- **O22.90 Venous complication in pregnancy, unspecified, unspecified trimester** Ⓜ♀
- **O22.91 Venous complication in pregnancy, unspecified, first trimester** Ⓜ♀
- **O22.92 Venous complication in pregnancy, unspecified, second trimester** Ⓜ♀
- **O22.93 Venous complication in pregnancy, unspecified, third trimester** Ⓜ♀

√4ᵗʰ **O23 Infections of genitourinary tract in pregnancy**

Use additional code to identify organism (B95.-, B96.-)

EXCLUDES 2   gonococcal infections complicating pregnancy, childbirth and the puerperium (O98.2)
- infections with a predominantly sexual mode of transmission NOS complicating pregnancy, childbirth and the puerperium (O98.3)
- syphilis complicating pregnancy, childbirth and the puerperium (O98.1)
- tuberculosis of genitourinary system complicating pregnancy, childbirth and the puerperium (O98.0)
- venereal disease NOS complicating pregnancy, childbirth and the puerperium (O98.3)

AHA: 2018,2Q,20

√5ᵗʰ **O23.0 Infections of kidney in pregnancy**

Pyelonephritis in pregnancy

- **O23.00 Infections of kidney in pregnancy, unspecified trimester** Ⓜ♀
- **O23.01 Infections of kidney in pregnancy, first trimester** Ⓜ♀
- **O23.02 Infections of kidney in pregnancy, second trimester** Ⓜ♀
- **O23.03 Infections of kidney in pregnancy, third trimester** Ⓜ♀

√5ᵗʰ **O23.1 Infections of bladder in pregnancy**

- **O23.10 Infections of bladder in pregnancy, unspecified trimester** Ⓜ♀
- **O23.11 Infections of bladder in pregnancy, first trimester** Ⓜ♀
- **O23.12 Infections of bladder in pregnancy, second trimester** Ⓜ♀
- **O23.13 Infections of bladder in pregnancy, third trimester** Ⓜ♀

√5ᵗʰ **O23.2 Infections of urethra in pregnancy**

- **O23.20 Infections of urethra in pregnancy, unspecified trimester** Ⓜ♀
- **O23.21 Infections of urethra in pregnancy, first trimester** Ⓜ♀
- **O23.22 Infections of urethra in pregnancy, second trimester** Ⓜ♀
- **O23.23 Infections of urethra in pregnancy, third trimester** Ⓜ♀

√5ᵗʰ **O23.3 Infections of other parts of urinary tract in pregnancy**

- **O23.30 Infections of other parts of urinary tract in pregnancy, unspecified trimester** Ⓜ♀
- **O23.31 Infections of other parts of urinary tract in pregnancy, first trimester** Ⓜ♀
- **O23.32 Infections of other parts of urinary tract in pregnancy, second trimester** Ⓜ♀
- **O23.33 Infections of other parts of urinary tract in pregnancy, third trimester** Ⓜ♀

Ⓝ Newborn: 0   Ⓟ Pediatric: 0-17   Ⓜ Maternity: 12-55   Ⓐ Adult: 15-124   🄲🄷 Comorbidity High   🄲🄻 Comorbidity Low   🄽🄲🄳🅇 Noncancer Dx   🄿🄳🅇 Primary Dx

856   ICD-10-CM 2020

✓5th **O23.4** **Unspecified infection of urinary tract in pregnancy**

    O23.40 **Unspecified infection of urinary tract in pregnancy, unspecified trimester** Ⓜ♀

    O23.41 **Unspecified infection of urinary tract in pregnancy, first trimester** Ⓜ♀

    O23.42 **Unspecified infection of urinary tract in pregnancy, second trimester** Ⓜ♀

    O23.43 **Unspecified infection of urinary tract in pregnancy, third trimester** Ⓜ♀

✓5th **O23.5** **Infections of the genital tract in pregnancy**

    ✓6th **O23.51** **Infection of cervix in pregnancy**

        O23.511 **Infections of cervix in pregnancy, first trimester** Ⓜ♀

        O23.512 **Infections of cervix in pregnancy, second trimester** Ⓜ♀

        O23.513 **Infections of cervix in pregnancy, third trimester** Ⓜ♀

        O23.519 **Infections of cervix in pregancy, unspecified trimester** Ⓜ♀

    ✓6th **O23.52** **Salpingo-oophoritis in pregnancy**

        Oophoritis in pregnancy

        Salpingitis in pregnancy

        O23.521 **Salpingo-oophoritis in pregnancy, first trimester** Ⓜ♀

        O23.522 **Salpingo-oophoritis in pregnancy, second trimester** Ⓜ♀

        O23.523 **Salpingo-oophoritis in pregnancy, third trimester** Ⓜ♀

        O23.529 **Salpingo-oophoritis in pregnancy, unspecified trimester** Ⓜ♀

    ✓6th **O23.59** **Infection of other part of genital tract in pregnancy**

        O23.591 **Infection of other part of genital tract in pregnancy, first trimester** Ⓜ♀

        O23.592 **Infection of other part of genital tract in pregnancy, second trimester** Ⓜ♀

        O23.593 **Infection of other part of genital tract in pregnancy, third trimester** Ⓜ♀

        O23.599 **Infection of other part of genital tract in pregnancy, unspecified trimester** Ⓜ♀

✓5th **O23.9** **Unspecified genitourinary tract infection in pregnancy**

    Genitourinary tract infection in pregnancy NOS

    O23.90 **Unspecified genitourinary tract infection in pregnancy, unspecified trimester** Ⓜ♀

    O23.91 **Unspecified genitourinary tract infection in pregnancy, first trimester** Ⓜ♀

    O23.92 **Unspecified genitourinary tract infection in pregnancy, second trimester** Ⓜ♀

    O23.93 **Unspecified genitourinary tract infection in pregnancy, third trimester** Ⓜ♀

✓4th **O24** **Diabetes mellitus in pregnancy, childbirth and the puerperium**

✓5th **O24.0** **Pre-existing type 1 diabetes mellitus, in pregnancy, childbirth and the puerperium**

    Juvenile onset diabetes mellitus, in pregnancy, childbirth and the puerperium

    Ketosis-prone diabetes mellitus in pregnancy, childbirth and the puerperium

    Use additional code from category E10 to further identify any manifestations

    ✓6th **O24.01** **Pre-existing type 1 diabetes mellitus, in pregnancy**

        O24.011 **Pre-existing type 1 diabetes mellitus, in pregnancy, first trimester** Ⓜ♀

        O24.012 **Pre-existing type 1 diabetes mellitus, in pregnancy, second trimester** Ⓜ♀

        O24.013 **Pre-existing type 1 diabetes mellitus, in pregnancy, third trimester** Ⓜ♀

        O24.019 **Pre-existing type 1 diabetes mellitus, in pregnancy, unspecified trimester** Ⓜ♀

    O24.02 **Pre-existing type 1 diabetes mellitus, in childbirth** Ⓜ♀

    O24.03 **Pre-existing type 1 diabetes mellitus, in the puerperium** Ⓜ♀

✓5th **O24.1** **Pre-existing type 2 diabetes mellitus, in pregnancy, childbirth and the puerperium**

    Insulin-resistant diabetes mellitus in pregnancy, childbirth and the puerperium

    Use additional code (for):

        from category E11 to further identify any manifestations

        long-term (current) use of insulin (Z79.4)

    ✓6th **O24.11** **Pre-existing type 2 diabetes mellitus, in pregnancy**

        O24.111 **Pre-existing type 2 diabetes mellitus, in pregnancy, first trimester** Ⓜ♀

        O24.112 **Pre-existing type 2 diabetes mellitus, in pregnancy, second trimester** Ⓜ♀

        O24.113 **Pre-existing type 2 diabetes mellitus, in pregnancy, third trimester** Ⓜ♀

        O24.119 **Pre-existing type 2 diabetes mellitus, in pregnancy, unspecified trimester** Ⓜ♀

    O24.12 **Pre-existing type 2 diabetes mellitus, in childbirth** Ⓜ♀

    O24.13 **Pre-existing type 2 diabetes mellitus, in the puerperium** Ⓜ♀

✓5th **O24.3** **Unspecified pre-existing diabetes mellitus in pregnancy, childbirth and the puerperium**

    Use additional code (for):

        from category E11 to further identify any manifestation

        long-term (current) use of insulin (Z79.4)

    ✓6th **O24.31** **Unspecified pre-existing diabetes mellitus in pregnancy**

        O24.311 **Unspecified pre-existing diabetes mellitus in pregnancy, first trimester** Ⓜ♀

        O24.312 **Unspecified pre-existing diabetes mellitus in pregnancy, second trimester** Ⓜ♀

        O24.313 **Unspecified pre-existing diabetes mellitus in pregnancy, third trimester** Ⓜ♀

        O24.319 **Unspecified pre-existing diabetes mellitus in pregnancy, unspecified trimester** Ⓜ♀

    O24.32 **Unspecified pre-existing diabetes mellitus in childbirth** Ⓜ♀

    O24.33 **Unspecified pre-existing diabetes mellitus in the puerperium** Ⓜ♀

✓5th **O24.4** **Gestational diabetes mellitus**

    Diabetes mellitus arising in pregnancy

    Gestational diabetes mellitus NOS

    AHA: 2016,4Q,50; 2015,4Q,34

    ✓6th **O24.41** **Gestational diabetes mellitus in pregnancy**

        O24.410 **Gestational diabetes mellitus in pregnancy, diet controlled** Ⓜ♀

        O24.414 **Gestational diabetes mellitus in pregnancy, insulin controlled** Ⓜ♀

        O24.415 **Gestational diabetes mellitus in pregnancy, controlled by oral hypoglycemic drugs** Ⓜ♀

            Gestational diabetes mellitus in pregnancy, controlled by oral antidiabetic drugs

        O24.419 **Gestational diabetes mellitus in pregnancy, unspecified control** Ⓜ♀

    ✓6th **O24.42** **Gestational diabetes mellitus in childbirth**

        AHA: 2016,1Q,5

        O24.420 **Gestational diabetes mellitus in childbirth, diet controlled** Ⓜ♀

        O24.424 **Gestational diabetes mellitus in childbirth, insulin controlled** Ⓜ♀

        O24.425 **Gestational diabetes mellitus in childbirth, controlled by oral hypoglycemic drugs** Ⓜ♀

            Gestational diabetes mellitus in childbirth, controlled by oral antidiabetic drugs

✅ Additional Character Required   ✓x7th Placeholder Alert   Manifestation   Unspecified Dx   ►◄ Revised Text   ● New Code   ▲ Revised Title

ICD-10-CM 2020

857

O24.429 Gestational diabetes mellitus in childbirth, unspecified control Ⓜ♀

✓6ᵗʰ **O24.43 Gestational diabetes mellitus in the puerperium**

    O24.430 Gestational diabetes mellitus in the puerperium, diet controlled Ⓜ♀

    O24.434 Gestational diabetes mellitus in the puerperium, insulin controlled Ⓜ♀

    O24.435 Gestational diabetes mellitus in puerperium, controlled by oral hypoglycemic drugs Ⓜ♀
        Gestational diabetes mellitus in puerperium, controlled by oral antidiabetic drugs

    O24.439 Gestational diabetes mellitus in the puerperium, unspecified control Ⓜ♀

✓5ᵗʰ **O24.8 Other pre-existing diabetes mellitus in pregnancy, childbirth, and the puerperium**
    Use additional code (for):
       from categories E08, E09 and E13 to further identify any manifestation
       long-term (current) use of insulin (Z79.4)

    ✓6ᵗʰ **O24.81 Other pre-existing diabetes mellitus in pregnancy**

        O24.811 Other pre-existing diabetes mellitus in pregnancy, first trimester Ⓜ♀

        O24.812 Other pre-existing diabetes mellitus in pregnancy, second trimester Ⓜ♀

        O24.813 Other pre-existing diabetes mellitus in pregnancy, third trimester Ⓜ♀

        O24.819 Other pre-existing diabetes mellitus in pregnancy, unspecified trimester ♀

    O24.82 Other pre-existing diabetes mellitus in childbirth Ⓜ♀

    O24.83 Other pre-existing diabetes mellitus in the puerperium Ⓜ♀

✓5ᵗʰ **O24.9 Unspecified diabetes mellitus in pregnancy, childbirth and the puerperium**
    Use additional code for long-term (current) use of insulin (Z79.4)

    ✓6ᵗʰ **O24.91 Unspecified diabetes mellitus in pregnancy**

        O24.911 Unspecified diabetes mellitus in pregnancy, first trimester Ⓜ♀

        O24.912 Unspecified diabetes mellitus in pregnancy, second trimester Ⓜ♀

        O24.913 Unspecified diabetes mellitus in pregnancy, third trimester Ⓜ♀

        O24.919 Unspecified diabetes mellitus in pregnancy, unspecified trimester Ⓜ♀

    O24.92 Unspecified diabetes mellitus in childbirth Ⓜ♀

    O24.93 Unspecified diabetes mellitus in the puerperium Ⓜ♀

✓4ᵗʰ **O25 Malnutrition in pregnancy, childbirth and the puerperium**

    ✓5ᵗʰ **O25.1 Malnutrition in pregnancy**

        O25.10 Malnutrition in pregnancy, unspecified trimester ♀

        O25.11 Malnutrition in pregnancy, first trimester Ⓜ♀

        O25.12 Malnutrition in pregnancy, second trimester Ⓜ♀

        O25.13 Malnutrition in pregnancy, third trimester Ⓜ♀

    O25.2 Malnutrition in childbirth Ⓜ♀

    O25.3 Malnutrition in the puerperium Ⓜ♀

✓4ᵗʰ **O26 Maternal care for other conditions predominantly related to pregnancy**

    ✓5ᵗʰ **O26.0 Excessive weight gain in pregnancy**
       EXCLUDES 2   gestational edema (O12.0, O12.2)

        O26.00 Excessive weight gain in pregnancy, unspecified trimester Ⓜ♀

        O26.01 Excessive weight gain in pregnancy, first trimester Ⓜ♀

        O26.02 Excessive weight gain in pregnancy, second trimester Ⓜ♀

        O26.03 Excessive weight gain in pregnancy, third trimester Ⓜ♀

    ✓5ᵗʰ **O26.1 Low weight gain in pregnancy**

        O26.10 Low weight gain in pregnancy, unspecified trimester Ⓜ♀

        O26.11 Low weight gain in pregnancy, first trimester Ⓜ♀

        O26.12 Low weight gain in pregnancy, second trimester Ⓜ♀

        O26.13 Low weight gain in pregnancy, third trimester Ⓜ♀

    ✓5ᵗʰ **O26.2 Pregnancy care for patient with recurrent pregnancy loss**

        O26.20 Pregnancy care for patient with recurrent pregnancy loss, unspecified trimester Ⓜ♀

        O26.21 Pregnancy care for patient with recurrent pregnancy loss, first trimester Ⓜ♀

        O26.22 Pregnancy care for patient with recurrent pregnancy loss, second trimester Ⓜ♀

        O26.23 Pregnancy care for patient with recurrent pregnancy loss, third trimester Ⓜ♀

    ✓5ᵗʰ **O26.3 Retained intrauterine contraceptive device in pregnancy**

        O26.30 Retained intrauterine contraceptive device in pregnancy, unspecified trimester Ⓜ♀

        O26.31 Retained intrauterine contraceptive device in pregnancy, first trimester Ⓜ♀

        O26.32 Retained intrauterine contraceptive device in pregnancy, second trimester Ⓜ♀

        O26.33 Retained intrauterine contraceptive device in pregnancy, third trimester Ⓜ♀

    ✓5ᵗʰ **O26.4 Herpes gestationis**
       DEF: Rare skin disorder of unknown origin that appears on the abdomen in the second and third trimester as intensely itchy blisters that spread to other sites.

        O26.40 Herpes gestationis, unspecified trimester Ⓜ♀

        O26.41 Herpes gestationis, first trimester Ⓜ♀

        O26.42 Herpes gestationis, second trimester Ⓜ♀

        O26.43 Herpes gestationis, third trimester Ⓜ♀

    ✓5ᵗʰ **O26.5 Maternal hypotension syndrome**
       Supine hypotensive syndrome

        O26.50 Maternal hypotension syndrome, unspecified trimester Ⓜ♀

        O26.51 Maternal hypotension syndrome, first trimester Ⓜ♀

        O26.52 Maternal hypotension syndrome, second trimester Ⓜ♀

        O26.53 Maternal hypotension syndrome, third trimester Ⓜ♀

    ✓5ᵗʰ **O26.6 Liver and biliary tract disorders in pregnancy, childbirth and the puerperium**
       Use additional code to identify the specific disorder
       EXCLUDES 2   hepatorenal syndrome following labor and delivery (O90.4)

       ✓6ᵗʰ **O26.61 Liver and biliary tract disorders in pregnancy**

        O26.611 Liver and biliary tract disorders in pregnancy, first trimester Ⓜ♀

        O26.612 Liver and biliary tract disorders in pregnancy, second trimester Ⓜ♀

        O26.613 Liver and biliary tract disorders in pregnancy, third trimester Ⓜ♀

        O26.619 Liver and biliary tract disorders in pregnancy, unspecified trimester Ⓜ♀

       O26.62 Liver and biliary tract disorders in childbirth Ⓜ♀

       O26.63 Liver and biliary tract disorders in the puerperium Ⓜ♀

√5ᵗʰ **O26.7 Subluxation of symphysis (pubis) in pregnancy, childbirth and the puerperium**

> *EXCLUDES 1*   traumatic separation of symphysis (pubis) during childbirth (O71.6)

√6ᵗʰ **O26.71 Subluxation of symphysis (pubis) in** pregnancy

O26.711 Subluxation of symphysis (pubis) in pregnancy, first trimester   Ⅿ♀

O26.712 Subluxation of symphysis (pubis) in pregnancy, second trimester   Ⅿ♀

O26.713 Subluxation of symphysis (pubis) in pregnancy, third trimester   Ⅿ♀

O26.719 Subluxation of symphysis (pubis) in pregnancy, unspecified trimester   Ⅿ♀

O26.72 Subluxation of symphysis (pubis) in childbirth   Ⅿ♀

O26.73 Subluxation of symphysis (pubis) in the puerperium   Ⅿ♀

√5ᵗʰ **O26.8 Other specified pregnancy related conditions**

√6ᵗʰ **O26.81 Pregnancy related exhaustion and fatigue**

O26.811 Pregnancy related exhaustion and fatigue, first trimester   Ⅿ♀

O26.812 Pregnancy related exhaustion and fatigue, second trimester   Ⅿ♀

O26.813 Pregnancy related exhaustion and fatigue, third trimester   Ⅿ♀

O26.819 Pregnancy related exhaustion and fatigue, unspecified trimester   Ⅿ♀

√6ᵗʰ **O26.82 Pregnancy related peripheral neuritis**

O26.821 Pregnancy related peripheral neuritis, first trimester   Ⅿ♀

O26.822 Pregnancy related peripheral neuritis, second trimester   Ⅿ♀

O26.823 Pregnancy related peripheral neuritis, third trimester   Ⅿ♀

O26.829 Pregnancy related peripheral neuritis, unspecified trimester   Ⅿ♀

√6ᵗʰ **O26.83 Pregnancy related renal disease**

Use additional code to identify the specific disorder

O26.831 Pregnancy related renal disease, first trimester   Ⅿ♀

O26.832 Pregnancy related renal disease, second trimester   Ⅿ♀

O26.833 Pregnancy related renal disease, third trimester   Ⅿ♀

O26.839 Pregnancy related renal disease, unspecified trimester   Ⅿ♀

√6ᵗʰ **O26.84 Uterine size-date discrepancy complicating pregnancy**

> *EXCLUDES 1*   encounter for suspected problem with fetal growth ruled out (Z03.74)

O26.841 Uterine size-date discrepancy, first trimester   Ⅿ♀

O26.842 Uterine size-date discrepancy, second trimester   Ⅿ♀

O26.843 Uterine size-date discrepancy, third trimester   Ⅿ♀

O26.849 Uterine size-date discrepancy, unspecified trimester   Ⅿ♀

√6ᵗʰ **O26.85 Spotting complicating pregnancy**

O26.851 Spotting complicating pregnancy, first trimester   Ⅿ♀

O26.852 Spotting complicating pregnancy, second trimester   Ⅿ♀

O26.853 Spotting complicating pregnancy, third trimester   Ⅿ♀

O26.859 Spotting complicating pregnancy, unspecified trimester   Ⅿ♀

O26.86 Pruritic urticarial papules and plaques of pregnancy (PUPPP)   Ⅿ♀

Polymorphic eruption of pregnancy

√6ᵗʰ **O26.87 Cervical shortening**

> *EXCLUDES 1*   encounter for suspected cervical shortening ruled out (Z03.75)

DEF: Cervix that has shortened to less than 25 mm before the 24th week of pregnancy. A shortened cervix is a warning sign for impending premature delivery and is treated by cervical cerclage placement or progesterone.

O26.872 Cervical shortening, second trimester   Ⅿ♀

O26.873 Cervical shortening, third trimester   Ⅿ♀

O26.879 Cervical shortening, unspecified trimester   Ⅿ♀

√6ᵗʰ **O26.89 Other specified pregnancy related conditions**

AHA: 2015,3Q,40

O26.891 Other specified pregnancy related conditions, first trimester   Ⅿ♀

O26.892 Other specified pregnancy related conditions, second trimester   Ⅿ♀

O26.893 Other specified pregnancy related conditions, third trimester   Ⅿ♀

O26.899 Other specified pregnancy related conditions, unspecified trimester   Ⅿ♀

√5ᵗʰ **O26.9 Pregnancy related conditions, unspecified**

O26.90 Pregnancy related conditions, unspecified, unspecified trimester   Ⅿ♀

O26.91 Pregnancy related conditions, unspecified, first trimester   Ⅿ♀

O26.92 Pregnancy related conditions, unspecified, second trimester   Ⅿ♀

O26.93 Pregnancy related conditions, unspecified, third trimester   Ⅿ♀

√4ᵗʰ **O28 Abnormal findings on antenatal screening of mother**

> *EXCLUDES 1*   diagnostic findings classified elsewhere — see Alphabetical Index

O28.0 Abnormal hematological finding on antenatal screening of mother   Ⅿ♀

O28.1 Abnormal biochemical finding on antenatal screening of mother   Ⅿ♀

O28.2 Abnormal cytological finding on antenatal screening of mother   Ⅿ♀

O28.3 Abnormal ultrasonic finding on antenatal screening of mother   Ⅿ♀

O28.4 Abnormal radiological finding on antenatal screening of mother   Ⅿ♀

O28.5 Abnormal chromosomal and genetic finding on antenatal screening of mother   Ⅿ♀

O28.8 Other abnormal findings on antenatal screening of mother   Ⅿ♀

O28.9 Unspecified abnormal findings on antenatal screening of mother   Ⅿ♀

√4ᵗʰ **O29 Complications of anesthesia during pregnancy**

> *INCLUDES*   maternal complications arising from the administration of a general, regional or local anesthetic, analgesic or other sedation during pregnancy

Use additional code, if necessary, to identify the complication

> *EXCLUDES 2*   complications of anesthesia during labor and delivery (O74.-)
> complications of anesthesia during the puerperium (O89.-)

√5ᵗʰ **O29.0 Pulmonary complications of anesthesia during pregnancy**

√6ᵗʰ **O29.01 Aspiration pneumonitis due to anesthesia during pregnancy**

Inhalation of stomach contents or secretions NOS due to anesthesia during pregnancy

Mendelson's syndrome due to anesthesia during pregnancy

O29.011 Aspiration pneumonitis due to anesthesia during pregnancy, first trimester   Ⅿ♀

O29.012 Aspiration pneumonitis due to anesthesia during pregnancy, second trimester   Ⅿ♀

O29.013 Aspiration pneumonitis due to anesthesia during pregnancy, third trimester   Ⅿ♀

✔ Additional Character Required   √x7ᵗʰ Placeholder Alert   Manifestation   Unspecified Dx   ►◄ Revised Text   ● New Code   ▲ Revised Title

ICD-10-CM 2020   **859**

O29.019 Aspiration pneumonitis due to anesthesia during pregnancy, unspecified trimester Ⓜ♀

✓6ᵗʰ **O29.02** Pressure collapse of lung due to anesthesia during pregnancy

O29.021 Pressure collapse of lung due to anesthesia during pregnancy, first trimester Ⓜ♀

O29.022 Pressure collapse of lung due to anesthesia during pregnancy, second trimester Ⓜ♀

O29.023 Pressure collapse of lung due to anesthesia during pregnancy, third trimester Ⓜ♀

O29.029 Pressure collapse of lung due to anesthesia during pregnancy, unspecified trimester Ⓜ♀

✓6ᵗʰ **O29.09** Other pulmonary complications of anesthesia during pregnancy

O29.091 Other pulmonary complications of anesthesia during pregnancy, first trimester Ⓜ♀

O29.092 Other pulmonary complications of anesthesia during pregnancy, second trimester Ⓜ♀

O29.093 Other pulmonary complications of anesthesia during pregnancy, third trimester Ⓜ♀

O29.099 Other pulmonary complications of anesthesia during pregnancy, unspecified trimester Ⓜ♀

✓5ᵗʰ **O29.1** Cardiac complications of anesthesia during pregnancy

✓6ᵗʰ **O29.11** Cardiac arrest due to anesthesia during pregnancy

O29.111 Cardiac arrest due to anesthesia during pregnancy, first trimester Ⓜ♀

O29.112 Cardiac arrest due to anesthesia during pregnancy, second trimester Ⓜ♀

O29.113 Cardiac arrest due to anesthesia during pregnancy, third trimester Ⓜ♀

O29.119 Cardiac arrest due to anesthesia during pregnancy, unspecified trimester Ⓜ♀

✓6ᵗʰ **O29.12** Cardiac failure due to anesthesia during pregnancy

O29.121 Cardiac failure due to anesthesia during pregnancy, first trimester Ⓜ♀

O29.122 Cardiac failure due to anesthesia during pregnancy, second trimester Ⓜ♀

O29.123 Cardiac failure due to anesthesia during pregnancy, third trimester Ⓜ♀

O29.129 Cardiac failure due to anesthesia during pregnancy, unspecified trimester Ⓜ♀

✓6ᵗʰ **O29.19** Other cardiac complications of anesthesia during pregnancy

O29.191 Other cardiac complications of anesthesia during pregnancy, first trimester Ⓜ♀

O29.192 Other cardiac complications of anesthesia during pregnancy, second trimester Ⓜ♀

O29.193 Other cardiac complications of anesthesia during pregnancy, third trimester Ⓜ♀

O29.199 Other cardiac complications of anesthesia during pregnancy, unspecified trimester Ⓜ♀

✓5ᵗʰ **O29.2** Central nervous system complications of anesthesia during pregnancy

✓6ᵗʰ **O29.21** Cerebral anoxia due to anesthesia during pregnancy

O29.211 Cerebral anoxia due to anesthesia during pregnancy, first trimester Ⓜ♀

O29.212 Cerebral anoxia due to anesthesia during pregnancy, second trimester Ⓜ♀

O29.213 Cerebral anoxia due to anesthesia during pregnancy, third trimester Ⓜ♀

O29.219 Cerebral anoxia due to anesthesia during pregnancy, unspecified trimester Ⓜ♀

✓6ᵗʰ **O29.29** Other central nervous system complications of anesthesia during pregnancy

O29.291 Other central nervous system complications of anesthesia during pregnancy, first trimester Ⓜ♀

O29.292 Other central nervous system complications of anesthesia during pregnancy, second trimester Ⓜ♀

O29.293 Other central nervous system complications of anesthesia during pregnancy, third trimester Ⓜ♀

O29.299 Other central nervous system complications of anesthesia during pregnancy, unspecified trimester Ⓜ♀

✓5ᵗʰ **O29.3** Toxic reaction to local anesthesia during pregnancy

✓6ᵗʰ **O29.3X** Toxic reaction to local anesthesia during pregnancy

O29.3X1 Toxic reaction to local anesthesia during pregnancy, first trimester Ⓜ♀

O29.3X2 Toxic reaction to local anesthesia during pregnancy, second trimester Ⓜ♀

O29.3X3 Toxic reaction to local anesthesia during pregnancy, third trimester Ⓜ♀

O29.3X9 Toxic reaction to local anesthesia during pregnancy, unspecified trimester Ⓜ♀

✓5ᵗʰ **O29.4** Spinal and epidural anesthesia induced headache during pregnancy

O29.40 Spinal and epidural anesthesia induced headache during pregnancy, unspecified trimester Ⓜ♀

O29.41 Spinal and epidural anesthesia induced headache during pregnancy, first trimester Ⓜ♀

O29.42 Spinal and epidural anesthesia induced headache during pregnancy, second trimester Ⓜ♀

O29.43 Spinal and epidural anesthesia induced headache during pregnancy, third trimester Ⓜ♀

✓5ᵗʰ **O29.5** Other complications of spinal and epidural anesthesia during pregnancy

✓6ᵗʰ **O29.5X** Other complications of spinal and epidural anesthesia during pregnancy

O29.5X1 Other complications of spinal and epidural anesthesia during pregnancy, first trimester Ⓜ♀

O29.5X2 Other complications of spinal and epidural anesthesia during pregnancy, second trimester Ⓜ♀

O29.5X3 Other complications of spinal and epidural anesthesia during pregnancy, third trimester Ⓜ♀

O29.5X9 Other complications of spinal and epidural anesthesia during pregnancy, unspecified trimester Ⓜ♀

✓5ᵗʰ **O29.6** Failed or difficult intubation for anesthesia during pregnancy

     O29.60 Failed or difficult intubation for anesthesia during pregnancy, unspecified trimester   Ⓜ♀

     O29.61 Failed or difficult intubation for anesthesia during pregnancy, first trimester   Ⓜ♀

     O29.62 Failed or difficult intubation for anesthesia during pregnancy, second trimester   Ⓜ♀

     O29.63 Failed or difficult intubation for anesthesia during pregnancy, third trimester   Ⓜ♀

✓5ᵗʰ **O29.8** Other complications of anesthesia during pregnancy

     ✓6ᵗʰ **O29.8X** Other complications of anesthesia during pregnancy

         O29.8X1 Other complications of anesthesia during pregnancy, first trimester   Ⓜ♀

         O29.8X2 Other complications of anesthesia during pregnancy, second trimester   Ⓜ♀

         O29.8X3 Other complications of anesthesia during pregnancy, third trimester   Ⓜ♀

         O29.8X9 Other complications of anesthesia during pregnancy, unspecified trimester   Ⓜ♀

✓5ᵗʰ **O29.9** Unspecified complication of anesthesia during pregnancy

     O29.90 Unspecified complication of anesthesia during pregnancy, unspecified trimester   Ⓜ♀

     O29.91 Unspecified complication of anesthesia during pregnancy, first trimester   Ⓜ♀

     O29.92 Unspecified complication of anesthesia during pregnancy, second trimester   Ⓜ♀

     O29.93 Unspecified complication of anesthesia during pregnancy, third trimester   Ⓜ♀

Maternal care related to the fetus and amniotic cavity and possible delivery problems (O30-O48)

✓4ᵗʰ **O30 Multiple gestation**

Code also any complications specific to multiple gestation
AHA: 2016,4Q,51

✓5ᵗʰ **O30.0** Twin pregnancy

     ✓6ᵗʰ **O30.00** Twin pregnancy, unspecified number of placenta and unspecified number of amniotic sacs

         O30.001 Twin pregnancy, unspecified number of placenta and unspecified number of amniotic sacs, first trimester   Ⓜ♀

         O30.002 Twin pregnancy, unspecified number of placenta and unspecified number of amniotic sacs, second trimester   Ⓜ♀

         O30.003 Twin pregnancy, unspecified number of placenta and unspecified number of amniotic sacs, third trimester   Ⓜ♀

         O30.009 Twin pregnancy, unspecified number of placenta and unspecified number of amniotic sacs, unspecified trimester   Ⓜ♀

     ✓6ᵗʰ **O30.01** Twin pregnancy, monochorionic/monoamniotic

Twin pregnancy, one placenta, one amniotic sac

EXCLUDES 1   conjoined twins (O30.02-)

Twin Gestation – Monochorionic/Monoamniotic

- 1 Chorionic sac
- 1 Amniotic sac
- 2 Fetuses
- 2 Umbilical cords
- 1 Placenta

         O30.011 Twin pregnancy, monochorionic/monoamniotic, first trimester   Ⓜ♀

         O30.012 Twin pregnancy, monochorionic/monoamniotic, second trimester   Ⓜ♀

         O30.013 Twin pregnancy, monochorionic/monoamniotic, third trimester   Ⓜ♀

         O30.019 Twin pregnancy, monochorionic/monoamniotic, unspecified trimester   Ⓜ♀

     ✓6ᵗʰ **O30.02** Conjoined twin pregnancy

         O30.021 Conjoined twin pregnancy, first trimester   Ⓜ♀

         O30.022 Conjoined twin pregnancy, second trimester   Ⓜ♀

         O30.023 Conjoined twin pregnancy, third trimester   Ⓜ♀

         O30.029 Conjoined twin pregnancy, unspecified trimester   Ⓜ♀

     ✓6ᵗʰ **O30.03** Twin pregnancy, monochorionic/diamniotic

Twin pregnancy, one placenta, two amniotic sacs

Twin Gestation – Monochorionic/Diamniotic

- 1 Chorionic sac
- 2 Amniotic sacs
- 2 Fetuses
- 2 Umbilical cords
- 1 Placenta

         O30.031 Twin pregnancy, monochorionic/diamniotic, first trimester   Ⓜ♀

         O30.032 Twin pregnancy, monochorionic/diamniotic, second trimester   Ⓜ♀

         O30.033 Twin pregnancy, monochorionic/diamniotic, third trimester   Ⓜ♀

         O30.039 Twin pregnancy, monochorionic/diamniotic, unspecified trimester   Ⓜ♀

✔ Additional Character Required   ✓x7ᵗʰ Placeholder Alert   Manifestation   Unspecified Dx   ►◄ Revised Text   ● New Code   ▲ Revised Title

ICD-10-CM 2020   **861**

✓6ᵗʰ **O30.04 Twin pregnancy,** dichorionic/diamniotic

Twin pregnancy, two placentae, two amniotic sacs

Twin Gestation – Dichorionic/Diamniotic

- 2 Chorionic sacs
- 2 Amniotic sacs
- 2 Fetuses
- 2 Umbilical cords
- 2 Placentas

O30.041 **Twin pregnancy, dichorionic/diamniotic,** first **trimester**   Ⓜ♀

O30.042 **Twin pregnancy, dichorionic/diamniotic,** second trimester   Ⓜ♀

O30.043 **Twin pregnancy, dichorionic/diamniotic,** third **trimester**   Ⓜ♀

O30.049 **Twin pregnancy, dichorionic/diamniotic, unspecified trimester**   Ⓜ♀

✓6ᵗʰ **O30.09 Twin pregnancy,** unable to determine number **of placenta and number of amniotic sacs**

O30.091 **Twin pregnancy, unable to determine number of placenta and number of amniotic sacs,** first trimester   Ⓜ♀

O30.092 **Twin pregnancy, unable to determine number of placenta and number of amniotic sacs,** second trimester   Ⓜ♀

O30.093 **Twin pregnancy, unable to determine number of placenta and number of amniotic sacs,** third trimester   Ⓜ♀

O30.099 **Twin pregnancy, unable to determine number of placenta and number of amniotic sacs, unspecified trimester**   Ⓜ♀

✓5ᵗʰ **O30.1** Triplet **pregnancy**

✓6ᵗʰ **O30.10 Triplet pregnancy, unspecified number of placenta and unspecified number of amniotic sacs**
AHA: 2016,2Q,8

O30.101 **Triplet pregnancy, unspecified number of placenta and unspecified number of amniotic sacs,** first **trimester**   Ⓜ♀

O30.102 **Triplet pregnancy, unspecified number of placenta and unspecified number of amniotic sacs,** second **trimester**   Ⓜ♀

O30.103 **Triplet pregnancy, unspecified number of placenta and unspecified number of amniotic sacs,** third **trimester**   Ⓜ♀

O30.109 **Triplet pregnancy, unspecified number of placenta and unspecified number of amniotic sacs, unspecified trimester**   Ⓜ♀

✓6ᵗʰ **O30.11 Triplet pregnancy with** two or more monochorionic **fetuses**

O30.111 **Triplet pregnancy with two or more monochorionic fetuses,** first trimester   Ⓜ♀

O30.112 **Triplet pregnancy with two or more monochorionic fetuses,** second trimester   Ⓜ♀

O30.113 **Triplet pregnancy with two or more monochorionic fetuses,** third trimester   Ⓜ♀

O30.119 **Triplet pregnancy with two or more monochorionic fetuses, unspecified trimester**   Ⓜ♀

✓6ᵗʰ **O30.12 Triplet pregnancy with** two or more monoamniotic **fetuses**

O30.121 **Triplet pregnancy with two or more monoamniotic fetuses,** first trimester   Ⓜ♀

O30.122 **Triplet pregnancy with two or more monoamniotic fetuses,** second trimester   Ⓜ♀

O30.123 **Triplet pregnancy with two or more monoamniotic fetuses,** third trimester   Ⓜ♀

O30.129 **Triplet pregnancy with two or more monoamniotic fetuses, unspecified trimester**   Ⓜ♀

✓6ᵗʰ **O30.13 Triplet pregnancy, trichorionic/triamniotic**
AHA: 2018,4Q,22

O30.131 **Triplet pregnancy, trichorionic/triamniotic,** first trimester   Ⓜ♀

O30.132 **Triplet pregnancy, trichorionic/triamniotic,** second trimester   Ⓜ♀

O30.133 **Triplet pregnancy, trichorionic/triamniotic,** third trimester   Ⓜ♀

O30.139 **Triplet pregnancy, trichorionic/triamniotic, unspecified trimester**   Ⓜ♀

✓6ᵗʰ **O30.19 Triplet pregnancy,** unable to determine number **of placenta and number of amniotic sacs**

O30.191 **Triplet pregnancy, unable to determine number of placenta and number of amniotic sacs,** first trimester   Ⓜ♀

O30.192 **Triplet pregnancy, unable to determine number of placenta and number of amniotic sacs,** second trimester   Ⓜ♀

O30.193 **Triplet pregnancy, unable to determine number of placenta and number of amniotic sacs,** third trimester   Ⓜ♀

O30.199 **Triplet pregnancy, unable to determine number of placenta and number of amniotic sacs, unspecified trimester**   Ⓜ♀

✓5ᵗʰ **O30.2** Quadruplet **pregnancy**

✓6ᵗʰ **O30.20 Quadruplet pregnancy, unspecified number of placenta and unspecified number of amniotic sacs**

O30.201 **Quadruplet pregnancy, unspecified number of placenta and unspecified number of amniotic sacs,** first trimester   Ⓜ♀

O30.202 **Quadruplet pregnancy, unspecified number of placenta and unspecified number of amniotic sacs,** second trimester   Ⓜ♀

O30.203 **Quadruplet pregnancy, unspecified number of placenta and unspecified number of amniotic sacs,** third trimester   Ⓜ♀

O30.209 **Quadruplet pregnancy, unspecified number of placenta and unspecified number of amniotic sacs, unspecified trimester**   Ⓜ♀

✓6ᵗʰ **O30.21** **Quadruplet pregnancy with** two or more monochorionic fetuses

    O30.211 **Quadruplet pregnancy with two or more monochorionic fetuses, first trimester** Ⓜ♀

    O30.212 **Quadruplet pregnancy with two or more monochorionic fetuses, second trimester** Ⓜ♀

    O30.213 **Quadruplet pregnancy with two or more monochorionic fetuses, third trimester** Ⓜ♀

    O30.219 **Quadruplet pregnancy with two or more monochorionic fetuses, unspecified trimester** Ⓜ♀

✓6ᵗʰ **O30.22** **Quadruplet pregnancy with** two or more monoamniotic fetuses

    O30.221 **Quadruplet pregnancy with two or more monoamniotic fetuses, first trimester** Ⓜ♀

    O30.222 **Quadruplet pregnancy with two or more monoamniotic fetuses, second trimester** Ⓜ♀

    O30.223 **Quadruplet pregnancy with two or more monoamniotic fetuses, third trimester** Ⓜ♀

    O30.229 **Quadruplet pregnancy with two or more monoamniotic fetuses, unspecified trimester** Ⓜ♀

✓6ᵗʰ **O30.23** **Quadruplet pregnancy, quadrachorionic/quadra-amniotic**
    AHA: 2018,4Q,22

    O30.231 **Quadruplet pregnancy, quadrachorionic/quadra-amniotic, first trimester** Ⓜ♀

    O30.232 **Quadruplet pregnancy, quadrachorionic/quadra-amniotic, second trimester** Ⓜ♀

    O30.233 **Quadruplet pregnancy, quadrachorionic/quadra-amniotic, third trimester** Ⓜ♀

    O30.239 **Quadruplet pregnancy, quadrachorionic/quadra-amniotic, unspecified trimester** Ⓜ♀

✓6ᵗʰ **O30.29** **Quadruplet pregnancy,** unable to determine number **of placenta and number of amniotic sacs**

    O30.291 **Quadruplet pregnancy, unable to determine number of placenta and number of amniotic sacs, first trimester** Ⓜ♀

    O30.292 **Quadruplet pregnancy, unable to determine number of placenta and number of amniotic sacs, second trimester** Ⓜ♀

    O30.293 **Quadruplet pregnancy, unable to determine number of placenta and number of amniotic sacs, third trimester** Ⓜ♀

    O30.299 **Quadruplet pregnancy, unable to determine number of placenta and number of amniotic sacs, unspecified trimester** Ⓜ♀

✓5ᵗʰ **O30.8** **Other specified multiple gestation**
    Multiple gestation pregnancy greater then quadruplets

✓6ᵗʰ **O30.80** **Other specified multiple gestation, unspecified number of placenta and unspecified number of amniotic sacs**

    O30.801 **Other specified multiple gestation, unspecified number of placenta and unspecified number of amniotic sacs, first trimester** Ⓜ♀

    O30.802 **Other specified multiple gestation, unspecified number of placenta and unspecified number of amniotic sacs, second trimester** Ⓜ♀

    O30.803 **Other specified multiple gestation, unspecified number of placenta and unspecified number of amniotic sacs, third trimester** Ⓜ♀

    O30.809 **Other specified multiple gestation, unspecified number of placenta and unspecified number of amniotic sacs, unspecified trimester** Ⓜ♀

✓6ᵗʰ **O30.81** **Other specified multiple gestation with** two or more monochorionic fetuses

    O30.811 **Other specified multiple gestation with two or more monochorionic fetuses, first trimester** Ⓜ♀

    O30.812 **Other specified multiple gestation with two or more monochorionic fetuses, second trimester** Ⓜ♀

    O30.813 **Other specified multiple gestation with two or more monochorionic fetuses, third trimester** Ⓜ♀

    O30.819 **Other specified multiple gestation with two or more monochorionic fetuses, unspecified trimester** Ⓜ♀

✓6ᵗʰ **O30.82** **Other specified multiple gestation with** two or more monoamniotic fetuses

    O30.821 **Other specified multiple gestation with two or more monoamniotic fetuses, first trimester** Ⓜ♀

    O30.822 **Other specified multiple gestation with two or more monoamniotic fetuses, second trimester** Ⓜ♀

    O30.823 **Other specified multiple gestation with two or more monoamniotic fetuses, third trimester** Ⓜ♀

    O30.829 **Other specified multiple gestation with two or more monoamniotic fetuses, unspecified trimester** Ⓜ♀

✓6ᵗʰ **O30.83** **Other specified multiple gestation,** number of chorions and amnions are both equal to the number of fetuses
    Pentachorionic, penta-amniotic pregnancy (quintuplets)
    Hexachorionic, hexa-amniotic pregnancy (sextuplets)
    Heptachorionic, hepta-amniotic pregnancy (septuplets)
    AHA: 2018,4Q,22

    O30.831 **Other specified multiple gestation, number of chorions and amnions are both equal to the number of fetuses, first trimester** Ⓜ♀

    O30.832 **Other specified multiple gestation, number of chorions and amnions are both equal to the number of fetuses, second trimester** Ⓜ♀

    O30.833 **Other specified multiple gestation, number of chorions and amnions are both equal to the number of fetuses, third trimester** Ⓜ♀

    O30.839 **Other specified multiple gestation, number of chorions and amnions are both equal to the number of fetuses, unspecified trimester** Ⓜ♀

✓6ᵗʰ **O30.89** **Other specified multiple gestation,** unable to determine number **of placenta and number of amniotic sacs**

    O30.891 **Other specified multiple gestation, unable to determine number of placenta and number of amniotic sacs, first trimester** Ⓜ♀

    O30.892 **Other specified multiple gestation, unable to determine number of placenta and number of amniotic sacs, second trimester** Ⓜ♀

☑ Additional Character Required   ✓x7ᵗʰ Placeholder Alert   Manifestation   Unspecified Dx   ▶◀ Revised Text   ● New Code   ▲ Revised Title

ICD-10-CM 2020   863

O30.893 Other specified multiple gestation, unable to determine number of placenta and number of amniotic sacs, third trimester Ⓜ♀

O30.899 Other specified multiple gestation, unable to determine number of placenta and number of amniotic sacs, unspecified trimester Ⓜ♀

√5ᵗʰ **O30.9 Multiple gestation, unspecified**

Multiple pregnancy NOS

O30.90 Multiple gestation, unspecified, unspecified trimester Ⓜ♀

O30.91 Multiple gestation, unspecified, first trimester Ⓜ♀

O30.92 Multiple gestation, unspecified, second trimester Ⓜ♀

O30.93 Multiple gestation, unspecified, third trimester Ⓜ♀

√4ᵗʰ **O31 Complications specific to multiple gestation**

EXCLUDES 2   delayed delivery of second twin, triplet, etc. (O63.2)
malpresentation of one fetus or more (O32.9)
placental transfusion syndromes (O43.0-)

AHA: 2012,4Q,107

One of the following 7th characters is to be assigned to each code under category O31. 7th character 0 is for single gestations and multiple gestations where the fetus is unspecified. 7th characters 1 through 9 are for cases of multiple gestations to identify the fetus for which the code applies. The appropriate code from category O30, Multiple gestation, must also be assigned when assigning a code from category O31 that has a 7th character of 1 through 9.
0   not applicable or unspecified
1   fetus 1
2   fetus 2
3   fetus 3
4   fetus 4
5   fetus 5
9   other fetus

√5ᵗʰ **O31.0 Papyraceous fetus**

Fetus compressus
DEF: Fetus that has died, but remains in utero for weeks before delivery, becoming compacted and mummified in appearance, with skin resembling parchment. Occurs most commonly in multigestational pregnancies. **Synonym(s):** paper doll fetus.

√x7ᵗʰ **O31.00** Papyraceous fetus, unspecified trimester Ⓜ♀

√x7ᵗʰ **O31.01** Papyraceous fetus, first trimester Ⓜ♀

√x7ᵗʰ **O31.02** Papyraceous fetus, second trimester Ⓜ♀

√x7ᵗʰ **O31.03** Papyraceous fetus, third trimester Ⓜ♀

√5ᵗʰ **O31.1 Continuing pregnancy after spontaneous abortion of one fetus or more**

√x7ᵗʰ **O31.10** Continuing pregnancy after spontaneous abortion of one fetus or more, unspecified trimester Ⓜ♀

√x7ᵗʰ **O31.11** Continuing pregnancy after spontaneous abortion of one fetus or more, first trimester Ⓜ♀

√x7ᵗʰ **O31.12** Continuing pregnancy after spontaneous abortion of one fetus or more, second trimester Ⓜ♀

√x7ᵗʰ **O31.13** Continuing pregnancy after spontaneous abortion of one fetus or more, third trimester Ⓜ♀

√5ᵗʰ **O31.2 Continuing pregnancy after intrauterine death of one fetus or more**

√x7ᵗʰ **O31.20** Continuing pregnancy after intrauterine death of one fetus or more, unspecified trimester Ⓜ♀

√x7ᵗʰ **O31.21** Continuing pregnancy after intrauterine death of one fetus or more, first trimester Ⓜ♀

√x7ᵗʰ **O31.22** Continuing pregnancy after intrauterine death of one fetus or more, second trimester Ⓜ♀

√x7ᵗʰ **O31.23** Continuing pregnancy after intrauterine death of one fetus or more, third trimester Ⓜ♀

√5ᵗʰ **O31.3 Continuing pregnancy after elective fetal reduction of one fetus or more**

Continuing pregnancy after selective termination of one fetus or more

√x7ᵗʰ **O31.30** Continuing pregnancy after elective fetal reduction of one fetus or more, unspecified trimester Ⓜ♀

√x7ᵗʰ **O31.31** Continuing pregnancy after elective fetal reduction of one fetus or more, first trimester Ⓜ♀

√x7ᵗʰ **O31.32** Continuing pregnancy after elective fetal reduction of one fetus or more, second trimester Ⓜ♀

√x7ᵗʰ **O31.33** Continuing pregnancy after elective fetal reduction of one fetus or more, third trimester Ⓜ♀

√5ᵗʰ **O31.8 Other complications specific to multiple gestation**

√6ᵗʰ **O31.8X** Other complications specific to multiple gestation

√7ᵗʰ **O31.8X1** Other complications specific to multiple gestation, first trimester Ⓜ♀

√7ᵗʰ **O31.8X2** Other complications specific to multiple gestation, second trimester Ⓜ♀

√7ᵗʰ **O31.8X3** Other complications specific to multiple gestation, third trimester Ⓜ♀

√7ᵗʰ **O31.8X9** Other complications specific to multiple gestation, unspecified trimester Ⓜ♀

√4ᵗʰ **O32 Maternal care for malpresentation of fetus**

INCLUDES   the listed conditions as a reason for observation, hospitalization or other obstetric care of the mother, or for cesarean delivery before onset of labor

EXCLUDES 1   malpresentation of fetus with obstructed labor (O64.-)

AHA: 2012,4Q,107

One of the following 7th characters is to be assigned to each code under category O32. 7th character 0 is for single gestations and multiple gestations where the fetus is unspecified. 7th characters 1 through 9 are for cases of multiple gestations to identify the fetus for which the code applies. The appropriate code from category O30, Multiple gestation, must also be assigned when assigning a code from category O32 that has a 7th character of 1 through 9.
0   not applicable or unspecified
1   fetus 1
2   fetus 2
3   fetus 3
4   fetus 4
5   fetus 5
9   other fetus

√x7ᵗʰ **O32.0** Maternal care for unstable lie Ⓜ♀

√x7ᵗʰ **O32.1** Maternal care for breech presentation Ⓜ♀

Maternal care for buttocks presentation
Maternal care for complete breech
Maternal care for frank breech
EXCLUDES 1   footling presentation (O32.8)
incomplete breech (O32.8)
DEF: Fetus presentation in a longitudinal lie with the buttocks or feet closest to birth canal that may require external cephalic version or cesarean delivery.

√x7ᵗʰ **O32.2** Maternal care for transverse and oblique lie Ⓜ♀

Maternal care for oblique presentation
Maternal care for transverse presentation

√x7ᵗʰ **O32.3** Maternal care for face, brow and chin presentation Ⓜ♀

√x7ᵗʰ **O32.4** Maternal care for high head at term Ⓜ♀

Maternal care for failure of head to enter pelvic brim

√x7ᵗʰ **O32.6** Maternal care for compound presentation Ⓜ♀

√x7ᵗʰ **O32.8** Maternal care for other malpresentation of fetus Ⓜ♀

Maternal care for footling presentation
Maternal care for incomplete breech

√x7ᵗʰ **O32.9** **Maternal care for malpresentation of fetus,** Ⓜ♀
unspecified

Fetal Malpresentation

Breech

Mother's pelvis

Shoulder
(arm prolapse)

Compound
(extremity together with head)

Face
(mentum)

Oblique

√4ᵗʰ **O33** **Maternal care for disproportion**

> INCLUDES   the listed conditions as a reason for observation, hospitalization or other obstetric care of the mother, or for cesarean delivery before onset of labor
> EXCLUDES 1   *disproportion with obstructed labor (O65-O66)*

O33.0 **Maternal care for disproportion due to** deformity Ⓜ♀
of maternal pelvic bones
> Maternal care for disproportion due to pelvic deformity causing disproportion NOS

O33.1 **Maternal care for disproportion due to** generally Ⓜ♀
contracted pelvis
> Maternal care for disproportion due to contracted pelvis NOS causing disproportion

O33.2 **Maternal care for disproportion due to** inlet Ⓜ♀
contraction of pelvis
> Maternal care for disproportion due to inlet contraction (pelvis) causing disproportion

√x7ᵗʰ **O33.3** **Maternal care for disproportion due to** outlet Ⓜ♀
contraction of pelvis
> Maternal care for disproportion due to mid-cavity contraction (pelvis)
> Maternal care for disproportion due to outlet contraction (pelvis)

> One of the following 7th characters is to be assigned to code O33.3. 7th character Ø is for single gestations and multiple gestations where the fetus is unspecified. 7th characters 1 through 9 are for cases of multiple gestations to identify the fetus for which the code applies. The appropriate code from category O30, Multiple gestation, must also be assigned when assigning code O33.3 with a 7th character of 1 through 9.
> Ø   not applicable or unspecified
> 1   fetus 1
> 2   fetus 2
> 3   fetus 3
> 4   fetus 4
> 5   fetus 5
> 9   other fetus

√x7ᵗʰ **O33.4** **Maternal care for disproportion of mixed** Ⓜ♀
maternal and fetal origin

> One of the following 7th characters is to be assigned to code O33.4. 7th character Ø is for single gestations and multiple gestations where the fetus is unspecified. 7th characters 1 through 9 are for cases of multiple gestations to identify the fetus for which the code applies. The appropriate code from category O30, Multiple gestation, must also be assigned when assigning code O33.4 with a 7th character of 1 through 9.
> Ø   not applicable or unspecified
> 1   fetus 1
> 2   fetus 2
> 3   fetus 3
> 4   fetus 4
> 5   fetus 5
> 9   other fetus

√x7ᵗʰ **O33.5** **Maternal care for disproportion due to unusually** Ⓜ♀
large fetus
> Maternal care for disproportion due to disproportion of fetal origin with normally formed fetus
> Maternal care for disproportion due to fetal disproportion NOS

> One of the following 7th characters is to be assigned to code O33.5. 7th character Ø is for single gestations and multiple gestations where the fetus is unspecified. 7th characters 1 through 9 are for cases of multiple gestations to identify the fetus for which the code applies. The appropriate code from category O30, Multiple gestation, must also be assigned when assigning code O33.5 with a 7th character of 1 through 9.
> Ø   not applicable or unspecified
> 1   fetus 1
> 2   fetus 2
> 3   fetus 3
> 4   fetus 4
> 5   fetus 5
> 9   other fetus

√x7ᵗʰ **O33.6** **Maternal care for disproportion due to** Ⓜ♀
hydrocephalic fetus

> One of the following 7th characters is to be assigned to code O33.6. 7th character Ø is for single gestations and multiple gestations where the fetus is unspecified. 7th characters 1 through 9 are for cases of multiple gestations to identify the fetus for which the code applies. The appropriate code from category O30, Multiple gestation, must also be assigned when assigning code O33.6 with a 7th character of 1 through 9.
> Ø   not applicable or unspecified
> 1   fetus 1
> 2   fetus 2
> 3   fetus 3
> 4   fetus 4
> 5   fetus 5
> 9   other fetus

√x7ᵗʰ **O33.7** **Maternal care for disproportion due to other fetal** Ⓜ♀
deformities
> Maternal care for disproportion due to fetal ascites
> Maternal care for disproportion due to fetal hydrops
> Maternal care for disproportion due to fetal meningomyelocele
> Maternal care for disproportion due to fetal sacral teratoma
> Maternal care for disproportion due to fetal tumor
> EXCLUDES 1   *obstructed labor due to other fetal deformities (O66.3)*

> **AHA:** 2016,4Q,51

> One of the following 7th characters is to be assigned to code O33.7. 7th character Ø is for single gestations and multiple gestations where the fetus is unspecified. 7th characters 1 through 9 are for cases of multiple gestations to identify the fetus for which the code applies. The appropriate code from category O30, Multiple gestation, must also be assigned when assigning code O33.7 with a 7th character of 1 through 9.
> Ø   not applicable or unspecified
> 1   fetus 1
> 2   fetus 2
> 3   fetus 3
> 4   fetus 4
> 5   fetus 5
> 9   other fetus

O33.8 **Maternal care for disproportion of other origin** Ⓜ♀

O33.9 **Maternal care for disproportion, unspecified** Ⓜ♀
> Maternal care for disproportion due to cephalopelvic disproportion NOS
> Maternal care for disproportion due to fetopelvic disproportion NOS

Chapter 15. Pregnancy, Childbirth and the Puerperium

✓4ᵗʰ **O34 Maternal care for abnormality of pelvic organs**

INCLUDES   the listed conditions as a reason for hospitalization or other obstetric care of the mother, or for cesarean delivery before onset of labor

Code first any associated obstructed labor (O65.5)

Use additional code for specific condition

✓5ᵗʰ **O34.0 Maternal care for congenital malformation of uterus**

Maternal care for double uterus

Maternal care for uterus bicornis

O34.00 Maternal care for unspecified congenital malformation of uterus, unspecified trimester Ⓜ♀

O34.01 Maternal care for unspecified congenital malformation of uterus, first trimester Ⓜ♀

O34.02 Maternal care for unspecified congenital malformation of uterus, second trimester Ⓜ♀

O34.03 Maternal care for unspecified congenital malformation of uterus, third trimester Ⓜ♀

✓5ᵗʰ **O34.1 Maternal care for benign tumor of corpus uteri**

EXCLUDES 2   maternal care for benign tumor of cervix (O34.4-)

maternal care for malignant neoplasm of uterus (O9A.1-)

O34.10 Maternal care for benign tumor of corpus uteri, unspecified trimester Ⓜ♀

O34.11 Maternal care for benign tumor of corpus uteri, first trimester Ⓜ♀

O34.12 Maternal care for benign tumor of corpus uteri, second trimester Ⓜ♀

O34.13 Maternal care for benign tumor of corpus uteri, third trimester Ⓜ♀

✓5ᵗʰ **O34.2 Maternal care due to uterine scar from previous surgery**

AHA: 2016,4Q,76

✓6ᵗʰ **O34.21 Maternal care for scar from previous cesarean delivery**

AHA: 2018,3Q,23; 2016,4Q,51-52

O34.211 Maternal care for low transverse scar from previous cesarean delivery Ⓜ♀

O34.212 Maternal care for vertical scar from previous cesarean delivery Ⓜ♀

Maternal care for classical scar from previous cesarean delivery

O34.219 Maternal care for unspecified type scar from previous cesarean delivery Ⓜ♀

O34.29 Maternal care due to uterine scar from other previous surgery Ⓜ♀

Maternal care due to uterine scar from other transmural uterine incision

✓5ᵗʰ **O34.3 Maternal care for cervical incompetence**

Maternal care for cerclage with or without cervical incompetence

Maternal care for Shirodkar suture with or without cervical incompetence

DEF: Inadequate functioning of the cervix marked by abnormal widening during pregnancy and causing premature birth or miscarriage.

O34.30 Maternal care for cervical incompetence, unspecified trimester Ⓜ♀

O34.31 Maternal care for cervical incompetence, first trimester Ⓜ♀

O34.32 Maternal care for cervical incompetence, second trimester Ⓜ♀

O34.33 Maternal care for cervical incompetence, third trimester Ⓜ♀

✓5ᵗʰ **O34.4 Maternal care for other abnormalities of cervix**

O34.40 Maternal care for other abnormalities of cervix, unspecified trimester Ⓜ♀

O34.41 Maternal care for other abnormalities of cervix, first trimester Ⓜ♀

O34.42 Maternal care for other abnormalities of cervix, second trimester Ⓜ♀

O34.43 Maternal care for other abnormalities of cervix, third trimester Ⓜ♀

✓5ᵗʰ **O34.5 Maternal care for other abnormalities of gravid uterus**

✓6ᵗʰ **O34.51 Maternal care for incarceration of gravid uterus**

O34.511 Maternal care for incarceration of gravid uterus, first trimester Ⓜ♀

O34.512 Maternal care for incarceration of gravid uterus, second trimester Ⓜ♀

O34.513 Maternal care for incarceration of gravid uterus, third trimester Ⓜ♀

O34.519 Maternal care for incarceration of gravid uterus, unspecified trimester Ⓜ♀

✓6ᵗʰ **O34.52 Maternal care for prolapse of gravid uterus**

O34.521 Maternal care for prolapse of gravid uterus, first trimester Ⓜ♀

O34.522 Maternal care for prolapse of gravid uterus, second trimester Ⓜ♀

O34.523 Maternal care for prolapse of gravid uterus, third trimester Ⓜ♀

O34.529 Maternal care for prolapse of gravid uterus, unspecified trimester Ⓜ♀

✓6ᵗʰ **O34.53 Maternal care for retroversion of gravid uterus**

O34.531 Maternal care for retroversion of gravid uterus, first trimester Ⓜ♀

O34.532 Maternal care for retroversion of gravid uterus, second trimester Ⓜ♀

O34.533 Maternal care for retroversion of gravid uterus, third trimester Ⓜ♀

O34.539 Maternal care for retroversion of gravid uterus, unspecified trimester Ⓜ♀

✓6ᵗʰ **O34.59 Maternal care for other abnormalities of gravid uterus**

O34.591 Maternal care for other abnormalities of gravid uterus, first trimester Ⓜ♀

O34.592 Maternal care for other abnormalities of gravid uterus, second trimester Ⓜ♀

O34.593 Maternal care for other abnormalities of gravid uterus, third trimester Ⓜ♀

O34.599 Maternal care for other abnormalities of gravid uterus, unspecified trimester Ⓜ♀

✓5ᵗʰ **O34.6 Maternal care for abnormality of vagina**

EXCLUDES 2   maternal care for vaginal varices in pregnancy (O22.1-)

O34.60 Maternal care for abnormality of vagina, unspecified trimester Ⓜ♀

O34.61 Maternal care for abnormality of vagina, first trimester Ⓜ♀

O34.62 Maternal care for abnormality of vagina, second trimester Ⓜ♀

O34.63 Maternal care for abnormality of vagina, third trimester Ⓜ♀

✓5ᵗʰ **O34.7 Maternal care for abnormality of vulva and perineum**

EXCLUDES 2   maternal care for perineal and vulval varices in pregnancy (O22.1-)

O34.70 Maternal care for abnormality of vulva and perineum, unspecified trimester Ⓜ♀

O34.71 Maternal care for abnormality of vulva and perineum, first trimester Ⓜ♀

O34.72 Maternal care for abnormality of vulva and perineum, second trimester Ⓜ♀

O34.73 Maternal care for abnormality of vulva and perineum, third trimester Ⓜ♀

✓5ᵗʰ **O34.8 Maternal care for other abnormalities of pelvic organs**

O34.80 Maternal care for other abnormalities of pelvic organs, unspecified trimester Ⓜ♀

O34.81 Maternal care for other abnormalities of pelvic organs, first trimester Ⓜ♀

O34.82 Maternal care for other abnormalities of pelvic organs, second trimester Ⓜ♀

Ⓝ Newborn: 0   Ⓟ Pediatric: 0-17   Ⓜ Maternity: 12-55   Ⓐ Adult: 15-124   CH Comorbidity High   CL Comorbidity Low   NCDx Noncancer Dx   PDx Primary Dx

866   ICD-10-CM 2020

O34.83 Maternal care for other abnormalities of pelvic organs, third trimester ⓜ♀

✓5ᵗʰ **O34.9** Maternal care for abnormality of pelvic organ, unspecified

O34.90 Maternal care for abnormality of pelvic organ, unspecified, unspecified trimester ⓜ♀

O34.91 Maternal care for abnormality of pelvic organ, unspecified, first trimester ⓜ♀

O34.92 Maternal care for abnormality of pelvic organ, unspecified, second trimester ⓜ♀

O34.93 Maternal care for abnormality of pelvic organ, unspecified, third trimester ⓜ♀

✓4ᵗʰ **O35** Maternal care for known or suspected fetal abnormality and damage

INCLUDES   the listed conditions in the fetus as a reason for hospitalization or other obstetric care to the mother, or for termination of pregnancy

Code also any associated maternal condition

EXCLUDES 1   encounter for suspected maternal and fetal conditions ruled out (Z03.7-)

One of the following 7th characters is to be assigned to each code under category O35. 7th character 0 is for single gestations and multiple gestations where the fetus is unspecified. 7th characters 1 through 9 are for cases of multiple gestations to identify the fetus for which the code applies. The appropriate code from category O30, Multiple gestation, must also be assigned when assigning a code from category O35 that has a 7th character of 1 through 9.

   0   not applicable or unspecified
   1   fetus 1
   2   fetus 2
   3   fetus 3
   4   fetus 4
   5   fetus 5
   9   other fetus

✓x7ᵗʰ **O35.0** Maternal care for (suspected) central nervous system malformation in fetus ⓜ♀
     Maternal care for fetal anencephaly
     Maternal care for fetal hydrocephalus
     Maternal care for fetal spina bifida
     EXCLUDES 2   chromosomal abnormality in fetus (O35.1)

✓x7ᵗʰ **O35.1** Maternal care for (suspected) chromosomal abnormality in fetus ⓜ♀

✓x7ᵗʰ **O35.2** Maternal care for (suspected) hereditary disease in fetus ⓜ♀
     EXCLUDES 2   chromosomal abnormality in fetus (O35.1)

✓x7ᵗʰ **O35.3** Maternal care for (suspected) damage to fetus from viral disease in mother ⓜ♀
     Maternal care for damage to fetus from maternal cytomegalovirus infection
     Maternal care for damage to fetus from maternal rubella

✓x7ᵗʰ **O35.4** Maternal care for (suspected) damage to fetus from alcohol ⓜ♀

✓x7ᵗʰ **O35.5** Maternal care for (suspected) damage to fetus by drugs ⓜ♀
     Maternal care for damage to fetus from drug addiction

✓x7ᵗʰ **O35.6** Maternal care for (suspected) damage to fetus by radiation ⓜ♀

✓x7ᵗʰ **O35.7** Maternal care for (suspected) damage to fetus by other medical procedures ⓜ♀
     Maternal care for damage to fetus by amniocentesis
     Maternal care for damage to fetus by biopsy procedures
     Maternal care for damage to fetus by hematological investigation
     Maternal care for damage to fetus by intrauterine contraceptive device
     Maternal care for damage to fetus by intrauterine surgery

✓x7ᵗʰ **O35.8** Maternal care for other (suspected) fetal abnormality and damage ⓜ♀
     Maternal care for damage to fetus from maternal listeriosis
     Maternal care for damage to fetus from maternal toxoplasmosis

✓x7ᵗʰ **O35.9** Maternal care for (suspected) fetal abnormality and damage, unspecified ⓜ♀

✓4ᵗʰ **O36** Maternal care for other fetal problems

INCLUDES   the listed conditions in the fetus as a reason for hospitalization or other obstetric care of the mother, or for termination of pregnancy

EXCLUDES 1   encounter for suspected maternal and fetal conditions ruled out (Z03.7-)
     placental transfusion syndromes (O43.0-)

EXCLUDES 2   labor and delivery complicated by fetal stress (O77.-)

AHA: 2015,3Q,40

One of the following 7th characters is to be assigned to each code under category O36. 7th character 0 is for single gestations and multiple gestations where the fetus is unspecified. 7th characters 1 through 9 are for cases of multiple gestations to identify the fetus for which the code applies. The appropriate code from category O30, Multiple gestation, must also be assigned when assigning a code from category O36 that has a 7th character of 1 through 9.

   0   not applicable or unspecified
   1   fetus 1
   2   fetus 2
   3   fetus 3
   4   fetus 4
   5   fetus 5
   9   other fetus

✓5ᵗʰ **O36.0** Maternal care for rhesus isoimmunization
     Maternal care for Rh incompatibility (with hydrops fetalis)

✓6ᵗʰ **O36.01** Maternal care for anti-D [Rh] antibodies
     AHA: 2014,4Q,17

✓7ᵗʰ **O36.011** Maternal care for anti-D [Rh] antibodies, first trimester ⓜ♀

✓7ᵗʰ **O36.012** Maternal care for anti-D [Rh] antibodies, second trimester ⓜ♀

✓7ᵗʰ **O36.013** Maternal care for anti-D [Rh] antibodies, third trimester ⓜ♀

✓7ᵗʰ **O36.019** Maternal care for anti-D [Rh] antibodies, unspecified trimester ⓜ♀

✓6ᵗʰ **O36.09** Maternal care for other rhesus isoimmunization

✓7ᵗʰ **O36.091** Maternal care for other rhesus isoimmunization, first trimester ⓜ♀

✓7ᵗʰ **O36.092** Maternal care for other rhesus isoimmunization, second trimester ⓜ♀

✓7ᵗʰ **O36.093** Maternal care for other rhesus isoimmunization, third trimester ⓜ♀

✓7ᵗʰ **O36.099** Maternal care for other rhesus isoimmunization, unspecified trimester ⓜ♀

✓5ᵗʰ **O36.1** Maternal care for other isoimmunization
     Maternal care for ABO isoimmunization

✓6ᵗʰ **O36.11** Maternal care for Anti-A sensitization
     Maternal care for isoimmunization NOS (with hydrops fetalis)

✓7ᵗʰ **O36.111** Maternal care for Anti-A sensitization, first trimester ⓜ♀

✓7ᵗʰ **O36.112** Maternal care for Anti-A sensitization, second trimester ⓜ♀

✓7ᵗʰ **O36.113** Maternal care for Anti-A sensitization, third trimester ⓜ♀

✓7ᵗʰ **O36.119** Maternal care for Anti-A sensitization, unspecified trimester ⓜ♀

✓6ᵗʰ **O36.19** Maternal care for other isoimmunization
     Maternal care for Anti-B sensitization

✓7ᵗʰ **O36.191** Maternal care for other isoimmunization, first trimester ⓜ♀

✓7ᵗʰ **O36.192** Maternal care for other isoimmunization, second trimester ⓜ♀

✓7ᵗʰ **O36.193** Maternal care for other isoimmunization, third trimester ⓜ♀

✓7ᵗʰ **O36.199** Maternal care for other isoimmunization, unspecified trimester ⓜ♀

✅ Additional Character Required   ✓x7ᵗʰ Placeholder Alert   Manifestation   Unspecified Dx   ►◄ Revised Text   ● New Code   ▲ Revised Title

ICD-10-CM 2020   867

√5ᵗʰ **O36.2　Maternal care for hydrops fetalis**

Maternal care for hydrops fetalis NOS

Maternal care for hydrops fetalis not associated with isoimmunization

EXCLUDES 1　hydrops fetalis associated with ABO isoimmunization (O36.1-)

hydrops fetalis associated with rhesus isoimmunization (O36.0-)

DEF: Hydrops fetalis: Abnormal fluid buildup in at least two of the following fetal organ spaces: the skin (edema), abdomen (ascites), around the heart (pericardia effusion), and around the lung (pleural effusion). Fluid accumulation may also occur in the mother as polyhydramnios and edema of the placenta.

√x7ᵗʰ **O36.20　Maternal care for hydrops fetalis, unspecified trimester**　Ⓜ♀

√x7ᵗʰ **O36.21　Maternal care for hydrops fetalis, first trimester**　Ⓜ♀

√x7ᵗʰ **O36.22　Maternal care for hydrops fetalis, second trimester**　Ⓜ♀

√x7ᵗʰ **O36.23　Maternal care for hydrops fetalis, third trimester**　Ⓜ♀

√x7ᵗʰ **O36.4　Maternal care for intrauterine death**　Ⓜ♀

Maternal care for intrauterine fetal death NOS

Maternal care for intrauterine fetal death after completion of 20 weeks of gestation

Maternal care for late fetal death

Maternal care for missed delivery

EXCLUDES 1　missed abortion (O02.1)

stillbirth (P95)

√5ᵗʰ **O36.5　Maternal care for known or suspected poor fetal growth**

√6ᵗʰ **O36.51　Maternal care for known or suspected placental insufficiency**

√7ᵗʰ **O36.511　Maternal care for known or suspected placental insufficiency, first trimester**　Ⓜ♀

√7ᵗʰ **O36.512　Maternal care for known or suspected placental insufficiency, second trimester**　Ⓜ♀

√7ᵗʰ **O36.513　Maternal care for known or suspected placental insufficiency, third trimester**　Ⓜ♀

√7ᵗʰ **O36.519　Maternal care for known or suspected placental insufficiency, unspecified trimester**　Ⓜ♀

√6ᵗʰ **O36.59　Maternal care for other known or suspected poor fetal growth**

Maternal care for known or suspected light-for-dates NOS

Maternal care for known or suspected small-for-dates NOS

√7ᵗʰ **O36.591　Maternal care for other known or suspected poor fetal growth, first trimester**　Ⓜ♀

√7ᵗʰ **O36.592　Maternal care for other known or suspected poor fetal growth, second trimester**　Ⓜ♀

√7ᵗʰ **O36.593　Maternal care for other known or suspected poor fetal growth, third trimester**　Ⓜ♀

√7ᵗʰ **O36.599　Maternal care for other known or suspected poor fetal growth, unspecified trimester**　Ⓜ♀

√5ᵗʰ **O36.6　Maternal care for excessive fetal growth**

Maternal care for known or suspected large-for-dates

√x7ᵗʰ **O36.60　Maternal care for excessive fetal growth, unspecified trimester**　Ⓜ♀

√x7ᵗʰ **O36.61　Maternal care for excessive fetal growth, first trimester**　Ⓜ♀

√x7ᵗʰ **O36.62　Maternal care for excessive fetal growth, second trimester**　Ⓜ♀

√x7ᵗʰ **O36.63　Maternal care for excessive fetal growth, third trimester**　Ⓜ♀

√5ᵗʰ **O36.7　Maternal care for viable fetus in abdominal pregnancy**

√x7ᵗʰ **O36.70　Maternal care for viable fetus in abdominal pregnancy, unspecified trimester**　Ⓜ♀

√x7ᵗʰ **O36.71　Maternal care for viable fetus in abdominal pregnancy, first trimester**　Ⓜ♀

√x7ᵗʰ **O36.72　Maternal care for viable fetus in abdominal pregnancy, second trimester**　Ⓜ♀

√x7ᵗʰ **O36.73　Maternal care for viable fetus in abdominal pregnancy, third trimester**　Ⓜ♀

√5ᵗʰ **O36.8　Maternal care for other specified fetal problems**

√x7ᵗʰ **O36.80　Pregnancy with inconclusive fetal viability**　Ⓜ♀

Encounter to determine fetal viability of pregnancy

AHA: 2019,2Q,29

√6ᵗʰ **O36.81　Decreased fetal movements**

√7ᵗʰ **O36.812　Decreased fetal movements, second trimester**　Ⓜ♀

√7ᵗʰ **O36.813　Decreased fetal movements, third trimester**　Ⓜ♀

√7ᵗʰ **O36.819　Decreased fetal movements, unspecified trimester**　Ⓜ♀

√6ᵗʰ **O36.82　Fetal anemia and thrombocytopenia**

√7ᵗʰ **O36.821　Fetal anemia and thrombocytopenia, first trimester**　Ⓜ♀

√7ᵗʰ **O36.822　Fetal anemia and thrombocytopenia, second trimester**　Ⓜ♀

√7ᵗʰ **O36.823　Fetal anemia and thrombocytopenia, third trimester**　Ⓜ♀

√7ᵗʰ **O36.829　Fetal anemia and thrombocytopenia, unspecified trimester**　Ⓜ♀

√6ᵗʰ **O36.83　Maternal care for abnormalities of the fetal heart rate or rhythm**

▶Maternal care for depressed fetal heart rate tones◀

▶Maternal care for fetal bradycardia◀

▶Maternal care for fetal heart rate abnormal variability◀

▶Maternal care for fetal heart rate decelerations◀

▶Maternal care for fetal heart rate irregularity◀

▶Maternal care for fetal tachycardia◀

▶Maternal care for non-reassuring fetal heart rate or rhythm◀

AHA: 2017,4Q,20

√7ᵗʰ **O36.831　Maternal care for abnormalities of the fetal heart rate or rhythm, first trimester**　Ⓜ♀

√7ᵗʰ **O36.832　Maternal care for abnormalities of the fetal heart rate or rhythm, second trimester**　Ⓜ♀

√7ᵗʰ **O36.833　Maternal care for abnormalities of the fetal heart rate or rhythm, third trimester**　Ⓜ♀

√7ᵗʰ **O36.839　Maternal care for abnormalities of the fetal heart rate or rhythm, unspecified trimester**　Ⓜ♀

√6ᵗʰ **O36.89　Maternal care for other specified fetal problems**

√7ᵗʰ **O36.891　Maternal care for other specified fetal problems, first trimester**　Ⓜ♀

√7ᵗʰ **O36.892　Maternal care for other specified fetal problems, second trimester**　Ⓜ♀

√7ᵗʰ **O36.893　Maternal care for other specified fetal problems, third trimester**　Ⓜ♀

√7ᵗʰ **O36.899　Maternal care for other specified fetal problems, unspecified trimester**　Ⓜ♀

√5ᵗʰ **O36.9　Maternal care for fetal problem, unspecified**

√x7ᵗʰ **O36.90　Maternal care for fetal problem, unspecified, unspecified trimester**　Ⓜ♀

√x7ᵗʰ **O36.91　Maternal care for fetal problem, unspecified, first trimester**　Ⓜ♀

√x7ᵗʰ **O36.92　Maternal care for fetal problem, unspecified, second trimester**　Ⓜ♀

√x7ᵗʰ **O36.93　Maternal care for fetal problem, unspecified, third trimester**　Ⓜ♀

Ⓝ Newborn: 0　Ⓟ Pediatric: 0-17　Ⓜ Maternity: 12-55　Ⓐ Adult: 15-124　CH Comorbidity High　CL Comorbidity Low　NCDx Noncancer Dx　PDx Primary Dx

868　　ICD-10-CM 2020

☑4ᵗʰ **O40 Polyhydramnios**

INCLUDES   hydramnios

EXCLUDES 1   encounter for suspected maternal and fetal conditions ruled out (Z03.7-)

AHA: 2016,1Q,4

DEF: Excess amniotic fluid surrounding the fetus, typically defined as a total fluid volume of greater than 24.0 cc.

> One of the following 7th characters is to be assigned to each code under category O40. 7th character 0 is for single gestations and multiple gestations where the fetus is unspecified. 7th characters 1 through 9 are for cases of multiple gestations to identify the fetus for which the code applies. The appropriate code from category O30, Multiple gestation, must also be assigned when assigning a code from category O40 that has a 7th character of 1 through 9.
> 0   not applicable or unspecified
> 1   fetus 1
> 2   fetus 2
> 3   fetus 3
> 4   fetus 4
> 5   fetus 5
> 9   other fetus

☑x7ᵗʰ **O40.1 Polyhydramnios,** first trimester   Ⓜ ♀

☑x7ᵗʰ **O40.2 Polyhydramnios,** second trimester   Ⓜ ♀

☑x7ᵗʰ **O40.3 Polyhydramnios,** third trimester   Ⓜ ♀

☑x7ᵗʰ **O40.9 Polyhydramnios,** unspecified trimester   Ⓜ ♀

☑4ᵗʰ **O41 Other disorders of amniotic fluid and membranes**

EXCLUDES 1   encounter for suspected maternal and fetal conditions ruled out (Z03.7-)

> One of the following 7th characters is to be assigned to each code under category O41. 7th character 0 is for single gestations and multiple gestations where the fetus is unspecified. 7th characters 1 through 9 are for cases of multiple gestations to identify the fetus for which the code applies. The appropriate code from category O30, Multiple gestation, must also be assigned when assigning a code from category O41 that has a 7th character of 1 through 9.
> 0   not applicable or unspecified
> 1   fetus 1
> 2   fetus 2
> 3   fetus 3
> 4   fetus 4
> 5   fetus 5
> 9   other fetus

☑5ᵗʰ **O41.0 Oligohydramnios**

Oligohydramnios without rupture of membranes

DEF: Low amniotic fluid, occurring most frequently in the last trimester.

☑x7ᵗʰ **O41.00 Oligohydramnios,** unspecified trimester   Ⓜ ♀

☑x7ᵗʰ **O41.01 Oligohydramnios,** first trimester   Ⓜ ♀

☑x7ᵗʰ **O41.02 Oligohydramnios,** second trimester   Ⓜ ♀

☑x7ᵗʰ **O41.03 Oligohydramnios,** third trimester   Ⓜ ♀

☑5ᵗʰ **O41.1 Infection of amniotic sac and membranes**

☑6ᵗʰ **O41.10 Infection of amniotic sac and membranes, unspecified**

☑7ᵗʰ **O41.101 Infection of amniotic sac and membranes, unspecified,** first trimester   Ⓜ ♀

☑7ᵗʰ **O41.102 Infection of amniotic sac and membranes, unspecified,** second trimester   Ⓜ ♀

☑7ᵗʰ **O41.103 Infection of amniotic sac and membranes, unspecified,** third trimester   Ⓜ ♀

☑7ᵗʰ **O41.109 Infection of amniotic sac and membranes, unspecified,** unspecified trimester   Ⓜ ♀

☑6ᵗʰ **O41.12 Chorioamnionitis**

AHA: 2019,2Q,34

☑7ᵗʰ **O41.121 Chorioamnionitis,** first trimester   Ⓜ ♀

☑7ᵗʰ **O41.122 Chorioamnionitis,** second trimester   Ⓜ ♀

☑7ᵗʰ **O41.123 Chorioamnionitis,** third trimester   Ⓜ ♀

☑7ᵗʰ **O41.129 Chorioamnionitis,** unspecified trimester   Ⓜ ♀

☑6ᵗʰ **O41.14 Placentitis**

☑7ᵗʰ **O41.141 Placentitis,** first trimester   Ⓜ ♀

☑7ᵗʰ **O41.142 Placentitis,** second trimester   Ⓜ ♀

☑7ᵗʰ **O41.143 Placentitis,** third trimester   Ⓜ ♀

☑7ᵗʰ **O41.149 Placentitis,** unspecified trimester   Ⓜ ♀

☑5ᵗʰ **O41.8 Other specified disorders of amniotic fluid and membranes**

☑6ᵗʰ **O41.8X Other specified disorders of amniotic fluid and membranes**

☑7ᵗʰ **O41.8X1 Other specified disorders of amniotic fluid and membranes,** first trimester   Ⓜ ♀

☑7ᵗʰ **O41.8X2 Other specified disorders of amniotic fluid and membranes,** second trimester   Ⓜ ♀

☑7ᵗʰ **O41.8X3 Other specified disorders of amniotic fluid and membranes,** third trimester   Ⓜ ♀

☑7ᵗʰ **O41.8X9 Other specified disorders of amniotic fluid and membranes,** unspecified trimester   Ⓜ ♀

☑5ᵗʰ **O41.9 Disorder of amniotic fluid and membranes, unspecified**

☑x7ᵗʰ **O41.90 Disorder of amniotic fluid and membranes, unspecified, unspecified trimester**   Ⓜ ♀

☑x7ᵗʰ **O41.91 Disorder of amniotic fluid and membranes, unspecified,** first trimester   Ⓜ ♀

☑x7ᵗʰ **O41.92 Disorder of amniotic fluid and membranes, unspecified,** second trimester   Ⓜ ♀

☑x7ᵗʰ **O41.93 Disorder of amniotic fluid and membranes, unspecified,** third trimester   Ⓜ ♀

☑4ᵗʰ **O42 Premature rupture of membranes**

AHA: 2016,1Q,3

☑5ᵗʰ **O42.0 Premature rupture of membranes,** onset of labor within 24 hours of rupture

O42.00 Premature rupture of membranes, onset of labor within 24 hours of rupture, unspecified weeks of gestation   Ⓜ ♀

☑6ᵗʰ **O42.01 Preterm premature rupture of membranes, onset of labor within 24 hours of rupture**

Premature rupture of membranes before 37 completed weeks of gestation

O42.011 Preterm premature rupture of membranes, onset of labor within 24 hours of rupture, first trimester   Ⓜ ♀

O42.012 Preterm premature rupture of membranes, onset of labor within 24 hours of rupture, second trimester   Ⓜ ♀

O42.013 Preterm premature rupture of membranes, onset of labor within 24 hours of rupture, third trimester   Ⓜ ♀

O42.019 Preterm premature rupture of membranes, onset of labor within 24 hours of rupture, unspecified trimester   Ⓜ ♀

O42.02 Full-term premature rupture of membranes, onset of labor within 24 hours of rupture   Ⓜ ♀

Premature rupture of membranes at or after 37 completed weeks of gestation, onset of labor within 24 hours of rupture

☑5ᵗʰ **O42.1 Premature rupture of membranes,** onset of labor more than 24 hours following rupture

AHA: 2016,1Q,5

O42.10 Premature rupture of membranes, onset of labor more than 24 hours following rupture, unspecified weeks of gestation   Ⓜ ♀

☑6ᵗʰ **O42.11 Preterm premature rupture of membranes, onset of labor more than 24 hours following rupture**

Premature rupture of membranes before 37 completed weeks of gestation

O42.111 Preterm premature rupture of membranes, onset of labor more than 24 hours following rupture, first trimester   Ⓜ ♀

☑ Additional Character Required   ☑x7ᵗʰ Placeholder Alert   Manifestation   Unspecified Dx   ►◄ Revised Text   ● New Code   ▲ Revised Title

ICD-10-CM 2020   869

O42.112 **Preterm premature rupture of membranes, onset of labor more than 24 hours following rupture,** second trimester Ⓜ♀

O42.113 **Preterm premature rupture of membranes, onset of labor more than 24 hours following rupture,** third trimester Ⓜ♀

O42.119 **Preterm premature rupture of membranes, onset of labor more than 24 hours following rupture, unspecified trimester** Ⓜ♀

O42.12 **Full-term premature rupture of membranes, onset of labor more than 24 hours following rupture** Ⓜ♀
  Premature rupture of membranes at or after 37 completed weeks of gestation, onset of labor more than 24 hours following rupture

O42.9 **Premature rupture of membranes,** unspecified as to length of time between rupture and onset of labor

  O42.90 **Premature rupture of membranes, unspecified as to length of time between rupture and onset of labor, unspecified weeks of gestation** Ⓜ♀

  O42.91 **Preterm premature rupture of membranes, unspecified as to length of time between rupture and onset of labor**
    Premature rupture of membranes before 37 completed weeks of gestation

    O42.911 **Preterm premature rupture of membranes, unspecified as to length of time between rupture and onset of labor,** first trimester Ⓜ♀

    O42.912 **Preterm premature rupture of membranes, unspecified as to length of time between rupture and onset of labor,** second trimester Ⓜ♀

    O42.913 **Preterm premature rupture of membranes, unspecified as to length of time between rupture and onset of labor,** third trimester Ⓜ♀

    O42.919 **Preterm premature rupture of membranes, unspecified as to length of time between rupture and onset of labor, unspecified trimester** Ⓜ♀

  O42.92 **Full-term premature rupture of membranes, unspecified as to length of time between rupture and onset of labor** Ⓜ♀
    Premature rupture of membranes at or after 37 completed weeks of gestation, unspecified as to length of time between rupture and onset of labor

O43 **Placental disorders**
  EXCLUDES 2: maternal care for poor fetal growth due to placental insufficiency (O36.5-)
  placenta previa (O44.-)
  placental polyp (O90.89)
  placentitis (O41.14-)
  premature separation of placenta [abruptio placentae] (O45.-)

  O43.0 **Placental transfusion syndromes**

    O43.01 **Fetomaternal placental transfusion syndrome**
      Maternofetal placental transfusion syndrome

      O43.011 **Fetomaternal placental transfusion syndrome,** first trimester Ⓜ♀

      O43.012 **Fetomaternal placental transfusion syndrome,** second trimester Ⓜ♀

      O43.013 **Fetomaternal placental transfusion syndrome,** third trimester Ⓜ♀

      O43.019 **Fetomaternal placental transfusion syndrome, unspecified trimester** Ⓜ♀

    O43.02 **Fetus-to-fetus placental transfusion syndrome**
      DEF: Condition in which an imbalance in amniotic fluid occurs due to uneven blood flow between twins sharing a placenta.

Twin to Twin Transfusion Syndrome (TTTS)

Healthy twins   Twins with TTTS

      O43.021 **Fetus-to-fetus placental transfusion syndrome,** first trimester Ⓜ♀

      O43.022 **Fetus-to-fetus placental transfusion syndrome,** second trimester Ⓜ♀

      O43.023 **Fetus-to-fetus placental transfusion syndrome,** third trimester Ⓜ♀

      O43.029 **Fetus-to-fetus placental transfusion syndrome, unspecified trimester** Ⓜ♀

  O43.1 **Malformation of placenta**

    O43.10 **Malformation of placenta, unspecified**
      Abnormal placenta NOS

      O43.101 **Malformation of placenta, unspecified,** first trimester Ⓜ♀

      O43.102 **Malformation of placenta, unspecified,** second trimester Ⓜ♀

      O43.103 **Malformation of placenta, unspecified,** third trimester Ⓜ♀

      O43.109 **Malformation of placenta, unspecified, unspecified trimester** Ⓜ♀

    O43.11 **Circumvallate placenta**

      O43.111 **Circumvallate placenta,** first trimester Ⓜ♀

      O43.112 **Circumvallate placenta,** second trimester Ⓜ♀

      O43.113 **Circumvallate placenta,** third trimester Ⓜ♀

      O43.119 **Circumvallate placenta, unspecified trimester** Ⓜ♀

    O43.12 **Velamentous insertion of umbilical cord**

      O43.121 **Velamentous insertion of umbilical cord,** first trimester Ⓜ♀

      O43.122 **Velamentous insertion of umbilical cord,** second trimester Ⓜ♀

      O43.123 **Velamentous insertion of umbilical cord,** third trimester Ⓜ♀

      O43.129 **Velamentous insertion of umbilical cord, unspecified trimester** Ⓜ♀

    O43.19 **Other malformation of placenta**

      O43.191 **Other malformation of placenta,** first trimester Ⓜ♀

      O43.192 **Other malformation of placenta,** second trimester Ⓜ♀

      O43.193 **Other malformation of placenta,** third trimester Ⓜ♀

      O43.199 **Other malformation of placenta, unspecified trimester** Ⓜ♀

Chapter 15. Pregnancy, Childbirth and the Puerperium

✓5ᵗʰ **O43.2 Morbidly adherent placenta**

Code also associated third stage postpartum hemorrhage, if applicable (O72.0)

EXCLUDES 1   retained placenta (O73.-)

✓6ᵗʰ **O43.21 Placenta accreta**

DEF: Condition where the placenta adheres too deeply to the uterine wall; often associated with placenta previa.

O43.211 Placenta accreta, first trimester Ⓜ♀

O43.212 Placenta accreta, second trimester Ⓜ♀

O43.213 Placenta accreta, third trimester Ⓜ♀

O43.219 Placenta accreta, unspecified trimester Ⓜ♀

✓6ᵗʰ **O43.22 Placenta increta**

DEF: Condition where the placenta adheres too deeply to the uterine wall and penetrates the muscle; often associated with placenta previa.

O43.221 Placenta increta, first trimester Ⓜ♀

O43.222 Placenta increta, second trimester Ⓜ♀

O43.223 Placenta increta, third trimester Ⓜ♀

O43.229 Placenta increta, unspecified trimester Ⓜ♀

✓6ᵗʰ **O43.23 Placenta percreta**

DEF: Condition where the placenta attaches through the uterine muscle and may invade other organs, resulting in antenatal complications, premature delivery, retention of all or a portion of the placenta, or postpartum bleeding.

O43.231 Placenta percreta, first trimester Ⓜ♀

O43.232 Placenta percreta, second trimester Ⓜ♀

O43.233 Placenta percreta, third trimester Ⓜ♀

O43.239 Placenta percreta, unspecified trimester Ⓜ♀

✓5ᵗʰ **O43.8 Other placental disorders**

✓6ᵗʰ **O43.81 Placental infarction**

O43.811 Placental infarction, first trimester Ⓜ♀

O43.812 Placental infarction, second trimester Ⓜ♀

O43.813 Placental infarction, third trimester Ⓜ♀

O43.819 Placental infarction, unspecified trimester Ⓜ♀

✓6ᵗʰ **O43.89 Other placental disorders**

Placental dysfunction

O43.891 Other placental disorders, first trimester Ⓜ♀

O43.892 Other placental disorders, second trimester Ⓜ♀

O43.893 Other placental disorders, third trimester Ⓜ♀

O43.899 Other placental disorders, unspecified trimester Ⓜ♀

✓5ᵗʰ **O43.9 Unspecified placental disorder**

O43.90 Unspecified placental disorder, unspecified trimester Ⓜ♀

O43.91 Unspecified placental disorder, first trimester Ⓜ♀

O43.92 Unspecified placental disorder, second trimester Ⓜ♀

O43.93 Unspecified placental disorder, third trimester Ⓜ♀

✓4ᵗʰ **O44 Placenta previa**

AHA: 2016,4Q,52-53

DEF: Placenta implanted in the lower segment of the uterus, which commonly causes hemorrhage in the last trimester of pregnancy.

✓5ᵗʰ **O44.0 Complete placenta previa NOS or without hemorrhage**

Placenta previa NOS

O44.00 Complete placenta previa NOS or without hemorrhage, unspecified trimester Ⓜ♀

O44.01 Complete placenta previa NOS or without hemorrhage, first trimester Ⓜ♀

O44.02 Complete placenta previa NOS or without hemorrhage, second trimester Ⓜ♀

O44.03 Complete placenta previa NOS or without hemorrhage, third trimester Ⓜ♀

✓5ᵗʰ **O44.1 Complete placenta previa with hemorrhage**

EXCLUDES 1   labor and delivery complicated by hemorrhage from vasa previa (O69.4)

O44.10 Complete placenta previa with hemorrhage, unspecified trimester Ⓜ♀

O44.11 Complete placenta previa with hemorrhage, first trimester Ⓜ♀

O44.12 Complete placenta previa with hemorrhage, second trimester Ⓜ♀

O44.13 Complete placenta previa with hemorrhage, third trimester Ⓜ♀

✓5ᵗʰ **O44.2 Partial placenta previa without hemorrhage**

Marginal placenta previa, NOS or without hemorrhage

O44.20 Partial placenta previa NOS or without hemorrhage, unspecified trimester Ⓜ♀

O44.21 Partial placenta previa NOS or without hemorrhage, first trimester Ⓜ♀

O44.22 Partial placenta previa NOS or without hemorrhage, second trimester Ⓜ♀

O44.23 Partial placenta previa NOS or without hemorrhage, third trimester Ⓜ♀

✓5ᵗʰ **O44.3 Partial placenta previa with hemorrhage**

Marginal placenta previa with hemorrhage

O44.30 Partial placenta previa with hemorrhage, unspecified trimester Ⓜ♀

O44.31 Partial placenta previa with hemorrhage, first trimester Ⓜ♀

O44.32 Partial placenta previa with hemorrhage, second trimester Ⓜ♀

O44.33 Partial placenta previa with hemorrhage, third trimester Ⓜ♀

✓5ᵗʰ **O44.4 Low lying placenta NOS or without hemorrhage**

Low implantation of placenta NOS or without hemorrhage

O44.40 Low lying placenta NOS or without hemorrhage, unspecified trimester Ⓜ♀

O44.41 Low lying placenta NOS or without hemorrhage, first trimester Ⓜ♀

O44.42 Low lying placenta NOS or without hemorrhage, second trimester Ⓜ♀

O44.43 Low lying placenta NOS or without hemorrhage, third trimester Ⓜ♀

✓5ᵗʰ **O44.5 Low lying placenta with hemorrhage**

Low implantation of placenta with hemorrhage

O44.50 Low lying placenta with hemorrhage, unspecified trimester Ⓜ♀

O44.51 Low lying placenta with hemorrhage, first trimester Ⓜ♀

O44.52 Low lying placenta with hemorrhage, second trimester Ⓜ♀

O44.53 Low lying placenta with hemorrhage, third trimester Ⓜ♀

✓4ᵗʰ **O45 Premature separation of placenta [abruptio placentae]**

✓5ᵗʰ **O45.0 Premature separation of placenta with coagulation defect**

✓6ᵗʰ **O45.00 Premature separation of placenta with coagulation defect, unspecified**

O45.001 Premature separation of placenta with coagulation defect, unspecified, first trimester Ⓜ♀

O45.002 Premature separation of placenta with coagulation defect, unspecified, second trimester Ⓜ♀

O45.003 Premature separation of placenta with coagulation defect, unspecified, third trimester Ⓜ♀

O45.009 Premature separation of placenta with coagulation defect, unspecified, unspecified trimester Ⓜ♀

☑ Additional Character Required   ✓x7ᵗʰ Placeholder Alert   Manifestation   Unspecified Dx   ▶◀ Revised Text   ● New Code   ▲ Revised Title

ICD-10-CM 2020   871

Chapter 15. Pregnancy, Childbirth and the Puerperium

√6ᵗʰ **O45.01** **Premature separation of placenta with afibrinogenemia**
Premature separation of placenta with hypofibrinogenemia

O45.011 Premature separation of placenta with afibrinogenemia, first trimester   M ♀

O45.012 Premature separation of placenta with afibrinogenemia, second trimester   M ♀

O45.013 Premature separation of placenta with afibrinogenemia, third trimester   M ♀

O45.019 Premature separation of placenta with afibrinogenemia, unspecified trimester   M ♀

√6ᵗʰ **O45.02** **Premature separation of placenta with disseminated intravascular coagulation**

O45.021 Premature separation of placenta with disseminated intravascular coagulation, first trimester   M ♀

O45.022 Premature separation of placenta with disseminated intravascular coagulation, second trimester   M ♀

O45.023 Premature separation of placenta with disseminated intravascular coagulation, third trimester   M ♀

O45.029 Premature separation of placenta with disseminated intravascular coagulation, unspecified trimester   M ♀

√6ᵗʰ **O45.09** **Premature separation of placenta with other coagulation defect**

O45.091 Premature separation of placenta with other coagulation defect, first trimester   M ♀

O45.092 Premature separation of placenta with other coagulation defect, second trimester   M ♀

O45.093 Premature separation of placenta with other coagulation defect, third trimester   M ♀

O45.099 Premature separation of placenta with other coagulation defect, unspecified trimester   M ♀

√5ᵗʰ **O45.8** **Other premature separation of placenta**

√6ᵗʰ **O45.8X** **Other premature separation of placenta**

O45.8X1 Other premature separation of placenta, first trimester   M ♀

O45.8X2 Other premature separation of placenta, second trimester   M ♀

O45.8X3 Other premature separation of placenta, third trimester   M ♀

O45.8X9 Other premature separation of placenta, unspecified trimester   M ♀

√5ᵗʰ **O45.9** **Premature separation of placenta, unspecified**
Abruptio placentae NOS

O45.90 Premature separation of placenta, unspecified, unspecified trimester   M ♀

O45.91 Premature separation of placenta, unspecified, first trimester   M ♀

O45.92 Premature separation of placenta, unspecified, second trimester   M ♀

O45.93 Premature separation of placenta, unspecified, third trimester   M ♀

√4ᵗʰ **O46** **Antepartum hemorrhage, not elsewhere classified**

EXCLUDES 1   hemorrhage in early pregnancy (O20.-)
intrapartum hemorrhage NEC (O67.-)
placenta previa (O44.-)
premature separation of placenta [abruptio placentae] (O45.-)

DEF: Uterine hemorrhage prior to delivery that is not related to placenta previa or abruptio placentae.

√5ᵗʰ **O46.0** **Antepartum hemorrhage with coagulation defect**

√6ᵗʰ **O46.00** **Antepartum hemorrhage with coagulation defect, unspecified**

O46.001 Antepartum hemorrhage with coagulation defect, unspecified, first trimester   M ♀

O46.002 Antepartum hemorrhage with coagulation defect, unspecified, second trimester   M ♀

O46.003 Antepartum hemorrhage with coagulation defect, unspecified, third trimester   M ♀

O46.009 Antepartum hemorrhage with coagulation defect, unspecified, unspecified trimester   M ♀

√6ᵗʰ **O46.01** **Antepartum hemorrhage with afibrinogenemia**
Antepartum hemorrhage with hypofibrinogenemia

O46.011 Antepartum hemorrhage with afibrinogenemia, first trimester   M ♀

O46.012 Antepartum hemorrhage with afibrinogenemia, second trimester   M ♀

O46.013 Antepartum hemorrhage with afibrinogenemia, third trimester   M ♀

O46.019 Antepartum hemorrhage with afibrinogenemia, unspecified trimester   M ♀

√6ᵗʰ **O46.02** **Antepartum hemorrhage with disseminated intravascular coagulation**

O46.021 Antepartum hemorrhage with disseminated intravascular coagulation, first trimester   M ♀

O46.022 Antepartum hemorrhage with disseminated intravascular coagulation, second trimester   M ♀

O46.023 Antepartum hemorrhage with disseminated intravascular coagulation, third trimester   M ♀

O46.029 Antepartum hemorrhage with disseminated intravascular coagulation, unspecified trimester   M ♀

√6ᵗʰ **O46.09** **Antepartum hemorrhage with other coagulation defect**

O46.091 Antepartum hemorrhage with other coagulation defect, first trimester   M ♀

O46.092 Antepartum hemorrhage with other coagulation defect, second trimester   M ♀

O46.093 Antepartum hemorrhage with other coagulation defect, third trimester   M ♀

O46.099 Antepartum hemorrhage with other coagulation defect, unspecified trimester   M ♀

√5ᵗʰ **O46.8** **Other antepartum hemorrhage**

√6ᵗʰ **O46.8X** **Other antepartum hemorrhage**

O46.8X1 Other antepartum hemorrhage, first trimester   M ♀

O46.8X2 Other antepartum hemorrhage, second trimester   M ♀

O46.8X3 Other antepartum hemorrhage, third trimester   M ♀

O46.8X9 Other antepartum hemorrhage, unspecified trimester   M ♀

√5ᵗʰ **O46.9** **Antepartum hemorrhage, unspecified**

O46.90 Antepartum hemorrhage, unspecified, unspecified trimester   M ♀

O46.91 Antepartum hemorrhage, unspecified, first trimester   M ♀

N Newborn: 0   P Pediatric: 0-17   M Maternity: 12-55   A Adult: 15-124   CH Comorbidity High   CL Comorbidity Low   NCDx Noncancer Dx   PDx Primary Dx

872   ICD-10-CM 2020

O46.92 **Antepartum hemorrhage, unspecified, second trimester** Ⓜ ♀

O46.93 **Antepartum hemorrhage, unspecified, third trimester** Ⓜ ♀

✓4ᵗʰ **O47** **False labor**

　INCLUDES　Braxton Hicks contractions
　　　　　threatened labor
　EXCLUDES 1　preterm labor (O60.-)

✓5ᵗʰ **O47.0** **False labor** before 37 completed weeks of gestation

O47.00 **False labor before 37 completed weeks of gestation, unspecified trimester** Ⓜ ♀

O47.02 **False labor before 37 completed weeks of gestation, second trimester** Ⓜ ♀

O47.03 **False labor before 37 completed weeks of gestation, third trimester** Ⓜ ♀

O47.1 **False labor** at or after 37 completed weeks of gestation Ⓜ ♀

O47.9 **False labor, unspecified** Ⓜ ♀

✓4ᵗʰ **O48** **Late pregnancy**

O48.0 **Post-term pregnancy** Ⓜ ♀
Pregnancy over 40 completed weeks to 42 completed weeks gestation

O48.1 **Prolonged pregnancy** Ⓜ ♀
Pregnancy which has advanced beyond 42 completed weeks gestation
AHA: 2016,1Q,5

Complications of labor and delivery (O60-O77)

✓4ᵗʰ **O60** **Preterm labor**

　INCLUDES　onset (spontaneous) of labor before 37 completed weeks of gestation
　EXCLUDES 1　false labor (O47.0-)
　　　　　threatened labor NOS (O47.0-)

✓5ᵗʰ **O60.0** **Preterm labor** without delivery

O60.00 **Preterm labor without delivery, unspecified trimester** Ⓜ ♀

O60.02 **Preterm labor without delivery,** second trimester Ⓜ ♀

O60.03 **Preterm labor without delivery,** third trimester Ⓜ ♀

✓5ᵗʰ **O60.1** **Preterm labor** with preterm delivery
AHA: 2016,2Q,10

One of the following 7th characters is to be assigned to each code under subcategory O60.1. 7th character Ø is for single gestations and multiple gestations where the fetus is unspecified. 7th characters 1 through 9 are for cases of multiple gestations to identify the fetus for which the code applies. The appropriate code from category O30, Multiple gestation, must also be assigned when assigning a code from subcategory O60.1 that has a 7th character of 1 through 9.
Ø　not applicable or unspecified
1　fetus 1
2　fetus 2
3　fetus 3
4　fetus 4
5　fetus 5
9　other fetus

✓x7ᵗʰ **O60.10** **Preterm labor with preterm delivery, unspecified trimester** Ⓜ ♀
Preterm labor with delivery NOS

✓x7ᵗʰ **O60.12** **Preterm labor** second trimester **with preterm delivery** second trimester Ⓜ ♀

✓x7ᵗʰ **O60.13** **Preterm labor** second trimester **with preterm delivery** third trimester Ⓜ ♀

✓x7ᵗʰ **O60.14** **Preterm labor** third trimester **with preterm delivery** third trimester Ⓜ ♀

✓5ᵗʰ **O60.2** **Term delivery with preterm labor**

One of the following 7th characters is to be assigned to each code under subcategory O60.2. 7th character Ø is for single gestations and multiple gestations where the fetus is unspecified. 7th characters 1 through 9 are for cases of multiple gestations to identify the fetus for which the code applies. The appropriate code from category O30, Multiple gestation, must also be assigned when assigning a code from subcategory O60.2 that has a 7th character of 1 through 9.
Ø　not applicable or unspecified
1　fetus 1
2　fetus 2
3　fetus 3
4　fetus 4
5　fetus 5
9　other fetus

✓x7ᵗʰ **O60.20** **Term delivery with preterm labor, unspecified trimester** Ⓜ ♀

✓x7ᵗʰ **O60.22** **Term delivery with preterm labor,** second trimester Ⓜ ♀

✓x7ᵗʰ **O60.23** **Term delivery with preterm labor,** third trimester Ⓜ ♀

✓4ᵗʰ **O61** **Failed induction of labor**

O61.0 **Failed** medical **induction of labor** Ⓜ ♀
Failed induction (of labor) by oxytocin
Failed induction (of labor) by prostaglandins

O61.1 **Failed** instrumental **induction of labor** Ⓜ ♀
Failed mechanical induction (of labor)
Failed surgical induction (of labor)

O61.8 **Other failed induction of labor** Ⓜ ♀

O61.9 **Failed induction of labor, unspecified** Ⓜ ♀

✓4ᵗʰ **O62** **Abnormalities of forces of labor**
DEF: Uterine inertia: Weak or poorly coordinated contractions of the uterus during labor.

O62.0 **Primary inadequate contractions** Ⓜ ♀
Failure of cervical dilatation
Primary hypotonic uterine dysfunction
Uterine inertia during latent phase of labor

O62.1 **Secondary uterine inertia** Ⓜ ♀
Arrested active phase of labor
Secondary hypotonic uterine dysfunction

O62.2 **Other uterine inertia** Ⓜ ♀
Atony of uterus without hemorrhage
Atony of uterus NOS
Desultory labor
Hypotonic uterine dysfunction NOS
Irregular labor
Poor contractions
Slow slope active phase of labor
Uterine inertia NOS
　EXCLUDES 1　atony of uterus with hemorrhage (postpartum) (O72.1)
　　　　　postpartum atony of uterus without hemorrhage (O75.89)
DEF: Uterine atony: Failure of the uterine muscles to contract after the fetus and placenta are delivered.

O62.3 **Precipitate labor** Ⓜ ♀
DEF: Rapid labor with delivery occurring in three hours or less from the onset of contractions.

O62.4 **Hypertonic, incoordinate, and prolonged uterine contractions** Ⓜ ♀
Cervical spasm
Contraction ring dystocia
Dyscoordinate labor
Hour-glass contraction of uterus
Hypertonic uterine dysfunction
Incoordinate uterine action
Tetanic contractions
Uterine dystocia NOS
Uterine spasm
　EXCLUDES 1　dystocia (fetal) (maternal) NOS (O66.9)

O62.8 **Other abnormalities of forces of labor** Ⓜ ♀

O62.9 **Abnormality of forces of labor, unspecified** Ⓜ ♀

Chapter 15. Pregnancy, Childbirth and the Puerperium (side margin)

O63–O67.9 (side margin)

✓4ᵗʰ **O63 Long labor**

O63.0 Prolonged first stage (of labor)   Ⓜ ♀

O63.1 Prolonged second stage (of labor)   Ⓜ ♀

O63.2 Delayed delivery of second twin, triplet, etc.   Ⓜ ♀

O63.9 Long labor, unspecified   Ⓜ ♀
Prolonged labor NOS

✓4ᵗʰ **O64 Obstructed labor due to malposition and malpresentation of fetus**

One of the following 7th characters is to be assigned to each code under category O64. 7th character 0 is for single gestations and multiple gestations where the fetus is unspecified. 7th characters 1 through 9 are for cases of multiple gestations to identify the fetus for which the code applies. The appropriate code from category O30, Multiple gestation, must also be assigned when assigning a code from category O64 that has a 7th character of 1 through 9.

0   not applicable or unspecified
1   fetus 1
2   fetus 2
3   fetus 3
4   fetus 4
5   fetus 5
9   other fetus

Fetal Malposition

Breech

Mother's pelvis

Shoulder (arm prolapse)

Compound (extremity together with head)

Face (mentum)

Oblique

✓x7ᵗʰ **O64.0** Obstructed labor due to incomplete rotation of fetal head   Ⓜ ♀
Deep transverse arrest
Obstructed labor due to persistent occipitoiliac (position)
Obstructed labor due to persistent occipitoposterior (position)
Obstructed labor due to persistent occipitosacral (position)
Obstructed labor due to persistent occipitotransverse (position)

✓x7ᵗʰ **O64.1** Obstructed labor due to breech presentation   Ⓜ ♀
Obstructed labor due to buttocks presentation
Obstructed labor due to complete breech presentation
Obstructed labor due to frank breech presentation

✓x7ᵗʰ **O64.2** Obstructed labor due to face presentation   Ⓜ ♀
Obstructed labor due to chin presentation

✓x7ᵗʰ **O64.3** Obstructed labor due to brow presentation   Ⓜ ♀

✓x7ᵗʰ **O64.4** Obstructed labor due to shoulder presentation   Ⓜ ♀
Prolapsed arm
EXCLUDES 1   impacted shoulders (O66.0)
shoulder dystocia (O66.0)

✓x7ᵗʰ **O64.5** Obstructed labor due to compound presentation   Ⓜ ♀

✓x7ᵗʰ **O64.8** Obstructed labor due to other malposition and malpresentation   Ⓜ ♀
Obstructed labor due to footling presentation
Obstructed labor due to incomplete breech presentation

✓x7ᵗʰ **O64.9** Obstructed labor due to malposition and malpresentation, unspecified   Ⓜ ♀

✓4ᵗʰ **O65 Obstructed labor due to maternal pelvic abnormality**

O65.0 Obstructed labor due to deformed pelvis   Ⓜ ♀

O65.1 Obstructed labor due to generally contracted pelvis   Ⓜ ♀

O65.2 Obstructed labor due to pelvic inlet contraction   Ⓜ ♀

O65.3 Obstructed labor due to pelvic outlet and mid-cavity contraction   Ⓜ ♀

O65.4 Obstructed labor due to fetopelvic disproportion, unspecified   Ⓜ ♀
EXCLUDES 1   dystocia due to abnormality of fetus (O66.2-O66.3)

O65.5 Obstructed labor due to abnormality of maternal pelvic organs   Ⓜ ♀
Obstructed labor due to conditions listed in O34.-
Use additional code to identify abnormality of pelvic organs O34.-

O65.8 Obstructed labor due to other maternal pelvic abnormalities   Ⓜ ♀

O65.9 Obstructed labor due to maternal pelvic abnormality, unspecified   Ⓜ ♀

✓4ᵗʰ **O66 Other obstructed labor**

O66.0 Obstructed labor due to shoulder dystocia   Ⓜ ♀
Impacted shoulders
DEF: Obstructed labor due to impacted fetal shoulders. It is an emergency condition that may require cesarean section, forceps delivery, vacuum extraction, or symphysiotomy.

O66.1 Obstructed labor due to locked twins   Ⓜ ♀

O66.2 Obstructed labor due to unusually large fetus   Ⓜ ♀

O66.3 Obstructed labor due to other abnormalities of fetus   Ⓜ ♀
Dystocia due to fetal ascites
Dystocia due to fetal hydrops
Dystocia due to fetal meningomyelocele
Dystocia due to fetal sacral teratoma
Dystocia due to fetal tumor
Dystocia due to hydrocephalic fetus
Use additional code to identify cause of obstruction

✓5ᵗʰ **O66.4** Failed trial of labor

O66.40 Failed trial of labor, unspecified   Ⓜ ♀

O66.41 Failed attempted vaginal birth after previous cesarean delivery   Ⓜ ♀
Code first rupture of uterus, if applicable (O71.0-, O71.1)

O66.5 Attempted application of vacuum extractor and forceps   Ⓜ ♀
Attempted application of vacuum or forceps, with subsequent delivery by forceps or cesarean delivery

O66.6 Obstructed labor due to other multiple fetuses   Ⓜ ♀

O66.8 Other specified obstructed labor   Ⓜ ♀
Use additional code to identify cause of obstruction

O66.9 Obstructed labor, unspecified   Ⓜ ♀
Dystocia NOS
Fetal dystocia NOS
Maternal dystocia NOS

✓4ᵗʰ **O67 Labor and delivery complicated by intrapartum hemorrhage, not elsewhere classified**
EXCLUDES 1   antepartum hemorrhage NEC (O46.-)
placenta previa (O44.-)
premature separation of placenta [abruptio placentae] (O45.-)
EXCLUDES 2   postpartum hemorrhage (O72.-)

O67.0 Intrapartum hemorrhage with coagulation defect   Ⓜ ♀
Intrapartum hemorrhage (excessive) associated with afibrinogenemia
Intrapartum hemorrhage (excessive) associated with disseminated intravascular coagulation
Intrapartum hemorrhage (excessive) associated with hyperfibrinolysis
Intrapartum hemorrhage (excessive) associated with hypofibrinogenemia

O67.8 Other intrapartum hemorrhage   Ⓜ ♀
Excessive intrapartum hemorrhage

O67.9 Intrapartum hemorrhage, unspecified   Ⓜ ♀

Ⓝ Newborn: 0   Ⓟ Pediatric: 0-17   Ⓜ Maternity: 12-55   Ⓐ Adult: 15-124   CH Comorbidity High   CL Comorbidity Low   NCDx Noncancer Dx   PDx Primary Dx

874   ICD-10-CM 2020

O68 Labor and delivery complicated by abnormality of fetal acid-base balance   Ⓜ ♀

Fetal acidemia complicating labor and delivery

Fetal acidosis complicating labor and delivery

Fetal alkalosis complicating labor and delivery

Fetal metabolic acidemia complicating labor and delivery

EXCLUDES 1   *fetal stress NOS (O77.9)*

labor and delivery complicated by electrocardiographic evidence of fetal stress (O77.8)

labor and delivery complicated by ultrasonic evidence of fetal stress (O77.8)

EXCLUDES 2   *abnormality in fetal heart rate or rhythm (O76)*

labor and delivery complicated by meconium in amniotic fluid (O77.0)

✓4ᵗʰ **O69 Labor and delivery complicated by umbilical cord complications**

AHA: 2016,1Q,5

One of the following 7th characters is to be assigned to each code under category O69. 7th character Ø is for single gestations and multiple gestations where the fetus is unspecified. 7th characters 1 through 9 are for cases of multiple gestations to identify the fetus for which the code applies. The appropriate code from category O3Ø, Multiple gestation, must also be assigned when assigning a code from category O69 that has a 7th character of 1 through 9.

Ø   not applicable or unspecified

1   fetus 1

2   fetus 2

3   fetus 3

4   fetus 4

5   fetus 5

9   other fetus

✓x7ᵗʰ **O69.Ø Labor and delivery complicated by** prolapse of cord   Ⓜ ♀

DEF: Abnormal presentation of the fetus marked by a protruding umbilical cord during labor. It can cause fetal death.

✓x7ᵗʰ **O69.1 Labor and delivery complicated by** cord around neck, with compression   Ⓜ ♀

EXCLUDES 1   *labor and delivery complicated by cord around neck, without compression (O69.81)*

✓x7ᵗʰ **O69.2 Labor and delivery complicated by** other cord entanglement, with compression   Ⓜ ♀

Labor and delivery complicated by compression of cord NOS

Labor and delivery complicated by entanglement of cords of twins in monoamniotic sac

Labor and delivery complicated by knot in cord

EXCLUDES 1   *labor and delivery complicated by other cord entanglement, without compression (O69.82)*

✓x7ᵗʰ **O69.3 Labor and delivery complicated by** short cord   Ⓜ ♀

✓x7ᵗʰ **O69.4 Labor and delivery complicated by** vasa previa   Ⓜ ♀

Labor and delivery complicated by hemorrhage from vasa previa

✓x7ᵗʰ **O69.5 Labor and delivery complicated by** vascular lesion of cord   Ⓜ ♀

Labor and delivery complicated by cord bruising

Labor and delivery complicated by cord hematoma

Labor and delivery complicated by thrombosis of umbilical vessels

✓5ᵗʰ **O69.8 Labor and delivery complicated by other cord complications**

✓x7ᵗʰ **O69.81 Labor and delivery complicated by** cord around neck, without compression   Ⓜ ♀

AHA: 2016,1Q,5

✓x7ᵗʰ **O69.82 Labor and delivery complicated by** other cord entanglement, without compression   Ⓜ ♀

✓x7ᵗʰ **O69.89 Labor and delivery complicated by other** cord complications   Ⓜ ♀

✓x7ᵗʰ **O69.9 Labor and delivery complicated by** cord complication, unspecified   Ⓜ ♀

✓4ᵗʰ **O7Ø Perineal laceration during delivery**

INCLUDES   episiotomy extended by laceration

EXCLUDES 1   *obstetric high vaginal laceration alone (O71.4)*

AHA: 2016,2Q,34; 2016,1Q,3-4,5

O7Ø.Ø First degree perineal laceration during delivery   Ⓜ ♀

Perineal laceration, rupture or tear involving fourchette during delivery

Perineal laceration, rupture or tear involving labia during delivery

Perineal laceration, rupture or tear involving skin during delivery

Perineal laceration, rupture or tear involving vagina during delivery

Perineal laceration, rupture or tear involving vulva during delivery

Slight perineal laceration, rupture or tear during delivery

O7Ø.1 Second degree perineal laceration during delivery   Ⓜ ♀

Perineal laceration, rupture or tear during delivery as in O7Ø.Ø, also involving pelvic floor

Perineal laceration, rupture or tear during delivery as in O7Ø.Ø, also involving perineal muscles

Perineal laceration, rupture or tear during delivery as in O7Ø.Ø, also involving vaginal muscles

EXCLUDES 1   *perineal laceration involving anal sphincter (O7Ø.2)*

✓5ᵗʰ **O7Ø.2 Third degree** perineal laceration during delivery

Perineal laceration, rupture or tear during delivery as in O7Ø.1, also involving anal sphincter

Perineal laceration, rupture or tear during delivery as in O7Ø.1, also involving rectovaginal septum

Perineal laceration, rupture or tear during delivery as in O7Ø.1, also involving sphincter NOS

EXCLUDES 1   *anal sphincter tear during delivery without third degree perineal laceration (O7Ø.4)*

perineal laceration involving anal or rectal mucosa (O7Ø.3)

AHA: 2016,4Q,53-54

O7Ø.2Ø Third degree perineal laceration during delivery, unspecified   Ⓜ ♀

O7Ø.21 Third degree perineal laceration during delivery, IIIa   Ⓜ ♀

Third degree perineal laceration during delivery with less than 50% of external anal sphincter (EAS) thickness torn

O7Ø.22 Third degree perineal laceration during delivery, IIIb   Ⓜ ♀

Third degree perineal laceration during delivery with more than 50% external anal sphincter (EAS) thickness torn

O7Ø.23 Third degree perineal laceration during delivery, IIIc   Ⓜ ♀

Third degree perineal laceration during delivery with both external anal sphincter (EAS) and internal anal sphincter (IAS) torn

O7Ø.3 Fourth degree perineal laceration during delivery   Ⓜ ♀

Perineal laceration, rupture or tear during delivery as in O7Ø.2, also involving anal mucosa

Perineal laceration, rupture or tear during delivery as in O7Ø.2, also involving rectal mucosa

O7Ø.4 Anal sphincter tear complicating delivery, not associated with third degree laceration   Ⓜ ♀

EXCLUDES 1   *anal sphincter tear with third degree perineal laceration (O7Ø.2)*

O7Ø.9 Perineal laceration during delivery, unspecified   Ⓜ ♀

✓4ᵗʰ **O71 Other obstetric trauma**

INCLUDES   obstetric damage from instruments

✓5ᵗʰ **O71.Ø Rupture of uterus (spontaneous)** before onset of labor

EXCLUDES 1   *disruption of (current) cesarean delivery wound (O9Ø.Ø)*

laceration of uterus, NEC (O71.81)

O71.ØØ Rupture of uterus before onset of labor, unspecified trimester   Ⓜ ♀

O71.Ø2 Rupture of uterus before onset of labor, second trimester   Ⓜ ♀

O71.Ø3 Rupture of uterus before onset of labor, third trimester   Ⓜ ♀

✔ Additional Character Required   ✓x7ᵗʰ Placeholder Alert   Manifestation   Unspecified Dx   ▶◀ Revised Text   ● New Code   ▲ Revised Title

ICD-10-CM 2020   875

O71.1 Rupture of uterus during labor   Ⓜ♀

Rupture of uterus not stated as occurring before onset of labor

EXCLUDES 1   *disruption of cesarean delivery wound (O90.0)*

laceration of uterus, NEC (O71.81)

O71.2 Postpartum inversion of uterus   Ⓜ♀

O71.3 Obstetric laceration of cervix   Ⓜ♀

Annular detachment of cervix

O71.4 Obstetric high vaginal laceration **alone**   Ⓜ♀

Laceration of vaginal wall without perineal laceration

EXCLUDES 1   *obstetric high vaginal laceration with perineal laceration (O70.-)*

AHA: 2016,1Q,5

O71.5 Other obstetric injury to pelvic organs   Ⓜ♀

Obstetric injury to bladder

Obstetric injury to urethra

EXCLUDES 2   *obstetric periurethral trauma (O71.82)*

AHA: 2014,4Q,18

O71.6 Obstetric damage to pelvic joints and ligaments   Ⓜ♀

Obstetric avulsion of inner symphyseal cartilage

Obstetric damage to coccyx

Obstetric traumatic separation of symphysis (pubis)

O71.7 Obstetric hematoma of pelvis   Ⓜ♀

Obstetric hematoma of perineum

Obstetric hematoma of vagina

Obstetric hematoma of vulva

✓5ᵗʰ **O71.8 Other specified obstetric trauma**

O71.81 Laceration of uterus, not elsewhere classified   Ⓜ♀

O71.82 Other specified trauma to perineum and vulva   Ⓜ♀

Obstetric periurethral trauma

AHA: 2016,1Q,4; 2014,4Q,18

O71.89 Other specified obstetric trauma   Ⓜ♀

O71.9 Obstetric trauma, unspecified   Ⓜ♀

✓4ᵗʰ **O72 Postpartum hemorrhage**

INCLUDES   hemorrhage after delivery of fetus or infant

O72.0 Third-stage hemorrhage   Ⓜ♀

Hemorrhage associated with retained, trapped or adherent placenta

Retained placenta NOS

Code also type of adherent placenta (O43.2-)

O72.1 Other immediate **postpartum hemorrhage**   Ⓜ♀

Hemorrhage following delivery of placenta

Postpartum hemorrhage (atonic) NOS

Uterine atony with hemorrhage

EXCLUDES 1   *uterine atony NOS (O62.2)*

uterine atony without hemorrhage (O62.2)

postpartum atony of uterus without hemorrhage (O75.89)

AHA: 2016,1Q,4

DEF: Uterine atony: Failure of the uterine muscles to contract after the fetus and placenta are delivered.

O72.2 Delayed and secondary postpartum hemorrhage   Ⓜ♀

Hemorrhage associated with retained portions of placenta or membranes after the first 24 hours following delivery of placenta

Retained products of conception NOS, following delivery

O72.3 Postpartum coagulation defects   Ⓜ♀

Postpartum afibrinogenemia

Postpartum fibrinolysis

✓4ᵗʰ **O73 Retained placenta and membranes, without hemorrhage**

EXCLUDES 1   *placenta accreta (O43.21-)*

placenta increta (O43.22-)

placenta percreta (O43.23-)

DEF: Postpartum condition resulting from failure to expel placental membrane tissues due to failed contractions of the uterine wall.

O73.0 Retained placenta without hemorrhage   Ⓜ♀

Adherent placenta, without hemorrhage

Trapped placenta without hemorrhage

O73.1 Retained portions of placenta and membranes, **without hemorrhage**   Ⓜ♀

Retained products of conception following delivery, without hemorrhage

✓4ᵗʰ **O74 Complications of anesthesia during labor and delivery**

INCLUDES   maternal complications arising from the administration of a general, regional or local anesthetic, analgesic or other sedation during labor and delivery

Use additional code, if applicable, to identify specific complication

O74.0 Aspiration pneumonitis due to anesthesia during labor and delivery   Ⓜ♀

Inhalation of stomach contents or secretions NOS due to anesthesia during labor and delivery

Mendelson's syndrome due to anesthesia during labor and delivery

O74.1 Other pulmonary **complications of anesthesia during labor and delivery**   Ⓜ♀

O74.2 Cardiac complications of anesthesia during labor and delivery   Ⓜ♀

O74.3 Central nervous system complications of anesthesia during labor and delivery   Ⓜ♀

O74.4 Toxic reaction to local anesthesia during labor and delivery   Ⓜ♀

O74.5 Spinal and epidural anesthesia-induced headache during labor and delivery   Ⓜ♀

O74.6 Other complications of spinal and epidural **anesthesia during labor and delivery**   Ⓜ♀

O74.7 Failed or difficult intubation for anesthesia during labor and delivery   Ⓜ♀

O74.8 Other complications of anesthesia during labor and delivery   Ⓜ♀

O74.9 Complication of anesthesia during labor and delivery, unspecified   Ⓜ♀

✓4ᵗʰ **O75 Other complications of labor and delivery, not elsewhere classified**

EXCLUDES 2   *puerperal (postpartum) infection (O86.-)*

puerperal (postpartum) sepsis (O85)

O75.0 Maternal distress during labor and delivery   Ⓜ♀

O75.1 Shock during or following labor and delivery   Ⓜ♀

Obstetric shock following labor and delivery

O75.2 Pyrexia during labor, not elsewhere classified   Ⓜ♀

O75.3 Other infection during labor   Ⓜ♀

Sepsis during labor

Use additional code (B95-B97), to identify infectious agent

O75.4 Other complications of obstetric surgery and procedures   Ⓜ♀

Cardiac arrest following obstetric surgery or procedures

Cardiac failure following obstetric surgery or procedures

Cerebral anoxia following obstetric surgery or procedures

Pulmonary edema following obstetric surgery or procedures

Use additional code to identify specific complication

EXCLUDES 2   *complications of anesthesia during labor and delivery (O74.-)*

disruption of obstetrical (surgical) wound (O90.0-O90.1)

hematoma of obstetrical (surgical) wound (O90.2)

infection of obstetrical (surgical) wound (O86.0-)

O75.5 Delayed delivery after artificial rupture of membranes   Ⓜ♀

✓5ᵗʰ **O75.8 Other specified complications of labor and delivery**

O75.81 Maternal exhaustion complicating labor and delivery   Ⓜ♀

O75.82 Onset (spontaneous) of labor after 37 completed weeks of gestation but before 39 completed weeks gestation, with delivery by (planned) cesarean section   Ⓜ♀

Delivery by (planned) cesarean section occurring after 37 completed weeks of gestation but before 39 completed weeks gestation due to (spontaneous) onset of labor

Code first to specify reason for planned cesarean section such as:

cephalopelvic disproportion (normally formed fetus) (O33.9)

previous cesarean delivery (O34.21)

O75.89 Other specified complications of labor and delivery   Ⓜ♀

Ⓝ Newborn: 0   Ⓟ Pediatric: 0-17   Ⓜ Maternity: 12-55   Ⓐ Adult: 15-124   CH Comorbidity High   CL Comorbidity Low   NCDx Noncancer Dx   PDx Primary Dx

876   ICD-10-CM 2020

O75.9 Complication of labor and delivery, unspecified　Ⓜ♀

O76 **Abnormality in fetal heart rate and rhythm complicating labor and delivery**　Ⓜ♀
- Depressed fetal heart rate tones complicating labor and delivery
- Fetal bradycardia complicating labor and delivery
- Fetal heart rate decelerations complicating labor and delivery
- Fetal heart rate irregularity complicating labor and delivery
- Fetal heart rate abnormal variability complicating labor and delivery
- Fetal tachycardia complicating labor and delivery
- Non-reassuring fetal heart rate or rhythm complicating labor and delivery

> EXCLUDES 1　fetal stress NOS (O77.9)
> labor and delivery complicated by electrocardiographic evidence of fetal stress (O77.8)
> labor and delivery complicated by ultrasonic evidence of fetal stress (O77.8)
>
> EXCLUDES 2　fetal metabolic acidemia (O68)
> other fetal stress (O77.Ø-O77.1)

AHA: 2013,4Q,118

✓4ᵗʰ O77 **Other fetal stress complicating labor and delivery**

O77.Ø Labor and delivery complicated by meconium in amniotic fluid　Ⓜ♀
AHA: 2013,4Q,117-118

O77.1 Fetal stress in labor or delivery due to drug administration　Ⓜ♀

O77.8 Labor and delivery complicated by other evidence of fetal stress　Ⓜ♀
- Labor and delivery complicated by electrocardiographic evidence of fetal stress
- Labor and delivery complicated by ultrasonic evidence of fetal stress

> EXCLUDES 1　abnormality of fetal acid-base balance (O68)
> abnormality in fetal heart rate or rhythm (O76)
> fetal metabolic acidemia (O68)

O77.9 Labor and delivery complicated by fetal stress, unspecified　Ⓜ♀

> EXCLUDES 1　abnormality of fetal acid-base balance (O68)
> abnormality in fetal heart rate or rhythm (O76)
> fetal metabolic acidemia (O68)

Encounter for delivery (O8Ø-O82)

O8Ø **Encounter for full-term uncomplicated delivery**　Ⓜ♀

> NOTE　Delivery requiring minimal or no assistance, with or without episiotomy, without fetal manipulation [e.g., rotation version] or instrumentation [forceps] of a spontaneous, cephalic, vaginal, full-term, single, live-born infant. This code is for use as a single diagnosis code and is not to be used with any other code from chapter 15.

Use additional code to indicate outcome of delivery (Z37.Ø)
AHA: 2016,4Q,150; 2014,2Q,9

O82 **Encounter for cesarean delivery without indication**　Ⓜ♀
Use additional code to indicate outcome of delivery (Z37.Ø)

Complications predominantly related to the puerperium (O85-O92)

> EXCLUDES 2　mental and behavioral disorders associated with the puerperium (F53.-)
> obstetrical tetanus (A34)
> puerperal osteomalacia (M83.Ø)

O85 **Puerperal sepsis**　Ⓜ♀
- Postpartum sepsis
- Puerperal peritonitis
- Puerperal pyemia
Use additional code (B95-B97), to identify infectious agent
Use additional code (R65.2-) to identify severe sepsis, if applicable

> EXCLUDES 1　fever of unknown origin following delivery (O86.4)
> genital tract infection following delivery (O86.1-)
> obstetric pyemic and septic embolism (O88.3-)
> puerperal septic thrombophlebitis (O86.81)
> urinary tract infection following delivery (O86.2-)
>
> EXCLUDES 2　sepsis during labor (O75.3)

AHA: 2018,4Q,23

✓4ᵗʰ O86 **Other puerperal infections**
Use additional code (B95-B97), to identify infectious agent

> EXCLUDES 2　infection during labor (O75.3)
> obstetrical tetanus (A34)

✓5ᵗʰ O86.Ø Infection of obstetric surgical wound
- Infected cesarean delivery wound following delivery
- Infected perineal repair following delivery

> EXCLUDES 1　complications of procedures, not elsewhere classified (T81.4-)
> postprocedural fever NOS (R50.82)
> postprocedural retroperitoneal abscess (K68.11)

AHA: 2018,4Q,22-23,62

O86.ØØ Infection of obstetric surgical wound, unspecified　Ⓜ♀

O86.Ø1 Infection of obstetric surgical wound, superficial incisional site　Ⓜ♀
- Subcutaneous abscess following an obstetrical procedure
- Stitch abscess following an obstetrical procedure

O86.Ø2 Infection of obstetric surgical wound, deep incisional site　Ⓜ♀
- Intramuscular abscess following an obstetrical procedure
- ▶Sub-fascial abscess following an obstetrical procedure◀

O86.Ø3 Infection of obstetric surgical wound, organ and space site　Ⓜ♀
- Intraabdominal abscess following an obstetrical procedure
- Subphrenic abscess following an obstetrical procedure

O86.Ø4 Sepsis following an obstetrical procedure　Ⓜ♀
Use additional code to identify the sepsis
AHA: 2019,2Q,39

O86.Ø9 Infection of obstetric surgical wound, other surgical site　Ⓜ♀

✓5ᵗʰ O86.1 Other infection of genital tract following delivery

O86.11 Cervicitis following delivery　Ⓜ♀

O86.12 Endometritis following delivery　Ⓜ♀

O86.13 Vaginitis following delivery　Ⓜ♀

O86.19 Other infection of genital tract following delivery　Ⓜ♀

✓5ᵗʰ O86.2 Urinary tract infection following delivery

O86.2Ø Urinary tract infection following delivery, unspecified　Ⓜ♀
Puerperal urinary tract infection NOS

O86.21 Infection of kidney following delivery　Ⓜ♀

O86.22 Infection of bladder following delivery　Ⓜ♀
Infection of urethra following delivery

O86.29 Other urinary tract infection following delivery　Ⓜ♀

O86.4 Pyrexia of unknown origin following delivery　Ⓜ♀
- Puerperal infection NOS following delivery
- Puerperal pyrexia NOS following delivery

> EXCLUDES 2　pyrexia during labor (O75.2)

DEF: Fever of unknown origin experienced by the mother after childbirth.

✓5ᵗʰ O86.8 Other specified puerperal infections

O86.81 Puerperal septic thrombophlebitis　Ⓜ♀

O86.89 Other specified puerperal infections　Ⓜ♀

✓4ᵗʰ O87 **Venous complications and hemorrhoids in the puerperium**

> INCLUDES　venous complications in labor, delivery and the puerperium
>
> EXCLUDES 2　obstetric embolism (O88.-)
> puerperal septic thrombophlebitis (O86.81)
> venous complications in pregnancy (O22.-)

O87.Ø Superficial thrombophlebitis in the puerperium　Ⓜ♀
- Puerperal phlebitis NOS
- Puerperal thrombosis NOS

O87.1 Deep phlebothrombosis in the puerperium Ⓜ♀

    Deep vein thrombosis, postpartum

    Pelvic thrombophlebitis, postpartum

    Use additional code to identify the deep vein thrombosis (I82.4-, I82.5-, I82.62-. I82.72-)

    Use additional code, if applicable, for associated long-term (current) use of anticoagulants (Z79.01)

O87.2 Hemorrhoids in the puerperium Ⓜ♀

O87.3 Cerebral venous thrombosis in the puerperium Ⓜ♀

    Cerebrovenous sinus thrombosis in the puerperium

O87.4 Varicose veins of lower extremity in the puerperium Ⓜ♀

O87.8 Other venous complications in the puerperium Ⓜ♀

    Genital varices in the puerperium

O87.9 Venous complication in the puerperium, unspecified Ⓜ♀

    Puerperal phlebopathy NOS

✓4ᵗʰ **O88 Obstetric embolism**

    EXCLUDES 1   *embolism complicating abortion NOS (O03.2)*

        embolism complicating ectopic or molar pregnancy (O08.2)

        embolism complicating failed attempted abortion (O07.2)

        embolism complicating induced abortion (O04.7)

        embolism complicating spontaneous abortion (O03.2, O03.7)

✓5ᵗʰ **O88.0 Obstetric air embolism**

    DEF: Sudden blocking of the pulmonary artery or right ventricle with air or nitrogen bubbles.

    ✓6ᵗʰ **O88.01 Obstetric air embolism in pregnancy**

        O88.011 Air embolism in pregnancy, first trimester Ⓜ♀

        O88.012 Air embolism in pregnancy, second trimester Ⓜ♀

        O88.013 Air embolism in pregnancy, third trimester Ⓜ♀

        O88.019 Air embolism in pregnancy, unspecified trimester Ⓜ♀

    O88.02 Air embolism in childbirth Ⓜ♀

    O88.03 Air embolism in the puerperium Ⓜ♀

✓5ᵗʰ **O88.1 Amniotic fluid embolism**

    Anaphylactoid syndrome in pregnancy

    ✓6ᵗʰ **O88.11 Amniotic fluid embolism in pregnancy**

        O88.111 Amniotic fluid embolism in pregnancy, first trimester Ⓜ♀

        O88.112 Amniotic fluid embolism in pregnancy, second trimester Ⓜ♀

        O88.113 Amniotic fluid embolism in pregnancy, third trimester Ⓜ♀

        O88.119 Amniotic fluid embolism in pregnancy, unspecified trimester Ⓜ♀

    O88.12 Amniotic fluid embolism in childbirth Ⓜ♀

    O88.13 Amniotic fluid embolism in the puerperium Ⓜ♀

✓5ᵗʰ **O88.2 Obstetric thromboembolism**

    ✓6ᵗʰ **O88.21 Thromboembolism in pregnancy**

        Obstetric (pulmonary) embolism NOS

        O88.211 Thromboembolism in pregnancy, first trimester Ⓜ♀

        O88.212 Thromboembolism in pregnancy, second trimester Ⓜ♀

        O88.213 Thromboembolism in pregnancy, third trimester Ⓜ♀

        O88.219 Thromboembolism in pregnancy, unspecified trimester Ⓜ♀

    O88.22 Thromboembolism in childbirth Ⓜ♀

    O88.23 Thromboembolism in the puerperium Ⓜ♀

        Puerperal (pulmonary) embolism NOS

✓5ᵗʰ **O88.3 Obstetric pyemic and septic embolism**

    ✓6ᵗʰ **O88.31 Pyemic and septic embolism in pregnancy**

        O88.311 Pyemic and septic embolism in pregnancy, first trimester Ⓜ♀

        O88.312 Pyemic and septic embolism in pregnancy, second trimester Ⓜ♀

        O88.313 Pyemic and septic embolism in pregnancy, third trimester Ⓜ♀

        O88.319 Pyemic and septic embolism in pregnancy, unspecified trimester Ⓜ♀

    O88.32 Pyemic and septic embolism in childbirth Ⓜ♀

    O88.33 Pyemic and septic embolism in the puerperium Ⓜ♀

✓5ᵗʰ **O88.8 Other obstetric embolism**

    Obstetric fat embolism

    ✓6ᵗʰ **O88.81 Other embolism in pregnancy**

        O88.811 Other embolism in pregnancy, first trimester Ⓜ♀

        O88.812 Other embolism in pregnancy, second trimester Ⓜ♀

        O88.813 Other embolism in pregnancy, third trimester Ⓜ♀

        O88.819 Other embolism in pregnancy, unspecified trimester Ⓜ♀

    O88.82 Other embolism in childbirth Ⓜ♀

    O88.83 Other embolism in the puerperium Ⓜ♀

✓4ᵗʰ **O89 Complications of anesthesia during the puerperium**

    INCLUDES   maternal complications arising from the administration of a general, regional or local anesthetic, analgesic or other sedation during the puerperium

    Use additional code, if applicable, to identify specific complication

✓5ᵗʰ **O89.0 Pulmonary complications of anesthesia during the puerperium**

    O89.01 Aspiration pneumonitis due to anesthesia during the puerperium Ⓜ♀

        Inhalation of stomach contents or secretions NOS due to anesthesia during the puerperium

        Mendelson's syndrome due to anesthesia during the puerperium

    O89.09 Other pulmonary complications of anesthesia during the puerperium Ⓜ♀

O89.1 Cardiac complications of anesthesia during the puerperium Ⓜ♀

O89.2 Central nervous system complications of anesthesia during the puerperium Ⓜ♀

O89.3 Toxic reaction to local anesthesia during the puerperium Ⓜ♀

O89.4 Spinal and epidural anesthesia-induced headache during the puerperium Ⓜ♀

O89.5 Other complications of spinal and epidural anesthesia during the puerperium Ⓜ♀

O89.6 Failed or difficult intubation for anesthesia during the puerperium Ⓜ♀

O89.8 Other complications of anesthesia during the puerperium Ⓜ♀

O89.9 Complication of anesthesia during the puerperium, unspecified Ⓜ♀

✓4ᵗʰ **O90 Complications of the puerperium, not elsewhere classified**

O90.0 Disruption of cesarean delivery wound Ⓜ♀

    Dehiscence of cesarean delivery wound

    EXCLUDES 1   *rupture of uterus (spontaneous) before onset of labor (O71.0-)*

        rupture of uterus during labor (O71.1)

O90.1 Disruption of perineal obstetric wound Ⓜ♀

    Disruption of wound of episiotomy

    Disruption of wound of perineal laceration

    Secondary perineal tear

O90.2 Hematoma of obstetric wound Ⓜ♀

O90.3 Peripartum cardiomyopathy Ⓜ♀

    Conditions in I42- arising during pregnancy and the puerperium

    EXCLUDES 1   *pre-existing heart disease complicating pregnancy and the puerperium (O99.4-)*

    DEF: Any structural or functional abnormality of the ventricular myocardium. It is a noninflammatory disease of obscure or unknown etiology with onset during the postpartum period.

O90.4 Postpartum acute kidney failure Ⓜ♀

    Hepatorenal syndrome following labor and delivery

O90.5 Postpartum thyroiditis Ⓜ♀

Ⓝ Newborn: 0   Ⓟ Pediatric: 0-17   Ⓜ Maternity: 12-55   Ⓐ Adult: 15-124   CH Comorbidity High   CL Comorbidity Low   NCDx Noncancer Dx   PDx Primary Dx

878   ICD-10-CM 2020

O90.6 **Postpartum mood disturbance** Ⓜ♀

    Postpartum blues
    Postpartum dysphoria
    Postpartum sadness
    EXCLUDES 1   *postpartum depression (F53.Ø)*
          puerperal psychosis (F53.1)

√5ᵗʰ **O90.8** **Other complications of the puerperium, not elsewhere classified**

  O90.81   **Anemia of the puerperium** Ⓜ♀

      Postpartum anemia NOS
      EXCLUDES 1   *pre-existing anemia complicating the puerperium (O99.Ø3)*

  O90.89   **Other complications of the puerperium, not elsewhere classified** Ⓜ♀
      Placental polyp

  O90.9 **Complication of the puerperium, unspecified** Ⓜ♀

√4ᵗʰ **O91** **Infections of breast associated with pregnancy, the puerperium and lactation**
    Use additional code to identify infection

√5ᵗʰ **O91.Ø** **Infection of nipple associated with pregnancy, the puerperium and lactation**

  √6ᵗʰ **O91.01**   **Infection of nipple associated with** pregnancy
      Gestational abscess of nipple

    O91.011   **Infection of nipple associated with pregnancy, first trimester** Ⓜ♀

    O91.012   **Infection of nipple associated with pregnancy, second trimester** Ⓜ♀

    O91.013   **Infection of nipple associated with pregnancy, third trimester** Ⓜ♀

    O91.019   **Infection of nipple associated with pregnancy, unspecified trimester** Ⓜ♀

  O91.02   **Infection of nipple associated with the** puerperium Ⓜ♀
      Puerperal abscess of nipple

  O91.03   **Infection of nipple associated with** lactation Ⓜ♀
      Abscess of nipple associated with lactation

√5ᵗʰ **O91.1** **Abscess of breast associated with pregnancy, the puerperium and lactation**

  √6ᵗʰ **O91.11**   **Abscess of breast associated with** pregnancy
      Gestational mammary abscess
      Gestational purulent mastitis
      Gestational subareolar abscess

    O91.111   **Abscess of breast associated with pregnancy, first trimester** Ⓜ♀

    O91.112   **Abscess of breast associated with pregnancy, second trimester** Ⓜ♀

    O91.113   **Abscess of breast associated with pregnancy, third trimester** Ⓜ♀

    O91.119   **Abscess of breast associated with pregnancy, unspecified trimester** Ⓜ♀

  O91.12   **Abscess of breast associated with the** puerperium Ⓜ♀
      Puerperal mammary abscess
      Puerperal purulent mastitis
      Puerperal subareolar abscess

  O91.13   **Abscess of breast associated with** lactation Ⓜ♀
      Mammary abscess associated with lactation
      Purulent mastitis associated with lactation
      Subareolar abscess associated with lactation

√5ᵗʰ **O91.2** **Nonpurulent mastitis associated with pregnancy, the puerperium and lactation**

  √6ᵗʰ **O91.21**   **Nonpurulent mastitis associated with** pregnancy
      Gestational interstitial mastitis
      Gestational lymphangitis of breast
      Gestational mastitis NOS
      Gestational parenchymatous mastitis

    O91.211   **Nonpurulent mastitis associated with pregnancy, first trimester** Ⓜ♀

    O91.212   **Nonpurulent mastitis associated with pregnancy, second trimester** Ⓜ♀

    O91.213   **Nonpurulent mastitis associated with pregnancy, third trimester** Ⓜ♀

    O91.219   **Nonpurulent mastitis associated with pregnancy, unspecified trimester** Ⓜ♀

  O91.22   **Nonpurulent mastitis associated with the** puerperium Ⓜ♀
      Puerperal interstitial mastitis
      Puerperal lymphangitis of breast
      Puerperal mastitis NOS
      Puerperal parenchymatous mastitis

  O91.23   **Nonpurulent mastitis associated with** lactation Ⓜ♀
      Interstitial mastitis associated with lactation
      Lymphangitis of breast associated with lactation
      Mastitis NOS associated with lactation
      Parenchymatous mastitis associated with lactation

√4ᵗʰ **O92** **Other disorders of breast and disorders of lactation associated with pregnancy and the puerperium**

√5ᵗʰ **O92.Ø** **Retracted nipple associated with pregnancy, the puerperium, and lactation**

  √6ᵗʰ **O92.01**   **Retracted nipple associated with** pregnancy

    O92.011   **Retracted nipple associated with pregnancy, first trimester** Ⓜ♀

    O92.012   **Retracted nipple associated with pregnancy, second trimester** Ⓜ♀

    O92.013   **Retracted nipple associated with pregnancy, third trimester** Ⓜ♀

    O92.019   **Retracted nipple associated with pregnancy, unspecified trimester** Ⓜ♀

  O92.02   **Retracted nipple associated with the** puerperium Ⓜ♀

  O92.03   **Retracted nipple associated with** lactation Ⓜ♀

√5ᵗʰ **O92.1** **Cracked nipple associated with pregnancy, the puerperium, and lactation**
    Fissure of nipple, gestational or puerperal

  √6ᵗʰ **O92.11**   **Cracked nipple associated with** pregnancy

    O92.111   **Cracked nipple associated with pregnancy, first trimester** Ⓜ♀

    O92.112   **Cracked nipple associated with pregnancy, second trimester** Ⓜ♀

    O92.113   **Cracked nipple associated with pregnancy, third trimester** Ⓜ♀

    O92.119   **Cracked nipple associated with pregnancy, unspecified trimester** Ⓜ♀

  O92.12   **Cracked nipple associated with the** puerperium Ⓜ♀

  O92.13   **Cracked nipple associated with** lactation Ⓜ♀

√5ᵗʰ **O92.2** **Other and unspecified disorders of breast associated with pregnancy and the puerperium**

  O92.20   **Unspecified disorder of breast associated with pregnancy and the puerperium** Ⓜ♀

  O92.29   **Other disorders of breast associated with pregnancy and the puerperium** Ⓜ♀

O92.3 **Agalactia** Ⓜ♀
    Primary agalactia
    EXCLUDES 1   *elective agalactia (O92.5)*
          secondary agalactia (O92.5)
          therapeutic agalactia (O92.5)
    DEF: Absence of milk secretion in a female after delivery.

O92.4 **Hypogalactia** Ⓜ♀

☑ Additional Character Required   √7ᵗʰ Placeholder Alert   Manifestation   Unspecified Dx   ▶◀ Revised Text   ● New Code   ▲ Revised Title

O92.5 Suppressed lactation Ⓜ♀
  Elective agalactia
  Secondary agalactia
  Therapeutic agalactia
  EXCLUDES 1 primary agalactia (O92.3)

O92.6 Galactorrhea Ⓜ♀
  DEF: Excessive or persistent milk secretion by the breast that may occur in the absence of nursing.

✓5ᵗʰ **O92.7 Other and unspecified disorders of lactation**
  O92.70 Unspecified disorders of lactation Ⓜ♀
  O92.79 Other disorders of lactation Ⓜ♀
    Puerperal galactocele

Other obstetric conditions, not elsewhere classified (O94-O9A)

O94 Sequelae of complication of pregnancy, childbirth, and the puerperium Ⓜ♀
  NOTE This category is to be used to indicate conditions in O00-O77.-, O85-O94 and O98-O9A.- as the cause of late effects. The sequelae include conditions specified as such, or as late effects, which may occur at any time after the puerperium
  Code first condition resulting from (sequela) of complication of pregnancy, childbirth, and the puerperium

✓4ᵗʰ **O98 Maternal infectious and parasitic diseases classifiable elsewhere but complicating pregnancy, childbirth and the puerperium**
  INCLUDES the listed conditions when complicating the pregnant state, when aggravated by the pregnancy, or as a reason for obstetric care
  Use additional code (Chapter 1), to identify specific infectious or parasitic disease
  EXCLUDES 2 herpes gestationis (O26.4-)
    infectious carrier state (O99.82-, O99.83-)
    obstetrical tetanus (A34)
    puerperal infection (O86.-)
    puerperal sepsis (O85)
    when the reason for maternal care is that the disease is known or suspected to have affected the fetus (O35-O36)

✓5ᵗʰ **O98.0 Tuberculosis complicating pregnancy, childbirth and the puerperium**
  Conditions in A15-A19
  ✓6ᵗʰ **O98.01 Tuberculosis complicating pregnancy**
    O98.011 Tuberculosis complicating pregnancy, first trimester Ⓜ♀
    O98.012 Tuberculosis complicating pregnancy, second trimester Ⓜ♀
    O98.013 Tuberculosis complicating pregnancy, third trimester Ⓜ♀
    O98.019 Tuberculosis complicating pregnancy, unspecified trimester Ⓜ♀
  O98.02 Tuberculosis complicating childbirth Ⓜ♀
  O98.03 Tuberculosis complicating the puerperium Ⓜ♀

✓5ᵗʰ **O98.1 Syphilis complicating pregnancy, childbirth and the puerperium**
  Conditions in A50-A53
  ✓6ᵗʰ **O98.11 Syphilis complicating pregnancy**
    O98.111 Syphilis complicating pregnancy, first trimester Ⓜ♀
    O98.112 Syphilis complicating pregnancy, second trimester Ⓜ♀
    O98.113 Syphilis complicating pregnancy, third trimester Ⓜ♀
    O98.119 Syphilis complicating pregnancy, unspecified trimester Ⓜ♀
  O98.12 Syphilis complicating childbirth Ⓜ♀
  O98.13 Syphilis complicating the puerperium Ⓜ♀

✓5ᵗʰ **O98.2 Gonorrhea complicating pregnancy, childbirth and the puerperium**
  Conditions in A54.-
  ✓6ᵗʰ **O98.21 Gonorrhea complicating pregnancy**
    O98.211 Gonorrhea complicating pregnancy, first trimester Ⓜ♀
    O98.212 Gonorrhea complicating pregnancy, second trimester Ⓜ♀

O98.213 Gonorrhea complicating pregnancy, third trimester Ⓜ♀
O98.219 Gonorrhea complicating pregnancy, unspecified trimester Ⓜ♀
O98.22 Gonorrhea complicating childbirth Ⓜ♀
O98.23 Gonorrhea complicating the puerperium Ⓜ♀

✓5ᵗʰ **O98.3 Other infections with a predominantly sexual mode of transmission complicating pregnancy, childbirth and the puerperium**
  Conditions in A55-A64
  ✓6ᵗʰ **O98.31 Other infections with a predominantly sexual mode of transmission complicating pregnancy**
    O98.311 Other infections with a predominantly sexual mode of transmission complicating pregnancy, first trimester Ⓜ♀
    O98.312 Other infections with a predominantly sexual mode of transmission complicating pregnancy, second trimester Ⓜ♀
    O98.313 Other infections with a predominantly sexual mode of transmission complicating pregnancy, third trimester Ⓜ♀
    O98.319 Other infections with a predominantly sexual mode of transmission complicating pregnancy, unspecified trimester Ⓜ♀
  O98.32 Other infections with a predominantly sexual mode of transmission complicating childbirth Ⓜ♀
  O98.33 Other infections with a predominantly sexual mode of transmission complicating the puerperium Ⓜ♀

✓5ᵗʰ **O98.4 Viral hepatitis complicating pregnancy, childbirth and the puerperium**
  Conditions in B15-B19
  ✓6ᵗʰ **O98.41 Viral hepatitis complicating pregnancy**
    O98.411 Viral hepatitis complicating pregnancy, first trimester Ⓜ♀
    O98.412 Viral hepatitis complicating pregnancy, second trimester Ⓜ♀
    O98.413 Viral hepatitis complicating pregnancy, third trimester Ⓜ♀
    O98.419 Viral hepatitis complicating pregnancy, unspecified trimester Ⓜ♀
  O98.42 Viral hepatitis complicating childbirth Ⓜ♀
  O98.43 Viral hepatitis complicating the puerperium Ⓜ♀

✓5ᵗʰ **O98.5 Other viral diseases complicating pregnancy, childbirth and the puerperium**
  Conditions in A80-B09, B25-B34, R87.81-, R87.82-
    EXCLUDES 1 human immunodeficiency virus [HIV] disease complicating pregnancy, childbirth and the puerperium (O98.7-)
  ✓6ᵗʰ **O98.51 Other viral diseases complicating pregnancy**
    O98.511 Other viral diseases complicating pregnancy, first trimester Ⓜ♀
    O98.512 Other viral diseases complicating pregnancy, second trimester Ⓜ♀
    O98.513 Other viral diseases complicating pregnancy, third trimester Ⓜ♀
    O98.519 Other viral diseases complicating pregnancy, unspecified trimester Ⓜ♀
  O98.52 Other viral diseases complicating childbirth Ⓜ♀
  O98.53 Other viral diseases complicating the puerperium Ⓜ♀

✓5ᵗʰ **O98.6 Protozoal diseases complicating pregnancy, childbirth and the puerperium**
  Conditions in B50-B64
  ✓6ᵗʰ **O98.61 Protozoal diseases complicating pregnancy**
    O98.611 Protozoal diseases complicating pregnancy, first trimester Ⓜ♀

O98.612 **Protozoal diseases complicating pregnancy, second trimester** Ⓜ♀

O98.613 **Protozoal diseases complicating pregnancy, third trimester** Ⓜ♀

O98.619 **Protozoal diseases complicating pregnancy, unspecified trimester** Ⓜ♀

O98.62 **Protozoal diseases complicating childbirth** Ⓜ♀

O98.63 **Protozoal diseases complicating the puerperium** Ⓜ♀

✓5ᵗʰ O98.7 Human immunodeficiency virus [HIV] disease **complicating pregnancy, childbirth and the puerperium**
    Use additional code to identify the type of HIV disease:
    acquired immune deficiency syndrome (AIDS) (B20)
    asymptomatic HIV status (Z21)
    HIV positive NOS (Z21)
    symptomatic HIV disease (B20)

✓6ᵗʰ O98.71 **Human immunodeficiency virus [HIV] disease complicating** pregnancy

O98.711 **Human immunodeficiency virus [HIV] disease complicating pregnancy,** first trimester Ⓜ♀

O98.712 **Human immunodeficiency virus [HIV] disease complicating pregnancy, second trimester** Ⓜ♀

O98.713 **Human immunodeficiency virus [HIV] disease complicating pregnancy,** third trimester Ⓜ♀

O98.719 **Human immunodeficiency virus [HIV] disease complicating pregnancy, unspecified trimester** Ⓜ♀

O98.72 **Human immunodeficiency virus [HIV] disease complicating** childbirth Ⓜ♀

O98.73 **Human immunodeficiency virus [HIV] disease complicating the** puerperium Ⓜ♀

✓5ᵗʰ O98.8 **Other maternal infectious and parasitic diseases complicating pregnancy, childbirth and the puerperium**

✓6ᵗʰ O98.81 **Other maternal infectious and parasitic diseases complicating** pregnancy

O98.811 **Other maternal infectious and parasitic diseases complicating pregnancy,** first trimester Ⓜ♀

O98.812 **Other maternal infectious and parasitic diseases complicating pregnancy,** second trimester Ⓜ♀

O98.813 **Other maternal infectious and parasitic diseases complicating pregnancy,** third trimester Ⓜ♀

O98.819 **Other maternal infectious and parasitic diseases complicating pregnancy, unspecified trimester** Ⓜ♀

O98.82 **Other maternal infectious and parasitic diseases complicating** childbirth Ⓜ♀

O98.83 **Other maternal infectious and parasitic diseases complicating the** puerperium Ⓜ♀

✓5ᵗʰ O98.9 **Unspecified maternal infectious and parasitic disease complicating pregnancy, childbirth and the puerperium**

✓6ᵗʰ O98.91 **Unspecified maternal infectious and parasitic disease complicating** pregnancy

O98.911 **Unspecified maternal infectious and parasitic disease complicating pregnancy,** first trimester Ⓜ♀

O98.912 **Unspecified maternal infectious and parasitic disease complicating pregnancy,** second trimester Ⓜ♀

O98.913 **Unspecified maternal infectious and parasitic disease complicating pregnancy,** third trimester Ⓜ♀

O98.919 **Unspecified maternal infectious and parasitic disease complicating pregnancy, unspecified trimester** Ⓜ♀

O98.92 **Unspecified maternal infectious and parasitic disease complicating** childbirth Ⓜ♀

O98.93 **Unspecified maternal infectious and parasitic disease complicating the** puerperium Ⓜ♀

✓4ᵗʰ O99 **Other maternal diseases classifiable elsewhere but complicating pregnancy, childbirth and the puerperium**
    [INCLUDES] conditions which complicate the pregnant state, are aggravated by the pregnancy or are a main reason for obstetric care
    Use additional code to identify specific condition
    EXCLUDES 2 when the reason for maternal care is that the condition is known or suspected to have affected the fetus (O35-O36)

✓5ᵗʰ O99.0 Anemia **complicating pregnancy, childbirth and the puerperium**
    Conditions in D50-D64
    EXCLUDES 1 anemia arising in the puerperium (O90.81)
    postpartum anemia NOS (O90.81)

✓6ᵗʰ O99.01 **Anemia complicating** pregnancy
    AHA: 2016,1Q,4

O99.011 **Anemia complicating pregnancy,** first trimester Ⓜ♀

O99.012 **Anemia complicating pregnancy,** second trimester Ⓜ♀

O99.013 **Anemia complicating pregnancy,** third trimester Ⓜ♀

O99.019 **Anemia complicating pregnancy, unspecified trimester** Ⓜ♀

O99.02 **Anemia complicating** childbirth Ⓜ♀

O99.03 **Anemia complicating the** puerperium Ⓜ♀
    EXCLUDES 1 postpartum anemia not pre-existing prior to delivery (O90.81)

✓5ᵗʰ O99.1 **Other diseases of the** blood and blood-forming organs and **certain disorders** involving the immune mechanism **complicating pregnancy, childbirth and the puerperium**
    Conditions in D65-D89
    EXCLUDES 1 hemorrhage with coagulation defects (O45.-, O46.0-, O67.0, O72.3)

✓6ᵗʰ O99.11 **Other diseases of the blood and blood-forming organs and certain disorders involving the immune mechanism complicating** pregnancy

O99.111 **Other diseases of the blood and blood-forming organs and certain disorders involving the immune mechanism complicating pregnancy,** first trimester Ⓜ♀

O99.112 **Other diseases of the blood and blood-forming organs and certain disorders involving the immune mechanism complicating pregnancy,** second trimester Ⓜ♀

O99.113 **Other diseases of the blood and blood-forming organs and certain disorders involving the immune mechanism complicating pregnancy,** third trimester Ⓜ♀

O99.119 **Other diseases of the blood and blood-forming organs and certain disorders involving the immune mechanism complicating pregnancy, unspecified trimester** Ⓜ♀

O99.12 **Other diseases of the blood and blood-forming organs and certain disorders involving the immune mechanism complicating** childbirth Ⓜ♀

O99.13 **Other diseases of the blood and blood-forming organs and certain disorders involving the immune mechanism complicating the** puerperium Ⓜ♀

✓5ᵗʰ O99.2 Endocrine, nutritional and metabolic diseases complicating pregnancy, childbirth and the puerperium
Conditions in E00-E88
EXCLUDES 2   diabetes mellitus (O24.-)
malnutrition (O25.-)
postpartum thyroiditis (O90.5)

✓6ᵗʰ O99.21 Obesity complicating pregnancy, childbirth, and the puerperium
Use additional code to identify the type of obesity (E66.-)
AHA: 2018,4Q,80
O99.210 Obesity complicating pregnancy, unspecified trimester   M ♀
O99.211 Obesity complicating pregnancy, first trimester   M ♀
O99.212 Obesity complicating pregnancy, second trimester   M ♀
O99.213 Obesity complicating pregnancy, third trimester   M ♀
O99.214 Obesity complicating childbirth   M ♀
O99.215 Obesity complicating the puerperium   M ♀

✓6ᵗʰ O99.28 Other endocrine, nutritional and metabolic diseases complicating pregnancy, childbirth and the puerperium
O99.280 Endocrine, nutritional and metabolic diseases complicating pregnancy, unspecified trimester   M ♀
O99.281 Endocrine, nutritional and metabolic diseases complicating pregnancy, first trimester   M ♀
O99.282 Endocrine, nutritional and metabolic diseases complicating pregnancy, second trimester   M ♀
O99.283 Endocrine, nutritional and metabolic diseases complicating pregnancy, third trimester   M ♀
O99.284 Endocrine, nutritional and metabolic diseases complicating childbirth   M ♀
O99.285 Endocrine, nutritional and metabolic diseases complicating the puerperium   M ♀

✓5ᵗʰ O99.3 Mental disorders and diseases of the nervous system complicating pregnancy, childbirth and the puerperium

✓6ᵗʰ O99.31 Alcohol use complicating pregnancy, childbirth, and the puerperium
Use additional code(s) from F10 to identify manifestations of the alcohol use
O99.310 Alcohol use complicating pregnancy, unspecified trimester   M ♀
O99.311 Alcohol use complicating pregnancy, first trimester   M ♀
O99.312 Alcohol use complicating pregnancy, second trimester   M ♀
O99.313 Alcohol use complicating pregnancy, third trimester   M ♀
O99.314 Alcohol use complicating childbirth   M ♀
O99.315 Alcohol use complicating the puerperium   M ♀

✓6ᵗʰ O99.32 Drug use complicating pregnancy, childbirth, and the puerperium
Use additional code(s) from F11-F16 and F18-F19 to identify manifestations of the drug use
AHA: 2018,4Q,69-70; 2018,2Q,10
O99.320 Drug use complicating pregnancy, unspecified trimester   M ♀
O99.321 Drug use complicating pregnancy, first trimester   M ♀
O99.322 Drug use complicating pregnancy, second trimester   M ♀
O99.323 Drug use complicating pregnancy, third trimester   M ♀

O99.324 Drug use complicating childbirth   M ♀
O99.325 Drug use complicating the puerperium   M ♀

✓6ᵗʰ O99.33 Tobacco use disorder complicating pregnancy, childbirth, and the puerperium
Smoking complicating pregnancy, childbirth, and the puerperium
Use additional code from category F17 to identify type of tobacco nicotine dependence
O99.330 Smoking (tobacco) complicating pregnancy, unspecified trimester   M ♀
O99.331 Smoking (tobacco) complicating pregnancy, first trimester   M ♀
O99.332 Smoking (tobacco) complicating pregnancy, second trimester   M ♀
O99.333 Smoking (tobacco) complicating pregnancy, third trimester   M ♀
O99.334 Smoking (tobacco) complicating childbirth   M ♀
O99.335 Smoking (tobacco) complicating the puerperium   M ♀

✓6ᵗʰ O99.34 Other mental disorders complicating pregnancy, childbirth, and the puerperium
▶Conditions in F01-F09, F20-F99 and F54-F99◀
EXCLUDES 2   postpartum mood disturbance (O90.6)
postnatal psychosis (F53.1)
puerperal psychosis (F53.1)
O99.340 Other mental disorders complicating pregnancy, unspecified trimester   M ♀
O99.341 Other mental disorders complicating pregnancy, first trimester   M ♀
O99.342 Other mental disorders complicating pregnancy, second trimester   M ♀
O99.343 Other mental disorders complicating pregnancy, third trimester   M ♀
O99.344 Other mental disorders complicating childbirth   M ♀
O99.345 Other mental disorders complicating the puerperium   M ♀
AHA: 2018,4Q,8

✓6ᵗʰ O99.35 Diseases of the nervous system complicating pregnancy, childbirth, and the puerperium
Conditions in G00-G99
EXCLUDES 2   pregnancy related peripheral neuritis (O26.8-)
O99.350 Diseases of the nervous system complicating pregnancy, unspecified trimester   M ♀
O99.351 Diseases of the nervous system complicating pregnancy, first trimester   M ♀
O99.352 Diseases of the nervous system complicating pregnancy, second trimester   M ♀
O99.353 Diseases of the nervous system complicating pregnancy, third trimester   M ♀
O99.354 Diseases of the nervous system complicating childbirth   M ♀
O99.355 Diseases of the nervous system complicating the puerperium   M ♀

✓5th O99.4 Diseases of the circulatory system complicating pregnancy, childbirth and the puerperium
Conditions in I00-I99
> EXCLUDES 1   peripartum cardiomyopathy (O90.3)
> EXCLUDES 2   hypertensive disorders (O10-O16)
> obstetric embolism (O88.-)
> venous complications and cerebrovenous sinus thrombosis in labor, childbirth and the puerperium (O87.-)
> venous complications and cerebrovenous sinus thrombosis in pregnancy (O22.-)

AHA: 2016,2Q,8

✓6th O99.41 Diseases of the circulatory system complicating pregnancy
- **O99.411 Diseases of the circulatory system complicating pregnancy, first trimester**   M ♀
- **O99.412 Diseases of the circulatory system complicating pregnancy, second trimester**   M ♀
- **O99.413 Diseases of the circulatory system complicating pregnancy, third trimester**   M ♀
- **O99.419 Diseases of the circulatory system complicating pregnancy, unspecified trimester**   M ♀

O99.42 Diseases of the circulatory system complicating childbirth   M ♀
O99.43 Diseases of the circulatory system complicating the puerperium   M ♀

✓5th O99.5 Diseases of the respiratory system complicating pregnancy, childbirth and the puerperium
Conditions in J00-J99

✓6th O99.51 Diseases of the respiratory system complicating pregnancy
- **O99.511 Diseases of the respiratory system complicating pregnancy, first trimester**   M ♀
- **O99.512 Diseases of the respiratory system complicating pregnancy, second trimester**   M ♀
- **O99.513 Diseases of the respiratory system complicating pregnancy, third trimester**   M ♀
- **O99.519 Diseases of the respiratory system complicating pregnancy, unspecified trimester**   M ♀

O99.52 Diseases of the respiratory system complicating childbirth   M ♀
O99.53 Diseases of the respiratory system complicating the puerperium   M ♀

✓5th O99.6 Diseases of the digestive system complicating pregnancy, childbirth and the puerperium
Conditions in K00-K93
> EXCLUDES 2   hemorrhoids in pregnancy (O22.4-)
> liver and biliary tract disorders in pregnancy, childbirth and the puerperium (O26.6-)

✓6th O99.61 Diseases of the digestive system complicating pregnancy
AHA: 2016,1Q,4
- **O99.611 Diseases of the digestive system complicating pregnancy, first trimester**   M ♀
- **O99.612 Diseases of the digestive system complicating pregnancy, second trimester**   M ♀
- **O99.613 Diseases of the digestive system complicating pregnancy, third trimester**   M ♀
- **O99.619 Diseases of the digestive system complicating pregnancy, unspecified trimester**   M ♀

O99.62 Diseases of the digestive system complicating childbirth   M ♀
O99.63 Diseases of the digestive system complicating the puerperium   M ♀

✓5th O99.7 Diseases of the skin and subcutaneous tissue complicating pregnancy, childbirth and the puerperium
Conditions in L00-L99
> EXCLUDES 2   herpes gestationis (O26.4)
> pruritic urticarial papules and plaques of pregnancy (PUPPP) (O26.86)

✓6th O99.71 Diseases of the skin and subcutaneous tissue complicating pregnancy
- **O99.711 Diseases of the skin and subcutaneous tissue complicating pregnancy, first trimester**   M ♀
- **O99.712 Diseases of the skin and subcutaneous tissue complicating pregnancy, second trimester**   M ♀
- **O99.713 Diseases of the skin and subcutaneous tissue complicating pregnancy, third trimester**   M ♀
- **O99.719 Diseases of the skin and subcutaneous tissue complicating pregnancy, unspecified trimester**   M ♀

O99.72 Diseases of the skin and subcutaneous tissue complicating childbirth   M ♀
O99.73 Diseases of the skin and subcutaneous tissue complicating the puerperium   M ♀

✓5th O99.8 Other specified diseases and conditions complicating pregnancy, childbirth and the puerperium
Conditions in D00-D48, H00-H95, M00-N99, and Q00-Q99
Use additional code to identify condition
> EXCLUDES 2   genitourinary infections in pregnancy (O23.-)
> infection of genitourinary tract following delivery ►(O86.1-O86.4)◄
> malignant neoplasm complicating pregnancy, childbirth and the puerperium (O9A.1-)
> maternal care for known or suspected abnormality of maternal pelvic organs (O34.-)
> postpartum acute kidney failure (O90.4)
> traumatic injuries in pregnancy (O9A.2-)

✓6th O99.81 Abnormal glucose complicating pregnancy, childbirth and the puerperium
> EXCLUDES 1   gestational diabetes (O24.4-)
- **O99.810 Abnormal glucose complicating pregnancy**   M ♀
- **O99.814 Abnormal glucose complicating childbirth**   M ♀
- **O99.815 Abnormal glucose complicating the puerperium**   M ♀

✓6th O99.82 Streptococcus B carrier state complicating pregnancy, childbirth and the puerperium
> EXCLUDES 1   carrier of streptococcus group B (GBS) in a nonpregnant woman (Z22.330)
DEF: *Streptococcus* group B colonization: Bacteria normally found in the vagina or lower intestine of many healthy adult women that may infect the fetus during childbirth, causing mental or physical handicaps or death. Women who test positive for *streptococcus* Group B during pregnancy are considered a "colonized" status and are treated with IV antibiotics at the time of delivery and may also be treated with oral antibiotics during the pregnancy.
- **O99.820 Streptococcus B carrier state complicating pregnancy**   M ♀
- **O99.824 Streptococcus B carrier state complicating childbirth**   M ♀
  AHA: 2019,2Q,8
- **O99.825 Streptococcus B carrier state complicating the puerperium**   M ♀

✓6th O99.83 Other infection carrier state complicating pregnancy, childbirth and the puerperium
Use additional code to identify the carrier state (Z22.-)
- **O99.830 Other infection carrier state complicating pregnancy**   M ♀
- **O99.834 Other infection carrier state complicating childbirth**   M ♀
- **O99.835 Other infection carrier state complicating the puerperium**   M ♀

✔ Additional Character Required   ✔x7th Placeholder Alert   Manifestation   Unspecified Dx   ►◄ Revised Text   ● New Code   ▲ Revised Title

ICD-10-CM 2020   883

√6ᵗʰ **O99.84** Bariatric surgery status **complicating pregnancy, childbirth and the puerperium**

Gastric banding status complicating pregnancy, childbirth and the puerperium

Gastric bypass status for obesity complicating pregnancy, childbirth and the puerperium

Obesity surgery status complicating pregnancy, childbirth and the puerperium

O99.840 Bariatric surgery status M ♀
complicating pregnancy, unspecified trimester

O99.841 Bariatric surgery status M ♀
complicating pregnancy, first **trimester**

O99.842 Bariatric surgery status M ♀
complicating pregnancy, second trimester

O99.843 Bariatric surgery status M ♀
complicating pregnancy, third **trimester**

O99.844 Bariatric surgery status M ♀
complicating childbirth

O99.845 Bariatric surgery status M ♀
complicating the puerperium

O99.89 Other specified diseases and conditions M ♀
complicating pregnancy, childbirth and the puerperium

√4ᵗʰ **O9A** **Maternal malignant neoplasms, traumatic injuries and abuse classifiable elsewhere but complicating pregnancy, childbirth and the puerperium**

√5ᵗʰ **O9A.1** Malignant neoplasm **complicating pregnancy, childbirth and the puerperium**

Conditions in C00-C96

Use additional code to identify neoplasm

> **EXCLUDES 2** *maternal care for benign tumor of corpus uteri (O34.1-)*
> *maternal care for benign tumor of cervix (O34.4-)*

AHA: 2015,3Q,19

√6ᵗʰ **O9A.11** **Malignant neoplasm complicating** pregnancy

O9A.111 Malignant neoplasm M ♀
complicating pregnancy, first **trimester**

O9A.112 Malignant neoplasm M ♀
complicating pregnancy, second trimester

O9A.113 Malignant neoplasm M ♀
complicating pregnancy, third **trimester**

O9A.119 Malignant neoplasm M ♀
complicating pregnancy, unspecified trimester

O9A.12 Malignant neoplasm complicating M ♀
childbirth

O9A.13 Malignant neoplasm complicating the M ♀
puerperium

√5ᵗʰ **O9A.2** Injury, poisoning and certain other consequences of external causes **complicating pregnancy, childbirth and the puerperium**

Conditions in S00-T88, except T74 and T76

Use additional code(s) to identify the injury or poisoning

> **EXCLUDES 2** *physical, sexual and psychological abuse complicating pregnancy, childbirth and the puerperium (O9A.3-, O9A.4-, O9A.5-)*

√6ᵗʰ **O9A.21** **Injury, poisoning and certain other consequences of external causes complicating** pregnancy

O9A.211 Injury, poisoning and certain M ♀
other consequences of external causes complicating pregnancy, first trimester

O9A.212 Injury, poisoning and certain M ♀
other consequences of external causes complicating pregnancy, second trimester

O9A.213 Injury, poisoning and certain M ♀
other consequences of external causes complicating pregnancy, third trimester

O9A.219 Injury, poisoning and certain M ♀
other consequences of external causes complicating pregnancy, unspecified trimester

O9A.22 Injury, poisoning and certain other M ♀
consequences of external causes complicating childbirth

O9A.23 Injury, poisoning and certain other M ♀
consequences of external causes complicating the puerperium

√5ᵗʰ **O9A.3** Physical abuse **complicating pregnancy, childbirth and the puerperium**

Conditions in T74.11 or T76.11

Use additional code (if applicable):
to identify any associated current injury due to physical abuse
to identify the perpetrator of abuse (Y07.-)

> **EXCLUDES 2** *sexual abuse complicating pregnancy, childbirth and the puerperium (O9A.4)*

√6ᵗʰ **O9A.31** **Physical abuse complicating** pregnancy

O9A.311 Physical abuse complicating M ♀
pregnancy, first trimester

O9A.312 Physical abuse complicating M ♀
pregnancy, second trimester

O9A.313 Physical abuse complicating M ♀
pregnancy, third trimester

O9A.319 Physical abuse complicating M ♀
pregnancy, unspecified trimester

O9A.32 Physical abuse complicating childbirth M ♀

O9A.33 Physical abuse complicating the M ♀
puerperium

√5ᵗʰ **O9A.4** Sexual abuse **complicating pregnancy, childbirth and the puerperium**

Conditions in T74.21 or T76.21

Use additional code (if applicable):
to identify any associated current injury due to sexual abuse
to identify the perpetrator of abuse (Y07.-)

√6ᵗʰ **O9A.41** **Sexual abuse complicating** pregnancy

O9A.411 Sexual abuse complicating M ♀
pregnancy, first trimester

O9A.412 Sexual abuse complicating M ♀
pregnancy, second trimester

O9A.413 Sexual abuse complicating M ♀
pregnancy, third trimester

O9A.419 Sexual abuse complicating M ♀
pregnancy, unspecified trimester

O9A.42 Sexual abuse complicating childbirth M ♀

O9A.43 Sexual abuse complicating the M ♀
puerperium

√5ᵗʰ **O9A.5** Psychological abuse **complicating pregnancy, childbirth and the puerperium**

Conditions in T74.31 or T76.31

Use additional code to identify the perpetrator of abuse (Y07.-)

√6ᵗʰ **O9A.51** **Psychological abuse complicating** pregnancy

O9A.511 Psychological abuse M ♀
complicating pregnancy, first trimester

O9A.512 Psychological abuse M ♀
complicating pregnancy, second trimester

O9A.513 Psychological abuse M ♀
complicating pregnancy, third trimester

O9A.519 Psychological abuse M ♀
complicating pregnancy, unspecified trimester

O9A.52 Psychological abuse complicating M ♀
childbirth

O9A.53 Psychological abuse complicating the M ♀
puerperium

Chapter 16. Certain Conditions Originating in the Perinatal Period (P00–P96)

Chapter-specific Guidelines with Coding Examples

The chapter-specific guidelines from the ICD-10-CM Official Guidelines for Coding and Reporting have been provided below. Along with these guidelines are coding examples, contained in the shaded boxes, that have been developed to help illustrate the coding and/or sequencing guidance found in these guidelines.

For coding and reporting purposes the perinatal period is defined as before birth through the 28th day following birth. The following guidelines are provided for reporting purposes

a. General Perinatal Rules

1) Use of chapter 16 codes

Codes in this chapter are never for use on the maternal record. Codes from Chapter 15, the obstetric chapter, are never permitted on the newborn record. Chapter 16 codes may be used throughout the life of the patient if the condition is still present.

2) Principal diagnosis for birth record

When coding the birth episode in a newborn record, assign a code from category Z38, Liveborn infants according to place of birth and type of delivery, as the principal diagnosis. A code from category Z38 is assigned only once, to a newborn at the time of birth. If a newborn is transferred to another institution, a code from category Z38 should not be used at the receiving hospital.

A code from category Z38 is used only on the newborn record, not on the mother's record.

3) Use of codes from other chapters with codes from chapter 16

Codes from other chapters may be used with codes from chapter 16 if the codes from the other chapters provide more specific detail. Codes for signs and symptoms may be assigned when a definitive diagnosis has not been established. If the reason for the encounter is a perinatal condition, the code from chapter 16 should be sequenced first.

4) Use of chapter 16 codes after the perinatal period

Should a condition originate in the perinatal period, and continue throughout the life of the patient, the perinatal code should continue to be used regardless of the patient's age.

> A 7-year-old patient with history of birth injury that resulted in Erb's palsy is seen for subscapularis release.
>
> **P14.0**   **Erb's paralysis due to birth injury**
>
> *Explanation:* Although in this instance Erb's palsy is specifically related to a birth injury, it has not resolved and continues to be a health concern. A perinatal code is appropriate even though this patient is beyond the perinatal period.

5) Birth process or community acquired conditions

If a newborn has a condition that may be either due to the birth process or community acquired and the documentation does not indicate which it is, the default is due to the birth process and the code from Chapter 16 should be used. If the condition is community-acquired, a code from Chapter 16 should not be assigned.

6) Code all clinically significant conditions

All clinically significant conditions noted on routine newborn examination should be coded. A condition is clinically significant if it requires:

clinical evaluation; or

therapeutic treatment; or

diagnostic procedures; or

extended length of hospital stay; or

increased nursing care and/or monitoring; or

has implications for future health care needs

Note: The perinatal guidelines listed above are the same as the general coding guidelines for "additional diagnoses", except for the final point regarding implications for future health care needs. Codes should be assigned for conditions that have been specified by the provider as having implications for future health care needs.

b. Observation and Evaluation of Newborns for Suspected Conditions not Found

1) Use of Z05 codes

Assign a code from category Z05, Observation and evaluation of newborns and infants for suspected conditions ruled out, to identify those instances when a healthy newborn is evaluated for a suspected condition that is determined after study not to be present. Do not use a code from category Z05 when the patient has identified signs or symptoms of a suspected problem; in such cases code the sign or symptom.

2) Z05 on other than the birth record

A code from category Z05 may also be assigned as a principal or first-listed code for readmissions or encounters when the code from category Z38 code no longer applies. Codes from category Z05 are for use only for healthy newborns and infants for which no condition after study is found to be present.

3) Z05 on a birth record

A code from category Z05 is to be used as a secondary code after the code from category Z38, Liveborn infants according to place of birth and type of delivery.

c. Coding additional perinatal diagnoses

1) Assigning codes for conditions that require treatment

Assign codes for conditions that require treatment or further investigation, prolong the length of stay, or require resource utilization.

2) Codes for conditions specified as having implications for future health care needs

Assign codes for conditions that have been specified by the provider as having implications for future health care needs.

Note: This guideline should not be used for adult patients.

d. Prematurity and fetal growth retardation

Providers utilize different criteria in determining prematurity. A code for prematurity should not be assigned unless it is documented. Assignment of codes in categories P05, Disorders of newborn related to slow fetal growth and fetal malnutrition, and P07, Disorders of newborn related to short gestation and low birth weight, not elsewhere classified, should be based on the recorded birth weight and estimated gestational age.

When both birth weight and gestational age are available, two codes from category P07 should be assigned, with the code for birth weight sequenced before the code for gestational age.

e. Low birth weight and immaturity status

Codes from category P07, Disorders of newborn related to short gestation and low birth weight, not elsewhere classified, are for use for a child or adult who was premature or had a low birth weight as a newborn and this is affecting the patient's current health status.

See Section I.C.21. Factors influencing health status and contact with health services, Status.

> A 35-year-old patient, who weighed 659 grams at birth, is seen for heart disease documented as being a consequence of the low birth weight.
>
> **I51.9**   **Heart disease, unspecified**
>
> **P07.02**   **Extremely low birth weight newborn, 500–749 grams**
>
> *Explanation:* A code from subcategories P07.0- and P07.1- is appropriate, regardless of the age of the patient, as long as the documentation provides a clear link between the patient's current illness and the low birth weight.

f. **Bacterial sepsis of newborn**

Category P36, Bacterial sepsis of newborn, includes congenital sepsis. If a perinate is documented as having sepsis without documentation of congenital or community acquired, the default is congenital and a code from category P36 should be assigned. If the P36 code includes the causal organism, an additional code from category B95, Streptococcus, Staphylococcus, and Enterococcus as the cause of diseases classified elsewhere, or B96, Other bacterial agents as the cause of diseases classified elsewhere, should not be assigned. If the P36 code does not include the causal organism, assign an additional code from category B96. If applicable, use additional codes to identify severe sepsis (R65.2-) and any associated acute organ dysfunction.

> A full-term infant born 7 days ago developed severe sepsis within 48 hours of discharge. The infant was readmitted. Cultures were taken, which came back positive for *E. coli*. The infant was stabilized and will now be transferred to a pediatric home health agency for an additional 2 weeks of IV antibiotic therapy administration.
>
> **P36.4**   **Sepsis of newborn due to Escherichia coli**
>
> **R65.2Ø**   **Severe sepsis without septic shock**
>
> *Explanation:* When the provider documentation does not specify whether sepsis in the newborn/perinate is congenital or community-acquired, the default code is from category P36 and the condition is assumed to be congenital. A code from chapter 1, "Certain Infectious and Parasitic Diseases," is not required as the sepsis code is a combination code that includes the organism.

g. **Stillbirth**

Code P95, Stillbirth, is only for use in institutions that maintain separate records for stillbirths. No other code should be used with P95. Code P95 should not be used on the mother's record.

Chapter 16. Certain Conditions Originating in the Perinatal Period (P00-P96)

NOTE   Codes from this chapter are for use on newborn records only, never on maternal records

INCLUDES   conditions that have their origin in the fetal or perinatal period (before birth through the first 28 days after birth) even if morbidity occurs later

EXCLUDES 2   congenital malformations, deformations and chromosomal abnormalities (Q00-Q99)
endocrine, nutritional and metabolic diseases (E00-E88)
injury, poisoning and certain other consequences of external causes (S00-T88)
neoplasms (C00-D49)
tetanus neonatorum (A33)

This chapter contains the following blocks:

P00-P04   Newborn affected by maternal factors and by complications of pregnancy, labor, and delivery
P05-P08   Disorders of newborn related to length of gestation and fetal growth
P09   Abnormal findings on neonatal screening
P10-P15   Birth trauma
P19-P29   Respiratory and cardiovascular disorders specific to the perinatal period
P35-P39   Infections specific to the perinatal period
P50-P61   Hemorrhagic and hematological disorders of newborn
P70-P74   Transitory endocrine and metabolic disorders specific to newborn
P76-P78   Digestive system disorders of newborn
P80-P83   Conditions involving the integument and temperature regulation of newborn
P84   Other problems with newborn
P90-P96   Other disorders originating in the perinatal period

Newborn affected by maternal factors and by complications of pregnancy, labor, and delivery (P00-P04)

NOTE   These codes are for use when the listed maternal conditions are specified as the cause of confirmed morbidity or potential morbidity which have their origin in the perinatal period (before birth through the first 28 days after birth).

AHA: 2016,4Q,54-55

√4ᵗʰ **P00**   **Newborn affected by** maternal conditions **that may be unrelated to present pregnancy**
   Code first any current condition in newborn
   EXCLUDES 2   encounter for observation of newborn for suspected diseases and conditions ruled out (Z05.-)
     newborn affected by maternal complications of pregnancy (P01.-)
     newborn affected by maternal endocrine and metabolic disorders (P70-P74)
     newborn affected by noxious substances transmitted via placenta or breast milk (P04.-)

   P00.0   **Newborn affected by maternal** hypertensive **disorders**
     Newborn affected by maternal conditions classifiable to O10-O11, O13-O16

   P00.1   **Newborn affected by maternal** renal and urinary tract **diseases**
     Newborn affected by maternal conditions classifiable to N00-N39

   P00.2   **Newborn affected by maternal** infectious and parasitic **diseases**
     Newborn affected by maternal infectious disease classifiable to A00-B99, J09 and J10
     EXCLUDES 1   maternal genital tract or other localized infections (P00.8)
     EXCLUDES 2   infections specific to the perinatal period (P35-P39)
     AHA: 2019,2Q,10; 2015,3Q,20

   P00.3   **Newborn affected by other maternal** circulatory and respiratory **diseases**
     Newborn affected by maternal conditions classifiable to I00-I99, J00-J99, Q20-Q34 and not included in P00.0, P00.2

   P00.4   **Newborn affected by maternal** nutritional **disorders**
     Newborn affected by maternal disorders classifiable to E40-E64
     Maternal malnutrition NOS

   P00.5   **Newborn affected by maternal** injury
     Newborn affected by maternal conditions classifiable to O9A.2-

   P00.6   **Newborn affected by** surgical procedure on mother
     Newborn affected by amniocentesis
     EXCLUDES 1   Cesarean delivery for present delivery (P03.4)
       damage to placenta from amniocentesis, Cesarean delivery or surgical induction (P02.1)
       previous surgery to uterus or pelvic organs (P03.89)
     EXCLUDES 2   newborn affected by complication of (fetal) intrauterine procedure (P96.5)

   P00.7   **Newborn affected by other medical procedures on mother, not elsewhere classified**
     Newborn affected by radiation to mother
     EXCLUDES 1   damage to placenta from amniocentesis, cesarean delivery or surgical induction (P02.1)
       newborn affected by other complications of labor and delivery (P03.-)

√5ᵗʰ   **P00.8**   **Newborn affected by other maternal conditions**
     P00.81   **Newborn affected by** periodontal disease **in mother**
     P00.89   **Newborn affected by other maternal conditions**
       Newborn affected by conditions classifiable to T80-T88
       Newborn affected by maternal genital tract or other localized infections
       Newborn affected by maternal systemic lupus erythematosus
       AHA: 2019,2Q,9

   P00.9   **Newborn affected by unspecified maternal condition**

√4ᵗʰ **P01**   **Newborn affected by** maternal complications of pregnancy
   Code first any current condition in newborn
   EXCLUDES 2   encounter for observation of newborn for suspected diseases and conditions ruled out (Z05.-)

   P01.0   **Newborn affected by** incompetent cervix
   P01.1   **Newborn affected by** premature rupture of membranes
   P01.2   **Newborn affected by** oligohydramnios
     EXCLUDES 1   oligohydramnios due to premature rupture of membranes (P01.1)
     DEF: Oligohydramnios: Low amniotic fluid level, resulting in underdeveloped organs in the fetus.

   P01.3   **Newborn affected by** polyhydramnios
     Newborn affected by hydramnios
     DEF: Polyhydramnios: Excess amniotic fluid surrounding the fetus, typically defined as a total fluid volume of greater than 24.0 cc.

   P01.4   **Newborn affected by** ectopic pregnancy
     Newborn affected by abdominal pregnancy

   P01.5   **Newborn affected by** multiple pregnancy
     Newborn affected by triplet (pregnancy)
     Newborn affected by twin (pregnancy)

   P01.6   **Newborn affected by** maternal death

   P01.7   **Newborn affected by** malpresentation before labor
     Newborn affected by breech presentation before labor
     Newborn affected by external version before labor
     Newborn affected by face presentation before labor
     Newborn affected by transverse lie before labor
     Newborn affected by unstable lie before labor

   P01.8   **Newborn affected by other maternal complications of pregnancy**
   P01.9   **Newborn affected by maternal complication of pregnancy, unspecified**

√4ᵗʰ **P02**   **Newborn affected by complications of** placenta, cord and membranes
   Code first any current condition in newborn
   EXCLUDES 2   encounter for observation of newborn for suspected diseases and conditions ruled out (Z05.-)

   P02.0   **Newborn affected by** placenta previa
     DEF: Placenta developed in the lower segment of the uterus that can cause hemorrhaging leading to preterm delivery.

   P02.1   **Newborn affected by other forms of placental** separation and hemorrhage
     Newborn affected by abruptio placenta
     Newborn affected by accidental hemorrhage
     Newborn affected by antepartum hemorrhage
     Newborn affected by damage to placenta from amniocentesis, cesarean delivery or surgical induction
     Newborn affected by maternal blood loss
     Newborn affected by premature separation of placenta

√5ᵗʰ   **P02.2**   **Newborn affected by other and unspecified** morphological and functional abnormalities **of placenta**
     P02.20   **Newborn affected by unspecified morphological and functional abnormalities of placenta**

Chapter 16. Certain Conditions Originating in the Perinatal Period

P02.29   **Newborn affected by other morphological and functional abnormalities of placenta**
Newborn affected by placental dysfunction
Newborn affected by placental infarction
Newborn affected by placental insufficiency

P02.3   **Newborn affected by** placental transfusion syndromes
Newborn affected by placental and cord abnormalities resulting in twin-to-twin or other transplacental transfusion

P02.4   **Newborn affected by** prolapsed cord

P02.5   **Newborn affected by other compression of umbilical cord**
Newborn affected by umbilical cord (tightly) around neck
Newborn affected by entanglement of umbilical cord
Newborn affected by knot in umbilical cord

✓5ᵗʰ **P02.6**   **Newborn affected by other and unspecified** conditions of umbilical cord

     P02.60   **Newborn affected by unspecified conditions of umbilical cord**

     P02.69   **Newborn affected by other conditions of umbilical cord**
Newborn affected by short umbilical cord
Newborn affected by vasa previa
EXCLUDES 1   *newborn affected by single umbilical artery (Q27.0)*

✓5ᵗʰ **P02.7**   **Newborn affected by** chorioamnionitis
AHA: 2018,4Q,23-24
DEF: Inflammation of the fetal membranes due to maternal infection characterized by fetal tachycardia, respiratory distress, apnea, weak cries, and poor sucking.

     P02.70   **Newborn affected by** fetal inflammatory response syndrome
Newborn affected by FIRS

     P02.78   **Newborn affected by other conditions from chorioamnionitis**
Newborn affected by amnionitis
Newborn affected by membranitis
Newborn affected by placentitis

P02.8   **Newborn affected by other abnormalities of membranes**

P02.9   **Newborn affected by abnormality of membranes, unspecified**

✓4ᵗʰ **P03**   **Newborn affected by other complications of** labor and delivery
Code first any current condition in newborn
EXCLUDES 2   *encounter for observation of newborn for suspected diseases and conditions ruled out (Z05.-)*

P03.0   **Newborn affected by** breech delivery and extraction

P03.1   **Newborn affected by other** malpresentation, malposition and disproportion **during labor and delivery**
Newborn affected by contracted pelvis
Newborn affected by conditions classifiable to O64-O66
Newborn affected by persistent occipitoposterior
Newborn affected by transverse lie

P03.2   **Newborn affected by** forceps **delivery**

Forceps Assisted Birth

Forceps extractor

P03.3   **Newborn affected by delivery by** vacuum extractor [ventouse]

Vacuum Assisted Birth

Vacuum extractor

P03.4   **Newborn affected by** Cesarean **delivery**

P03.5   **Newborn affected by** precipitate **delivery**
Newborn affected by rapid second stage

P03.6   **Newborn affected by** abnormal uterine contractions
Newborn affected by conditions classifiable to O62.-, except O62.3
Newborn affected by hypertonic labor
Newborn affected by uterine inertia

✓5ᵗʰ **P03.8**   **Newborn affected by other specified complications of labor and delivery**

     ✓6ᵗʰ **P03.81**   **Newborn affected by** abnormality in fetal (intrauterine) heart rate or rhythm
EXCLUDES 1   *neonatal cardiac dysrhythmia (P29.1-)*

         P03.810   **Newborn affected by abnormality in fetal (intrauterine) heart rate or rhythm** before the onset of labor

         P03.811   **Newborn affected by abnormality in fetal (intrauterine) heart rate or rhythm** during labor

         P03.819   **Newborn affected by abnormality in fetal (intrauterine) heart rate or rhythm, unspecified as to time of onset**

     P03.82   Meconium passage **during delivery**
EXCLUDES 1   *meconium aspiration (P24.00, P24.01)*
meconium staining (P96.83)
DEF: Fetal intestinal activity that increases in response to a fetomaternal distressed state during delivery. The anal sphincter relaxes and meconium is passed into the amniotic fluid.

     P03.89   **Newborn affected by other specified complications of labor and delivery**
Newborn affected by abnormality of maternal soft tissues
Newborn affected by conditions classifiable to O60-O75 and by procedures used in labor and delivery not included in P02.- and P03.0-P03.6
Newborn affected by induction of labor

P03.9   **Newborn affected by complication of labor and delivery, unspecified**

✓4ᵗʰ **P04**   **Newborn affected by** noxious substances transmitted via placenta or breast milk
INCLUDES   nonteratogenic effects of substances transmitted via placenta
EXCLUDES 2   *congenital malformations (Q00-Q99)*
encounter for observation of newborn for suspected diseases and conditions ruled out (Z05.-)
neonatal jaundice from excessive hemolysis due to drugs or toxins transmitted from mother (P58.4)
newborn in contact with and (suspected) exposures hazardous to health not transmitted via placenta or breast milk (Z77.-)

P04.0   **Newborn affected by maternal** anesthesia and analgesia **in pregnancy, labor and delivery**
Newborn affected by reactions and intoxications from maternal opiates and tranquilizers administered for procedures during pregnancy or labor and delivery
EXCLUDES 2   *newborn affected by other maternal medication (P04.1-)*

☑5ᵗʰ P04.1 Newborn affected by other maternal medication
Code first withdrawal symptoms from maternal use of drugs of addiction, if applicable (P96.1)
EXCLUDES 1 *dysmorphism due to warfarin (Q86.2)*
fetal hydantoin syndrome (Q86.1)
EXCLUDES 2 *maternal anesthesia and analgesia in pregnancy, labor and delivery (P04.0)*
maternal use of drugs of addiction (P04.4-)
AHA: 2018,4Q,24-25

P04.11 Newborn affected by maternal antineoplastic chemotherapy
P04.12 Newborn affected by maternal cytotoxic drugs
P04.13 Newborn affected by maternal use of anticonvulsants
P04.14 Newborn affected by maternal use of opiates
P04.15 Newborn affected by maternal use of antidepressants
P04.16 Newborn affected by maternal use of amphetamines
P04.17 Newborn affected by maternal use of sedative-hypnotics
P04.1A Newborn affected by maternal use of anxiolytics
P04.18 Newborn affected by other maternal medication
P04.19 Newborn affected by maternal use of unspecified medication

P04.2 Newborn affected by maternal use of tobacco
Newborn affected by exposure in utero to tobacco smoke
EXCLUDES 2 *newborn exposure to environmental tobacco smoke (P96.81)*

P04.3 Newborn affected by maternal use of alcohol
EXCLUDES 1 *fetal alcohol syndrome (Q86.0)*

☑5ᵗʰ P04.4 Newborn affected by maternal use of drugs of addiction
AHA: 2018,4Q,25
P04.40 Newborn affected by maternal use of unspecified drugs of addiction
P04.41 Newborn affected by maternal use of cocaine "Crack baby"
P04.42 Newborn affected by maternal use of hallucinogens
EXCLUDES 2 *newborn affected by other maternal medication (P04.1-)*
P04.49 Newborn affected by maternal use of other drugs of addiction
EXCLUDES 2 *newborn affected by maternal anesthesia and analgesia (P04.0)*
withdrawal symptoms from maternal use of drugs of addiction (P96.1)

P04.5 Newborn affected by maternal use of nutritional chemical substances
P04.6 Newborn affected by maternal exposure to environmental chemical substances
☑5ᵗʰ P04.8 Newborn affected by other maternal noxious substances
AHA: 2018,4Q,25
P04.81 Newborn affected by maternal use of cannabis
P04.89 Newborn affected by other maternal noxious substances
P04.9 Newborn affected by maternal noxious substance, unspecified

Disorders of newborn related to length of gestation and fetal growth (P05-P08)

☑4ᵗʰ P05 Disorders of newborn related to slow fetal growth and fetal malnutrition
AHA: 2016,4Q,55-56
☑5ᵗʰ P05.0 Newborn light for gestational age
Newborn light-for-dates
Weight below but length above 10th percentile for gestational age
P05.00 Newborn light for gestational age, unspecified weight
P05.01 Newborn light for gestational age, less than 500 grams
P05.02 Newborn light for gestational age, 500-749 grams
P05.03 Newborn light for gestational age, 750-999 grams
P05.04 Newborn light for gestational age, 1000-1249 grams
P05.05 Newborn light for gestational age, 1250-1499 grams

P05.06 Newborn light for gestational age, 1500-1749 grams
P05.07 Newborn light for gestational age, 1750-1999 grams
P05.08 Newborn light for gestational age, 2000-2499 grams
P05.09 Newborn light for gestational age, 2500 grams and over
Newborn light for gestational age, other

☑5ᵗʰ P05.1 Newborn small for gestational age
Newborn small-and-light-for-dates
Newborn small-for-dates
Weight and length below 10th percentile for gestational age
P05.10 Newborn small for gestational age, unspecified weight
P05.11 Newborn small for gestational age, less than 500 grams
P05.12 Newborn small for gestational age, 500-749 grams
P05.13 Newborn small for gestational age, 750-999 grams
P05.14 Newborn small for gestational age, 1000-1249 grams
P05.15 Newborn small for gestational age, 1250-1499 grams
P05.16 Newborn small for gestational age, 1500-1749 grams
P05.17 Newborn small for gestational age, 1750-1999 grams
P05.18 Newborn small for gestational age, 2000-2499 grams
P05.19 Newborn small for gestational age, other
Newborn small for gestational age, 2500 grams and over

P05.2 Newborn affected by fetal (intrauterine) malnutrition not light or small for gestational age
Infant, not light or small for gestational age, showing signs of fetal malnutrition, such as dry, peeling skin and loss of subcutaneous tissue
EXCLUDES 1 *newborn affected by fetal malnutrition with light for gestational age (P05.0-)*
newborn affected by fetal malnutrition with small for gestational age (P05.1-)

P05.9 Newborn affected by slow intrauterine growth, unspecified
Newborn affected by fetal growth retardation NOS

☑4ᵗʰ P07 Disorders of newborn related to short gestation and low birth weight, not elsewhere classified
NOTE When both birth weight and gestational age of the newborn are available, both should be coded with birth weight sequenced before gestational age
INCLUDES the listed conditions, without further specification, as the cause of morbidity or additional care, in newborn

☑5ᵗʰ P07.0 Extremely low birth weight newborn
Newborn birth weight 999 g. or less
EXCLUDES 1 *low birth weight due to slow fetal growth and fetal malnutrition (P05.-)*
P07.00 Extremely low birth weight newborn, unspecified weight
P07.01 Extremely low birth weight newborn, less than 500 grams
P07.02 Extremely low birth weight newborn, 500-749 grams
P07.03 Extremely low birth weight newborn, 750-999 grams

☑5ᵗʰ P07.1 Other low birth weight newborn
Newborn birth weight 1000-2499 g.
EXCLUDES 1 *low birth weight due to slow fetal growth and fetal malnutrition (P05.-)*
P07.10 Other low birth weight newborn, unspecified weight
P07.14 Other low birth weight newborn, 1000-1249 grams
P07.15 Other low birth weight newborn, 1250-1499 grams
P07.16 Other low birth weight newborn, 1500-1749 grams
P07.17 Other low birth weight newborn, 1750-1999 grams
P07.18 Other low birth weight newborn, 2000-2499 grams

Chapter 16. Certain Conditions Originating in the Perinatal Period

P07.2 Extreme immaturity of newborn
Less than 28 completed weeks (less than 196 completed days) of gestation.

P07.20 Extreme immaturity of newborn, unspecified weeks of gestation
Gestational age less than 28 completed weeks NOS

P07.21 Extreme immaturity of newborn, gestational age less than 23 completed weeks
Extreme immaturity of newborn, gestational age less than 23 weeks, 0 days

P07.22 Extreme immaturity of newborn, gestational age 23 completed weeks
Extreme immaturity of newborn, gestational age 23 weeks, 0 days through 23 weeks, 6 days

P07.23 Extreme immaturity of newborn, gestational age 24 completed weeks
Extreme immaturity of newborn, gestational age 24 weeks, 0 days through 24 weeks, 6 days

P07.24 Extreme immaturity of newborn, gestational age 25 completed weeks
Extreme immaturity of newborn, gestational age 25 weeks, 0 days through 25 weeks, 6 days

P07.25 Extreme immaturity of newborn, gestational age 26 completed weeks
Extreme immaturity of newborn, gestational age 26 weeks, 0 days through 26 weeks, 6 days

P07.26 Extreme immaturity of newborn, gestational age 27 completed weeks
Extreme immaturity of newborn, gestational age 27 weeks, 0 days through 27 weeks, 6 days

P07.3 Preterm [premature] newborn [other]
28 completed weeks or more but less than 37 completed weeks (196 completed days but less than 259 completed days) of gestation
Prematurity NOS
AHA: 2017,3Q,26

P07.30 Preterm newborn, unspecified weeks of gestation

P07.31 Preterm newborn, gestational age 28 completed weeks
Preterm newborn, gestational age 28 weeks, 0 days through 28 weeks, 6 days

P07.32 Preterm newborn, gestational age 29 completed weeks
Preterm newborn, gestational age 29 weeks, 0 days through 29 weeks, 6 days

P07.33 Preterm newborn, gestational age 30 completed weeks
Preterm newborn, gestational age 30 weeks, 0 days through 30 weeks, 6 days

P07.34 Preterm newborn, gestational age 31 completed weeks
Preterm newborn, gestational age 31 weeks, 0 days through 31 weeks, 6 days

P07.35 Preterm newborn, gestational age 32 completed weeks
Preterm newborn, gestational age 32 weeks, 0 days through 32 weeks, 6 days

P07.36 Preterm newborn, gestational age 33 completed weeks
Preterm newborn, gestational age 33 weeks, 0 days through 33 weeks, 6 days

P07.37 Preterm newborn, gestational age 34 completed weeks
Preterm newborn, gestational age 34 weeks, 0 days through 34 weeks, 6 days

P07.38 Preterm newborn, gestational age 35 completed weeks
Preterm newborn, gestational age 35 weeks, 0 days through 35 weeks, 6 days

P07.39 Preterm newborn, gestational age 36 completed weeks
Preterm newborn, gestational age 36 weeks, 0 days through 36 weeks, 6 days

P08 Disorders of newborn related to long gestation and high birth weight
NOTE: When both birth weight and gestational age of the newborn are available, priority of assignment should be given to birth weight
INCLUDES: the listed conditions, without further specification, as causes of morbidity or additional care, in newborn

P08.0 Exceptionally large newborn baby
Usually implies a birth weight of 4500 g. or more
EXCLUDES 1: syndrome of infant of diabetic mother (P70.1)
syndrome of infant of mother with gestational diabetes (P70.0)

P08.1 Other heavy for gestational age newborn
Other newborn heavy- or large-for-dates regardless of period of gestation
Usually implies a birth weight of 4000 g. to 4499 g.
EXCLUDES 1: newborn with a birth weight of 4500 or more (P08.0)
syndrome of infant of diabetic mother (P70.1)
syndrome of infant of mother with gestational diabetes (P70.0).

P08.2 Late newborn, not heavy for gestational age
AHA: 2014,1Q,14

P08.21 Post-term newborn
Newborn with gestation period over 40 completed weeks to 42 completed weeks

P08.22 Prolonged gestation of newborn
Newborn with gestation period over 42 completed weeks (294 days or more), not heavy- or large-for-dates.
Postmaturity NOS

Abnormal findings on neonatal screening (P09)

P09 Abnormal findings on neonatal screening
Use additional code to identify signs, symptoms and conditions associated with the screening
EXCLUDES 2: nonspecific serologic evidence of human immunodeficiency virus [HIV] (R75)

Birth trauma (P10-P15)

P10 Intracranial laceration and hemorrhage due to birth injury
EXCLUDES 1: intracranial hemorrhage of newborn NOS (P52.9)
intracranial hemorrhage of newborn due to anoxia or hypoxia (P52.-)
nontraumatic intracranial hemorrhage of newborn (P52.-)

P10.0 Subdural hemorrhage due to birth injury
Subdural hematoma (localized) due to birth injury
EXCLUDES 1: subdural hemorrhage accompanying tentorial tear (P10.4)

P10.1 Cerebral hemorrhage due to birth injury

P10.2 Intraventricular hemorrhage due to birth injury

P10.3 Subarachnoid hemorrhage due to birth injury

P10.4 Tentorial tear due to birth injury

P10.8 Other intracranial lacerations and hemorrhages due to birth injury

P10.9 Unspecified intracranial laceration and hemorrhage due to birth injury

P11 Other birth injuries to central nervous system

P11.0 Cerebral edema due to birth injury

P11.1 Other specified brain damage due to birth injury

P11.2 Unspecified brain damage due to birth injury

P11.3 Birth injury to facial nerve
Facial palsy due to birth injury

P11.4 Birth injury to other cranial nerves

P11.5 Birth injury to spine and spinal cord
Fracture of spine due to birth injury

P11.9 Birth injury to central nervous system, unspecified

☑4ᵗʰ **P12 Birth injury to** scalp

Birth Injuries to Scalp

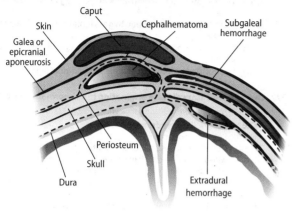

P12.0 **Cephalhematoma due to birth injury**
DEF: Condition that occurs in a neonate when blood vessels between the skull and periosteum rupture and blood collects in the subperiosteal space (below the periosteum). It is typically caused by prolonged labor or trauma due to instrument-assisted delivery (e.g., forceps, vacuum extraction), although in rare circumstances, it may indicate a linear skull fracture with intracranial hemorrhage.

P12.1 Chignon **(from vacuum extraction) due to birth injury**
DEF: Artificial swelling of the scalp that occurs when a collection of interstitial fluid and blood forms in the area of the scalp where the suction cup was applied during a vacuum-assisted delivery.

P12.2 **Epicranial subaponeurotic hemorrhage due to birth injury**
Subgaleal hemorrhage

P12.3 Bruising of scalp **due to birth injury**

P12.4 **Injury of scalp of newborn due to** monitoring equipment
Sampling incision of scalp of newborn
Scalp clip (electrode) injury of newborn

☑5ᵗʰ P12.8 **Other birth injuries to scalp**

P12.81 **Caput succedaneum**
DEF: Swelling of the scalp as a result of pressure being exerted on the head from the vaginal walls, uterus, or instrumentation used in assisting a delivery (e.g., vacuum).

P12.89 **Other birth injuries to scalp**

P12.9 **Birth injury to scalp, unspecified**

☑4ᵗʰ **P13 Birth injury to** skeleton
EXCLUDES 2 birth injury to spine (P11.5)

P13.0 Fracture of skull **due to birth injury**

P13.1 **Other birth injuries to skull**
EXCLUDES 1 cephalhematoma (P12.0)

P13.2 **Birth injury to** femur

P13.3 **Birth injury to other long bones**

P13.4 Fracture of clavicle **due to birth injury**

P13.8 **Birth injuries to other parts of skeleton**

P13.9 **Birth injury to skeleton, unspecified**

☑4ᵗʰ **P14 Birth injury to** peripheral nervous system

P14.0 Erb's paralysis **due to birth injury**
DEF: Erb's paralysis: Most common type of brachial plexus (peripheral nerve) injury in a neonate that involves nerve damage at the level of C5-C6. **Synonym(s):** Erb's palsy

P14.1 Klumpke's paralysis **due to birth injury**

P14.2 Phrenic nerve paralysis **due to birth injury**

P14.3 **Other brachial plexus birth injuries**

P14.8 **Birth injuries to other parts of peripheral nervous system**

P14.9 **Birth injury to peripheral nervous system, unspecified**

☑4ᵗʰ **P15 Other birth injuries**

P15.0 **Birth injury to** liver
Rupture of liver due to birth injury

P15.1 **Birth injury to** spleen
Rupture of spleen due to birth injury

P15.2 Sternomastoid **injury due to birth injury**

P15.3 **Birth injury to** eye
Subconjunctival hemorrhage due to birth injury
Traumatic glaucoma due to birth injury

P15.4 **Birth injury to** face
Facial congestion due to birth injury

P15.5 **Birth injury to** external genitalia

P15.6 Subcutaneous fat necrosis **due to birth injury**

P15.8 **Other specified birth injuries**
TIP: Use for any injury of newborn from scalpel.

P15.9 **Birth injury, unspecified**

Respiratory and cardiovascular disorders specific to the perinatal period (P19-P29)

☑4ᵗʰ **P19 Metabolic acidemia in newborn**
INCLUDES metabolic acidemia in newborn

P19.0 **Metabolic acidemia in newborn first noted** before onset of labor

P19.1 **Metabolic acidemia in newborn first noted** during labor

P19.2 **Metabolic acidemia noted** at birth

P19.9 **Metabolic acidemia, unspecified**

☑4ᵗʰ **P22 Respiratory distress of newborn**
EXCLUDES 1 *respiratory arrest of newborn (P28.81)*
respiratory failure of newborn NOS (P28.5)
AHA: 2019,2Q,29

P22.0 **Respiratory distress syndrome of newborn**
Cardiorespiratory distress syndrome of newborn
Hyaline membrane disease
Idiopathic respiratory distress syndrome [IRDS or RDS] of newborn
Pulmonary hypoperfusion syndrome
Respiratory distress syndrome, type I
EXCLUDES 2 ▶*respiratory arrest of newborn (P28.81)*◀
▶*respiratory failure of newborn NOS (P28.5)*◀
AHA: 2019,2Q,29
DEF: Severe chest contractions upon air intake and expiratory grunting. The infant appears blue due to oxygen deficiency and has a rapid respiratory rate, formerly called hyaline membrane disease.

P22.1 **Transient tachypnea of newborn**
Idiopathic tachypnea of newborn
Respiratory distress syndrome, type II
Wet lung syndrome
DEF: Rapid, labored breathing of a newborn. It is a short-term problem that begins after birth and lasts about three days.

P22.8 **Other respiratory distress of newborn**
EXCLUDES 1 ▶*respiratory arrest of newborn (P28.81)*◀
▶*respiratory failure of newborn NOS (P28.5)*◀

P22.9 **Respiratory distress of newborn, unspecified**
EXCLUDES 1 ▶*respiratory arrest of newborn (P28.81)*◀
▶*respiratory failure of newborn NOS (P28.5)*◀

☑4ᵗʰ **P23 Congenital pneumonia**
INCLUDES infective pneumonia acquired in utero or during birth
EXCLUDES 1 neonatal pneumonia resulting from aspiration (P24.-)

P23.0 **Congenital pneumonia due to** viral agent
Use additional code (B97) to identify organism
EXCLUDES 1 congenital rubella pneumonitis (P35.0)

P23.1 **Congenital pneumonia due to** Chlamydia

P23.2 **Congenital pneumonia due to** staphylococcus

P23.3 **Congenital pneumonia due to** streptococcus, group B

P23.4 **Congenital pneumonia due to** Escherichia coli

P23.5 **Congenital pneumonia due to** Pseudomonas

P23.6 **Congenital pneumonia due to other bacterial agents**
Congenital pneumonia due to Hemophilus influenzae
Congenital pneumonia due to Klebsiella pneumoniae
Congenital pneumonia due to Mycoplasma
Congenital pneumonia due to Streptococcus, except group B
Use additional code (B95-B96) to identify organism

P23.8 **Congenital pneumonia due to other organisms**

P23.9 **Congenital pneumonia, unspecified**

Chapter 16. Certain Conditions Originating in the Perinatal Period *(left margin)*

✓4ᵗʰ **P24 Neonatal aspiration**

INCLUDES   aspiration in utero and during delivery

✓5ᵗʰ **P24.0 Meconium aspiration**

EXCLUDES 1   meconium passage (without aspiration) during delivery (P03.82)
meconium staining (P96.83)

DEF: Meconium in the trachea or seen on chest x-ray after birth.

P24.00 Meconium aspiration without respiratory symptoms
Meconium aspiration NOS

P24.01 Meconium aspiration with respiratory symptoms
Meconium aspiration pneumonia
Meconium aspiration pneumonitis
Meconium aspiration syndrome NOS
Use additional code to identify any secondary pulmonary hypertension, if applicable (I27.2-)
DEF: Aspiration of fetal intestinal material during or prior to delivery. If is usually a complication of placental insufficiency, causing pneumonitis and bronchial obstruction (inflammatory reaction of lungs).

✓5ᵗʰ **P24.1 Neonatal aspiration of (clear)** amniotic fluid and mucus
Neonatal aspiration of liquor (amnii)

P24.10 Neonatal aspiration of (clear) amniotic fluid and mucus without respiratory symptoms
Neonatal aspiration of amniotic fluid and mucus NOS

P24.11 Neonatal aspiration of (clear) amniotic fluid and mucus with respiratory symptoms
Neonatal aspiration of amniotic fluid and mucus with pneumonia
Neonatal aspiration of amniotic fluid and mucus with pneumonitis
Use additional code to identify any secondary pulmonary hypertension, if applicable (I27.2-)

✓5ᵗʰ **P24.2 Neonatal aspiration of** blood

P24.20 Neonatal aspiration of blood without respiratory symptoms
Neonatal aspiration of blood NOS

P24.21 Neonatal aspiration of blood with respiratory symptoms
Neonatal aspiration of blood with pneumonia
Neonatal aspiration of blood with pneumonitis
Use additional code to identify any secondary pulmonary hypertension, if applicable (I27.2-)

✓5ᵗʰ **P24.3 Neonatal aspiration of** milk and regurgitated food
Neonatal aspiration of stomach contents

P24.30 Neonatal aspiration of milk and regurgitated food without respiratory symptoms
Neonatal aspiration of milk and regurgitated food NOS

P24.31 Neonatal aspiration of milk and regurgitated food with respiratory symptoms
Neonatal aspiration of milk and regurgitated food with pneumonia
Neonatal aspiration of milk and regurgitated food with pneumonitis
Use additional code to identify any secondary pulmonary hypertension, if applicable (I27.2-)

✓5ᵗʰ **P24.8 Other neonatal aspiration**

P24.80 Other neonatal aspiration without respiratory symptoms
Neonatal aspiration NEC

P24.81 Other neonatal aspiration with respiratory symptoms
Neonatal aspiration pneumonia NEC
Neonatal aspiration with pneumonitis NEC
Neonatal aspiration with pneumonia NOS
Neonatal aspiration with pneumonitis NOS
Use additional code to identify any secondary pulmonary hypertension, if applicable (I27.2-)

P24.9 Neonatal aspiration, unspecified

✓4ᵗʰ **P25 Interstitial emphysema and related conditions originating in the perinatal period**

P25.0 Interstitial emphysema originating in the perinatal period
P25.1 Pneumothorax originating in the perinatal period
P25.2 Pneumomediastinum originating in the perinatal period
P25.3 Pneumopericardium originating in the perinatal period
P25.8 Other conditions related to interstitial emphysema originating in the perinatal period

✓4ᵗʰ **P26 Pulmonary hemorrhage originating in the perinatal period**

EXCLUDES 1   acute idiopathic hemorrhage in infants over 28 days old (R04.81)

P26.0 Tracheobronchial hemorrhage originating in the perinatal period

P26.1 Massive pulmonary hemorrhage originating in the perinatal period

P26.8 Other pulmonary hemorrhages originating in the perinatal period

P26.9 Unspecified pulmonary hemorrhage originating in the perinatal period

✓4ᵗʰ **P27 Chronic respiratory disease originating in the perinatal period**

EXCLUDES 2   respiratory distress of newborn (P22.0-P22.9)

P27.0 Wilson-Mikity syndrome
Pulmonary dysmaturity
DEF: Pulmonary insufficiency in newborn babies, especially those with low birth weight. Rapid onset of hypercapnia and cyanosis occur during the first month of life frequently resulting in death.

P27.1 Bronchopulmonary dysplasia originating in the perinatal period

P27.8 Other chronic respiratory diseases originating in the perinatal period
Congenital pulmonary fibrosis
Ventilator lung in newborn

P27.9 Unspecified chronic respiratory disease originating in the perinatal period

✓4ᵗʰ **P28 Other respiratory conditions originating in the perinatal period**

EXCLUDES 1   congenital malformations of the respiratory system (Q30-Q34)

P28.0 Primary atelectasis of newborn
Primary failure to expand terminal respiratory units
Pulmonary hypoplasia associated with short gestation
Pulmonary immaturity NOS

✓5ᵗʰ **P28.1 Other and unspecified atelectasis of newborn**

P28.10 Unspecified atelectasis of newborn
Atelectasis of newborn NOS

P28.11 Resorption atelectasis without respiratory distress syndrome
EXCLUDES 1   resorption atelectasis with respiratory distress syndrome (P22.0)

P28.19 Other atelectasis of newborn
Partial atelectasis of newborn
Secondary atelectasis of newborn

P28.2 Cyanotic attacks of newborn
EXCLUDES 1   apnea of newborn (P28.3-P28.4)

P28.3 Primary sleep apnea of newborn
Central sleep apnea of newborn
Obstructive sleep apnea of newborn
Sleep apnea of newborn NOS
DEF: Unexplained cessation of breathing when a neonate makes no respiratory effort for 20 seconds or longer or when a neonate's breathing cessation is accompanied by cyanosis, bradycardia, or hypotonia.

P28.4 Other apnea of newborn
Apnea of prematurity
Obstructive apnea of newborn
EXCLUDES 1   obstructive sleep apnea of newborn (P28.3)

P28.5 Respiratory failure of newborn
EXCLUDES 1   respiratory arrest of newborn (P28.81)
respiratory distress of newborn (P22.0-)
AHA: 2019,2Q,29

✓5ᵗʰ **P28.8 Other specified respiratory conditions of newborn**

P28.81 Respiratory arrest of newborn

P28.89 Other specified respiratory conditions of newborn
Congenital laryngeal stridor
Sniffles in newborn
Snuffles in newborn
EXCLUDES 1   early congenital syphilitic rhinitis (A50.05)

P28.9 Respiratory condition of newborn, unspecified
Respiratory depression in newborn

✓4ᵗʰ **P29 Cardiovascular disorders originating in the perinatal period**

EXCLUDES 1   congenital malformations of the circulatory system (Q20-Q28)

P29.0 Neonatal cardiac failure

✓5ᵗʰ **P29.1 Neonatal cardiac dysrhythmia**

P29.11 Neonatal tachycardia

P29.12 Neonatal bradycardia

P29.2 Neonatal hypertension

N Newborn: 0   P Pediatric: 0-17   M Maternity: 12-55   A Adult: 15-124   CH Comorbidity High   CL Comorbidity Low   NCDx Noncancer Dx   PDx Primary Dx

892   ICD-10-CM 2020

√5ᵗʰ **P29.3 Persistent fetal circulation**
    AHA: 2017,4Q,20-21
    P29.30 Pulmonary hypertension of newborn
        Persistent pulmonary hypertension of newborn
        DEF: Condition that occurs when pressure within the pulmonary artery is elevated and vascular resistance is observed in the lungs.
    P29.38 Other persistent fetal circulation
        Delayed closure of ductus arteriosus

P29.4 Transient myocardial ischemia in newborn

√5ᵗʰ **P29.8 Other cardiovascular disorders originating in the perinatal period**
    P29.81 Cardiac arrest of newborn
    P29.89 Other cardiovascular disorders originating in the perinatal period
        AHA: 2014,4Q,23

P29.9 Cardiovascular disorder originating in the perinatal period, unspecified

Infections specific to the perinatal period (P35-P39)

Infections acquired in utero, during birth via the umbilicus, or during the first 28 days after birth

EXCLUDES 2   *asymptomatic human immunodeficiency virus [HIV] infection status (Z21)*
      congenital gonococcal infection (A54.-)
      congenital pneumonia (P23.-)
      congenital syphilis (A50.-)
      human immunodeficiency virus [HIV] disease (B20)
      infant botulism (A48.51)
      infectious diseases not specific to the perinatal period (A00-B99, J09, J10.-)
      intestinal infectious disease (A00-A09)
      laboratory evidence of human immunodeficiency virus [HIV] (R75)
      tetanus neonatorum (A33)

√4ᵗʰ **P35 Congenital viral diseases**
    INCLUDES   infections acquired in utero or during birth
    P35.0 Congenital rubella syndrome
        Congenital rubella pneumonitis
    P35.1 Congenital cytomegalovirus infection
    P35.2 Congenital herpesviral [herpes simplex] infection
    P35.3 Congenital viral hepatitis
    P35.4 Congenital Zika virus disease
        Use additional code to identify manifestations of congenital Zika virus disease
        AHA: 2018,4Q,25-26
    P35.8 Other congenital viral diseases
        Congenital varicella [chickenpox]
    P35.9 Congenital viral disease, unspecified

√4ᵗʰ **P36 Bacterial sepsis of newborn**
    INCLUDES   congenital sepsis
    Use additional code(s), if applicable, to identify severe sepsis (R65.2-) and associated acute organ dysfunction(s)
    P36.0 Sepsis of newborn due to streptococcus, group B
√5ᵗʰ   **P36.1 Sepsis of newborn due to other and unspecified streptococci**
        P36.10 Sepsis of newborn due to unspecified streptococci
        P36.19 Sepsis of newborn due to other streptococci
    P36.2 Sepsis of newborn due to Staphylococcus aureus
√5ᵗʰ   **P36.3 Sepsis of newborn due to other and unspecified staphylococci**
        P36.30 Sepsis of newborn due to unspecified staphylococci
        P36.39 Sepsis of newborn due to other staphylococci
    P36.4 Sepsis of newborn due to Escherichia coli
    P36.5 Sepsis of newborn due to anaerobes
    P36.8 Other bacterial sepsis of newborn
        Use additional code from category B96 to identify organism
    P36.9 Bacterial sepsis of newborn, unspecified

√4ᵗʰ **P37 Other congenital infectious and parasitic diseases**
    EXCLUDES 2   *congenital syphilis (A50.-)*
        infectious neonatal diarrhea (A00-A09)
        necrotizing enterocolitis in newborn (P77.-)
        noninfectious neonatal diarrhea (P78.3)
        ophthalmia neonatorum due to gonococcus (A54.31)
        tetanus neonatorum (A33)
    P37.0 Congenital tuberculosis
    P37.1 Congenital toxoplasmosis
        Hydrocephalus due to congenital toxoplasmosis
    P37.2 Neonatal (disseminated) listeriosis

P37.3 Congenital falciparum malaria
P37.4 Other congenital malaria
P37.5 Neonatal candidiasis
P37.8 Other specified congenital infectious and parasitic diseases
P37.9 Congenital infectious or parasitic disease, unspecified

√4ᵗʰ **P38 Omphalitis of newborn**
    EXCLUDES 1   *omphalitis not of newborn (L08.82)*
        tetanus omphalitis (A33)
        umbilical hemorrhage of newborn (P51.-)
    DEF: Omphalitis: Infection and inflammation of the umbilical stump, often due to bacteria that can spread beyond the umbilical stump to the fascia, muscle, or even the umbilical vessels.
    P38.1 Omphalitis with mild hemorrhage
    P38.9 Omphalitis without hemorrhage
        Omphalitis of newborn NOS

√4ᵗʰ **P39 Other infections specific to the perinatal period**
    Use additional code to identify organism or specific infection
    P39.0 Neonatal infective mastitis
        EXCLUDES 1   *breast engorgement of newborn (P83.4)*
            noninfective mastitis of newborn (P83.4)
    P39.1 Neonatal conjunctivitis and dacryocystitis
        Neonatal chlamydial conjunctivitis
        Ophthalmia neonatorum NOS
        EXCLUDES 1   *gonococcal conjunctivitis (A54.31)*
    P39.2 Intra-amniotic infection affecting newborn, not elsewhere classified
    P39.3 Neonatal urinary tract infection
    P39.4 Neonatal skin infection
        Neonatal pyoderma
        EXCLUDES 1   *pemphigus neonatorum (L00)*
            staphylococcal scalded skin syndrome (L00)
    P39.8 Other specified infections specific to the perinatal period
    P39.9 Infection specific to the perinatal period, unspecified

Hemorrhagic and hematological disorders of newborn (P50-P61)

EXCLUDES 1   *congenital stenosis and stricture of bile ducts (Q44.3)*
      Crigler-Najjar syndrome (E80.5)
      Dubin-Johnson syndrome (E80.6)
      Gilbert syndrome (E80.4)
      hereditary hemolytic anemias (D55-D58)

√4ᵗʰ **P50 Newborn affected by intrauterine (fetal) blood loss**
    EXCLUDES 1   *congenital anemia from intrauterine (fetal) blood loss (P61.3)*
    P50.0 Newborn affected by intrauterine (fetal) blood loss from vasa previa
    P50.1 Newborn affected by intrauterine (fetal) blood loss from ruptured cord
    P50.2 Newborn affected by intrauterine (fetal) blood loss from placenta
    P50.3 Newborn affected by hemorrhage into co-twin
    P50.4 Newborn affected by hemorrhage into maternal circulation
    P50.5 Newborn affected by intrauterine (fetal) blood loss from cut end of co-twin's cord
    P50.8 Newborn affected by other intrauterine (fetal) blood loss
    P50.9 Newborn affected by intrauterine (fetal) blood loss, unspecified
        Newborn affected by fetal hemorrhage NOS

√4ᵗʰ **P51 Umbilical hemorrhage of newborn**
    EXCLUDES 1   *omphalitis with mild hemorrhage (P38.1)*
        umbilical hemorrhage from cut end of co-twins cord (P50.5)
    P51.0 Massive umbilical hemorrhage of newborn
    P51.8 Other umbilical hemorrhages of newborn
        Slipped umbilical ligature NOS
    P51.9 Umbilical hemorrhage of newborn, unspecified

√4ᵗʰ **P52 Intracranial nontraumatic hemorrhage of newborn**
    INCLUDES   intracranial hemorrhage due to anoxia or hypoxia
    EXCLUDES 1   *intracranial hemorrhage due to birth injury (P10.-)*
        intracranial hemorrhage due to other injury (S06.-)
    P52.0 Intraventricular (nontraumatic) hemorrhage, grade 1, of newborn
        Subependymal hemorrhage (without intraventricular extension)
        Bleeding into germinal matrix

Chapter 16. Certain Conditions Originating in the Perinatal Period

P52.1   Intraventricular (nontraumatic) hemorrhage, grade 2, **of newborn**
Subependymal hemorrhage with intraventricular extension
Bleeding into ventricle

✓5ᵗʰ **P52.2   Intraventricular (nontraumatic) hemorrhage,** grade 3 and grade 4, **of newborn**

P52.21   Intraventricular (nontraumatic) hemorrhage, grade 3, **of newborn**
Subependymal hemorrhage with intraventricular extension with enlargement of ventricle

P52.22   Intraventricular (nontraumatic) hemorrhage, grade 4, **of newborn**
Bleeding into cerebral cortex
Subependymal hemorrhage with intracerebral extension

P52.3   Unspecified intraventricular (nontraumatic) hemorrhage of newborn

P52.4   Intracerebral (nontraumatic) hemorrhage of newborn

P52.5   Subarachnoid (nontraumatic) hemorrhage of newborn

P52.6   Cerebellar (nontraumatic) and posterior fossa hemorrhage of newborn

P52.8   Other intracranial (nontraumatic) hemorrhages of newborn

P52.9   Intracranial (nontraumatic) hemorrhage of newborn, unspecified

P53   Hemorrhagic disease of newborn
Vitamin K deficiency of newborn

✓4ᵗʰ **P54   Other neonatal hemorrhages**
EXCLUDES 1   *newborn affected by (intrauterine) blood loss (P50.-)*
pulmonary hemorrhage originating in the perinatal period (P26.-)

P54.0   Neonatal hematemesis
EXCLUDES 1   *neonatal hematemesis due to swallowed maternal blood (P78.2)*

P54.1   Neonatal melena
EXCLUDES 1   *neonatal melena due to swallowed maternal blood (P78.2)*

P54.2   Neonatal rectal hemorrhage

P54.3   Other neonatal gastrointestinal hemorrhage

P54.4   Neonatal adrenal hemorrhage

P54.5   Neonatal cutaneous hemorrhage
Neonatal bruising
Neonatal ecchymoses
Neonatal petechiae
Neonatal superficial hematomata
EXCLUDES 2   *bruising of scalp due to birth injury (P12.3)*
cephalhematoma due to birth injury (P12.0)

P54.6   Neonatal vaginal hemorrhage   ♀
Neonatal pseudomenses

P54.8   Other specified neonatal hemorrhages

P54.9   Neonatal hemorrhage, unspecified

✓4ᵗʰ **P55   Hemolytic disease of newborn**

P55.0   Rh isoimmunization of newborn
DEF: Incompatible Rh fetal-maternal blood grouping that prematurely destroys red blood cells. Symptoms include jaundice, asphyxia, pulmonary hypertension, edema, respiratory distress, kernicterus, and coagulopathies. It is detected by a Coombs test.

P55.1   ABO isoimmunization of newborn
AHA: 2015,3Q,20

P55.8   Other hemolytic diseases of newborn
AHA: 2018,3Q,24

P55.9   Hemolytic disease of newborn, unspecified

✓4ᵗʰ **P56   Hydrops fetalis due to hemolytic disease**
EXCLUDES 1   *hydrops fetalis NOS (P83.2)*

P56.0   Hydrops fetalis due to isoimmunization

✓5ᵗʰ **P56.9   Hydrops fetalis due to other and unspecified hemolytic disease**

P56.90   Hydrops fetalis due to unspecified hemolytic disease

P56.99   Hydrops fetalis due to other hemolytic disease

✓4ᵗʰ **P57   Kernicterus**

P57.0   Kernicterus due to isoimmunization
DEF: Complication of erythroblastosis fetalis associated with severe neural symptoms, high blood bilirubin levels, and nerve cell destruction. It results in bilirubin-pigmented gray matter of the central nervous system.

P57.8   Other specified kernicterus
EXCLUDES 1   *Crigler-Najjar syndrome (E80.5)*

P57.9   Kernicterus, unspecified

✓4ᵗʰ **P58   Neonatal jaundice due to other excessive hemolysis**
EXCLUDES 1   *jaundice due to isoimmunization (P55-P57)*

P58.0   Neonatal jaundice due to bruising

P58.1   Neonatal jaundice due to bleeding

P58.2   Neonatal jaundice due to infection

P58.3   Neonatal jaundice due to polycythemia

✓5ᵗʰ **P58.4   Neonatal jaundice due to** drugs or toxins **transmitted from mother or given to newborn**
Code first poisoning due to drug or toxin, if applicable (T36-T65 with fifth or sixth character 1-4 or 6)
Use additional code for adverse effect, if applicable, to identify drug (T36-T50 with fifth or sixth character 5)

P58.41   Neonatal jaundice due to drugs or toxins transmitted from mother

P58.42   Neonatal jaundice due to drugs or toxins given to newborn

P58.5   Neonatal jaundice due to swallowed maternal blood

P58.8   Neonatal jaundice due to other specified excessive hemolysis

P58.9   Neonatal jaundice due to excessive hemolysis, unspecified

✓4ᵗʰ **P59   Neonatal jaundice from other and unspecified causes**
EXCLUDES 1   *jaundice due to inborn errors of metabolism (E70-E88)*
kernicterus (P57.-)

P59.0   Neonatal jaundice associated with preterm delivery
Hyperbilirubinemia of prematurity
Jaundice due to delayed conjugation associated with preterm delivery

P59.1   Inspissated bile syndrome
DEF: Biliary obstruction in newborn resulting from obstruction of outflow tract.

✓5ᵗʰ **P59.2   Neonatal jaundice from other and unspecified** hepatocellular damage
EXCLUDES 1   *congenital viral hepatitis (P35.3)*

P59.20   Neonatal jaundice from unspecified hepatocellular damage

P59.29   Neonatal jaundice from other hepatocellular damage
Neonatal giant cell hepatitis
Neonatal (idiopathic) hepatitis

P59.3   Neonatal jaundice from breast milk inhibitor

P59.8   Neonatal jaundice from other specified causes

P59.9   Neonatal jaundice, unspecified
Neonatal physiological jaundice (intense)(prolonged) NOS
AHA: 2015,3Q,20

P60   Disseminated intravascular coagulation of newborn
Defibrination syndrome of newborn

✓4ᵗʰ **P61   Other perinatal hematological disorders**
EXCLUDES 1   *transient hypogammaglobulinemia of infancy (D80.7)*

P61.0   Transient neonatal thrombocytopenia
Neonatal thrombocytopenia due to exchange transfusion
Neonatal thrombocytopenia due to idiopathic maternal thrombocytopenia
Neonatal thrombocytopenia due to isoimmunization
DEF: Temporary decrease in blood platelets of a newborn that is secondary to placental insufficiency.

P61.1   Polycythemia neonatorum
DEF: Abnormal increase of total red blood cells of a newborn that results in hyperviscosity, which slows the flow of blood through small blood vessels.

P61.2   Anemia of prematurity

P61.3   Congenital anemia from fetal blood loss

P61.4   Other congenital anemias, not elsewhere classified
Congenital anemia NOS

P61.5   Transient neonatal neutropenia
EXCLUDES 1   *congenital neutropenia (nontransient) (D70.0)*
DEF: Low blood neutrophil counts of newborn that occurs due to maternal hypertension, sepsis, twin-twin transfusion, alloimmunization, and hemolytic disease.

P61.6   Other transient neonatal disorders of coagulation

P61.8   Other specified perinatal hematological disorders

P61.9   Perinatal hematological disorder, unspecified

Transitory endocrine and metabolic disorders specific to newborn (P70-P74)

INCLUDES   transitory endocrine and metabolic disturbances caused by the infant's response to maternal endocrine and metabolic factors, or its adjustment to extrauterine environment

AHA: 2018,2Q,6

✓4ᵗʰ **P70 Transitory disorders of carbohydrate metabolism specific to newborn**

P70.0 Syndrome of infant of mother with gestational diabetes
Newborn (with hypoglycemia) affected by maternal gestational diabetes
> EXCLUDES 1   newborn (with hypoglycemia) affected by maternal (pre-existing) diabetes mellitus (P70.1)
> syndrome of infant of a diabetic mother (P70.1)

P70.1 Syndrome of infant of a diabetic mother
Newborn (with hypoglycemia) affected by maternal (pre-existing) diabetes mellitus
> EXCLUDES 1   newborn (with hypoglycemia) affected by maternal gestational diabetes (P70.0)
> syndrome of infant of mother with gestational diabetes (P70.0)

P70.2 Neonatal diabetes mellitus

P70.3 Iatrogenic neonatal hypoglycemia

P70.4 Other neonatal hypoglycemia
Transitory neonatal hypoglycemia

P70.8 Other transitory disorders of carbohydrate metabolism of newborn

P70.9 Transitory disorder of carbohydrate metabolism of newborn, unspecified

✓4ᵗʰ **P71 Transitory neonatal disorders of calcium and magnesium metabolism**

P71.0 Cow's milk hypocalcemia in newborn

P71.1 Other neonatal hypocalcemia
> EXCLUDES 1   neonatal hypoparathyroidism (P71.4)

P71.2 Neonatal hypomagnesemia

P71.3 Neonatal tetany without calcium or magnesium deficiency
Neonatal tetany NOS

P71.4 Transitory neonatal hypoparathyroidism

P71.8 Other transitory neonatal disorders of calcium and magnesium metabolism
AHA: 2016,4Q,54

P71.9 Transitory neonatal disorder of calcium and magnesium metabolism, unspecified

✓4ᵗʰ **P72 Other transitory neonatal endocrine disorders**
> EXCLUDES 1   congenital hypothyroidism with or without goiter (E03.0-E03.1)
> dyshormogenetic goiter (E07.1)
> Pendred's syndrome (E07.1)

P72.0 Neonatal goiter, not elsewhere classified
Transitory congenital goiter with normal functioning

P72.1 Transitory neonatal hyperthyroidism
Neonatal thyrotoxicosis

P72.2 Other transitory neonatal disorders of thyroid function, not elsewhere classified
Transitory neonatal hypothyroidism

P72.8 Other specified transitory neonatal endocrine disorders

P72.9 Transitory neonatal endocrine disorder, unspecified

✓4ᵗʰ **P74 Other transitory neonatal electrolyte and metabolic disturbances**
AHA: 2018,4Q,26-27

P74.0 Late metabolic acidosis of newborn
> EXCLUDES 1   (fetal) metabolic acidosis of newborn (P19)

P74.1 Dehydration of newborn

✓5ᵗʰ **P74.2 Disturbances of sodium balance of newborn**

    P74.21 Hypernatremia of newborn

    P74.22 Hyponatremia of newborn

✓5ᵗʰ **P74.3 Disturbances of potassium balance of newborn**

    P74.31 Hyperkalemia of newborn

    P74.32 Hypokalemia of newborn

✓5ᵗʰ **P74.4 Other transitory electrolyte disturbances of newborn**

    P74.41 Alkalosis of newborn
    Hyperbicarbonatemia

✓6ᵗʰ **P74.42 Disturbances of chlorine balance of newborn**

    P74.421 Hyperchloremia of newborn
    Hyperchloremic metabolic acidosis
> EXCLUDES 2   late metabolic acidosis of the newborn ▶(P74.0)◀

    P74.422 Hypochloremia of newborn

    P74.49 Other transitory electrolyte disturbance of newborn

P74.5 Transitory tyrosinemia of newborn

P74.6 Transitory hyperammonemia of newborn

P74.8 Other transitory metabolic disturbances of newborn
Amino-acid metabolic disorders described as transitory

P74.9 Transitory metabolic disturbance of newborn, unspecified

Digestive system disorders of newborn (P76-P78)

✓4ᵗʰ **P76 Other intestinal obstruction of newborn**

P76.0 Meconium plug syndrome
Meconium ileus NOS
> EXCLUDES 1   meconium ileus in cystic fibrosis (E84.11)
DEF: Meconium obstruction of a newborn's intestines, resulting from unusually thick or hard meconium.

P76.1 Transitory ileus of newborn
> EXCLUDES 1   Hirschsprung's disease (Q43.1)

P76.2 Intestinal obstruction due to inspissated milk

P76.8 Other specified intestinal obstruction of newborn
> EXCLUDES 1   intestinal obstruction classifiable to K56.-

P76.9 Intestinal obstruction of newborn, unspecified

✓4ᵗʰ **P77 Necrotizing enterocolitis of newborn**
DEF: Serious intestinal infection and inflammation in preterm infants. Severity is measured by stages and may progress to life-threatening perforation or peritonitis. Resection surgical treatment may be necessary.

P77.1 Stage 1 necrotizing enterocolitis in newborn
Necrotizing enterocolitis without pneumatosis, without perforation
DEF: Broad-spectrum symptoms with nonspecific signs, including feeding intolerance, abdominal distention, bradycardia, and metabolic abnormalities.

P77.2 Stage 2 necrotizing enterocolitis in newborn
Necrotizing enterocolitis with pneumatosis, without perforation
DEF: Radiographic confirmation of necrotizing enterocolitis showing intestinal dilatation, fixed loops of bowels, pneumatosis intestinalis, metabolic acidosis, and thrombocytopenia.

P77.3 Stage 3 necrotizing enterocolitis in newborn
Necrotizing enterocolitis with perforation
Necrotizing enterocolitis with pneumatosis and perforation
DEF: Advanced stage in which an infant demonstrates signs of bowel perforation, septic shock, metabolic acidosis, ascites, disseminated intravascular coagulopathy, and neutropenia.

P77.9 Necrotizing enterocolitis in newborn, unspecified
Necrotizing enterocolitis in newborn, NOS

✓4ᵗʰ **P78 Other perinatal digestive system disorders**
> EXCLUDES 1   cystic fibrosis (E84.0-E84.9)
> neonatal gastrointestinal hemorrhages (P54.0-P54.3)

P78.0 Perinatal intestinal perforation
Meconium peritonitis

P78.1 Other neonatal peritonitis
Neonatal peritonitis NOS

P78.2 Neonatal hematemesis and melena due to swallowed maternal blood

P78.3 Noninfective neonatal diarrhea
Neonatal diarrhea NOS

✓5ᵗʰ **P78.8 Other specified perinatal digestive system disorders**

    P78.81 Congenital cirrhosis (of liver)

    P78.82 Peptic ulcer of newborn

    P78.83 Newborn esophageal reflux
    Neonatal esophageal reflux

    P78.84 Gestational alloimmune liver disease
    GALD
    Neonatal hemochromatosis
> EXCLUDES 1   hemochromatosis (E83.11-)
    AHA: 2017,4Q,21
    DEF: Severe hepatic injury with onset during fetal development with manifestations beginning during fetal life. It is due to maternal antibodies to fetal hepatic cells (hepatocytes) that cross the placenta into the fetal circulation, causing hepatic cell necrosis.

    P78.89 Other specified perinatal digestive system disorders

P78.9 Perinatal digestive system disorder, unspecified

✓ Additional Character Required   ✓x7ᵗʰ Placeholder Alert   Manifestation   Unspecified Dx   ▶◀ Revised Text   ● New Code   ▲ Revised Title

ICD-10-CM 2020   895

Chapter 16. Certain Conditions Originating in the Perinatal Period

Conditions involving the integument and temperature regulation of newborn (P80-P83)

☑4ᵗʰ P80 Hypothermia of newborn
DEF: Decrease in newborn body temperature due to their larger ratio of surface area to body weight, thin skin with blood vessels close to the surface, and a limited amount of subcutaneous fat.

P80.0 Cold injury syndrome
Severe and usually chronic hypothermia associated with a pink flushed appearance, edema and neurological and biochemical abnormalities.
EXCLUDES 1 *mild hypothermia of newborn (P80.8)*

P80.8 Other hypothermia of newborn
Mild hypothermia of newborn

P80.9 Hypothermia of newborn, unspecified

☑4ᵗʰ P81 Other disturbances of temperature regulation of newborn

P81.0 Environmental hyperthermia of newborn

P81.8 Other specified disturbances of temperature regulation of newborn

P81.9 Disturbance of temperature regulation of newborn, unspecified
Fever of newborn NOS

☑4ᵗʰ P83 Other conditions of integument specific to newborn
EXCLUDES 1 *congenital malformations of skin and integument (Q80-Q84)*
hydrops fetalis due to hemolytic disease (P56.-)
neonatal skin infection (P39.4)
staphylococcal scalded skin syndrome (L00)
EXCLUDES 2 *cradle cap (L21.0)*
diaper [napkin] dermatitis (L22)

P83.0 Sclerema neonatorum
DEF: Diffuse, rapidly progressing white, waxy, nonpitting hardening of tissue, usually of legs and feet that is life-threatening. It is found in preterm or debilitated infants. Etiology is unknown.

P83.1 Neonatal erythema toxicum

P83.2 Hydrops fetalis not due to hemolytic disease
Hydrops fetalis NOS
DEF: Severe, life-threatening problem of a newborn characterized by severe edema of the entire body. It is unrelated to immune response.

☑5ᵗʰ P83.3 Other and unspecified edema specific to newborn
P83.30 Unspecified edema specific to newborn
P83.39 Other edema specific to newborn

P83.4 Breast engorgement of newborn
Noninfective mastitis of newborn

P83.5 Congenital hydrocele ♂
DEF: Hydrocele: Serous fluid that collects in the tunica vaginalis of the scrotum along the spermatic cord in males.

P83.6 Umbilical polyp of newborn

☑5ᵗʰ P83.8 Other specified conditions of integument specific to newborn
AHA: 2017,4Q,21-22
P83.81 Umbilical granuloma
EXCLUDES 2 *granulomatous disorder of the skin and subcutaneous tissue, unspecified (L92.9)*
P83.88 Other specified conditions of integument specific to newborn
Bronze baby syndrome
Neonatal scleroderma
Urticaria neonatorum

P83.9 Condition of the integument specific to newborn, unspecified

Other problems with newborn (P84)

P84 Other problems with newborn
Acidemia of newborn
Acidosis of newborn
Anoxia of newborn NOS
Asphyxia of newborn NOS
Hypercapnia of newborn
Hypoxemia of newborn
Hypoxia of newborn NOS
Mixed metabolic and respiratory acidosis of newborn
EXCLUDES 1 *intracranial hemorrhage due to anoxia or hypoxia (P52.-)*
hypoxic ischemic encephalopathy [HIE] (P91.6-)
late metabolic acidosis of newborn (P74.0)

Other disorders originating in the perinatal period (P90-P96)

P90 Convulsions of newborn
EXCLUDES 1 *benign myoclonic epilepsy in infancy (G40.3-)*
benign neonatal convulsions (familial) (G40.3-)

☑4ᵗʰ P91 Other disturbances of cerebral status of newborn
P91.0 Neonatal cerebral ischemia
P91.1 Acquired periventricular cysts of newborn
P91.2 Neonatal cerebral leukomalacia
Periventricular leukomalacia
P91.3 Neonatal cerebral irritability
P91.4 Neonatal cerebral depression
P91.5 Neonatal coma
☑5ᵗʰ P91.6 Hypoxic ischemic encephalopathy [HIE]
EXCLUDES 1 *neonatal cerebral depression (P91.4)*
neonatal cerebral irritability (P91.3)
neonatal coma (P91.5)
AHA: 2017,4Q,22
P91.60 Hypoxic ischemic encephalopathy [HIE], unspecified
P91.61 Mild hypoxic ischemic encephalopathy [HIE]
P91.62 Moderate hypoxic ischemic encephalopathy [HIE]
P91.63 Severe hypoxic ischemic encephalopathy [HIE]
☑5ᵗʰ P91.8 Other specified disturbances of cerebral status of newborn
AHA: 2017,4Q,22
☑6ᵗʰ P91.81 Neonatal encephalopathy
P91.811 Neonatal encephalopathy in diseases classified elsewhere
Code first underlying condition, if known, such as:
congenital cirrhosis (of liver) (P78.81)
intracranial nontraumatic hemorrhage of newborn (P52.-)
kernicterus (P57.-)
P91.819 Neonatal encephalopathy, unspecified
P91.88 Other specified disturbances of cerebral status of newborn
P91.9 Disturbance of cerebral status of newborn, unspecified

☑4ᵗʰ P92 Feeding problems of newborn
EXCLUDES 1 *eating disorders (F50.-)*
feeding problems in child over 28 days old (R63.3)
AHA: 2016,3Q,19
☑5ᵗʰ P92.0 Vomiting of newborn
EXCLUDES 1 *vomiting of child over 28 days old (R11.-)*
P92.01 Bilious vomiting of newborn
EXCLUDES 1 *bilious vomiting in child over 28 days old (R11.14)*
P92.09 Other vomiting of newborn
EXCLUDES 1 *regurgitation of food in newborn (P92.1)*
P92.1 Regurgitation and rumination of newborn
P92.2 Slow feeding of newborn
P92.3 Underfeeding of newborn
P92.4 Overfeeding of newborn
P92.5 Neonatal difficulty in feeding at breast
AHA: 2017,1Q,28
P92.6 Failure to thrive in newborn
EXCLUDES 1 *failure to thrive in child over 28 days old (R62.51)*
P92.8 Other feeding problems of newborn
P92.9 Feeding problem of newborn, unspecified

☑4ᵗʰ P93 Reactions and intoxications due to drugs administered to newborn
INCLUDES reactions and intoxications due to drugs administered to fetus affecting newborn
EXCLUDES 1 *jaundice due to drugs or toxins transmitted from mother or given to newborn (P58.4-)*
reactions and intoxications from maternal opiates, tranquilizers and other medication (P04.0-P04.1, P04.4-)
withdrawal symptoms from maternal use of drugs of addiction (P96.1)
withdrawal symptoms from therapeutic use of drugs in newborn (P96.2)
P93.0 Grey baby syndrome
Grey syndrome from chloramphenicol administration in newborn

P93.8 **Other reactions and intoxications due to drugs administered to newborn**
Use additional code for adverse effect, if applicable, to identify drug (T36-T50 with fifth or sixth character 5)

√4ᵗʰ P94 Disorders of muscle tone of newborn

P94.0 Transient neonatal myasthenia gravis
　EXCLUDES 1　myasthenia gravis (G70.0)

P94.1 Congenital hypertonia

P94.2 Congenital hypotonia
Floppy baby syndrome, unspecified

P94.8 Other disorders of muscle tone of newborn

P94.9 Disorder of muscle tone of newborn, unspecified

P95 Stillbirth
Deadborn fetus NOS
Fetal death of unspecified cause
Stillbirth NOS
　EXCLUDES 1　maternal care for intrauterine death (O36.4)
　　　　missed abortion (O02.1)
　　　　outcome of delivery, stillbirth (Z37.1, Z37.3, Z37.4, Z37.7)

√4ᵗʰ P96 Other conditions originating in the perinatal period

P96.0 Congenital renal failure
Uremia of newborn

P96.1 Neonatal withdrawal symptoms from maternal use of drugs of addiction
Drug withdrawal syndrome in infant of dependent mother
Neonatal abstinence syndrome
　EXCLUDES 1　reactions and intoxications from maternal opiates and tranquilizers administered during labor and delivery (P04.0)
　AHA: 2018,4Q,24-25

P96.2 Withdrawal symptoms from therapeutic use of drugs in newborn

P96.3 Wide cranial sutures of newborn
Neonatal craniotabes

P96.5 Complication to newborn due to (fetal) intrauterine procedure
　EXCLUDES 2　newborn affected by amniocentesis (P00.6)

√5ᵗʰ P96.8 Other specified conditions originating in the perinatal period

P96.81 Exposure to (parental) (environmental) tobacco smoke in the perinatal period
　EXCLUDES 2　newborn affected by in utero exposure to tobacco (P04.2)
　　　　exposure to environmental tobacco smoke after the perinatal period (Z77.22)

P96.82 Delayed separation of umbilical cord

P96.83 Meconium staining
　EXCLUDES 1　meconium aspiration (P24.00, P24.01)
　　　　meconium passage during delivery (P03.82)
　DEF: Meconium passed in utero causing discoloration on the fetal skin and nails or on the umbilicus. This staining may be incidental or may be an indicator of significant fetal stress that could affect outcomes.

P96.89 Other specified conditions originating in the perinatal period
Use additional code to specify condition

P96.9 Condition originating in the perinatal period, unspecified
Congenital debility NOS

Chapter 17. Congenital Malformations, Deformations and Chromosomal Abnormalities (Q00–Q99)

Chapter-specific Guidelines with Coding Examples

The chapter-specific guidelines from the ICD-10-CM Official Guidelines for Coding and Reporting have been provided below. Along with these guidelines are coding examples, contained in the shaded boxes, that have been developed to help illustrate the coding and/or sequencing guidance found in these guidelines.

Assign an appropriate code(s) from categories Q00–Q99, Congenital malformations, deformations, and chromosomal abnormalities when a malformation/deformation or chromosomal abnormality is documented. A malformation/deformation/or chromosomal abnormality may be the principal/first-listed diagnosis on a record or a secondary diagnosis.

When a malformation/deformation/or chromosomal abnormality does not have a unique code assignment, assign additional code(s) for any manifestations that may be present.

When the code assignment specifically identifies the malformation/deformation/or chromosomal abnormality, manifestations that are an inherent component of the anomaly should not be coded separately. Additional codes should be assigned for manifestations that are not an inherent component.

8-day-old infant with tetralogy of Fallot and pulmonary stenosis

Q21.3   **Tetralogy of Fallot**

Explanation: Pulmonary stenosis is inherent in the disease process of tetralogy of Fallot. When the code assignment specifically identifies the malformation/deformation/or chromosomal abnormality, manifestations that are inherent components of the anomaly should not be coded separately.

7-month-old infant with Down syndrome and common atrioventricular canal

Q90.9   **Down syndrome, unspecified**

Q21.2   **Atrioventricular septal defect**

Explanation: While a common atrioventricular canal is often associated with patients with Down syndrome, this manifestation is not an inherent component and may be reported separately. When the code assignment specifically identifies the anomaly, manifestations that are inherent components of the condition should not be coded separately. Additional codes should be assigned for manifestations that are not inherent components.

Codes from Chapter 17 may be used throughout the life of the patient. If a congenital malformation or deformity has been corrected, a personal history code should be used to identify the history of the malformation or deformity. Although present at birth, **a** malformation/deformation/or chromosomal abnormality may not be identified until later in life. Whenever the condition is diagnosed by the **provider**, it is appropriate to assign a code from codes Q00-Q99. For the birth admission, the appropriate code from category Z38, Liveborn infants, according to place of birth and type of delivery, should be sequenced as the principal diagnosis, followed by any congenital anomaly codes, Q00- Q99.

Three-year-old with history of corrected ventricular septal defect

Z87.74   **Personal history of (corrected) congenital malformations of heart and circulatory system**

Explanation: If a congenital malformation or deformity has been corrected, a personal history code should be used to identify the history of the malformation or deformity.

Forty-year-old man with headaches diagnosed with congenital arteriovenous malformation by brain scan

Q28.2   **Arteriovenous malformation of cerebral vessels**

Explanation: Although present at birth, malformations may not be identified until later in life. Whenever the condition is diagnosed by the physician, it is appropriate to assign a code from the range Q00–Q99.

Chapter 17. Congenital Malformations, Deformations and Chromosomal Abnormalities (Q00-Q99)

NOTE   Codes from this chapter are not for use on maternal records
EXCLUDES 2 *inborn errors of metabolism (E70-E88)*

This chapter contains the following blocks:
Q00-Q07   Congenital malformations of the nervous system
Q10-Q18   Congenital malformations of eye, ear, face and neck
Q20-Q28   Congenital malformations of the circulatory system
Q30-Q34   Congenital malformations of the respiratory system
Q35-Q37   Cleft lip and cleft palate
Q38-Q45   Other congenital malformations of the digestive system
Q50-Q56   Congenital malformations of genital organs
Q60-Q64   Congenital malformations of the urinary system
Q65-Q79   Congenital malformations and deformations of the musculoskeletal system
Q80-Q89   Other congenital malformations
Q90-Q99   Chromosomal abnormalities, not elsewhere classified

Congenital malformations of the nervous system (Q00-Q07)

✓4ᵗʰ **Q00   Anencephaly and similar malformations**

  Q00.0   Anencephaly
      Acephaly
      Acrania
      Amyelencephaly
      Hemianencephaly
      Hemicephaly
  Q00.1   Craniorachischisis
  Q00.2   Iniencephaly

✓4ᵗʰ **Q01   Encephalocele**
  INCLUDES   Arnold-Chiari syndrome, type III
            encephalocystocele
            encephalomyelocele
            hydroencephalocele
            hydromeningocele, cranial
            meningocele, cerebral
            meningoencephalocele
  EXCLUDES 1 *Meckel-Gruber syndrome (Q61.9)*
  DEF: Congenital protrusion of brain tissue through a defect in the skull.
  Q01.0   Frontal encephalocele
  Q01.1   Nasofrontal encephalocele
  Q01.2   Occipital encephalocele
  Q01.8   Encephalocele of other sites
  Q01.9   Encephalocele, unspecified

Q02   Microcephaly
  INCLUDES   hydromicrocephaly
            micrencephalon
  ►Code first, if applicable, congenital Zika virus disease◄
  Use additional code, if applicable, to identify congenital Zika virus disease
  EXCLUDES 1 *Meckel-Gruber syndrome (Q61.9)*
  AHA: 2018,4Q,26
  DEF: Congenital disorder in which the head circumference is more than two standard deviations below the mean for age, sex, race, and gestation and associated with a decreased life expectancy.

✓4ᵗʰ **Q03   Congenital hydrocephalus**
  INCLUDES   hydrocephalus in newborn
  EXCLUDES 1 *Arnold-Chiari syndrome, type II (Q07.0-)*
            acquired hydrocephalus (G91.-)
            hydrocephalus due to congenital toxoplasmosis (P37.1)
            hydrocephalus with spina bifida (Q05.0-Q05.4)
  DEF: Hydrocephalus: Abnormal buildup of cerebrospinal fluid in the brain causing dilation of the ventricles.

Congenital Hydrocephalus

Pressure

Normal ventricles   Hydrocephalic ventricles

  Q03.0   Malformations of aqueduct of Sylvius
      Anomaly of aqueduct of Sylvius
      Obstruction of aqueduct of Sylvius, congenital
      Stenosis of aqueduct of Sylvius
  Q03.1   Atresia of foramina of Magendie and Luschka
      Dandy-Walker syndrome
  Q03.8   Other congenital hydrocephalus
  Q03.9   Congenital hydrocephalus, unspecified

✓4ᵗʰ **Q04   Other congenital malformations of brain**
  EXCLUDES 1 *cyclopia (Q87.0)*
            macrocephaly (Q75.3)
  Q04.0   Congenital malformations of corpus callosum
      Agenesis of corpus callosum
  Q04.1   Arhinencephaly
  Q04.2   Holoprosencephaly
  Q04.3   Other reduction deformities of brain
      Absence of part of brain
      Agenesis of part of brain
      Agyria
      Aplasia of part of brain
      Hydranencephaly
      Hypoplasia of part of brain
      Lissencephaly
      Microgyria
      Pachygyria
      EXCLUDES 1 *congenital malformations of corpus callosum (Q04.0)*
  Q04.4   Septo-optic dysplasia of brain
  Q04.5   Megalencephaly
  Q04.6   Congenital cerebral cysts
      Porencephaly
      Schizencephaly
      EXCLUDES 1 *acquired porencephalic cyst (G93.0)*
  Q04.8   Other specified congenital malformations of brain
      Arnold-Chiari syndrome, type IV
      Macrogyria
  Q04.9   Congenital malformation of brain, unspecified
      Congenital anomaly NOS of brain
      Congenital deformity NOS of brain
      Congenital disease or lesion NOS of brain
      Multiple anomalies NOS of brain, congenital

✓4ᵗʰ Q05 Spina bifida

> INCLUDES   hydromeningocele (spinal)
> meningocele (spinal)
> meningomyelocele
> myelocele
> myelomeningocele
> rachischisis
> spina bifida (aperta)(cystica)
> syringomyelocele

Use additional code for any associated paraplegia (paraparesis) (G82.2-)

> EXCLUDES 1   Arnold-Chiari syndrome, type II (Q07.0-)
> spina bifida occulta (Q76.0)

DEF: Lack of closure in the vertebral column with protrusion of the spinal cord through the defect, often in the lumbosacral area. This condition can be recognized by the presence of alpha-fetoproteins in the amniotic fluid.

Spina Bifida

Spina bifida occulta   Meningocele   Myelomeningocele

- **Q05.0** Cervical **spina bifida** with hydrocephalus
- **Q05.1** Thoracic **spina bifida** with hydrocephalus
  - Dorsal spina bifida with hydrocephalus
  - Thoracolumbar spina bifida with hydrocephalus
- **Q05.2** Lumbar **spina bifida** with hydrocephalus
  - Lumbosacral spina bifida with hydrocephalus
- **Q05.3** Sacral **spina bifida** with hydrocephalus
- **Q05.4** Unspecified spina bifida with hydrocephalus
- **Q05.5** Cervical **spina bifida** without hydrocephalus
- **Q05.6** Thoracic **spina bifida** without hydrocephalus
  - Dorsal spina bifida NOS
  - Thoracolumbar spina bifida NOS
- **Q05.7** Lumbar **spina bifida** without hydrocephalus
  - Lumbosacral spina bifida NOS
- **Q05.8** Sacral **spina bifida** without hydrocephalus
- **Q05.9** Spina bifida, unspecified

✓4ᵗʰ Q06 Other congenital malformations of spinal cord

- **Q06.0** Amyelia
- **Q06.1** Hypoplasia and dysplasia of spinal cord
  - Atelomyelia
  - Myelatelia
  - Myelodysplasia of spinal cord
- **Q06.2** Diastematomyelia
  - **DEF:** Rare congenital anomaly often associated with spina bifida. The spinal cord is separated into longitudinal halves by a bony, cartilaginous or fibrous septum, each half surrounded by a dural sac.
- **Q06.3** Other congenital cauda equina malformations
- **Q06.4** Hydromyelia
  - Hydrorachis
- **Q06.8** Other specified congenital malformations of spinal cord
- **Q06.9** Congenital malformation of spinal cord, unspecified
  - Congenital anomaly NOS of spinal cord
  - Congenital deformity NOS of spinal cord
  - Congenital disease or lesion NOS of spinal cord

✓4ᵗʰ Q07 Other congenital malformations of nervous system

> EXCLUDES 2   congenital central alveolar hypoventilation syndrome (G47.35)
> familial dysautonomia [Riley-Day] (G90.1)
> neurofibromatosis (nonmalignant) (Q85.0-)

✓5ᵗʰ Q07.0 Arnold-Chiari syndrome

Arnold-Chiari syndrome, type II

> EXCLUDES 1   Arnold-Chiari syndrome, type III (Q01.-)
> Arnold-Chiari syndrome, type IV (Q04.8)

DEF: Congenital malformation of the brain in which the cerebellum protrudes through the foramen magnum into the spinal canal.

- **Q07.00** **Arnold-Chiari syndrome** without spina bifida or hydrocephalus
- **Q07.01** **Arnold-Chiari syndrome** with spina bifida
- **Q07.02** **Arnold-Chiari syndrome** with hydrocephalus
- **Q07.03** **Arnold-Chiari syndrome** with spina bifida and hydrocephalus

- **Q07.8** Other specified congenital malformations of nervous system
  - Agenesis of nerve
  - Displacement of brachial plexus
  - Jaw-winking syndrome
  - Marcus Gunn's syndrome
- **Q07.9** Congenital malformation of nervous system, unspecified
  - Congenital anomaly NOS of nervous system
  - Congenital deformity NOS of nervous system
  - Congenital disease or lesion NOS of nervous system

Congenital malformations of eye, ear, face and neck (Q10-Q18)

> EXCLUDES 2   cleft lip and cleft palate (Q35-Q37)
> congenital malformation of cervical spine (Q05.0, Q05.5, Q67.5, Q76.0-Q76.4)
> congenital malformation of larynx (Q31.-)
> congenital malformation of lip NEC (Q38.0)
> congenital malformation of nose (Q30.-)
> congenital malformation of parathyroid gland (Q89.2)
> congenital malformation of thyroid gland (Q89.2)

✓4ᵗʰ Q10 Congenital malformations of eyelid, lacrimal apparatus and orbit

> EXCLUDES 1   cryptophthalmos NOS (Q11.2)
> cryptophthalmos syndrome (Q87.0)

- **Q10.0** Congenital ptosis
  - **DEF:** Congenital drooping of the eyelid. Ptosis is mostly idiopathic, but may occur genetically.
- **Q10.1** Congenital ectropion
- **Q10.2** Congenital entropion
- **Q10.3** Other congenital malformations of eyelid
  - Ablepharon
  - Blepharophimosis, congenital
  - Coloboma of eyelid
  - Congenital absence or agenesis of cilia
  - Congenital absence or agenesis of eyelid
  - Congenital accessory eyelid
  - Congenital accessory eye muscle
  - Congenital malformation of eyelid NOS
- **Q10.4** Absence and agenesis of lacrimal apparatus
  - Congenital absence of punctum lacrimale
- **Q10.5** Congenital stenosis and stricture of lacrimal duct
- **Q10.6** Other congenital malformations of lacrimal apparatus
  - Congenital malformation of lacrimal apparatus NOS
- **Q10.7** Congenital malformation of orbit

✓4ᵗʰ Q11 Anophthalmos, microphthalmos and macrophthalmos

- **Q11.0** Cystic eyeball
- **Q11.1** Other anophthalmos
  - Anophthalmos NOS
  - Agenesis of eye
  - Aplasia of eye
- **Q11.2** Microphthalmos
  - Cryptophthalmos NOS
  - Dysplasia of eye
  - Hypoplasia of eye
  - Rudimentary eye
  > EXCLUDES 1   cryptophthalmos syndrome (Q87.0)
- **Q11.3** Macrophthalmos
  > EXCLUDES 1   macrophthalmos in congenital glaucoma (Q15.0)

✓4ᵗʰ Q12 Congenital lens malformations

- **Q12.0** Congenital cataract

Chapter 17. Congenital Malformations, Deformations and Chromosomal Abnormalities

Q12.1–Q18.1

Q12.1   **Congenital** displaced lens
Q12.2   Coloboma of lens

Coloboma of Lens

Coloboma

Q12.3   **Congenital** aphakia
Q12.4   Spherophakia
Q12.8   Other congenital lens malformations
     Microphakia
Q12.9   Congenital lens malformation, unspecified

✓4ᵗʰ **Q13**   Congenital malformations of anterior segment of eye

Q13.0   Coloboma of iris
     Coloboma NOS
     DEF: Defective or absent section of ocular tissue that may present as mild cupping or a small pit in the ocular disc due to extensive defects in the iris, ciliary body, choroids, and retina.

Q13.1   Absence of iris
     Aniridia
     Use additional code for associated glaucoma (H42)
     DEF: Incompletely formed or absent iris. It affects both eyes and is a dominant trait.

Q13.2   Other congenital malformations of iris
     Anisocoria, congenital
     Atresia of pupil
     Congenital malformation of iris NOS
     Corectopia

Q13.3   Congenital corneal opacity

Q13.4   Other congenital corneal malformations
     Congenital malformation of cornea NOS
     Microcornea
     Peter's anomaly

Q13.5   Blue sclera

✓5ᵗʰ **Q13.8**   Other congenital malformations of anterior segment of eye

     Q13.81   Rieger's anomaly
         Use additional code for associated glaucoma (H42)

     Q13.89   Other congenital malformations of anterior segment of eye

Q13.9   Congenital malformation of anterior segment of eye, unspecified

✓4ᵗʰ **Q14**   Congenital malformations of posterior segment of eye

     EXCLUDES 2   *optic nerve hypoplasia (H47.03-)*

Q14.0   Congenital malformation of vitreous humor
     Congenital vitreous opacity

Q14.1   Congenital malformation of retina
     Congenital retinal aneurysm

Q14.2   Congenital malformation of optic disc
     Coloboma of optic disc

Q14.3   Congenital malformation of choroid

Q14.8   Other congenital malformations of posterior segment of eye
     Coloboma of the fundus

Q14.9   Congenital malformation of posterior segment of eye, unspecified

✓4ᵗʰ **Q15**   Other congenital malformations of eye

     EXCLUDES 1   *congenital nystagmus (H55.01)*
         ocular albinism (E70.31-)
         optic nerve hypoplasia (H47.03-)
         retinitis pigmentosa (H35.52)

Q15.0   Congenital glaucoma
     Axenfeld's anomaly
     Buphthalmos
     Glaucoma of childhood
     Glaucoma of newborn
     Hydrophthalmos
     Keratoglobus, congenital, with glaucoma
     Macrocornea with glaucoma
     Macrophthalmos in congenital glaucoma
     Megalocornea with glaucoma

Q15.8   Other specified congenital malformations of eye

Q15.9   Congenital malformation of eye, unspecified
     Congenital anomaly of eye
     Congenital deformity of eye

✓4ᵗʰ **Q16**   Congenital malformations of ear causing impairment of hearing

     EXCLUDES 1   *congenital deafness (H90.-)*

Q16.0   Congenital absence of (ear) auricle

Q16.1   Congenital absence, atresia and stricture of auditory canal (external)
     Congenital atresia or stricture of osseous meatus

Q16.2   Absence of eustachian tube

Q16.3   Congenital malformation of ear ossicles
     Congenital fusion of ear ossicles

Q16.4   Other congenital malformations of middle ear
     Congenital malformation of middle ear NOS

Q16.5   Congenital malformation of inner ear
     Congenital anomaly of membranous labyrinth
     Congenital anomaly of organ of Corti

Q16.9   Congenital malformation of ear causing impairment of hearing, unspecified
     Congenital absence of ear NOS

✓4ᵗʰ **Q17**   Other congenital malformations of ear

     EXCLUDES 1   *congenital malformations of ear with impairment of hearing (Q16.0-Q16.9)*
         preauricular sinus (Q18.1)

Q17.0   Accessory auricle
     Accessory tragus
     Polyotia
     Preauricular appendage or tag
     Supernumerary ear
     Supernumerary lobule

Q17.1   Macrotia
     DEF: Birth defect characterized by abnormal enlargement of the pinna of the ear.

Q17.2   Microtia

Q17.3   Other misshapen ear
     Pointed ear

Q17.4   Misplaced ear
     Low-set ears
     EXCLUDES 1   *cervical auricle (Q18.2)*

Q17.5   Prominent ear
     Bat ear

Q17.8   Other specified congenital malformations of ear
     Congenital absence of lobe of ear

Q17.9   Congenital malformation of ear, unspecified
     Congenital anomaly of ear NOS

✓4ᵗʰ **Q18**   Other congenital malformations of face and neck

     EXCLUDES 1   *cleft lip and cleft palate (Q35-Q37)*
         conditions classified to Q67.0-Q67.4
         congenital malformations of skull and face bones (Q75.-)
         cyclopia (Q87.0)
         dentofacial anomalies [including malocclusion] (M26.-)
         malformation syndromes affecting facial appearance (Q87.0)
         persistent thyroglossal duct (Q89.2)

Q18.0   Sinus, fistula and cyst of branchial cleft
     Branchial vestige

Q18.1   Preauricular sinus and cyst
     Fistula of auricle, congenital
     Cervicoaural fistula

Ⓝ Newborn: 0   Ⓟ Pediatric: 0-17   Ⓜ Maternity: 12-55   Ⓐ Adult: 15-124   CH Comorbidity High   CL Comorbidity Low   NCDx Noncancer Dx   PDx Primary Dx

902   ICD-10-CM 2020

Q18.2 Other branchial cleft malformations
Branchial cleft malformation NOS
Cervical auricle
Otocephaly

Q18.3 Webbing of neck
Pterygium colli
DEF: Congenital malformation characterized by a thick, triangular skinfold that stretches from the lateral side of the neck across the shoulder. It is associated with genetic conditions such as Turner's and Noonan's syndromes.

Q18.4 Macrostomia
DEF: Rare congenital craniofacial bilateral or unilateral anomaly of the mouth due to malformed maxillary and mandibular processes. It results in an abnormally large mouth extending toward the ear.

Q18.5 Microstomia

Q18.6 Macrocheilia
Hypertrophy of lip, congenital

Q18.7 Microcheilia

Q18.8 Other specified congenital malformations of face and neck
Medial cyst of face and neck
Medial fistula of face and neck
Medial sinus of face and neck

Q18.9 Congenital malformation of face and neck, unspecified
Congenital anomaly NOS of face and neck

Congenital malformations of the circulatory system (Q20-Q28)

☑4ᵗʰ Q20 Congenital malformations of cardiac chambers and connections
    EXCLUDES 1   dextrocardia with situs inversus (Q89.3)
                   mirror-image atrial arrangement with situs inversus (Q89.3)

Q20.0 Common arterial trunk
Persistent truncus arteriosus
    EXCLUDES 1   aortic septal defect (Q21.4)

Q20.1 Double outlet right ventricle
Taussig-Bing syndrome

Q20.2 Double outlet left ventricle

Q20.3 Discordant ventriculoarterial connection
Dextrotransposition of aorta
Transposition of great vessels (complete)

Q20.4 Double inlet ventricle
Common ventricle
Cor triloculare biatriatum
Single ventricle

Q20.5 Discordant atrioventricular connection
Corrected transposition
Levotransposition
Ventricular inversion

Q20.6 Isomerism of atrial appendages
Isomerism of atrial appendages with asplenia or polysplenia

Q20.8 Other congenital malformations of cardiac chambers and connections
Cor binoculare

Q20.9 Congenital malformation of cardiac chambers and connections, unspecified

☑4ᵗʰ Q21 Congenital malformations of cardiac septa
    EXCLUDES 1   acquired cardiac septal defect (I51.0)

Q21.0 Ventricular septal defect
Roger's disease

Ventricular Septal Defect

Q21.1 Atrial septal defect
Coronary sinus defect
Patent or persistent foramen ovale
Patent or persistent ostium secundum defect (type II)
Patent or persistent sinus venosus defect

Atrial Septal Defect

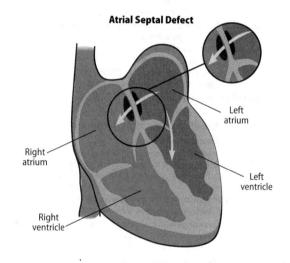

Q21.2   Atrioventricular **septal defect**
> Common atrioventricular canal
> Endocardial cushion defect
> Ostium primum atrial septal defect (type I)

Atrioventricular Septal Defect

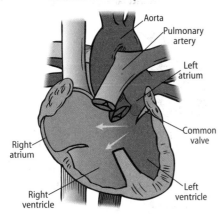

Q21.3   Tetralogy of Fallot
> Ventricular septal defect with pulmonary stenosis or atresia, dextroposition of aorta and hypertrophy of right ventricle.
> **AHA:** 2014,3Q,16
> **TIP:** Do not assign an additional code for obstruction of right ventricular outflow tract muscle bundles in a patient with tetralogy of Fallot, as this is an inherent component of the disease.

Q21.4   Aortopulmonary septal **defect**
> Aortic septal defect
> Aortopulmonary window

Q21.8   **Other congenital malformations of cardiac septa**
> Eisenmenger's defect
> Pentalogy of Fallot
> Code also if applicable:
> > Eisenmenger's complex (I27.83)
> > Eisenmenger's syndrome (I27.83)

Q21.9   **Congenital malformation of cardiac septum, unspecified**
> Septal (heart) defect NOS

☑4ᵗʰ **Q22**   **Congenital malformations of** pulmonary and tricuspid valves

Q22.0   Pulmonary **valve** atresia

Q22.1   **Congenital** pulmonary **valve** stenosis
> **DEF:** Stenosis of the opening between the pulmonary artery and right ventricle, causing obstructed blood outflow from the right ventricle.

Q22.2   **Congenital** pulmonary **valve** insufficiency
> Congenital pulmonary valve regurgitation

Q22.3   **Other congenital malformations of pulmonary valve**
> Congenital malformation of pulmonary valve NOS
> Supernumerary cusps of pulmonary valve

Q22.4   **Congenital** tricuspid stenosis
> Congenital tricuspid atresia

Q22.5   Ebstein's anomaly
> **DEF:** Malformation of the tricuspid valve characterized by septal and posterior leaflets attaching to the wall of the right ventricle. Ebstein's anomaly causes the right ventricle to fuse with the atrium into a large right atrium and a small ventricle and leads to heart failure and abnormal cardiac rhythm.

Q22.6   Hypoplastic right heart syndrome

Q22.8   **Other congenital malformations of tricuspid valve**

Q22.9   **Congenital malformation of tricuspid valve, unspecified**

☑4ᵗʰ **Q23**   **Congenital malformations of** aortic and mitral valves

Q23.0   **Congenital** stenosis **of aortic valve**
> Congenital aortic atresia
> Congenital aortic stenosis NOS
> > **EXCLUDES 1**   *congenital stenosis of aortic valve in hypoplastic left heart syndrome (Q23.4)*
> > *congenital subaortic stenosis (Q24.4)*
> > *supravalvular aortic stenosis (congenital) (Q25.3)*

Q23.1   **Congenital** insufficiency **of** aortic **valve**
> Bicuspid aortic valve
> Congenital aortic insufficiency

Q23.2   **Congenital** mitral stenosis
> Congenital mitral atresia
> **DEF:** Congenital stenosis of the mitral valve orifice between the left atrium and ventricle, at the supravalvular, valvular, or subvalvular levels, causing obstruction to left ventricular filling.

Q23.3   **Congenital** mitral insufficiency

Q23.4   Hypoplastic left heart syndrome

Q23.8   **Other congenital malformations of aortic and mitral valves**

Q23.9   **Congenital malformation of aortic and mitral valves, unspecified**

☑4ᵗʰ **Q24**   **Other congenital malformations of** heart
> **EXCLUDES 1**   *endocardial fibroelastosis (I42.4)*

Q24.0   Dextrocardia
> **EXCLUDES 1**   *dextrocardia with situs inversus (Q89.3)*
> > *isomerism of atrial appendages (with asplenia or polysplenia) (Q20.6)*
> > *mirror-image atrial arrangement with situs inversus (Q89.3)*
> **DEF:** Congenital condition in which the heart is located on the right side of the chest rather than in its normal position on the left.

Q24.1   **Levocardia**

Q24.2   **Cor triatriatum**

Q24.3   **Pulmonary infundibular stenosis**
> Subvalvular pulmonic stenosis

Q24.4   **Congenital subaortic stenosis**
> **DEF:** Congenital heart defect characterized by stenosis of the left ventricular outflow tract due to a fibrous tissue ring or septal hypertrophy below the aortic valve.

Q24.5   **Malformation of coronary vessels**
> Congenital coronary (artery) aneurysm

Q24.6   **Congenital heart block**

Q24.8   **Other specified congenital malformations of heart**
> Congenital diverticulum of left ventricle
> Congenital malformation of myocardium
> Congenital malformation of pericardium
> Malposition of heart
> Uhl's disease

Q24.9   **Congenital malformation of heart, unspecified**
> Congenital anomaly of heart
> Congenital disease of heart

☑4ᵗʰ **Q25**   **Congenital malformations of** great arteries

Q25.0   Patent ductus arteriosus
> Patent ductus Botallo
> Persistent ductus arteriosus
> **DEF:** Condition in which the normal channel between the pulmonary artery and the aorta fails to close at birth, causing arterial blood to recirculate in the lungs and inhibiting the blood supply to the aorta. **Synonym(s):** PDA.

Patent Ductus Arteriosus

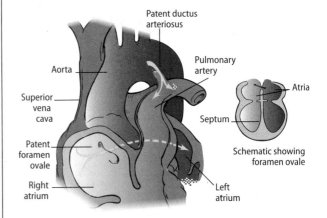

Schematic showing foramen ovale

Q25.1   Coarctation **of** aorta
> Coarctation of aorta (preductal) (postductal)
> Stenosis of aorta
> **AHA:** 2016,4Q,56-57

N Newborn: 0   P Pediatric: 0-17   M Maternity: 12-55   A Adult: 15-124   CH Comorbidity High   CL Comorbidity Low   NCDx Noncancer Dx   PDx Primary Dx

904   ICD-10-CM 2020

✓5ᵗʰ **Q25.2** Atresia of aorta
> AHA: 2016,4Q,56-57

    Q25.21 **Interruption of aortic arch**
> Atresia of aortic arch

    Q25.29 **Other atresia of aorta**
> Atresia of aorta

Q25.3 Supravalvular **aortic stenosis**
> *EXCLUDES 1*   *congenital aortic stenosis NOS (Q23.0)*
>   *congenital stenosis of aortic valve (Q23.0)*

✓5ᵗʰ **Q25.4** **Other congenital malformations of aorta**
> *EXCLUDES 1*   *hypoplasia of aorta in hypoplastic left heart*
>   *syndrome (Q23.4)*
> AHA: 2016,4Q,57

    Q25.40 **Congenital malformation of aorta unspecified**

    Q25.41 **Absence and aplasia of aorta**

    Q25.42 **Hypoplasia of aorta**

    Q25.43 **Congenital aneurysm of aorta**
> Congenital aneurysm of aortic root
> Congenital aneurysm of aortic sinus

    Q25.44 **Congenital dilation of aorta**

    Q25.45 **Double aortic arch**
> Vascular ring of aorta

Aortic Arch Anomalies

Normal aortic arch

Double aortic arch

Right aortic arch

    Q25.46 **Tortuous aortic arch**
> Persistent convolutions of aortic arch

    Q25.47 **Right aortic arch**
> Persistent right aortic arch

    Q25.48 **Anomalous origin of subclavian artery**

    Q25.49 **Other congenital malformations of aorta**
> Aortic arch
> Bovine arch

Q25.5 Atresia of pulmonary **artery**

Q25.6 Stenosis of pulmonary **artery**
> Supravalvular pulmonary stenosis

✓5ᵗʰ **Q25.7** **Other congenital malformations of pulmonary artery**

    Q25.71 **Coarctation of pulmonary artery**

    Q25.72 **Congenital pulmonary arteriovenous malformation**
> Congenital pulmonary arteriovenous aneurysm

    Q25.79 **Other congenital malformations of pulmonary artery**
> Aberrant pulmonary artery
> Agenesis of pulmonary artery
> Congenital aneurysm of pulmonary artery
> Congenital anomaly of pulmonary artery
> Hypoplasia of pulmonary artery

Q25.8 **Other congenital malformations of other great arteries**

Q25.9 **Congenital malformation of great arteries, unspecified**

✓4ᵗʰ **Q26** **Congenital malformations of great veins**

    Q26.0 **Congenital stenosis of vena cava**
> Congenital stenosis of vena cava (inferior)(superior)

    Q26.1 **Persistent left superior vena cava**

    Q26.2 **Total anomalous pulmonary venous connection**
> Total anomalous pulmonary venous return [TAPVR], subdiaphragmatic
> Total anomalous pulmonary venous return [TAPVR], supradiaphragmatic

    Q26.3 **Partial anomalous pulmonary venous connection**
> Partial anomalous pulmonary venous return

    Q26.4 **Anomalous pulmonary venous connection, unspecified**

    Q26.5 **Anomalous portal venous connection**

    Q26.6 **Portal vein-hepatic artery fistula**

    Q26.8 **Other congenital malformations of great veins**
> Absence of vena cava (inferior) (superior)
> Azygos continuation of inferior vena cava
> Persistent left posterior cardinal vein
> Scimitar syndrome

    Q26.9 **Congenital malformation of great vein, unspecified**
> Congenital anomaly of vena cava (inferior) (superior) NOS

✓4ᵗʰ **Q27** **Other congenital malformations of peripheral vascular system**
> *EXCLUDES 2*   *anomalies of cerebral and precerebral vessels (Q28.0-Q28.3)*
>   *anomalies of coronary vessels (Q24.5)*
>   *anomalies of pulmonary artery (Q25.5-Q25.7)*
>   *congenital retinal aneurysm (Q14.1)*
>   *hemangioma and lymphangioma (D18.-)*

    Q27.0 **Congenital absence and hypoplasia of umbilical artery**
> Single umbilical artery

    Q27.1 **Congenital renal artery stenosis**

    Q27.2 **Other congenital malformations of renal artery**
> Congenital malformation of renal artery NOS
> Multiple renal arteries

✓5ᵗʰ **Q27.3** **Arteriovenous malformation (peripheral)**
> Arteriovenous aneurysm
> *EXCLUDES 1*   *acquired arteriovenous aneurysm (I77.0)*
> *EXCLUDES 2*   *arteriovenous malformation of cerebral vessels (Q28.2)*
>   *arteriovenous malformation of precerebral vessels (Q28.0)*
> **DEF:** Arteriovenous malformation: Connecting passage between an artery and a vein.

    Q27.30 **Arteriovenous malformation, site unspecified**

    Q27.31 **Arteriovenous malformation of vessel of upper limb**

    Q27.32 **Arteriovenous malformation of vessel of lower limb**

    Q27.33 **Arteriovenous malformation of digestive system vessel**
> AHA: 2018,3Q,21

    Q27.34 **Arteriovenous malformation of renal vessel**

    Q27.39 **Arteriovenous malformation, other site**

    Q27.4 **Congenital phlebectasia**

    Q27.8 **Other specified congenital malformations of peripheral vascular system**
> Absence of peripheral vascular system
> Atresia of peripheral vascular system
> Congenital aneurysm (peripheral)
> Congenital stricture, artery
> Congenital varix
> *EXCLUDES 1*   *arteriovenous malformation (Q27.3-)*

    Q27.9 **Congenital malformation of peripheral vascular system, unspecified**
> Anomaly of artery or vein NOS

✓4ᵗʰ **Q28** **Other congenital malformations of circulatory system**
> *EXCLUDES 1*   *congenital aneurysm NOS (Q27.8)*
>   *congenital coronary aneurysm (Q24.5)*
>   *ruptured cerebral arteriovenous malformation (I60.8)*
>   *ruptured malformation of precerebral vessels (I72.0)*
> *EXCLUDES 2*   *congenital peripheral aneurysm (Q27.8)*
>   *congenital pulmonary aneurysm (Q25.79)*
>   *congenital retinal aneurysm (Q14.1)*

    Q28.0 **Arteriovenous malformation of precerebral vessels**
> Congenital arteriovenous precerebral aneurysm (nonruptured)

    Q28.1 **Other malformations of precerebral vessels**
> Congenital malformation of precerebral vessels NOS
> Congenital precerebral aneurysm (nonruptured)

Q28.2 Arteriovenous **malformation of** cerebral **vessels**
Arteriovenous malformation of brain NOS
Congenital arteriovenous cerebral aneurysm (nonruptured)

Q28.3 **Other malformations of cerebral vessels**
Congenital cerebral aneurysm (nonruptured)
Congenital malformation of cerebral vessels NOS
Developmental venous anomaly

Q28.8 **Other specified congenital malformations of circulatory system**
Congenital aneurysm, specified site NEC
Spinal vessel anomaly

Q28.9 **Congenital malformation of circulatory system, unspecified**

Congenital malformations of the respiratory system (Q30-Q34)

☑4ᵗʰ **Q30** **Congenital malformations of** nose
EXCLUDES 1   *congenital deviation of nasal septum (Q67.4)*

Q30.0 **Choanal** atresia
Atresia of nares (anterior) (posterior)
Congenital stenosis of nares (anterior) (posterior)

Q30.1 Agenesis **and underdevelopment of nose**
Congenital absent of nose

Q30.2 Fissured, notched and cleft **nose**

Q30.3 **Congenital** perforated **nasal septum**

Q30.8 **Other congenital malformations of nose**
Accessory nose
Congenital anomaly of nasal sinus wall

Q30.9 **Congenital malformation of nose, unspecified**

☑4ᵗʰ **Q31** **Congenital malformations of** larynx
EXCLUDES 1   *congenital laryngeal stridor NOS (P28.89)*

Q31.0 Web **of larynx**
Glottic web of larynx
Subglottic web of larynx
Web of larynx NOS
DEF: Congenital malformation of the larynx marked by thin, translucent, or thick fibrotic membrane-like structure between the vocal folds. It is characterized by shortness of breath and stridor.

Q31.1 **Congenital** subglottic stenosis

Q31.2 **Laryngeal** hypoplasia

Q31.3 Laryngocele

Q31.5 **Congenital** laryngomalacia

Q31.8 **Other congenital malformations of larynx**
Absence of larynx
Agenesis of larynx
Atresia of larynx
Congenital cleft thyroid cartilage
Congenital fissure of epiglottis
Congenital stenosis of larynx NEC
Posterior cleft of cricoid cartilage

Q31.9 **Congenital malformation of larynx, unspecified**

☑4ᵗʰ **Q32** **Congenital malformations of** trachea and bronchus
EXCLUDES 1   *congenital bronchiectasis (Q33.4)*

Q32.0 **Congenital** tracheomalacia

Q32.1 **Other congenital malformations of trachea**
Atresia of trachea
Congenital anomaly of tracheal cartilage
Congenital dilatation of trachea
Congenital malformation of trachea
Congenital stenosis of trachea
Congenital tracheocele

Q32.2 **Congenital** bronchomalacia

Q32.3 **Congenital** stenosis of bronchus

Q32.4 **Other congenital malformations of bronchus**
Absence of bronchus
Agenesis of bronchus
Atresia of bronchus
Congenital diverticulum of bronchus
Congenital malformation of bronchus NOS

☑4ᵗʰ **Q33** **Congenital malformations of** lung

Q33.0 **Congenital** cystic **lung**
Congenital cystic lung disease
Congenital honeycomb lung
Congenital polycystic lung disease
EXCLUDES 1   *cystic fibrosis (E84.0)*
cystic lung disease, acquired or unspecified (J98.4)

Q33.1 Accessory **lobe of lung**
Azygos lobe (fissured), lung

Q33.2 Sequestration **of lung**

Q33.3 Agenesis **of lung**
Congenital absence of lung (lobe)

Q33.4 **Congenital** bronchiectasis

Q33.5 Ectopic **tissue in lung**

Q33.6 **Congenital** hypoplasia and dysplasia **of lung**
EXCLUDES 1   *pulmonary hypoplasia associated with short gestation (P28.0)*

Q33.8 **Other congenital malformations of lung**

Q33.9 **Congenital malformation of lung, unspecified**

☑4ᵗʰ **Q34** **Other congenital malformations of** respiratory system
EXCLUDES 2   *congenital central alveolar hypoventilation syndrome (G47.35)*

Q34.0 **Anomaly of** pleura

Q34.1 **Congenital cyst of** mediastinum

Q34.8 **Other specified congenital malformations of respiratory system**
Atresia of nasopharynx

Q34.9 **Congenital malformation of respiratory system, unspecified**
Congenital absence of respiratory system
Congenital anomaly of respiratory system NOS

Cleft lip and cleft palate (Q35-Q37)

Use additional code to identify associated malformation of the nose (Q30.2)
EXCLUDES 1   *Robin's syndrome (Q87.0)*

☑4ᵗʰ **Q35** **Cleft** palate
INCLUDES   fissure of palate
palatoschisis
EXCLUDES 1   *cleft palate with cleft lip (Q37.-)*
DEF: Congenital fissure or defect of the roof of the mouth opening to the nasal cavity due to failure of embryonic cells to fuse completely.

Cleft Palate

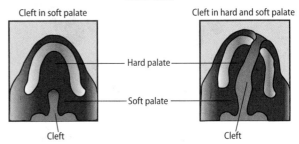

Cleft in soft palate   Cleft in hard and soft palate

Hard palate
Soft palate
Cleft   Cleft

Q35.1 **Cleft** hard **palate**

Q35.3 **Cleft** soft **palate**

Q35.5 **Cleft** hard **palate** with cleft soft palate

Q35.7 **Cleft** uvula

Q35.9 **Cleft palate, unspecified**
Cleft palate NOS

N Newborn: 0   P Pediatric: 0-17   M Maternity: 12-55   A Adult: 15-124   CH Comorbidity High   CL Comorbidity Low   NCDx Noncancer Dx   PDx Primary Dx

906   ICD-10-CM 2020

✓4ᵗʰ Q36 Cleft lip

> **INCLUDES**
> cheiloschisis
> congenital fissure of lip
> harelip
> labium leporinum
> **EXCLUDES 1** cleft lip with cleft palate (Q37.-)
> **DEF:** Congenital fissure or opening in the upper lip due to failure of embryonic cells to fuse completely.

Cleft Lip

Unilateral incomplete   Unilateral complete   Bilateral complete

- **Q36.0 Cleft lip, bilateral**
- **Q36.1 Cleft lip, median**
- **Q36.9 Cleft lip, unilateral**
  Cleft lip NOS

✓4ᵗʰ Q37 Cleft palate with cleft lip

> **INCLUDES** cheilopalatoschisis

- **Q37.0 Cleft hard palate with bilateral cleft lip**
- **Q37.1 Cleft hard palate with unilateral cleft lip**
  Cleft hard palate with cleft lip NOS
- **Q37.2 Cleft soft palate with bilateral cleft lip**
- **Q37.3 Cleft soft palate with unilateral cleft lip**
  Cleft soft palate with cleft lip NOS
- **Q37.4 Cleft hard and soft palate with bilateral cleft lip**
- **Q37.5 Cleft hard and soft palate with unilateral cleft lip**
  Cleft hard and soft palate with cleft lip NOS
- **Q37.8 Unspecified cleft palate with bilateral cleft lip**
- **Q37.9 Unspecified cleft palate with unilateral cleft lip**
  Cleft palate with cleft lip NOS

Other congenital malformations of the digestive system (Q38-Q45)

✓4ᵗʰ Q38 Other congenital malformations of tongue, mouth and pharynx

> **EXCLUDES 1** dentofacial anomalies (M26.-)
> macrostomia (Q18.4)
> microstomia (Q18.5)

- **Q38.0 Congenital malformations of lips, not elsewhere classified**
  Congenital fistula of lip
  Congenital malformation of lip NOS
  Van der Woude's syndrome
  > **EXCLUDES 1** cleft lip (Q36.-)
  > cleft lip with cleft palate (Q37.-)
  > macrocheilia (Q18.6)
  > microcheilia (Q18.7)
- **Q38.1 Ankyloglossia**
  Tongue tie
- **Q38.2 Macroglossia**
  Congenital hypertrophy of tongue
- **Q38.3 Other congenital malformations of tongue**
  Aglossia
  Bifid tongue
  Congenital adhesion of tongue
  Congenital fissure of tongue
  Congenital malformation of tongue NOS
  Double tongue
  Hypoglossia
  Hypoplasia of tongue
  Microglossia
- **Q38.4 Congenital malformations of salivary glands and ducts**
  Atresia of salivary glands and ducts
  Congenital absence of salivary glands and ducts
  Congenital accessory salivary glands and ducts
  Congenital fistula of salivary gland

- **Q38.5 Congenital malformations of palate, not elsewhere classified**
  Congenital absence of uvula
  Congenital malformation of palate NOS
  Congenital high arched palate
  > **EXCLUDES 1** cleft palate (Q35.-)
  > cleft palate with cleft lip (Q37.-)
- **Q38.6 Other congenital malformations of mouth**
  Congenital malformation of mouth NOS
- **Q38.7 Congenital pharyngeal pouch**
  Congenital diverticulum of pharynx
  > **EXCLUDES 1** pharyngeal pouch syndrome (D82.1)
- **Q38.8 Other congenital malformations of pharynx**
  Congenital malformation of pharynx NOS
  Imperforate pharynx

✓4ᵗʰ Q39 Congenital malformations of esophagus

- **Q39.0 Atresia of esophagus without fistula**
  Atresia of esophagus NOS
- **Q39.1 Atresia of esophagus with tracheo-esophageal fistula**
  Atresia of esophagus with broncho-esophageal fistula
- **Q39.2 Congenital tracheo-esophageal fistula without atresia**
  Congenital tracheo-esophageal fistula NOS
- **Q39.3 Congenital stenosis and stricture of esophagus**
- **Q39.4 Esophageal web**
- **Q39.5 Congenital dilatation of esophagus**
  Congenital cardiospasm
- **Q39.6 Congenital diverticulum of esophagus**
  Congenital esophageal pouch
- **Q39.8 Other congenital malformations of esophagus**
  Congenital absence of esophagus
  Congenital displacement of esophagus
  Congenital duplication of esophagus
- **Q39.9 Congenital malformation of esophagus, unspecified**

✓4ᵗʰ Q40 Other congenital malformations of upper alimentary tract

- **Q40.0 Congenital hypertrophic pyloric stenosis**
  Congenital or infantile constriction
  Congenital or infantile hypertrophy
  Congenital or infantile spasm
  Congenital or infantile stenosis
  Congenital or infantile stricture
- **Q40.1 Congenital hiatus hernia**
  Congenital displacement of cardia through esophageal hiatus
  > **EXCLUDES 1** congenital diaphragmatic hernia (Q79.0)
- **Q40.2 Other specified congenital malformations of stomach**
  Congenital displacement of stomach
  Congenital diverticulum of stomach
  Congenital hourglass stomach
  Congenital duplication of stomach
  Megalogastria
  Microgastria
- **Q40.3 Congenital malformation of stomach, unspecified**
- **Q40.8 Other specified congenital malformations of upper alimentary tract**
- **Q40.9 Congenital malformation of upper alimentary tract, unspecified**
  Congenital anomaly of upper alimentary tract
  Congenital deformity of upper alimentary tract

✓4ᵗʰ Q41 Congenital absence, atresia and stenosis of small intestine

> **INCLUDES** congenital obstruction, occlusion or stricture of small intestine or intestine NOS
> **EXCLUDES 1** cystic fibrosis with intestinal manifestation (E84.11)
> meconium ileus NOS (without cystic fibrosis) (P76.0)

- **Q41.0 Congenital absence, atresia and stenosis of duodenum**
- **Q41.1 Congenital absence, atresia and stenosis of jejunum**
  Apple peel syndrome
  Imperforate jejunum
- **Q41.2 Congenital absence, atresia and stenosis of ileum**
- **Q41.8 Congenital absence, atresia and stenosis of other specified parts of small intestine**
- **Q41.9 Congenital absence, atresia and stenosis of small intestine, part unspecified**
  Congenital absence, atresia and stenosis of intestine NOS

✓4ᵗʰ Q42 Congenital absence, atresia and stenosis of large intestine

> **INCLUDES** congenital obstruction, occlusion and stricture of large intestine

- **Q42.0 Congenital absence, atresia and stenosis of rectum with fistula**

☑ Additional Character Required   ✓x7ᵗʰ Placeholder Alert   Manifestation   Unspecified Dx   ►◄ Revised Text   ● New Code   ▲ Revised Title

ICD-10-CM 2020   **907**

Q42.1 Congenital absence, atresia and stenosis of rectum without fistula

     Imperforate rectum

Q42.2 Congenital absence, atresia and stenosis of anus with fistula

Q42.3 Congenital absence, atresia and stenosis of anus without fistula

     Imperforate anus

Q42.8 Congenital absence, atresia and stenosis of other parts of large intestine

Q42.9 Congenital absence, atresia and stenosis of large intestine, part unspecified

☑4ᵗʰ Q43 Other congenital malformations of intestine

Q43.0 Meckel's diverticulum (displaced) (hypertrophic)

     Persistent omphalomesenteric duct

     Persistent vitelline duct

     DEF: Congenital, abnormal remnant of embryonic digestive system development that leaves a sacculation or outpouching from the wall of the small intestine near the terminal part of the ileum made of acid-secreting tissue as in the stomach.

Q43.1 Hirschsprung's disease

     Aganglionosis

     Congenital (aganglionic) megacolon

     DEF: Congenital enlargement or dilation of the colon, with the absence of nerve cells in a segment of colon distally that causes the inability to defecate.

Q43.2 Other congenital functional disorders of colon

     Congenital dilatation of colon

Q43.3 Congenital malformations of intestinal fixation

     Congenital omental, anomalous adhesions [bands]

     Congenital peritoneal adhesions [bands]

     Incomplete rotation of cecum and colon

     Insufficient rotation of cecum and colon

     Jackson's membrane

     Malrotation of colon

     Rotation failure of cecum and colon

     Universal mesentery

Q43.4 Duplication of intestine

Q43.5 Ectopic anus

Q43.6 Congenital fistula of rectum and anus

     EXCLUDES 1   congenital fistula of anus with absence, atresia and stenosis (Q42.2)

           congenital fistula of rectum with absence, atresia and stenosis (Q42.0)

           congenital rectovaginal fistula (Q52.2)

           congenital urethrorectal fistula (Q64.73)

           pilonidal fistula or sinus (L05.-)

Q43.7 Persistent cloaca

     Cloaca NOS

Q43.8 Other specified congenital malformations of intestine

     Congenital blind loop syndrome

     Congenital diverticulitis, colon

     Congenital diverticulum, intestine

     Dolichocolon

     Megaloappendix

     Megaloduodenum

     Microcolon

     Transposition of appendix

     Transposition of colon

     Transposition of intestine

     AHA: 2013,2Q,31

Q43.9 Congenital malformation of intestine, unspecified

☑4ᵗʰ Q44 Congenital malformations of gallbladder, bile ducts and liver

Q44.0 Agenesis, aplasia and hypoplasia of gallbladder

     Congenital absence of gallbladder

Q44.1 Other congenital malformations of gallbladder

     Congenital malformation of gallbladder NOS

     Intrahepatic gallbladder

Q44.2 Atresia of bile ducts

Q44.3 Congenital stenosis and stricture of bile ducts

Q44.4 Choledochal cyst

Q44.5 Other congenital malformations of bile ducts

     Accessory hepatic duct

     Biliary duct duplication

     Congenital malformation of bile duct NOS

     Cystic duct duplication

Q44.6 Cystic disease of liver

     Fibrocystic disease of liver

Q44.7 Other congenital malformations of liver

     Accessory liver

     Alagille's syndrome

     Congenital absence of liver

     Congenital hepatomegaly

     Congenital malformation of liver NOS

☑4ᵗʰ Q45 Other congenital malformations of digestive system

     EXCLUDES 2   congenital diaphragmatic hernia (Q79.0)

           congenital hiatus hernia (Q40.1)

Q45.0 Agenesis, aplasia and hypoplasia of pancreas

     Congenital absence of pancreas

Q45.1 Annular pancreas

Q45.2 Congenital pancreatic cyst

Q45.3 Other congenital malformations of pancreas and pancreatic duct

     Accessory pancreas

     Congenital malformation of pancreas or pancreatic duct NOS

     EXCLUDES 1   congenital diabetes mellitus (E10.-)

           cystic fibrosis (E84.0-E84.9)

           fibrocystic disease of pancreas (E84.-)

           neonatal diabetes mellitus (P70.2)

Q45.8 Other specified congenital malformations of digestive system

     Absence (complete) (partial) of alimentary tract NOS

     Duplication of digestive system

     Malposition, congenital of digestive system

Q45.9 Congenital malformation of digestive system, unspecified

     Congenital anomaly of digestive system

     Congenital deformity of digestive system

Congenital malformations of genital organs (Q50-Q56)

     EXCLUDES 1   androgen insensitivity syndrome (E34.5-)

           syndromes associated with anomalies in the number and form of chromosomes (Q90-Q99)

☑4ᵗʰ Q50 Congenital malformations of ovaries, fallopian tubes and broad ligaments

   ☑5ᵗʰ Q50.0 Congenital absence of ovary

       EXCLUDES 1   Turner's syndrome (Q96.-)

     Q50.01 Congenital absence of ovary, unilateral   ♀

     Q50.02 Congenital absence of ovary, bilateral   ♀

   Q50.1 Developmental ovarian cyst   ♀

   Q50.2 Congenital torsion of ovary   ♀

   ☑5ᵗʰ Q50.3 Other congenital malformations of ovary

     Q50.31 Accessory ovary   ♀

     Q50.32 Ovarian streak

         46, XX with streak gonads

     Q50.39 Other congenital malformation of ovary   ♀

         Congenital malformation of ovary NOS

   Q50.4 Embryonic cyst of fallopian tube   ♀

     Fimbrial cyst

   Q50.5 Embryonic cyst of broad ligament   ♀

     Epoophoron cyst

     Parovarian cyst

   Q50.6 Other congenital malformations of fallopian tube and broad ligament   ♀

     Absence of fallopian tube and broad ligament

     Accessory fallopian tube and broad ligament

     Atresia of fallopian tube and broad ligament

     Congenital malformation of fallopian tube or broad ligament NOS

☑4ᵗʰ Q51 Congenital malformations of uterus and cervix

   Q51.0 Agenesis and aplasia of uterus   ♀

     Congenital absence of uterus

   ☑5ᵗʰ Q51.1 Doubling of uterus with doubling of cervix and vagina

     Q51.10 Doubling of uterus with doubling of cervix and vagina without obstruction   ♀

         Doubling of uterus with doubling of cervix and vagina NOS

     Q51.11 Doubling of uterus with doubling of cervix and vagina with obstruction   ♀

Ⓝ Newborn: 0   Ⓟ Pediatric: 0-17   Ⓜ Maternity: 12-55   Ⓐ Adult: 15-124   🄲🄷 Comorbidity High   🄲🄻 Comorbidity Low   🄽🄲🄳🅇 Noncancer Dx   🄿🄳🅇 Primary Dx

908   ICD-10-CM 2020

√5ᵗʰ **Q51.2 Other doubling of uterus**
Doubling of uterus NOS
Septate uterus
AHA: 2018,4Q,27

Q51.20 Other doubling of uterus, unspecified ♀
Septate uterus, unspecified

Q51.21 Other complete doubling of uterus ♀
Complete septate uterus

Q51.22 Other partial doubling of uterus ♀
Partial septate uterus

Q51.28 Other doubling of uterus, other specified ♀
Septate uterus, other specified

Q51.3 Bicornate uterus ♀
Bicornate uterus, complete or partial

Q51.4 Unicornate uterus ♀
Unicornate uterus with or without a separate uterine horn
Uterus with only one functioning horn

Q51.5 Agenesis and aplasia of cervix ♀
Congenital absence of cervix

Q51.6 Embryonic cyst of cervix ♀

Q51.7 Congenital fistulae between uterus and digestive and urinary tracts ♀

√5ᵗʰ **Q51.8 Other congenital malformations of uterus and cervix**

√6ᵗʰ **Q51.81 Other congenital malformations of uterus**

Q51.810 Arcuate uterus ♀
Arcuatus uterus

Q51.811 Hypoplasia of uterus ♀

Q51.818 Other congenital malformations of uterus ♀
Müllerian anomaly of uterus NEC

√6ᵗʰ **Q51.82 Other congenital malformations of cervix**

Q51.820 Cervical duplication ♀

Q51.821 Hypoplasia of cervix ♀

Q51.828 Other congenital malformations of cervix ♀

Q51.9 Congenital malformation of uterus and cervix, unspecified ♀

√4ᵗʰ **Q52 Other congenital malformations of female genitalia**

Q52.0 Congenital absence of vagina ♀
Vaginal agenesis, total or partial

√5ᵗʰ **Q52.1 Doubling of vagina**
EXCLUDES 1   doubling of vagina with doubling of uterus and cervix (Q51.1-)

Q52.10 Doubling of vagina, unspecified ♀
Septate vagina NOS

Q52.11 Transverse vaginal septum ♀

√6ᵗʰ **Q52.12 Longitudinal vaginal septum**
AHA: 2016,4Q,58-59

Q52.120 Longitudinal vaginal septum, nonobstructing ♀

Q52.121 Longitudinal vaginal septum, obstructing, right side ♀

Q52.122 Longitudinal vaginal septum, obstructing, left side ♀

Q52.123 Longitudinal vaginal septum, microperforate, right side ♀

Q52.124 Longitudinal vaginal septum, microperforate, left side ♀

Q52.129 Other and unspecified longitudinal vaginal septum ♀

Q52.2 Congenital rectovaginal fistula ♀
EXCLUDES 1   cloaca (Q43.7)

Q52.3 Imperforate hymen ♀
DEF: Obstructive anomaly of vagina, characterized by complete closure of the membranous fold around the external opening of the vagina, obstructing the vaginal introitus.

Q52.4 Other congenital malformations of vagina ♀
Canal of Nuck cyst, congenital
Congenital malformation of vagina NOS
Embryonic vaginal cyst
Gartner's duct cyst

Q52.5 Fusion of labia ♀

Q52.6 Congenital malformation of clitoris ♀

√5ᵗʰ **Q52.7 Other and unspecified congenital malformations of vulva**

Q52.70 Unspecified congenital malformations of vulva ♀
Congenital malformation of vulva NOS

Q52.71 Congenital absence of vulva ♀

Q52.79 Other congenital malformations of vulva ♀
Congenital cyst of vulva

Q52.8 Other specified congenital malformations of female genitalia ♀

Q52.9 Congenital malformation of female genitalia, unspecified ♀

√4ᵗʰ **Q53 Undescended and ectopic testicle**

√5ᵗʰ **Q53.0 Ectopic testis**

Q53.00 Ectopic testis, unspecified ♂

Q53.01 Ectopic testis, unilateral ♂

Q53.02 Ectopic testes, bilateral ♂

√5ᵗʰ **Q53.1 Undescended testicle, unilateral**
AHA: 2017,4Q,22-23

Q53.10 Unspecified undescended testicle, unilateral ♂

√6ᵗʰ **Q53.11 Abdominal testis, unilateral**

Q53.111 Unilateral intraabdominal testis ♂

Q53.112 Unilateral inguinal testis ♂

Q53.12 Ectopic perineal testis, unilateral ♂

Q53.13 Unilateral high scrotal testis ♂

√5ᵗʰ **Q53.2 Undescended testicle, bilateral**
AHA: 2017,4Q,22-23

Q53.20 Undescended testicle, unspecified, bilateral ♂

√6ᵗʰ **Q53.21 Abdominal testis, bilateral**

Q53.211 Bilateral intraabdominal testes ♂

Q53.212 Bilateral inguinal testes ♂

Q53.22 Ectopic perineal testis, bilateral ♂

Q53.23 Bilateral high scrotal testes ♂

Q53.9 Undescended testicle, unspecified ♂
Cryptorchism NOS

√4ᵗʰ **Q54 Hypospadias**
EXCLUDES 1   epispadias (Q64.0)
DEF: Abnormal opening of the urethra on the ventral (underside) surface of the penis.

Hypospadias

- Balanic (glanular, coronal) hypospadias
- Subcoronal hypospadias
- Penile hypospadias
- Scrotal hypospadias
- Scrotum
- Penile raphe
- Penoscrotal hypospadias
- Scrotal raphe
- Perineal hypospadias

Hypospadias (ventral view)

Q54.0 Hypospadias, balanic ♂
Hypospadias, coronal
Hypospadias, glandular

Q54.1 Hypospadias, penile ♂

Q54.2 Hypospadias, penoscrotal ♂

Q54.3 Hypospadias, perineal ♂

Q54.4 Congenital chordee ♂
Chordee without hypospadias

Chapter 17. Congenital Malformations, Deformations and Chromosomal Abnormalities

Q51.2–Q54.4

Q54.8 Other hypospadias ♂

Hypospadias with intersex state

Q54.9 Hypospadias, unspecified ♂

✓4ᵗʰ **Q55 Other congenital malformations of** male genital organs

EXCLUDES 1   congenital hydrocele (P83.5)

hypospadias (Q54.-)

Q55.0 Absence and aplasia of testis ♂

Monorchism

Q55.1 Hypoplasia of testis and scrotum ♂

Fusion of testes

✓5ᵗʰ **Q55.2 Other and unspecified congenital malformations of** testis and scrotum

Q55.20 Unspecified congenital malformations of testis and scrotum ♂

Congenital malformation of testis or scrotum NOS

Q55.21 Polyorchism ♂

DEF: Congenital anomaly in which there are more than two testes.

Q55.22 Retractile testis ♂

Q55.23 Scrotal transposition ♂

Q55.29 Other congenital malformations of testis and scrotum ♂

Q55.3 Atresia of vas deferens ♂

Code first any associated cystic fibrosis (E84.-)

Q55.4 Other congenital malformations of vas deferens, epididymis, seminal vesicles and prostate ♂

Absence or aplasia of prostate

Absence or aplasia of spermatic cord

Congenital malformation of vas deferens, epididymis, seminal vesicles or prostate NOS

Q55.5 Congenital absence and aplasia of penis ♂

✓5ᵗʰ **Q55.6 Other congenital malformations of** penis

Q55.61 Curvature of penis (lateral) ♂

Q55.62 Hypoplasia of penis ♂

Micropenis

Q55.63 Congenital torsion of penis ♂

EXCLUDES 1   acquired torsion of penis (N48.82)

Q55.64 Hidden penis ♂

Buried penis

Concealed penis

EXCLUDES 1   acquired buried penis (N48.83)

Q55.69 Other congenital malformation of penis ♂

Congenital malformation of penis NOS

Q55.7 Congenital vasocutaneous fistula ♂

Q55.8 Other specified congenital malformations of male genital organs ♂

Q55.9 Congenital malformation of male genital organ, unspecified ♂

Congenital anomaly of male genital organ

Congenital deformity of male genital organ

✓4ᵗʰ **Q56 Indeterminate sex and pseudohermaphroditism**

EXCLUDES 1   46, XX true hermaphrodite (Q99.1)

androgen insensitivity syndrome (E34.5-)

chimera 46, XX/46, XY true hermaphrodite (Q99.0)

female pseudohermaphroditism with adrenocortical disorder (E25.-)

pseudohermaphroditism with specified chromosomal anomaly (Q96-Q99)

pure gonadal dysgenesis (Q99.1)

DEF: Indeterminate sex: External genitalia that is nondescript, lacking the physical appearance specific to either sex.

DEF: Pseudohermaphroditism: Presence of gonads of one sex and external genitalia of another sex.

Q56.0 Hermaphroditism, not elsewhere classified

Ovotestis

Q56.1 Male pseudohermaphroditism, not elsewhere classified ♂

46, XY with streak gonads

Male pseudohermaphroditism NOS

Q56.2 Female pseudohermaphroditism, not elsewhere classified ♀

Female pseudohermaphroditism NOS

Q56.3 Pseudohermaphroditism, unspecified

Q56.4 Indeterminate sex, unspecified

Ambiguous genitalia

Congenital malformations of the urinary system (Q60-Q64)

✓4ᵗʰ **Q60 Renal agenesis and other** reduction defects of kidney

INCLUDES   congenital absence of kidney

congenital atrophy of kidney

infantile atrophy of kidney

Q60.0 Renal agenesis, unilateral

Q60.1 Renal agenesis, bilateral

Q60.2 Renal agenesis, unspecified

Q60.3 Renal hypoplasia, unilateral

Q60.4 Renal hypoplasia, bilateral

Q60.5 Renal hypoplasia, unspecified

Q60.6 Potter's syndrome

✓4ᵗʰ **Q61 Cystic kidney disease**

EXCLUDES 1   acquired cyst of kidney (N28.1)

Potter's syndrome (Q60.6)

✓5ᵗʰ **Q61.0 Congenital renal** cyst

Q61.00 Congenital renal cyst, unspecified

Cyst of kidney NOS (congenital)

Q61.01 Congenital single renal cyst

Q61.02 Congenital multiple renal cysts

✓5ᵗʰ **Q61.1 Polycystic kidney, infantile type**

Polycystic kidney, autosomal recessive

Q61.11 Cystic dilatation of collecting ducts

Q61.19 Other polycystic kidney, infantile type

Q61.2 Polycystic kidney, adult type

Polycystic kidney, autosomal dominant

Q61.3 Polycystic kidney, unspecified

AHA: 2016,3Q,22

Q61.4 Renal dysplasia

Multicystic dysplastic kidney

Multicystic kidney (development)

Multicystic kidney disease

Multicystic renal dysplasia

EXCLUDES 1   polycystic kidney disease (Q61.11-Q61.3)

Q61.5 Medullary cystic kidney

Nephronopthisis

Sponge kidney NOS

DEF: Sponge kidney: Dilated collecting tubules that are usually asymptomatic. Calcinosis in tubules may cause renal insufficiency.

Q61.8 Other cystic kidney diseases

Fibrocystic kidney

Fibrocystic renal degeneration or disease

Q61.9 Cystic kidney disease, unspecified

Meckel-Gruber syndrome

✓4ᵗʰ **Q62 Congenital obstructive defects of** renal pelvis **and congenital malformations of** ureter

Q62.0 Congenital hydronephrosis

✓5ᵗʰ **Q62.1 Congenital** occlusion of ureter

Atresia and stenosis of ureter

Q62.10 Congenital occlusion of ureter, unspecified

Q62.11 Congenital occlusion of ureteropelvic junction

Q62.12 Congenital occlusion of ureterovesical orifice

Q62.2 Congenital megaureter

Congenital dilatation of ureter

✓5ᵗʰ **Q62.3 Other obstructive defects of renal pelvis and ureter**

Q62.31 Congenital ureterocele, orthotopic

Q62.32 Cecoureterocele

Ectopic ureterocele

Q62.39 Other obstructive defects of renal pelvis and ureter

Ureteropelvic junction obstruction NOS

Q62.4 Agenesis of ureter

Congenital absence ureter

Q62.5 Duplication of ureter

Accessory ureter

Double ureter

✓5ᵗʰ **Q62.6 Malposition of** ureter

Q62.60 Malposition of ureter, unspecified

Q62.61 Deviation of ureter

Q62.62 Displacement of ureter

Ⓝ Newborn: 0   Ⓟ Pediatric: 0-17   Ⓜ Maternity: 12-55   Ⓐ Adult: 15-124   CH Comorbidity High   CL Comorbidity Low   NCDx Noncancer Dx   PDx Primary Dx

910

ICD-10-CM 2020

Q62.63   Anomalous implantation of ureter
Ectopia of ureter
Ectopic ureter

Q62.69   Other malposition of ureter

Q62.7   Congenital vesico-uretero-renal reflux

Q62.8   Other congenital malformations of ureter
Anomaly of ureter NOS

✓4ᵗʰ **Q63**   Other congenital malformations of kidney

> EXCLUDES 1   congenital nephrotic syndrome (N04.-)

Q63.0   Accessory kidney

Q63.1   Lobulated, fused and horseshoe kidney

Q63.2   Ectopic kidney
Congenital displaced kidney
Malrotation of kidney

Q63.3   Hyperplastic and giant kidney
Compensatory hypertrophy of kidney

Q63.8   Other specified congenital malformations of kidney
Congenital renal calculi

Q63.9   Congenital malformation of kidney, unspecified

✓4ᵗʰ **Q64**   Other congenital malformations of urinary system

Q64.0   Epispadias

> EXCLUDES 1   hypospadias (Q54.-)

Epispadias

Normal external urethral orifice

Glans penis

Foreskin (retracted)

Epispadias

Epispadias (dorsal view)

✓5ᵗʰ **Q64.1**   Exstrophy of urinary bladder

Q64.10   Exstrophy of urinary bladder, unspecified
Ectopia vesicae

Q64.11   Supravesical fissure of urinary bladder

Q64.12   Cloacal exstrophy of urinary bladder

Q64.19   Other exstrophy of urinary bladder
Extroversion of bladder

Q64.2   Congenital posterior urethral valves

✓5ᵗʰ **Q64.3**   Other atresia and stenosis of urethra and bladder neck

Q64.31   Congenital bladder neck obstruction
Congenital obstruction of vesicourethral orifice

Q64.32   Congenital stricture of urethra

Q64.33   Congenital stricture of urinary meatus

Q64.39   Other atresia and stenosis of urethra and bladder neck
Atresia and stenosis of urethra and bladder neck NOS

Q64.4   Malformation of urachus
Cyst of urachus
Patent urachus
Prolapse of urachus

Q64.5   Congenital absence of bladder and urethra

Q64.6   Congenital diverticulum of bladder

✓5ᵗʰ **Q64.7**   Other and unspecified congenital malformations of bladder and urethra

> EXCLUDES 1   congenital prolapse of bladder (mucosa) (Q79.4)

Q64.70   Unspecified congenital malformation of bladder and urethra
Malformation of bladder or urethra NOS

Q64.71   Congenital prolapse of urethra

Q64.72   Congenital prolapse of urinary meatus

Q64.73   Congenital urethrorectal fistula

Q64.74   Double urethra

Q64.75   Double urinary meatus

Q64.79   Other congenital malformations of bladder and urethra

Q64.8   Other specified congenital malformations of urinary system

Q64.9   Congenital malformation of urinary system, unspecified
Congenital anomaly NOS of urinary system
Congenital deformity NOS of urinary system

Congenital malformations and deformations of the musculoskeletal system (Q65-Q79)

✓4ᵗʰ **Q65**   Congenital deformities of hip

> EXCLUDES 1   clicking hip (R29.4)

✓5ᵗʰ **Q65.0**   Congenital dislocation of hip, unilateral

Q65.00   Congenital dislocation of unspecified hip, unilateral

Q65.01   Congenital dislocation of right hip, unilateral

Q65.02   Congenital dislocation of left hip, unilateral

Q65.1   Congenital dislocation of hip, bilateral

Q65.2   Congenital dislocation of hip, unspecified

✓5ᵗʰ **Q65.3**   Congenital partial dislocation of hip, unilateral

Q65.30   Congenital partial dislocation of unspecified hip, unilateral

Q65.31   Congenital partial dislocation of right hip, unilateral

Q65.32   Congenital partial dislocation of left hip, unilateral

Q65.4   Congenital partial dislocation of hip, bilateral

Q65.5   Congenital partial dislocation of hip, unspecified

Q65.6   Congenital unstable hip
Congenital dislocatable hip

✓5ᵗʰ **Q65.8**   Other congenital deformities of hip

Q65.81   Congenital coxa valga

Q65.82   Congenital coxa vara

Q65.89   Other specified congenital deformities of hip
Anteversion of femoral neck
Congenital acetabular dysplasia

Q65.9   Congenital deformity of hip, unspecified

✓4ᵗʰ **Q66**   Congenital deformities of feet

> EXCLUDES 1   reduction defects of feet (Q72.-)
> valgus deformities (acquired) (M21.0-)
> varus deformities (acquired) (M21.1-)

▲ ✓5ᵗʰ **Q66.0**   Congenital talipes equinovarus

● **Q66.00**   Congenital talipes equinovarus, unspecified foot

● **Q66.01**   Congenital talipes equinovarus, right foot

● **Q66.02**   Congenital talipes equinovarus, left foot

▲ ✓5ᵗʰ **Q66.1**   Congenital talipes calcaneovarus

● **Q66.10**   Congenital talipes calcaneovarus, unspecified foot

● **Q66.11**   Congenital talipes calcaneovarus, right foot

● **Q66.12**   Congenital talipes calcaneovarus, left foot

✓5ᵗʰ **Q66.2**   Congenital metatarsus (primus) varus

> AHA: 2016,4Q,59

▲ ✓6ᵗʰ **Q66.21**   Congenital metatarsus primus varus

● **Q66.211**   Congenital metatarsus primus varus, right foot

● **Q66.212**   Congenital metatarsus primus varus, left foot

● **Q66.219**   Congenital metatarsus primus varus, unspecified foot

▲ ✓6ᵗʰ **Q66.22**   Congenital metatarsus adductus
Congenital metatarsus varus

● **Q66.221**   Congenital metatarsus adductus, right foot

● **Q66.222**   Congenital metatarsus adductus, left foot

● **Q66.229**   Congenital metatarsus adductus, unspecified foot

▲ ✓5ᵗʰ **Q66.3**   Other congenital varus deformities of feet
Hallux varus, congenital

● **Q66.30**   Other congenital varus deformities of feet, unspecified foot

● **Q66.31**   Other congenital varus deformities of feet, right foot

● **Q66.32**   Other congenital varus deformities of feet, left foot

▲ ✓5ᵗʰ **Q66.4**   Congenital talipes calcaneovalgus

● **Q66.40**   Congenital talipes calcaneovalgus, unspecified foot

● **Q66.41**   Congenital talipes calcaneovalgus, right foot

● **Q66.42**   Congenital talipes calcaneovalgus, left foot

✓ Additional Character Required   ✓x7ᵗʰ Placeholder Alert   Manifestation   Unspecified Dx   ▶◀ Revised Text   ● New Code   ▲ Revised Title

ICD-10-CM 2020   911

Q66.5 Congenital pes planus
Congenital flat foot
Congenital rigid flat foot
Congenital spastic (everted) flat foot
EXCLUDES 1 pes planus, acquired (M21.4)
Q66.50 Congenital pes planus, unspecified foot
Q66.51 Congenital pes planus, right foot
Q66.52 Congenital pes planus, left foot
Q66.6 Other congenital valgus deformities of feet
Congenital metatarsus valgus
Q66.7 Congenital pes cavus
Q66.70 Congenital pes cavus, unspecified foot
Q66.71 Congenital pes cavus, right foot
Q66.72 Congenital pes cavus, left foot
Q66.8 Other congenital deformities of feet
Q66.80 Congenital vertical talus deformity, unspecified foot
Q66.81 Congenital vertical talus deformity, right foot
Q66.82 Congenital vertical talus deformity, left foot
Q66.89 Other specified congenital deformities of feet
Congenital asymmetric talipes
Congenital clubfoot NOS
Congenital talipes NOS
Congenital tarsal coalition
Hammer toe, congenital
DEF: Clubfoot: Congenital anomaly of the foot with the heel elevated and rotated outward and the toes pointing inward.
Q66.9 Congenital deformity of feet, unspecified
Q66.90 Congenital deformity of feet, unspecified, unspecified foot
Q66.91 Congenital deformity of feet, unspecified, right foot
Q66.92 Congenital deformity of feet, unspecified, left foot

Q67 Congenital musculoskeletal deformities of head, face, spine and chest
EXCLUDES 1 congenital malformation syndromes classified to Q87.- Potter's syndrome (Q60.6)
Q67.0 Congenital facial asymmetry
Q67.1 Congenital compression facies
Q67.2 Dolichocephaly
Q67.3 Plagiocephaly
Q67.4 Other congenital deformities of skull, face and jaw
Congenital depressions in skull
Congenital hemifacial atrophy or hypertrophy
Deviation of nasal septum, congenital
Squashed or bent nose, congenital
EXCLUDES 1 dentofacial anomalies [including malocclusion] (M26.-)
syphilitic saddle nose (A50.5)
DEF: Deviated septum: Condition in which the nasal septum, a thin wall composed of cartilage and bone that separates the two nostrils, is crooked or displaced from the midline.
Q67.5 Congenital deformity of spine
Congenital postural scoliosis
Congenital scoliosis NOS
EXCLUDES 1 infantile idiopathic scoliosis (M41.0)
scoliosis due to congenital bony malformation (Q76.3)
AHA: 2014,4Q,26
Q67.6 Pectus excavatum
Congenital funnel chest
Q67.7 Pectus carinatum
Congenital pigeon chest
Q67.8 Other congenital deformities of chest
Congenital deformity of chest wall NOS

Q68 Other congenital musculoskeletal deformities
EXCLUDES 1 reduction defects of limb(s) (Q71-Q73)
EXCLUDES 2 congenital myotonic chondrodystrophy (G71.13)
Q68.0 Congenital deformity of sternocleidomastoid muscle
Congenital contracture of sternocleidomastoid (muscle)
Congenital (sternomastoid) torticollis
Sternomastoid tumor (congenital)

Q68.1 Congenital deformity of finger(s) and hand
Congenital clubfinger
Spade-like hand (congenital)
Q68.2 Congenital deformity of knee
Congenital dislocation of knee
Congenital genu recurvatum
Q68.3 Congenital bowing of femur
EXCLUDES 1 anteversion of femur (neck) (Q65.89)
Q68.4 Congenital bowing of tibia and fibula
Q68.5 Congenital bowing of long bones of leg, unspecified
Q68.6 Discoid meniscus
Q68.8 Other specified congenital musculoskeletal deformities
Congenital deformity of clavicle
Congenital deformity of elbow
Congenital deformity of forearm
Congenital deformity of scapula
Congenital deformity of wrist
Congenital dislocation of elbow
Congenital dislocation of shoulder
Congenital dislocation of wrist

Q69 Polydactyly
Q69.0 Accessory finger(s)
Q69.1 Accessory thumb(s)
Q69.2 Accessory toe(s)
Accessory hallux
Q69.9 Polydactyly, unspecified
Supernumerary digit(s) NOS

Q70 Syndactyly
Q70.0 Fused fingers
Complex syndactyly of fingers with synostosis
Q70.00 Fused fingers, unspecified hand
Q70.01 Fused fingers, right hand
Q70.02 Fused fingers, left hand
Q70.03 Fused fingers, bilateral
Q70.1 Webbed fingers
Simple syndactyly of fingers without synostosis
Q70.10 Webbed fingers, unspecified hand
Q70.11 Webbed fingers, right hand
Q70.12 Webbed fingers, left hand
Q70.13 Webbed fingers, bilateral
Q70.2 Fused toes
Complex syndactyly of toes with synostosis
Q70.20 Fused toes, unspecified foot
Q70.21 Fused toes, right foot
Q70.22 Fused toes, left foot
Q70.23 Fused toes, bilateral
Q70.3 Webbed toes
Simple syndactyly of toes without synostosis
Q70.30 Webbed toes, unspecified foot
Q70.31 Webbed toes, right foot
Q70.32 Webbed toes, left foot
Q70.33 Webbed toes, bilateral
Q70.4 Polysyndactyly, unspecified
EXCLUDES 1 specified syndactyly of hand and feet — code to specified conditions (Q70.0-Q70.3-)
Q70.9 Syndactyly, unspecified
Symphalangy NOS

Q71 Reduction defects of upper limb
Q71.0 Congenital complete absence of upper limb
Q71.00 Congenital complete absence of unspecified upper limb
Q71.01 Congenital complete absence of right upper limb
Q71.02 Congenital complete absence of left upper limb
Q71.03 Congenital complete absence of upper limb, bilateral
Q71.1 Congenital absence of upper arm and forearm with hand present
Q71.10 Congenital absence of unspecified upper arm and forearm with hand present
Q71.11 Congenital absence of right upper arm and forearm with hand present
Q71.12 Congenital absence of left upper arm and forearm with hand present
Q71.13 Congenital absence of upper arm and forearm with hand present, bilateral

√5ᵗʰ **Q71.2** Congenital absence of both forearm and hand

    Q71.20 Congenital absence of both forearm and hand, unspecified upper limb

    Q71.21 Congenital absence of both forearm and hand, right upper limb

    Q71.22 Congenital absence of both forearm and hand, left upper limb

    Q71.23 Congenital absence of both forearm and hand, bilateral

√5ᵗʰ **Q71.3** Congenital absence of hand and finger

    Q71.30 Congenital absence of unspecified hand and finger

    Q71.31 Congenital absence of right hand and finger

    Q71.32 Congenital absence of left hand and finger

    Q71.33 Congenital absence of hand and finger, bilateral

√5ᵗʰ **Q71.4** Longitudinal reduction defect of radius

    Clubhand (congenital)
    Radial clubhand

    Q71.40 Longitudinal reduction defect of unspecified radius

    Q71.41 Longitudinal reduction defect of right radius

    Q71.42 Longitudinal reduction defect of left radius

    Q71.43 Longitudinal reduction defect of radius, bilateral

√5ᵗʰ **Q71.5** Longitudinal reduction defect of ulna

    Q71.50 Longitudinal reduction defect of unspecified ulna

    Q71.51 Longitudinal reduction defect of right ulna

    Q71.52 Longitudinal reduction defect of left ulna

    Q71.53 Longitudinal reduction defect of ulna, bilateral

√5ᵗʰ **Q71.6** Lobster-claw hand

    Q71.60 Lobster-claw hand, unspecified hand

    Q71.61 Lobster-claw right hand

    Q71.62 Lobster-claw left hand

    Q71.63 Lobster-claw hand, bilateral

√5ᵗʰ **Q71.8** Other reduction defects of upper limb

    √6ᵗʰ **Q71.81** Congenital shortening of upper limb

        Q71.811 Congenital shortening of right upper limb

        Q71.812 Congenital shortening of left upper limb

        Q71.813 Congenital shortening of upper limb, bilateral

        Q71.819 Congenital shortening of unspecified upper limb

    √6ᵗʰ **Q71.89** Other reduction defects of upper limb

        Q71.891 Other reduction defects of right upper limb

        Q71.892 Other reduction defects of left upper limb

        Q71.893 Other reduction defects of upper limb, bilateral

        Q71.899 Other reduction defects of unspecified upper limb

√5ᵗʰ **Q71.9** Unspecified reduction defect of upper limb

    Q71.90 Unspecified reduction defect of unspecified upper limb

    Q71.91 Unspecified reduction defect of right upper limb

    Q71.92 Unspecified reduction defect of left upper limb

    Q71.93 Unspecified reduction defect of upper limb, bilateral

√4ᵗʰ **Q72** Reduction defects of lower limb

√5ᵗʰ **Q72.0** Congenital complete absence of lower limb

    Q72.00 Congenital complete absence of unspecified lower limb

    Q72.01 Congenital complete absence of right lower limb

    Q72.02 Congenital complete absence of left lower limb

    Q72.03 Congenital complete absence of lower limb, bilateral

√5ᵗʰ **Q72.1** Congenital absence of thigh and lower leg with foot present

    Q72.10 Congenital absence of unspecified thigh and lower leg with foot present

    Q72.11 Congenital absence of right thigh and lower leg with foot present

    Q72.12 Congenital absence of left thigh and lower leg with foot present

    Q72.13 Congenital absence of thigh and lower leg with foot present, bilateral

√5ᵗʰ **Q72.2** Congenital absence of both lower leg and foot

    Q72.20 Congenital absence of both lower leg and foot, unspecified lower limb

    Q72.21 Congenital absence of both lower leg and foot, right lower limb

    Q72.22 Congenital absence of both lower leg and foot, left lower limb

    Q72.23 Congenital absence of both lower leg and foot, bilateral

√5ᵗʰ **Q72.3** Congenital absence of foot and toe(s)

    Q72.30 Congenital absence of unspecified foot and toe(s)

    Q72.31 Congenital absence of right foot and toe(s)

    Q72.32 Congenital absence of left foot and toe(s)

    Q72.33 Congenital absence of foot and toe(s), bilateral

√5ᵗʰ **Q72.4** Longitudinal reduction defect of femur

    Proximal femoral focal deficiency

    Q72.40 Longitudinal reduction defect of unspecified femur

    Q72.41 Longitudinal reduction defect of right femur

    Q72.42 Longitudinal reduction defect of left femur

    Q72.43 Longitudinal reduction defect of femur, bilateral

√5ᵗʰ **Q72.5** Longitudinal reduction defect of tibia

    Q72.50 Longitudinal reduction defect of unspecified tibia

    Q72.51 Longitudinal reduction defect of right tibia

    Q72.52 Longitudinal reduction defect of left tibia

    Q72.53 Longitudinal reduction defect of tibia, bilateral

√5ᵗʰ **Q72.6** Longitudinal reduction defect of fibula

    Q72.60 Longitudinal reduction defect of unspecified fibula

    Q72.61 Longitudinal reduction defect of right fibula

    Q72.62 Longitudinal reduction defect of left fibula

    Q72.63 Longitudinal reduction defect of fibula, bilateral

√5ᵗʰ **Q72.7** Split foot

    Q72.70 Split foot, unspecified lower limb

    Q72.71 Split foot, right lower limb

    Q72.72 Split foot, left lower limb

    Q72.73 Split foot, bilateral

√5ᵗʰ **Q72.8** Other reduction defects of lower limb

    √6ᵗʰ **Q72.81** Congenital shortening of lower limb

        Q72.811 Congenital shortening of right lower limb

        Q72.812 Congenital shortening of left lower limb

        Q72.813 Congenital shortening of lower limb, bilateral

        Q72.819 Congenital shortening of unspecified lower limb

    √6ᵗʰ **Q72.89** Other reduction defects of lower limb

        Q72.891 Other reduction defects of right lower limb

        Q72.892 Other reduction defects of left lower limb

        Q72.893 Other reduction defects of lower limb, bilateral

        Q72.899 Other reduction defects of unspecified lower limb

√5ᵗʰ **Q72.9** Unspecified reduction defect of lower limb

    Q72.90 Unspecified reduction defect of unspecified lower limb

    Q72.91 Unspecified reduction defect of right lower limb

    Q72.92 Unspecified reduction defect of left lower limb

    Q72.93 Unspecified reduction defect of lower limb, bilateral

√4ᵗʰ **Q73** Reduction defects of unspecified limb

    Q73.0 Congenital absence of unspecified limb(s)

        Amelia NOS

    Q73.1 Phocomelia, unspecified limb(s)

        Phocomelia NOS

    Q73.8 Other reduction defects of unspecified limb(s)

        Longitudinal reduction deformity of unspecified limb(s)
        Ectromelia of limb NOS
        Hemimelia of limb NOS
        Reduction defect of limb NOS

✔ Additional Character Required   √x7ᵗʰ Placeholder Alert   Manifestation   Unspecified Dx   ►◄ Revised Text   ● New Code   ▲ Revised Title

✓4th **Q74 Other congenital malformations of limb(s)**

EXCLUDES 1   *polydactyly (Q69.-)*
reduction defect of limb (Q71-Q73)
syndactyly (Q70.-)

Q74.0 Other congenital malformations of upper limb(s), including shoulder girdle
Accessory carpal bones
Cleidocranial dysostosis
Congenital pseudarthrosis of clavicle
Macrodactylia (fingers)
Madelung's deformity
Radioulnar synostosis
Sprengel's deformity
Triphalangeal thumb

Q74.1 Congenital malformation of knee
Congenital absence of patella
Congenital dislocation of patella
Congenital genu valgum
Congenital genu varum
Rudimentary patella
EXCLUDES 1   *congenital dislocation of knee (Q68.2)*
congenital genu recurvatum (Q68.2)
nail patella syndrome (Q87.2)

Q74.2 Other congenital malformations of lower limb(s), including pelvic girdle
Congenital fusion of sacroiliac joint
Congenital malformation of ankle joint
Congenital malformation of sacroiliac joint
EXCLUDES 1   *anteversion of femur (neck) (Q65.89)*

Q74.3 Arthrogryposis multiplex congenita

Q74.8 Other specified congenital malformations of limb(s)

Q74.9 Unspecified congenital malformation of limb(s)
Congenital anomaly of limb(s) NOS

✓4th **Q75 Other congenital malformations of skull and face bones**

EXCLUDES 1   *congenital malformation of face NOS (Q18.-)*
congenital malformation syndromes classified to Q87.-
dentofacial anomalies [including malocclusion] (M26.-)
musculoskeletal deformities of head and face (Q67.0-Q67.4)
skull defects associated with congenital anomalies of brain such as:
anencephaly (Q00.0)
encephalocele (Q01.-)
hydrocephalus (Q03.-)
microcephaly (Q02)

Q75.0 Craniosynostosis
Acrocephaly
Imperfect fusion of skull
Oxycephaly
Trigonocephaly
DEF: Congenital condition in which one or more of the cranial sutures fuse prematurely, creating a deformed or aberrant head shape.

Q75.1 Craniofacial dysostosis
Crouzon's disease

Q75.2 Hypertelorism

Q75.3 Macrocephaly

Q75.4 Mandibulofacial dysostosis
Franceschetti syndrome
Treacher Collins syndrome

Q75.5 Oculomandibular dysostosis

Q75.8 Other specified congenital malformations of skull and face bones
Absence of skull bone, congenital
Congenital deformity of forehead
Platybasia

Q75.9 Congenital malformation of skull and face bones, unspecified
Congenital anomaly of face bones NOS
Congenital anomaly of skull NOS

✓4th **Q76 Congenital malformations of spine and bony thorax**

EXCLUDES 1   *congenital musculoskeletal deformities of spine and chest (Q67.5-Q67.8)*

Q76.0 Spina bifida occulta
EXCLUDES 1   *meningocele (spinal) (Q05.-)*
spina bifida (aperta) (cystica) (Q05.-)

Q76.1 Klippel-Feil syndrome
Cervical fusion syndrome

Q76.2 Congenital spondylolisthesis
Congenital spondylolysis
EXCLUDES 1   *spondylolisthesis (acquired) (M43.1-)*
spondylolysis (acquired) (M43.0-)

Q76.3 Congenital scoliosis due to congenital bony malformation
Hemivertebra fusion or failure of segmentation with scoliosis

✓5th **Q76.4 Other congenital malformations of spine, not associated with scoliosis**

✓6th **Q76.41 Congenital kyphosis**

Q76.411 Congenital kyphosis, occipito-atlanto-axial region
Q76.412 Congenital kyphosis, cervical region
Q76.413 Congenital kyphosis, cervicothoracic region
Q76.414 Congenital kyphosis, thoracic region
Q76.415 Congenital kyphosis, thoracolumbar region
Q76.419 Congenital kyphosis, unspecified region

✓6th **Q76.42 Congenital lordosis**

Q76.425 Congenital lordosis, thoracolumbar region
Q76.426 Congenital lordosis, lumbar region
Q76.427 Congenital lordosis, lumbosacral region
Q76.428 Congenital lordosis, sacral and sacrococcygeal region
Q76.429 Congenital lordosis, unspecified region

Q76.49 Other congenital malformations of spine, not associated with scoliosis
Congenital absence of vertebra NOS
Congenital fusion of spine NOS
Congenital malformation of lumbosacral (joint) (region) NOS
Congenital malformation of spine NOS
Hemivertebra NOS
Malformation of spine NOS
Platyspondylisis NOS
Supernumerary vertebra NOS

Q76.5 Cervical rib
Supernumerary rib in cervical region

Q76.6 Other congenital malformations of ribs
Accessory rib
Congenital absence of rib
Congenital fusion of ribs
Congenital malformation of ribs NOS
EXCLUDES 1   *short rib syndrome (Q77.2)*

Q76.7 Congenital malformation of sternum
Congenital absence of sternum
Sternum bifidum

Q76.8 Other congenital malformations of bony thorax

Q76.9 Congenital malformation of bony thorax, unspecified

✓4th **Q77 Osteochondrodysplasia with defects of growth of tubular bones and spine**
EXCLUDES 1   *mucopolysaccharidosis (E76.0-E76.3)*
EXCLUDES 2   *congenital myotonic chondrodystrophy (G71.13)*

Q77.0 Achondrogenesis
Hypochondrogenesis

Q77.1 Thanatophoric short stature

Q77.2 Short rib syndrome
Asphyxiating thoracic dysplasia [Jeune]

Q77.3 Chondrodysplasia punctata
EXCLUDES 1   *Rhizomelic chondrodysplasia punctata (E71.43)*

Q77.4 Achondroplasia
Hypochondroplasia
Osteosclerosis congenita

Q77.5 Diastrophic dysplasia

Q77.6 Chondroectodermal dysplasia
Ellis-van Creveld syndrome

Q77.7 Spondyloepiphyseal dysplasia

Q77.8 Other osteochondrodysplasia with defects of growth of tubular bones and spine

Q77.9 Osteochondrodysplasia with defects of growth of tubular bones and spine, unspecified

✓4ᵗʰ **Q78** **Other osteochondrodysplasias**

     EXCLUDES 2   *congenital myotonic chondrodystrophy (G71.13)*

   Q78.0 **Osteogenesis imperfecta**
     Fragilitas ossium
     Osteopsathyrosis

   Q78.1 **Polyostotic fibrous dysplasia**
     Albright(-McCune)(-Sternberg) syndrome

   Q78.2 **Osteopetrosis**
     Albers-Schönberg syndrome
     Osteosclerosis NOS
     DEF: Rare congenital condition in which the bones are excessively dense, resulting from a discrepancy in the formation and breakdown of bone.

   Q78.3 **Progressive diaphyseal dysplasia**
     Camurati-Engelmann syndrome

   Q78.4 **Enchondromatosis**
     Maffucci's syndrome
     Ollier's disease

   Q78.5 **Metaphyseal dysplasia**
     Pyle's syndrome

   Q78.6 **Multiple congenital exostoses**
     Diaphyseal aclasis

   Q78.8 **Other specified osteochondrodysplasias**
     Osteopoikilosis

   Q78.9 **Osteochondrodysplasia, unspecified**
     Chondrodystrophy NOS
     Osteodystrophy NOS

✓4ᵗʰ **Q79** **Congenital malformations of musculoskeletal system, not elsewhere classified**

     EXCLUDES 2   *congenital (sternomastoid) torticollis (Q68.0)*

   Q79.0 **Congenital diaphragmatic hernia**
     EXCLUDES 1   *congenital hiatus hernia (Q40.1)*

   Q79.1 **Other congenital malformations of diaphragm**
     Absence of diaphragm
     Congenital malformation of diaphragm NOS
     Eventration of diaphragm

   Q79.2 **Exomphalos**
     Omphalocele
     EXCLUDES 1   *umbilical hernia (K42.-)*

   Q79.3 **Gastroschisis**

Gastroschisis

     Herniated small bowel (gastroschisis)

     Rectus abdominus m.

     Umbilicus

     skin

     distal   proximal

     Defect

   Q79.4 **Prune belly syndrome**
     Congenital prolapse of bladder mucosa
     Eagle-Barrett syndrome

   ✓5ᵗʰ **Q79.5** **Other congenital malformations of abdominal wall**
     EXCLUDES 1   *umbilical hernia (K42.-)*

     Q79.51 **Congenital hernia of bladder**

     Q79.59 **Other congenital malformations of abdominal wall**

▲ ✓5ᵗʰ **Q79.6** **Ehlers-Danlos syndromes**
     DEF: Connective tissue disorder that causes hyperextended skin and joints and results in fragile blood vessels with bleeding, poor wound healing, and subcutaneous pseudotumors.

  ●   **Q79.60** **Ehlers-Danlos syndrome, unspecified**

  ●   **Q79.61** **Classical Ehlers-Danlos syndrome**
       Classical EDS (cEDS)

  ●   **Q79.62** **Hypermobile Ehlers-Danlos syndrome**
       Hypermobile EDS (hEDS)

●   **Q79.63** **Vascular Ehlers-Danlos syndrome**
       Vascular EDS (vEDS)

●   **Q79.69** **Other Ehlers-Danlos syndromes**

   Q79.8 **Other congenital malformations of musculoskeletal system**
     Absence of muscle
     Absence of tendon
     Accessory muscle
     Amyotrophia congenita
     Congenital constricting bands
     Congenital shortening of tendon
     Poland syndrome

   Q79.9 **Congenital malformation of musculoskeletal system, unspecified**
     Congenital anomaly of musculoskeletal system NOS
     Congenital deformity of musculoskeletal system NOS

Other congenital malformations (Q80-Q89)

✓4ᵗʰ **Q80** **Congenital ichthyosis**

     EXCLUDES 1   *Refsum's disease (G60.1)*
     DEF: Excessive production of skin cells resulting in red, dry, scaly skin.

   Q80.0 **Ichthyosis vulgaris**

   Q80.1 **X-linked ichthyosis**

   Q80.2 **Lamellar ichthyosis**
     Collodion baby

   Q80.3 **Congenital bullous ichthyosiform erythroderma**

   Q80.4 **Harlequin fetus**

   Q80.8 **Other congenital ichthyosis**

   Q80.9 **Congenital ichthyosis, unspecified**

✓4ᵗʰ **Q81** **Epidermolysis bullosa**

   Q81.0 **Epidermolysis bullosa simplex**
     EXCLUDES 1   *Cockayne's syndrome ▶(Q87.19)◀*

   Q81.1 **Epidermolysis bullosa letalis**
     Herlitz' syndrome

   Q81.2 **Epidermolysis bullosa dystrophica**

   Q81.8 **Other epidermolysis bullosa**

   Q81.9 **Epidermolysis bullosa, unspecified**

✓4ᵗʰ **Q82** **Other congenital malformations of skin**

     EXCLUDES 1   *acrodermatitis enteropathica (E83.2)*
         congenital erythropoietic porphyria (E80.0)
         pilonidal cyst or sinus (L05.-)
         Sturge-Weber (-Dimitri) syndrome (Q85.8)

   Q82.0 **Hereditary lymphedema**

   Q82.1 **Xeroderma pigmentosum**

   Q82.2 **Congenital cutaneous mastocytosis**
     Congenital diffuse cutaneous mastocytosis
     Congenital maculopapular cutaneous mastocytosis
     Congenital urticaria pigmentosa
     EXCLUDES 1   *cutaneous mastocytosis NOS (D47.01)*
         diffuse cutaneous mastocytosis (with onset after newborn period) (D47.01)
         malignant mastocytosis (C96.2-)
         systemic mastocytosis (D47.02)
         urticaria pigmentosa (non-congenital) (with onset after newborn period) (D47.01)

     AHA: 2017,4Q,5

   Q82.3 **Incontinentia pigmenti**

   Q82.4 **Ectodermal dysplasia (anhidrotic)**
     EXCLUDES 1   *Ellis-van Creveld syndrome (Q77.6)*

☑ Additional Character Required   ✓x7ᵗʰ Placeholder Alert   Manifestation   Unspecified Dx   ▶◀ Revised Text   ● New Code   ▲ Revised Title

ICD-10-CM 2020   915

Q82.5   Congenital non-neoplastic nevus
Birthmark NOS
Flammeus Nevus
Portwine Nevus
Sanguineous Nevus
Strawberry Nevus
Vascular Nevus NOS
Verrucous Nevus
EXCLUDES 2   *araneus nevus (I78.1)*
Café au lait spots (L81.3)
lentigo (L81.4)
melanocytic nevus (D22.-)
nevus NOS (D22.-)
pigmented nevus (D22.-)
spider nevus (I78.1)
stellar nevus (I78.1)

Q82.6   Congenital sacral dimple
Parasacral dimple
EXCLUDES 2   *pilonidal cyst with abscess (L05.01)*
pilonidal cyst without abscess (L05.91)
AHA: 2016,4Q,60

Q82.8   Other specified congenital malformations of skin
Abnormal palmar creases
Accessory skin tags
Benign familial pemphigus [Hailey-Hailey]
Congenital poikiloderma
Cutis laxa (hyperelastica)
Dermatoglyphic anomalies
Inherited keratosis palmaris et plantaris
Keratosis follicularis [Darier-White]
EXCLUDES 1   *Ehlers-Danlos syndrome ►(Q79.6-)◄*
AHA: 2016,1Q,17

Q82.9   Congenital malformation of skin, unspecified

☑4ᵗʰ **Q83   Congenital malformations of breast**
EXCLUDES 2   *absence of pectoral muscle (Q79.8)*
hypoplasia of breast (N64.82)
micromastia (N64.82)

Q83.0   Congenital absence of breast with absent nipple

Q83.1   Accessory breast
Supernumerary breast

Q83.2   Absent nipple

Q83.3   Accessory nipple
Supernumerary nipple

Q83.8   Other congenital malformations of breast

Q83.9   Congenital malformation of breast, unspecified

☑4ᵗʰ **Q84   Other congenital malformations of integument**

Q84.0   Congenital alopecia
Congenital atrichosis

Q84.1   Congenital morphological disturbances of hair, not elsewhere classified
Beaded hair
Monilethrix
Pili annulati
EXCLUDES 1   *Menkes' kinky hair syndrome (E83.0)*

Q84.2   Other congenital malformations of hair
Congenital hypertrichosis
Congenital malformation of hair NOS
Persistent lanugo

Q84.3   Anonychia
EXCLUDES 1   *nail patella syndrome (Q87.2)*

Q84.4   Congenital leukonychia

Q84.5   Enlarged and hypertrophic nails
Congenital onychauxis
Pachyonychia

Q84.6   Other congenital malformations of nails
Congenital clubnail
Congenital koilonychia
Congenital malformation of nail NOS

Q84.8   Other specified congenital malformations of integument
Aplasia cutis congenita

Q84.9   Congenital malformation of integument, unspecified
Congenital anomaly of integument NOS
Congenital deformity of integument NOS

☑4ᵗʰ **Q85   Phakomatoses, not elsewhere classified**
EXCLUDES 1   *ataxia telangiectasia [Louis-Bar] (G11.3)*
familial dysautonomia [Riley-Day] (G90.1)

☑5ᵗʰ **Q85.0   Neurofibromatosis (nonmalignant)**

Q85.00   Neurofibromatosis, unspecified

Q85.01   Neurofibromatosis, type 1
Von Recklinghausen disease

Q85.02   Neurofibromatosis, type 2
Acoustic neurofibromatosis
DEF: Inherited condition with cutaneous lesions, benign tumors of peripheral nerves, and bilateral 8th nerve masses.

Q85.03   Schwannomatosis
DEF: Genetic mutation (SMARCB1/INI1) causing multiple benign tumors along the nerve pathways, except on the 8th cranial (vestibular) nerve.

Q85.09   Other neurofibromatosis

Q85.1   Tuberous sclerosis
Bourneville's disease
Epiloia

Q85.8   Other phakomatoses, not elsewhere classified
Peutz-Jeghers Syndrome
Sturge-Weber(-Dimitri) syndrome
von Hippel-Lindau syndrome
EXCLUDES 1   *Meckel-Gruber syndrome (Q61.9)*

Q85.9   Phakomatosis, unspecified
Hamartosis NOS

☑4ᵗʰ **Q86   Congenital malformation syndromes due to known exogenous causes, not elsewhere classified**
EXCLUDES 2   *iodine-deficiency-related hypothyroidism (E00-E02)*
nonteratogenic effects of substances transmitted via placenta or breast milk (P04.-)

Q86.0   Fetal alcohol syndrome (dysmorphic)

Q86.1   Fetal hydantoin syndrome
Meadow's syndrome

Q86.2   Dysmorphism due to warfarin

Q86.8   Other congenital malformation syndromes due to known exogenous causes

☑4ᵗʰ **Q87   Other specified congenital malformation syndromes affecting multiple systems**
Use additional code(s) to identify all associated manifestations

Q87.0   Congenital malformation syndromes predominantly affecting facial appearance
Acrocephalopolysyndactyly
Acrocephalosyndactyly [Apert]
Cryptophthalmos syndrome
Cyclopia
Goldenhar syndrome
Moebius syndrome
Oro-facial-digital syndrome
Robin syndrome
Whistling face

▲   ☑5ᵗʰ **Q87.1   Congenital malformation syndromes predominantly associated with short stature**
~~Aarskog syndrome~~
~~Cockayne syndrome~~
~~De Lange syndrome~~
~~Dubowitz syndrome~~
~~Noonan syndrome~~
~~Prader-Willi syndrome~~
~~Robinow-Silverman-Smith syndrome~~
~~Russell-Silver syndrome~~
~~Seckel syndrome~~
EXCLUDES 1   *Ellis-van Creveld syndrome (Q77.6)*
Smith-Lemli-Opitz syndrome (E78.72)

●   **Q87.11   Prader-Willi syndrome**

●   **Q87.19   Other congenital malformation syndromes predominantly associated with short stature**
Aarskog syndrome
Cockayne syndrome
De Lange syndrome
Dubowitz syndrome
Noonan syndrome
Robinow-Silverman-Smith syndrome
Russell-Silver syndrome
Seckel syndrome

Q87.2 Congenital malformation syndromes predominantly involving limbs
Holt-Oram syndrome
Klippel-Trenaunay-Weber syndrome
Nail patella syndrome
Rubinstein-Taybi syndrome
Sirenomelia syndrome
Thrombocytopenia with absent radius [TAR] syndrome
VATER syndrome

Q87.3 Congenital malformation syndromes involving early overgrowth
Beckwith-Wiedemann syndrome
Sotos syndrome
Weaver syndrome

✓5ᵗʰ Q87.4 Marfan's syndrome
DEF: Disorder that affects the connective tissue of multiple systems, including disproportionally long or abnormal bone structure and eye and cardiovascular complications.

Q87.40 Marfan's syndrome, unspecified
✓6ᵗʰ Q87.41 Marfan's syndrome with cardiovascular manifestations
Q87.410 Marfan's syndrome with aortic dilation
Q87.418 Marfan's syndrome with other cardiovascular manifestations
Q87.42 Marfan's syndrome with ocular manifestations
Q87.43 Marfan's syndrome with skeletal manifestation

Q87.5 Other congenital malformation syndromes with other skeletal changes

✓5ᵗʰ Q87.8 Other specified congenital malformation syndromes, not elsewhere classified
EXCLUDES 1 Zellweger syndrome (E71.510)

Q87.81 Alport syndrome
Use additional code to identify stage of chronic kidney disease (N18.1-N18.6)
Q87.82 Arterial tortuosity syndrome
AHA: 2016,4Q,60-61
Q87.89 Other specified congenital malformation syndromes, not elsewhere classified
Laurence-Moon (-Bardet)-Biedl syndrome

✓4ᵗʰ Q89 Other congenital malformations, not elsewhere classified

✓5ᵗʰ Q89.0 Congenital absence and malformations of spleen
EXCLUDES 1 isomerism of atrial appendages (with asplenia or polysplenia) (Q20.6)

Q89.01 Asplenia (congenital)
Q89.09 Congenital malformations of spleen
Congenital splenomegaly

Q89.1 Congenital malformations of adrenal gland
EXCLUDES 1 adrenogenital disorders (E25.-)
congenital adrenal hyperplasia (E25.0)

Q89.2 Congenital malformations of other endocrine glands
Congenital malformation of parathyroid or thyroid gland
Persistent thyroglossal duct
Thyroglossal cyst
EXCLUDES 1 congenital goiter (E03.0)
congenital hypothyroidism (E03.1)

Q89.3 Situs inversus
Dextrocardia with situs inversus
Mirror-image atrial arrangement with situs inversus
Situs inversus or transversus abdominalis
Situs inversus or transversus thoracis
Transposition of abdominal viscera
Transposition of thoracic viscera
EXCLUDES 1 dextrocardia NOS (Q24.0)
DEF: Congenital anomaly in which the internal thoracic and abdominal organs are transposed laterally and found on the opposite side from the normal position.

Q89.4 Conjoined twins
Craniopagus
Dicephaly
Pygopagus
Thoracopagus

Q89.7 Multiple congenital malformations, not elsewhere classified
Multiple congenital anomalies NOS
Multiple congenital deformities NOS
EXCLUDES 1 congenital malformation syndromes affecting multiple systems (Q87.-)

Q89.8 Other specified congenital malformations
Use additional code(s) to identify all associated manifestations
Q89.9 Congenital malformation, unspecified
Congenital anomaly NOS
Congenital deformity NOS

Chromosomal abnormalities, not elsewhere classified (Q90-Q99)

EXCLUDES 2 mitochondrial metabolic disorders (E88.4-)

✓4ᵗʰ Q90 Down syndrome
Use additional code(s) to identify any associated physical conditions and degree of intellectual disabilities (F70-F79)
Q90.0 Trisomy 21, nonmosaicism (meiotic nondisjunction)
Q90.1 Trisomy 21, mosaicism (mitotic nondisjunction)
Q90.2 Trisomy 21, translocation
Q90.9 Down syndrome, unspecified
Trisomy 21 NOS

✓4ᵗʰ Q91 Trisomy 18 and Trisomy 13
Q91.0 Trisomy 18, nonmosaicism (meiotic nondisjunction)
Q91.1 Trisomy 18, mosaicism (mitotic nondisjunction)
Q91.2 Trisomy 18, translocation
Q91.3 Trisomy 18, unspecified
Q91.4 Trisomy 13, nonmosaicism (meiotic nondisjunction)
Q91.5 Trisomy 13, mosaicism (mitotic nondisjunction)
Q91.6 Trisomy 13, translocation
Q91.7 Trisomy 13, unspecified

✓4ᵗʰ Q92 Other trisomies and partial trisomies of the autosomes, not elsewhere classified
INCLUDES unbalanced translocations and insertions
EXCLUDES 1 trisomies of chromosomes 13, 18, 21 (Q90-Q91)
Q92.0 Whole chromosome trisomy, nonmosaicism (meiotic nondisjunction)
Q92.1 Whole chromosome trisomy, mosaicism (mitotic nondisjunction)
Q92.2 Partial trisomy
Less than whole arm duplicated
Whole arm or more duplicated
EXCLUDES 1 partial trisomy due to unbalanced translocation (Q92.5)
Q92.5 Duplications with other complex rearrangements
Partial trisomy due to unbalanced translocations
Code also any associated deletions due to unbalanced translocations, inversions and insertions (Q93.7)
✓5ᵗʰ Q92.6 Marker chromosomes
Trisomies due to dicentrics
Trisomies due to extra rings
Trisomies due to isochromosomes
Individual with marker heterochromatin
Q92.61 Marker chromosomes in normal individual
Q92.62 Marker chromosomes in abnormal individual
Q92.7 Triploidy and polyploidy
Q92.8 Other specified trisomies and partial trisomies of autosomes
Duplications identified by fluorescence in situ hybridization (FISH)
Duplications identified by in situ hybridization (ISH)
Duplications seen only at prometaphase
Q92.9 Trisomy and partial trisomy of autosomes, unspecified

✓4ᵗʰ Q93 Monosomies and deletions from the autosomes, not elsewhere classified
Q93.0 Whole chromosome monosomy, nonmosaicism (meiotic nondisjunction)
Q93.1 Whole chromosome monosomy, mosaicism (mitotic nondisjunction)
Q93.2 Chromosome replaced with ring, dicentric or isochromosome
Q93.3 Deletion of short arm of chromosome 4
Wolff-Hirschorn syndrome
Q93.4 Deletion of short arm of chromosome 5
Cri-du-chat syndrome
✓5ᵗʰ Q93.5 Other deletions of part of a chromosome
AHA: 2018,4Q,28
Q93.51 Angelman syndrome
Q93.59 Other deletions of part of a chromosome

Q93.7 Deletions with other complex rearrangements
Deletions due to unbalanced translocations, inversions and insertions
Code also any associated duplications due to unbalanced translocations, inversions and insertions (Q92.5)

✓5ᵗʰ **Q93.8 Other deletions from the autosomes**

  Q93.81 Velo-cardio-facial syndrome
Deletion 22q11.2
DEF: Microdeletion syndrome affecting multiple organs characterized by a cleft palate, heart defects, an elongated face with almond-shaped eyes, wide nose, small ears, weak immune system, weak musculature, hypothyroidism, short stature, and scoliosis. The deletion occurs at q11.2 on the long arm of the chromosome 22.

  Q93.82 Williams syndrome
AHA: 2018,4Q,28-29

  Q93.88 Other microdeletions
Miller-Dieker syndrome
Smith-Magenis syndrome

  Q93.89 Other deletions from the autosomes
Deletions identified by fluorescence in situ hybridization (FISH)
Deletions identified by in situ hybridization (ISH)
Deletions seen only at prometaphase

Q93.9 Deletion from autosomes, unspecified

✓4ᵗʰ **Q95 Balanced rearrangements and structural markers, not elsewhere classified**
INCLUDES Robertsonian and balanced reciprocal translocations and insertions

Q95.0 Balanced translocation and insertion in normal individual
Q95.1 Chromosome inversion in normal individual
Q95.2 Balanced autosomal rearrangement in abnormal individual
Q95.3 Balanced sex/autosomal rearrangement in abnormal individual
Q95.5 Individual with autosomal fragile site
Q95.8 Other balanced rearrangements and structural markers
Q95.9 Balanced rearrangement and structural marker, unspecified

✓4ᵗʰ **Q96 Turner's syndrome**
EXCLUDES 1 Noonan syndrome ▶(Q87.19)◀

Q96.0 Karyotype 45, X ♀
Q96.1 Karyotype 46, X iso (Xq) ♀
Karyotype 46, isochromosome Xq
Q96.2 Karyotype 46, X with abnormal sex chromosome, except iso (Xq) ♀
Karyotype 46, X with abnormal sex chromosome, except isochromosome Xq
Q96.3 Mosaicism, 45, X/46, XX or XY ♀
Q96.4 Mosaicism, 45, X/other cell line(s) with abnormal sex chromosome ♀
Q96.8 Other variants of Turner's syndrome ♀
Q96.9 Turner's syndrome, unspecified ♀

✓4ᵗʰ **Q97 Other sex chromosome abnormalities, female phenotype, not elsewhere classified**
EXCLUDES 1 Turner's syndrome (Q96.-)

Q97.0 Karyotype 47, XXX ♀
Q97.1 Female with more than three X chromosomes ♀
Q97.2 Mosaicism, lines with various numbers of X chromosomes ♀
Q97.3 Female with 46, XY karyotype ♀
Q97.8 Other specified sex chromosome abnormalities, female phenotype ♀
Q97.9 Sex chromosome abnormality, female phenotype, unspecified ♀

✓4ᵗʰ **Q98 Other sex chromosome abnormalities, male phenotype, not elsewhere classified**
Q98.0 Klinefelter syndrome karyotype 47, XXY ♂
Q98.1 Klinefelter syndrome, male with more than two X chromosomes ♂
Q98.3 Other male with 46, XX karyotype ♂
Q98.4 Klinefelter syndrome, unspecified ♂
Q98.5 Karyotype 47, XYY
Q98.6 Male with structurally abnormal sex chromosome ♂
Q98.7 Male with sex chromosome mosaicism ♂

Q98.8 Other specified sex chromosome abnormalities, male phenotype ♂
Q98.9 Sex chromosome abnormality, male phenotype, unspecified ♂

✓4ᵗʰ **Q99 Other chromosome abnormalities, not elsewhere classified**
Q99.0 Chimera 46, XX/46, XY
Chimera 46, XX/46, XY true hermaphrodite
Q99.1 46, XX true hermaphrodite
46, XX with streak gonads
46, XY with streak gonads
Pure gonadal dysgenesis
Q99.2 Fragile X chromosome
Fragile X syndrome
Q99.8 Other specified chromosome abnormalities
Q99.9 Chromosomal abnormality, unspecified

Chapter 18. Symptoms, Signs and Abnormal Clinical and Laboratory Findings, Not Elsewhere Classified (R00–R99)

Chapter-specific Guidelines with Coding Examples

The chapter-specific guidelines from the ICD-10-CM Official Guidelines for Coding and Reporting have been provided below. Along with these guidelines are coding examples, contained in the shaded boxes, that have been developed to help illustrate the coding and/or sequencing guidance found in these guidelines.

Chapter 18 includes symptoms, signs, abnormal results of clinical or other investigative procedures, and ill-defined conditions regarding which no diagnosis classifiable elsewhere is recorded. Signs and symptoms that point to a specific diagnosis have been assigned to a category in other chapters of the classification.

a. Use of symptom codes

Codes that describe symptoms and signs are acceptable for reporting purposes when a related definitive diagnosis has not been established (confirmed) by the provider.

Chest pain of unknown origin

R07.9   **Chest pain, unspecified**

Explanation: Codes that describe symptoms such as chest pain are acceptable for reporting purposes when the provider has not established (confirmed) a related definitive diagnosis.

b. Use of a symptom code with a definitive diagnosis code

Codes for signs and symptoms may be reported in addition to a related definitive diagnosis when the sign or symptom is not routinely associated with that diagnosis, such as the various signs and symptoms associated with complex syndromes. The definitive diagnosis code should be sequenced before the symptom code.

Signs or symptoms that are associated routinely with a disease process should not be assigned as additional codes, unless otherwise instructed by the classification.

Pneumonia with hemoptysis

J18.9   **Pneumonia, unspecified organism**

R04.2   **Hemoptysis**

Explanation: Codes for signs and symptoms may be reported in addition to a related definitive diagnosis when the sign or symptom is not routinely associated with that diagnosis.

Parkinson's disease noted with shuffling gait and weakness

G20   **Parkinson's disease**

Explanation: Codes for signs and symptoms routinely associated with a disease process should not be assigned unless the classification instructs otherwise. Shuffling or abnormal gait patterns as well as weakness are inherent symptoms of Parkinson's disease.

c. Combination codes that include symptoms

ICD-10-CM contains a number of combination codes that identify both the definitive diagnosis and common symptoms of that diagnosis. When using one of these combination codes, an additional code should not be assigned for the symptom.

Acute gastritis with hemorrhage

K29.01   **Acute gastritis with bleeding**

Explanation: When a combination code identifies both the definitive diagnosis and the symptom, an additional code should not be assigned for the symptom.

d. Repeated falls

Code R29.6, Repeated falls, is for use for encounters when a patient has recently fallen and the reason for the fall is being investigated.

Code Z91.81, History of falling, is for use when a patient has fallen in the past and is at risk for future falls. When appropriate, both codes R29.6 and Z91.81 may be assigned together.

e. Coma scale

The coma scale codes (R40.2-) can be used in conjunction with traumatic brain injury codes, acute cerebrovascular disease or sequelae of cerebrovascular disease codes. These codes are primarily for use by trauma registries, but they may be used in any setting where this information is collected. The coma scale may also be used to assess the status of the central nervous system for other non-trauma conditions, such as monitoring patients in the intensive care unit regardless of medical condition. The coma scale codes should be sequenced after the diagnosis code(s).

These codes, one from each subcategory, are needed to complete the scale. The 7th character indicates when the scale was recorded. The 7th character should match for all three codes.

At a minimum, report the initial score documented on presentation at your facility. This may be a score from the emergency medicine technician (EMT) or in the emergency department. If desired, a facility may choose to capture multiple coma scale scores.

Assign code R40.24, Glasgow coma scale, total score, when only the total score is documented in the medical record and not the individual score(s).

Do not report codes for individual or total Glasgow coma scale scores for a patient with a medically induced coma or a sedated patient.

See Section I.B.14 for coma scale documentation by clinicians other than patient's provider

A 23-year-old male was found unresponsive due to a skull fracture with concussion and loss of consciousness of unknown duration resulting from an unidentified injury. He was admitted to the hospital, placed on ventilator support, and remained unresponsive. Four weeks following the event, he is sent home with home care and on a home ventilator. He remains unresponsive to all stimuli.

S02.0XXD   **Fracture of vault of skull, subsequent encounter for fracture with routine healing**

S06.0X9D   **Concussion with loss of consciousness of unspecified duration, subsequent encounter**

R40.2114   **Coma scale, eyes open, never, 24 hours or more after hospital admission**

R40.2214   **Coma scale, best verbal response, none, 24 hours or more after hospital admission**

R40.2314   **Coma scale, best motor response, none, 24 hours or more after hospital admission**

Z99.11   **Dependence on respirator [ventilator] status**

Explanation: When individual scores for the Glasgow coma scale are documented, codes from each category are needed to complete the scale. The seventh character 4 indicates that the scores were recorded 24 hours or more after hospital admission. Assign a code from subcategory R40.24- Glasgow coma scale, total score, when only the total and not individual score(s) is documented. Coma scale scores, when coded, should be sequenced after any associated fracture of the skull or intracranial injury.

f. Functional quadriplegia

GUIDELINE HAS BEEN DELETED EFFECTIVE OCTOBER 1, 2017

g. SIRS due to non-infectious process

The systemic inflammatory response syndrome (SIRS) can develop as a result of certain non-infectious disease processes, such as trauma, malignant neoplasm, or pancreatitis. When SIRS is documented with a noninfectious condition, and no subsequent infection is documented, the code for the underlying condition, such as an injury, should be assigned, followed by code R65.10, Systemic inflammatory response syndrome (SIRS) of non-infectious origin without acute organ dysfunction, or code R65.11, Systemic inflammatory response syndrome (SIRS) of non-infectious origin with acute organ dysfunction. If an associated acute organ dysfunction is documented, the appropriate code(s) for the specific type of organ dysfunction(s) should be assigned in addition to code R65.11. If acute organ dysfunction is documented, but it cannot be determined if the acute organ dysfunction is associated with SIRS or due to another condition (e.g., directly due to the trauma), the provider should be queried

Systemic inflammatory response syndrome (SIRS) due to acute gallstone pancreatitis

K85.10   **Biliary acute pancreatitis without necrosis or infection**

R65.10   **Systemic inflammatory response syndrome [SIRS] of non-infectious origin without acute organ dysfunction**

Explanation: When SIRS is documented with a noninfectious condition without subsequent infection documented, the code for the underlying condition such as pancreatitis should be assigned followed by the appropriate code for SIRS of noninfectious origin, either with or without associated organ dysfunction.

h. Death NOS

Code R99, Ill-defined and unknown cause of mortality, is only for use in the very limited circumstance when a patient who has already died is brought into an emergency department or other healthcare facility and is pronounced dead upon arrival. It does not represent the discharge disposition of death.

i. NIHSS stroke scale

The NIH stroke scale (NIHSS) codes (R29.7- -) can be used in conjunction with acute stroke codes (I63) to identify the patient's neurological status and the severity of the stroke. The stroke scale codes should be sequenced after the acute stroke diagnosis code(s).

At a minimum, report the initial score documented. If desired, a facility may choose to capture multiple stroke scale scores.

See Section I.B.14 for NIHSS stroke scale documentation by clinicians other than patient's provider

Chapter 18. Symptoms, Signs and Abnormal Clinical and Laboratory Findings, Not Elsewhere Classified (R00-R99)

NOTE This chapter includes symptoms, signs, abnormal results of clinical or other investigative procedures, and ill-defined conditions regarding which no diagnosis classifiable elsewhere is recorded.

Signs and symptoms that point rather definitely to a given diagnosis have been assigned to a category in other chapters of the classification. In general, categories in this chapter include the less well-defined conditions and symptoms that, without the necessary study of the case to establish a final diagnosis, point perhaps equally to two or more diseases or to two or more systems of the body. Practically all categories in the chapter could be designated 'not otherwise specified', 'unknown etiology' or 'transient'. The Alphabetical Index should be consulted to determine which symptoms and signs are to be allocated here and which to other chapters. The residual subcategories, numbered .8, are generally provided for other relevant symptoms that cannot be allocated elsewhere in the classification.

The conditions and signs or symptoms included in categories R00-R94 consist of:

(a) cases for which no more specific diagnosis can be made even after all the facts bearing on the case have been investigated;

(b) signs or symptoms existing at the time of initial encounter that proved to be transient and whose causes could not be determined;

(c) provisional diagnosis in a patient who failed to return for further investigation or care;

(d) cases referred elsewhere for investigation or treatment before the diagnosis was made;

(e) cases in which a more precise diagnosis was not available for any other reason;

(f) certain symptoms, for which supplementary information is provided, that represent important problems in medical care in their own right.

EXCLUDES 2   *abnormal findings on antenatal screening of mother (O28.-)*
certain conditions originating in the perinatal period (P04-P96)
signs and symptoms classified in the body system chapters
signs and symptoms of breast (N63, N64.5)

AHA: 2017,1Q,6,7

This chapter contains the following blocks:

R00-R09   Symptoms and signs involving the circulatory and respiratory systems
R10-R19   Symptoms and signs involving the digestive system and abdomen
R20-R23   Symptoms and signs involving the skin and subcutaneous tissue
R25-R29   Symptoms and signs involving the nervous and musculoskeletal systems
R30-R39   Symptoms and signs involving the genitourinary system
R40-R46   Symptoms and signs involving cognition, perception, emotional state and behavior
R47-R49   Symptoms and signs involving speech and voice
R50-R69   General symptoms and signs
R70-R79   Abnormal findings on examination of blood, without diagnosis
R80-R82   Abnormal findings on examination of urine, without diagnosis
R83-R89   Abnormal findings on examination of other body fluids, substances and tissues, without diagnosis
R90-R94   Abnormal findings on diagnostic imaging and in function studies, without diagnosis
R97   Abnormal tumor markers
R99   Ill-defined and unknown cause of mortality

Symptoms and signs involving the circulatory and respiratory systems (R00-R09)

✓4ᵗʰ **R00 Abnormalities of heart beat**
    EXCLUDES 1   *abnormalities originating in the perinatal period (P29.1-)*
    EXCLUDES 2   *specified arrhythmias (I47-I49)*

   R00.0 Tachycardia, unspecified
     Rapid heart beat
     Sinoauricular tachycardia NOS
     Sinus [sinusal] tachycardia NOS
     EXCLUDES 1   *neonatal tachycardia (P29.11)*
             paroxysmal tachycardia (I47.-)
     DEF: Excessively rapid heart rate of more than 100 beats per minute.

   R00.1 Bradycardia, unspecified   CH CL
     Sinoatrial bradycardia
     Sinus bradycardia
     Slow heart beat
     Vagal bradycardia
     Use additional code for adverse effect, if applicable, to identify drug (T36-T50 with fifth or sixth character 5)
     EXCLUDES 1   *neonatal bradycardia (P29.12)*
     DEF: Slowed heartbeat, usually defined as a rate fewer than 60 beats per minute. Heart rhythm may be slow as a result of a congenital defect or an acquired problem.

   R00.2 Palpitations
     Awareness of heart beat

   R00.8 Other abnormalities of heart beat

   R00.9 Unspecified abnormalities of heart beat

✓4ᵗʰ **R01 Cardiac murmurs and other cardiac sounds**
    EXCLUDES 1   *cardiac murmurs and sounds originating in the perinatal period (P29.8)*

   R01.0 Benign and innocent cardiac murmurs
     Functional cardiac murmur

   R01.1 Cardiac murmur, unspecified
     Cardiac bruit NOS
     Heart murmur NOS
     Systolic murmur NOS

   R01.2 Other cardiac sounds
     Cardiac dullness, increased or decreased
     Precordial friction

✓4ᵗʰ **R03 Abnormal blood-pressure reading, without diagnosis**

   R03.0 Elevated blood-pressure reading, without diagnosis of hypertension
     NOTE   This category is to be used to record an episode of elevated blood pressure in a patient in whom no formal diagnosis of hypertension has been made, or as an isolated incidental finding.

   R03.1 Nonspecific low blood-pressure reading
     EXCLUDES 1   *hypotension (I95.-)*
             maternal hypotension syndrome (O26.5-)
             neurogenic orthostatic hypotension (G90.3)

✓4ᵗʰ **R04 Hemorrhage from respiratory passages**

   R04.0 Epistaxis
     Hemorrhage from nose
     Nosebleed

   R04.1 Hemorrhage from throat
     EXCLUDES 2   *hemoptysis (R04.2)*

   R04.2 Hemoptysis
     Blood-stained sputum
     Cough with hemorrhage
     AHA: 2013,4Q,118

✓5ᵗʰ **R04.8 Hemorrhage from other sites in respiratory passages**

     R04.81 Acute idiopathic pulmonary hemorrhage in infants   P
         AIPHI
         Acute idiopathic hemorrhage in infants over 28 days old
         EXCLUDES 1   *perinatal pulmonary hemorrhage (P26.-)*
                von Willebrand's disease (D68.0)

     R04.89 Hemorrhage from other sites in respiratory passages
         Pulmonary hemorrhage NOS

   R04.9 Hemorrhage from respiratory passages, unspecified

R05 Cough
    EXCLUDES 1   *cough with hemorrhage (R04.2)*
             smoker's cough (J41.0)
    AHA: 2016,2Q,33

✓4th R06 Abnormalities of breathing

EXCLUDES 1   *acute respiratory distress syndrome (J80)*
           respiratory arrest (R09.2)
           respiratory arrest of newborn (P28.81)
           respiratory distress syndrome of newborn (P22.-)
           respiratory failure (J96.-)
           respiratory failure of newborn (P28.5)

✓5th R06.0 Dyspnea

EXCLUDES 1   *tachypnea NOS (R06.82)*
           transient tachypnea of newborn (P22.1)

R06.00 Dyspnea, unspecified
      AHA: 2017,1Q,26

R06.01 Orthopnea

R06.02 Shortness of breath

R06.03 Acute respiratory distress
      AHA: 2017,4Q,23

R06.09 Other forms of dyspnea

R06.1 Stridor

EXCLUDES 1   *congenital laryngeal stridor (P28.89)*
           laryngismus (stridulus) (J38.5)

DEF: Certain type of wheezing described as a loud, constant, musical sound produced when breathing with an obstructed airway, like the inspiratory sound heard when laryngeal or esophageal obstruction is present.

R06.2 Wheezing

EXCLUDES 1   *asthma (J45.-)*

AHA: 2016,2Q,33

DEF: High-pitched whistling sound during breathing due to stenosis of the respiratory passageway. Wheezing is associated with asthma, sleep apnea, bronchiectasis, bronchiolitis, COPD, and pleural effusion.

R06.3 Periodic breathing
Cheyne-Stokes breathing

R06.4 Hyperventilation

EXCLUDES 1   *psychogenic hyperventilation (F45.8)*

R06.5 Mouth breathing

EXCLUDES 2   *dry mouth NOS (R68.2)*

R06.6 Hiccough

EXCLUDES 1   *psychogenic hiccough (F45.8)*

R06.7 Sneezing

✓5th R06.8 Other abnormalities of breathing

R06.81 Apnea, not elsewhere classified
Apnea NOS

EXCLUDES 1   *apnea (of) newborn (P28.4)*
           sleep apnea (G47.3-)
           sleep apnea of newborn (primary) (P28.3)

R06.82 Tachypnea, not elsewhere classified
Tachypnea NOS

EXCLUDES 1   *transitory tachypnea of newborn (P22.1)*

R06.83 Snoring

R06.89 Other abnormalities of breathing
Breath-holding (spells)
Sighing

R06.9 Unspecified abnormalities of breathing

✓4th R07 Pain in throat and chest

EXCLUDES 1   *epidemic myalgia (B33.0)*
EXCLUDES 2   *jaw pain R68.84*
           pain in breast (N64.4)

R07.0 Pain in throat

EXCLUDES 1   *chronic sore throat (J31.2)*
           sore throat (acute) NOS (J02.9)
EXCLUDES 2   *dysphagia (R13.1-)*
           pain in neck (M54.2)

R07.1 Chest pain on breathing
Painful respiration

R07.2 Precordial pain
DEF: Pain felt in the anterior (front) chest wall over the region of the heart. This type of pain is generally felt slightly to the left of the sternum, but may also extend into the surrounding chest wall region.

✓5th R07.8 Other chest pain

R07.81 Pleurodynia
Pleurodynia NOS

EXCLUDES 1   *epidemic pleurodynia (B33.0)*

R07.82 Intercostal pain

R07.89 Other chest pain
Anterior chest-wall pain NOS

R07.9 Chest pain, unspecified

✓4th R09 Other symptoms and signs involving the circulatory and respiratory system

EXCLUDES 1   *acute respiratory distress syndrome (J80)*
           respiratory arrest of newborn (P28.81)
           respiratory distress syndrome of newborn (P22.0)
           respiratory failure (J96.-)
           respiratory failure of newborn (P28.5)

✓5th R09.0 Asphyxia and hypoxemia

EXCLUDES 1   *asphyxia due to carbon monoxide (T58.-)*
           asphyxia due to foreign body in respiratory tract (T17.-)
           birth (intrauterine) asphyxia (P84)
           hyperventilation (R06.4)
           traumatic asphyxia (T71.-)
EXCLUDES 2   *hypercapnia (R06.89)*

R09.01 Asphyxia
DEF: Interference of oxygen intake due to obstruction or injury of airways resulting in a lack of oxygen perfusion to the tissues or excessive carbon dioxide in the blood. Can cause unconsciousness or death.

R09.02 Hypoxemia
DEF: Insufficient oxygen in the arterial blood resulting in inadequate delivery of oxygen to the body tissues.

R09.1 Pleurisy

EXCLUDES 1   *pleurisy with effusion (J90)*

R09.2 Respiratory arrest
Cardiorespiratory failure

EXCLUDES 1   *cardiac arrest (I46.-)*
           respiratory arrest of newborn (P28.81)
           respiratory distress of newborn (P22.0)
           respiratory failure (J96.-)
           respiratory failure of newborn (P28.5)
           respiratory insufficiency (R06.89)
           respiratory insufficiency of newborn (P28.5)

R09.3 Abnormal sputum
Abnormal amount of sputum
Abnormal color of sputum
Abnormal odor of sputum
Excessive sputum

EXCLUDES 1   *blood-stained sputum (R04.2)*

✓5th R09.8 Other specified symptoms and signs involving the circulatory and respiratory systems

R09.81 Nasal congestion

R09.82 Postnasal drip

R09.89 Other specified symptoms and signs involving the circulatory and respiratory systems
Abnormal chest percussion
Bruit (arterial)
Chest tympany
Choking sensation
Feeling of foreign body in throat
Friction sounds in chest
Rales
Weak pulse

EXCLUDES 2   *foreign body in throat (T17.2-)*
           wheezing (R06.2)

Symptoms and signs involving the digestive system and abdomen (R10-R19)

EXCLUDES 2   congenital or infantile pylorospasm (Q40.0)
      gastrointestinal hemorrhage (K92.0-K92.2)
      intestinal obstruction (K56.-)
      newborn gastrointestinal hemorrhage (P54.0-P54.3)
      newborn intestinal obstruction (P76.-)
      pylorospasm (K31.3)
      signs and symptoms involving the urinary system (R30-R39)
      symptoms referable to female genital organs (N94.-)
      symptoms referable to male genital organs (N48-N50)

✓4ᵗʰ **R10   Abdominal and pelvic pain**
   EXCLUDES 1   renal colic (N23)
   EXCLUDES 2   dorsalgia (M54.-)
      flatulence and related conditions (R14.-)
   TIP: Codes from category R10 may be assigned concurrently with a G89 code for pain if needed to describe the site of the pain.

   R10.0   Acute abdomen
      Severe abdominal pain (generalized) (with abdominal rigidity)
      EXCLUDES 1   abdominal rigidity NOS (R19.3)
        generalized abdominal pain NOS (R10.84)
        localized abdominal pain (R10.1-R10.3-)

✓5ᵗʰ   **R10.1   Pain localized to upper abdomen**
     R10.10   **Upper abdominal pain, unspecified**
     R10.11   **Right upper quadrant pain**
     R10.12   **Left upper quadrant pain**
     R10.13   **Epigastric pain**
        Dyspepsia
        EXCLUDES 1   functional dyspepsia (K30)

Abdominal Pain

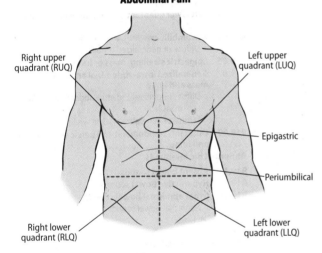

Right upper quadrant (RUQ)
Left upper quadrant (LUQ)
Epigastric
Periumbilical
Right lower quadrant (RLQ)
Left lower quadrant (LLQ)

   R10.2   Pelvic and perineal pain
     EXCLUDES 1   vulvodynia (N94.81)

✓5ᵗʰ   **R10.3   Pain localized to other parts of lower abdomen**
     R10.30   **Lower abdominal pain, unspecified**
     R10.31   **Right lower quadrant pain**
     R10.32   **Left lower quadrant pain**
     R10.33   **Periumbilical pain**

✓5ᵗʰ   **R10.8   Other abdominal pain**
    ✓6ᵗʰ   **R10.81**   **Abdominal tenderness**
       Abdominal tenderness NOS
       R10.811   **Right upper quadrant abdominal tenderness**
       R10.812   **Left upper quadrant abdominal tenderness**
       R10.813   **Right lower quadrant abdominal tenderness**
       R10.814   **Left lower quadrant abdominal tenderness**
       R10.815   **Periumbilic abdominal tenderness**
       R10.816   **Epigastric abdominal tenderness**
       R10.817   **Generalized abdominal tenderness**
       R10.819   **Abdominal tenderness, unspecified site**

    ✓6ᵗʰ   **R10.82**   **Rebound abdominal tenderness**
       R10.821   **Right upper quadrant rebound abdominal tenderness**
       R10.822   **Left upper quadrant rebound abdominal tenderness**
       R10.823   **Right lower quadrant rebound abdominal tenderness**
       R10.824   **Left lower quadrant rebound abdominal tenderness**
       R10.825   **Periumbilic rebound abdominal tenderness**
       R10.826   **Epigastric rebound abdominal tenderness**
       R10.827   **Generalized rebound abdominal tenderness**
       R10.829   **Rebound abdominal tenderness, unspecified site**

     R10.83   **Colic**   P
       Colic NOS
       Infantile colic
       EXCLUDES 1   colic in adult and child over 12 months old (R10.84)
       DEF: Inconsolable crying in an otherwise well-fed and healthy infant for more than three hours a day, three days a week, for more than three weeks.

     R10.84   **Generalized abdominal pain**
       EXCLUDES 1   generalized abdominal pain associated with acute abdomen (R10.0)

   R10.9   Unspecified abdominal pain

✓4ᵗʰ **R11   Nausea and vomiting**
   EXCLUDES 1   cyclical vomiting associated with migraine (G43.A-)
      excessive vomiting in pregnancy (O21.-)
      hematemesis (K92.0)
      neonatal hematemesis (P54.0)
      newborn vomiting (P92.0-)
      psychogenic vomiting (F50.89)
      vomiting associated with bulimia nervosa (F50.2)
      vomiting following gastrointestinal surgery (K91.0)
   AHA: 2017,1Q,28
   TIP: Assign a code from this category along with K31.89 Other diseases of stomach and duodenum, to describe cyclical vomiting not due to migraine.

   R11.0   Nausea
      Nausea NOS
      Nausea without vomiting

✓5ᵗʰ   **R11.1   Vomiting**
     R11.10   **Vomiting, unspecified**
       Vomiting NOS
     R11.11   **Vomiting without nausea**
     R11.12   **Projectile vomiting**
     R11.13   **Vomiting of fecal matter**
     R11.14   **Bilious vomiting**
       Bilious emesis
     R11.15   **Cyclical vomiting syndrome unrelated to migraine**
       Cyclic vomiting syndrome NOS
       Persistent vomiting
       EXCLUDES 1   cyclical vomiting in migraine (G43.A-)
       EXCLUDES 2   bulimia nervosa (F50.2)
        diabetes mellitus due to underlying condition (E08.-)

   R11.2   Nausea with vomiting, unspecified
      Persistent nausea with vomiting NOS

   R12   Heartburn
   EXCLUDES 1   dyspepsia NOS (R10.13)
      functional dyspepsia (K30)

✓4ᵗʰ **R13   Aphagia and dysphagia**
   R13.0   Aphagia
      Inability to swallow
      EXCLUDES 1   psychogenic aphagia (F50.9)

✓ Additional Character Required   ✓×7ᵗʰ Placeholder Alert   Manifestation   Unspecified Dx   ►◄ Revised Text   ● New Code   ▲ Revised Title

ICD-10-CM 2020   923

✓5ᵗʰ **R13.1 Dysphagia**

Code first, if applicable, dysphagia following cerebrovascular disease (I69. with final characters -91)

EXCLUDES 1   *psychogenic dysphagia (F45.8)*

Swallowing Function

Oral phase

Oropharyngeal phase

Pharyngeal phase

Pharyngoesophageal phase

R13.10 Dysphagia, unspecified
Difficulty in swallowing NOS

R13.11 Dysphagia, oral phase

R13.12 Dysphagia, oropharyngeal phase

R13.13 Dysphagia, pharyngeal phase

R13.14 Dysphagia, pharyngoesophageal phase

R13.19 Other dysphagia
Cervical dysphagia
Neurogenic dysphagia

✓4ᵗʰ **R14 Flatulence and related conditions**

EXCLUDES 1   *psychogenic aerophagy (F45.8)*

R14.0 Abdominal distension (gaseous)
Bloating
Tympanites (abdominal) (intestinal)

R14.1 Gas pain

R14.2 Eructation

R14.3 Flatulence

✓4ᵗʰ **R15 Fecal incontinence**

INCLUDES   encopresis NOS

EXCLUDES 1   *fecal incontinence of nonorganic origin (F98.1)*

R15.0 Incomplete defecation

EXCLUDES 1   *constipation (K59.0-)*
fecal impaction (K56.41)

R15.1 Fecal smearing
Fecal soiling

R15.2 Fecal urgency

R15.9 Full incontinence of feces
Fecal incontinence NOS

✓4ᵗʰ **R16 Hepatomegaly and splenomegaly, not elsewhere classified**

R16.0 Hepatomegaly, not elsewhere classified
Hepatomegaly NOS

R16.1 Splenomegaly, not elsewhere classified
Splenomegaly NOS

R16.2 Hepatomegaly with splenomegaly, not elsewhere classified
Hepatosplenomegaly NOS

R17 Unspecified jaundice

EXCLUDES 1   *neonatal jaundice (P55, P57-P59)*

✓4ᵗʰ **R18 Ascites**

INCLUDES   fluid in peritoneal cavity

EXCLUDES 1   *ascites in alcoholic cirrhosis (K70.31)*
ascites in alcoholic hepatitis (K70.11)
ascites in toxic liver disease with chronic active hepatitis (K71.51)

DEF: Abnormal accumulation of free fluid in the abdominal cavity, causing distention and tightness in addition to shortness of breath as the fluid accumulates. Ascites is usually an underlying disorder and can be a manifestation of any number of diseases.

R18.0 Malignant ascites
Code first malignancy, such as:
malignant neoplasm of ovary (C56.-)
secondary malignant neoplasm of retroperitoneum and peritoneum (C78.6)

R18.8 Other ascites
Ascites NOS
Peritoneal effusion (chronic)
AHA: 2018,1Q,4

✓4ᵗʰ **R19 Other symptoms and signs involving the digestive system and abdomen**

EXCLUDES 1   *acute abdomen (R10.0)*

✓5ᵗʰ **R19.0 Intra-abdominal and pelvic swelling, mass and lump**

EXCLUDES 1   *abdominal distension (gaseous) (R14.-)*
ascites (R18.-)

R19.00 Intra-abdominal and pelvic swelling, mass and lump, unspecified site

R19.01 Right upper quadrant abdominal swelling, mass and lump

R19.02 Left upper quadrant abdominal swelling, mass and lump

R19.03 Right lower quadrant abdominal swelling, mass and lump

R19.04 Left lower quadrant abdominal swelling, mass and lump

R19.05 Periumbilic swelling, mass or lump
Diffuse or generalized umbilical swelling or mass

R19.06 Epigastric swelling, mass or lump

R19.07 Generalized intra-abdominal and pelvic swelling, mass and lump
Diffuse or generalized intra-abdominal swelling or mass NOS
Diffuse or generalized pelvic swelling or mass NOS

R19.09 Other intra-abdominal and pelvic swelling, mass and lump

✓5ᵗʰ **R19.1 Abnormal bowel sounds**

R19.11 Absent bowel sounds

R19.12 Hyperactive bowel sounds

R19.15 Other abnormal bowel sounds
Abnormal bowel sounds NOS

R19.2 Visible peristalsis
Hyperperistalsis
DEF: Visible movements of muscular attempts to move food through the digestive tract due to pyloric obstruction, stomach obstruction, or intestinal obstruction.

✓5ᵗʰ **R19.3 Abdominal rigidity**

EXCLUDES 1   *abdominal rigidity with severe abdominal pain (R10.0)*

R19.30 Abdominal rigidity, unspecified site

R19.31 Right upper quadrant abdominal rigidity

R19.32 Left upper quadrant abdominal rigidity

R19.33 Right lower quadrant abdominal rigidity

R19.34 Left lower quadrant abdominal rigidity

R19.35 Periumbilic abdominal rigidity

R19.36 Epigastric abdominal rigidity

R19.37 Generalized abdominal rigidity

R19.4 Change in bowel habit

EXCLUDES 1   *constipation (K59.0-)*
functional diarrhea (K59.1)

N Newborn: 0   P Pediatric: 0-17   M Maternity: 12-55   A Adult: 15-124   CH Comorbidity High   CL Comorbidity Low   NCDx Noncancer Dx   PDx Primary Dx

924   ICD-10-CM 2020

R19.5 Other fecal abnormalities
Abnormal stool color
Bulky stools
Mucus in stools
Occult blood in feces
Occult blood in stools
EXCLUDES 1   *melena (K92.1)*
    neonatal melena (P54.1)
AHA: 2019,1Q,32

R19.6 Halitosis

R19.7 Diarrhea, unspecified
Diarrhea NOS
EXCLUDES 1   *functional diarrhea (K59.1)*
    neonatal diarrhea (P78.3)
    psychogenic diarrhea (F45.8)

R19.8 Other specified symptoms and signs involving the digestive system and abdomen

Symptoms and signs involving the skin and subcutaneous tissue (R20-R23)

EXCLUDES 2   *symptoms relating to breast (N64.4-N64.5)*

✓4ᵗʰ **R20 Disturbances of skin sensation**
EXCLUDES 1   *dissociative anesthesia and sensory loss (F44.6)*
    psychogenic disturbances (F45.8)

R20.0 Anesthesia of skin

R20.1 Hypoesthesia of skin

R20.2 Paresthesia of skin
Formication
Pins and needles
Tingling skin
EXCLUDES 1   *acroparesthesia (I73.8)*

R20.3 Hyperesthesia

R20.8 Other disturbances of skin sensation

R20.9 Unspecified disturbances of skin sensation

R21 Rash and other nonspecific skin eruption
INCLUDES   rash NOS
EXCLUDES 1   *specified type of rash — code to condition*
    vesicular eruption (R23.8)

✓4ᵗʰ **R22 Localized swelling, mass and lump of skin and subcutaneous tissue**
INCLUDES   subcutaneous nodules (localized)(superficial)
EXCLUDES 1   *abnormal findings on diagnostic imaging (R90-R93)*
    edema (R60.-)
    enlarged lymph nodes (R59.-)
    localized adiposity (E65)
    swelling of joint (M25.4-)

R22.0 Localized swelling, mass and lump, head

R22.1 Localized swelling, mass and lump, neck

R22.2 Localized swelling, mass and lump, trunk
EXCLUDES 1   *intra-abdominal or pelvic mass and lump (R19.0-)*
    intra-abdominal or pelvic swelling (R19.0-)
EXCLUDES 2   *breast mass and lump (N63)*

✓5ᵗʰ **R22.3 Localized swelling, mass and lump, upper limb**
  R22.30 Localized swelling, mass and lump, unspecified upper limb
  R22.31 Localized swelling, mass and lump, right upper limb
  R22.32 Localized swelling, mass and lump, left upper limb
  R22.33 Localized swelling, mass and lump, upper limb, bilateral

✓5ᵗʰ **R22.4 Localized swelling, mass and lump, lower limb**
  R22.40 Localized swelling, mass and lump, unspecified lower limb
  R22.41 Localized swelling, mass and lump, right lower limb
  R22.42 Localized swelling, mass and lump, left lower limb
  R22.43 Localized swelling, mass and lump, lower limb, bilateral

R22.9 Localized swelling, mass and lump, unspecified

✓4ᵗʰ **R23 Other skin changes**

R23.0 Cyanosis
EXCLUDES 1   *acrocyanosis (I73.8)*
    cyanotic attacks of newborn (P28.2)
DEF: Bluish or purplish discoloration of the skin due to an inadequate oxygen blood level.

R23.1 Pallor
Clammy skin

R23.2 Flushing
Excessive blushing
Code first, if applicable, menopausal and female climacteric states (N95.1)

R23.3 Spontaneous ecchymoses
Petechiae
EXCLUDES 1   *ecchymoses of newborn (P54.5)*
    purpura (D69.-)

R23.4 Changes in skin texture
Desquamation of skin
Induration of skin
Scaling of skin
EXCLUDES 1   *epidermal thickening NOS (L85.9)*

R23.8 Other skin changes

R23.9 Unspecified skin changes

Symptoms and signs involving the nervous and musculoskeletal systems (R25-R29)

✓4ᵗʰ **R25 Abnormal involuntary movements**
EXCLUDES 1   *specific movement disorders (G20-G26)*
    stereotyped movement disorders (F98.4)
    tic disorders (F95.-)

R25.0 Abnormal head movements

R25.1 Tremor, unspecified
EXCLUDES 1   *chorea NOS (G25.5)*
    essential tremor (G25.0)
    hysterical tremor (F44.4)
    intention tremor (G25.2)

R25.2 Cramp and spasm
EXCLUDES 2   *carpopedal spasm (R29.0)*
    charley-horse (M62.831)
    infantile spasms (G40.4-)
    muscle spasm of back (M62.830)
    muscle spasm of calf (M62.831)

R25.3 Fasciculation
Twitching NOS

R25.8 Other abnormal involuntary movements

R25.9 Unspecified abnormal involuntary movements

✓4ᵗʰ **R26 Abnormalities of gait and mobility**
EXCLUDES 1   *ataxia NOS (R27.0)*
    hereditary ataxia (G11.-)
    locomotor (syphilitic) ataxia (A52.11)
    immobility syndrome (paraplegic) (M62.3)
TIP: Assign when the abnormality of gait or mobility is not integral to a known diagnosis.

R26.0 Ataxic gait
Staggering gait

R26.1 Paralytic gait
Spastic gait

R26.2 Difficulty in walking, not elsewhere classified
EXCLUDES 1   *falling (R29.6)*
    unsteadiness on feet (R26.81)
AHA: 2016,2Q,7

✓5ᵗʰ **R26.8 Other abnormalities of gait and mobility**
  R26.81 Unsteadiness on feet
  R26.89 Other abnormalities of gait and mobility

R26.9 Unspecified abnormalities of gait and mobility

✓4ᵗʰ **R27 Other lack of coordination**
EXCLUDES 1   *ataxic gait (R26.0)*
    hereditary ataxia (G11.-)
    vertigo NOS (R42)

R27.0 Ataxia, unspecified
EXCLUDES 1   *ataxia following cerebrovascular disease (I69. with final characters -93)*

R27.8 Other lack of coordination

R27.9 Unspecified lack of coordination

Chapter 18. Symptoms, Signs and Abnormal Clinical and Laboratory Findings

✓4ᵗʰ **R29**   **Other symptoms and signs involving the nervous and musculoskeletal systems**

   R29.0   **Tetany**
Carpopedal spasm
> *EXCLUDES 1*   *hysterical tetany (F44.5)*
> *neonatal tetany (P71.3)*
> *parathyroid tetany (E20.9)*
> *post-thyroidectomy tetany (E89.2)*

DEF: Calcium or other mineral imbalance causing voluntary muscles such as hands, feet, or larynx to spasm rhythmically.

   R29.1   **Meningismus**

   R29.2   **Abnormal reflex**
> *EXCLUDES 2*   *abnormal pupillary reflex (H57.0)*
> *hyperactive gag reflex (J39.2)*
> *vasovagal reaction or syncope (R55)*

   R29.3   **Abnormal posture**

   R29.4   **Clicking hip**
> *EXCLUDES 1*   *congenital deformities of hip (Q65.-)*

   R29.5   **Transient paralysis**
Code first any associated spinal cord injury (S14.0, S14.1-, S24.0, S24.1-, S34.0-, S34.1-)
> *EXCLUDES 1*   *transient ischemic attack (G45.9)*

   R29.6   **Repeated falls**
Falling
Tendency to fall
> *EXCLUDES 2*   *at risk for falling (Z91.81)*
> *history of falling (Z91.81)*

AHA: 2016,2Q,6

✓5ᵗʰ **R29.7**   **National Institutes of Health Stroke Scale (NIHSS) score**
Code first the type of cerebral infarction (I63.-)
AHA: 2016,4Q,61-62
TIP: These codes are intended to be used as secondary codes following the code for the stroke. Code assignment for the NIHSS may be based on documentation from nonprovider clinicians (i.e., other qualified healthcare practitioners legally accountable for establishing the patient's diagnosis).

    ✓6ᵗʰ **R29.70**   **NIHSS** score 0-9
      R29.700   **NIHSS score 0**
      R29.701   **NIHSS score 1**
      R29.702   **NIHSS score 2**
      R29.703   **NIHSS score 3**
      R29.704   **NIHSS score 4**
      R29.705   **NIHSS score 5**
      R29.706   **NIHSS score 6**
      R29.707   **NIHSS score 7**
      R29.708   **NIHSS score 8**
      R29.709   **NIHSS score 9**

    ✓6ᵗʰ **R29.71**   **NIHSS** score 10-19
      R29.710   **NIHSS score 10**
      R29.711   **NIHSS score 11**
      R29.712   **NIHSS score 12**
      R29.713   **NIHSS score 13**
      R29.714   **NIHSS score 14**
      R29.715   **NIHSS score 15**
      R29.716   **NIHSS score 16**
      R29.717   **NIHSS score 17**
      R29.718   **NIHSS score 18**
      R29.719   **NIHSS score 19**

    ✓6ᵗʰ **R29.72**   **NIHSS** score 20-29
      R29.720   **NIHSS score 20**
      R29.721   **NIHSS score 21**
      R29.722   **NIHSS score 22**
      R29.723   **NIHSS score 23**
      R29.724   **NIHSS score 24**
      R29.725   **NIHSS score 25**
      R29.726   **NIHSS score 26**
      R29.727   **NIHSS score 27**
      R29.728   **NIHSS score 28**
      R29.729   **NIHSS score 29**

    ✓6ᵗʰ **R29.73**   **NIHSS** score 30-39
      R29.730   **NIHSS score 30**
      R29.731   **NIHSS score 31**
      R29.732   **NIHSS score 32**
      R29.733   **NIHSS score 33**
      R29.734   **NIHSS score 34**
      R29.735   **NIHSS score 35**
      R29.736   **NIHSS score 36**

      R29.737   **NIHSS score 37**
      R29.738   **NIHSS score 38**
      R29.739   **NIHSS score 39**

    ✓6ᵗʰ **R29.74**   **NIHSS** score 40-42
      R29.740   **NIHSS score 40**
      R29.741   **NIHSS score 41**
      R29.742   **NIHSS score 42**

✓5ᵗʰ **R29.8**   **Other symptoms and signs involving the nervous and musculoskeletal systems**

   ✓6ᵗʰ **R29.81**   **Other symptoms and signs involving the nervous system**
     R29.810   **Facial weakness**
Facial droop
> *EXCLUDES 1*   *Bell's palsy (G51.0)*
> *facial weakness following cerebrovascular disease (I69. with final characters -92)*

     R29.818   **Other symptoms and signs involving the nervous system**

   ✓6ᵗʰ **R29.89**   **Other symptoms and signs involving the musculoskeletal system**
> *EXCLUDES 2*   *pain in limb (M79.6-)*

     R29.890   **Loss of height**
> *EXCLUDES 1*   *osteoporosis (M80-M81)*

     R29.891   **Ocular torticollis**
> *EXCLUDES 1*   *congenital (sternomastoid) torticollis Q68.0*
> *psychogenic torticollis (F45.8)*
> *spasmodic torticollis (G24.3)*
> *torticollis due to birth injury (P15.8)*
> *torticollis NOS M43.6*

DEF: Abnormal head posture as a result of a contracted state of cervical muscles to correct a visual disturbance, either double vision or a visual field defect.

     R29.898   **Other symptoms and signs involving the musculoskeletal system**

✓5ᵗʰ **R29.9**   **Unspecified symptoms and signs involving the nervous and musculoskeletal systems**

   R29.90   **Unspecified symptoms and signs involving the nervous system**

   R29.91   **Unspecified symptoms and signs involving the musculoskeletal system**

Symptoms and signs involving the genitourinary system (R30-R39)

✓4ᵗʰ **R30**   **Pain associated with micturition**
> *EXCLUDES 1*   *psychogenic pain associated with micturition (F45.8)*

   R30.0   **Dysuria**
Strangury

   R30.1   **Vesical tenesmus**
DEF: Feeling of a full bladder even when there is little or no urine in the bladder.

   R30.9   **Painful micturition, unspecified**
Painful urination NOS

✓4ᵗʰ **R31**   **Hematuria**
> *EXCLUDES 1*   *hematuria included with underlying conditions, such as:*
> *acute cystitis with hematuria (N30.01)*
> *recurrent and persistent hematuria in glomerular diseases (N02.-)*

AHA: 2017,1Q,17

   R31.0   **Gross hematuria**

   R31.1   **Benign essential microscopic hematuria**

✓5ᵗʰ **R31.2**   **Other microscopic hematuria**
AHA: 2016,4Q,62

   R31.21   **Asymptomatic microscopic hematuria**
AMH

   R31.29   **Other microscopic hematuria**

   R31.9   **Hematuria, unspecified**

Ⓝ Newborn: 0   Ⓟ Pediatric: 0-17   Ⓜ Maternity: 12-55   Ⓐ Adult: 15-124   ᶜᴴ Comorbidity High   ᶜᴸ Comorbidity Low   ᴺᶜᴰˣ Noncancer Dx   ᴾᴰˣ Primary Dx

926   ICD-10-CM 2020

R32 Unspecified urinary incontinence
Enuresis NOS
EXCLUDES 1   *functional urinary incontinence (R39.81)*
nonorganic enuresis (F98.0)
stress incontinence and other specified urinary incontinence (N39.3-N39.4-)
urinary incontinence associated with cognitive impairment (R39.81)

✓4ᵗʰ R33 Retention of urine
EXCLUDES 1   *psychogenic retention of urine (F45.8)*
R33.0 Drug induced retention of urine
Use additional code for adverse effect, if applicable, to identify drug (T36-T50 with fifth or sixth character 5)
R33.8 Other retention of urine
Code first, if applicable, any causal condition, such as:
enlarged prostate (N40.1)
AHA: 2018,4Q,55
R33.9 Retention of urine, unspecified

R34 Anuria and oliguria
EXCLUDES 1   *anuria and oliguria complicating abortion or ectopic or molar pregnancy (O00-O07, O08.4)*
anuria and oliguria complicating pregnancy (O26.83-)
anuria and oliguria complicating the puerperium (O90.4)

✓4ᵗʰ R35 Polyuria
Code first, if applicable, any causal condition, such as:
enlarged prostate (N40.1)
EXCLUDES 1   *psychogenic polyuria (F45.8)*
R35.0 Frequency of micturition
R35.1 Nocturia
R35.8 Other polyuria
Polyuria NOS

✓4ᵗʰ R36 Urethral discharge
R36.0 Urethral discharge without blood
R36.1 Hematospermia ♂
R36.9 Urethral discharge, unspecified
Penile discharge NOS
Urethrorrhea

R37 Sexual dysfunction, unspecified

✓4ᵗʰ R39 Other and unspecified symptoms and signs involving the genitourinary system
R39.0 Extravasation of urine
✓5ᵗʰ R39.1 Other difficulties with micturition
Code first, if applicable, any causal condition, such as:
enlarged prostate (N40.1)
R39.11 Hesitancy of micturition
R39.12 Poor urinary stream
Weak urinary steam
R39.13 Splitting of urinary stream
R39.14 Feeling of incomplete bladder emptying
R39.15 Urgency of urination
EXCLUDES 1   *urge incontinence (N39.41, N39.46)*
R39.16 Straining to void
✓6ᵗʰ R39.19 Other difficulties with micturition
AHA: 2016,4Q,63
R39.191 Need to immediately re-void
R39.192 Position dependent micturition
R39.198 Other difficulties with micturition
R39.2 Extrarenal uremia
Prerenal uremia
EXCLUDES 1   *uremia NOS (N19)*
✓5ᵗʰ R39.8 Other symptoms and signs involving the genitourinary system
AHA: 2017,4Q,22-23
R39.81 Functional urinary incontinence
Urinary incontinence due to cognitive impairment, or severe physical disability or immobility
EXCLUDES 1   *stress incontinence and other specified urinary incontinence (N39.3-N39.4-)*
urinary incontinence NOS (R32)
R39.82 Chronic bladder pain
AHA: 2016,4Q,64
R39.83 Unilateral non-palpable testicle ♂
R39.84 Bilateral non-palpable testicles ♂

R39.89 Other symptoms and signs involving the genitourinary system
R39.9 Unspecified symptoms and signs involving the genitourinary system

Symptoms and signs involving cognition, perception, emotional state and behavior (R40-R46)

EXCLUDES 2   *symptoms and signs constituting part of a pattern of mental disorder (F01-F99)*

✓4ᵗʰ R40 Somnolence, stupor and coma
EXCLUDES 1   *neonatal coma (P91.5)*
somnolence, stupor and coma in diabetes (E08-E13)
somnolence, stupor and coma in hepatic failure (K72.-)
somnolence, stupor and coma in hypoglycemia (nondiabetic) (E15)
R40.0 Somnolence
Drowsiness
EXCLUDES 1   *coma (R40.2-)*
R40.1 Stupor
Catatonic stupor
Semicoma
EXCLUDES 1   *catatonic schizophrenia (F20.2)*
coma (R40.2-)
depressive stupor (F31-F33)
dissociative stupor (F44.2)
manic stupor (F30.2)
✓5ᵗʰ R40.2 Coma
Code first any associated:
fracture of skull (S02.-)
intracranial injury (S06.-)
NOTE One code from each subcategory, R40.21-R40.23, is required to complete the coma scale
AHA: 2019,2Q,12; 2018,4Q,70; 2017,4Q,23-25,95; 2015,2Q,17; 2014,1Q,19
TIP: Codes for individual (R40.21-, R40.22, R40.23-) or total (R40.24-) coma scale scores may be assigned based on medical record documentation from clinicians who are not the patient's provider.
TIP: It is not appropriate to assign individual (R40.21-, R40.22-, R40.23-) or total (R40.24-) coma scale score codes for patients who are sedated or in medically induced comas.
R40.20 Unspecified coma NC Dx
Coma NOS
Unconsciousness NOS
TIP: This code would be viewed by Medicare as a questionable admission if used as the admitting diagnosis for a hospice encounter.
✓6ᵗʰ R40.21 Coma scale, eyes open
The following appropriate 7th character is to be added to subcategory R40.21-, R40.22-, R40.23-, and R40.24-.
0   unspecified time
1   in the field [EMT or ambulance]
2   at arrival to emergency department
3   at hospital admission
4   24 hours or more after hospital admission
✓7ᵗʰ R40.211 Coma scale, eyes open, never
Coma scale eye opening score of 1
✓7ᵗʰ R40.212 Coma scale, eyes open, to pain
Coma scale eye opening score of 2
✓7ᵗʰ R40.213 Coma scale, eyes open, to sound
Coma scale eye opening score of 3
✓7ᵗʰ R40.214 Coma scale, eyes open, spontaneous
Coma scale eye opening score of 4
✓6ᵗʰ R40.22 Coma scale, best verbal response
✓7ᵗʰ R40.221 Coma scale, best verbal response, none
Coma scale verbal score of 1
✓7ᵗʰ R40.222 Coma scale, best verbal response, incomprehensible words
Coma scale verbal score of 2
Incomprehensible sounds (2-5 years of age)
Moans/grunts to pain; restless (< 2 years old)

√7th **R40.223 Coma scale, best verbal response, inappropriate words**
Coma scale verbal score of 3
Inappropriate crying or screaming (< 2 years of age)
Screaming (2-5 years of age)

√7th **R40.224 Coma scale, best verbal response, confused conversation**
Coma scale verbal score of 4
Inappropriate words (2-5 years of age)
Irritable cries (< 2 years of age)

√7th **R40.225 Coma scale, best verbal response, oriented**
Coma scale verbal score of 5
Cooing or babbling or crying appropriately (< 2 years of age)
Uses appropriate words (2-5 years of age)

√6th **R40.23 Coma scale, best motor response**

√7th **R40.231 Coma scale, best motor response, none**
Coma scale motor score of 1

√7th **R40.232 Coma scale, best motor response, extension**
Abnormal extensor posturing to pain or noxious stimuli (< 2 years of age)
Coma scale motor score of 2
Extensor posturing to pain or noxious stimuli (2-5 years of age)

√7th **R40.233 Coma scale, best motor response, abnormal flexion**
Abnormal flexure posturing to pain or noxious stimuli (2-5 years of age)
Coma scale motor score of 3
Flexion/decorticate posturing (< 2 years of age)

√7th **R40.234 Coma scale, best motor response, flexion withdrawal**
Coma scale motor score of 4
Withdraws from pain or noxious stimuli (2-5 years of age)

√7th **R40.235 Coma scale, best motor response, localizes pain**
Coma scale motor score of 5
Localizes pain (2-5 years of age)
Withdraws to touch (< 2 years of age)

√7th **R40.236 Coma scale, best motor response, obeys commands**
Coma scale motor score of 6
Normal or spontaneous movement (< 2 years of age)
Obeys commands (2-5 years of age)

√6th **R40.24 Glasgow coma scale, total score**
NOTE Assign a code from subcategory R40.24, when only the total coma score is documented
AHA: 2016,4Q,64-65

√7th **R40.241 Glasgow coma scale score 13-15**
√7th **R40.242 Glasgow coma scale score 9-12**
√7th **R40.243 Glasgow coma scale score 3-8**
√7th **R40.244 Other coma, without documented Glasgow coma scale score, or with partial score reported**

R40.3 Persistent vegetative state
DEF: Persistent wakefulness without consciousness due to a nonfunctioning cerebral cortex.

R40.4 Transient alteration of awareness

√4th **R41 Other symptoms and signs involving cognitive functions and awareness**
EXCLUDES 1 dissociative [conversion] disorders (F44.-)
mild cognitive impairment, so stated (G31.84)

R41.0 Disorientation, unspecified
Confusion NOS
Delirium NOS
AHA: 2019,2Q,34

R41.1 Anterograde amnesia
R41.2 Retrograde amnesia

R41.3 Other amnesia
Amnesia NOS
Memory loss NOS
EXCLUDES 1 amnestic disorder due to known physiologic condition (F04)
amnestic syndrome due to psychoactive substance use (F10-F19 with 5th character .6)
mild memory disturbance due to known physiological condition (F06.8)
transient global amnesia (G45.4)

R41.4 Neurologic neglect syndrome
Asomatognosia
Hemi-akinesia
Hemi-inattention
Hemispatial neglect
Left-sided neglect
Sensory neglect
Visuospatial neglect
EXCLUDES 1 visuospatial deficit (R41.842)

√5th **R41.8 Other symptoms and signs involving cognitive functions and awareness**
R41.81 Age-related cognitive decline A
Senility NOS
R41.82 Altered mental status, unspecified
Change in mental status NOS
EXCLUDES 1 altered level of consciousness (R40.-)
altered mental status due to known condition — code to condition
delirium NOS (R41.0)
AHA: 2012,4Q,97
R41.83 Borderline intellectual functioning
IQ level 71 to 84
EXCLUDES 1 intellectual disabilities (F70-F79)
√6th **R41.84 Other specified cognitive deficit**
EXCLUDES 1 cognitive deficits as sequelae of cerebrovascular disease (I69.01-, I69.11-, I69.21-, I69.31-, I69.81-, I69.91-)
R41.840 Attention and concentration deficit
EXCLUDES 1 attention-deficit hyperactivity disorders (F90.-)
R41.841 Cognitive communication deficit
R41.842 Visuospatial deficit
R41.843 Psychomotor deficit
R41.844 Frontal lobe and executive function deficit
R41.89 Other symptoms and signs involving cognitive functions and awareness
Anosognosia
R41.9 Unspecified symptoms and signs involving cognitive functions and awareness
Unspecified neurocognitive disorder

R42 Dizziness and giddiness
Light-headedness
Vertigo NOS
EXCLUDES 1 vertiginous syndromes (H81.-)
vertigo from infrasound (T75.23)

√4th **R43 Disturbances of smell and taste**
R43.0 Anosmia
DEF: Permanent or transient absence of smell that may be congenital or acquired.
R43.1 Parosmia
DEF: Abnormal perception of smell usually triggered by environmental odors.
R43.2 Parageusia
DEF: Abnormal perception of taste.
R43.8 Other disturbances of smell and taste
Mixed disturbance of smell and taste
R43.9 Unspecified disturbances of smell and taste

R44 Other symptoms and signs involving general sensations and perceptions

   EXCLUDES 1   alcoholic hallucinations (F1.5)

           hallucinations in drug psychosis (F11-F19 with .5)

           hallucinations in mood disorders with psychotic symptoms (F30.2, F31.5, F32.3, F33.3)

           hallucinations in schizophrenia, schizotypal and delusional disorders (F20-F29)

   EXCLUDES 2   disturbances of skin sensation (R20.-)

- R44.0 **Auditory** hallucinations
- R44.1 **Visual** hallucinations
- R44.2 **Other hallucinations**
- R44.3 **Hallucinations, unspecified**
- R44.8 **Other symptoms and signs involving general sensations and perceptions**
- R44.9 **Unspecified symptoms and signs involving general sensations and perceptions**

R45 Symptoms and signs involving emotional state

- R45.0 **Nervousness**
  - Nervous tension
- R45.1 **Restlessness and agitation**
- R45.2 **Unhappiness**
- R45.3 **Demoralization and apathy**
  -   *EXCLUDES 1*   anhedonia (R45.84)
- R45.4 **Irritability and anger**
- R45.5 **Hostility**
- R45.6 **Violent behavior**
- R45.7 **State of emotional shock and stress, unspecified**
- R45.8 **Other symptoms and signs involving emotional state**
  - R45.81 **Low self-esteem**
  - R45.82 **Worries**
  - R45.83 **Excessive crying of child, adolescent or adult**
    -   *EXCLUDES 1*   excessive crying of infant (baby) R68.11
  - R45.84 **Anhedonia**
  - R45.85 **Homicidal and suicidal ideations**
    -   *EXCLUDES 1*   suicide attempt (T14.91)
    - R45.850 **Homicidal ideations**
    - R45.851 **Suicidal ideations**
      - **DEF:** Thoughts of committing suicide but no actual attempt of suicide has been made.
  - R45.86 **Emotional lability**
  - R45.87 **Impulsiveness**
  - R45.89 **Other symptoms and signs involving emotional state**

R46 Symptoms and signs involving appearance and behavior

   EXCLUDES 1   appearance and behavior in schizophrenia, schizotypal and delusional disorders (F20-F29)

           mental and behavioral disorders (F01-F99)

- R46.0 **Very low level of personal hygiene**
- R46.1 **Bizarre personal appearance**
- R46.2 **Strange and inexplicable behavior**
- R46.3 **Overactivity**
- R46.4 **Slowness and poor responsiveness**
  -   *EXCLUDES 1*   stupor (R40.1)
- R46.5 **Suspiciousness and marked evasiveness**
- R46.6 **Undue concern and preoccupation with stressful events**
- R46.7 **Verbosity and circumstantial detail obscuring reason for contact**
- R46.8 **Other symptoms and signs involving appearance and behavior**
  - R46.81 **Obsessive-compulsive behavior**
    -   *EXCLUDES 1*   obsessive-compulsive disorder (F42-)
  - R46.89 **Other symptoms and signs involving appearance and behavior**

Symptoms and signs involving speech and voice (R47-R49)

R47 Speech disturbances, not elsewhere classified

   EXCLUDES 1   autism (F84.0)

           cluttering (F80.81)

           specific developmental disorders of speech and language (F80.-)

           stuttering (F80.81)

- R47.0 **Dysphasia and aphasia**
  - R47.01 **Aphasia**
    -   *EXCLUDES 1*   aphasia following cerebrovascular disease (I69. with final characters -20)
    -          progressive isolated aphasia (G31.01)
  - R47.02 **Dysphasia**
    -   *EXCLUDES 1*   dysphasia following cerebrovascular disease (I69. with final characters -21)
- R47.1 **Dysarthria and anarthria**
  -   *EXCLUDES 1*   dysarthria following cerebrovascular disease (I69. with final characters -22)
- R47.8 **Other speech disturbances**
  -   *EXCLUDES 1*   dysarthria following cerebrovascular disease (I69. with final characters -28)
  - R47.81 **Slurred speech**
  - R47.82 ***Fluency disorder in conditions classified elsewhere***
    - Stuttering in conditions classified elsewhere
    - Code first underlying disease or condition, such as:
    - Parkinson's disease (G20)
    -   *EXCLUDES 1*   adult onset fluency disorder (F98.5)
    -          childhood onset fluency disorder (F80.81)
    -          fluency disorder (stuttering) following cerebrovascular disease (I69. with final characters -23)
  - R47.89 **Other speech disturbances**
- R47.9 **Unspecified speech disturbances**

R48 Dyslexia and other symbolic dysfunctions, not elsewhere classified

   EXCLUDES 1   specific developmental disorders of scholastic skills (F81.-)

- R48.0 **Dyslexia and alexia**
- R48.1 **Agnosia**
  - Astereognosia (astereognosis)
  - Autotopagnosia
  -   *EXCLUDES 1*   visual object agnosia (R48.3)
  - **DEF:** Inability to recognize common things such as faces, objects, smells, or voices.
- R48.2 **Apraxia**
  -   *EXCLUDES 1*   apraxia following cerebrovascular disease (I69. with final characters -90)
- R48.3 **Visual agnosia**
  - Prosopagnosia
  - Simultanagnosia (asimultagnosia)
- R48.8 **Other symbolic dysfunctions**
  - Acalculia
  - Agraphia
  - **AHA:** 2017,1Q,27
  - **TIP:** Assign to indicate echolalia. May be assigned along with F84.0 Autistic disorder, to provide additional information about symptoms being addressed by treatment that are not integral to autism.
- R48.9 **Unspecified symbolic dysfunctions**

R49 Voice and resonance disorders

   EXCLUDES 1   psychogenic voice and resonance disorders (F44.4)

- R49.0 **Dysphonia**
  - Hoarseness
- R49.1 **Aphonia**
  - Loss of voice
- R49.2 **Hypernasality and hyponasality**
  - R49.21 **Hypernasality**
  - R49.22 **Hyponasality**
- R49.8 **Other voice and resonance disorders**
- R49.9 **Unspecified voice and resonance disorder**
  - Change in voice NOS
  - Resonance disorder NOS

☑ Additional Character Required   ✓x7ᵗʰ Placeholder Alert   Manifestation   Unspecified Dx   ►◄ Revised Text   ● New Code   ▲ Revised Title

ICD-10-CM 2020   929

Chapter 18. Symptoms, Signs and Abnormal Clinical and Laboratory Findings

General symptoms and signs (R50-R69)

✓4ᵗʰ R50 Fever of other and unknown origin
EXCLUDES 1 chills without fever (R68.83)
febrile convulsions (R56.0-)
fever of unknown origin during labor (O75.2)
fever of unknown origin in newborn (P81.9)
hypothermia due to illness (R68.0)
malignant hyperthermia due to anesthesia (T88.3)
puerperal pyrexia NOS (O86.4)

R50.2 Drug induced fever
Use additional code for adverse effect, if applicable, to identify drug (T36-T50 with fifth or sixth character 5)
EXCLUDES 1 postvaccination (postimmunization) fever (R50.83)

✓5ᵗʰ R50.8 Other specified fever
R50.81 Fever presenting with conditions classified elsewhere
Code first underlying condition when associated fever is present, such as with:
leukemia (C91-C95)
neutropenia (D70.-)
sickle-cell disease (D57.-)
AHA: 2014,4Q,22

R50.82 Postprocedural fever
EXCLUDES 1 postprocedural infection (T81.4-)
posttransfusion fever (R50.84)
postvaccination (postimmunization) fever (R50.83)

R50.83 Postvaccination fever
Postimmunization fever

R50.84 Febrile nonhemolytic transfusion reaction
FNHTR
Posttransfusion fever

R50.9 Fever, unspecified
Fever NOS
Fever of unknown origin [FUO]
Fever with chills
Fever with rigors
Hyperpyrexia NOS
Persistent fever
Pyrexia NOS

R51 Headache
Facial pain NOS
EXCLUDES 1 atypical face pain (G50.1)
migraine and other headache syndromes (G43-G44)
trigeminal neuralgia (G50.0)

R52 Pain, unspecified
Acute pain NOS
Generalized pain NOS
Pain NOS
EXCLUDES 1 acute and chronic pain, not elsewhere classified (G89.-)
localized pain, unspecified type — code to pain by site, such as:
abdomen pain (R10.-)
back pain (M54.9)
breast pain (N64.4)
chest pain (R07.1-R07.9)
ear pain (H92.0-)
eye pain (H57.1)
headache (R51)
joint pain (M25.5-)
limb pain (M79.6-)
lumbar region pain (M54.5)
pelvic and perineal pain (R10.2)
renal colic (N23)
shoulder pain (M25.51-)
spine pain (M54.-)
throat pain (R07.0)
tongue pain (K14.6)
tooth pain (K08.8)
pain disorders exclusively related to psychological factors (F45.41)

✓4ᵗʰ R53 Malaise and fatigue
R53.0 Neoplastic (malignant) related fatigue
Code first associated neoplasm

R53.1 Weakness
Asthenia NOS
EXCLUDES 1 age-related weakness (R54)
muscle weakness (M62.8-)
sarcopenia (M62.84)
senile asthenia (R54)
AHA: 2017,1Q,7; 2015,1Q,25

R53.2 Functional quadriplegia
Complete immobility due to severe physical disability or frailty
EXCLUDES 1 frailty NOS (R54)
hysterical paralysis (F44.4)
immobility syndrome (M62.3)
neurologic quadriplegia (G82.5-)
quadriplegia (G82.50)
AHA: 2016,2Q,6
DEF: Inability to move due to a nonphysiological condition, such as dementia. The patient has no mental ability to move independently.
TIP: Functional quadriplegia is not considered an integral component of Alzheimer's dementia and may be coded with G30 and F02.80-.

✓5ᵗʰ R53.8 Other malaise and fatigue
EXCLUDES 1 combat exhaustion and fatigue (F43.0)
congenital debility (P96.9)
exhaustion and fatigue due to excessive exertion (T73.3)
exhaustion and fatigue due to exposure (T73.2)
exhaustion and fatigue due to heat (T67.-)
exhaustion and fatigue due to pregnancy (O26.8-)
exhaustion and fatigue due to recurrent depressive episode (F33)
exhaustion and fatigue due to senile debility (R54)

R53.81 Other malaise `NC Dx`
Chronic debility
Debility NOS
General physical deterioration
Malaise NOS
Nervous debility
EXCLUDES 1 age-related physical debility (R54)
TIP: This code would be viewed by Medicare as a questionable admission if used as the admitting diagnosis for a hospice encounter.

R53.82 Chronic fatigue, unspecified
Chronic fatigue syndrome NOS
EXCLUDES 1 postviral fatigue syndrome (G93.3)

R53.83 Other fatigue
Fatigue NOS
Lack of energy
Lethargy
Tiredness
EXCLUDES 2 exhaustion and fatigue due to depressive episode (F32.-)

R54 Age-related physical debility `NC Dx` `A`
Frailty
Old age
Senescence
Senile asthenia
Senile debility
EXCLUDES 1 age-related cognitive decline (R41.81)
sarcopenia (M62.84)
senile psychosis (F03)
senility NOS (R41.81)
TIP: This code would be viewed by Medicare as a questionable admission if used as the admitting diagnosis for a hospice encounter.

R55 Syncope and collapse
Blackout
Fainting
Vasovagal attack
> EXCLUDES 1   *cardiogenic shock (R57.0)*
> *carotid sinus syncope (G90.01)*
> *heat syncope (T67.1)*
> *neurocirculatory asthenia (F45.8)*
> *neurogenic orthostatic hypotension (G90.3)*
> *orthostatic hypotension (I95.1)*
> *postprocedural shock (T81.1-)*
> *psychogenic syncope (F48.8)*
> *shock NOS (R57.9)*
> *shock complicating or following abortion or ectopic or molar pregnancy (O00-O07, O08.3)*
> *shock complicating or following labor and delivery (O75.1)*
> *Stokes-Adams attack (I45.9)*
> *unconsciousness NOS (R40.2-)*

✓4th R56 Convulsions, not elsewhere classified
> EXCLUDES 1   *dissociative convulsions and seizures (F44.5)*
> *epileptic convulsions and seizures (G40.-)*
> *newborn convulsions and seizures (P90)*

✓5th R56.0 Febrile convulsions
R56.00 Simple febrile convulsions
Febrile convulsion NOS
Febrile seizure NOS
R56.01 Complex febrile convulsions
Atypical febrile seizure
Complex febrile seizure
Complicated febrile seizure
> EXCLUDES 1   *status epilepticus (G40.901)*

R56.1 Post traumatic seizures
> EXCLUDES 1   *post traumatic epilepsy (G40.-)*

R56.9 Unspecified convulsions
Convulsion disorder
Fit NOS
Recurrent convulsions
Seizure(s) (convulsive) NOS
AHA: 2019,1Q,19

✓4th R57 Shock, not elsewhere classified
> EXCLUDES 1   *anaphylactic shock NOS (T78.2)*
> *anaphylactic reaction or shock due to adverse food reaction (T78.0-)*
> *anaphylactic shock due to adverse effect of correct drug or medicament properly administered (T88.6)*
> *anaphylactic shock due to serum (T80.5-)*
> *anesthetic shock (T88.3)*
> *electric shock (T75.4)*
> *obstetric shock (O75.1)*
> *postprocedural shock (T81.1-)*
> *psychic shock (F43.0)*
> *shock complicating or following ectopic or molar pregnancy (O00-O07, O08.3)*
> *shock due to lightning (T75.01)*
> *traumatic shock (T79.4)*
> *toxic shock syndrome (A48.3)*

R57.0 Cardiogenic shock
> EXCLUDES 2   *septic shock (R65.21)*

DEF: Associated with myocardial infarction, cardiac tamponade, and massive pulmonary embolism. Symptoms include mental confusion, reduced blood pressure, tachycardia, pallor, and cold, clammy skin.

R57.1 Hypovolemic shock
AHA: 2019,2Q,7

R57.8 Other shock
R57.9 Shock, unspecified
Failure of peripheral circulation NOS

R58 Hemorrhage, not elsewhere classified
Hemorrhage NOS
> EXCLUDES 1   *hemorrhage included with underlying conditions, such as:*
> *acute duodenal ulcer with hemorrhage (K26.0)*
> *acute gastritis with bleeding (K29.01)*
> *ulcerative enterocolitis with rectal bleeding (K51.01)*

✓4th R59 Enlarged lymph nodes
> INCLUDES   swollen glands
> EXCLUDES 1   *acute lymphadenitis (L04.-)*
> *chronic lymphadenitis (I88.1)*
> *lymphadenitis NOS (I88.9)*
> *mesenteric (acute) (chronic) lymphadenitis (I88.0)*

R59.0 Localized enlarged lymph nodes
R59.1 Generalized enlarged lymph nodes
Lymphadenopathy NOS
R59.9 Enlarged lymph nodes, unspecified

✓4th R60 Edema, not elsewhere classified
> EXCLUDES 1   *angioneurotic edema (T78.3)*
> *ascites (R18.-)*
> *cerebral edema (G93.6)*
> *cerebral edema due to birth injury (P11.0)*
> *edema of larynx (J38.4)*
> *edema of nasopharynx (J39.2)*
> *edema of pharynx (J39.2)*
> *gestational edema (O12.0-)*
> *hereditary edema (Q82.0)*
> *hydrops fetalis NOS (P83.2)*
> *hydrothorax (J94.8)*
> *hydrops fetalis NOS (P83.2)*
> *newborn edema (P83.3)*
> *pulmonary edema (J81.-)*

R60.0 Localized edema
R60.1 Generalized edema
> EXCLUDES 2   *nutritional edema (E40-E46)*

R60.9 Edema, unspecified
Fluid retention NOS

R61 Generalized hyperhidrosis
Excessive sweating
Night sweats
Secondary hyperhidrosis
Code first, if applicable, menopausal and female climacteric states (N95.1)
> EXCLUDES 1   *focal (primary) (secondary) hyperhidrosis (L74.5-)*
> *Frey's syndrome (L74.52)*
> *localized (primary) (secondary) hyperhidrosis (L74.5-)*

✓4th R62 Lack of expected normal physiological development in childhood and adults
> EXCLUDES 1   *delayed puberty (E30.0)*
> *gonadal dysgenesis (Q99.1)*
> *hypopituitarism (E23.0)*

R62.0 Delayed milestone in childhood   P
Delayed attainment of expected physiological developmental stage
Late talker
Late walker

✓5th R62.5 Other and unspecified lack of expected normal physiological development in childhood
> EXCLUDES 1   *HIV disease resulting in failure to thrive (B20)*
> *physical retardation due to malnutrition (E45)*

R62.50 Unspecified lack of expected normal physiological development in childhood
Infantilism NOS
R62.51 Failure to thrive (child)   P
Failure to gain weight
> EXCLUDES 1   *failure to thrive in child under 28 days old (P92.6)*

AHA: 2018,4Q,82
DEF: Organic failure to thrive (FTT): Acute or chronic illness that interferes with nutritional intake, absorption, metabolism excretion, and energy requirements.
DEF: Nonorganic failure to thrive (FTT): Symptom of neglect or abuse.
R62.52 Short stature (child)
Lack of growth
Physical retardation
Short stature NOS
> EXCLUDES 1   *short stature due to endocrine disorder (E34.3)*

R62.59 Other lack of expected normal physiological development in childhood

☑ Additional Character Required   ✓x7th Placeholder Alert   Manifestation   Unspecified Dx   ►◄ Revised Text   ● New Code   ▲ Revised Title

ICD-10-CM 2020   931

R62.7   Adult failure to thrive   NC Dx   A

> **TIP:** This code would be viewed by Medicare as a questionable admission if used as the admitting diagnosis for a hospice encounter.

✓4ᵗʰ **R63   Symptoms and signs concerning food and fluid intake**

> EXCLUDES 1   bulimia NOS (F50.2)
> ~~eating disorders of nonorganic origin (F50.-)~~
> ~~malnutrition (E40-E46)~~

R63.0   Anorexia

> Loss of appetite
> EXCLUDES 1   anorexia nervosa (F50.0-)
> loss of appetite of nonorganic origin (F50.89)
> **AHA:** 2018,4Q,82
> **TIP:** Assign an additional code from category Z68 when BMI is documented. BMI can be based on documentation from clinicians who are not the patient's provider.

R63.1   Polydipsia

> Excessive thirst

R63.2   Polyphagia

> Excessive eating
> Hyperalimentation NOS

R63.3   Feeding difficulties

> Feeding problem (elderly) (infant) NOS
> Picky eater
> EXCLUDES 1   eating disorders (F50.-)
> feeding problems of newborn (P92.-)
> infant feeding disorder of nonorganic origin (F98.2-)
> **AHA:** 2017,1Q,28; 2016,3Q,19

R63.4   Abnormal weight loss

> **AHA:** 2018,4Q,82
> **TIP:** Assign an additional code from category Z68 when BMI is documented. BMI can be based on documentation from clinicians who are not the patient's provider.

R63.5   Abnormal weight gain

> EXCLUDES 1   excessive weight gain in pregnancy (O26.0-)
> obesity (E66.-)
> **AHA:** 2018,4Q,82
> **TIP:** Assign an additional code from category Z68 when BMI is documented. BMI can be based on documentation from clinicians who are not the patient's provider.

R63.6   Underweight

> Use additional code to identify body mass index (BMI), if known (Z68.-)
> EXCLUDES 1   abnormal weight loss (R63.4)
> anorexia nervosa (F50.0-)
> malnutrition (E40-E46)
> **AHA:** 2018,4Q,82

R63.8   Other symptoms and signs concerning food and fluid intake

R64   Cachexia

> Wasting syndrome
> Code first underlying condition, if known
> EXCLUDES 1   abnormal weight loss (R63.4)
> nutritional marasmus (E41)
> **AHA:** 2018,4Q,82; 2017,3Q,24
> **TIP:** Assign code E41 when emaciated or emaciation is documented in relation to malnutrition.

✓4ᵗʰ **R65   Symptoms and signs specifically associated with systemic inflammation and infection**

> **AHA:** 2019,2Q,38
> **TIP:** When documentation states SIRS with an infection, assign only a code for the infection. ICD-10-CM does not offer a code for SIRS due to infectious process. If sepsis is suspected, query the provider.

✓5ᵗʰ **R65.1   Systemic inflammatory response syndrome [SIRS] of non-infectious origin**

> Code first underlying condition, such as:
> heatstroke ►(T67.0-)◄
> injury and trauma (S00-T88)
> EXCLUDES 1   sepsis — code to infection
> severe sepsis (R65.2)

R65.10   Systemic inflammatory response syndrome [SIRS] of non-infectious origin without acute organ dysfunction

> Systemic inflammatory response syndrome (SIRS) NOS
> **AHA:** 2019,2Q,24

R65.11   Systemic inflammatory response syndrome [SIRS] of non-infectious origin with acute organ dysfunction

> Use additional code to identify specific acute organ dysfunction, such as:
> acute kidney failure (N17.-)
> acute respiratory failure (J96.0-)
> critical illness myopathy (G72.81)
> critical illness polyneuropathy (G62.81)
> disseminated intravascular coagulopathy [DIC] (D65)
> encephalopathy (metabolic) (septic) (G93.41)
> hepatic failure (K72.0-)

✓5ᵗʰ **R65.2   Severe sepsis**

> Infection with associated acute organ dysfunction
> Sepsis with acute organ dysfunction
> Sepsis with multiple organ dysfunction
> Systemic inflammatory response syndrome due to infectious process with acute organ dysfunction
> Code first underlying infection, such as:
> infection following a procedure (T81.4-)
> infections following infusion, transfusion and therapeutic injection (T80.2-)
> puerperal sepsis (O85)
> sepsis following complete or unspecified spontaneous abortion (O03.87)
> sepsis following ectopic and molar pregnancy (O08.82)
> sepsis following incomplete spontaneous abortion (O03.37)
> sepsis following (induced) termination of pregnancy (O04.87)
> sepsis NOS (A41.9)
> Use additional code to identify specific acute organ dysfunction, such as:
> acute kidney failure (N17.-)
> acute respiratory failure (J96.0-)
> critical illness myopathy (G72.81)
> critical illness polyneuropathy (G62.81)
> disseminated intravascular coagulopathy [DIC] (D65)
> encephalopathy (metabolic) (septic) (G93.41)
> hepatic failure (K72.0-)
> **AHA:** 2018,4Q,62-63; 2017,4Q,98-99; 2016,3Q,8

R65.20   Severe sepsis without septic shock

> Severe sepsis NOS
> **AHA:** 2016,3Q,14; 2013,4Q,119

R65.21   Severe sepsis with septic shock

> **AHA:** 2018,4Q,63

✓4ᵗʰ **R68   Other general symptoms and signs**

R68.0   Hypothermia, not associated with low environmental temperature

> EXCLUDES 1   hypothermia NOS (accidental) (T68)
> hypothermia due to anesthesia (T88.51)
> hypothermia due to low environmental temperature (T68)
> newborn hypothermia (P80.-)

✓5ᵗʰ **R68.1   Nonspecific symptoms peculiar to infancy**

> EXCLUDES 1   colic, infantile (R10.83)
> neonatal cerebral irritability (P91.3)
> teething syndrome (K00.7)

R68.11   Excessive crying of infant (baby)   P

> EXCLUDES 1   excessive crying of child, adolescent, or adult (R45.83)

R68.12   Fussy infant (baby)   P

> Irritable infant

R68.13   Apparent life threatening event in infant (ALTE)   P

> Apparent life threatening event in newborn
> Brief resolved unexplained event (BRUE)
> Code first confirmed diagnosis, if known
> Use additional code(s) for associated signs and symptoms if no confirmed diagnosis established, or if signs and symptoms are not associated routinely with confirmed diagnosis, or provide additional information for cause of ALTE

R68.19   Other nonspecific symptoms peculiar to infancy   P

N Newborn: 0   P Pediatric: 0-17   M Maternity: 12-55   A Adult: 15-124   CH Comorbidity High   CL Comorbidity Low   NC Dx Noncancer Dx   PDx Primary Dx

932   ICD-10-CM 2020

R68.2 **Dry mouth, unspecified**
   EXCLUDES 1   *dry mouth due to dehydration (E86.Ø)*
       dry mouth due to sicca syndrome [Sjögren] (M35.Ø-)
       salivary gland hyposecretion (K11.7)

R68.3 **Clubbing of fingers**
   Clubbing of nails
   EXCLUDES 1   *congenital clubfinger (Q68.1)*
   DEF: Enlarged soft tissue of the distal fingers that usually occurs in heart and lung diseases.

☑5ᵗʰ R68.8 **Other general symptoms and signs**

   R68.81 **Early satiety**
      DEF: Premature feeling of being full after eating only a small amount of food. The mechanism of satiety is multifactorial.

   R68.82 **Decreased libido**   A
      Decreased sexual desire

   R68.83 **Chills (without fever)**
      Chills NOS
      EXCLUDES 1   *chills with fever (R5Ø.9)*

   R68.84 **Jaw pain**
      Mandibular pain
      Maxilla pain
      EXCLUDES 1   *temporomandibular joint arthralgia (M26.62-)*

   R68.89 **Other general symptoms and signs**

R69 **Illness, unspecified**
   Unknown and unspecified cases of morbidity

Abnormal findings on examination of blood, without diagnosis (R70-R79)

EXCLUDES 2   *abnormal findings on antenatal screening of mother (O28.-)*
      abnormalities of lipids (E78.-)
      abnormalities of platelets and thrombocytes (D69.-)
      abnormalities of white blood cells classified elsewhere (D70-D72)
      coagulation hemorrhagic disorders (D65-D68)
      diagnostic abnormal findings classified elsewhere — see Alphabetical Index
      hemorrhagic and hematological disorders of newborn (P5Ø-P61)

☑4ᵗʰ R70 **Elevated erythrocyte sedimentation rate and abnormality of plasma viscosity**
   R70.Ø **Elevated erythrocyte sedimentation rate**
   R70.1 **Abnormal plasma viscosity**

☑4ᵗʰ R71 **Abnormality of red blood cells**
   EXCLUDES 1   *anemias (D5Ø-D64)*
      anemia of premature infant (P61.2)
      benign (familial) polycythemia (D75.Ø)
      congenital anemias (P61.2-P61.4)
      newborn anemia due to isoimmunization (P55.-)
      polycythemia neonatorum (P61.1)
      polycythemia NOS (D75.1)
      polycythemia vera (D45)
      secondary polycythemia (D75.1)

   R71.Ø **Precipitous drop in hematocrit**
      Drop (precipitous) in hemoglobin
      Drop in hematocrit

   R71.8 **Other abnormality of red blood cells**
      Abnormal red-cell morphology NOS
      Abnormal red-cell volume NOS
      Anisocytosis
      Poikilocytosis

☑4ᵗʰ R73 **Elevated blood glucose level**
   EXCLUDES 1   *diabetes mellitus (E08-E13)*
      diabetes mellitus in pregnancy, childbirth and the puerperium (O24.-)
      neonatal disorders (P70.Ø-P70.2)
      postsurgical hypoinsulinemia (E89.1)

   ☑5ᵗʰ R73.Ø **Abnormal glucose**
      EXCLUDES 1   *abnormal glucose in pregnancy (O99.81-)*
        diabetes mellitus (E08-E13)
        dysmetabolic syndrome X (E88.81)
        gestational diabetes (O24.4-)
        glycosuria (R81)
        hypoglycemia (E16.2)

     R73.Ø1 **Impaired fasting glucose**
       Elevated fasting glucose

     R73.Ø2 **Impaired glucose tolerance (oral)**
       Elevated glucose tolerance

     R73.Ø3 **Prediabetes**
       Latent diabetes
       AHA: 2016,4Q,65

     R73.Ø9 **Other abnormal glucose**
       Abnormal glucose NOS
       Abnormal non-fasting glucose tolerance

   R73.9 **Hyperglycemia, unspecified**

☑4ᵗʰ R74 **Abnormal serum enzyme levels**
   R74.Ø **Nonspecific elevation of levels of transaminase and lactic acid dehydrogenase [LDH]**

   R74.8 **Abnormal levels of other serum enzymes**
      Abnormal level of acid phosphatase
      Abnormal level of alkaline phosphatase
      Abnormal level of amylase
      Abnormal level of lipase [triacylglycerol lipase]
      AHA: 2019,2Q,6

   R74.9 **Abnormal serum enzyme level, unspecified**

R75 **Inconclusive laboratory evidence of human immunodeficiency virus [HIV]**
   Nonconclusive HIV-test finding in infants
   EXCLUDES 1   *asymptomatic human immunodeficiency virus [HIV] infection status (Z21)*
      human immunodeficiency virus [HIV] disease (B20)

☑4ᵗʰ R76 **Other abnormal immunological findings in serum**
   R76.Ø **Raised antibody titer**
      EXCLUDES 1   *isoimmunization in pregnancy (O36.Ø-O36.1)*
        isoimmunization affecting newborn (P55.-)

   ☑5ᵗʰ R76.1 **Nonspecific reaction to test for tuberculosis**

     R76.11 **Nonspecific reaction to tuberculin skin test without active tuberculosis**
       Abnormal result of Mantoux test
       PPD positive
       Tuberculin (skin test) positive
       Tuberculin (skin test) reactor
       EXCLUDES 1   *nonspecific reaction to cell mediated immunity measurement of gamma interferon antigen response without active tuberculosis (R76.12)*

     R76.12 **Nonspecific reaction to cell mediated immunity measurement of gamma interferon antigen response without active tuberculosis**
       Nonspecific reaction to QuantiFERON-TB test (QFT) without active tuberculosis
       EXCLUDES 1   *nonspecific reaction to tuberculin skin test without active tuberculosis (R76.11)*
        positive tuberculin skin test (R76.11)

   R76.8 **Other specified abnormal immunological findings in serum**
      Raised level of immunoglobulins NOS

   R76.9 **Abnormal immunological finding in serum, unspecified**

☑4ᵗʰ R77 **Other abnormalities of plasma proteins**
   EXCLUDES 1   *disorders of plasma-protein metabolism (E88.Ø-)*
   R77.Ø **Abnormality of albumin**
   R77.1 **Abnormality of globulin**
      Hyperglobulinemia NOS
   R77.2 **Abnormality of alphafetoprotein**
   R77.8 **Other specified abnormalities of plasma proteins**

R77.9   Abnormality of plasma protein, unspecified
AHA: 2019,2Q,6

✓4ᵗʰ **R78   Findings of drugs and other substances, not normally found in blood**
Use additional code to identify the any retained foreign body, if applicable (Z18.-)
EXCLUDES 1   *mental or behavioral disorders due to psychoactive substance use (F10-F19)*

R78.0   Finding of alcohol in blood
Use additional external cause code (Y90.-), for detail regarding alcohol level

R78.1   Finding of opiate drug in blood

R78.2   Finding of cocaine in blood

R78.3   Finding of hallucinogen in blood

R78.4   Finding of other drugs of addictive potential in blood

R78.5   Finding of other psychotropic drug in blood

R78.6   Finding of steroid agent in blood

✓5ᵗʰ **R78.7   Finding of abnormal level of heavy metals in blood**

R78.71   Abnormal lead level in blood
EXCLUDES 1   *lead poisoning (T56.0-)*

R78.79   Finding of abnormal level of heavy metals in blood

✓5ᵗʰ **R78.8   Finding of other specified substances, not normally found in blood**

R78.81   Bacteremia
EXCLUDES 1   *sepsis — code to specified infection*
DEF: Laboratory finding of bacteria in the blood in the absence of two or more signs of sepsis. Transient in nature, it can progress to septicemia with a severe infectious process.

R78.89   Finding of other specified substances, not normally found in blood
Finding of abnormal level of lithium in blood

R78.9   Finding of unspecified substance, not normally found in blood

✓4ᵗʰ **R79   Other abnormal findings of blood chemistry**
Use additional code to identify any retained foreign body, if applicable (Z18.-)
EXCLUDES 1   *asymptomatic hyperuricemia (E79.0)*
hyperglycemia NOS (R73.9)
hypoglycemia NOS (E16.2)
neonatal hypoglycemia (P70.3-P70.4)
specific findings indicating disorder of amino-acid metabolism (E70-E72)
specific findings indicating disorder of carbohydrate metabolism (E73-E74)
specific findings indicating disorder of lipid metabolism (E75.-)

R79.0   Abnormal level of blood mineral
Abnormal blood level of cobalt
Abnormal blood level of copper
Abnormal blood level of iron
Abnormal blood level of magnesium
Abnormal blood level of mineral NEC
Abnormal blood level of zinc
EXCLUDES 1   *abnormal level of lithium (R78.89)*
disorders of mineral metabolism (E83.-)
neonatal hypomagnesemia (P71.2)
nutritional mineral deficiency (E58-E61)

R79.1   Abnormal coagulation profile
Abnormal or prolonged bleeding time
Abnormal or prolonged coagulation time
Abnormal or prolonged partial thromboplastin time [PTT]
Abnormal or prolonged prothrombin time [PT]
EXCLUDES 1   *coagulation defects (D68.-)*
EXCLUDES 2   *abnormality of fluid, electrolyte or acid-base balance (E86-E87)*

✓5ᵗʰ **R79.8   Other specified abnormal findings of blood chemistry**

R79.81   Abnormal blood-gas level

R79.82   Elevated C-reactive protein [CRP]

R79.89   Other specified abnormal findings of blood chemistry
AHA: 2019,2Q,6

R79.9   Abnormal finding of blood chemistry, unspecified

Abnormal findings on examination of urine, without diagnosis (R80-R82)

EXCLUDES 1   *abnormal findings on antenatal screening of mother (O28.-)*
diagnostic abnormal findings classified elsewhere — see Alphabetical Index
specific findings indicating disorder of amino-acid metabolism (E70-E72)
specific findings indicating disorder of carbohydrate metabolism (E73-E74)

✓4ᵗʰ **R80   Proteinuria**
EXCLUDES 1   *gestational proteinuria (O12.1-)*

R80.0   Isolated proteinuria
Idiopathic proteinuria
EXCLUDES 1   *isolated proteinuria with specific morphological lesion (N06.-)*

R80.1   Persistent proteinuria, unspecified

R80.2   Orthostatic proteinuria, unspecified
Postural proteinuria

R80.3   Bence Jones proteinuria

R80.8   Other proteinuria

R80.9   Proteinuria, unspecified
Albuminuria NOS

R81   Glycosuria
EXCLUDES 1   *renal glycosuria (E74.8)*

✓4ᵗʰ **R82   Other and unspecified abnormal findings in urine**
INCLUDES   chromoabnormalities in urine
Use additional code to identify any retained foreign body, if applicable (Z18.-)
EXCLUDES 2   *hematuria (R31.-)*

R82.0   Chyluria
EXCLUDES 1   *filarial chyluria (B74.-)*

R82.1   Myoglobinuria

R82.2   Biliuria

R82.3   Hemoglobinuria
EXCLUDES 1   *hemoglobinuria due to hemolysis from external causes NEC (D59.6)*
hemoglobinuria due to paroxysmal nocturnal [Marchiafava-Micheli] (D59.5)
DEF: Free hemoglobin in blood due to rapid hemolysis of red blood cells. Causes include burns, crushed injury, sickle cell anemia, thalassemia, parasitic infections, or kidney infections.

R82.4   Acetonuria
Ketonuria
DEF: Excessive excretion of acetone in urine that commonly occurs in diabetic acidosis.

R82.5   Elevated urine levels of drugs, medicaments and biological substances
Elevated urine levels of catecholamines
Elevated urine levels of indoleacetic acid
Elevated urine levels of 17-ketosteroids
Elevated urine levels of steroids

R82.6   Abnormal urine levels of substances chiefly nonmedicinal as to source
Abnormal urine level of heavy metals

✓5ᵗʰ **R82.7   Abnormal findings on microbiological examination of urine**
EXCLUDES 1   *colonization status (Z22.-)*
AHA: 2016,4Q,65

R82.71   Bacteriuria

R82.79   Other abnormal findings on microbiological examination of urine
Positive culture findings of urine

▲ ✓5ᵗʰ **R82.8   Abnormal findings on cytological and histological examination of urine**

● **R82.81   Pyuria**
Sterile pyuria

● **R82.89   Other abnormal findings on cytological and histological examination of urine**

✓5ᵗʰ **R82.9   Other and unspecified abnormal findings in urine**

R82.90   Unspecified abnormal findings in urine

R82.91   **Other chromoabnormalities of urine**
Chromoconversion (dipstick)
Idiopathic dipstick converts positive for blood with no cellular forms in sediment
> *EXCLUDES 1*   *hemoglobinuria (R82.3)*
>   *myoglobinuria (R82.1)*

✓6ᵗʰ **R82.99**   **Other abnormal findings in urine**
AHA: 2018,4Q,29-30

R82.991   **Hypocitraturia**

R82.992   **Hyperoxaluria**
> *EXCLUDES 1*   *primary hyperoxaluria (E72.53)*

R82.993   **Hyperuricosuria**

R82.994   **Hypercalciuria**
Idiopathic hypercalciuria

R82.998   **Other abnormal findings in urine**
Cells and casts in urine
Crystalluria
Melanuria

Abnormal findings on examination of other body fluids, substances and tissues, without diagnosis (R83-R89)

> *EXCLUDES 1*   *abnormal findings on antenatal screening of mother (O28.-)*
>   *diagnostic abnormal findings classified elsewhere — see Alphabetical Index*
> *EXCLUDES 2*   *abnormal findings on examination of blood, without diagnosis (R70-R79)*
>   *abnormal findings on examination of urine, without diagnosis (R80-R82)*
>   *abnormal tumor markers (R97.-)*

✓4ᵗʰ **R83**   **Abnormal findings in cerebrospinal fluid**

Cerebrospinal Fluid

Ventricles

Cerebrospinal fluid

Spinal cord

R83.0   **Abnormal level of enzymes in cerebrospinal fluid**

R83.1   **Abnormal level of hormones in cerebrospinal fluid**

R83.2   **Abnormal level of other drugs, medicaments and biological substances in cerebrospinal fluid**

R83.3   **Abnormal level of substances chiefly nonmedicinal as to source in cerebrospinal fluid**

R83.4   **Abnormal immunological findings in cerebrospinal fluid**

R83.5   **Abnormal microbiological findings in cerebrospinal fluid**
Positive culture findings in cerebrospinal fluid
> *EXCLUDES 1*   *colonization status (Z22.-)*

R83.6   **Abnormal cytological findings in cerebrospinal fluid**

R83.8   **Other abnormal findings in cerebrospinal fluid**
Abnormal chromosomal findings in cerebrospinal fluid

R83.9   **Unspecified abnormal finding in cerebrospinal fluid**

✓4ᵗʰ **R84**   **Abnormal findings in specimens from respiratory organs and thorax**
> *INCLUDES*   abnormal findings in bronchial washings
>   abnormal findings in nasal secretions
>   abnormal findings in pleural fluid
>   abnormal findings in sputum
>   abnormal findings in throat scrapings
> *EXCLUDES 1*   *blood-stained sputum (R04.2)*

R84.0   **Abnormal level of enzymes in specimens from respiratory organs and thorax**

R84.1   **Abnormal level of hormones in specimens from respiratory organs and thorax**

R84.2   **Abnormal level of other drugs, medicaments and biological substances in specimens from respiratory organs and thorax**

R84.3   **Abnormal level of substances chiefly nonmedicinal as to source in specimens from respiratory organs and thorax**

R84.4   **Abnormal immunological findings in specimens from respiratory organs and thorax**

R84.5   **Abnormal microbiological findings in specimens from respiratory organs and thorax**
Positive culture findings in specimens from respiratory organs and thorax
> *EXCLUDES 1*   *colonization status (Z22.-)*

R84.6   **Abnormal cytological findings in specimens from respiratory organs and thorax**

R84.7   **Abnormal histological findings in specimens from respiratory organs and thorax**

R84.8   **Other abnormal findings in specimens from respiratory organs and thorax**
Abnormal chromosomal findings in specimens from respiratory organs and thorax

R84.9   **Unspecified abnormal finding in specimens from respiratory organs and thorax**

✓4ᵗʰ **R85**   **Abnormal findings in specimens from digestive organs and abdominal cavity**
> *INCLUDES*   abnormal findings in peritoneal fluid
>   abnormal findings in saliva
> *EXCLUDES 1*   *cloudy peritoneal dialysis effluent (R88.0)*
>   *fecal abnormalities (R19.5)*

R85.0   **Abnormal level of enzymes in specimens from digestive organs and abdominal cavity**

R85.1   **Abnormal level of hormones in specimens from digestive organs and abdominal cavity**

R85.2   **Abnormal level of other drugs, medicaments and biological substances in specimens from digestive organs and abdominal cavity**

R85.3   **Abnormal level of substances chiefly nonmedicinal as to source in specimens from digestive organs and abdominal cavity**

R85.4   **Abnormal immunological findings in specimens from digestive organs and abdominal cavity**

R85.5   **Abnormal microbiological findings in specimens from digestive organs and abdominal cavity**
Positive culture findings in specimens from digestive organs and abdominal cavity
> *EXCLUDES 1*   *colonization status (Z22.-)*

✓5ᵗʰ R85.6 Abnormal cytological findings in specimens from digestive organs and abdominal cavity

    ✓6ᵗʰ R85.61 Abnormal cytologic smear of anus

        EXCLUDES 1   *abnormal cytological findings in specimens from other digestive organs and abdominal cavity (R85.69)*

        anal intraepithelial neoplasia I [AIN I] (K62.82)

        anal intraepithelial neoplasia II [AIN II] (K62.82)

        anal intraepithelial neoplasia III [AIN III] (D01.3)

        carcinoma in situ of anus (histologically confirmed) (D01.3)

        dysplasia (mild) (moderate) of anus (histologically confirmed) (K62.82)

        severe dysplasia of anus (histologically confirmed) (D01.3)

        EXCLUDES 2   *anal high risk human papillomavirus (HPV) DNA test positive (R85.81)*

        anal low risk human papillomavirus (HPV) DNA test positive (R85.82)

        R85.610 Atypical squamous cells of undetermined significance on cytologic smear of anus [ASC-US]

        R85.611 Atypical squamous cells cannot exclude high grade squamous intraepithelial lesion on cytologic smear of anus [ASC-H]

        R85.612 Low grade squamous intraepithelial lesion on cytologic smear of anus [LGSIL]

        R85.613 High grade squamous intraepithelial lesion on cytologic smear of anus [HGSIL]

        R85.614 Cytologic evidence of malignancy on smear of anus

        R85.615 Unsatisfactory cytologic smear of anus

        Inadequate sample of cytologic smear of anus

        R85.616 Satisfactory anal smear but lacking transformation zone

        R85.618 Other abnormal cytological findings on specimens from anus

        R85.619 Unspecified abnormal cytological findings in specimens from anus

        Abnormal anal cytology NOS

        Atypical glandular cells of anus NOS

    R85.69 Abnormal cytological findings in specimens from other digestive organs and abdominal cavity

  R85.7 Abnormal histological findings in specimens from digestive organs and abdominal cavity

✓5ᵗʰ R85.8 Other abnormal findings in specimens from digestive organs and abdominal cavity

    R85.81 Anal high risk human papillomavirus [HPV] DNA test positive

        EXCLUDES 1   *anogenital warts due to human papillomavirus (HPV) (A63.0)*

        condyloma acuminatum (A63.0)

    R85.82 Anal low risk human papillomavirus [HPV] DNA test positive

        Use additional code for associated human papillomavirus (B97.7)

    R85.89 Other abnormal findings in specimens from digestive organs and abdominal cavity

        Abnormal chromosomal findings in specimens from digestive organs and abdominal cavity

  R85.9 Unspecified abnormal finding in specimens from digestive organs and abdominal cavity

✓4ᵗʰ R86 Abnormal findings in specimens from male genital organs

    INCLUDES   abnormal findings in prostatic secretions

    abnormal findings in semen, seminal fluid

    abnormal spermatozoa

    EXCLUDES 1   *azoospermia (N46.0-)*

    oligospermia (N46.1-)

  R86.0 Abnormal level of enzymes in specimens from male genital organs   ♂

  R86.1 Abnormal level of hormones in specimens from male genital organs   ♂

  R86.2 Abnormal level of other drugs, medicaments and biological substances in specimens from male genital organs   ♂

  R86.3 Abnormal level of substances chiefly nonmedicinal as to source in specimens from male genital organs   ♂

  R86.4 Abnormal immunological findings in specimens from male genital organs   ♂

  R86.5 Abnormal microbiological findings in specimens from male genital organs   ♂

    Positive culture findings in specimens from male genital organs

    EXCLUDES 1   *colonization status (Z22.-)*

  R86.6 Abnormal cytological findings in specimens from male genital organs   ♂

  R86.7 Abnormal histological findings in specimens from male genital organs   ♂

  R86.8 Other abnormal findings in specimens from male genital organs   ♂

    Abnormal chromosomal findings in specimens from male genital organs

  R86.9 Unspecified abnormal finding in specimens from male genital organs   ♂

✓4ᵗʰ R87 Abnormal findings in specimens from female genital organs

    INCLUDES   abnormal findings in secretion and smears from cervix uteri

    abnormal findings in secretion and smears from vagina

    abnormal findings in secretion and smears from vulva

  R87.0 Abnormal level of enzymes in specimens from female genital organs   ♀

  R87.1 Abnormal level of hormones in specimens from female genital organs   ♀

  R87.2 Abnormal level of other drugs, medicaments and biological substances in specimens from female genital organs   ♀

  R87.3 Abnormal level of substances chiefly nonmedicinal as to source in specimens from female genital organs   ♀

  R87.4 Abnormal immunological findings in specimens from female genital organs   ♀

  R87.5 Abnormal microbiological findings in specimens from female genital organs   ♀

    Positive culture findings in specimens from female genital organs

    EXCLUDES 1   *colonization status (Z22.-)*

✓5ᵗʰ R87.6 Abnormal cytological findings in specimens from female genital organs

    ✓6ᵗʰ R87.61 Abnormal cytological findings in specimens from cervix uteri

        EXCLUDES 1   *abnormal cytological findings in specimens from other female genital organs (R87.69)*

        abnormal cytological findings in specimens from vagina (R87.62-)

        carcinoma in situ of cervix uteri (histologically confirmed) (D06.-)

        cervical intraepithelial neoplasia I [CIN I] (N87.0)

        cervical intraepithelial neoplasia II [CIN II] (N87.1)

        cervical intraepithelial neoplasia III [CIN III] (D06.-)

        dysplasia (mild) (moderate) of cervix uteri (histologically confirmed) (N87.-)

        severe dysplasia of cervix uteri (histologically confirmed) (D06.-)

        EXCLUDES 2   *cervical high risk human papillomavirus (HPV) DNA test positive (R87.810)*

        cervical low risk human papillomavirus (HPV) DNA test positive (R87.820)

        R87.610 Atypical squamous cells of undetermined significance on cytologic smear of cervix [ASC-US]   ♀

        R87.611 Atypical squamous cells cannot exclude high grade squamous intraepithelial lesion on cytologic smear of cervix [ASC-H]   ♀

Ⓝ Newborn: 0   Ⓟ Pediatric: 0-17   Ⓜ Maternity: 12-55   Ⓐ Adult: 15-124   **CH** Comorbidity High   **CL** Comorbidity Low   **NCDx** Noncancer Dx   **PDx** Primary Dx

936   ICD-10-CM 2020

R87.612 Low grade squamous intraepithelial lesion on cytologic smear of cervix [LGSIL] ♀

R87.613 High grade squamous intraepithelial lesion on cytologic smear of cervix [HGSIL] ♀

R87.614 Cytologic evidence of malignancy on smear of cervix ♀

R87.615 Unsatisfactory cytologic smear of cervix ♀
     Inadequate sample of cytologic smear of cervix

R87.616 Satisfactory cervical smear but lacking transformation zone ♀

R87.618 Other abnormal cytological findings on specimens from cervix uteri ♀

R87.619 Unspecified abnormal cytological findings in specimens from cervix uteri ♀
     Abnormal cervical cytology NOS
     Abnormal Papanicolaou smear of cervix NOS
     Abnormal thin preparation smear of cervix NOS
     Atypical endocervical cells of cervix NOS
     Atypical endometrial cells of cervix NOS
     Atypical glandular cells of cervix NOS

✓6ᵗʰ R87.62 Abnormal cytological findings in specimens from vagina
     Use additional code to identify acquired absence of uterus and cervix, if applicable (Z90.71-)
     EXCLUDES 1   abnormal cytological findings in specimens from cervix uteri (R87.61-)
               abnormal cytological findings in specimens from other female genital organs (R87.69)
               carcinoma in situ of vagina (histologically confirmed) (D07.2)
               dysplasia (mild) (moderate) of vagina (histologically confirmed) (N89.-)
               severe dysplasia of vagina (histologically confirmed) (D07.2)
               vaginal intraepithelial neoplasia I [VAIN I] (N89.0)
               vaginal intraepithelial neoplasia II [VAIN II] (N89.1)
               vaginal intraepithelial neoplasia III [VAIN III] (D07.2)
     EXCLUDES 2   vaginal high risk human papillomavirus (HPV) DNA test positive (R87.811)
               vaginal low risk human papillomavirus (HPV) DNA test positive (R87.821)

R87.620 Atypical squamous cells of undetermined significance on cytologic smear of vagina [ASC-US] ♀

R87.621 Atypical squamous cells cannot exclude high grade squamous intraepithelial lesion on cytologic smear of vagina [ASC-H] ♀

R87.622 Low grade squamous intraepithelial lesion on cytologic smear of vagina [LGSIL] ♀

R87.623 High grade squamous intraepithelial lesion on cytologic smear of vagina [HGSIL] ♀

R87.624 Cytologic evidence of malignancy on smear of vagina ♀

R87.625 Unsatisfactory cytologic smear of vagina ♀
     Inadequate sample of cytologic smear of vagina

R87.628 Other abnormal cytological findings on specimens from vagina ♀

R87.629 Unspecified abnormal cytological findings in specimens from vagina ♀
     Abnormal Papanicolaou smear of vagina NOS
     Abnormal thin preparation smear of vagina NOS
     Abnormal vaginal cytology NOS
     Atypical endocervical cells of vagina NOS
     Atypical endometrial cells of vagina NOS
     Atypical glandular cells of vagina NOS

R87.69 Abnormal cytological findings in specimens from other female genital organs ♀
     Abnormal cytological findings in specimens from female genital organs NOS
     EXCLUDES 1   dysplasia of vulva (histologically confirmed) (N90.0-N90.3)

R87.7 Abnormal histological findings in specimens from female genital organs ♀
     EXCLUDES 1   carcinoma in situ (histologically confirmed) of female genital organs (D06-D07.3)
               cervical intraepithelial neoplasia I [CIN I] (N87.0)
               cervical intraepithelial neoplasia II [CIN II] (N87.1)
               cervical intraepithelial neoplasia III [CIN III] (D06.-)
               dysplasia (mild) (moderate) of cervix uteri (histologically confirmed) (N87.-)
               dysplasia (mild) (moderate) of vagina (histologically confirmed) (N89.-)
               severe dysplasia of cervix uteri (histologically confirmed) (D06.-)
               severe dysplasia of vagina (histologically confirmed) (D07.2)
               vaginal intraepithelial neoplasia I [VAIN I] (N89.0)
               vaginal intraepithelial neoplasia II [VAIN II] (N89.1)
               vaginal intraepithelial neoplasia III [VAIN III] (D07.2)

✓5ᵗʰ R87.8 Other abnormal findings in specimens from female genital organs

✓6ᵗʰ R87.81 High risk human papillomavirus [HPV] DNA test positive from female genital organs
     EXCLUDES 1   anogenital warts due to human papillomavirus (HPV) (A63.0)
               condyloma acuminatum (A63.0)

R87.810 Cervical high risk human papillomavirus [HPV] DNA test positive ♀

R87.811 Vaginal high risk human papillomavirus [HPV] DNA test positive ♀

✓6ᵗʰ R87.82 Low risk human papillomavirus [HPV] DNA test positive from female genital organs
     Use additional code for associated human papillomavirus (B97.7)

R87.820 Cervical low risk human papillomavirus [HPV] DNA test positive ♀

R87.821 Vaginal low risk human papillomavirus [HPV] DNA test positive ♀

R87.89 Other abnormal findings in specimens from female genital organs ♀
     Abnormal chromosomal findings in specimens from female genital organs

R87.9 Unspecified abnormal finding in specimens from female genital organs ♀

✓4ᵗʰ R88 Abnormal findings in other body fluids and substances

R88.0 Cloudy (hemodialysis) (peritoneal) dialysis effluent

R88.8 Abnormal findings in other body fluids and substances

✓4ᵗʰ R89 Abnormal findings in specimens from other organs, systems and tissues
     INCLUDES   abnormal findings in nipple discharge
             abnormal findings in synovial fluid
             abnormal findings in wound secretions

R89.0 Abnormal level of enzymes in specimens from other organs, systems and tissues

---

☑ Additional Character Required   ✓x7ᵗʰ Placeholder Alert   Manifestation   Unspecified Dx   ►◄ Revised Text   ● New Code   ▲ Revised Title

R89.1 Abnormal level of hormones in specimens from other organs, systems and tissues

R89.2 Abnormal level of other drugs, medicaments and biological substances in specimens from other organs, systems and tissues

R89.3 Abnormal level of substances chiefly nonmedicinal as to source in specimens from other organs, systems and tissues

R89.4 Abnormal immunological findings in specimens from other organs, systems and tissues

R89.5 Abnormal microbiological findings in specimens from other organs, systems and tissues

> Positive culture findings in specimens from other organs, systems and tissues
>
> EXCLUDES 1   colonization status (Z22.-)

R89.6 Abnormal cytological findings in specimens from other organs, systems and tissues

R89.7 Abnormal histological findings in specimens from other organs, systems and tissues

R89.8 Other abnormal findings in specimens from other organs, systems and tissues

> Abnormal chromosomal findings in specimens from other organs, systems and tissues

R89.9 Unspecified abnormal finding in specimens from other organs, systems and tissues

Abnormal findings on diagnostic imaging and in function studies, without diagnosis (R90-R94)

INCLUDES   nonspecific abnormal findings on diagnostic imaging by computerized axial tomography [CAT scan]

nonspecific abnormal findings on diagnostic imaging by magnetic resonance imaging [MRI][NMR]

nonspecific abnormal findings on diagnostic imaging by positron emission tomography [PET scan]

nonspecific abnormal findings on diagnostic imaging by thermography

nonspecific abnormal findings on diagnostic imaging by ultrasound [echogram]

nonspecific abnormal findings on diagnostic imaging by X-ray examination

EXCLUDES 1   abnormal findings on antenatal screening of mother (O28.-)

diagnostic abnormal findings classified elsewhere — see Alphabetical Index

✓4ᵗʰ R90 Abnormal findings on diagnostic imaging of central nervous system

R90.0 Intracranial space-occupying lesion found on diagnostic imaging of central nervous system

✓5ᵗʰ R90.8 Other abnormal findings on diagnostic imaging of central nervous system

R90.81 Abnormal echoencephalogram

R90.82 White matter disease, unspecified

R90.89 Other abnormal findings on diagnostic imaging of central nervous system

> Other cerebrovascular abnormality found on diagnostic imaging of central nervous system

✓4ᵗʰ R91 Abnormal findings on diagnostic imaging of lung

R91.1 Solitary pulmonary nodule

> Coin lesion lung
>
> Solitary pulmonary nodule, subsegmental branch of the bronchial tree

R91.8 Other nonspecific abnormal finding of lung field

> Lung mass NOS found on diagnostic imaging of lung
>
> Pulmonary infiltrate NOS
>
> Shadow, lung

✓4ᵗʰ R92 Abnormal and inconclusive findings on diagnostic imaging of breast

R92.0 Mammographic microcalcification found on diagnostic imaging of breast

> EXCLUDES 2   mammographic calcification (calculus) found on diagnostic imaging of breast (R92.1)
>
> DEF: Calcium and cellular debris deposits in the breast that cannot be felt but can be detected on a mammogram. The deposits can be a sign of cancer, benign conditions, or changes in the breast tissue as a result of inflammation, injury, or an obstructed duct.

R92.1 Mammographic calcification found on diagnostic imaging of breast

> Mammographic calculus found on diagnostic imaging of breast

R92.2 Inconclusive mammogram

> Dense breasts NOS
>
> Inconclusive mammogram NEC
>
> Inconclusive mammography due to dense breasts
>
> Inconclusive mammography NEC
>
> AHA: 2015,1Q,24

R92.8 Other abnormal and inconclusive findings on diagnostic imaging of breast

✓4ᵗʰ R93 Abnormal findings on diagnostic imaging of other body structures

R93.0 Abnormal findings on diagnostic imaging of skull and head, not elsewhere classified

> EXCLUDES 1   intracranial space-occupying lesion found on diagnostic imaging (R90.0)

R93.1 Abnormal findings on diagnostic imaging of heart and coronary circulation

> Abnormal echocardiogram NOS
>
> Abnormal heart shadow

R93.2 Abnormal findings on diagnostic imaging of liver and biliary tract

> Nonvisualization of gallbladder

R93.3 Abnormal findings on diagnostic imaging of other parts of digestive tract

✓5ᵗʰ R93.4 Abnormal findings on diagnostic imaging of urinary organs

> EXCLUDES 2   hypertrophy of kidney (N28.81)
>
> AHA: 2016,4Q,66

R93.41 Abnormal radiologic findings on diagnostic imaging of renal pelvis, ureter, or bladder

> Filling defect of bladder found on diagnostic imaging
>
> Filling defect of renal pelvis found on diagnostic imaging
>
> Filling defect of ureter found on diagnostic imaging

✓6ᵗʰ R93.42 Abnormal radiologic findings on diagnostic imaging of kidney

R93.421 Abnormal radiologic findings on diagnostic imaging of right kidney

R93.422 Abnormal radiologic findings on diagnostic imaging of left kidney

R93.429 Abnormal radiologic findings on diagnostic imaging of unspecified kidney

R93.49 Abnormal radiologic findings on diagnostic imaging of other urinary organs

R93.5 Abnormal findings on diagnostic imaging of other abdominal regions, including retroperitoneum

R93.6 Abnormal findings on diagnostic imaging of limbs

> EXCLUDES 2   abnormal finding in skin and subcutaneous tissue (R93.8-)

R93.7 Abnormal findings on diagnostic imaging of other parts of musculoskeletal system

> EXCLUDES 2   abnormal findings on diagnostic imaging of skull (R93.0)

✓5ᵗʰ R93.8 Abnormal findings on diagnostic imaging of other specified body structures

> AHA: 2018,4Q,30

✓6ᵗʰ R93.81 Abnormal radiologic findings on diagnostic imaging of testis

R93.811 Abnormal radiologic findings on diagnostic imaging of right testicle ♂

R93.812 Abnormal radiologic findings on diagnostic imaging of left testicle ♂

R93.813 Abnormal radiologic findings on diagnostic imaging of testicles, bilateral ♂

R93.819 Abnormal radiologic findings on diagnostic imaging of unspecified testicle ♂

R93.89 Abnormal findings on diagnostic imaging of other specified body structures

> Abnormal finding by radioisotope localization of placenta
>
> Abnormal radiological finding in skin and subcutaneous tissue
>
> Mediastinal shift

R93.9 Diagnostic imaging inconclusive due to excess body fat of patient

N Newborn: 0   P Pediatric: 0-17   M Maternity: 12-55   A Adult: 15-124   CH Comorbidity High   CL Comorbidity Low   NCDx Noncancer Dx   PDx Primary Dx

938   ICD-10-CM 2020

☑4ᵗʰ **R94　Abnormal results of function studies**

[INCLUDES]　abnormal results of radionuclide [radioisotope] uptake studies

abnormal results of scintigraphy

☑5ᵗʰ **R94.0　Abnormal results of function studies of** central nervous system

　R94.01　Abnormal electroencephalogram [EEG]

　R94.02　Abnormal brain scan

　R94.09　Abnormal results of other function studies of central nervous system

☑5ᵗʰ **R94.1　Abnormal results of function studies of** peripheral nervous system and special senses

　☑6ᵗʰ **R94.11　Abnormal results of function studies of** eye

　　R94.110　Abnormal electro-oculogram [EOG]

　　R94.111　Abnormal electroretinogram [ERG]
　　　　Abnormal retinal function study

　　R94.112　Abnormal visually evoked potential [VEP]

　　R94.113　Abnormal oculomotor **study**

　　R94.118　Abnormal results of other function studies of eye

　☑6ᵗʰ **R94.12　Abnormal results of function studies of** ear and other special senses
　　AHA: 2016,3Q,17

　　R94.120　Abnormal auditory **function study**

　　R94.121　Abnormal vestibular **function study**

　　R94.128　Abnormal results of other function studies of ear and other special senses

　☑6ᵗʰ **R94.13　Abnormal results of function studies of** peripheral nervous system

　　R94.130　Abnormal response to nerve stimulation, unspecified

　　R94.131　Abnormal electromyogram [EMG]
　　　　EXCLUDES 1　electromyogram of eye (R94.113)

　　R94.138　Abnormal results of other function studies of peripheral nervous system

R94.2　Abnormal results of pulmonary function **studies**
　　Reduced ventilatory capacity
　　Reduced vital capacity

☑5ᵗʰ **R94.3　Abnormal results of** cardiovascular function **studies**

　R94.30　Abnormal result of cardiovascular function study, unspecified

　R94.31　Abnormal electrocardiogram [ECG] [EKG]
　　　EXCLUDES 1　long QT syndrome (I45.81)

　R94.39　Abnormal result of other cardiovascular function study
　　　Abnormal electrophysiological intracardiac studies
　　　Abnormal phonocardiogram
　　　Abnormal vectorcardiogram

R94.4　Abnormal results of kidney function **studies**
　　Abnormal renal function test

R94.5　Abnormal results of liver function **studies**

R94.6　Abnormal results of thyroid function **studies**

R94.7　Abnormal results of other endocrine function studies
　　EXCLUDES 2　abnormal glucose (R73.0-)

R94.8　Abnormal results of function studies of other organs and systems
　　Abnormal basal metabolic rate [BMR]
　　Abnormal bladder function test
　　Abnormal splenic function test

Abnormal tumor markers (R97)

☑4ᵗʰ **R97　Abnormal tumor markers**

Elevated tumor associated antigens [TAA]

Elevated tumor specific antigens [TSA]

R97.0　Elevated carcinoembryonic antigen [CEA]

R97.1　Elevated cancer antigen 125 [CA 125]

☑5ᵗʰ **R97.2　Elevated prostate specific antigen [PSA]**

　AHA: 2016,4Q,66

　R97.20　Elevated prostate specific antigen [PSA]　Ⓐ ♂

　R97.21　Rising PSA following treatment for malignant neoplasm of prostate　Ⓐ ♂

R97.8　Other abnormal tumor markers

III-defined and unknown cause of mortality (R99)

R99　III-defined and unknown cause of mortality
　Death (unexplained) NOS
　Unspecified cause of mortality

Chapter 18. Symptoms, Signs and Abnormal Clinical and Laboratory Findings

R94–R99

☑ Additional Character Required　　☑x7ᵗʰ Placeholder Alert　　Manifestation　　Unspecified Dx　　►◄ Revised Text　　● New Code　　▲ Revised Title

ICD-10-CM 2020

939

Chapter 19. Injury, Poisoning and Certain Other Consequences of External Causes (S00–T88)

Chapter-specific Guidelines with Coding Examples

The chapter-specific guidelines from the ICD-10-CM Official Guidelines for Coding and Reporting have been provided below. Along with these guidelines are coding examples, contained in the shaded boxes, that have been developed to help illustrate the coding and/or sequencing guidance found in these guidelines.

a. Application of 7th characters in Chapter 19

Most categories in chapter 19 have a 7th character requirement for each applicable code. Most categories in this chapter have three 7th character values (with the exception of fractures): A, initial encounter, D, subsequent encounter and S, sequela. Categories for traumatic fractures have additional 7th character values. While the patient may be seen by a new or different provider over the course of treatment for an injury, assignment of the 7th character is based on whether the patient is undergoing active treatment and not whether the provider is seeing the patient for the first time.

For complication codes, active treatment refers to treatment for the condition described by the code, even though it may be related to an earlier precipitating problem. For example, code T84.50XA, Infection and inflammatory reaction due to unspecified internal joint prosthesis, initial encounter, is used when active treatment is provided for the infection, even though the condition relates to the prosthetic device, implant or graft that was placed at a previous encounter.

7th character "A", initial encounter is used for each encounter where the patient is receiving active treatment for the condition.

7th character "D" subsequent encounter is used for encounters after the patient has completed active treatment of the condition and is receiving routine care for the condition during the healing or recovery phase.

> Patient was admitted to home health for continued therapy following acute care stay to treat a nondisplaced fracture to the distal pole of the right scaphoid bone due to a fall from skateboard onto the sidewalk.
>
> **S62.014D**   **Nondisplaced fracture of distal pole of navicular [scaphoid] bone of right wrist, subsequent encounter for fracture with routine healing**
>
> **V00.131D**   **Fall from skateboard, subsequent encounter**
>
> *Explanation:* The fracture is coded with the seventh character D, as routine care is being provided in the recovery phase within this home health setting. The external cause code, V00.131D, describes the cause of the injury and may be applied for each encounter involving treatment for the fracture. Activity codes, place-of-occurrence codes, and external cause status codes are used only once, at the initial encounter for treatment, and are not required for this environment.

The aftercare Z codes should not be used for aftercare for conditions such as injuries or poisonings, where 7th characters are provided to identify subsequent care. For example, for aftercare of an injury, assign the acute injury code with the 7th character "D" (subsequent encounter).

7th character "S", sequela, is for use for complications or conditions that arise as a direct result of a condition, such as scar formation after a burn. The scars are sequelae of the burn. When using 7th character "S", it is necessary to use both the injury code that precipitated the sequela and the code for the sequela itself. The "S" is added only to the injury code, not the sequela code. The 7th character "S" identifies the injury responsible for the sequela. The specific type of sequela (e.g. scar) is sequenced first, followed by the injury code.

See Section I.B.10 Sequelae, (Late Effects)

> Patient with a history of a nondisplaced fracture to the distal pole of the right scaphoid bone due to a fall from a skateboard is admitted for evaluation of arthritis to the right wrist that has developed as a consequence of the traumatic fracture.
>
> **M12.531**   **Traumatic arthropathy, right wrist**
>
> **S62.014S**   **Nondisplaced fracture of distal pole of navicular [scaphoid] bone of right wrist, sequela**
>
> **V00.131S**   **Fall from skateboard, sequela**
>
> *Explanation:* The code identifying the specific sequela condition (traumatic arthritis) should be coded first followed by the injury that instigated the development of the sequela (fracture). The scaphoid fracture injury code is given a 7th character S for sequela to represent its role as the inciting injury. The fracture has healed and is not being managed or treated on this admit and therefore is not applicable as a first listed or principal diagnosis. However, it is directly related to the development of the arthritis and should be appended as a secondary code to signify this cause and effect relationship.

b. Coding of injuries

When coding injuries, assign separate codes for each injury unless a combination code is provided, in which case the combination code is assigned. Codes from category T07, Unspecified multiple injuries should not be assigned in the inpatient setting unless information for a more specific code is not available. Traumatic injury codes (S00-T14.9) are not to be used for normal, healing surgical wounds or to identify complications of surgical wounds.

> A 76-year-old man fell from a ladder, resulting in a right humerus fracture, laceration of the right forearm, and laceration of the left shin. Lacerations required sutures, and the humerus fracture was casted. All injuries are healing well.
>
> **S42.301D**   **Unspecified fracture of shaft of humerus, right arm, subsequent encounter for fracture with routine healing**
>
> **S51.811D**   **Laceration without foreign body of right forearm, subsequent encounter**
>
> **S81.812D**   **Laceration without foreign body, left lower leg, subsequent encounter**
>
> **W11.XXXD**   **Fall on and from ladder, subsequent encounter**
>
> *Explanation:* Each injury is coded separately. The seventh character D should be assigned for the fracture, which is healing in the recovery phase. The lacerations are coded with the seventh character D as these wounds are not complicated and are healing well, requiring no wound care. An external cause code reports the cause of the injuries.

The code for the most serious injury, as determined by the provider and the focus of treatment, is sequenced first.

1) Superficial injuries

Superficial injuries such as abrasions or contusions are not coded when associated with more severe injuries of the same site.

2) Primary injury with damage to nerves/blood vessels

When a primary injury results in minor damage to peripheral nerves or blood vessels, the primary injury is sequenced first with additional code(s) for injuries to nerves and spinal cord (such as category S04), and/or injury to blood vessels (such as category S15). When the primary injury is to the blood vessels or nerves, that injury should be sequenced first.

3) Iatrogenic injuries

Injury codes from Chapter 19 should not be assigned for injuries that occur during, or as a result of, a medical intervention. Assign the appropriate complication code(s).

c. Coding of traumatic fractures

The principles of multiple coding of injuries should be followed in coding fractures. Fractures of specified sites are coded individually by site in accordance with both the provisions within categories S02, S12, S22, S32, S42, S49, S52, S59, S62, S72, S79, S82, S89, S92 and the level of detail furnished by medical record content.

A fracture not indicated as open or closed should be coded to closed. A fracture not indicated whether displaced or not displaced should be coded to displaced.

More specific guidelines are as follows:

1) Initial vs. subsequent encounter for fractures

Traumatic fractures are coded using the appropriate 7th character for initial encounter (A, B, C) for each encounter where the patient is receiving active treatment for the fracture. The appropriate 7th character for initial encounter should also be assigned for a patient who delayed seeking treatment for the fracture or nonunion.

Fractures are coded using the appropriate 7th character for subsequent care for encounters after the patient has completed active treatment of the fracture and is receiving routine care for the fracture during the healing or recovery phase.

Care for complications of surgical treatment for fracture repairs during the healing or recovery phase should be coded with the appropriate complication codes.

Care of complications of fractures, such as malunion and nonunion, should be reported with the appropriate 7th character for subsequent care with nonunion (K, M, N,) or subsequent care with malunion (P, Q, R).

Malunion/nonunion: The appropriate 7th character for initial encounter should also be assigned for a patient who delayed seeking treatment for the fracture or nonunion.

Female patient fell during a hiking excursion almost six months ago and until recently did not feel she needed to seek medical attention for her left ankle pain; x-rays show nonunion of lateral malleolus and surgery has been scheduled

S82.62XA	**Displaced fracture of lateral malleolus of left fibula, initial encounter for closed fracture**
WØ1.ØXXA	**Fall on same level from slipping, tripping and stumbling without subsequent striking against object, initial encounter**
Y92.821	**Forest as place of occurrence of the external cause**
Y93.Ø1	**Activity, walking, marching and hiking**
Y99.8	**Other external cause status**

Explanation: A seventh character of A is used for the lateral malleolus nonunion fracture to signify that the fracture is receiving active treatment. The delayed care for the fracture has resulted in a nonunion, but capturing the nonunion in the seventh character is trumped by the provision of active care.

The open fracture designations in the assignment of the 7th character for fractures of the forearm, femur and lower leg, including ankle are based on the Gustilo open fracture classification. When the Gustilo classification type is not specified for an open fracture, the 7th character for open fracture type I or II should be assigned (B, E, H, M, Q).

A code from category M8Ø, not a traumatic fracture code, should be used for any patient with known osteoporosis who suffers a fracture, even if the patient had a minor fall or trauma, if that fall or trauma would not usually break a normal, healthy bone.

See Section I.C.13. Osteoporosis.

The aftercare Z codes should not be used for aftercare for traumatic fractures. For aftercare of a traumatic fracture, assign the acute fracture code with the appropriate 7th character.

2) Multiple fractures sequencing

Multiple fractures are sequenced in accordance with the severity of the fracture.

3) Physeal fractures

For physeal fractures, assign only the code identifying the type of physeal fracture. Do not assign a separate code to identify the specific bone that is fractured.

d. Coding of burns and corrosions

The ICD-10-CM makes a distinction between burns and corrosions. The burn codes are for thermal burns, except sunburns, that come from a heat source, such as a fire or hot appliance. The burn codes are also for burns resulting from electricity and radiation. Corrosions are burns due to chemicals. The guidelines are the same for burns and corrosions.

Current burns (T2Ø-T25) are classified by depth, extent and by agent (X code). Burns are classified by depth as first degree (erythema), second degree (blistering), and third degree (full-thickness involvement). Burns of the eye and internal organs (T26-T28) are classified by site, but not by degree.

1) Sequencing of burn and related condition codes

Sequence first the code that reflects the highest degree of burn when more than one burn is present.

a. When the reason for the admission or encounter is for treatment of external multiple burns, sequence first the code that reflects the burn of the highest degree.

b. When a patient has both internal and external burns, the circumstances of admission govern the selection of the principal diagnosis or first-listed diagnosis.

c. When a patient is admitted for burn injuries and other related conditions such as smoke inhalation and/or respiratory failure, the circumstances of admission govern the selection of the principal or first-listed diagnosis

Patient is admitted following hospitalization for multiple third-degree burns to both hands and severe smoke inhalation when a candle lit her bedroom curtains on fire. The burns require frequent and complex wound care three times a day. The patient continues with shortness of breath and poor endurance due to smoke inhalation. She is recovering well from the smoke inhalation with normal SpO2 levels, nebulizer treatments, and use of oxygen.

T23.391A	**Burn of third degree of multiple sites of right wrist and hand, initial encounter**
T23.392A	**Burn of third degree of multiple sites of left wrist and hand, initial encounter**
X08.8XXA	**Exposure to other specified smoke, fire and flames, initial encounter**
T59.811D	**Toxic effect of smoke, accidental (unintentional), subsequent encounter**
J7Ø.5	**Respiratory conditions due to smoke inhalation**

Explanation: Based upon provider orders and documentation, the burns are complex and require the most intense care and therefore are coded first. The seventh character A is used for both burns as they remain open with complex active treatment. Because the respiratory condition resulting from smoke inhalation is resolving well and the patient is now in the recovery phase for this condition, the seventh character D is assigned for subsequent episode for the toxic-effect code. For the external cause code X08.8-, the seventh character A is assigned because the resulting burns remain an initial encounter.

2) Burns of the same anatomic site

Classify burns of the same anatomic site and on the same side but of different degrees to the subcategory identifying the highest degree recorded in the diagnosis (e.g., for second and third degree burns of right thigh, assign only code T24.311-).

3) Non-healing burns

Non-healing burns are coded as acute burns.

Necrosis of burned skin should be coded as a non-healed burn.

4) Infected burn

For any documented infected burn site, use an additional code for the infection.

Patient is admitted and has a third-degree burn to the left anterior thigh, which the provider reports is infected with pseudomonas. The patient is ordered 4 weeks of IV antibiotics.

T24.312A	**Burn of third degree of left thigh, initial encounter**
B96.5	**Pseudomonas (aeruginosa) (mallei) (pseudomallei) as the cause of diseases classified elsewhere**
Z45.2	**Encounter for adjustment and management of vascular access device**
Z79.2	**Long term (current) use of antibiotics**

Explanation: This burn is infected, and the organism is identified as pseudomonas. ICD-10-CM guidelines indicate to code first the burn and use an additional code to report the infection. Because active treatment, in the form of antibiotic administration, is being provided for the infected burn, the seventh character A is appropriate for this encounter.

5) Assign separate codes for each burn site

When coding burns, assign separate codes for each burn site. Category T3Ø, Burn and corrosion, body region unspecified is extremely vague and should rarely be used.

Codes for burns of "multiple sites" should only be assigned when the medical record documentation does not specify the individual sites.

Patient is admitted with third-degree burns of the scalp as well as second-degree burns to the back of the right hand. The burns continue to drain heavily with frequent need for debridement.

T2Ø.35XA	**Burn of third degree of scalp [any part], initial encounter**
T23.261A	**Burn of second degree of back of right hand, initial encounter**

Explanation: Since burns to the hand and scalp are classified to two different three-digit categories, both burns may be reported as they represent distinct sites. The seventh character A is used as the burns continue to require active treatment with heavy drainage present and a need for frequent debridement.

6) Burns and corrosions classified according to extent of body surface involved

Assign codes from category T31, Burns classified according to extent of body surface involved, or T32, Corrosions classified according to extent of body surface involved, when the site of the burn is not specified or when there is a need for additional data. It is advisable to use category T31 as additional coding when needed to provide data for evaluating burn mortality, such as that needed by burn units. It is also advisable to use category T31 as an additional code for reporting purposes when there is mention of a third-degree burn involving 20 percent or more of the body surface.

Categories T31 and T32 are based on the classic "rule of nines" in estimating body surface involved: head and neck are assigned nine percent, each arm nine percent, each leg 18 percent, the anterior trunk 18 percent, posterior trunk 18 percent, and genitalia one percent. Providers may change these percentage assignments where necessary to accommodate infants and children who have proportionately larger heads than adults, and patients who have large buttocks, thighs, or abdomen that involve burns.

> Patient seen for dressing change after he accidentally spilled acetic acid on himself two days ago. The second-degree burns to his right thigh, covering about 3 percent of his body surface, are healing appropriately.
>
> **T54.2X1D**   **Toxic effect of corrosive acids and acid-like substances, accidental (unintentional), subsequent encounter**
>
> **T24.611D**   **Corrosion of second degree of right thigh, subsequent encounter**
>
> **T32.0**   **Corrosions involving less than 10% of body surface**
>
> *Explanation:* Code T32.0 provides additional information as to how much of the patient's body was affected by the corrosive substance.

7) Encounters for treatment of sequela of burns

Encounters for the treatment of the late effects of burns or corrosions (i.e., scars or joint contractures) should be coded with a burn or corrosion code with the 7th character "S" for sequela.

8) Sequelae with a late effect code and current burn

When appropriate, both a code for a current burn or corrosion with 7th character "A" or "D" and a burn or corrosion code with 7th character "S" may be assigned on the same record (when both a current burn and sequelae of an old burn exist). Burns and corrosions do not heal at the same rate and a current healing wound may still exist with sequela of a healed burn or corrosion.

See Section I.B.10 Sequela (Late Effects)

> Female patient seen for second-degree burn to the left ear; that is healing well with no current treatment orders. She also has significant scarring on her left elbow from a third-degree burn from childhood.
>
> **T20.212D**   **Burn of second degree of left ear [any part, except ear drum], subsequent encounter**
>
> **L90.5**   **Scar conditions and fibrosis of skin**
>
> **T22.322S**   **Burn of third degree of left elbow, sequela**
>
> *Explanation:* The patient is being seen for management of a current second-degree burn, which is reflected in the code by appending the seventh character D, indicating that active treatment is no longer needed and the burn is in the recovery phase of healing. The elbow scarring is a sequela of a previous third-degree burn. The sequela condition precedes the original burn injury, which is appended with a seventh character of S.

9) Use of an external cause code with burns and corrosions

An external cause code should be used with burns and corrosions to identify the source and intent of the burn, as well as the place where it occurred.

e. Adverse effects, poisoning, underdosing and toxic effects

Codes in categories T36-T65 are combination codes that include the substance that was taken as well as the intent. No additional external cause code is required for poisonings, toxic effects, adverse effects and underdosing codes.

1) Do not code directly from the Table of Drugs

Do not code directly from the Table of Drugs and Chemicals. Always refer back to the Tabular List.

2) Use as many codes as necessary to describe

Use as many codes as necessary to describe completely all drugs, medicinal or biological substances.

3) If the same code would describe the causative agent

If the same code would describe the causative agent for more than one adverse reaction, poisoning, toxic effect or underdosing, assign the code only once.

4) If two or more drugs, medicinal or biological substances

If two or more drugs, medicinal or biological substances are **taken**, code each individually unless a combination code is listed in the Table of Drugs and Chemicals.

If multiple unspecified drugs, medicinal or biological substances were taken, assign the appropriate code from subcategory T50.91, Poisoning by, adverse effect of and underdosing of multiple unspecified drugs, medicaments and biological substances.

5) The occurrence of drug toxicity is classified in ICD-10-CM as follows:

(a) Adverse effect

When coding an adverse effect of a drug that has been correctly prescribed and properly administered, assign the appropriate code for the nature of the adverse effect followed by the appropriate code for the adverse effect of the drug (T36-T50). The code for the drug should have a 5th or 6th character "5" (for example T36.0X5-) Examples of the nature of an adverse effect are tachycardia, delirium, gastrointestinal hemorrhaging, vomiting, hypokalemia, hepatitis, renal failure, or respiratory failure.

(b) Poisoning

When coding a poisoning or reaction to the improper use of a medication (e.g., overdose, wrong substance given or taken in error, wrong route of administration), first assign the appropriate code from categories T36-T50. The poisoning codes have an associated intent as their 5th or 6th character (accidental, intentional self-harm, assault and undetermined. If the intent of the poisoning is unknown or unspecified, code the intent as accidental intent. The undetermined intent is only for use if the documentation in the record specifies that the intent cannot be determined. Use additional code(s) for all manifestations of poisonings.

If there is also a diagnosis of abuse or dependence of the substance, the abuse or dependence is assigned as an additional code.

Examples of poisoning include:

(i) Error was made in drug prescription

Errors made in drug prescription or in the administration of the drug by provider, nurse, patient, or other person.

(ii) Overdose of a drug intentionally taken

If an overdose of a drug was intentionally taken or administered and resulted in drug toxicity, it would be coded as a poisoning.

(iii) Nonprescribed drug taken with correctly prescribed and properly administered drug

If a nonprescribed drug or medicinal agent was taken in combination with a correctly prescribed and properly administered drug, any drug toxicity or other reaction resulting from the interaction of the two drugs would be classified as a poisoning.

(iv) Interaction of drug(s) and alcohol

When a reaction results from the interaction of a drug(s) and alcohol, this would be classified as poisoning.

See Section I.C.4. if poisoning is the result of insulin pump malfunctions.

(c) Underdosing

Underdosing refers to taking less of a medication than is prescribed by a provider or a manufacturer's instruction. Discontinuing the use of a prescribed medication on the patient's own initiative (not directed by the patient's provider) is also classified as an underdosing. For underdosing, assign the code from categories T36-T50 (fifth or sixth character "6").

Codes for underdosing should never be assigned as principal or first-listed codes. If a patient has a relapse or exacerbation of the medical condition for which the drug is prescribed because of the reduction in dose, then the medical condition itself should be coded.

Noncompliance (Z91.12-, Z91.13- and Z91.14-) or complication of care (Y63.6-Y63.9) codes are to be used with an underdosing code to indicate intent, if known.

> Patient admitted for atrial fibrillation with history of chronic atrial fibrillation for which she is prescribed amiodarone. Financial concerns have left the patient unable to pay for her prescriptions and she has been skipping her amiodarone dose every other day to offset the cost.
>
> **I48.20**   **Chronic atrial fibrillation, unspecified**
>
> **T46.2X6A**   **Underdosing of other antidysrhythmic drugs, initial encounter**
>
> **Z91.120**   **Patient's intentional underdosing of medication regimen due to financial hardship**

Explanation: By skipping her amiodarone pill every other day, the patient's atrial fibrillation returned. The condition for which the drug was being taken is reported first, followed by an underdosing code to show that the patient was not adhering to her prescription regiment. The Z code helps elaborate on the patient's social and/or economic circumstances that led to the patient taking less then what she was prescribed.

(d) Toxic effects

When a harmful substance is ingested or comes in contact with a person, this is classified as a toxic effect. The toxic effect codes are in categories T51-T65.

Toxic effect codes have an associated intent: accidental, intentional self-harm, assault and undetermined.

f. Adult and child abuse, neglect and other maltreatment

Sequence first the appropriate code from categories T74.- (Adult and child abuse, neglect and other maltreatment, confirmed) or T76.- (Adult and child abuse, neglect and other maltreatment, suspected) for abuse, neglect and other maltreatment, followed by any accompanying mental health or injury code(s).

If the documentation in the medical record states abuse or neglect it is coded as confirmed (T74.-). It is coded as suspected if it is documented as suspected (T76.-).

For cases of confirmed abuse or neglect an external cause code from the assault section (X92-Y09) should be added to identify the cause of any physical injuries. A perpetrator code (Y07) should be added when the perpetrator of the abuse is known. For suspected cases of abuse or neglect, do not report external cause or perpetrator code.

If a suspected case of abuse, neglect or mistreatment is ruled out during an encounter code Z04.71, Encounter for examination and observation following alleged physical adult abuse, ruled out, or code Z04.72, Encounter for examination and observation following alleged child physical abuse, ruled out, should be used, not a code from T76.

If a suspected case of alleged rape or sexual abuse is ruled out during an encounter code Z04.41, Encounter for examination and observation following alleged adult rape or code Z04.42, Encounter for examination and observation following alleged child rape, should be used, not a code from T76.

If a suspected case of forced sexual exploitation or forced labor exploitation is ruled out during an encounter, code Z04.81, Encounter for examination and observation of victim following forced sexual exploitation, or code Z04.82, Encounter for examination and observation of victim following forced labor exploitation, should be used, not a code from T76.

See Section I.C.15. Abuse in a pregnant patient.

g. Complications of care

1) General guidelines for complications of care

(a) Documentation of complications of care

See Section I.B.16. for information on documentation of complications of care.

2) Pain due to medical devices

Pain associated with devices, implants or grafts left in a surgical site (for example painful hip prosthesis) is assigned to the appropriate code(s) found in Chapter 19, Injury, poisoning, and certain other consequences of external causes. Specific codes for pain due to medical devices are found in the T code section of the ICD-10-CM. Use additional code(s) from category G89 to identify acute or chronic pain due to presence of the device, implant or graft (G89.18 or G89.28).

A patient with multiple sclerosis has an implanted pain pump in the upper right buttock. The provider notes indicate chronic pain of the lower back due to placement of pain pump.

T85.848D	Pain due to other internal prosthetic devices, implants and grafts, subsequent encounter
M54.5	Low back pain
G89.28	Other chronic postprocedural pain
G35	Multiple sclerosis

Explanation: As the pain is a complication of the implanted pain pump, the complication code is sequenced first. The seventh character D is used, as caregivers in the post-acute care setting will be monitoring this chronic pain condition but not providing active treatment. The T code does not fully describe the site or type of pain, and additional codes should be assigned for these.

3) Transplant complications

(a) Transplant complications other than kidney

Codes under category T86, Complications of transplanted organs and tissues, are for use for both complications and rejection of transplanted organs. A transplant complication code is only assigned if the complication affects the function of the transplanted organ. Two codes are required to fully describe a transplant complication: the appropriate code from category T86 and a secondary code that identifies the complication.

Pre-existing conditions or conditions that develop after the transplant are not coded as complications unless they affect the function of the transplanted organs.

See I.C.21. for transplant organ removal status

See I.C.2. for malignant neoplasm associated with transplanted organ.

(b) Kidney transplant complications

Patients who have undergone kidney transplant may still have some form of chronic kidney disease (CKD) because the kidney transplant may not fully restore kidney function. Code T86.1- should be assigned for documented complications of a kidney transplant, such as transplant failure or rejection or other transplant complication. Code T86.1- should not be assigned for post kidney transplant patients who have chronic kidney (CKD) unless a transplant complication such as transplant failure or rejection is documented. If the documentation is unclear as to whether the patient has a complication of the transplant, query the provider.

Conditions that affect the function of the transplanted kidney, other than CKD, should be assigned a code from subcategory T86.1, Complications of transplanted organ, Kidney, and a secondary code that identifies the complication.

For patients with CKD following a kidney transplant, but who do not have a complication such as failure or rejection, *see section I.C.14. Chronic kidney disease and kidney transplant status.*

Patient seen for chronic kidney disease stage 2; history of successful kidney transplant with no complications identified

N18.2	**Chronic kidney disease, stage 2 (mild)**
Z94.0	**Kidney transplant status**

Explanation: This patient's stage 2 CKD is not indicated as being due to the transplanted kidney but instead is just the residual disease the patient had prior to the transplant.

4) Complication codes that include the external cause

As with certain other T codes, some of the complications of care codes have the external cause included in the code. The code includes the nature of the complication as well as the type of procedure that caused the complication. No external cause code indicating the type of procedure is necessary for these codes.

5) Complications of care codes within the body system chapters

Intraoperative and postprocedural complication codes are found within the body system chapters with codes specific to the organs and structures of that body system. These codes should be sequenced first, followed by a code(s) for the specific complication, if applicable.

Complication codes from the body system chapters should be assigned for intraoperative and postprocedural complications (e.g., the appropriate complication code from chapter 9 would be assigned for a vascular intraoperative or postprocedural complication) unless the complication is specifically indexed to a T code in chapter 19.

Muscle/Tendon Table

ICD-10-CM categorizes certain muscles and tendons in the upper and lower extremities by their action (e.g., extension, flexion), their anatomical location (e.g., posterior, anterior), and/or whether they are intrinsic or extrinsic to a certain anatomical area. The Muscle/Tendon Table is provided at the beginning of chapters 13 and 19 as a resource to help users when code selection depends on one or more of these characteristics. Please note that this table is not all-inclusive, and proper code assignment should be based on the provider's documentation.

Body Region	Muscle	Extensor Tendon	Flexor Tendon	Other Tendon
Shoulder				
	Deltoid	Posterior deltoid	Anterior deltoid	
	Rotator cuff			
	Infraspinatus			Infraspinatus
	Subscapularis			Subscapularis
	Supraspinatus			Supraspinatus
	Teres minor			Teres minor
	Teres major	Teres major		
Upper arm				
	Anterior muscles			
	Biceps brachii — long head		Biceps brachii — long head	
	Biceps brachii — short head		Biceps brachii — short head	
	Brachialis		Brachialis	
	Coracobrachialis		Coracobrachialis	
	Posterior muscles			
	Triceps brachii	Triceps brachii		
Forearm				
	Anterior muscles			
	Flexors			
	Deep			
	Flexor digitorum profundus		Flexor digitorum profundus	
	Flexor pollicis longus		Flexor pollicis longus	
	Intermediate			
	Flexor digitorum superficialis		Flexor digitorum superficialis	
	Superficial			
	Flexor carpi radialis		Flexor carpi radialis	
	Flexor carpi ulnaris		Flexor carpi ulnaris	
	Palmaris longus		Palmaris longus	
	Pronators			
	Pronator quadratus			Pronator quadratus
	Pronator teres			Pronator teres
	Posterior muscles			
	Extensors			
	Deep			
	Abductor pollicis longus			Abductor pollicis longus
	Extensor indicis	Extensor indicis		
	Extensor pollicis brevis	Extensor pollicis brevis		
	Extensor pollicis longus	Extensor pollicis longus		
	Superficial			
	Brachioradialis			Brachioradialis
	Extensor carpi radialis brevis	Extensor carpi radialis brevis		
	Extensor carpi radialis longus	Extensor carpi radialis longus		
	Extensor carpi ulnaris	Extensor carpi ulnaris		
	Extensor digiti minimi	Extensor digiti minimi		
	Extensor digitorum	Extensor digitorum		
	Anconeus	Anconeus		
	Supinator			Supinator

Body Region	Muscle	Extensor Tendon	Flexor Tendon	Other Tendon
Hand				
Extrinsic — attach to a site in the forearm as well as a site in the hand with action related to hand movement at the wrist				
	Extensor carpi radialis brevis	Extensor carpi radialis brevis		
	Extensor carpi radialis longus	Extensor carpie radialis longus		
	Extensor carpi ulnaris	Extensor carpi ulnaris		
	Flexor carpi radialis		Flexor carpi radialis	
	Flexor carpi ulnaris		Flexor carpi ulnaris	
	Flexor digitorum superficialis		Flexor digitorum superficialis	
	Palmaris longus		Palmaris longus	
Extrinsic — attach to a site in the forearm as well as a site in the hand with action in the hand related to finger movement				
	Adductor pollicis longus			Adductor pollicis longus
	Extensor digiti minimi	Extensor digiti minimi		
	Extensor digitorum	Extensor digitorum		
	Extensor indicis	Extensor indicis		
	Flexor digitorum profundus		Flexor digitorum profundus	
	Flexor digitorum superficialis		Flexor digitorum superficialis	
Extrinsic — attach to a site in the forearm as well as a site in the hand with action in the hand related to thumb movement				
	Extensor pollicis brevis	Extensor pollicis brevis		
	Extensor pollicis longus	Extensor pollicis longus		
	Flexor pollicis longus		Flexor pollicis longus	
Intrinsic — found within the hand only				
	Adductor pollicis			Adductor pollicis
	Dorsal interossei	Dorsal interossei	Dorsal interossei	
	Lumbricals	Lumbricals	Lumbricals	
	Palmaris brevis			Palmaris brevis
	Palmar interossei	Palmar interossei	Palmar interossei	
	Hypothenar muscles			
	Abductor digiti minimi			Abductor digiti minimi
	Flexor digiti minimi brevis		Flexor digiti minimi brevis	
	Oppenens digiti minimi		Oppenens digiti minimi	
	Thenar muscles			
	Abductor pollicis brevis			Abductor pollicis brevis
	Flexor pollicis brevis		Flexor pollicis brevis	
	Oppenens pollicis		Oppenens pollicis	
Thigh				
	Anterior muscles			
	Iliopsoas		Iliopsoas	
	Pectineus		Pectineus	
	Quadriceps	Quadriceps		
	Rectus femoris	Rectus femoris — Extends knee	Rectus femoris — Flexes hip	
	Vastus intermedius	Vastus intermedius		
	Vastus lateralis	Vastus lateralis		
	Vastus medialis	Vastus medialis		
	Sartorius		Sartorius	
	Medial muscles			
	Adductor brevis			Adductor brevis
	Adductor longus			Adductor longus
	Adductor magnus			Adductor magnus
	Gracilis			Gracilis
	Obturator externus			Obturator externus
	Posterior muscles			
	Hamstring	Hamstring — Extends hip	Hamstring — Flexes knee	
	Biceps femoris	Biceps femoris	Biceps femoris	
	Semimembranosus	Semimembranosus	Semimembranosus	
	Semitendinosus	Semitendinosus	Semitendinosus	

Body Region	Muscle	Extensor Tendon	Flexor Tendon	Other Tendon
Lower leg				
	Anterior muscles			
	Extensor digitorum longus	Extensor digitorum longus		
	Extensor hallucis longus	Extensor hallucis longus		
	Fibularis (peroneus) tertius	Fibularis (peroneus) tertius		
	Tibialis anterior	Tibialis anterior		Tibialis anterior
	Lateral muscles			
	Fibularis (peroneus) brevis		Fibularis (peroneus) brevis	
	Fibularis (peroneus) longus		Fibularis (peroneus) longus	
	Posterior muscles			
	Deep			
	Flexor digitorum longus		Flexor digitorum longus	
	Flexor hallucis longus		Flexor hallucis longus	
	Popliteus		Popliteus	
	Tibialis posterior		Tibialis posterior	
	Superficial			
	Gastrocnemius		Gastrocnemius	
	Plantaris		Plantaris	
	Soleus		Soleus	
				Calcaneal (Achilles)
Ankle/Foot				
Extrinsic — attach to a site in the lower leg as well as a site in the foot with action related to foot movement at the ankle				
	Plantaris		Plantaris	
	Soleus		Soleus	
	Tibialis anterior	Tibialis anterior		
	Tibialis posterior		Tibialis posterior	
Extrinsic — attach to a site in the lower leg as well as a site in the foot with action in the foot related to toe movement				
	Extensor digitorum longus	Extensor digitorum longus		
	Extensor hallicus longus	Extensor hallicus longus		
	Flexor digitorum longus		Flexor digitorum longus	
	Flexor hallucis longus		Flexor hallucis longus	
Intrinsic — found within the ankle/foot only				
	Dorsal muscles			
	Extensor digitorum brevis	Extensor digitorum brevis		
	Extensor hallucis brevis	Extensor hallucis brevis		
	Plantar muscles			
	Abductor digiti minimi		Abductor digiti minimi	
	Abductor hallucis		Abductor hallucis	
	Dorsal interossei	Dorsal interossei	Dorsal interossei	
	Flexor digiti minimi brevis		Flexor digiti minimi brevis	
	Flexor digitorum brevis		Flexor digitorum brevis	
	Flexor hallucis brevis		Flexor hallucis brevis	
	Lumbricals	Lumbricals	Lumbricals	
	Quadratus plantae		Quadratus plantae	
	Plantar interossei	Plantar interossei	Plantar interossei	

Chapter 19. Injury, Poisoning and Certain Other Consequences of External Causes (S00-T88)

NOTE Use secondary code(s) from Chapter 20, External causes of morbidity, to indicate cause of injury. Codes within the T section that include the external cause do not require an additional external cause code.

Use additional code to identify any retained foreign body, if applicable (Z18.-)

EXCLUDES 1   birth trauma (P1Ø-P15)
            obstetric trauma (O7Ø-O71)

NOTE The chapter uses the S-section for coding different types of injuries related to single body regions and the T-section to cover injuries to unspecified body regions as well as poisoning and certain other consequences of external causes.

AHA: 2016,2Q,3-7; 2015,4Q,35-38; 2015,3Q,37-39,40; 2015,2Q,6; 2015,1Q,3-21
TIP: The specific site of an injury can be determined from the radiology report when authenticated by a radiologist and available at the time of code assignment.

This chapter contains the following blocks:

S00-S09	Injuries to the head
S10-S19	Injuries to the neck
S20-S29	Injuries to the thorax
S30-S39	Injuries to the abdomen, lower back, lumbar spine, pelvis and external genitals
S40-S49	Injuries to the shoulder and upper arm
S50-S59	Injuries to the elbow and forearm
S60-S69	Injuries to the wrist, hand and fingers
S70-S79	Injuries to the hip and thigh
S80-S89	Injuries to the knee and lower leg
S90-S99	Injuries to the ankle and foot
T07	Injuries involving multiple body regions
T14	Injury of unspecified body region
T15-T19	Effects of foreign body entering through natural orifice
T20-T25	Burns and corrosions of external body surface, specified by site
T26-T28	Burns and corrosions confined to eye and internal organs
T3Ø-T32	Burns and corrosions of multiple and unspecified body regions
T33-T34	Frostbite
T36-T5Ø	Poisoning by, adverse effect of and underdosing of drugs, medicaments and biological substances
T51-T65	Toxic effects of substances chiefly nonmedicinal as to source
T66-T78	Other and unspecified effects of external causes
T79	Certain early complications of trauma
T8Ø-T88	Complications of surgical and medical care, not elsewhere classified

Injuries to the head (S00-S09)

INCLUDES injuries of ear
            injuries of eye
            injuries of face [any part]
            injuries of gum
            injuries of jaw
            injuries of oral cavity
            injuries of palate
            injuries of periocular area
            injuries of scalp
            injuries of temporomandibular joint area
            injuries of tongue
            injuries of tooth

Code also for any associated infection

EXCLUDES 2   burns and corrosions (T20-T32)
            effects of foreign body in ear (T16)
            effects of foreign body in larynx (T17.3)
            effects of foreign body in mouth NOS (T18.Ø)
            effects of foreign body in nose (T17.Ø-T17.1)
            effects of foreign body in pharynx (T17.2)
            effects of foreign body on external eye (T15.-)
            frostbite (T33-T34)
            insect bite or sting, venomous (T63.4)

✓4ᵗʰ S00 Superficial injury of head

    EXCLUDES 1   diffuse cerebral contusion (S06.2-)
                     focal cerebral contusion (S06.3-)
                     injury of eye and orbit (S05.-)
                     open wound of head (S01.-)

> The appropriate 7th character is to be added to each code from category S00.
> A   initial encounter
> D   subsequent encounter
> S   sequela

    ✓5ᵗʰ S00.0 Superficial injury of scalp

        ✓x7ᵗʰ S00.00 Unspecified superficial injury of scalp

        ✓x7ᵗʰ S00.01 Abrasion of scalp

        ✓x7ᵗʰ S00.02 Blister (nonthermal) of scalp

        ✓x7ᵗʰ S00.03 Contusion of scalp
                 Bruise of scalp
                 Hematoma of scalp

        ✓x7ᵗʰ S00.04 External constriction of part of scalp

        ✓x7ᵗʰ S00.05 Superficial foreign body of scalp
                 Splinter in the scalp

        ✓x7ᵗʰ S00.06 Insect bite (nonvenomous) of scalp

        ✓x7ᵗʰ S00.07 Other superficial bite of scalp
           EXCLUDES 1   open bite of scalp (S01.05)

    ✓5ᵗʰ S00.1 Contusion of eyelid and periocular area
         Black eye
        EXCLUDES 2   contusion of eyeball and orbital tissues (S05.1)

        ✓x7ᵗʰ S00.10 Contusion of unspecified eyelid and periocular area

        ✓x7ᵗʰ S00.11 Contusion of right eyelid and periocular area

        ✓x7ᵗʰ S00.12 Contusion of left eyelid and periocular area

    ✓5ᵗʰ S00.2 Other and unspecified superficial injuries of eyelid and periocular area
        EXCLUDES 2   superficial injury of conjunctiva and cornea (S05.Ø-)

        ✓6ᵗʰ S00.20 Unspecified superficial injury of eyelid and periocular area

            ✓7ᵗʰ S00.201 Unspecified superficial injury of right eyelid and periocular area

            ✓7ᵗʰ S00.202 Unspecified superficial injury of left eyelid and periocular area

            ✓7ᵗʰ S00.209 Unspecified superficial injury of unspecified eyelid and periocular area

        ✓6ᵗʰ S00.21 Abrasion of eyelid and periocular area

            ✓7ᵗʰ S00.211 Abrasion of right eyelid and periocular area

            ✓7ᵗʰ S00.212 Abrasion of left eyelid and periocular area

            ✓7ᵗʰ S00.219 Abrasion of unspecified eyelid and periocular area

        ✓6ᵗʰ S00.22 Blister (nonthermal) of eyelid and periocular area

            ✓7ᵗʰ S00.221 Blister (nonthermal) of right eyelid and periocular area

            ✓7ᵗʰ S00.222 Blister (nonthermal) of left eyelid and periocular area

            ✓7ᵗʰ S00.229 Blister (nonthermal) of unspecified eyelid and periocular area

        ✓6ᵗʰ S00.24 External constriction of eyelid and periocular area

            ✓7ᵗʰ S00.241 External constriction of right eyelid and periocular area

            ✓7ᵗʰ S00.242 External constriction of left eyelid and periocular area

            ✓7ᵗʰ S00.249 External constriction of unspecified eyelid and periocular area

        ✓6ᵗʰ S00.25 Superficial foreign body of eyelid and periocular area
             Splinter of eyelid and periocular area
           EXCLUDES 2   retained foreign body in eyelid (H02.81-)

            ✓7ᵗʰ S00.251 Superficial foreign body of right eyelid and periocular area

            ✓7ᵗʰ S00.252 Superficial foreign body of left eyelid and periocular area

            ✓7ᵗʰ S00.259 Superficial foreign body of unspecified eyelid and periocular area

        ✓6ᵗʰ S00.26 Insect bite (nonvenomous) of eyelid and periocular area

            ✓7ᵗʰ S00.261 Insect bite (nonvenomous) of right eyelid and periocular area

            ✓7ᵗʰ S00.262 Insect bite (nonvenomous) of left eyelid and periocular area

            ✓7ᵗʰ S00.269 Insect bite (nonvenomous) of unspecified eyelid and periocular area

        ✓6ᵗʰ S00.27 Other superficial bite of eyelid and periocular area
           EXCLUDES 1   open bite of eyelid and periocular area (S01.15)

            ✓7ᵗʰ S00.271 Other superficial bite of right eyelid and periocular area

            ✓7ᵗʰ S00.272 Other superficial bite of left eyelid and periocular area

            ✓7ᵗʰ S00.279 Other superficial bite of unspecified eyelid and periocular area

    ✓5ᵗʰ S00.3 Superficial injury of nose

        ✓x7ᵗʰ S00.30 Unspecified superficial injury of nose

        ✓x7ᵗʰ S00.31 Abrasion of nose

        ✓x7ᵗʰ S00.32 Blister (nonthermal) of nose

✓x7ᵗʰ **S00.33** Contusion of nose
    Bruise of nose
    Hematoma of nose

✓x7ᵗʰ **S00.34** External constriction of nose

✓x7ᵗʰ **S00.35** Superficial foreign body of nose
    Splinter in the nose

✓x7ᵗʰ **S00.36** Insect bite (nonvenomous) of nose

✓x7ᵗʰ **S00.37** Other superficial bite of nose
    EXCLUDES 1   open bite of nose (S01.25)

✓5ᵗʰ **S00.4** Superficial injury of ear

  ✓6ᵗʰ **S00.40** Unspecified superficial injury of ear

    ✓7ᵗʰ **S00.401** Unspecified superficial injury of right ear

    ✓7ᵗʰ **S00.402** Unspecified superficial injury of left ear

    ✓7ᵗʰ **S00.409** Unspecified superficial injury of unspecified ear

  ✓6ᵗʰ **S00.41** Abrasion of ear

    ✓7ᵗʰ **S00.411** Abrasion of right ear

    ✓7ᵗʰ **S00.412** Abrasion of left ear

    ✓7ᵗʰ **S00.419** Abrasion of unspecified ear

  ✓6ᵗʰ **S00.42** Blister (nonthermal) of ear

    ✓7ᵗʰ **S00.421** Blister (nonthermal) of right ear

    ✓7ᵗʰ **S00.422** Blister (nonthermal) of left ear

    ✓7ᵗʰ **S00.429** Blister (nonthermal) of unspecified ear

  ✓6ᵗʰ **S00.43** Contusion of ear
     Bruise of ear
     Hematoma of ear

    ✓7ᵗʰ **S00.431** Contusion of right ear

    ✓7ᵗʰ **S00.432** Contusion of left ear

    ✓7ᵗʰ **S00.439** Contusion of unspecified ear

  ✓6ᵗʰ **S00.44** External constriction of ear

    ✓7ᵗʰ **S00.441** External constriction of right ear

    ✓7ᵗʰ **S00.442** External constriction of left ear

    ✓7ᵗʰ **S00.449** External constriction of unspecified ear

  ✓6ᵗʰ **S00.45** Superficial foreign body of ear
     Splinter in the ear

    ✓7ᵗʰ **S00.451** Superficial foreign body of right ear

    ✓7ᵗʰ **S00.452** Superficial foreign body of left ear

    ✓7ᵗʰ **S00.459** Superficial foreign body of unspecified ear

  ✓6ᵗʰ **S00.46** Insect bite (nonvenomous) of ear

    ✓7ᵗʰ **S00.461** Insect bite (nonvenomous) of right ear

    ✓7ᵗʰ **S00.462** Insect bite (nonvenomous) of left ear

    ✓7ᵗʰ **S00.469** Insect bite (nonvenomous) of unspecified ear

  ✓6ᵗʰ **S00.47** Other superficial bite of ear
     EXCLUDES 1   open bite of ear (S01.35)

    ✓7ᵗʰ **S00.471** Other superficial bite of right ear

    ✓7ᵗʰ **S00.472** Other superficial bite of left ear

    ✓7ᵗʰ **S00.479** Other superficial bite of unspecified ear

✓5ᵗʰ **S00.5** Superficial injury of lip and oral cavity

  ✓6ᵗʰ **S00.50** Unspecified superficial injury of lip and oral cavity

    ✓7ᵗʰ **S00.501** Unspecified superficial injury of lip

    ✓7ᵗʰ **S00.502** Unspecified superficial injury of oral cavity

  ✓6ᵗʰ **S00.51** Abrasion of lip and oral cavity

    ✓7ᵗʰ **S00.511** Abrasion of lip

    ✓7ᵗʰ **S00.512** Abrasion of oral cavity

  ✓6ᵗʰ **S00.52** Blister (nonthermal) of lip and oral cavity

    ✓7ᵗʰ **S00.521** Blister (nonthermal) of lip

    ✓7ᵗʰ **S00.522** Blister (nonthermal) of oral cavity

  ✓6ᵗʰ **S00.53** Contusion of lip and oral cavity

    ✓7ᵗʰ **S00.531** Contusion of lip
      Bruise of lip
      Hematoma of lip

    ✓7ᵗʰ **S00.532** Contusion of oral cavity
      Bruise of oral cavity
      Hematoma of oral cavity

  ✓6ᵗʰ **S00.54** External constriction of lip and oral cavity

    ✓7ᵗʰ **S00.541** External constriction of lip

    ✓7ᵗʰ **S00.542** External constriction of oral cavity

  ✓6ᵗʰ **S00.55** Superficial foreign body of lip and oral cavity

    ✓7ᵗʰ **S00.551** Superficial foreign body of lip
      Splinter of lip and oral cavity

    ✓7ᵗʰ **S00.552** Superficial foreign body of oral cavity
      Splinter of lip and oral cavity

  ✓6ᵗʰ **S00.56** Insect bite (nonvenomous) of lip and oral cavity

    ✓7ᵗʰ **S00.561** Insect bite (nonvenomous) of lip

    ✓7ᵗʰ **S00.562** Insect bite (nonvenomous) of oral cavity

  ✓6ᵗʰ **S00.57** Other superficial bite of lip and oral cavity

    ✓7ᵗʰ **S00.571** Other superficial bite of lip
      EXCLUDES 1   open bite of lip (S01.551)

    ✓7ᵗʰ **S00.572** Other superficial bite of oral cavity
      EXCLUDES 1   open bite of oral cavity (S01.552)

✓5ᵗʰ **S00.8** Superficial injury of other parts of head
    Superficial injuries of face [any part]

  ✓x7ᵗʰ **S00.80** Unspecified superficial injury of other part of head

  ✓x7ᵗʰ **S00.81** Abrasion of other part of head

  ✓x7ᵗʰ **S00.82** Blister (nonthermal) of other part of head

  ✓x7ᵗʰ **S00.83** Contusion of other part of head
     Bruise of other part of head
     Hematoma of other part of head

  ✓x7ᵗʰ **S00.84** External constriction of other part of head

  ✓x7ᵗʰ **S00.85** Superficial foreign body of other part of head
     Splinter in other part of head

  ✓x7ᵗʰ **S00.86** Insect bite (nonvenomous) of other part of head

  ✓x7ᵗʰ **S00.87** Other superficial bite of other part of head
     EXCLUDES 1   open bite of other part of head (S01.85)

✓5ᵗʰ **S00.9** Superficial injury of unspecified part of head

  ✓x7ᵗʰ **S00.90** Unspecified superficial injury of unspecified part of head

  ✓x7ᵗʰ **S00.91** Abrasion of unspecified part of head

  ✓x7ᵗʰ **S00.92** Blister (nonthermal) of unspecified part of head

  ✓x7ᵗʰ **S00.93** Contusion of unspecified part of head
     Bruise of head
     Hematoma of head

  ✓x7ᵗʰ **S00.94** External constriction of unspecified part of head

  ✓x7ᵗʰ **S00.95** Superficial foreign body of unspecified part of head
     Splinter of head

  ✓x7ᵗʰ **S00.96** Insect bite (nonvenomous) of unspecified part of head

  ✓x7ᵗʰ **S00.97** Other superficial bite of unspecified part of head
     EXCLUDES 1   open bite of head (S01.95)

✓4ᵗʰ **S01** Open wound of head
    Code also any associated:
     injury of cranial nerve (S04.-)
     injury of muscle and tendon of head (S09.1-)
     intracranial injury (S06.-)
     wound infection
    EXCLUDES 1   open skull fracture (S02.- with 7th character B)
    EXCLUDES 2   injury of eye and orbit (S05.-)
           traumatic amputation of part of head (S08.-)

    The appropriate 7th character is to be added to each code from category S01.
    A   initial encounter
    D   subsequent encounter
    S   sequela

✓5ᵗʰ **S01.0** Open wound of scalp
    EXCLUDES 1   avulsion of scalp (S08.0)

  ✓x7ᵗʰ **S01.00** Unspecified open wound of scalp

  ✓x7ᵗʰ **S01.01** Laceration without foreign body of scalp

  ✓x7ᵗʰ **S01.02** Laceration with foreign body of scalp

  ✓x7ᵗʰ **S01.03** Puncture wound without foreign body of scalp

  ✓x7ᵗʰ **S01.04** Puncture wound with foreign body of scalp

  ✓x7ᵗʰ **S01.05** Open bite of scalp
     Bite of scalp NOS
     EXCLUDES 1   superficial bite of scalp (S00.06, S00.07-)

✔ Additional Character Required   ✓x7ᵗʰ Placeholder Alert   Manifestation   Unspecified Dx   ▶◀ Revised Text   ● New Code   ▲ Revised Title

ICD-10-CM 2020   949

√5ᵗʰ **S01.1** **Open wound of** eyelid and periocular area

Open wound of eyelid and periocular area with or without involvement of lacrimal passages

√6ᵗʰ **S01.10** **Unspecified open wound of eyelid and periocular area**

√7ᵗʰ **S01.101** **Unspecified open wound of** right **eyelid and periocular area**

√7ᵗʰ **S01.102** **Unspecified open wound of** left **eyelid and periocular area**

√7ᵗʰ **S01.109** **Unspecified open wound of unspecified eyelid and periocular area**

√6ᵗʰ **S01.11** Laceration without foreign body **of eyelid and periocular area**

√7ᵗʰ **S01.111** **Laceration without foreign body of** right **eyelid and periocular area**

√7ᵗʰ **S01.112** **Laceration without foreign body of** left **eyelid and periocular area**

√7ᵗʰ **S01.119** **Laceration without foreign body of unspecified eyelid and periocular area**

√6ᵗʰ **S01.12** Laceration with foreign body **of eyelid and periocular area**

√7ᵗʰ **S01.121** **Laceration with foreign body of** right **eyelid and periocular area**

√7ᵗʰ **S01.122** **Laceration with foreign body of** left **eyelid and periocular area**

√7ᵗʰ **S01.129** **Laceration with foreign body of unspecified eyelid and periocular area**

√6ᵗʰ **S01.13** Puncture wound without foreign body **of eyelid and periocular area**

√7ᵗʰ **S01.131** **Puncture wound without foreign body of** right **eyelid and periocular area**

√7ᵗʰ **S01.132** **Puncture wound without foreign body of** left **eyelid and periocular area**

√7ᵗʰ **S01.139** **Puncture wound without foreign body of unspecified eyelid and periocular area**

√6ᵗʰ **S01.14** Puncture wound with foreign body **of eyelid and periocular area**

√7ᵗʰ **S01.141** **Puncture wound with foreign body of** right **eyelid and periocular area**

√7ᵗʰ **S01.142** **Puncture wound with foreign body of** left **eyelid and periocular area**

√7ᵗʰ **S01.149** **Puncture wound with foreign body of unspecified eyelid and periocular area**

√6ᵗʰ **S01.15** Open bite **of eyelid and periocular area**

Bite of eyelid and periocular area NOS

EXCLUDES 1   superficial bite of eyelid and periocular area (S00.26, S00.27)

√7ᵗʰ **S01.151** **Open bite of** right **eyelid and periocular area**

√7ᵗʰ **S01.152** **Open bite of** left **eyelid and periocular area**

√7ᵗʰ **S01.159** **Open bite of unspecified eyelid and periocular area**

√5ᵗʰ **S01.2** **Open wound of** nose

√x7ᵗʰ **S01.20** **Unspecified open wound of nose**

√x7ᵗʰ **S01.21** Laceration without foreign body **of nose**

√x7ᵗʰ **S01.22** Laceration with foreign body **of nose**

√x7ᵗʰ **S01.23** Puncture wound without foreign body **of nose**

√x7ᵗʰ **S01.24** Puncture wound with foreign body **of nose**

√x7ᵗʰ **S01.25** Open bite **of nose**

Bite of nose NOS

EXCLUDES 1   superficial bite of nose (S00.36, S00.37)

√5ᵗʰ **S01.3** **Open wound of** ear

√6ᵗʰ **S01.30** **Unspecified open wound of ear**

√7ᵗʰ **S01.301** **Unspecified open wound of** right **ear**

√7ᵗʰ **S01.302** **Unspecified open wound of** left **ear**

√7ᵗʰ **S01.309** **Unspecified open wound of unspecified ear**

√6ᵗʰ **S01.31** Laceration without foreign body **of ear**

√7ᵗʰ **S01.311** **Laceration without foreign body of** right **ear**

√7ᵗʰ **S01.312** **Laceration without foreign body of** left **ear**

√7ᵗʰ **S01.319** **Laceration without foreign body of unspecified ear**

√6ᵗʰ **S01.32** Laceration with foreign body **of ear**

√7ᵗʰ **S01.321** **Laceration with foreign body of** right **ear**

√7ᵗʰ **S01.322** **Laceration with foreign body of** left **ear**

√7ᵗʰ **S01.329** **Laceration with foreign body of unspecified ear**

√6ᵗʰ **S01.33** Puncture wound without foreign body **of ear**

√7ᵗʰ **S01.331** **Puncture wound without foreign body of** right **ear**

√7ᵗʰ **S01.332** **Puncture wound without foreign body of** left **ear**

√7ᵗʰ **S01.339** **Puncture wound without foreign body of unspecified ear**

√6ᵗʰ **S01.34** Puncture wound with foreign body **of ear**

√7ᵗʰ **S01.341** **Puncture wound with foreign body of** right **ear**

√7ᵗʰ **S01.342** **Puncture wound with foreign body of** left **ear**

√7ᵗʰ **S01.349** **Puncture wound with foreign body of unspecified ear**

√6ᵗʰ **S01.35** Open bite **of ear**

Bite of ear NOS

EXCLUDES 1   superficial bite of ear (S00.46, S00.47)

√7ᵗʰ **S01.351** **Open bite of** right **ear**

√7ᵗʰ **S01.352** **Open bite of** left **ear**

√7ᵗʰ **S01.359** **Open bite of unspecified ear**

√5ᵗʰ **S01.4** **Open wound of** cheek and temporomandibular area

√6ᵗʰ **S01.40** **Unspecified open wound of cheek and temporomandibular area**

√7ᵗʰ **S01.401** **Unspecified open wound of** right **cheek and temporomandibular area**

√7ᵗʰ **S01.402** **Unspecified open wound of** left **cheek and temporomandibular area**

√7ᵗʰ **S01.409** **Unspecified open wound of unspecified cheek and temporomandibular area**

√6ᵗʰ **S01.41** Laceration without foreign body **of cheek and temporomandibular area**

√7ᵗʰ **S01.411** **Laceration without foreign body of** right **cheek and temporomandibular area**

√7ᵗʰ **S01.412** **Laceration without foreign body of** left **cheek and temporomandibular area**

√7ᵗʰ **S01.419** **Laceration without foreign body of unspecified cheek and temporomandibular area**

√6ᵗʰ **S01.42** Laceration with foreign body **of cheek and temporomandibular area**

√7ᵗʰ **S01.421** **Laceration with foreign body of** right **cheek and temporomandibular area**

√7ᵗʰ **S01.422** **Laceration with foreign body of** left **cheek and temporomandibular area**

√7ᵗʰ **S01.429** **Laceration with foreign body of unspecified cheek and temporomandibular area**

√6ᵗʰ **S01.43** Puncture wound without foreign body **of cheek and temporomandibular area**

√7ᵗʰ **S01.431** **Puncture wound without foreign body of** right **cheek and temporomandibular area**

√7ᵗʰ **S01.432** **Puncture wound without foreign body of** left **cheek and temporomandibular area**

√7ᵗʰ **S01.439** **Puncture wound without foreign body of unspecified cheek and temporomandibular area**

√6ᵗʰ **S01.44** Puncture wound with foreign body **of cheek and temporomandibular area**

√7ᵗʰ **S01.441** **Puncture wound with foreign body of** right **cheek and temporomandibular area**

√7ᵗʰ **S01.442** **Puncture wound with foreign body of** left **cheek and temporomandibular area**

√7ᵗʰ **S01.449** **Puncture wound with foreign body of unspecified cheek and temporomandibular area**

√6ᵗʰ **S01.45** Open bite **of cheek and temporomandibular area**

Bite of cheek and temporomandibular area NOS

EXCLUDES 2   superficial bite of cheek and temporomandibular area (S00.86, S00.87)

√7ᵗʰ **S01.451** **Open bite of** right **cheek and temporomandibular area**

√7ᵗʰ **S01.452** **Open bite of** left **cheek and temporomandibular area**

√7ᵗʰ **S01.459** **Open bite of unspecified cheek and temporomandibular area**

N Newborn: 0   P Pediatric: 0-17   M Maternity: 12-55   A Adult: 15-124   CH Comorbidity High   CL Comorbidity Low   NCDx Noncancer Dx   PDx Primary Dx

950   ICD-10-CM 2020

√5th **S01.5 Open wound of lip and oral cavity**
  EXCLUDES 2 tooth dislocation (S03.2)
  tooth fracture (S02.5)
  √6th **S01.50 Unspecified open wound of lip and oral cavity**
    √7th **S01.501 Unspecified open wound of lip**
    √7th **S01.502 Unspecified open wound of oral cavity**
  √6th **S01.51 Laceration of lip and oral cavity without foreign body**
    √7th **S01.511 Laceration without foreign body of lip**
    √7th **S01.512 Laceration without foreign body of oral cavity**
  √6th **S01.52 Laceration of lip and oral cavity with foreign body**
    √7th **S01.521 Laceration with foreign body of lip**
    √7th **S01.522 Laceration with foreign body of oral cavity**
  √6th **S01.53 Puncture wound of lip and oral cavity without foreign body**
    √7th **S01.531 Puncture wound without foreign body of lip**
    √7th **S01.532 Puncture wound without foreign body of oral cavity**
  √6th **S01.54 Puncture wound of lip and oral cavity with foreign body**
    √7th **S01.541 Puncture wound with foreign body of lip**
    √7th **S01.542 Puncture wound with foreign body of oral cavity**
  √6th **S01.55 Open bite of lip and oral cavity**
    √7th **S01.551 Open bite of lip**
      Bite of lip NOS
      EXCLUDES 1 superficial bite of lip (S00.571)
    √7th **S01.552 Open bite of oral cavity**
      Bite of oral cavity NOS
      EXCLUDES 1 superficial bite of oral cavity (S00.572)
√5th **S01.8 Open wound of other parts of head**
  √x7th **S01.80 Unspecified open wound of other part of head**
  √x7th **S01.81 Laceration without foreign body of other part of head**
  √x7th **S01.82 Laceration with foreign body of other part of head**
  √x7th **S01.83 Puncture wound without foreign body of other part of head**
  √x7th **S01.84 Puncture wound with foreign body of other part of head**
  √x7th **S01.85 Open bite of other part of head**
    Bite of other part of head NOS
    EXCLUDES 1 superficial bite of other part of head (S00.87)
√5th **S01.9 Open wound of unspecified part of head**
  √x7th **S01.90 Unspecified open wound of unspecified part of head**
  √x7th **S01.91 Laceration without foreign body of unspecified part of head**
  √x7th **S01.92 Laceration with foreign body of unspecified part of head**
  √x7th **S01.93 Puncture wound without foreign body of unspecified part of head**
  √x7th **S01.94 Puncture wound with foreign body of unspecified part of head**
  √x7th **S01.95 Open bite of unspecified part of head**
    Bite of head NOS
    EXCLUDES 1 superficial bite of head NOS (S00.97)

√4th **S02 Fracture of skull and facial bones**
  NOTE A fracture not indicated as open or closed should be coded to closed.
  Code also any associated intracranial injury (S06.-)
  AHA: 2017,1Q,42; 2016,4Q,66-67
  The appropriate 7th character is to be added to each code from category S02.
  A initial encounter for closed fracture
  B initial encounter for open fracture
  D subsequent encounter for fracture with routine healing
  G subsequent encounter for fracture with delayed healing
  K subsequent encounter for fracture with nonunion
  S sequela
  √x7th **S02.0 Fracture of vault of skull**
    Fracture of frontal bone
    Fracture of parietal bone
  √5th **S02.1 Fracture of base of skull**
    EXCLUDES 1 orbit NOS (S02.8)
    EXCLUDES 2 ►lateral orbital wall (S02.84-)◄
      ►medial orbital wall (S02.83-)◄
      orbital floor (S02.3-)
    √6th **S02.10 Unspecified fracture of base of skull**
      √7th **S02.101 Fracture of base of skull, right side**
      √7th **S02.102 Fracture of base of skull, left side**
      √7th **S02.109 Fracture of base of skull, unspecified side**
    √6th **S02.11 Fracture of occiput**
      √7th **S02.110 Type I occipital condyle fracture, unspecified side**
      √7th **S02.111 Type II occipital condyle fracture, unspecified side**
      √7th **S02.112 Type III occipital condyle fracture, unspecified side**
      √7th **S02.113 Unspecified occipital condyle fracture**
      √7th **S02.118 Other fracture of occiput, unspecified side**
      √7th **S02.119 Unspecified fracture of occiput**
      √7th **S02.11A Type I occipital condyle fracture, right side**
      √7th **S02.11B Type I occipital condyle fracture, left side**
      √7th **S02.11C Type II occipital condyle fracture, right side**
      √7th **S02.11D Type II occipital condyle fracture, left side**
      √7th **S02.11E Type III occipital condyle fracture, right side**
      √7th **S02.11F Type III occipital condyle fracture, left side**
      √7th **S02.11G Other fracture of occiput, right side**
      √7th **S02.11H Other fracture of occiput, left side**
    √6th **S02.12 Fracture of orbital roof**
      √7th **S02.121 Fracture of orbital roof, right side**
      √7th **S02.122 Fracture of orbital roof, left side**
      √7th **S02.129 Fracture of orbital roof, unspecified side**
    √x7th **S02.19 Other fracture of base of skull**
      Fracture of anterior fossa of base of skull
      Fracture of ethmoid sinus
      Fracture of frontal sinus
      Fracture of middle fossa of base of skull
      Fracture of orbital roof
      Fracture of posterior fossa of base of skull
      Fracture of sphenoid
      Fracture of temporal bone
  √x7th **S02.2 Fracture of nasal bones**
  √5th **S02.3 Fracture of orbital floor**
    ►Fracture of inferior orbital wall◄
    EXCLUDES 1 orbit NOS ►(S02.85)◄
    EXCLUDES 2 ►lateral orbital wall (S02.84-)◄
      ►medial orbital wall (S02.83-)◄
      orbital roof (S02.1-)
    √x7th **S02.30 Fracture of orbital floor, unspecified side**
    √x7th **S02.31 Fracture of orbital floor, right side**
    √x7th **S02.32 Fracture of orbital floor, left side**

√5ᵗʰ **S02.4** **Fracture of** malar, maxillary and zygoma bones
  Fracture of superior maxilla
  Fracture of upper jaw (bone)
  Fracture of zygomatic process of temporal bone

√6ᵗʰ **S02.40** **Fracture of malar, maxillary and zygoma bones, unspecified**
  √7ᵗʰ **S02.400** Malar fracture, unspecified side
  √7ᵗʰ **S02.401** Maxillary fracture, unspecified side
  √7ᵗʰ **S02.402** Zygomatic fracture, unspecified side
  √7ᵗʰ **S02.40A** Malar fracture, right side
  √7ᵗʰ **S02.40B** Malar fracture, left side
  √7ᵗʰ **S02.40C** Maxillary fracture, right side
  √7ᵗʰ **S02.40D** Maxillary fracture, left side
  √7ᵗʰ **S02.40E** Zygomatic fracture, right side
  √7ᵗʰ **S02.40F** Zygomatic fracture, left side

√6ᵗʰ **S02.41** **LeFort fracture**
  DEF: Named for Rene Le Fort, these fractures describe different combinations of multiple fractures that occur from significant force to the midface. A common denominator in all three types of LeFort fractures is fracture of the pterygoid processes, which are two bony plates resembling wings that extend downward from the sphenoid bone.

LeFort Fracture Types

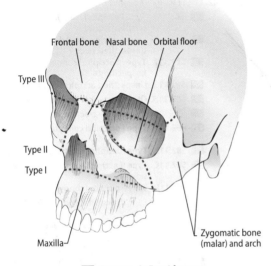

Frontal bone   Nasal bone   Orbital floor
Type III
Type II
Type I
Maxilla
Zygomatic bone (malar) and arch

  √7ᵗʰ **S02.411** LeFort I fracture
  √7ᵗʰ **S02.412** LeFort II fracture
  √7ᵗʰ **S02.413** LeFort III fracture

√x7ᵗʰ **S02.42** **Fracture of** alveolus of maxilla

√x7ᵗʰ **S02.5** **Fracture of** tooth (traumatic)
  Broken tooth
  EXCLUDES 1 cracked tooth (nontraumatic) (K03.81)

√5ᵗʰ **S02.6** **Fracture of** mandible
  Fracture of lower jaw (bone)

√6ᵗʰ **S02.60** **Fracture of mandible, unspecified**
  √7ᵗʰ **S02.600** Fracture of unspecified part of body of mandible, unspecified side
  √7ᵗʰ **S02.601** Fracture of unspecified part of body of right mandible
  √7ᵗʰ **S02.602** Fracture of unspecified part of body of left mandible
  √7ᵗʰ **S02.609** Fracture of mandible, unspecified

√6ᵗʰ **S02.61** **Fracture of** condylar process **of mandible**
  √7ᵗʰ **S02.610** Fracture of condylar process of mandible, unspecified side
  √7ᵗʰ **S02.611** Fracture of condylar process of right mandible
  √7ᵗʰ **S02.612** Fracture of condylar process of left mandible

√6ᵗʰ **S02.62** **Fracture of** subcondylar process **of mandible**
  √7ᵗʰ **S02.620** Fracture of subcondylar process of mandible, unspecified side

  √7ᵗʰ **S02.621** Fracture of subcondylar process of right mandible
  √7ᵗʰ **S02.622** Fracture of subcondylar process of left mandible

√6ᵗʰ **S02.63** **Fracture of** coronoid process **of mandible**
  √7ᵗʰ **S02.630** Fracture of coronoid process of mandible, unspecified side
  √7ᵗʰ **S02.631** Fracture of coronoid process of right mandible
  √7ᵗʰ **S02.632** Fracture of coronoid process of left mandible

√6ᵗʰ **S02.64** **Fracture of** ramus **of mandible**
  √7ᵗʰ **S02.640** Fracture of ramus of mandible, unspecified side
  √7ᵗʰ **S02.641** Fracture of ramus of right mandible
  √7ᵗʰ **S02.642** Fracture of ramus of left mandible

√6ᵗʰ **S02.65** **Fracture of** angle **of mandible**
  √7ᵗʰ **S02.650** Fracture of angle of mandible, unspecified side
  √7ᵗʰ **S02.651** Fracture of angle of right mandible
  √7ᵗʰ **S02.652** Fracture of angle of left mandible

√x7ᵗʰ **S02.66** **Fracture of** symphysis **of mandible**

√6ᵗʰ **S02.67** **Fracture of** alveolus **of mandible**
  √7ᵗʰ **S02.670** Fracture of alveolus of mandible, unspecified side
  √7ᵗʰ **S02.671** Fracture of alveolus of right mandible
  √7ᵗʰ **S02.672** Fracture of alveolus of left mandible

√x7ᵗʰ **S02.69** **Fracture of mandible of other specified site**

√5ᵗʰ **S02.8** **Fractures of other specified skull and facial bones**
  Fracture of orbit NOS
  Fracture of palate
  EXCLUDES 1 fracture of orbital floor (S02.3-)
            fracture of orbital roof (S02.1-)
  EXCLUDES 2 ▶fracture of orbital floor (S02.3-)◀
            ▶fracture of orbital roof (S02.12-)◀

√x7ᵗʰ **S02.80** **Fracture of other specified skull and facial bones, unspecified side**
√x7ᵗʰ **S02.81** **Fracture of other specified skull and facial bones,** right **side**
√x7ᵗʰ **S02.82** **Fracture of other specified skull and facial bones,** left **side**

√6ᵗʰ **S02.83** **Fracture of** medial orbital wall
  EXCLUDES 2 orbital floor (S02.3-)
            orbital roof (S02.12-)
  √7ᵗʰ **S02.831** Fracture of medial orbital wall, right side
  √7ᵗʰ **S02.832** Fracture of medial orbital wall, left side
  √7ᵗʰ **S02.839** Fracture of medial orbital wall, unspecified side

√6ᵗʰ **S02.84** **Fracture of** lateral orbital wall
  EXCLUDES 2 orbital floor (S02.3-)
            orbital roof (S02.12-)
  √7ᵗʰ **S02.841** Fracture of lateral orbital wall, right side
  √7ᵗʰ **S02.842** Fracture of lateral orbital wall, left side
  √7ᵗʰ **S02.849** Fracture of lateral orbital wall, unspecified side

√x7ᵗʰ **S02.85** **Fracture of orbit, unspecified**
  Fracture of orbit NOS
  Fracture of orbit wall NOS
  EXCLUDES 1 lateral orbital wall (S02.84-)
            medial orbital wall (S02.83-)
            orbital floor (S02.3-)
            orbital roof (S02.12-)

√5ᵗʰ **S02.9** **Fracture of unspecified skull and facial bones**
  √x7ᵗʰ **S02.91** Unspecified fracture of skull
  √x7ᵗʰ **S02.92** Unspecified fracture of facial bones

☑4ᵗʰ **S03 Dislocation and sprain of joints and ligaments of head**

    INCLUDES   avulsion of joint (capsule) or ligament of head
                  laceration of cartilage, joint (capsule) or ligament of head
                  sprain of cartilage, joint (capsule) or ligament of head
                  traumatic hemarthrosis of joint or ligament of head
                  traumatic rupture of joint or ligament of head
                  traumatic subluxation of joint or ligament of head
                  traumatic tear of joint or ligament of head

    Code also any associated open wound
    EXCLUDES 2   strain of muscle or tendon of head (S09.1)

> The appropriate 7th character is to be added to each code from category S03.
> A   initial encounter
> D   subsequent encounter
> S   sequela

  ☑5ᵗʰ **S03.0 Dislocation of jaw**

      Dislocation of jaw (cartilage) (meniscus)
      Dislocation of mandible
      Dislocation of temporomandibular (joint)
      AHA: 2016,4Q,67

    ✓x7ᵗʰ **S03.00 Dislocation of jaw, unspecified side**
    ✓x7ᵗʰ **S03.01 Dislocation of jaw, right side**
    ✓x7ᵗʰ **S03.02 Dislocation of jaw, left side**
    ✓x7ᵗʰ **S03.03 Dislocation of jaw, bilateral**

  ✓x7ᵗʰ **S03.1 Dislocation of septal cartilage of nose**

  ✓x7ᵗʰ **S03.2 Dislocation of tooth**

  ☑5ᵗʰ **S03.4 Sprain of jaw**

      Sprain of temporomandibular (joint) (ligament)
      AHA: 2016,4Q,67

    ✓x7ᵗʰ **S03.40 Sprain of jaw, unspecified side**
    ✓x7ᵗʰ **S03.41 Sprain of jaw, right side**
    ✓x7ᵗʰ **S03.42 Sprain of jaw, left side**
    ✓x7ᵗʰ **S03.43 Sprain of jaw, bilateral**

  ✓x7ᵗʰ **S03.8 Sprain of joints and ligaments of other parts of head**

  ✓x7ᵗʰ **S03.9 Sprain of joints and ligaments of unspecified parts of head**

☑4ᵗʰ **S04 Injury of cranial nerve**

    The selection of side should be based on the side of the body being affected
    Code first any associated intracranial injury (S06.-)
    Code also any associated:
      open wound of head (S01.-)
      skull fracture (S02.-)

> The appropriate 7th character is to be added to each code from category S04.
> A   initial encounter
> D   subsequent encounter
> S   sequela

  ☑5ᵗʰ **S04.0 Injury of optic nerve and pathways**

      Use additional code to identify any visual field defect or blindness (H53.4-, H54.-)

    ☑6ᵗʰ **S04.01 Injury of optic nerve**

      Injury of 2nd cranial nerve

      ✓7ᵗʰ **S04.011 Injury of optic nerve, right eye**
      ✓7ᵗʰ **S04.012 Injury of optic nerve, left eye**
      ✓7ᵗʰ **S04.019 Injury of optic nerve, unspecified eye**
        Injury of optic nerve NOS

    ✓x7ᵗʰ **S04.02 Injury of optic chiasm**

    ☑6ᵗʰ **S04.03 Injury of optic tract and pathways**

      Injury of optic radiation

      ✓7ᵗʰ **S04.031 Injury of optic tract and pathways, right side**
      ✓7ᵗʰ **S04.032 Injury of optic tract and pathways, left side**
      ✓7ᵗʰ **S04.039 Injury of optic tract and pathways, unspecified side**
        Injury of optic tract and pathways NOS

    ☑6ᵗʰ **S04.04 Injury of visual cortex**

      ✓7ᵗʰ **S04.041 Injury of visual cortex, right side**
      ✓7ᵗʰ **S04.042 Injury of visual cortex, left side**
      ✓7ᵗʰ **S04.049 Injury of visual cortex, unspecified side**
        Injury of visual cortex NOS

  ☑5ᵗʰ **S04.1 Injury of oculomotor nerve**

      Injury of 3rd cranial nerve

    ✓7ᵗʰ **S04.10 Injury of oculomotor nerve, unspecified side**
    ✓7ᵗʰ **S04.11 Injury of oculomotor nerve, right side**
    ✓7ᵗʰ **S04.12 Injury of oculomotor nerve, left side**

  ☑5ᵗʰ **S04.2 Injury of trochlear nerve**

      Injury of 4th cranial nerve

    ✓7ᵗʰ **S04.20 Injury of trochlear nerve, unspecified side**
    ✓7ᵗʰ **S04.21 Injury of trochlear nerve, right side**
    ✓7ᵗʰ **S04.22 Injury of trochlear nerve, left side**

  ☑5ᵗʰ **S04.3 Injury of trigeminal nerve**

      Injury of 5th cranial nerve

    ✓7ᵗʰ **S04.30 Injury of trigeminal nerve, unspecified side**
    ✓7ᵗʰ **S04.31 Injury of trigeminal nerve, right side**
    ✓7ᵗʰ **S04.32 Injury of trigeminal nerve, left side**

  ☑5ᵗʰ **S04.4 Injury of abducent nerve**

      Injury of 6th cranial nerve

    ✓7ᵗʰ **S04.40 Injury of abducent nerve, unspecified side**
    ✓7ᵗʰ **S04.41 Injury of abducent nerve, right side**
    ✓7ᵗʰ **S04.42 Injury of abducent nerve, left side**

  ☑5ᵗʰ **S04.5 Injury of facial nerve**

      Injury of 7th cranial nerve

    ✓7ᵗʰ **S04.50 Injury of facial nerve, unspecified side**
    ✓7ᵗʰ **S04.51 Injury of facial nerve, right side**
    ✓7ᵗʰ **S04.52 Injury of facial nerve, left side**

  ☑5ᵗʰ **S04.6 Injury of acoustic nerve**

      Injury of auditory nerve
      Injury of 8th cranial nerve

    ✓7ᵗʰ **S04.60 Injury of acoustic nerve, unspecified side**
    ✓7ᵗʰ **S04.61 Injury of acoustic nerve, right side**
    ✓7ᵗʰ **S04.62 Injury of acoustic nerve, left side**

  ☑5ᵗʰ **S04.7 Injury of accessory nerve**

      Injury of 11th cranial nerve

    ✓7ᵗʰ **S04.70 Injury of accessory nerve, unspecified side**
    ✓7ᵗʰ **S04.71 Injury of accessory nerve, right side**
    ✓7ᵗʰ **S04.72 Injury of accessory nerve, left side**

  ☑5ᵗʰ **S04.8 Injury of other cranial nerves**

    ☑6ᵗʰ **S04.81 Injury of olfactory [1st] nerve**

      ✓7ᵗʰ **S04.811 Injury of olfactory [1st] nerve, right side**
      ✓7ᵗʰ **S04.812 Injury of olfactory [1st] nerve, left side**
      ✓7ᵗʰ **S04.819 Injury of olfactory [1st] nerve, unspecified side**

    ☑6ᵗʰ **S04.89 Injury of other cranial nerves**

      Injury of vagus [10th] nerve

      ✓7ᵗʰ **S04.891 Injury of other cranial nerves, right side**
      ✓7ᵗʰ **S04.892 Injury of other cranial nerves, left side**
      ✓7ᵗʰ **S04.899 Injury of other cranial nerves, unspecified side**

  ✓x7ᵗʰ **S04.9 Injury of unspecified cranial nerve**

☑4ᵗʰ **S05 Injury of eye and orbit**

    INCLUDES   open wound of eye and orbit
    EXCLUDES 2   2nd cranial [optic] nerve injury (S04.0-)
                 3rd cranial [oculomotor] nerve injury (S04.1-)
                 open wound of eyelid and periocular area (S01.1-)
                 orbital bone fracture (S02.1-, S02.3-, S02.8-)
                 superficial injury of eyelid (S00.1-S00.2)

> The appropriate 7th character is to be added to each code from category S05.
> A   initial encounter
> D   subsequent encounter
> S   sequela

  ☑5ᵗʰ **S05.0 Injury of conjunctiva and corneal abrasion without foreign body**

    EXCLUDES 1   foreign body in conjunctival sac (T15.1)
                 foreign body in cornea (T15.0)

    ✓x7ᵗʰ **S05.00 Injury of conjunctiva and corneal abrasion without foreign body, unspecified eye**

☑ Additional Character Required   ✓x7ᵗʰ Placeholder Alert   Manifestation   Unspecified Dx   ▶◀ Revised Text   ● New Code   ▲ Revised Title

Chapter 19. Injury, Poisoning and Certain Other Consequences of External Causes

✓x7ᵗʰ **S05.01** **Injury of conjunctiva and corneal abrasion without foreign body,** right **eye**

✓x7ᵗʰ **S05.02** **Injury of conjunctiva and corneal abrasion without foreign body,** left **eye**

✓5ᵗʰ **S05.1** **Contusion** of eyeball and orbital tissues

Traumatic hyphema

EXCLUDES 2 *black eye NOS (S00.1)*

contusion of eyelid and periocular area (S00.1)

✓x7ᵗʰ **S05.10** **Contusion of eyeball and orbital tissues, unspecified eye**

✓x7ᵗʰ **S05.11** **Contusion of eyeball and orbital tissues,** right **eye**

✓x7ᵗʰ **S05.12** **Contusion of eyeball and orbital tissues,** left **eye**

✓5ᵗʰ **S05.2** **Ocular laceration and rupture** with prolapse or loss of intraocular tissue

✓x7ᵗʰ **S05.20** **Ocular laceration and rupture with prolapse or loss of intraocular tissue, unspecified eye**

✓x7ᵗʰ **S05.21** **Ocular laceration and rupture with prolapse or loss of intraocular tissue,** right **eye**

✓x7ᵗʰ **S05.22** **Ocular laceration and rupture with prolapse or loss of intraocular tissue,** left **eye**

✓5ᵗʰ **S05.3** **Ocular laceration** without prolapse or loss of intraocular tissue

Laceration of eye NOS

DEF: Tear in ocular tissue without displacing structures that is due to blunt trauma. It is characterized by pain, redness, and decreased vision.

✓x7ᵗʰ **S05.30** **Ocular laceration without prolapse or loss of intraocular tissue, unspecified eye**

✓x7ᵗʰ **S05.31** **Ocular laceration without prolapse or loss of intraocular tissue,** right **eye**

✓x7ᵗʰ **S05.32** **Ocular laceration without prolapse or loss of intraocular tissue,** left **eye**

✓5ᵗʰ **S05.4** **Penetrating wound** of orbit with or without foreign body

EXCLUDES 2 *retained (old) foreign body following penetrating wound in orbit (H05.5-)*

✓x7ᵗʰ **S05.40** **Penetrating wound of orbit with or without foreign body, unspecified eye**

✓x7ᵗʰ **S05.41** **Penetrating wound of orbit with or without foreign body,** right **eye**

✓x7ᵗʰ **S05.42** **Penetrating wound of orbit with or without foreign body,** left **eye**

✓5ᵗʰ **S05.5** **Penetrating wound with foreign body** of eyeball

EXCLUDES 2 *retained (old) intraocular foreign body (H44.6-, H44.7)*

✓x7ᵗʰ **S05.50** **Penetrating wound with foreign body of unspecified eyeball**

✓x7ᵗʰ **S05.51** **Penetrating wound with foreign body of** right **eyeball**

✓x7ᵗʰ **S05.52** **Penetrating wound with foreign body of** left **eyeball**

✓5ᵗʰ **S05.6** **Penetrating wound without foreign body** of eyeball

Ocular penetration NOS

✓x7ᵗʰ **S05.60** **Penetrating wound without foreign body of unspecified eyeball**

✓x7ᵗʰ **S05.61** **Penetrating wound without foreign body of** right **eyeball**

✓x7ᵗʰ **S05.62** **Penetrating wound without foreign body of** left **eyeball**

✓5ᵗʰ **S05.7** **Avulsion of eye**

Traumatic enucleation

✓x7ᵗʰ **S05.70** **Avulsion of unspecified eye**

✓x7ᵗʰ **S05.71** **Avulsion of** right **eye**

✓x7ᵗʰ **S05.72** **Avulsion of** left **eye**

✓5ᵗʰ **S05.8** **Other injuries of eye and orbit**

Lacrimal duct injury

✓6ᵗʰ **S05.8X** **Other injuries of eye and orbit**

✓7ᵗʰ **S05.8X1** **Other injuries of** right **eye and orbit**

✓7ᵗʰ **S05.8X2** **Other injuries of** left **eye and orbit**

✓7ᵗʰ **S05.8X9** **Other injuries of unspecified eye and orbit**

✓5ᵗʰ **S05.9** **Unspecified injury of eye and orbit**

Injury of eye NOS

✓x7ᵗʰ **S05.90** **Unspecified injury of unspecified eye and orbit**

✓x7ᵗʰ **S05.91** **Unspecified injury of** right **eye and orbit**

✓x7ᵗʰ **S05.92** **Unspecified injury of** left **eye and orbit**

✓4ᵗʰ **S06** **Intracranial injury**

NOTE 7th characters D and S do not apply to codes in category S06 with 6th character 7 – death due to brain injury prior to regaining consciousness, or 8 – death due to other cause prior to regaining consciousness.

INCLUDES traumatic brain injury

Code also any associated:

open wound of head (S01.-)

skull fracture (S02.-)

EXCLUDES 1 *head injury NOS (S09.90)*

AHA: 2017,4Q,25; 2017,1Q,42; 2015,3Q,37

TIP: Do not assign Z87.820 Personal history of traumatic brain injury, when residual conditions persist after an intracranial injury. The codes for the residual conditions should be first listed, followed by a code from category S06 using seventh character S to identify sequelae.

The appropriate 7th character is to be added to each code from category S06.

A initial encounter

D subsequent encounter

S sequela

✓5ᵗʰ **S06.0** **Concussion**

Commotio cerebri

EXCLUDES 1 *concussion with other intracranial injuries classified in subcategories S06.1- to S06.6- , S06.81- and S06.82- — code to specified intracranial injury*

AHA: 2016,4Q,67-68

✓6ᵗʰ **S06.0X** **Concussion**

✓7ᵗʰ **S06.0X0** **Concussion** without loss of consciousness

✓7ᵗʰ **S06.0X1** **Concussion with loss of consciousness of** 30 minutes or less

✓7ᵗʰ **S06.0X9** **Concussion with loss of consciousness of unspecified duration**

Concussion NOS

✓5ᵗʰ **S06.1** **Traumatic cerebral edema**

Diffuse traumatic cerebral edema

Focal traumatic cerebral edema

✓6ᵗʰ **S06.1X** **Traumatic** cerebral edema

✓7ᵗʰ **S06.1X0** **Traumatic cerebral edema** without loss of consciousness

✓7ᵗʰ **S06.1X1** **Traumatic cerebral edema with loss of consciousness of** 30 minutes or less

✓7ᵗʰ **S06.1X2** **Traumatic cerebral edema with loss of consciousness of** 31 minutes to 59 minutes

✓7ᵗʰ **S06.1X3** **Traumatic cerebral edema with loss of consciousness of** 1 hour to 5 hours 59 minutes

✓7ᵗʰ **S06.1X4** **Traumatic cerebral edema with loss of consciousness of** 6 hours to 24 hours

✓7ᵗʰ **S06.1X5** **Traumatic cerebral edema with loss of consciousness** greater than 24 hours with return to pre-existing conscious level

✓7ᵗʰ **S06.1X6** **Traumatic cerebral edema with loss of consciousness** greater than 24 hours without return to pre-existing conscious level with patient surviving   NC Dx

✓7ᵗʰ **S06.1X7** **Traumatic cerebral edema with loss of consciousness of** any duration with death due to brain injury prior to regaining consciousness

✓7ᵗʰ **S06.1X8** **Traumatic cerebral edema with loss of consciousness of** any duration with death due to **other** cause prior to regaining consciousness

✓7ᵗʰ **S06.1X9** **Traumatic cerebral edema with loss of consciousness of unspecified duration**

Traumatic cerebral edema NOS

✓5ᵗʰ **S06.2** **Diffuse traumatic brain injury**

Diffuse axonal brain injury

EXCLUDES 1 *traumatic diffuse cerebral edema (S06.1X-)*

✓6ᵗʰ **S06.2X** **Diffuse traumatic brain injury**

✓7ᵗʰ **S06.2X0** **Diffuse traumatic brain injury** without loss of consciousness

✓7ᵗʰ **S06.2X1** **Diffuse traumatic brain injury with loss of consciousness of** 30 minutes or less

N Newborn: 0 P Pediatric: 0-17 M Maternity: 12-55 A Adult: 15-124 CH Comorbidity High CL Comorbidity Low NCDx Noncancer Dx PDx Primary Dx

954 ICD-10-CM 2020

√7ᵗʰ **S06.2X2** **Diffuse traumatic brain injury with loss of consciousness of** 31 minutes to 59 minutes

√7ᵗʰ **S06.2X3** **Diffuse traumatic brain injury with loss of consciousness of** 1 hour to 5 hours 59 minutes

√7ᵗʰ **S06.2X4** **Diffuse traumatic brain injury with loss of consciousness of** 6 hours to 24 hours

S06.2X5 **Diffuse traumatic brain injury with loss of consciousness** greater than 24 hours with return to pre-existing conscious levels

√7ᵗʰ **S06.2X6** **Diffuse traumatic brain injury with loss of consciousness** greater than 24 hours without return to pre-existing conscious level with patient surviving NC Dx

√7ᵗʰ **S06.2X7** **Diffuse traumatic brain injury with loss of consciousness of** any duration with death due to brain injury prior to regaining consciousness

√7ᵗʰ **S06.2X8** **Diffuse traumatic brain injury with loss of consciousness of** any duration with death due to other cause prior to regaining consciousness

√7ᵗʰ **S06.2X9** **Diffuse traumatic brain injury with loss of consciousness of unspecified duration**
Diffuse traumatic brain injury NOS

√5ᵗʰ **S06.3** Focal traumatic brain injury
EXCLUDES 1 any condition classifiable to S06.4-S06.6
focal cerebral edema (S06.1)

√6ᵗʰ **S06.30** **Unspecified focal traumatic brain injury**

√7ᵗʰ **S06.300** **Unspecified focal traumatic brain injury** without loss of consciousness

√7ᵗʰ **S06.301** **Unspecified focal traumatic brain injury with loss of consciousness of** 30 minutes or less

√7ᵗʰ **S06.302** **Unspecified focal traumatic brain injury with loss of consciousness of** 31 minutes to 59 minutes

√7ᵗʰ **S06.303** **Unspecified focal traumatic brain injury with loss of consciousness of** 1 hour to 5 hours 59 minutes

√7ᵗʰ **S06.304** **Unspecified focal traumatic brain injury with loss of consciousness of** 6 hours to 24 hours

√7ᵗʰ **S06.305** **Unspecified focal traumatic brain injury with loss of consciousness** greater than 24 hours with return to pre-existing conscious level

√7ᵗʰ **S06.306** **Unspecified focal traumatic brain injury with loss of consciousness** greater than 24 hours without return to pre-existing conscious level with patient surviving NC Dx

√7ᵗʰ **S06.307** **Unspecified focal traumatic brain injury with loss of consciousness of** any duration with death due to brain injury prior to regaining consciousness

√7ᵗʰ **S06.308** **Unspecified focal traumatic brain injury with loss of consciousness of** any duration with death due to other cause prior to regaining consciousness

√7ᵗʰ **S06.309** **Unspecified focal traumatic brain injury with loss of consciousness of unspecified duration**
Unspecified focal traumatic brain injury NOS

√6ᵗʰ **S06.31** **Contusion and laceration of** right cerebrum

√7ᵗʰ **S06.310** **Contusion and laceration of right cerebrum** without loss of consciousness

√7ᵗʰ **S06.311** **Contusion and laceration of right cerebrum with loss of consciousness of** 30 minutes or less

√7ᵗʰ **S06.312** **Contusion and laceration of right cerebrum with loss of consciousness of** 31 minutes to 59 minutes

√7ᵗʰ **S06.313** **Contusion and laceration of right cerebrum with loss of consciousness of** 1 hour to 5 hours 59 minutes

√7ᵗʰ **S06.314** **Contusion and laceration of right cerebrum with loss of consciousness of** 6 hours to 24 hours

√7ᵗʰ **S06.315** **Contusion and laceration of right cerebrum with loss of consciousness** greater than 24 hours with return to pre-existing conscious level

√7ᵗʰ **S06.316** **Contusion and laceration of right cerebrum with loss of consciousness** greater than 24 hours without return to pre-existing conscious level with patient surviving NC Dx

√7ᵗʰ **S06.317** **Contusion and laceration of right cerebrum with loss of consciousness of** any duration with death due to brain injury prior to regaining consciousness

√7ᵗʰ **S06.318** **Contusion and laceration of right cerebrum with loss of consciousness of** any duration with death due to other cause prior to regaining consciousness

√7ᵗʰ **S06.319** **Contusion and laceration of right cerebrum with loss of consciousness of unspecified duration**
Contusion and laceration of right cerebrum NOS

√6ᵗʰ **S06.32** **Contusion and laceration of** left cerebrum

√7ᵗʰ **S06.320** **Contusion and laceration of left cerebrum** without loss of consciousness

√7ᵗʰ **S06.321** **Contusion and laceration of left cerebrum with loss of consciousness of** 30 minutes or less

√7ᵗʰ **S06.322** **Contusion and laceration of left cerebrum with loss of consciousness of** 31 minutes to 59 minutes

√7ᵗʰ **S06.323** **Contusion and laceration of left cerebrum with loss of consciousness of** 1 hour to 5 hours 59 minutes

√7ᵗʰ **S06.324** **Contusion and laceration of left cerebrum with loss of consciousness of** 6 hours to 24 hours

√7ᵗʰ **S06.325** **Contusion and laceration of left cerebrum with loss of consciousness** greater than 24 hours with return to pre-existing conscious level

√7ᵗʰ **S06.326** **Contusion and laceration of left cerebrum with loss of consciousness** greater than 24 hours without return to pre-existing conscious level with patient surviving NC Dx

√7ᵗʰ **S06.327** **Contusion and laceration of left cerebrum with loss of consciousness of** any duration with death due to brain injury prior to regaining consciousness

√7ᵗʰ **S06.328** **Contusion and laceration of left cerebrum with loss of consciousness of** any duration with death due to other cause prior to regaining consciousness

√7ᵗʰ **S06.329** **Contusion and laceration of left cerebrum with loss of consciousness of unspecified duration**
Contusion and laceration of left cerebrum NOS

√6ᵗʰ **S06.33** **Contusion and laceration of cerebrum, unspecified**

√7ᵗʰ **S06.330** **Contusion and laceration of cerebrum, unspecified,** without loss of consciousness

√7ᵗʰ **S06.331** **Contusion and laceration of cerebrum, unspecified, with loss of consciousness of** 30 minutes or less

√7ᵗʰ **S06.332** **Contusion and laceration of cerebrum, unspecified, with loss of consciousness of** 31 minutes to 59 minutes

√7ᵗʰ **S06.333** **Contusion and laceration of cerebrum, unspecified, with loss of consciousness of** 1 hour to 5 hours 59 minutes

√7ᵗʰ **S06.334** **Contusion and laceration of cerebrum, unspecified, with loss of consciousness of** 6 hours to 24 hours

√7ᵗʰ **S06.335** **Contusion and laceration of cerebrum, unspecified, with loss of consciousness** greater than 24 hours with return to pre-existing conscious level

√7ᵗʰ **S06.336 Contusion and laceration of cerebrum, unspecified, with loss of consciousness** greater than 24 hours without return to pre-existing conscious level with patient surviving NC Dx

√7ᵗʰ **S06.337 Contusion and laceration of cerebrum, unspecified, with loss of consciousness of** any duration with death due to brain injury prior to regaining consciousness

√7ᵗʰ **S06.338 Contusion and laceration of cerebrum, unspecified, with loss of consciousness of** any duration with death due to **other** cause prior to regaining consciousness

√7ᵗʰ **S06.339 Contusion and laceration of cerebrum, unspecified, with loss of consciousness of unspecified duration**
Contusion and laceration of cerebrum NOS

√6ᵗʰ **S06.34 Traumatic hemorrhage of** right cerebrum
Traumatic intracerebral hemorrhage and hematoma of right cerebrum

√7ᵗʰ **S06.340 Traumatic hemorrhage of right cerebrum** without loss of consciousness

√7ᵗʰ **S06.341 Traumatic hemorrhage of right cerebrum with loss of consciousness of** 30 minutes or less

√7ᵗʰ **S06.342 Traumatic hemorrhage of right cerebrum with loss of consciousness of** 31 minutes to 59 minutes

√7ᵗʰ **S06.343 Traumatic hemorrhage of right cerebrum with loss of consciousness of** 1 hours to 5 hours 59 minutes

√7ᵗʰ **S06.344 Traumatic hemorrhage of right cerebrum with loss of consciousness of** 6 hours to 24 hours

√7ᵗʰ **S06.345 Traumatic hemorrhage of right cerebrum with loss of consciousness** greater than 24 hours with return to pre-existing conscious level

√7ᵗʰ **S06.346 Traumatic hemorrhage of right cerebrum with loss of consciousness** greater than 24 hours without return to pre-existing conscious level with patient surviving NC Dx

√7ᵗʰ **S06.347 Traumatic hemorrhage of right cerebrum with loss of consciousness of** any duration with death due to brain injury prior to regaining consciousness

√7ᵗʰ **S06.348 Traumatic hemorrhage of right cerebrum with loss of consciousness of** any duration with death due to **other** cause prior to regaining consciousness

√7ᵗʰ **S06.349 Traumatic hemorrhage of right cerebrum with loss of consciousness of unspecified duration**
Traumatic hemorrhage of right cerebrum NOS

√6ᵗʰ **S06.35 Traumatic hemorrhage of** left cerebrum
Traumatic intracerebral hemorrhage and hematoma of left cerebrum

√7ᵗʰ **S06.350 Traumatic hemorrhage of left cerebrum** without loss of consciousness

√7ᵗʰ **S06.351 Traumatic hemorrhage of left cerebrum with loss of consciousness of** 30 minutes or less

√7ᵗʰ **S06.352 Traumatic hemorrhage of left cerebrum with loss of consciousness of** 31 minutes to 59 minutes

√7ᵗʰ **S06.353 Traumatic hemorrhage of left cerebrum with loss of consciousness of** 1 hours to 5 hours 59 minutes

√7ᵗʰ **S06.354 Traumatic hemorrhage of left cerebrum with loss of consciousness of** 6 hours to 24 hours

√7ᵗʰ **S06.355 Traumatic hemorrhage of left cerebrum with loss of consciousness** greater than 24 hours with return to pre-existing conscious level

√7ᵗʰ **S06.356 Traumatic hemorrhage of left cerebrum with loss of consciousness** greater than 24 hours without return to pre-existing conscious level with patient surviving NC Dx

√7ᵗʰ **S06.357 Traumatic hemorrhage of left cere...** with loss of consciousness of any du... with death due to brain injury pri... regaining consciousness

√7ᵗʰ **S06.358 Traumatic hemorrhage of left cere...** with loss of consciousness of any du... with death due to **other** cause pri... regaining consciousness

√7ᵗʰ **S06.359 Traumatic hemorrhage of left cere...** with loss of consciousness of unspe... duration
Traumatic hemorrhage of left cere... NOS

√6ᵗʰ **S06.36 Traumatic hemorrhage of cerebrum, unspe...**
Traumatic intracerebral hemorrhage and hema... unspecified

√7ᵗʰ **S06.360 Traumatic hemorrhage of cerebru...** unspecified, without loss of consciousness

√7ᵗʰ **S06.361 Traumatic hemorrhage of cerebru...** unspecified, with loss of consciou... of 30 minutes or less

√7ᵗʰ **S06.362 Traumatic hemorrhage of cerebru...** unspecified, with loss of consciou... of 31 minutes to 59 minutes

√7ᵗʰ **S06.363 Traumatic hemorrhage of cerebru...** unspecified, with loss of consciou... of 1 hours to 5 hours 59 minutes

√7ᵗʰ **S06.364 Traumatic hemorrhage of cerebru...** unspecified, with loss of consciou... of 6 hours to 24 hours

√7ᵗʰ **S06.365 Traumatic hemorrhage of cerebru...** unspecified, with loss of consciou... greater than 24 hours with return t... pre-existing conscious level

√7ᵗʰ **S06.366 Traumatic hemorrhage of cerebrum, unspecified, with loss of consciousness** greater than 24 hours without return to pre-existing conscious level with patient surviving

√7ᵗʰ **S06.367 Traumatic hemorrhage of cerebru...** unspecified, with loss of consciousn... of any duration with death due to b... injury prior to regaining consciousn...

√7ᵗʰ **S06.368 Traumatic hemorrhage of cerebru...** unspecified, with loss of consciousn... of any duration with death due to o... cause prior to regaining consciousn...

√7ᵗʰ **S06.369 Traumatic hemorrhage of cerebru...** unspecified, with loss of consciousn... of unspecified duration
Traumatic hemorrhage of cerebrum...

√6ᵗʰ **S06.37 Contusion, laceration, and hemorrhage of** cerebellum

√7ᵗʰ **S06.370 Contusion, laceration, and hemorrh...** of cerebellum without loss of consciousness

√7ᵗʰ **S06.371 Contusion, laceration, and hemorrh...** of cerebellum with loss of consciou... of 30 minutes or less

√7ᵗʰ **S06.372 Contusion, laceration, and hemorrh...** of cerebellum with loss of consciou... of 31 minutes to 59 minutes

√7ᵗʰ **S06.373 Contusion, laceration, and hemorrh...** of cerebellum with loss of consciou... of 1 hour to 5 hours 59 minutes

√7ᵗʰ **S06.374 Contusion, laceration, and hemorrh...** of cerebellum with loss of consciou... of 6 hours to 24 hours

√7ᵗʰ **S06.375 Contusion, laceration, and hemorrh...** of cerebellum with loss of consciou... greater than 24 hours with return to pre-existing conscious level

√7ᵗʰ **S06.376 Contusion, laceration, and hemorrhage of cerebellum with loss of consciousness** greater than 24 hours without return to pre-existing conscious level with patient surviving

√7ᵗʰ **S06.377 Contusion, laceration, and hemorrh...** of cerebellum with loss of consciousn... of any duration with death due to bra... injury prior to regaining consciousne...

N Newborn: 0   P Pediatric: 0-17   M Maternity: 12-55   A Adult: 15-124   CH Comorbidity High   CL Comorbidity Low   NC Dx Noncancer Dx   PDx Primar...

956   ICD-10-CM 2

☑7ᵗʰ **S06.378** **Contusion, laceration, and hemorrhage of cerebellum with loss of consciousness of** any duration with death due to **other cause prior to regaining consciousness**

☑7ᵗʰ **S06.379** **Contusion, laceration, and hemorrhage of cerebellum with loss of consciousness of unspecified duration**
Contusion, laceration, and hemorrhage of cerebellum NOS

☑6ᵗʰ **S06.38** **Contusion, laceration, and hemorrhage of brainstem**

☑7ᵗʰ **S06.380** **Contusion, laceration, and hemorrhage of brainstem** without loss of consciousness

☑7ᵗʰ **S06.381** **Contusion, laceration, and hemorrhage of brainstem with loss of consciousness of** 30 minutes or less

☑7ᵗʰ **S06.382** **Contusion, laceration, and hemorrhage of brainstem with loss of consciousness of** 31 minutes to 59 minutes

☑7ᵗʰ **S06.383** **Contusion, laceration, and hemorrhage of brainstem with loss of consciousness of** 1 hour to 5 hours 59 minutes

☑7ᵗʰ **S06.384** **Contusion, laceration, and hemorrhage of brainstem with loss of consciousness of** 6 hours to 24 hours

☑7ᵗʰ **S06.385** **Contusion, laceration, and hemorrhage of brainstem with loss of consciousness** greater than 24 hours with return to pre-existing conscious level

☑7ᵗʰ **S06.386** **Contusion, laceration, and hemorrhage of brainstem with loss of consciousness** greater than 24 hours without return to pre-existing conscious level with patient surviving   NC Dx

☑7ᵗʰ **S06.387** **Contusion, laceration, and hemorrhage of brainstem with loss of consciousness of** any duration with death due to brain injury prior to regaining consciousness

☑7ᵗʰ **S06.388** **Contusion, laceration, and hemorrhage of brainstem with loss of consciousness of** any duration with death due to **other cause prior to regaining consciousness**

☑7ᵗʰ **S06.389** **Contusion, laceration, and hemorrhage of brainstem with loss of consciousness of unspecified duration**
Contusion, laceration, and hemorrhage of brainstem NOS

☑5ᵗʰ **S06.4** **Epidural hemorrhage**
Extradural hemorrhage NOS
Extradural hemorrhage (traumatic)
DEF: Epidural space: Space between the endosteum of the cranium (skull) and the dura mater, the outermost layer of a three-layer membrane that covers the brain.

☑6ᵗʰ **S06.4X** **Epidural hemorrhage**

☑7ᵗʰ **S06.4X0** **Epidural hemorrhage** without loss of consciousness

☑7ᵗʰ **S06.4X1** **Epidural hemorrhage with loss of consciousness of** 30 minutes or less

☑7ᵗʰ **S06.4X2** **Epidural hemorrhage with loss of consciousness of** 31 minutes to 59 minutes

☑7ᵗʰ **S06.4X3** **Epidural hemorrhage with loss of consciousness of** 1 hour to 5 hours 59 minutes

☑7ᵗʰ **S06.4X4** **Epidural hemorrhage with loss of consciousness of** 6 hours to 24 hours

☑7ᵗʰ **S06.4X5** **Epidural hemorrhage with loss of consciousness** greater than 24 hours with return to pre-existing conscious level

☑7ᵗʰ **S06.4X6** **Epidural hemorrhage with loss of consciousness** greater than 24 hours without return to pre-existing conscious level with patient surviving   NC Dx

☑7ᵗʰ **S06.4X7** **Epidural hemorrhage with loss of consciousness of** any duration with death due to brain injury prior to regaining consciousness

☑7ᵗʰ **S06.4X8** **Epidural hemorrhage with loss of consciousness of** any duration with death due to **other causes prior to regaining consciousness**

☑7ᵗʰ **S06.4X9** **Epidural hemorrhage with loss of consciousness of unspecified duration**
Epidural hemorrhage NOS

☑5ᵗʰ **S06.5** **Traumatic subdural hemorrhage**
DEF: Subdural: Potential space between the dura mater and arachnoid membrane around the brain.

☑6ᵗʰ **S06.5X** **Traumatic subdural hemorrhage**

☑7ᵗʰ **S06.5X0** **Traumatic subdural hemorrhage** without loss of consciousness

☑7ᵗʰ **S06.5X1** **Traumatic subdural hemorrhage with loss of consciousness of** 30 minutes or less

☑7ᵗʰ **S06.5X2** **Traumatic subdural hemorrhage with loss of consciousness of** 31 minutes to 59 minutes

☑7ᵗʰ **S06.5X3** **Traumatic subdural hemorrhage with loss of consciousness of** 1 hour to 5 hours 59 minutes

☑7ᵗʰ **S06.5X4** **Traumatic subdural hemorrhage with loss of consciousness of** 6 hours to 24 hours

☑7ᵗʰ **S06.5X5** **Traumatic subdural hemorrhage with loss of consciousness** greater than 24 hours with return to pre-existing conscious level

☑7ᵗʰ **S06.5X6** **Traumatic subdural hemorrhage with loss of consciousness** greater than 24 hours without return to pre-existing conscious level with patient surviving   NC Dx

☑7ᵗʰ **S06.5X7** **Traumatic subdural hemorrhage with loss of consciousness of** any duration with death due to brain injury before regaining consciousness

☑7ᵗʰ **S06.5X8** **Traumatic subdural hemorrhage with loss of consciousness of** any duration with death due to **other cause before regaining consciousness**

☑7ᵗʰ **S06.5X9** **Traumatic subdural hemorrhage with loss of consciousness of unspecified duration**
Traumatic subdural hemorrhage NOS

☑5ᵗʰ **S06.6** **Traumatic subarachnoid hemorrhage**
DEF: Subarachnoid: Space located between the arachnoid membrane and the pia mater that contains cerebrospinal fluid.

☑6ᵗʰ **S06.6X** **Traumatic subarachnoid hemorrhage**

☑7ᵗʰ **S06.6X0** **Traumatic subarachnoid hemorrhage** without loss of consciousness

☑7ᵗʰ **S06.6X1** **Traumatic subarachnoid hemorrhage with loss of consciousness of** 30 minutes or less

☑7ᵗʰ **S06.6X2** **Traumatic subarachnoid hemorrhage with loss of consciousness of** 31 minutes to 59 minutes

☑7ᵗʰ **S06.6X3** **Traumatic subarachnoid hemorrhage with loss of consciousness of** 1 hour to 5 hours 59 minutes

☑7ᵗʰ **S06.6X4** **Traumatic subarachnoid hemorrhage with loss of consciousness of** 6 hours to 24 hours

☑7ᵗʰ **S06.6X5** **Traumatic subarachnoid hemorrhage with loss of consciousness** greater than 24 hours with return to pre-existing conscious level

☑7ᵗʰ **S06.6X6** **Traumatic subarachnoid hemorrhage with loss of consciousness** greater than 24 hours without return to pre-existing conscious level with patient surviving   NC Dx

☑7ᵗʰ **S06.6X7** **Traumatic subarachnoid hemorrhage with loss of consciousness of** any duration with death due to brain injury prior to regaining consciousness

☑7ᵗʰ **S06.6X8** **Traumatic subarachnoid hemorrhage with loss of consciousness of** any duration with death due to **other cause prior to regaining consciousness**

Chapter 19. Injury, Poisoning and Certain Other Consequences of External Causes

✓7ᵗʰ **S06.6X9 Traumatic subarachnoid hemorrhage with loss of consciousness of unspecified duration**
Traumatic subarachnoid hemorrhage NOS

✓5ᵗʰ **S06.8 Other specified intracranial injuries**

✓6ᵗʰ **S06.81 Injury of** right internal carotid artery, **intracranial portion, not elsewhere classified**

✓7ᵗʰ **S06.810 Injury of right internal carotid artery, intracranial portion, not elsewhere classified** without loss of consciousness

✓7ᵗʰ **S06.811 Injury of right internal carotid artery, intracranial portion, not elsewhere classified with loss of consciousness of** 30 minutes or less

✓7ᵗʰ **S06.812 Injury of right internal carotid artery, intracranial portion, not elsewhere classified with loss of consciousness of** 31 minutes to 59 minutes

✓7ᵗʰ **S06.813 Injury of right internal carotid artery, intracranial portion, not elsewhere classified with loss of consciousness of** 1 hour to 5 hours 59 minutes

✓7ᵗʰ **S06.814 Injury of right internal carotid artery, intracranial portion, not elsewhere classified with loss of consciousness of** 6 hours to 24 hours

✓7ᵗʰ **S06.815 Injury of right internal carotid artery, intracranial portion, not elsewhere classified with loss of consciousness** greater than 24 hours with return to pre-existing conscious level

✓7ᵗʰ **S06.816 Injury of right internal carotid artery, intracranial portion, not elsewhere classified with loss of consciousness** greater than 24 hours without return to pre-existing conscious level with patient surviving   NC Dx

✓7ᵗʰ **S06.817 Injury of right internal carotid artery, intracranial portion, not elsewhere classified with loss of consciousness of** any duration with death due to brain injury prior to regaining consciousness

✓7ᵗʰ **S06.818 Injury of right internal carotid artery, intracranial portion, not elsewhere classified with loss of consciousness of** any duration with death due to **other** cause prior to regaining consciousness

✓7ᵗʰ **S06.819 Injury of right internal carotid artery, intracranial portion, not elsewhere classified with loss of consciousness of unspecified duration**
Injury of right internal carotid artery, intracranial portion, not elsewhere classified NOS

✓6ᵗʰ **S06.82 Injury of** left internal carotid artery, **intracranial portion, not elsewhere classified**

✓7ᵗʰ **S06.820 Injury of left internal carotid artery, intracranial portion, not elsewhere classified** without loss of consciousness

✓7ᵗʰ **S06.821 Injury of left internal carotid artery, intracranial portion, not elsewhere classified with loss of consciousness of** 30 minutes or less

✓7ᵗʰ **S06.822 Injury of left internal carotid artery, intracranial portion, not elsewhere classified with loss of consciousness of** 31 minutes to 59 minutes

✓7ᵗʰ **S06.823 Injury of left internal carotid artery, intracranial portion, not elsewhere classified with loss of consciousness of** 1 hour to 5 hours 59 minutes

✓7ᵗʰ **S06.824 Injury of left internal carotid artery, intracranial portion, not elsewhere classified with loss of consciousness of** 6 hours to 24 hours

✓7ᵗʰ **S06.825 Injury of left internal carotid artery, intracranial portion, not elsewhere classified with loss of consciousness** greater than 24 hours with return to pre-existing conscious level

✓7ᵗʰ **S06.826 Injury of left internal carotid artery, intracranial portion, not elsewhere classified with** loss of consciousness greater than 24 hours without return to pre-existing conscious level with patient surviving   NC Dx

✓7ᵗʰ **S06.827 Injury of left internal carotid artery, intracranial portion, not elsewhere classified with loss of consciousness of** any duration with death due to brain injury prior to regaining consciousness

✓7ᵗʰ **S06.828 Injury of left internal carotid artery, intracranial portion, not elsewhere classified with loss of consciousness of** any duration with death due to **other** cause prior to regaining consciousness

✓7ᵗʰ **S06.829 Injury of left internal carotid artery, intracranial portion, not elsewhere classified with loss of consciousness of unspecified duration**
Injury of left internal carotid artery, intracranial portion, not elsewhere classified NOS

✓6ᵗʰ **S06.89 Other specified intracranial injury**
EXCLUDES 1   concussion (S06.0X-)

✓7ᵗʰ **S06.890 Other specified intracranial injury** without loss of consciousness

✓7ᵗʰ **S06.891 Other specified intracranial injury with loss of consciousness of** 30 minutes or less

✓7ᵗʰ **S06.892 Other specified intracranial injury with loss of consciousness of** 31 minutes to 59 minutes

✓7ᵗʰ **S06.893 Other specified intracranial injury with loss of consciousness of** 1 hour to 5 hours 59 minutes

✓7ᵗʰ **S06.894 Other specified intracranial injury with loss of consciousness of** 6 hours to 24 hours

✓7ᵗʰ **S06.895 Other specified intracranial injury with loss of consciousness** greater than 24 hours with return to pre-existing conscious level

✓7ᵗʰ **S06.896 Other specified intracranial injury with loss of consciousness** greater than 24 hours without return to pre-existing conscious level with patient surviving   NC Dx

✓7ᵗʰ **S06.897 Other specified intracranial injury with loss of consciousness of** any duration with death due to brain injury prior to regaining consciousness

✓7ᵗʰ **S06.898 Other specified intracranial injury with loss of consciousness of** any duration with death due to **other** cause prior to regaining consciousness

✓7ᵗʰ **S06.899 Other specified intracranial injury with loss of consciousness of unspecified duration**

✓5ᵗʰ **S06.9 Unspecified intracranial injury**
Brain injury NOS
Head injury NOS with loss of consciousness
Traumatic brain injury NOS
EXCLUDES 1   conditions classifiable to S06.0- to S06.8- code to specified intracranial injury
head injury NOS (S09.90)

✓6ᵗʰ **S06.9X Unspecified intracranial injury**

✓7ᵗʰ **S06.9X0 Unspecified intracranial injury** without loss of consciousness

✓7ᵗʰ **S06.9X1 Unspecified intracranial injury with loss of consciousness of** 30 minutes or less

✓7ᵗʰ **S06.9X2 Unspecified intracranial injury with loss of consciousness of** 31 minutes to 59 minutes

✓7ᵗʰ **S06.9X3 Unspecified intracranial injury with loss of consciousness of** 1 hour to 5 hours 59 minutes

✓7ᵗʰ **S06.9X4 Unspecified intracranial injury with loss of consciousness of** 6 hours to 24 hours

N Newborn: 0   P Pediatric: 0-17   M Maternity: 12-55   A Adult: 15-124   CH Comorbidity High   CL Comorbidity Low   NC Dx Noncancer Dx   PDx Primary Dx

958   ICD-10-CM 2020

√7ᵗʰ **S06.9X5** **Unspecified intracranial injury with loss of consciousness** greater than 24 hours **with return to pre-existing conscious level**

√7ᵗʰ **S06.9X6** **Unspecified intracranial injury with loss of consciousness** greater than 24 hours without return to pre-existing conscious level with patient surviving   NC Dx

√7ᵗʰ **S06.9X7** **Unspecified intracranial injury with loss of consciousness of** any duration **with death due to brain injury prior to regaining consciousness**

√7ᵗʰ **S06.9X8** **Unspecified intracranial injury with loss of consciousness of** any duration **with death due to** other **cause prior to regaining consciousness**

√7ᵗʰ **S06.9X9** **Unspecified intracranial injury with loss of consciousness of unspecified duration**

√4ᵗʰ **S07** **Crushing injury of head**

Use additional code for all associated injuries, such as:
   intracranial injuries (S06.-)
   skull fractures (S02.-)

The appropriate 7th character is to be added to each code from category S07.
   A   initial encounter
   D   subsequent encounter
   S   sequela

√x7ᵗʰ **S07.0** **Crushing injury of** face

√x7ᵗʰ **S07.1** **Crushing injury of** skull

√x7ᵗʰ **S07.8** **Crushing injury of other parts of head**

√x7ᵗʰ **S07.9** **Crushing injury of head, part unspecified**

√4ᵗʰ **S08** **Avulsion and traumatic amputation of part of head**

An amputation not identified as partial or complete should be coded to complete

The appropriate 7th character is to be added to each code from category S08.
   A   initial encounter
   D   subsequent encounter
   S   sequela

√x7ᵗʰ **S08.0** **Avulsion of** scalp

√5ᵗʰ **S08.1** **Traumatic amputation of** ear

√6ᵗʰ **S08.11** Complete **traumatic amputation of ear**

√7ᵗʰ **S08.111** **Complete traumatic amputation of** right **ear**

√7ᵗʰ **S08.112** **Complete traumatic amputation of** left **ear**

√7ᵗʰ **S08.119** **Complete traumatic amputation of unspecified ear**

√6ᵗʰ **S08.12** Partial **traumatic amputation of ear**

√7ᵗʰ **S08.121** **Partial traumatic amputation of** right **ear**

√7ᵗʰ **S08.122** **Partial traumatic amputation of** left **ear**

√7ᵗʰ **S08.129** **Partial traumatic amputation of unspecified ear**

√5ᵗʰ **S08.8** **Traumatic amputation of other parts of head**

√6ᵗʰ **S08.81** **Traumatic amputation of** nose

√7ᵗʰ **S08.811** Complete **traumatic amputation of nose**

√7ᵗʰ **S08.812** Partial **traumatic amputation of nose**

√x7ᵗʰ **S08.89** **Traumatic amputation of other parts of head**

√4ᵗʰ **S09** **Other and unspecified injuries of head**

The appropriate 7th character is to be added to each code from category S09.
   A   initial encounter
   D   subsequent encounter
   S   sequela

√x7ᵗʰ **S09.0** **Injury of** blood vessels **of head, not elsewhere classified**

EXCLUDES 1   injury of cerebral blood vessels (S06.-)
           injury of precerebral blood vessels (S15.-)

√5ᵗʰ **S09.1** **Injury of** muscle and tendon **of head**

Code also any associated open wound (S01.-)

EXCLUDES 2   sprain to joints and ligament of head (S03.9)

√7ᵗʰ **S09.10** **Unspecified injury of muscle and tendon of head**

Injury of muscle and tendon of head NOS

√x7ᵗʰ **S09.11** **Strain of muscle and tendon of head**

√x7ᵗʰ **S09.12** **Laceration of muscle and tendon of head**

√x7ᵗʰ **S09.19** **Other specified injury of muscle and tendon of head**

√5ᵗʰ **S09.2** **Traumatic rupture of** ear drum

EXCLUDES 1   traumatic rupture of ear drum due to blast injury (S09.31-)

√x7ᵗʰ **S09.20** **Traumatic rupture of unspecified ear drum**

√x7ᵗʰ **S09.21** **Traumatic rupture of** right **ear drum**

√x7ᵗʰ **S09.22** **Traumatic rupture of** left **ear drum**

√5ᵗʰ **S09.3** **Other specified and unspecified injury of middle and inner ear**

EXCLUDES 1   injury to ear NOS (S09.91-)

EXCLUDES 2   injury to external ear (S00.4-, S01.3-, S08.1-)

√6ᵗʰ **S09.30** **Unspecified injury of** middle and inner ear

√7ᵗʰ **S09.301** **Unspecified injury of** right **middle and inner ear**

√7ᵗʰ **S09.302** **Unspecified injury of** left **middle and inner ear**

√7ᵗʰ **S09.309** **Unspecified injury of unspecified middle and inner ear**

√6ᵗʰ **S09.31** **Primary** blast injury **of ear**

Blast injury of ear NOS

√7ᵗʰ **S09.311** **Primary blast injury of** right **ear**

√7ᵗʰ **S09.312** **Primary blast injury of** left **ear**

√7ᵗʰ **S09.313** **Primary blast injury of ear,** bilateral

√7ᵗʰ **S09.319** **Primary blast injury of unspecified ear**

√6ᵗʰ **S09.39** **Other specified injury of middle and inner ear**

Secondary blast injury to ear

√7ᵗʰ **S09.391** **Other specified injury of** right **middle and inner ear**

√7ᵗʰ **S09.392** **Other specified injury of** left **middle and inner ear**

√7ᵗʰ **S09.399** **Other specified injury of unspecified middle and inner ear**

√x7ᵗʰ **S09.8** **Other specified injuries of head**

√5ᵗʰ **S09.9** **Unspecified injury of face and head**

√x7ᵗʰ **S09.90** **Unspecified injury of** head

Head injury NOS

EXCLUDES 1   brain injury NOS (S06.9-)
           head injury NOS with loss of consciousness (S06.9-)
           intracranial injury NOS (S06.9-)

√x7ᵗʰ **S09.91** **Unspecified injury of** ear

Injury of ear NOS

√x7ᵗʰ **S09.92** **Unspecified injury of** nose

Injury of nose NOS

√x7ᵗʰ **S09.93** **Unspecified injury of** face

Injury of face NOS

AHA: 2019,2Q,23

✓ Additional Character Required   √x7ᵗʰ Placeholder Alert   Manifestation   Unspecified Dx   ►◄ Revised Text   ● New Code   ▲ Revised Title

Injuries to the neck (S10-S19)

INCLUDES injuries of nape
injuries of supraclavicular region
injuries of throat

EXCLUDES 2 burns and corrosions (T20-T32)
effects of foreign body in esophagus (T18.1)
effects of foreign body in larynx (T17.3)
effects of foreign body in pharynx (T17.2)
effects of foreign body in trachea (T17.4)
frostbite (T33-T34)
insect bite or sting, venomous (T63.4)

✓4ᵗʰ **S10 Superficial injury of neck**

The appropriate 7th character is to be added to each code from category S10.
A   initial encounter
D   subsequent encounter
S   sequela

✓x7ᵗʰ **S10.0 Contusion of throat**
Contusion of cervical esophagus
Contusion of larynx
Contusion of pharynx
Contusion of trachea

✓5ᵗʰ **S10.1 Other and unspecified superficial injuries of throat**
✓x7ᵗʰ **S10.10 Unspecified superficial injuries of throat**
✓x7ᵗʰ **S10.11 Abrasion of throat**
✓x7ᵗʰ **S10.12 Blister (nonthermal) of throat**
✓x7ᵗʰ **S10.14 External constriction of part of throat**
✓x7ᵗʰ **S10.15 Superficial foreign body of throat**
Splinter in the throat
✓x7ᵗʰ **S10.16 Insect bite (nonvenomous) of throat**
✓x7ᵗʰ **S10.17 Other superficial bite of throat**
EXCLUDES 1 open bite of throat (S11.85)

✓5ᵗʰ **S10.8 Superficial injury of other specified parts of neck**
✓x7ᵗʰ **S10.80 Unspecified superficial injury of other specified part of neck**
✓x7ᵗʰ **S10.81 Abrasion of other specified part of neck**
✓x7ᵗʰ **S10.82 Blister (nonthermal) of other specified part of neck**
✓x7ᵗʰ **S10.83 Contusion of other specified part of neck**
✓x7ᵗʰ **S10.84 External constriction of other specified part of neck**
✓x7ᵗʰ **S10.85 Superficial foreign body of other specified part of neck**
Splinter in other specified part of neck
✓x7ᵗʰ **S10.86 Insect bite of other specified part of neck**
✓x7ᵗʰ **S10.87 Other superficial bite of other specified part of neck**
EXCLUDES 1 open bite of other specified parts of neck (S11.85)

✓5ᵗʰ **S10.9 Superficial injury of unspecified part of neck**
✓x7ᵗʰ **S10.90 Unspecified superficial injury of unspecified part of neck**
✓x7ᵗʰ **S10.91 Abrasion of unspecified part of neck**
✓x7ᵗʰ **S10.92 Blister (nonthermal) of unspecified part of neck**
✓x7ᵗʰ **S10.93 Contusion of unspecified part of neck**
✓x7ᵗʰ **S10.94 External constriction of unspecified part of neck**
✓x7ᵗʰ **S10.95 Superficial foreign body of unspecified part of neck**
✓x7ᵗʰ **S10.96 Insect bite of unspecified part of neck**
✓x7ᵗʰ **S10.97 Other superficial bite of unspecified part of neck**

✓4ᵗʰ **S11 Open wound of neck**
Code also any associated:
spinal cord injury (S14.0, S14.1-)
wound infection
EXCLUDES 2 open fracture of vertebra (S12.- with 7th character B)

The appropriate 7th character is to be added to each code from category S11.
A   initial encounter
D   subsequent encounter
S   sequela

✓5ᵗʰ **S11.0 Open wound of larynx and trachea**
✓6ᵗʰ **S11.01 Open wound of larynx**
EXCLUDES 2 open wound of vocal cord (S11.03)
✓7ᵗʰ **S11.011 Laceration without foreign body of larynx**

✓7ᵗʰ **S11.012 Laceration with foreign body of larynx**
✓7ᵗʰ **S11.013 Puncture wound without foreign body of larynx**
✓7ᵗʰ **S11.014 Puncture wound with foreign body of larynx**
✓7ᵗʰ **S11.015 Open bite of larynx**
Bite of larynx NOS
✓7ᵗʰ **S11.019 Unspecified open wound of larynx**
✓6ᵗʰ **S11.02 Open wound of trachea**
Open wound of cervical trachea
Open wound of trachea NOS
EXCLUDES 2 open wound of thoracic trachea (S27.5-)
✓7ᵗʰ **S11.021 Laceration without foreign body of trachea**
✓7ᵗʰ **S11.022 Laceration with foreign body of trachea**
✓7ᵗʰ **S11.023 Puncture wound without foreign body of trachea**
✓7ᵗʰ **S11.024 Puncture wound with foreign body of trachea**
✓7ᵗʰ **S11.025 Open bite of trachea**
Bite of trachea NOS
✓7ᵗʰ **S11.029 Unspecified open wound of trachea**
✓6ᵗʰ **S11.03 Open wound of vocal cord**
✓7ᵗʰ **S11.031 Laceration without foreign body of vocal cord**
✓7ᵗʰ **S11.032 Laceration with foreign body of vocal cord**
✓7ᵗʰ **S11.033 Puncture wound without foreign body of vocal cord**
✓7ᵗʰ **S11.034 Puncture wound with foreign body of vocal cord**
✓7ᵗʰ **S11.035 Open bite of vocal cord**
Bite of vocal cord NOS
✓7ᵗʰ **S11.039 Unspecified open wound of vocal cord**

✓5ᵗʰ **S11.1 Open wound of thyroid gland**
✓x7ᵗʰ **S11.10 Unspecified open wound of thyroid gland**
✓x7ᵗʰ **S11.11 Laceration without foreign body of thyroid gland**
✓x7ᵗʰ **S11.12 Laceration with foreign body of thyroid gland**
✓x7ᵗʰ **S11.13 Puncture wound without foreign body of thyroid gland**
✓x7ᵗʰ **S11.14 Puncture wound with foreign body of thyroid gland**
✓x7ᵗʰ **S11.15 Open bite of thyroid gland**
Bite of thyroid gland NOS

✓5ᵗʰ **S11.2 Open wound of pharynx and cervical esophagus**
EXCLUDES 1 open wound of esophagus NOS (S27.8-)
✓x7ᵗʰ **S11.20 Unspecified open wound of pharynx and cervical esophagus**
✓x7ᵗʰ **S11.21 Laceration without foreign body of pharynx and cervical esophagus**
✓x7ᵗʰ **S11.22 Laceration with foreign body of pharynx and cervical esophagus**
✓x7ᵗʰ **S11.23 Puncture wound without foreign body of pharynx and cervical esophagus**
✓x7ᵗʰ **S11.24 Puncture wound with foreign body of pharynx and cervical esophagus**
✓x7ᵗʰ **S11.25 Open bite of pharynx and cervical esophagus**
Bite of pharynx and cervical esophagus NOS

✓5ᵗʰ **S11.8 Open wound of other specified parts of neck**
✓x7ᵗʰ **S11.80 Unspecified open wound of other specified part of neck**
✓x7ᵗʰ **S11.81 Laceration without foreign body of other specified part of neck**
✓x7ᵗʰ **S11.82 Laceration with foreign body of other specified part of neck**
✓x7ᵗʰ **S11.83 Puncture wound without foreign body of other specified part of neck**
✓x7ᵗʰ **S11.84 Puncture wound with foreign body of other specified part of neck**
✓x7ᵗʰ **S11.85 Open bite of other specified part of neck**
Bite of other specified part of neck NOS
EXCLUDES 1 superficial bite of other specified part of neck (S10.87)
✓x7ᵗʰ **S11.89 Other open wound of other specified part of neck**

✓5ᵗʰ **S11.9 Open wound of unspecified part of neck**
✓x7ᵗʰ **S11.90 Unspecified open wound of unspecified part of neck**

✓x7ᵗʰ **S11.91** Laceration without foreign body of unspecified part of neck

✓x7ᵗʰ **S11.92** Laceration with foreign body of unspecified part of neck

✓x7ᵗʰ **S11.93** Puncture wound without foreign body of unspecified part of neck

✓x7ᵗʰ **S11.94** Puncture wound with foreign body of unspecified part of neck

✓x7ᵗʰ **S11.95** Open bite of unspecified part of neck
Bite of neck NOS
EXCLUDES 1 superficial bite of neck (S10.97)

✓4ᵗʰ **S12** **Fracture of cervical vertebra and other parts of neck**

NOTE A fracture not indicated as displaced or nondisplaced should be coded to displaced.
A fracture not indicated as open or closed should be coded to closed.

INCLUDES fracture of cervical neural arch
fracture of cervical spine
fracture of cervical spinous process
fracture of cervical transverse process
fracture of cervical vertebral arch
fracture of neck

Code first any associated cervical spinal cord injury (S14.0, S14.1-)
AHA: 2018,2Q,12; 2015,3Q,37-39
TIP: The term "improper alignment" is not synonymous with malunion or nonunion of a fracture when noted in provider documentation.

The appropriate 7th character is to be added to all codes from subcategories S12.0-S12.6.
A   initial encounter for closed fracture
B   initial encounter for open fracture
D   subsequent encounter for fracture with routine healing
G   subsequent encounter for fracture with delayed healing
K   subsequent encounter for fracture with nonunion
S   sequela

✓5ᵗʰ **S12.0** **Fracture of first cervical vertebra**
Atlas
✓6ᵗʰ **S12.00** Unspecified fracture of first cervical vertebra
✓7ᵗʰ **S12.000** Unspecified displaced fracture of first cervical vertebra
✓7ᵗʰ **S12.001** Unspecified nondisplaced fracture of first cervical vertebra
✓x7ᵗʰ **S12.01** Stable burst fracture of first cervical vertebra
✓x7ᵗʰ **S12.02** Unstable burst fracture of first cervical vertebra
✓6ᵗʰ **S12.03** Posterior arch fracture of first cervical vertebra
✓7ᵗʰ **S12.030** Displaced posterior arch fracture of first cervical vertebra
✓7ᵗʰ **S12.031** Nondisplaced posterior arch fracture of first cervical vertebra
✓6ᵗʰ **S12.04** Lateral mass fracture of first cervical vertebra
✓7ᵗʰ **S12.040** Displaced lateral mass fracture of first cervical vertebra
✓7ᵗʰ **S12.041** Nondisplaced lateral mass fracture of first cervical vertebra
✓6ᵗʰ **S12.09** Other fracture of first cervical vertebra
✓7ᵗʰ **S12.090** Other displaced fracture of first cervical vertebra
✓7ᵗʰ **S12.091** Other nondisplaced fracture of first cervical vertebra

✓5ᵗʰ **S12.1** **Fracture of second cervical vertebra**
Axis
✓6ᵗʰ **S12.10** Unspecified fracture of second cervical vertebra
✓7ᵗʰ **S12.100** Unspecified displaced fracture of second cervical vertebra
✓7ᵗʰ **S12.101** Unspecified nondisplaced fracture of second cervical vertebra
✓6ᵗʰ **S12.11** Type II dens fracture
✓7ᵗʰ **S12.110** Anterior displaced Type II dens fracture
✓7ᵗʰ **S12.111** Posterior displaced Type II dens fracture
✓7ᵗʰ **S12.112** Nondisplaced Type II dens fracture
✓6ᵗʰ **S12.12** Other dens fracture
✓7ᵗʰ **S12.120** Other displaced dens fracture
✓7ᵗʰ **S12.121** Other nondisplaced dens fracture

✓6ᵗʰ **S12.13** Unspecified traumatic spondylolisthesis of second cervical vertebra
✓7ᵗʰ **S12.130** Unspecified traumatic displaced spondylolisthesis of second cervical vertebra
✓7ᵗʰ **S12.131** Unspecified traumatic nondisplaced spondylolisthesis of second cervical vertebra
✓x7ᵗʰ **S12.14** Type III traumatic spondylolisthesis of second cervical vertebra
✓6ᵗʰ **S12.15** Other traumatic spondylolisthesis of second cervical vertebra
✓7ᵗʰ **S12.150** Other traumatic displaced spondylolisthesis of second cervical vertebra
✓7ᵗʰ **S12.151** Other traumatic nondisplaced spondylolisthesis of second cervical vertebra
✓6ᵗʰ **S12.19** Other fracture of second cervical vertebra
✓7ᵗʰ **S12.190** Other displaced fracture of second cervical vertebra
✓7ᵗʰ **S12.191** Other nondisplaced fracture of second cervical vertebra

✓5ᵗʰ **S12.2** **Fracture of third cervical vertebra**
✓6ᵗʰ **S12.20** Unspecified fracture of third cervical vertebra
✓7ᵗʰ **S12.200** Unspecified displaced fracture of third cervical vertebra
✓7ᵗʰ **S12.201** Unspecified nondisplaced fracture of third cervical vertebra
✓6ᵗʰ **S12.23** Unspecified traumatic spondylolisthesis of third cervical vertebra
✓7ᵗʰ **S12.230** Unspecified traumatic displaced spondylolisthesis of third cervical vertebra
✓7ᵗʰ **S12.231** Unspecified traumatic nondisplaced spondylolisthesis of third cervical vertebra
✓x7ᵗʰ **S12.24** Type III traumatic spondylolisthesis of third cervical vertebra
✓6ᵗʰ **S12.25** Other traumatic spondylolisthesis of third cervical vertebra
✓7ᵗʰ **S12.250** Other traumatic displaced spondylolisthesis of third cervical vertebra
✓7ᵗʰ **S12.251** Other traumatic nondisplaced spondylolisthesis of third cervical vertebra
✓6ᵗʰ **S12.29** Other fracture of third cervical vertebra
✓7ᵗʰ **S12.290** Other displaced fracture of third cervical vertebra
✓7ᵗʰ **S12.291** Other nondisplaced fracture of third cervical vertebra

✓5ᵗʰ **S12.3** **Fracture of fourth cervical vertebra**
✓6ᵗʰ **S12.30** Unspecified fracture of fourth cervical vertebra
✓7ᵗʰ **S12.300** Unspecified displaced fracture of fourth cervical vertebra
✓7ᵗʰ **S12.301** Unspecified nondisplaced fracture of fourth cervical vertebra
✓6ᵗʰ **S12.33** Unspecified traumatic spondylolisthesis of fourth cervical vertebra
✓7ᵗʰ **S12.330** Unspecified traumatic displaced spondylolisthesis of fourth cervical vertebra
✓7ᵗʰ **S12.331** Unspecified traumatic nondisplaced spondylolisthesis of fourth cervical vertebra
✓x7ᵗʰ **S12.34** Type III traumatic spondylolisthesis of fourth cervical vertebra
✓6ᵗʰ **S12.35** Other traumatic spondylolisthesis of fourth cervical vertebra
✓7ᵗʰ **S12.350** Other traumatic displaced spondylolisthesis of fourth cervical vertebra
✓7ᵗʰ **S12.351** Other traumatic nondisplaced spondylolisthesis of fourth cervical vertebra
✓6ᵗʰ **S12.39** Other fracture of fourth cervical vertebra
✓7ᵗʰ **S12.390** Other displaced fracture of fourth cervical vertebra
✓7ᵗʰ **S12.391** Other nondisplaced fracture of fourth cervical vertebra

☑5ʰ S12.4 Fracture of fifth cervical vertebra

  ☑6ʰ S12.40 Unspecified fracture of fifth cervical vertebra

    ☑7ʰ S12.400 Unspecified displaced fracture of fifth cervical vertebra

    ☑7ʰ S12.401 Unspecified nondisplaced fracture of fifth cervical vertebra

  ☑6ʰ S12.43 Unspecified traumatic spondylolisthesis of fifth cervical vertebra

    ☑7ʰ S12.430 Unspecified traumatic displaced spondylolisthesis of fifth cervical vertebra

    ☑7ʰ S12.431 Unspecified traumatic nondisplaced spondylolisthesis of fifth cervical vertebra

  ☑x7ʰ S12.44 Type III traumatic spondylolisthesis of fifth cervical vertebra

  ☑6ʰ S12.45 Other traumatic spondylolisthesis of fifth cervical vertebra

    ☑7ʰ S12.450 Other traumatic displaced spondylolisthesis of fifth cervical vertebra

    ☑7ʰ S12.451 Other traumatic nondisplaced spondylolisthesis of fifth cervical vertebra

  ☑6ʰ S12.49 Other fracture of fifth cervical vertebra

    ☑7ʰ S12.490 Other displaced fracture of fifth cervical vertebra

    ☑7ʰ S12.491 Other nondisplaced fracture of fifth cervical vertebra

☑5ʰ S12.5 Fracture of sixth cervical vertebra

  ☑6ʰ S12.50 Unspecified fracture of sixth cervical vertebra

    ☑7ʰ S12.500 Unspecified displaced fracture of sixth cervical vertebra

    ☑7ʰ S12.501 Unspecified nondisplaced fracture of sixth cervical vertebra

  ☑6ʰ S12.53 Unspecified traumatic spondylolisthesis of sixth cervical vertebra

    ☑7ʰ S12.530 Unspecified traumatic displaced spondylolisthesis of sixth cervical vertebra

    ☑7ʰ S12.531 Unspecified traumatic nondisplaced spondylolisthesis of sixth cervical vertebra

  ☑x7ʰ S12.54 Type III traumatic spondylolisthesis of sixth cervical vertebra

  ☑6ʰ S12.55 Other traumatic spondylolisthesis of sixth cervical vertebra

    ☑7ʰ S12.550 Other traumatic displaced spondylolisthesis of sixth cervical vertebra

    ☑7ʰ S12.551 Other traumatic nondisplaced spondylolisthesis of sixth cervical vertebra

  ☑6ʰ S12.59 Other fracture of sixth cervical vertebra

    ☑7ʰ S12.590 Other displaced fracture of sixth cervical vertebra

    ☑7ʰ S12.591 Other nondisplaced fracture of sixth cervical vertebra

☑5ʰ S12.6 Fracture of seventh cervical vertebra

  ☑6ʰ S12.60 Unspecified fracture of seventh cervical vertebra

    ☑7ʰ S12.600 Unspecified displaced fracture of seventh cervical vertebra

    ☑7ʰ S12.601 Unspecified nondisplaced fracture of seventh cervical vertebra

  ☑6ʰ S12.63 Unspecified traumatic spondylolisthesis of seventh cervical vertebra

    ☑7ʰ S12.630 Unspecified traumatic displaced spondylolisthesis of seventh cervical vertebra

    ☑7ʰ S12.631 Unspecified traumatic nondisplaced spondylolisthesis of seventh cervical vertebra

  ☑x7ʰ S12.64 Type III traumatic spondylolisthesis of seventh cervical vertebra

  ☑6ʰ S12.65 Other traumatic spondylolisthesis of seventh cervical vertebra

    ☑7ʰ S12.650 Other traumatic displaced spondylolisthesis of seventh cervical vertebra

    ☑7ʰ S12.651 Other traumatic nondisplaced spondylolisthesis of seventh cervical vertebra

  ☑6ʰ S12.69 Other fracture of seventh cervical vertebra

    ☑7ʰ S12.690 Other displaced fracture of seventh cervical vertebra

    ☑7ʰ S12.691 Other nondisplaced fracture of seventh cervical vertebra

☑x7ʰ S12.8 Fracture of other parts of neck

  Hyoid bone
  Larynx
  Thyroid cartilage
  Trachea

  The appropriate 7th character is to be added to code S12.8.
  A initial encounter
  D subsequent encounter
  S sequela

☑x7ʰ S12.9 Fracture of neck, unspecified

  Fracture of neck NOS
  Fracture of cervical spine NOS
  Fracture of cervical vertebra NOS

  The appropriate 7th character is to be added to code S12.9.
  A initial encounter
  D subsequent encounter
  S sequela

☑4ʰ S13 Dislocation and sprain of joints and ligaments at neck level

  INCLUDES avulsion of joint or ligament at neck level
    laceration of cartilage, joint or ligament at neck level
    sprain of cartilage, joint or ligament at neck level
    traumatic hemarthrosis of joint or ligament at neck level
    traumatic rupture of joint or ligament at neck level
    traumatic subluxation of joint or ligament at neck level
    traumatic tear of joint or ligament at neck level
  Code also any associated open wound
  EXCLUDES 2 strain of muscle or tendon at neck level (S16.1)

  The appropriate 7th character is to be added to each code from category S13.
  A initial encounter
  D subsequent encounter
  S sequela

☑x7ʰ S13.0 Traumatic rupture of cervical intervertebral disc

  EXCLUDES 1 rupture or displacement (nontraumatic) of cervical intervertebral disc NOS (M50.-)

☑5ʰ S13.1 Subluxation and dislocation of cervical vertebrae

  Code also any associated:
    open wound of neck (S11.-)
    spinal cord injury (S14.1-)
  EXCLUDES 2 fracture of cervical vertebrae (S12.0-S12.3-)

  ☑6ʰ S13.10 Subluxation and dislocation of unspecified cervical vertebrae

    ☑7ʰ S13.100 Subluxation of unspecified cervical vertebrae

    ☑7ʰ S13.101 Dislocation of unspecified cervical vertebrae

  ☑6ʰ S13.11 Subluxation and dislocation of C0/C1 cervical vertebrae

    Subluxation and dislocation of atlantooccipital joint
    Subluxation and dislocation of atloidooccipital joint
    Subluxation and dislocation of occipitoatloid joint

    ☑7ʰ S13.110 Subluxation of C0/C1 cervical vertebrae

    ☑7ʰ S13.111 Dislocation of C0/C1 cervical vertebrae

  ☑6ʰ S13.12 Subluxation and dislocation of C1/C2 cervical vertebrae

    Subluxation and dislocation of atlantoaxial joint

    ☑7ʰ S13.120 Subluxation of C1/C2 cervical vertebrae

    ☑7ʰ S13.121 Dislocation of C1/C2 cervical vertebrae

  ☑6ʰ S13.13 Subluxation and dislocation of C2/C3 cervical vertebrae

    ☑7ʰ S13.130 Subluxation of C2/C3 cervical vertebrae

    ☑7ʰ S13.131 Dislocation of C2/C3 cervical vertebrae

  ☑6ʰ S13.14 Subluxation and dislocation of C3/C4 cervical vertebrae

    ☑7ʰ S13.140 Subluxation of C3/C4 cervical vertebrae

    ☑7ʰ S13.141 Dislocation of C3/C4 cervical vertebrae

  ☑6ʰ S13.15 Subluxation and dislocation of C4/C5 cervical vertebrae

    ☑7ʰ S13.150 Subluxation of C4/C5 cervical vertebrae

    ☑7ʰ S13.151 Dislocation of C4/C5 cervical vertebrae

N Newborn: 0   P Pediatric: 0-17   M Maternity: 12-55   A Adult: 15-124   CH Comorbidity High   CL Comorbidity Low   NC Dx Noncancer Dx   PDx Primary Dx

962

ICD-10-CM 2020

S13.16 Subluxation and dislocation of C5/C6 cervical vertebrae
- **S13.160** Subluxation of C5/C6 cervical vertebrae
- **S13.161** Dislocation of C5/C6 cervical vertebrae

S13.17 Subluxation and dislocation of C6/C7 cervical vertebrae
- **S13.170** Subluxation of C6/C7 cervical vertebrae
- **S13.171** Dislocation of C6/C7 cervical vertebrae

S13.18 Subluxation and dislocation of C7/T1 cervical vertebrae
- **S13.180** Subluxation of C7/T1 cervical vertebrae
- **S13.181** Dislocation of C7/T1 cervical vertebrae

S13.2 Dislocation of other and unspecified parts of neck
- **S13.20** Dislocation of unspecified parts of neck
- **S13.29** Dislocation of other parts of neck

S13.4 Sprain of ligaments of cervical spine
> Sprain of anterior longitudinal (ligament), cervical
> Sprain of atlanto-axial (joints)
> Sprain of atlanto-occipital (joints)
> Whiplash injury of cervical spine

S13.5 Sprain of thyroid region
> Sprain of cricoarytenoid (joint) (ligament)
> Sprain of cricothyroid (joint) (ligament)
> Sprain of thyroid cartilage

S13.8 Sprain of joints and ligaments of other parts of neck

S13.9 Sprain of joints and ligaments of unspecified parts of neck

S14 Injury of nerves and spinal cord at neck level

> **NOTE** Code to highest level of cervical cord injury

> Code also any associated:
> fracture of cervical vertebra (S12.0- — S12.6-.)
> open wound of neck (S11.-)
> transient paralysis (R29.5)

> The appropriate 7th character is to be added to each code from category S14.
> A initial encounter
> D subsequent encounter
> S sequela

S14.0 Concussion and edema of cervical spinal cord

S14.1 Other and unspecified injuries of cervical spinal cord
- **S14.10** Unspecified injury of cervical spinal cord
  - **S14.101** Unspecified injury at C1 level of cervical spinal cord
  - **S14.102** Unspecified injury at C2 level of cervical spinal cord
  - **S14.103** Unspecified injury at C3 level of cervical spinal cord
  - **S14.104** Unspecified injury at C4 level of cervical spinal cord
  - **S14.105** Unspecified injury at C5 level of cervical spinal cord
  - **S14.106** Unspecified injury at C6 level of cervical spinal cord
  - **S14.107** Unspecified injury at C7 level of cervical spinal cord
  - **S14.108** Unspecified injury at C8 level of cervical spinal cord
  - **S14.109** Unspecified injury at unspecified level of cervical spinal cord
    > Injury of cervical spinal cord NOS
- **S14.11** Complete lesion of cervical spinal cord
  - **S14.111** Complete lesion at C1 level of cervical spinal cord
  - **S14.112** Complete lesion at C2 level of cervical spinal cord
  - **S14.113** Complete lesion at C3 level of cervical spinal cord
  - **S14.114** Complete lesion at C4 level of cervical spinal cord
  - **S14.115** Complete lesion at C5 level of cervical spinal cord
  - **S14.116** Complete lesion at C6 level of cervical spinal cord
  - **S14.117** Complete lesion at C7 level of cervical spinal cord
  - **S14.118** Complete lesion at C8 level of cervical spinal cord

- **S14.119** Complete lesion at unspecified level of cervical spinal cord
- **S14.12** Central cord syndrome of cervical spinal cord
  - **S14.121** Central cord syndrome at C1 level of cervical spinal cord
  - **S14.122** Central cord syndrome at C2 level of cervical spinal cord
  - **S14.123** Central cord syndrome at C3 level of cervical spinal cord
  - **S14.124** Central cord syndrome at C4 level of cervical spinal cord
  - **S14.125** Central cord syndrome at C5 level of cervical spinal cord
  - **S14.126** Central cord syndrome at C6 level of cervical spinal cord
  - **S14.127** Central cord syndrome at C7 level of cervical spinal cord
  - **S14.128** Central cord syndrome at C8 level of cervical spinal cord
  - **S14.129** Central cord syndrome at unspecified level of cervical spinal cord
- **S14.13** Anterior cord syndrome of cervical spinal cord
  - **S14.131** Anterior cord syndrome at C1 level of cervical spinal cord
  - **S14.132** Anterior cord syndrome at C2 level of cervical spinal cord
  - **S14.133** Anterior cord syndrome at C3 level of cervical spinal cord
  - **S14.134** Anterior cord syndrome at C4 level of cervical spinal cord
  - **S14.135** Anterior cord syndrome at C5 level of cervical spinal cord
  - **S14.136** Anterior cord syndrome at C6 level of cervical spinal cord
  - **S14.137** Anterior cord syndrome at C7 level of cervical spinal cord
  - **S14.138** Anterior cord syndrome at C8 level of cervical spinal cord
  - **S14.139** Anterior cord syndrome at unspecified level of cervical spinal cord
- **S14.14** Brown-Séquard syndrome of cervical spinal cord
  - **S14.141** Brown-Séquard syndrome at C1 level of cervical spinal cord
  - **S14.142** Brown-Séquard syndrome at C2 level of cervical spinal cord
  - **S14.143** Brown-Séquard syndrome at C3 level of cervical spinal cord
  - **S14.144** Brown-Séquard syndrome at C4 level of cervical spinal cord
  - **S14.145** Brown-Séquard syndrome at C5 level of cervical spinal cord
  - **S14.146** Brown-Séquard syndrome at C6 level of cervical spinal cord
  - **S14.147** Brown-Séquard syndrome at C7 level of cervical spinal cord
  - **S14.148** Brown-Séquard syndrome at C8 level of cervical spinal cord
  - **S14.149** Brown-Séquard syndrome at unspecified level of cervical spinal cord
- **S14.15** Other incomplete lesions of cervical spinal cord
  > Incomplete lesion of cervical spinal cord NOS
  > Posterior cord syndrome of cervical spinal cord
  - **S14.151** Other incomplete lesion at C1 level of cervical spinal cord
  - **S14.152** Other incomplete lesion at C2 level of cervical spinal cord
  - **S14.153** Other incomplete lesion at C3 level of cervical spinal cord
  - **S14.154** Other incomplete lesion at C4 level of cervical spinal cord
  - **S14.155** Other incomplete lesion at C5 level of cervical spinal cord
  - **S14.156** Other incomplete lesion at C6 level of cervical spinal cord
  - **S14.157** Other incomplete lesion at C7 level of cervical spinal cord
  - **S14.158** Other incomplete lesion at C8 level of cervical spinal cord
  - **S14.159** Other incomplete lesion at unspecified level of cervical spinal cord

S14.2 Injury of nerve root of cervical spine

S14.3 Injury of brachial plexus

Chapter 19. Injury, Poisoning and Certain Other Consequences of External Causes

√x7ᵗʰ **S14.4** **Injury of** peripheral nerves of neck

√x7ᵗʰ **S14.5** **Injury of** cervical sympathetic nerves

√x7ᵗʰ **S14.8** **Injury of other specified nerves of neck**

√x7ᵗʰ **S14.9** **Injury of unspecified nerves of neck**

√4ᵗʰ **S15** **Injury of blood vessels at neck level**

    Code also any associated open wound (S11.-)

> The appropriate 7th character is to be added to each code from category S15.
> A   initial encounter
> D   subsequent encounter
> S   sequela

√6ᵗʰ **S15.0** **Injury of** carotid artery **of neck**

    Injury of carotid artery (common) (external) (internal, extracranial portion)
    Injury of carotid artery NOS

    EXCLUDES 1   injury of internal carotid artery, intracranial portion (S06.8)

√6ᵗʰ **S15.00** **Unspecified injury of carotid artery**

  √7ᵗʰ **S15.001** **Unspecified injury of** right **carotid artery**

  √7ᵗʰ **S15.002** **Unspecified injury of** left **carotid artery**

  √7ᵗʰ **S15.009** **Unspecified injury of unspecified carotid artery**

√6ᵗʰ **S15.01** Minor laceration **of carotid artery**

    Incomplete transection of carotid artery
    Laceration of carotid artery NOS
    Superficial laceration of carotid artery

  √7ᵗʰ **S15.011** **Minor laceration of** right **carotid artery**

  √7ᵗʰ **S15.012** **Minor laceration of** left **carotid artery**

  √7ᵗʰ **S15.019** **Minor laceration of unspecified carotid artery**

√6ᵗʰ **S15.02** Major laceration **of carotid artery**

    Complete transection of carotid artery
    Traumatic rupture of carotid artery

  √7ᵗʰ **S15.021** **Major laceration of** right **carotid artery**

  √7ᵗʰ **S15.022** **Major laceration of** left **carotid artery**

  √7ᵗʰ **S15.029** **Major laceration of unspecified carotid artery**

√6ᵗʰ **S15.09** **Other specified injury of carotid artery**

  √7ᵗʰ **S15.091** **Other specified injury of** right **carotid artery**

  √7ᵗʰ **S15.092** **Other specified injury of** left **carotid artery**

  √7ᵗʰ **S15.099** **Other specified injury of unspecified carotid artery**

√5ᵗʰ **S15.1** **Injury of** vertebral artery

√6ᵗʰ **S15.10** **Unspecified injury of vertebral artery**

  √7ᵗʰ **S15.101** **Unspecified injury of** right **vertebral artery**

  √7ᵗʰ **S15.102** **Unspecified injury of** left **vertebral artery**

  √7ᵗʰ **S15.109** **Unspecified injury of unspecified vertebral artery**

√6ᵗʰ **S15.11** Minor laceration **of vertebral artery**

    Incomplete transection of vertebral artery
    Laceration of vertebral artery NOS
    Superficial laceration of vertebral artery

  √7ᵗʰ **S15.111** **Minor laceration of** right **vertebral artery**

  √7ᵗʰ **S15.112** **Minor laceration of** left **vertebral artery**

  √7ᵗʰ **S15.119** **Minor laceration of unspecified vertebral artery**

√6ᵗʰ **S15.12** Major laceration **of vertebral artery**

    Complete transection of vertebral artery
    Traumatic rupture of vertebral artery

  √7ᵗʰ **S15.121** **Major laceration of** right **vertebral artery**

  √7ᵗʰ **S15.122** **Major laceration of** left **vertebral artery**

  √7ᵗʰ **S15.129** **Major laceration of unspecified vertebral artery**

√6ᵗʰ **S15.19** **Other specified injury of vertebral artery**

  √7ᵗʰ **S15.191** **Other specified injury of** right **vertebral artery**

  √7ᵗʰ **S15.192** **Other specified injury of** left **vertebral artery**

  √7ᵗʰ **S15.199** **Other specified injury of unspecified vertebral artery**

√5ᵗʰ **S15.2** **Injury of** external jugular vein

√6ᵗʰ **S15.20** **Unspecified injury of external jugular vein**

  √7ᵗʰ **S15.201** **Unspecified injury of** right **external jugular vein**

  √7ᵗʰ **S15.202** **Unspecified injury of** left **external jugular vein**

  √7ᵗʰ **S15.209** **Unspecified injury of unspecified external jugular vein**

√6ᵗʰ **S15.21** Minor laceration **of external jugular vein**

    Incomplete transection of external jugular vein
    Laceration of external jugular vein NOS
    Superficial laceration of external jugular vein

  √7ᵗʰ **S15.211** **Minor laceration of** right **external jugular vein**

  √7ᵗʰ **S15.212** **Minor laceration of** left **external jugular vein**

  √7ᵗʰ **S15.219** **Minor laceration of unspecified external jugular vein**

√6ᵗʰ **S15.22** Major laceration **of external jugular vein**

    Complete transection of external jugular vein
    Traumatic rupture of external jugular vein

  √7ᵗʰ **S15.221** **Major laceration of** right **external jugular vein**

  √7ᵗʰ **S15.222** **Major laceration of** left **external jugular vein**

  √7ᵗʰ **S15.229** **Major laceration of unspecified external jugular vein**

√6ᵗʰ **S15.29** **Other specified injury of external jugular vein**

  √7ᵗʰ **S15.291** **Other specified injury of** right **external jugular vein**

  √7ᵗʰ **S15.292** **Other specified injury of** left **external jugular vein**

  √7ᵗʰ **S15.299** **Other specified injury of unspecified external jugular vein**

√5ᵗʰ **S15.3** **Injury of** internal jugular vein

√6ᵗʰ **S15.30** **Unspecified injury of internal jugular vein**

  √7ᵗʰ **S15.301** **Unspecified injury of** right **internal jugular vein**

  √7ᵗʰ **S15.302** **Unspecified injury of** left **internal jugular vein**

  √7ᵗʰ **S15.309** **Unspecified injury of unspecified internal jugular vein**

√6ᵗʰ **S15.31** Minor laceration **of internal jugular vein**

    Incomplete transection of internal jugular vein
    Laceration of internal jugular vein NOS
    Superficial laceration of internal jugular vein

  √7ᵗʰ **S15.311** **Minor laceration of** right **internal jugular vein**

  √7ᵗʰ **S15.312** **Minor laceration of** left **internal jugular vein**

  √7ᵗʰ **S15.319** **Minor laceration of unspecified internal jugular vein**

√6ᵗʰ **S15.32** Major laceration **of internal jugular vein**

    Complete transection of internal jugular vein
    Traumatic rupture of internal jugular vein

  √7ᵗʰ **S15.321** **Major laceration of** right **internal jugular vein**

  √7ᵗʰ **S15.322** **Major laceration of** left **internal jugular vein**

  √7ᵗʰ **S15.329** **Major laceration of unspecified internal jugular vein**

√6ᵗʰ **S15.39** **Other specified injury of internal jugular vein**

  √7ᵗʰ **S15.391** **Other specified injury of** right **internal jugular vein**

  √7ᵗʰ **S15.392** **Other specified injury of** left **internal jugular vein**

  √7ᵗʰ **S15.399** **Other specified injury of unspecified internal jugular vein**

√x7ᵗʰ **S15.8** **Injury of other specified blood vessels at neck level**

√x7ᵗʰ **S15.9** **Injury of unspecified blood vessel at neck level**

Ⓝ Newborn: 0   Ⓟ Pediatric: 0-17   Ⓜ Maternity: 12-55   Ⓐ Adult: 15-124   CH Comorbidity High   CL Comorbidity Low   NCDx Noncancer Dx   PDx Primary Dx

964   ICD-10-CM 2020

✓4ᵗʰ **S16 Injury of muscle, fascia and tendon at neck level**

> Code also any associated open wound (S11.-)
>
> EXCLUDES 2   *sprain of joint or ligament at neck level (S13.9)*
>
> The appropriate 7th character is to be added to each code from category S16.
> A   initial encounter
> D   subsequent encounter
> S   sequela

✓x7ᵗʰ **S16.1 Strain of muscle, fascia and tendon at neck level**

✓x7ᵗʰ **S16.2 Laceration of muscle, fascia and tendon at neck level**

✓x7ᵗʰ **S16.8 Other specified injury of muscle, fascia and tendon at neck level**

✓x7ᵗʰ **S16.9 Unspecified injury of muscle, fascia and tendon at neck level**

✓4ᵗʰ **S17 Crushing injury of neck**

> Use additional code for all associated injuries, such as:
>   injury of blood vessels (S15.-)
>   open wound of neck (S11.-)
>   spinal cord injury (S14.0, S14.1-)
>   vertebral fracture (S12.0- — S12.3-)
>
> The appropriate 7th character is to be added to each code from category S17.
> A   initial encounter
> D   subsequent encounter
> S   sequela

✓x7ᵗʰ **S17.0 Crushing injury of larynx and trachea**

✓x7ᵗʰ **S17.8 Crushing injury of other specified parts of neck**

✓x7ᵗʰ **S17.9 Crushing injury of neck, part unspecified**

✓4ᵗʰ **S19 Other specified and unspecified injuries of neck**

> The appropriate 7th character is to be added to each code from category S19.
> A   initial encounter
> D   subsequent encounter
> S   sequela

✓5ᵗʰ **S19.8 Other specified injuries of neck**

✓x7ᵗʰ **S19.80 Other specified injuries of unspecified part of neck**

✓x7ᵗʰ **S19.81 Other specified injuries of larynx**

✓x7ᵗʰ **S19.82 Other specified injuries of cervical trachea**

> EXCLUDES 2   *other specified injury of thoracic trachea (S27.5-)*

✓x7ᵗʰ **S19.83 Other specified injuries of vocal cord**

✓x7ᵗʰ **S19.84 Other specified injuries of thyroid gland**

✓x7ᵗʰ **S19.85 Other specified injuries of pharynx and cervical esophagus**

✓x7ᵗʰ **S19.89 Other specified injuries of other specified part of neck**

✓x7ᵗʰ **S19.9 Unspecified injury of neck**

Injuries to the thorax (S20-S29)

INCLUDES   injuries of breast
            injuries of chest (wall)
            injuries of interscapular area

EXCLUDES 2 *burns and corrosions (T20-T32)*
            effects of foreign body in bronchus (T17.5)
            effects of foreign body in esophagus (T18.1)
            effects of foreign body in lung (T17.8)
            effects of foreign body in trachea (T17.4)
            frostbite (T33-T34)
            injuries of axilla
            injuries of clavicle
            injuries of scapular region
            injuries of shoulder
            insect bite or sting, venomous (T63.4)

✓4ᵗʰ **S20 Superficial injury of thorax**

> The appropriate 7th character is to be added to each code from category S20.
> A   initial encounter
> D   subsequent encounter
> S   sequela

✓5ᵗʰ **S20.0 Contusion of breast**

✓x7ᵗʰ **S20.00 Contusion of breast, unspecified breast**

✓x7ᵗʰ **S20.01 Contusion of right breast**

✓x7ᵗʰ **S20.02 Contusion of left breast**

✓5ᵗʰ **S20.1 Other and unspecified superficial injuries of breast**

✓6ᵗʰ **S20.10 Unspecified superficial injuries of breast**

✓7ᵗʰ **S20.101 Unspecified superficial injuries of breast, right breast**

✓7ᵗʰ **S20.102 Unspecified superficial injuries of breast, left breast**

✓7ᵗʰ **S20.109 Unspecified superficial injuries of breast, unspecified breast**

✓6ᵗʰ **S20.11 Abrasion of breast**

✓7ᵗʰ **S20.111 Abrasion of breast, right breast**

✓7ᵗʰ **S20.112 Abrasion of breast, left breast**

✓7ᵗʰ **S20.119 Abrasion of breast, unspecified breast**

✓6ᵗʰ **S20.12 Blister (nonthermal) of breast**

✓7ᵗʰ **S20.121 Blister (nonthermal) of breast, right breast**

✓7ᵗʰ **S20.122 Blister (nonthermal) of breast, left breast**

✓7ᵗʰ **S20.129 Blister (nonthermal) of breast, unspecified breast**

✓6ᵗʰ **S20.14 External constriction of part of breast**

✓7ᵗʰ **S20.141 External constriction of part of breast, right breast**

✓7ᵗʰ **S20.142 External constriction of part of breast, left breast**

✓7ᵗʰ **S20.149 External constriction of part of breast, unspecified breast**

✓6ᵗʰ **S20.15 Superficial foreign body of breast**

> Splinter in the breast

✓7ᵗʰ **S20.151 Superficial foreign body of breast, right breast**

✓7ᵗʰ **S20.152 Superficial foreign body of breast, left breast**

✓7ᵗʰ **S20.159 Superficial foreign body of breast, unspecified breast**

✓6ᵗʰ **S20.16 Insect bite (nonvenomous) of breast**

✓7ᵗʰ **S20.161 Insect bite (nonvenomous) of breast, right breast**

✓7ᵗʰ **S20.162 Insect bite (nonvenomous) of breast, left breast**

✓7ᵗʰ **S20.169 Insect bite (nonvenomous) of breast, unspecified breast**

✓6ᵗʰ **S20.17 Other superficial bite of breast**

> EXCLUDES 1   *open bite of breast (S21.05-)*

✓7ᵗʰ **S20.171 Other superficial bite of breast, right breast**

✓7ᵗʰ **S20.172 Other superficial bite of breast, left breast**

✓7ᵗʰ **S20.179 Other superficial bite of breast, unspecified breast**

✓5ᵗʰ **S20.2 Contusion of thorax**

✓x7ᵗʰ **S20.20 Contusion of thorax, unspecified**

✓6ᵗʰ **S20.21 Contusion of front wall of thorax**

✓7ᵗʰ **S20.211 Contusion of right front wall of thorax**

✓7ᵗʰ **S20.212 Contusion of left front wall of thorax**

✓7ᵗʰ **S20.219 Contusion of unspecified front wall of thorax**

✓6ᵗʰ **S20.22 Contusion of back wall of thorax**

✓7ᵗʰ **S20.221 Contusion of right back wall of thorax**

✓7ᵗʰ **S20.222 Contusion of left back wall of thorax**

✓7ᵗʰ **S20.229 Contusion of unspecified back wall of thorax**

✓5ᵗʰ **S20.3 Other and unspecified superficial injuries of front wall of thorax**

✓6ᵗʰ **S20.30 Unspecified superficial injuries of front wall of thorax**

✓7ᵗʰ **S20.301 Unspecified superficial injuries of right front wall of thorax**

✓7ᵗʰ **S20.302 Unspecified superficial injuries of left front wall of thorax**

✓7ᵗʰ **S20.309 Unspecified superficial injuries of unspecified front wall of thorax**

✓6ᵗʰ **S20.31 Abrasion of front wall of thorax**

✓7ᵗʰ **S20.311 Abrasion of right front wall of thorax**

✓7ᵗʰ **S20.312 Abrasion of left front wall of thorax**

✓7ᵗʰ **S20.319 Abrasion of unspecified front wall of thorax**

☑ Additional Character Required   ✓x7ᵗʰ Placeholder Alert   Manifestation   Unspecified Dx   ▶◀ Revised Text   ● New Code   ▲ Revised Title

√6ᵗʰ **S20.32** Blister (nonthermal) of front wall of thorax
- √7ᵗʰ **S20.321** Blister (nonthermal) of right front wall of thorax
- √7ᵗʰ **S20.322** Blister (nonthermal) of left front wall of thorax
- √7ᵗʰ **S20.329** Blister (nonthermal) of unspecified front wall of thorax

√6ᵗʰ **S20.34** External constriction of front wall of thorax
- √7ᵗʰ **S20.341** External constriction of right front wall of thorax
- √7ᵗʰ **S20.342** External constriction of left front wall of thorax
- √7ᵗʰ **S20.349** External constriction of unspecified front wall of thorax

√6ᵗʰ **S20.35** Superficial foreign body of front wall of thorax
Splinter in front wall of thorax
- √7ᵗʰ **S20.351** Superficial foreign body of right front wall of thorax
- √7ᵗʰ **S20.352** Superficial foreign body of left front wall of thorax
- √7ᵗʰ **S20.359** Superficial foreign body of unspecified front wall of thorax

√6ᵗʰ **S20.36** Insect bite (nonvenomous) of front wall of thorax
- √7ᵗʰ **S20.361** Insect bite (nonvenomous) of right front wall of thorax
- √7ᵗʰ **S20.362** Insect bite (nonvenomous) of left front wall of thorax
- √7ᵗʰ **S20.369** Insect bite (nonvenomous) of unspecified front wall of thorax

√6ᵗʰ **S20.37** Other superficial bite of front wall of thorax
- EXCLUDES 1   open bite of front wall of thorax (S21.15)
- √7ᵗʰ **S20.371** Other superficial bite of right front wall of thorax
- √7ᵗʰ **S20.372** Other superficial bite of left front wall of thorax
- √7ᵗʰ **S20.379** Other superficial bite of unspecified front wall of thorax

√5ᵗʰ **S20.4** Other and unspecified superficial injuries of back wall of thorax

√6ᵗʰ **S20.40** Unspecified superficial injuries of back wall of thorax
- √7ᵗʰ **S20.401** Unspecified superficial injuries of right back wall of thorax
- √7ᵗʰ **S20.402** Unspecified superficial injuries of left back wall of thorax
- √7ᵗʰ **S20.409** Unspecified superficial injuries of unspecified back wall of thorax

√6ᵗʰ **S20.41** Abrasion of back wall of thorax
- √7ᵗʰ **S20.411** Abrasion of right back wall of thorax
- √7ᵗʰ **S20.412** Abrasion of left back wall of thorax
- √7ᵗʰ **S20.419** Abrasion of unspecified back wall of thorax

√6ᵗʰ **S20.42** Blister (nonthermal) of back wall of thorax
- √7ᵗʰ **S20.421** Blister (nonthermal) of right back wall of thorax
- √7ᵗʰ **S20.422** Blister (nonthermal) of left back wall of thorax
- √7ᵗʰ **S20.429** Blister (nonthermal) of unspecified back wall of thorax

√6ᵗʰ **S20.44** External constriction of back wall of thorax
- √7ᵗʰ **S20.441** External constriction of right back wall of thorax
- √7ᵗʰ **S20.442** External constriction of left back wall of thorax
- √7ᵗʰ **S20.449** External constriction of unspecified back wall of thorax

√6ᵗʰ **S20.45** Superficial foreign body of back wall of thorax
Splinter of back wall of thorax
- √7ᵗʰ **S20.451** Superficial foreign body of right back wall of thorax
- √7ᵗʰ **S20.452** Superficial foreign body of left back wall of thorax
- √7ᵗʰ **S20.459** Superficial foreign body of unspecified back wall of thorax

√6ᵗʰ **S20.46** Insect bite (nonvenomous) of back wall of thorax
- √7ᵗʰ **S20.461** Insect bite (nonvenomous) of right back wall of thorax
- √7ᵗʰ **S20.462** Insect bite (nonvenomous) of left back wall of thorax

---

- √7ᵗʰ **S20.469** Insect bite (nonvenomous) of unspecified back wall of thorax

√6ᵗʰ **S20.47** Other superficial bite of back wall of thorax
- EXCLUDES 1   open bite of back wall of thorax (S21.25)
- √7ᵗʰ **S20.471** Other superficial bite of right back wall of thorax
- √7ᵗʰ **S20.472** Other superficial bite of left back wall of thorax
- √7ᵗʰ **S20.479** Other superficial bite of unspecified back wall of thorax

√5ᵗʰ **S20.9** Superficial injury of unspecified parts of thorax
- EXCLUDES 1   contusion of thorax NOS (S20.20)

√x7ᵗʰ **S20.90** Unspecified superficial injury of unspecified parts of thorax
Superficial injury of thoracic wall NOS

√x7ᵗʰ **S20.91** Abrasion of unspecified parts of thorax

√x7ᵗʰ **S20.92** Blister (nonthermal) of unspecified parts of thorax

√x7ᵗʰ **S20.94** External constriction of unspecified parts of thorax

√x7ᵗʰ **S20.95** Superficial foreign body of unspecified parts of thorax
Splinter in thorax NOS

√x7ᵗʰ **S20.96** Insect bite (nonvenomous) of unspecified parts of thorax

√x7ᵗʰ **S20.97** Other superficial bite of unspecified parts of thorax
- EXCLUDES 1   open bite of thorax NOS (S21.95)

√4ᵗʰ **S21** **Open wound of thorax**
Code also any associated injury, such as:
injury of heart (S26.-)
injury of intrathoracic organs (S27.-)
rib fracture (S22.3-, S22.4-)
spinal cord injury (S24.0-, S24.1-)
traumatic hemopneumothorax (S27.3)
traumatic hemothorax (S27.1)
traumatic pneumothorax (S27.0)
wound infection
- EXCLUDES 1   traumatic amputation (partial) of thorax (S28.1)

The appropriate 7th character is to be added to each code from category S21.
- A   initial encounter
- D   subsequent encounter
- S   sequela

√5ᵗʰ **S21.0** Open wound of breast

√6ᵗʰ **S21.00** Unspecified open wound of breast
- √7ᵗʰ **S21.001** Unspecified open wound of right breast
- √7ᵗʰ **S21.002** Unspecified open wound of left breast
- √7ᵗʰ **S21.009** Unspecified open wound of unspecified breast

√6ᵗʰ **S21.01** Laceration without foreign body of breast
- √7ᵗʰ **S21.011** Laceration without foreign body of right breast
- √7ᵗʰ **S21.012** Laceration without foreign body of left breast
- √7ᵗʰ **S21.019** Laceration without foreign body of unspecified breast

√6ᵗʰ **S21.02** Laceration with foreign body of breast
- √7ᵗʰ **S21.021** Laceration with foreign body of right breast
- √7ᵗʰ **S21.022** Laceration with foreign body of left breast
- √7ᵗʰ **S21.029** Laceration with foreign body of unspecified breast

√6ᵗʰ **S21.03** Puncture wound without foreign body of breast
- √7ᵗʰ **S21.031** Puncture wound without foreign body of right breast
- √7ᵗʰ **S21.032** Puncture wound without foreign body of left breast
- √7ᵗʰ **S21.039** Puncture wound without foreign body of unspecified breast

√6ᵗʰ **S21.04** Puncture wound with foreign body of breast
- √7ᵗʰ **S21.041** Puncture wound with foreign body of right breast
- √7ᵗʰ **S21.042** Puncture wound with foreign body of left breast
- √7ᵗʰ **S21.049** Puncture wound with foreign body of unspecified breast

√6ᵗʰ **S21.Ø5** Open bite of breast

     Bite of breast NOS

     EXCLUDES 1   *superficial bite of breast (S2Ø.17)*

     √7ᵗʰ **S21.Ø51** Open bite of right breast

     √7ᵗʰ **S21.Ø52** Open bite of left breast

     √7ᵗʰ **S21.Ø59** Open bite of unspecified breast

√5ᵗʰ **S21.1** Open wound of front wall of thorax without penetration into thoracic cavity

     Open wound of chest without penetration into thoracic cavity

   √6ᵗʰ **S21.1Ø** Unspecified open wound of front wall of thorax without penetration into thoracic cavity

     √7ᵗʰ **S21.1Ø1** Unspecified open wound of right front wall of thorax without penetration into thoracic cavity

     √7ᵗʰ **S21.1Ø2** Unspecified open wound of left front wall of thorax without penetration into thoracic cavity

     √7ᵗʰ **S21.1Ø9** Unspecified open wound of unspecified front wall of thorax without penetration into thoracic cavity

   √6ᵗʰ **S21.11** Laceration without foreign body of front wall of thorax without penetration into thoracic cavity

     √7ᵗʰ **S21.111** Laceration without foreign body of right front wall of thorax without penetration into thoracic cavity

     √7ᵗʰ **S21.112** Laceration without foreign body of left front wall of thorax without penetration into thoracic cavity

     √7ᵗʰ **S21.119** Laceration without foreign body of unspecified front wall of thorax without penetration into thoracic cavity

   √6ᵗʰ **S21.12** Laceration with foreign body of front wall of thorax without penetration into thoracic cavity

     √7ᵗʰ **S21.121** Laceration with foreign body of right front wall of thorax without penetration into thoracic cavity

     √7ᵗʰ **S21.122** Laceration with foreign body of left front wall of thorax without penetration into thoracic cavity

     √7ᵗʰ **S21.129** Laceration with foreign body of unspecified front wall of thorax without penetration into thoracic cavity

   √6ᵗʰ **S21.13** Puncture wound without foreign body of front wall of thorax without penetration into thoracic cavity

     √7ᵗʰ **S21.131** Puncture wound without foreign body of right front wall of thorax without penetration into thoracic cavity

     √7ᵗʰ **S21.132** Puncture wound without foreign body of left front wall of thorax without penetration into thoracic cavity

     √7ᵗʰ **S21.139** Puncture wound without foreign body of unspecified front wall of thorax without penetration into thoracic cavity

   √6ᵗʰ **S21.14** Puncture wound with foreign body of front wall of thorax without penetration into thoracic cavity

     √7ᵗʰ **S21.141** Puncture wound with foreign body of right front wall of thorax without penetration into thoracic cavity

     √7ᵗʰ **S21.142** Puncture wound with foreign body of left front wall of thorax without penetration into thoracic cavity

     √7ᵗʰ **S21.149** Puncture wound with foreign body of unspecified front wall of thorax without penetration into thoracic cavity

   √6ᵗʰ **S21.15** Open bite of front wall of thorax without penetration into thoracic cavity

     Bite of front wall of thorax NOS

     EXCLUDES 1   *superficial bite of front wall of thorax (S2Ø.37)*

     √7ᵗʰ **S21.151** Open bite of right front wall of thorax without penetration into thoracic cavity

     √7ᵗʰ **S21.152** Open bite of left front wall of thorax without penetration into thoracic cavity

     √7ᵗʰ **S21.159** Open bite of unspecified front wall of thorax without penetration into thoracic cavity

√5ᵗʰ **S21.2** Open wound of back wall of thorax without penetration into thoracic cavity

   √6ᵗʰ **S21.2Ø** Unspecified open wound of back wall of thorax without penetration into thoracic cavity

     √7ᵗʰ **S21.2Ø1** Unspecified open wound of right back wall of thorax without penetration into thoracic cavity

     √7ᵗʰ **S21.2Ø2** Unspecified open wound of left back wall of thorax without penetration into thoracic cavity

     √7ᵗʰ **S21.2Ø9** Unspecified open wound of unspecified back wall of thorax without penetration into thoracic cavity

   √6ᵗʰ **S21.21** Laceration without foreign body of back wall of thorax without penetration into thoracic cavity

     √7ᵗʰ **S21.211** Laceration without foreign body of right back wall of thorax without penetration into thoracic cavity

     √7ᵗʰ **S21.212** Laceration without foreign body of left back wall of thorax without penetration into thoracic cavity

     √7ᵗʰ **S21.219** Laceration without foreign body of unspecified back wall of thorax without penetration into thoracic cavity

   √6ᵗʰ **S21.22** Laceration with foreign body of back wall of thorax without penetration into thoracic cavity

     √7ᵗʰ **S21.221** Laceration with foreign body of right back wall of thorax without penetration into thoracic cavity

     √7ᵗʰ **S21.222** Laceration with foreign body of left back wall of thorax without penetration into thoracic cavity

     √7ᵗʰ **S21.229** Laceration with foreign body of unspecified back wall of thorax without penetration into thoracic cavity

   √6ᵗʰ **S21.23** Puncture wound without foreign body of back wall of thorax without penetration into thoracic cavity

     √7ᵗʰ **S21.231** Puncture wound without foreign body of right back wall of thorax without penetration into thoracic cavity

     √7ᵗʰ **S21.232** Puncture wound without foreign body of left back wall of thorax without penetration into thoracic cavity

     √7ᵗʰ **S21.239** Puncture wound without foreign body of unspecified back wall of thorax without penetration into thoracic cavity

   √6ᵗʰ **S21.24** Puncture wound with foreign body of back wall of thorax without penetration into thoracic cavity

     √7ᵗʰ **S21.241** Puncture wound with foreign body of right back wall of thorax without penetration into thoracic cavity

     √7ᵗʰ **S21.242** Puncture wound with foreign body of left back wall of thorax without penetration into thoracic cavity

     √7ᵗʰ **S21.249** Puncture wound with foreign body of unspecified back wall of thorax without penetration into thoracic cavity

   √6ᵗʰ **S21.25** Open bite of back wall of thorax without penetration into thoracic cavity

     Bite of back wall of thorax NOS

     EXCLUDES 1   *superficial bite of back wall of thorax (S2Ø.47)*

     √7ᵗʰ **S21.251** Open bite of right back wall of thorax without penetration into thoracic cavity

     √7ᵗʰ **S21.252** Open bite of left back wall of thorax without penetration into thoracic cavity

     √7ᵗʰ **S21.259** Open bite of unspecified back wall of thorax without penetration into thoracic cavity

√5ᵗʰ **S21.3** Open wound of front wall of thorax with penetration into thoracic cavity

     Open wound of chest with penetration into thoracic cavity

   √6ᵗʰ **S21.3Ø** Unspecified open wound of front wall of thorax with penetration into thoracic cavity

     √7ᵗʰ **S21.3Ø1** Unspecified open wound of right front wall of thorax with penetration into thoracic cavity

     √7ᵗʰ **S21.3Ø2** Unspecified open wound of left front wall of thorax with penetration into thoracic cavity

     √7ᵗʰ **S21.3Ø9** Unspecified open wound of unspecified front wall of thorax with penetration into thoracic cavity

   √6ᵗʰ **S21.31** Laceration without foreign body of front wall of thorax with penetration into thoracic cavity

     √7ᵗʰ **S21.311** Laceration without foreign body of right front wall of thorax with penetration into thoracic cavity

     √7ᵗʰ **S21.312** Laceration without foreign body of left front wall of thorax with penetration into thoracic cavity

---

√✔ Additional Character Required   √x7ᵗʰ Placeholder Alert   Manifestation   Unspecified Dx   ►◄ Revised Text   ● New Code   ▲ Revised Title

√7ᵗʰ **S21.319** Laceration without foreign body of unspecified front wall of thorax with penetration into thoracic cavity

√6ᵗʰ **S21.32** Laceration with foreign body of front wall of thorax with penetration into thoracic cavity

√7ᵗʰ **S21.321** Laceration with foreign body of right front wall of thorax with penetration into thoracic cavity

√7ᵗʰ **S21.322** Laceration with foreign body of left front wall of thorax with penetration into thoracic cavity

√7ᵗʰ **S21.329** Laceration with foreign body of unspecified front wall of thorax with penetration into thoracic cavity

√6ᵗʰ **S21.33** Puncture wound without foreign body of front wall of thorax with penetration into thoracic cavity

√7ᵗʰ **S21.331** Puncture wound without foreign body of right front wall of thorax with penetration into thoracic cavity

√7ᵗʰ **S21.332** Puncture wound without foreign body of left front wall of thorax with penetration into thoracic cavity

√7ᵗʰ **S21.339** Puncture wound without foreign body of unspecified front wall of thorax with penetration into thoracic cavity

√6ᵗʰ **S21.34** Puncture wound with foreign body of front wall of thorax with penetration into thoracic cavity

√7ᵗʰ **S21.341** Puncture wound with foreign body of right front wall of thorax with penetration into thoracic cavity

√7ᵗʰ **S21.342** Puncture wound with foreign body of left front wall of thorax with penetration into thoracic cavity

√7ᵗʰ **S21.349** Puncture wound with foreign body of unspecified front wall of thorax with penetration into thoracic cavity

√6ᵗʰ **S21.35** Open bite of front wall of thorax with penetration into thoracic cavity

     EXCLUDES 1   *superficial bite of front wall of thorax (S20.37)*

√7ᵗʰ **S21.351** Open bite of right front wall of thorax with penetration into thoracic cavity

√7ᵗʰ **S21.352** Open bite of left front wall of thorax with penetration into thoracic cavity

√7ᵗʰ **S21.359** Open bite of unspecified front wall of thorax with penetration into thoracic cavity

√5ᵗʰ **S21.4** Open wound of back wall of thorax with penetration into thoracic cavity

√6ᵗʰ **S21.40** Unspecified open wound of back wall of thorax with penetration into thoracic cavity

√7ᵗʰ **S21.401** Unspecified open wound of right back wall of thorax with penetration into thoracic cavity

√7ᵗʰ **S21.402** Unspecified open wound of left back wall of thorax with penetration into thoracic cavity

√7ᵗʰ **S21.409** Unspecified open wound of unspecified back wall of thorax with penetration into thoracic cavity

√6ᵗʰ **S21.41** Laceration without foreign body of back wall of thorax with penetration into thoracic cavity

√7ᵗʰ **S21.411** Laceration without foreign body of right back wall of thorax with penetration into thoracic cavity

√7ᵗʰ **S21.412** Laceration without foreign body of left back wall of thorax with penetration into thoracic cavity

√7ᵗʰ **S21.419** Laceration without foreign body of unspecified back wall of thorax with penetration into thoracic cavity

√6ᵗʰ **S21.42** Laceration with foreign body of back wall of thorax with penetration into thoracic cavity

√7ᵗʰ **S21.421** Laceration with foreign body of right back wall of thorax with penetration into thoracic cavity

√7ᵗʰ **S21.422** Laceration with foreign body of left back wall of thorax with penetration into thoracic cavity

√7ᵗʰ **S21.429** Laceration with foreign body of unspecified back wall of thorax with penetration into thoracic cavity

√6ᵗʰ **S21.43** Puncture wound without foreign body of back wall of thorax with penetration into thoracic cavity

√7ᵗʰ **S21.431** Puncture wound without foreign body of right back wall of thorax with penetration into thoracic cavity

√7ᵗʰ **S21.432** Puncture wound without foreign body of left back wall of thorax with penetration into thoracic cavity

√7ᵗʰ **S21.439** Puncture wound without foreign body of unspecified back wall of thorax with penetration into thoracic cavity

√6ᵗʰ **S21.44** Puncture wound with foreign body of back wall of thorax with penetration into thoracic cavity

√7ᵗʰ **S21.441** Puncture wound with foreign body of right back wall of thorax with penetration into thoracic cavity

√7ᵗʰ **S21.442** Puncture wound with foreign body of left back wall of thorax with penetration into thoracic cavity

√7ᵗʰ **S21.449** Puncture wound with foreign body of unspecified back wall of thorax with penetration into thoracic cavity

√6ᵗʰ **S21.45** Open bite of back wall of thorax with penetration into thoracic cavity

     Bite of back wall of thorax NOS

     EXCLUDES 1   *superficial bite of back wall of thorax (S20.47)*

√7ᵗʰ **S21.451** Open bite of right back wall of thorax with penetration into thoracic cavity

√7ᵗʰ **S21.452** Open bite of left back wall of thorax with penetration into thoracic cavity

√7ᵗʰ **S21.459** Open bite of unspecified back wall of thorax with penetration into thoracic cavity

√5ᵗʰ **S21.9** Open wound of unspecified part of thorax

     Open wound of thoracic wall NOS

√x7ᵗʰ **S21.90** Unspecified open wound of unspecified part of thorax

√x7ᵗʰ **S21.91** Laceration without foreign body of unspecified part of thorax

√x7ᵗʰ **S21.92** Laceration with foreign body of unspecified part of thorax

√x7ᵗʰ **S21.93** Puncture wound without foreign body of unspecified part of thorax

√x7ᵗʰ **S21.94** Puncture wound with foreign body of unspecified part of thorax

√x7ᵗʰ **S21.95** Open bite of unspecified part of thorax

     EXCLUDES 1   *superficial bite of thorax (S20.97)*

√4ᵗʰ **S22** Fracture of rib(s), sternum and thoracic spine

     NOTE   A fracture not indicated as displaced or nondisplaced should be coded to displaced

            A fracture not indicated as open or closed should be coded to closed

     INCLUDES   fracture of thoracic neural arch
            fracture of thoracic spinous process
            fracture of thoracic transverse process
            fracture of thoracic vertebra
            fracture of thoracic vertebral arch

Code first any associated:
     injury of intrathoracic organ (S27.-)
     spinal cord injury (S24.0-, S24.1-)

     EXCLUDES 1   *transection of thorax (S28.1)*
     EXCLUDES 2   *fracture of clavicle (S42.0-)*
                     fracture of scapula (S42.1-)

AHA: 2018,2Q,12; 2015,3Q,37-39

TIP: The term "improper alignment" is not synonymous with malunion or nonunion of a fracture when noted in provider documentation.

The appropriate 7th character is to be added to each code from category S22.
A   initial encounter for closed fracture
B   initial encounter for open fracture
D   subsequent encounter for fracture with routine healing
G   subsequent encounter for fracture with delayed healing
K   subsequent encounter for fracture with nonunion
S   sequela

√5ᵗʰ **S22.0** Fracture of thoracic vertebra

√6ᵗʰ **S22.00** Fracture of unspecified thoracic vertebra

√7ᵗʰ **S22.000** Wedge compression fracture of unspecified thoracic vertebra

N Newborn: 0   **P** Pediatric: 0-17   **M** Maternity: 12-55   **A** Adult: 15-124   **CH** Comorbidity High   **CL** Comorbidity Low   **NCDx** Noncancer Dx   **PDx** Primary Dx

968   ICD-10-CM 2020

√7ᵗʰ **S22.001** Stable burst fracture of unspecified thoracic vertebra

√7ᵗʰ **S22.002** Unstable burst fracture of unspecified thoracic vertebra

√7ᵗʰ **S22.008** Other fracture of unspecified thoracic vertebra

√7ᵗʰ **S22.009** Unspecified fracture of unspecified thoracic vertebra

√6ᵗʰ **S22.01** Fracture of first thoracic vertebra

√7ᵗʰ **S22.010** Wedge compression fracture of first thoracic vertebra

√7ᵗʰ **S22.011** Stable burst fracture of first thoracic vertebra

√7ᵗʰ **S22.012** Unstable burst fracture of first thoracic vertebra

√7ᵗʰ **S22.018** Other fracture of first thoracic vertebra

√7ᵗʰ **S22.019** Unspecified fracture of first thoracic vertebra

√6ᵗʰ **S22.02** Fracture of second thoracic vertebra

√7ᵗʰ **S22.020** Wedge compression fracture of second thoracic vertebra

√7ᵗʰ **S22.021** Stable burst fracture of second thoracic vertebra

√7ᵗʰ **S22.022** Unstable burst fracture of second thoracic vertebra

√7ᵗʰ **S22.028** Other fracture of second thoracic vertebra

√7ᵗʰ **S22.029** Unspecified fracture of second thoracic vertebra

√6ᵗʰ **S22.03** Fracture of third thoracic vertebra

√7ᵗʰ **S22.030** Wedge compression fracture of third thoracic vertebra

√7ᵗʰ **S22.031** Stable burst fracture of third thoracic vertebra

√7ᵗʰ **S22.032** Unstable burst fracture of third thoracic vertebra

√7ᵗʰ **S22.038** Other fracture of third thoracic vertebra

√7ᵗʰ **S22.039** Unspecified fracture of third thoracic vertebra

√6ᵗʰ **S22.04** Fracture of fourth thoracic vertebra

√7ᵗʰ **S22.040** Wedge compression fracture of fourth thoracic vertebra

√7ᵗʰ **S22.041** Stable burst fracture of fourth thoracic vertebra

√7ᵗʰ **S22.042** Unstable burst fracture of fourth thoracic vertebra

√7ᵗʰ **S22.048** Other fracture of fourth thoracic vertebra

√7ᵗʰ **S22.049** Unspecified fracture of fourth thoracic vertebra

√6ᵗʰ **S22.05** Fracture of T5-T6 vertebra

√7ᵗʰ **S22.050** Wedge compression fracture of T5-T6 vertebra

√7ᵗʰ **S22.051** Stable burst fracture of T5-T6 vertebra

√7ᵗʰ **S22.052** Unstable burst fracture of T5-T6 vertebra

√7ᵗʰ **S22.058** Other fracture of T5-T6 vertebra

√7ᵗʰ **S22.059** Unspecified fracture of T5-T6 vertebra

√6ᵗʰ **S22.06** Fracture of T7-T8 vertebra

√7ᵗʰ **S22.060** Wedge compression fracture of T7-T8 vertebra

√7ᵗʰ **S22.061** Stable burst fracture of T7-T8 vertebra

√7ᵗʰ **S22.062** Unstable burst fracture of T7-T8 vertebra

√7ᵗʰ **S22.068** Other fracture of T7-T8 thoracic vertebra

√7ᵗʰ **S22.069** Unspecified fracture of T7-T8 vertebra

√6ᵗʰ **S22.07** Fracture of T9-T10 vertebra

√7ᵗʰ **S22.070** Wedge compression fracture of T9-T10 vertebra

√7ᵗʰ **S22.071** Stable burst fracture of T9-T10 vertebra

√7ᵗʰ **S22.072** Unstable burst fracture of T9-T10 vertebra

√7ᵗʰ **S22.078** Other fracture of T9-T10 vertebra

√7ᵗʰ **S22.079** Unspecified fracture of T9-T10 vertebra

√6ᵗʰ **S22.08** Fracture of T11-T12 vertebra

√7ᵗʰ **S22.080** Wedge compression fracture of T11-T12 vertebra

√7ᵗʰ **S22.081** Stable burst fracture of T11-T12 vertebra

√7ᵗʰ **S22.082** Unstable burst fracture of T11-T12 vertebra

√7ᵗʰ **S22.088** Other fracture of T11-T12 vertebra

√7ᵗʰ **S22.089** Unspecified fracture of T11-T12 vertebra

√5ᵗʰ **S22.2** Fracture of sternum

DEF: Break in flat bone (breast bone) in the anterior thorax caused by blunt trauma to the anterior chest.

√x7ᵗʰ **S22.20** Unspecified fracture of sternum

√x7ᵗʰ **S22.21** Fracture of manubrium

√x7ᵗʰ **S22.22** Fracture of body of sternum

√x7ᵗʰ **S22.23** Sternal manubrial dissociation

√x7ᵗʰ **S22.24** Fracture of xiphoid process

√5ᵗʰ **S22.3** Fracture of one rib

√x7ᵗʰ **S22.31** Fracture of one rib, right side

√x7ᵗʰ **S22.32** Fracture of one rib, left side

√x7ᵗʰ **S22.39** Fracture of one rib, unspecified side

√5ᵗʰ **S22.4** Multiple fractures of ribs

Fractures of two or more ribs

EXCLUDES 1   flail chest (S22.5-)

√x7ᵗʰ **S22.41** Multiple fractures of ribs, right side

√x7ᵗʰ **S22.42** Multiple fractures of ribs, left side

√x7ᵗʰ **S22.43** Multiple fractures of ribs, bilateral

√x7ᵗʰ **S22.49** Multiple fractures of ribs, unspecified side

√x7ᵗʰ **S22.5** Flail chest

√x7ᵗʰ **S22.9** Fracture of bony thorax, part unspecified

√4ᵗʰ **S23** Dislocation and sprain of joints and ligaments of thorax

INCLUDES   avulsion of joint or ligament of thorax

laceration of cartilage, joint or ligament of thorax

sprain of cartilage, joint or ligament of thorax

traumatic hemarthrosis of joint or ligament of thorax

traumatic rupture of joint or ligament of thorax

traumatic subluxation of joint or ligament of thorax

traumatic tear of joint or ligament of thorax

Code also any associated open wound

EXCLUDES 2   dislocation, sprain of sternoclavicular joint (S43.2, S43.6)

strain of muscle or tendon of thorax (S29.01-)

The appropriate 7th character is to be added to each code from category S23.
A   initial encounter
D   subsequent encounter
S   sequela

√x7ᵗʰ **S23.0** Traumatic rupture of thoracic intervertebral disc

EXCLUDES 1   rupture or displacement (nontraumatic) of thoracic intervertebral disc NOS (M51.- with fifth character 4)

√5ᵗʰ **S23.1** Subluxation and dislocation of thoracic vertebra

Code also any associated:
open wound of thorax (S21.-)
spinal cord injury (S24.0-, S24.1-)
EXCLUDES 2   fracture of thoracic vertebrae (S22.0-)

√6ᵗʰ **S23.10** Subluxation and dislocation of unspecified thoracic vertebra

√7ᵗʰ **S23.100** Subluxation of unspecified thoracic vertebra

√7ᵗʰ **S23.101** Dislocation of unspecified thoracic vertebra

√6ᵗʰ **S23.11** Subluxation and dislocation of T1/T2 thoracic vertebra

√7ᵗʰ **S23.110** Subluxation of T1/T2 thoracic vertebra

√7ᵗʰ **S23.111** Dislocation of T1/T2 thoracic vertebra

√6ᵗʰ **S23.12** Subluxation and dislocation of T2/T3-T3/T4 thoracic vertebra

√7ᵗʰ **S23.120** Subluxation of T2/T3 thoracic vertebra

√7ᵗʰ **S23.121** Dislocation of T2/T3 thoracic vertebra

√7ᵗʰ **S23.122** Subluxation of T3/T4 thoracic vertebra

√7ᵗʰ **S23.123** Dislocation of T3/T4 thoracic vertebra

√6ᵗʰ **S23.13** Subluxation and dislocation of T4/T5-T5/T6 thoracic vertebra

√7ᵗʰ **S23.130** Subluxation of T4/T5 thoracic vertebra

√7ᵗʰ **S23.131** Dislocation of T4/T5 thoracic vertebra

√7ᵗʰ **S23.132** Subluxation of T5/T6 thoracic vertebra

√7ᵗʰ **S23.133** Dislocation of T5/T6 thoracic vertebra

✓6ᵗʰ **S23.14** Subluxation and dislocation of T6/T7-T7/T8 thoracic vertebra
- ✓7ᵗʰ **S23.140** Subluxation of T6/T7 thoracic vertebra
- ✓7ᵗʰ **S23.141** Dislocation of T6/T7 thoracic vertebra
- ✓7ᵗʰ **S23.142** Subluxation of T7/T8 thoracic vertebra
- ✓7ᵗʰ **S23.143** Dislocation of T7/T8 thoracic vertebra

✓6ᵗʰ **S23.15** Subluxation and dislocation of T8/T9-T9/T10 thoracic vertebra
- ✓7ᵗʰ **S23.150** Subluxation of T8/T9 thoracic vertebra
- ✓7ᵗʰ **S23.151** Dislocation of T8/T9 thoracic vertebra
- ✓7ᵗʰ **S23.152** Subluxation of T9/T10 thoracic vertebra
- ✓7ᵗʰ **S23.153** Dislocation of T9/T10 thoracic vertebra

✓6ᵗʰ **S23.16** Subluxation and dislocation of T10/T11-T11/T12 thoracic vertebra
- ✓7ᵗʰ **S23.160** Subluxation of T10/T11 thoracic vertebra
- ✓7ᵗʰ **S23.161** Dislocation of T10/T11 thoracic vertebra
- ✓7ᵗʰ **S23.162** Subluxation of T11/T12 thoracic vertebra
- ✓7ᵗʰ **S23.163** Dislocation of T11/T12 thoracic vertebra

✓6ᵗʰ **S23.17** Subluxation and dislocation of T12/L1 thoracic vertebra
- ✓7ᵗʰ **S23.170** Subluxation of T12/L1 thoracic vertebra
- ✓7ᵗʰ **S23.171** Dislocation of T12/L1 thoracic vertebra

✓5ᵗʰ **S23.2** Dislocation of other and unspecified parts of thorax
- ✓x7ᵗʰ **S23.20** Dislocation of unspecified part of thorax
- ✓x7ᵗʰ **S23.29** Dislocation of other parts of thorax

✓x7ᵗʰ **S23.3** Sprain of ligaments of thoracic spine

✓5ᵗʰ **S23.4** Sprain of ribs and sternum
- ✓x7ᵗʰ **S23.41** Sprain of ribs
- ✓6ᵗʰ **S23.42** Sprain of sternum
  - ✓7ᵗʰ **S23.420** Sprain of sternoclavicular (joint) (ligament)
  - ✓7ᵗʰ **S23.421** Sprain of chondrosternal joint
  - ✓7ᵗʰ **S23.428** Other sprain of sternum
  - ✓7ᵗʰ **S23.429** Unspecified sprain of sternum

✓x7ᵗʰ **S23.8** Sprain of other specified parts of thorax

✓x7ᵗʰ **S23.9** Sprain of unspecified parts of thorax

✓4ᵗʰ **S24** Injury of nerves and spinal cord at thorax level

NOTE Code to highest level of thoracic spinal cord injury.

Injuries to the spinal cord (S24.0 and S24.1) refer to the cord level and not bone level injury, and can affect nerve roots at and below the level given.

Code also any associated:
fracture of thoracic vertebra (S22.0-)
open wound of thorax (S21.-)
transient paralysis (R29.5)
EXCLUDES 2 injury of brachial plexus (S14.3)

The appropriate 7th character is to be added to each code from category S24.
A initial encounter
D subsequent encounter
S sequela

✓x7ᵗʰ **S24.0** Concussion and edema of thoracic spinal cord

✓5ᵗʰ **S24.1** Other and unspecified injuries of thoracic spinal cord
- ✓6ᵗʰ **S24.10** Unspecified injury of thoracic spinal cord
  - ✓7ᵗʰ **S24.101** Unspecified injury at T1 level of thoracic spinal cord
  - ✓7ᵗʰ **S24.102** Unspecified injury at T2-T6 level of thoracic spinal cord
  - ✓7ᵗʰ **S24.103** Unspecified injury at T7-T10 level of thoracic spinal cord
  - ✓7ᵗʰ **S24.104** Unspecified injury at T11-T12 level of thoracic spinal cord
  - ✓7ᵗʰ **S24.109** Unspecified injury at unspecified level of thoracic spinal cord
    Injury of thoracic spinal cord NOS
- ✓6ᵗʰ **S24.11** Complete lesion of thoracic spinal cord
  - ✓7ᵗʰ **S24.111** Complete lesion at T1 level of thoracic spinal cord
  - ✓7ᵗʰ **S24.112** Complete lesion at T2-T6 level of thoracic spinal cord
  - ✓7ᵗʰ **S24.113** Complete lesion at T7-T10 level of thoracic spinal cord

  - ✓7ᵗʰ **S24.114** Complete lesion at T11-T12 level of thoracic spinal cord
  - ✓7ᵗʰ **S24.119** Complete lesion at unspecified level of thoracic spinal cord

✓6ᵗʰ **S24.13** Anterior cord syndrome of thoracic spinal cord
- ✓7ᵗʰ **S24.131** Anterior cord syndrome at T1 level of thoracic spinal cord
- ✓7ᵗʰ **S24.132** Anterior cord syndrome at T2-T6 level of thoracic spinal cord
- ✓7ᵗʰ **S24.133** Anterior cord syndrome at T7-T10 level of thoracic spinal cord
- ✓7ᵗʰ **S24.134** Anterior cord syndrome at T11-T12 level of thoracic spinal cord
- ✓7ᵗʰ **S24.139** Anterior cord syndrome at unspecified level of thoracic spinal cord

✓6ᵗʰ **S24.14** Brown-Séquard syndrome of thoracic spinal cord
- ✓7ᵗʰ **S24.141** Brown-Séquard syndrome at T1 level of thoracic spinal cord
- ✓7ᵗʰ **S24.142** Brown-Séquard syndrome at T2-T6 level of thoracic spinal cord
- ✓7ᵗʰ **S24.143** Brown-Séquard syndrome at T7-T10 level of thoracic spinal cord
- ✓7ᵗʰ **S24.144** Brown-Séquard syndrome at T11-T12 level of thoracic spinal cord
- ✓7ᵗʰ **S24.149** Brown-Séquard syndrome at unspecified level of thoracic spinal cord

✓6ᵗʰ **S24.15** Other incomplete lesions of thoracic spinal cord
Incomplete lesion of thoracic spinal cord NOS
Posterior cord syndrome of thoracic spinal cord
- ✓7ᵗʰ **S24.151** Other incomplete lesion at T1 level of thoracic spinal cord
- ✓7ᵗʰ **S24.152** Other incomplete lesion at T2-T6 level of thoracic spinal cord
- ✓7ᵗʰ **S24.153** Other incomplete lesion at T7-T10 level of thoracic spinal cord
- ✓7ᵗʰ **S24.154** Other incomplete lesion at T11-T12 level of thoracic spinal cord
- ✓7ᵗʰ **S24.159** Other incomplete lesion at unspecified level of thoracic spinal cord

✓x7ᵗʰ **S24.2** Injury of nerve root of thoracic spine

✓x7ᵗʰ **S24.3** Injury of peripheral nerves of thorax

✓x7ᵗʰ **S24.4** Injury of thoracic sympathetic nervous system
Injury of cardiac plexus
Injury of esophageal plexus
Injury of pulmonary plexus
Injury of stellate ganglion
Injury of thoracic sympathetic ganglion

✓x7ᵗʰ **S24.8** Injury of other specified nerves of thorax

✓x7ᵗʰ **S24.9** Injury of unspecified nerve of thorax

✓4ᵗʰ **S25** Injury of blood vessels of thorax
Code also any associated open wound (S21.-)

The appropriate 7th character is to be added to each code from category S25.
A initial encounter
D subsequent encounter
S sequela

✓5ᵗʰ **S25.0** Injury of thoracic aorta
Injury of aorta NOS
- ✓x7ᵗʰ **S25.00** Unspecified injury of thoracic aorta
- ✓x7ᵗʰ **S25.01** Minor laceration of thoracic aorta
  Incomplete transection of thoracic aorta
  Laceration of thoracic aorta NOS
  Superficial laceration of thoracic aorta
- ✓x7ᵗʰ **S25.02** Major laceration of thoracic aorta
  Complete transection of thoracic aorta
  Traumatic rupture of thoracic aorta
- ✓x7ᵗʰ **S25.09** Other specified injury of thoracic aorta

✓5ᵗʰ **S25.1** Injury of innominate or subclavian artery
- ✓6ᵗʰ **S25.10** Unspecified injury of innominate or subclavian artery
  - ✓7ᵗʰ **S25.101** Unspecified injury of right innominate or subclavian artery
  - ✓7ᵗʰ **S25.102** Unspecified injury of left innominate or subclavian artery
  - ✓7ᵗʰ **S25.109** Unspecified injury of unspecified innominate or subclavian artery

√6ᵗʰ **S25.11** Minor laceration of innominate or subclavian artery

Incomplete transection of innominate or subclavian artery

Laceration of innominate or subclavian artery NOS

Superficial laceration of innominate or subclavian artery

√7ᵗʰ **S25.111** Minor laceration of right innominate or subclavian artery

√7ᵗʰ **S25.112** Minor laceration of left innominate or subclavian artery

√7ᵗʰ **S25.119** Minor laceration of unspecified innominate or subclavian artery

√6ᵗʰ **S25.12** Major laceration of innominate or subclavian artery

Complete transection of innominate or subclavian artery

Traumatic rupture of innominate or subclavian artery

√7ᵗʰ **S25.121** Major laceration of right innominate or subclavian artery

√7ᵗʰ **S25.122** Major laceration of left innominate or subclavian artery

√7ᵗʰ **S25.129** Major laceration of unspecified innominate or subclavian artery

√6ᵗʰ **S25.19** Other specified injury of innominate or subclavian artery

√7ᵗʰ **S25.191** Other specified injury of right innominate or subclavian artery

√7ᵗʰ **S25.192** Other specified injury of left innominate or subclavian artery

√7ᵗʰ **S25.199** Other specified injury of unspecified innominate or subclavian artery

√5ᵗʰ **S25.2** Injury of superior vena cava

Injury of vena cava NOS

√x7ᵗʰ **S25.20** Unspecified injury of superior vena cava

√x7ᵗʰ **S25.21** Minor laceration of superior vena cava

Incomplete transection of superior vena cava

Laceration of superior vena cava NOS

Superficial laceration of superior vena cava

√x7ᵗʰ **S25.22** Major laceration of superior vena cava

Complete transection of superior vena cava

Traumatic rupture of superior vena cava

√x7ᵗʰ **S25.29** Other specified injury of superior vena cava

√5ᵗʰ **S25.3** Injury of innominate or subclavian vein

√6ᵗʰ **S25.30** Unspecified injury of innominate or subclavian vein

√7ᵗʰ **S25.301** Unspecified injury of right innominate or subclavian vein

√7ᵗʰ **S25.302** Unspecified injury of left innominate or subclavian vein

√7ᵗʰ **S25.309** Unspecified injury of unspecified innominate or subclavian vein

√6ᵗʰ **S25.31** Minor laceration of innominate or subclavian vein

Incomplete transection of innominate or subclavian vein

Laceration of innominate or subclavian vein NOS

Superficial laceration of innominate or subclavian vein

√7ᵗʰ **S25.311** Minor laceration of right innominate or subclavian vein

√7ᵗʰ **S25.312** Minor laceration of left innominate or subclavian vein

√7ᵗʰ **S25.319** Minor laceration of unspecified innominate or subclavian vein

√6ᵗʰ **S25.32** Major laceration of innominate or subclavian vein

Complete transection of innominate or subclavian vein

Traumatic rupture of innominate or subclavian vein

√7ᵗʰ **S25.321** Major laceration of right innominate or subclavian vein

√7ᵗʰ **S25.322** Major laceration of left innominate or subclavian vein

√7ᵗʰ **S25.329** Major laceration of unspecified innominate or subclavian vein

√6ᵗʰ **S25.39** Other specified injury of innominate or subclavian vein

√7ᵗʰ **S25.391** Other specified injury of right innominate or subclavian vein

√7ᵗʰ **S25.392** Other specified injury of left innominate or subclavian vein

√7ᵗʰ **S25.399** Other specified injury of unspecified innominate or subclavian vein

√5ᵗʰ **S25.4** Injury of pulmonary blood vessels

√6ᵗʰ **S25.40** Unspecified injury of pulmonary blood vessels

√7ᵗʰ **S25.401** Unspecified injury of right pulmonary blood vessels

√7ᵗʰ **S25.402** Unspecified injury of left pulmonary blood vessels

√7ᵗʰ **S25.409** Unspecified injury of unspecified pulmonary blood vessels

√6ᵗʰ **S25.41** Minor laceration of pulmonary blood vessels

Incomplete transection of pulmonary blood vessels

Laceration of pulmonary blood vessels NOS

Superficial laceration of pulmonary blood vessels

√7ᵗʰ **S25.411** Minor laceration of right pulmonary blood vessels

√7ᵗʰ **S25.412** Minor laceration of left pulmonary blood vessels

√7ᵗʰ **S25.419** Minor laceration of unspecified pulmonary blood vessels

√6ᵗʰ **S25.42** Major laceration of pulmonary blood vessels

Complete transection of pulmonary blood vessels

Traumatic rupture of pulmonary blood vessels

√7ᵗʰ **S25.421** Major laceration of right pulmonary blood vessels

√7ᵗʰ **S25.422** Major laceration of left pulmonary blood vessels

√7ᵗʰ **S25.429** Major laceration of unspecified pulmonary blood vessels

√6ᵗʰ **S25.49** Other specified injury of pulmonary blood vessels

√7ᵗʰ **S25.491** Other specified injury of right pulmonary blood vessels

√7ᵗʰ **S25.492** Other specified injury of left pulmonary blood vessels

√7ᵗʰ **S25.499** Other specified injury of unspecified pulmonary blood vessels

√5ᵗʰ **S25.5** Injury of intercostal blood vessels

√6ᵗʰ **S25.50** Unspecified injury of intercostal blood vessels

√7ᵗʰ **S25.501** Unspecified injury of intercostal blood vessels, right side

√7ᵗʰ **S25.502** Unspecified injury of intercostal blood vessels, left side

√7ᵗʰ **S25.509** Unspecified injury of intercostal blood vessels, unspecified side

√6ᵗʰ **S25.51** Laceration of intercostal blood vessels

√7ᵗʰ **S25.511** Laceration of intercostal blood vessels, right side

√7ᵗʰ **S25.512** Laceration of intercostal blood vessels, left side

√7ᵗʰ **S25.519** Laceration of intercostal blood vessels, unspecified side

√6ᵗʰ **S25.59** Other specified injury of intercostal blood vessels

√7ᵗʰ **S25.591** Other specified injury of intercostal blood vessels, right side

√7ᵗʰ **S25.592** Other specified injury of intercostal blood vessels, left side

√7ᵗʰ **S25.599** Other specified injury of intercostal blood vessels, unspecified side

√5ᵗʰ **S25.8** Injury of other blood vessels of thorax

Injury of azygos vein

Injury of mammary artery or vein

√6ᵗʰ **S25.80** Unspecified injury of other blood vessels of thorax

√7ᵗʰ **S25.801** Unspecified injury of other blood vessels of thorax, right side

√7ᵗʰ **S25.802** Unspecified injury of other blood vessels of thorax, left side

√7ᵗʰ **S25.809** Unspecified injury of other blood vessels of thorax, unspecified side

√6ᵗʰ **S25.81** Laceration of other blood vessels of thorax

√7ᵗʰ **S25.811** Laceration of other blood vessels of thorax, right side

√7ᵗʰ **S25.812** Laceration of other blood vessels of thorax, left side

√7ᵗʰ **S25.819** Laceration of other blood vessels of thorax, unspecified side

√6ᵗʰ **S25.89** Other specified injury of other blood vessels of thorax

√7ᵗʰ **S25.891** Other specified injury of other blood vessels of thorax, right side

√7ᵗʰ **S25.892** Other specified injury of other blood vessels of thorax, left side

---

☑ Additional Character Required   √x7ᵗʰ Placeholder Alert   Manifestation   Unspecified Dx   ▶◀ Revised Text   ● New Code   ▲ Revised Title

Chapter 19. Injury, Poisoning and Certain Other Consequences of External Causes

√7ᵗʰ **S25.899** **Other specified injury of other blood vessels of thorax, unspecified side**

√5ᵗʰ **S25.9** **Injury of unspecified blood vessel of thorax**

√x7ᵗʰ **S25.90** **Unspecified injury of unspecified blood vessel of thorax**

√x7ᵗʰ **S25.91** Laceration of unspecified blood vessel of thorax

√x7ᵗʰ **S25.99** **Other specified injury of unspecified blood vessel of thorax**

√4ᵗʰ **S26** **Injury of heart**

Code also any associated:
open wound of thorax (S21.-)
traumatic hemopneumothorax (S27.2)
traumatic hemothorax (S27.1)
traumatic pneumothorax (S27.0)

The appropriate 7th character is to be added to each code from category S26.
A   initial encounter
D   subsequent encounter
S   sequela

√5ᵗʰ **S26.0** **Injury of heart** with hemopericardium

TIP: Do not assign for hemopericardium that is not due to trauma or that has occurred as a result of an intra- or postoperative complication.

√x7ᵗʰ **S26.00** **Unspecified injury of heart with hemopericardium**

√x7ᵗʰ **S26.01** Contusion of heart with hemopericardium

√6ᵗʰ **S26.02** Laceration of heart with hemopericardium

√7ᵗʰ **S26.020** Mild laceration of heart with hemopericardium
Laceration of heart without penetration of heart chamber

√7ᵗʰ **S26.021** Moderate laceration of heart with hemopericardium
Laceration of heart with penetration of heart chamber

√7ᵗʰ **S26.022** Major laceration of heart with hemopericardium
Laceration of heart with penetration of multiple heart chambers

√x7ᵗʰ **S26.09** **Other injury of heart with hemopericardium**

√5ᵗʰ **S26.1** **Injury of heart** without hemopericardium

√x7ᵗʰ **S26.10** **Unspecified injury of heart without hemopericardium**

√x7ᵗʰ **S26.11** Contusion of heart without hemopericardium

√x7ᵗʰ **S26.12** Laceration of heart without hemopericardium

√x7ᵗʰ **S26.19** Other injury of heart without hemopericardium

√5ᵗʰ **S26.9** **Injury of heart, unspecified with or without hemopericardium**

√x7ᵗʰ **S26.90** **Unspecified injury of heart, unspecified with or without hemopericardium**

√x7ᵗʰ **S26.91** Contusion of heart, unspecified with or without hemopericardium
DEF: Bruising within the heart muscle, with no mention of an open wound, usually caused by blunt chest trauma in motor vehicle accidents, falling from great heights, or receiving CPR.

√x7ᵗʰ **S26.92** Laceration of heart, unspecified with or without hemopericardium
Laceration of heart NOS
AHA: 2019,2Q,24

√x7ᵗʰ **S26.99** **Other injury of heart, unspecified with or without hemopericardium**

√4ᵗʰ **S27** **Injury of other and unspecified intrathoracic organs**

Code also any associated open wound of thorax (S21.-)

EXCLUDES 2   injury of cervical esophagus (S10-S19)
injury of trachea (cervical) (S10-S19)

The appropriate 7th character is to be added to each code from category S27.
A   initial encounter
D   subsequent encounter
S   sequela

√x7ᵗʰ **S27.0** **Traumatic pneumothorax**
EXCLUDES 1   spontaneous pneumothorax (J93.-)

√x7ᵗʰ **S27.1** **Traumatic hemothorax**

√x7ᵗʰ **S27.2** **Traumatic hemopneumothorax**

√5ᵗʰ **S27.3** **Other and unspecified injuries of** lung

√6ᵗʰ **S27.30** **Unspecified injury of lung**

√7ᵗʰ **S27.301** **Unspecified injury of lung,** unilateral

√7ᵗʰ **S27.302** **Unspecified injury of lung,** bilateral

√7ᵗʰ **S27.309** **Unspecified injury of lung, unspecified**

√6ᵗʰ **S27.31** Primary blast **injury of lung**
Blast injury of lung NOS

√7ᵗʰ **S27.311** **Primary blast injury of lung,** unilateral

√7ᵗʰ **S27.312** **Primary blast injury of lung,** bilateral

√7ᵗʰ **S27.319** **Primary blast injury of lung, unspecified**

√6ᵗʰ **S27.32** Contusion **of lung**
DEF: Bruising of the lung without mention of an open wound.

√7ᵗʰ **S27.321** **Contusion of lung,** unilateral

√7ᵗʰ **S27.322** **Contusion of lung,** bilateral

√7ᵗʰ **S27.329** **Contusion of lung, unspecified**

√6ᵗʰ **S27.33** Laceration **of lung**

√7ᵗʰ **S27.331** **Laceration of lung,** unilateral

√7ᵗʰ **S27.332** **Laceration of lung,** bilateral

√7ᵗʰ **S27.339** **Laceration of lung, unspecified**

√6ᵗʰ **S27.39** **Other injuries of lung**
Secondary blast injury of lung

√7ᵗʰ **S27.391** **Other injuries of lung,** unilateral

√7ᵗʰ **S27.392** **Other injuries of lung,** bilateral

√7ᵗʰ **S27.399** **Other injuries of lung, unspecified**

√5ᵗʰ **S27.4** **Injury of** bronchus

√6ᵗʰ **S27.40** **Unspecified injury of bronchus**

√7ᵗʰ **S27.401** **Unspecified injury of bronchus,** unilateral

√7ᵗʰ **S27.402** **Unspecified injury of bronchus,** bilateral

√7ᵗʰ **S27.409** **Unspecified injury of bronchus, unspecified**

√6ᵗʰ **S27.41** Primary blast **injury of bronchus**
Blast injury of bronchus NOS

√7ᵗʰ **S27.411** **Primary blast injury of bronchus,** unilateral

√7ᵗʰ **S27.412** **Primary blast injury of bronchus,** bilateral

√7ᵗʰ **S27.419** **Primary blast injury of bronchus, unspecified**

√6ᵗʰ **S27.42** Contusion **of bronchus**

√7ᵗʰ **S27.421** **Contusion of bronchus,** unilateral

√7ᵗʰ **S27.422** **Contusion of bronchus,** bilateral

√7ᵗʰ **S27.429** **Contusion of bronchus, unspecified**

√6ᵗʰ **S27.43** Laceration **of bronchus**

√7ᵗʰ **S27.431** **Laceration of bronchus,** unilateral

√7ᵗʰ **S27.432** **Laceration of bronchus,** bilateral

√7ᵗʰ **S27.439** **Laceration of bronchus, unspecified**

√6ᵗʰ **S27.49** **Other injury of bronchus**
Secondary blast injury of bronchus

√7ᵗʰ **S27.491** **Other injury of bronchus,** unilateral

√7ᵗʰ **S27.492** **Other injury of bronchus,** bilateral

√7ᵗʰ **S27.499** **Other injury of bronchus, unspecified**

√5ᵗʰ **S27.5** **Injury of** thoracic trachea

√x7ᵗʰ **S27.50** **Unspecified injury of thoracic trachea**

√x7ᵗʰ **S27.51** Primary blast **injury of thoracic trachea**
Blast injury of thoracic trachea NOS

√x7ᵗʰ **S27.52** Contusion **of thoracic trachea**

√x7ᵗʰ **S27.53** Laceration **of thoracic trachea**

√x7ᵗʰ **S27.59** **Other injury of thoracic trachea**
Secondary blast injury of thoracic trachea

√5ᵗʰ **S27.6** **Injury of** pleura

√x7ᵗʰ **S27.60** **Unspecified injury of pleura**

√x7ᵗʰ **S27.63** Laceration **of pleura**

√x7ᵗʰ **S27.69** **Other injury of pleura**

√5ᵗʰ **S27.8** **Injury of other specified intrathoracic organs**

√6ᵗʰ **S27.80** **Injury of** diaphragm

√7ᵗʰ **S27.802** Contusion **of diaphragm**

√7ᵗʰ **S27.803** Laceration **of diaphragm**

√7ᵗʰ **S27.808** **Other injury of diaphragm**

N Newborn: 0   P Pediatric: 0-17   M Maternity: 12-55   A Adult: 15-124   CH Comorbidity High   CL Comorbidity Low   NCDx Noncancer Dx   PDx Primary Dx

972   ICD-10-CM 2020

√6ᵗʰ **S27.809** Unspecified injury of diaphragm

√6ᵗʰ **S27.81** **Injury of** esophagus (thoracic part)

    √7ᵗʰ **S27.812** Contusion **of esophagus (thoracic part)**

    √7ᵗʰ **S27.813** Laceration **of esophagus (thoracic part)**

    √7ᵗʰ **S27.818** **Other injury of esophagus (thoracic part)**

    √7ᵗʰ **S27.819** **Unspecified injury of esophagus (thoracic part)**

√6ᵗʰ **S27.89** **Injury of other specified intrathoracic organs**

    Injury of lymphatic thoracic duct

    Injury of thymus gland

    √7ᵗʰ **S27.892** Contusion **of other specified intrathoracic organs**

    √7ᵗʰ **S27.893** Laceration **of other specified intrathoracic organs**

    √7ᵗʰ **S27.898** **Other injury of other specified intrathoracic organs**

    √7ᵗʰ **S27.899** **Unspecified injury of other specified intrathoracic organs**

√x7ᵗʰ **S27.9** **Injury of unspecified intrathoracic organ**

√4ᵗʰ **S28** **Crushing injury of thorax, and traumatic amputation of part of thorax**

> The appropriate 7th character is to be added to each code from category S28.
> A   initial encounter
> D   subsequent encounter
> S   sequela

√x7ᵗʰ **S28.0** **Crushed chest**

    Use additional code for all associated injuries

    EXCLUDES 1   flail chest (S22.5)

√x7ᵗʰ **S28.1** **Traumatic amputation (partial) of** part of thorax, except breast

√5ᵗʰ **S28.2** **Traumatic amputation of** breast

    √6ᵗʰ **S28.21** Complete **traumatic amputation of breast**

        Traumatic amputation of breast NOS

        √7ᵗʰ **S28.211** **Complete traumatic amputation of** right **breast**

        √7ᵗʰ **S28.212** **Complete traumatic amputation of** left **breast**

        √7ᵗʰ **S28.219** **Complete traumatic amputation of unspecified breast**

    √6ᵗʰ **S28.22** Partial **traumatic amputation of breast**

        √7ᵗʰ **S28.221** **Partial traumatic amputation of** right **breast**

        √7ᵗʰ **S28.222** **Partial traumatic amputation of** left **breast**

        √7ᵗʰ **S28.229** **Partial traumatic amputation of unspecified breast**

√4ᵗʰ **S29** **Other and unspecified injuries of thorax**

    Code also any associated open wound (S21.-)

> The appropriate 7th character is to be added to each code from category S29.
> A   initial encounter
> D   subsequent encounter
> S   sequela

√5ᵗʰ **S29.0** **Injury of muscle and tendon at thorax level**

    √6ᵗʰ **S29.00** **Unspecified injury of muscle and tendon of thorax**

        √7ᵗʰ **S29.001** **Unspecified injury of muscle and tendon of** front **wall of thorax**

        √7ᵗʰ **S29.002** **Unspecified injury of muscle and tendon of** back **wall of thorax**

        √7ᵗʰ **S29.009** **Unspecified injury of muscle and tendon of unspecified wall of thorax**

    √6ᵗʰ **S29.01** Strain **of muscle and tendon of thorax**

        √7ᵗʰ **S29.011** **Strain of muscle and tendon of** front **wall of thorax**

        √7ᵗʰ **S29.012** **Strain of muscle and tendon of** back **wall of thorax**

        √7ᵗʰ **S29.019** **Strain of muscle and tendon of unspecified wall of thorax**

    √6ᵗʰ **S29.02** Laceration **of muscle and tendon of thorax**

        √7ᵗʰ **S29.021** **Laceration of muscle and tendon of** front **wall of thorax**

        √7ᵗʰ **S29.022** **Laceration of muscle and tendon of** back **wall of thorax**

        √7ᵗʰ **S29.029** **Laceration of muscle and tendon of unspecified wall of thorax**

√7ᵗʰ **S29.09** **Other injury of muscle and tendon of thorax**

    √7ᵗʰ **S29.091** **Other injury of muscle and tendon of** front **wall of thorax**

    √7ᵗʰ **S29.092** **Other injury of muscle and tendon of** back **wall of thorax**

    √7ᵗʰ **S29.099** **Other injury of muscle and tendon of unspecified wall of thorax**

√x7ᵗʰ **S29.8** **Other specified injuries of thorax**

√x7ᵗʰ **S29.9** **Unspecified injury of thorax**

Injuries to the abdomen, lower back, lumbar spine, pelvis and external genitals (S30-S39)

INCLUDES   injuries to the abdominal wall
           injuries to the anus
           injuries to the buttock
           injuries to the external genitalia
           injuries to the flank
           injuries to the groin

EXCLUDES 2   burns and corrosions (T20-T32)
           effects of foreign body in anus and rectum (T18.5)
           effects of foreign body in genitourinary tract (T19.-)
           effects of foreign body in stomach, small intestine and colon (T18.2-T18.4)
           frostbite (T33-T34)
           insect bite or sting, venomous (T63.4)

√4ᵗʰ **S30** **Superficial injury of abdomen, lower back, pelvis and external genitals**

    EXCLUDES 2   superficial injury of hip (S70.-)

> The appropriate 7th character is to be added to each code from category S30.
> A   initial encounter
> D   subsequent encounter
> S   sequela

√x7ᵗʰ **S30.0** **Contusion of lower back and pelvis**

    Contusion of buttock

√x7ᵗʰ **S30.1** **Contusion of abdominal wall**

    Contusion of flank

    Contusion of groin

√5ᵗʰ **S30.2** **Contusion of** external genital organs

    √6ᵗʰ **S30.20** **Contusion of unspecified external genital organ**

        √7ᵗʰ **S30.201** **Contusion of unspecified external genital organ,** male ♂

        √7ᵗʰ **S30.202** **Contusion of unspecified external genital organ,** female ♀

    √x7ᵗʰ **S30.21** **Contusion of** penis ♂

    √x7ᵗʰ **S30.22** **Contusion of** scrotum and testes ♂

    √x7ᵗʰ **S30.23** **Contusion of** vagina and vulva ♀

√x7ᵗʰ **S30.3** **Contusion of** anus

√5ᵗʰ **S30.8** **Other superficial injuries of abdomen, lower back, pelvis and external genitals**

    √6ᵗʰ **S30.81** Abrasion **of abdomen, lower back, pelvis and external genitals**

        √7ᵗʰ **S30.810** **Abrasion of** lower back and pelvis

        √7ᵗʰ **S30.811** **Abrasion of** abdominal wall

        √7ᵗʰ **S30.812** **Abrasion of** penis ♂

        √7ᵗʰ **S30.813** **Abrasion of** scrotum and testes ♂

        √7ᵗʰ **S30.814** **Abrasion of** vagina and vulva ♀

        √7ᵗʰ **S30.815** **Abrasion of unspecified** external genital organs, male ♂

        √7ᵗʰ **S30.816** **Abrasion of unspecified** external genital organs, female ♀

        √7ᵗʰ **S30.817** **Abrasion of** anus

    √6ᵗʰ **S30.82** Blister (nonthermal) **of abdomen, lower back, pelvis and external genitals**

        √7ᵗʰ **S30.820** **Blister (nonthermal) of** lower back and pelvis

        √7ᵗʰ **S30.821** **Blister (nonthermal) of** abdominal wall

        √7ᵗʰ **S30.822** **Blister (nonthermal) of** penis ♂

        √7ᵗʰ **S30.823** **Blister (nonthermal) of** scrotum and testes ♂

        √7ᵗʰ **S30.824** **Blister (nonthermal) of** vagina and vulva ♀

☑ Additional Character Required   √x7ᵗʰ Placeholder Alert   Manifestation   Unspecified Dx   ▶◀ Revised Text   ● New Code   ▲ Revised Title

ICD-10-CM 2020   973

√7ᵗʰ **S30.825** **Blister (nonthermal) of unspecified** external genital organs, male   ♂

√7ᵗʰ **S30.826** **Blister (nonthermal) of unspecified** external genital organs, female   ♀

√7ᵗʰ **S30.827** **Blister (nonthermal) of** anus

√6ᵗʰ **S30.84** External constriction of abdomen, lower back, pelvis and external genitals

√7ᵗʰ **S30.840** **External constriction of** lower back and pelvis

√7ᵗʰ **S30.841** **External constriction of** abdominal wall

√7ᵗʰ **S30.842** **External constriction of** penis   ♂

Hair tourniquet syndrome of penis
Use additional cause code to identify the constricting item (W49.0-)

√7ᵗʰ **S30.843** **External constriction of** scrotum and testes   ♂

√7ᵗʰ **S30.844** **External constriction of** vagina and vulva   ♀

√7ᵗʰ **S30.845** **External constriction of unspecified** external genital organs, male   ♂

√7ᵗʰ **S30.846** **External constriction of unspecified** external genital organs, female   ♀

√6ᵗʰ **S30.85** Superficial foreign body of abdomen, lower back, pelvis and external genitals

Splinter in the abdomen, lower back, pelvis and external genitals

√7ᵗʰ **S30.850** **Superficial foreign body of** lower back and pelvis

√7ᵗʰ **S30.851** **Superficial foreign body of** abdominal wall

√7ᵗʰ **S30.852** **Superficial foreign body of** penis   ♂

√7ᵗʰ **S30.853** **Superficial foreign body of** scrotum and testes   ♂

√7ᵗʰ **S30.854** **Superficial foreign body of** vagina and vulva   ♀

√7ᵗʰ **S30.855** **Superficial foreign body of unspecified** external genital organs, male   ♂

√7ᵗʰ **S30.856** **Superficial foreign body of unspecified** external genital organs, female   ♀

√7ᵗʰ **S30.857** **Superficial foreign body of** anus

√6ᵗʰ **S30.86** Insect bite (nonvenomous) of abdomen, lower back, pelvis and external genitals

√7ᵗʰ **S30.860** **Insect bite (nonvenomous) of** lower back and pelvis

√7ᵗʰ **S30.861** **Insect bite (nonvenomous) of** abdominal wall

√7ᵗʰ **S30.862** **Insect bite (nonvenomous) of** penis   ♂

√7ᵗʰ **S30.863** **Insect bite (nonvenomous) of** scrotum and testes   ♂

√7ᵗʰ **S30.864** **Insect bite (nonvenomous) of** vagina and vulva   ♀

√7ᵗʰ **S30.865** **Insect bite (nonvenomous) of unspecified** external genital organs, male   ♂

√7ᵗʰ **S30.866** **Insect bite (nonvenomous) of unspecified** external genital organs, female   ♀

√7ᵗʰ **S30.867** **Insect bite (nonvenomous) of** anus

√6ᵗʰ **S30.87** Other superficial bite of abdomen, lower back, pelvis and external genitals

EXCLUDES 1   open bite of abdomen, lower back, pelvis and external genitals (S31.05, S31.15, S31.25, S31.35, S31.45, S31.55)

√7ᵗʰ **S30.870** **Other superficial bite of** lower back and pelvis

√7ᵗʰ **S30.871** **Other superficial bite of** abdominal wall

√7ᵗʰ **S30.872** **Other superficial bite of** penis   ♂

√7ᵗʰ **S30.873** **Other superficial bite of** scrotum and testes   ♂

√7ᵗʰ **S30.874** **Other superficial bite of** vagina and vulva   ♀

√7ᵗʰ **S30.875** **Other superficial bite of unspecified** external genital organs, male   ♂

√7ᵗʰ **S30.876** **Other superficial bite of unspecified** external genital organs, female   ♀

√7ᵗʰ **S30.877** **Other superficial bite of** anus

√5ᵗʰ **S30.9** Unspecified superficial injury of abdomen, lower back, pelvis and external genitals

√x7ᵗʰ **S30.91** **Unspecified superficial injury of** lower back and pelvis

√x7ᵗʰ **S30.92** **Unspecified superficial injury of** abdominal wall

√x7ᵗʰ **S30.93** **Unspecified superficial injury of** penis   ♂

√x7ᵗʰ **S30.94** **Unspecified superficial injury of** scrotum and testes   ♂

√x7ᵗʰ **S30.95** **Unspecified superficial injury of** vagina and vulva   ♀

√x7ᵗʰ **S30.96** **Unspecified superficial injury of unspecified** external genital organs, male   ♂

√x7ᵗʰ **S30.97** **Unspecified superficial injury of unspecified** external genital organs, female   ♀

√x7ᵗʰ **S30.98** **Unspecified superficial injury of** anus

√4ᵗʰ **S31** Open wound of abdomen, lower back, pelvis and external genitals

Code also any associated:
spinal cord injury (S24.0, S24.1-, S34.0-, S34.1-)
wound infection

EXCLUDES 1   traumatic amputation of part of abdomen, lower back and pelvis (S38.2-, S38.3)

EXCLUDES 2   open wound of hip (S71.00-S71.02)
open fracture of pelvis (S32.1- – S32.9 with 7th character B)

The appropriate 7th character is to be added to each code from category S31.
A   initial encounter
D   subsequent encounter
S   sequela

√5ᵗʰ **S31.0** Open wound of lower back and pelvis

√6ᵗʰ **S31.00** **Unspecified open wound of lower back and pelvis**

√7ᵗʰ **S31.000** **Unspecified open wound of lower back and pelvis** without penetration into retroperitoneum

Unspecified open wound of lower back and pelvis NOS

√7ᵗʰ **S31.001** **Unspecified open wound of lower back and pelvis** with penetration into retroperitoneum

√6ᵗʰ **S31.01** Laceration without foreign body of lower back and pelvis

√7ᵗʰ **S31.010** **Laceration without foreign body of lower back and pelvis** without penetration into retroperitoneum

Laceration without foreign body of lower back and pelvis NOS

√7ᵗʰ **S31.011** **Laceration without foreign body of lower back and pelvis** with penetration into retroperitoneum

√6ᵗʰ **S31.02** Laceration with foreign body of lower back and pelvis

√7ᵗʰ **S31.020** **Laceration with foreign body of lower back and pelvis** without penetration into retroperitoneum

Laceration with foreign body of lower back and pelvis NOS

√7ᵗʰ **S31.021** **Laceration with foreign body of lower back and pelvis** with penetration into retroperitoneum

√6ᵗʰ **S31.03** Puncture wound without foreign body of lower back and pelvis

√7ᵗʰ **S31.030** **Puncture wound without foreign body of lower back and pelvis** without penetration into retroperitoneum

Puncture wound without foreign body of lower back and pelvis NOS

√7ᵗʰ **S31.031** **Puncture wound without foreign body of lower back and pelvis** with penetration into retroperitoneum

N Newborn: 0   **P** Pediatric: 0-17   **M** Maternity: 12-55   **A** Adult: 15-124   **CH** Comorbidity High   **CL** Comorbidity Low   **NCDx** Noncancer Dx   **PDx** Primary Dx

974   ICD-10-CM 2020

√6ᵗʰ **S31.04** Puncture wound with foreign body of lower back and pelvis

√7ᵗʰ **S31.040** Puncture wound with foreign body of lower back and pelvis without penetration into retroperitoneum

Puncture wound with foreign body of lower back and pelvis NOS

√7ᵗʰ **S31.041** Puncture wound with foreign body of lower back and pelvis with penetration into retroperitoneum

√6ᵗʰ **S31.05** Open bite of lower back and pelvis

Bite of lower back and pelvis NOS

EXCLUDES 1   *superficial bite of lower back and pelvis (S30.860, S30.870)*

√7ᵗʰ **S31.050** Open bite of lower back and pelvis without penetration into retroperitoneum

Open bite of lower back and pelvis NOS

√7ᵗʰ **S31.051** Open bite of lower back and pelvis with penetration into retroperitoneum

√5ᵗʰ **S31.1** Open wound of abdominal wall without penetration into peritoneal cavity

Open wound of abdominal wall NOS

EXCLUDES 2   *open wound of abdominal wall with penetration into peritoneal cavity (S31.6-)*

√6ᵗʰ **S31.10** Unspecified open wound of abdominal wall without penetration into peritoneal cavity

√7ᵗʰ **S31.100** Unspecified open wound of abdominal wall, right upper quadrant without penetration into peritoneal cavity

√7ᵗʰ **S31.101** Unspecified open wound of abdominal wall, left upper quadrant without penetration into peritoneal cavity

√7ᵗʰ **S31.102** Unspecified open wound of abdominal wall, epigastric region without penetration into peritoneal cavity

√7ᵗʰ **S31.103** Unspecified open wound of abdominal wall, right lower quadrant without penetration into peritoneal cavity

√7ᵗʰ **S31.104** Unspecified open wound of abdominal wall, left lower quadrant without penetration into peritoneal cavity

√7ᵗʰ **S31.105** Unspecified open wound of abdominal wall, periumbilic region without penetration into peritoneal cavity

√7ᵗʰ **S31.109** Unspecified open wound of abdominal wall, unspecified quadrant without penetration into peritoneal cavity

Unspecified open wound of abdominal wall NOS

√6ᵗʰ **S31.11** Laceration without foreign body of abdominal wall without penetration into peritoneal cavity

√7ᵗʰ **S31.110** Laceration without foreign body of abdominal wall, right upper quadrant without penetration into peritoneal cavity

√7ᵗʰ **S31.111** Laceration without foreign body of abdominal wall, left upper quadrant without penetration into peritoneal cavity

√7ᵗʰ **S31.112** Laceration without foreign body of abdominal wall, epigastric region without penetration into peritoneal cavity

√7ᵗʰ **S31.113** Laceration without foreign body of abdominal wall, right lower quadrant without penetration into peritoneal cavity

√7ᵗʰ **S31.114** Laceration without foreign body of abdominal wall, left lower quadrant without penetration into peritoneal cavity

√7ᵗʰ **S31.115** Laceration without foreign body of abdominal wall, periumbilic region without penetration into peritoneal cavity

√7ᵗʰ **S31.119** Laceration without foreign body of abdominal wall, unspecified quadrant without penetration into peritoneal cavity

√6ᵗʰ **S31.12** Laceration with foreign body of abdominal wall without penetration into peritoneal cavity

√7ᵗʰ **S31.120** Laceration of abdominal wall with foreign body, right upper quadrant without penetration into peritoneal cavity

√7ᵗʰ **S31.121** Laceration of abdominal wall with foreign body, left upper quadrant without penetration into peritoneal cavity

√7ᵗʰ **S31.122** Laceration of abdominal wall with foreign body, epigastric region without penetration into peritoneal cavity

√7ᵗʰ **S31.123** Laceration of abdominal wall with foreign body, right lower quadrant without penetration into peritoneal cavity

√7ᵗʰ **S31.124** Laceration of abdominal wall with foreign body, left lower quadrant without penetration into peritoneal cavity

√7ᵗʰ **S31.125** Laceration of abdominal wall with foreign body, periumbilic region without penetration into peritoneal cavity

√7ᵗʰ **S31.129** Laceration of abdominal wall with foreign body, unspecified quadrant without penetration into peritoneal cavity

√6ᵗʰ **S31.13** Puncture wound of abdominal wall without foreign body without penetration into peritoneal cavity

√7ᵗʰ **S31.130** Puncture wound of abdominal wall without foreign body, right upper quadrant without penetration into peritoneal cavity

√7ᵗʰ **S31.131** Puncture wound of abdominal wall without foreign body, left upper quadrant without penetration into peritoneal cavity

√7ᵗʰ **S31.132** Puncture wound of abdominal wall without foreign body, epigastric region without penetration into peritoneal cavity

√7ᵗʰ **S31.133** Puncture wound of abdominal wall without foreign body, right lower quadrant without penetration into peritoneal cavity

√7ᵗʰ **S31.134** Puncture wound of abdominal wall without foreign body, left lower quadrant without penetration into peritoneal cavity

√7ᵗʰ **S31.135** Puncture wound of abdominal wall without foreign body, periumbilic region without penetration into peritoneal cavity

√7ᵗʰ **S31.139** Puncture wound of abdominal wall without foreign body, unspecified quadrant without penetration into peritoneal cavity

√6ᵗʰ **S31.14** Puncture wound of abdominal wall with foreign body without penetration into peritoneal cavity

√7ᵗʰ **S31.140** Puncture wound of abdominal wall with foreign body, right upper quadrant without penetration into peritoneal cavity

√7ᵗʰ **S31.141** Puncture wound of abdominal wall with foreign body, left upper quadrant without penetration into peritoneal cavity

√7ᵗʰ **S31.142** Puncture wound of abdominal wall with foreign body, epigastric region without penetration into peritoneal cavity

√7ᵗʰ **S31.143** Puncture wound of abdominal wall with foreign body, right lower quadrant without penetration into peritoneal cavity

√7ᵗʰ **S31.144** Puncture wound of abdominal wall with foreign body, left lower quadrant without penetration into peritoneal cavity

√7ᵗʰ **S31.145** Puncture wound of abdominal wall with foreign body, periumbilic region without penetration into peritoneal cavity

√7ᵗʰ **S31.149** Puncture wound of abdominal wall with foreign body, unspecified quadrant without penetration into peritoneal cavity

√6ᵗʰ **S31.15** Open bite of abdominal wall without penetration into peritoneal cavity

Bite of abdominal wall NOS

EXCLUDES 1   *superficial bite of abdominal wall (S30.871)*

√7ᵗʰ **S31.150** Open bite of abdominal wall, right upper quadrant without penetration into peritoneal cavity

☑ Additional Character Required   √x7ᵗʰ Placeholder Alert   Manifestation   Unspecified Dx   ▶◀ Revised Text   ● New Code   ▲ Revised Title

ICD-10-CM 2020   975

Chapter 19. Injury, Poisoning and Certain Other Consequences of External Causes

    ✓7ᵗʰ **S31.151**   Open bite of abdominal wall, left upper quadrant without penetration into peritoneal cavity

    ✓7ᵗʰ **S31.152**   Open bite of abdominal wall, epigastric region without penetration into peritoneal cavity

    ✓7ᵗʰ **S31.153**   Open bite of abdominal wall, right lower quadrant without penetration into peritoneal cavity

    ✓7ᵗʰ **S31.154**   Open bite of abdominal wall, left lower quadrant without penetration into peritoneal cavity

    ✓7ᵗʰ **S31.155**   Open bite of abdominal wall, periumbilic region without penetration into peritoneal cavity

    ✓7ᵗʰ **S31.159**   Open bite of abdominal wall, unspecified quadrant without penetration into peritoneal cavity

✓5ᵗʰ **S31.2**   Open wound of penis

  ✓x7ᵗʰ **S31.20**   Unspecified open wound of penis ♂

  ✓x7ᵗʰ **S31.21** ·   Laceration without foreign body of penis ♂

  ✓x7ᵗʰ **S31.22**   Laceration with foreign body of penis ♂

  ✓x7ᵗʰ **S31.23**   Puncture wound without foreign body of penis ♂

  ✓x7ᵗʰ **S31.24**   Puncture wound with foreign body of penis ♂

  ✓x7ᵗʰ **S31.25**   Open bite of penis ♂

       Bite of penis NOS
         EXCLUDES 1   superficial bite of penis (S30.862, S30.872)

✓5ᵗʰ **S31.3**   Open wound of scrotum and testes

  ✓x7ᵗʰ **S31.30**   Unspecified open wound of scrotum and testes ♂

  ✓x7ᵗʰ **S31.31**   Laceration without foreign body of scrotum and testes ♂

  ✓x7ᵗʰ **S31.32**   Laceration with foreign body of scrotum and testes ♂

  ✓x7ᵗʰ **S31.33**   Puncture wound without foreign body of scrotum and testes ♂

  ✓x7ᵗʰ **S31.34**   Puncture wound with foreign body of scrotum and testes ♂

  ✓x7ᵗʰ **S31.35**   Open bite of scrotum and testes ♂

       Bite of scrotum and testes NOS
         EXCLUDES 1   superficial bite of scrotum and testes (S30.863, S30.873)

✓5ᵗʰ **S31.4**   Open wound of vagina and vulva

     EXCLUDES 1   injury to vagina and vulva during delivery (O70.-, O71.4)

  ✓x7ᵗʰ **S31.40**   Unspecified open wound of vagina and vulva ♀

  ✓x7ᵗʰ **S31.41**   Laceration without foreign body of vagina and vulva ♀

  ✓x7ᵗʰ **S31.42**   Laceration with foreign body of vagina and vulva ♀

  ✓x7ᵗʰ **S31.43**   Puncture wound without foreign body of vagina and vulva ♀

  ✓x7ᵗʰ **S31.44** ·   Puncture wound with foreign body of vagina and vulva ♀

  ✓x7ᵗʰ **S31.45**   Open bite of vagina and vulva ♀

       Bite of vagina and vulva NOS
         EXCLUDES 1   superficial bite of vagina and vulva (S30.864, S30.874)

✓5ᵗʰ **S31.5**   Open wound of unspecified external genital organs

     EXCLUDES 1   traumatic amputation of external genital organs (S38.21, S38.22)

  ✓6ᵗʰ **S31.50**   Unspecified open wound of unspecified external genital organs

    ✓7ᵗʰ **S31.501**   Unspecified open wound of unspecified external genital organs, male ♂

    ✓7ᵗʰ **S31.502**   Unspecified open wound of unspecified external genital organs, female ♀

  ✓6ᵗʰ **S31.51**   Laceration without foreign body of unspecified external genital organs

    ✓7ᵗʰ **S31.511**   Laceration without foreign body of unspecified external genital organs, male ♂

    ✓7ᵗʰ **S31.512**   Laceration without foreign body of unspecified external genital organs, female ♀

  ✓6ᵗʰ **S31.52**   Laceration with foreign body of unspecified external genital organs

    ✓7ᵗʰ **S31.521**   Laceration with foreign body of unspecified external genital organs, male ♂

    ✓7ᵗʰ **S31.522**   Laceration with foreign body of unspecified external genital organs, female ♀

  ✓6ᵗʰ **S31.53**   Puncture wound without foreign body of unspecified external genital organs

    ✓7ᵗʰ **S31.531**   Puncture wound without foreign body of unspecified external genital organs, male ♂

    ✓7ᵗʰ **S31.532**   Puncture wound without foreign body of unspecified external genital organs, female ♀

  ✓6ᵗʰ **S31.54**   Puncture wound with foreign body of unspecified external genital organs

    ✓7ᵗʰ **S31.541**   Puncture wound with foreign body of unspecified external genital organs, male ♂

    ✓7ᵗʰ **S31.542**   Puncture wound with foreign body of unspecified external genital organs, female ♀

  ✓6ᵗʰ **S31.55**   Open bite of unspecified external genital organs

       Bite of unspecified external genital organs NOS
         EXCLUDES 1   superficial bite of unspecified external genital organs (S30.865, S30.866, S30.875, S30.876)

    ✓7ᵗʰ **S31.551**   Open bite of unspecified external genital organs, male ♂

    ✓7ᵗʰ **S31.552**   Open bite of unspecified external genital organs, female ♀

✓5ᵗʰ **S31.6**   Open wound of abdominal wall with penetration into peritoneal cavity

  ✓6ᵗʰ **S31.60**   Unspecified open wound of abdominal wall with penetration into peritoneal cavity

    ✓7ᵗʰ **S31.600**   Unspecified open wound of abdominal wall, right upper quadrant with penetration into peritoneal cavity

    ✓7ᵗʰ **S31.601**   Unspecified open wound of abdominal wall, left upper quadrant with penetration into peritoneal cavity

    ✓7ᵗʰ **S31.602**   Unspecified open wound of abdominal wall, epigastric region with penetration into peritoneal cavity

    ✓7ᵗʰ **S31.603**   Unspecified open wound of abdominal wall, right lower quadrant with penetration into peritoneal cavity

    ✓7ᵗʰ **S31.604**   Unspecified open wound of abdominal wall, left lower quadrant with penetration into peritoneal cavity

    ✓7ᵗʰ **S31.605**   Unspecified open wound of abdominal wall, periumbilic region with penetration into peritoneal cavity

    ✓7ᵗʰ **S31.609**   Unspecified open wound of abdominal wall, unspecified quadrant with penetration into peritoneal cavity

  ✓6ᵗʰ **S31.61**   Laceration without foreign body of abdominal wall with penetration into peritoneal cavity

    ✓7ᵗʰ **S31.610**   Laceration without foreign body of abdominal wall, right upper quadrant with penetration into peritoneal cavity

    ✓7ᵗʰ **S31.611**   Laceration without foreign body of abdominal wall, left upper quadrant with penetration into peritoneal cavity

    ✓7ᵗʰ **S31.612**   Laceration without foreign body of abdominal wall, epigastric region with penetration into peritoneal cavity

    ✓7ᵗʰ **S31.613**   Laceration without foreign body of abdominal wall, right lower quadrant with penetration into peritoneal cavity

    ✓7ᵗʰ **S31.614**   Laceration without foreign body of abdominal wall, left lower quadrant with penetration into peritoneal cavity

    ✓7ᵗʰ **S31.615**   Laceration without foreign body of abdominal wall, periumbilic region with penetration into peritoneal cavity

N Newborn: 0   **P** Pediatric: 0-17   **M** Maternity: 12-55   **A** Adult: 15-124   **CH** Comorbidity High   **CL** Comorbidity Low   **NCDx** Noncancer Dx   **PDx** Primary Dx

976   ICD-10-CM 2020

√7ᵗʰ **S31.619** Laceration without foreign body of abdominal wall, unspecified quadrant with penetration into peritoneal cavity

√6ᵗʰ **S31.62** Laceration with foreign body of abdominal wall with penetration into peritoneal cavity

√7ᵗʰ **S31.620** Laceration with foreign body of abdominal wall, right upper quadrant with penetration into peritoneal cavity

√7ᵗʰ **S31.621** Laceration with foreign body of abdominal wall, left upper quadrant with penetration into peritoneal cavity

√7ᵗʰ **S31.622** Laceration with foreign body of abdominal wall, epigastric region with penetration into peritoneal cavity

√7ᵗʰ **S31.623** Laceration with foreign body of abdominal wall, right lower quadrant with penetration into peritoneal cavity

√7ᵗʰ **S31.624** Laceration with foreign body of abdominal wall, left lower quadrant with penetration into peritoneal cavity

√7ᵗʰ **S31.625** Laceration with foreign body of abdominal wall, periumbilic region with penetration into peritoneal cavity

√7ᵗʰ **S31.629** Laceration with foreign body of abdominal wall, unspecified quadrant with penetration into peritoneal cavity

√6ᵗʰ **S31.63** Puncture wound without foreign body of abdominal wall with penetration into peritoneal cavity

√7ᵗʰ **S31.630** Puncture wound without foreign body of abdominal wall, right upper quadrant with penetration into peritoneal cavity

√7ᵗʰ **S31.631** Puncture wound without foreign body of abdominal wall, left upper quadrant with penetration into peritoneal cavity

√7ᵗʰ **S31.632** Puncture wound without foreign body of abdominal wall, epigastric region with penetration into peritoneal cavity

√7ᵗʰ **S31.633** Puncture wound without foreign body of abdominal wall, right lower quadrant with penetration into peritoneal cavity

√7ᵗʰ **S31.634** Puncture wound without foreign body of abdominal wall, left lower quadrant with penetration into peritoneal cavity

√7ᵗʰ **S31.635** Puncture wound without foreign body of abdominal wall, periumbilic region with penetration into peritoneal cavity

√7ᵗʰ **S31.639** Puncture wound without foreign body of abdominal wall, unspecified quadrant with penetration into peritoneal cavity

√6ᵗʰ **S31.64** Puncture wound with foreign body of abdominal wall with penetration into peritoneal cavity

√7ᵗʰ **S31.640** Puncture wound with foreign body of abdominal wall, right upper quadrant with penetration into peritoneal cavity

√7ᵗʰ **S31.641** Puncture wound with foreign body of abdominal wall, left upper quadrant with penetration into peritoneal cavity

√7ᵗʰ **S31.642** Puncture wound with foreign body of abdominal wall, epigastric region with penetration into peritoneal cavity

√7ᵗʰ **S31.643** Puncture wound with foreign body of abdominal wall, right lower quadrant with penetration into peritoneal cavity

√7ᵗʰ **S31.644** Puncture wound with foreign body of abdominal wall, left lower quadrant with penetration into peritoneal cavity

√7ᵗʰ **S31.645** Puncture wound with foreign body of abdominal wall, periumbilic region with penetration into peritoneal cavity

√7ᵗʰ **S31.649** Puncture wound with foreign body of abdominal wall, unspecified quadrant with penetration into peritoneal cavity

√6ᵗʰ **S31.65** Open bite of abdominal wall with penetration into peritoneal cavity

EXCLUDES 1 superficial bite of abdominal wall (S30.861, S30.871)

√7ᵗʰ **S31.650** Open bite of abdominal wall, right upper quadrant with penetration into peritoneal cavity

√7ᵗʰ **S31.651** Open bite of abdominal wall, left upper quadrant with penetration into peritoneal cavity

√7ᵗʰ **S31.652** Open bite of abdominal wall, epigastric region with penetration into peritoneal cavity

√7ᵗʰ **S31.653** Open bite of abdominal wall, right lower quadrant with penetration into peritoneal cavity

√7ᵗʰ **S31.654** Open bite of abdominal wall, left lower quadrant with penetration into peritoneal cavity

√7ᵗʰ **S31.655** Open bite of abdominal wall, periumbilic region with penetration into peritoneal cavity

√7ᵗʰ **S31.659** Open bite of abdominal wall, unspecified quadrant with penetration into peritoneal cavity

√5ᵗʰ **S31.8** Open wound of other parts of abdomen, lower back and pelvis

√6ᵗʰ **S31.80** Open wound of unspecified buttock

√7ᵗʰ **S31.801** Laceration without foreign body of unspecified buttock

√7ᵗʰ **S31.802** Laceration with foreign body of unspecified buttock

√7ᵗʰ **S31.803** Puncture wound without foreign body of unspecified buttock

√7ᵗʰ **S31.804** Puncture wound with foreign body of unspecified buttock

√7ᵗʰ **S31.805** Open bite of unspecified buttock

Bite of buttock NOS

EXCLUDES 1 superficial bite of buttock (S30.870)

√7ᵗʰ **S31.809** Unspecified open wound of unspecified buttock

√6ᵗʰ **S31.81** Open wound of right buttock

√7ᵗʰ **S31.811** Laceration without foreign body of right buttock

√7ᵗʰ **S31.812** Laceration with foreign body of right buttock

√7ᵗʰ **S31.813** Puncture wound without foreign body of right buttock

√7ᵗʰ **S31.814** Puncture wound with foreign body of right buttock

√7ᵗʰ **S31.815** Open bite of right buttock

Bite of right buttock NOS

EXCLUDES 1 superficial bite of buttock (S30.870)

√7ᵗʰ **S31.819** Unspecified open wound of right buttock

√6ᵗʰ **S31.82** Open wound of left buttock

√7ᵗʰ **S31.821** Laceration without foreign body of left buttock

√7ᵗʰ **S31.822** Laceration with foreign body of left buttock

√7ᵗʰ **S31.823** Puncture wound without foreign body of left buttock

√7ᵗʰ **S31.824** Puncture wound with foreign body of left buttock

√7ᵗʰ **S31.825** Open bite of left buttock

Bite of left buttock NOS

EXCLUDES 1 superficial bite of buttock (S30.870)

√7ᵗʰ **S31.829** Unspecified open wound of left buttock

√6ᵗʰ **S31.83** Open wound of anus

√7ᵗʰ **S31.831** Laceration without foreign body of anus

√7ᵗʰ **S31.832** Laceration with foreign body of anus

√7ᵗʰ **S31.833** Puncture wound without foreign body of anus

√7ᵗʰ **S31.834** Puncture wound with foreign body of anus

√7ᵗʰ **S31.835** Open bite of anus

Bite of anus NOS

EXCLUDES 1 superficial bite of anus (S30.877)

√7ᵗʰ **S31.839** Unspecified open wound of anus

☑ Additional Character Required √×7ᵗʰ Placeholder Alert Manifestation Unspecified Dx ▶◀ Revised Text ● New Code ▲ Revised Title

ICD-10-CM 2020 977

☑4ᵗʰ S32 Fracture of lumbar spine and pelvis

> **NOTE**   A fracture not indicated as displaced or nondisplaced should be coded to displaced.
>
> A fracture not indicated as opened or closed should be coded to closed.

> **INCLUDES**   fracture of lumbosacral neural arch
> fracture of lumbosacral spinous process
> fracture of lumbosacral transverse process
> fracture of lumbosacral vertebra
> fracture of lumbosacral vertebral arch

Code first any associated spinal cord and spinal nerve injury (S34.-)

EXCLUDES 1   transection of abdomen (S38.3)

EXCLUDES 2   fracture of hip NOS (S72.0-)

AHA: 2018,2Q,12; 2015,3Q,37-39; 2012,4Q,93

TIP: The term "improper alignment" is not synonymous with malunion or nonunion of a fracture when noted in provider documentation.

> The appropriate 7th character is to be added to each code from category S32.
> A   initial encounter for closed fracture
> B   initial encounter for open fracture
> D   subsequent encounter for fracture with routine healing
> G   subsequent encounter for fracture with delayed healing
> K   subsequent encounter for fracture with nonunion
> S   sequela

☑5ᵗʰ S32.0 Fracture of lumbar vertebra

Fracture of lumbar spine NOS

   ☑6ᵗʰ S32.00 Fracture of unspecified lumbar vertebra

     ☑7ᵗʰ S32.000 Wedge compression **fracture of unspecified lumbar vertebra**

     ☑7ᵗʰ S32.001 Stable burst **fracture of unspecified lumbar vertebra**

     ☑7ᵗʰ S32.002 Unstable burst **fracture of unspecified lumbar vertebra**

     ☑7ᵗʰ S32.008 Other fracture of unspecified lumbar vertebra

     ☑7ᵗʰ S32.009 Unspecified fracture of unspecified lumbar vertebra

   ☑6ᵗʰ S32.01 Fracture of first lumbar vertebra

     ☑7ᵗʰ S32.010 Wedge compression **fracture of first lumbar vertebra**

     ☑7ᵗʰ S32.011 Stable burst **fracture of first lumbar vertebra**

     ☑7ᵗʰ S32.012 Unstable burst **fracture of first lumbar vertebra**

     ☑7ᵗʰ S32.018 Other fracture of first lumbar vertebra

     ☑7ᵗʰ S32.019 Unspecified fracture of first lumbar vertebra

   ☑6ᵗʰ S32.02 Fracture of second lumbar vertebra

     ☑7ᵗʰ S32.020 Wedge compression **fracture of second lumbar vertebra**

     ☑7ᵗʰ S32.021 Stable burst **fracture of second lumbar vertebra**

     ☑7ᵗʰ S32.022 Unstable burst **fracture of second lumbar vertebra**

     ☑7ᵗʰ S32.028 Other fracture of second lumbar vertebra

     ☑7ᵗʰ S32.029 Unspecified fracture of second lumbar vertebra

   ☑6ᵗʰ S32.03 Fracture of third lumbar vertebra

     ☑7ᵗʰ S32.030 Wedge compression **fracture of third lumbar vertebra**

     ☑7ᵗʰ S32.031 Stable burst **fracture of third lumbar vertebra**

     ☑7ᵗʰ S32.032 Unstable burst **fracture of third lumbar vertebra**

     ☑7ᵗʰ S32.038 Other fracture of third lumbar vertebra

     ☑7ᵗʰ S32.039 Unspecified fracture of third lumbar vertebra

   ☑6ᵗʰ S32.04 Fracture of fourth lumbar vertebra

     ☑7ᵗʰ S32.040 Wedge compression **fracture of fourth lumbar vertebra**

     ☑7ᵗʰ S32.041 Stable burst **fracture of fourth lumbar vertebra**

     ☑7ᵗʰ S32.042 Unstable burst **fracture of fourth lumbar vertebra**

     ☑7ᵗʰ S32.048 Other fracture of fourth lumbar vertebra

     ☑7ᵗʰ S32.049 Unspecified fracture of fourth lumbar vertebra

   ☑6ᵗʰ S32.05 Fracture of fifth lumbar vertebra

     ☑7ᵗʰ S32.050 Wedge compression **fracture of fifth lumbar vertebra**

     ☑7ᵗʰ S32.051 Stable burst **fracture of fifth lumbar vertebra**

     ☑7ᵗʰ S32.052 Unstable burst **fracture of fifth lumbar vertebra**

     ☑7ᵗʰ S32.058 Other fracture of fifth lumbar vertebra

     ☑7ᵗʰ S32.059 Unspecified fracture of fifth lumbar vertebra

☑5ᵗʰ S32.1 Fracture of sacrum

> **NOTE**   For vertical fractures, code to most medial fracture extension
>
> Use two codes if both a vertical and transverse fracture are present

Code also any associated fracture of pelvic ring (S32.8-)

   ☑x7ᵗʰ S32.10 Unspecified fracture of sacrum

   ☑6ᵗʰ S32.11 Zone I fracture of sacrum

     Vertical sacral ala fracture of sacrum

Vertical Sacral Fracture Zones

     ☑7ᵗʰ S32.110 Nondisplaced **Zone I fracture of sacrum**

     ☑7ᵗʰ S32.111 Minimally displaced **Zone I fracture of sacrum**

     ☑7ᵗʰ S32.112 Severely displaced **Zone I fracture of sacrum**

     ☑7ᵗʰ S32.119 Unspecified **Zone I fracture of sacrum**

   ☑6ᵗʰ S32.12 Zone II fracture of sacrum

     Vertical foraminal region fracture of sacrum

     ☑7ᵗʰ S32.120 Nondisplaced **Zone II fracture of sacrum**

     ☑7ᵗʰ S32.121 Minimally displaced **Zone II fracture of sacrum**

     ☑7ᵗʰ S32.122 Severely displaced **Zone II fracture of sacrum**

     ☑7ᵗʰ S32.129 Unspecified **Zone II fracture of sacrum**

   ☑6ᵗʰ S32.13 Zone III fracture of sacrum

     Vertical fracture into spinal canal region of sacrum

     ☑7ᵗʰ S32.130 Nondisplaced **Zone III fracture of sacrum**

     ☑7ᵗʰ S32.131 Minimally displaced **Zone III fracture of sacrum**

     ☑7ᵗʰ S32.132 Severely displaced **Zone III fracture of sacrum**

☑ Newborn: 0   ☑ Pediatric: 0-17   ☑ Maternity: 12-55   ☑ Adult: 15-124   **CH** Comorbidity High   **CL** Comorbidity Low   **NCDx** Noncancer Dx   **PDx** Primary Dx

978   ICD-10-CM 2020

☑7ᵗʰ **S32.139** Unspecified Zone III fracture of sacrum

Transverse Sacral Fracture Types

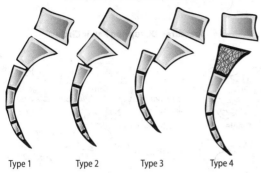

Type 1   Type 2   Type 3   Type 4

✓x7ᵗʰ **S32.14** Type 1 fracture of sacrum
Transverse flexion fracture of sacrum without displacement

✓x7ᵗʰ **S32.15** Type 2 fracture of sacrum
Transverse flexion fracture of sacrum with posterior displacement

✓x7ᵗʰ **S32.16** Type 3 fracture of sacrum
Transverse extension fracture of sacrum with anterior displacement

✓x7ᵗʰ **S32.17** Type 4 fracture of sacrum
Transverse segmental comminution of upper sacrum

✓x7ᵗʰ **S32.19** Other fracture of sacrum

✓x7ᵗʰ **S32.2** Fracture of coccyx

✓5ᵗʰ **S32.3** Fracture of ilium

> **EXCLUDES 1** *fracture of ilium with associated disruption of pelvic ring (S32.8-)*

✓6ᵗʰ **S32.30** Unspecified fracture of ilium
    ✓7ᵗʰ **S32.301** Unspecified fracture of right ilium
    ✓7ᵗʰ **S32.302** Unspecified fracture of left ilium
    ✓7ᵗʰ **S32.309** Unspecified fracture of unspecified ilium

✓6ᵗʰ **S32.31** Avulsion fracture of ilium
    ✓7ᵗʰ **S32.311** Displaced avulsion fracture of right ilium
    ✓7ᵗʰ **S32.312** Displaced avulsion fracture of left ilium
    ✓7ᵗʰ **S32.313** Displaced avulsion fracture of unspecified ilium
    ✓7ᵗʰ **S32.314** Nondisplaced avulsion fracture of right ilium
    ✓7ᵗʰ **S32.315** Nondisplaced avulsion fracture of left ilium
    ✓7ᵗʰ **S32.316** Nondisplaced avulsion fracture of unspecified ilium

✓6ᵗʰ **S32.39** Other fracture of ilium
    ✓7ᵗʰ **S32.391** Other fracture of right ilium
    ✓7ᵗʰ **S32.392** Other fracture of left ilium
    ✓7ᵗʰ **S32.399** Other fracture of unspecified ilium

✓5ᵗʰ **S32.4** Fracture of acetabulum
Code also any associated fracture of pelvic ring (S32.8-)
AHA: 2016, 3Q, 16

✓6ᵗʰ **S32.40** Unspecified fracture of acetabulum
    ✓7ᵗʰ **S32.401** Unspecified fracture of right acetabulum
    ✓7ᵗʰ **S32.402** Unspecified fracture of left acetabulum
    ✓7ᵗʰ **S32.409** Unspecified fracture of unspecified acetabulum

✓6ᵗʰ **S32.41** Fracture of anterior wall of acetabulum
    ✓7ᵗʰ **S32.411** Displaced fracture of anterior wall of right acetabulum
    ✓7ᵗʰ **S32.412** Displaced fracture of anterior wall of left acetabulum
    ✓7ᵗʰ **S32.413** Displaced fracture of anterior wall of unspecified acetabulum
    ✓7ᵗʰ **S32.414** Nondisplaced fracture of anterior wall of right acetabulum
    ✓7ᵗʰ **S32.415** Nondisplaced fracture of anterior wall of left acetabulum

✓7ᵗʰ **S32.416** Nondisplaced fracture of anterior wall of unspecified acetabulum

✓6ᵗʰ **S32.42** Fracture of posterior wall of acetabulum
    ✓7ᵗʰ **S32.421** Displaced fracture of posterior wall of right acetabulum
    ✓7ᵗʰ **S32.422** Displaced fracture of posterior wall of left acetabulum
    ✓7ᵗʰ **S32.423** Displaced fracture of posterior wall of unspecified acetabulum
    ✓7ᵗʰ **S32.424** Nondisplaced fracture of posterior wall of right acetabulum
    ✓7ᵗʰ **S32.425** Nondisplaced fracture of posterior wall of left acetabulum
    ✓7ᵗʰ **S32.426** Nondisplaced fracture of posterior wall of unspecified acetabulum

✓6ᵗʰ **S32.43** Fracture of anterior column [iliopubic] of acetabulum
    ✓7ᵗʰ **S32.431** Displaced fracture of anterior column [iliopubic] of right acetabulum
    ✓7ᵗʰ **S32.432** Displaced fracture of anterior column [iliopubic] of left acetabulum
    ✓7ᵗʰ **S32.433** Displaced fracture of anterior column [iliopubic] of unspecified acetabulum
    ✓7ᵗʰ **S32.434** Nondisplaced fracture of anterior column [iliopubic] of right acetabulum
    ✓7ᵗʰ **S32.435** Nondisplaced fracture of anterior column [iliopubic] of left acetabulum
    ✓7ᵗʰ **S32.436** Nondisplaced fracture of anterior column [iliopubic] of unspecified acetabulum

✓6ᵗʰ **S32.44** Fracture of posterior column [ilioischial] of acetabulum
    ✓7ᵗʰ **S32.441** Displaced fracture of posterior column [ilioischial] of right acetabulum
    ✓7ᵗʰ **S32.442** Displaced fracture of posterior column [ilioischial] of left acetabulum
    ✓7ᵗʰ **S32.443** Displaced fracture of posterior column [ilioischial] of unspecified acetabulum
    ✓7ᵗʰ **S32.444** Nondisplaced fracture of posterior column [ilioischial] of right acetabulum
    ✓7ᵗʰ **S32.445** Nondisplaced fracture of posterior column [ilioischial] of left acetabulum
    ✓7ᵗʰ **S32.446** Nondisplaced fracture of posterior column [ilioischial] of unspecified acetabulum

✓6ᵗʰ **S32.45** Transverse fracture of acetabulum
    ✓7ᵗʰ **S32.451** Displaced transverse fracture of right acetabulum
    ✓7ᵗʰ **S32.452** Displaced transverse fracture of left acetabulum
    ✓7ᵗʰ **S32.453** Displaced transverse fracture of unspecified acetabulum
    ✓7ᵗʰ **S32.454** Nondisplaced transverse fracture of right acetabulum
    ✓7ᵗʰ **S32.455** Nondisplaced transverse fracture of left acetabulum
    ✓7ᵗʰ **S32.456** Nondisplaced transverse fracture of unspecified acetabulum

✓6ᵗʰ **S32.46** Associated transverse-posterior fracture of acetabulum
    ✓7ᵗʰ **S32.461** Displaced associated transverse-posterior fracture of right acetabulum
    ✓7ᵗʰ **S32.462** Displaced associated transverse-posterior fracture of left acetabulum
    ✓7ᵗʰ **S32.463** Displaced associated transverse-posterior fracture of unspecified acetabulum
    ✓7ᵗʰ **S32.464** Nondisplaced associated transverse-posterior fracture of right acetabulum
    ✓7ᵗʰ **S32.465** Nondisplaced associated transverse-posterior fracture of left acetabulum
    ✓7ᵗʰ **S32.466** Nondisplaced associated transverse-posterior fracture of unspecified acetabulum

✓6ᵗʰ **S32.47** Fracture of medial wall of acetabulum
    ✓7ᵗʰ **S32.471** Displaced fracture of medial wall of right acetabulum
    ✓7ᵗʰ **S32.472** Displaced fracture of medial wall of left acetabulum
    ✓7ᵗʰ **S32.473** Displaced fracture of medial wall of unspecified acetabulum
    ✓7ᵗʰ **S32.474** Nondisplaced fracture of medial wall of right acetabulum

☑ Additional Character Required   ✓x7ᵗʰ Placeholder Alert   Manifestation   Unspecified Dx   ▶◀ Revised Text   ● New Code   ▲ Revised Title

ICD-10-CM 2020   979

Chapter 19. Injury, Poisoning and Certain Other Consequences of External Causes

√7ᵗʰ **S32.475** Nondisplaced **fracture of medial wall of** left **acetabulum**

√7ᵗʰ **S32.476** Nondisplaced **fracture of medial wall of** unspecified acetabulum

√6ᵗʰ **S32.48** Dome fracture **of acetabulum**

   √7ᵗʰ **S32.481** Displaced **dome fracture of** right **acetabulum**

   √7ᵗʰ **S32.482** Displaced **dome fracture of** left **acetabulum**

   √7ᵗʰ **S32.483** Displaced **dome fracture of unspecified acetabulum**

   √7ᵗʰ **S32.484** Nondisplaced **dome fracture of** right **acetabulum**

   √7ᵗʰ **S32.485** Nondisplaced **dome fracture of** left **acetabulum**

   √7ᵗʰ **S32.486** Nondisplaced **dome fracture of unspecified acetabulum**

√6ᵗʰ **S32.49** Other specified fracture of acetabulum

   √7ᵗʰ **S32.491** Other specified fracture of right acetabulum

   √7ᵗʰ **S32.492** Other specified fracture of left acetabulum

   √7ᵗʰ **S32.499** Other specified fracture of unspecified acetabulum

√5ᵗʰ **S32.5** Fracture of pubis

   EXCLUDES 1 *fracture of pubis with associated disruption of pelvic ring (S32.8-)*

   √6ᵗʰ **S32.50** Unspecified fracture of pubis

      √7ᵗʰ **S32.501** Unspecified fracture of right pubis

      √7ᵗʰ **S32.502** Unspecified fracture of left pubis

      √7ᵗʰ **S32.509** Unspecified fracture of unspecified pubis

   √6ᵗʰ **S32.51** Fracture of superior rim of pubis

      √7ᵗʰ **S32.511** Fracture of superior rim of right pubis

      √7ᵗʰ **S32.512** Fracture of superior rim of left pubis

      √7ᵗʰ **S32.519** Fracture of superior rim of unspecified pubis

   √6ᵗʰ **S32.59** Other specified fracture of pubis

      √7ᵗʰ **S32.591** Other specified fracture of right pubis

      √7ᵗʰ **S32.592** Other specified fracture of left pubis

      √7ᵗʰ **S32.599** Other specified fracture of unspecified pubis

√5ᵗʰ **S32.6** Fracture of ischium

   EXCLUDES 1 *fracture of ischium with associated disruption of pelvic ring (S32.8-)*

   √6ᵗʰ **S32.60** Unspecified fracture of ischium

      √7ᵗʰ **S32.601** Unspecified fracture of right ischium

      √7ᵗʰ **S32.602** Unspecified fracture of left ischium

      √7ᵗʰ **S32.609** Unspecified fracture of unspecified ischium

   √6ᵗʰ **S32.61** Avulsion fracture of ischium

      √7ᵗʰ **S32.611** Displaced avulsion fracture of right ischium

      √7ᵗʰ **S32.612** Displaced avulsion fracture of left ischium

      √7ᵗʰ **S32.613** Displaced avulsion fracture of unspecified ischium

      √7ᵗʰ **S32.614** Nondisplaced avulsion fracture of right ischium

      √7ᵗʰ **S32.615** Nondisplaced avulsion fracture of left ischium

      √7ᵗʰ **S32.616** Nondisplaced avulsion fracture of unspecified ischium

   √6ᵗʰ **S32.69** Other specified fracture of ischium

      √7ᵗʰ **S32.691** Other specified fracture of right ischium

      √7ᵗʰ **S32.692** Other specified fracture of left ischium

      √7ᵗʰ **S32.699** Other specified fracture of unspecified ischium

√5ᵗʰ **S32.8** **Fracture of other parts of pelvis**

   Code also any associated:
      fracture of acetabulum (S32.4-)
      sacral fracture (S32.1-)

Fractures Disrupting Pelvic Circle

Pelvic circle — Stable

Unstable (two-place fracture)

Iliac crest · Anterior superior iliac spine · Ischial spine · Acetabulum · Femur · Ilium · L5 · Sacrum · Coccyx · Pubis · Ischium · Pubic symphysis · **Pelvic Bones**

   √6ᵗʰ **S32.81** Multiple fractures of pelvis with disruption of pelvic ring

      Multiple pelvic fractures with disruption of pelvic circle

      √7ᵗʰ **S32.810** Multiple fractures of pelvis with stable disruption of pelvic ring

      √7ᵗʰ **S32.811** Multiple fractures of pelvis with unstable disruption of pelvic ring

   √x7ᵗʰ **S32.82** Multiple fractures of pelvis without disruption of pelvic ring

      Multiple pelvic fractures without disruption of pelvic circle

   √x7ᵗʰ **S32.89** Fracture of other parts of pelvis

√x7ᵗʰ **S32.9** **Fracture of unspecified parts of lumbosacral spine and pelvis**

   Fracture of lumbosacral spine NOS
   Fracture of pelvis NOS
   AHA: 2012,4Q,93

√4ᵗʰ **S33** **Dislocation and sprain of joints and ligaments of lumbar spine and pelvis**

   INCLUDES avulsion of joint or ligament of lumbar spine and pelvis
      laceration of cartilage, joint or ligament of lumbar spine and pelvis
      sprain of cartilage, joint or ligament of lumbar spine and pelvis
      traumatic hemarthrosis of joint or ligament of lumbar spine and pelvis
      traumatic rupture of joint or ligament of lumbar spine and pelvis
      traumatic subluxation of joint or ligament of lumbar spine and pelvis
      traumatic tear of joint or ligament of lumbar spine and pelvis

   Code also any associated open wound

   EXCLUDES 1 *nontraumatic rupture or displacement of lumbar intervertebral disc NOS (M51.-)*
      obstetric damage to pelvic joints and ligaments (O71.6)

   EXCLUDES 2 *dislocation and sprain of joints and ligaments of hip (S73.-)*
      strain of muscle of lower back and pelvis (S39.Ø1-)

   The appropriate 7th character is to be added to each code from category S33.
   A   initial encounter
   D   subsequent encounter
   S   sequela

√x7ᵗʰ **S33.Ø** **Traumatic rupture of lumbar intervertebral disc**

   EXCLUDES 1 *rupture or displacement (nontraumatic) of lumbar intervertebral disc NOS (M51.- with fifth character 6)*

Ⓝ Newborn: 0   Ⓟ Pediatric: 0-17   Ⓜ Maternity: 12-55   Ⓐ Adult: 15-124   ᴄᴴ Comorbidity High   ᴄᴸ Comorbidity Low   ɴᴄ ᴅˣ Noncancer Dx   ᴾᴰˣ Primary Dx

980

ICD-10-CM 2020

S32.475–S33.Ø

√5ᵗʰ **S33.1** **Subluxation and dislocation of** lumbar vertebra

> Code also any associated:
> open wound of abdomen, lower back and pelvis (S31)
> spinal cord injury (S24.0, S24.1-, S34.0-, S34.1-)
> EXCLUDES 2   fracture of lumbar vertebrae (S32.0-)

√6ᵗʰ **S33.10** **Subluxation and dislocation of unspecified lumbar vertebra**

√7ᵗʰ **S33.100** Subluxation of unspecified lumbar vertebra

√7ᵗʰ **S33.101** Dislocation of unspecified lumbar vertebra

√6ᵗʰ **S33.11** **Subluxation and dislocation of** L1/L2 **lumbar vertebra**

√7ᵗʰ **S33.110** Subluxation of L1/L2 lumbar vertebra

√7ᵗʰ **S33.111** Dislocation of L1/L2 lumbar vertebra

√6ᵗʰ **S33.12** **Subluxation and dislocation of** L2/L3 **lumbar vertebra**

√7ᵗʰ **S33.120** Subluxation of L2/L3 lumbar vertebra

√7ᵗʰ **S33.121** Dislocation of L2/L3 lumbar vertebra

√6ᵗʰ **S33.13** **Subluxation and dislocation of** L3/L4 **lumbar vertebra**

√7ᵗʰ **S33.130** Subluxation of L3/L4 lumbar vertebra

√7ᵗʰ **S33.131** Dislocation of L3/L4 lumbar vertebra

√6ᵗʰ **S33.14** **Subluxation and dislocation of** L4/L5 **lumbar vertebra**

√7ᵗʰ **S33.140** Subluxation of L4/L5 lumbar vertebra

√7ᵗʰ **S33.141** Dislocation of L4/L5 lumbar vertebra

√x7ᵗʰ **S33.2** **Dislocation of** sacroiliac and sacrococcygeal joint

√5ᵗʰ **S33.3** **Dislocation of other and unspecified parts of lumbar spine and pelvis**

√x7ᵗʰ **S33.30** **Dislocation of unspecified parts of lumbar spine and pelvis**

√x7ᵗʰ **S33.39** **Dislocation of other parts of lumbar spine and pelvis**

√x7ᵗʰ **S33.4** **Traumatic rupture of** symphysis pubis

√x7ᵗʰ **S33.5** **Sprain of ligaments of** lumbar spine

√x7ᵗʰ **S33.6** **Sprain of** sacroiliac joint

√x7ᵗʰ **S33.8** **Sprain of other parts of lumbar spine and pelvis**

√x7ᵗʰ **S33.9** **Sprain of unspecified parts of lumbar spine and pelvis**

√4ᵗʰ **S34** **Injury of lumbar and sacral spinal cord and nerves at abdomen, lower back and pelvis level**

> **NOTE**   Code to highest level of lumbar cord injury.
> Injuries to the spinal cord (S34.0 and S34.1) refer to the cord level and not bone level injury, and can affect nerve roots at and below the level given.

> Code also any associated:
> fracture of vertebra (S22.0-, S32.0-)
> open wound of abdomen, lower back and pelvis (S31.-)
> transient paralysis (R29.5)

> The appropriate 7th character is to be added to each code from category S34.
> A   initial encounter
> D   subsequent encounter
> S   sequela

√5ᵗʰ **S34.0** **Concussion and edema** of lumbar and sacral spinal cord

√x7ᵗʰ **S34.01** **Concussion and edema of** lumbar spinal cord

√x7ᵗʰ **S34.02** **Concussion and edema of** sacral spinal cord

> Concussion and edema of conus medullaris

√5ᵗʰ **S34.1** **Other and unspecified injury of lumbar and sacral spinal cord**

√6ᵗʰ **S34.10** **Unspecified injury to lumbar spinal cord**

√7ᵗʰ **S34.101** **Unspecified injury to** L1 level **of lumbar spinal cord**

> Unspecified injury to lumbar spinal cord level 1

√7ᵗʰ **S34.102** **Unspecified injury to** L2 level **of lumbar spinal cord**

> Unspecified injury to lumbar spinal cord level 2

√7ᵗʰ **S34.103** **Unspecified injury to** L3 level **of lumbar spinal cord**

> Unspecified injury to lumbar spinal cord level 3

√7ᵗʰ **S34.104** **Unspecified injury to** L4 level **of lumbar spinal cord**

> Unspecified injury to lumbar spinal cord level 4

√7ᵗʰ **S34.105** **Unspecified injury to** L5 level **of lumbar spinal cord**

> Unspecified injury to lumbar spinal cord level 5

√7ᵗʰ **S34.109** **Unspecified injury to unspecified level of lumbar spinal cord**

√6ᵗʰ **S34.11** **Complete lesion** of lumbar spinal cord

√7ᵗʰ **S34.111** **Complete lesion of** L1 level **of lumbar spinal cord**

> Complete lesion of lumbar spinal cord level 1

√7ᵗʰ **S34.112** **Complete lesion of** L2 level **of lumbar spinal cord**

> Complete lesion of lumbar spinal cord level 2

√7ᵗʰ **S34.113** **Complete lesion of** L3 level **of lumbar spinal cord**

> Complete lesion of lumbar spinal cord level 3

√7ᵗʰ **S34.114** **Complete lesion of** L4 level **of lumbar spinal cord**

> Complete lesion of lumbar spinal cord level 4

√7ᵗʰ **S34.115** **Complete lesion of** L5 level **of lumbar spinal cord**

> Complete lesion of lumbar spinal cord level 5

√7ᵗʰ **S34.119** **Complete lesion of unspecified level of lumbar spinal cord**

√6ᵗʰ **S34.12** **Incomplete lesion** of lumbar spinal cord

√7ᵗʰ **S34.121** **Incomplete lesion of** L1 level **of lumbar spinal cord**

> Incomplete lesion of lumbar spinal cord level 1

√7ᵗʰ **S34.122** **Incomplete lesion of** L2 level **of lumbar spinal cord**

> Incomplete lesion of lumbar spinal cord level 2

√7ᵗʰ **S34.123** **Incomplete lesion of** L3 level **of lumbar spinal cord**

> Incomplete lesion of lumbar spinal cord level 3

√7ᵗʰ **S34.124** **Incomplete lesion of** L4 level **of lumbar spinal cord**

> Incomplete lesion of lumbar spinal cord level 4

√7ᵗʰ **S34.125** **Incomplete lesion of** L5 level **of lumbar spinal cord**

> Incomplete lesion of lumbar spinal cord level 5

√7ᵗʰ **S34.129** **Incomplete lesion of unspecified level of lumbar spinal cord**

√6ᵗʰ **S34.13** **Other and unspecified injury to sacral spinal cord**

> Other injury to conus medullaris

√7ᵗʰ **S34.131** **Complete lesion of sacral spinal cord**

> Complete lesion of conus medullaris

√7ᵗʰ **S34.132** **Incomplete lesion of sacral spinal cord**

> Incomplete lesion of conus medullaris

√7ᵗʰ **S34.139** **Unspecified injury to sacral spinal cord**

> Unspecified injury of conus medullaris

√5ᵗʰ **S34.2** **Injury of nerve root of lumbar and sacral spine**

√x7ᵗʰ **S34.21** **Injury of nerve root of** lumbar spine

√x7ᵗʰ **S34.22** **Injury of nerve root of** sacral spine

√x7ᵗʰ **S34.3** **Injury of cauda equina**

√x7ᵗʰ **S34.4** **Injury of lumbosacral plexus**

√x7ᵗʰ **S34.5** **Injury of lumbar, sacral and pelvic sympathetic nerves**

> Injury of celiac ganglion or plexus
> Injury of hypogastric plexus
> Injury of mesenteric plexus (inferior) (superior)
> Injury of splanchnic nerve

√x7ᵗʰ **S34.6** **Injury of peripheral nerve(s) at abdomen, lower back and pelvis level**

√x7ᵗʰ **S34.8** **Injury of other nerves at abdomen, lower back and pelvis level**

| ☑ Additional Character Required | √x7ᵗʰ Placeholder Alert | Manifestation | Unspecified Dx | ▶◀ Revised Text | ● New Code | ▲ Revised Title |

√x 7th **S34.9** **Injury of unspecified nerves at abdomen, lower back and pelvis level**

√4th **S35** **Injury of blood vessels at abdomen, lower back and pelvis level**

Code also any associated open wound (S31.-)

The appropriate 7th character is to be added to each code from category S35.
A   initial encounter
D   subsequent encounter
S   sequela

√5th **S35.0** **Injury of** abdominal aorta

EXCLUDES 1   injury of aorta NOS (S25.Ø)

√x 7th **S35.00** **Unspecified injury of abdominal aorta**

√x 7th **S35.01** Minor laceration **of abdominal aorta**

Incomplete transection of abdominal aorta
Laceration of abdominal aorta NOS
Superficial laceration of abdominal aorta

√x 7th **S35.02** Major laceration **of abdominal aorta**

Complete transection of abdominal aorta
Traumatic rupture of abdominal aorta

√x 7th **S35.09** **Other injury of abdominal aorta**

√5th **S35.1** **Injury of** inferior vena cava

Injury of hepatic vein

EXCLUDES 1   injury of vena cava NOS (S25.2)

√x 7th **S35.10** **Unspecified injury of inferior vena cava**

√x 7th **S35.11** Minor laceration **of inferior vena cava**

Incomplete transection of inferior vena cava
Laceration of inferior vena cava NOS
Superficial laceration of inferior vena cava

√x 7th **S35.12** Major laceration **of inferior vena cava**

Complete transection of inferior vena cava
Traumatic rupture of inferior vena cava

√x 7th **S35.19** **Other injury of inferior vena cava**

√5th **S35.2** **Injury of celiac or mesenteric artery and branches**

√6th **S35.21** **Injury of** celiac artery

√7th **S35.211** Minor laceration **of celiac artery**

Incomplete transection of celiac artery
Laceration of celiac artery NOS
Superficial laceration of celiac artery

√7th **S35.212** Major laceration **of celiac artery**

Complete transection of celiac artery
Traumatic rupture of celiac artery

√7th **S35.218** **Other injury of celiac artery**

√7th **S35.219** **Unspecified injury of celiac artery**

√6th **S35.22** **Injury of** superior mesenteric artery

√7th **S35.221** Minor laceration **of superior mesenteric artery**

Incomplete transection of superior mesenteric artery
Laceration of superior mesenteric artery NOS
Superficial laceration of superior mesenteric artery

√7th **S35.222** Major laceration **of superior mesenteric artery**

Complete transection of superior mesenteric artery
Traumatic rupture of superior mesenteric artery

√7th **S35.228** **Other injury of superior mesenteric artery**

√7th **S35.229** **Unspecified injury of superior mesenteric artery**

√6th **S35.23** **Injury of** inferior mesenteric artery

√7th **S35.231** Minor laceration **of inferior mesenteric artery**

Incomplete transection of inferior mesenteric artery
Laceration of inferior mesenteric artery NOS
Superficial laceration of inferior mesenteric artery

√7th **S35.232** Major laceration **of inferior mesenteric artery**

Complete transection of inferior mesenteric artery
Traumatic rupture of inferior mesenteric artery

√7th **S35.238** **Other injury of inferior mesenteric artery**

√7th **S35.239** **Unspecified injury of inferior mesenteric artery**

√6th **S35.29** **Injury of** branches of celiac and mesenteric artery

Injury of gastric artery
Injury of gastroduodenal artery
Injury of hepatic artery
Injury of splenic artery

√7th **S35.291** Minor laceration **of branches of celiac and mesenteric artery**

Incomplete transection of branches of celiac and mesenteric artery
Laceration of branches of celiac and mesenteric artery NOS
Superficial laceration of branches of celiac and mesenteric artery

√7th **S35.292** Major laceration **of branches of celiac and mesenteric artery**

Complete transection of branches of celiac and mesenteric artery
Traumatic rupture of branches of celiac and mesenteric artery

√7th **S35.298** **Other injury of branches of celiac and mesenteric artery**

√7th **S35.299** **Unspecified injury of branches of celiac and mesenteric artery**

√5th **S35.3** **Injury of portal or splenic vein and branches**

√6th **S35.31** **Injury of** portal vein

√7th **S35.311** Laceration **of portal vein**

√7th **S35.318** **Other specified injury of portal vein**

√7th **S35.319** **Unspecified injury of portal vein**

√6th **S35.32** **Injury of** splenic vein

√7th **S35.321** Laceration **of splenic vein**

√7th **S35.328** **Other specified injury of splenic vein**

√7th **S35.329** **Unspecified injury of splenic vein**

√6th **S35.33** **Injury of** superior mesenteric vein

√7th **S35.331** Laceration **of superior mesenteric vein**

√7th **S35.338** **Other specified injury of superior mesenteric vein**

√7th **S35.339** **Unspecified injury of superior mesenteric vein**

√6th **S35.34** **Injury of** inferior mesenteric vein

√7th **S35.341** Laceration **of inferior mesenteric vein**

√7th **S35.348** **Other specified injury of inferior mesenteric vein**

√7th **S35.349** **Unspecified injury of inferior mesenteric vein**

√5th **S35.4** **Injury of** renal blood vessels

√6th **S35.40** **Unspecified injury of renal blood vessel**

√7th **S35.401** **Unspecified injury of** right **renal** artery

√7th **S35.402** **Unspecified injury of** left **renal** artery

√7th **S35.403** **Unspecified injury of unspecified renal artery**

√7th **S35.404** **Unspecified injury of** right **renal** vein

√7th **S35.405** **Unspecified injury of** left **renal** vein

√7th **S35.406** **Unspecified injury of unspecified renal vein**

√6th **S35.41** Laceration **of renal blood vessel**

√7th **S35.411** Laceration **of** right **renal** artery

√7th **S35.412** Laceration **of** left **renal** artery

√7th **S35.413** Laceration **of unspecified renal artery**

√7th **S35.414** Laceration **of** right **renal** vein

√7th **S35.415** Laceration **of** left **renal** vein

√7th **S35.416** Laceration **of unspecified renal vein**

√6th **S35.49** **Other specified injury of renal blood vessel**

√7th **S35.491** **Other specified injury of** right **renal** artery

√7th **S35.492** **Other specified injury of** left **renal** artery

√7ᵗʰ **S35.493** Other specified injury of unspecified renal artery

√7ᵗʰ **S35.494** Other specified injury of right renal vein

√7ᵗʰ **S35.495** Other specified injury of left renal vein

√7ᵗʰ **S35.496** Other specified injury of unspecified renal vein

√6ᵗʰ **S35.5** Injury of iliac blood vessels

√x7ᵗʰ **S35.50** Injury of unspecified iliac blood vessel(s)

√6ᵗʰ **S35.51** Injury of iliac artery or vein

Injury of hypogastric artery or vein

√7ᵗʰ **S35.511** Injury of right iliac artery

√7ᵗʰ **S35.512** Injury of left iliac artery

√7ᵗʰ **S35.513** Injury of unspecified iliac artery

√7ᵗʰ **S35.514** Injury of right iliac vein

√7ᵗʰ **S35.515** Injury of left iliac vein

√7ᵗʰ **S35.516** Injury of unspecified iliac vein

√6ᵗʰ **S35.53** Injury of uterine artery or vein

√7ᵗʰ **S35.531** Injury of right uterine artery ♀

√7ᵗʰ **S35.532** Injury of left uterine artery ♀

√7ᵗʰ **S35.533** Injury of unspecified uterine artery ♀

√7ᵗʰ **S35.534** Injury of right uterine vein ♀

√7ᵗʰ **S35.535** Injury of left uterine vein ♀

√7ᵗʰ **S35.536** Injury of unspecified uterine vein ♀

√x7ᵗʰ **S35.59** Injury of other iliac blood vessels

√5ᵗʰ **S35.8** Injury of other blood vessels at abdomen, lower back and pelvis level

Injury of ovarian artery or vein

√6ᵗʰ **S35.8X** Injury of other blood vessels at abdomen, lower back and pelvis level

√7ᵗʰ **S35.8X1** Laceration of other blood vessels at abdomen, lower back and pelvis level

√7ᵗʰ **S35.8X8** Other specified injury of other blood vessels at abdomen, lower back and pelvis level

√7ᵗʰ **S35.8X9** Unspecified injury of other blood vessels at abdomen, lower back and pelvis level

√5ᵗʰ **S35.9** Injury of unspecified blood vessel at abdomen, lower back and pelvis level

√x7ᵗʰ **S35.90** Unspecified injury of unspecified blood vessel at abdomen, lower back and pelvis level

√x7ᵗʰ **S35.91** Laceration of unspecified blood vessel at abdomen, lower back and pelvis level

√x7ᵗʰ **S35.99** Other specified injury of unspecified blood vessel at abdomen, lower back and pelvis level

√4ᵗʰ **S36 Injury of intra-abdominal organs**

Code also any associated open wound (S31.-)

TIP: Code only the most severe injury reported when assigning a code for intra-abdominal injury; a laceration is more severe than a contusion.

The appropriate 7th character is to be added to each code from category S36.
A   initial encounter
D   subsequent encounter
S   sequela

√5ᵗʰ **S36.0** Injury of spleen

AHA: 2015,2Q,36; 2015,1Q,10

√x7ᵗʰ **S36.00** Unspecified injury of spleen

√6ᵗʰ **S36.02** Contusion of spleen

√7ᵗʰ **S36.020** Minor contusion of spleen

Contusion of spleen less than 2 cm

√7ᵗʰ **S36.021** Major contusion of spleen

Contusion of spleen greater than 2 cm

√7ᵗʰ **S36.029** Unspecified contusion of spleen

√6ᵗʰ **S36.03** Laceration of spleen

√7ᵗʰ **S36.030** Superficial (capsular) laceration of spleen

Laceration of spleen less than 1 cm
Minor laceration of spleen

√7ᵗʰ **S36.031** Moderate laceration of spleen

Laceration of spleen 1 to 3 cm

√7ᵗʰ **S36.032** Major laceration of spleen

Avulsion of spleen
Laceration of spleen greater than 3 cm
Massive laceration of spleen
Multiple moderate lacerations of spleen
Stellate laceration of spleen

√7ᵗʰ **S36.039** Unspecified laceration of spleen

√x7ᵗʰ **S36.09** Other injury of spleen

√5ᵗʰ **S36.1** Injury of liver and gallbladder and bile duct

√6ᵗʰ **S36.11** Injury of liver

√7ᵗʰ **S36.112** Contusion of liver

√7ᵗʰ **S36.113** Laceration of liver, unspecified degree

√7ᵗʰ **S36.114** Minor laceration of liver

Laceration involving capsule only, or, without significant involvement of hepatic parenchyma [i.e., less than 1 cm deep]

√7ᵗʰ **S36.115** Moderate laceration of liver

Laceration involving parenchyma but without major disruption of parenchyma [i.e., less than 10 cm long and less than 3 cm deep]

√7ᵗʰ **S36.116** Major laceration of liver

Laceration with significant disruption of hepatic parenchyma [i.e., greater than 10 cm long and 3 cm deep]
Multiple moderate lacerations, with or without hematoma
Stellate laceration of liver

√7ᵗʰ **S36.118** Other injury of liver

√7ᵗʰ **S36.119** Unspecified injury of liver

√6ᵗʰ **S36.12** Injury of gallbladder

√7ᵗʰ **S36.122** Contusion of gallbladder

√7ᵗʰ **S36.123** Laceration of gallbladder

√7ᵗʰ **S36.128** Other injury of gallbladder

√7ᵗʰ **S36.129** Unspecified injury of gallbladder

√x7ᵗʰ **S36.13** Injury of bile duct

√5ᵗʰ **S36.2** Injury of pancreas

√6ᵗʰ **S36.20** Unspecified injury of pancreas

√7ᵗʰ **S36.200** Unspecified injury of head of pancreas

√7ᵗʰ **S36.201** Unspecified injury of body of pancreas

√7ᵗʰ **S36.202** Unspecified injury of tail of pancreas

√7ᵗʰ **S36.209** Unspecified injury of unspecified part of pancreas

√6ᵗʰ **S36.22** Contusion of pancreas

√7ᵗʰ **S36.220** Contusion of head of pancreas

√7ᵗʰ **S36.221** Contusion of body of pancreas

√7ᵗʰ **S36.222** Contusion of tail of pancreas

√7ᵗʰ **S36.229** Contusion of unspecified part of pancreas

√6ᵗʰ **S36.23** Laceration of pancreas, unspecified degree

√7ᵗʰ **S36.230** Laceration of head of pancreas, unspecified degree

√7ᵗʰ **S36.231** Laceration of body of pancreas, unspecified degree

√7ᵗʰ **S36.232** Laceration of tail of pancreas, unspecified degree

√7ᵗʰ **S36.239** Laceration of unspecified part of pancreas, unspecified degree

√6ᵗʰ **S36.24** Minor laceration of pancreas

√7ᵗʰ **S36.240** Minor laceration of head of pancreas

√7ᵗʰ **S36.241** Minor laceration of body of pancreas

√7ᵗʰ **S36.242** Minor laceration of tail of pancreas

√7ᵗʰ **S36.249** Minor laceration of unspecified part of pancreas

√6ᵗʰ **S36.25** Moderate laceration of pancreas

√7ᵗʰ **S36.250** Moderate laceration of head of pancreas

√7ᵗʰ **S36.251** Moderate laceration of body of pancreas

√7ᵗʰ **S36.252** Moderate laceration of tail of pancreas

√7ᵗʰ **S36.259** Moderate laceration of unspecified part of pancreas

✔️ Additional Character Required   √x7ᵗʰ Placeholder Alert   Manifestation   Unspecified Dx   ▶◀ Revised Text   ● New Code   ▲ Revised Title

ICD-10-CM 2020   983

√6ᵗʰ **S36.26** Major laceration of pancreas
- √7ᵗʰ **S36.260** Major laceration of head of pancreas
- √7ᵗʰ **S36.261** Major laceration of body of pancreas
- √7ᵗʰ **S36.262** Major laceration of tail of pancreas
- √7ᵗʰ **S36.269** Major laceration of unspecified part of pancreas

√6ᵗʰ **S36.29** Other injury of pancreas
- √7ᵗʰ **S36.290** Other injury of head of pancreas
- √7ᵗʰ **S36.291** Other injury of body of pancreas
- √7ᵗʰ **S36.292** Other injury of tail of pancreas
- √7ᵗʰ **S36.299** Other injury of unspecified part of pancreas

√5ᵗʰ **S36.3** Injury of stomach
- √x7ᵗʰ **S36.30** Unspecified injury of stomach
- √x7ᵗʰ **S36.32** Contusion of stomach
- √x7ᵗʰ **S36.33** Laceration of stomach
- √x7ᵗʰ **S36.39** Other injury of stomach

√5ᵗʰ **S36.4** Injury of small intestine
- √6ᵗʰ **S36.40** Unspecified injury of small intestine
  - √7ᵗʰ **S36.400** Unspecified injury of duodenum
  - √7ᵗʰ **S36.408** Unspecified injury of other part of small intestine
  - √7ᵗʰ **S36.409** Unspecified injury of unspecified part of small intestine
- √6ᵗʰ **S36.41** Primary blast injury of small intestine
  - Blast injury of small intestine NOS
  - √7ᵗʰ **S36.410** Primary blast injury of duodenum
  - √7ᵗʰ **S36.418** Primary blast injury of other part of small intestine
  - √7ᵗʰ **S36.419** Primary blast injury of unspecified part of small intestine
- √6ᵗʰ **S36.42** Contusion of small intestine
  - √7ᵗʰ **S36.420** Contusion of duodenum
  - √7ᵗʰ **S36.428** Contusion of other part of small intestine
  - √7ᵗʰ **S36.429** Contusion of unspecified part of small intestine
- √6ᵗʰ **S36.43** Laceration of small intestine
  - √7ᵗʰ **S36.430** Laceration of duodenum
  - √7ᵗʰ **S36.438** Laceration of other part of small intestine
  - √7ᵗʰ **S36.439** Laceration of unspecified part of small intestine
- √6ᵗʰ **S36.49** Other injury of small intestine
  - √7ᵗʰ **S36.490** Other injury of duodenum
  - √7ᵗʰ **S36.498** Other injury of other part of small intestine
  - √7ᵗʰ **S36.499** Other injury of unspecified part of small intestine

√5ᵗʰ **S36.5** Injury of colon
- EXCLUDES 2   injury of rectum (S36.6-)
- √6ᵗʰ **S36.50** Unspecified injury of colon
  - √7ᵗʰ **S36.500** Unspecified injury of ascending [right] colon
  - √7ᵗʰ **S36.501** Unspecified injury of transverse colon
  - √7ᵗʰ **S36.502** Unspecified injury of descending [left] colon
  - √7ᵗʰ **S36.503** Unspecified injury of sigmoid colon
  - √7ᵗʰ **S36.508** Unspecified injury of other part of colon
  - √7ᵗʰ **S36.509** Unspecified injury of unspecified part of colon
- √6ᵗʰ **S36.51** Primary blast injury of colon
  - Blast injury of colon NOS
  - √7ᵗʰ **S36.510** Primary blast injury of ascending [right] colon
  - √7ᵗʰ **S36.511** Primary blast injury of transverse colon
  - √7ᵗʰ **S36.512** Primary blast injury of descending [left] colon
  - √7ᵗʰ **S36.513** Primary blast injury of sigmoid colon
  - √7ᵗʰ **S36.518** Primary blast injury of other part of colon
  - √7ᵗʰ **S36.519** Primary blast injury of unspecified part of colon
- √6ᵗʰ **S36.52** Contusion of colon
  - √7ᵗʰ **S36.520** Contusion of ascending [right] colon
  - √7ᵗʰ **S36.521** Contusion of transverse colon
  - √7ᵗʰ **S36.522** Contusion of descending [left] colon
  - √7ᵗʰ **S36.523** Contusion of sigmoid colon
  - √7ᵗʰ **S36.528** Contusion of other part of colon
  - √7ᵗʰ **S36.529** Contusion of unspecified part of colon
- √6ᵗʰ **S36.53** Laceration of colon
  - √7ᵗʰ **S36.530** Laceration of ascending [right] colon
  - √7ᵗʰ **S36.531** Laceration of transverse colon
  - √7ᵗʰ **S36.532** Laceration of descending [left] colon
  - √7ᵗʰ **S36.533** Laceration of sigmoid colon
  - √7ᵗʰ **S36.538** Laceration of other part of colon
  - √7ᵗʰ **S36.539** Laceration of unspecified part of colon
- √6ᵗʰ **S36.59** Other injury of colon
  - Secondary blast injury of colon
  - √7ᵗʰ **S36.590** Other injury of ascending [right] colon
  - √7ᵗʰ **S36.591** Other injury of transverse colon
  - √7ᵗʰ **S36.592** Other injury of descending [left] colon
  - √7ᵗʰ **S36.593** Other injury of sigmoid colon
  - √7ᵗʰ **S36.598** Other injury of other part of colon
  - √7ᵗʰ **S36.599** Other injury of unspecified part of colon

√5ᵗʰ **S36.6** Injury of rectum
- √x7ᵗʰ **S36.60** Unspecified injury of rectum
- √x7ᵗʰ **S36.61** Primary blast injury of rectum
  - Blast injury of rectum NOS
- √x7ᵗʰ **S36.62** Contusion of rectum
- √x7ᵗʰ **S36.63** Laceration of rectum
- √x7ᵗʰ **S36.69** Other injury of rectum
  - Secondary blast injury of rectum

√5ᵗʰ **S36.8** Injury of other intra-abdominal organs
- √x7ᵗʰ **S36.81** Injury of peritoneum
- √6ᵗʰ **S36.89** Injury of other intra-abdominal organs
  - Injury of retroperitoneum
  - √7ᵗʰ **S36.892** Contusion of other intra-abdominal organs
  - √7ᵗʰ **S36.893** Laceration of other intra-abdominal organs
  - √7ᵗʰ **S36.898** Other injury of other intra-abdominal organs
  - √7ᵗʰ **S36.899** Unspecified injury of other intra-abdominal organs

√5ᵗʰ **S36.9** Injury of unspecified intra-abdominal organ
- √x7ᵗʰ **S36.90** Unspecified injury of unspecified intra-abdominal organ
- √x7ᵗʰ **S36.92** Contusion of unspecified intra-abdominal organ
- √x7ᵗʰ **S36.93** Laceration of unspecified intra-abdominal organ
- √x7ᵗʰ **S36.99** Other injury of unspecified intra-abdominal organ

√4ᵗʰ **S37** Injury of urinary and pelvic organs
- Code also any associated open wound (S31.-)
- EXCLUDES 1   obstetric trauma to pelvic organs (O71.-)
- EXCLUDES 2   injury of peritoneum (S36.81)
  - injury of retroperitoneum (S36.89-)

The appropriate 7th character is to be added to each code from category S37.
A initial encounter
D subsequent encounter
S sequela

√5ᵗʰ **S37.0** Injury of kidney
- EXCLUDES 2   acute kidney injury (nontraumatic) (N17.9)
- √6ᵗʰ **S37.00** Unspecified injury of kidney
  - √7ᵗʰ **S37.001** Unspecified injury of right kidney
  - √7ᵗʰ **S37.002** Unspecified injury of left kidney
  - √7ᵗʰ **S37.009** Unspecified injury of unspecified kidney
- √6ᵗʰ **S37.01** Minor contusion of kidney
  - Contusion of kidney less than 2 cm
  - Contusion of kidney NOS
  - √7ᵗʰ **S37.011** Minor contusion of right kidney
  - √7ᵗʰ **S37.012** Minor contusion of left kidney
  - √7ᵗʰ **S37.019** Minor contusion of unspecified kidney

✓6ᵗʰ **S37.02** Major contusion of kidney
      Contusion of kidney greater than 2 cm
    ✓7ᵗʰ **S37.021** Major contusion of right kidney
    ✓7ᵗʰ **S37.022** Major contusion of left kidney
    ✓7ᵗʰ **S37.029** Major contusion of unspecified kidney

✓6ᵗʰ **S37.03** Laceration of kidney, unspecified degree
    ✓7ᵗʰ **S37.031** Laceration of right kidney, unspecified degree
    ✓7ᵗʰ **S37.032** Laceration of left kidney, unspecified degree
    ✓7ᵗʰ **S37.039** Laceration of unspecified kidney, unspecified degree

✓6ᵗʰ **S37.04** Minor laceration of kidney
      Laceration of kidney less than 1 cm
    ✓7ᵗʰ **S37.041** Minor laceration of right kidney
    ✓7ᵗʰ **S37.042** Minor laceration of left kidney
    ✓7ᵗʰ **S37.049** Minor laceration of unspecified kidney

✓6ᵗʰ **S37.05** Moderate laceration of kidney
      Laceration of kidney 1 to 3 cm
    ✓7ᵗʰ **S37.051** Moderate laceration of right kidney
    ✓7ᵗʰ **S37.052** Moderate laceration of left kidney
    ✓7ᵗʰ **S37.059** Moderate laceration of unspecified kidney

✓6ᵗʰ **S37.06** Major laceration of kidney
      Avulsion of kidney
      Laceration of kidney greater than 3 cm
      Massive laceration of kidney
      Multiple moderate lacerations of kidney
      Stellate laceration of kidney
    ✓7ᵗʰ **S37.061** Major laceration of right kidney
    ✓7ᵗʰ **S37.062** Major laceration of left kidney
    ✓7ᵗʰ **S37.069** Major laceration of unspecified kidney

✓6ᵗʰ **S37.09** Other injury of kidney
    ✓7ᵗʰ **S37.091** Other injury of right kidney
    ✓7ᵗʰ **S37.092** Other injury of left kidney
    ✓7ᵗʰ **S37.099** Other injury of unspecified kidney

✓5ᵗʰ **S37.1** Injury of ureter
  ✓x7ᵗʰ **S37.10** Unspecified injury of ureter
  ✓x7ᵗʰ **S37.12** Contusion of ureter
  ✓x7ᵗʰ **S37.13** Laceration of ureter
  ✓x7ᵗʰ **S37.19** Other injury of ureter

✓5ᵗʰ **S37.2** Injury of bladder
  ✓x7ᵗʰ **S37.20** Unspecified injury of bladder
  ✓x7ᵗʰ **S37.22** Contusion of bladder
  ✓x7ᵗʰ **S37.23** Laceration of bladder
  ✓x7ᵗʰ **S37.29** Other injury of bladder

✓5ᵗʰ **S37.3** Injury of urethra
  ✓x7ᵗʰ **S37.30** Unspecified injury of urethra
  ✓x7ᵗʰ **S37.32** Contusion of urethra
  ✓x7ᵗʰ **S37.33** Laceration of urethra
  ✓x7ᵗʰ **S37.39** Other injury of urethra

✓5ᵗʰ **S37.4** Injury of ovary
  ✓6ᵗʰ **S37.40** Unspecified injury of ovary
    ✓7ᵗʰ **S37.401** Unspecified injury of ovary, unilateral ♀
    ✓7ᵗʰ **S37.402** Unspecified injury of ovary, bilateral ♀
    ✓7ᵗʰ **S37.409** Unspecified injury of ovary, unspecified ♀
  ✓6ᵗʰ **S37.42** Contusion of ovary
    ✓7ᵗʰ **S37.421** Contusion of ovary, unilateral ♀
    ✓7ᵗʰ **S37.422** Contusion of ovary, bilateral ♀
    ✓7ᵗʰ **S37.429** Contusion of ovary, unspecified ♀
  ✓6ᵗʰ **S37.43** Laceration of ovary
    ✓7ᵗʰ **S37.431** Laceration of ovary, unilateral ♀
    ✓7ᵗʰ **S37.432** Laceration of ovary, bilateral ♀
    ✓7ᵗʰ **S37.439** Laceration of ovary, unspecified ♀

✓6ᵗʰ **S37.49** Other injury of ovary
    ✓7ᵗʰ **S37.491** Other injury of ovary, unilateral ♀
    ✓7ᵗʰ **S37.492** Other injury of ovary, bilateral ♀
    ✓7ᵗʰ **S37.499** Other injury of ovary, unspecified ♀

✓5ᵗʰ **S37.5** Injury of fallopian tube
  ✓6ᵗʰ **S37.50** Unspecified injury of fallopian tube
    ✓7ᵗʰ **S37.501** Unspecified injury of fallopian tube, unilateral ♀
    ✓7ᵗʰ **S37.502** Unspecified injury of fallopian tube, bilateral ♀
    ✓7ᵗʰ **S37.509** Unspecified injury of fallopian tube, unspecified ♀
  ✓6ᵗʰ **S37.51** Primary blast injury of fallopian tube
      Blast injury of fallopian tube NOS
    ✓7ᵗʰ **S37.511** Primary blast injury of fallopian tube, unilateral ♀
    ✓7ᵗʰ **S37.512** Primary blast injury of fallopian tube, bilateral ♀
    ✓7ᵗʰ **S37.519** Primary blast injury of fallopian tube, unspecified ♀
  ✓6ᵗʰ **S37.52** Contusion of fallopian tube
    ✓7ᵗʰ **S37.521** Contusion of fallopian tube, unilateral ♀
    ✓7ᵗʰ **S37.522** Contusion of fallopian tube, bilateral ♀
    ✓7ᵗʰ **S37.529** Contusion of fallopian tube, unspecified ♀
  ✓6ᵗʰ **S37.53** Laceration of fallopian tube
    ✓7ᵗʰ **S37.531** Laceration of fallopian tube, unilateral ♀
    ✓7ᵗʰ **S37.532** Laceration of fallopian tube, bilateral ♀
    ✓7ᵗʰ **S37.539** Laceration of fallopian tube, unspecified ♀
  ✓6ᵗʰ **S37.59** Other injury of fallopian tube
      Secondary blast injury of fallopian tube
    ✓7ᵗʰ **S37.591** Other injury of fallopian tube, unilateral ♀
    ✓7ᵗʰ **S37.592** Other injury of fallopian tube, bilateral ♀
    ✓7ᵗʰ **S37.599** Other injury of fallopian tube, unspecified ♀

✓5ᵗʰ **S37.6** Injury of uterus
    EXCLUDES 1   injury to gravid uterus (O9A.2-)
               injury to uterus during delivery (O71.-)
  ✓x7ᵗʰ **S37.60** Unspecified injury of uterus ♀
  ✓x7ᵗʰ **S37.62** Contusion of uterus ♀
  ✓x7ᵗʰ **S37.63** Laceration of uterus ♀
  ✓x7ᵗʰ **S37.69** Other injury of uterus ♀

✓5ᵗʰ **S37.8** Injury of other urinary and pelvic organs
  ✓6ᵗʰ **S37.81** Injury of adrenal gland
    ✓7ᵗʰ **S37.812** Contusion of adrenal gland
    ✓7ᵗʰ **S37.813** Laceration of adrenal gland
    ✓7ᵗʰ **S37.818** Other injury of adrenal gland
    ✓7ᵗʰ **S37.819** Unspecified injury of adrenal gland
  ✓6ᵗʰ **S37.82** Injury of prostate
    ✓7ᵗʰ **S37.822** Contusion of prostate ♂
    ✓7ᵗʰ **S37.823** Laceration of prostate ♂
    ✓7ᵗʰ **S37.828** Other injury of prostate ♂
    ✓7ᵗʰ **S37.829** Unspecified injury of prostate ♂
  ✓6ᵗʰ **S37.89** Injury of other urinary and pelvic organ
    ✓7ᵗʰ **S37.892** Contusion of other urinary and pelvic organ
    ✓7ᵗʰ **S37.893** Laceration of other urinary and pelvic organ
    ✓7ᵗʰ **S37.898** Other injury of other urinary and pelvic organ
    ✓7ᵗʰ **S37.899** Unspecified injury of other urinary and pelvic organ

✓5ᵗʰ **S37.9** Injury of unspecified urinary and pelvic organ
  ✓x7ᵗʰ **S37.90** Unspecified injury of unspecified urinary and pelvic organ
  ✓x7ᵗʰ **S37.92** Contusion of unspecified urinary and pelvic organ

---

✅ Additional Character Required   ✓x7ᵗʰ Placeholder Alert   Manifestation   Unspecified Dx   ▶◀ Revised Text   ● New Code   ▲ Revised Title

√x7ᵗʰ **S37.93** Laceration of unspecified urinary and pelvic organ

√x7ᵗʰ **S37.99** Other injury of unspecified urinary and pelvic organ

√4ᵗʰ **S38 Crushing injury and traumatic amputation of abdomen, lower back, pelvis and external genitals**

> **NOTE** An amputation not identified as partial or complete should be coded to complete

> The appropriate 7th character is to be added to each code from category S38.
> A initial encounter
> D subsequent encounter
> S sequela

√5ᵗʰ **S38.0 Crushing injury of external genital organs**

> Use additional code for any associated injuries

√6ᵗʰ **S38.00 Crushing injury of unspecified external genital organs**

√7ᵗʰ **S38.001** Crushing injury of unspecified external genital organs, male ♂

√7ᵗʰ **S38.002** Crushing injury of unspecified external genital organs, female ♀

√x7ᵗʰ **S38.01 Crushing injury of penis** ♂

√x7ᵗʰ **S38.02 Crushing injury of scrotum and testis** ♂

√x7ᵗʰ **S38.03 Crushing injury of vulva** ♀

√x7ᵗʰ **S38.1 Crushing injury of abdomen, lower back, and pelvis**

> Use additional code for all associated injuries, such as:
> fracture of thoracic or lumbar spine and pelvis (S22.0-, S32.-)
> injury to intra-abdominal organs (S36.-)
> injury to urinary and pelvic organs (S37.-)
> open wound of abdominal wall (S31.-)
> spinal cord injury (S34.0, S34.1-)
> EXCLUDES 2   crushing injury of external genital organs (S38.0-)

√5ᵗʰ **S38.2 Traumatic amputation of external genital organs**

√6ᵗʰ **S38.21 Traumatic amputation of female external genital organs**

> Traumatic amputation of clitoris
> Traumatic amputation of labium (majus) (minus)
> Traumatic amputation of vulva

√7ᵗʰ **S38.211** Complete traumatic amputation of female external genital organs ♀

√7ᵗʰ **S38.212** Partial traumatic amputation of female external genital organs ♀

√6ᵗʰ **S38.22 Traumatic amputation of penis**

√7ᵗʰ **S38.221** Complete traumatic amputation of penis ♂

√7ᵗʰ **S38.222** Partial traumatic amputation of penis ♂

√6ᵗʰ **S38.23 Traumatic amputation of scrotum and testis**

√7ᵗʰ **S38.231** Complete traumatic amputation of scrotum and testis ♂

√7ᵗʰ **S38.232** Partial traumatic amputation of scrotum and testis ♂

√x7ᵗʰ **S38.3 Transection (partial) of abdomen**

√4ᵗʰ **S39 Other and unspecified injuries of abdomen, lower back, pelvis and external genitals**

> Code also any associated open wound (S31.-)
> EXCLUDES 2   sprain of joints and ligaments of lumbar spine and pelvis (S33.-)

> The appropriate 7th character is to be added to each code from category S39.
> A initial encounter
> D subsequent encounter
> S sequela

√5ᵗʰ **S39.0 Injury of muscle, fascia and tendon of abdomen, lower back and pelvis**

√6ᵗʰ **S39.00 Unspecified injury of muscle, fascia and tendon of abdomen, lower back and pelvis**

√7ᵗʰ **S39.001** Unspecified injury of muscle, fascia and tendon of abdomen

√7ᵗʰ **S39.002** Unspecified injury of muscle, fascia and tendon of lower back

√7ᵗʰ **S39.003** Unspecified injury of muscle, fascia and tendon of pelvis

√6ᵗʰ **S39.01 Strain of muscle, fascia and tendon of abdomen, lower back and pelvis**

√7ᵗʰ **S39.011** Strain of muscle, fascia and tendon of abdomen

√7ᵗʰ **S39.012** Strain of muscle, fascia and tendon of lower back

√7ᵗʰ **S39.013** Strain of muscle, fascia and tendon of pelvis

√6ᵗʰ **S39.02 Laceration of muscle, fascia and tendon of abdomen, lower back and pelvis**

√7ᵗʰ **S39.021** Laceration of muscle, fascia and tendon of abdomen

√7ᵗʰ **S39.022** Laceration of muscle, fascia and tendon of lower back

√7ᵗʰ **S39.023** Laceration of muscle, fascia and tendon of pelvis

√6ᵗʰ **S39.09 Other injury of muscle, fascia and tendon of abdomen, lower back and pelvis**

√7ᵗʰ **S39.091** Other injury of muscle, fascia and tendon of abdomen

√7ᵗʰ **S39.092** Other injury of muscle, fascia and tendon of lower back

√7ᵗʰ **S39.093** Other injury of muscle, fascia and tendon of pelvis

√5ᵗʰ **S39.8 Other specified injuries of abdomen, lower back, pelvis and external genitals**

√x7ᵗʰ **S39.81** Other specified injuries of abdomen

√x7ᵗʰ **S39.82** Other specified injuries of lower back

√x7ᵗʰ **S39.83** Other specified injuries of pelvis

√6ᵗʰ **S39.84** Other specified injuries of external genitals

√7ᵗʰ **S39.840** Fracture of corpus cavernosum penis ♂

√7ᵗʰ **S39.848** Other specified injuries of external genitals

√5ᵗʰ **S39.9 Unspecified injury of abdomen, lower back, pelvis and external genitals**

√x7ᵗʰ **S39.91** Unspecified injury of abdomen

√x7ᵗʰ **S39.92** Unspecified injury of lower back

√x7ᵗʰ **S39.93** Unspecified injury of pelvis

√x7ᵗʰ **S39.94** Unspecified injury of external genitals

Injuries to the shoulder and upper arm (S40-S49)

INCLUDES   injuries of axilla
injuries of scapular region

EXCLUDES 2   burns and corrosions (T20-T32)
frostbite (T33-T34)
injuries of elbow (S50-S59)
insect bite or sting, venomous (T63.4)

√4ᵗʰ **S40 Superficial injury of shoulder and upper arm**

> The appropriate 7th character is to be added to each code from category S40.
> A initial encounter
> D subsequent encounter
> S sequela

√5ᵗʰ **S40.0 Contusion of shoulder and upper arm**

√6ᵗʰ **S40.01 Contusion of shoulder**

√7ᵗʰ **S40.011** Contusion of right shoulder

√7ᵗʰ **S40.012** Contusion of left shoulder

√7ᵗʰ **S40.019** Contusion of unspecified shoulder

√6ᵗʰ **S40.02 Contusion of upper arm**

√7ᵗʰ **S40.021** Contusion of right upper arm

√7ᵗʰ **S40.022** Contusion of left upper arm

√7ᵗʰ **S40.029** Contusion of unspecified upper arm

√5ᵗʰ **S40.2 Other superficial injuries of shoulder**

√6ᵗʰ **S40.21 Abrasion of shoulder**

√7ᵗʰ **S40.211** Abrasion of right shoulder

√7ᵗʰ **S40.212** Abrasion of left shoulder

√7ᵗʰ **S40.219** Abrasion of unspecified shoulder

√6ᵗʰ **S40.22 Blister (nonthermal) of shoulder**

√7ᵗʰ **S40.221** Blister (nonthermal) of right shoulder

√7ᵗʰ **S40.222** Blister (nonthermal) of left shoulder

√7ᵗʰ **S40.229** Blister (nonthermal) of unspecified shoulder

√6ᵗʰ **S40.24** External constriction **of shoulder**

    √7ᵗʰ **S40.241** **External constriction of** right **shoulder**

    √7ᵗʰ **S40.242** **External constriction of** left **shoulder**

    √7ᵗʰ **S40.249** **External constriction of unspecified shoulder**

√6ᵗʰ **S40.25** **Superficial** foreign body **of shoulder**

    Splinter in the shoulder

    √7ᵗʰ **S40.251** **Superficial foreign body of** right **shoulder**

    √7ᵗʰ **S40.252** **Superficial foreign body of** left **shoulder**

    √7ᵗʰ **S40.259** **Superficial foreign body of unspecified shoulder**

√6ᵗʰ **S40.26** Insect bite (nonvenomous) **of shoulder**

    √7ᵗʰ **S40.261** **Insect bite (nonvenomous) of** right **shoulder**

    √7ᵗʰ **S40.262** **Insect bite (nonvenomous) of** left **shoulder**

    √7ᵗʰ **S40.269** **Insect bite (nonvenomous) of unspecified shoulder**

√6ᵗʰ **S40.27** **Other superficial** bite **of shoulder**

    EXCLUDES 1   open bite of shoulder (S41.05)

    √7ᵗʰ **S40.271** **Other superficial bite of** right **shoulder**

    √7ᵗʰ **S40.272** **Other superficial bite of** left **shoulder**

    √7ᵗʰ **S40.279** **Other superficial bite of unspecified shoulder**

√5ᵗʰ **S40.8** **Other superficial injuries of** upper arm

√6ᵗʰ **S40.81** Abrasion **of upper arm**

    √7ᵗʰ **S40.811** **Abrasion of** right **upper arm**

    √7ᵗʰ **S40.812** **Abrasion of** left **upper arm**

    √7ᵗʰ **S40.819** **Abrasion of unspecified upper arm**

√6ᵗʰ **S40.82** Blister (nonthermal) **of upper arm**

    √7ᵗʰ **S40.821** **Blister (nonthermal) of** right **upper arm**

    √7ᵗʰ **S40.822** **Blister (nonthermal) of** left **upper arm**

    √7ᵗʰ **S40.829** **Blister (nonthermal) of unspecified upper arm**

√6ᵗʰ **S40.84** External constriction **of upper arm**

    √7ᵗʰ **S40.841** **External constriction of** right **upper arm**

    √7ᵗʰ **S40.842** **External constriction of** left **upper arm**

    √7ᵗʰ **S40.849** **External constriction of unspecified upper arm**

√6ᵗʰ **S40.85** **Superficial** foreign body **of upper arm**

    Splinter in the upper arm

    √7ᵗʰ **S40.851** **Superficial foreign body of** right **upper arm**

    √7ᵗʰ **S40.852** **Superficial foreign body of** left **upper arm**

    √7ᵗʰ **S40.859** **Superficial foreign body of unspecified upper arm**

√6ᵗʰ **S40.86** Insect bite (nonvenomous) **of upper arm**

    √7ᵗʰ **S40.861** **Insect bite (nonvenomous) of** right **upper arm**

    √7ᵗʰ **S40.862** **Insect bite (nonvenomous) of** left **upper arm**

    √7ᵗʰ **S40.869** **Insect bite (nonvenomous) of unspecified upper arm**

√6ᵗʰ **S40.87** **Other superficial** bite **of upper arm**

    EXCLUDES 1   open bite of upper arm (S41.14)

    EXCLUDES 2   other superficial bite of shoulder (S40.27-)

    √7ᵗʰ **S40.871** **Other superficial bite of** right **upper arm**

    √7ᵗʰ **S40.872** **Other superficial bite of** left **upper arm**

    √7ᵗʰ **S40.879** **Other superficial bite of unspecified upper arm**

√5ᵗʰ **S40.9** **Unspecified superficial injury of shoulder and upper arm**

√6ᵗʰ **S40.91** **Unspecified superficial injury of** shoulder

    √7ᵗʰ **S40.911** **Unspecified superficial injury of** right **shoulder**

    √7ᵗʰ **S40.912** **Unspecified superficial injury of** left **shoulder**

    √7ᵗʰ **S40.919** **Unspecified superficial injury of unspecified shoulder**

√6ᵗʰ **S40.92** **Unspecified superficial injury of** upper arm

    √7ᵗʰ **S40.921** **Unspecified superficial injury of** right **upper arm**

    √7ᵗʰ **S40.922** **Unspecified superficial injury of** left **upper arm**

√4ᵗʰ **S41** **Open wound of shoulder and upper arm**

    Code also any associated wound infection

    EXCLUDES 1   traumatic amputation of shoulder and upper arm (S48.-)

    EXCLUDES 2   open fracture of shoulder and upper arm (S42.- with 7th character B or C)

    The appropriate 7th character is to be added to each code from category S41.
    A   initial encounter
    D   subsequent encounter
    S   sequela

√5ᵗʰ **S41.0** **Open wound of** shoulder

√6ᵗʰ **S41.00** **Unspecified open wound of shoulder**

    √7ᵗʰ **S41.001** **Unspecified open wound of** right **shoulder**

    √7ᵗʰ **S41.002** **Unspecified open wound of** left **shoulder**

    √7ᵗʰ **S41.009** **Unspecified open wound of unspecified shoulder**

√6ᵗʰ **S41.01** Laceration without foreign body **of shoulder**

    √7ᵗʰ **S41.011** **Laceration without foreign body of** right **shoulder**

    √7ᵗʰ **S41.012** **Laceration without foreign body of** left **shoulder**

    √7ᵗʰ **S41.019** **Laceration without foreign body of unspecified shoulder**

√6ᵗʰ **S41.02** Laceration with foreign body **of shoulder**

    √7ᵗʰ **S41.021** **Laceration with foreign body of** right **shoulder**

    √7ᵗʰ **S41.022** **Laceration with foreign body of** left **shoulder**

    √7ᵗʰ **S41.029** **Laceration with foreign body of unspecified shoulder**

√6ᵗʰ **S41.03** Puncture wound without foreign body **of shoulder**

    √7ᵗʰ **S41.031** **Puncture wound without foreign body of** right **shoulder**

    √7ᵗʰ **S41.032** **Puncture wound without foreign body of** left **shoulder**

    √7ᵗʰ **S41.039** **Puncture wound without foreign body of unspecified shoulder**

√6ᵗʰ **S41.04** Puncture wound with foreign body **of shoulder**

    √7ᵗʰ **S41.041** **Puncture wound with foreign body of** right **shoulder**

    √7ᵗʰ **S41.042** **Puncture wound with foreign body of** left **shoulder**

    √7ᵗʰ **S41.049** **Puncture wound with foreign body of unspecified shoulder**

√6ᵗʰ **S41.05** Open bite **of shoulder**

    Bite of shoulder NOS

    EXCLUDES 1   superficial bite of shoulder (S40.27)

    √7ᵗʰ **S41.051** **Open bite of** right **shoulder**

    √7ᵗʰ **S41.052** **Open bite of** left **shoulder**

    √7ᵗʰ **S41.059** **Open bite of unspecified shoulder**

√5ᵗʰ **S41.1** **Open wound of** upper arm

√6ᵗʰ **S41.10** **Unspecified open wound of upper arm**

    AHA: 2016,3Q,24

    √7ᵗʰ **S41.101** **Unspecified open wound of** right **upper arm**

    √7ᵗʰ **S41.102** **Unspecified open wound of** left **upper arm**

    √7ᵗʰ **S41.109** **Unspecified open wound of unspecified upper arm**

√6ᵗʰ **S41.11** Laceration without foreign body **of upper arm**

    √7ᵗʰ **S41.111** **Laceration without foreign body of** right **upper arm**

    √7ᵗʰ **S41.112** **Laceration without foreign body of** left **upper arm**

    √7ᵗʰ **S41.119** **Laceration without foreign body of unspecified upper arm**

√6ᵗʰ **S41.12** Laceration with foreign body **of upper arm**

    √7ᵗʰ **S41.121** **Laceration with foreign body of** right **upper arm**

    √7ᵗʰ **S41.122** **Laceration with foreign body of** left **upper arm**

    √7ᵗʰ **S41.129** **Laceration with foreign body of unspecified upper arm**

✔ Additional Character Required   √x7ᵗʰ Placeholder Alert   Manifestation   Unspecified Dx   ▶◀ Revised Text   ● New Code   ▲ Revised Title

ICD-10-CM 2020   987

✓6ᵗʰ **S41.13** Puncture wound without foreign body of upper arm
    AHA: 2016,3Q,24
  ✓7ᵗʰ **S41.131** Puncture wound without foreign body of right upper arm
  ✓7ᵗʰ **S41.132** Puncture wound without foreign body of left upper arm
  ✓7ᵗʰ **S41.139** Puncture wound without foreign body of unspecified upper arm

✓6ᵗʰ **S41.14** Puncture wound with foreign body of upper arm
    AHA: 2016,3Q,24
  ✓7ᵗʰ **S41.141** Puncture wound with foreign body of right upper arm
  ✓7ᵗʰ **S41.142** Puncture wound with foreign body of left upper arm
  ✓7ᵗʰ **S41.149** Puncture wound with foreign body of unspecified upper arm

✓6ᵗʰ **S41.15** Open bite of upper arm
    Bite of upper arm NOS
    EXCLUDES 1 superficial bite of upper arm (S40.87)
  ✓7ᵗʰ **S41.151** Open bite of right upper arm
  ✓7ᵗʰ **S41.152** Open bite of left upper arm
  ✓7ᵗʰ **S41.159** Open bite of unspecified upper arm

✓4ᵗʰ **S42** Fracture of shoulder and upper arm
  NOTE A fracture not indicated as displaced or nondisplaced should be coded to displaced
      A fracture not indicated as open or closed should be coded to closed
  EXCLUDES 1 traumatic amputation of shoulder and upper arm (S48.-)
  AHA: 2018,2Q,12; 2015,3Q,37-39
  DEF: Diaphysis: Central shaft of a long bone.
  DEF: Epiphysis: Proximal and distal rounded ends of a long bone, communicates with the joint.
  DEF: Metaphysis: Section of a long bone located between the epiphysis and diaphysis at the proximal and distal ends.
  DEF: Physis (growth plate): Narrow zone of cartilaginous tissue between the epiphysis and metaphysis at each end of a long bone. In childhood, proliferation of cells in this zone lengthens the bone. As the bone matures, this area thins, ossification eventually fusing into solid bone and growth stops. **Synonyms:** Epiphyseal plate.
  TIP: The term "improper alignment" is not synonymous with malunion or nonunion of a fracture when noted in provider documentation.

The appropriate 7th character is to be added to all codes from category S42 [unless otherwise indicated].
A   initial encounter for closed fracture
B   initial encounter for open fracture
D   subsequent encounter for fracture with routine healing
G   subsequent encounter for fracture with delayed healing
K   subsequent encounter for fracture with nonunion
P   subsequent encounter for fracture with malunion
S   sequela

✓5ᵗʰ **S42.0** Fracture of clavicle
  ✓6ᵗʰ **S42.00** Fracture of unspecified part of clavicle
    ✓7ᵗʰ **S42.001** Fracture of unspecified part of right clavicle
    ✓7ᵗʰ **S42.002** Fracture of unspecified part of left clavicle
    ✓7ᵗʰ **S42.009** Fracture of unspecified part of unspecified clavicle
      AHA: 2012,4Q,93
  ✓6ᵗʰ **S42.01** Fracture of sternal end of clavicle
    ✓7ᵗʰ **S42.011** Anterior displaced fracture of sternal end of right clavicle
    ✓7ᵗʰ **S42.012** Anterior displaced fracture of sternal end of left clavicle
    ✓7ᵗʰ **S42.013** Anterior displaced fracture of sternal end of unspecified clavicle
      Displaced fracture of sternal end of clavicle NOS
    ✓7ᵗʰ **S42.014** Posterior displaced fracture of sternal end of right clavicle
    ✓7ᵗʰ **S42.015** Posterior displaced fracture of sternal end of left clavicle
    ✓7ᵗʰ **S42.016** Posterior displaced fracture of sternal end of unspecified clavicle
    ✓7ᵗʰ **S42.017** Nondisplaced fracture of sternal end of right clavicle

    ✓7ᵗʰ **S42.018** Nondisplaced fracture of sternal end of left clavicle
    ✓7ᵗʰ **S42.019** Nondisplaced fracture of sternal end of unspecified clavicle
  ✓6ᵗʰ **S42.02** Fracture of shaft of clavicle
    ✓7ᵗʰ **S42.021** Displaced fracture of shaft of right clavicle
    ✓7ᵗʰ **S42.022** Displaced fracture of shaft of left clavicle
    ✓7ᵗʰ **S42.023** Displaced fracture of shaft of unspecified clavicle
    ✓7ᵗʰ **S42.024** Nondisplaced fracture of shaft of right clavicle
    ✓7ᵗʰ **S42.025** Nondisplaced fracture of shaft of left clavicle
    ✓7ᵗʰ **S42.026** Nondisplaced fracture of shaft of unspecified clavicle
  ✓6ᵗʰ **S42.03** Fracture of lateral end of clavicle
    Fracture of acromial end of clavicle
    ✓7ᵗʰ **S42.031** Displaced fracture of lateral end of right clavicle
    ✓7ᵗʰ **S42.032** Displaced fracture of lateral end of left clavicle
    ✓7ᵗʰ **S42.033** Displaced fracture of lateral end of unspecified clavicle
    ✓7ᵗʰ **S42.034** Nondisplaced fracture of lateral end of right clavicle
    ✓7ᵗʰ **S42.035** Nondisplaced fracture of lateral end of left clavicle
    ✓7ᵗʰ **S42.036** Nondisplaced fracture of lateral end of unspecified clavicle

✓5ᵗʰ **S42.1** Fracture of scapula
  ✓6ᵗʰ **S42.10** Fracture of unspecified part of scapula
    ✓7ᵗʰ **S42.101** Fracture of unspecified part of scapula, right shoulder
    ✓7ᵗʰ **S42.102** Fracture of unspecified part of scapula, left shoulder
    ✓7ᵗʰ **S42.109** Fracture of unspecified part of scapula, unspecified shoulder
  ✓6ᵗʰ **S42.11** Fracture of body of scapula
    ✓7ᵗʰ **S42.111** Displaced fracture of body of scapula, right shoulder
    ✓7ᵗʰ **S42.112** Displaced fracture of body of scapula, left shoulder
    ✓7ᵗʰ **S42.113** Displaced fracture of body of scapula, unspecified shoulder
    ✓7ᵗʰ **S42.114** Nondisplaced fracture of body of scapula, right shoulder
    ✓7ᵗʰ **S42.115** Nondisplaced fracture of body of scapula, left shoulder
    ✓7ᵗʰ **S42.116** Nondisplaced fracture of body of scapula, unspecified shoulder
  ✓6ᵗʰ **S42.12** Fracture of acromial process
    ✓7ᵗʰ **S42.121** Displaced fracture of acromial process, right shoulder
    ✓7ᵗʰ **S42.122** Displaced fracture of acromial process, left shoulder
    ✓7ᵗʰ **S42.123** Displaced fracture of acromial process, unspecified shoulder
    ✓7ᵗʰ **S42.124** Nondisplaced fracture of acromial process, right shoulder
    ✓7ᵗʰ **S42.125** Nondisplaced fracture of acromial process, left shoulder
    ✓7ᵗʰ **S42.126** Nondisplaced fracture of acromial process, unspecified shoulder
  ✓6ᵗʰ **S42.13** Fracture of coracoid process
    ✓7ᵗʰ **S42.131** Displaced fracture of coracoid process, right shoulder
    ✓7ᵗʰ **S42.132** Displaced fracture of coracoid process, left shoulder
    ✓7ᵗʰ **S42.133** Displaced fracture of coracoid process, unspecified shoulder
    ✓7ᵗʰ **S42.134** Nondisplaced fracture of coracoid process, right shoulder
    ✓7ᵗʰ **S42.135** Nondisplaced fracture of coracoid process, left shoulder
    ✓7ᵗʰ **S42.136** Nondisplaced fracture of coracoid process, unspecified shoulder
  ✓6ᵗʰ **S42.14** Fracture of glenoid cavity of scapula
    ✓7ᵗʰ **S42.141** Displaced fracture of glenoid cavity of scapula, right shoulder

√7ᵗʰ **S42.142** Displaced fracture of glenoid cavity of scapula, left shoulder

√7ᵗʰ **S42.143** Displaced fracture of glenoid cavity of scapula, unspecified shoulder

√7ᵗʰ **S42.144** Nondisplaced fracture of glenoid cavity of scapula, right shoulder

√7ᵗʰ **S42.145** Nondisplaced fracture of glenoid cavity of scapula, left shoulder

√7ᵗʰ **S42.146** Nondisplaced fracture of glenoid cavity of scapula, unspecified shoulder

√6ᵗʰ **S42.15** Fracture of neck of scapula

√7ᵗʰ **S42.151** Displaced fracture of neck of scapula, right shoulder

√7ᵗʰ **S42.152** Displaced fracture of neck of scapula, left shoulder

√7ᵗʰ **S42.153** Displaced fracture of neck of scapula, unspecified shoulder

√7ᵗʰ **S42.154** Nondisplaced fracture of neck of scapula, right shoulder

√7ᵗʰ **S42.155** Nondisplaced fracture of neck of scapula, left shoulder

√7ᵗʰ **S42.156** Nondisplaced fracture of neck of scapula, unspecified shoulder

√6ᵗʰ **S42.19** Fracture of other part of scapula

√7ᵗʰ **S42.191** Fracture of other part of scapula, right shoulder

√7ᵗʰ **S42.192** Fracture of other part of scapula, left shoulder

√7ᵗʰ **S42.199** Fracture of other part of scapula, unspecified shoulder

√5ᵗʰ **S42.2** Fracture of upper end of humerus

Fracture of proximal end of humerus
EXCLUDES 2   fracture of shaft of humerus (S42.3-)
     physeal fracture of upper end of humerus (S49.0-)

√6ᵗʰ **S42.20** Unspecified fracture of upper end of humerus

√7ᵗʰ **S42.201** Unspecified fracture of upper end of right humerus

√7ᵗʰ **S42.202** Unspecified fracture of upper end of left humerus

√7ᵗʰ **S42.209** Unspecified fracture of upper end of unspecified humerus

√6ᵗʰ **S42.21** Unspecified fracture of surgical neck of humerus

Fracture of neck of humerus NOS

√7ᵗʰ **S42.211** Unspecified displaced fracture of surgical neck of right humerus

√7ᵗʰ **S42.212** Unspecified displaced fracture of surgical neck of left humerus

√7ᵗʰ **S42.213** Unspecified displaced fracture of surgical neck of unspecified humerus

√7ᵗʰ **S42.214** Unspecified nondisplaced fracture of surgical neck of right humerus

√7ᵗʰ **S42.215** Unspecified nondisplaced fracture of surgical neck of left humerus

√7ᵗʰ **S42.216** Unspecified nondisplaced fracture of surgical neck of unspecified humerus

√6ᵗʰ **S42.22** 2-part fracture of surgical neck of humerus

√7ᵗʰ **S42.221** 2-part displaced fracture of surgical neck of right humerus

√7ᵗʰ **S42.222** 2-part displaced fracture of surgical neck of left humerus

√7ᵗʰ **S42.223** 2-part displaced fracture of surgical neck of unspecified humerus

√7ᵗʰ **S42.224** 2-part nondisplaced fracture of surgical neck of right humerus

√7ᵗʰ **S42.225** 2-part nondisplaced fracture of surgical neck of left humerus

√7ᵗʰ **S42.226** 2-part nondisplaced fracture of surgical neck of unspecified humerus

√6ᵗʰ **S42.23** 3-part fracture of surgical neck of humerus

√7ᵗʰ **S42.231** 3-part fracture of surgical neck of right humerus

√7ᵗʰ **S42.232** 3-part fracture of surgical neck of left humerus

√7ᵗʰ **S42.239** 3-part fracture of surgical neck of unspecified humerus

√6ᵗʰ **S42.24** 4-part fracture of surgical neck of humerus

√7ᵗʰ **S42.241** 4-part fracture of surgical neck of right humerus

√7ᵗʰ **S42.242** 4-part fracture of surgical neck of left humerus

√7ᵗʰ **S42.249** 4-part fracture of surgical neck of unspecified humerus

√6ᵗʰ **S42.25** Fracture of greater tuberosity of humerus

√7ᵗʰ **S42.251** Displaced fracture of greater tuberosity of right humerus

√7ᵗʰ **S42.252** Displaced fracture of greater tuberosity of left humerus

√7ᵗʰ **S42.253** Displaced fracture of greater tuberosity of unspecified humerus

√7ᵗʰ **S42.254** Nondisplaced fracture of greater tuberosity of right humerus

√7ᵗʰ **S42.255** Nondisplaced fracture of greater tuberosity of left humerus

√7ᵗʰ **S42.256** Nondisplaced fracture of greater tuberosity of unspecified humerus

√6ᵗʰ **S42.26** Fracture of lesser tuberosity of humerus

√7ᵗʰ **S42.261** Displaced fracture of lesser tuberosity of right humerus

√7ᵗʰ **S42.262** Displaced fracture of lesser tuberosity of left humerus

√7ᵗʰ **S42.263** Displaced fracture of lesser tuberosity of unspecified humerus

√7ᵗʰ **S42.264** Nondisplaced fracture of lesser tuberosity of right humerus

√7ᵗʰ **S42.265** Nondisplaced fracture of lesser tuberosity of left humerus

√7ᵗʰ **S42.266** Nondisplaced fracture of lesser tuberosity of unspecified humerus

√6ᵗʰ **S42.27** Torus fracture of upper end of humerus

The appropriate 7th character is to be added to all codes in subcategory S42.27
A   initial encounter for closed fracture
D   subsequent encounter for fracture with routine healing
G   subsequent encounter for fracture with delayed healing
K   subsequent encounter for fracture with nonunion
P   subsequent encounter for fracture with malunion
S   sequela

√7ᵗʰ **S42.271** Torus fracture of upper end of right humerus

√7ᵗʰ **S42.272** Torus fracture of upper end of left humerus

√7ᵗʰ **S42.279** Torus fracture of upper end of unspecified humerus

√6ᵗʰ **S42.29** Other fracture of upper end of humerus

Fracture of anatomical neck of humerus
Fracture of articular head of humerus
AHA: 2019,1Q,18

√7ᵗʰ **S42.291** Other displaced fracture of upper end of right humerus

√7ᵗʰ **S42.292** Other displaced fracture of upper end of left humerus

√7ᵗʰ **S42.293** Other displaced fracture of upper end of unspecified humerus

√7ᵗʰ **S42.294** Other nondisplaced fracture of upper end of right humerus

√7ᵗʰ **S42.295** Other nondisplaced fracture of upper end of left humerus

√7ᵗʰ **S42.296** Other nondisplaced fracture of upper end of unspecified humerus

√5ᵗʰ **S42.3** Fracture of shaft of humerus

Fracture of humerus NOS
Fracture of upper arm NOS
EXCLUDES 2   physeal fractures of upper end of humerus (S49.0-)
     physeal fractures of lower end of humerus (S49.1-)

√6ᵗʰ **S42.30** Unspecified fracture of shaft of humerus

√7ᵗʰ **S42.301** Unspecified fracture of shaft of humerus, right arm

√7ᵗʰ **S42.302** Unspecified fracture of shaft of humerus, left arm

√7ᵗʰ **S42.309** Unspecified fracture of shaft of humerus, unspecified arm

✓6ᵗʰ **S42.31** Greenstick **fracture of shaft of humerus**

> The appropriate 7th character is to be added to all codes in subcategory S42.31
> A   initial encounter for closed fracture
> D   subsequent encounter for fracture with routine healing
> G   subsequent encounter for fracture with delayed healing
> K   subsequent encounter for fracture with nonunion
> P   subsequent encounter for fracture with malunion
> S   sequela

     ✓7ᵗʰ **S42.311** **Greenstick fracture of shaft of humerus,** right **arm**

     ✓7ᵗʰ **S42.312** **Greenstick fracture of shaft of humerus,** left **arm**

     ✓7ᵗʰ **S42.319** **Greenstick fracture of shaft of humerus, unspecified arm**

✓6ᵗʰ **S42.32** Transverse **fracture of shaft of humerus**

     ✓7ᵗʰ **S42.321** Displaced **transverse fracture of shaft of humerus,** right **arm**

     ✓7ᵗʰ **S42.322** Displaced **transverse fracture of shaft of humerus,** left **arm**

     ✓7ᵗʰ **S42.323** Displaced **transverse fracture of shaft of humerus, unspecified arm**

     ✓7ᵗʰ **S42.324** Nondisplaced **transverse fracture of shaft of humerus,** right **arm**

     ✓7ᵗʰ **S42.325** Nondisplaced **transverse fracture of shaft of humerus,** left **arm**

     ✓7ᵗʰ **S42.326** Nondisplaced **transverse fracture of shaft of humerus, unspecified arm**

✓6ᵗʰ **S42.33** Oblique **fracture of shaft of humerus**

     ✓7ᵗʰ **S42.331** Displaced **oblique fracture of shaft of humerus,** right **arm**

     ✓7ᵗʰ **S42.332** Displaced **oblique fracture of shaft of humerus,** left **arm**

     ✓7ᵗʰ **S42.333** Displaced **oblique fracture of shaft of humerus, unspecified arm**

     ✓7ᵗʰ **S42.334** Nondisplaced **oblique fracture of shaft of humerus,** right **arm**

     ✓7ᵗʰ **S42.335** Nondisplaced **oblique fracture of shaft of humerus,** left **arm**

     ✓7ᵗʰ **S42.336** Nondisplaced **oblique fracture of shaft of humerus, unspecified arm**

✓6ᵗʰ **S42.34** Spiral **fracture of shaft of humerus**

     ✓7ᵗʰ **S42.341** Displaced **spiral fracture of shaft of humerus,** right **arm**

     ✓7ᵗʰ **S42.342** Displaced **spiral fracture of shaft of humerus,** left **arm**

     ✓7ᵗʰ **S42.343** Displaced **spiral fracture of shaft of humerus, unspecified arm**

     ✓7ᵗʰ **S42.344** Nondisplaced **spiral fracture of shaft of humerus,** right **arm**

     ✓7ᵗʰ **S42.345** Nondisplaced **spiral fracture of shaft of humerus,** left **arm**

     ✓7ᵗʰ **S42.346** Nondisplaced **spiral fracture of shaft of humerus, unspecified arm**

✓6ᵗʰ **S42.35** Comminuted **fracture of shaft of humerus**

     ✓7ᵗʰ **S42.351** Displaced **comminuted fracture of shaft of humerus,** right **arm**

     ✓7ᵗʰ **S42.352** Displaced **comminuted fracture of shaft of humerus,** left **arm**

     ✓7ᵗʰ **S42.353** Displaced **comminuted fracture of shaft of humerus, unspecified arm**

     ✓7ᵗʰ **S42.354** Nondisplaced **comminuted fracture of shaft of humerus,** right **arm**

     ✓7ᵗʰ **S42.355** Nondisplaced **comminuted fracture of shaft of humerus,** left **arm**

     ✓7ᵗʰ **S42.356** Nondisplaced **comminuted fracture of shaft of humerus, unspecified arm**

✓6ᵗʰ **S42.36** Segmental **fracture of shaft of humerus**

     ✓7ᵗʰ **S42.361** Displaced **segmental fracture of shaft of humerus,** right **arm**

     ✓7ᵗʰ **S42.362** Displaced **segmental fracture of shaft of humerus,** left **arm**

     ✓7ᵗʰ **S42.363** Displaced **segmental fracture of shaft of humerus, unspecified arm**

     ✓7ᵗʰ **S42.364** Nondisplaced **segmental fracture of shaft of humerus,** right **arm**

     ✓7ᵗʰ **S42.365** Nondisplaced **segmental fracture of shaft of humerus,** left **arm**

     ✓7ᵗʰ **S42.366** Nondisplaced **segmental fracture of shaft of humerus, unspecified arm**

✓6ᵗʰ **S42.39** Other **fracture of shaft of humerus**

     ✓7ᵗʰ **S42.391** Other fracture of shaft of right humerus

     ✓7ᵗʰ **S42.392** Other fracture of shaft of left humerus

     ✓7ᵗʰ **S42.399** Other fracture of shaft of unspecified humerus

✓5ᵗʰ **S42.4** **Fracture of** lower end **of humerus**

     Fracture of distal end of humerus

     EXCLUDES 2   *fracture of shaft of humerus (S42.3-)*

                       physeal fracture of lower end of humerus (S49.1-)

✓6ᵗʰ **S42.40** Unspecified **fracture of lower end of humerus**

     Fracture of elbow NOS

     ✓7ᵗʰ **S42.401** **Unspecified fracture of lower end of** right **humerus**

     ✓7ᵗʰ **S42.402** **Unspecified fracture of lower end of** left **humerus**

     ✓7ᵗʰ **S42.409** **Unspecified fracture of lower end of unspecified humerus**

✓6ᵗʰ **S42.41** Simple supracondylar **fracture** without intercondylar **fracture of humerus**

     ✓7ᵗʰ **S42.411** Displaced **simple supracondylar fracture without intercondylar fracture of** right **humerus**

     ✓7ᵗʰ **S42.412** Displaced **simple supracondylar fracture without intercondylar fracture of** left **humerus**

     ✓7ᵗʰ **S42.413** Displaced **simple supracondylar fracture without intercondylar fracture of unspecified humerus**

     ✓7ᵗʰ **S42.414** Nondisplaced **simple supracondylar fracture without intercondylar fracture of** right **humerus**

     ✓7ᵗʰ **S42.415** Nondisplaced **simple supracondylar fracture without intercondylar fracture of** left **humerus**

     ✓7ᵗʰ **S42.416** Nondisplaced **simple supracondylar fracture without intercondylar fracture of unspecified humerus**

✓6ᵗʰ **S42.42** Comminuted supracondylar **fracture** without intercondylar **fracture of humerus**

     ✓7ᵗʰ **S42.421** Displaced **comminuted supracondylar fracture without intercondylar fracture of** right **humerus**

     ✓7ᵗʰ **S42.422** Displaced **comminuted supracondylar fracture without intercondylar fracture of** left **humerus**

     ✓7ᵗʰ **S42.423** Displaced **comminuted supracondylar fracture without intercondylar fracture of unspecified humerus**

     ✓7ᵗʰ **S42.424** Nondisplaced **comminuted supracondylar fracture without intercondylar fracture of** right **humerus**

     ✓7ᵗʰ **S42.425** Nondisplaced **comminuted supracondylar fracture without intercondylar fracture of** left **humerus**

     ✓7ᵗʰ **S42.426** Nondisplaced **comminuted supracondylar fracture without intercondylar fracture of unspecified humerus**

✓6ᵗʰ **S42.43** Fracture (avulsion) of lateral epicondyle **of humerus**

     ✓7ᵗʰ **S42.431** Displaced **fracture (avulsion) of lateral epicondyle of** right **humerus**

     ✓7ᵗʰ **S42.432** Displaced **fracture (avulsion) of lateral epicondyle of** left **humerus**

     ✓7ᵗʰ **S42.433** Displaced **fracture (avulsion) of lateral epicondyle of unspecified humerus**

     ✓7ᵗʰ **S42.434** Nondisplaced **fracture (avulsion) of lateral epicondyle of** right **humerus**

     ✓7ᵗʰ **S42.435** Nondisplaced **fracture (avulsion) of lateral epicondyle of** left **humerus**

     ✓7ᵗʰ **S42.436** Nondisplaced **fracture (avulsion) of lateral epicondyle of unspecified humerus**

✓6ᵗʰ **S42.44** Fracture (avulsion) of medial epicondyle **of humerus**

     ✓7ᵗʰ **S42.441** Displaced **fracture (avulsion) of medial epicondyle of** right **humerus**

     ✓7ᵗʰ **S42.442** Displaced **fracture (avulsion) of medial epicondyle of** left **humerus**

     ✓7ᵗʰ **S42.443** Displaced **fracture (avulsion) of medial epicondyle of unspecified humerus**

Ⓝ Newborn: 0   Ⓟ Pediatric: 0-17   Ⓜ Maternity: 12-55   Ⓐ Adult: 15-124   **CH** Comorbidity High   **CL** Comorbidity Low   **NCDx** Noncancer Dx   **PDx** Primary Dx

990   ICD-10-CM 2020

√7ᵗʰ **S42.444** Nondisplaced fracture (avulsion) of medial epicondyle of right humerus

√7ᵗʰ **S42.445** Nondisplaced fracture (avulsion) of medial epicondyle of left humerus

√7ᵗʰ **S42.446** Nondisplaced fracture (avulsion) of medial epicondyle of unspecified humerus

√7ᵗʰ **S42.447** Incarcerated fracture (avulsion) of medial epicondyle of right humerus

√7ᵗʰ **S42.448** Incarcerated fracture (avulsion) of medial epicondyle of left humerus

√7ᵗʰ **S42.449** Incarcerated fracture (avulsion) of medial epicondyle of unspecified humerus

√6ᵗʰ **S42.45** Fracture of lateral condyle of humerus

Fracture of capitellum of humerus

√7ᵗʰ **S42.451** Displaced fracture of lateral condyle of right humerus

√7ᵗʰ **S42.452** Displaced fracture of lateral condyle of left humerus

√7ᵗʰ **S42.453** Displaced fracture of lateral condyle of unspecified humerus

√7ᵗʰ **S42.454** Nondisplaced fracture of lateral condyle of right humerus

√7ᵗʰ **S42.455** Nondisplaced fracture of lateral condyle of left humerus

√7ᵗʰ **S42.456** Nondisplaced fracture of lateral condyle of unspecified humerus

√6ᵗʰ **S42.46** Fracture of medial condyle of humerus

Trochlea fracture of humerus

√7ᵗʰ **S42.461** Displaced fracture of medial condyle of right humerus

√7ᵗʰ **S42.462** Displaced fracture of medial condyle of left humerus

√7ᵗʰ **S42.463** Displaced fracture of medial condyle of unspecified humerus

√7ᵗʰ **S42.464** Nondisplaced fracture of medial condyle of right humerus

√7ᵗʰ **S42.465** Nondisplaced fracture of medial condyle of left humerus

√7ᵗʰ **S42.466** Nondisplaced fracture of medial condyle of unspecified humerus

√6ᵗʰ **S42.47** Transcondylar fracture of humerus

√7ᵗʰ **S42.471** Displaced transcondylar fracture of right humerus

√7ᵗʰ **S42.472** Displaced transcondylar fracture of left humerus

√7ᵗʰ **S42.473** Displaced transcondylar fracture of unspecified humerus

√7ᵗʰ **S42.474** Nondisplaced transcondylar fracture of right humerus

√7ᵗʰ **S42.475** Nondisplaced transcondylar fracture of left humerus

√7ᵗʰ **S42.476** Nondisplaced transcondylar fracture of unspecified humerus

√6ᵗʰ **S42.48** Torus fracture of lower end of humerus

> The appropriate 7th character is to be added to all codes in subcategory S42.48.
> A   initial encounter for closed fracture
> D   subsequent encounter for fracture with routine healing
> G   subsequent encounter for fracture with delayed healing
> K   subsequent encounter for fracture with nonunion
> P   subsequent encounter for fracture with malunion
> S   sequela

√7ᵗʰ **S42.481** Torus fracture of lower end of right humerus

√7ᵗʰ **S42.482** Torus fracture of lower end of left humerus

√7ᵗʰ **S42.489** Torus fracture of lower end of unspecified humerus

√6ᵗʰ **S42.49** Other fracture of lower end of humerus

√7ᵗʰ **S42.491** Other displaced fracture of lower end of right humerus

√7ᵗʰ **S42.492** Other displaced fracture of lower end of left humerus

√7ᵗʰ **S42.493** Other displaced fracture of lower end of unspecified humerus

√7ᵗʰ **S42.494** Other nondisplaced fracture of lower end of right humerus

√7ᵗʰ **S42.495** Other nondisplaced fracture of lower end of left humerus

√7ᵗʰ **S42.496** Other nondisplaced fracture of lower end of unspecified humerus

√5ᵗʰ **S42.9** Fracture of shoulder girdle, part unspecified

Fracture of shoulder NOS

√x7ᵗʰ **S42.90** Fracture of unspecified shoulder girdle, part unspecified

√x7ᵗʰ **S42.91** Fracture of right shoulder girdle, part unspecified

√x7ᵗʰ **S42.92** Fracture of left shoulder girdle, part unspecified

√4ᵗʰ **S43** Dislocation and sprain of joints and ligaments of shoulder girdle

INCLUDES	avulsion of joint or ligament of shoulder girdle
	laceration of cartilage, joint or ligament of shoulder girdle
	sprain of cartilage, joint or ligament of shoulder girdle
	traumatic hemarthrosis of joint or ligament of shoulder girdle
	traumatic rupture of joint or ligament of shoulder girdle
	traumatic subluxation of joint or ligament of shoulder girdle
	traumatic tear of joint or ligament of shoulder girdle

Code also any associated open wound

EXCLUDES 2   *strain of muscle, fascia and tendon of shoulder and upper arm (S46.-)*

> The appropriate 7th character is to be added to each code from category S43.
> A   initial encounter
> D   subsequent encounter
> S   sequela

√5ᵗʰ **S43.0** Subluxation and dislocation of shoulder joint

Dislocation of glenohumeral joint

Subluxation of glenohumeral joint

√6ᵗʰ **S43.00** Unspecified subluxation and dislocation of shoulder joint

Dislocation of humerus NOS

Subluxation of humerus NOS

√7ᵗʰ **S43.001** Unspecified subluxation of right shoulder joint

√7ᵗʰ **S43.002** Unspecified subluxation of left shoulder joint

√7ᵗʰ **S43.003** Unspecified subluxation of unspecified shoulder joint

√7ᵗʰ **S43.004** Unspecified dislocation of right shoulder joint

√7ᵗʰ **S43.005** Unspecified dislocation of left shoulder joint

√7ᵗʰ **S43.006** Unspecified dislocation of unspecified shoulder joint

√6ᵗʰ **S43.01** Anterior subluxation and dislocation of humerus

√7ᵗʰ **S43.011** Anterior subluxation of right humerus

√7ᵗʰ **S43.012** Anterior subluxation of left humerus

√7ᵗʰ **S43.013** Anterior subluxation of unspecified humerus

√7ᵗʰ **S43.014** Anterior dislocation of right humerus

√7ᵗʰ **S43.015** Anterior dislocation of left humerus

√7ᵗʰ **S43.016** Anterior dislocation of unspecified humerus

√6ᵗʰ **S43.02** Posterior subluxation and dislocation of humerus

√7ᵗʰ **S43.021** Posterior subluxation of right humerus

√7ᵗʰ **S43.022** Posterior subluxation of left humerus

√7ᵗʰ **S43.023** Posterior subluxation of unspecified humerus

√7ᵗʰ **S43.024** Posterior dislocation of right humerus

√7ᵗʰ **S43.025** Posterior dislocation of left humerus

√7ᵗʰ **S43.026** Posterior dislocation of unspecified humerus

√6ᵗʰ **S43.03** Inferior subluxation and dislocation of humerus

√7ᵗʰ **S43.031** Inferior subluxation of right humerus

√7ᵗʰ **S43.032** Inferior subluxation of left humerus

√7ᵗʰ **S43.033** Inferior subluxation of unspecified humerus

√7ᵗʰ **S43.034** Inferior dislocation of right humerus

√7ᵗʰ **S43.035** Inferior dislocation of left humerus

√7ᵗʰ **S43.036** Inferior dislocation of unspecified humerus

☑ Additional Character Required   √x7ᵗʰ Placeholder Alert   Manifestation   Unspecified Dx   ►◄ Revised Text   ● New Code   ▲ Revised Title

ICD-10-CM 2020   991

√6ᵗʰ **S43.08** Other subluxation and dislocation of shoulder joint

    √7ᵗʰ **S43.081** Other subluxation of right shoulder joint

    √7ᵗʰ **S43.082** Other subluxation of left shoulder joint

    √7ᵗʰ **S43.083** Other subluxation of unspecified shoulder joint

    √7ᵗʰ **S43.084** Other dislocation of right shoulder joint

    √7ᵗʰ **S43.085** Other dislocation of left shoulder joint

    √7ᵗʰ **S43.086** Other dislocation of unspecified shoulder joint

√5ᵗʰ **S43.1** Subluxation and dislocation of acromioclavicular joint

   √6ᵗʰ **S43.10** Unspecified dislocation of acromioclavicular joint

    √7ᵗʰ **S43.101** Unspecified dislocation of right acromioclavicular joint

    √7ᵗʰ **S43.102** Unspecified dislocation of left acromioclavicular joint

    √7ᵗʰ **S43.109** Unspecified dislocation of unspecified acromioclavicular joint

   √6ᵗʰ **S43.11** Subluxation of acromioclavicular joint

    √7ᵗʰ **S43.111** Subluxation of right acromioclavicular joint

    √7ᵗʰ **S43.112** Subluxation of left acromioclavicular joint

    √7ᵗʰ **S43.119** Subluxation of unspecified acromioclavicular joint

   √6ᵗʰ **S43.12** Dislocation of acromioclavicular joint, 100%-200% displacement

    √7ᵗʰ **S43.121** Dislocation of right acromioclavicular joint, 100%-200% displacement

    √7ᵗʰ **S43.122** Dislocation of left acromioclavicular joint, 100%-200% displacement

    √7ᵗʰ **S43.129** Dislocation of unspecified acromioclavicular joint, 100%-200% displacement

   √6ᵗʰ **S43.13** Dislocation of acromioclavicular joint, greater than 200% displacement

    √7ᵗʰ **S43.131** Dislocation of right acromioclavicular joint, greater than 200% displacement

    √7ᵗʰ **S43.132** Dislocation of left acromioclavicular joint, greater than 200% displacement

    √7ᵗʰ **S43.139** Dislocation of unspecified acromioclavicular joint, greater than 200% displacement

   √6ᵗʰ **S43.14** Inferior dislocation of acromioclavicular joint

    √7ᵗʰ **S43.141** Inferior dislocation of right acromioclavicular joint

    √7ᵗʰ **S43.142** Inferior dislocation of left acromioclavicular joint

    √7ᵗʰ **S43.149** Inferior dislocation of unspecified acromioclavicular joint

   √6ᵗʰ **S43.15** Posterior dislocation of acromioclavicular joint

    √7ᵗʰ **S43.151** Posterior dislocation of right acromioclavicular joint

    √7ᵗʰ **S43.152** Posterior dislocation of left acromioclavicular joint

    √7ᵗʰ **S43.159** Posterior dislocation of unspecified acromioclavicular joint

√5ᵗʰ **S43.2** Subluxation and dislocation of sternoclavicular joint

   √6ᵗʰ **S43.20** Unspecified subluxation and dislocation of sternoclavicular joint

    √7ᵗʰ **S43.201** Unspecified subluxation of right sternoclavicular joint

    √7ᵗʰ **S43.202** Unspecified subluxation of left sternoclavicular joint

    √7ᵗʰ **S43.203** Unspecified subluxation of unspecified sternoclavicular joint

    √7ᵗʰ **S43.204** Unspecified dislocation of right sternoclavicular joint

    √7ᵗʰ **S43.205** Unspecified dislocation of left sternoclavicular joint

    √7ᵗʰ **S43.206** Unspecified dislocation of unspecified sternoclavicular joint

   √6ᵗʰ **S43.21** Anterior subluxation and dislocation of sternoclavicular joint

    √7ᵗʰ **S43.211** Anterior subluxation of right sternoclavicular joint

    √7ᵗʰ **S43.212** Anterior subluxation of left sternoclavicular joint

    √7ᵗʰ **S43.213** Anterior subluxation of unspecified sternoclavicular joint

    √7ᵗʰ **S43.214** Anterior dislocation of right sternoclavicular joint

    √7ᵗʰ **S43.215** Anterior dislocation of left sternoclavicular joint

    √7ᵗʰ **S43.216** Anterior dislocation of unspecified sternoclavicular joint

   √6ᵗʰ **S43.22** Posterior subluxation and dislocation of sternoclavicular joint

    √7ᵗʰ **S43.221** Posterior subluxation of right sternoclavicular joint

    √7ᵗʰ **S43.222** Posterior subluxation of left sternoclavicular joint

    √7ᵗʰ **S43.223** Posterior subluxation of unspecified sternoclavicular joint

    √7ᵗʰ **S43.224** Posterior dislocation of right sternoclavicular joint

    √7ᵗʰ **S43.225** Posterior dislocation of left sternoclavicular joint

    √7ᵗʰ **S43.226** Posterior dislocation of unspecified sternoclavicular joint

√5ᵗʰ **S43.3** Subluxation and dislocation of other and unspecified parts of shoulder girdle

   √6ᵗʰ **S43.30** Subluxation and dislocation of unspecified parts of shoulder girdle

    Dislocation of shoulder girdle NOS

    Subluxation of shoulder girdle NOS

    √7ᵗʰ **S43.301** Subluxation of unspecified parts of right shoulder girdle

    √7ᵗʰ **S43.302** Subluxation of unspecified parts of left shoulder girdle

    √7ᵗʰ **S43.303** Subluxation of unspecified parts of unspecified shoulder girdle

    √7ᵗʰ **S43.304** Dislocation of unspecified parts of right shoulder girdle

    √7ᵗʰ **S43.305** Dislocation of unspecified parts of left shoulder girdle

    √7ᵗʰ **S43.306** Dislocation of unspecified parts of unspecified shoulder girdle

   √6ᵗʰ **S43.31** Subluxation and dislocation of scapula

    √7ᵗʰ **S43.311** Subluxation of right scapula

    √7ᵗʰ **S43.312** Subluxation of left scapula

    √7ᵗʰ **S43.313** Subluxation of unspecified scapula

    √7ᵗʰ **S43.314** Dislocation of right scapula

    √7ᵗʰ **S43.315** Dislocation of left scapula

    √7ᵗʰ **S43.316** Dislocation of unspecified scapula

   √6ᵗʰ **S43.39** Subluxation and dislocation of other parts of shoulder girdle

    √7ᵗʰ **S43.391** Subluxation of other parts of right shoulder girdle

    √7ᵗʰ **S43.392** Subluxation of other parts of left shoulder girdle

    √7ᵗʰ **S43.393** Subluxation of other parts of unspecified shoulder girdle

    √7ᵗʰ **S43.394** Dislocation of other parts of right shoulder girdle

    √7ᵗʰ **S43.395** Dislocation of other parts of left shoulder girdle

    √7ᵗʰ **S43.396** Dislocation of other parts of unspecified shoulder girdle

√5ᵗʰ **S43.4** Sprain of shoulder joint

   √6ᵗʰ **S43.40** Unspecified sprain of shoulder joint

    √7ᵗʰ **S43.401** Unspecified sprain of right shoulder joint

    √7ᵗʰ **S43.402** Unspecified sprain of left shoulder joint

    √7ᵗʰ **S43.409** Unspecified sprain of unspecified shoulder joint

   √6ᵗʰ **S43.41** Sprain of coracohumeral (ligament)

    √7ᵗʰ **S43.411** Sprain of right coracohumeral (ligament)

    √7ᵗʰ **S43.412** Sprain of left coracohumeral (ligament)

    √7ᵗʰ **S43.419** Sprain of unspecified coracohumeral (ligament)

   √6ᵗʰ **S43.42** Sprain of rotator cuff capsule

    EXCLUDES 1   rotator cuff syndrome (complete) (incomplete), not specified as traumatic (M75.1-)

    EXCLUDES 2   injury of tendon of rotator cuff (S46.0-)

    √7ᵗʰ **S43.421** Sprain of right rotator cuff capsule

    √7ᵗʰ **S43.422** Sprain of left rotator cuff capsule

    √7ᵗʰ **S43.429** Sprain of unspecified rotator cuff capsule

Ⓝ Newborn: 0   Ⓟ Pediatric: 0-17   Ⓜ Maternity: 12-55   Ⓐ Adult: 15-124   **CH** Comorbidity High   **CL** Comorbidity Low   **NCDx** Noncancer Dx   **PDx** Primary Dx

992   ICD-10-CM 2020

√6ᵗʰ **S43.43** Superior glenoid labrum **lesion**
SLAP lesion
AHA: 2019,2Q,26
DEF: Detachment injury of the superior aspect of the glenoid labrum, which is the ring of fibrocartilage attached to the rim of the glenoid cavity of the scapula.

√7ᵗʰ **S43.431** Superior glenoid labrum lesion of right shoulder

√7ᵗʰ **S43.432** Superior glenoid labrum lesion of left shoulder

√7ᵗʰ **S43.439** Superior glenoid labrum lesion of unspecified shoulder

√6ᵗʰ **S43.49** Other sprain of shoulder joint

√7ᵗʰ **S43.491** Other sprain of right shoulder joint

√7ᵗʰ **S43.492** Other sprain of left shoulder joint

√7ᵗʰ **S43.499** Other sprain of unspecified shoulder joint

√5ᵗʰ **S43.5** Sprain of acromioclavicular joint
Sprain of acromioclavicular ligament

√x7ᵗʰ **S43.50** Sprain of unspecified acromioclavicular joint

√x7ᵗʰ **S43.51** Sprain of right acromioclavicular joint

√x7ᵗʰ **S43.52** Sprain of left acromioclavicular joint

√5ᵗʰ **S43.6** Sprain of sternoclavicular joint

√x7ᵗʰ **S43.60** Sprain of unspecified sternoclavicular joint

√x7ᵗʰ **S43.61** Sprain of right sternoclavicular joint

√x7ᵗʰ **S43.62** Sprain of left sternoclavicular joint

√5ᵗʰ **S43.8** Sprain of other specified parts of shoulder girdle

√x7ᵗʰ **S43.80** Sprain of other specified parts of unspecified shoulder girdle

√x7ᵗʰ **S43.81** Sprain of other specified parts of right shoulder girdle

√x7ᵗʰ **S43.82** Sprain of other specified parts of left shoulder girdle

√5ᵗʰ **S43.9** Sprain of unspecified parts of shoulder girdle

√x7ᵗʰ **S43.90** Sprain of unspecified parts of unspecified shoulder girdle
Sprain of shoulder girdle NOS

√x7ᵗʰ **S43.91** Sprain of unspecified parts of right shoulder girdle

√x7ᵗʰ **S43.92** Sprain of unspecified parts of left shoulder girdle

√4ᵗʰ **S44** Injury of nerves at shoulder and upper arm level
Code also any associated open wound (S41.-)
EXCLUDES 2   injury of brachial plexus (S14.3-)

The appropriate 7th character is to be added to each code from category S44.
A   initial encounter
D   subsequent encounter
S   sequela

√5ᵗʰ **S44.0** Injury of ulnar nerve at upper arm level
EXCLUDES 1   ulnar nerve NOS (S54.0)

√x7ᵗʰ **S44.00** Injury of ulnar nerve at upper arm level, unspecified arm

√x7ᵗʰ **S44.01** Injury of ulnar nerve at upper arm level, right arm

√x7ᵗʰ **S44.02** Injury of ulnar nerve at upper arm level, left arm

√5ᵗʰ **S44.1** Injury of median nerve at upper arm level
EXCLUDES 1   median nerve NOS (S54.1)

√x7ᵗʰ **S44.10** Injury of median nerve at upper arm level, unspecified arm

√x7ᵗʰ **S44.11** Injury of median nerve at upper arm level, right arm

√x7ᵗʰ **S44.12** Injury of median nerve at upper arm level, left arm

√5ᵗʰ **S44.2** Injury of radial nerve at upper arm level
EXCLUDES 1   radial nerve NOS (S54.2)

√x7ᵗʰ **S44.20** Injury of radial nerve at upper arm level, unspecified arm

√x7ᵗʰ **S44.21** Injury of radial nerve at upper arm level, right arm

√x7ᵗʰ **S44.22** Injury of radial nerve at upper arm level, left arm

√5ᵗʰ **S44.3** Injury of axillary nerve

√x7ᵗʰ **S44.30** Injury of axillary nerve, unspecified arm

√x7ᵗʰ **S44.31** Injury of axillary nerve, right arm

√x7ᵗʰ **S44.32** Injury of axillary nerve, left arm

√5ᵗʰ **S44.4** Injury of musculocutaneous nerve

√x7ᵗʰ **S44.40** Injury of musculocutaneous nerve, unspecified arm

√x7ᵗʰ **S44.41** Injury of musculocutaneous nerve, right arm

√x7ᵗʰ **S44.42** Injury of musculocutaneous nerve, left arm

√5ᵗʰ **S44.5** Injury of cutaneous sensory nerve at shoulder and upper arm level

√x7ᵗʰ **S44.50** Injury of cutaneous sensory nerve at shoulder and upper arm level, unspecified arm

√x7ᵗʰ **S44.51** Injury of cutaneous sensory nerve at shoulder and upper arm level, right arm

√x7ᵗʰ **S44.52** Injury of cutaneous sensory nerve at shoulder and upper arm level, left arm

√5ᵗʰ **S44.8** Injury of other nerves at shoulder and upper arm level

√6ᵗʰ **S44.8X** Injury of other nerves at shoulder and upper arm level

√7ᵗʰ **S44.8X1** Injury of other nerves at shoulder and upper arm level, right arm

√7ᵗʰ **S44.8X2** Injury of other nerves at shoulder and upper arm level, left arm

√7ᵗʰ **S44.8X9** Injury of other nerves at shoulder and upper arm level, unspecified arm

√5ᵗʰ **S44.9** Injury of unspecified nerve at shoulder and upper arm level

√x7ᵗʰ **S44.90** Injury of unspecified nerve at shoulder and upper arm level, unspecified arm

√x7ᵗʰ **S44.91** Injury of unspecified nerve at shoulder and upper arm level, right arm

√x7ᵗʰ **S44.92** Injury of unspecified nerve at shoulder and upper arm level, left arm

√4ᵗʰ **S45** Injury of blood vessels at shoulder and upper arm level
Code also any associated open wound (S41.-)
EXCLUDES 2   injury of subclavian artery (S25.1)
      injury of subclavian vein (S25.3)

The appropriate 7th character is to be added to each code from category S45.
A   initial encounter
D   subsequent encounter
S   sequela

√5ᵗʰ **S45.0** Injury of axillary artery

√6ᵗʰ **S45.00** Unspecified injury of axillary artery

√7ᵗʰ **S45.001** Unspecified injury of axillary artery, right side

√7ᵗʰ **S45.002** Unspecified injury of axillary artery, left side

√7ᵗʰ **S45.009** Unspecified injury of axillary artery, unspecified side

√6ᵗʰ **S45.01** Laceration of axillary artery

√7ᵗʰ **S45.011** Laceration of axillary artery, right side

√7ᵗʰ **S45.012** Laceration of axillary artery, left side

√7ᵗʰ **S45.019** Laceration of axillary artery, unspecified side

√6ᵗʰ **S45.09** Other specified injury of axillary artery

√7ᵗʰ **S45.091** Other specified injury of axillary artery, right side

√7ᵗʰ **S45.092** Other specified injury of axillary artery, left side

√7ᵗʰ **S45.099** Other specified injury of axillary artery, unspecified side

√5ᵗʰ **S45.1** Injury of brachial artery

√6ᵗʰ **S45.10** Unspecified injury of brachial artery

√7ᵗʰ **S45.101** Unspecified injury of brachial artery, right side

√7ᵗʰ **S45.102** Unspecified injury of brachial artery, left side

√7ᵗʰ **S45.109** Unspecified injury of brachial artery, unspecified side

√6ᵗʰ **S45.11** Laceration of brachial artery

√7ᵗʰ **S45.111** Laceration of brachial artery, right side

√7ᵗʰ **S45.112** Laceration of brachial artery, left side

√7ᵗʰ **S45.119** Laceration of brachial artery, unspecified side

√6ᵗʰ **S45.19** Other specified injury of brachial artery

√7ᵗʰ **S45.191** Other specified injury of brachial artery, right side

√7ᵗʰ **S45.192** Other specified injury of brachial artery, left side

√7ᵗʰ **S45.199** Other specified injury of brachial artery, unspecified side

✓ Additional Character Required   √x7ᵗʰ Placeholder Alert   Manifestation   Unspecified Dx   ►◄ Revised Text   ● New Code   ▲ Revised Title

ICD-10-CM 2020   993

✓5ᵗʰ **S45.2** Injury of axillary or brachial vein

  ✓6ᵗʰ **S45.20** Unspecified injury of axillary or brachial vein

    ✓7ᵗʰ **S45.201** Unspecified injury of axillary or brachial vein, right side

    ✓7ᵗʰ **S45.202** Unspecified injury of axillary or brachial vein, left side

    ✓7ᵗʰ **S45.209** Unspecified injury of axillary or brachial vein, unspecified side

  ✓6ᵗʰ **S45.21** Laceration of axillary or brachial vein

    ✓7ᵗʰ **S45.211** Laceration of axillary or brachial vein, right side

    ✓7ᵗʰ **S45.212** Laceration of axillary or brachial vein, left side

    ✓7ᵗʰ **S45.219** Laceration of axillary or brachial vein, unspecified side

  ✓6ᵗʰ **S45.29** Other specified injury of axillary or brachial vein

    ✓7ᵗʰ **S45.291** Other specified injury of axillary or brachial vein, right side

    ✓7ᵗʰ **S45.292** Other specified injury of axillary or brachial vein, left side

    ✓7ᵗʰ **S45.299** Other specified injury of axillary or brachial vein, unspecified side

✓5ᵗʰ **S45.3** Injury of superficial vein at shoulder and upper arm level

  ✓6ᵗʰ **S45.30** Unspecified injury of superficial vein at shoulder and upper arm level

    ✓7ᵗʰ **S45.301** Unspecified injury of superficial vein at shoulder and upper arm level, right arm

    ✓7ᵗʰ **S45.302** Unspecified injury of superficial vein at shoulder and upper arm level, left arm

    ✓7ᵗʰ **S45.309** Unspecified injury of superficial vein at shoulder and upper arm level, unspecified arm

  ✓6ᵗʰ **S45.31** Laceration of superficial vein at shoulder and upper arm level

    ✓7ᵗʰ **S45.311** Laceration of superficial vein at shoulder and upper arm level, right arm

    ✓7ᵗʰ **S45.312** Laceration of superficial vein at shoulder and upper arm level, left arm

    ✓7ᵗʰ **S45.319** Laceration of superficial vein at shoulder and upper arm level, unspecified arm

  ✓6ᵗʰ **S45.39** Other specified injury of superficial vein at shoulder and upper arm level

    ✓7ᵗʰ **S45.391** Other specified injury of superficial vein at shoulder and upper arm level, right arm

    ✓7ᵗʰ **S45.392** Other specified injury of superficial vein at shoulder and upper arm level, left arm

    ✓7ᵗʰ **S45.399** Other specified injury of superficial vein at shoulder and upper arm level, unspecified arm

✓5ᵗʰ **S45.8** Injury of other specified blood vessels at shoulder and upper arm level

  ✓6ᵗʰ **S45.80** Unspecified injury of other specified blood vessels at shoulder and upper arm level

    ✓7ᵗʰ **S45.801** Unspecified injury of other specified blood vessels at shoulder and upper arm level, right arm

    ✓7ᵗʰ **S45.802** Unspecified injury of other specified blood vessels at shoulder and upper arm level, left arm

    ✓7ᵗʰ **S45.809** Unspecified injury of other specified blood vessels at shoulder and upper arm level, unspecified arm

  ✓6ᵗʰ **S45.81** Laceration of other specified blood vessels at shoulder and upper arm level

    ✓7ᵗʰ **S45.811** Laceration of other specified blood vessels at shoulder and upper arm level, right arm

    ✓7ᵗʰ **S45.812** Laceration of other specified blood vessels at shoulder and upper arm level, left arm

    ✓7ᵗʰ **S45.819** Laceration of other specified blood vessels at shoulder and upper arm level, unspecified arm

  ✓6ᵗʰ **S45.89** Other specified injury of other specified blood vessels at shoulder and upper arm level

    ✓7ᵗʰ **S45.891** Other specified injury of other specified blood vessels at shoulder and upper arm level, right arm

    ✓7ᵗʰ **S45.892** Other specified injury of other specified blood vessels at shoulder and upper arm level, left arm

    ✓7ᵗʰ **S45.899** Other specified injury of other specified blood vessels at shoulder and upper arm level, unspecified arm

✓5ᵗʰ **S45.9** Injury of unspecified blood vessel at shoulder and upper arm level

  ✓6ᵗʰ **S45.90** Unspecified injury of unspecified blood vessel at shoulder and upper arm level

    ✓7ᵗʰ **S45.901** Unspecified injury of unspecified blood vessel at shoulder and upper arm level, right arm

    ✓7ᵗʰ **S45.902** Unspecified injury of unspecified blood vessel at shoulder and upper arm level, left arm

    ✓7ᵗʰ **S45.909** Unspecified injury of unspecified blood vessel at shoulder and upper arm level, unspecified arm

  ✓6ᵗʰ **S45.91** Laceration of unspecified blood vessel at shoulder and upper arm level

    ✓7ᵗʰ **S45.911** Laceration of unspecified blood vessel at shoulder and upper arm level, right arm

    ✓7ᵗʰ **S45.912** Laceration of unspecified blood vessel at shoulder and upper arm level, left arm

    ✓7ᵗʰ **S45.919** Laceration of unspecified blood vessel at shoulder and upper arm level, unspecified arm

  ✓6ᵗʰ **S45.99** Other specified injury of unspecified blood vessel at shoulder and upper arm level

    ✓7ᵗʰ **S45.991** Other specified injury of unspecified blood vessel at shoulder and upper arm level, right arm

    ✓7ᵗʰ **S45.992** Other specified injury of unspecified blood vessel at shoulder and upper arm level, left arm

    ✓7ᵗʰ **S45.999** Other specified injury of unspecified blood vessel at shoulder and upper arm level, unspecified arm

✓4ᵗʰ **S46** Injury of muscle, fascia and tendon at shoulder and upper arm level

Code also any associated open wound (S41.-)

EXCLUDES 2   *injury of muscle, fascia and tendon at elbow (S56.-)*

          sprain of joints and ligaments of shoulder girdle (S43.9)

TIP: Refer to the Muscle/Tendon table at the beginning of this chapter.

> The appropriate 7th character is to be added to each code from category S46.
> A   initial encounter
> D   subsequent encounter
> S   sequela

✓5ᵗʰ **S46.0** Injury of muscle(s) and tendon(s) of the rotator cuff of shoulder

  ✓6ᵗʰ **S46.00** Unspecified injury of muscle(s) and tendon(s) of the rotator cuff of shoulder

    ✓7ᵗʰ **S46.001** Unspecified injury of muscle(s) and tendon(s) of the rotator cuff of right shoulder

    ✓7ᵗʰ **S46.002** Unspecified injury of muscle(s) and tendon(s) of the rotator cuff of left shoulder

    ✓7ᵗʰ **S46.009** Unspecified injury of muscle(s) and tendon(s) of the rotator cuff of unspecified shoulder

  ✓6ᵗʰ **S46.01** Strain of muscle(s) and tendon(s) of the rotator cuff of shoulder

    ✓7ᵗʰ **S46.011** Strain of muscle(s) and tendon(s) of the rotator cuff of right shoulder

    ✓7ᵗʰ **S46.012** Strain of muscle(s) and tendon(s) of the rotator cuff of left shoulder

    ✓7ᵗʰ **S46.019** Strain of muscle(s) and tendon(s) of the rotator cuff of unspecified shoulder

  ✓6ᵗʰ **S46.02** Laceration of muscle(s) and tendon(s) of the rotator cuff of shoulder

    ✓7ᵗʰ **S46.021** Laceration of muscle(s) and tendon(s) of the rotator cuff of right shoulder

    ✓7ᵗʰ **S46.022** Laceration of muscle(s) and tendon(s) of the rotator cuff of left shoulder

    ✓7ᵗʰ **S46.029** Laceration of muscle(s) and tendon(s) of the rotator cuff of unspecified shoulder

  ✓6ᵗʰ **S46.09** Other injury of muscle(s) and tendon(s) of the rotator cuff of shoulder

    ✓7ᵗʰ **S46.091** Other injury of muscle(s) and tendon(s) of the rotator cuff of right shoulder

    ✓7ᵗʰ **S46.092** Other injury of muscle(s) and tendon(s) of the rotator cuff of left shoulder

Ⓝ Newborn: 0   Ⓟ Pediatric: 0-17   Ⓜ Maternity: 12-55   Ⓐ Adult: 15-124   CH Comorbidity High   CL Comorbidity Low   NCDx Noncancer Dx   PDx Primary Dx

994   ICD-10-CM 2020

✓7ᵗʰ **S46.099** Other injury of muscle(s) and tendon(s) of the rotator cuff of unspecified shoulder

✓5ᵗʰ **S46.1** Injury of muscle, fascia and tendon of long head of biceps
- ✓6ᵗʰ **S46.10** Unspecified injury of muscle, fascia and tendon of long head of biceps
  - ✓7ᵗʰ **S46.101** Unspecified injury of muscle, fascia and tendon of long head of biceps, right arm
  - ✓7ᵗʰ **S46.102** Unspecified injury of muscle, fascia and tendon of long head of biceps, left arm
  - ✓7ᵗʰ **S46.109** Unspecified injury of muscle, fascia and tendon of long head of biceps, unspecified arm
- ✓6ᵗʰ **S46.11** Strain of muscle, fascia and tendon of long head of biceps
  - **AHA:** 2019,2Q,27
  - ✓7ᵗʰ **S46.111** Strain of muscle, fascia and tendon of long head of biceps, right arm
  - ✓7ᵗʰ **S46.112** Strain of muscle, fascia and tendon of long head of biceps, left arm
  - ✓7ᵗʰ **S46.119** Strain of muscle, fascia and tendon of long head of biceps, unspecified arm
- ✓6ᵗʰ **S46.12** Laceration of muscle, fascia and tendon of long head of biceps
  - ✓7ᵗʰ **S46.121** Laceration of muscle, fascia and tendon of long head of biceps, right arm
  - ✓7ᵗʰ **S46.122** Laceration of muscle, fascia and tendon of long head of biceps, left arm
  - ✓7ᵗʰ **S46.129** Laceration of muscle, fascia and tendon of long head of biceps, unspecified arm
- ✓6ᵗʰ **S46.19** Other injury of muscle, fascia and tendon of long head of biceps
  - ✓7ᵗʰ **S46.191** Other injury of muscle, fascia and tendon of long head of biceps, right arm
  - ✓7ᵗʰ **S46.192** Other injury of muscle, fascia and tendon of long head of biceps, left arm
  - ✓7ᵗʰ **S46.199** Other injury of muscle, fascia and tendon of long head of biceps, unspecified arm

✓5ᵗʰ **S46.2** Injury of muscle, fascia and tendon of other parts of biceps
- ✓6ᵗʰ **S46.20** Unspecified injury of muscle, fascia and tendon of other parts of biceps
  - ✓7ᵗʰ **S46.201** Unspecified injury of muscle, fascia and tendon of other parts of biceps, right arm
  - ✓7ᵗʰ **S46.202** Unspecified injury of muscle, fascia and tendon of other parts of biceps, left arm
  - ✓7ᵗʰ **S46.209** Unspecified injury of muscle, fascia and tendon of other parts of biceps, unspecified arm
- ✓6ᵗʰ **S46.21** Strain of muscle, fascia and tendon of other parts of biceps
  - ✓7ᵗʰ **S46.211** Strain of muscle, fascia and tendon of other parts of biceps, right arm
  - ✓7ᵗʰ **S46.212** Strain of muscle, fascia and tendon of other parts of biceps, left arm
  - ✓7ᵗʰ **S46.219** Strain of muscle, fascia and tendon of other parts of biceps, unspecified arm
- ✓6ᵗʰ **S46.22** Laceration of muscle, fascia and tendon of other parts of biceps
  - ✓7ᵗʰ **S46.221** Laceration of muscle, fascia and tendon of other parts of biceps, right arm
  - ✓7ᵗʰ **S46.222** Laceration of muscle, fascia and tendon of other parts of biceps, left arm
  - ✓7ᵗʰ **S46.229** Laceration of muscle, fascia and tendon of other parts of biceps, unspecified arm
- ✓6ᵗʰ **S46.29** Other injury of muscle, fascia and tendon of other parts of biceps
  - ✓7ᵗʰ **S46.291** Other injury of muscle, fascia and tendon of other parts of biceps, right arm
  - ✓7ᵗʰ **S46.292** Other injury of muscle, fascia and tendon of other parts of biceps, left arm
  - ✓7ᵗʰ **S46.299** Other injury of muscle, fascia and tendon of other parts of biceps, unspecified arm

✓5ᵗʰ **S46.3** Injury of muscle, fascia and tendon of triceps
- ✓6ᵗʰ **S46.30** Unspecified injury of muscle, fascia and tendon of triceps
  - ✓7ᵗʰ **S46.301** Unspecified injury of muscle, fascia and tendon of triceps, right arm
  - ✓7ᵗʰ **S46.302** Unspecified injury of muscle, fascia and tendon of triceps, left arm
  - ✓7ᵗʰ **S46.309** Unspecified injury of muscle, fascia and tendon of triceps, unspecified arm

- ✓6ᵗʰ **S46.31** Strain of muscle, fascia and tendon of triceps
  - ✓7ᵗʰ **S46.311** Strain of muscle, fascia and tendon of triceps, right arm
  - ✓7ᵗʰ **S46.312** Strain of muscle, fascia and tendon of triceps, left arm
  - ✓7ᵗʰ **S46.319** Strain of muscle, fascia and tendon of triceps, unspecified arm
- ✓6ᵗʰ **S46.32** Laceration of muscle, fascia and tendon of triceps
  - ✓7ᵗʰ **S46.321** Laceration of muscle, fascia and tendon of triceps, right arm
  - ✓7ᵗʰ **S46.322** Laceration of muscle, fascia and tendon of triceps, left arm
  - ✓7ᵗʰ **S46.329** Laceration of muscle, fascia and tendon of triceps, unspecified arm
- ✓6ᵗʰ **S46.39** Other injury of muscle, fascia and tendon of triceps
  - ✓7ᵗʰ **S46.391** Other injury of muscle, fascia and tendon of triceps, right arm
  - ✓7ᵗʰ **S46.392** Other injury of muscle, fascia and tendon of triceps, left arm
  - ✓7ᵗʰ **S46.399** Other injury of muscle, fascia and tendon of triceps, unspecified arm

✓5ᵗʰ **S46.8** Injury of other muscles, fascia and tendons at shoulder and upper arm level
- ✓6ᵗʰ **S46.80** Unspecified injury of other muscles, fascia and tendons at shoulder and upper arm level
  - ✓7ᵗʰ **S46.801** Unspecified injury of other muscles, fascia and tendons at shoulder and upper arm level, right arm
  - ✓7ᵗʰ **S46.802** Unspecified injury of other muscles, fascia and tendons at shoulder and upper arm level, left arm
  - ✓7ᵗʰ **S46.809** Unspecified injury of other muscles, fascia and tendons at shoulder and upper arm level, unspecified arm
- ✓6ᵗʰ **S46.81** Strain of other muscles, fascia and tendons at shoulder and upper arm level
  - ✓7ᵗʰ **S46.811** Strain of other muscles, fascia and tendons at shoulder and upper arm level, right arm
  - ✓7ᵗʰ **S46.812** Strain of other muscles, fascia and tendons at shoulder and upper arm level, left arm
  - ✓7ᵗʰ **S46.819** Strain of other muscles, fascia and tendons at shoulder and upper arm level, unspecified arm
- ✓6ᵗʰ **S46.82** Laceration of other muscles, fascia and tendons at shoulder and upper arm level
  - ✓7ᵗʰ **S46.821** Laceration of other muscles, fascia and tendons at shoulder and upper arm level, right arm
  - ✓7ᵗʰ **S46.822** Laceration of other muscles, fascia and tendons at shoulder and upper arm level, left arm
  - ✓7ᵗʰ **S46.829** Laceration of other muscles, fascia and tendons at shoulder and upper arm level, unspecified arm
- ✓6ᵗʰ **S46.89** Other injury of other muscles, fascia and tendons at shoulder and upper arm level
  - ✓7ᵗʰ **S46.891** Other injury of other muscles, fascia and tendons at shoulder and upper arm level, right arm
  - ✓7ᵗʰ **S46.892** Other injury of other muscles, fascia and tendons at shoulder and upper arm level, left arm
  - ✓7ᵗʰ **S46.899** Other injury of other muscles, fascia and tendons at shoulder and upper arm level, unspecified arm

✓5ᵗʰ **S46.9** Injury of unspecified muscle, fascia and tendon at shoulder and upper arm level
- ✓6ᵗʰ **S46.90** Unspecified injury of unspecified muscle, fascia and tendon at shoulder and upper arm level
  - ✓7ᵗʰ **S46.901** Unspecified injury of unspecified muscle, fascia and tendon at shoulder and upper arm level, right arm
  - ✓7ᵗʰ **S46.902** Unspecified injury of unspecified muscle, fascia and tendon at shoulder and upper arm level, left arm
  - ✓7ᵗʰ **S46.909** Unspecified injury of unspecified muscle, fascia and tendon at shoulder and upper arm level, unspecified arm

✔ Additional Character Required   ✓ₓ7ᵗʰ Placeholder Alert   Manifestation   Unspecified Dx   ▶◀ Revised Text   ● New Code   ▲ Revised Title

ICD-10-CM 2020   995

√6ᵗʰ **S46.91** Strain of unspecified muscle, fascia and tendon at shoulder and upper arm level

√7ᵗʰ **S46.911** Strain of unspecified muscle, fascia and tendon at shoulder and upper arm level, right arm

√7ᵗʰ **S46.912** Strain of unspecified muscle, fascia and tendon at shoulder and upper arm level, left arm

√7ᵗʰ **S46.919** Strain of unspecified muscle, fascia and tendon at shoulder and upper arm level, unspecified arm

√6ᵗʰ **S46.92** Laceration of unspecified muscle, fascia and tendon at shoulder and upper arm level

√7ᵗʰ **S46.921** Laceration of unspecified muscle, fascia and tendon at shoulder and upper arm level, right arm

√7ᵗʰ **S46.922** Laceration of unspecified muscle, fascia and tendon at shoulder and upper arm level, left arm

√7ᵗʰ **S46.929** Laceration of unspecified muscle, fascia and tendon at shoulder and upper arm level, unspecified arm

√6ᵗʰ **S46.99** Other injury of unspecified muscle, fascia and tendon at shoulder and upper arm level

√7ᵗʰ **S46.991** Other injury of unspecified muscle, fascia and tendon at shoulder and upper arm level, right arm

√7ᵗʰ **S46.992** Other injury of unspecified muscle, fascia and tendon at shoulder and upper arm level, left arm

√7ᵗʰ **S46.999** Other injury of unspecified muscle, fascia and tendon at shoulder and upper arm level, unspecified arm

√4ᵗʰ **S47** **Crushing injury of shoulder and upper arm**

Use additional code for all associated injuries

EXCLUDES 2   crushing injury of elbow (S57.0-)

The appropriate 7th character is to be added to each code from category S47.
A   initial encounter
D   subsequent encounter
S   sequela

√x7ᵗʰ **S47.1** Crushing injury of right shoulder and upper arm

√x7ᵗʰ **S47.2** Crushing injury of left shoulder and upper arm

√x7ᵗʰ **S47.9** Crushing injury of shoulder and upper arm, unspecified arm

√4ᵗʰ **S48** **Traumatic amputation of shoulder and upper arm**

An amputation not identified as partial or complete should be coded to complete

EXCLUDES 1   traumatic amputation at elbow level (S58.0)

The appropriate 7th character is to be added to each code from category S48.
A   initial encounter
D   subsequent encounter
S   sequela

√5ᵗʰ **S48.0** Traumatic amputation at shoulder joint

√6ᵗʰ **S48.01** Complete traumatic amputation at shoulder joint

√7ᵗʰ **S48.011** Complete traumatic amputation at right shoulder joint

√7ᵗʰ **S48.012** Complete traumatic amputation at left shoulder joint

√7ᵗʰ **S48.019** Complete traumatic amputation at unspecified shoulder joint

√6ᵗʰ **S48.02** Partial traumatic amputation at shoulder joint

√7ᵗʰ **S48.021** Partial traumatic amputation at right shoulder joint

√7ᵗʰ **S48.022** Partial traumatic amputation at left shoulder joint

√7ᵗʰ **S48.029** Partial traumatic amputation at unspecified shoulder joint

√5ᵗʰ **S48.1** Traumatic amputation at level between shoulder and elbow

√6ᵗʰ **S48.11** Complete traumatic amputation at level between shoulder and elbow

√7ᵗʰ **S48.111** Complete traumatic amputation at level between right shoulder and elbow

√7ᵗʰ **S48.112** Complete traumatic amputation at level between left shoulder and elbow

√7ᵗʰ **S48.119** Complete traumatic amputation at level between unspecified shoulder and elbow

√6ᵗʰ **S48.12** Partial traumatic amputation at level between shoulder and elbow

√7ᵗʰ **S48.121** Partial traumatic amputation at level between right shoulder and elbow

√7ᵗʰ **S48.122** Partial traumatic amputation at level between left shoulder and elbow

√7ᵗʰ **S48.129** Partial traumatic amputation at level between unspecified shoulder and elbow

√5ᵗʰ **S48.9** Traumatic amputation of shoulder and upper arm, level unspecified

√6ᵗʰ **S48.91** Complete traumatic amputation of shoulder and upper arm, level unspecified

√7ᵗʰ **S48.911** Complete traumatic amputation of right shoulder and upper arm, level unspecified

√7ᵗʰ **S48.912** Complete traumatic amputation of left shoulder and upper arm, level unspecified

√7ᵗʰ **S48.919** Complete traumatic amputation of unspecified shoulder and upper arm, level unspecified

√6ᵗʰ **S48.92** Partial traumatic amputation of shoulder and upper arm, level unspecified

√7ᵗʰ **S48.921** Partial traumatic amputation of right shoulder and upper arm, level unspecified

√7ᵗʰ **S48.922** Partial traumatic amputation of left shoulder and upper arm, level unspecified

√7ᵗʰ **S48.929** Partial traumatic amputation of unspecified shoulder and upper arm, level unspecified

√4ᵗʰ **S49** **Other and unspecified injuries of shoulder and upper arm**

AHA: 2018,2Q,12; 2018,1Q,3

TIP: The term "improper alignment" is not synonymous with malunion or nonunion of a fracture when noted in provider documentation.

The appropriate 7th character is to be added to each code from subcategories S49.0 and S49.1.
A   initial encounter for closed fracture
D   subsequent encounter for fracture with routine healing
G   subsequent encounter for fracture with delayed healing
K   subsequent encounter for fracture with nonunion
P   subsequent encounter for fracture with malunion
S   sequela

√5ᵗʰ **S49.0** Physeal fracture of upper end of humerus

√6ᵗʰ **S49.00** Unspecified physeal fracture of upper end of humerus

√7ᵗʰ **S49.001** Unspecified physeal fracture of upper end of humerus, right arm

√7ᵗʰ **S49.002** Unspecified physeal fracture of upper end of humerus, left arm

√7ᵗʰ **S49.009** Unspecified physeal fracture of upper end of humerus, unspecified arm

√6ᵗʰ **S49.01** Salter-Harris Type I physeal fracture of upper end of humerus

√7ᵗʰ **S49.011** Salter-Harris Type I physeal fracture of upper end of humerus, right arm

√7ᵗʰ **S49.012** Salter-Harris Type I physeal fracture of upper end of humerus, left arm

√7ᵗʰ **S49.019** Salter-Harris Type I physeal fracture of upper end of humerus, unspecified arm

√6ᵗʰ **S49.02** Salter-Harris Type II physeal fracture of upper end of humerus

√7ᵗʰ **S49.021** Salter-Harris Type II physeal fracture of upper end of humerus, right arm

√7ᵗʰ **S49.022** Salter-Harris Type II physeal fracture of upper end of humerus, left arm

√7ᵗʰ **S49.029** Salter-Harris Type II physeal fracture of upper end of humerus, unspecified arm

√6ᵗʰ **S49.03** Salter-Harris Type III physeal fracture of upper end of humerus

√7ᵗʰ **S49.031** Salter-Harris Type III physeal fracture of upper end of humerus, right arm

√7ᵗʰ **S49.032** Salter-Harris Type III physeal fracture of upper end of humerus, left arm

√7ᵗʰ **S49.039** Salter-Harris Type III physeal fracture of upper end of humerus, unspecified arm

√6ᵗʰ **S49.04** Salter-Harris Type IV physeal fracture of upper end of humerus

√7ᵗʰ **S49.041** Salter-Harris Type IV physeal fracture of upper end of humerus, right arm

N Newborn: 0   P Pediatric: 0-17   M Maternity: 12-55   A Adult: 15-124   CH Comorbidity High   CL Comorbidity Low   NCDx Noncancer Dx   PDx Primary Dx

996   ICD-10-CM 2020

☑7ᵗʰ **S49.042** Salter-Harris Type IV physeal fracture of upper end of humerus, left arm

☑7ᵗʰ **S49.049** Salter-Harris Type IV physeal fracture of upper end of humerus, unspecified arm

☑6ᵗʰ **S49.09** Other physeal fracture of upper end of humerus

☑7ᵗʰ **S49.091** Other physeal fracture of upper end of humerus, right arm

☑7ᵗʰ **S49.092** Other physeal fracture of upper end of humerus, left arm

☑7ᵗʰ **S49.099** Other physeal fracture of upper end of humerus, unspecified arm

☑5ᵗʰ **S49.1** Physeal fracture of lower end of humerus

☑6ᵗʰ **S49.10** Unspecified physeal fracture of lower end of humerus

☑7ᵗʰ **S49.101** Unspecified physeal fracture of lower end of humerus, right arm

☑7ᵗʰ **S49.102** Unspecified physeal fracture of lower end of humerus, left arm

☑7ᵗʰ **S49.109** Unspecified physeal fracture of lower end of humerus, unspecified arm

☑6ᵗʰ **S49.11** Salter-Harris Type I physeal fracture of lower end of humerus

☑7ᵗʰ **S49.111** Salter-Harris Type I physeal fracture of lower end of humerus, right arm

☑7ᵗʰ **S49.112** Salter-Harris Type I physeal fracture of lower end of humerus, left arm

☑7ᵗʰ **S49.119** Salter-Harris Type I physeal fracture of lower end of humerus, unspecified arm

☑6ᵗʰ **S49.12** Salter-Harris Type II physeal fracture of lower end of humerus

☑7ᵗʰ **S49.121** Salter-Harris Type II physeal fracture of lower end of humerus, right arm

☑7ᵗʰ **S49.122** Salter-Harris Type II physeal fracture of lower end of humerus, left arm

☑7ᵗʰ **S49.129** Salter-Harris Type II physeal fracture of lower end of humerus, unspecified arm

☑6ᵗʰ **S49.13** Salter-Harris Type III physeal fracture of lower end of humerus

☑7ᵗʰ **S49.131** Salter-Harris Type III physeal fracture of lower end of humerus, right arm

☑7ᵗʰ **S49.132** Salter-Harris Type III physeal fracture of lower end of humerus, left arm

☑7ᵗʰ **S49.139** Salter-Harris Type III physeal fracture of lower end of humerus, unspecified arm

☑6ᵗʰ **S49.14** Salter-Harris Type IV physeal fracture of lower end of humerus

☑7ᵗʰ **S49.141** Salter-Harris Type IV physeal fracture of lower end of humerus, right arm

☑7ᵗʰ **S49.142** Salter-Harris Type IV physeal fracture of lower end of humerus, left arm

☑7ᵗʰ **S49.149** Salter-Harris Type IV physeal fracture of lower end of humerus, unspecified arm

☑6ᵗʰ **S49.19** Other physeal fracture of lower end of humerus

☑7ᵗʰ **S49.191** Other physeal fracture of lower end of humerus, right arm

☑7ᵗʰ **S49.192** Other physeal fracture of lower end of humerus, left arm

☑7ᵗʰ **S49.199** Other physeal fracture of lower end of humerus, unspecified arm

☑5ᵗʰ **S49.8** Other specified injuries of shoulder and upper arm

> The appropriate 7th character is to be added to each code in subcategory S49.8.
> A   initial encounter
> D   subsequent encounter
> S   sequela

☑x7ᵗʰ **S49.80** Other specified injuries of shoulder and upper arm, unspecified arm

☑x7ᵗʰ **S49.81** Other specified injuries of right shoulder and upper arm

☑x7ᵗʰ **S49.82** Other specified injuries of left shoulder and upper arm

☑5ᵗʰ **S49.9** Unspecified injury of shoulder and upper arm

> The appropriate 7th character is to be added to each code in subcategory S49.9.
> A   initial encounter
> D   subsequent encounter
> S   sequela

☑x7ᵗʰ **S49.90** Unspecified injury of shoulder and upper arm, unspecified arm

☑x7ᵗʰ **S49.91** Unspecified injury of right shoulder and upper arm

☑x7ᵗʰ **S49.92** Unspecified injury of left shoulder and upper arm

Injuries to the elbow and forearm (S50-S59)

EXCLUDES 2   burns and corrosions (T20-T32)
frostbite (T33-T34)
injuries of wrist and hand (S60-S69)
insect bite or sting, venomous (T63.4)

☑4ᵗʰ **S50** **Superficial injury of elbow and forearm**

EXCLUDES 2   superficial injury of wrist and hand (S60.-)

> The appropriate 7th character is to be added to each code from category S50.
> A   initial encounter
> D   subsequent encounter
> S   sequela

☑5ᵗʰ **S50.0** Contusion of elbow

☑x7ᵗʰ **S50.00** Contusion of unspecified elbow

☑x7ᵗʰ **S50.01** Contusion of right elbow

☑x7ᵗʰ **S50.02** Contusion of left elbow

☑5ᵗʰ **S50.1** Contusion of forearm

☑x7ᵗʰ **S50.10** Contusion of unspecified forearm

☑x7ᵗʰ **S50.11** Contusion of right forearm

☑x7ᵗʰ **S50.12** Contusion of left forearm

☑5ᵗʰ **S50.3** Other superficial injuries of elbow

☑6ᵗʰ **S50.31** Abrasion of elbow

☑7ᵗʰ **S50.311** Abrasion of right elbow

☑7ᵗʰ **S50.312** Abrasion of left elbow

☑7ᵗʰ **S50.319** Abrasion of unspecified elbow

☑6ᵗʰ **S50.32** Blister (nonthermal) of elbow

☑7ᵗʰ **S50.321** Blister (nonthermal) of right elbow

☑7ᵗʰ **S50.322** Blister (nonthermal) of left elbow

☑7ᵗʰ **S50.329** Blister (nonthermal) of unspecified elbow

☑6ᵗʰ **S50.34** External constriction of elbow

☑7ᵗʰ **S50.341** External constriction of right elbow

☑7ᵗʰ **S50.342** External constriction of left elbow

☑7ᵗʰ **S50.349** External constriction of unspecified elbow

☑6ᵗʰ **S50.35** Superficial foreign body of elbow

> Splinter in the elbow

☑7ᵗʰ **S50.351** Superficial foreign body of right elbow

☑7ᵗʰ **S50.352** Superficial foreign body of left elbow

☑7ᵗʰ **S50.359** Superficial foreign body of unspecified elbow

☑6ᵗʰ **S50.36** Insect bite (nonvenomous) of elbow

☑7ᵗʰ **S50.361** Insect bite (nonvenomous) of right elbow

☑7ᵗʰ **S50.362** Insect bite (nonvenomous) of left elbow

☑7ᵗʰ **S50.369** Insect bite (nonvenomous) of unspecified elbow

☑6ᵗʰ **S50.37** Other superficial bite of elbow

EXCLUDES 1   open bite of elbow (S51.05)

☑7ᵗʰ **S50.371** Other superficial bite of right elbow

☑7ᵗʰ **S50.372** Other superficial bite of left elbow

☑7ᵗʰ **S50.379** Other superficial bite of unspecified elbow

☑5ᵗʰ **S50.8** Other superficial injuries of forearm

☑6ᵗʰ **S50.81** Abrasion of forearm

☑7ᵗʰ **S50.811** Abrasion of right forearm

☑7ᵗʰ **S50.812** Abrasion of left forearm

☑7ᵗʰ **S50.819** Abrasion of unspecified forearm

☑6ᵗʰ **S50.82** Blister (nonthermal) of forearm

☑7ᵗʰ **S50.821** Blister (nonthermal) of right forearm

☑7ᵗʰ **S50.822** Blister (nonthermal) of left forearm

☑7ᵗʰ **S50.829** Blister (nonthermal) of unspecified forearm

☑6ᵗʰ **S50.84** External constriction of forearm

☑7ᵗʰ **S50.841** External constriction of right forearm

☑7ᵗʰ **S50.842** External constriction of left forearm

☑7ᵗʰ **S50.849** External constriction of unspecified forearm

☑ Additional Character Required   ☑x7ᵗʰ Placeholder Alert   Manifestation   Unspecified Dx   ▶◀ Revised Text   ● New Code   ▲ Revised Title

ICD-10-CM 2020   **997**

Chapter 19. Injury, Poisoning and Certain Other Consequences of External Causes

✓6ᵗʰ **S50.85** **Superficial foreign body of forearm**
Splinter in the forearm

     ✓7ᵗʰ **S50.851** **Superficial foreign body of right forearm**

     ✓7ᵗʰ **S50.852** **Superficial foreign body of left forearm**

     ✓7ᵗʰ **S50.859** **Superficial foreign body of unspecified forearm**

✓6ᵗʰ **S50.86** **Insect bite (nonvenomous) of forearm**

     ✓7ᵗʰ **S50.861** **Insect bite (nonvenomous) of right forearm**

     ✓7ᵗʰ **S50.862** **Insect bite (nonvenomous) of left forearm**

     ✓7ᵗʰ **S50.869** **Insect bite (nonvenomous) of unspecified forearm**

✓6ᵗʰ **S50.87** **Other superficial bite of forearm**
     EXCLUDES 1   open bite of forearm (S51.85)

     ✓7ᵗʰ **S50.871** **Other superficial bite of right forearm**

     ✓7ᵗʰ **S50.872** **Other superficial bite of left forearm**

     ✓7ᵗʰ **S50.879** **Other superficial bite of unspecified forearm**

✓5ᵗʰ **S50.9** **Unspecified superficial injury of elbow and forearm**

     ✓6ᵗʰ **S50.90** **Unspecified superficial injury of elbow**

         ✓7ᵗʰ **S50.901** **Unspecified superficial injury of right elbow**

         ✓7ᵗʰ **S50.902** **Unspecified superficial injury of left elbow**

         ✓7ᵗʰ **S50.909** **Unspecified superficial injury of unspecified elbow**

     ✓6ᵗʰ **S50.91** **Unspecified superficial injury of forearm**

         ✓7ᵗʰ **S50.911** **Unspecified superficial injury of right forearm**

         ✓7ᵗʰ **S50.912** **Unspecified superficial injury of left forearm**

         ✓7ᵗʰ **S50.919** **Unspecified superficial injury of unspecified forearm**

✓4ᵗʰ **S51** **Open wound of elbow and forearm**
Code also any associated wound infection
     EXCLUDES 1   open fracture of elbow and forearm (S52.- with open fracture 7th character)
                 traumatic amputation of elbow and forearm (S58.-)
     EXCLUDES 2   open wound of wrist and hand (S61.-)

The appropriate 7th character is to be added to each code from category S51.
A   initial encounter
D   subsequent encounter
S   sequela

     ✓5ᵗʰ **S51.0** **Open wound of elbow**

     ✓6ᵗʰ **S51.00** **Unspecified open wound of elbow**

         ✓7ᵗʰ **S51.001** **Unspecified open wound of right elbow**
             AHA: 2012,4Q,108

         ✓7ᵗʰ **S51.002** **Unspecified open wound of left elbow**

         ✓7ᵗʰ **S51.009** **Unspecified open wound of unspecified elbow**
             Open wound of elbow NOS

     ✓6ᵗʰ **S51.01** **Laceration without foreign body of elbow**

         ✓7ᵗʰ **S51.011** **Laceration without foreign body of right elbow**

         ✓7ᵗʰ **S51.012** **Laceration without foreign body of left elbow**

         ✓7ᵗʰ **S51.019** **Laceration without foreign body of unspecified elbow**

     ✓6ᵗʰ **S51.02** **Laceration with foreign body of elbow**

         ✓7ᵗʰ **S51.021** **Laceration with foreign body of right elbow**

         ✓7ᵗʰ **S51.022** **Laceration with foreign body of left elbow**

         ✓7ᵗʰ **S51.029** **Laceration with foreign body of unspecified elbow**

     ✓6ᵗʰ **S51.03** **Puncture wound without foreign body of elbow**

         ✓7ᵗʰ **S51.031** **Puncture wound without foreign body of right elbow**

         ✓7ᵗʰ **S51.032** **Puncture wound without foreign body of left elbow**

         ✓7ᵗʰ **S51.039** **Puncture wound without foreign body of unspecified elbow**

     ✓6ᵗʰ **S51.04** **Puncture wound with foreign body of elbow**

         ✓7ᵗʰ **S51.041** **Puncture wound with foreign body of right elbow**

         ✓7ᵗʰ **S51.042** **Puncture wound with foreign body of left elbow**

         ✓7ᵗʰ **S51.049** **Puncture wound with foreign body of unspecified elbow**

     ✓6ᵗʰ **S51.05** **Open bite of elbow**
         Bite of elbow NOS
           EXCLUDES 1   superficial bite of elbow (S50.36, S50.37)

         ✓7ᵗʰ **S51.051** **Open bite, right elbow**

         ✓7ᵗʰ **S51.052** **Open bite, left elbow**

         ✓7ᵗʰ **S51.059** **Open bite, unspecified elbow**

✓5ᵗʰ **S51.8** **Open wound of forearm**
     EXCLUDES 2   open wound of elbow (S51.0-)

     ✓6ᵗʰ **S51.80** **Unspecified open wound of forearm**
         AHA: 2016,3Q,24

         ✓7ᵗʰ **S51.801** **Unspecified open wound of right forearm**

         ✓7ᵗʰ **S51.802** **Unspecified open wound of left forearm**

         ✓7ᵗʰ **S51.809** **Unspecified open wound of unspecified forearm**
             Open wound of forearm NOS

     ✓6ᵗʰ **S51.81** **Laceration without foreign body of forearm**

         ✓7ᵗʰ **S51.811** **Laceration without foreign body of right forearm**

         ✓7ᵗʰ **S51.812** **Laceration without foreign body of left forearm**

         ✓7ᵗʰ **S51.819** **Laceration without foreign body of unspecified forearm**

     ✓6ᵗʰ **S51.82** **Laceration with foreign body of forearm**

         ✓7ᵗʰ **S51.821** **Laceration with foreign body of right forearm**

         ✓7ᵗʰ **S51.822** **Laceration with foreign body of left forearm**

         ✓7ᵗʰ **S51.829** **Laceration with foreign body of unspecified forearm**

     ✓6ᵗʰ **S51.83** **Puncture wound without foreign body of forearm**
         AHA: 2016,3Q,24

         ✓7ᵗʰ **S51.831** **Puncture wound without foreign body of right forearm**

         ✓7ᵗʰ **S51.832** **Puncture wound without foreign body of left forearm**

         ✓7ᵗʰ **S51.839** **Puncture wound without foreign body of unspecified forearm**

     ✓6ᵗʰ **S51.84** **Puncture wound with foreign body of forearm**
         AHA: 2016,3Q,24

         ✓7ᵗʰ **S51.841** **Puncture wound with foreign body of right forearm**

         ✓7ᵗʰ **S51.842** **Puncture wound with foreign body of left forearm**

         ✓7ᵗʰ **S51.849** **Puncture wound with foreign body of unspecified forearm**

     ✓6ᵗʰ **S51.85** **Open bite of forearm**
         Bite of forearm NOS
           EXCLUDES 1   superficial bite of forearm (S50.86, S50.87)

         ✓7ᵗʰ **S51.851** **Open bite of right forearm**

         ✓7ᵗʰ **S51.852** **Open bite of left forearm**

         ✓7ᵗʰ **S51.859** **Open bite of unspecified forearm**

N Newborn: 0   P Pediatric: 0-17   M Maternity: 12-55   A Adult: 15-124   CH Comorbidity High   CL Comorbidity Low   NCDx Noncancer Dx   PDx Primary Dx

998   ICD-10-CM 2020

☑4ᵗʰ **S52 Fracture of forearm**

> **NOTE**   A fracture not indicated as displaced or nondisplaced should be coded to displaced.
>
> A fracture not indicated as open or closed should be coded to closed.
>
> The open fracture designations are based on the Gustilo open fracture classification.

> **EXCLUDES 1**   traumatic amputation of forearm (S58.-)
>
> **EXCLUDES 2**   fracture at wrist and hand level (S62.-)

AHA: 2018,2Q,12; 2016,1Q,33; 2015,3Q,37-39

DEF: Diaphysis: Central shaft of a long bone.

DEF: Epiphysis: Proximal and distal rounded ends of a long bone, communicates with the joint.

DEF: Metaphysis: Section of a long bone located between the epiphysis and diaphysis at the proximal and distal ends.

DEF: Physis (growth plate): Narrow zone of cartilaginous tissue between the epiphysis and metaphysis at each end of a long bone. In childhood, proliferation of cells in this zone lengthens the bone. As the bone matures, this area thins, ossification eventually fusing into solid bone and growth stops. *Synonyms: Epiphyseal plate.*

TIP: The term "improper alignment" is not synonymous with malunion or nonunion of a fracture when noted in provider documentation.

> The appropriate 7th character is to be added to all codes from category S52 [unless otherwise indicated].
>
> A   initial encounter for closed fracture
>
> B   initial encounter for open fracture type I or II
>
>   initial encounter for open fracture NOS
>
> C   initial encounter for open fracture type IIIA, IIIB, or IIIC
>
> D   subsequent encounter for closed fracture with routine healing
>
> E   subsequent encounter for open fracture type I or II with routine healing
>
> F   subsequent encounter for open fracture type IIIA, IIIB, or IIIC with routine healing
>
> G   subsequent encounter for closed fracture with delayed healing
>
> H   subsequent encounter for open fracture type I or II with delayed healing
>
> J   subsequent encounter for open fracture type IIIA, IIIB, or IIIC with delayed healing
>
> K   subsequent encounter for closed fracture with nonunion
>
> M   subsequent encounter for open fracture type I or II with nonunion
>
> N   subsequent encounter for open fracture type IIIA, IIIB, or IIIC with nonunion
>
> P   subsequent encounter for closed fracture with malunion
>
> Q   subsequent encounter for open fracture type I or II with malunion
>
> R   subsequent encounter for open fracture type IIIA, IIIB, or IIIC with malunion
>
> S   sequela

☑5ᵗʰ **S52.0 Fracture of upper end of ulna**

Fracture of proximal end of ulna

> **EXCLUDES 2**   fracture of elbow NOS (S42.40-)
>
> fractures of shaft of ulna (S52.2-)

☑6ᵗʰ **S52.00 Unspecified fracture of upper end of ulna**

☑7ᵗʰ **S52.001** Unspecified fracture of upper end of right ulna

☑7ᵗʰ **S52.002** Unspecified fracture of upper end of left ulna

☑7ᵗʰ **S52.009** Unspecified fracture of upper end of unspecified ulna

☑6ᵗʰ **S52.01 Torus fracture of upper end of ulna**

> The appropriate 7th character is to be added to all codes in subcategory S52.01
>
> A   initial encounter for closed fracture
>
> D   subsequent encounter for fracture with routine healing
>
> G   subsequent encounter for fracture with delayed healing
>
> K   subsequent encounter for fracture with nonunion
>
> P   subsequent encounter for fracture with malunion
>
> S   sequela

☑7ᵗʰ **S52.011** Torus fracture of upper end of right ulna

☑7ᵗʰ **S52.012** Torus fracture of upper end of left ulna

☑7ᵗʰ **S52.019** Torus fracture of upper end of unspecified ulna

☑6ᵗʰ **S52.02 Fracture of olecranon process without intraarticular extension of ulna**

☑7ᵗʰ **S52.021** Displaced fracture of olecranon process without intraarticular extension of right ulna

☑7ᵗʰ **S52.022** Displaced fracture of olecranon process without intraarticular extension of left ulna

☑7ᵗʰ **S52.023** Displaced fracture of olecranon process without intraarticular extension of unspecified ulna

☑7ᵗʰ **S52.024** Nondisplaced fracture of olecranon process without intraarticular extension of right ulna

☑7ᵗʰ **S52.025** Nondisplaced fracture of olecranon process without intraarticular extension of left ulna

☑7ᵗʰ **S52.026** Nondisplaced fracture of olecranon process without intraarticular extension of unspecified ulna

☑6ᵗʰ **S52.03 Fracture of olecranon process with intraarticular extension of ulna**

☑7ᵗʰ **S52.031** Displaced fracture of olecranon process with intraarticular extension of right ulna

☑7ᵗʰ **S52.032** Displaced fracture of olecranon process with intraarticular extension of left ulna

☑7ᵗʰ **S52.033** Displaced fracture of olecranon process with intraarticular extension of unspecified ulna

☑7ᵗʰ **S52.034** Nondisplaced fracture of olecranon process with intraarticular extension of right ulna

☑7ᵗʰ **S52.035** Nondisplaced fracture of olecranon process with intraarticular extension of left ulna

☑7ᵗʰ **S52.036** Nondisplaced fracture of olecranon process with intraarticular extension of unspecified ulna

☑6ᵗʰ **S52.04 Fracture of coronoid process of ulna**

☑7ᵗʰ **S52.041** Displaced fracture of coronoid process of right ulna

☑7ᵗʰ **S52.042** Displaced fracture of coronoid process of left ulna

☑7ᵗʰ **S52.043** Displaced fracture of coronoid process of unspecified ulna

☑7ᵗʰ **S52.044** Nondisplaced fracture of coronoid process of right ulna

☑7ᵗʰ **S52.045** Nondisplaced fracture of coronoid process of left ulna

☑7ᵗʰ **S52.046** Nondisplaced fracture of coronoid process of unspecified ulna

☑6ᵗʰ **S52.09 Other fracture of upper end of ulna**

☑7ᵗʰ **S52.091** Other fracture of upper end of right ulna

☑7ᵗʰ **S52.092** Other fracture of upper end of left ulna

☑7ᵗʰ **S52.099** Other fracture of upper end of unspecified ulna

☑5ᵗʰ **S52.1 Fracture of upper end of radius**

Fracture of proximal end of radius

> **EXCLUDES 2**   physeal fractures of upper end of radius (S59.2-)
>
> fracture of shaft of radius (S52.3-)

☑6ᵗʰ **S52.10 Unspecified fracture of upper end of radius**

☑7ᵗʰ **S52.101** Unspecified fracture of upper end of right radius

☑7ᵗʰ **S52.102** Unspecified fracture of upper end of left radius

☑7ᵗʰ **S52.109** Unspecified fracture of upper end of unspecified radius

☑ Additional Character Required   ☑x7ᵗʰ Placeholder Alert   Manifestation   Unspecified Dx   ▶◀ Revised Text   ● New Code   ▲ Revised Title

ICD-10-CM 2020

999

√6ᵗʰ **S52.11**   **Torus** fracture of upper end of radius

> The appropriate 7th character is to be added to all codes in subcategory S52.11
> A   initial encounter for closed fracture
> D   subsequent encounter for fracture with routine healing
> G   subsequent encounter for fracture with delayed healing
> K   subsequent encounter for fracture with nonunion
> P   subsequent encounter for fracture with malunion
> S   sequela

    √7ᵗʰ **S52.111**   **Torus** fracture of upper end of right radius

    √7ᵗʰ **S52.112**   **Torus** fracture of upper end of left radius

    √7ᵗʰ **S52.119**   **Torus** fracture of upper end of unspecified radius

√6ᵗʰ **S52.12**   Fracture of head of radius

    √7ᵗʰ **S52.121**   **Displaced** fracture of head of right radius

    √7ᵗʰ **S52.122**   **Displaced** fracture of head of left radius

    √7ᵗʰ **S52.123**   **Displaced** fracture of head of unspecified radius

    √7ᵗʰ **S52.124**   **Nondisplaced** fracture of head of right radius

    √7ᵗʰ **S52.125**   **Nondisplaced** fracture of head of left radius

    √7ᵗʰ **S52.126**   **Nondisplaced** fracture of head of unspecified radius

√6ᵗʰ **S52.13**   Fracture of neck of radius

    √7ᵗʰ **S52.131**   **Displaced** fracture of neck of right radius

    √7ᵗʰ **S52.132**   **Displaced** fracture of neck of left radius

    √7ᵗʰ **S52.133**   **Displaced** fracture of neck of unspecified radius

    √7ᵗʰ **S52.134**   **Nondisplaced** fracture of neck of right radius

    √7ᵗʰ **S52.135**   **Nondisplaced** fracture of neck of left radius

    √7ᵗʰ **S52.136**   **Nondisplaced** fracture of neck of unspecified radius

√6ᵗʰ **S52.18**   Other fracture of upper end of radius

    √7ᵗʰ **S52.181**   **Other** fracture of upper end of right radius

    √7ᵗʰ **S52.182**   **Other** fracture of upper end of left radius

    √7ᵗʰ **S52.189**   **Other** fracture of upper end of unspecified radius

√5ᵗʰ **S52.2**   Fracture of shaft of ulna

√6ᵗʰ **S52.20**   **Unspecified** fracture of shaft of ulna

> Fracture of ulna NOS

    √7ᵗʰ **S52.201**   **Unspecified** fracture of shaft of right ulna

    √7ᵗʰ **S52.202**   **Unspecified** fracture of shaft of left ulna

    √7ᵗʰ **S52.209**   **Unspecified** fracture of shaft of unspecified ulna

√6ᵗʰ **S52.21**   **Greenstick** fracture of shaft of ulna

> The appropriate 7th character is to be added to all codes in subcategory S52.21
> A   initial encounter for closed fracture
> D   subsequent encounter for fracture with routine healing
> G   subsequent encounter for fracture with delayed healing
> K   subsequent encounter for fracture with nonunion
> P   subsequent encounter for fracture with malunion
> S   sequela

    √7ᵗʰ **S52.211**   **Greenstick** fracture of shaft of right ulna

    √7ᵗʰ **S52.212**   **Greenstick** fracture of shaft of left ulna

    √7ᵗʰ **S52.219**   **Greenstick** fracture of shaft of unspecified ulna

√6ᵗʰ **S52.22**   **Transverse** fracture of shaft of ulna

    √7ᵗʰ **S52.221**   **Displaced** transverse fracture of shaft of right ulna

    √7ᵗʰ **S52.222**   **Displaced** transverse fracture of shaft of left ulna

    √7ᵗʰ **S52.223**   **Displaced** transverse fracture of shaft of unspecified ulna

    √7ᵗʰ **S52.224**   **Nondisplaced** transverse fracture of shaft of right ulna

    √7ᵗʰ **S52.225**   **Nondisplaced** transverse fracture of shaft of left ulna

    √7ᵗʰ **S52.226**   **Nondisplaced** transverse fracture of shaft of unspecified ulna

√6ᵗʰ **S52.23**   **Oblique** fracture of shaft of ulna

    √7ᵗʰ **S52.231**   **Displaced** oblique fracture of shaft of right ulna

    √7ᵗʰ **S52.232**   **Displaced** oblique fracture of shaft of left ulna

    √7ᵗʰ **S52.233**   **Displaced** oblique fracture of shaft of unspecified ulna

    √7ᵗʰ **S52.234**   **Nondisplaced** oblique fracture of shaft of right ulna

    √7ᵗʰ **S52.235**   **Nondisplaced** oblique fracture of shaft of left ulna

    √7ᵗʰ **S52.236**   **Nondisplaced** oblique fracture of shaft of unspecified ulna

√6ᵗʰ **S52.24**   **Spiral** fracture of shaft of ulna

    √7ᵗʰ **S52.241**   **Displaced** spiral fracture of shaft of ulna, right arm

    √7ᵗʰ **S52.242**   **Displaced** spiral fracture of shaft of ulna, left arm

    √7ᵗʰ **S52.243**   **Displaced** spiral fracture of shaft of ulna, unspecified arm

    √7ᵗʰ **S52.244**   **Nondisplaced** spiral fracture of shaft of ulna, right arm

    √7ᵗʰ **S52.245**   **Nondisplaced** spiral fracture of shaft of ulna, left arm

    √7ᵗʰ **S52.246**   **Nondisplaced** spiral fracture of shaft of ulna, unspecified arm

√6ᵗʰ **S52.25**   **Comminuted** fracture of shaft of ulna

    √7ᵗʰ **S52.251**   **Displaced** comminuted fracture of shaft of ulna, right arm

    √7ᵗʰ **S52.252**   **Displaced** comminuted fracture of shaft of ulna, left arm

    √7ᵗʰ **S52.253**   **Displaced** comminuted fracture of shaft of ulna, unspecified arm

    √7ᵗʰ **S52.254**   **Nondisplaced** comminuted fracture of shaft of ulna, right arm

    √7ᵗʰ **S52.255**   **Nondisplaced** comminuted fracture of shaft of ulna, left arm

    √7ᵗʰ **S52.256**   **Nondisplaced** comminuted fracture of shaft of ulna, unspecified arm

√6ᵗʰ **S52.26**   **Segmental** fracture of shaft of ulna

    √7ᵗʰ **S52.261**   **Displaced** segmental fracture of shaft of ulna, right arm

    √7ᵗʰ **S52.262**   **Displaced** segmental fracture of shaft of ulna, left arm

    √7ᵗʰ **S52.263**   **Displaced** segmental fracture of shaft of ulna, unspecified arm

    √7ᵗʰ **S52.264**   **Nondisplaced** segmental fracture of shaft of ulna, right arm

    √7ᵗʰ **S52.265**   **Nondisplaced** segmental fracture of shaft of ulna, left arm

    √7ᵗʰ **S52.266**   **Nondisplaced** segmental fracture of shaft of ulna, unspecified arm

√6ᵗʰ **S52.27**   **Monteggia's** fracture of ulna

> Fracture of upper shaft of ulna with dislocation of radial head

    √7ᵗʰ **S52.271**   **Monteggia's** fracture of right ulna

    √7ᵗʰ **S52.272**   **Monteggia's** fracture of left ulna

    √7ᵗʰ **S52.279**   **Monteggia's** fracture of unspecified ulna

√6ᵗʰ **S52.28**   **Bent bone** of ulna

    √7ᵗʰ **S52.281**   **Bent bone** of right ulna

    √7ᵗʰ **S52.282**   **Bent bone** of left ulna

    √7ᵗʰ **S52.283**   **Bent bone** of unspecified ulna

√6ᵗʰ **S52.29**   **Other** fracture of shaft of ulna

    √7ᵗʰ **S52.291**   **Other** fracture of shaft of right ulna

    √7ᵗʰ **S52.292**   **Other** fracture of shaft of left ulna

    √7ᵗʰ **S52.299**   **Other** fracture of shaft of unspecified ulna

√5ᵗʰ **S52.3**   Fracture of shaft of radius

√6ᵗʰ **S52.30**   **Unspecified** fracture of shaft of radius

    √7ᵗʰ **S52.301**   **Unspecified** fracture of shaft of right radius

Ⓝ Newborn: 0   Ⓟ Pediatric: 0-17   Ⓜ Maternity: 12-55   Ⓐ Adult: 15-124   CH Comorbidity High   CL Comorbidity Low   NCDx Noncancer Dx   PDx Primary Dx

1000   ICD-10-CM 2020

√7ᵗʰ **S52.302** Unspecified fracture of shaft of left radius

√7ᵗʰ **S52.309** Unspecified fracture of shaft of unspecified radius

√6ᵗʰ **S52.31** Greenstick fracture of shaft of radius

> The appropriate 7th character is to be added to all codes in subcategory S52.31.
> A initial encounter for closed fracture
> D subsequent encounter for fracture with routine healing
> G subsequent encounter for fracture with delayed healing
> K subsequent encounter for fracture with nonunion
> P subsequent encounter for fracture with malunion
> S sequela

√7ᵗʰ **S52.311** Greenstick fracture of shaft of radius, right arm

√7ᵗʰ **S52.312** Greenstick fracture of shaft of radius, left arm

√7ᵗʰ **S52.319** Greenstick fracture of shaft of radius, unspecified arm

√6ᵗʰ **S52.32** Transverse fracture of shaft of radius

√7ᵗʰ **S52.321** Displaced transverse fracture of shaft of right radius

√7ᵗʰ **S52.322** Displaced transverse fracture of shaft of left radius

√7ᵗʰ **S52.323** Displaced transverse fracture of shaft of unspecified radius

√7ᵗʰ **S52.324** Nondisplaced transverse fracture of shaft of right radius

√7ᵗʰ **S52.325** Nondisplaced transverse fracture of shaft of left radius

√7ᵗʰ **S52.326** Nondisplaced transverse fracture of shaft of unspecified radius

√6ᵗʰ **S52.33** Oblique fracture of shaft of radius

√7ᵗʰ **S52.331** Displaced oblique fracture of shaft of right radius

√7ᵗʰ **S52.332** Displaced oblique fracture of shaft of left radius

√7ᵗʰ **S52.333** Displaced oblique fracture of shaft of unspecified radius

√7ᵗʰ **S52.334** Nondisplaced oblique fracture of shaft of right radius

√7ᵗʰ **S52.335** Nondisplaced oblique fracture of shaft of left radius

√7ᵗʰ **S52.336** Nondisplaced oblique fracture of shaft of unspecified radius

√6ᵗʰ **S52.34** Spiral fracture of shaft of radius

√7ᵗʰ **S52.341** Displaced spiral fracture of shaft of radius, right arm

√7ᵗʰ **S52.342** Displaced spiral fracture of shaft of radius, left arm

√7ᵗʰ **S52.343** Displaced spiral fracture of shaft of radius, unspecified arm

√7ᵗʰ **S52.344** Nondisplaced spiral fracture of shaft of radius, right arm

√7ᵗʰ **S52.345** Nondisplaced spiral fracture of shaft of radius, left arm

√7ᵗʰ **S52.346** Nondisplaced spiral fracture of shaft of radius, unspecified arm

√6ᵗʰ **S52.35** Comminuted fracture of shaft of radius

√7ᵗʰ **S52.351** Displaced comminuted fracture of shaft of radius, right arm

√7ᵗʰ **S52.352** Displaced comminuted fracture of shaft of radius, left arm

√7ᵗʰ **S52.353** Displaced comminuted fracture of shaft of radius, unspecified arm

√7ᵗʰ **S52.354** Nondisplaced comminuted fracture of shaft of radius, right arm

√7ᵗʰ **S52.355** Nondisplaced comminuted fracture of shaft of radius, left arm

√7ᵗʰ **S52.356** Nondisplaced comminuted fracture of shaft of radius, unspecified arm

√6ᵗʰ **S52.36** Segmental fracture of shaft of radius

√7ᵗʰ **S52.361** Displaced segmental fracture of shaft of radius, right arm

√7ᵗʰ **S52.362** Displaced segmental fracture of shaft of radius, left arm

√7ᵗʰ **S52.363** Displaced segmental fracture of shaft of radius, unspecified arm

√7ᵗʰ **S52.364** Nondisplaced segmental fracture of shaft of radius, right arm

√7ᵗʰ **S52.365** Nondisplaced segmental fracture of shaft of radius, left arm

√7ᵗʰ **S52.366** Nondisplaced segmental fracture of shaft of radius, unspecified arm

√6ᵗʰ **S52.37** Galeazzi's fracture

> Fracture of lower shaft of radius with radioulnar joint dislocation

√7ᵗʰ **S52.371** Galeazzi's fracture of right radius

√7ᵗʰ **S52.372** Galeazzi's fracture of left radius

√7ᵗʰ **S52.379** Galeazzi's fracture of unspecified radius

√6ᵗʰ **S52.38** Bent bone of radius

√7ᵗʰ **S52.381** Bent bone of right radius

√7ᵗʰ **S52.382** Bent bone of left radius

√7ᵗʰ **S52.389** Bent bone of unspecified radius

√6ᵗʰ **S52.39** Other fracture of shaft of radius

√7ᵗʰ **S52.391** Other fracture of shaft of radius, right arm

√7ᵗʰ **S52.392** Other fracture of shaft of radius, left arm

√7ᵗʰ **S52.399** Other fracture of shaft of radius, unspecified arm

√5ᵗʰ **S52.5** Fracture of lower end of radius

> Fracture of distal end of radius
> **EXCLUDES 2** physeal fractures of lower end of radius (S59.2-)
> **DEF:** Fracture of the distal end of the radius above the wrist, most commonly caused by a fall onto an outstretched hand.

√6ᵗʰ **S52.50** Unspecified fracture of the lower end of radius

√7ᵗʰ **S52.501** Unspecified fracture of the lower end of right radius

√7ᵗʰ **S52.502** Unspecified fracture of the lower end of left radius

√7ᵗʰ **S52.509** Unspecified fracture of the lower end of unspecified radius

√6ᵗʰ **S52.51** Fracture of radial styloid process

√7ᵗʰ **S52.511** Displaced fracture of right radial styloid process

√7ᵗʰ **S52.512** Displaced fracture of left radial styloid process

√7ᵗʰ **S52.513** Displaced fracture of unspecified radial styloid process

√7ᵗʰ **S52.514** Nondisplaced fracture of right radial styloid process

√7ᵗʰ **S52.515** Nondisplaced fracture of left radial styloid process

√7ᵗʰ **S52.516** Nondisplaced fracture of unspecified radial styloid process

√6ᵗʰ **S52.52** Torus fracture of lower end of radius

> The appropriate 7th character is to be added to all codes in subcategory S52.52.
> A initial encounter for closed fracture
> D subsequent encounter for fracture with routine healing
> G subsequent encounter for fracture with delayed healing
> K subsequent encounter for fracture with nonunion
> P subsequent encounter for fracture with malunion
> S sequela

√7ᵗʰ **S52.521** Torus fracture of lower end of right radius

√7ᵗʰ **S52.522** Torus fracture of lower end of left radius

√7ᵗʰ **S52.529** Torus fracture of lower end of unspecified radius

√6ᵗʰ **S52.53** Colles' fracture

> **AHA:** 2016,2Q,4
> **DEF:** Fracture of the radius at the wrist in which the distal fragment is pushed posteriorly. The dorsal angulation of the fragment results in the wrist cocking up.

√7ᵗʰ **S52.531** Colles' fracture of right radius

√7ᵗʰ **S52.532** Colles' fracture of left radius

√7ᵗʰ **S52.539** Colles' fracture of unspecified radius

☑ Additional Character Required   √x7ᵗʰ Placeholder Alert   Manifestation   Unspecified Dx   ►◄ Revised Text   ● New Code   ▲ Revised Title

ICD-10-CM 2020

1001

√6ᵗʰ **S52.54** Smith's fracture
- √7ᵗʰ **S52.541** Smith's fracture of right radius
- √7ᵗʰ **S52.542** Smith's fracture of left radius
- √7ᵗʰ **S52.549** Smith's fracture of unspecified radius

√6ᵗʰ **S52.55** Other extraarticular fracture of lower end of radius
- √7ᵗʰ **S52.551** Other extraarticular fracture of lower end of right radius
- √7ᵗʰ **S52.552** Other extraarticular fracture of lower end of left radius
- √7ᵗʰ **S52.559** Other extraarticular fracture of lower end of unspecified radius

√6ᵗʰ **S52.56** Barton's fracture
- √7ᵗʰ **S52.561** Barton's fracture of right radius
- √7ᵗʰ **S52.562** Barton's fracture of left radius
- √7ᵗʰ **S52.569** Barton's fracture of unspecified radius

√6ᵗʰ **S52.57** Other intraarticular fracture of lower end of radius
- √7ᵗʰ **S52.571** Other intraarticular fracture of lower end of right radius
- √7ᵗʰ **S52.572** Other intraarticular fracture of lower end of left radius
- √7ᵗʰ **S52.579** Other intraarticular fracture of lower end of unspecified radius

√6ᵗʰ **S52.59** Other fractures of lower end of radius
- √7ᵗʰ **S52.591** Other fractures of lower end of right radius
- √7ᵗʰ **S52.592** Other fractures of lower end of left radius
- √7ᵗʰ **S52.599** Other fractures of lower end of unspecified radius

√5ᵗʰ **S52.6** Fracture of lower end of ulna

√6ᵗʰ **S52.60** Unspecified fracture of lower end of ulna
- √7ᵗʰ **S52.601** Unspecified fracture of lower end of right ulna
- √7ᵗʰ **S52.602** Unspecified fracture of lower end of left ulna
- √7ᵗʰ **S52.609** Unspecified fracture of lower end of unspecified ulna

√6ᵗʰ **S52.61** Fracture of ulna styloid process
- √7ᵗʰ **S52.611** Displaced fracture of right ulna styloid process
- √7ᵗʰ **S52.612** Displaced fracture of left ulna styloid process
- √7ᵗʰ **S52.613** Displaced fracture of unspecified ulna styloid process
- √7ᵗʰ **S52.614** Nondisplaced fracture of right ulna styloid process
- √7ᵗʰ **S52.615** Nondisplaced fracture of left ulna styloid process
- √7ᵗʰ **S52.616** Nondisplaced fracture of unspecified ulna styloid process

√6ᵗʰ **S52.62** Torus fracture of lower end of ulna

> The appropriate 7th character is to be added to all codes in subcategory S52.62.
> A initial encounter for closed fracture
> D subsequent encounter for fracture with routine healing
> G subsequent encounter for fracture with delayed healing
> K subsequent encounter for fracture with nonunion
> P subsequent encounter for fracture with malunion
> S sequela

- √7ᵗʰ **S52.621** Torus fracture of lower end of right ulna
- √7ᵗʰ **S52.622** Torus fracture of lower end of left ulna
- √7ᵗʰ **S52.629** Torus fracture of lower end of unspecified ulna

√6ᵗʰ **S52.69** Other fracture of lower end of ulna
- √7ᵗʰ **S52.691** Other fracture of lower end of right ulna
- √7ᵗʰ **S52.692** Other fracture of lower end of left ulna
- √7ᵗʰ **S52.699** Other fracture of lower end of unspecified ulna

√5ᵗʰ **S52.9** Unspecified fracture of forearm
- √x7ᵗʰ **S52.90** Unspecified fracture of unspecified forearm
- √x7ᵗʰ **S52.91** Unspecified fracture of right forearm
- √x7ᵗʰ **S52.92** Unspecified fracture of left forearm

√4ᵗʰ **S53 Dislocation and sprain of joints and ligaments of elbow**

INCLUDES avulsion of joint or ligament of elbow
laceration of cartilage, joint or ligament of elbow
sprain of cartilage, joint or ligament of elbow
traumatic hemarthrosis of joint or ligament of elbow
traumatic rupture of joint or ligament of elbow
traumatic subluxation of joint or ligament of elbow
traumatic tear of joint or ligament of elbow

Code also any associated open wound

EXCLUDES 2 *strain of muscle, fascia and tendon at forearm level (S56.-)*

> The appropriate 7th character is to be added to each code from category S53.
> A initial encounter
> D subsequent encounter
> S sequela

√5ᵗʰ **S53.0** Subluxation and dislocation of radial head
Dislocation of radiohumeral joint
Subluxation of radiohumeral joint
EXCLUDES 1 *Monteggia's fracture-dislocation (S52.27-)*

√6ᵗʰ **S53.00** Unspecified subluxation and dislocation of radial head
- √7ᵗʰ **S53.001** Unspecified subluxation of right radial head
- √7ᵗʰ **S53.002** Unspecified subluxation of left radial head
- √7ᵗʰ **S53.003** Unspecified subluxation of unspecified radial head
- √7ᵗʰ **S53.004** Unspecified dislocation of right radial head
- √7ᵗʰ **S53.005** Unspecified dislocation of left radial head
- √7ᵗʰ **S53.006** Unspecified dislocation of unspecified radial head

√6ᵗʰ **S53.01** Anterior subluxation and dislocation of radial head
Anteriomedial subluxation and dislocation of radial head
- √7ᵗʰ **S53.011** Anterior subluxation of right radial head
- √7ᵗʰ **S53.012** Anterior subluxation of left radial head
- √7ᵗʰ **S53.013** Anterior subluxation of unspecified radial head
- √7ᵗʰ **S53.014** Anterior dislocation of right radial head
- √7ᵗʰ **S53.015** Anterior dislocation of left radial head
- √7ᵗʰ **S53.016** Anterior dislocation of unspecified radial head

√6ᵗʰ **S53.02** Posterior subluxation and dislocation of radial head
Posteriolateral subluxation and dislocation of radial head
- √7ᵗʰ **S53.021** Posterior subluxation of right radial head
- √7ᵗʰ **S53.022** Posterior subluxation of left radial head
- √7ᵗʰ **S53.023** Posterior subluxation of unspecified radial head
- √7ᵗʰ **S53.024** Posterior dislocation of right radial head
- √7ᵗʰ **S53.025** Posterior dislocation of left radial head
- √7ᵗʰ **S53.026** Posterior dislocation of unspecified radial head

√6ᵗʰ **S53.03** Nursemaid's elbow
- √7ᵗʰ **S53.031** Nursemaid's elbow, right elbow
- √7ᵗʰ **S53.032** Nursemaid's elbow, left elbow
- √7ᵗʰ **S53.033** Nursemaid's elbow, unspecified elbow

√6ᵗʰ **S53.09** Other subluxation and dislocation of radial head
- √7ᵗʰ **S53.091** Other subluxation of right radial head
- √7ᵗʰ **S53.092** Other subluxation of left radial head
- √7ᵗʰ **S53.093** Other subluxation of unspecified radial head
- √7ᵗʰ **S53.094** Other dislocation of right radial head
- √7ᵗʰ **S53.095** Other dislocation of left radial head
- √7ᵗʰ **S53.096** Other dislocation of unspecified radial head

√5ᵗʰ **S53.1** Subluxation and dislocation of ulnohumeral joint
Subluxation and dislocation of elbow NOS
EXCLUDES 1 *dislocation of radial head alone (S53.0-)*

√6ᵗʰ **S53.10** Unspecified subluxation and dislocation of ulnohumeral joint
- √7ᵗʰ **S53.101** Unspecified subluxation of right ulnohumeral joint

√7ᵗʰ **S53.102** Unspecified subluxation of left ulnohumeral joint

√7ᵗʰ **S53.103** Unspecified subluxation of unspecified ulnohumeral joint

√7ᵗʰ **S53.104** Unspecified dislocation of right ulnohumeral joint

√7ᵗʰ **S53.105** Unspecified dislocation of left ulnohumeral joint

√7ᵗʰ **S53.106** Unspecified dislocation of unspecified ulnohumeral joint

√6ᵗʰ **S53.11** Anterior subluxation and dislocation of ulnohumeral joint

√7ᵗʰ **S53.111** Anterior subluxation of right ulnohumeral joint

√7ᵗʰ **S53.112** Anterior subluxation of left ulnohumeral joint

√7ᵗʰ **S53.113** Anterior subluxation of unspecified ulnohumeral joint

√7ᵗʰ **S53.114** Anterior dislocation of right ulnohumeral joint
     AHA: 2012,4Q,108

√7ᵗʰ **S53.115** Anterior dislocation of left ulnohumeral joint

√7ᵗʰ **S53.116** Anterior dislocation of unspecified ulnohumeral joint

√6ᵗʰ **S53.12** Posterior subluxation and dislocation of ulnohumeral joint

√7ᵗʰ **S53.121** Posterior subluxation of right ulnohumeral joint

√7ᵗʰ **S53.122** Posterior subluxation of left ulnohumeral joint

√7ᵗʰ **S53.123** Posterior subluxation of unspecified ulnohumeral joint

√7ᵗʰ **S53.124** Posterior dislocation of right ulnohumeral joint

√7ᵗʰ **S53.125** Posterior dislocation of left ulnohumeral joint

√7ᵗʰ **S53.126** Posterior dislocation of unspecified ulnohumeral joint

√6ᵗʰ **S53.13** Medial subluxation and dislocation of ulnohumeral joint

√7ᵗʰ **S53.131** Medial subluxation of right ulnohumeral joint

√7ᵗʰ **S53.132** Medial subluxation of left ulnohumeral joint

√7ᵗʰ **S53.133** Medial subluxation of unspecified ulnohumeral joint

√7ᵗʰ **S53.134** Medial dislocation of right ulnohumeral joint

√7ᵗʰ **S53.135** Medial dislocation of left ulnohumeral joint

√7ᵗʰ **S53.136** Medial dislocation of unspecified ulnohumeral joint

√6ᵗʰ **S53.14** Lateral subluxation and dislocation of ulnohumeral joint

√7ᵗʰ **S53.141** Lateral subluxation of right ulnohumeral joint

√7ᵗʰ **S53.142** Lateral subluxation of left ulnohumeral joint

√7ᵗʰ **S53.143** Lateral subluxation of unspecified ulnohumeral joint

√7ᵗʰ **S53.144** Lateral dislocation of right ulnohumeral joint

√7ᵗʰ **S53.145** Lateral dislocation of left ulnohumeral joint

√7ᵗʰ **S53.146** Lateral dislocation of unspecified ulnohumeral joint

√6ᵗʰ **S53.19** Other subluxation and dislocation of ulnohumeral joint

√7ᵗʰ **S53.191** Other subluxation of right ulnohumeral joint

√7ᵗʰ **S53.192** Other subluxation of left ulnohumeral joint

√7ᵗʰ **S53.193** Other subluxation of unspecified ulnohumeral joint

√7ᵗʰ **S53.194** Other dislocation of right ulnohumeral joint

√7ᵗʰ **S53.195** Other dislocation of left ulnohumeral joint

√7ᵗʰ **S53.196** Other dislocation of unspecified ulnohumeral joint

√5ᵗʰ **S53.2** Traumatic rupture of radial collateral ligament
     EXCLUDES 1   sprain of radial collateral ligament NOS (S53.43-)

√x7ᵗʰ **S53.20** Traumatic rupture of unspecified radial collateral ligament

√x7ᵗʰ **S53.21** Traumatic rupture of right radial collateral ligament

√x7ᵗʰ **S53.22** Traumatic rupture of left radial collateral ligament

√5ᵗʰ **S53.3** Traumatic rupture of ulnar collateral ligament
     EXCLUDES 1   sprain of ulnar collateral ligament (S53.44-)

√x7ᵗʰ **S53.30** Traumatic rupture of unspecified ulnar collateral ligament

√x7ᵗʰ **S53.31** Traumatic rupture of right ulnar collateral ligament

√x7ᵗʰ **S53.32** Traumatic rupture of left ulnar collateral ligament

√5ᵗʰ **S53.4** Sprain of elbow
     EXCLUDES 2   traumatic rupture of radial collateral ligament (S53.2-)
                      traumatic rupture of ulnar collateral ligament (S53.3-)

√6ᵗʰ **S53.40** Unspecified sprain of elbow

√7ᵗʰ **S53.401** Unspecified sprain of right elbow

√7ᵗʰ **S53.402** Unspecified sprain of left elbow

√7ᵗʰ **S53.409** Unspecified sprain of unspecified elbow
     Sprain of elbow NOS

√6ᵗʰ **S53.41** Radiohumeral (joint) sprain

√7ᵗʰ **S53.411** Radiohumeral (joint) sprain of right elbow

√7ᵗʰ **S53.412** Radiohumeral (joint) sprain of left elbow

√7ᵗʰ **S53.419** Radiohumeral (joint) sprain of unspecified elbow

√6ᵗʰ **S53.42** Ulnohumeral (joint) sprain

√7ᵗʰ **S53.421** Ulnohumeral (joint) sprain of right elbow

√7ᵗʰ **S53.422** Ulnohumeral (joint) sprain of left elbow

√7ᵗʰ **S53.429** Ulnohumeral (joint) sprain of unspecified elbow

√6ᵗʰ **S53.43** Radial collateral ligament sprain

√7ᵗʰ **S53.431** Radial collateral ligament sprain of right elbow

√7ᵗʰ **S53.432** Radial collateral ligament sprain of left elbow

√7ᵗʰ **S53.439** Radial collateral ligament sprain of unspecified elbow

√6ᵗʰ **S53.44** Ulnar collateral ligament sprain

√7ᵗʰ **S53.441** Ulnar collateral ligament sprain of right elbow

√7ᵗʰ **S53.442** Ulnar collateral ligament sprain of left elbow

√7ᵗʰ **S53.449** Ulnar collateral ligament sprain of unspecified elbow

√6ᵗʰ **S53.49** Other sprain of elbow

√7ᵗʰ **S53.491** Other sprain of right elbow

√7ᵗʰ **S53.492** Other sprain of left elbow

√7ᵗʰ **S53.499** Other sprain of unspecified elbow

√4ᵗʰ **S54** Injury of nerves at forearm level
     Code also any associated open wound (S51.-)
     EXCLUDES 2   injury of nerves at wrist and hand level (S64.-)

     The appropriate 7th character is to be added to each code from category S54.
     A   initial encounter
     D   subsequent encounter
     S   sequela

√5ᵗʰ **S54.0** Injury of ulnar nerve at forearm level
     Injury of ulnar nerve NOS

√x7ᵗʰ **S54.00** Injury of ulnar nerve at forearm level, unspecified arm

√x7ᵗʰ **S54.01** Injury of ulnar nerve at forearm level, right arm

√x7ᵗʰ **S54.02** Injury of ulnar nerve at forearm level, left arm

√5ᵗʰ **S54.1** Injury of median nerve at forearm level
     Injury of median nerve NOS

√x7ᵗʰ **S54.10** Injury of median nerve at forearm level, unspecified arm

√x7ᵗʰ **S54.11** Injury of median nerve at forearm level, right arm

√x7ᵗʰ **S54.12** Injury of median nerve at forearm level, left arm

✓5ᵗʰ S54.2   Injury of radial nerve at forearm level
> Injury of radial nerve NOS

> **✓x7ᵗʰ S54.20   Injury of radial nerve at forearm level, unspecified arm**

> **✓x7ᵗʰ S54.21   Injury of radial nerve at forearm level, right arm**

> **✓x7ᵗʰ S54.22   Injury of radial nerve at forearm level, left arm**

✓5ᵗʰ S54.3   Injury of cutaneous sensory nerve at forearm level

> **✓x7ᵗʰ S54.30   Injury of cutaneous sensory nerve at forearm level, unspecified arm**

> **✓x7ᵗʰ S54.31   Injury of cutaneous sensory nerve at forearm level, right arm**

> **✓x7ᵗʰ S54.32   Injury of cutaneous sensory nerve at forearm level, left arm**

✓5ᵗʰ S54.8   Injury of other nerves at forearm level

> **✓6ᵗʰ S54.8X   Injury of other nerves at forearm level**

>> **✓7ᵗʰ S54.8X1   Injury of other nerves at forearm level, right arm**

>> **✓7ᵗʰ S54.8X2   Injury of other nerves at forearm level, left arm**

>> **✓7ᵗʰ S54.8X9   Injury of other nerves at forearm level, unspecified arm**

✓5ᵗʰ S54.9   Injury of unspecified nerve at forearm level

> **✓x7ᵗʰ S54.90   Injury of unspecified nerve at forearm level, unspecified arm**

> **✓x7ᵗʰ S54.91   Injury of unspecified nerve at forearm level, right arm**

> **✓x7ᵗʰ S54.92   Injury of unspecified nerve at forearm level, left arm**

✓4ᵗʰ S55   Injury of blood vessels at forearm level
> Code also any associated open wound (S51.-)
> **EXCLUDES 2**   injury of blood vessels at wrist and hand level (S65.-)
> injury of brachial vessels (S45.1-S45.2)

> The appropriate 7th character is to be added to each code from category S55.
> A   initial encounter
> D   subsequent encounter
> S   sequela

✓5ᵗʰ S55.0   Injury of ulnar artery at forearm level

> **✓6ᵗʰ S55.00   Unspecified injury of ulnar artery at forearm level**

>> **✓7ᵗʰ S55.001   Unspecified injury of ulnar artery at forearm level, right arm**

>> **✓7ᵗʰ S55.002   Unspecified injury of ulnar artery at forearm level, left arm**

>> **✓7ᵗʰ S55.009   Unspecified injury of ulnar artery at forearm level, unspecified arm**

> **✓6ᵗʰ S55.01   Laceration of ulnar artery at forearm level**

>> **✓7ᵗʰ S55.011   Laceration of ulnar artery at forearm level, right arm**

>> **✓7ᵗʰ S55.012   Laceration of ulnar artery at forearm level, left arm**

>> **✓7ᵗʰ S55.019   Laceration of ulnar artery at forearm level, unspecified arm**

> **✓6ᵗʰ S55.09   Other specified injury of ulnar artery at forearm level**

>> **✓7ᵗʰ S55.091   Other specified injury of ulnar artery at forearm level, right arm**

>> **✓7ᵗʰ S55.092   Other specified injury of ulnar artery at forearm level, left arm**

>> **✓7ᵗʰ S55.099   Other specified injury of ulnar artery at forearm level, unspecified arm**

✓5ᵗʰ S55.1   Injury of radial artery at forearm level

> **✓6ᵗʰ S55.10   Unspecified injury of radial artery at forearm level**

>> **✓7ᵗʰ S55.101   Unspecified injury of radial artery at forearm level, right arm**

>> **✓7ᵗʰ S55.102   Unspecified injury of radial artery at forearm level, left arm**

>> **✓7ᵗʰ S55.109   Unspecified injury of radial artery at forearm level, unspecified arm**

> **✓6ᵗʰ S55.11   Laceration of radial artery at forearm level**

>> **✓7ᵗʰ S55.111   Laceration of radial artery at forearm level, right arm**

>> **✓7ᵗʰ S55.112   Laceration of radial artery at forearm level, left arm**

>> **✓7ᵗʰ S55.119   Laceration of radial artery at forearm level, unspecified arm**

> **✓6ᵗʰ S55.19   Other specified injury of radial artery at forearm level**

>> **✓7ᵗʰ S55.191   Other specified injury of radial artery at forearm level, right arm**

>> **✓7ᵗʰ S55.192   Other specified injury of radial artery at forearm level, left arm**

>> **✓7ᵗʰ S55.199   Other specified injury of radial artery at forearm level, unspecified arm**

✓5ᵗʰ S55.2   Injury of vein at forearm level

> **✓6ᵗʰ S55.20   Unspecified injury of vein at forearm level**

>> **✓7ᵗʰ S55.201   Unspecified injury of vein at forearm level, right arm**

>> **✓7ᵗʰ S55.202   Unspecified injury of vein at forearm level, left arm**

>> **✓7ᵗʰ S55.209   Unspecified injury of vein at forearm level, unspecified arm**

> **✓6ᵗʰ S55.21   Laceration of vein at forearm level**

>> **✓7ᵗʰ S55.211   Laceration of vein at forearm level, right arm**

>> **✓7ᵗʰ S55.212   Laceration of vein at forearm level, left arm**

>> **✓7ᵗʰ S55.219   Laceration of vein at forearm level, unspecified arm**

> **✓6ᵗʰ S55.29   Other specified injury of vein at forearm level**

>> **✓7ᵗʰ S55.291   Other specified injury of vein at forearm level, right arm**

>> **✓7ᵗʰ S55.292   Other specified injury of vein at forearm level, left arm**

>> **✓7ᵗʰ S55.299   Other specified injury of vein at forearm level, unspecified arm**

✓5ᵗʰ S55.8   Injury of other blood vessels at forearm level

> **✓6ᵗʰ S55.80   Unspecified injury of other blood vessels at forearm level**

>> **✓7ᵗʰ S55.801   Unspecified injury of other blood vessels at forearm level, right arm**

>> **✓7ᵗʰ S55.802   Unspecified injury of other blood vessels at forearm level, left arm**

>> **✓7ᵗʰ S55.809   Unspecified injury of other blood vessels at forearm level, unspecified arm**

> **✓6ᵗʰ S55.81   Laceration of other blood vessels at forearm level**

>> **✓7ᵗʰ S55.811   Laceration of other blood vessels at forearm level, right arm**

>> **✓7ᵗʰ S55.812   Laceration of other blood vessels at forearm level, left arm**

>> **✓7ᵗʰ S55.819   Laceration of other blood vessels at forearm level, unspecified arm**

> **✓6ᵗʰ S55.89   Other specified injury of other blood vessels at forearm level**

>> **✓7ᵗʰ S55.891   Other specified injury of other blood vessels at forearm level, right arm**

>> **✓7ᵗʰ S55.892   Other specified injury of other blood vessels at forearm level, left arm**

>> **✓7ᵗʰ S55.899   Other specified injury of other blood vessels at forearm level, unspecified arm**

✓5ᵗʰ S55.9   Injury of unspecified blood vessel at forearm level

> **✓6ᵗʰ S55.90   Unspecified injury of unspecified blood vessel at forearm level**

>> **✓7ᵗʰ S55.901   Unspecified injury of unspecified blood vessel at forearm level, right arm**

>> **✓7ᵗʰ S55.902   Unspecified injury of unspecified blood vessel at forearm level, left arm**

>> **✓7ᵗʰ S55.909   Unspecified injury of unspecified blood vessel at forearm level, unspecified arm**

> **✓6ᵗʰ S55.91   Laceration of unspecified blood vessel at forearm level**

>> **✓7ᵗʰ S55.911   Laceration of unspecified blood vessel at forearm level, right arm**

>> **✓7ᵗʰ S55.912   Laceration of unspecified blood vessel at forearm level, left arm**

>> **✓7ᵗʰ S55.919   Laceration of unspecified blood vessel at forearm level, unspecified arm**

> **✓6ᵗʰ S55.99   Other specified injury of unspecified blood vessel at forearm level**

>> **✓7ᵗʰ S55.991   Other specified injury of unspecified blood vessel at forearm level, right arm**

>> **✓7ᵗʰ S55.992   Other specified injury of unspecified blood vessel at forearm level, left arm**

>> **✓7ᵗʰ S55.999   Other specified injury of unspecified blood vessel at forearm level, unspecified arm**

√4ᵗʰ **S56 Injury of muscle, fascia and tendon at forearm level**

Code also any associated open wound (S51.-)

EXCLUDES 2   injury of muscle, fascia and tendon at or below wrist (S66.-)
           sprain of joints and ligaments of elbow (S53.4-)

TIP: Refer to the Muscle/Tendon table at the beginning of this chapter.

The appropriate 7th character is to be added to each code from category S56.
- A   initial encounter
- D   subsequent encounter
- S   sequela

√5ᵗʰ **S56.0 Injury of flexor muscle, fascia and tendon of thumb at forearm level**

     √6ᵗʰ **S56.00 Unspecified injury of flexor muscle, fascia and tendon of thumb at forearm level**

         √7ᵗʰ **S56.001** Unspecified injury of flexor muscle, fascia and tendon of right thumb at forearm level

         √7ᵗʰ **S56.002** Unspecified injury of flexor muscle, fascia and tendon of left thumb at forearm level

         √7ᵗʰ **S56.009** Unspecified injury of flexor muscle, fascia and tendon of unspecified thumb at forearm level

     √6ᵗʰ **S56.01 Strain of flexor muscle, fascia and tendon of thumb at forearm level**

         √7ᵗʰ **S56.011** Strain of flexor muscle, fascia and tendon of right thumb at forearm level

         √7ᵗʰ **S56.012** Strain of flexor muscle, fascia and tendon of left thumb at forearm level

         √7ᵗʰ **S56.019** Strain of flexor muscle, fascia and tendon of unspecified thumb at forearm level

     √6ᵗʰ **S56.02 Laceration of flexor muscle, fascia and tendon of thumb at forearm level**

         √7ᵗʰ **S56.021** Laceration of flexor muscle, fascia and tendon of right thumb at forearm level

         √7ᵗʰ **S56.022** Laceration of flexor muscle, fascia and tendon of left thumb at forearm level

         √7ᵗʰ **S56.029** Laceration of flexor muscle, fascia and tendon of unspecified thumb at forearm level

     √6ᵗʰ **S56.09 Other injury of flexor muscle, fascia and tendon of thumb at forearm level**

         √7ᵗʰ **S56.091** Other injury of flexor muscle, fascia and tendon of right thumb at forearm level

         √7ᵗʰ **S56.092** Other injury of flexor muscle, fascia and tendon of left thumb at forearm level

         √7ᵗʰ **S56.099** Other injury of flexor muscle, fascia and tendon of unspecified thumb at forearm level

√5ᵗʰ **S56.1 Injury of flexor muscle, fascia and tendon of other and unspecified finger at forearm level**

     √6ᵗʰ **S56.10 Unspecified injury of flexor muscle, fascia and tendon of other and unspecified finger at forearm level**

         √7ᵗʰ **S56.101** Unspecified injury of flexor muscle, fascia and tendon of right index finger at forearm level

         √7ᵗʰ **S56.102** Unspecified injury of flexor muscle, fascia and tendon of left index finger at forearm level

         √7ᵗʰ **S56.103** Unspecified injury of flexor muscle, fascia and tendon of right middle finger at forearm level

         √7ᵗʰ **S56.104** Unspecified injury of flexor muscle, fascia and tendon of left middle finger at forearm level

         √7ᵗʰ **S56.105** Unspecified injury of flexor muscle, fascia and tendon of right ring finger at forearm level

         √7ᵗʰ **S56.106** Unspecified injury of flexor muscle, fascia and tendon of left ring finger at forearm level

         √7ᵗʰ **S56.107** Unspecified injury of flexor muscle, fascia and tendon of right little finger at forearm level

         √7ᵗʰ **S56.108** Unspecified injury of flexor muscle, fascia and tendon of left little finger at forearm level

         √7ᵗʰ **S56.109** Unspecified injury of flexor muscle, fascia and tendon of unspecified finger at forearm level

     √6ᵗʰ **S56.11 Strain of flexor muscle, fascia and tendon of other and unspecified finger at forearm level**

         √7ᵗʰ **S56.111** Strain of flexor muscle, fascia and tendon of right index finger at forearm level

         √7ᵗʰ **S56.112** Strain of flexor muscle, fascia and tendon of left index finger at forearm level

         √7ᵗʰ **S56.113** Strain of flexor muscle, fascia and tendon of right middle finger at forearm level

         √7ᵗʰ **S56.114** Strain of flexor muscle, fascia and tendon of left middle finger at forearm level

         √7ᵗʰ **S56.115** Strain of flexor muscle, fascia and tendon of right ring finger at forearm level

         √7ᵗʰ **S56.116** Strain of flexor muscle, fascia and tendon of left ring finger at forearm level

         √7ᵗʰ **S56.117** Strain of flexor muscle, fascia and tendon of right little finger at forearm level

         √7ᵗʰ **S56.118** Strain of flexor muscle, fascia and tendon of left little finger at forearm level

         √7ᵗʰ **S56.119** Strain of flexor muscle, fascia and tendon of finger of unspecified finger at forearm level

     √6ᵗʰ **S56.12 Laceration of flexor muscle, fascia and tendon of other and unspecified finger at forearm level**

         √7ᵗʰ **S56.121** Laceration of flexor muscle, fascia and tendon of right index finger at forearm level

         √7ᵗʰ **S56.122** Laceration of flexor muscle, fascia and tendon of left index finger at forearm level

         √7ᵗʰ **S56.123** Laceration of flexor muscle, fascia and tendon of right middle finger at forearm level

         √7ᵗʰ **S56.124** Laceration of flexor muscle, fascia and tendon of left middle finger at forearm level

         √7ᵗʰ **S56.125** Laceration of flexor muscle, fascia and tendon of right ring finger at forearm level

         √7ᵗʰ **S56.126** Laceration of flexor muscle, fascia and tendon of left ring finger at forearm level

         √7ᵗʰ **S56.127** Laceration of flexor muscle, fascia and tendon of right little finger at forearm level

         √7ᵗʰ **S56.128** Laceration of flexor muscle, fascia and tendon of left little finger at forearm level

         √7ᵗʰ **S56.129** Laceration of flexor muscle, fascia and tendon of unspecified finger at forearm level

     √6ᵗʰ **S56.19 Other injury of flexor muscle, fascia and tendon of other and unspecified finger at forearm level**

         √7ᵗʰ **S56.191** Other injury of flexor muscle, fascia and tendon of right index finger at forearm level

         √7ᵗʰ **S56.192** Other injury of flexor muscle, fascia and tendon of left index finger at forearm level

         √7ᵗʰ **S56.193** Other injury of flexor muscle, fascia and tendon of right middle finger at forearm level

         √7ᵗʰ **S56.194** Other injury of flexor muscle, fascia and tendon of left middle finger at forearm level

         √7ᵗʰ **S56.195** Other injury of flexor muscle, fascia and tendon of right ring finger at forearm level

         √7ᵗʰ **S56.196** Other injury of flexor muscle, fascia and tendon of left ring finger at forearm level

         √7ᵗʰ **S56.197** Other injury of flexor muscle, fascia and tendon of right little finger at forearm level

         √7ᵗʰ **S56.198** Other injury of flexor muscle, fascia and tendon of left little finger at forearm level

         √7ᵗʰ **S56.199** Other injury of flexor muscle, fascia and tendon of unspecified finger at forearm level

√5ᵗʰ **S56.2 Injury of other flexor muscle, fascia and tendon at forearm level**

     √6ᵗʰ **S56.20 Unspecified injury of other flexor muscle, fascia and tendon at forearm level**

         √7ᵗʰ **S56.201** Unspecified injury of other flexor muscle, fascia and tendon at forearm level, right arm

√ Additional Character Required   √x7ᵗʰ Placeholder Alert   Manifestation   Unspecified Dx   ►◄ Revised Text   ● New Code   ▲ Revised Title

ICD-10-CM 2020   1005

✓7ᵗʰ **S56.202** Unspecified injury of other flexor muscle, fascia and tendon at forearm level, *left arm*

✓7ᵗʰ **S56.209** Unspecified injury of other flexor muscle, fascia and tendon at forearm level, unspecified arm

✓6ᵗʰ **S56.21** Strain of other flexor muscle, fascia and tendon at forearm level

     ✓7ᵗʰ **S56.211** Strain of other flexor muscle, fascia and tendon at forearm level, *right arm*

     ✓7ᵗʰ **S56.212** Strain of other flexor muscle, fascia and tendon at forearm level, *left arm*

     ✓7ᵗʰ **S56.219** Strain of other flexor muscle, fascia and tendon at forearm level, unspecified arm

✓6ᵗʰ **S56.22** Laceration of other flexor muscle, fascia and tendon at forearm level

     ✓7ᵗʰ **S56.221** Laceration of other flexor muscle, fascia and tendon at forearm level, *right arm*

     ✓7ᵗʰ **S56.222** Laceration of other flexor muscle, fascia and tendon at forearm level, *left arm*

     ✓7ᵗʰ **S56.229** Laceration of other flexor muscle, fascia and tendon at forearm level, unspecified arm

✓6ᵗʰ **S56.29** Other injury of other flexor muscle, fascia and tendon at forearm level

     ✓7ᵗʰ **S56.291** Other injury of other flexor muscle, fascia and tendon at forearm level, *right arm*

     ✓7ᵗʰ **S56.292** Other injury of other flexor muscle, fascia and tendon at forearm level, *left arm*

     ✓7ᵗʰ **S56.299** Other injury of other flexor muscle, fascia and tendon at forearm level, unspecified arm

✓5ᵗʰ **S56.3** Injury of *extensor or abductor* muscles, fascia and tendons of *thumb* at forearm level

✓6ᵗʰ **S56.30** Unspecified injury of extensor or abductor muscles, fascia and tendons of thumb at forearm level

     ✓7ᵗʰ **S56.301** Unspecified injury of extensor or abductor muscles, fascia and tendons of *right thumb* at forearm level

     ✓7ᵗʰ **S56.302** Unspecified injury of extensor or abductor muscles, fascia and tendons of *left thumb* at forearm level

     ✓7ᵗʰ **S56.309** Unspecified injury of extensor or abductor muscles, fascia and tendons of unspecified thumb at forearm level

✓6ᵗʰ **S56.31** Strain of extensor or abductor muscles, fascia and tendons of thumb at forearm level

     ✓7ᵗʰ **S56.311** Strain of extensor or abductor muscles, fascia and tendons of *right thumb* at forearm level

     ✓7ᵗʰ **S56.312** Strain of extensor or abductor muscles, fascia and tendons of *left thumb* at forearm level

     ✓7ᵗʰ **S56.319** Strain of extensor or abductor muscles, fascia and tendons of unspecified thumb at forearm level

✓6ᵗʰ **S56.32** Laceration of extensor or abductor muscles, fascia and tendons of thumb at forearm level

     ✓7ᵗʰ **S56.321** Laceration of extensor or abductor muscles, fascia and tendons of *right thumb* at forearm level

     ✓7ᵗʰ **S56.322** Laceration of extensor or abductor muscles, fascia and tendons of *left thumb* at forearm level

     ✓7ᵗʰ **S56.329** Laceration of extensor or abductor muscles, fascia and tendons of unspecified thumb at forearm level

✓6ᵗʰ **S56.39** Other injury of extensor or abductor muscles, fascia and tendons of thumb at forearm level

     ✓7ᵗʰ **S56.391** Other injury of extensor or abductor muscles, fascia and tendons of *right thumb* at forearm level

     ✓7ᵗʰ **S56.392** Other injury of extensor or abductor muscles, fascia and tendons of *left thumb* at forearm level

     ✓7ᵗʰ **S56.399** Other injury of extensor or abductor muscles, fascia and tendons of unspecified thumb at forearm level

✓5ᵗʰ **S56.4** Injury of *extensor* muscle, fascia and tendon of other and unspecified *finger* at forearm level

✓6ᵗʰ **S56.40** Unspecified injury of extensor muscle, fascia and tendon of other and unspecified finger at forearm level

     ✓7ᵗʰ **S56.401** Unspecified injury of extensor muscle, fascia and tendon of *right index finger* at forearm level

     ✓7ᵗʰ **S56.402** Unspecified injury of extensor muscle, fascia and tendon of *left index finger* at forearm level

     ✓7ᵗʰ **S56.403** Unspecified injury of extensor muscle, fascia and tendon of *right middle finger* at forearm level

     ✓7ᵗʰ **S56.404** Unspecified injury of extensor muscle, fascia and tendon of *left middle finger* at forearm level

     ✓7ᵗʰ **S56.405** Unspecified injury of extensor muscle, fascia and tendon of *right ring finger* at forearm level

     ✓7ᵗʰ **S56.406** Unspecified injury of extensor muscle, fascia and tendon of *left ring finger* at forearm level

     ✓7ᵗʰ **S56.407** Unspecified injury of extensor muscle, fascia and tendon of *right little finger* at forearm level

     ✓7ᵗʰ **S56.408** Unspecified injury of extensor muscle, fascia and tendon of *left little finger* at forearm level

     ✓7ᵗʰ **S56.409** Unspecified injury of extensor muscle, fascia and tendon of unspecified finger at forearm level

✓6ᵗʰ **S56.41** Strain of extensor muscle, fascia and tendon of other and unspecified finger at forearm level

     ✓7ᵗʰ **S56.411** Strain of extensor muscle, fascia and tendon of *right index finger* at forearm level

     ✓7ᵗʰ **S56.412** Strain of extensor muscle, fascia and tendon of *left index finger* at forearm level

     ✓7ᵗʰ **S56.413** Strain of extensor muscle, fascia and tendon of *right middle finger* at forearm level

     ✓7ᵗʰ **S56.414** Strain of extensor muscle, fascia and tendon of *left middle finger* at forearm level

     ✓7ᵗʰ **S56.415** Strain of extensor muscle, fascia and tendon of *right ring finger* at forearm level

     ✓7ᵗʰ **S56.416** Strain of extensor muscle, fascia and tendon of *left ring finger* at forearm level

     ✓7ᵗʰ **S56.417** Strain of extensor muscle, fascia and tendon of *right little finger* at forearm level

     ✓7ᵗʰ **S56.418** Strain of extensor muscle, fascia and tendon of *left little finger* at forearm level

     ✓7ᵗʰ **S56.419** Strain of extensor muscle, fascia and tendon of finger, unspecified finger at forearm level

✓6ᵗʰ **S56.42** Laceration of extensor muscle, fascia and tendon of other and unspecified finger at forearm level

     ✓7ᵗʰ **S56.421** Laceration of extensor muscle, fascia and tendon of *right index finger* at forearm level

     ✓7ᵗʰ **S56.422** Laceration of extensor muscle, fascia and tendon of *left index finger* at forearm level

     ✓7ᵗʰ **S56.423** Laceration of extensor muscle, fascia and tendon of *right middle finger* at forearm level

     ✓7ᵗʰ **S56.424** Laceration of extensor muscle, fascia and tendon of *left middle finger* at forearm level

     ✓7ᵗʰ **S56.425** Laceration of extensor muscle, fascia and tendon of *right ring finger* at forearm level

     ✓7ᵗʰ **S56.426** Laceration of extensor muscle, fascia and tendon of *left ring finger* at forearm level

     ✓7ᵗʰ **S56.427** Laceration of extensor muscle, fascia and tendon of *right little finger* at forearm level

     ✓7ᵗʰ **S56.428** Laceration of extensor muscle, fascia and tendon of *left little finger* at forearm level

---

N Newborn: 0   P Pediatric: 0-17   M Maternity: 12-55   A Adult: 15-124   CH Comorbidity High   CL Comorbidity Low   NCDx Noncancer Dx   PDx Primary Dx

√7ᵗʰ **S56.429** Laceration of extensor muscle, fascia and tendon of unspecified finger at forearm level

√6ᵗʰ **S56.49** Other injury of extensor muscle, fascia and tendon of other and unspecified finger at forearm level

√7ᵗʰ **S56.491** Other injury of extensor muscle, fascia and tendon of right index finger at forearm level

√7ᵗʰ **S56.492** Other injury of extensor muscle, fascia and tendon of left index finger at forearm level

√7ᵗʰ **S56.493** Other injury of extensor muscle, fascia and tendon of right middle finger at forearm level

√7ᵗʰ **S56.494** Other injury of extensor muscle, fascia and tendon of left middle finger at forearm level

√7ᵗʰ **S56.495** Other injury of extensor muscle, fascia and tendon of right ring finger at forearm level

√7ᵗʰ **S56.496** Other injury of extensor muscle, fascia and tendon of left ring finger at forearm level

√7ᵗʰ **S56.497** Other injury of extensor muscle, fascia and tendon of right little finger at forearm level

√7ᵗʰ **S56.498** Other injury of extensor muscle, fascia and tendon of left little finger at forearm level

√7ᵗʰ **S56.499** Other injury of extensor muscle, fascia and tendon of unspecified finger at forearm level

√5ᵗʰ **S56.5** Injury of other extensor muscle, fascia and tendon at forearm level

√6ᵗʰ **S56.50** Unspecified injury of other extensor muscle, fascia and tendon at forearm level

√7ᵗʰ **S56.501** Unspecified injury of other extensor muscle, fascia and tendon at forearm level, right arm

√7ᵗʰ **S56.502** Unspecified injury of other extensor muscle, fascia and tendon at forearm level, left arm

√7ᵗʰ **S56.509** Unspecified injury of other extensor muscle, fascia and tendon at forearm level, unspecified arm

√6ᵗʰ **S56.51** Strain of other extensor muscle, fascia and tendon at forearm level

√7ᵗʰ **S56.511** Strain of other extensor muscle, fascia and tendon at forearm level, right arm

√7ᵗʰ **S56.512** Strain of other extensor muscle, fascia and tendon at forearm level, left arm

√7ᵗʰ **S56.519** Strain of other extensor muscle, fascia and tendon at forearm level, unspecified arm

√6ᵗʰ **S56.52** Laceration of other extensor muscle, fascia and tendon at forearm level

√7ᵗʰ **S56.521** Laceration of other extensor muscle, fascia and tendon at forearm level, right arm

√7ᵗʰ **S56.522** Laceration of other extensor muscle, fascia and tendon at forearm level, left arm

√7ᵗʰ **S56.529** Laceration of other extensor muscle, fascia and tendon at forearm level, unspecified arm

√6ᵗʰ **S56.59** Other injury of other extensor muscle, fascia and tendon at forearm level

√7ᵗʰ **S56.591** Other injury of other extensor muscle, fascia and tendon at forearm level, right arm

√7ᵗʰ **S56.592** Other injury of other extensor muscle, fascia and tendon at forearm level, left arm

√7ᵗʰ **S56.599** Other injury of other extensor muscle, fascia and tendon at forearm level, unspecified arm

√5ᵗʰ **S56.8** Injury of other muscles, fascia and tendons at forearm level

√6ᵗʰ **S56.80** Unspecified injury of other muscles, fascia and tendons at forearm level

√7ᵗʰ **S56.801** Unspecified injury of other muscles, fascia and tendons at forearm level, right arm

√7ᵗʰ **S56.802** Unspecified injury of other muscles, fascia and tendons at forearm level, left arm

√7ᵗʰ **S56.809** Unspecified injury of other muscles, fascia and tendons at forearm level, unspecified arm

√6ᵗʰ **S56.81** Strain of other muscles, fascia and tendons at forearm level

√7ᵗʰ **S56.811** Strain of other muscles, fascia and tendons at forearm level, right arm

√7ᵗʰ **S56.812** Strain of other muscles, fascia and tendons at forearm level, left arm

√7ᵗʰ **S56.819** Strain of other muscles, fascia and tendons at forearm level, unspecified arm

√6ᵗʰ **S56.82** Laceration of other muscles, fascia and tendons at forearm level

√7ᵗʰ **S56.821** Laceration of other muscles, fascia and tendons at forearm level, right arm

√7ᵗʰ **S56.822** Laceration of other muscles, fascia and tendons at forearm level, left arm

√7ᵗʰ **S56.829** Laceration of other muscles, fascia and tendons at forearm level, unspecified arm

√6ᵗʰ **S56.89** Other injury of other muscles, fascia and tendons at forearm level

√7ᵗʰ **S56.891** Other injury of other muscles, fascia and tendons at forearm level, right arm

√7ᵗʰ **S56.892** Other injury of other muscles, fascia and tendons at forearm level, left arm

√7ᵗʰ **S56.899** Other injury of other muscles, fascia and tendons at forearm level, unspecified arm

√5ᵗʰ **S56.9** Injury of unspecified muscles, fascia and tendons at forearm level

√6ᵗʰ **S56.90** Unspecified injury of unspecified muscles, fascia and tendons at forearm level

√7ᵗʰ **S56.901** Unspecified injury of unspecified muscles, fascia and tendons at forearm level, right arm

√7ᵗʰ **S56.902** Unspecified injury of unspecified muscles, fascia and tendons at forearm level, left arm

√7ᵗʰ **S56.909** Unspecified injury of unspecified muscles, fascia and tendons at forearm level, unspecified arm

√6ᵗʰ **S56.91** Strain of unspecified muscles, fascia and tendons at forearm level

√7ᵗʰ **S56.911** Strain of unspecified muscles, fascia and tendons at forearm level, right arm

√7ᵗʰ **S56.912** Strain of unspecified muscles, fascia and tendons at forearm level, left arm

√7ᵗʰ **S56.919** Strain of unspecified muscles, fascia and tendons at forearm level, unspecified arm

√6ᵗʰ **S56.92** Laceration of unspecified muscles, fascia and tendons at forearm level

√7ᵗʰ **S56.921** Laceration of unspecified muscles, fascia and tendons at forearm level, right arm

√7ᵗʰ **S56.922** Laceration of unspecified muscles, fascia and tendons at forearm level, left arm

√7ᵗʰ **S56.929** Laceration of unspecified muscles, fascia and tendons at forearm level, unspecified arm

√6ᵗʰ **S56.99** Other injury of unspecified muscles, fascia and tendons at forearm level

√7ᵗʰ **S56.991** Other injury of unspecified muscles, fascia and tendons at forearm level, right arm

√7ᵗʰ **S56.992** Other injury of unspecified muscles, fascia and tendons at forearm level, left arm

√7ᵗʰ **S56.999** Other injury of unspecified muscles, fascia and tendons at forearm level, unspecified arm

√4ᵗʰ **S57** **Crushing injury** of elbow and forearm

Use additional code(s) for all associated injuries

EXCLUDES 2   crushing injury of wrist and hand (S67.-)

The appropriate 7th character is to be added to each code from category S57.
A   initial encounter
D   subsequent encounter
S   sequela

√5ᵗʰ **S57.0** Crushing injury of elbow

√x7ᵗʰ **S57.00** Crushing injury of unspecified elbow

√x7ᵗʰ **S57.01** Crushing injury of right elbow

√x7ᵗʰ **S57.02** Crushing injury of left elbow

✓5ᵗʰ S57.8   Crushing injury of forearm

    ✓x7ᵗʰ **S57.80   Crushing injury of unspecified forearm**

    ✓x7ᵗʰ **S57.81   Crushing injury of right forearm**

    ✓x7ᵗʰ **S57.82   Crushing injury of left forearm**

✓4ᵗʰ S58   Traumatic amputation of elbow and forearm

An amputation not identified as partial or complete should be coded to complete

    EXCLUDES 1   *traumatic amputation of wrist and hand (S68.-)*

The appropriate 7th character is to be added to each code from category S58.
A   initial encounter
D   subsequent encounter
S   sequela

✓5ᵗʰ S58.0   Traumatic amputation at elbow level

    ✓6ᵗʰ **S58.01   Complete traumatic amputation at elbow level**

       ✓7ᵗʰ **S58.011   Complete traumatic amputation at elbow level, right arm**

       ✓7ᵗʰ **S58.012   Complete traumatic amputation at elbow level, left arm**

       ✓7ᵗʰ **S58.019   Complete traumatic amputation at elbow level, unspecified arm**

    ✓6ᵗʰ **S58.02   Partial traumatic amputation at elbow level**

       ✓7ᵗʰ **S58.021   Partial traumatic amputation at elbow level, right arm**

       ✓7ᵗʰ **S58.022   Partial traumatic amputation at elbow level, left arm**

       ✓7ᵗʰ **S58.029   Partial traumatic amputation at elbow level, unspecified arm**

✓5ᵗʰ S58.1   Traumatic amputation at level between elbow and wrist

    ✓6ᵗʰ **S58.11   Complete traumatic amputation at level between elbow and wrist**

       ✓7ᵗʰ **S58.111   Complete traumatic amputation at level between elbow and wrist, right arm**

       ✓7ᵗʰ **S58.112   Complete traumatic amputation at level between elbow and wrist, left arm**

       ✓7ᵗʰ **S58.119   Complete traumatic amputation at level between elbow and wrist, unspecified arm**

    ✓6ᵗʰ **S58.12   Partial traumatic amputation at level between elbow and wrist**

       ✓7ᵗʰ **S58.121   Partial traumatic amputation at level between elbow and wrist, right arm**

       ✓7ᵗʰ **S58.122   Partial traumatic amputation at level between elbow and wrist, left arm**

       ✓7ᵗʰ **S58.129   Partial traumatic amputation at level between elbow and wrist, unspecified arm**

✓5ᵗʰ S58.9   Traumatic amputation of forearm, level unspecified

    EXCLUDES 1   *traumatic amputation of wrist (S68.-)*

    ✓6ᵗʰ **S58.91   Complete traumatic amputation of forearm, level unspecified**

       ✓7ᵗʰ **S58.911   Complete traumatic amputation of right forearm, level unspecified**

       ✓7ᵗʰ **S58.912   Complete traumatic amputation of left forearm, level unspecified**

       ✓7ᵗʰ **S58.919   Complete traumatic amputation of unspecified forearm, level unspecified**

    ✓6ᵗʰ **S58.92   Partial traumatic amputation of forearm, level unspecified**

       ✓7ᵗʰ **S58.921   Partial traumatic amputation of right forearm, level unspecified**

       ✓7ᵗʰ **S58.922   Partial traumatic amputation of left forearm, level unspecified**

       ✓7ᵗʰ **S58.929   Partial traumatic amputation of unspecified forearm, level unspecified**

✓4ᵗʰ S59   Other and unspecified injuries of elbow and forearm

    EXCLUDES 2   *other and unspecified injuries of wrist and hand (S69.-)*

AHA: 2018,2Q,12; 2018,1Q,3; 2015,3Q,37-39

TIP: The term "improper alignment" is not synonymous with malunion or nonunion of a fracture when noted in provider documentation.

The appropriate 7th character is to be added to each code from subcategories S59.0, S59.1, and S59.2.
A   initial encounter for closed fracture
D   subsequent encounter for fracture with routine healing
G   subsequent encounter for fracture with delayed healing
K   subsequent encounter for fracture with nonunion
P   subsequent encounter for fracture with malunion
S   sequela

✓5ᵗʰ S59.0   Physeal fracture of lower end of ulna

    ✓6ᵗʰ **S59.00   Unspecified physeal fracture of lower end of ulna**

       ✓7ᵗʰ **S59.001   Unspecified physeal fracture of lower end of ulna, right arm**

       ✓7ᵗʰ **S59.002   Unspecified physeal fracture of lower end of ulna, left arm**

       ✓7ᵗʰ **S59.009   Unspecified physeal fracture of lower end of ulna, unspecified arm**

    ✓6ᵗʰ **S59.01   Salter-Harris Type I physeal fracture of lower end of ulna**

       ✓7ᵗʰ **S59.011   Salter-Harris Type I physeal fracture of lower end of ulna, right arm**

       ✓7ᵗʰ **S59.012   Salter-Harris Type I physeal fracture of lower end of ulna, left arm**

       ✓7ᵗʰ **S59.019   Salter-Harris Type I physeal fracture of lower end of ulna, unspecified arm**

    ✓6ᵗʰ **S59.02   Salter-Harris Type II physeal fracture of lower end of ulna**

       ✓7ᵗʰ **S59.021   Salter-Harris Type II physeal fracture of lower end of ulna, right arm**

       ✓7ᵗʰ **S59.022   Salter-Harris Type II physeal fracture of lower end of ulna, left arm**

       ✓7ᵗʰ **S59.029   Salter-Harris Type II physeal fracture of lower end of ulna, unspecified arm**

    ✓6ᵗʰ **S59.03   Salter-Harris Type III physeal fracture of lower end of ulna**

       ✓7ᵗʰ **S59.031   Salter-Harris Type III physeal fracture of lower end of ulna, right arm**

       ✓7ᵗʰ **S59.032   Salter-Harris Type III physeal fracture of lower end of ulna, left arm**

       ✓7ᵗʰ **S59.039   Salter-Harris Type III physeal fracture of lower end of ulna, unspecified arm**

    ✓6ᵗʰ **S59.04   Salter-Harris Type IV physeal fracture of lower end of ulna**

       ✓7ᵗʰ **S59.041   Salter-Harris Type IV physeal fracture of lower end of ulna, right arm**

       ✓7ᵗʰ **S59.042   Salter-Harris Type IV physeal fracture of lower end of ulna, left arm**

       ✓7ᵗʰ **S59.049   Salter-Harris Type IV physeal fracture of lower end of ulna, unspecified arm**

    ✓6ᵗʰ **S59.09   Other physeal fracture of lower end of ulna**

       ✓7ᵗʰ **S59.091   Other physeal fracture of lower end of ulna, right arm**

       ✓7ᵗʰ **S59.092   Other physeal fracture of lower end of ulna, left arm**

       ✓7ᵗʰ **S59.099   Other physeal fracture of lower end of ulna, unspecified arm**

✓5ᵗʰ S59.1   Physeal fracture of upper end of radius

    ✓6ᵗʰ **S59.10   Unspecified physeal fracture of upper end of radius**

       ✓7ᵗʰ **S59.101   Unspecified physeal fracture of upper end of radius, right arm**

       ✓7ᵗʰ **S59.102   Unspecified physeal fracture of upper end of radius, left arm**

       ✓7ᵗʰ **S59.109   Unspecified physeal fracture of upper end of radius, unspecified arm**

    ✓6ᵗʰ **S59.11   Salter-Harris Type I physeal fracture of upper end of radius**

       ✓7ᵗʰ **S59.111   Salter-Harris Type I physeal fracture of upper end of radius, right arm**

       ✓7ᵗʰ **S59.112   Salter-Harris Type I physeal fracture of upper end of radius, left arm**

       ✓7ᵗʰ **S59.119   Salter-Harris Type I physeal fracture of upper end of radius, unspecified arm**

    ✓6ᵗʰ **S59.12   Salter-Harris Type II physeal fracture of upper end of radius**

       ✓7ᵗʰ **S59.121   Salter-Harris Type II physeal fracture of upper end of radius, right arm**

√7ᵗʰ **S59.122** Salter-Harris Type II physeal fracture of upper end of radius, left arm

√7ᵗʰ **S59.129** Salter-Harris Type II physeal fracture of upper end of radius, unspecified arm

√6ᵗʰ **S59.13** Salter-Harris Type III physeal fracture of upper end of radius

    √7ᵗʰ **S59.131** Salter-Harris Type III physeal fracture of upper end of radius, right arm

    √7ᵗʰ **S59.132** Salter-Harris Type III physeal fracture of upper end of radius, left arm

    √7ᵗʰ **S59.139** Salter-Harris Type III physeal fracture of upper end of radius, unspecified arm

√6ᵗʰ **S59.14** Salter-Harris Type IV physeal fracture of upper end of radius

    √7ᵗʰ **S59.141** Salter-Harris Type IV physeal fracture of upper end of radius, right arm

    √7ᵗʰ **S59.142** Salter-Harris Type IV physeal fracture of upper end of radius, left arm

    √7ᵗʰ **S59.149** Salter-Harris Type IV physeal fracture of upper end of radius, unspecified arm

√6ᵗʰ **S59.19** Other physeal fracture of upper end of radius

    √7ᵗʰ **S59.191** Other physeal fracture of upper end of radius, right arm

    √7ᵗʰ **S59.192** Other physeal fracture of upper end of radius, left arm

    √7ᵗʰ **S59.199** Other physeal fracture of upper end of radius, unspecified arm

√5ᵗʰ **S59.2 Physeal fracture of** lower end of radius

√6ᵗʰ **S59.20** Unspecified physeal fracture of lower end of radius

    √7ᵗʰ **S59.201** Unspecified physeal fracture of lower end of radius, right arm

    √7ᵗʰ **S59.202** Unspecified physeal fracture of lower end of radius, left arm

    √7ᵗʰ **S59.209** Unspecified physeal fracture of lower end of radius, unspecified arm

√6ᵗʰ **S59.21** Salter-Harris Type I physeal fracture of lower end of radius

    √7ᵗʰ **S59.211** Salter-Harris Type I physeal fracture of lower end of radius, right arm

    √7ᵗʰ **S59.212** Salter-Harris Type I physeal fracture of lower end of radius, left arm

    √7ᵗʰ **S59.219** Salter-Harris Type I physeal fracture of lower end of radius, unspecified arm

√6ᵗʰ **S59.22** Salter-Harris Type II physeal fracture of lower end of radius

    √7ᵗʰ **S59.221** Salter-Harris Type II physeal fracture of lower end of radius, right arm

    √7ᵗʰ **S59.222** Salter-Harris Type II physeal fracture of lower end of radius, left arm

    √7ᵗʰ **S59.229** Salter-Harris Type II physeal fracture of lower end of radius, unspecified arm

√6ᵗʰ **S59.23** Salter-Harris Type III physeal fracture of lower end of radius

    √7ᵗʰ **S59.231** Salter-Harris Type III physeal fracture of lower end of radius, right arm

    √7ᵗʰ **S59.232** Salter-Harris Type III physeal fracture of lower end of radius, left arm

    √7ᵗʰ **S59.239** Salter-Harris Type III physeal fracture of lower end of radius, unspecified arm

√6ᵗʰ **S59.24** Salter-Harris Type IV physeal fracture of lower end of radius

    √7ᵗʰ **S59.241** Salter-Harris Type IV physeal fracture of lower end of radius, right arm

    √7ᵗʰ **S59.242** Salter-Harris Type IV physeal fracture of lower end of radius, left arm

    √7ᵗʰ **S59.249** Salter-Harris Type IV physeal fracture of lower end of radius, unspecified arm

√6ᵗʰ **S59.29** Other physeal fracture of lower end of radius

    √7ᵗʰ **S59.291** Other physeal fracture of lower end of radius, right arm

    √7ᵗʰ **S59.292** Other physeal fracture of lower end of radius, left arm

    √7ᵗʰ **S59.299** Other physeal fracture of lower end of radius, unspecified arm

√5ᵗʰ **S59.8 Other specified injuries of elbow and forearm**

The appropriate 7th character is to be added to each code in subcategory S59.8.
A   initial encounter
D   subsequent encounter
S   sequela

√6ᵗʰ **S59.80** Other specified injuries of elbow

    √7ᵗʰ **S59.801** Other specified injuries of right elbow

    √7ᵗʰ **S59.802** Other specified injuries of left elbow

    √7ᵗʰ **S59.809** Other specified injuries of unspecified elbow

√6ᵗʰ **S59.81** Other specified injuries of forearm

    √7ᵗʰ **S59.811** Other specified injuries right forearm

    √7ᵗʰ **S59.812** Other specified injuries left forearm

    √7ᵗʰ **S59.819** Other specified injuries unspecified forearm

√5ᵗʰ **S59.9 Unspecified injury of elbow and forearm**

The appropriate 7th character is to be added to each code in subcategory S59.8.
A   initial encounter
D   subsequent encounter
S   sequela

√6ᵗʰ **S59.90** Unspecified injury of elbow

    √7ᵗʰ **S59.901** Unspecified injury of right elbow

    √7ᵗʰ **S59.902** Unspecified injury of left elbow

    √7ᵗʰ **S59.909** Unspecified injury of unspecified elbow

√6ᵗʰ **S59.91** Unspecified injury of forearm

    √7ᵗʰ **S59.911** Unspecified injury of right forearm

    √7ᵗʰ **S59.912** Unspecified injury of left forearm

    √7ᵗʰ **S59.919** Unspecified injury of unspecified forearm

Injuries to the wrist, hand and fingers (S60-S69)

EXCLUDES 2   *burns and corrosions (T20-T32)*
frostbite (T33-T34)
insect bite or sting, venomous (T63.4)

√4ᵗʰ **S60 Superficial injury of wrist, hand and fingers**

The appropriate 7th character is to be added to each code from category S60.
A   initial encounter
D   subsequent encounter
S   sequela

√5ᵗʰ **S60.0 Contusion of** finger without damage to nail

    EXCLUDES 1   *contusion involving nail (matrix) (S60.1)*

√x7ᵗʰ **S60.00** Contusion of unspecified finger without damage to nail
       Contusion of finger(s) NOS

√6ᵗʰ **S60.01** Contusion of thumb without damage to nail

    √7ᵗʰ **S60.011** Contusion of right thumb without damage to nail

    √7ᵗʰ **S60.012** Contusion of left thumb without damage to nail

    √7ᵗʰ **S60.019** Contusion of unspecified thumb without damage to nail

√6ᵗʰ **S60.02** Contusion of index finger without damage to nail

    √7ᵗʰ **S60.021** Contusion of right index finger without damage to nail

    √7ᵗʰ **S60.022** Contusion of left index finger without damage to nail

    √7ᵗʰ **S60.029** Contusion of unspecified index finger without damage to nail

√6ᵗʰ **S60.03** Contusion of middle finger without damage to nail

    √7ᵗʰ **S60.031** Contusion of right middle finger without damage to nail

    √7ᵗʰ **S60.032** Contusion of left middle finger without damage to nail

    √7ᵗʰ **S60.039** Contusion of unspecified middle finger without damage to nail

√6ᵗʰ **S60.04** Contusion of ring finger without damage to nail

    √7ᵗʰ **S60.041** Contusion of right ring finger without damage to nail

    √7ᵗʰ **S60.042** Contusion of left ring finger without damage to nail

    √7ᵗʰ **S60.049** Contusion of unspecified ring finger without damage to nail

✔ Additional Character Required   √x7ᵗʰ Placeholder Alert   Manifestation   Unspecified Dx   ►◄ Revised Text   ● New Code   ▲ Revised Title

ICD-10-CM 2020   **1009**

Chapter 19. Injury, Poisoning and Certain Other Consequences of External Causes

S60.05–S60.449

√6ᵗʰ **S60.05** Contusion of little finger without damage to nail
- √7ᵗʰ **S60.051** Contusion of right little finger without damage to nail
- √7ᵗʰ **S60.052** Contusion of left little finger without damage to nail
- √7ᵗʰ **S60.059** Contusion of unspecified little finger without damage to nail

√5ᵗʰ **S60.1** Contusion of finger with damage to nail
- √x7ᵗʰ **S60.10** Contusion of unspecified finger with damage to nail

√6ᵗʰ **S60.11** Contusion of thumb with damage to nail
- √7ᵗʰ **S60.111** Contusion of right thumb with damage to nail
- √7ᵗʰ **S60.112** Contusion of left thumb with damage to nail
- √7ᵗʰ **S60.119** Contusion of unspecified thumb with damage to nail

√6ᵗʰ **S60.12** Contusion of index finger with damage to nail
- √7ᵗʰ **S60.121** Contusion of right index finger with damage to nail
- √7ᵗʰ **S60.122** Contusion of left index finger with damage to nail
- √7ᵗʰ **S60.129** Contusion of unspecified index finger with damage to nail

√6ᵗʰ **S60.13** Contusion of middle finger with damage to nail
- √7ᵗʰ **S60.131** Contusion of right middle finger with damage to nail
- √7ᵗʰ **S60.132** Contusion of left middle finger with damage to nail
- √7ᵗʰ **S60.139** Contusion of unspecified middle finger with damage to nail

√6ᵗʰ **S60.14** Contusion of ring finger with damage to nail
- √7ᵗʰ **S60.141** Contusion of right ring finger with damage to nail
- √7ᵗʰ **S60.142** Contusion of left ring finger with damage to nail
- √7ᵗʰ **S60.149** Contusion of unspecified ring finger with damage to nail

√6ᵗʰ **S60.15** Contusion of little finger with damage to nail
- √7ᵗʰ **S60.151** Contusion of right little finger with damage to nail
- √7ᵗʰ **S60.152** Contusion of left little finger with damage to nail
- √7ᵗʰ **S60.159** Contusion of unspecified little finger with damage to nail

√5ᵗʰ **S60.2** Contusion of wrist and hand
   EXCLUDES 2   contusion of fingers (S60.0-, S60.1-)

√6ᵗʰ **S60.21** Contusion of wrist
- √7ᵗʰ **S60.211** Contusion of right wrist
- √7ᵗʰ **S60.212** Contusion of left wrist
- √7ᵗʰ **S60.219** Contusion of unspecified wrist

√6ᵗʰ **S60.22** Contusion of hand
- √7ᵗʰ **S60.221** Contusion of right hand
- √7ᵗʰ **S60.222** Contusion of left hand
- √7ᵗʰ **S60.229** Contusion of unspecified hand

√5ᵗʰ **S60.3** Other superficial injuries of thumb

√6ᵗʰ **S60.31** Abrasion of thumb
- √7ᵗʰ **S60.311** Abrasion of right thumb
- √7ᵗʰ **S60.312** Abrasion of left thumb
- √7ᵗʰ **S60.319** Abrasion of unspecified thumb

√6ᵗʰ **S60.32** Blister (nonthermal) of thumb
- √7ᵗʰ **S60.321** Blister (nonthermal) of right thumb
- √7ᵗʰ **S60.322** Blister (nonthermal) of left thumb
- √7ᵗʰ **S60.329** Blister (nonthermal) of unspecified thumb

√6ᵗʰ **S60.34** External constriction of thumb
Hair tourniquet syndrome of thumb
Use additional cause code to identify the constricting item (W49.0-)
- √7ᵗʰ **S60.341** External constriction of right thumb
- √7ᵗʰ **S60.342** External constriction of left thumb
- √7ᵗʰ **S60.349** External constriction of unspecified thumb

√6ᵗʰ **S60.35** Superficial foreign body of thumb
Splinter in the thumb
- √7ᵗʰ **S60.351** Superficial foreign body of right thumb
- √7ᵗʰ **S60.352** Superficial foreign body of left thumb
- √7ᵗʰ **S60.359** Superficial foreign body of unspecified thumb

√6ᵗʰ **S60.36** Insect bite (nonvenomous) of thumb
- √7ᵗʰ **S60.361** Insect bite (nonvenomous) of right thumb
- √7ᵗʰ **S60.362** Insect bite (nonvenomous) of left thumb
- √7ᵗʰ **S60.369** Insect bite (nonvenomous) of unspecified thumb

√6ᵗʰ **S60.37** Other superficial bite of thumb
   EXCLUDES 1   open bite of thumb (S61.05-, S61.15-)
- √7ᵗʰ **S60.371** Other superficial bite of right thumb
- √7ᵗʰ **S60.372** Other superficial bite of left thumb
- √7ᵗʰ **S60.379** Other superficial bite of unspecified thumb

√6ᵗʰ **S60.39** Other superficial injuries of thumb
- √7ᵗʰ **S60.391** Other superficial injuries of right thumb
- √7ᵗʰ **S60.392** Other superficial injuries of left thumb
- √7ᵗʰ **S60.399** Other superficial injuries of unspecified thumb

√5ᵗʰ **S60.4** Other superficial injuries of other fingers

√6ᵗʰ **S60.41** Abrasion of fingers
- √7ᵗʰ **S60.410** Abrasion of right index finger
- √7ᵗʰ **S60.411** Abrasion of left index finger
- √7ᵗʰ **S60.412** Abrasion of right middle finger
- √7ᵗʰ **S60.413** Abrasion of left middle finger
- √7ᵗʰ **S60.414** Abrasion of right ring finger
- √7ᵗʰ **S60.415** Abrasion of left ring finger
- √7ᵗʰ **S60.416** Abrasion of right little finger
- √7ᵗʰ **S60.417** Abrasion of left little finger
- √7ᵗʰ **S60.418** Abrasion of other finger
  Abrasion of specified finger with unspecified laterality
- √7ᵗʰ **S60.419** Abrasion of unspecified finger

√6ᵗʰ **S60.42** Blister (nonthermal) of fingers
- √7ᵗʰ **S60.420** Blister (nonthermal) of right index finger
- √7ᵗʰ **S60.421** Blister (nonthermal) of left index finger
- √7ᵗʰ **S60.422** Blister (nonthermal) of right middle finger
- √7ᵗʰ **S60.423** Blister (nonthermal) of left middle finger
- √7ᵗʰ **S60.424** Blister (nonthermal) of right ring finger
- √7ᵗʰ **S60.425** Blister (nonthermal) of left ring finger
- √7ᵗʰ **S60.426** Blister (nonthermal) of right little finger
- √7ᵗʰ **S60.427** Blister (nonthermal) of left little finger
- √7ᵗʰ **S60.428** Blister (nonthermal) of other finger
  Blister (nonthermal) of specified finger with unspecified laterality
- √7ᵗʰ **S60.429** Blister (nonthermal) of unspecified finger

√6ᵗʰ **S60.44** External constriction of fingers
Hair tourniquet syndrome of finger
Use additional cause code to identify the constricting item (W49.0-)
- √7ᵗʰ **S60.440** External constriction of right index finger
- √7ᵗʰ **S60.441** External constriction of left index finger
- √7ᵗʰ **S60.442** External constriction of right middle finger
- √7ᵗʰ **S60.443** External constriction of left middle finger
- √7ᵗʰ **S60.444** External constriction of right ring finger
- √7ᵗʰ **S60.445** External constriction of left ring finger
- √7ᵗʰ **S60.446** External constriction of right little finger
- √7ᵗʰ **S60.447** External constriction of left little finger
- √7ᵗʰ **S60.448** External constriction of other finger
  External constriction of specified finger with unspecified laterality
- √7ᵗʰ **S60.449** External constriction of unspecified finger

N Newborn: 0   P Pediatric: 0-17   M Maternity: 12-55   A Adult: 15-124   CH Comorbidity High   CL Comorbidity Low   NCDx Noncancer Dx   PDx Primary Dx

1010   ICD-10-CM 2020

✓6th **S60.45** **Superficial** foreign body **of fingers**
Splinter in the finger(s)
    ✓7th **S60.450** **Superficial foreign body of** right index finger
    ✓7th **S60.451** **Superficial foreign body of** left index finger
    ✓7th **S60.452** **Superficial foreign body of** right middle finger
    ✓7th **S60.453** **Superficial foreign body of** left middle finger
    ✓7th **S60.454** **Superficial foreign body of** right ring finger
    ✓7th **S60.455** **Superficial foreign body of** left ring **finger**
    ✓7th **S60.456** **Superficial foreign body of** right little finger
    ✓7th **S60.457** **Superficial foreign body of** left little finger
    ✓7th **S60.458** **Superficial foreign body of other finger**
Superficial foreign body of specified finger with unspecified laterality
    ✓7th **S60.459** **Superficial foreign body of unspecified finger**

✓6th **S60.46** **Insect bite** (nonvenomous) **of fingers**
    ✓7th **S60.460** **Insect bite (nonvenomous) of** right index finger
    ✓7th **S60.461** **Insect bite (nonvenomous) of** left index finger
    ✓7th **S60.462** **Insect bite (nonvenomous) of** right middle **finger**
    ✓7th **S60.463** **Insect bite (nonvenomous) of** left middle finger
    ✓7th **S60.464** **Insect bite (nonvenomous) of** right ring finger
    ✓7th **S60.465** **Insect bite (nonvenomous) of** left ring finger
    ✓7th **S60.466** **Insect bite (nonvenomous) of** right little finger
    ✓7th **S60.467** **Insect bite (nonvenomous) of** left little finger
    ✓7th **S60.468** **Insect bite (nonvenomous) of other finger**
Insect bite (nonvenomous) of specified finger with unspecified laterality
    ✓7th **S60.469** **Insect bite (nonvenomous) of unspecified finger**

✓6th **S60.47** **Other superficial** bite **of fingers**
    EXCLUDES 1   *open bite of fingers (S61.25-, S61.35-)*
    ✓7th **S60.470** **Other superficial bite of** right index **finger**
    ✓7th **S60.471** **Other superficial bite of** left index **finger**
    ✓7th **S60.472** **Other superficial bite of** right middle finger
    ✓7th **S60.473** **Other superficial bite of** left middle **finger**
    ✓7th **S60.474** **Other superficial bite of** right ring **finger**
    ✓7th **S60.475** **Other superficial bite of** left ring **finger**
    ✓7th **S60.476** **Other superficial bite of** right little **finger**
    ✓7th **S60.477** **Other superficial bite of** left little **finger**
    ✓7th **S60.478** **Other superficial bite of other finger**
Other superficial bite of specified finger with unspecified laterality
    ✓7th **S60.479** **Other superficial bite of unspecified finger**

✓5th **S60.5** **Other superficial injuries of** hand
    EXCLUDES 2   *superficial injuries of fingers (S60.3-, S60.4-)*

✓6th **S60.51** **Abrasion** of hand
    ✓7th **S60.511** **Abrasion of** right **hand**
    ✓7th **S60.512** **Abrasion of** left **hand**
    ✓7th **S60.519** **Abrasion of unspecified hand**

✓6th **S60.52** **Blister** (nonthermal) **of hand**
    ✓7th **S60.521** **Blister (nonthermal) of** right **hand**
    ✓7th **S60.522** **Blister (nonthermal) of** left **hand**
    ✓7th **S60.529** **Blister (nonthermal) of unspecified hand**

✓6th **S60.54** **External constriction of hand**
    ✓7th **S60.541** **External constriction of** right **hand**
    ✓7th **S60.542** **External constriction of** left **hand**
    ✓7th **S60.549** **External constriction of unspecified hand**

✓6th **S60.55** **Superficial** foreign body **of hand**
Splinter in the hand
    ✓7th **S60.551** **Superficial foreign body of** right **hand**
    ✓7th **S60.552** **Superficial foreign body of** left **hand**
    ✓7th **S60.559** **Superficial foreign body of unspecified hand**

✓6th **S60.56** **Insect bite** (nonvenomous) **of hand**
    ✓7th **S60.561** **Insect bite (nonvenomous) of** right **hand**
    ✓7th **S60.562** **Insect bite (nonvenomous) of** left **hand**
    ✓7th **S60.569** **Insect bite (nonvenomous) of unspecified hand**

✓6th **S60.57** **Other superficial** bite **of hand**
    EXCLUDES 1   *open bite of hand (S61.45-)*
    ✓7th **S60.571** **Other superficial bite of hand of** right **hand**
    ✓7th **S60.572** **Other superficial bite of hand of** left **hand**
    ✓7th **S60.579** **Other superficial bite of hand of unspecified hand**

✓5th **S60.8** **Other superficial injuries of** wrist

✓6th **S60.81** **Abrasion** of wrist
    ✓7th **S60.811** **Abrasion of** right **wrist**
    ✓7th **S60.812** **Abrasion of** left **wrist**
    ✓7th **S60.819** **Abrasion of unspecified wrist**

✓6th **S60.82** **Blister** (nonthermal) **of wrist**
    ✓7th **S60.821** **Blister (nonthermal) of** right **wrist**
    ✓7th **S60.822** **Blister (nonthermal) of** left **wrist**
    ✓7th **S60.829** **Blister (nonthermal) of unspecified wrist**

✓6th **S60.84** **External constriction of wrist**
    ✓7th **S60.841** **External constriction of** right **wrist**
    ✓7th **S60.842** **External constriction of** left **wrist**
    ✓7th **S60.849** **External constriction of unspecified wrist**

✓6th **S60.85** **Superficial** foreign body **of wrist**
Splinter in the wrist
    ✓7th **S60.851** **Superficial foreign body of** right **wrist**
    ✓7th **S60.852** **Superficial foreign body of** left **wrist**
    ✓7th **S60.859** **Superficial foreign body of unspecified wrist**

✓6th **S60.86** **Insect bite** (nonvenomous) **of wrist**
    ✓7th **S60.861** **Insect bite (nonvenomous) of** right **wrist**
    ✓7th **S60.862** **Insect bite (nonvenomous) of** left **wrist**
    ✓7th **S60.869** **Insect bite (nonvenomous) of unspecified wrist**

✓6th **S60.87** **Other superficial** bite **of wrist**
    EXCLUDES 1   *open bite of wrist (S61.55)*
    ✓7th **S60.871** **Other superficial bite of** right **wrist**
    ✓7th **S60.872** **Other superficial bite of** left **wrist**
    ✓7th **S60.879** **Other superficial bite of unspecified wrist**

✓5th **S60.9** **Unspecified superficial injury of wrist, hand and fingers**

✓6th **S60.91** **Unspecified superficial injury of** wrist
    ✓7th **S60.911** **Unspecified superficial injury of** right **wrist**
    ✓7th **S60.912** **Unspecified superficial injury of** left **wrist**
    ✓7th **S60.919** **Unspecified superficial injury of unspecified wrist**

✓6th **S60.92** **Unspecified superficial injury of** hand
    ✓7th **S60.921** **Unspecified superficial injury of** right **hand**
    ✓7th **S60.922** **Unspecified superficial injury of** left **hand**
    ✓7th **S60.929** **Unspecified superficial injury of unspecified hand**

✓6th **S60.93** **Unspecified superficial injury of** thumb
    ✓7th **S60.931** **Unspecified superficial injury of** right **thumb**
    ✓7th **S60.932** **Unspecified superficial injury of** left **thumb**
    ✓7th **S60.939** **Unspecified superficial injury of unspecified thumb**

✓6th **S60.94** **Unspecified superficial injury of other** fingers
    ✓7th **S60.940** **Unspecified superficial injury of** right index finger
    ✓7th **S60.941** **Unspecified superficial injury of** left index finger

---

√7ᵗʰ **S60.942** Unspecified superficial injury of right middle finger

√7ᵗʰ **S60.943** Unspecified superficial injury of left middle finger

√7ᵗʰ **S60.944** Unspecified superficial injury of right ring finger

√7ᵗʰ **S60.945** Unspecified superficial injury of left ring finger

√7ᵗʰ **S60.946** Unspecified superficial injury of right little finger

√7ᵗʰ **S60.947** Unspecified superficial injury of left little finger

√7ᵗʰ **S60.948** Unspecified superficial injury of other finger

Unspecified superficial injury of specified finger with unspecified laterality

√7ᵗʰ **S60.949** Unspecified superficial injury of unspecified finger

√4ᵗʰ **S61** **Open wound of wrist, hand and fingers**

Code also any associated wound infection

EXCLUDES 1 open fracture of wrist, hand and finger (S62.- with 7th character B)

traumatic amputation of wrist and hand (S68.-)

The appropriate 7th character is to be added to each code from category S61.
A initial encounter
D subsequent encounter
S sequela

√5ᵗʰ **S61.0** **Open wound of thumb without damage to nail**

EXCLUDES 1 open wound of thumb with damage to nail (S61.1-)

√6ᵗʰ **S61.00** Unspecified open wound of thumb without damage to nail

√7ᵗʰ **S61.001** Unspecified open wound of right thumb without damage to nail

√7ᵗʰ **S61.002** Unspecified open wound of left thumb without damage to nail

√7ᵗʰ **S61.009** Unspecified open wound of unspecified thumb without damage to nail

√6ᵗʰ **S61.01** Laceration without foreign body of thumb without damage to nail

√7ᵗʰ **S61.011** Laceration without foreign body of right thumb without damage to nail

√7ᵗʰ **S61.012** Laceration without foreign body of left thumb without damage to nail

√7ᵗʰ **S61.019** Laceration without foreign body of unspecified thumb without damage to nail

√6ᵗʰ **S61.02** Laceration with foreign body of thumb without damage to nail

√7ᵗʰ **S61.021** Laceration with foreign body of right thumb without damage to nail

√7ᵗʰ **S61.022** Laceration with foreign body of left thumb without damage to nail

√7ᵗʰ **S61.029** Laceration with foreign body of unspecified thumb without damage to nail

√6ᵗʰ **S61.03** Puncture wound without foreign body of thumb without damage to nail

√7ᵗʰ **S61.031** Puncture wound without foreign body of right thumb without damage to nail

√7ᵗʰ **S61.032** Puncture wound without foreign body of left thumb without damage to nail

√7ᵗʰ **S61.039** Puncture wound without foreign body of unspecified thumb without damage to nail

√6ᵗʰ **S61.04** Puncture wound with foreign body of thumb without damage to nail

√7ᵗʰ **S61.041** Puncture wound with foreign body of right thumb without damage to nail

√7ᵗʰ **S61.042** Puncture wound with foreign body of left thumb without damage to nail

√7ᵗʰ **S61.049** Puncture wound with foreign body of unspecified thumb without damage to nail

√6ᵗʰ **S61.05** Open bite of thumb without damage to nail

Bite of thumb NOS

EXCLUDES 1 superficial bite of thumb (S60.36-, S60.37-)

√7ᵗʰ **S61.051** Open bite of right thumb without damage to nail

√7ᵗʰ **S61.052** Open bite of left thumb without damage to nail

√7ᵗʰ **S61.059** Open bite of unspecified thumb without damage to nail

√5ᵗʰ **S61.1** **Open wound of thumb with damage to nail**

√6ᵗʰ **S61.10** Unspecified open wound of thumb with damage to nail

√7ᵗʰ **S61.101** Unspecified open wound of right thumb with damage to nail

√7ᵗʰ **S61.102** Unspecified open wound of left thumb with damage to nail

√7ᵗʰ **S61.109** Unspecified open wound of unspecified thumb with damage to nail

√6ᵗʰ **S61.11** Laceration without foreign body of thumb with damage to nail

√7ᵗʰ **S61.111** Laceration without foreign body of right thumb with damage to nail

√7ᵗʰ **S61.112** Laceration without foreign body of left thumb with damage to nail

√7ᵗʰ **S61.119** Laceration without foreign body of unspecified thumb with damage to nail

√6ᵗʰ **S61.12** Laceration with foreign body of thumb with damage to nail

√7ᵗʰ **S61.121** Laceration with foreign body of right thumb with damage to nail

√7ᵗʰ **S61.122** Laceration with foreign body of left thumb with damage to nail

√7ᵗʰ **S61.129** Laceration with foreign body of unspecified thumb with damage to nail

√6ᵗʰ **S61.13** Puncture wound without foreign body of thumb with damage to nail

√7ᵗʰ **S61.131** Puncture wound without foreign body of right thumb with damage to nail

√7ᵗʰ **S61.132** Puncture wound without foreign body of left thumb with damage to nail

√7ᵗʰ **S61.139** Puncture wound without foreign body of unspecified thumb with damage to nail

√6ᵗʰ **S61.14** Puncture wound with foreign body of thumb with damage to nail

√7ᵗʰ **S61.141** Puncture wound with foreign body of right thumb with damage to nail

√7ᵗʰ **S61.142** Puncture wound with foreign body of left thumb with damage to nail

√7ᵗʰ **S61.149** Puncture wound with foreign body of unspecified thumb with damage to nail

√6ᵗʰ **S61.15** Open bite of thumb with damage to nail

Bite of thumb with damage to nail NOS

EXCLUDES 1 superficial bite of thumb (S60.36-, S60.37-)

√7ᵗʰ **S61.151** Open bite of right thumb with damage to nail

√7ᵗʰ **S61.152** Open bite of left thumb with damage to nail

√7ᵗʰ **S61.159** Open bite of unspecified thumb with damage to nail

√5ᵗʰ **S61.2** **Open wound of other finger without damage to nail**

EXCLUDES 1 open wound of finger involving nail (matrix) (S61.3-)

EXCLUDES 2 open wound of thumb without damage to nail (S61.0-)

√6ᵗʰ **S61.20** Unspecified open wound of other finger without damage to nail

√7ᵗʰ **S61.200** Unspecified open wound of right index finger without damage to nail

√7ᵗʰ **S61.201** Unspecified open wound of left index finger without damage to nail

√7ᵗʰ **S61.202** Unspecified open wound of right middle finger without damage to nail

√7ᵗʰ **S61.203** Unspecified open wound of left middle finger without damage to nail

√7ᵗʰ **S61.204** Unspecified open wound of right ring finger without damage to nail

√7ᵗʰ **S61.205** Unspecified open wound of left ring finger without damage to nail

√7ᵗʰ **S61.206** Unspecified open wound of right little finger without damage to nail

√7ᵗʰ **S61.207** Unspecified open wound of left little finger without damage to nail

√7ᵗʰ **S61.208** Unspecified open wound of other finger without damage to nail

Unspecified open wound of specified finger with unspecified laterality without damage to nail

√7ᵗʰ **S61.209** Unspecified open wound of unspecified finger without damage to nail

N Newborn: 0   P Pediatric: 0-17   M Maternity: 12-55   A Adult: 15-124   CH Comorbidity High   CL Comorbidity Low   NCDx Noncancer Dx   PDx Primary Dx

1012   ICD-10-CM 2020

√6ᵗʰ **S61.21** Laceration without foreign body of finger without damage to nail

  √7ᵗʰ **S61.210** Laceration without foreign body of right index finger without damage to nail

  √7ᵗʰ **S61.211** Laceration without foreign body of left index finger without damage to nail

  √7ᵗʰ **S61.212** Laceration without foreign body of right middle finger without damage to nail

  √7ᵗʰ **S61.213** Laceration without foreign body of left middle finger without damage to nail

  √7ᵗʰ **S61.214** Laceration without foreign body of right ring finger without damage to nail

  √7ᵗʰ **S61.215** Laceration without foreign body of left ring finger without damage to nail

  √7ᵗʰ **S61.216** Laceration without foreign body of right little finger without damage to nail

  √7ᵗʰ **S61.217** Laceration without foreign body of left little finger without damage to nail

  √7ᵗʰ **S61.218** Laceration without foreign body of other finger without damage to nail

    Laceration without foreign body of specified finger with unspecified laterality without damage to nail

  √7ᵗʰ **S61.219** Laceration without foreign body of unspecified finger without damage to nail

√6ᵗʰ **S61.22** Laceration with foreign body of finger without damage to nail

  √7ᵗʰ **S61.220** Laceration with foreign body of right index finger without damage to nail

  √7ᵗʰ **S61.221** Laceration with foreign body of left index finger without damage to nail

  √7ᵗʰ **S61.222** Laceration with foreign body of right middle finger without damage to nail

  √7ᵗʰ **S61.223** Laceration with foreign body of left middle finger without damage to nail

  √7ᵗʰ **S61.224** Laceration with foreign body of right ring finger without damage to nail

  √7ᵗʰ **S61.225** Laceration with foreign body of left ring finger without damage to nail

  √7ᵗʰ **S61.226** Laceration with foreign body of right little finger without damage to nail

  √7ᵗʰ **S61.227** Laceration with foreign body of left little finger without damage to nail

  √7ᵗʰ **S61.228** Laceration with foreign body of other finger without damage to nail

    Laceration with foreign body of specified finger with unspecified laterality without damage to nail

  √7ᵗʰ **S61.229** Laceration with foreign body of unspecified finger without damage to nail

√6ᵗʰ **S61.23** Puncture wound without foreign body of finger without damage to nail

  √7ᵗʰ **S61.230** Puncture wound without foreign body of right index finger without damage to nail

  √7ᵗʰ **S61.231** Puncture wound without foreign body of left index finger without damage to nail

  √7ᵗʰ **S61.232** Puncture wound without foreign body of right middle finger without damage to nail

  √7ᵗʰ **S61.233** Puncture wound without foreign body of left middle finger without damage to nail

  √7ᵗʰ **S61.234** Puncture wound without foreign body of right ring finger without damage to nail

  √7ᵗʰ **S61.235** Puncture wound without foreign body of left ring finger without damage to nail

  √7ᵗʰ **S61.236** Puncture wound without foreign body of right little finger without damage to nail

  √7ᵗʰ **S61.237** Puncture wound without foreign body of left little finger without damage to nail

  √7ᵗʰ **S61.238** Puncture wound without foreign body of other finger without damage to nail

    Puncture wound without foreign body of specified finger with unspecified laterality without damage to nail

  √7ᵗʰ **S61.239** Puncture wound without foreign body of unspecified finger without damage to nail

√6ᵗʰ **S61.24** Puncture wound with foreign body of finger without damage to nail

  √7ᵗʰ **S61.240** Puncture wound with foreign body of right index finger without damage to nail

√7ᵗʰ **S61.241** Puncture wound with foreign body of left index finger without damage to nail

√7ᵗʰ **S61.242** Puncture wound with foreign body of right middle finger without damage to nail

√7ᵗʰ **S61.243** Puncture wound with foreign body of left middle finger without damage to nail

√7ᵗʰ **S61.244** Puncture wound with foreign body of right ring finger without damage to nail

√7ᵗʰ **S61.245** Puncture wound with foreign body of left ring finger without damage to nail

√7ᵗʰ **S61.246** Puncture wound with foreign body of right little finger without damage to nail

√7ᵗʰ **S61.247** Puncture wound with foreign body of left little finger without damage to nail

√7ᵗʰ **S61.248** Puncture wound with foreign body of other finger without damage to nail

  Puncture wound with foreign body of specified finger with unspecified laterality without damage to nail

√7ᵗʰ **S61.249** Puncture wound with foreign body of unspecified finger without damage to nail

√6ᵗʰ **S61.25** Open bite of finger without damage to nail

  Bite of finger without damage to nail NOS

  EXCLUDES 1 superficial bite of finger (S60.46-, S60.47-)

√7ᵗʰ **S61.250** Open bite of right index finger without damage to nail

√7ᵗʰ **S61.251** Open bite of left index finger without damage to nail

√7ᵗʰ **S61.252** Open bite of right middle finger without damage to nail

√7ᵗʰ **S61.253** Open bite of left middle finger without damage to nail

√7ᵗʰ **S61.254** Open bite of right ring finger without damage to nail

√7ᵗʰ **S61.255** Open bite of left ring finger without damage to nail

√7ᵗʰ **S61.256** Open bite of right little finger without damage to nail

√7ᵗʰ **S61.257** Open bite of left little finger without damage to nail

√7ᵗʰ **S61.258** Open bite of other finger without damage to nail

  Open bite of specified finger with unspecified laterality without damage to nail

√7ᵗʰ **S61.259** Open bite of unspecified finger without damage to nail

√5ᵗʰ **S61.3** Open wound of other finger with damage to nail

  √6ᵗʰ **S61.30** Unspecified open wound of finger with damage to nail

    √7ᵗʰ **S61.300** Unspecified open wound of right index finger with damage to nail

    √7ᵗʰ **S61.301** Unspecified open wound of left index finger with damage to nail

    √7ᵗʰ **S61.302** Unspecified open wound of right middle finger with damage to nail

    √7ᵗʰ **S61.303** Unspecified open wound of left middle finger with damage to nail

    √7ᵗʰ **S61.304** Unspecified open wound of right ring finger with damage to nail

    √7ᵗʰ **S61.305** Unspecified open wound of left ring finger with damage to nail

    √7ᵗʰ **S61.306** Unspecified open wound of right little finger with damage to nail

    √7ᵗʰ **S61.307** Unspecified open wound of left little finger with damage to nail

    √7ᵗʰ **S61.308** Unspecified open wound of other finger with damage to nail

      Unspecified open wound of specified finger with unspecified laterality with damage to nail

    √7ᵗʰ **S61.309** Unspecified open wound of unspecified finger with damage to nail

  √6ᵗʰ **S61.31** Laceration without foreign body of finger with damage to nail

    √7ᵗʰ **S61.310** Laceration without foreign body of right index finger with damage to nail

    √7ᵗʰ **S61.311** Laceration without foreign body of left index finger with damage to nail

✔ Additional Character Required   √ˣ7ᵗʰ Placeholder Alert   Manifestation   Unspecified Dx   ►◄ Revised Text   ● New Code   ▲ Revised Title

ICD-10-CM 2020

1013

√7ᵗʰ **S61.312** Laceration without foreign body of right middle finger with damage to nail

√7ᵗʰ **S61.313** Laceration without foreign body of left middle finger with damage to nail

√7ᵗʰ **S61.314** Laceration without foreign body of right ring finger with damage to nail

√7ᵗʰ **S61.315** Laceration without foreign body of left ring finger with damage to nail

√7ᵗʰ **S61.316** Laceration without foreign body of right little finger with damage to nail

√7ᵗʰ **S61.317** Laceration without foreign body of left little finger with damage to nail

√7ᵗʰ **S61.318** Laceration without foreign body of other finger with damage to nail

Laceration without foreign body of specified finger with unspecified laterality with damage to nail

√7ᵗʰ **S61.319** Laceration without foreign body of unspecified finger with damage to nail

√6ᵗʰ **S61.32** Laceration with foreign body of finger with damage to nail

√7ᵗʰ **S61.320** Laceration with foreign body of right index finger with damage to nail

√7ᵗʰ **S61.321** Laceration with foreign body of left index finger with damage to nail

√7ᵗʰ **S61.322** Laceration with foreign body of right middle finger with damage to nail

√7ᵗʰ **S61.323** Laceration with foreign body of left middle finger with damage to nail

√7ᵗʰ **S61.324** Laceration with foreign body of right ring finger with damage to nail

√7ᵗʰ **S61.325** Laceration with foreign body of left ring finger with damage to nail

√7ᵗʰ **S61.326** Laceration with foreign body of right little finger with damage to nail

√7ᵗʰ **S61.327** Laceration with foreign body of left little finger with damage to nail

√7ᵗʰ **S61.328** Laceration with foreign body of other finger with damage to nail

Laceration with foreign body of specified finger with unspecified laterality with damage to nail

√7ᵗʰ **S61.329** Laceration with foreign body of unspecified finger with damage to nail

√6ᵗʰ **S61.33** Puncture wound without foreign body of finger with damage to nail

√7ᵗʰ **S61.330** Puncture wound without foreign body of right index finger with damage to nail

√7ᵗʰ **S61.331** Puncture wound without foreign body of left index finger with damage to nail

√7ᵗʰ **S61.332** Puncture wound without foreign body of right middle finger with damage to nail

√7ᵗʰ **S61.333** Puncture wound without foreign body of left middle finger with damage to nail

√7ᵗʰ **S61.334** Puncture wound without foreign body of right ring finger with damage to nail

√7ᵗʰ **S61.335** Puncture wound without foreign body of left ring finger with damage to nail

√7ᵗʰ **S61.336** Puncture wound without foreign body of right little finger with damage to nail

√7ᵗʰ **S61.337** Puncture wound without foreign body of left little finger with damage to nail

√7ᵗʰ **S61.338** Puncture wound without foreign body of other finger with damage to nail

Puncture wound without foreign body of specified finger with unspecified laterality with damage to nail

√7ᵗʰ **S61.339** Puncture wound without foreign body of unspecified finger with damage to nail

√6ᵗʰ **S61.34** Puncture wound with foreign body of finger with damage to nail

√7ᵗʰ **S61.340** Puncture wound with foreign body of right index finger with damage to nail

√7ᵗʰ **S61.341** Puncture wound with foreign body of left index finger with damage to nail

√7ᵗʰ **S61.342** Puncture wound with foreign body of right middle finger with damage to nail

√7ᵗʰ **S61.343** Puncture wound with foreign body of left middle finger with damage to nail

√7ᵗʰ **S61.344** Puncture wound with foreign body of right ring finger with damage to nail

√7ᵗʰ **S61.345** Puncture wound with foreign body of left ring finger with damage to nail

√7ᵗʰ **S61.346** Puncture wound with foreign body of right little finger with damage to nail

√7ᵗʰ **S61.347** Puncture wound with foreign body of left little finger with damage to nail

√7ᵗʰ **S61.348** Puncture wound with foreign body of other finger with damage to nail

Puncture wound with foreign body of specified finger with unspecified laterality with damage to nail

√7ᵗʰ **S61.349** Puncture wound with foreign body of unspecified finger with damage to nail

√6ᵗʰ **S61.35** Open bite of finger with damage to nail

Bite of finger with damage to nail NOS

EXCLUDES 1 superficial bite of finger (S60.46-, S60.47-)

√7ᵗʰ **S61.350** Open bite of right index finger with damage to nail

√7ᵗʰ **S61.351** Open bite of left index finger with damage to nail

√7ᵗʰ **S61.352** Open bite of right middle finger with damage to nail

√7ᵗʰ **S61.353** Open bite of left middle finger with damage to nail

√7ᵗʰ **S61.354** Open bite of right ring finger with damage to nail

√7ᵗʰ **S61.355** Open bite of left ring finger with damage to nail

√7ᵗʰ **S61.356** Open bite of right little finger with damage to nail

√7ᵗʰ **S61.357** Open bite of left little finger with damage to nail

√7ᵗʰ **S61.358** Open bite of other finger with damage to nail

Open bite of specified finger with unspecified laterality with damage to nail

√7ᵗʰ **S61.359** Open bite of unspecified finger with damage to nail

√5ᵗʰ **S61.4** Open wound of hand

√6ᵗʰ **S61.40** Unspecified open wound of hand

√7ᵗʰ **S61.401** Unspecified open wound of right hand

√7ᵗʰ **S61.402** Unspecified open wound of left hand

√7ᵗʰ **S61.409** Unspecified open wound of unspecified hand

√6ᵗʰ **S61.41** Laceration without foreign body of hand

√7ᵗʰ **S61.411** Laceration without foreign body of right hand

√7ᵗʰ **S61.412** Laceration without foreign body of left hand

√7ᵗʰ **S61.419** Laceration without foreign body of unspecified hand

√6ᵗʰ **S61.42** Laceration with foreign body of hand

√7ᵗʰ **S61.421** Laceration with foreign body of right hand

√7ᵗʰ **S61.422** Laceration with foreign body of left hand

√7ᵗʰ **S61.429** Laceration with foreign body of unspecified hand

√6ᵗʰ **S61.43** Puncture wound without foreign body of hand

√7ᵗʰ **S61.431** Puncture wound without foreign body of right hand

√7ᵗʰ **S61.432** Puncture wound without foreign body of left hand

√7ᵗʰ **S61.439** Puncture wound without foreign body of unspecified hand

√6ᵗʰ **S61.44** Puncture wound with foreign body of hand

√7ᵗʰ **S61.441** Puncture wound with foreign body of right hand

√7ᵗʰ **S61.442** Puncture wound with foreign body of left hand

√7ᵗʰ **S61.449** Puncture wound with foreign body of unspecified hand

√6ᵗʰ **S61.45** Open bite of hand

Bite of hand NOS

EXCLUDES 1 superficial bite of hand (S60.56-, S60.57-)

√7ᵗʰ **S61.451** Open bite of right hand

√7ᵗʰ **S61.452** Open bite of left hand

√7ᵗʰ **S61.459** Open bite of unspecified hand

Ⓝ Newborn: 0 Ⓟ Pediatric: 0-17 Ⓜ Maternity: 12-55 Ⓐ Adult: 15-124 **CH** Comorbidity High **CL** Comorbidity Low **NCDx** Noncancer Dx **PDx** Primary Dx

1014 ICD-10-CM 2020

√5ᵗʰ **S61.5** Open wound of wrist

  √6ᵗʰ **S61.50** Unspecified open wound of wrist

    √7ᵗʰ **S61.501** Unspecified open wound of right wrist

    √7ᵗʰ **S61.502** Unspecified open wound of left wrist

    √7ᵗʰ **S61.509** Unspecified open wound of unspecified wrist

  √6ᵗʰ **S61.51** Laceration without foreign body of wrist

    √7ᵗʰ **S61.511** Laceration without foreign body of right wrist

    √7ᵗʰ **S61.512** Laceration without foreign body of left wrist

    √7ᵗʰ **S61.519** Laceration without foreign body of unspecified wrist

  √6ᵗʰ **S61.52** Laceration with foreign body of wrist

    √7ᵗʰ **S61.521** Laceration with foreign body of right wrist

    √7ᵗʰ **S61.522** Laceration with foreign body of left wrist

    √7ᵗʰ **S61.529** Laceration with foreign body of unspecified wrist

  √6ᵗʰ **S61.53** Puncture wound without foreign body of wrist

    √7ᵗʰ **S61.531** Puncture wound without foreign body of right wrist

    √7ᵗʰ **S61.532** Puncture wound without foreign body of left wrist

    √7ᵗʰ **S61.539** Puncture wound without foreign body of unspecified wrist

  √6ᵗʰ **S61.54** Puncture wound with foreign body of wrist

    √7ᵗʰ **S61.541** Puncture wound with foreign body of right wrist

    √7ᵗʰ **S61.542** Puncture wound with foreign body of left wrist

    √7ᵗʰ **S61.549** Puncture wound with foreign body of unspecified wrist

  √6ᵗʰ **S61.55** Open bite of wrist

    Bite of wrist NOS

    EXCLUDES 1   superficial bite of wrist (S60.86-, S60.87-)

    √7ᵗʰ **S61.551** Open bite of right wrist

    √7ᵗʰ **S61.552** Open bite of left wrist

    √7ᵗʰ **S61.559** Open bite of unspecified wrist

√4ᵗʰ **S62 Fracture at wrist and hand level**

  NOTE   A fracture not indicated as displaced or nondisplaced should be coded to displaced

    A fracture not indicated as open or closed should be coded to closed

  EXCLUDES 1   traumatic amputation of wrist and hand (S68.-)

  EXCLUDES 2   fracture of distal parts of ulna and radius (S52.-)

  AHA: 2018,2Q,12; 2015,3Q,37-39

  TIP: The term "improper alignment" is not synonymous with malunion or nonunion of a fracture when noted in provider documentation.

The appropriate 7th character is to be added to each code from category S62.

A   initial encounter for closed fracture
B   initial encounter for open fracture
D   subsequent encounter for fracture with routine healing
G   subsequent encounter for fracture with delayed healing
K   subsequent encounter for fracture with nonunion
P   subsequent encounter for fracture with malunion
S   sequela

√5ᵗʰ **S62.0** Fracture of navicular [scaphoid] bone of wrist

  √6ᵗʰ **S62.00** Unspecified fracture of navicular [scaphoid] bone of wrist

    √7ᵗʰ **S62.001** Unspecified fracture of navicular [scaphoid] bone of right wrist

    √7ᵗʰ **S62.002** Unspecified fracture of navicular [scaphoid] bone of left wrist

      AHA: 2012,4Q,106

    √7ᵗʰ **S62.009** Unspecified fracture of navicular [scaphoid] bone of unspecified wrist

  √6ᵗʰ **S62.01** Fracture of distal pole of navicular [scaphoid] bone of wrist

    Fracture of volar tuberosity of navicular [scaphoid] bone of wrist

    √7ᵗʰ **S62.011** Displaced fracture of distal pole of navicular [scaphoid] bone of right wrist

    √7ᵗʰ **S62.012** Displaced fracture of distal pole of navicular [scaphoid] bone of left wrist

    √7ᵗʰ **S62.013** Displaced fracture of distal pole of navicular [scaphoid] bone of unspecified wrist

    √7ᵗʰ **S62.014** Nondisplaced fracture of distal pole of navicular [scaphoid] bone of right wrist

    √7ᵗʰ **S62.015** Nondisplaced fracture of distal pole of navicular [scaphoid] bone of left wrist

    √7ᵗʰ **S62.016** Nondisplaced fracture of distal pole of navicular [scaphoid] bone of unspecified wrist

  √6ᵗʰ **S62.02** Fracture of middle third of navicular [scaphoid] bone of wrist

    √7ᵗʰ **S62.021** Displaced fracture of middle third of navicular [scaphoid] bone of right wrist

    √7ᵗʰ **S62.022** Displaced fracture of middle third of navicular [scaphoid] bone of left wrist

    √7ᵗʰ **S62.023** Displaced fracture of middle third of navicular [scaphoid] bone of unspecified wrist

    √7ᵗʰ **S62.024** Nondisplaced fracture of middle third of navicular [scaphoid] bone of right wrist

    √7ᵗʰ **S62.025** Nondisplaced fracture of middle third of navicular [scaphoid] bone of left wrist

    √7ᵗʰ **S62.026** Nondisplaced fracture of middle third of navicular [scaphoid] bone of unspecified wrist

  √6ᵗʰ **S62.03** Fracture of proximal third of navicular [scaphoid] bone of wrist

    √7ᵗʰ **S62.031** Displaced fracture of proximal third of navicular [scaphoid] bone of right wrist

    √7ᵗʰ **S62.032** Displaced fracture of proximal third of navicular [scaphoid] bone of left wrist

    √7ᵗʰ **S62.033** Displaced fracture of proximal third of navicular [scaphoid] bone of unspecified wrist

    √7ᵗʰ **S62.034** Nondisplaced fracture of proximal third of navicular [scaphoid] bone of right wrist

    √7ᵗʰ **S62.035** Nondisplaced fracture of proximal third of navicular [scaphoid] bone of left wrist

    √7ᵗʰ **S62.036** Nondisplaced fracture of proximal third of navicular [scaphoid] bone of unspecified wrist

√5ᵗʰ **S62.1** Fracture of other and unspecified carpal bone(s)

  EXCLUDES 2   fracture of scaphoid of wrist (S62.0-)

  √6ᵗʰ **S62.10** Fracture of unspecified carpal bone

    Fracture of wrist NOS

    √7ᵗʰ **S62.101** Fracture of unspecified carpal bone, right wrist

    √7ᵗʰ **S62.102** Fracture of unspecified carpal bone, left wrist

      AHA: 2012,4Q,95

    √7ᵗʰ **S62.109** Fracture of unspecified carpal bone, unspecified wrist

  √6ᵗʰ **S62.11** Fracture of triquetrum [cuneiform] bone of wrist

    √7ᵗʰ **S62.111** Displaced fracture of triquetrum [cuneiform] bone, right wrist

    √7ᵗʰ **S62.112** Displaced fracture of triquetrum [cuneiform] bone, left wrist

    √7ᵗʰ **S62.113** Displaced fracture of triquetrum [cuneiform] bone, unspecified wrist

    √7ᵗʰ **S62.114** Nondisplaced fracture of triquetrum [cuneiform] bone, right wrist

    √7ᵗʰ **S62.115** Nondisplaced fracture of triquetrum [cuneiform] bone, left wrist

    √7ᵗʰ **S62.116** Nondisplaced fracture of triquetrum [cuneiform] bone, unspecified wrist

  √6ᵗʰ **S62.12** Fracture of lunate [semilunar]

    √7ᵗʰ **S62.121** Displaced fracture of lunate [semilunar], right wrist

    √7ᵗʰ **S62.122** Displaced fracture of lunate [semilunar], left wrist

    √7ᵗʰ **S62.123** Displaced fracture of lunate [semilunar], unspecified wrist

    √7ᵗʰ **S62.124** Nondisplaced fracture of lunate [semilunar], right wrist

    √7ᵗʰ **S62.125** Nondisplaced fracture of lunate [semilunar], left wrist

    √7ᵗʰ **S62.126** Nondisplaced fracture of lunate [semilunar], unspecified wrist

  √6ᵗʰ **S62.13** Fracture of capitate [os magnum] bone

    √7ᵗʰ **S62.131** Displaced fracture of capitate [os magnum] bone, right wrist

✔ Additional Character Required   √x7ᵗʰ Placeholder Alert   Manifestation   Unspecified Dx   ►◄ Revised Text   ● New Code   ▲ Revised Title

ICD-10-CM 2020   1015

    ☑7ᵗʰ **S62.132** Displaced fracture of capitate [os magnum] bone, left wrist

    ☑7ᵗʰ **S62.133** Displaced fracture of capitate [os magnum] bone, unspecified wrist

    ☑7ᵗʰ **S62.134** Nondisplaced fracture of capitate [os magnum] bone, right wrist

    ☑7ᵗʰ **S62.135** Nondisplaced fracture of capitate [os magnum] bone, left wrist

    ☑7ᵗʰ **S62.136** Nondisplaced fracture of capitate [os magnum] bone, unspecified wrist

☑6ᵗʰ **S62.14** Fracture of body of hamate [unciform] bone

    Fracture of hamate [unciform] bone NOS

    ☑7ᵗʰ **S62.141** Displaced fracture of body of hamate [unciform] bone, right wrist

    ☑7ᵗʰ **S62.142** Displaced fracture of body of hamate [unciform] bone, left wrist

    ☑7ᵗʰ **S62.143** Displaced fracture of body of hamate [unciform] bone, unspecified wrist

    ☑7ᵗʰ **S62.144** Nondisplaced fracture of body of hamate [unciform] bone, right wrist

    ☑7ᵗʰ **S62.145** Nondisplaced fracture of body of hamate [unciform] bone, left wrist

    ☑7ᵗʰ **S62.146** Nondisplaced fracture of body of hamate [unciform] bone, unspecified wrist

☑6ᵗʰ **S62.15** Fracture of hook process of hamate [unciform] bone

    Fracture of unciform process of hamate [unciform] bone

    ☑7ᵗʰ **S62.151** Displaced fracture of hook process of hamate [unciform] bone, right wrist

    ☑7ᵗʰ **S62.152** Displaced fracture of hook process of hamate [unciform] bone, left wrist

    ☑7ᵗʰ **S62.153** Displaced fracture of hook process of hamate [unciform] bone, unspecified wrist

    ☑7ᵗʰ **S62.154** Nondisplaced fracture of hook process of hamate [unciform] bone, right wrist

    ☑7ᵗʰ **S62.155** Nondisplaced fracture of hook process of hamate [unciform] bone, left wrist

    ☑7ᵗʰ **S62.156** Nondisplaced fracture of hook process of hamate [unciform] bone, unspecified wrist

☑6ᵗʰ **S62.16** Fracture of pisiform

    ☑7ᵗʰ **S62.161** Displaced fracture of pisiform, right wrist

    ☑7ᵗʰ **S62.162** Displaced fracture of pisiform, left wrist

    ☑7ᵗʰ **S62.163** Displaced fracture of pisiform, unspecified wrist

    ☑7ᵗʰ **S62.164** Nondisplaced fracture of pisiform, right wrist

    ☑7ᵗʰ **S62.165** Nondisplaced fracture of pisiform, left wrist

    ☑7ᵗʰ **S62.166** Nondisplaced fracture of pisiform, unspecified wrist

☑6ᵗʰ **S62.17** Fracture of trapezium [larger multangular]

    ☑7ᵗʰ **S62.171** Displaced fracture of trapezium [larger multangular], right wrist

    ☑7ᵗʰ **S62.172** Displaced fracture of trapezium [larger multangular], left wrist

    ☑7ᵗʰ **S62.173** Displaced fracture of trapezium [larger multangular], unspecified wrist

    ☑7ᵗʰ **S62.174** Nondisplaced fracture of trapezium [larger multangular], right wrist

    ☑7ᵗʰ **S62.175** Nondisplaced fracture of trapezium [larger multangular], left wrist

    ☑7ᵗʰ **S62.176** Nondisplaced fracture of trapezium [larger multangular], unspecified wrist

☑6ᵗʰ **S62.18** Fracture of trapezoid [smaller multangular]

    ☑7ᵗʰ **S62.181** Displaced fracture of trapezoid [smaller multangular], right wrist

    ☑7ᵗʰ **S62.182** Displaced fracture of trapezoid [smaller multangular], left wrist

    ☑7ᵗʰ **S62.183** Displaced fracture of trapezoid [smaller multangular], unspecified wrist

    ☑7ᵗʰ **S62.184** Nondisplaced fracture of trapezoid [smaller multangular], right wrist

    ☑7ᵗʰ **S62.185** Nondisplaced fracture of trapezoid [smaller multangular], left wrist

    ☑7ᵗʰ **S62.186** Nondisplaced fracture of trapezoid [smaller multangular], unspecified wrist

☑5ᵗʰ **S62.2** Fracture of first metacarpal bone

☑6ᵗʰ **S62.20** Unspecified fracture of first metacarpal bone

    ☑7ᵗʰ **S62.201** Unspecified fracture of first metacarpal bone, right hand

    ☑7ᵗʰ **S62.202** Unspecified fracture of first metacarpal bone, left hand

    ☑7ᵗʰ **S62.209** Unspecified fracture of first metacarpal bone, unspecified hand

☑6ᵗʰ **S62.21** Bennett's fracture

    DEF: Intra-articular, two-part fracture at the base of the first metacarpal bone (thumb) on the ulnar side at the carpometacarpal (CMC) joint.

    ☑7ᵗʰ **S62.211** Bennett's fracture, right hand

    ☑7ᵗʰ **S62.212** Bennett's fracture, left hand

    ☑7ᵗʰ **S62.213** Bennett's fracture, unspecified hand

☑6ᵗʰ **S62.22** Rolando's fracture

    DEF: Comminuted, three part intra-articular fracture at the base of the thumb metacarpal.

    ☑7ᵗʰ **S62.221** Displaced Rolando's fracture, right hand

    ☑7ᵗʰ **S62.222** Displaced Rolando's fracture, left hand

    ☑7ᵗʰ **S62.223** Displaced Rolando's fracture, unspecified hand

    ☑7ᵗʰ **S62.224** Nondisplaced Rolando's fracture, right hand

    ☑7ᵗʰ **S62.225** Nondisplaced Rolando's fracture, left hand

    ☑7ᵗʰ **S62.226** Nondisplaced Rolando's fracture, unspecified hand

☑6ᵗʰ **S62.23** Other fracture of base of first metacarpal bone

    ☑7ᵗʰ **S62.231** Other displaced fracture of base of first metacarpal bone, right hand

    ☑7ᵗʰ **S62.232** Other displaced fracture of base of first metacarpal bone, left hand

    ☑7ᵗʰ **S62.233** Other displaced fracture of base of first metacarpal bone, unspecified hand

    ☑7ᵗʰ **S62.234** Other nondisplaced fracture of base of first metacarpal bone, right hand

    ☑7ᵗʰ **S62.235** Other nondisplaced fracture of base of first metacarpal bone, left hand

    ☑7ᵗʰ **S62.236** Other nondisplaced fracture of base of first metacarpal bone, unspecified hand

☑6ᵗʰ **S62.24** Fracture of shaft of first metacarpal bone

    ☑7ᵗʰ **S62.241** Displaced fracture of shaft of first metacarpal bone, right hand

    ☑7ᵗʰ **S62.242** Displaced fracture of shaft of first metacarpal bone, left hand

    ☑7ᵗʰ **S62.243** Displaced fracture of shaft of first metacarpal bone, unspecified hand

    ☑7ᵗʰ **S62.244** Nondisplaced fracture of shaft of first metacarpal bone, right hand

    ☑7ᵗʰ **S62.245** Nondisplaced fracture of shaft of first metacarpal bone, left hand

    ☑7ᵗʰ **S62.246** Nondisplaced fracture of shaft of first metacarpal bone, unspecified hand

☑6ᵗʰ **S62.25** Fracture of neck of first metacarpal bone

    ☑7ᵗʰ **S62.251** Displaced fracture of neck of first metacarpal bone, right hand

    ☑7ᵗʰ **S62.252** Displaced fracture of neck of first metacarpal bone, left hand

    ☑7ᵗʰ **S62.253** Displaced fracture of neck of first metacarpal bone, unspecified hand

    ☑7ᵗʰ **S62.254** Nondisplaced fracture of neck of first metacarpal bone, right hand

    ☑7ᵗʰ **S62.255** Nondisplaced fracture of neck of first metacarpal bone, left hand

    ☑7ᵗʰ **S62.256** Nondisplaced fracture of neck of first metacarpal bone, unspecified hand

☑6ᵗʰ **S62.29** Other fracture of first metacarpal bone

    ☑7ᵗʰ **S62.291** Other fracture of first metacarpal bone, right hand

    ☑7ᵗʰ **S62.292** Other fracture of first metacarpal bone, left hand

    ☑7ᵗʰ **S62.299** Other fracture of first metacarpal bone, unspecified hand

☑5ᵗʰ **S62.3** Fracture of other and unspecified metacarpal bone

    EXCLUDES 2   fracture of first metacarpal bone (S62.2-)

☑6ᵗʰ **S62.30** Unspecified fracture of other metacarpal bone

    ☑7ᵗʰ **S62.300** Unspecified fracture of second metacarpal bone, right hand

N Newborn: 0   P Pediatric: 0-17   M Maternity: 12-55   A Adult: 15-124   CH Comorbidity High   CL Comorbidity Low   NCDx Noncancer Dx   PDx Primary Dx

1016   ICD-10-CM 2020

√7ᵗʰ **S62.301** Unspecified fracture of second metacarpal bone, left hand

√7ᵗʰ **S62.302** Unspecified fracture of third metacarpal bone, right hand

√7ᵗʰ **S62.303** Unspecified fracture of third metacarpal bone, left hand

√7ᵗʰ **S62.304** Unspecified fracture of fourth metacarpal bone, right hand

√7ᵗʰ **S62.305** Unspecified fracture of fourth metacarpal bone, left hand

√7ᵗʰ **S62.306** Unspecified fracture of fifth metacarpal bone, right hand

√7ᵗʰ **S62.307** Unspecified fracture of fifth metacarpal bone, left hand

√7ᵗʰ **S62.308** Unspecified fracture of other metacarpal bone

    Unspecified fracture of specified metacarpal bone with unspecified laterality

√7ᵗʰ **S62.309** Unspecified fracture of unspecified metacarpal bone

√6ᵗʰ **S62.31** Displaced fracture of base of other metacarpal bone

√7ᵗʰ **S62.310** Displaced fracture of base of second metacarpal bone, right hand

√7ᵗʰ **S62.311** Displaced fracture of base of second metacarpal bone, left hand

√7ᵗʰ **S62.312** Displaced fracture of base of third metacarpal bone, right hand

√7ᵗʰ **S62.313** Displaced fracture of base of third metacarpal bone, left hand

√7ᵗʰ **S62.314** Displaced fracture of base of fourth metacarpal bone, right hand

√7ᵗʰ **S62.315** Displaced fracture of base of fourth metacarpal bone, left hand

√7ᵗʰ **S62.316** Displaced fracture of base of fifth metacarpal bone, right hand

√7ᵗʰ **S62.317** Displaced fracture of base of fifth metacarpal bone, left hand

√7ᵗʰ **S62.318** Displaced fracture of base of other metacarpal bone

    Displaced fracture of base of specified metacarpal bone with unspecified laterality

√7ᵗʰ **S62.319** Displaced fracture of base of unspecified metacarpal bone

√6ᵗʰ **S62.32** Displaced fracture of shaft of other metacarpal bone

√7ᵗʰ **S62.320** Displaced fracture of shaft of second metacarpal bone, right hand

√7ᵗʰ **S62.321** Displaced fracture of shaft of second metacarpal bone, left hand

√7ᵗʰ **S62.322** Displaced fracture of shaft of third metacarpal bone, right hand

√7ᵗʰ **S62.323** Displaced fracture of shaft of third metacarpal bone, left hand

√7ᵗʰ **S62.324** Displaced fracture of shaft of fourth metacarpal bone, right hand

√7ᵗʰ **S62.325** Displaced fracture of shaft of fourth metacarpal bone, left hand

√7ᵗʰ **S62.326** Displaced fracture of shaft of fifth metacarpal bone, right hand

√7ᵗʰ **S62.327** Displaced fracture of shaft of fifth metacarpal bone, left hand

√7ᵗʰ **S62.328** Displaced fracture of shaft of other metacarpal bone

    Displaced fracture of shaft of specified metacarpal bone with unspecified laterality

√7ᵗʰ **S62.329** Displaced fracture of shaft of unspecified metacarpal bone

√6ᵗʰ **S62.33** Displaced fracture of neck of other metacarpal bone

√7ᵗʰ **S62.330** Displaced fracture of neck of second metacarpal bone, right hand

√7ᵗʰ **S62.331** Displaced fracture of neck of second metacarpal bone, left hand

√7ᵗʰ **S62.332** Displaced fracture of neck of third metacarpal bone, right hand

√7ᵗʰ **S62.333** Displaced fracture of neck of third metacarpal bone, left hand

√7ᵗʰ **S62.334** Displaced fracture of neck of fourth metacarpal bone, right hand

√7ᵗʰ **S62.335** Displaced fracture of neck of fourth metacarpal bone, left hand

√7ᵗʰ **S62.336** Displaced fracture of neck of fifth metacarpal bone, right hand

√7ᵗʰ **S62.337** Displaced fracture of neck of fifth metacarpal bone, left hand

√7ᵗʰ **S62.338** Displaced fracture of neck of other metacarpal bone

    Displaced fracture of neck of specified metacarpal bone with unspecified laterality

√7ᵗʰ **S62.339** Displaced fracture of neck of unspecified metacarpal bone

√6ᵗʰ **S62.34** Nondisplaced fracture of base of other metacarpal bone

√7ᵗʰ **S62.340** Nondisplaced fracture of base of second metacarpal bone, right hand

√7ᵗʰ **S62.341** Nondisplaced fracture of base of second metacarpal bone, left hand

√7ᵗʰ **S62.342** Nondisplaced fracture of base of third metacarpal bone, right hand

√7ᵗʰ **S62.343** Nondisplaced fracture of base of third metacarpal bone, left hand

√7ᵗʰ **S62.344** Nondisplaced fracture of base of fourth metacarpal bone, right hand

√7ᵗʰ **S62.345** Nondisplaced fracture of base of fourth metacarpal bone, left hand

√7ᵗʰ **S62.346** Nondisplaced fracture of base of fifth metacarpal bone, right hand

√7ᵗʰ **S62.347** Nondisplaced fracture of base of fifth metacarpal bone, left hand

√7ᵗʰ **S62.348** Nondisplaced fracture of base of other metacarpal bone

    Nondisplaced fracture of base of specified metacarpal bone with unspecified laterality

√7ᵗʰ **S62.349** Nondisplaced fracture of base of unspecified metacarpal bone

√6ᵗʰ **S62.35** Nondisplaced fracture of shaft of other metacarpal bone

√7ᵗʰ **S62.350** Nondisplaced fracture of shaft of second metacarpal bone, right hand

√7ᵗʰ **S62.351** Nondisplaced fracture of shaft of second metacarpal bone, left hand

√7ᵗʰ **S62.352** Nondisplaced fracture of shaft of third metacarpal bone, right hand

√7ᵗʰ **S62.353** Nondisplaced fracture of shaft of third metacarpal bone, left hand

√7ᵗʰ **S62.354** Nondisplaced fracture of shaft of fourth metacarpal bone, right hand

√7ᵗʰ **S62.355** Nondisplaced fracture of shaft of fourth metacarpal bone, left hand

√7ᵗʰ **S62.356** Nondisplaced fracture of shaft of fifth metacarpal bone, right hand

√7ᵗʰ **S62.357** Nondisplaced fracture of shaft of fifth metacarpal bone, left hand

√7ᵗʰ **S62.358** Nondisplaced fracture of shaft of other metacarpal bone

    Nondisplaced fracture of shaft of specified metacarpal bone with unspecified laterality

√7ᵗʰ **S62.359** Nondisplaced fracture of shaft of unspecified metacarpal bone

√6ᵗʰ **S62.36** Nondisplaced fracture of neck of other metacarpal bone

√7ᵗʰ **S62.360** Nondisplaced fracture of neck of second metacarpal bone, right hand

√7ᵗʰ **S62.361** Nondisplaced fracture of neck of second metacarpal bone, left hand

√7ᵗʰ **S62.362** Nondisplaced fracture of neck of third metacarpal bone, right hand

√7ᵗʰ **S62.363** Nondisplaced fracture of neck of third metacarpal bone, left hand

√7ᵗʰ **S62.364** Nondisplaced fracture of neck of fourth metacarpal bone, right hand

√7ᵗʰ **S62.365** Nondisplaced fracture of neck of fourth metacarpal bone, left hand

√7ᵗʰ **S62.366** Nondisplaced fracture of neck of fifth metacarpal bone, right hand

√7ᵗʰ **S62.367** Nondisplaced fracture of neck of fifth metacarpal bone, left hand

---

☑ Additional Character Required   √x7ᵗʰ Placeholder Alert   Manifestation   Unspecified Dx   ▶◀ Revised Text   ● New Code   ▲ Revised Title

✓7ᵗʰ **S62.368 Nondisplaced fracture of neck of other metacarpal bone**
Nondisplaced fracture of neck of specified metacarpal bone with unspecified laterality

✓7ᵗʰ **S62.369 Nondisplaced fracture of neck of unspecified metacarpal bone**

✓6ᵗʰ **S62.39 Other fracture of other metacarpal bone**

✓7ᵗʰ **S62.390 Other fracture of** second **metacarpal bone,** right **hand**

✓7ᵗʰ **S62.391 Other fracture of** second **metacarpal bone,** left **hand**

✓7ᵗʰ **S62.392 Other fracture of** third **metacarpal bone,** right **hand**

✓7ᵗʰ **S62.393 Other fracture of** third **metacarpal bone,** left **hand**

✓7ᵗʰ **S62.394 Other fracture of** fourth **metacarpal bone,** right **hand**

✓7ᵗʰ **S62.395 Other fracture of** fourth **metacarpal bone,** left **hand**

✓7ᵗʰ **S62.396 Other fracture of** fifth **metacarpal bone,** right **hand**

✓7ᵗʰ **S62.397 Other fracture of** fifth **metacarpal bone,** left **hand**

✓7ᵗʰ **S62.398 Other fracture of other metacarpal bone**
Other fracture of specified metacarpal bone with unspecified laterality

✓7ᵗʰ **S62.399 Other fracture of unspecified metacarpal bone**

✓5ᵗʰ **S62.5 Fracture of** thumb

✓6ᵗʰ **S62.50 Fracture of unspecified phalanx of thumb**

✓7ᵗʰ **S62.501 Fracture of unspecified phalanx of** right **thumb**

✓7ᵗʰ **S62.502 Fracture of unspecified phalanx of** left **thumb**

✓7ᵗʰ **S62.509 Fracture of unspecified phalanx of unspecified thumb**

✓6ᵗʰ **S62.51 Fracture of** proximal phalanx **of thumb**

✓7ᵗʰ **S62.511** Displaced **fracture of proximal phalanx of** right **thumb**

✓7ᵗʰ **S62.512** Displaced **fracture of proximal phalanx of** left **thumb**

✓7ᵗʰ **S62.513** Displaced **fracture of proximal phalanx of unspecified thumb**

✓7ᵗʰ **S62.514** Nondisplaced **fracture of proximal phalanx of** right **thumb**

✓7ᵗʰ **S62.515** Nondisplaced **fracture of proximal phalanx of** left **thumb**

✓7ᵗʰ **S62.516** Nondisplaced **fracture of proximal phalanx of unspecified thumb**

✓6ᵗʰ **S62.52 Fracture of** distal phalanx **of thumb**

✓7ᵗʰ **S62.521** Displaced **fracture of distal phalanx of** right **thumb**

✓7ᵗʰ **S62.522** Displaced **fracture of distal phalanx of** left **thumb**

✓7ᵗʰ **S62.523** Displaced **fracture of distal phalanx of unspecified thumb**

✓7ᵗʰ **S62.524** Nondisplaced **fracture of distal phalanx of** right **thumb**

✓7ᵗʰ **S62.525** Nondisplaced **fracture of distal phalanx of** left **thumb**

✓7ᵗʰ **S62.526** Nondisplaced **fracture of distal phalanx of unspecified thumb**

✓5ᵗʰ **S62.6 Fracture of other and unspecified** finger(s)
EXCLUDES 2 fracture of thumb (S62.5-)

✓6ᵗʰ **S62.60 Fracture of unspecified phalanx of finger**

✓7ᵗʰ **S62.600 Fracture of unspecified phalanx of** right index **finger**

✓7ᵗʰ **S62.601 Fracture of unspecified phalanx of** left index **finger**

✓7ᵗʰ **S62.602 Fracture of unspecified phalanx of** right middle **finger**

✓7ᵗʰ **S62.603 Fracture of unspecified phalanx of** left middle **finger**

✓7ᵗʰ **S62.604 Fracture of unspecified phalanx of** right ring **finger**

✓7ᵗʰ **S62.605 Fracture of unspecified phalanx of** left ring **finger**

✓7ᵗʰ **S62.606 Fracture of unspecified phalanx of** right little **finger**

✓7ᵗʰ **S62.607 Fracture of unspecified phalanx of** left little **finger**

✓7ᵗʰ **S62.608 Fracture of unspecified phalanx of other finger**
Fracture of unspecified phalanx of specified finger with unspecified laterality

✓7ᵗʰ **S62.609 Fracture of unspecified phalanx of unspecified finger**

✓6ᵗʰ **S62.61 Displaced fracture of** proximal phalanx **of finger**

✓7ᵗʰ **S62.610 Displaced fracture of proximal phalanx of** right index **finger**

✓7ᵗʰ **S62.611 Displaced fracture of proximal phalanx of** left index **finger**

✓7ᵗʰ **S62.612 Displaced fracture of proximal phalanx of** right middle **finger**

✓7ᵗʰ **S62.613 Displaced fracture of proximal phalanx of** left middle **finger**

✓7ᵗʰ **S62.614 Displaced fracture of proximal phalanx of** right ring **finger**

✓7ᵗʰ **S62.615 Displaced fracture of proximal phalanx of** left ring **finger**

✓7ᵗʰ **S62.616 Displaced fracture of proximal phalanx of** right little **finger**

✓7ᵗʰ **S62.617 Displaced fracture of proximal phalanx of** left little **finger**

✓7ᵗʰ **S62.618 Displaced fracture of proximal phalanx of other finger**
Displaced fracture of proximal phalanx of specified finger with unspecified laterality

✓7ᵗʰ **S62.619 Displaced fracture of proximal phalanx of unspecified finger**

✓6ᵗʰ **S62.62 Displaced fracture of** middle phalanx **of finger**

✓7ᵗʰ **S62.620 Displaced fracture of middle phalanx of** right index **finger**

✓7ᵗʰ **S62.621 Displaced fracture of middle phalanx of** left index **finger**

✓7ᵗʰ **S62.622 Displaced fracture of middle phalanx of** right middle **finger**

✓7ᵗʰ **S62.623 Displaced fracture of middle phalanx of** left middle **finger**

✓7ᵗʰ **S62.624 Displaced fracture of middle phalanx of** right ring **finger**

✓7ᵗʰ **S62.625 Displaced fracture of middle phalanx of** left ring **finger**

✓7ᵗʰ **S62.626 Displaced fracture of middle phalanx of** right little **finger**

✓7ᵗʰ **S62.627 Displaced fracture of middle phalanx of** left little **finger**

✓7ᵗʰ **S62.628 Displaced fracture of middle phalanx of other finger**
Displaced fracture of middle phalanx of specified finger with unspecified laterality

✓7ᵗʰ **S62.629 Displaced fracture of middle phalanx of unspecified finger**

✓6ᵗʰ **S62.63 Displaced fracture of** distal phalanx **of finger**

✓7ᵗʰ **S62.630 Displaced fracture of distal phalanx of** right index **finger**

✓7ᵗʰ **S62.631 Displaced fracture of distal phalanx of** left index **finger**

✓7ᵗʰ **S62.632 Displaced fracture of distal phalanx of** right middle **finger**

✓7ᵗʰ **S62.633 Displaced fracture of distal phalanx of** left middle **finger**

✓7ᵗʰ **S62.634 Displaced fracture of distal phalanx of** right ring **finger**

✓7ᵗʰ **S62.635 Displaced fracture of distal phalanx of** left ring **finger**

✓7ᵗʰ **S62.636 Displaced fracture of distal phalanx of** right little **finger**

✓7ᵗʰ **S62.637 Displaced fracture of distal phalanx of** left little **finger**

✓7ᵗʰ **S62.638 Displaced fracture of distal phalanx of other finger**
Displaced fracture of distal phalanx of specified finger with unspecified laterality

✓7ᵗʰ **S62.639 Displaced fracture of distal phalanx of unspecified finger**

√6ᵗʰ **S62.64** Nondisplaced fracture of proximal phalanx of finger

√7ᵗʰ **S62.640** Nondisplaced fracture of proximal phalanx of right index finger

√7ᵗʰ **S62.641** Nondisplaced fracture of proximal phalanx of left index finger

√7ᵗʰ **S62.642** Nondisplaced fracture of proximal phalanx of right middle finger

√7ᵗʰ **S62.643** Nondisplaced fracture of proximal phalanx of left middle finger

√7ᵗʰ **S62.644** Nondisplaced fracture of proximal phalanx of right ring finger

√7ᵗʰ **S62.645** Nondisplaced fracture of proximal phalanx of left ring finger

√7ᵗʰ **S62.646** Nondisplaced fracture of proximal phalanx of right little finger

√7ᵗʰ **S62.647** Nondisplaced fracture of proximal phalanx of left little finger

√7ᵗʰ **S62.648** Nondisplaced fracture of proximal phalanx of other finger

Nondisplaced fracture of proximal phalanx of specified finger with unspecified laterality

√7ᵗʰ **S62.649** Nondisplaced fracture of proximal phalanx of unspecified finger

√6ᵗʰ **S62.65** Nondisplaced fracture of middle phalanx of finger

√7ᵗʰ **S62.650** Nondisplaced fracture of middle phalanx of right index finger

√7ᵗʰ **S62.651** Nondisplaced fracture of middle phalanx of left index finger

√7ᵗʰ **S62.652** Nondisplaced fracture of middle phalanx of right middle finger

√7ᵗʰ **S62.653** Nondisplaced fracture of middle phalanx of left middle finger

√7ᵗʰ **S62.654** Nondisplaced fracture of middle phalanx of right ring finger

√7ᵗʰ **S62.655** Nondisplaced fracture of middle phalanx of left ring finger

√7ᵗʰ **S62.656** Nondisplaced fracture of middle phalanx of right little finger

√7ᵗʰ **S62.657** Nondisplaced fracture of middle phalanx of left little finger

√7ᵗʰ **S62.658** Nondisplaced fracture of middle phalanx of other finger

Nondisplaced fracture of middle phalanx of specified finger with unspecified laterality

√7ᵗʰ **S62.659** Nondisplaced fracture of middle phalanx of unspecified finger

√6ᵗʰ **S62.66** Nondisplaced fracture of distal phalanx of finger

√7ᵗʰ **S62.660** Nondisplaced fracture of distal phalanx of right index finger

√7ᵗʰ **S62.661** Nondisplaced fracture of distal phalanx of left index finger

√7ᵗʰ **S62.662** Nondisplaced fracture of distal phalanx of right middle finger

√7ᵗʰ **S62.663** Nondisplaced fracture of distal phalanx of left middle finger

√7ᵗʰ **S62.664** Nondisplaced fracture of distal phalanx of right ring finger

√7ᵗʰ **S62.665** Nondisplaced fracture of distal phalanx of left ring finger

√7ᵗʰ **S62.666** Nondisplaced fracture of distal phalanx of right little finger

√7ᵗʰ **S62.667** Nondisplaced fracture of distal phalanx of left little finger

√7ᵗʰ **S62.668** Nondisplaced fracture of distal phalanx of other finger

Nondisplaced fracture of distal phalanx of specified finger with unspecified laterality

√7ᵗʰ **S62.669** Nondisplaced fracture of distal phalanx of unspecified finger

√5ᵗʰ **S62.9** Unspecified fracture of wrist and hand

√x7ᵗʰ **S62.90** Unspecified fracture of unspecified wrist and hand

√x7ᵗʰ **S62.91** Unspecified fracture of right wrist and hand

√x7ᵗʰ **S62.92** Unspecified fracture of left wrist and hand

√4ᵗʰ **S63** Dislocation and sprain of joints and ligaments at wrist and hand level

INCLUDES avulsion of joint or ligament at wrist and hand level

laceration of cartilage, joint or ligament at wrist and hand level

sprain of cartilage, joint or ligament at wrist and hand level

traumatic hemarthrosis of joint or ligament at wrist and hand level

traumatic rupture of joint or ligament at wrist and hand level

traumatic subluxation of joint or ligament at wrist and hand level

traumatic tear of joint or ligament at wrist and hand level

Code also any associated open wound

EXCLUDES 2 *strain of muscle, fascia and tendon of wrist and hand (S66.-)*

The appropriate 7th character is to be added to each code from category S63.
A initial encounter
D subsequent encounter
S sequela

√5ᵗʰ **S63.0** Subluxation and dislocation of wrist and hand joints

√6ᵗʰ **S63.00** Unspecified subluxation and dislocation of wrist and hand

Dislocation of carpal bone NOS
Dislocation of distal end of radius NOS
Subluxation of carpal bone NOS
Subluxation of distal end of radius NOS

√7ᵗʰ **S63.001** Unspecified subluxation of right wrist and hand

√7ᵗʰ **S63.002** Unspecified subluxation of left wrist and hand

√7ᵗʰ **S63.003** Unspecified subluxation of unspecified wrist and hand

√7ᵗʰ **S63.004** Unspecified dislocation of right wrist and hand

√7ᵗʰ **S63.005** Unspecified dislocation of left wrist and hand

√7ᵗʰ **S63.006** Unspecified dislocation of unspecified wrist and hand

√6ᵗʰ **S63.01** Subluxation and dislocation of distal radioulnar joint

√7ᵗʰ **S63.011** Subluxation of distal radioulnar joint of right wrist

√7ᵗʰ **S63.012** Subluxation of distal radioulnar joint of left wrist

√7ᵗʰ **S63.013** Subluxation of distal radioulnar joint of unspecified wrist

√7ᵗʰ **S63.014** Dislocation of distal radioulnar joint of right wrist

√7ᵗʰ **S63.015** Dislocation of distal radioulnar joint of left wrist

√7ᵗʰ **S63.016** Dislocation of distal radioulnar joint of unspecified wrist

√6ᵗʰ **S63.02** Subluxation and dislocation of radiocarpal joint

√7ᵗʰ **S63.021** Subluxation of radiocarpal joint of right wrist

√7ᵗʰ **S63.022** Subluxation of radiocarpal joint of left wrist

√7ᵗʰ **S63.023** Subluxation of radiocarpal joint of unspecified wrist

√7ᵗʰ **S63.024** Dislocation of radiocarpal joint of right wrist

√7ᵗʰ **S63.025** Dislocation of radiocarpal joint of left wrist

√7ᵗʰ **S63.026** Dislocation of radiocarpal joint of unspecified wrist

√6ᵗʰ **S63.03** Subluxation and dislocation of midcarpal joint

√7ᵗʰ **S63.031** Subluxation of midcarpal joint of right wrist

√7ᵗʰ **S63.032** Subluxation of midcarpal joint of left wrist

√7ᵗʰ **S63.033** Subluxation of midcarpal joint of unspecified wrist

√7ᵗʰ **S63.034** Dislocation of midcarpal joint of right wrist

√7ᵗʰ **S63.035** Dislocation of midcarpal joint of left wrist

√7ᵗʰ **S63.036** Dislocation of midcarpal joint of unspecified wrist

✔ Additional Character Required √x7ᵗʰ Placeholder Alert Manifestation Unspecified Dx ►◄ Revised Text ● New Code ▲ Revised Title

ICD-10-CM 2020 **1019**

✓6ᵗʰ **S63.04** **Subluxation and dislocation of** carpometacarpal joint of thumb
    EXCLUDES 2 *interphalangeal subluxation and dislocation of thumb (S63.1-)*
✓7ᵗʰ **S63.041** Subluxation of carpometacarpal joint of right thumb
✓7ᵗʰ **S63.042** Subluxation of carpometacarpal joint of left thumb
✓7ᵗʰ **S63.043** Subluxation of carpometacarpal joint of unspecified thumb
✓7ᵗʰ **S63.044** Dislocation of carpometacarpal joint of right thumb
✓7ᵗʰ **S63.045** Dislocation of carpometacarpal joint of left thumb
✓7ᵗʰ **S63.046** Dislocation of carpometacarpal joint of unspecified thumb

✓6ᵗʰ **S63.05** **Subluxation and dislocation of other carpometacarpal joint**
    EXCLUDES 2 *subluxation and dislocation of carpometacarpal joint of thumb (S63.04-)*
✓7ᵗʰ **S63.051** Subluxation of other carpometacarpal joint of right hand
✓7ᵗʰ **S63.052** Subluxation of other carpometacarpal joint of left hand
✓7ᵗʰ **S63.053** Subluxation of other carpometacarpal joint of unspecified hand
✓7ᵗʰ **S63.054** Dislocation of other carpometacarpal joint of right hand
✓7ᵗʰ **S63.055** Dislocation of other carpometacarpal joint of left hand
✓7ᵗʰ **S63.056** Dislocation of other carpometacarpal joint of unspecified hand

✓6ᵗʰ **S63.06** **Subluxation and dislocation of** metacarpal (bone), proximal end
✓7ᵗʰ **S63.061** Subluxation of metacarpal (bone), proximal end of right hand
✓7ᵗʰ **S63.062** Subluxation of metacarpal (bone), proximal end of left hand
✓7ᵗʰ **S63.063** Subluxation of metacarpal (bone), proximal end of unspecified hand
✓7ᵗʰ **S63.064** Dislocation of metacarpal (bone), proximal end of right hand
✓7ᵗʰ **S63.065** Dislocation of metacarpal (bone), proximal end of left hand
✓7ᵗʰ **S63.066** Dislocation of metacarpal (bone), proximal end of unspecified hand

✓6ᵗʰ **S63.07** **Subluxation and dislocation of** distal end of ulna
✓7ᵗʰ **S63.071** Subluxation of distal end of right ulna
✓7ᵗʰ **S63.072** Subluxation of distal end of left ulna
✓7ᵗʰ **S63.073** Subluxation of distal end of unspecified ulna
✓7ᵗʰ **S63.074** Dislocation of distal end of right ulna
✓7ᵗʰ **S63.075** Dislocation of distal end of left ulna
✓7ᵗʰ **S63.076** Dislocation of distal end of unspecified ulna

✓6ᵗʰ **S63.09** **Other subluxation and dislocation of wrist and hand**
✓7ᵗʰ **S63.091** Other subluxation of right wrist and hand
✓7ᵗʰ **S63.092** Other subluxation of left wrist and hand
✓7ᵗʰ **S63.093** Other subluxation of unspecified wrist and hand
✓7ᵗʰ **S63.094** Other dislocation of right wrist and hand
✓7ᵗʰ **S63.095** Other dislocation of left wrist and hand
✓7ᵗʰ **S63.096** Other dislocation of unspecified wrist and hand

✓5ᵗʰ **S63.1** **Subluxation and dislocation of** thumb
✓6ᵗʰ **S63.10** **Unspecified subluxation and dislocation of thumb**
✓7ᵗʰ **S63.101** Unspecified subluxation of right thumb
✓7ᵗʰ **S63.102** Unspecified subluxation of left thumb
✓7ᵗʰ **S63.103** Unspecified subluxation of unspecified thumb
✓7ᵗʰ **S63.104** Unspecified dislocation of right thumb
✓7ᵗʰ **S63.105** Unspecified dislocation of left thumb
✓7ᵗʰ **S63.106** Unspecified dislocation of unspecified thumb

✓6ᵗʰ **S63.11** **Subluxation and dislocation of** metacarpophalangeal joint of thumb
✓7ᵗʰ **S63.111** Subluxation of metacarpophalangeal joint of right thumb

✓7ᵗʰ **S63.112** Subluxation of metacarpophalangeal joint of left thumb
✓7ᵗʰ **S63.113** Subluxation of metacarpophalangeal joint of unspecified thumb
✓7ᵗʰ **S63.114** Dislocation of metacarpophalangeal joint of right thumb
✓7ᵗʰ **S63.115** Dislocation of metacarpophalangeal joint of left thumb
✓7ᵗʰ **S63.116** Dislocation of metacarpophalangeal joint of unspecified thumb

✓6ᵗʰ **S63.12** **Subluxation and dislocation of** interphalangeal joint of thumb
✓7ᵗʰ **S63.121** Subluxation of interphalangeal joint of right thumb
✓7ᵗʰ **S63.122** Subluxation of interphalangeal joint of left thumb
✓7ᵗʰ **S63.123** Subluxation of interphalangeal joint of unspecified thumb
✓7ᵗʰ **S63.124** Dislocation of interphalangeal joint of right thumb
✓7ᵗʰ **S63.125** Dislocation of interphalangeal joint of left thumb
✓7ᵗʰ **S63.126** Dislocation of interphalangeal joint of unspecified thumb

✓5ᵗʰ **S63.2** **Subluxation and dislocation of other** finger(s)
    EXCLUDES 2 *subluxation and dislocation of thumb (S63.1-)*
✓6ᵗʰ **S63.20** **Unspecified subluxation of other finger**
✓7ᵗʰ **S63.200** Unspecified subluxation of right index finger
✓7ᵗʰ **S63.201** Unspecified subluxation of left index finger
✓7ᵗʰ **S63.202** Unspecified subluxation of right middle finger
✓7ᵗʰ **S63.203** Unspecified subluxation of left middle finger
✓7ᵗʰ **S63.204** Unspecified subluxation of right ring finger
✓7ᵗʰ **S63.205** Unspecified subluxation of left ring finger
✓7ᵗʰ **S63.206** Unspecified subluxation of right little finger
✓7ᵗʰ **S63.207** Unspecified subluxation of left little finger
✓7ᵗʰ **S63.208** Unspecified subluxation of other finger
    Unspecified subluxation of specified finger with unspecified laterality
✓7ᵗʰ **S63.209** Unspecified subluxation of unspecified finger

✓6ᵗʰ **S63.21** **Subluxation of** metacarpophalangeal joint of finger
✓7ᵗʰ **S63.210** Subluxation of metacarpophalangeal joint of right index finger
✓7ᵗʰ **S63.211** Subluxation of metacarpophalangeal joint of left index finger
✓7ᵗʰ **S63.212** Subluxation of metacarpophalangeal joint of right middle finger
✓7ᵗʰ **S63.213** Subluxation of metacarpophalangeal joint of left middle finger
✓7ᵗʰ **S63.214** Subluxation of metacarpophalangeal joint of right ring finger
✓7ᵗʰ **S63.215** Subluxation of metacarpophalangeal joint of left ring finger
✓7ᵗʰ **S63.216** Subluxation of metacarpophalangeal joint of right little finger
✓7ᵗʰ **S63.217** Subluxation of metacarpophalangeal joint of left little finger
✓7ᵗʰ **S63.218** Subluxation of metacarpophalangeal joint of other finger
    Subluxation of metacarpophalangeal joint of specified finger with unspecified laterality
✓7ᵗʰ **S63.219** Subluxation of metacarpophalangeal joint of unspecified finger

✓6ᵗʰ **S63.22** **Subluxation of unspecified** interphalangeal joint of finger
✓7ᵗʰ **S63.220** Subluxation of unspecified interphalangeal joint of right index finger
✓7ᵗʰ **S63.221** Subluxation of unspecified interphalangeal joint of left index finger
✓7ᵗʰ **S63.222** Subluxation of unspecified interphalangeal joint of right middle finger
✓7ᵗʰ **S63.223** Subluxation of unspecified interphalangeal joint of left middle finger

√7th **S63.224** Subluxation of unspecified interphalangeal joint of right ring finger

√7th **S63.225** Subluxation of unspecified interphalangeal joint of left ring finger

√7th **S63.226** Subluxation of unspecified interphalangeal joint of right little finger

√7th **S63.227** Subluxation of unspecified interphalangeal joint of left little finger

√7th **S63.228** Subluxation of unspecified interphalangeal joint of other finger
       Subluxation of unspecified interphalangeal joint of specified finger with unspecified laterality

√7th **S63.229** Subluxation of unspecified interphalangeal joint of unspecified finger

√6th **S63.23** Subluxation of proximal interphalangeal joint of finger

√7th **S63.230** Subluxation of proximal interphalangeal joint of right index finger

√7th **S63.231** Subluxation of proximal interphalangeal joint of left index finger

√7th **S63.232** Subluxation of proximal interphalangeal joint of right middle finger

√7th **S63.233** Subluxation of proximal interphalangeal joint of left middle finger

√7th **S63.234** Subluxation of proximal interphalangeal joint of right ring finger

√7th **S63.235** Subluxation of proximal interphalangeal joint of left ring finger

√7th **S63.236** Subluxation of proximal interphalangeal joint of right little finger

√7th **S63.237** Subluxation of proximal interphalangeal joint of left little finger

√7th **S63.238** Subluxation of proximal interphalangeal joint of other finger
       Subluxation of proximal interphalangeal joint of specified finger with unspecified laterality

√7th **S63.239** Subluxation of proximal interphalangeal joint of unspecified finger

√6th **S63.24** Subluxation of distal interphalangeal joint of finger

√7th **S63.240** Subluxation of distal interphalangeal joint of right index finger

√7th **S63.241** Subluxation of distal interphalangeal joint of left index finger

√7th **S63.242** Subluxation of distal interphalangeal joint of right middle finger

√7th **S63.243** Subluxation of distal interphalangeal joint of left middle finger

√7th **S63.244** Subluxation of distal interphalangeal joint of right ring finger

√7th **S63.245** Subluxation of distal interphalangeal joint of left ring finger

√7th **S63.246** Subluxation of distal interphalangeal joint of right little finger

√7th **S63.247** Subluxation of distal interphalangeal joint of left little finger

√7th **S63.248** Subluxation of distal interphalangeal joint of other finger
       Subluxation of distal interphalangeal joint of specified finger with unspecified laterality

√7th **S63.249** Subluxation of distal interphalangeal joint of unspecified finger

√6th **S63.25** Unspecified dislocation of other finger

√7th **S63.250** Unspecified dislocation of right index finger

√7th **S63.251** Unspecified dislocation of left index finger

√7th **S63.252** Unspecified dislocation of right middle finger

√7th **S63.253** Unspecified dislocation of left middle finger

√7th **S63.254** Unspecified dislocation of right ring finger

√7th **S63.255** Unspecified dislocation of left ring finger

√7th **S63.256** Unspecified dislocation of right little finger

√7th **S63.257** Unspecified dislocation of left little finger

√7th **S63.258** Unspecified dislocation of other finger
       Unspecified dislocation of specified finger with unspecified laterality

√7th **S63.259** Unspecified dislocation of unspecified finger
       Unspecified dislocation of unspecified finger with unspecified laterality

√6th **S63.26** Dislocation of metacarpophalangeal joint of finger

√7th **S63.260** Dislocation of metacarpophalangeal joint of right index finger

√7th **S63.261** Dislocation of metacarpophalangeal joint of left index finger

√7th **S63.262** Dislocation of metacarpophalangeal joint of right middle finger

√7th **S63.263** Dislocation of metacarpophalangeal joint of left middle finger

√7th **S63.264** Dislocation of metacarpophalangeal joint of right ring finger

√7th **S63.265** Dislocation of metacarpophalangeal joint of left ring finger

√7th **S63.266** Dislocation of metacarpophalangeal joint of right little finger

√7th **S63.267** Dislocation of metacarpophalangeal joint of left little finger

√7th **S63.268** Dislocation of metacarpophalangeal joint of other finger
       Dislocation of metacarpophalangeal joint of specified finger with unspecified laterality

√7th **S63.269** Dislocation of metacarpophalangeal joint of unspecified finger

√6th **S63.27** Dislocation of unspecified interphalangeal joint of finger

√7th **S63.270** Dislocation of unspecified interphalangeal joint of right index finger

√7th **S63.271** Dislocation of unspecified interphalangeal joint of left index finger

√7th **S63.272** Dislocation of unspecified interphalangeal joint of right middle finger

√7th **S63.273** Dislocation of unspecified interphalangeal joint of left middle finger

√7th **S63.274** Dislocation of unspecified interphalangeal joint of right ring finger

√7th **S63.275** Dislocation of unspecified interphalangeal joint of left ring finger

√7th **S63.276** Dislocation of unspecified interphalangeal joint of right little finger

√7th **S63.277** Dislocation of unspecified interphalangeal joint of left little finger

√7th **S63.278** Dislocation of unspecified interphalangeal joint of other finger
       Dislocation of unspecified interphalangeal joint of specified finger with unspecified laterality

√7th **S63.279** Dislocation of unspecified interphalangeal joint of unspecified finger
       Dislocation of unspecified interphalangeal joint of unspecified finger without specified laterality

√6th **S63.28** Dislocation of proximal interphalangeal joint of finger

√7th **S63.280** Dislocation of proximal interphalangeal joint of right index finger

√7th **S63.281** Dislocation of proximal interphalangeal joint of left index finger

√7th **S63.282** Dislocation of proximal interphalangeal joint of right middle finger

√7th **S63.283** Dislocation of proximal interphalangeal joint of left middle finger

√7th **S63.284** Dislocation of proximal interphalangeal joint of right ring finger

√7th **S63.285** Dislocation of proximal interphalangeal joint of left ring finger

√7th **S63.286** Dislocation of proximal interphalangeal joint of right little finger

√7th **S63.287** Dislocation of proximal interphalangeal joint of left little finger

☑ Additional Character Required   √x7th Placeholder Alert   Manifestation   Unspecified Dx   ►◄ Revised Text   ● New Code   ▲ Revised Title

ICD-10-CM 2020   1021

☑7ᵗʰ **S63.288 Dislocation of proximal interphalangeal joint of other finger**
Dislocation of proximal interphalangeal joint of specified finger with unspecified laterality

☑7ᵗʰ **S63.289 Dislocation of proximal interphalangeal joint of unspecified finger**

☑6ᵗʰ **S63.29 Dislocation of** distal interphalangeal joint **of finger**

☑7ᵗʰ **S63.290 Dislocation of distal interphalangeal joint of** right index **finger**

☑7ᵗʰ **S63.291 Dislocation of distal interphalangeal joint of** left index **finger**

☑7ᵗʰ **S63.292 Dislocation of distal interphalangeal joint of** right middle **finger**

☑7ᵗʰ **S63.293 Dislocation of distal interphalangeal joint of** left middle **finger**

☑7ᵗʰ **S63.294 Dislocation of distal interphalangeal joint of** right ring **finger**

☑7ᵗʰ **S63.295 Dislocation of distal interphalangeal joint of** left ring **finger**

☑7ᵗʰ **S63.296 Dislocation of distal interphalangeal joint of** right little **finger**

☑7ᵗʰ **S63.297 Dislocation of distal interphalangeal joint of** left little **finger**

☑7ᵗʰ **S63.298 Dislocation of distal interphalangeal joint of other finger**
Dislocation of distal interphalangeal joint of specified finger with unspecified laterality

☑7ᵗʰ **S63.299 Dislocation of distal interphalangeal joint of unspecified finger**

☑5ᵗʰ **S63.3 Traumatic rupture of** ligament of wrist

☑6ᵗʰ **S63.30 Traumatic rupture of unspecified ligament of wrist**

☑7ᵗʰ **S63.301 Traumatic rupture of unspecified ligament of** right **wrist**

☑7ᵗʰ **S63.302 Traumatic rupture of unspecified ligament of** left **wrist**

☑7ᵗʰ **S63.309 Traumatic rupture of unspecified ligament of unspecified wrist**

☑6ᵗʰ **S63.31 Traumatic rupture of** collateral **ligament of wrist**

☑7ᵗʰ **S63.311 Traumatic rupture of collateral ligament of** right **wrist**

☑7ᵗʰ **S63.312 Traumatic rupture of collateral ligament of** left **wrist**

☑7ᵗʰ **S63.319 Traumatic rupture of collateral ligament of unspecified wrist**

☑6ᵗʰ **S63.32 Traumatic rupture of** radiocarpal ligament

☑7ᵗʰ **S63.321 Traumatic rupture of** right **radiocarpal ligament**

☑7ᵗʰ **S63.322 Traumatic rupture of** left **radiocarpal ligament**

☑7ᵗʰ **S63.329 Traumatic rupture of unspecified radiocarpal ligament**

☑6ᵗʰ **S63.33 Traumatic rupture of** ulnocarpal (palmar) ligament

☑7ᵗʰ **S63.331 Traumatic rupture of** right **ulnocarpal (palmar) ligament**

☑7ᵗʰ **S63.332 Traumatic rupture of** left **ulnocarpal (palmar) ligament**

☑7ᵗʰ **S63.339 Traumatic rupture of unspecified ulnocarpal (palmar) ligament**

☑6ᵗʰ **S63.39 Traumatic rupture of other ligament of wrist**

☑7ᵗʰ **S63.391 Traumatic rupture of other ligament of** right **wrist**

☑7ᵗʰ **S63.392 Traumatic rupture of other ligament of** left **wrist**

☑7ᵗʰ **S63.399 Traumatic rupture of other ligament of unspecified wrist**

☑5ᵗʰ **S63.4 Traumatic rupture of ligament of finger at** metacarpophalangeal and interphalangeal joint(s)

☑6ᵗʰ **S63.40 Traumatic rupture of unspecified ligament of finger at metacarpophalangeal and interphalangeal joint**

☑7ᵗʰ **S63.400 Traumatic rupture of unspecified ligament of** right index **finger at metacarpophalangeal and interphalangeal joint**

☑7ᵗʰ **S63.401 Traumatic rupture of unspecified ligament of** left index **finger at metacarpophalangeal and interphalangeal joint**

☑7ᵗʰ **S63.402 Traumatic rupture of unspecified ligament of** right middle **finger at metacarpophalangeal and interphalangeal joint**

☑7ᵗʰ **S63.403 Traumatic rupture of unspecified ligament of** left middle **finger at metacarpophalangeal and interphalangeal joint**

☑7ᵗʰ **S63.404 Traumatic rupture of unspecified ligament of** right ring **finger at metacarpophalangeal and interphalangeal joint**

☑7ᵗʰ **S63.405 Traumatic rupture of unspecified ligament of** left ring **finger at metacarpophalangeal and interphalangeal joint**

☑7ᵗʰ **S63.406 Traumatic rupture of unspecified ligament of** right little **finger at metacarpophalangeal and interphalangeal joint**

☑7ᵗʰ **S63.407 Traumatic rupture of unspecified ligament of** left little **finger at metacarpophalangeal and interphalangeal joint**

☑7ᵗʰ **S63.408 Traumatic rupture of unspecified ligament of other finger at metacarpophalangeal and interphalangeal joint**
Traumatic rupture of unspecified ligament of specified finger with unspecified laterality at metacarpophalangeal and interphalangeal joint

☑7ᵗʰ **S63.409 Traumatic rupture of unspecified ligament of unspecified finger at metacarpophalangeal and interphalangeal joint**

☑6ᵗʰ **S63.41 Traumatic rupture of** collateral ligament **of finger at metacarpophalangeal and interphalangeal joint**

☑7ᵗʰ **S63.410 Traumatic rupture of collateral ligament of** right index **finger at metacarpophalangeal and interphalangeal joint**

☑7ᵗʰ **S63.411 Traumatic rupture of collateral ligament of** left index **finger at metacarpophalangeal and interphalangeal joint**

☑7ᵗʰ **S63.412 Traumatic rupture of collateral ligament of** right middle **finger at metacarpophalangeal and interphalangeal joint**

☑7ᵗʰ **S63.413 Traumatic rupture of collateral ligament of** left middle **finger at metacarpophalangeal and interphalangeal joint**

☑7ᵗʰ **S63.414 Traumatic rupture of collateral ligament of** right ring **finger at metacarpophalangeal and interphalangeal joint**

☑7ᵗʰ **S63.415 Traumatic rupture of collateral ligament of** left ring **finger at metacarpophalangeal and interphalangeal joint**

☑7ᵗʰ **S63.416 Traumatic rupture of collateral ligament of** right little **finger at metacarpophalangeal and interphalangeal joint**

☑7ᵗʰ **S63.417 Traumatic rupture of collateral ligament of** left little **finger at metacarpophalangeal and interphalangeal joint**

☑7ᵗʰ **S63.418 Traumatic rupture of collateral ligament of other finger at metacarpophalangeal and interphalangeal joint**
Traumatic rupture of collateral ligament of specified finger with unspecified laterality at metacarpophalangeal and interphalangeal joint

☑7ᵗʰ **S63.419 Traumatic rupture of collateral ligament of unspecified finger at metacarpophalangeal and interphalangeal joint**

Ⓝ Newborn: 0   Ⓟ Pediatric: 0-17   Ⓜ Maternity: 12-55   Ⓐ Adult: 15-124   CH Comorbidity High   CL Comorbidity Low   NCDx Noncancer Dx   PDx Primary Dx

1022   ICD-10-CM 2020

√6ᵗʰ **S63.42** Traumatic rupture of palmar ligament of finger at metacarpophalangeal and interphalangeal joint

√7ᵗʰ **S63.420** Traumatic rupture of palmar ligament of right index finger at metacarpophalangeal and interphalangeal joint

√7ᵗʰ **S63.421** Traumatic rupture of palmar ligament of left index finger at metacarpophalangeal and interphalangeal joint

√7ᵗʰ **S63.422** Traumatic rupture of palmar ligament of right middle finger at metacarpophalangeal and interphalangeal joint

√7ᵗʰ **S63.423** Traumatic rupture of palmar ligament of left middle finger at metacarpophalangeal and interphalangeal joint

√7ᵗʰ **S63.424** Traumatic rupture of palmar ligament of right ring finger at metacarpophalangeal and interphalangeal joint

√7ᵗʰ **S63.425** Traumatic rupture of palmar ligament of left ring finger at metacarpophalangeal and interphalangeal joint

√7ᵗʰ **S63.426** Traumatic rupture of palmar ligament of right little finger at metacarpophalangeal and interphalangeal joint

√7ᵗʰ **S63.427** Traumatic rupture of palmar ligament of left little finger at metacarpophalangeal and interphalangeal joint

√7ᵗʰ **S63.428** Traumatic rupture of palmar ligament of other finger at metacarpophalangeal and interphalangeal joint
  Traumatic rupture of palmar ligament of specified finger with unspecified laterality at metacarpophalangeal and interphalangeal joint

√7ᵗʰ **S63.429** Traumatic rupture of palmar ligament of unspecified finger at metacarpophalangeal and interphalangeal joint

√6ᵗʰ **S63.43** Traumatic rupture of volar plate of finger at metacarpophalangeal and interphalangeal joint

√7ᵗʰ **S63.430** Traumatic rupture of volar plate of right index finger at metacarpophalangeal and interphalangeal joint

√7ᵗʰ **S63.431** Traumatic rupture of volar plate of left index finger at metacarpophalangeal and interphalangeal joint

√7ᵗʰ **S63.432** Traumatic rupture of volar plate of right middle finger at metacarpophalangeal and interphalangeal joint

√7ᵗʰ **S63.433** Traumatic rupture of volar plate of left middle finger at metacarpophalangeal and interphalangeal joint

√7ᵗʰ **S63.434** Traumatic rupture of volar plate of right ring finger at metacarpophalangeal and interphalangeal joint

√7ᵗʰ **S63.435** Traumatic rupture of volar plate of left ring finger at metacarpophalangeal and interphalangeal joint

√7ᵗʰ **S63.436** Traumatic rupture of volar plate of right little finger at metacarpophalangeal and interphalangeal joint

√7ᵗʰ **S63.437** Traumatic rupture of volar plate of left little finger at metacarpophalangeal and interphalangeal joint

√7ᵗʰ **S63.438** Traumatic rupture of volar plate of other finger at metacarpophalangeal and interphalangeal joint
  Traumatic rupture of volar plate of specified finger with unspecified laterality at metacarpophalangeal and interphalangeal joint

√7ᵗʰ **S63.439** Traumatic rupture of volar plate of unspecified finger at metacarpophalangeal and interphalangeal joint

√6ᵗʰ **S63.49** Traumatic rupture of other ligament of finger at metacarpophalangeal and interphalangeal joint

√7ᵗʰ **S63.490** Traumatic rupture of other ligament of right index finger at metacarpophalangeal and interphalangeal joint

√7ᵗʰ **S63.491** Traumatic rupture of other ligament of left index finger at metacarpophalangeal and interphalangeal joint

√7ᵗʰ **S63.492** Traumatic rupture of other ligament of right middle finger at metacarpophalangeal and interphalangeal joint

√7ᵗʰ **S63.493** Traumatic rupture of other ligament of left middle finger at metacarpophalangeal and interphalangeal joint

√7ᵗʰ **S63.494** Traumatic rupture of other ligament of right ring finger at metacarpophalangeal and interphalangeal joint

√7ᵗʰ **S63.495** Traumatic rupture of other ligament of left ring finger at metacarpophalangeal and interphalangeal joint

√7ᵗʰ **S63.496** Traumatic rupture of other ligament of right little finger at metacarpophalangeal and interphalangeal joint

√7ᵗʰ **S63.497** Traumatic rupture of other ligament of left little finger at metacarpophalangeal and interphalangeal joint

√7ᵗʰ **S63.498** Traumatic rupture of other ligament of other finger at metacarpophalangeal and interphalangeal joint
  Traumatic rupture of ligament of specified finger with unspecified laterality at metacarpophalangeal and interphalangeal joint

√7ᵗʰ **S63.499** Traumatic rupture of other ligament of unspecified finger at metacarpophalangeal and interphalangeal joint

√5ᵗʰ **S63.5** Other and unspecified sprain of wrist

√6ᵗʰ **S63.50** Unspecified sprain of wrist

√7ᵗʰ **S63.501** Unspecified sprain of right wrist

√7ᵗʰ **S63.502** Unspecified sprain of left wrist

√7ᵗʰ **S63.509** Unspecified sprain of unspecified wrist

√6ᵗʰ **S63.51** Sprain of carpal (joint)

√7ᵗʰ **S63.511** Sprain of carpal joint of right wrist

√7ᵗʰ **S63.512** Sprain of carpal joint of left wrist

√7ᵗʰ **S63.519** Sprain of carpal joint of unspecified wrist

√6ᵗʰ **S63.52** Sprain of radiocarpal joint
  EXCLUDES 1 *traumatic rupture of radiocarpal ligament (S63.32-)*

√7ᵗʰ **S63.521** Sprain of radiocarpal joint of right wrist

√7ᵗʰ **S63.522** Sprain of radiocarpal joint of left wrist

√7ᵗʰ **S63.529** Sprain of radiocarpal joint of unspecified wrist

√6ᵗʰ **S63.59** Other specified sprain of wrist

√7ᵗʰ **S63.591** Other specified sprain of right wrist

√7ᵗʰ **S63.592** Other specified sprain of left wrist

√7ᵗʰ **S63.599** Other specified sprain of unspecified wrist

√5ᵗʰ **S63.6** Other and unspecified sprain of finger(s)
  EXCLUDES 1 *traumatic rupture of ligament of finger at metacarpophalangeal and interphalangeal joint(s) (S63.4-)*

√6ᵗʰ **S63.60** Unspecified sprain of thumb

√7ᵗʰ **S63.601** Unspecified sprain of right thumb

√7ᵗʰ **S63.602** Unspecified sprain of left thumb

√7ᵗʰ **S63.609** Unspecified sprain of unspecified thumb

√6ᵗʰ **S63.61** Unspecified sprain of other and unspecified finger(s)

√7ᵗʰ **S63.610** Unspecified sprain of right index finger

√7ᵗʰ **S63.611** Unspecified sprain of left index finger

√7ᵗʰ **S63.612** Unspecified sprain of right middle finger

√7ᵗʰ **S63.613** Unspecified sprain of left middle finger

√7ᵗʰ **S63.614** Unspecified sprain of right ring finger

√7ᵗʰ **S63.615** Unspecified sprain of left ring finger

√7ᵗʰ **S63.616** Unspecified sprain of right little finger

√7ᵗʰ **S63.617** Unspecified sprain of left little finger

√7ᵗʰ **S63.618 Unspecified sprain of other finger**
Unspecified sprain of specified finger with unspecified laterality

√7ᵗʰ **S63.619 Unspecified sprain of unspecified finger**

√6ᵗʰ **S63.62 Sprain of** interphalangeal joint of thumb

√7ᵗʰ **S63.621 Sprain of interphalangeal joint of** right **thumb**

√7ᵗʰ **S63.622 Sprain of interphalangeal joint of** left **thumb**

√7ᵗʰ **S63.629 Sprain of interphalangeal joint of unspecified thumb**

√6ᵗʰ **S63.63 Sprain of** interphalangeal joint **of other and unspecified** finger(s)

√7ᵗʰ **S63.630 Sprain of interphalangeal joint of** right index **finger**

√7ᵗʰ **S63.631 Sprain of interphalangeal joint of** left index **finger**

√7ᵗʰ **S63.632 Sprain of interphalangeal joint of** right middle **finger**

√7ᵗʰ **S63.633 Sprain of interphalangeal joint of** left middle **finger**

√7ᵗʰ **S63.634 Sprain of interphalangeal joint of** right ring **finger**

√7ᵗʰ **S63.635 Sprain of interphalangeal joint of** left ring **finger**

√7ᵗʰ **S63.636 Sprain of interphalangeal joint of** right little **finger**

√7ᵗʰ **S63.637 Sprain of interphalangeal joint of** left little **finger**

√7ᵗʰ **S63.638 Sprain of interphalangeal joint of other finger**

√7ᵗʰ **S63.639 Sprain of interphalangeal joint of unspecified finger**

√6ᵗʰ **S63.64 Sprain of** metacarpophalangeal joint of thumb

√7ᵗʰ **S63.641 Sprain of metacarpophalangeal joint of** right **thumb**

√7ᵗʰ **S63.642 Sprain of metacarpophalangeal joint of** left **thumb**

√7ᵗʰ **S63.649 Sprain of metacarpophalangeal joint of unspecified thumb**

√6ᵗʰ **S63.65 Sprain of** metacarpophalangeal joint **of other and unspecified** finger(s)

√7ᵗʰ **S63.650 Sprain of metacarpophalangeal joint of** right index **finger**

√7ᵗʰ **S63.651 Sprain of metacarpophalangeal joint of** left index **finger**

√7ᵗʰ **S63.652 Sprain of metacarpophalangeal joint of** right middle **finger**

√7ᵗʰ **S63.653 Sprain of metacarpophalangeal joint of** left middle **finger**

√7ᵗʰ **S63.654 Sprain of metacarpophalangeal joint of** right ring **finger**

√7ᵗʰ **S63.655 Sprain of metacarpophalangeal joint of** left ring **finger**

√7ᵗʰ **S63.656 Sprain of metacarpophalangeal joint of** right little **finger**

√7ᵗʰ **S63.657 Sprain of metacarpophalangeal joint of** left little **finger**

√7ᵗʰ **S63.658 Sprain of metacarpophalangeal joint of other finger**
Sprain of metacarpophalangeal joint of specified finger with unspecified laterality

√7ᵗʰ **S63.659 Sprain of metacarpophalangeal joint of unspecified finger**

√6ᵗʰ **S63.68 Other sprain of** thumb

√7ᵗʰ **S63.681 Other sprain of** right **thumb**

√7ᵗʰ **S63.682 Other sprain of** left **thumb**

√7ᵗʰ **S63.689 Other sprain of unspecified thumb**

√6ᵗʰ **S63.69 Other sprain of other and unspecified** finger(s)

√7ᵗʰ **S63.690 Other sprain of** right index **finger**

√7ᵗʰ **S63.691 Other sprain of** left index **finger**

√7ᵗʰ **S63.692 Other sprain of** right middle **finger**

√7ᵗʰ **S63.693 Other sprain of** left middle **finger**

√7ᵗʰ **S63.694 Other sprain of** right ring **finger**

√7ᵗʰ **S63.695 Other sprain of** left ring **finger**

√7ᵗʰ **S63.696 Other sprain of** right little **finger**

√7ᵗʰ **S63.697 Other sprain of** left little **finger**

√7ᵗʰ **S63.698 Other sprain of other finger**
Other sprain of specified finger with unspecified laterality

√7ᵗʰ **S63.699 Other sprain of unspecified finger**

√5ᵗʰ **S63.8 Sprain of other part of wrist and hand**

√6ᵗʰ **S63.8X Sprain of other part of wrist and hand**

√7ᵗʰ **S63.8X1 Sprain of other part of** right **wrist and hand**

√7ᵗʰ **S63.8X2 Sprain of other part of** left **wrist and hand**

√7ᵗʰ **S63.8X9 Sprain of other part of unspecified wrist and hand**

√5ᵗʰ **S63.9 Sprain of unspecified part of wrist and hand**

√x7ᵗʰ **S63.90 Sprain of unspecified part of unspecified wrist and hand**

√x7ᵗʰ **S63.91 Sprain of unspecified part of** right **wrist and hand**

√x7ᵗʰ **S63.92 Sprain of unspecified part of** left **wrist and hand**

√4ᵗʰ **S64 Injury of nerves at wrist and hand level**

Code also any associated open wound (S61.-)

The appropriate 7th character is to be added to each code from category S64.
A   initial encounter
D   subsequent encounter
S   sequela

√5ᵗʰ **S64.0 Injury of** ulnar **nerve at wrist and hand level**

√x7ᵗʰ **S64.00 Injury of ulnar nerve at wrist and hand level of unspecified arm**

√x7ᵗʰ **S64.01 Injury of ulnar nerve at wrist and hand level of** right **arm**

√x7ᵗʰ **S64.02 Injury of ulnar nerve at wrist and hand level of** left **arm**

√5ᵗʰ **S64.1 Injury of** median **nerve at wrist and hand level**

√x7ᵗʰ **S64.10 Injury of median nerve at wrist and hand level of unspecified arm**

√x7ᵗʰ **S64.11 Injury of median nerve at wrist and hand level of** right **arm**

√x7ᵗʰ **S64.12 Injury of median nerve at wrist and hand level of** left **arm**

√5ᵗʰ **S64.2 Injury of** radial **nerve at wrist and hand level**

√x7ᵗʰ **S64.20 Injury of radial nerve at wrist and hand level of unspecified arm**

√x7ᵗʰ **S64.21 Injury of radial nerve at wrist and hand level of** right **arm**

√x7ᵗʰ **S64.22 Injury of radial nerve at wrist and hand level of** left **arm**

√5ᵗʰ **S64.3 Injury of** digital nerve **of** thumb

√x7ᵗʰ **S64.30 Injury of digital nerve of unspecified thumb**

√x7ᵗʰ **S64.31 Injury of digital nerve of** right **thumb**

√x7ᵗʰ **S64.32 Injury of digital nerve of** left **thumb**

√5ᵗʰ **S64.4 Injury of** digital nerve **of other and unspecified** finger

√x7ᵗʰ **S64.40 Injury of digital nerve of unspecified finger**

√6ᵗʰ **S64.49 Injury of digital nerve of other finger**

√7ᵗʰ **S64.490 Injury of digital nerve of** right index **finger**

√7ᵗʰ **S64.491 Injury of digital nerve of** left index **finger**

√7ᵗʰ **S64.492 Injury of digital nerve of** right middle **finger**

√7ᵗʰ **S64.493 Injury of digital nerve of** left middle **finger**

√7ᵗʰ **S64.494 Injury of digital nerve of** right ring **finger**

√7ᵗʰ **S64.495 Injury of digital nerve of** left ring **finger**

√7ᵗʰ **S64.496 Injury of digital nerve of** right little **finger**

√7ᵗʰ **S64.497 Injury of digital nerve of** left little **finger**

√7ᵗʰ **S64.498 Injury of digital nerve of other finger**
Injury of digital nerve of specified finger with unspecified laterality

√5ᵗʰ **S64.8 Injury of other nerves at wrist and hand level**

√6ᵗʰ **S64.8X Injury of other nerves at wrist and hand level**

√7ᵗʰ **S64.8X1 Injury of other nerves at wrist and hand level of** right **arm**

√7ᵗʰ **S64.8X2 Injury of other nerves at wrist and hand level of** left **arm**

√7ᵗʰ **S64.8X9 Injury of other nerves at wrist and hand level of unspecified arm**

N Newborn: 0   **P** Pediatric: 0-17   **M** Maternity: 12-55   **A** Adult: 15-124   **CH** Comorbidity High   **CL** Comorbidity Low   **NCDx** Noncancer Dx   **PDx** Primary Dx

1024

ICD-10-CM 2020

√5ᵗʰ **S64.9 Injury of unspecified nerve at wrist and hand level**

√x7ᵗʰ **S64.90 Injury of unspecified nerve at wrist and hand level of unspecified arm**

√x7ᵗʰ **S64.91 Injury of unspecified nerve at wrist and hand level of right arm**

√x7ᵗʰ **S64.92 Injury of unspecified nerve at wrist and hand level of left arm**

√4ᵗʰ **S65 Injury of blood vessels at wrist and hand level**

Code also any associated open wound (S61.-)

The appropriate 7th character is to be added to each code from category S65.
A   initial encounter
D   subsequent encounter
S   sequela

√5ᵗʰ **S65.0 Injury of ulnar artery at wrist and hand level**

√6ᵗʰ **S65.00 Unspecified injury of ulnar artery at wrist and hand level**

√7ᵗʰ **S65.001 Unspecified injury of ulnar artery at wrist and hand level of right arm**

√7ᵗʰ **S65.002 Unspecified injury of ulnar artery at wrist and hand level of left arm**

√7ᵗʰ **S65.009 Unspecified injury of ulnar artery at wrist and hand level of unspecified arm**

√6ᵗʰ **S65.01 Laceration of ulnar artery at wrist and hand level**

√7ᵗʰ **S65.011 Laceration of ulnar artery at wrist and hand level of right arm**

√7ᵗʰ **S65.012 Laceration of ulnar artery at wrist and hand level of left arm**

√7ᵗʰ **S65.019 Laceration of ulnar artery at wrist and hand level of unspecified arm**

√6ᵗʰ **S65.09 Other specified injury of ulnar artery at wrist and hand level**

√7ᵗʰ **S65.091 Other specified injury of ulnar artery at wrist and hand level of right arm**

√7ᵗʰ **S65.092 Other specified injury of ulnar artery at wrist and hand level of left arm**

√7ᵗʰ **S65.099 Other specified injury of ulnar artery at wrist and hand level of unspecified arm**

√5ᵗʰ **S65.1 Injury of radial artery at wrist and hand level**

√6ᵗʰ **S65.10 Unspecified injury of radial artery at wrist and hand level**

√7ᵗʰ **S65.101 Unspecified injury of radial artery at wrist and hand level of right arm**

√7ᵗʰ **S65.102 Unspecified injury of radial artery at wrist and hand level of left arm**

√7ᵗʰ **S65.109 Unspecified injury of radial artery at wrist and hand level of unspecified arm**

√6ᵗʰ **S65.11 Laceration of radial artery at wrist and hand level**

√7ᵗʰ **S65.111 Laceration of radial artery at wrist and hand level of right arm**

√7ᵗʰ **S65.112 Laceration of radial artery at wrist and hand level of left arm**

√7ᵗʰ **S65.119 Laceration of radial artery at wrist and hand level of unspecified arm**

√6ᵗʰ **S65.19 Other specified injury of radial artery at wrist and hand level**

√7ᵗʰ **S65.191 Other specified injury of radial artery at wrist and hand level of right arm**

√7ᵗʰ **S65.192 Other specified injury of radial artery at wrist and hand level of left arm**

√7ᵗʰ **S65.199 Other specified injury of radial artery at wrist and hand level of unspecified arm**

√5ᵗʰ **S65.2 Injury of superficial palmar arch**

√6ᵗʰ **S65.20 Unspecified injury of superficial palmar arch**

√7ᵗʰ **S65.201 Unspecified injury of superficial palmar arch of right hand**

√7ᵗʰ **S65.202 Unspecified injury of superficial palmar arch of left hand**

√7ᵗʰ **S65.209 Unspecified injury of superficial palmar arch of unspecified hand**

√6ᵗʰ **S65.21 Laceration of superficial palmar arch**

√7ᵗʰ **S65.211 Laceration of superficial palmar arch of right hand**

√7ᵗʰ **S65.212 Laceration of superficial palmar arch of left hand**

√7ᵗʰ **S65.219 Laceration of superficial palmar arch of unspecified hand**

√6ᵗʰ **S65.29 Other specified injury of superficial palmar arch**

√7ᵗʰ **S65.291 Other specified injury of superficial palmar arch of right hand**

√7ᵗʰ **S65.292 Other specified injury of superficial palmar arch of left hand**

√7ᵗʰ **S65.299 Other specified injury of superficial palmar arch of unspecified hand**

√5ᵗʰ **S65.3 Injury of deep palmar arch**

√6ᵗʰ **S65.30 Unspecified injury of deep palmar arch**

√7ᵗʰ **S65.301 Unspecified injury of deep palmar arch of right hand**

√7ᵗʰ **S65.302 Unspecified injury of deep palmar arch of left hand**

√7ᵗʰ **S65.309 Unspecified injury of deep palmar arch of unspecified hand**

√6ᵗʰ **S65.31 Laceration of deep palmar arch**

√7ᵗʰ **S65.311 Laceration of deep palmar arch of right hand**

√7ᵗʰ **S65.312 Laceration of deep palmar arch of left hand**

√7ᵗʰ **S65.319 Laceration of deep palmar arch of unspecified hand**

√6ᵗʰ **S65.39 Other specified injury of deep palmar arch**

√7ᵗʰ **S65.391 Other specified injury of deep palmar arch of right hand**

√7ᵗʰ **S65.392 Other specified injury of deep palmar arch of left hand**

√7ᵗʰ **S65.399 Other specified injury of deep palmar arch of unspecified hand**

√5ᵗʰ **S65.4 Injury of blood vessel of thumb**

√6ᵗʰ **S65.40 Unspecified injury of blood vessel of thumb**

√7ᵗʰ **S65.401 Unspecified injury of blood vessel of right thumb**

√7ᵗʰ **S65.402 Unspecified injury of blood vessel of left thumb**

√7ᵗʰ **S65.409 Unspecified injury of blood vessel of unspecified thumb**

√6ᵗʰ **S65.41 Laceration of blood vessel of thumb**

√7ᵗʰ **S65.411 Laceration of blood vessel of right thumb**

√7ᵗʰ **S65.412 Laceration of blood vessel of left thumb**

√7ᵗʰ **S65.419 Laceration of blood vessel of unspecified thumb**

√6ᵗʰ **S65.49 Other specified injury of blood vessel of thumb**

√7ᵗʰ **S65.491 Other specified injury of blood vessel of right thumb**

√7ᵗʰ **S65.492 Other specified injury of blood vessel of left thumb**

√7ᵗʰ **S65.499 Other specified injury of blood vessel of unspecified thumb**

√5ᵗʰ **S65.5 Injury of blood vessel of other and unspecified finger**

√6ᵗʰ **S65.50 Unspecified injury of blood vessel of other and unspecified finger**

√7ᵗʰ **S65.500 Unspecified injury of blood vessel of right index finger**

√7ᵗʰ **S65.501 Unspecified injury of blood vessel of left index finger**

√7ᵗʰ **S65.502 Unspecified injury of blood vessel of right middle finger**

√7ᵗʰ **S65.503 Unspecified injury of blood vessel of left middle finger**

√7ᵗʰ **S65.504 Unspecified injury of blood vessel of right ring finger**

√7ᵗʰ **S65.505 Unspecified injury of blood vessel of left ring finger**

√7ᵗʰ **S65.506 Unspecified injury of blood vessel of right little finger**

√7ᵗʰ **S65.507 Unspecified injury of blood vessel of left little finger**

√7ᵗʰ **S65.508 Unspecified injury of blood vessel of other finger**

Unspecified injury of blood vessel of specified finger with unspecified laterality

√7ᵗʰ **S65.509 Unspecified injury of blood vessel of unspecified finger**

√6ᵗʰ **S65.51 Laceration of blood vessel of other and unspecified finger**

√7ᵗʰ **S65.510 Laceration of blood vessel of right index finger**

✓ Additional Character Required   √x7ᵗʰ Placeholder Alert   Manifestation   Unspecified Dx   ►◄ Revised Text   ● New Code   ▲ Revised Title

ICD-10-CM 2020   1025

√7ᵗʰ **S65.511** **Laceration of blood vessel** of left index finger

√7ᵗʰ **S65.512** **Laceration of blood vessel of** right middle finger

√7ᵗʰ **S65.513** **Laceration of blood vessel of** left middle finger

√7ᵗʰ **S65.514** **Laceration of blood vessel of** right ring finger

√7ᵗʰ **S65.515** **Laceration of blood vessel of** left ring finger

√7ᵗʰ **S65.516** **Laceration of blood vessel of** right little finger

√7ᵗʰ **S65.517** **Laceration of blood vessel of** left little finger

√7ᵗʰ **S65.518** **Laceration of blood vessel of other finger**
Laceration of blood vessel of specified finger with unspecified laterality

√7ᵗʰ **S65.519** **Laceration of blood vessel of unspecified finger**

√6ᵗʰ **S65.59** **Other specified injury of blood vessel of other and unspecified finger**

√7ᵗʰ **S65.590** **Other specified injury of blood vessel of** right index **finger**

√7ᵗʰ **S65.591** **Other specified injury of blood vessel of** left index **finger**

√7ᵗʰ **S65.592** **Other specified injury of blood vessel of** right middle **finger**

√7ᵗʰ **S65.593** **Other specified injury of blood vessel of** left middle **finger**

√7ᵗʰ **S65.594** **Other specified injury of blood vessel of** right ring **finger**

√7ᵗʰ **S65.595** **Other specified injury of blood vessel of** left ring **finger**

√7ᵗʰ **S65.596** **Other specified injury of blood vessel of** right little **finger**

√7ᵗʰ **S65.597** **Other specified injury of blood vessel of** left little **finger**

√7ᵗʰ **S65.598** **Other specified injury of blood vessel of other finger**
Other specified injury of blood vessel of specified finger with unspecified laterality

√7ᵗʰ **S65.599** **Other specified injury of blood vessel of unspecified finger**

√5ᵗʰ **S65.8** **Injury of other blood vessels at** wrist and hand level

√6ᵗʰ **S65.80** **Unspecified injury of other blood vessels at wrist and hand level**

√7ᵗʰ **S65.801** **Unspecified injury of other blood vessels at wrist and hand level of right arm**

√7ᵗʰ **S65.802** **Unspecified injury of other blood vessels at wrist and hand level of left arm**

√7ᵗʰ **S65.809** **Unspecified injury of other blood vessels at wrist and hand level of unspecified arm**

√6ᵗʰ **S65.81** **Laceration of other blood vessels at wrist and hand level**

√7ᵗʰ **S65.811** **Laceration of other blood vessels at wrist and hand level of** right arm

√7ᵗʰ **S65.812** **Laceration of other blood vessels at wrist and hand level of** left arm

√7ᵗʰ **S65.819** **Laceration of other blood vessels at wrist and hand level of unspecified arm**

√6ᵗʰ **S65.89** **Other specified injury of other blood vessels at wrist and hand level**

√7ᵗʰ **S65.891** **Other specified injury of other blood vessels at wrist and hand level of** right arm

√7ᵗʰ **S65.892** **Other specified injury of other blood vessels at wrist and hand level of** left arm

√7ᵗʰ **S65.899** **Other specified injury of other blood vessels at wrist and hand level of unspecified arm**

√5ᵗʰ **S65.9** **Injury of unspecified blood vessel at** wrist and hand level

√6ᵗʰ **S65.90** **Unspecified injury of unspecified blood vessel at wrist and hand level**

√7ᵗʰ **S65.901** **Unspecified injury of unspecified blood vessel at wrist and hand level of** right arm

√7ᵗʰ **S65.902** **Unspecified injury of unspecified blood vessel at wrist and hand level of** left arm

√7ᵗʰ **S65.909** **Unspecified injury of unspecified blood vessel at wrist and hand level of unspecified arm**

√6ᵗʰ **S65.91** **Laceration** of unspecified blood vessel at wrist and hand level

√7ᵗʰ **S65.911** **Laceration of unspecified blood vessel at wrist and hand level of** right arm

√7ᵗʰ **S65.912** **Laceration of unspecified blood vessel at wrist and hand level of** left arm

√7ᵗʰ **S65.919** **Laceration of unspecified blood vessel at wrist and hand level of unspecified arm**

√6ᵗʰ **S65.99** **Other specified injury of unspecified blood vessel at wrist and hand level**

√7ᵗʰ **S65.991** **Other specified injury of unspecified blood vessel at wrist and hand of** right arm

√7ᵗʰ **S65.992** **Other specified injury of unspecified blood vessel at wrist and hand of** left arm

√7ᵗʰ **S65.999** **Other specified injury of unspecified blood vessel at wrist and hand of unspecified arm**

√4ᵗʰ **S66** **Injury of muscle, fascia and tendon at wrist and hand level**
Code also any associated open wound (S61.-)
EXCLUDES 2   *sprain of joints and ligaments of wrist and hand (S63.-)*
TIP: Refer to the Muscle/Tendon table at the beginning of this chapter.

The appropriate 7th character is to be added to each code from category S66.
A   initial encounter
D   subsequent encounter
S   sequela

√5ᵗʰ **S66.0** **Injury of** long flexor **muscle, fascia and tendon of** thumb **at wrist and hand level**

√6ᵗʰ **S66.00** **Unspecified injury of long flexor muscle, fascia and tendon of thumb at wrist and hand level**

√7ᵗʰ **S66.001** **Unspecified injury of long flexor muscle, fascia and tendon of** right **thumb at wrist and hand level**

√7ᵗʰ **S66.002** **Unspecified injury of long flexor muscle, fascia and tendon of** left **thumb at wrist and hand level**

√7ᵗʰ **S66.009** **Unspecified injury of long flexor muscle, fascia and tendon of unspecified thumb at wrist and hand level**

√6ᵗʰ **S66.01** **Strain** of long flexor muscle, fascia and tendon of thumb at wrist and hand level

√7ᵗʰ **S66.011** **Strain of long flexor muscle, fascia and tendon of** right **thumb at wrist and hand level**

√7ᵗʰ **S66.012** **Strain of long flexor muscle, fascia and tendon of** left **thumb at wrist and hand level**

√7ᵗʰ **S66.019** **Strain of long flexor muscle, fascia and tendon of unspecified thumb at wrist and hand level**

√6ᵗʰ **S66.02** **Laceration** of long flexor muscle, fascia and tendon of thumb at wrist and hand level

√7ᵗʰ **S66.021** **Laceration of long flexor muscle, fascia and tendon of** right **thumb at wrist and hand level**

√7ᵗʰ **S66.022** **Laceration of long flexor muscle, fascia and tendon of** left **thumb at wrist and hand level**

√7ᵗʰ **S66.029** **Laceration of long flexor muscle, fascia and tendon of unspecified thumb at wrist and hand level**

√6ᵗʰ **S66.09** **Other specified injury of long flexor muscle, fascia and tendon of thumb at wrist and hand level**

√7ᵗʰ **S66.091** **Other specified injury of long flexor muscle, fascia and tendon of** right **thumb at wrist and hand level**

√7ᵗʰ **S66.092** **Other specified injury of long flexor muscle, fascia and tendon of** left **thumb at wrist and hand level**

√7ᵗʰ **S66.099** **Other specified injury of long flexor muscle, fascia and tendon of unspecified thumb at wrist and hand level**

√5ᵗʰ **S66.1** **Injury of** flexor **muscle, fascia and tendon of other and unspecified** finger **at wrist and hand level**
EXCLUDES 2   *injury of long flexor muscle, fascia and tendon of thumb at wrist and hand level (S66.0-)*

√6ᵗʰ **S66.10** **Unspecified injury of flexor muscle, fascia and tendon of other and unspecified finger at wrist and hand level**

√7ᵗʰ **S66.100** **Unspecified injury of flexor muscle, fascia and tendon of** right index **finger at wrist and hand level**

N Newborn: 0   P Pediatric: 0-17   M Maternity: 12-55   A Adult: 15-124   CH Comorbidity High   CL Comorbidity Low   NCDx Noncancer Dx   PDx Primary Dx

1026   ICD-10-CM 2020

√7ᵗʰ **S66.101** Unspecified injury of flexor muscle, fascia and tendon of left index finger at wrist and hand level

√7ᵗʰ **S66.102** Unspecified injury of flexor muscle, fascia and tendon of right middle finger at wrist and hand level

√7ᵗʰ **S66.103** Unspecified injury of flexor muscle, fascia and tendon of left middle finger at wrist and hand level

√7ᵗʰ **S66.104** Unspecified injury of flexor muscle, fascia and tendon of right ring finger at wrist and hand level

√7ᵗʰ **S66.105** Unspecified injury of flexor muscle, fascia and tendon of left ring finger at wrist and hand level

√7ᵗʰ **S66.106** Unspecified injury of flexor muscle, fascia and tendon of right little finger at wrist and hand level

√7ᵗʰ **S66.107** Unspecified injury of flexor muscle, fascia and tendon of left little finger at wrist and hand level

√7ᵗʰ **S66.108** Unspecified injury of flexor muscle, fascia and tendon of other finger at wrist and hand level

    Unspecified injury of flexor muscle, fascia and tendon of specified finger with unspecified laterality at wrist and hand level

√7ᵗʰ **S66.109** Unspecified injury of flexor muscle, fascia and tendon of unspecified finger at wrist and hand level

√6ᵗʰ **S66.11** Strain of flexor muscle, fascia and tendon of other and unspecified finger at wrist and hand level

√7ᵗʰ **S66.110** Strain of flexor muscle, fascia and tendon of right index finger at wrist and hand level

√7ᵗʰ **S66.111** Strain of flexor muscle, fascia and tendon of left index finger at wrist and hand level

√7ᵗʰ **S66.112** Strain of flexor muscle, fascia and tendon of right middle finger at wrist and hand level

√7ᵗʰ **S66.113** Strain of flexor muscle, fascia and tendon of left middle finger at wrist and hand level

√7ᵗʰ **S66.114** Strain of flexor muscle, fascia and tendon of right ring finger at wrist and hand level

√7ᵗʰ **S66.115** Strain of flexor muscle, fascia and tendon of left ring finger at wrist and hand level

√7ᵗʰ **S66.116** Strain of flexor muscle, fascia and tendon of right little finger at wrist and hand level

√7ᵗʰ **S66.117** Strain of flexor muscle, fascia and tendon of left little finger at wrist and hand level

√7ᵗʰ **S66.118** Strain of flexor muscle, fascia and tendon of other finger at wrist and hand level

    Strain of flexor muscle, fascia and tendon of specified finger with unspecified laterality at wrist and hand level

√7ᵗʰ **S66.119** Strain of flexor muscle, fascia and tendon of unspecified finger at wrist and hand level

√6ᵗʰ **S66.12** Laceration of flexor muscle, fascia and tendon of other and unspecified finger at wrist and hand level

√7ᵗʰ **S66.120** Laceration of flexor muscle, fascia and tendon of right index finger at wrist and hand level

√7ᵗʰ **S66.121** Laceration of flexor muscle, fascia and tendon of left index finger at wrist and hand level

√7ᵗʰ **S66.122** Laceration of flexor muscle, fascia and tendon of right middle finger at wrist and hand level

√7ᵗʰ **S66.123** Laceration of flexor muscle, fascia and tendon of left middle finger at wrist and hand level

√7ᵗʰ **S66.124** Laceration of flexor muscle, fascia and tendon of right ring finger at wrist and hand level

√7ᵗʰ **S66.125** Laceration of flexor muscle, fascia and tendon of left ring finger at wrist and hand level

√7ᵗʰ **S66.126** Laceration of flexor muscle, fascia and tendon of right little finger at wrist and hand level

√7ᵗʰ **S66.127** Laceration of flexor muscle, fascia and tendon of left little finger at wrist and hand level

√7ᵗʰ **S66.128** Laceration of flexor muscle, fascia and tendon of other finger at wrist and hand level

    Laceration of flexor muscle, fascia and tendon of specified finger with unspecified laterality at wrist and hand level

√7ᵗʰ **S66.129** Laceration of flexor muscle, fascia and tendon of unspecified finger at wrist and hand level

√6ᵗʰ **S66.19** Other injury of flexor muscle, fascia and tendon of other and unspecified finger at wrist and hand level

√7ᵗʰ **S66.190** Other injury of flexor muscle, fascia and tendon of right index finger at wrist and hand level

√7ᵗʰ **S66.191** Other injury of flexor muscle, fascia and tendon of left index finger at wrist and hand level

√7ᵗʰ **S66.192** Other injury of flexor muscle, fascia and tendon of right middle finger at wrist and hand level

√7ᵗʰ **S66.193** Other injury of flexor muscle, fascia and tendon of left middle finger at wrist and hand level

√7ᵗʰ **S66.194** Other injury of flexor muscle, fascia and tendon of right ring finger at wrist and hand level

√7ᵗʰ **S66.195** Other injury of flexor muscle, fascia and tendon of left ring finger at wrist and hand level

√7ᵗʰ **S66.196** Other injury of flexor muscle, fascia and tendon of right little finger at wrist and hand level

√7ᵗʰ **S66.197** Other injury of flexor muscle, fascia and tendon of left little finger at wrist and hand level

√7ᵗʰ **S66.198** Other injury of flexor muscle, fascia and tendon of other finger at wrist and hand level

    Other injury of flexor muscle, fascia and tendon of specified finger with unspecified laterality at wrist and hand level

√7ᵗʰ **S66.199** Other injury of flexor muscle, fascia and tendon of unspecified finger at wrist and hand level

√5ᵗʰ **S66.2** Injury of extensor muscle, fascia and tendon of thumb at wrist and hand level

√6ᵗʰ **S66.20** Unspecified injury of extensor muscle, fascia and tendon of thumb at wrist and hand level

√7ᵗʰ **S66.201** Unspecified injury of extensor muscle, fascia and tendon of right thumb at wrist and hand level

√7ᵗʰ **S66.202** Unspecified injury of extensor muscle, fascia and tendon of left thumb at wrist and hand level

√7ᵗʰ **S66.209** Unspecified injury of extensor muscle, fascia and tendon of unspecified thumb at wrist and hand level

√6ᵗʰ **S66.21** Strain of extensor muscle, fascia and tendon of thumb at wrist and hand level

√7ᵗʰ **S66.211** Strain of extensor muscle, fascia and tendon of right thumb at wrist and hand level

√7ᵗʰ **S66.212** Strain of extensor muscle, fascia and tendon of left thumb at wrist and hand level

√7ᵗʰ **S66.219** Strain of extensor muscle, fascia and tendon of unspecified thumb at wrist and hand level

√6ᵗʰ **S66.22** Laceration of extensor muscle, fascia and tendon of thumb at wrist and hand level

√7ᵗʰ **S66.221** Laceration of extensor muscle, fascia and tendon of right thumb at wrist and hand level

√7ᵗʰ **S66.222** Laceration of extensor muscle, fascia and tendon of left thumb at wrist and hand level

√7ᵗʰ **S66.229** Laceration of extensor muscle, fascia and tendon of unspecified thumb at wrist and hand level

☑ Additional Character Required   √x7ᵗʰ Placeholder Alert   Manifestation   Unspecified Dx   ▶◀ Revised Text   ● New Code   ▲ Revised Title

ICD-10-CM 2020   1027

√6ᵗʰ **S66.29** **Other specified injury of extensor muscle, fascia and tendon of thumb at wrist and hand level**

√7ᵗʰ **S66.291** Other specified injury of extensor muscle, fascia and tendon of right thumb at wrist and hand level

√7ᵗʰ **S66.292** Other specified injury of extensor muscle, fascia and tendon of left thumb at wrist and hand level

√7ᵗʰ **S66.299** Other specified injury of extensor muscle, fascia and tendon of unspecified thumb at wrist and hand level

√5ᵗʰ **S66.3** **Injury of extensor muscle, fascia and tendon of other and unspecified finger at wrist and hand level**

> EXCLUDES 2   *injury of extensor muscle, fascia and tendon of thumb at wrist and hand level (S66.2-)*

√6ᵗʰ **S66.30** **Unspecified injury of extensor muscle, fascia and tendon of other and unspecified finger at wrist and hand level**

√7ᵗʰ **S66.300** Unspecified injury of extensor muscle, fascia and tendon of right index finger at wrist and hand level

√7ᵗʰ **S66.301** Unspecified injury of extensor muscle, fascia and tendon of left index finger at wrist and hand level

√7ᵗʰ **S66.302** Unspecified injury of extensor muscle, fascia and tendon of right middle finger at wrist and hand level

√7ᵗʰ **S66.303** Unspecified injury of extensor muscle, fascia and tendon of left middle finger at wrist and hand level

√7ᵗʰ **S66.304** Unspecified injury of extensor muscle, fascia and tendon of right ring finger at wrist and hand level

√7ᵗʰ **S66.305** Unspecified injury of extensor muscle, fascia and tendon of left ring finger at wrist and hand level

√7ᵗʰ **S66.306** Unspecified injury of extensor muscle, fascia and tendon of right little finger at wrist and hand level

√7ᵗʰ **S66.307** Unspecified injury of extensor muscle, fascia and tendon of left little finger at wrist and hand level

√7ᵗʰ **S66.308** Unspecified injury of extensor muscle, fascia and tendon of other finger at wrist and hand level

> Unspecified injury of extensor muscle, fascia and tendon of specified finger with unspecified laterality at wrist and hand level

√7ᵗʰ **S66.309** Unspecified injury of extensor muscle, fascia and tendon of unspecified finger at wrist and hand level

√6ᵗʰ **S66.31** **Strain of extensor muscle, fascia and tendon of other and unspecified finger at wrist and hand level**

√7ᵗʰ **S66.310** Strain of extensor muscle, fascia and tendon of right index finger at wrist and hand level

√7ᵗʰ **S66.311** Strain of extensor muscle, fascia and tendon of left index finger at wrist and hand level

√7ᵗʰ **S66.312** Strain of extensor muscle, fascia and tendon of right middle finger at wrist and hand level

√7ᵗʰ **S66.313** Strain of extensor muscle, fascia and tendon of left middle finger at wrist and hand level

√7ᵗʰ **S66.314** Strain of extensor muscle, fascia and tendon of right ring finger at wrist and hand level

√7ᵗʰ **S66.315** Strain of extensor muscle, fascia and tendon of left ring finger at wrist and hand level

√7ᵗʰ **S66.316** Strain of extensor muscle, fascia and tendon of right little finger at wrist and hand level

√7ᵗʰ **S66.317** Strain of extensor muscle, fascia and tendon of left little finger at wrist and hand level

√7ᵗʰ **S66.318** Strain of extensor muscle, fascia and tendon of other finger at wrist and hand level

> Strain of extensor muscle, fascia and tendon of specified finger with unspecified laterality at wrist and hand level

√7ᵗʰ **S66.319** Strain of extensor muscle, fascia and tendon of unspecified finger at wrist and hand level

√6ᵗʰ **S66.32** **Laceration of extensor muscle, fascia and tendon of other and unspecified finger at wrist and hand level**

√7ᵗʰ **S66.320** Laceration of extensor muscle, fascia and tendon of right index finger at wrist and hand level

√7ᵗʰ **S66.321** Laceration of extensor muscle, fascia and tendon of left index finger at wrist and hand level

√7ᵗʰ **S66.322** Laceration of extensor muscle, fascia and tendon of right middle finger at wrist and hand level

√7ᵗʰ **S66.323** Laceration of extensor muscle, fascia and tendon of left middle finger at wrist and hand level

√7ᵗʰ **S66.324** Laceration of extensor muscle, fascia and tendon of right ring finger at wrist and hand level

√7ᵗʰ **S66.325** Laceration of extensor muscle, fascia and tendon of left ring finger at wrist and hand level

√7ᵗʰ **S66.326** Laceration of extensor muscle, fascia and tendon of right little finger at wrist and hand level

√7ᵗʰ **S66.327** Laceration of extensor muscle, fascia and tendon of left little finger at wrist and hand level

√7ᵗʰ **S66.328** Laceration of extensor muscle, fascia and tendon of other finger at wrist and hand level

> Laceration of extensor muscle, fascia and tendon of specified finger with unspecified laterality at wrist and hand level

√7ᵗʰ **S66.329** Laceration of extensor muscle, fascia and tendon of unspecified finger at wrist and hand level

√6ᵗʰ **S66.39** **Other injury of extensor muscle, fascia and tendon of other and unspecified finger at wrist and hand level**

√7ᵗʰ **S66.390** Other injury of extensor muscle, fascia and tendon of right index finger at wrist and hand level

√7ᵗʰ **S66.391** Other injury of extensor muscle, fascia and tendon of left index finger at wrist and hand level

√7ᵗʰ **S66.392** Other injury of extensor muscle, fascia and tendon of right middle finger at wrist and hand level

√7ᵗʰ **S66.393** Other injury of extensor muscle, fascia and tendon of left middle finger at wrist and hand level

√7ᵗʰ **S66.394** Other injury of extensor muscle, fascia and tendon of right ring finger at wrist and hand level

√7ᵗʰ **S66.395** Other injury of extensor muscle, fascia and tendon of left ring finger at wrist and hand level

√7ᵗʰ **S66.396** Other injury of extensor muscle, fascia and tendon of right little finger at wrist and hand level

√7ᵗʰ **S66.397** Other injury of extensor muscle, fascia and tendon of left little finger at wrist and hand level

√7ᵗʰ **S66.398** Other injury of extensor muscle, fascia and tendon of other finger at wrist and hand level

> Other injury of extensor muscle, fascia and tendon of specified finger with unspecified laterality at wrist and hand level

√7ᵗʰ **S66.399** Other injury of extensor muscle, fascia and tendon of unspecified finger at wrist and hand level

✓5th **S66.4 Injury of** intrinsic muscle, fascia and tendon of thumb **at wrist and hand level**

  ✓6th **S66.40 Unspecified injury of intrinsic muscle, fascia and tendon of thumb at wrist and hand level**

    ✓7th **S66.401 Unspecified injury of intrinsic muscle, fascia and tendon of** right **thumb at wrist and hand level**

    ✓7th **S66.402 Unspecified injury of intrinsic muscle, fascia and tendon of** left **thumb at wrist and hand level**

    ✓7th **S66.409 Unspecified injury of intrinsic muscle, fascia and tendon of unspecified thumb at wrist and hand level**

  ✓6th **S66.41 Strain of** intrinsic muscle, fascia and tendon of **thumb at wrist and hand level**

    ✓7th **S66.411 Strain of intrinsic muscle, fascia and tendon of** right **thumb at wrist and hand level**

    ✓7th **S66.412 Strain of intrinsic muscle, fascia and tendon of** left **thumb at wrist and hand level**

    ✓7th **S66.419 Strain of intrinsic muscle, fascia and tendon of unspecified thumb at wrist and hand level**

  ✓6th **S66.42 Laceration of** intrinsic muscle, fascia and tendon of **thumb at wrist and hand level**

    ✓7th **S66.421 Laceration of intrinsic muscle, fascia and tendon of** right **thumb at wrist and hand level**

    ✓7th **S66.422 Laceration of intrinsic muscle, fascia and tendon of** left **thumb at wrist and hand level**

    ✓7th **S66.429 Laceration of intrinsic muscle, fascia and tendon of unspecified thumb at wrist and hand level**

  ✓6th **S66.49 Other specified injury of intrinsic muscle, fascia and tendon of thumb at wrist and hand level**

    ✓7th **S66.491 Other specified injury of intrinsic muscle, fascia and tendon of** right **thumb at wrist and hand level**

    ✓7th **S66.492 Other specified injury of intrinsic muscle, fascia and tendon of** left **thumb at wrist and hand level**

    ✓7th **S66.499 Other specified injury of intrinsic muscle, fascia and tendon of unspecified thumb at wrist and hand level**

✓5th **S66.5 Injury of** intrinsic muscle, fascia and tendon of other and unspecified finger **at wrist and hand level**

    EXCLUDES 2   injury of intrinsic muscle, fascia and tendon of thumb at wrist and hand level (S66.4-)

  ✓6th **S66.50 Unspecified injury of intrinsic muscle, fascia and tendon of other and unspecified finger at wrist and hand level**

    ✓7th **S66.500 Unspecified injury of intrinsic muscle, fascia and tendon of** right index **finger at wrist and hand level**

    ✓7th **S66.501 Unspecified injury of intrinsic muscle, fascia and tendon of** left index **finger at wrist and hand level**

    ✓7th **S66.502 Unspecified injury of intrinsic muscle, fascia and tendon of** right middle **finger at wrist and hand level**

    ✓7th **S66.503 Unspecified injury of intrinsic muscle, fascia and tendon of** left middle **finger at wrist and hand level**

    ✓7th **S66.504 Unspecified injury of intrinsic muscle, fascia and tendon of** right ring **finger at wrist and hand level**

    ✓7th **S66.505 Unspecified injury of intrinsic muscle, fascia and tendon of** left ring **finger at wrist and hand level**

    ✓7th **S66.506 Unspecified injury of intrinsic muscle, fascia and tendon of** right little **finger at wrist and hand level**

    ✓7th **S66.507 Unspecified injury of intrinsic muscle, fascia and tendon of** left little **finger at wrist and hand level**

    ✓7th **S66.508 Unspecified injury of intrinsic muscle, fascia and tendon of other finger at wrist and hand level**

      Unspecified injury of intrinsic muscle, fascia and tendon of specified finger with unspecified laterality at wrist and hand level

    ✓7th **S66.509 Unspecified injury of intrinsic muscle, fascia and tendon of unspecified finger at wrist and hand level**

  ✓6th **S66.51 Strain of** intrinsic muscle, fascia and tendon of other and unspecified finger at wrist and hand level

    ✓7th **S66.510 Strain of intrinsic muscle, fascia and tendon of** right index **finger at wrist and hand level**

    ✓7th **S66.511 Strain of intrinsic muscle, fascia and tendon of** left index **finger at wrist and hand level**

    ✓7th **S66.512 Strain of intrinsic muscle, fascia and tendon of** right middle **finger at wrist and hand level**

    ✓7th **S66.513 Strain of intrinsic muscle, fascia and tendon of** left middle **finger at wrist and hand level**

    ✓7th **S66.514 Strain of intrinsic muscle, fascia and tendon of** right ring **finger at wrist and hand level**

    ✓7th **S66.515 Strain of intrinsic muscle, fascia and tendon of** left ring **finger at wrist and hand level**

    ✓7th **S66.516 Strain of intrinsic muscle, fascia and tendon of** right little **finger at wrist and hand level**

    ✓7th **S66.517 Strain of intrinsic muscle, fascia and tendon of** left little **finger at wrist and hand level**

    ✓7th **S66.518 Strain of intrinsic muscle, fascia and tendon of other finger at wrist and hand level**

      Strain of intrinsic muscle, fascia and tendon of specified finger with unspecified laterality at wrist and hand level

    ✓7th **S66.519 Strain of intrinsic muscle, fascia and tendon of unspecified finger at wrist and hand level**

  ✓6th **S66.52 Laceration of** intrinsic muscle, fascia and tendon of other and unspecified finger at wrist and hand level

    ✓7th **S66.520 Laceration of intrinsic muscle, fascia and tendon of** right index **finger at wrist and hand level**

    ✓7th **S66.521 Laceration of intrinsic muscle, fascia and tendon of** left index **finger at wrist and hand level**

    ✓7th **S66.522 Laceration of intrinsic muscle, fascia and tendon of** right middle **finger at wrist and hand level**

    ✓7th **S66.523 Laceration of intrinsic muscle, fascia and tendon of** left middle **finger at wrist and hand level**

    ✓7th **S66.524 Laceration of intrinsic muscle, fascia and tendon of** right ring **finger at wrist and hand level**

    ✓7th **S66.525 Laceration of intrinsic muscle, fascia and tendon of** left ring **finger at wrist and hand level**

    ✓7th **S66.526 Laceration of intrinsic muscle, fascia and tendon of** right little **finger at wrist and hand level**

    ✓7th **S66.527 Laceration of intrinsic muscle, fascia and tendon of** left little **finger at wrist and hand level**

    ✓7th **S66.528 Laceration of intrinsic muscle, fascia and tendon of other finger at wrist and hand level**

      Laceration of intrinsic muscle, fascia and tendon of specified finger with unspecified laterality at wrist and hand level

    ✓7th **S66.529 Laceration of intrinsic muscle, fascia and tendon of unspecified finger at wrist and hand level**

☑ Additional Character Required   ✓x7th Placeholder Alert   Manifestation   Unspecified Dx   ▶◀ Revised Text   ● New Code   ▲ Revised Title

ICD-10-CM 2020   1029

√6ᵗʰ **S66.59** **Other injury of intrinsic muscle, fascia and tendon of other and unspecified finger at wrist and hand level**

√7ᵗʰ **S66.590** Other injury of intrinsic muscle, fascia and tendon of right index finger at wrist and hand level

√7ᵗʰ **S66.591** Other injury of intrinsic muscle, fascia and tendon of left index finger at wrist and hand level

√7ᵗʰ **S66.592** Other injury of intrinsic muscle, fascia and tendon of right middle finger at wrist and hand level

√7ᵗʰ **S66.593** Other injury of intrinsic muscle, fascia and tendon of left middle finger at wrist and hand level

√7ᵗʰ **S66.594** Other injury of intrinsic muscle, fascia and tendon of right ring finger at wrist and hand level

√7ᵗʰ **S66.595** Other injury of intrinsic muscle, fascia and tendon of left ring finger at wrist and hand level

√7ᵗʰ **S66.596** Other injury of intrinsic muscle, fascia and tendon of right little finger at wrist and hand level

√7ᵗʰ **S66.597** Other injury of intrinsic muscle, fascia and tendon of left little finger at wrist and hand level

√7ᵗʰ **S66.598** Other injury of intrinsic muscle, fascia and tendon of other finger at wrist and hand level

Other injury of intrinsic muscle, fascia and tendon of specified finger with unspecified laterality at wrist and hand level

√7ᵗʰ **S66.599** Other injury of intrinsic muscle, fascia and tendon of unspecified finger at wrist and hand level

√5ᵗʰ **S66.8** **Injury of other specified muscles, fascia and tendons at wrist and hand level**

√6ᵗʰ **S66.80** Unspecified injury of other specified muscles, fascia and tendons at wrist and hand level

√7ᵗʰ **S66.801** Unspecified injury of other specified muscles, fascia and tendons at wrist and hand level, right hand

√7ᵗʰ **S66.802** Unspecified injury of other specified muscles, fascia and tendons at wrist and hand level, left hand

√7ᵗʰ **S66.809** Unspecified injury of other specified muscles, fascia and tendons at wrist and hand level, unspecified hand

√6ᵗʰ **S66.81** Strain of other specified muscles, fascia and tendons at wrist and hand level

√7ᵗʰ **S66.811** Strain of other specified muscles, fascia and tendons at wrist and hand level, right hand

√7ᵗʰ **S66.812** Strain of other specified muscles, fascia and tendons at wrist and hand level, left hand

√7ᵗʰ **S66.819** Strain of other specified muscles, fascia and tendons at wrist and hand level, unspecified hand

√6ᵗʰ **S66.82** Laceration of other specified muscles, fascia and tendons at wrist and hand level

√7ᵗʰ **S66.821** Laceration of other specified muscles, fascia and tendons at wrist and hand level, right hand

√7ᵗʰ **S66.822** Laceration of other specified muscles, fascia and tendons at wrist and hand level, left hand

√7ᵗʰ **S66.829** Laceration of other specified muscles, fascia and tendons at wrist and hand level, unspecified hand

√6ᵗʰ **S66.89** Other injury of other specified muscles, fascia and tendons at wrist and hand level

√7ᵗʰ **S66.891** Other injury of other specified muscles, fascia and tendons at wrist and hand level, right hand

√7ᵗʰ **S66.892** Other injury of other specified muscles, fascia and tendons at wrist and hand level, left hand

√7ᵗʰ **S66.899** Other injury of other specified muscles, fascia and tendons at wrist and hand level, unspecified hand

√5ᵗʰ **S66.9** **Injury of unspecified muscle, fascia and tendon at wrist and hand level**

√6ᵗʰ **S66.90** Unspecified injury of unspecified muscle, fascia and tendon at wrist and hand level

√7ᵗʰ **S66.901** Unspecified injury of unspecified muscle, fascia and tendon at wrist and hand level, right hand

√7ᵗʰ **S66.902** Unspecified injury of unspecified muscle, fascia and tendon at wrist and hand level, left hand

√7ᵗʰ **S66.909** Unspecified injury of unspecified muscle, fascia and tendon at wrist and hand level, unspecified hand

√6ᵗʰ **S66.91** Strain of unspecified muscle, fascia and tendon at wrist and hand level

√7ᵗʰ **S66.911** Strain of unspecified muscle, fascia and tendon at wrist and hand level, right hand

√7ᵗʰ **S66.912** Strain of unspecified muscle, fascia and tendon at wrist and hand level, left hand

√7ᵗʰ **S66.919** Strain of unspecified muscle, fascia and tendon at wrist and hand level, unspecified hand

√6ᵗʰ **S66.92** Laceration of unspecified muscle, fascia and tendon at wrist and hand level

√7ᵗʰ **S66.921** Laceration of unspecified muscle, fascia and tendon at wrist and hand level, right hand

√7ᵗʰ **S66.922** Laceration of unspecified muscle, fascia and tendon at wrist and hand level, left hand

√7ᵗʰ **S66.929** Laceration of unspecified muscle, fascia and tendon at wrist and hand level, unspecified hand

√6ᵗʰ **S66.99** Other injury of unspecified muscle, fascia and tendon at wrist and hand level

√7ᵗʰ **S66.991** Other injury of unspecified muscle, fascia and tendon at wrist and hand level, right hand

√7ᵗʰ **S66.992** Other injury of unspecified muscle, fascia and tendon at wrist and hand level, left hand

√7ᵗʰ **S66.999** Other injury of unspecified muscle, fascia and tendon at wrist and hand level, unspecified hand

√4ᵗʰ **S67** **Crushing injury of wrist, hand and fingers**

Use additional code for all associated injuries, such as:
  fracture of wrist and hand (S62.-)
  open wound of wrist and hand (S61.-)

The appropriate 7th character is to be added to each code from category S67.
A   initial encounter
D   subsequent encounter
S   sequela

√5ᵗʰ **S67.0** **Crushing injury of thumb**

√x7ᵗʰ **S67.00** Crushing injury of unspecified thumb

√x7ᵗʰ **S67.01** Crushing injury of right thumb

√x7ᵗʰ **S67.02** Crushing injury of left thumb

√5ᵗʰ **S67.1** **Crushing injury of other and unspecified finger(s)**

EXCLUDES 2   crushing injury of thumb (S67.0-)

√x7ᵗʰ **S67.10** Crushing injury of unspecified finger(s)

√6ᵗʰ **S67.19** Crushing injury of other finger(s)

√7ᵗʰ **S67.190** Crushing injury of right index finger

√7ᵗʰ **S67.191** Crushing injury of left index finger

√7ᵗʰ **S67.192** Crushing injury of right middle finger

√7ᵗʰ **S67.193** Crushing injury of left middle finger

√7ᵗʰ **S67.194** Crushing injury of right ring finger

√7ᵗʰ **S67.195** Crushing injury of left ring finger

√7ᵗʰ **S67.196** Crushing injury of right little finger

√7ᵗʰ **S67.197** Crushing injury of left little finger

√7ᵗʰ **S67.198** Crushing injury of other finger

Crushing injury of specified finger with unspecified laterality

√5ᵗʰ **S67.2** **Crushing injury of hand**

EXCLUDES 2   crushing injury of fingers (S67.1-)
              crushing injury of thumb (S67.0-)

√x7ᵗʰ **S67.20** Crushing injury of unspecified hand

N Newborn: 0   P Pediatric: 0-17   M Maternity: 12-55   A Adult: 15-124   CH Comorbidity High   CL Comorbidity Low   NCDx Noncancer Dx   PDx Primary Dx

1030   ICD-10-CM 2020

✓x 7ᵗʰ   **S67.21**   **Crushing injury of** right **hand**

✓x 7ᵗʰ   **S67.22**   **Crushing injury of** left **hand**

✓ 5ᵗʰ   **S67.3**   **Crushing injury of** wrist

     ✓x 7ᵗʰ   **S67.30**   **Crushing injury of unspecified wrist**

     ✓x 7ᵗʰ   **S67.31**   **Crushing injury of** right **wrist**

     ✓x 7ᵗʰ   **S67.32**   **Crushing injury of** left **wrist**

✓ 5ᵗʰ   **S67.4**   **Crushing injury of** wrist and hand

     EXCLUDES 1   crushing injury of hand alone (S67.2-)

                     crushing injury of wrist alone (S67.3-)

     EXCLUDES 2   crushing injury of fingers (S67.1-)

                     crushing injury of thumb (S67.0-)

     ✓x 7ᵗʰ   **S67.40**   **Crushing injury of unspecified wrist and hand**

     ✓x 7ᵗʰ   **S67.41**   **Crushing injury of** right **wrist and hand**

     ✓x 7ᵗʰ   **S67.42**   **Crushing injury of** left **wrist and hand**

✓ 5ᵗʰ   **S67.9**   **Crushing injury of unspecified part(s) of wrist, hand and fingers**

     ✓x 7ᵗʰ   **S67.90**   **Crushing injury of unspecified part(s) of unspecified wrist, hand and fingers**

     ✓x 7ᵗʰ   **S67.91**   **Crushing injury of unspecified part(s) of** right **wrist, hand and fingers**

     ✓x 7ᵗʰ   **S67.92**   **Crushing injury of unspecified part(s) of** left **wrist, hand and fingers**

✓ 4ᵗʰ   **S68**   **Traumatic amputation of wrist, hand and fingers**

     An amputation not identified as partial or complete should be coded to complete.

     The appropriate 7th character is to be added to each code from category S68.
     A   initial encounter
     D   subsequent encounter
     S   sequela

✓ 5ᵗʰ   **S68.0**   **Traumatic** metacarpophalangeal **amputation of** thumb

     Traumatic amputation of thumb NOS

     ✓ 6ᵗʰ   **S68.01**   Complete **traumatic metacarpophalangeal amputation of thumb**

         ✓ 7ᵗʰ   **S68.011**   **Complete traumatic metacarpophalangeal amputation of** right **thumb**

         ✓ 7ᵗʰ   **S68.012**   **Complete traumatic metacarpophalangeal amputation of** left **thumb**

         ✓ 7ᵗʰ   **S68.019**   **Complete traumatic metacarpophalangeal amputation of unspecified thumb**

     ✓ 6ᵗʰ   **S68.02**   Partial **traumatic metacarpophalangeal amputation of thumb**

         ✓ 7ᵗʰ   **S68.021**   **Partial traumatic metacarpophalangeal amputation of** right **thumb**

         ✓ 7ᵗʰ   **S68.022**   **Partial traumatic metacarpophalangeal amputation of** left **thumb**

         ✓ 7ᵗʰ   **S68.029**   **Partial traumatic metacarpophalangeal amputation of unspecified thumb**

✓ 5ᵗʰ   **S68.1**   **Traumatic** metacarpophalangeal **amputation of other and unspecified** finger

     Traumatic amputation of finger NOS

     EXCLUDES 2   traumatic metacarpophalangeal amputation of thumb (S68.0-)

     ✓ 6ᵗʰ   **S68.11**   Complete **traumatic metacarpophalangeal amputation of other and unspecified finger**

         ✓ 7ᵗʰ   **S68.110**   **Complete traumatic metacarpophalangeal amputation of** right index **finger**

         ✓ 7ᵗʰ   **S68.111**   **Complete traumatic metacarpophalangeal amputation of** left index **finger**

         ✓ 7ᵗʰ   **S68.112**   **Complete traumatic metacarpophalangeal amputation of** right middle **finger**

         ✓ 7ᵗʰ   **S68.113**   **Complete traumatic metacarpophalangeal amputation of** left middle **finger**

         ✓ 7ᵗʰ   **S68.114**   **Complete traumatic metacarpophalangeal amputation of** right ring **finger**

         ✓ 7ᵗʰ   **S68.115**   **Complete traumatic metacarpophalangeal amputation of** left ring **finger**

         ✓ 7ᵗʰ   **S68.116**   **Complete traumatic metacarpophalangeal amputation of** right little **finger**

         ✓ 7ᵗʰ   **S68.117**   **Complete traumatic metacarpophalangeal amputation of** left little **finger**

         ✓ 7ᵗʰ   **S68.118**   **Complete traumatic metacarpophalangeal amputation of other finger**

            Complete traumatic metacarpophalangeal amputation of specified finger with unspecified laterality

         ✓ 7ᵗʰ   **S68.119**   **Complete traumatic metacarpophalangeal amputation of unspecified finger**

     ✓ 6ᵗʰ   **S68.12**   Partial **traumatic metacarpophalangeal amputation of other and unspecified finger**

         ✓ 7ᵗʰ   **S68.120**   **Partial traumatic metacarpophalangeal amputation of** right index **finger**

         ✓ 7ᵗʰ   **S68.121**   **Partial traumatic metacarpophalangeal amputation of** left index **finger**

         ✓ 7ᵗʰ   **S68.122**   **Partial traumatic metacarpophalangeal amputation of** right middle **finger**

         ✓ 7ᵗʰ   **S68.123**   **Partial traumatic metacarpophalangeal amputation of** left middle **finger**

         ✓ 7ᵗʰ   **S68.124**   **Partial traumatic metacarpophalangeal amputation of** right ring **finger**

         ✓ 7ᵗʰ   **S68.125**   **Partial traumatic metacarpophalangeal amputation of** left ring **finger**

         ✓ 7ᵗʰ   **S68.126**   **Partial traumatic metacarpophalangeal amputation of** right little **finger**

         ✓ 7ᵗʰ   **S68.127**   **Partial traumatic metacarpophalangeal amputation of** left little **finger**

         ✓ 7ᵗʰ   **S68.128**   **Partial traumatic metacarpophalangeal amputation of other finger**

            Partial traumatic metacarpophalangeal amputation of specified finger with unspecified laterality

         ✓ 7ᵗʰ   **S68.129**   **Partial traumatic metacarpophalangeal amputation of unspecified finger**

✓ 5ᵗʰ   **S68.4**   **Traumatic amputation of** hand at wrist level

     Traumatic amputation of hand NOS

     Traumatic amputation of wrist

     ✓ 6ᵗʰ   **S68.41**   Complete **traumatic amputation of hand at wrist level**

         ✓ 7ᵗʰ   **S68.411**   **Complete traumatic amputation of** right **hand at wrist level**

         ✓ 7ᵗʰ   **S68.412**   **Complete traumatic amputation of** left **hand at wrist level**

         ✓ 7ᵗʰ   **S68.419**   **Complete traumatic amputation of unspecified hand at wrist level**

     ✓ 6ᵗʰ   **S68.42**   Partial **traumatic amputation of hand at wrist level**

         ✓ 7ᵗʰ   **S68.421**   **Partial traumatic amputation of** right **hand at wrist level**

         ✓ 7ᵗʰ   **S68.422**   **Partial traumatic amputation of** left **hand at wrist level**

         ✓ 7ᵗʰ   **S68.429**   **Partial traumatic amputation of unspecified hand at wrist level**

✓ 5ᵗʰ   **S68.5**   **Traumatic** transphalangeal **amputation of** thumb

     Traumatic interphalangeal joint amputation of thumb

     ✓ 6ᵗʰ   **S68.51**   Complete **traumatic transphalangeal amputation of thumb**

         ✓ 7ᵗʰ   **S68.511**   **Complete traumatic transphalangeal amputation of** right **thumb**

         ✓ 7ᵗʰ   **S68.512**   **Complete traumatic transphalangeal amputation of** left **thumb**

         ✓ 7ᵗʰ   **S68.519**   **Complete traumatic transphalangeal amputation of unspecified thumb**

     ✓ 6ᵗʰ   **S68.52**   Partial **traumatic transphalangeal amputation of thumb**

         ✓ 7ᵗʰ   **S68.521**   **Partial traumatic transphalangeal amputation of** right **thumb**

         ✓ 7ᵗʰ   **S68.522**   **Partial traumatic transphalangeal amputation of** left **thumb**

         ✓ 7ᵗʰ   **S68.529**   **Partial traumatic transphalangeal amputation of unspecified thumb**

✓ 5ᵗʰ   **S68.6**   **Traumatic** transphalangeal **amputation of other and unspecified** finger

     ✓ 6ᵗʰ   **S68.61**   Complete **traumatic transphalangeal amputation of other and unspecified finger(s)**

         ✓ 7ᵗʰ   **S68.610**   **Complete traumatic transphalangeal amputation of** right index **finger**

✓ Additional Character Required   ✓x 7ᵗʰ Placeholder Alert   Manifestation   Unspecified Dx   ▶◀ Revised Text   ● New Code   ▲ Revised Title

ICD-10-CM 2020   1031

✓7ᵗʰ **S68.611 Complete traumatic transphalangeal amputation of** left index **finger**

✓7ᵗʰ **S68.612 Complete traumatic transphalangeal amputation of** right middle **finger**

✓7ᵗʰ **S68.613 Complete traumatic transphalangeal amputation of** left middle **finger**

✓7ᵗʰ **S68.614 Complete traumatic transphalangeal amputation of** right ring **finger**

✓7ᵗʰ **S68.615 Complete traumatic transphalangeal amputation of** left ring **finger**

✓7ᵗʰ **S68.616 Complete traumatic transphalangeal amputation of** right little **finger**

✓7ᵗʰ **S68.617 Complete traumatic transphalangeal amputation of** left little **finger**

✓7ᵗʰ **S68.618 Complete traumatic transphalangeal amputation of other finger**
Complete traumatic transphalangeal amputation of specified finger with unspecified laterality

✓7ᵗʰ **S68.619 Complete traumatic transphalangeal amputation of unspecified finger**

✓6ᵗʰ **S68.62 Partial traumatic transphalangeal amputation of other and unspecified finger**

✓7ᵗʰ **S68.620 Partial traumatic transphalangeal amputation of** right index **finger**

✓7ᵗʰ **S68.621 Partial traumatic transphalangeal amputation of** left index **finger**

✓7ᵗʰ **S68.622 Partial traumatic transphalangeal amputation of** right middle **finger**

✓7ᵗʰ **S68.623 Partial traumatic transphalangeal amputation of** left middle **finger**

✓7ᵗʰ **S68.624 Partial traumatic transphalangeal amputation of** right ring **finger**

✓7ᵗʰ **S68.625 Partial traumatic transphalangeal amputation of** left ring **finger**

✓7ᵗʰ **S68.626 Partial traumatic transphalangeal amputation of** right little **finger**

✓7ᵗʰ **S68.627 Partial traumatic transphalangeal amputation of** left little **finger**

✓7ᵗʰ **S68.628 Partial traumatic transphalangeal amputation of other finger**
Partial traumatic transphalangeal amputation of specified finger with unspecified laterality

✓7ᵗʰ **S68.629 Partial traumatic transphalangeal amputation of unspecified finger**

✓5ᵗʰ **S68.7 Traumatic** transmetacarpal **amputation of** hand

✓6ᵗʰ **S68.71 Complete traumatic transmetacarpal amputation of hand**

✓7ᵗʰ **S68.711 Complete traumatic transmetacarpal amputation of** right hand

✓7ᵗʰ **S68.712 Complete traumatic transmetacarpal amputation of** left hand

✓7ᵗʰ **S68.719 Complete traumatic transmetacarpal amputation of** unspecified hand

✓6ᵗʰ **S68.72 Partial traumatic transmetacarpal amputation of hand**

✓7ᵗʰ **S68.721 Partial traumatic transmetacarpal amputation of** right hand

✓7ᵗʰ **S68.722 Partial traumatic transmetacarpal amputation of** left hand

✓7ᵗʰ **S68.729 Partial traumatic transmetacarpal amputation of** unspecified hand

✓4ᵗʰ **S69 Other and unspecified injuries of wrist, hand and finger(s)**

The appropriate 7th character is to be added to each code from category S69.
A initial encounter
D subsequent encounter
S sequela

✓5ᵗʰ **S69.8 Other specified injuries of wrist, hand and finger(s)**

✓x7ᵗʰ **S69.80 Other specified injuries of unspecified wrist, hand and finger(s)**

✓x7ᵗʰ **S69.81 Other specified injuries of** right **wrist, hand and finger(s)**

✓x7ᵗʰ **S69.82 Other specified injuries of** left **wrist, hand and finger(s)**

✓5ᵗʰ **S69.9 Unspecified injury of wrist, hand and finger(s)**

✓x7ᵗʰ **S69.90 Unspecified injury of unspecified wrist, hand and finger(s)**

✓x7ᵗʰ **S69.91 Unspecified injury of** right **wrist, hand and finger(s)**

✓x7ᵗʰ **S69.92 Unspecified injury of** left **wrist, hand and finger(s)**

Injuries to the hip and thigh (S70-S79)

EXCLUDES 2   burns and corrosions (T20-T32)
frostbite (T33-T34)
snake bite (T63.0-)
venomous insect bite or sting (T63.4-)

✓4ᵗʰ **S70 Superficial injury of hip and thigh**

The appropriate 7th character is to be added to each code from category S70.
A initial encounter
D subsequent encounter
S sequela

✓5ᵗʰ **S70.0 Contusion of** hip

✓x7ᵗʰ **S70.00 Contusion of unspecified hip**

✓x7ᵗʰ **S70.01 Contusion of** right **hip**

✓x7ᵗʰ **S70.02 Contusion of** left **hip**

✓5ᵗʰ **S70.1 Contusion of** thigh

✓x7ᵗʰ **S70.10 Contusion of unspecified thigh**

✓x7ᵗʰ **S70.11 Contusion of** right **thigh**

✓x7ᵗʰ **S70.12 Contusion of** left **thigh**

✓5ᵗʰ **S70.2 Other superficial injuries of** hip

✓6ᵗʰ **S70.21 Abrasion of hip**

✓7ᵗʰ **S70.211 Abrasion,** right **hip**

✓7ᵗʰ **S70.212 Abrasion,** left **hip**

✓7ᵗʰ **S70.219 Abrasion, unspecified hip**

✓6ᵗʰ **S70.22 Blister (nonthermal) of hip**

✓7ᵗʰ **S70.221 Blister (nonthermal),** right **hip**

✓7ᵗʰ **S70.222 Blister (nonthermal),** left **hip**

✓7ᵗʰ **S70.229 Blister (nonthermal), unspecified hip**

✓6ᵗʰ **S70.24 External constriction of hip**

✓7ᵗʰ **S70.241 External constriction,** right **hip**

✓7ᵗʰ **S70.242 External constriction,** left **hip**

✓7ᵗʰ **S70.249 External constriction, unspecified hip**

✓6ᵗʰ **S70.25 Superficial** foreign body **of hip**
Splinter in the hip

✓7ᵗʰ **S70.251 Superficial foreign body,** right **hip**

✓7ᵗʰ **S70.252 Superficial foreign body,** left **hip**

✓7ᵗʰ **S70.259 Superficial foreign body, unspecified hip**

✓6ᵗʰ **S70.26 Insect bite (nonvenomous) of hip**

✓7ᵗʰ **S70.261 Insect bite (nonvenomous),** right **hip**

✓7ᵗʰ **S70.262 Insect bite (nonvenomous),** left **hip**

✓7ᵗʰ **S70.269 Insect bite (nonvenomous), unspecified hip**

✓6ᵗʰ **S70.27 Other superficial** bite **of hip**
EXCLUDES 1   open bite of hip (S71.05-)

✓7ᵗʰ **S70.271 Other superficial bite of hip,** right **hip**

✓7ᵗʰ **S70.272 Other superficial bite of hip,** left **hip**

✓7ᵗʰ **S70.279 Other superficial bite of hip, unspecified hip**

✓5ᵗʰ **S70.3 Other superficial injuries of** thigh

✓6ᵗʰ **S70.31 Abrasion of thigh**

✓7ᵗʰ **S70.311 Abrasion,** right **thigh**

✓7ᵗʰ **S70.312 Abrasion,** left **thigh**

✓7ᵗʰ **S70.319 Abrasion, unspecified thigh**

✓6ᵗʰ **S70.32 Blister (nonthermal) of thigh**

✓7ᵗʰ **S70.321 Blister (nonthermal),** right **thigh**

✓7ᵗʰ **S70.322 Blister (nonthermal),** left **thigh**

✓7ᵗʰ **S70.329 Blister (nonthermal), unspecified thigh**

✓6ᵗʰ **S70.34 External constriction of thigh**

✓7ᵗʰ **S70.341 External constriction,** right **thigh**

✓7ᵗʰ **S70.342 External constriction,** left **thigh**

✓7ᵗʰ **S70.349 External constriction, unspecified thigh**

✓6ᵗʰ **S70.35 Superficial** foreign body **of thigh**
Splinter in the thigh

✓7ᵗʰ **S70.351 Superficial foreign body,** right **thigh**

✓7ᵗʰ **S70.352 Superficial foreign body,** left **thigh**

√7ᵗʰ **S70.359** Superficial foreign body, unspecified thigh

√6ᵗʰ **S70.36** Insect bite (nonvenomous) of thigh

    √7ᵗʰ **S70.361** Insect bite (nonvenomous), right thigh

    √7ᵗʰ **S70.362** Insect bite (nonvenomous), left thigh

    √7ᵗʰ **S70.369** Insect bite (nonvenomous), unspecified thigh

√6ᵗʰ **S70.37** Other superficial bite of thigh

    EXCLUDES 1   open bite of thigh (S71.15)

    √7ᵗʰ **S70.371** Other superficial bite of right thigh

    √7ᵗʰ **S70.372** Other superficial bite of left thigh

    √7ᵗʰ **S70.379** Other superficial bite of unspecified thigh

√5ᵗʰ **S70.9** Unspecified superficial injury of hip and thigh

√6ᵗʰ **S70.91** Unspecified superficial injury of hip

    √7ᵗʰ **S70.911** Unspecified superficial injury of right hip

    √7ᵗʰ **S70.912** Unspecified superficial injury of left hip

    √7ᵗʰ **S70.919** Unspecified superficial injury of unspecified hip

√6ᵗʰ **S70.92** Unspecified superficial injury of thigh

    √7ᵗʰ **S70.921** Unspecified superficial injury of right thigh

    √7ᵗʰ **S70.922** Unspecified superficial injury of left thigh

    √7ᵗʰ **S70.929** Unspecified superficial injury of unspecified thigh

√4ᵗʰ **S71** Open wound of hip and thigh

Code also any associated wound infection

EXCLUDES 1   open fracture of hip and thigh (S72.-)

            traumatic amputation of hip and thigh (S78.-)

EXCLUDES 2   bite of venomous animal (T63.-)

            open wound of ankle, foot and toes (S91.-)

            open wound of knee and lower leg (S81.-)

> The appropriate 7th character is to be added to each code from category S71.
> A   initial encounter
> D   subsequent encounter
> S   sequela

√5ᵗʰ **S71.0** Open wound of hip

√6ᵗʰ **S71.00** Unspecified open wound of hip

    √7ᵗʰ **S71.001** Unspecified open wound, right hip

    √7ᵗʰ **S71.002** Unspecified open wound, left hip

    √7ᵗʰ **S71.009** Unspecified open wound, unspecified hip

√6ᵗʰ **S71.01** Laceration without foreign body of hip

    √7ᵗʰ **S71.011** Laceration without foreign body, right hip

    √7ᵗʰ **S71.012** Laceration without foreign body, left hip

    √7ᵗʰ **S71.019** Laceration without foreign body, unspecified hip

√6ᵗʰ **S71.02** Laceration with foreign body of hip

    √7ᵗʰ **S71.021** Laceration with foreign body, right hip

    √7ᵗʰ **S71.022** Laceration with foreign body, left hip

    √7ᵗʰ **S71.029** Laceration with foreign body, unspecified hip

√6ᵗʰ **S71.03** Puncture wound without foreign body of hip

    √7ᵗʰ **S71.031** Puncture wound without foreign body, right hip

    √7ᵗʰ **S71.032** Puncture wound without foreign body, left hip

    √7ᵗʰ **S71.039** Puncture wound without foreign body, unspecified hip

√6ᵗʰ **S71.04** Puncture wound with foreign body of hip

    √7ᵗʰ **S71.041** Puncture wound with foreign body, right hip

    √7ᵗʰ **S71.042** Puncture wound with foreign body, left hip

    √7ᵗʰ **S71.049** Puncture wound with foreign body, unspecified hip

√6ᵗʰ **S71.05** Open bite of hip

Bite of hip NOS

    EXCLUDES 1   superficial bite of hip (S70.26, S70.27)

    √7ᵗʰ **S71.051** Open bite, right hip

    √7ᵗʰ **S71.052** Open bite, left hip

    √7ᵗʰ **S71.059** Open bite, unspecified hip

√5ᵗʰ **S71.1** Open wound of thigh

√6ᵗʰ **S71.10** Unspecified open wound of thigh

AHA: 2016,3Q,24

    √7ᵗʰ **S71.101** Unspecified open wound, right thigh

    √7ᵗʰ **S71.102** Unspecified open wound, left thigh

    √7ᵗʰ **S71.109** Unspecified open wound, unspecified thigh

√6ᵗʰ **S71.11** Laceration without foreign body of thigh

    √7ᵗʰ **S71.111** Laceration without foreign body, right thigh

    √7ᵗʰ **S71.112** Laceration without foreign body, left thigh

    √7ᵗʰ **S71.119** Laceration without foreign body, unspecified thigh

√6ᵗʰ **S71.12** Laceration with foreign body of thigh

    √7ᵗʰ **S71.121** Laceration with foreign body, right thigh

    √7ᵗʰ **S71.122** Laceration with foreign body, left thigh

    √7ᵗʰ **S71.129** Laceration with foreign body, unspecified thigh

√6ᵗʰ **S71.13** Puncture wound without foreign body of thigh

AHA: 2016,3Q,24

    √7ᵗʰ **S71.131** Puncture wound without foreign body, right thigh

    √7ᵗʰ **S71.132** Puncture wound without foreign body, left thigh

    √7ᵗʰ **S71.139** Puncture wound without foreign body, unspecified thigh

√6ᵗʰ **S71.14** Puncture wound with foreign body of thigh

AHA: 2016,3Q,24

    √7ᵗʰ **S71.141** Puncture wound with foreign body, right thigh

    √7ᵗʰ **S71.142** Puncture wound with foreign body, left thigh

    √7ᵗʰ **S71.149** Puncture wound with foreign body, unspecified thigh

√6ᵗʰ **S71.15** Open bite of thigh

Bite of thigh NOS

    EXCLUDES 1   superficial bite of thigh (S70.37-)

    √7ᵗʰ **S71.151** Open bite, right thigh

    √7ᵗʰ **S71.152** Open bite, left thigh

    √7ᵗʰ **S71.159** Open bite, unspecified thigh

☑ Additional Character Required   √x7ᵗʰ Placeholder Alert   Manifestation   Unspecified Dx   ►◄ Revised Text   ● New Code   ▲ Revised Title

✓4ᵗʰ **S72 Fracture of femur**

NOTE: A fracture not indicated as displaced or nondisplaced should be coded to displaced.

A fracture not indicated as open or closed should be coded to closed.

The open fracture designations are based on the Gustilo open fracture classification.

EXCLUDES 1 traumatic amputation of hip and thigh (S78.-)
EXCLUDES 2 fracture of lower leg and ankle (S82.-)
fracture of foot (S92.-)
periprosthetic fracture of prosthetic implant of hip (M97.0-)

AHA: 2018,2Q,12; 2016,1Q,33; 2015,3Q,37-39; 2015,1Q,17; 2013,4Q,128
DEF: Diaphysis: Central shaft of a long bone.
DEF: Epiphysis: Proximal and distal rounded ends of a long bone communicates with the joint.
DEF: Metaphysis: Section of a long bone located between the epiphysis and diaphysis at the proximal and distal ends.
DEF: Physis (growth plate): Narrow zone of cartilaginous tissue between the epiphysis and metaphysis at each end of a long bone. In childhood, proliferation of cells in this zone lengthens the bone. As the bone matures, this area thins, ossification eventually fusing into solid bone and growth stops. *Synonyms: Epiphyseal plate.*
TIP: The term "improper alignment" is not synonymous with malunion or nonunion of a fracture when noted in provider documentation.

The appropriate 7th character is to be added to all codes from category S72 [unless otherwise indicated].
A   initial encounter for closed fracture
B   initial encounter for open fracture type I or II
    initial encounter for open fracture NOS
C   initial encounter for open fracture type IIIA, IIIB, or IIIC
D   subsequent encounter for closed fracture with routine healing
E   subsequent encounter for open fracture type I or II with routine healing
F   subsequent encounter for open fracture type IIIA, IIIB, or IIIC with routine healing
G   subsequent encounter for closed fracture with delayed healing
H   subsequent encounter for open fracture type I or II with delayed healing
J   subsequent encounter for open fracture type IIIA, IIIB, or IIIC with delayed healing
K   subsequent encounter for closed fracture with nonunion
M   subsequent encounter for open fracture type I or II with nonunion
N   subsequent encounter for open fracture type IIIA, IIIB, or IIIC with nonunion
P   subsequent encounter for closed fracture with malunion
Q   subsequent encounter for open fracture type I or II with malunion
R   subsequent encounter for open fracture type IIIA, IIIB, or IIIC with malunion
S   sequela

✓5ᵗʰ **S72.0 Fracture of head and neck of femur**
EXCLUDES 2 physeal fracture of upper end of femur (S79.0-)
AHA: 2016,3Q,16

✓6ᵗʰ **S72.00 Fracture of unspecified part of neck of femur**
Fracture of hip NOS
Fracture of neck of femur NOS
✓7ᵗʰ **S72.001 Fracture of unspecified part of neck of right femur**
✓7ᵗʰ **S72.002 Fracture of unspecified part of neck of left femur**
✓7ᵗʰ **S72.009 Fracture of unspecified part of neck of unspecified femur**

✓6ᵗʰ **S72.01 Unspecified intracapsular fracture of femur**
Subcapital fracture of femur
✓7ᵗʰ **S72.011 Unspecified intracapsular fracture of right femur**
✓7ᵗʰ **S72.012 Unspecified intracapsular fracture of left femur**
✓7ᵗʰ **S72.019 Unspecified intracapsular fracture of unspecified femur**

✓6ᵗʰ **S72.02 Fracture of epiphysis (separation) (upper) of femur**
Transepiphyseal fracture of femur
EXCLUDES 1 capital femoral epiphyseal fracture (pediatric) of femur (S79.01-)
Salter-Harris Type I physeal fracture of upper end of femur (S79.01-)
✓7ᵗʰ **S72.021 Displaced fracture of epiphysis (separation) (upper) of right femur**

✓7ᵗʰ **S72.022 Displaced fracture of epiphysis (separation) (upper) of left femur**
✓7ᵗʰ **S72.023 Displaced fracture of epiphysis (separation) (upper) of unspecified femur**
✓7ᵗʰ **S72.024 Nondisplaced fracture of epiphysis (separation) (upper) of right femur**
✓7ᵗʰ **S72.025 Nondisplaced fracture of epiphysis (separation) (upper) of left femur**
✓7ᵗʰ **S72.026 Nondisplaced fracture of epiphysis (separation) (upper) of unspecified femur**

✓6ᵗʰ **S72.03 Midcervical fracture of femur**
Transcervical fracture of femur NOS
✓7ᵗʰ **S72.031 Displaced midcervical fracture of right femur**
✓7ᵗʰ **S72.032 Displaced midcervical fracture of left femur**
✓7ᵗʰ **S72.033 Displaced midcervical fracture of unspecified femur**
✓7ᵗʰ **S72.034 Nondisplaced midcervical fracture of right femur**
✓7ᵗʰ **S72.035 Nondisplaced midcervical fracture of left femur**
✓7ᵗʰ **S72.036 Nondisplaced midcervical fracture of unspecified femur**

✓6ᵗʰ **S72.04 Fracture of base of neck of femur**
Cervicotrochanteric fracture of femur
✓7ᵗʰ **S72.041 Displaced fracture of base of neck of right femur**
✓7ᵗʰ **S72.042 Displaced fracture of base of neck of left femur**
✓7ᵗʰ **S72.043 Displaced fracture of base of neck of unspecified femur**
✓7ᵗʰ **S72.044 Nondisplaced fracture of base of neck of right femur**
✓7ᵗʰ **S72.045 Nondisplaced fracture of base of neck of left femur**
✓7ᵗʰ **S72.046 Nondisplaced fracture of base of neck of unspecified femur**

✓6ᵗʰ **S72.05 Unspecified fracture of head of femur**
Fracture of head of femur NOS
✓7ᵗʰ **S72.051 Unspecified fracture of head of right femur**
✓7ᵗʰ **S72.052 Unspecified fracture of head of left femur**
✓7ᵗʰ **S72.059 Unspecified fracture of head of unspecified femur**

✓6ᵗʰ **S72.06 Articular fracture of head of femur**
✓7ᵗʰ **S72.061 Displaced articular fracture of head of right femur**
✓7ᵗʰ **S72.062 Displaced articular fracture of head of left femur**
✓7ᵗʰ **S72.063 Displaced articular fracture of head of unspecified femur**
✓7ᵗʰ **S72.064 Nondisplaced articular fracture of head of right femur**
✓7ᵗʰ **S72.065 Nondisplaced articular fracture of head of left femur**
✓7ᵗʰ **S72.066 Nondisplaced articular fracture of head of unspecified femur**

✓6ᵗʰ **S72.09 Other fracture of head and neck of femur**
✓7ᵗʰ **S72.091 Other fracture of head and neck of right femur**
✓7ᵗʰ **S72.092 Other fracture of head and neck of left femur**
✓7ᵗʰ **S72.099 Other fracture of head and neck of unspecified femur**

✓5ᵗʰ **S72.1 Pertrochanteric fracture**
AHA: 2016,3Q,16
✓6ᵗʰ **S72.10 Unspecified trochanteric fracture of femur**
Fracture of trochanter NOS
✓7ᵗʰ **S72.101 Unspecified trochanteric fracture of right femur**
✓7ᵗʰ **S72.102 Unspecified trochanteric fracture of left femur**
✓7ᵗʰ **S72.109 Unspecified trochanteric fracture of unspecified femur**

✓6ᵗʰ **S72.11 Fracture of greater trochanter of femur**
✓7ᵗʰ **S72.111 Displaced fracture of greater trochanter of right femur**
✓7ᵗʰ **S72.112 Displaced fracture of greater trochanter of left femur**

√7ᵗʰ **S72.113** Displaced fracture of greater trochanter of unspecified femur

√7ᵗʰ **S72.114** Nondisplaced fracture of greater trochanter of right femur

√7ᵗʰ **S72.115** Nondisplaced fracture of greater trochanter of left femur

√7ᵗʰ **S72.116** Nondisplaced fracture of greater trochanter of unspecified femur

√6ᵗʰ **S72.12** Fracture of lesser trochanter of femur

√7ᵗʰ **S72.121** Displaced fracture of lesser trochanter of right femur

√7ᵗʰ **S72.122** Displaced fracture of lesser trochanter of left femur

√7ᵗʰ **S72.123** Displaced fracture of lesser trochanter of unspecified femur

√7ᵗʰ **S72.124** Nondisplaced fracture of lesser trochanter of right femur

√7ᵗʰ **S72.125** Nondisplaced fracture of lesser trochanter of left femur

√7ᵗʰ **S72.126** Nondisplaced fracture of lesser trochanter of unspecified femur

√6ᵗʰ **S72.13** Apophyseal fracture of femur

> EXCLUDES 1   chronic (nontraumatic) slipped upper femoral epiphysis (M93.0-)

√7ᵗʰ **S72.131** Displaced apophyseal fracture of right femur

√7ᵗʰ **S72.132** Displaced apophyseal fracture of left femur

√7ᵗʰ **S72.133** Displaced apophyseal fracture of unspecified femur

√7ᵗʰ **S72.134** Nondisplaced apophyseal fracture of right femur

√7ᵗʰ **S72.135** Nondisplaced apophyseal fracture of left femur

√7ᵗʰ **S72.136** Nondisplaced apophyseal fracture of unspecified femur

√6ᵗʰ **S72.14** Intertrochanteric fracture of femur

√7ᵗʰ **S72.141** Displaced intertrochanteric fracture of right femur

√7ᵗʰ **S72.142** Displaced intertrochanteric fracture of left femur

√7ᵗʰ **S72.143** Displaced intertrochanteric fracture of unspecified femur

√7ᵗʰ **S72.144** Nondisplaced intertrochanteric fracture of right femur

√7ᵗʰ **S72.145** Nondisplaced intertrochanteric fracture of left femur

√7ᵗʰ **S72.146** Nondisplaced intertrochanteric fracture of unspecified femur

√5ᵗʰ **S72.2** Subtrochanteric fracture of femur

√x7ᵗʰ **S72.21** Displaced subtrochanteric fracture of right femur

√x7ᵗʰ **S72.22** Displaced subtrochanteric fracture of left femur

√x7ᵗʰ **S72.23** Displaced subtrochanteric fracture of unspecified femur

√x7ᵗʰ **S72.24** Nondisplaced subtrochanteric fracture of right femur

√x7ᵗʰ **S72.25** Nondisplaced subtrochanteric fracture of left femur

√x7ᵗʰ **S72.26** Nondisplaced subtrochanteric fracture of unspecified femur

√5ᵗʰ **S72.3** Fracture of shaft of femur

√6ᵗʰ **S72.30** Unspecified fracture of shaft of femur

√7ᵗʰ **S72.301** Unspecified fracture of shaft of right femur

√7ᵗʰ **S72.302** Unspecified fracture of shaft of left femur

√7ᵗʰ **S72.309** Unspecified fracture of shaft of unspecified femur

√6ᵗʰ **S72.32** Transverse fracture of shaft of femur

√7ᵗʰ **S72.321** Displaced transverse fracture of shaft of right femur

√7ᵗʰ **S72.322** Displaced transverse fracture of shaft of left femur

√7ᵗʰ **S72.323** Displaced transverse fracture of shaft of unspecified femur

√7ᵗʰ **S72.324** Nondisplaced transverse fracture of shaft of right femur

√7ᵗʰ **S72.325** Nondisplaced transverse fracture of shaft of left femur

√7ᵗʰ **S72.326** Nondisplaced transverse fracture of shaft of unspecified femur

√6ᵗʰ **S72.33** Oblique fracture of shaft of femur

√7ᵗʰ **S72.331** Displaced oblique fracture of shaft of right femur

√7ᵗʰ **S72.332** Displaced oblique fracture of shaft of left femur

√7ᵗʰ **S72.333** Displaced oblique fracture of shaft of unspecified femur

√7ᵗʰ **S72.334** Nondisplaced oblique fracture of shaft of right femur

√7ᵗʰ **S72.335** Nondisplaced oblique fracture of shaft of left femur

√7ᵗʰ **S72.336** Nondisplaced oblique fracture of shaft of unspecified femur

√6ᵗʰ **S72.34** Spiral fracture of shaft of femur

√7ᵗʰ **S72.341** Displaced spiral fracture of shaft of right femur

√7ᵗʰ **S72.342** Displaced spiral fracture of shaft of left femur

√7ᵗʰ **S72.343** Displaced spiral fracture of shaft of unspecified femur

√7ᵗʰ **S72.344** Nondisplaced spiral fracture of shaft of right femur

√7ᵗʰ **S72.345** Nondisplaced spiral fracture of shaft of left femur

√7ᵗʰ **S72.346** Nondisplaced spiral fracture of shaft of unspecified femur

√6ᵗʰ **S72.35** Comminuted fracture of shaft of femur

√7ᵗʰ **S72.351** Displaced comminuted fracture of shaft of right femur

√7ᵗʰ **S72.352** Displaced comminuted fracture of shaft of left femur

√7ᵗʰ **S72.353** Displaced comminuted fracture of shaft of unspecified femur

√7ᵗʰ **S72.354** Nondisplaced comminuted fracture of shaft of right femur

√7ᵗʰ **S72.355** Nondisplaced comminuted fracture of shaft of left femur

√7ᵗʰ **S72.356** Nondisplaced comminuted fracture of shaft of unspecified femur

√6ᵗʰ **S72.36** Segmental fracture of shaft of femur

√7ᵗʰ **S72.361** Displaced segmental fracture of shaft of right femur

√7ᵗʰ **S72.362** Displaced segmental fracture of shaft of left femur

√7ᵗʰ **S72.363** Displaced segmental fracture of shaft of unspecified femur

√7ᵗʰ **S72.364** Nondisplaced segmental fracture of shaft of right femur

√7ᵗʰ **S72.365** Nondisplaced segmental fracture of shaft of left femur

√7ᵗʰ **S72.366** Nondisplaced segmental fracture of shaft of unspecified femur

√6ᵗʰ **S72.39** Other fracture of shaft of femur

√7ᵗʰ **S72.391** Other fracture of shaft of right femur

√7ᵗʰ **S72.392** Other fracture of shaft of left femur

√7ᵗʰ **S72.399** Other fracture of shaft of unspecified femur

√5ᵗʰ **S72.4** Fracture of lower end of femur

Fracture of distal end of femur

> EXCLUDES 2   fracture of shaft of femur (S72.3-)
> physeal fracture of lower end of femur (S79.1-)

AHA: 2016,4Q,42

√6ᵗʰ **S72.40** Unspecified fracture of lower end of femur

AHA: 2018,1Q,21; 2016,4Q,42

√7ᵗʰ **S72.401** Unspecified fracture of lower end of right femur

√7ᵗʰ **S72.402** Unspecified fracture of lower end of left femur

√7ᵗʰ **S72.409** Unspecified fracture of lower end of unspecified femur

√6ᵗʰ **S72.41** Unspecified condyle fracture of lower end of femur

Condyle fracture of femur NOS

√7ᵗʰ **S72.411** Displaced unspecified condyle fracture of lower end of right femur

√7ᵗʰ **S72.412** Displaced unspecified condyle fracture of lower end of left femur

√7ᵗʰ **S72.413** Displaced unspecified condyle fracture of lower end of unspecified femur

√7ᵗʰ **S72.414** Nondisplaced unspecified condyle fracture of lower end of right femur

---

☑ Additional Character Required   √x7ᵗʰ Placeholder Alert   Manifestation   Unspecified Dx   ►◄ Revised Text   ● New Code   ▲ Revised Title

ICD-10-CM 2020   1035

Chapter 19. Injury, Poisoning and Certain Other Consequences of External Causes

√7ᵗʰ **S72.415** Nondisplaced unspecified condyle fracture of lower end of left femur

√7ᵗʰ **S72.416** Nondisplaced unspecified condyle fracture of lower end of unspecified femur

√6ᵗʰ **S72.42** Fracture of lateral condyle of femur

√7ᵗʰ **S72.421** Displaced fracture of lateral condyle of right femur

√7ᵗʰ **S72.422** Displaced fracture of lateral condyle of left femur

√7ᵗʰ **S72.423** Displaced fracture of lateral condyle of unspecified femur

√7ᵗʰ **S72.424** Nondisplaced fracture of lateral condyle of right femur

√7ᵗʰ **S72.425** Nondisplaced fracture of lateral condyle of left femur

√7ᵗʰ **S72.426** Nondisplaced fracture of lateral condyle of unspecified femur

√6ᵗʰ **S72.43** Fracture of medial condyle of femur

√7ᵗʰ **S72.431** Displaced fracture of medial condyle of right femur

√7ᵗʰ **S72.432** Displaced fracture of medial condyle of left femur

√7ᵗʰ **S72.433** Displaced fracture of medial condyle of unspecified femur

√7ᵗʰ **S72.434** Nondisplaced fracture of medial condyle of right femur

√7ᵗʰ **S72.435** Nondisplaced fracture of medial condyle of left femur

√7ᵗʰ **S72.436** Nondisplaced fracture of medial condyle of unspecified femur

√6ᵗʰ **S72.44** Fracture of lower epiphysis (separation) of femur

> **EXCLUDES 1**   Salter-Harris Type I physeal fracture of lower end of femur (S79.11-)

√7ᵗʰ **S72.441** Displaced fracture of lower epiphysis (separation) of right femur

√7ᵗʰ **S72.442** Displaced fracture of lower epiphysis (separation) of left femur

√7ᵗʰ **S72.443** Displaced fracture of lower epiphysis (separation) of unspecified femur

√7ᵗʰ **S72.444** Nondisplaced fracture of lower epiphysis (separation) of right femur

√7ᵗʰ **S72.445** Nondisplaced fracture of lower epiphysis (separation) of left femur

√7ᵗʰ **S72.446** Nondisplaced fracture of lower epiphysis (separation) of unspecified femur

√6ᵗʰ **S72.45** Supracondylar fracture without intracondylar extension of lower end of femur

Supracondylar fracture of lower end of femur NOS

> **EXCLUDES 1**   supracondylar fracture with intracondylar extension of lower end of femur (S72.46-)

√7ᵗʰ **S72.451** Displaced supracondylar fracture without intracondylar extension of lower end of right femur

√7ᵗʰ **S72.452** Displaced supracondylar fracture without intracondylar extension of lower end of left femur

√7ᵗʰ **S72.453** Displaced supracondylar fracture without intracondylar extension of lower end of unspecified femur

√7ᵗʰ **S72.454** Nondisplaced supracondylar fracture without intracondylar extension of lower end of right femur

√7ᵗʰ **S72.455** Nondisplaced supracondylar fracture without intracondylar extension of lower end of left femur

√7ᵗʰ **S72.456** Nondisplaced supracondylar fracture without intracondylar extension of lower end of unspecified femur

√6ᵗʰ **S72.46** Supracondylar fracture with intracondylar extension of lower end of femur

> **EXCLUDES 1**   supracondylar fracture without intracondylar extension of lower end of femur (S72.45-)

√7ᵗʰ **S72.461** Displaced supracondylar fracture with intracondylar extension of lower end of right femur

√7ᵗʰ **S72.462** Displaced supracondylar fracture with intracondylar extension of lower end of left femur

√7ᵗʰ **S72.463** Displaced supracondylar fracture with intracondylar extension of lower end of unspecified femur

√7ᵗʰ **S72.464** Nondisplaced supracondylar fracture with intracondylar extension of lower end of right femur

√7ᵗʰ **S72.465** Nondisplaced supracondylar fracture with intracondylar extension of lower end of left femur

√7ᵗʰ **S72.466** Nondisplaced supracondylar fracture with intracondylar extension of lower end of unspecified femur

√6ᵗʰ **S72.47** Torus fracture of lower end of femur

> The appropriate 7th character is to be added to all codes in subcategory S72.47.
> A   initial encounter for closed fracture
> D   subsequent encounter for fracture with routine healing
> G   subsequent encounter for fracture with delayed healing
> K   subsequent encounter for fracture with nonunion
> P   subsequent encounter for fracture with malunion
> S   sequela

√7ᵗʰ **S72.471** Torus fracture of lower end of right femur

√7ᵗʰ **S72.472** Torus fracture of lower end of left femur

√7ᵗʰ **S72.479** Torus fracture of lower end of unspecified femur

√6ᵗʰ **S72.49** Other fracture of lower end of femur

√7ᵗʰ **S72.491** Other fracture of lower end of right femur

√7ᵗʰ **S72.492** Other fracture of lower end of left femur

√7ᵗʰ **S72.499** Other fracture of lower end of unspecified femur

√5ᵗʰ **S72.8** Other fracture of femur

√6ᵗʰ **S72.8X** Other fracture of femur

√7ᵗʰ **S72.8X1** Other fracture of right femur

√7ᵗʰ **S72.8X2** Other fracture of left femur

√7ᵗʰ **S72.8X9** Other fracture of unspecified femur

√5ᵗʰ **S72.9** Unspecified fracture of femur

Fracture of thigh NOS

Fracture of upper leg NOS

> **EXCLUDES 1**   fracture of hip NOS (S72.00-, S72.01-)

√x7ᵗʰ **S72.90** Unspecified fracture of unspecified femur

      AHA: 2012,4Q,93

√x7ᵗʰ **S72.91** Unspecified fracture of right femur

√x7ᵗʰ **S72.92** Unspecified fracture of left femur

√4ᵗʰ **S73** Dislocation and sprain of joint and ligaments of hip

> **INCLUDES**   avulsion of joint or ligament of hip
> laceration of cartilage, joint or ligament of hip
> sprain of cartilage, joint or ligament of hip
> traumatic hemarthrosis of joint or ligament of hip
> traumatic rupture of joint or ligament of hip
> traumatic subluxation of joint or ligament of hip
> traumatic tear of joint or ligament of hip

Code also any associated open wound

> **EXCLUDES 2**   strain of muscle, fascia and tendon of hip and thigh (S76.-)

> The appropriate 7th character is to be added to each code from category S73.
> A   initial encounter
> D   subsequent encounter
> S   sequela

√5ᵗʰ **S73.0** Subluxation and dislocation of hip

> **EXCLUDES 2**   dislocation and subluxation of hip prosthesis (T84.020, T84.021)

√6ᵗʰ **S73.00** Unspecified subluxation and dislocation of hip

Dislocation of hip NOS

Subluxation of hip NOS

√7ᵗʰ **S73.001** Unspecified subluxation of right hip

√7ᵗʰ **S73.002** Unspecified subluxation of left hip

√7ᵗʰ **S73.003** Unspecified subluxation of unspecified hip

√7ᵗʰ **S73.004** Unspecified dislocation of right hip

√7ᵗʰ **S73.005** Unspecified dislocation of left hip

N Newborn: 0   P Pediatric: 0-17   M Maternity: 12-55   A Adult: 15-124   CH Comorbidity High   CL Comorbidity Low   NCDx Noncancer Dx   PDx Primary Dx

1036   ICD-10-CM 2020

√7ᵗʰ **S73.006** Unspecified dislocation of unspecified hip

√6ᵗʰ **S73.01** Posterior subluxation and dislocation of hip

    √7ᵗʰ **S73.011** Posterior subluxation of right hip

    √7ᵗʰ **S73.012** Posterior subluxation of left hip

    √7ᵗʰ **S73.013** Posterior subluxation of unspecified hip

    √7ᵗʰ **S73.014** Posterior dislocation of right hip

    √7ᵗʰ **S73.015** Posterior dislocation of left hip

    √7ᵗʰ **S73.016** Posterior dislocation of unspecified hip

√6ᵗʰ **S73.02** Obturator subluxation and dislocation of hip

    √7ᵗʰ **S73.021** Obturator subluxation of right hip

    √7ᵗʰ **S73.022** Obturator subluxation of left hip

    √7ᵗʰ **S73.023** Obturator subluxation of unspecified hip

    √7ᵗʰ **S73.024** Obturator dislocation of right hip

    √7ᵗʰ **S73.025** Obturator dislocation of left hip

    √7ᵗʰ **S73.026** Obturator dislocation of unspecified hip

√6ᵗʰ **S73.03** Other anterior subluxation and dislocation of hip

    √7ᵗʰ **S73.031** Other anterior subluxation of right hip

    √7ᵗʰ **S73.032** Other anterior subluxation of left hip

    √7ᵗʰ **S73.033** Other anterior subluxation of unspecified hip

    √7ᵗʰ **S73.034** Other anterior dislocation of right hip

    √7ᵗʰ **S73.035** Other anterior dislocation of left hip

    √7ᵗʰ **S73.036** Other anterior dislocation of unspecified hip

√6ᵗʰ **S73.04** Central subluxation and dislocation of hip

    √7ᵗʰ **S73.041** Central subluxation of right hip

    √7ᵗʰ **S73.042** Central subluxation of left hip

    √7ᵗʰ **S73.043** Central subluxation of unspecified hip

    √7ᵗʰ **S73.044** Central dislocation of right hip

    √7ᵗʰ **S73.045** Central dislocation of left hip

    √7ᵗʰ **S73.046** Central dislocation of unspecified hip

√5ᵗʰ **S73.1** Sprain of hip

    AHA: 2014,4Q,25

√6ᵗʰ **S73.10** Unspecified sprain of hip

    √7ᵗʰ **S73.101** Unspecified sprain of right hip

    √7ᵗʰ **S73.102** Unspecified sprain of left hip

    √7ᵗʰ **S73.109** Unspecified sprain of unspecified hip

√6ᵗʰ **S73.11** Iliofemoral ligament sprain of hip

    √7ᵗʰ **S73.111** Iliofemoral ligament sprain of right hip

    √7ᵗʰ **S73.112** Iliofemoral ligament sprain of left hip

    √7ᵗʰ **S73.119** Iliofemoral ligament sprain of unspecified hip

√6ᵗʰ **S73.12** Ischiocapsular (ligament) sprain of hip

    √7ᵗʰ **S73.121** Ischiocapsular ligament sprain of right hip

    √7ᵗʰ **S73.122** Ischiocapsular ligament sprain of left hip

    √7ᵗʰ **S73.129** Ischiocapsular ligament sprain of unspecified hip

√6ᵗʰ **S73.19** Other sprain of hip

    √7ᵗʰ **S73.191** Other sprain of right hip

    √7ᵗʰ **S73.192** Other sprain of left hip

    √7ᵗʰ **S73.199** Other sprain of unspecified hip

√4ᵗʰ **S74** Injury of nerves at hip and thigh level

    Code also any associated open wound (S71.-)

    EXCLUDES 2   injury of nerves at ankle and foot level (S94.-)

                injury of nerves at lower leg level (S84.-)

> The appropriate 7th character is to be added to each code from category S74.
> A   initial encounter
> D   subsequent encounter
> S   sequela

√5ᵗʰ **S74.0** Injury of sciatic nerve at hip and thigh level

    √x7ᵗʰ **S74.00** Injury of sciatic nerve at hip and thigh level, unspecified leg

    √x7ᵗʰ **S74.01** Injury of sciatic nerve at hip and thigh level, right leg

    √x7ᵗʰ **S74.02** Injury of sciatic nerve at hip and thigh level, left leg

√5ᵗʰ **S74.1** Injury of femoral nerve at hip and thigh level

    √x7ᵗʰ **S74.10** Injury of femoral nerve at hip and thigh level, unspecified leg

    √x7ᵗʰ **S74.11** Injury of femoral nerve at hip and thigh level, right leg

    √x7ᵗʰ **S74.12** Injury of femoral nerve at hip and thigh level, left leg

√5ᵗʰ **S74.2** Injury of cutaneous sensory nerve at hip and thigh level

    √x7ᵗʰ **S74.20** Injury of cutaneous sensory nerve at hip and thigh level, unspecified leg

    √x7ᵗʰ **S74.21** Injury of cutaneous sensory nerve at hip and thigh level, right leg

    √x7ᵗʰ **S74.22** Injury of cutaneous sensory nerve at hip and thigh level, left leg

√5ᵗʰ **S74.8** Injury of other nerves at hip and thigh level

    √6ᵗʰ **S74.8X** Injury of other nerves at hip and thigh level

       √7ᵗʰ **S74.8X1** Injury of other nerves at hip and thigh level, right leg

       √7ᵗʰ **S74.8X2** Injury of other nerves at hip and thigh level, left leg

       √7ᵗʰ **S74.8X9** Injury of other nerves at hip and thigh level, unspecified leg

√5ᵗʰ **S74.9** Injury of unspecified nerve at hip and thigh level

    √x7ᵗʰ **S74.90** Injury of unspecified nerve at hip and thigh level, unspecified leg

    √x7ᵗʰ **S74.91** Injury of unspecified nerve at hip and thigh level, right leg

    √x7ᵗʰ **S74.92** Injury of unspecified nerve at hip and thigh level, left leg

√4ᵗʰ **S75** Injury of blood vessels at hip and thigh level

    Code also any associated open wound (S71.-)

    EXCLUDES 2   injury of blood vessels at lower leg level (S85.-)

                injury of popliteal artery (S85.0)

> The appropriate 7th character is to be added to each code from category S75.
> A   initial encounter
> D   subsequent encounter
> S   sequela

√5ᵗʰ **S75.0** Injury of femoral artery

    √6ᵗʰ **S75.00** Unspecified injury of femoral artery

       √7ᵗʰ **S75.001** Unspecified injury of femoral artery, right leg

       √7ᵗʰ **S75.002** Unspecified injury of femoral artery, left leg

       √7ᵗʰ **S75.009** Unspecified injury of femoral artery, unspecified leg

    √6ᵗʰ **S75.01** Minor laceration of femoral artery

       Incomplete transection of femoral artery

       Laceration of femoral artery NOS

       Superficial laceration of femoral artery

       √7ᵗʰ **S75.011** Minor laceration of femoral artery, right leg

       √7ᵗʰ **S75.012** Minor laceration of femoral artery, left leg

       √7ᵗʰ **S75.019** Minor laceration of femoral artery, unspecified leg

    √6ᵗʰ **S75.02** Major laceration of femoral artery

       Complete transection of femoral artery

       Traumatic rupture of femoral artery

       √7ᵗʰ **S75.021** Major laceration of femoral artery, right leg

       √7ᵗʰ **S75.022** Major laceration of femoral artery, left leg

       √7ᵗʰ **S75.029** Major laceration of femoral artery, unspecified leg

    √6ᵗʰ **S75.09** Other specified injury of femoral artery

       √7ᵗʰ **S75.091** Other specified injury of femoral artery, right leg

       √7ᵗʰ **S75.092** Other specified injury of femoral artery, left leg

       √7ᵗʰ **S75.099** Other specified injury of femoral artery, unspecified leg

√5ᵗʰ **S75.1** Injury of femoral vein at hip and thigh level

    √6ᵗʰ **S75.10** Unspecified injury of femoral vein at hip and thigh level

       √7ᵗʰ **S75.101** Unspecified injury of femoral vein at hip and thigh level, right leg

✔ Additional Character Required   √x7ᵗʰ Placeholder Alert   Manifestation   Unspecified Dx   ►◄ Revised Text   ● New Code   ▲ Revised Title

ICD-10-CM 2020   1037

      ✓7ᵗʰ **S75.102** Unspecified injury of femoral vein at hip and thigh level, left leg

      ✓7ᵗʰ **S75.109** Unspecified injury of femoral vein at hip and thigh level, unspecified leg

  ✓6ᵗʰ **S75.11** Minor laceration of femoral vein at hip and thigh level

      Incomplete transection of femoral vein at hip and thigh level

      Laceration of femoral vein at hip and thigh level NOS

      Superficial laceration of femoral vein at hip and thigh level

      ✓7ᵗʰ **S75.111** Minor laceration of femoral vein at hip and thigh level, right leg

      ✓7ᵗʰ **S75.112** Minor laceration of femoral vein at hip and thigh level, left leg

      ✓7ᵗʰ **S75.119** Minor laceration of femoral vein at hip and thigh level, unspecified leg

  ✓6ᵗʰ **S75.12** Major laceration of femoral vein at hip and thigh level

      Complete transection of femoral vein at hip and thigh level

      Traumatic rupture of femoral vein at hip and thigh level

      ✓7ᵗʰ **S75.121** Major laceration of femoral vein at hip and thigh level, right leg

      ✓7ᵗʰ **S75.122** Major laceration of femoral vein at hip and thigh level, left leg

      ✓7ᵗʰ **S75.129** Major laceration of femoral vein at hip and thigh level, unspecified leg

  ✓6ᵗʰ **S75.19** Other specified injury of femoral vein at hip and thigh level

      ✓7ᵗʰ **S75.191** Other specified injury of femoral vein at hip and thigh level, right leg

      ✓7ᵗʰ **S75.192** Other specified injury of femoral vein at hip and thigh level, left leg

      ✓7ᵗʰ **S75.199** Other specified injury of femoral vein at hip and thigh level, unspecified leg

✓5ᵗʰ **S75.2** Injury of greater saphenous vein at hip and thigh level

    EXCLUDES 1   greater saphenous vein NOS (S85.3)

  ✓6ᵗʰ **S75.20** Unspecified injury of greater saphenous vein at hip and thigh level

      ✓7ᵗʰ **S75.201** Unspecified injury of greater saphenous vein at hip and thigh level, right leg

      ✓7ᵗʰ **S75.202** Unspecified injury of greater saphenous vein at hip and thigh level, left leg

      ✓7ᵗʰ **S75.209** Unspecified injury of greater saphenous vein at hip and thigh level, unspecified leg

  ✓6ᵗʰ **S75.21** Minor laceration of greater saphenous vein at hip and thigh level

      Incomplete transection of greater saphenous vein at hip and thigh level

      Laceration of greater saphenous vein at hip and thigh level NOS

      Superficial laceration of greater saphenous vein at hip and thigh level

      ✓7ᵗʰ **S75.211** Minor laceration of greater saphenous vein at hip and thigh level, right leg

      ✓7ᵗʰ **S75.212** Minor laceration of greater saphenous vein at hip and thigh level, left leg

      ✓7ᵗʰ **S75.219** Minor laceration of greater saphenous vein at hip and thigh level, unspecified leg

  ✓6ᵗʰ **S75.22** Major laceration of greater saphenous vein at hip and thigh level

      Complete transection of greater saphenous vein at hip and thigh level

      Traumatic rupture of greater saphenous vein at hip and thigh level

      ✓7ᵗʰ **S75.221** Major laceration of greater saphenous vein at hip and thigh level, right leg

      ✓7ᵗʰ **S75.222** Major laceration of greater saphenous vein at hip and thigh level, left leg

      ✓7ᵗʰ **S75.229** Major laceration of greater saphenous vein at hip and thigh level, unspecified leg

  ✓6ᵗʰ **S75.29** Other specified injury of greater saphenous vein at hip and thigh level

      ✓7ᵗʰ **S75.291** Other specified injury of greater saphenous vein at hip and thigh level, right leg

      ✓7ᵗʰ **S75.292** Other specified injury of greater saphenous vein at hip and thigh level, left leg

      ✓7ᵗʰ **S75.299** Other specified injury of greater saphenous vein at hip and thigh level, unspecified leg

✓5ᵗʰ **S75.8** Injury of other blood vessels at hip and thigh level

  ✓6ᵗʰ **S75.80** Unspecified injury of other blood vessels at hip and thigh level

      ✓7ᵗʰ **S75.801** Unspecified injury of other blood vessels at hip and thigh level, right leg

      ✓7ᵗʰ **S75.802** Unspecified injury of other blood vessels at hip and thigh level, left leg

      ✓7ᵗʰ **S75.809** Unspecified injury of other blood vessels at hip and thigh level, unspecified leg

  ✓6ᵗʰ **S75.81** Laceration of other blood vessels at hip and thigh level

      ✓7ᵗʰ **S75.811** Laceration of other blood vessels at hip and thigh level, right leg

      ✓7ᵗʰ **S75.812** Laceration of other blood vessels at hip and thigh level, left leg

      ✓7ᵗʰ **S75.819** Laceration of other blood vessels at hip and thigh level, unspecified leg

  ✓6ᵗʰ **S75.89** Other specified injury of other blood vessels at hip and thigh level

      ✓7ᵗʰ **S75.891** Other specified injury of other blood vessels at hip and thigh level, right leg

      ✓7ᵗʰ **S75.892** Other specified injury of other blood vessels at hip and thigh level, left leg

      ✓7ᵗʰ **S75.899** Other specified injury of other blood vessels at hip and thigh level, unspecified leg

✓5ᵗʰ **S75.9** Injury of unspecified blood vessel at hip and thigh level

  ✓6ᵗʰ **S75.90** Unspecified injury of unspecified blood vessel at hip and thigh level

      ✓7ᵗʰ **S75.901** Unspecified injury of unspecified blood vessel at hip and thigh level, right leg

      ✓7ᵗʰ **S75.902** Unspecified injury of unspecified blood vessel at hip and thigh level, left leg

      ✓7ᵗʰ **S75.909** Unspecified injury of unspecified blood vessel at hip and thigh level, unspecified leg

  ✓6ᵗʰ **S75.91** Laceration of unspecified blood vessel at hip and thigh level

      ✓7ᵗʰ **S75.911** Laceration of unspecified blood vessel at hip and thigh level, right leg

      ✓7ᵗʰ **S75.912** Laceration of unspecified blood vessel at hip and thigh level, left leg

      ✓7ᵗʰ **S75.919** Laceration of unspecified blood vessel at hip and thigh level, unspecified leg

  ✓6ᵗʰ **S75.99** Other specified injury of unspecified blood vessel at hip and thigh level

      ✓7ᵗʰ **S75.991** Other specified injury of unspecified blood vessel at hip and thigh level, right leg

      ✓7ᵗʰ **S75.992** Other specified injury of unspecified blood vessel at hip and thigh level, left leg

      ✓7ᵗʰ **S75.999** Other specified injury of unspecified blood vessel at hip and thigh level, unspecified leg

✓4ᵗʰ **S76** Injury of muscle, fascia and tendon at hip and thigh level

    Code also any associated open wound (S71.-)

    EXCLUDES 2   injury of muscle, fascia and tendon at lower leg level (S86)

                  sprain of joint and ligament of hip (S73.1)

    TIP: Refer to the Muscle/Tendon table at the beginning of this chapter.

    The appropriate 7th character is to be added to each code from category S76.
    A   initial encounter
    D   subsequent encounter
    S   sequela

  ✓5ᵗʰ **S76.0** Injury of muscle, fascia and tendon of hip

    ✓6ᵗʰ **S76.00** Unspecified injury of muscle, fascia and tendon of hip

      ✓7ᵗʰ **S76.001** Unspecified injury of muscle, fascia and tendon of right hip

      ✓7ᵗʰ **S76.002** Unspecified injury of muscle, fascia and tendon of left hip

      ✓7ᵗʰ **S76.009** Unspecified injury of muscle, fascia and tendon of unspecified hip

N Newborn: 0   **P** Pediatric: 0-17   **M** Maternity: 12-55   **A** Adult: 15-124   **CH** Comorbidity High   **CL** Comorbidity Low   **NCDx** Noncancer Dx   **PDx** Primary Dx

1038   ICD-10-CM 2020

√6ᵗʰ **S76.01** Strain of muscle, fascia and tendon of hip
> √7ᵗʰ **S76.011** Strain of muscle, fascia and tendon of right hip
> √7ᵗʰ **S76.012** Strain of muscle, fascia and tendon of left hip
> √7ᵗʰ **S76.019** Strain of muscle, fascia and tendon of unspecified hip

√6ᵗʰ **S76.02** Laceration of muscle, fascia and tendon of hip
> √7ᵗʰ **S76.021** Laceration of muscle, fascia and tendon of right hip
> √7ᵗʰ **S76.022** Laceration of muscle, fascia and tendon of left hip
> √7ᵗʰ **S76.029** Laceration of muscle, fascia and tendon of unspecified hip

√6ᵗʰ **S76.09** Other specified injury of muscle, fascia and tendon of hip
> √7ᵗʰ **S76.091** Other specified injury of muscle, fascia and tendon of right hip
> √7ᵗʰ **S76.092** Other specified injury of muscle, fascia and tendon of left hip
> √7ᵗʰ **S76.099** Other specified injury of muscle, fascia and tendon of unspecified hip

√5ᵗʰ **S76.1** Injury of quadriceps muscle, fascia and tendon
> Injury of patellar ligament (tendon)

√6ᵗʰ **S76.10** Unspecified injury of quadriceps muscle, fascia and tendon
> √7ᵗʰ **S76.101** Unspecified injury of right quadriceps muscle, fascia and tendon
> √7ᵗʰ **S76.102** Unspecified injury of left quadriceps muscle, fascia and tendon
> √7ᵗʰ **S76.109** Unspecified injury of unspecified quadriceps muscle, fascia and tendon

√6ᵗʰ **S76.11** Strain of quadriceps muscle, fascia and tendon
> √7ᵗʰ **S76.111** Strain of right quadriceps muscle, fascia and tendon
> √7ᵗʰ **S76.112** Strain of left quadriceps muscle, fascia and tendon
> √7ᵗʰ **S76.119** Strain of unspecified quadriceps muscle, fascia and tendon

√6ᵗʰ **S76.12** Laceration of quadriceps muscle, fascia and tendon
> √7ᵗʰ **S76.121** Laceration of right quadriceps muscle, fascia and tendon
> √7ᵗʰ **S76.122** Laceration of left quadriceps muscle, fascia and tendon
> √7ᵗʰ **S76.129** Laceration of unspecified quadriceps muscle, fascia and tendon

√6ᵗʰ **S76.19** Other specified injury of quadriceps muscle, fascia and tendon
> √7ᵗʰ **S76.191** Other specified injury of right quadriceps muscle, fascia and tendon
> √7ᵗʰ **S76.192** Other specified injury of left quadriceps muscle, fascia and tendon
> √7ᵗʰ **S76.199** Other specified injury of unspecified quadriceps muscle, fascia and tendon

√5ᵗʰ **S76.2** Injury of adductor muscle, fascia and tendon of thigh
√6ᵗʰ **S76.20** Unspecified injury of adductor muscle, fascia and tendon of thigh
> √7ᵗʰ **S76.201** Unspecified injury of adductor muscle, fascia and tendon of right thigh
> √7ᵗʰ **S76.202** Unspecified injury of adductor muscle, fascia and tendon of left thigh
> √7ᵗʰ **S76.209** Unspecified injury of adductor muscle, fascia and tendon of unspecified thigh

√6ᵗʰ **S76.21** Strain of adductor muscle, fascia and tendon of thigh
> √7ᵗʰ **S76.211** Strain of adductor muscle, fascia and tendon of right thigh
> √7ᵗʰ **S76.212** Strain of adductor muscle, fascia and tendon of left thigh
> √7ᵗʰ **S76.219** Strain of adductor muscle, fascia and tendon of unspecified thigh

√6ᵗʰ **S76.22** Laceration of adductor muscle, fascia and tendon of thigh
> √7ᵗʰ **S76.221** Laceration of adductor muscle, fascia and tendon of right thigh
> √7ᵗʰ **S76.222** Laceration of adductor muscle, fascia and tendon of left thigh
> √7ᵗʰ **S76.229** Laceration of adductor muscle, fascia and tendon of unspecified thigh

√6ᵗʰ **S76.29** Other injury of adductor muscle, fascia and tendon of thigh
> √7ᵗʰ **S76.291** Other injury of adductor muscle, fascia and tendon of right thigh
> √7ᵗʰ **S76.292** Other injury of adductor muscle, fascia and tendon of left thigh
> √7ᵗʰ **S76.299** Other injury of adductor muscle, fascia and tendon of unspecified thigh

√5ᵗʰ **S76.3** Injury of muscle, fascia and tendon of the posterior muscle group at thigh level
√6ᵗʰ **S76.30** Unspecified injury of muscle, fascia and tendon of the posterior muscle group at thigh level
> √7ᵗʰ **S76.301** Unspecified injury of muscle, fascia and tendon of the posterior muscle group at thigh level, right thigh
> √7ᵗʰ **S76.302** Unspecified injury of muscle, fascia and tendon of the posterior muscle group at thigh level, left thigh
> √7ᵗʰ **S76.309** Unspecified injury of muscle, fascia and tendon of the posterior muscle group at thigh level, unspecified thigh

√6ᵗʰ **S76.31** Strain of muscle, fascia and tendon of the posterior muscle group at thigh level
> √7ᵗʰ **S76.311** Strain of muscle, fascia and tendon of the posterior muscle group at thigh level, right thigh
> √7ᵗʰ **S76.312** Strain of muscle, fascia and tendon of the posterior muscle group at thigh level, left thigh
> √7ᵗʰ **S76.319** Strain of muscle, fascia and tendon of the posterior muscle group at thigh level, unspecified thigh

√6ᵗʰ **S76.32** Laceration of muscle, fascia and tendon of the posterior muscle group at thigh level
> √7ᵗʰ **S76.321** Laceration of muscle, fascia and tendon of the posterior muscle group at thigh level, right thigh
> √7ᵗʰ **S76.322** Laceration of muscle, fascia and tendon of the posterior muscle group at thigh level, left thigh
> √7ᵗʰ **S76.329** Laceration of muscle, fascia and tendon of the posterior muscle group at thigh level, unspecified thigh

√6ᵗʰ **S76.39** Other specified injury of muscle, fascia and tendon of the posterior muscle group at thigh level
> √7ᵗʰ **S76.391** Other specified injury of muscle, fascia and tendon of the posterior muscle group at thigh level, right thigh
> √7ᵗʰ **S76.392** Other specified injury of muscle, fascia and tendon of the posterior muscle group at thigh level, left thigh
> √7ᵗʰ **S76.399** Other specified injury of muscle, fascia and tendon of the posterior muscle group at thigh level, unspecified thigh

√5ᵗʰ **S76.8** Injury of other specified muscles, fascia and tendons at thigh level
√6ᵗʰ **S76.80** Unspecified injury of other specified muscles, fascia and tendons at thigh level
> √7ᵗʰ **S76.801** Unspecified injury of other specified muscles, fascia and tendons at thigh level, right thigh
> √7ᵗʰ **S76.802** Unspecified injury of other specified muscles, fascia and tendons at thigh level, left thigh
> √7ᵗʰ **S76.809** Unspecified injury of other specified muscles, fascia and tendons at thigh level, unspecified thigh

√6ᵗʰ **S76.81** Strain of other specified muscles, fascia and tendons at thigh level
> √7ᵗʰ **S76.811** Strain of other specified muscles, fascia and tendons at thigh level, right thigh
> √7ᵗʰ **S76.812** Strain of other specified muscles, fascia and tendons at thigh level, left thigh
> √7ᵗʰ **S76.819** Strain of other specified muscles, fascia and tendons at thigh level, unspecified thigh

√6ᵗʰ **S76.82** Laceration of other specified muscles, fascia and tendons at thigh level
> √7ᵗʰ **S76.821** Laceration of other specified muscles, fascia and tendons at thigh level, right thigh
> √7ᵗʰ **S76.822** Laceration of other specified muscles, fascia and tendons at thigh level, left thigh

☑ Additional Character Required   √x7ᵗʰ Placeholder Alert   Manifestation   Unspecified Dx   ►◄ Revised Text   ● New Code   ▲ Revised Title

ICD-10-CM 2020   **1039**

√7ᵗʰ **S76.829** Laceration of other specified muscles, fascia and tendons at thigh level, unspecified thigh

√6ᵗʰ **S76.89** Other injury of other specified muscles, fascia and tendons at thigh level

√7ᵗʰ **S76.891** Other injury of other specified muscles, fascia and tendons at thigh level, right thigh

√7ᵗʰ **S76.892** Other injury of other specified muscles, fascia and tendons at thigh level, left thigh

√7ᵗʰ **S76.899** Other injury of other specified muscles, fascia and tendons at thigh level, unspecified thigh

√5ᵗʰ **S76.9** Injury of unspecified muscles, fascia and tendons at thigh level

√6ᵗʰ **S76.90** Unspecified injury of unspecified muscles, fascia and tendons at thigh level

√7ᵗʰ **S76.901** Unspecified injury of unspecified muscles, fascia and tendons at thigh level, right thigh

√7ᵗʰ **S76.902** Unspecified injury of unspecified muscles, fascia and tendons at thigh level, left thigh

√7ᵗʰ **S76.909** Unspecified injury of unspecified muscles, fascia and tendons at thigh level, unspecified thigh

√6ᵗʰ **S76.91** Strain of unspecified muscles, fascia and tendons at thigh level

√7ᵗʰ **S76.911** Strain of unspecified muscles, fascia and tendons at thigh level, right thigh

√7ᵗʰ **S76.912** Strain of unspecified muscles, fascia and tendons at thigh level, left thigh

√7ᵗʰ **S76.919** Strain of unspecified muscles, fascia and tendons at thigh level, unspecified thigh

√6ᵗʰ **S76.92** Laceration of unspecified muscles, fascia and tendons at thigh level

√7ᵗʰ **S76.921** Laceration of unspecified muscles, fascia and tendons at thigh level, right thigh

√7ᵗʰ **S76.922** Laceration of unspecified muscles, fascia and tendons at thigh level, left thigh

√7ᵗʰ **S76.929** Laceration of unspecified muscles, fascia and tendons at thigh level, unspecified thigh

√6ᵗʰ **S76.99** Other specified injury of unspecified muscles, fascia and tendons at thigh level

√7ᵗʰ **S76.991** Other specified injury of unspecified muscles, fascia and tendons at thigh level, right thigh

√7ᵗʰ **S76.992** Other specified injury of unspecified muscles, fascia and tendons at thigh level, left thigh

√7ᵗʰ **S76.999** Other specified injury of unspecified muscles, fascia and tendons at thigh level, unspecified thigh

√4ᵗʰ **S77 Crushing injury of hip and thigh**

Use additional code(s) for all associated injuries

EXCLUDES 2   crushing injury of ankle and foot (S97.-)
crushing injury of lower leg (S87.-)

The appropriate 7th character is to be added to each code from category S77.
A   initial encounter
D   subsequent encounter
S   sequela

√5ᵗʰ **S77.0** Crushing injury of hip

√x7ᵗʰ **S77.00** Crushing injury of unspecified hip

√x7ᵗʰ **S77.01** Crushing injury of right hip

√x7ᵗʰ **S77.02** Crushing injury of left hip

√5ᵗʰ **S77.1** Crushing injury of thigh

√x7ᵗʰ **S77.10** Crushing injury of unspecified thigh

√x7ᵗʰ **S77.11** Crushing injury of right thigh

√x7ᵗʰ **S77.12** Crushing injury of left thigh

√5ᵗʰ **S77.2** Crushing injury of hip with thigh

√x7ᵗʰ **S77.20** Crushing injury of unspecified hip with thigh

√x7ᵗʰ **S77.21** Crushing injury of right hip with thigh

√x7ᵗʰ **S77.22** Crushing injury of left hip with thigh

√4ᵗʰ **S78 Traumatic amputation of hip and thigh**

An amputation not identified as partial or complete should be coded to complete

EXCLUDES 1   traumatic amputation of knee (S88.0-)

The appropriate 7th character is to be added to each code from category S78.
A   initial encounter
D   subsequent encounter
S   sequela

√5ᵗʰ **S78.0** Traumatic amputation at hip joint

√6ᵗʰ **S78.01** Complete traumatic amputation at hip joint

√7ᵗʰ **S78.011** Complete traumatic amputation at right hip joint

√7ᵗʰ **S78.012** Complete traumatic amputation at left hip joint

√7ᵗʰ **S78.019** Complete traumatic amputation at unspecified hip joint

√6ᵗʰ **S78.02** Partial traumatic amputation at hip joint

√7ᵗʰ **S78.021** Partial traumatic amputation at right hip joint

√7ᵗʰ **S78.022** Partial traumatic amputation at left hip joint

√7ᵗʰ **S78.029** Partial traumatic amputation at unspecified hip joint

√5ᵗʰ **S78.1** Traumatic amputation at level between hip and knee

EXCLUDES 1   traumatic amputation of knee (S88.0-)

√6ᵗʰ **S78.11** Complete traumatic amputation at level between hip and knee

√7ᵗʰ **S78.111** Complete traumatic amputation at level between right hip and knee

√7ᵗʰ **S78.112** Complete traumatic amputation at level between left hip and knee

√7ᵗʰ **S78.119** Complete traumatic amputation at level between unspecified hip and knee

√6ᵗʰ **S78.12** Partial traumatic amputation at level between hip and knee

√7ᵗʰ **S78.121** Partial traumatic amputation at level between right hip and knee

√7ᵗʰ **S78.122** Partial traumatic amputation at level between left hip and knee

√7ᵗʰ **S78.129** Partial traumatic amputation at level between unspecified hip and knee

√5ᵗʰ **S78.9** Traumatic amputation of hip and thigh, level unspecified

√6ᵗʰ **S78.91** Complete traumatic amputation of hip and thigh, level unspecified

√7ᵗʰ **S78.911** Complete traumatic amputation of right hip and thigh, level unspecified

√7ᵗʰ **S78.912** Complete traumatic amputation of left hip and thigh, level unspecified

√7ᵗʰ **S78.919** Complete traumatic amputation of unspecified hip and thigh, level unspecified

√6ᵗʰ **S78.92** Partial traumatic amputation of hip and thigh, level unspecified

√7ᵗʰ **S78.921** Partial traumatic amputation of right hip and thigh, level unspecified

√7ᵗʰ **S78.922** Partial traumatic amputation of left hip and thigh, level unspecified

√7ᵗʰ **S78.929** Partial traumatic amputation of unspecified hip and thigh, level unspecified

√4th S79 Other and unspecified injuries of hip and thigh

NOTE A fracture not indicated as open or closed should be coded to closed

AHA: 2018,2Q,12; 2018,1Q,3; 2015,3Q,37-39
TIP: The term "improper alignment" is not synonymous with malunion or nonunion of a fracture when noted in provider documentation.

The appropriate 7th character is to be added to each code from subcategories S79.0 and S79.1.
A initial encounter for closed fracture
D subsequent encounter for fracture with routine healing
G subsequent encounter for fracture with delayed healing
K subsequent encounter for fracture with nonunion
P subsequent encounter for fracture with malunion
S sequela

√5th S79.0 Physeal fracture of upper end of femur

EXCLUDES 1 apophyseal fracture of upper end of femur (S72.13-)
nontraumatic slipped upper femoral epiphysis (M93.0-)

√6th **S79.00** Unspecified physeal fracture of upper end of femur
- √7th **S79.001** Unspecified physeal fracture of upper end of right femur
- √7th **S79.002** Unspecified physeal fracture of upper end of left femur
- √7th **S79.009** Unspecified physeal fracture of upper end of unspecified femur

√6th **S79.01** Salter-Harris Type I physeal fracture of upper end of femur
Acute on chronic slipped capital femoral epiphysis (traumatic)
Acute slipped capital femoral epiphysis (traumatic)
Capital femoral epiphyseal fracture
EXCLUDES 1 chronic slipped upper femoral epiphysis (nontraumatic) (M93.02-)
- √7th **S79.011** Salter-Harris Type I physeal fracture of upper end of right femur
- √7th **S79.012** Salter-Harris Type I physeal fracture of upper end of left femur
- √7th **S79.019** Salter-Harris Type I physeal fracture of upper end of unspecified femur

√6th **S79.09** Other physeal fracture of upper end of femur
- √7th **S79.091** Other physeal fracture of upper end of right femur
- √7th **S79.092** Other physeal fracture of upper end of left femur
- √7th **S79.099** Other physeal fracture of upper end of unspecified femur

√5th S79.1 Physeal fracture of lower end of femur

√6th **S79.10** Unspecified physeal fracture of lower end of femur
- √7th **S79.101** Unspecified physeal fracture of lower end of right femur
- √7th **S79.102** Unspecified physeal fracture of lower end of left femur
- √7th **S79.109** Unspecified physeal fracture of lower end of unspecified femur

√6th **S79.11** Salter-Harris Type I physeal fracture of lower end of femur
- √7th **S79.111** Salter-Harris Type I physeal fracture of lower end of right femur
- √7th **S79.112** Salter-Harris Type I physeal fracture of lower end of left femur
- √7th **S79.119** Salter-Harris Type I physeal fracture of lower end of unspecified femur

√6th **S79.12** Salter-Harris Type II physeal fracture of lower end of femur
- √7th **S79.121** Salter-Harris Type II physeal fracture of lower end of right femur
- √7th **S79.122** Salter-Harris Type II physeal fracture of lower end of left femur
- √7th **S79.129** Salter-Harris Type II physeal fracture of lower end of unspecified femur

√6th **S79.13** Salter-Harris Type III physeal fracture of lower end of femur
- √7th **S79.131** Salter-Harris Type III physeal fracture of lower end of right femur
- √7th **S79.132** Salter-Harris Type III physeal fracture of lower end of left femur
- √7th **S79.139** Salter-Harris Type III physeal fracture of lower end of unspecified femur

√6th **S79.14** Salter-Harris Type IV physeal fracture of lower end of femur
- √7th **S79.141** Salter-Harris Type IV physeal fracture of lower end of right femur
- √7th **S79.142** Salter-Harris Type IV physeal fracture of lower end of left femur
- √7th **S79.149** Salter-Harris Type IV physeal fracture of lower end of unspecified femur

√6th **S79.19** Other physeal fracture of lower end of femur
- √7th **S79.191** Other physeal fracture of lower end of right femur
- √7th **S79.192** Other physeal fracture of lower end of left femur
- √7th **S79.199** Other physeal fracture of lower end of unspecified femur

√5th S79.8 Other specified injuries of hip and thigh

The appropriate 7th character is to be added to each code in subcategory S79.8.
A initial encounter
D subsequent encounter
S sequela

√6th **S79.81** Other specified injuries of hip
- √7th **S79.811** Other specified injuries of right hip
- √7th **S79.812** Other specified injuries of left hip
- √7th **S79.819** Other specified injuries of unspecified hip

√6th **S79.82** Other specified injuries of thigh
- √7th **S79.821** Other specified injuries of right thigh
- √7th **S79.822** Other specified injuries of left thigh
- √7th **S79.829** Other specified injuries of unspecified thigh

√5th S79.9 Unspecified injury of hip and thigh

The appropriate 7th character is to be added to each code in subcategory S79.9.
A initial encounter
D subsequent encounter
S sequela

√6th **S79.91** Unspecified injury of hip
- √7th **S79.911** Unspecified injury of right hip
- √7th **S79.912** Unspecified injury of left hip
- √7th **S79.919** Unspecified injury of unspecified hip

√6th **S79.92** Unspecified injury of thigh
- √7th **S79.921** Unspecified injury of right thigh
- √7th **S79.922** Unspecified injury of left thigh
- √7th **S79.929** Unspecified injury of unspecified thigh

Injuries to the knee and lower leg (S80-S89)

EXCLUDES 2 burns and corrosions (T20-T32)
frostbite (T33-T34)
injuries of ankle and foot, except fracture of ankle and malleolus (S90-S99)
insect bite or sting, venomous (T63.4)

√4th S80 Superficial injury of knee and lower leg

EXCLUDES 2 superficial injury of ankle and foot (S90.-)

The appropriate 7th character is to be added to each code from category S80.
A initial encounter
D subsequent encounter
S sequela

√5th S80.0 Contusion of knee
- √x7th **S80.00** Contusion of unspecified knee
- √x7th **S80.01** Contusion of right knee
- √x7th **S80.02** Contusion of left knee

√5th S80.1 Contusion of lower leg
- √x7th **S80.10** Contusion of unspecified lower leg
- √x7th **S80.11** Contusion of right lower leg
- √x7th **S80.12** Contusion of left lower leg

√5th S80.2 Other superficial injuries of knee
√6th **S80.21** Abrasion of knee
- √7th **S80.211** Abrasion, right knee
- √7th **S80.212** Abrasion, left knee
- √7th **S80.219** Abrasion, unspecified knee

✓6ᵗʰ **S80.22** Blister (nonthermal) of knee
- ✓7ᵗʰ **S80.221** Blister (nonthermal), right knee
- ✓7ᵗʰ **S80.222** Blister (nonthermal), left knee
- ✓7ᵗʰ **S80.229** Blister (nonthermal), unspecified knee

✓6ᵗʰ **S80.24** External constriction of knee
- ✓7ᵗʰ **S80.241** External constriction, right knee
- ✓7ᵗʰ **S80.242** External constriction, left knee
- ✓7ᵗʰ **S80.249** External constriction, unspecified knee

✓6ᵗʰ **S80.25** Superficial foreign body of knee
  Splinter in the knee
- ✓7ᵗʰ **S80.251** Superficial foreign body, right knee
- ✓7ᵗʰ **S80.252** Superficial foreign body, left knee
- ✓7ᵗʰ **S80.259** Superficial foreign body, unspecified knee

✓6ᵗʰ **S80.26** Insect bite (nonvenomous) of knee
- ✓7ᵗʰ **S80.261** Insect bite (nonvenomous), right knee
- ✓7ᵗʰ **S80.262** Insect bite (nonvenomous), left knee
- ✓7ᵗʰ **S80.269** Insect bite (nonvenomous), unspecified knee

✓6ᵗʰ **S80.27** Other superficial bite of knee
  EXCLUDES 1   open bite of knee (S81.05-)
- ✓7ᵗʰ **S80.271** Other superficial bite of right knee
- ✓7ᵗʰ **S80.272** Other superficial bite of left knee
- ✓7ᵗʰ **S80.279** Other superficial bite of unspecified knee

✓5ᵗʰ **S80.8** Other superficial injuries of lower leg

✓6ᵗʰ **S80.81** Abrasion of lower leg
- ✓7ᵗʰ **S80.811** Abrasion, right lower leg
- ✓7ᵗʰ **S80.812** Abrasion, left lower leg
- ✓7ᵗʰ **S80.819** Abrasion, unspecified lower leg

✓6ᵗʰ **S80.82** Blister (nonthermal) of lower leg
- ✓7ᵗʰ **S80.821** Blister (nonthermal), right lower leg
- ✓7ᵗʰ **S80.822** Blister (nonthermal), left lower leg
- ✓7ᵗʰ **S80.829** Blister (nonthermal), unspecified lower leg

✓6ᵗʰ **S80.84** External constriction of lower leg
- ✓7ᵗʰ **S80.841** External constriction, right lower leg
- ✓7ᵗʰ **S80.842** External constriction, left lower leg
- ✓7ᵗʰ **S80.849** External constriction, unspecified lower leg

✓6ᵗʰ **S80.85** Superficial foreign body of lower leg
  Splinter in the lower leg
- ✓7ᵗʰ **S80.851** Superficial foreign body, right lower leg
- ✓7ᵗʰ **S80.852** Superficial foreign body, left lower leg
- ✓7ᵗʰ **S80.859** Superficial foreign body, unspecified lower leg

✓6ᵗʰ **S80.86** Insect bite (nonvenomous) of lower leg
- ✓7ᵗʰ **S80.861** Insect bite (nonvenomous), right lower leg
- ✓7ᵗʰ **S80.862** Insect bite (nonvenomous), left lower leg
- ✓7ᵗʰ **S80.869** Insect bite (nonvenomous), unspecified lower leg

✓6ᵗʰ **S80.87** Other superficial bite of lower leg
  EXCLUDES 1   open bite of lower leg (S81.85-)
- ✓7ᵗʰ **S80.871** Other superficial bite, right lower leg
- ✓7ᵗʰ **S80.872** Other superficial bite, left lower leg
- ✓7ᵗʰ **S80.879** Other superficial bite, unspecified lower leg

✓5ᵗʰ **S80.9** Unspecified superficial injury of knee and lower leg

✓6ᵗʰ **S80.91** Unspecified superficial injury of knee
- ✓7ᵗʰ **S80.911** Unspecified superficial injury of right knee
- ✓7ᵗʰ **S80.912** Unspecified superficial injury of left knee
- ✓7ᵗʰ **S80.919** Unspecified superficial injury of unspecified knee

✓6ᵗʰ **S80.92** Unspecified superficial injury of lower leg
- ✓7ᵗʰ **S80.921** Unspecified superficial injury of right lower leg
- ✓7ᵗʰ **S80.922** Unspecified superficial injury of left lower leg
- ✓7ᵗʰ **S80.929** Unspecified superficial injury of unspecified lower leg

✓4ᵗʰ **S81 Open wound of knee and lower leg**
  Code also any associated wound infection
  EXCLUDES 1   open fracture of knee and lower leg (S82.-)
             traumatic amputation of lower leg (S88.-)
  EXCLUDES 2   open wound of ankle and foot (S91.-)

  The appropriate 7th character is to be added to each code from category S81.
  A initial encounter
  D subsequent encounter
  S sequela

✓5ᵗʰ **S81.0** Open wound of knee

✓6ᵗʰ **S81.00** Unspecified open wound of knee
- ✓7ᵗʰ **S81.001** Unspecified open wound, right knee
- ✓7ᵗʰ **S81.002** Unspecified open wound, left knee
- ✓7ᵗʰ **S81.009** Unspecified open wound, unspecified knee

✓6ᵗʰ **S81.01** Laceration without foreign body of knee
- ✓7ᵗʰ **S81.011** Laceration without foreign body, right knee
- ✓7ᵗʰ **S81.012** Laceration without foreign body, left knee
- ✓7ᵗʰ **S81.019** Laceration without foreign body, unspecified knee

✓6ᵗʰ **S81.02** Laceration with foreign body of knee
- ✓7ᵗʰ **S81.021** Laceration with foreign body, right knee
- ✓7ᵗʰ **S81.022** Laceration with foreign body, left knee
- ✓7ᵗʰ **S81.029** Laceration with foreign body, unspecified knee

✓6ᵗʰ **S81.03** Puncture wound without foreign body of knee
- ✓7ᵗʰ **S81.031** Puncture wound without foreign body, right knee
- ✓7ᵗʰ **S81.032** Puncture wound without foreign body, left knee
- ✓7ᵗʰ **S81.039** Puncture wound without foreign body, unspecified knee

✓6ᵗʰ **S81.04** Puncture wound with foreign body of knee
- ✓7ᵗʰ **S81.041** Puncture wound with foreign body, right knee
- ✓7ᵗʰ **S81.042** Puncture wound with foreign body, left knee
- ✓7ᵗʰ **S81.049** Puncture wound with foreign body, unspecified knee

✓6ᵗʰ **S81.05** Open bite of knee
  Bite of knee NOS
  EXCLUDES 1   superficial bite of knee (S80.27-)
- ✓7ᵗʰ **S81.051** Open bite, right knee
- ✓7ᵗʰ **S81.052** Open bite, left knee
- ✓7ᵗʰ **S81.059** Open bite, unspecified knee

✓5ᵗʰ **S81.8** Open wound of lower leg

✓6ᵗʰ **S81.80** Unspecified open wound of lower leg
  AHA: 2016,3Q,24
- ✓7ᵗʰ **S81.801** Unspecified open wound, right lower leg
- ✓7ᵗʰ **S81.802** Unspecified open wound, left lower leg
- ✓7ᵗʰ **S81.809** Unspecified open wound, unspecified lower leg

✓6ᵗʰ **S81.81** Laceration without foreign body of lower leg
- ✓7ᵗʰ **S81.811** Laceration without foreign body, right lower leg
- ✓7ᵗʰ **S81.812** Laceration without foreign body, left lower leg
- ✓7ᵗʰ **S81.819** Laceration without foreign body, unspecified lower leg

✓6ᵗʰ **S81.82** Laceration with foreign body of lower leg
- ✓7ᵗʰ **S81.821** Laceration with foreign body, right lower leg
- ✓7ᵗʰ **S81.822** Laceration with foreign body, left lower leg
- ✓7ᵗʰ **S81.829** Laceration with foreign body, unspecified lower leg

✓6ᵗʰ **S81.83** Puncture wound without foreign body of lower leg
  AHA: 2016,3Q,24
- ✓7ᵗʰ **S81.831** Puncture wound without foreign body, right lower leg
- ✓7ᵗʰ **S81.832** Puncture wound without foreign body, left lower leg

N Newborn: 0   **P** Pediatric: 0-17   **M** Maternity: 12-55   **A** Adult: 15-124   **CH** Comorbidity High   **CL** Comorbidity Low   **NC Dx** Noncancer Dx   **PDx** Primary Dx

1042   ICD-10-CM 2020

√7ᵗʰ **S81.839** Puncture wound without foreign body, unspecified lower leg

√6ᵗʰ **S81.84** Puncture wound with foreign body of lower leg

　　AHA: 2016,3Q,24

√7ᵗʰ **S81.841** Puncture wound with foreign body, right lower leg

√7ᵗʰ **S81.842** Puncture wound with foreign body, left lower leg

√7ᵗʰ **S81.849** Puncture wound with foreign body, unspecified lower leg

√6ᵗʰ **S81.85** Open bite of lower leg

　　Bite of lower leg NOS

　　EXCLUDES 1　superficial bite of lower leg (S80.86-, S80.87-)

√7ᵗʰ **S81.851** Open bite, right lower leg

√7ᵗʰ **S81.852** Open bite, left lower leg

√7ᵗʰ **S81.859** Open bite, unspecified lower leg

√4ᵗʰ **S82** Fracture of lower leg, including ankle

　　NOTE　A fracture not indicated as displaced or nondisplaced should be coded to displaced

　　　　A fracture not indicated as open or closed should be coded to closed

　　　　The open fracture designations are based on the Gustilo open fracture classification.

　　INCLUDES　fracture of malleolus

　　EXCLUDES 1　traumatic amputation of lower leg (S88.-)

　　EXCLUDES 2　fracture of foot, except ankle (S92.-)

　　　　periprosthetic fracture of prosthetic implant of knee (M97.0-)

　　AHA: 2018,2Q,12; 2016,1Q,33; 2015,3Q,37-39

　　DEF: Diaphysis: Central shaft of a long bone.

　　DEF: Epiphysis: Proximal and distal rounded ends of a long bone, communicates with the joint.

　　DEF: Metaphysis: Section of a long bone located between the epiphysis and diaphysis at the proximal and distal ends.

　　DEF: Physis (growth plate): Narrow zone of cartilaginous tissue between the epiphysis and metaphysis at each end of a long bone. In childhood, proliferation of cells in this zone lengthens the bone. As the bone matures, this area thins, ossification eventually fusing into solid bone and growth stops. *Synonyms: Epiphyseal plate.*

　　TIP: The term "improper alignment" is not synonymous with malunion or nonunion of a fracture when noted in provider documentation.

The appropriate 7th character is to be added to all codes from category S82 [unless otherwise indicated].

A　initial encounter for closed fracture

B　initial encounter for open fracture type I or II
　　initial encounter for open fracture NOS

C　initial encounter for open fracture type IIIA, IIIB, or IIIC

D　subsequent encounter for closed fracture with routine healing

E　subsequent encounter for open fracture type I or II with routine healing

F　subsequent encounter for open fracture type IIIA, IIIB, or IIIC with routine healing

G　subsequent encounter for closed fracture with delayed healing

H　subsequent encounter for open fracture type I or II with delayed healing

J　subsequent encounter for open fracture type IIIA, IIIB, or IIIC with delayed healing

K　subsequent encounter for closed fracture with nonunion

M　subsequent encounter for open fracture type I or II with nonunion

N　subsequent encounter for open fracture type IIIA, IIIB, or IIIC with nonunion

P　subsequent encounter for closed fracture with malunion

Q　subsequent encounter for open fracture type I or II with malunion

R　subsequent encounter for open fracture type IIIA, IIIB, or IIIC with malunion

S　sequela

√5ᵗʰ **S82.0** Fracture of patella

　　Knee cap

√6ᵗʰ **S82.00** Unspecified fracture of patella

√7ᵗʰ **S82.001** Unspecified fracture of right patella

√7ᵗʰ **S82.002** Unspecified fracture of left patella

√7ᵗʰ **S82.009** Unspecified fracture of unspecified patella

√6ᵗʰ **S82.01** Osteochondral fracture of patella

√7ᵗʰ **S82.011** Displaced osteochondral fracture of right patella

√7ᵗʰ **S82.012** Displaced osteochondral fracture of left patella

√7ᵗʰ **S82.013** Displaced osteochondral fracture of unspecified patella

√7ᵗʰ **S82.014** Nondisplaced osteochondral fracture of right patella

√7ᵗʰ **S82.015** Nondisplaced osteochondral fracture of left patella

√7ᵗʰ **S82.016** Nondisplaced osteochondral fracture of unspecified patella

√6ᵗʰ **S82.02** Longitudinal fracture of patella

√7ᵗʰ **S82.021** Displaced longitudinal fracture of right patella

√7ᵗʰ **S82.022** Displaced longitudinal fracture of left patella

√7ᵗʰ **S82.023** Displaced longitudinal fracture of unspecified patella

√7ᵗʰ **S82.024** Nondisplaced longitudinal fracture of right patella

√7ᵗʰ **S82.025** Nondisplaced longitudinal fracture of left patella

√7ᵗʰ **S82.026** Nondisplaced longitudinal fracture of unspecified patella

√6ᵗʰ **S82.03** Transverse fracture of patella

√7ᵗʰ **S82.031** Displaced transverse fracture of right patella

√7ᵗʰ **S82.032** Displaced transverse fracture of left patella

√7ᵗʰ **S82.033** Displaced transverse fracture of unspecified patella

√7ᵗʰ **S82.034** Nondisplaced transverse fracture of right patella

√7ᵗʰ **S82.035** Nondisplaced transverse fracture of left patella

√7ᵗʰ **S82.036** Nondisplaced transverse fracture of unspecified patella

√6ᵗʰ **S82.04** Comminuted fracture of patella

√7ᵗʰ **S82.041** Displaced comminuted fracture of right patella

√7ᵗʰ **S82.042** Displaced comminuted fracture of left patella

√7ᵗʰ **S82.043** Displaced comminuted fracture of unspecified patella

√7ᵗʰ **S82.044** Nondisplaced comminuted fracture of right patella

√7ᵗʰ **S82.045** Nondisplaced comminuted fracture of left patella

√7ᵗʰ **S82.046** Nondisplaced comminuted fracture of unspecified patella

√6ᵗʰ **S82.09** Other fracture of patella

√7ᵗʰ **S82.091** Other fracture of right patella

√7ᵗʰ **S82.092** Other fracture of left patella

√7ᵗʰ **S82.099** Other fracture of unspecified patella

√5ᵗʰ **S82.1** Fracture of upper end of tibia

　　Fracture of proximal end of tibia

　　EXCLUDES 2　fracture of shaft of tibia (S82.2-)

　　　　physeal fracture of upper end of tibia (S89.0-)

√6ᵗʰ **S82.10** Unspecified fracture of upper end of tibia

√7ᵗʰ **S82.101** Unspecified fracture of upper end of right tibia

√7ᵗʰ **S82.102** Unspecified fracture of upper end of left tibia

√7ᵗʰ **S82.109** Unspecified fracture of upper end of unspecified tibia

√6ᵗʰ **S82.11** Fracture of tibial spine

√7ᵗʰ **S82.111** Displaced fracture of right tibial spine

√7ᵗʰ **S82.112** Displaced fracture of left tibial spine

√7ᵗʰ **S82.113** Displaced fracture of unspecified tibial spine

√7ᵗʰ **S82.114** Nondisplaced fracture of right tibial spine

√7ᵗʰ **S82.115** Nondisplaced fracture of left tibial spine

√7ᵗʰ **S82.116** Nondisplaced fracture of unspecified tibial spine

√6ᵗʰ **S82.12** Fracture of lateral condyle of tibia

√7ᵗʰ **S82.121** Displaced fracture of lateral condyle of right tibia

√7ᵗʰ **S82.122** Displaced fracture of lateral condyle of left tibia

√7ᵗʰ **S82.123** Displaced **fracture of lateral condyle of unspecified tibia**

√7ᵗʰ **S82.124** Nondisplaced **fracture of lateral condyle of** right **tibia**

√7ᵗʰ **S82.125** Nondisplaced **fracture of lateral condyle of** left **tibia**

√7ᵗʰ **S82.126** Nondisplaced **fracture of lateral condyle of unspecified tibia**

√6ᵗʰ **S82.13** **Fracture of** medial condyle of tibia

√7ᵗʰ **S82.131** Displaced **fracture of medial condyle of** right **tibia**

√7ᵗʰ **S82.132** Displaced **fracture of medial condyle of** left **tibia**

√7ᵗʰ **S82.133** Displaced **fracture of medial condyle of unspecified tibia**

√7ᵗʰ **S82.134** Nondisplaced **fracture of medial condyle of** right **tibia**

√7ᵗʰ **S82.135** Nondisplaced **fracture of medial condyle of** left **tibia**

√7ᵗʰ **S82.136** Nondisplaced **fracture of medial condyle of unspecified tibia**

√6ᵗʰ **S82.14** **Bicondylar fracture of tibia**

Fracture of tibial plateau NOS

√7ᵗʰ **S82.141** Displaced **bicondylar fracture of** right **tibia**

√7ᵗʰ **S82.142** Displaced **bicondylar fracture of** left **tibia**

√7ᵗʰ **S82.143** Displaced **bicondylar fracture of unspecified tibia**

√7ᵗʰ **S82.144** Nondisplaced **bicondylar fracture of** right **tibia**

√7ᵗʰ **S82.145** Nondisplaced **bicondylar fracture of** left **tibia**

√7ᵗʰ **S82.146** Nondisplaced **bicondylar fracture of unspecified tibia**

√6ᵗʰ **S82.15** **Fracture of** tibial tuberosity

√7ᵗʰ **S82.151** Displaced **fracture of** right **tibial tuberosity**

√7ᵗʰ **S82.152** Displaced **fracture of** left **tibial tuberosity**

√7ᵗʰ **S82.153** Displaced **fracture of unspecified tibial tuberosity**

√7ᵗʰ **S82.154** Nondisplaced **fracture of** right **tibial tuberosity**

√7ᵗʰ **S82.155** Nondisplaced **fracture of** left **tibial tuberosity**

√7ᵗʰ **S82.156** Nondisplaced **fracture of unspecified tibial tuberosity**

√6ᵗʰ **S82.16** **Torus fracture of upper end of tibia**

The appropriate 7th character is to be added to all codes in subcategory S82.16.
A   initial encounter for closed fracture
D   subsequent encounter for fracture with routine healing
G   subsequent encounter for fracture with delayed healing
K   subsequent encounter for fracture with nonunion
P   subsequent encounter for fracture with malunion
S   sequela

√7ᵗʰ **S82.161** **Torus fracture of upper end of** right **tibia**

√7ᵗʰ **S82.162** **Torus fracture of upper end of** left **tibia**

√7ᵗʰ **S82.169** **Torus fracture of upper end of unspecified tibia**

√6ᵗʰ **S82.19** **Other fracture of upper end of tibia**

√7ᵗʰ **S82.191** **Other fracture of upper end of** right **tibia**

√7ᵗʰ **S82.192** **Other fracture of upper end of** left **tibia**

√7ᵗʰ **S82.199** **Other fracture of upper end of unspecified tibia**

√5ᵗʰ **S82.2** **Fracture of** shaft of tibia

√6ᵗʰ **S82.20** **Unspecified fracture of shaft of tibia**

Fracture of tibia NOS

√7ᵗʰ **S82.201** **Unspecified fracture of shaft of** right **tibia**

√7ᵗʰ **S82.202** **Unspecified fracture of shaft of** left **tibia**

√7ᵗʰ **S82.209** **Unspecified fracture of shaft of unspecified tibia**

√6ᵗʰ **S82.22** **Transverse fracture of shaft of tibia**

√7ᵗʰ **S82.221** Displaced **transverse fracture of shaft of** right **tibia**

√7ᵗʰ **S82.222** Displaced **transverse fracture of shaft of** left **tibia**

√7ᵗʰ **S82.223** Displaced **transverse fracture of shaft of unspecified tibia**

√7ᵗʰ **S82.224** Nondisplaced **transverse fracture of shaft of** right **tibia**

√7ᵗʰ **S82.225** Nondisplaced **transverse fracture of shaft of** left **tibia**

√7ᵗʰ **S82.226** Nondisplaced **transverse fracture of shaft of unspecified tibia**

√6ᵗʰ **S82.23** Oblique **fracture of shaft of tibia**

√7ᵗʰ **S82.231** Displaced **oblique fracture of shaft of** right **tibia**

√7ᵗʰ **S82.232** Displaced **oblique fracture of shaft of** left **tibia**

√7ᵗʰ **S82.233** Displaced **oblique fracture of shaft of unspecified tibia**

√7ᵗʰ **S82.234** Nondisplaced **oblique fracture of shaft of** right **tibia**

√7ᵗʰ **S82.235** Nondisplaced **oblique fracture of shaft of** left **tibia**

√7ᵗʰ **S82.236** Nondisplaced **oblique fracture of shaft of unspecified tibia**

√6ᵗʰ **S82.24** Spiral **fracture of shaft of tibia**

Toddler fracture

√7ᵗʰ **S82.241** Displaced **spiral fracture of shaft of** right **tibia**

√7ᵗʰ **S82.242** Displaced **spiral fracture of shaft of** left **tibia**

√7ᵗʰ **S82.243** Displaced **spiral fracture of shaft of unspecified tibia**

√7ᵗʰ **S82.244** Nondisplaced **spiral fracture of shaft of** right **tibia**

√7ᵗʰ **S82.245** Nondisplaced **spiral fracture of shaft of** left **tibia**

√7ᵗʰ **S82.246** Nondisplaced **spiral fracture of shaft of unspecified tibia**

√6ᵗʰ **S82.25** Comminuted **fracture of shaft of tibia**

√7ᵗʰ **S82.251** Displaced **comminuted fracture of shaft of** right **tibia**

√7ᵗʰ **S82.252** Displaced **comminuted fracture of shaft of** left **tibia**

√7ᵗʰ **S82.253** Displaced **comminuted fracture of shaft of unspecified tibia**

√7ᵗʰ **S82.254** Nondisplaced **comminuted fracture of shaft of** right **tibia**

√7ᵗʰ **S82.255** Nondisplaced **comminuted fracture of shaft of** left **tibia**

√7ᵗʰ **S82.256** Nondisplaced **comminuted fracture of shaft of unspecified tibia**

√6ᵗʰ **S82.26** Segmental **fracture of shaft of tibia**

√7ᵗʰ **S82.261** Displaced **segmental fracture of shaft of** right **tibia**

√7ᵗʰ **S82.262** Displaced **segmental fracture of shaft of** left **tibia**

√7ᵗʰ **S82.263** Displaced **segmental fracture of shaft of unspecified tibia**

√7ᵗʰ **S82.264** Nondisplaced **segmental fracture of shaft of** right **tibia**

√7ᵗʰ **S82.265** Nondisplaced **segmental fracture of shaft of** left **tibia**

√7ᵗʰ **S82.266** Nondisplaced **segmental fracture of shaft of unspecified tibia**

√6ᵗʰ **S82.29** Other **fracture of shaft of tibia**

√7ᵗʰ **S82.291** **Other fracture of shaft of** right **tibia**

√7ᵗʰ **S82.292** **Other fracture of shaft of** left **tibia**

√7ᵗʰ **S82.299** **Other fracture of shaft of unspecified tibia**

√5ᵗʰ **S82.3** **Fracture of** lower end of tibia

EXCLUDES 1   *bimalleolar fracture of lower leg (S82.84-)*
fracture of medial malleolus alone (S82.5-)
Maisonneuve's fracture (S82.86-)
pilon fracture of distal tibia (S82.87-)
trimalleolar fractures of lower leg (S82.85-)

√6ᵗʰ **S82.30** **Unspecified fracture of lower end of tibia**

√7ᵗʰ **S82.301** **Unspecified fracture of lower end of** right **tibia**

√7ᵗʰ **S82.302** **Unspecified fracture of lower end of** left **tibia**

N Newborn: 0   **P** Pediatric: 0-17   **M** Maternity: 12-55   **A** Adult: 15-124   **CH** Comorbidity High   **CL** Comorbidity Low   **NCDx** Noncancer Dx   **PDx** Primary Dx

1044   ICD-10-CM 2020

√7ᵗʰ **S82.309** Unspecified fracture of lower end of unspecified tibia

√6ᵗʰ **S82.31** Torus fracture of lower end of tibia

> The appropriate 7th character is to be added to all codes in subcategory S82.31.
> A   initial encounter for closed fracture
> D   subsequent encounter for fracture with routine healing
> G   subsequent encounter for fracture with delayed healing
> K   subsequent encounter for fracture with nonunion
> P   subsequent encounter for fracture with malunion
> S   sequela

√7ᵗʰ **S82.311** Torus fracture of lower end of right tibia

√7ᵗʰ **S82.312** Torus fracture of lower end of left tibia

√7ᵗʰ **S82.319** Torus fracture of lower end of unspecified tibia

√6ᵗʰ **S82.39** Other fracture of lower end of tibia

    AHA: 2015,1Q,25

√7ᵗʰ **S82.391** Other fracture of lower end of right tibia

√7ᵗʰ **S82.392** Other fracture of lower end of left tibia

√7ᵗʰ **S82.399** Other fracture of lower end of unspecified tibia

√5ᵗʰ **S82.4** Fracture of shaft of fibula

    EXCLUDES 2   fracture of lateral malleolus alone (S82.6-)

√6ᵗʰ **S82.40** Unspecified fracture of shaft of fibula

√7ᵗʰ **S82.401** Unspecified fracture of shaft of right fibula

√7ᵗʰ **S82.402** Unspecified fracture of shaft of left fibula

√7ᵗʰ **S82.409** Unspecified fracture of shaft of unspecified fibula

√6ᵗʰ **S82.42** Transverse fracture of shaft of fibula

√7ᵗʰ **S82.421** Displaced transverse fracture of shaft of right fibula

√7ᵗʰ **S82.422** Displaced transverse fracture of shaft of left fibula

√7ᵗʰ **S82.423** Displaced transverse fracture of shaft of unspecified fibula

√7ᵗʰ **S82.424** Nondisplaced transverse fracture of shaft of right fibula

√7ᵗʰ **S82.425** Nondisplaced transverse fracture of shaft of left fibula

√7ᵗʰ **S82.426** Nondisplaced transverse fracture of shaft of unspecified fibula

√6ᵗʰ **S82.43** Oblique fracture of shaft of fibula

√7ᵗʰ **S82.431** Displaced oblique fracture of shaft of right fibula

√7ᵗʰ **S82.432** Displaced oblique fracture of shaft of left fibula

√7ᵗʰ **S82.433** Displaced oblique fracture of shaft of unspecified fibula

√7ᵗʰ **S82.434** Nondisplaced oblique fracture of shaft of right fibula

√7ᵗʰ **S82.435** Nondisplaced oblique fracture of shaft of left fibula

√7ᵗʰ **S82.436** Nondisplaced oblique fracture of shaft of unspecified fibula

√6ᵗʰ **S82.44** Spiral fracture of shaft of fibula

√7ᵗʰ **S82.441** Displaced spiral fracture of shaft of right fibula

√7ᵗʰ **S82.442** Displaced spiral fracture of shaft of left fibula

√7ᵗʰ **S82.443** Displaced spiral fracture of shaft of unspecified fibula

√7ᵗʰ **S82.444** Nondisplaced spiral fracture of shaft of right fibula

√7ᵗʰ **S82.445** Nondisplaced spiral fracture of shaft of left fibula

√7ᵗʰ **S82.446** Nondisplaced spiral fracture of shaft of unspecified fibula

√6ᵗʰ **S82.45** Comminuted fracture of shaft of fibula

√7ᵗʰ **S82.451** Displaced comminuted fracture of shaft of right fibula

√7ᵗʰ **S82.452** Displaced comminuted fracture of shaft of left fibula

√7ᵗʰ **S82.453** Displaced comminuted fracture of shaft of unspecified fibula

√7ᵗʰ **S82.454** Nondisplaced comminuted fracture of shaft of right fibula

√7ᵗʰ **S82.455** Nondisplaced comminuted fracture of shaft of left fibula

√7ᵗʰ **S82.456** Nondisplaced comminuted fracture of shaft of unspecified fibula

√6ᵗʰ **S82.46** Segmental fracture of shaft of fibula

√7ᵗʰ **S82.461** Displaced segmental fracture of shaft of right fibula

√7ᵗʰ **S82.462** Displaced segmental fracture of shaft of left fibula

√7ᵗʰ **S82.463** Displaced segmental fracture of shaft of unspecified fibula

√7ᵗʰ **S82.464** Nondisplaced segmental fracture of shaft of right fibula

√7ᵗʰ **S82.465** Nondisplaced segmental fracture of shaft of left fibula

√7ᵗʰ **S82.466** Nondisplaced segmental fracture of shaft of unspecified fibula

√6ᵗʰ **S82.49** Other fracture of shaft of fibula

√7ᵗʰ **S82.491** Other fracture of shaft of right fibula

√7ᵗʰ **S82.492** Other fracture of shaft of left fibula

√7ᵗʰ **S82.499** Other fracture of shaft of unspecified fibula

√5ᵗʰ **S82.5** Fracture of medial malleolus

    EXCLUDES 1   pilon fracture of distal tibia (S82.87-)
                 Salter-Harris type III of lower end of tibia (S89.13-)
                 Salter-Harris type IV of lower end of tibia (S89.14-)

√x7ᵗʰ **S82.51** Displaced fracture of medial malleolus of right tibia

√x7ᵗʰ **S82.52** Displaced fracture of medial malleolus of left tibia

√x7ᵗʰ **S82.53** Displaced fracture of medial malleolus of unspecified tibia

√x7ᵗʰ **S82.54** Nondisplaced fracture of medial malleolus of right tibia

√x7ᵗʰ **S82.55** Nondisplaced fracture of medial malleolus of left tibia

√x7ᵗʰ **S82.56** Nondisplaced fracture of medial malleolus of unspecified tibia

√5ᵗʰ **S82.6** Fracture of lateral malleolus

    EXCLUDES 1   pilon fracture of distal tibia (S82.87-)

√x7ᵗʰ **S82.61** Displaced fracture of lateral malleolus of right fibula

√x7ᵗʰ **S82.62** Displaced fracture of lateral malleolus of left fibula

√x7ᵗʰ **S82.63** Displaced fracture of lateral malleolus of unspecified fibula

√x7ᵗʰ **S82.64** Nondisplaced fracture of lateral malleolus of right fibula

√x7ᵗʰ **S82.65** Nondisplaced fracture of lateral malleolus of left fibula

√x7ᵗʰ **S82.66** Nondisplaced fracture of lateral malleolus of unspecified fibula

√5ᵗʰ **S82.8** Other fractures of lower leg

√6ᵗʰ **S82.81** Torus fracture of upper end of fibula

> The appropriate 7th character is to be added to all codes in subcategory S82.81
> A   initial encounter for closed fracture
> D   subsequent encounter for fracture with routine healing
> G   subsequent encounter for fracture with delayed healing
> K   subsequent encounter for fracture with nonunion
> P   subsequent encounter for fracture with malunion
> S   sequela

√7ᵗʰ **S82.811** Torus fracture of upper end of right fibula

√7ᵗʰ **S82.812** Torus fracture of upper end of left fibula

√7ᵗʰ **S82.819** Torus fracture of upper end of unspecified fibula

---

☑ Additional Character Required   √x7ᵗʰ Placeholder Alert   Manifestation   Unspecified Dx   ▶◀ Revised Text   ● New Code   ▲ Revised Title

√6ᵗʰ **S82.82**   Torus **fracture of** lower end of fibula

> The appropriate 7th character is to be added to all codes in subcategory S82.82.
> A   initial encounter for closed fracture
> D   subsequent encounter for fracture with routine healing
> G   subsequent encounter for fracture with delayed healing
> K   subsequent encounter for fracture with nonunion
> P   subsequent encounter for fracture with malunion
> S   sequela

   √7ᵗʰ **S82.821**   Torus fracture of lower end of right fibula
   √7ᵗʰ **S82.822**   Torus fracture of lower end of left fibula
   √7ᵗʰ **S82.829**   Torus fracture of lower end of unspecified fibula

√6ᵗʰ **S82.83**   Other fracture of upper and lower end of fibula
   AHA: 2015,1Q,25
   √7ᵗʰ **S82.831**   Other fracture of upper and lower end of right fibula
   √7ᵗʰ **S82.832**   Other fracture of upper and lower end of left fibula
   √7ᵗʰ **S82.839**   Other fracture of upper and lower end of unspecified fibula

√6ᵗʰ **S82.84**   Bimalleolar **fracture of lower leg**

Right Bimalleolar Fracture

- Patella
- Tibial plateau
- Tibial tubercle
- Fibula
- Tibia
- Fracture medial malleolus
- Fracture lateral malleolus
- Talus
- Medial (tibial) malleolus
- Lateral (fibular) malleolus

   √7ᵗʰ **S82.841**   Displaced bimalleolar fracture of right lower leg
   √7ᵗʰ **S82.842**   Displaced bimalleolar fracture of left lower leg
   √7ᵗʰ **S82.843**   Displaced bimalleolar fracture of unspecified lower leg
   √7ᵗʰ **S82.844**   Nondisplaced bimalleolar fracture of right lower leg
   √7ᵗʰ **S82.845**   Nondisplaced bimalleolar fracture of left lower leg
   √7ᵗʰ **S82.846**   Nondisplaced bimalleolar fracture of unspecified lower leg

√6ᵗʰ **S82.85**   Trimalleolar **fracture of lower leg**
   √7ᵗʰ **S82.851**   Displaced trimalleolar fracture of right lower leg
   √7ᵗʰ **S82.852**   Displaced trimalleolar fracture of left lower leg
   √7ᵗʰ **S82.853**   Displaced trimalleolar fracture of unspecified lower leg
   √7ᵗʰ **S82.854**   Nondisplaced trimalleolar fracture of right lower leg
   √7ᵗʰ **S82.855**   Nondisplaced trimalleolar fracture of left lower leg

---

   √7ᵗʰ **S82.856**   Nondisplaced trimalleolar fracture of unspecified lower leg

√6ᵗʰ **S82.86**   Maisonneuve's **fracture**
   √7ᵗʰ **S82.861**   Displaced Maisonneuve's fracture of right leg
   √7ᵗʰ **S82.862**   Displaced Maisonneuve's fracture of left leg
   √7ᵗʰ **S82.863**   Displaced Maisonneuve's fracture of unspecified leg
   √7ᵗʰ **S82.864**   Nondisplaced Maisonneuve's fracture of right leg
   √7ᵗʰ **S82.865**   Nondisplaced Maisonneuve's fracture of left leg
   √7ᵗʰ **S82.866**   Nondisplaced Maisonneuve's fracture of unspecified leg

√6ᵗʰ **S82.87**   Pilon **fracture of tibia**
   √7ᵗʰ **S82.871**   Displaced pilon fracture of right tibia
   √7ᵗʰ **S82.872**   Displaced pilon fracture of left tibia
   √7ᵗʰ **S82.873**   Displaced pilon fracture of unspecified tibia
   √7ᵗʰ **S82.874**   Nondisplaced pilon fracture of right tibia
   √7ᵗʰ **S82.875**   Nondisplaced pilon fracture of left tibia
   √7ᵗʰ **S82.876**   Nondisplaced pilon fracture of unspecified tibia

√6ᵗʰ **S82.89**   Other fractures of lower leg
   Fracture of ankle NOS
   √7ᵗʰ **S82.891**   Other fracture of right lower leg
   √7ᵗʰ **S82.892**   Other fracture of left lower leg
   √7ᵗʰ **S82.899**   Other fracture of unspecified lower leg

√5ᵗʰ **S82.9**   Unspecified fracture of lower leg
   √x7ᵗʰ **S82.90**   Unspecified fracture of unspecified lower leg
   √x7ᵗʰ **S82.91**   Unspecified fracture of right lower leg
   √x7ᵗʰ **S82.92**   Unspecified fracture of left lower leg

√4ᵗʰ **S83**   **Dislocation and sprain of joints and ligaments of knee**

   INCLUDES   avulsion of joint or ligament of knee
      laceration of cartilage, joint or ligament of knee
      sprain of cartilage, joint or ligament of knee
      traumatic hemarthrosis of joint or ligament of knee
      traumatic rupture of joint or ligament of knee
      traumatic subluxation of joint or ligament of knee
      traumatic tear of joint or ligament of knee

   Code also any associated open wound
   EXCLUDES 1   derangement of patella (M22.Ø-M22.3)
      injury of patellar ligament (tendon) (S76.1-)
      internal derangement of knee (M23.-)
      old dislocation of knee (M23.8X)
      pathological dislocation of knee (M24.36)
      recurrent dislocation of knee (M22.Ø)
   EXCLUDES 2   strain of muscle, fascia and tendon of lower leg (S86.-)

> The appropriate 7th character is to be added to each code from category S83.
> A   initial encounter
> D   subsequent encounter
> S   sequela

√5ᵗʰ **S83.Ø**   Subluxation and dislocation of patella
   √6ᵗʰ **S83.ØØ**   Unspecified subluxation and dislocation of patella
     √7ᵗʰ **S83.ØØ1**   Unspecified subluxation of right patella
     √7ᵗʰ **S83.ØØ2**   Unspecified subluxation of left patella
     √7ᵗʰ **S83.ØØ3**   Unspecified subluxation of unspecified patella
     √7ᵗʰ **S83.ØØ4**   Unspecified dislocation of right patella
     √7ᵗʰ **S83.ØØ5**   Unspecified dislocation of left patella
     √7ᵗʰ **S83.ØØ6**   Unspecified dislocation of unspecified patella
   √6ᵗʰ **S83.Ø1**   Lateral subluxation and dislocation of patella
     √7ᵗʰ **S83.Ø11**   Lateral subluxation of right patella
     √7ᵗʰ **S83.Ø12**   Lateral subluxation of left patella
     √7ᵗʰ **S83.Ø13**   Lateral subluxation of unspecified patella
     √7ᵗʰ **S83.Ø14**   Lateral dislocation of right patella
     √7ᵗʰ **S83.Ø15**   Lateral dislocation of left patella
     √7ᵗʰ **S83.Ø16**   Lateral dislocation of unspecified patella

√6ᵗʰ **S83.09**   Other subluxation and dislocation of patella
- √7ᵗʰ **S83.091** Other subluxation of right patella
- √7ᵗʰ **S83.092** Other subluxation of left patella
- **S83.093** Other subluxation of unspecified patella
- √7ᵗʰ **S83.094** Other dislocation of right patella
- √7ᵗʰ **S83.095** Other dislocation of left patella
- √7ᵗʰ **S83.096** Other dislocation of unspecified patella

√5ᵗʰ **S83.1**   Subluxation and dislocation of knee

     EXCLUDES 2   instability of knee prosthesis (T84.022, T84.023)

√6ᵗʰ **S83.10**   Unspecified subluxation and dislocation of knee
- √7ᵗʰ **S83.101** Unspecified subluxation of right knee
- √7ᵗʰ **S83.102** Unspecified subluxation of left knee
- √7ᵗʰ **S83.103** Unspecified subluxation of unspecified knee
- √7ᵗʰ **S83.104** Unspecified dislocation of right knee
- √7ᵗʰ **S83.105** Unspecified dislocation of left knee
- √7ᵗʰ **S83.106** Unspecified dislocation of unspecified knee

√6ᵗʰ **S83.11**   Anterior subluxation and dislocation of proximal end of tibia

     Posterior subluxation and dislocation of distal end of femur
- √7ᵗʰ **S83.111** Anterior subluxation of proximal end of tibia, right knee
- √7ᵗʰ **S83.112** Anterior subluxation of proximal end of tibia, left knee
- **S83.113** Anterior subluxation of proximal end of tibia, unspecified knee
- √7ᵗʰ **S83.114** Anterior dislocation of proximal end of tibia, right knee
- √7ᵗʰ **S83.115** Anterior dislocation of proximal end of tibia, left knee
- **S83.116** Anterior dislocation of proximal end of tibia, unspecified knee

√6ᵗʰ **S83.12**   Posterior subluxation and dislocation of proximal end of tibia

     Anterior dislocation of distal end of femur
- √7ᵗʰ **S83.121** Posterior subluxation of proximal end of tibia, right knee
- √7ᵗʰ **S83.122** Posterior subluxation of proximal end of tibia, left knee
- **S83.123** Posterior subluxation of proximal end of tibia, unspecified knee
- √7ᵗʰ **S83.124** Posterior dislocation of proximal end of tibia, right knee
- √7ᵗʰ **S83.125** Posterior dislocation of proximal end of tibia, left knee
- **S83.126** Posterior dislocation of proximal end of tibia, unspecified knee

√6ᵗʰ **S83.13**   Medial subluxation and dislocation of proximal end of tibia
- √7ᵗʰ **S83.131** Medial subluxation of proximal end of tibia, right knee
- √7ᵗʰ **S83.132** Medial subluxation of proximal end of tibia, left knee
- **S83.133** Medial subluxation of proximal end of tibia, unspecified knee
- √7ᵗʰ **S83.134** Medial dislocation of proximal end of tibia, right knee
- √7ᵗʰ **S83.135** Medial dislocation of proximal end of tibia, left knee
- **S83.136** Medial dislocation of proximal end of tibia, unspecified knee

√6ᵗʰ **S83.14**   Lateral subluxation and dislocation of proximal end of tibia
- √7ᵗʰ **S83.141** Lateral subluxation of proximal end of tibia, right knee
- √7ᵗʰ **S83.142** Lateral subluxation of proximal end of tibia, left knee
- **S83.143** Lateral subluxation of proximal end of tibia, unspecified knee
- √7ᵗʰ **S83.144** Lateral dislocation of proximal end of tibia, right knee
- √7ᵗʰ **S83.145** Lateral dislocation of proximal end of tibia, left knee
- **S83.146** Lateral dislocation of proximal end of tibia, unspecified knee

√6ᵗʰ **S83.19**   Other subluxation and dislocation of knee
- √7ᵗʰ **S83.191** Other subluxation of right knee
- √7ᵗʰ **S83.192** Other subluxation of left knee
- √7ᵗʰ **S83.193** Other subluxation of unspecified knee
- √7ᵗʰ **S83.194** Other dislocation of right knee
- √7ᵗʰ **S83.195** Other dislocation of left knee
- √7ᵗʰ **S83.196** Other dislocation of unspecified knee

√5ᵗʰ **S83.2**   Tear of meniscus, current injury

     EXCLUDES 1   old bucket-handle tear (M23.2)

     AHA: 2019, 2Q, 26

√6ᵗʰ **S83.20**   Tear of unspecified meniscus, current injury

     Tear of meniscus of knee NOS
- √7ᵗʰ **S83.200** Bucket-handle tear of unspecified meniscus, current injury, right knee
- √7ᵗʰ **S83.201** Bucket-handle tear of unspecified meniscus, current injury, left knee
- √7ᵗʰ **S83.202** Bucket-handle tear of unspecified meniscus, current injury, unspecified knee
- √7ᵗʰ **S83.203** Other tear of unspecified meniscus, current injury, right knee
- √7ᵗʰ **S83.204** Other tear of unspecified meniscus, current injury, left knee
- √7ᵗʰ **S83.205** Other tear of unspecified meniscus, current injury, unspecified knee
- √7ᵗʰ **S83.206** Unspecified tear of unspecified meniscus, current injury, right knee
- √7ᵗʰ **S83.207** Unspecified tear of unspecified meniscus, current injury, left knee
- √7ᵗʰ **S83.209** Unspecified tear of unspecified meniscus, current injury, unspecified knee

√6ᵗʰ **S83.21**   Bucket-handle tear of medial meniscus, current injury
- √7ᵗʰ **S83.211** Bucket-handle tear of medial meniscus, current injury, right knee
- √7ᵗʰ **S83.212** Bucket-handle tear of medial meniscus, current injury, left knee
- √7ᵗʰ **S83.219** Bucket-handle tear of medial meniscus, current injury, unspecified knee

√6ᵗʰ **S83.22**   Peripheral tear of medial meniscus, current injury
- √7ᵗʰ **S83.221** Peripheral tear of medial meniscus, current injury, right knee
- √7ᵗʰ **S83.222** Peripheral tear of medial meniscus, current injury, left knee
- √7ᵗʰ **S83.229** Peripheral tear of medial meniscus, current injury, unspecified knee

√6ᵗʰ **S83.23**   Complex tear of medial meniscus, current injury
- √7ᵗʰ **S83.231** Complex tear of medial meniscus, current injury, right knee
- √7ᵗʰ **S83.232** Complex tear of medial meniscus, current injury, left knee
- √7ᵗʰ **S83.239** Complex tear of medial meniscus, current injury, unspecified knee

√6ᵗʰ **S83.24**   Other tear of medial meniscus, current injury
- √7ᵗʰ **S83.241** Other tear of medial meniscus, current injury, right knee
- √7ᵗʰ **S83.242** Other tear of medial meniscus, current injury, left knee
- √7ᵗʰ **S83.249** Other tear of medial meniscus, current injury, unspecified knee

√6ᵗʰ **S83.25**   Bucket-handle tear of lateral meniscus, current injury
- √7ᵗʰ **S83.251** Bucket-handle tear of lateral meniscus, current injury, right knee
- √7ᵗʰ **S83.252** Bucket-handle tear of lateral meniscus, current injury, left knee
- √7ᵗʰ **S83.259** Bucket-handle tear of lateral meniscus, current injury, unspecified knee

√6ᵗʰ **S83.26**   Peripheral tear of lateral meniscus, current injury
- √7ᵗʰ **S83.261** Peripheral tear of lateral meniscus, current injury, right knee
- √7ᵗʰ **S83.262** Peripheral tear of lateral meniscus, current injury, left knee
- √7ᵗʰ **S83.269** Peripheral tear of lateral meniscus, current injury, unspecified knee

√6ᵗʰ **S83.27**   Complex tear of lateral meniscus, current injury
- √7ᵗʰ **S83.271** Complex tear of lateral meniscus, current injury, right knee
- √7ᵗʰ **S83.272** Complex tear of lateral meniscus, current injury, left knee
- √7ᵗʰ **S83.279** Complex tear of lateral meniscus, current injury, unspecified knee

---

✔ Additional Character Required   √x7ᵗʰ Placeholder Alert   Manifestation   Unspecified Dx   ▶◀ Revised Text   ● New Code   ▲ Revised Title

√6ᵗʰ **S83.28** Other tear of lateral meniscus, current injury

 √7ᵗʰ **S83.281** Other tear of lateral meniscus, current injury, right knee

 √7ᵗʰ **S83.282** Other tear of lateral meniscus, current injury, left knee

 √7ᵗʰ **S83.289** Other tear of lateral meniscus, current injury, unspecified knee

√5ᵗʰ **S83.3** Tear of articular cartilage of knee, current

 √x7ᵗʰ **S83.30** Tear of articular cartilage of unspecified knee, current

 √x7ᵗʰ **S83.31** Tear of articular cartilage of right knee, current

 √x7ᵗʰ **S83.32** Tear of articular cartilage of left knee, current

√5ᵗʰ **S83.4** Sprain of collateral ligament of knee

 √6ᵗʰ **S83.40** Sprain of unspecified collateral ligament of knee

 √7ᵗʰ **S83.401** Sprain of unspecified collateral ligament of right knee

 √7ᵗʰ **S83.402** Sprain of unspecified collateral ligament of left knee

 √7ᵗʰ **S83.409** Sprain of unspecified collateral ligament of unspecified knee

 √6ᵗʰ **S83.41** Sprain of medial collateral ligament of knee

 Sprain of tibial collateral ligament

 √7ᵗʰ **S83.411** Sprain of medial collateral ligament of right knee

 √7ᵗʰ **S83.412** Sprain of medial collateral ligament of left knee

 √7ᵗʰ **S83.419** Sprain of medial collateral ligament of unspecified knee

 √6ᵗʰ **S83.42** Sprain of lateral collateral ligament of knee

 Sprain of fibular collateral ligament

 √7ᵗʰ **S83.421** Sprain of lateral collateral ligament of right knee

 √7ᵗʰ **S83.422** Sprain of lateral collateral ligament of left knee

 √7ᵗʰ **S83.429** Sprain of lateral collateral ligament of unspecified knee

√5ᵗʰ **S83.5** Sprain of cruciate ligament of knee

 AHA: 2016,2Q,3

 √6ᵗʰ **S83.50** Sprain of unspecified cruciate ligament of knee

 √7ᵗʰ **S83.501** Sprain of unspecified cruciate ligament of right knee

 √7ᵗʰ **S83.502** Sprain of unspecified cruciate ligament of left knee

 √7ᵗʰ **S83.509** Sprain of unspecified cruciate ligament of unspecified knee

 √6ᵗʰ **S83.51** Sprain of anterior cruciate ligament of knee

 √7ᵗʰ **S83.511** Sprain of anterior cruciate ligament of right knee

 √7ᵗʰ **S83.512** Sprain of anterior cruciate ligament of left knee

 √7ᵗʰ **S83.519** Sprain of anterior cruciate ligament of unspecified knee

 √6ᵗʰ **S83.52** Sprain of posterior cruciate ligament of knee

 √7ᵗʰ **S83.521** Sprain of posterior cruciate ligament of right knee

 √7ᵗʰ **S83.522** Sprain of posterior cruciate ligament of left knee

 √7ᵗʰ **S83.529** Sprain of posterior cruciate ligament of unspecified knee

√5ᵗʰ **S83.6** Sprain of the superior tibiofibular joint and ligament

 √x7ᵗʰ **S83.60** Sprain of the superior tibiofibular joint and ligament, unspecified knee

 √x7ᵗʰ **S83.61** Sprain of the superior tibiofibular joint and ligament, right knee

 √x7ᵗʰ **S83.62** Sprain of the superior tibiofibular joint and ligament, left knee

√5ᵗʰ **S83.8** Sprain of other specified parts of knee

 √6ᵗʰ **S83.8X** Sprain of other specified parts of knee

 √7ᵗʰ **S83.8X1** Sprain of other specified parts of right knee

 √7ᵗʰ **S83.8X2** Sprain of other specified parts of left knee

 √7ᵗʰ **S83.8X9** Sprain of other specified parts of unspecified knee

√5ᵗʰ **S83.9** Sprain of unspecified site of knee

 √x7ᵗʰ **S83.90** Sprain of unspecified site of unspecified knee

 √x7ᵗʰ **S83.91** Sprain of unspecified site of right knee

 √x7ᵗʰ **S83.92** Sprain of unspecified site of left knee

√4ᵗʰ **S84** Injury of nerves at lower leg level

 Code also any associated open wound (S81.-)

 EXCLUDES 2 injury of nerves at ankle and foot level (S94.-)

 The appropriate 7th character is to be added to each code from category S84.
 A initial encounter
 D subsequent encounter
 S sequela

√5ᵗʰ **S84.0** Injury of tibial nerve at lower leg level

 √x7ᵗʰ **S84.00** Injury of tibial nerve at lower leg level, unspecified leg

 √x7ᵗʰ **S84.01** Injury of tibial nerve at lower leg level, right leg

 √x7ᵗʰ **S84.02** Injury of tibial nerve at lower leg level, left leg

√5ᵗʰ **S84.1** Injury of peroneal nerve at lower leg level

 √x7ᵗʰ **S84.10** Injury of peroneal nerve at lower leg level, unspecified leg

 √x7ᵗʰ **S84.11** Injury of peroneal nerve at lower leg level, right leg

 √x7ᵗʰ **S84.12** Injury of peroneal nerve at lower leg level, left leg

√5ᵗʰ **S84.2** Injury of cutaneous sensory nerve at lower leg level

 √x7ᵗʰ **S84.20** Injury of cutaneous sensory nerve at lower leg level, unspecified leg

 √x7ᵗʰ **S84.21** Injury of cutaneous sensory nerve at lower leg level, right leg

 √x7ᵗʰ **S84.22** Injury of cutaneous sensory nerve at lower leg level, left leg

√5ᵗʰ **S84.8** Injury of other nerves at lower leg level

 √6ᵗʰ **S84.80** Injury of other nerves at lower leg level

 √7ᵗʰ **S84.801** Injury of other nerves at lower leg level, right leg

 √7ᵗʰ **S84.802** Injury of other nerves at lower leg level, left leg

 √7ᵗʰ **S84.809** Injury of other nerves at lower leg level, unspecified leg

√5ᵗʰ **S84.9** Injury of unspecified nerve at lower leg level

 √x7ᵗʰ **S84.90** Injury of unspecified nerve at lower leg level, unspecified leg

 √x7ᵗʰ **S84.91** Injury of unspecified nerve at lower leg level, right leg

 √x7ᵗʰ **S84.92** Injury of unspecified nerve at lower leg level, left leg

√4ᵗʰ **S85** Injury of blood vessels at lower leg level

 Code also any associated open wound (S81.-)

 EXCLUDES 2 injury of blood vessels at ankle and foot level (S95.-)

 The appropriate 7th character is to be added to each code from category S85.
 A initial encounter
 D subsequent encounter
 S sequela

√5ᵗʰ **S85.0** Injury of popliteal artery

 √6ᵗʰ **S85.00** Unspecified injury of popliteal artery

 √7ᵗʰ **S85.001** Unspecified injury of popliteal artery, right leg

 √7ᵗʰ **S85.002** Unspecified injury of popliteal artery, left leg

 √7ᵗʰ **S85.009** Unspecified injury of popliteal artery, unspecified leg

 √6ᵗʰ **S85.01** Laceration of popliteal artery

 √7ᵗʰ **S85.011** Laceration of popliteal artery, right leg

 √7ᵗʰ **S85.012** Laceration of popliteal artery, left leg

 √7ᵗʰ **S85.019** Laceration of popliteal artery, unspecified leg

 √6ᵗʰ **S85.09** Other specified injury of popliteal artery

 √7ᵗʰ **S85.091** Other specified injury of popliteal artery, right leg

 √7ᵗʰ **S85.092** Other specified injury of popliteal artery, left leg

 √7ᵗʰ **S85.099** Other specified injury of popliteal artery, unspecified leg

√5ᵗʰ **S85.1** Injury of tibial artery

 √6ᵗʰ **S85.10** Unspecified injury of unspecified tibial artery

 Injury of tibial artery NOS

 √7ᵗʰ **S85.101** Unspecified injury of unspecified tibial artery, right leg

 √7ᵗʰ **S85.102** Unspecified injury of unspecified tibial artery, left leg

✓7ᵗʰ **S85.109** Unspecified injury of unspecified tibial artery, unspecified leg

✓6ᵗʰ **S85.11** Laceration of unspecified tibial artery

    ✓7ᵗʰ **S85.111** Laceration of unspecified tibial artery, right leg

    ✓7ᵗʰ **S85.112** Laceration of unspecified tibial artery, left leg

    ✓7ᵗʰ **S85.119** Laceration of unspecified tibial artery, unspecified leg

✓6ᵗʰ **S85.12** Other specified injury of unspecified tibial artery

    ✓7ᵗʰ **S85.121** Other specified injury of unspecified tibial artery, right leg

    ✓7ᵗʰ **S85.122** Other specified injury of unspecified tibial artery, left leg

    ✓7ᵗʰ **S85.129** Other specified injury of unspecified tibial artery, unspecified leg

✓6ᵗʰ **S85.13** Unspecified injury of anterior tibial artery

    ✓7ᵗʰ **S85.131** Unspecified injury of anterior tibial artery, right leg

    ✓7ᵗʰ **S85.132** Unspecified injury of anterior tibial artery, left leg

    ✓7ᵗʰ **S85.139** Unspecified injury of anterior tibial artery, unspecified leg

✓6ᵗʰ **S85.14** Laceration of anterior tibial artery

    ✓7ᵗʰ **S85.141** Laceration of anterior tibial artery, right leg

    ✓7ᵗʰ **S85.142** Laceration of anterior tibial artery, left leg

    ✓7ᵗʰ **S85.149** Laceration of anterior tibial artery, unspecified leg

✓6ᵗʰ **S85.15** Other specified injury of anterior tibial artery

    ✓7ᵗʰ **S85.151** Other specified injury of anterior tibial artery, right leg

    ✓7ᵗʰ **S85.152** Other specified injury of anterior tibial artery, left leg

    ✓7ᵗʰ **S85.159** Other specified injury of anterior tibial artery, unspecified leg

✓6ᵗʰ **S85.16** Unspecified injury of posterior tibial artery

    ✓7ᵗʰ **S85.161** Unspecified injury of posterior tibial artery, right leg

    ✓7ᵗʰ **S85.162** Unspecified injury of posterior tibial artery, left leg

    ✓7ᵗʰ **S85.169** Unspecified injury of posterior tibial artery, unspecified leg

✓6ᵗʰ **S85.17** Laceration of posterior tibial artery

    ✓7ᵗʰ **S85.171** Laceration of posterior tibial artery, right leg

    ✓7ᵗʰ **S85.172** Laceration of posterior tibial artery, left leg

    ✓7ᵗʰ **S85.179** Laceration of posterior tibial artery, unspecified leg

✓6ᵗʰ **S85.18** Other specified injury of posterior tibial artery

    ✓7ᵗʰ **S85.181** Other specified injury of posterior tibial artery, right leg

    ✓7ᵗʰ **S85.182** Other specified injury of posterior tibial artery, left leg

    ✓7ᵗʰ **S85.189** Other specified injury of posterior tibial artery, unspecified leg

✓5ᵗʰ **S85.2** Injury of peroneal artery

✓6ᵗʰ **S85.20** Unspecified injury of peroneal artery

    ✓7ᵗʰ **S85.201** Unspecified injury of peroneal artery, right leg

    ✓7ᵗʰ **S85.202** Unspecified injury of peroneal artery, left leg

    ✓7ᵗʰ **S85.209** Unspecified injury of peroneal artery, unspecified leg

✓6ᵗʰ **S85.21** Laceration of peroneal artery

    ✓7ᵗʰ **S85.211** Laceration of peroneal artery, right leg

    ✓7ᵗʰ **S85.212** Laceration of peroneal artery, left leg

    ✓7ᵗʰ **S85.219** Laceration of peroneal artery, unspecified leg

✓6ᵗʰ **S85.29** Other specified injury of peroneal artery

    ✓7ᵗʰ **S85.291** Other specified injury of peroneal artery, right leg

    ✓7ᵗʰ **S85.292** Other specified injury of peroneal artery, left leg

    ✓7ᵗʰ **S85.299** Other specified injury of peroneal artery, unspecified leg

✓5ᵗʰ **S85.3** Injury of greater saphenous vein at lower leg level

    Injury of greater saphenous vein NOS

    Injury of saphenous vein NOS

✓6ᵗʰ **S85.30** Unspecified injury of greater saphenous vein at lower leg level

    ✓7ᵗʰ **S85.301** Unspecified injury of greater saphenous vein at lower leg level, right leg

    ✓7ᵗʰ **S85.302** Unspecified injury of greater saphenous vein at lower leg level, left leg

    ✓7ᵗʰ **S85.309** Unspecified injury of greater saphenous vein at lower leg level, unspecified leg

✓6ᵗʰ **S85.31** Laceration of greater saphenous vein at lower leg level

    ✓7ᵗʰ **S85.311** Laceration of greater saphenous vein at lower leg level, right leg

    ✓7ᵗʰ **S85.312** Laceration of greater saphenous vein at lower leg level, left leg

    ✓7ᵗʰ **S85.319** Laceration of greater saphenous vein at lower leg level, unspecified leg

✓6ᵗʰ **S85.39** Other specified injury of greater saphenous vein at lower leg level

    ✓7ᵗʰ **S85.391** Other specified injury of greater saphenous vein at lower leg level, right leg

    ✓7ᵗʰ **S85.392** Other specified injury of greater saphenous vein at lower leg level, left leg

    ✓7ᵗʰ **S85.399** Other specified injury of greater saphenous vein at lower leg level, unspecified leg

✓5ᵗʰ **S85.4** Injury of lesser saphenous vein at lower leg level

✓6ᵗʰ **S85.40** Unspecified injury of lesser saphenous vein at lower leg level

    ✓7ᵗʰ **S85.401** Unspecified injury of lesser saphenous vein at lower leg level, right leg

    ✓7ᵗʰ **S85.402** Unspecified injury of lesser saphenous vein at lower leg level, left leg

    ✓7ᵗʰ **S85.409** Unspecified injury of lesser saphenous vein at lower leg level, unspecified leg

✓6ᵗʰ **S85.41** Laceration of lesser saphenous vein at lower leg level

    ✓7ᵗʰ **S85.411** Laceration of lesser saphenous vein at lower leg level, right leg

    ✓7ᵗʰ **S85.412** Laceration of lesser saphenous vein at lower leg level, left leg

    ✓7ᵗʰ **S85.419** Laceration of lesser saphenous vein at lower leg level, unspecified leg

✓6ᵗʰ **S85.49** Other specified injury of lesser saphenous vein at lower leg level

    ✓7ᵗʰ **S85.491** Other specified injury of lesser saphenous vein at lower leg level, right leg

    ✓7ᵗʰ **S85.492** Other specified injury of lesser saphenous vein at lower leg level, left leg

    ✓7ᵗʰ **S85.499** Other specified injury of lesser saphenous vein at lower leg level, unspecified leg

✓5ᵗʰ **S85.5** Injury of popliteal vein

✓6ᵗʰ **S85.50** Unspecified injury of popliteal vein

    ✓7ᵗʰ **S85.501** Unspecified injury of popliteal vein, right leg

    ✓7ᵗʰ **S85.502** Unspecified injury of popliteal vein, left leg

    ✓7ᵗʰ **S85.509** Unspecified injury of popliteal vein, unspecified leg

✓6ᵗʰ **S85.51** Laceration of popliteal vein

    ✓7ᵗʰ **S85.511** Laceration of popliteal vein, right leg

    ✓7ᵗʰ **S85.512** Laceration of popliteal vein, left leg

    ✓7ᵗʰ **S85.519** Laceration of popliteal vein, unspecified leg

✓6ᵗʰ **S85.59** Other specified injury of popliteal vein

    ✓7ᵗʰ **S85.591** Other specified injury of popliteal vein, right leg

    ✓7ᵗʰ **S85.592** Other specified injury of popliteal vein, left leg

    ✓7ᵗʰ **S85.599** Other specified injury of popliteal vein, unspecified leg

✓5ᵗʰ **S85.8** Injury of other blood vessels at lower leg level

✓6ᵗʰ **S85.80** Unspecified injury of other blood vessels at lower leg level

    ✓7ᵗʰ **S85.801** Unspecified injury of other blood vessels at lower leg level, right leg

    ✓7ᵗʰ **S85.802** Unspecified injury of other blood vessels at lower leg level, left leg

☑ Additional Character Required   ✓ˣ7ᵗʰ Placeholder Alert   Manifestation   Unspecified Dx   ▶◀ Revised Text   ● New Code   ▲ Revised Title

ICD-10-CM 2020   **1049**

√7ᵗʰ **S85.809** Unspecified injury of other blood vessels at lower leg level, unspecified leg

√6ᵗʰ **S85.81** Laceration of other blood vessels at lower leg level

   √7ᵗʰ **S85.811** Laceration of other blood vessels at lower leg level, right leg

   √7ᵗʰ **S85.812** Laceration of other blood vessels at lower leg level, left leg

   √7ᵗʰ **S85.819** Laceration of other blood vessels at lower leg level, unspecified leg

√6ᵗʰ **S85.89** Other specified injury of other blood vessels at lower leg level

   √7ᵗʰ **S85.891** Other specified injury of other blood vessels at lower leg level, right leg

   √7ᵗʰ **S85.892** Other specified injury of other blood vessels at lower leg level, left leg

   √7ᵗʰ **S85.899** Other specified injury of other blood vessels at lower leg level, unspecified leg

√5ᵗʰ **S85.9** Injury of unspecified blood vessel at lower leg level

√6ᵗʰ **S85.90** Unspecified injury of unspecified blood vessel at lower leg level

   √7ᵗʰ **S85.901** Unspecified injury of unspecified blood vessel at lower leg level, right leg

   √7ᵗʰ **S85.902** Unspecified injury of unspecified blood vessel at lower leg level, left leg

   √7ᵗʰ **S85.909** Unspecified injury of unspecified blood vessel at lower leg level, unspecified leg

√6ᵗʰ **S85.91** Laceration of unspecified blood vessel at lower leg level

   √7ᵗʰ **S85.911** Laceration of unspecified blood vessel at lower leg level, right leg

   √7ᵗʰ **S85.912** Laceration of unspecified blood vessel at lower leg level, left leg

   √7ᵗʰ **S85.919** Laceration of unspecified blood vessel at lower leg level, unspecified leg

√6ᵗʰ **S85.99** Other specified injury of unspecified blood vessel at lower leg level

   √7ᵗʰ **S85.991** Other specified injury of unspecified blood vessel at lower leg level, right leg

   √7ᵗʰ **S85.992** Other specified injury of unspecified blood vessel at lower leg level, left leg

   √7ᵗʰ **S85.999** Other specified injury of unspecified blood vessel at lower leg level, unspecified leg

√4ᵗʰ **S86** Injury of muscle, fascia and tendon at lower leg level

Code also any associated open wound (S81.-)

EXCLUDES 2   *injury of muscle, fascia and tendon at ankle (S96.-)*
injury of patellar ligament (tendon) (S76.1-)
sprain of joints and ligaments of knee (S83.-)

TIP: Refer to the Muscle/Tendon table at the beginning of this chapter.

The appropriate 7th character is to be added to each code from category S86.
A   initial encounter
D   subsequent encounter
S   sequela

√5ᵗʰ **S86.0** Injury of Achilles tendon

√6ᵗʰ **S86.00** Unspecified injury of Achilles tendon

   √7ᵗʰ **S86.001** Unspecified injury of right Achilles tendon

   √7ᵗʰ **S86.002** Unspecified injury of left Achilles tendon

   √7ᵗʰ **S86.009** Unspecified injury of unspecified Achilles tendon

√6ᵗʰ **S86.01** Strain of Achilles tendon

   √7ᵗʰ **S86.011** Strain of right Achilles tendon

   √7ᵗʰ **S86.012** Strain of left Achilles tendon

   √7ᵗʰ **S86.019** Strain of unspecified Achilles tendon

√6ᵗʰ **S86.02** Laceration of Achilles tendon

   √7ᵗʰ **S86.021** Laceration of right Achilles tendon

   √7ᵗʰ **S86.022** Laceration of left Achilles tendon

   √7ᵗʰ **S86.029** Laceration of unspecified Achilles tendon

√6ᵗʰ **S86.09** Other specified injury of Achilles tendon

   √7ᵗʰ **S86.091** Other specified injury of right Achilles tendon

   √7ᵗʰ **S86.092** Other specified injury of left Achilles tendon

   √7ᵗʰ **S86.099** Other specified injury of unspecified Achilles tendon

√5ᵗʰ **S86.1** Injury of other muscle(s) and tendon(s) of posterior muscle group at lower leg level

√6ᵗʰ **S86.10** Unspecified injury of other muscle(s) and tendon(s) of posterior muscle group at lower leg level

   √7ᵗʰ **S86.101** Unspecified injury of other muscle(s) and tendon(s) of posterior muscle group at lower leg level, right leg

   √7ᵗʰ **S86.102** Unspecified injury of other muscle(s) and tendon(s) of posterior muscle group at lower leg level, left leg

   √7ᵗʰ **S86.109** Unspecified injury of other muscle(s) and tendon(s) of posterior muscle group at lower leg level, unspecified leg

√6ᵗʰ **S86.11** Strain of other muscle(s) and tendon(s) of posterior muscle group at lower leg level

   √7ᵗʰ **S86.111** Strain of other muscle(s) and tendon(s) of posterior muscle group at lower leg level, right leg

   √7ᵗʰ **S86.112** Strain of other muscle(s) and tendon(s) of posterior muscle group at lower leg level, left leg

   √7ᵗʰ **S86.119** Strain of other muscle(s) and tendon(s) of posterior muscle group at lower leg level, unspecified leg

√6ᵗʰ **S86.12** Laceration of other muscle(s) and tendon(s) of posterior muscle group at lower leg level

   √7ᵗʰ **S86.121** Laceration of other muscle(s) and tendon(s) of posterior muscle group at lower leg level, right leg

   √7ᵗʰ **S86.122** Laceration of other muscle(s) and tendon(s) of posterior muscle group at lower leg level, left leg

   √7ᵗʰ **S86.129** Laceration of other muscle(s) and tendon(s) of posterior muscle group at lower leg level, unspecified leg

√6ᵗʰ **S86.19** Other injury of other muscle(s) and tendon(s) of posterior muscle group at lower leg level

   √7ᵗʰ **S86.191** Other injury of other muscle(s) and tendon(s) of posterior muscle group at lower leg level, right leg

   √7ᵗʰ **S86.192** Other injury of other muscle(s) and tendon(s) of posterior muscle group at lower leg level, left leg

   √7ᵗʰ **S86.199** Other injury of other muscle(s) and tendon(s) of posterior muscle group at lower leg level, unspecified leg

√5ᵗʰ **S86.2** Injury of muscle(s) and tendon(s) of anterior muscle group at lower leg level

√6ᵗʰ **S86.20** Unspecified injury of muscle(s) and tendon(s) of anterior muscle group at lower leg level

   √7ᵗʰ **S86.201** Unspecified injury of muscle(s) and tendon(s) of anterior muscle group at lower leg level, right leg

   √7ᵗʰ **S86.202** Unspecified injury of muscle(s) and tendon(s) of anterior muscle group at lower leg level, left leg

   √7ᵗʰ **S86.209** Unspecified injury of muscle(s) and tendon(s) of anterior muscle group at lower leg level, unspecified leg

√6ᵗʰ **S86.21** Strain of muscle(s) and tendon(s) of anterior muscle group at lower leg level

   √7ᵗʰ **S86.211** Strain of muscle(s) and tendon(s) of anterior muscle group at lower leg level, right leg

   √7ᵗʰ **S86.212** Strain of muscle(s) and tendon(s) of anterior muscle group at lower leg level, left leg

   √7ᵗʰ **S86.219** Strain of muscle(s) and tendon(s) of anterior muscle group at lower leg level, unspecified leg

√6ᵗʰ **S86.22** Laceration of muscle(s) and tendon(s) of anterior muscle group at lower leg level

   √7ᵗʰ **S86.221** Laceration of muscle(s) and tendon(s) of anterior muscle group at lower leg level, right leg

   √7ᵗʰ **S86.222** Laceration of muscle(s) and tendon(s) of anterior muscle group at lower leg level, left leg

   √7ᵗʰ **S86.229** Laceration of muscle(s) and tendon(s) of anterior muscle group at lower leg level, unspecified leg

√6ᵗʰ **S86.29** Other injury of muscle(s) and tendon(s) of anterior muscle group at lower leg level
- √7ᵗʰ **S86.291** Other injury of muscle(s) and tendon(s) of anterior muscle group at lower leg level, right leg
- √7ᵗʰ **S86.292** Other injury of muscle(s) and tendon(s) of anterior muscle group at lower leg level, left leg
- √7ᵗʰ **S86.299** Other injury of muscle(s) and tendon(s) of anterior muscle group at lower leg level, unspecified leg

√5ᵗʰ **S86.3** Injury of muscle(s) and tendon(s) of peroneal muscle group at lower leg level
- √6ᵗʰ **S86.30** Unspecified injury of muscle(s) and tendon(s) of peroneal muscle group at lower leg level
  - √7ᵗʰ **S86.301** Unspecified injury of muscle(s) and tendon(s) of peroneal muscle group at lower leg level, right leg
  - √7ᵗʰ **S86.302** Unspecified injury of muscle(s) and tendon(s) of peroneal muscle group at lower leg level, left leg
  - √7ᵗʰ **S86.309** Unspecified injury of muscle(s) and tendon(s) of peroneal muscle group at lower leg level, unspecified leg
- √6ᵗʰ **S86.31** Strain of muscle(s) and tendon(s) of peroneal muscle group at lower leg level
  - √7ᵗʰ **S86.311** Strain of muscle(s) and tendon(s) of peroneal muscle group at lower leg level, right leg
  - √7ᵗʰ **S86.312** Strain of muscle(s) and tendon(s) of peroneal muscle group at lower leg level, left leg
  - √7ᵗʰ **S86.319** Strain of muscle(s) and tendon(s) of peroneal muscle group at lower leg level, unspecified leg
- √6ᵗʰ **S86.32** Laceration of muscle(s) and tendon(s) of peroneal muscle group at lower leg level
  - √7ᵗʰ **S86.321** Laceration of muscle(s) and tendon(s) of peroneal muscle group at lower leg level, right leg
  - √7ᵗʰ **S86.322** Laceration of muscle(s) and tendon(s) of peroneal muscle group at lower leg level, left leg
  - √7ᵗʰ **S86.329** Laceration of muscle(s) and tendon(s) of peroneal muscle group at lower leg level, unspecified leg
- √6ᵗʰ **S86.39** Other injury of muscle(s) and tendon(s) of peroneal muscle group at lower leg level
  - √7ᵗʰ **S86.391** Other injury of muscle(s) and tendon(s) of peroneal muscle group at lower leg level, right leg
  - √7ᵗʰ **S86.392** Other injury of muscle(s) and tendon(s) of peroneal muscle group at lower leg level, left leg
  - √7ᵗʰ **S86.399** Other injury of muscle(s) and tendon(s) of peroneal muscle group at lower leg level, unspecified leg

√5ᵗʰ **S86.8** Injury of other muscles and tendons at lower leg level
- √6ᵗʰ **S86.80** Unspecified injury of other muscles and tendons at lower leg level
  - √7ᵗʰ **S86.801** Unspecified injury of other muscle(s) and tendon(s) at lower leg level, right leg
  - √7ᵗʰ **S86.802** Unspecified injury of other muscle(s) and tendon(s) at lower leg level, left leg
  - √7ᵗʰ **S86.809** Unspecified injury of other muscle(s) and tendon(s) at lower leg level, unspecified leg
- √6ᵗʰ **S86.81** Strain of other muscles and tendons at lower leg level
  - √7ᵗʰ **S86.811** Strain of other muscle(s) and tendon(s) at lower leg level, right leg
  - √7ᵗʰ **S86.812** Strain of other muscle(s) and tendon(s) at lower leg level, left leg
  - √7ᵗʰ **S86.819** Strain of other muscle(s) and tendon(s) at lower leg level, unspecified leg
- √6ᵗʰ **S86.82** Laceration of other muscles and tendons at lower leg level
  - √7ᵗʰ **S86.821** Laceration of other muscle(s) and tendon(s) at lower leg level, right leg
  - √7ᵗʰ **S86.822** Laceration of other muscle(s) and tendon(s) at lower leg level, left leg
  - √7ᵗʰ **S86.829** Laceration of other muscle(s) and tendon(s) at lower leg level, unspecified leg

√6ᵗʰ **S86.89** Other injury of other muscles and tendons at lower leg level
- √7ᵗʰ **S86.891** Other injury of other muscle(s) and tendon(s) at lower leg level, right leg
- √7ᵗʰ **S86.892** Other injury of other muscle(s) and tendon(s) at lower leg level, left leg
- √7ᵗʰ **S86.899** Other injury of other muscle(s) and tendon(s) at lower leg level, unspecified leg

√5ᵗʰ **S86.9** Injury of unspecified muscle and tendon at lower leg level
- √6ᵗʰ **S86.90** Unspecified injury of unspecified muscle and tendon at lower leg level
  - √7ᵗʰ **S86.901** Unspecified injury of unspecified muscle(s) and tendon(s) at lower leg level, right leg
  - √7ᵗʰ **S86.902** Unspecified injury of unspecified muscle(s) and tendon(s) at lower leg level, left leg
  - √7ᵗʰ **S86.909** Unspecified injury of unspecified muscle(s) and tendon(s) at lower leg level, unspecified leg
- √6ᵗʰ **S86.91** Strain of unspecified muscle and tendon at lower leg level
  - √7ᵗʰ **S86.911** Strain of unspecified muscle(s) and tendon(s) at lower leg level, right leg
  - √7ᵗʰ **S86.912** Strain of unspecified muscle(s) and tendon(s) at lower leg level, left leg
  - √7ᵗʰ **S86.919** Strain of unspecified muscle(s) and tendon(s) at lower leg level, unspecified leg
- √6ᵗʰ **S86.92** Laceration of unspecified muscle and tendon at lower leg level
  - √7ᵗʰ **S86.921** Laceration of unspecified muscle(s) and tendon(s) at lower leg level, right leg
  - √7ᵗʰ **S86.922** Laceration of unspecified muscle(s) and tendon(s) at lower leg level, left leg
  - √7ᵗʰ **S86.929** Laceration of unspecified muscle(s) and tendon(s) at lower leg level, unspecified leg
- √6ᵗʰ **S86.99** Other injury of unspecified muscle and tendon at lower leg level
  - √7ᵗʰ **S86.991** Other injury of unspecified muscle(s) and tendon(s) at lower leg level, right leg
  - √7ᵗʰ **S86.992** Other injury of unspecified muscle(s) and tendon(s) at lower leg level, left leg
  - √7ᵗʰ **S86.999** Other injury of unspecified muscle(s) and tendon(s) at lower leg level, unspecified leg

√4ᵗʰ **S87** Crushing injury of lower leg

Use additional code(s) for all associated injuries

EXCLUDES 2   crushing injury of ankle and foot (S97.-)

The appropriate 7th character is to be added to each code from category S87.
A   initial encounter
D   subsequent encounter
S   sequela

√5ᵗʰ **S87.0** Crushing injury of knee
- √x7ᵗʰ **S87.00** Crushing injury of unspecified knee
- √x7ᵗʰ **S87.01** Crushing injury of right knee
- √x7ᵗʰ **S87.02** Crushing injury of left knee

√5ᵗʰ **S87.8** Crushing injury of lower leg
- √x7ᵗʰ **S87.80** Crushing injury of unspecified lower leg
- √x7ᵗʰ **S87.81** Crushing injury of right lower leg
- √x7ᵗʰ **S87.82** Crushing injury of left lower leg

√4ᵗʰ **S88** Traumatic amputation of lower leg

An amputation not identified as partial or complete should be coded to complete

EXCLUDES 1   traumatic amputation of ankle and foot (S98.-)

The appropriate 7th character is to be added to each code from category S88.
A   initial encounter
D   subsequent encounter
S   sequela

√5ᵗʰ **S88.0** Traumatic amputation at knee level
- √6ᵗʰ **S88.01** Complete traumatic amputation at knee level
  - √7ᵗʰ **S88.011** Complete traumatic amputation at knee level, right lower leg

✓ Additional Character Required   √x7ᵗʰ Placeholder Alert   Manifestation   Unspecified Dx   ▶◀ Revised Text   ● New Code   ▲ Revised Title

ICD-10-CM 2020   1051

Chapter 19. Injury, Poisoning and Certain Other Consequences of External Causes (side margin)

    ☑7ᵗʰ **S88.012** Complete traumatic amputation at knee level, left lower leg

    ☑7ᵗʰ **S88.019** Complete traumatic amputation at knee level, unspecified lower leg

  ☑6ᵗʰ **S88.02** Partial traumatic amputation at knee level

    ☑7ᵗʰ **S88.021** Partial traumatic amputation at knee level, right lower leg

    ☑7ᵗʰ **S88.022** Partial traumatic amputation at knee level, left lower leg

    ☑7ᵗʰ **S88.029** Partial traumatic amputation at knee level, unspecified lower leg

☑5ᵗʰ **S88.1** Traumatic amputation at level between knee and ankle

  ☑6ᵗʰ **S88.11** Complete traumatic amputation at level between knee and ankle

    ☑7ᵗʰ **S88.111** Complete traumatic amputation at level between knee and ankle, right lower leg

    ☑7ᵗʰ **S88.112** Complete traumatic amputation at level between knee and ankle, left lower leg

    ☑7ᵗʰ **S88.119** Complete traumatic amputation at level between knee and ankle, unspecified lower leg

  ☑6ᵗʰ **S88.12** Partial traumatic amputation at level between knee and ankle

    ☑7ᵗʰ **S88.121** Partial traumatic amputation at level between knee and ankle, right lower leg

    ☑7ᵗʰ **S88.122** Partial traumatic amputation at level between knee and ankle, left lower leg

    ☑7ᵗʰ **S88.129** Partial traumatic amputation at level between knee and ankle, unspecified lower leg

☑5ᵗʰ **S88.9** Traumatic amputation of lower leg, level unspecified

  ☑6ᵗʰ **S88.91** Complete traumatic amputation of lower leg, level unspecified

    ☑7ᵗʰ **S88.911** Complete traumatic amputation of right lower leg, level unspecified

    ☑7ᵗʰ **S88.912** Complete traumatic amputation of left lower leg, level unspecified

    ☑7ᵗʰ **S88.919** Complete traumatic amputation of unspecified lower leg, level unspecified

  ☑6ᵗʰ **S88.92** Partial traumatic amputation of lower leg, level unspecified

    ☑7ᵗʰ **S88.921** Partial traumatic amputation of right lower leg, level unspecified

    ☑7ᵗʰ **S88.922** Partial traumatic amputation of left lower leg, level unspecified

    ☑7ᵗʰ **S88.929** Partial traumatic amputation of unspecified lower leg, level unspecified

☑4ᵗʰ **S89** Other and unspecified injuries of lower leg

   NOTE   A fracture not indicated as open or closed should be coded to closed.

   EXCLUDES 2   other and unspecified injuries of ankle and foot (S99.-)

   AHA: 2018,2Q,12; 2018,1Q,3; 2015,3Q,37-39

   TIP: The term "improper alignment" is not synonymous with malunion or nonunion of a fracture when noted in provider documentation.

   The appropriate 7th character is to be added to each code from subcategories S89.0, S89.1, S89.2, and S89.3.
   A   initial encounter for closed fracture
   D   subsequent encounter for fracture with routine healing
   G   subsequent encounter for fracture with delayed healing
   K   subsequent encounter for fracture with nonunion
   P   subsequent encounter for fracture with malunion
   S   sequela

☑5ᵗʰ **S89.0** Physeal fracture of upper end of tibia

  ☑6ᵗʰ **S89.00** Unspecified physeal fracture of upper end of tibia

    ☑7ᵗʰ **S89.001** Unspecified physeal fracture of upper end of right tibia

    ☑7ᵗʰ **S89.002** Unspecified physeal fracture of upper end of left tibia

    ☑7ᵗʰ **S89.009** Unspecified physeal fracture of upper end of unspecified tibia

  ☑6ᵗʰ **S89.01** Salter-Harris Type I physeal fracture of upper end of tibia

    ☑7ᵗʰ **S89.011** Salter-Harris Type I physeal fracture of upper end of right tibia

    ☑7ᵗʰ **S89.012** Salter-Harris Type I physeal fracture of upper end of left tibia

    ☑7ᵗʰ **S89.019** Salter-Harris Type I physeal fracture of upper end of unspecified tibia

  ☑6ᵗʰ **S89.02** Salter-Harris Type II physeal fracture of upper end of tibia

    ☑7ᵗʰ **S89.021** Salter-Harris Type II physeal fracture of upper end of right tibia

    ☑7ᵗʰ **S89.022** Salter-Harris Type II physeal fracture of upper end of left tibia

    ☑7ᵗʰ **S89.029** Salter-Harris Type II physeal fracture of upper end of unspecified tibia

  ☑6ᵗʰ **S89.03** Salter-Harris Type III physeal fracture of upper end of tibia

    ☑7ᵗʰ **S89.031** Salter-Harris Type III physeal fracture of upper end of right tibia

    ☑7ᵗʰ **S89.032** Salter-Harris Type III physeal fracture of upper end of left tibia

    ☑7ᵗʰ **S89.039** Salter-Harris Type III physeal fracture of upper end of unspecified tibia

  ☑6ᵗʰ **S89.04** Salter-Harris Type IV physeal fracture of upper end of tibia

    ☑7ᵗʰ **S89.041** Salter-Harris Type IV physeal fracture of upper end of right tibia

    ☑7ᵗʰ **S89.042** Salter-Harris Type IV physeal fracture of upper end of left tibia

    ☑7ᵗʰ **S89.049** Salter-Harris Type IV physeal fracture of upper end of unspecified tibia

  ☑6ᵗʰ **S89.09** Other physeal fracture of upper end of tibia

    ☑7ᵗʰ **S89.091** Other physeal fracture of upper end of right tibia

    ☑7ᵗʰ **S89.092** Other physeal fracture of upper end of left tibia

    ☑7ᵗʰ **S89.099** Other physeal fracture of upper end of unspecified tibia

☑5ᵗʰ **S89.1** Physeal fracture of lower end of tibia

  ☑6ᵗʰ **S89.10** Unspecified physeal fracture of lower end of tibia

    ☑7ᵗʰ **S89.101** Unspecified physeal fracture of lower end of right tibia

    ☑7ᵗʰ **S89.102** Unspecified physeal fracture of lower end of left tibia

    ☑7ᵗʰ **S89.109** Unspecified physeal fracture of lower end of unspecified tibia

  ☑6ᵗʰ **S89.11** Salter-Harris Type I physeal fracture of lower end of tibia

    ☑7ᵗʰ **S89.111** Salter-Harris Type I physeal fracture of lower end of right tibia

    ☑7ᵗʰ **S89.112** Salter-Harris Type I physeal fracture of lower end of left tibia

    ☑7ᵗʰ **S89.119** Salter-Harris Type I physeal fracture of lower end of unspecified tibia

  ☑6ᵗʰ **S89.12** Salter-Harris Type II physeal fracture of lower end of tibia

    ☑7ᵗʰ **S89.121** Salter-Harris Type II physeal fracture of lower end of right tibia

    ☑7ᵗʰ **S89.122** Salter-Harris Type II physeal fracture of lower end of left tibia

    ☑7ᵗʰ **S89.129** Salter-Harris Type II physeal fracture of lower end of unspecified tibia

  ☑6ᵗʰ **S89.13** Salter-Harris Type III physeal fracture of lower end of tibia

    EXCLUDES 1   fracture of medial malleolus (adult) (S82.5-)

    ☑7ᵗʰ **S89.131** Salter-Harris Type III physeal fracture of lower end of right tibia

    ☑7ᵗʰ **S89.132** Salter-Harris Type III physeal fracture of lower end of left tibia

    ☑7ᵗʰ **S89.139** Salter-Harris Type III physeal fracture of lower end of unspecified tibia

  ☑6ᵗʰ **S89.14** Salter-Harris Type IV physeal fracture of lower end of tibia

    EXCLUDES 1   fracture of medial malleolus (adult) (S82.5-)

    ☑7ᵗʰ **S89.141** Salter-Harris Type IV physeal fracture of lower end of right tibia

    ☑7ᵗʰ **S89.142** Salter-Harris Type IV physeal fracture of lower end of left tibia

    ☑7ᵗʰ **S89.149** Salter-Harris Type IV physeal fracture of lower end of unspecified tibia

  ☑6ᵗʰ **S89.19** Other physeal fracture of lower end of tibia

    ☑7ᵗʰ **S89.191** Other physeal fracture of lower end of right tibia

    ☑7ᵗʰ **S89.192** Other physeal fracture of lower end of left tibia

    ☑7ᵗʰ **S89.199** Other physeal fracture of lower end of unspecified tibia

N Newborn: 0   P Pediatric: 0-17   M Maternity: 12-55   A Adult: 15-124   CH Comorbidity High   CL Comorbidity Low   NCDx Noncancer Dx   PDx Primary Dx

1052   ICD-10-CM 2020

√5ᵗʰ **S89.2** **Physeal fracture of** upper end of fibula

    √6ᵗʰ **S89.20** **Unspecified physeal fracture of upper end of fibula**

       √7ᵗʰ **S89.201** **Unspecified physeal fracture of upper end of** right **fibula**

       √7ᵗʰ **S89.202** **Unspecified physeal fracture of upper end of** left **fibula**

       √7ᵗʰ **S89.209** **Unspecified physeal fracture of upper end of unspecified fibula**

    √6ᵗʰ **S89.21** Salter-Harris Type I **physeal fracture of upper end of fibula**

       √7ᵗʰ **S89.211** **Salter-Harris Type I physeal fracture of upper end of** right **fibula**

       √7ᵗʰ **S89.212** **Salter-Harris Type I physeal fracture of upper end of** left **fibula**

       √7ᵗʰ **S89.219** **Salter-Harris Type I physeal fracture of upper end of unspecified fibula**

    √6ᵗʰ **S89.22** Salter-Harris Type II **physeal fracture of upper end of fibula**

       √7ᵗʰ **S89.221** **Salter-Harris Type II physeal fracture of upper end of** right **fibula**

       √7ᵗʰ **S89.222** **Salter-Harris Type II physeal fracture of upper end of** left **fibula**

       √7ᵗʰ **S89.229** **Salter-Harris Type II physeal fracture of upper end of unspecified fibula**

    √6ᵗʰ **S89.29** **Other physeal fracture of upper end of fibula**

       √7ᵗʰ **S89.291** **Other physeal fracture of upper end of** right **fibula**

       √7ᵗʰ **S89.292** **Other physeal fracture of upper end of** left **fibula**

       √7ᵗʰ **S89.299** **Other physeal fracture of upper end of unspecified fibula**

√5ᵗʰ **S89.3** **Physeal fracture of** lower end of fibula

    √6ᵗʰ **S89.30** **Unspecified physeal fracture of lower end of fibula**

       √7ᵗʰ **S89.301** **Unspecified physeal fracture of lower end of** right **fibula**

       √7ᵗʰ **S89.302** **Unspecified physeal fracture of lower end of** left **fibula**

       √7ᵗʰ **S89.309** **Unspecified physeal fracture of lower end of unspecified fibula**

    √6ᵗʰ **S89.31** Salter-Harris Type I **physeal fracture of lower end of fibula**

       √7ᵗʰ **S89.311** **Salter-Harris Type I physeal fracture of lower end of** right **fibula**

       √7ᵗʰ **S89.312** **Salter-Harris Type I physeal fracture of lower end of** left **fibula**

       √7ᵗʰ **S89.319** **Salter-Harris Type I physeal fracture of lower end of unspecified fibula**

    √6ᵗʰ **S89.32** Salter-Harris Type II **physeal fracture of lower end of fibula**

       √7ᵗʰ **S89.321** **Salter-Harris Type II physeal fracture of lower end of** right **fibula**

       √7ᵗʰ **S89.322** **Salter-Harris Type II physeal fracture of lower end of** left **fibula**

       √7ᵗʰ **S89.329** **Salter-Harris Type II physeal fracture of lower end of unspecified fibula**

    √6ᵗʰ **S89.39** **Other physeal fracture of lower end of fibula**

       √7ᵗʰ **S89.391** **Other physeal fracture of lower end of right fibula**

       √7ᵗʰ **S89.392** **Other physeal fracture of lower end of left fibula**

       √7ᵗʰ **S89.399** **Other physeal fracture of lower end of unspecified fibula**

√5ᵗʰ **S89.8** **Other specified injuries of lower leg**

> The appropriate 7th character is to be added to each code in subcategory S89.8.
> A   initial encounter
> D   subsequent encounter
> S   sequela

    √x7ᵗʰ **S89.80** **Other specified injuries of unspecified lower leg**

    √x7ᵗʰ **S89.81** **Other specified injuries of** right **lower leg**

    √x7ᵗʰ **S89.82** **Other specified injuries of** left **lower leg**

√5ᵗʰ **S89.9** **Unspecified injury of lower** leg

> The appropriate 7th character is to be added to each code in subcategory S89.9.
> A   initial encounter
> D   subsequent encounter
> S   sequela

    √x7ᵗʰ **S89.90** **Unspecified injury of unspecified lower leg**

    √x7ᵗʰ **S89.91** **Unspecified injury of** right **lower leg**

    √x7ᵗʰ **S89.92** **Unspecified injury of** left **lower leg**

Injuries to the ankle and foot (S90-S99)

EXCLUDES 2   burns and corrosions (T20-T32)
              fracture of ankle and malleolus (S82.-)
              frostbite (T33-T34)
              insect bite or sting, venomous (T63.4)

√4ᵗʰ **S90** **Superficial injury of ankle, foot and toes**

> The appropriate 7th character is to be added to each code from category S90.
> A   initial encounter
> D   subsequent encounter
> S   sequela

    √5ᵗʰ **S90.0** **Contusion of** ankle

       √x7ᵗʰ **S90.00** **Contusion of unspecified ankle**

       √x7ᵗʰ **S90.01** **Contusion of** right **ankle**

       √x7ᵗʰ **S90.02** **Contusion of** left **ankle**

    √5ᵗʰ **S90.1** **Contusion of** toe without damage to nail

       √6ᵗʰ **S90.11** **Contusion of** great **toe without damage to nail**

          √7ᵗʰ **S90.111** **Contusion of** right **great toe without damage to nail**

          √7ᵗʰ **S90.112** **Contusion of** left **great toe without damage to nail**

          √7ᵗʰ **S90.119** **Contusion of unspecified great toe without damage to nail**

       √6ᵗʰ **S90.12** **Contusion of** lesser **toe without damage to nail**

          √7ᵗʰ **S90.121** **Contusion of** right **lesser toe(s) without damage to nail**

          √7ᵗʰ **S90.122** **Contusion of** left **lesser toe(s) without damage to nail**

          √7ᵗʰ **S90.129** **Contusion of unspecified lesser toe(s) without damage to nail**
               Contusion of toe NOS

    √5ᵗʰ **S90.2** **Contusion of** toe with damage to nail

       √6ᵗʰ **S90.21** **Contusion of** great **toe with damage to nail**

          √7ᵗʰ **S90.211** **Contusion of** right **great toe with damage to nail**

          √7ᵗʰ **S90.212** **Contusion of** left **great toe with damage to nail**

          √7ᵗʰ **S90.219** **Contusion of unspecified great toe with damage to nail**

       √6ᵗʰ **S90.22** **Contusion of** lesser **toe with damage to nail**

          √7ᵗʰ **S90.221** **Contusion of** right **lesser toe(s) with damage to nail**

          √7ᵗʰ **S90.222** **Contusion of** left **lesser toe(s) with damage to nail**

          √7ᵗʰ **S90.229** **Contusion of unspecified lesser toe(s) with damage to nail**

    √5ᵗʰ **S90.3** **Contusion of** foot

       EXCLUDES 2   contusion of toes (S90.1-, S90.2-)

       √x7ᵗʰ **S90.30** **Contusion of unspecified foot**
               Contusion of foot NOS

       √x7ᵗʰ **S90.31** **Contusion of** right **foot**

       √x7ᵗʰ **S90.32** **Contusion of** left **foot**

    √5ᵗʰ **S90.4** **Other superficial injuries of** toe

       √6ᵗʰ **S90.41** Abrasion **of toe**

          √7ᵗʰ **S90.411** **Abrasion,** right great **toe**

          √7ᵗʰ **S90.412** **Abrasion,** left great **toe**

          √7ᵗʰ **S90.413** **Abrasion, unspecified great toe**

          √7ᵗʰ **S90.414** **Abrasion,** right lesser **toe(s)**

          √7ᵗʰ **S90.415** **Abrasion,** left lesser **toe(s)**

          √7ᵗʰ **S90.416** **Abrasion, unspecified lesser toe(s)**

       √6ᵗʰ **S90.42** Blister (nonthermal) **of toe**

          √7ᵗʰ **S90.421** **Blister (nonthermal),** right great **toe**

          √7ᵗʰ **S90.422** **Blister (nonthermal),** left great **toe**

          √7ᵗʰ **S90.423** **Blister (nonthermal), unspecified great toe**

          √7ᵗʰ **S90.424** **Blister (nonthermal),** right lesser **toe(s)**

          √7ᵗʰ **S90.425** **Blister (nonthermal),** left lesser **toe(s)**

          √7ᵗʰ **S90.426** **Blister (nonthermal), unspecified lesser toe(s)**

✔ Additional Character Required   √x7ᵗʰ Placeholder Alert   Manifestation   Unspecified Dx   ▶◀ Revised Text   ● New Code   ▲ Revised Title

ICD-10-CM 2020   **1053**

√6ᵗʰ **S90.44** **External constriction** of toe
  Hair tourniquet syndrome of toe
    √7ᵗʰ **S90.441** **External constriction,** right great **toe**
    √7ᵗʰ **S90.442** **External constriction,** left great **toe**
    √7ᵗʰ **S90.443** **External constriction, unspecified great toe**
    √7ᵗʰ **S90.444** **External constriction,** right lesser **toe(s)**
    √7ᵗʰ **S90.445** **External constriction,** left lesser **toe(s)**
    √7ᵗʰ **S90.446** **External constriction, unspecified lesser toe(s)**

√6ᵗʰ **S90.45** **Superficial** foreign body **of toe**
  Splinter in the toe
    √7ᵗʰ **S90.451** **Superficial foreign body,** right great **toe**
    √7ᵗʰ **S90.452** **Superficial foreign body,** left great **toe**
    √7ᵗʰ **S90.453** **Superficial foreign body, unspecified great toe**
    √7ᵗʰ **S90.454** **Superficial foreign body,** right lesser **toe(s)**
    √7ᵗʰ **S90.455** **Superficial foreign body,** left lesser **toe(s)**
    √7ᵗʰ **S90.456** **Superficial foreign body, unspecified lesser toe(s)**

√6ᵗʰ **S90.46** **Insect bite** (nonvenomous) of toe
    √7ᵗʰ **S90.461** **Insect bite (nonvenomous),** right great **toe**
    √7ᵗʰ **S90.462** **Insect bite (nonvenomous),** left great **toe**
    √7ᵗʰ **S90.463** **Insect bite (nonvenomous), unspecified great toe**
    √7ᵗʰ **S90.464** **Insect bite (nonvenomous),** right lesser **toe(s)**
    √7ᵗʰ **S90.465** **Insect bite (nonvenomous),** left lesser **toe(s)**
    √7ᵗʰ **S90.466** **Insect bite (nonvenomous), unspecified lesser toe(s)**

√6ᵗʰ **S90.47** **Other superficial** bite **of toe**
    EXCLUDES 1   *open bite of toe (S91.15-, S91.25-)*
    √7ᵗʰ **S90.471** **Other superficial bite of** right great **toe**
    √7ᵗʰ **S90.472** **Other superficial bite of** left great **toe**
    √7ᵗʰ **S90.473** **Other superficial bite of unspecified great toe**
    √7ᵗʰ **S90.474** **Other superficial bite of** right lesser **toe(s)**
    √7ᵗʰ **S90.475** **Other superficial bite of** left lesser **toe(s)**
    √7ᵗʰ **S90.476** **Other superficial bite of unspecified lesser toe(s)**

√5ᵗʰ **S90.5** **Other superficial injuries of** ankle

√6ᵗʰ **S90.51** **Abrasion** of ankle
    √7ᵗʰ **S90.511** **Abrasion,** right **ankle**
    √7ᵗʰ **S90.512** **Abrasion,** left **ankle**
    √7ᵗʰ **S90.519** **Abrasion, unspecified ankle**

√6ᵗʰ **S90.52** **Blister** (nonthermal) of ankle
    √7ᵗʰ **S90.521** **Blister (nonthermal),** right **ankle**
    √7ᵗʰ **S90.522** **Blister (nonthermal),** left **ankle**
    √7ᵗʰ **S90.529** **Blister (nonthermal), unspecified ankle**

√6ᵗʰ **S90.54** **External constriction** of ankle
    √7ᵗʰ **S90.541** **External constriction,** right **ankle**
    √7ᵗʰ **S90.542** **External constriction,** left **ankle**
    √7ᵗʰ **S90.549** **External constriction, unspecified ankle**

√6ᵗʰ **S90.55** **Superficial** foreign body **of ankle**
  Splinter in the ankle
    √7ᵗʰ **S90.551** **Superficial foreign body,** right **ankle**
    √7ᵗʰ **S90.552** **Superficial foreign body,** left **ankle**
    √7ᵗʰ **S90.559** **Superficial foreign body, unspecified ankle**

√6ᵗʰ **S90.56** **Insect bite** (nonvenomous) of ankle
    √7ᵗʰ **S90.561** **Insect bite (nonvenomous),** right **ankle**
    √7ᵗʰ **S90.562** **Insect bite (nonvenomous),** left **ankle**
    √7ᵗʰ **S90.569** **Insect bite (nonvenomous), unspecified ankle**

√6ᵗʰ **S90.57** **Other superficial** bite **of ankle**
    EXCLUDES 1   *open bite of ankle (S91.05-)*
    √7ᵗʰ **S90.571** **Other superficial bite of ankle,** right **ankle**
    √7ᵗʰ **S90.572** **Other superficial bite of ankle,** left **ankle**

    √7ᵗʰ **S90.579** **Other superficial bite of ankle, unspecified ankle**

√5ᵗʰ **S90.8** **Other superficial injuries of** foot

√6ᵗʰ **S90.81** **Abrasion** of foot
    √7ᵗʰ **S90.811** **Abrasion,** right **foot**
    √7ᵗʰ **S90.812** **Abrasion,** left **foot**
    √7ᵗʰ **S90.819** **Abrasion, unspecified foot**

√6ᵗʰ **S90.82** **Blister** (nonthermal) of foot
    √7ᵗʰ **S90.821** **Blister (nonthermal),** right **foot**
    √7ᵗʰ **S90.822** **Blister (nonthermal),** left **foot**
    √7ᵗʰ **S90.829** **Blister (nonthermal), unspecified foot**

√6ᵗʰ **S90.84** **External constriction** of foot
    √7ᵗʰ **S90.841** **External constriction,** right **foot**
    √7ᵗʰ **S90.842** **External constriction,** left **foot**
    √7ᵗʰ **S90.849** **External constriction, unspecified foot**

√6ᵗʰ **S90.85** **Superficial** foreign body **of foot**
  Splinter in the foot
    √7ᵗʰ **S90.851** **Superficial foreign body,** right **foot**
    √7ᵗʰ **S90.852** **Superficial foreign body,** left **foot**
    √7ᵗʰ **S90.859** **Superficial foreign body, unspecified foot**

√6ᵗʰ **S90.86** **Insect bite** (nonvenomous) of foot
    √7ᵗʰ **S90.861** **Insect bite (nonvenomous),** right **foot**
    √7ᵗʰ **S90.862** **Insect bite (nonvenomous),** left **foot**
    √7ᵗʰ **S90.869** **Insect bite (nonvenomous), unspecified foot**

√6ᵗʰ **S90.87** **Other superficial** bite **of foot**
    EXCLUDES 1   *open bite of foot (S91.35-)*
    √7ᵗʰ **S90.871** **Other superficial bite of** right **foot**
    √7ᵗʰ **S90.872** **Other superficial bite of** left **foot**
    √7ᵗʰ **S90.879** **Other superficial bite of unspecified foot**

√5ᵗʰ **S90.9** **Unspecified superficial injury of ankle, foot and toe**

√6ᵗʰ **S90.91** **Unspecified superficial injury of** ankle
    √7ᵗʰ **S90.911** **Unspecified superficial injury of** right **ankle**
    √7ᵗʰ **S90.912** **Unspecified superficial injury of** left **ankle**
    √7ᵗʰ **S90.919** **Unspecified superficial injury of unspecified ankle**

√6ᵗʰ **S90.92** **Unspecified superficial injury of** foot
    √7ᵗʰ **S90.921** **Unspecified superficial injury of** right **foot**
    √7ᵗʰ **S90.922** **Unspecified superficial injury of** left **foot**
    √7ᵗʰ **S90.929** **Unspecified superficial injury of unspecified foot**

√6ᵗʰ **S90.93** **Unspecified superficial injury of** toes
    √7ᵗʰ **S90.931** **Unspecified superficial injury of** right great **toe**
    √7ᵗʰ **S90.932** **Unspecified superficial injury of** left great **toe**
    √7ᵗʰ **S90.933** **Unspecified superficial injury of unspecified great toe**
    √7ᵗʰ **S90.934** **Unspecified superficial injury of** right lesser **toe(s)**
    √7ᵗʰ **S90.935** **Unspecified superficial injury of** left lesser **toe(s)**
    √7ᵗʰ **S90.936** **Unspecified superficial injury of unspecified lesser toe(s)**

√4ᵗʰ **S91** **Open wound of ankle, foot and toes**
  Code also any associated wound infection
    EXCLUDES 1   *open fracture of ankle, foot and toes (S92.- with 7th character B)*
                  traumatic amputation of ankle and foot (S98.-)

  The appropriate 7th character is to be added to each code from category S91.
  A   initial encounter
  D   subsequent encounter
  S   sequela

√5ᵗʰ **S91.0** **Open wound of** ankle

√6ᵗʰ **S91.00** **Unspecified open wound of ankle**
    √7ᵗʰ **S91.001** **Unspecified open wound,** right **ankle**
    √7ᵗʰ **S91.002** **Unspecified open wound,** left **ankle**
    √7ᵗʰ **S91.009** **Unspecified open wound, unspecified ankle**

√6ᵗʰ **S91.01** Laceration without foreign body of ankle

   √7ᵗʰ **S91.011** Laceration without foreign body, right ankle

   √7ᵗʰ **S91.012** Laceration without foreign body, left ankle

   √7ᵗʰ **S91.019** Laceration without foreign body, unspecified ankle

√6ᵗʰ **S91.02** Laceration with foreign body of ankle

   √7ᵗʰ **S91.021** Laceration with foreign body, right ankle

   √7ᵗʰ **S91.022** Laceration with foreign body, left ankle

   √7ᵗʰ **S91.029** Laceration with foreign body, unspecified ankle

√6ᵗʰ **S91.03** Puncture wound without foreign body of ankle

   √7ᵗʰ **S91.031** Puncture wound without foreign body, right ankle

   √7ᵗʰ **S91.032** Puncture wound without foreign body, left ankle

   √7ᵗʰ **S91.039** Puncture wound without foreign body, unspecified ankle

√6ᵗʰ **S91.04** Puncture wound with foreign body of ankle

   √7ᵗʰ **S91.041** Puncture wound with foreign body, right ankle

   √7ᵗʰ **S91.042** Puncture wound with foreign body, left ankle

   √7ᵗʰ **S91.049** Puncture wound with foreign body, unspecified ankle

√6ᵗʰ **S91.05** Open bite of ankle

   EXCLUDES 1   superficial bite of ankle (S90.56-, S90.57-)

   √7ᵗʰ **S91.051** Open bite, right ankle

   √7ᵗʰ **S91.052** Open bite, left ankle

   √7ᵗʰ **S91.059** Open bite, unspecified ankle

√5ᵗʰ **S91.1** Open wound of toe without damage to nail

√6ᵗʰ **S91.10** Unspecified open wound of toe without damage to nail

   √7ᵗʰ **S91.101** Unspecified open wound of right great toe without damage to nail

   √7ᵗʰ **S91.102** Unspecified open wound of left great toe without damage to nail

   √7ᵗʰ **S91.103** Unspecified open wound of unspecified great toe without damage to nail

   √7ᵗʰ **S91.104** Unspecified open wound of right lesser toe(s) without damage to nail

   √7ᵗʰ **S91.105** Unspecified open wound of left lesser toe(s) without damage to nail

   √7ᵗʰ **S91.106** Unspecified open wound of unspecified lesser toe(s) without damage to nail

   √7ᵗʰ **S91.109** Unspecified open wound of unspecified toe(s) without damage to nail

√6ᵗʰ **S91.11** Laceration without foreign body of toe without damage to nail

   √7ᵗʰ **S91.111** Laceration without foreign body of right great toe without damage to nail

   √7ᵗʰ **S91.112** Laceration without foreign body of left great toe without damage to nail

   √7ᵗʰ **S91.113** Laceration without foreign body of unspecified great toe without damage to nail

   √7ᵗʰ **S91.114** Laceration without foreign body of right lesser toe(s) without damage to nail

   √7ᵗʰ **S91.115** Laceration without foreign body of left lesser toe(s) without damage to nail

   √7ᵗʰ **S91.116** Laceration without foreign body of unspecified lesser toe(s) without damage to nail

   √7ᵗʰ **S91.119** Laceration without foreign body of unspecified toe without damage to nail

√6ᵗʰ **S91.12** Laceration with foreign body of toe without damage to nail

   √7ᵗʰ **S91.121** Laceration with foreign body of right great toe without damage to nail

   √7ᵗʰ **S91.122** Laceration with foreign body of left great toe without damage to nail

   √7ᵗʰ **S91.123** Laceration with foreign body of unspecified great toe without damage to nail

   √7ᵗʰ **S91.124** Laceration with foreign body of right lesser toe(s) without damage to nail

   √7ᵗʰ **S91.125** Laceration with foreign body of left lesser toe(s) without damage to nail

   √7ᵗʰ **S91.126** Laceration with foreign body of unspecified lesser toe(s) without damage to nail

   √7ᵗʰ **S91.129** Laceration with foreign body of unspecified toe(s) without damage to nail

√6ᵗʰ **S91.13** Puncture wound without foreign body of toe without damage to nail

   √7ᵗʰ **S91.131** Puncture wound without foreign body of right great toe without damage to nail

   √7ᵗʰ **S91.132** Puncture wound without foreign body of left great toe without damage to nail

   √7ᵗʰ **S91.133** Puncture wound without foreign body of unspecified great toe without damage to nail

   √7ᵗʰ **S91.134** Puncture wound without foreign body of right lesser toe(s) without damage to nail

   √7ᵗʰ **S91.135** Puncture wound without foreign body of left lesser toe(s) without damage to nail

   √7ᵗʰ **S91.136** Puncture wound without foreign body of unspecified lesser toe(s) without damage to nail

   √7ᵗʰ **S91.139** Puncture wound without foreign body of unspecified toe(s) without damage to nail

√6ᵗʰ **S91.14** Puncture wound with foreign body of toe without damage to nail

   √7ᵗʰ **S91.141** Puncture wound with foreign body of right great toe without damage to nail

   √7ᵗʰ **S91.142** Puncture wound with foreign body of left great toe without damage to nail

   √7ᵗʰ **S91.143** Puncture wound with foreign body of unspecified great toe without damage to nail

   √7ᵗʰ **S91.144** Puncture wound with foreign body of right lesser toe(s) without damage to nail

   √7ᵗʰ **S91.145** Puncture wound with foreign body of left lesser toe(s) without damage to nail

   √7ᵗʰ **S91.146** Puncture wound with foreign body of unspecified lesser toe(s) without damage to nail

   √7ᵗʰ **S91.149** Puncture wound with foreign body of unspecified toe(s) without damage to nail

√6ᵗʰ **S91.15** Open bite of toe without damage to nail

   Bite of toe NOS

   EXCLUDES 1   superficial bite of toe (S90.46-, S90.47-)

   √7ᵗʰ **S91.151** Open bite of right great toe without damage to nail

   √7ᵗʰ **S91.152** Open bite of left great toe without damage to nail

   √7ᵗʰ **S91.153** Open bite of unspecified great toe without damage to nail

   √7ᵗʰ **S91.154** Open bite of right lesser toe(s) without damage to nail

   √7ᵗʰ **S91.155** Open bite of left lesser toe(s) without damage to nail

   √7ᵗʰ **S91.156** Open bite of unspecified lesser toe(s) without damage to nail

   √7ᵗʰ **S91.159** Open bite of unspecified toe(s) without damage to nail

√5ᵗʰ **S91.2** Open wound of toe with damage to nail

√6ᵗʰ **S91.20** Unspecified open wound of toe with damage to nail

   √7ᵗʰ **S91.201** Unspecified open wound of right great toe with damage to nail

   √7ᵗʰ **S91.202** Unspecified open wound of left great toe with damage to nail

   √7ᵗʰ **S91.203** Unspecified open wound of unspecified great toe with damage to nail

   √7ᵗʰ **S91.204** Unspecified open wound of right lesser toe(s) with damage to nail

   √7ᵗʰ **S91.205** Unspecified open wound of left lesser toe(s) with damage to nail

   √7ᵗʰ **S91.206** Unspecified open wound of unspecified lesser toe(s) with damage to nail

   √7ᵗʰ **S91.209** Unspecified open wound of unspecified toe(s) with damage to nail

√6ᵗʰ **S91.21** Laceration without foreign body of toe with damage to nail

   √7ᵗʰ **S91.211** Laceration without foreign body of right great toe with damage to nail

   √7ᵗʰ **S91.212** Laceration without foreign body of left great toe with damage to nail

   √7ᵗʰ **S91.213** Laceration without foreign body of unspecified great toe with damage to nail

☑ Additional Character Required   √x7ᵗʰ Placeholder Alert   **Manifestation**   Unspecified Dx   ▶◀ Revised Text   ● New Code   ▲ Revised Title

ICD-10-CM 2020   **1055**

Chapter 19. Injury, Poisoning and Certain Other Consequences of External Causes

✓7ᵗʰ **S91.214** Laceration without foreign body of right lesser toe(s) with damage to nail

✓7ᵗʰ **S91.215** Laceration without foreign body of left lesser toe(s) with damage to nail

✓7ᵗʰ **S91.216** Laceration without foreign body of unspecified lesser toe(s) with damage to nail

✓7ᵗʰ **S91.219** Laceration without foreign body of unspecified toe(s) with damage to nail

✓6ᵗʰ **S91.22** Laceration with foreign body of toe with damage to nail

✓7ᵗʰ **S91.221** Laceration with foreign body of right great toe with damage to nail

✓7ᵗʰ **S91.222** Laceration with foreign body of left great toe with damage to nail

✓7ᵗʰ **S91.223** Laceration with foreign body of unspecified great toe with damage to nail

✓7ᵗʰ **S91.224** Laceration with foreign body of right lesser toe(s) with damage to nail

✓7ᵗʰ **S91.225** Laceration with foreign body of left lesser toe(s) with damage to nail

✓7ᵗʰ **S91.226** Laceration with foreign body of unspecified lesser toe(s) with damage to nail

✓7ᵗʰ **S91.229** Laceration with foreign body of unspecified toe(s) with damage to nail

✓6ᵗʰ **S91.23** Puncture wound without foreign body of toe with damage to nail

✓7ᵗʰ **S91.231** Puncture wound without foreign body of right great toe with damage to nail

✓7ᵗʰ **S91.232** Puncture wound without foreign body of left great toe with damage to nail

✓7ᵗʰ **S91.233** Puncture wound without foreign body of unspecified great toe with damage to nail

✓7ᵗʰ **S91.234** Puncture wound without foreign body of right lesser toe(s) with damage to nail

✓7ᵗʰ **S91.235** Puncture wound without foreign body of left lesser toe(s) with damage to nail

✓7ᵗʰ **S91.236** Puncture wound without foreign body of unspecified lesser toe(s) with damage to nail

✓7ᵗʰ **S91.239** Puncture wound without foreign body of unspecified toe(s) with damage to nail

✓6ᵗʰ **S91.24** Puncture wound with foreign body of toe with damage to nail

✓7ᵗʰ **S91.241** Puncture wound with foreign body of right great toe with damage to nail

✓7ᵗʰ **S91.242** Puncture wound with foreign body of left great toe with damage to nail

✓7ᵗʰ **S91.243** Puncture wound with foreign body of unspecified great toe with damage to nail

✓7ᵗʰ **S91.244** Puncture wound with foreign body of right lesser toe(s) with damage to nail

✓7ᵗʰ **S91.245** Puncture wound with foreign body of left lesser toe(s) with damage to nail

✓7ᵗʰ **S91.246** Puncture wound with foreign body of unspecified lesser toe(s) with damage to nail

✓7ᵗʰ **S91.249** Puncture wound with foreign body of unspecified toe(s) with damage to nail

✓6ᵗʰ **S91.25** Open bite of toe with damage to nail

Bite of toe with damage to nail NOS

EXCLUDES 1   superficial bite of toe (S90.46-, S90.47-)

✓7ᵗʰ **S91.251** Open bite of right great toe with damage to nail

✓7ᵗʰ **S91.252** Open bite of left great toe with damage to nail

✓7ᵗʰ **S91.253** Open bite of unspecified great toe with damage to nail

✓7ᵗʰ **S91.254** Open bite of right lesser toe(s) with damage to nail

✓7ᵗʰ **S91.255** Open bite of left lesser toe(s) with damage to nail

✓7ᵗʰ **S91.256** Open bite of unspecified lesser toe(s) with damage to nail

✓7ᵗʰ **S91.259** Open bite of unspecified toe(s) with damage to nail

✓5ᵗʰ **S91.3** Open wound of foot

✓6ᵗʰ **S91.30** Unspecified open wound of foot

✓7ᵗʰ **S91.301** Unspecified open wound, right foot

✓7ᵗʰ **S91.302** Unspecified open wound, left foot

✓7ᵗʰ **S91.309** Unspecified open wound, unspecified foot

✓6ᵗʰ **S91.31** Laceration without foreign body of foot

✓7ᵗʰ **S91.311** Laceration without foreign body, right foot

✓7ᵗʰ **S91.312** Laceration without foreign body, left foot

✓7ᵗʰ **S91.319** Laceration without foreign body, unspecified foot

✓6ᵗʰ **S91.32** Laceration with foreign body of foot

✓7ᵗʰ **S91.321** Laceration with foreign body, right foot

✓7ᵗʰ **S91.322** Laceration with foreign body, left foot

✓7ᵗʰ **S91.329** Laceration with foreign body, unspecified foot

✓6ᵗʰ **S91.33** Puncture wound without foreign body of foot

✓7ᵗʰ **S91.331** Puncture wound without foreign body, right foot

✓7ᵗʰ **S91.332** Puncture wound without foreign body, left foot

✓7ᵗʰ **S91.339** Puncture wound without foreign body, unspecified foot

✓6ᵗʰ **S91.34** Puncture wound with foreign body of foot

✓7ᵗʰ **S91.341** Puncture wound with foreign body, right foot

✓7ᵗʰ **S91.342** Puncture wound with foreign body, left foot

✓7ᵗʰ **S91.349** Puncture wound with foreign body, unspecified foot

✓6ᵗʰ **S91.35** Open bite of foot

EXCLUDES 1   superficial bite of foot (S90.86-, S90.87-)

✓7ᵗʰ **S91.351** Open bite, right foot

✓7ᵗʰ **S91.352** Open bite, left foot

✓7ᵗʰ **S91.359** Open bite, unspecified foot

✓4ᵗʰ **S92** Fracture of foot and toe, except ankle

NOTE   A fracture not indicated as displaced or nondisplaced should be coded to displaced

A fracture not indicated as open or closed should be coded to closed.

EXCLUDES 1   traumatic amputation of ankle and foot (S98.-)

EXCLUDES 2   fracture of ankle (S82.-)

fracture of malleolus (S82.-)

AHA: 2018,2Q,12; 2015,3Q,37-39

TIP: The term "improper alignment" is not synonymous with malunion or nonunion of a fracture when noted in provider documentation.

The appropriate 7th character is to be added to each code from category S92.
A   initial encounter for closed fracture
B   initial encounter for open fracture
D   subsequent encounter for fracture with routine healing
G   subsequent encounter for fracture with delayed healing
K   subsequent encounter for fracture with nonunion
P   subsequent encounter for fracture with malunion
S   sequela

✓5ᵗʰ **S92.0** Fracture of calcaneus

Heel bone
Os calcis

EXCLUDES 2   physeal fracture of calcaneus (S99.0-)

✓6ᵗʰ **S92.00** Unspecified fracture of calcaneus

✓7ᵗʰ **S92.001** Unspecified fracture of right calcaneus

✓7ᵗʰ **S92.002** Unspecified fracture of left calcaneus

✓7ᵗʰ **S92.009** Unspecified fracture of unspecified calcaneus

✓6ᵗʰ **S92.01** Fracture of body of calcaneus

✓7ᵗʰ **S92.011** Displaced fracture of body of right calcaneus

✓7ᵗʰ **S92.012** Displaced fracture of body of left calcaneus

✓7ᵗʰ **S92.013** Displaced fracture of body of unspecified calcaneus

✓7ᵗʰ **S92.014** Nondisplaced fracture of body of right calcaneus

✓7ᵗʰ **S92.015** Nondisplaced fracture of body of left calcaneus

✓7ᵗʰ **S92.016** Nondisplaced fracture of body of unspecified calcaneus

N Newborn: 0   P Pediatric: 0-17   M Maternity: 12-55   A Adult: 15-124   CH Comorbidity High   CL Comorbidity Low   NC Dx Noncancer Dx   PDx Primary Dx

1056   ICD-10-CM 2020

√6ᵗʰ **S92.02** **Fracture of** anterior process **of calcaneus**

    √7ᵗʰ **S92.021** Displaced **fracture of anterior process of** right **calcaneus**

    √7ᵗʰ **S92.022** Displaced **fracture of anterior process of** left **calcaneus**

    √7ᵗʰ **S92.023** Displaced **fracture of anterior process of** unspecified **calcaneus**

    √7ᵗʰ **S92.024** Nondisplaced **fracture of anterior process of** right **calcaneus**

    √7ᵗʰ **S92.025** Nondisplaced **fracture of anterior process of** left **calcaneus**

    √7ᵗʰ **S92.026** Nondisplaced **fracture of anterior process of** unspecified **calcaneus**

√6ᵗʰ **S92.03** Avulsion **fracture of** tuberosity **of calcaneus**

    √7ᵗʰ **S92.031** Displaced **avulsion fracture of tuberosity of** right **calcaneus**

    √7ᵗʰ **S92.032** Displaced **avulsion fracture of tuberosity of** left **calcaneus**

    √7ᵗʰ **S92.033** Displaced **avulsion fracture of tuberosity of** unspecified **calcaneus**

    √7ᵗʰ **S92.034** Nondisplaced **avulsion fracture of tuberosity of** right **calcaneus**

    √7ᵗʰ **S92.035** Nondisplaced **avulsion fracture of tuberosity of** left **calcaneus**

    √7ᵗʰ **S92.036** Nondisplaced **avulsion fracture of tuberosity of unspecified calcaneus**

√6ᵗʰ **S92.04** **Other fracture of** tuberosity **of calcaneus**

    √7ᵗʰ **S92.041** Displaced **other fracture of tuberosity of** right **calcaneus**

    √7ᵗʰ **S92.042** Displaced **other fracture of tuberosity of** left **calcaneus**

    √7ᵗʰ **S92.043** Displaced **other fracture of tuberosity of** unspecified **calcaneus**

    √7ᵗʰ **S92.044** Nondisplaced **other fracture of tuberosity of** right **calcaneus**

    √7ᵗʰ **S92.045** Nondisplaced **other fracture of tuberosity of** left **calcaneus**

    √7ᵗʰ **S92.046** Nondisplaced **other fracture of tuberosity of unspecified calcaneus**

√6ᵗʰ **S92.05** **Other** extraarticular **fracture of calcaneus**

    √7ᵗʰ **S92.051** Displaced **other extraarticular fracture of** right **calcaneus**

    √7ᵗʰ **S92.052** Displaced **other extraarticular fracture of** left **calcaneus**

    √7ᵗʰ **S92.053** Displaced **other extraarticular fracture of** unspecified **calcaneus**

    √7ᵗʰ **S92.054** Nondisplaced **other extraarticular fracture of** right **calcaneus**

    √7ᵗʰ **S92.055** Nondisplaced **other extraarticular fracture of** left **calcaneus**

    √7ᵗʰ **S92.056** Nondisplaced **other extraarticular fracture of unspecified calcaneus**

√6ᵗʰ **S92.06** Intraarticular **fracture of calcaneus**

    √7ᵗʰ **S92.061** Displaced **intraarticular fracture of** right **calcaneus**

    √7ᵗʰ **S92.062** Displaced **intraarticular fracture of** left **calcaneus**

    √7ᵗʰ **S92.063** Displaced **intraarticular fracture of** unspecified **calcaneus**

    √7ᵗʰ **S92.064** Nondisplaced **intraarticular fracture of** right **calcaneus**

    √7ᵗʰ **S92.065** Nondisplaced **intraarticular fracture of** left **calcaneus**

    √7ᵗʰ **S92.066** Nondisplaced **intraarticular fracture of** unspecified **calcaneus**

√5ᵗʰ **S92.1** **Fracture of** talus

    Astragalus

    √6ᵗʰ **S92.10** **Unspecified fracture of talus**

      √7ᵗʰ **S92.101** **Unspecified fracture of** right **talus**

      √7ᵗʰ **S92.102** **Unspecified fracture of** left **talus**

      √7ᵗʰ **S92.109** **Unspecified fracture of unspecified talus**

    √6ᵗʰ **S92.11** **Fracture of** neck **of talus**

      √7ᵗʰ **S92.111** Displaced **fracture of neck of** right **talus**

      √7ᵗʰ **S92.112** Displaced **fracture of neck of** left **talus**

      √7ᵗʰ **S92.113** Displaced **fracture of neck of unspecified talus**

      √7ᵗʰ **S92.114** Nondisplaced **fracture of neck of** right **talus**

      √7ᵗʰ **S92.115** Nondisplaced **fracture of neck of** left **talus**

      √7ᵗʰ **S92.116** Nondisplaced **fracture of neck of unspecified talus**

    √6ᵗʰ **S92.12** **Fracture of** body **of talus**

      √7ᵗʰ **S92.121** Displaced **fracture of body of** right **talus**

      √7ᵗʰ **S92.122** Displaced **fracture of body of** left **talus**

      √7ᵗʰ **S92.123** Displaced **fracture of body of unspecified talus**

      √7ᵗʰ **S92.124** Nondisplaced **fracture of body of** right **talus**

      √7ᵗʰ **S92.125** Nondisplaced **fracture of body of** left **talus**

      √7ᵗʰ **S92.126** Nondisplaced **fracture of body of unspecified talus**

    √6ᵗʰ **S92.13** **Fracture of** posterior process **of talus**

      √7ᵗʰ **S92.131** Displaced **fracture of posterior process of** right **talus**

      √7ᵗʰ **S92.132** Displaced **fracture of posterior process of** left **talus**

      √7ᵗʰ **S92.133** Displaced **fracture of posterior process of** unspecified **talus**

      √7ᵗʰ **S92.134** Nondisplaced **fracture of posterior process of** right **talus**

      √7ᵗʰ **S92.135** Nondisplaced **fracture of posterior process of** left **talus**

      √7ᵗʰ **S92.136** Nondisplaced **fracture of posterior process of unspecified talus**

    √6ᵗʰ **S92.14** **Dome fracture of talus**

      EXCLUDES 1   osteochondritis dissecans (M93.2)

      √7ᵗʰ **S92.141** Displaced **dome fracture of** right **talus**

      √7ᵗʰ **S92.142** Displaced **dome fracture of** left **talus**

      √7ᵗʰ **S92.143** Displaced **dome fracture of unspecified talus**

      √7ᵗʰ **S92.144** Nondisplaced **dome fracture of** right **talus**

      √7ᵗʰ **S92.145** Nondisplaced **dome fracture of** left **talus**

      √7ᵗʰ **S92.146** Nondisplaced **dome fracture of unspecified talus**

    √6ᵗʰ **S92.15** Avulsion **fracture (chip fracture) of talus**

      √7ᵗʰ **S92.151** Displaced **avulsion fracture (chip fracture) of** right **talus**

      √7ᵗʰ **S92.152** Displaced **avulsion fracture (chip fracture) of** left **talus**

      √7ᵗʰ **S92.153** Displaced **avulsion fracture (chip fracture) of** unspecified **talus**

      √7ᵗʰ **S92.154** Nondisplaced **avulsion fracture (chip fracture) of** right **talus**

      √7ᵗʰ **S92.155** Nondisplaced **avulsion fracture (chip fracture) of** left **talus**

      √7ᵗʰ **S92.156** Nondisplaced **avulsion fracture (chip fracture) of unspecified talus**

    √6ᵗʰ **S92.19** **Other fracture of talus**

      √7ᵗʰ **S92.191** **Other fracture of** right **talus**

      √7ᵗʰ **S92.192** **Other fracture of** left **talus**

      √7ᵗʰ **S92.199** **Other fracture of unspecified talus**

√5ᵗʰ **S92.2** **Fracture of other and unspecified tarsal bone(s)**

    √6ᵗʰ **S92.20** **Fracture of unspecified tarsal bone(s)**

      √7ᵗʰ **S92.201** **Fracture of unspecified tarsal bone(s) of** right **foot**

      √7ᵗʰ **S92.202** **Fracture of unspecified tarsal bone(s) of** left **foot**

      √7ᵗʰ **S92.209** **Fracture of unspecified tarsal bone(s) of unspecified foot**

    √6ᵗʰ **S92.21** **Fracture of** cuboid **bone**

      √7ᵗʰ **S92.211** Displaced **fracture of cuboid bone of** right **foot**

      √7ᵗʰ **S92.212** Displaced **fracture of cuboid bone of** left **foot**

      √7ᵗʰ **S92.213** Displaced **fracture of cuboid bone of** unspecified **foot**

      √7ᵗʰ **S92.214** Nondisplaced **fracture of cuboid bone of** right **foot**

      √7ᵗʰ **S92.215** Nondisplaced **fracture of cuboid bone of** left **foot**

      √7ᵗʰ **S92.216** Nondisplaced **fracture of cuboid bone of unspecified foot**

    √6ᵗʰ **S92.22** **Fracture of** lateral cuneiform

      √7ᵗʰ **S92.221** Displaced **fracture of lateral cuneiform of** right **foot**

☑ Additional Character Required   √x7ᵗʰ Placeholder Alert   Manifestation   Unspecified Dx   ▶◀ Revised Text   ● New Code   ▲ Revised Title

ICD-10-CM 2020   **1057**

√7ᵗʰ **S92.222** Displaced fracture of lateral cuneiform of left foot

√7ᵗʰ **S92.223** Displaced fracture of lateral cuneiform of unspecified foot

√7ᵗʰ S92.224 Nondisplaced fracture of lateral cuneiform of right foot

√7ᵗʰ S92.225 Nondisplaced fracture of lateral cuneiform of left foot

√7ᵗʰ **S92.226** Nondisplaced fracture of lateral cuneiform of unspecified foot

√6ᵗʰ **S92.23** Fracture of intermediate cuneiform

   √7ᵗʰ S92.231 Displaced fracture of intermediate cuneiform of right foot

   √7ᵗʰ S92.232 Displaced fracture of intermediate cuneiform of left foot

   √7ᵗʰ **S92.233** Displaced fracture of intermediate cuneiform of unspecified foot

   √7ᵗʰ S92.234 Nondisplaced fracture of intermediate cuneiform of right foot

   √7ᵗʰ S92.235 Nondisplaced fracture of intermediate cuneiform of left foot

   √7ᵗʰ **S92.236** Nondisplaced fracture of intermediate cuneiform of unspecified foot

√6ᵗʰ **S92.24** Fracture of medial cuneiform

   √7ᵗʰ S92.241 Displaced fracture of medial cuneiform of right foot

   √7ᵗʰ S92.242 Displaced fracture of medial cuneiform of left foot

   √7ᵗʰ **S92.243** Displaced fracture of medial cuneiform of unspecified foot

   √7ᵗʰ S92.244 Nondisplaced fracture of medial cuneiform of right foot

   √7ᵗʰ S92.245 Nondisplaced fracture of medial cuneiform of left foot

   √7ᵗʰ **S92.246** Nondisplaced fracture of medial cuneiform of unspecified foot

√6ᵗʰ **S92.25** Fracture of navicular [scaphoid] of foot

   √7ᵗʰ S92.251 Displaced fracture of navicular [scaphoid] of right foot

   √7ᵗʰ S92.252 Displaced fracture of navicular [scaphoid] of left foot

   √7ᵗʰ **S92.253** Displaced fracture of navicular [scaphoid] of unspecified foot

   √7ᵗʰ S92.254 Nondisplaced fracture of navicular [scaphoid] of right foot

   √7ᵗʰ S92.255 Nondisplaced fracture of navicular [scaphoid] of left foot

   √7ᵗʰ **S92.256** Nondisplaced fracture of navicular [scaphoid] of unspecified foot

√5ᵗʰ **S92.3** Fracture of metatarsal bone(s)

   EXCLUDES 2   physeal fracture of metatarsal (S99.1-)

   AHA: 2018,1Q,3

√6ᵗʰ **S92.30** Fracture of unspecified metatarsal bone(s)

   √7ᵗʰ **S92.301** Fracture of unspecified metatarsal bone(s), right foot

   √7ᵗʰ **S92.302** Fracture of unspecified metatarsal bone(s), left foot

   √7ᵗʰ **S92.309** Fracture of unspecified metatarsal bone(s), unspecified foot

√6ᵗʰ **S92.31** Fracture of first metatarsal bone

   √7ᵗʰ S92.311 Displaced fracture of first metatarsal bone, right foot

   √7ᵗʰ S92.312 Displaced fracture of first metatarsal bone, left foot

   √7ᵗʰ **S92.313** Displaced fracture of first metatarsal bone, unspecified foot

   √7ᵗʰ S92.314 Nondisplaced fracture of first metatarsal bone, right foot

   √7ᵗʰ S92.315 Nondisplaced fracture of first metatarsal bone, left foot

   √7ᵗʰ **S92.316** Nondisplaced fracture of first metatarsal bone, unspecified foot

√6ᵗʰ **S92.32** Fracture of second metatarsal bone

   √7ᵗʰ S92.321 Displaced fracture of second metatarsal bone, right foot

   √7ᵗʰ S92.322 Displaced fracture of second metatarsal bone, left foot

   √7ᵗʰ **S92.323** Displaced fracture of second metatarsal bone, unspecified foot

   √7ᵗʰ S92.324 Nondisplaced fracture of second metatarsal bone, right foot

√7ᵗʰ S92.325 Nondisplaced fracture of second metatarsal bone, left foot

√7ᵗʰ S92.326 Nondisplaced fracture of second metatarsal bone, unspecified foot

√6ᵗʰ **S92.33** Fracture of third metatarsal bone

   √7ᵗʰ S92.331 Displaced fracture of third metatarsal bone, right foot

   √7ᵗʰ S92.332 Displaced fracture of third metatarsal bone, left foot

   √7ᵗʰ S92.333 Displaced fracture of third metatarsal bone, unspecified foot

   √7ᵗʰ S92.334 Nondisplaced fracture of third metatarsal bone, right foot

   √7ᵗʰ S92.335 Nondisplaced fracture of third metatarsal bone, left foot

   √7ᵗʰ **S92.336** Nondisplaced fracture of third metatarsal bone, unspecified foot

√6ᵗʰ **S92.34** Fracture of fourth metatarsal bone

   √7ᵗʰ S92.341 Displaced fracture of fourth metatarsal bone, right foot

   √7ᵗʰ S92.342 Displaced fracture of fourth metatarsal bone, left foot

   √7ᵗʰ S92.343 Displaced fracture of fourth metatarsal bone, unspecified foot

   √7ᵗʰ S92.344 Nondisplaced fracture of fourth metatarsal bone, right foot

   √7ᵗʰ S92.345 Nondisplaced fracture of fourth metatarsal bone, left foot

   √7ᵗʰ S92.346 Nondisplaced fracture of fourth metatarsal bone, unspecified foot

√6ᵗʰ **S92.35** Fracture of fifth metatarsal bone

   √7ᵗʰ S92.351 Displaced fracture of fifth metatarsal bone, right foot

   √7ᵗʰ S92.352 Displaced fracture of fifth metatarsal bone, left foot

   √7ᵗʰ S92.353 Displaced fracture of fifth metatarsal bone, unspecified foot

   √7ᵗʰ S92.354 Nondisplaced fracture of fifth metatarsal bone, right foot

   √7ᵗʰ S92.355 Nondisplaced fracture of fifth metatarsal bone, left foot

   √7ᵗʰ **S92.356** Nondisplaced fracture of fifth metatarsal bone, unspecified foot

√5ᵗʰ **S92.4** Fracture of great toe

   EXCLUDES 2   physeal fracture of phalanx of toe (S99.2-)

√6ᵗʰ **S92.40** Unspecified fracture of great toe

   √7ᵗʰ **S92.401** Displaced unspecified fracture of right great toe

   √7ᵗʰ **S92.402** Displaced unspecified fracture of left great toe

   √7ᵗʰ **S92.403** Displaced unspecified fracture of unspecified great toe

   √7ᵗʰ **S92.404** Nondisplaced unspecified fracture of right great toe

   √7ᵗʰ **S92.405** Nondisplaced unspecified fracture of left great toe

   √7ᵗʰ **S92.406** Nondisplaced unspecified fracture of unspecified great toe

√6ᵗʰ **S92.41** Fracture of proximal phalanx of great toe

   √7ᵗʰ S92.411 Displaced fracture of proximal phalanx of right great toe

   √7ᵗʰ S92.412 Displaced fracture of proximal phalanx of left great toe

   √7ᵗʰ **S92.413** Displaced fracture of proximal phalanx of unspecified great toe

   √7ᵗʰ S92.414 Nondisplaced fracture of proximal phalanx of right great toe

   √7ᵗʰ S92.415 Nondisplaced fracture of proximal phalanx of left great toe

   √7ᵗʰ **S92.416** Nondisplaced fracture of proximal phalanx of unspecified great toe

√6ᵗʰ **S92.42** Fracture of distal phalanx of great toe

   √7ᵗʰ S92.421 Displaced fracture of distal phalanx of right great toe

   √7ᵗʰ S92.422 Displaced fracture of distal phalanx of left great toe

   √7ᵗʰ **S92.423** Displaced fracture of distal phalanx of unspecified great toe

   √7ᵗʰ S92.424 Nondisplaced fracture of distal phalanx of right great toe

---

N Newborn: 0   P Pediatric: 0-17   M Maternity: 12-55   A Adult: 15-124   CH Comorbidity High   CL Comorbidity Low   NCDx Noncancer Dx   PDx Primary Dx

1058   ICD-10-CM 2020

√7ᵗʰ **S92.425** Nondisplaced fracture of distal phalanx of left great toe

√7ᵗʰ **S92.426** Nondisplaced fracture of distal phalanx of unspecified great toe

√6ᵗʰ **S92.49** Other fracture of great toe

√7ᵗʰ **S92.491** Other fracture of right great toe

√7ᵗʰ **S92.492** Other fracture of left great toe

√7ᵗʰ **S92.499** Other fracture of unspecified great toe

√5ᵗʰ **S92.5** Fracture of lesser toe(s)

    EXCLUDES 2   physeal fracture of phalanx of toe (S99.2-)

√6ᵗʰ **S92.50** Unspecified fracture of lesser toe(s)

√7ᵗʰ **S92.501** Displaced unspecified fracture of right lesser toe(s)

√7ᵗʰ **S92.502** Displaced unspecified fracture of left lesser toe(s)

√7ᵗʰ **S92.503** Displaced unspecified fracture of unspecified lesser toe(s)

√7ᵗʰ **S92.504** Nondisplaced unspecified fracture of right lesser toe(s)

√7ᵗʰ **S92.505** Nondisplaced unspecified fracture of left lesser toe(s)

√7ᵗʰ **S92.506** Nondisplaced unspecified fracture of unspecified lesser toe(s)

√6ᵗʰ **S92.51** Fracture of proximal phalanx of lesser toe(s)

√7ᵗʰ **S92.511** Displaced fracture of proximal phalanx of right lesser toe(s)

√7ᵗʰ **S92.512** Displaced fracture of proximal phalanx of left lesser toe(s)

√7ᵗʰ **S92.513** Displaced fracture of proximal phalanx of unspecified lesser toe(s)

√7ᵗʰ **S92.514** Nondisplaced fracture of proximal phalanx of right lesser toe(s)

√7ᵗʰ **S92.515** Nondisplaced fracture of proximal phalanx of left lesser toe(s))

√7ᵗʰ **S92.516** Nondisplaced fracture of proximal phalanx of unspecified lesser toe(s)

√6ᵗʰ **S92.52** Fracture of middle phalanx of lesser toe(s)

√7ᵗʰ **S92.521** Displaced fracture of middle phalanx of right lesser toe(s)

√7ᵗʰ **S92.522** Displaced fracture of middle phalanx of left lesser toe(s)

√7ᵗʰ **S92.523** Displaced fracture of middle phalanx of unspecified lesser toe(s)

√7ᵗʰ **S92.524** Nondisplaced fracture of middle phalanx of right lesser toe(s)

√7ᵗʰ **S92.525** Nondisplaced fracture of middle phalanx of left lesser toe(s)

√7ᵗʰ **S92.526** Nondisplaced fracture of middle phalanx of unspecified lesser toe(s)

√6ᵗʰ **S92.53** Fracture of distal phalanx of lesser toe(s)

√7ᵗʰ **S92.531** Displaced fracture of distal phalanx of right lesser toe(s)

√7ᵗʰ **S92.532** Displaced fracture of distal phalanx of left lesser toe(s)

√7ᵗʰ **S92.533** Displaced fracture of distal phalanx of unspecified lesser toe(s)

√7ᵗʰ **S92.534** Nondisplaced fracture of distal phalanx of right lesser toe(s)

√7ᵗʰ **S92.535** Nondisplaced fracture of distal phalanx of left lesser toe(s)

√7ᵗʰ **S92.536** Nondisplaced fracture of distal phalanx of unspecified lesser toe(s)

√6ᵗʰ **S92.59** Other fracture of lesser toe(s)

√7ᵗʰ **S92.591** Other fracture of right lesser toe(s)

√7ᵗʰ **S92.592** Other fracture of left lesser toe(s)

√7ᵗʰ **S92.599** Other fracture of unspecified lesser toe(s)

√5ᵗʰ **S92.8** Other fracture of foot, except ankle

√6ᵗʰ **S92.81** Other fracture of foot

    Sesamoid fracture of foot

    AHA: 2016,4Q,68

√7ᵗʰ **S92.811** Other fracture of right foot

√7ᵗʰ **S92.812** Other fracture of left foot

√7ᵗʰ **S92.819** Other fracture of unspecified foot

√5ᵗʰ **S92.9** Unspecified fracture of foot and toe

√6ᵗʰ **S92.90** Unspecified fracture of foot

√7ᵗʰ **S92.901** Unspecified fracture of right foot

√7ᵗʰ **S92.902** Unspecified fracture of left foot

√7ᵗʰ **S92.909** Unspecified fracture of unspecified foot

√6ᵗʰ **S92.91** Unspecified fracture of toe

√7ᵗʰ **S92.911** Unspecified fracture of right toe(s)

√7ᵗʰ **S92.912** Unspecified fracture of left toe(s)

√7ᵗʰ **S92.919** Unspecified fracture of unspecified toe(s)

√4ᵗʰ **S93** Dislocation and sprain of joints and ligaments at ankle, foot and toe level

    INCLUDES   avulsion of joint or ligament of ankle, foot and toe

       laceration of cartilage, joint or ligament of ankle, foot and toe

       sprain of cartilage, joint or ligament of ankle, foot and toe

       traumatic hemarthrosis of joint or ligament of ankle, foot and toe

       traumatic rupture of joint or ligament of ankle, foot and toe

       traumatic subluxation of joint or ligament of ankle, foot and toe

       traumatic tear of joint or ligament of ankle, foot and toe

Code also any associated open wound

    EXCLUDES 2   strain of muscle and tendon of ankle and foot (S96.-)

> The appropriate 7th character is to be added to each code from category S93.
> A   initial encounter
> D   subsequent encounter
> S   sequela

√5ᵗʰ **S93.0** Subluxation and dislocation of ankle joint

    Subluxation and dislocation of astragalus

    Subluxation and dislocation of fibula, lower end

    Subluxation and dislocation of talus

    Subluxation and dislocation of tibia, lower end

√x7ᵗʰ **S93.01** Subluxation of right ankle joint

√x7ᵗʰ **S93.02** Subluxation of left ankle joint

√x7ᵗʰ **S93.03** Subluxation of unspecified ankle joint

√x7ᵗʰ **S93.04** Dislocation of right ankle joint

√x7ᵗʰ **S93.05** Dislocation of left ankle joint

√x7ᵗʰ **S93.06** Dislocation of unspecified ankle joint

√5ᵗʰ **S93.1** Subluxation and dislocation of toe

√6ᵗʰ **S93.10** Unspecified subluxation and dislocation of toe

    Dislocation of toe NOS

    Subluxation of toe NOS

√7ᵗʰ **S93.101** Unspecified subluxation of right toe(s)

√7ᵗʰ **S93.102** Unspecified subluxation of left toe(s)

√7ᵗʰ **S93.103** Unspecified subluxation of unspecified toe(s)

√7ᵗʰ **S93.104** Unspecified dislocation of right toe(s)

√7ᵗʰ **S93.105** Unspecified dislocation of left toe(s)

√7ᵗʰ **S93.106** Unspecified dislocation of unspecified toe(s)

√6ᵗʰ **S93.11** Dislocation of interphalangeal joint

√7ᵗʰ **S93.111** Dislocation of interphalangeal joint of right great toe

√7ᵗʰ **S93.112** Dislocation of interphalangeal joint of left great toe

√7ᵗʰ **S93.113** Dislocation of interphalangeal joint of unspecified great toe

√7ᵗʰ **S93.114** Dislocation of interphalangeal joint of right lesser toe(s)

√7ᵗʰ **S93.115** Dislocation of interphalangeal joint of left lesser toe(s)

√7ᵗʰ **S93.116** Dislocation of interphalangeal joint of unspecified lesser toe(s)

√7ᵗʰ **S93.119** Dislocation of interphalangeal joint of unspecified toe(s)

√6ᵗʰ **S93.12** Dislocation of metatarsophalangeal joint

√7ᵗʰ **S93.121** Dislocation of metatarsophalangeal joint of right great toe

√7ᵗʰ **S93.122** Dislocation of metatarsophalangeal joint of left great toe

√7ᵗʰ **S93.123** Dislocation of metatarsophalangeal joint of unspecified great toe

√7ᵗʰ **S93.124** Dislocation of metatarsophalangeal joint of right lesser toe(s)

√7ᵗʰ **S93.125** Dislocation of metatarsophalangeal joint of left lesser toe(s)

✅ Additional Character Required   √x7ᵗʰ Placeholder Alert   Manifestation   Unspecified Dx   ▶◀ Revised Text   ● New Code   ▲ Revised Title

ICD-10-CM 2020   1059

√7ᵗʰ **S93.126** Dislocation of metatarsophalangeal joint of unspecified lesser toe(s)

√7ᵗʰ **S93.129** Dislocation of metatarsophalangeal joint of unspecified toe(s)

√6ᵗʰ **S93.13** Subluxation of interphalangeal joint

√7ᵗʰ **S93.131** Subluxation of interphalangeal joint of right great toe

√7ᵗʰ **S93.132** Subluxation of interphalangeal joint of left great toe

√7ᵗʰ **S93.133** Subluxation of interphalangeal joint of unspecified great toe

√7ᵗʰ **S93.134** Subluxation of interphalangeal joint of right lesser toe(s)

√7ᵗʰ **S93.135** Subluxation of interphalangeal joint of left lesser toe(s)

√7ᵗʰ **S93.136** Subluxation of interphalangeal joint of unspecified lesser toe(s)

√7ᵗʰ **S93.139** Subluxation of interphalangeal joint of unspecified toe(s)

√6ᵗʰ **S93.14** Subluxation of metatarsophalangeal joint

√7ᵗʰ **S93.141** Subluxation of metatarsophalangeal joint of right great toe

√7ᵗʰ **S93.142** Subluxation of metatarsophalangeal joint of left great toe

√7ᵗʰ **S93.143** Subluxation of metatarsophalangeal joint of unspecified great toe

√7ᵗʰ **S93.144** Subluxation of metatarsophalangeal joint of right lesser toe(s)

√7ᵗʰ **S93.145** Subluxation of metatarsophalangeal joint of left lesser toe(s)

√7ᵗʰ **S93.146** Subluxation of metatarsophalangeal joint of unspecified lesser toe(s)

√7ᵗʰ **S93.149** Subluxation of metatarsophalangeal joint of unspecified toe(s)

√5ᵗʰ **S93.3** Subluxation and dislocation of foot

EXCLUDES 2   *dislocation of toe (S93.1-)*

√6ᵗʰ **S93.30** Unspecified subluxation and dislocation of foot

Dislocation of foot NOS
Subluxation of foot NOS

√7ᵗʰ **S93.301** Unspecified subluxation of right foot

√7ᵗʰ **S93.302** Unspecified subluxation of left foot

√7ᵗʰ **S93.303** Unspecified subluxation of unspecified foot

√7ᵗʰ **S93.304** Unspecified dislocation of right foot

√7ᵗʰ **S93.305** Unspecified dislocation of left foot

√7ᵗʰ **S93.306** Unspecified dislocation of unspecified foot

√6ᵗʰ **S93.31** Subluxation and dislocation of tarsal joint

√7ᵗʰ **S93.311** Subluxation of tarsal joint of right foot

√7ᵗʰ **S93.312** Subluxation of tarsal joint of left foot

√7ᵗʰ **S93.313** Subluxation of tarsal joint of unspecified foot

√7ᵗʰ **S93.314** Dislocation of tarsal joint of right foot

√7ᵗʰ **S93.315** Dislocation of tarsal joint of left foot

√7ᵗʰ **S93.316** Dislocation of tarsal joint of unspecified foot

√6ᵗʰ **S93.32** Subluxation and dislocation of tarsometatarsal joint

√7ᵗʰ **S93.321** Subluxation of tarsometatarsal joint of right foot

√7ᵗʰ **S93.322** Subluxation of tarsometatarsal joint of left foot

√7ᵗʰ **S93.323** Subluxation of tarsometatarsal joint of unspecified foot

√7ᵗʰ **S93.324** Dislocation of tarsometatarsal joint of right foot

√7ᵗʰ **S93.325** Dislocation of tarsometatarsal joint of left foot

√7ᵗʰ **S93.326** Dislocation of tarsometatarsal joint of unspecified foot

√6ᵗʰ **S93.33** Other subluxation and dislocation of foot

√7ᵗʰ **S93.331** Other subluxation of right foot

√7ᵗʰ **S93.332** Other subluxation of left foot

√7ᵗʰ **S93.333** Other subluxation of unspecified foot

√7ᵗʰ **S93.334** Other dislocation of right foot

√7ᵗʰ **S93.335** Other dislocation of left foot

√7ᵗʰ **S93.336** Other dislocation of unspecified foot

√5ᵗʰ **S93.4** Sprain of ankle

EXCLUDES 2   *injury of Achilles tendon (S86.0-)*

√6ᵗʰ **S93.40** Sprain of unspecified ligament of ankle

Sprain of ankle NOS
Sprained ankle NOS

√7ᵗʰ **S93.401** Sprain of unspecified ligament of right ankle

√7ᵗʰ **S93.402** Sprain of unspecified ligament of left ankle

√7ᵗʰ **S93.409** Sprain of unspecified ligament of unspecified ankle

√6ᵗʰ **S93.41** Sprain of calcaneofibular ligament

√7ᵗʰ **S93.411** Sprain of calcaneofibular ligament of right ankle

√7ᵗʰ **S93.412** Sprain of calcaneofibular ligament of left ankle

√7ᵗʰ **S93.419** Sprain of calcaneofibular ligament of unspecified ankle

√6ᵗʰ **S93.42** Sprain of deltoid ligament

√7ᵗʰ **S93.421** Sprain of deltoid ligament of right ankle

√7ᵗʰ **S93.422** Sprain of deltoid ligament of left ankle

√7ᵗʰ **S93.429** Sprain of deltoid ligament of unspecified ankle

√6ᵗʰ **S93.43** Sprain of tibiofibular ligament

√7ᵗʰ **S93.431** Sprain of tibiofibular ligament of right ankle

√7ᵗʰ **S93.432** Sprain of tibiofibular ligament of left ankle

√7ᵗʰ **S93.439** Sprain of tibiofibular ligament of unspecified ankle

√6ᵗʰ **S93.49** Sprain of other ligament of ankle

Sprain of internal collateral ligament
Sprain of talofibular ligament

√7ᵗʰ **S93.491** Sprain of other ligament of right ankle

√7ᵗʰ **S93.492** Sprain of other ligament of left ankle

√7ᵗʰ **S93.499** Sprain of other ligament of unspecified ankle

√5ᵗʰ **S93.5** Sprain of toe

√6ᵗʰ **S93.50** Unspecified sprain of toe

√7ᵗʰ **S93.501** Unspecified sprain of right great toe

√7ᵗʰ **S93.502** Unspecified sprain of left great toe

√7ᵗʰ **S93.503** Unspecified sprain of unspecified great toe

√7ᵗʰ **S93.504** Unspecified sprain of right lesser toe(s)

√7ᵗʰ **S93.505** Unspecified sprain of left lesser toe(s)

√7ᵗʰ **S93.506** Unspecified sprain of unspecified lesser toe(s)

√7ᵗʰ **S93.509** Unspecified sprain of unspecified toe(s)

√6ᵗʰ **S93.51** Sprain of interphalangeal joint of toe

√7ᵗʰ **S93.511** Sprain of interphalangeal joint of right great toe

√7ᵗʰ **S93.512** Sprain of interphalangeal joint of left great toe

√7ᵗʰ **S93.513** Sprain of interphalangeal joint of unspecified great toe

√7ᵗʰ **S93.514** Sprain of interphalangeal joint of right lesser toe(s)

√7ᵗʰ **S93.515** Sprain of interphalangeal joint of left lesser toe(s)

√7ᵗʰ **S93.516** Sprain of interphalangeal joint of unspecified lesser toe(s)

√7ᵗʰ **S93.519** Sprain of interphalangeal joint of unspecified toe(s)

√6ᵗʰ **S93.52** Sprain of metatarsophalangeal joint of toe

√7ᵗʰ **S93.521** Sprain of metatarsophalangeal joint of right great toe

√7ᵗʰ **S93.522** Sprain of metatarsophalangeal joint of left great toe

√7ᵗʰ **S93.523** Sprain of metatarsophalangeal joint of unspecified great toe

√7ᵗʰ **S93.524** Sprain of metatarsophalangeal joint of right lesser toe(s)

√7ᵗʰ **S93.525** Sprain of metatarsophalangeal joint of left lesser toe(s)

√7ᵗʰ **S93.526** Sprain of metatarsophalangeal joint of unspecified lesser toe(s)

√7ᵗʰ **S93.529** Sprain of metatarsophalangeal joint of unspecified toe(s)

N Newborn: 0   P Pediatric: 0-17   M Maternity: 12-55   A Adult: 15-124   CH Comorbidity High   CL Comorbidity Low   NCDx Noncancer Dx   PDx Primary Dx

1060   ICD-10-CM 2020

☑5ᵗʰ **S93.6 Sprain of** foot

> EXCLUDES 2   *sprain of metatarsophalangeal joint of toe (S93.52-)*
> *sprain of toe (S93.5-)*

    ☑6ᵗʰ **S93.60 Unspecified sprain of foot**
- ☑7ᵗʰ **S93.601** Unspecified sprain of right foot
- ☑7ᵗʰ **S93.602** Unspecified sprain of left foot
- ☑7ᵗʰ **S93.609** Unspecified sprain of unspecified foot

    ☑6ᵗʰ **S93.61 Sprain of** tarsal ligament **of foot**
- ☑7ᵗʰ **S93.611** Sprain of tarsal ligament of right foot
- ☑7ᵗʰ **S93.612** Sprain of tarsal ligament of left foot
- ☑7ᵗʰ **S93.619** Sprain of tarsal ligament of unspecified foot

    ☑6ᵗʰ **S93.62 Sprain of** tarsometatarsal ligament **of foot**
- ☑7ᵗʰ **S93.621** Sprain of tarsometatarsal ligament of right foot
- ☑7ᵗʰ **S93.622** Sprain of tarsometatarsal ligament of left foot
- ☑7ᵗʰ **S93.629** Sprain of tarsometatarsal ligament of unspecified foot

    ☑6ᵗʰ **S93.69 Other sprain of foot**
- ☑7ᵗʰ **S93.691** Other sprain of right foot .
- ☑7ᵗʰ **S93.692** Other sprain of left foot
- ☑7ᵗʰ **S93.699** Other sprain of unspecified foot

☑4ᵗʰ **S94 Injury of nerves at ankle and foot level**

Code also any associated open wound (S91.-)

> The appropriate 7th character is to be added to each code from category S94.
> A   initial encounter
> D   subsequent encounter
> S   sequela

    ☑5ᵗʰ **S94.0 Injury of** lateral plantar **nerve**
- ☑ₓ7ᵗʰ **S94.00** Injury of lateral plantar nerve, unspecified leg
- ☑ₓ7ᵗʰ **S94.01** Injury of lateral plantar nerve, right leg
- ☑ₓ7ᵗʰ **S94.02** Injury of lateral plantar nerve, left leg

    ☑5ᵗʰ **S94.1 Injury of** medial plantar **nerve**
- ☑ₓ7ᵗʰ **S94.10** Injury of medial plantar nerve, unspecified leg
- ☑ₓ7ᵗʰ **S94.11** Injury of medial plantar nerve, right leg
- ☑ₓ7ᵗʰ **S94.12** Injury of medial plantar nerve, left leg

    ☑5ᵗʰ **S94.2 Injury of** deep peroneal **nerve at ankle and foot level**

Injury of terminal, lateral branch of deep peroneal nerve
- ☑ₓ7ᵗʰ **S94.20** Injury of deep peroneal nerve at ankle and foot level, unspecified leg
- ☑ₓ7ᵗʰ **S94.21** Injury of deep peroneal nerve at ankle and foot level, right leg
- ☑ₓ7ᵗʰ **S94.22** Injury of deep peroneal nerve at ankle and foot level, left leg

    ☑5ᵗʰ **S94.3 Injury of** cutaneous sensory **nerve at ankle and foot level**
- ☑ₓ7ᵗʰ **S94.30** Injury of cutaneous sensory nerve at ankle and foot level, unspecified leg
- ☑ₓ7ᵗʰ **S94.31** Injury of cutaneous sensory nerve at ankle and foot level, right leg
- ☑ₓ7ᵗʰ **S94.32** Injury of cutaneous sensory nerve at ankle and foot level, left leg

    ☑5ᵗʰ **S94.8 Injury of other nerves at ankle and foot level**
- ☑6ᵗʰ **S94.8X** Injury of other nerves at ankle and foot level
  - ☑7ᵗʰ **S94.8X1** Injury of other nerves at ankle and foot level, right leg
  - ☑7ᵗʰ **S94.8X2** Injury of other nerves at ankle and foot level, left leg
  - ☑7ᵗʰ **S94.8X9** Injury of other nerves at ankle and foot level, unspecified leg

    ☑5ᵗʰ **S94.9 Injury of unspecified nerve at ankle and foot level**
- ☑ₓ7ᵗʰ **S94.90** Injury of unspecified nerve at ankle and foot level, unspecified leg
- ☑ₓ7ᵗʰ **S94.91** Injury of unspecified nerve at ankle and foot level, right leg
- ☑ₓ7ᵗʰ **S94.92** Injury of unspecified nerve at ankle and foot level, left leg

☑4ᵗʰ **S95 Injury of blood vessels at ankle and foot level**

Code also any associated open wound (S91.-)

> EXCLUDES 2   *injury of posterior tibial artery and vein (S85.1-, S85.8-)*

> The appropriate 7th character is to be added to each code from category S95.
> A   initial encounter
> D   subsequent encounter
> S   sequela

    ☑5ᵗʰ **S95.0 Injury of** dorsal artery **of foot**
- ☑6ᵗʰ **S95.00** Unspecified injury of dorsal artery of foot
  - ☑7ᵗʰ **S95.001** Unspecified injury of dorsal artery of right foot
  - ☑7ᵗʰ **S95.002** Unspecified injury of dorsal artery of left foot
  - ☑7ᵗʰ **S95.009** Unspecified injury of dorsal artery of unspecified foot
- ☑6ᵗʰ **S95.01** Laceration **of dorsal artery of foot**
  - ☑7ᵗʰ **S95.011** Laceration of dorsal artery of right foot
  - ☑7ᵗʰ **S95.012** Laceration of dorsal artery of left foot
  - ☑7ᵗʰ **S95.019** Laceration of dorsal artery of unspecified foot
- ☑6ᵗʰ **S95.09** Other specified injury of dorsal artery of foot
  - ☑7ᵗʰ **S95.091** Other specified injury of dorsal artery of right foot
  - ☑7ᵗʰ **S95.092** Other specified injury of dorsal artery of left foot
  - ☑7ᵗʰ **S95.099** Other specified injury of dorsal artery of unspecified foot

    ☑5ᵗʰ **S95.1 Injury of** plantar artery **of foot**
- ☑6ᵗʰ **S95.10** Unspecified injury of plantar artery of foot
  - ☑7ᵗʰ **S95.101** Unspecified injury of plantar artery of right foot
  - ☑7ᵗʰ **S95.102** Unspecified injury of plantar artery of left foot
  - ☑7ᵗʰ **S95.109** Unspecified injury of plantar artery of unspecified foot
- ☑6ᵗʰ **S95.11** Laceration **of plantar artery of foot**
  - ☑7ᵗʰ **S95.111** Laceration of plantar artery of right foot
  - ☑7ᵗʰ **S95.112** Laceration of plantar artery of left foot
  - ☑7ᵗʰ **S95.119** Laceration of plantar artery of unspecified foot
- ☑6ᵗʰ **S95.19** Other specified injury of plantar artery of foot
  - ☑7ᵗʰ **S95.191** Other specified injury of plantar artery of right foot
  - ☑7ᵗʰ **S95.192** Other specified injury of plantar artery of left foot
  - ☑7ᵗʰ **S95.199** Other specified injury of plantar artery of unspecified foot

    ☑5ᵗʰ **S95.2 Injury of** dorsal vein **of foot**
- ☑6ᵗʰ **S95.20** Unspecified injury of dorsal vein of foot
  - ☑7ᵗʰ **S95.201** Unspecified injury of dorsal vein of right foot
  - ☑7ᵗʰ **S95.202** Unspecified injury of dorsal vein of left foot
  - ☑7ᵗʰ **S95.209** Unspecified injury of dorsal vein of unspecified foot
- ☑6ᵗʰ **S95.21** Laceration **of dorsal vein of foot**
  - ☑7ᵗʰ **S95.211** Laceration of dorsal vein of right foot
  - ☑7ᵗʰ **S95.212** Laceration of dorsal vein of left foot
  - ☑7ᵗʰ **S95.219** Laceration of dorsal vein of unspecified foot
- ☑6ᵗʰ **S95.29** Other specified injury of dorsal vein of foot
  - ☑7ᵗʰ **S95.291** Other specified injury of dorsal vein of right foot
  - ☑7ᵗʰ **S95.292** Other specified injury of dorsal vein of left foot
  - ☑7ᵗʰ **S95.299** Other specified injury of dorsal vein of unspecified foot

    ☑5ᵗʰ **S95.8 Injury of other blood vessels at ankle and foot level**
- ☑6ᵗʰ **S95.80** Unspecified injury of other blood vessels at ankle and foot level
  - ☑7ᵗʰ **S95.801** Unspecified injury of other blood vessels at ankle and foot level, right leg
  - ☑7ᵗʰ **S95.802** Unspecified injury of other blood vessels at ankle and foot level, left leg
  - ☑7ᵗʰ **S95.809** Unspecified injury of other blood vessels at ankle and foot level, unspecified leg

---

☑ Additional Character Required   ☑ₓ7ᵗʰ Placeholder Alert   Manifestation   Unspecified Dx   ▶◀ Revised Text   ● New Code   ▲ Revised Title

√6ᵗʰ **S95.81** Laceration of other blood vessels at ankle and foot level

    √7ᵗʰ **S95.811** Laceration of other blood vessels at ankle and foot level, right leg

    √7ᵗʰ **S95.812** Laceration of other blood vessels at ankle and foot level, left leg

    √7ᵗʰ **S95.819** Laceration of other blood vessels at ankle and foot level, unspecified leg

√6ᵗʰ **S95.89** Other specified injury of other blood vessels at ankle and foot level

    √7ᵗʰ **S95.891** Other specified injury of other blood vessels at ankle and foot level, right leg

    √7ᵗʰ **S95.892** Other specified injury of other blood vessels at ankle and foot level, left leg

    √7ᵗʰ **S95.899** Other specified injury of other blood vessels at ankle and foot level, unspecified leg

√5ᵗʰ **S95.9** Injury of unspecified blood vessel at ankle and foot level

√6ᵗʰ **S95.90** Unspecified injury of unspecified blood vessel at ankle and foot level

    √7ᵗʰ **S95.901** Unspecified injury of unspecified blood vessel at ankle and foot level, right leg

    √7ᵗʰ **S95.902** Unspecified injury of unspecified blood vessel at ankle and foot level, left leg

    √7ᵗʰ **S95.909** Unspecified injury of unspecified blood vessel at ankle and foot level, unspecified leg

√6ᵗʰ **S95.91** Laceration of unspecified blood vessel at ankle and foot level

    √7ᵗʰ **S95.911** Laceration of unspecified blood vessel at ankle and foot level, right leg

    √7ᵗʰ **S95.912** Laceration of unspecified blood vessel at ankle and foot level, left leg

    √7ᵗʰ **S95.919** Laceration of unspecified blood vessel at ankle and foot level, unspecified leg

√6ᵗʰ **S95.99** Other specified injury of unspecified blood vessel at ankle and foot level

    √7ᵗʰ **S95.991** Other specified injury of unspecified blood vessel at ankle and foot level, right leg

    √7ᵗʰ **S95.992** Other specified injury of unspecified blood vessel at ankle and foot level, left leg

    √7ᵗʰ **S95.999** Other specified injury of unspecified blood vessel at ankle and foot level, unspecified leg

√4ᵗʰ **S96 Injury of muscle and tendon at ankle and foot level**

    Code also any associated open wound (S91.-)

    EXCLUDES 2   injury of Achilles tendon (S86.0-)

          sprain of joints and ligaments of ankle and foot (S93.-)

    TIP: Refer to the Muscle/Tendon table at the beginning of this chapter.

    The appropriate 7th character is to be added to each code from category S96.
    A   initial encounter
    D   subsequent encounter
    S   sequela

√5ᵗʰ **S96.0** Injury of muscle and tendon of long flexor muscle of toe at ankle and foot level

√6ᵗʰ **S96.00** Unspecified injury of muscle and tendon of long flexor muscle of toe at ankle and foot level

    √7ᵗʰ **S96.001** Unspecified injury of muscle and tendon of long flexor muscle of toe at ankle and foot level, right foot

    √7ᵗʰ **S96.002** Unspecified injury of muscle and tendon of long flexor muscle of toe at ankle and foot level, left foot

    √7ᵗʰ **S96.009** Unspecified injury of muscle and tendon of long flexor muscle of toe at ankle and foot level, unspecified foot

√6ᵗʰ **S96.01** Strain of muscle and tendon of long flexor muscle of toe at ankle and foot level

    √7ᵗʰ **S96.011** Strain of muscle and tendon of long flexor muscle of toe at ankle and foot level, right foot

    √7ᵗʰ **S96.012** Strain of muscle and tendon of long flexor muscle of toe at ankle and foot level, left foot

    √7ᵗʰ **S96.019** Strain of muscle and tendon of long flexor muscle of toe at ankle and foot level, unspecified foot

√6ᵗʰ **S96.02** Laceration of muscle and tendon of long flexor muscle of toe at ankle and foot level

    √7ᵗʰ **S96.021** Laceration of muscle and tendon of long flexor muscle of toe at ankle and foot level, right foot

    √7ᵗʰ **S96.022** Laceration of muscle and tendon of long flexor muscle of toe at ankle and foot level, left foot

    √7ᵗʰ **S96.029** Laceration of muscle and tendon of long flexor muscle of toe at ankle and foot level, unspecified foot

√6ᵗʰ **S96.09** Other injury of muscle and tendon of long flexor muscle of toe at ankle and foot level

    √7ᵗʰ **S96.091** Other injury of muscle and tendon of long flexor muscle of toe at ankle and foot level, right foot

    √7ᵗʰ **S96.092** Other injury of muscle and tendon of long flexor muscle of toe at ankle and foot level, left foot

    √7ᵗʰ **S96.099** Other injury of muscle and tendon of long flexor muscle of toe at ankle and foot level, unspecified foot

√5ᵗʰ **S96.1** Injury of muscle and tendon of long extensor muscle of toe at ankle and foot level

√6ᵗʰ **S96.10** Unspecified injury of muscle and tendon of long extensor muscle of toe at ankle and foot level

    √7ᵗʰ **S96.101** Unspecified injury of muscle and tendon of long extensor muscle of toe at ankle and foot level, right foot

    √7ᵗʰ **S96.102** Unspecified injury of muscle and tendon of long extensor muscle of toe at ankle and foot level, left foot

    √7ᵗʰ **S96.109** Unspecified injury of muscle and tendon of long extensor muscle of toe at ankle and foot level, unspecified foot

√6ᵗʰ **S96.11** Strain of muscle and tendon of long extensor muscle of toe at ankle and foot level

    √7ᵗʰ **S96.111** Strain of muscle and tendon of long extensor muscle of toe at ankle and foot level, right foot

    √7ᵗʰ **S96.112** Strain of muscle and tendon of long extensor muscle of toe at ankle and foot level, left foot

    √7ᵗʰ **S96.119** Strain of muscle and tendon of long extensor muscle of toe at ankle and foot level, unspecified foot

√6ᵗʰ **S96.12** Laceration of muscle and tendon of long extensor muscle of toe at ankle and foot level

    √7ᵗʰ **S96.121** Laceration of muscle and tendon of long extensor muscle of toe at ankle and foot level, right foot

    √7ᵗʰ **S96.122** Laceration of muscle and tendon of long extensor muscle of toe at ankle and foot level, left foot

    √7ᵗʰ **S96.129** Laceration of muscle and tendon of long extensor muscle of toe at ankle and foot level, unspecified foot

√6ᵗʰ **S96.19** Other specified injury of muscle and tendon of long extensor muscle of toe at ankle and foot level

    √7ᵗʰ **S96.191** Other specified injury of muscle and tendon of long extensor muscle of toe at ankle and foot level, right foot

    √7ᵗʰ **S96.192** Other specified injury of muscle and tendon of long extensor muscle of toe at ankle and foot level, left foot

    √7ᵗʰ **S96.199** Other specified injury of muscle and tendon of long extensor muscle of toe at ankle and foot level, unspecified foot

√5ᵗʰ **S96.2** Injury of intrinsic muscle and tendon at ankle and foot level

√6ᵗʰ **S96.20** Unspecified injury of intrinsic muscle and tendon at ankle and foot level

    √7ᵗʰ **S96.201** Unspecified injury of intrinsic muscle and tendon at ankle and foot level, right foot

    √7ᵗʰ **S96.202** Unspecified injury of intrinsic muscle and tendon at ankle and foot level, left foot

    √7ᵗʰ **S96.209** Unspecified injury of intrinsic muscle and tendon at ankle and foot level, unspecified foot

√6ᵗʰ **S96.21** Strain of intrinsic muscle and tendon at ankle and foot level

    √7ᵗʰ **S96.211** Strain of intrinsic muscle and tendon at ankle and foot level, right foot

    √7ᵗʰ **S96.212** Strain of intrinsic muscle and tendon at ankle and foot level, left foot

N Newborn: 0   P Pediatric: 0-17   M Maternity: 12-55   A Adult: 15-124   CH Comorbidity High   CL Comorbidity Low   NCDx Noncancer Dx   PDx Primary Dx

1062   ICD-10-CM 2020

√7ᵗʰ **S96.219** Strain of intrinsic muscle and tendon at ankle and foot level, unspecified foot

√6ᵗʰ **S96.22** Laceration of intrinsic muscle and tendon at ankle and foot level

    √7ᵗʰ **S96.221** Laceration of intrinsic muscle and tendon at ankle and foot level, right foot

    √7ᵗʰ **S96.222** Laceration of intrinsic muscle and tendon at ankle and foot level, left foot

    √7ᵗʰ **S96.229** Laceration of intrinsic muscle and tendon at ankle and foot level, unspecified foot

√6ᵗʰ **S96.29** Other specified injury of intrinsic muscle and tendon at ankle and foot level

    √7ᵗʰ **S96.291** Other specified injury of intrinsic muscle and tendon at ankle and foot level, right foot

    √7ᵗʰ **S96.292** Other specified injury of intrinsic muscle and tendon at ankle and foot level, left foot

    √7ᵗʰ **S96.299** Other specified injury of intrinsic muscle and tendon at ankle and foot level, unspecified foot

√5ᵗʰ **S96.8** Injury of other specified muscles and tendons at ankle and foot level

√6ᵗʰ **S96.80** Unspecified injury of other specified muscles and tendons at ankle and foot level

    √7ᵗʰ **S96.801** Unspecified injury of other specified muscles and tendons at ankle and foot level, right foot

    √7ᵗʰ **S96.802** Unspecified injury of other specified muscles and tendons at ankle and foot level, left foot

    √7ᵗʰ **S96.809** Unspecified injury of other specified muscles and tendons at ankle and foot level, unspecified foot

√6ᵗʰ **S96.81** Strain of other specified muscles and tendons at ankle and foot level

    √7ᵗʰ **S96.811** Strain of other specified muscles and tendons at ankle and foot level, right foot

    √7ᵗʰ **S96.812** Strain of other specified muscles and tendons at ankle and foot level, left foot

    √7ᵗʰ **S96.819** Strain of other specified muscles and tendons at ankle and foot level, unspecified foot

√6ᵗʰ **S96.82** Laceration of other specified muscles and tendons at ankle and foot level

    √7ᵗʰ **S96.821** Laceration of other specified muscles and tendons at ankle and foot level, right foot

    √7ᵗʰ **S96.822** Laceration of other specified muscles and tendons at ankle and foot level, left foot

    √7ᵗʰ **S96.829** Laceration of other specified muscles and tendons at ankle and foot level, unspecified foot

√6ᵗʰ **S96.89** Other specified injury of other specified muscles and tendons at ankle and foot level

    √7ᵗʰ **S96.891** Other specified injury of other specified muscles and tendons at ankle and foot level, right foot

    √7ᵗʰ **S96.892** Other specified injury of other specified muscles and tendons at ankle and foot level, left foot

    √7ᵗʰ **S96.899** Other specified injury of other specified muscles and tendons at ankle and foot level, unspecified foot

√5ᵗʰ **S96.9** Injury of unspecified muscle and tendon at ankle and foot level

√6ᵗʰ **S96.90** Unspecified injury of unspecified muscle and tendon at ankle and foot level

    √7ᵗʰ **S96.901** Unspecified injury of unspecified muscle and tendon at ankle and foot level, right foot

    √7ᵗʰ **S96.902** Unspecified injury of unspecified muscle and tendon at ankle and foot level, left foot

    √7ᵗʰ **S96.909** Unspecified injury of unspecified muscle and tendon at ankle and foot level, unspecified foot

√6ᵗʰ **S96.91** Strain of unspecified muscle and tendon at ankle and foot level

    √7ᵗʰ **S96.911** Strain of unspecified muscle and tendon at ankle and foot level, right foot

    √7ᵗʰ **S96.912** Strain of unspecified muscle and tendon at ankle and foot level, left foot

    √7ᵗʰ **S96.919** Strain of unspecified muscle and tendon at ankle and foot level, unspecified foot

√6ᵗʰ **S96.92** Laceration of unspecified muscle and tendon at ankle and foot level

    √7ᵗʰ **S96.921** Laceration of unspecified muscle and tendon at ankle and foot level, right foot

    √7ᵗʰ **S96.922** Laceration of unspecified muscle and tendon at ankle and foot level, left foot

    √7ᵗʰ **S96.929** Laceration of unspecified muscle and tendon at ankle and foot level, unspecified foot

√6ᵗʰ **S96.99** Other specified injury of unspecified muscle and tendon at ankle and foot level

    √7ᵗʰ **S96.991** Other specified injury of unspecified muscle and tendon at ankle and foot level, right foot

    √7ᵗʰ **S96.992** Other specified injury of unspecified muscle and tendon at ankle and foot level, left foot

    √7ᵗʰ **S96.999** Other specified injury of unspecified muscle and tendon at ankle and foot level, unspecified foot

√4ᵗʰ **S97** Crushing injury of ankle and foot

Use additional code(s) for all associated injuries

> The appropriate 7th character is to be added to each code from category S97.
> A   initial encounter
> D   subsequent encounter
> S   sequela

√5ᵗʰ **S97.0** Crushing injury of ankle

    √x7ᵗʰ **S97.00** Crushing injury of unspecified ankle

    √x7ᵗʰ **S97.01** Crushing injury of right ankle

    √x7ᵗʰ **S97.02** Crushing injury of left ankle

√5ᵗʰ **S97.1** Crushing injury of toe

√6ᵗʰ **S97.10** Crushing injury of unspecified toe(s)

    √7ᵗʰ **S97.101** Crushing injury of unspecified right toe(s)

    √7ᵗʰ **S97.102** Crushing injury of unspecified left toe(s)

    √7ᵗʰ **S97.109** Crushing injury of unspecified toe(s)

      Crushing injury of toe NOS

√6ᵗʰ **S97.11** Crushing injury of great toe

    √7ᵗʰ **S97.111** Crushing injury of right great toe

    √7ᵗʰ **S97.112** Crushing injury of left great toe

    √7ᵗʰ **S97.119** Crushing injury of unspecified great toe

√6ᵗʰ **S97.12** Crushing injury of lesser toe(s)

    √7ᵗʰ **S97.121** Crushing injury of right lesser toe(s)

    √7ᵗʰ **S97.122** Crushing injury of left lesser toe(s)

    √7ᵗʰ **S97.129** Crushing injury of unspecified lesser toe(s)

√5ᵗʰ **S97.8** Crushing injury of foot

    √x7ᵗʰ **S97.80** Crushing injury of unspecified foot

      Crushing injury of foot NOS

    √x7ᵗʰ **S97.81** Crushing injury of right foot

    √x7ᵗʰ **S97.82** Crushing injury of left foot

√4ᵗʰ **S98** Traumatic amputation of ankle and foot

An amputation not identified as partial or complete should be coded to complete

> The appropriate 7th character is to be added to each code from category S98.
> A   initial encounter
> D   subsequent encounter
> S   sequela

√5ᵗʰ **S98.0** Traumatic amputation of foot at ankle level

√6ᵗʰ **S98.01** Complete traumatic amputation of foot at ankle level

    √7ᵗʰ **S98.011** Complete traumatic amputation of right foot at ankle level

    √7ᵗʰ **S98.012** Complete traumatic amputation of left foot at ankle level

    √7ᵗʰ **S98.019** Complete traumatic amputation of unspecified foot at ankle level

√6ᵗʰ **S98.02** Partial traumatic amputation of foot at ankle level

    √7ᵗʰ **S98.021** Partial traumatic amputation of right foot at ankle level

    √7ᵗʰ **S98.022** Partial traumatic amputation of left foot at ankle level

---

☑ Additional Character Required   √x7ᵗʰ Placeholder Alert   Manifestation   Unspecified Dx   ►◄ Revised Text   ● New Code   ▲ Revised Title

Chapter 19. Injury, Poisoning and Certain Other Consequences of External Causes

√7ᵗ **S98.029** Partial traumatic amputation of unspecified foot at ankle level

√5ᵗ **S98.1** Traumatic amputation of one toe

√6ᵗ **S98.11** Complete traumatic amputation of great toe

√7ᵗ **S98.111** Complete traumatic amputation of right great toe

√7ᵗ **S98.112** Complete traumatic amputation of left great toe

√7ᵗ **S98.119** Complete traumatic amputation of unspecified great toe

√6ᵗ **S98.12** Partial traumatic amputation of great toe

√7ᵗ **S98.121** Partial traumatic amputation of right great toe

√7ᵗ **S98.122** Partial traumatic amputation of left great toe

√7ᵗ **S98.129** Partial traumatic amputation of unspecified great toe

√6ᵗ **S98.13** Complete traumatic amputation of one lesser toe

Traumatic amputation of toe NOS

√7ᵗ **S98.131** Complete traumatic amputation of one right lesser toe

√7ᵗ **S98.132** Complete traumatic amputation of one left lesser toe

√7ᵗ **S98.139** Complete traumatic amputation of one unspecified lesser toe

√6ᵗ **S98.14** Partial traumatic amputation of one lesser toe

√7ᵗ **S98.141** Partial traumatic amputation of one right lesser toe

√7ᵗ **S98.142** Partial traumatic amputation of one left lesser toe

√7ᵗ **S98.149** Partial traumatic amputation of one unspecified lesser toe

√5ᵗ **S98.2** Traumatic amputation of two or more lesser toes

√6ᵗ **S98.21** Complete traumatic amputation of two or more lesser toes

√7ᵗ **S98.211** Complete traumatic amputation of two or more right lesser toes

√7ᵗ **S98.212** Complete traumatic amputation of two or more left lesser toes

√7ᵗ **S98.219** Complete traumatic amputation of two or more unspecified lesser toes

√6ᵗ **S98.22** Partial traumatic amputation of two or more lesser toes

√7ᵗ **S98.221** Partial traumatic amputation of two or more right lesser toes

√7ᵗ **S98.222** Partial traumatic amputation of two or more left lesser toes

√7ᵗ **S98.229** Partial traumatic amputation of two or more unspecified lesser toes

√5ᵗ **S98.3** Traumatic amputation of midfoot

√6ᵗ **S98.31** Complete traumatic amputation of midfoot

√7ᵗ **S98.311** Complete traumatic amputation of right midfoot

√7ᵗ **S98.312** Complete traumatic amputation of left midfoot

√7ᵗ **S98.319** Complete traumatic amputation of unspecified midfoot

√6ᵗ **S98.32** Partial traumatic amputation of midfoot

√7ᵗ **S98.321** Partial traumatic amputation of right midfoot

√7ᵗ **S98.322** Partial traumatic amputation of left midfoot

√7ᵗ **S98.329** Partial traumatic amputation of unspecified midfoot

√5ᵗ **S98.9** Traumatic amputation of foot, level unspecified

√6ᵗ **S98.91** Complete traumatic amputation of foot, level unspecified

√7ᵗ **S98.911** Complete traumatic amputation of right foot, level unspecified

√7ᵗ **S98.912** Complete traumatic amputation of left foot, level unspecified

√7ᵗ **S98.919** Complete traumatic amputation of unspecified foot, level unspecified

√6ᵗ **S98.92** Partial traumatic amputation of foot, level unspecified

√7ᵗ **S98.921** Partial traumatic amputation of right foot, level unspecified

√7ᵗ **S98.922** Partial traumatic amputation of left foot, level unspecified

√7ᵗ **S98.929** Partial traumatic amputation of unspecified foot, level unspecified

√4ᵗ **S99** Other and unspecified injuries of ankle and foot

AHA: 2018,2Q,12; 2018,1Q,3; 2016,4Q,68-69

TIP: The term "improper alignment" is not synonymous with malunion or nonunion of a fracture when noted in provider documentation.

√5ᵗ **S99.0** Physeal fracture of calcaneus

The appropriate 7th character is to be added to each code from subcategory S99.0.
A   initial encounter for closed fracture
B   initial encounter for open fracture
D   subsequent encounter for fracture with routine healing
G   subsequent encounter for fracture with delayed healing
K   subsequent encounter for fracture with nonunion
P   subsequent encounter for fracture with malunion
S   sequela

√6ᵗ **S99.00** Unspecified physeal fracture of calcaneus

√7ᵗ **S99.001** Unspecified physeal fracture of right calcaneus

√7ᵗ **S99.002** Unspecified physeal fracture of left calcaneus

√7ᵗ **S99.009** Unspecified physeal fracture of unspecified calcaneus

√6ᵗ **S99.01** Salter-Harris Type I physeal fracture of calcaneus

√7ᵗ **S99.011** Salter-Harris Type I physeal fracture of right calcaneus

√7ᵗ **S99.012** Salter-Harris Type I physeal fracture of left calcaneus

√7ᵗ **S99.019** Salter-Harris Type I physeal fracture of unspecified calcaneus

√6ᵗ **S99.02** Salter-Harris Type II physeal fracture of calcaneus

√7ᵗ **S99.021** Salter-Harris Type II physeal fracture of right calcaneus

√7ᵗ **S99.022** Salter-Harris Type II physeal fracture of left calcaneus

√7ᵗ **S99.029** Salter-Harris Type II physeal fracture of unspecified calcaneus

√6ᵗ **S99.03** Salter-Harris Type III physeal fracture of calcaneus

√7ᵗ **S99.031** Salter-Harris Type III physeal fracture of right calcaneus

√7ᵗ **S99.032** Salter-Harris Type III physeal fracture of left calcaneus

√7ᵗ **S99.039** Salter-Harris Type III physeal fracture of unspecified calcaneus

√6ᵗ **S99.04** Salter-Harris Type IV physeal fracture of calcaneus

√7ᵗ **S99.041** Salter-Harris Type IV physeal fracture of right calcaneus

√7ᵗ **S99.042** Salter-Harris Type IV physeal fracture of left calcaneus

√7ᵗ **S99.049** Salter-Harris Type IV physeal fracture of unspecified calcaneus

√6ᵗ **S99.09** Other physeal fracture of calcaneus

√7ᵗ **S99.091** Other physeal fracture of right calcaneus

√7ᵗ **S99.092** Other physeal fracture of left calcaneus

√7ᵗ **S99.099** Other physeal fracture of unspecified calcaneus

√5ᵗ **S99.1** Physeal fracture of metatarsal

The appropriate 7th character is to be added to each code from subcategory S99.1
A   initial encounter for closed fracture
B   initial encounter for open fracture
D   subsequent encounter for fracture with routine healing
G   subsequent encounter for fracture with delayed healing
K   subsequent encounter for fracture with nonunion
P   subsequent encounter for fracture with malunion
S   sequela

√6ᵗ **S99.10** Unspecified physeal fracture of metatarsal

√7ᵗ **S99.101** Unspecified physeal fracture of right metatarsal

√7ᵗ **S99.102** Unspecified physeal fracture of left metatarsal

√7ᵗ **S99.109** Unspecified physeal fracture of unspecified metatarsal

√6ᵗ **S99.11** Salter-Harris Type I physeal fracture of metatarsal

√7ᵗ **S99.111** Salter-Harris Type I physeal fracture of right metatarsal

Ⓝ Newborn: 0   Ⓟ Pediatric: 0-17   Ⓜ Maternity: 12-55   Ⓐ Adult: 15-124   CH Comorbidity High   CL Comorbidity Low   NCDx Noncancer Dx   PDx Primary Dx

1064   ICD-10-CM 2020

☑7ᵗʰ **S99.112** Salter-Harris Type I physeal fracture of left metatarsal

☑7ᵗʰ **S99.119** Salter-Harris Type I physeal fracture of unspecified metatarsal

☑6ᵗʰ **S99.12** Salter-Harris Type II physeal fracture of metatarsal

☑7ᵗʰ **S99.121** Salter-Harris Type II physeal fracture of right metatarsal

☑7ᵗʰ **S99.122** Salter-Harris Type II physeal fracture of left metatarsal

☑7ᵗʰ **S99.129** Salter-Harris Type II physeal fracture of unspecified metatarsal

☑6ᵗʰ **S99.13** Salter-Harris Type III physeal fracture of metatarsal

☑7ᵗʰ **S99.131** Salter-Harris Type III physeal fracture of right metatarsal

☑7ᵗʰ **S99.132** Salter-Harris Type III physeal fracture of left metatarsal

☑7ᵗʰ **S99.139** Salter-Harris Type III physeal fracture of unspecified metatarsal

☑6ᵗʰ **S99.14** Salter-Harris Type IV physeal fracture of metatarsal

☑7ᵗʰ **S99.141** Salter-Harris Type IV physeal fracture of right metatarsal

☑7ᵗʰ **S99.142** Salter-Harris Type IV physeal fracture of left metatarsal

☑7ᵗʰ **S99.149** Salter-Harris Type IV physeal fracture of unspecified metatarsal

☑6ᵗʰ **S99.19** Other physeal fracture of metatarsal

☑7ᵗʰ **S99.191** Other physeal fracture of right metatarsal

☑7ᵗʰ **S99.192** Other physeal fracture of left metatarsal

☑7ᵗʰ **S99.199** Other physeal fracture of unspecified metatarsal

☑5ᵗʰ **S99.2** Physeal fracture of phalanx of toe

> The appropriate 7th character is to be added to each code from subcategories S99.2.
> A   initial encounter for closed fracture
> B   initial encounter for open fracture
> D   subsequent encounter for fracture with routine healing
> G   subsequent encounter for fracture with delayed healing
> K   subsequent encounter for fracture with nonunion
> P   subsequent encounter for fracture with malunion
> S   sequela

☑6ᵗʰ **S99.20** Unspecified physeal fracture of phalanx of toe

☑7ᵗʰ **S99.201** Unspecified physeal fracture of phalanx of right toe

☑7ᵗʰ **S99.202** Unspecified physeal fracture of phalanx of left toe

☑7ᵗʰ **S99.209** Unspecified physeal fracture of phalanx of unspecified toe

☑6ᵗʰ **S99.21** Salter-Harris Type I physeal fracture of phalanx of toe

☑7ᵗʰ **S99.211** Salter-Harris Type I physeal fracture of phalanx of right toe

☑7ᵗʰ **S99.212** Salter-Harris Type I physeal fracture of phalanx of left toe

☑7ᵗʰ **S99.219** Salter-Harris Type I physeal fracture of phalanx of unspecified toe

☑6ᵗʰ **S99.22** Salter-Harris Type II physeal fracture of phalanx of toe

☑7ᵗʰ **S99.221** Salter-Harris Type II physeal fracture of phalanx of right toe

☑7ᵗʰ **S99.222** Salter-Harris Type II physeal fracture of phalanx of left toe

☑7ᵗʰ **S99.229** Salter-Harris Type II physeal fracture of phalanx of unspecified toe

☑6ᵗʰ **S99.23** Salter-Harris Type III physeal fracture of phalanx of toe

☑7ᵗʰ **S99.231** Salter-Harris Type III physeal fracture of phalanx of right toe

☑7ᵗʰ **S99.232** Salter-Harris Type III physeal fracture of phalanx of left toe

☑7ᵗʰ **S99.239** Salter-Harris Type III physeal fracture of phalanx of unspecified toe

☑6ᵗʰ **S99.24** Salter-Harris Type IV physeal fracture of phalanx of toe

☑7ᵗʰ **S99.241** Salter-Harris Type IV physeal fracture of phalanx of right toe

☑7ᵗʰ **S99.242** Salter-Harris Type IV physeal fracture of phalanx of left toe

☑7ᵗʰ **S99.249** Salter-Harris Type IV physeal fracture of phalanx of unspecified toe

☑6ᵗʰ **S99.29** Other physeal fracture of phalanx of toe

☑7ᵗʰ **S99.291** Other physeal fracture of phalanx of right toe

☑7ᵗʰ **S99.292** Other physeal fracture of phalanx of left toe

☑7ᵗʰ **S99.299** Other physeal fracture of phalanx of unspecified toe

☑5ᵗʰ **S99.8** Other specified injuries of ankle and foot

> The appropriate 7th character is to be added to each code from subcategory S99.8.
> A   initial encounter
> D   subsequent encounter
> S   sequela

☑6ᵗʰ **S99.81** Other specified injuries of ankle

☑7ᵗʰ **S99.811** Other specified injuries of right ankle

☑7ᵗʰ **S99.812** Other specified injuries of left ankle

☑7ᵗʰ **S99.819** Other specified injuries of unspecified ankle

☑6ᵗʰ **S99.82** Other specified injuries of foot

☑7ᵗʰ **S99.821** Other specified injuries of right foot

☑7ᵗʰ **S99.822** Other specified injuries of left foot

☑7ᵗʰ **S99.829** Other specified injuries of unspecified foot

☑5ᵗʰ **S99.9** Unspecified injury of ankle and foot

> The appropriate 7th character is to be added to each code from subcategory S99.9.
> A   initial encounter
> D   subsequent encounter
> S   sequela

☑6ᵗʰ **S99.91** Unspecified injury of ankle

☑7ᵗʰ **S99.911** Unspecified injury of right ankle

☑7ᵗʰ **S99.912** Unspecified injury of left ankle

☑7ᵗʰ **S99.919** Unspecified injury of unspecified ankle

☑6ᵗʰ **S99.92** Unspecified injury of foot

☑7ᵗʰ **S99.921** Unspecified injury of right foot

☑7ᵗʰ **S99.922** Unspecified injury of left foot

☑7ᵗʰ **S99.929** Unspecified injury of unspecified foot

INJURY, POISONING AND CERTAIN OTHER CONSEQUENCES OF EXTERNAL CAUSES (T07-T88)

Injuries involving multiple body regions (T07)

> **EXCLUDES 1**   burns and corrosions (T20-T32)
> frostbite (T33-T34)
> insect bite or sting, venomous (T63.4)
> sunburn (L55.-)

☑x7ᵗʰ **T07** **Unspecified multiple injuries**

> **EXCLUDES 1**   injury NOS (T14.90)

AHA: 2017,4Q,26

> The appropriate 7th character is to be added to code T07.
> A   initial encounter
> D   subsequent encounter
> S   sequela

Injury of unspecified body region (T14)

☑4ᵗʰ **T14** **Injury of unspecified body region**

> **EXCLUDES 1**   multiple unspecified injuries (T07)

AHA: 2017,4Q,26

> The appropriate 7th character is to be added to each code from category T14.
> A   initial encounter
> D   subsequent encounter
> S   sequela

☑x7ᵗʰ **T14.8** **Other injury of unspecified body region**

Abrasion NOS
Contusion NOS
Crush injury NOS
Fracture NOS
Skin injury NOS
Vascular injury NOS
Wound NOS

☑ Additional Character Required   ☑x7ᵗʰ Placeholder Alert   Manifestation   Unspecified Dx   ▶◀ Revised Text   ● New Code   ▲ Revised Title

ICD-10-CM 2020   **1065**

☑5ᵗʰ **T14.9 Unspecified injury**

    ☑x7ᵗʰ **T14.90 Injury, unspecified**

        Injury NOS

    ☑x7ᵗʰ **T14.91 Suicide attempt**

        Attempted suicide NOS

Effects of foreign body entering through natural orifice (T15-T19)

EXCLUDES 2   foreign body accidentally left in operation wound (T81.5-)
        foreign body in penetrating wound — see open wound by body region
        residual foreign body in soft tissue (M79.5)
        splinter, without open wound — see superficial injury by body region

☑4ᵗʰ **T15 Foreign body on external eye**

    EXCLUDES 2   foreign body in penetrating wound of orbit and eye ball (S05.4-, S05.5-)
        open wound of eyelid and periocular area (S01.1-)
        retained foreign body in eyelid (H02.8-)
        retained (old) foreign body in penetrating wound of orbit and eye ball (H05.5-, H44.6-, H44.7-)
        superficial foreign body of eyelid and periocular area (S00.25-)

> The appropriate 7th character is to be added to each code from category T15.
> A initial encounter
> D subsequent encounter
> S sequela

  ☑5ᵗʰ **T15.0 Foreign body in cornea**

    ☑x7ᵗʰ **T15.00 Foreign body in cornea, unspecified eye**

    ☑x7ᵗʰ **T15.01 Foreign body in cornea, right eye**

    ☑x7ᵗʰ **T15.02 Foreign body in cornea, left eye**

  ☑5ᵗʰ **T15.1 Foreign body in conjunctival sac**

    ☑x7ᵗʰ **T15.10 Foreign body in conjunctival sac, unspecified eye**

    ☑x7ᵗʰ **T15.11 Foreign body in conjunctival sac, right eye**

    ☑x7ᵗʰ **T15.12 Foreign body in conjunctival sac, left eye**

  ☑5ᵗʰ **T15.8 Foreign body in other and multiple parts of external eye**

    Foreign body in lacrimal punctum

    ☑x7ᵗʰ **T15.80 Foreign body in other and multiple parts of external eye, unspecified eye**

    ☑x7ᵗʰ **T15.81 Foreign body in other and multiple parts of external eye, right eye**

    ☑x7ᵗʰ **T15.82 Foreign body in other and multiple parts of external eye, left eye**

  ☑5ᵗʰ **T15.9 Foreign body on external eye, part unspecified**

    ☑x7ᵗʰ **T15.90 Foreign body on external eye, part unspecified, unspecified eye**

    ☑x7ᵗʰ **T15.91 Foreign body on external eye, part unspecified, right eye**

    ☑x7ᵗʰ **T15.92 Foreign body on external eye, part unspecified, left eye**

☑4ᵗʰ **T16 Foreign body in ear**

    INCLUDES   foreign body in auditory canal

> The appropriate 7th character is to be added to each code from category T16.
> A initial encounter
> D subsequent encounter
> S sequela

  ☑x7ᵗʰ **T16.1 Foreign body in right ear**

  ☑x7ᵗʰ **T16.2 Foreign body in left ear**

  ☑x7ᵗʰ **T16.9 Foreign body in ear, unspecified ear**

☑4ᵗʰ **T17 Foreign body in respiratory tract**

> The appropriate 7th character is to be added to each code from category T17.
> A initial encounter
> D subsequent encounter
> S sequela

  ☑x7ᵗʰ **T17.0 Foreign body in nasal sinus**

  ☑x7ᵗʰ **T17.1 Foreign body in nostril**

    Foreign body in nose NOS

☑5ᵗʰ **T17.2 Foreign body in pharynx**

    Foreign body in nasopharynx
    Foreign body in throat NOS

  ☑6ᵗʰ **T17.20 Unspecified foreign body in pharynx**

    ☑7ᵗʰ **T17.200 Unspecified foreign body in pharynx causing asphyxiation**

    ☑7ᵗʰ **T17.208 Unspecified foreign body in pharynx causing other injury**

  ☑6ᵗʰ **T17.21 Gastric contents in pharynx**

    Aspiration of gastric contents into pharynx
    Vomitus in pharynx

    ☑7ᵗʰ **T17.210 Gastric contents in pharynx causing asphyxiation**

    ☑7ᵗʰ **T17.218 Gastric contents in pharynx causing other injury**

  ☑6ᵗʰ **T17.22 Food in pharynx**

    Bones in pharynx
    Seeds in pharynx

    ☑7ᵗʰ **T17.220 Food in pharynx causing asphyxiation**

    ☑7ᵗʰ **T17.228 Food in pharynx causing other injury**

  ☑6ᵗʰ **T17.29 Other foreign object in pharynx**

    ☑7ᵗʰ **T17.290 Other foreign object in pharynx causing asphyxiation**

    ☑7ᵗʰ **T17.298 Other foreign object in pharynx causing other injury**

☑5ᵗʰ **T17.3 Foreign body in larynx**

  ☑6ᵗʰ **T17.30 Unspecified foreign body in larynx**

    ☑7ᵗʰ **T17.300 Unspecified foreign body in larynx causing asphyxiation**

    ☑7ᵗʰ **T17.308 Unspecified foreign body in larynx causing other injury**

  ☑6ᵗʰ **T17.31 Gastric contents in larynx**

    Aspiration of gastric contents into larynx
    Vomitus in larynx

    ☑7ᵗʰ **T17.310 Gastric contents in larynx causing asphyxiation**

    ☑7ᵗʰ **T17.318 Gastric contents in larynx causing other injury**

  ☑6ᵗʰ **T17.32 Food in larynx**

    Bones in larynx
    Seeds in larynx

    ☑7ᵗʰ **T17.320 Food in larynx causing asphyxiation**

    ☑7ᵗʰ **T17.328 Food in larynx causing other injury**

  ☑6ᵗʰ **T17.39 Other foreign object in larynx**

    ☑7ᵗʰ **T17.390 Other foreign object in larynx causing asphyxiation**

    ☑7ᵗʰ **T17.398 Other foreign object in larynx causing other injury**

☑5ᵗʰ **T17.4 Foreign body in trachea**

  ☑6ᵗʰ **T17.40 Unspecified foreign body in trachea**

    ☑7ᵗʰ **T17.400 Unspecified foreign body in trachea causing asphyxiation**

    ☑7ᵗʰ **T17.408 Unspecified foreign body in trachea causing other injury**

  ☑6ᵗʰ **T17.41 Gastric contents in trachea**

    Aspiration of gastric contents into trachea
    Vomitus in trachea

    ☑7ᵗʰ **T17.410 Gastric contents in trachea causing asphyxiation**

    ☑7ᵗʰ **T17.418 Gastric contents in trachea causing other injury**

  ☑6ᵗʰ **T17.42 Food in trachea**

    Bones in trachea
    Seeds in trachea

    ☑7ᵗʰ **T17.420 Food in trachea causing asphyxiation**

    ☑7ᵗʰ **T17.428 Food in trachea causing other injury**

  ☑6ᵗʰ **T17.49 Other foreign object in trachea**

    ☑7ᵗʰ **T17.490 Other foreign object in trachea causing asphyxiation**

    ☑7ᵗʰ **T17.498 Other foreign object in trachea causing other injury**

☑5ᵗʰ **T17.5 Foreign body in bronchus**

  ☑6ᵗʰ **T17.50 Unspecified foreign body in bronchus**

    ☑7ᵗʰ **T17.500 Unspecified foreign body in bronchus causing asphyxiation**

✓7ᵗʰ **T17.508 Unspecified foreign body in bronchus causing other injury**

✓6ᵗʰ **T17.51 Gastric contents in bronchus**

Aspiration of gastric contents into bronchus
Vomitus in bronchus

✓7ᵗʰ **T17.510 Gastric contents in bronchus causing asphyxiation**

✓7ᵗʰ **T17.518 Gastric contents in bronchus causing other injury**

✓6ᵗʰ **T17.52 Food in bronchus**

Bones in bronchus
Seeds in bronchus

✓7ᵗʰ **T17.520 Food in bronchus causing asphyxiation**

✓7ᵗʰ **T17.528 Food in bronchus causing other injury**

✓6ᵗʰ **T17.59 Other foreign object in bronchus**

✓7ᵗʰ **T17.590 Other foreign object in bronchus causing asphyxiation**

✓7ᵗʰ **T17.598 Other foreign object in bronchus causing other injury**

✓5ᵗʰ **T17.8 Foreign body in other parts of respiratory tract**

Foreign body in bronchioles
Foreign body in lung

✓6ᵗʰ **T17.80 Unspecified foreign body in other parts of respiratory tract**

✓7ᵗʰ **T17.800 Unspecified foreign body in other parts of respiratory tract causing asphyxiation**

✓7ᵗʰ **T17.808 Unspecified foreign body in other parts of respiratory tract causing other injury**

✓6ᵗʰ **T17.81 Gastric contents in other parts of respiratory tract**

Aspiration of gastric contents into other parts of respiratory tract
Vomitus in other parts of respiratory tract

✓7ᵗʰ **T17.810 Gastric contents in other parts of respiratory tract causing asphyxiation**

✓7ᵗʰ **T17.818 Gastric contents in other parts of respiratory tract causing other injury**

✓6ᵗʰ **T17.82 Food in other parts of respiratory tract**

Bones in other parts of respiratory tract
Seeds in other parts of respiratory tract

✓7ᵗʰ **T17.820 Food in other parts of respiratory tract causing asphyxiation**

✓7ᵗʰ **T17.828 Food in other parts of respiratory tract causing other injury**

✓6ᵗʰ **T17.89 Other foreign object in other parts of respiratory tract**

✓7ᵗʰ **T17.890 Other foreign object in other parts of respiratory tract causing asphyxiation**

✓7ᵗʰ **T17.898 Other foreign object in other parts of respiratory tract causing other injury**

✓5ᵗʰ **T17.9 Foreign body in respiratory tract, part unspecified**

✓6ᵗʰ **T17.90 Unspecified foreign body in respiratory tract, part unspecified**

✓7ᵗʰ **T17.900 Unspecified foreign body in respiratory tract, part unspecified causing asphyxiation**

✓7ᵗʰ **T17.908 Unspecified foreign body in respiratory tract, part unspecified causing other injury**

✓6ᵗʰ **T17.91 Gastric contents in respiratory tract, part unspecified**

Aspiration of gastric contents into respiratory tract, part unspecified
Vomitus in trachea respiratory tract, part unspecified

✓7ᵗʰ **T17.910 Gastric contents in respiratory tract, part unspecified causing asphyxiation**

✓7ᵗʰ **T17.918 Gastric contents in respiratory tract, part unspecified causing other injury**

✓6ᵗʰ **T17.92 Food in respiratory tract, part unspecified**

Bones in respiratory tract, part unspecified
Seeds in respiratory tract, part unspecified

✓7ᵗʰ **T17.920 Food in respiratory tract, part unspecified causing asphyxiation**

✓7ᵗʰ **T17.928 Food in respiratory tract, part unspecified causing other injury**

✓6ᵗʰ **T17.99 Other foreign object in respiratory tract, part unspecified**

✓7ᵗʰ **T17.990 Other foreign object in respiratory tract, part unspecified in causing asphyxiation**

✓7ᵗʰ **T17.998 Other foreign object in respiratory tract, part unspecified causing other injury**

✓4ᵗʰ **T18 Foreign body in alimentary tract**

EXCLUDES 2   foreign body in pharynx (T17.2-)

The appropriate 7th character is to be added to each code from category T18.
A   initial encounter
D   subsequent encounter
S   sequela

✓x7ᵗʰ **T18.0 Foreign body in mouth**

✓5ᵗʰ **T18.1 Foreign body in esophagus**

EXCLUDES 2   foreign body in respiratory tract (T17.-)

✓6ᵗʰ **T18.10 Unspecified foreign body in esophagus**

✓7ᵗʰ **T18.100 Unspecified foreign body in esophagus causing compression of trachea**

Unspecified foreign body in esophagus causing obstruction of respiration

✓7ᵗʰ **T18.108 Unspecified foreign body in esophagus causing other injury**

✓6ᵗʰ **T18.11 Gastric contents in esophagus**

Vomitus in esophagus

✓7ᵗʰ **T18.110 Gastric contents in esophagus causing compression of trachea**

Gastric contents in esophagus causing obstruction of respiration

✓7ᵗʰ **T18.118 Gastric contents in esophagus causing other injury**

✓6ᵗʰ **T18.12 Food in esophagus**

Bones in esophagus
Seeds in esophagus

✓7ᵗʰ **T18.120 Food in esophagus causing compression of trachea**

Food in esophagus causing obstruction of respiration

✓7ᵗʰ **T18.128 Food in esophagus causing other injury**

✓6ᵗʰ **T18.19 Other foreign object in esophagus**

AHA: 2015,1Q,23

✓7ᵗʰ **T18.190 Other foreign object in esophagus causing compression of trachea**

Other foreign body in esophagus causing obstruction of respiration

✓7ᵗʰ **T18.198 Other foreign object in esophagus causing other injury**

✓x7ᵗʰ **T18.2 Foreign body in stomach**

✓x7ᵗʰ **T18.3 Foreign body in small intestine**

✓x7ᵗʰ **T18.4 Foreign body in colon**

✓x7ᵗʰ **T18.5 Foreign body in anus and rectum**

Foreign body in rectosigmoid (junction)

✓x7ᵗʰ **T18.8 Foreign body in other parts of alimentary tract**

✓x7ᵗʰ **T18.9 Foreign body of alimentary tract, part unspecified**

Foreign body in digestive system NOS
Swallowed foreign body NOS

✓4ᵗʰ **T19 Foreign body in genitourinary tract**

EXCLUDES 2   complications due to implanted mesh (T83.7-)
mechanical complications of contraceptive device (intrauterine) (vaginal) (T83.3-)
presence of contraceptive device (intrauterine) (vaginal) (Z97.5)

The appropriate 7th character is to be added to each code from category T19.
A   initial encounter
D   subsequent encounter
S   sequela

✓x7ᵗʰ **T19.0 Foreign body in urethra**

✓x7ᵗʰ **T19.1 Foreign body in bladder**

✓x7ᵗʰ **T19.2 Foreign body in vulva and vagina**   ♀

✓x7ᵗʰ **T19.3 Foreign body in uterus**   ♀

✓x7ᵗʰ **T19.4 Foreign body in penis**   ♂

✓x7ᵗʰ **T19.8 Foreign body in other parts of genitourinary tract**

✓x7ᵗʰ **T19.9 Foreign body in genitourinary tract, part unspecified**

BURNS AND CORROSIONS (T20-T32)

INCLUDES
burns (thermal) from electrical heating appliances
burns (thermal) from electricity
burns (thermal) from flame
burns (thermal) from friction
burns (thermal) from hot air and hot gases
burns (thermal) from hot objects
burns (thermal) from lightning
burns (thermal) from radiation
chemical burn [corrosion] (external) (internal)
scalds

EXCLUDES 2
erythema [dermatitis] ab igne (L59.0)
radiation-related disorders of the skin and subcutaneous tissue
(L55-L59)
sunburn (L55.-)

AHA: 2016,2Q,4
TIP: Burn wound treatment is considered active care and reported with 7th character A.

Burns and corrosions of external body surface, specified by site (T20-T25)

INCLUDES
burns and corrosions of first degree [erythema]
burns and corrosions of second degree [blisters] [epidermal loss]
burns and corrosions of third degree [deep necrosis of underlying tissue] [full-thickness skin loss]
Use additional code from category T31 or T32 to identify extent of body surface involved

√4ᵗʰ **T20 Burn and corrosion of head, face, and neck**

     EXCLUDES 2
       burn and corrosion of ear drum (T28.41, T28.91)
       burn and corrosion of eye and adnexa (T26.-)
       burn and corrosion of mouth and pharynx (T28.0)

     AHA: 2015,1Q,18-19

> The appropriate 7th character is to be added to each code from category T20.
> A   initial encounter
> D   subsequent encounter
> S   sequela

√5ᵗʰ **T20.0 Burn of unspecified degree of head, face, and neck**
     Use additional external cause code to identify the source, place and intent of the burn (X00-X19, X75-X77, X96-X98, Y92)

     √x7ᵗʰ **T20.00 Burn of unspecified degree of head, face, and neck, unspecified site**

     √6ᵗʰ **T20.01 Burn of unspecified degree of ear [any part, except ear drum]**
       EXCLUDES 2   burn of ear drum (T28.41-)

       √7ᵗʰ **T20.011 Burn of unspecified degree of right ear [any part, except ear drum]**

       √7ᵗʰ **T20.012 Burn of unspecified degree of left ear [any part, except ear drum]**

       √7ᵗʰ **T20.019 Burn of unspecified degree of unspecified ear [any part, except ear drum]**

     √x7ᵗʰ **T20.02 Burn of unspecified degree of lip(s)**

     √x7ᵗʰ **T20.03 Burn of unspecified degree of chin**

     √x7ᵗʰ **T20.04 Burn of unspecified degree of nose (septum)**

     √x7ᵗʰ **T20.05 Burn of unspecified degree of scalp [any part]**

     √x7ᵗʰ **T20.06 Burn of unspecified degree of forehead and cheek**

     √x7ᵗʰ **T20.07 Burn of unspecified degree of neck**

     √x7ᵗʰ **T20.09 Burn of unspecified degree of multiple sites of head, face, and neck**

√5ᵗʰ **T20.1 Burn of first degree of head, face, and neck**
     Use additional external cause code to identify the source, place and intent of the burn (X00-X19, X75-X77, X96-X98, Y92)

     √x7ᵗʰ **T20.10 Burn of first degree of head, face, and neck, unspecified site**

     √6ᵗʰ **T20.11 Burn of first degree of ear [any part, except ear drum]**
       EXCLUDES 2   burn of ear drum (T28.41-)

       √7ᵗʰ **T20.111 Burn of first degree of right ear [any part, except ear drum]**

       √7ᵗʰ **T20.112 Burn of first degree of left ear [any part, except ear drum]**

       √7ᵗʰ **T20.119 Burn of first degree of unspecified ear [any part, except ear drum]**

     √x7ᵗʰ **T20.12 Burn of first degree of lip(s)**

     √x7ᵗʰ **T20.13 Burn of first degree of chin**

     √x7ᵗʰ **T20.14 Burn of first degree of nose (septum)**

     √x7ᵗʰ **T20.15 Burn of first degree of scalp [any part]**

     √x7ᵗʰ **T20.16 Burn of first degree of forehead and cheek**

     √x7ᵗʰ **T20.17 Burn of first degree of neck**

     √x7ᵗʰ **T20.19 Burn of first degree of multiple sites of head, face, and neck**

Degree of Burns

Epidermis
Dermis
Subcutaneous

Normal   First Degree Burn

Epidermis
Dermis
Subcutaneous

Second Degree Burn   Third Degree Burn

√5ᵗʰ **T20.2 Burn of second degree of head, face, and neck**
     Use additional external cause code to identify the source, place and intent of the burn (X00-X19, X75-X77, X96-X98, Y92)

     √x7ᵗʰ **T20.20 Burn of second degree of head, face, and neck, unspecified site**

     √6ᵗʰ **T20.21 Burn of second degree of ear [any part, except ear drum]**
       EXCLUDES 2   burn of ear drum (T28.41-)

       √7ᵗʰ **T20.211 Burn of second degree of right ear [any part, except ear drum]**

       √7ᵗʰ **T20.212 Burn of second degree of left ear [any part, except ear drum]**

       √7ᵗʰ **T20.219 Burn of second degree of unspecified ear [any part, except ear drum]**

     √x7ᵗʰ **T20.22 Burn of second degree of lip(s)**

     √x7ᵗʰ **T20.23 Burn of second degree of chin**

     √x7ᵗʰ **T20.24 Burn of second degree of nose (septum)**

     √x7ᵗʰ **T20.25 Burn of second degree of scalp [any part]**

     √x7ᵗʰ **T20.26 Burn of second degree of forehead and cheek**

     √x7ᵗʰ **T20.27 Burn of second degree of neck**

     √x7ᵗʰ **T20.29 Burn of second degree of multiple sites of head, face, and neck**

√5ᵗʰ **T20.3 Burn of third degree of head, face, and neck**
     Use additional external cause code to identify the source, place and intent of the burn (X00-X19, X75-X77, X96-X98, Y92)

     √x7ᵗʰ **T20.30 Burn of third degree of head, face, and neck, unspecified site**

     √6ᵗʰ **T20.31 Burn of third degree of ear [any part, except ear drum]**
       EXCLUDES 2   burn of ear drum (T28.41-)
       AHA: 2015,1Q,18

       √7ᵗʰ **T20.311 Burn of third degree of right ear [any part, except ear drum]**

       √7ᵗʰ **T20.312 Burn of third degree of left ear [any part, except ear drum]**

       √7ᵗʰ **T20.319 Burn of third degree of unspecified ear [any part, except ear drum]**

     √x7ᵗʰ **T20.32 Burn of third degree of lip(s)**

     √x7ᵗʰ **T20.33 Burn of third degree of chin**

     √x7ᵗʰ **T20.34 Burn of third degree of nose (septum)**

     √x7ᵗʰ **T20.35 Burn of third degree of scalp [any part]**

     √x7ᵗʰ **T20.36 Burn of third degree of forehead and cheek**

     √x7ᵗʰ **T20.37 Burn of third degree of neck**

√x7ᵗʰ **T20.39** **Burn of third degree of** multiple sites **of head, face, and neck**

√5ᵗʰ **T20.4** **Corrosion of unspecified degree of head, face, and neck**
Code first (T51-T65) to identify chemical and intent
Use additional external cause code to identify place (Y92)

√x7ᵗʰ **T20.40** **Corrosion of unspecified degree of head, face, and neck, unspecified site**

√6ᵗʰ **T20.41** **Corrosion of unspecified degree of** ear [any part, except ear drum]
EXCLUDES 2   corrosion of ear drum (T28.91-)

√7ᵗʰ **T20.411** **Corrosion of unspecified degree of** right **ear [any part, except ear drum]**

√7ᵗʰ **T20.412** **Corrosion of unspecified degree of** left **ear [any part, except ear drum]**

√7ᵗʰ **T20.419** **Corrosion of unspecified degree of** unspecified **ear [any part, except ear drum]**

√x7ᵗʰ **T20.42** **Corrosion of unspecified degree of** lip(s)

√x7ᵗʰ **T20.43** **Corrosion of unspecified degree of** chin

√x7ᵗʰ **T20.44** **Corrosion of unspecified degree of** nose **(septum)**

√x7ᵗʰ **T20.45** **Corrosion of unspecified degree of** scalp **[any part]**

√x7ᵗʰ **T20.46** **Corrosion of unspecified degree of** forehead and cheek

√x7ᵗʰ **T20.47** **Corrosion of unspecified degree of** neck

√x7ᵗʰ **T20.49** **Corrosion of unspecified degree of** multiple sites **of head, face, and neck**

√5ᵗʰ **T20.5** **Corrosion of** first degree **of head, face, and neck**
Code first (T51-T65) to identify chemical and intent
Use additional external cause code to identify place (Y92)

√x7ᵗʰ **T20.50** **Corrosion of first degree of head, face, and neck, unspecified site**

√6ᵗʰ **T20.51** **Corrosion of first degree of** ear **[any part, except ear drum]**
EXCLUDES 2   corrosion of ear drum (T28.91-)

√7ᵗʰ **T20.511** **Corrosion of first degree of** right **ear [any part, except ear drum]**

√7ᵗʰ **T20.512** **Corrosion of first degree of** left **ear [any part, except ear drum]**

√7ᵗʰ **T20.519** **Corrosion of first degree of unspecified ear [any part, except ear drum]**

√x7ᵗʰ **T20.52** **Corrosion of first degree of** lip(s)

√x7ᵗʰ **T20.53** **Corrosion of first degree of** chin

√x7ᵗʰ **T20.54** **Corrosion of first degree of** nose **(septum)**

√x7ᵗʰ **T20.55** **Corrosion of first degree of** scalp **[any part]**

√x7ᵗʰ **T20.56** **Corrosion of first degree of** forehead and cheek

√x7ᵗʰ **T20.57** **Corrosion of first degree of** neck

√x7ᵗʰ **T20.59** **Corrosion of first degree of** multiple sites **of head, face, and neck**

√5ᵗʰ **T20.6** **Corrosion of** second degree **of head, face, and neck**
Code first (T51-T65) to identify chemical and intent
Use additional external cause code to identify place (Y92)

√x7ᵗʰ **T20.60** **Corrosion of second degree of head, face, and neck, unspecified site**

√6ᵗʰ **T20.61** **Corrosion of second degree of** ear **[any part, except ear drum]**
EXCLUDES 2   corrosion of ear drum (T28.91-)

√7ᵗʰ **T20.611** **Corrosion of second degree of** right **ear [any part, except ear drum]**

√7ᵗʰ **T20.612** **Corrosion of second degree of** left **ear [any part, except ear drum]**

√7ᵗʰ **T20.619** **Corrosion of second degree of unspecified ear [any part, except ear drum]**

√x7ᵗʰ **T20.62** **Corrosion of second degree of** lip(s)

√x7ᵗʰ **T20.63** **Corrosion of second degree of** chin

√x7ᵗʰ **T20.64** **Corrosion of second degree of** nose **(septum)**

√x7ᵗʰ **T20.65** **Corrosion of second degree of** scalp **[any part]**

√x7ᵗʰ **T20.66** **Corrosion of second degree of** forehead and cheek

√x7ᵗʰ **T20.67** **Corrosion of second degree of** neck

√x7ᵗʰ **T20.69** **Corrosion of second degree of** multiple sites **of head, face, and neck**

√6ᵗʰ **T20.7** **Corrosion of** third degree **of head, face, and neck**
Code first (T51-T65) to identify chemical and intent
Use additional external cause code to identify place (Y92)

√x7ᵗʰ **T20.70** **Corrosion of third degree of head, face, and neck, unspecified site**

√6ᵗʰ **T20.71** **Corrosion of third degree of** ear **[any part, except ear drum]**
EXCLUDES 2   corrosion of ear drum (T28.91-)

√7ᵗʰ **T20.711** **Corrosion of third degree of** right **ear [any part, except ear drum]**

√7ᵗʰ **T20.712** **Corrosion of third degree of** left **ear [any part, except ear drum]**

√7ᵗʰ **T20.719** **Corrosion of third degree of unspecified ear [any part, except ear drum]**

√x7ᵗʰ **T20.72** **Corrosion of third degree of** lip(s)

√x7ᵗʰ **T20.73** **Corrosion of third degree of** chin

√x7ᵗʰ **T20.74** **Corrosion of third degree of** nose **(septum)**

√x7ᵗʰ **T20.75** **Corrosion of third degree of** scalp **[any part]**

√x7ᵗʰ **T20.76** **Corrosion of third degree of** forehead and cheek

√x7ᵗʰ **T20.77** **Corrosion of third degree of** neck

√x7ᵗʰ **T20.79** **Corrosion of third degree of** multiple sites **of head, face, and neck**

√4ᵗʰ **T21** **Burn and corrosion of trunk**
INCLUDES   burns and corrosion of hip region
EXCLUDES 2   burns and corrosion of axilla (T22.- with fifth character 4)
burns and corrosion of scapular region (T22.- with fifth character 6)
burns and corrosion of shoulder (T22.- with fifth character 5)

The appropriate 7th character is to be added to each code from category T21.
A   initial encounter
D   subsequent encounter
S   sequela

√5ᵗʰ **T21.0** **Burn of unspecified degree of trunk**
Use additional external cause code to identify the source, place and intent of the burn (X00-X19, X75-X77, X96-X98, Y92)

√x7ᵗʰ **T21.00** **Burn of unspecified degree of trunk, unspecified site**

√x7ᵗʰ **T21.01** **Burn of unspecified degree of** chest wall
Burn of unspecified degree of breast

√x7ᵗʰ **T21.02** **Burn of unspecified degree of** abdominal wall
Burn of unspecified degree of flank
Burn of unspecified degree of groin

√x7ᵗʰ **T21.03** **Burn of unspecified degree of** upper back
Burn of unspecified degree of interscapular region

√x7ᵗʰ **T21.04** **Burn of unspecified degree of** lower back

√x7ᵗʰ **T21.05** **Burn of unspecified degree of** buttock
Burn of unspecified degree of anus

√x7ᵗʰ **T21.06** **Burn of unspecified degree of** male genital region   ♂
Burn of unspecified degree of penis
Burn of unspecified degree of scrotum
Burn of unspecified degree of testis

√x7ᵗʰ **T21.07** **Burn of unspecified degree of** female genital region   ♀
Burn of unspecified degree of labium (majus) (minus)
Burn of unspecified degree of perineum
Burn of unspecified degree of vulva
EXCLUDES 2   burn of vagina (T28.3)

√x7ᵗʰ **T21.09** **Burn of unspecified degree of other site of trunk**

√5ᵗʰ **T21.1** **Burn of** first degree **of trunk**
Use additional external cause code to identify the source, place and intent of the burn (X00-X19, X75-X77, X96-X98, Y92)

√x7ᵗʰ **T21.10** **Burn of first degree of trunk, unspecified site**

√x7ᵗʰ **T21.11** **Burn of first degree of** chest wall
Burn of first degree of breast

√x7ᵗʰ **T21.12** **Burn of first degree of** abdominal wall
Burn of first degree of flank
Burn of first degree of groin

√x7ᵗʰ **T21.13** **Burn of first degree of** upper back
Burn of first degree of interscapular region

√x7ᵗʰ **T21.14** **Burn of first degree of** lower back

√x7ᵗʰ **T21.15** **Burn of first degree of** buttock
Burn of first degree of anus

☑ Additional Character Required   √x7ᵗʰ Placeholder Alert   Manifestation   Unspecified Dx   ▶◀ Revised Text   ● New Code   ▲ Revised Title

ICD-10-CM 2020   1069

✓x7ᵗʰ **T21.16** **Burn of first degree of** male genital region ♂
Burn of first degree of penis
Burn of first degree of scrotum
Burn of first degree of testis

✓x7ᵗʰ **T21.17** **Burn of first degree of** female genital region ♀
Burn of first degree of labium (majus) (minus)
Burn of first degree of perineum
Burn of first degree of vulva
EXCLUDES 2   burn of vagina (T28.3)

✓x7ᵗʰ **T21.19** **Burn of first degree of other site of trunk**

✓5ᵗʰ **T21.2** **Burn of** second degree **of trunk**
Use additional external cause code to identify the source, place and intent of the burn (X00-X19, X75-X77, X96-X98, Y92)

✓x7ᵗʰ **T21.20** **Burn of second degree of trunk, unspecified site**

✓x7ᵗʰ **T21.21** **Burn of second degree of** chest wall
Burn of second degree of breast

✓x7ᵗʰ **T21.22** **Burn of second degree of** abdominal wall
Burn of second degree of flank
Burn of second degree of groin

✓x7ᵗʰ **T21.23** **Burn of second degree of** upper back
Burn of second degree of interscapular region

✓x7ᵗʰ **T21.24** **Burn of second degree of** lower back

✓x7ᵗʰ **T21.25** **Burn of second degree of** buttock
Burn of second degree of anus

✓x7ᵗʰ **T21.26** **Burn of second degree of** male genital region ♂
Burn of second degree of penis
Burn of second degree of scrotum
Burn of second degree of testis

✓x7ᵗʰ **T21.27** **Burn of second degree of** female genital region ♀
Burn of second degree of labium (majus) (minus)
Burn of second degree of perineum
Burn of second degree of vulva
EXCLUDES 2   burn of vagina (T28.3)

✓x7ᵗʰ **T21.29** **Burn of second degree of other site of trunk**

✓5ᵗʰ **T21.3** **Burn of** third degree **of trunk**
Use additional external cause code to identify the source, place and intent of the burn (X00-X19, X75-X77, X96-X98, Y92)

✓x7ᵗʰ **T21.30** **Burn of third degree of trunk, unspecified site**

✓x7ᵗʰ **T21.31** **Burn of third degree of** chest wall
Burn of third degree of breast
AHA: 2016,2Q,5

✓x7ᵗʰ **T21.32** **Burn of third degree of** abdominal wall
Burn of third degree of flank
Burn of third degree of groin

✓x7ᵗʰ **T21.33** **Burn of third degree of** upper back
Burn of third degree of interscapular region

✓x7ᵗʰ **T21.34** **Burn of third degree of** lower back

✓x7ᵗʰ **T21.35** **Burn of third degree of** buttock
Burn of third degree of anus

✓x7ᵗʰ **T21.36** **Burn of third degree of** male genital region ♂
Burn of third degree of penis
Burn of third degree of scrotum
Burn of third degree of testis

✓x7ᵗʰ **T21.37** **Burn of third degree of** female genital region ♀
Burn of third degree of labium (majus) (minus)
Burn of third degree of perineum
Burn of third degree of vulva
EXCLUDES 2   burn of vagina (T28.3)

✓x7ᵗʰ **T21.39** **Burn of third degree of other site of trunk**

✓5ᵗʰ **T21.4** **Corrosion of unspecified degree of trunk**
Code first (T51-T65) to identify chemical and intent
Use additional external cause code to identify place (Y92)

✓x7ᵗʰ **T21.40** **Corrosion of unspecified degree of trunk, unspecified site**

✓x7ᵗʰ **T21.41** **Corrosion of unspecified degree of** chest wall
Corrosion of unspecified degree of breast

✓x7ᵗʰ **T21.42** **Corrosion of unspecified degree of** abdominal wall
Corrosion of unspecified degree of flank
Corrosion of unspecified degree of groin

✓x7ᵗʰ **T21.43** **Corrosion of unspecified degree of** upper back
Corrosion of unspecified degree of interscapular region

✓x7ᵗʰ **T21.44** **Corrosion of unspecified degree of** lower back

✓x7ᵗʰ **T21.45** **Corrosion of unspecified degree of** buttock
Corrosion of unspecified degree of anus

✓x7ᵗʰ **T21.46** **Corrosion of unspecified degree of** male genital region ♂
Corrosion of unspecified degree of penis
Corrosion of unspecified degree of scrotum
Corrosion of unspecified degree of testis

✓x7ᵗʰ **T21.47** **Corrosion of unspecified degree of** female genital region ♀
Corrosion of unspecified degree of labium (majus) (minus)
Corrosion of unspecified degree of perineum
Corrosion of unspecified degree of vulva
EXCLUDES 2   corrosion of vagina (T28.8)

✓x7ᵗʰ **T21.49** **Corrosion of unspecified degree of other site of trunk**

✓5ᵗʰ **T21.5** **Corrosion of** first degree **of trunk**
Code first (T51-T65) to identify chemical and intent
Use additional external cause code to identify place (Y92)

✓x7ᵗʰ **T21.50** **Corrosion of first degree of trunk, unspecified site**

✓x7ᵗʰ **T21.51** **Corrosion of first degree of** chest wall
Corrosion of first degree of breast

✓x7ᵗʰ **T21.52** **Corrosion of first degree of** abdominal wall
Corrosion of first degree of flank
Corrosion of first degree of groin

✓x7ᵗʰ **T21.53** **Corrosion of first degree of** upper back
Corrosion of first degree of interscapular region

✓x7ᵗʰ **T21.54** **Corrosion of first degree of** lower back

✓x7ᵗʰ **T21.55** **Corrosion of first degree of** buttock
Corrosion of first degree of anus

✓x7ᵗʰ **T21.56** **Corrosion of first degree of** male genital region ♂
Corrosion of first degree of penis
Corrosion of first degree of scrotum
Corrosion of first degree of testis

✓x7ᵗʰ **T21.57** **Corrosion of first degree of** female genital region ♀
Corrosion of first degree of labium (majus) (minus)
Corrosion of first degree of perineum
Corrosion of first degree of vulva
EXCLUDES 2   corrosion of vagina (T28.8)

✓x7ᵗʰ **T21.59** **Corrosion of first degree of other site of trunk**

✓5ᵗʰ **T21.6** **Corrosion of** second degree **of trunk**
Code first (T51-T65) to identify chemical and intent
Use additional external cause code to identify place (Y92)

✓x7ᵗʰ **T21.60** **Corrosion of second degree of trunk, unspecified site**

✓x7ᵗʰ **T21.61** **Corrosion of second degree of** chest wall
Corrosion of second degree of breast

✓x7ᵗʰ **T21.62** **Corrosion of second degree of** abdominal wall
Corrosion of second degree of flank
Corrosion of second degree of groin

✓x7ᵗʰ **T21.63** **Corrosion of second degree of** upper back
Corrosion of second degree of interscapular region

✓x7ᵗʰ **T21.64** **Corrosion of second degree of** lower back

✓x7ᵗʰ **T21.65** **Corrosion of second degree of** buttock
Corrosion of second degree of anus

✓x7ᵗʰ **T21.66** **Corrosion of second degree of** male genital region ♂
Corrosion of second degree of penis
Corrosion of second degree of scrotum
Corrosion of second degree of testis

√x7ᵗʰ **T21.67** **Corrosion of second degree of** female genital region ♀
    Corrosion of second degree of labium (majus) (minus)
    Corrosion of second degree of perineum
    Corrosion of second degree of vulva
    EXCLUDES 2   corrosion of vagina (T28.8)

√x7ᵗʰ **T21.69** **Corrosion of second degree of other site of trunk**

√5ᵗʰ **T21.7** **Corrosion of** third degree **of trunk**
    Code first (T51-T65) to identify chemical and intent
    Use additional external cause code to identify place (Y92)

√x7ᵗʰ **T21.70** **Corrosion of third degree of trunk, unspecified site**

√x7ᵗʰ **T21.71** **Corrosion of third degree of** chest wall
    Corrosion of third degree of breast

√x7ᵗʰ **T21.72** **Corrosion of third degree of** abdominal wall
    Corrosion of third degree of flank
    Corrosion of third degree of groin

√x7ᵗʰ **T21.73** **Corrosion of third degree of** upper back
    Corrosion of third degree of interscapular region

√x7ᵗʰ **T21.74** **Corrosion of third degree of** lower back

√x7ᵗʰ **T21.75** **Corrosion of third degree of** buttock
    Corrosion of third degree of anus

√x7ᵗʰ **T21.76** **Corrosion of third degree of** male genital region ♂
    Corrosion of third degree of penis
    Corrosion of third degree of scrotum
    Corrosion of third degree of testis

√x7ᵗʰ **T21.77** **Corrosion of third degree of** female genital region ♀
    Corrosion of third degree of labium (majus) (minus)
    Corrosion of third degree of perineum
    Corrosion of third degree of vulva
    EXCLUDES 2   corrosion of vagina (T28.8)

√x7ᵗʰ **T21.79** **Corrosion of third degree of other site of trunk**

√4ᵗʰ **T22** **Burn and corrosion of shoulder and upper limb, except wrist and hand**
    EXCLUDES 2   burn and corrosion of interscapular region (T21.-)
              burn and corrosion of wrist and hand (T23.-)

> The appropriate 7th character is to be added to each code from category T22.
> A   initial encounter
> D   subsequent encounter
> S   sequela

√5ᵗʰ **T22.0** **Burn of unspecified degree of shoulder and upper limb, except wrist and hand**
    Use additional external cause code to identify the source, place and intent of the burn (X00-X19, X75-X77, X96-X98, Y92)

√x7ᵗʰ **T22.00** **Burn of unspecified degree of shoulder and upper limb, except wrist and hand, unspecified site**

√6ᵗʰ **T22.01** **Burn of unspecified degree of** forearm

√7ᵗʰ **T22.011** **Burn of unspecified degree of** right forearm

√7ᵗʰ **T22.012** **Burn of unspecified degree of** left forearm

√7ᵗʰ **T22.019** **Burn of unspecified degree of unspecified forearm**

√6ᵗʰ **T22.02** **Burn of unspecified degree of** elbow

√7ᵗʰ **T22.021** **Burn of unspecified degree of** right elbow

√7ᵗʰ **T22.022** **Burn of unspecified degree of** left elbow

√7ᵗʰ **T22.029** **Burn of unspecified degree of unspecified elbow**

√6ᵗʰ **T22.03** **Burn of unspecified degree of** upper arm

√7ᵗʰ **T22.031** **Burn of unspecified degree of** right upper arm

√7ᵗʰ **T22.032** **Burn of unspecified degree of** left upper arm

√7ᵗʰ **T22.039** **Burn of unspecified degree of unspecified upper arm**

√6ᵗʰ **T22.04** **Burn of unspecified degree of** axilla

√7ᵗʰ **T22.041** **Burn of unspecified degree of** right axilla

√7ᵗʰ **T22.042** **Burn of unspecified degree of** left axilla

√7ᵗʰ **T22.049** **Burn of unspecified degree of unspecified axilla**

√6ᵗʰ **T22.05** **Burn of unspecified degree of** shoulder

√7ᵗʰ **T22.051** **Burn of unspecified degree of** right shoulder

√7ᵗʰ **T22.052** **Burn of unspecified degree of** left shoulder

√7ᵗʰ **T22.059** **Burn of unspecified degree of unspecified shoulder**

√6ᵗʰ **T22.06** **Burn of unspecified degree of** scapular region

√7ᵗʰ **T22.061** **Burn of unspecified degree of** right scapular region

√7ᵗʰ **T22.062** **Burn of unspecified degree of** left scapular region

√7ᵗʰ **T22.069** **Burn of unspecified degree of unspecified scapular region**

√6ᵗʰ **T22.09** **Burn of unspecified degree of** multiple sites **of shoulder and upper limb, except wrist and hand**

√7ᵗʰ **T22.091** **Burn of unspecified degree of multiple sites of** right **shoulder and upper limb, except wrist and hand**

√7ᵗʰ **T22.092** **Burn of unspecified degree of multiple sites of** left **shoulder and upper limb, except wrist and hand**

√7ᵗʰ **T22.099** **Burn of unspecified degree of multiple sites of unspecified shoulder and upper limb, except wrist and hand**

√5ᵗʰ **T22.1** **Burn of** first degree **of shoulder and upper limb, except wrist and hand**
    Use additional external cause code to identify the source, place and intent of the burn (X00-X19, X75-X77, X96-X98, Y92)

√x7ᵗʰ **T22.10** **Burn of first degree of shoulder and upper limb, except wrist and hand, unspecified site**

√6ᵗʰ **T22.11** **Burn of first degree of** forearm

√7ᵗʰ **T22.111** **Burn of first degree of** right forearm

√7ᵗʰ **T22.112** **Burn of first degree of** left forearm

√7ᵗʰ **T22.119** **Burn of first degree of unspecified forearm**

√6ᵗʰ **T22.12** **Burn of first degree of** elbow

√7ᵗʰ **T22.121** **Burn of first degree of** right elbow

√7ᵗʰ **T22.122** **Burn of first degree of** left elbow

√7ᵗʰ **T22.129** **Burn of first degree of unspecified elbow**

√6ᵗʰ **T22.13** **Burn of first degree of** upper arm

√7ᵗʰ **T22.131** **Burn of first degree of** right upper arm

√7ᵗʰ **T22.132** **Burn of first degree of** left upper arm

√7ᵗʰ **T22.139** **Burn of first degree of unspecified upper arm**

√6ᵗʰ **T22.14** **Burn of first degree of** axilla

√7ᵗʰ **T22.141** **Burn of first degree of** right axilla

√7ᵗʰ **T22.142** **Burn of first degree of** left axilla

√7ᵗʰ **T22.149** **Burn of first degree of unspecified axilla**

√6ᵗʰ **T22.15** **Burn of first degree of** shoulder

√7ᵗʰ **T22.151** **Burn of first degree of** right shoulder

√7ᵗʰ **T22.152** **Burn of first degree of** left shoulder

√7ᵗʰ **T22.159** **Burn of first degree of unspecified shoulder**

√6ᵗʰ **T22.16** **Burn of first degree of** scapular region

√7ᵗʰ **T22.161** **Burn of first degree of** right scapular region

√7ᵗʰ **T22.162** **Burn of first degree of** left scapular region

√7ᵗʰ **T22.169** **Burn of first degree of unspecified scapular region**

√6ᵗʰ **T22.19** **Burn of first degree of** multiple sites **of shoulder and upper limb, except wrist and hand**

√7ᵗʰ **T22.191** **Burn of first degree of multiple sites of** right **shoulder and upper limb, except wrist and hand**

√7ᵗʰ **T22.192** **Burn of first degree of multiple sites of** left **shoulder and upper limb, except wrist and hand**

√7ᵗʰ **T22.199** **Burn of first degree of multiple sites of unspecified shoulder and upper limb, except wrist and hand**

√5ᵗʰ **T22.2** **Burn of** second degree **of shoulder and upper limb, except wrist and hand**
    Use additional external cause code to identify the source, place and intent of the burn (X00-X19, X75-X77, X96-X98, Y92)

√x7ᵗʰ **T22.20** **Burn of second degree of shoulder and upper limb, except wrist and hand, unspecified site**

√6ᵗʰ **T22.21** **Burn of second degree of** forearm

√7ᵗʰ **T22.211** **Burn of second degree of** right forearm

√7ᵗʰ **T22.212** **Burn of second degree of** left forearm

| ☑ Additional Character Required | √x7ᵗʰ Placeholder Alert | Manifestation | Unspecified Dx | ▶◀ Revised Text | ● New Code | ▲ Revised Title |

ICD-10-CM 2020   1071

√7ᵗʰ **T22.219** Burn of second degree of unspecified forearm
√6ᵗʰ **T22.22** Burn of second degree of elbow
　√7ᵗʰ **T22.221** Burn of second degree of right elbow
　√7ᵗʰ **T22.222** Burn of second degree of left elbow
　√7ᵗʰ **T22.229** Burn of second degree of unspecified elbow
√6ᵗʰ **T22.23** Burn of second degree of upper arm
　√7ᵗʰ **T22.231** Burn of second degree of right upper arm
　√7ᵗʰ **T22.232** Burn of second degree of left upper arm
　√7ᵗʰ **T22.239** Burn of second degree of unspecified upper arm
√6ᵗʰ **T22.24** Burn of second degree of axilla
　√7ᵗʰ **T22.241** Burn of second degree of right axilla
　√7ᵗʰ **T22.242** Burn of second degree of left axilla
　√7ᵗʰ **T22.249** Burn of second degree of unspecified axilla
√6ᵗʰ **T22.25** Burn of second degree of shoulder
　√7ᵗʰ **T22.251** Burn of second degree of right shoulder
　√7ᵗʰ **T22.252** Burn of second degree of left shoulder
　√7ᵗʰ **T22.259** Burn of second degree of unspecified shoulder
√6ᵗʰ **T22.26** Burn of second degree of scapular region
　√7ᵗʰ **T22.261** Burn of second degree of right scapular region
　√7ᵗʰ **T22.262** Burn of second degree of left scapular region
　√7ᵗʰ **T22.269** Burn of second degree of unspecified scapular region
√6ᵗʰ **T22.29** Burn of second degree of multiple sites of shoulder and upper limb, except wrist and hand
　√7ᵗʰ **T22.291** Burn of second degree of multiple sites of right shoulder and upper limb, except wrist and hand
　√7ᵗʰ **T22.292** Burn of second degree of multiple sites of left shoulder and upper limb, except wrist and hand
　√7ᵗʰ **T22.299** Burn of second degree of multiple sites of unspecified shoulder and upper limb, except wrist and hand
√5ᵗʰ **T22.3** Burn of third degree of shoulder and upper limb, except wrist and hand
　Use additional external cause code to identify the source, place and intent of the burn (X00-X19, X75-X77, X96-X98, Y92)
√x7ᵗʰ **T22.30** Burn of third degree of shoulder and upper limb, except wrist and hand, unspecified site
√6ᵗʰ **T22.31** Burn of third degree of forearm
　√7ᵗʰ **T22.311** Burn of third degree of right forearm
　√7ᵗʰ **T22.312** Burn of third degree of left forearm
　√7ᵗʰ **T22.319** Burn of third degree of unspecified forearm
√6ᵗʰ **T22.32** Burn of third degree of elbow
　√7ᵗʰ **T22.321** Burn of third degree of right elbow
　√7ᵗʰ **T22.322** Burn of third degree of left elbow
　√7ᵗʰ **T22.329** Burn of third degree of unspecified elbow
√6ᵗʰ **T22.33** Burn of third degree of upper arm
　√7ᵗʰ **T22.331** Burn of third degree of right upper arm
　√7ᵗʰ **T22.332** Burn of third degree of left upper arm
　√7ᵗʰ **T22.339** Burn of third degree of unspecified upper arm
√6ᵗʰ **T22.34** Burn of third degree of axilla
　√7ᵗʰ **T22.341** Burn of third degree of right axilla
　√7ᵗʰ **T22.342** Burn of third degree of left axilla
　√7ᵗʰ **T22.349** Burn of third degree of unspecified axilla
√6ᵗʰ **T22.35** Burn of third degree of shoulder
　√7ᵗʰ **T22.351** Burn of third degree of right shoulder
　√7ᵗʰ **T22.352** Burn of third degree of left shoulder
　√7ᵗʰ **T22.359** Burn of third degree of unspecified shoulder
√6ᵗʰ **T22.36** Burn of third degree of scapular region
　√7ᵗʰ **T22.361** Burn of third degree of right scapular region
　√7ᵗʰ **T22.362** Burn of third degree of left scapular region

√7ᵗʰ **T22.369** Burn of third degree of unspecified scapular region
√6ᵗʰ **T22.39** Burn of third degree of multiple sites of shoulder and upper limb, except wrist and hand
　√7ᵗʰ **T22.391** Burn of third degree of multiple sites of right shoulder and upper limb, except wrist and hand
　√7ᵗʰ **T22.392** Burn of third degree of multiple sites of left shoulder and upper limb, except wrist and hand
　√7ᵗʰ **T22.399** Burn of third degree of multiple sites of unspecified shoulder and upper limb, except wrist and hand
√5ᵗʰ **T22.4** Corrosion of unspecified degree of shoulder and upper limb, except wrist and hand
　Code first (T51-T65) to identify chemical and intent
　Use additional external cause code to identify place (Y92)
√x7ᵗʰ **T22.40** Corrosion of unspecified degree of shoulder and upper limb, except wrist and hand, unspecified site
√6ᵗʰ **T22.41** Corrosion of unspecified degree of forearm
　√7ᵗʰ **T22.411** Corrosion of unspecified degree of right forearm
　√7ᵗʰ **T22.412** Corrosion of unspecified degree of left forearm
　√7ᵗʰ **T22.419** Corrosion of unspecified degree of unspecified forearm
√6ᵗʰ **T22.42** Corrosion of unspecified degree of elbow
　√7ᵗʰ **T22.421** Corrosion of unspecified degree of right elbow
　√7ᵗʰ **T22.422** Corrosion of unspecified degree of left elbow
　√7ᵗʰ **T22.429** Corrosion of unspecified degree of unspecified elbow
√6ᵗʰ **T22.43** Corrosion of unspecified degree of upper arm
　√7ᵗʰ **T22.431** Corrosion of unspecified degree of right upper arm
　√7ᵗʰ **T22.432** Corrosion of unspecified degree of left upper arm
　√7ᵗʰ **T22.439** Corrosion of unspecified degree of unspecified upper arm
√6ᵗʰ **T22.44** Corrosion of unspecified degree of axilla
　√7ᵗʰ **T22.441** Corrosion of unspecified degree of right axilla
　√7ᵗʰ **T22.442** Corrosion of unspecified degree of left axilla
　√7ᵗʰ **T22.449** Corrosion of unspecified degree of unspecified axilla
√6ᵗʰ **T22.45** Corrosion of unspecified degree of shoulder
　√7ᵗʰ **T22.451** Corrosion of unspecified degree of right shoulder
　√7ᵗʰ **T22.452** Corrosion of unspecified degree of left shoulder
　√7ᵗʰ **T22.459** Corrosion of unspecified degree of unspecified shoulder
√6ᵗʰ **T22.46** Corrosion of unspecified degree of scapular region
　√7ᵗʰ **T22.461** Corrosion of unspecified degree of right scapular region
　√7ᵗʰ **T22.462** Corrosion of unspecified degree of left scapular region
　√7ᵗʰ **T22.469** Corrosion of unspecified degree of unspecified scapular region
√6ᵗʰ **T22.49** Corrosion of unspecified degree of multiple sites of shoulder and upper limb, except wrist and hand
　√7ᵗʰ **T22.491** Corrosion of unspecified degree of multiple sites of right shoulder and upper limb, except wrist and hand
　√7ᵗʰ **T22.492** Corrosion of unspecified degree of multiple sites of left shoulder and upper limb, except wrist and hand
　√7ᵗʰ **T22.499** Corrosion of unspecified degree of multiple sites of unspecified shoulder and upper limb, except wrist and hand
√5ᵗʰ **T22.5** Corrosion of first degree of shoulder and upper limb, except wrist and hand
　Code first (T51-T65) to identify chemical and intent
　Use additional external cause code to identify place (Y92)
√x7ᵗʰ **T22.50** Corrosion of first degree of shoulder and upper limb, except wrist and hand unspecified site
√6ᵗʰ **T22.51** Corrosion of first degree of forearm
　√7ᵗʰ **T22.511** Corrosion of first degree of right forearm
　√7ᵗʰ **T22.512** Corrosion of first degree of left forearm

√6ᵗʰ **T22.519** Corrosion of first degree of unspecified forearm

√6ᵗʰ **T22.52** Corrosion of first degree of elbow
- √7ᵗʰ **T22.521** Corrosion of first degree of right elbow
- √7ᵗʰ **T22.522** Corrosion of first degree of left elbow
- √7ᵗʰ **T22.529** Corrosion of first degree of unspecified elbow

√6ᵗʰ **T22.53** Corrosion of first degree of upper arm
- √7ᵗʰ **T22.531** Corrosion of first degree of right upper arm
- √7ᵗʰ **T22.532** Corrosion of first degree of left upper arm
- √7ᵗʰ **T22.539** Corrosion of first degree of unspecified upper arm

√6ᵗʰ **T22.54** Corrosion of first degree of axilla
- √7ᵗʰ **T22.541** Corrosion of first degree of right axilla
- √7ᵗʰ **T22.542** Corrosion of first degree of left axilla
- √7ᵗʰ **T22.549** Corrosion of first degree of unspecified axilla

√6ᵗʰ **T22.55** Corrosion of first degree of shoulder
- √7ᵗʰ **T22.551** Corrosion of first degree of right shoulder
- √7ᵗʰ **T22.552** Corrosion of first degree of left shoulder
- √7ᵗʰ **T22.559** Corrosion of first degree of unspecified shoulder

√6ᵗʰ **T22.56** Corrosion of first degree of scapular region
- √7ᵗʰ **T22.561** Corrosion of first degree of right scapular region
- √7ᵗʰ **T22.562** Corrosion of first degree of left scapular region
- √7ᵗʰ **T22.569** Corrosion of first degree of unspecified scapular region

√6ᵗʰ **T22.59** Corrosion of first degree of multiple sites of shoulder and upper limb, except wrist and hand
- √7ᵗʰ **T22.591** Corrosion of first degree of multiple sites of right shoulder and upper limb, except wrist and hand
- √7ᵗʰ **T22.592** Corrosion of first degree of multiple sites of left shoulder and upper limb, except wrist and hand
- √7ᵗʰ **T22.599** Corrosion of first degree of multiple sites of unspecified shoulder and upper limb, except wrist and hand

√5ᵗʰ **T22.6** Corrosion of second degree of shoulder and upper limb, except wrist and hand
Code first (T51-T65) to identify chemical and intent
Use additional external cause code to identify place (Y92)

√x7ᵗʰ **T22.60** Corrosion of second degree of shoulder and upper limb, except wrist and hand, unspecified site

√6ᵗʰ **T22.61** Corrosion of second degree of forearm
- √7ᵗʰ **T22.611** Corrosion of second degree of right forearm
- √7ᵗʰ **T22.612** Corrosion of second degree of left forearm
- √7ᵗʰ **T22.619** Corrosion of second degree of unspecified forearm

√6ᵗʰ **T22.62** Corrosion of second degree of elbow
- √7ᵗʰ **T22.621** Corrosion of second degree of right elbow
- √7ᵗʰ **T22.622** Corrosion of second degree of left elbow
- √7ᵗʰ **T22.629** Corrosion of second degree of unspecified elbow

√6ᵗʰ **T22.63** Corrosion of second degree of upper arm
- √7ᵗʰ **T22.631** Corrosion of second degree of right upper arm
- √7ᵗʰ **T22.632** Corrosion of second degree of left upper arm
- √7ᵗʰ **T22.639** Corrosion of second degree of unspecified upper arm

√6ᵗʰ **T22.64** Corrosion of second degree of axilla
- √7ᵗʰ **T22.641** Corrosion of second degree of right axilla
- √7ᵗʰ **T22.642** Corrosion of second degree of left axilla
- √7ᵗʰ **T22.649** Corrosion of second degree of unspecified axilla

√6ᵗʰ **T22.65** Corrosion of second degree of shoulder
- √7ᵗʰ **T22.651** Corrosion of second degree of right shoulder
- √7ᵗʰ **T22.652** Corrosion of second degree of left shoulder
- √7ᵗʰ **T22.659** Corrosion of second degree of unspecified shoulder

√6ᵗʰ **T22.66** Corrosion of second degree of scapular region
- √7ᵗʰ **T22.661** Corrosion of second degree of right scapular region
- √7ᵗʰ **T22.662** Corrosion of second degree of left scapular region
- √7ᵗʰ **T22.669** Corrosion of second degree of unspecified scapular region

√6ᵗʰ **T22.69** Corrosion of second degree of multiple sites of shoulder and upper limb, except wrist and hand
- √7ᵗʰ **T22.691** Corrosion of second degree of multiple sites of right shoulder and upper limb, except wrist and hand
- √7ᵗʰ **T22.692** Corrosion of second degree of multiple sites of left shoulder and upper limb, except wrist and hand
- √7ᵗʰ **T22.699** Corrosion of second degree of multiple sites of unspecified shoulder and upper limb, except wrist and hand

√5ᵗʰ **T22.7** Corrosion of third degree of shoulder and upper limb, except wrist and hand
Code first (T51-T65) to identify chemical and intent
Use additional external cause code to identify place (Y92)

√x7ᵗʰ **T22.70** Corrosion of third degree of shoulder and upper limb, except wrist and hand, unspecified site

√6ᵗʰ **T22.71** Corrosion of third degree of forearm
- √7ᵗʰ **T22.711** Corrosion of third degree of right forearm
- √7ᵗʰ **T22.712** Corrosion of third degree of left forearm
- √7ᵗʰ **T22.719** Corrosion of third degree of unspecified forearm

√6ᵗʰ **T22.72** Corrosion of third degree of elbow
- √7ᵗʰ **T22.721** Corrosion of third degree of right elbow
- √7ᵗʰ **T22.722** Corrosion of third degree of left elbow
- √7ᵗʰ **T22.729** Corrosion of third degree of unspecified elbow

√6ᵗʰ **T22.73** Corrosion of third degree of upper arm
- √7ᵗʰ **T22.731** Corrosion of third degree of right upper arm
- √7ᵗʰ **T22.732** Corrosion of third degree of left upper arm
- √7ᵗʰ **T22.739** Corrosion of third degree of unspecified upper arm

√6ᵗʰ **T22.74** Corrosion of third degree of axilla
- √7ᵗʰ **T22.741** Corrosion of third degree of right axilla
- √7ᵗʰ **T22.742** Corrosion of third degree of left axilla
- √7ᵗʰ **T22.749** Corrosion of third degree of unspecified axilla

√6ᵗʰ **T22.75** Corrosion of third degree of shoulder
- √7ᵗʰ **T22.751** Corrosion of third degree of right shoulder
- √7ᵗʰ **T22.752** Corrosion of third degree of left shoulder
- √7ᵗʰ **T22.759** Corrosion of third degree of unspecified shoulder

√6ᵗʰ **T22.76** Corrosion of third degree of scapular region
- √7ᵗʰ **T22.761** Corrosion of third degree of right scapular region
- √7ᵗʰ **T22.762** Corrosion of third degree of left scapular region
- √7ᵗʰ **T22.769** Corrosion of third degree of unspecified scapular region

√6ᵗʰ **T22.79** Corrosion of third degree of multiple sites of shoulder and upper limb, except wrist and hand
- √7ᵗʰ **T22.791** Corrosion of third degree of multiple sites of right shoulder and upper limb, except wrist and hand
- √7ᵗʰ **T22.792** Corrosion of third degree of multiple sites of left shoulder and upper limb, except wrist and hand
- √7ᵗʰ **T22.799** Corrosion of third degree of multiple sites of unspecified shoulder and upper limb, except wrist and hand

Chapter 19. Injury, Poisoning and Certain Other Consequences of External Causes

✓4ᵗʰ **T23 Burn and corrosion of wrist and hand**

     AHA: 2015, 1Q, 19

> The appropriate 7th character is to be added to each code from category T23.
> A   initial encounter
> D   subsequent encounter
> S   sequela

✓5ᵗʰ **T23.0 Burn of unspecified degree of wrist and hand**

     Use additional external cause code to identify the source, place and intent of the burn (X00-X19, X75-X77, X96-X98, Y92)

   ✓6ᵗʰ **T23.00 Burn of unspecified degree of hand, unspecified site**

     ✓7ᵗʰ **T23.001** Burn of unspecified degree of right hand, unspecified site

     ✓7ᵗʰ **T23.002** Burn of unspecified degree of left hand, unspecified site

     ✓7ᵗʰ **T23.009** Burn of unspecified degree of unspecified hand, unspecified site

   ✓6ᵗʰ **T23.01 Burn of unspecified degree of thumb (nail)**

     ✓7ᵗʰ **T23.011** Burn of unspecified degree of right thumb (nail)

     ✓7ᵗʰ **T23.012** Burn of unspecified degree of left thumb (nail)

     ✓7ᵗʰ **T23.019** Burn of unspecified degree of unspecified thumb (nail)

   ✓6ᵗʰ **T23.02 Burn of unspecified degree of single finger (nail) except thumb**

     ✓7ᵗʰ **T23.021** Burn of unspecified degree of single right finger (nail) except thumb

     ✓7ᵗʰ **T23.022** Burn of unspecified degree of single left finger (nail) except thumb

     ✓7ᵗʰ **T23.029** Burn of unspecified degree of unspecified single finger (nail) except thumb

   ✓6ᵗʰ **T23.03 Burn of unspecified degree of multiple fingers (nail), not including thumb**

     ✓7ᵗʰ **T23.031** Burn of unspecified degree of multiple right fingers (nail), not including thumb

     ✓7ᵗʰ **T23.032** Burn of unspecified degree of multiple left fingers (nail), not including thumb

     ✓7ᵗʰ **T23.039** Burn of unspecified degree of unspecified multiple fingers (nail), not including thumb

   ✓6ᵗʰ **T23.04 Burn of unspecified degree of multiple fingers (nail), including thumb**

     ✓7ᵗʰ **T23.041** Burn of unspecified degree of multiple right fingers (nail), including thumb

     ✓7ᵗʰ **T23.042** Burn of unspecified degree of multiple left fingers (nail), including thumb

     ✓7ᵗʰ **T23.049** Burn of unspecified degree of unspecified multiple fingers (nail), including thumb

   ✓6ᵗʰ **T23.05 Burn of unspecified degree of palm**

     ✓7ᵗʰ **T23.051** Burn of unspecified degree of right palm

     ✓7ᵗʰ **T23.052** Burn of unspecified degree of left palm

     ✓7ᵗʰ **T23.059** Burn of unspecified degree of unspecified palm

   ✓6ᵗʰ **T23.06 Burn of unspecified degree of back of hand**

     ✓7ᵗʰ **T23.061** Burn of unspecified degree of back of right hand

     ✓7ᵗʰ **T23.062** Burn of unspecified degree of back of left hand

     ✓7ᵗʰ **T23.069** Burn of unspecified degree of back of unspecified hand

   ✓6ᵗʰ **T23.07 Burn of unspecified degree of wrist**

     ✓7ᵗʰ **T23.071** Burn of unspecified degree of right wrist

     ✓7ᵗʰ **T23.072** Burn of unspecified degree of left wrist

     ✓7ᵗʰ **T23.079** Burn of unspecified degree of unspecified wrist

   ✓6ᵗʰ **T23.09 Burn of unspecified degree of multiple sites of wrist and hand**

     ✓7ᵗʰ **T23.091** Burn of unspecified degree of multiple sites of right wrist and hand

     ✓7ᵗʰ **T23.092** Burn of unspecified degree of multiple sites of left wrist and hand

     ✓7ᵗʰ **T23.099** Burn of unspecified degree of multiple sites of unspecified wrist and hand

✓5ᵗʰ **T23.1 Burn of first degree of wrist and hand**

     Use additional external cause code to identify the source, place and intent of the burn (X00-X19, X75-X77, X96-X98, Y92)

   ✓6ᵗʰ **T23.10 Burn of first degree of hand, unspecified site**

     ✓7ᵗʰ **T23.101** Burn of first degree of right hand, unspecified site

     ✓7ᵗʰ **T23.102** Burn of first degree of left hand, unspecified site

     ✓7ᵗʰ **T23.109** Burn of first degree of unspecified hand, unspecified site

   ✓6ᵗʰ **T23.11 Burn of first degree of thumb (nail)**

     ✓7ᵗʰ **T23.111** Burn of first degree of right thumb (nail)

     ✓7ᵗʰ **T23.112** Burn of first degree of left thumb (nail)

     ✓7ᵗʰ **T23.119** Burn of first degree of unspecified thumb (nail)

   ✓6ᵗʰ **T23.12 Burn of first degree of single finger (nail) except thumb**

     ✓7ᵗʰ **T23.121** Burn of first degree of single right finger (nail) except thumb

     ✓7ᵗʰ **T23.122** Burn of first degree of single left finger (nail) except thumb

     ✓7ᵗʰ **T23.129** Burn of first degree of unspecified single finger (nail) except thumb

   ✓6ᵗʰ **T23.13 Burn of first degree of multiple fingers (nail), not including thumb**

     ✓7ᵗʰ **T23.131** Burn of first degree of multiple right fingers (nail), not including thumb

     ✓7ᵗʰ **T23.132** Burn of first degree of multiple left fingers (nail), not including thumb

     ✓7ᵗʰ **T23.139** Burn of first degree of unspecified multiple fingers (nail), not including thumb

   ✓6ᵗʰ **T23.14 Burn of first degree of multiple fingers (nail), including thumb**

     ✓7ᵗʰ **T23.141** Burn of first degree of multiple right fingers (nail), including thumb

     ✓7ᵗʰ **T23.142** Burn of first degree of multiple left fingers (nail), including thumb

     ✓7ᵗʰ **T23.149** Burn of first degree of unspecified multiple fingers (nail), including thumb

   ✓6ᵗʰ **T23.15 Burn of first degree of palm**

     ✓7ᵗʰ **T23.151** Burn of first degree of right palm

     ✓7ᵗʰ **T23.152** Burn of first degree of left palm

     ✓7ᵗʰ **T23.159** Burn of first degree of unspecified palm

   ✓6ᵗʰ **T23.16 Burn of first degree of back of hand**

     ✓7ᵗʰ **T23.161** Burn of first degree of back of right hand

     ✓7ᵗʰ **T23.162** Burn of first degree of back of left hand

     ✓7ᵗʰ **T23.169** Burn of first degree of back of unspecified hand

   ✓6ᵗʰ **T23.17 Burn of first degree of wrist**

     ✓7ᵗʰ **T23.171** Burn of first degree of right wrist

     ✓7ᵗʰ **T23.172** Burn of first degree of left wrist

     ✓7ᵗʰ **T23.179** Burn of first degree of unspecified wrist

   ✓6ᵗʰ **T23.19 Burn of first degree of multiple sites of wrist and hand**

     ✓7ᵗʰ **T23.191** Burn of first degree of multiple sites of right wrist and hand

     ✓7ᵗʰ **T23.192** Burn of first degree of multiple sites of left wrist and hand

     ✓7ᵗʰ **T23.199** Burn of first degree of multiple sites of unspecified wrist and hand

✓5ᵗʰ **T23.2 Burn of second degree of wrist and hand**

     Use additional external cause code to identify the source, place and intent of the burn (X00-X19, X75-X77, X96-X98, Y92)

   ✓6ᵗʰ **T23.20 Burn of second degree of hand, unspecified site**

     ✓7ᵗʰ **T23.201** Burn of second degree of right hand, unspecified site

     ✓7ᵗʰ **T23.202** Burn of second degree of left hand, unspecified site

     ✓7ᵗʰ **T23.209** Burn of second degree of unspecified hand, unspecified site

   ✓6ᵗʰ **T23.21 Burn of second degree of thumb (nail)**

     ✓7ᵗʰ **T23.211** Burn of second degree of right thumb (nail)

     ✓7ᵗʰ **T23.212** Burn of second degree of left thumb (nail)

     ✓7ᵗʰ **T23.219** Burn of second degree of unspecified thumb (nail)

N Newborn: 0   P Pediatric: 0-17   M Maternity: 12-55   A Adult: 15-124   CH Comorbidity High   CL Comorbidity Low   NCDx Noncancer Dx   PDx Primary Dx

1074   ICD-10-CM 2020

√6ᵗʰ **T23.22** **Burn of second degree of** single finger (nail) except thumb
- √7ᵗʰ **T23.221** Burn of second degree of single right finger (nail) except thumb
- √7ᵗʰ **T23.222** Burn of second degree of single left finger (nail) except thumb
- √7ᵗʰ **T23.229** Burn of second degree of unspecified single finger (nail) except thumb

√6ᵗʰ **T23.23** **Burn of second degree of** multiple fingers (nail), not including thumb
- √7ᵗʰ **T23.231** Burn of second degree of multiple right fingers (nail), not including thumb
- √7ᵗʰ **T23.232** Burn of second degree of multiple left fingers (nail), not including thumb
- √7ᵗʰ **T23.239** Burn of second degree of unspecified multiple fingers (nail), not including thumb

√6ᵗʰ **T23.24** **Burn of second degree of** multiple fingers (nail), including thumb
- √7ᵗʰ **T23.241** Burn of second degree of multiple right fingers (nail), including thumb
- √7ᵗʰ **T23.242** Burn of second degree of multiple left fingers (nail), including thumb
- √7ᵗʰ **T23.249** Burn of second degree of unspecified multiple fingers (nail), including thumb

√6ᵗʰ **T23.25** **Burn of second degree of** palm
- √7ᵗʰ **T23.251** Burn of second degree of right palm
- √7ᵗʰ **T23.252** Burn of second degree of left palm
- √7ᵗʰ **T23.259** Burn of second degree of unspecified palm

√6ᵗʰ **T23.26** **Burn of second degree of back of** hand
- √7ᵗʰ **T23.261** Burn of second degree of back of right hand
- √7ᵗʰ **T23.262** Burn of second degree of back of left hand
- √7ᵗʰ **T23.269** Burn of second degree of back of unspecified hand

√6ᵗʰ **T23.27** **Burn of second degree of** wrist
- √7ᵗʰ **T23.271** Burn of second degree of right wrist
- √7ᵗʰ **T23.272** Burn of second degree of left wrist
- √7ᵗʰ **T23.279** Burn of second degree of unspecified wrist

√6ᵗʰ **T23.29** **Burn of second degree of** multiple sites of wrist and hand
- √7ᵗʰ **T23.291** Burn of second degree of multiple sites of right wrist and hand
- √7ᵗʰ **T23.292** Burn of second degree of multiple sites of left wrist and hand
- √7ᵗʰ **T23.299** Burn of second degree of multiple sites of unspecified wrist and hand

√5ᵗʰ **T23.3** **Burn of** third degree **of wrist and hand**
> Use additional external cause code to identify the source, place and intent of the burn (X00-X19, X75-X77, X96-X98, Y92)

√6ᵗʰ **T23.30** **Burn of third degree of hand, unspecified site**
> **AHA:** 2016,2Q,5
- √7ᵗʰ **T23.301** Burn of third degree of right hand, unspecified site
- √7ᵗʰ **T23.302** Burn of third degree of left hand, unspecified site
- √7ᵗʰ **T23.309** Burn of third degree of unspecified hand, unspecified site

√6ᵗʰ **T23.31** **Burn of third degree of** thumb (nail)
- √7ᵗʰ **T23.311** Burn of third degree of right thumb (nail)
- √7ᵗʰ **T23.312** Burn of third degree of left thumb (nail)
- √7ᵗʰ **T23.319** Burn of third degree of unspecified thumb (nail)

√6ᵗʰ **T23.32** **Burn of third degree of** single finger (nail) except thumb
- √7ᵗʰ **T23.321** Burn of third degree of single right finger (nail) except thumb
- √7ᵗʰ **T23.322** Burn of third degree of single left finger (nail) except thumb
- √7ᵗʰ **T23.329** Burn of third degree of unspecified single finger (nail) except thumb

√6ᵗʰ **T23.33** **Burn of third degree of** multiple fingers (nail), not including thumb
- √7ᵗʰ **T23.331** Burn of third degree of multiple right fingers (nail), not including thumb
- √7ᵗʰ **T23.332** Burn of third degree of multiple left fingers (nail), not including thumb

√6ᵗʰ **T23.339** Burn of third degree of unspecified multiple fingers (nail), not including thumb

√6ᵗʰ **T23.34** **Burn of third degree of** multiple fingers (nail), including thumb
- √7ᵗʰ **T23.341** Burn of third degree of multiple right fingers (nail), including thumb
- √7ᵗʰ **T23.342** Burn of third degree of multiple left fingers (nail), including thumb
- √7ᵗʰ **T23.349** Burn of third degree of unspecified multiple fingers (nail), including thumb

√6ᵗʰ **T23.35** **Burn of third degree of** palm
- √7ᵗʰ **T23.351** Burn of third degree of right palm
- √7ᵗʰ **T23.352** Burn of third degree of left palm
- √7ᵗʰ **T23.359** Burn of third degree of unspecified palm

√6ᵗʰ **T23.36** **Burn of third degree of** back of hand
- √7ᵗʰ **T23.361** Burn of third degree of back of right hand
- √7ᵗʰ **T23.362** Burn of third degree of back of left hand
- √7ᵗʰ **T23.369** Burn of third degree of back of unspecified hand

√6ᵗʰ **T23.37** **Burn of third degree of** wrist
- √7ᵗʰ **T23.371** Burn of third degree of right wrist
- √7ᵗʰ **T23.372** Burn of third degree of left wrist
- √7ᵗʰ **T23.379** Burn of third degree of unspecified wrist

√6ᵗʰ **T23.39** **Burn of third degree of** multiple sites of wrist and hand
- √7ᵗʰ **T23.391** Burn of third degree of multiple sites of right wrist and hand
- √7ᵗʰ **T23.392** Burn of third degree of multiple sites of left wrist and hand
- √7ᵗʰ **T23.399** Burn of third degree of multiple sites of unspecified wrist and hand

√5ᵗʰ **T23.4** **Corrosion of unspecified degree of wrist and hand**
> Code first (T51-T65) to identify chemical and intent
> Use additional external cause code to identify place (Y92)

√6ᵗʰ **T23.40** **Corrosion of unspecified degree of hand, unspecified site**
- √7ᵗʰ **T23.401** Corrosion of unspecified degree of right hand, unspecified site
- √7ᵗʰ **T23.402** Corrosion of unspecified degree of left hand, unspecified site
- √7ᵗʰ **T23.409** Corrosion of unspecified degree of unspecified hand, unspecified site

√6ᵗʰ **T23.41** **Corrosion of unspecified degree of** thumb (nail)
- √7ᵗʰ **T23.411** Corrosion of unspecified degree of right thumb (nail)
- √7ᵗʰ **T23.412** Corrosion of unspecified degree of left thumb (nail)
- √7ᵗʰ **T23.419** Corrosion of unspecified degree of unspecified thumb (nail)

√6ᵗʰ **T23.42** **Corrosion of unspecified degree of** single finger (nail) except thumb
- √7ᵗʰ **T23.421** Corrosion of unspecified degree of single right finger (nail) except thumb
- √7ᵗʰ **T23.422** Corrosion of unspecified degree of single left finger (nail) except thumb
- √7ᵗʰ **T23.429** Corrosion of unspecified degree of unspecified single finger (nail) except thumb

√6ᵗʰ **T23.43** **Corrosion of unspecified degree of** multiple fingers (nail), not including thumb
- √7ᵗʰ **T23.431** Corrosion of unspecified degree of multiple right fingers (nail), not including thumb
- √7ᵗʰ **T23.432** Corrosion of unspecified degree of multiple left fingers (nail), not including thumb
- √7ᵗʰ **T23.439** Corrosion of unspecified degree of unspecified multiple fingers (nail), not including thumb

√6ᵗʰ **T23.44** **Corrosion of unspecified degree of** multiple fingers (nail), including thumb
- √7ᵗʰ **T23.441** Corrosion of unspecified degree of multiple right fingers (nail), including thumb
- √7ᵗʰ **T23.442** Corrosion of unspecified degree of multiple left fingers (nail), including thumb

☑ Additional Character Required   √x7ᵗʰ Placeholder Alert   Manifestation   Unspecified Dx   ►◄ Revised Text   ● New Code   ▲ Revised Title

ICD-10-CM 2020   **1075**

Chapter 19. Injury, Poisoning and Certain Other Consequences of External Causes

√7ᵗʰ **T23.449** Corrosion of unspecified degree of unspecified multiple fingers (nail), including thumb

√6ᵗʰ **T23.45** Corrosion of unspecified degree of palm
- √7ᵗʰ **T23.451** Corrosion of unspecified degree of right palm
- √7ᵗʰ **T23.452** Corrosion of unspecified degree of left palm
- √7ᵗʰ **T23.459** Corrosion of unspecified degree of unspecified palm

√6ᵗʰ **T23.46** Corrosion of unspecified degree of back of hand
- √7ᵗʰ **T23.461** Corrosion of unspecified degree of back of right hand
- √7ᵗʰ **T23.462** Corrosion of unspecified degree of back of left hand
- √7ᵗʰ **T23.469** Corrosion of unspecified degree of back of unspecified hand

√6ᵗʰ **T23.47** Corrosion of unspecified degree of wrist
- √7ᵗʰ **T23.471** Corrosion of unspecified degree of right wrist
- √7ᵗʰ **T23.472** Corrosion of unspecified degree of left wrist
- √7ᵗʰ **T23.479** Corrosion of unspecified degree of unspecified wrist

√6ᵗʰ **T23.49** Corrosion of unspecified degree of multiple sites of wrist and hand
- √7ᵗʰ **T23.491** Corrosion of unspecified degree of multiple sites of right wrist and hand
- √7ᵗʰ **T23.492** Corrosion of unspecified degree of multiple sites of left wrist and hand
- √7ᵗʰ **T23.499** Corrosion of unspecified degree of multiple sites of unspecified wrist and hand

√5ᵗʰ **T23.5** Corrosion of first degree of wrist and hand
Code first (T51-T65) to identify chemical and intent
Use additional external cause code to identify place (Y92)

√6ᵗʰ **T23.50** Corrosion of first degree of hand, unspecified site
- √7ᵗʰ **T23.501** Corrosion of first degree of right hand, unspecified site
- √7ᵗʰ **T23.502** Corrosion of first degree of left hand, unspecified site
- √7ᵗʰ **T23.509** Corrosion of first degree of unspecified hand, unspecified site

√6ᵗʰ **T23.51** Corrosion of first degree of thumb (nail)
- √7ᵗʰ **T23.511** Corrosion of first degree of right thumb (nail)
- √7ᵗʰ **T23.512** Corrosion of first degree of left thumb (nail)
- √7ᵗʰ **T23.519** Corrosion of first degree of unspecified thumb (nail)

√6ᵗʰ **T23.52** Corrosion of first degree of single finger (nail) except thumb
- √7ᵗʰ **T23.521** Corrosion of first degree of single right finger (nail) except thumb
- √7ᵗʰ **T23.522** Corrosion of first degree of single left finger (nail) except thumb
- √7ᵗʰ **T23.529** Corrosion of first degree of unspecified single finger (nail) except thumb

√6ᵗʰ **T23.53** Corrosion of first degree of multiple fingers (nail), not including thumb
- √7ᵗʰ **T23.531** Corrosion of first degree of multiple right fingers (nail), not including thumb
- √7ᵗʰ **T23.532** Corrosion of first degree of multiple left fingers (nail), not including thumb
- √7ᵗʰ **T23.539** Corrosion of first degree of unspecified multiple fingers (nail), not including thumb

√6ᵗʰ **T23.54** Corrosion of first degree of multiple fingers (nail), including thumb
- √7ᵗʰ **T23.541** Corrosion of first degree of multiple right fingers (nail), including thumb
- √7ᵗʰ **T23.542** Corrosion of first degree of multiple left fingers (nail), including thumb
- √7ᵗʰ **T23.549** Corrosion of first degree of unspecified multiple fingers (nail), including thumb

√6ᵗʰ **T23.55** Corrosion of first degree of palm
- √7ᵗʰ **T23.551** Corrosion of first degree of right palm
- √7ᵗʰ **T23.552** Corrosion of first degree of left palm
- √7ᵗʰ **T23.559** Corrosion of first degree of unspecified palm

√6ᵗʰ **T23.56** Corrosion of first degree of back of hand
- √7ᵗʰ **T23.561** Corrosion of first degree of back of right hand
- √7ᵗʰ **T23.562** Corrosion of first degree of back of left hand
- √7ᵗʰ **T23.569** Corrosion of first degree of back of unspecified hand

√6ᵗʰ **T23.57** Corrosion of first degree of wrist
- √7ᵗʰ **T23.571** Corrosion of first degree of right wrist
- √7ᵗʰ **T23.572** Corrosion of first degree of left wrist
- √7ᵗʰ **T23.579** Corrosion of first degree of unspecified wrist

√6ᵗʰ **T23.59** Corrosion of first degree of multiple sites of wrist and hand
- √7ᵗʰ **T23.591** Corrosion of first degree of multiple sites of right wrist and hand
- √7ᵗʰ **T23.592** Corrosion of first degree of multiple sites of left wrist and hand
- √7ᵗʰ **T23.599** Corrosion of first degree of multiple sites of unspecified wrist and hand

√5ᵗʰ **T23.6** Corrosion of second degree of wrist and hand
Code first (T51-T65) to identify chemical and intent
Use additional external cause code to identify place (Y92)

√6ᵗʰ **T23.60** Corrosion of second degree of hand, unspecified site
- √7ᵗʰ **T23.601** Corrosion of second degree of right hand, unspecified site
- √7ᵗʰ **T23.602** Corrosion of second degree of left hand, unspecified site
- √7ᵗʰ **T23.609** Corrosion of second degree of unspecified hand, unspecified site

√6ᵗʰ **T23.61** Corrosion of second degree of thumb (nail)
- √7ᵗʰ **T23.611** Corrosion of second degree of right thumb (nail)
- √7ᵗʰ **T23.612** Corrosion of second degree of left thumb (nail)
- √7ᵗʰ **T23.619** Corrosion of second degree of unspecified thumb (nail)

√6ᵗʰ **T23.62** Corrosion of second degree of single finger (nail) except thumb
- √7ᵗʰ **T23.621** Corrosion of second degree of single right finger (nail) except thumb
- √7ᵗʰ **T23.622** Corrosion of second degree of single left finger (nail) except thumb
- √7ᵗʰ **T23.629** Corrosion of second degree of unspecified single finger (nail) except thumb

√6ᵗʰ **T23.63** Corrosion of second degree of multiple fingers (nail), not including thumb
- √7ᵗʰ **T23.631** Corrosion of second degree of multiple right fingers (nail), not including thumb
- √7ᵗʰ **T23.632** Corrosion of second degree of multiple left fingers (nail), not including thumb
- √7ᵗʰ **T23.639** Corrosion of second degree of unspecified multiple fingers (nail), not including thumb

√6ᵗʰ **T23.64** Corrosion of second degree of multiple fingers (nail), including thumb
- √7ᵗʰ **T23.641** Corrosion of second degree of multiple right fingers (nail), including thumb
- √7ᵗʰ **T23.642** Corrosion of second degree of multiple left fingers (nail), including thumb
- √7ᵗʰ **T23.649** Corrosion of second degree of unspecified multiple fingers (nail), including thumb

√6ᵗʰ **T23.65** Corrosion of second degree of palm
- √7ᵗʰ **T23.651** Corrosion of second degree of right palm
- √7ᵗʰ **T23.652** Corrosion of second degree of left palm
- √7ᵗʰ **T23.659** Corrosion of second degree of unspecified palm

√6ᵗʰ **T23.66** Corrosion of second degree of back of hand
- √7ᵗʰ **T23.661** Corrosion of second degree back of right hand
- √7ᵗʰ **T23.662** Corrosion of second degree back of left hand
- √7ᵗʰ **T23.669** Corrosion of second degree back of unspecified hand

√6ᵗʰ **T23.67** Corrosion of second degree of wrist
- √7ᵗʰ **T23.671** Corrosion of second degree of right wrist
- √7ᵗʰ **T23.672** Corrosion of second degree of left wrist
- √7ᵗʰ **T23.679** Corrosion of second degree of unspecified wrist

√6ᵗʰ **T23.69** **Corrosion of second degree of** multiple sites **of wrist and hand**

√7ᵗʰ **T23.691** Corrosion of second degree of multiple sites of right **wrist and hand**

√7ᵗʰ **T23.692** Corrosion of second degree of multiple sites of left **wrist and hand**

√7ᵗʰ **T23.699** Corrosion of second degree of multiple sites of unspecified wrist and hand

√5ᵗʰ **T23.7** **Corrosion of** third degree **of wrist and hand**

Code first (T51-T65) to identify chemical and intent
Use additional external cause code to identify place (Y92)

√6ᵗʰ **T23.70** **Corrosion of third degree of hand, unspecified site**

√7ᵗʰ **T23.701** Corrosion of third degree of right **hand, unspecified site**

√7ᵗʰ **T23.702** Corrosion of third degree of left **hand, unspecified site**

√7ᵗʰ **T23.709** Corrosion of third degree of unspecified **hand, unspecified site**

√6ᵗʰ **T23.71** **Corrosion of third degree of** thumb **(nail)**

√7ᵗʰ **T23.711** Corrosion of third degree of right **thumb (nail)**

√7ᵗʰ **T23.712** Corrosion of third degree of left **thumb (nail)**

√7ᵗʰ **T23.719** Corrosion of third degree of unspecified **thumb (nail)**

√6ᵗʰ **T23.72** **Corrosion of third degree of** single finger **(nail) except thumb**

√7ᵗʰ **T23.721** Corrosion of third degree of single right **finger (nail) except thumb**

√7ᵗʰ **T23.722** Corrosion of third degree of single left **finger (nail) except thumb**

√7ᵗʰ **T23.729** Corrosion of third degree of unspecified single finger (nail) except thumb

√6ᵗʰ **T23.73** **Corrosion of third degree of** multiple fingers **(nail), not including thumb**

√7ᵗʰ **T23.731** Corrosion of third degree of multiple right **fingers (nail), not including thumb**

√7ᵗʰ **T23.732** Corrosion of third degree of multiple left **fingers (nail), not including thumb**

√7ᵗʰ **T23.739** Corrosion of third degree of unspecified multiple fingers (nail), not including thumb

√6ᵗʰ **T23.74** **Corrosion of third degree of** multiple fingers **(nail), including thumb**

√7ᵗʰ **T23.741** Corrosion of third degree of multiple right **fingers (nail), including thumb**

√7ᵗʰ **T23.742** Corrosion of third degree of multiple left **fingers (nail), including thumb**

√7ᵗʰ **T23.749** Corrosion of third degree of unspecified multiple fingers (nail), including thumb

√6ᵗʰ **T23.75** **Corrosion of third degree of** palm

√7ᵗʰ **T23.751** Corrosion of third degree of right **palm**

√7ᵗʰ **T23.752** Corrosion of third degree of left **palm**

√7ᵗʰ **T23.759** Corrosion of third degree of unspecified palm

√6ᵗʰ **T23.76** **Corrosion of third degree of** back of hand

√7ᵗʰ **T23.761** Corrosion of third degree of back of right **hand**

√7ᵗʰ **T23.762** Corrosion of third degree of back of left **hand**

√7ᵗʰ **T23.769** Corrosion of third degree back of unspecified hand

√6ᵗʰ **T23.77** **Corrosion of third degree of** wrist

√7ᵗʰ **T23.771** Corrosion of third degree of right **wrist**

√7ᵗʰ **T23.772** Corrosion of third degree of left **wrist**

√7ᵗʰ **T23.779** Corrosion of third degree of unspecified wrist

√6ᵗʰ **T23.79** **Corrosion of third degree of** multiple sites **of wrist and hand**

√7ᵗʰ **T23.791** Corrosion of third degree of multiple sites of right **wrist and hand**

√7ᵗʰ **T23.792** Corrosion of third degree of multiple sites of left **wrist and hand**

√7ᵗʰ **T23.799** Corrosion of third degree of multiple sites of unspecified wrist and hand

√4ᵗʰ **T24** **Burn and corrosion of lower limb, except ankle and foot**

EXCLUDES 2   *burn and corrosion of ankle and foot (T25.-)*
burn and corrosion of hip region (T21.-)

The appropriate 7th character is to be added to each code from category T24.
A   initial encounter
D   subsequent encounter
S   sequela

√5ᵗʰ **T24.0** **Burn of unspecified degree of lower limb, except ankle and foot**

Use additional external cause code to identify the source, place and intent of the burn (X00-X19, X75-X77, X96-X98, Y92)

√6ᵗʰ **T24.00** **Burn of unspecified degree of unspecified site of lower limb, except ankle and foot**

√7ᵗʰ **T24.001** Burn of unspecified degree of unspecified site of right **lower limb, except ankle and foot**

√7ᵗʰ **T24.002** Burn of unspecified degree of unspecified site of left **lower limb, except ankle and foot**

√7ᵗʰ **T24.009** Burn of unspecified degree of unspecified site of unspecified lower limb, except ankle and foot

√6ᵗʰ **T24.01** **Burn of unspecified degree of** thigh

√7ᵗʰ **T24.011** Burn of unspecified degree of right **thigh**

√7ᵗʰ **T24.012** Burn of unspecified degree of left **thigh**

√7ᵗʰ **T24.019** Burn of unspecified degree of unspecified **thigh**

√6ᵗʰ **T24.02** **Burn of unspecified degree of** knee

√7ᵗʰ **T24.021** Burn of unspecified degree of right **knee**

√7ᵗʰ **T24.022** Burn of unspecified degree of left **knee**

√7ᵗʰ **T24.029** Burn of unspecified degree of unspecified **knee**

√6ᵗʰ **T24.03** **Burn of unspecified degree of** lower leg

√7ᵗʰ **T24.031** Burn of unspecified degree of right **lower leg**

√7ᵗʰ **T24.032** Burn of unspecified degree of left **lower leg**

√7ᵗʰ **T24.039** Burn of unspecified degree of unspecified **lower leg**

√6ᵗʰ **T24.09** **Burn of unspecified degree of** multiple sites **of lower limb, except ankle and foot**

√7ᵗʰ **T24.091** Burn of unspecified degree of multiple sites of right **lower limb, except ankle and foot**

√7ᵗʰ **T24.092** Burn of unspecified degree of multiple sites of left **lower limb, except ankle and foot**

√7ᵗʰ **T24.099** Burn of unspecified degree of multiple sites of unspecified lower limb, except ankle and foot

√5ᵗʰ **T24.1** **Burn of** first degree **of lower limb, except ankle and foot**

Use additional external cause code to identify the source, place and intent of the burn (X00-X19, X75-X77, X96-X98, Y92)

√6ᵗʰ **T24.10** **Burn of first degree of unspecified site of lower limb, except ankle and foot**

√7ᵗʰ **T24.101** Burn of first degree of unspecified site of right **lower limb, except ankle and foot**

√7ᵗʰ **T24.102** Burn of first degree of unspecified site of left **lower limb, except ankle and foot**

√7ᵗʰ **T24.109** Burn of first degree of unspecified site of unspecified lower limb, except ankle and foot

√6ᵗʰ **T24.11** **Burn of first degree of** thigh

√7ᵗʰ **T24.111** Burn of first degree of right **thigh**

√7ᵗʰ **T24.112** Burn of first degree of left **thigh**

√7ᵗʰ **T24.119** Burn of first degree of unspecified **thigh**

√6ᵗʰ **T24.12** **Burn of first degree of** knee

√7ᵗʰ **T24.121** Burn of first degree of right **knee**

√7ᵗʰ **T24.122** Burn of first degree of left **knee**

√7ᵗʰ **T24.129** Burn of first degree of unspecified **knee**

√6ᵗʰ **T24.13** **Burn of first degree of** lower leg

√7ᵗʰ **T24.131** Burn of first degree of right **lower leg**

√7ᵗʰ **T24.132** Burn of first degree of left **lower leg**

√7ᵗʰ **T24.139** Burn of first degree of unspecified lower leg

---

☑ Additional Character Required   √xⁿ Placeholder Alert   Manifestation   Unspecified Dx   ►◄ Revised Text   ● New Code   ▲ Revised Title

√6ᵗʰ **T24.19** **Burn of first degree of** multiple sites **of lower limb, except ankle and foot**

    √7ᵗʰ **T24.191** Burn of first degree of multiple sites of right lower limb, except ankle and foot

    √7ᵗʰ **T24.192** Burn of first degree of multiple sites of left lower limb, except ankle and foot

    √7ᵗʰ **T24.199** Burn of first degree of multiple sites of unspecified lower limb, except ankle and foot

√5ᵗʰ **T24.2** **Burn of** second degree **of lower limb, except ankle and foot**

    Use additional external cause code to identify the source, place and intent of the burn (X00-X19, X75-X77, X96-X98, Y92)

    √6ᵗʰ **T24.20** **Burn of second degree of unspecified site of lower limb, except ankle and foot**

      √7ᵗʰ **T24.201** Burn of second degree of unspecified site of right lower limb, except ankle and foot

      √7ᵗʰ **T24.202** Burn of second degree of unspecified site of left lower limb, except ankle and foot

      √7ᵗʰ **T24.209** Burn of second degree of unspecified site of unspecified lower limb, except ankle and foot

    √6ᵗʰ **T24.21** **Burn of second degree of** thigh

      √7ᵗʰ **T24.211** Burn of second degree of right thigh

      √7ᵗʰ **T24.212** Burn of second degree of left thigh

      √7ᵗʰ **T24.219** Burn of second degree of unspecified thigh

    √6ᵗʰ **T24.22** **Burn of second degree of** knee

      √7ᵗʰ **T24.221** Burn of second degree of right knee

      √7ᵗʰ **T24.222** Burn of second degree of left knee

      √7ᵗʰ **T24.229** Burn of second degree of unspecified knee

    √6ᵗʰ **T24.23** **Burn of second degree of** lower leg

      √7ᵗʰ **T24.231** Burn of second degree of right lower leg

      √7ᵗʰ **T24.232** Burn of second degree of left lower leg

      √7ᵗʰ **T24.239** Burn of second degree of unspecified lower leg

    √6ᵗʰ **T24.29** **Burn of second degree of** multiple sites **of lower limb, except ankle and foot**

      √7ᵗʰ **T24.291** Burn of second degree of multiple sites of right lower limb, except ankle and foot

      √7ᵗʰ **T24.292** Burn of second degree of multiple sites of left lower limb, except ankle and foot

      √7ᵗʰ **T24.299** Burn of second degree of multiple sites of unspecified lower limb, except ankle and foot

√5ᵗʰ **T24.3** **Burn of** third degree **of lower limb, except ankle and foot**

    Use additional external cause code to identify the source, place and intent of the burn (X00-X19, X75-X77, X96-X98, Y92)

    √6ᵗʰ **T24.30** **Burn of third degree of unspecified site of lower limb, except ankle and foot**

      √7ᵗʰ **T24.301** Burn of third degree of unspecified site of right lower limb, except ankle and foot

      √7ᵗʰ **T24.302** Burn of third degree of unspecified site of left lower limb, except ankle and foot

      √7ᵗʰ **T24.309** Burn of third degree of unspecified site of unspecified lower limb, except ankle and foot

    √6ᵗʰ **T24.31** **Burn of third degree of** thigh

      √7ᵗʰ **T24.311** Burn of third degree of right thigh

      √7ᵗʰ **T24.312** Burn of third degree of left thigh

      √7ᵗʰ **T24.319** Burn of third degree of unspecified thigh

    √6ᵗʰ **T24.32** **Burn of third degree of** knee

      √7ᵗʰ **T24.321** Burn of third degree of right knee

      √7ᵗʰ **T24.322** Burn of third degree of left knee

      √7ᵗʰ **T24.329** Burn of third degree of unspecified knee

    √6ᵗʰ **T24.33** **Burn of third degree of** lower leg

      √7ᵗʰ **T24.331** Burn of third degree of right lower leg

      √7ᵗʰ **T24.332** Burn of third degree of left lower leg

      √7ᵗʰ **T24.339** Burn of third degree of unspecified lower leg

    √6ᵗʰ **T24.39** **Burn of third degree of** multiple sites **of lower limb, except ankle and foot**

      AHA: 2016,2Q,4

      √7ᵗʰ **T24.391** Burn of third degree of multiple sites of right lower limb, except ankle and foot

      √7ᵗʰ **T24.392** Burn of third degree of multiple sites of left lower limb, except ankle and foot

      √7ᵗʰ **T24.399** Burn of third degree of multiple sites of unspecified lower limb, except ankle and foot

√5ᵗʰ **T24.4** **Corrosion of unspecified degree of lower limb, except ankle and foot**

    Code first (T51-T65) to identify chemical and intent

    Use additional external cause code to identify place (Y92)

    √6ᵗʰ **T24.40** **Corrosion of unspecified degree of unspecified site of lower limb, except ankle and foot**

      √7ᵗʰ **T24.401** Corrosion of unspecified degree of unspecified site of right lower limb, except ankle and foot

      √7ᵗʰ **T24.402** Corrosion of unspecified degree of unspecified site of left lower limb, except ankle and foot

      √7ᵗʰ **T24.409** Corrosion of unspecified degree of unspecified site of unspecified lower limb, except ankle and foot

    √6ᵗʰ **T24.41** **Corrosion of unspecified degree of** thigh

      √7ᵗʰ **T24.411** Corrosion of unspecified degree of right thigh

      √7ᵗʰ **T24.412** Corrosion of unspecified degree of left thigh

      √7ᵗʰ **T24.419** Corrosion of unspecified degree of unspecified thigh

    √6ᵗʰ **T24.42** **Corrosion of unspecified degree of** knee

      √7ᵗʰ **T24.421** Corrosion of unspecified degree of right knee

      √7ᵗʰ **T24.422** Corrosion of unspecified degree of left knee

      √7ᵗʰ **T24.429** Corrosion of unspecified degree of unspecified knee

    √6ᵗʰ **T24.43** **Corrosion of unspecified degree of** lower leg

      √7ᵗʰ **T24.431** Corrosion of unspecified degree of right lower leg

      √7ᵗʰ **T24.432** Corrosion of unspecified degree of left lower leg

      √7ᵗʰ **T24.439** Corrosion of unspecified degree of unspecified lower leg

    √6ᵗʰ **T24.49** **Corrosion of unspecified degree of** multiple sites **of lower limb, except ankle and foot**

      √7ᵗʰ **T24.491** Corrosion of unspecified degree of multiple sites of right lower limb, except ankle and foot

      √7ᵗʰ **T24.492** Corrosion of unspecified degree of multiple sites of left lower limb, except ankle and foot

      √7ᵗʰ **T24.499** Corrosion of unspecified degree of multiple sites of unspecified lower limb, except ankle and foot

√5ᵗʰ **T24.5** **Corrosion of** first degree **of lower limb, except ankle and foot**

    Code first (T51-T65) to identify chemical and intent

    Use additional external cause code to identify place (Y92)

    √6ᵗʰ **T24.50** **Corrosion of first degree of unspecified site of lower limb, except ankle and foot**

      √7ᵗʰ **T24.501** Corrosion of first degree of unspecified site of right lower limb, except ankle and foot

      √7ᵗʰ **T24.502** Corrosion of first degree of unspecified site of left lower limb, except ankle and foot

      √7ᵗʰ **T24.509** Corrosion of first degree of unspecified site of unspecified lower limb, except ankle and foot

    √6ᵗʰ **T24.51** **Corrosion of first degree of** thigh

      √7ᵗʰ **T24.511** Corrosion of first degree of right thigh

      √7ᵗʰ **T24.512** Corrosion of first degree of left thigh

      √7ᵗʰ **T24.519** Corrosion of first degree of unspecified thigh

    √6ᵗʰ **T24.52** **Corrosion of first degree of** knee

      √7ᵗʰ **T24.521** Corrosion of first degree of right knee

      √7ᵗʰ **T24.522** Corrosion of first degree of left knee

      √7ᵗʰ **T24.529** Corrosion of first degree of unspecified knee

    √6ᵗʰ **T24.53** **Corrosion of first degree of** lower leg

      √7ᵗʰ **T24.531** Corrosion of first degree of right lower leg

      √7ᵗʰ **T24.532** Corrosion of first degree of left lower leg

      √7ᵗʰ **T24.539** Corrosion of first degree of unspecified lower leg

✓6th **T24.59** **Corrosion of first degree of** multiple sites **of lower limb, except ankle and foot**

    ✓7th **T24.591** **Corrosion of first degree of multiple sites of** right **lower limb, except ankle and foot**

    ✓7th **T24.592** **Corrosion of first degree of multiple sites of** left **lower limb, except ankle and foot**

    ✓7th **T24.599** **Corrosion of first degree of multiple sites of unspecified lower limb, except ankle and foot**

✓5th **T24.6** **Corrosion of** second degree **of lower limb, except ankle and foot**

    Code first (T51-T65) to identify chemical and intent

    Use additional external cause code to identify place (Y92)

✓6th **T24.60** **Corrosion of second degree of unspecified site of lower limb, except ankle and foot**

    ✓7th **T24.601** **Corrosion of second degree of unspecified site of** right **lower limb, except ankle and foot**

    ✓7th **T24.602** **Corrosion of second degree of unspecified site of** left **lower limb, except ankle and foot**

    ✓7th **T24.609** **Corrosion of second degree of unspecified site of unspecified lower limb, except ankle and foot**

✓6th **T24.61** **Corrosion of second degree of** thigh

    ✓7th **T24.611** **Corrosion of second degree of** right **thigh**

    ✓7th **T24.612** **Corrosion of second degree of** left **thigh**

    ✓7th **T24.619** **Corrosion of second degree of unspecified thigh**

✓6th **T24.62** **Corrosion of second degree of** knee

    ✓7th **T24.621** **Corrosion of second degree of** right **knee**

    ✓7th **T24.622** **Corrosion of second degree of** left **knee**

    ✓7th **T24.629** **Corrosion of second degree of unspecified knee**

✓6th **T24.63** **Corrosion of second degree of** lower leg

    ✓7th **T24.631** **Corrosion of second degree of** right **lower leg**

    ✓7th **T24.632** **Corrosion of second degree of** left **lower leg**

    ✓7th **T24.639** **Corrosion of second degree of unspecified lower leg**

✓6th **T24.69** **Corrosion of second degree of** multiple sites **of lower limb, except ankle and foot**

    ✓7th **T24.691** **Corrosion of second degree of multiple sites of** right **lower limb, except ankle and foot**

    ✓7th **T24.692** **Corrosion of second degree of multiple sites of** left **lower limb, except ankle and foot**

    ✓7th **T24.699** **Corrosion of second degree of multiple sites of unspecified lower limb, except ankle and foot**

✓5th **T24.7** **Corrosion of** third degree **of lower limb, except ankle and foot**

    Code first (T51-T65) to identify chemical and intent

    Use additional external cause code to identify place (Y92)

✓6th **T24.70** **Corrosion of third degree of unspecified site of lower limb, except ankle and foot**

    ✓7th **T24.701** **Corrosion of third degree of unspecified site of** right **lower limb, except ankle and foot**

    ✓7th **T24.702** **Corrosion of third degree of unspecified site of** left **lower limb, except ankle and foot**

    ✓7th **T24.709** **Corrosion of third degree of unspecified site of unspecified lower limb, except ankle and foot**

✓6th **T24.71** **Corrosion of third degree of** thigh

    ✓7th **T24.711** **Corrosion of third degree of** right **thigh**

    ✓7th **T24.712** **Corrosion of third degree of** left **thigh**

    ✓7th **T24.719** **Corrosion of third degree of unspecified thigh**

✓6th **T24.72** **Corrosion of third degree of** knee

    ✓7th **T24.721** **Corrosion of third degree of** right **knee**

    ✓7th **T24.722** **Corrosion of third degree of** left **knee**

    ✓7th **T24.729** **Corrosion of third degree of unspecified knee**

✓6th **T24.73** **Corrosion of third degree of** lower leg

    ✓7th **T24.731** **Corrosion of third degree of** right **lower leg**

✓7th **T24.732** **Corrosion of third degree of** left **lower leg**

✓7th **T24.739** **Corrosion of third degree of unspecified lower leg**

✓6th **T24.79** **Corrosion of third degree of** multiple sites **of lower limb, except ankle and foot**

    ✓7th **T24.791** **Corrosion of third degree of multiple sites of** right **lower limb, except ankle and foot**

    ✓7th **T24.792** **Corrosion of third degree of multiple sites of** left **lower limb, except ankle and foot**

    ✓7th **T24.799** **Corrosion of third degree of multiple sites of unspecified lower limb, except ankle and foot**

✓4th **T25** **Burn and corrosion of ankle and foot**

> The appropriate 7th character is to be added to each code from category T25.
> A   initial encounter
> D   subsequent encounter
> S   sequela

✓5th **T25.0** **Burn of unspecified degree of ankle and foot**

    Use additional external cause code to identify the source, place and intent of the burn (X00-X19, X75-X77, X96-X98, Y92)

✓6th **T25.01** **Burn of unspecified degree of** ankle

    ✓7th **T25.011** **Burn of unspecified degree of** right **ankle**

    ✓7th **T25.012** **Burn of unspecified degree of** left **ankle**

    ✓7th **T25.019** **Burn of unspecified degree of unspecified ankle**

✓6th **T25.02** **Burn of unspecified degree of** foot

    EXCLUDES 2   *burn of unspecified degree of toe(s) (nail) (T25.03-)*

    ✓7th **T25.021** **Burn of unspecified degree of** right **foot**

    ✓7th **T25.022** **Burn of unspecified degree of** left **foot**

    ✓7th **T25.029** **Burn of unspecified degree of unspecified foot**

✓6th **T25.03** **Burn of unspecified degree of** toe(s) (nail)

    ✓7th **T25.031** **Burn of unspecified degree of** right **toe(s) (nail)**

    ✓7th **T25.032** **Burn of unspecified degree of** left **toe(s) (nail)**

    ✓7th **T25.039** **Burn of unspecified degree of unspecified toe(s) (nail)**

✓6th **T25.09** **Burn of unspecified degree of** multiple sites **of ankle and foot**

    ✓7th **T25.091** **Burn of unspecified degree of multiple sites of** right **ankle and foot**

    ✓7th **T25.092** **Burn of unspecified degree of multiple sites of** left **ankle and foot**

    ✓7th **T25.099** **Burn of unspecified degree of multiple sites of unspecified ankle and foot**

✓5th **T25.1** **Burn of** first degree **of ankle and foot**

    Use additional external cause code to identify the source, place and intent of the burn (X00-X19, X75-X77, X96-X98, Y92)

✓6th **T25.11** **Burn of first degree of** ankle

    ✓7th **T25.111** **Burn of first degree of** right **ankle**

    ✓7th **T25.112** **Burn of first degree of** left **ankle**

    ✓7th **T25.119** **Burn of first degree of unspecified ankle**

✓6th **T25.12** **Burn of first degree of** foot

    EXCLUDES 2   *burn of first degree of toe(s) (nail) (T25.13-)*

    ✓7th **T25.121** **Burn of first degree of** right **foot**

    ✓7th **T25.122** **Burn of first degree of** left **foot**

    ✓7th **T25.129** **Burn of first degree of unspecified foot**

✓6th **T25.13** **Burn of first degree of** toe(s) (nail)

    ✓7th **T25.131** **Burn of first degree of** right **toe(s) (nail)**

    ✓7th **T25.132** **Burn of first degree of** left **toe(s) (nail)**

    ✓7th **T25.139** **Burn of first degree of unspecified toe(s) (nail)**

✓6th **T25.19** **Burn of first degree of** multiple sites **of ankle and foot**

    ✓7th **T25.191** **Burn of first degree of multiple sites of** right **ankle and foot**

    ✓7th **T25.192** **Burn of first degree of multiple sites of** left **ankle and foot**

    ✓7th **T25.199** **Burn of first degree of multiple sites of unspecified ankle and foot**

✓ Additional Character Required   ✓x7th Placeholder Alert   Manifestation   Unspecified Dx   ▶◀ Revised Text   ● New Code   ▲ Revised Title

√5ᵗʰ **T25.2 Burn of second degree of ankle and foot**

Use additional external cause code to identify the source, place and intent of the burn (X00-X19, X75-X77, X96-X98, Y92)

√6ᵗʰ **T25.21 Burn of second degree of ankle**

√7ᵗʰ **T25.211** Burn of second degree of right ankle

√7ᵗʰ **T25.212** Burn of second degree of left ankle

√7ᵗʰ **T25.219** Burn of second degree of unspecified ankle

√6ᵗʰ **T25.22 Burn of second degree of foot**

EXCLUDES 2 burn of second degree of toe(s) (nail) (T25.23-)

√7ᵗʰ **T25.221** Burn of second degree of right foot

√7ᵗʰ **T25.222** Burn of second degree of left foot

√7ᵗʰ **T25.229** Burn of second degree of unspecified foot

√6ᵗʰ **T25.23 Burn of second degree of toe(s) (nail)**

√7ᵗʰ **T25.231** Burn of second degree of right toe(s) (nail)

√7ᵗʰ **T25.232** Burn of second degree of left toe(s) (nail)

√7ᵗʰ **T25.239** Burn of second degree of unspecified toe(s) (nail)

√6ᵗʰ **T25.29 Burn of second degree of multiple sites of ankle and foot**

√7ᵗʰ **T25.291** Burn of second degree of multiple sites of right ankle and foot

√7ᵗʰ **T25.292** Burn of second degree of multiple sites of left ankle and foot

√7ᵗʰ **T25.299** Burn of second degree of multiple sites of unspecified ankle and foot

√5ᵗʰ **T25.3 Burn of third degree of ankle and foot**

Use additional external cause code to identify the source, place and intent of the burn (X00-X19, X75-X77, X96-X98, Y92)

√6ᵗʰ **T25.31 Burn of third degree of ankle**

√7ᵗʰ **T25.311** Burn of third degree of right ankle

√7ᵗʰ **T25.312** Burn of third degree of left ankle

√7ᵗʰ **T25.319** Burn of third degree of unspecified ankle

√6ᵗʰ **T25.32 Burn of third degree of foot**

EXCLUDES 2 burn of third degree of toe(s) (nail) (T25.33-)

√7ᵗʰ **T25.321** Burn of third degree of right foot

√7ᵗʰ **T25.322** Burn of third degree of left foot

√7ᵗʰ **T25.329** Burn of third degree of unspecified foot

√6ᵗʰ **T25.33 Burn of third degree of toe(s) (nail)**

√7ᵗʰ **T25.331** Burn of third degree of right toe(s) (nail)

√7ᵗʰ **T25.332** Burn of third degree of left toe(s) (nail)

√7ᵗʰ **T25.339** Burn of third degree of unspecified toe(s) (nail)

√6ᵗʰ **T25.39 Burn of third degree of multiple sites of ankle and foot**

√7ᵗʰ **T25.391** Burn of third degree of multiple sites of right ankle and foot

√7ᵗʰ **T25.392** Burn of third degree of multiple sites of left ankle and foot

√7ᵗʰ **T25.399** Burn of third degree of multiple sites of unspecified ankle and foot

√5ᵗʰ **T25.4 Corrosion of unspecified degree of ankle and foot**

Code first (T51-T65) to identify chemical and intent

Use additional external cause code to identify place (Y92)

√6ᵗʰ **T25.41 Corrosion of unspecified degree of ankle**

√7ᵗʰ **T25.411** Corrosion of unspecified degree of right ankle

√7ᵗʰ **T25.412** Corrosion of unspecified degree of left ankle

√7ᵗʰ **T25.419** Corrosion of unspecified degree of unspecified ankle

√6ᵗʰ **T25.42 Corrosion of unspecified degree of foot**

EXCLUDES 2 corrosion of unspecified degree of toe(s) (nail) (T25.43-)

√7ᵗʰ **T25.421** Corrosion of unspecified degree of right foot

√7ᵗʰ **T25.422** Corrosion of unspecified degree of left foot

√7ᵗʰ **T25.429** Corrosion of unspecified degree of unspecified foot

√6ᵗʰ **T25.43 Corrosion of unspecified degree of toe(s) (nail)**

√7ᵗʰ **T25.431** Corrosion of unspecified degree of right toe(s) (nail)

√7ᵗʰ **T25.432** Corrosion of unspecified degree of left toe(s) (nail)

√7ᵗʰ **T25.439** Corrosion of unspecified degree of unspecified toe(s) (nail)

√6ᵗʰ **T25.49 Corrosion of unspecified degree of multiple sites of ankle and foot**

√7ᵗʰ **T25.491** Corrosion of unspecified degree of multiple sites of right ankle and foot

√7ᵗʰ **T25.492** Corrosion of unspecified degree of multiple sites of left ankle and foot

√7ᵗʰ **T25.499** Corrosion of unspecified degree of multiple sites of unspecified ankle and foot

√5ᵗʰ **T25.5 Corrosion of first degree of ankle and foot**

Code first (T51-T65) to identify chemical and intent

Use additional external cause code to identify place (Y92)

√6ᵗʰ **T25.51 Corrosion of first degree of ankle**

√7ᵗʰ **T25.511** Corrosion of first degree of right ankle

√7ᵗʰ **T25.512** Corrosion of first degree of left ankle

√7ᵗʰ **T25.519** Corrosion of first degree of unspecified ankle

√6ᵗʰ **T25.52 Corrosion of first degree of foot**

EXCLUDES 2 corrosion of first degree of toe(s) (nail) (T25.53-)

√7ᵗʰ **T25.521** Corrosion of first degree of right foot

√7ᵗʰ **T25.522** Corrosion of first degree of left foot

√7ᵗʰ **T25.529** Corrosion of first degree of unspecified foot

√6ᵗʰ **T25.53 Corrosion of first degree of toe(s) (nail)**

√7ᵗʰ **T25.531** Corrosion of first degree of right toe(s) (nail)

√7ᵗʰ **T25.532** Corrosion of first degree of left toe(s) (nail)

√7ᵗʰ **T25.539** Corrosion of first degree of unspecified toe(s) (nail)

√6ᵗʰ **T25.59 Corrosion of first degree of multiple sites of ankle and foot**

√7ᵗʰ **T25.591** Corrosion of first degree of multiple sites of right ankle and foot

√7ᵗʰ **T25.592** Corrosion of first degree of multiple sites of left ankle and foot

√7ᵗʰ **T25.599** Corrosion of first degree of multiple sites of unspecified ankle and foot

√5ᵗʰ **T25.6 Corrosion of second degree of ankle and foot**

Code first (T51-T65) to identify chemical and intent

Use additional external cause code to identify place (Y92)

√6ᵗʰ **T25.61 Corrosion of second degree of ankle**

√7ᵗʰ **T25.611** Corrosion of second degree of right ankle

√7ᵗʰ **T25.612** Corrosion of second degree of left ankle

√7ᵗʰ **T25.619** Corrosion of second degree of unspecified ankle

√6ᵗʰ **T25.62 Corrosion of second degree of foot**

EXCLUDES 2 corrosion of second degree of toe(s) (nail) (T25.63-)

√7ᵗʰ **T25.621** Corrosion of second degree of right foot

√7ᵗʰ **T25.622** Corrosion of second degree of left foot

√7ᵗʰ **T25.629** Corrosion of second degree of unspecified foot

√6ᵗʰ **T25.63 Corrosion of second degree of toe(s) (nail)**

√7ᵗʰ **T25.631** Corrosion of second degree of right toe(s) (nail)

√7ᵗʰ **T25.632** Corrosion of second degree of left toe(s) (nail)

√7ᵗʰ **T25.639** Corrosion of second degree of unspecified toe(s) (nail)

√6ᵗʰ **T25.69 Corrosion of second degree of multiple sites of ankle and foot**

√7ᵗʰ **T25.691** Corrosion of second degree of right ankle and foot

√7ᵗʰ **T25.692** Corrosion of second degree of left ankle and foot

√7ᵗʰ **T25.699** Corrosion of second degree of unspecified ankle and foot

N Newborn: 0 P Pediatric: 0-17 M Maternity: 12-55 A Adult: 15-124 CH Comorbidity High CL Comorbidity Low NCDx Noncancer Dx PDx Primary Dx

1080 ICD-10-CM 2020

√5ᵗʰ **T25.7** Corrosion of third degree of ankle and foot

> Code first (T51-T65) to identify chemical and intent
> Use additional external cause code to identify place (Y92)

√6ᵗʰ **T25.71** Corrosion of third degree of ankle

√7ᵗʰ **T25.711** Corrosion of third degree of right ankle

√7ᵗʰ **T25.712** Corrosion of third degree of left ankle

√7ᵗʰ **T25.719** Corrosion of third degree of unspecified ankle

√6ᵗʰ **T25.72** Corrosion of third degree of foot

> EXCLUDES 2 corrosion of third degree of toe(s) (nail) (T25.73-)

√7ᵗʰ **T25.721** Corrosion of third degree of right foot

√7ᵗʰ **T25.722** Corrosion of third degree of left foot

√7ᵗʰ **T25.729** Corrosion of third degree of unspecified foot

√6ᵗʰ **T25.73** Corrosion of third degree of toe(s) (nail)

√7ᵗʰ **T25.731** Corrosion of third degree of right toe(s) (nail)

√7ᵗʰ **T25.732** Corrosion of third degree of left toe(s) (nail)

√7ᵗʰ **T25.739** Corrosion of third degree of unspecified toe(s) (nail)

√6ᵗʰ **T25.79** Corrosion of third degree of multiple sites of ankle and foot

√7ᵗʰ **T25.791** Corrosion of third degree of multiple sites of right ankle and foot

√7ᵗʰ **T25.792** Corrosion of third degree of multiple sites of left ankle and foot

√7ᵗʰ **T25.799** Corrosion of third degree of multiple sites of unspecified ankle and foot

Burns and corrosions confined to eye and internal organs (T26-T28)

√4ᵗʰ **T26** Burn and corrosion confined to eye and adnexa

> The appropriate 7th character is to be added to each code from category T26.
> A initial encounter
> D subsequent encounter
> S sequela

√5ᵗʰ **T26.0** Burn of eyelid and periocular area

> Use additional external cause code to identify the source, place and intent of the burn (X00-X19, X75-X77, X96-X98, Y92)

√7ᵗʰ **T26.00** Burn of unspecified eyelid and periocular area

√7ᵗʰ **T26.01** Burn of right eyelid and periocular area

√7ᵗʰ **T26.02** Burn of left eyelid and periocular area

√5ᵗʰ **T26.1** Burn of cornea and conjunctival sac

> Use additional external cause code to identify the source, place and intent of the burn (X00-X19, X75-X77, X96-X98, Y92)

√7ᵗʰ **T26.10** Burn of cornea and conjunctival sac, unspecified eye

√7ᵗʰ **T26.11** Burn of cornea and conjunctival sac, right eye

√7ᵗʰ **T26.12** Burn of cornea and conjunctival sac, left eye

√5ᵗʰ **T26.2** Burn with resulting rupture and destruction of eyeball

> Use additional external cause code to identify the source, place and intent of the burn (X00-X19, X75-X77, X96-X98, Y92)

√7ᵗʰ **T26.20** Burn with resulting rupture and destruction of unspecified eyeball

√7ᵗʰ **T26.21** Burn with resulting rupture and destruction of right eyeball

√7ᵗʰ **T26.22** Burn with resulting rupture and destruction of left eyeball

√5ᵗʰ **T26.3** Burns of other specified parts of eye and adnexa

> Use additional external cause code to identify the source, place and intent of the burn (X00-X19, X75-X77, X96-X98, Y92)

√7ᵗʰ **T26.30** Burns of other specified parts of unspecified eye and adnexa

√7ᵗʰ **T26.31** Burns of other specified parts of right eye and adnexa

√7ᵗʰ **T26.32** Burns of other specified parts of left eye and adnexa

√5ᵗʰ **T26.4** Burn of eye and adnexa, part unspecified

> Use additional external cause code to identify the source, place and intent of the burn (X00-X19, X75-X77, X96-X98, Y92)

√7ᵗʰ **T26.40** Burn of unspecified eye and adnexa, part unspecified

√7ᵗʰ **T26.41** Burn of right eye and adnexa, part unspecified

√7ᵗʰ **T26.42** Burn of left eye and adnexa, part unspecified

√5ᵗʰ **T26.5** Corrosion of eyelid and periocular area

> Code first (T51-T65) to identify chemical and intent
> Use additional external cause code to identify place (Y92)

√7ᵗʰ **T26.50** Corrosion of unspecified eyelid and periocular area

√7ᵗʰ **T26.51** Corrosion of right eyelid and periocular area

√7ᵗʰ **T26.52** Corrosion of left eyelid and periocular area

√5ᵗʰ **T26.6** Corrosion of cornea and conjunctival sac

> Code first (T51-T65) to identify chemical and intent
> Use additional external cause code to identify place (Y92)

√7ᵗʰ **T26.60** Corrosion of cornea and conjunctival sac, unspecified eye

√7ᵗʰ **T26.61** Corrosion of cornea and conjunctival sac, right eye

√7ᵗʰ **T26.62** Corrosion of cornea and conjunctival sac, left eye

√5ᵗʰ **T26.7** Corrosion with resulting rupture and destruction of eyeball

> Code first (T51-T65) to identify chemical and intent
> Use additional external cause code to identify place (Y92)

√7ᵗʰ **T26.70** Corrosion with resulting rupture and destruction of unspecified eyeball

√7ᵗʰ **T26.71** Corrosion with resulting rupture and destruction of right eyeball

√7ᵗʰ **T26.72** Corrosion with resulting rupture and destruction of left eyeball

√5ᵗʰ **T26.8** Corrosions of other specified parts of eye and adnexa

> Code first (T51-T65) to identify chemical and intent
> Use additional external cause code to identify place (Y92)

√7ᵗʰ **T26.80** Corrosions of other specified parts of unspecified eye and adnexa

√7ᵗʰ **T26.81** Corrosions of other specified parts of right eye and adnexa

√7ᵗʰ **T26.82** Corrosions of other specified parts of left eye and adnexa

√5ᵗʰ **T26.9** Corrosion of eye and adnexa, part unspecified

> Code first (T51-T65) to identify chemical and intent
> Use additional external cause code to identify place (Y92)

√7ᵗʰ **T26.90** Corrosion of unspecified eye and adnexa, part unspecified

√7ᵗʰ **T26.91** Corrosion of right eye and adnexa, part unspecified

√7ᵗʰ **T26.92** Corrosion of left eye and adnexa, part unspecified

√4ᵗʰ **T27** Burn and corrosion of respiratory tract

> Use additional external cause code to identify the source and intent of the burn (X00-X19, X75-X77, X96-X98)
> Use additional external cause code to identify place (Y92)

> The appropriate 7th character is to be added to each code from category T27.
> A initial encounter
> D subsequent encounter
> S sequela

√7ᵗʰ **T27.0** Burn of larynx and trachea

√7ᵗʰ **T27.1** Burn involving larynx and trachea with lung

√7ᵗʰ **T27.2** Burn of other parts of respiratory tract

> Burn of thoracic cavity

√7ᵗʰ **T27.3** Burn of respiratory tract, part unspecified

√7ᵗʰ **T27.4** Corrosion of larynx and trachea

> Code first (T51-T65) to identify chemical and intent

√7ᵗʰ **T27.5** Corrosion involving larynx and trachea with lung

> ▶Code first (T51-T65) to identify chemical and intent◀

√7ᵗʰ **T27.6** Corrosion of other parts of respiratory tract

> Code first (T51-T65) to identify chemical and intent

√7ᵗʰ **T27.7** Corrosion of respiratory tract, part unspecified

> Code first (T51-T65) to identify chemical and intent

√4ᵗʰ **T28** Burn and corrosion of other internal organs

> Use additional external cause code to identify the source and intent of the burn (X00-X19, X75-X77, X96-X98)
> Use additional external cause code to identify place (Y92)

> The appropriate 7th character is to be added to each code from category T28.
> A initial encounter
> D subsequent encounter
> S sequela

√7ᵗʰ **T28.0** Burn of mouth and pharynx

√7ᵗʰ **T28.1** Burn of esophagus

✅ Additional Character Required √7ᵗʰ Placeholder Alert Manifestation Unspecified Dx ▶◀ Revised Text ● New Code ▲ Revised Title

ICD-10-CM 2020 1081

✓x 7ᵗʰ **T28.2** Burn of other parts of alimentary tract

✓x 7ᵗʰ **T28.3** Burn of internal genitourinary organs

✓ 5ᵗʰ **T28.4** Burns of other and unspecified internal organs
> Code first (T51-T65) to identify chemical and intent

 ✓x 7ᵗʰ **T28.40** Burn of unspecified internal organ

 ✓ 6ᵗʰ **T28.41** Burn of ear drum

   ✓ 7ᵗʰ **T28.411** Burn of right ear drum

   ✓ 7ᵗʰ **T28.412** Burn of left ear drum

   ✓ 7ᵗʰ **T28.419** Burn of unspecified ear drum

 ✓x 7ᵗʰ **T28.49** Burn of other internal organ

✓x 7ᵗʰ **T28.5** Corrosion of mouth and pharynx
> Code first (T51-T65) to identify chemical and intent

✓x 7ᵗʰ **T28.6** Corrosion of esophagus
> Code first (T51-T65) to identify chemical and intent

✓x 7ᵗʰ **T28.7** Corrosion of other parts of alimentary tract
> Code first (T51-T65) to identify chemical and intent

✓x 7ᵗʰ **T28.8** Corrosion of internal genitourinary organs
> Code first (T51-T65) to identify chemical and intent

✓ 5ᵗʰ **T28.9** Corrosions of other and unspecified internal organs
> Code first (T51-T65) to identify chemical and intent

 ✓x 7ᵗʰ **T28.90** Corrosions of unspecified internal organs

 ✓ 6ᵗʰ **T28.91** Corrosions of ear drum

   ✓ 7ᵗʰ **T28.911** Corrosions of right ear drum

   ✓ 7ᵗʰ **T28.912** Corrosions of left ear drum

   ✓ 7ᵗʰ **T28.919** Corrosions of unspecified ear drum

 ✓x 7ᵗʰ **T28.99** Corrosions of other internal organs

Burns and corrosions of multiple and unspecified body regions (T30-T32)

✓ 4ᵗʰ **T30** Burn and corrosion, body region unspecified

 T30.0 Burn of unspecified body region, unspecified degree
> This code is not for inpatient use. Code to specified site and degree of burns
> Burn NOS
> Multiple burns NOS

 T30.4 Corrosion of unspecified body region, unspecified degree
> This code is not for inpatient use. Code to specified site and degree of corrosion
> Corrosion NOS
> Multiple corrosion NOS

✓ 4ᵗʰ **T31** Burns classified according to extent of body surface involved

 NOTE This category is to be used as the primary code only when the site of the burn is unspecified. It should be used as a supplementary code with categories T20-T25 when the site is specified.

 T31.0 Burns involving less than 10% of body surface

✓ 5ᵗʰ **T31.1** Burns involving 10-19% of body surface

 T31.10 Burns involving 10-19% of body surface with 0% to 9% third degree burns
> Burns involving 10-19% of body surface NOS

 T31.11 Burns involving 10-19% of body surface with 10-19% third degree burns

✓ 5ᵗʰ **T31.2** Burns involving 20-29% of body surface

 T31.20 Burns involving 20-29% of body surface with 0% to 9% third degree burns
> Burns involving 20-29% of body surface NOS

 T31.21 Burns involving 20-29% of body surface with 10-19% third degree burns

 T31.22 Burns involving 20-29% of body surface with 20-29% third degree burns

✓ 5ᵗʰ **T31.3** Burns involving 30-39% of body surface

 T31.30 Burns involving 30-39% of body surface with 0% to 9% third degree burns
> Burns involving 30-39% of body surface NOS

 T31.31 Burns involving 30-39% of body surface with 10-19% third degree burns

 T31.32 Burns involving 30-39% of body surface with 20-29% third degree burns

 T31.33 Burns involving 30-39% of body surface with 30-39% third degree burns

✓ 5ᵗʰ **T31.4** Burns involving 40-49% of body surface

 T31.40 Burns involving 40-49% of body surface with 0% to 9% third degree burns
> Burns involving 40-49% of body surface NOS

 T31.41 Burns involving 40-49% of body surface with 10-19% third degree burns

 T31.42 Burns involving 40-49% of body surface with 20-29% third degree burns

 T31.43 Burns involving 40-49% of body surface with 30-39% third degree burns

 T31.44 Burns involving 40-49% of body surface with 40-49% third degree burns

✓ 5ᵗʰ **T31.5** Burns involving 50-59% of body surface

 T31.50 Burns involving 50-59% of body surface with 0% to 9% third degree burns
> Burns involving 50-59% of body surface NOS

 T31.51 Burns involving 50-59% of body surface with 10-19% third degree burns

 T31.52 Burns involving 50-59% of body surface with 20-29% third degree burns

 T31.53 Burns involving 50-59% of body surface with 30-39% third degree burns

 T31.54 Burns involving 50-59% of body surface with 40-49% third degree burns

 T31.55 Burns involving 50-59% of body surface with 50-59% third degree burns

✓ 5ᵗʰ **T31.6** Burns involving 60-69% of body surface

 T31.60 Burns involving 60-69% of body surface with 0% to 9% third degree burns
> Burns involving 60-69% of body surface NOS

 T31.61 Burns involving 60-69% of body surface with 10-19% third degree burns

 T31.62 Burns involving 60-69% of body surface with 20-29% third degree burns

 T31.63 Burns involving 60-69% of body surface with 30-39% third degree burns

 T31.64 Burns involving 60-69% of body surface with 40-49% third degree burns

 T31.65 Burns involving 60-69% of body surface with 50-59% third degree burns

 T31.66 Burns involving 60-69% of body surface with 60-69% third degree burns

✓ 5ᵗʰ **T31.7** Burns involving 70-79% of body surface

 T31.70 Burns involving 70-79% of body surface with 0% to 9% third degree burns
> Burns involving 70-79% of body surface NOS

 T31.71 Burns involving 70-79% of body surface with 10-19% third degree burns

 T31.72 Burns involving 70-79% of body surface with 20-29% third degree burns

 T31.73 Burns involving 70-79% of body surface with 30-39% third degree burns

 T31.74 Burns involving 70-79% of body surface with 40-49% third degree burns

 T31.75 Burns involving 70-79% of body surface with 50-59% third degree burns

 T31.76 Burns involving 70-79% of body surface with 60-69% third degree burns

 T31.77 Burns involving 70-79% of body surface with 70-79% third degree burns

✓ 5ᵗʰ **T31.8** Burns involving 80-89% of body surface

 T31.80 Burns involving 80-89% of body surface with 0% to 9% third degree burns
> Burns involving 80-89% of body surface NOS

 T31.81 Burns involving 80-89% of body surface with 10-19% third degree burns

 T31.82 Burns involving 80-89% of body surface with 20-29% third degree burns

 T31.83 Burns involving 80-89% of body surface with 30-39% third degree burns

 T31.84 Burns involving 80-89% of body surface with 40-49% third degree burns

 T31.85 Burns involving 80-89% of body surface with 50-59% third degree burns

 T31.86 Burns involving 80-89% of body surface with 60-69% third degree burns

 T31.87 Burns involving 80-89% of body surface with 70-79% third degree burns

 T31.88 Burns involving 80-89% of body surface with 80-89% third degree burns

✓5ᵗʰ **T31.9**   **Burns involving** 90% or more **of body surface**

    T31.90   **Burns involving 90% or more of body surface with 0% to 9% third degree burns**
       Burns involving 90% or more of body surface NOS

    T31.91   **Burns involving 90% or more of body surface with 10-19% third degree burns**

    T31.92   **Burns involving 90% or more of body surface with 20-29% third degree burns**

    T31.93   **Burns involving 90% or more of body surface with 30-39% third degree burns**

    T31.94   **Burns involving 90% or more of body surface with 40-49% third degree burns**

    T31.95   **Burns involving 90% or more of body surface with 50-59% third degree burns**

    T31.96   **Burns involving 90% or more of body surface with 60-69% third degree burns**

    T31.97   **Burns involving 90% or more of body surface with 70-79% third degree burns**

    T31.98   **Burns involving 90% or more of body surface with 80-89% third degree burns**

    T31.99   **Burns involving 90% or more of body surface with 90% or more third degree burns**

Rule of Nines Estimation of Total Body Surface Burned

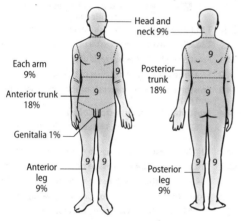

Head and neck 9%
Each arm 9%
Anterior trunk 18%
Genitalia 1%
Anterior leg 9%
Posterior trunk 18%
Posterior leg 9%

✓4ᵗʰ **T32**   **Corrosions** classified according to extent of body surface involved

NOTE   This category is to be used as the primary code only when the site of the corrosion is unspecified. It may be used as a supplementary code with categories T20-T25 when the site is specified.

T32.0   **Corrosions involving** less than 10% **of body surface**

✓5ᵗʰ **T32.1**   **Corrosions involving** 10-19% **of body surface**

    T32.10   **Corrosions involving 10-19% of body surface with 0% to 9% third degree corrosion**
       Corrosions involving 10-19% of body surface NOS

    T32.11   **Corrosions involving 10-19% of body surface with 10-19% third degree corrosion**

✓5ᵗʰ **T32.2**   **Corrosions involving** 20-29% **of body surface**

    T32.20   **Corrosions involving 20-29% of body surface with 0% to 9% third degree corrosion**

    T32.21   **Corrosions involving 20-29% of body surface with 10-19% third degree corrosion**

    T32.22   **Corrosions involving 20-29% of body surface with 20-29% third degree corrosion**

✓5ᵗʰ **T32.3**   **Corrosions involving** 30-39% **of body surface**

    T32.30   **Corrosions involving 30-39% of body surface with 0% to 9% third degree corrosion**

    T32.31   **Corrosions involving 30-39% of body surface with 10-19% third degree corrosion**

    T32.32   **Corrosions involving 30-39% of body surface with 20-29% third degree corrosion**

    T32.33   **Corrosions involving 30-39% of body surface with 30-39% third degree corrosion**

✓5ᵗʰ **T32.4**   **Corrosions involving** 40-49% **of body surface**

    T32.40   **Corrosions involving 40-49% of body surface with 0% to 9% third degree corrosion**

    T32.41   **Corrosions involving 40-49% of body surface with 10-19% third degree corrosion**

    T32.42   **Corrosions involving 40-49% of body surface with 20-29% third degree corrosion**

    T32.43   **Corrosions involving 40-49% of body surface with 30-39% third degree corrosion**

    T32.44   **Corrosions involving 40-49% of body surface with 40-49% third degree corrosion**

✓5ᵗʰ **T32.5**   **Corrosions involving** 50-59% **of body surface**

    T32.50   **Corrosions involving 50-59% of body surface with 0% to 9% third degree corrosion**

    T32.51   **Corrosions involving 50-59% of body surface with 10-19% third degree corrosion**

    T32.52   **Corrosions involving 50-59% of body surface with 20-29% third degree corrosion**

    T32.53   **Corrosions involving 50-59% of body surface with 30-39% third degree corrosion**

    T32.54   **Corrosions involving 50-59% of body surface with 40-49% third degree corrosion**

    T32.55   **Corrosions involving 50-59% of body surface with 50-59% third degree corrosion**

✓5ᵗʰ **T32.6**   **Corrosions involving** 60-69% **of body surface**

    T32.60   **Corrosions involving 60-69% of body surface with 0% to 9% third degree corrosion**

    T32.61   **Corrosions involving 60-69% of body surface with 10-19% third degree corrosion**

    T32.62   **Corrosions involving 60-69% of body surface with 20-29% third degree corrosion**

    T32.63   **Corrosions involving 60-69% of body surface with 30-39% third degree corrosion**

    T32.64   **Corrosions involving 60-69% of body surface with 40-49% third degree corrosion**

    T32.65   **Corrosions involving 60-69% of body surface with 50-59% third degree corrosion**

    T32.66   **Corrosions involving 60-69% of body surface with 60-69% third degree corrosion**

✓5ᵗʰ **T32.7**   **Corrosions involving** 70-79% **of body surface**

    T32.70   **Corrosions involving 70-79% of body surface with 0% to 9% third degree corrosion**

    T32.71   **Corrosions involving 70-79% of body surface with 10-19% third degree corrosion**

    T32.72   **Corrosions involving 70-79% of body surface with 20-29% third degree corrosion**

    T32.73   **Corrosions involving 70-79% of body surface with 30-39% third degree corrosion**

    T32.74   **Corrosions involving 70-79% of body surface with 40-49% third degree corrosion**

    T32.75   **Corrosions involving 70-79% of body surface with 50-59% third degree corrosion**

    T32.76   **Corrosions involving 70-79% of body surface with 60-69% third degree corrosion**

    T32.77   **Corrosions involving 70-79% of body surface with 70-79% third degree corrosion**

✓5ᵗʰ **T32.8**   **Corrosions involving** 80-89% **of body surface**

    T32.80   **Corrosions involving 80-89% of body surface with 0% to 9% third degree corrosion**

    T32.81   **Corrosions involving 80-89% of body surface with 10-19% third degree corrosion**

    T32.82   **Corrosions involving 80-89% of body surface with 20-29% third degree corrosion**

    T32.83   **Corrosions involving 80-89% of body surface with 30-39% third degree corrosion**

    T32.84   **Corrosions involving 80-89% of body surface with 40-49% third degree corrosion**

    T32.85   **Corrosions involving 80-89% of body surface with 50-59% third degree corrosion**

    T32.86   **Corrosions involving 80-89% of body surface with 60-69% third degree corrosion**

    T32.87   **Corrosions involving 80-89% of body surface with 70-79% third degree corrosion**

    T32.88   **Corrosions involving 80-89% of body surface with 80-89% third degree corrosion**

✓5ᵗʰ **T32.9**   **Corrosions involving** 90% or more **of body surface**

    T32.90   **Corrosions involving 90% or more of body surface with 0% to 9% third degree corrosion**

    T32.91   **Corrosions involving 90% or more of body surface with 10-19% third degree corrosion**

    T32.92   **Corrosions involving 90% or more of body surface with 20-29% third degree corrosion**

    T32.93   **Corrosions involving 90% or more of body surface with 30-39% third degree corrosion**

    T32.94   **Corrosions involving 90% or more of body surface with 40-49% third degree corrosion**

    T32.95   **Corrosions involving 90% or more of body surface with 50-59% third degree corrosion**

✔ Additional Character Required   ✔x7ᵗʰ Placeholder Alert   Manifestation   Unspecified Dx   ►◄ Revised Text   ● New Code   ▲ Revised Title

T32.96   Corrosions involving 90% or more of body surface with 60-69% third degree corrosion

T32.97   Corrosions involving 90% or more of body surface with 70-79% third degree corrosion

T32.98   Corrosions involving 90% or more of body surface with 80-89% third degree corrosion

T32.99   Corrosions involving 90% or more of body surface with 90% or more third degree corrosion

Frostbite (T33-T34)

EXCLUDES 2   *hypothermia and other effects of reduced temperature (T68, T69.-)*

√4ᵗʰ **T33**   Superficial **frostbite**

> INCLUDES   frostbite with partial thickness skin loss

> The appropriate 7th character is to be added to each code from category T33.
> A   initial encounter
> D   subsequent encounter
> S   sequela

√5ᵗʰ   **T33.0**   Superficial frostbite of head

     √6ᵗʰ   **T33.01**   Superficial frostbite of ear

         √7ᵗʰ   **T33.011**   Superficial frostbite of right ear

         √7ᵗʰ   **T33.012**   Superficial frostbite of left ear

         √7ᵗʰ   **T33.019**   Superficial frostbite of unspecified ear

     √x7ᵗʰ   **T33.02**   Superficial frostbite of nose

     √x7ᵗʰ   **T33.09**   Superficial frostbite of other part of head

√x7ᵗʰ   **T33.1**   Superficial frostbite of neck

√x7ᵗʰ   **T33.2**   Superficial frostbite of thorax

√x7ᵗʰ   **T33.3**   Superficial frostbite of abdominal wall, lower back and pelvis

√5ᵗʰ   **T33.4**   Superficial frostbite of arm

> EXCLUDES 2   *superficial frostbite of wrist and hand (T33.5-)*

     √x7ᵗʰ   **T33.40**   Superficial frostbite of unspecified arm

     √x7ᵗʰ   **T33.41**   Superficial frostbite of right arm

     √x7ᵗʰ   **T33.42**   Superficial frostbite of left arm

√5ᵗʰ   **T33.5**   Superficial frostbite of wrist, hand, and fingers

     √6ᵗʰ   **T33.51**   Superficial frostbite of wrist

         √7ᵗʰ   **T33.511**   Superficial frostbite of right wrist

         √7ᵗʰ   **T33.512**   Superficial frostbite of left wrist

         √7ᵗʰ   **T33.519**   Superficial frostbite of unspecified wrist

     √6ᵗʰ   **T33.52**   Superficial frostbite of hand

>   EXCLUDES 2   *superficial frostbite of fingers (T33.53-)*

         √7ᵗʰ   **T33.521**   Superficial frostbite of right hand

         √7ᵗʰ   **T33.522**   Superficial frostbite of left hand

         √7ᵗʰ   **T33.529**   Superficial frostbite of unspecified hand

     √6ᵗʰ   **T33.53**   Superficial frostbite of finger(s)

         √7ᵗʰ   **T33.531**   Superficial frostbite of right finger(s)

         √7ᵗʰ   **T33.532**   Superficial frostbite of left finger(s)

         √7ᵗʰ   **T33.539**   Superficial frostbite of unspecified finger(s)

√5ᵗʰ   **T33.6**   Superficial frostbite of hip and thigh

     √x7ᵗʰ   **T33.60**   Superficial frostbite of unspecified hip and thigh

     √x7ᵗʰ   **T33.61**   Superficial frostbite of right hip and thigh

     √x7ᵗʰ   **T33.62**   Superficial frostbite of left hip and thigh

√5ᵗʰ   **T33.7**   Superficial frostbite of knee and lower leg

> EXCLUDES 2   *superficial frostbite of ankle and foot (T33.8-)*

     √x7ᵗʰ   **T33.70**   Superficial frostbite of unspecified knee and lower leg

     √x7ᵗʰ   **T33.71**   Superficial frostbite of right knee and lower leg

     √x7ᵗʰ   **T33.72**   Superficial frostbite of left knee and lower leg

√5ᵗʰ   **T33.8**   Superficial frostbite of ankle, foot, and toe(s)

     √6ᵗʰ   **T33.81**   Superficial frostbite of ankle

         √7ᵗʰ   **T33.811**   Superficial frostbite of right ankle

         √7ᵗʰ   **T33.812**   Superficial frostbite of left ankle

         √7ᵗʰ   **T33.819**   Superficial frostbite of unspecified ankle

     √6ᵗʰ   **T33.82**   Superficial frostbite of foot

         √7ᵗʰ   **T33.821**   Superficial frostbite of right foot

         √7ᵗʰ   **T33.822**   Superficial frostbite of left foot

         √7ᵗʰ   **T33.829**   Superficial frostbite of unspecified foot

     √6ᵗʰ   **T33.83**   Superficial frostbite of toe(s)

         √7ᵗʰ   **T33.831**   Superficial frostbite of right toe(s)

         √7ᵗʰ   **T33.832**   Superficial frostbite of left toe(s)

         √7ᵗʰ   **T33.839**   Superficial frostbite of unspecified toe(s)

√5ᵗʰ   **T33.9**   Superficial frostbite of other and unspecified sites

     √x7ᵗʰ   **T33.90**   Superficial frostbite of unspecified sites

         Superficial frostbite NOS

     √x7ᵗʰ   **T33.99**   Superficial frostbite of other sites

         Superficial frostbite of leg NOS

         Superficial frostbite of trunk NOS

√4ᵗʰ **T34**   Frostbite with tissue necrosis

> The appropriate 7th character is to be added to each code from category T34.
> A   initial encounter
> D   subsequent encounter
> S   sequela

√5ᵗʰ   **T34.0**   Frostbite with tissue necrosis of head

     √6ᵗʰ   **T34.01**   Frostbite with tissue necrosis of ear

         √7ᵗʰ   **T34.011**   Frostbite with tissue necrosis of right ear

         √7ᵗʰ   **T34.012**   Frostbite with tissue necrosis of left ear

         √7ᵗʰ   **T34.019**   Frostbite with tissue necrosis of unspecified ear

     √x7ᵗʰ   **T34.02**   Frostbite with tissue necrosis of nose

     √x7ᵗʰ   **T34.09**   Frostbite with tissue necrosis of other part of head

√x7ᵗʰ   **T34.1**   Frostbite with tissue necrosis of neck

√x7ᵗʰ   **T34.2**   Frostbite with tissue necrosis of thorax

√x7ᵗʰ   **T34.3**   Frostbite with tissue necrosis of abdominal wall, lower back and pelvis

√5ᵗʰ   **T34.4**   Frostbite with tissue necrosis of arm

> EXCLUDES 2   *frostbite with tissue necrosis of wrist and hand (T34.5-)*

     √x7ᵗʰ   **T34.40**   Frostbite with tissue necrosis of unspecified arm

     √x7ᵗʰ   **T34.41**   Frostbite with tissue necrosis of right arm

     √x7ᵗʰ   **T34.42**   Frostbite with tissue necrosis of left arm

√5ᵗʰ   **T34.5**   Frostbite with tissue necrosis of wrist, hand, and finger(s)

     √6ᵗʰ   **T34.51**   Frostbite with tissue necrosis of wrist

         √7ᵗʰ   **T34.511**   Frostbite with tissue necrosis of right wrist

         √7ᵗʰ   **T34.512**   Frostbite with tissue necrosis of left wrist

         √7ᵗʰ   **T34.519**   Frostbite with tissue necrosis of unspecified wrist

     √6ᵗʰ   **T34.52**   Frostbite with tissue necrosis of hand

>   EXCLUDES 2   *frostbite with tissue necrosis of finger(s) (T34.53-)*

         √7ᵗʰ   **T34.521**   Frostbite with tissue necrosis of right hand

         √7ᵗʰ   **T34.522**   Frostbite with tissue necrosis of left hand

         √7ᵗʰ   **T34.529**   Frostbite with tissue necrosis of unspecified hand

     √6ᵗʰ   **T34.53**   Frostbite with tissue necrosis of finger(s)

         √7ᵗʰ   **T34.531**   Frostbite with tissue necrosis of right finger(s)

         √7ᵗʰ   **T34.532**   Frostbite with tissue necrosis of left finger(s)

         √7ᵗʰ   **T34.539**   Frostbite with tissue necrosis of unspecified finger(s)

√5ᵗʰ   **T34.6**   Frostbite with tissue necrosis of hip and thigh

     √x7ᵗʰ   **T34.60**   Frostbite with tissue necrosis of unspecified hip and thigh

     √x7ᵗʰ   **T34.61**   Frostbite with tissue necrosis of right hip and thigh

     √x7ᵗʰ   **T34.62**   Frostbite with tissue necrosis of left hip and thigh

√5ᵗʰ   **T34.7**   Frostbite with tissue necrosis of knee and lower leg

> EXCLUDES 2   *frostbite with tissue necrosis of ankle and foot (T34.8-)*

     √x7ᵗʰ   **T34.70**   Frostbite with tissue necrosis of unspecified knee and lower leg

     √x7ᵗʰ   **T34.71**   Frostbite with tissue necrosis of right knee and lower leg

     √x7ᵗʰ   **T34.72**   Frostbite with tissue necrosis of left knee and lower leg

N Newborn: 0   P Pediatric: 0-17   M Maternity: 12-55   A Adult: 15-124   CH Comorbidity High   CL Comorbidity Low   NCDx Noncancer Dx   PDx Primary Dx

1084   ICD-10-CM 2020

√5ᵗʰ **T34.8** Frostbite with tissue necrosis of ankle, foot, and toe(s)
  √6ᵗʰ **T34.81** Frostbite with tissue necrosis of ankle
    √7ᵗʰ **T34.811** Frostbite with tissue necrosis of right ankle
    √7ᵗʰ **T34.812** Frostbite with tissue necrosis of left ankle
    √7ᵗʰ **T34.819** Frostbite with tissue necrosis of unspecified ankle
  √6ᵗʰ **T34.82** Frostbite with tissue necrosis of foot
    √7ᵗʰ **T34.821** Frostbite with tissue necrosis of right foot
    √7ᵗʰ **T34.822** Frostbite with tissue necrosis of left foot
    √7ᵗʰ **T34.829** Frostbite with tissue necrosis of unspecified foot
  √6ᵗʰ **T34.83** Frostbite with tissue necrosis of toe(s)
    √7ᵗʰ **T34.831** Frostbite with tissue necrosis of right toe(s)
    √7ᵗʰ **T34.832** Frostbite with tissue necrosis of left toe(s)
    √7ᵗʰ **T34.839** Frostbite with tissue necrosis of unspecified toe(s)
√5ᵗʰ **T34.9** Frostbite with tissue necrosis of other and unspecified sites
  √x7ᵗʰ **T34.90** Frostbite with tissue necrosis of unspecified sites
    Frostbite with tissue necrosis NOS
  √x7ᵗʰ **T34.99** Frostbite with tissue necrosis of other sites
    Frostbite with tissue necrosis of leg NOS
    Frostbite with tissue necrosis of trunk NOS

Poisoning by, adverse effects of and underdosing of drugs, medicaments and biological substances (T36-T50)

INCLUDES adverse effect of correct substance properly administered
poisoning by overdose of substance
poisoning by wrong substance given or taken in error
underdosing by (inadvertently) (deliberately) taking less substance than prescribed or instructed

Code first, for adverse effects, the nature of the adverse effect, such as:
adverse effect NOS (T88.7)
aspirin gastritis (K29.-)
blood disorders (D56-D76)
contact dermatitis (L23-L25)
dermatitis due to substances taken internally (L27.-)
nephropathy (N14.0-N14.2)

NOTE The drug giving rise to the adverse effect should be identified by use of codes from categories T36-T50 with fifth or sixth character 5.

Use additional code(s) to specify:
manifestations of poisoning
underdosing or failure in dosage during medical and surgical care (Y63.6, Y63.8-Y63.9)
underdosing of medication regimen (Z91.12-, Z91.13-)
EXCLUDES 1 toxic reaction to local anesthesia in pregnancy (O29.3-)
EXCLUDES 2 abuse and dependence of psychoactive substances (F10-F19)
abuse of non-dependence-producing substances (F55.-)
drug reaction and poisoning affecting newborn (P00-P96)
pathological drug intoxication (inebriation) (F10-F19)

AHA: 2018,4Q,71; 2016,2Q,8; 2015,3Q,22
TIP: Assign any condition resulting from a poisoning, toxic effect, or adverse effect, followed by the appropriate code from categories T36–T50 while the resulting effects of the poisoning, toxic effect, or adverse effect remains unresolved and requires treatment.
TIP: When the intent of a poisoning is not specified, the intent should be coded as accidental.

√4ᵗʰ **T36** Poisoning by, adverse effect of and underdosing of systemic antibiotics
  EXCLUDES 1 antineoplastic antibiotics (T45.1-)
  locally applied antibiotic NEC (T49.0)
  topically used antibiotic for ear, nose and throat (T49.6)
  topically used antibiotic for eye (T49.5)

The appropriate 7th character is to be added to each code from category T36.
A initial encounter
D subsequent encounter
S sequela

√5ᵗʰ **T36.0** Poisoning by, adverse effect of and underdosing of penicillins
  √6ᵗʰ **T36.0X** Poisoning by, adverse effect of and underdosing of penicillins
    √7ᵗʰ **T36.0X1** Poisoning by penicillins, accidental (unintentional)
      Poisoning by penicillins NOS
    √7ᵗʰ **T36.0X2** Poisoning by penicillins, intentional self-harm
    √7ᵗʰ **T36.0X3** Poisoning by penicillins, assault

    √7ᵗʰ **T36.0X4** Poisoning by penicillins, undetermined
    √7ᵗʰ **T36.0X5** Adverse effect of penicillins
    √7ᵗʰ **T36.0X6** Underdosing of penicillins
√5ᵗʰ **T36.1** Poisoning by, adverse effect of and underdosing of cephalosporins and other beta-lactam antibiotics
  √6ᵗʰ **T36.1X** Poisoning by, adverse effect of and underdosing of cephalosporins and other beta-lactam antibiotics
    √7ᵗʰ **T36.1X1** Poisoning by cephalosporins and other beta-lactam antibiotics, accidental (unintentional)
      Poisoning by cephalosporins and other beta-lactam antibiotics NOS
    √7ᵗʰ **T36.1X2** Poisoning by cephalosporins and other beta-lactam antibiotics, intentional self-harm
    √7ᵗʰ **T36.1X3** Poisoning by cephalosporins and other beta-lactam antibiotics, assault
    √7ᵗʰ **T36.1X4** Poisoning by cephalosporins and other beta-lactam antibiotics, undetermined
    √7ᵗʰ **T36.1X5** Adverse effect of cephalosporins and other beta-lactam antibiotics
    √7ᵗʰ **T36.1X6** Underdosing of cephalosporins and other beta-lactam antibiotics
√5ᵗʰ **T36.2** Poisoning by, adverse effect of and underdosing of chloramphenicol group
  √6ᵗʰ **T36.2X** Poisoning by, adverse effect of and underdosing of chloramphenicol group
    √7ᵗʰ **T36.2X1** Poisoning by chloramphenicol group, accidental (unintentional)
      Poisoning by chloramphenicol group NOS
    √7ᵗʰ **T36.2X2** Poisoning by chloramphenicol group, intentional self-harm
    √7ᵗʰ **T36.2X3** Poisoning by chloramphenicol group, assault
    √7ᵗʰ **T36.2X4** Poisoning by chloramphenicol group, undetermined
    √7ᵗʰ **T36.2X5** Adverse effect of chloramphenicol group
    √7ᵗʰ **T36.2X6** Underdosing of chloramphenicol group
√5ᵗʰ **T36.3** Poisoning by, adverse effect of and underdosing of macrolides
  √6ᵗʰ **T36.3X** Poisoning by, adverse effect of and underdosing of macrolides
    √7ᵗʰ **T36.3X1** Poisoning by macrolides, accidental (unintentional)
      Poisoning by macrolides NOS
    √7ᵗʰ **T36.3X2** Poisoning by macrolides, intentional self-harm
    √7ᵗʰ **T36.3X3** Poisoning by macrolides, assault
    √7ᵗʰ **T36.3X4** Poisoning by macrolides, undetermined
    √7ᵗʰ **T36.3X5** Adverse effect of macrolides
    √7ᵗʰ **T36.3X6** Underdosing of macrolides
√5ᵗʰ **T36.4** Poisoning by, adverse effect of and underdosing of tetracyclines
  √6ᵗʰ **T36.4X** Poisoning by, adverse effect of and underdosing of tetracyclines
    √7ᵗʰ **T36.4X1** Poisoning by tetracyclines, accidental (unintentional)
      Poisoning by tetracyclines NOS
    √7ᵗʰ **T36.4X2** Poisoning by tetracyclines, intentional self-harm
    √7ᵗʰ **T36.4X3** Poisoning by tetracyclines, assault
    √7ᵗʰ **T36.4X4** Poisoning by tetracyclines, undetermined
    √7ᵗʰ **T36.4X5** Adverse effect of tetracyclines
    √7ᵗʰ **T36.4X6** Underdosing of tetracyclines
√5ᵗʰ **T36.5** Poisoning by, adverse effect of and underdosing of aminoglycosides
  Poisoning by, adverse effect of and underdosing of streptomycin
  √6ᵗʰ **T36.5X** Poisoning by, adverse effect of and underdosing of aminoglycosides
    √7ᵗʰ **T36.5X1** Poisoning by aminoglycosides, accidental (unintentional)
      Poisoning by aminoglycosides NOS
    √7ᵗʰ **T36.5X2** Poisoning by aminoglycosides, intentional self-harm
    √7ᵗʰ **T36.5X3** Poisoning by aminoglycosides, assault
    √7ᵗʰ **T36.5X4** Poisoning by aminoglycosides, undetermined
    √7ᵗʰ **T36.5X5** Adverse effect of aminoglycosides

✓7th **T36.5X6** Underdosing of aminoglycosides

✓5th **T36.6** Poisoning by, adverse effect of and underdosing of rifampicins
  ✓6th **T36.6X** Poisoning by, adverse effect of and underdosing of rifampicins
    ✓7th **T36.6X1** Poisoning by rifampicins, accidental (unintentional)
      Poisoning by rifampicins NOS
    ✓7th **T36.6X2** Poisoning by rifampicins, intentional self-harm
    ✓7th **T36.6X3** Poisoning by rifampicins, assault
    ✓7th **T36.6X4** Poisoning by rifampicins, undetermined
    ✓7th **T36.6X5** Adverse effect of rifampicins
    ✓7th **T36.6X6** Underdosing of rifampicins

✓5th **T36.7** Poisoning by, adverse effect of and underdosing of antifungal antibiotics, systemically used
  ✓6th **T36.7X** Poisoning by, adverse effect of and underdosing of antifungal antibiotics, systemically used
    ✓7th **T36.7X1** Poisoning by antifungal antibiotics, systemically used, accidental (unintentional)
      Poisoning by antifungal antibiotics, systemically used NOS
    ✓7th **T36.7X2** Poisoning by antifungal antibiotics, systemically used, intentional self-harm
    ✓7th **T36.7X3** Poisoning by antifungal antibiotics, systemically used, assault
    ✓7th **T36.7X4** Poisoning by antifungal antibiotics, systemically used, undetermined
    ✓7th **T36.7X5** Adverse effect of antifungal antibiotics, systemically used
    ✓7th **T36.7X6** Underdosing of antifungal antibiotics, systemically used

✓5th **T36.8** Poisoning by, adverse effect of and underdosing of other systemic antibiotics
  ✓6th **T36.8X** Poisoning by, adverse effect of and underdosing of other systemic antibiotics
    AHA: 2017,1Q,39
    ✓7th **T36.8X1** Poisoning by other systemic antibiotics, accidental (unintentional)
      Poisoning by other systemic antibiotics NOS
    ✓7th **T36.8X2** Poisoning by other systemic antibiotics, intentional self-harm
    ✓7th **T36.8X3** Poisoning by other systemic antibiotics, assault
    ✓7th **T36.8X4** Poisoning by other systemic antibiotics, undetermined
    ✓7th **T36.8X5** Adverse effect of other systemic antibiotics
    ✓7th **T36.8X6** Underdosing of other systemic antibiotics

✓5th **T36.9** Poisoning by, adverse effect of and underdosing of unspecified systemic antibiotic
  ✓x7th **T36.91** Poisoning by unspecified systemic antibiotic, accidental (unintentional)
    Poisoning by systemic antibiotic NOS
  ✓x7th **T36.92** Poisoning by unspecified systemic antibiotic, intentional self-harm
  ✓x7th **T36.93** Poisoning by unspecified systemic antibiotic, assault
  ✓x7th **T36.94** Poisoning by unspecified systemic antibiotic, undetermined
  ✓x7th **T36.95** Adverse effect of unspecified systemic antibiotic
  ✓x7th **T36.96** Underdosing of unspecified systemic antibiotic

✓4th **T37** Poisoning by, adverse effect of and underdosing of other systemic anti-infectives and antiparasitics
  EXCLUDES 1 anti-infectives topically used for ear, nose and throat (T49.6-)
    anti-infectives topically used for eye (T49.5-)
    locally applied anti-infectives NEC (T49.0-)

  The appropriate 7th character is to be added to each code from category T37.
  A initial encounter
  D subsequent encounter
  S sequela

✓5th **T37.0** Poisoning by, adverse effect of and underdosing of sulfonamides
  ✓6th **T37.0X** Poisoning by, adverse effect of and underdosing of sulfonamides
    ✓7th **T37.0X1** Poisoning by sulfonamides, accidental (unintentional)
      Poisoning by sulfonamides NOS
    ✓7th **T37.0X2** Poisoning by sulfonamides, intentional self-harm
    ✓7th **T37.0X3** Poisoning by sulfonamides, assault
    ✓7th **T37.0X4** Poisoning by sulfonamides, undetermined
    ✓7th **T37.0X5** Adverse effect of sulfonamides
    ✓7th **T37.0X6** Underdosing of sulfonamides

✓5th **T37.1** Poisoning by, adverse effect of and underdosing of antimycobacterial drugs
  EXCLUDES 1 rifampicins (T36.6-)
    streptomycin (T36.5-)
  ✓6th **T37.1X** Poisoning by, adverse effect of and underdosing of antimycobacterial drugs
    ✓7th **T37.1X1** Poisoning by antimycobacterial drugs, accidental (unintentional)
      Poisoning by antimycobacterial drugs NOS
    ✓7th **T37.1X2** Poisoning by antimycobacterial drugs, intentional self-harm
    ✓7th **T37.1X3** Poisoning by antimycobacterial drugs, assault
    ✓7th **T37.1X4** Poisoning by antimycobacterial drugs, undetermined
    ✓7th **T37.1X5** Adverse effect of antimycobacterial drugs
    ✓7th **T37.1X6** Underdosing of antimycobacterial drugs

✓5th **T37.2** Poisoning by, adverse effect of and underdosing of antimalarials and drugs acting on other blood protozoa
  EXCLUDES 1 hydroxyquinoline derivatives (T37.8-)
  ✓6th **T37.2X** Poisoning by, adverse effect of and underdosing of antimalarials and drugs acting on other blood protozoa
    ✓7th **T37.2X1** Poisoning by antimalarials and drugs acting on other blood protozoa, accidental (unintentional)
      Poisoning by antimalarials and drugs acting on other blood protozoa NOS
    ✓7th **T37.2X2** Poisoning by antimalarials and drugs acting on other blood protozoa, intentional self-harm
    ✓7th **T37.2X3** Poisoning by antimalarials and drugs acting on other blood protozoa, assault
    ✓7th **T37.2X4** Poisoning by antimalarials and drugs acting on other blood protozoa, undetermined
    ✓7th **T37.2X5** Adverse effect of antimalarials and drugs acting on other blood protozoa
    ✓7th **T37.2X6** Underdosing of antimalarials and drugs acting on other blood protozoa

✓5th **T37.3** Poisoning by, adverse effect of and underdosing of other antiprotozoal drugs
  ✓6th **T37.3X** Poisoning by, adverse effect of and underdosing of other antiprotozoal drugs
    ✓7th **T37.3X1** Poisoning by other antiprotozoal drugs, accidental (unintentional)
      Poisoning by other antiprotozoal drugs NOS
    ✓7th **T37.3X2** Poisoning by other antiprotozoal drugs, intentional self-harm
    ✓7th **T37.3X3** Poisoning by other antiprotozoal drugs, assault
    ✓7th **T37.3X4** Poisoning by other antiprotozoal drugs, undetermined
    ✓7th **T37.3X5** Adverse effect of other antiprotozoal drugs

✓7th **T37.3X6** Underdosing of other antiprotozoal drugs

✓5th **T37.4** Poisoning by, adverse effect of and underdosing of anthelminthics

✓6th **T37.4X** Poisoning by, adverse effect of and underdosing of anthelminthics

✓7th **T37.4X1** Poisoning by anthelminthics, accidental (unintentional)
Poisoning by anthelminthics NOS

✓7th **T37.4X2** Poisoning by anthelminthics, intentional self-harm

✓7th **T37.4X3** Poisoning by anthelminthics, assault

✓7th **T37.4X4** Poisoning by anthelminthics, undetermined

✓7th **T37.4X5** Adverse effect of anthelminthics

✓7th **T37.4X6** Underdosing of anthelminthics

✓5th **T37.5** Poisoning by, adverse effect of and underdosing of antiviral drugs

EXCLUDES 1   amantadine (T42.8-)
cytarabine (T45.1-)

✓6th **T37.5X** Poisoning by, adverse effect of and underdosing of antiviral drugs

✓7th **T37.5X1** Poisoning by antiviral drugs, accidental (unintentional)
Poisoning by antiviral drugs NOS

✓7th **T37.5X2** Poisoning by antiviral drugs, intentional self-harm

✓7th **T37.5X3** Poisoning by antiviral drugs, assault

✓7th **T37.5X4** Poisoning by antiviral drugs, undetermined

✓7th **T37.5X5** Adverse effect of antiviral drugs

✓7th **T37.5X6** Underdosing of antiviral drugs

✓5th **T37.8** Poisoning by, adverse effect of and underdosing of other specified systemic anti-infectives and antiparasitics
Poisoning by, adverse effect of and underdosing of hydroxyquinoline derivatives

EXCLUDES 1   antimalarial drugs (T37.2-)

✓6th **T37.8X** Poisoning by, adverse effect of and underdosing of other specified systemic anti-infectives and antiparasitics

✓7th **T37.8X1** Poisoning by other specified systemic anti-infectives and antiparasitics, accidental (unintentional)
Poisoning by other specified systemic anti-infectives and antiparasitics NOS

✓7th **T37.8X2** Poisoning by other specified systemic anti-infectives and antiparasitics, intentional self-harm

✓7th **T37.8X3** Poisoning by other specified systemic anti-infectives and antiparasitics, assault

✓7th **T37.8X4** Poisoning by other specified systemic anti-infectives and antiparasitics, undetermined

✓7th **T37.8X5** Adverse effect of other specified systemic anti-infectives and antiparasitics

✓7th **T37.8X6** Underdosing of other specified systemic anti-infectives and antiparasitics

✓5th **T37.9** Poisoning by, adverse effect of and underdosing of unspecified systemic anti-infective and antiparasitics

✓x7th **T37.91** Poisoning by unspecified systemic anti-infective and antiparasitics, accidental (unintentional)
Poisoning by, adverse effect of and underdosing of systemic anti-infective and antiparasitics NOS

✓x7th **T37.92** Poisoning by unspecified systemic anti-infective and antiparasitics, intentional self-harm

✓x7th **T37.93** Poisoning by unspecified systemic anti-infective and antiparasitics, assault

✓x7th **T37.94** Poisoning by unspecified systemic anti-infective and antiparasitics, undetermined

✓x7th **T37.95** Adverse effect of unspecified systemic anti-infective and antiparasitic

✓x7th **T37.96** Underdosing of unspecified systemic anti-infectives and antiparasitics

✓4th **T38** Poisoning by, adverse effect of and underdosing of hormones and their synthetic substitutes and antagonists, not elsewhere classified

EXCLUDES 1   mineralocorticoids and their antagonists (T50.0-)
oxytocic hormones (T48.0-)
parathyroid hormones and derivatives (T50.9-)

The appropriate 7th character is to be added to each code from category T38.
A   initial encounter
D   subsequent encounter
S   sequela

✓5th **T38.0** Poisoning by, adverse effect of and underdosing of glucocorticoids and synthetic analogues

EXCLUDES 1   glucocorticoids, topically used (T49.-)

✓6th **T38.0X** Poisoning by, adverse effect of and underdosing of glucocorticoids and synthetic analogues

✓7th **T38.0X1** Poisoning by glucocorticoids and synthetic analogues, accidental (unintentional)
Poisoning by glucocorticoids and synthetic analogues NOS

✓7th **T38.0X2** Poisoning by glucocorticoids and synthetic analogues, intentional self-harm

✓7th **T38.0X3** Poisoning by glucocorticoids and synthetic analogues, assault

✓7th **T38.0X4** Poisoning by glucocorticoids and synthetic analogues, undetermined

✓7th **T38.0X5** Adverse effect of glucocorticoids and synthetic analogues

✓7th **T38.0X6** Underdosing of glucocorticoids and synthetic analogues

✓5th **T38.1** Poisoning by, adverse effect of and underdosing of thyroid hormones and substitutes

✓6th **T38.1X** Poisoning by, adverse effect of and underdosing of thyroid hormones and substitutes

✓7th **T38.1X1** Poisoning by thyroid hormones and substitutes, accidental (unintentional)
Poisoning by thyroid hormones and substitutes NOS

✓7th **T38.1X2** Poisoning by thyroid hormones and substitutes, intentional self-harm

✓7th **T38.1X3** Poisoning by thyroid hormones and substitutes, assault

✓7th **T38.1X4** Poisoning by thyroid hormones and substitutes, undetermined

✓7th **T38.1X5** Adverse effect of thyroid hormones and substitutes

✓7th **T38.1X6** Underdosing of thyroid hormones and substitutes

✓5th **T38.2** Poisoning by, adverse effect of and underdosing of antithyroid drugs

✓6th **T38.2X** Poisoning by, adverse effect of and underdosing of antithyroid drugs

✓7th **T38.2X1** Poisoning by antithyroid drugs, accidental (unintentional)
Poisoning by antithyroid drugs NOS

✓7th **T38.2X2** Poisoning by antithyroid drugs, intentional self-harm

✓7th **T38.2X3** Poisoning by antithyroid drugs, assault

✓7th **T38.2X4** Poisoning by antithyroid drugs, undetermined

✓7th **T38.2X5** Adverse effect of antithyroid drugs

✓7th **T38.2X6** Underdosing of antithyroid drugs

✓5th **T38.3** Poisoning by, adverse effect of and underdosing of insulin and oral hypoglycemic [antidiabetic] drugs

✓6th **T38.3X** Poisoning by, adverse effect of and underdosing of insulin and oral hypoglycemic [antidiabetic] drugs

✓7th **T38.3X1** Poisoning by insulin and oral hypoglycemic [antidiabetic] drugs, accidental (unintentional)
Poisoning by insulin and oral hypoglycemic [antidiabetic] drugs NOS

✓7th **T38.3X2** Poisoning by insulin and oral hypoglycemic [antidiabetic] drugs, intentional self-harm

✓7th **T38.3X3** Poisoning by insulin and oral hypoglycemic [antidiabetic] drugs, assault

√7ᵗʰ **T38.3X4 Poisoning by insulin and oral hypoglycemic [antidiabetic] drugs,** undetermined

√7ᵗʰ **T38.3X5** Adverse effect **of insulin and oral hypoglycemic [antidiabetic] drugs**

√7ᵗʰ **T38.3X6** Underdosing **of insulin and oral hypoglycemic [antidiabetic] drugs**

√5ᵗʰ **T38.4 Poisoning by, adverse effect of and underdosing of oral contraceptives**
  Poisoning by, adverse effect of and underdosing of multiple- and single-ingredient oral contraceptive preparations

√6ᵗʰ **T38.4X Poisoning by, adverse effect of and underdosing of** oral contraceptives

√7ᵗʰ **T38.4X1 Poisoning by oral contraceptives,** accidental **(unintentional)**
  Poisoning by oral contraceptives NOS

√7ᵗʰ **T38.4X2 Poisoning by oral contraceptives,** intentional self-harm

√7ᵗʰ **T38.4X3 Poisoning by oral contraceptives,** assault

√7ᵗʰ **T38.4X4 Poisoning by oral contraceptives,** undetermined

√7ᵗʰ **T38.4X5** Adverse effect **of oral contraceptives**

√7ᵗʰ **T38.4X6** Underdosing **of oral contraceptives**

√5ᵗʰ **T38.5 Poisoning by, adverse effect of and underdosing of other estrogens and progestogens**
  Poisoning by, adverse effect of and underdosing of estrogens and progestogens mixtures and substitutes

√6ᵗʰ **T38.5X Poisoning by, adverse effect of and underdosing of other estrogens and progestogens**

√7ᵗʰ **T38.5X1 Poisoning by other estrogens and progestogens,** accidental **(unintentional)**
  Poisoning by other estrogens and progestogens NOS

√7ᵗʰ **T38.5X2 Poisoning by other estrogens and progestogens,** intentional self-harm

√7ᵗʰ **T38.5X3 Poisoning by other estrogens and progestogens,** assault

√7ᵗʰ **T38.5X4 Poisoning by other estrogens and progestogens,** undetermined

√7ᵗʰ **T38.5X5** Adverse effect **of other estrogens and progestogens**

√7ᵗʰ **T38.5X6** Underdosing **of other estrogens and progestogens**

√5ᵗʰ **T38.6 Poisoning by, adverse effect of and underdosing of antigonadotrophins, antiestrogens, antiandrogens, not elsewhere classified**
  Poisoning by, adverse effect of and underdosing of tamoxifen

√6ᵗʰ **T38.6X Poisoning by, adverse effect of and underdosing of** antigonadotrophins, antiestrogens, antiandrogens, **not elsewhere classified**

√7ᵗʰ **T38.6X1 Poisoning by antigonadotrophins, antiestrogens, antiandrogens, not elsewhere classified,** accidental **(unintentional)**
  Poisoning by antigonadotrophins, antiestrogens, antiandrogens, not elsewhere classified NOS

√7ᵗʰ **T38.6X2 Poisoning by antigonadotrophins, antiestrogens, antiandrogens, not elsewhere classified,** intentional self-harm

√7ᵗʰ **T38.6X3 Poisoning by antigonadotrophins, antiestrogens, antiandrogens, not elsewhere classified,** assault

√7ᵗʰ **T38.6X4 Poisoning by antigonadotrophins, antiestrogens, antiandrogens, not elsewhere classified,** undetermined

√7ᵗʰ **T38.6X5** Adverse effect **of antigonadotrophins, antiestrogens, antiandrogens, not elsewhere classified**

√7ᵗʰ **T38.6X6** Underdosing **of antigonadotrophins, antiestrogens, antiandrogens, not elsewhere classified**

√5ᵗʰ **T38.7 Poisoning by, adverse effect of and underdosing of androgens and anabolic congeners**

√6ᵗʰ **T38.7X Poisoning by, adverse effect of and underdosing of** androgens and anabolic congeners

√7ᵗʰ **T38.7X1 Poisoning by androgens and anabolic congeners,** accidental **(unintentional)**
  Poisoning by androgens and anabolic congeners NOS

√7ᵗʰ **T38.7X2 Poisoning by androgens and anabolic congeners,** intentional self-harm

√7ᵗʰ **T38.7X3 Poisoning by androgens and anabolic congeners,** assault

√7ᵗʰ **T38.7X4 Poisoning by androgens and anabolic congeners,** undetermined

√7ᵗʰ **T38.7X5** Adverse effect **of androgens and anabolic congeners**

√7ᵗʰ **T38.7X6** Underdosing **of androgens and anabolic congeners**

√5ᵗʰ **T38.8 Poisoning by, adverse effect of and underdosing of other and unspecified hormones and synthetic substitutes**

√6ᵗʰ **T38.80 Poisoning by, adverse effect of and underdosing of unspecified hormones and synthetic substitutes**

√7ᵗʰ **T38.801 Poisoning by unspecified hormones and synthetic substitutes,** accidental **(unintentional)**
  Poisoning by unspecified hormones and synthetic substitutes NOS

√7ᵗʰ **T38.802 Poisoning by unspecified hormones and synthetic substitutes,** intentional self-harm

√7ᵗʰ **T38.803 Poisoning by unspecified hormones and synthetic substitutes,** assault

√7ᵗʰ **T38.804 Poisoning by unspecified hormones and synthetic substitutes,** undetermined

√7ᵗʰ **T38.805** Adverse effect **of unspecified hormones and synthetic substitutes**

√7ᵗʰ **T38.806** Underdosing **of unspecified hormones and synthetic substitutes**

√6ᵗʰ **T38.81 Poisoning by, adverse effect of and underdosing of** anterior pituitary [adenohypophyseal] hormones

√7ᵗʰ **T38.811 Poisoning by anterior pituitary [adenohypophyseal] hormones,** accidental **(unintentional)**
  Poisoning by anterior pituitary [adenohypophyseal] hormones NOS

√7ᵗʰ **T38.812 Poisoning by anterior pituitary [adenohypophyseal] hormones,** intentional self-harm

√7ᵗʰ **T38.813 Poisoning by anterior pituitary [adenohypophyseal] hormones,** assault

√7ᵗʰ **T38.814 Poisoning by anterior pituitary [adenohypophyseal] hormones,** undetermined

√7ᵗʰ **T38.815** Adverse effect **of anterior pituitary [adenohypophyseal] hormones**

√7ᵗʰ **T38.816** Underdosing **of anterior pituitary [adenohypophyseal] hormones**

√6ᵗʰ **T38.89 Poisoning by, adverse effect of and underdosing of other hormones and synthetic substitutes**

√7ᵗʰ **T38.891 Poisoning by other hormones and synthetic substitutes,** accidental **(unintentional)**
  Poisoning by other hormones and synthetic substitutes NOS

√7ᵗʰ **T38.892 Poisoning by other hormones and synthetic substitutes,** intentional self-harm

√7ᵗʰ **T38.893 Poisoning by other hormones and synthetic substitutes,** assault

√7ᵗʰ **T38.894 Poisoning by other hormones and synthetic substitutes,** undetermined

√7ᵗʰ **T38.895** Adverse effect **of other hormones and synthetic substitutes**

√7ᵗʰ **T38.896** Underdosing **of other hormones and synthetic substitutes**

√5ᵗʰ **T38.9 Poisoning by, adverse effect of and underdosing of other and unspecified hormone antagonists**

√6ᵗʰ **T38.90 Poisoning by, adverse effect of and underdosing of unspecified hormone antagonists**

√7ᵗʰ **T38.901 Poisoning by unspecified hormone antagonists,** accidental **(unintentional)**
  Poisoning by unspecified hormone antagonists NOS

√7ᵗʰ **T38.902 Poisoning by unspecified hormone antagonists,** intentional self-harm

√7ᵗʰ **T38.903 Poisoning by unspecified hormone antagonists,** assault

√7ᵗʰ **T38.904 Poisoning by unspecified hormone antagonists,** undetermined

√7ᵗʰ **T38.905** Adverse effect **of unspecified hormone antagonists**

√7ᵗʰ **T38.906** Underdosing of unspecified hormone antagonists

√6ᵗʰ **T38.99** Poisoning by, adverse effect of and underdosing of other hormone antagonists

√7ᵗʰ **T38.991** Poisoning by other hormone antagonists, accidental (unintentional)
Poisoning by other hormone antagonists NOS

√7ᵗʰ **T38.992** Poisoning by other hormone antagonists, intentional self-harm

√7ᵗʰ **T38.993** Poisoning by other hormone antagonists, assault

√7ᵗʰ **T38.994** Poisoning by other hormone antagonists, undetermined

√7ᵗʰ **T38.995** Adverse effect of other hormone antagonists

√7ᵗʰ **T38.996** Underdosing of other hormone antagonists

√4ᵗʰ **T39** Poisoning by, adverse effect of and underdosing of nonopioid analgesics, antipyretics and antirheumatics

The appropriate 7th character is to be added to each code from category T39.
A initial encounter
D subsequent encounter
S sequela

√5ᵗʰ **T39.0** Poisoning by, adverse effect of and underdosing of salicylates

√6ᵗʰ **T39.01** Poisoning by, adverse effect of and underdosing of aspirin
Poisoning by, adverse effect of and underdosing of acetylsalicylic acid

√7ᵗʰ **T39.011** Poisoning by aspirin, accidental (unintentional)

√7ᵗʰ **T39.012** Poisoning by aspirin, intentional self-harm

√7ᵗʰ **T39.013** Poisoning by aspirin, assault

√7ᵗʰ **T39.014** Poisoning by aspirin, undetermined

√7ᵗʰ **T39.015** Adverse effect of aspirin
AHA: 2016,1Q,15

√7ᵗʰ **T39.016** Underdosing of aspirin

√6ᵗʰ **T39.09** Poisoning by, adverse effect of and underdosing of other salicylates

√7ᵗʰ **T39.091** Poisoning by salicylates, accidental (unintentional)
Poisoning by salicylates NOS

√7ᵗʰ **T39.092** Poisoning by salicylates, intentional self-harm

√7ᵗʰ **T39.093** Poisoning by salicylates, assault

√7ᵗʰ **T39.094** Poisoning by salicylates, undetermined

√7ᵗʰ **T39.095** Adverse effect of salicylates

√7ᵗʰ **T39.096** Underdosing of salicylates

√5ᵗʰ **T39.1** Poisoning by, adverse effect of and underdosing of 4-Aminophenol derivatives

√6ᵗʰ **T39.1X** Poisoning by, adverse effect of and underdosing of 4-Aminophenol derivatives

√7ᵗʰ **T39.1X1** Poisoning by 4-Aminophenol derivatives, accidental (unintentional)
Poisoning by 4-Aminophenol derivatives NOS

√7ᵗʰ **T39.1X2** Poisoning by 4-Aminophenol derivatives, intentional self-harm

√7ᵗʰ **T39.1X3** Poisoning by 4-Aminophenol derivatives, assault

√7ᵗʰ **T39.1X4** Poisoning by 4-Aminophenol derivatives, undetermined

√7ᵗʰ **T39.1X5** Adverse effect of 4-Aminophenol derivatives

√7ᵗʰ **T39.1X6** Underdosing of 4-Aminophenol derivatives

√5ᵗʰ **T39.2** Poisoning by, adverse effect of and underdosing of pyrazolone derivatives

√6ᵗʰ **T39.2X** Poisoning by, adverse effect of and underdosing of pyrazolone derivatives

√7ᵗʰ **T39.2X1** Poisoning by pyrazolone derivatives, accidental (unintentional)
Poisoning by pyrazolone derivatives NOS

√7ᵗʰ **T39.2X2** Poisoning by pyrazolone derivatives, intentional self-harm

√7ᵗʰ **T39.2X3** Poisoning by pyrazolone derivatives, assault

√7ᵗʰ **T39.2X4** Poisoning by pyrazolone derivatives, undetermined

√7ᵗʰ **T39.2X5** Adverse effect of pyrazolone derivatives

√7ᵗʰ **T39.2X6** Underdosing of pyrazolone derivatives

√5ᵗʰ **T39.3** Poisoning by, adverse effect of and underdosing of other nonsteroidal anti-inflammatory drugs [NSAID]

√6ᵗʰ **T39.31** Poisoning by, adverse effect of and underdosing of propionic acid derivatives
Poisoning by, adverse effect of and underdosing of fenoprofen
Poisoning by, adverse effect of and underdosing of flurbiprofen
Poisoning by, adverse effect of and underdosing of ibuprofen
Poisoning by, adverse effect of and underdosing of ketoprofen
Poisoning by, adverse effect of and underdosing of naproxen
Poisoning by, adverse effect of and underdosing of oxaprozin

√7ᵗʰ **T39.311** Poisoning by propionic acid derivatives, accidental (unintentional)

√7ᵗʰ **T39.312** Poisoning by propionic acid derivatives, intentional self-harm

√7ᵗʰ **T39.313** Poisoning by propionic acid derivatives, assault

√7ᵗʰ **T39.314** Poisoning by propionic acid derivatives, undetermined

√7ᵗʰ **T39.315** Adverse effect of propionic acid derivatives

√7ᵗʰ **T39.316** Underdosing of propionic acid derivatives

√6ᵗʰ **T39.39** Poisoning by, adverse effect of and underdosing of other nonsteroidal anti-inflammatory drugs [NSAID]

√7ᵗʰ **T39.391** Poisoning by other nonsteroidal anti-inflammatory drugs [NSAID], accidental (unintentional)
Poisoning by other nonsteroidal anti-inflammatory drugs NOS

√7ᵗʰ **T39.392** Poisoning by other nonsteroidal anti-inflammatory drugs [NSAID], intentional self-harm

√7ᵗʰ **T39.393** Poisoning by other nonsteroidal anti-inflammatory drugs [NSAID], assault

√7ᵗʰ **T39.394** Poisoning by other nonsteroidal anti-inflammatory drugs [NSAID], undetermined

√7ᵗʰ **T39.395** Adverse effect of other nonsteroidal anti-inflammatory drugs [NSAID]

√7ᵗʰ **T39.396** Underdosing of other nonsteroidal anti-inflammatory drugs [NSAID]

√5ᵗʰ **T39.4** Poisoning by, adverse effect of and underdosing of antirheumatics, not elsewhere classified
EXCLUDES 1 poisoning by, adverse effect of and underdosing of glucocorticoids (T38.0-)
poisoning by, adverse effect of and underdosing of salicylates (T39.0-)

√6ᵗʰ **T39.4X** Poisoning by, adverse effect of and underdosing of antirheumatics, not elsewhere classified

√7ᵗʰ **T39.4X1** Poisoning by antirheumatics, not elsewhere classified, accidental (unintentional)
Poisoning by antirheumatics, not elsewhere classified NOS

√7ᵗʰ **T39.4X2** Poisoning by antirheumatics, not elsewhere classified, intentional self-harm

√7ᵗʰ **T39.4X3** Poisoning by antirheumatics, not elsewhere classified, assault

√7ᵗʰ **T39.4X4** Poisoning by antirheumatics, not elsewhere classified, undetermined

√7ᵗʰ **T39.4X5** Adverse effect of antirheumatics, not elsewhere classified

√7ᵗʰ **T39.4X6** Underdosing of antirheumatics, not elsewhere classified

Chapter 19. Injury, Poisoning and Certain Other Consequences of External Causes

T39.8–T40.692

✓5ᵗʰ **T39.8** Poisoning by, adverse effect of and underdosing of other nonopioid analgesics and antipyretics, not elsewhere classified

  ✓6ᵗʰ **T39.8X** Poisoning by, adverse effect of and underdosing of other nonopioid analgesics and antipyretics, not elsewhere classified

    ✓7ᵗʰ **T39.8X1** Poisoning by other nonopioid analgesics and antipyretics, not elsewhere classified, accidental (unintentional)
      Poisoning by other nonopioid analgesics and antipyretics, not elsewhere classified NOS

    ✓7ᵗʰ **T39.8X2** Poisoning by other nonopioid analgesics and antipyretics, not elsewhere classified, intentional self-harm

    ✓7ᵗʰ **T39.8X3** Poisoning by other nonopioid analgesics and antipyretics, not elsewhere classified, assault

    ✓7ᵗʰ **T39.8X4** Poisoning by other nonopioid analgesics and antipyretics, not elsewhere classified, undetermined

    ✓7ᵗʰ **T39.8X5** Adverse effect of other nonopioid analgesics and antipyretics, not elsewhere classified

    ✓7ᵗʰ **T39.8X6** Underdosing of other nonopioid analgesics and antipyretics, not elsewhere classified

✓5ᵗʰ **T39.9** Poisoning by, adverse effect of and underdosing of unspecified nonopioid analgesic, antipyretic and antirheumatic

  ✓✗7ᵗʰ **T39.91** Poisoning by unspecified nonopioid analgesic, antipyretic and antirheumatic, accidental (unintentional)
    Poisoning by nonopioid analgesic, antipyretic and antirheumatic NOS

  ✓✗7ᵗʰ **T39.92** Poisoning by unspecified nonopioid analgesic, antipyretic and antirheumatic, intentional self-harm

  ✓✗7ᵗʰ **T39.93** Poisoning by unspecified nonopioid analgesic, antipyretic and antirheumatic, assault

  ✓✗7ᵗʰ **T39.94** Poisoning by unspecified nonopioid analgesic, antipyretic and antirheumatic, undetermined

  ✓✗7ᵗʰ **T39.95** Adverse effect of unspecified nonopioid analgesic, antipyretic and antirheumatic

  ✓✗7ᵗʰ **T39.96** Underdosing of unspecified nonopioid analgesic, antipyretic and antirheumatic

✓4ᵗʰ **T40** Poisoning by, adverse effect of and underdosing of narcotics and psychodysleptics [hallucinogens]

  EXCLUDES 2   drug dependence and related mental and behavioral disorders due to psychoactive substance use (F10.-F19.-)

> The appropriate 7th character is to be added to each code from category T40.
> A initial encounter
> D subsequent encounter
> S sequela

✓5ᵗʰ **T40.0** Poisoning by, adverse effect of and underdosing of opium

  ✓6ᵗʰ **T40.0X** Poisoning by, adverse effect of and underdosing of opium

    ✓7ᵗʰ **T40.0X1** Poisoning by opium, accidental (unintentional)
      Poisoning by opium NOS

    ✓7ᵗʰ **T40.0X2** Poisoning by opium, intentional self-harm

    ✓7ᵗʰ **T40.0X3** Poisoning by opium, assault

    ✓7ᵗʰ **T40.0X4** Poisoning by opium, undetermined

    ✓7ᵗʰ **T40.0X5** Adverse effect of opium

    ✓7ᵗʰ **T40.0X6** Underdosing of opium

✓5ᵗʰ **T40.1** Poisoning by and adverse effect of heroin

  ✓6ᵗʰ **T40.1X** Poisoning by and adverse effect of heroin

    ✓7ᵗʰ **T40.1X1** Poisoning by heroin, accidental (unintentional)
      Poisoning by heroin NOS

    ✓7ᵗʰ **T40.1X2** Poisoning by heroin, intentional self-harm

    ✓7ᵗʰ **T40.1X3** Poisoning by heroin, assault

    ✓7ᵗʰ **T40.1X4** Poisoning by heroin, undetermined

✓5ᵗʰ **T40.2** Poisoning by, adverse effect of and underdosing of other opioids

  ✓6ᵗʰ **T40.2X** Poisoning by, adverse effect of and underdosing of other opioids

    ✓7ᵗʰ **T40.2X1** Poisoning by other opioids, accidental (unintentional)
      Poisoning by other opioids NOS

    ✓7ᵗʰ **T40.2X2** Poisoning by other opioids, intentional self-harm

    ✓7ᵗʰ **T40.2X3** Poisoning by other opioids, assault

    ✓7ᵗʰ **T40.2X4** Poisoning by other opioids, undetermined

    ✓7ᵗʰ **T40.2X5** Adverse effect of other opioids

    ✓7ᵗʰ **T40.2X6** Underdosing of other opioids

✓5ᵗʰ **T40.3** Poisoning by, adverse effect of and underdosing of methadone

  ✓6ᵗʰ **T40.3X** Poisoning by, adverse effect of and underdosing of methadone

    ✓7ᵗʰ **T40.3X1** Poisoning by methadone, accidental (unintentional)
      Poisoning by methadone NOS

    ✓7ᵗʰ **T40.3X2** Poisoning by methadone, intentional self-harm

    ✓7ᵗʰ **T40.3X3** Poisoning by methadone, assault

    ✓7ᵗʰ **T40.3X4** Poisoning by methadone, undetermined

    ✓7ᵗʰ **T40.3X5** Adverse effect of methadone

    ✓7ᵗʰ **T40.3X6** Underdosing of methadone

✓5ᵗʰ **T40.4** Poisoning by, adverse effect of and underdosing of other synthetic narcotics

  ✓6ᵗʰ **T40.4X** Poisoning by, adverse effect of and underdosing of other synthetic narcotics

    ✓7ᵗʰ **T40.4X1** Poisoning by other synthetic narcotics, accidental (unintentional)
      Poisoning by other synthetic narcotics NOS

    ✓7ᵗʰ **T40.4X2** Poisoning by other synthetic narcotics, intentional self-harm

    ✓7ᵗʰ **T40.4X3** Poisoning by other synthetic narcotics, assault

    ✓7ᵗʰ **T40.4X4** Poisoning by other synthetic narcotics, undetermined

    ✓7ᵗʰ **T40.4X5** Adverse effect of other synthetic narcotics

    ✓7ᵗʰ **T40.4X6** Underdosing of other synthetic narcotics

✓5ᵗʰ **T40.5** Poisoning by, adverse effect of and underdosing of cocaine

  ✓6ᵗʰ **T40.5X** Poisoning by, adverse effect of and underdosing of cocaine

    ✓7ᵗʰ **T40.5X1** Poisoning by cocaine, accidental (unintentional)
      Poisoning by cocaine NOS
      AHA: 2016,2Q,8

    ✓7ᵗʰ **T40.5X2** Poisoning by cocaine, intentional self-harm

    ✓7ᵗʰ **T40.5X3** Poisoning by cocaine, assault

    ✓7ᵗʰ **T40.5X4** Poisoning by cocaine, undetermined

    ✓7ᵗʰ **T40.5X5** Adverse effect of cocaine

    ✓7ᵗʰ **T40.5X6** Underdosing of cocaine

✓5ᵗʰ **T40.6** Poisoning by, adverse effect of and underdosing of other and unspecified narcotics

  ✓6ᵗʰ **T40.60** Poisoning by, adverse effect of and underdosing of unspecified narcotics

    ✓7ᵗʰ **T40.601** Poisoning by unspecified narcotics, accidental (unintentional)
      Poisoning by narcotics NOS

    ✓7ᵗʰ **T40.602** Poisoning by unspecified narcotics, intentional self-harm

    ✓7ᵗʰ **T40.603** Poisoning by unspecified narcotics, assault

    ✓7ᵗʰ **T40.604** Poisoning by unspecified narcotics, undetermined

    ✓7ᵗʰ **T40.605** Adverse effect of unspecified narcotics

    ✓7ᵗʰ **T40.606** Underdosing of unspecified narcotics

  ✓6ᵗʰ **T40.69** Poisoning by, adverse effect of and underdosing of other narcotics

    ✓7ᵗʰ **T40.691** Poisoning by other narcotics, accidental (unintentional)
      Poisoning by other narcotics NOS

    ✓7ᵗʰ **T40.692** Poisoning by other narcotics, intentional self-harm

✓7ᵗʰ **T40.693** Poisoning by other narcotics, assault

✓7ᵗʰ **T40.694** Poisoning by other narcotics, undetermined

✓7ᵗʰ **T40.695** Adverse effect of other narcotics

✓7ᵗʰ **T40.696** Underdosing of other narcotics

✓5ᵗʰ **T40.7** Poisoning by, adverse effect of and underdosing of cannabis (derivatives)

✓6ᵗʰ **T40.7X** Poisoning by, adverse effect of and underdosing of cannabis (derivatives)

✓7ᵗʰ **T40.7X1** Poisoning by cannabis (derivatives), accidental (unintentional)
Poisoning by cannabis NOS

✓7ᵗʰ **T40.7X2** Poisoning by cannabis (derivatives), intentional self-harm

✓7ᵗʰ **T40.7X3** Poisoning by cannabis (derivatives), assault

✓7ᵗʰ **T40.7X4** Poisoning by cannabis (derivatives), undetermined

✓7ᵗʰ **T40.7X5** Adverse effect of cannabis (derivatives)

✓7ᵗʰ **T40.7X6** Underdosing of cannabis (derivatives)

✓5ᵗʰ **T40.8** Poisoning by and adverse effect of lysergide [LSD]

✓6ᵗʰ **T40.8X** Poisoning by and adverse effect of lysergide [LSD]

✓7ᵗʰ **T40.8X1** Poisoning by lysergide [LSD], accidental (unintentional)
Poisoning by lysergide [LSD] NOS

✓7ᵗʰ **T40.8X2** Poisoning by lysergide [LSD], intentional self-harm

✓7ᵗʰ **T40.8X3** Poisoning by lysergide [LSD], assault

✓7ᵗʰ **T40.8X4** Poisoning by lysergide [LSD], undetermined

✓5ᵗʰ **T40.9** Poisoning by, adverse effect of and underdosing of other and unspecified psychodysleptics [hallucinogens]

✓6ᵗʰ **T40.90** Poisoning by, adverse effect of and underdosing of unspecified psychodysleptics [hallucinogens]

✓7ᵗʰ **T40.901** Poisoning by unspecified psychodysleptics [hallucinogens], accidental (unintentional)

✓7ᵗʰ **T40.902** Poisoning by unspecified psychodysleptics [hallucinogens], intentional self-harm

✓7ᵗʰ **T40.903** Poisoning by unspecified psychodysleptics [hallucinogens], assault

✓7ᵗʰ **T40.904** Poisoning by unspecified psychodysleptics [hallucinogens], undetermined

✓7ᵗʰ **T40.905** Adverse effect of unspecified psychodysleptics [hallucinogens]

✓7ᵗʰ **T40.906** Underdosing of unspecified psychodysleptics [hallucinogens]

✓6ᵗʰ **T40.99** Poisoning by, adverse effect of and underdosing of other psychodysleptics [hallucinogens]

✓7ᵗʰ **T40.991** Poisoning by other psychodysleptics [hallucinogens], accidental (unintentional)
Poisoning by other psychodysleptics [hallucinogens] NOS

✓7ᵗʰ **T40.992** Poisoning by other psychodysleptics [hallucinogens], intentional self-harm

✓7ᵗʰ **T40.993** Poisoning by other psychodysleptics [hallucinogens], assault

✓7ᵗʰ **T40.994** Poisoning by other psychodysleptics [hallucinogens], undetermined

✓7ᵗʰ **T40.995** Adverse effect of other psychodysleptics [hallucinogens]

✓7ᵗʰ **T40.996** Underdosing of other psychodysleptics [hallucinogens]

✓4ᵗʰ **T41** Poisoning by, adverse effect of and underdosing of anesthetics and therapeutic gases

EXCLUDES 1　benzodiazepines (T42.4-)
cocaine (T40.5-)
complications of anesthesia during labor and delivery (O74.-)
complications of anesthesia during pregnancy (O29.-)
complications of anesthesia during the puerperium (O89.-)
opioids (T40.0-T40.2-)

The appropriate 7th character is to be added to each code from category T41.
A initial encounter
D subsequent encounter
S sequela

✓5ᵗʰ **T41.0** Poisoning by, adverse effect of and underdosing of inhaled anesthetics
EXCLUDES 1　oxygen (T41.5-)

✓6ᵗʰ **T41.0X** Poisoning by, adverse effect of and underdosing of inhaled anesthetics

✓7ᵗʰ **T41.0X1** Poisoning by inhaled anesthetics, accidental (unintentional)
Poisoning by inhaled anesthetics NOS

✓7ᵗʰ **T41.0X2** Poisoning by inhaled anesthetics, intentional self-harm

✓7ᵗʰ **T41.0X3** Poisoning by inhaled anesthetics, assault

✓7ᵗʰ **T41.0X4** Poisoning by inhaled anesthetics, undetermined

✓7ᵗʰ **T41.0X5** Adverse effect of inhaled anesthetics

✓7ᵗʰ **T41.0X6** Underdosing of inhaled anesthetics

✓5ᵗʰ **T41.1** Poisoning by, adverse effect of and underdosing of intravenous anesthetics
Poisoning by, adverse effect of and underdosing of thiobarbiturates

✓6ᵗʰ **T41.1X** Poisoning by, adverse effect of and underdosing of intravenous anesthetics

✓7ᵗʰ **T41.1X1** Poisoning by intravenous anesthetics, accidental (unintentional)
Poisoning by intravenous anesthetics NOS

✓7ᵗʰ **T41.1X2** Poisoning by intravenous anesthetics, intentional self-harm

✓7ᵗʰ **T41.1X3** Poisoning by intravenous anesthetics, assault

✓7ᵗʰ **T41.1X4** Poisoning by intravenous anesthetics, undetermined

✓7ᵗʰ **T41.1X5** Adverse effect of intravenous anesthetics

✓7ᵗʰ **T41.1X6** Underdosing of intravenous anesthetics

✓5ᵗʰ **T41.2** Poisoning by, adverse effect of and underdosing of other and unspecified general anesthetics

✓6ᵗʰ **T41.20** Poisoning by, adverse effect of and underdosing of unspecified general anesthetics

✓7ᵗʰ **T41.201** Poisoning by unspecified general anesthetics, accidental (unintentional)
Poisoning by general anesthetics NOS

✓7ᵗʰ **T41.202** Poisoning by unspecified general anesthetics, intentional self-harm

✓7ᵗʰ **T41.203** Poisoning by unspecified general anesthetics, assault

✓7ᵗʰ **T41.204** Poisoning by unspecified general anesthetics, undetermined

✓7ᵗʰ **T41.205** Adverse effect of unspecified general anesthetics
AHA: 2016,4Q,73

✓7ᵗʰ **T41.206** Underdosing of unspecified general anesthetics

✓6ᵗʰ **T41.29** Poisoning by, adverse effect of and underdosing of other general anesthetics

✓7ᵗʰ **T41.291** Poisoning by other general anesthetics, accidental (unintentional)
Poisoning by other general anesthetics NOS

✓7ᵗʰ **T41.292** Poisoning by other general anesthetics, intentional self-harm

✓7ᵗʰ **T41.293** Poisoning by other general anesthetics, assault

✓7ᵗʰ **T41.294** Poisoning by other general anesthetics, undetermined

✓7ᵗʰ **T41.295** Adverse effect of other general anesthetics

✓7ᵗʰ **T41.296** Underdosing of other general anesthetics

√5ᵗʰ **T41.3** **Poisoning by, adverse effect of and underdosing of local anesthetics**
Cocaine (topical)
    EXCLUDES 2   *poisoning by cocaine used as a central nervous system stimulant (T40.5X1-T40.5X4)*

   √6ᵗʰ **T41.3X** **Poisoning by, adverse effect of and underdosing of local anesthetics**

     √7ᵗʰ **T41.3X1** **Poisoning by local anesthetics,** accidental **(unintentional)**
Poisoning by local anesthetics NOS

     √7ᵗʰ **T41.3X2** **Poisoning by local anesthetics,** intentional self-harm

     √7ᵗʰ **T41.3X3** **Poisoning by local anesthetics,** assault

     √7ᵗʰ **T41.3X4** **Poisoning by local anesthetics,** undetermined

     √7ᵗʰ **T41.3X5** Adverse effect **of local anesthetics**

     √7ᵗʰ **T41.3X6** Underdosing **of local anesthetics**

√5ᵗʰ **T41.4** **Poisoning by, adverse effect of and underdosing of unspecified anesthetic**

   √x7ᵗʰ **T41.41** **Poisoning by unspecified anesthetic,** accidental **(unintentional)**
Poisoning by anesthetic NOS

   √x7ᵗʰ **T41.42** **Poisoning by unspecified anesthetic,** intentional self-harm

   √x7ᵗʰ **T41.43** **Poisoning by unspecified anesthetic,** assault

   √x7ᵗʰ **T41.44** **Poisoning by unspecified anesthetic,** undetermined

   √x7ᵗʰ **T41.45** Adverse effect **of unspecified anesthetic**

   √x7ᵗʰ **T41.46** Underdosing **of unspecified anesthetics**

√5ᵗʰ **T41.5** **Poisoning by, adverse effect of and underdosing of therapeutic gases**

   √6ᵗʰ **T41.5X** **Poisoning by, adverse effect of and underdosing of therapeutic gases**

     √7ᵗʰ **T41.5X1** **Poisoning by therapeutic gases,** accidental **(unintentional)**
Poisoning by therapeutic gases NOS

     √7ᵗʰ **T41.5X2** **Poisoning by therapeutic gases,** intentional self-harm

     √7ᵗʰ **T41.5X3** **Poisoning by therapeutic gases,** assault

     √7ᵗʰ **T41.5X4** **Poisoning by therapeutic gases,** undetermined

     √7ᵗʰ **T41.5X5** Adverse effect **of therapeutic gases**

     √7ᵗʰ **T41.5X6** Underdosing **of therapeutic gases**

√4ᵗʰ **T42** **Poisoning by, adverse effect of and underdosing of antiepileptic, sedative- hypnotic and antiparkinsonism drugs**
    EXCLUDES 2   *drug dependence and related mental and behavioral disorders due to psychoactive substance use (F10.- – F19.-)*

> The appropriate 7th character is to be added to each code from category T42.
> A   initial encounter
> D   subsequent encounter
> S   sequela

  √5ᵗʰ **T42.0** **Poisoning by, adverse effect of and underdosing of hydantoin derivatives**

   √6ᵗʰ **T42.0X** **Poisoning by, adverse effect of and underdosing of hydantoin derivatives**

     √7ᵗʰ **T42.0X1** **Poisoning by hydantoin derivatives,** accidental **(unintentional)**
Poisoning by hydantoin derivatives NOS

     √7ᵗʰ **T42.0X2** **Poisoning by hydantoin derivatives,** intentional self-harm

     √7ᵗʰ **T42.0X3** **Poisoning by hydantoin derivatives,** assault

     √7ᵗʰ **T42.0X4** **Poisoning by hydantoin derivatives,** undetermined

     √7ᵗʰ **T42.0X5** Adverse effect **of hydantoin derivatives**

     √7ᵗʰ **T42.0X6** Underdosing **of hydantoin derivatives**

  √5ᵗʰ **T42.1** **Poisoning by, adverse effect of and underdosing of iminostilbenes**
Poisoning by, adverse effect of and underdosing of carbamazepine

   √6ᵗʰ **T42.1X** **Poisoning by, adverse effect of and underdosing of iminostilbenes**

     √7ᵗʰ **T42.1X1** **Poisoning by iminostilbenes,** accidental **(unintentional)**
Poisoning by iminostilbenes NOS

     √7ᵗʰ **T42.1X2** **Poisoning by iminostilbenes,** intentional self-harm

     √7ᵗʰ **T42.1X3** **Poisoning by iminostilbenes,** assault

     √7ᵗʰ **T42.1X4** **Poisoning by iminostilbenes,** undetermined

     √7ᵗʰ **T42.1X5** Adverse effect **of iminostilbenes**

     √7ᵗʰ **T42.1X6** Underdosing **of iminostilbenes**

  √5ᵗʰ **T42.2** **Poisoning by, adverse effect of and underdosing of succinimides and oxazolidinediones**

   √6ᵗʰ **T42.2X** **Poisoning by, adverse effect of and underdosing of succinimides and oxazolidinediones**

     √7ᵗʰ **T42.2X1** **Poisoning by succinimides and oxazolidinediones,** accidental **(unintentional)**
Poisoning by succinimides and oxazolidinediones NOS

     √7ᵗʰ **T42.2X2** **Poisoning by succinimides and oxazolidinediones,** intentional self-harm

     √7ᵗʰ **T42.2X3** **Poisoning by succinimides and oxazolidinediones,** assault

     √7ᵗʰ **T42.2X4** **Poisoning by succinimides and oxazolidinediones,** undetermined

     √7ᵗʰ **T42.2X5** Adverse effect **of succinimides and oxazolidinediones**

     √7ᵗʰ **T42.2X6** Underdosing **of succinimides and oxazolidinediones**

  √5ᵗʰ **T42.3** **Poisoning by, adverse effect of and underdosing of barbiturates**
    EXCLUDES 1   *poisoning by, adverse effect of and underdosing of thiobarbiturates (T41.1-)*

   √6ᵗʰ **T42.3X** **Poisoning by, adverse effect of and underdosing of barbiturates**

     √7ᵗʰ **T42.3X1** **Poisoning by barbiturates,** accidental **(unintentional)**
Poisoning by barbiturates NOS

     √7ᵗʰ **T42.3X2** **Poisoning by barbiturates,** intentional self-harm

     √7ᵗʰ **T42.3X3** **Poisoning by barbiturates,** assault

     √7ᵗʰ **T42.3X4** **Poisoning by barbiturates,** undetermined

     √7ᵗʰ **T42.3X5** Adverse effect **of barbiturates**

     √7ᵗʰ **T42.3X6** Underdosing **of barbiturates**

  √5ᵗʰ **T42.4** **Poisoning by, adverse effect of and underdosing of benzodiazepines**

   √6ᵗʰ **T42.4X** **Poisoning by, adverse effect of and underdosing of benzodiazepines**

     √7ᵗʰ **T42.4X1** **Poisoning by benzodiazepines,** accidental **(unintentional)**
Poisoning by benzodiazepines NOS

     √7ᵗʰ **T42.4X2** **Poisoning by benzodiazepines,** intentional self-harm

     √7ᵗʰ **T42.4X3** **Poisoning by benzodiazepines,** assault

     √7ᵗʰ **T42.4X4** **Poisoning by benzodiazepines,** undetermined

     √7ᵗʰ **T42.4X5** Adverse effect **of benzodiazepines**

     √7ᵗʰ **T42.4X6** Underdosing **of benzodiazepines**

  √5ᵗʰ **T42.5** **Poisoning by, adverse effect of and underdosing of mixed antiepileptics**

   √6ᵗʰ **T42.5X** **Poisoning by, adverse effect of and underdosing of antiepileptics**

     √7ᵗʰ **T42.5X1** **Poisoning by mixed antiepileptics,** accidental **(unintentional)**
Poisoning by mixed antiepileptics NOS

     √7ᵗʰ **T42.5X2** **Poisoning by mixed antiepileptics,** intentional self-harm

     √7ᵗʰ **T42.5X3** **Poisoning by mixed antiepileptics,** assault

     √7ᵗʰ **T42.5X4** **Poisoning by mixed antiepileptics,** undetermined

     √7ᵗʰ **T42.5X5** Adverse effect **of mixed antiepileptics**

     √7ᵗʰ **T42.5X6** Underdosing **of mixed antiepileptics**

☑5ᵗʰ **T42.6** **Poisoning by, adverse effect of and underdosing of other antiepileptic and sedative-hypnotic drugs**
Poisoning by, adverse effect of and underdosing of methaqualone
Poisoning by, adverse effect of and underdosing of valproic acid
EXCLUDES 1 *poisoning by, adverse effect of and underdosing of carbamazepine (T42.1-)*

    ☑6ᵗʰ **T42.6X** **Poisoning by, adverse effect of and underdosing of other antiepileptic and sedative-hypnotic drugs**

        ☑7ᵗʰ **T42.6X1** **Poisoning by other antiepileptic and sedative-hypnotic drugs, accidental (unintentional)**
Poisoning by other antiepileptic and sedative-hypnotic drugs NOS

        ☑7ᵗʰ **T42.6X2** **Poisoning by other antiepileptic and sedative-hypnotic drugs, intentional self-harm**

        ☑7ᵗʰ **T42.6X3** **Poisoning by other antiepileptic and sedative-hypnotic drugs, assault**

        ☑7ᵗʰ **T42.6X4** **Poisoning by other antiepileptic and sedative-hypnotic drugs, undetermined**

        ☑7ᵗʰ **T42.6X5** **Adverse effect of other antiepileptic and sedative-hypnotic drugs**

        ☑7ᵗʰ **T42.6X6** **Underdosing of other antiepileptic and sedative-hypnotic drugs**

☑5ᵗʰ **T42.7** **Poisoning by, adverse effect of and underdosing of unspecified antiepileptic and sedative-hypnotic drugs**

    ☑x7ᵗʰ **T42.71** **Poisoning by unspecified antiepileptic and sedative-hypnotic drugs, accidental (unintentional)**
Poisoning by antiepileptic and sedative-hypnotic drugs NOS

    ☑x7ᵗʰ **T42.72** **Poisoning by unspecified antiepileptic and sedative-hypnotic drugs, intentional self-harm**

    ☑x7ᵗʰ **T42.73** **Poisoning by unspecified antiepileptic and sedative-hypnotic drugs, assault**

    ☑x7ᵗʰ **T42.74** **Poisoning by unspecified antiepileptic and sedative-hypnotic drugs, undetermined**

    ☑x7ᵗʰ **T42.75** **Adverse effect of unspecified antiepileptic and sedative-hypnotic drugs**

    ☑x7ᵗʰ **T42.76** **Underdosing of unspecified antiepileptic and sedative-hypnotic drugs**

☑5ᵗʰ **T42.8** **Poisoning by, adverse effect of and underdosing of antiparkinsonism drugs and other central muscle-tone depressants**
Poisoning by, adverse effect of and underdosing of amantadine

    ☑6ᵗʰ **T42.8X** **Poisoning by, adverse effect of and underdosing of antiparkinsonism drugs and other central muscle-tone depressants**

        ☑7ᵗʰ **T42.8X1** **Poisoning by antiparkinsonism drugs and other central muscle-tone depressants, accidental (unintentional)**
Poisoning by antiparkinsonism drugs and other central muscle-tone depressants NOS

        ☑7ᵗʰ **T42.8X2** **Poisoning by antiparkinsonism drugs and other central muscle-tone depressants, intentional self-harm**

        ☑7ᵗʰ **T42.8X3** **Poisoning by antiparkinsonism drugs and other central muscle-tone depressants, assault**

        ☑7ᵗʰ **T42.8X4** **Poisoning by antiparkinsonism drugs and other central muscle-tone depressants, undetermined**

        ☑7ᵗʰ **T42.8X5** **Adverse effect of antiparkinsonism drugs and other central muscle-tone depressants**

        ☑7ᵗʰ **T42.8X6** **Underdosing of antiparkinsonism drugs and other central muscle-tone depressants**

☑4ᵗʰ **T43** **Poisoning by, adverse effect of and underdosing of psychotropic drugs, not elsewhere classified**
    EXCLUDES 1 *appetite depressants (T50.5-)*
        barbiturates (T42.3-)
        benzodiazepines (T42.4-)
        methaqualone (T42.6-)
        psychodysleptics [hallucinogens] (T40.7-T40.9-)
    EXCLUDES 2 *drug dependence and related mental and behavioral disorders due to psychoactive substance use (F10.- – F19.-)*

The appropriate 7th character is to be added to each code from category T43.
A initial encounter
D subsequent encounter
S sequela

☑5ᵗʰ **T43.0** **Poisoning by, adverse effect of and underdosing of tricyclic and tetracyclic antidepressants**

    ☑6ᵗʰ **T43.01** **Poisoning by, adverse effect of and underdosing of tricyclic antidepressants**

        ☑7ᵗʰ **T43.011** **Poisoning by tricyclic antidepressants, accidental (unintentional)**
Poisoning by tricyclic antidepressants NOS

        ☑7ᵗʰ **T43.012** **Poisoning by tricyclic antidepressants, intentional self-harm**

        ☑7ᵗʰ **T43.013** **Poisoning by tricyclic antidepressants, assault**

        ☑7ᵗʰ **T43.014** **Poisoning by tricyclic antidepressants, undetermined**

        ☑7ᵗʰ **T43.015** **Adverse effect of tricyclic antidepressants**

        ☑7ᵗʰ **T43.016** **Underdosing of tricyclic antidepressants**

    ☑6ᵗʰ **T43.02** **Poisoning by, adverse effect of and underdosing of tetracyclic antidepressants**

        ☑7ᵗʰ **T43.021** **Poisoning by tetracyclic antidepressants, accidental (unintentional)**
Poisoning by tetracyclic antidepressants NOS

        ☑7ᵗʰ **T43.022** **Poisoning by tetracyclic antidepressants, intentional self-harm**

        ☑7ᵗʰ **T43.023** **Poisoning by tetracyclic antidepressants, assault**

        ☑7ᵗʰ **T43.024** **Poisoning by tetracyclic antidepressants, undetermined**

        ☑7ᵗʰ **T43.025** **Adverse effect of tetracyclic antidepressants**

        ☑7ᵗʰ **T43.026** **Underdosing of tetracyclic antidepressants**

☑5ᵗʰ **T43.1** **Poisoning by, adverse effect of and underdosing of monoamine-oxidase-inhibitor antidepressants**

    ☑6ᵗʰ **T43.1X** **Poisoning by, adverse effect of and underdosing of monoamine-oxidase-inhibitor antidepressants**

        ☑7ᵗʰ **T43.1X1** **Poisoning by monoamine-oxidase-inhibitor antidepressants, accidental (unintentional)**
Poisoning by monoamine-oxidase-inhibitor antidepressants NOS

        ☑7ᵗʰ **T43.1X2** **Poisoning by monoamine-oxidase-inhibitor antidepressants, intentional self-harm**

        ☑7ᵗʰ **T43.1X3** **Poisoning by monoamine-oxidase-inhibitor antidepressants, assault**

        ☑7ᵗʰ **T43.1X4** **Poisoning by monoamine-oxidase-inhibitor antidepressants, undetermined**

        ☑7ᵗʰ **T43.1X5** **Adverse effect of monoamine-oxidase-inhibitor antidepressants**

        ☑7ᵗʰ **T43.1X6** **Underdosing of monoamine-oxidase-inhibitor antidepressants**

☑5ᵗʰ **T43.2** **Poisoning by, adverse effect of and underdosing of other and unspecified antidepressants**

    ☑6ᵗʰ **T43.20** **Poisoning by, adverse effect of and underdosing of unspecified antidepressants**

        ☑7ᵗʰ **T43.201** **Poisoning by unspecified antidepressants, accidental (unintentional)**
Poisoning by antidepressants NOS

        ☑7ᵗʰ **T43.202** **Poisoning by unspecified antidepressants, intentional self-harm**

☑7ᵗʰ **T43.203** **Poisoning by unspecified antidepressants, assault**

☑7ᵗʰ **T43.204** **Poisoning by unspecified antidepressants, undetermined**

☑7ᵗʰ **T43.205** Adverse effect of unspecified antidepressants

Antidepressant discontinuation syndrome

☑7ᵗʰ **T43.206** Underdosing of unspecified antidepressants

☑6ᵗʰ **T43.21** **Poisoning by, adverse effect of and underdosing of selective serotonin and norepinephrine reuptake inhibitors**

Poisoning by, adverse effect of and underdosing of SSNRI antidepressants

☑7ᵗʰ **T43.211** **Poisoning by selective serotonin and norepinephrine reuptake inhibitors, accidental (unintentional)**

☑7ᵗʰ **T43.212** **Poisoning by selective serotonin and norepinephrine reuptake inhibitors, intentional self-harm**

☑7ᵗʰ **T43.213** **Poisoning by selective serotonin and norepinephrine reuptake inhibitors, assault**

☑7ᵗʰ **T43.214** **Poisoning by selective serotonin and norepinephrine reuptake inhibitors, undetermined**

☑7ᵗʰ **T43.215** Adverse effect of selective serotonin and norepinephrine reuptake inhibitors

☑7ᵗʰ **T43.216** Underdosing of selective serotonin and norepinephrine reuptake inhibitors

☑6ᵗʰ **T43.22** **Poisoning by, adverse effect of and underdosing of selective serotonin reuptake inhibitors**

Poisoning by, adverse effect of and underdosing of SSRI antidepressants

☑7ᵗʰ **T43.221** **Poisoning by selective serotonin reuptake inhibitors, accidental (unintentional)**

☑7ᵗʰ **T43.222** **Poisoning by selective serotonin reuptake inhibitors, intentional self-harm**

☑7ᵗʰ **T43.223** **Poisoning by selective serotonin reuptake inhibitors, assault**

☑7ᵗʰ **T43.224** **Poisoning by selective serotonin reuptake inhibitors, undetermined**

☑7ᵗʰ **T43.225** Adverse effect of selective serotonin reuptake inhibitors

☑7ᵗʰ **T43.226** Underdosing of selective serotonin reuptake inhibitors

☑6ᵗʰ **T43.29** **Poisoning by, adverse effect of and underdosing of other antidepressants**

☑7ᵗʰ **T43.291** **Poisoning by other antidepressants, accidental (unintentional)**

Poisoning by other antidepressants NOS

☑7ᵗʰ **T43.292** **Poisoning by other antidepressants, intentional self-harm**

☑7ᵗʰ **T43.293** **Poisoning by other antidepressants, assault**

☑7ᵗʰ **T43.294** **Poisoning by other antidepressants, undetermined**

☑7ᵗʰ **T43.295** Adverse effect of other antidepressants

☑7ᵗʰ **T43.296** Underdosing of other antidepressants

☑5ᵗʰ **T43.3** **Poisoning by, adverse effect of and underdosing of phenothiazine antipsychotics and neuroleptics**

☑6ᵗʰ **T43.3X** **Poisoning by, adverse effect of and underdosing of phenothiazine antipsychotics and neuroleptics**

☑7ᵗʰ **T43.3X1** **Poisoning by phenothiazine antipsychotics and neuroleptics, accidental (unintentional)**

Poisoning by phenothiazine antipsychotics and neuroleptics NOS

☑7ᵗʰ **T43.3X2** **Poisoning by phenothiazine antipsychotics and neuroleptics, intentional self-harm**

☑7ᵗʰ **T43.3X3** **Poisoning by phenothiazine antipsychotics and neuroleptics, assault**

☑7ᵗʰ **T43.3X4** **Poisoning by phenothiazine antipsychotics and neuroleptics, undetermined**

☑7ᵗʰ **T43.3X5** Adverse effect of phenothiazine antipsychotics and neuroleptics

☑7ᵗʰ **T43.3X6** Underdosing of phenothiazine antipsychotics and neuroleptics

☑5ᵗʰ **T43.4** **Poisoning by, adverse effect of and underdosing of butyrophenone and thiothixene neuroleptics**

☑6ᵗʰ **T43.4X** **Poisoning by, adverse effect of and underdosing of butyrophenone and thiothixene neuroleptics**

☑7ᵗʰ **T43.4X1** **Poisoning by butyrophenone and thiothixene neuroleptics, accidental (unintentional)**

Poisoning by butyrophenone and thiothixene neuroleptics NOS

☑7ᵗʰ **T43.4X2** **Poisoning by butyrophenone and thiothixene neuroleptics, intentional self-harm**

☑7ᵗʰ **T43.4X3** **Poisoning by butyrophenone and thiothixene neuroleptics, assault**

☑7ᵗʰ **T43.4X4** **Poisoning by butyrophenone and thiothixene neuroleptics, undetermined**

☑7ᵗʰ **T43.4X5** Adverse effect of butyrophenone and thiothixene neuroleptics

☑7ᵗʰ **T43.4X6** Underdosing of butyrophenone and thiothixene neuroleptics

☑5ᵗʰ **T43.5** **Poisoning by, adverse effect of and underdosing of other and unspecified antipsychotics and neuroleptics**

EXCLUDES 1   *poisoning by, adverse effect of and underdosing of rauwolfia (T46.5-)*

☑6ᵗʰ **T43.50** **Poisoning by, adverse effect of and underdosing of unspecified antipsychotics and neuroleptics**

☑7ᵗʰ **T43.501** **Poisoning by unspecified antipsychotics and neuroleptics, accidental (unintentional)**

Poisoning by antipsychotics and neuroleptics NOS

☑7ᵗʰ **T43.502** **Poisoning by unspecified antipsychotics and neuroleptics, intentional self-harm**

☑7ᵗʰ **T43.503** **Poisoning by unspecified antipsychotics and neuroleptics, assault**

☑7ᵗʰ **T43.504** **Poisoning by unspecified antipsychotics and neuroleptics, undetermined**

☑7ᵗʰ **T43.505** Adverse effect of unspecified antipsychotics and neuroleptics

☑7ᵗʰ **T43.506** Underdosing of unspecified antipsychotics and neuroleptics

☑6ᵗʰ **T43.59** **Poisoning by, adverse effect of and underdosing of other antipsychotics and neuroleptics**

AHA: 2017,1Q,40

☑7ᵗʰ **T43.591** **Poisoning by other antipsychotics and neuroleptics, accidental (unintentional)**

Poisoning by other antipsychotics and neuroleptics NOS

☑7ᵗʰ **T43.592** **Poisoning by other antipsychotics and neuroleptics, intentional self-harm**

☑7ᵗʰ **T43.593** **Poisoning by other antipsychotics and neuroleptics, assault**

☑7ᵗʰ **T43.594** **Poisoning by other antipsychotics and neuroleptics, undetermined**

☑7ᵗʰ **T43.595** Adverse effect of other antipsychotics and neuroleptics

☑7ᵗʰ **T43.596** Underdosing of other antipsychotics and neuroleptics

☑5ᵗʰ **T43.6** **Poisoning by, adverse effect of and underdosing of psychostimulants**

EXCLUDES 1   *poisoning by, adverse effect of and underdosing of cocaine (T40.5-)*

☑6ᵗʰ **T43.60** **Poisoning by, adverse effect of and underdosing of unspecified psychostimulant**

☑7ᵗʰ **T43.601** **Poisoning by unspecified psychostimulants, accidental (unintentional)**

Poisoning by psychostimulants NOS

☑7ᵗʰ **T43.602** **Poisoning by unspecified psychostimulants, intentional self-harm**

☑7ᵗʰ **T43.603** **Poisoning by unspecified psychostimulants, assault**

☑7ᵗʰ **T43.604** **Poisoning by unspecified psychostimulants, undetermined**

☑7ᵗʰ **T43.605** Adverse effect of unspecified psychostimulants

☑7ᵗʰ **T43.606** Underdosing of unspecified psychostimulants

Ⓝ Newborn: 0   Ⓟ Pediatric: 0-17   Ⓜ Maternity: 12-55   Ⓐ Adult: 15-124   CH Comorbidity High   CL Comorbidity Low   NCDx Noncancer Dx   PDx Primary Dx

1094   ICD-10-CM 2020

√6ᵗʰ **T43.61** **Poisoning by, adverse effect of and underdosing of** caffeine

   √7ᵗʰ **T43.611** **Poisoning by caffeine, accidental (unintentional)**
      Poisoning by caffeine NOS

   √7ᵗʰ **T43.612** **Poisoning by caffeine, intentional self-harm**

   √7ᵗʰ **T43.613** **Poisoning by caffeine, assault**

   √7ᵗʰ **T43.614** **Poisoning by caffeine, undetermined**

   √7ᵗʰ **T43.615** Adverse effect of caffeine

   √7ᵗʰ **T43.616** Underdosing of caffeine

√6ᵗʰ **T43.62** **Poisoning by, adverse effect of and underdosing of** amphetamines
   Poisoning by, adverse effect of and underdosing of methamphetamines

   √7ᵗʰ **T43.621** **Poisoning by amphetamines, accidental (unintentional)**
      Poisoning by amphetamines NOS

   √7ᵗʰ **T43.622** **Poisoning by amphetamines, intentional self-harm**

   √7ᵗʰ **T43.623** **Poisoning by amphetamines, assault**

   √7ᵗʰ **T43.624** **Poisoning by amphetamines, undetermined**

   √7ᵗʰ **T43.625** Adverse effect of amphetamines

   √7ᵗʰ **T43.626** Underdosing of amphetamines

√6ᵗʰ **T43.63** **Poisoning by, adverse effect of and underdosing of** methylphenidate

   √7ᵗʰ **T43.631** **Poisoning by methylphenidate, accidental (unintentional)**
      Poisoning by methylphenidate NOS

   √7ᵗʰ **T43.632** **Poisoning by methylphenidate, intentional self-harm**

   √7ᵗʰ **T43.633** **Poisoning by methylphenidate, assault**

   √7ᵗʰ **T43.634** **Poisoning by methylphenidate, undetermined**

   √7ᵗʰ **T43.635** Adverse effect of methylphenidate

   √7ᵗʰ **T43.636** Underdosing of methylphenidate

√6ᵗʰ **T43.64** **Poisoning by** ecstasy
   Poisoning by MDMA
   Poisoning by 3,4-methylenedioxymethamphetamine
   AHA: 2018,4Q,30-31

   √7ᵗʰ **T43.641** **Poisoning by ecstasy, accidental (unintentional)**
      Poisoning by ecstasy NOS

   √7ᵗʰ **T43.642** **Poisoning by ecstasy, intentional self-harm**

   √7ᵗʰ **T43.643** **Poisoning by ecstasy, assault**

   √7ᵗʰ **T43.644** **Poisoning by ecstasy, undetermined**

√6ᵗʰ **T43.69** **Poisoning by, adverse effect of and underdosing of other psychostimulants**

   √7ᵗʰ **T43.691** **Poisoning by other psychostimulants, accidental (unintentional)**
      Poisoning by other psychostimulants NOS

   √7ᵗʰ **T43.692** **Poisoning by other psychostimulants, intentional self-harm**

   √7ᵗʰ **T43.693** **Poisoning by other psychostimulants, assault**

   √7ᵗʰ **T43.694** **Poisoning by other psychostimulants, undetermined**

   √7ᵗʰ **T43.695** Adverse effect of other psychostimulants

   √7ᵗʰ **T43.696** Underdosing of other psychostimulants

√5ᵗʰ **T43.8** **Poisoning by, adverse effect of and underdosing of other psychotropic drugs**

√6ᵗʰ **T43.8X** **Poisoning by, adverse effect of and underdosing of other psychotropic drugs**

   √7ᵗʰ **T43.8X1** **Poisoning by other psychotropic drugs, accidental (unintentional)**
      Poisoning by other psychotropic drugs NOS

   √7ᵗʰ **T43.8X2** **Poisoning by other psychotropic drugs, intentional self-harm**

   √7ᵗʰ **T43.8X3** **Poisoning by other psychotropic drugs, assault**

   √7ᵗʰ **T43.8X4** **Poisoning by other psychotropic drugs, undetermined**

   √7ᵗʰ **T43.8X5** Adverse effect of other psychotropic drugs

   √7ᵗʰ **T43.8X6** Underdosing of other psychotropic drugs

√5ᵗʰ **T43.9** **Poisoning by, adverse effect of and underdosing of unspecified psychotropic drug**

   √x7ᵗʰ **T43.91** **Poisoning by unspecified psychotropic drug, accidental (unintentional)**
      Poisoning by psychotropic drug NOS

   √x7ᵗʰ **T43.92** **Poisoning by unspecified psychotropic drug, intentional self-harm**

   √x7ᵗʰ **T43.93** **Poisoning by unspecified psychotropic drug, assault**

   √x7ᵗʰ **T43.94** **Poisoning by unspecified psychotropic drug, undetermined**

   √x7ᵗʰ **T43.95** Adverse effect of unspecified psychotropic drug

   √x7ᵗʰ **T43.96** Underdosing of unspecified psychotropic drug

√4ᵗʰ **T44** **Poisoning by, adverse effect of and underdosing of drugs primarily affecting the autonomic nervous system**

   The appropriate 7th character is to be added to each code from category T44.
   A initial encounter
   D subsequent encounter
   S sequela

√5ᵗʰ **T44.0** **Poisoning by, adverse effect of and underdosing of anticholinesterase agents**

√6ᵗʰ **T44.0X** **Poisoning by, adverse effect of and underdosing of** anticholinesterase agents

   √7ᵗʰ **T44.0X1** **Poisoning by anticholinesterase agents, accidental (unintentional)**
      Poisoning by anticholinesterase agents NOS

   √7ᵗʰ **T44.0X2** **Poisoning by anticholinesterase agents, intentional self-harm**

   √7ᵗʰ **T44.0X3** **Poisoning by anticholinesterase agents, assault**

   √7ᵗʰ **T44.0X4** **Poisoning by anticholinesterase agents, undetermined**

   √7ᵗʰ **T44.0X5** Adverse effect of anticholinesterase agents

   √7ᵗʰ **T44.0X6** Underdosing of anticholinesterase agents

√5ᵗʰ **T44.1** **Poisoning by, adverse effect of and underdosing of other parasympathomimetics [cholinergics]**

√6ᵗʰ **T44.1X** **Poisoning by, adverse effect of and underdosing of other parasympathomimetics [cholinergics]**

   √7ᵗʰ **T44.1X1** **Poisoning by other parasympathomimetics [cholinergics], accidental (unintentional)**
      Poisoning by other parasympathomimetics [cholinergics] NOS

   √7ᵗʰ **T44.1X2** **Poisoning by other parasympathomimetics [cholinergics], intentional self-harm**

   √7ᵗʰ **T44.1X3** **Poisoning by other parasympathomimetics [cholinergics], assault**

   √7ᵗʰ **T44.1X4** **Poisoning by other parasympathomimetics [cholinergics], undetermined**

   √7ᵗʰ **T44.1X5** Adverse effect of other parasympathomimetics [cholinergics]

   √7ᵗʰ **T44.1X6** Underdosing of other parasympathomimetics [cholinergics]

√5ᵗʰ **T44.2** **Poisoning by, adverse effect of and underdosing of ganglionic blocking drugs**

√6ᵗʰ **T44.2X** **Poisoning by, adverse effect of and underdosing of** ganglionic blocking drugs

   √7ᵗʰ **T44.2X1** **Poisoning by ganglionic blocking drugs, accidental (unintentional)**
      Poisoning by ganglionic blocking drugs NOS

   √7ᵗʰ **T44.2X2** **Poisoning by ganglionic blocking drugs, intentional self-harm**

   √7ᵗʰ **T44.2X3** **Poisoning by ganglionic blocking drugs, assault**

   √7ᵗʰ **T44.2X4** **Poisoning by ganglionic blocking drugs, undetermined**

   √7ᵗʰ **T44.2X5** Adverse effect of ganglionic blocking drugs

   √7ᵗʰ **T44.2X6** Underdosing of ganglionic blocking drugs

☑ Additional Character Required   √x7ᵗʰ Placeholder Alert   Manifestation   Unspecified Dx   ▶◀ Revised Text   ● New Code   ▲ Revised Title

ICD-10-CM 2020   **1095**

✓5ᵗʰ **T44.3 Poisoning by, adverse effect of and underdosing of other parasympatholytics [anticholinergics and antimuscarinics] and spasmolytics**

     Poisoning by, adverse effect of and underdosing of papaverine

     ✓6ᵗʰ **T44.3X Poisoning by, adverse effect of and underdosing of other parasympatholytics [anticholinergics and antimuscarinics] and spasmolytics**

       ✓7ᵗʰ **T44.3X1 Poisoning by other parasympatholytics [anticholinergics and antimuscarinics] and spasmolytics, accidental (unintentional)**

         Poisoning by other parasympatholytics [anticholinergics and antimuscarinics] and spasmolytics NOS

       ✓7ᵗʰ **T44.3X2 Poisoning by other parasympatholytics [anticholinergics and antimuscarinics] and spasmolytics, intentional self-harm**

       ✓7ᵗʰ **T44.3X3 Poisoning by other parasympatholytics [anticholinergics and antimuscarinics] and spasmolytics, assault**

       ✓7ᵗʰ **T44.3X4 Poisoning by other parasympatholytics [anticholinergics and antimuscarinics] and spasmolytics, undetermined**

       ✓7ᵗʰ **T44.3X5 Adverse effect of other parasympatholytics [anticholinergics and antimuscarinics] and spasmolytics**

       ✓7ᵗʰ **T44.3X6 Underdosing of other parasympatholytics [anticholinergics and antimuscarinics] and spasmolytics**

✓5ᵗʰ **T44.4 Poisoning by, adverse effect of and underdosing of predominantly alpha-adrenoreceptor agonists**

     Poisoning by, adverse effect of and underdosing of metaraminol

     ✓6ᵗʰ **T44.4X Poisoning by, adverse effect of and underdosing of predominantly alpha-adrenoreceptor agonists**

       ✓7ᵗʰ **T44.4X1 Poisoning by predominantly alpha-adrenoreceptor agonists, accidental (unintentional)**

         Poisoning by predominantly alpha-adrenoreceptor agonists NOS

       ✓7ᵗʰ **T44.4X2 Poisoning by predominantly alpha-adrenoreceptor agonists, intentional self-harm**

       ✓7ᵗʰ **T44.4X3 Poisoning by predominantly alpha-adrenoreceptor agonists, assault**

       ✓7ᵗʰ **T44.4X4 Poisoning by predominantly alpha-adrenoreceptor agonists, undetermined**

       ✓7ᵗʰ **T44.4X5 Adverse effect of predominantly alpha-adrenoreceptor agonists**

       ✓7ᵗʰ **T44.4X6 Underdosing of predominantly alpha-adrenoreceptor agonists**

✓5ᵗʰ **T44.5 Poisoning by, adverse effect of and underdosing of predominantly beta-adrenoreceptor agonists**

     EXCLUDES 1   *poisoning by, adverse effect of and underdosing of beta-adrenoreceptor agonists used in asthma therapy (T48.6-)*

     ✓6ᵗʰ **T44.5X Poisoning by, adverse effect of and underdosing of predominantly beta-adrenoreceptor agonists**

       ✓7ᵗʰ **T44.5X1 Poisoning by predominantly beta-adrenoreceptor agonists, accidental (unintentional)**

         Poisoning by predominantly beta-adrenoreceptor agonists NOS

       ✓7ᵗʰ **T44.5X2 Poisoning by predominantly beta-adrenoreceptor agonists, intentional self-harm**

       ✓7ᵗʰ **T44.5X3 Poisoning by predominantly beta-adrenoreceptor agonists, assault**

       ✓7ᵗʰ **T44.5X4 Poisoning by predominantly beta-adrenoreceptor agonists, undetermined**

       ✓7ᵗʰ **T44.5X5 Adverse effect of predominantly beta-adrenoreceptor agonists**

       ✓7ᵗʰ **T44.5X6 Underdosing of predominantly beta-adrenoreceptor agonists**

✓5ᵗʰ **T44.6 Poisoning by, adverse effect of and underdosing of alpha-adrenoreceptor antagonists**

     EXCLUDES 1   *poisoning by, adverse effect of and underdosing of ergot alkaloids (T48.0)*

     ✓6ᵗʰ **T44.6X Poisoning by, adverse effect of and underdosing of alpha-adrenoreceptor antagonists**

       ✓7ᵗʰ **T44.6X1 Poisoning by alpha-adrenoreceptor antagonists, accidental (unintentional)**

         Poisoning by alpha-adrenoreceptor antagonists NOS

       ✓7ᵗʰ **T44.6X2 Poisoning by alpha-adrenoreceptor antagonists, intentional self-harm**

       ✓7ᵗʰ **T44.6X3 Poisoning by alpha-adrenoreceptor antagonists, assault**

       ✓7ᵗʰ **T44.6X4 Poisoning by alpha-adrenoreceptor antagonists, undetermined**

       ✓7ᵗʰ **T44.6X5 Adverse effect of alpha-adrenoreceptor antagonists**

       ✓7ᵗʰ **T44.6X6 Underdosing of alpha-adrenoreceptor antagonists**

✓5ᵗʰ **T44.7 Poisoning by, adverse effect of and underdosing of beta-adrenoreceptor antagonists**

     ✓6ᵗʰ **T44.7X Poisoning by, adverse effect of and underdosing of beta-adrenoreceptor antagonists**

       ✓7ᵗʰ **T44.7X1 Poisoning by beta-adrenoreceptor antagonists, accidental (unintentional)**

         Poisoning by beta-adrenoreceptor antagonists NOS

       ✓7ᵗʰ **T44.7X2 Poisoning by beta-adrenoreceptor antagonists, intentional self-harm**

       ✓7ᵗʰ **T44.7X3 Poisoning by beta-adrenoreceptor antagonists, assault**

       ✓7ᵗʰ **T44.7X4 Poisoning by beta-adrenoreceptor antagonists, undetermined**

       ✓7ᵗʰ **T44.7X5 Adverse effect of beta-adrenoreceptor antagonists**

       ✓7ᵗʰ **T44.7X6 Underdosing of beta-adrenoreceptor antagonists**

✓5ᵗʰ **T44.8 Poisoning by, adverse effect of and underdosing of centrally-acting and adrenergic-neuron- blocking agents**

     EXCLUDES 1   *poisoning by, adverse effect of and underdosing of clonidine (T46.5)*

              poisoning by, adverse effect of and underdosing of guanethidine (T46.5)

     ✓6ᵗʰ **T44.8X Poisoning by, adverse effect of and underdosing of centrally-acting and adrenergic- neuron-blocking agents**

       ✓7ᵗʰ **T44.8X1 Poisoning by centrally-acting and adrenergic-neuron-blocking agents, accidental (unintentional)**

         Poisoning by centrally-acting and adrenergic-neuron-blocking agents NOS

       ✓7ᵗʰ **T44.8X2 Poisoning by centrally-acting and adrenergic-neuron-blocking agents, intentional self-harm**

       ✓7ᵗʰ **T44.8X3 Poisoning by centrally-acting and adrenergic-neuron-blocking agents, assault**

       ✓7ᵗʰ **T44.8X4 Poisoning by centrally-acting and adrenergic-neuron-blocking agents, undetermined**

       ✓7ᵗʰ **T44.8X5 Adverse effect of centrally-acting and adrenergic-neuron-blocking agents**

       ✓7ᵗʰ **T44.8X6 Underdosing of centrally-acting and adrenergic-neuron-blocking agents**

✓5ᵗʰ **T44.9 Poisoning by, adverse effect of and underdosing of other and unspecified drugs primarily affecting the autonomic nervous system**

     Poisoning by, adverse effect of and underdosing of drug stimulating both alpha and beta-adrenoreceptors

     ✓6ᵗʰ **T44.90 Poisoning by, adverse effect of and underdosing of unspecified drugs primarily affecting the autonomic nervous system**

       ✓7ᵗʰ **T44.901 Poisoning by unspecified drugs primarily affecting the autonomic nervous system, accidental (unintentional)**

         Poisoning by unspecified drugs primarily affecting the autonomic nervous system NOS

       ✓7ᵗʰ **T44.902 Poisoning by unspecified drugs primarily affecting the autonomic nervous system, intentional self-harm**

N Newborn: 0   P Pediatric: 0-17   M Maternity: 12-55   A Adult: 15-124   CH Comorbidity High   CL Comorbidity Low   NCDx Noncancer Dx   PDx Primary Dx

1096   ICD-10-CM 2020

✓7th **T44.903** Poisoning by unspecified drugs primarily affecting the autonomic nervous system, assault

✓7th **T44.904** Poisoning by unspecified drugs primarily affecting the autonomic nervous system, undetermined

✓7th **T44.905** Adverse effect of unspecified drugs primarily affecting the autonomic nervous system

✓7th **T44.906** Underdosing of unspecified drugs primarily affecting the autonomic nervous system

✓6th **T44.99** Poisoning by, adverse effect of and underdosing of other drugs primarily affecting the autonomic nervous system

✓7th **T44.991** Poisoning by other drug primarily affecting the autonomic nervous system, accidental (unintentional)

Poisoning by other drugs primarily affecting the autonomic nervous system NOS

✓7th **T44.992** Poisoning by other drug primarily affecting the autonomic nervous system, intentional self-harm

✓7th **T44.993** Poisoning by other drug primarily affecting the autonomic nervous system, assault

✓7th **T44.994** Poisoning by other drug primarily affecting the autonomic nervous system, undetermined

✓7th **T44.995** Adverse effect of other drug primarily affecting the autonomic nervous system

✓7th **T44.996** Underdosing of other drug primarily affecting the autonomic nervous system

✓4th **T45** Poisoning by, adverse effect of and underdosing of primarily systemic and hematological agents, not elsewhere classified

The appropriate 7th character is to be added to each code from category T45.
A   initial encounter
D   subsequent encounter
S   sequela

✓5th **T45.0** Poisoning by, adverse effect of and underdosing of antiallergic and antiemetic drugs

EXCLUDES 1   poisoning by, adverse effect of and underdosing of phenothiazine-based neuroleptics (T43.3)

✓6th **T45.0X** Poisoning by, adverse effect of and underdosing of antiallergic and antiemetic drugs

✓7th **T45.0X1** Poisoning by antiallergic and antiemetic drugs, accidental (unintentional)

Poisoning by antiallergic and antiemetic drugs NOS

✓7th **T45.0X2** Poisoning by antiallergic and antiemetic drugs, intentional self-harm

✓7th **T45.0X3** Poisoning by antiallergic and antiemetic drugs, assault

✓7th **T45.0X4** Poisoning by antiallergic and antiemetic drugs, undetermined

✓7th **T45.0X5** Adverse effect of antiallergic and antiemetic drugs

✓7th **T45.0X6** Underdosing of antiallergic and antiemetic drugs

✓5th **T45.1** Poisoning by, adverse effect of and underdosing of antineoplastic and immunosuppressive drugs

EXCLUDES 1   poisoning by, adverse effect of and underdosing of tamoxifen (T38.6)

AHA: 2019,1Q,17,20; 2014,4Q,22

✓6th **T45.1X** Poisoning by, adverse effect of and underdosing of antineoplastic and immunosuppressive drugs

✓7th **T45.1X1** Poisoning by antineoplastic and immunosuppressive drugs, accidental (unintentional)

Poisoning by antineoplastic and immunosuppressive drugs NOS

✓7th **T45.1X2** Poisoning by antineoplastic and immunosuppressive drugs, intentional self-harm

✓7th **T45.1X3** Poisoning by antineoplastic and immunosuppressive drugs, assault

✓7th **T45.1X4** Poisoning by antineoplastic and immunosuppressive drugs, undetermined

✓7th **T45.1X5** Adverse effect of antineoplastic and immunosuppressive drugs

AHA: 2019,2Q,24,28

✓7th **T45.1X6** Underdosing of antineoplastic and immunosuppressive drugs

✓5th **T45.2** Poisoning by, adverse effect of and underdosing of vitamins

EXCLUDES 2   poisoning by, adverse effect of and underdosing of iron (T45.4)

poisoning by, adverse effect of and underdosing of nicotinic acid (derivatives) (T46.7)

poisoning by, adverse effect of and underdosing of vitamin K (T45.7)

✓6th **T45.2X** Poisoning by, adverse effect of and underdosing of vitamins

✓7th **T45.2X1** Poisoning by vitamins, accidental (unintentional)

Poisoning by vitamins NOS

✓7th **T45.2X2** Poisoning by vitamins, intentional self-harm

✓7th **T45.2X3** Poisoning by vitamins, assault

✓7th **T45.2X4** Poisoning by vitamins, undetermined

✓7th **T45.2X5** Adverse effect of vitamins

✓7th **T45.2X6** Underdosing of vitamins

EXCLUDES 1   vitamin deficiencies (E50-E56)

✓5th **T45.3** Poisoning by, adverse effect of and underdosing of enzymes

✓6th **T45.3X** Poisoning by, adverse effect of and underdosing of enzymes

✓7th **T45.3X1** Poisoning by enzymes, accidental (unintentional)

Poisoning by enzymes NOS

✓7th **T45.3X2** Poisoning by enzymes, intentional self-harm

✓7th **T45.3X3** Poisoning by enzymes, assault

✓7th **T45.3X4** Poisoning by enzymes, undetermined

✓7th **T45.3X5** Adverse effect of enzymes

✓7th **T45.3X6** Underdosing of enzymes

✓5th **T45.4** Poisoning by, adverse effect of and underdosing of iron and its compounds

✓6th **T45.4X** Poisoning by, adverse effect of and underdosing of iron and its compounds

✓7th **T45.4X1** Poisoning by iron and its compounds, accidental (unintentional)

Poisoning by iron and its compounds NOS

✓7th **T45.4X2** Poisoning by iron and its compounds, intentional self-harm

✓7th **T45.4X3** Poisoning by iron and its compounds, assault

✓7th **T45.4X4** Poisoning by iron and its compounds, undetermined

✓7th **T45.4X5** Adverse effect of iron and its compounds

✓7th **T45.4X6** Underdosing of iron and its compounds

EXCLUDES 1   iron deficiency (E61.1)

✓5th **T45.5** Poisoning by, adverse effect of and underdosing of anticoagulants and antithrombotic drugs

✓6th **T45.51** Poisoning by, adverse effect of and underdosing of anticoagulants

✓7th **T45.511** Poisoning by anticoagulants, accidental (unintentional)

Poisoning by anticoagulants NOS

✓7th **T45.512** Poisoning by anticoagulants, intentional self-harm

✓7th **T45.513** Poisoning by anticoagulants, assault

✓7th **T45.514** Poisoning by anticoagulants, undetermined

✓7th **T45.515** Adverse effect of anticoagulants

AHA: 2016,1Q,14; 2013,2Q,34

✓7th **T45.516** Underdosing of anticoagulants

☑ Additional Character Required   ✓x7th Placeholder Alert   Manifestation   Unspecified Dx   ▶◀ Revised Text   ● New Code   ▲ Revised Title

√6ᵗʰ T45.52 Poisoning by, adverse effect of and underdosing of antithrombotic drugs
Poisoning by, adverse effect of and underdosing of antiplatelet drugs

> EXCLUDES 2 poisoning by, adverse effect of and underdosing of aspirin (T39.Ø1-)
> poisoning by, adverse effect of and underdosing of acetylsalicylic acid (T39.Ø1-)

- **√7ᵗʰ T45.521 Poisoning by antithrombotic drugs, accidental (unintentional)**
  Poisoning by antithrombotic drug NOS
- **√7ᵗʰ T45.522 Poisoning by antithrombotic drugs, intentional self-harm**
- **√7ᵗʰ T45.523 Poisoning by antithrombotic drugs, assault**
- **√7ᵗʰ T45.524 Poisoning by antithrombotic drugs, undetermined**
- **√7ᵗʰ T45.525 Adverse effect of antithrombotic drugs**
  AHA: 2016,1Q,15
- **√7ᵗʰ T45.526 Underdosing of antithrombotic drugs**

√5ᵗʰ T45.6 Poisoning by, adverse effect of and underdosing of fibrinolysis-affecting drugs

- **√6ᵗʰ T45.6Ø Poisoning by, adverse effect of and underdosing of unspecified fibrinolysis-affecting drugs**
  - **√7ᵗʰ T45.6Ø1 Poisoning by unspecified fibrinolysis-affecting drugs, accidental (unintentional)**
    Poisoning by fibrinolysis-affecting drug NOS
  - **√7ᵗʰ T45.6Ø2 Poisoning by unspecified fibrinolysis-affecting drugs, intentional self-harm**
  - **√7ᵗʰ T45.6Ø3 Poisoning by unspecified fibrinolysis-affecting drugs, assault**
  - **√7ᵗʰ T45.6Ø4 Poisoning by unspecified fibrinolysis-affecting drugs, undetermined**
  - **√7ᵗʰ T45.6Ø5 Adverse effect of unspecified fibrinolysis-affecting drugs**
  - **√7ᵗʰ T45.6Ø6 Underdosing of unspecified fibrinolysis-affecting drugs**
- **√6ᵗʰ T45.61 Poisoning by, adverse effect of and underdosing of** thrombolytic drugs
  - **√7ᵗʰ T45.611 Poisoning by thrombolytic drug, accidental (unintentional)**
    Poisoning by thrombolytic drug NOS
  - **√7ᵗʰ T45.612 Poisoning by thrombolytic drug, intentional self-harm**
  - **√7ᵗʰ T45.613 Poisoning by thrombolytic drug, assault**
  - **√7ᵗʰ T45.614 Poisoning by thrombolytic drug, undetermined**
  - **√7ᵗʰ T45.615 Adverse effect of thrombolytic drugs**
    AHA: 2017,2Q,9
  - **√7ᵗʰ T45.616 Underdosing of thrombolytic drugs**
- **√6ᵗʰ T45.62 Poisoning by, adverse effect of and underdosing of** hemostatic drugs
  - **√7ᵗʰ T45.621 Poisoning by hemostatic drug, accidental (unintentional)**
    Poisoning by hemostatic drug NOS
  - **√7ᵗʰ T45.622 Poisoning by hemostatic drug, intentional self-harm**
  - **√7ᵗʰ T45.623 Poisoning by hemostatic drug, assault**
  - **√7ᵗʰ T45.624 Poisoning by hemostatic drug, undetermined**
  - **√7ᵗʰ T45.625 Adverse effect of hemostatic drug**
  - **√7ᵗʰ T45.626 Underdosing of hemostatic drugs**
- **√6ᵗʰ T45.69 Poisoning by, adverse effect of and underdosing of other** fibrinolysis-affecting drugs
  - **√7ᵗʰ T45.691 Poisoning by other fibrinolysis-affecting drugs, accidental (unintentional)**
    Poisoning by other fibrinolysis-affecting drug NOS
  - **√7ᵗʰ T45.692 Poisoning by other fibrinolysis-affecting drugs, intentional self-harm**
  - **√7ᵗʰ T45.693 Poisoning by other fibrinolysis-affecting drugs, assault**
  - **√7ᵗʰ T45.694 Poisoning by other fibrinolysis-affecting drugs, undetermined**

- **√7ᵗʰ T45.695 Adverse effect of other fibrinolysis-affecting drugs**
- **√7ᵗʰ T45.696 Underdosing of other fibrinolysis-affecting drugs**

√5ᵗʰ T45.7 Poisoning by, adverse effect of and underdosing of anticoagulant antagonists, vitamin K and other coagulants

- **√6ᵗʰ T45.7X Poisoning by, adverse effect of and underdosing of** anticoagulant antagonists, vitamin K and other coagulants
  - **√7ᵗʰ T45.7X1 Poisoning by anticoagulant antagonists, vitamin K and other coagulants, accidental (unintentional)**
    Poisoning by anticoagulant antagonists, vitamin K and other coagulants NOS
  - **√7ᵗʰ T45.7X2 Poisoning by anticoagulant antagonists, vitamin K and other coagulants, intentional self-harm**
  - **√7ᵗʰ T45.7X3 Poisoning by anticoagulant antagonists, vitamin K and other coagulants, assault**
  - **√7ᵗʰ T45.7X4 Poisoning by anticoagulant antagonists, vitamin K and other coagulants, undetermined**
  - **√7ᵗʰ T45.7X5 Adverse effect of anticoagulant antagonists, vitamin K and other coagulants**
  - **√7ᵗʰ T45.7X6 Underdosing of anticoagulant antagonist, vitamin K and other coagulants**
    > EXCLUDES 1 vitamin K deficiency (E56.1)

√5ᵗʰ T45.8 Poisoning by, adverse effect of and underdosing of other primarily systemic and hematological agents
Poisoning by, adverse effect of and underdosing of liver preparations and other antianemic agents
Poisoning by, adverse effect of and underdosing of natural blood and blood products
Poisoning by, adverse effect of and underdosing of plasma substitute

> EXCLUDES 2 poisoning by, adverse effect of and underdosing of immunoglobulin (T5Ø.Z1)
> poisoning by, adverse effect of and underdosing of iron (T45.4)
> transfusion reactions (T8Ø.-)

- **√6ᵗʰ T45.8X Poisoning by, adverse effect of and underdosing of other primarily systemic and hematological agents**
  - **√7ᵗʰ T45.8X1 Poisoning by other primarily systemic and hematological agents, accidental (unintentional)**
    Poisoning by other primarily systemic and hematological agents NOS
  - **√7ᵗʰ T45.8X2 Poisoning by other primarily systemic and hematological agents, intentional self-harm**
  - **√7ᵗʰ T45.8X3 Poisoning by other primarily systemic and hematological agents, assault**
  - **√7ᵗʰ T45.8X4 Poisoning by other primarily systemic and hematological agents, undetermined**
  - **√7ᵗʰ T45.8X5 Adverse effect of other primarily systemic and hematological agents**
    AHA: 2016,4Q,42
  - **√7ᵗʰ T45.8X6 Underdosing of other primarily systemic and hematological agents**

√5ᵗʰ T45.9 Poisoning by, adverse effect of and underdosing of unspecified primarily systemic and hematological agent

- **√x7ᵗʰ T45.91 Poisoning by unspecified primarily systemic and hematological agent, accidental (unintentional)**
  Poisoning by primarily systemic and hematological agent NOS
- **√x7ᵗʰ T45.92 Poisoning by unspecified primarily systemic and hematological agent, intentional self-harm**
- **√x7ᵗʰ T45.93 Poisoning by unspecified primarily systemic and hematological agent, assault**
- **√x7ᵗʰ T45.94 Poisoning by unspecified primarily systemic and hematological agent, undetermined**
- **√x7ᵗʰ T45.95 Adverse effect of unspecified primarily systemic and hematological agent**
- **√x7ᵗʰ T45.96 Underdosing of unspecified primarily systemic and hematological agent**

√4ᵗʰ **T46** **Poisoning by, adverse effect of and underdosing of agents primarily affecting the cardiovascular system**
    EXCLUDES 1   poisoning by, adverse effect of and underdosing of metaraminol (T44.4)

The appropriate 7th character is to be added to each code from category T46.
A   initial encounter
D   subsequent encounter
S   sequela

√5ᵗʰ **T46.0** **Poisoning by, adverse effect of and underdosing of cardiac-stimulant glycosides and drugs of similar action**
   √6ᵗʰ **T46.0X** **Poisoning by, adverse effect of and underdosing of** cardiac-stimulant glycosides and drugs of similar action
    √7ᵗʰ **T46.0X1** **Poisoning by cardiac-stimulant glycosides and drugs of similar action,** accidental **(unintentional)**
      Poisoning by cardiac-stimulant glycosides and drugs of similar action NOS
    √7ᵗʰ **T46.0X2** **Poisoning by cardiac-stimulant glycosides and drugs of similar action,** intentional self-harm
    √7ᵗʰ **T46.0X3** **Poisoning by cardiac-stimulant glycosides and drugs of similar action,** assault
    √7ᵗʰ **T46.0X4** **Poisoning by cardiac-stimulant glycosides and drugs of similar action, undetermined**
    √7ᵗʰ **T46.0X5** Adverse effect **of cardiac-stimulant glycosides and drugs of similar action**
    √7ᵗʰ **T46.0X6** Underdosing **of cardiac-stimulant glycosides and drugs of similar action**

√5ᵗʰ **T46.1** **Poisoning by, adverse effect of and underdosing of calcium-channel blockers**
   √6ᵗʰ **T46.1X** **Poisoning by, adverse effect of and underdosing of** calcium-channel blockers
    √7ᵗʰ **T46.1X1** **Poisoning by calcium-channel blockers,** accidental **(unintentional)**
      Poisoning by calcium-channel blockers NOS
    √7ᵗʰ **T46.1X2** **Poisoning by calcium-channel blockers,** intentional self-harm
    √7ᵗʰ **T46.1X3** **Poisoning by calcium-channel blockers,** assault
    √7ᵗʰ **T46.1X4** **Poisoning by calcium-channel blockers,** undetermined
    √7ᵗʰ **T46.1X5** Adverse effect **of calcium-channel blockers**
    √7ᵗʰ **T46.1X6** Underdosing **of calcium-channel blockers**

√5ᵗʰ **T46.2** **Poisoning by, adverse effect of and underdosing of other antidysrhythmic drugs, not elsewhere classified**
    EXCLUDES 1   poisoning by, adverse effect of and underdosing of beta-adrenoreceptor antagonists (T44.7-)
   √6ᵗʰ **T46.2X** **Poisoning by, adverse effect of and underdosing of other antidysrhythmic drugs**
    √7ᵗʰ **T46.2X1** **Poisoning by other antidysrhythmic drugs,** accidental **(unintentional)**
      Poisoning by other antidysrhythmic drugs NOS
    √7ᵗʰ **T46.2X2** **Poisoning by other antidysrhythmic drugs,** intentional self-harm
    √7ᵗʰ **T46.2X3** **Poisoning by other antidysrhythmic drugs,** assault
    √7ᵗʰ **T46.2X4** **Poisoning by other antidysrhythmic drugs,** undetermined
    √7ᵗʰ **T46.2X5** Adverse effect **of other antidysrhythmic drugs**
    √7ᵗʰ **T46.2X6** Underdosing **of other antidysrhythmic drugs**

√5ᵗʰ **T46.3** **Poisoning by, adverse effect of and underdosing of coronary vasodilators**
   Poisoning by, adverse effect of and underdosing of dipyridamole
    EXCLUDES 1   poisoning by, adverse effect of and underdosing of calcium-channel blockers (T46.1)
   √6ᵗʰ **T46.3X** **Poisoning by, adverse effect of and underdosing of** coronary vasodilators
    √7ᵗʰ **T46.3X1** **Poisoning by coronary vasodilators,** accidental **(unintentional)**
      Poisoning by coronary vasodilators NOS
    √7ᵗʰ **T46.3X2** **Poisoning by coronary vasodilators,** intentional self-harm
    √7ᵗʰ **T46.3X3** **Poisoning by coronary vasodilators,** assault

    √7ᵗʰ **T46.3X4** **Poisoning by coronary vasodilators, undetermined**
    √7ᵗʰ **T46.3X5** Adverse effect **of coronary vasodilators**
    √7ᵗʰ **T46.3X6** Underdosing **of coronary vasodilators**

√5ᵗʰ **T46.4** **Poisoning by, adverse effect of and underdosing of angiotensin-converting-enzyme inhibitors**
   √6ᵗʰ **T46.4X** **Poisoning by, adverse effect of and underdosing of** angiotensin-converting-enzyme inhibitors
    √7ᵗʰ **T46.4X1** **Poisoning by angiotensin-converting-enzyme inhibitors,** accidental **(unintentional)**
      Poisoning by angiotensin-converting-enzyme inhibitors NOS
    √7ᵗʰ **T46.4X2** **Poisoning by angiotensin-converting-enzyme inhibitors,** intentional self-harm
    √7ᵗʰ **T46.4X3** **Poisoning by angiotensin-converting-enzyme inhibitors,** assault
    √7ᵗʰ **T46.4X4** **Poisoning by angiotensin-converting-enzyme inhibitors, undetermined**
    √7ᵗʰ **T46.4X5** Adverse effect **of angiotensin-converting-enzyme inhibitors**
    √7ᵗʰ **T46.4X6** Underdosing **of angiotensin-converting-enzyme inhibitors**

√5ᵗʰ **T46.5** **Poisoning by, adverse effect of and underdosing of other antihypertensive drugs**
    EXCLUDES 2   poisoning by, adverse effect of and underdosing of beta-adrenoreceptor antagonists (T44.7)
      poisoning by, adverse effect of and underdosing of calcium-channel blockers (T46.1)
      poisoning by, adverse effect of and underdosing of diuretics (T50.0-T50.2)
   √6ᵗʰ **T46.5X** **Poisoning by, adverse effect of and underdosing of other antihypertensive drugs**
    √7ᵗʰ **T46.5X1** **Poisoning by other antihypertensive drugs,** accidental **(unintentional)**
      Poisoning by other antihypertensive drugs NOS
    √7ᵗʰ **T46.5X2** **Poisoning by other antihypertensive drugs,** intentional self-harm
    √7ᵗʰ **T46.5X3** **Poisoning by other antihypertensive drugs,** assault
    √7ᵗʰ **T46.5X4** **Poisoning by other antihypertensive drugs,** undetermined
    √7ᵗʰ **T46.5X5** Adverse effect **of other antihypertensive drugs**
    √7ᵗʰ **T46.5X6** Underdosing **of other antihypertensive drugs**

√5ᵗʰ **T46.6** **Poisoning by, adverse effect of and underdosing of antihyperlipidemic and antiarteriosclerotic drugs**
   √6ᵗʰ **T46.6X** **Poisoning by, adverse effect of and underdosing of** antihyperlipidemic and antiarteriosclerotic drugs
    √7ᵗʰ **T46.6X1** **Poisoning by antihyperlipidemic and antiarteriosclerotic drugs,** accidental **(unintentional)**
      Poisoning by antihyperlipidemic and antiarteriosclerotic drugs NOS
    √7ᵗʰ **T46.6X2** **Poisoning by antihyperlipidemic and antiarteriosclerotic drugs,** intentional self-harm
    √7ᵗʰ **T46.6X3** **Poisoning by antihyperlipidemic and antiarteriosclerotic drugs,** assault
    √7ᵗʰ **T46.6X4** **Poisoning by antihyperlipidemic and antiarteriosclerotic drugs,** undetermined
    √7ᵗʰ **T46.6X5** Adverse effect **of antihyperlipidemic and antiarteriosclerotic drugs**
    √7ᵗʰ **T46.6X6** Underdosing **of antihyperlipidemic and antiarteriosclerotic drugs**

✓5ᵗʰ **T46.7 Poisoning by, adverse effect of and underdosing of peripheral vasodilators**
Poisoning by, adverse effect of and underdosing of nicotinic acid (derivatives)
EXCLUDES 1 *poisoning by, adverse effect of and underdosing of papaverine (T44.3)*

✓6ᵗʰ **T46.7X Poisoning by, adverse effect of and underdosing of peripheral vasodilators**
✓7ᵗʰ **T46.7X1 Poisoning by peripheral vasodilators, accidental (unintentional)**
Poisoning by peripheral vasodilators NOS
✓7ᵗʰ **T46.7X2 Poisoning by peripheral vasodilators, intentional self-harm**
✓7ᵗʰ **T46.7X3 Poisoning by peripheral vasodilators, assault**
✓7ᵗʰ **T46.7X4 Poisoning by peripheral vasodilators, undetermined**
✓7ᵗʰ **T46.7X5 Adverse effect of peripheral vasodilators**
✓7ᵗʰ **T46.7X6 Underdosing of peripheral vasodilators**

✓5ᵗʰ **T46.8 Poisoning by, adverse effect of and underdosing of antivaricose drugs, including sclerosing agents**
✓6ᵗʰ **T46.8X Poisoning by, adverse effect of and underdosing of antivaricose drugs, including sclerosing agents**
✓7ᵗʰ **T46.8X1 Poisoning by antivaricose drugs, including sclerosing agents, accidental (unintentional)**
Poisoning by antivaricose drugs, including sclerosing agents NOS
✓7ᵗʰ **T46.8X2 Poisoning by antivaricose drugs, including sclerosing agents, intentional self-harm**
✓7ᵗʰ **T46.8X3 Poisoning by antivaricose drugs, including sclerosing agents, assault**
✓7ᵗʰ **T46.8X4 Poisoning by antivaricose drugs, including sclerosing agents, undetermined**
✓7ᵗʰ **T46.8X5 Adverse effect of antivaricose drugs, including sclerosing agents**
✓7ᵗʰ **T46.8X6 Underdosing of antivaricose drugs, including sclerosing agents**

✓5ᵗʰ **T46.9 Poisoning by, adverse effect of and underdosing of other and unspecified agents primarily affecting the cardiovascular system**
✓6ᵗʰ **T46.90 Poisoning by, adverse effect of and underdosing of unspecified agents primarily affecting the cardiovascular system**
✓7ᵗʰ **T46.901 Poisoning by unspecified agents primarily affecting the cardiovascular system, accidental (unintentional)**
✓7ᵗʰ **T46.902 Poisoning by unspecified agents primarily affecting the cardiovascular system, intentional self-harm**
✓7ᵗʰ **T46.903 Poisoning by unspecified agents primarily affecting the cardiovascular system, assault**
✓7ᵗʰ **T46.904 Poisoning by unspecified agents primarily affecting the cardiovascular system, undetermined**
✓7ᵗʰ **T46.905 Adverse effect of unspecified agents primarily affecting the cardiovascular system**
✓7ᵗʰ **T46.906 Underdosing of unspecified agents primarily affecting the cardiovascular system**
✓6ᵗʰ **T46.99 Poisoning by, adverse effect of and underdosing of other agents primarily affecting the cardiovascular system**
✓7ᵗʰ **T46.991 Poisoning by other agents primarily affecting the cardiovascular system, accidental (unintentional)**
✓7ᵗʰ **T46.992 Poisoning by other agents primarily affecting the cardiovascular system, intentional self-harm**
✓7ᵗʰ **T46.993 Poisoning by other agents primarily affecting the cardiovascular system, assault**
✓7ᵗʰ **T46.994 Poisoning by other agents primarily affecting the cardiovascular system, undetermined**
✓7ᵗʰ **T46.995 Adverse effect of other agents primarily affecting the cardiovascular system**
✓7ᵗʰ **T46.996 Underdosing of other agents primarily affecting the cardiovascular system**

✓4ᵗʰ **T47 Poisoning by, adverse effect of and underdosing of agents primarily affecting the gastrointestinal system**
The appropriate 7th character is to be added to each code from category T47.
A initial encounter
D subsequent encounter
S sequela

✓5ᵗʰ **T47.0 Poisoning by, adverse effect of and underdosing of histamine H2-receptor blockers**
✓6ᵗʰ **T47.0X Poisoning by, adverse effect of and underdosing of histamine H2-receptor blockers**
✓7ᵗʰ **T47.0X1 Poisoning by histamine H2-receptor blockers, accidental (unintentional)**
Poisoning by histamine H2-receptor blockers NOS
✓7ᵗʰ **T47.0X2 Poisoning by histamine H2-receptor blockers, intentional self-harm**
✓7ᵗʰ **T47.0X3 Poisoning by histamine H2-receptor blockers, assault**
✓7ᵗʰ **T47.0X4 Poisoning by histamine H2-receptor blockers, undetermined**
✓7ᵗʰ **T47.0X5 Adverse effect of histamine H2-receptor blockers**
✓7ᵗʰ **T47.0X6 Underdosing of histamine H2-receptor blockers**

✓5ᵗʰ **T47.1 Poisoning by, adverse effect of and underdosing of other antacids and anti-gastric-secretion drugs**
✓6ᵗʰ **T47.1X Poisoning by, adverse effect of and underdosing of other antacids and anti-gastric-secretion drugs**
✓7ᵗʰ **T47.1X1 Poisoning by other antacids and anti-gastric-secretion drugs, accidental (unintentional)**
Poisoning by other antacids and anti-gastric-secretion drugs NOS
✓7ᵗʰ **T47.1X2 Poisoning by other antacids and anti-gastric-secretion drugs, intentional self-harm**
✓7ᵗʰ **T47.1X3 Poisoning by other antacids and anti-gastric-secretion drugs, assault**
✓7ᵗʰ **T47.1X4 Poisoning by other antacids and anti-gastric-secretion drugs, undetermined**
✓7ᵗʰ **T47.1X5 Adverse effect of other antacids and anti-gastric-secretion drugs**
✓7ᵗʰ **T47.1X6 Underdosing of other antacids and anti-gastric-secretion drugs**

✓5ᵗʰ **T47.2 Poisoning by, adverse effect of and underdosing of stimulant laxatives**
✓6ᵗʰ **T47.2X Poisoning by, adverse effect of and underdosing of stimulant laxatives**
✓7ᵗʰ **T47.2X1 Poisoning by stimulant laxatives, accidental (unintentional)**
Poisoning by stimulant laxatives NOS
✓7ᵗʰ **T47.2X2 Poisoning by stimulant laxatives, intentional self-harm**
✓7ᵗʰ **T47.2X3 Poisoning by stimulant laxatives, assault**
✓7ᵗʰ **T47.2X4 Poisoning by stimulant laxatives, undetermined**
✓7ᵗʰ **T47.2X5 Adverse effect of stimulant laxatives**
✓7ᵗʰ **T47.2X6 Underdosing of stimulant laxatives**

✓5ᵗʰ **T47.3 Poisoning by, adverse effect of and underdosing of saline and osmotic laxatives**
✓6ᵗʰ **T47.3X Poisoning by and adverse effect of saline and osmotic laxatives**
✓7ᵗʰ **T47.3X1 Poisoning by saline and osmotic laxatives, accidental (unintentional)**
Poisoning by saline and osmotic laxatives NOS
✓7ᵗʰ **T47.3X2 Poisoning by saline and osmotic laxatives, intentional self-harm**
✓7ᵗʰ **T47.3X3 Poisoning by saline and osmotic laxatives, assault**
✓7ᵗʰ **T47.3X4 Poisoning by saline and osmotic laxatives, undetermined**
✓7ᵗʰ **T47.3X5 Adverse effect of saline and osmotic laxatives**
✓7ᵗʰ **T47.3X6 Underdosing of saline and osmotic laxatives**

√5ᵗʰ **T47.4 Poisoning by, adverse effect of and underdosing of other laxatives**

√6ᵗʰ **T47.4X Poisoning by, adverse effect of and underdosing of other laxatives**

√7ᵗʰ **T47.4X1 Poisoning by other laxatives, accidental (unintentional)**
Poisoning by other laxatives NOS

√7ᵗʰ **T47.4X2 Poisoning by other laxatives, intentional self-harm**

√7ᵗʰ **T47.4X3 Poisoning by other laxatives, assault**

√7ᵗʰ **T47.4X4 Poisoning by other laxatives, undetermined**

√7ᵗʰ **T47.4X5 Adverse effect of other laxatives**

√7ᵗʰ **T47.4X6 Underdosing of other laxatives**

√5ᵗʰ **T47.5 Poisoning by, adverse effect of and underdosing of digestants**

√6ᵗʰ **T47.5X Poisoning by, adverse effect of and underdosing of digestants**

√7ᵗʰ **T47.5X1 Poisoning by digestants, accidental (unintentional)**
Poisoning by digestants NOS

√7ᵗʰ **T47.5X2 Poisoning by digestants, intentional self-harm**

√7ᵗʰ **T47.5X3 Poisoning by digestants, assault**

√7ᵗʰ **T47.5X4 Poisoning by digestants, undetermined**

√7ᵗʰ **T47.5X5 Adverse effect of digestants**

√7ᵗʰ **T47.5X6 Underdosing of digestants**

√5ᵗʰ **T47.6 Poisoning by, adverse effect of and underdosing of antidiarrheal drugs**

EXCLUDES 2   *poisoning by, adverse effect of and underdosing of systemic antibiotics and other anti-infectives (T36-T37)*

√6ᵗʰ **T47.6X Poisoning by, adverse effect of and underdosing of antidiarrheal drugs**

√7ᵗʰ **T47.6X1 Poisoning by antidiarrheal drugs, accidental (unintentional)**
Poisoning by antidiarrheal drugs NOS

√7ᵗʰ **T47.6X2 Poisoning by antidiarrheal drugs, intentional self-harm**

√7ᵗʰ **T47.6X3 Poisoning by antidiarrheal drugs, assault**

√7ᵗʰ **T47.6X4 Poisoning by antidiarrheal drugs, undetermined**

√7ᵗʰ **T47.6X5 Adverse effect of antidiarrheal drugs**

√7ᵗʰ **T47.6X6 Underdosing of antidiarrheal drugs**

√5ᵗʰ **T47.7 Poisoning by, adverse effect of and underdosing of emetics**

√6ᵗʰ **T47.7X Poisoning by, adverse effect of and underdosing of emetics**

√7ᵗʰ **T47.7X1 Poisoning by emetics, accidental (unintentional)**
Poisoning by emetics NOS

√7ᵗʰ **T47.7X2 Poisoning by emetics, intentional self-harm**

√7ᵗʰ **T47.7X3 Poisoning by emetics, assault**

√7ᵗʰ **T47.7X4 Poisoning by emetics, undetermined**

√7ᵗʰ **T47.7X5 Adverse effect of emetics**

√7ᵗʰ **T47.7X6 Underdosing of emetics**

√5ᵗʰ **T47.8 Poisoning by, adverse effect of and underdosing of other agents primarily affecting gastrointestinal system**

√6ᵗʰ **T47.8X Poisoning by, adverse effect of and underdosing of other agents primarily affecting gastrointestinal system**

√7ᵗʰ **T47.8X1 Poisoning by other agents primarily affecting gastrointestinal system, accidental (unintentional)**
Poisoning by other agents primarily affecting gastrointestinal system NOS

√7ᵗʰ **T47.8X2 Poisoning by other agents primarily affecting gastrointestinal system, intentional self-harm**

√7ᵗʰ **T47.8X3 Poisoning by other agents primarily affecting gastrointestinal system, assault**

√7ᵗʰ **T47.8X4 Poisoning by other agents primarily affecting gastrointestinal system, undetermined**

√7ᵗʰ **T47.8X5 Adverse effect of other agents primarily affecting gastrointestinal system**

√7ᵗʰ **T47.8X6 Underdosing of other agents primarily affecting gastrointestinal system**

√5ᵗʰ **T47.9 Poisoning by, adverse effect of and underdosing of unspecified agents primarily affecting the gastrointestinal system**

√x7ᵗʰ **T47.91 Poisoning by unspecified agents primarily affecting the gastrointestinal system, accidental (unintentional)**
Poisoning by agents primarily affecting the gastrointestinal system NOS

√x7ᵗʰ **T47.92 Poisoning by unspecified agents primarily affecting the gastrointestinal system, intentional self-harm**

√x7ᵗʰ **T47.93 Poisoning by unspecified agents primarily affecting the gastrointestinal system, assault**

√x7ᵗʰ **T47.94 Poisoning by unspecified agents primarily affecting the gastrointestinal system, undetermined**

√x7ᵗʰ **T47.95 Adverse effect of unspecified agents primarily affecting the gastrointestinal system**

√x7ᵗʰ **T47.96 Underdosing of unspecified agents primarily affecting the gastrointestinal system**

√4ᵗʰ **T48 Poisoning by, adverse effect of and underdosing of agents primarily acting on smooth and skeletal muscles and the respiratory system**

The appropriate 7th character is to be added to each code from category T48.
A   initial encounter
D   subsequent encounter
S   sequela

√5ᵗʰ **T48.0 Poisoning by, adverse effect of and underdosing of oxytocic drugs**

EXCLUDES 1   *poisoning by, adverse effect of and underdosing of estrogens, progestogens and antagonists (T38.4-T38.6)*

√6ᵗʰ **T48.0X Poisoning by, adverse effect of and underdosing of oxytocic drugs**

√7ᵗʰ **T48.0X1 Poisoning by oxytocic drugs, accidental (unintentional)**
Poisoning by oxytocic drugs NOS

√7ᵗʰ **T48.0X2 Poisoning by oxytocic drugs, intentional self-harm**

√7ᵗʰ **T48.0X3 Poisoning by oxytocic drugs, assault**

√7ᵗʰ **T48.0X4 Poisoning by oxytocic drugs, undetermined**

√7ᵗʰ **T48.0X5 Adverse effect of oxytocic drugs**

√7ᵗʰ **T48.0X6 Underdosing of oxytocic drugs**

√5ᵗʰ **T48.1 Poisoning by, adverse effect of and underdosing of skeletal muscle relaxants [neuromuscular blocking agents]**

√6ᵗʰ **T48.1X Poisoning by, adverse effect of and underdosing of skeletal muscle relaxants [neuromuscular blocking agents]**

√7ᵗʰ **T48.1X1 Poisoning by skeletal muscle relaxants [neuromuscular blocking agents], accidental (unintentional)**
Poisoning by skeletal muscle relaxants [neuromuscular blocking agents] NOS

√7ᵗʰ **T48.1X2 Poisoning by skeletal muscle relaxants [neuromuscular blocking agents], intentional self-harm**

√7ᵗʰ **T48.1X3 Poisoning by skeletal muscle relaxants [neuromuscular blocking agents], assault**

√7ᵗʰ **T48.1X4 Poisoning by skeletal muscle relaxants [neuromuscular blocking agents], undetermined**

√7ᵗʰ **T48.1X5 Adverse effect of skeletal muscle relaxants [neuromuscular blocking agents]**

√7ᵗʰ **T48.1X6 Underdosing of skeletal muscle relaxants [neuromuscular blocking agents]**

√5ᵗʰ **T48.2 Poisoning by, adverse effect of and underdosing of other and unspecified drugs acting on muscles**

√6ᵗʰ **T48.20 Poisoning by, adverse effect of and underdosing of unspecified drugs acting on muscles**

√7ᵗʰ **T48.201 Poisoning by unspecified drugs acting on muscles, accidental (unintentional)**
Poisoning by unspecified drugs acting on muscles NOS

√7ᵗʰ **T48.202 Poisoning by unspecified drugs acting on muscles, intentional self-harm**

√7ᵗʰ **T48.203 Poisoning by unspecified drugs acting on muscles, assault**

√7ᵗʰ **T48.204 Poisoning by unspecified drugs acting on muscles, undetermined**

Chapter 19. Injury, Poisoning and Certain Other Consequences of External Causes

T47.4–T48.204

√7ᵗʰ **T48.205** Adverse effect of unspecified drugs acting on muscles

√7ᵗʰ **T48.206** Underdosing of unspecified drugs acting on muscles

√6ᵗʰ **T48.29** Poisoning by, adverse effect of and underdosing of other drugs acting on muscles

 √7ᵗʰ **T48.291** Poisoning by other drugs acting on muscles, accidental (unintentional)
 Poisoning by other drugs acting on muscles NOS

 √7ᵗʰ **T48.292** Poisoning by other drugs acting on muscles, intentional self-harm

 √7ᵗʰ **T48.293** Poisoning by other drugs acting on muscles, assault

 √7ᵗʰ **T48.294** Poisoning by other drugs acting on muscles, undetermined

 √7ᵗʰ **T48.295** Adverse effect of other drugs acting on muscles

 √7ᵗʰ **T48.296** Underdosing of other drugs acting on muscles

√5ᵗʰ **T48.3** Poisoning by, adverse effect of and underdosing of antitussives

 √6ᵗʰ **T48.3X** Poisoning by, adverse effect of and underdosing of antitussives

 √7ᵗʰ **T48.3X1** Poisoning by antitussives, accidental (unintentional)
 Poisoning by antitussives NOS

 √7ᵗʰ **T48.3X2** Poisoning by antitussives, intentional self-harm

 √7ᵗʰ **T48.3X3** Poisoning by antitussives, assault

 √7ᵗʰ **T48.3X4** Poisoning by antitussives, undetermined

 √7ᵗʰ **T48.3X5** Adverse effect of antitussives

 √7ᵗʰ **T48.3X6** Underdosing of antitussives

√5ᵗʰ **T48.4** Poisoning by, adverse effect of and underdosing of expectorants

 √6ᵗʰ **T48.4X** Poisoning by, adverse effect of and underdosing of expectorants

 √7ᵗʰ **T48.4X1** Poisoning by expectorants, accidental (unintentional)
 Poisoning by expectorants NOS

 √7ᵗʰ **T48.4X2** Poisoning by expectorants, intentional self-harm

 √7ᵗʰ **T48.4X3** Poisoning by expectorants, assault

 √7ᵗʰ **T48.4X4** Poisoning by expectorants, undetermined

 √7ᵗʰ **T48.4X5** Adverse effect of expectorants

 √7ᵗʰ **T48.4X6** Underdosing of expectorants

√5ᵗʰ **T48.5** Poisoning by, adverse effect of and underdosing of other anti-common-cold drugs
 Poisoning by, adverse effect of and underdosing of decongestants

 EXCLUDES 2 poisoning by, adverse effect of and underdosing of antipyretics, NEC (T39.9-)
 poisoning by, adverse effect of and underdosing of non-steroidal antiinflammatory drugs (T39.3-)
 poisoning by, adverse effect of and underdosing of salicylates (T39.0-)

 √6ᵗʰ **T48.5X** Poisoning by, adverse effect of and underdosing of other anti-common-cold drugs

 √7ᵗʰ **T48.5X1** Poisoning by other anti-common-cold drugs, accidental (unintentional)
 Poisoning by other anti-common-cold drugs NOS

 √7ᵗʰ **T48.5X2** Poisoning by other anti-common-cold drugs, intentional self-harm

 √7ᵗʰ **T48.5X3** Poisoning by other anti-common-cold drugs, assault

 √7ᵗʰ **T48.5X4** Poisoning by other anti-common-cold drugs, undetermined

 √7ᵗʰ **T48.5X5** Adverse effect of other anti-common-cold drugs

 √7ᵗʰ **T48.5X6** Underdosing of other anti-common-cold drugs

√5ᵗʰ **T48.6** Poisoning by, adverse effect of and underdosing of antiasthmatics, not elsewhere classified
 Poisoning by, adverse effect of and underdosing of beta-adrenoreceptor agonists used in asthma therapy

 EXCLUDES 1 poisoning by, adverse effect of and underdosing of anterior pituitary [adenohypophyseal] hormones (T38.8)
 poisoning by, adverse effect of and underdosing of beta-adrenoreceptor agonists not used in asthma therapy (T44.5)

 √6ᵗʰ **T48.6X** Poisoning by, adverse effect of and underdosing of antiasthmatics

 √7ᵗʰ **T48.6X1** Poisoning by antiasthmatics, accidental (unintentional)
 Poisoning by antiasthmatics NOS

 √7ᵗʰ **T48.6X2** Poisoning by antiasthmatics, intentional self-harm

 √7ᵗʰ **T48.6X3** Poisoning by antiasthmatics, assault

 √7ᵗʰ **T48.6X4** Poisoning by antiasthmatics, undetermined

 √7ᵗʰ **T48.6X5** Adverse effect of antiasthmatics

 √7ᵗʰ **T48.6X6** Underdosing of antiasthmatics

√5ᵗʰ **T48.9** Poisoning by, adverse effect of and underdosing of other and unspecified agents primarily acting on the respiratory system

 √6ᵗʰ **T48.90** Poisoning by, adverse effect of and underdosing of unspecified agents primarily acting on the respiratory system

 √7ᵗʰ **T48.901** Poisoning by unspecified agents primarily acting on the respiratory system, accidental (unintentional)

 √7ᵗʰ **T48.902** Poisoning by unspecified agents primarily acting on the respiratory system, intentional self-harm

 √7ᵗʰ **T48.903** Poisoning by unspecified agents primarily acting on the respiratory system, assault

 √7ᵗʰ **T48.904** Poisoning by unspecified agents primarily acting on the respiratory system, undetermined

 √7ᵗʰ **T48.905** Adverse effect of unspecified agents primarily acting on the respiratory system

 √7ᵗʰ **T48.906** Underdosing of unspecified agents primarily acting on the respiratory system

 √6ᵗʰ **T48.99** Poisoning by, adverse effect of and underdosing of other agents primarily acting on the respiratory system

 √7ᵗʰ **T48.991** Poisoning by other agents primarily acting on the respiratory system, accidental (unintentional)

 √7ᵗʰ **T48.992** Poisoning by other agents primarily acting on the respiratory system, intentional self-harm

 √7ᵗʰ **T48.993** Poisoning by other agents primarily acting on the respiratory system, assault

 √7ᵗʰ **T48.994** Poisoning by other agents primarily acting on the respiratory system, undetermined

 √7ᵗʰ **T48.995** Adverse effect of other agents primarily acting on the respiratory system

 √7ᵗʰ **T48.996** Underdosing of other agents primarily acting on the respiratory system

N Newborn: 0 | P Pediatric: 0-17 | M Maternity: 12-55 | A Adult: 15-124 | CH Comorbidity High | CL Comorbidity Low | NCDx Noncancer Dx | PDx Primary Dx

1102 | ICD-10-CM 2020

√4ᵗʰ **T49 Poisoning by, adverse effect of and underdosing of topical agents primarily affecting skin and mucous membrane and by ophthalmological, otorhinolaryngological and dental drugs**

INCLUDES poisoning by, adverse effect of and underdosing of glucocorticoids, topically used

The appropriate 7th character is to be added to each code from category T49.
A   initial encounter
D   subsequent encounter
S   sequela

√5ᵗʰ **T49.0 Poisoning by, adverse effect of and underdosing of local antifungal, anti-infective and anti-inflammatory drugs**

√6ᵗʰ **T49.0X Poisoning by, adverse effect of and underdosing of** local antifungal, anti-infective and anti-inflammatory drugs

√7ᵗʰ **T49.0X1 Poisoning by local antifungal, anti-infective and anti-inflammatory drugs,** accidental **(unintentional)**
Poisoning by local antifungal, anti-infective and anti-inflammatory drugs NOS

√7ᵗʰ **T49.0X2 Poisoning by local antifungal, anti-infective and anti-inflammatory drugs,** intentional self-harm

√7ᵗʰ **T49.0X3 Poisoning by local antifungal, anti-infective and anti-inflammatory drugs,** assault

√7ᵗʰ **T49.0X4 Poisoning by local antifungal, anti-infective and anti-inflammatory drugs,** undetermined

√7ᵗʰ **T49.0X5 Adverse effect of local antifungal, anti-infective and anti-inflammatory drugs**

√7ᵗʰ **T49.0X6 Underdosing of local antifungal, anti-infective and anti-inflammatory drugs**

√5ᵗʰ **T49.1 Poisoning by, adverse effect of and underdosing of antipruritics**

√6ᵗʰ **T49.1X Poisoning by, adverse effect of and underdosing of** antipruritics

√7ᵗʰ **T49.1X1 Poisoning by antipruritics,** accidental **(unintentional)**
Poisoning by antipruritics NOS

√7ᵗʰ **T49.1X2 Poisoning by antipruritics,** intentional self-harm

√7ᵗʰ **T49.1X3 Poisoning by antipruritics,** assault

√7ᵗʰ **T49.1X4 Poisoning by antipruritics,** undetermined

√7ᵗʰ **T49.1X5 Adverse effect of antipruritics**

√7ᵗʰ **T49.1X6 Underdosing of antipruritics**

√5ᵗʰ **T49.2 Poisoning by, adverse effect of and underdosing of local astringents and local detergents**

√6ᵗʰ **T49.2X Poisoning by, adverse effect of and underdosing of** local astringents and local detergents

√7ᵗʰ **T49.2X1 Poisoning by local astringents and local detergents,** accidental **(unintentional)**
Poisoning by local astringents and local detergents NOS

√7ᵗʰ **T49.2X2 Poisoning by local astringents and local detergents,** intentional self-harm

√7ᵗʰ **T49.2X3 Poisoning by local astringents and local detergents,** assault

√7ᵗʰ **T49.2X4 Poisoning by local astringents and local detergents,** undetermined

√7ᵗʰ **T49.2X5 Adverse effect of local astringents and local detergents**

√7ᵗʰ **T49.2X6 Underdosing of local astringents and local detergents**

√5ᵗʰ **T49.3 Poisoning by, adverse effect of and underdosing of emollients, demulcents and protectants**

√6ᵗʰ **T49.3X Poisoning by, adverse effect of and underdosing of** emollients, demulcents and protectants

√7ᵗʰ **T49.3X1 Poisoning by emollients, demulcents and protectants,** accidental **(unintentional)**
Poisoning by emollients, demulcents and protectants NOS

√7ᵗʰ **T49.3X2 Poisoning by emollients, demulcents and protectants,** intentional self-harm

√7ᵗʰ **T49.3X3 Poisoning by emollients, demulcents and protectants,** assault

√7ᵗʰ **T49.3X4 Poisoning by emollients, demulcents and protectants,** undetermined

√7ᵗʰ **T49.3X5 Adverse effect of emollients, demulcents and protectants**

√7ᵗʰ **T49.3X6 Underdosing of emollients, demulcents and protectants**

√5ᵗʰ **T49.4 Poisoning by, adverse effect of and underdosing of keratolytics, keratoplastics, and other hair treatment drugs and preparations**

√6ᵗʰ **T49.4X Poisoning by, adverse effect of and underdosing of** keratolytics, keratoplastics, and other hair treatment drugs and preparations

√7ᵗʰ **T49.4X1 Poisoning by keratolytics, keratoplastics, and other hair treatment drugs and preparations,** accidental **(unintentional)**
Poisoning by keratolytics, keratoplastics, and other hair treatment drugs and preparations NOS

√7ᵗʰ **T49.4X2 Poisoning by keratolytics, keratoplastics, and other hair treatment drugs and preparations,** intentional self-harm

√7ᵗʰ **T49.4X3 Poisoning by keratolytics, keratoplastics, and other hair treatment drugs and preparations,** assault

√7ᵗʰ **T49.4X4 Poisoning by keratolytics, keratoplastics, and other hair treatment drugs and preparations,** undetermined

√7ᵗʰ **T49.4X5 Adverse effect of keratolytics, keratoplastics, and other hair treatment drugs and preparations**

√7ᵗʰ **T49.4X6 Underdosing of keratolytics, keratoplastics, and other hair treatment drugs and preparations**

√5ᵗʰ **T49.5 Poisoning by, adverse effect of and underdosing of ophthalmological drugs and preparations**

√6ᵗʰ **T49.5X Poisoning by, adverse effect of and underdosing of** ophthalmological drugs and preparations

√7ᵗʰ **T49.5X1 Poisoning by ophthalmological drugs and preparations,** accidental **(unintentional)**
Poisoning by ophthalmological drugs and preparations NOS

√7ᵗʰ **T49.5X2 Poisoning by ophthalmological drugs and preparations,** intentional self-harm

√7ᵗʰ **T49.5X3 Poisoning by ophthalmological drugs and preparations,** assault

√7ᵗʰ **T49.5X4 Poisoning by ophthalmological drugs and preparations,** undetermined

√7ᵗʰ **T49.5X5 Adverse effect of ophthalmological drugs and preparations**

√7ᵗʰ **T49.5X6 Underdosing of ophthalmological drugs and preparations**

√5ᵗʰ **T49.6 Poisoning by, adverse effect of and underdosing of otorhinolaryngological drugs and preparations**

√6ᵗʰ **T49.6X Poisoning by, adverse effect of and underdosing of** otorhinolaryngological drugs and preparations

√7ᵗʰ **T49.6X1 Poisoning by otorhinolaryngological drugs and preparations,** accidental **(unintentional)**
Poisoning by otorhinolaryngological drugs and preparations NOS

√7ᵗʰ **T49.6X2 Poisoning by otorhinolaryngological drugs and preparations,** intentional self-harm

√7ᵗʰ **T49.6X3 Poisoning by otorhinolaryngological drugs and preparations,** assault

√7ᵗʰ **T49.6X4 Poisoning by otorhinolaryngological drugs and preparations,** undetermined

√7ᵗʰ **T49.6X5 Adverse effect of otorhinolaryngological drugs and preparations**

√7ᵗʰ **T49.6X6 Underdosing of otorhinolaryngological drugs and preparations**

√5ᵗʰ **T49.7 Poisoning by, adverse effect of and underdosing of dental drugs, topically applied**

√6ᵗʰ **T49.7X Poisoning by, adverse effect of and underdosing of** dental drugs, topically applied

√7ᵗʰ **T49.7X1 Poisoning by dental drugs, topically applied,** accidental **(unintentional)**
Poisoning by dental drugs, topically applied NOS

√7ᵗʰ **T49.7X2 Poisoning by dental drugs, topically applied,** intentional self-harm

√7ᵗʰ **T49.7X3 Poisoning by dental drugs, topically applied,** assault

√7ᵗʰ **T49.7X4 Poisoning by dental drugs, topically applied,** undetermined

✓ Additional Character Required   √x7ᵗʰ Placeholder Alert   Manifestation   Unspecified Dx   ▶◀ Revised Text   ● New Code   ▲ Revised Title

☑7ᵗʰ **T49.7X5** Adverse effect of dental drugs, topically applied

☑7ᵗʰ **T49.7X6** Underdosing of dental drugs, topically applied

☑5ᵗʰ **T49.8** Poisoning by, adverse effect of and underdosing of other topical agents

Poisoning by, adverse effect of and underdosing of spermicides

☑6ᵗʰ **T49.8X** Poisoning by, adverse effect of and underdosing of other topical agents

☑7ᵗʰ **T49.8X1** Poisoning by other topical agents, accidental (unintentional)

Poisoning by other topical agents NOS

☑7ᵗʰ **T49.8X2** Poisoning by other topical agents, intentional self-harm

☑7ᵗʰ **T49.8X3** Poisoning by other topical agents, assault

☑7ᵗʰ **T49.8X4** Poisoning by other topical agents, undetermined

☑7ᵗʰ **T49.8X5** Adverse effect of other topical agents

☑7ᵗʰ **T49.8X6** Underdosing of other topical agents

☑5ᵗʰ **T49.9** Poisoning by, adverse effect of and underdosing of unspecified topical agent

☑x7ᵗʰ **T49.91** Poisoning by unspecified topical agent, accidental (unintentional)

☑x7ᵗʰ **T49.92** Poisoning by unspecified topical agent, intentional self-harm

☑x7ᵗʰ **T49.93** Poisoning by unspecified topical agent, assault

☑x7ᵗʰ **T49.94** Poisoning by unspecified topical agent, undetermined

☑x7ᵗʰ **T49.95** Adverse effect of unspecified topical agent

☑x7ᵗʰ **T49.96** Underdosing of unspecified topical agent

☑4ᵗʰ **T50** Poisoning by, adverse effect of and underdosing of diuretics and other and unspecified drugs, medicaments and biological substances

The appropriate 7th character is to be added to each code from category T50.
A   initial encounter
D   subsequent encounter
S   sequela

☑5ᵗʰ **T50.0** Poisoning by, adverse effect of and underdosing of mineralocorticoids and their antagonists

☑6ᵗʰ **T50.0X** Poisoning by, adverse effect of and underdosing of mineralocorticoids and their antagonists

☑7ᵗʰ **T50.0X1** Poisoning by mineralocorticoids and their antagonists, accidental (unintentional)

Poisoning by mineralocorticoids and their antagonists NOS

☑7ᵗʰ **T50.0X2** Poisoning by mineralocorticoids and their antagonists, intentional self-harm

☑7ᵗʰ **T50.0X3** Poisoning by mineralocorticoids and their antagonists, assault

☑7ᵗʰ **T50.0X4** Poisoning by mineralocorticoids and their antagonists, undetermined

☑7ᵗʰ **T50.0X5** Adverse effect of mineralocorticoids and their antagonists

☑7ᵗʰ **T50.0X6** Underdosing of mineralocorticoids and their antagonists

☑5ᵗʰ **T50.1** Poisoning by, adverse effect of and underdosing of loop [high-ceiling] diuretics

☑6ᵗʰ **T50.1X** Poisoning by, adverse effect of and underdosing of loop [high-ceiling] diuretics

☑7ᵗʰ **T50.1X1** Poisoning by loop [high-ceiling] diuretics, accidental (unintentional)

Poisoning by loop [high-ceiling] diuretics NOS

☑7ᵗʰ **T50.1X2** Poisoning by loop [high-ceiling] diuretics, intentional self-harm

☑7ᵗʰ **T50.1X3** Poisoning by loop [high-ceiling] diuretics, assault

☑7ᵗʰ **T50.1X4** Poisoning by loop [high-ceiling] diuretics, undetermined

☑7ᵗʰ **T50.1X5** Adverse effect of loop [high-ceiling] diuretics

☑7ᵗʰ **T50.1X6** Underdosing of loop [high-ceiling] diuretics

☑5ᵗʰ **T50.2** Poisoning by, adverse effect of and underdosing of carbonic-anhydrase inhibitors, benzothiadiazides and other diuretics

Poisoning by, adverse effect of and underdosing of acetazolamide

☑6ᵗʰ **T50.2X** Poisoning by, adverse effect of and underdosing of carbonic-anhydrase inhibitors, benzothiadiazides and other diuretics

☑7ᵗʰ **T50.2X1** Poisoning by carbonic-anhydrase inhibitors, benzothiadiazides and other diuretics, accidental (unintentional)

Poisoning by carbonic-anhydrase inhibitors, benzothiadiazides and other diuretics NOS

☑7ᵗʰ **T50.2X2** Poisoning by carbonic-anhydrase inhibitors, benzothiadiazides and other diuretics, intentional self-harm

☑7ᵗʰ **T50.2X3** Poisoning by carbonic-anhydrase inhibitors, benzothiadiazides and other diuretics, assault

☑7ᵗʰ **T50.2X4** Poisoning by carbonic-anhydrase inhibitors, benzothiadiazides and other diuretics, undetermined

☑7ᵗʰ **T50.2X5** Adverse effect of carbonic-anhydrase inhibitors, benzothiadiazides and other diuretics

☑7ᵗʰ **T50.2X6** Underdosing of carbonic-anhydrase inhibitors, benzothiadiazides and other diuretics

☑5ᵗʰ **T50.3** Poisoning by, adverse effect of and underdosing of electrolytic, caloric and water-balance agents

Poisoning by, adverse effect of and underdosing of oral rehydration salts

☑6ᵗʰ **T50.3X** Poisoning by, adverse effect of and underdosing of electrolytic, caloric and water-balance agents

☑7ᵗʰ **T50.3X1** Poisoning by electrolytic, caloric and water-balance agents, accidental (unintentional)

Poisoning by electrolytic, caloric and water-balance agents NOS

☑7ᵗʰ **T50.3X2** Poisoning by electrolytic, caloric and water-balance agents, intentional self-harm

☑7ᵗʰ **T50.3X3** Poisoning by electrolytic, caloric and water-balance agents, assault

☑7ᵗʰ **T50.3X4** Poisoning by electrolytic, caloric and water-balance agents, undetermined

☑7ᵗʰ **T50.3X5** Adverse effect of electrolytic, caloric and water-balance agents

☑7ᵗʰ **T50.3X6** Underdosing of electrolytic, caloric and water-balance agents

☑5ᵗʰ **T50.4** Poisoning by, adverse effect of and underdosing of drugs affecting uric acid metabolism

☑6ᵗʰ **T50.4X** Poisoning by, adverse effect of and underdosing of drugs affecting uric acid metabolism

☑7ᵗʰ **T50.4X1** Poisoning by drugs affecting uric acid metabolism, accidental (unintentional)

Poisoning by drugs affecting uric acid metabolism NOS

☑7ᵗʰ **T50.4X2** Poisoning by drugs affecting uric acid metabolism, intentional self-harm

☑7ᵗʰ **T50.4X3** Poisoning by drugs affecting uric acid metabolism, assault

☑7ᵗʰ **T50.4X4** Poisoning by drugs affecting uric acid metabolism, undetermined

☑7ᵗʰ **T50.4X5** Adverse effect of drugs affecting uric acid metabolism

☑7ᵗʰ **T50.4X6** Underdosing of drugs affecting uric acid metabolism

☑5ᵗʰ **T50.5** Poisoning by, adverse effect of and underdosing of appetite depressants

☑6ᵗʰ **T50.5X** Poisoning by, adverse effect of and underdosing of appetite depressants

☑7ᵗʰ **T50.5X1** Poisoning by appetite depressants, accidental (unintentional)

Poisoning by appetite depressants NOS

☑7ᵗʰ **T50.5X2** Poisoning by appetite depressants, intentional self-harm

☑7ᵗʰ **T50.5X3** Poisoning by appetite depressants, assault

☑7ᵗʰ **T50.5X4** Poisoning by appetite depressants, undetermined

☑7ᵗʰ **T50.5X5** Adverse effect of appetite depressants

Ⓝ Newborn: 0   Ⓟ Pediatric: 0-17   Ⓜ Maternity: 12-55   Ⓐ Adult: 15-124   CH Comorbidity High   CL Comorbidity Low   NCDx Noncancer Dx   PDx Primary Dx

1104   ICD-10-CM 2020

√5ᵗʰ **T50.5X6** Underdosing of appetite depressants

√5ᵗʰ **T50.6** **Poisoning by, adverse effect of and underdosing of antidotes and chelating agents**
    Poisoning by, adverse effect of and underdosing of alcohol deterrents

    √6ᵗʰ **T50.6X** **Poisoning by, adverse effect of and underdosing of** antidotes and chelating agents

      √7ᵗʰ **T50.6X1** **Poisoning by antidotes and chelating agents,** accidental **(unintentional)**
         Poisoning by antidotes and chelating agents NOS

      √7ᵗʰ **T50.6X2** **Poisoning by antidotes and chelating agents,** intentional self-harm

      √7ᵗʰ **T50.6X3** **Poisoning by antidotes and chelating agents,** assault

      √7ᵗʰ **T50.6X4** **Poisoning by antidotes and chelating agents,** undetermined

      √7ᵗʰ **T50.6X5** Adverse effect **of antidotes and chelating agents**

      √7ᵗʰ **T50.6X6** Underdosing **of antidotes and chelating agents**

√5ᵗʰ **T50.7** **Poisoning by, adverse effect of and underdosing of analeptics and opioid receptor antagonists**

    √6ᵗʰ **T50.7X** **Poisoning by, adverse effect of and underdosing of** analeptics and opioid receptor antagonists

      √7ᵗʰ **T50.7X1** **Poisoning by analeptics and opioid receptor antagonists,** accidental **(unintentional)**
         Poisoning by analeptics and opioid receptor antagonists NOS

      √7ᵗʰ **T50.7X2** **Poisoning by analeptics and opioid receptor antagonists,** intentional self-harm

      √7ᵗʰ **T50.7X3** **Poisoning by analeptics and opioid receptor antagonists,** assault

      √7ᵗʰ **T50.7X4** **Poisoning by analeptics and opioid receptor antagonists,** undetermined

      √7ᵗʰ **T50.7X5** Adverse effect **of analeptics and opioid receptor antagonists**

      √7ᵗʰ **T50.7X6** Underdosing **of analeptics and opioid receptor antagonists**

√5ᵗʰ **T50.8** **Poisoning by, adverse effect of and underdosing of diagnostic agents**

    √6ᵗʰ **T50.8X** **Poisoning by, adverse effect of and underdosing of** diagnostic agents

      √7ᵗʰ **T50.8X1** **Poisoning by diagnostic agents,** accidental **(unintentional)**
         Poisoning by diagnostic agents NOS

      √7ᵗʰ **T50.8X2** **Poisoning by diagnostic agents,** intentional self-harm

      √7ᵗʰ **T50.8X3** **Poisoning by diagnostic agents,** assault

      √7ᵗʰ **T50.8X4** **Poisoning by diagnostic agents,** undetermined

      √7ᵗʰ **T50.8X5** Adverse effect **of diagnostic agents**

      √7ᵗʰ **T50.8X6** Underdosing **of diagnostic agents**

√5ᵗʰ **T50.A** **Poisoning by, adverse effect of and underdosing of bacterial vaccines**

    √6ᵗʰ **T50.A1** **Poisoning by, adverse effect of and underdosing of** pertussis vaccine, including combinations with a pertussis component

      √7ᵗʰ **T50.A11** **Poisoning by pertussis vaccine, including combinations with a pertussis component,** accidental **(unintentional)**

      √7ᵗʰ **T50.A12** **Poisoning by pertussis vaccine, including combinations with a pertussis component,** intentional self-harm

      √7ᵗʰ **T50.A13** **Poisoning by pertussis vaccine, including combinations with a pertussis component,** assault

      √7ᵗʰ **T50.A14** **Poisoning by pertussis vaccine, including combinations with a pertussis component,** undetermined

      √7ᵗʰ **T50.A15** Adverse effect **of pertussis vaccine, including combinations with a pertussis component**

      √7ᵗʰ **T50.A16** Underdosing **of pertussis vaccine, including combinations with a pertussis component**

√6ᵗʰ **T50.A2** **Poisoning by, adverse effect of and underdosing of** mixed bacterial vaccines without a pertussis component

    √7ᵗʰ **T50.A21** **Poisoning by mixed bacterial vaccines without a pertussis component,** accidental **(unintentional)**

    √7ᵗʰ **T50.A22** **Poisoning by mixed bacterial vaccines without a pertussis component,** intentional self-harm

    √7ᵗʰ **T50.A23** **Poisoning by mixed bacterial vaccines without a pertussis component,** assault

    √7ᵗʰ **T50.A24** **Poisoning by mixed bacterial vaccines without a pertussis component,** undetermined

    √7ᵗʰ **T50.A25** Adverse effect **of mixed bacterial vaccines without a pertussis component**

    √7ᵗʰ **T50.A26** Underdosing **of mixed bacterial vaccines without a pertussis component**

√6ᵗʰ **T50.A9** **Poisoning by, adverse effect of and underdosing of other bacterial vaccines**

    √7ᵗʰ **T50.A91** **Poisoning by other bacterial vaccines,** accidental **(unintentional)**

    √7ᵗʰ **T50.A92** **Poisoning by other bacterial vaccines,** intentional self-harm

    √7ᵗʰ **T50.A93** **Poisoning by other bacterial vaccines,** assault

    √7ᵗʰ **T50.A94** **Poisoning by other bacterial vaccines,** undetermined

    √7ᵗʰ **T50.A95** Adverse effect **of other bacterial vaccines**

    √7ᵗʰ **T50.A96** Underdosing **of other bacterial vaccines**

√5ᵗʰ **T50.B** **Poisoning by, adverse effect of and underdosing of viral vaccines**

    √6ᵗʰ **T50.B1** **Poisoning by, adverse effect of and underdosing of** smallpox vaccines

      √7ᵗʰ **T50.B11** **Poisoning by smallpox vaccines,** accidental **(unintentional)**

      √7ᵗʰ **T50.B12** **Poisoning by smallpox vaccines,** intentional self-harm

      √7ᵗʰ **T50.B13** **Poisoning by smallpox vaccines,** assault

      √7ᵗʰ **T50.B14** **Poisoning by smallpox vaccines,** undetermined

      √7ᵗʰ **T50.B15** Adverse effect **of smallpox vaccines**

      √7ᵗʰ **T50.B16** Underdosing **of smallpox vaccines**

    √6ᵗʰ **T50.B9** **Poisoning by, adverse effect of and underdosing of other viral vaccines**

      √7ᵗʰ **T50.B91** **Poisoning by other viral vaccines,** accidental **(unintentional)**

      √7ᵗʰ **T50.B92** **Poisoning by other viral vaccines,** intentional self-harm

      √7ᵗʰ **T50.B93** **Poisoning by other viral vaccines,** assault

      √7ᵗʰ **T50.B94** **Poisoning by other viral vaccines,** undetermined

      √7ᵗʰ **T50.B95** Adverse effect **of other viral vaccines**

      √7ᵗʰ **T50.B96** Underdosing **of other viral vaccines**

√5ᵗʰ **T50.Z** **Poisoning by, adverse effect of and underdosing of other vaccines and biological substances**

    √6ᵗʰ **T50.Z1** **Poisoning by, adverse effect of and underdosing of** immunoglobulin

      √7ᵗʰ **T50.Z11** **Poisoning by immunoglobulin,** accidental **(unintentional)**

      √7ᵗʰ **T50.Z12** **Poisoning by immunoglobulin,** intentional self-harm

      √7ᵗʰ **T50.Z13** **Poisoning by immunoglobulin,** assault

      √7ᵗʰ **T50.Z14** **Poisoning by immunoglobulin,** undetermined

      √7ᵗʰ **T50.Z15** Adverse effect **of immunoglobulin**

      √7ᵗʰ **T50.Z16** Underdosing **of immunoglobulin**

    √6ᵗʰ **T50.Z9** **Poisoning by, adverse effect of and underdosing of other vaccines and biological substances**

      √7ᵗʰ **T50.Z91** **Poisoning by other vaccines and biological substances,** accidental **(unintentional)**

      √7ᵗʰ **T50.Z92** **Poisoning by other vaccines and biological substances,** intentional self-harm

      √7ᵗʰ **T50.Z93** **Poisoning by other vaccines and biological substances,** assault

      √7ᵗʰ **T50.Z94** **Poisoning by other vaccines and biological substances,** undetermined

      √7ᵗʰ **T50.Z95** Adverse effect **of other vaccines and biological substances**

✔ Additional Character Required   √x7ᵗʰ Placeholder Alert   Manifestation   Unspecified Dx   ▶◀ Revised Text   ● New Code   ▲ Revised Title

ICD-10-CM 2020   **1105**

√7ᵗʰ **T50.Z96** Underdosing of other vaccines and biological substances

√5ᵗʰ **T50.9** Poisoning by, adverse effect of and underdosing of other and unspecified drugs, medicaments and biological substances

AHA: 2016,1Q,38; 2015,1Q,21

√6ᵗʰ **T50.90** Poisoning by, adverse effect of and underdosing of unspecified drugs, medicaments and biological substances

√7ᵗʰ **T50.901** Poisoning by unspecified drugs, medicaments and biological substances, accidental (unintentional)

√7ᵗʰ **T50.902** Poisoning by unspecified drugs, medicaments and biological substances, intentional self-harm

√7ᵗʰ **T50.903** Poisoning by unspecified drugs, medicaments and biological substances, assault

√7ᵗʰ **T50.904** Poisoning by unspecified drugs, medicaments and biological substances, undetermined

√7ᵗʰ **T50.905** Adverse effect of unspecified drugs, medicaments and biological substances

√7ᵗʰ **T50.906** Underdosing of unspecified drugs, medicaments and biological substances

√6ᵗʰ **T50.91** Poisoning by, adverse effect of and underdosing of multiple unspecified drugs, medicaments and biological substances

Multiple drug ingestion NOS

Code also any specific drugs, medicaments and biological substances

√7ᵗʰ **T50.911** Poisoning by multiple unspecified drugs, medicaments and biological substances, accidental (unintentional)

√7ᵗʰ **T50.912** Poisoning by multiple unspecified drugs, medicaments and biological substances, intentional self-harm

√7ᵗʰ **T50.913** Poisoning by multiple unspecified drugs, medicaments and biological substances, assault

√7ᵗʰ **T50.914** Poisoning by multiple unspecified drugs, medicaments and biological substances, undetermined

√7ᵗʰ **T50.915** Adverse effect of multiple unspecified drugs, medicaments and biological substances

√7ᵗʰ **T50.916** Underdosing of multiple unspecified drugs, medicaments and biological substances

√6ᵗʰ **T50.99** Poisoning by, adverse effect of and underdosing of other drugs, medicaments and biological substances

√7ᵗʰ **T50.991** Poisoning by other drugs, medicaments and biological substances, accidental (unintentional)

√7ᵗʰ **T50.992** Poisoning by other drugs, medicaments and biological substances, intentional self-harm

√7ᵗʰ **T50.993** Poisoning by other drugs, medicaments and biological substances, assault

√7ᵗʰ **T50.994** Poisoning by other drugs, medicaments and biological substances, undetermined

√7ᵗʰ **T50.995** Adverse effect of other drugs, medicaments and biological substances

√7ᵗʰ **T50.996** Underdosing of other drugs, medicaments and biological substances

Toxic effects of substances chiefly nonmedicinal as to source (T51-T65)

NOTE   When no intent is indicated code to accidental. Undetermined intent is only for use when there is specific documentation in the record that the intent of the toxic effect cannot be determined.

Use additional code(s) for all associated manifestations of toxic effect, such as:
personal history of foreign body fully removed (Z87.821)
respiratory conditions due to external agents (J60-J70)
to identify any retained foreign body, if applicable (Z18.-)

EXCLUDES 1   contact with and (suspected) exposure to toxic substances (Z77.-)

AHA: 2017,1Q,39-40

TIP: Assign any condition resulting from a poisoning, toxic effect, or adverse effect, followed by the appropriate code from categories T51–T65 while the resulting effects of the poisoning, toxic effect, or adverse effect remain unresolved and require treatment.

√4ᵗʰ **T51 Toxic effect of alcohol**

The appropriate 7th character is to be added to each code from category T51.
A   initial encounter
D   subsequent encounter
S   sequela

√5ᵗʰ **T51.0** Toxic effect of ethanol

Toxic effect of ethyl alcohol

EXCLUDES 2   acute alcohol intoxication or "hangover" effects (F10.129, F10.229, F10.929)
drunkenness (F10.129, F10.229, F10.929)
pathological alcohol intoxication (F10.129, F10.229, F10.929)

√6ᵗʰ **T51.0X** Toxic effect of ethanol

√7ᵗʰ **T51.0X1** Toxic effect of ethanol, accidental (unintentional)

Toxic effect of ethanol NOS

√7ᵗʰ **T51.0X2** Toxic effect of ethanol, intentional self-harm

√7ᵗʰ **T51.0X3** Toxic effect of ethanol, assault

√7ᵗʰ **T51.0X4** Toxic effect of ethanol, undetermined

√5ᵗʰ **T51.1** Toxic effect of methanol

Toxic effect of methyl alcohol

√6ᵗʰ **T51.1X** Toxic effect of methanol

√7ᵗʰ **T51.1X1** Toxic effect of methanol, accidental (unintentional)

Toxic effect of methanol NOS

√7ᵗʰ **T51.1X2** Toxic effect of methanol, intentional self-harm

√7ᵗʰ **T51.1X3** Toxic effect of methanol, assault

√7ᵗʰ **T51.1X4** Toxic effect of methanol, undetermined

√5ᵗʰ **T51.2** Toxic effect of 2-Propanol

Toxic effect of isopropyl alcohol

√6ᵗʰ **T51.2X** Toxic effect of 2-Propanol

√7ᵗʰ **T51.2X1** Toxic effect of 2-Propanol, accidental (unintentional)

Toxic effect of 2-Propanol NOS

√7ᵗʰ **T51.2X2** Toxic effect of 2-Propanol, intentional self-harm

√7ᵗʰ **T51.2X3** Toxic effect of 2-Propanol, assault

√7ᵗʰ **T51.2X4** Toxic effect of 2-Propanol, undetermined

√5ᵗʰ **T51.3** Toxic effect of fusel oil

Toxic effect of amyl alcohol
Toxic effect of butyl [1-butanol] alcohol
Toxic effect of propyl [1-propanol] alcohol

√6ᵗʰ **T51.3X** Toxic effect of fusel oil

√7ᵗʰ **T51.3X1** Toxic effect of fusel oil, accidental (unintentional)

Toxic effect of fusel oil NOS

√7ᵗʰ **T51.3X2** Toxic effect of fusel oil, intentional self-harm

√7ᵗʰ **T51.3X3** Toxic effect of fusel oil, assault

√7ᵗʰ **T51.3X4** Toxic effect of fusel oil, undetermined

√5ᵗʰ **T51.8** Toxic effect of other alcohols

√6ᵗʰ **T51.8X** Toxic effect of other alcohols

√7ᵗʰ **T51.8X1** Toxic effect of other alcohols, accidental (unintentional)

Toxic effect of other alcohols NOS

N Newborn: 0   P Pediatric: 0-17   M Maternity: 12-55   A Adult: 15-124   CH Comorbidity High   CL Comorbidity Low   NCDx Noncancer Dx   PDx Primary Dx

1106   ICD-10-CM 2020

√7th **T51.8X2** **Toxic effect of other alcohols,** intentional self-harm

√7th **T51.8X3** **Toxic effect of other alcohols,** assault

√7th **T51.8X4** **Toxic effect of other alcohols,** undetermined

√5th **T51.9** **Toxic effect of unspecified alcohol**

√x7th **T51.91** **Toxic effect of unspecified alcohol,** accidental (unintentional)

√x7th **T51.92** **Toxic effect of unspecified alcohol,** intentional self-harm

√x7th **T51.93** **Toxic effect of unspecified alcohol,** assault

√x7th **T51.94** **Toxic effect of unspecified alcohol,** undetermined

√4th **T52** **Toxic effect of organic solvents**

> **EXCLUDES 1**   halogen derivatives of aliphatic and aromatic hydrocarbons (T53.-)

> The appropriate 7th character is to be added to each code from category T52.
> A   initial encounter
> D   subsequent encounter
> S   sequela

√5th **T52.0** **Toxic effects of petroleum products**

Toxic effects of ether petroleum
Toxic effects of gasoline [petrol]
Toxic effects of kerosene [paraffin oil]
Toxic effects of naphtha petroleum
Toxic effects of paraffin wax
Toxic effects of spirit petroleum

√6th **T52.0X** **Toxic effects of** petroleum products

√7th **T52.0X1** **Toxic effect of petroleum products,** accidental (unintentional)
Toxic effects of petroleum products NOS

√7th **T52.0X2** **Toxic effect of petroleum products,** intentional self-harm

√7th **T52.0X3** **Toxic effect of petroleum products,** assault

√7th **T52.0X4** **Toxic effect of petroleum products,** undetermined

√5th **T52.1** **Toxic effects of benzene**

> **EXCLUDES 1**   homologues of benzene (T52.2)
> nitroderivatives and aminoderivatives of benzene and its homologues (T65.3)

√6th **T52.1X** **Toxic effects of** benzene

√7th **T52.1X1** **Toxic effect of benzene,** accidental (unintentional)
Toxic effects of benzene NOS

√7th **T52.1X2** **Toxic effect of benzene,** intentional self-harm

√7th **T52.1X3** **Toxic effect of benzene,** assault

√7th **T52.1X4** **Toxic effect of benzene,** undetermined

√5th **T52.2** **Toxic effects of homologues of benzene**

Toxic effects of toluene [methylbenzene]
Toxic effects of xylene [dimethylbenzene]

√6th **T52.2X** **Toxic effects of** homologues of benzene

√7th **T52.2X1** **Toxic effect of homologues of benzene,** accidental (unintentional)
Toxic effects of homologues of benzene NOS

√7th **T52.2X2** **Toxic effect of homologues of benzene,** intentional self-harm

√7th **T52.2X3** **Toxic effect of homologues of benzene,** assault

√7th **T52.2X4** **Toxic effect of homologues of benzene,** undetermined

√5th **T52.3** **Toxic effects of glycols**

√6th **T52.3X** **Toxic effects of** glycols

√7th **T52.3X1** **Toxic effect of glycols,** accidental (unintentional)
Toxic effects of glycols NOS

√7th **T52.3X2** **Toxic effect of glycols,** intentional self-harm

√7th **T52.3X3** **Toxic effect of glycols,** assault

√7th **T52.3X4** **Toxic effect of glycols,** undetermined

√5th **T52.4** **Toxic effects of ketones**

√6th **T52.4X** **Toxic effects of** ketones

√7th **T52.4X1** **Toxic effect of ketones,** accidental (unintentional)
Toxic effects of ketones NOS

√7th **T52.4X2** **Toxic effect of ketones,** intentional self-harm

√7th **T52.4X3** **Toxic effect of ketones,** assault

√7th **T52.4X4** **Toxic effect of ketones,** undetermined

√5th **T52.8** **Toxic effects of other organic solvents**

√6th **T52.8X** **Toxic effects of other organic solvents**

√7th **T52.8X1** **Toxic effect of other organic solvents,** accidental (unintentional)
Toxic effects of other organic solvents NOS

√7th **T52.8X2** **Toxic effect of other organic solvents,** intentional self-harm

√7th **T52.8X3** **Toxic effect of other organic solvents,** assault

√7th **T52.8X4** **Toxic effect of other organic solvents,** undetermined

√5th **T52.9** **Toxic effects of unspecified organic solvent**

√x7th **T52.91** **Toxic effect of unspecified organic solvent,** accidental (unintentional)

√x7th **T52.92** **Toxic effect of unspecified organic solvent,** intentional self-harm

√x7th **T52.93** **Toxic effect of unspecified organic solvent,** assault

√x7th **T52.94** **Toxic effect of unspecified organic solvent,** undetermined

√4th **T53** **Toxic effect of halogen derivatives of aliphatic and aromatic hydrocarbons**

> The appropriate 7th character is to be added to each code from category T53.
> A   initial encounter
> D   subsequent encounter
> S   sequela

√5th **T53.0** **Toxic effects of carbon tetrachloride**

Toxic effects of tetrachloromethane

√6th **T53.0X** **Toxic effects of** carbon tetrachloride

√7th **T53.0X1** **Toxic effect of carbon tetrachloride,** accidental (unintentional)
Toxic effects of carbon tetrachloride NOS

√7th **T53.0X2** **Toxic effect of carbon tetrachloride,** intentional self-harm

√7th **T53.0X3** **Toxic effect of carbon tetrachloride,** assault

√7th **T53.0X4** **Toxic effect of carbon tetrachloride,** undetermined

√5th **T53.1** **Toxic effects of chloroform**

Toxic effects of trichloromethane

√6th **T53.1X** **Toxic effects of** chloroform

√7th **T53.1X1** **Toxic effect of chloroform,** accidental (unintentional)
Toxic effects of chloroform NOS

√7th **T53.1X2** **Toxic effect of chloroform,** intentional self-harm

√7th **T53.1X3** **Toxic effect of chloroform,** assault

√7th **T53.1X4** **Toxic effect of chloroform,** undetermined

√5th **T53.2** **Toxic effects of trichloroethylene**

Toxic effects of trichloroethene

√6th **T53.2X** **Toxic effects of** trichloroethylene

√7th **T53.2X1** **Toxic effect of trichloroethylene,** accidental (unintentional)
Toxic effects of trichloroethylene NOS

√7th **T53.2X2** **Toxic effect of trichloroethylene,** intentional self-harm

√7th **T53.2X3** **Toxic effect of trichloroethylene,** assault

√7th **T53.2X4** **Toxic effect of trichloroethylene,** undetermined

√5th **T53.3** **Toxic effects of tetrachloroethylene**

Toxic effects of perchloroethylene
Toxic effect of tetrachloroethene

√6th **T53.3X** **Toxic effects of** tetrachloroethylene

√7th **T53.3X1** **Toxic effect of tetrachloroethylene,** accidental (unintentional)
Toxic effects of tetrachloroethylene NOS

☑ Additional Character Required   √x7th Placeholder Alert   Manifestation   Unspecified Dx   ▶◀ Revised Text   ● New Code   ▲ Revised Title

ICD-10-CM 2020   1107

√7ᵗʰ **T53.3X2** **Toxic effect of tetrachloroethylene,** intentional self-harm

√7ᵗʰ **T53.3X3** **Toxic effect of tetrachloroethylene,** assault

√7ᵗʰ **T53.3X4** **Toxic effect of tetrachloroethylene,** undetermined

√5ᵗʰ **T53.4** **Toxic effects of dichloromethane**
Toxic effects of methylene chloride

√6ᵗʰ **T53.4X** **Toxic effects of** dichloromethane

√7ᵗʰ **T53.4X1** **Toxic effect of dichloromethane,** accidental (**unintentional**)
Toxic effects of dichloromethane NOS

√7ᵗʰ **T53.4X2** **Toxic effect of dichloromethane,** intentional self-harm

√7ᵗʰ **T53.4X3** **Toxic effect of dichloromethane,** assault

√7ᵗʰ **T53.4X4** **Toxic effect of dichloromethane,** undetermined

√5ᵗʰ **T53.5** **Toxic effects of chlorofluorocarbons**

√6ᵗʰ **T53.5X** **Toxic effects of** chlorofluorocarbons

√7ᵗʰ **T53.5X1** **Toxic effect of chlorofluorocarbons,** accidental (**unintentional**)
Toxic effects of chlorofluorocarbons NOS

√7ᵗʰ **T53.5X2** **Toxic effect of chlorofluorocarbons,** intentional self-harm

√7ᵗʰ **T53.5X3** **Toxic effect of chlorofluorocarbons,** assault

√7ᵗʰ **T53.5X4** **Toxic effect of chlorofluorocarbons,** undetermined

√5ᵗʰ **T53.6** **Toxic effects of other halogen derivatives of aliphatic hydrocarbons**

√6ᵗʰ **T53.6X** **Toxic effects of** other halogen derivatives of aliphatic hydrocarbons

√7ᵗʰ **T53.6X1** **Toxic effect of other halogen derivatives of aliphatic hydrocarbons,** accidental (**unintentional**)
Toxic effects of other halogen derivatives of aliphatic hydrocarbons NOS

√7ᵗʰ **T53.6X2** **Toxic effect of other halogen derivatives of aliphatic hydrocarbons,** intentional self-harm

√7ᵗʰ **T53.6X3** **Toxic effect of other halogen derivatives of aliphatic hydrocarbons,** assault

√7ᵗʰ **T53.6X4** **Toxic effect of other halogen derivatives of aliphatic hydrocarbons,** undetermined

√5ᵗʰ **T53.7** **Toxic effects of other halogen derivatives of aromatic hydrocarbons**

√6ᵗʰ **T53.7X** **Toxic effects of** other halogen derivatives of aromatic hydrocarbons

√7ᵗʰ **T53.7X1** **Toxic effect of other halogen derivatives of aromatic hydrocarbons,** accidental (**unintentional**)
Toxic effects of other halogen derivatives of aromatic hydrocarbons NOS

√7ᵗʰ **T53.7X2** **Toxic effect of other halogen derivatives of aromatic hydrocarbons,** intentional self-harm

√7ᵗʰ **T53.7X3** **Toxic effect of other halogen derivatives of aromatic hydrocarbons,** assault

√7ᵗʰ **T53.7X4** **Toxic effect of other halogen derivatives of aromatic hydrocarbons,** undetermined

√5ᵗʰ **T53.9** **Toxic effects of unspecified halogen derivatives of aliphatic and aromatic hydrocarbons**

√x7ᵗʰ **T53.91** **Toxic effect of unspecified halogen derivatives of aliphatic and aromatic hydrocarbons,** accidental (**unintentional**)

√x7ᵗʰ **T53.92** **Toxic effect of unspecified halogen derivatives of aliphatic and aromatic hydrocarbons,** intentional self-harm

√x7ᵗʰ **T53.93** **Toxic effect of unspecified halogen derivatives of aliphatic and aromatic hydrocarbons,** assault

√x7ᵗʰ **T53.94** **Toxic effect of unspecified halogen derivatives of aliphatic and aromatic hydrocarbons,** undetermined

√4ᵗʰ **T54** **Toxic effect of corrosive substances**

> The appropriate 7th character is to be added to each code from category T54.
> A initial encounter
> D subsequent encounter
> S sequela

√5ᵗʰ **T54.0** **Toxic effects of phenol and phenol homologues**

√6ᵗʰ **T54.0X** **Toxic effects of** phenol and phenol homologues

√7ᵗʰ **T54.0X1** **Toxic effect of phenol and phenol homologues,** accidental (**unintentional**)
Toxic effects of phenol and phenol homologues NOS

√7ᵗʰ **T54.0X2** **Toxic effect of phenol and phenol homologues,** intentional self-harm

√7ᵗʰ **T54.0X3** **Toxic effect of phenol and phenol homologues,** assault

√7ᵗʰ **T54.0X4** **Toxic effect of phenol and phenol homologues,** undetermined

√5ᵗʰ **T54.1** **Toxic effects of other corrosive organic compounds**

√6ᵗʰ **T54.1X** **Toxic effects of other corrosive organic compounds**

√7ᵗʰ **T54.1X1** **Toxic effect of other corrosive organic compounds,** accidental (**unintentional**)
Toxic effects of other corrosive organic compounds NOS

√7ᵗʰ **T54.1X2** **Toxic effect of other corrosive organic compounds,** intentional self-harm

√7ᵗʰ **T54.1X3** **Toxic effect of other corrosive organic compounds,** assault

√7ᵗʰ **T54.1X4** **Toxic effect of other corrosive organic compounds,** undetermined

√5ᵗʰ **T54.2** **Toxic effects of corrosive acids and acid-like substances**
Toxic effects of hydrochloric acid
Toxic effects of sulfuric acid

√6ᵗʰ **T54.2X** **Toxic effects of** corrosive acids and acid-like substances

√7ᵗʰ **T54.2X1** **Toxic effect of corrosive acids and acid-like substances,** accidental (**unintentional**)
Toxic effects of corrosive acids and acid-like substances NOS

√7ᵗʰ **T54.2X2** **Toxic effect of corrosive acids and acid-like substances,** intentional self-harm

√7ᵗʰ **T54.2X3** **Toxic effect of corrosive acids and acid-like substances,** assault

√7ᵗʰ **T54.2X4** **Toxic effect of corrosive acids and acid-like substances,** undetermined

√5ᵗʰ **T54.3** **Toxic effects of corrosive alkalis and alkali-like substances**
Toxic effects of potassium hydroxide
Toxic effects of sodium hydroxide

√6ᵗʰ **T54.3X** **Toxic effects of** corrosive alkalis and alkali-like substances

√7ᵗʰ **T54.3X1** **Toxic effect of corrosive alkalis and alkali-like substances,** accidental (**unintentional**)
Toxic effects of corrosive alkalis and alkali-like substances NOS

√7ᵗʰ **T54.3X2** **Toxic effect of corrosive alkalis and alkali-like substances,** intentional self-harm

√7ᵗʰ **T54.3X3** **Toxic effect of corrosive alkalis and alkali-like substances,** assault

√7ᵗʰ **T54.3X4** **Toxic effect of corrosive alkalis and alkali-like substances,** undetermined

√5ᵗʰ **T54.9** **Toxic effects of unspecified corrosive substance**

√x7ᵗʰ **T54.91** **Toxic effect of unspecified corrosive substance,** accidental (**unintentional**)

√x7ᵗʰ **T54.92** **Toxic effect of unspecified corrosive substance,** intentional self-harm

√x7ᵗʰ **T54.93** **Toxic effect of unspecified corrosive substance,** assault

√x7ᵗʰ **T54.94** **Toxic effect of unspecified corrosive substance,** undetermined

Ⓝ Newborn: 0   Ⓟ Pediatric: 0-17   Ⓜ Maternity: 12-55   Ⓐ Adult: 15-124   CH Comorbidity High   CL Comorbidity Low   NCDx Noncancer Dx   PDx Primary Dx

1108

ICD-10-CM 2020

✓4ᵗʰ **T55 Toxic effect of soaps and detergents**

> The appropriate 7th character is to be added to each code from category T55.
> A   initial encounter
> D   subsequent encounter
> S   sequela

  ✓5ᵗʰ **T55.0 Toxic effect of soaps**

    ✓6ᵗʰ **T55.0X Toxic effect of soaps**

      ✓7ᵗʰ **T55.0X1 Toxic effect of soaps, accidental (unintentional)**
        Toxic effect of soaps NOS

      ✓7ᵗʰ **T55.0X2 Toxic effect of soaps, intentional self-harm**

      ✓7ᵗʰ **T55.0X3 Toxic effect of soaps, assault**

      ✓7ᵗʰ **T55.0X4 Toxic effect of soaps, undetermined**

  ✓5ᵗʰ **T55.1 Toxic effect of detergents**

    ✓6ᵗʰ **T55.1X Toxic effect of detergents**

      ✓7ᵗʰ **T55.1X1 Toxic effect of detergents, accidental (unintentional)**
        Toxic effect of detergents NOS

      ✓7ᵗʰ **T55.1X2 Toxic effect of detergents, intentional self-harm**

      ✓7ᵗʰ **T55.1X3 Toxic effect of detergents, assault**

      ✓7ᵗʰ **T55.1X4 Toxic effect of detergents, undetermined**

✓4ᵗʰ **T56 Toxic effect of metals**

> INCLUDES   toxic effects of fumes and vapors of metals
>   toxic effects of metals from all sources, except medicinal substances

Use additional code to identify any retained metal foreign body, if applicable (Z18.0-, T18.1-)

> EXCLUDES 1   arsenic and its compounds (T57.0)
>   manganese and its compounds (T57.2)

> The appropriate 7th character is to be added to each code from category T56.
> A   initial encounter
> D   subsequent encounter
> S   sequela

  ✓5ᵗʰ **T56.0 Toxic effects of lead and its compounds**

    ✓6ᵗʰ **T56.0X Toxic effects of lead and its compounds**

      ✓7ᵗʰ **T56.0X1 Toxic effect of lead and its compounds, accidental (unintentional)**
        Toxic effects of lead and its compounds NOS

      ✓7ᵗʰ **T56.0X2 Toxic effect of lead and its compounds, intentional self-harm**

      ✓7ᵗʰ **T56.0X3 Toxic effect of lead and its compounds, assault**

      ✓7ᵗʰ **T56.0X4 Toxic effect of lead and its compounds, undetermined**

  ✓5ᵗʰ **T56.1 Toxic effects of mercury and its compounds**

    ✓6ᵗʰ **T56.1X Toxic effects of mercury and its compounds**

      ✓7ᵗʰ **T56.1X1 Toxic effect of mercury and its compounds, accidental (unintentional)**
        Toxic effects of mercury and its compounds NOS

      ✓7ᵗʰ **T56.1X2 Toxic effect of mercury and its compounds, intentional self-harm**

      ✓7ᵗʰ **T56.1X3 Toxic effect of mercury and its compounds, assault**

      ✓7ᵗʰ **T56.1X4 Toxic effect of mercury and its compounds, undetermined**

  ✓5ᵗʰ **T56.2 Toxic effects of chromium and its compounds**

    ✓6ᵗʰ **T56.2X Toxic effects of chromium and its compounds**

      ✓7ᵗʰ **T56.2X1 Toxic effect of chromium and its compounds, accidental (unintentional)**
        Toxic effects of chromium and its compounds NOS

      ✓7ᵗʰ **T56.2X2 Toxic effect of chromium and its compounds, intentional self-harm**

      ✓7ᵗʰ **T56.2X3 Toxic effect of chromium and its compounds, assault**

      ✓7ᵗʰ **T56.2X4 Toxic effect of chromium and its compounds, undetermined**

  ✓5ᵗʰ **T56.3 Toxic effects of cadmium and its compounds**

    ✓6ᵗʰ **T56.3X Toxic effects of cadmium and its compounds**

      ✓7ᵗʰ **T56.3X1 Toxic effects of cadmium and its compounds, accidental (unintentional)**
        Toxic effects of cadmium and its compounds NOS

      ✓7ᵗʰ **T56.3X2 Toxic effects of cadmium and its compounds, intentional self-harm**

      ✓7ᵗʰ **T56.3X3 Toxic effects of cadmium and its compounds, assault**

      ✓7ᵗʰ **T56.3X4 Toxic effects of cadmium and its compounds, undetermined**

  ✓5ᵗʰ **T56.4 Toxic effects of copper and its compounds**

    ✓6ᵗʰ **T56.4X Toxic effects of copper and its compounds**

      ✓7ᵗʰ **T56.4X1 Toxic effect of copper and its compounds, accidental (unintentional)**
        Toxic effects of copper and its compounds NOS

      ✓7ᵗʰ **T56.4X2 Toxic effect of copper and its compounds, intentional self-harm**

      ✓7ᵗʰ **T56.4X3 Toxic effect of copper and its compounds, assault**

      ✓7ᵗʰ **T56.4X4 Toxic effect of copper and its compounds, undetermined**

  ✓5ᵗʰ **T56.5 Toxic effects of zinc and its compounds**

    ✓6ᵗʰ **T56.5X Toxic effects of zinc and its compounds**

      ✓7ᵗʰ **T56.5X1 Toxic effect of zinc and its compounds, accidental (unintentional)**
        Toxic effect of zinc and its compounds NOS

      ✓7ᵗʰ **T56.5X2 Toxic effect of zinc and its compounds, intentional self-harm**

      ✓7ᵗʰ **T56.5X3 Toxic effect of zinc and its compounds, assault**

      ✓7ᵗʰ **T56.5X4 Toxic effect of zinc and its compounds, undetermined**

  ✓5ᵗʰ **T56.6 Toxic effects of tin and its compounds**

    ✓6ᵗʰ **T56.6X Toxic effects of tin and its compounds**

      ✓7ᵗʰ **T56.6X1 Toxic effect of tin and its compounds, accidental (unintentional)**
        Toxic effects of tin and its compounds NOS

      ✓7ᵗʰ **T56.6X2 Toxic effect of tin and its compounds, intentional self-harm**

      ✓7ᵗʰ **T56.6X3 Toxic effect of tin and its compounds, assault**

      ✓7ᵗʰ **T56.6X4 Toxic effect of tin and its compounds, undetermined**

  ✓5ᵗʰ **T56.7 Toxic effects of beryllium and its compounds**

    ✓6ᵗʰ **T56.7X Toxic effects of beryllium and its compounds**

      ✓7ᵗʰ **T56.7X1 Toxic effect of beryllium and its compounds, accidental (unintentional)**
        Toxic effects of beryllium and its compounds NOS

      ✓7ᵗʰ **T56.7X2 Toxic effect of beryllium and its compounds, intentional self-harm**

      ✓7ᵗʰ **T56.7X3 Toxic effect of beryllium and its compounds, assault**

      ✓7ᵗʰ **T56.7X4 Toxic effect of beryllium and its compounds, undetermined**

  ✓5ᵗʰ **T56.8 Toxic effects of other metals**

    ✓6ᵗʰ **T56.81 Toxic effect of thallium**

      ✓7ᵗʰ **T56.811 Toxic effect of thallium, accidental (unintentional)**
        Toxic effect of thallium NOS

      ✓7ᵗʰ **T56.812 Toxic effect of thallium, intentional self-harm**

      ✓7ᵗʰ **T56.813 Toxic effect of thallium, assault**

      ✓7ᵗʰ **T56.814 Toxic effect of thallium, undetermined**

    ✓6ᵗʰ **T56.89 Toxic effects of other metals**

      ✓7ᵗʰ **T56.891 Toxic effects of other metals, accidental (unintentional)**
        Toxic effects of other metals NOS

      ✓7ᵗʰ **T56.892 Toxic effects of other metals, intentional self-harm**

      ✓7ᵗʰ **T56.893 Toxic effects of other metals, assault**

      ✓7ᵗʰ **T56.894 Toxic effect of other metals, undetermined**

✓ Additional Character Required   ✓ˣ⁷ᵗʰ Placeholder Alert   Manifestation   Unspecified Dx   ▶◀ Revised Text   ● New Code   ▲ Revised Title

ICD-10-CM 2020   1109

Chapter 19. Injury, Poisoning and Certain Other Consequences of External Causes

√5ᵗʰ **T56.9 Toxic effects of unspecified metal**

√x7ᵗʰ **T56.91** Toxic effect of unspecified metal, accidental (unintentional)

√x7ᵗʰ **T56.92** Toxic effect of unspecified metal, intentional self-harm

√x7ᵗʰ **T56.93** Toxic effect of unspecified metal, assault

√x7ᵗʰ **T56.94** Toxic effect of unspecified metal, undetermined

√4ᵗʰ **T57 Toxic effect of other inorganic substances**

The appropriate 7th character is to be added to each code from category T57.
A initial encounter
D subsequent encounter
S sequela

√5ᵗʰ **T57.0 Toxic effect of arsenic and its compounds**

√6ᵗʰ **T57.0X** Toxic effect of arsenic and its compounds

√7ᵗʰ **T57.0X1** Toxic effect of arsenic and its compounds, accidental (unintentional)
Toxic effect of arsenic and its compounds NOS

√7ᵗʰ **T57.0X2** Toxic effect of arsenic and its compounds, intentional self-harm

√7ᵗʰ **T57.0X3** Toxic effect of arsenic and its compounds, assault

√7ᵗʰ **T57.0X4** Toxic effect of arsenic and its compounds, undetermined

√5ᵗʰ **T57.1 Toxic effect of phosphorus and its compounds**

EXCLUDES 1 organophosphate insecticides (T60.0)

√6ᵗʰ **T57.1X** Toxic effect of phosphorus and its compounds

√7ᵗʰ **T57.1X1** Toxic effect of phosphorus and its compounds, accidental (unintentional)
Toxic effect of phosphorus and its compounds NOS

√7ᵗʰ **T57.1X2** Toxic effect of phosphorus and its compounds, intentional self-harm

√7ᵗʰ **T57.1X3** Toxic effect of phosphorus and its compounds, assault

√7ᵗʰ **T57.1X4** Toxic effect of phosphorus and its compounds, undetermined

√5ᵗʰ **T57.2 Toxic effect of manganese and its compounds**

√6ᵗʰ **T57.2X** Toxic effect of manganese and its compounds

√7ᵗʰ **T57.2X1** Toxic effect of manganese and its compounds, accidental (unintentional)
Toxic effect of manganese and its compounds NOS

√7ᵗʰ **T57.2X2** Toxic effect of manganese and its compounds, intentional self-harm

√7ᵗʰ **T57.2X3** Toxic effect of manganese and its compounds, assault

√7ᵗʰ **T57.2X4** Toxic effect of manganese and its compounds, undetermined

√5ᵗʰ **T57.3 Toxic effect of hydrogen cyanide**

√6ᵗʰ **T57.3X** Toxic effect of hydrogen cyanide

√7ᵗʰ **T57.3X1** Toxic effect of hydrogen cyanide, accidental (unintentional)
Toxic effect of hydrogen cyanide NOS

√7ᵗʰ **T57.3X2** Toxic effect of hydrogen cyanide, intentional self-harm

√7ᵗʰ **T57.3X3** Toxic effect of hydrogen cyanide, assault

√7ᵗʰ **T57.3X4** Toxic effect of hydrogen cyanide, undetermined

√5ᵗʰ **T57.8 Toxic effect of other specified inorganic substances**

√6ᵗʰ **T57.8X** Toxic effect of other specified inorganic substances

√7ᵗʰ **T57.8X1** Toxic effect of other specified inorganic substances, accidental (unintentional)
Toxic effect of other specified inorganic substances NOS

√7ᵗʰ **T57.8X2** Toxic effect of other specified inorganic substances, intentional self-harm

√7ᵗʰ **T57.8X3** Toxic effect of other specified inorganic substances, assault

√7ᵗʰ **T57.8X4** Toxic effect of other specified inorganic substances, undetermined

√5ᵗʰ **T57.9 Toxic effect of unspecified inorganic substance**

√x7ᵗʰ **T57.91** Toxic effect of unspecified inorganic substance, accidental (unintentional)

√x7ᵗʰ **T57.92** Toxic effect of unspecified inorganic substance, intentional self-harm

√x7ᵗʰ **T57.93** Toxic effect of unspecified inorganic substance, assault

√x7ᵗʰ **T57.94** Toxic effect of unspecified inorganic substance, undetermined

√4ᵗʰ **T58 Toxic effect of carbon monoxide**

INCLUDES asphyxiation from carbon monoxide
toxic effect of carbon monoxide from all sources

The appropriate 7th character is to be added to each code from category T58.
A initial encounter
D subsequent encounter
S sequela

√5ᵗʰ **T58.0 Toxic effect of carbon monoxide from motor vehicle exhaust**

Toxic effect of exhaust gas from gas engine
Toxic effect of exhaust gas from motor pump

√x7ᵗʰ **T58.01** Toxic effect of carbon monoxide from motor vehicle exhaust, accidental (unintentional)

√x7ᵗʰ **T58.02** Toxic effect of carbon monoxide from motor vehicle exhaust, intentional self-harm

√x7ᵗʰ **T58.03** Toxic effect of carbon monoxide from motor vehicle exhaust, assault

√x7ᵗʰ **T58.04** Toxic effect of carbon monoxide from motor vehicle exhaust, undetermined

√5ᵗʰ **T58.1 Toxic effect of carbon monoxide from utility gas**

Toxic effect of acetylene
Toxic effect of gas NOS used for lighting, heating, cooking
Toxic effect of water gas

√x7ᵗʰ **T58.11** Toxic effect of carbon monoxide from utility gas, accidental (unintentional)

√x7ᵗʰ **T58.12** Toxic effect of carbon monoxide from utility gas, intentional self-harm

√x7ᵗʰ **T58.13** Toxic effect of carbon monoxide from utility gas, assault

√x7ᵗʰ **T58.14** Toxic effect of carbon monoxide from utility gas, undetermined

√5ᵗʰ **T58.2 Toxic effect of carbon monoxide from incomplete combustion of other domestic fuels**

Toxic effect of carbon monoxide from incomplete combustion of coal, coke, kerosene, wood

√6ᵗʰ **T58.2X** Toxic effect of carbon monoxide from incomplete combustion of other domestic fuels

√7ᵗʰ **T58.2X1** Toxic effect of carbon monoxide from incomplete combustion of other domestic fuels, accidental (unintentional)

√7ᵗʰ **T58.2X2** Toxic effect of carbon monoxide from incomplete combustion of other domestic fuels, intentional self-harm

√7ᵗʰ **T58.2X3** Toxic effect of carbon monoxide from incomplete combustion of other domestic fuels, assault

√7ᵗʰ **T58.2X4** Toxic effect of carbon monoxide from incomplete combustion of other domestic fuels, undetermined

√5ᵗʰ **T58.8 Toxic effect of carbon monoxide from other source**

Toxic effect of carbon monoxide from blast furnace gas
Toxic effect of carbon monoxide from fuels in industrial use
Toxic effect of carbon monoxide from kiln vapor

√6ᵗʰ **T58.8X** Toxic effect of carbon monoxide from other source

√7ᵗʰ **T58.8X1** Toxic effect of carbon monoxide from other source, accidental (unintentional)

√7ᵗʰ **T58.8X2** Toxic effect of carbon monoxide from other source, intentional self-harm

√7ᵗʰ **T58.8X3** Toxic effect of carbon monoxide from other source, assault

√7ᵗʰ **T58.8X4** Toxic effect of carbon monoxide from other source, undetermined

√5ᵗʰ **T58.9 Toxic effect of carbon monoxide from unspecified source**

√x7ᵗʰ **T58.91** Toxic effect of carbon monoxide from unspecified source, accidental (unintentional)

√x7ᵗʰ **T58.92** Toxic effect of carbon monoxide from unspecified source, intentional self-harm

√x7ᵗʰ **T58.93** Toxic effect of carbon monoxide from unspecified source, assault

√x7ᵗʰ **T58.94** Toxic effect of carbon monoxide from unspecified source, undetermined

✓4ᵗʰ **T59 Toxic effect of other gases, fumes and vapors**

> INCLUDES   aerosol propellants
> EXCLUDES 1   *chlorofluorocarbons (T53.5)*

> The appropriate 7th character is to be added to each code from category T59.
> A   initial encounter
> D   subsequent encounter
> S   sequela

✓5ᵗʰ **T59.0 Toxic effect of nitrogen oxides**

   ✓6ᵗʰ **T59.0X Toxic effect of** nitrogen oxides

     ✓7ᵗʰ **T59.0X1 Toxic effect of nitrogen oxides,** accidental (unintentional)
       Toxic effect of nitrogen oxides NOS

     ✓7ᵗʰ **T59.0X2 Toxic effect of nitrogen oxides,** intentional self-harm

     ✓7ᵗʰ **T59.0X3 Toxic effect of nitrogen oxides,** assault

     ✓7ᵗʰ **T59.0X4 Toxic effect of nitrogen oxides,** undetermined

✓5ᵗʰ **T59.1 Toxic effect of sulfur dioxide**

   ✓6ᵗʰ **T59.1X Toxic effect of** sulfur dioxide

     ✓7ᵗʰ **T59.1X1 Toxic effect of sulfur dioxide,** accidental (unintentional)
       Toxic effect of sulfur dioxide NOS

     ✓7ᵗʰ **T59.1X2 Toxic effect of sulfur dioxide,** intentional self-harm

     ✓7ᵗʰ **T59.1X3 Toxic effect of sulfur dioxide,** assault

     ✓7ᵗʰ **T59.1X4 Toxic effect of sulfur dioxide,** undetermined

✓5ᵗʰ **T59.2 Toxic effect of formaldehyde**

   ✓6ᵗʰ **T59.2X Toxic effect of** formaldehyde

     ✓7ᵗʰ **T59.2X1 Toxic effect of formaldehyde,** accidental (unintentional)
       Toxic effect of formaldehyde NOS

     ✓7ᵗʰ **T59.2X2 Toxic effect of formaldehyde,** intentional self-harm

     ✓7ᵗʰ **T59.2X3 Toxic effect of formaldehyde,** assault

     ✓7ᵗʰ **T59.2X4 Toxic effect of formaldehyde,** undetermined

✓5ᵗʰ **T59.3 Toxic effect of lacrimogenic gas**

   Toxic effect of tear gas

   ✓6ᵗʰ **T59.3X Toxic effect of** lacrimogenic gas

     ✓7ᵗʰ **T59.3X1 Toxic effect of lacrimogenic gas,** accidental (unintentional)
       Toxic effect of lacrimogenic gas NOS

     ✓7ᵗʰ **T59.3X2 Toxic effect of lacrimogenic gas,** intentional self-harm

     ✓7ᵗʰ **T59.3X3 Toxic effect of lacrimogenic gas,** assault

     ✓7ᵗʰ **T59.3X4 Toxic effect of lacrimogenic gas,** undetermined

✓5ᵗʰ **T59.4 Toxic effect of chlorine gas**

   ✓6ᵗʰ **T59.4X Toxic effect of** chlorine gas

     ✓7ᵗʰ **T59.4X1 Toxic effect of chlorine gas,** accidental (unintentional)
       Toxic effect of chlorine gas NOS

     ✓7ᵗʰ **T59.4X2 Toxic effect of chlorine gas,** intentional self-harm

     ✓7ᵗʰ **T59.4X3 Toxic effect of chlorine gas,** assault

     ✓7ᵗʰ **T59.4X4 Toxic effect of chlorine gas,** undetermined

✓5ᵗʰ **T59.5 Toxic effect of fluorine gas and hydrogen fluoride**

   ✓6ᵗʰ **T59.5X Toxic effect of** fluorine gas and hydrogen fluoride

     ✓7ᵗʰ **T59.5X1 Toxic effect of fluorine gas and hydrogen fluoride,** accidental (unintentional)
       Toxic effect of fluorine gas and hydrogen fluoride NOS

     ✓7ᵗʰ **T59.5X2 Toxic effect of fluorine gas and hydrogen fluoride,** intentional self-harm

     ✓7ᵗʰ **T59.5X3 Toxic effect of fluorine gas and hydrogen fluoride,** assault

     ✓7ᵗʰ **T59.5X4 Toxic effect of fluorine gas and hydrogen fluoride,** undetermined

✓5ᵗʰ **T59.6 Toxic effect of hydrogen sulfide**

   ✓6ᵗʰ **T59.6X Toxic effect of** hydrogen sulfide

     ✓7ᵗʰ **T59.6X1 Toxic effect of hydrogen sulfide,** accidental (unintentional)
       Toxic effect of hydrogen sulfide NOS

     ✓7ᵗʰ **T59.6X2 Toxic effect of hydrogen sulfide,** intentional self-harm

     ✓7ᵗʰ **T59.6X3 Toxic effect of hydrogen sulfide,** assault

     ✓7ᵗʰ **T59.6X4 Toxic effect of hydrogen sulfide,** undetermined

✓5ᵗʰ **T59.7 Toxic effect of carbon dioxide**

   ✓6ᵗʰ **T59.7X Toxic effect of** carbon dioxide

     ✓7ᵗʰ **T59.7X1 Toxic effect of carbon dioxide,** accidental (unintentional)
       Toxic effect of carbon dioxide NOS

     ✓7ᵗʰ **T59.7X2 Toxic effect of carbon dioxide,** intentional self-harm

     ✓7ᵗʰ **T59.7X3 Toxic effect of carbon dioxide,** assault

     ✓7ᵗʰ **T59.7X4 Toxic effect of carbon dioxide,** undetermined

✓5ᵗʰ **T59.8 Toxic effect of other specified gases, fumes and vapors**

   ✓6ᵗʰ **T59.81 Toxic effect of** smoke

     Smoke inhalation
     EXCLUDES 2   *toxic effect of cigarette (tobacco) smoke (T65.22-)*

     ✓7ᵗʰ **T59.811 Toxic effect of smoke,** accidental (unintentional)
       Toxic effect of smoke NOS
       AHA: 2013,4Q,121

     ✓7ᵗʰ **T59.812 Toxic effect of smoke,** intentional self-harm

     ✓7ᵗʰ **T59.813 Toxic effect of smoke,** assault

     ✓7ᵗʰ **T59.814 Toxic effect of smoke,** undetermined

   ✓6ᵗʰ **T59.89 Toxic effect of other specified gases, fumes and vapors**

     ✓7ᵗʰ **T59.891 Toxic effect of other specified gases, fumes and vapors,** accidental (unintentional)

     ✓7ᵗʰ **T59.892 Toxic effect of other specified gases, fumes and vapors,** intentional self-harm

     ✓7ᵗʰ **T59.893 Toxic effect of other specified gases, fumes and vapors,** assault

     ✓7ᵗʰ **T59.894 Toxic effect of other specified gases, fumes and vapors,** undetermined

✓5ᵗʰ **T59.9 Toxic effect of unspecified gases, fumes and vapors**

   ✓x7ᵗʰ **T59.91 Toxic effect of unspecified gases, fumes and vapors,** accidental (unintentional)

   ✓x7ᵗʰ **T59.92 Toxic effect of unspecified gases, fumes and vapors,** intentional self-harm

   ✓x7ᵗʰ **T59.93 Toxic effect of unspecified gases, fumes and vapors,** assault

   ✓x7ᵗʰ **T59.94 Toxic effect of unspecified gases, fumes and vapors,** undetermined

✓4ᵗʰ **T60 Toxic effect of pesticides**

> INCLUDES   toxic effect of wood preservatives

> The appropriate 7th character is to be added to each code from category T60.
> A   initial encounter
> D   subsequent encounter
> S   sequela

✓5ᵗʰ **T60.0 Toxic effect of organophosphate and carbamate insecticides**

   ✓6ᵗʰ **T60.0X Toxic effect of** organophosphate and carbamate insecticides

     ✓7ᵗʰ **T60.0X1 Toxic effect of organophosphate and carbamate insecticides,** accidental (unintentional)
       Toxic effect of organophosphate and carbamate insecticides NOS

     ✓7ᵗʰ **T60.0X2 Toxic effect of organophosphate and carbamate insecticides,** intentional self-harm

     ✓7ᵗʰ **T60.0X3 Toxic effect of organophosphate and carbamate insecticides,** assault

     ✓7ᵗʰ **T60.0X4 Toxic effect of organophosphate and carbamate insecticides,** undetermined

✔ Additional Character Required   ✓x7ᵗʰ Placeholder Alert   Manifestation   Unspecified Dx   ►◄ Revised Text   ● New Code   ▲ Revised Title

ICD-10-CM 2020   **1111**

Chapter 19. Injury, Poisoning and Certain Other Consequences of External Causes

✓5ᵗʰ **T60.1 Toxic effect of halogenated insecticides**
    EXCLUDES 1   *chlorinated hydrocarbon (T53.-)*
  ✓6ᵗʰ **T60.1X Toxic effect of** halogenated insecticides
    ✓7ᵗʰ **T60.1X1 Toxic effect of halogenated insecticides, accidental (unintentional)**
      Toxic effect of halogenated insecticides NOS
    ✓7ᵗʰ **T60.1X2 Toxic effect of halogenated insecticides, intentional self-harm**
    ✓7ᵗʰ **T60.1X3 Toxic effect of halogenated insecticides, assault**
    ✓7ᵗʰ **T60.1X4 Toxic effect of halogenated insecticides, undetermined**

✓5ᵗʰ **T60.2 Toxic effect of other insecticides**
  ✓6ᵗʰ **T60.2X Toxic effect of** other insecticides
    ✓7ᵗʰ **T60.2X1 Toxic effect of other insecticides, accidental (unintentional)**
      Toxic effect of other insecticides NOS
    ✓7ᵗʰ **T60.2X2 Toxic effect of other insecticides, intentional self-harm**
    ✓7ᵗʰ **T60.2X3 Toxic effect of other insecticides, assault**
    ✓7ᵗʰ **T60.2X4 Toxic effect of other insecticides, undetermined**

✓5ᵗʰ **T60.3 Toxic effect of herbicides and fungicides**
  ✓6ᵗʰ **T60.3X Toxic effect of** herbicides and fungicides
    ✓7ᵗʰ **T60.3X1 Toxic effect of herbicides and fungicides, accidental (unintentional)**
      Toxic effect of herbicides and fungicides NOS
    ✓7ᵗʰ **T60.3X2 Toxic effect of herbicides and fungicides, intentional self-harm**
    ✓7ᵗʰ **T60.3X3 Toxic effect of herbicides and fungicides, assault**
    ✓7ᵗʰ **T60.3X4 Toxic effect of herbicides and fungicides, undetermined**

✓5ᵗʰ **T60.4 Toxic effect of rodenticides**
    EXCLUDES 1   *strychnine and its salts (T65.1)*
          thallium (T56.81-)
  ✓6ᵗʰ **T60.4X Toxic effect of** rodenticides
    ✓7ᵗʰ **T60.4X1 Toxic effect of rodenticides, accidental (unintentional)**
      Toxic effect of rodenticides NOS
    ✓7ᵗʰ **T60.4X2 Toxic effect of rodenticides, intentional self-harm**
    ✓7ᵗʰ **T60.4X3 Toxic effect of rodenticides, assault**
    ✓7ᵗʰ **T60.4X4 Toxic effect of rodenticides, undetermined**

✓5ᵗʰ **T60.8 Toxic effect of other pesticides**
  ✓6ᵗʰ **T60.8X Toxic effect of other pesticides**
    ✓7ᵗʰ **T60.8X1 Toxic effect of other pesticides, accidental (unintentional)**
      Toxic effect of other pesticides NOS
    ✓7ᵗʰ **T60.8X2 Toxic effect of other pesticides, intentional self-harm**
    ✓7ᵗʰ **T60.8X3 Toxic effect of other pesticides, assault**
    ✓7ᵗʰ **T60.8X4 Toxic effect of other pesticides, undetermined**

✓5ᵗʰ **T60.9 Toxic effect of unspecified pesticide**
  ✓x7ᵗʰ **T60.91 Toxic effect of unspecified pesticide, accidental (unintentional)**
  ✓x7ᵗʰ **T60.92 Toxic effect of unspecified pesticide, intentional self-harm**
  ✓x7ᵗʰ **T60.93 Toxic effect of unspecified pesticide, assault**
  ✓x7ᵗʰ **T60.94 Toxic effect of unspecified pesticide, undetermined**

✓4ᵗʰ **T61 Toxic effect of noxious substances eaten as seafood**
    EXCLUDES 1   *allergic reaction to food, such as:*
        anaphylactic reaction or shock due to adverse food reaction (T78.0-)
        bacterial foodborne intoxications (A05.-)
        dermatitis (L23.6, L25.4, L27.2)
        food protein-induced enterocolitis syndrome (K52.21)
        food protein-induced enteropathy (K52.22)
        gastroenteritis (noninfective) (K52.29)
      toxic effect of aflatoxin and other mycotoxins (T64)
      toxic effect of cyanides (T65.0-)
      toxic effect of harmful algae bloom (T65.82-)
      toxic effect of hydrogen cyanide (T57.3-)
      toxic effect of mercury (T56.1-)
      toxic effect of red tide (T65.82-)

> The appropriate 7th character is to be added to each code from category T61.
> A   initial encounter
> D   subsequent encounter
> S   sequela

✓5ᵗʰ **T61.0 Ciguatera fish poisoning**
  ✓x7ᵗʰ **T61.01 Ciguatera fish poisoning, accidental (unintentional)**
  ✓x7ᵗʰ **T61.02 Ciguatera fish poisoning, intentional self-harm**
  ✓x7ᵗʰ **T61.03 Ciguatera fish poisoning, assault**
  ✓x7ᵗʰ **T61.04 Ciguatera fish poisoning, undetermined**

✓5ᵗʰ **T61.1 Scombroid fish poisoning**
    Histamine-like syndrome
  ✓x7ᵗʰ **T61.11 Scombroid fish poisoning, accidental (unintentional)**
  ✓x7ᵗʰ **T61.12 Scombroid fish poisoning, intentional self-harm**
  ✓x7ᵗʰ **T61.13 Scombroid fish poisoning, assault**
  ✓x7ᵗʰ **T61.14 Scombroid fish poisoning, undetermined**

✓5ᵗʰ **T61.7 Other fish and shellfish poisoning**
  ✓6ᵗʰ **T61.77 Other fish poisoning**
    ✓7ᵗʰ **T61.771 Other fish poisoning, accidental (unintentional)**
    ✓7ᵗʰ **T61.772 Other fish poisoning, intentional self-harm**
    ✓7ᵗʰ **T61.773 Other fish poisoning, assault**
    ✓7ᵗʰ **T61.774 Other fish poisoning, undetermined**
  ✓6ᵗʰ **T61.78 Other shellfish poisoning**
    ✓7ᵗʰ **T61.781 Other shellfish poisoning, accidental (unintentional)**
    ✓7ᵗʰ **T61.782 Other shellfish poisoning, intentional self-harm**
    ✓7ᵗʰ **T61.783 Other shellfish poisoning, assault**
    ✓7ᵗʰ **T61.784 Other shellfish poisoning, undetermined**

✓5ᵗʰ **T61.8 Toxic effect of other seafood**
  ✓6ᵗʰ **T61.8X Toxic effect of other seafood**
    ✓7ᵗʰ **T61.8X1 Toxic effect of other seafood, accidental (unintentional)**
    ✓7ᵗʰ **T61.8X2 Toxic effect of other seafood, intentional self-harm**
    ✓7ᵗʰ **T61.8X3 Toxic effect of other seafood, assault**
    ✓7ᵗʰ **T61.8X4 Toxic effect of other seafood, undetermined**

✓5ᵗʰ **T61.9 Toxic effect of unspecified seafood**
  ✓x7ᵗʰ **T61.91 Toxic effect of unspecified seafood, accidental (unintentional)**
  ✓x7ᵗʰ **T61.92 Toxic effect of unspecified seafood, intentional self-harm**
  ✓x7ᵗʰ **T61.93 Toxic effect of unspecified seafood, assault**
  ✓x7ᵗʰ **T61.94 Toxic effect of unspecified seafood, undetermined**

☑4ᵗʰ **T62 Toxic effect of other noxious substances eaten as food**

     EXCLUDES 1   *allergic reaction to food, such as:*
         anaphylactic shock (reaction) due to adverse food reaction
         (T78.0-)
         bacterial food borne intoxications (A05.-)
         dermatitis (L23.6, L25.4, L27.2)
         food protein-induced enterocolitis syndrome (K52.21)
         food protein-induced enteropathy (K52.22)
         gastroenteritis (noninfective) (K52.29)
         toxic effect of aflatoxin and other mycotoxins (T64)
         toxic effect of cyanides (T65.0-)
         toxic effect of hydrogen cyanide (T57.3-)
         toxic effect of mercury (T56.1-)

     The appropriate 7th character is to be added to each code from category T62.
     A   initial encounter
     D   subsequent encounter
     S   sequela

☑5ᵗʰ **T62.0 Toxic effect of ingested mushrooms**

    ☑6ᵗʰ **T62.0X Toxic effect of** ingested mushrooms
       ☑7ᵗʰ **T62.0X1 Toxic effect of ingested mushrooms, accidental (unintentional)**
          Toxic effect of ingested mushrooms NOS
       ☑7ᵗʰ **T62.0X2 Toxic effect of ingested mushrooms, intentional self-harm**
       ☑7ᵗʰ **T62.0X3 Toxic effect of ingested mushrooms, assault**
       ☑7ᵗʰ **T62.0X4 Toxic effect of ingested mushrooms, undetermined**

☑5ᵗʰ **T62.1 Toxic effect of ingested berries**

    ☑6ᵗʰ **T62.1X Toxic effect of** ingested berries
       ☑7ᵗʰ **T62.1X1 Toxic effect of ingested berries, accidental (unintentional)**
          Toxic effect of ingested berries NOS
       ☑7ᵗʰ **T62.1X2 Toxic effect of ingested berries, intentional self-harm**
       ☑7ᵗʰ **T62.1X3 Toxic effect of ingested berries,** assault
       ☑7ᵗʰ **T62.1X4 Toxic effect of ingested berries, undetermined**

☑5ᵗʰ **T62.2 Toxic effect of other ingested (parts of) plant(s)**

    ☑6ᵗʰ **T62.2X Toxic effect of** other ingested **(parts of)** plant(s)
       ☑7ᵗʰ **T62.2X1 Toxic effect of other ingested (parts of) plant(s), accidental (unintentional)**
          Toxic effect of other ingested (parts of) plant(s) NOS
       ☑7ᵗʰ **T62.2X2 Toxic effect of other ingested (parts of) plant(s),** intentional self-harm
       ☑7ᵗʰ **T62.2X3 Toxic effect of other ingested (parts of) plant(s),** assault
       ☑7ᵗʰ **T62.2X4 Toxic effect of other ingested (parts of) plant(s),** undetermined

☑5ᵗʰ **T62.8 Toxic effect of other specified noxious substances eaten as food**

    ☑6ᵗʰ **T62.8X Toxic effect of other specified noxious substances eaten as food**
       ☑7ᵗʰ **T62.8X1 Toxic effect of other specified noxious substances eaten as food,** accidental **(unintentional)**
          Toxic effect of other specified noxious substances eaten as food NOS
       ☑7ᵗʰ **T62.8X2 Toxic effect of other specified noxious substances eaten as food,** intentional self-harm
       ☑7ᵗʰ **T62.8X3 Toxic effect of other specified noxious substances eaten as food,** assault
       ☑7ᵗʰ **T62.8X4 Toxic effect of other specified noxious substances eaten as food,** undetermined

☑5ᵗʰ **T62.9 Toxic effect of unspecified noxious substance eaten as food**

    ☑x7ᵗʰ **T62.91 Toxic effect of unspecified noxious substance eaten as food,** accidental **(unintentional)**
          Toxic effect of unspecified noxious substance eaten as food NOS
    ☑x7ᵗʰ **T62.92 Toxic effect of unspecified noxious substance eaten as food,** intentional self-harm
    ☑x7ᵗʰ **T62.93 Toxic effect of unspecified noxious substance eaten as food,** assault
    ☑x7ᵗʰ **T62.94 Toxic effect of unspecified noxious substance eaten as food,** undetermined

☑4ᵗʰ **T63 Toxic effect of contact with venomous animals and plants**

     INCLUDES   bite or touch of venomous animal
         pricked or stuck by thorn or leaf
     EXCLUDES 2   *ingestion of toxic animal or plant (T61.-, T62.-)*

     The appropriate 7th character is to be added to each code from category T63.
     A   initial encounter
     D   subsequent encounter
     S   sequela

☑5ᵗʰ **T63.0 Toxic effect of** snake venom

    ☑6ᵗʰ **T63.00 Toxic effect of** unspecified snake venom
       ☑7ᵗʰ **T63.001 Toxic effect of unspecified snake venom, accidental (unintentional)**
          Toxic effect of unspecified snake venom NOS
       ☑7ᵗʰ **T63.002 Toxic effect of unspecified snake venom, intentional self-harm**
       ☑7ᵗʰ **T63.003 Toxic effect of unspecified snake venom, assault**
       ☑7ᵗʰ **T63.004 Toxic effect of unspecified snake venom, undetermined**

    ☑6ᵗʰ **T63.01 Toxic effect of** rattlesnake **venom**
       ☑7ᵗʰ **T63.011 Toxic effect of rattlesnake venom, accidental (unintentional)**
          Toxic effect of rattlesnake venom NOS
       ☑7ᵗʰ **T63.012 Toxic effect of rattlesnake venom, intentional self-harm**
       ☑7ᵗʰ **T63.013 Toxic effect of rattlesnake venom,** assault
       ☑7ᵗʰ **T63.014 Toxic effect of rattlesnake venom, undetermined**

    ☑6ᵗʰ **T63.02 Toxic effect of** coral snake **venom**
       ☑7ᵗʰ **T63.021 Toxic effect of coral snake venom, accidental (unintentional)**
          Toxic effect of coral snake venom NOS
       ☑7ᵗʰ **T63.022 Toxic effect of coral snake venom, intentional self-harm**
       ☑7ᵗʰ **T63.023 Toxic effect of coral snake venom,** assault
       ☑7ᵗʰ **T63.024 Toxic effect of coral snake venom, undetermined**

    ☑6ᵗʰ **T63.03 Toxic effect of** taipan **venom**
       ☑7ᵗʰ **T63.031 Toxic effect of taipan venom,** accidental **(unintentional)**
          Toxic effect of taipan venom NOS
       ☑7ᵗʰ **T63.032 Toxic effect of taipan venom,** intentional self-harm
       ☑7ᵗʰ **T63.033 Toxic effect of taipan venom,** assault
       ☑7ᵗʰ **T63.034 Toxic effect of taipan venom, undetermined**

    ☑6ᵗʰ **T63.04 Toxic effect of** cobra **venom**
       ☑7ᵗʰ **T63.041 Toxic effect of cobra venom,** accidental **(unintentional)**
          Toxic effect of cobra venom NOS
       ☑7ᵗʰ **T63.042 Toxic effect of cobra venom,** intentional self-harm
       ☑7ᵗʰ **T63.043 Toxic effect of cobra venom,** assault
       ☑7ᵗʰ **T63.044 Toxic effect of cobra venom, undetermined**

    ☑6ᵗʰ **T63.06 Toxic effect of venom of** other North and South American snake
       ☑7ᵗʰ **T63.061 Toxic effect of venom of other North and South American snake,** accidental **(unintentional)**
          Toxic effect of venom of other North and South American snake NOS
       ☑7ᵗʰ **T63.062 Toxic effect of venom of other North and South American snake,** intentional self-harm
       ☑7ᵗʰ **T63.063 Toxic effect of venom of other North and South American snake,** assault
       ☑7ᵗʰ **T63.064 Toxic effect of venom of other North and South American snake,** undetermined

    ☑6ᵗʰ **T63.07 Toxic effect of venom of** other Australian snake
       ☑7ᵗʰ **T63.071 Toxic effect of venom of other Australian snake,** accidental **(unintentional)**
          Toxic effect of venom of other Australian snake NOS
       ☑7ᵗʰ **T63.072 Toxic effect of venom of other Australian snake,** intentional self-harm

√7ᵗʰ **T63.073 Toxic effect of venom of other Australian snake,** assault

√7ᵗʰ **T63.074 Toxic effect of venom of other Australian snake,** undetermined

√6ᵗʰ **T63.08 Toxic effect of venom of** other African and Asian snake

√7ᵗʰ **T63.081 Toxic effect of venom of other African and Asian snake,** accidental **(unintentional)**
　　Toxic effect of venom of other African and Asian snake NOS

√7ᵗʰ **T63.082 Toxic effect of venom of other African and Asian snake,** intentional self-harm

√7ᵗʰ **T63.083 Toxic effect of venom of other African and Asian snake,** assault

√7ᵗʰ **T63.084 Toxic effect of venom of other African and Asian snake,** undetermined

√6ᵗʰ **T63.09 Toxic effect of venom of** other snake

√7ᵗʰ **T63.091 Toxic effect of venom of other snake,** accidental **(unintentional)**
　　Toxic effect of venom of other snake NOS

√7ᵗʰ **T63.092 Toxic effect of venom of other snake,** intentional self-harm

√7ᵗʰ **T63.093 Toxic effect of venom of other snake,** assault

√7ᵗʰ **T63.094 Toxic effect of venom of other snake,** undetermined

√5ᵗʰ **T63.1 Toxic effect of venom of other reptiles**

√6ᵗʰ **T63.11 Toxic effect of venom of** gila monster

√7ᵗʰ **T63.111 Toxic effect of venom of gila monster,** accidental **(unintentional)**
　　Toxic effect of venom of gila monster NOS

√7ᵗʰ **T63.112 Toxic effect of venom of gila monster,** intentional self-harm

√7ᵗʰ **T63.113 Toxic effect of venom of gila monster,** assault

√7ᵗʰ **T63.114 Toxic effect of venom of gila monster,** undetermined

√6ᵗʰ **T63.12 Toxic effect of venom of other venomous lizard**

√7ᵗʰ **T63.121 Toxic effect of venom of other venomous lizard,** accidental **(unintentional)**
　　Toxic effect of venom of other venomous lizard NOS

√7ᵗʰ **T63.122 Toxic effect of venom of other venomous lizard,** intentional self-harm

√7ᵗʰ **T63.123 Toxic effect of venom of other venomous lizard,** assault

√7ᵗʰ **T63.124 Toxic effect of venom of other venomous lizard,** undetermined

√6ᵗʰ **T63.19 Toxic effect of venom of other reptiles**

√7ᵗʰ **T63.191 Toxic effect of venom of other reptiles,** accidental **(unintentional)**
　　Toxic effect of venom of other reptiles NOS

√7ᵗʰ **T63.192 Toxic effect of venom of other reptiles,** intentional self-harm

√7ᵗʰ **T63.193 Toxic effect of venom of other reptiles,** assault

√7ᵗʰ **T63.194 Toxic effect of venom of other reptiles,** undetermined

√5ᵗʰ **T63.2 Toxic effect of venom of scorpion**

√6ᵗʰ **T63.2X Toxic effect of** venom of scorpion

√7ᵗʰ **T63.2X1 Toxic effect of venom of scorpion,** accidental **(unintentional)**
　　Toxic effect of venom of scorpion NOS

√7ᵗʰ **T63.2X2 Toxic effect of venom of scorpion,** intentional self-harm

√7ᵗʰ **T63.2X3 Toxic effect of venom of scorpion,** assault

√7ᵗʰ **T63.2X4 Toxic effect of venom of scorpion,** undetermined

√5ᵗʰ **T63.3 Toxic effect of** venom of spider

√6ᵗʰ **T63.30 Toxic effect of unspecified spider venom**

√7ᵗʰ **T63.301 Toxic effect of unspecified spider venom,** accidental **(unintentional)**

√7ᵗʰ **T63.302 Toxic effect of unspecified spider venom,** intentional self-harm

√7ᵗʰ **T63.303 Toxic effect of unspecified spider venom,** assault

√7ᵗʰ **T63.304 Toxic effect of unspecified spider venom,** undetermined

√6ᵗʰ **T63.31 Toxic effect of venom of** black widow **spider**

√7ᵗʰ **T63.311 Toxic effect of venom of black widow spider,** accidental **(unintentional)**

√7ᵗʰ **T63.312 Toxic effect of venom of black widow spider,** intentional self-harm

√7ᵗʰ **T63.313 Toxic effect of venom of black widow spider,** assault

√7ᵗʰ **T63.314 Toxic effect of venom of black widow spider,** undetermined

√6ᵗʰ **T63.32 Toxic effect of venom of** tarantula

√7ᵗʰ **T63.321 Toxic effect of venom of tarantula,** accidental **(unintentional)**

√7ᵗʰ **T63.322 Toxic effect of venom of tarantula,** intentional self-harm

√7ᵗʰ **T63.323 Toxic effect of venom of tarantula,** assault

√7ᵗʰ **T63.324 Toxic effect of venom of tarantula,** undetermined

√6ᵗʰ **T63.33 Toxic effect of venom of** brown recluse **spider**

√7ᵗʰ **T63.331 Toxic effect of venom of brown recluse spider,** accidental **(unintentional)**

√7ᵗʰ **T63.332 Toxic effect of venom of brown recluse spider,** intentional self-harm

√7ᵗʰ **T63.333 Toxic effect of venom of brown recluse spider,** assault

√7ᵗʰ **T63.334 Toxic effect of venom of brown recluse spider,** undetermined

√6ᵗʰ **T63.39 Toxic effect of venom of other spider**

√7ᵗʰ **T63.391 Toxic effect of venom of other spider,** accidental **(unintentional)**

√7ᵗʰ **T63.392 Toxic effect of venom of other spider,** intentional self-harm

√7ᵗʰ **T63.393 Toxic effect of venom of other spider,** assault

√7ᵗʰ **T63.394 Toxic effect of venom of other spider,** undetermined

√5ᵗʰ **T63.4 Toxic effect of venom of other arthropods**

√6ᵗʰ **T63.41 Toxic effect of venom of** centipedes and venomous millipedes

√7ᵗʰ **T63.411 Toxic effect of venom of centipedes and venomous millipedes,** accidental **(unintentional)**

√7ᵗʰ **T63.412 Toxic effect of venom of centipedes and venomous millipedes,** intentional self-harm

√7ᵗʰ **T63.413 Toxic effect of venom of centipedes and venomous millipedes,** assault

√7ᵗʰ **T63.414 Toxic effect of venom of centipedes and venomous millipedes,** undetermined

√6ᵗʰ **T63.42 Toxic effect of venom of** ants

√7ᵗʰ **T63.421 Toxic effect of venom of ants,** accidental **(unintentional)**

√7ᵗʰ **T63.422 Toxic effect of venom of ants,** intentional self-harm

√7ᵗʰ **T63.423 Toxic effect of venom of ants,** assault

√7ᵗʰ **T63.424 Toxic effect of venom of ants,** undetermined

√6ᵗʰ **T63.43 Toxic effect of venom of** caterpillars

√7ᵗʰ **T63.431 Toxic effect of venom of caterpillars,** accidental **(unintentional)**

√7ᵗʰ **T63.432 Toxic effect of venom of caterpillars,** intentional self-harm

√7ᵗʰ **T63.433 Toxic effect of venom of caterpillars,** assault

√7ᵗʰ **T63.434 Toxic effect of venom of caterpillars,** undetermined

√6ᵗʰ **T63.44 Toxic effect of venom of** bees

√7ᵗʰ **T63.441 Toxic effect of venom of bees,** accidental **(unintentional)**

√7ᵗʰ **T63.442 Toxic effect of venom of bees,** intentional self-harm

√7ᵗʰ **T63.443 Toxic effect of venom of bees,** assault

√7ᵗʰ **T63.444 Toxic effect of venom of bees,** undetermined

√6ᵗʰ **T63.45 Toxic effect of venom of** hornets

√7ᵗʰ **T63.451 Toxic effect of venom of hornets,** accidental **(unintentional)**

√7ᵗʰ **T63.452 Toxic effect of venom of hornets,** intentional self-harm

√7ᵗʰ **T63.453 Toxic effect of venom of hornets,** assault

√7ᵗʰ **T63.454** Toxic effect of venom of hornets, undetermined

√6ᵗʰ **T63.46** **Toxic effect of venom of** wasps
Toxic effect of yellow jacket

√7ᵗʰ **T63.461** Toxic effect of venom of wasps, accidental (unintentional)

√7ᵗʰ **T63.462** Toxic effect of venom of wasps, intentional self-harm

√7ᵗʰ **T63.463** Toxic effect of venom of wasps, assault

√7ᵗʰ **T63.464** Toxic effect of venom of wasps, undetermined

√6ᵗʰ **T63.48** **Toxic effect of venom of other arthropod**

√7ᵗʰ **T63.481** Toxic effect of venom of other arthropod, accidental (unintentional)

√7ᵗʰ **T63.482** Toxic effect of venom of other arthropod, intentional self-harm

√7ᵗʰ **T63.483** Toxic effect of venom of other arthropod, assault

√7ᵗʰ **T63.484** Toxic effect of venom of other arthropod, undetermined

√5ᵗʰ **T63.5** **Toxic effect of contact with** venomous fish

EXCLUDES 2   *poisoning by ingestion of fish (T61.-)*

√6ᵗʰ **T63.51** **Toxic effect of contact with** stingray

√7ᵗʰ **T63.511** Toxic effect of contact with stingray, accidental (unintentional)

√7ᵗʰ **T63.512** Toxic effect of contact with stingray, intentional self-harm

√7ᵗʰ **T63.513** Toxic effect of contact with stingray, assault

√7ᵗʰ **T63.514** Toxic effect of contact with stingray, undetermined

√6ᵗʰ **T63.59** **Toxic effect of contact with other venomous fish**

√7ᵗʰ **T63.591** Toxic effect of contact with other venomous fish, accidental (unintentional)

√7ᵗʰ **T63.592** Toxic effect of contact with other venomous fish, intentional self-harm

√7ᵗʰ **T63.593** Toxic effect of contact with other venomous fish, assault

√7ᵗʰ **T63.594** Toxic effect of contact with other venomous fish, undetermined

√5ᵗʰ **T63.6** **Toxic effect of contact with other** venomous marine animals

EXCLUDES 1   *sea-snake venom (T63.09)*

EXCLUDES 2   *poisoning by ingestion of shellfish (T61.78-)*

√6ᵗʰ **T63.61** **Toxic effect of contact with** Portugese Man-o-war
Toxic effect of contact with bluebottle

√7ᵗʰ **T63.611** Toxic effect of contact with Portugese Man-o-war, accidental (unintentional)

√7ᵗʰ **T63.612** Toxic effect of contact with Portugese Man-o-war, intentional self-harm

√7ᵗʰ **T63.613** Toxic effect of contact with Portugese Man-o-war, assault

√7ᵗʰ **T63.614** Toxic effect of contact with Portugese Man-o-war, undetermined

√6ᵗʰ **T63.62** **Toxic effect of contact with other jellyfish**

√7ᵗʰ **T63.621** Toxic effect of contact with other jellyfish, accidental (unintentional)

√7ᵗʰ **T63.622** Toxic effect of contact with other jellyfish, intentional self-harm

√7ᵗʰ **T63.623** Toxic effect of contact with other jellyfish, assault

√7ᵗʰ **T63.624** Toxic effect of contact with other jellyfish, undetermined

√6ᵗʰ **T63.63** **Toxic effect of contact with** sea anemone

√7ᵗʰ **T63.631** Toxic effect of contact with sea anemone, accidental (unintentional)

√7ᵗʰ **T63.632** Toxic effect of contact with sea anemone, intentional self-harm

√7ᵗʰ **T63.633** Toxic effect of contact with sea anemone, assault

√7ᵗʰ **T63.634** Toxic effect of contact with sea anemone, undetermined

√6ᵗʰ **T63.69** **Toxic effect of contact with other venomous marine animals**

√7ᵗʰ **T63.691** Toxic effect of contact with other venomous marine animals, accidental (unintentional)

√7ᵗʰ **T63.692** Toxic effect of contact with other venomous marine animals, intentional self harm

√7ᵗʰ **T63.693** Toxic effect of contact with other venomous marine animals, assault

√7ᵗʰ **T63.694** Toxic effect of contact with other venomous marine animals, undetermined

√5ᵗʰ **T63.7** **Toxic effect of contact with** venomous plant

√6ᵗʰ **T63.71** **Toxic effect of contact with venomous** marine plant

√7ᵗʰ **T63.711** Toxic effect of contact with venomous marine plant, accidental (unintentional)

√7ᵗʰ **T63.712** Toxic effect of contact with venomous marine plant, intentional self-harm

√7ᵗʰ **T63.713** Toxic effect of contact with venomous marine plant, assault

√7ᵗʰ **T63.714** Toxic effect of contact with venomous marine plant, undetermined

√6ᵗʰ **T63.79** **Toxic effect of contact with other venomous plant**

√7ᵗʰ **T63.791** Toxic effect of contact with other venomous plant, accidental (unintentional)

√7ᵗʰ **T63.792** Toxic effect of contact with other venomous plant, intentional self-harm

√7ᵗʰ **T63.793** Toxic effect of contact with other venomous plant, assault

√7ᵗʰ **T63.794** Toxic effect of contact with other venomous plant, undetermined

√5ᵗʰ **T63.8** **Toxic effect of contact with other venomous animals**

√6ᵗʰ **T63.81** **Toxic effect of contact with venomous** frog

EXCLUDES 1   *contact with nonvenomous frog (W62.0)*

√7ᵗʰ **T63.811** Toxic effect of contact with venomous frog, accidental (unintentional)

√7ᵗʰ **T63.812** Toxic effect of contact with venomous frog, intentional self-harm

√7ᵗʰ **T63.813** Toxic effect of contact with venomous frog, assault

√7ᵗʰ **T63.814** Toxic effect of contact with venomous frog, undetermined

√6ᵗʰ **T63.82** **Toxic effect of contact with venomous** toad

EXCLUDES 1   *contact with nonvenomous toad (W62.1)*

√7ᵗʰ **T63.821** Toxic effect of contact with venomous toad, accidental (unintentional)

√7ᵗʰ **T63.822** Toxic effect of contact with venomous toad, intentional self-harm

√7ᵗʰ **T63.823** Toxic effect of contact with venomous toad, assault

√7ᵗʰ **T63.824** Toxic effect of contact with venomous toad, undetermined

√6ᵗʰ **T63.83** **Toxic effect of contact with other venomous amphibian**

EXCLUDES 1   *contact with nonvenomous amphibian (W62.9)*

√7ᵗʰ **T63.831** Toxic effect of contact with other venomous amphibian, accidental (unintentional)

√7ᵗʰ **T63.832** Toxic effect of contact with other venomous amphibian, intentional self-harm

√7ᵗʰ **T63.833** Toxic effect of contact with other venomous amphibian, assault

√7ᵗʰ **T63.834** Toxic effect of contact with other venomous amphibian, undetermined

√6ᵗʰ **T63.89** **Toxic effect of contact with other venomous animals**

√7ᵗʰ **T63.891** Toxic effect of contact with other venomous animals, accidental (unintentional)

√7ᵗʰ **T63.892** Toxic effect of contact with other venomous animals, intentional self-harm

√7ᵗʰ **T63.893** Toxic effect of contact with other venomous animals, assault

√7ᵗʰ **T63.894** Toxic effect of contact with other venomous animals, undetermined

√5ᵗʰ **T63.9** **Toxic effect of contact with unspecified venomous animal**

√x7ᵗʰ **T63.91** Toxic effect of contact with unspecified venomous animal, accidental (unintentional)

√x7ᵗʰ **T63.92** Toxic effect of contact with unspecified venomous animal, intentional self-harm

√x7ᵗʰ **T63.93** Toxic effect of contact with unspecified venomous animal, assault

√x7ᵗʰ **T63.94** Toxic effect of contact with unspecified venomous animal, undetermined

Chapter 19. Injury, Poisoning and Certain Other Consequences of External Causes

✔4ᵗʰ **T64** **Toxic effect of aflatoxin and other mycotoxin food contaminants**

> The appropriate 7th character is to be added to each code from category T64.
> A   initial encounter
> D   subsequent encounter
> S   sequela

✔5ᵗʰ **T64.0** **Toxic effect of** aflatoxin

    ✔x7ᵗʰ **T64.01** **Toxic effect of aflatoxin,** accidental (unintentional)

    ✔x7ᵗʰ **T64.02** **Toxic effect of aflatoxin,** intentional self-harm

    ✔x7ᵗʰ **T64.03** **Toxic effect of aflatoxin,** assault

    ✔x7ᵗʰ **T64.04** **Toxic effect of aflatoxin,** undetermined

✔5ᵗʰ **T64.8** **Toxic effect of other mycotoxin food contaminants**

    ✔x7ᵗʰ **T64.81** **Toxic effect of other mycotoxin food contaminants,** accidental (unintentional)

    ✔x7ᵗʰ **T64.82** **Toxic effect of other mycotoxin food contaminants,** intentional self-harm

    ✔x7ᵗʰ **T64.83** **Toxic effect of other mycotoxin food contaminants,** assault

    ✔x7ᵗʰ **T64.84** **Toxic effect of other mycotoxin food contaminants,** undetermined

✔4ᵗʰ **T65** **Toxic effect of other and unspecified substances**

> The appropriate 7th character is to be added to each code from category T65.
> A   initial encounter
> D   subsequent encounter
> S   sequela

✔5ᵗʰ **T65.0** **Toxic effect of cyanides**

     EXCLUDES 1   *hydrogen cyanide (T57.3-)*

    ✔6ᵗʰ **T65.0X** **Toxic effect of** cyanides

        ✔7ᵗʰ **T65.0X1** **Toxic effect of cyanides,** accidental (unintentional)
             Toxic effect of cyanides NOS

        ✔7ᵗʰ **T65.0X2** **Toxic effect of cyanides,** intentional self-harm

        ✔7ᵗʰ **T65.0X3** **Toxic effect of cyanides,** assault

        ✔7ᵗʰ **T65.0X4** **Toxic effect of cyanides,** undetermined

✔5ᵗʰ **T65.1** **Toxic effect of strychnine and its salts**

    ✔6ᵗʰ **T65.1X** **Toxic effect of** strychnine and its salts

        ✔7ᵗʰ **T65.1X1** **Toxic effect of strychnine and its salts,** accidental (unintentional)
             Toxic effect of strychnine and its salts NOS

        ✔7ᵗʰ **T65.1X2** **Toxic effect of strychnine and its salts,** intentional self-harm

        ✔7ᵗʰ **T65.1X3** **Toxic effect of strychnine and its salts,** assault

        ✔7ᵗʰ **T65.1X4** **Toxic effect of strychnine and its salts,** undetermined

✔5ᵗʰ **T65.2** **Toxic effect of tobacco and nicotine**

     EXCLUDES 2   *nicotine dependence (F17.-)*

    ✔6ᵗʰ **T65.21** **Toxic effect of** chewing tobacco

        ✔7ᵗʰ **T65.211** **Toxic effect of chewing tobacco,** accidental (unintentional)
             Toxic effect of chewing tobacco NOS

        ✔7ᵗʰ **T65.212** **Toxic effect of chewing tobacco,** intentional self-harm

        ✔7ᵗʰ **T65.213** **Toxic effect of chewing tobacco,** assault

        ✔7ᵗʰ **T65.214** **Toxic effect of chewing tobacco,** undetermined

    ✔6ᵗʰ **T65.22** **Toxic effect of** tobacco cigarettes

         Toxic effect of tobacco smoke
         Use additional code for exposure to second hand tobacco smoke (Z57.31, Z77.22)

        ✔7ᵗʰ **T65.221** **Toxic effect of tobacco cigarettes,** accidental (unintentional)
             Toxic effect of tobacco cigarettes NOS

        ✔7ᵗʰ **T65.222** **Toxic effect of tobacco cigarettes,** intentional self-harm

        ✔7ᵗʰ **T65.223** **Toxic effect of tobacco cigarettes,** assault

        ✔7ᵗʰ **T65.224** **Toxic effect of tobacco cigarettes,** undetermined

    ✔6ᵗʰ **T65.29** **Toxic effect of other tobacco and nicotine**

        ✔7ᵗʰ **T65.291** **Toxic effect of other tobacco and nicotine,** accidental (unintentional)
             Toxic effect of other tobacco and nicotine NOS

        ✔7ᵗʰ **T65.292** **Toxic effect of other tobacco and nicotine,** intentional self-harm

        ✔7ᵗʰ **T65.293** **Toxic effect of other tobacco and nicotine,** assault

        ✔7ᵗʰ **T65.294** **Toxic effect of other tobacco and nicotine,** undetermined

✔5ᵗʰ **T65.3** **Toxic effect of nitroderivatives and aminoderivatives of benzene and its homologues**

     Toxic effect of anilin [benzenamine]
     Toxic effect of nitrobenzene
     Toxic effect of trinitrotoluene

    ✔6ᵗʰ **T65.3X** **Toxic effect of** nitroderivatives and aminoderivatives of benzene and its homologues

        ✔7ᵗʰ **T65.3X1** **Toxic effect of nitroderivatives and aminoderivatives of benzene and its homologues,** accidental (unintentional)
             Toxic effect of nitroderivatives and aminoderivatives of benzene and its homologues NOS

        ✔7ᵗʰ **T65.3X2** **Toxic effect of nitroderivatives and aminoderivatives of benzene and its homologues,** intentional self-harm

        ✔7ᵗʰ **T65.3X3** **Toxic effect of nitroderivatives and aminoderivatives of benzene and its homologues,** assault

        ✔7ᵗʰ **T65.3X4** **Toxic effect of nitroderivatives and aminoderivatives of benzene and its homologues,** undetermined

✔5ᵗʰ **T65.4** **Toxic effect of carbon disulfide**

    ✔6ᵗʰ **T65.4X** **Toxic effect of** carbon disulfide

        ✔7ᵗʰ **T65.4X1** **Toxic effect of carbon disulfide,** accidental (unintentional)
             Toxic effect of carbon disulfide NOS

        ✔7ᵗʰ **T65.4X2** **Toxic effect of carbon disulfide,** intentional self-harm

        ✔7ᵗʰ **T65.4X3** **Toxic effect of carbon disulfide,** assault

        ✔7ᵗʰ **T65.4X4** **Toxic effect of carbon disulfide,** undetermined

✔5ᵗʰ **T65.5** **Toxic effect of nitroglycerin and other nitric acids and esters**

     Toxic effect of 1,2,3-Propanetriol trinitrate

    ✔6ᵗʰ **T65.5X** **Toxic effect of** nitroglycerin and other nitric acids and esters

        ✔7ᵗʰ **T65.5X1** **Toxic effect of nitroglycerin and other nitric acids and esters,** accidental (unintentional)
             Toxic effect of nitroglycerin and other nitric acids and esters NOS

        ✔7ᵗʰ **T65.5X2** **Toxic effect of nitroglycerin and other nitric acids and esters,** intentional self-harm

        ✔7ᵗʰ **T65.5X3** **Toxic effect of nitroglycerin and other nitric acids and esters,** assault

        ✔7ᵗʰ **T65.5X4** **Toxic effect of nitroglycerin and other nitric acids and esters,** undetermined

✔5ᵗʰ **T65.6** **Toxic effect of paints and dyes, not elsewhere classified**

    ✔6ᵗʰ **T65.6X** **Toxic effect of** paints and dyes, **not elsewhere classified**

        ✔7ᵗʰ **T65.6X1** **Toxic effect of paints and dyes, not elsewhere classified,** accidental (unintentional)
             Toxic effect of paints and dyes NOS

        ✔7ᵗʰ **T65.6X2** **Toxic effect of paints and dyes, not elsewhere classified,** intentional self-harm

        ✔7ᵗʰ **T65.6X3** **Toxic effect of paints and dyes, not elsewhere classified,** assault

        ✔7ᵗʰ **T65.6X4** **Toxic effect of paints and dyes, not elsewhere classified,** undetermined

✔5ᵗʰ **T65.8** **Toxic effect of other specified substances**

    ✔6ᵗʰ **T65.81** **Toxic effect of** latex

        ✔7ᵗʰ **T65.811** **Toxic effect of latex,** accidental (unintentional)
             Toxic effect of latex NOS

        ✔7ᵗʰ **T65.812** **Toxic effect of latex,** intentional self-harm

        ✔7ᵗʰ **T65.813** **Toxic effect of latex,** assault

Ⓝ Newborn: 0   Ⓟ Pediatric: 0-17   Ⓜ Maternity: 12-55   Ⓐ Adult: 15-124   CH Comorbidity High   CL Comorbidity Low   NCDx Noncancer Dx   PDx Primary Dx

1116   ICD-10-CM 2020

✓7th **T65.814** **Toxic effect of latex,** undetermined

✓6th **T65.82** **Toxic effect of harmful** algae and algae toxins

    Toxic effect of (harmful) algae bloom NOS
    Toxic effect of blue-green algae bloom
    Toxic effect of brown tide
    Toxic effect of cyanobacteria bloom
    Toxic effect of Florida red tide
    Toxic effect of pfiesteria piscicida
    Toxic effect of red tide

    ✓7th **T65.821** **Toxic effect of harmful algae and algae toxins,** accidental **(unintentional)**
        Toxic effect of harmful algae and algae toxins NOS

    ✓7th **T65.822** **Toxic effect of harmful algae and algae toxins,** intentional self-harm

    ✓7th **T65.823** **Toxic effect of harmful algae and algae toxins,** assault

    ✓7th **T65.824** **Toxic effect of harmful algae and algae toxins,** undetermined

✓6th **T65.83** **Toxic effect of** fiberglass

    ✓7th **T65.831** **Toxic effect of fiberglass,** accidental **(unintentional)**
        Toxic effect of fiberglass NOS

    ✓7th **T65.832** **Toxic effect of fiberglass,** intentional self-harm

    ✓7th **T65.833** **Toxic effect of fiberglass,** assault

    ✓7th **T65.834** **Toxic effect of fiberglass,** undetermined

✓6th **T65.89** **Toxic effect of other specified substances**

    ✓7th **T65.891** **Toxic effect of other specified substances,** accidental **(unintentional)**
        Toxic effect of other specified substances NOS
        AHA: 2018,1Q,5

    ✓7th **T65.892** **Toxic effect of other specified substances,** intentional self-harm

    ✓7th **T65.893** **Toxic effect of other specified substances,** assault

    ✓7th **T65.894** **Toxic effect of other specified substances,** undetermined

✓5th **T65.9** **Toxic effect of unspecified substance**

    ✓x7th **T65.91** **Toxic effect of unspecified substance,** accidental **(unintentional)**
        Poisoning NOS

    ✓x7th **T65.92** **Toxic effect of unspecified substance,** intentional self-harm

    ✓x7th **T65.93** **Toxic effect of unspecified substance,** assault

    ✓x7th **T65.94** **Toxic effect of unspecified substance,** undetermined

Other and unspecified effects of external causes (T66-T78)

✓x7th **T66** **Radiation sickness, unspecified**

    EXCLUDES 1   *specified adverse effects of radiation, such as:*
        burns (T20-T31)
        leukemia (C91-C95)
        radiation gastroenteritis and colitis (K52.0)
        radiation pneumonitis (J70.0)
        radiation related disorders of the skin and subcutaneous tissue (L55-L59)
        radiation sunburn (L55.-)

    The appropriate 7th character is to be added to code T66.
    A initial encounter
    D subsequent encounter
    S sequela

✓4th **T67** **Effects of heat and light**

    EXCLUDES 1   *erythema [dermatitis] ab igne (L59.0)*
        malignant hyperpyrexia due to anesthesia (T88.3)
        radiation-related disorders of the skin and subcutaneous tissue (L55-L59)

    EXCLUDES 2   *burns (T20-T31)*
        sunburn (L55.-)
        sweat disorder due to heat (L74-L75)

    The appropriate 7th character is to be added to each code from category T67.
    A initial encounter
    D subsequent encounter
    S sequela

    ✓5th **T67.0** **Heatstroke and sunstroke**

        ~~Heat apoplexy~~
        ~~Heat pyrexia~~
        ~~Siriasis~~
        ~~Thermoplegia~~
        Use additional code(s) to identify any associated complications of heatstroke, such as:
        coma and stupor (R40.-)
        ▶rhabdomyolysis (M62.82)◀
        systemic inflammatory response syndrome (R65.1-)
        DEF: Headache, vertigo, cramps, and elevated body temperature due to prolonged exposure to high environmental temperatures that requires emergency intervention.

        ✓x7th **T67.01** **Heatstroke and sunstroke**
            Heat apoplexy
            Heat pyrexia
            Siriasis
            Thermoplegia

        ✓x7th **T67.02** **Exertional** heatstroke

        ✓x7th **T67.09** **Other heatstroke and sunstroke**

    ✓x7th **T67.1** **Heat** syncope
        Heat collapse

    ✓x7th **T67.2** **Heat** cramp

    ✓x7th **T67.3** **Heat exhaustion,** anhydrotic
        Heat prostration due to water depletion
        EXCLUDES 1   *heat exhaustion due to salt depletion (T67.4)*

    ✓x7th **T67.4** **Heat exhaustion** due to salt depletion
        Heat prostration due to salt (and water) depletion

    ✓x7th **T67.5** **Heat exhaustion, unspecified**
        Heat prostration NOS

    ✓x7th **T67.6** **Heat** fatigue, transient

    ✓x7th **T67.7** **Heat** edema

    ✓x7th **T67.8** **Other effects of heat and light**

    ✓x7th **T67.9** **Effect of heat and light, unspecified**

✓x7th **T68** **Hypothermia**

    Accidental hypothermia
    Hypothermia NOS
    Use additional code to identify source of exposure:
        exposure to excessive cold of man-made origin (W93)
        exposure to excessive cold of natural origin (X31)
    EXCLUDES 1   *hypothermia following anesthesia (T88.51)*
        hypothermia not associated with low environmental temperature (R68.0)
        hypothermia of newborn (P80.-)

    EXCLUDES 2   *frostbite (T33-T34)*

    The appropriate 7th character is to be added to code T68.
    A initial encounter
    D subsequent encounter
    S sequela

☑ Additional Character Required   ✓x7th Placeholder Alert   Manifestation   Unspecified Dx   ▶◀ Revised Text   ● New Code   ▲ Revised Title

ICD-10-CM 2020   1117

✓4ᵗʰ T69 Other effects of reduced temperature

Use additional code to identify source of exposure:
     exposure to excessive cold of man-made origin (W93)
     exposure to excessive cold of natural origin (X31)

EXCLUDES 2   frostbite (T33-T34)

The appropriate 7th character is to be added to each code from category T69.
A   initial encounter
D   subsequent encounter
S   sequela

✓5ᵗʰ T69.0 Immersion hand and foot

✓6ᵗʰ T69.01 Immersion hand

     ✓7ᵗʰ T69.011 Immersion hand, right hand
     ✓7ᵗʰ T69.012 Immersion hand, left hand
     ✓7ᵗʰ T69.019 Immersion hand, unspecified hand

✓6ᵗʰ T69.02 Immersion foot

Trench foot
     ✓7ᵗʰ T69.021 Immersion foot, right foot
     ✓7ᵗʰ T69.022 Immersion foot, left foot
     ✓7ᵗʰ T69.029 Immersion foot, unspecified foot

✓x7ᵗʰ T69.1 Chilblains

DEF: Red, swollen, itchy skin primarily affecting the fingers and toes, nose and ears, and legs. Chilblains follows damp-cold exposure, and can also be associated with pruritus and a burning feeling.

✓x7ᵗʰ T69.8 Other specified effects of reduced temperature

✓x7ᵗʰ T69.9 Effect of reduced temperature, unspecified

✓4ᵗʰ T70 Effects of air pressure and water pressure

The appropriate 7th character is to be added to each code from category T70.
A   initial encounter
D   subsequent encounter
S   sequela

✓x7ᵗʰ T70.0 Otitic barotrauma

Aero-otitis media
Effects of change in ambient atmospheric pressure or water pressure on ears

✓x7ᵗʰ T70.1 Sinus barotrauma

Aerosinusitis
Effects of change in ambient atmospheric pressure on sinuses

✓5ᵗʰ T70.2 Other and unspecified effects of high altitude

EXCLUDES 2   polycythemia due to high altitude (D75.1)

     ✓x7ᵗʰ T70.20 Unspecified effects of high altitude

     ✓x7ᵗʰ T70.29 Other effects of high altitude
         Alpine sickness
         Anoxia due to high altitude
         Barotrauma NOS
         Hypobaropathy
         Mountain sickness

✓x7ᵗʰ T70.3 Caisson disease [decompression sickness]

Compressed-air disease
Diver's palsy or paralysis
DEF: Rapid reduction in air pressure while breathing compressed air. Symptoms include skin lesions, joint pains, and respiratory and neurological problems.

✓x7ᵗʰ T70.4 Effects of high-pressure fluids

Hydraulic jet injection (industrial)
Pneumatic jet injection (industrial)
Traumatic jet injection (industrial)

✓x7ᵗʰ T70.8 Other effects of air pressure and water pressure

✓x7ᵗʰ T70.9 Effect of air pressure and water pressure, unspecified

✓4ᵗʰ T71 Asphyxiation

Mechanical suffocation
Traumatic suffocation

EXCLUDES 1   acute respiratory distress (syndrome) (J80)
     anoxia due to high altitude (T70.2)
     asphyxia NOS (R09.01)
     asphyxia from carbon monoxide (T58.-)
     asphyxia from inhalation of food or foreign body (T17.-)
     asphyxia from other gases, fumes and vapors (T59.-)
     respiratory distress (syndrome) in newborn (P22.-)

The appropriate 7th character is to be added to each code from category T71.
A   initial encounter
D   subsequent encounter
S   sequela

✓5ᵗʰ T71.1 Asphyxiation due to mechanical threat to breathing

Suffocation due to mechanical threat to breathing

✓6ᵗʰ T71.11 Asphyxiation due to smothering under pillow

     ✓7ᵗʰ T71.111 Asphyxiation due to smothering under pillow, accidental
         Asphyxiation due to smothering under pillow NOS
     ✓7ᵗʰ T71.112 Asphyxiation due to smothering under pillow, intentional self-harm
     ✓7ᵗʰ T71.113 Asphyxiation due to smothering under pillow, assault
     ✓7ᵗʰ T71.114 Asphyxiation due to smothering under pillow, undetermined

✓6ᵗʰ T71.12 Asphyxiation due to plastic bag

     ✓7ᵗʰ T71.121 Asphyxiation due to plastic bag, accidental
         Asphyxiation due to plastic bag NOS
     ✓7ᵗʰ T71.122 Asphyxiation due to plastic bag, intentional self-harm
     ✓7ᵗʰ T71.123 Asphyxiation due to plastic bag, assault
     ✓7ᵗʰ T71.124 Asphyxiation due to plastic bag, undetermined

✓6ᵗʰ T71.13 Asphyxiation due to being trapped in bed linens

     ✓7ᵗʰ T71.131 Asphyxiation due to being trapped in bed linens, accidental
         Asphyxiation due to being trapped in bed linens NOS
     ✓7ᵗʰ T71.132 Asphyxiation due to being trapped in bed linens, intentional self-harm
     ✓7ᵗʰ T71.133 Asphyxiation due to being trapped in bed linens, assault
     ✓7ᵗʰ T71.134 Asphyxiation due to being trapped in bed linens, undetermined

✓6ᵗʰ T71.14 Asphyxiation due to smothering under another person's body (in bed)

     ✓7ᵗʰ T71.141 Asphyxiation due to smothering under another person's body (in bed), accidental
         Asphyxiation due to smothering under another person's body (in bed) NOS
     ✓7ᵗʰ T71.143 Asphyxiation due to smothering under another person's body (in bed), assault
     ✓7ᵗʰ T71.144 Asphyxiation due to smothering under another person's body (in bed), undetermined

✓6ᵗʰ T71.15 Asphyxiation due to smothering in furniture

     ✓7ᵗʰ T71.151 Asphyxiation due to smothering in furniture, accidental
         Asphyxiation due to smothering in furniture NOS
     ✓7ᵗʰ T71.152 Asphyxiation due to smothering in furniture, intentional self-harm
     ✓7ᵗʰ T71.153 Asphyxiation due to smothering in furniture, assault
     ✓7ᵗʰ T71.154 Asphyxiation due to smothering in furniture, undetermined

N Newborn: 0   P Pediatric: 0-17   M Maternity: 12-55   A Adult: 15-124   CH Comorbidity High   CL Comorbidity Low   NCDx Noncancer Dx   PDx Primary Dx

1118   ICD-10-CM 2020

☑6ᵗʰ **T71.16** **Asphyxiation due to** hanging

Hanging by window shade cord
Use additional code for any associated injuries, such as:
  crushing injury of neck (S17.-)
  fracture of cervical vertebrae (S12.0-S12.2-)
  open wound of neck (S11.-)

  ☑7ᵗʰ **T71.161** **Asphyxiation due to hanging,** accidental
    Asphyxiation due to hanging NOS
    Hanging NOS

  ☑7ᵗʰ **T71.162** **Asphyxiation due to hanging,** intentional self-harm

  ☑7ᵗʰ **T71.163** **Asphyxiation due to hanging,** assault

  ☑7ᵗʰ **T71.164** **Asphyxiation due to hanging,** undetermined

☑6ᵗʰ **T71.19** **Asphyxiation due to mechanical threat to breathing due to other causes**

  ☑7ᵗʰ **T71.191** **Asphyxiation due to mechanical threat to breathing due to other causes,** accidental
    Asphyxiation due to other causes NOS

  ☑7ᵗʰ **T71.192** **Asphyxiation due to mechanical threat to breathing due to other causes,** intentional self-harm

  ☑7ᵗʰ **T71.193** **Asphyxiation due to mechanical threat to breathing due to other causes,** assault

  ☑7ᵗʰ **T71.194** **Asphyxiation due to mechanical threat to breathing due to other causes,** undetermined

☑5ᵗʰ **T71.2** **Asphyxiation due to** systemic oxygen deficiency due to low oxygen content in ambient air

Suffocation due to systemic oxygen deficiency due to low oxygen content in ambient air

  ☑x7ᵗʰ **T71.20** **Asphyxiation due to systemic oxygen deficiency due to low oxygen content in ambient air due to unspecified cause**

  ☑x7ᵗʰ **T71.21** **Asphyxiation due to** cave-in or falling earth
    Use additional code for any associated cataclysm (X34-X38)

☑6ᵗʰ **T71.22** **Asphyxiation due to** being trapped in a car trunk

  ☑7ᵗʰ **T71.221** **Asphyxiation due to being trapped in a car trunk,** accidental

  ☑7ᵗʰ **T71.222** **Asphyxiation due to being trapped in a car trunk,** intentional self-harm

  ☑7ᵗʰ **T71.223** **Asphyxiation due to being trapped in a car trunk,** assault

  ☑7ᵗʰ **T71.224** **Asphyxiation due to being trapped in a car trunk,** undetermined

☑6ᵗʰ **T71.23** **Asphyxiation due to being** trapped in a (discarded) refrigerator

  ☑7ᵗʰ **T71.231** **Asphyxiation due to being trapped in a (discarded) refrigerator,** accidental

  ☑7ᵗʰ **T71.232** **Asphyxiation due to being trapped in a (discarded) refrigerator,** intentional self-harm

  ☑7ᵗʰ **T71.233** **Asphyxiation due to being trapped in a (discarded) refrigerator,** assault

  ☑7ᵗʰ **T71.234** **Asphyxiation due to being trapped in a (discarded) refrigerator,** undetermined

  ☑x7ᵗʰ **T71.29** **Asphyxiation due to being trapped in other low oxygen environment**

☑x7ᵗʰ **T71.9** **Asphyxiation due to unspecified cause**

Suffocation (by strangulation) due to unspecified cause
Suffocation NOS
Systemic oxygen deficiency due to low oxygen content in ambient air due to unspecified cause
Systemic oxygen deficiency due to mechanical threat to breathing due to unspecified cause
Traumatic asphyxia NOS

☑4ᵗʰ **T73** **Effects of other deprivation**

The appropriate 7th character is to be added to each code from category T73.
A initial encounter
D subsequent encounter
S sequela

☑x7ᵗʰ **T73.0** **Starvation**
  Deprivation of food

☑x7ᵗʰ **T73.1** **Deprivation of water**

☑x7ᵗʰ **T73.2** **Exhaustion due to exposure**

☑x7ᵗʰ **T73.3** **Exhaustion due to excessive exertion**
  Exhaustion due to overexertion

☑x7ᵗʰ **T73.8** **Other effects of deprivation**

☑x7ᵗʰ **T73.9** **Effect of deprivation, unspecified**

☑4ᵗʰ **T74** **Adult and child abuse, neglect and other maltreatment,** confirmed

Use additional code, if applicable, to identify any associated current injury
Use additional external cause code to identify perpetrator, if known (Y07.-)

EXCLUDES 1   abuse and maltreatment in pregnancy (O9A.3-, O9A.4-, O9A.5-)
        adult and child maltreatment, suspected (T76.-)

The appropriate 7th character is to be added to each code from category T74.
A initial encounter
D subsequent encounter
S sequela

☑5ᵗʰ **T74.0** **Neglect or abandonment, confirmed**

  ☑x7ᵗʰ **T74.01** Adult **neglect or abandonment, confirmed** Ⓐ

  ☑x7ᵗʰ **T74.02** Child **neglect or abandonment, confirmed** Ⓟ

☑5ᵗʰ **T74.1** **Physical abuse, confirmed**

  EXCLUDES 2 sexual abuse (T74.2-)

  ☑x7ᵗʰ **T74.11** Adult **physical abuse, confirmed** Ⓐ

  ☑x7ᵗʰ **T74.12** Child **physical abuse, confirmed** Ⓟ
    EXCLUDES 2 shaken infant syndrome (T74.4)

☑5ᵗʰ **T74.2** **Sexual abuse, confirmed**
  Rape, confirmed
  Sexual assault, confirmed

  ☑x7ᵗʰ **T74.21** Adult **sexual abuse, confirmed** Ⓐ

  ☑x7ᵗʰ **T74.22** Child **sexual abuse, confirmed** Ⓟ

☑5ᵗʰ **T74.3** **Psychological abuse, confirmed**
  Bullying and intimidation, confirmed
  Intimidation through social media, confirmed

  ☑x7ᵗʰ **T74.31** Adult **psychological abuse, confirmed** Ⓐ

  ☑x7ᵗʰ **T74.32** Child **psychological abuse, confirmed** Ⓟ

☑x7ᵗʰ **T74.4** **Shaken infant syndrome** Ⓟ

☑5ᵗʰ **T74.5** **Forced sexual exploitation, confirmed**
  AHA: 2018,4Q,32-33,65

  ☑x7ᵗʰ **T74.51** Adult **forced sexual exploitation, confirmed** Ⓐ

  ☑x7ᵗʰ **T74.52** Child **sexual exploitation, confirmed** Ⓟ

☑5ᵗʰ **T74.6** **Forced labor exploitation, confirmed**
  AHA: 2018,4Q,32-33,65

  ☑x7ᵗʰ **T74.61** Adult **forced labor exploitation, confirmed** Ⓐ

  ☑x7ᵗʰ **T74.62** Child **forced labor exploitation, confirmed** Ⓟ

☑5ᵗʰ **T74.9** **Unspecified maltreatment, confirmed**

  ☑x7ᵗʰ **T74.91** **Unspecified** adult **maltreatment, confirmed** Ⓐ

  ☑x7ᵗʰ **T74.92** **Unspecified** child **maltreatment, confirmed** Ⓟ

☑4ᵗʰ **T75** **Other and unspecified effects of other external causes**

  EXCLUDES 1 adverse effects NEC (T78.-)
  EXCLUDES 2 burns (electric) (T20-T31)

The appropriate 7th character is to be added to each code from category T75.
A initial encounter
D subsequent encounter
S sequela

☑5ᵗʰ **T75.0** **Effects of lightning**
  Struck by lightning

  ☑x7ᵗʰ **T75.00** **Unspecified effects of lightning**
    Struck by lightning NOS

  ☑x7ᵗʰ **T75.01** **Shock due to being struck by lightning**

  ☑x7ᵗʰ **T75.09** **Other effects of lightning**
    Use additional code for other effects of lightning

☑ Additional Character Required   ☑x7ᵗʰ Placeholder Alert   Manifestation   Unspecified Dx   ▶◀ Revised Text   ● New Code   ▲ Revised Title

ICD-10-CM 2020   1119

Chapter 19. Injury, Poisoning and Certain Other Consequences of External Causes

√x7ᵗʰ **T75.1** **Unspecified effects of drowning and nonfatal submersion**
Immersion
EXCLUDES 1   *specified effects of drowning — code to effects*

√5ᵗʰ **T75.2** **Effects of vibration**

√x7ᵗʰ **T75.20** **Unspecified effects of vibration**

√x7ᵗʰ **T75.21** **Pneumatic hammer syndrome**

√x7ᵗʰ **T75.22** **Traumatic vasospastic syndrome**

√x7ᵗʰ **T75.23** **Vertigo from infrasound**
EXCLUDES 1   *vertigo NOS (R42)*

√x7ᵗʰ **T75.29** **Other effects of vibration**

√x7ᵗʰ **T75.3** **Motion sickness**
Airsickness
Seasickness
Travel sickness
Use additional external cause code to identify vehicle or type of motion (Y92.81-, Y93.5-)

√x7ᵗʰ **T75.4** **Electrocution**
Shock from electric current
Shock from electroshock gun (taser)

√5ᵗʰ **T75.8** **Other specified effects of external causes**

√x7ᵗʰ **T75.81** **Effects of abnormal gravitation [G] forces**

√x7ᵗʰ **T75.82** **Effects of weightlessness**

√x7ᵗʰ **T75.89** **Other specified effects of external causes**

√4ᵗʰ **T76** **Adult and child abuse, neglect and other maltreatment,** suspected
Use additional code, if applicable, to identify any associated current injury
EXCLUDES 1   *adult and child maltreatment, confirmed (T74.-)*
suspected abuse and maltreatment in pregnancy (O9A.3-, O9A.4-, O9A.5-)
suspected adult physical abuse, ruled out (Z04.71)
suspected adult sexual abuse, ruled out (Z04.41)
suspected child physical abuse, ruled out (Z04.72)
suspected child sexual abuse, ruled out (Z04.42)
AHA: 2018,4Q,72

The appropriate 7th character is to be added to each code from category T76.
A   initial encounter
D   subsequent encounter
S   sequela

√5ᵗʰ **T76.0** **Neglect or abandonment, suspected**

√x7ᵗʰ **T76.01** **Adult neglect or abandonment, suspected**   A

√x7ᵗʰ **T76.02** **Child neglect or abandonment, suspected**   P

√5ᵗʰ **T76.1** **Physical abuse, suspected**

√x7ᵗʰ **T76.11** **Adult physical abuse, suspected**   A

√x7ᵗʰ **T76.12** **Child physical abuse, suspected**   P
AHA: 2019,2Q,12

√5ᵗʰ **T76.2** **Sexual abuse, suspected**
Rape, suspected
EXCLUDES 1   *alleged abuse, ruled out (Z04.7)*

√x7ᵗʰ **T76.21** **Adult sexual abuse, suspected**   A

√x7ᵗʰ **T76.22** **Child sexual abuse, suspected**   P

√5ᵗʰ **T76.3** **Psychological abuse, suspected**
Bullying and intimidation, suspected
Intimidation through social media, suspected

√x7ᵗʰ **T76.31** **Adult psychological abuse, suspected**   A

√x7ᵗʰ **T76.32** **Child psychological abuse, suspected**   P

√5ᵗʰ **T76.5** **Forced sexual exploitation, suspected**
AHA: 2018,4Q,32-33,65

√x7ᵗʰ **T76.51** **Adult forced sexual exploitation, suspected**   A

√x7ᵗʰ **T76.52** **Child sexual exploitation, suspected**   P

√5ᵗʰ **T76.6** **Forced labor exploitation, suspected**
AHA: 2018,4Q,32-33,65

√x7ᵗʰ **T76.61** **Adult forced labor exploitation, suspected**   A

√x7ᵗʰ **T76.62** **Child forced labor exploitation, suspected**   P

√5ᵗʰ **T76.9** **Unspecified maltreatment, suspected**

√x7ᵗʰ **T76.91** **Unspecified adult maltreatment, suspected**   A

√x7ᵗʰ **T76.92** **Unspecified child maltreatment, suspected**   P

√4ᵗʰ **T78** **Adverse effects, not elsewhere classified**
EXCLUDES 2   *complications of surgical and medical care NEC (T80-T88)*
TIP: Do not assign to indicate previous, resolved allergic reactions or the presence of drug and other allergies; use a code from category Z88 Allergy status to drugs, medicaments and biological substances, to report status only.

The appropriate 7th character is to be added to each code from category T78.
A   initial encounter
D   subsequent encounter
S   sequela

√5ᵗʰ **T78.0** **Anaphylactic reaction due to food**
Anaphylactic reaction due to adverse food reaction
Anaphylactic shock or reaction due to nonpoisonous foods
Anaphylactoid reaction due to food

√x7ᵗʰ **T78.00** **Anaphylactic reaction due to unspecified food**

√x7ᵗʰ **T78.01** **Anaphylactic reaction due to peanuts**

√x7ᵗʰ **T78.02** **Anaphylactic reaction due to shellfish (crustaceans)**

√x7ᵗʰ **T78.03** **Anaphylactic reaction due to other fish**

√x7ᵗʰ **T78.04** **Anaphylactic reaction due to fruits and vegetables**

√x7ᵗʰ **T78.05** **Anaphylactic reaction due to tree nuts and seeds**
EXCLUDES 2   *anaphylactic reaction due to peanuts (T78.01)*

√x7ᵗʰ **T78.06** **Anaphylactic reaction due to food additives**

√x7ᵗʰ **T78.07** **Anaphylactic reaction due to milk and dairy products**

√x7ᵗʰ **T78.08** **Anaphylactic reaction due to eggs**

√x7ᵗʰ **T78.09** **Anaphylactic reaction due to other food products**

√x7ᵗʰ **T78.1** **Other adverse food reactions, not elsewhere classified**
Use additional code to identify the type of reaction, if applicable
EXCLUDES 1   *anaphylactic reaction or shock due to adverse food reaction (T78.0-)*
anaphylactic reaction due to food (T78.0-)
bacterial food borne intoxications (A05.-)
EXCLUDES 2   *allergic and dietetic gastroenteritis and colitis (K52.29)*
allergic rhinitis due to food (J30.5)
dermatitis due to food in contact with skin (L23.6, L24.6, L25.4)
dermatitis due to ingested food (L27.2)
food protein-induced enterocolitis syndrome (K52.21)
food protein-induced enteropathy (K52.22)

√x7ᵗʰ **T78.2** **Anaphylactic shock, unspecified**
Allergic shock
Anaphylactic reaction
Anaphylaxis
EXCLUDES 1   *anaphylactic reaction or shock due to adverse effect of correct medicinal substance properly administered (T88.6)*
anaphylactic reaction or shock due to adverse food reaction (T78.0-)
anaphylactic reaction or shock due to serum (T80.5-)

√x7ᵗʰ **T78.3** **Angioneurotic edema**
Allergic angioedema
Giant urticaria
Quincke's edema
EXCLUDES 1   *serum urticaria (T80.6-)*
urticaria (L50.-)

✓5ᵗʰ **T78.4 Other and unspecified allergy**

     EXCLUDES 1   specified types of allergic reaction such as:
          allergic diarrhea (K52.29)
          allergic gastroenteritis and colitis (K52.29)
          dermatitis (L23-L25, L27.-)
          food protein-induced enterocolitis syndrome
            (K52.21)
          food protein-induced enteropathy (K52.22)
          hay fever (J30.1)

     ✓x7ᵗʰ **T78.40 Allergy, unspecified**
         Allergic reaction NOS
         Hypersensitivity NOS

     ✓x7ᵗʰ **T78.41 Arthus phenomenon**
         Arthus reaction

     ✓x7ᵗʰ **T78.49 Other allergy**

✓x7ᵗʰ **T78.8 Other adverse effects, not elsewhere classified**

Certain early complications of trauma (T79)

✓4ᵗʰ **T79 Certain early complications of trauma, not elsewhere classified**

     EXCLUDES 2   *acute respiratory distress syndrome (J80)*
         complications occurring during or following medical
           procedures (T80-T88)
         complications of surgical and medical care NEC (T80-T88)
         newborn respiratory distress syndrome (P22.0)

The appropriate 7th character is to be added to each code from category T79.
A   initial encounter
D   subsequent encounter
S   sequela

✓x7ᵗʰ **T79.0 Air embolism (traumatic)**

     EXCLUDES 1   *air embolism complicating abortion or ectopic or*
          molar pregnancy (O00-O07, O08.2)
         air embolism complicating pregnancy, childbirth and
          the puerperium (O88.0)
         air embolism following infusion, transfusion, and
          therapeutic injection (T80.0)
         air embolism following procedure NEC (T81.7-)
     DEF: Arterial or venous obstruction due to the introduction of air bubbles into the blood vessels following surgery or trauma.

✓x7ᵗʰ **T79.1 Fat embolism (traumatic)**

     EXCLUDES 1   *fat embolism complicating:*
         abortion or ectopic or molar pregnancy (O00-O07, O08.2)
         pregnancy, childbirth and the puerperium (O88.8)
     DEF: Arterial blockage due to the entrance of fat into the circulatory system after a fracture of the large bones or administration of corticosteroids.

✓x7ᵗʰ **T79.2 Traumatic secondary and recurrent hemorrhage and seroma**

✓x7ᵗʰ **T79.4 Traumatic shock**

     Shock (immediate) (delayed) following injury
     EXCLUDES 1   *anaphylactic shock due to adverse food reaction (T78.0-)*
         anaphylactic shock due to correct medicinal substance properly administered (T88.6)
         anaphylactic shock due to serum (T80.5-)
         anaphylactic shock NOS (T78.2)
         anesthetic shock (T88.2)
         electric shock (T75.4)
         nontraumatic shock NEC (R57.-)
         obstetric shock (O75.1)
         postprocedural shock (T81.1-)
         septic shock (R65.21)
         shock complicating abortion or ectopic or molar pregnancy (O00-O07, O08.3)
         shock due to lightning (T75.01)
         shock NOS (R57.9)

✓x7ᵗʰ **T79.5 Traumatic anuria**
     Crush syndrome
     Renal failure following crushing

✓x7ᵗʰ **T79.6 Traumatic ischemia of muscle**
     Traumatic rhabdomyolysis
     Volkmann's ischemic contracture
     EXCLUDES 2   *anterior tibial syndrome (M76.8)*
         compartment syndrome (traumatic) (T79.A-)
         nontraumatic ischemia of muscle (M62.2-)
     AHA: 2019,2Q,12

✓x7ᵗʰ **T79.7 Traumatic subcutaneous emphysema**
     EXCLUDES 1   *emphysema NOS (J43)*
         emphysema (subcutaneous) resulting from a procedure (T81.82)

✓5ᵗʰ **T79.A Traumatic compartment syndrome**
     EXCLUDES 1   *fibromyalgia (M79.7)*
         nontraumatic compartment syndrome (M79.A-)
         ~~*traumatic ischemic infarction of muscle (T79.6)*~~
     EXCLUDES 2   ►*traumatic ischemic infarction of muscle (T79.6)*◄
     DEF: Compression of nerves and blood vessels within an enclosed muscle space due to previous trauma, which leads to impaired blood flow and muscle and nerve damage.

     ✓x7ᵗʰ **T79.A0 Compartment syndrome, unspecified**
         Compartment syndrome NOS

     ✓6ᵗʰ **T79.A1 Traumatic compartment syndrome of upper extremity**
         Traumatic compartment syndrome of shoulder, arm, forearm, wrist, hand, and fingers
         ✓7ᵗʰ **T79.A11 Traumatic compartment syndrome of right upper extremity**
         ✓7ᵗʰ **T79.A12 Traumatic compartment syndrome of left upper extremity**
         ✓7ᵗʰ **T79.A19 Traumatic compartment syndrome of unspecified upper extremity**

     ✓6ᵗʰ **T79.A2 Traumatic compartment syndrome of lower extremity**
         Traumatic compartment syndrome of hip, buttock, thigh, leg, foot, and toes
         ✓7ᵗʰ **T79.A21 Traumatic compartment syndrome of right lower extremity**
         ✓7ᵗʰ **T79.A22 Traumatic compartment syndrome of left lower extremity**
         ✓7ᵗʰ **T79.A29 Traumatic compartment syndrome of unspecified lower extremity**

     ✓x7ᵗʰ **T79.A3 Traumatic compartment syndrome of abdomen**
     ✓x7ᵗʰ **T79.A9 Traumatic compartment syndrome of other sites**

✓x7ᵗʰ **T79.8 Other early complications of trauma**
✓x7ᵗʰ **T79.9 Unspecified early complication of trauma**

✓ Additional Character Required   ✓x7ᵗʰ Placeholder Alert   Manifestation   Unspecified Dx   ►◄ Revised Text   ● New Code   ▲ Revised Title

ICD-10-CM 2020   1121

Complications of surgical and medical care, not elsewhere classified (T80-T88)

Use additional code for adverse effect, if applicable, to identify drug (T36-T50 with fifth or sixth character 5)

Use additional code(s) to identify the specified condition resulting from the complication

Use additional code to identify devices involved and details of circumstances (Y62-Y82)

EXCLUDES 2   *any encounters with medical care for postprocedural conditions in which no complications are present, such as:*
    artificial opening status (Z93.-)
    closure of external stoma (Z43.-)
    fitting and adjustment of external prosthetic device (Z44.-)
  burns and corrosions from local applications and irradiation (T20-T32)
  complications of surgical procedures during pregnancy, childbirth and the puerperium (O00-O9A)
  mechanical complication of respirator [ventilator] (J95.850)
  poisoning and toxic effects of drugs and chemicals (T36-T65 with fifth or sixth character 1-4 or 6)
  postprocedural fever (R50.82)
  specified complications classified elsewhere, such as:
    cerebrospinal fluid leak from spinal puncture (G97.0)
    colostomy malfunction (K94.0-)
    disorders of fluid and electrolyte imbalance (E86-E87)
    functional disturbances following cardiac surgery (I97.0-I97.1)
    intraoperative and postprocedural complications of specified body systems (D78.-, E36.-, E89.-, G97.3-, G97.4, H59.3-, H59.-, H95.2-, H95.3, I97.4-, J95.6-, J95.7, K91.6-, L76.-, M96.-, N99.-)
    ostomy complications (J95.0-, K94.-, N99.5-)
    postgastric surgery syndromes (K91.1)
    postlaminectomy syndrome NEC (M96.1)
    postmastectomy lymphedema syndrome (I97.2)
    postsurgical blind-loop syndrome (K91.2)
    ventilator associated pneumonia (J95.851)

AHA: 2015,1Q,15

✔4ᵗʰ **T80** **Complications following infusion, transfusion and therapeutic injection**

    INCLUDES   complications following perfusion
    EXCLUDES 2   *bone marrow transplant rejection (T86.01)*
    febrile nonhemolytic transfusion reaction (R50.84)
    fluid overload due to transfusion (E87.71)
    posttransfusion purpura (D69.51)
    transfusion associated circulatory overload (TACO) (E87.71)
    transfusion (red blood cell) associated hemochromatosis (E83.111)
    transfusion related acute lung injury (TRALI) (J95.84)

> The appropriate 7th character is to be added to each code from category T80.
> A   initial encounter
> D   subsequent encounter
> S   sequela

✔x7ᵗʰ **T80.0** **Air embolism** following infusion, transfusion and therapeutic injection

✔x7ᵗʰ **T80.1** **Vascular complications** following infusion, transfusion and therapeutic injection
    Use additional code to identify the vascular complication
    EXCLUDES 2   *extravasation of vesicant agent (T80.81-)*
    infiltration of vesicant agent (T80.81-)
    postprocedural vascular complications (T81.7-)
    vascular complications specified as due to prosthetic devices, implants and grafts (T82.8-, T83.8-, T84.8-, T85.8-)

✔5ᵗʰ **T80.2** **Infections** following infusion, transfusion and therapeutic injection
    Use additional code to identify the specific infection, such as: sepsis (A41.9)
    Use additional code (R65.2-) to identify severe sepsis, if applicable
    EXCLUDES 2   *infections specified as due to prosthetic devices, implants and grafts (T82.6-T82.7, T83.5-T83.6, T84.5-T84.7, T85.7)*
    postprocedural infections (T81.4-)

AHA: 2018,4Q,62

✔6ᵗʰ **T80.21** **Infection** due to central venous catheter

    Infection due to pulmonary artery catheter (Swan-Ganz catheter)

    AHA: 2019,1Q,13-14

    TIP: Provider documentation needs to support that an existing, unresolved infection is directly linked to the central venous catheter.

    TIP: Only centrally placed catheters are captured with this subcategory. Infections resulting from catheters that are not central lines, including those used for hemodialysis, should be coded to T82.7-.

    ✔7ᵗʰ **T80.211** **Bloodstream infection** due to central venous catheter
        Catheter-related bloodstream infection (CRBSI) NOS
        Central line-associated bloodstream infection (CLABSI)
        Bloodstream infection due to Hickman catheter
        Bloodstream infection due to peripherally inserted central catheter (PICC)
        Bloodstream infection due to portacath (port-a-cath)
        Bloodstream infection due to pulmonary artery catheter
        Bloodstream infection due to triple lumen catheter
        Bloodstream infection due to umbilical venous catheter
        AHA: 2019,1Q,13,14; 2018,4Q,89

    ✔7ᵗʰ **T80.212** **Local infection** due to central venous catheter
        Exit or insertion site infection
        Local infection due to Hickman catheter
        Local infection due to peripherally inserted central catheter (PICC)
        Local infection due to portacath (port-a-cath)
        Local infection due to pulmonary artery catheter
        Local infection due to triple lumen catheter
        Local infection due to umbilical venous catheter
        Port or reservoir infection
        Tunnel infection

    ✔7ᵗʰ **T80.218** **Other infection** due to central venous catheter
        Other central line-associated infection
        Other infection due to Hickman catheter
        Other infection due to peripherally inserted central catheter (PICC)
        Other infection due to portacath (port-a-cath)
        Other infection due to pulmonary artery catheter
        Other infection due to triple lumen catheter
        Other infection due to umbilical venous catheter

Ⓝ Newborn: 0   Ⓟ Pediatric: 0-17   Ⓜ Maternity: 12-55   Ⓐ Adult: 15-124   CH Comorbidity High   CL Comorbidity Low   NCDx Noncancer Dx   PDx Primary Dx

1122   ICD-10-CM 2020

✓7ᵗʰ **T80.219 Unspecified infection due to central venous catheter**
Central line-associated infection NOS
Unspecified infection due to Hickman catheter
Unspecified infection due to peripherally inserted central catheter (PICC)
Unspecified infection due to portacath (port-a-cath)
Unspecified infection due to pulmonary artery catheter
Unspecified infection due to triple lumen catheter
Unspecified infection due to umbilical venous catheter

✓x7ᵗʰ **T80.22 Acute infection following transfusion, infusion, or injection of blood and blood products**

✓x7ᵗʰ **T80.29 Infection following other infusion, transfusion and therapeutic injection**

✓5ᵗʰ **T80.3 ABO incompatibility reaction due to transfusion of blood or blood products**
EXCLUDES 1 *minor blood group antigens reactions (Duffy) (E) (K) (Kell) (Kidd) (Lewis) (M) (N) (P) (S) (T80.A-)*

✓x7ᵗʰ **T80.30 ABO incompatibility reaction due to transfusion of blood or blood products, unspecified**
ABO incompatibility blood transfusion NOS
Reaction to ABO incompatibility from transfusion NOS

✓6ᵗʰ **T80.31 ABO incompatibility with hemolytic transfusion reaction**
✓7ᵗʰ **T80.310 ABO incompatibility with acute hemolytic transfusion reaction**
ABO incompatibility with hemolytic transfusion reaction less than 24 hours after transfusion
Acute hemolytic transfusion reaction (AHTR) due to ABO incompatibility

✓7ᵗʰ **T80.311 ABO incompatibility with delayed hemolytic transfusion reaction**
ABO incompatibility with hemolytic transfusion reaction 24 hours or more after transfusion
Delayed hemolytic transfusion reaction (DHTR) due to ABO incompatibility

✓7ᵗʰ **T80.319 ABO incompatibility with hemolytic transfusion reaction, unspecified**
ABO incompatibility with hemolytic transfusion reaction at unspecified time after transfusion
Hemolytic transfusion reaction (HTR) due to ABO incompatibility NOS

✓x7ᵗʰ **T80.39 Other ABO incompatibility reaction due to transfusion of blood or blood products**
Delayed serologic transfusion reaction (DSTR) from ABO incompatibility
Other ABO incompatible blood transfusion
Other reaction to ABO incompatible blood transfusion

✓5ᵗʰ **T80.4 Rh incompatibility reaction due to transfusion of blood or blood products**
Reaction due to incompatibility of Rh antigens (C) (c) (D) (E) (e)

✓x7ᵗʰ **T80.40 Rh incompatibility reaction due to transfusion of blood or blood products, unspecified**
Reaction due to Rh factor in transfusion NOS
Rh incompatible blood transfusion NOS

✓6ᵗʰ **T80.41 Rh incompatibility with hemolytic transfusion reaction**
✓7ᵗʰ **T80.410 Rh incompatibility with acute hemolytic transfusion reaction**
Acute hemolytic transfusion reaction (AHTR) due to Rh incompatibility
Rh incompatibility with hemolytic transfusion reaction less than 24 hours after transfusion

✓7ᵗʰ **T80.411 Rh incompatibility with delayed hemolytic transfusion reaction**
Delayed hemolytic transfusion reaction (DHTR) due to Rh incompatibility
Rh incompatibility with hemolytic transfusion reaction 24 hours or more after transfusion

✓7ᵗʰ **T80.419 Rh incompatibility with hemolytic transfusion reaction, unspecified**
Rh incompatibility with hemolytic transfusion reaction at unspecified time after transfusion
Hemolytic transfusion reaction (HTR) due to Rh incompatibility NOS

✓x7ᵗʰ **T80.49 Other Rh incompatibility reaction due to transfusion of blood or blood products**
Delayed serologic transfusion reaction (DSTR) from Rh incompatibility
Other reaction to Rh incompatible blood transfusion

✓5ᵗʰ **T80.A Non-ABO incompatibility reaction due to transfusion of blood or blood products**
Reaction due to incompatibility of minor antigens (Duffy) (Kell) (Kidd) (Lewis) (M) (N) (P) (S)

✓x7ᵗʰ **T80.A0 Non-ABO incompatibility reaction due to transfusion of blood or blood products, unspecified**
Non-ABO antigen incompatibility reaction from transfusion NOS

✓6ᵗʰ **T80.A1 Non-ABO incompatibility with hemolytic transfusion reaction**
✓7ᵗʰ **T80.A10 Non-ABO incompatibility with acute hemolytic transfusion reaction**
Acute hemolytic transfusion reaction (AHTR) due to non-ABO incompatibility
Non-ABO incompatibility with hemolytic transfusion reaction less than 24 hours after transfusion

✓7ᵗʰ **T80.A11 Non-ABO incompatibility with delayed hemolytic transfusion reaction**
Delayed hemolytic transfusion reaction (DHTR) due to non-ABO incompatibility
Non-ABO incompatibility with hemolytic transfusion reaction 24 or more hours after transfusion

✓7ᵗʰ **T80.A19 Non-ABO incompatibility with hemolytic transfusion reaction, unspecified**
Hemolytic transfusion reaction (HTR) due to non-ABO incompatibility NOS
Non-ABO incompatibility with hemolytic transfusion reaction at unspecified time after transfusion

✓x7ᵗʰ **T80.A9 Other non-ABO incompatibility reaction due to transfusion of blood or blood products**
Delayed serologic transfusion reaction (DSTR) from non-ABO incompatibility
Other reaction to non-ABO incompatible blood transfusion

✓5ᵗʰ **T80.5 Anaphylactic reaction due to serum**
Allergic shock due to serum
Anaphylactic shock due to serum
Anaphylactoid reaction due to serum
Anaphylaxis due to serum
EXCLUDES 1 *ABO incompatibility reaction due to transfusion of blood or blood products (T80.3-)*
allergic reaction or shock NOS (T78.2)
anaphylactic reaction or shock NOS (T78.2)
anaphylactic reaction or shock due to adverse effect of correct medicinal substance properly administered (T88.6)
other serum reaction (T80.6-)
DEF: Life-threatening hypersensitivity to a foreign serum causing respiratory distress, vascular collapse, and shock.

✓x7ᵗʰ **T80.51 Anaphylactic reaction due to administration of blood and blood products**

✓x7ᵗʰ **T80.52 Anaphylactic reaction due to vaccination**

✓x7ᵗʰ **T80.59 Anaphylactic reaction due to other serum**

✓5ᵗʰ **T80.6   Other serum reactions**

Intoxiation by serum
Protein sickness
Serum rash
Serum sickness
Serum urticaria

EXCLUDES 2   *serum hepatitis (B16-B19)*

DEF: Serum sickness: Hypersensitivity to a foreign serum that causes fever, hives, swelling, and lymphadenopathy.

✓x7ᵗʰ **T80.61   Other serum reaction due to administration of blood and blood products**

✓x7ᵗʰ **T80.62   Other serum reaction due to vaccination**

✓x7ᵗʰ **T80.69   Other serum reaction due to other serum**

Code also, if applicable, arthropathy in hypersensitivity reactions classified elsewhere (M36.4)

✓5ᵗʰ **T80.8   Other complications following infusion, transfusion and therapeutic injection**

✓6ᵗʰ **T80.81   Extravasation of vesicant agent**

Infiltration of vesicant agent

✓7ᵗʰ **T80.810   Extravasation of vesicant antineoplastic chemotherapy**

Infiltration of vesicant antineoplastic chemotherapy

✓7ᵗʰ **T80.818   Extravasation of other vesicant agent**

Infiltration of other vesicant agent

✓x7ᵗʰ **T80.89   Other complications following infusion, transfusion and therapeutic injection**

Delayed serologic transfusion reaction (DSTR), unspecified incompatibility

Use additional code to identify graft-versus-host reaction, if applicable, (D89.81-)

✓5ᵗʰ **T80.9   Unspecified complication following infusion, transfusion and therapeutic injection**

✓x7ᵗʰ **T80.90   Unspecified complication following infusion and therapeutic injection**

✓6ᵗʰ **T80.91   Hemolytic transfusion reaction, unspecified incompatibility**

EXCLUDES 1   *ABO incompatibility with hemolytic transfusion reaction (T80.31-)*
non-ABO incompatibility with hemolytic transfusion reaction (T80.A1-)
Rh incompatibility with hemolytic transfusion reaction (T80.41-)

✓7ᵗʰ **T80.910   Acute hemolytic transfusion reaction, unspecified incompatibility**

✓7ᵗʰ **T80.911   Delayed hemolytic transfusion reaction, unspecified incompatibility**

✓7ᵗʰ **T80.919   Hemolytic transfusion reaction, unspecified incompatibility, unspecified as acute or delayed**

Hemolytic transfusion reaction NOS

✓x7ᵗʰ **T80.92   Unspecified transfusion reaction**

Transfusion reaction NOS

✓4ᵗʰ **T81   Complications of procedures, not elsewhere classified**

Use additional code for adverse effect, if applicable, to identify drug (T36-T50 with fifth or sixth character 5)

EXCLUDES 2   *complications following immunization (T88.0-T88.1)*
complications following infusion, transfusion and therapeutic injection (T80.-)
complications of transplanted organs and tissue (T86.-)
specified complications classified elsewhere, such as:
complication of prosthetic devices, implants and grafts (T82-T85)
dermatitis due to drugs and medicaments (L23.3, L24.4, L25.1, L27.0-L27.1)
endosseous dental implant failure (M27.6-)
floppy iris syndrome (IFIS) (intraoperative) (H21.81)
intraoperative and postprocedural complications of specific body system (D78.-, E36.-, E89.-, G97.3, G97.4, H59.3-, H59.-, H95.2-, H95.3, I97.4-, I97.5, J95, K91.-, L76.-, M96.-, N99.-)
ostomy complications (J95.0-, K94.-, N99.5-)
plateau iris syndrome (post-iridectomy) (postprocedural) H21.82
poisoning and toxic effects of drugs and chemicals (T36-T65 with fifth or sixth character 1-4 or 6)

AHA: 2019,2Q,21

The appropriate 7th character is to be added to each code from category T81.
A   initial encounter
D   subsequent encounter
S   sequela

✓5ᵗʰ **T81.1   Postprocedural shock**

Shock during or resulting from a procedure, not elsewhere classified

EXCLUDES 1   *anaphylactic shock due to correct substance properly administered (T88.6)*
anaphylactic shock due to serum (T80.5-)
anaphylactic shock NOS (T78.2)
anesthetic shock (T88.2)
electric shock (T75.4)
obstetric shock (O75.1)
septic shock (R65.21)
shock following abortion or ectopic or molar pregnancy (O00-O07, O08.3)
traumatic shock (T79.4)

✓x7ᵗʰ **T81.10   Postprocedural shock unspecified**

Collapse NOS during or resulting from a procedure, not elsewhere classified
Postprocedural failure of peripheral circulation
Postprocedural shock NOS

✓x7ᵗʰ **T81.11   Postprocedural cardiogenic shock**

✓x7ᵗʰ **T81.12   Postprocedural septic shock**

Postprocedural endotoxic shock resulting from a procedure, not elsewhere classified
Postprocedural gram-negative shock resulting from a procedure, not elsewhere classified
Code first underlying infection
Use additional code, to identify any associated acute organ dysfunction, if applicable

AHA: 2018,4Q,63

✓x7ᵗʰ **T81.19   Other postprocedural shock**

Postprocedural hypovolemic shock

✓5ᵗʰ **T81.3   Disruption of wound, not elsewhere classified**

Disruption of any suture materials or other closure methods

EXCLUDES 1   *breakdown (mechanical) of permanent sutures (T85.612)*
displacement of permanent sutures (T85.622)
disruption of cesarean delivery wound (O90.0)
disruption of perineal obstetric wound (O90.1)
mechanical complication of permanent sutures NEC (T85.692)

AHA: 2014,1Q,23

✓x7ᵗʰ **T81.30   Disruption of wound, unspecified**

Disruption of wound NOS

N Newborn: 0   P Pediatric: 0-17   M Maternity: 12-55   A Adult: 15-124   CH Comorbidity High   CL Comorbidity Low   NCDx Noncancer Dx   PDx Primary Dx

1124

ICD-10-CM 2020

✓x7ᵗʰ **T81.31** **Disruption of** external operation **(surgical) wound, not elsewhere classified**
- Dehiscence of operation wound NOS
- Disruption of operation wound NOS
- Disruption or dehiscence of closure of cornea
- Disruption or dehiscence of closure of mucosa
- Disruption or dehiscence of closure of skin and subcutaneous tissue
- Full-thickness skin disruption or dehiscence
- Superficial disruption or dehiscence of operation wound

     EXCLUDES 1   dehiscence of amputation stump (T87.81)

✓x7ᵗʰ **T81.32** **Disruption of** internal operation **(surgical) wound, not elsewhere classified**
- Deep disruption or dehiscence of operation wound NOS
- Disruption or dehiscence of closure of internal organ or other internal tissue
- Disruption or dehiscence of closure of muscle or muscle flap
- Disruption or dehiscence of closure of ribs or rib cage
- Disruption or dehiscence of closure of skull or craniotomy
- Disruption or dehiscence of closure of sternum or sternotomy
- Disruption or dehiscence of closure of tendon or ligament
- Disruption or dehiscence of closure of superficial or muscular fascia

     AHA: 2017,3Q,4

✓x7ᵗʰ **T81.33** **Disruption of** traumatic injury **wound** repair
- Disruption or dehiscence of closure of traumatic laceration (external) (internal)

✓5ᵗʰ **T81.4** **Infection following a procedure**
- Wound abscess following a procedure
- Use additional code to identify infection
- Use additional code (R65.2-) to identify severe sepsis, if applicable

     EXCLUDES 2   bleb associated endophthalmitis (H59.4-)
             infection due to infusion, transfusion and therapeutic injection (T80.2-)
             infection due to prosthetic devices, implants and grafts (T82.6-T82.7, T83.5-T83.6, T84.5-T84.7, T85.7)
             obstetric surgical wound infection (O86.0-)
             postprocedural fever NOS (R50.82)
             postprocedural retroperitoneal abscess (K68.11)

     AHA: 2018,4Q,33-34,62; 2014,1Q,23

✓x7ᵗʰ **T81.40** **Infection following a procedure, unspecified**

✓x7ᵗʰ **T81.41** **Infection following a procedure,** superficial incisional surgical site
- Subcutaneous abscess following a procedure
- Stitch abscess following a procedure

✓x7ᵗʰ **T81.42** **Infection following a procedure,** deep incisional surgical site
- Intra-muscular abscess following a procedure

✓x7ᵗʰ **T81.43** **Infection following a procedure,** organ and space surgical site
- Intra-abdominal abscess following a procedure
- Subphrenic abscess following a procedure

✓x7ᵗʰ **T81.44** Sepsis **following a procedure**
- Use additional code to identify the sepsis

✓x7ᵗʰ **T81.49** **Infection following a procedure, other surgical site**

✓5ᵗʰ **T81.5** **Complications of** foreign body accidentally left in body following procedure
     AHA: 2014,4Q,24

✓6ᵗʰ **T81.50** **Unspecified complication of foreign body accidentally left in body following procedure**

✓7ᵗʰ **T81.500** **Unspecified complication of foreign body accidentally left in body following** surgical operation

✓7ᵗʰ **T81.501** **Unspecified complication of foreign body accidentally left in body following** infusion or transfusion

✓7ᵗʰ **T81.502** **Unspecified complication of foreign body accidentally left in body following** kidney dialysis

✓7ᵗʰ **T81.503** **Unspecified complication of foreign body accidentally left in body following** injection or immunization

✓7ᵗʰ **T81.504** **Unspecified complication of foreign body accidentally left in body following** endoscopic examination

✓7ᵗʰ **T81.505** **Unspecified complication of foreign body accidentally left in body following** heart catheterization

✓7ᵗʰ **T81.506** **Unspecified complication of foreign body accidentally left in body following** aspiration, puncture or other catheterization

✓7ᵗʰ **T81.507** **Unspecified complication of foreign body accidentally left in body following** removal of catheter or packing

✓7ᵗʰ **T81.508** **Unspecified complication of foreign body accidentally left in body following** other procedure

✓7ᵗʰ **T81.509** **Unspecified complication of foreign body accidentally left in body following** unspecified procedure

✓6ᵗʰ **T81.51** Adhesions **due to foreign body accidentally left in body following procedure**

✓7ᵗʰ **T81.510** **Adhesions due to foreign body accidentally left in body following** surgical operation

✓7ᵗʰ **T81.511** **Adhesions due to foreign body accidentally left in body following** infusion or transfusion

✓7ᵗʰ **T81.512** **Adhesions due to foreign body accidentally left in body following** kidney dialysis

✓7ᵗʰ **T81.513** **Adhesions due to foreign body accidentally left in body following** injection or immunization

✓7ᵗʰ **T81.514** **Adhesions due to foreign body accidentally left in body following** endoscopic examination

✓7ᵗʰ **T81.515** **Adhesions due to foreign body accidentally left in body following** heart catheterization

✓7ᵗʰ **T81.516** **Adhesions due to foreign body accidentally left in body following** aspiration, puncture or other catheterization

✓7ᵗʰ **T81.517** **Adhesions due to foreign body accidentally left in body following** removal of catheter or packing

✓7ᵗʰ **T81.518** **Adhesions due to foreign body accidentally left in body following** other procedure

✓7ᵗʰ **T81.519** **Adhesions due to foreign body accidentally left in body following** unspecified procedure

✓6ᵗʰ **T81.52** Obstruction **due to foreign body accidentally left in body following procedure**

✓7ᵗʰ **T81.520** **Obstruction due to foreign body accidentally left in body following** surgical operation

✓7ᵗʰ **T81.521** **Obstruction due to foreign body accidentally left in body following** infusion or transfusion

✓7ᵗʰ **T81.522** **Obstruction due to foreign body accidentally left in body following** kidney dialysis

✓7ᵗʰ **T81.523** **Obstruction due to foreign body accidentally left in body following** injection or immunization

✓7ᵗʰ **T81.524** **Obstruction due to foreign body accidentally left in body following** endoscopic examination

✓7ᵗʰ **T81.525** **Obstruction due to foreign body accidentally left in body following** heart catheterization

✓7ᵗʰ **T81.526** **Obstruction due to foreign body accidentally left in body following** aspiration, puncture or other catheterization

✓7ᵗʰ **T81.527** **Obstruction due to foreign body accidentally left in body following** removal of catheter or packing

✓7ᵗʰ **T81.528** **Obstruction due to foreign body accidentally left in body following** other procedure

☑ Additional Character Required   ✓x7ᵗʰ Placeholder Alert   Manifestation   Unspecified Dx   ▶◀ Revised Text   ● New Code   ▲ Revised Title

ICD-10-CM 2020   **1125**

✓7ᵗʰ T81.529 Obstruction due to foreign body accidentally left in body following unspecified procedure

✓6ᵗʰ T81.53 Perforation due to foreign body accidentally left in body following procedure

✓7ᵗʰ T81.530 Perforation due to foreign body accidentally left in body following surgical operation

✓7ᵗʰ T81.531 Perforation due to foreign body accidentally left in body following infusion or transfusion

✓7ᵗʰ T81.532 Perforation due to foreign body accidentally left in body following kidney dialysis

✓7ᵗʰ T81.533 Perforation due to foreign body accidentally left in body following injection or immunization

✓7ᵗʰ T81.534 Perforation due to foreign body accidentally left in body following endoscopic examination

✓7ᵗʰ T81.535 Perforation due to foreign body accidentally left in body following heart catheterization

✓7ᵗʰ T81.536 Perforation due to foreign body accidentally left in body following aspiration, puncture or other catheterization

✓7ᵗʰ T81.537 Perforation due to foreign body accidentally left in body following removal of catheter or packing

✓7ᵗʰ T81.538 Perforation due to foreign body accidentally left in body following other procedure

✓7ᵗʰ T81.539 Perforation due to foreign body accidentally left in body following unspecified procedure

✓6ᵗʰ T81.59 Other complications of foreign body accidentally left in body following procedure

> EXCLUDES 2   obstruction or perforation due to prosthetic devices and implants intentionally left in body (T82.0-T82.5, T83.0-T83.4, T83.7, T84.0-T84.4, T85.0-T85.6)

✓7ᵗʰ T81.590 Other complications of foreign body accidentally left in body following surgical operation

✓7ᵗʰ T81.591 Other complications of foreign body accidentally left in body following infusion or transfusion

✓7ᵗʰ T81.592 Other complications of foreign body accidentally left in body following kidney dialysis

✓7ᵗʰ T81.593 Other complications of foreign body accidentally left in body following injection or immunization

✓7ᵗʰ T81.594 Other complications of foreign body accidentally left in body following endoscopic examination

✓7ᵗʰ T81.595 Other complications of foreign body accidentally left in body following heart catheterization

✓7ᵗʰ T81.596 Other complications of foreign body accidentally left in body following aspiration, puncture or other catheterization

✓7ᵗʰ T81.597 Other complications of foreign body accidentally left in body following removal of catheter or packing

✓7ᵗʰ T81.598 Other complications of foreign body accidentally left in body following other procedure

✓7ᵗʰ T81.599 Other complications of foreign body accidentally left in body following unspecified procedure

✓5ᵗʰ T81.6 Acute reaction to foreign substance accidentally left during a procedure

> EXCLUDES 2   complications of foreign body accidentally left in body cavity or operation wound following procedure (T81.5-)

✓x7ᵗʰ T81.60 Unspecified acute reaction to foreign substance accidentally left during a procedure

✓x7ᵗʰ T81.61 Aseptic peritonitis due to foreign substance accidentally left during a procedure
Chemical peritonitis

✓x7ᵗʰ T81.69 Other acute reaction to foreign substance accidentally left during a procedure

✓5ᵗʰ T81.7 Vascular complications following a procedure, not elsewhere classified
Air embolism following procedure NEC
Phlebitis or thrombophlebitis resulting from a procedure

> EXCLUDES 1   embolism complicating abortion or ectopic or molar pregnancy (O00-O07, O08.2)
> embolism complicating pregnancy, childbirth and the puerperium (O88.-)
> traumatic embolism (T79.0)

> EXCLUDES 2   embolism due to prosthetic devices, implants and grafts (T82.8-, T83.81, T84.8-, T85.81-)
> embolism following infusion, transfusion and therapeutic injection (T80.0)

AHA: 2019,2Q,22

✓6ᵗʰ T81.71 Complication of artery following a procedure, not elsewhere classified

✓7ᵗʰ T81.710 Complication of mesenteric artery following a procedure, not elsewhere classified

✓7ᵗʰ T81.711 Complication of renal artery following a procedure, not elsewhere classified

✓7ᵗʰ T81.718 Complication of other artery following a procedure, not elsewhere classified
AHA: 2019,2Q,21-22

✓7ᵗʰ T81.719 Complication of unspecified artery following a procedure, not elsewhere classified

✓x7ᵗʰ T81.72 Complication of vein following a procedure, not elsewhere classified

✓5ᵗʰ T81.8 Other complications of procedures, not elsewhere classified

> EXCLUDES 2   hypothermia following anesthesia (T88.51)
> malignant hyperpyrexia due to anesthesia (T88.3)

✓x7ᵗʰ T81.81 Complication of inhalation therapy

✓x7ᵗʰ T81.82 Emphysema (subcutaneous) resulting from a procedure

✓x7ᵗʰ T81.83 Persistent postprocedural fistula
AHA: 2017,3Q,3-4

✓x7ᵗʰ T81.89 Other complications of procedures, not elsewhere classified

Non-healing ✗ wound

Use additional code to specify complication, such as: postprocedural delirium (F05)
AHA: 2014,1Q,23

✓x7ᵗʰ T81.9 Unspecified complication of procedure

✓4ᵗʰ T82 Complications of cardiac and vascular prosthetic devices, implants and grafts

> EXCLUDES 2   failure and rejection of transplanted organs and tissue (T86.-)

The appropriate 7th character is to be added to each code from category T82.
A   initial encounter
D   subsequent encounter
S   sequela

✓5ᵗʰ T82.0 Mechanical complication of heart valve prosthesis
Mechanical complication of artificial heart valve

> EXCLUDES 1   mechanical complication of biological heart valve graft (T82.22-)

✓x7ᵗʰ T82.01 Breakdown (mechanical) of heart valve prosthesis

✓x7ᵗʰ T82.02 Displacement of heart valve prosthesis
Malposition of heart valve prosthesis

✓x7ᵗʰ T82.03 Leakage of heart valve prosthesis

✓x7ᵗʰ T82.09 Other mechanical complication of heart valve prosthesis
Obstruction (mechanical) of heart valve prosthesis
Perforation of heart valve prosthesis
Protrusion of heart valve prosthesis

✓5ᵗʰ T82.1 Mechanical complication of cardiac electronic device

✓6ᵗʰ T82.11 Breakdown (mechanical) of cardiac electronic device

✓7ᵗʰ T82.110 Breakdown (mechanical) of cardiac electrode

✓7ᵗʰ T82.111 Breakdown (mechanical) of cardiac pulse generator (battery)

√7ᵗʰ **T82.118** **Breakdown (mechanical) of other cardiac electronic device**

√7ᵗʰ **T82.119** **Breakdown (mechanical) of unspecified cardiac electronic device**

√6ᵗʰ **T82.12** Displacement **of cardiac electronic device**

    Malposition of cardiac electronic device

√7ᵗʰ **T82.120** **Displacement of** cardiac electrode

√7ᵗʰ **T82.121** **Displacement of cardiac** pulse generator (battery)

√7ᵗʰ **T82.128** **Displacement of other cardiac electronic device**

√7ᵗʰ **T82.129** **Displacement of unspecified cardiac electronic device**

√6ᵗʰ **T82.19** **Other mechanical complication of cardiac electronic device**

    Leakage of cardiac electronic device

    Obstruction of cardiac electronic device

    Perforation of cardiac electronic device

    Protrusion of cardiac electronic device

√7ᵗʰ **T82.190** **Other mechanical complication of** cardiac electrode

√7ᵗʰ **T82.191** **Other mechanical complication of cardiac** pulse generator (battery)

√7ᵗʰ **T82.198** **Other mechanical complication of other cardiac electronic device**

√7ᵗʰ **T82.199** **Other mechanical complication of unspecified cardiac device**

√5ᵗʰ **T82.2** **Mechanical complication of coronary artery bypass graft and biological heart valve graft**

    EXCLUDES 1   *mechanical complication of artificial heart valve prosthesis (T82.0-)*

√6ᵗʰ **T82.21** **Mechanical complication of** coronary artery bypass graft

√7ᵗʰ **T82.211** **Breakdown (mechanical) of coronary artery bypass graft**

√7ᵗʰ **T82.212** **Displacement of coronary artery bypass graft**

    Malposition of coronary artery bypass graft

√7ᵗʰ **T82.213** **Leakage of coronary artery bypass graft**

√7ᵗʰ **T82.218** **Other mechanical complication of coronary artery bypass graft**

    Obstruction, mechanical of coronary artery bypass graft

    Perforation of coronary artery bypass graft

    Protrusion of coronary artery bypass graft

√6ᵗʰ **T82.22** **Mechanical complication of** biological heart valve graft

√7ᵗʰ **T82.221** **Breakdown (mechanical) of biological heart valve graft**

√7ᵗʰ **T82.222** **Displacement of biological heart valve graft**

    Malposition of biological heart valve graft

√7ᵗʰ **T82.223** **Leakage of biological heart valve graft**

√7ᵗʰ **T82.228** **Other mechanical complication of biological heart valve graft**

    Obstruction of biological heart valve graft

    Perforation of biological heart valve graft

    Protrusion of biological heart valve graft

√5ᵗʰ **T82.3** **Mechanical complication of other vascular grafts**

√6ᵗʰ **T82.31** Breakdown (mechanical) of other vascular grafts

√7ᵗʰ **T82.310** **Breakdown (mechanical) of** aortic (bifurcation) graft (replacement)

√7ᵗʰ **T82.311** **Breakdown (mechanical) of** carotid arterial graft (bypass)

√7ᵗʰ **T82.312** **Breakdown (mechanical) of** femoral arterial graft (bypass)

√7ᵗʰ **T82.318** **Breakdown (mechanical) of other vascular grafts**

√7ᵗʰ **T82.319** **Breakdown (mechanical) of unspecified vascular grafts**

√6ᵗʰ **T82.32** Displacement **of other vascular grafts**

    Malposition of other vascular grafts

√7ᵗʰ **T82.320** **Displacement of** aortic (bifurcation) graft (replacement)

√7ᵗʰ **T82.321** **Displacement of** carotid arterial graft (bypass)

√7ᵗʰ **T82.322** **Displacement of** femoral arterial graft (bypass)

√7ᵗʰ **T82.328** **Displacement of other vascular grafts**

√7ᵗʰ **T82.329** **Displacement of unspecified vascular grafts**

√6ᵗʰ **T82.33** **Leakage of other vascular grafts**

√7ᵗʰ **T82.330** **Leakage of** aortic (bifurcation) graft (replacement)

√7ᵗʰ **T82.331** **Leakage of** carotid arterial graft (bypass)

√7ᵗʰ **T82.332** **Leakage of** femoral arterial graft (bypass)

√7ᵗʰ **T82.338** **Leakage of other vascular grafts**

√7ᵗʰ **T82.339** **Leakage of unspecified vascular graft**

√6ᵗʰ **T82.39** **Other mechanical complication of other vascular grafts**

    Obstruction (mechanical) of other vascular grafts

    Perforation of other vascular grafts

    Protrusion of other vascular grafts

√7ᵗʰ **T82.390** **Other mechanical complication of** aortic (bifurcation) graft (replacement)

√7ᵗʰ **T82.391** **Other mechanical complication of** carotid arterial graft (bypass)

√7ᵗʰ **T82.392** **Other mechanical complication of** femoral arterial graft (bypass)

√7ᵗʰ **T82.398** **Other mechanical complication of other vascular grafts**

√7ᵗʰ **T82.399** **Other mechanical complication of unspecified vascular grafts**

√5ᵗʰ **T82.4** **Mechanical complication of** vascular dialysis catheter

    Mechanical complication of hemodialysis catheter

    EXCLUDES 1   *mechanical complication of intraperitoneal dialysis catheter (T85.62)*

√x7ᵗʰ **T82.41** Breakdown (mechanical) of vascular dialysis catheter

√x7ᵗʰ **T82.42** Displacement **of vascular dialysis catheter**

    Malposition of vascular dialysis catheter

√x7ᵗʰ **T82.43** Leakage **of vascular dialysis catheter**

√x7ᵗʰ **T82.49** **Other complication of vascular dialysis catheter**

    Obstruction (mechanical) of vascular dialysis catheter

    Perforation of vascular dialysis catheter

    Protrusion of vascular dialysis catheter

√5ᵗʰ **T82.5** **Mechanical complication of other cardiac and vascular devices and implants**

    EXCLUDES 2   *mechanical complication of epidural and subdural infusion catheter (T85.61)*

√6ᵗʰ **T82.51** **Breakdown (mechanical) of other cardiac and vascular devices and implants**

√7ᵗʰ **T82.510** **Breakdown (mechanical) of** surgically created arteriovenous fistula

√7ᵗʰ **T82.511** **Breakdown (mechanical) of** surgically created arteriovenous shunt

√7ᵗʰ **T82.512** **Breakdown (mechanical) of** artificial heart

√7ᵗʰ **T82.513** **Breakdown (mechanical) of** balloon (counterpulsation) device

√7ᵗʰ **T82.514** **Breakdown (mechanical) of** infusion catheter

√7ᵗʰ **T82.515** **Breakdown (mechanical) of** umbrella device

√7ᵗʰ **T82.518** **Breakdown (mechanical) of other cardiac and vascular devices and implants**

√7ᵗʰ **T82.519** **Breakdown (mechanical) of unspecified cardiac and vascular devices and implants**

√6ᵗʰ **T82.52** Displacement **of other cardiac and vascular devices and implants**

    Malposition of other cardiac and vascular devices and implants

√7ᵗʰ **T82.520** **Displacement of** surgically created arteriovenous fistula

√7ᵗʰ **T82.521** **Displacement of** surgically created arteriovenous shunt

√7ᵗʰ **T82.522** **Displacement of** artificial heart

√7ᵗʰ **T82.523** **Displacement of** balloon (counterpulsation) device

√7ᵗʰ **T82.524** **Displacement of** infusion catheter

√7ᵗʰ **T82.525** **Displacement of** umbrella device

√7ᵗʰ **T82.528** **Displacement of other cardiac and vascular devices and implants**

√7ᵗʰ **T82.529** **Displacement of unspecified cardiac and vascular devices and implants**

√6ᵗʰ **T82.53** Leakage **of other cardiac and vascular devices and implants**

√7ᵗʰ **T82.530** **Leakage of** surgically created arteriovenous fistula

✔ Additional Character Required   √x7ᵗʰ Placeholder Alert   Manifestation   Unspecified Dx   ►◄ Revised Text   ● New Code   ▲ Revised Title

ICD-10-CM 2020   1127

T82.118–T82.530

Chapter 19. Injury, Poisoning and Certain Other Consequences of External Causes

☑7ᵗʰ **T82.531** **Leakage of** surgically created arteriovenous shunt

☑7ᵗʰ **T82.532** **Leakage of** artificial heart

☑7ᵗʰ **T82.533** **Leakage of** balloon (counterpulsation) device

☑7ᵗʰ **T82.534** **Leakage of** infusion catheter

☑7ᵗʰ **T82.535** **Leakage of** umbrella device

☑7ᵗʰ **T82.538** **Leakage of other cardiac and vascular devices and implants**

☑7ᵗʰ **T82.539** **Leakage of unspecified cardiac and vascular devices and implants**

☑6ᵗʰ **T82.59** **Other mechanical complication of other cardiac and vascular devices and implants**

Obstruction (mechanical) of other cardiac and vascular devices and implants

Perforation of other cardiac and vascular devices and implants

Protrusion of other cardiac and vascular devices and implants

☑7ᵗʰ **T82.590** **Other mechanical complication of** surgically created arteriovenous fistula

☑7ᵗʰ **T82.591** **Other mechanical complication of** surgically created arteriovenous shunt

☑7ᵗʰ **T82.592** **Other mechanical complication of** artificial heart

☑7ᵗʰ **T82.593** **Other mechanical complication of** balloon (counterpulsation) device

☑7ᵗʰ **T82.594** **Other mechanical complication of** infusion catheter

☑7ᵗʰ **T82.595** **Other mechanical complication of** umbrella device

☑7ᵗʰ **T82.598** **Other mechanical complication of other cardiac and vascular devices and implants**

☑7ᵗʰ **T82.599** **Other mechanical complication of unspecified cardiac and vascular devices and implants**

☑x7ᵗʰ **T82.6** **Infection and inflammatory reaction due to cardiac valve prosthesis**

Use additional code to identify infection

☑x7ᵗʰ **T82.7** **Infection and inflammatory reaction due to other cardiac and vascular devices, implants and grafts**

Use additional code to identify infection

AHA: 2019,1Q,13-14

TIP: Assign this code for infections and/or cellulitis resulting from catheters that are not centrally placed (e.g., midline catheters).

☑5ᵗʰ **T82.8** **Other specified complications of cardiac and vascular prosthetic devices, implants and grafts**

AHA: 2016,4Q,70

☑6ᵗʰ **T82.81** **Embolism due to cardiac and vascular prosthetic devices, implants and grafts**

☑7ᵗʰ **T82.817** **Embolism due to** cardiac prosthetic devices, implants and grafts

☑7ᵗʰ **T82.818** **Embolism due to** vascular prosthetic devices, implants and grafts

☑6ᵗʰ **T82.82** **Fibrosis due to cardiac and vascular prosthetic devices, implants and grafts**

☑7ᵗʰ **T82.827** **Fibrosis due to** cardiac prosthetic devices, implants and grafts

☑7ᵗʰ **T82.828** **Fibrosis due** vascular prosthetic devices, implants and grafts

☑6ᵗʰ **T82.83** **Hemorrhage due to cardiac and vascular prosthetic devices, implants and grafts**

☑7ᵗʰ **T82.837** **Hemorrhage due to** cardiac prosthetic devices, implants and grafts

☑7ᵗʰ **T82.838** **Hemorrhage due to** vascular prosthetic devices, implants and grafts

☑6ᵗʰ **T82.84** **Pain due to cardiac and vascular prosthetic devices, implants and grafts**

☑7ᵗʰ **T82.847** **Pain due to** cardiac prosthetic devices, implants and grafts

☑7ᵗʰ **T82.848** **Pain due to** vascular prosthetic devices, implants and grafts

☑6ᵗʰ **T82.85** **Stenosis due to cardiac and vascular prosthetic devices, implants and grafts**

☑7ᵗʰ **T82.855** **Stenosis of** coronary artery stent

In-stent stenosis (restenosis) of coronary artery stent

Restenosis of coronary artery stent

☑7ᵗʰ **T82.856** **Stenosis of** peripheral vascular stent

In-stent stenosis (restenosis) of peripheral vascular stent

Restenosis of peripheral vascular stent

☑7ᵗʰ **T82.857** **Stenosis of other** cardiac **prosthetic devices, implants and grafts**

☑7ᵗʰ **T82.858** **Stenosis of other** vascular **prosthetic devices, implants and grafts**

☑6ᵗʰ **T82.86** **Thrombosis of cardiac and vascular prosthetic devices, implants and grafts**

☑7ᵗʰ **T82.867** **Thrombosis due to** cardiac **prosthetic devices, implants and grafts**

☑7ᵗʰ **T82.868** **Thrombosis due to** vascular **prosthetic devices, implants and grafts**

☑6ᵗʰ **T82.89** **Other specified complication of cardiac and vascular prosthetic devices, implants and grafts**

☑7ᵗʰ **T82.897** **Other specified complication of** cardiac **prosthetic devices, implants and grafts**

AHA: 2019,2Q,33

☑7ᵗʰ **T82.898** **Other specified complication of** vascular **prosthetic devices, implants and grafts**

☑x7ᵗʰ **T82.9** **Unspecified complication of cardiac and vascular prosthetic device, implant and graft**

☑4ᵗʰ **T83** **Complications of genitourinary prosthetic devices, implants and grafts**

EXCLUDES 2   failure and rejection of transplanted organs and tissue (T86.-)

AHA: 2016,4Q,70-71

TIP: Use to report treatment for a urinary device complication; do not assign a code from category Z46.6 Encounter for fitting and adjustment of urinary device, when a complication of the urinary device is the focus of treatment.

The appropriate 7th character is to be added to each code from category T83.
A   initial encounter
D   subsequent encounter
S   sequela

☑5ᵗʰ **T83.0** **Mechanical complication of** urinary catheter

EXCLUDES 2   complications of stoma of urinary tract (N99.5-)

☑6ᵗʰ **T83.01** **Breakdown (mechanical) of** urinary catheter

☑7ᵗʰ **T83.010** **Breakdown (mechanical) of** cystostomy **catheter**

☑7ᵗʰ **T83.011** **Breakdown (mechanical) of** indwelling urethral **catheter**

☑7ᵗʰ **T83.012** **Breakdown (mechanical) of** nephrostomy **catheter**

☑7ᵗʰ **T83.018** **Breakdown (mechanical) of other urinary catheter**

Breakdown (mechanical) of Hopkins catheter

Breakdown (mechanical) of ileostomy catheter

Breakdown (mechanical) urostomy catheter

☑6ᵗʰ **T83.02** **Displacement of urinary catheter**

Malposition of urinary catheter

☑7ᵗʰ **T83.020** **Displacement of** cystostomy **catheter**

☑7ᵗʰ **T83.021** **Displacement of** indwelling urethral **catheter**

☑7ᵗʰ **T83.022** **Displacement of** nephrostomy **catheter**

☑7ᵗʰ **T83.028** **Displacement of other urinary catheter**

Displacement of Hopkins catheter

Displacement of ileostomy catheter

Displacement of urostomy catheter

☑6ᵗʰ **T83.03** **Leakage of urinary catheter**

☑7ᵗʰ **T83.030** **Leakage of** cystostomy **catheter**

☑7ᵗʰ **T83.031** **Leakage of** indwelling urethral **catheter**

☑7ᵗʰ **T83.032** **Leakage of** nephrostomy **catheter**

☑7ᵗʰ **T83.038** **Leakage of other urinary catheter**

Leakage of Hopkins catheter

Leakage of ileostomy catheter

Leakage of urostomy catheter

☑6ᵗʰ **T83.09** **Other mechanical complication of urinary catheter**

Obstruction (mechanical) of urinary catheter

Perforation of urinary catheter

Protrusion of urinary catheter

☑7ᵗʰ **T83.090** **Other mechanical complication of** cystostomy **catheter**

N Newborn: 0   P Pediatric: 0-17   M Maternity: 12-55   A Adult: 15-124   CH Comorbidity High   CL Comorbidity Low   NCDx Noncancer Dx   PDx Primary Dx

1128   ICD-10-CM 2020

√7ᵗʰ T83.091 Other mechanical complication of indwelling urethral catheter

√7ᵗʰ T83.092 Other mechanical complication of nephrostomy catheter

√7ᵗʰ T83.098 Other mechanical complication of other urinary catheter

Other mechanical complication of Hopkins catheter

Other mechanical complication of ileostomy catheter

Other mechanical complication of urostomy catheter

√5ᵗʰ T83.1 Mechanical complication of other urinary devices and implants

√6ᵗʰ T83.11 Breakdown (mechanical) of other urinary devices and implants

√7ᵗʰ T83.110 Breakdown (mechanical) of urinary electronic stimulator device

    EXCLUDES 2 breakdown (mechanical) of electrode (lead) for sacral nerve neurostimulator (T85.111)

    breakdown (mechanical) of implanted electronic sacral neurostimulator, pulse generator or receiver (T85.113)

√7ᵗʰ T83.111 Breakdown (mechanical) of implanted urinary sphincter

√7ᵗʰ T83.112 Breakdown (mechanical) of indwelling ureteral stent

√7ᵗʰ T83.113 Breakdown (mechanical) of other urinary stents

Breakdown (mechanical) of ileal conduit stent

Breakdown (mechanical) of nephroureteral stent

√7ᵗʰ T83.118 Breakdown (mechanical) of other urinary devices and implants

√6ᵗʰ T83.12 Displacement of other urinary devices and implants

Malposition of other urinary devices and implants

√7ᵗʰ T83.120 Displacement of urinary electronic stimulator device

    EXCLUDES 2 displacement of electrode (lead) for sacral nerve neurostimulator (T85.121)

    displacement of implanted electronic sacral neurostimulator, pulse generator or receiver (T85.123)

√7ᵗʰ T83.121 Displacement of implanted urinary sphincter

√7ᵗʰ T83.122 Displacement of indwelling ureteral stent

√7ᵗʰ T83.123 Displacement of other urinary stents

Displacement of ileal conduit stent

Displacement of nephroureteral stent

√7ᵗʰ T83.128 Displacement of other urinary devices and implants

√6ᵗʰ T83.19 Other mechanical complication of other urinary devices and implants

Leakage of other urinary devices and implants

Obstruction (mechanical) of other urinary devices and implants

Perforation of other urinary devices and implants

Protrusion of other urinary devices and implants

√7ᵗʰ T83.190 Other mechanical complication of urinary electronic stimulator device

    EXCLUDES 2 other mechanical complication of electrode (lead) for sacral nerve neurostimulator (T85.191)

    other mechanical complication of implanted electronic sacral neurostimulator, pulse generator or receiver (T85.193)

√7ᵗʰ T83.191 Other mechanical complication of implanted urinary sphincter

√7ᵗʰ T83.192 Other mechanical complication of indwelling ureteral stent

√7ᵗʰ T83.193 Other mechanical complication of other urinary stent

Other mechanical complication of ileal conduit stent

Other mechanical complication of nephroureteral stent

√7ᵗʰ T83.198 Other mechanical complication of other urinary devices and implants

√5ᵗʰ T83.2 Mechanical complication of graft of urinary organ

√x7ᵗʰ T83.21 Breakdown (mechanical) of graft of urinary organ

√x7ᵗʰ T83.22 Displacement of graft of urinary organ

Malposition of graft of urinary organ

√x7ᵗʰ T83.23 Leakage of graft of urinary organ

√x7ᵗʰ T83.24 Erosion of graft of urinary organ

√x7ᵗʰ T83.25 Exposure of graft of urinary organ

√x7ᵗʰ T83.29 Other mechanical complication of graft of urinary organ

Obstruction (mechanical) of graft of urinary organ

Perforation of graft of urinary organ

Protrusion of graft of urinary organ

√5ᵗʰ T83.3 Mechanical complication of intrauterine contraceptive device

√x7ᵗʰ T83.31 Breakdown (mechanical) of intrauterine contraceptive device ♀

√x7ᵗʰ T83.32 Displacement of intrauterine contraceptive device ♀

Malposition of intrauterine contraceptive device

Missing string of intrauterine contraceptive device

AHA: 2018,1Q,5

√x7ᵗʰ T83.39 Other mechanical complication of intrauterine contraceptive device ♀

Leakage of intrauterine contraceptive device

Obstruction (mechanical) of intrauterine contraceptive device

Perforation of intrauterine contraceptive device

Protrusion of intrauterine contraceptive device

√5ᵗʰ T83.4 Mechanical complication of other prosthetic devices, implants and grafts of genital tract

√6ᵗʰ T83.41 Breakdown (mechanical) of other prosthetic devices, implants and grafts of genital tract

√7ᵗʰ T83.410 Breakdown (mechanical) of implanted penile prosthesis ♂

Breakdown (mechanical) of penile prosthesis cylinder

Breakdown (mechanical) of penile prosthesis pump

Breakdown (mechanical) of penile prosthesis reservoir

√7ᵗʰ T83.411 Breakdown (mechanical) of implanted testicular prosthesis

√7ᵗʰ T83.418 Breakdown (mechanical) of other prosthetic devices, implants and grafts of genital tract

√6ᵗʰ T83.42 Displacement of other prosthetic devices, implants and grafts of genital tract

Malposition of other prosthetic devices, implants and grafts of genital tract

√7ᵗʰ T83.420 Displacement of implanted penile prosthesis ♂

Displacement of penile prosthesis cylinder

Displacement of penile prosthesis pump

Displacement of penile prosthesis reservoir

√7ᵗʰ T83.421 Displacement of implanted testicular prosthesis

√7ᵗʰ T83.428 Displacement of other prosthetic devices, implants and grafts of genital tract

AHA: 2018,1Q,5

✔ Additional Character Required   √x7ᵗʰ Placeholder Alert   Manifestation   Unspecified Dx   ►◄ Revised Text   ● New Code   ▲ Revised Title

ICD-10-CM 2020   1129

Chapter 19. Injury, Poisoning and Certain Other Consequences of External Causes

☑6ᵗʰ **T83.49 Other mechanical complication of other prosthetic devices, implants and grafts of genital tract**
Leakage of other prosthetic devices, implants and grafts of genital tract
Obstruction, mechanical of other prosthetic devices, implants and grafts of genital tract
Perforation of other prosthetic devices, implants and grafts of genital tract
Protrusion of other prosthetic devices, implants and grafts of genital tract

     ☑7ᵗʰ **T83.490 Other mechanical complication of** implanted penile prosthesis   ♂
Other mechanical complication of penile prosthesis cylinder
Other mechanical complication of penile prosthesis pump
Other mechanical complication of penile prosthesis reservoir

     ☑7ᵗʰ **T83.491 Other mechanical complication of** implanted testicular prosthesis

     ☑7ᵗʰ **T83.498 Other mechanical complication of other prosthetic devices, implants and grafts of genital tract**

☑5ᵗʰ **T83.5 Infection and inflammatory reaction due to prosthetic device, implant and graft in** urinary system
Use additional code to identify infection

     ☑6ᵗʰ **T83.51 Infection and inflammatory reaction due to** urinary catheter
       EXCLUDES 2 complications of stoma of urinary tract (N99.5-)

     ☑7ᵗʰ **T83.510 Infection and inflammatory reaction due to** cystostomy **catheter**

     ☑7ᵗʰ **T83.511 Infection and inflammatory reaction due to** indwelling urethral **catheter**

     ☑7ᵗʰ **T83.512 Infection and inflammatory reaction due to** nephrostomy **catheter**

     ☑7ᵗʰ **T83.518 Infection and inflammatory reaction due to other urinary catheter**
Infection and inflammatory reaction due to Hopkins catheter
Infection and inflammatory reaction due to ileostomy catheter
Infection and inflammatory reaction due to urostomy catheter

     ☑6ᵗʰ **T83.59 Infection and inflammatory reaction due to** prosthetic device, implant and graft **in urinary system**

     ☑7ᵗʰ **T83.590 Infection and inflammatory reaction due to implanted urinary** neurostimulation device
       EXCLUDES 2 infection and inflammatory reaction due to electrode lead of sacral nerve neurostimulator (T85.732)
infection and inflammatory reaction due to pulse generator or receiver of sacral nerve neurostimulator (T85.734)

     ☑7ᵗʰ **T83.591 Infection and inflammatory reaction due to** implanted urinary sphincter

     ☑7ᵗʰ **T83.592 Infection and inflammatory reaction due to** indwelling ureteral stent

     ☑7ᵗʰ **T83.593 Infection and inflammatory reaction due to other urinary stents**
Infection and inflammatory reaction due to ileal conduit stents
Infection and inflammatory reaction due to nephroureteral stent

     ☑7ᵗʰ **T83.598 Infection and inflammatory reaction due to other prosthetic device, implant and graft in urinary system**

☑5ᵗʰ **T83.6 Infection and inflammatory reaction due to prosthetic device, implant and graft in** genital tract
Use additional code to identify infection

     ☑x7ᵗʰ **T83.61 Infection and inflammatory reaction due to** implanted penile prosthesis
Infection and inflammatory reaction due to penile prosthesis cylinder
Infection and inflammatory reaction due to penile prosthesis pump
Infection and inflammatory reaction due to penile prosthesis reservoir

     ☑x7ᵗʰ **T83.62 Infection and inflammatory reaction due to** implanted testicular prosthesis

     ☑x7ᵗʰ **T83.69 Infection and inflammatory reaction due to other prosthetic device, implant and graft in genital tract**

☑5ᵗʰ **T83.7 Complications due to** implanted mesh and other prosthetic materials

     ☑6ᵗʰ **T83.71 Erosion of implanted mesh and other prosthetic materials**

     ☑7ᵗʰ **T83.711 Erosion of implanted** vaginal **mesh to surrounding organ or tissue**   ♀
Erosion of implanted vaginal mesh into pelvic floor muscles

     ☑7ᵗʰ **T83.712 Erosion of implanted** urethral **mesh to surrounding organ or tissue**
Erosion of implanted female urethral sling
Erosion of implanted male urethral sling
Erosion of implanted urethral mesh into pelvic floor muscles

     ☑7ᵗʰ **T83.713 Erosion of implanted** urethral bulking agent **to surrounding organ or tissue**

     ☑7ᵗʰ **T83.714 Erosion of implanted** ureteral bulking agent **to surrounding organ or tissue**

     ☑7ᵗʰ **T83.718 Erosion of other implanted mesh to organ or tissue**

     ☑7ᵗʰ **T83.719 Erosion of other prosthetic materials to surrounding organ or tissue**

     ☑6ᵗʰ **T83.72 Exposure of implanted mesh and other prosthetic materials into surrounding organ or tissue**
Extrusion of implanted mesh

     ☑7ᵗʰ **T83.721 Exposure of implanted** vaginal **mesh into** vagina   ♀
Exposure of implanted vaginal mesh through vaginal wall

     ☑7ᵗʰ **T83.722 Exposure of implanted** urethral mesh **into** urethra
Exposure of implanted female urethral sling
Exposure of implanted male urethral sling
Exposure of implanted urethral mesh through urethral wall

     ☑7ᵗʰ **T83.723 Exposure of implanted** urethral bulking agent **into** urethra

     ☑7ᵗʰ **T83.724 Exposure of implanted** ureteral bulking agent **into** ureter

     ☑7ᵗʰ **T83.728 Exposure of** other implanted mesh **into organ or tissue**

     ☑7ᵗʰ **T83.729 Exposure of** other prosthetic materials **into organ or tissue**

     ☑x7ᵗʰ **T83.79 Other specified complications due to other genitourinary prosthetic materials**

☑5ᵗʰ **T83.8 Other specified complications of** genitourinary prosthetic devices, implants and grafts

     ☑x7ᵗʰ **T83.81 Embolism due to genitourinary prosthetic devices, implants and grafts**

     ☑x7ᵗʰ **T83.82 Fibrosis due to genitourinary prosthetic devices, implants and grafts**

     ☑x7ᵗʰ **T83.83 Hemorrhage due to genitourinary prosthetic devices, implants and grafts**

     ☑x7ᵗʰ **T83.84 Pain due to genitourinary prosthetic devices, implants and grafts**

     ☑x7ᵗʰ **T83.85 Stenosis due to genitourinary prosthetic devices, implants and grafts**

     ☑x7ᵗʰ **T83.86 Thrombosis due to genitourinary prosthetic devices, implants and grafts**

     ☑x7ᵗʰ **T83.89 Other specified complication of genitourinary prosthetic devices, implants and grafts**

☑x7ᵗʰ **T83.9 Unspecified complication of genitourinary prosthetic device, implant and graft**

Ⓝ Newborn: 0   Ⓟ Pediatric: 0-17   Ⓜ Maternity: 12-55   Ⓐ Adult: 15-124   **CH** Comorbidity High   **CL** Comorbidity Low   **NCDx** Noncancer Dx   **PDx** Primary Dx

1130   ICD-10-CM 2020

✓4ᵗʰ **T84 Complications of internal orthopedic prosthetic devices, implants and grafts**

EXCLUDES 2   *failure and rejection of transplanted organs and tissues (T86.-)*
fracture of bone following insertion of orthopedic implant, joint prosthesis or bone plate (M96.6)

The appropriate 7th character is to be added to each code from category T84.
A   initial encounter
D   subsequent encounter
S   sequela

✓5ᵗʰ **T84.0 Mechanical complication of** internal joint prosthesis

✓6ᵗʰ **T84.01 Broken internal joint prosthesis**
Breakage (fracture) of prosthetic joint
Broken prosthetic joint implant
EXCLUDES 1 *periprosthetic joint implant fracture (M97-)*
AHA: 2016,4Q,42

✓7ᵗʰ **T84.010 Broken internal** right hip **prosthesis**
✓7ᵗʰ **T84.011 Broken internal** left hip **prosthesis**
✓7ᵗʰ **T84.012 Broken internal** right knee **prosthesis**
✓7ᵗʰ **T84.013 Broken internal** left knee **prosthesis**
✓7ᵗʰ **T84.018 Broken internal joint prosthesis, other site**
Use additional code to identify the joint (Z96.6-)
✓7ᵗʰ **T84.019 Broken internal joint prosthesis, unspecified site**

✓6ᵗʰ **T84.02 Dislocation** of internal joint prosthesis
Instability of internal joint prosthesis
Subluxation of internal joint prosthesis
AHA: 2019,2Q,27

✓7ᵗʰ **T84.020 Dislocation of internal** right hip **prosthesis**
✓7ᵗʰ **T84.021 Dislocation of internal** left hip **prosthesis**
✓7ᵗʰ **T84.022 Instability of internal** right knee **prosthesis**
✓7ᵗʰ **T84.023 Instability of internal** left knee **prosthesis**
✓7ᵗʰ **T84.028 Dislocation of other internal joint prosthesis**
Use additional code to identify the joint (Z96.6-)
✓7ᵗʰ **T84.029 Dislocation of unspecified internal joint prosthesis**

✓6ᵗʰ **T84.03 Mechanical loosening** of internal prosthetic joint
Aseptic loosening of prosthetic joint
✓7ᵗʰ **T84.030 Mechanical loosening of internal** right hip **prosthetic joint**
✓7ᵗʰ **T84.031 Mechanical loosening of internal** left hip **prosthetic joint**
✓7ᵗʰ **T84.032 Mechanical loosening of internal** right knee **prosthetic joint**
✓7ᵗʰ **T84.033 Mechanical loosening of internal** left knee **prosthetic joint**
✓7ᵗʰ **T84.038 Mechanical loosening of other internal prosthetic joint**
Use additional code to identify the joint (Z96.6-)
✓7ᵗʰ **T84.039 Mechanical loosening of unspecified internal prosthetic joint**

✓6ᵗʰ **T84.05 Periprosthetic osteolysis** of internal prosthetic joint
Use additional code to identify major osseous defect, if applicable (M89.7-)
✓7ᵗʰ **T84.050 Periprosthetic osteolysis of internal prosthetic** right hip joint
✓7ᵗʰ **T84.051 Periprosthetic osteolysis of internal prosthetic** left hip joint
✓7ᵗʰ **T84.052 Periprosthetic osteolysis of internal prosthetic** right knee joint
✓7ᵗʰ **T84.053 Periprosthetic osteolysis of internal prosthetic** left knee joint
✓7ᵗʰ **T84.058 Periprosthetic osteolysis of other internal prosthetic joint**
Use additional code to identify the joint (Z96.6-)
✓7ᵗʰ **T84.059 Periprosthetic osteolysis of unspecified internal prosthetic joint**

✓6ᵗʰ **T84.06 Wear of articular bearing surface** of internal prosthetic joint
✓7ᵗʰ **T84.060 Wear of articular bearing surface of internal prosthetic** right hip joint
✓7ᵗʰ **T84.061 Wear of articular bearing surface of internal prosthetic** left hip joint
✓7ᵗʰ **T84.062 Wear of articular bearing surface of internal prosthetic** right knee joint
✓7ᵗʰ **T84.063 Wear of articular bearing surface of internal prosthetic** left knee joint
✓7ᵗʰ **T84.068 Wear of articular bearing surface of other internal prosthetic joint**
Use additional code to identify the joint (Z96.6-)
✓7ᵗʰ **T84.069 Wear of articular bearing surface of unspecified internal prosthetic joint**

✓6ᵗʰ **T84.09 Other mechanical complication** of internal joint prosthesis
Prosthetic joint implant failure NOS
AHA: 2019,1Q,20
✓7ᵗʰ **T84.090 Other mechanical complication of internal** right hip prosthesis
✓7ᵗʰ **T84.091 Other mechanical complication of internal** left hip prosthesis
✓7ᵗʰ **T84.092 Other mechanical complication of internal** right knee prosthesis
✓7ᵗʰ **T84.093 Other mechanical complication of internal** left knee prosthesis
✓7ᵗʰ **T84.098 Other mechanical complication of other internal joint prosthesis**
Use additional code to identify the joint (Z96.6-)
✓7ᵗʰ **T84.099 Other mechanical complication of unspecified internal joint prosthesis**

✓5ᵗʰ **T84.1 Mechanical complication of** internal fixation device of bones of limb
EXCLUDES 2 *mechanical complication of internal fixation device of bones of feet (T84.2-)*
mechanical complication of internal fixation device of bones of fingers (T84.2-)
mechanical complication of internal fixation device of bones of hands (T84.2-)
mechanical complication of internal fixation device of bones of toes (T84.2-)

✓6ᵗʰ **T84.11 Breakdown** (mechanical) of internal fixation device of bones of limb
✓7ᵗʰ **T84.110 Breakdown (mechanical) of internal fixation device of** right humerus
✓7ᵗʰ **T84.111 Breakdown (mechanical) of internal fixation device of** left humerus
✓7ᵗʰ **T84.112 Breakdown (mechanical) of internal fixation device of bone of** right forearm
✓7ᵗʰ **T84.113 Breakdown (mechanical) of internal fixation device of bone of** left forearm
✓7ᵗʰ **T84.114 Breakdown (mechanical) of internal fixation device of** right femur
✓7ᵗʰ **T84.115 Breakdown (mechanical) of internal fixation device of** left femur
✓7ᵗʰ **T84.116 Breakdown (mechanical) of internal fixation device of bone of** right lower leg
✓7ᵗʰ **T84.117 Breakdown (mechanical) of internal fixation device of bone of** left lower leg
✓7ᵗʰ **T84.119 Breakdown (mechanical) of internal fixation device of unspecified bone of limb**

✓6ᵗʰ **T84.12 Displacement** of internal fixation device of bones of limb
Malposition of internal fixation device of bones of limb
✓7ᵗʰ **T84.120 Displacement of internal fixation device of** right humerus
✓7ᵗʰ **T84.121 Displacement of internal fixation device of** left humerus
✓7ᵗʰ **T84.122 Displacement of internal fixation device of bone of** right forearm
✓7ᵗʰ **T84.123 Displacement of internal fixation device of bone of** left forearm
✓7ᵗʰ **T84.124 Displacement of internal fixation device of** right femur
✓7ᵗʰ **T84.125 Displacement of internal fixation device of** left femur

√7ᵗʰ **T84.126** Displacement of internal fixation device of bone of right lower leg

√7ᵗʰ **T84.127** Displacement of internal fixation device of bone of left lower leg

√7ᵗʰ **T84.129** Displacement of internal fixation device of unspecified bone of limb

√6ᵗʰ **T84.19** Other mechanical complication of internal fixation device of bones of limb

    Obstruction (mechanical) of internal fixation device of bones of limb

    Perforation of internal fixation device of bones of limb

    Protrusion of internal fixation device of bones of limb

√7ᵗʰ **T84.190** Other mechanical complication of internal fixation device of right humerus

√7ᵗʰ **T84.191** Other mechanical complication of internal fixation device of left humerus

√7ᵗʰ **T84.192** Other mechanical complication of internal fixation device of bone of right forearm

√7ᵗʰ **T84.193** Other mechanical complication of internal fixation device of bone of left forearm

√7ᵗʰ **T84.194** Other mechanical complication of internal fixation device of right femur

√7ᵗʰ **T84.195** Other mechanical complication of internal fixation device of left femur

√7ᵗʰ **T84.196** Other mechanical complication of internal fixation device of bone of right lower leg

√7ᵗʰ **T84.197** Other mechanical complication of internal fixation device of bone of left lower leg

√7ᵗʰ **T84.199** Other mechanical complication of internal fixation device of unspecified bone of limb

√5ᵗʰ **T84.2** Mechanical complication of internal fixation device of other bones

√6ᵗʰ **T84.21** Breakdown (mechanical) of internal fixation device of other bones

√7ᵗʰ **T84.210** Breakdown (mechanical) of internal fixation device of bones of hand and fingers

√7ᵗʰ **T84.213** Breakdown (mechanical) of internal fixation device of bones of foot and toes

√7ᵗʰ **T84.216** Breakdown (mechanical) of internal fixation device of vertebrae

√7ᵗʰ **T84.218** Breakdown (mechanical) of internal fixation device of other bones

√6ᵗʰ **T84.22** Displacement of internal fixation device of other bones

    Malposition of internal fixation device of other bones

√7ᵗʰ **T84.220** Displacement of internal fixation device of bones of hand and fingers

√7ᵗʰ **T84.223** Displacement of internal fixation device of bones of foot and toes

√7ᵗʰ **T84.226** Displacement of internal fixation device of vertebrae

√7ᵗʰ **T84.228** Displacement of internal fixation device of other bones

√6ᵗʰ **T84.29** Other mechanical complication of internal fixation device of other bones

    Obstruction (mechanical) of internal fixation device of other bones

    Perforation of internal fixation device of other bones

    Protrusion of internal fixation device of other bones

√7ᵗʰ **T84.290** Other mechanical complication of internal fixation device of bones of hand and fingers

√7ᵗʰ **T84.293** Other mechanical complication of internal fixation device of bones of foot and toes

√7ᵗʰ **T84.296** Other mechanical complication of internal fixation device of vertebrae

√7ᵗʰ **T84.298** Other mechanical complication of internal fixation device of other bones

√5ᵗʰ **T84.3** Mechanical complication of other bone devices, implants and grafts

    EXCLUDES 2   other complications of bone graft (T86.83-)

√6ᵗʰ **T84.31** Breakdown (mechanical) of other bone devices, implants and grafts

√7ᵗʰ **T84.310** Breakdown (mechanical) of electronic bone stimulator

√7ᵗʰ **T84.318** Breakdown (mechanical) of other bone devices, implants and grafts

√6ᵗʰ **T84.32** Displacement of other bone devices, implants and grafts

    Malposition of other bone devices, implants and grafts

√7ᵗʰ **T84.320** Displacement of electronic bone stimulator

√7ᵗʰ **T84.328** Displacement of other bone devices, implants and grafts

    AHA: 2014,4Q,28

√6ᵗʰ **T84.39** Other mechanical complication of other bone devices, implants and grafts

    Obstruction (mechanical) of other bone devices, implants and grafts

    Perforation of other bone devices, implants and grafts

    Protrusion of other bone devices, implants and grafts

√7ᵗʰ **T84.390** Other mechanical complication of electronic bone stimulator

√7ᵗʰ **T84.398** Other mechanical complication of other bone devices, implants and grafts

√5ᵗʰ **T84.4** Mechanical complication of other internal orthopedic devices, implants and grafts

√6ᵗʰ **T84.41** Breakdown (mechanical) of other internal orthopedic devices, implants and grafts

√7ᵗʰ **T84.410** Breakdown (mechanical) of muscle and tendon graft

√7ᵗʰ **T84.418** Breakdown (mechanical) of other internal orthopedic devices, implants and grafts

√6ᵗʰ **T84.42** Displacement of other internal orthopedic devices, implants and grafts

    Malposition of other internal orthopedic devices, implants and grafts

√7ᵗʰ **T84.420** Displacement of muscle and tendon graft

√7ᵗʰ **T84.428** Displacement of other internal orthopedic devices, implants and grafts

√6ᵗʰ **T84.49** Other mechanical complication of other internal orthopedic devices, implants and grafts

    Mechanical complication of other internal orthopedic devices, implants and grafts NOS

    Obstruction (mechanical) of other internal orthopedic devices, implants and grafts

    Perforation of other internal orthopedic devices, implants and grafts

    Protrusion of other internal orthopedic devices, implants and grafts

√7ᵗʰ **T84.490** Other mechanical complication of muscle and tendon graft

√7ᵗʰ **T84.498** Other mechanical complication of other internal orthopedic devices, implants and grafts

√5ᵗʰ **T84.5** Infection and inflammatory reaction due to internal joint prosthesis

    Use additional code to identify infection

    AHA: 2015,1Q,16

√x7ᵗʰ **T84.50** Infection and inflammatory reaction due to unspecified internal joint prosthesis

√x7ᵗʰ **T84.51** Infection and inflammatory reaction due to internal right hip prosthesis

√x7ᵗʰ **T84.52** Infection and inflammatory reaction due to internal left hip prosthesis

√x7ᵗʰ **T84.53** Infection and inflammatory reaction due to internal right knee prosthesis

√x7ᵗʰ **T84.54** Infection and inflammatory reaction due to internal left knee prosthesis

√x7ᵗʰ **T84.59** Infection and inflammatory reaction due to other internal joint prosthesis

√5ᵗʰ **T84.6** Infection and inflammatory reaction due to internal fixation device

    Use additional code to identify infection

√x7ᵗʰ **T84.60** Infection and inflammatory reaction due to internal fixation device of unspecified site

√6ᵗʰ **T84.61** Infection and inflammatory reaction due to internal fixation device of arm

√7ᵗʰ **T84.610** Infection and inflammatory reaction due to internal fixation device of right humerus

√7ᵗʰ **T84.611** Infection and inflammatory reaction due to internal fixation device of left humerus

√7ᵗʰ **T84.612** Infection and inflammatory reaction due to internal fixation device of right radius

Ⓝ Newborn: 0   Ⓟ Pediatric: 0-17   Ⓜ Maternity: 12-55   Ⓐ Adult: 15-124   CH Comorbidity High   CL Comorbidity Low   NCDx Noncancer Dx   PDx Primary Dx

1132   ICD-10-CM 2020

☑7ᵗʰ **T84.613** Infection and inflammatory reaction due to internal fixation device of left radius

☑7ᵗʰ **T84.614** Infection and inflammatory reaction due to internal fixation device of right ulna

☑7ᵗʰ **T84.615** Infection and inflammatory reaction due to internal fixation device of left ulna

☑7ᵗʰ **T84.619** Infection and inflammatory reaction due to internal fixation device of unspecified bone of arm

√6ᵗʰ **T84.62** Infection and inflammatory reaction due to internal fixation device of leg

☑7ᵗʰ **T84.620** Infection and inflammatory reaction due to internal fixation device of right femur

☑7ᵗʰ **T84.621** Infection and inflammatory reaction due to internal fixation device of left femur

☑7ᵗʰ **T84.622** Infection and inflammatory reaction due to internal fixation device of right tibia

☑7ᵗʰ **T84.623** Infection and inflammatory reaction due to internal fixation device of left tibia

☑7ᵗʰ **T84.624** Infection and inflammatory reaction due to internal fixation device of right fibula

☑7ᵗʰ **T84.625** Infection and inflammatory reaction due to internal fixation device of left fibula

☑7ᵗʰ **T84.629** Infection and inflammatory reaction due to internal fixation device of unspecified bone of leg

√x7ᵗʰ **T84.63** Infection and inflammatory reaction due to internal fixation device of spine

√x7ᵗʰ **T84.69** Infection and inflammatory reaction due to internal fixation device of other site

√x7ᵗʰ **T84.7** Infection and inflammatory reaction due to other internal orthopedic prosthetic devices, implants and grafts
Use additional code to identify infection

√5ᵗʰ **T84.8** Other specified complications of internal orthopedic prosthetic devices, implants and grafts

√x7ᵗʰ **T84.81** Embolism due to internal orthopedic prosthetic devices, implants and grafts

√x7ᵗʰ **T84.82** Fibrosis due to internal orthopedic prosthetic devices, implants and grafts

√x7ᵗʰ **T84.83** Hemorrhage due to internal orthopedic prosthetic devices, implants and grafts

√x7ᵗʰ **T84.84** Pain due to internal orthopedic prosthetic devices, implants and grafts

√x7ᵗʰ **T84.85** Stenosis due to internal orthopedic prosthetic devices, implants and grafts

√x7ᵗʰ **T84.86** Thrombosis due to internal orthopedic prosthetic devices, implants and grafts

√x7ᵗʰ **T84.89** Other specified complication of internal orthopedic prosthetic devices, implants and grafts

√x7ᵗʰ **T84.9** Unspecified complication of internal orthopedic prosthetic device, implant and graft

√4ᵗʰ **T85** Complications of other internal prosthetic devices, implants and grafts

EXCLUDES 2   *failure and rejection of transplanted organs and tissue (T86.-)*

AHA: 2016,4Q,71-72

The appropriate 7th character is to be added to each code from category T85.
A   initial encounter
D   subsequent encounter
S   sequela

√5ᵗʰ **T85.0** Mechanical complication of ventricular intracranial (communicating) shunt

√x7ᵗʰ **T85.01** Breakdown (mechanical) of ventricular intracranial (communicating) shunt

√x7ᵗʰ **T85.02** Displacement of ventricular intracranial (communicating) shunt
Malposition of ventricular intracranial (communicating) shunt

√x7ᵗʰ **T85.03** Leakage of ventricular intracranial (communicating) shunt

√x7ᵗʰ **T85.09** Other mechanical complication of ventricular intracranial (communicating) shunt
Obstruction (mechanical) of ventricular intracranial (communicating) shunt
Perforation of ventricular intracranial (communicating) shunt
Protrusion of ventricular intracranial (communicating) shunt

√5ᵗʰ **T85.1** Mechanical complication of implanted electronic stimulator of nervous system

√6ᵗʰ **T85.11** Breakdown (mechanical) of implanted electronic stimulator of nervous system

☑7ᵗʰ **T85.110** Breakdown (mechanical) of implanted electronic neurostimulator of brain electrode (lead)

☑7ᵗʰ **T85.111** Breakdown (mechanical) of implanted electronic neurostimulator of peripheral nerve electrode (lead)
Breakdown of electrode (lead) for cranial nerve neurostimulators
Breakdown of electrode (lead) for gastric neurostimulator
Breakdown of electrode (lead) for sacral nerve neurostimulator
Breakdown of electrode (lead) for vagal nerve neurostimulators

☑7ᵗʰ **T85.112** Breakdown (mechanical) of implanted electronic neurostimulator of spinal cord electrode (lead)

☑7ᵗʰ **T85.113** Breakdown (mechanical) of implanted electronic neurostimulator, generator
Breakdown (mechanical) of implanted electronic neurostimulator generator, brain, peripheral, gastric, spinal
Breakdown (mechanical) of implanted electronic sacral neurostimulator, pulse generator or receiver

☑7ᵗʰ **T85.118** Breakdown (mechanical) of other implanted electronic stimulator of nervous system

√6ᵗʰ **T85.12** Displacement of implanted electronic stimulator of nervous system
Malposition of implanted electronic stimulator of nervous system

☑7ᵗʰ **T85.120** Displacement of implanted electronic neurostimulator of brain electrode (lead)

☑7ᵗʰ **T85.121** Displacement of implanted electronic neurostimulator of peripheral nerve electrode (lead)
Displacement of electrode (lead) for cranial nerve neurostimulators
Displacement of electrode (lead) for gastric neurostimulator
Displacement of electrode (lead) for sacral nerve neurostimulator
Displacement of electrode (lead) for vagal nerve neurostimulators

☑7ᵗʰ **T85.122** Displacement of implanted electronic neurostimulator of spinal cord electrode (lead)

☑7ᵗʰ **T85.123** Displacement of implanted electronic neurostimulator, generator
Displacement of implanted electronic neurostimulator generator, brain, peripheral, gastric, spinal
Displacement of implanted electronic sacral neurostimulator, pulse generator or receiver

☑7ᵗʰ **T85.128** Displacement of other implanted electronic stimulator of nervous system

√6ᵗʰ **T85.19** Other mechanical complication of implanted electronic stimulator of nervous system
Leakage of implanted electronic stimulator of nervous system
Obstruction (mechanical) of implanted electronic stimulator of nervous system
Perforation of implanted electronic stimulator of nervous system
Protrusion of implanted electronic stimulator of nervous system

☑7ᵗʰ **T85.190** Other mechanical complication of implanted electronic neurostimulator of brain electrode (lead)

☑ Additional Character Required   √x7ᵗʰ Placeholder Alert   Manifestation   Unspecified Dx   ►◄ Revised Text   ● New Code   ▲ Revised Title

☑7ᵗʰ **T85.191** **Other mechanical complication of implanted electronic neurostimulator of** peripheral nerve electrode (lead)

Other mechanical complication of electrode (lead) for cranial nerve neurostimulators

Other mechanical complication of electrode (lead) for gastric neurostimulator

Other mechanical complication of electrode (lead) for sacral nerve neurostimulator

Other mechanical complication of electrode (lead) for vagal nerve neurostimulators

☑7ᵗʰ **T85.192** **Other mechanical complication of implanted electronic neurostimulator of** spinal cord electrode (lead)

☑7ᵗʰ **T85.193** **Other mechanical complication of implanted electronic neurostimulator,** generator

Other mechanical complication of implanted electronic neurostimulator generator, brain, peripheral, gastric, spinal

Other mechanical complication of implanted electronic sacral neurostimulator, pulse generator or receiver

☑7ᵗʰ **T85.199** **Other mechanical complication of other implanted electronic stimulator of nervous system**

☑5ᵗʰ **T85.2** **Mechanical complication of** intraocular lens

☑ₓ7ᵗʰ **T85.21** **Breakdown (mechanical) of intraocular lens**

☑ₓ7ᵗʰ **T85.22** **Displacement of intraocular lens**

Malposition of intraocular lens

☑ₓ7ᵗʰ **T85.29** **Other mechanical complication of intraocular lens**

Obstruction (mechanical) of intraocular lens

Perforation of intraocular lens

Protrusion of intraocular lens

☑5ᵗʰ **T85.3** **Mechanical complication of other ocular prosthetic devices, implants and grafts**

EXCLUDES 2   other complications of corneal graft (T86.84-)

☑6ᵗʰ **T85.31** **Breakdown (mechanical) of other ocular prosthetic devices, implants and grafts**

☑7ᵗʰ **T85.310** **Breakdown (mechanical) of prosthetic orbit of** right eye

☑7ᵗʰ **T85.311** **Breakdown (mechanical) of prosthetic orbit of** left eye

☑7ᵗʰ **T85.318** **Breakdown (mechanical) of other ocular prosthetic devices, implants and grafts**

☑6ᵗʰ **T85.32** **Displacement of other ocular prosthetic devices, implants and grafts**

Malposition of other ocular prosthetic devices, implants and grafts

☑7ᵗʰ **T85.320** **Displacement of prosthetic orbit of** right eye

☑7ᵗʰ **T85.321** **Displacement of prosthetic orbit of** left eye

☑7ᵗʰ **T85.328** **Displacement of other ocular prosthetic devices, implants and grafts**

☑6ᵗʰ **T85.39** **Other mechanical complication of other ocular prosthetic devices, implants and grafts**

Obstruction (mechanical) of other ocular prosthetic devices, implants and grafts

Perforation of other ocular prosthetic devices, implants and grafts

Protrusion of other ocular prosthetic devices, implants and grafts

☑7ᵗʰ **T85.390** **Other mechanical complication of prosthetic orbit of** right eye

☑7ᵗʰ **T85.391** **Other mechanical complication of prosthetic orbit of** left eye

☑7ᵗʰ **T85.398** **Other mechanical complication of other ocular prosthetic devices, implants and grafts**

☑5ᵗʰ **T85.4** **Mechanical complication of** breast prosthesis and implant

☑ₓ7ᵗʰ **T85.41** **Breakdown (mechanical) of breast prosthesis and implant**

☑ₓ7ᵗʰ **T85.42** **Displacement of breast prosthesis and implant**

Malposition of breast prosthesis and implant

☑ₓ7ᵗʰ **T85.43** **Leakage of breast prosthesis and implant**

☑ₓ7ᵗʰ **T85.44** **Capsular contracture of breast implant**

☑ₓ7ᵗʰ **T85.49** **Other mechanical complication of breast prosthesis and implant**

Obstruction (mechanical) of breast prosthesis and implant

Perforation of breast prosthesis and implant

Protrusion of breast prosthesis and implant

☑5ᵗʰ **T85.5** **Mechanical complication of** gastrointestinal prosthetic devices, implants and grafts

☑6ᵗʰ **T85.51** **Breakdown (mechanical) of gastrointestinal prosthetic devices, implants and grafts**

☑7ᵗʰ **T85.510** **Breakdown (mechanical) of** bile duct prosthesis

☑7ᵗʰ **T85.511** **Breakdown (mechanical) of** esophageal anti-reflux **device**

☑7ᵗʰ **T85.518** **Breakdown (mechanical) of other gastrointestinal prosthetic devices, implants and grafts**

☑6ᵗʰ **T85.52** **Displacement of gastrointestinal prosthetic devices, implants and grafts**

Malposition of gastrointestinal prosthetic devices, implants and grafts

☑7ᵗʰ **T85.520** **Displacement of** bile duct prosthesis

☑7ᵗʰ **T85.521** **Displacement of** esophageal anti-reflux **device**

☑7ᵗʰ **T85.528** **Displacement of other gastrointestinal prosthetic devices, implants and grafts**

☑6ᵗʰ **T85.59** **Other mechanical complication of gastrointestinal prosthetic devices, implants and**

Obstruction, mechanical of gastrointestinal prosthetic devices, implants and grafts

Perforation of gastrointestinal prosthetic devices, implants and grafts

Protrusion of gastrointestinal prosthetic devices, implants and grafts

☑7ᵗʰ **T85.590** **Other mechanical complication of** bile duct **prosthesis**

☑7ᵗʰ **T85.591** **Other mechanical complication of** esophageal anti-reflux **device**

☑7ᵗʰ **T85.598** **Other mechanical complication of other gastrointestinal prosthetic devices, implants and grafts**

☑5ᵗʰ **T85.6** **Mechanical complication of other specified internal and external prosthetic devices, implants and grafts**

☑6ᵗʰ **T85.61** **Breakdown (mechanical) of other specified internal prosthetic devices, implants and grafts**

☑7ᵗʰ **T85.610** **Breakdown (mechanical) of** cranial or spinal infusion catheter

Breakdown (mechanical) of epidural infusion catheter

Breakdown (mechanical) of intrathecal infusion catheter

Breakdown (mechanical) of subarachnoid infusion catheter

Breakdown (mechanical) of subdural infusion catheter

☑7ᵗʰ **T85.611** **Breakdown (mechanical) of** intraperitoneal dialysis catheter

EXCLUDES 1   mechanical complication of vascular dialysis catheter (T82.4-)

☑7ᵗʰ **T85.612** **Breakdown (mechanical) of** permanent sutures

EXCLUDES 1   mechanical complication of permanent (wire) suture used in bone repair (T84.1-T84.2)

Ⓝ Newborn: 0   Ⓟ Pediatric: 0-17   Ⓜ Maternity: 12-55   Ⓐ Adult: 15-124   CH Comorbidity High   CL Comorbidity Low   NCDx Noncancer Dx   PDx Primary Dx

1134   ICD-10-CM 2020

√7ᵗʰ **T85.613 Breakdown (mechanical) of** artificial skin graft and decellularized allodermis

Failure of artificial skin graft and decellularized allodermis

Non-adherence of artificial skin graft and decellularized allodermis

Poor incorporation of artificial skin graft and decellularized allodermis

Shearing of artificial skin graft and decellularized allodermis

√7ᵗʰ **T85.614 Breakdown (mechanical) of** insulin pump

√7ᵗʰ **T85.615 Breakdown (mechanical) of other nervous system device, implant or graft**

Breakdown (mechanical) of intrathecal infusion pump

√7ᵗʰ **T85.618 Breakdown (mechanical) of other specified internal prosthetic devices, implants and grafts**

√6ᵗʰ **T85.62 Displacement of other specified internal prosthetic devices, implants and grafts**

Malposition of other specified internal prosthetic devices, implants and grafts

√7ᵗʰ **T85.620 Displacement of** cranial or spinal infusion catheter

Displacement of epidural infusion catheter

Displacement of intrathecal infusion catheter

Displacement of subarachnoid infusion catheter

Displacement of subdural infusion catheter

√7ᵗʰ **T85.621 Displacement of** intraperitoneal dialysis catheter

EXCLUDES 1   mechanical complication of vascular dialysis catheter (T82.4-)

√7ᵗʰ **T85.622 Displacement of** permanent sutures

EXCLUDES 1   mechanical complication of permanent (wire) suture used in bone repair (T84.1-T84.2)

√7ᵗʰ **T85.623 Displacement of** artificial skin graft and decellularized allodermis

Dislodgement of artificial skin graft and decellularized allodermis

√7ᵗʰ **T85.624 Displacement of** insulin pump

√7ᵗʰ **T85.625 Displacement of other nervous system device, implant or graft**

Displacement of intrathecal infusion pump

√7ᵗʰ **T85.628 Displacement of other specified internal prosthetic devices, implants and grafts**

√6ᵗʰ **T85.63 Leakage of other specified internal prosthetic devices, implants and grafts**

√7ᵗʰ **T85.630 Leakage of** cranial or spinal infusion catheter

Leakage of epidural infusion catheter

Leakage of intrathecal infusion catheter infusion catheter

Leakage of subdural infusion catheter

Leakage of subarachnoid infusion catheter

√7ᵗʰ **T85.631 Leakage of** intraperitoneal dialysis catheter

EXCLUDES 1   mechanical complication of vascular dialysis catheter (T82.4)

√7ᵗʰ **T85.633 Leakage of** insulin pump

√7ᵗʰ **T85.635 Leakage of other nervous system device, implant or graft**

Leakage of intrathecal infusion pump

√7ᵗʰ **T85.638 Leakage of other specified internal prosthetic devices, implants and grafts**

√6ᵗʰ **T85.69 Other mechanical complication of other specified internal prosthetic devices, implants and grafts**

Obstruction, mechanical of other specified internal prosthetic devices, implants and grafts

Perforation of other specified internal prosthetic devices, implants and grafts

Protrusion of other specified internal prosthetic devices, implants and grafts

√7ᵗʰ **T85.690 Other mechanical complication of** cranial or spinal infusion catheter

Other mechanical complication of epidural infusion catheter

Other mechanical complication of intrathecal infusion catheter

Other mechanical complication of subarachnoid infusion catheter

Other mechanical complication of subdural infusion catheter

√7ᵗʰ **T85.691 Other mechanical complication of intraperitoneal dialysis catheter**

EXCLUDES 1   mechanical complication of vascular dialysis catheter (T82.4)

√7ᵗʰ **T85.692 Other mechanical complication of permanent sutures**

EXCLUDES 1   mechanical complication of permanent (wire) suture used in bone repair (T84.1-T84.2)

√7ᵗʰ **T85.693 Other mechanical complication of artificial skin graft and decellularized allodermis**

√7ᵗʰ **T85.694 Other mechanical complication of** insulin pump

√7ᵗʰ **T85.695 Other mechanical complication of other nervous system device, implant or graft**

Other mechanical complication of intrathecal infusion pump

√7ᵗʰ **T85.698 Other mechanical complication of other specified internal prosthetic devices, implants and grafts**

Mechanical complication of nonabsorbable surgical material NOS

√5ᵗʰ **T85.7 Infection and inflammatory reaction due to other internal prosthetic devices, implants and grafts**

Use additional code to identify infection

√x7ᵗʰ **T85.71 Infection and inflammatory reaction due to** peritoneal dialysis catheter

√x7ᵗʰ **T85.72 Infection and inflammatory reaction due to** insulin pump

√6ᵗʰ **T85.73 Infection and inflammatory reaction due to** nervous system **devices, implants and graft**

√7ᵗʰ **T85.730 Infection and inflammatory reaction due to** ventricular intracranial (communicating) shunt

√7ᵗʰ **T85.731 Infection and inflammatory reaction due to implanted electronic neurostimulator of** brain, electrode (lead)

√7ᵗʰ **T85.732 Infection and inflammatory reaction due to implanted electronic neurostimulator of** peripheral nerve, electrode (lead)

Infection and inflammatory reaction due to electrode (lead) for cranial nerve neurostimulators

Infection and inflammatory reaction due to electrode (lead) for gastric neurostimulator

Infection and inflammatory reaction due to electrode (lead) for sacral nerve neurostimulator

Infection and inflammatory reaction due to electrode (lead) for vagal nerve neurostimulators

√7ᵗʰ **T85.733 Infection and inflammatory reaction due to implanted electronic neurostimulator of** spinal cord, electrode (lead)

√7ᵗʰ **T85.734 Infection and inflammatory reaction due to implanted electronic neurostimulator, generator**

Generator pocket infection

☑ Additional Character Required   √x7ᵗʰ Placeholder Alert   Manifestation   Unspecified Dx   ▶◀ Revised Text   ● New Code   ▲ Revised Title

ICD-10-CM 2020   1135

Chapter 19. Injury, Poisoning and Certain Other Consequences of External Causes

✓7ᵗʰ **T85.735** **Infection and inflammatory reaction due to cranial or spinal infusion catheter**

Infection and inflammatory reaction due to epidural catheter

Infection and inflammatory reaction due to intrathecal infusion catheter

Infection and inflammatory reaction due to subarachnoid catheter

Infection and inflammatory reaction due to subdural catheter

✓7ᵗʰ **T85.738** **Infection and inflammatory reaction due to other nervous system device, implant or graft**

Infection and inflammatory reaction due to intrathecal infusion pump

✓x7ᵗʰ **T85.79** **Infection and inflammatory reaction due to other internal prosthetic devices, implants and grafts**

✓5ᵗʰ **T85.8** **Other specified complications of internal prosthetic devices, implants and grafts, not elsewhere classified**

✓6ᵗʰ **T85.81** **Embolism due to internal prosthetic devices, implants and grafts, not elsewhere classified**

✓7ᵗʰ **T85.810** **Embolism due to nervous system prosthetic devices, implants and grafts**

✓7ᵗʰ **T85.818** **Embolism due to other internal prosthetic devices, implants and grafts**

✓6ᵗʰ **T85.82** **Fibrosis due to internal prosthetic devices, implants and grafts, not elsewhere classified**

✓7ᵗʰ **T85.820** **Fibrosis due to nervous system prosthetic devices, implants and grafts**

✓7ᵗʰ **T85.828** **Fibrosis due to other internal prosthetic devices, implants and grafts**

✓6ᵗʰ **T85.83** **Hemorrhage due to internal prosthetic devices, implants and grafts, not elsewhere classified**

✓7ᵗʰ **T85.830** **Hemorrhage due to nervous system prosthetic devices, implants and grafts**

✓7ᵗʰ **T85.838** **Hemorrhage due to other internal prosthetic devices, implants and grafts**

✓6ᵗʰ **T85.84** **Pain due to internal prosthetic devices, implants and grafts, not elsewhere classified**

✓7ᵗʰ **T85.840** **Pain due to nervous system prosthetic devices, implants and grafts**

✓7ᵗʰ **T85.848** **Pain due to other internal prosthetic devices, implants and grafts**

✓6ᵗʰ **T85.85** **Stenosis due to internal prosthetic devices, implants and grafts, not elsewhere classified**

✓7ᵗʰ **T85.850** **Stenosis due to nervous system prosthetic devices, implants and grafts**

✓7ᵗʰ **T85.858** **Stenosis due to other internal prosthetic devices, implants and grafts**

✓6ᵗʰ **T85.86** **Thrombosis due to internal prosthetic devices, implants and grafts, not elsewhere classified**

✓7ᵗʰ **T85.860** **Thrombosis due to nervous system prosthetic devices, implants and grafts**

✓7ᵗʰ **T85.868** **Thrombosis due to other internal prosthetic devices, implants and grafts**

✓6ᵗʰ **T85.89** **Other specified complication of internal prosthetic devices, implants and grafts, not elsewhere classified**

Erosion or breakdown of subcutaneous device pocket

✓7ᵗʰ **T85.890** **Other specified complication of nervous system prosthetic devices, implants and grafts**

✓7ᵗʰ **T85.898** **Other specified complication of other internal prosthetic devices, implants and grafts**

✓x7ᵗʰ **T85.9** **Unspecified complication of internal prosthetic device, implant and graft**

Complication of internal prosthetic device, implant and graft NOS

✓4ᵗʰ **T86** **Complications of transplanted organs and tissue**

Use additional code to identify other transplant complications, such as:
graft-versus-host disease (D89.81-)
malignancy associated with organ transplant (C80.2)
post-transplant lymphoproliferative disorders (PTLD) (D47.Z1)

TIP: A nonmalignancy associated complication in a transplanted organ should be directly indicated in provider documentation.

✓5ᵗʰ **T86.0** **Complications of bone marrow transplant**

T86.00 **Unspecified complication of bone marrow transplant**

T86.01 **Bone marrow transplant rejection**

T86.02 **Bone marrow transplant failure**

T86.03 **Bone marrow transplant infection**

T86.09 **Other complications of bone marrow transplant**

✓5ᵗʰ **T86.1** **Complications of kidney transplant**

T86.10 **Unspecified complication of kidney transplant**

T86.11 **Kidney transplant rejection**

T86.12 **Kidney transplant failure**
AHA: 2013,1Q,24

T86.13 **Kidney transplant infection**
Use additional code to specify infection

T86.19 **Other complication of kidney transplant**
AHA: 2019,2Q,7

✓5ᵗʰ **T86.2** **Complications of heart transplant**

EXCLUDES 1   complication of:
artificial heart device (T82.5)
heart-lung transplant (T86.3)

T86.20 **Unspecified complication of heart transplant**

T86.21 **Heart transplant rejection**

T86.22 **Heart transplant failure**

T86.23 **Heart transplant infection**
Use additional code to specify infection

✓6ᵗʰ **T86.29** **Other complications of heart transplant**

T86.290 **Cardiac allograft vasculopathy**

EXCLUDES 1   atherosclerosis of coronary arteries (I25.75-, I25.76-, I25.81-)

T86.298 **Other complications of heart transplant**

✓5ᵗʰ **T86.3** **Complications of heart-lung transplant**

T86.30 **Unspecified complication of heart-lung transplant**

T86.31 **Heart-lung transplant rejection**

T86.32 **Heart-lung transplant failure**

T86.33 **Heart-lung transplant infection**
Use additional code to specify infection

T86.39 **Other complications of heart-lung transplant**

✓5ᵗʰ **T86.4** **Complications of liver transplant**

T86.40 **Unspecified complication of liver transplant**

T86.41 **Liver transplant rejection**

T86.42 **Liver transplant failure**

T86.43 **Liver transplant infection**
Use additional code to identify infection, such as: cytomegalovirus (CMV) infection (B25.-)

T86.49 **Other complications of liver transplant**

T86.5 **Complications of stem cell transplant**

Complications from stem cells from peripheral blood
Complications from stem cells from umbilical cord

✓5ᵗʰ **T86.8** **Complications of other transplanted organs and tissues**

✓6ᵗʰ **T86.81** **Complications of lung transplant**

EXCLUDES 1   complication of heart-lung transplant (T86.3-)

T86.810 **Lung transplant rejection**

T86.811 **Lung transplant failure**

T86.812 **Lung transplant infection**
Use additional code to specify infection

T86.818 **Other complications of lung transplant**
AHA: 2019,2Q,6

T86.819 **Unspecified complication of lung transplant**

✓6ᵗʰ **T86.82** **Complications of skin graft (allograft) (autograft)**

EXCLUDES 2   complication of artificial skin graft (T85.693)

T86.820 **Skin graft (allograft) rejection**

T86.821 **Skin graft (allograft) (autograft) failure**

T86.822 **Skin graft (allograft) (autograft) infection**
Use additional code to specify infection

T86.828 **Other complications of skin graft (allograft) (autograft)**

T86.829 **Unspecified complication of skin graft (allograft) (autograft)**

✓6ᵗʰ **T86.83** **Complications of bone graft**

EXCLUDES 2   mechanical complications of bone graft (T84.3-)

T86.830 **Bone graft rejection**

T86.831 **Bone graft failure**

T86.832 **Bone graft infection**
Use additional code to specify infection

T86.838 **Other complications of bone graft**

T86.839 **Unspecified complication of bone graft**

√6ᵗʰ **T86.84 Complications of corneal transplant**
> EXCLUDES 2   *mechanical complications of corneal graft (T85.3-)*

T86.840 Corneal transplant rejection
T86.841 Corneal transplant failure
T86.842 Corneal transplant infection
> Use additional code to specify infection

T86.848 Other complications of corneal transplant
T86.849 Unspecified complication of corneal transplant

√6ᵗʰ **T86.85 Complication of intestine transplant**
T86.850 Intestine transplant rejection
T86.851 Intestine transplant failure
T86.852 Intestine transplant infection
> Use additional code to specify infection

T86.858 Other complications of intestine transplant
T86.859 Unspecified complication of intestine transplant

√6ᵗʰ **T86.89 Complications of other transplanted tissue**
> Transplant failure or rejection of pancreas

T86.890 Other transplanted tissue rejection
T86.891 Other transplanted tissue failure
T86.892 Other transplanted tissue infection
> Use additional code to specify infection

T86.898 Other complications of other transplanted tissue
T86.899 Unspecified complication of other transplanted tissue

√5ᵗʰ **T86.9 Complication of unspecified transplanted organ and tissue**
T86.90 Unspecified complication of unspecified transplanted organ and tissue
T86.91 Unspecified transplanted organ and tissue rejection
T86.92 Unspecified transplanted organ and tissue failure
T86.93 Unspecified transplanted organ and tissue infection
> Use additional code to specify infection

T86.99 Other complications of unspecified transplanted organ and tissue

√4ᵗʰ **T87 Complications peculiar to reattachment and amputation**

√5ᵗʰ **T87.0 Complications of reattached (part of) upper extremity**
√6ᵗʰ **T87.0X Complications of reattached (part of) upper extremity**
T87.0X1 Complications of reattached (part of) right upper extremity
T87.0X2 Complications of reattached (part of) left upper extremity
T87.0X9 Complications of reattached (part of) unspecified upper extremity

√5ᵗʰ **T87.1 Complications of reattached (part of) lower extremity**
√6ᵗʰ **T87.1X Complications of reattached (part of) lower extremity**
T87.1X1 Complications of reattached (part of) right lower extremity
T87.1X2 Complications of reattached (part of) left lower extremity
T87.1X9 Complications of reattached (part of) unspecified lower extremity

T87.2 Complications of other reattached body part
√5ᵗʰ **T87.3 Neuroma of amputation stump**
> **DEF:** Non-neoplastic tumor generated at the proximal end of severed, partially transected, or injured nerve following amputation.

T87.30 Neuroma of amputation stump, unspecified extremity
T87.31 Neuroma of amputation stump, right upper extremity
T87.32 Neuroma of amputation stump, left upper extremity
T87.33 Neuroma of amputation stump, right lower extremity
T87.34 Neuroma of amputation stump, left lower extremity

√5ᵗʰ **T87.4 Infection of amputation stump**
T87.40 Infection of amputation stump, unspecified extremity
T87.41 Infection of amputation stump, right upper extremity
T87.42 Infection of amputation stump, left upper extremity
T87.43 Infection of amputation stump, right lower extremity

T87.44 Infection of amputation stump, left lower extremity
√5ᵗʰ **T87.5 Necrosis of amputation stump**
T87.50 Necrosis of amputation stump, unspecified extremity
T87.51 Necrosis of amputation stump, right upper extremity
T87.52 Necrosis of amputation stump, left upper extremity
T87.53 Necrosis of amputation stump, right lower extremity
T87.54 Necrosis of amputation stump, left lower extremity

√5ᵗʰ **T87.8 Other complications of amputation stump**
> **TIP:** An ulcer (such as pressure ulcer, diabetic ulcer, or other) is generally not considered a complication of the amputation stump. Code the ulcer by site and etiology.

T87.81 Dehiscence of amputation stump
T87.89 Other complications of amputation stump
> Amputation stump contracture
> Amputation stump contracture of next proximal joint
> Amputation stump flexion
> Amputation stump edema
> Amputation stump hematoma
> EXCLUDES 2   *phantom limb syndrome (G54.6-G54.7)*

T87.9 Unspecified complications of amputation stump

√4ᵗʰ **T88 Other complications of surgical and medical care, not elsewhere classified**
> EXCLUDES 2   *complication following infusion, transfusion and therapeutic injection (T80.-)*
> *complication following procedure NEC (T81.-)*
> *complications of anesthesia in labor and delivery (O74.-)*
> *complications of anesthesia in pregnancy (O29.-)*
> *complications of anesthesia in puerperium (O89.-)*
> *complications of devices, implants and grafts (T82-T85)*
> *complications of obstetric surgery and procedure (O75.4)*
> *dermatitis due to drugs and medicaments (L23.3, L24.4, L25.1, L27.0-L27.1)*
> *poisoning and toxic effects of drugs and chemicals (T36-T65 with fifth or sixth character 1-4 or 6)*
> *specified complications classified elsewhere*

> The appropriate 7th character is to be added to each code from category T88.
> A   initial encounter
> D   subsequent encounter
> S   sequela

√x7ᵗʰ **T88.0 Infection following immunization**
> Sepsis following immunization
> **AHA:** 2018,4Q,62-63

√x7ᵗʰ **T88.1 Other complications following immunization, not elsewhere classified**
> Generalized vaccinia
> Rash following immunization
> EXCLUDES 1   *vaccinia not from vaccine (B08.011)*
> EXCLUDES 2   *anaphylactic shock due to serum (T80.5-)*
> *other serum reactions (T80.6-)*
> *postimmunization arthropathy (M02.2)*
> *postimmunization encephalitis (G04.02)*
> *postimmunization fever (R50.83)*

√x7ᵗʰ **T88.2 Shock due to anesthesia**
> Use additional code for adverse effect, if applicable, to identify drug (T41.- with fifth or sixth character 5)
> EXCLUDES 1   *complications of anesthesia (in):*
> *labor and delivery (O74.-)*
> *postprocedural shock NOS (T81.1-)*
> *pregnancy (O29.-)*
> *puerperium (O89.-)*

√x7ᵗʰ **T88.3 Malignant hyperthermia due to anesthesia**
> Use additional code for adverse effect, if applicable, to identify drug (T41.- with fifth or sixth character 5)

√x7ᵗʰ **T88.4 Failed or difficult intubation**
√5ᵗʰ **T88.5 Other complications of anesthesia**
> Use additional code for adverse effect, if applicable, to identify drug (T41.- with fifth or sixth character 5)
√x7ᵗʰ **T88.51 Hypothermia following anesthesia**

√x7ᵗʰ **T88.52** **Failed moderate sedation during procedure**

Failed conscious sedation during procedure

EXCLUDES 2   *personal history of failed moderate sedation (Z92.83)*

√x7ᵗʰ **T88.53** **Unintended awareness under general anesthesia during procedure**

EXCLUDES 2   *personal history of unintended awareness under general anesthesia (Z92.84)*

AHA: 2016,4Q,72-73

√x7ᵗʰ **T88.59** **Other complications of anesthesia**

√x7ᵗʰ **T88.6** **Anaphylactic reaction due to adverse effect of correct drug or medicament properly administered**

Anaphylactic shock due to adverse effect of correct drug or medicament properly administered

Anaphylactoid reaction NOS

Use additional code for adverse effect, if applicable, to identify drug (T36-T50 with fifth or sixth character 5)

EXCLUDES 1   *anaphylactic reaction due to serum (T80.5-)*

anaphylactic shock or reaction due to adverse food reaction (T78.0-)

√x7ᵗʰ **T88.7** **Unspecified adverse effect of drug or medicament**

Drug hypersensitivity NOS

Drug reaction NOS

Use additional code for adverse effect, if applicable, to identify drug (T36-T50 with fifth or sixth character 5)

EXCLUDES 1   *specified adverse effects of drugs and medicaments (A00-R94 and T80-T88.6, T88.8)*

√x7ᵗʰ **T88.8** **Other specified complications of surgical and medical care, not elsewhere classified**

Use additional code to identify the complication

√x7ᵗʰ **T88.9** **Complication of surgical and medical care, unspecified**

N Newborn: 0   P Pediatric: 0-17   M Maternity: 12-55   A Adult: 15-124   CH Comorbidity High   CL Comorbidity Low   NC Dx Noncancer Dx   PDx Primary Dx

1138   ICD-10-CM 2020

Chapter 20. External Causes of Morbidity (V00–Y99)

Chapter-specific Guidelines with Coding Examples

The chapter-specific guidelines from the ICD-10-CM Official Guidelines for Coding and Reporting have been provided below. Along with these guidelines are coding examples, contained in the shaded boxes, that have been developed to help illustrate the coding and/or sequencing guidance found in these guidelines.

The external causes of morbidity codes should never be sequenced as the first-listed or principal diagnosis.

External cause codes are intended to provide data for injury research and evaluation of injury prevention strategies. These codes capture how the injury or health condition happened (cause), the intent (unintentional or accidental; or intentional, such as suicide or assault), the place where the event occurred, the activity of the patient at the time of the event, and the person's status (e.g., civilian, military).

There is no national requirement for mandatory ICD-10-CM external cause code reporting. Unless a provider is subject to a state-based external cause code reporting mandate or these codes are required by a particular payer, reporting of ICD-10-CM codes in Chapter 20, External Causes of Morbidity, is not required. In the absence of a mandatory reporting requirement, providers are encouraged to voluntarily report external cause codes, as they provide valuable data for injury research and evaluation of injury prevention strategies.

a. General external cause coding guidelines

1) Used with any code in the range of A00.0–T88.9, Z00–Z99

An external cause code may be used with any code in the range of A00.0-T88.9, Z00-Z99, classification that represents a health condition due to an external cause. Though they are most applicable to injuries, they are also valid for use with such things as infections or diseases due to an external source, and other health conditions, such as a heart attack that occurs during strenuous physical activity.

> Patient has bilateral sensorineural hearing loss due to history of exposure to loud noise over 100 dB for a period of greater than 10 years as a sound technician for a band.
>
> **H90.3**   **Sensorineural hearing loss, bilateral**
>
> **W42.9XXS**   **Exposure to other noise, sequela**
>
> *Explanation:* The hearing loss is due to noise exposure. An external cause code identifies the noise as the cause. The seventh character S is used in this case as the hearing loss is a residual effect of the exposure.

2) External cause code used for length of treatment

Assign the external cause code, with the appropriate 7th character (initial encounter, subsequent encounter or sequela) for each encounter for which the injury or condition is being treated.

Most categories in chapter 20 have a 7th character requirement for each applicable code. Most categories in this chapter have three 7th character values: A, initial encounter, D, subsequent encounter and S, sequela. While the patient may be seen by a new or different provider over the course of treatment for an injury or condition, assignment of the 7th character for external cause should match the 7th character of the code assigned for the associated injury or condition for the encounter.

3) Use the full range of external cause codes

Use the full range of external cause codes to completely describe the cause, the intent, the place of occurrence, and if applicable, the activity of the patient at the time of the event, and the patient's status, for all injuries, and other health conditions due to an external cause.

4) Assign as many external cause codes as necessary

Assign as many external cause codes as necessary to fully explain each cause. If only one external code can be recorded, assign the code most related to the principal diagnosis.

5) The selection of the appropriate external cause code

The selection of the appropriate external cause code is guided by the Alphabetic Index of External Causes and by Inclusion and Exclusion notes in the Tabular List.

6) External cause code can never be a principal diagnosis

An external cause code can never be a principal (first-listed) diagnosis.

7) Combination external cause codes

Certain of the external cause codes are combination codes that identify sequential events that result in an injury, such as a fall which results in striking against an object. The injury may be due to either event or both.

The combination external cause code used should correspond to the sequence of events regardless of which caused the most serious injury.

> An 86-year-old patient fell and hit his head against the nightstand. He went to the local ER and returned the same day with a diagnosis of scalp contusion.
>
> **S00.03XD**   **Contusion of scalp, subsequent encounter**
>
> **W01.190D**   **Fall on same level from slipping, tripping, and stumbling with subsequent striking against furniture, subsequent encounter**
>
> *Explanation:* Combination external cause codes identify sequential events that result in an injury, such as a fall resulting in striking against an object. The injury may be due to either or both events.

8) No external cause code needed in certain circumstances

No external cause code from Chapter 20 is needed if the external cause and intent are included in a code from another chapter (e.g. T36.0X1-Poisoning by penicillins, accidental (unintentional)).

b. Place of occurrence guideline

Codes from category Y92, Place of occurrence of the external cause, are secondary codes for use after other external cause codes to identify the location of the patient at the time of injury or other condition.

Generally, a place of occurrence code is assigned only once, at the initial encounter for treatment. However, in the rare instance that a new injury occurs during hospitalization, an additional place of occurrence code may be assigned. No 7th characters are used for Y92.

Do not use place of occurrence code Y92.9 if the place is not stated or is not applicable.

c. Activity code

Assign a code from category Y93, Activity code, to describe the activity of the patient at the time the injury or other health condition occurred.

An activity code is used only once, at the initial encounter for treatment. Only one code from Y93 should be recorded on a medical record.

The activity codes are not applicable to poisonings, adverse effects, misadventures or sequela.

Do not assign Y93.9, Unspecified activity, if the activity is not stated.

A code from category Y93 is appropriate for use with external cause and intent codes if identifying the activity provides additional information about the event.

d. Place of occurrence, activity, and status codes used with other external cause code

When applicable, place of occurrence, activity, and external cause status codes are sequenced after the main external cause code(s). Regardless of the number of external cause codes assigned, there should be only one place of occurrence code, one activity code, and one external cause status code assigned to an encounter. However, in the rare instance that a new injury occurs during hospitalization, an additional place of occurrence code may be assigned.

e. If the reporting format limits the number of external cause codes

If the reporting format limits the number of external cause codes that can be used in reporting clinical data, report the code for the cause/intent most related to the principal diagnosis. If the format permits, capture of additional external cause codes, the cause/intent, including medical misadventures, of the additional events should be reported rather than the codes for place, activity, or external status.

f. Multiple external cause coding guidelines

More than one external cause code is required to fully describe the external cause of an illness or injury. The assignment of external cause codes should be sequenced in the following priority:

If two or more events cause separate injuries, an external cause code should be assigned for each cause. The first-listed external cause code will be selected in the following order:

External codes for child and adult abuse take priority over all other external cause codes.

See Section I.C.19., Child and Adult abuse guidelines.

External cause codes for terrorism events take priority over all other external cause codes except child and adult abuse.

External cause codes for cataclysmic events take priority over all other external cause codes except child and adult abuse and terrorism.

External cause codes for transport accidents take priority over all other external cause codes except cataclysmic events, child and adult abuse and terrorism.

Activity and external cause status codes are assigned following all causal (intent) external cause codes.

The first-listed external cause code should correspond to the cause of the most serious diagnosis due to an assault, accident, or self-harm, following the order of hierarchy listed above.

> A 70-year-old male was cleaning his basement and accidentally discharged a handgun, resulting in a gunshot wound to his left foot. As he was attempting to go up his stairs to seek help, he fell backwards and sustained a left hip fracture. The GSW is currently being treated with a wound VAC.
>
> **S91.332A**   **Puncture wound without foreign body, left foot, initial encounter**
>
> **W32.0XXA**   **Accidental handgun discharge, initial encounter**
>
> **S72.002D**   **Fracture of unspecified part of neck of left femur, subsequent encounter for closed fracture with routine healing**
>
> **W10.8XXD**   **Fall (on) (from) other stairs and steps, subsequent encounter**
>
> *Explanation:* If one or more events cause separate injuries, each injury and the appropriate external cause code should be assigned. The left foot wound requires active treatment with a VAC dressing and should be coded with seventh character A.

g. Child and adult abuse guideline

Adult and child abuse, neglect and maltreatment are classified as assault. Any of the assault codes may be used to indicate the external cause of any injury resulting from the confirmed abuse.

For confirmed cases of abuse, neglect and maltreatment, when the perpetrator is known, a code from Y07, Perpetrator of maltreatment and neglect, should accompany any other assault codes.

See Section I.C.19. Adult and child abuse, neglect and other maltreatment

h. Unknown or undetermined intent guideline

If the intent (accident, self-harm, assault) of the cause of an injury or other condition is unknown or unspecified, code the intent as accidental intent. All transport accident categories assume accidental intent.

1) Use of undetermined intent

External cause codes for events of undetermined intent are only for use if the documentation in the record specifies that the intent cannot be determined.

i. Sequelae (late effects) of external cause guidelines

1) Sequelae external cause codes

Sequela are reported using the external cause code with the 7th character "S" for sequela. These codes should be used with any report of a late effect or sequela resulting from a previous injury.

See Section I.B.10 Sequela (Late Effects)

2) Sequela external cause code with a related current injury

A sequela external cause code should never be used with a related current nature of injury code.

3) Use of sequela external cause codes for subsequent visits

Use a late effect external cause code for subsequent visits when a late effect of the initial injury is being treated. Do not use a late effect external cause code for subsequent visits for follow-up care (e.g., to assess healing, to receive rehabilitative therapy) of the injury when no late effect of the injury has been documented.

j. Terrorism guidelines

1) Cause of injury identified by the Federal Government (FBI) as terrorism

When the cause of an injury is identified by the Federal Government (FBI) as terrorism, the first-listed external cause code should be a code from category Y38, Terrorism. The definition of terrorism employed by the FBI is found at the inclusion note at the beginning of category Y38. Use additional code for place of occurrence (Y92.-). More than one Y38 code may be assigned if the injury is the result of more than one mechanism of terrorism.

2) Cause of an injury is suspected to be the result of terrorism

When the cause of an injury is suspected to be the result of terrorism a code from category Y38 should not be assigned. Suspected cases should be classified as assault.

3) Code Y38.9, Terrorism, secondary effects

Assign code Y38.9, Terrorism, secondary effects, for conditions occurring subsequent to the terrorist event. This code should not be assigned for conditions that are due to the initial terrorist act.

It is acceptable to assign code Y38.9 with another code from Y38 if there is an injury due to the initial terrorist event and an injury that is a subsequent result of the terrorist event.

k. External cause status

A code from category Y99, External cause status, should be assigned whenever any other external cause code is assigned for an encounter, including an Activity code, except for the events noted below. Assign a code from category Y99, External cause status, to indicate the work status of the person at the time the event occurred. The status code indicates whether the event occurred during military activity, whether a non-military person was at work, whether an individual including a student or volunteer was involved in a non-work activity at the time of the causal event.

A code from Y99, External cause status, should be assigned, when applicable, with other external cause codes, such as transport accidents and falls. The external cause status codes are not applicable to poisonings, adverse effects, misadventures or late effects.

Do not assign a code from category Y99 if no other external cause codes (cause, activity) are applicable for the encounter.

An external cause status code is used only once, at the initial encounter for treatment. Only one code from Y99 should be recorded on a medical record.

Do not assign code Y99.9, Unspecified external cause status, if the status is not stated.

Chapter 20. External Causes of Morbidity (V00-Y99)

NOTE This chapter permits the classification of environmental events and circumstances as the cause of injury, and other adverse effects. Where a code from this section is applicable, it is intended that it shall be used secondary to a code from another chapter of the Classification indicating the nature of the condition. Most often, the condition will be classifiable to Chapter 19, Injury, poisoning and certain other consequences of external causes (S00-T88). Other conditions that may be stated to be due to external causes are classified in Chapters I to XVIII. For these conditions, codes from Chapter 20 should be used to provide additional information as to the cause of the condition.

AHA: 2018,4Q,58-60

This chapter contains the following blocks:

V00-X58	Accidents
V00-V99	Transport accidents
V00-V09	Pedestrian injured in transport accident
V10-V19	Pedal cycle rider injured in transport accident
V20-V29	Motorcycle rider injured in transport accident
V30-V39	Occupant of three-wheeled motor vehicle injured in transport accident
V40-V49	Car occupant injured in transport accident
V50-V59	Occupant of pick-up truck or van injured in transport accident
V60-V69	Occupant of heavy transport vehicle injured in transport accident
V70-V79	Bus occupant injured in transport accident
V80-V89	Other land transport accidents
V90-V94	Water transport accidents
V95-V97	Air and space transport accidents
V98-V99	Other and unspecified transport accidents
W00-X58	Other external causes of accidental injury
W00-W19	Slipping, tripping, stumbling and falls
W20-W49	Exposure to inanimate mechanical forces
W50-W64	Exposure to animate mechanical forces
W65-W74	Accidental non-transport drowning and submersion
W85-W99	Exposure to electric current, radiation and extreme ambient air temperature and pressure
X00-X08	Exposure to smoke, fire and flames
X10-X19	Contact with heat and hot substances
X30-X39	Exposure to forces of nature
X50	Overexertion and strenuous or repetitive movements
X52-X58	Accidental exposure to other specified factors
X71-X83	Intentional self-harm
X92-Y09	Assault
Y21-Y33	Event of undetermined intent
Y35-Y38	Legal intervention, operations of war, military operations, and terrorism
Y62-Y84	Complications of medical and surgical care
Y62-Y69	Misadventures to patients during surgical and medical care
Y70-Y82	Medical devices associated with adverse incidents in diagnostic and therapeutic use
Y83-Y84	Surgical and other medical procedures as the cause of abnormal reaction of the patient, or of later complication, without mention of misadventure at the time of the procedure
Y90-Y99	Supplementary factors related to causes of morbidity classified elsewhere

ACCIDENTS (V00-X58)

AHA: 2018,2Q,7-8

Transport accidents (V00-V99)

NOTE This section is structured in 12 groups. Those relating to land transport accidents (V00-V89) reflect the victim's mode of transport and are subdivided to identify the victim's 'counterpart' or the type of event. The vehicle of which the injured person is an occupant is identified in the first two characters since it is seen as the most important factor to identify for prevention purposes. A transport accident is one in which the vehicle involved must be moving or running or in use for transport purposes at the time of the accident.

Use additional code to identify:
airbag injury (W22.1)
type of street or road (Y92.4-)
use of cellular telephone and other electronic equipment at the time of the transport accident (Y93.C-)

EXCLUDES 1 agricultural vehicles in stationary use or maintenance (W31.-)
assault by crashing of motor vehicle (Y03.-)
automobile or motor cycle in stationary use or maintenance — code to type of accident
crashing of motor vehicle, undetermined intent (Y32)
intentional self-harm by crashing of motor vehicle (X82)

EXCLUDES 2 transport accidents due to cataclysm (X34-X38)

NOTE Definitions related to transport accidents:

(a) A transport accident (V00-V99) is any accident involving a device designed primarily for, or used at the time primarily for, conveying persons or good from one place to another.

(b) A public highway [trafficway] or street is the entire width between property lines (or other boundary lines) of land open to the public as a matter of right or custom for purposes of moving persons or property from one place to another. A roadway is that part of the public highway designed, improved and customarily used for vehicular traffic.

(c) A traffic accident is any vehicle accident occurring on the public highway [i.e. originating on, terminating on, or involving a vehicle partially on the highway]. A vehicle accident is assumed to have occurred on the public highway unless another place is specified, except in the case of accidents involving only off-road motor vehicles, which are classified as nontraffic accidents unless the contrary is stated.

(d) A nontraffic accident is any vehicle accident that occurs entirely in any place other than a public highway.

(e) A pedestrian is any person involved in an accident who was not at the time of the accident riding in or on a motor vehicle, railway train, streetcar or animal-drawn or other vehicle, or on a pedal cycle or animal. This includes, a person changing a tire, working on a parked car, or a person on foot. It also includes the user of a pedestrian conveyance such as a baby stroller, ice-skates, skis, sled, roller skates, a skateboard, nonmotorized or motorized wheelchair, motorized mobility scooter, or nonmotorized scooter.

(f) A driver is an occupant of a transport vehicle who is operating or intending to operate it.

(g) A passenger is any occupant of a transport vehicle other than the driver, except a person traveling on the outside of the vehicle.

(h) A person on the outside of a vehicle is any person being transported by a vehicle but not occupying the space normally reserved for the driver or passengers, or the space intended for the transport of property. This includes a person travelling on the bodywork, bumper, fender, roof, running board or step of a vehicle, as well as, hanging on the outside of the vehicle.

(i) A pedal cycle is any land transport vehicle operated solely by nonmotorized pedals including a bicycle or tricycle.

(j) A pedal cyclist is any person riding a pedal cycle or in a sidecar or trailer attached to a pedal cycle.

(k) A motorcycle is a two-wheeled motor vehicle with one or two riding saddles and sometimes with a third wheel for the support of a sidecar. The sidecar is considered part of the motorcycle. This includes a moped, motor scooter, or motorized bicycle.

(l) A motorcycle rider is any person riding a motorcycle or in a sidecar or trailer attached to the motorcycle.

(m) A three-wheeled motor vehicle is a motorized tricycle designed primarily for on-road use. This includes a motor-driven tricycle, a motorized rickshaw, or a three-wheeled motor car.

(n) A car [automobile] is a four-wheeled motor vehicle designed primarily for carrying up to 7 persons. A trailer being towed by the car is considered part of the car. It does not include a van or minivan — see definition (o).

(o) A pick-up truck or van is a four or six-wheeled motor vehicle designed for carrying passengers as well as property or cargo weighing less than the local limit for classification as a heavy goods vehicle, and not requiring a special driver's license. This includes a minivan and a sport-utility vehicle (SUV).

(p) A heavy transport vehicle is a motor vehicle designed primarily for carrying property, meeting local criteria for classification as a heavy goods vehicle in terms of weight and requiring a special driver's license.

(q) A bus (coach) is a motor vehicle designed or adapted primarily for carrying more than 10 passengers, and requiring a special driver's license.

(r) A railway train or railway vehicle is any device, with or without freight or passenger cars couple to it, designed for traffic on a railway track. This includes subterranean (subways) or elevated trains.

(s) A streetcar, is a device designed and used primarily for transporting passengers within a municipality, running on rails, usually subject to normal traffic control signals, and operated principally on a right-of-way that forms part of the roadway. This includes a tram or trolley that runs on rails. A trailer being towed by a streetcar is considered part of the streetcar.

(t) A special vehicle mainly used on industrial premises is a motor vehicle designed primarily for use within the buildings and premises of industrial or commercial establishments. This includes battery-powered airport passenger vehicles or baggage/mail trucks, forklifts, coal-cars in a coal mine, logging cars and trucks used in mines or quarries.

(u) A special vehicle mainly used in agriculture is a motor vehicle designed specifically for use in farming and agriculture (horticulture), to work the land, tend and harvest crops and transport materials on the farm. This includes harvesters, farm machinery and tractor and trailers.

(v) A special construction vehicle is a motor vehicle designed specifically for use on construction and demolition sites. This includes bulldozers, diggers, earth levellers, dump trucks, backhoes, front-end loaders, pavers, and mechanical shovels.

(w) A special all-terrain vehicle is a motor vehicle of special design to enable it to negotiate over rough or soft terrain, snow or sand. Examples of special design are high construction, special wheels and tires, tracks, and support on a cushion of air. This includes snow mobiles, All-terrain vehicles (ATV), and dune buggies. It does not include passenger vehicle designated as Sport Utility Vehicles. (SUV)

(x) A watercraft is any device designed for transporting passengers or goods on water. This includes motor or sailboats, ships, and hovercraft.

(y) An aircraft is any device for transporting passengers or goods in the air. This includes hot-air balloons, gliders, helicopters and airplanes.

(z) A military vehicle is any motorized vehicle operating on a public roadway owned by the military and being operated by a member of the military.

Pedestrian injured in transport accident (V00-V09)

INCLUDES   person changing tire on transport vehicle
person examining engine of vehicle broken down in (on side of) road

EXCLUDES 1   *fall due to non-transport collision with other person (W03)*
pedestrian on foot falling (slipping) on ice and snow (W00.-)
struck or bumped by another person (W51)

The appropriate 7th character is to be added to each code from categories V00-V09.
A   initial encounter
D   subsequent encounter
S   sequela

√4ᵗʰ **V00**   **Pedestrian conveyance accident**
Use additional place of occurrence and activity external cause codes, if known (Y92.-, Y93.-)
   EXCLUDES 1   *collision with another person without fall (W51)*
fall due to person on foot colliding with another person on foot (W03)
fall from non-moving wheelchair, nonmotorized scooter and motorized mobility scooter without collision (W05.-)
pedestrian (conveyance) collision with other land transport vehicle (V01-V09)
pedestrian on foot falling (slipping) on ice and snow (W00.-)

√5ᵗʰ **V00.0**   **Pedestrian on foot injured in collision with pedestrian conveyance**
√x7ᵗʰ   **V00.01**   **Pedestrian on foot injured in collision with roller-skater**
√x7ᵗʰ   **V00.02**   **Pedestrian on foot injured in collision with skateboarder**
√x7ᵗʰ   **V00.09**   **Pedestrian on foot injured in collision with other pedestrian conveyance**

√5ᵗʰ **V00.1**   **Rolling-type pedestrian conveyance accident**
   EXCLUDES 1   *accident with baby stroller (V00.82-)*
accident with motorized mobility scooter (V00.83-)
accident with wheelchair (powered) (V00.81-)

√6ᵗʰ   **V00.11**   **In-line roller-skate accident**
√7ᵗʰ   **V00.111**   **Fall from in-line roller-skates**
√7ᵗʰ   **V00.112**   **In-line roller-skater colliding with stationary object**
√7ᵗʰ   **V00.118**   **Other in-line roller-skate accident**
     EXCLUDES 1   *roller-skater collision with other land transport vehicle (V01-V09 with 5th character 1)*

√6ᵗʰ   **V00.12**   **Non-in-line roller-skate accident**
√7ᵗʰ   **V00.121**   **Fall from non-in-line roller-skates**
√7ᵗʰ   **V00.122**   **Non-in-line roller-skater colliding with stationary object**
√7ᵗʰ   **V00.128**   **Other non-in-line roller-skating accident**
     EXCLUDES 1   *roller-skater collision with other land transport vehicle (V01-V09 with 5th character 1)*

√6ᵗʰ   **V00.13**   **Skateboard accident**
√7ᵗʰ   **V00.131**   **Fall from skateboard**
√7ᵗʰ   **V00.132**   **Skateboarder colliding with stationary object**
√7ᵗʰ   **V00.138**   **Other skateboard accident**
     EXCLUDES 1   *skateboarder collision with other land transport vehicle (V01-V09 with 5th character 2)*

√6ᵗʰ   **V00.14**   **Scooter (nonmotorized) accident**
     EXCLUDES 1   *motor scooter accident (V20-V29)*
√7ᵗʰ   **V00.141**   **Fall from scooter (nonmotorized)**
√7ᵗʰ   **V00.142**   **Scooter (nonmotorized) colliding with stationary object**
√7ᵗʰ   **V00.148**   **Other scooter (nonmotorized) accident**
     EXCLUDES 1   *scooter (nonmotorized) collision with other land transport vehicle (V01-V09 with fifth character 9)*

√6ᵗʰ   **V00.15**   **Heelies accident**
Rolling shoe
Wheeled shoe
Wheelies accident
√7ᵗʰ   **V00.151**   **Fall from heelies**
√7ᵗʰ   **V00.152**   **Heelies colliding with stationary object**
√7ᵗʰ   **V00.158**   **Other heelies accident**

√6ᵗʰ   **V00.18**   **Accident on other rolling-type pedestrian conveyance**
√7ᵗʰ   **V00.181**   **Fall from other rolling-type pedestrian conveyance**
√7ᵗʰ   **V00.182**   **Pedestrian on other rolling-type pedestrian conveyance colliding with stationary object**
√7ᵗʰ   **V00.188**   **Other accident on other rolling-type pedestrian conveyance**

√5ᵗʰ **V00.2**   **Gliding-type pedestrian conveyance accident**
√6ᵗʰ   **V00.21**   **Ice-skates accident**
√7ᵗʰ   **V00.211**   **Fall from ice-skates**
√7ᵗʰ   **V00.212**   **Ice-skater colliding with stationary object**
√7ᵗʰ   **V00.218**   **Other ice-skates accident**
     EXCLUDES 1   *ice-skater collision with other land transport vehicle (V01-V09 with 5th character 9)*

√6ᵗʰ   **V00.22**   **Sled accident**
√7ᵗʰ   **V00.221**   **Fall from sled**
√7ᵗʰ   **V00.222**   **Sledder colliding with stationary object**
√7ᵗʰ   **V00.228**   **Other sled accident**
     EXCLUDES 1   *sled collision with other land transport vehicle (V01-V09 with 5th character 9)*

√6ᵗʰ   **V00.28**   **Other gliding-type pedestrian conveyance accident**
√7ᵗʰ   **V00.281**   **Fall from other gliding-type pedestrian conveyance**
√7ᵗʰ   **V00.282**   **Pedestrian on other gliding-type pedestrian conveyance colliding with stationary object**
√7ᵗʰ   **V00.288**   **Other accident on other gliding-type pedestrian conveyance**
     EXCLUDES 1   *gliding-type pedestrian conveyance collision with other land transport vehicle (V01-V09 with 5th character 9)*

√5ᵗʰ **V00.3**   **Flat-bottomed pedestrian conveyance accident**
√6ᵗʰ   **V00.31**   **Snowboard accident**
√7ᵗʰ   **V00.311**   **Fall from snowboard**
√7ᵗʰ   **V00.312**   **Snowboarder colliding with stationary object**

√7ᵗʰ **V00.318 Other snowboard accident**
> EXCLUDES 1   *snowboarder collision with other land transport vehicle (V01-V09 with 5th character 9)*

√6ᵗʰ **V00.32 Snow-ski accident**
> √7ᵗʰ **V00.321 Fall from snow-skis**
> √7ᵗʰ **V00.322 Snow-skier colliding with stationary object**
> √7ᵗʰ **V00.328 Other snow-ski accident**
> > EXCLUDES 1   *snow-skier collision with other land transport vehicle (V01-V09 with 5th character 9)*

√6ᵗʰ **V00.38 Other flat-bottomed pedestrian conveyance accident**
> √7ᵗʰ **V00.381 Fall from other flat-bottomed pedestrian conveyance**
> √7ᵗʰ **V00.382 Pedestrian on other flat-bottomed pedestrian conveyance colliding with stationary object**
> √7ᵗʰ **V00.388 Other accident on other flat-bottomed pedestrian conveyance**

√5ᵗʰ **V00.8 Accident on other pedestrian conveyance**
> √6ᵗʰ **V00.81 Accident with wheelchair (powered)**
> > √7ᵗʰ **V00.811 Fall from moving wheelchair (powered)**
> > > EXCLUDES 1   *fall from non-moving wheelchair (W05.0)*
> > √7ᵗʰ **V00.812 Wheelchair (powered) colliding with stationary object**
> > √7ᵗʰ **V00.818 Other accident with wheelchair (powered)**
> √6ᵗʰ **V00.82 Accident with baby stroller**
> > √7ᵗʰ **V00.821 Fall from baby stroller**
> > √7ᵗʰ **V00.822 Baby stroller colliding with stationary object**
> > √7ᵗʰ **V00.828 Other accident with baby stroller**
> √6ᵗʰ **V00.83 Accident with motorized mobility scooter**
> > √7ᵗʰ **V00.831 Fall from motorized mobility scooter**
> > > EXCLUDES 1   *fall from non-moving motorized mobility scooter (W05.2)*
> > √7ᵗʰ **V00.832 Motorized mobility scooter colliding with stationary object**
> > √7ᵗʰ **V00.838 Other accident with motorized mobility scooter**
> √6ᵗʰ **V00.89 Accident on other pedestrian conveyance**
> > √7ᵗʰ **V00.891 Fall from other pedestrian conveyance**
> > √7ᵗʰ **V00.892 Pedestrian on other pedestrian conveyance colliding with stationary object**
> > √7ᵗʰ **V00.898 Other accident on other pedestrian conveyance**
> > > EXCLUDES 1   *other pedestrian (conveyance) collision with other land transport vehicle (V01-V09 with 5th character 9)*

√4ᵗʰ **V01 Pedestrian injured in collision with pedal cycle**
> √5ᵗʰ **V01.0 Pedestrian injured in collision with pedal cycle in nontraffic accident**
> > √x7ᵗʰ **V01.00 Pedestrian on foot injured in collision with pedal cycle in nontraffic accident**
> > > Pedestrian NOS injured in collision with pedal cycle in nontraffic accident
> > √x7ᵗʰ **V01.01 Pedestrian on roller-skates injured in collision with pedal cycle in nontraffic accident**
> > √x7ᵗʰ **V01.02 Pedestrian on skateboard injured in collision with pedal cycle in nontraffic accident**

√x7ᵗʰ **V01.09 Pedestrian with other conveyance injured in collision with pedal cycle in nontraffic accident**
> Pedestrian with baby stroller injured in collision with pedal cycle in nontraffic accident
> Pedestrian on ice-skates injured in collision with pedal cycle in nontraffic accident
> Pedestrian on nonmotorized scooter injured in collision with pedal cycle in nontraffic accident
> Pedestrian on sled injured in collision with pedal cycle in nontraffic accident
> Pedestrian on snowboard injured in collision with pedal cycle in nontraffic accident
> Pedestrian on snow-skis injured in collision with pedal cycle in nontraffic accident
> Pedestrian in wheelchair (powered) injured in collision with pedal cycle in nontraffic accident
> Pedestrian in motorized mobility scooter injured in collision with pedal cycle in nontraffic accident

√5ᵗʰ **V01.1 Pedestrian injured in collision with pedal cycle in traffic accident**
> √x7ᵗʰ **V01.10 Pedestrian on foot injured in collision with pedal cycle in traffic accident**
> > Pedestrian NOS injured in collision with pedal cycle in traffic accident
> √x7ᵗʰ **V01.11 Pedestrian on roller-skates injured in collision with pedal cycle in traffic accident**
> √x7ᵗʰ **V01.12 Pedestrian on skateboard injured in collision with pedal cycle in traffic accident**
> √x7ᵗʰ **V01.19 Pedestrian with other conveyance injured in collision with pedal cycle in traffic accident**
> > Pedestrian with baby stroller injured in collision with pedal cycle in traffic accident
> > Pedestrian on ice-skates injured in collision with pedal cycle in traffic accident
> > Pedestrian on nonmotorized scooter injured in collision with pedal cycle in traffic accident
> > Pedestrian on sled injured in collision with pedal cycle in traffic accident
> > Pedestrian on snowboard injured in collision with pedal cycle in traffic accident
> > Pedestrian on snow-skis injured in collision with pedal cycle in traffic accident
> > Pedestrian in wheelchair (powered) injured in collision with pedal cycle in traffic accident
> > Pedestrian in motorized mobility scooter injured in collision with pedal cycle in traffic accident

√5ᵗʰ **V01.9 Pedestrian injured in collision with pedal cycle, unspecified whether traffic or nontraffic accident**
> √x7ᵗʰ **V01.90 Pedestrian on foot injured in collision with pedal cycle, unspecified whether traffic or nontraffic accident**
> > Pedestrian NOS injured in collision with pedal cycle, unspecified whether traffic or nontraffic accident
> √x7ᵗʰ **V01.91 Pedestrian on roller-skates injured in collision with pedal cycle, unspecified whether traffic or nontraffic accident**
> √x7ᵗʰ **V01.92 Pedestrian on skateboard injured in collision with pedal cycle, unspecified whether traffic or nontraffic accident**

☑ Additional Character Required   √x7ᵗʰ Placeholder Alert   Manifestation   Unspecified Dx   ►◄ Revised Text   ● New Code   ▲ Revised Title

√x7ᵗʰ **V01.99 Pedestrian with other conveyance injured in collision with pedal cycle, unspecified whether traffic or nontraffic accident**

Pedestrian with baby stroller injured in collision with pedal cycle, unspecified whether traffic or nontraffic accident

Pedestrian on ice-skates injured in collision with pedal cycle unspecified, whether traffic or nontraffic accident

Pedestrian on nonmotorized scooter injured in collision with pedal cycle, unspecified whether traffic or nontraffic accident

Pedestrian on sled injured in collision with pedal cycle unspecified, whether traffic or nontraffic accident

Pedestrian on snowboard injured in collision with pedal cycle, unspecified whether traffic or nontraffic accident

Pedestrian on snow-skis injured in collision with pedal cycle, unspecified whether traffic or nontraffic accident

Pedestrian in wheelchair (powered) injured in collision with pedal cycle, unspecified whether traffic or nontraffic accident

Pedestrian in motorized mobility scooter injured in collision with pedal cycle, unspecified whether traffic or nontraffic accident

√4ᵗʰ **V02 Pedestrian injured in collision with two- or three-wheeled motor vehicle**

√5ᵗʰ **V02.0 Pedestrian injured in collision with two- or three-wheeled motor vehicle in nontraffic accident**

√x7ᵗʰ **V02.00 Pedestrian on foot injured in collision with two- or three-wheeled motor vehicle in nontraffic accident**

Pedestrian NOS injured in collision with two- or three-wheeled motor vehicle in nontraffic accident

√x7ᵗʰ **V02.01 Pedestrian on roller-skates injured in collision with two- or three-wheeled motor vehicle in nontraffic accident**

√x7ᵗʰ **V02.02 Pedestrian on skateboard injured in collision with two- or three-wheeled motor vehicle in nontraffic accident**

√x7ᵗʰ **V02.09 Pedestrian with other conveyance injured in collision with two- or three-wheeled motor vehicle in nontraffic accident**

Pedestrian with baby stroller injured in collision with two- or three-wheeled motor vehicle in nontraffic accident

Pedestrian on ice-skates injured in collision with two- or three-wheeled motor vehicle in nontraffic accident

Pedestrian on nonmotorized scooter injured in collision with two- or three-wheeled motor vehicle in nontraffic accident

Pedestrian on sled injured in collision with two- or three-wheeled motor vehicle in nontraffic accident

Pedestrian on snowboard injured in collision with two- or three-wheeled motor vehicle in nontraffic accident

Pedestrian on snow-skis injured in collision with two- or three-wheeled motor vehicle in nontraffic accident

Pedestrian in wheelchair (powered) injured in collision with two- or three-wheeled motor vehicle in nontraffic accident

Pedestrian in motorized mobility scooter injured in collision with two- or three-wheeled motor vehicle in nontraffic accident

√5ᵗʰ **V02.1 Pedestrian injured in collision with two- or three-wheeled motor vehicle in traffic accident**

√x7ᵗʰ **V02.10 Pedestrian on foot injured in collision with two- or three-wheeled motor vehicle in traffic accident**

Pedestrian NOS injured in collision with two- or three-wheeled motor vehicle in traffic accident

√x7ᵗʰ **V02.11 Pedestrian on roller-skates injured in collision with two- or three-wheeled motor vehicle in traffic accident**

√x7ᵗʰ **V02.12 Pedestrian on skateboard injured in collision with two- or three-wheeled motor vehicle in traffic accident**

√x7ᵗʰ **V02.19 Pedestrian with other conveyance injured in collision with two- or three-wheeled motor vehicle in traffic accident**

Pedestrian with baby stroller injured in collision with two- or three-wheeled motor vehicle in traffic accident

Pedestrian on ice-skates injured in collision with two- or three-wheeled motor vehicle in traffic accident

Pedestrian on nonmotorized scooter injured in collision with two- or three-wheeled motor vehicle in traffic accident

Pedestrian on sled injured in collision with two- or three-wheeled motor vehicle in traffic accident

Pedestrian on snowboard injured in collision with two- or three-wheeled motor vehicle in traffic accident

Pedestrian on snow-skis injured in collision with two- or three-wheeled motor vehicle in traffic accident

Pedestrian in wheelchair (powered) injured in collision with two- or three-wheeled motor vehicle in traffic accident

Pedestrian in motorized mobility scooter injued in collision with two- or three-wheeled motor vehicle in traffic accident

√5ᵗʰ **V02.9 Pedestrian injured in collision with two- or three-wheeled motor vehicle, unspecified whether traffic or nontraffic accident**

√x7ᵗʰ **V02.90 Pedestrian on foot injured in collision with two- or three-wheeled motor vehicle, unspecified whether traffic or nontraffic accident**

Pedestrian NOS injured in collision with two- or three-wheeled motor vehicle, unspecified whether traffic or nontraffic accident

√x7ᵗʰ **V02.91 Pedestrian on roller-skates injured in collision with two- or three-wheeled motor vehicle, unspecified whether traffic or nontraffic accident**

√x7ᵗʰ **V02.92 Pedestrian on skateboard injured in collision with two- or three-wheeled motor vehicle, unspecified whether traffic or nontraffic accident**

√x7ᵗʰ **V02.99 Pedestrian with other conveyance injured in collision with two- or three-wheeled motor vehicle, unspecified whether traffic or nontraffic accident**

Pedestrian with baby stroller injured in collision with two- or three-wheeled motor vehicle, unspecified whether traffic or nontraffic accident

Pedestrian on ice-skates injured in collision with two- or three-wheeled motor vehicle, unspecified whether traffic or nontraffic accident

Pedestrian on nonmotorized scooter injured in collision with two- or three-wheeled motor vehicle, unspecified whether traffic or nontraffic accident

Pedestrian on sled injured in collision with two- or three-wheeled motor vehicle, unspecified whether traffic or nontraffic accident

Pedestrian on snowboard injured in collision with two- or three-wheeled motor vehicle, unspecified whether traffic or nontraffic accident

Pedestrian on snow-skis injured in collision with two- or three-wheeled motor vehicle, unspecified whether traffic or nontraffic accident

Pedestrian in wheelchair (powered) injured in collision with two- or three-wheeled motor vehicle, unspecified whether traffic or nontraffic accident

Pedestrian in motorized mobility scooter injured in collision with two- or three wheeled motor vehicle, unspecified whether traffic or nontraffic accident

√4ᵗʰ **V03 Pedestrian injured in collision with car, pick-up truck or van**

√5ᵗʰ **V03.0 Pedestrian injured in collision with car, pick-up truck or van in nontraffic accident**

√x7ᵗʰ **V03.00 Pedestrian on foot injured in collision with car, pick-up truck or van in nontraffic accident**

Pedestrian NOS injured in collision with car, pick-up truck or van in nontraffic accident

√x7ᵗʰ **V03.01 Pedestrian on roller-skates injured in collision with car, pick-up truck or van in nontraffic accident**

✓x7th **V03.02** Pedestrian on skateboard injured in collision with car, pick-up truck or van in nontraffic accident

✓x7th **V03.09** Pedestrian with other conveyance injured in collision with car, pick-up truck or van in nontraffic accident

Pedestrian with baby stroller injured in collision with car, pick-up truck or van in nontraffic accident

Pedestrian on ice-skates injured in collision with car, pick-up truck or van in nontraffic accident

Pedestrian on nonmotorized scooter injured in collision with car, pick-up truck or van in nontraffic accident

Pedestrian on sled injured in collision with car, pick-up truck or van in nontraffic accident

Pedestrian on snowboard injured in collision with car, pick-up truck or van in nontraffic accident

Pedestrian on snow-skis injured in collision with car, pick-up truck or van in nontraffic accident

Pedestrian in wheelchair (powered) injured in collision with car, pick-up truck or van in nontraffic accident

Pedestrian in motorized mobility scooter injured in collision with car, pick-up truck or van in nontraffic accident

✓5th **V03.1** Pedestrian injured in collision with car, pick-up truck or van in traffic accident

✓x7th **V03.10** Pedestrian on foot injured in collision with car, pick-up truck or van in traffic accident

Pedestrian NOS injured in collision with car, pick-up truck or van in traffic accident

✓x7th **V03.11** Pedestrian on roller-skates injured in collision with car, pick-up truck or van in traffic accident

✓x7th **V03.12** Pedestrian on skateboard injured in collision with car, pick-up truck or van in traffic accident

✓x7th **V03.19** Pedestrian with other conveyance injured in collision with car, pick-up truck or van in traffic accident

Pedestrian with baby stroller injured in collision with car, pick-up truck or van in traffic accident

Pedestrian on ice-skates injured in collision with car, pick-up truck or van in traffic accident

Pedestrian on nonmotorized scooter injured in collision with car, pick-up truck or van in nontraffic accident

Pedestrian on sled injured in collision with car, pick-up truck or van in traffic accident

Pedestrian on snowboard injured in collision with car, pick-up truck or van in traffic accident

Pedestrian on snow-skis injured in collision with car, pick-up truck or van in traffic accident

Pedestrian in wheelchair (powered) injured in collision with car, pick-up truck or van in traffic accident

Pedestrian in motorized mobility scooter injured in collision with car, pick-up truck or van in nontraffic accident

✓5th **V03.9** Pedestrian injured in collision with car, pick-up truck or van, unspecified whether traffic or nontraffic accident

✓x7th **V03.90** Pedestrian on foot injured in collision with car, pick-up truck or van, unspecified whether traffic or nontraffic accident

Pedestrian NOS injured in collision with car, pick-up truck or van, unspecified whether traffic or nontraffic accident

✓x7th **V03.91** Pedestrian on roller-skates injured in collision with car, pick-up truck or van, unspecified whether traffic or nontraffic accident

✓x7th **V03.92** Pedestrian on skateboard injured in collision with car, pick-up truck or van, unspecified whether traffic or nontraffic accident

✓x7th **V03.99** Pedestrian with other conveyance injured in collision with car, pick-up truck or van, unspecified whether traffic or nontraffic accident

Pedestrian with baby stroller injured in collision with car, pick-up truck or van, unspecified whether traffic or nontraffic accident

Pedestrian on ice-skates injured in collision with car, pick-up truck or van, unspecified whether traffic or nontraffic accident

Pedestrian on nonmotorized scooter injured in collision with car, pick-up truck or van, unspecified whether traffic or nontraffic accident

Pedestrian on sled injured in collision with car, pick-up truck or van in traffic accident

Pedestrian on snowboard injured in collision with car, pick-up truck or van, unspecified whether traffic or nontraffic accident

Pedestrian on snow-skis injured in collision with car, pick-up truck or van, unspecified whether traffic or nontraffic accident

Pedestrian in wheelchair (powered) injured in collision with car, pick-up truck or van, unspecified whether traffic or nontraffic accident

Pedestrian in motorized mobility scooter injured in collision with car, pick-up truck or van, unspecified whether traffic or nontraffic accident

✓4th **V04** Pedestrian injured in collision with heavy transport vehicle or bus

EXCLUDES 1   pedestrian injured in collision with military vehicle (V09.01, V09.21)

✓5th **V04.0** Pedestrian injured in collision with heavy transport vehicle or bus in nontraffic accident

✓x7th **V04.00** Pedestrian on foot injured in collision with heavy transport vehicle or bus in nontraffic accident

Pedestrian NOS injured in collision with heavy transport vehicle or bus in nontraffic accident

✓x7th **V04.01** Pedestrian on roller-skates injured in collision with heavy transport vehicle or bus in nontraffic accident

✓x7th **V04.02** Pedestrian on skateboard injured in collision with heavy transport vehicle or bus in nontraffic accident

✓x7th **V04.09** Pedestrian with other conveyance injured in collision with heavy transport vehicle or bus in nontraffic accident

Pedestrian with baby stroller injured in collision with heavy transport vehicle or bus in nontraffic accident

Pedestrian on ice-skates injured in collision with heavy transport vehicle or bus in nontraffic accident

Pedestrian on nonmotorized scooter injured in collision with heavy transport vehicle or bus in nontraffic accident

Pedestrian on sled injured in collision with heavy transport vehicle or bus in nontraffic accident

Pedestrian on snowboard injured in collision with heavy transport vehicle or bus in nontraffic accident

Pedestrian on snow-skis injured in collision with heavy transport vehicle or bus in nontraffic accident

Pedestrian in wheelchair (powered) injured in collision with heavy transport vehicle or bus in nontraffic accident

Pedestrian in motorized mobility scooter injured in collision with heavy transport vehicle or bus in nontraffic accident

✓5th **V04.1** Pedestrian injured in collision with heavy transport vehicle or bus in traffic accident

✓x7th **V04.10** Pedestrian on foot injured in collision with heavy transport vehicle or bus in traffic accident

Pedestrian NOS injured in collision with heavy transport vehicle or bus in traffic accident

✓x7th **V04.11** Pedestrian on roller-skates injured in collision with heavy transport vehicle or bus in traffic accident

✓x7th **V04.12** Pedestrian on skateboard injured in collision with heavy transport vehicle or bus in traffic accident

✓ Additional Character Required   ✓x7th Placeholder Alert   Manifestation   Unspecified Dx   ▶◀ Revised Text   ● New Code   ▲ Revised Title

ICD-10-CM 2020   1145

Chapter 20. External Causes of Morbidity

√x7ᵗʰ **V04.19 Pedestrian with other conveyance injured in collision with heavy transport vehicle or bus in traffic accident**
Pedestrian with baby stroller injured in collision with heavy transport vehicle or bus in traffic accident
Pedestrian on ice-skates injured in collision with heavy transport vehicle or bus in traffic accident
Pedestrian on nonmotorized scooter injured in collision with heavy transport vehicle or bus in traffic accident
Pedestrian on sled injured in collision with heavy transport vehicle or bus in traffic accident
Pedestrian on snowboard injured in collision with heavy transport vehicle or bus in traffic accident
Pedestrian on snow-skis injured in collision with heavy transport vehicle or bus in traffic accident
Pedestrian in wheelchair (powered) injured in collision with heavy transport vehicle or bus in traffic accident
Pedestrian in motorized mobility scooter injured in collision with heavy transport vehicle or bus in traffic accident

√5ᵗʰ **V04.9 Pedestrian injured in collision with heavy transport vehicle or bus, unspecified whether traffic or nontraffic accident**

√x7ᵗʰ **V04.90 Pedestrian on foot injured in collision with heavy transport vehicle or bus, unspecified whether traffic or nontraffic accident**
Pedestrian NOS injured in collision with heavy transport vehicle or bus, unspecified whether traffic or nontraffic accident

√x7ᵗʰ **V04.91 Pedestrian on roller-skates injured in collision with heavy transport vehicle or bus, unspecified whether traffic or nontraffic accident**

√x7ᵗʰ **V04.92 Pedestrian on skateboard injured in collision with heavy transport vehicle or bus, unspecified whether traffic or nontraffic accident**

√x7ᵗʰ **V04.99 Pedestrian with other conveyance injured in collision with heavy transport vehicle or bus, unspecified whether traffic or nontraffic accident**
Pedestrian with baby stroller injured in collision with heavy transport vehicle or bus, unspecified whether traffic or nontraffic accident
Pedestrian on ice-skates injured in collision with heavy transport vehicle or bus, unspecified whether traffic or nontraffic accident
Pedestrian on nonmotorized scooter injured in collision with heavy transport vehicle or bus, unspecified whether traffic or nontraffic accident
Pedestrian on sled injured in collision with heavy transport vehicle or bus, unspecified whether traffic or nontraffic accident
Pedestrian on snowboard injured in collision with heavy transport vehicle or bus, unspecified whether traffic or nontraffic accident
Pedestrian on snow-skis injured in collision with heavy transport vehicle or bus, unspecified whether traffic or nontraffic accident
Pedestrian in wheelchair (powered) injured in collision with heavy transport vehicle or bus, unspecified whether traffic or nontraffic accident
Pedestrian in motorized mobility scooter injured in collision with heavy transport vehicle or bus, unspecified whether traffic or nontraffic accident

√4ᵗʰ **V05 Pedestrian injured in collision with railway train or railway vehicle**

√5ᵗʰ **V05.0 Pedestrian injured in collision with railway train or railway vehicle in nontraffic accident**

√x7ᵗʰ **V05.00 Pedestrian on foot injured in collision with railway train or railway vehicle in nontraffic accident**
Pedestrian NOS injured in collision with railway train or railway vehicle in nontraffic accident

√x7ᵗʰ **V05.01 Pedestrian on roller-skates injured in collision with railway train or railway vehicle in nontraffic accident**

√x7ᵗʰ **V05.02 Pedestrian on skateboard injured in collision with railway train or railway vehicle in nontraffic accident**

√x7ᵗʰ **V05.09 Pedestrian with other conveyance injured in collision with railway train or railway vehicle in nontraffic accident**
Pedestrian with baby stroller injured in collision with railway train or railway vehicle in nontraffic accident
Pedestrian on ice-skates injured in collision with railway train or railway vehicle in nontraffic accident
Pedestrian on nonmotorized scooter injured in collision with railway train or railway vehicle in nontraffic accident
Pedestrian on sled injured in collision with railway train or railway vehicle in nontraffic accident
Pedestrian on snowboard injured in collision with railway train or railway vehicle in nontraffic accident
Pedestrian on snow-skis injured in collision with railway train or railway vehicle in nontraffic accident
Pedestrian in wheelchair (powered) injured in collision with railway train or railway vehicle in nontraffic accident
Pedestrian in motorized mobility scooter injured in collision with railway train or railway vehicle in nontraffic accident

√5ᵗʰ **V05.1 Pedestrian injured in collision with railway train or railway vehicle in traffic accident**

√x7ᵗʰ **V05.10 Pedestrian on foot injured in collision with railway train or railway vehicle in traffic accident**
Pedestrian NOS injured in collision with railway train or railway vehicle in traffic accident

√x7ᵗʰ **V05.11 Pedestrian on roller-skates injured in collision with railway train or railway vehicle in traffic accident**

√x7ᵗʰ **V05.12 Pedestrian on skateboard injured in collision with railway train or railway vehicle in traffic accident**

√x7ᵗʰ **V05.19 Pedestrian with other conveyance injured in collision with railway train or railway vehicle in traffic accident**
Pedestrian with baby stroller injured in collision with railway train or railway vehicle in traffic accident
Pedestrian on ice-skates injured in collision with railway train or railway vehicle in traffic accident
Pedestrian on nonmotorized scooter injured in collision with railway train or railway vehicle in traffic accident
Pedestrian on sled injured in collision with railway train or railway vehicle in traffic accident
Pedestrian on snowboard injured in collision with railway train or railway vehicle in traffic accident
Pedestrian on snow-skis injured in collision with railway train or railway vehicle in traffic accident
Pedestrian in wheelchair (powered) injured in collision with railway train or railway vehicle in traffic accident
Pedestrian in motorized mobility scooter injured in collision with railway train or railway vehicle in traffic accident

√5ᵗʰ **V05.9 Pedestrian injured in collision with railway train or railway vehicle, unspecified whether traffic or nontraffic accident**

√x7ᵗʰ **V05.90 Pedestrian on foot injured in collision with railway train or railway vehicle, unspecified whether traffic or nontraffic accident**
Pedestrian NOS injured in collision with railway train or railway vehicle, unspecified whether traffic or nontraffic accident

√x7ᵗʰ **V05.91 Pedestrian on roller-skates injured in collision with railway train or railway vehicle, unspecified whether traffic or nontraffic accident**

√x7ᵗʰ **V05.92 Pedestrian on skateboard injured in collision with railway train or railway vehicle, unspecified whether traffic or nontraffic accident**

N Newborn: 0   P Pediatric: 0-17   M Maternity: 12-55   A Adult: 15-124   CH Comorbidity High   CL Comorbidity Low   NCDx Noncancer Dx   PDx Primary Dx

1146   ICD-10-CM 2020

V04.19–V05.92

✓x7ᵗʰ **V05.99** **Pedestrian with other conveyance injured in collision with railway train or railway vehicle, unspecified whether traffic or nontraffic accident**

Pedestrian with baby stroller injured in collision with railway train or railway vehicle, unspecified whether traffic or nontraffic

Pedestrian on ice-skates injured in collision with railway train or railway vehicle, unspecified whether traffic or nontraffic

Pedestrian on nonmotorized scooter injured in collision with railway train or railway vehicle, unspecified whether traffic or nontraffic

Pedestrian on sled injured in collision with railway train or railway vehicle, unspecified whether traffic or nontraffic

Pedestrian on snowboard injured in collision with railway train or railway vehicle, unspecified whether traffic or nontraffic

Pedestrian on snow-skis injured in collision with railway train or railway vehicle, unspecified whether traffic or nontraffic

Pedestrian in wheelchair (powered) injured in collision with railway train or railway vehicle, unspecified whether traffic or nontraffic

Pedestrian in motorized mobility scooter injured in collision with railway train or railway vehicle, unspecified whether traffic or nontraffic

✓4ᵗʰ **V06** **Pedestrian injured in collision with other nonmotor vehicle**

INCLUDES   collision with animal-drawn vehicle, animal being ridden, nonpowered streetcar

EXCLUDES 1   pedestrian injured in collision with pedestrian conveyance (V00.0-)

✓5ᵗʰ **V06.0** **Pedestrian injured in collision with other nonmotor vehicle in nontraffic accident**

✓x7ᵗʰ **V06.00** **Pedestrian on foot injured in collision with other nonmotor vehicle in nontraffic accident**

Pedestrian NOS injured in collision with other nonmotor vehicle in nontraffic accident

✓x7ᵗʰ **V06.01** **Pedestrian on roller-skates injured in collision with other nonmotor vehicle in nontraffic accident**

✓x7ᵗʰ **V06.02** **Pedestrian on skateboard injured in collision with other nonmotor vehicle in nontraffic accident**

✓x7ᵗʰ **V06.09** **Pedestrian with other conveyance injured in collision with other nonmotor vehicle in nontraffic accident**

Pedestrian with baby stroller injured in collision with other nonmotor vehicle in nontraffic accident

Pedestrian on ice-skates injured in collision with other nonmotor vehicle in nontraffic accident

Pedestrian on nonmotorized scooter injured in collision with other nonmotor vehicle in nontraffic accident

Pedestrian on sled injured in collision with other nonmotor vehicle in nontraffic accident

Pedestrian on snowboard injured in collision with other nonmotor vehicle in nontraffic accident

Pedestrian on snow-skis injured in collision with other nonmotor vehicle in nontraffic accident

Pedestrian in wheelchair (powered) injured in collision with other nonmotor vehicle in nontraffic accident

Pedestrian in motorized mobility scooter injured in collision with other nonmotor vehicle in nontraffic accident

✓5ᵗʰ **V06.1** **Pedestrian injured in collision with other nonmotor vehicle in traffic accident**

✓x7ᵗʰ **V06.10** **Pedestrian on foot injured in collision with other nonmotor vehicle in traffic accident**

Pedestrian NOS injured in collision with other nonmotor vehicle in traffic accident

✓x7ᵗʰ **V06.11** **Pedestrian on roller-skates injured in collision with other nonmotor vehicle in traffic accident**

✓x7ᵗʰ **V06.12** **Pedestrian on skateboard injured in collision with other nonmotor vehicle in traffic accident**

✓x7ᵗʰ **V06.19** **Pedestrian with other conveyance injured in collision with other nonmotor vehicle in traffic accident**

Pedestrian with baby stroller injured in collision with other nonmotor vehicle in nontraffic accident

Pedestrian on ice-skates injured in collision with other nonmotor vehicle in traffic accident

Pedestrian on nonmotorized scooter injured in collision with other nonmotor vehicle in traffic accident

Pedestrian on sled injured in collision with other nonmotor vehicle in traffic accident

Pedestrian on snowboard injured in collision with other nonmotor vehicle in traffic accident

Pedestrian on snow-skis injured in collision with other nonmotor vehicle in traffic accident

Pedestrian in wheelchair (powered) injured in collision with other nonmotor vehicle in traffic accident

Pedestrian in motorized mobility scooter injured in collision with other nonmotor vehicle in traffic accident

✓5ᵗʰ **V06.9** **Pedestrian injured in collision with other nonmotor vehicle, unspecified whether traffic or nontraffic accident**

✓x7ᵗʰ **V06.90** **Pedestrian on foot injured in collision with other nonmotor vehicle, unspecified whether traffic or nontraffic accident**

Pedestrian NOS injured in collision with other nonmotor vehicle, unspecified whether traffic or nontraffic accident

✓x7ᵗʰ **V06.91** **Pedestrian on roller-skates injured in collision with other nonmotor vehicle, unspecified whether traffic or nontraffic accident**

✓x7ᵗʰ **V06.92** **Pedestrian on skateboard injured in collision with other nonmotor vehicle, unspecified whether traffic or nontraffic accident**

✓x7ᵗʰ **V06.99** **Pedestrian with other conveyance injured in collision with other nonmotor vehicle, unspecified whether traffic or nontraffic accident**

Pedestrian with baby stroller injured in collision with other nonmotor vehicle, unspecified whether traffic or nontraffic accident

Pedestrian on ice-skates injured in collision with other nonmotor vehicle, unspecified whether traffic or nontraffic accident

Pedestrian on nonmotorized scooter injured in collision with other nonmotor vehicle, unspecified whether traffic or nontraffic accident

Pedestrian on sled injured in collision with other nonmotor vehicle, unspecified whether traffic or nontraffic accident

Pedestrian on snowboard injured in collision with other nonmotor vehicle, unspecified whether traffic or nontraffic accident

Pedestrian on snow-skis injured in collision with other nonmotor vehicle, unspecified whether traffic or nontraffic accident

Pedestrian in wheelchair (powered) injured in collision with other nonmotor vehicle, unspecified whether traffic or nontraffic accident

Pedestrian in motorized mobility scooter injured in collision with other nonmotorized vehicle, unspecified whether traffic or nontraffic accident

✓4ᵗʰ **V09** **Pedestrian injured in other and unspecified transport accidents**

✓5ᵗʰ **V09.0** **Pedestrian injured in nontraffic accident involving other and unspecified motor vehicles**

✓x7ᵗʰ **V09.00** **Pedestrian injured in nontraffic accident involving unspecified motor vehicles**

✓x7ᵗʰ **V09.01** **Pedestrian injured in nontraffic accident involving military vehicle**

✓x7ᵗʰ **V09.09** **Pedestrian injured in nontraffic accident involving other motor vehicles**

Pedestrian injured in nontraffic accident by special vehicle

✓x7ᵗʰ **V09.1** **Pedestrian injured in unspecified nontraffic accident**

✓5ᵗʰ **V09.2** **Pedestrian injured in traffic accident involving other and unspecified motor vehicles**

✓x7ᵗʰ **V09.20** **Pedestrian injured in traffic accident involving unspecified motor vehicles**

✓x7ᵗʰ **V09.21** **Pedestrian injured in traffic accident involving military vehicle**

✓ Additional Character Required   ✓x7ᵗʰ Placeholder Alert   Manifestation   Unspecified Dx   ▶◀ Revised Text   ● New Code   ▲ Revised Title

ICD-10-CM 2020

1147

V05.99–V09.21

✓x7ᵗʰ V09.29 **Pedestrian injured in traffic accident involving other motor vehicles**

✓x7ᵗʰ **V09.3** **Pedestrian injured in unspecified traffic accident**

✓x7ᵗʰ **V09.9** **Pedestrian injured in unspecified transport accident**

Pedal cycle rider injured in transport accident (V10-V19)

INCLUDES any non-motorized vehicle, excluding an animal-drawn vehicle, or a sidecar or trailer attached to the pedal cycle

EXCLUDES 2 rupture of pedal cycle tire (W37.0)

The appropriate 7th character is to be added to each code from categories V10-V19.
A   initial encounter
D   subsequent encounter
S   sequela

✓4ᵗʰ **V10** **Pedal cycle rider injured in collision with pedestrian or animal**

EXCLUDES 1 pedal cycle rider collision with animal-drawn vehicle or animal being ridden (V16.-)

✓x7ᵗʰ **V10.0** **Pedal cycle driver injured in collision with pedestrian or animal in nontraffic accident**

✓x7ᵗʰ **V10.1** **Pedal cycle passenger injured in collision with pedestrian or animal in nontraffic accident**

✓x7ᵗʰ **V10.2** **Unspecified pedal cyclist injured in collision with pedestrian or animal in nontraffic accident**

✓x7ᵗʰ **V10.3** **Person boarding or alighting a pedal cycle injured in collision with pedestrian or animal**

✓x7ᵗʰ **V10.4** **Pedal cycle driver injured in collision with pedestrian or animal in traffic accident**

✓x7ᵗʰ **V10.5** **Pedal cycle passenger injured in collision with pedestrian or animal in traffic accident**

✓x7ᵗʰ **V10.9** **Unspecified pedal cyclist injured in collision with pedestrian or animal in traffic accident**

✓4ᵗʰ **V11** **Pedal cycle rider injured in collision with other pedal cycle**

✓x7ᵗʰ **V11.0** **Pedal cycle driver injured in collision with other pedal cycle in nontraffic accident**

✓x7ᵗʰ **V11.1** **Pedal cycle passenger injured in collision with other pedal cycle in nontraffic accident**

✓x7ᵗʰ **V11.2** **Unspecified pedal cyclist injured in collision with other pedal cycle in nontraffic accident**

✓x7ᵗʰ **V11.3** **Person boarding or alighting a pedal cycle injured in collision with other pedal cycle**

✓x7ᵗʰ **V11.4** **Pedal cycle driver injured in collision with other pedal cycle in traffic accident**

✓x7ᵗʰ **V11.5** **Pedal cycle passenger injured in collision with other pedal cycle in traffic accident**

✓x7ᵗʰ **V11.9** **Unspecified pedal cyclist injured in collision with other pedal cycle in traffic accident**

✓4ᵗʰ **V12** **Pedal cycle rider injured in collision with two- or three-wheeled motor vehicle**

✓x7ᵗʰ **V12.0** **Pedal cycle driver injured in collision with two- or three-wheeled motor vehicle in nontraffic accident**

✓x7ᵗʰ **V12.1** **Pedal cycle passenger injured in collision with two- or three-wheeled motor vehicle in nontraffic accident**

✓x7ᵗʰ **V12.2** **Unspecified pedal cyclist injured in collision with two- or three-wheeled motor vehicle in nontraffic accident**

✓x7ᵗʰ **V12.3** **Person boarding or alighting a pedal cycle injured in collision with two- or three-wheeled motor vehicle**

✓x7ᵗʰ **V12.4** **Pedal cycle driver injured in collision with two- or three-wheeled motor vehicle in traffic accident**

✓x7ᵗʰ **V12.5** **Pedal cycle passenger injured in collision with two- or three-wheeled motor vehicle in traffic accident**

✓x7ᵗʰ **V12.9** **Unspecified pedal cyclist injured in collision with two- or three-wheeled motor vehicle in traffic accident**

✓4ᵗʰ **V13** **Pedal cycle rider injured in collision with car, pick-up truck or van**

✓x7ᵗʰ **V13.0** **Pedal cycle driver injured in collision with car, pick-up truck or van in nontraffic accident**

✓x7ᵗʰ **V13.1** **Pedal cycle passenger injured in collision with car, pick-up truck or van in nontraffic accident**

✓x7ᵗʰ **V13.2** **Unspecified pedal cyclist injured in collision with car, pick-up truck or van in nontraffic accident**

✓x7ᵗʰ **V13.3** **Person boarding or alighting a pedal cycle injured in collision with car, pick-up truck or van**

✓x7ᵗʰ **V13.4** **Pedal cycle driver injured in collision with car, pick-up truck or van in traffic accident**

✓x7ᵗʰ **V13.5** **Pedal cycle passenger injured in collision with car, pick-up truck or van in traffic accident**

✓x7ᵗʰ **V13.9** **Unspecified pedal cyclist injured in collision with car, pick-up truck or van in traffic accident**

✓4ᵗʰ **V14** **Pedal cycle rider injured in collision with heavy transport vehicle or bus**

EXCLUDES 1 pedal cycle rider injured in collision with military vehicle (V19.81)

✓x7ᵗʰ **V14.0** **Pedal cycle driver injured in collision with heavy transport vehicle or bus in nontraffic accident**

✓x7ᵗʰ **V14.1** **Pedal cycle passenger injured in collision with heavy transport vehicle or bus in nontraffic accident**

✓x7ᵗʰ **V14.2** **Unspecified pedal cyclist injured in collision with heavy transport vehicle or bus in nontraffic accident**

✓x7ᵗʰ **V14.3** **Person boarding or alighting a pedal cycle injured in collision with heavy transport vehicle or bus**

✓x7ᵗʰ **V14.4** **Pedal cycle driver injured in collision with heavy transport vehicle or bus in traffic accident**

✓x7ᵗʰ **V14.5** **Pedal cycle passenger injured in collision with heavy transport vehicle or bus in traffic accident**

✓x7ᵗʰ **V14.9** **Unspecified pedal cyclist injured in collision with heavy transport vehicle or bus in traffic accident**

✓4ᵗʰ **V15** **Pedal cycle rider injured in collision with railway train or railway vehicle**

✓x7ᵗʰ **V15.0** **Pedal cycle driver injured in collision with railway train or railway vehicle in nontraffic accident**

✓x7ᵗʰ **V15.1** **Pedal cycle passenger injured in collision with railway train or railway vehicle in nontraffic accident**

✓x7ᵗʰ **V15.2** **Unspecified pedal cyclist injured in collision with railway train or railway vehicle in nontraffic accident**

✓x7ᵗʰ **V15.3** **Person boarding or alighting a pedal cycle injured in collision with railway train or railway vehicle**

✓x7ᵗʰ **V15.4** **Pedal cycle driver injured in collision with railway train or railway vehicle in traffic accident**

✓x7ᵗʰ **V15.5** **Pedal cycle passenger injured in collision with railway train or railway vehicle in traffic accident**

✓x7ᵗʰ **V15.9** **Unspecified pedal cyclist injured in collision with railway train or railway vehicle in traffic accident**

✓4ᵗʰ **V16** **Pedal cycle rider injured in collision with other nonmotor vehicle**

INCLUDES collision with animal-drawn vehicle, animal being ridden, streetcar

✓x7ᵗʰ **V16.0** **Pedal cycle driver injured in collision with other nonmotor vehicle in nontraffic accident**

✓x7ᵗʰ **V16.1** **Pedal cycle passenger injured in collision with other nonmotor vehicle in nontraffic accident**

✓x7ᵗʰ **V16.2** **Unspecified pedal cyclist injured in collision with other nonmotor vehicle in nontraffic accident**

✓x7ᵗʰ **V16.3** **Person boarding or alighting a pedal cycle injured in collision with other nonmotor vehicle in nontraffic accident**

✓x7ᵗʰ **V16.4** **Pedal cycle driver injured in collision with other nonmotor vehicle in traffic accident**

✓x7ᵗʰ **V16.5** **Pedal cycle passenger injured in collision with other nonmotor vehicle in traffic accident**

✓x7ᵗʰ **V16.9** **Unspecified pedal cyclist injured in collision with other nonmotor vehicle in traffic accident**

✓4ᵗʰ **V17** **Pedal cycle rider injured in collision with fixed or stationary object**

✓x7ᵗʰ **V17.0** **Pedal cycle driver injured in collision with fixed or stationary object in nontraffic accident**

✓x7ᵗʰ **V17.1** **Pedal cycle passenger injured in collision with fixed or stationary object in nontraffic accident**

✓x7ᵗʰ **V17.2** **Unspecified pedal cyclist injured in collision with fixed or stationary object in nontraffic accident**

✓x7ᵗʰ **V17.3** **Person boarding or alighting a pedal cycle injured in collision with fixed or stationary object**

✓x7ᵗʰ **V17.4** **Pedal cycle driver injured in collision with fixed or stationary object in traffic accident**

✓x7ᵗʰ **V17.5** **Pedal cycle passenger injured in collision with fixed or stationary object in traffic accident**

✓x7ᵗʰ **V17.9** **Unspecified pedal cyclist injured in collision with fixed or stationary object in traffic accident**

✓4ᵗʰ **V18** **Pedal cycle rider injured in noncollision transport accident**

INCLUDES fall or thrown from pedal cycle (without antecedent collision)
overturning pedal cycle NOS
overturning pedal cycle without collision

✓x7ᵗʰ **V18.0** **Pedal cycle driver injured in noncollision transport accident in nontraffic accident**

✓x7ᵗʰ **V18.1** **Pedal cycle passenger injured in noncollision transport accident in nontraffic accident**

✓x7ᵗʰ **V18.2** **Unspecified pedal cyclist injured in noncollision transport accident in nontraffic accident**

✓x7ᵗʰ **V18.3** **Person boarding or alighting a pedal cycle injured in noncollision transport accident**

√x7ᵗʰ **V18.4** Pedal cycle driver injured in noncollision transport accident in traffic accident

√x7ᵗʰ **V18.5** Pedal cycle passenger injured in noncollision transport accident in traffic accident

√x7ᵗʰ **V18.9** Unspecified pedal cyclist injured in noncollision transport accident in traffic accident

√4ᵗʰ **V19** Pedal cycle rider injured in other and unspecified transport accidents

√5ᵗʰ **V19.0** Pedal cycle driver injured in collision with other and unspecified motor vehicles in nontraffic accident

√x7ᵗʰ **V19.00** Pedal cycle driver injured in collision with unspecified motor vehicles in nontraffic accident

√x7ᵗʰ **V19.09** Pedal cycle driver injured in collision with other motor vehicles in nontraffic accident

√5ᵗʰ **V19.1** Pedal cycle passenger injured in collision with other and unspecified motor vehicles in nontraffic accident

√x7ᵗʰ **V19.10** Pedal cycle passenger injured in collision with unspecified motor vehicles in nontraffic accident

√x7ᵗʰ **V19.19** Pedal cycle passenger injured in collision with other motor vehicles in nontraffic accident

√5ᵗʰ **V19.2** Unspecified pedal cyclist injured in collision with other and unspecified motor vehicles in nontraffic accident

√x7ᵗʰ **V19.20** Unspecified pedal cyclist injured in collision with unspecified motor vehicles in nontraffic accident
Pedal cycle collision NOS, nontraffic

√x7ᵗʰ **V19.29** Unspecified pedal cyclist injured in collision with other motor vehicles in nontraffic accident

√x7ᵗʰ **V19.3** Pedal cyclist (driver) (passenger) injured in unspecified nontraffic accident
Pedal cycle accident NOS, nontraffic
Pedal cyclist injured in nontraffic accident NOS

√5ᵗʰ **V19.4** Pedal cycle driver injured in collision with other and unspecified motor vehicles in traffic accident

√x7ᵗʰ **V19.40** Pedal cycle driver injured in collision with unspecified motor vehicles in traffic accident

√x7ᵗʰ **V19.49** Pedal cycle driver injured in collision with other motor vehicles in traffic accident

√5ᵗʰ **V19.5** Pedal cycle passenger injured in collision with other and unspecified motor vehicles in traffic accident

√x7ᵗʰ **V19.50** Pedal cycle passenger injured in collision with unspecified motor vehicles in traffic accident

√x7ᵗʰ **V19.59** Pedal cycle passenger injured in collision with other motor vehicles in traffic accident

√5ᵗʰ **V19.6** Unspecified pedal cyclist injured in collision with other and unspecified motor vehicles in traffic accident

√x7ᵗʰ **V19.60** Unspecified pedal cyclist injured in collision with unspecified motor vehicles in traffic accident
Pedal cycle collision NOS (traffic)

√x7ᵗʰ **V19.69** Unspecified pedal cyclist injured in collision with other motor vehicles in traffic accident

√5ᵗʰ **V19.8** Pedal cyclist (driver) (passenger) injured in other specified transport accidents

√x7ᵗʰ **V19.81** Pedal cyclist (driver) (passenger) injured in transport accident with military vehicle

√x7ᵗʰ **V19.88** Pedal cyclist (driver) (passenger) injured in other specified transport accidents

√x7ᵗʰ **V19.9** Pedal cyclist (driver) (passenger) injured in unspecified traffic accident
Pedal cycle accident NOS

Motorcycle rider injured in transport accident (V20-V29)

INCLUDES moped
motorcycle with sidecar
motorized bicycle
motor scooter

EXCLUDES 1 three-wheeled motor vehicle (V30-V39)

The appropriate 7th character is to be added to each code from categories V20-V29.
A initial encounter
D subsequent encounter
S sequela

√4ᵗʰ **V20** Motorcycle rider injured in collision with pedestrian or animal

EXCLUDES 1 motorcycle rider collision with animal-drawn vehicle or animal being ridden (V26.-)

√x7ᵗʰ **V20.0** Motorcycle driver injured in collision with pedestrian or animal in nontraffic accident

√x7ᵗʰ **V20.1** Motorcycle passenger injured in collision with pedestrian or animal in nontraffic accident

√x7ᵗʰ **V20.2** Unspecified motorcycle rider injured in collision with pedestrian or animal in nontraffic accident

√x7ᵗʰ **V20.3** Person boarding or alighting a motorcycle injured in collision with pedestrian or animal

√x7ᵗʰ **V20.4** Motorcycle driver injured in collision with pedestrian or animal in traffic accident

√x7ᵗʰ **V20.5** Motorcycle passenger injured in collision with pedestrian or animal in traffic accident

√x7ᵗʰ **V20.9** Unspecified motorcycle rider injured in collision with pedestrian or animal in traffic accident

√4ᵗʰ **V21** Motorcycle rider injured in collision with pedal cycle

√x7ᵗʰ **V21.0** Motorcycle driver injured in collision with pedal cycle in nontraffic accident

√x7ᵗʰ **V21.1** Motorcycle passenger injured in collision with pedal cycle in nontraffic accident

√x7ᵗʰ **V21.2** Unspecified motorcycle rider injured in collision with pedal cycle in nontraffic accident

√x7ᵗʰ **V21.3** Person boarding or alighting a motorcycle injured in collision with pedal cycle

√x7ᵗʰ **V21.4** Motorcycle driver injured in collision with pedal cycle in traffic accident

√x7ᵗʰ **V21.5** Motorcycle passenger injured in collision with pedal cycle in traffic accident

√x7ᵗʰ **V21.9** Unspecified motorcycle rider injured in collision with pedal cycle in traffic accident

√4ᵗʰ **V22** Motorcycle rider injured in collision with two- or three-wheeled motor vehicle

√x7ᵗʰ **V22.0** Motorcycle driver injured in collision with two- or three-wheeled motor vehicle in nontraffic accident

√x7ᵗʰ **V22.1** Motorcycle passenger injured in collision with two- or three-wheeled motor vehicle in nontraffic accident

√x7ᵗʰ **V22.2** Unspecified motorcycle rider injured in collision with two- or three-wheeled motor vehicle in nontraffic accident

√x7ᵗʰ **V22.3** Person boarding or alighting a motorcycle injured in collision with two- or three-wheeled motor vehicle

√x7ᵗʰ **V22.4** Motorcycle driver injured in collision with two- or three-wheeled motor vehicle in traffic accident

√x7ᵗʰ **V22.5** Motorcycle passenger injured in collision with two- or three-wheeled motor vehicle in traffic accident

√x7ᵗʰ **V22.9** Unspecified motorcycle rider injured in collision with two- or three-wheeled motor vehicle in traffic accident

√4ᵗʰ **V23** Motorcycle rider injured in collision with car, pick-up truck or van

√x7ᵗʰ **V23.0** Motorcycle driver injured in collision with car, pick-up truck or van in nontraffic accident

√x7ᵗʰ **V23.1** Motorcycle passenger injured in collision with car, pick-up truck or van in nontraffic accident

√x7ᵗʰ **V23.2** Unspecified motorcycle rider injured in collision with car, pick-up truck or van in nontraffic accident

√x7ᵗʰ **V23.3** Person boarding or alighting a motorcycle injured in collision with car, pick-up truck or van

√x7ᵗʰ **V23.4** Motorcycle driver injured in collision with car, pick-up truck or van in traffic accident

√x7ᵗʰ **V23.5** Motorcycle passenger injured in collision with car, pick-up truck or van in traffic accident

√x7ᵗʰ **V23.9** Unspecified motorcycle rider injured in collision with car, pick-up truck or van in traffic accident

√4ᵗʰ **V24** Motorcycle rider injured in collision with heavy transport vehicle or bus

EXCLUDES 1 motorcycle rider injured in collision with military vehicle (V29.81)

√x7ᵗʰ **V24.0** Motorcycle driver injured in collision with heavy transport vehicle or bus in nontraffic accident

√x7ᵗʰ **V24.1** Motorcycle passenger injured in collision with heavy transport vehicle or bus in nontraffic accident

√x7ᵗʰ **V24.2** Unspecified motorcycle rider injured in collision with heavy transport vehicle or bus in nontraffic accident

√x7ᵗʰ **V24.3** Person boarding or alighting a motorcycle injured in collision with heavy transport vehicle or bus

√x7ᵗʰ **V24.4** Motorcycle driver injured in collision with heavy transport vehicle or bus in traffic accident

√x7ᵗʰ **V24.5** Motorcycle passenger injured in collision with heavy transport vehicle or bus in traffic accident

√x7ᵗʰ **V24.9** Unspecified motorcycle rider injured in collision with heavy transport vehicle or bus in traffic accident

√4ᵗʰ **V25** Motorcycle rider injured in collision with railway train or railway vehicle

√x7ᵗʰ **V25.0** Motorcycle driver injured in collision with railway train or railway vehicle in nontraffic accident

√x7ᵗʰ **V25.1** Motorcycle passenger injured in collision with railway train or railway vehicle in nontraffic accident

✓ Additional Character Required   √x7ᵗʰ Placeholder Alert   Manifestation   Unspecified Dx   ►◄ Revised Text   ● New Code   ▲ Revised Title

ICD-10-CM 2020   1149

✓x7th V25.2 Unspecified motorcycle rider injured in collision with railway train or railway vehicle in nontraffic accident

✓x7th V25.3 Person boarding or alighting a motorcycle injured in collision with railway train or railway vehicle

✓x7th V25.4 Motorcycle driver injured in collision with railway train or railway vehicle in traffic accident

✓x7th V25.5 Motorcycle passenger injured in collision with railway train or railway vehicle in traffic accident

✓x7th V25.9 Unspecified motorcycle rider injured in collision with railway train or railway vehicle in traffic accident

✓4th V26 Motorcycle rider injured in collision with other nonmotor vehicle
> INCLUDES collision with animal-drawn vehicle, animal being ridden, streetcar

✓x7th V26.0 Motorcycle driver injured in collision with other nonmotor vehicle in nontraffic accident

✓x7th V26.1 Motorcycle passenger injured in collision with other nonmotor vehicle in nontraffic accident

✓x7th V26.2 Unspecified motorcycle rider injured in collision with other nonmotor vehicle in nontraffic accident

✓x7th V26.3 Person boarding or alighting a motorcycle injured in collision with other nonmotor vehicle

✓x7th V26.4 Motorcycle driver injured in collision with other nonmotor vehicle in traffic accident

✓x7th V26.5 Motorcycle passenger injured in collision with other nonmotor vehicle in traffic accident

✓x7th V26.9 Unspecified motorcycle rider injured in collision with other nonmotor vehicle in traffic accident

✓4th V27 Motorcycle rider injured in collision with fixed or stationary object

✓x7th V27.0 Motorcycle driver injured in collision with fixed or stationary object in nontraffic accident

✓x7th V27.1 Motorcycle passenger injured in collision with fixed or stationary object in nontraffic accident

✓x7th V27.2 Unspecified motorcycle rider injured in collision with fixed or stationary object in nontraffic accident

✓x7th V27.3 Person boarding or alighting a motorcycle injured in collision with fixed or stationary object

✓x7th V27.4 Motorcycle driver injured in collision with fixed or stationary object in traffic accident

✓x7th V27.5 Motorcycle passenger injured in collision with fixed or stationary object in traffic accident

✓x7th V27.9 Unspecified motorcycle rider injured in collision with fixed or stationary object in traffic accident

✓4th V28 Motorcycle rider injured in noncollision transport accident
> INCLUDES fall or thrown from motorcycle (without antecedent collision)
> overturning motorcycle NOS
> overturning motorcycle without collision

✓x7th V28.0 Motorcycle driver injured in noncollision transport accident in nontraffic accident

✓x7th V28.1 Motorcycle passenger injured in noncollision transport accident in nontraffic accident

✓x7th V28.2 Unspecified motorcycle rider injured in noncollision transport accident in nontraffic accident

✓x7th V28.3 Person boarding or alighting a motorcycle injured in noncollision transport accident

✓x7th V28.4 Motorcycle driver injured in noncollision transport accident in traffic accident

✓x7th V28.5 Motorcycle passenger injured in noncollision transport accident in traffic accident

✓x7th V28.9 Unspecified motorcycle rider injured in noncollision transport accident in traffic accident

✓4th V29 Motorcycle rider injured in other and unspecified transport accidents

✓5th V29.0 Motorcycle driver injured in collision with other and unspecified motor vehicles in nontraffic accident

> **✓x7th V29.00** Motorcycle driver injured in collision with unspecified motor vehicles in nontraffic accident

> **✓x7th V29.09** Motorcycle driver injured in collision with other motor vehicles in nontraffic accident

✓5th V29.1 Motorcycle passenger injured in collision with other and unspecified motor vehicles in nontraffic accident

> **✓x7th V29.10** Motorcycle passenger injured in collision with unspecified motor vehicles in nontraffic accident

> **✓x7th V29.19** Motorcycle passenger injured in collision with other motor vehicles in nontraffic accident

✓5th V29.2 Unspecified motorcycle rider injured in collision with other and unspecified motor vehicles in nontraffic accident

> **✓x7th V29.20** Unspecified motorcycle rider injured in collision with unspecified motor vehicles in nontraffic accident
> Motorcycle collision NOS, nontraffic

> **✓x7th V29.29** Unspecified motorcycle rider injured in collision with other motor vehicles in nontraffic accident

✓5th V29.3 Motorcycle rider (driver) (passenger) injured in unspecified nontraffic accident
> Motorcycle accident NOS, nontraffic
> Motorcycle rider injured in nontraffic accident NOS

✓5th V29.4 Motorcycle driver injured in collision with other and unspecified motor vehicles in traffic accident

> **✓x7th V29.40** Motorcycle driver injured in collision with unspecified motor vehicles in traffic accident

> **✓x7th V29.49** Motorcycle driver injured in collision with other motor vehicles in traffic accident

✓5th V29.5 Motorcycle passenger injured in collision with other and unspecified motor vehicles in traffic accident

> **✓x7th V29.50** Motorcycle passenger injured in collision with unspecified motor vehicles in traffic accident

> **✓x7th V29.59** Motorcycle passenger injured in collision with other motor vehicles in traffic accident

✓5th V29.6 Unspecified motorcycle rider injured in collision with other and unspecified motor vehicles in traffic accident

> **✓x7th V29.60** Unspecified motorcycle rider injured in collision with unspecified motor vehicles in traffic accident
> Motorcycle collision NOS (traffic)

> **✓x7th V29.69** Unspecified motorcycle rider injured in collision with other motor vehicles in traffic accident

✓5th V29.8 Motorcycle rider (driver) (passenger) injured in other specified transport accidents

> **✓x7th V29.81** Motorcycle rider (driver) (passenger) injured in transport accident with military vehicle

> **✓x7th V29.88** Motorcycle rider (driver) (passenger) injured in other specified transport accidents

✓x7th V29.9 Motorcycle rider (driver) (passenger) injured in unspecified traffic accident
> Motorcycle accident NOS

Occupant of three-wheeled motor vehicle injured in transport accident (V30-V39)

> INCLUDES motorized tricycle
> motorized rickshaw
> three-wheeled motor car
> EXCLUDES 1 all-terrain vehicles (V86.-)
> motorcycle with sidecar (V20-V29)
> vehicle designed primarily for off-road use (V86.-)

The appropriate 7th character is to be added to each code from categories V30-V39.
A initial encounter
D subsequent encounter
S sequela

✓4th V30 Occupant of three-wheeled motor vehicle injured in collision with pedestrian or animal
> EXCLUDES 1 three-wheeled motor vehicle collision with animal-drawn vehicle or animal being ridden (V36.-)

✓x7th V30.0 Driver of three-wheeled motor vehicle injured in collision with pedestrian or animal in nontraffic accident

✓x7th V30.1 Passenger in three-wheeled motor vehicle injured in collision with pedestrian or animal in nontraffic accident

✓x7th V30.2 Person on outside of three-wheeled motor vehicle injured in collision with pedestrian or animal in nontraffic accident

✓x7th V30.3 Unspecified occupant of three-wheeled motor vehicle injured in collision with pedestrian or animal in nontraffic accident

✓x7th V30.4 Person boarding or alighting a three-wheeled motor vehicle injured in collision with pedestrian or animal

✓x7th V30.5 Driver of three-wheeled motor vehicle injured in collision with pedestrian or animal in traffic accident

✓x7th V30.6 Passenger in three-wheeled motor vehicle injured in collision with pedestrian or animal in traffic accident

✓x7th V30.7 Person on outside of three-wheeled motor vehicle injured in collision with pedestrian or animal in traffic accident

✓x7th V30.9 Unspecified occupant of three-wheeled motor vehicle injured in collision with pedestrian or animal in traffic accident

✓4th V31 Occupant of three-wheeled motor vehicle injured in collision with pedal cycle

✓x7th V31.0 Driver of three-wheeled motor vehicle injured in collision with pedal cycle in nontraffic accident

√x7ᵗʰ **V31.1** Passenger in three-wheeled motor vehicle injured in collision with pedal cycle in nontraffic accident

√x7ᵗʰ **V31.2** Person on outside of three-wheeled motor vehicle injured in collision with pedal cycle in nontraffic accident

√x7ᵗʰ **V31.3** Unspecified occupant of three-wheeled motor vehicle injured in collision with pedal cycle in nontraffic accident

√x7ᵗʰ **V31.4** Person boarding or alighting a three-wheeled motor vehicle injured in collision with pedal cycle

√x7ᵗʰ **V31.5** Driver of three-wheeled motor vehicle injured in collision with pedal cycle in traffic accident

√x7ᵗʰ **V31.6** Passenger in three-wheeled motor vehicle injured in collision with pedal cycle in traffic accident

√x7ᵗʰ **V31.7** Person on outside of three-wheeled motor vehicle injured in collision with pedal cycle in traffic accident

√x7ᵗʰ **V31.9** Unspecified occupant of three-wheeled motor vehicle injured in collision with pedal cycle in traffic accident

√4ᵗʰ **V32** Occupant of three-wheeled motor vehicle injured in collision with two- or three-wheeled motor vehicle

√x7ᵗʰ **V32.0** Driver of three-wheeled motor vehicle injured in collision with two- or three-wheeled motor vehicle in nontraffic accident

√x7ᵗʰ **V32.1** Passenger in three-wheeled motor vehicle injured in collision with two- or three-wheeled motor vehicle in nontraffic accident

√x7ᵗʰ **V32.2** Person on outside of three-wheeled motor vehicle injured in collision with two- or three-wheeled motor vehicle in nontraffic accident

√x7ᵗʰ **V32.3** Unspecified occupant of three-wheeled motor vehicle injured in collision with two- or three-wheeled motor vehicle in nontraffic accident

√x7ᵗʰ **V32.4** Person boarding or alighting a three-wheeled motor vehicle injured in collision with two- or three-wheeled motor vehicle

√x7ᵗʰ **V32.5** Driver of three-wheeled motor vehicle injured in collision with two- or three-wheeled motor vehicle in traffic accident

√x7ᵗʰ **V32.6** Passenger in three-wheeled motor vehicle injured in collision with two- or three-wheeled motor vehicle in traffic accident

√x7ᵗʰ **V32.7** Person on outside of three-wheeled motor vehicle injured in collision with two- or three-wheeled motor vehicle in traffic accident

√x7ᵗʰ **V32.9** Unspecified occupant of three-wheeled motor vehicle injured in collision with two- or three-wheeled motor vehicle in traffic accident

√4ᵗʰ **V33** Occupant of three-wheeled motor vehicle injured in collision with car, pick-up truck or van

√x7ᵗʰ **V33.0** Driver of three-wheeled motor vehicle injured in collision with car, pick-up truck or van in nontraffic accident

√x7ᵗʰ **V33.1** Passenger in three-wheeled motor vehicle injured in collision with car, pick-up truck or van in nontraffic accident

√x7ᵗʰ **V33.2** Person on outside of three-wheeled motor vehicle injured in collision with car, pick-up truck or van in nontraffic accident

√x7ᵗʰ **V33.3** Unspecified occupant of three-wheeled motor vehicle injured in collision with car, pick-up truck or van in nontraffic accident

√x7ᵗʰ **V33.4** Person boarding or alighting a three-wheeled motor vehicle injured in collision with car, pick-up truck or van

√x7ᵗʰ **V33.5** Driver of three-wheeled motor vehicle injured in collision with car, pick-up truck or van in traffic accident

√x7ᵗʰ **V33.6** Passenger in three-wheeled motor vehicle injured in collision with car, pick-up truck or van in traffic accident

√x7ᵗʰ **V33.7** Person on outside of three-wheeled motor vehicle injured in collision with car, pick-up truck or van in traffic accident

√x7ᵗʰ **V33.9** Unspecified occupant of three-wheeled motor vehicle injured in collision with car, pick-up truck or van in traffic accident

√4ᵗʰ **V34** Occupant of three-wheeled motor vehicle injured in collision with heavy transport vehicle or bus

EXCLUDES 1   occupant of three-wheeled motor vehicle injured in collision with military vehicle (V39.81)

√x7ᵗʰ **V34.0** Driver of three-wheeled motor vehicle injured in collision with heavy transport vehicle or bus in nontraffic accident

√x7ᵗʰ **V34.1** Passenger in three-wheeled motor vehicle injured in collision with heavy transport vehicle or bus in nontraffic accident

√x7ᵗʰ **V34.2** Person on outside of three-wheeled motor vehicle injured in collision with heavy transport vehicle or bus in nontraffic accident

√x7ᵗʰ **V34.3** Unspecified occupant of three-wheeled motor vehicle injured in collision with heavy transport vehicle or bus in nontraffic accident

√x7ᵗʰ **V34.4** Person boarding or alighting a three-wheeled motor vehicle injured in collision with heavy transport vehicle or bus

√x7ᵗʰ **V34.5** Driver of three-wheeled motor vehicle injured in collision with heavy transport vehicle or bus in traffic accident

√x7ᵗʰ **V34.6** Passenger in three-wheeled motor vehicle injured in collision with heavy transport vehicle or bus in traffic accident

√x7ᵗʰ **V34.7** Person on outside of three-wheeled motor vehicle injured in collision with heavy transport vehicle or bus in traffic accident

√x7ᵗʰ **V34.9** Unspecified occupant of three-wheeled motor vehicle injured in collision with heavy transport vehicle or bus in traffic accident

√4ᵗʰ **V35** Occupant of three-wheeled motor vehicle injured in collision with railway train or railway vehicle

√x7ᵗʰ **V35.0** Driver of three-wheeled motor vehicle injured in collision with railway train or railway vehicle in nontraffic accident

√x7ᵗʰ **V35.1** Passenger in three-wheeled motor vehicle injured in collision with railway train or railway vehicle in nontraffic accident

√x7ᵗʰ **V35.2** Person on outside of three-wheeled motor vehicle injured in collision with railway train or railway vehicle in nontraffic accident

√x7ᵗʰ **V35.3** Unspecified occupant of three-wheeled motor vehicle injured in collision with railway train or railway vehicle in nontraffic accident

√x7ᵗʰ **V35.4** Person boarding or alighting a three-wheeled motor vehicle injured in collision with railway train or railway vehicle

√x7ᵗʰ **V35.5** Driver of three-wheeled motor vehicle injured in collision with railway train or railway vehicle in traffic accident

√x7ᵗʰ **V35.6** Passenger in three-wheeled motor vehicle injured in collision with railway train or railway vehicle in traffic accident

√x7ᵗʰ **V35.7** Person on outside of three-wheeled motor vehicle injured in collision with railway train or railway vehicle in traffic accident

√x7ᵗʰ **V35.9** Unspecified occupant of three-wheeled motor vehicle injured in collision with railway train or railway vehicle in traffic accident

√4ᵗʰ **V36** Occupant of three-wheeled motor vehicle injured in collision with other nonmotor vehicle

INCLUDES   collision with animal-drawn vehicle, animal being ridden, streetcar

√x7ᵗʰ **V36.0** Driver of three-wheeled motor vehicle injured in collision with other nonmotor vehicle in nontraffic accident

√x7ᵗʰ **V36.1** Passenger in three-wheeled motor vehicle injured in collision with other nonmotor vehicle in nontraffic accident

√x7ᵗʰ **V36.2** Person on outside of three-wheeled motor vehicle injured in collision with other nonmotor vehicle in nontraffic accident

√x7ᵗʰ **V36.3** Unspecified occupant of three-wheeled motor vehicle injured in collision with other nonmotor vehicle in nontraffic accident

√x7ᵗʰ **V36.4** Person boarding or alighting a three-wheeled motor vehicle injured in collision with other nonmotor vehicle

√x7ᵗʰ **V36.5** Driver of three-wheeled motor vehicle injured in collision with other nonmotor vehicle in traffic accident

√x7ᵗʰ **V36.6** Passenger in three-wheeled motor vehicle injured in collision with other nonmotor vehicle in traffic accident

√x7ᵗʰ **V36.7** Person on outside of three-wheeled motor vehicle injured in collision with other nonmotor vehicle in traffic accident

√x7ᵗʰ **V36.9** Unspecified occupant of three-wheeled motor vehicle injured in collision with other nonmotor vehicle in traffic accident

√4ᵗʰ **V37** Occupant of three-wheeled motor vehicle injured in collision with fixed or stationary object

√x7ᵗʰ **V37.0** Driver of three-wheeled motor vehicle injured in collision with fixed or stationary object in nontraffic accident

√x7ᵗʰ **V37.1** Passenger in three-wheeled motor vehicle injured in collision with fixed or stationary object in nontraffic accident

√x7ᵗʰ **V37.2** Person on outside of three-wheeled motor vehicle injured in collision with fixed or stationary object in nontraffic accident

√x7ᵗʰ **V37.3** Unspecified occupant of three-wheeled motor vehicle injured in collision with fixed or stationary object in nontraffic accident

√x7ᵗʰ **V37.4** Person boarding or alighting a three-wheeled motor vehicle injured in collision with fixed or stationary object

√x7ᵗʰ **V37.5** Driver of three-wheeled motor vehicle injured in collision with fixed or stationary object in traffic accident

√x7ᵗʰ **V37.6** Passenger in three-wheeled motor vehicle injured in collision with fixed or stationary object in traffic accident

√x7ᵗʰ **V37.7** Person on outside of three-wheeled motor vehicle injured in collision with fixed or stationary object in traffic accident

√x7ᵗʰ **V37.9** Unspecified occupant of three-wheeled motor vehicle injured in collision with fixed or stationary object in traffic accident

✔ Additional Character Required   √x7ᵗʰ Placeholder Alert   Manifestation   Unspecified Dx   ▶◀ Revised Text   ● New Code   ▲ Revised Title

ICD-10-CM 2020   1151

Chapter 20. External Causes of Morbidity

V38–V41.9

√4ᵗʰ **V38** **Occupant of three-wheeled motor vehicle injured in noncollision transport accident**

INCLUDES   fall or thrown from three-wheeled motor vehicle
overturning of three-wheeled motor vehicle NOS
overturning of three-wheeled motor vehicle without collision

√x7ᵗʰ **V38.0** Driver of three-wheeled motor vehicle injured in noncollision transport accident in nontraffic accident

√x7ᵗʰ **V38.1** Passenger in three-wheeled motor vehicle injured in noncollision transport accident in nontraffic accident

√x7ᵗʰ **V38.2** Person on outside of three-wheeled motor vehicle injured in noncollision transport accident in nontraffic accident

√x7ᵗʰ **V38.3** Unspecified occupant of three-wheeled motor vehicle injured in noncollision transport accident in nontraffic accident

√x7ᵗʰ **V38.4** Person boarding or alighting a three-wheeled motor vehicle injured in noncollision transport accident

√x7ᵗʰ **V38.5** Driver of three-wheeled motor vehicle injured in noncollision transport accident in traffic accident

√x7ᵗʰ **V38.6** Passenger in three-wheeled motor vehicle injured in noncollision transport accident in traffic accident

√x7ᵗʰ **V38.7** Person on outside of three-wheeled motor vehicle injured in noncollision transport accident in traffic accident

√x7ᵗʰ **V38.9** Unspecified occupant of three-wheeled motor vehicle injured in noncollision transport accident in traffic accident

√4ᵗʰ **V39** **Occupant of three-wheeled motor vehicle injured in other and unspecified transport accidents**

√5ᵗʰ **V39.0** Driver of three-wheeled motor vehicle injured in collision with other and unspecified motor vehicles in nontraffic accident

√x7ᵗʰ **V39.00** Driver of three-wheeled motor vehicle injured in collision with unspecified motor vehicles in nontraffic accident

√x7ᵗʰ **V39.09** Driver of three-wheeled motor vehicle injured in collision with other motor vehicles in nontraffic accident

√5ᵗʰ **V39.1** Passenger in three-wheeled motor vehicle injured in collision with other and unspecified motor vehicles in nontraffic accident

√x7ᵗʰ **V39.10** Passenger in three-wheeled motor vehicle injured in collision with unspecified motor vehicles in nontraffic accident

√x7ᵗʰ **V39.19** Passenger in three-wheeled motor vehicle injured in collision with other motor vehicles in nontraffic accident

√5ᵗʰ **V39.2** Unspecified occupant of three-wheeled motor vehicle injured in collision with other and unspecified motor vehicles in nontraffic accident

√x7ᵗʰ **V39.20** Unspecified occupant of three-wheeled motor vehicle injured in collision with unspecified motor vehicles in nontraffic accident
Collision NOS involving three-wheeled motor vehicle, nontraffic

√x7ᵗʰ **V39.29** Unspecified occupant of three-wheeled motor vehicle injured in collision with other motor vehicles in nontraffic accident

√x7ᵗʰ **V39.3** Occupant (driver) (passenger) of three-wheeled motor vehicle injured in unspecified nontraffic accident
Accident NOS involving three-wheeled motor vehicle, nontraffic
Occupant of three-wheeled motor vehicle injured in nontraffic accident NOS

√5ᵗʰ **V39.4** Driver of three-wheeled motor vehicle injured in collision with other and unspecified motor vehicles in traffic accident

√x7ᵗʰ **V39.40** Driver of three-wheeled motor vehicle injured in collision with unspecified motor vehicles in traffic accident

√x7ᵗʰ **V39.49** Driver of three-wheeled motor vehicle injured in collision with other motor vehicles in traffic accident

√5ᵗʰ **V39.5** Passenger in three-wheeled motor vehicle injured in collision with other and unspecified motor vehicles in traffic accident

√x7ᵗʰ **V39.50** Passenger in three-wheeled motor vehicle injured in collision with unspecified motor vehicles in traffic accident

√x7ᵗʰ **V39.59** Passenger in three-wheeled motor vehicle injured in collision with other motor vehicles in traffic accident

√5ᵗʰ **V39.6** Unspecified occupant of three-wheeled motor vehicle injured in collision with other and unspecified motor vehicles in traffic accident

√x7ᵗʰ **V39.60** Unspecified occupant of three-wheeled motor vehicle injured in collision with unspecified motor vehicles in traffic accident
Collision NOS involving three-wheeled motor vehicle (traffic)

√x7ᵗʰ **V39.69** Unspecified occupant of three-wheeled motor vehicle injured in collision with other motor vehicles in traffic accident

√5ᵗʰ **V39.8** Occupant (driver) (passenger) of three-wheeled motor vehicle injured in other specified transport accidents

√x7ᵗʰ **V39.81** Occupant (driver) (passenger) of three-wheeled motor vehicle injured in transport accident with military vehicle

√x7ᵗʰ **V39.89** Occupant (driver) (passenger) of three-wheeled motor vehicle injured in other specified transport accidents

√x7ᵗʰ **V39.9** Occupant (driver) (passenger) of three-wheeled motor vehicle injured in unspecified traffic accident
Accident NOS involving three-wheeled motor vehicle

Car occupant injured in transport accident (V40-V49)

INCLUDES   a four-wheeled motor vehicle designed primarily for carrying passengers
automobile (pulling a trailer or camper)

EXCLUDES 1   bus (V50-V59)
minibus (V50-V59)
minivan (V50-V59)
motorcoach (V70-V79)
pick-up truck (V50-V59)
sport utility vehicle (SUV) (V50-V59)

The appropriate 7th character is to be added to each code from categories V40-V49.
A   initial encounter
D   subsequent encounter
S   sequela

√4ᵗʰ **V40** **Car occupant injured in collision with pedestrian or animal**

EXCLUDES 1   car collision with animal-drawn vehicle or animal being ridden (V46.-)

√x7ᵗʰ **V40.0** Car driver injured in collision with pedestrian or animal in nontraffic accident

√x7ᵗʰ **V40.1** Car passenger injured in collision with pedestrian or animal in nontraffic accident

√x7ᵗʰ **V40.2** Person on outside of car injured in collision with pedestrian or animal in nontraffic accident

√x7ᵗʰ **V40.3** Unspecified car occupant injured in collision with pedestrian or animal in nontraffic accident

√x7ᵗʰ **V40.4** Person boarding or alighting a car injured in collision with pedestrian or animal

√x7ᵗʰ **V40.5** Car driver injured in collision with pedestrian or animal in traffic accident

√x7ᵗʰ **V40.6** Car passenger injured in collision with pedestrian or animal in traffic accident

√x7ᵗʰ **V40.7** Person on outside of car injured in collision with pedestrian or animal in traffic accident

√x7ᵗʰ **V40.9** Unspecified car occupant injured in collision with pedestrian or animal in traffic accident

√4ᵗʰ **V41** **Car occupant injured in collision with pedal cycle**

√x7ᵗʰ **V41.0** Car driver injured in collision with pedal cycle in nontraffic accident

√x7ᵗʰ **V41.1** Car passenger injured in collision with pedal cycle in nontraffic accident

√x7ᵗʰ **V41.2** Person on outside of car injured in collision with pedal cycle in nontraffic accident

√x7ᵗʰ **V41.3** Unspecified car occupant injured in collision with pedal cycle in nontraffic accident

√x7ᵗʰ **V41.4** Person boarding or alighting a car injured in collision with pedal cycle

√x7ᵗʰ **V41.5** Car driver injured in collision with pedal cycle in traffic accident

√x7ᵗʰ **V41.6** Car passenger injured in collision with pedal cycle in traffic accident

√x7ᵗʰ **V41.7** Person on outside of car injured in collision with pedal cycle in traffic accident

√x7ᵗʰ **V41.9** Unspecified car occupant injured in collision with pedal cycle in traffic accident

Ⓝ Newborn: 0   Ⓟ Pediatric: 0-17   Ⓜ Maternity: 12-55   Ⓐ Adult: 15-124   CH Comorbidity High   CL Comorbidity Low   NCDx Noncancer Dx   PDx Primary Dx

1152   ICD-10-CM 2020

✓4ᵗʰ **V42** **Car occupant injured in collision with two- or three-wheeled motor vehicle**

✓x7ᵗʰ **V42.0** Car driver injured in collision with two- or three-wheeled motor vehicle in nontraffic accident

✓x7ᵗʰ **V42.1** Car passenger injured in collision with two- or three-wheeled motor vehicle in nontraffic accident

✓x7ᵗʰ **V42.2** Person on outside of car injured in collision with two- or three-wheeled motor vehicle in nontraffic accident

✓x7ᵗʰ **V42.3** Unspecified car occupant injured in collision with two- or three-wheeled motor vehicle in nontraffic accident

✓x7ᵗʰ **V42.4** Person boarding or alighting a car injured in collision with two- or three-wheeled motor vehicle

✓x7ᵗʰ **V42.5** Car driver injured in collision with two- or three-wheeled motor vehicle in traffic accident

✓x7ᵗʰ **V42.6** Car passenger injured in collision with two- or three-wheeled motor vehicle in traffic accident

✓x7ᵗʰ **V42.7** Person on outside of car injured in collision with two- or three-wheeled motor vehicle in traffic accident

✓x7ᵗʰ **V42.9** Unspecified car occupant injured in collision with two- or three-wheeled motor vehicle in traffic accident

✓4ᵗʰ **V43** **Car occupant injured in collision with car, pick-up truck or van**

✓5ᵗʰ **V43.0** Car driver injured in collision with car, pick-up truck or van in nontraffic accident

✓x7ᵗʰ **V43.01** Car driver injured in collision with sport utility vehicle in nontraffic accident

✓x7ᵗʰ **V43.02** Car driver injured in collision with other type car in nontraffic accident

✓x7ᵗʰ **V43.03** Car driver injured in collision with pick-up truck in nontraffic accident

✓x7ᵗʰ **V43.04** Car driver injured in collision with van in nontraffic accident

✓5ᵗʰ **V43.1** Car passenger injured in collision with car, pick-up truck or van in nontraffic accident

✓x7ᵗʰ **V43.11** Car passenger injured in collision with sport utility vehicle in nontraffic accident

✓x7ᵗʰ **V43.12** Car passenger injured in collision with other type car in nontraffic accident

✓x7ᵗʰ **V43.13** Car passenger injured in collision with pick-up truck in nontraffic accident

✓x7ᵗʰ **V43.14** Car passenger injured in collision with van in nontraffic accident

✓5ᵗʰ **V43.2** Person on outside of car injured in collision with car, pick-up truck or van in nontraffic accident

✓x7ᵗʰ **V43.21** Person on outside of car injured in collision with sport utility vehicle in nontraffic accident

✓x7ᵗʰ **V43.22** Person on outside of car injured in collision with other type car in nontraffic accident

✓x7ᵗʰ **V43.23** Person on outside of car injured in collision with pick-up truck in nontraffic accident

✓x7ᵗʰ **V43.24** Person on outside of car injured in collision with van in nontraffic accident

✓5ᵗʰ **V43.3** Unspecified car occupant injured in collision with car, pick-up truck or van in nontraffic accident

✓x7ᵗʰ **V43.31** Unspecified car occupant injured in collision with sport utility vehicle in nontraffic accident

✓x7ᵗʰ **V43.32** Unspecified car occupant injured in collision with other type car in nontraffic accident

✓x7ᵗʰ **V43.33** Unspecified car occupant injured in collision with pick-up truck in nontraffic accident

✓x7ᵗʰ **V43.34** Unspecified car occupant injured in collision with van in nontraffic accident

✓5ᵗʰ **V43.4** Person boarding or alighting a car injured in collision with car, pick-up truck or van

✓x7ᵗʰ **V43.41** Person boarding or alighting a car injured in collision with sport utility vehicle

✓x7ᵗʰ **V43.42** Person boarding or alighting a car injured in collision with other type car

✓x7ᵗʰ **V43.43** Person boarding or alighting a car injured in collision with pick-up truck

✓x7ᵗʰ **V43.44** Person boarding or alighting a car injured in collision with van

✓5ᵗʰ **V43.5** Car driver injured in collision with car, pick-up truck or van in traffic accident

✓x7ᵗʰ **V43.51** Car driver injured in collision with sport utility vehicle in traffic accident

✓x7ᵗʰ **V43.52** Car driver injured in collision with other type car in traffic accident

✓x7ᵗʰ **V43.53** Car driver injured in collision with pick-up truck in traffic accident

✓x7ᵗʰ **V43.54** Car driver injured in collision with van in traffic accident

✓5ᵗʰ **V43.6** Car passenger injured in collision with car, pick-up truck or van in traffic accident

✓x7ᵗʰ **V43.61** Car passenger injured in collision with sport utility vehicle in traffic accident

✓x7ᵗʰ **V43.62** Car passenger injured in collision with other type car in traffic accident

✓x7ᵗʰ **V43.63** Car passenger injured in collision with pick-up truck in traffic accident

✓x7ᵗʰ **V43.64** Car passenger injured in collision with van in traffic accident

✓5ᵗʰ **V43.7** Person on outside of car injured in collision with car, pick-up truck or van in traffic accident

✓x7ᵗʰ **V43.71** Person on outside of car injured in collision with sport utility vehicle in traffic accident

✓x7ᵗʰ **V43.72** Person on outside of car injured in collision with other type car in traffic accident

✓x7ᵗʰ **V43.73** Person on outside of car injured in collision with pick-up truck in traffic accident

✓x7ᵗʰ **V43.74** Person on outside of car injured in collision with van in traffic accident

✓5ᵗʰ **V43.9** Unspecified car occupant injured in collision with car, pick-up truck or van in traffic accident

✓x7ᵗʰ **V43.91** Unspecified car occupant injured in collision with sport utility vehicle in traffic accident

✓x7ᵗʰ **V43.92** Unspecified car occupant injured in collision with other type car in traffic accident

✓x7ᵗʰ **V43.93** Unspecified car occupant injured in collision with pick-up truck in traffic accident

✓x7ᵗʰ **V43.94** Unspecified car occupant injured in collision with van in traffic accident

✓4ᵗʰ **V44** **Car occupant injured in collision with heavy transport vehicle or bus**

EXCLUDES 1   car occupant injured in collision with military vehicle (V49.81)

✓x7ᵗʰ **V44.0** Car driver injured in collision with heavy transport vehicle or bus in nontraffic accident

✓x7ᵗʰ **V44.1** Car passenger injured in collision with heavy transport vehicle or bus in nontraffic accident

✓x7ᵗʰ **V44.2** Person on outside of car injured in collision with heavy transport vehicle or bus in nontraffic accident

✓x7ᵗʰ **V44.3** Unspecified car occupant injured in collision with heavy transport vehicle or bus in nontraffic accident

✓x7ᵗʰ **V44.4** Person boarding or alighting a car injured in collision with heavy transport vehicle or bus

✓x7ᵗʰ **V44.5** Car driver injured in collision with heavy transport vehicle or bus in traffic accident

✓x7ᵗʰ **V44.6** Car passenger injured in collision with heavy transport vehicle or bus in traffic accident

✓x7ᵗʰ **V44.7** Person on outside of car injured in collision with heavy transport vehicle or bus in traffic accident

✓x7ᵗʰ **V44.9** Unspecified car occupant injured in collision with heavy transport vehicle or bus in traffic accident

✓4ᵗʰ **V45** **Car occupant injured in collision with railway train or railway vehicle**

✓x7ᵗʰ **V45.0** Car driver injured in collision with railway train or railway vehicle in nontraffic accident

✓x7ᵗʰ **V45.1** Car passenger injured in collision with railway train or railway vehicle in nontraffic accident

✓x7ᵗʰ **V45.2** Person on outside of car injured in collision with railway train or railway vehicle in nontraffic accident

✓x7ᵗʰ **V45.3** Unspecified car occupant injured in collision with railway train or railway vehicle in nontraffic accident

✓x7ᵗʰ **V45.4** Person boarding or alighting a car injured in collision with railway train or railway vehicle

✓x7ᵗʰ **V45.5** Car driver injured in collision with railway train or railway vehicle in traffic accident

✓x7ᵗʰ **V45.6** Car passenger injured in collision with railway train or railway vehicle in traffic accident

✓x7ᵗʰ **V45.7** Person on outside of car injured in collision with railway train or railway vehicle in traffic accident

✓x7ᵗʰ **V45.9** Unspecified car occupant injured in collision with railway train or railway vehicle in traffic accident

✓4ᵗʰ **V46** **Car occupant injured in collision with other nonmotor vehicle**

INCLUDES   collision with animal-drawn vehicle, animal being ridden, streetcar

✓x7ᵗʰ **V46.0** Car driver injured in collision with other nonmotor vehicle in nontraffic accident

✓x7ᵗʰ **V46.1** Car passenger injured in collision with other nonmotor vehicle in nontraffic accident

✓x7ᵗʰ **V46.2** Person on outside of car injured in collision with other nonmotor vehicle in nontraffic accident

Chapter 20. External Causes of Morbidity (side tab)

V46.3–V51.5 (side tab)

✓x7ᵗʰ **V46.3** Unspecified car occupant injured in collision with other nonmotor vehicle in nontraffic accident

✓x7ᵗʰ **V46.4** Person boarding or alighting a car injured in collision with other nonmotor vehicle

✓x7ᵗʰ **V46.5** Car driver injured in collision with other nonmotor vehicle in traffic accident

✓x7ᵗʰ **V46.6** Car passenger injured in collision with other nonmotor vehicle in traffic accident

✓x7ᵗʰ **V46.7** Person on outside of car injured in collision with other nonmotor vehicle in traffic accident

✓x7ᵗʰ **V46.9** Unspecified car occupant injured in collision with other nonmotor vehicle in traffic accident

✓4ᵗʰ **V47 Car occupant injured in collision with fixed or stationary object**

     AHA: 2016,4Q,73

✓x7ᵗʰ **V47.0** Car driver injured in collision with fixed or stationary object in nontraffic accident

✓x7ᵗʰ **V47.1** Car passenger injured in collision with fixed or stationary object in nontraffic accident

✓x7ᵗʰ **V47.2** Person on outside of car injured in collision with fixed or stationary object in nontraffic accident

✓x7ᵗʰ **V47.3** Unspecified car occupant injured in collision with fixed or stationary object in nontraffic accident

✓x7ᵗʰ **V47.4** Person boarding or alighting a car injured in collision with fixed or stationary object

✓x7ᵗʰ **V47.5** Car driver injured in collision with fixed or stationary object in traffic accident

✓x7ᵗʰ **V47.6** Car passenger injured in collision with fixed or stationary object in traffic accident

✓x7ᵗʰ **V47.7** Person on outside of car injured in collision with fixed or stationary object in traffic accident

✓x7ᵗʰ **V47.9** Unspecified car occupant injured in collision with fixed or stationary object in traffic accident

✓4ᵗʰ **V48 Car occupant injured in noncollision transport accident**

     INCLUDES   overturning car NOS
                  overturning car without collision

✓x7ᵗʰ **V48.0** Car driver injured in noncollision transport accident in nontraffic accident

✓x7ᵗʰ **V48.1** Car passenger injured in noncollision transport accident in nontraffic accident

✓x7ᵗʰ **V48.2** Person on outside of car injured in noncollision transport accident in nontraffic accident

✓x7ᵗʰ **V48.3** Unspecified car occupant injured in noncollision transport accident in nontraffic accident

✓x7ᵗʰ **V48.4** Person boarding or alighting a car injured in noncollision transport accident

✓x7ᵗʰ **V48.5** Car driver injured in noncollision transport accident in traffic accident

✓x7ᵗʰ **V48.6** Car passenger injured in noncollision transport accident in traffic accident

✓x7ᵗʰ **V48.7** Person on outside of car injured in noncollision transport accident in traffic accident

✓x7ᵗʰ **V48.9** Unspecified car occupant injured in noncollision transport accident in traffic accident

✓4ᵗʰ **V49 Car occupant injured in other and unspecified transport accidents**

✓5ᵗʰ **V49.0** Driver injured in collision with other and unspecified motor vehicles in nontraffic accident

     ✓x7ᵗʰ **V49.00** Driver injured in collision with unspecified motor vehicles in nontraffic accident

     ✓x7ᵗʰ **V49.09** Driver injured in collision with other motor vehicles in nontraffic accident

✓5ᵗʰ **V49.1** Passenger injured in collision with other and unspecified motor vehicles in nontraffic accident

     ✓x7ᵗʰ **V49.10** Passenger injured in collision with unspecified motor vehicles in nontraffic accident

     ✓x7ᵗʰ **V49.19** Passenger injured in collision with other motor vehicles in nontraffic accident

✓5ᵗʰ **V49.2** Unspecified car occupant injured in collision with other and unspecified motor vehicles in nontraffic accident

     ✓x7ᵗʰ **V49.20** Unspecified car occupant injured in collision with unspecified motor vehicles in nontraffic accident
           Car collision NOS, nontraffic

     ✓x7ᵗʰ **V49.29** Unspecified car occupant injured in collision with other motor vehicles in nontraffic accident

✓x7ᵗʰ **V49.3** Car occupant (driver) (passenger) injured in unspecified nontraffic accident
       Car accident NOS, nontraffic
       Car occupant injured in nontraffic accident NOS

✓5ᵗʰ **V49.4** Driver injured in collision with other and unspecified motor vehicles in traffic accident

     ✓x7ᵗʰ **V49.40** Driver injured in collision with unspecified motor vehicles in traffic accident

     ✓x7ᵗʰ **V49.49** Driver injured in collision with other motor vehicles in traffic accident

✓5ᵗʰ **V49.5** Passenger injured in collision with other and unspecified motor vehicles in traffic accident

     ✓x7ᵗʰ **V49.50** Passenger injured in collision with unspecified motor vehicles in traffic accident

     ✓x7ᵗʰ **V49.59** Passenger injured in collision with other motor vehicles in traffic accident

✓5ᵗʰ **V49.6** Unspecified car occupant injured in collision with other and unspecified motor vehicles in traffic accident

     ✓x7ᵗʰ **V49.60** Unspecified car occupant injured in collision with unspecified motor vehicles in traffic accident
           Car collision NOS (traffic)

     ✓x7ᵗʰ **V49.69** Unspecified car occupant injured in collision with other motor vehicles in traffic accident

✓5ᵗʰ **V49.8** Car occupant (driver) (passenger) injured in other specified transport accidents

     ✓x7ᵗʰ **V49.81** Car occupant (driver) (passenger) injured in transport accident with military vehicle

     ✓x7ᵗʰ **V49.88** Car occupant (driver) (passenger) injured in other specified transport accidents

✓x7ᵗʰ **V49.9** Car occupant (driver) (passenger) injured in unspecified traffic accident
       Car accident NOS

Occupant of pick-up truck or van injured in transport accident (V50-V59)

INCLUDES   a four or six wheel motor vehicle designed primarily for carrying passengers and property but weighing less than the local limit for classification as a heavy goods vehicle
           minibus
           minivan
           sport utility vehicle (SUV)
           truck
           van

EXCLUDES 1   *heavy transport vehicle (V60-V69)*

The appropriate 7th character is to be added to each code from categories V50-V59.
A   initial encounter
D   subsequent encounter
S   sequela

✓4ᵗʰ **V50 Occupant of pick-up truck or van injured in collision with pedestrian or animal**

     EXCLUDES 1   *pick-up truck or van collision with animal-drawn vehicle or animal being ridden (V56.-)*

✓x7ᵗʰ **V50.0** Driver of pick-up truck or van injured in collision with pedestrian or animal in nontraffic accident

✓x7ᵗʰ **V50.1** Passenger in pick-up truck or van injured in collision with pedestrian or animal in nontraffic accident

✓x7ᵗʰ **V50.2** Person on outside of pick-up truck or van injured in collision with pedestrian or animal in nontraffic accident

✓x7ᵗʰ **V50.3** Unspecified occupant of pick-up truck or van injured in collision with pedestrian or animal in nontraffic accident

✓x7ᵗʰ **V50.4** Person boarding or alighting a pick-up truck or van injured in collision with pedestrian or animal

✓x7ᵗʰ **V50.5** Driver of pick-up truck or van injured in collision with pedestrian or animal in traffic accident

✓x7ᵗʰ **V50.6** Passenger in pick-up truck or van injured in collision with pedestrian or animal in traffic accident

✓x7ᵗʰ **V50.7** Person on outside of pick-up truck or van injured in collision with pedestrian or animal in traffic accident

✓x7ᵗʰ **V50.9** Unspecified occupant of pick-up truck or van injured in collision with pedestrian or animal in traffic accident

✓4ᵗʰ **V51 Occupant of pick-up truck or van injured in collision with pedal cycle**

✓x7ᵗʰ **V51.0** Driver of pick-up truck or van injured in collision with pedal cycle in nontraffic accident

✓x7ᵗʰ **V51.1** Passenger in pick-up truck or van injured in collision with pedal cycle in nontraffic accident

✓x7ᵗʰ **V51.2** Person on outside of pick-up truck or van injured in collision with pedal cycle in nontraffic accident

✓x7ᵗʰ **V51.3** Unspecified occupant of pick-up truck or van injured in collision with pedal cycle in nontraffic accident

✓x7ᵗʰ **V51.4** Person boarding or alighting a pick-up truck or van injured in collision with pedal cycle

✓x7ᵗʰ **V51.5** Driver of pick-up truck or van injured in collision with pedal cycle in traffic accident

N Newborn: 0   P Pediatric: 0-17   M Maternity: 12-55   A Adult: 15-124   CH Comorbidity High   CL Comorbidity Low   NCDx Noncancer Dx   PDx Primary Dx

1154   ICD-10-CM 2020

√x7ᵗʰ **V51.6** Passenger in pick-up truck or van injured in collision with pedal cycle in traffic accident

√x7ᵗʰ **V51.7** Person on outside of pick-up truck or van injured in collision with pedal cycle in traffic accident

√x7ᵗʰ **V51.9** Unspecified occupant of pick-up truck or van injured in collision with pedal cycle in traffic accident

√4ᵗʰ **V52 Occupant of pick-up truck or van injured in collision with two- or three-wheeled motor vehicle**

√x7ᵗʰ **V52.0** Driver of pick-up truck or van injured in collision with two- or three-wheeled motor vehicle in nontraffic accident

√x7ᵗʰ **V52.1** Passenger in pick-up truck or van injured in collision with two- or three-wheeled motor vehicle in nontraffic accident

√x7ᵗʰ **V52.2** Person on outside of pick-up truck or van injured in collision with two- or three-wheeled motor vehicle in nontraffic accident

√x7ᵗʰ **V52.3** Unspecified occupant of pick-up truck or van injured in collision with two- or three-wheeled motor vehicle in nontraffic accident

√x7ᵗʰ **V52.4** Person boarding or alighting a pick-up truck or van injured in collision with two- or three-wheeled motor vehicle

√x7ᵗʰ **V52.5** Driver of pick-up truck or van injured in collision with two- or three-wheeled motor vehicle in traffic accident

√x7ᵗʰ **V52.6** Passenger in pick-up truck or van injured in collision with two- or three-wheeled motor vehicle in traffic accident

√x7ᵗʰ **V52.7** Person on outside of pick-up truck or van injured in collision with two- or three-wheeled motor vehicle in traffic accident

√x7ᵗʰ **V52.9** Unspecified occupant of pick-up truck or van injured in collision with two- or three-wheeled motor vehicle in traffic accident

√4ᵗʰ **V53 Occupant of pick-up truck or van injured in collision with car, pick-up truck or van**

√x7ᵗʰ **V53.0** Driver of pick-up truck or van injured in collision with car, pick-up truck or van in nontraffic accident

√x7ᵗʰ **V53.1** Passenger in pick-up truck or van injured in collision with car, pick-up truck or van in nontraffic accident

√x7ᵗʰ **V53.2** Person on outside of pick-up truck or van injured in collision with car, pick-up truck or van in nontraffic accident

√x7ᵗʰ **V53.3** Unspecified occupant of pick-up truck or van injured in collision with car, pick-up truck or van in nontraffic accident

√x7ᵗʰ **V53.4** Person boarding or alighting a pick-up truck or van injured in collision with car, pick-up truck or van

√x7ᵗʰ **V53.5** Driver of pick-up truck or van injured in collision with car, pick-up truck or van in traffic accident

√x7ᵗʰ **V53.6** Passenger in pick-up truck or van injured in collision with car, pick-up truck or van in traffic accident

√x7ᵗʰ **V53.7** Person on outside of pick-up truck or van injured in collision with car, pick-up truck or van in traffic accident

√x7ᵗʰ **V53.9** Unspecified occupant of pick-up truck or van injured in collision with car, pick-up truck or van in traffic accident

√4ᵗʰ **V54 Occupant of pick-up truck or van injured in collision with heavy transport vehicle or bus**

EXCLUDES 1   occupant of pick-up truck or van injured in collision with military vehicle (V59.81)

√x7ᵗʰ **V54.0** Driver of pick-up truck or van injured in collision with heavy transport vehicle or bus in nontraffic accident

√x7ᵗʰ **V54.1** Passenger in pick-up truck or van injured in collision with heavy transport vehicle or bus in nontraffic accident

√x7ᵗʰ **V54.2** Person on outside of pick-up truck or van injured in collision with heavy transport vehicle or bus in nontraffic accident

√x7ᵗʰ **V54.3** Unspecified occupant of pick-up truck or van injured in collision with heavy transport vehicle or bus in nontraffic accident

√x7ᵗʰ **V54.4** Person boarding or alighting a pick-up truck or van injured in collision with heavy transport vehicle or bus

√x7ᵗʰ **V54.5** Driver of pick-up truck or van injured in collision with heavy transport vehicle or bus in traffic accident

√x7ᵗʰ **V54.6** Passenger in pick-up truck or van injured in collision with heavy transport vehicle or bus in traffic accident

√x7ᵗʰ **V54.7** Person on outside of pick-up truck or van injured in collision with heavy transport vehicle or bus in traffic accident

√x7ᵗʰ **V54.9** Unspecified occupant of pick-up truck or van injured in collision with heavy transport vehicle or bus in traffic accident

√4ᵗʰ **V55 Occupant of pick-up truck or van injured in collision with railway train or railway vehicle**

√x7ᵗʰ **V55.0** Driver of pick-up truck or van injured in collision with railway train or railway vehicle in nontraffic accident

√x7ᵗʰ **V55.1** Passenger in pick-up truck or van injured in collision with railway train or railway vehicle in nontraffic accident

√x7ᵗʰ **V55.2** Person on outside of pick-up truck or van injured in collision with railway train or railway vehicle in nontraffic accident

√x7ᵗʰ **V55.3** Unspecified occupant of pick-up truck or van injured in collision with railway train or railway vehicle in nontraffic accident

√x7ᵗʰ **V55.4** Person boarding or alighting a pick-up truck or van injured in collision with railway train or railway vehicle

√x7ᵗʰ **V55.5** Driver of pick-up truck or van injured in collision with railway train or railway vehicle in traffic accident

√x7ᵗʰ **V55.6** Passenger in pick-up truck or van injured in collision with railway train or railway vehicle in traffic accident

√x7ᵗʰ **V55.7** Person on outside of pick-up truck or van injured in collision with railway train or railway vehicle in traffic accident

√x7ᵗʰ **V55.9** Unspecified occupant of pick-up truck or van injured in collision with railway train or railway vehicle in traffic accident

√4ᵗʰ **V56 Occupant of pick-up truck or van injured in collision with other nonmotor vehicle**

INCLUDES   collision with animal-drawn vehicle, animal being ridden, streetcar

√x7ᵗʰ **V56.0** Driver of pick-up truck or van injured in collision with other nonmotor vehicle in nontraffic accident

√x7ᵗʰ **V56.1** Passenger in pick-up truck or van injured in collision with other nonmotor vehicle in nontraffic accident

√x7ᵗʰ **V56.2** Person on outside of pick-up truck or van injured in collision with other nonmotor vehicle in nontraffic accident

√x7ᵗʰ **V56.3** Unspecified occupant of pick-up truck or van injured in collision with other nonmotor vehicle in nontraffic accident

√x7ᵗʰ **V56.4** Person boarding or alighting a pick-up truck or van injured in collision with other nonmotor vehicle

√x7ᵗʰ **V56.5** Driver of pick-up truck or van injured in collision with other nonmotor vehicle in traffic accident

√x7ᵗʰ **V56.6** Passenger in pick-up truck or van injured in collision with other nonmotor vehicle in traffic accident

√x7ᵗʰ **V56.7** Person on outside of pick-up truck or van injured in collision with other nonmotor vehicle in traffic accident

√x7ᵗʰ **V56.9** Unspecified occupant of pick-up truck or van injured in collision with other nonmotor vehicle in traffic accident

√4ᵗʰ **V57 Occupant of pick-up truck or van injured in collision with fixed or stationary object**

√x7ᵗʰ **V57.0** Driver of pick-up truck or van injured in collision with fixed or stationary object in nontraffic accident

√x7ᵗʰ **V57.1** Passenger in pick-up truck or van injured in collision with fixed or stationary object in nontraffic accident

√x7ᵗʰ **V57.2** Person on outside of pick-up truck or van injured in collision with fixed or stationary object in nontraffic accident

√x7ᵗʰ **V57.3** Unspecified occupant of pick-up truck or van injured in collision with fixed or stationary object in nontraffic accident

√x7ᵗʰ **V57.4** Person boarding or alighting a pick-up truck or van injured in collision with fixed or stationary object

√x7ᵗʰ **V57.5** Driver of pick-up truck or van injured in collision with fixed or stationary object in traffic accident

√x7ᵗʰ **V57.6** Passenger in pick-up truck or van injured in collision with fixed or stationary object in traffic accident

√x7ᵗʰ **V57.7** Person on outside of pick-up truck or van injured in collision with fixed or stationary object in traffic accident

√x7ᵗʰ **V57.9** Unspecified occupant of pick-up truck or van injured in collision with fixed or stationary object in traffic accident

√4ᵗʰ **V58 Occupant of pick-up truck or van injured in noncollision transport accident**

INCLUDES   overturning pick-up truck or van NOS
overturning pick-up truck or van without collision

√x7ᵗʰ **V58.0** Driver of pick-up truck or van injured in noncollision transport accident in nontraffic accident

√x7ᵗʰ **V58.1** Passenger in pick-up truck or van injured in noncollision transport accident in nontraffic accident

√x7ᵗʰ **V58.2** Person on outside of pick-up truck or van injured in noncollision transport accident in nontraffic accident

√x7ᵗʰ **V58.3** Unspecified occupant of pick-up truck or van injured in noncollision transport accident in nontraffic accident

√x7ᵗʰ **V58.4** Person boarding or alighting a pick-up truck or van injured in noncollision transport accident

√x7ᵗʰ **V58.5** Driver of pick-up truck or van injured in noncollision transport accident in traffic accident

√x7ᵗʰ **V58.6** Passenger in pick-up truck or van injured in noncollision transport accident in traffic accident

√x7ᵗʰ **V58.7** Person on outside of pick-up truck or van injured in noncollision transport accident in traffic accident

√x7ᵗʰ **V58.9** Unspecified occupant of pick-up truck or van injured in noncollision transport accident in traffic accident

---

☑ Additional Character Required   √x7ᵗʰ Placeholder Alert   Manifestation   Unspecified Dx   ►◄ Revised Text   ● New Code   ▲ Revised Title

ICD-10-CM 2020   1155

✓4ᵗʰ **V59 Occupant of pick-up truck or van injured in other and unspecified transport accidents**

  ✓5ᵗʰ **V59.0** Driver of pick-up truck or van injured in collision with other and unspecified motor vehicles in nontraffic accident

    ✓x7ᵗʰ **V59.00** Driver of pick-up truck or van injured in collision with unspecified motor vehicles in nontraffic accident

    ✓x7ᵗʰ **V59.09** Driver of pick-up truck or van injured in collision with other motor vehicles in nontraffic accident

  ✓5ᵗʰ **V59.1** Passenger in pick-up truck or van injured in collision with other and unspecified motor vehicles in nontraffic accident

    ✓x7ᵗʰ **V59.10** Passenger in pick-up truck or van injured in collision with unspecified motor vehicles in nontraffic accident

    ✓x7ᵗʰ **V59.19** Passenger in pick-up truck or van injured in collision with other motor vehicles in nontraffic accident

  ✓5ᵗʰ **V59.2** Unspecified occupant of pick-up truck or van injured in collision with other and unspecified motor vehicles in nontraffic accident

    ✓x7ᵗʰ **V59.20** Unspecified occupant of pick-up truck or van injured in collision with unspecified motor vehicles in nontraffic accident

      Collision NOS involving pick-up truck or van, nontraffic

    ✓x7ᵗʰ **V59.29** Unspecified occupant of pick-up truck or van injured in collision with other motor vehicles in nontraffic accident

    ✓x7ᵗʰ **V59.3** Occupant (driver) (passenger) of pick-up truck or van injured in unspecified nontraffic accident

      Accident NOS involving pick-up truck or van, nontraffic
      Occupant of pick-up truck or van injured in nontraffic accident NOS

  ✓5ᵗʰ **V59.4** Driver of pick-up truck or van injured in collision with other and unspecified motor vehicles in traffic accident

    ✓x7ᵗʰ **V59.40** Driver of pick-up truck or van injured in collision with unspecified motor vehicles in traffic accident

    ✓x7ᵗʰ **V59.49** Driver of pick-up truck or van injured in collision with other motor vehicles in traffic accident

  ✓5ᵗʰ **V59.5** Passenger in pick-up truck or van injured in collision with other and unspecified motor vehicles in traffic accident

    ✓x7ᵗʰ **V59.50** Passenger in pick-up truck or van injured in collision with unspecified motor vehicles in traffic accident

    ✓x7ᵗʰ **V59.59** Passenger in pick-up truck or van injured in collision with other motor vehicles in traffic accident

  ✓5ᵗʰ **V59.6** Unspecified occupant of pick-up truck or van injured in collision with other and unspecified motor vehicles in traffic accident

    ✓x7ᵗʰ **V59.60** Unspecified occupant of pick-up truck or van injured in collision with unspecified motor vehicles in traffic accident

      Collision NOS involving pick-up truck or van (traffic)

    ✓x7ᵗʰ **V59.69** Unspecified occupant of pick-up truck or van injured in collision with other motor vehicles in traffic accident

  ✓5ᵗʰ **V59.8** Occupant (driver) (passenger) of pick-up truck or van injured in other specified transport accidents

    ✓x7ᵗʰ **V59.81** Occupant (driver) (passenger) of pick-up truck or van injured in transport accident with military vehicle

    ✓x7ᵗʰ **V59.88** Occupant (driver) (passenger) of pick-up truck or van injured in other specified transport accidents

    ✓x7ᵗʰ **V59.9** Occupant (driver) (passenger) of pick-up truck or van injured in unspecified traffic accident

      Accident NOS involving pick-up truck or van

Occupant of heavy transport vehicle injured in transport accident (V60-V69)

INCLUDES 18 wheeler
armored car
panel truck

EXCLUDES 1 *bus*
motorcoach

The appropriate 7th character is to be added to each code from categories V60-V69.
A   initial encounter
D   subsequent encounter
S   sequela

✓4ᵗʰ **V60 Occupant of heavy transport vehicle injured in collision with pedestrian or animal**

    EXCLUDES 1 *heavy transport vehicle collision with animal-drawn vehicle or animal being ridden (V66.-)*

  ✓x7ᵗʰ **V60.0** Driver of heavy transport vehicle injured in collision with pedestrian or animal in nontraffic accident

  ✓x7ᵗʰ **V60.1** Passenger in heavy transport vehicle injured in collision with pedestrian or animal in nontraffic accident

  ✓x7ᵗʰ **V60.2** Person on outside of heavy transport vehicle injured in collision with pedestrian or animal in nontraffic accident

  ✓x7ᵗʰ **V60.3** Unspecified occupant of heavy transport vehicle injured in collision with pedestrian or animal in nontraffic accident

  ✓x7ᵗʰ **V60.4** Person boarding or alighting a heavy transport vehicle injured in collision with pedestrian or animal

  ✓x7ᵗʰ **V60.5** Driver of heavy transport vehicle injured in collision with pedestrian or animal in traffic accident

  ✓x7ᵗʰ **V60.6** Passenger in heavy transport vehicle injured in collision with pedestrian or animal in traffic accident

  ✓x7ᵗʰ **V60.7** Person on outside of heavy transport vehicle injured in collision with pedestrian or animal in traffic accident

  ✓x7ᵗʰ **V60.9** Unspecified occupant of heavy transport vehicle injured in collision with pedestrian or animal in traffic accident

✓4ᵗʰ **V61 Occupant of heavy transport vehicle injured in collision with pedal cycle**

  ✓x7ᵗʰ **V61.0** Driver of heavy transport vehicle injured in collision with pedal cycle in nontraffic accident

  ✓x7ᵗʰ **V61.1** Passenger in heavy transport vehicle injured in collision with pedal cycle in nontraffic accident

  ✓x7ᵗʰ **V61.2** Person on outside of heavy transport vehicle injured in collision with pedal cycle in nontraffic accident

  ✓x7ᵗʰ **V61.3** Unspecified occupant of heavy transport vehicle injured in collision with pedal cycle in nontraffic accident

  ✓x7ᵗʰ **V61.4** Person boarding or alighting a heavy transport vehicle injured in collision with pedal cycle while boarding or alighting

  ✓x7ᵗʰ **V61.5** Driver of heavy transport vehicle injured in collision with pedal cycle in traffic accident

  ✓x7ᵗʰ **V61.6** Passenger in heavy transport vehicle injured in collision with pedal cycle in traffic accident

  ✓x7ᵗʰ **V61.7** Person on outside of heavy transport vehicle injured in collision with pedal cycle in traffic accident

  ✓x7ᵗʰ **V61.9** Unspecified occupant of heavy transport vehicle injured in collision with pedal cycle in traffic accident

✓4ᵗʰ **V62 Occupant of heavy transport vehicle injured in collision with two- or three-wheeled motor vehicle**

  ✓x7ᵗʰ **V62.0** Driver of heavy transport vehicle injured in collision with two- or three-wheeled motor vehicle in nontraffic accident

  ✓x7ᵗʰ **V62.1** Passenger in heavy transport vehicle injured in collision with two- or three-wheeled motor vehicle in nontraffic accident

  ✓x7ᵗʰ **V62.2** Person on outside of heavy transport vehicle injured in collision with two- or three-wheeled motor vehicle in nontraffic accident

  ✓x7ᵗʰ **V62.3** Unspecified occupant of heavy transport vehicle injured in collision with two- or three-wheeled motor vehicle in nontraffic accident

  ✓x7ᵗʰ **V62.4** Person boarding or alighting a heavy transport vehicle injured in collision with two- or three-wheeled motor vehicle

  ✓x7ᵗʰ **V62.5** Driver of heavy transport vehicle injured in collision with two- or three-wheeled motor vehicle in traffic accident

  ✓x7ᵗʰ **V62.6** Passenger in heavy transport vehicle injured in collision with two- or three-wheeled motor vehicle in traffic accident

  ✓x7ᵗʰ **V62.7** Person on outside of heavy transport vehicle injured in collision with two- or three-wheeled motor vehicle in traffic accident

  ✓x7ᵗʰ **V62.9** Unspecified occupant of heavy transport vehicle injured in collision with two- or three-wheeled motor vehicle in traffic accident

Ⓝ Newborn: 0   Ⓟ Pediatric: 0-17   Ⓜ Maternity: 12-55   Ⓐ Adult: 15-124   CH Comorbidity High   CL Comorbidity Low   NCDx Noncancer Dx   PDx Primary Dx

1156   ICD-10-CM 2020

✓4th **V63 Occupant of heavy transport vehicle injured in collision with car, pick-up truck or van**

✓x7th **V63.0** Driver of heavy transport vehicle injured in collision with car, pick-up truck or van in nontraffic accident

✓x7th **V63.1** Passenger in heavy transport vehicle injured in collision with car, pick-up truck or van in nontraffic accident

✓x7th **V63.2** Person on outside of heavy transport vehicle injured in collision with car, pick-up truck or van in nontraffic accident

✓x7th **V63.3** Unspecified occupant of heavy transport vehicle injured in collision with car, pick-up truck or van in nontraffic accident

✓x7th **V63.4** Person boarding or alighting a heavy transport vehicle injured in collision with car, pick-up truck or van

✓x7th **V63.5** Driver of heavy transport vehicle injured in collision with car, pick-up truck or van in traffic accident

✓x7th **V63.6** Passenger in heavy transport vehicle injured in collision with car, pick-up truck or van in traffic accident

✓x7th **V63.7** Person on outside of heavy transport vehicle injured in collision with car, pick-up truck or van in traffic accident

✓x7th **V63.9** Unspecified occupant of heavy transport vehicle injured in collision with car, pick-up truck or van in traffic accident

✓4th **V64 Occupant of heavy transport vehicle injured in collision with heavy transport vehicle or bus**

> **EXCLUDES 1** occupant of heavy transport vehicle injured in collision with military vehicle (V69.81)

✓x7th **V64.0** Driver of heavy transport vehicle injured in collision with heavy transport vehicle or bus in nontraffic accident

✓x7th **V64.1** Passenger in heavy transport vehicle injured in collision with heavy transport vehicle or bus in nontraffic accident

✓x7th **V64.2** Person on outside of heavy transport vehicle injured in collision with heavy transport vehicle or bus in nontraffic accident

✓x7th **V64.3** Unspecified occupant of heavy transport vehicle injured in collision with heavy transport vehicle or bus in nontraffic accident

✓x7th **V64.4** Person boarding or alighting a heavy transport vehicle injured in collision with heavy transport vehicle or bus while boarding or alighting

✓x7th **V64.5** Driver of heavy transport vehicle injured in collision with heavy transport vehicle or bus in traffic accident

✓x7th **V64.6** Passenger in heavy transport vehicle injured in collision with heavy transport vehicle or bus in traffic accident

✓x7th **V64.7** Person on outside of heavy transport vehicle injured in collision with heavy transport vehicle or bus in traffic accident

✓x7th **V64.9** Unspecified occupant of heavy transport vehicle injured in collision with heavy transport vehicle or bus in traffic accident

✓4th **V65 Occupant of heavy transport vehicle injured in collision with railway train or railway vehicle**

✓x7th **V65.0** Driver of heavy transport vehicle injured in collision with railway train or railway vehicle in nontraffic accident

✓x7th **V65.1** Passenger in heavy transport vehicle injured in collision with railway train or railway vehicle in nontraffic accident

✓x7th **V65.2** Person on outside of heavy transport vehicle injured in collision with railway train or railway vehicle in nontraffic accident

✓x7th **V65.3** Unspecified occupant of heavy transport vehicle injured in collision with railway train or railway vehicle in nontraffic accident

✓x7th **V65.4** Person boarding or alighting a heavy transport vehicle injured in collision with railway train or railway vehicle

✓x7th **V65.5** Driver of heavy transport vehicle injured in collision with railway train or railway vehicle in traffic accident

✓x7th **V65.6** Passenger in heavy transport vehicle injured in collision with railway train or railway vehicle in traffic accident

✓x7th **V65.7** Person on outside of heavy transport vehicle injured in collision with railway train or railway vehicle in traffic accident

✓x7th **V65.9** Unspecified occupant of heavy transport vehicle injured in collision with railway train or railway vehicle in traffic accident

✓4th **V66 Occupant of heavy transport vehicle injured in collision with other nonmotor vehicle**

> **INCLUDES** collision with animal-drawn vehicle, animal being ridden, streetcar

✓x7th **V66.0** Driver of heavy transport vehicle injured in collision with other nonmotor vehicle in nontraffic accident

✓x7th **V66.1** Passenger in heavy transport vehicle injured in collision with other nonmotor vehicle in nontraffic accident

✓x7th **V66.2** Person on outside of heavy transport vehicle injured in collision with other nonmotor vehicle in nontraffic accident

✓x7th **V66.3** Unspecified occupant of heavy transport vehicle injured in collision with other nonmotor vehicle in nontraffic accident

✓x7th **V66.4** Person boarding or alighting a heavy transport vehicle injured in collision with other nonmotor vehicle

✓x7th **V66.5** Driver of heavy transport vehicle injured in collision with other nonmotor vehicle in traffic accident

✓x7th **V66.6** Passenger in heavy transport vehicle injured in collision with other nonmotor vehicle in traffic accident

✓x7th **V66.7** Person on outside of heavy transport vehicle injured in collision with other nonmotor vehicle in traffic accident

✓x7th **V66.9** Unspecified occupant of heavy transport vehicle injured in collision with other nonmotor vehicle in traffic accident

✓4th **V67 Occupant of heavy transport vehicle injured in collision with fixed or stationary object**

✓x7th **V67.0** Driver of heavy transport vehicle injured in collision with fixed or stationary object in nontraffic accident

✓x7th **V67.1** Passenger in heavy transport vehicle injured in collision with fixed or stationary object in nontraffic accident

✓x7th **V67.2** Person on outside of heavy transport vehicle injured in collision with fixed or stationary object in nontraffic accident

✓x7th **V67.3** Unspecified occupant of heavy transport vehicle injured in collision with fixed or stationary object in nontraffic accident

✓x7th **V67.4** Person boarding or alighting a heavy transport vehicle injured in collision with fixed or stationary object

✓x7th **V67.5** Driver of heavy transport vehicle injured in collision with fixed or stationary object in traffic accident

✓x7th **V67.6** Passenger in heavy transport vehicle injured in collision with fixed or stationary object in traffic accident

✓x7th **V67.7** Person on outside of heavy transport vehicle injured in collision with fixed or stationary object in traffic accident

✓x7th **V67.9** Unspecified occupant of heavy transport vehicle injured in collision with fixed or stationary object in traffic accident

✓4th **V68 Occupant of heavy transport vehicle injured in noncollision transport accident**

> **INCLUDES** overturning heavy transport vehicle NOS
> overturning heavy transport vehicle without collision

✓x7th **V68.0** Driver of heavy transport vehicle injured in noncollision transport accident in nontraffic accident

✓x7th **V68.1** Passenger in heavy transport vehicle injured in noncollision transport accident in nontraffic accident

✓x7th **V68.2** Person on outside of heavy transport vehicle injured in noncollision transport accident in nontraffic accident

✓x7th **V68.3** Unspecified occupant of heavy transport vehicle injured in noncollision transport accident in nontraffic accident

✓x7th **V68.4** Person boarding or alighting a heavy transport vehicle injured in noncollision transport accident

✓x7th **V68.5** Driver of heavy transport vehicle injured in noncollision transport accident in traffic accident

✓x7th **V68.6** Passenger in heavy transport vehicle injured in noncollision transport accident in traffic accident

✓x7th **V68.7** Person on outside of heavy transport vehicle injured in noncollision transport accident in traffic accident

✓x7th **V68.9** Unspecified occupant of heavy transport vehicle injured in noncollision transport accident in traffic accident

✓4th **V69 Occupant of heavy transport vehicle injured in other and unspecified transport accidents**

✓5th **V69.0** Driver of heavy transport vehicle injured in collision with other and unspecified motor vehicles in nontraffic accident

✓x7th **V69.00** Driver of heavy transport vehicle injured in collision with unspecified motor vehicles in nontraffic accident

✓x7th **V69.09** Driver of heavy transport vehicle injured in collision with other motor vehicles in nontraffic accident

✓5th **V69.1** Passenger in heavy transport vehicle injured in collision with other and unspecified motor vehicles in nontraffic accident

✓x7th **V69.10** Passenger in heavy transport vehicle injured in collision with unspecified motor vehicles in nontraffic accident

✓x7th **V69.19** Passenger in heavy transport vehicle injured in collision with other motor vehicles in nontraffic accident

✓5th **V69.2** Unspecified occupant of heavy transport vehicle injured in collision with other and unspecified motor vehicles in nontraffic accident

✓x7th **V69.20** Unspecified occupant of heavy transport vehicle injured in collision with unspecified motor vehicles in nontraffic accident

> Collision NOS involving heavy transport vehicle, nontraffic

---

✓ Additional Character Required   ✓x7th Placeholder Alert   Manifestation   Unspecified Dx   ▶◀ Revised Text   ● New Code   ▲ Revised Title

√x7ᵗʰ **V69.29** Unspecified occupant of heavy transport vehicle injured in collision with other motor vehicles in nontraffic accident

√x7ᵗʰ **V69.3** Occupant (driver) (passenger) of heavy transport vehicle injured in unspecified nontraffic accident
Accident NOS involving heavy transport vehicle, nontraffic
Occupant of heavy transport vehicle injured in nontraffic accident NOS

√5ᵗʰ **V69.4** Driver of heavy transport vehicle injured in collision with other and unspecified motor vehicles in traffic accident

√x7ᵗʰ **V69.40** Driver of heavy transport vehicle injured in collision with unspecified motor vehicles in traffic accident

√x7ᵗʰ **V69.49** Driver of heavy transport vehicle injured in collision with other motor vehicles in traffic accident

√5ᵗʰ **V69.5** Passenger in heavy transport vehicle injured in collision with other and unspecified motor vehicles in traffic accident

√x7ᵗʰ **V69.50** Passenger in heavy transport vehicle injured in collision with unspecified motor vehicles in traffic accident

√x7ᵗʰ **V69.59** Passenger in heavy transport vehicle injured in collision with other motor vehicles in traffic accident

√5ᵗʰ **V69.6** Unspecified occupant of heavy transport vehicle injured in collision with other and unspecified motor vehicles in traffic accident

√x7ᵗʰ **V69.60** Unspecified occupant of heavy transport vehicle injured in collision with unspecified motor vehicles in traffic accident
Collision NOS involving heavy transport vehicle (traffic)

√x7ᵗʰ **V69.69** Unspecified occupant of heavy transport vehicle injured in collision with other motor vehicles in traffic accident

√5ᵗʰ **V69.8** Occupant (driver) (passenger) of heavy transport vehicle injured in other specified transport accidents

√x7ᵗʰ **V69.81** Occupant (driver) (passenger) of heavy transport vehicle injured in transport accidents with military vehicle

√x7ᵗʰ **V69.88** Occupant (driver) (passenger) of heavy transport vehicle injured in other specified transport accidents

√x7ᵗʰ **V69.9** Occupant (driver) (passenger) of heavy transport vehicle injured in unspecified traffic accident
Accident NOS involving heavy transport vehicle

Bus occupant injured in transport accident (V70–V79)

INCLUDES   motorcoach
EXCLUDES 1 minibus (V50-V59)

The appropriate 7th character is to be added to each code from categories V70-V79.
A   initial encounter
D   subsequent encounter
S   sequela

√4ᵗʰ **V70** Bus occupant injured in collision with pedestrian or animal

EXCLUDES 1 bus collision with animal-drawn vehicle or animal being ridden (V76.-)

√x7ᵗʰ **V70.0** Driver of bus injured in collision with pedestrian or animal in nontraffic accident

√x7ᵗʰ **V70.1** Passenger on bus injured in collision with pedestrian or animal in nontraffic accident

√x7ᵗʰ **V70.2** Person on outside of bus injured in collision with pedestrian or animal in nontraffic accident

√x7ᵗʰ **V70.3** Unspecified occupant of bus injured in collision with pedestrian or animal in nontraffic accident

√x7ᵗʰ **V70.4** Person boarding or alighting from bus injured in collision with pedestrian or animal

√x7ᵗʰ **V70.5** Driver of bus injured in collision with pedestrian or animal in traffic accident

√x7ᵗʰ **V70.6** Passenger on bus injured in collision with pedestrian or animal in traffic accident

√x7ᵗʰ **V70.7** Person on outside of bus injured in collision with pedestrian or animal in traffic accident

√x7ᵗʰ **V70.9** Unspecified occupant of bus injured in collision with pedestrian or animal in traffic accident

√4ᵗʰ **V71** Bus occupant injured in collision with pedal cycle

√x7ᵗʰ **V71.0** Driver of bus injured in collision with pedal cycle in nontraffic accident

√x7ᵗʰ **V71.1** Passenger on bus injured in collision with pedal cycle in nontraffic accident

√x7ᵗʰ **V71.2** Person on outside of bus injured in collision with pedal cycle in nontraffic accident

√x7ᵗʰ **V71.3** Unspecified occupant of bus injured in collision with pedal cycle in nontraffic accident

√x7ᵗʰ **V71.4** Person boarding or alighting from bus injured in collision with pedal cycle

√x7ᵗʰ **V71.5** Driver of bus injured in collision with pedal cycle in traffic accident

√x7ᵗʰ **V71.6** Passenger on bus injured in collision with pedal cycle in traffic accident

√x7ᵗʰ **V71.7** Person on outside of bus injured in collision with pedal cycle in traffic accident

√x7ᵗʰ **V71.9** Unspecified occupant of bus injured in collision with pedal cycle in traffic accident

√4ᵗʰ **V72** Bus occupant injured in collision with two- or three-wheeled motor vehicle

√x7ᵗʰ **V72.0** Driver of bus injured in collision with two- or three-wheeled motor vehicle in nontraffic accident

√x7ᵗʰ **V72.1** Passenger on bus injured in collision with two- or three-wheeled motor vehicle in nontraffic accident

√x7ᵗʰ **V72.2** Person on outside of bus injured in collision with two- or three-wheeled motor vehicle in nontraffic accident

√x7ᵗʰ **V72.3** Unspecified occupant of bus injured in collision with two- or three-wheeled motor vehicle in nontraffic accident

√x7ᵗʰ **V72.4** Person boarding or alighting from bus injured in collision with two- or three-wheeled motor vehicle

√x7ᵗʰ **V72.5** Driver of bus injured in collision with two- or three-wheeled motor vehicle in traffic accident

√x7ᵗʰ **V72.6** Passenger on bus injured in collision with two- or three-wheeled motor vehicle in traffic accident

√x7ᵗʰ **V72.7** Person on outside of bus injured in collision with two- or three-wheeled motor vehicle in traffic accident

√x7ᵗʰ **V72.9** Unspecified occupant of bus injured in collision with two- or three-wheeled motor vehicle in traffic accident

√4ᵗʰ **V73** Bus occupant injured in collision with car, pick-up truck or van

√x7ᵗʰ **V73.0** Driver of bus injured in collision with car, pick-up truck or van in nontraffic accident

√x7ᵗʰ **V73.1** Passenger on bus injured in collision with car, pick-up truck or van in nontraffic accident

√x7ᵗʰ **V73.2** Person on outside of bus injured in collision with car, pick-up truck or van in nontraffic accident

√x7ᵗʰ **V73.3** Unspecified occupant of bus injured in collision with car, pick-up truck or van in nontraffic accident

√x7ᵗʰ **V73.4** Person boarding or alighting from bus injured in collision with car, pick-up truck or van

√x7ᵗʰ **V73.5** Driver of bus injured in collision with car, pick-up truck or van in traffic accident

√x7ᵗʰ **V73.6** Passenger on bus injured in collision with car, pick-up truck or van in traffic accident

√x7ᵗʰ **V73.7** Person on outside of bus injured in collision with car, pick-up truck or van in traffic accident

√x7ᵗʰ **V73.9** Unspecified occupant of bus injured in collision with car, pick-up truck or van in traffic accident

√4ᵗʰ **V74** Bus occupant injured in collision with heavy transport vehicle or bus

EXCLUDES 1 bus occupant injured in collision with military vehicle (V79.81)

√x7ᵗʰ **V74.0** Driver of bus injured in collision with heavy transport vehicle or bus in nontraffic accident

√x7ᵗʰ **V74.1** Passenger on bus injured in collision with heavy transport vehicle or bus in nontraffic accident

√x7ᵗʰ **V74.2** Person on outside of bus injured in collision with heavy transport vehicle or bus in nontraffic accident

√x7ᵗʰ **V74.3** Unspecified occupant of bus injured in collision with heavy transport vehicle or bus in nontraffic accident

√x7ᵗʰ **V74.4** Person boarding or alighting from bus injured in collision with heavy transport vehicle or bus

√x7ᵗʰ **V74.5** Driver of bus injured in collision with heavy transport vehicle or bus in traffic accident

√x7ᵗʰ **V74.6** Passenger on bus injured in collision with heavy transport vehicle or bus in traffic accident

√x7ᵗʰ **V74.7** Person on outside of bus injured in collision with heavy transport vehicle or bus in traffic accident

√x7ᵗʰ **V74.9** Unspecified occupant of bus injured in collision with heavy transport vehicle or bus in traffic accident

√4ᵗʰ **V75** Bus occupant injured in collision with railway train or railway vehicle

√x7ᵗʰ **V75.0** Driver of bus injured in collision with railway train or railway vehicle in nontraffic accident

√x7ᵗʰ **V75.1** Passenger on bus injured in collision with railway train or railway vehicle in nontraffic accident

√x7ᵗʰ **V75.2** Person on outside of bus injured in collision with railway train or railway vehicle in nontraffic accident

☑x7ᵗʰ **V75.3** Unspecified occupant of bus injured in collision with railway train or railway vehicle in nontraffic accident

☑x7ᵗʰ **V75.4** Person boarding or alighting from bus injured in collision with railway train or railway vehicle

☑x7ᵗʰ **V75.5** Driver of bus injured in collision with railway train or railway vehicle in traffic accident

☑x7ᵗʰ **V75.6** Passenger on bus injured in collision with railway train or railway vehicle in traffic accident

☑x7ᵗʰ **V75.7** Person on outside of bus injured in collision with railway train or railway vehicle in traffic accident

☑x7ᵗʰ **V75.9** Unspecified occupant of bus injured in collision with railway train or railway vehicle in traffic accident

☑4ᵗʰ **V76 Bus occupant injured in collision with other nonmotor vehicle**

> **INCLUDES** collision with animal-drawn vehicle, animal being ridden, streetcar

☑x7ᵗʰ **V76.0** Driver of bus injured in collision with other nonmotor vehicle in nontraffic accident

☑x7ᵗʰ **V76.1** Passenger on bus injured in collision with other nonmotor vehicle in nontraffic accident

☑x7ᵗʰ **V76.2** Person on outside of bus injured in collision with other nonmotor vehicle in nontraffic accident

☑x7ᵗʰ **V76.3** Unspecified occupant of bus injured in collision with other nonmotor vehicle in nontraffic accident

☑x7ᵗʰ **V76.4** Person boarding or alighting from bus injured in collision with other nonmotor vehicle

☑x7ᵗʰ **V76.5** Driver of bus injured in collision with other nonmotor vehicle in traffic accident

☑x7ᵗʰ **V76.6** Passenger on bus injured in collision with other nonmotor vehicle in traffic accident

☑x7ᵗʰ **V76.7** Person on outside of bus injured in collision with other nonmotor vehicle in traffic accident

☑x7ᵗʰ **V76.9** Unspecified occupant of bus injured in collision with other nonmotor vehicle in traffic accident

☑4ᵗʰ **V77 Bus occupant injured in collision with fixed or stationary object**

☑x7ᵗʰ **V77.0** Driver of bus injured in collision with fixed or stationary object in nontraffic accident

☑x7ᵗʰ **V77.1** Passenger on bus injured in collision with fixed or stationary object in nontraffic accident

☑x7ᵗʰ **V77.2** Person on outside of bus injured in collision with fixed or stationary object in nontraffic accident

☑x7ᵗʰ **V77.3** Unspecified occupant of bus injured in collision with fixed or stationary object in nontraffic accident

☑x7ᵗʰ **V77.4** Person boarding or alighting from bus injured in collision with fixed or stationary object

☑x7ᵗʰ **V77.5** Driver of bus injured in collision with fixed or stationary object in traffic accident

☑x7ᵗʰ **V77.6** Passenger on bus injured in collision with fixed or stationary object in traffic accident

☑x7ᵗʰ **V77.7** Person on outside of bus injured in collision with fixed or stationary object in traffic accident

☑x7ᵗʰ **V77.9** Unspecified occupant of bus injured in collision with fixed or stationary object in traffic accident

☑4ᵗʰ **V78 Bus occupant injured in noncollision transport accident**

> **INCLUDES** overturning bus NOS
> overturning bus without collision

☑x7ᵗʰ **V78.0** Driver of bus injured in noncollision transport accident in nontraffic accident

☑x7ᵗʰ **V78.1** Passenger on bus injured in noncollision transport accident in nontraffic accident

☑x7ᵗʰ **V78.2** Person on outside of bus injured in noncollision transport accident in nontraffic accident

☑x7ᵗʰ **V78.3** Unspecified occupant of bus injured in noncollision transport accident in nontraffic accident

☑x7ᵗʰ **V78.4** Person boarding or alighting from bus injured in noncollision transport accident

☑x7ᵗʰ **V78.5** Driver of bus injured in noncollision transport accident in traffic accident

☑x7ᵗʰ **V78.6** Passenger on bus injured in noncollision transport accident in traffic accident

☑x7ᵗʰ **V78.7** Person on outside of bus injured in noncollision transport accident in traffic accident

☑x7ᵗʰ **V78.9** Unspecified occupant of bus injured in noncollision transport accident in traffic accident

☑4ᵗʰ **V79 Bus occupant injured in other and unspecified transport accidents**

☑5ᵗʰ **V79.0** Driver of bus injured in collision with other and unspecified motor vehicles in nontraffic accident

☑x7ᵗʰ **V79.00** Driver of bus injured in collision with unspecified motor vehicles in nontraffic accident

☑x7ᵗʰ **V79.09** Driver of bus injured in collision with other motor vehicles in nontraffic accident

☑5ᵗʰ **V79.1** Passenger on bus injured in collision with other and unspecified motor vehicles in nontraffic accident

☑x7ᵗʰ **V79.10** Passenger on bus injured in collision with unspecified motor vehicles in nontraffic accident

☑x7ᵗʰ **V79.19** Passenger on bus injured in collision with other motor vehicles in nontraffic accident

☑5ᵗʰ **V79.2** Unspecified bus occupant injured in collision with other and unspecified motor vehicles in nontraffic accident

☑x7ᵗʰ **V79.20** Unspecified bus occupant injured in collision with unspecified motor vehicles in nontraffic accident

> Bus collision NOS, nontraffic

☑x7ᵗʰ **V79.29** Unspecified bus occupant injured in collision with other motor vehicles in nontraffic accident

☑x7ᵗʰ **V79.3** Bus occupant (driver) (passenger) injured in unspecified nontraffic accident

> Bus accident NOS, nontraffic
> Bus occupant injured in nontraffic accident NOS

☑5ᵗʰ **V79.4** Driver of bus injured in collision with other and unspecified motor vehicles in traffic accident

☑x7ᵗʰ **V79.40** Driver of bus injured in collision with unspecified motor vehicles in traffic accident

☑x7ᵗʰ **V79.49** Driver of bus injured in collision with other motor vehicles in traffic accident

☑5ᵗʰ **V79.5** Passenger on bus injured in collision with other and unspecified motor vehicles in traffic accident

☑x7ᵗʰ **V79.50** Passenger on bus injured in collision with unspecified motor vehicles in traffic accident

☑x7ᵗʰ **V79.59** Passenger on bus injured in collision with other motor vehicles in traffic accident

☑5ᵗʰ **V79.6** Unspecified bus occupant injured in collision with other and unspecified motor vehicles in traffic accident

☑x7ᵗʰ **V79.60** Unspecified bus occupant injured in collision with unspecified motor vehicles in traffic accident

> Bus collision NOS (traffic)

☑x7ᵗʰ **V79.69** Unspecified bus occupant injured in collision with other motor vehicles in traffic accident

☑5ᵗʰ **V79.8** Bus occupant (driver) (passenger) injured in other specified transport accidents

☑x7ᵗʰ **V79.81** Bus occupant (driver) (passenger) injured in transport accidents with military vehicle

☑x7ᵗʰ **V79.88** Bus occupant (driver) (passenger) injured in other specified transport accidents

☑x7ᵗʰ **V79.9** Bus occupant (driver) (passenger) injured in unspecified traffic accident

> Bus accident NOS

Other land transport accidents (V80-V89)

> The appropriate 7th character is to be added to each code from categories V80-V89.
> A initial encounter
> D subsequent encounter
> S sequela

☑4ᵗʰ **V80 Animal-rider or occupant of animal-drawn vehicle injured in transport accident**

☑5ᵗʰ **V80.0** Animal-rider or occupant of animal drawn vehicle injured by fall from or being thrown from animal or animal-drawn vehicle in noncollision accident

☑6ᵗʰ **V80.01** Animal-rider injured by fall from or being thrown from animal in noncollision accident

☑7ᵗʰ **V80.010** Animal-rider injured by fall from or being thrown from horse in noncollision accident

☑7ᵗʰ **V80.018** Animal-rider injured by fall from or being thrown from other animal in noncollision accident

☑x7ᵗʰ **V80.02** Occupant of animal-drawn vehicle injured by fall from or being thrown from animal-drawn vehicle in noncollision accident

> Overturning animal-drawn vehicle NOS
> Overturning animal-drawn vehicle without collision

☑5ᵗʰ **V80.1** Animal-rider or occupant of animal-drawn vehicle injured in collision with pedestrian or animal

> **EXCLUDES 1** animal-rider or animal-drawn vehicle collision with animal-drawn vehicle or animal being ridden (V80.7)

☑x7ᵗʰ **V80.11** Animal-rider injured in collision with pedestrian or animal

☑x7ᵗʰ **V80.12** Occupant of animal-drawn vehicle injured in collision with pedestrian or animal

☑ Additional Character Required   ☑x7ᵗʰ Placeholder Alert   Manifestation   Unspecified Dx   ►◄ Revised Text   ● New Code   ▲ Revised Title

ICD-10-CM 2020   1159

Chapter 20. External Causes of Morbidity

☑5ᵗʰ **V80.2** **Animal-rider or occupant of animal-drawn vehicle injured in collision with** pedal cycle

☑x7ᵗʰ **V80.21** Animal-rider injured in collision with pedal cycle

☑x7ᵗʰ **V80.22** Occupant of animal-drawn vehicle injured in collision with pedal cycle

☑5ᵗʰ **V80.3** **Animal-rider or occupant of animal-drawn vehicle injured in collision with** two- or three-wheeled motor vehicle

☑x7ᵗʰ **V80.31** Animal-rider injured in collision with two- or three-wheeled motor vehicle

☑x7ᵗʰ **V80.32** Occupant of animal-drawn vehicle injured in collision with two- or three-wheeled motor vehicle

☑5ᵗʰ **V80.4** **Animal-rider or occupant of animal-drawn vehicle injured in collision with** car, pick-up truck, van, heavy transport vehicle or bus

     EXCLUDES 1   *animal-rider injured in collision with military vehicle (V80.910)*

             occupant of animal-drawn vehicle injured in collision with military vehicle (V80.920)

☑x7ᵗʰ **V80.41** Animal-rider injured in collision with car, pick-up truck, van, heavy transport vehicle or bus

☑x7ᵗʰ **V80.42** Occupant of animal-drawn vehicle injured in collision with car, pick-up truck, van, heavy transport vehicle or bus

☑5ᵗʰ **V80.5** **Animal-rider or occupant of animal-drawn vehicle injured in collision with other specified motor vehicle**

☑x7ᵗʰ **V80.51** Animal-rider injured in collision with other specified motor vehicle

☑x7ᵗʰ **V80.52** Occupant of animal-drawn vehicle injured in collision with other specified motor vehicle

☑5ᵗʰ **V80.6** **Animal-rider or occupant of animal-drawn vehicle injured in collision with** railway train or railway vehicle

☑x7ᵗʰ **V80.61** Animal-rider injured in collision with railway train or railway vehicle

☑x7ᵗʰ **V80.62** Occupant of animal-drawn vehicle injured in collision with railway train or railway vehicle

☑5ᵗʰ **V80.7** **Animal-rider or occupant of animal-drawn vehicle injured in collision with other nonmotor vehicles**

☑6ᵗʰ **V80.71** Animal-rider or occupant of animal-drawn vehicle injured in collision with animal being ridden

☑7ᵗʰ **V80.710** Animal-rider injured in collision with other animal being ridden

☑7ᵗʰ **V80.711** Occupant of animal-drawn vehicle injured in collision with animal being ridden

☑6ᵗʰ **V80.72** Animal-rider or occupant of animal-drawn vehicle injured in collision with other animal-drawn vehicle

☑7ᵗʰ **V80.720** Animal-rider injured in collision with animal-drawn vehicle

☑7ᵗʰ **V80.721** Occupant of animal-drawn vehicle injured in collision with other animal-drawn vehicle

☑6ᵗʰ **V80.73** Animal-rider or occupant of animal-drawn vehicle injured in collision with streetcar

☑7ᵗʰ **V80.730** Animal-rider injured in collision with streetcar

☑7ᵗʰ **V80.731** Occupant of animal-drawn vehicle injured in collision with streetcar

☑6ᵗʰ **V80.79** Animal-rider or occupant of animal-drawn vehicle injured in collision with other nonmotor vehicles

☑7ᵗʰ **V80.790** Animal-rider injured in collision with other nonmotor vehicles

☑7ᵗʰ **V80.791** Occupant of animal-drawn vehicle injured in collision with other nonmotor vehicles

☑5ᵗʰ **V80.8** **Animal-rider or occupant of animal-drawn vehicle injured in collision with** fixed or stationary object

☑x7ᵗʰ **V80.81** Animal-rider injured in collision with fixed or stationary object

☑x7ᵗʰ **V80.82** Occupant of animal-drawn vehicle injured in collision with fixed or stationary object

☑5ᵗʰ **V80.9** **Animal-rider or occupant of animal-drawn vehicle injured in other and unspecified transport accidents**

☑6ᵗʰ **V80.91** Animal-rider injured in other and unspecified transport accidents

☑7ᵗʰ **V80.910** Animal-rider injured in transport accident with military vehicle

☑7ᵗʰ **V80.918** Animal-rider injured in other transport accident

☑7ᵗʰ **V80.919** Animal-rider injured in unspecified transport accident

         Animal rider accident NOS

☑6ᵗʰ **V80.92** Occupant of animal-drawn vehicle injured in other and unspecified transport accidents

☑7ᵗʰ **V80.920** Occupant of animal-drawn vehicle injured in transport accident with military vehicle

☑7ᵗʰ **V80.928** Occupant of animal-drawn vehicle injured in other transport accident

☑7ᵗʰ **V80.929** Occupant of animal-drawn vehicle injured in unspecified transport accident

         Animal-drawn vehicle accident NOS

☑4ᵗʰ **V81** **Occupant of railway train or railway vehicle injured in transport accident**

     INCLUDES   derailment of railway train or railway vehicle

              person on outside of train

     EXCLUDES 1   *streetcar (V82.-)*

☑x7ᵗʰ **V81.0** **Occupant of railway train or railway vehicle injured in collision with motor vehicle** in nontraffic accident

       EXCLUDES 1   *occupant of railway train or railway vehicle injured due to collision with military vehicle (V81.83)*

☑x7ᵗʰ **V81.1** **Occupant of railway train or railway vehicle injured in collision with motor vehicle** in traffic accident

       EXCLUDES 1   *occupant of railway train or railway vehicle injured due to collision with military vehicle (V81.83)*

☑x7ᵗʰ **V81.2** **Occupant of railway train or railway vehicle injured in collision with or** hit by rolling stock

☑x7ᵗʰ **V81.3** **Occupant of railway train or railway vehicle injured in collision with other object**

       Railway collision NOS

☑x7ᵗʰ **V81.4** **Person injured** while boarding or alighting **from railway train or railway vehicle**

☑x7ᵗʰ **V81.5** **Occupant of railway train or railway vehicle injured by** fall in railway train **or railway vehicle**

☑x7ᵗʰ **V81.6** **Occupant of railway train or railway vehicle injured by** fall from railway train **or railway vehicle**

☑x7ᵗʰ **V81.7** **Occupant of railway train or railway vehicle injured in** derailment without antecedent collision

☑5ᵗʰ **V81.8** **Occupant of railway train or railway vehicle injured in other specified railway accidents**

☑x7ᵗʰ **V81.81** Occupant of railway train or railway vehicle injured due to explosion or fire on train

☑x7ᵗʰ **V81.82** Occupant of railway train or railway vehicle injured due to object falling onto train

         Occupant of railway train or railway vehicle injured due to falling earth onto train

         Occupant of railway train or railway vehicle injured due to falling rocks onto train

         Occupant of railway train or railway vehicle injured due to falling snow onto train

         Occupant of railway train or railway vehicle injured due to falling trees onto train

☑x7ᵗʰ **V81.83** Occupant of railway train or railway vehicle injured due to collision with military vehicle

☑x7ᵗʰ **V81.89** Occupant of railway train or railway vehicle injured due to other specified railway accident

☑x7ᵗʰ **V81.9** **Occupant of railway train or railway vehicle injured in unspecified railway accident**

       Railway accident NOS

☑4ᵗʰ **V82** **Occupant of powered streetcar injured in transport accident**

     INCLUDES   interurban electric car

              person on outside of streetcar

              tram (car)

              trolley (car)

     EXCLUDES 1   *bus (V70-V79)*

              motorcoach (V70-V79)

              nonpowered streetcar (V76.-)

              train (V81.-)

☑x7ᵗʰ **V82.0** **Occupant of streetcar injured in collision with motor vehicle** in nontraffic accident

☑x7ᵗʰ **V82.1** **Occupant of streetcar injured in collision with motor vehicle** in traffic accident

☑x7ᵗʰ **V82.2** **Occupant of streetcar injured in collision with or** hit by rolling stock

☑x7ᵗʰ **V82.3** **Occupant of streetcar injured in collision with other object**

       EXCLUDES 1   *collision with animal-drawn vehicle or animal being ridden (V82.8)*

☑x7ᵗʰ **V82.4** **Person injured** while boarding or alighting **from streetcar**

☒ Newborn: 0   ☒ Pediatric: 0-17   ☒ Maternity: 12-55   ☒ Adult: 15-124   **CH** Comorbidity High   **CL** Comorbidity Low   **NCDx** Noncancer Dx   **PDx** Primary Dx

1160   ICD-10-CM 2020

V82.5 Occupant of streetcar injured by fall in streetcar
> EXCLUDES 1 *fall in streetcar:*
> *while boarding or alighting (V82.4)*
> *with antecedent collision (V82.0-V82.3)*

V82.6 Occupant of streetcar injured by fall from streetcar
> EXCLUDES 1 *fall from streetcar:*
> *while boarding or alighting (V82.4)*
> *with antecedent collision (V82.0-V82.3)*

V82.7 Occupant of streetcar injured in derailment without antecedent collision
> EXCLUDES 1 *occupant of streetcar injured in derailment with antecedent collision (V82.0-V82.3)*

V82.8 Occupant of streetcar injured in other specified transport accidents
> Streetcar collision with military vehicle
> Streetcar collision with train or nonmotor vehicles

V82.9 Occupant of streetcar injured in unspecified traffic accident
> Streetcar accident NOS

V83 Occupant of special vehicle mainly used on industrial premises injured in transport accident
> INCLUDES battery-powered airport passenger vehicle
> battery-powered truck (baggage) (mail)
> coal-car in mine
> forklift (truck)
> logging car
> self-propelled industrial truck
> station baggage truck (powered)
> tram, truck, or tub (powered) in mine or quarry
> EXCLUDES 1 *special construction vehicles (V85.-)*
> *special industrial vehicle in stationary use or maintenance (W31.-)*

V83.0 Driver of special industrial vehicle injured in traffic accident

V83.1 Passenger of special industrial vehicle injured in traffic accident

V83.2 Person on outside of special industrial vehicle injured in traffic accident

V83.3 Unspecified occupant of special industrial vehicle injured in traffic accident

V83.4 Person injured while boarding or alighting from special industrial vehicle

V83.5 Driver of special industrial vehicle injured in nontraffic accident

V83.6 Passenger of special industrial vehicle injured in nontraffic accident

V83.7 Person on outside of special industrial vehicle injured in nontraffic accident

V83.9 Unspecified occupant of special industrial vehicle injured in nontraffic accident
> Special-industrial-vehicle accident NOS

V84 Occupant of special vehicle mainly used in agriculture injured in transport accident
> INCLUDES self-propelled farm machinery
> tractor (and trailer)
> EXCLUDES 1 *animal-powered farm machinery accident (W30.8-)*
> *contact with combine harvester (W30.0)*
> *special agricultural vehicle in stationary use or maintenance (W30.-)*

V84.0 Driver of special agricultural vehicle injured in traffic accident

V84.1 Passenger of special agricultural vehicle injured in traffic accident

V84.2 Person on outside of special agricultural vehicle injured in traffic accident

V84.3 Unspecified occupant of special agricultural vehicle injured in traffic accident

V84.4 Person injured while boarding or alighting from special agricultural vehicle

V84.5 Driver of special agricultural vehicle injured in nontraffic accident

V84.6 Passenger of special agricultural vehicle injured in nontraffic accident

V84.7 Person on outside of special agricultural vehicle injured in nontraffic accident

V84.9 Unspecified occupant of special agricultural vehicle injured in nontraffic accident
> Special-agricultural vehicle accident NOS

V85 Occupant of special construction vehicle injured in transport accident
> INCLUDES bulldozer
> digger
> dump truck
> earth-leveller
> mechanical shovel
> road-roller
> EXCLUDES 1 *special industrial vehicle (V83.-)*
> *special construction vehicle in stationary use or maintenance (W31.-)*

V85.0 Driver of special construction vehicle injured in traffic accident

V85.1 Passenger of special construction vehicle injured in traffic accident

V85.2 Person on outside of special construction vehicle injured in traffic accident

V85.3 Unspecified occupant of special construction vehicle injured in traffic accident

V85.4 Person injured while boarding or alighting from special construction vehicle

V85.5 Driver of special construction vehicle injured in nontraffic accident

V85.6 Passenger of special construction vehicle injured in nontraffic accident

V85.7 Person on outside of special construction vehicle injured in nontraffic accident

V85.9 Unspecified occupant of special construction vehicle injured in nontraffic accident
> Special-construction-vehicle accident NOS

V86 Occupant of special all-terrain or other off-road motor vehicle, injured in transport accident
> EXCLUDES 1 *special all-terrain vehicle in stationary use or maintenance (W31.-)*
> *sport-utility vehicle (V50-V59)*
> *three-wheeled motor vehicle designed for on-road use (V30-V39)*

AHA: 2017,4Q,26

V86.0 Driver of special all-terrain or other off-road motor vehicle injured in traffic accident

V86.01 Driver of ambulance or fire engine injured in traffic accident

V86.02 Driver of snowmobile injured in traffic accident

V86.03 Driver of dune buggy injured in traffic accident

V86.04 Driver of military vehicle injured in traffic accident

V86.05 Driver of 3- or 4- wheeled all-terrain vehicle (ATV) injured in traffic accident

V86.06 Driver of dirt bike or motor/cross bike injured in traffic accident

V86.09 Driver of other special all-terrain or other off-road motor vehicle injured in traffic accident
> ~~Driver of dirt bike injured in traffic accident~~
> Driver of go cart injured in traffic accident
> Driver of golf cart injured in traffic accident

V86.1 Passenger of special all-terrain or other off-road motor vehicle injured in traffic accident

V86.11 Passenger of ambulance or fire engine injured in traffic accident

V86.12 Passenger of snowmobile injured in traffic accident

V86.13 Passenger of dune buggy injured in traffic accident

V86.14 Passenger of military vehicle injured in traffic accident

V86.15 Passenger of 3- or 4- wheeled all-terrain vehicle (ATV) injured in traffic accident

V86.16 Passenger of dirt bike or motor/cross bike injured in traffic accident

V86.19 Passenger of other special all-terrain or other off-road motor vehicle injured in traffic accident
> ~~Passenger of dirt bike injured in traffic accident~~
> Passenger of go cart injured in traffic accident
> Passenger of golf cart injured in traffic accident

V86.2 Person on outside of special all-terrain or other off-road motor vehicle injured in traffic accident

V86.21 Person on outside of ambulance or fire engine injured in traffic accident

V86.22 Person on outside of snowmobile injured in traffic accident

V86.23 Person on outside of dune buggy injured in traffic accident

Chapter 20. External Causes of Morbidity

V82.5–V86.23

Chapter 20. External Causes of Morbidity

☑x7ᵗʰ **V86.24** Person on outside of military vehicle injured in traffic accident

☑x7ᵗʰ **V86.25** Person on outside of 3- or 4- wheeled all-terrain vehicle (ATV) injured in traffic accident

☑x7ᵗʰ **V86.26** Person on outside of dirt bike or motor/cross bike injured in traffic accident

☑x7ᵗʰ **V86.29** Person on outside of other special all-terrain or other off-road motor vehicle injured in traffic accident

~~Person on outside of dirt bike injured in traffic accident~~

Person on outside of go cart in traffic accident

Person on outside of golf cart injured in traffic accident

☑5ᵗʰ **V86.3** Unspecified occupant of special all-terrain or other off-road motor vehicle injured in traffic accident

☑x7ᵗʰ **V86.31** Unspecified occupant of ambulance or fire engine injured in traffic accident

☑x7ᵗʰ **V86.32** Unspecified occupant of snowmobile injured in traffic accident

☑x7ᵗʰ **V86.33** Unspecified occupant of dune buggy injured in traffic accident

☑x7ᵗʰ **V86.34** Unspecified occupant of military vehicle injured in traffic accident

☑x7ᵗʰ **V86.35** Unspecified occupant of 3- or 4- wheeled all-terrain vehicle (ATV) injured in traffic accident

☑x7ᵗʰ **V86.36** Unspecified occupant of dirt bike or motor/cross bike injured in traffic accident

☑x7ᵗʰ **V86.39** Unspecified occupant of other special all-terrain or other off-road motor vehicle injured in traffic accident

~~Unspecified occupant of dirt bike injured in traffic accident~~

Unspecified occupant of go cart injured in traffic accident

Unspecified occupant of golf cart injured in traffic accident

☑5ᵗʰ **V86.4** Person injured while boarding or alighting from special all-terrain or other off-road motor vehicle

☑x7ᵗʰ **V86.41** Person injured while boarding or alighting from ambulance or fire engine

☑x7ᵗʰ **V86.42** Person injured while boarding or alighting from snowmobile

☑x7ᵗʰ **V86.43** Person injured while boarding or alighting from dune buggy

☑x7ᵗʰ **V86.44** Person injured while boarding or alighting from military vehicle

☑x7ᵗʰ **V86.45** Person injured while boarding or alighting from a 3- or 4- wheeled all-terrain vehicle (ATV)

☑x7ᵗʰ **V86.46** Person injured while boarding or alighting from a dirt bike or motor/cross bike

☑x7ᵗʰ **V86.49** Person injured while boarding or alighting from other special all-terrain or other off-road motor vehicle

~~Person injured while boarding or alighting from dirt bike~~

Person injured while boarding or alighting from go cart

Person injured while boarding or alighting from golf cart

☑5ᵗʰ **V86.5** Driver of special all-terrain or other off-road motor vehicle injured in nontraffic accident

☑x7ᵗʰ **V86.51** Driver of ambulance or fire engine injured in nontraffic accident

☑x7ᵗʰ **V86.52** Driver of snowmobile injured in nontraffic accident

☑x7ᵗʰ **V86.53** Driver of dune buggy injured in nontraffic accident

☑x7ᵗʰ **V86.54** Driver of military vehicle injured in nontraffic accident

☑x7ᵗʰ **V86.55** Driver of 3- or 4- wheeled all-terrain vehicle (ATV) injured in nontraffic accident

☑x7ᵗʰ **V86.56** Driver of dirt bike or motor/cross bike injured in nontraffic accident

☑x7ᵗʰ **V86.59** Driver of other special all-terrain or other off-road motor vehicle injured in nontraffic accident

~~Driver of dirt bike injured in nontraffic accident~~

Driver of go cart injured in nontraffic accident

Driver of golf cart injured in nontraffic accident

☑5ᵗʰ **V86.6** Passenger of special all-terrain or other off-road motor vehicle injured in nontraffic accident

☑x7ᵗʰ **V86.61** Passenger of ambulance or fire engine injured in nontraffic accident

☑x7ᵗʰ **V86.62** Passenger of snowmobile injured in nontraffic accident

☑x7ᵗʰ **V86.63** Passenger of dune buggy injured in nontraffic accident

☑x7ᵗʰ **V86.64** Passenger of military vehicle injured in nontraffic accident

☑x7ᵗʰ **V86.65** Passenger of 3- or 4- wheeled all-terrain vehicle (ATV) injured in nontraffic accident

☑x7ᵗʰ **V86.66** Passenger of dirt bike or motor/cross bike injured in nontraffic accident

☑x7ᵗʰ **V86.69** Passenger of other special all-terrain or other off-road motor vehicle injured in nontraffic accident

~~Passenger of dirt bike injured in nontraffic accident~~

Passenger of go cart injured in nontraffic accident

Passenger of golf cart injured in nontraffic accident

☑5ᵗʰ **V86.7** Person on outside of special all-terrain or other off-road motor vehicle injured in nontraffic accident

☑x7ᵗʰ **V86.71** Person on outside of ambulance or fire engine injured in nontraffic accident

☑x7ᵗʰ **V86.72** Person on outside of snowmobile injured in nontraffic accident

☑x7ᵗʰ **V86.73** Person on outside of dune buggy injured in nontraffic accident

☑x7ᵗʰ **V86.74** Person on outside of military vehicle injured in nontraffic accident

☑x7ᵗʰ **V86.75** Person on outside of 3- or 4- wheeled all-terrain vehicle (ATV) injured in nontraffic accident

☑x7ᵗʰ **V86.76** Person on outside of dirt bike or motor/cross bike injured in nontraffic accident

☑x7ᵗʰ **V86.79** Person on outside of other special all-terrain or other off-road motor vehicles injured in nontraffic accident

~~Person on outside of dirt bike injured in nontraffic accident~~

Person on outside of go cart injured in nontraffic accident

Person on outside of golf cart injured in nontraffic accident

☑5ᵗʰ **V86.9** Unspecified occupant of special all-terrain or other off-road motor vehicle injured in nontraffic accident

☑x7ᵗʰ **V86.91** Unspecified occupant of ambulance or fire engine injured in nontraffic accident

☑x7ᵗʰ **V86.92** Unspecified occupant of snowmobile injured in nontraffic accident

☑x7ᵗʰ **V86.93** Unspecified occupant of dune buggy injured in nontraffic accident

☑x7ᵗʰ **V86.94** Unspecified occupant of military vehicle injured in nontraffic accident

☑x7ᵗʰ **V86.95** Unspecified occupant of 3- or 4- wheeled all-terrain vehicle (ATV) injured in nontraffic accident

☑x7ᵗʰ **V86.96** Unspecified occupant of dirt bike or motor/cross bike injured in nontraffic accident

☑x7ᵗʰ **V86.99** Unspecified occupant of other special all-terrain or other off-road motor vehicle injured in nontraffic accident

Off-road motor-vehicle accident NOS

Other motor-vehicle accident NOS

Unspecified occupant of go cart injured in nontraffic accident

Unspecified occupant of golf cart injured in nontraffic accident

☑4ᵗʰ **V87** Traffic accident of specified type but victim's mode of transport unknown

EXCLUDES 1 collision involving:
     pedal cycle (V10-V19)
     pedestrian (V01-V09)

☑x7ᵗʰ **V87.0** Person injured in collision between car and two- or three-wheeled powered vehicle (traffic)

☑x7ᵗʰ **V87.1** Person injured in collision between other motor vehicle and two- or three-wheeled motor vehicle (traffic)

☑x7ᵗʰ **V87.2** Person injured in collision between car and pick-up truck or van (traffic)

☑x7ᵗʰ **V87.3** Person injured in collision between car and bus (traffic)

☑x7ᵗʰ **V87.4** Person injured in collision between car and heavy transport vehicle (traffic)

☑x7ᵗʰ **V87.5** Person injured in collision between heavy transport vehicle and bus (traffic)

☑x7ᵗʰ **V87.6** Person injured in collision between railway train or railway vehicle and car (traffic)

☑x7ᵗʰ **V87.7** Person injured in collision between other specified motor vehicles (traffic)

Ⓝ Newborn: 0   Ⓟ Pediatric: 0-17   Ⓜ Maternity: 12-55   Ⓐ Adult: 15-124   ᴄʜ Comorbidity High   ᴄʟ Comorbidity Low   ɴᴄᴅˣ Noncancer Dx   ᴘᴅˣ Primary Dx

1162   ICD-10-CM 2020

☑x7ᵗʰ **V87.8** Person injured in other specified noncollision transport accidents involving motor vehicle (traffic)

☑x7ᵗʰ **V87.9** Person injured in other specified (collision)(noncollision) transport accidents involving nonmotor vehicle (traffic)

☑4ᵗʰ **V88** Nontraffic accident of specified type but victim's mode of transport unknown

   EXCLUDES 1   collision involving:
      pedal cycle (V10-V19)
      pedestrian (V01-V09)

☑x7ᵗʰ **V88.0** Person injured in collision between car and two- or three-wheeled motor vehicle, nontraffic

☑x7ᵗʰ **V88.1** Person injured in collision between other motor vehicle and two- or three-wheeled motor vehicle, nontraffic

☑x7ᵗʰ **V88.2** Person injured in collision between car and pick-up truck or van, nontraffic

☑x7ᵗʰ **V88.3** Person injured in collision between car and bus, nontraffic

☑x7ᵗʰ **V88.4** Person injured in collision between car and heavy transport vehicle, nontraffic

☑x7ᵗʰ **V88.5** Person injured in collision between heavy transport vehicle and bus, nontraffic

☑x7ᵗʰ **V88.6** Person injured in collision between railway train or railway vehicle and car, nontraffic

☑x7ᵗʰ **V88.7** Person injured in collision between other specified motor vehicle, nontraffic

☑x7ᵗʰ **V88.8** Person injured in other specified noncollision transport accidents involving motor vehicle, nontraffic

☑x7ᵗʰ **V88.9** Person injured in other specified (collision)(noncollision) transport accidents involving nonmotor vehicle, nontraffic

☑4ᵗʰ **V89** Motor- or nonmotor-vehicle accident, type of vehicle unspecified

☑x7ᵗʰ **V89.0** Person injured in unspecified motor-vehicle accident, nontraffic
    Motor-vehicle accident NOS, nontraffic

☑x7ᵗʰ **V89.1** Person injured in unspecified nonmotor-vehicle accident, nontraffic
    Nonmotor-vehicle accident NOS (nontraffic)

☑x7ᵗʰ **V89.2** Person injured in unspecified motor-vehicle accident, traffic
    Motor-vehicle accident [MVA] NOS
    Road (traffic) accident [RTA] NOS

☑x7ᵗʰ **V89.3** Person injured in unspecified nonmotor-vehicle accident, traffic
    Nonmotor-vehicle traffic accident NOS

☑x7ᵗʰ **V89.9** Person injured in unspecified vehicle accident
    Collision NOS

Water transport accidents (V90-V94)

The appropriate 7th character is to be added to each code from categories V90-V94.
A   initial encounter
D   subsequent encounter
S   sequela

☑4ᵗʰ **V90** Drowning and submersion due to accident to watercraft

   EXCLUDES 1   civilian water transport accident involving military watercraft (V94.81-)
      fall into water not from watercraft (W16.-)
      military watercraft accident in military or war operations (Y36.0-, Y37.0-)
      water-transport-related drowning or submersion without accident to watercraft (V92.-)

☑5ᵗʰ **V90.0** Drowning and submersion due to watercraft overturning

☑x7ᵗʰ **V90.00** Drowning and submersion due to merchant ship overturning

☑x7ᵗʰ **V90.01** Drowning and submersion due to passenger ship overturning
    Drowning and submersion due to Ferry-boat overturning
    Drowning and submersion due to Liner overturning

☑x7ᵗʰ **V90.02** Drowning and submersion due to fishing boat overturning

☑x7ᵗʰ **V90.03** Drowning and submersion due to other powered watercraft overturning
    Drowning and submersion due to Hovercraft (on open water) overturning
    Drowning and submersion due to Jet ski overturning

☑x7ᵗʰ **V90.04** Drowning and submersion due to sailboat overturning

☑x7ᵗʰ **V90.05** Drowning and submersion due to canoe or kayak overturning

☑x7ᵗʰ **V90.06** Drowning and submersion due to (nonpowered) inflatable craft overturning

☑x7ᵗʰ **V90.08** Drowning and submersion due to other unpowered watercraft overturning
    Drowning and submersion due to windsurfer overturning

☑x7ᵗʰ **V90.09** Drowning and submersion due to unspecified watercraft overturning
    Drowning and submersion due to boat NOS overturning
    Drowning and submersion due to ship NOS overturning
    Drowning and submersion due to watercraft NOS overturning

☑5ᵗʰ **V90.1** Drowning and submersion due to watercraft sinking

☑x7ᵗʰ **V90.10** Drowning and submersion due to merchant ship sinking

☑x7ᵗʰ **V90.11** Drowning and submersion due to passenger ship sinking
    Drowning and submersion due to Ferry-boat sinking
    Drowning and submersion due to Liner sinking

☑x7ᵗʰ **V90.12** Drowning and submersion due to fishing boat sinking

☑x7ᵗʰ **V90.13** Drowning and submersion due to other powered watercraft sinking
    Drowning and submersion due to Hovercraft (on open water) sinking
    Drowning and submersion due to Jet ski sinking

☑x7ᵗʰ **V90.14** Drowning and submersion due to sailboat sinking

☑x7ᵗʰ **V90.15** Drowning and submersion due to canoe or kayak sinking

☑x7ᵗʰ **V90.16** Drowning and submersion due to (nonpowered) inflatable craft sinking

☑x7ᵗʰ **V90.18** Drowning and submersion due to other unpowered watercraft sinking

☑x7ᵗʰ **V90.19** Drowning and submersion due to unspecified watercraft sinking
    Drowning and submersion due to boat NOS sinking
    Drowning and submersion due to ship NOS sinking
    Drowning and submersion due to watercraft NOS sinking

☑5ᵗʰ **V90.2** Drowning and submersion due to falling or jumping from burning watercraft

☑x7ᵗʰ **V90.20** Drowning and submersion due to falling or jumping from burning merchant ship

☑x7ᵗʰ **V90.21** Drowning and submersion due to falling or jumping from burning passenger ship
    Drowning and submersion due to falling or jumping from burning Ferry-boat
    Drowning and submersion due to falling or jumping from burning Liner

☑x7ᵗʰ **V90.22** Drowning and submersion due to falling or jumping from burning fishing boat

☑x7ᵗʰ **V90.23** Drowning and submersion due to falling or jumping from other burning powered watercraft
    Drowning and submersion due to falling and jumping from burning Hovercraft (on open water)
    Drowning and submersion due to falling and jumping from burning Jet ski

☑x7ᵗʰ **V90.24** Drowning and submersion due to falling or jumping from burning sailboat

☑x7ᵗʰ **V90.25** Drowning and submersion due to falling or jumping from burning canoe or kayak

☑x7ᵗʰ **V90.26** Drowning and submersion due to falling or jumping from burning (nonpowered) inflatable craft

☑x7ᵗʰ **V90.27** Drowning and submersion due to falling or jumping from burning water-skis

☑x7ᵗʰ **V90.28** Drowning and submersion due to falling or jumping from other burning unpowered watercraft
    Drowning and submersion due to falling and jumping from burning surf-board
    Drowning and submersion due to falling and jumping from burning windsurfer

☑ Additional Character Required   ☑x7ᵗʰ Placeholder Alert   Manifestation   Unspecified Dx   ▶◀ Revised Text   ● New Code   ▲ Revised Title

ICD-10-CM 2020   **1163**

✓x7th **V90.29** **Drowning and submersion due to falling or jumping from unspecified burning watercraft**

Drowning and submersion due to falling or jumping from burning boat NOS

Drowning and submersion due to falling or jumping from burning ship NOS

Drowning and submersion due to falling or jumping from burning watercraft NOS

✓5th **V90.3** **Drowning and submersion due to** falling or jumping from crushed watercraft

✓x7th **V90.30** **Drowning and submersion due to falling or jumping from crushed** merchant ship

✓x7th **V90.31** **Drowning and submersion due to falling or jumping from crushed** passenger ship

Drowning and submersion due to falling and jumping from crushed Ferry boat

Drowning and submersion due to falling and jumping from crushed Liner

✓x7th **V90.32** **Drowning and submersion due to falling or jumping from crushed** fishing boat

✓x7th **V90.33** **Drowning and submersion due to falling or jumping from other crushed** powered **watercraft**

Drowning and submersion due to falling and jumping from crushed Hovercraft

Drowning and submersion due to falling and jumping from crushed Jet ski

✓x7th **V90.34** **Drowning and submersion due to falling or jumping from crushed** sailboat

✓x7th **V90.35** **Drowning and submersion due to falling or jumping from crushed** canoe or kayak

✓x7th **V90.36** **Drowning and submersion due to falling or jumping from crushed (nonpowered)** inflatable craft

✓x7th **V90.37** **Drowning and submersion due to falling or jumping from crushed** water-skis

✓x7th **V90.38** **Drowning and submersion due to falling or jumping from other crushed** unpowered **watercraft**

Drowning and submersion due to falling and jumping from crushed surf-board

Drowning and submersion due to falling and jumping from crushed windsurfer

✓x7th **V90.39** **Drowning and submersion due to falling or jumping from crushed unspecified watercraft**

Drowning and submersion due to falling and jumping from crushed boat NOS

Drowning and submersion due to falling and jumping from crushed ship NOS

Drowning and submersion due to falling and jumping from crushed watercraft NOS

✓5th **V90.8** **Drowning and submersion due to other accident to watercraft**

✓x7th **V90.80** **Drowning and submersion due to other accident to** merchant ship

✓x7th **V90.81** **Drowning and submersion due to other accident to** passenger ship

Drowning and submersion due to other accident to Ferry-boat

Drowning and submersion due to other accident to Liner

✓x7th **V90.82** **Drowning and submersion due to other accident to** fishing boat

✓x7th **V90.83** **Drowning and submersion due to other accident to other** powered **watercraft**

Drowning and submersion due to other accident to Hovercraft (on open water)

Drowning and submersion due to other accident to Jet ski

✓x7th **V90.84** **Drowning and submersion due to other accident to** sailboat

✓x7th **V90.85** **Drowning and submersion due to other accident to** canoe or kayak

✓x7th **V90.86** **Drowning and submersion due to other accident to (nonpowered)** inflatable craft

✓x7th **V90.87** **Drowning and submersion due to other accident to** water-skis

✓x7th **V90.88** **Drowning and submersion due to other accident to other** unpowered **watercraft**

Drowning and submersion due to other accident to surf-board

Drowning and submersion due to other accident to windsurfer

✓x7th **V90.89** **Drowning and submersion due to other accident to unspecified watercraft**

Drowning and submersion due to other accident to boat NOS

Drowning and submersion due to other accident to ship NOS

Drowning and submersion due to other accident to watercraft NOS

✓4th **V91** **Other injury due to accident to watercraft**

INCLUDES   any injury except drowning and submersion as a result of an accident to watercraft

EXCLUDES 1   *civilian water transport accident involving military watercraft (V94.81-)*

military watercraft accident in military or war operations (Y36, Y37.-)

EXCLUDES 2   *drowning and submersion due to accident to watercraft (V90.-)*

✓5th **V91.0** **Burn due to watercraft on fire**

EXCLUDES 1   *burn from localized fire or explosion on board ship without accident to watercraft (V93.-)*

✓x7th **V91.00** **Burn due to** merchant ship **on fire**

✓x7th **V91.01** **Burn due to** passenger ship **on fire**

Burn due to Ferry-boat on fire

Burn due to Liner on fire

✓x7th **V91.02** **Burn due to** fishing boat **on fire**

✓x7th **V91.03** **Burn due to other** powered **watercraft on fire**

Burn due to Hovercraft (on open water) on fire

Burn due to Jet ski on fire

✓x7th **V91.04** **Burn due to** sailboat **on fire**

✓x7th **V91.05** **Burn due to** canoe or kayak **on fire**

✓x7th **V91.06** **Burn due to (nonpowered)** inflatable craft **on fire**

✓x7th **V91.07** **Burn due to** water-skis **on fire**

✓x7th **V91.08** **Burn due to other** unpowered **watercraft on fire**

✓x7th **V91.09** **Burn due to unspecified watercraft on fire**

Burn due to boat NOS on fire

Burn due to ship NOS on fire

Burn due to watercraft NOS on fire

✓5th **V91.1** **Crushed between watercraft and other watercraft or other object due to collision**

Crushed by lifeboat after abandoning ship in a collision

NOTE   Select the specified type of watercraft that the victim was on at the time of the collision

✓x7th **V91.10** **Crushed between** merchant ship **and other watercraft or other object due to collision**

✓x7th **V91.11** **Crushed between** passenger ship **and other watercraft or other object due to collision**

Crushed between Ferry-boat and other watercraft or other object due to collision

Crushed between Liner and other watercraft or other object due to collision

✓x7th **V91.12** **Crushed between** fishing boat **and other watercraft or other object due to collision**

✓x7th **V91.13** **Crushed between other** powered **watercraft and other watercraft or other object due to collision**

Crushed between Hovercraft (on open water) and other watercraft or other object due to collision

Crushed between Jet ski and other watercraft or other object due to collision

✓x7th **V91.14** **Crushed between** sailboat **and other watercraft or other object due to collision**

✓x7th **V91.15** **Crushed between** canoe or kayak **and other watercraft or other object due to collision**

✓x7th **V91.16** **Crushed between (nonpowered)** inflatable craft **and other watercraft or other object due to collision**

N Newborn: 0   P Pediatric: 0-17   M Maternity: 12-55   A Adult: 15-124   CH Comorbidity High   CL Comorbidity Low   NCDx Noncancer Dx   PDx Primary Dx

1164   ICD-10-CM 2020

√x7ᵗʰ **V91.18** **Crushed between other** unpowered **watercraft and other watercraft or other object due to collision**
     Crushed between surfboard and other watercraft or other object due to collision
     Crushed between windsurfer and other watercraft or other object due to collision

√x7ᵗʰ **V91.19** **Crushed between unspecified watercraft and other watercraft or other object due to collision**
     Crushed between boat NOS and other watercraft or other object due to collision
     Crushed between ship NOS and other watercraft or other object due to collision
     Crushed between watercraft NOS and other watercraft or other object due to collision

√5ᵗʰ **V91.2** **Fall due to collision between watercraft and other watercraft or other object**
     Fall while remaining on watercraft after collision

> **NOTE** Select the specified type of watercraft that the victim was on at the time of the collision

> **EXCLUDES 1** crushed between watercraft and other watercraft and other object due to collision (V91.1-)
> drowning and submersion due to falling from crushed watercraft (V90.3-)

√x7ᵗʰ **V91.20** **Fall due to collision between** merchant ship **and other watercraft or other object**

√x7ᵗʰ **V91.21** **Fall due to collision between** passenger ship **and other watercraft or other object**
     Fall due to collision between Ferry-boat and other watercraft or other object
     Fall due to collision between Liner and other watercraft or other object

√x7ᵗʰ **V91.22** **Fall due to collision between** fishing boat **and other watercraft or other object**

√x7ᵗʰ **V91.23** **Fall due to collision between other** powered **watercraft and other watercraft or other object**
     Fall due to collision between Hovercraft (on open water) and other watercraft or other object
     Fall due to collision between Jet ski and other watercraft or other object

√x7ᵗʰ **V91.24** **Fall due to collision between** sailboat **and other watercraft or other object**

√x7ᵗʰ **V91.25** **Fall due to collision between** canoe or kayak **and other watercraft or other object**

√x7ᵗʰ **V91.26** **Fall due to collision between (nonpowered)** inflatable craft **and other watercraft or other object**

√x7ᵗʰ **V91.29** **Fall due to collision between unspecified watercraft and other watercraft or other object**
     Fall due to collision between boat NOS and other watercraft or other object
     Fall due to collision between ship NOS and other watercraft or other object
     Fall due to collision between watercraft NOS and other watercraft or other object

√5ᵗʰ **V91.3** **Hit or struck by falling object due to accident to watercraft**
     Hit or struck by falling object (part of damaged watercraft or other object) after falling or jumping from damaged watercraft

> **EXCLUDES 2** drowning or submersion due to fall or jumping from damaged watercraft (V90.2-, V90.3-)

√x7ᵗʰ **V91.30** **Hit or struck by falling object due to accident to** merchant ship

√x7ᵗʰ **V91.31** **Hit or struck by falling object due to accident to** passenger ship
     Hit or struck by falling object due to accident to Ferry-boat
     Hit or struck by falling object due to accident to Liner

√x7ᵗʰ **V91.32** **Hit or struck by falling object due to accident to** fishing boat

√x7ᵗʰ **V91.33** **Hit or struck by falling object due to accident to other** powered **watercraft**
     Hit or struck by falling object due to accident to Hovercraft (on open water)
     Hit or struck by falling object due to accident to Jet ski

√x7ᵗʰ **V91.34** **Hit or struck by falling object due to accident to** sailboat

√x7ᵗʰ **V91.35** **Hit or struck by falling object due to accident to** canoe or kayak

√x7ᵗʰ **V91.36** **Hit or struck by falling object due to accident to (nonpowered)** inflatable craft

√x7ᵗʰ **V91.37** **Hit or struck by falling object due to accident to** water-skis
     Hit by water-skis after jumping off of waterskis

√x7ᵗʰ **V91.38** **Hit or struck by falling object due to accident to other** unpowered **watercraft**
     Hit or struck by surf-board after falling off damaged surf-board
     Hit or struck by object after falling off damaged windsurfer

√x7ᵗʰ **V91.39** **Hit or struck by falling object due to accident to unspecified watercraft**
     Hit or struck by falling object due to accident to boat NOS
     Hit or struck by falling object due to accident to ship NOS
     Hit or struck by falling object due to accident to watercraft NOS

√5ᵗʰ **V91.8** **Other injury due to other accident to watercraft**

√x7ᵗʰ **V91.80** **Other injury due to other accident to** merchant ship

√x7ᵗʰ **V91.81** **Other injury due to other accident to** passenger ship
     Other injury due to other accident to Ferry-boat
     Other injury due to other accident to Liner

√x7ᵗʰ **V91.82** **Other injury due to other accident to** fishing boat

√x7ᵗʰ **V91.83** **Other injury due to other accident to other** powered **watercraft**
     Other injury due to other accident to Hovercraft (on open water)
     Other injury due to other accident to Jet ski

√x7ᵗʰ **V91.84** **Other injury due to other accident to** sailboat

√x7ᵗʰ **V91.85** **Other injury due to other accident to** canoe or kayak

√x7ᵗʰ **V91.86** **Other injury due to other accident to (nonpowered)** inflatable craft

√x7ᵗʰ **V91.87** **Other injury due to other accident to** water-skis

√x7ᵗʰ **V91.88** **Other injury due to other accident to other** unpowered **watercraft**
     Other injury due to other accident to surf-board
     Other injury due to other accident to windsurfer

√x7ᵗʰ **V91.89** **Other injury due to other accident to unspecified watercraft**
     Other injury due to other accident to boat NOS
     Other injury due to other accident to ship NOS
     Other injury due to other accident to watercraft NOS

√4ᵗʰ **V92** **Drowning and submersion due to accident on board watercraft, without accident to watercraft**

> **EXCLUDES 1** civilian water transport accident involving military watercraft (V94.81-)
> drowning or submersion due to accident to watercraft (V90-V91)
> drowning or submersion of diver who voluntarily jumps from boat not involved in an accident (W16.711, W16.721)
> fall into water without watercraft (W16.-)
> military watercraft accident in military or war operations (Y36, Y37)

√5ᵗʰ **V92.0** **Drowning and submersion due to** fall off **watercraft**
     Drowning and submersion due to fall from gangplank of watercraft
     Drowning and submersion due to fall overboard watercraft

> **EXCLUDES 2** hitting head on object or bottom of body of water due to fall from watercraft (V94.0-)

√x7ᵗʰ **V92.00** **Drowning and submersion due to fall off** merchant ship

√x7ᵗʰ **V92.01** **Drowning and submersion due to fall off** passenger ship
     Drowning and submersion due to fall off Ferry-boat
     Drowning and submersion due to fall off Liner

√x7ᵗʰ **V92.02** **Drowning and submersion due to fall off** fishing boat

√x7ᵗʰ **V92.03** **Drowning and submersion due to fall off other** powered **watercraft**
     Drowning and submersion due to fall off Hovercraft (on open water)
     Drowning and submersion due to fall off Jet ski

√x7ᵗʰ **V92.04** **Drowning and submersion due to fall off** sailboat

√x7ᵗʰ **V92.05** **Drowning and submersion due to fall off** canoe or kayak

√x7ᵗʰ **V92.06** **Drowning and submersion due to fall off (nonpowered)** inflatable craft

√x7ᵗʰ **V92.07** **Drowning and submersion due to fall off** water-skis

> **EXCLUDES 1** *drowning and submersion due to falling off burning water-skis (V90.27)*
> *drowning and submersion due to falling off crushed water-skis (V90.37)*
> *hit by boat while water-skiing NOS (V94.X)*

√x7ᵗʰ **V92.08** **Drowning and submersion due to fall off other** unpowered **watercraft**

Drowning and submersion due to fall off surf-board
Drowning and submersion due to fall off windsurfer

> **EXCLUDES 1** *drowning and submersion due to fall off burning unpowered watercraft (V90.28)*
> *drowning and submersion due to fall off crushed unpowered watercraft (V90.38)*
> *drowning and submersion due to fall off damaged unpowered watercraft (V90.88)*
> *drowning and submersion due to rider of nonpowered watercraft being hit by other watercraft (V94.-)*
> *other injury due to rider of nonpowered watercraft being hit by other watercraft (V94.-)*

√x7ᵗʰ **V92.09** **Drowning and submersion due to fall off unspecified watercraft**

Drowning and submersion due to fall off boat NOS
Drowning and submersion due to fall off ship
Drowning and submersion due to fall off watercraft NOS

√5ᵗʰ **V92.1** **Drowning and submersion due to being** thrown overboard **by motion of watercraft**

> **EXCLUDES 1** *drowning and submersion due to fall off surf-board (V92.08)*
> *drowning and submersion due to fall off water-skis (V92.07)*
> *drowning and submersion due to fall off windsurfer (V92.08)*

√x7ᵗʰ **V92.10** **Drowning and submersion due to being thrown overboard by motion of** merchant ship

√x7ᵗʰ **V92.11** **Drowning and submersion due to being thrown overboard by motion of** passenger ship

Drowning and submersion due to being thrown overboard by motion of Ferry-boat
Drowning and submersion due to being thrown overboard by motion of Liner

√x7ᵗʰ **V92.12** **Drowning and submersion due to being thrown overboard by motion of** fishing boat

√x7ᵗʰ **V92.13** **Drowning and submersion due to being thrown overboard by motion of other** powered **watercraft**

Drowning and submersion due to being thrown overboard by motion of Hovercraft

√x7ᵗʰ **V92.14** **Drowning and submersion due to being thrown overboard by motion of** sailboat

√x7ᵗʰ **V92.15** **Drowning and submersion due to being thrown overboard by motion of** canoe or kayak

√x7ᵗʰ **V92.16** **Drowning and submersion due to being thrown overboard by motion of (nonpowered)** inflatable craft

√x7ᵗʰ **V92.19** **Drowning and submersion due to being thrown overboard by motion of unspecified watercraft**

Drowning and submersion due to being thrown overboard by motion of boat NOS
Drowning and submersion due to being thrown overboard by motion of ship NOS
Drowning and submersion due to being thrown overboard by motion of watercraft NOS

√5ᵗʰ **V92.2** **Drowning and submersion due to being** washed overboard **from watercraft**

Code first any associated cataclysm (X37.0-)

√x7ᵗʰ **V92.20** **Drowning and submersion due to being washed overboard from** merchant ship

√x7ᵗʰ **V92.21** **Drowning and submersion due to being washed overboard from** passenger ship

Drowning and submersion due to being washed overboard from Ferry-boat
Drowning and submersion due to being washed overboard from Liner

√x7ᵗʰ **V92.22** **Drowning and submersion due to being washed overboard from** fishing boat

√x7ᵗʰ **V92.23** **Drowning and submersion due to being washed overboard from other** powered **watercraft**

Drowning and submersion due to being washed overboard from Hovercraft (on open water)
Drowning and submersion due to being washed overboard from Jet ski

√x7ᵗʰ **V92.24** **Drowning and submersion due to being washed overboard from** sailboat

√x7ᵗʰ **V92.25** **Drowning and submersion due to being washed overboard from** canoe or kayak

√x7ᵗʰ **V92.26** **Drowning and submersion due to being washed overboard from (nonpowered)** inflatable craft

√x7ᵗʰ **V92.27** **Drowning and submersion due to being washed overboard from** water-skis

> **EXCLUDES 1** *drowning and submersion due to fall off water-skis (V92.07)*

√x7ᵗʰ **V92.28** **Drowning and submersion due to being washed overboard from other** unpowered **watercraft**

Drowning and submersion due to being washed overboard from surf-board
Drowning and submersion due to being washed overboard from windsurfer

√x7ᵗʰ **V92.29** **Drowning and submersion due to being washed overboard from unspecified watercraft**

Drowning and submersion due to being washed overboard from boat NOS
Drowning and submersion due to being washed overboard from ship NOS
Drowning and submersion due to being washed overboard from watercraft NOS

√4ᵗʰ **V93** **Other injury due to accident on board watercraft, without accident to watercraft**

> **EXCLUDES 1** *civilian water transport accident involving military watercraft (V94.81-)*
> *other injury due to accident to watercraft (V91.-)*
> *military watercraft accident in military or war operations (Y36, Y37.-)*
>
> **EXCLUDES 2** *drowning and submersion due to accident on board watercraft, without accident to watercraft (V92.-)*

√5ᵗʰ **V93.0** **Burn due to localized fire on board watercraft**

> **EXCLUDES 1** *burn due to watercraft on fire (V91.0-)*

√x7ᵗʰ **V93.00** **Burn due to localized fire on board** merchant vessel

√x7ᵗʰ **V93.01** **Burn due to localized fire on board** passenger vessel

Burn due to localized fire on board Ferry-boat
Burn due to localized fire on board Liner

√x7ᵗʰ **V93.02** **Burn due to localized fire on board** fishing boat

√x7ᵗʰ **V93.03** **Burn due to localized fire on board other** powered **watercraft**

Burn due to localized fire on board Hovercraft
Burn due to localized fire on board Jet ski

√x7ᵗʰ **V93.04** **Burn due to localized fire on board** sailboat

√x7ᵗʰ **V93.09** **Burn due to localized fire on board unspecified watercraft**

Burn due to localized fire on board boat NOS
Burn due to localized fire on board ship NOS
Burn due to localized fire on board watercraft NOS

√5ᵗʰ **V93.1** **Other burn on board watercraft**

Burn due to source other than fire on board watercraft

> **EXCLUDES 1** *burn due to watercraft on fire (V91.0-)*

√x7ᵗʰ **V93.10** **Other burn on board** merchant vessel

√x7ᵗʰ **V93.11** **Other burn on board** passenger vessel

Other burn on board Ferry-boat
Other burn on board Liner

√x7ᵗʰ **V93.12** **Other burn on board** fishing boat

√x7ᵗʰ **V93.13** **Other burn on board other** powered **watercraft**

Other burn on board Hovercraft
Other burn on board Jet ski

√x7ᵗʰ **V93.14** **Other burn on board** sailboat

✓x7ᵗʰ **V93.19** **Other burn on board unspecified watercraft**
Other burn on board boat NOS
Other burn on board ship NOS
Other burn on board watercraft NOS

✓5ᵗʰ **V93.2** **Heat exposure on board watercraft**
> EXCLUDES 1   *exposure to man-made heat not aboard watercraft (W92)*
> *exposure to natural heat while on board watercraft (X30)*
> *exposure to sunlight while on board watercraft (X32)*
> EXCLUDES 2   *burn due to fire on board watercraft (V93.0-)*

✓x7ᵗʰ **V93.20** **Heat exposure on board** merchant ship

✓x7ᵗʰ **V93.21** **Heat exposure on board** passenger ship
Heat exposure on board Ferry-boat
Heat exposure on board Liner

✓x7ᵗʰ **V93.22** **Heat exposure on board** fishing boat

✓x7ᵗʰ **V93.23** **Heat exposure on board other** powered **watercraft**
Heat exposure on board hovercraft

✓x7ᵗʰ **V93.24** **Heat exposure on board** sailboat

✓x7ᵗʰ **V93.29** **Heat exposure on board unspecified watercraft**
Heat exposure on board boat NOS
Heat exposure on board ship NOS
Heat exposure on board watercraft NOS

✓5ᵗʰ **V93.3** **Fall on board watercraft**
> EXCLUDES 1   *fall due to collision of watercraft (V91.2-)*

✓x7ᵗʰ **V93.30** **Fall on board** merchant ship

✓x7ᵗʰ **V93.31** **Fall on board** passenger ship
Fall on board Ferry-boat
Fall on board Liner

✓x7ᵗʰ **V93.32** **Fall on board** fishing boat

✓x7ᵗʰ **V93.33** **Fall on board other** powered **watercraft**
Fall on board Hovercraft (on open water)
Fall on board Jet ski

✓x7ᵗʰ **V93.34** **Fall on board** sailboat

✓x7ᵗʰ **V93.35** **Fall on board** canoe or kayak

✓x7ᵗʰ **V93.36** **Fall on board (nonpowered)** inflatable craft

✓x7ᵗʰ **V93.38** **Fall on board other** unpowered **watercraft**

✓x7ᵗʰ **V93.39** **Fall on board unspecified watercraft**
Fall on board boat NOS
Fall on board ship NOS
Fall on board watercraft NOS

✓5ᵗʰ **V93.4** **Struck by falling object on board watercraft**
Hit by falling object on board watercraft
> EXCLUDES 1   *struck by falling object due to accident to watercraft (V91.3)*

✓x7ᵗʰ **V93.40** **Struck by falling object on** merchant ship

✓x7ᵗʰ **V93.41** **Struck by falling object on** passenger ship
Struck by falling object on Ferry-boat
Struck by falling object on Liner

✓x7ᵗʰ **V93.42** **Struck by falling object on** fishing boat

✓x7ᵗʰ **V93.43** **Struck by falling object on other** powered **watercraft**
Struck by falling object on Hovercraft

✓x7ᵗʰ **V93.44** **Struck by falling object on** sailboat

✓x7ᵗʰ **V93.48** **Struck by falling object on other** unpowered **watercraft**

✓x7ᵗʰ **V93.49** **Struck by falling object on unspecified watercraft**

✓5ᵗʰ **V93.5** **Explosion on board watercraft**
Boiler explosion on steamship
> EXCLUDES 2   *fire on board watercraft (V93.0-)*

✓x7ᵗʰ **V93.50** **Explosion on board** merchant ship

✓x7ᵗʰ **V93.51** **Explosion on board** passenger ship
Explosion on board Ferry-boat
Explosion on board Liner

✓x7ᵗʰ **V93.52** **Explosion on board** fishing boat

✓x7ᵗʰ **V93.53** **Explosion on board other** powered **watercraft**
Explosion on board Hovercraft
Explosion on board Jet ski

✓x7ᵗʰ **V93.54** **Explosion on board** sailboat

✓x7ᵗʰ **V93.59** **Explosion on board unspecified watercraft**
Explosion on board boat NOS
Explosion on board ship NOS
Explosion on board watercraft NOS

✓5ᵗʰ **V93.6** **Machinery accident on board watercraft**
> EXCLUDES 1   *machinery explosion on board watercraft (V93.4-)*
> *machinery fire on board watercraft (V93.0-)*

✓x7ᵗʰ **V93.60** **Machinery accident on board** merchant ship

✓x7ᵗʰ **V93.61** **Machinery accident on board** passenger ship
Machinery accident on board Ferry-boat
Machinery accident on board Liner

✓x7ᵗʰ **V93.62** **Machinery accident on board** fishing boat

✓x7ᵗʰ **V93.63** **Machinery accident on board other** powered **watercraft**
Machinery accident on board Hovercraft

✓x7ᵗʰ **V93.64** **Machinery accident on board** sailboat

✓x7ᵗʰ **V93.69** **Machinery accident on board unspecified watercraft**
Machinery accident on board boat NOS
Machinery accident on board ship NOS
Machinery accident on board watercraft NOS

✓5ᵗʰ **V93.8** **Other injury due to other accident on board watercraft**
Accidental poisoning by gases or fumes on watercraft

✓x7ᵗʰ **V93.80** **Other injury due to other accident on board** merchant ship

✓x7ᵗʰ **V93.81** **Other injury due to other accident on board** passenger ship
Other injury due to other accident on board Ferry-boat
Other injury due to other accident on board Liner

✓x7ᵗʰ **V93.82** **Other injury due to other accident on board** fishing boat

✓x7ᵗʰ **V93.83** **Other injury due to other accident on board other** powered **watercraft**
Other injury due to other accident on board Hovercraft
Other injury due to other accident on board Jet ski

✓x7ᵗʰ **V93.84** **Other injury due to other accident on board** sailboat

✓x7ᵗʰ **V93.85** **Other injury due to other accident on board** canoe or kayak

✓x7ᵗʰ **V93.86** **Other injury due to other accident on board (nonpowered)** inflatable craft

✓x7ᵗʰ **V93.87** **Other injury due to other accident on board** water-skis
Hit or struck by object while waterskiing

✓x7ᵗʰ **V93.88** **Other injury due to other accident on board other** unpowered **watercraft**
Hit or struck by object while surfing
Hit or struck by object while on board windsurfer

✓x7ᵗʰ **V93.89** **Other injury due to other accident on board unspecified watercraft**
Other injury due to other accident on board boat NOS
Other injury due to other accident on board ship NOS
Other injury due to other accident on board watercraft NOS

✓4ᵗʰ **V94** **Other and unspecified water transport accidents**
> EXCLUDES 1   *military watercraft accidents in military or war operations (Y36, Y37)*

✓x7ᵗʰ **V94.0** **Hitting object or bottom of body of water due to fall from watercraft**
> EXCLUDES 2   *drowning and submersion due to fall from watercraft (V92.0-)*

✓5ᵗʰ **V94.1** **Bather struck by watercraft**
Swimmer hit by watercraft

✓x7ᵗʰ **V94.11** **Bather struck by** powered **watercraft**

✓x7ᵗʰ **V94.12** **Bather struck by** nonpowered **watercraft**

✓5ᵗʰ **V94.2** **Rider of nonpowered watercraft struck by other watercraft**

✓x7ᵗʰ **V94.21** **Rider of nonpowered watercraft struck by other** nonpowered **watercraft**
Canoer hit by other nonpowered watercraft
Surfer hit by other nonpowered watercraft
Windsurfer hit by other nonpowered watercraft

Chapter 20. External Causes of Morbidity

V93.19–V94.21

✓x7ᵗʰ **V94.22 Rider of nonpowered watercraft struck by** powered **watercraft**
  Canoer hit by motorboat
  Surfer hit by motorboat
  Windsurfer hit by motorboat

✓5ᵗʰ **V94.3 Injury to rider of (inflatable) watercraft being pulled behind other watercraft**

✓x7ᵗʰ **V94.31 Injury to rider of (inflatable)** recreational **watercraft being pulled behind other watercraft**
  Injury to rider of inner-tube pulled behind motor boat

✓x7ᵗʰ **V94.32 Injury to rider of** non-recreational **watercraft being pulled behind other watercraft**
  Injury to occupant of dingy being pulled behind boat or ship
  Injury to occupant of life-raft being pulled behind boat or ship

✓x7ᵗʰ **V94.4 Injury to barefoot water-skier**
  Injury to person being pulled behind boat or ship

✓5ᵗʰ **V94.8 Other water transport accident**

✓6ᵗʰ **V94.81 Water transport accident involving military watercraft**

✓7ᵗʰ **V94.810 Civilian watercraft involved in water transport accident with military watercraft**
  Passenger on civilian watercraft injured due to accident with military watercraft

✓7ᵗʰ **V94.811 Civilian in water injured by military watercraft**

✓7ᵗʰ **V94.818 Other water transport accident involving military watercraft**

✓x7ᵗʰ **V94.89 Other water transport accident**

✓x7ᵗʰ **V94.9 Unspecified water transport accident**
  Water transport accident NOS

Air and space transport accidents (V95-V97)

EXCLUDES 1 *military aircraft accidents in military or war operations (Y36, Y37)*

The appropriate 7th character is to be added to each code from categories V95-V97.
A initial encounter
D subsequent encounter
S sequela

✓4ᵗʰ **V95 Accident to powered aircraft causing injury to occupant**

✓5ᵗʰ **V95.0** Helicopter **accident injuring occupant**

✓x7ᵗʰ **V95.00 Unspecified helicopter accident injuring occupant**

✓x7ᵗʰ **V95.01 Helicopter** crash **injuring occupant**

✓x7ᵗʰ **V95.02** Forced landing **of helicopter injuring occupant**

✓x7ᵗʰ **V95.03 Helicopter** collision **injuring occupant**
  Helicopter collision with any object, fixed, movable or moving

✓x7ᵗʰ **V95.04 Helicopter** fire **injuring occupant**

✓x7ᵗʰ **V95.05 Helicopter** explosion **injuring occupant**

✓x7ᵗʰ **V95.09 Other helicopter accident injuring occupant**

✓5ᵗʰ **V95.1** Ultralight, microlight or powered-glider **accident injuring occupant**

✓x7ᵗʰ **V95.10 Unspecified ultralight, microlight or powered-glider accident injuring occupant**

✓x7ᵗʰ **V95.11 Ultralight, microlight or powered-glider** crash **injuring occupant**

✓x7ᵗʰ **V95.12** Forced landing **of ultralight, microlight or powered-glider injuring occupant**

✓x7ᵗʰ **V95.13 Ultralight, microlight or powered-glider** collision **injuring occupant**
  Ultralight, microlight or powered-glider collision with any object, fixed, movable or moving

✓x7ᵗʰ **V95.14 Ultralight, microlight or powered-glider** fire **injuring occupant**

✓x7ᵗʰ **V95.15 Ultralight, microlight or powered-glider** explosion **injuring occupant**

✓x7ᵗʰ **V95.19 Other ultralight, microlight or powered-glider accident injuring occupant**

✓5ᵗʰ **V95.2 Other private fixed-wing aircraft accident injuring occupant**

✓x7ᵗʰ **V95.20 Unspecified accident to other private fixed-wing aircraft, injuring occupant**

✓x7ᵗʰ **V95.21 Other private fixed-wing aircraft crash injuring occupant**

✓x7ᵗʰ **V95.22** Forced landing **of other private fixed-wing aircraft injuring occupant**

✓x7ᵗʰ **V95.23 Other private fixed-wing aircraft** collision **injuring occupant**
  Other private fixed-wing aircraft collision with any object, fixed, movable or moving

✓x7ᵗʰ **V95.24 Other private fixed-wing aircraft** fire **injuring occupant**

✓x7ᵗʰ **V95.25 Other private fixed-wing aircraft** explosion **injuring occupant**

✓x7ᵗʰ **V95.29 Other accident to other private fixed-wing aircraft injuring occupant**

✓5ᵗʰ **V95.3** Commercial fixed-wing **aircraft accident injuring occupant**

✓x7ᵗʰ **V95.30 Unspecified accident to commercial fixed-wing aircraft injuring occupant**

✓x7ᵗʰ **V95.31 Commercial fixed-wing aircraft** crash **injuring occupant**

✓x7ᵗʰ **V95.32** Forced landing **of commercial fixed-wing aircraft injuring occupant**

✓x7ᵗʰ **V95.33 Commercial fixed-wing aircraft** collision **injuring occupant**
  Commercial fixed-wing aircraft collision with any object, fixed, movable or moving

✓x7ᵗʰ **V95.34 Commercial fixed-wing aircraft** fire **injuring occupant**

✓x7ᵗʰ **V95.35 Commercial fixed-wing aircraft** explosion **injuring occupant**

✓x7ᵗʰ **V95.39 Other accident to commercial fixed-wing aircraft injuring occupant**

✓5ᵗʰ **V95.4** Spacecraft **accident injuring occupant**

✓x7ᵗʰ **V95.40 Unspecified spacecraft accident injuring occupant**

✓x7ᵗʰ **V95.41 Spacecraft** crash **injuring occupant**

✓x7ᵗʰ **V95.42** Forced landing **of spacecraft injuring occupant**

✓x7ᵗʰ **V95.43 Spacecraft** collision **injuring occupant**
  Spacecraft collision with any object, fixed, moveable or moving

✓x7ᵗʰ **V95.44 Spacecraft** fire **injuring occupant**

✓x7ᵗʰ **V95.45 Spacecraft** explosion **injuring occupant**

✓x7ᵗʰ **V95.49 Other spacecraft accident injuring occupant**

✓x7ᵗʰ **V95.8 Other powered aircraft accidents injuring occupant**

✓x7ᵗʰ **V95.9 Unspecified aircraft accident injuring occupant**
  Aircraft accident NOS
  Air transport accident NOS

✓4ᵗʰ **V96 Accident to nonpowered aircraft causing injury to occupant**

✓5ᵗʰ **V96.0** Balloon **accident injuring occupant**

✓x7ᵗʰ **V96.00 Unspecified balloon accident injuring occupant**

✓x7ᵗʰ **V96.01 Balloon** crash **injuring occupant**

✓x7ᵗʰ **V96.02** Forced landing **of balloon injuring occupant**

✓x7ᵗʰ **V96.03 Balloon** collision **injuring occupant**
  Balloon collision with any object, fixed, moveable or moving

✓x7ᵗʰ **V96.04 Balloon** fire **injuring occupant**

✓x7ᵗʰ **V96.05 Balloon** explosion **injuring occupant**

✓x7ᵗʰ **V96.09 Other balloon accident injuring occupant**

✓5ᵗʰ **V96.1** Hang-glider **accident injuring occupant**

✓x7ᵗʰ **V96.10 Unspecified hang-glider accident injuring occupant**

✓x7ᵗʰ **V96.11 Hang-glider** crash **injuring occupant**

✓x7ᵗʰ **V96.12** Forced landing **of hang-glider injuring occupant**

✓x7ᵗʰ **V96.13 Hang-glider** collision **injuring occupant**
  Hang-glider collision with any object, fixed, moveable or moving

✓x7ᵗʰ **V96.14 Hang-glider** fire **injuring occupant**

✓x7ᵗʰ **V96.15 Hang-glider** explosion **injuring occupant**

✓x7ᵗʰ **V96.19 Other hang-glider accident injuring occupant**

✓5ᵗʰ **V96.2** Glider (nonpowered) **accident injuring occupant**

✓x7ᵗʰ **V96.20 Unspecified glider (nonpowered) accident injuring occupant**

✓x7ᵗʰ **V96.21 Glider (nonpowered)** crash **injuring occupant**

✓x7ᵗʰ **V96.22** Forced landing **of glider (nonpowered) injuring occupant**

☑x7ᵗʰ **V96.23** **Glider (nonpowered) collision injuring occupant**
> Glider (nonpowered) collision with any object, fixed, moveable or moving

☑x7ᵗʰ **V96.24** **Glider (nonpowered) fire injuring occupant**

☑x7ᵗʰ **V96.25** **Glider (nonpowered) explosion injuring occupant**

☑x7ᵗʰ **V96.29** **Other glider (nonpowered) accident injuring occupant**

☑x7ᵗʰ **V96.8** **Other nonpowered-aircraft accidents injuring occupant**
> Kite carrying a person accident injuring occupant

☑x7ᵗʰ **V96.9** **Unspecified nonpowered-aircraft accident injuring occupant**
> Nonpowered-aircraft accident NOS

☑4ᵗʰ **V97** **Other specified air transport accidents**

☑x7ᵗʰ **V97.0** **Occupant of aircraft injured in other specified air transport accidents**
> Fall in, on or from aircraft in air transport accident
> > EXCLUDES 1   *accident while boarding or alighting aircraft (V97.1)*

☑x7ᵗʰ **V97.1** **Person injured while boarding or alighting from aircraft**

☑5ᵗʰ **V97.2** **Parachutist accident**

☑x7ᵗʰ **V97.21** **Parachutist entangled in object**
> Parachutist landing in tree

☑x7ᵗʰ **V97.22** **Parachutist injured on landing**

☑x7ᵗʰ **V97.29** **Other parachutist accident**

☑5ᵗʰ **V97.3** **Person on ground injured in air transport accident**

☑x7ᵗʰ **V97.31** **Hit by object falling from aircraft**
> Hit by crashing aircraft
> Injured by aircraft hitting house
> Injured by aircraft hitting car

☑x7ᵗʰ **V97.32** **Injured by rotating propeller**

☑x7ᵗʰ **V97.33** **Sucked into jet engine**

☑x7ᵗʰ **V97.39** **Other injury to person on ground due to air transport accident**

☑5ᵗʰ **V97.8** **Other air transport accidents, not elsewhere classified**
> > EXCLUDES 1   *aircraft accident NOS (V95.9)*
> > *exposure to changes in air pressure during ascent or descent (W94.-)*

☑6ᵗʰ **V97.81** **Air transport accident involving military aircraft**

☑7ᵗʰ **V97.810** **Civilian aircraft involved in air transport accident with military aircraft**
> Passenger in civilian aircraft injured due to accident with military aircraft

☑7ᵗʰ **V97.811** **Civilian injured by military aircraft**

☑7ᵗʰ **V97.818** **Other air transport accident involving military aircraft**

☑x7ᵗʰ **V97.89** **Other air transport accidents, not elsewhere classified**
> Injury from machinery on aircraft

Other and unspecified transport accidents (V98-V99)

EXCLUDES 1   *vehicle accident, type of vehicle unspecified (V89.-)*

The appropriate 7th character is to be added to each code from categories V98-V99.
A   initial encounter
D   subsequent encounter
S   sequela

☑4ᵗʰ **V98** **Other specified transport accidents**

☑x7ᵗʰ **V98.0** **Accident to, on or involving cable-car, not on rails**
> Caught or dragged by cable-car, not on rails
> Fall or jump from cable-car, not on rails
> Object thrown from or in cable-car, not on rails

☑x7ᵗʰ **V98.1** **Accident to, on or involving land-yacht**

☑x7ᵗʰ **V98.2** **Accident to, on or involving ice yacht**

☑x7ᵗʰ **V98.3** **Accident to, on or involving ski lift**
> Accident to, on or involving ski chair-lift
> Accident to, on or involving ski-lift with gondola

☑x7ᵗʰ **V98.8** **Other specified transport accidents**

☑x7ᵗʰ **V99** **Unspecified transport accident**

OTHER EXTERNAL CAUSES OF ACCIDENTAL INJURY (W00-X58)

Slipping, tripping, stumbling and falls (W00-W19)

EXCLUDES 1   *assault involving a fall (Y01-Y02)*
fall from animal (V80.-)
fall (in) (from) machinery (in operation) (W28-W31)
fall (in) (from) transport vehicle (V01-V99)
intentional self-harm involving a fall (X80-X81)

EXCLUDES 2   *at risk for fall (history of fall) Z91.81*
fall (in) (from) burning building (X00.-)
fall into fire (X00-X04, X08)

The appropriate 7th character is to be added to each code from categories W00-W19.
A   initial encounter
D   subsequent encounter
S   sequela

☑4ᵗʰ **W00** **Fall due to ice and snow**
> > INCLUDES   pedestrian on foot falling (slipping) on ice and snow
> > EXCLUDES 1   *fall on (from) ice and snow involving pedestrian conveyance (V00.-)*
> > *fall from stairs and steps not due to ice and snow (W10.-)*
>
> AHA: 2016,2Q,4

☑x7ᵗʰ **W00.0** **Fall on same level due to ice and snow**

☑x7ᵗʰ **W00.1** **Fall from stairs and steps due to ice and snow**

☑x7ᵗʰ **W00.2** **Other fall from one level to another due to ice and snow**

☑x7ᵗʰ **W00.9** **Unspecified fall due to ice and snow**

☑4ᵗʰ **W01** **Fall on same level from slipping, tripping and stumbling**
> > INCLUDES   fall on moving sidewalk
> > EXCLUDES 1   *fall due to bumping (striking) against object (W18.0-)*
> > *fall in shower or bathtub (W18.2-)*
> > *fall on same level NOS (W18.30)*
> > *fall on same level from slipping, tripping and stumbling due to ice or snow (W00.0)*
> > *fall off or from toilet (W18.1-)*
> > *slipping, tripping and stumbling NOS (W18.40)*
> > *slipping, tripping and stumbling without falling (W18.4-)*

☑x7ᵗʰ **W01.0** **Fall on same level from slipping, tripping and stumbling without subsequent striking against object**
> Falling over animal

☑5ᵗʰ **W01.1** **Fall on same level from slipping, tripping and stumbling with subsequent striking against object**

☑x7ᵗʰ **W01.10** **Fall on same level from slipping, tripping and stumbling with subsequent striking against unspecified object**

☑6ᵗʰ **W01.11** **Fall on same level from slipping, tripping and stumbling with subsequent striking against sharp object**

☑7ᵗʰ **W01.110** **Fall on same level from slipping, tripping and stumbling with subsequent striking against sharp glass**

☑7ᵗʰ **W01.111** **Fall on same level from slipping, tripping and stumbling with subsequent striking against power tool or machine**

☑7ᵗʰ **W01.118** **Fall on same level from slipping, tripping and stumbling with subsequent striking against other sharp object**

☑7ᵗʰ **W01.119** **Fall on same level from slipping, tripping and stumbling with subsequent striking against unspecified sharp object**

☑6ᵗʰ **W01.19** **Fall on same level from slipping, tripping and stumbling with subsequent striking against other object**

☑7ᵗʰ **W01.190** **Fall on same level from slipping, tripping and stumbling with subsequent striking against furniture**

☑7ᵗʰ **W01.198** **Fall on same level from slipping, tripping and stumbling with subsequent striking against other object**

Chapter 20. External Causes of Morbidity

W03–W16.212

☑x7ᵗʰ W03   **Other fall on same level due to collision with another person**
> Fall due to non-transport collision with other person
> **EXCLUDES 1**   *collision with another person without fall (W51)*
> *crushed or pushed by a crowd or human stampede (W52)*
> *fall involving pedestrian conveyance (V00-V09)*
> *fall due to ice or snow (W00)*
> *fall on same level NOS (W18.30)*
> **AHA:** 2012,4Q,108

☑x7ᵗʰ W04   **Fall while being carried or supported by other persons**
> Accidentally dropped while being carried

☑4ᵗʰ W05   **Fall from non-moving wheelchair, nonmotorized scooter and motorized mobility scooter**
> **EXCLUDES 1**   *fall from moving wheelchair (powered) (V00.811)*
> *fall from moving motorized mobility scooter (V00.831)*
> *fall from nonmotorized scooter (V00.141)*

> **☑x7ᵗʰ W05.0**   **Fall from non-moving** wheelchair
> **AHA:** 2019,2Q,27

> **☑x7ᵗʰ W05.1**   **Fall from non-moving** nonmotorized scooter

> **☑x7ᵗʰ W05.2**   **Fall from non-moving** motorized mobility scooter

☑x7ᵗʰ W06   **Fall from bed**

☑x7ᵗʰ W07   **Fall from chair**

☑x7ᵗʰ W08   **Fall from other furniture**

☑4ᵗʰ W09   **Fall on and from playground equipment**
> **EXCLUDES 1**   *fall involving recreational machinery (W31)*

> **☑x7ᵗʰ W09.0**   **Fall on or from playground slide**

> **☑x7ᵗʰ W09.1**   **Fall from playground swing**

> **☑x7ᵗʰ W09.2**   **Fall on or from jungle gym**

> **☑x7ᵗʰ W09.8**   **Fall on or from other playground equipment**

☑4ᵗʰ W10   **Fall on and from stairs and steps**
> **EXCLUDES 1**   *Fall from stairs and steps due to ice and snow (W00.1)*

> **☑x7ᵗʰ W10.0**   **Fall (on)(from) escalator**

> **☑x7ᵗʰ W10.1**   **Fall (on)(from) sidewalk curb**

> **☑x7ᵗʰ W10.2**   **Fall (on)(from) incline**
> Fall (on) (from) ramp

> **☑x7ᵗʰ W10.8**   **Fall (on) (from) other stairs and steps**

> **☑x7ᵗʰ W10.9**   **Fall (on) (from) unspecified stairs and steps**

☑x7ᵗʰ W11   **Fall on and from ladder**

☑x7ᵗʰ W12   **Fall on and from scaffolding**

☑4ᵗʰ W13   **Fall from, out of or through building or structure**

> **☑x7ᵗʰ W13.0**   **Fall from, out of or through balcony**
> Fall from, out of or through railing

> **☑x7ᵗʰ W13.1**   **Fall from, out of or through bridge**

> **☑x7ᵗʰ W13.2**   **Fall from, out of or through roof**

> **☑x7ᵗʰ W13.3**   **Fall through floor**

> **☑x7ᵗʰ W13.4**   **Fall from, out of or through window**
> **EXCLUDES 2**   *fall with subsequent striking against sharp glass (W01.110)*

> **☑x7ᵗʰ W13.8**   **Fall from, out of or through other building or structure**
> Fall from, out of or through viaduct
> Fall from, out of or through wall
> Fall from, out of or through flag-pole

> **☑x7ᵗʰ W13.9**   **Fall from, out of or through building, not otherwise specified**
> **EXCLUDES 1**   *collapse of a building or structure (W20.-)*
> *fall or jump from burning building or structure (X00.-)*

☑x7ᵗʰ W14   **Fall from tree**

☑x7ᵗʰ W15   **Fall from cliff**

☑4ᵗʰ W16   **Fall, jump or diving into water**
> **EXCLUDES 1**   *accidental non-watercraft drowning and submersion not involving fall (W65-W74)*
> *effects of air pressure from diving (W94.-)*
> *fall into water from watercraft (V90-V94)*
> *hitting an object or against bottom when falling from watercraft (V94.0)*
> **EXCLUDES 2**   *striking or hitting diving board (W21.4)*

> **☑5ᵗʰ W16.0**   **Fall into** swimming pool
> Fall into swimming pool NOS
> **EXCLUDES 1**   *fall into empty swimming pool (W17.3)*

>> **☑6ᵗʰ W16.01**   **Fall into swimming pool** striking water surface
>>> **☑7ᵗʰ W16.011**   **Fall into swimming pool striking water surface causing** drowning and submersion
>>> **EXCLUDES 1**   *drowning and submersion while in swimming pool without fall (W67)*

>>> **☑7ᵗʰ W16.012**   **Fall into swimming pool striking water surface causing other injury**

>> **☑6ᵗʰ W16.02**   **Fall into swimming pool** striking bottom
>>> **☑7ᵗʰ W16.021**   **Fall into swimming pool striking bottom causing** drowning and submersion
>>> **EXCLUDES 1**   *drowning and submersion while in swimming pool without fall (W67)*

>>> **☑7ᵗʰ W16.022**   **Fall into swimming pool striking bottom causing other injury**

>> **☑6ᵗʰ W16.03**   **Fall into swimming pool** striking wall
>>> **☑7ᵗʰ W16.031**   **Fall into swimming pool striking wall causing** drowning and submersion
>>> **EXCLUDES 1**   *drowning and submersion while in swimming pool without fall (W67)*

>>> **☑7ᵗʰ W16.032**   **Fall into swimming pool striking wall causing other injury**

> **☑5ᵗʰ W16.1**   **Fall into** natural body of water
> Fall into lake
> Fall into open sea
> Fall into river
> Fall into stream

>> **☑6ᵗʰ W16.11**   **Fall into natural body of water** striking water surface
>>> **☑7ᵗʰ W16.111**   **Fall into natural body of water striking water surface causing** drowning and submersion
>>> **EXCLUDES 1**   *drowning and submersion while in natural body of water without fall (W69)*

>>> **☑7ᵗʰ W16.112**   **Fall into natural body of water striking water surface causing other injury**

>> **☑6ᵗʰ W16.12**   **Fall into natural body of water** striking bottom
>>> **☑7ᵗʰ W16.121**   **Fall into natural body of water striking bottom causing** drowning and submersion
>>> **EXCLUDES 1**   *drowning and submersion while in natural body of water without fall (W69)*

>>> **☑7ᵗʰ W16.122**   **Fall into natural body of water striking bottom causing other injury**

>> **☑6ᵗʰ W16.13**   **Fall into natural body of water** striking side
>>> **☑7ᵗʰ W16.131**   **Fall into natural body of water striking side causing** drowning and submersion
>>> **EXCLUDES 1**   *drowning and submersion while in natural body of water without fall (W69)*

>>> **☑7ᵗʰ W16.132**   **Fall into natural body of water striking side causing other injury**

> **☑5ᵗʰ W16.2**   **Fall in (into)** filled bathtub or bucket of water
>> **☑6ᵗʰ W16.21**   **Fall in (into)** filled bathtub
>>> **EXCLUDES 1**   *fall into empty bathtub (W18.2)*

>>> **☑7ᵗʰ W16.211**   **Fall in (into) filled bathtub causing** drowning and submersion
>>> **EXCLUDES 1**   *drowning and submersion while in filled bathtub without fall (W65)*

>>> **☑7ᵗʰ W16.212**   **Fall in (into) filled bathtub causing other injury**

N Newborn: 0   **P** Pediatric: 0-17   **M** Maternity: 12-55   **A** Adult: 15-124   **CH** Comorbidity High   **CL** Comorbidity Low   **NCDx** Noncancer Dx   **PDx** Primary Dx

1170   ICD-10-CM 2020

√6ᵗʰ **W16.22 Fall in (into)** bucket of water

    √7ᵗʰ **W16.221 Fall in (into) bucket of water causing** drowning and submersion

    √7ᵗʰ **W16.222 Fall in (into) bucket of water causing** other injury

√5ᵗʰ **W16.3 Fall into other water**

   Fall into fountain
   Fall into reservoir

√6ᵗʰ **W16.31 Fall into other water** striking water surface

    √7ᵗʰ **W16.311 Fall into other water striking water surface causing** drowning and submersion

     EXCLUDES 1   *drowning and submersion while in other water without fall (W73)*

    √7ᵗʰ **W16.312 Fall into other water striking water surface causing other injury**

√6ᵗʰ **W16.32 Fall into other water** striking bottom

    √7ᵗʰ **W16.321 Fall into other water striking bottom causing** drowning and submersion

     EXCLUDES 1   *drowning and submersion while in other water without fall (W73)*

    √7ᵗʰ **W16.322 Fall into other water striking bottom causing other injury**

√6ᵗʰ **W16.33 Fall into other water** striking wall

    √7ᵗʰ **W16.331 Fall into other water striking wall causing** drowning and submersion

     EXCLUDES 1   *drowning and submersion while in other water without fall (W73)*

    √7ᵗʰ **W16.332 Fall into other water striking wall causing other injury**

√5ᵗʰ **W16.4 Fall into unspecified water**

   √x7ᵗʰ **W16.41 Fall into unspecified water causing** drowning and submersion

   √x7ᵗʰ **W16.42 Fall into unspecified water causing other injury**

√5ᵗʰ **W16.5 Jumping or diving into** swimming pool

√6ᵗʰ **W16.51 Jumping or diving into swimming pool** striking water surface

    √7ᵗʰ **W16.511 Jumping or diving into swimming pool striking water surface causing** drowning and submersion

     EXCLUDES 1   *drowning and submersion while in swimming pool without jumping or diving (W67)*

    √7ᵗʰ **W16.512 Jumping or diving into swimming pool striking water surface causing other injury**

√6ᵗʰ **W16.52 Jumping or diving into swimming pool** striking bottom

    √7ᵗʰ **W16.521 Jumping or diving into swimming pool striking bottom causing** drowning and submersion

     EXCLUDES 1   *drowning and submersion while in swimming pool without jumping or diving (W67)*

    √7ᵗʰ **W16.522 Jumping or diving into swimming pool striking bottom causing other injury**

√6ᵗʰ **W16.53 Jumping or diving into swimming pool** striking wall

    √7ᵗʰ **W16.531 Jumping or diving into swimming pool striking wall causing** drowning and submersion

     EXCLUDES 1   *drowning and submersion while in swimming pool without jumping or diving (W67)*

    √7ᵗʰ **W16.532 Jumping or diving into swimming pool striking wall causing other injury**

√5ᵗʰ **W16.6 Jumping or diving into** natural body of water

   Jumping or diving into lake
   Jumping or diving into open sea
   Jumping or diving into river
   Jumping or diving into stream

√6ᵗʰ **W16.61 Jumping or diving into natural body of water** striking water surface

    √7ᵗʰ **W16.611 Jumping or diving into natural body of water striking water surface causing** drowning and submersion

     EXCLUDES 1   *drowning and submersion while in natural body of water without jumping or diving (W69)*

    √7ᵗʰ **W16.612 Jumping or diving into natural body of water striking water surface causing other injury**

√6ᵗʰ **W16.62 Jumping or diving into natural body of water** striking bottom

    √7ᵗʰ **W16.621 Jumping or diving into natural body of water striking bottom causing** drowning and submersion

     EXCLUDES 1   *drowning and submersion while in natural body of water without jumping or diving (W69)*

    √7ᵗʰ **W16.622 Jumping or diving into natural body of water striking bottom causing other injury**

√5ᵗʰ **W16.7 Jumping or diving** from boat

   EXCLUDES 1   *fall from boat into water — see watercraft accident (V90-V94)*

√6ᵗʰ **W16.71 Jumping or diving from boat** striking water surface

    √7ᵗʰ **W16.711 Jumping or diving from boat striking water surface causing** drowning and submersion

    √7ᵗʰ **W16.712 Jumping or diving from boat striking water surface causing other injury**

√6ᵗʰ **W16.72 Jumping or diving from boat** striking bottom

    √7ᵗʰ **W16.721 Jumping or diving from boat striking bottom causing** drowning and submersion

    √7ᵗʰ **W16.722 Jumping or diving from boat striking bottom causing other injury**

√5ᵗʰ **W16.8 Jumping or diving into** other water

   Jumping or diving into fountain
   Jumping or diving into reservoir

√6ᵗʰ **W16.81 Jumping or diving into other water** striking water surface

    √7ᵗʰ **W16.811 Jumping or diving into other water striking water surface causing** drowning and submersion

     EXCLUDES 1   *drowning and submersion while in other water without jumping or diving (W73)*

    √7ᵗʰ **W16.812 Jumping or diving into other water striking water surface causing other injury**

√6ᵗʰ **W16.82 Jumping or diving into other water** striking bottom

    √7ᵗʰ **W16.821 Jumping or diving into other water striking bottom causing** drowning and submersion

     EXCLUDES 1   *drowning and submersion while in other water without jumping or diving (W73)*

    √7ᵗʰ **W16.822 Jumping or diving into other water striking bottom causing other injury**

√6ᵗʰ **W16.83 Jumping or diving into other water** striking wall

    √7ᵗʰ **W16.831 Jumping or diving into other water striking wall causing** drowning and submersion

     EXCLUDES 1   *drowning and submersion while in other water without jumping or diving (W73)*

    √7ᵗʰ **W16.832 Jumping or diving into other water striking wall causing other injury**

Chapter 20. External Causes of Morbidity

√5ᵗʰ **W16.9 Jumping or diving into unspecified water**

√x7ᵗʰ **W16.91 Jumping or diving into unspecified water causing drowning and submersion**

√x7ᵗʰ **W16.92 Jumping or diving into unspecified water causing other injury**

√4ᵗʰ **W17 Other fall from one level to another**

√x7ᵗʰ **W17.0 Fall into well**

√x7ᵗʰ **W17.1 Fall into storm drain or manhole**

√x7ᵗʰ **W17.2 Fall into hole**

Fall into pit

√x7ᵗʰ **W17.3 Fall into empty swimming pool**

EXCLUDES 1   *fall into filled swimming pool (W16.0-)*

√x7ᵗʰ **W17.4 Fall from dock**

√5ᵗʰ **W17.8 Other fall from one level to another**

√x7ᵗʰ **W17.81 Fall down embankment (hill)**

√x7ᵗʰ **W17.82 Fall from (out of) grocery cart**

Fall due to grocery cart tipping over

√x7ᵗʰ **W17.89 Other fall from one level to another**

Fall from cherry picker

Fall from lifting device

Fall from mobile elevated work platform [MEWP]

Fall from sky lift

AHA: 2015,2Q,6

√4ᵗʰ **W18 Other slipping, tripping and stumbling and falls**

√5ᵗʰ **W18.0 Fall due to bumping against object**

Striking against object with subsequent fall

EXCLUDES 1   *fall on same level due to slipping, tripping, or stumbling with subsequent striking against object (W01.1-)*

√x7ᵗʰ **W18.00 Striking against unspecified object with subsequent fall**

√x7ᵗʰ **W18.01 Striking against sports equipment with subsequent fall**

√x7ᵗʰ **W18.02 Striking against glass with subsequent fall**

√x7ᵗʰ **W18.09 Striking against other object with subsequent fall**

√5ᵗʰ **W18.1 Fall from or off toilet**

√x7ᵗʰ **W18.11 Fall from or off toilet without subsequent striking against object**

Fall from (off) toilet NOS

√x7ᵗʰ **W18.12 Fall from or off toilet with subsequent striking against object**

√x7ᵗʰ **W18.2 Fall in (into) shower or empty bathtub**

EXCLUDES 1   *fall in full bathtub causing drowning or submersion (W16.21-)*

√5ᵗʰ **W18.3 Other and unspecified fall on same level**

√x7ᵗʰ **W18.30 Fall on same level, unspecified**

√x7ᵗʰ **W18.31 Fall on same level due to stepping on an object**

Fall on same level due to stepping on an animal

EXCLUDES 1   *slipping, tripping and stumbling without fall due to stepping on animal (W18.41)*

√x7ᵗʰ **W18.39 Other fall on same level**

√5ᵗʰ **W18.4 Slipping, tripping and stumbling without falling**

EXCLUDES 1   *collision with another person without fall (W51)*

√x7ᵗʰ **W18.40 Slipping, tripping and stumbling without falling, unspecified**

√x7ᵗʰ **W18.41 Slipping, tripping and stumbling without falling due to stepping on object**

Slipping, tripping and stumbling without falling due to stepping on animal

EXCLUDES 1   *slipping, tripping and stumbling with fall due to stepping on animal (W18.31)*

√x7ᵗʰ **W18.42 Slipping, tripping and stumbling without falling due to stepping into hole or opening**

√x7ᵗʰ **W18.43 Slipping, tripping and stumbling without falling due to stepping from one level to another**

√x7ᵗʰ **W18.49 Other slipping, tripping and stumbling without falling**

√x7ᵗʰ **W19 Unspecified fall**

Accidental fall NOS

AHA: 2012,4Q,95

Exposure to inanimate mechanical forces (W20-W49)

EXCLUDES 1   *assault (X92-Y09)*

contact or collision with animals or persons (W50-W64)

exposure to inanimate mechanical forces involving military or war operations (Y36.-, Y37.-)

intentional self-harm (X71-X83)

The appropriate 7th character is to be added to each code from categories W20-W49.

A   initial encounter

D   subsequent encounter

S   sequela

√4ᵗʰ **W20 Struck by thrown, projected or falling object**

Code first any associated:

cataclysm (X34-X39)

lightning strike (T75.00)

EXCLUDES 1   *falling object in machinery accident (W24, W28-W31)*

falling object in transport accident (V01-V99)

object set in motion by explosion (W35-W40)

object set in motion by firearm (W32-W34)

struck by thrown sports equipment (W21.-)

√x7ᵗʰ **W20.0 Struck by falling object in cave-in**

EXCLUDES 2   *asphyxiation due to cave-in (T71.21)*

√x7ᵗʰ **W20.1 Struck by object due to collapse of building**

EXCLUDES 1   *struck by object due to collapse of burning building (X00.2, X02.2)*

√x7ᵗʰ **W20.8 Other cause of strike by thrown, projected or falling object**

EXCLUDES 1   *struck by thrown sports equipment (W21.-)*

√4ᵗʰ **W21 Striking against or struck by sports equipment**

EXCLUDES 1   *assault with sports equipment (Y08.0-)*

striking against or struck by sports equipment with subsequent fall (W18.01)

√5ᵗʰ **W21.0 Struck by hit or thrown ball**

√x7ᵗʰ **W21.00 Struck by hit or thrown ball, unspecified type**

√x7ᵗʰ **W21.01 Struck by football**

√x7ᵗʰ **W21.02 Struck by soccer ball**

√x7ᵗʰ **W21.03 Struck by baseball**

√x7ᵗʰ **W21.04 Struck by golf ball**

√x7ᵗʰ **W21.05 Struck by basketball**

√x7ᵗʰ **W21.06 Struck by volleyball**

√x7ᵗʰ **W21.07 Struck by softball**

√x7ᵗʰ **W21.09 Struck by other hit or thrown ball**

√5ᵗʰ **W21.1 Struck by bat, racquet or club**

√x7ᵗʰ **W21.11 Struck by baseball bat**

√x7ᵗʰ **W21.12 Struck by tennis racquet**

√x7ᵗʰ **W21.13 Struck by golf club**

√x7ᵗʰ **W21.19 Struck by other bat, racquet or club**

√5ᵗʰ **W21.2 Struck by hockey stick or puck**

√6ᵗʰ **W21.21 Struck by hockey stick**

√7ᵗʰ **W21.210 Struck by ice hockey stick**

√7ᵗʰ **W21.211 Struck by field hockey stick**

√6ᵗʰ **W21.22 Struck by hockey puck**

√7ᵗʰ **W21.220 Struck by ice hockey puck**

√7ᵗʰ **W21.221 Struck by field hockey puck**

√5ᵗʰ **W21.3 Struck by sports foot wear**

√x7ᵗʰ **W21.31 Struck by shoe cleats**

Stepped on by shoe cleats

√x7ᵗʰ **W21.32 Struck by skate blades**

Skated over by skate blades

√x7ᵗʰ **W21.39 Struck by other sports foot wear**

√x7ᵗʰ **W21.4 Striking against diving board**

Use additional code for subsequent falling into water, if applicable (W16.-)

√5ᵗʰ **W21.8 Striking against or struck by other sports equipment**

√x7ᵗʰ **W21.81 Striking against or struck by football helmet**

√x7ᵗʰ **W21.89 Striking against or struck by other sports equipment**

√x7ᵗʰ **W21.9 Striking against or struck by unspecified sports equipment**

N Newborn: 0   P Pediatric: 0-17   M Maternity: 12-55   A Adult: 15-124   CH Comorbidity High   CL Comorbidity Low   NCDx Noncancer Dx   PDx Primary Dx

1172   ICD-10-CM 2020

☑4ᵗʰ **W22 Striking against or struck by other objects**
    EXCLUDES 1   *striking against or struck by object with subsequent fall (W18.Ø9)*

  ☑5ᵗʰ **W22.Ø Striking against** stationary object
      EXCLUDES 1   *striking against stationary sports equipment (W21.8)*

    ✓x7ᵗʰ **W22.Ø1 Walked into** wall
    ✓x7ᵗʰ **W22.Ø2 Walked into** lamppost
    ✓x7ᵗʰ **W22.Ø3 Walked into** furniture

    ☑6ᵗʰ **W22.Ø4 Striking against wall of** swimming pool
      ✓7ᵗʰ **W22.Ø41 Striking against wall of swimming pool causing** drowning and submersion
        EXCLUDES 1   *drowning and submersion while swimming without striking against wall (W67)*
      ✓7ᵗʰ **W22.Ø42 Striking against wall of swimming pool causing other injury**

    ✓x7ᵗʰ **W22.Ø9 Striking against other stationary object**

  ☑5ᵗʰ **W22.1 Striking against or struck by** automobile airbag
    ✓x7ᵗʰ **W22.1Ø Striking against or struck by unspecified automobile airbag**
    ✓x7ᵗʰ **W22.11 Striking against or struck by** driver side **automobile airbag**
    ✓x7ᵗʰ **W22.12 Striking against or struck by** front passenger side **automobile airbag**
    ✓x7ᵗʰ **W22.19 Striking against or struck by other automobile airbag**

  ✓x7ᵗʰ **W22.8 Striking against or struck by other objects**
    Striking against or struck by object NOS
    EXCLUDES 1   *struck by thrown, projected or falling object (W2Ø.-)*

☑4ᵗʰ **W23 Caught, crushed, jammed or pinched in or between objects**
    EXCLUDES 1   *injury caused by cutting or piercing instruments (W25-W27)*
             injury caused by firearms malfunction (W32.1, W33.1-, W34.1-)
             injury caused by lifting and transmission devices (W24.-)
             injury caused by machinery (W28-W31)
             injury caused by nonpowered hand tools (W27.-)
             injury caused by transport vehicle being used as a means of transportation (VØ1-V99)
             injury caused by struck by thrown, projected or falling object (W2Ø.-)

  ✓x7ᵗʰ **W23.Ø Caught, crushed, jammed, or pinched between** moving objects
  ✓x7ᵗʰ **W23.1 Caught, crushed, jammed, or pinched between** stationary objects

☑4ᵗʰ **W24 Contact with lifting and transmission devices, not elsewhere classified**
    EXCLUDES 1   *transport accidents (VØ1-V99)*

  ✓x7ᵗʰ **W24.Ø Contact with lifting devices, not elsewhere classified**
    Contact with chain hoist
    Contact with drive belt
    Contact with pulley (block)

  ✓x7ᵗʰ **W24.1 Contact with transmission devices, not elsewhere classified**
    Contact with transmission belt or cable

☑4ᵗʰ **W25 Contact with sharp glass**
    Code first any associated:
    injury due to flying glass from explosion or firearm discharge (W32-W4Ø)
    transport accident (VØØ-V99)
    EXCLUDES 1   *fall on same level due to slipping, tripping and stumbling with subsequent striking against sharp glass ►(WØ1.11Ø)◄*
             striking against sharp glass with subsequent fall (W18.Ø2)
    EXCLUDES 2   *glass embedded in skin (W45)*

☑4ᵗʰ **W26 Contact with other sharp objects**
    EXCLUDES 2   *sharp object(s) embedded in skin (W45)*
    AHA: 2016,4Q,73

  ✓x7ᵗʰ **W26.Ø Contact with knife**
    EXCLUDES 1   *contact with electric knife (W29.1)*

  ✓x7ᵗʰ **W26.1 Contact with sword or dagger**

  ✓x7ᵗʰ **W26.2 Contact with edge of stiff paper**
    Paper cut

  ✓x7ᵗʰ **W26.8 Contact with other sharp object(s), not elsewhere classified**
    Contact with tin can lid

  ✓x7ᵗʰ **W26.9 Contact with unspecified sharp object(s)**

☑4ᵗʰ **W27 Contact with nonpowered hand tool**

  ✓x7ᵗʰ **W27.Ø Contact with** workbench tool
    Contact with auger
    Contact with axe
    Contact with chisel
    Contact with handsaw
    Contact with screwdriver

  ✓x7ᵗʰ **W27.1 Contact with** garden tool
    Contact with hoe
    Contact with nonpowered lawn mower
    Contact with pitchfork
    Contact with rake

  ✓x7ᵗʰ **W27.2 Contact with** scissors

  ✓x7ᵗʰ **W27.3 Contact with** needle **(sewing)**
    EXCLUDES 1   *contact with hypodermic needle (W46.-)*

  ✓x7ᵗʰ **W27.4 Contact with** kitchen utensil
    Contact with fork
    Contact with ice-pick
    Contact with can-opener NOS

  ✓x7ᵗʰ **W27.5 Contact with** paper-cutter

  ✓x7ᵗʰ **W27.8 Contact with other nonpowered hand tool**
    Contact with nonpowered sewing machine
    Contact with shovel

✓x7ᵗʰ **W28 Contact with powered lawn mower**
    Powered lawn mower (commercial) (residential)
    EXCLUDES 1   *contact with nonpowered lawn mower (W27.1)*
    EXCLUDES 2   *exposure to electric current (W86.-)*

☑4ᵗʰ **W29 Contact with other powered hand tools and household machinery**
    EXCLUDES 1   *contact with commercial machinery (W31.82)*
             contact with hot household appliance (X15)
             contact with nonpowered hand tool (W27.-)
             exposure to electric current (W86)

  ✓x7ᵗʰ **W29.Ø Contact with powered kitchen appliance**
    Contact with blender
    Contact with can-opener
    Contact with garbage disposal
    Contact with mixer

  ✓x7ᵗʰ **W29.1 Contact with electric knife**

  ✓x7ᵗʰ **W29.2 Contact with other powered household machinery**
    Contact with electric fan
    Contact with powered dryer (clothes) (powered) (spin)
    Contact with washing-machine
    Contact with sewing machine

  ✓x7ᵗʰ **W29.3 Contact with powered garden and outdoor hand tools and machinery**
    Contact with chainsaw
    Contact with edger
    Contact with garden cultivator (tiller)
    Contact with hedge trimmer
    Contact with other powered garden tool
    EXCLUDES 1   *contact with powered lawn mower (W28)*

  ✓x7ᵗʰ **W29.4 Contact with nail gun**

  ✓x7ᵗʰ **W29.8 Contact with other powered hand tools and household machinery**
    Contact with do-it-yourself tool NOS

☑4ᵗʰ **W30 Contact with agricultural machinery**
    INCLUDES   animal-powered farm machine
    EXCLUDES 1   *agricultural transport vehicle accident (VØ1-V99)*
             explosion of grain store (W4Ø.8)
             exposure to electric current (W86.-)

  ✓x7ᵗʰ **W30.Ø Contact with combine harvester**
    Contact with reaper
    Contact with thresher

  ✓x7ᵗʰ **W30.1 Contact with power take-off devices (PTO)**

  ✓x7ᵗʰ **W30.2 Contact with hay derrick**

  ✓x7ᵗʰ **W30.3 Contact with grain storage elevator**
    EXCLUDES 1   *explosion of grain store (W4Ø.8)*

☑ Additional Character Required   ✓x7ᵗʰ Placeholder Alert   Manifestation   Unspecified Dx   ►◄ Revised Text   ● New Code   ▲ Revised Title

Chapter 20. External Causes of Morbidity

✓5ᵗʰ **W30.8 Contact with other specified agricultural machinery**

✓x7ᵗʰ **W30.81 Contact with agricultural transport vehicle in stationary use**

Contact with agricultural transport vehicle under repair, not on public roadway

EXCLUDES 1   *agricultural transport vehicle accident (V01-V99)*

✓x7ᵗʰ **W30.89 Contact with other specified agricultural machinery**

✓x7ᵗʰ **W30.9 Contact with unspecified agricultural machinery**

Contact with farm machinery NOS

✓4ᵗʰ **W31 Contact with other and unspecified machinery**

EXCLUDES 1   *contact with agricultural machinery (W30.-)*

contact with machinery in transport under own power or being towed by a vehicle (V01-V99)

exposure to electric current (W86)

✓x7ᵗʰ **W31.0 Contact with mining and earth-drilling machinery**

Contact with bore or drill (land) (seabed)

Contact with shaft hoist

Contact with shaft lift

Contact with undercutter

✓x7ᵗʰ **W31.1 Contact with metalworking machines**

Contact with abrasive wheel

Contact with forging machine

Contact with lathe

Contact with mechanical shears

Contact with metal drilling machine

Contact with milling machine

Contact with power press

Contact with rolling-mill

Contact with metal sawing machine

✓x7ᵗʰ **W31.2 Contact with powered woodworking and forming machines**

Contact with band saw

Contact with bench saw

Contact with circular saw

Contact with molding machine

Contact with overhead plane

Contact with powered saw

Contact with radial saw

Contact with sander

EXCLUDES 1   *nonpowered woodworking tools (W27.0)*

✓x7ᵗʰ **W31.3 Contact with prime movers**

Contact with gas turbine

Contact with internal combustion engine

Contact with steam engine

Contact with water driven turbine

✓5ᵗʰ **W31.8 Contact with other specified machinery**

✓x7ᵗʰ **W31.81 Contact with recreational machinery**

Contact with roller coaster

✓x7ᵗʰ **W31.82 Contact with other commercial machinery**

Contact with commercial electric fan

Contact with commercial kitchen appliances

Contact with commercial powered dryer (clothes) (powered) (spin)

Contact with commercial washing-machine

Contact with commercial sewing machine

EXCLUDES 1   *contact with household machinery (W29.-)*

contact with powered lawn mower (W28)

✓x7ᵗʰ **W31.83 Contact with special construction vehicle in stationary use**

Contact with special construction vehicle under repair, not on public roadway

EXCLUDES 1   *special construction vehicle accident (V01-V99)*

✓x7ᵗʰ **W31.89 Contact with other specified machinery**

✓x7ᵗʰ **W31.9 Contact with unspecified machinery**

Contact with machinery NOS

✓4ᵗʰ **W32 Accidental handgun discharge and malfunction**

INCLUDES   accidental discharge and malfunction of gun for single hand use

accidental discharge and malfunction of pistol

accidental discharge and malfunction of revolver

handgun discharge and malfunction NOS

EXCLUDES 1   *accidental airgun discharge and malfunction (W34.010, W34.110)*

accidental BB gun discharge and malfunction (W34.010, W34.110)

accidental pellet gun discharge and malfunction (W34.010, W34.110)

accidental shotgun discharge and malfunction (W33.01, W33.11)

assault by handgun discharge (X93)

handgun discharge involving legal intervention (Y35.0-)

handgun discharge involving military or war operations (Y36.4-)

intentional self-harm by handgun discharge (X72)

Very pistol discharge and malfunction (W34.09, W34.19)

✓x7ᵗʰ **W32.0 Accidental handgun discharge**

✓x7ᵗʰ **W32.1 Accidental handgun malfunction**

Injury due to explosion of handgun (parts)

Injury due to malfunction of mechanism or component of handgun

Injury due to recoil of handgun

Powder burn from handgun

✓4ᵗʰ **W33 Accidental rifle, shotgun and larger firearm discharge and malfunction**

INCLUDES   rifle, shotgun and larger firearm discharge and malfunction NOS

EXCLUDES 1   *accidental airgun discharge and malfunction (W34.010, W34.110)*

accidental BB gun discharge and malfunction (W34.010, W34.110)

accidental handgun discharge and malfunction (W32.-)

accidental pellet gun discharge and malfunction (W34.010, W34.110)

assault by rifle, shotgun and larger firearm discharge (X94)

firearm discharge involving legal intervention (Y35.0-)

firearm discharge involving military or war operations (Y36.4-)

intentional self-harm by rifle, shotgun and larger firearm discharge (X73)

✓5ᵗʰ **W33.0 Accidental rifle, shotgun and larger firearm discharge**

✓x7ᵗʰ **W33.00 Accidental discharge of unspecified larger firearm**

Discharge of unspecified larger firearm NOS

✓x7ᵗʰ **W33.01 Accidental discharge of shotgun**

Discharge of shotgun NOS

✓x7ᵗʰ **W33.02 Accidental discharge of hunting rifle**

Discharge of hunting rifle NOS

✓x7ᵗʰ **W33.03 Accidental discharge of machine gun**

Discharge of machine gun NOS

✓x7ᵗʰ **W33.09 Accidental discharge of other larger firearm**

Discharge of other larger firearm NOS

✓5ᵗʰ **W33.1 Accidental rifle, shotgun and larger firearm malfunction**

Injury due to explosion of rifle, shotgun and larger firearm (parts)

Injury due to malfunction of mechanism or component of rifle, shotgun and larger firearm

Injury due to piercing, cutting, crushing or pinching due to (by) slide trigger mechanism, scope or other gun part

Injury due to recoil of rifle, shotgun and larger firearm

Powder burn from rifle, shotgun and larger firearm

✓x7ᵗʰ **W33.10 Accidental malfunction of unspecified larger firearm**

Malfunction of unspecified larger firearm NOS

✓x7ᵗʰ **W33.11 Accidental malfunction of shotgun**

Malfunction of shotgun NOS

✓x7ᵗʰ **W33.12 Accidental malfunction of hunting rifle**

Malfunction of hunting rifle NOS

✓x7ᵗʰ **W33.13 Accidental malfunction of machine gun**

Malfunction of machine gun NOS

☑x7ᵗʰ **W33.19** **Accidental malfunction of other larger firearm**
     Malfunction of other larger firearm NOS

☑4ᵗʰ **W34** **Accidental discharge and malfunction from other and unspecified firearms and guns**

   ☑5ᵗʰ **W34.0** **Accidental discharge from other and unspecified firearms and guns**

     ☑x7ᵗʰ **W34.00** **Accidental discharge from unspecified firearms or gun**
       Discharge from firearm NOS
       Gunshot wound NOS
       Shot NOS

     ☑6ᵗʰ **W34.01** **Accidental discharge of gas, air or spring-operated guns**

       ☑7ᵗʰ **W34.010** **Accidental discharge of airgun**
         Accidental discharge of BB gun
         Accidental discharge of pellet gun

       ☑7ᵗʰ **W34.011** **Accidental discharge of paintball gun**
         Accidental injury due to paintball discharge

       ☑7ᵗʰ **W34.018** **Accidental discharge of other gas, air or spring-operated gun**

     ☑x7ᵗʰ **W34.09** **Accidental discharge from other specified firearms**
       Accidental discharge from Very pistol [flare]

   ☑5ᵗʰ **W34.1** **Accidental malfunction from other and unspecified firearms and guns**

     ☑x7ᵗʰ **W34.10** **Accidental malfunction from unspecified firearms or gun**
       Firearm malfunction NOS

     ☑6ᵗʰ **W34.11** **Accidental malfunction of gas, air or spring-operated guns**

       ☑7ᵗʰ **W34.110** **Accidental malfunction of airgun**
         Accidental malfunction of BB gun
         Accidental malfunction of pellet gun

       ☑7ᵗʰ **W34.111** **Accidental malfunction of paintball gun**
         Accidental injury due to paintball gun malfunction

       ☑7ᵗʰ **W34.118** **Accidental malfunction of other gas, air or spring-operated gun**

     ☑x7ᵗʰ **W34.19** **Accidental malfunction from other specified firearms**
       Accidental malfunction from Very pistol [flare]

☑x7ᵗʰ **W35** **Explosion and rupture of boiler**
   EXCLUDES 1   explosion and rupture of boiler on watercraft (V93.4)

☑4ᵗʰ **W36** **Explosion and rupture of gas cylinder**

   ☑x7ᵗʰ **W36.1** **Explosion and rupture of aerosol can**

   ☑x7ᵗʰ **W36.2** **Explosion and rupture of air tank**

   ☑x7ᵗʰ **W36.3** **Explosion and rupture of pressurized-gas tank**

   ☑x7ᵗʰ **W36.8** **Explosion and rupture of other gas cylinder**

   ☑x7ᵗʰ **W36.9** **Explosion and rupture of unspecified gas cylinder**

☑4ᵗʰ **W37** **Explosion and rupture of pressurized tire, pipe or hose**

   ☑x7ᵗʰ **W37.0** **Explosion of bicycle tire**

   ☑x7ᵗʰ **W37.8** **Explosion and rupture of other pressurized tire, pipe or hose**

☑x7ᵗʰ **W38** **Explosion and rupture of other specified pressurized devices**

☑x7ᵗʰ **W39** **Discharge of firework**

☑4ᵗʰ **W40** **Explosion of other materials**
   EXCLUDES 1   assault by explosive material (X96)
       explosion involving legal intervention (Y35.1-)
       explosion involving military or war operations (Y36.0-, Y36.2-)
       intentional self-harm by explosive material (X75)

   ☑x7ᵗʰ **W40.0** **Explosion of blasting material**
     Explosion of blasting cap
     Explosion of detonator
     Explosion of dynamite
     Explosion of explosive (any) used in blasting operations

   ☑x7ᵗʰ **W40.1** **Explosion of explosive gases**
     Explosion of acetylene
     Explosion of butane
     Explosion of coal gas
     Explosion in mine NOS
     Explosion of explosive gas
     Explosion of fire damp
     Explosion of gasoline fumes
     Explosion of methane
     Explosion of propane

   ☑x7ᵗʰ **W40.8** **Explosion of other specified explosive materials**
     Explosion in dump NOS
     Explosion in factory NOS
     Explosion in grain store
     Explosion in munitions
     EXCLUDES 1   explosion involving legal intervention (Y35.1-)
       explosion involving military or war operations (Y36.0-, Y36.2-)

   ☑x7ᵗʰ **W40.9** **Explosion of unspecified explosive materials**
     Explosion NOS

☑4ᵗʰ **W42** **Exposure to noise**

   ☑x7ᵗʰ **W42.0** **Exposure to supersonic waves**

   ☑x7ᵗʰ **W42.9** **Exposure to other noise**
     Exposure to sound waves NOS

☑4ᵗʰ **W45** **Foreign body or object entering through skin**
   INCLUDES   foreign body or object embedded in skin
       nail embedded in skin
   EXCLUDES 2   contact with hand tools (nonpowered) (powered) (W27-W29)
       contact with other sharp objects (W26.-)
       contact with sharp glass (W25.-)
       struck by objects (W20-W22)

   ☑x7ᵗʰ **W45.0** **Nail entering through skin**

   ☑x7ᵗʰ **W45.8** **Other foreign body or object entering through skin**
     Splinter in skin NOS

☑4ᵗʰ **W46** **Contact with hypodermic needle**

   ☑x7ᵗʰ **W46.0** **Contact with hypodermic needle**
     Hypodermic needle stick NOS

   ☑x7ᵗʰ **W46.1** **Contact with contaminated hypodermic needle**

☑4ᵗʰ **W49** **Exposure to other inanimate mechanical forces**
   INCLUDES   exposure to abnormal gravitational [G] forces
       exposure to inanimate mechanical forces NEC
   EXCLUDES 1   exposure to inanimate mechanical forces involving military or war operations (Y36.-, Y37.-)

   ☑5ᵗʰ **W49.0** **Item causing external constriction**

     ☑x7ᵗʰ **W49.01** **Hair causing external constriction**

     ☑x7ᵗʰ **W49.02** **String or thread causing external constriction**

     ☑x7ᵗʰ **W49.03** **Rubber band causing external constriction**

     ☑x7ᵗʰ **W49.04** **Ring or other jewelry causing external constriction**

     ☑x7ᵗʰ **W49.09** **Other specified item causing external constriction**

   ☑x7ᵗʰ **W49.9** **Exposure to other inanimate mechanical forces**

Exposure to animate mechanical forces (W50-W64)

   EXCLUDES 1   toxic effect of contact with venomous animals and plants (T63.-)

The appropriate 7th character is to be added to each code from categories W50-W64.
A   initial encounter
D   subsequent encounter
S   sequela

☑4ᵗʰ **W50** **Accidental hit, strike, kick, twist, bite or scratch by another person**
   INCLUDES   hit, strike, kick, twist, bite, or scratch by another person NOS
   EXCLUDES 1   assault by bodily force (Y04)
       struck by objects (W20-W22)

   ☑x7ᵗʰ **W50.0** **Accidental hit or strike by another person**
     Hit or strike by another person NOS

   ☑x7ᵗʰ **W50.1** **Accidental kick by another person**
     Kick by another person NOS

   ☑x7ᵗʰ **W50.2** **Accidental twist by another person**
     Twist by another person NOS

☑ Additional Character Required   ☑x7ᵗʰ Placeholder Alert   Manifestation   Unspecified Dx   ▶◀ Revised Text   ● New Code   ▲ Revised Title

ICD-10-CM 2020   1175

W33.19–W50.2

√x7ᵗʰ **W50.3 Accidental** bite **by another person**
     Human bite
     Bite by another person NOS

√x7ᵗʰ **W50.4 Accidental** scratch **by another person**
     Scratch by another person NOS

√x7ᵗʰ **W51 Accidental striking against or bumped into by another person**
     EXCLUDES 1   *assault by striking against or bumping into by another person (Y04.2)*
                    fall due to collision with another person (W03)

√x7ᵗʰ **W52 Crushed, pushed or stepped on by crowd or human stampede**
     Crushed, pushed or stepped on by crowd or human stampede with or without fall

√4ᵗʰ **W53 Contact with rodent**
     INCLUDES   contact with saliva, feces or urine of rodent

√5ᵗʰ **W53.0 Contact with** mouse
     √x7ᵗʰ **W53.01 Bitten by mouse**
     √x7ᵗʰ **W53.09 Other contact with mouse**

√5ᵗʰ **W53.1 Contact with** rat
     √x7ᵗʰ **W53.11 Bitten by rat**
     √x7ᵗʰ **W53.19 Other contact with rat**

√5ᵗʰ **W53.2 Contact with** squirrel
     √x7ᵗʰ **W53.21 Bitten by squirrel**
     √x7ᵗʰ **W53.29 Other contact with squirrel**

√5ᵗʰ **W53.8 Contact with other rodent**
     √x7ᵗʰ **W53.81 Bitten by other rodent**
     √x7ᵗʰ **W53.89 Other contact with other rodent**

√4ᵗʰ **W54 Contact with dog**
     INCLUDES   contact with saliva, feces or urine of dog

√x7ᵗʰ **W54.0 Bitten by dog**

√x7ᵗʰ **W54.1 Struck by dog**
     Knocked over by dog

√x7ᵗʰ **W54.8 Other contact with dog**

√4ᵗʰ **W55 Contact with other mammals**
     INCLUDES   contact with saliva, feces or urine of mammal
     EXCLUDES 1   *animal being ridden — see transport accidents*
                 bitten or struck by dog (W54)
                 bitten or struck by rodent (W53.-)
                 contact with marine mammals (W56.-)

√5ᵗʰ **W55.0 Contact with** cat
     √x7ᵗʰ **W55.01 Bitten by cat**
     √x7ᵗʰ **W55.03 Scratched by cat**
     √x7ᵗʰ **W55.09 Other contact with cat**

√5ᵗʰ **W55.1 Contact with** horse
     √x7ᵗʰ **W55.11 Bitten by horse**
     √x7ᵗʰ **W55.12 Struck by horse**
     √x7ᵗʰ **W55.19 Other contact with horse**

√5ᵗʰ **W55.2 Contact with** cow
     Contact with bull
     √x7ᵗʰ **W55.21 Bitten by cow**
     √x7ᵗʰ **W55.22 Struck by cow**
          Gored by bull
     √x7ᵗʰ **W55.29 Other contact with cow**

√5ᵗʰ **W55.3 Contact with other hoof stock**
     Contact with goats
     Contact with sheep
     √x7ᵗʰ **W55.31 Bitten by other hoof stock**
     √x7ᵗʰ **W55.32 Struck by other hoof stock**
          Gored by goat
          Gored by ram
     √x7ᵗʰ **W55.39 Other contact with other hoof stock**

√5ᵗʰ **W55.4 Contact with** pig
     √x7ᵗʰ **W55.41 Bitten by pig**
     √x7ᵗʰ **W55.42 Struck by pig**
     √x7ᵗʰ **W55.49 Other contact with pig**

√5ᵗʰ **W55.5 Contact with** raccoon
     √x7ᵗʰ **W55.51 Bitten by raccoon**

√x7ᵗʰ **W55.52 Struck by raccoon**
√x7ᵗʰ **W55.59 Other contact with raccoon**

√5ᵗʰ **W55.8 Contact with other mammals**
     √x7ᵗʰ **W55.81 Bitten by other mammals**
     √x7ᵗʰ **W55.82 Struck by other mammals**
     √x7ᵗʰ **W55.89 Other contact with other mammals**

√4ᵗʰ **W56 Contact with nonvenomous marine animal**
     EXCLUDES 1   *contact with venomous marine animal (T63.-)*

√5ᵗʰ **W56.0 Contact with** dolphin
     √x7ᵗʰ **W56.01 Bitten by dolphin**
     √x7ᵗʰ **W56.02 Struck by dolphin**
     √x7ᵗʰ **W56.09 Other contact with dolphin**

√5ᵗʰ **W56.1 Contact with** sea lion
     √x7ᵗʰ **W56.11 Bitten by sea lion**
     √x7ᵗʰ **W56.12 Struck by sea lion**
     √x7ᵗʰ **W56.19 Other contact with sea lion**

√5ᵗʰ **W56.2 Contact with** orca
     Contact with killer whale
     √x7ᵗʰ **W56.21 Bitten by orca**
     √x7ᵗʰ **W56.22 Struck by orca**
     √x7ᵗʰ **W56.29 Other contact with orca**

√5ᵗʰ **W56.3 Contact with other marine mammals**
     √x7ᵗʰ **W56.31 Bitten by other marine mammals**
     √x7ᵗʰ **W56.32 Struck by other marine mammals**
     √x7ᵗʰ **W56.39 Other contact with other marine mammals**

√5ᵗʰ **W56.4 Contact with** shark
     √x7ᵗʰ **W56.41 Bitten by shark**
     √x7ᵗʰ **W56.42 Struck by shark**
     √x7ᵗʰ **W56.49 Other contact with shark**

√5ᵗʰ **W56.5 Contact with other fish**
     √x7ᵗʰ **W56.51 Bitten by other fish**
     √x7ᵗʰ **W56.52 Struck by other fish**
     √x7ᵗʰ **W56.59 Other contact with other fish**

√5ᵗʰ **W56.8 Contact with other nonvenomous marine animals**
     √x7ᵗʰ **W56.81 Bitten by other nonvenomous marine animals**
     √x7ᵗʰ **W56.82 Struck by other nonvenomous marine animals**
     √x7ᵗʰ **W56.89 Other contact with other nonvenomous marine animals**

√x7ᵗʰ **W57 Bitten or stung by nonvenomous insect and other nonvenomous arthropods**
     EXCLUDES 1   *contact with venomous insects and arthropods (T63.2-, T63.3-, T63.4-)*

√4ᵗʰ **W58 Contact with crocodile or alligator**
√5ᵗʰ **W58.0 Contact with** alligator
     √x7ᵗʰ **W58.01 Bitten by alligator**
     √x7ᵗʰ **W58.02 Struck by alligator**
     √x7ᵗʰ **W58.03 Crushed by alligator**
     √x7ᵗʰ **W58.09 Other contact with alligator**

√5ᵗʰ **W58.1 Contact with** crocodile
     √x7ᵗʰ **W58.11 Bitten by crocodile**
     √x7ᵗʰ **W58.12 Struck by crocodile**
     √x7ᵗʰ **W58.13 Crushed by crocodile**
     √x7ᵗʰ **W58.19 Other contact with crocodile**

√4ᵗʰ **W59 Contact with other nonvenomous reptiles**
     EXCLUDES 1   *contact with venomous reptile (T63.0-, T63.1-)*

√5ᵗʰ **W59.0 Contact with nonvenomous** lizards
     √x7ᵗʰ **W59.01 Bitten by nonvenomous lizards**
     √x7ᵗʰ **W59.02 Struck by nonvenomous lizards**
     √x7ᵗʰ **W59.09 Other contact with nonvenomous lizards**
          Exposure to nonvenomous lizards

√5ᵗʰ **W59.1 Contact with nonvenomous** snakes
     √x7ᵗʰ **W59.11 Bitten by nonvenomous snake**
     √x7ᵗʰ **W59.12 Struck by nonvenomous snake**
     √x7ᵗʰ **W59.13 Crushed by nonvenomous snake**
     √x7ᵗʰ **W59.19 Other contact with nonvenomous snake**

✓5ᵗʰ **W59.2** **Contact with** turtles
> *EXCLUDES 1*   contact with tortoises (W59.8-)

✓x7ᵗʰ **W59.21** **Bitten by turtle**

✓x7ᵗʰ **W59.22** **Struck by turtle**

✓x7ᵗʰ **W59.29** **Other contact with turtle**
> Exposure to turtles

✓5ᵗʰ **W59.8** **Contact with other nonvenomous reptiles**

✓x7ᵗʰ **W59.81** **Bitten by other nonvenomous reptiles**

✓x7ᵗʰ **W59.82** **Struck by other nonvenomous reptiles**

✓x7ᵗʰ **W59.83** **Crushed by other nonvenomous reptiles**

✓x7ᵗʰ **W59.89** **Other contact with other nonvenomous reptiles**

✓x7ᵗʰ **W60** **Contact with nonvenomous plant thorns and spines and sharp leaves**
> *EXCLUDES 1*   contact with venomous plants (T63.7-)

✓4ᵗʰ **W61** **Contact with birds (domestic) (wild)**
> *INCLUDES*   contact with excreta of birds

✓5ᵗʰ **W61.0** **Contact with** parrot

✓x7ᵗʰ **W61.01** **Bitten by parrot**

✓x7ᵗʰ **W61.02** **Struck by parrot**

✓x7ᵗʰ **W61.09** **Other contact with parrot**
> Exposure to parrots

✓5ᵗʰ **W61.1** **Contact with** macaw

✓x7ᵗʰ **W61.11** **Bitten by macaw**

✓x7ᵗʰ **W61.12** **Struck by macaw**

✓x7ᵗʰ **W61.19** **Other contact with macaw**
> Exposure to macaws

✓5ᵗʰ **W61.2** **Contact with other** psittacines

✓x7ᵗʰ **W61.21** **Bitten by other psittacines**

✓x7ᵗʰ **W61.22** **Struck by other psittacines**

✓x7ᵗʰ **W61.29** **Other contact with other psittacines**
> Exposure to other psittacines

✓5ᵗʰ **W61.3** **Contact with** chicken

✓x7ᵗʰ **W61.32** **Struck by chicken**

✓x7ᵗʰ **W61.33** **Pecked by chicken**

✓x7ᵗʰ **W61.39** **Other contact with chicken**
> Exposure to chickens

✓5ᵗʰ **W61.4** **Contact with** turkey

✓x7ᵗʰ **W61.42** **Struck by turkey**

✓x7ᵗʰ **W61.43** **Pecked by turkey**

✓x7ᵗʰ **W61.49** **Other contact with turkey**

✓5ᵗʰ **W61.5** **Contact with** goose

✓x7ᵗʰ **W61.51** **Bitten by goose**

✓x7ᵗʰ **W61.52** **Struck by goose**

✓x7ᵗʰ **W61.59** **Other contact with goose**

✓5ᵗʰ **W61.6** **Contact with** duck

✓x7ᵗʰ **W61.61** **Bitten by duck**

✓x7ᵗʰ **W61.62** **Struck by duck**

✓x7ᵗʰ **W61.69** **Other contact with duck**

✓5ᵗʰ **W61.9** **Contact with other birds**

✓x7ᵗʰ **W61.91** **Bitten by other birds**

✓x7ᵗʰ **W61.92** **Struck by other birds**

✓x7ᵗʰ **W61.99** **Other contact with other birds**
> Contact with bird NOS

✓4ᵗʰ **W62** **Contact with nonvenomous amphibians**
> *EXCLUDES 1*   contact with venomous amphibians (T63.81-R63.83)

✓x7ᵗʰ **W62.0** **Contact with nonvenomous** frogs

✓x7ᵗʰ **W62.1** **Contact with nonvenomous** toads

✓x7ᵗʰ **W62.9** **Contact with other nonvenomous amphibians**

✓x7ᵗʰ **W64** **Exposure to other animate mechanical forces**
> *INCLUDES*   exposure to nonvenomous animal NOS
> *EXCLUDES 1*   contact with venomous animal (T63.-)

Accidental non-transport drowning and submersion (W65-W74)

> *EXCLUDES 1*   accidental drowning and submersion due to fall into water (W16.-)
> accidental drowning and submersion due to water transport accident (V90.-, V92.-)
> *EXCLUDES 2*   accidental drowning and submersion due to cataclysm (X34-X39)

> The appropriate 7th character is to be added to each code from categories W65-W74.
> A   initial encounter
> D   subsequent encounter
> S   sequela

✓x7ᵗʰ **W65** **Accidental drowning and submersion while in** bath-tub
> *EXCLUDES 1*   accidental drowning and submersion due to fall in (into) bathtub (W16.211)

✓x7ᵗʰ **W67** **Accidental drowning and submersion while in** swimming-pool
> *EXCLUDES 1*   accidental drowning and submersion due to fall into swimming pool (W16.011, W16.021, W16.031)
> accidental drowning and submersion due to striking into wall of swimming pool (W22.041)

✓x7ᵗʰ **W69** **Accidental drowning and submersion while in** natural water
> Accidental drowning and submersion while in lake
> Accidental drowning and submersion while in open sea
> Accidental drowning and submersion while in river
> Accidental drowning and submersion while in stream
> *EXCLUDES 1*   accidental drowning and submersion due to fall into natural body of water (W16.111, W16.121, W16.131)

✓x7ᵗʰ **W73** **Other specified cause of accidental non-transport drowning and submersion**
> Accidental drowning and submersion while in quenching tank
> Accidental drowning and submersion while in reservoir
> *EXCLUDES 1*   accidental drowning and submersion due to fall into other water (W16.311, W16.321, W16.331)

✓x7ᵗʰ **W74** **Unspecified cause of accidental drowning and submersion**
> Drowning NOS

Exposure to electric current, radiation and extreme ambient air temperature and pressure (W85-W99)

> *EXCLUDES 1*   exposure to:
> failure in dosage of radiation or temperature during surgical and medical care (Y63.2-Y63.5)
> lightning (T75.0-)
> natural cold (X31)
> natural heat (X30)
> natural radiation NOS (X39)
> radiological procedure and radiotherapy (Y84.2)
> sunlight (X32)

AHA: 2018,2Q,7-8

> The appropriate 7th character is to be added to each code from categories W85-W99.
> A   initial encounter
> D   subsequent encounter
> S   sequela

✓x7ᵗʰ **W85** **Exposure to electric transmission lines**
> Broken power line

✓4ᵗʰ **W86** **Exposure to other specified electric current**

✓x7ᵗʰ **W86.0** **Exposure to domestic wiring and appliances**

✓x7ᵗʰ **W86.1** **Exposure to industrial wiring, appliances and electrical machinery**
> Exposure to conductors
> Exposure to control apparatus
> Exposure to electrical equipment and machinery
> Exposure to transformers

✓x7ᵗʰ **W86.8** **Exposure to other electric current**
> Exposure to wiring and appliances in or on farm (not farmhouse)
> Exposure to wiring and appliances outdoors
> Exposure to wiring and appliances in or on public building
> Exposure to wiring and appliances in or on residential institutions
> Exposure to wiring and appliances in or on schools

✓4ᵗʰ **W88** **Exposure to ionizing radiation**
> *EXCLUDES 1*   exposure to sunlight (X32)

✓x7ᵗʰ **W88.0** **Exposure to** X-rays

✓x7ᵗʰ **W88.1** **Exposure to** radioactive isotopes

✓ Additional Character Required   ✓x7ᵗʰ Placeholder Alert   Manifestation   Unspecified Dx   ►◄ Revised Text   ● New Code   ▲ Revised Title

ICD-10-CM 2020   1177

Chapter 20. External Causes of Morbidity

√x7ᵗʰ **W88.8 Exposure to other ionizing radiation**

√4ᵗʰ **W89 Exposure to man-made visible and ultraviolet light**
> INCLUDES exposure to welding light (arc)
> EXCLUDES 1 exposure to sunlight (X32)

√x7ᵗʰ **W89.0 Exposure to welding light (arc)**

√x7ᵗʰ **W89.1 Exposure to tanning bed**

√x7ᵗʰ **W89.8 Exposure to other man-made visible and ultraviolet light**

√x7ᵗʰ **W89.9 Exposure to unspecified man-made visible and ultraviolet light**

√4ᵗʰ **W90 Exposure to other nonionizing radiation**
> EXCLUDES 1 exposure to sunlight (X32)
> AHA: 2019,1Q,21

√x7ᵗʰ **W90.0 Exposure to radiofrequency**

√x7ᵗʰ **W90.1 Exposure to infrared radiation**

√x7ᵗʰ **W90.2 Exposure to laser radiation**

√x7ᵗʰ **W90.8 Exposure to other nonionizing radiation**

√x7ᵗʰ **W92 Exposure to excessive heat of man-made origin**

√4ᵗʰ **W93 Exposure to excessive cold of man-made origin**

√5ᵗʰ **W93.0 Contact with or inhalation of dry ice**

√x7ᵗʰ **W93.01 Contact with dry ice**

√x7ᵗʰ **W93.02 Inhalation of dry ice**

√5ᵗʰ **W93.1 Contact with or inhalation of liquid air**

√x7ᵗʰ **W93.11 Contact with liquid air**
> Contact with liquid hydrogen
> Contact with liquid nitrogen

√x7ᵗʰ **W93.12 Inhalation of liquid air**
> Inhalation of liquid hydrogen
> Inhalation of liquid nitrogen

√x7ᵗʰ **W93.2 Prolonged exposure in deep freeze unit or refrigerator**

√x7ᵗʰ **W93.8 Exposure to other excessive cold of man-made origin**

√4ᵗʰ **W94 Exposure to high and low air pressure and changes in air pressure**

√x7ᵗʰ **W94.0 Exposure to prolonged high air pressure**

√5ᵗʰ **W94.1 Exposure to prolonged low air pressure**

√x7ᵗʰ **W94.11 Exposure to residence or prolonged visit at high altitude**

√x7ᵗʰ **W94.12 Exposure to other prolonged low air pressure**

√5ᵗʰ **W94.2 Exposure to rapid changes in air pressure during ascent**

√x7ᵗʰ **W94.21 Exposure to reduction in atmospheric pressure while surfacing from deep-water diving**

√x7ᵗʰ **W94.22 Exposure to reduction in atmospheric pressure while surfacing from underground**

√x7ᵗʰ **W94.23 Exposure to sudden change in air pressure in aircraft during ascent**

√x7ᵗʰ **W94.29 Exposure to other rapid changes in air pressure during ascent**

√5ᵗʰ **W94.3 Exposure to rapid changes in air pressure during descent**

√x7ᵗʰ **W94.31 Exposure to sudden change in air pressure in aircraft during descent**

√x7ᵗʰ **W94.32 Exposure to high air pressure from rapid descent in water**

√x7ᵗʰ **W94.39 Exposure to other rapid changes in air pressure during descent**

√x7ᵗʰ **W99 Exposure to other man-made environmental factors**

Exposure to smoke, fire and flames (X00-X08)

> EXCLUDES 1 arson (X97)
> EXCLUDES 2 explosions (W35-W40)
> lightning (T75.0-)
> transport accident (V01-V99)
> AHA: 2018,2Q,7-8

> The appropriate 7th character is to be added to each code from categories X00-X08.
> A   initial encounter
> D   subsequent encounter
> S   sequela

√4ᵗʰ **X00 Exposure to uncontrolled fire in building or structure**
> INCLUDES conflagration in building or structure
> Code first any associated cataclysm
> EXCLUDES 2 exposure to ignition or melting of nightwear (X05)
> exposure to ignition or melting of other clothing and apparel (X06.-)
> exposure to other specified smoke, fire and flames (X08.-)
> AHA: 2016,2Q,5

√x7ᵗʰ **X00.0 Exposure to flames in uncontrolled fire in building or structure**

√x7ᵗʰ **X00.1 Exposure to smoke in uncontrolled fire in building or structure**

√x7ᵗʰ **X00.2 Injury due to collapse of burning building or structure in uncontrolled fire**
> EXCLUDES 1 injury due to collapse of building not on fire (W20.1)

√x7ᵗʰ **X00.3 Fall from burning building or structure in uncontrolled fire**

√x7ᵗʰ **X00.4 Hit by object from burning building or structure in uncontrolled fire**
> AHA: 2016,2Q,4

√x7ᵗʰ **X00.5 Jump from burning building or structure in uncontrolled fire**

√x7ᵗʰ **X00.8 Other exposure to uncontrolled fire in building or structure**

√4ᵗʰ **X01 Exposure to uncontrolled fire, not in building or structure**
> INCLUDES exposure to forest fire

√x7ᵗʰ **X01.0 Exposure to flames in uncontrolled fire, not in building or structure**

√x7ᵗʰ **X01.1 Exposure to smoke in uncontrolled fire, not in building or structure**

√x7ᵗʰ **X01.3 Fall due to uncontrolled fire, not in building or structure**

√x7ᵗʰ **X01.4 Hit by object due to uncontrolled fire, not in building or structure**

√x7ᵗʰ **X01.8 Other exposure to uncontrolled fire, not in building or structure**

√4ᵗʰ **X02 Exposure to controlled fire in building or structure**
> INCLUDES exposure to fire in fireplace
> exposure to fire in stove

√x7ᵗʰ **X02.0 Exposure to flames in controlled fire in building or structure**

√x7ᵗʰ **X02.1 Exposure to smoke in controlled fire in building or structure**

√x7ᵗʰ **X02.2 Injury due to collapse of burning building or structure in controlled fire**
> EXCLUDES 1 injury due to collapse of building not on fire (W20.1)

√x7ᵗʰ **X02.3 Fall from burning building or structure in controlled fire**

√x7ᵗʰ **X02.4 Hit by object from burning building or structure in controlled fire**

√x7ᵗʰ **X02.5 Jump from burning building or structure in controlled fire**

√x7ᵗʰ **X02.8 Other exposure to controlled fire in building or structure**

√4ᵗʰ **X03 Exposure to controlled fire, not in building or structure**
> INCLUDES exposure to bon fire
> exposure to camp-fire
> exposure to trash fire

√x7ᵗʰ **X03.0 Exposure to flames in controlled fire, not in building or structure**

√x7ᵗʰ **X03.1 Exposure to smoke in controlled fire, not in building or structure**

√x7ᵗʰ **X03.3 Fall due to controlled fire, not in building or structure**

√x7ᵗʰ **X03.4 Hit by object due to controlled fire, not in building or structure**

√x7ᵗʰ **X03.8 Other exposure to controlled fire, not in building or structure**

N Newborn: 0   P Pediatric: 0-17   M Maternity: 12-55   A Adult: 15-124   CH Comorbidity High   CL Comorbidity Low   NCDx Noncancer Dx   PDx Primary Dx

1178   ICD–10–CM 2020

√x7ᵗʰ **X04 Exposure to ignition of highly flammable material**

> Exposure to ignition of gasoline
> Exposure to ignition of kerosene
> Exposure to ignition of petrol
> EXCLUDES 2   exposure to ignition or melting of nightwear (X05)
>
> exposure to ignition or melting of other clothing and apparel (X06)
>
> **AHA:** 2016,2Q,4

√x7ᵗʰ **X05 Exposure to ignition or melting of nightwear**

> EXCLUDES 2   exposure to uncontrolled fire in building or structure (X00.-)
>
> exposure to uncontrolled fire, not in building or structure (X01.-)
>
> exposure to controlled fire in building or structure (X02.-)
> exposure to controlled fire, not in building or structure (X03.-)
> exposure to ignition of highly flammable materials (X04.-)

√4ᵗʰ **X06 Exposure to ignition or melting of other clothing and apparel**

> EXCLUDES 2   exposure to uncontrolled fire in building or structure (X00.-)
>
> exposure to uncontrolled fire, not in building or structure (X01.-)
>
> exposure to controlled fire in building or structure (X02.-)
> exposure to controlled fire, not in building or structure (X03.-)
> exposure to ignition of highly flammable materials (X04.-)

√x7ᵗʰ **X06.0 Exposure to ignition of plastic jewelry**

√x7ᵗʰ **X06.1 Exposure to melting of plastic jewelry**

√x7ᵗʰ **X06.2 Exposure to ignition of other clothing and apparel**

√x7ᵗʰ **X06.3 Exposure to melting of other clothing and apparel**

√4ᵗʰ **X08 Exposure to other specified smoke, fire and flames**

√5ᵗʰ **X08.0 Exposure to bed fire**

> Exposure to mattress fire

√x7ᵗʰ **X08.00 Exposure to bed fire due to unspecified burning material**

√x7ᵗʰ **X08.01 Exposure to bed fire due to burning cigarette**

√x7ᵗʰ **X08.09 Exposure to bed fire due to other burning material**

√5ᵗʰ **X08.1 Exposure to sofa fire**

√x7ᵗʰ **X08.10 Exposure to sofa fire due to unspecified burning material**

√x7ᵗʰ **X08.11 Exposure to sofa fire due to burning cigarette**

√x7ᵗʰ **X08.19 Exposure to sofa fire due to other burning material**

√5ᵗʰ **X08.2 Exposure to other furniture fire**

√x7ᵗʰ **X08.20 Exposure to other furniture fire due to unspecified burning material**

√x7ᵗʰ **X08.21 Exposure to other furniture fire due to burning cigarette**

√x7ᵗʰ **X08.29 Exposure to other furniture fire due to other burning material**

√x7ᵗʰ **X08.8 Exposure to other specified smoke, fire and flames**

Contact with heat and hot substances (X10-X19)

> EXCLUDES 1   exposure to excessive natural heat (X30)
> exposure to fire and flames (X00-X08)
>
> **AHA:** 2018,2Q,7-8
>
> The appropriate 7th character is to be added to each code from categories X10-X19.
> A   initial encounter
> D   subsequent encounter
> S   sequela

√4ᵗʰ **X10 Contact with hot drinks, food, fats and cooking oils**

√x7ᵗʰ **X10.0 Contact with hot drinks**

√x7ᵗʰ **X10.1 Contact with hot food**

√x7ᵗʰ **X10.2 Contact with fats and cooking oils**

√4ᵗʰ **X11 Contact with hot tap-water**

> INCLUDES   contact with boiling tap-water
> contact with boiling water NOS
> EXCLUDES 1   contact with water heated on stove (X12)

√x7ᵗʰ **X11.0 Contact with hot water in bath or tub**

> EXCLUDES 1   contact with running hot water in bath or tub (X11.1)

√x7ᵗʰ **X11.1 Contact with running hot water**

> Contact with hot water running out of hose
> Contact with hot water running out of tap

√x7ᵗʰ **X11.8 Contact with other hot tap-water**

> Contact with hot water in bucket
> Contact with hot tap-water NOS

√x7ᵗʰ **X12 Contact with other hot fluids**

> Contact with water heated on stove
> EXCLUDES 1   hot (liquid) metals (X18)

√4ᵗʰ **X13 Contact with steam and other hot vapors**

√x7ᵗʰ **X13.0 Inhalation of steam and other hot vapors**

√x7ᵗʰ **X13.1 Other contact with steam and other hot vapors**

√4ᵗʰ **X14 Contact with hot air and other hot gases**

√x7ᵗʰ **X14.0 Inhalation of hot air and gases**

√x7ᵗʰ **X14.1 Other contact with hot air and other hot gases**

√4ᵗʰ **X15 Contact with hot household appliances**

> EXCLUDES 1   contact with heating appliances (X16)
> contact with powered household appliances (W29.-)
> exposure to controlled fire in building or structure due to household appliance (X02.8)
> exposure to household appliances electrical current (W86.0)

√x7ᵗʰ **X15.0 Contact with hot stove (kitchen)**

√x7ᵗʰ **X15.1 Contact with hot toaster**

√x7ᵗʰ **X15.2 Contact with hotplate**

√x7ᵗʰ **X15.3 Contact with hot saucepan or skillet**

√x7ᵗʰ **X15.8 Contact with other hot household appliances**

> Contact with cooker
> Contact with kettle
> Contact with light bulbs

√x7ᵗʰ **X16 Contact with hot heating appliances, radiators and pipes**

> EXCLUDES 1   contact with powered appliances (W29.-)
> exposure to controlled fire in building or structure due to appliance (X02.8)
> exposure to industrial appliances electrical current (W86.1)

√x7ᵗʰ **X17 Contact with hot engines, machinery and tools**

> EXCLUDES 1   contact with hot heating appliances, radiators and pipes (X16)
> contact with hot household appliances (X15)

√x7ᵗʰ **X18 Contact with other hot metals**

> Contact with liquid metal

√x7ᵗʰ **X19 Contact with other heat and hot substances**

> EXCLUDES 1   objects that are not normally hot, e.g., an object made hot by a house fire (X00-X08)

Exposure to forces of nature (X30-X39)

> **AHA:** 2018,2Q,7-8
>
> The appropriate 7th character is to be added to each code from categories X30-X39.
> A   initial encounter
> D   subsequent encounter
> S   sequela

√x7ᵗʰ **X30 Exposure to excessive natural heat**

> Exposure to excessive heat as the cause of sunstroke
> Exposure to heat NOS
> EXCLUDES 1   excessive heat of man-made origin (W92)
> exposure to man-made radiation (W89)
> exposure to sunlight (X32)
> exposure to tanning bed (W89)

√x7ᵗʰ **X31 Exposure to excessive natural cold**

> Excessive cold as the cause of chilblains NOS
> Excessive cold as the cause of immersion foot or hand
> Exposure to cold NOS
> Exposure to weather conditions
> EXCLUDES 1   cold of man-made origin (W93.-)
> contact with or inhalation of dry ice (W93.-)
> contact with or inhalation of liquefied gas (W93.-)

√x7ᵗʰ **X32 Exposure to sunlight**

> EXCLUDES 1   man-made radiation (tanning bed) (W89)
> EXCLUDES 2   radiation-related disorders of the skin and subcutaneous tissue (L55-L59)

☑ Additional Character Required   √x7ᵗʰ Placeholder Alert   Manifestation   Unspecified Dx   ▶◀ Revised Text   ● New Code   ▲ Revised Title

√x7ᵗʰ **X34 Earthquake**
> EXCLUDES 2   *tidal wave (tsunami) due to earthquake (X37.41)*

√x7ᵗʰ **X35 Volcanic eruption**
> EXCLUDES 2   *tidal wave (tsunami) due to volcanic eruption (X37.41)*

√4ᵗʰ **X36 Avalanche, landslide and other earth movements**
> INCLUDES   victim of mudslide of cataclysmic nature
> EXCLUDES 1   *earthquake (X34)*
> EXCLUDES 2   *transport accident involving collision with avalanche or landslide not in motion (V01-V99)*

√x7ᵗʰ **X36.0 Collapse of dam or man-made structure causing earth movement**

√x7ᵗʰ **X36.1 Avalanche, landslide, or mudslide**

√4ᵗʰ **X37 Cataclysmic storm**

√x7ᵗʰ **X37.0 Hurricane**
> Storm surge
> Typhoon

√x7ᵗʰ **X37.1 Tornado**
> Cyclone
> Twister

√x7ᵗʰ **X37.2 Blizzard (snow)(ice)**

√x7ᵗʰ **X37.3 Dust storm**

√5ᵗʰ **X37.4 Tidalwave**

> √x7ᵗʰ **X37.41 Tidal wave due to earthquake or volcanic eruption**
> > Tidal wave NOS
> > Tsunami

> √x7ᵗʰ **X37.42 Tidal wave due to storm**

> √x7ᵗʰ **X37.43 Tidal wave due to landslide**

√x7ᵗʰ **X37.8 Other cataclysmic storms**
> Cloudburst
> Torrential rain
> > EXCLUDES 2   *flood (X38)*

√x7ᵗʰ **X37.9 Unspecified cataclysmic storm**
> Storm NOS
> > EXCLUDES 1   *collapse of dam or man-made structure causing earth movement (X36.0)*

√x7ᵗʰ **X38 Flood**
> Flood arising from remote storm
> Flood of cataclysmic nature arising from melting snow
> Flood resulting directly from storm
> > EXCLUDES 1   *collapse of dam or man-made structure causing earth movement (X36.0)*
> > *tidal wave NOS (X37.41)*
> > *tidal wave caused by storm (X37.42)*

√4ᵗʰ **X39 Exposure to other forces of nature**

√5ᵗʰ **X39.0 Exposure to natural radiation**
> > EXCLUDES 1   *contact with and (suspected) exposure to radon and other naturally occurring radiation (Z77.123)*
> > *exposure to man-made radiation (W88-W90)*
> > *exposure to sunlight (X32)*

> √x7ᵗʰ **X39.01 Exposure to radon**

> √x7ᵗʰ **X39.08 Exposure to other natural radiation**

√x7ᵗʰ **X39.8 Other exposure to forces of nature**

Overexertion and strenuous or repetitive movements (X50)

√4ᵗʰ **X50 Overexertion and strenuous or repetitive movements**
> **AHA:** 2018,2Q,7-8; 2016,4Q,73-74
>
> The appropriate 7th character is to be added to each code from category X50.
> A   initial encounter
> D   subsequent encounter
> S   sequela

√x7ᵗʰ **X50.0 Overexertion from strenuous movement or load**
> Lifting heavy objects
> Lifting weights

√x7ᵗʰ **X50.1 Overexertion from prolonged static or awkward postures**
> Prolonged bending
> Prolonged kneeling
> Prolonged reaching
> Prolonged sitting
> Prolonged standing
> Prolonged twisting
> Static bending
> Static kneeling
> Static reaching
> Static sitting
> Static standing
> Static twisting

√x7ᵗʰ **X50.3 Overexertion from repetitive movements**
> Use of hand as hammer
> > EXCLUDES 2   *overuse from prolonged static or awkward postures (X50.1)*

√x7ᵗʰ **X50.9 Other and unspecified overexertion or strenuous movements or postures**
> Contact pressure
> Contact stress

Accidental exposure to other specified factors (X52-X58)

AHA: 2018,2Q,7-8

> The appropriate 7th character is to be added to each code from categories X52-X58.
> A   initial encounter
> D   subsequent encounter
> S   sequela

√x7ᵗʰ **X52 Prolonged stay in weightless environment**
> Weightlessness in spacecraft (simulator)

√x7ᵗʰ **X58 Exposure to other specified factors**
> Accident NOS
> Exposure NOS

Intentional self-harm (X71-X83)

Purposely self-inflicted injury
Suicide (attempted)

> The appropriate 7th character is to be added to each code from categories X71-X83.
> A   initial encounter
> D   subsequent encounter
> S   sequela

√4ᵗʰ **X71 Intentional self-harm by drowning and submersion**

√x7ᵗʰ **X71.0 Intentional self-harm by drowning and submersion while in bathtub**

√x7ᵗʰ **X71.1 Intentional self-harm by drowning and submersion while in swimming pool**

√x7ᵗʰ **X71.2 Intentional self-harm by drowning and submersion after jump into swimming pool**

√x7ᵗʰ **X71.3 Intentional self-harm by drowning and submersion in natural water**

√x7ᵗʰ **X71.8 Other intentional self-harm by drowning and submersion**

√x7ᵗʰ **X71.9 Intentional self-harm by drowning and submersion, unspecified**

√x7ᵗʰ **X72 Intentional self-harm by handgun discharge**
> Intentional self-harm by gun for single hand use
> Intentional self-harm by pistol
> Intentional self-harm by revolver
> > EXCLUDES 1   *Very pistol (X74.8)*

√4ᵗʰ **X73 Intentional self-harm by rifle, shotgun and larger firearm discharge**
> EXCLUDES 1   *airgun (X74.01)*

√x7ᵗʰ **X73.0 Intentional self-harm by shotgun discharge**

√x7ᵗʰ **X73.1 Intentional self-harm by hunting rifle discharge**

√x7ᵗʰ **X73.2 Intentional self-harm by machine gun discharge**

√x7ᵗʰ **X73.8 Intentional self-harm by other larger firearm discharge**

√x7ᵗʰ **X73.9 Intentional self-harm by unspecified larger firearm discharge**

✓4th **X74** **Intentional self-harm by other and unspecified firearm and gun discharge**

  ✓5th **X74.0** **Intentional self-harm by** gas, air or spring-operated guns

    ✓x7th **X74.01** **Intentional self-harm by** airgun

        Intentional self-harm by BB gun discharge
        Intentional self-harm by pellet gun discharge

    ✓x7th **X74.02** **Intentional self-harm by** paintball gun

    ✓x7th **X74.09** **Intentional self-harm by other gas, air or spring-operated gun**

  ✓x7th **X74.8** **Intentional self-harm by other firearm discharge**

    Intentional self-harm by Very pistol [flare] discharge

  ✓x7th **X74.9** **Intentional self-harm by unspecified firearm discharge**

✓x7th **X75** **Intentional self-harm by explosive material**

✓x7th **X76** **Intentional self-harm by smoke, fire and flames**

✓4th **X77** **Intentional self-harm by steam, hot vapors and hot objects**

  ✓x7th **X77.0** **Intentional self-harm by** steam or hot vapors

  ✓x7th **X77.1** **Intentional self-harm by** hot tap water

  ✓x7th **X77.2** **Intentional self-harm by other hot fluids**

  ✓x7th **X77.3** **Intentional self-harm by** hot household appliances

  ✓x7th **X77.8** **Intentional self-harm by other hot objects**

  ✓x7th **X77.9** **Intentional self-harm by unspecified hot objects**

✓4th **X78** **Intentional self-harm by sharp object**

  ✓x7th **X78.0** **Intentional self-harm by sharp** glass

  ✓x7th **X78.1** **Intentional self-harm by** knife

  ✓x7th **X78.2** **Intentional self-harm by** sword or dagger

  ✓x7th **X78.8** **Intentional self-harm by other sharp object**

  ✓x7th **X78.9** **Intentional self-harm by unspecified sharp object**

✓x7th **X79** **Intentional self-harm by blunt object**

✓x7th **X80** **Intentional self-harm by jumping from a high place**

  Intentional fall from one level to another

✓4th **X81** **Intentional self-harm by jumping or lying in front of moving object**

  ✓x7th **X81.0** **Intentional self-harm by jumping or lying in front of** motor vehicle

  ✓x7th **X81.1** **Intentional self-harm by jumping or lying in front of (subway)** train

  ✓x7th **X81.8** **Intentional self-harm by jumping or lying in front of other moving object**

✓4th **X82** **Intentional self-harm by crashing of motor vehicle**

  ✓x7th **X82.0** **Intentional collision of motor vehicle with other motor vehicle**

  ✓x7th **X82.1** **Intentional collision of motor vehicle with** train

  ✓x7th **X82.2** **Intentional collision of motor vehicle with** tree

  ✓x7th **X82.8** **Other intentional self-harm by crashing of motor vehicle**

✓4th **X83** **Intentional self-harm by other specified means**

  EXCLUDES 1   *intentional self-harm by poisoning or contact with toxic substance — see Table of Drugs and Chemicals*

  ✓x7th **X83.0** **Intentional self-harm by** crashing of aircraft

  ✓x7th **X83.1** **Intentional self-harm by** electrocution

  ✓x7th **X83.2** **Intentional self-harm by** exposure to extremes of cold

  ✓x7th **X83.8** **Intentional self-harm by other specified means**

Assault (X92-Y09)

INCLUDES   homicide
        injuries inflicted by another person with intent to injure or kill, by any means

EXCLUDES 1   *injuries due to legal intervention (Y35.-)*
        injuries due to operations of war (Y36.-)
        injuries due to terrorism (Y38.-)

The appropriate 7th character is to be added to each code from categories X92-Y04 and Y08.
  A   initial encounter
  D   subsequent encounter
  S   sequela

✓4th **X92** **Assault by drowning and submersion**

  ✓x7th **X92.0** **Assault by drowning and submersion while in** bathtub

  ✓x7th **X92.1** **Assault by drowning and submersion while in** swimming pool

  ✓x7th **X92.2** **Assault by drowning and submersion** after push into swimming pool

  ✓x7th **X92.3** **Assault by drowning and submersion** in natural water

  ✓x7th **X92.8** **Other assault by drowning and submersion**

  ✓x7th **X92.9** **Assault by drowning and submersion, unspecified**

✓x7th **X93** **Assault by** handgun **discharge**

  Assault by discharge of gun for single hand use
  Assault by discharge of pistol
  Assault by discharge of revolver
  EXCLUDES 1   *Very pistol (X95.8)*

✓4th **X94** **Assault by** rifle, shotgun and larger firearm **discharge**

  EXCLUDES 1   *airgun (X95.01)*

  ✓x7th **X94.0** **Assault by** shotgun

  ✓x7th **X94.1** **Assault by** hunting rifle

  ✓x7th **X94.2** **Assault by** machine gun

  ✓x7th **X94.8** **Assault by other larger firearm discharge**

  ✓x7th **X94.9** **Assault by unspecified larger firearm discharge**

✓4th **X95** **Assault by other and unspecified firearm and gun discharge**

  ✓5th **X95.0** **Assault by** gas, air or spring-operated **guns**

    ✓x7th **X95.01** **Assault by** airgun **discharge**

        Assault by BB gun discharge
        Assault by pellet gun discharge

    ✓x7th **X95.02** **Assault by** paintball gun **discharge**

    ✓x7th **X95.09** **Assault by other gas, air or spring-operated gun**

  ✓x7th **X95.8** **Assault by other firearm discharge**

    Assault by Very pistol [flare] discharge

  ✓x7th **X95.9** **Assault by unspecified firearm discharge**

✓4th **X96** **Assault by explosive material**

  EXCLUDES 1   *incendiary device (X97)*
        terrorism involving explosive material (Y38.2-)

  ✓x7th **X96.0** **Assault by** antipersonnel **bomb**

    EXCLUDES 1   *antipersonnel bomb use in military or war (Y36.2-)*

  ✓x7th **X96.1** **Assault by** gasoline **bomb**

  ✓x7th **X96.2** **Assault by** letter **bomb**

  ✓x7th **X96.3** **Assault by** fertilizer **bomb**

  ✓x7th **X96.4** **Assault by** pipe **bomb**

  ✓x7th **X96.8** **Assault by other specified explosive**

  ✓x7th **X96.9** **Assault by unspecified explosive**

✓x7th **X97** **Assault by smoke, fire and flames**

  Assault by arson
  Assault by cigarettes
  Assault by incendiary device

✓4th **X98** **Assault by steam, hot vapors and hot objects**

  ✓x7th **X98.0** **Assault by** steam or hot vapors

  ✓x7th **X98.1** **Assault by** hot tap water

  ✓x7th **X98.2** **Assault by** hot fluids

  ✓x7th **X98.3** **Assault by** hot household appliances

  ✓x7th **X98.8** **Assault by other hot** objects

  ✓x7th **X98.9** **Assault by unspecified hot objects**

✓4th **X99** **Assault by sharp object**

  EXCLUDES 1   *assault by strike by sports equipment (Y08.0-)*

  ✓x7th **X99.0** **Assault by sharp** glass

  ✓x7th **X99.1** **Assault by** knife

  ✓x7th **X99.2** **Assault by** sword or dagger

  ✓x7th **X99.8** **Assault by other sharp object**

  ✓x7th **X99.9** **Assault by unspecified sharp object**

    Assault by stabbing NOS

✓x7th **Y00** **Assault by blunt object**

  EXCLUDES 1   *assault by strike by sports equipment (Y08.0-)*

✓x7th **Y01** **Assault by pushing from high place**

✓4th **Y02** **Assault by pushing or placing victim in front of moving object**

  ✓x7th **Y02.0** **Assault by pushing or placing victim in front of** motor vehicle

  ✓x7th **Y02.1** **Assault by pushing or placing victim in front of (subway)** train

  ✓x7th **Y02.8** **Assault by pushing or placing victim in front of other** moving object

---

Chapter 20. External Causes of Morbidity

✓4ᵗʰ **Y03** **Assault by crashing of motor vehicle**

     ✓x7ᵗʰ **Y03.0** **Assault by being hit or run over by motor vehicle**

     ✓x7ᵗʰ **Y03.8** **Other assault by crashing of motor vehicle**

✓4ᵗʰ **Y04** **Assault by bodily force**

     EXCLUDES 1   assault by:
                 submersion (X92.-)
                 use of weapon (X93-X95, X99, Y00)

     ✓x7ᵗʰ **Y04.0** **Assault by unarmed brawl or fight**

     ✓x7ᵗʰ **Y04.1** **Assault by human bite**

     ✓x7ᵗʰ **Y04.2** **Assault by strike against or bumped into by another person**

     ✓x7ᵗʰ **Y04.8** **Assault by other bodily force**

          Assault by bodily force NOS

✓4ᵗʰ **Y07** **Perpetrator of assault, maltreatment and neglect**

     NOTE   Codes from this category are for use only in cases of confirmed abuse (T74.-)

           Selection of the correct perpetrator code is based on the relationship between the perpetrator and the victim

     INCLUDES   perpetrator of abandonment
                perpetrator of emotional neglect
                perpetrator of mental cruelty
                perpetrator of physical abuse
                perpetrator of physical neglect
                perpetrator of sexual abuse
                perpetrator of torture

     ✓5ᵗʰ **Y07.0** **Spouse or partner, perpetrator of maltreatment and neglect**

          Spouse or partner, perpetrator of maltreatment and neglect against spouse or partner

        Y07.01 **Husband, perpetrator of maltreatment and neglect**

        Y07.02 **Wife, perpetrator of maltreatment and neglect**

        Y07.03 **Male partner, perpetrator of maltreatment and neglect**

        Y07.04 **Female partner, perpetrator of maltreatment and neglect**

     ✓5ᵗʰ **Y07.1** **Parent (adoptive) (biological), perpetrator of maltreatment and neglect**

        Y07.11 **Biological father, perpetrator of maltreatment and neglect**

        Y07.12 **Biological mother, perpetrator of maltreatment and neglect**

        Y07.13 **Adoptive father, perpetrator of maltreatment and neglect**

        Y07.14 **Adoptive mother, perpetrator of maltreatment and neglect**

     ✓5ᵗʰ **Y07.4** **Other family member, perpetrator of maltreatment and neglect**

       ✓6ᵗʰ **Y07.41** **Sibling, perpetrator of maltreatment and neglect**

          EXCLUDES 1   stepsibling, perpetrator of maltreatment and neglect (Y07.435, Y07.436)

          Y07.410 **Brother, perpetrator of maltreatment and neglect**

          Y07.411 **Sister, perpetrator of maltreatment and neglect**

       ✓6ᵗʰ **Y07.42** **Foster parent, perpetrator of maltreatment and neglect**

          Y07.420 **Foster father, perpetrator of maltreatment and neglect**

          Y07.421 **Foster mother, perpetrator of maltreatment and neglect**

       ✓6ᵗʰ **Y07.43** **Stepparent or stepsibling, perpetrator of maltreatment and neglect**

          Y07.430 **Stepfather, perpetrator of maltreatment and neglect**

          Y07.432 **Male friend of parent (co-residing in household), perpetrator of maltreatment and neglect**

          Y07.433 **Stepmother, perpetrator of maltreatment and neglect**

          Y07.434 **Female friend of parent (co-residing in household), perpetrator of maltreatment and neglect**

          Y07.435 **Stepbrother, perpetrator or maltreatment and neglect**

          Y07.436 **Stepsister, perpetrator of maltreatment and neglect**

       ✓6ᵗʰ **Y07.49** **Other family member, perpetrator of maltreatment and neglect**

          Y07.490 **Male cousin, perpetrator of maltreatment and neglect**

          Y07.491 **Female cousin, perpetrator of maltreatment and neglect**

          Y07.499 **Other family member, perpetrator of maltreatment and neglect**

     ✓5ᵗʰ **Y07.5** **Non-family member, perpetrator of maltreatment and neglect**

        Y07.50 **Unspecified non-family member, perpetrator of maltreatment and neglect**

       ✓6ᵗʰ **Y07.51** **Daycare provider, perpetrator of maltreatment and neglect**

          Y07.510 **At-home childcare provider, perpetrator of maltreatment and neglect**

          Y07.511 **Daycare center childcare provider, perpetrator of maltreatment and neglect**

          Y07.512 **At-home adultcare provider, perpetrator of maltreatment and neglect**

          Y07.513 **Adultcare center provider, perpetrator of maltreatment and neglect**

          Y07.519 **Unspecified daycare provider, perpetrator of maltreatment and neglect**

       ✓6ᵗʰ **Y07.52** **Healthcare provider, perpetrator of maltreatment and neglect**

          Y07.521 **Mental health provider, perpetrator of maltreatment and neglect**

          Y07.528 **Other therapist or healthcare provider, perpetrator of maltreatment and neglect**

            Nurse perpetrator of maltreatment and neglect

            Occupational therapist perpetrator of maltreatment and neglect

            Physical therapist perpetrator of maltreatment and neglect

            Speech therapist perpetrator of maltreatment and neglect

          Y07.529 **Unspecified healthcare provider, perpetrator of maltreatment and neglect**

        Y07.53 **Teacher or instructor, perpetrator of maltreatment and neglect**

          Coach, perpetrator of maltreatment and neglect

        Y07.59 **Other non-family member, perpetrator of maltreatment and neglect**

     Y07.6 **Multiple perpetrators of maltreatment and neglect**
        AHA: 2018,4Q,32

     Y07.9 **Unspecified perpetrator of maltreatment and neglect**

✓4ᵗʰ **Y08** **Assault by other specified means**

     ✓5ᵗʰ **Y08.0** **Assault by strike by sport equipment**

       ✓x7ᵗʰ **Y08.01** **Assault by strike by hockey stick**

       ✓x7ᵗʰ **Y08.02** **Assault by strike by baseball bat**

       ✓x7ᵗʰ **Y08.09** **Assault by strike by other specified type of sport equipment**

     ✓5ᵗʰ **Y08.8** **Assault by other specified means**

       ✓x7ᵗʰ **Y08.81** **Assault by crashing of aircraft**

       ✓x7ᵗʰ **Y08.89** **Assault by other specified means**

     Y09 **Assault by unspecified means**

        Assassination (attempted) NOS
        Homicide (attempted) NOS
        Manslaughter (attempted) NOS
        Murder (attempted) NOS

Event of undetermined intent (Y21-Y33)

Undetermined intent is only for use when there is specific documentation in the record that the intent of the injury cannot be determined. If no such documentation is present, code to accidental (unintentional).

The appropriate 7th character is to be added to each code from categories Y21-Y33.
A   initial encounter
D   subsequent encounter
S   sequela

✓4ᵗʰ **Y21** **Drowning and submersion, undetermined intent**

     ✓x7ᵗʰ **Y21.0** **Drowning and submersion while in bathtub, undetermined intent**

     ✓x7ᵗʰ **Y21.1** **Drowning and submersion after fall into bathtub, undetermined intent**

N Newborn: 0   P Pediatric: 0-17   M Maternity: 12-55   A Adult: 15-124   CH Comorbidity High   CL Comorbidity Low   NC Dx Noncancer Dx   PDx Primary Dx

1182   ICD-10-CM 2020

✓x7ᵗʰ **Y21.2** **Drowning and submersion** while in swimming pool, undetermined intent

✓x7ᵗʰ **Y21.3** **Drowning and submersion** after fall into swimming pool, undetermined intent

✓x7ᵗʰ **Y21.4** **Drowning and submersion** in natural water, undetermined intent

✓x7ᵗʰ **Y21.8** **Other drowning and submersion, undetermined intent**

✓x7ᵗʰ **Y21.9** **Unspecified drowning and submersion, undetermined intent**

✓x7ᵗʰ **Y22** Handgun **discharge, undetermined intent**

> Discharge of gun for single hand use, undetermined intent
> Discharge of pistol, undetermined intent
> Discharge of revolver, undetermined intent
> EXCLUDES 2   Very pistol (Y24.8)

✓4ᵗʰ **Y23** **Rifle, shotgun and larger firearm** discharge, undetermined intent

> EXCLUDES 2   airgun (Y24.0)

✓x7ᵗʰ **Y23.0** Shotgun **discharge, undetermined intent**

✓x7ᵗʰ **Y23.1** Hunting rifle **discharge, undetermined intent**

✓x7ᵗʰ **Y23.2** Military firearm **discharge, undetermined intent**

✓x7ᵗʰ **Y23.3** Machine gun **discharge, undetermined intent**

✓x7ᵗʰ **Y23.8** **Other larger firearm discharge, undetermined intent**

✓x7ᵗʰ **Y23.9** **Unspecified larger firearm discharge, undetermined intent**

✓4ᵗʰ **Y24** **Other and unspecified firearm discharge, undetermined intent**

✓x7ᵗʰ **Y24.0** Airgun **discharge, undetermined intent**

> BB gun discharge, undetermined intent
> Pellet gun discharge, undetermined intent

✓x7ᵗʰ **Y24.8** **Other firearm discharge, undetermined intent**

> Paintball gun discharge, undetermined intent
> Very pistol [flare] discharge, undetermined intent

✓x7ᵗʰ **Y24.9** **Unspecified firearm discharge, undetermined intent**

✓x7ᵗʰ **Y25** **Contact with explosive material, undetermined intent**

✓x7ᵗʰ **Y26** **Exposure to smoke, fire and flames, undetermined intent**

✓4ᵗʰ **Y27** **Contact with steam, hot vapors and hot objects, undetermined intent**

✓x7ᵗʰ **Y27.0** **Contact with** steam **and hot** vapors, **undetermined intent**

✓x7ᵗʰ **Y27.1** **Contact with hot** tap water, **undetermined intent**

✓x7ᵗʰ **Y27.2** **Contact with hot** fluids, **undetermined intent**

✓x7ᵗʰ **Y27.3** **Contact with hot** household appliance, **undetermined intent**

✓x7ᵗʰ **Y27.8** **Contact with other hot** objects, **undetermined intent**

✓x7ᵗʰ **Y27.9** **Contact with unspecified hot objects, undetermined intent**

✓4ᵗʰ **Y28** **Contact with sharp object, undetermined intent**

✓x7ᵗʰ **Y28.0** **Contact with sharp** glass, **undetermined intent**

✓x7ᵗʰ **Y28.1** **Contact with** knife, **undetermined intent**

✓x7ᵗʰ **Y28.2** **Contact with** sword or dagger, **undetermined intent**

✓x7ᵗʰ **Y28.8** **Contact with other sharp object, undetermined intent**

✓x7ᵗʰ **Y28.9** **Contact with unspecified sharp object, undetermined intent**

✓x7ᵗʰ **Y29** **Contact with blunt object, undetermined intent**

✓x7ᵗʰ **Y30** **Falling, jumping or pushed from a high place, undetermined intent**

> Victim falling from one level to another, undetermined intent

✓x7ᵗʰ **Y31** **Falling, lying or running before or into moving object, undetermined intent**

✓x7ᵗʰ **Y32** **Crashing of motor vehicle, undetermined intent**

✓x7ᵗʰ **Y33** **Other specified events, undetermined intent**

Legal intervention, operations of war, military operations, and terrorism (Y35-Y38)

> The appropriate 7th character is to be added to each code from categories Y35-Y38.
> A   initial encounter
> D   subsequent encounter
> S   sequela

✓4ᵗʰ **Y35** **Legal intervention**

> INCLUDES   any injury sustained as a result of an encounter with any law enforcement official, serving in any capacity at the time of the encounter, whether on-duty or off-duty. Includes injury to law enforcement official, suspect and bystander

✓5ᵗʰ **Y35.0** **Legal intervention involving** firearm discharge

✓6ᵗʰ **Y35.00** **Legal intervention involving unspecified firearm discharge**

> Legal intervention involving gunshot wound
> Legal intervention involving shot NOS

✓7ᵗʰ **Y35.001** **Legal intervention involving unspecified firearm discharge,** law enforcement official **injured**

✓7ᵗʰ **Y35.002** **Legal intervention involving unspecified firearm discharge,** bystander **injured**

✓7ᵗʰ **Y35.003** **Legal intervention involving unspecified firearm discharge,** suspect **injured**

✓7ᵗʰ **Y35.009** **Legal intervention involving unspecified firearm discharge, unspecified person injured**

✓6ᵗʰ **Y35.01** **Legal intervention involving injury by** machine gun

✓7ᵗʰ **Y35.011** **Legal intervention involving injury by machine gun,** law enforcement official **injured**

✓7ᵗʰ **Y35.012** **Legal intervention involving injury by machine gun,** bystander **injured**

✓7ᵗʰ **Y35.013** **Legal intervention involving injury by machine gun,** suspect **injured**

✓7ᵗʰ **Y35.019** **Legal intervention involving injury by machine gun, unspecified person injured**

✓6ᵗʰ **Y35.02** **Legal intervention involving injury by** handgun

✓7ᵗʰ **Y35.021** **Legal intervention involving injury by handgun,** law enforcement official **injured**

✓7ᵗʰ **Y35.022** **Legal intervention involving injury by handgun,** bystander **injured**

✓7ᵗʰ **Y35.023** **Legal intervention involving injury by handgun,** suspect **injured**

✓7ᵗʰ **Y35.029** **Legal intervention involving injury by handgun, unspecified person injured**

✓6ᵗʰ **Y35.03** **Legal intervention involving injury by** rifle pellet

✓7ᵗʰ **Y35.031** **Legal intervention involving injury by rifle pellet,** law enforcement official **injured**

✓7ᵗʰ **Y35.032** **Legal intervention involving injury by rifle pellet,** bystander **injured**

✓7ᵗʰ **Y35.033** **Legal intervention involving injury by rifle pellet,** suspect **injured**

✓7ᵗʰ **Y35.039** **Legal intervention involving injury by rifle pellet, unspecified person injured**

✓6ᵗʰ **Y35.04** **Legal intervention involving injury by** rubber bullet

✓7ᵗʰ **Y35.041** **Legal intervention involving injury by rubber bullet,** law enforcement official **injured**

✓7ᵗʰ **Y35.042** **Legal intervention involving injury by rubber bullet,** bystander **injured**

✓7ᵗʰ **Y35.043** **Legal intervention involving injury by rubber bullet,** suspect **injured**

✓7ᵗʰ **Y35.049** **Legal intervention involving injury by rubber bullet, unspecified person injured**

✓6ᵗʰ **Y35.09** **Legal intervention involving other firearm discharge**

✓7ᵗʰ **Y35.091** **Legal intervention involving other firearm discharge,** law enforcement official **injured**

✓7ᵗʰ **Y35.092** **Legal intervention involving other firearm discharge,** bystander **injured**

✓7ᵗʰ **Y35.093** **Legal intervention involving other firearm discharge,** suspect **injured**

✓7ᵗʰ **Y35.099** **Legal intervention involving other firearm discharge, unspecified person injured**

√5ᵗʰ **Y35.1** **Legal intervention involving** explosives

√6ᵗʰ **Y35.10** **Legal intervention involving unspecified explosives**

√7ᵗʰ **Y35.101** **Legal intervention involving unspecified explosives,** law enforcement official **injured**

√7ᵗʰ **Y35.102** **Legal intervention involving unspecified explosives,** bystander **injured**

√7ᵗʰ **Y35.103** **Legal intervention involving unspecified explosives,** suspect **injured**

√7ᵗʰ **Y35.109** **Legal intervention involving unspecified explosives, unspecified person injured**

√6ᵗʰ **Y35.11** **Legal intervention involving injury by** dynamite

√7ᵗʰ **Y35.111** **Legal intervention involving injury by dynamite,** law enforcement official **injured**

√7ᵗʰ **Y35.112** **Legal intervention involving injury by dynamite,** bystander **injured**

√7ᵗʰ **Y35.113** **Legal intervention involving injury by dynamite,** suspect **injured**

√7ᵗʰ **Y35.119** **Legal intervention involving injury by dynamite, unspecified person injured**

√6ᵗʰ **Y35.12** **Legal intervention involving injury by** explosive shell

√7ᵗʰ **Y35.121** **Legal intervention involving injury by explosive shell,** law enforcement official **injured**

√7ᵗʰ **Y35.122** **Legal intervention involving injury by explosive shell,** bystander **injured**

√7ᵗʰ **Y35.123** **Legal intervention involving injury by explosive shell,** suspect **injured**

√7ᵗʰ **Y35.129** **Legal intervention involving injury by explosive shell, unspecified person injured**

√6ᵗʰ **Y35.19** **Legal intervention involving other explosives**

Legal intervention involving injury by grenade
Legal intervention involving injury by mortar bomb

√7ᵗʰ **Y35.191** **Legal intervention involving other explosives,** law enforcement official **injured**

√7ᵗʰ **Y35.192** **Legal intervention involving other explosives,** bystander **injured**

√7ᵗʰ **Y35.193** **Legal intervention involving other explosives,** suspect **injured**

√7ᵗʰ **Y35.199** **Legal intervention involving other explosives, unspecified person injured**

√5ᵗʰ **Y35.2** **Legal intervention involving** gas

Legal intervention involving asphyxiation by gas
Legal intervention involving poisoning by gas

√6ᵗʰ **Y35.20** **Legal intervention involving unspecified gas**

√7ᵗʰ **Y35.201** **Legal intervention involving unspecified gas,** law enforcement official **injured**

√7ᵗʰ **Y35.202** **Legal intervention involving unspecified gas,** bystander **injured**

√7ᵗʰ **Y35.203** **Legal intervention involving unspecified gas,** suspect **injured**

√7ᵗʰ **Y35.209** **Legal intervention involving unspecified gas, unspecified person injured**

√6ᵗʰ **Y35.21** **Legal intervention involving injury by** tear gas

√7ᵗʰ **Y35.211** **Legal intervention involving injury by tear gas,** law enforcement official **injured**

√7ᵗʰ **Y35.212** **Legal intervention involving injury by tear gas,** bystander **injured**

√7ᵗʰ **Y35.213** **Legal intervention involving injury by tear gas,** suspect **injured**

√7ᵗʰ **Y35.219** **Legal intervention involving injury by tear gas, unspecified person injured**

√6ᵗʰ **Y35.29** **Legal intervention involving other gas**

√7ᵗʰ **Y35.291** **Legal intervention involving other gas,** law enforcement official **injured**

√7ᵗʰ **Y35.292** **Legal intervention involving other gas,** bystander **injured**

√7ᵗʰ **Y35.293** **Legal intervention involving other gas,** suspect **injured**

√7ᵗʰ **Y35.299** **Legal intervention involving other gas, unspecified person injured**

√5ᵗʰ **Y35.3** **Legal intervention involving** blunt objects

Legal intervention involving being hit or struck by blunt object

√6ᵗʰ **Y35.30** **Legal intervention involving unspecified blunt objects**

√7ᵗʰ **Y35.301** **Legal intervention involving unspecified blunt objects,** law enforcement official **injured**

√7ᵗʰ **Y35.302** **Legal intervention involving unspecified blunt objects,** bystander **injured**

√7ᵗʰ **Y35.303** **Legal intervention involving unspecified blunt objects,** suspect **injured**

√7ᵗʰ **Y35.309** **Legal intervention involving unspecified blunt objects, unspecified person injured**

√6ᵗʰ **Y35.31** **Legal intervention involving** baton

√7ᵗʰ **Y35.311** **Legal intervention involving baton,** law enforcement official **injured**

√7ᵗʰ **Y35.312** **Legal intervention involving baton,** bystander **injured**

√7ᵗʰ **Y35.313** **Legal intervention involving baton,** suspect **injured**

√7ᵗʰ **Y35.319** **Legal intervention involving baton, unspecified person injured**

√6ᵗʰ **Y35.39** **Legal intervention involving other blunt objects**

√7ᵗʰ **Y35.391** **Legal intervention involving other blunt objects,** law enforcement official **injured**

√7ᵗʰ **Y35.392** **Legal intervention involving other blunt objects,** bystander **injured**

√7ᵗʰ **Y35.393** **Legal intervention involving other blunt objects,** suspect **injured**

√7ᵗʰ **Y35.399** **Legal intervention involving other blunt objects, unspecified person injured**

√5ᵗʰ **Y35.4** **Legal intervention involving** sharp objects

Legal intervention involving being cut by sharp objects
Legal intervention involving being stabbed by sharp objects

√6ᵗʰ **Y35.40** **Legal intervention involving unspecified sharp objects**

√7ᵗʰ **Y35.401** **Legal intervention involving unspecified sharp objects,** law enforcement official **injured**

√7ᵗʰ **Y35.402** **Legal intervention involving unspecified sharp objects,** bystander **injured**

√7ᵗʰ **Y35.403** **Legal intervention involving unspecified sharp objects,** suspect **injured**

√7ᵗʰ **Y35.409** **Legal intervention involving unspecified sharp objects, unspecified person injured**

√6ᵗʰ **Y35.41** **Legal intervention involving** bayonet

√7ᵗʰ **Y35.411** **Legal intervention involving bayonet,** law enforcement official **injured**

√7ᵗʰ **Y35.412** **Legal intervention involving bayonet,** bystander **injured**

√7ᵗʰ **Y35.413** **Legal intervention involving bayonet,** suspect **injured**

√7ᵗʰ **Y35.419** **Legal intervention involving bayonet, unspecified person injured**

√6ᵗʰ **Y35.49** **Legal intervention involving other sharp objects**

√7ᵗʰ **Y35.491** **Legal intervention involving other sharp objects,** law enforcement official **injured**

√7ᵗʰ **Y35.492** **Legal intervention involving other sharp objects,** bystander **injured**

√7ᵗʰ **Y35.493** **Legal intervention involving other sharp objects,** suspect **injured**

√7ᵗʰ **Y35.499** **Legal intervention involving other sharp objects, unspecified person injured**

√5ᵗʰ **Y35.8** **Legal intervention involving other specified means**

√6ᵗʰ **Y35.81** **Legal intervention involving** manhandling

√7ᵗʰ **Y35.811** **Legal intervention involving manhandling,** law enforcement official **injured**

√7ᵗʰ **Y35.812** **Legal intervention involving manhandling,** bystander **injured**

√7ᵗʰ **Y35.813** **Legal intervention involving manhandling,** suspect **injured**

√7ᵗʰ **Y35.819** **Legal intervention involving manhandling, unspecified person injured**

√6ᵗʰ **Y35.83** **Legal intervention involving a** conducted energy device

Electroshock device (taser)
Stun gun

√7ᵗʰ **Y35.831** **Legal intervention involving a conducted energy device,** law enforcement official **injured**

☑7ᵗʰ **Y35.832** **Legal intervention involving a conducted energy device,** bystander **injured**

☑7ᵗʰ **Y35.833** **Legal intervention involving a conducted energy device,** suspect **injured**

☑7ᵗʰ **Y35.839** **Legal intervention involving a conducted energy device, unspecified person injured**

√6ᵗʰ **Y35.89** **Legal intervention involving other specified means**

☑7ᵗʰ **Y35.891** **Legal intervention involving other specified means,** law enforcement official **injured**

☑7ᵗʰ **Y35.892** **Legal intervention involving other specified means,** bystander **injured**

☑7ᵗʰ **Y35.893** **Legal intervention involving other specified means,** suspect **injured**

AHA: 2018,1Q,5

√5ᵗʰ **Y35.9** **Legal intervention, means unspecified**

√x7ᵗʰ **Y35.91** **Legal intervention, means unspecified,** law enforcement official **injured**

√x7ᵗʰ **Y35.92** **Legal intervention, means unspecified,** bystander **injured**

√x7ᵗʰ **Y35.93** **Legal intervention, means unspecified,** suspect **injured**

√x7ᵗʰ **Y35.99** **Legal intervention, means unspecified, unspecified person injured**

☑4ᵗʰ **Y36** **Operations of war**

INCLUDES   injuries to military personnel and civilians caused by war, civil insurrection, and peacekeeping missions

EXCLUDES 1   injury to military personnel occurring during peacetime military operations (Y37.-)

military vehicles involved in transport accidents with non-military vehicle during peacetime (V09.01, V09.21, V19.81, V29.81, V39.81, V49.81, V59.81, V69.81, V79.81)

AHA: 2014,3Q,4

√5ᵗʰ **Y36.0** **War operations involving** explosion of marine weapons

√6ᵗʰ **Y36.00** **War operations involving explosion of unspecified marine weapon**

War operations involving underwater blast NOS

☑7ᵗʰ **Y36.000** **War operations involving explosion of unspecified marine weapon,** military personnel

☑7ᵗʰ **Y36.001** **War operations involving explosion of unspecified marine weapon,** civilian

√6ᵗʰ **Y36.01** **War operations involving explosion of** depth-charge

☑7ᵗʰ **Y36.010** **War operations involving explosion of depth-charge,** military personnel

☑7ᵗʰ **Y36.011** **War operations involving explosion of depth-charge,** civilian

√6ᵗʰ **Y36.02** **War operations involving explosion of** marine mine

War operations involving explosion of marine mine, at sea or in harbor

☑7ᵗʰ **Y36.020** **War operations involving explosion of marine mine,** military personnel

☑7ᵗʰ **Y36.021** **War operations involving explosion of marine mine,** civilian

√6ᵗʰ **Y36.03** **War operations involving explosion of** sea-based artillery shell

☑7ᵗʰ **Y36.030** **War operations involving explosion of sea-based artillery shell,** military personnel

☑7ᵗʰ **Y36.031** **War operations involving explosion of sea-based artillery shell,** civilian

√6ᵗʰ **Y36.04** **War operations involving explosion of** torpedo

☑7ᵗʰ **Y36.040** **War operations involving explosion of torpedo,** military personnel

☑7ᵗʰ **Y36.041** **War operations involving explosion of torpedo,** civilian

√6ᵗʰ **Y36.05** **War operations involving** accidental detonation of onboard marine weapons

☑7ᵗʰ **Y36.050** **War operations involving accidental detonation of onboard marine weapons,** military personnel

☑7ᵗʰ **Y36.051** **War operations involving accidental detonation of onboard marine weapons,** civilian

√6ᵗʰ **Y36.09** **War operations involving explosion of other marine weapons**

☑7ᵗʰ **Y36.090** **War operations involving explosion of other marine weapons,** military personnel

☑7ᵗʰ **Y36.091** **War operations involving explosion of other marine weapons,** civilian

√5ᵗʰ **Y36.1** **War operations involving** destruction of aircraft

√6ᵗʰ **Y36.10** **War operations involving unspecified destruction of aircraft**

☑7ᵗʰ **Y36.100** **War operations involving unspecified destruction of aircraft,** military personnel

☑7ᵗʰ **Y36.101** **War operations involving unspecified destruction of aircraft,** civilian

√6ᵗʰ **Y36.11** **War operations involving destruction of aircraft due to** enemy fire or explosives

War operations involving destruction of aircraft due to air to air missile

War operations involving destruction of aircraft due to explosive placed on aircraft

War operations involving destruction of aircraft due to rocket propelled grenade [RPG]

War operations involving destruction of aircraft due to small arms fire

War operations involving destruction of aircraft due to surface to air missile

☑7ᵗʰ **Y36.110** **War operations involving destruction of aircraft due to enemy fire or explosives,** military personnel

☑7ᵗʰ **Y36.111** **War operations involving destruction of aircraft due to enemy fire or explosives,** civilian

√6ᵗʰ **Y36.12** **War operations involving destruction of aircraft due to** collision with other aircraft

☑7ᵗʰ **Y36.120** **War operations involving destruction of aircraft due to collision with other aircraft,** military personnel

☑7ᵗʰ **Y36.121** **War operations involving destruction of aircraft due to collision with other aircraft,** civilian

√6ᵗʰ **Y36.13** **War operations involving destruction of aircraft due to** onboard fire

☑7ᵗʰ **Y36.130** **War operations involving destruction of aircraft due to onboard fire,** military personnel

☑7ᵗʰ **Y36.131** **War operations involving destruction of aircraft due to onboard fire,** civilian

√6ᵗʰ **Y36.14** **War operations involving destruction of aircraft due to** accidental detonation of onboard munitions and explosives

☑7ᵗʰ **Y36.140** **War operations involving destruction of aircraft due to accidental detonation of onboard munitions and explosives,** military personnel

☑7ᵗʰ **Y36.141** **War operations involving destruction of aircraft due to accidental detonation of onboard munitions and explosives,** civilian

√6ᵗʰ **Y36.19** **War operations involving other destruction of aircraft**

☑7ᵗʰ **Y36.190** **War operations involving other destruction of aircraft,** military personnel

☑7ᵗʰ **Y36.191** **War operations involving other destruction of aircraft,** civilian

√5ᵗʰ **Y36.2** **War operations involving other explosions and fragments**

EXCLUDES 1   war operations involving explosion of aircraft (Y36.1-)

war operations involving explosion of marine weapons (Y36.0-)

war operations involving explosion of nuclear weapons (Y36.5-)

war operations involving explosion occurring after cessation of hostilities (Y36.8-)

√6ᵗʰ **Y36.20** **War operations involving unspecified explosion and fragments**

War operations involving air blast NOS

War operations involving blast NOS

War operations involving blast fragments NOS

War operations involving blast wave NOS

War operations involving blast wind NOS

War operations involving explosion NOS

War operations involving explosion of bomb NOS

☑7ᵗʰ **Y36.200** **War operations involving unspecified explosion and fragments,** military personnel

☑7ᵗʰ **Y36.201** **War operations involving unspecified explosion and fragments,** civilian

☑ Additional Character Required   √x7ᵗʰ Placeholder Alert   Manifestation   Unspecified Dx   ▶◀ Revised Text   ● New Code   ▲ Revised Title

ICD-10-CM 2020   1185

Chapter 20. External Causes of Morbidity

Y36.21–Y36.441

√6ᵗʰ **Y36.21 War operations involving explosion of** aerial bomb

√7ᵗʰ **Y36.210 War operations involving explosion of aerial bomb,** military personnel

√7ᵗʰ **Y36.211 War operations involving explosion of aerial bomb,** civilian

√6ᵗʰ **Y36.22 War operations involving explosion of** guided missile

√7ᵗʰ **Y36.220 War operations involving explosion of guided missile,** military personnel

√7ᵗʰ **Y36.221 War operations involving explosion of guided missile,** civilian

√6ᵗʰ **Y36.23 War operations involving explosion of** improvised explosive device [IED]

War operations involving explosion of person-borne improvised explosive device [IED]

War operations involving explosion of vehicle-borne improvised explosive device [IED]

War operations involving explosion of roadside improvised explosive device [IED]

√7ᵗʰ **Y36.230 War operations involving explosion of improvised explosive device [IED],** military personnel

√7ᵗʰ **Y36.231 War operations involving explosion of improvised explosive device [IED],** civilian

√6ᵗʰ **Y36.24 War operations involving explosion due to** accidental detonation and discharge of own munitions or munitions launch device

√7ᵗʰ **Y36.240 War operations involving explosion due to accidental detonation and discharge of own munitions or munitions launch device,** military personnel

√7ᵗʰ **Y36.241 War operations involving explosion due to accidental detonation and discharge of own munitions or munitions launch device,** civilian

√6ᵗʰ **Y36.25 War operations involving** fragments from munitions

√7ᵗʰ **Y36.250 War operations involving fragments from munitions,** military personnel

√7ᵗʰ **Y36.251 War operations involving fragments from munitions,** civilian

√6ᵗʰ **Y36.26 War operations involving fragments of** improvised explosive device [IED]

War operations involving fragments of person-borne improvised explosive device [IED]

War operations involving fragments of vehicle-borne improvised explosive device [IED]

War operations involving fragments of roadside improvised explosive device [IED]

√7ᵗʰ **Y36.260 War operations involving fragments of improvised explosive device [IED],** military personnel

√7ᵗʰ **Y36.261 War operations involving fragments of improvised explosive device [IED],** civilian

√6ᵗʰ **Y36.27 War operations involving** fragments from weapons

√7ᵗʰ **Y36.270 War operations involving fragments from weapons,** military personnel

√7ᵗʰ **Y36.271 War operations involving fragments from weapons,** civilian

√6ᵗʰ **Y36.29 War operations involving other explosions and fragments**

War operations involving explosion of grenade

War operations involving explosions of land mine

War operations involving shrapnel NOS

√7ᵗʰ **Y36.290 War operations involving other explosions and fragments,** military personnel

√7ᵗʰ **Y36.291 War operations involving other explosions and fragments,** civilian

√5ᵗʰ **Y36.3 War operations involving** fires, conflagrations and hot substances

War operations involving smoke, fumes, and heat from fires, conflagrations and hot substances

EXCLUDES 1 *war operations involving fires and conflagrations aboard military aircraft (Y36.1-)*

war operations involving fires and conflagrations aboard military watercraft (Y36.0-)

war operations involving fires and conflagrations caused indirectly by conventional weapons (Y36.2-)

war operations involving fires and thermal effects of nuclear weapons (Y36.53-)

√6ᵗʰ **Y36.30 War operations involving unspecified fire, conflagration and hot substance**

√7ᵗʰ **Y36.300 War operations involving unspecified fire, conflagration and hot substance,** military personnel

√7ᵗʰ **Y36.301 War operations involving unspecified fire, conflagration and hot substance,** civilian

√6ᵗʰ **Y36.31 War operations involving** gasoline bomb

War operations involving incendiary bomb

War operations involving petrol bomb

√7ᵗʰ **Y36.310 War operations involving gasoline bomb,** military personnel

√7ᵗʰ **Y36.311 War operations involving gasoline bomb,** civilian

√6ᵗʰ **Y36.32 War operations involving** incendiary bullet

√7ᵗʰ **Y36.320 War operations involving incendiary bullet,** military personnel

√7ᵗʰ **Y36.321 War operations involving incendiary bullet,** civilian

√6ᵗʰ **Y36.33 War operations involving** flamethrower

√7ᵗʰ **Y36.330 War operations involving flamethrower,** military personnel

√7ᵗʰ **Y36.331 War operations involving flamethrower,** civilian

√6ᵗʰ **Y36.39 War operations involving other fires, conflagrations and hot substances**

√7ᵗʰ **Y36.390 War operations involving other fires, conflagrations and hot substances,** military personnel

√7ᵗʰ **Y36.391 War operations involving other fires, conflagrations and hot substances,** civilian

√5ᵗʰ **Y36.4 War operations involving firearm discharge and other forms of conventional warfare**

√6ᵗʰ **Y36.41 War operations involving** rubber bullets

√7ᵗʰ **Y36.410 War operations involving rubber bullets,** military personnel

√7ᵗʰ **Y36.411 War operations involving rubber bullets,** civilian

√6ᵗʰ **Y36.42 War operations involving** firearms pellets

√7ᵗʰ **Y36.420 War operations involving firearms pellets,** military personnel

√7ᵗʰ **Y36.421 War operations involving firearms pellets,** civilian

√6ᵗʰ **Y36.43 War operations involving other firearms discharge**

War operations involving bullets NOS

EXCLUDES 1 *war operations involving munitions fragments (Y36.25-)*

war operations involving incendiary bullets (Y36.32-)

√7ᵗʰ **Y36.430 War operations involving other firearms discharge,** military personnel

√7ᵗʰ **Y36.431 War operations involving other firearms discharge,** civilian

√6ᵗʰ **Y36.44 War operations involving** unarmed hand to hand combat

EXCLUDES 1 *war operations involving combat using blunt or piercing object (Y36.45-)*

war operations involving intentional restriction of air and airway (Y36.46-)

war operations involving unintentional restriction of air and airway (Y36.47-)

√7ᵗʰ **Y36.440 War operations involving unarmed hand to hand combat,** military personnel

√7ᵗʰ **Y36.441 War operations involving unarmed hand to hand combat,** civilian

Ⓝ Newborn: 0   Ⓟ Pediatric: 0-17   Ⓜ Maternity: 12-55   Ⓐ Adult: 15-124   CH Comorbidity High   CL Comorbidity Low   NC Dx Noncancer Dx   PDx Primary Dx

1186   ICD-10-CM 2020

√6th **Y36.45** **War operations involving combat using** blunt or piercing object

   √7th **Y36.450** **War operations involving combat using blunt or piercing object,** military personnel

   √7th **Y36.451** **War operations involving combat using blunt or piercing object,** civilian

√6th **Y36.46** **War operations involving** intentional restriction of air and airway

   √7th **Y36.460** **War operations involving intentional restriction of air and airway,** military personnel

   √7th **Y36.461** **War operations involving intentional restriction of air and airway,** civilian

√6th **Y36.47** **War operations involving** unintentional restriction of air and airway

   √7th **Y36.470** **War operations involving unintentional restriction of air and airway,** military personnel

   √7th **Y36.471** **War operations involving unintentional restriction of air and airway,** civilian

√6th **Y36.49** **War operations involving other forms of conventional warfare**

   √7th **Y36.490** **War operations involving other forms of conventional warfare,** military personnel

   √7th **Y36.491** **War operations involving other forms of conventional warfare,** civilian

√5th **Y36.5** **War operations involving** nuclear weapons

   War operations involving dirty bomb NOS

√6th **Y36.50** **War operations involving unspecified effect of nuclear weapon**

   √7th **Y36.500** **War operations involving unspecified effect of nuclear weapon,** military personnel

   √7th **Y36.501** **War operations involving unspecified effect of nuclear weapon,** civilian

√6th **Y36.51** **War operations involving** direct blast **effect of nuclear weapon**

   War operations involving blast pressure of nuclear weapon

   √7th **Y36.510** **War operations involving direct blast effect of nuclear weapon,** military personnel

   √7th **Y36.511** **War operations involving direct blast effect of nuclear weapon,** civilian

√6th **Y36.52** **War operations involving** indirect blast **effect of nuclear weapon**

   War operations involving being thrown by blast of nuclear weapon

   War operations involving being struck or crushed by blast debris of nuclear weapon

   √7th **Y36.520** **War operations involving indirect blast effect of nuclear weapon,** military personnel

   √7th **Y36.521** **War operations involving indirect blast effect of nuclear weapon,** civilian

√6th **Y36.53** **War operations involving** thermal radiation **effect of nuclear weapon**

   War operations involving direct heat from nuclear weapon

   War operation involving fireball effects from nuclear weapon

   √7th **Y36.530** **War operations involving thermal radiation effect of nuclear weapon,** military personnel

   √7th **Y36.531** **War operations involving thermal radiation effect of nuclear weapon,** civilian

√6th **Y36.54** **War operation involving** nuclear radiation **effects of nuclear weapon**

   War operation involving acute radiation exposure from nuclear weapon

   War operation involving exposure to immediate ionizing radiation from nuclear weapon

   War operation involving fallout exposure from nuclear weapon

   War operation involving secondary effects of nuclear weapons

   √7th **Y36.540** **War operation involving nuclear radiation effects of nuclear weapon,** military personnel

   √7th **Y36.541** **War operation involving nuclear radiation effects of nuclear weapon,** civilian

√6th **Y36.59** **War operation involving other effects of nuclear weapons**

   √7th **Y36.590** **War operation involving other effects of nuclear weapons,** military personnel

   √7th **Y36.591** **War operation involving other effects of nuclear weapons,** civilian

√5th **Y36.6** **War operations involving biological weapons**

√6th **Y36.6X** **War operations involving** biological weapons

   √7th **Y36.6X0** **War operations involving biological weapons,** military personnel

   √7th **Y36.6X1** **War operations involving biological weapons,** civilian

√5th **Y36.7** **War operations involving chemical weapons and other forms of unconventional warfare**

   EXCLUDES 1   war operations involving incendiary devices (Y36.3-, Y36.5-)

√6th **Y36.7X** **War operations involving** chemical weapons and other forms of unconventional warfare

   √7th **Y36.7X0** **War operations involving chemical weapons and other forms of unconventional warfare,** military personnel

   √7th **Y36.7X1** **War operations involving chemical weapons and other forms of unconventional warfare,** civilian

√5th **Y36.8** **War operations occurring** after cessation of hostilities

   War operations classifiable to categories Y36.0-Y36.8 but occurring after cessation of hostilities

√6th **Y36.81** **Explosion of** mine **placed during war operations but exploding after cessation of hostilities**

   √7th **Y36.810** **Explosion of mine placed during war operations but exploding after cessation of hostilities,** military personnel

   √7th **Y36.811** **Explosion of mine placed during war operations but exploding after cessation of hostilities,** civilian

√6th **Y36.82** **Explosion of** bomb **placed during war operations but exploding after cessation of hostilities**

   √7th **Y36.820** **Explosion of bomb placed during war operations but exploding after cessation of hostilities,** military personnel

   √7th **Y36.821** **Explosion of bomb placed during war operations but exploding after cessation of hostilities,** civilian

√6th **Y36.88** **Other war operations occurring after cessation of hostilities**

   √7th **Y36.880** **Other war operations occurring after cessation of hostilities,** military personnel

   √7th **Y36.881** **Other war operations occurring after cessation of hostilities,** civilian

√6th **Y36.89** **Unspecified war operations occurring after cessation of hostilities**

   √7th **Y36.890** **Unspecified war operations occurring after cessation of hostilities,** military personnel

   √7th **Y36.891** **Unspecified war operations occurring after cessation of hostilities,** civilian

√5th **Y36.9** **Other and unspecified war operations**

   √x7th **Y36.90** **War operations, unspecified**

   √x7th **Y36.91** **War operations involving unspecified** weapon of mass destruction [WMD]

   √x7th **Y36.92** **War operations involving** friendly fire

---

☑ Additional Character Required   √x7th Placeholder Alert   Manifestation   Unspecified Dx   ▶◀ Revised Text   ● New Code   ▲ Revised Title

✓4ᵗʰ **Y37 Military operations**

INCLUDES   injuries to military personnel and civilians occurring during peacetime on military property and during routine military exercises and operations

EXCLUDES 1   *military aircraft involved in aircraft accident with civilian aircraft (V97.81-)*
military vehicles involved in transport accident with civilian vehicle (V09.01, V09.21, V19.81, V29.81, V39.81, V49.81, V59.81, V69.81, V79.81)
military watercraft involved in water transport accident with civilian watercraft (V94.81-)
war operations (Y36.-)

✓5ᵗʰ **Y37.0   Military operations involving** explosion of marine weapons

 ✓6ᵗʰ **Y37.00   Military operations involving explosion of unspecified marine weapon**
  Military operations involving underwater blast NOS
  ✓7ᵗʰ **Y37.000   Military operations involving explosion of unspecified marine weapon,** military personnel
  ✓7ᵗʰ **Y37.001   Military operations involving explosion of unspecified marine weapon,** civilian

 ✓6ᵗʰ **Y37.01   Military operations involving explosion of** depth-charge
  ✓7ᵗʰ **Y37.010   Military operations involving explosion of depth-charge,** military personnel
  ✓7ᵗʰ **Y37.011   Military operations involving explosion of depth-charge,** civilian

 ✓6ᵗʰ **Y37.02   Military operations involving explosion of** marine mine
  Military operations involving explosion of marine mine, at sea or in harbor
  ✓7ᵗʰ **Y37.020   Military operations involving explosion of marine mine,** military personnel
  ✓7ᵗʰ **Y37.021   Military operations involving explosion of marine mine,** civilian

 ✓6ᵗʰ **Y37.03   Military operations involving explosion of** sea-based artillery shell
  ✓7ᵗʰ **Y37.030   Military operations involving explosion of sea-based artillery shell,** military personnel
  ✓7ᵗʰ **Y37.031   Military operations involving explosion of sea-based artillery shell,** civilian

 ✓6ᵗʰ **Y37.04   Military operations involving explosion of** torpedo
  ✓7ᵗʰ **Y37.040   Military operations involving explosion of torpedo,** military personnel
  ✓7ᵗʰ **Y37.041   Military operations involving explosion of torpedo,** civilian

 ✓6ᵗʰ **Y37.05   Military operations involving accidental detonation of** onboard marine weapons
  ✓7ᵗʰ **Y37.050   Military operations involving accidental detonation of onboard marine weapons,** military personnel
  ✓7ᵗʰ **Y37.051   Military operations involving accidental detonation of onboard marine weapons,** civilian

 ✓6ᵗʰ **Y37.09   Military operations involving explosion of other marine weapons**
  ✓7ᵗʰ **Y37.090   Military operations involving explosion of other marine weapons,** military personnel
  ✓7ᵗʰ **Y37.091   Military operations involving explosion of other marine weapons,** civilian

✓5ᵗʰ **Y37.1   Military operations involving** destruction of aircraft

 ✓6ᵗʰ **Y37.10   Military operations involving unspecified destruction of aircraft**
  ✓7ᵗʰ **Y37.100   Military operations involving unspecified destruction of aircraft,** military personnel
  ✓7ᵗʰ **Y37.101   Military operations involving unspecified destruction of aircraft,** civilian

 ✓6ᵗʰ **Y37.11   Military operations involving destruction of aircraft** due to enemy fire or explosives
  Military operations involving destruction of aircraft due to air to air missile
  Military operations involving destruction of aircraft due to explosive placed on aircraft
  Military operations involving destruction of aircraft due to rocket propelled grenade [RPG]
  Military operations involving destruction of aircraft due to small arms fire
  Military operations involving destruction of aircraft due to surface to air missile
  ✓7ᵗʰ **Y37.110   Military operations involving destruction of aircraft due to enemy fire or explosives,** military personnel
  ✓7ᵗʰ **Y37.111   Military operations involving destruction of aircraft due to enemy fire or explosives,** civilian

 ✓6ᵗʰ **Y37.12   Military operations involving destruction of aircraft** due to collision with other aircraft
  ✓7ᵗʰ **Y37.120   Military operations involving destruction of aircraft due to collision with other aircraft,** military personnel
  ✓7ᵗʰ **Y37.121   Military operations involving destruction of aircraft due to collision with other aircraft,** civilian

 ✓6ᵗʰ **Y37.13   Military operations involving destruction of aircraft** due to onboard fire
  ✓7ᵗʰ **Y37.130   Military operations involving destruction of aircraft due to onboard fire,** military personnel
  ✓7ᵗʰ **Y37.131   Military operations involving destruction of aircraft due to onboard fire,** civilian

 ✓6ᵗʰ **Y37.14   Military operations involving destruction of aircraft due to** accidental detonation of onboard munitions and explosives
  ✓7ᵗʰ **Y37.140   Military operations involving destruction of aircraft due to accidental detonation of onboard munitions and explosives,** military personnel
  ✓7ᵗʰ **Y37.141   Military operations involving destruction of aircraft due to accidental detonation of onboard munitions and explosives,** civilian

 ✓6ᵗʰ **Y37.19   Military operations involving other destruction of aircraft**
  ✓7ᵗʰ **Y37.190   Military operations involving other destruction of aircraft,** military personnel
  ✓7ᵗʰ **Y37.191   Military operations involving other destruction of aircraft,** civilian

✓5ᵗʰ **Y37.2   Military operations involving** other explosions and fragments

 EXCLUDES 1   *military operations involving explosion of aircraft (Y37.1-)*
  military operations involving explosion of marine weapons (Y37.0-)
  military operations involving explosion of nuclear weapons (Y37.5-)

 ✓6ᵗʰ **Y37.20   Military operations involving unspecified explosion and fragments**
  Military operations involving air blast NOS
  Military operations involving blast NOS
  Military operations involving blast fragments NOS
  Military operations involving blast wave NOS
  Military operations involving blast wind NOS
  Military operations involving explosion NOS
  Military operations involving explosion of bomb NOS
  ✓7ᵗʰ **Y37.200   Military operations involving unspecified explosion and fragments,** military personnel
  ✓7ᵗʰ **Y37.201   Military operations involving unspecified explosion and fragments,** civilian

 ✓6ᵗʰ **Y37.21   Military operations involving explosion of** aerial bomb
  ✓7ᵗʰ **Y37.210   Military operations involving explosion of aerial bomb,** military personnel
  ✓7ᵗʰ **Y37.211   Military operations involving explosion of aerial bomb,** civilian

 ✓6ᵗʰ **Y37.22   Military operations involving explosion of** guided missile
  ✓7ᵗʰ **Y37.220   Military operations involving explosion of guided missile,** military personnel

√7ᵗʰ **Y37.221** Military operations involving explosion of guided missile, civilian

√6ᵗʰ **Y37.23** Military operations involving explosion of improvised explosive device [IED]
Military operations involving explosion of person-borne improvised explosive device [IED]
Military operations involving explosion of vehicle-borne improvised explosive device [IED]
Military operations involving explosion of roadside improvised explosive device [IED]

√7ᵗʰ **Y37.230** Military operations involving explosion of improvised explosive device [IED], military personnel

√7ᵗʰ **Y37.231** Military operations involving explosion of improvised explosive device [IED], civilian

√6ᵗʰ **Y37.24** Military operations involving explosion due to accidental detonation and discharge of own munitions or munitions launch device

√7ᵗʰ **Y37.240** Military operations involving explosion due to accidental detonation and discharge of own munitions or munitions launch device, military personnel

√7ᵗʰ **Y37.241** Military operations involving explosion due to accidental detonation and discharge of own munitions or munitions launch device, civilian

√6ᵗʰ **Y37.25** Military operations involving fragments from munitions

√7ᵗʰ **Y37.250** Military operations involving fragments from munitions, military personnel

√7ᵗʰ **Y37.251** Military operations involving fragments from munitions, civilian

√6ᵗʰ **Y37.26** Military operations involving fragments of improvised explosive device [IED]
Military operations involving fragments of person-borne improvised explosive device [IED]
Military operations involving fragments of vehicle-borne improvised explosive device [IED]
Military operations involving fragments of roadside improvised explosive device [IED]

√7ᵗʰ **Y37.260** Military operations involving fragments of improvised explosive device [IED], military personnel

√7ᵗʰ **Y37.261** Military operations involving fragments of improvised explosive device [IED], civilian

√6ᵗʰ **Y37.27** Military operations involving fragments from weapons

√7ᵗʰ **Y37.270** Military operations involving fragments from weapons, military personnel

√7ᵗʰ **Y37.271** Military operations involving fragments from weapons, civilian

√6ᵗʰ **Y37.29** Military operations involving other explosions and fragments
Military operations involving explosion of grenade
Military operations involving explosions of land mine
Military operations involving shrapnel NOS

√7ᵗʰ **Y37.290** Military operations involving other explosions and fragments, military personnel

√7ᵗʰ **Y37.291** Military operations involving other explosions and fragments, civilian

√5ᵗʰ **Y37.3** Military operations involving fires, conflagrations and hot substances
Military operations involving smoke, fumes, and heat from fires, conflagrations and hot substances
EXCLUDES 1 *military operations involving fires and conflagrations aboard military aircraft (Y37.1-)*
military operations involving fires and conflagrations aboard military watercraft (Y37.0-)
military operations involving fires and conflagrations caused indirectly by conventional weapons (Y37.2-)
military operations involving fires and thermal effects of nuclear weapons (Y36.53-)

√6ᵗʰ **Y37.30** Military operations involving unspecified fire, conflagration and hot substance

√7ᵗʰ **Y37.300** Military operations involving unspecified fire, conflagration and hot substance, military personnel

√7ᵗʰ **Y37.301** Military operations involving unspecified fire, conflagration and hot substance, civilian

√6ᵗʰ **Y37.31** Military operations involving gasoline bomb
Military operations involving incendiary bomb
Military operations involving petrol bomb

√7ᵗʰ **Y37.310** Military operations involving gasoline bomb, military personnel

√7ᵗʰ **Y37.311** Military operations involving gasoline bomb, civilian

√6ᵗʰ **Y37.32** Military operations involving incendiary bullet

√7ᵗʰ **Y37.320** Military operations involving incendiary bullet, military personnel

√7ᵗʰ **Y37.321** Military operations involving incendiary bullet, civilian

√6ᵗʰ **Y37.33** Military operations involving flamethrower

√7ᵗʰ **Y37.330** Military operations involving flamethrower, military personnel

√7ᵗʰ **Y37.331** Military operations involving flamethrower, civilian

√6ᵗʰ **Y37.39** Military operations involving other fires, conflagrations and hot substances

√7ᵗʰ **Y37.390** Military operations involving other fires, conflagrations and hot substances, military personnel

√7ᵗʰ **Y37.391** Military operations involving other fires, conflagrations and hot substances, civilian

√5ᵗʰ **Y37.4** Military operations involving firearm discharge and other forms of conventional warfare

√6ᵗʰ **Y37.41** Military operations involving rubber bullets

√7ᵗʰ **Y37.410** Military operations involving rubber bullets, military personnel

√7ᵗʰ **Y37.411** Military operations involving rubber bullets, civilian

√6ᵗʰ **Y37.42** Military operations involving firearms pellets

√7ᵗʰ **Y37.420** Military operations involving firearms pellets, military personnel

√7ᵗʰ **Y37.421** Military operations involving firearms pellets, civilian

√6ᵗʰ **Y37.43** Military operations involving other firearms discharge
Military operations involving bullets NOS
EXCLUDES 1 *military operations involving munitions fragments (Y37.25-)*
military operations involving incendiary bullets (Y37.32-)

√7ᵗʰ **Y37.430** Military operations involving other firearms discharge, military personnel

√7ᵗʰ **Y37.431** Military operations involving other firearms discharge, civilian

√6ᵗʰ **Y37.44** Military operations involving unarmed hand to hand combat
EXCLUDES 1 *military operations involving combat using blunt or piercing object (Y37.45-)*
military operations involving intentional restriction of air and airway (Y37.46-)
military operations involving unintentional restriction of air and airway (Y37.47-)

√7ᵗʰ **Y37.440** Military operations involving unarmed hand to hand combat, military personnel

√7ᵗʰ **Y37.441** Military operations involving unarmed hand to hand combat, civilian

√6ᵗʰ **Y37.45** Military operations involving combat using blunt or piercing object

√7ᵗʰ **Y37.450** Military operations involving combat using blunt or piercing object, military personnel

√7ᵗʰ **Y37.451** Military operations involving combat using blunt or piercing object, civilian

√6ᵗʰ **Y37.46** Military operations involving intentional restriction of air and airway

√7ᵗʰ **Y37.460** Military operations involving intentional restriction of air and airway, military personnel

√7ᵗʰ **Y37.461** Military operations involving intentional restriction of air and airway, civilian

✔ Additional Character Required   √x7ᵗʰ Placeholder Alert   Manifestation   Unspecified Dx   ▶◀ Revised Text   ● New Code   ▲ Revised Title

ICD-10-CM 2020   1189

✓6ᵗʰ **Y37.47** **Military operations involving** unintentional restriction of air and airway

     ✓7ᵗʰ **Y37.470** **Military operations involving unintentional restriction of air and airway,** military personnel

     ✓7ᵗʰ **Y37.471** **Military operations involving unintentional restriction of air and airway,** civilian

✓6ᵗʰ **Y37.49** **Military operations involving other forms of conventional warfare**

     ✓7ᵗʰ **Y37.490** **Military operations involving other forms of conventional warfare,** military personnel

     ✓7ᵗʰ **Y37.491** **Military operations involving other forms of conventional warfare,** civilian

✓5ᵗʰ **Y37.5** **Military operations involving** nuclear weapons

     Military operation involving dirty bomb NOS

✓6ᵗʰ **Y37.50** **Military operations involving unspecified effect of nuclear weapon**

     ✓7ᵗʰ **Y37.500** **Military operations involving unspecified effect of nuclear weapon,** military personnel

     ✓7ᵗʰ **Y37.501** **Military operations involving unspecified effect of nuclear weapon,** civilian

✓6ᵗʰ **Y37.51** **Military operations involving** direct blast effect **of nuclear weapon**

     Military operations involving blast pressure of nuclear weapon

     ✓7ᵗʰ **Y37.510** **Military operations involving direct blast effect of nuclear weapon,** military personnel

     ✓7ᵗʰ **Y37.511** **Military operations involving direct blast effect of nuclear weapon,** civilian

✓6ᵗʰ **Y37.52** **Military operations involving** indirect blast effect **of nuclear weapon**

     Military operations involving being thrown by blast of nuclear weapon

     Military operations involving being struck or crushed by blast debris of nuclear weapon

     ✓7ᵗʰ **Y37.520** **Military operations involving indirect blast effect of nuclear weapon,** military personnel

     ✓7ᵗʰ **Y37.521** **Military operations involving indirect blast effect of nuclear weapon,** civilian

✓6ᵗʰ **Y37.53** **Military operations involving** thermal radiation effect of nuclear weapon

     Military operations involving direct heat from nuclear weapon

     Military operation involving fireball effects from nuclear weapon

     ✓7ᵗʰ **Y37.530** **Military operations involving thermal radiation effect of nuclear weapon,** military personnel

     ✓7ᵗʰ **Y37.531** **Military operations involving thermal radiation effect of nuclear weapon,** civilian

✓6ᵗʰ **Y37.54** **Military operation involving** nuclear radiation effects of nuclear weapon

     Military operation involving acute radiation exposure from nuclear weapon

     Military operation involving exposure to immediate ionizing radiation from nuclear weapon

     Military operation involving fallout exposure from nuclear weapon

     Military operation involving secondary effects of nuclear weapons

     ✓7ᵗʰ **Y37.540** **Military operation involving nuclear radiation effects of nuclear weapon,** military personnel

     ✓7ᵗʰ **Y37.541** **Military operation involving nuclear radiation effects of nuclear weapon,** civilian

✓6ᵗʰ **Y37.59** **Military operation involving other effects of nuclear weapons**

     ✓7ᵗʰ **Y37.590** **Military operation involving other effects of nuclear weapons,** military personnel

     ✓7ᵗʰ **Y37.591** **Military operation involving other effects of nuclear weapons,** civilian

✓5ᵗʰ **Y37.6** **Military operations involving** biological weapons

✓6ᵗʰ **Y37.6X** **Military operations involving biological weapons**

     ✓7ᵗʰ **Y37.6X0** **Military operations involving biological weapons,** military personnel

✓7ᵗʰ **Y37.6X1** **Military operations involving biological weapons,** civilian

✓5ᵗʰ **Y37.7** **Military operations involving chemical weapons and other forms of unconventional warfare**

     EXCLUDES 1   military operations involving incendiary devices (Y36.3-, Y36.5-)

✓6ᵗʰ **Y37.7X** **Military operations involving** chemical weapons and other forms of unconventional warfare

     ✓7ᵗʰ **Y37.7X0** **Military operations involving chemical weapons and other forms of unconventional warfare,** military personnel

     ✓7ᵗʰ **Y37.7X1** **Military operations involving chemical weapons and other forms of unconventional warfare,** civilian

✓5ᵗʰ **Y37.9** **Other and unspecified military operations**

     ✓x7ᵗʰ **Y37.90** **Military operations, unspecified**

     ✓x7ᵗʰ **Y37.91** **Military operations involving unspecified** weapon of mass destruction [WMD]

     ✓x7ᵗʰ **Y37.92** **Military operations involving** friendly fire

✓4ᵗʰ **Y38** **Terrorism**

     NOTE   These codes are for use to identify injuries resulting from the unlawful use of force or violence against persons or property to intimidate or coerce a Government, the civilian population, or any segment thereof, in furtherance of political or social objective

     Use additional code for place of occurrence (Y92.-)

✓5ᵗʰ **Y38.0** **Terrorism involving explosion of marine weapons**

     Terrorism involving depth-charge

     Terrorism involving marine mine

     Terrorism involving mine NOS, at sea or in harbor

     Terrorism involving sea-based artillery shell

     Terrorism involving torpedo

     Terrorism involving underwater blast

✓6ᵗʰ **Y38.0X** **Terrorism involving explosion of** marine weapons

     ✓7ᵗʰ **Y38.0X1** **Terrorism involving explosion of marine weapons,** public safety official **injured**

     ✓7ᵗʰ **Y38.0X2** **Terrorism involving explosion of marine weapons,** civilian **injured**

     ✓7ᵗʰ **Y38.0X3** **Terrorism involving explosion of marine weapons,** terrorist **injured**

✓5ᵗʰ **Y38.1** **Terrorism involving destruction of aircraft**

     Terrorism involving aircraft burned

     Terrorism involving aircraft exploded

     Terrorism involving aircraft being shot down

     Terrorism involving aircraft used as a weapon

✓6ᵗʰ **Y38.1X** **Terrorism involving** destruction of aircraft

     ✓7ᵗʰ **Y38.1X1** **Terrorism involving destruction of aircraft,** public safety official **injured**

     ✓7ᵗʰ **Y38.1X2** **Terrorism involving destruction of aircraft,** civilian **injured**

     ✓7ᵗʰ **Y38.1X3** **Terrorism involving destruction of aircraft,** terrorist **injured**

✓5ᵗʰ **Y38.2** **Terrorism involving other explosions and fragments**

     Terrorism involving antipersonnel (fragments) bomb

     Terrorism involving blast NOS

     Terrorism involving explosion NOS

     Terrorism involving explosion of breech block

     Terrorism involving explosion of cannon block

     Terrorism involving explosion (fragments) of artillery shell

     Terrorism involving explosion (fragments) of bomb

     Terrorism involving explosion (fragments) of grenade

     Terrorism involving explosion (fragments) of guided missile

     Terrorism involving explosion (fragments) of land mine

     Terrorism involving explosion of mortar bomb

     Terrorism involving explosion of munitions

     Terrorism involving explosion (fragments) of rocket

     Terrorism involving explosion (fragments) of shell

     Terrorism involving shrapnel

     Terrorism involving mine NOS, on land

     EXCLUDES 1   terrorism involving explosion of nuclear weapon (Y38.5)

         terrorism involving suicide bomber (Y38.81)

✓6ᵗʰ **Y38.2X** **Terrorism involving other explosions and fragments**

     ✓7ᵗʰ **Y38.2X1** **Terrorism involving other explosions and fragments,** public safety official **injured**

✓7ᵗʰ **Y38.2X2** **Terrorism involving other explosions and fragments,** civilian **injured**

✓7ᵗʰ **Y38.2X3** **Terrorism involving other explosions and fragments,** terrorist **injured**

✓5ᵗʰ **Y38.3** **Terrorism involving fires, conflagration and hot substances**

Terrorism involving conflagration NOS

Terrorism involving fire NOS

Terrorism involving petrol bomb

EXCLUDES 1　*terrorism involving fire or heat of nuclear weapon (Y38.5)*

✓6ᵗʰ **Y38.3X** **Terrorism involving** fires, conflagration and hot substances

✓7ᵗʰ **Y38.3X1** **Terrorism involving fires, conflagration and hot substances,** public safety official **injured**

✓7ᵗʰ **Y38.3X2** **Terrorism involving fires, conflagration and hot substances,** civilian **injured**

✓7ᵗʰ **Y38.3X3** **Terrorism involving fires, conflagration and hot substances,** terrorist **injured**

✓5ᵗʰ **Y38.4** **Terrorism involving firearms**

Terrorism involving carbine bullet

Terrorism involving machine gun bullet

Terrorism involving pellets (shotgun)

Terrorism involving pistol bullet

Terrorism involving rifle bullet

Terrorism involving rubber (rifle) bullet

✓6ᵗʰ **Y38.4X** **Terrorism involving** firearms

✓7ᵗʰ **Y38.4X1** **Terrorism involving firearms,** public safety official **injured**

✓7ᵗʰ **Y38.4X2** **Terrorism involving firearms,** civilian **injured**

✓7ᵗʰ **Y38.4X3** **Terrorism involving firearms,** terrorist **injured**

✓5ᵗʰ **Y38.5** **Terrorism involving nuclear weapons**

Terrorism involving blast effects of nuclear weapon

Terrorism involving exposure to ionizing radiation from nuclear weapon

Terrorism involving fireball effect of nuclear weapon

Terrorism involving heat from nuclear weapon

✓6ᵗʰ **Y38.5X** **Terrorism involving** nuclear weapons

✓7ᵗʰ **Y38.5X1** **Terrorism involving nuclear weapons,** public safety official **injured**

✓7ᵗʰ **Y38.5X2** **Terrorism involving nuclear weapons,** civilian **injured**

✓7ᵗʰ **Y38.5X3** **Terrorism involving nuclear weapons,** terrorist **injured**

✓5ᵗʰ **Y38.6** **Terrorism involving biological weapons**

Terrorism involving anthrax

Terrorism involving cholera

Terrorism involving smallpox

✓6ᵗʰ **Y38.6X** **Terrorism involving** biological weapons

✓7ᵗʰ **Y38.6X1** **Terrorism involving biological weapons,** public safety official **injured**

✓7ᵗʰ **Y38.6X2** **Terrorism involving biological weapons,** civilian **injured**

✓7ᵗʰ **Y38.6X3** **Terrorism involving biological weapons,** terrorist **injured**

✓5ᵗʰ **Y38.7** **Terrorism involving chemical weapons**

Terrorism involving gases, fumes, chemicals

Terrorism involving hydrogen cyanide

Terrorism involving phosgene

Terrorism involving sarin

✓6ᵗʰ **Y38.7X** **Terrorism involving** chemical weapons

✓7ᵗʰ **Y38.7X1** **Terrorism involving chemical weapons,** public safety official **injured**

✓7ᵗʰ **Y38.7X2** **Terrorism involving chemical weapons,** civilian **injured**

✓7ᵗʰ **Y38.7X3** **Terrorism involving chemical weapons,** terrorist **injured**

✓5ᵗʰ **Y38.8** **Terrorism involving other and unspecified means**

✓x7ᵗʰ **Y38.80** **Terrorism involving unspecified means**

Terrorism NOS

✓6ᵗʰ **Y38.81** **Terrorism involving** suicide bomber

✓7ᵗʰ **Y38.811** **Terrorism involving suicide bomber,** public safety official **injured**

✓7ᵗʰ **Y38.812** **Terrorism involving suicide bomber,** civilian **injured**

✓6ᵗʰ **Y38.89** **Terrorism involving other means**

Terrorism involving drowning and submersion

Terrorism involving lasers

Terrorism involving piercing or stabbing instruments

✓7ᵗʰ **Y38.891** **Terrorism involving other means,** public safety official **injured**

✓7ᵗʰ **Y38.892** **Terrorism involving other means,** civilian **injured**

✓7ᵗʰ **Y38.893** **Terrorism involving other means,** terrorist **injured**

✓5ᵗʰ **Y38.9** **Terrorism, secondary effects**

NOTE　This code is for use to identify conditions occurring subsequent to a terrorist attack not those that are due to the initial terrorist attack

✓6ᵗʰ **Y38.9X** **Terrorism,** secondary effects

✓7ᵗʰ **Y38.9X1** **Terrorism, secondary effects,** public safety official **injured**

✓7ᵗʰ **Y38.9X2** **Terrorism, secondary effects,** civilian **injured**

COMPLICATIONS OF MEDICAL AND SURGICAL CARE (Y62-Y84)

INCLUDES　complications of medical devices

surgical and medical procedures as the cause of abnormal reaction of the patient, or of later complication, without mention of misadventure at the time of the procedure

Misadventures to patients during surgical and medical care (Y62-Y69)

EXCLUDES 1　*surgical and medical procedures as the cause of abnormal reaction of the patient, without mention of misadventure at the time of the procedure (Y83-Y84)*

EXCLUDES 2　*breakdown or malfunctioning of medical device (during procedure) (after implantation) (ongoing use) (Y70-Y82)*

✓4ᵗʰ **Y62** **Failure of sterile precautions during surgical and medical care**

Y62.0 **Failure of sterile precautions during surgical operation**

Y62.1 **Failure of sterile precautions during infusion or transfusion**

Y62.2 **Failure of sterile precautions during kidney dialysis and other perfusion**

Y62.3 **Failure of sterile precautions during injection or immunization**

Y62.4 **Failure of sterile precautions during endoscopic examination**

Y62.5 **Failure of sterile precautions during heart catheterization**

Y62.6 **Failure of sterile precautions during aspiration, puncture and other catheterization**

Y62.8 **Failure of sterile precautions during other surgical and medical care**

Y62.9 **Failure of sterile precautions during unspecified surgical and medical care**

✓4ᵗʰ **Y63** **Failure in dosage during surgical and medical care**

EXCLUDES 2　*accidental overdose of drug or wrong drug given in error (T36-T50)*

Y63.0 **Excessive amount of blood or other fluid given during transfusion or infusion**

Y63.1 **Incorrect dilution of fluid used during infusion**

Y63.2 **Overdose of radiation given during therapy**

Y63.3 **Inadvertent exposure of patient to radiation during medical care**

Y63.4 **Failure in dosage in electroshock or insulin-shock therapy**

Y63.5 **Inappropriate temperature in local application and packing**

Y63.6 **Underdosing and nonadministration of necessary drug, medicament or biological substance**

AHA: 2018,4Q,72

Y63.8 **Failure in dosage during other surgical and medical care**

AHA: 2018,4Q,72

Y63.9 **Failure in dosage during unspecified surgical and medical care**

AHA: 2018,4Q,72

✓4ᵗʰ **Y64** **Contaminated medical or biological substances**

Y64.0 **Contaminated medical or biological substance, transfused or infused**

Y64.1 **Contaminated medical or biological substance, injected or used for immunization**

Y64.8 **Contaminated medical or biological substance administered by other means**

✓ Additional Character Required　　✓x7ᵗʰ Placeholder Alert　　Manifestation　　Unspecified Dx　　▶◀ Revised Text　　● New Code　　▲ Revised Title

ICD-10-CM 2020　　　　　　　　　　　　　　　　　　　　　　　　　　　　　　　　　　　　　　1191

Chapter 20. External Causes of Morbidity

Y64.9–Y78.1

Y64.9   **Contaminated medical or biological substance administered by unspecified means**
     Administered contaminated medical or biological substance NOS

✓4ᵗʰ **Y65**   **Other misadventures during surgical and medical care**

Y65.0   **Mismatched blood in transfusion**

Y65.1   **Wrong fluid used in infusion**

Y65.2   **Failure in suture or ligature during surgical operation**

Y65.3   **Endotracheal tube wrongly placed during anesthetic procedure**

Y65.4   **Failure to introduce or to remove other tube or instrument**

✓5ᵗʰ **Y65.5**   **Performance of** wrong procedure **(operation)**

Y65.51   **Performance of wrong procedure (operation) on** correct patient
     Wrong device implanted into correct surgical site
     EXCLUDES 1   *performance of correct procedure (operation) on wrong side or body part (Y65.53)*

Y65.52   **Performance of procedure (operation) on** patient not scheduled for surgery
     Performance of procedure (operation) intended for another patient
     Performance of procedure (operation) on wrong patient

Y65.53   **Performance of correct procedure (operation) on** wrong side or body part
     Performance of correct procedure (operation) on wrong side
     Performance of correct procedure (operation) on wrong site

Y65.8   **Other specified misadventures during surgical and medical care**
     AHA: 2019,2Q,23-24

Y66   **Nonadministration of surgical and medical care**
     Premature cessation of surgical and medical care
     EXCLUDES 1   *DNR status (Z66)*
         palliative care (Z51.5)

Y69   **Unspecified misadventure during surgical and medical care**

Medical devices associated with adverse incidents in diagnostic and therapeutic use (Y70-Y82)

INCLUDES   breakdown or malfunction of medical devices (during use) (after implantation) (ongoing use)

EXCLUDES 2   *later complications following use of medical devices without breakdown or malfunctioning of device (Y83-Y84)*
misadventure to patients during surgical and medical care, classifiable to (Y62-Y69)
surgical and other medical procedures as the cause of abnormal reaction of the patient, or of later complication, without mention of misadventure at the time of the procedure (Y83-Y84)

✓4ᵗʰ **Y70**   **Anesthesiology** devices associated with adverse incidents

Y70.0   Diagnostic and monitoring **anesthesiology devices associated with adverse incidents**

Y70.1   Therapeutic (nonsurgical) and rehabilitative **anesthesiology devices associated with adverse incidents**

Y70.2   Prosthetic and other implants, **materials and accessory anesthesiology devices associated with adverse incidents**

Y70.3   Surgical instruments, **materials and anesthesiology devices (including sutures) associated with adverse incidents**

Y70.8   Miscellaneous anesthesiology devices associated with adverse incidents, not elsewhere classified

✓4ᵗʰ **Y71**   **Cardiovascular** devices associated with adverse incidents

Y71.0   Diagnostic and monitoring **cardiovascular devices associated with adverse incidents**

Y71.1   Therapeutic (nonsurgical) and rehabilitative **cardiovascular devices associated with adverse incidents**

Y71.2   Prosthetic and other implants, **materials and accessory cardiovascular devices associated with adverse incidents**

Y71.3   Surgical instruments, **materials and cardiovascular devices (including sutures) associated with adverse incidents**

Y71.8   Miscellaneous cardiovascular devices associated with adverse incidents, not elsewhere classified

✓4ᵗʰ **Y72**   **Otorhinolaryngological** devices associated with adverse incidents

Y72.0   Diagnostic and monitoring **otorhinolaryngological devices associated with adverse incidents**

Y72.1   Therapeutic (nonsurgical) and rehabilitative **otorhinolaryngological devices associated with adverse incidents**

Y72.2   Prosthetic and other implants, **materials and accessory otorhinolaryngological devices associated with adverse incidents**

Y72.3   Surgical instruments, **materials and otorhinolaryngological devices (including sutures) associated with adverse incidents**

Y72.8   Miscellaneous otorhinolaryngological devices associated with adverse incidents, not elsewhere classified

✓4ᵗʰ **Y73**   **Gastroenterology and urology** devices associated with adverse incidents

Y73.0   Diagnostic and monitoring **gastroenterology and urology devices associated with adverse incidents**

Y73.1   Therapeutic (nonsurgical) and rehabilitative **gastroenterology and urology devices associated with adverse incidents**

Y73.2   Prosthetic and other implants, **materials and accessory gastroenterology and urology devices associated with adverse incidents**

Y73.3   Surgical instruments, materials and gastroenterology and urology devices (including sutures) associated with adverse incidents

Y73.8   Miscellaneous gastroenterology and urology devices associated with adverse incidents, not elsewhere classified

✓4ᵗʰ **Y74**   **General hospital and personal-use devices associated with adverse incidents**

Y74.0   Diagnostic and monitoring **general hospital and personal-use devices associated with adverse incidents**

Y74.1   Therapeutic (nonsurgical) and rehabilitative **general hospital and personal-use devices associated with adverse incidents**

Y74.2   Prosthetic and other implants, **materials and accessory general hospital and personal-use devices associated with adverse incidents**

Y74.3   Surgical instruments, **materials and general hospital and personal-use devices (including sutures) associated with adverse incidents**

Y74.8   Miscellaneous general hospital and personal-use devices associated with adverse incidents, not elsewhere classified

✓4ᵗʰ **Y75**   **Neurological** devices associated with adverse incidents

Y75.0   Diagnostic and monitoring **neurological devices associated with adverse incidents**

Y75.1   Therapeutic (nonsurgical) and rehabilitative **neurological devices associated with adverse incidents**

Y75.2   Prosthetic and other implants, **materials and neurological devices associated with adverse incidents**

Y75.3   Surgical instruments, **materials and neurological devices (including sutures) associated with adverse incidents**

Y75.8   Miscellaneous neurological devices associated with adverse incidents, not elsewhere classified

✓4ᵗʰ **Y76**   **Obstetric and gynecological** devices associated with adverse incidents

Y76.0   Diagnostic and monitoring **obstetric and gynecological devices associated with adverse incidents**   ♀

Y76.1   Therapeutic (nonsurgical) and rehabilitative **obstetric and gynecological devices associated with adverse incidents**   ♀

Y76.2   Prosthetic and other implants, **materials and accessory obstetric and gynecological devices associated with adverse incidents**   ♀

Y76.3   Surgical instruments, **materials and obstetric and gynecological devices (including sutures) associated with adverse incidents**   ♀

Y76.8   Miscellaneous obstetric and gynecological devices associated with adverse incidents, not elsewhere classified   ♀

✓4ᵗʰ **Y77**   **Ophthalmic** devices associated with adverse incidents

Y77.0   Diagnostic and monitoring **ophthalmic devices associated with adverse incidents**

Y77.1   Therapeutic (nonsurgical) and rehabilitative **ophthalmic devices associated with adverse incidents**

Y77.2   Prosthetic and other implants, **materials and accessory ophthalmic devices associated with adverse incidents**

Y77.3   Surgical instruments, **materials and ophthalmic devices (including sutures) associated with adverse incidents**

Y77.8   Miscellaneous ophthalmic devices associated with adverse incidents, not elsewhere classified

✓4ᵗʰ **Y78**   **Radiological** devices associated with adverse incidents

Y78.0   Diagnostic and monitoring **radiological devices associated with adverse incidents**

Y78.1   Therapeutic (nonsurgical) and rehabilitative **radiological devices associated with adverse incidents**

N Newborn: 0   P Pediatric: 0-17   M Maternity: 12-55   A Adult: 15-124   CH Comorbidity High   CL Comorbidity Low   NCDx Noncancer Dx   PDx Primary Dx

1192   ICD-10-CM 2020

Y78.2 Prosthetic and other implants, **materials and accessory radiological devices associated with adverse incidents**

Y78.3 Surgical instruments, **materials and radiological devices (including sutures) associated with adverse incidents**

Y78.8 **Miscellaneous radiological devices associated with adverse incidents, not elsewhere classified**

√4ᵗʰ **Y79** Orthopedic **devices associated with adverse incidents**

Y79.0 Diagnostic and monitoring **orthopedic devices associated with adverse incidents**

Y79.1 Therapeutic (**nonsurgical**) and rehabilitative **orthopedic devices associated with adverse incidents**

Y79.2 Prosthetic and other implants, **materials and accessory orthopedic devices associated with adverse incidents**

Y79.3 Surgical instruments, **materials and orthopedic devices (including sutures) associated with adverse incidents**

Y79.8 **Miscellaneous orthopedic devices associated with adverse incidents, not elsewhere classified**

√4ᵗʰ **Y80** Physical medicine **devices associated with adverse incidents**

Y80.0 Diagnostic and monitoring **physical medicine devices associated with adverse incidents**

Y80.1 Therapeutic (**nonsurgical**) and rehabilitative **physical medicine devices associated with adverse incidents**

Y80.2 Prosthetic and other implants, **materials and accessory physical medicine devices associated with adverse incidents**

Y80.3 Surgical instruments, **materials and physical medicine devices (including sutures) associated with adverse incidents**

Y80.8 **Miscellaneous physical medicine devices associated with adverse incidents, not elsewhere classified**

√4ᵗʰ **Y81** General- and plastic-surgery **devices associated with adverse incidents**

Y81.0 Diagnostic and monitoring **general- and plastic-surgery devices associated with adverse incidents**

Y81.1 Therapeutic (**nonsurgical**) and rehabilitative **general- and plastic-surgery devices associated with adverse incidents**

Y81.2 Prosthetic and other implants, **materials and accessory general- and plastic-surgery devices associated with adverse incidents**

Y81.3 Surgical instruments, **materials and general- and plastic-surgery devices (including sutures) associated with adverse incidents**

Y81.8 **Miscellaneous general- and plastic-surgery devices associated with adverse incidents, not elsewhere classified**

√4ᵗʰ **Y82** **Other and unspecified medical devices associated with adverse incidents**

Y82.8 **Other medical devices associated with adverse incidents**

Y82.9 **Unspecified medical devices associated with adverse incidents**

Surgical and other medical procedures as the cause of abnormal reaction of the patient, or of later complication, without mention of misadventure at the time of the procedure (Y83-Y84)

EXCLUDES 1   misadventures to patients during surgical and medical care, classifiable to (Y62-Y69)

EXCLUDES 2   breakdown or malfunctioning of medical device (during procedure) (after implantation) (ongoing use) (Y70-Y82)

√4ᵗʰ **Y83** Surgical operation **and other** surgical procedures **as the cause of abnormal reaction of the patient, or of later complication, without mention of misadventure at the time of the procedure**

Y83.0 **Surgical operation** with transplant of whole organ **as the cause of abnormal reaction of the patient, or of later complication, without mention of misadventure at the time of the procedure**

Y83.1 **Surgical operation** with implant of artificial internal device **as the cause of abnormal reaction of the patient, or of later complication, without mention of misadventure at the time of the procedure**

Y83.2 **Surgical operation** with anastomosis, bypass or graft **as the cause of abnormal reaction of the patient, or of later complication, without mention of misadventure at the time of the procedure**

Y83.3 **Surgical operation** with formation of external stoma **as the cause of abnormal reaction of the patient, or of later complication, without mention of misadventure at the time of the procedure**

Y83.4 **Other reconstructive surgery as the cause of abnormal reaction of the patient, or of later complication, without mention of misadventure at the time of the procedure**

Y83.5 Amputation of limb(s) **as the cause of abnormal reaction of the patient, or of later complication, without mention of misadventure at the time of the procedure**

Y83.6 Removal of other organ (partial) (total) **as the cause of abnormal reaction of the patient, or of later complication, without mention of misadventure at the time of the procedure**

Y83.8 **Other surgical procedures as the cause of abnormal reaction of the patient, or of later complication, without mention of misadventure at the time of the procedure**

Y83.9 **Surgical procedure, unspecified as the cause of abnormal reaction of the patient, or of later complication, without mention of misadventure at the time of the procedure**

√4ᵗʰ **Y84** **Other medical procedures as the cause of abnormal reaction of the patient, or of later complication, without mention of misadventure at the time of the procedure**

Y84.0 Cardiac catheterization **as the cause of abnormal reaction of the patient, or of later complication, without mention of misadventure at the time of the procedure**

Y84.1 Kidney dialysis **as the cause of abnormal reaction of the patient, or of later complication, without mention of misadventure at the time of the procedure**

Y84.2 Radiological procedure and radiotherapy **as the cause of abnormal reaction of the patient, or of later complication, without mention of misadventure at the time of the procedure**

AHA: 2019,1Q,21; 2017,1Q,33

Y84.3 Shock therapy **as the cause of abnormal reaction of the patient, or of later complication, without mention of misadventure at the time of the procedure**

Y84.4 Aspiration of fluid **as the cause of abnormal reaction of the patient, or of later complication, without mention of misadventure at the time of the procedure**

Y84.5 Insertion of gastric or duodenal sound **as the cause of abnormal reaction of the patient, or of later complication, without mention of misadventure at the time of the procedure**

Y84.6 Urinary catheterization **as the cause of abnormal reaction of the patient, or of later complication, without mention of misadventure at the time of the procedure**

Y84.7 Blood-sampling **as the cause of abnormal reaction of the patient, or of later complication, without mention of misadventure at the time of the procedure**

Y84.8 **Other medical procedures as the cause of abnormal reaction of the patient, or of later complication, without mention of misadventure at the time of the procedure**

AHA: 2014,4Q,24

Y84.9 **Medical procedure, unspecified as the cause of abnormal reaction of the patient, or of later complication, without mention of misadventure at the time of the procedure**

Supplementary factors related to causes of morbidity classified elsewhere (Y90-Y99)

NOTE   These categories may be used to provide supplementary information concerning causes of morbidity. They are not to be used for single-condition coding.

√4ᵗʰ **Y90** **Evidence of alcohol involvement determined by blood alcohol level**

Code first any associated alcohol related disorders (F10)

Y90.0 **Blood alcohol level of** less than 20 mg/100 ml

Y90.1 **Blood alcohol level of** 20-39 mg/100 ml

Y90.2 **Blood alcohol level of** 40-59 mg/100 ml

Y90.3 **Blood alcohol level of** 60-79 mg/100 ml

Y90.4 **Blood alcohol level of** 80-99 mg/100 ml

Y90.5 **Blood alcohol level of** 100-119 mg/100 ml

Y90.6 **Blood alcohol level of** 120-199 mg/100 ml

Y90.7 **Blood alcohol level of** 200-239 mg/100 ml

Y90.8 **Blood alcohol level of** 240 mg/100 ml or more

Y90.9 **Presence of alcohol in blood, level not specified**

☑ Additional Character Required   √x7ᵗʰ Placeholder Alert   Manifestation   Unspecified Dx   ▶◀ Revised Text   ● New Code   ▲ Revised Title

ICD-10-CM 2020   1193

Chapter 20. External Causes of Morbidity   Y78.2–Y90.9

Chapter 20. External Causes of Morbidity

☑4ᵗʰ **Y92 Place of occurrence of the external cause**

The following category is for use, when relevant, to identify the place of occurrence of the external cause. Use in conjunction with an activity code.

Place of occurrence should be recorded only at the initial encounter for treatment

☑5ᵗʰ **Y92.Ø Non-institutional (private) residence as the place of occurrence of the external cause**

> EXCLUDES 1   *abandoned or derelict house (Y92.89)*
> *home under construction but not yet occupied (Y92.6-)*
> *institutional place of residence (Y92.1-)*

☑6ᵗʰ **Y92.ØØ Unspecified non-institutional (private) residence as the place of occurrence of the external cause**

Y92.ØØØ Kitchen of unspecified non-institutional (private) residence as the place of occurrence of the external cause

Y92.ØØ1 Dining room of unspecified non-institutional (private) residence as the place of occurrence of the external cause

Y92.ØØ2 Bathroom of unspecified non-institutional (private) residence single-family (private) house as the place of occurrence of the external cause

Y92.ØØ3 Bedroom of unspecified non-institutional (private) residence as the place of occurrence of the external cause

Y92.ØØ7 Garden or yard of unspecified non-institutional (private) residence as the place of occurrence of the external cause

Y92.ØØ8 Other place in unspecified non-institutional (private) residence as the place of occurrence of the external cause

Y92.ØØ9 Unspecified place in unspecified non-institutional (private) residence as the place of occurrence of the external cause

> Home (NOS) as the place of occurrence of the external cause

☑6ᵗʰ **Y92.Ø1 Single-family non-institutional (private) house as the place of occurrence of the external cause**

Farmhouse as the place of occurrence of the external cause

> EXCLUDES 1   *barn (Y92.71)*
> *chicken coop or hen house (Y92.72)*
> *farm field (Y92.73)*
> *orchard (Y92.74)*
> *single family mobile home or trailer (Y92.Ø2-)*
> *slaughter house (Y92.86)*

Y92.Ø1Ø Kitchen of single-family (private) house as the place of occurrence of the external cause

Y92.Ø11 Dining room of single-family (private) house as the place of occurrence of the external cause

Y92.Ø12 Bathroom of single-family (private) house as the place of occurrence of the external cause

Y92.Ø13 Bedroom of single-family (private) house as the place of occurrence of the external cause

Y92.Ø14 Private driveway to single-family (private) house as the place of occurrence of the external cause

Y92.Ø15 Private garage of single-family (private) house as the place of occurrence of the external cause

Y92.Ø16 Swimming-pool in single-family (private) house or garden as the place of occurrence of the external cause

Y92.Ø17 Garden or yard in single-family (private) house as the place of occurrence of the external cause

Y92.Ø18 Other place in single-family (private) house as the place of occurrence of the external cause

Y92.Ø19 Unspecified place in single-family (private) house as the place of occurrence of the external cause

☑6ᵗʰ **Y92.Ø2 Mobile home as the place of occurrence of the external cause**

Y92.Ø2Ø Kitchen in mobile home as the place of occurrence of the external cause

Y92.Ø21 Dining room in mobile home as the place of occurrence of the external cause

Y92.Ø22 Bathroom in mobile home as the place of occurrence of the external cause

Y92.Ø23 Bedroom in mobile home as the place of occurrence of the external cause

Y92.Ø24 Driveway of mobile home as the place of occurrence of the external cause

Y92.Ø25 Garage of mobile home as the place of occurrence of the external cause

Y92.Ø26 Swimming-pool of mobile home as the place of occurrence of the external cause

Y92.Ø27 Garden or yard of mobile home as the place of occurrence of the external cause

Y92.Ø28 Other place in mobile home as the place of occurrence of the external cause

Y92.Ø29 Unspecified place in mobile home as the place of occurrence of the external cause

☑6ᵗʰ **Y92.Ø3 Apartment as the place of occurrence of the external cause**

Condominium as the place of occurrence of the external cause

Co-op apartment as the place of occurrence of the external cause

Y92.Ø3Ø Kitchen in apartment as the place of occurrence of the external cause

Y92.Ø31 Bathroom in apartment as the place of occurrence of the external cause

Y92.Ø32 Bedroom in apartment as the place of occurrence of the external cause

Y92.Ø38 Other place in apartment as the place of occurrence of the external cause

Y92.Ø39 Unspecified place in apartment as the place of occurrence of the external cause

☑6ᵗʰ **Y92.Ø4 Boarding-house as the place of occurrence of the external cause**

Y92.Ø4Ø Kitchen in boarding-house as the place of occurrence of the external cause

Y92.Ø41 Bathroom in boarding-house as the place of occurrence of the external cause

Y92.Ø42 Bedroom in boarding-house as the place of occurrence of the external cause

Y92.Ø43 Driveway of boarding-house as the place of occurrence of the external cause

Y92.Ø44 Garage of boarding-house as the place of occurrence of the external cause

Y92.Ø45 Swimming-pool of boarding-house as the place of occurrence of the external cause

Y92.Ø46 Garden or yard of boarding-house as the place of occurrence of the external cause

Y92.Ø48 Other place in boarding-house as the place of occurrence of the external cause

Y92.Ø49 Unspecified place in boarding-house as the place of occurrence of the external cause

☑6ᵗʰ **Y92.Ø9 Other non-institutional residence as the place of occurrence of the external cause**

> AHA: 2017,2Q,10

Y92.Ø9Ø Kitchen in other non-institutional residence as the place of occurrence of the external cause

Y92.Ø91 Bathroom in other non-institutional residence as the place of occurrence of the external cause

Y92.Ø92 Bedroom in other non-institutional residence as the place of occurrence of the external cause

Y92.Ø93 Driveway of other non-institutional residence as the place of occurrence of the external cause

Y92.Ø94 Garage of other non-institutional residence as the place of occurrence of the external cause

Y92.Ø95 Swimming-pool of other non-institutional residence as the place of occurrence of the external cause

Y92.Ø96 Garden or yard of other non-institutional residence as the place of occurrence of the external cause

Y92.Ø98   Other place in other non-institutional residence as the place of occurrence of the external cause

Y92.Ø99   Unspecified place in other non-institutional residence as the place of occurrence of the external cause

✓5ᵗʰ   **Y92.1**   Institutional (nonprivate) residence as the place of occurrence of the external cause

Y92.1Ø   Unspecified residential institution as the place of occurrence of the external cause

✓6ᵗʰ   **Y92.11**   Children's home and orphanage as the place of occurrence of the external cause

Y92.11Ø   Kitchen in children's home and orphanage as the place of occurrence of the external cause

Y92.111   Bathroom in children's home and orphanage as the place of occurrence of the external cause

Y92.112   Bedroom in children's home and orphanage as the place of occurrence of the external cause

Y92.113   Driveway of children's home and orphanage as the place of occurrence of the external cause

Y92.114   Garage of children's home and orphanage as the place of occurrence of the external cause

Y92.115   Swimming-pool of children's home and orphanage as the place of occurrence of the external cause

Y92.116   Garden or yard of children's home and orphanage as the place of occurrence of the external cause

Y92.118   Other place in children's home and orphanage as the place of occurrence of the external cause

Y92.119   Unspecified place in children's home and orphanage as the place of occurrence of the external cause

✓6ᵗʰ   **Y92.12**   Nursing home as the place of occurrence of the external cause

Home for the sick as the place of occurrence of the external cause

Hospice as the place of occurrence of the external cause

AHA: 2017,2Q,10

Y92.12Ø   Kitchen in nursing home as the place of occurrence of the external cause

Y92.121   Bathroom in nursing home as the place of occurrence of the external cause

Y92.122   Bedroom in nursing home as the place of occurrence of the external cause

Y92.123   Driveway of nursing home as the place of occurrence of the external cause

Y92.124   Garage of nursing home as the place of occurrence of the external cause

Y92.125   Swimming-pool of nursing home as the place of occurrence of the external cause

Y92.126   Garden or yard of nursing home as the place of occurrence of the external cause

Y92.128   Other place in nursing home as the place of occurrence of the external cause

Y92.129   Unspecified place in nursing home as the place of occurrence of the external cause

✓6ᵗʰ   **Y92.13**   Military base as the place of occurrence of the external cause

EXCLUDES 1   military training grounds (Y92.84)

Y92.13Ø   Kitchen on military base as the place of occurrence of the external cause

Y92.131   Mess hall on military base as the place of occurrence of the external cause

Y92.133   Barracks on military base as the place of occurrence of the external cause

Y92.135   Garage on military base as the place of occurrence of the external cause

Y92.136   Swimming-pool on military base as the place of occurrence of the external cause

Y92.137   Garden or yard on military base as the place of occurrence of the external cause

Y92.138   Other place on military base as the place of occurrence of the external cause

Y92.139   Unspecified place military base as the place of occurrence of the external cause

✓6ᵗʰ   **Y92.14**   Prison as the place of occurrence of the external cause

Y92.14Ø   Kitchen in prison as the place of occurrence of the external cause

Y92.141   Dining room in prison as the place of occurrence of the external cause

Y92.142   Bathroom in prison as the place of occurrence of the external cause

Y92.143   Cell of prison as the place of occurrence of the external cause

Y92.146   Swimming-pool of prison as the place of occurrence of the external cause

Y92.147   Courtyard of prison as the place of occurrence of the external cause

Y92.148   Other place in prison as the place of occurrence of the external cause

Y92.149   Unspecified place in prison as the place of occurrence of the external cause

✓6ᵗʰ   **Y92.15**   Reform school as the place of occurrence of the external cause

Y92.15Ø   Kitchen in reform school as the place of occurrence of the external cause

Y92.151   Dining room in reform school as the place of occurrence of the external cause

Y92.152   Bathroom in reform school as the place of occurrence of the external cause

Y92.153   Bedroom in reform school as the place of occurrence of the external cause

Y92.154   Driveway of reform school as the place of occurrence of the external cause

Y92.155   Garage of reform school as the place of occurrence of the external cause

Y92.156   Swimming-pool of reform school as the place of occurrence of the external cause

Y92.157   Garden or yard of reform school as the place of occurrence of the external cause

Y92.158   Other place in reform school as the place of occurrence of the external cause

Y92.159   Unspecified place in reform school as the place of occurrence of the external cause

✓6ᵗʰ   **Y92.16**   School dormitory as the place of occurrence of the external cause

EXCLUDES 1   reform school as the place of occurrence of the external cause (Y92.15-)

school buildings and grounds as the place of occurrence of the external cause (Y92.2-)

school sports and athletic areas as the place of occurrence of the external cause (Y92.3-)

Y92.16Ø   Kitchen in school dormitory as the place of occurrence of the external cause

Y92.161   Dining room in school dormitory as the place of occurrence of the external cause

Y92.162   Bathroom in school dormitory as the place of occurrence of the external cause

Y92.163   Bedroom in school dormitory as the place of occurrence of the external cause

Y92.168   Other place in school dormitory as the place of occurrence of the external cause

Y92.169   Unspecified place in school dormitory as the place of occurrence of the external cause

✓6ᵗʰ   **Y92.19**   Other specified residential institution as the place of occurrence of the external cause

AHA: 2017,2Q,10

Y92.19Ø   Kitchen in other specified residential institution as the place of occurrence of the external cause

Y92.191   Dining room in other specified residential institution as the place of occurrence of the external cause

Y92.192   Bathroom in other specified residential institution as the place of occurrence of the external cause

Y92.193   Bedroom in other specified residential institution as the place of occurrence of the external cause

Y92.194   Driveway of other specified residential institution as the place of occurrence of the external cause

Y92.195 **Garage** of other specified residential institution as the place of occurrence of the external cause

Y92.196 **Pool** of other specified residential institution as the place of occurrence of the external cause

Y92.197 **Garden or yard** of other specified residential institution as the place of occurrence of the external cause

Y92.198 **Other place** in other specified residential institution as the place of occurrence of the external cause

Y92.199 **Unspecified place** in other specified residential institution as the place of occurrence of the external cause

√5ᵗʰ Y92.2 **School, other institution and public administrative area** as the place of occurrence of the external cause

Building and adjacent grounds used by the general public or by a particular group of the public

EXCLUDES 1 *building under construction as the place of occurrence of the external cause (Y92.6)*

residential institution as the place of occurrence of the external cause (Y92.1)

school dormitory as the place of occurrence of the external cause (Y92.16-)

sports and athletics area of schools as the place of occurrence of the external cause (Y92.3-)

√6ᵗʰ Y92.21 **School (private) (public) (state)** as the place of occurrence of the external cause

Y92.210 **Daycare center** as the place of occurrence of the external cause

Y92.211 **Elementary school** as the place of occurrence of the external cause

Kindergarten as the place of occurrence of the external cause

Y92.212 **Middle school** as the place of occurrence of the external cause

Y92.213 **High school** as the place of occurrence of the external cause

AHA: 2012,4Q,108

Y92.214 **College** as the place of occurrence of the external cause

University as the place of occurrence of the external cause

Y92.215 **Trade school** as the place of occurrence of the external cause

Y92.218 **Other school** as the place of occurrence of the external cause

Y92.219 **Unspecified school** as the place of occurrence of the external cause

Y92.22 **Religious institution** as the place of occurrence of the external cause

Church as the place of occurrence of the external cause

Mosque as the place of occurrence of the external cause

Synagogue as the place of occurrence of the external cause

√6ᵗʰ Y92.23 **Hospital** as the place of occurrence of the external cause

EXCLUDES 1 *ambulatory (outpatient) health services establishments (Y92.53-)*

home for the sick as the place of occurrence of the external cause (Y92.12-)

hospice as the place of occurrence of the external cause (Y92.12-)

nursing home as the place of occurrence of the external cause (Y92.12-)

Y92.230 **Patient room** in hospital as the place of occurrence of the external cause

Y92.231 **Patient bathroom** in hospital as the place of occurrence of the external cause

Y92.232 **Corridor** of hospital as the place of occurrence of the external cause

Y92.233 **Cafeteria** of hospital as the place of occurrence of the external cause

Y92.234 **Operating room** of hospital as the place of occurrence of the external cause

Y92.238 **Other place** in hospital as the place of occurrence of the external cause

Y92.239 **Unspecified place** in hospital as the place of occurrence of the external cause

√6ᵗʰ Y92.24 **Public administrative building** as the place of occurrence of the external cause

Y92.240 **Courthouse** as the place of occurrence of the external cause

Y92.241 **Library** as the place of occurrence of the external cause

Y92.242 **Post office** as the place of occurrence of the external cause

Y92.243 **City hall** as the place of occurrence of the external cause

Y92.248 **Other** public administrative building as the place of occurrence of the external cause

√6ᵗʰ Y92.25 **Cultural building** as the place of occurrence of the external cause

Y92.250 **Art Gallery** as the place of occurrence of the external cause

Y92.251 **Museum** as the place of occurrence of the external cause

Y92.252 **Music hall** as the place of occurrence of the external cause

Y92.253 **Opera house** as the place of occurrence of the external cause

Y92.254 **Theater (live)** as the place of occurrence of the external cause

Y92.258 **Other cultural public building** as the place of occurrence of the external cause

Y92.26 **Movie house or cinema** as the place of occurrence of the external cause

Y92.29 **Other specified public building** as the place of occurrence of the external cause

Assembly hall as the place of occurrence of the external cause

Clubhouse as the place of occurrence of the external cause

√5ᵗʰ Y92.3 **Sports and athletics area** as the place of occurrence of the external cause

√6ᵗʰ Y92.31 **Athletic court** as the place of occurrence of the external cause

EXCLUDES 1 *tennis court in private home or garden (Y92.09)*

Y92.310 **Basketball court** as the place of occurrence of the external cause

Y92.311 **Squash court** as the place of occurrence of the external cause

Y92.312 **Tennis court** as the place of occurrence of the external cause

Y92.318 **Other athletic court** as the place of occurrence of the external cause

√6ᵗʰ Y92.32 **Athletic field** as the place of occurrence of the external cause

Y92.320 **Baseball field** as the place of occurrence of the external cause

Y92.321 **Football field** as the place of occurrence of the external cause

Y92.322 **Soccer field** as the place of occurrence of the external cause

Y92.328 **Other athletic field** as the place of occurrence of the external cause

Cricket field as the place of occurrence of the external cause

Hockey field as the place of occurrence of the external cause

√6ᵗʰ Y92.33 **Skating rink** as the place of occurrence of the external cause

Y92.330 **Ice skating rink (indoor) (outdoor)** as the place of occurrence of the external cause

Y92.331 **Roller skating rink** as the place of occurrence of the external cause

Y92.34 **Swimming pool (public)** as the place of occurrence of the external cause

EXCLUDES 1 *swimming pool in private home or garden (Y92.016)*

Y92.39 Other specified sports and athletic area as the place of occurrence of the external cause

Golf-course as the place of occurrence of the external cause

Gymnasium as the place of occurrence of the external cause

Riding-school as the place of occurrence of the external cause

Stadium as the place of occurrence of the external cause

√5ᵗʰ **Y92.4** Street, highway and other paved roadways as the place of occurrence of the external cause

EXCLUDES 1   *private driveway of residence (Y92.014, Y92.024, Y92.043, Y92.093, Y92.113, Y92.123, Y92.154, Y92.194)*

√6ᵗʰ **Y92.41** Street and highway as the place of occurrence of the external cause

Y92.410 Unspecified street and highway as the place of occurrence of the external cause

Road NOS as the place of occurrence of the external cause

Y92.411 Interstate highway as the place of occurrence of the external cause

Freeway as the place of occurrence of the external cause

Motorway as the place of occurrence of the external cause

Y92.412 Parkway as the place of occurrence of the external cause

Y92.413 State road as the place of occurrence of the external cause

Y92.414 Local residential or business street as the place of occurrence of the external cause

Y92.415 Exit ramp or entrance ramp of street or highway as the place of occurrence of the external cause

√6ᵗʰ **Y92.48** Other paved roadways as the place of occurrence of the external cause

Y92.480 Sidewalk as the place of occurrence of the external cause

Y92.481 Parking lot as the place of occurrence of the external cause

Y92.482 Bike path as the place of occurrence of the external cause

Y92.488 Other paved roadways as the place of occurrence of the external cause

√5ᵗʰ **Y92.5** Trade and service area as the place of occurrence of the external cause

EXCLUDES 1   *garage in private home (Y92.015)*

schools and other public administration buildings (Y92.2-)

√6ᵗʰ **Y92.51** Private commercial establishments as the place of occurrence of the external cause

Y92.510 Bank as the place of occurrence of the external cause

Y92.511 Restaurant or café as the place of occurrence of the external cause

Y92.512 Supermarket, store or market as the place of occurrence of the external cause

Y92.513 Shop (commercial) as the place of occurrence of the external cause

√6ᵗʰ **Y92.52** Service areas as the place of occurrence of the external cause

Y92.520 Airport as the place of occurrence of the external cause

Y92.521 Bus station as the place of occurrence of the external cause

Y92.522 Railway station as the place of occurrence of the external cause

Y92.523 Highway rest stop as the place of occurrence of the external cause

Y92.524 Gas station as the place of occurrence of the external cause

Petroleum station as the place of occurrence of the external cause

Service station as the place of occurrence of the external cause

√6ᵗʰ **Y92.53** Ambulatory health services establishments as the place of occurrence of the external cause

Y92.530 Ambulatory surgery center as the place of occurrence of the external cause

Outpatient surgery center, including that connected with a hospital as the place of occurrence of the external cause

Same day surgery center, including that connected with a hospital as the place of occurrence of the external cause

Y92.531 Health care provider office as the place of occurrence of the external cause

Physician office as the place of occurrence of the external cause

Y92.532 Urgent care center as the place of occurrence of the external cause

Y92.538 Other ambulatory health services establishments as the place of occurrence of the external cause

AHA: 2019,1Q,21

Y92.59 Other trade areas as the place of occurrence of the external cause

Office building as the place of occurrence of the external cause

Casino as the place of occurrence of the external cause

Garage (commercial) as the place of occurrence of the external cause

Hotel as the place of occurrence of the external cause

Radio or television station as the place of occurrence of the external cause

Shopping mall as the place of occurrence of the external cause

Warehouse as the place of occurrence of the external cause

√5ᵗʰ **Y92.6** Industrial and construction area as the place of occurrence of the external cause

Y92.61 Building [any] under construction as the place of occurrence of the external cause

Y92.62 Dock or shipyard as the place of occurrence of the external cause

Dockyard as the place of occurrence of the external cause

Dry dock as the place of occurrence of the external cause

Shipyard as the place of occurrence of the external cause

Y92.63 Factory as the place of occurrence of the external cause

Factory building as the place of occurrence of the external cause

Factory premises as the place of occurrence of the external cause

Industrial yard as the place of occurrence of the external cause

Y92.64 Mine or pit as the place of occurrence of the external cause

Mine as the place of occurrence of the external cause

Y92.65 Oil rig as the place of occurrence of the external cause

Pit (coal) (gravel) (sand) as the place of occurrence of the external cause

Y92.69 Other specified industrial and construction area as the place of occurrence of the external cause

Gasworks as the place of occurrence of the external cause

Power-station (coal) (nuclear) (oil) as the place of occurrence of the external cause

Tunnel under construction as the place of occurrence of the external cause

Workshop as the place of occurrence of the external cause

√5ᵗʰ **Y92.7** Farm as the place of occurrence of the external cause

Ranch as the place of occurrence of the external cause

EXCLUDES 1   *farmhouse and home premises of farm (Y92.01-)*

Y92.71 Barn as the place of occurrence of the external cause

Chapter 20. External Causes of Morbidity

Y92.72   Chicken coop as the place of occurrence of the external cause
> Hen house as the place of occurrence of the external cause

Y92.73   Farm field as the place of occurrence of the external cause

Y92.74   Orchard as the place of occurrence of the external cause

Y92.79   Other farm location as the place of occurrence of the external cause

✓5ᵗʰ **Y92.8**   Other places as the place of occurrence of the external cause

✓6ᵗʰ **Y92.81**   Transport vehicle as the place of occurrence of the external cause
> EXCLUDES 1   transport accidents (V00-V99)

Y92.810   Car as the place of occurrence of the external cause

Y92.811   Bus as the place of occurrence of the external cause

Y92.812   Truck as the place of occurrence of the external cause

Y92.813   Airplane as the place of occurrence of the external cause

Y92.814   Boat as the place of occurrence of the external cause

Y92.815   Train as the place of occurrence of the external cause

Y92.816   Subway car as the place of occurrence of the external cause

Y92.818   Other transport vehicle as the place of occurrence of the external cause

✓6ᵗʰ **Y92.82**   Wilderness area

Y92.820   Desert as the place of occurrence of the external cause

Y92.821   Forest as the place of occurrence of the external cause

Y92.828   Other wilderness area as the place of occurrence of the external cause
> Swamp as the place of occurrence of the external cause
> Mountain as the place of occurrence of the external cause
> Marsh as the place of occurrence of the external cause
> Prairie as the place of occurrence of the external cause

✓6ᵗʰ **Y92.83**   Recreation area as the place of occurrence of the external cause

Y92.830   Public park as the place of occurrence of the external cause

Y92.831   Amusement park as the place of occurrence of the external cause

Y92.832   Beach as the place of occurrence of the external cause
> Seashore as the place of occurrence of the external cause

Y92.833   Campsite as the place of occurrence of the external cause

Y92.834   Zoological garden (Zoo) as the place of occurrence of the external cause

Y92.838   Other recreation area as the place of occurrence of the external cause

Y92.84   Military training ground as the place of occurrence of the external cause

Y92.85   Railroad track as the place of occurrence of the external cause

Y92.86   Slaughter house as the place of occurrence of the external cause

Y92.89   Other specified places as the place of occurrence of the external cause
> Derelict house as the place of occurrence of the external cause

Y92.9   Unspecified place or not applicable

✓4ᵗʰ **Y93**   **Activity codes**

NOTE   Category Y93 is provided for use to indicate the activity of the person seeking healthcare for an injury or health condition, such as a heart attack while shoveling snow, which resulted from, or was contributed to, by the activity. These codes are appropriate for use for both acute injuries, such as those from chapter 19, and conditions that are due to the long-term, cumulative effects of an activity, such as those from chapter 13. They are also appropriate for use with external cause codes for cause and intent if identifying the activity provides additional information on the event. These codes should be used in conjunction with codes for external cause status (Y99) and place of occurrence (Y92).

This section contains the following broad activity categories:

Y93.0   Activities involving walking and running
Y93.1   Activities involving water and water craft
Y93.2   Activities involving ice and snow
Y93.3   Activities involving climbing, rappelling, and jumping off
Y93.4   Activities involving dancing and other rhythmic movement
Y93.5   Activities involving other sports and athletics played individually
Y93.6   Activities involving other sports and athletics played as a team or group
Y93.7   Activities involving other specified sports and athletics
Y93.A   Activities involving other cardiorespiratory exercise
Y93.B   Activities involving other muscle strengthening exercises
Y93.C   Activities involving computer technology and electronic devices
Y93.D   Activities involving arts and handcrafts
Y93.E   Activities involving personal hygiene and interior property and clothing maintenance
Y93.F   Activities involving caregiving
Y93.G   Activities involving food preparation, cooking and grilling
Y93.H   Activities involving exterior property and land maintenance, building and construction
Y93.I   Activities involving roller coasters and other types of external motion
Y93.J   Activities involving playing musical instrument
Y93.K   Activities involving animal care
Y93.8   Activities, other specified
Y93.9   Activity, unspecified

✓5ᵗʰ **Y93.0**   **Activities involving walking and running**
> EXCLUDES 1   activity, walking an animal (Y93.K1)
>   activity, walking or running on a treadmill (Y93.A1)

Y93.01   Activity, walking, marching and hiking
> Activity, walking, marching and hiking on level or elevated terrain
> EXCLUDES 1   activity, mountain climbing (Y93.31)

Y93.02   Activity, running

✓5ᵗʰ **Y93.1**   **Activities involving water and water craft**
> EXCLUDES 1   activities involving ice (Y93.2-)

Y93.11   Activity, swimming

Y93.12   Activity, springboard and platform diving

Y93.13   Activity, water polo

Y93.14   Activity, water aerobics and water exercise

Y93.15   Activity, underwater diving and snorkeling
> Activity, SCUBA diving

Y93.16   Activity, rowing, canoeing, kayaking, rafting and tubing
> Activity, canoeing, kayaking, rafting and tubing in calm and turbulent water

Y93.17   Activity, water skiing and wake boarding

Y93.18   Activity, surfing, windsurfing and boogie boarding
> Activity, water sliding

Y93.19   Activity, other involving water and watercraft
> Activity involving water NOS
> Activity, parasailing
> Activity, water survival training and testing

N Newborn: 0   P Pediatric: 0-17   M Maternity: 12-55   A Adult: 15-124   CH Comorbidity High   CL Comorbidity Low   NCDx Noncancer Dx   PDx Primary Dx

1198   ICD-10-CM 2020

√5ᵗʰ **Y93.2 Activities involving ice and snow**

EXCLUDES 1   *activity, shoveling ice and snow (Y93.H1)*

Y93.21 Activity, ice skating
Activity, figure skating (singles) (pairs)
Activity, ice dancing
EXCLUDES 1   *activity, ice hockey (Y93.22)*

Y93.22 Activity, ice hockey

Y93.23 Activity, snow (alpine) (downhill) skiing, snowboarding, sledding, tobogganing and snow tubing
EXCLUDES 1   *activity, cross country skiing (Y93.24)*

Y93.24 Activity, cross country skiing
Activity, nordic skiing

Y93.29 Activity, other involving ice and snow
Activity involving ice and snow NOS

√5ᵗʰ **Y93.3 Activities involving climbing, rappelling and jumping off**

EXCLUDES 1   *activity, hiking on level or elevated terrain (Y93.01)*
activity, jumping rope (Y93.56)
activity, trampoline jumping (Y93.44)

Y93.31 Activity, mountain climbing, rock climbing and wall climbing

Y93.32 Activity, rappelling

Y93.33 Activity, BASE jumping
Activity, Building, Antenna, Span, Earth jumping

Y93.34 Activity, bungee jumping

Y93.35 Activity, hang gliding

Y93.39 Activity, other involving climbing, rappelling and jumping off

√5ᵗʰ **Y93.4 Activities involving dancing and other rhythmic movement**

EXCLUDES 1   *activity, martial arts (Y93.75)*

Y93.41 Activity, dancing
AHA: 2012,4Q,108

Y93.42 Activity, yoga

Y93.43 Activity, gymnastics
Activity, rhythmic gymnastics
EXCLUDES 1   *activity, trampolining (Y93.44)*

Y93.44 Activity, trampolining

Y93.45 Activity, cheerleading

Y93.49 Activity, other involving dancing and other rhythmic movements

√5ᵗʰ **Y93.5 Activities involving other sports and athletics played individually**

EXCLUDES 1   *activity, dancing (Y93.41)*
activity, gymnastic (Y93.43)
activity, trampolining (Y93.44)
activity, yoga (Y93.42)

Y93.51 Activity, roller skating (inline) and skateboarding

Y93.52 Activity, horseback riding

Y93.53 Activity, golf

Y93.54 Activity, bowling

Y93.55 Activity, bike riding

Y93.56 Activity, jumping rope

Y93.57 Activity, non-running track and field events
EXCLUDES 1   *activity, running (any form) (Y93.02)*

Y93.59 Activity, other involving other sports and athletics played individually
EXCLUDES 1   *activities involving climbing, rappelling, and jumping (Y93.3-)*
activities involving ice and snow (Y93.2-)
activities involving walking and running (Y93.0-)
activities involving water and watercraft (Y93.1-)

√5ᵗʰ **Y93.6 Activities involving other sports and athletics played as a team or group**

EXCLUDES 1   *activity, ice hockey (Y93.22)*
activity, water polo (Y93.13)

Y93.61 Activity, American tackle football
Activity, football NOS

Y93.62 Activity, American flag or touch football

Y93.63 Activity, rugby

Y93.64 Activity, baseball
Activity, softball

Y93.65 Activity, lacrosse and field hockey

Y93.66 Activity, soccer

Y93.67 Activity, basketball

Y93.68 Activity, volleyball (beach) (court)

Y93.6A Activity, physical games generally associated with school recess, summer camp and children
Activity, capture the flag
Activity, dodge ball
Activity, four square
Activity, kickball

Y93.69 Activity, other involving other sports and athletics played as a team or group
Activity, cricket

√5ᵗʰ **Y93.7 Activities involving other specified sports and athletics**

Y93.71 Activity, boxing

Y93.72 Activity, wrestling

Y93.73 Activity, racquet and hand sports
Activity, handball
Activity, racquetball
Activity, squash
Activity, tennis

Y93.74 Activity, frisbee
Activity, ultimate frisbee

Y93.75 Activity, martial arts
Activity, combatives

Y93.79 Activity, other specified sports and athletics
EXCLUDES 1   *sports and athletics activities specified in categories Y93.0-Y93.6*

√5ᵗʰ **Y93.A Activities involving other cardiorespiratory exercise**
Activities involving physical training

Y93.A1 Activity, exercise machines primarily for cardiorespiratory conditioning
Activity, elliptical and stepper machines
Activity, stationary bike
Activity, treadmill

Y93.A2 Activity, calisthenics
Activity, jumping jacks
Activity, warm up and cool down

Y93.A3 Activity, aerobic and step exercise

Y93.A4 Activity, circuit training

Y93.A5 Activity, obstacle course
Activity, challenge course
Activity, confidence course

Y93.A6 Activity, grass drills
Activity, guerilla drills

Y93.A9 Activity, other involving cardiorespiratory exercise
EXCLUDES 1   *activities involving cardiorespiratory exercise specified in categories Y93.0-Y93.7*

√5ᵗʰ **Y93.B Activities involving other muscle strengthening exercises**

Y93.B1 Activity, exercise machines primarily for muscle strengthening

Y93.B2 Activity, push-ups, pull-ups, sit-ups

Y93.B3 Activity, free weights
Activity, barbells
Activity, dumbbells

Y93.B4 Activity, pilates

Y93.B9 Activity, other involving muscle strengthening exercises
EXCLUDES 1   *activities involving muscle strengthening specified in categories Y93.0-Y93.A*

√5ᵗʰ **Y93.C Activities involving computer technology and electronic devices**
EXCLUDES 1   *activity, electronic musical keyboard or instruments (Y93.J-)*

Y93.C1 Activity, computer keyboarding
Activity, electronic game playing using keyboard or other stationary device

Y93.C2 Activity, hand held interactive electronic device
Activity, cellular telephone and communication device
Activity, electronic game playing using interactive device
EXCLUDES 1   *activity, electronic game playing using keyboard or other stationary device (Y93.C1)*

Y93.C9 Activity, other involving computer technology and electronic devices

√5ᵗʰ **Y93.D Activities involving arts and handcrafts**
EXCLUDES 1   *activities involving playing musical instrument (Y93.J-)*

Y93.D1 Activity, knitting and crocheting

☑ Additional Character Required   √x7ᵗʰ Placeholder Alert   Manifestation   Unspecified Dx   ▶◀ Revised Text   ● New Code   ▲ Revised Title

Chapter 20. External Causes of Morbidity

Y93.D2   **Activity,** sewing
Y93.D3   **Activity,** furniture building and finishing
     Activity, furniture repair
Y93.D9   **Activity, other involving arts and handcrafts**
✓5ᵗʰ **Y93.E**   **Activities involving personal hygiene and interior property and clothing maintenance**
     EXCLUDES 1   *activities involving cooking and grilling (Y93.G-)*
         activities involving exterior property and land maintenance, building and construction (Y93.H-)
         activities involving caregiving (Y93.F-)
         activity, dishwashing (Y93.G1)
         activity, food preparation (Y93.G1)
         activity, gardening (Y93.H2)
Y93.E1   **Activity,** personal bathing and showering
Y93.E2   **Activity,** laundry
Y93.E3   **Activity,** vacuuming
Y93.E4   **Activity,** ironing
Y93.E5   **Activity,** floor mopping and cleaning
Y93.E6   **Activity,** residential relocation
     Activity, packing up and unpacking involved in moving to a new residence
Y93.E8   **Activity, other personal hygiene**
Y93.E9   **Activity, other interior property and clothing maintenance**
✓5ᵗʰ **Y93.F**   **Activities involving** caregiving
     Activity involving the provider of caregiving
Y93.F1   **Activity, caregiving,** bathing
Y93.F2   **Activity, caregiving,** lifting
Y93.F9   **Activity, other caregiving**
✓5ᵗʰ **Y93.G**   **Activities involving food preparation, cooking and grilling**
Y93.G1   **Activity,** food preparation and clean up
     Activity, dishwashing
Y93.G2   **Activity,** grilling and smoking food
Y93.G3   **Activity,** cooking and baking
     Activity, use of stove, oven and microwave oven
Y93.G9   **Activity, other involving cooking and grilling**
✓5ᵗʰ **Y93.H**   **Activities involving exterior property and land maintenance, building and construction**
Y93.H1   **Activity,** digging, shoveling and raking
     Activity, dirt digging
     Activity, raking leaves
     Activity, snow shoveling
Y93.H2   **Activity,** gardening and landscaping
     Activity, pruning, trimming shrubs, weeding
Y93.H3   **Activity,** building and construction
Y93.H9   **Activity, other involving exterior property and land maintenance, building and construction**
✓5ᵗʰ **Y93.I**   **Activities involving roller coasters and other types of external motion**
Y93.I1   **Activity,** rollercoaster riding
Y93.I9   **Activity, other involving external motion**
✓5ᵗʰ **Y93.J**   **Activities involving playing musical instrument**
     Activity involving playing electric musical instrument
Y93.J1   **Activity,** piano **playing**
     Activity, musical keyboard (electronic) playing
Y93.J2   **Activity,** drum and other percussion instrument **playing**
Y93.J3   **Activity,** string instrument **playing**
Y93.J4   **Activity,** winds and brass instrument **playing**
✓5ᵗʰ **Y93.K**   **Activities involving animal care**
     EXCLUDES 1   *activity, horseback riding (Y93.52)*
Y93.K1   **Activity,** walking **an animal**
Y93.K2   **Activity,** milking **an animal**
Y93.K3   **Activity,** grooming and shearing **an animal**
Y93.K9   **Activity, other involving animal care**
✓5ᵗʰ **Y93.8**   **Activities, other specified**
Y93.81   **Activity,** refereeing **a sports activity**
Y93.82   **Activity,** spectator **at an event**
Y93.83   **Activity,** rough housing and horseplay
Y93.84   **Activity,** sleeping

Y93.85   **Activity,** choking game
     Activity, blackout game
     Activity, fainting game
     Activity, pass out game
     AHA: 2016,4Q,74-76
Y93.89   **Activity, other specified**
Y93.9   **Activity, unspecified**
Y95   **Nosocomial condition**
     AHA: 2013,4Q,119
✓4ᵗʰ **Y99**   **External cause status**
     NOTE   A single code from category Y99 should be used in conjunction with the external cause code(s) assigned to a record to indicate the status of the person at the time the event occurred.
Y99.0   **Civilian activity done for income or pay**
     Civilian activity done for financial or other compensation
     EXCLUDES 1   *military activity (Y99.1)*
         volunteer activity (Y99.2)
Y99.1   **Military activity**
     EXCLUDES 1   *activity of off duty military personnel (Y99.8)*
Y99.2   **Volunteer activity**
     EXCLUDES 1   *activity of child or other family member assisting in compensated work of other family member (Y99.8)*
Y99.8   **Other external cause status**
     Activity NEC
     Activity of child or other family member assisting in compensated work of other family member
     Hobby not done for income
     Leisure activity
     Off-duty activity of military personnel
     Recreation or sport not for income or while a student
     Student activity
     EXCLUDES 1   *civilian activity done for income or compensation (Y99.0)*
         military activity (Y99.1)
     AHA: 2012,4Q,108
Y99.9   **Unspecified external cause status**

N Newborn: 0   P Pediatric: 0-17   M Maternity: 12-55   A Adult: 15-124   CH Comorbidity High   CL Comorbidity Low   NC Dx Noncancer Dx   PDx Primary Dx

1200   ICD-10-CM 2020

Chapter 21. Factors Influencing Health Status and Contact with Health Services (Z00–Z99)

Chapter-specific Guidelines with Coding Examples

The chapter-specific guidelines from the ICD-10-CM Official Guidelines for Coding and Reporting have been provided below. Along with these guidelines are coding examples, contained in the shaded boxes, that have been developed to help illustrate the coding and/or sequencing guidance found in these guidelines.

Note: The chapter-specific guidelines provide additional information about the use of Z codes for specified encounters.

a. Use of Z Codes in any healthcare setting

Z codes are for use in any healthcare setting. Z codes may be used as either a first-listed (principal diagnosis code in the inpatient setting) or secondary code, depending on the circumstances of the encounter. Certain Z codes may only be used as first-listed or principal diagnosis.

> Patient with middle lobe lung cancer admitted for observation and discontinuation of chemotherapy
>
> **Z51.11   Encounter for antineoplastic chemotherapy**
>
> **C34.2   Malignant neoplasm of middle lobe, bronchus or lung**
>
> *Explanation:* A Z code can be used as first-listed in this situation based on guidelines in this chapter as well as chapter 2, "Neoplasms."

b. Z Codes indicate a reason for an encounter

Z codes are not procedure codes. A corresponding procedure code must accompany a Z code to describe any procedure performed.

c. Categories of Z Codes

1) Contact/exposure

Category Z20 indicates contact with, and suspected exposure to, communicable diseases. These codes are for patients who do not show any sign or symptom of a disease but are suspected to have been exposed to it by close personal contact with an infected individual or are in an area where a disease is epidemic.

Category Z77, Other contact with and (suspected) exposures hazardous to health, indicates contact with and suspected exposures hazardous to health.

Contact/exposure codes may be used as a first-listed code to explain an encounter for testing, or, more commonly, as a secondary code to identify a potential risk.

2) Inoculations and vaccinations

Code Z23 is for encounters for inoculations and vaccinations. It indicates that a patient is being seen to receive a prophylactic inoculation against a disease. Procedure codes are required to identify the actual administration of the injection and the type(s) of immunizations given. Code Z23 may be used as a secondary code if the inoculation is given as a routine part of preventive health care, such as a well-baby visit.

3) Status

Status codes indicate that a patient is either a carrier of a disease or has the sequelae or residual of a past disease or condition. This includes such things as the presence of prosthetic or mechanical devices resulting from past treatment. A status code is informative, because the status may affect the course of treatment and its outcome. A status code is distinct from a history code. The history code indicates that the patient no longer has the condition.

A status code should not be used with a diagnosis code from one of the body system chapters, if the diagnosis code includes the information provided by the status code. For example, code Z94.1, Heart transplant status, should not be used with a code from subcategory T86.2, Complications of heart transplant. The status code does not provide additional information. The complication code indicates that the patient is a heart transplant patient.

For encounters for weaning from a mechanical ventilator, assign a code from subcategory J96.1, Chronic respiratory failure, followed by code Z99.11, Dependence on respirator [ventilator] status.

The status Z codes/categories are:

Z14   Genetic carrier

Genetic carrier status indicates that a person carries a gene, associated with a particular disease, which may be passed to offspring who may develop that disease. The person does not have the disease and is not at risk of developing the disease.

Z15   Genetic susceptibility to disease

Genetic susceptibility indicates that a person has a gene that increases the risk of that person developing the disease.

Codes from category Z15 should not be used as principal or first-listed codes. If the patient has the condition to which he/she is susceptible, and that condition is the reason for the encounter, the code for the current condition should be sequenced first. If the patient is being seen for follow-up after completed treatment for this condition, and the condition no longer exists, a follow-up code should be sequenced first, followed by the appropriate personal history and genetic susceptibility codes. If the purpose of the encounter is genetic counseling associated with procreative management, code Z31.5, Encounter for genetic counseling, should be assigned as the first-listed code, followed by a code from category Z15. Additional codes should be assigned for any applicable family or personal history.

Z16   Resistance to antimicrobial drugs

This code indicates that a patient has a condition that is resistant to antimicrobial drug treatment. Sequence the infection code first.

Z17   Estrogen receptor status

Z18   Retained foreign body fragments

Z19   Hormone sensitivity malignancy status

Z21   Asymptomatic HIV infection status

This code indicates that a patient has tested positive for HIV but has manifested no signs or symptoms of the disease.

Z22   Carrier of infectious disease

Carrier status indicates that a person harbors the specific organisms of a disease without manifest symptoms and is capable of transmitting the infection.

Z28.3   Underimmunization status

Z33.1   Pregnant state, incidental

This code is a secondary code only for use when the pregnancy is in no way complicating the reason for visit. Otherwise, a code from the obstetric chapter is required.

Z66   Do not resuscitate

This code may be used when it is documented by the provider that a patient is on do not resuscitate status at any time during the stay.

Z67   Blood type

Z68   Body mass index (BMI)

BMI codes should only be assigned when **there is an associated, reportable diagnosis (such as obesity).** Do not assign BMI codes during pregnancy.

See Section I.B.14 for BMI documentation by clinicians other than the patient's provider.

Z74.01   Bed confinement status

Z76.82   Awaiting organ transplant status

Z78   Other specified health status

Code Z78.1, Physical restraint status, may be used when it is documented by the provider that a patient has been put in restraints during the current encounter. Please note that this code should not be reported when it is documented by the provider that a patient is temporarily restrained during a procedure.

Z79   Long-term (current) drug therapy

Codes from this category indicate a patient's continuous use of a prescribed drug (including such things as aspirin therapy) for the long-term treatment of a condition or for prophylactic use. It is not for use for patients who have addictions to drugs. This subcategory is not for use of medications for detoxification or maintenance programs to prevent withdrawal symptoms in patients with drug dependence (e.g., methadone maintenance for opiate dependence). Assign the appropriate code for the drug dependence instead.

Assign a code from Z79 if the patient is receiving a medication for an extended period as a prophylactic measure (such as for the prevention of deep vein thrombosis) or as treatment of a chronic condition (such as arthritis) or a disease requiring a lengthy course of treatment (such as cancer). Do not assign a code from category Z79 for medication being administered for a brief period of time to treat an acute illness or injury (such as a course of antibiotics to treat acute bronchitis).

Z88	Allergy status to drugs, medicaments and biological substances

Except: Z88.9, Allergy status to unspecified drugs, medicaments and biological substances status

Z89	Acquired absence of limb
Z90	Acquired absence of organs, not elsewhere classified
Z91.0-	Allergy status, other than to drugs and biological substances
Z92.82	Status post administration of tPA (rtPA) in a different facility within the last 24 hours prior to admission to a current facility

Assign code Z92.82, Status post administration of tPA (rtPA) in a different facility within the last 24 hours prior to admission to current facility, as a secondary diagnosis when a patient is received by transfer into a facility and documentation indicates they were administered tissue plasminogen activator (tPA) within the last 24 hours prior to admission to the current facility.

This guideline applies even if the patient is still receiving the tPA at the time they are received into the current facility.

The appropriate code for the condition for which the tPA was administered (such as cerebrovascular disease or myocardial infarction) should be assigned first.

Code Z92.82 is only applicable to the receiving facility record and not to the transferring facility record.

Z93	Artificial opening status
Z94	Transplanted organ and tissue status
Z95	Presence of cardiac and vascular implants and grafts
Z96	Presence of other functional implants
Z97	Presence of other devices
Z98	Other postprocedural states

Assign code Z98.85, Transplanted organ removal status, to indicate that a transplanted organ has been previously removed. This code should not be assigned for the encounter in which the transplanted organ is removed. The complication necessitating removal of the transplant organ should be assigned for that encounter.

See section I.C19. for information on the coding of organ transplant complications.

Z99	Dependence on enabling machines and devices, not elsewhere classified

Note: Categories Z89-Z90 and Z93-Z99 are for use only if there are no complications or malfunctions of the organ or tissue replaced, the amputation site or the equipment on which the patient is dependent..

4) History (of)

There are two types of history Z codes, personal and family. Personal history codes explain a patient's past medical condition that no longer exists and is not receiving any treatment, but that has the potential for recurrence, and therefore may require continued monitoring.

Family history codes are for use when a patient has a family member(s) who has had a particular disease that causes the patient to be at higher risk of also contracting the disease.

Personal history codes may be used in conjunction with follow-up codes and family history codes may be used in conjunction with screening codes to explain the need for a test or procedure. History codes are also acceptable on any medical record regardless of the reason for visit. A history of an illness, even if no longer present, is important information that may alter the type of treatment ordered.

The history Z code categories are:

Z80	Family history of primary malignant neoplasm
Z81	Family history of mental and behavioral disorders
Z82	Family history of certain disabilities and chronic diseases (leading to disablement)
Z83	Family history of other specific disorders
Z84	Family history of other conditions
Z85	Personal history of malignant neoplasm
Z86	Personal history of certain other diseases

Z87	Personal history of other diseases and conditions
Z91.4-	Personal history of psychological trauma, not elsewhere classified
Z91.5	Personal history of self-harm
Z91.81	History of falling
Z91.82	Personal history of military deployment
Z92	Personal history of medical treatment

Except: Z92.0, Personal history of contraception

Except: Z92.82, Status post administration of tPA (rtPA) in a different facility within the last 24 hours prior to admission to a current facility

5) Screening

Screening is the testing for disease or disease precursors in seemingly well individuals so that early detection and treatment can be provided for those who test positive for the disease (e.g., screening mammogram).

The testing of a person to rule out or confirm a suspected diagnosis because the patient has some sign or symptom is a diagnostic examination, not a screening. In these cases, the sign or symptom is used to explain the reason for the test.

A screening code may be a first-listed code if the reason for the visit is specifically the screening exam. It may also be used as an additional code if the screening is done during an office visit for other health problems. A screening code is not necessary if the screening is inherent to a routine examination, such as a pap smear done during a routine pelvic examination.

Should a condition be discovered during the screening then the code for the condition may be assigned as an additional diagnosis.

The Z code indicates that a screening exam is planned. A procedure code is required to confirm that the screening was performed.

The screening Z codes/categories:

Z11	Encounter for screening for infectious and parasitic diseases
Z12	Encounter for screening for malignant neoplasms
Z13	Encounter for screening for other diseases and disorders

Except: Z13.9, Encounter for screening, unspecified

Z36	Encounter for antenatal screening for mother

6) Observation

There are three observation Z code categories. They are for use in very limited circumstances when a person is being observed for a suspected condition that is ruled out. The observation codes are not for use if an injury or illness or any signs or symptoms related to the suspected condition are present. In such cases the diagnosis/symptom code is used with the corresponding external cause code.

The observation codes are to be used as principal diagnosis only. The only exception to this is when the principal diagnosis is required to be a code from category Z38, Liveborn infants according to place of birth and type of delivery. Then a code from category Z05, Encounter for observation and evaluation of newborn for suspected diseases and conditions ruled out, is sequenced after the Z38 code. Additional codes may be used in addition to the observation code but only if they are unrelated to the suspected condition being observed.

Codes from subcategory Z03.7, Encounter for suspected maternal and fetal conditions ruled out, may either be used as a first-listed or as an additional code assignment depending on the case. They are for use in very limited circumstances on a maternal record when an encounter is for a suspected maternal or fetal condition that is ruled out during that encounter (for example, a maternal or fetal condition may be suspected due to an abnormal test result). These codes should not be used when the condition is confirmed. In those cases, the confirmed condition should be coded. In addition, these codes are not for use if an illness or any signs or symptoms related to the suspected condition or problem are present. In such cases the diagnosis/symptom code is used.

Additional codes may be used in addition to the code from subcategory Z03.7, but only if they are unrelated to the suspected condition being evaluated.

Codes from subcategory Z03.7 may not be used for encounters for antenatal screening of mother. *See Section I.C.21. Screening.*

For encounters for suspected fetal condition that are inconclusive following testing and evaluation, assign the appropriate code from category O35, O36, O40 or O41.

The observation Z code categories:

Z03   Encounter for medical observation for suspected diseases and conditions ruled out

Z04   Encounter for examination and observation for other reasons
      Except: Z04.9, Encounter for examination and observation for unspecified reason

Z05   Encounter for observation and evaluation of newborn for suspected diseases and conditions ruled out

7) Aftercare

Aftercare visit codes cover situations when the initial treatment of a disease has been performed and the patient requires continued care during the healing or recovery phase, or for the long-term consequences of the disease. The aftercare Z code should not be used if treatment is directed at a current, acute disease. The diagnosis code is to be used in these cases. Exceptions to this rule are codes Z51.0, Encounter for antineoplastic radiation therapy, and codes from subcategory Z51.1, Encounter for antineoplastic chemotherapy and immunotherapy. These codes are to be first-listed, followed by the diagnosis code when a patient's encounter is solely to receive radiation therapy, chemotherapy, or immunotherapy for the treatment of a neoplasm. If the reason for the encounter is more than one type of antineoplastic therapy, code Z51.0 and a code from subcategory Z51.1 may be assigned together, in which case one of these codes would be reported as a secondary diagnosis.

The aftercare Z codes should also not be used for aftercare for injuries. For aftercare of an injury, assign the acute injury code with the appropriate 7th character (for subsequent encounter).

The aftercare codes are generally first-listed to explain the specific reason for the encounter. An aftercare code may be used as an additional code when some type of aftercare is provided in addition to the reason for admission and no diagnosis code is applicable. An example of this would be the closure of a colostomy during an encounter for treatment of another condition.

Aftercare codes should be used in conjunction with other aftercare codes or diagnosis codes to provide better detail on the specifics of an aftercare encounter visit, unless otherwise directed by the classification. The sequencing of multiple aftercare codes depends on the circumstances of the encounter.

Certain aftercare Z code categories need a secondary diagnosis code to describe the resolving condition or sequelae. For others, the condition is included in the code title.

Additional Z code aftercare category terms include fitting and adjustment, and attention to artificial openings.

Status Z codes may be used with aftercare Z codes to indicate the nature of the aftercare. For example code Z95.1, Presence of aortocoronary bypass graft, may be used with code Z48.812, Encounter for surgical aftercare following surgery on the circulatory system, to indicate the surgery for which the aftercare is being performed. A status code should not be used when the aftercare code indicates the type of status, such as using Z43.0, Encounter for attention to tracheostomy, with Z93.0, Tracheostomy status.

The aftercare Z category/codes:

Z42   Encounter for plastic and reconstructive surgery following medical procedure or healed injury

Z43   Encounter for attention to artificial openings

Z44   Encounter for fitting and adjustment of external prosthetic device

Z45   Encounter for adjustment and management of implanted device

Z46   Encounter for fitting and adjustment of other devices

Z47   Orthopedic aftercare

Z48   Encounter for other postprocedural aftercare

Z49   Encounter for care involving renal dialysis

Z51   Encounter for other aftercare and medical care

Patient admitted post right total knee replacement for physical therapy

Z47.1   Aftercare following joint replacement surgery

Z96.651   Presence of right artificial knee joint

Explanation: An elective joint replacement, that is one done by choice and not to correct a fracture or other injury, should reported by the post-acute care provider by using code Z47.1. Guidelines for the assignment of Z47.1 include instructions to "use additional code to identify the joint."

8) Follow-up

The follow-up codes are used to explain continuing surveillance following completed treatment of a disease, condition, or injury. They imply that the condition has been fully treated and no longer exists. They should not be confused with aftercare codes, or injury codes with a 7th character for subsequent encounter, that explain ongoing care of a healing condition or its sequelae. Follow-up codes may be used in conjunction with history codes to provide the full picture of the healed condition and its treatment. The follow-up code is sequenced first, followed by the history code.

A follow-up code may be used to explain multiple visits. Should a condition be found to have recurred on the follow-up visit, then the diagnosis code for the condition should be assigned in place of the follow-up code.

The follow-up Z code categories:

Z08   Encounter for follow-up examination after completed treatment for malignant neoplasm

Z09   Encounter for follow-up examination after completed treatment for conditions other than malignant neoplasm

Z39   Encounter for maternal postpartum care and examination

9) Donor

Codes in category Z52, Donors of organs and tissues, are used for living individuals who are donating blood or other body tissue. These codes are only for individuals donating for others, not for self-donations. They are not used to identify cadaveric donations.

10) Counseling

Counseling Z codes are used when a patient or family member receives assistance in the aftermath of an illness or injury, or when support is required in coping with family or social problems.

The counseling Z codes/categories:

Z30.0-   Encounter for general counseling and advice on contraception

Z31.5   Encounter for procreative genetic counseling

Z31.6-   Encounter for general counseling and advice on procreation

Z32.2   Encounter for childbirth instruction

Z32.3   Encounter for childcare instruction

Z69   Encounter for mental health services for victim and perpetrator of abuse

Z70   Counseling related to sexual attitude, behavior and orientation

Z71   Persons encountering health services for other counseling and medical advice, not elsewhere classified

Note: Code Z71.84, Encounter for health counseling related to travel, is to be used for health risk and safety counseling for future travel purposes.

Z76.81   Expectant mother prebirth pediatrician visit

11) Encounters for obstetrical and reproductive services

See Section I.C.15. Pregnancy, Childbirth, and the Puerperium, for further instruction on the use of these codes.

Z codes for pregnancy are for use in those circumstances when none of the problems or complications included in the codes from the Obstetrics chapter exist (a routine prenatal visit or postpartum care). Codes in category Z34, Encounter for supervision of normal pregnancy, are always first-listed and are not to be used with any other code from the OB chapter.

Codes in category Z3A, Weeks of gestation, may be assigned to provide additional information about the pregnancy. Category Z3A codes should not be assigned for pregnancies with abortive outcomes (categories O00-O08), elective termination of pregnancy (code Z33.2), nor for postpartum conditions, as category Z3A is not applicable to these conditions. The date of the admission should be used to determine weeks of gestation for inpatient admissions that encompass more than one gestational week.

The outcome of delivery, category Z37, should be included on all maternal delivery records. It is always a secondary code. Codes in category Z37 should not be used on the newborn record.

Z codes for family planning (contraceptive) or procreative management and counseling should be included on an obstetric record either during the pregnancy or the postpartum stage, if applicable.

Z codes/categories for obstetrical and reproductive services:

Z30	Encounter for contraceptive management
Z31	Encounter for procreative management
Z32.2	Encounter for childbirth instruction
Z32.3	Encounter for childcare instruction
Z33	Pregnant state
Z34	Encounter for supervision of normal pregnancy
Z36	Encounter for antenatal screening of mother
Z3A	Weeks of gestation
Z37	Outcome of delivery
Z39	Encounter for maternal postpartum care and examination
Z76.81	Expectant mother prebirth pediatrician visit

12) Newborns and infants

See Section I.C.16. Newborn (Perinatal) Guidelines, for further instruction on the use of these codes.

Newborn Z codes/categories:

Z76.1	Encounter for health supervision and care of foundling
Z00.1-	Encounter for routine child health examination
Z38	Liveborn infants according to place of birth and type of delivery

13) Routine and administrative examinations

The Z codes allow for the description of encounters for routine examinations, such as, a general check-up, or, examinations for administrative purposes, such as, a pre-employment physical. The codes are not to be used if the examination is for diagnosis of a suspected condition or for treatment purposes. In such cases the diagnosis code is used. During a routine exam, should a diagnosis or condition be discovered, it should be coded as an additional code. Pre-existing and chronic conditions and history codes may also be included as additional codes as long as the examination is for administrative purposes and not focused on any particular condition.

Some of the codes for routine health examinations distinguish between "with" and "without" abnormal findings. Code assignment depends on the information that is known at the time the encounter is being coded. For example, if no abnormal findings were found during the examination, but the encounter is being coded before test results are back, it is acceptable to assign the code for "without abnormal findings." When assigning a code for "with abnormal findings," additional code(s) should be assigned to identify the specific abnormal finding(s).

Pre-operative examination and pre-procedural laboratory examination Z codes are for use only in those situations when a patient is being cleared for a procedure or surgery and no treatment is given.

The Z codes/categories for routine and administrative examinations:

Z00	Encounter for general examination without complaint, suspected or reported diagnosis
Z01	Encounter for other special examination without complaint, suspected or reported diagnosis
Z02	Encounter for administrative examination
	Except: Z02.9, Encounter for administrative examinations, unspecified
Z32.0-	Encounter for pregnancy test

14) Miscellaneous Z codes

The miscellaneous Z codes capture a number of other health care encounters that do not fall into one of the other categories. Certain of these codes identify the reason for the encounter; others are for use as additional codes that provide useful information on circumstances that may affect a patient's care and treatment.

Patient has Asperger's syndrome and wanders.

F84.5   Asperger's syndrome

Z91.83   Wandering in diseases classified elsewhere

Explanation: Code Z91.83 is a miscellaneous Z code that provides additional insight into this patient's Asperger's diagnosis. Care provided to an Asperger's patient who wanders or elopes may be different than for an Asperger's patient who does not wander.

Prophylactic organ removal

For encounters specifically for prophylactic removal of an organ (such as prophylactic removal of breasts due to a genetic susceptibility to cancer or a family history of cancer), the principal or first-listed code should be a code from category Z40, Encounter for prophylactic surgery, followed by the appropriate codes to identify the associated risk factor (such as genetic susceptibility or family history).

If the patient has a malignancy of one site and is having prophylactic removal at another site to prevent either a new primary malignancy or metastatic disease, a code for the malignancy should also be assigned in addition to a code from subcategory Z40.0, Encounter for prophylactic surgery for risk factors related to malignant neoplasms. A Z40.0 code should not be assigned if the patient is having organ removal for treatment of a malignancy, such as the removal of the testes for the treatment of prostate cancer.

Miscellaneous Z codes/categories:

Z28	Immunization not carried out
	Except: Z28.3, Underimmunization status
Z29	Encounter for other prophylactic measures
Z40	Encounter for prophylactic surgery
Z41	Encounter for procedures for purposes other than remedying health state
	Except: Z41.9, Encounter for procedure for purposes other than remedying health state, unspecified
Z53	Persons encountering health services for specific procedures and treatment, not carried out
Z55	Problems related to education and literacy
Z56	Problems related to employment and unemployment
Z57	Occupational exposure to risk factors
Z58	Problems related to physical environment
Z59	Problems related to housing and economic circumstances
Z60	Problems related to social environment
Z62	Problems related to upbringing
Z63	Other problems related to primary support group, including family circumstances
Z64	Problems related to certain psychosocial circumstances
Z65	Problems related to other psychosocial circumstances
Z72	Problems related to lifestyle
	Note: These codes should be assigned only when the documentation specifies that the patient has an associated problem
Z73	Problems related to life management difficulty
Z74	Problems related to care provider dependency
	Except: Z74.01, Bed confinement status
Z75	Problems related to medical facilities and other health care
Z76.0	Encounter for issue of repeat prescription
Z76.3	Healthy person accompanying sick person
Z76.4	Other boarder to healthcare facility
Z76.5	Malingerer [conscious simulation]
Z91.1-	Patient's noncompliance with medical treatment and regimen
Z91.83	Wandering in diseases classified elsewhere
Z91.84-	Oral health risk factors
Z91.89	Other specified personal risk factors, not elsewhere classified

See Section I.B.14 for Z55-Z65 Persons with potential health hazards related to socioeconomic and psychosocial circumstances, documentation by clinicians other than the patient's provider

15) Nonspecific Z codes

Certain Z codes are so non-specific, or potentially redundant with other codes in the classification, that there can be little justification for their use in the inpatient setting. Their use in the outpatient setting should be limited to those instances when there is no further documentation to permit more precise coding. Otherwise, any sign or symptom or any other reason for visit that is captured in another code should be used.

Nonspecific Z codes/categories:

Z02.9	Encounter for administrative examinations, unspecified
Z04.9	Encounter for examination and observation for unspecified reason
Z13.9	Encounter for screening, unspecified
Z41.9	Encounter for procedure for purposes other than remedying health state, unspecified
Z52.9	Donor of unspecified organ or tissue

Z86.59   Personal history of other mental and behavioral disorders

Z88.9   Allergy status to unspecified drugs, medicaments and biological substances status

Z92.0   Personal history of contraception

16) Z codes that may only be principal/first-listed diagnosis

The following Z codes/categories may only be reported as the principal/first-listed diagnosis, except when there are multiple encounters on the same day and the medical records for the encounters are combined:

Z00   Encounter for general examination without complaint, suspected or reported diagnosis
  Except: Z00.6

Z01   Encounter for other special examination without complaint, suspected or reported diagnosis

Z02   Encounter for administrative examination

Z03   Encounter for medical observation for suspected diseases and conditions ruled out

Z04   Encounter for examination and observation for other reasons

Z33.2   Encounter for elective termination of pregnancy

Z31.81   Encounter for male factor infertility in female patient

Z31.82   Encounter for Rh incompatibility status

Z31.83   Encounter for assisted reproductive fertility procedure cycle

Z31.84   Encounter for fertility preservation procedure

Z34   Encounter for supervision of normal pregnancy

Z39   Encounter for maternal postpartum care and examination

Z38   Liveborn infants according to place of birth and type of delivery

Z40   Encounter for prophylactic surgery

Z42   Encounter for plastic and reconstructive surgery following medical procedure or healed injury

Z51.0   Encounter for antineoplastic radiation therapy

Z51.1-   Encounter for antineoplastic chemotherapy and immunotherapy

Z52   Donors of organs and tissues
  Except: Z52.9, Donor of unspecified organ or tissue

Z76.1   Encounter for health supervision and care of foundling

Z76.2   Encounter for health supervision and care of other healthy infant and child

Z99.12   Encounter for respirator [ventilator] dependence during power failure

Chapter 21. Factors Influencing Health Status and Contact With Health Services (Z00-Z99)

NOTE   Z codes represent reasons for encounters. A corresponding procedure code must accompany a Z code if a procedure is performed. Categories Z00-Z99 are provided for occasions when circumstances other than a disease, injury or external cause classifiable to categories A00-Y89 are recorded as "diagnoses" or "problems." This can arise in two main ways:

(a) When a person who may or may not be sick encounters the health services for some specific purpose, such as to receive limited care or service for a current condition, to donate an organ or tissue, to receive prophylactic vaccination (immunization), or to discuss a problem which is in itself not a disease or injury.

(b) When some circumstance or problem is present which influences the person's health status but is not in itself a current illness or injury.

AHA: 2018,4Q,60-61

This chapter contains the following blocks:

Z00-Z13	Persons encountering health services for examinations
Z14-Z15	Genetic carrier and genetic susceptibility to disease
Z16	Resistance to antimicrobial drugs
Z17	Estrogen receptor status
Z18	Retained foreign body fragments
Z19	Hormone sensitivity malignancy status
Z20-Z29	Persons with potential health hazards related to communicable diseases
Z30-Z39	Persons encountering health services in circumstances related to reproduction
Z40-Z53	Encounters for other specific health care
Z55-Z65	Persons with potential health hazards related to socioeconomic and psychosocial circumstances
Z66	Do not resuscitate status
Z67	Blood type
Z68	Body mass index (BMI)
Z69-Z76	Persons encountering health services in other circumstances
Z77-Z99	Persons with potential health hazards related to family and personal history and certain conditions influencing health status

Persons encountering health services for examinations (Z00-Z13)

NOTE   Nonspecific abnormal findings disclosed at the time of these examinations are classified to categories R70-R94.

EXCLUDES 1   examinations related to pregnancy and reproduction (Z30-Z36, Z39.-)

√4ᵗʰ Z00 Encounter for general examination without complaint, suspected or reported diagnosis

     EXCLUDES 1   encounter for examination for administrative purposes (Z02.-)

     EXCLUDES 2   encounter for pre-procedural examinations (Z01.81-)

                 special screening examinations (Z11-Z13)

     AHA: 2017,4Q,95

√5ᵗʰ Z00.0 Encounter for general adult medical examination

     Encounter for adult periodic examination (annual) (physical) and any associated laboratory and radiologic examinations

     EXCLUDES 1   encounter for examination of sign or symptom — code to sign or symptom

                 general health check-up of infant or child (Z00.12-)

Z00.00 Encounter for general adult medical examination without abnormal findings   **PDx** **A**

     Encounter for adult health check-up NOS

     AHA: 2016,1Q,36

Z00.01 Encounter for general adult medical examination with abnormal findings   **PDx** **A**

     Use additional code to identify abnormal findings

     AHA: 2016,1Q,35-36

√5ᵗʰ Z00.1 Encounter for newborn, infant and child health examinations

√6ᵗʰ Z00.11 Newborn health examination

     Health check for child under 29 days old

     Use additional code to identify any abnormal findings

     EXCLUDES 1   health check for child over 28 days old (Z00.12-)

Z00.110 Health examination for newborn under 8 days old   **PDx** **N**

     Health check for newborn under 8 days old

Z00.111 Health examination for newborn 8 to 28 days old   **PDx** **N**

     Health check for newborn 8 to 28 days old

     Newborn weight check

√6ᵗʰ Z00.12 Encounter for routine child **health examination**

     Health check (routine) for child over 28 days old

     Immunizations appropriate for age

     Routine developmental screening of infant or child

     Routine vison and hearing testing

     EXCLUDES 1   health check for child under 29 days old (Z00.11-)

                 health supervision of foundling or other healthy infant or child (Z76.1-Z76.2)

                 newborn health examination (Z00.11-)

     AHA: 2018,4Q,36

Z00.121 Encounter for routine child health examination with abnormal findings   **PDx** **P**

     Use additional code to identify abnormal findings

     AHA: 2016,1Q,34-35

Z00.129 Encounter for routine child health examination without abnormal findings   **PDx** **P**

     Encounter for routine child health examination NOS

     AHA: 2016,1Q,34

Z00.2 Encounter for examination for period of rapid growth in childhood   **PDx** **P**

Z00.3 Encounter for examination for adolescent development **state**   **PDx** **P**

     Encounter for puberty development state

Z00.5 Encounter for examination of potential donor of organ and tissue   **PDx**

Z00.6 Encounter for examination for normal comparison and control in clinical research program   **PDx**

     Examination of participant or control in clinical research program

√5ᵗʰ Z00.7 Encounter for examination for period of delayed growth in childhood

Z00.70 Encounter for examination for period of delayed growth in childhood without abnormal findings   **PDx** **P**

Z00.71 Encounter for examination for period of delayed growth in childhood with abnormal findings   **PDx** **P**

     Use additional code to identify abnormal findings

Z00.8 Encounter for other general examination   **PDx**

     Encounter for health examination in population surveys

√4ᵗʰ Z01 Encounter for other special examination **without complaint, suspected or reported diagnosis**

     INCLUDES   routine examination of specific system

     NOTE   Codes from category Z01 represent the reason for the encounter. A separate procedure code is required to identify any examinations or procedures performed

     EXCLUDES 1   encounter for examination for administrative purposes (Z02.-)

                 encounter for examination for suspected conditions, proven not to exist (Z03.-)

                 encounter for laboratory and radiologic examinations as a component of general medical examinations (Z00.0-)

                 encounter for laboratory, radiologic and imaging examinations for sign(s) and symptom(s) — code to the sign(s) or symptom(s)

     EXCLUDES 2   screening examinations (Z11-Z13)

√5ᵗʰ Z01.0 Encounter for examination of eyes and vision

     EXCLUDES 1   examination for driving license (Z02.4)

Z01.00 Encounter for examination of eyes and vision without abnormal findings   **PDx**

     Encounter for examination of eyes and vision NOS

Z01.01 Encounter for examination of eyes and vision with abnormal findings   **PDx**

     Use additional code to identify abnormal findings

     AHA: 2016,4Q,21

N Newborn: 0   **P** Pediatric: 0-17   **M** Maternity: 12-55   **A** Adult: 15-124   **CH** Comorbidity High   **CL** Comorbidity Low   **NCDx** Noncancer Dx   **PDx** Primary Dx

1206   ICD-10-CM 2020

● ☑6ᵗʰ **Z01.02 Encounter for examination of eyes and vision following failed vision screening**

EXCLUDES 1   *examination for examination of eyes and vision with abnormal findings (Z01.01)*

examination for examination of eyes and vision without abnormal findings (Z01.00)

● **Z01.020 Encounter for examination of eyes and vision following failed vision screening without abnormal findings** PDx

● **Z01.021 Encounter for examination of eyes and vision following failed vision screening with abnormal findings** PDx

Use additional code to identify abnormal findings

☑5ᵗʰ **Z01.1 Encounter for examination of ears and hearing**

Z01.10 Encounter for examination of ears and hearing without abnormal findings PDx

Encounter for examination of ears and hearing NOS

AHA: 2016,4Q,24

☑6ᵗʰ **Z01.11 Encounter for examination of ears and hearing with abnormal findings**

AHA: 2016,3Q,17-18

Z01.110 Encounter for hearing examination following failed hearing screening PDx

Z01.118 Encounter for examination of ears and hearing with other abnormal findings PDx

Use additional code to identify abnormal findings

Z01.12 Encounter for hearing conservation and treatment PDx

☑5ᵗʰ **Z01.2 Encounter for dental examination and cleaning**

Z01.20 Encounter for dental examination and cleaning without abnormal findings PDx

Encounter for dental examination and cleaning NOS

Z01.21 Encounter for dental examination and cleaning with abnormal findings PDx

Use additional code to identify abnormal findings

☑5ᵗʰ **Z01.3 Encounter for examination of blood pressure**

Z01.30 Encounter for examination of blood pressure without abnormal findings PDx

Encounter for examination of blood pressure NOS

Z01.31 Encounter for examination of blood pressure with abnormal findings PDx

Use additional code to identify abnormal findings

☑5ᵗʰ **Z01.4 Encounter for gynecological examination**

EXCLUDES 2   *pregnancy examination or test (Z32.0-)*

routine examination for contraceptive maintenance (Z30.4-)

☑6ᵗʰ **Z01.41 Encounter for routine gynecological examination**

Encounter for general gynecological examination with or without cervical smear

Encounter for gynecological examination (general) (routine) NOS

Encounter for pelvic examination (annual) (periodic)

Use additional code:

for screening for human papillomavirus, if applicable, (Z11.51)

for screening vaginal pap smear, if applicable (Z12.72)

to identify acquired absence of uterus, if applicable (Z90.71-)

EXCLUDES 1   *gynecologic examination status-post hysterectomy for malignant condition (Z08)*

screening cervical pap smear not a part of a routine gynecological examination (Z12.4)

Z01.411 Encounter for gynecological examination (general) (routine) with abnormal findings PDx ♀

Use additional code to identify abnormal findings

Z01.419 Encounter for gynecological examination (general) (routine) without abnormal findings PDx ♀

Z01.42 Encounter for cervical smear to confirm findings of recent normal smear following initial abnormal smear PDx ♀

☑5ᵗʰ **Z01.8 Encounter for other specified special examinations**

☑6ᵗʰ **Z01.81 Encounter for preprocedural examinations**

Encounter for preoperative examinations

Encounter for radiological and imaging examinations as part of preprocedural examination

Z01.810 Encounter for preprocedural cardiovascular examination PDx

Z01.811 Encounter for preprocedural respiratory examination PDx

Z01.812 Encounter for preprocedural laboratory examination PDx

Blood and urine tests prior to treatment or procedure

Z01.818 Encounter for other preprocedural examination PDx

Encounter for preprocedural examination NOS

Encounter for examinations prior to antineoplastic chemotherapy

Z01.82 Encounter for allergy testing PDx

EXCLUDES 1   *encounter for antibody response examination (Z01.84)*

Z01.83 Encounter for blood typing PDx

Encounter for Rh typing

Z01.84 Encounter for antibody response examination PDx

Encounter for immunity status testing

EXCLUDES 1   *encounter for allergy testing (Z01.82)*

Z01.89 Encounter for other specified special examinations PDx

☑4ᵗʰ **Z02 Encounter for administrative examination**

Z02.0 Encounter for examination for admission to educational institution PDx

Encounter for examination for admission to preschool (education)

Encounter for examination for re-admission to school following illness or medical treatment

Z02.1 Encounter for pre-employment examination PDx

Z02.2 Encounter for examination for admission to residential institution PDx

EXCLUDES 1   *examination for admission to prison (Z02.89)*

☑ Additional Character Required   ☑x7ᵗʰ Placeholder Alert   Manifestation   Unspecified Dx   ▶◀ Revised Text   ● New Code   ▲ Revised Title

ICD-10-CM 2020   **1207**

Z02.3 **Encounter for examination for** recruitment to armed forces `PDx`

Z02.4 **Encounter for examination for** driving license `PDx`

Z02.5 **Encounter for examination for** participation in sport `PDx`
　　EXCLUDES 1　blood-alcohol and blood-drug test (Z02.83)

Z02.6 **Encounter for examination for** insurance purposes `PDx`

✓5ᵗʰ **Z02.7** **Encounter for** issue of medical certificate
　　EXCLUDES 1　encounter for general medical examination (Z00–Z01, Z02.0–Z02.6, Z02.8–Z02.9)

　　Z02.71 **Encounter for** disability determination `PDx`
　　　Encounter for issue of medical certificate of incapacity
　　　Encounter for issue of medical certificate of invalidity

　　Z02.79 **Encounter for issue of other medical certificate** `PDx`

✓5ᵗʰ **Z02.8** **Encounter for other administrative examinations**

　　Z02.81 **Encounter for** paternity testing `PDx`

　　Z02.82 **Encounter for** adoption services `PDx`

　　Z02.83 **Encounter for** blood-alcohol and blood-drug test `PDx`
　　　Use additional code for findings of alcohol or drugs in blood (R78.-)

　　Z02.89 **Encounter for other administrative examinations** `PDx`
　　　Encounter for examination for admission to prison
　　　Encounter for examination for admission to summer camp
　　　Encounter for immigration examination
　　　Encounter for naturalization examination
　　　Encounter for premarital examination
　　　EXCLUDES 1　health supervision of foundling or other healthy infant or child (Z76.1-Z76.2)

Z02.9 **Encounter for administrative examinations, unspecified** `PDx`

✓4ᵗʰ **Z03** **Encounter for** medical observation **for suspected diseases and conditions ruled out**
　This category is to be used when a person without a diagnosis is suspected of having an abnormal condition, without signs or symptoms, which requires study, but after examination and observation, is ruled out. This category is also for use for administrative and legal observation status.
　EXCLUDES 1　contact with and (suspected) exposures hazardous to health (Z77.-)
　　encounter for observation and evaluation of newborn for suspected diseases and conditions ruled out (Z05.-)
　　person with feared complaint in whom no diagnosis is made (Z71.1)
　　signs or symptoms under study — code to signs or symptoms
　AHA: 2018,2Q,7-8; 2017,4Q,27

Z03.6 **Encounter for observation for suspected** toxic effect from ingested substance **ruled out** `PDx`
　Encounter for observation for suspected adverse effect from drug
　Encounter for observation for suspected poisoning

✓5ᵗʰ **Z03.7** **Encounter for suspected** maternal and fetal conditions **ruled out**
　Encounter for suspected maternal and fetal conditions not found
　EXCLUDES 1　known or suspected fetal anomalies affecting management of mother, not ruled out (O26.-, O35.-, O36.-, O40.-, O41.-)

　　Z03.71 **Encounter for suspected problem with** amniotic cavity and membrane **ruled out** `PDx` M ♀
　　　Encounter for suspected oligohydramnios ruled out
　　　Encounter for suspected polyhydramnios ruled out

　　Z03.72 **Encounter for suspected** placental problem **ruled out** `PDx` M ♀

　　Z03.73 **Encounter for suspected** fetal anomaly **ruled out** `PDx` M ♀

　　Z03.74 **Encounter for suspected** problem with fetal growth **ruled out** `PDx` M ♀

　　Z03.75 **Encounter for suspected** cervical shortening **ruled out** `PDx` M ♀

　　Z03.79 **Encounter for other suspected maternal and fetal conditions ruled out** `PDx` M ♀

✓5ᵗʰ **Z03.8** **Encounter for** observation **for other suspected diseases and conditions ruled out**

✓6ᵗʰ **Z03.81** **Encounter for observation for suspected** exposure to biological agents **ruled out** `PDx`

　　Z03.810 **Encounter for observation for suspected exposure to** anthrax **ruled out** `PDx`

　　Z03.818 **Encounter for observation for suspected exposure to other biological agents ruled out** `PDx`

Z03.89 **Encounter for observation for other suspected diseases and conditions ruled out** `PDx`

✓4ᵗʰ **Z04** **Encounter for examination and observation for other reasons**
　INCLUDES　encounter for examination for medicolegal reasons
　This category is to be used when a person without a diagnosis is suspected of having an abnormal condition, without signs or symptoms, which requires study, but after examination and observation, is ruled-out. This category is also for use for administrative and legal observation status.
　AHA: 2018,2Q,7-8

Z04.1 **Encounter for examination and observation following** transport accident `PDx`
　EXCLUDES 1　encounter for examination and observation following work accident (Z04.2)
　AHA: 2019,2Q,11; 2018,2Q,8

Z04.2 **Encounter for examination and observation following** work accident `PDx`

Z04.3 **Encounter for examination and observation following other accident** `PDx`

✓5ᵗʰ **Z04.4** **Encounter for examination and observation following** alleged rape
　Encounter for examination and observation of victim following alleged rape
　Encounter for examination and observation of victim following alleged sexual abuse

　　Z04.41 **Encounter for examination and observation following alleged** adult rape `PDx` A
　　　Suspected adult rape, ruled out
　　　Suspected adult sexual abuse, ruled out

　　Z04.42 **Encounter for examination and observation following alleged** child rape `PDx` P
　　　Suspected child rape, ruled out
　　　Suspected child sexual abuse, ruled out

Z04.6 **Encounter for** general psychiatric examination, requested by authority `PDx`

✓5ᵗʰ **Z04.7** **Encounter for examination and observation following** alleged physical abuse

　　Z04.71 **Encounter for examination and observation following alleged** adult physical abuse `PDx` A
　　　Suspected adult physical abuse, ruled out
　　　EXCLUDES 1　confirmed case of adult physical abuse (T74.-)
　　　　encounter for examination and observation following alleged adult sexual abuse (Z04.41)
　　　　suspected case of adult physical abuse, not ruled out (T76.-)

　　Z04.72 **Encounter for examination and observation following alleged** child physical abuse `PDx` P
　　　Suspected child physical abuse, ruled out
　　　EXCLUDES 1　confirmed case of child physical abuse (T74.-)
　　　　encounter for examination and observation following alleged child sexual abuse (Z04.42)
　　　　suspected case of child physical abuse, not ruled out (T76.-)

✓5ᵗʰ **Z04.8** **Encounter for examination and observation for** other specified reasons
　Encounter for examination and observation for request for expert evidence
　AHA: 2018,4Q,32,35,72

　　Z04.81 **Encounter for examination and observation of** victim following forced sexual exploitation `PDx`

Z04.82   **Encounter for examination and observation of** victim following forced labor exploitation   `PDx`

Z04.89   **Encounter for examination and observation for** other specified reasons   `PDx`

Z04.9   **Encounter for examination and observation for** unspecified reason   `PDx`
     Encounter for observation NOS

`√4ᵗʰ` **Z05**   **Encounter for observation and evaluation of newborn for** suspected diseases and conditions ruled out
     This category is to be used for newborns, within the neonatal period (the first 28 days of life), who are suspected of having an abnormal condition, but without signs or symptoms, and which, after examination and observation, is ruled out.
     AHA: 2017,4Q,27; 2016,4Q,77

Z05.0   **Observation and evaluation of newborn for** suspected cardiac condition ruled out   `N`

Z05.1   **Observation and evaluation of newborn for** suspected infectious condition ruled out   `N`
     AHA: 2019,2Q,10

Z05.2   **Observation and evaluation of newborn for** suspected neurological condition ruled out   `N`

Z05.3   **Observation and evaluation of newborn for** suspected respiratory condition ruled out   `N`

`√5ᵗʰ` Z05.4   **Observation and evaluation of newborn for suspected** genetic, metabolic or immunologic condition ruled out

     Z05.41   **Observation and evaluation of newborn for suspected** genetic condition ruled out   `N`
         AHA: 2016,4Q,55

     Z05.42   **Observation and evaluation of newborn for suspected** metabolic condition ruled out   `N`

     Z05.43   **Observation and evaluation of newborn for suspected** immunologic condition ruled out   `N`

Z05.5   **Observation and evaluation of newborn for** suspected gastrointestinal condition ruled out   `N`

Z05.6   **Observation and evaluation of newborn for** suspected genitourinary condition ruled out   `N`

`√5ᵗʰ` Z05.7   **Observation and evaluation of newborn for suspected** skin, subcutaneous, musculoskeletal and connective tissue condition ruled out

     Z05.71   **Observation and evaluation of newborn for suspected** skin and subcutaneous tissue condition ruled out   `N`

     Z05.72   **Observation and evaluation of newborn for suspected** musculoskeletal condition ruled out   `N`

     Z05.73   **Observation and evaluation of newborn for suspected** connective tissue condition ruled out   `N`

Z05.8   **Observation and evaluation of newborn for other** specified suspected condition ruled out   `N`

Z05.9   **Observation and evaluation of newborn for** unspecified suspected condition ruled out   `N`

Z08   **Encounter for** follow-up examination after completed treatment for malignant neoplasm
     Medical surveillance following completed treatment
     Use additional code to identify any acquired absence of organs (Z90.-)
     Use additional code to identify the personal history of malignant neoplasm (Z85.-)
     `EXCLUDES 1`   *aftercare following medical care (Z43-Z49, Z51)*

Z09   **Encounter for** follow-up examination after completed treatment for conditions other than malignant neoplasm
     Medical surveillance following completed treatment
     Use additional code to identify any applicable history of disease code (Z86.-. Z87.-)
     `EXCLUDES 1`   *aftercare following medical care (Z43-Z49, Z51)*
               surveillance of contraception (Z30.4-)
               surveillance of prosthetic and other medical devices (Z44-Z46)
     AHA: 2017,1Q,9; 2015,1Q,8

`√4ᵗʰ` **Z11**   **Encounter for** screening for infectious and parasitic diseases
     Screening is the testing for disease or disease precursors in asymptomatic individuals so that early detection and treatment can be provided for those who test positive for the disease.
     `EXCLUDES 1`   *encounter for diagnostic examination — code to sign or symptom*

     Z11.0   **Encounter for screening for** intestinal infectious diseases

Z11.1   **Encounter for screening for** respiratory tuberculosis
     ►Encounter for screening for active tuberculosis disease◄

Z11.2   **Encounter for screening for** other bacterial diseases

Z11.3   **Encounter for screening for infections with a** predominantly sexual mode of transmission
     `EXCLUDES 2`   *encounter for screening for human immunodeficiency virus [HIV] (Z11.4)*
               encounter for screening for human papillomavirus (Z11.51)

Z11.4   **Encounter for screening for** human immunodeficiency virus [HIV]

`√5ᵗʰ` Z11.5   **Encounter for screening for** other viral diseases
     `EXCLUDES 2`   *encounter for screening for viral intestinal disease (Z11.0)*

     Z11.51   **Encounter for screening for** human papillomavirus (HPV)

     Z11.59   **Encounter for screening for** other viral diseases

Z11.6   **Encounter for screening for** other protozoal diseases and helminthiases
     `EXCLUDES 2`   *encounter for screening for protozoal intestinal disease (Z11.0)*

● Z11.7   **Encounter for testing for** latent tuberculosis infection

Z11.8   **Encounter for screening for** other infectious and parasitic diseases
     Encounter for screening for chlamydia
     Encounter for screening for rickettsial
     Encounter for screening for spirochetal
     Encounter for screening for mycoses

Z11.9   **Encounter for screening for** infectious and parasitic diseases, unspecified

`√4ᵗʰ` **Z12**   **Encounter for** screening for malignant neoplasms
     Screening is the testing for disease or disease precursors in asymptomatic individuals so that early detection and treatment can be provided for those who test positive for the disease.
     Use additional code to identify any family history of malignant neoplasm (Z80.-)
     `EXCLUDES 1`   *encounter for diagnostic examination — code to sign or symptom*

Z12.0   **Encounter for screening for malignant neoplasm of** stomach

`√5ᵗʰ` Z12.1   **Encounter for screening for malignant neoplasm of** intestinal tract
     AHA: 2017,1Q,8,9

     Z12.10   **Encounter for screening for malignant neoplasm of intestinal tract, unspecified**

     Z12.11   **Encounter for screening for malignant neoplasm of** colon
         Encounter for screening colonoscopy NOS
         AHA: 2019,1Q,32-33; 2018,1Q,6

     Z12.12   **Encounter for screening for malignant neoplasm of** rectum
         AHA: 2018,1Q,6

     Z12.13   **Encounter for screening for malignant neoplasm of** small intestine

Z12.2   **Encounter for screening for malignant neoplasm of** respiratory organs

`√5ᵗʰ` Z12.3   **Encounter for screening for malignant neoplasm of** breast

     Z12.31   **Encounter for screening** mammogram for malignant neoplasm of breast
         `EXCLUDES 1`   *inconclusive mammogram (R92.2)*
         AHA: 2015,1Q,24

     Z12.39   **Encounter for other screening for malignant neoplasm of breast**

Z12.4   **Encounter for screening for malignant neoplasm of** cervix   ♀
     Encounter for screening pap smear for malignant neoplasm of cervix
     `EXCLUDES 1`   *when screening is part of general gynecological examination (Z01.4-)*
     `EXCLUDES 2`   *encounter for screening for human papillomavirus (Z11.51)*

Z12.5   **Encounter for screening for malignant neoplasm of** prostate   ♂

Z12.6   **Encounter for screening for malignant neoplasm of** bladder

`√5ᵗʰ` Z12.7   **Encounter for screening for malignant neoplasm of other** genitourinary organs

     Z12.71   **Encounter for screening for malignant neoplasm of** testis   ♂

Z12.72 **Encounter for screening for malignant neoplasm of** vagina ♀

Vaginal pap smear status-post hysterectomy for non-malignant condition

Use additional code to identify acquired absence of uterus (Z90.71-)

> EXCLUDES 1 *vaginal pap smear status-post hysterectomy for malignant conditions (Z08)*

Z12.73 **Encounter for screening for malignant neoplasm of** ovary ♀

Z12.79 **Encounter for screening for malignant neoplasm of other genitourinary organs**

✓5ᵗʰ **Z12.8** **Encounter for screening for malignant neoplasm of other sites**

Z12.81 **Encounter for screening for malignant neoplasm of** oral cavity

Z12.82 **Encounter for screening for malignant neoplasm of** nervous system

Z12.83 **Encounter for screening for malignant neoplasm of** skin

Z12.89 **Encounter for screening for malignant neoplasm of other sites**

Z12.9 **Encounter for screening for malignant neoplasm, site unspecified**

✓4ᵗʰ **Z13** **Encounter for screening for other diseases and disorders**

Screening is the testing for disease or disease precursors in asymptomatic individuals so that early detection and treatment can be provided for those who test positive for the disease.

> EXCLUDES 1 *encounter for diagnostic examination — code to sign or symptom*

Z13.0 **Encounter for screening for diseases of the** blood and blood-forming organs **and certain disorders involving the** immune mechanism

Z13.1 **Encounter for screening for** diabetes mellitus

✓5ᵗʰ **Z13.2** **Encounter for screening for nutritional, metabolic and other endocrine disorders**

Z13.21 **Encounter for screening for** nutritional **disorder**

✓6ᵗʰ **Z13.22** **Encounter for screening for** metabolic **disorder**

Z13.220 **Encounter for screening for** lipoid **disorders**

Encounter for screening for cholesterol level

Encounter for screening for hypercholesterolemia

Encounter for screening for hyperlipidemia

Z13.228 **Encounter for screening for other metabolic disorders**

Z13.29 **Encounter for screening for other suspected endocrine disorder**

> EXCLUDES 1 *encounter for screening for diabetes mellitus (Z13.1)*

✓5ᵗʰ **Z13.3** **Encounter for screening examination for** mental health and behavioral **disorders**

AHA: 2018,4Q,35-36

Z13.30 **Encounter for screening examination for mental health and behavioral disorders, unspecified**

Z13.31 **Encounter for screening for** depression

Encounter for screening for depression, adult

Encounter for screening for depression for child or adolescent

Z13.32 **Encounter for screening for** maternal depression ♀

Encounter for screening for perinatal depression

Z13.39 **Encounter for screening examination for other mental health and behavioral disorders**

Encounter for screening for alcoholism

Encounter for screening for intellectual disabilities

✓5ᵗʰ **Z13.4** **Encounter for screening for certain** developmental **disorders in** childhood

Encounter for development testing of infant or child

Encounter for screening for developmental handicaps in early childhood

> EXCLUDES 2 *encounter for routine child health examination (Z00.12-)*

AHA: 2018,4Q,36

Z13.40 **Encounter for screening for unspecified developmental delays**

Z13.41 **Encounter for** autism **screening**

Z13.42 **Encounter for screening for** global developmental delays **(milestones)**

Encounter for screening for developmental handicaps in early childhood

Z13.49 **Encounter for screening for other developmental delays**

Z13.5 **Encounter for screening for** eye and ear **disorders**

> EXCLUDES 2 *encounter for general hearing examination (Z01.1-)*
> *encounter for general vision examination (Z01.0-)*

AHA: 2016,3Q,17

Z13.6 **Encounter for screening for** cardiovascular **disorders**

✓5ᵗʰ **Z13.7** **Encounter for screening for** genetic **and** chromosomal **anomalies**

> EXCLUDES 1 *genetic testing for procreative management (Z31.4-)*

Z13.71 **Encounter for nonprocreative screening for genetic disease carrier status**

Z13.79 **Encounter for other screening for genetic and chromosomal anomalies**

✓5ᵗʰ **Z13.8** **Encounter for screening for other specified diseases and disorders**

> EXCLUDES 2 *screening for malignant neoplasms (Z12.-)*

✓6ᵗʰ **Z13.81** **Encounter for screening for** digestive system **disorders**

Z13.810 **Encounter for screening for** upper gastrointestinal **disorder**

Z13.811 **Encounter for screening for** lower gastrointestinal **disorder**

> EXCLUDES 1 *encounter for screening for intestinal infectious disease (Z11.0)*

Z13.818 **Encounter for screening for other digestive system disorders**

✓6ᵗʰ **Z13.82** **Encounter for screening for** musculoskeletal **disorder**

Z13.820 **Encounter for screening for** osteoporosis

Z13.828 **Encounter for screening for other musculoskeletal disorder**

Z13.83 **Encounter for screening for** respiratory **disorder NEC**

> EXCLUDES 1 *encounter for screening for respiratory tuberculosis (Z11.1)*

Z13.84 **Encounter for screening for** dental **disorders**

✓6ᵗʰ **Z13.85** **Encounter for screening for** nervous system **disorders**

Z13.850 **Encounter for screening for** traumatic brain injury

Z13.858 **Encounter for screening for other nervous system disorders**

Z13.88 **Encounter for screening for disorder** due to exposure to contaminants

> EXCLUDES 1 *those exposed to contaminants without suspected disorders (Z57.-, Z77.-)*

Z13.89 **Encounter for screening for other disorder**

Encounter for screening for genitourinary disorders

Z13.9 **Encounter for screening, unspecified**

Genetic carrier and genetic susceptibility to disease (Z14-Z15)

✓4ᵗʰ **Z14** **Genetic carrier**

DEF: Individuals carrying a gene mutation associated with a certain disease that typically do not develop the disease but are able to pass the mutated genes to offspring.

✓5ᵗʰ **Z14.0** Hemophilia A **carrier**

Z14.01 Asymptomatic **hemophilia A carrier**

Z14.02 Symptomatic **hemophilia A carrier**

Z14.1 Cystic fibrosis **carrier**

Z14.8 **Genetic carrier of other disease**

N Newborn: 0   P Pediatric: 0-17   M Maternity: 12-55   A Adult: 15-124   CH Comorbidity High   CL Comorbidity Low   NCDx Noncancer Dx   PDx Primary Dx

1210
ICD-10-CM 2020

Chapter 21. Factors Influencing Health Status and Contact With Health Services

☑4ᵗʰ **Z15 Genetic susceptibility to disease**

INCLUDES confirmed abnormal gene

Use additional code, if applicable, for any associated family history of the disease (Z80-Z84)

EXCLUDES 1 *chromosomal anomalies (Q90-Q99)*

☑5ᵗʰ **Z15.0 Genetic susceptibility to malignant neoplasm**

Code first, if applicable, any current malignant neoplasm (C00-C75, C81-C96)

Use additional code, if applicable, for any personal history of malignant neoplasm (Z85.-)

Z15.01 Genetic susceptibility to malignant neoplasm of breast

TIP: May be assigned in addition to a code for aftercare following prophylactic mastectomy.

Z15.02 Genetic susceptibility to malignant neoplasm of ovary ♀

Z15.03 Genetic susceptibility to malignant neoplasm of prostate ♂

Z15.04 Genetic susceptibility to malignant neoplasm of endometrium ♀

Z15.09 Genetic susceptibility to other malignant neoplasm

☑5ᵗʰ **Z15.8 Genetic susceptibility to other disease**

Z15.81 Genetic susceptibility to multiple endocrine neoplasia [MEN]

EXCLUDES 1 *multiple endocrine neoplasia [MEN] syndromes (E31.2-)*

DEF: Group of conditions in which several endocrine glands grow excessively (such as in adenomatous hyperplasia) and/or develop benign or malignant tumors. Tumors and hyperplasia associated with MEN often produce excess hormones, which impede normal physiology. There is no comprehensive cure known for MEN syndrome. Treatment is directed at the hyperplasia or tumors in each individual gland. Tumors are usually surgically removed and oral medications or hormonal injections are used to correct hormone imbalances.

Z15.89 Genetic susceptibility to other disease

Resistance to antimicrobial drugs (Z16)

☑4ᵗʰ **Z16 Resistance to antimicrobial drugs**

NOTE The codes in this category are provided for use as additional codes to identify the resistance and non-responsiveness of a condition to antimicrobial drugs.

Code first the infection

EXCLUDES 1 *Methicillin resistant Staphylococcus aureus infection (A49.02)*

Methicillin resistant Staphylococcus aureus pneumonia (J15.212)

sepsis due to Methicillin resistant Staphylococcus aureus (A41.02)

☑5ᵗʰ **Z16.1 Resistance to beta lactam antibiotics**

Z16.10 Resistance to unspecified beta lactam antibiotics

Z16.11 Resistance to penicillins
Resistance to amoxicillin
Resistance to ampicillin

Z16.12 Extended spectrum beta lactamase (ESBL) resistance

EXCLUDES 2 *Methicillin resistant Staphylococcus aureus infection in diseases classified elsewhere (B95.62)*

Z16.19 Resistance to other specified beta lactam antibiotics
Resistance to cephalosporins

☑5ᵗʰ **Z16.2 Resistance to other antibiotics**

Z16.20 Resistance to unspecified antibiotic
Resistance to antibiotics NOS

Z16.21 Resistance to vancomycin

Z16.22 Resistance to vancomycin related antibiotics

Z16.23 Resistance to quinolones and fluoroquinolones

Z16.24 Resistance to multiple antibiotics

Z16.29 Resistance to other single specified antibiotic
Resistance to aminoglycosides
Resistance to macrolides
Resistance to sulfonamides
Resistance to tetracyclines

☑5ᵗʰ **Z16.3 Resistance to other antimicrobial drugs**

EXCLUDES 1 *resistance to antibiotics (Z16.1-, Z16.2-)*

Z16.30 Resistance to unspecified antimicrobial drugs
Drug resistance NOS

Z16.31 Resistance to antiparasitic drug(s)
Resistance to quinine and related compounds

Z16.32 Resistance to antifungal drug(s)

Z16.33 Resistance to antiviral drug(s)

☑6ᵗʰ **Z16.34 Resistance to antimycobacterial drug(s)**
Resistance to tuberculostatics

Z16.341 Resistance to single antimycobacterial drug
Resistance to antimycobacterial drug NOS

Z16.342 Resistance to multiple antimycobacterial drugs

Z16.35 Resistance to multiple antimicrobial drugs

EXCLUDES 1 *resistance to multiple antibiotics only (Z16.24)*

Z16.39 Resistance to other specified antimicrobial drug

Estrogen receptor status (Z17)

☑4ᵗʰ **Z17 Estrogen receptor status**

Code first malignant neoplasm of breast (C50.-)

DEF: Receptor status of breast cancer cells for the hormone estrogen that is used to help determine treatment and evaluate prognosis. ER+ breast cancer responds to hormone therapies while ER- breast cancer does not.

Z17.0 Estrogen receptor positive status [ER+]

Z17.1 Estrogen receptor negative status [ER-]

Retained foreign body fragments (Z18)

☑4ᵗʰ **Z18 Retained foreign body fragments**

INCLUDES embedded fragment (status)
embedded splinter (status)
retained foreign body status

EXCLUDES 1 *artificial joint prosthesis status (Z96.6-)*
foreign body accidentally left during a procedure (T81.5-)
foreign body entering through orifice (T15-T19)
in situ cardiac device (Z95.-)
organ or tissue replaced by means other than transplant (Z96.-, Z97.-)
organ or tissue replaced by transplant (Z94.-)
personal history of retained foreign body fully removed Z87.821
superficial foreign body (non-embedded splinter) — code to superficial foreign body, by site

DEF: Embedded or retained fragment, splinter, or foreign body, natural or synthetic that can cause infection.

☑5ᵗʰ **Z18.0 Retained radioactive fragments**

Z18.01 Retained depleted uranium fragments

Z18.09 Other retained radioactive fragments
Other retained depleted isotope fragments
Retained nontherapeutic radioactive fragments

☑5ᵗʰ **Z18.1 Retained metal fragments**

EXCLUDES 1 *retained radioactive metal fragments (Z18.01-Z18.09)*

Z18.10 Retained metal fragments, unspecified
Retained metal fragment NOS

Z18.11 Retained magnetic metal fragments

Z18.12 Retained nonmagnetic metal fragments

Z18.2 Retained plastic fragments
Acrylics fragments
Diethylhexyl phthalates fragments
Isocyanate fragments

☑5ᵗʰ **Z18.3 Retained organic fragments**

Z18.31 Retained animal quills or spines

Z18.32 Retained tooth

Z18.33 Retained wood fragments

Z18.39 Other retained organic fragments

☑5ᵗʰ **Z18.8 Other specified retained foreign body**

Z18.81 Retained glass fragments

Z18.83 Retained stone or crystalline fragments
Retained concrete or cement fragments

Z18.89 Other specified retained foreign body fragments

Z18.9 Retained foreign body fragments, unspecified material

Hormone sensitivity malignancy status (Z19)

☑4ᵗʰ Z19 Hormone sensitivity malignancy status
Code first malignant neoplasm — see Table of Neoplasms, by site, malignant
AHA: 2016,4Q,76

Z19.1 Hormone sensitive malignancy status

Z19.2 Hormone resistant malignancy status
Castrate resistant prostate malignancy status

Persons with potential health hazards related to communicable diseases (Z20-Z29)

☑4ᵗʰ Z20 Contact with and (suspected) exposure to communicable diseases
EXCLUDES 1 carrier of infectious disease (Z22.-)
diagnosed current infectious or parasitic disease — see Alphabetic Index
EXCLUDES 2 personal history of infectious and parasitic diseases (Z86.1-)

☑5ᵗʰ Z20.0 Contact with and (suspected) exposure to intestinal infectious diseases
Z20.01 Contact with and (suspected) exposure to intestinal infectious diseases due to Escherichia coli (E. coli)
Z20.09 Contact with and (suspected) exposure to other intestinal infectious diseases

Z20.1 Contact with and (suspected) exposure to tuberculosis

Z20.2 Contact with and (suspected) exposure to infections with a predominantly sexual mode of transmission

Z20.3 Contact with and (suspected) exposure to rabies

Z20.4 Contact with and (suspected) exposure to rubella

Z20.5 Contact with and (suspected) exposure to viral hepatitis

Z20.6 Contact with and (suspected) exposure to human immunodeficiency virus [HIV]
EXCLUDES 1 asymptomatic human immunodeficiency virus [HIV] HIV infection status (Z21)

Z20.7 Contact with and (suspected) exposure to pediculosis, acariasis and other infestations

☑5ᵗʰ Z20.8 Contact with and (suspected) exposure to other communicable diseases
☑6ᵗʰ Z20.81 Contact with and (suspected) exposure to other bacterial communicable diseases
Z20.810 Contact with and (suspected) exposure to anthrax
Z20.811 Contact with and (suspected) exposure to meningococcus
Z20.818 Contact with and (suspected) exposure to other bacterial communicable diseases
AHA: 2019,2Q,10

☑6ᵗʰ Z20.82 Contact with and (suspected) exposure to other viral communicable diseases
Z20.820 Contact with and (suspected) exposure to varicella
Z20.821 Contact with and (suspected) exposure to Zika virus
AHA: 2018,4Q,35,64
Z20.828 Contact with and (suspected) exposure to other viral communicable diseases

Z20.89 Contact with and (suspected) exposure to other communicable diseases

Z20.9 Contact with and (suspected) exposure to unspecified communicable disease

Z21 Asymptomatic human immunodeficiency virus [HIV] infection status
HIV positive NOS
Code first human immunodeficiency virus [HIV] disease complicating pregnancy, childbirth and the puerperium, if applicable (O98.7-)
EXCLUDES 1 acquired immunodeficiency syndrome (B20)
contact with human immunodeficiency virus [HIV] (Z20.6)
exposure to human immunodeficiency virus [HIV] (Z20.6)
human immunodeficiency virus [HIV] disease (B20)
inconclusive laboratory evidence of human immunodeficiency virus [HIV] (R75)
AHA: 2019,1Q,8-11
DEF: Phase of human immunodeficiency virus (HIV) infection with no clinical symptoms. This phase may last for 10 years or more.

☑4ᵗʰ Z22 Carrier of infectious disease
INCLUDES colonization status
suspected carrier
EXCLUDES 2 carrier of viral hepatitis (B18.-)

Z22.0 Carrier of typhoid

Z22.1 Carrier of other intestinal infectious diseases

Z22.2 Carrier of diphtheria

☑5ᵗʰ Z22.3 Carrier of other specified bacterial diseases
Z22.31 Carrier of bacterial disease due to meningococci
☑6ᵗʰ Z22.32 Carrier of bacterial disease due to staphylococci
Z22.321 Carrier or suspected carrier of Methicillin susceptible **Staphylococcus aureus**
MSSA colonization
Z22.322 Carrier or suspected carrier of Methicillin resistant **Staphylococcus aureus**
MRSA colonization
DEF: Carriers (colonization) of methicillin resistant *Staphylococcus aureus* (MRSA) have MRSA on their skin or in their body but do not exhibit signs of infection. These individuals are able to pass MRSA on to others who may develop an infection.

☑6ᵗʰ Z22.33 Carrier of bacterial disease due to streptococci
Z22.330 Carrier of Group B streptococcus
EXCLUDES 1 carrier of streptococcus group B (GBS) complicating pregnancy, childbirth and the puerperium (O99.82-)
Z22.338 Carrier of other streptococcus
Z22.39 Carrier of other specified bacterial diseases

Z22.4 Carrier of infections with a predominantly sexual mode of transmission

Z22.6 Carrier of human T-lymphotropic virus type-1 [HTLV-1] infection

Z22.7 Latent tuberculosis
Latent tuberculosis infection (LTBI)
EXCLUDES 1 nonspecific reaction to cell mediated immunity measurement of gamma interferon antigen response without active tuberculosis (R76.12)
nonspecific reaction to tuberculin skin test without active tuberculosis (R76.11)

Z22.8 Carrier of other infectious diseases

Z22.9 Carrier of infectious disease, unspecified

Z23 Encounter for immunization
Code first any routine childhood examination
NOTE Procedure codes are required to identify the types of immunizations given

☑4ᵗʰ Z28 Immunization not carried out and underimmunization status
INCLUDES vaccination not carried out

☑5ᵗʰ Z28.0 Immunization not carried out because of contraindication
DEF: Contraindication: Situation where a drug, surgery, or other procedure may negatively affect or cause harm to a patient.
Z28.01 Immunization not carried out because of acute illness **of patient**
Z28.02 Immunization not carried out because of chronic illness **or condition of patient**
Z28.03 Immunization not carried out because of immune compromised state **of patient**
Z28.04 Immunization not carried out because of patient allergy to vaccine or component
Z28.09 Immunization not carried out because of other contraindication

Z28.1 Immunization not carried out because of patient decision for reasons of belief or group pressure
Immunization not carried out because of religious belief

☑5ᵗʰ Z28.2 Immunization not carried out because of patient decision for other and unspecified **reason**
Z28.20 Immunization not carried out because of patient decision for unspecified reason
Z28.21 Immunization not carried out because of patient refusal
Z28.29 Immunization not carried out because of patient decision for other reason

Z28.3 Underimmunization status
Delinquent immunization status
Lapsed immunization schedule status

N Newborn: 0   **P** Pediatric: 0-17   **M** Maternity: 12-55   **A** Adult: 15-124   **CH** Comorbidity High   **CL** Comorbidity Low   **NCDx** Noncancer Dx   **PDx** Primary Dx

1212   ICD-10-CM 2020

✓5ᵗʰ **Z28.8 Immunization not carried out for other reason**

    Z28.81 Immunization not carried out due to patient having had the disease

    Z28.82 Immunization not carried out because of caregiver refusal

       Immunization not carried out because of guardian refusal

       Immunization not carried out because of parent refusal

       EXCLUDES 1   immunization not carried out because of caregiver refusal because of religious belief (Z28.1)

    Z28.83 Immunization not carried out due to unavailability of vaccine

       Delay in delivery of vaccine

       Lack of availability of vaccine

       Manufacturer delay of vaccine

       AHA: 2018,4Q,36

    Z28.89 Immunization not carried out for other reason

   Z28.9 Immunization not carried out for unspecified reason

✓4ᵗʰ **Z29 Encounter for other prophylactic measures**

    EXCLUDES 1   desensitization to allergens (Z51.6)

            prophylactic surgery (Z40.-)

    AHA: 2016,4Q,78-79

✓5ᵗʰ **Z29.1 Encounter for prophylactic immunotherapy**

       Encounter for administration of immunoglobulin

    Z29.11 Encounter for prophylactic immunotherapy for respiratory syncytial virus (RSV)

    Z29.12 Encounter for prophylactic antivenin

    Z29.13 Encounter for prophylactic Rho(D) immune globulin

    Z29.14 Encounter for prophylactic rabies immune globin

   Z29.3 Encounter for prophylactic fluoride administration

   Z29.8 Encounter for other specified prophylactic measures

   Z29.9 Encounter for prophylactic measures, unspecified

Persons encountering health services in circumstances related to reproduction (Z30-Z39)

✓4ᵗʰ **Z30 Encounter for contraceptive management**

    AHA: 2016,4Q,78

    DEF: Contraceptive management to prevent pregnancy. Methods include oral medications, intrauterine devices, and surgical procedures for males and females (sterilization).

✓5ᵗʰ **Z30.0 Encounter for general counseling and advice on** contraception

✓6ᵗʰ **Z30.01 Encounter for** initial prescription of contraceptives

       EXCLUDES 1   encounter for surveillance of contraceptives (Z30.4-)

    Z30.011 Encounter for initial prescription of contraceptive pills ♀

    Z30.012 Encounter for prescription of emergency contraception ♀

       Encounter for postcoital contraception

    Z30.013 Encounter for initial prescription of injectable contraceptive ♀

    Z30.014 Encounter for initial prescription of intrauterine contraceptive device ♀

       EXCLUDES 1   encounter for insertion of intrauterine contraceptive device (Z30.430, Z30.432)

    Z30.015 Encounter for initial prescription of vaginal ring hormonal contraceptive ♀

    Z30.016 Encounter for initial prescription of transdermal patch hormonal contraceptive device

    Z30.017 Encounter for initial prescription of implantable subdermal contraceptive

    Z30.018 Encounter for initial prescription of other contraceptives ♀

       Encounter for initial prescription of barrier contraception

       Encounter for initial prescription of diaphragm

    Z30.019 Encounter for initial prescription of contraceptives, unspecified ♀

   Z30.02 Counseling and instruction in natural family planning to avoid pregnancy

   Z30.09 Encounter for other general counseling and advice on contraception

       Encounter for family planning advice NOS

  Z30.2 Encounter for sterilization

✓5ᵗʰ **Z30.4 Encounter for** surveillance of contraceptives

   Z30.40 Encounter for surveillance of contraceptives, unspecified

   Z30.41 Encounter for surveillance of contraceptive pills ♀

       Encounter for repeat prescription for contraceptive pill

   Z30.42 Encounter for surveillance of injectable contraceptive ♀

✓6ᵗʰ **Z30.43 Encounter for surveillance of** intrauterine contraceptive device

    Z30.430 Encounter for insertion of intrauterine contraceptive device ♀

    Z30.431 Encounter for routine checking of intrauterine contraceptive device ♀

    Z30.432 Encounter for removal of intrauterine contraceptive device ♀

    Z30.433 Encounter for removal and reinsertion of intrauterine contraceptive device ♀

       Encounter for replacement of intrauterine contraceptive device

   Z30.44 Encounter for surveillance of vaginal ring hormonal contraceptive device ♀

   Z30.45 Encounter for surveillance of transdermal patch hormonal contraceptive device ♀

   Z30.46 Encounter for surveillance of implantable subdermal contraceptive ♀

       Encounter for checking, reinsertion or removal of implantable subdermal contraceptive

   Z30.49 Encounter for surveillance of other contraceptives ♀

       Encounter for surveillance of barrier contraception

       Encounter for surveillance of diaphragm

  Z30.8 Encounter for other contraceptive management

       Encounter for postvasectomy sperm count

       Encounter for routine examination for contraceptive maintenance

       EXCLUDES 1   sperm count following sterilization reversal (Z31.42)

             sperm count for fertility testing (Z31.41)

  Z30.9 Encounter for contraceptive management, unspecified

✓4ᵗʰ **Z31 Encounter for procreative management**

    EXCLUDES 1   complications associated with artificial fertilization (N98.-)

            female infertility (N97.-)

            male infertility (N46.-)

  Z31.0 Encounter for reversal of previous sterilization

✓5ᵗʰ **Z31.4 Encounter for** procreative investigation and testing

    EXCLUDES 1   postvasectomy sperm count (Z30.8)

   Z31.41 Encounter for fertility testing

       Encounter for fallopian tube patency testing

       Encounter for sperm count for fertility testing

   Z31.42 Aftercare following sterilization reversal

       Sperm count following sterilization reversal

✓6ᵗʰ **Z31.43 Encounter for genetic testing of** female for procreative management

       Use additional code for recurrent pregnancy loss, if applicable (N96, O26.2-)

       EXCLUDES 1   nonprocreative genetic testing (Z13.7-)

    Z31.430 Encounter of female for testing for genetic disease carrier status for procreative management ♀

    Z31.438 Encounter for other genetic testing of female for procreative management ♀

✓ Additional Character Required   ✓x7ᵗʰ Placeholder Alert   Manifestation   Unspecified Dx   ►◄ Revised Text   ● New Code   ▲ Revised Title

ICD-10-CM 2020   1213

Chapter 21. Factors Influencing Health Status and Contact With Health Services

Z31.44–Z36.82

√6ᵗʰ **Z31.44** **Encounter for genetic testing of male for procreative management**
> EXCLUDES 1   *nonprocreative genetic testing (Z13.7-)*

Z31.440 **Encounter of male for testing for genetic disease carrier status for procreative management** ♂

Z31.441 **Encounter for testing of male partner of patient with recurrent pregnancy loss** A ♂

Z31.448 **Encounter for other genetic testing of male for procreative management** A ♂

Z31.49 **Encounter for other procreative investigation and testing**

Z31.5 **Encounter for procreative genetic counseling**
AHA: 2017,4Q,27

√5ᵗʰ **Z31.6** **Encounter for general counseling and advice on procreation**

Z31.61 **Procreative counseling and advice using natural family planning**

Z31.62 **Encounter for fertility preservation counseling**
Encounter for fertility preservation counseling prior to cancer therapy
Encounter for fertility preservation counseling prior to surgical removal of gonads

Z31.69 **Encounter for other general counseling and advice on procreation**

Z31.7 **Encounter for procreative management and counseling for gestational carrier** ♀
> EXCLUDES 1   *pregnant state, gestational carrier (Z33.3)*
AHA: 2016,4Q,78

√5ᵗʰ **Z31.8** **Encounter for other procreative management**

Z31.81 **Encounter for male factor infertility in female patient** PDx ♀

Z31.82 **Encounter for Rh incompatibility status** ♀
AHA: 2015,3Q,40; 2014,4Q,17

Z31.83 **Encounter for assisted reproductive fertility procedure cycle** PDx ♀
Patient undergoing in vitro fertilization cycle
Use additional code to identify the type of infertility
> EXCLUDES 1   *pre-cycle diagnosis and testing — code to reason for encounter*

Z31.84 **Encounter for fertility preservation procedure** PDx
Encounter for fertility preservation procedure prior to cancer therapy
Encounter for fertility preservation procedure prior to surgical removal of gonads

Z31.89 **Encounter for other procreative management**

Z31.9 **Encounter for procreative management, unspecified**

√4ᵗʰ **Z32** **Encounter for pregnancy test and childbirth and childcare instruction**

√5ᵗʰ **Z32.0** **Encounter for pregnancy test**

Z32.00 **Encounter for pregnancy test, result unknown** ♀
Encounter for pregnancy test NOS

Z32.01 **Encounter for pregnancy test, result positive** M ♀

Z32.02 **Encounter for pregnancy test, result negative** ♀

Z32.2 **Encounter for childbirth instruction**

Z32.3 **Encounter for childcare instruction**
Encounter for prenatal or postpartum childcare instruction

√4ᵗʰ **Z33** **Pregnant state**

Z33.1 **Pregnant state, incidental** M ♀
Pregnant state NOS
> EXCLUDES 1   *complications of pregnancy (O00-O9A)*
> *pregnant state, gestational carrier (Z33.3)*

Z33.2 **Encounter for elective termination of pregnancy** PDx M ♀
> EXCLUDES 1   *early fetal death with retention of dead fetus (O02.1)*
> *late fetal death (O36.4)*
> *spontaneous abortion (O03)*

Z33.3 **Pregnant state, gestational carrier** M ♀
> EXCLUDES 1   *encounter for procreative management and counseling for gestational carrier (Z31.7)*
AHA: 2016,4Q,78

√4ᵗʰ **Z34** **Encounter for supervision of normal pregnancy**
> EXCLUDES 1   *any complication of pregnancy (O00-O9A)*
> *encounter for pregnancy test (Z32.0-)*
> *encounter for supervision of high risk pregnancy (O09.-)*
AHA: 2014,4Q,17

√5ᵗʰ **Z34.0** **Encounter for supervision of normal first pregnancy**

Z34.00 **Encounter for supervision of normal first pregnancy, unspecified trimester** PDx M ♀

Z34.01 **Encounter for supervision of normal first pregnancy, first trimester** PDx M ♀

Z34.02 **Encounter for supervision of normal first pregnancy, second trimester** PDx M ♀

Z34.03 **Encounter for supervision of normal first pregnancy, third trimester** PDx M ♀

√5ᵗʰ **Z34.8** **Encounter for supervision of other normal pregnancy**

Z34.80 **Encounter for supervision of other normal pregnancy, unspecified trimester** PDx M ♀

Z34.81 **Encounter for supervision of other normal pregnancy, first trimester** PDx M ♀

Z34.82 **Encounter for supervision of other normal pregnancy, second trimester** PDx M ♀

Z34.83 **Encounter for supervision of other normal pregnancy, third trimester** PDx M ♀

√5ᵗʰ **Z34.9** **Encounter for supervision of normal pregnancy, unspecified**

Z34.90 **Encounter for supervision of normal pregnancy, unspecified, unspecified trimester** PDx M ♀

Z34.91 **Encounter for supervision of normal pregnancy, unspecified, first trimester** PDx M ♀

Z34.92 **Encounter for supervision of normal pregnancy, unspecified, second trimester** PDx M ♀

Z34.93 **Encounter for supervision of normal pregnancy, unspecified, third trimester** PDx M ♀

√4ᵗʰ **Z36** **Encounter for antenatal screening of mother**
> INCLUDES   encounter for placental sample (taken vaginally)
> screening is the testing for disease or disease precursors in asymptomatic individuals so that early detection and treatment can be provided for those who test positive for the disease.
> EXCLUDES 1   *diagnostic examination — code to sign or symptom*
> *encounter for suspected maternal and fetal conditions ruled out (Z03.7-)*
> *suspected fetal condition affecting management of pregnancy — code to condition in Chapter 15*
> EXCLUDES 2   *abnormal findings on antenatal screening of mother (O28.-)*
> *genetic counseling and testing (Z31.43-, Z31.5)*
> *routine prenatal care (Z34)*
AHA: 2017,4Q,28

Z36.0 **Encounter for antenatal screening for chromosomal anomalies** M ♀

Z36.1 **Encounter for antenatal screening for raised alphafetoprotein level** M ♀
Encounter for antenatal screening for elevated maternal serum alphafetoprotein level
DEF: High levels of alpha-fetoprotein (AFP) that may indicate a possibility of spina bifida and other neural tube defects, anencephaly, or omphalocele in the fetus.

Z36.2 **Encounter for other antenatal screening follow-up** M ♀
Non-visualized anatomy on a previous scan

Z36.3 **Encounter for antenatal screening for malformations** M ♀
Screening for a suspected anomaly

Z36.4 **Encounter for antenatal screening for fetal growth retardation** M ♀
Intrauterine growth restriction (IUGR)/small-for-dates

Z36.5 **Encounter for antenatal screening for isoimmunization** M ♀

√5ᵗʰ **Z36.8** **Encounter for other antenatal screening**

Z36.81 **Encounter for antenatal screening for hydrops fetalis** M ♀
DEF: Hydrops fetalis: Abnormal accumulation of fluid in two or more parts of the fetus, such as ascites, effusion of the pleural or pericardial tissues, or edema.

Z36.82 **Encounter for antenatal screening for nuchal translucency** M ♀

Z36.83 Encounter for fetal screening for congenital cardiac abnormalities M ♀

Z36.84 Encounter for antenatal screening for fetal lung maturity M ♀

Z36.85 Encounter for antenatal screening for Streptococcus B M ♀

Z36.86 Encounter for antenatal screening for cervical length M ♀
Screening for risk of pre-term labor

Z36.87 Encounter for antenatal screening for uncertain dates M ♀

Z36.88 Encounter for antenatal screening for fetal macrosomia M ♀
Screening for large-for-dates

Z36.89 Encounter for other specified antenatal screening M ♀

Z36.8A Encounter for antenatal screening for other genetic defects M ♀

Z36.9 Encounter for antenatal screening, unspecified M ♀

√4th **Z3A Weeks of gestation**

NOTE Codes from category Z3A are for use, only on the maternal record, to indicate the weeks of gestation of the pregnancy, if known.

Code first complications of pregnancy, childbirth and the puerperium (O09-O9A)
AHA: 2019,2Q,11; 2016,2Q,34; 2014,3Q,17; 2014,2Q,9; 2013,2Q,33

√5th **Z3A.0 Weeks of gestation of pregnancy, unspecified or less than 10 weeks**

Z3A.00 Weeks of gestation of pregnancy not specified M ♀
Z3A.01 Less than 8 weeks gestation of pregnancy M ♀
Z3A.08 8 weeks gestation of pregnancy M ♀
Z3A.09 9 weeks gestation of pregnancy M ♀

√5th **Z3A.1 Weeks of gestation of pregnancy, weeks 10-19**
Z3A.10 10 weeks gestation of pregnancy M ♀
Z3A.11 11 weeks gestation of pregnancy M ♀
Z3A.12 12 weeks gestation of pregnancy M ♀
Z3A.13 13 weeks gestation of pregnancy M ♀
Z3A.14 14 weeks gestation of pregnancy M ♀
Z3A.15 15 weeks gestation of pregnancy M ♀
Z3A.16 16 weeks gestation of pregnancy M ♀
Z3A.17 17 weeks gestation of pregnancy M ♀
Z3A.18 18 weeks gestation of pregnancy M ♀
Z3A.19 19 weeks gestation of pregnancy M ♀

√5th **Z3A.2 Weeks of gestation of pregnancy, weeks 20-29**
Z3A.20 20 weeks gestation of pregnancy M ♀
Z3A.21 21 weeks gestation of pregnancy M ♀
Z3A.22 22 weeks gestation of pregnancy M ♀
Z3A.23 23 weeks gestation of pregnancy M ♀
Z3A.24 24 weeks gestation of pregnancy M ♀
Z3A.25 25 weeks gestation of pregnancy M ♀
Z3A.26 26 weeks gestation of pregnancy M ♀
Z3A.27 27 weeks gestation of pregnancy M ♀
Z3A.28 28 weeks gestation of pregnancy M ♀
Z3A.29 29 weeks gestation of pregnancy M ♀

√5th **Z3A.3 Weeks of gestation of pregnancy, weeks 30-39**
Z3A.30 30 weeks gestation of pregnancy M ♀
Z3A.31 31 weeks gestation of pregnancy M ♀
Z3A.32 32 weeks gestation of pregnancy M ♀
Z3A.33 33 weeks gestation of pregnancy M ♀
Z3A.34 34 weeks gestation of pregnancy M ♀
Z3A.35 35 weeks gestation of pregnancy M ♀
Z3A.36 36 weeks gestation of pregnancy M ♀
Z3A.37 37 weeks gestation of pregnancy M ♀
Z3A.38 38 weeks gestation of pregnancy M ♀
Z3A.39 39 weeks gestation of pregnancy M ♀

√5th **Z3A.4 Weeks of gestation of pregnancy, weeks 40 or greater**
AHA: 2014,4Q,23
Z3A.40 40 weeks gestation of pregnancy M ♀
Z3A.41 41 weeks gestation of pregnancy M ♀
Z3A.42 42 weeks gestation of pregnancy M ♀
Z3A.49 Greater than 42 weeks gestation of pregnancy M ♀

√4th **Z37 Outcome of delivery**
This category is intended for use as an additional code to identify the outcome of delivery on the mother's record. It is not for use on the newborn record.
EXCLUDES 1 stillbirth (P95)
Z37.0 Single live birth M ♀
AHA: 2016,2Q,34; 2014,2Q,9
Z37.1 Single stillbirth M ♀
Z37.2 Twins, both liveborn M ♀
Z37.3 Twins, one liveborn and one stillborn M ♀
Z37.4 Twins, both stillborn M ♀
√5th **Z37.5 Other multiple births, all liveborn**
Z37.50 Multiple births, unspecified, all liveborn M ♀
Z37.51 Triplets, all liveborn M ♀
Z37.52 Quadruplets, all liveborn M ♀
Z37.53 Quintuplets, all liveborn M ♀
Z37.54 Sextuplets, all liveborn M ♀
Z37.59 Other multiple births, all liveborn M ♀
√5th **Z37.6 Other multiple births, some liveborn**
Z37.60 Multiple births, unspecified, some liveborn M ♀
Z37.61 Triplets, some liveborn M ♀
Z37.62 Quadruplets, some liveborn M ♀
Z37.63 Quintuplets, some liveborn M ♀
Z37.64 Sextuplets, some liveborn M ♀
Z37.69 Other multiple births, some liveborn M ♀
Z37.7 Other multiple births, all stillborn M ♀
Z37.9 Outcome of delivery, unspecified M ♀
Multiple birth NOS
Single birth NOS

√4th **Z38 Liveborn infants according to place of birth and type of delivery**
This category is for use as the principal code on the initial record of a newborn baby. It is to be used for the initial birth record only. It is not to be used on the mother's record.
AHA: 2017,2Q,5-7; 2016,3Q,18; 2015,2Q,15
√5th **Z38.0 Single liveborn infant, born in hospital**
Single liveborn infant, born in birthing center or other health care facility
Z38.00 Single liveborn infant, delivered vaginally PDx N
Z38.01 Single liveborn infant, delivered by cesarean PDx N
Z38.1 Single liveborn infant, born outside hospital PDx N
Z38.2 Single liveborn infant, unspecified as to place of birth PDx N
Single liveborn infant NOS
√5th **Z38.3 Twin liveborn infant, born in hospital**
Z38.30 Twin liveborn infant, delivered vaginally PDx N
Z38.31 Twin liveborn infant, delivered by cesarean PDx N
Z38.4 Twin liveborn infant, born outside hospital PDx N
Z38.5 Twin liveborn infant, unspecified as to place of birth PDx N
√5th **Z38.6 Other multiple liveborn infant, born in hospital**
Z38.61 Triplet liveborn infant, delivered vaginally PDx N
Z38.62 Triplet liveborn infant, delivered by cesarean PDx N
Z38.63 Quadruplet liveborn infant, delivered vaginally PDx N
Z38.64 Quadruplet liveborn infant, delivered by cesarean PDx N
Z38.65 Quintuplet liveborn infant, delivered vaginally PDx N

Z38.66 Quintuplet **liveborn infant,** delivered by cesarean `PDx` `N`

Z38.68 **Other multiple liveborn infant,** delivered vaginally `PDx` `N`

Z38.69 **Other multiple liveborn infant,** delivered by cesarean `PDx` `N`

Z38.7 **Other multiple liveborn infant,** born outside hospital `PDx` `N`

Z38.8 **Other multiple liveborn infant, unspecified as to place of birth** `PDx` `N`

√4th **Z39 Encounter for maternal postpartum care and examination**

Z39.0 **Encounter for care and examination of mother** immediately after delivery `PDx` `M` ♀

Care and observation in uncomplicated cases when the delivery occurs outside a healthcare facility

EXCLUDES 1 *care for postpartum complication — see Alphabetic Index*

Z39.1 **Encounter for care and examination of** lactating mother `PDx` `M` ♀

Encounter for supervision of lactation

EXCLUDES 1 *disorders of lactation (O92.-)*

Z39.2 **Encounter for** routine postpartum **follow-up** `PDx` `M` ♀

Encounters for other specific health care (Z40-Z53)

Categories Z40-Z53 are intended for use to indicate a reason for care. They may be used for patients who have already been treated for a disease or injury, but who are receiving aftercare or prophylactic care, or care to consolidate the treatment, or to deal with a residual state

EXCLUDES 2 *follow-up examination for medical surveillance after treatment (Z08-Z09)*

√4th **Z40 Encounter for prophylactic surgery**

EXCLUDES 1 *organ donations (Z52.-)*

therapeutic organ removal — code to condition

DEF: Agent or treatment measure intended to prevent or ward off a disease condition.

√5th **Z40.0 Encounter for prophylactic surgery for** risk factors related to malignant neoplasms

Admission for prophylactic organ removal

Use additional code to identify risk factor

AHA: 2017,4Q,28-29

Z40.00 **Encounter for prophylactic removal of** unspecified organ `PDx`

Z40.01 **Encounter for prophylactic removal of** breast `PDx`

TIP: Use during the surgical encounter for removal of the breast; do not assign to indicate aftercare of prophylactic breast removal.

Z40.02 **Encounter for prophylactic removal of** ovary(s) `PDx` ♀

Encounter for prophylactic removal of ovary(s) and fallopian tube(s)

Z40.03 **Encounter for prophylactic removal of** fallopian tube(s) `PDx` ♀

Z40.09 **Encounter for prophylactic removal of** other organ `PDx`

Z40.8 **Encounter for other** prophylactic **surgery** `PDx`

Z40.9 **Encounter for prophylactic surgery, unspecified** `PDx`

√4th **Z41 Encounter for procedures for purposes other than remedying health state**

Z41.1 **Encounter for** cosmetic surgery

Encounter for cosmetic breast implant

Encounter for cosmetic procedure

EXCLUDES 1 *encounter for plastic and reconstructive surgery following medical procedure or healed injury (Z42.-)*

encounter for post-mastectomy breast implantation (Z42.1)

Z41.2 **Encounter for** routine and ritual male circumcision ♂

AHA: 2018,3Q,15

Z41.3 **Encounter for** ear piercing

Z41.8 **Encounter for other procedures for purposes other than remedying health state**

Z41.9 **Encounter for procedure for purposes other than remedying health state, unspecified**

√4th **Z42 Encounter for plastic and reconstructive surgery following medical procedure or healed injury**

EXCLUDES 1 *encounter for cosmetic plastic surgery (Z41.1)*

encounter for plastic surgery for treatment of current injury — code to relevent injury

Z42.1 **Encounter for** breast reconstruction following mastectomy `PDx` `A`

EXCLUDES 1 *deformity and disproportion of reconstructed breast (N65.1-)*

Z42.8 **Encounter for other plastic and reconstructive surgery following medical procedure or healed injury** `PDx`

AHA: 2017,1Q,42

√4th **Z43 Encounter for attention to artificial openings**

INCLUDES closure of artificial openings

passage of sounds or bougies through artificial openings

reforming artificial openings

removal of catheter from artificial openings

toilet or cleansing of artificial openings

EXCLUDES 1 *complications of external stoma (J95.0-, K94.-, N99.5-)*

EXCLUDES 2 *fitting and adjustment of prosthetic and other devices (Z44-Z46)*

AHA: 2019,2Q,33

TIP: Use only for routine care of the artificial opening.

Z43.0 **Encounter for attention to** tracheostomy

Z43.1 **Encounter for attention to** gastrostomy

EXCLUDES 2 *artificial opening status only, without need for care (Z93.-)*

Z43.2 **Encounter for attention to** ileostomy

Z43.3 **Encounter for attention to** colostomy

Z43.4 **Encounter for attention to other artificial** openings of digestive tract

Z43.5 **Encounter for attention to** cystostomy

Z43.6 **Encounter for attention to other artificial** openings of urinary tract

Encounter for attention to nephrostomy

Encounter for attention to ureterostomy

Encounter for attention to urethrostomy

Z43.7 **Encounter for attention to artificial** vagina

Z43.8 **Encounter for attention to other artificial openings**

Z43.9 **Encounter for attention to unspecified artificial opening**

√4th **Z44 Encounter for fitting and adjustment of external prosthetic device**

INCLUDES removal or replacement of external prosthetic device

EXCLUDES 1 *malfunction or other complications of device — see Alphabetical Index*

presence of prosthetic device (Z97.-)

√5th **Z44.0 Encounter for fitting and adjustment of** artificial arm

√6th Z44.00 **Encounter for fitting and adjustment of unspecified artificial arm**

Z44.001 **Encounter for fitting and adjustment of** unspecified right **artificial arm**

Z44.002 **Encounter for fitting and adjustment of** unspecified left **artificial arm**

Z44.009 **Encounter for fitting and adjustment of unspecified artificial arm, unspecified arm**

√6th Z44.01 **Encounter for fitting and adjustment of** complete **artificial arm**

Z44.011 **Encounter for fitting and adjustment of** complete right **artificial arm**

Z44.012 **Encounter for fitting and adjustment of** complete left **artificial arm**

Z44.019 **Encounter for fitting and adjustment of complete artificial arm, unspecified arm**

√6th Z44.02 **Encounter for fitting and adjustment of** partial **artificial arm**

Z44.021 **Encounter for fitting and adjustment of partial artificial** right **arm**

Z44.022 **Encounter for fitting and adjustment of partial artificial** left **arm**

Z44.029 **Encounter for fitting and adjustment of partial artificial arm, unspecified arm**

√5th **Z44.1 Encounter for fitting and adjustment of** artificial leg

√6th Z44.10 **Encounter for fitting and adjustment of unspecified artificial leg**

Z44.101 **Encounter for fitting and adjustment of** unspecified right **artificial leg**

Z44.102 **Encounter for fitting and adjustment of** unspecified left **artificial leg**

`N` Newborn: 0 `P` Pediatric: 0-17 `M` Maternity: 12-55 `A` Adult: 15-124 `CH` Comorbidity High `CL` Comorbidity Low `NCDx` Noncancer Dx `PDx` Primary Dx

1216 | ICD-10-CM 2020

Z44.109 Encounter for fitting and adjustment of unspecified artificial leg, unspecified leg

✓6ᵗʰ **Z44.11** Encounter for fitting and adjustment of complete artificial leg

Z44.111 Encounter for fitting and adjustment of complete right artificial leg

Z44.112 Encounter for fitting and adjustment of complete left artificial leg

Z44.119 Encounter for fitting and adjustment of complete artificial leg, unspecified leg

✓6ᵗʰ **Z44.12** Encounter for fitting and adjustment of partial artificial leg

Z44.121 Encounter for fitting and adjustment of partial artificial right leg

Z44.122 Encounter for fitting and adjustment of partial artificial left leg

Z44.129 Encounter for fitting and adjustment of partial artificial leg, unspecified leg

✓5ᵗʰ **Z44.2** Encounter for fitting and adjustment of artificial eye

> EXCLUDES 1   mechanical complication of ocular prosthesis (T85.3)

Z44.20 Encounter for fitting and adjustment of artificial eye, unspecified

Z44.21 Encounter for fitting and adjustment of artificial right eye

Z44.22 Encounter for fitting and adjustment of artificial left eye

✓5ᵗʰ **Z44.3** Encounter for fitting and adjustment of external breast prosthesis

> EXCLUDES 1   complications of breast implant (T85.4-)
>
> encounter for adjustment or removal of breast implant (Z45.81-)
>
> encounter for initial breast implant insertion for cosmetic breast augmentation (Z41.1)
>
> encounter for breast reconstruction following mastectomy (Z42.1)

Z44.30 Encounter for fitting and adjustment of external breast prosthesis, unspecified breast

Z44.31 Encounter for fitting and adjustment of external right breast prosthesis

Z44.32 Encounter for fitting and adjustment of external left breast prosthesis

Z44.8 Encounter for fitting and adjustment of other external prosthetic devices

Z44.9 Encounter for fitting and adjustment of unspecified external prosthetic device

✓4ᵗʰ **Z45** Encounter for adjustment and management of implanted device

> INCLUDES   removal or replacement of implanted device
>
> EXCLUDES 1   malfunction or other complications of device — see Alphabetical Index
>
> EXCLUDES 2   encounter for fitting and adjustment of non-implanted device (Z46.-)

✓5ᵗʰ **Z45.0** Encounter for adjustment and management of cardiac device

> **TIP:** Do not assign to indicate the presence of a pacemaker; these codes are reserved for indicating services provided to adjust the pacemaker rate, battery, and other management of the device, which generally are not performed by post-acute care providers.

✓6ᵗʰ **Z45.01** Encounter for adjustment and management of cardiac pacemaker

Encounter for adjustment and management of cardiac resynchronization therapy pacemaker (CRT-P)

> EXCLUDES 1   encounter for adjustment and management of automatic implantable cardiac defibrillator with synchronous cardiac pacemaker (Z45.02)

Z45.010 Encounter for checking and testing of cardiac pacemaker pulse generator [battery]

Encounter for replacing cardiac pacemaker pulse generator [battery]

Z45.018 Encounter for adjustment and management of other part of cardiac pacemaker

> EXCLUDES 1   ▶presence of other part of cardiac pacemaker (Z95.0)◄
>
> EXCLUDES 2   presence of prosthetic and other devices ▶(Z95.1-Z95.5, Z95.811-Z97)◄

Z45.02 Encounter for adjustment and management of automatic implantable cardiac defibrillator

Encounter for adjustment and management of automatic implantable cardiac defibrillator with synchronous cardiac pacemaker

Encounter for adjustment and management of cardiac resynchronization therapy defibrillator (CRT-D)

Z45.09 Encounter for adjustment and management of other cardiac device

Z45.1 Encounter for adjustment and management of infusion pump

Z45.2 Encounter for adjustment and management of vascular access device

Encounter for adjustment and management of vascular catheters

> EXCLUDES 1   encounter for adjustment and management of renal dialysis catheter (Z49.01)

AHA: 2018,3Q,20

TIP: This code is assigned if the service provided involves caring for or maintaining a device, observing for infection or adverse reaction, or teaching a caregiver how to administer the infusion. If the service includes the administration of the infusion, code the condition being treated rather than this aftercare code.

✓5ᵗʰ **Z45.3** Encounter for adjustment and management of implanted devices of the special senses

Z45.31 Encounter for adjustment and management of implanted visual substitution device

✓6ᵗʰ **Z45.32** Encounter for adjustment and management of implanted hearing device

> EXCLUDES 1   encounter for fitting and adjustment of hearing aide (Z46.1)

Z45.320 Encounter for adjustment and management of bone conduction device

Z45.321 Encounter for adjustment and management of cochlear device

Z45.328 Encounter for adjustment and management of other implanted hearing device

✓5ᵗʰ **Z45.4** Encounter for adjustment and management of implanted nervous system device

Z45.41 Encounter for adjustment and management of cerebrospinal fluid drainage device

Encounter for adjustment and management of cerebral ventricular (communicating) shunt

Z45.42 Encounter for adjustment and management of neurostimulator

▶Encounter for adjustment and management of brain neurostimulator◄

▶Encounter for adjustment and management of gastric neurostimulator◄

▶Encounter for adjustment and management of peripheral nerve neurostimulator◄

▶Encounter for adjustment and management of sacral nerve neurostimulator◄

▶Encounter for adjustment and management of spinal cord neurostimulator◄

▶Encounter for adjustment and management of vagus nerve neurostimulator◄

Z45.49 Encounter for adjustment and management of other implanted nervous system device

AHA: 2014,3Q,19

☑ Additional Character Required   ✓x7ᵗʰ Placeholder Alert   Manifestation   Unspecified Dx   ▶◄ Revised Text   ● New Code   ▲ Revised Title

ICD-10-CM 2020   **1217**

Chapter 21. Factors Influencing Health Status and Contact With Health Services

✓5ᵗʰ **Z45.8** **Encounter for adjustment and management of other implanted devices**

     ✓6ᵗʰ **Z45.81** **Encounter for adjustment or** removal of breast implant

         Encounter for elective implant exchange (different material) (different size)

         ▶Encounter removal of tissue expander with or without synchronous insertion of permanent implant◀

         EXCLUDES 1   complications of breast implant (T85.4-)

            encounter for initial breast implant insertion for cosmetic breast augmentation (Z41.1)

            encounter for breast reconstruction following mastectomy (Z42.1)

         Z45.811 **Encounter for adjustment or removal of** right **breast implant**

         Z45.812 **Encounter for adjustment or removal of** left **breast implant**

         Z45.819 **Encounter for adjustment or removal of unspecified breast implant**

     Z45.82 **Encounter for** adjustment or removal of myringotomy device **(stent) (tube)**

     Z45.89 **Encounter for adjustment and management of other implanted devices**

         AHA: 2014,4Q,26-28

Z45.9 **Encounter for adjustment and management of unspecified implanted device**

✓4ᵗʰ **Z46** **Encounter for fitting and adjustment of other devices**

     INCLUDES   removal or replacement of other device

     EXCLUDES 1   malfunction or other complications of device — see Alphabetical Index

     EXCLUDES 2   encounter for fitting and management of implanted devices (Z45.-)

         issue of repeat prescription only (Z76.0)

         presence of prosthetic and other devices (Z95-Z97)

Z46.0 **Encounter for fitting and adjustment of** spectacles and contact lenses

Z46.1 **Encounter for fitting and adjustment of** hearing aid

     EXCLUDES 1   encounter for adjustment and management of implanted hearing device (Z45.32-)

Z46.2 **Encounter for fitting and adjustment of other devices related to nervous system and special senses**

     EXCLUDES 2   encounter for adjustment and management of implanted nervous system device (Z45.4-)

         encounter for adjustment and management of implanted visual substitution device (Z45.31)

Z46.3 **Encounter for fitting and adjustment of** dental prosthetic device

     Encounter for fitting and adjustment of dentures

Z46.4 **Encounter for fitting and adjustment of** orthodontic device

✓5ᵗʰ **Z46.5** **Encounter for fitting and adjustment of other** gastrointestinal appliance and device

     EXCLUDES 1   encounter for attention to artificial openings of digestive tract (Z43.1-Z43.4)

     Z46.51 **Encounter for fitting and adjustment of** gastric lap band

     Z46.59 **Encounter for fitting and adjustment of other gastrointestinal appliance and device**

Z46.6 **Encounter for fitting and adjustment of** urinary device

     EXCLUDES 2   attention to artificial openings of urinary tract (Z43.5, Z43.6)

✓5ᵗʰ **Z46.8** **Encounter for fitting and adjustment of other specified devices**

     Z46.81 **Encounter for fitting and adjustment of** insulin pump

         Encounter for insulin pump instruction and training

         Encounter for insulin pump titration

     Z46.82 **Encounter for fitting and adjustment of** non-vascular catheter

     Z46.89 **Encounter for fitting and adjustment of other specified devices**

         Encounter for fitting and adjustment of wheelchair

Z46.9 **Encounter for fitting and adjustment of unspecified device**

✓4ᵗʰ **Z47** **Orthopedic aftercare**

     EXCLUDES 1   aftercare for healing fracture — code to fracture with 7th character D

Z47.1 **Aftercare following** joint replacement surgery   *OA NOT FX*

     Use additional code to identify the joint (Z96.6-)

Z47.2 **Encounter for removal of** internal fixation device

     EXCLUDES 1   encounter for adjustment of internal fixation device for fracture treatment — code to fracture with appropriate 7th character

         encounter for removal of external fixation device — code to fracture with 7th character D

         infection or inflammatory reaction to internal fixation device (T84.6-)

         mechanical complication of internal fixation device (T84.1-)

✓5ᵗʰ **Z47.3** **Aftercare following explantation of** joint prosthesis

     Aftercare following explantation of joint prosthesis, staged procedure

     Encounter for joint prosthesis insertion following prior explantation of joint prosthesis

     AHA: 2015,1Q,16

     TIP: Do not assign when a complication necessitating joint prosthesis explantation remains active or unresolved. When the complication remains, even in the presence of explantation of the prosthesis, assign the appropriate complication code.

     Z47.31 **Aftercare following explantation of** shoulder **joint prosthesis**

         EXCLUDES 1   acquired absence of shoulder joint following prior explantation of shoulder joint prosthesis (Z89.23-)

            shoulder joint prosthesis explantation status (Z89.23-)

     Z47.32 **Aftercare following explantation of** hip **joint prosthesis**

         EXCLUDES 1   acquired absence of hip joint following prior explantation of hip joint prosthesis (Z89.62-)

            hip joint prosthesis explantation status (Z89.62-)

     Z47.33 **Aftercare following explantation of** knee **joint prosthesis**

         EXCLUDES 1   acquired absence of knee joint following prior explantation of knee prosthesis (Z89.52-)

            knee joint prosthesis explantation status (Z89.52-)

✓5ᵗʰ **Z47.8** **Encounter for other orthopedic aftercare**

     Z47.81 **Encounter for orthopedic aftercare** following surgical amputation

         Use additional code to identify the limb amputated (Z89.-)

     Z47.82 **Encounter for orthopedic aftercare** following scoliosis surgery

     Z47.89 **Encounter for other orthopedic aftercare**

         AHA: 2015,1Q,8

         TIP: Do not assign this aftercare code for rehabilitation services following a total hip replacement due to a fracture. Since this fracture is now considered to be in the healing and recovery phase, assign first the appropriate injury code from category S72 with the seventh character of subsequent encounter, followed by a code from subcategory Z96.64 Presence of artificial hip joint.

N Newborn: 0   P Pediatric: 0-17   M Maternity: 12-55   A Adult: 15-124   CH Comorbidity High   CL Comorbidity Low   NCDx Noncancer Dx   PDx Primary Dx

1218   ICD-10-CM 2020

✔4th **Z48** **Encounter for other postprocedural aftercare**

> EXCLUDES 1   *encounter for aftercare following injury — code to Injury, by site, with appropriate 7th character for subsequent encounter*
> *encounter for follow-up examination after completed treatment (Z08-Z09)*
> EXCLUDES 2   *encounter for attention to artificial openings (Z43.-)*
> *encounter for fitting and adjustment of prosthetic and other devices (Z44-Z46)*
> AHA: 2015,4Q,38; 2015,1Q,6-7

✔5th **Z48.0** **Encounter for** attention to dressings, sutures and drains

> EXCLUDES 1   *encounter for planned postprocedural wound closure (Z48.1)*

     Z48.00 **Encounter for change or removal of** nonsurgical **wound** dressing
> Encounter for change or removal of wound dressing NOS

     Z48.01 **Encounter for change or removal of** surgical **wound** dressing
> AHA: 2019,2Q,33

     Z48.02 **Encounter for removal of** sutures
> Encounter for removal of staples

     Z48.03 **Encounter for change or removal of** drains
> AHA: 2019,2Q,33

   Z48.1 **Encounter for planned** postprocedural **wound closure**
> EXCLUDES 1   *encounter for attention to dressings and sutures (Z48.0-)*

✔5th **Z48.2** **Encounter for aftercare following** organ transplant

     Z48.21 **Encounter for aftercare following** heart **transplant**
     Z48.22 **Encounter for aftercare following** kidney **transplant**
     Z48.23 **Encounter for aftercare following** liver **transplant**
     Z48.24 **Encounter for aftercare following** lung **transplant**
   ✔6th **Z48.28** **Encounter for aftercare following** multiple **organ transplant**

       Z48.280 **Encounter for aftercare following** heart-lung **transplant**
       Z48.288 **Encounter for aftercare following** multiple **organ transplant**

   ✔6th **Z48.29** **Encounter for aftercare following other organ transplant**

       Z48.290 **Encounter for aftercare following** bone marrow **transplant**
       Z48.298 **Encounter for aftercare following other organ transplant**

   Z48.3 **Aftercare following** surgery for neoplasm
> Use additional code to identify the neoplasm

✔5th **Z48.8** **Encounter for other specified postprocedural aftercare**

   ✔6th **Z48.81** **Encounter for surgical aftercare following** surgery on specified body systems
> These codes identify the body system requiring aftercare. They are for use in conjunction with other aftercare codes to fully explain the aftercare encounter. The condition treated should also be coded if still present.
> EXCLUDES 1   *aftercare for injury — code the injury with 7th character D*
> *aftercare following surgery for neoplasm (Z48.3)*
> EXCLUDES 2   *aftercare following organ transplant (Z48.2-)*
> *orthopedic aftercare (Z47.-)*
> AHA: 2015,4Q,38

     Z48.810 **Encounter for surgical aftercare following surgery on the** sense organs
     Z48.811 **Encounter for surgical aftercare following surgery on the** nervous system
> EXCLUDES 2   *encounter for surgical aftercare following surgery on the sense organs (Z48.810)*
     Z48.812 **Encounter for surgical aftercare following surgery on the** circulatory system
> AHA: 2012,4Q,96
     Z48.813 **Encounter for surgical aftercare following surgery on the** respiratory system
> AHA: 2019,2Q,33
     Z48.814 **Encounter for surgical aftercare following surgery on the** teeth or oral cavity
     Z48.815 **Encounter for surgical aftercare following surgery on the** digestive system

     Z48.816 **Encounter for surgical aftercare following surgery on the** genitourinary system
> EXCLUDES 1   *encounter for aftercare following sterilization reversal (Z31.42)*
     Z48.817 **Encounter for surgical aftercare following surgery on the** skin and subcutaneous tissue

   Z48.89 **Encounter for other specified surgical aftercare**

✔4th **Z49** **Encounter for care involving renal dialysis**
> Code also associated end stage renal disease (N18.6)

✔5th **Z49.0** **Preparatory care for renal dialysis**
> Encounter for dialysis instruction and training

     Z49.01 **Encounter for fitting and adjustment of** extracorporeal dialysis catheter
> Removal or replacement of renal dialysis catheter
> Toilet or cleansing of renal dialysis catheter
     Z49.02 **Encounter for fitting and adjustment of** peritoneal dialysis catheter

✔5th **Z49.3** **Encounter for** adequacy testing for dialysis

     Z49.31 **Encounter for adequacy testing for** hemodialysis
     Z49.32 **Encounter for adequacy testing for** peritoneal dialysis
> Encounter for peritoneal equilibration test

✔4th **Z51** **Encounter for other aftercare and medical care**
> Code also condition requiring care
> EXCLUDES 1   *follow-up examination after treatment (Z08-Z09)*

   Z51.0 **Encounter for antineoplastic** radiation therapy   **PDx**
> AHA: 2017,4Q,103

✔5th **Z51.1** **Encounter for antineoplastic chemotherapy and immunotherapy**
> EXCLUDES 2   *encounter for chemotherapy and immunotherapy for nonneoplastic condition — code to condition*

     Z51.11 **Encounter for antineoplastic** chemotherapy   **PDx**
> AHA: 2015,3Q,19
     Z51.12 **Encounter for antineoplastic** immunotherapy   **PDx**

   Z51.5 **Encounter for** palliative care
> AHA: 2017,1Q,48
> TIP: Post-acute providers may assign as a primary diagnosis if the purpose of the admission is for palliative care.

   Z51.6 **Encounter for** desensitization to allergens
> AHA: 2016,4Q,77

✔5th **Z51.8** **Encounter for other specified aftercare**
> EXCLUDES 1   *holiday relief care (Z75.5)*

     Z51.81 **Encounter for** therapeutic drug level **monitoring**
> Code also any long-term (current) drug therapy (Z79.-)
> EXCLUDES 1   *encounter for blood-drug test for administrative or medicolegal reasons (Z02.83)*
> DEF: Drug monitoring: Measurement of the level of a specific drug in the body or measurement of a specific function to assess effectiveness of a drug.
     Z51.89 **Encounter for other specified aftercare**
> AHA: 2012,4Q,95-97

✔4th **Z52** **Donors of organs and tissues**
> INCLUDES   autologous and other living donors
> EXCLUDES 1   *cadaveric donor - omit code*
> *examination of potential donor (Z00.5)*
> AHA: 2012,4Q,99

✔5th **Z52.0** **Blood donor**

   ✔6th **Z52.00** **Unspecified blood donor**

     Z52.000 **Unspecified donor,** whole **blood**   **PDx**
     Z52.001 **Unspecified donor,** stem cells   **PDx**
     Z52.008 **Unspecified donor, other blood**   **PDx**

   ✔6th **Z52.01** **Autologous blood donor**

     Z52.010 **Autologous donor,** whole **blood**   **PDx**
     Z52.011 **Autologous donor,** stem cells   **PDx**
     Z52.018 **Autologous donor, other blood**   **PDx**

√6ᵗʰ **Z52.09** **Other blood donor**
Volunteer donor

Z52.090 **Other blood donor,** whole blood   PDx

Z52.091 **Other blood donor,** stem cells   PDx

Z52.098 **Other blood donor, other blood**   PDx

√5ᵗʰ **Z52.1** Skin **donor**

Z52.10 **Skin donor, unspecified**   PDx

Z52.11 **Skin donor,** autologous   PDx

Z52.19 **Skin donor, other**   PDx

√5ᵗʰ **Z52.2** Bone **donor**

Z52.20 **Bone donor, unspecified**   PDx

Z52.21 **Bone donor,** autologous   PDx

Z52.29 **Bone donor, other**   PDx

Z52.3 Bone marrow **donor**   PDx

Z52.4 Kidney **donor**   PDx

Z52.5 Cornea **donor**   PDx

Z52.6 Liver **donor**   PDx

√5ᵗʰ **Z52.8** **Donor of other specified organs or tissues**

√6ᵗʰ **Z52.81** Egg (Oocyte) **donor**

Z52.810 **Egg (Oocyte) donor** under age 35, anonymous **recipient**   PDx ♀
Egg donor under age 35 NOS

Z52.811 **Egg (Oocyte) donor** under age 35, designated **recipient**   PDx ♀

Z52.812 **Egg (Oocyte) donor** age 35 and over, anonymous **recipient**   PDx ♀
Egg donor age 35 and over NOS

Z52.813 **Egg (Oocyte) donor** age 35 and over, designated **recipient**   PDx ♀

Z52.819 **Egg (Oocyte) donor, unspecified**   PDx ♀

Z52.89 **Donor of other specified organs or tissues**   PDx

Z52.9 **Donor of unspecified organ or tissue**
Donor NOS

√4ᵗʰ **Z53** **Persons encountering health services for specific procedures and treatment, not carried out**

√5ᵗʰ **Z53.0** **Procedure and treatment not carried out because of contraindication**

Z53.01 **Procedure and treatment not carried out due to** patient smoking

Z53.09 **Procedure and treatment not carried out because of other contraindication**

Z53.1 **Procedure and treatment not carried out because of patient's decision for** reasons of belief and group pressure

√5ᵗʰ **Z53.2** **Procedure and treatment not carried out because of patient's decision for other and unspecified reasons**

Z53.20 **Procedure and treatment not carried out because of patient's decision for unspecified reasons**

Z53.21 **Procedure and treatment not carried out due to patient** leaving prior to being seen by health care provider

Z53.29 **Procedure and treatment not carried out because of patient's decision for other reasons**

√5ᵗʰ **Z53.3** **Procedure converted to open procedure**
AHA: 2016,4Q,79

Z53.31 Laparoscopic **surgical procedure converted to open procedure**

Z53.32 Thoracoscopic **surgical procedure converted to open procedure**

Z53.33 Arthroscopic **surgical procedure converted to open procedure**

Z53.39 **Other specified procedure converted to open procedure**

Z53.8 **Procedure and treatment not carried out for other reasons**

Z53.9 **Procedure and treatment not carried out, unspecified reason**

Persons with potential health hazards related to socioeconomic and psychosocial circumstances (Z55-Z65)

AHA: 2018,4Q,58,73; 2018,1Q,18

TIP: Because codes in these categories represent social information rather than medical diagnoses, they can be assigned based on documentation by nonphysician clinicians involved in the care of these patients.

√4ᵗʰ **Z55** **Problems related to education and literacy**

EXCLUDES 1   *disorders of psychological development (F80-F89)*

Z55.0 **Illiteracy and low-level literacy**

Z55.1 **Schooling unavailable and unattainable**

Z55.2 **Failed school examinations**

Z55.3 **Underachievement in school**

Z55.4 **Educational maladjustment and discord with teachers and classmates**

Z55.8 **Other problems related to education and literacy**
Problems related to inadequate teaching

Z55.9 **Problems related to education and literacy, unspecified**
Academic problems NOS

√4ᵗʰ **Z56** **Problems related to employment and unemployment**

EXCLUDES 2   *occupational exposure to risk factors (Z57.-)*
problems related to housing and economic circumstances (Z59.-)

Z56.0 **Unemployment, unspecified**

Z56.1 **Change of job**   A

Z56.2 **Threat of job loss**

Z56.3 **Stressful work schedule**

Z56.4 **Discord with boss and workmates**

Z56.5 **Uncongenial work environment**
Difficult conditions at work

Z56.6 **Other physical and mental strain related to work**

√5ᵗʰ **Z56.8** **Other problems related to employment**

Z56.81 **Sexual harassment on the job**

Z56.82 **Military deployment status**
Individual (civilian or military) currently deployed in theater or in support of military war, peacekeeping and humanitarian operations

Z56.89 **Other problems related to employment**

Z56.9 **Unspecified problems related to employment**
Occupational problems NOS

√4ᵗʰ **Z57** **Occupational exposure to risk factors**

Z57.0 **Occupational exposure to** noise

Z57.1 **Occupational exposure to** radiation

Z57.2 **Occupational exposure to** dust

√5ᵗʰ **Z57.3** **Occupational exposure to other air contaminants**

Z57.31 **Occupational exposure to environmental** tobacco smoke

EXCLUDES 2   *exposure to environmental tobacco smoke (Z77.22)*

Z57.39 **Occupational exposure to other air contaminants**

Z57.4 **Occupational exposure to** toxic agents in agriculture
Occupational exposure to solids, liquids, gases or vapors in agriculture

Z57.5 **Occupational exposure to** toxic agents in other industries
Occupational exposure to solids, liquids, gases or vapors in other industries

Z57.6 **Occupational exposure to** extreme temperature

Z57.7 **Occupational exposure to** vibration

Z57.8 **Occupational exposure to other risk factors**

Z57.9 **Occupational exposure to unspecified risk factor**

√4ᵗʰ **Z59** **Problems related to housing and economic circumstances**

EXCLUDES 2   *problems related to upbringing (Z62.-)*

Z59.0 **Homelessness**

Z59.1 **Inadequate housing**
Lack of heating
Restriction of space
Technical defects in home preventing adequate care
Unsatisfactory surroundings

EXCLUDES 1   *problems related to the natural and physical environment (Z77.1-)*

Z59.2 **Discord with neighbors, lodgers and landlord**

N Newborn: 0   P Pediatric: 0-17   M Maternity: 12-55   A Adult: 15-124   CH Comorbidity High   CL Comorbidity Low   NCDx Noncancer Dx   PDx Primary Dx

1220   ICD-10-CM 2020

Z59.3   **Problems related to living in residential institution**
Boarding-school resident
EXCLUDES 1   *institutional upbringing (Z62.2)*

Z59.4   **Lack of adequate food and safe drinking water**
Inadequate drinking water supply
EXCLUDES 1   *effects of hunger (T73.0)*
inappropriate diet or eating habits (Z72.4)
malnutrition (E40-E46)

Z59.5   **Extreme poverty**

Z59.6   **Low income**

Z59.7   **Insufficient social insurance and welfare support**

Z59.8   **Other problems related to housing and economic circumstances**
Foreclosure on loan
Isolated dwelling
Problems with creditors

Z59.9   **Problem related to housing and economic circumstances, unspecified**

✓4ᵗʰ **Z60**   **Problems related to social environment**

Z60.0   **Problems of adjustment to life-cycle transitions**
Empty nest syndrome
Phase of life problem
Problem with adjustment to retirement [pension]

Z60.2   **Problems related to living alone**

Z60.3   **Acculturation difficulty**
Problem with migration
Problem with social transplantation
DEF: Problem adapting to a different culture or environment not based on any coexisting mental disorder.

Z60.4   **Social exclusion and rejection**
Exclusion and rejection on the basis of personal characteristics, such as unusual physical appearance, illness or behavior.
EXCLUDES 1   *target of adverse discrimination such as for racial or religious reasons (Z60.5)*

Z60.5   **Target of (perceived) adverse discrimination and persecution**
EXCLUDES 1   *social exclusion and rejection (Z60.4)*

Z60.8   **Other problems related to social environment**

Z60.9   **Problem related to social environment, unspecified**

✓4ᵗʰ **Z62**   **Problems related to upbringing**
INCLUDES   current and past negative life events in childhood
current and past problems of a child related to upbringing
EXCLUDES 2   *maltreatment syndrome (T74.-)*
problems related to housing and economic circumstances (Z59.-)

Z62.0   **Inadequate parental supervision and control**

Z62.1   **Parental overprotection**

✓5ᵗʰ **Z62.2**   **Upbringing away from parents**
EXCLUDES 1   *problems with boarding school (Z59.3)*

Z62.21   **Child in welfare custody**   P
Child in care of non-parental family member
Child in foster care
EXCLUDES 2   *problem for parent due to child in welfare custody (Z63.5)*

Z62.22   **Institutional upbringing**
Child living in orphanage or group home

Z62.29   **Other upbringing away from parents**

Z62.3   **Hostility towards and scapegoating of child**   P

Z62.6   **Inappropriate (excessive) parental pressure**

✓5ᵗʰ **Z62.8**   **Other specified problems related to upbringing**

✓6ᵗʰ **Z62.81**   **Personal history of abuse in childhood**

Z62.810   **Personal history of physical and sexual abuse in childhood**
EXCLUDES 1   *current child physical abuse (T74.12, T76.12)*
current child sexual abuse (T74.22, T76.22)

Z62.811   **Personal history of psychological abuse in childhood**
EXCLUDES 1   *current child psychological abuse (T74.32, T76.32)*

Z62.812   **Personal history of neglect in childhood**
EXCLUDES 1   *current child neglect (T74.02, T76.02)*

Z62.813   **Personal history of forced labor or sexual exploitation in childhood**
AHA: 2018,4Q,32,35

Z62.819   **Personal history of unspecified abuse in childhood**
EXCLUDES 1   *current child abuse NOS (T74.92, T76.92)*

✓6ᵗʰ **Z62.82**   **Parent-child conflict**

Z62.820   **Parent-biological child conflict**
Parent-child problem NOS

Z62.821   **Parent-adopted child conflict**

Z62.822   **Parent-foster child conflict**

✓6ᵗʰ **Z62.89**   **Other specified problems related to upbringing**

Z62.890   **Parent-child estrangement NEC**

Z62.891   **Sibling rivalry**

Z62.898   **Other specified problems related to upbringing**

Z62.9   **Problem related to upbringing, unspecified**

✓4ᵗʰ **Z63**   **Other problems related to primary support group, including family circumstances**
EXCLUDES 2   *maltreatment syndrome (T74.-, T76)*
parent-child problems (Z62.-)
problems related to negative life events in childhood (Z62.-)
problems related to upbringing (Z62.-)

Z63.0   **Problems in relationship with spouse or partner**
Relationship distress with spouse or intimate partner
EXCLUDES 1   *counseling for spousal or partner abuse problems (Z69.1)*
counseling related to sexual attitude, behavior, and orientation (Z70.-)

Z63.1   **Problems in relationship with in-laws**

✓5ᵗʰ **Z63.3**   **Absence of family member**
EXCLUDES 1   *absence of family member due to disappearance and death (Z63.4)*
absence of family member due to separation and divorce (Z63.5)

Z63.31   **Absence of family member due to military deployment**
Individual or family affected by other family member being on military deployment
EXCLUDES 1   *family disruption due to return of family member from military deployment (Z63.71)*

Z63.32   **Other absence of family member**

Z63.4   **Disappearance and death of family member**
Assumed death of family member
Bereavement
AHA: 2014,1Q,25

Z63.5   **Disruption of family by separation and divorce**
Marital estrangement

Z63.6   **Dependent relative needing care at home**

✓5ᵗʰ **Z63.7**   **Other stressful life events affecting family and household**

Z63.71   **Stress on family due to return of family member from military deployment**
Individual or family affected by family member having returned from military deployment (current or past conflict)

Z63.72   **Alcoholism and drug addiction in family**

Z63.79   **Other stressful life events affecting family and household**
Anxiety (normal) about sick person in family
Health problems within family
Ill or disturbed family member
Isolated family

Z63.8   **Other specified problems related to primary support group**
Family discord NOS
Family estrangement NOS
High expressed emotional level within family
Inadequate family support NOS
Inadequate or distorted communication within family

Z63.9   **Problem related to primary support group, unspecified**
Relationship disorder NOS

✓4ᵗʰ **Z64**   **Problems related to certain psychosocial circumstances**

Z64.0   **Problems related to unwanted pregnancy**   ♀

Z64.1   **Problems related to multiparity**   ♀

Z64.4   **Discord with counselors**
Discord with probation officer
Discord with social worker

✓4th **Z65**   **Problems related to other psychosocial circumstances**

Z65.0   **Conviction in civil and criminal proceedings without imprisonment**

Z65.1   **Imprisonment and other incarceration**

Z65.2   **Problems related to release from prison**

Z65.3   **Problems related to other legal circumstances**
Arrest
Child custody or support proceedings
Litigation
Prosecution

Z65.4   **Victim of crime and terrorism**
Victim of torture

Z65.5   **Exposure to disaster, war and other hostilities**
EXCLUDES 1   *target of perceived discrimination or persecution (Z60.5)*

Z65.8   **Other specified problems related to psychosocial circumstances**
Religious or spiritual problem

Z65.9   **Problem related to unspecified psychosocial circumstances**

Do not resuscitate status (Z66)

Z66   **Do not resuscitate**
DNR status
DEF: Medical order written by a physician that instructs others not to perform cardiopulmonary resuscitation (CPR), intubation, or advanced life support (ACLS). It prevents unnecessary invasive treatment to prolong life should breathing stop or cardiac arrest occur.

Blood type (Z67)

✓4th **Z67**   **Blood type**
AHA: 2015,3Q,40

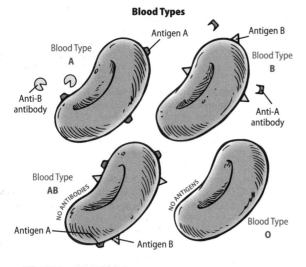

Blood Types

Antigen A

Antigen B

Blood Type A

Blood Type B

Anti-B antibody

Anti-A antibody

Blood Type AB

NO ANTIBODIES

NO ANTIGENS

Antigen A

Antigen B

Blood Type O

✓5th **Z67.1**   **Type A blood**

Z67.10   **Type A blood,** Rh positive
Z67.11   **Type A blood,** Rh negative

✓5th **Z67.2**   **Type B blood**

Z67.20   **Type B blood,** Rh positive
Z67.21   **Type B blood,** Rh negative

✓5th **Z67.3**   **Type AB blood**

Z67.30   **Type AB blood,** Rh positive
Z67.31   **Type AB blood,** Rh negative

✓5th **Z67.4**   **Type O blood**

Z67.40   **Type O blood,** Rh positive
Z67.41   **Type O blood,** Rh negative

✓5th **Z67.9**   **Unspecified blood type**

Z67.90   **Unspecified blood type,** Rh positive
Z67.91   **Unspecified blood type,** Rh negative

Body mass index [BMI] (Z68)

✓4th **Z68**   **Body mass index [BMI]**
Kilograms per meters squared

NOTE   ▶BMI adult codes are for use for persons 20 years of age or older◀

▶BMI pediatric codes are for use for persons 2-19 years of age.◀

▶These percentiles are based on the growth charts published by the Centers for Disease Control and Prevention (CDC)◀

AHA: 2018,4Q,73,77-83; 2017,1Q,39
DEF: Index used to help determine whether an individual is underweight, a healthy weight, overweight, or obese.
TIP: A BMI code may be assigned to support an associated condition based on medical record documentation from clinicians who are not the patient's provider.
TIP: In order to assign a BMI code, the associated condition must meet the definition of a reportable diagnosis for outpatient encounters, per section IV.J of the *ICD-10-CM Official Guidelines for Coding and Reporting.*

Z68.1   **Body mass index [BMI]** 19.9 or less, **adult**   A

✓5th **Z68.2**   **Body mass index [BMI]** 20-29, **adult**

Z68.20   **Body mass index [BMI]** 20.0-20.9, **adult**   A
Z68.21   **Body mass index [BMI]** 21.0-21.9, **adult**   A
Z68.22   **Body mass index [BMI]** 22.0-22.9, **adult**   A
Z68.23   **Body mass index [BMI]** 23.0-23.9, **adult**   A
Z68.24   **Body mass index [BMI]** 24.0-24.9, **adult**   A
Z68.25   **Body mass index [BMI]** 25.0-25.9, **adult**   A
Z68.26   **Body mass index [BMI]** 26.0-26.9, **adult**   A
Z68.27   **Body mass index [BMI]** 27.0-27.9, **adult**   A
Z68.28   **Body mass index [BMI]** 28.0-28.9, **adult**   A
Z68.29   **Body mass index [BMI]** 29.0-29.9, **adult**   A

✓5th **Z68.3**   **Body mass index [BMI]** 30-39, **adult**

Z68.30   **Body mass index [BMI]** 30.0-30.9, **adult**   A
Z68.31   **Body mass index [BMI]** 31.0-31.9, **adult**   A
Z68.32   **Body mass index [BMI]** 32.0-32.9, **adult**   A
Z68.33   **Body mass index [BMI]** 33.0-33.9, **adult**   A
Z68.34   **Body mass index [BMI]** 34.0-34.9, **adult**   A
Z68.35   **Body mass index [BMI]** 35.0-35.9, **adult**   A
Z68.36   **Body mass index [BMI]** 36.0-36.9, **adult**   A
Z68.37   **Body mass index [BMI]** 37.0-37.9, **adult**   A
Z68.38   **Body mass index [BMI]** 38.0-38.9, **adult**   A
Z68.39   **Body mass index [BMI]** 39.0-39.9, **adult**   A

✓5th **Z68.4**   **Body mass index [BMI]** 40 or greater, **adult**

Z68.41   **Body mass index [BMI]** 40.0-44.9, **adult**   A
Z68.42   **Body mass index [BMI]** 45.0-49.9, **adult**   A
Z68.43   **Body mass index [BMI]** 50.0-59.9, **adult**   A
Z68.44   **Body mass index [BMI]** 60.0-69.9, **adult**   A
Z68.45   **Body mass index [BMI]** 70 or greater, **adult**   A

✓5th **Z68.5**   **Body mass index [BMI]** pediatric
AHA: 2018,4Q,81-82

Z68.51   **Body mass index [BMI] pediatric,** less than 5th percentile for age
Z68.52   **Body mass index [BMI] pediatric,** 5th percentile to less than 85th percentile for age
Z68.53   **Body mass index [BMI] pediatric,** 85th percentile to less than 95th percentile for age
Z68.54   **Body mass index [BMI] pediatric,** greater than or equal to 95th percentile for age

Persons encountering health services in other circumstances (Z69-Z76)

✓4ᵗʰ **Z69 Encounter for mental health services for victim and perpetrator of abuse**

[INCLUDES] counseling for victims and perpetrators of abuse

✓5ᵗʰ **Z69.0 Encounter for mental health services for child abuse problems**

✓6ᵗʰ **Z69.01 Encounter for mental health services for parental child abuse**

Z69.010 Encounter for mental health services for victim of parental child abuse Ⓟ

Encounter for mental health services for victim of child abuse by parent

Encounter for mental health services for victim of child neglect by parent

Encounter for mental health services for victim of child psychological abuse by parent

Encounter for mental health services for victim of child sexual abuse by parent

Z69.011 Encounter for mental health services for perpetrator of parental child abuse

Encounter for mental health services for perpetrator of parental child neglect

Encounter for mental health services for perpetrator of parental child psychological abuse

Encounter for mental health services for perpetrator of parental child sexual abuse

[EXCLUDES 1] encounter for mental health services for non-parental child abuse (Z69.02-)

✓6ᵗʰ **Z69.02 Encounter for mental health services for non-parental child abuse**

Z69.020 Encounter for mental health services for victim of non-parental child abuse Ⓟ

Encounter for mental health services for victim of non-parental child neglect

Encounter for mental health services for victim of non-parental child psychological abuse

Encounter for mental health services for victim of non-parental child sexual abuse

Z69.021 Encounter for mental health services for perpetrator of non-parental child abuse

Encounter for mental health services for perpetrator of non-parental child neglect

Encounter for mental health services for perpetrator of non-parental child psychological abuse

Encounter for mental health services for perpetrator of non-parental child sexual abuse

✓5ᵗʰ **Z69.1 Encounter for mental health services for spousal or partner abuse problems**

Z69.11 Encounter for mental health services for victim of spousal or partner abuse

Encounter for mental health services for victim of spouse or partner neglect

Encounter for mental health services for victim of spouse or partner psychological abuse

Encounter for mental health services for victim of spouse or partner violence, physical

Z69.12 Encounter for mental health services for perpetrator of spousal or partner abuse

Encounter for mental health services for perpetrator of spouse or partner neglect

Encounter for mental health services for perpetrator of spouse or partner psychological abuse

Encounter for mental health services for perpetrator of spouse or partner violence, physical

Encounter for mental health services for perpetrator of spouse or partner violence, sexual

✓5ᵗʰ **Z69.8 Encounter for mental health services for victim or perpetrator of other abuse**

Z69.81 Encounter for mental health services for victim of other abuse

~~Encounter for mental health services for perpetrator of non-spousal adult abuse~~

Encounter for mental health services for victim of non-spousal adult abuse

Encounter for mental health services for victim of spouse or partner violence, sexual

Encounter for rape victim counseling

Z69.82 Encounter for mental health services for perpetrator of other abuse

▶Encounter for mental health services for perpetrator of non-spousal adult abuse◀

✓4ᵗʰ **Z70 Counseling related to sexual attitude, behavior and orientation**

[INCLUDES] encounter for mental health services for sexual attitude, behavior and orientation

[EXCLUDES 2] contraceptive or procreative counseling (Z30-Z31)

Z70.0 Counseling related to sexual attitude

Z70.1 Counseling related to patient's sexual behavior and orientation

Patient concerned regarding impotence

Patient concerned regarding non-responsiveness

Patient concerned regarding promiscuity

Patient concerned regarding sexual orientation

Z70.2 Counseling related to sexual behavior and orientation of third party

Advice sought regarding sexual behavior and orientation of child

Advice sought regarding sexual behavior and orientation of partner

Advice sought regarding sexual behavior and orientation of spouse

Z70.3 Counseling related to combined concerns regarding sexual attitude, behavior and orientation

Z70.8 Other sex counseling

Encounter for sex education

Z70.9 Sex counseling, unspecified

✓4ᵗʰ **Z71 Persons encountering health services for other counseling and medical advice, not elsewhere classified**

[EXCLUDES 2] contraceptive or procreation counseling (Z30-Z31)
sex counseling (Z70.-)

Z71.0 Person encountering health services to consult on behalf of another person

Person encountering health services to seek advice or treatment for non-attending third party

[EXCLUDES 2] anxiety (normal) about sick person in family (Z63.7)
expectant (adoptive) parent(s) pre-birth pediatrician visit (Z76.81)

Z71.1 Person with feared health complaint in whom no diagnosis is made

Person encountering health services with feared condition which was not demonstrated

Person encountering health services in which problem was normal state

"Worried well"

[EXCLUDES 1] medical observation for suspected diseases and conditions proven not to exist (Z03.-)

Z71.2 Person consulting for explanation of examination or test findings

Z71.3 Dietary counseling and surveillance

Use additional code for any associated underlying medical condition

Use additional code to identify body mass index (BMI), if known (Z68.-)

✅ Additional Character Required ✓x7ᵗʰ Placeholder Alert Manifestation Unspecified Dx ▶◀ Revised Text ● New Code ▲ Revised Title

ICD-10-CM 2020   1223

Chapter 21. Factors Influencing Health Status and Contact With Health Services

Z69–Z71.3

✓5ᵗʰ **Z71.4** Alcohol abuse **counseling and surveillance**
Use additional code for alcohol abuse or dependence (F10.-)

Z71.41 **Alcohol abuse counseling and surveillance of** alcoholic

Z71.42 **Counseling for** family member of alcoholic
Counseling for significant other, partner, or friend of alcoholic

✓5ᵗʰ **Z71.5** Drug abuse **counseling and surveillance**
Use additional code for drug abuse or dependence (F11-F16, F18-F19)

Z71.51 **Drug abuse counseling and surveillance of** drug abuser

Z71.52 **Counseling for** family member of drug abuser
Counseling for significant other, partner, or friend of drug abuser

Z71.6 Tobacco **abuse counseling**
Use additional code for nicotine dependence (F17.-)

Z71.7 Human immunodeficiency virus **[HIV] counseling**

✓5ᵗʰ **Z71.8** **Other specified counseling**
EXCLUDES 2   counseling for contraception (Z30.0-)
AHA: 2017,4Q,27

Z71.81 Spiritual or religious **counseling**

Z71.82 Exercise **counseling**

Z71.83 **Encounter for** nonprocreative genetic **counseling**
EXCLUDES 1   counseling for procreative genetics (Z31.5)
counseling for procreative management (Z31.6)

● **Z71.84** **Encounter for** health counseling related to travel
Encounter for health risk and safety counseling for (international) travel
Code also, if applicable, encounter for immunization (Z23)
EXCLUDES 2   encounter for administrative examination (Z02.-)
encounter for other special examination without complaint, suspected or reported diagnosis (Z01.-)

Z71.89 **Other specified counseling**

Z71.9 **Counseling, unspecified**
Encounter for medical advice NOS

✓4ᵗʰ **Z72** **Problems related to lifestyle**
EXCLUDES 2   problems related to life-management difficulty (Z73.-)
problems related to socioeconomic and psychosocial circumstances (Z55-Z65)

Z72.0 **Tobacco use**
Tobacco use NOS
EXCLUDES 1   history of tobacco dependence (Z87.891)
nicotine dependence (F17.2-)
tobacco dependence (F17.2-)
tobacco use during pregnancy (O99.33-)

Z72.3 **Lack of physical exercise**

Z72.4 **Inappropriate diet and eating habits**
EXCLUDES 1   behavioral eating disorders of infancy or childhood (F98.2-F98.3)
eating disorders (F50.-)
lack of adequate food (Z59.4)
malnutrition and other nutritional deficiencies (E40-E64)

✓5ᵗʰ **Z72.5** **High risk sexual behavior**
Promiscuity
EXCLUDES 1   paraphilias (F65)

Z72.51 **High risk** heterosexual **behavior**

Z72.52 **High risk** homosexual **behavior**

Z72.53 **High risk** bisexual **behavior**

Z72.6 **Gambling and betting**
EXCLUDES 1   compulsive or pathological gambling (F63.0)

✓5ᵗʰ **Z72.8** **Other problems related to lifestyle**

✓6ᵗʰ **Z72.81** **Antisocial behavior**
EXCLUDES 1   conduct disorders (F91.-)

Z72.810 Child and adolescent **antisocial behavior**   P
Antisocial behavior (child) (adolescent) without manifest psychiatric disorder
Delinquency NOS
Group delinquency
Offenses in the context of gang membership
Stealing in company with others
Truancy from school

Z72.811 Adult **antisocial behavior**   A
Adult antisocial behavior without manifest psychiatric disorder

✓6ᵗʰ **Z72.82** **Problems related to sleep**

Z72.820 **Sleep** deprivation
Lack of adequate sleep
EXCLUDES 1   insomnia (G47.0-)

Z72.821 Inadequate **sleep hygiene**
Bad sleep habits
Irregular sleep habits
Unhealthy sleep wake schedule
EXCLUDES 1   insomnia (F51.0-, G47.0-)

Z72.89 **Other problems related to lifestyle**
Self-damaging behavior

Z72.9 **Problem related to lifestyle, unspecified**

✓4ᵗʰ **Z73** **Problems related to life management difficulty**
EXCLUDES 2   problems related to socioeconomic and psychosocial circumstances (Z55-Z65)
DEF: State of emotional, mental, and physical exhaustion causing difficulties in managing personal, school, or work circumstances. It is usually due to prolonged stress or poor interpersonal relationship skills or parenting skills.

Z73.0 **Burn-out**

Z73.1 **Type A behavior pattern**

Z73.2 **Lack of relaxation and leisure**

Z73.3 **Stress, not elsewhere classified**
Physical and mental strain NOS
EXCLUDES 1   stress related to employment or unemployment (Z56.-)

Z73.4 **Inadequate social skills, not elsewhere classified**

Z73.5 **Social role conflict, not elsewhere classified**

Z73.6 **Limitation of activities due to disability**
EXCLUDES 1   care-provider dependency (Z74.-)

✓5ᵗʰ **Z73.8** **Other problems related to life management difficulty**

✓6ᵗʰ **Z73.81** **Behavioral insomnia of childhood**
DEF: Behaviors on the part of the child or caregivers that cause negative compliance with a child's sleep schedule resulting in lack of adequate sleep.

Z73.810 **Behavioral insomnia of childhood,** sleep-onset association **type**   P

Z73.811 **Behavioral insomnia of childhood,** limit setting **type**   P

Z73.812 **Behavioral insomnia of childhood,** combined **type**   P

Z73.819 **Behavioral insomnia of childhood, unspecified type**   P

Z73.82 **Dual sensory impairment**

Z73.89 **Other problems related to life management difficulty**

Z73.9 **Problem related to life management difficulty, unspecified**

✓4ᵗʰ **Z74** **Problems related to care provider dependency**
EXCLUDES 2   dependence on enabling machines or devices NEC (Z99.-)

✓5ᵗʰ **Z74.0** **Reduced mobility**

Z74.01 **Bed confinement status**
Bedridden

Z74.09 **Other reduced mobility**
Chair ridden
Reduced mobility NOS
EXCLUDES 2   wheelchair dependence (Z99.3)

Z74.1 **Need for assistance with** personal care

Z74.2 **Need for assistance at home and** no other household member able to render care

Z74.3   **Need for** continuous supervision

Z74.8   **Other problems related to care provider dependency**

Z74.9   **Problem related to care provider dependency, unspecified**

✓4ᵗʰ   **Z75**   **Problems related to medical facilities and other health care**

     Z75.0   **Medical services** not available in home
          EXCLUDES 1   no other household member able to render care
              (Z74.2)

     Z75.1   **Person** awaiting admission **to adequate facility elsewhere**

     Z75.2   **Other waiting period for investigation and treatment**

     Z75.3   **Unavailability** and inaccessibility of health-care facilities
          EXCLUDES 1   bed unavailable (Z75.1)

     Z75.4   **Unavailability** and inaccessibility of other helping agencies

     Z75.5   Holiday relief care

     Z75.8   **Other problems related to medical facilities and other health care**

     Z75.9   **Unspecified problem related to medical facilities and other health care**

✓4ᵗʰ   **Z76**   **Persons encountering health services in other circumstances**

     Z76.0   **Encounter for issue of repeat prescription**
          Encounter for issue of repeat prescription for appliance
          Encounter for issue of repeat prescription for medicaments
          Encounter for issue of repeat prescription for spectacles
          EXCLUDES 2   issue of medical certificate (Z02.7)
               repeat prescription for contraceptive (Z30.4-)

     Z76.1   **Encounter for health supervision and care of foundling**   PDx

     Z76.2   **Encounter for health supervision and care of other healthy infant and child**   PDx P
          Encounter for medical or nursing care or supervision of healthy infant under circumstances such as adverse socioeconomic conditions at home
          Encounter for medical or nursing care or supervision of healthy infant under circumstances such as awaiting foster or adoptive placement
          Encounter for medical or nursing care or supervision of healthy infant under circumstances such as maternal illness
          Encounter for medical or nursing care or supervision of healthy infant under circumstances such as number of children at home preventing or interfering with normal care

     Z76.3   **Healthy person accompanying sick person**

     Z76.4   **Other boarder to healthcare facility**
          EXCLUDES 1   homelessness (Z59.0)

     Z76.5   **Malingerer [conscious simulation]**
          Person feigning illness (with obvious motivation)
          EXCLUDES 1   factitious disorder (F68.1-, F68.A)
               peregrinating patient (F68.1-)
          DEF: Act of intentionally exaggerating an illness or disability in order to receive personal gain or to avoid punishment or responsibility.

✓5ᵗʰ   **Z76.8**   **Persons encountering health services in other specified circumstances**

     Z76.81   **Expectant parent(s) prebirth pediatrician visit**
          Pre-adoption pediatrician visit for adoptive parent(s)

     Z76.82   **Awaiting organ transplant status**
          Patient waiting for organ availability

     Z76.89   **Persons encountering health services in other specified circumstances**
          Persons encountering health services NOS
          AHA: 2014,2Q,10

Persons with potential health hazards related to family and personal history and certain conditions influencing health status (Z77-Z99)

Code also any follow-up examination (Z08-Z09)

✓4ᵗʰ   **Z77**   **Other contact with and (suspected) exposures hazardous to health**

     INCLUDES   contact with and (suspected) exposures to potential hazards to health
     EXCLUDES 2   contact with and (suspected) exposure to communicable diseases (Z20.-)
          exposure to (parental) (environmental) tobacco smoke in the perinatal period (P96.81)
          newborn affected by noxious substances transmitted via placenta or breast milk (P04.-)
          occupational exposure to risk factors (Z57.-)
          retained foreign body (Z18.-)
          retained foreign body fully removed (Z87.821)
          toxic effects of substances chiefly nonmedicinal as to source (T51-T65)

✓5ᵗʰ   **Z77.0**   **Contact with and (suspected) exposure to** hazardous, chiefly nonmedicinal, chemicals

     ✓6ᵗʰ   **Z77.01**   **Contact with and (suspected) exposure to hazardous** metals

          Z77.010   **Contact with and (suspected) exposure to** arsenic

          Z77.011   **Contact with and (suspected) exposure to** lead

          Z77.012   **Contact with and (suspected) exposure to** uranium
              EXCLUDES 1   retained depleted uranium fragments (Z18.01)

          Z77.018   **Contact with and (suspected) exposure to other hazardous metals**
              Contact with and (suspected) exposure to chromium compounds
              Contact with and (suspected) exposure to nickel dust

     ✓6ᵗʰ   **Z77.02**   **Contact with and (suspected) exposure to hazardous** aromatic compounds

          Z77.020   **Contact with and (suspected) exposure to** aromatic amines

          Z77.021   **Contact with and (suspected) exposure to** benzene

          Z77.028   **Contact with and (suspected) exposure to other hazardous aromatic compounds**
              Aromatic dyes NOS
              Polycyclic aromatic hydrocarbons

     ✓6ᵗʰ   **Z77.09**   **Contact with and (suspected) exposure to other hazardous, chiefly** nonmedicinal, chemicals

          Z77.090   **Contact with and (suspected) exposure to** asbestos

          Z77.098   **Contact with and (suspected) exposure to other hazardous, chiefly nonmedicinal, chemicals**
              Dyes NOS

✓5ᵗʰ   **Z77.1**   **Contact with and (suspected) exposure to** environmental pollution and hazards in the physical environment

     ✓6ᵗʰ   **Z77.11**   **Contact with and (suspected) exposure to** environmental pollution

          Z77.110   **Contact with and (suspected) exposure to** air **pollution**

          Z77.111   **Contact with and (suspected) exposure to** water **pollution**

          Z77.112   **Contact with and (suspected) exposure to** soil **pollution**

          Z77.118   **Contact with and (suspected) exposure to other environmental pollution**

     ✓6ᵗʰ   **Z77.12**   **Contact with and (suspected) exposure to** hazards in the physical environment

          Z77.120   **Contact with and (suspected) exposure to** mold **(toxic)**

✔ Additional Character Required   ✓x7ᵗʰ Placeholder Alert   Manifestation   Unspecified Dx   ►◄ Revised Text   ● New Code   ▲ Revised Title

Z77.121 Contact with and (suspected) exposure to harmful algae and algae toxins
Contact with and (suspected) exposure to (harmful) algae bloom NOS
Contact with and (suspected) exposure to blue-green algae bloom
Contact with and (suspected) exposure to brown tide
Contact with and (suspected) exposure to cyanobacteria bloom
Contact with and (suspected) exposure to Florida red tide
Contact with and (suspected) exposure to pfiesteria piscicida
Contact with and (suspected) exposure to red tide

Z77.122 Contact with and (suspected) exposure to noise

Z77.123 Contact with and (suspected) exposure to radon and other naturally occurring radiation
EXCLUDES 2 *radiation exposure as the cause of a confirmed condition (W88-W90, X39.0-)*
radiation sickness NOS (T66)

Z77.128 Contact with and (suspected) exposure to other hazards in the physical environment

√5ᵗʰ **Z77.2 Contact with and (suspected) exposure to other hazardous substances**

Z77.21 Contact with and (suspected) exposure to potentially hazardous body fluids

Z77.22 Contact with and (suspected) exposure to environmental tobacco smoke **(acute) (chronic)**
Exposure to second hand tobacco smoke (acute) (chronic)
Passive smoking (acute) (chronic)
EXCLUDES 1 *nicotine dependence (F17.-)*
tobacco use (Z72.0)
EXCLUDES 2 *occupational exposure to environmental tobacco smoke (Z57.31)*

Z77.29 Contact with and (suspected) exposure to other hazardous substances
AHA: 2016,2Q,33

Z77.9 Other contact with and (suspected) exposures hazardous to health

√4ᵗʰ **Z78 Other specified health status**
EXCLUDES 2 *asymptomatic human immunodeficiency virus [HIV] infection status (Z21)*
postprocedural status (Z93-Z99)
sex reassignment status (Z87.890)

Z78.0 Asymptomatic menopausal state 🅐 ♀
Menopausal state NOS
Postmenopausal status NOS
EXCLUDES 2 *symptomatic menopausal state (N95.1)*

Z78.1 Physical restraint status
EXCLUDES 1 *physical restraint due to a procedure — omit code*
DEF: Application of mechanical restraining devices or manual restraints to limit physical mobility of a patient.

Z78.9 Other specified health status

√4ᵗʰ **Z79 Long term (current) drug therapy**
INCLUDES long term (current) drug use for prophylactic purposes
Code also any therapeutic drug level monitoring (Z51.81)
EXCLUDES 2 *drug abuse and dependence (F11-F19)*
drug use complicating pregnancy, childbirth, and the puerperium (O99.32-)
long term (current) use of oral antidiabetic drugs (Z79.84)
long term (current) use of oral hypoglycemic drugs (Z79.84)
TIP: Do not assign when the focus of an encounter is due to the adverse effect or poisoning of a drug; use in the absence of current, unresolved complications.

√5ᵗʰ **Z79.0 Long term (current) use of anticoagulants and antithrombotics/antiplatelets**
EXCLUDES 2 *long term (current) use of aspirin (Z79.82)*

Z79.01 Long term (current) use of anticoagulants

Z79.02 Long term (current) use of antithrombotics/antiplatelets

Z79.1 Long term (current) use of non-steroidal anti-inflammatories **(NSAID)**
EXCLUDES 2 *long term (current) use of aspirin (Z79.82)*

Z79.2 Long term (current) use of antibiotics

Z79.3 Long term (current) use of hormonal contraceptives
Long term (current) use of birth control pill or patch

Z79.4 Long term (current) use of insulin
TIP: If the patient is using both oral hypoglycemic drugs and insulin for diabetes, assign only Z79.4 Long term (current) use of insulin.

√5ᵗʰ **Z79.5 Long term (current) use of steroids**

Z79.51 Long term (current) use of inhaled steroids

Z79.52 Long term (current) use of systemic steroids

√5ᵗʰ **Z79.8 Other long term (current) drug therapy**

√6ᵗʰ **Z79.81 Long term (current) use of agents affecting estrogen receptors and estrogen levels**
Code first, if applicable:
malignant neoplasm of breast (C50.-)
malignant neoplasm of prostate (C61)
Use additional code, if applicable, to identify:
estrogen receptor positive status (Z17.0)
family history of breast cancer (Z80.3)
genetic susceptibility to malignant neoplasm (cancer) (Z15.0-)
personal history of breast cancer (Z85.3)
personal history of prostate cancer (Z85.46)
postmenopausal status (Z78.0)
EXCLUDES 1 *hormone replacement therapy (Z79.890)*

Z79.810 Long term (current) use of selective estrogen receptor modulators (SERMs)
[handwritten: Tamoxifen]
Long term (current) use of raloxifene (Evista)
Long term (current) use of tamoxifen (Nolvadex)
Long term (current) use of toremifene (Fareston)

Z79.811 Long term (current) use of aromatase inhibitors
Long term (current) use of anastrozole (Arimidex)
Long term (current) use of exemestane (Aromasin)
Long term (current) use of letrozole (Femara)

Z79.818 Long term (current) use of other agents affecting estrogen receptors and estrogen levels
Long term (current) use of estrogen receptor downregulators
Long term (current) use of fulvestrant (Faslodex)
Long term (current) use of gonadotropin-releasing hormone (GnRH) agonist
Long term (current) use of goserelin acetate (Zoladex)
Long term (current) use of leuprolide acetate (leuprorelin) (Lupron)
Long term (current) use of megestrol acetate (Megace)

Z79.82 Long term (current) use of aspirin

Z79.83 Long term (current) use of bisphosphonates
AHA: 2016,4Q,42

Z79.84 Long term (current) use of oral hypoglycemic drugs
Long term (current) use of oral antidiabetic drugs
EXCLUDES 2 *long term (current) use of insulin (Z79.4)*
AHA: 2016,4Q,76
TIP: If the patient is using both oral hypoglycemic drugs and insulin for diabetes, assign only Z79.4 Long term (current) use of insulin.

√6ᵗʰ **Z79.89 Other long term (current) drug therapy**

Z79.890 Hormone replacement therapy

Z79.891   **Long term (current) use of** opiate analgesic
    Long term (current) use of methadone for pain management
    EXCLUDES 1   methodone use NOS (F11.9-)
      use of methodone for treatment of heroin addiction (F11.2-)

Z79.899   **Other long term (current) drug therapy**
    AHA: 2015,4Q,34; 2015,3Q,21

✓4ᵗʰ **Z80**   **Family history of primary malignant neoplasm**

Z80.0   **Family history of malignant neoplasm of** digestive organs
    Conditions classifiable to C15-C26
    AHA: 2018,1Q,6

Z80.1   **Family history of malignant neoplasm of** trachea, bronchus and lung
    Conditions classifiable to C33-C34

Z80.2   **Family history of malignant neoplasm of other respiratory and intrathoracic organs**
    Conditions classifiable to C30-C32, C37-C39

Z80.3   **Family history of malignant neoplasm of** breast
    Conditions classifiable to C50.-

✓5ᵗʰ **Z80.4**   **Family history of malignant neoplasm of genital organs**
    Conditions classifiable to C51-C63

    Z80.41   **Family history of malignant neoplasm of** ovary
    Z80.42   **Family history of malignant neoplasm of** prostate
    Z80.43   **Family history of malignant neoplasm of** testis
    Z80.49   **Family history of malignant neoplasm of other genital organs**

✓5ᵗʰ **Z80.5**   **Family history of malignant neoplasm of urinary tract**
    Conditions classifiable to C64-C68

    Z80.51   **Family history of malignant neoplasm of** kidney
    Z80.52   **Family history of malignant neoplasm of** bladder
    Z80.59   **Family history of malignant neoplasm of other urinary tract organ**

Z80.6   **Family history of** leukemia
    Conditions classifiable to C91-C95

Z80.7   **Family history of other malignant neoplasms of** lymphoid, hematopoietic and related tissues
    Conditions classifiable to C81-C90, C96.-

Z80.8   **Family history of malignant neoplasm of other organs or systems**
    Conditions classifiable to C00-C14, C40-C49, C69-C79

Z80.9   **Family history of malignant neoplasm, unspecified**
    Conditions classifiable to C80.1

✓4ᵗʰ **Z81**   **Family history of mental and behavioral disorders**

Z81.0   **Family history of** intellectual disabilities
    Conditions classifiable to F70-F79

Z81.1   **Family history of** alcohol abuse and dependence
    Conditions classifiable to F10.-

Z81.2   **Family history of** tobacco abuse and dependence
    Conditions classifiable to F17.-

Z81.3   **Family history of other psychoactive substance abuse and dependence**
    Conditions classifiable to F11-F16, F18-F19

Z81.4   **Family history of other substance abuse and dependence**
    Conditions classifiable to F55

Z81.8   **Family history of other mental and behavioral disorders**
    Conditions classifiable elsewhere in F01-F99

✓4ᵗʰ **Z82**   **Family history of certain disabilities and chronic diseases (leading to disablement)**

Z82.0   **Family history of** epilepsy **and other diseases of the nervous system**
    Conditions classifiable to G00-G99

Z82.1   **Family history of** blindness and visual loss
    Conditions classifiable to H54.-

Z82.2   **Family history of** deafness and hearing loss
    Conditions classifiable to H90-H91

Z82.3   **Family history of** stroke
    Conditions classifiable to I60-I64

✓5ᵗʰ **Z82.4**   **Family history of ischemic heart disease and other diseases of the circulatory system**
    Conditions classifiable to I00-I52, I65-I99

    Z82.41   **Family history of** sudden cardiac death
    Z82.49   **Family history of** ischemic heart disease **and other diseases of the circulatory system**

Z82.5   **Family history of** asthma **and other chronic lower respiratory diseases**
    Conditions classifiable to J40-J47
    EXCLUDES 2   family history of other diseases of the respiratory system (Z83.6)

✓5ᵗʰ **Z82.6**   **Family history of arthritis and other diseases of the musculoskeletal system and connective tissue**
    Conditions classifiable to M00-M99

    Z82.61   **Family history of** arthritis
    Z82.62   **Family history of** osteoporosis
    Z82.69   **Family history of other diseases of the musculoskeletal system and connective tissue**

✓5ᵗʰ **Z82.7**   **Family history of congenital malformations, deformations and chromosomal abnormalities**
    Conditions classifiable to Q00-Q99

    Z82.71   **Family history of** polycystic kidney
    Z82.79   **Family history of other congenital malformations, deformations and chromosomal abnormalities**

Z82.8   **Family history of other disabilities and chronic diseases leading to disablement, not elsewhere classified**

✓4ᵗʰ **Z83**   **Family history of other specific disorders**
    EXCLUDES 2   contact with and (suspected) exposure to communicable disease in the family (Z20.-)

Z83.0   **Family history of** human immunodeficiency virus **[HIV] disease**
    Conditions classifiable to B20

Z83.1   **Family history of other infectious and parasitic diseases**
    Conditions classifiable to A00-B19, B25-B94, B99

Z83.2   **Family history of diseases of the** blood and blood-forming organs **and certain disorders involving the immune mechanism**
    Conditions classifiable to D50-D89

Z83.3   **Family history of** diabetes mellitus
    Conditions classifiable to E08-E13

✓5ᵗʰ **Z83.4**   **Family history of other endocrine, nutritional and metabolic diseases**
    Conditions classifiable to E00-E07, E15-E88

    Z83.41   **Family history of** multiple endocrine neoplasia [MEN] syndrome
    Z83.42   **Family history of** familial hypercholesterolemia
      AHA: 2016,4Q,77

    ✓6ᵗʰ **Z83.43**   **Family history of other disorder of lipoprotein metabolism and other lipidemias**
      AHA: 2018,4Q,6,35

      Z83.430   **Family history of** elevated lipoprotein(a)
        Family history of elevated Lp(a)
      Z83.438   **Family history of other disorder of lipoprotein metabolism and other lipidemia**
        Family history of familial combined hyperlipidemia

    Z83.49   **Family history of other endocrine, nutritional and metabolic diseases**

✓5ᵗʰ **Z83.5**   **Family history of eye and ear disorders**

    ✓6ᵗʰ **Z83.51**   **Family history of** eye **disorders**
      Conditions classifiable to H00-H53, H55-H59
      EXCLUDES 2   family history of blindness and visual loss (Z82.1)

      Z83.511   **Family history of** glaucoma
      Z83.518   **Family history of other specified eye disorder**

    Z83.52   **Family history of** ear **disorders**
      Conditions classifiable to H60-H83, H92-H95
      EXCLUDES 2   family history of deafness and hearing loss (Z82.2)

Z83.6   **Family history of other diseases of the** respiratory system
    Conditions classifiable to J00-J39, J60-J99
    EXCLUDES 2   family history of asthma and other chronic lower respiratory diseases (Z82.5)

✓5ᵗʰ **Z83.7**   **Family history of diseases of the digestive system**
    Conditions classifiable to K00-K93

    Z83.71   **Family history of** colonic polyps
      EXCLUDES 2   family history of malignant neoplasm of digestive organs (Z80.0)

    Z83.79   **Family history of other diseases of the digestive system**

☑ Additional Character Required   ✓x7ᵗʰ Placeholder Alert   Manifestation   Unspecified Dx   ▶◀ Revised Text   ● New Code   ▲ Revised Title

ICD-10-CM 2020   1227

☑4ᵗʰ **Z84 Family history of other conditions**

Z84.0 Family history of diseases of the skin and subcutaneous tissue
Conditions classifiable to L00-L99

Z84.1 Family history of disorders of kidney and ureter
Conditions classifiable to N00-N29

Z84.2 Family history of other diseases of the genitourinary system
Conditions classifiable to N30-N99

Z84.3 Family history of consanguinity

☑5ᵗʰ **Z84.8 Family history of other specified conditions**

Z84.81 Family history of carrier of genetic disease

Z84.82 Family history of sudden infant death syndrome
Family history of SIDS
AHA: 2016,4Q,77

Z84.89 Family history of other specified conditions

☑4ᵗʰ **Z85 Personal history of malignant neoplasm**
Code first any follow-up examination after treatment of malignant neoplasm (Z08)
Use additional code to identify:
alcohol use and dependence (F10.-)
exposure to environmental tobacco smoke (Z77.22)
history of tobacco dependence (Z87.891)
occupational exposure to environmental tobacco smoke (Z57.31)
tobacco dependence (F17.-)
tobacco use (Z72.0)
EXCLUDES 2　personal history of benign neoplasm (Z86.01-)
　　　　　　personal history of carcinoma-in-situ (Z86.00-)
AHA: 2018,4Q,64

☑5ᵗʰ **Z85.0 Personal history of malignant neoplasm of** digestive organs
AHA: 2017,1Q,9

Z85.00 Personal history of malignant neoplasm of unspecified digestive organ

Z85.01 Personal history of malignant neoplasm of esophagus
Conditions classifiable to C15

☑6ᵗʰ **Z85.02 Personal history of malignant neoplasm of** stomach

Z85.020 Personal history of malignant carcinoid tumor **of stomach**
Conditions classifiable to C7A.092

Z85.028 Personal history of other malignant neoplasm of stomach
Conditions classifiable to C16

☑6ᵗʰ **Z85.03 Personal history of malignant neoplasm of** large intestine

Z85.030 Personal history of malignant carcinoid tumor **of large intestine**
Conditions classifiable to C7A.022-C7A.025, C7A.029

Z85.038 Personal history of other malignant neoplasm of large intestine
Conditions classifiable to C18

☑6ᵗʰ **Z85.04 Personal history of malignant neoplasm of** rectum, rectosigmoid junction, and anus

Z85.040 Personal history of malignant carcinoid tumor **of rectum**
Conditions classifiable to C7A.026

Z85.048 Personal history of other malignant neoplasm of rectum, rectosigmoid junction, and anus
Conditions classifiable to C19-C21

Z85.05 Personal history of malignant neoplasm of liver
Conditions classifiable to C22

☑6ᵗʰ **Z85.06 Personal history of malignant neoplasm of** small intestine

Z85.060 Personal history of malignant carcinoid tumor **of small intestine**
Conditions classifiable to C7A.01-

Z85.068 Personal history of other malignant neoplasm of small intestine
Conditions classifiable to C17

Z85.07 Personal history of malignant neoplasm of pancreas
Conditions classifiable to C25

Z85.09 Personal history of malignant neoplasm of other digestive organs

☑5ᵗʰ **Z85.1 Personal history of malignant neoplasm of** trachea, bronchus and lung

☑6ᵗʰ **Z85.11 Personal history of malignant neoplasm of** bronchus and lung

Z85.110 Personal history of malignant carcinoid tumor **of bronchus and lung**
Conditions classifiable to C7A.090

Z85.118 Personal history of other malignant neoplasm of bronchus and lung
Conditions classifiable to C34

Z85.12 Personal history of malignant neoplasm of trachea
Conditions classifiable to C33

☑5ᵗʰ **Z85.2 Personal history of malignant neoplasm of other** respiratory and intrathoracic organs

Z85.20 Personal history of malignant neoplasm of unspecified respiratory organ

Z85.21 Personal history of malignant neoplasm of larynx
Conditions classifiable to C32

Z85.22 Personal history of malignant neoplasm of nasal cavities, middle ear, and accessory sinuses
Conditions classifiable to C30-C31

☑6ᵗʰ **Z85.23 Personal history of malignant neoplasm of** thymus

Z85.230 Personal history of malignant carcinoid tumor **of thymus**
Conditions classifiable to C7A.091

Z85.238 Personal history of other malignant neoplasm of thymus
Conditions classifiable to C37

Z85.29 Personal history of malignant neoplasm of other respiratory and intrathoracic organs

Z85.3 Personal history of malignant neoplasm of breast
Conditions classifiable to C50.-

☑5ᵗʰ **Z85.4 Personal history of malignant neoplasm of** genital organs
Conditions classifiable to C51-C63

Z85.40 Personal history of malignant neoplasm of unspecified female **genital organ** ♀

Z85.41 Personal history of malignant neoplasm of cervix uteri ♀

Z85.42 Personal history of malignant neoplasm of other parts of uterus ♀

Z85.43 Personal history of malignant neoplasm of ovary ♀

Z85.44 Personal history of malignant neoplasm of other female **genital organs** ♀

Z85.45 Personal history of malignant neoplasm of unspecified male **genital organ** ♂

Z85.46 Personal history of malignant neoplasm of prostate ♂

Z85.47 Personal history of malignant neoplasm of testis ♂

Z85.48 Personal history of malignant neoplasm of epididymis ♂

Z85.49 Personal history of malignant neoplasm of other male **genital organs** ♂

☑5ᵗʰ **Z85.5 Personal history of malignant neoplasm of** urinary tract
Conditions classifiable to C64-C68

Z85.50 Personal history of malignant neoplasm of unspecified urinary tract organ

Z85.51 Personal history of malignant neoplasm of bladder

☑6ᵗʰ **Z85.52 Personal history of malignant neoplasm of** kidney
EXCLUDES 1　personal history of malignant neoplasm of renal pelvis (Z85.53)

Z85.520 Personal history of malignant carcinoid tumor **of kidney**
Conditions classifiable to C7A.093

Z85.528 Personal history of other malignant neoplasm of kidney
Conditions classifiable to C64

Z85.53 Personal history of malignant neoplasm of renal pelvis

Z85.54 Personal history of malignant neoplasm of ureter

Z85.59 Personal history of malignant neoplasm of other urinary tract organ

Z85.6 Personal history of leukemia
Conditions classifiable to C91-C95
EXCLUDES 1　leukemia in remission C91.0-C95.9 with 5th character 1

✓5ᵗʰ **Z85.7** **Personal history of other malignant neoplasms of lymphoid, hematopoietic and related tissues**

    Z85.71 **Personal history of** Hodgkin lymphoma
        Conditions classifiable to C81

    Z85.72 **Personal history of** non-Hodgkin lymphomas
        Conditions classifiable to C82-C85

    Z85.79 **Personal history of other malignant neoplasms of lymphoid, hematopoietic and related tissues**
        Conditions classifiable to C88-C90, C96
        EXCLUDES 1   *multiple myeloma in remission (C90.01)*
                   plasma cell leukemia in remission (C90.11)
                   plasmacytoma in remission (C90.21)

✓5ᵗʰ **Z85.8** **Personal history of malignant neoplasms of other organs and systems**
    Conditions classifiable to C00-C14, C40-C49, C69-C75, C7A.098, C76-C79

   ✓6ᵗʰ **Z85.81** **Personal history of malignant neoplasm of** lip, oral cavity, and pharynx

      Z85.810 **Personal history of malignant neoplasm of tongue**

      Z85.818 **Personal history of malignant neoplasm of other sites of lip, oral cavity, and pharynx**

      Z85.819 **Personal history of malignant neoplasm of unspecified site of lip, oral cavity, and pharynx**

   ✓6ᵗʰ **Z85.82** **Personal history of malignant neoplasm of** skin

      Z85.820 **Personal history of malignant** melanoma **of skin**
         Conditions classifiable to C43

      Z85.821 **Personal history of** Merkel cell carcinoma
         Conditions classifiable to C4A

      Z85.828 **Personal history of other malignant neoplasm of skin**
         Conditions classifiable to C44

   ✓6ᵗʰ **Z85.83** **Personal history of malignant neoplasm of** bone and soft tissue

      Z85.830 **Personal history of malignant neoplasm of** bone

      Z85.831 **Personal history of malignant neoplasm of** soft tissue
         EXCLUDES 2   *personal history of malignant neoplasm of skin (Z85.82-)*

   ✓6ᵗʰ **Z85.84** **Personal history of malignant neoplasm of** eye and nervous tissue

      Z85.840 **Personal history of malignant neoplasm of** eye

      Z85.841 **Personal history of malignant neoplasm of** brain

      Z85.848 **Personal history of malignant neoplasm of other parts of nervous tissue**

   ✓6ᵗʰ **Z85.85** **Personal history of malignant neoplasm of** endocrine glands

      Z85.850 **Personal history of malignant neoplasm of** thyroid

      Z85.858 **Personal history of malignant neoplasm of other endocrine glands**

    Z85.89 **Personal history of malignant neoplasm of other organs and systems**

  Z85.9 **Personal history of malignant neoplasm, unspecified**
    Conditions classifiable to C7A.00, C80.1

✓4ᵗʰ **Z86** **Personal history of certain other diseases**
    Code first any follow-up examination after treatment (Z09)

✓5ᵗʰ **Z86.0** **Personal history of in-situ and benign neoplasms and neoplasms of uncertain behavior**
    EXCLUDES 2   *personal history of malignant neoplasms (Z85.-)*
    AHA: 2017,1Q,9

   ✓6ᵗʰ **Z86.00** **Personal history of** in-situ neoplasm
      Conditions classifiable to D00-D09

      Z86.000 **Personal history of in-situ neoplasm of breast**
         ▶Conditions classifiable to D05◀

      Z86.001 **Personal history of in-situ neoplasm of** cervix uteri   ♀
         ▶Conditions classifiable to D06◀
         Personal history of cervical intraepithelial neoplasia III [CIN III]

●   **Z86.002** **Personal history of in-situ neoplasm of other and unspecified genital organs**
         Conditions classifiable to D07
         Personal history of high-grade prostatic intraepithelial neoplasia III [HGPIN III]
         Personal history of vaginal intraepithelial neoplasia III [VAIN III]
         Personal history of vulvar intraepithelial neoplasia III [VIN III]

●   **Z86.003** **Personal history of in-situ neoplasm of** oral cavity, esophagus and stomach
         Conditions classifiable to D00

●   **Z86.004** **Personal history of in-situ neoplasm of other and unspecified digestive organs**
         Conditions classifiable to D01
         Personal history of anal intraepithelial neoplasia (AIN III)

      Z86.005 **Personal history of in-situ neoplasm of** middle ear and respiratory system
         Conditions classifiable to D02

●   **Z86.006** **Personal history of** melanoma in-situ
         Conditions classifiable to D03
         EXCLUDES 2   *sites other than skin — code to personal history of in-situ neoplasm of the site*

      Z86.007 **Personal history of in-situ neoplasm of** skin
         Conditions classifiable to D04
         Personal history of carcinoma in situ of skin

      Z86.008 **Personal history of in-situ neoplasm of other site**
         ▶Conditions classifiable to D09◀
         ~~Personal history of vaginal intraepithelial neoplasia III [VAIN III]~~
         ~~Personal history of vulvar intraepithelial neoplasia III [VIN III]~~

   ✓6ᵗʰ **Z86.01** **Personal history of** benign neoplasm

      Z86.010 **Personal history of** colonic polyps
         AHA: 2017,1Q,14

      Z86.011 **Personal history of benign neoplasm of the** brain

      Z86.012 **Personal history of benign** carcinoid tumor

      Z86.018 **Personal history of other benign neoplasm**
         AHA: 2017,1Q,14

    Z86.03 **Personal history of** neoplasm of uncertain behavior

✓5ᵗʰ **Z86.1** **Personal history of** infectious and parasitic diseases
    Conditions classifiable to A00-B89, B99
    EXCLUDES 1   *personal history of infectious diseases specific to a body system*
                sequelae of infectious and parasitic diseases (B90-B94)

    Z86.11 **Personal history of** tuberculosis
    Z86.12 **Personal history of** poliomyelitis
    Z86.13 **Personal history of** malaria
    Z86.14 **Personal history of** Methicillin resistant Staphylococcus aureus **infection**
      Personal history of MRSA infection

    Z86.15 **Personal history of** latent tuberculosis **infection**

    Z86.19 **Personal history of other infectious and parasitic diseases**

Z86.2 **Personal history of diseases of the** blood and blood-forming organs **and certain disorders involving the** immune mechanism
    Conditions classifiable to D50-D89

✓5ᵗʰ **Z86.3** **Personal history of** endocrine, nutritional and metabolic diseases
    Conditions classifiable to E00-E88

    Z86.31 **Personal history of** diabetic foot ulcer
      EXCLUDES 2   *current diabetic foot ulcer (E08.621, E09.621, E10.621, E11.621, E13.621)*

    Z86.32 **Personal history of** gestational diabetes   ♀
      Personal history of conditions classifiable to O24.4-
      EXCLUDES 1   *gestational diabetes mellitus in current pregnancy (O24.4-)*

    Z86.39 **Personal history of other endocrine, nutritional and metabolic disease**

☑ Additional Character Required   ✓x7ᵗʰ Placeholder Alert   Manifestation   Unspecified Dx   ▶◀ Revised Text   ● New Code   ▲ Revised Title

✓5ᵗʰ **Z86.5** **Personal history of** mental and behavioral disorders
Conditions classifiable to F40-F59

Z86.51 **Personal history of** combat and operational stress reaction ▣A

Z86.59 **Personal history of other mental and behavioral disorders**

✓5ᵗʰ **Z86.6** **Personal history of diseases of the** nervous system and sense organs
Conditions classifiable to G00-G99, H00-H95

Z86.61 **Personal history of** infections of the central nervous system
Personal history of encephalitis
Personal history of meningitis

Z86.69 **Personal history of other diseases of the nervous system and sense organs**
AHA: 2016,4Q,24

✓5ᵗʰ **Z86.7** **Personal history of diseases of the** circulatory system
Conditions classifiable to I00-I99
EXCLUDES 2   old myocardial infarction (I25.2)
personal history of anaphylactic shock (Z87.892)
postmyocardial infarction syndrome (I24.1)

✓6ᵗʰ **Z86.71** **Personal history of** venous thrombosis and embolism

Z86.711 **Personal history of** pulmonary embolism
Z86.718 **Personal history of other venous thrombosis and embolism**

Z86.72 **Personal history of** thrombophlebitis

Z86.73 **Personal history of** transient ischemic attack **(TIA), and cerebral infarction without residual deficits**
Personal history of prolonged reversible ischemic neurological deficit (PRIND)
Personal history of stroke NOS without residual deficits
EXCLUDES 1   personal history of traumatic brain injury (Z87.820)
sequelae of cerebrovascular disease (I69.-)
AHA: 2012,4Q,92

Z86.74 **Personal history of** sudden cardiac arrest
Personal history of sudden cardiac death successfully resuscitated

Z86.79 **Personal history of other diseases of the circulatory system**

✓4ᵗʰ **Z87** **Personal history of other diseases and conditions**
Code first any follow-up examination after treatment (Z09)

✓5ᵗʰ **Z87.0** **Personal history of diseases of the** respiratory system
Conditions classifiable to J00-J99

Z87.01 **Personal history of** pneumonia **(recurrent)**
Z87.09 **Personal history of other diseases of the respiratory system**

✓5ᵗʰ **Z87.1** **Personal history of diseases of the** digestive system
Conditions classifiable to K00-K93

Z87.11 **Personal history of** peptic ulcer **disease**
Z87.19 **Personal history of other diseases of the digestive system**
AHA: 2017,1Q,14

Z87.2 **Personal history of diseases of the** skin and subcutaneous tissue
Conditions classifiable to L00-L99
EXCLUDES 2   personal history of diabetic foot ulcer (Z86.31)

✓5ᵗʰ **Z87.3** **Personal history of diseases of the** musculoskeletal system and connective tissue
Conditions classifiable to M00-M99
EXCLUDES 2   personal history of (healed) traumatic fracture (Z87.81)

✓6ᵗʰ **Z87.31** **Personal history of (healed)** nontraumatic fracture
TIP: Assign to indicate history of osteoporosis fractures that have resolved, even when a code from category M80 indicating current osteoporosis fracture is assigned.

Z87.310 **Personal history of (healed)** osteoporosis fracture
Personal history of (healed) fragility fracture
Personal history of (healed) collapsed vertebra due to osteoporosis
TIP: Assign for history of osteoporosis fractures that have resolved, even when a code from category M80 indicating current osteoporosis fracture is also reported.

Z87.311 **Personal history of (healed) other pathological fracture**
Personal history of (healed) collapsed vertebra NOS
EXCLUDES 2   personal history of osteoporosis fracture (Z87.310)

Z87.312 **Personal history of (healed)** stress fracture
Personal history of (healed) fatigue fracture

Z87.39 **Personal history of other diseases of the musculoskeletal system and connective tissue**

✓5ᵗʰ **Z87.4** **Personal history of diseases of the** genitourinary system
Conditions classifiable to N00-N99

✓6ᵗʰ **Z87.41** **Personal history of** dysplasia of the female genital tract
EXCLUDES 1   personal history of intraepithelial neoplasia III of female genital tract (Z86.001, Z86.008)
personal history of malignant neoplasm of female genital tract (Z85.40-Z85.44)

Z87.410 **Personal history of** cervical dysplasia ♀
Z87.411 **Personal history of** vaginal dysplasia ♀
Z87.412 **Personal history of** vulvar dysplasia ♀

Z87.42 **Personal history of other diseases of the** female **genital tract** ♀

✓6ᵗʰ **Z87.43** **Personal history of diseases of the** male genital organs

Z87.430 **Personal history of** prostatic dysplasia ♂
EXCLUDES 1   personal history of malignant neoplasm of prostate (Z85.46)

Z87.438 **Personal history of other diseases of** male **genital organs** ♂

✓6ᵗʰ **Z87.44** **Personal history of diseases of the** urinary system
EXCLUDES 1   personal history of malignant neoplasm of cervix uteri (Z85.41)

Z87.440 **Personal history of** urinary (tract) infections
Z87.441 **Personal history of** nephrotic syndrome
Z87.442 **Personal history of** urinary calculi
Personal history of kidney stones
Z87.448 **Personal history of other diseases of urinary system**

✓5ᵗʰ **Z87.5** **Personal history of complications of** pregnancy, childbirth and the puerperium
Conditions classifiable to O00-O9A
EXCLUDES 2   recurrent pregnancy loss (N96)

Z87.51 **Personal history of** pre-term labor ♀
EXCLUDES 1   current pregnancy with history of pre-term labor (O09.21-)

Z87.59 **Personal history of other complications of pregnancy, childbirth and the puerperium** ♀
Personal history of trophoblastic disease

✓5ᵗʰ **Z87.7** **Personal history of (corrected) congenital malformations**
Conditions classifiable to Q00-Q89 that have been repaired or corrected

     EXCLUDES 1   *congenital malformations that have been partially corrected or repair but which still require medical treatment — code to condition*

     EXCLUDES 2   *other postprocedural states (Z98.-)*
personal history of medical treatment (Z92.-)
presence of cardiac and vascular implants and grafts (Z95.-)
presence of other devices (Z97.-)
presence of other functional implants (Z96.-)
transplanted organ and tissue status (Z94.-)

✓6ᵗʰ **Z87.71** **Personal history of (corrected) congenital malformations of** genitourinary system

     Z87.710 **Personal history of (corrected) hypospadias** ♂

     Z87.718 **Personal history of other specified (corrected) congenital malformations of genitourinary system**

✓6ᵗʰ **Z87.72** **Personal history of (corrected) congenital malformations of** nervous system and sense organs

     Z87.720 **Personal history of (corrected) congenital malformations of** eye

     Z87.721 **Personal history of (corrected) congenital malformations of** ear

     Z87.728 **Personal history of other specified (corrected) congenital malformations of nervous system and sense organs**

✓6ᵗʰ **Z87.73** **Personal history of (corrected) congenital malformations of** digestive system

     Z87.730 **Personal history of (corrected)** cleft lip and palate

     Z87.738 **Personal history of other specified (corrected) congenital malformations of digestive system**

Z87.74 **Personal history of (corrected) congenital malformations of** heart and circulatory system

Z87.75 **Personal history of (corrected) congenital malformations of** respiratory system

Z87.76 **Personal history of (corrected) congenital malformations of** integument, limbs and musculoskeletal system

✓6ᵗʰ **Z87.79** **Personal history of other (corrected) congenital malformations**

     Z87.790 **Personal history of (corrected) congenital malformations of** face and neck

     Z87.798 **Personal history of other (corrected) congenital malformations**

✓5ᵗʰ **Z87.8** **Personal history of other specified conditions**

     EXCLUDES 2   *personal history of self harm (Z91.5)*

Z87.81 **Personal history of (healed)** traumatic fracture

     EXCLUDES 2   *personal history of (healed) nontraumatic fracture (Z87.31-)*

✓6ᵗʰ **Z87.82** **Personal history of other (healed)** physical injury and trauma
Conditions classifiable to S00-T88, except traumatic fractures

     Z87.820 **Personal history of** traumatic brain injury

       EXCLUDES 1   *personal history of transient ischemic attack (TIA), and cerebral infarction without residual deficits (Z86.73)*

     Z87.821 **Personal history of** retained foreign body fully removed

     Z87.828 **Personal history of other (healed) physical injury and trauma**

✓6ᵗʰ **Z87.89** **Personal history of other specified conditions**

     Z87.890 **Personal history of** sex reassignment

     Z87.891 **Personal history of** nicotine dependence

       EXCLUDES 1   *current nicotine dependence (F17.2-)*

     AHA: 2017,2Q,27

Z87.892 **Personal history of** anaphylaxis
Code also allergy status such as:
     allergy status to drugs, medicaments and biological substances (Z88.-)
     allergy status, other than to drugs and biological substances (Z91.0-)

Z87.898 **Personal history of other specified conditions**
     AHA: 2013,1Q,21

✓4ᵗʰ **Z88** **Allergy status to drugs, medicaments and biological substances**

     EXCLUDES 2   *allergy status, other than to drugs and biological substances (Z91.0-)*

     AHA: 2015,3Q,23

Z88.0 **Allergy status to** penicillin

Z88.1 **Allergy status to other antibiotic agents status**

Z88.2 **Allergy status to** sulfonamides **status**

Z88.3 **Allergy status to other anti-infective agents status**

Z88.4 **Allergy status to** anesthetic **agent status**

Z88.5 **Allergy status to** narcotic **agent status**

Z88.6 **Allergy status to** analgesic **agent status**

Z88.7 **Allergy status to** serum and vaccine **status**

Z88.8 **Allergy status to other drugs, medicaments and biological substances status**

Z88.9 **Allergy status to unspecified drugs, medicaments and biological substances status**

✓4ᵗʰ **Z89** **Acquired absence of limb**

     INCLUDES   amputation status
postprocedural loss of limb
post-traumatic loss of limb

     EXCLUDES 1   *acquired deformities of limbs (M20-M21)*
congenital absence of limbs (Q71-Q73)

✓5ᵗʰ **Z89.0** **Acquired absence of** thumb and other finger(s)

   ✓6ᵗʰ **Z89.01** **Acquired absence of** thumb

     Z89.011 **Acquired absence of** right **thumb**

     Z89.012 **Acquired absence of** left **thumb**

     Z89.019 **Acquired absence of unspecified thumb**

   ✓6ᵗʰ **Z89.02** **Acquired absence of other** finger(s)

     EXCLUDES 2   *acquired absence of thumb (Z89.01-)*

     Z89.021 **Acquired absence of** right **finger(s)**

     Z89.022 **Acquired absence of** left **finger(s)**

     Z89.029 **Acquired absence of unspecified finger(s)**

✓5ᵗʰ **Z89.1** **Acquired absence of** hand and wrist

   ✓6ᵗʰ **Z89.11** **Acquired absence of** hand

     Z89.111 **Acquired absence of** right **hand**

     Z89.112 **Acquired absence of** left **hand**

     Z89.119 **Acquired absence of unspecified hand**

   ✓6ᵗʰ **Z89.12** **Acquired absence of** wrist
Disarticulation at wrist

     Z89.121 **Acquired absence of** right **wrist**

     Z89.122 **Acquired absence of** left **wrist**

     Z89.129 **Acquired absence of unspecified wrist**

✓5ᵗʰ **Z89.2** **Acquired absence of** upper limb above wrist

   ✓6ᵗʰ **Z89.20** **Acquired absence of upper limb, unspecified level**

     Z89.201 **Acquired absence of** right **upper limb, unspecified level**

     Z89.202 **Acquired absence of** left **upper limb, unspecified level**

     Z89.209 **Acquired absence of unspecified upper limb, unspecified level**
Acquired absence of arm NOS

   ✓6ᵗʰ **Z89.21** **Acquired absence of** upper limb below elbow

     Z89.211 **Acquired absence of** right **upper limb below elbow**

     Z89.212 **Acquired absence of** left **upper limb below elbow**

     Z89.219 **Acquired absence of unspecified upper limb below elbow**

   ✓6ᵗʰ **Z89.22** **Acquired absence of** upper limb above elbow
Disarticulation at elbow

     Z89.221 **Acquired absence of** right **upper limb above elbow**

     Z89.222 **Acquired absence of** left **upper limb above elbow**

     Z89.229 **Acquired absence of unspecified upper limb above elbow**

✓ Additional Character Required   ✓x7ᵗʰ Placeholder Alert   Manifestation   Unspecified Dx   ▶◀ Revised Text   ● New Code   ▲ Revised Title

Chapter 21. Factors Influencing Health Status and Contact With Health Services

✓6th **Z89.23 Acquired absence of** shoulder

Acquired absence of shoulder joint following explantation of shoulder joint prosthesis, with or without presence of antibiotic-impregnated cement spacer

     Z89.231 Acquired absence of right **shoulder**
     Z89.232 Acquired absence of left **shoulder**
     Z89.239 Acquired absence of unspecified shoulder

✓5th **Z89.4 Acquired absence of** toe(s), foot, and ankle

   ✓6th **Z89.41 Acquired absence of** great toe

     Z89.411 Acquired absence of right **great toe**
     Z89.412 Acquired absence of left **great toe**
     Z89.419 Acquired absence of unspecified great toe

   ✓6th **Z89.42 Acquired absence of other** toe(s)

     EXCLUDES 2   *acquired absence of great toe (Z89.41-)*

     Z89.421 Acquired absence of other right **toe(s)**
     Z89.422 Acquired absence of other left **toe(s)**
     Z89.429 Acquired absence of other toe(s), unspecified side

   ✓6th **Z89.43 Acquired absence of** foot

     Z89.431 Acquired absence of right **foot**
     Z89.432 Acquired absence of left **foot**
     Z89.439 Acquired absence of unspecified foot

   ✓6th **Z89.44 Acquired absence of** ankle

     Disarticulation of ankle

     Z89.441 Acquired absence of right **ankle**
     Z89.442 Acquired absence of left **ankle**
     Z89.449 Acquired absence of unspecified ankle

✓5th **Z89.5 Acquired absence of leg below knee**

   ✓6th **Z89.51 Acquired absence of** leg below knee

     Z89.511 Acquired absence of right **leg below knee**
     Z89.512 Acquired absence of left **leg below knee**
     Z89.519 Acquired absence of unspecified leg below knee

   ✓6th **Z89.52 Acquired absence of** knee

Acquired absence of knee joint following explantation of knee joint prosthesis, with or without presence of antibiotic-impregnated cement spacer

     Z89.521 Acquired absence of right **knee**
     Z89.522 Acquired absence of left **knee**
     Z89.529 Acquired absence of unspecified knee

✓5th **Z89.6 Acquired absence of leg above knee**

   ✓6th **Z89.61 Acquired absence of** leg above knee

Acquired absence of leg NOS
Disarticulation at knee

     Z89.611 Acquired absence of right **leg above knee**
     Z89.612 Acquired absence of left **leg above knee**
     Z89.619 Acquired absence of unspecified leg above knee

   ✓6th **Z89.62 Acquired absence of** hip

Acquired absence of hip joint following explantation of hip joint prosthesis, with or without presence of antibiotic-impregnated cement spacer
Disarticulation at hip

     Z89.621 Acquired absence of right **hip joint**
     Z89.622 Acquired absence of left **hip joint**
     Z89.629 Acquired absence of unspecified hip joint

Z89.9 Acquired absence of limb, unspecified

✓4th **Z90 Acquired absence of organs, not elsewhere classified**

   INCLUDES   postprocedural or post-traumatic loss of body part NEC
   EXCLUDES 1   *congenital absence — see Alphabetical Index*
   EXCLUDES 2   *postprocedural absence of endocrine glands (E89.-)*

   ✓5th **Z90.0 Acquired absence of part of** head and neck

     Z90.01 Acquired absence of eye
     Z90.02 Acquired absence of larynx
     Z90.09 Acquired absence of other part of head and neck

Acquired absence of nose
     EXCLUDES 2   *teeth (K08.1)*

   ✓5th **Z90.1 Acquired absence of** breast and nipple

     Z90.10 Acquired absence of unspecified breast and nipple
     Z90.11 Acquired absence of right **breast and nipple**
     Z90.12 Acquired absence of left **breast and nipple**
     Z90.13 Acquired absence of bilateral **breasts and nipples**

Z90.2 Acquired absence of lung [part of]

Z90.3 Acquired absence of stomach [part of]

✓5th **Z90.4 Acquired absence of other specified parts of digestive tract**

   ✓6th **Z90.41 Acquired absence of** pancreas

Code also exocrine pancreatic insufficiency (K86.81)
Use additional code to identify any associated: diabetes mellitus, postpancreatectomy (E13.-) insulin use (Z79.4)

     Z90.410 Acquired total absence of pancreas
Acquired absence of pancreas NOS
     Z90.411 Acquired partial absence of pancreas

     Z90.49 Acquired absence of other specified parts of digestive tract

Z90.5 Acquired absence of kidney

Z90.6 Acquired absence of other parts of urinary tract
Acquired absence of bladder

✓5th **Z90.7 Acquired absence of** genital organ(s)

     EXCLUDES 1   *personal history of sex reassignment (Z87.890)*
     EXCLUDES 2   *female genital mutilation status (N90.81-)*

   ✓6th **Z90.71 Acquired absence of** cervix and uterus

     Z90.710 Acquired absence of both cervix and uterus   ♀
Acquired absence of uterus NOS
Status post total hysterectomy
     Z90.711 Acquired absence of uterus with remaining cervical stump   ♀
Status post partial hysterectomy with remaining cervical stump
     Z90.712 Acquired absence of cervix with remaining uterus   ♀

   ✓6th **Z90.72 Acquired absence of** ovaries

     Z90.721 Acquired absence of ovaries, unilateral   ♀
     Z90.722 Acquired absence of ovaries, bilateral   ♀

     Z90.79 Acquired absence of other genital organ(s)

✓5th **Z90.8 Acquired absence of other organs**

     Z90.81 Acquired absence of spleen
     Z90.89 Acquired absence of other organs

✓4th **Z91 Personal risk factors, not elsewhere classified**

   EXCLUDES 2   *contact with and (suspected) exposures hazardous to health (Z77.-)*
exposure to pollution and other problems related to physical environment (Z77.1-)
female genital mutilation status (N90.81-)
personal history of physical injury and trauma (Z87.81, Z87.82-)
occupational exposure to risk factors (Z57.-)

✓5th **Z91.0 Allergy status, other than to drugs and biological substances**

   EXCLUDES 2   *allergy status to drugs, medicaments, and biological substances (Z88.-)*

   ✓6th **Z91.01 Food allergy status**

     EXCLUDES 2   *food additives allergy status (Z91.02)*

     Z91.010 Allergy to peanuts
     Z91.011 Allergy to milk products
       EXCLUDES 1   *lactose intolerance (E73.-)*
     Z91.012 Allergy to eggs
     Z91.013 Allergy to seafood
Allergy to shellfish
Allergy to octopus or squid ink
     Z91.018 Allergy to other foods
Allergy to nuts other than peanuts

     Z91.02 Food additives allergy status

   ✓6th **Z91.03 Insect allergy status**

     Z91.030 Bee allergy status
     Z91.038 Other insect allergy status

   ✓6th **Z91.04 Nonmedicinal substance allergy status**

     Z91.040 Latex allergy status
Latex sensitivity status
     Z91.041 Radiographic dye allergy status
Allergy status to contrast media used for diagnostic X-ray procedure
     Z91.048 Other nonmedicinal substance allergy status

     Z91.09 Other allergy status, other than to drugs and biological substances

N Newborn: 0   P Pediatric: 0-17   M Maternity: 12-55   A Adult: 15-124   CH Comorbidity High   CL Comorbidity Low   NCDx Noncancer Dx   PDx Primary Dx

1232   ICD-10-CM 2020

...'s noncompliance with medical treatment and
...n

    Patient's noncompliance with dietary regimen
    Patient's intentional underdosing of medication **regimen**
      Code first underdosing of medication (T36-T50) with fifth or sixth character 6
        EXCLUDES 1   *adverse effect of prescribed drug taken as directed — code to adverse effect*
           poisoning (overdose) — code to poisoning
      AHA: 2018,4Q,72

Z91.120 Patient's intentional underdosing of medication regimen due to financial hardship
Z91.128 Patient's intentional underdosing of medication regimen for other reason

.13 Patient's unintentional underdosing of medication **regimen**
    Code first underdosing of medication (T36-T50) with fifth or sixth character 6
      EXCLUDES 1   *adverse effect of prescribed drug taken as directed — code to adverse effect*
           poisoning (overdose) — code to poisoning
    AHA: 2018,4Q,72

Z91.130 Patient's unintentional underdosing of medication regimen due to age-related debility
Z91.138 Patient's unintentional underdosing of medication regimen for other reason

Z91.14 Patient's other noncompliance with medication regimen
    Patient's underdosing of medication NOS
    AHA: 2018,4Q,72

Z91.15 Patient's noncompliance with renal dialysis
Z91.19 Patient's noncompliance with other medical treatment and regimen
    Nonadherence to medical treatment

4 Personal history of psychological trauma, not elsewhere classified

Z91.41 Personal history of adult abuse
    EXCLUDES 2   *personal history of abuse in childhood (Z62.81-)*

Z91.410 Personal history of adult physical and sexual **abuse** [A]
    EXCLUDES 1   *current adult physical abuse (T74.11, T76.11)*
          current adult sexual abuse (T74.21, T76.11)

Z91.411 Personal history of adult psychological **abuse** [A]
Z91.412 Personal history of adult neglect [A]
    EXCLUDES 1   *current adult neglect (T74.01, T76.01)*
Z91.419 Personal history of unspecified adult abuse [A]

Z91.42 Personal history of forced labor **or** sexual exploitation
    AHA: 2018,4Q,32,35

Z91.49 Other personal history of psychological trauma, not elsewhere classified

Z91.5 Personal history of self-harm
    Personal history of parasuicide
    Personal history of self-poisoning
    Personal history of suicide attempt

Z91.8 Other specified personal risk factors, not elsewhere classified

Z91.81 History of falling
    At risk for falling

Z91.82 Personal history of military deployment [A]
    Individual (civilian or military) with past history of military war, peacekeeping and humanitarian deployment (current or past conflict)
    Returned from military deployment

Z91.83 *Wandering in diseases classified elsewhere*
    Code first underlying disorder such as:
      Alzheimer's disease (G30.-)
      autism or pervasive developmental disorder (F84.-)
      intellectual disabilities (F70-F79)
      unspecified dementia with behavioral disturbance (F03.9-)

√6th **Z91.84 Oral health risk factors**
    AHA: 2017,4Q,29
    Z91.841 Risk for dental caries, low
    Z91.842 Risk for dental caries, moderate
    Z91.843 Risk for dental caries, high
    Z91.849 Unspecified risk for dental caries

Z91.89 Other specified personal risk factors, not elsewhere classified
    AHA: 2017,1Q,45

√4th **Z92 Personal history of medical treatment**
    EXCLUDES 2   *postprocedural states (Z98.-)*

Z92.0 Personal history of contraception
    EXCLUDES 1   *counseling or management of current contraceptive practices (Z30.-)*
          long term (current) use of contraception (Z79.3)
          presence of (intrauterine) contraceptive device (Z97.5)

√5th **Z92.2 Personal history of** drug therapy
    EXCLUDES 2   *long term (current) drug therapy (Z79.-)*

Z92.21 Personal history of antineoplastic chemotherapy
Z92.22 Personal history of monoclonal drug therapy
Z92.23 Personal history of estrogen therapy
√6th **Z92.24 Personal history of** steroid therapy
    Z92.240 Personal history of inhaled steroid therapy
    Z92.241 Personal history of systemic steroid therapy
      Personal history of steroid therapy NOS
Z92.25 Personal history of immunosupression therapy
    EXCLUDES 2   *personal history of steroid therapy (Z92.24)*
Z92.29 Personal history of other drug therapy

Z92.3 Personal history of irradiation
    Personal history of exposure to therapeutic radiation
    EXCLUDES 1   *exposure to radiation in the physical environment (Z77.12)*
          occupational exposure to radiation (Z57.1)

√5th **Z92.8 Personal history of other medical treatment**
Z92.81 Personal history of extracorporeal membrane oxygenation (ECMO)
Z92.82 Status post administration of tPA (rtPA) in a different facility within the last 24 hours prior to admission to current facility
    Code first condition requiring tPA administration, such as:
      acute cerebral infarction (I63.-)
      acute myocardial infarction (I21.-, I22.-)
    AHA: 2013,4Q,124

Z92.83 Personal history of failed moderate sedation
    Personal history of failed conscious sedation
    EXCLUDES 2   *failed moderate sedation during procedure (T88.52)*

Z92.84 Personal history of unintended awareness under general anesthesia
    EXCLUDES 2   *unintended awareness under general anesthesia during procedure (T88.53)*
    AHA: 2016,4Q,72-73,77

Z92.89 Personal history of other medical treatment

√4th **Z93 Artificial opening status**
    EXCLUDES 1   *artificial openings requiring attention or management (Z43.-)*
          complications of external stoma (J95.0-, K94.-, N99.5-)

Z93.0 Tracheostomy **status**
    AHA: 2013,4Q,129
Z93.1 Gastrostomy **status**
Z93.2 Ileostomy **status**
Z93.3 Colostomy **status**
Z93.4 Other artificial openings of gastrointestinal tract status
√5th **Z93.5** Cystostomy **status**
    Z93.50 Unspecified cystostomy status
    Z93.51 Cutaneous-vesicostomy **status**

Z93.52   Appendico-vesicostomy status

Z93.59   Other cystostomy status

Z93.6   Other artificial openings of urinary tract status
Nephrostomy status
Ureterostomy status
Urethrostomy status

Z93.8   Other artificial opening status

Z93.9   Artificial opening status, unspecified

√4th Z94   Transplanted organ and tissue status

INCLUDES   organ or tissue replaced by heterogenous or homogenous transplant

EXCLUDES 1   complications of transplanted organ or tissue — see Alphabetical Index

EXCLUDES 2   presence of vascular grafts (Z95.-)

Z94.0   Kidney transplant status

Z94.1   Heart transplant status

EXCLUDES 1   artificial heart status (Z95.812)
heart-valve replacement status (Z95.2-Z95.4)

Z94.2   Lung transplant status

Z94.3   Heart and lungs transplant status

Z94.4   Liver transplant status

Z94.5   Skin transplant status
Autogenous skin transplant status

Z94.6   Bone transplant status

Z94.7   Corneal transplant status

√5th Z94.8   Other transplanted organ and tissue status

Z94.81   Bone marrow transplant status

Z94.82   Intestine transplant status

Z94.83   Pancreas transplant status

Z94.84   Stem cells transplant status

Z94.89   Other transplanted organ and tissue status

Z94.9   Transplanted organ and tissue status, unspecified

√4th Z95   Presence of cardiac and vascular implants and grafts

EXCLUDES 2   complications of cardiac and vascular devices, implants and grafts (T82.-)

Z95.0   Presence of cardiac pacemaker
Presence of cardiac resynchronization therapy (CRT-P) pacemaker

EXCLUDES 1   adjustment or management of cardiac device (Z45.0-)
adjustment or management of cardiac pacemaker (Z45.0)
presence of automatic (implantable) cardiac defibrillator with synchronous cardiac pacemaker (Z95.810)

AHA: 2019,1Q,33

Z95.1   Presence of aortocoronary bypass graft
Presence of coronary artery bypass graft

Z95.2   Presence of prosthetic heart valve
Presence of heart valve NOS

Z95.3   Presence of xenogenic heart valve

Z95.4   Presence of other heart-valve replacement

Z95.5   Presence of coronary angioplasty implant and graft

EXCLUDES 1   coronary angioplasty status without implant and graft (Z98.61)

√5th Z95.8   Presence of other cardiac and vascular implants and grafts

√6th Z95.81   Presence of other cardiac implants and grafts

Z95.810   Presence of automatic (implantable) cardiac defibrillator
Presence of automatic (implantable) cardiac defibrillator with synchronous cardiac pacemaker
Presence of cardiac resynchronization therapy defibrillator (CRT-D)
Presence of cardioverter-defibrillator (ICD)

Z95.811   Presence of heart assist device

Z95.812   Presence of fully implantable artificial heart

Z95.818   Presence of other cardiac implants and grafts

√6th Z95.82   Presence of other vascular implan

Z95.820   Peripheral vascular angi with implants and grafts

EXCLUDES 1   peripheral v angiopl implant (Z98.62)

Z95.828   Presence of other vascula grafts
Presence of intravascular

Z95.9   Presence of cardiac and vascular implant and unspecified

√4th Z96   Presence of other functional implants

EXCLUDES 2   complications of internal prosthetic devices, grafts (T82-T85)
fitting and adjustment of prosthetic and othe (Z44-Z46)

Z96.0   Presence of urogenital implants

Z96.1   Presence of intraocular lens
Presence of pseudophakia

√5th Z96.2   Presence of otological and audiological implan

Z96.20   Presence of otological and audiologica unspecified

Z96.21   Cochlear implant status

Z96.22   Myringotomy tube(s) status

Z96.29   Presence of other otological and audio implants
Presence of bone-conduction hearing de
Presence of eustachian tube stent
Stapes replacement

Z96.3   Presence of artificial larynx

√5th Z96.4   Presence of endocrine implants

Z96.41   Presence of insulin pump (external) (inte

Z96.49   Presence of other endocrine implants

Z96.5   Presence of tooth-root and mandibular implants

√5th Z96.6   Presence of orthopedic joint implants

Z96.60   Presence of unspecified orthopedic joint

√6th Z96.61   Presence of artificial shoulder joint

Z96.611   Presence of right artificial shoul

Z96.612   Presence of left artificial should

Z96.619   Presence of unspecified artificial joint

√6th Z96.62   Presence of artificial elbow joint

Z96.621   Presence of right artificial elbow

Z96.622   Presence of left artificial elbow j

Z96.629   Presence of unspecified artificial joint

√6th Z96.63   Presence of artificial wrist joint

Z96.631   Presence of right artificial wrist j

Z96.632   Presence of left artificial wrist joi

Z96.639   Presence of unspecified artificial v joint

√6th Z96.64   Presence of artificial hip joint
Hip-joint replacement (partial) (total)

✳ TIP: For rehabilitation services following a total replacement due to a fracture, since this fracture considered to be in the healing and recovery p assign first the appropriate injury code from cat S72 with the seventh character of subsequent encounter, followed by this code.

Z96.641   Presence of right artificial hip joint

Z96.642   Presence of left artificial hip joint

Z96.643   Presence of artificial hip joint, bilat

Z96.649   Presence of unspecified artificial hip

√6th Z96.65   Presence of artificial knee joint

Z96.651   Presence of right artificial knee join

Z96.652   Presence of left artificial knee joint

Z96.653   Presence of artificial knee joint, bilat

Z96.659   Presence of unspecified artificial kne joint

√6th Z96.66   Presence of artificial ankle joint

Z96.661   Presence of right artificial ankle joint

Z96.662   Presence of left artificial ankle joint

Z96.669   Presence of unspecified artificial ank joint

√6th Z96.69   Presence of other orthopedic joint implants

Z96.691   Finger-joint replacement of right han

N Newborn: 0   P Pediatric: 0-17   M Maternity: 12-55   A Adult: 15-124   CH Comorbidity High   CL Comorbidity Low   NCDx Noncancer Dx   PDx Primar

1234   ICD-10-CM 2

Z96.692 **Finger-joint replacement of** left **hand**
Z96.693 **Finger-joint replacement,** bilateral
Z96.698 **Presence of other orthopedic joint implants**

Z96.7 **Presence of other bone and tendon implants**
Presence of skull plate

√5ᵗʰ Z96.8 **Presence of other specified functional implants**

Z96.81 **Presence of** artificial skin
Z96.82 **Presence of** neurostimulator
Presence of brain neurostimulator
Presence of gastric neurostimulator
Presence of peripheral nerve neurostimulator
Presence of sacral nerve neurostimulator
Presence of spinal cord neurostimulator
Presence of vagus nerve neurostimulator
Z96.89 **Presence of other specified functional implants**

Z96.9 **Presence of functional implant, unspecified**

√4ᵗʰ Z97 **Presence of other devices**
EXCLUDES 1 *complications of internal prosthetic devices, implants and grafts (T82-T85)*
~~fitting and adjustment of prosthetic and other devices (Z44-Z46)~~
EXCLUDES 2 ▶*fitting and adjustment of prosthetic and other devices (Z44-Z46)*◀
presence of cerebrospinal fluid drainage device (Z98.2)

Z97.0 **Presence of** artificial eye
√5ᵗʰ Z97.1 **Presence of** artificial limb (complete) (partial)

Z97.10 **Presence of artificial limb (complete) (partial), unspecified**
Z97.11 **Presence of artificial** right arm **(complete) (partial)**
Z97.12 **Presence of artificial** left arm **(complete) (partial)**
Z97.13 **Presence of artificial** right leg **(complete) (partial)**
Z97.14 **Presence of artificial** left leg **(complete) (partial)**
Z97.15 **Presence of artificial** arms, bilateral **(complete) (partial)**
Z97.16 **Presence of artificial** legs, bilateral **(complete) (partial)**

Z97.2 **Presence of** dental prosthetic device **(complete) (partial)**
Presence of dentures (complete) (partial)
Z97.3 **Presence of** spectacles and contact lenses
Z97.4 **Presence of** external hearing-aid
Z97.5 **Presence of (intrauterine)** contraceptive device   ♀
EXCLUDES 1 *checking, reinsertion or removal of implantable subdermal contraceptive (Z30.46)*
checking, reinsertion or removal of intrauterine contraceptive device (Z30.43-)

Z97.8 **Presence of other specified devices**

√4ᵗʰ Z98 **Other postprocedural states**
EXCLUDES 2 *aftercare (Z43-Z49, Z51)*
follow-up medical care (Z08-Z09)
postprocedural complication — see Alphabetical Index

Z98.0 **Intestinal bypass and anastomosis status**
EXCLUDES 2 *bariatric surgery status (Z98.84)*
gastric bypass status (Z98.84)
obesity surgery status (Z98.84)

Z98.1 **Arthrodesis status**
Z98.2 **Presence of cerebrospinal fluid drainage device**
Presence of CSF shunt
Z98.3 **Post therapeutic collapse of lung status**
Code first underlying disease
√6ᵗʰ Z98.4 **Cataract extraction status**
Use additional code to identify intraocular lens implant status (Z96.1)
EXCLUDES 1 *aphakia (H27.0)*
Z98.41 **Cataract extraction status,** right **eye**
Z98.42 **Cataract extraction status,** left **eye**
Z98.49 **Cataract extraction status, unspecified eye**
√5ᵗʰ Z98.5 **Sterilization status**
EXCLUDES 1 *female infertility (N97.-)*
male infertility (N46.-)
Z98.51 **Tubal ligation status**   ♀
Z98.52 **Vasectomy status**   🅐 ♂

√5ᵗʰ Z98.6 **Angioplasty status**
Z98.61 **Coronary angioplasty status**
EXCLUDES 1 *coronary angioplasty status with implant and graft (Z95.5)*
Z98.62 **Peripheral vascular angioplasty status**
EXCLUDES 1 *peripheral vascular angioplasty status with implant and graft (Z95.820)*
√5ᵗʰ Z98.8 **Other specified postprocedural states**
√6ᵗʰ Z98.81 **Dental procedure status**
Z98.810 **Dental sealant status**
Z98.811 **Dental restoration status**
Dental crown status
Dental fillings status
Z98.818 **Other dental procedure status**
Z98.82 **Breast implant status**
EXCLUDES 1 *breast implant removal status (Z98.86)*
Z98.83 **Filtering (vitreous) bleb after glaucoma surgery status**
EXCLUDES 1 *inflammation (infection) of postprocedural bleb (H59.4-)*
Z98.84 **Bariatric surgery status**
Gastric banding status
Gastric bypass status for obesity
Obesity surgery status
EXCLUDES 1 *bariatric surgery status complicating pregnancy, childbirth, or the puerperium (O99.84)*
EXCLUDES 2 *intestinal bypass and anastomosis status (Z98.0)*
Z98.85 **Transplanted organ removal status**
Transplanted organ previously removed due to complication, failure, rejection or infection
EXCLUDES 1 *encounter for removal of transplanted organ — code to complication of transplanted organ (T86.-)*
Z98.86 **Personal history of breast implant removal**
√6ᵗʰ Z98.87 **Personal history of** in utero procedure
Z98.870 **Personal history of in utero procedure** during pregnancy   ♀
EXCLUDES 2 *complications from in utero procedure for current pregnancy (O35.7)*
supervision of current pregnancy with history of in utero procedure during previous pregnancy (O09.82-)
Z98.871 **Personal history of in utero procedure** while a fetus
√6ᵗʰ Z98.89 **Other specified postprocedural states**
Z98.890 **Other specified postprocedural states**
Personal history of surgery, not elsewhere classified
Z98.891 **History of uterine scar from previous surgery**   ♀
EXCLUDES 1 *maternal care due to uterine scar from previous surgery (O34.2-)*
AHA: 2016,4Q,51-52,76

√4ᵗʰ Z99 **Dependence on enabling machines and devices, not elsewhere classified**
EXCLUDES 1 *cardiac pacemaker status (Z95.0)*
Z99.0 **Dependence on** aspirator
√5ᵗʰ Z99.1 **Dependence on** respirator
Dependence on ventilator
Z99.11 **Dependence on respirator [ventilator] status**
AHA: 2015,1Q,21
Z99.12 **Encounter for respirator [ventilator]** 𝗣𝗗𝘅
dependence during power failure
EXCLUDES 1 *mechanical complication of respirator [ventilator] (J95.850)*

Z99.2 Dependence on renal dialysis
    Hemodialysis status
    Peritoneal dialysis status
    Presence of arteriovenous shunt for dialysis
    Renal dialysis status NOS
    EXCLUDES 1   *encounter for fitting and adjustment of dialysis catheter (Z49.0-)*
    EXCLUDES 2   *noncompliance with renal dialysis (Z91.15)*
    AHA: 2016,1Q,12; 2013,4Q,125

Z99.3 Dependence on wheelchair
    Wheelchair confinement status
    Code first cause of dependence, such as:
      muscular dystrophy (G71.0-)
      obesity (E66.-)

✓5ᵗʰ **Z99.8 Dependence on other enabling machines and devices**

    Z99.81 Dependence on supplemental oxygen
        Dependence on long-term oxygen
        AHA: 2013,4Q,129

    Z99.89 Dependence on other enabling machines and devices
        Dependence on machine or device NOS

Appendixes

Appendix A: Valid 3-character ICD-10-CM Codes

A09	Infectious gastroenteritis and colitis, unspecified
A33	Tetanus neonatorum
A34	Obstetrical tetanus
A35	Other tetanus
A46	Erysipelas
A55	Chlamydial lymphogranuloma (venereum)
A57	Chancroid
A58	Granuloma inguinale
A64	Unspecified sexually transmitted disease
A65	Nonvenereal syphilis
A70	Chlamydia psittaci infections
A78	Q fever
A86	Unspecified viral encephalitis
A89	Unspecified viral infection of central nervous system
A90	Dengue fever [classical dengue]
A91	Dengue hemorrhagic fever
A94	Unspecified arthropod-borne viral fever
A99	Unspecified viral hemorrhagic fever
B03	Smallpox
B04	Monkeypox
B09	Unspecified viral infection characterized by skin and mucous membrane lesions
B20	Human immunodeficiency virus [HIV] disease
B49	Unspecified mycosis
B54	Unspecified malaria
B59	Pneumocystosis
B64	Unspecified protozoal disease
B72	Dracunculiasis
B75	Trichinellosis
B79	Trichuriasis
B80	Enterobiasis
B86	Scabies
B89	Unspecified parasitic disease
B91	Sequelae of poliomyelitis
B92	Sequelae of leprosy
C01	Malignant neoplasm of base of tongue
C07	Malignant neoplasm of parotid gland
C12	Malignant neoplasm of pyriform sinus
C19	Malignant neoplasm of rectosigmoid junction
C20	Malignant neoplasm of rectum
C23	Malignant neoplasm of gallbladder
C33	Malignant neoplasm of trachea
C37	Malignant neoplasm of thymus
C52	Malignant neoplasm of vagina
C55	Malignant neoplasm of uterus, part unspecified
C58	Malignant neoplasm of placenta
C61	Malignant neoplasm of prostate
C73	Malignant neoplasm of thyroid gland
D34	Benign neoplasm of thyroid gland
D45	Polycythemia vera
D62	Acute posthemorrhagic anemia
D65	Disseminated intravascular coagulation [defibrination syndrome]
D66	Hereditary factor VIII deficiency
D67	Hereditary factor IX deficiency
D71	Functional disorders of polymorphonuclear neutrophils
D77	Other disorders of blood and blood-forming organs in diseases classified elsewhere
E02	Subclinical iodine-deficiency hypothyroidism
E15	Nondiabetic hypoglycemic coma
E35	Disorders of endocrine glands in diseases classified elsewhere
E40	Kwashiorkor
E41	Nutritional marasmus
E42	Marasmic kwashiorkor
E43	Unspecified severe protein-calorie malnutrition
E45	Retarded development following protein-calorie malnutrition
E46	Unspecified protein-calorie malnutrition
E52	Niacin deficiency [pellagra]
E54	Ascorbic acid deficiency
E58	Dietary calcium deficiency
E59	Dietary selenium deficiency
E60	Dietary zinc deficiency
E65	Localized adiposity
E68	Sequelae of hyperalimentation
F04	Amnestic disorder due to known physiological condition
F05	Delirium due to known physiological condition
F09	Unspecified mental disorder due to known physiological condition
F21	Schizotypal disorder
F22	Delusional disorders
F23	Brief psychotic disorder
F24	Shared psychotic disorder
F28	Other psychotic disorder not due to a substance or known physiological condition
F29	Unspecified psychosis not due to a substance or known physiological condition
F39	Unspecified mood [affective] disorder
F54	Psychological and behavioral factors associated with disorders or diseases classified elsewhere
F59	Unspecified behavioral syndromes associated with physiological disturbances and physical factors
F66	Other sexual disorders
F69	Unspecified disorder of adult personality and behavior
F70	Mild intellectual disabilities
F71	Moderate intellectual disabilities
F72	Severe intellectual disabilities
F73	Profound intellectual disabilities
F78	Other intellectual disabilities
F79	Unspecified intellectual disabilities
F82	Specific developmental disorder of motor function
F88	Other disorders of psychological development
F89	Unspecified disorder of psychological development
F99	Mental disorder, not otherwise specified
G01	Meningitis in bacterial diseases classified elsewhere
G02	Meningitis in other infectious and parasitic diseases classified elsewhere
G07	Intracranial and intraspinal abscess and granuloma in diseases classified elsewhere
G08	Intracranial and intraspinal phlebitis and thrombophlebitis
G09	Sequelae of inflammatory diseases of central nervous system
G10	Huntington's disease
G14	Postpolio syndrome
G20	Parkinson's disease
G26	Extrapyramidal and movement disorders in diseases classified elsewhere
G35	Multiple sclerosis
G53	Cranial nerve disorders in diseases classified elsewhere
G55	Nerve root and plexus compressions in diseases classified elsewhere
G59	Mononeuropathy in diseases classified elsewhere
G63	Polyneuropathy in diseases classified elsewhere
G64	Other disorders of peripheral nervous system
G92	Toxic encephalopathy
G94	Other disorders of brain in diseases classified elsewhere
H22	Disorders of iris and ciliary body in diseases classified elsewhere
H28	Cataract in diseases classified elsewhere
H32	Chorioretinal disorders in diseases classified elsewhere
H36	Retinal disorders in diseases classified elsewhere
H42	Glaucoma in diseases classified elsewhere

I00	Rheumatic fever without heart involvement
I10	Essential (primary) hypertension
I32	Pericarditis in diseases classified elsewhere
I38	Endocarditis, valve unspecified
I39	Endocarditis and heart valve disorders in diseases classified elsewhere
I41	Myocarditis in diseases classified elsewhere
I43	Cardiomyopathy in diseases classified elsewhere
I52	Other heart disorders in diseases classified elsewhere
I76	Septic arterial embolism
I81	Portal vein thrombosis
I96	Gangrene, not elsewhere classified
J00	Acute nasopharyngitis (common cold)
J13	Pneumonia due to Streptococcus pneumoniae
J14	Pneumonia due to Hemophilus influenzae
J17	Pneumonia in diseases classified elsewhere
J22	Unspecified acute lower respiratory infection
J36	Peritonsillar abscess
J40	Bronchitis, not specified as acute or chronic
J42	Unspecified chronic bronchitis
J60	Coalworker's pneumoconiosis
J61	Pneumoconiosis due to asbestos and other mineral fibers
J64	Unspecified pneumoconiosis
J65	Pneumoconiosis associated with tuberculosis
J80	Acute respiratory distress syndrome
J82	Pulmonary eosinophilia, not elsewhere classified
J90	Pleural effusion, not elsewhere classified
J99	Respiratory disorders in diseases classified elsewhere
K23	Disorders of esophagus in diseases classified elsewhere
K30	Functional dyspepsia
K36	Other appendicitis
K37	Unspecified appendicitis
K67	Disorders of peritoneum in infectious diseases classified elsewhere
K77	Liver disorders in diseases classified elsewhere
K87	Disorders of gallbladder, biliary tract and pancreas in diseases classified elsewhere
L00	Staphylococcal scalded skin syndrome
L14	Bullous disorders in diseases classified elsewhere
L22	Diaper dermatitis
L26	Exfoliative dermatitis
L42	Pityriasis rosea
L45	Papulosquamous disorders in diseases classified elsewhere
L52	Erythema nodosum
L54	Erythema in diseases classified elsewhere
L62	Nail disorders in diseases classified elsewhere
L80	Vitiligo
L83	Acanthosis nigricans
L84	Corns and callosities
L86	Keratoderma in diseases classified elsewhere
L88	Pyoderma gangrenosum
L99	Other disorders of skin and subcutaneous tissue in diseases classified elsewhere
N08	Glomerular disorders in diseases classified elsewhere
N10	Acute tubulo-interstitial nephritis
N12	Tubulo-interstitial nephritis, not specified as acute or chronic
N16	Renal tubulo-interstitial disorders in diseases classified elsewhere

N19	Unspecified kidney failure
N22	Calculus of urinary tract in diseases classified elsewhere
N23	Unspecified renal colic
N29	Other disorders of kidney and ureter in diseases classified elsewhere
N33	Bladder disorders in diseases classified elsewhere
N37	Urethral disorders in diseases classified elsewhere
N51	Disorders of male genital organs in diseases classified elsewhere
N62	Hypertrophy of breast
N72	Inflammatory disease of cervix uteri
N74	Female pelvic inflammatory disorders in diseases classified elsewhere
N86	Erosion and ectropion of cervix uteri
N96	Recurrent pregnancy loss
O68	Labor and delivery complicated by abnormality of fetal acid-base balance
O76	Abnormality in fetal heart rate and rhythm complicating labor and delivery
O80	Encounter for full-term uncomplicated delivery
O82	Encounter for cesarean delivery without indication
O85	Puerperal sepsis
O94	Sequelae of complication of pregnancy, childbirth, and the puerperium
P09	Abnormal findings on neonatal screening
P53	Hemorrhagic disease of newborn
P60	Disseminated intravascular coagulation of newborn
P84	Other problems with newborn
P90	Convulsions of newborn
P95	Stillbirth
Q02	Microcephaly
R05	Cough
R12	Heartburn
R17	Unspecified jaundice
R21	Rash and other nonspecific skin eruption
R32	Unspecified urinary incontinence
R34	Anuria and oliguria
R37	Sexual dysfunction, unspecified
R42	Dizziness and giddiness
R51	Headache
R52	Pain, unspecified
R54	Age-related physical debility
R55	Syncope and collapse
R58	Hemorrhage, not elsewhere classified
R61	Generalized hyperhidrosis
R64	Cachexia
R69	Illness, unspecified
R75	Inconclusive laboratory evidence of human immunodeficiency virus [HIV]
R81	Glycosuria
R99	Ill-defined and unknown cause of mortality
Y09	Assault by unspecified means
Y66	Nonadministration of surgical and medical care
Y69	Unspecified misadventure during surgical and medical care
Y95	Nosocomial condition
Z08	Encounter for follow-up examination after completed treatment for malignant neoplasm
Z09	Encounter for follow-up examination after completed treatment for conditions other than malignant neoplasm
Z21	Asymptomatic human immunodeficiency virus [HIV] infection status
Z23	Encounter for immunization
Z66	Do not resuscitate

Appendix B: Pharmacology List 2020

This section enables the coder to quickly review drugs, drug actions, and indications that are often associated with overlooked or undocumented diagnoses. The coder should review the patient's medication record and know what condition the physician is treating with the prescribed medication based on documentation in the medical record. When documentation is lacking, the coder can reference this section to locate the drug, determine the drug action, confirm drug indications, and when necessary query the physician. When applicable, some of the drugs provided in this resource have also been mapped to their appropriate Z code for long-term drug use.

Drug	Z Code	Drug Action/Classification	Indications
A-Methapred [methylprednisolone sodium succinate]	Z79.52	Corticosteroid	Severe inflammation
Abilify [aripiprazole]		Antipsychotic	Depression, bipolar disorder, schizophrenia, autism symptoms
Abstral [fentanyl citrate]	Z79.891	Analgesic, narcotic	Breakthrough cancer pain
Acarbose [acarbose]	Z79.84	Oral hypoglycemic	Diabetes mellitus
Accupril [quinapril hydrochloride]		ACE inhibitor	Congestive heart failure; hypertension
Acetaminophen with codeine [acetaminophen/codeine phosphate]	Z79.891	Analgesic, narcotic	Pain, moderate to severe
Actemra [tocilizumab]		Antirheumatic	Rheumatoid arthritis
Actimmune [interferon gamma-1b]	Z79.899	Antineoplastic interferons; antiviral interferons	Chronic granulomatous disease; malignant osteopetrosis
Activella [estradiol/norethindrone acetate]	Z79.890	Estrogen therapy	Menopause symptoms; vaginal and vulvar atrophy; osteoporosis prevention
Actonel [risedronate sodium]	Z79.83	Biophosphonate	Decrease in bone loss in multiple myeloma patients; Paget's disease; hyperparathyroidism; osteoporosis
Actoplus Met [metformin hydrochloride/pioglitazone hydrochloride]	Z79.84	Oral hypoglycemic	Diabetes mellitus
Actos [pioglitazone hydrochloride]	Z79.84	Oral hypoglycemic	Diabetes mellitus
Aczone [dapsone]		Acne agent, topical	Acne vulgaris
Adalat CC [nifedipine]		Calcium channel blocker	Vasospastic angina; chronic stable angina; hypertension
Adderall XR [amphetamine aspartate and sulfate/dextroamphetamine saccharate and sulfate]		CNS stimulant	Attention deficit hyperactivity disorder (ADHD)
Admelog [insulin lispro]	Z79.4	Insulin	Diabetes mellitus
Advair [fluticasone propionate/salmeterol xinafoate]	Z79.51	Corticosteroid -inhaled; antiasthmatic	Prophylaxis and treatment of asthma and COPD
Advil [ibuprofen]	Z79.1	Nonsteroidal anti-inflammatory drug (NSAID)	Pain or fever relief
Aerospan HFA [flunisolide]	Z79.51	Corticosteroid -inhaled; antiasthmatic	Prophylaxis and treatment of asthma
Afrezza [human insulin recombinant]	Z79.4	Insulin -inhaled	Diabetes mellitus
Aggrastat [tirofiban hydrochloride]	Z79.02	Antiplatelet	Unstable angina; heart attacks
Aggrenox [aspirin/dipyridamole]	Z79.02	Antiplatelet	Lessening of the chance of heart attack or stroke
Aimovig [erenumab-aooe]		Antimigraine	Migraine headache
Airduo Respiclick [fluticasone propionate/salmeterol xinafoate]	Z79.51	Corticosteroid -- inhaled; antiasthmatic	Asthma
Aldactone [spironolactone]		Cardiovascular agent; antihypertensive agent; diuretic; electrolytic and renal agent	Severe heart failure; ascites associated with cirrhosis; hypokalemia
Aleve [naproxen sodium]	Z79.1	Nonsteroidal anti-inflammatory drug (NSAID)	Reduction of temporary aches and pains
Allegra allergy [fexofenadine hydrochloride]		Antihistamine	Seasonal allergic rhinitis
Allopurinol [allopurinol]		Antigout	Gouty arthritis, renal calculus, hyperuricemia, hyperuricemia secondary to leukemia, hyperuricemia secondary to lymphoma
Alora [estradiol]	Z79.890	Estrogen therapy	Menopause symptoms
Alphagan P [brimonidine tartrate]		Antiglaucoma agent (ophthalmic); antihypertensive, ocular	Open angle glaucoma or another condition in which pressure in the eye is too high (ocular hypertension)
Alprazolam [alprazolam]		Antianxiety; sedative/hypnotic	
Altabax [retapamulin]	Z79.2	Antibiotic, topical	Skin infections
Altace [ramipril]		ACE inhibitor	Congestive heart failure; hypertension
Altavera [ethinyl estradiol/levonorgestrel]	Z79.3	Contraceptive	Prevention of pregnancy
Alvesco [ciclesonide]	Z79.51	Corticosteroid -inhaled; antiasthmatic	Prophylaxis and treatment of asthma

Drug	Z Code	Drug Action/Classification	Indications
Alyacen [ethinyl estradiol/norethindrone]	Z79.3	Contraceptive	Prevention of pregnancy
Amaryl [glimepiride]	Z79.84	Oral hypoglycemic	Diabetes mellitus
Ambien [zolpidem tartrate]		CNS depressant; anoxiolytic/sedative/hypnotic	Insomnia
Amikacin [amikacin sulfate]	Z79.2	Antibiotic	Gram-negative bacterial infections such as Pseudomonas, Escherichia coli (E. coli), Proteus, Klebsiella-Enterobacter-Serratia
Amitriptyline HCl [amitriptyline hydrochloride]		Antidepressant	Depression
Amoxicillin [amoxicillin]	Z79.2	Antibiotic	Treatment of infections with a broad spectrum of bactericidal activity against many gram-positive and gram-negative micro-organisms; otitis media, gonorrhea, skin, respiratory, gastrointestinal, and genitourinary infections
Ampicillin [ampicillin sodium]	Z79.2	Antibiotic	Bacterial infections
Ampyra [dalfampridine]		Potassium channel blocker	Improvement in walking in patients with multiple sclerosis
Amrix [cyclobenzaprine hydrochloride]		Muscle relaxant	Adjunct to rest and physical therapy for muscle spasms
Anaprox DS [naproxen sodium]	Z79.1	Nonsteroidal anti-inflammatory drug (NSAID)	Pain, inflammation or fever relief
Anastrozole [anastrozole]	Z79.811	Aromatase inhibitor	Postmenopausal breast cancer
Ancef [cefazolin sodium]	Z79.2	Antibiotic	Respiratory tract infections due to Streptococcus pneumoniae, Klebsiella species, Haemophilus influenzae (H. influenzae), Staphylococcus aureus, and group A betahemolytic streptococci; urinary tract infections due to E. coli, Proteus mirabilis, Klebsiella species and some strains of Enterobacter and enterococci; skin and skin structure infections, biliary tract infections, bone and joint infections, genital infections, septicemia, and endocarditis
Androderm [testosterone]	Z79.890	Testosterone therapy -topical	Primary hypogonadism, hypogonadotropic hypogonadism
AndroGel [testosterone]	Z79.890	Testosterone therapy -topical	Primary hypogonadism, hypogonadotropic hypogonadism
Angeliq [drospirenone/estradiol]	Z79.890	Estrogen therapy	Menopause symptoms
Angiomax [bivalirudin]	Z79.01	Anticoagulant	Prevention of blood clots
Antabuse [disulfiram]		Alcohol treatment	Alcoholism
Antineoplastic/chemotherapy	Z79.899	Antineoplastic	Cancer
Apidra [insulin glulisine recombinant]	Z79.4	Insulin	Diabetes mellitus
Aranelle [ethinyl estradiol/norethindrone]	Z79.3	Contraceptive	Prevention of pregnancy; acne
Aranesp [darbepoetin alfa]		Erythropoiesis-stimulating agent (ESA)	Treatment of lower than normal blood cells (anemia) from disorders such as CKD and neoplasms
Argatroban [argatroban]	Z79.01	Anticoagulant	Prophylaxis and treatment of venous thrombosis in thrombocytopenia patients
Aricept [donepezil hydrochloride]		Acetylcholinesterase/cholinesterase inhibitors	Symptoms of mild to moderate Alzheimer's disease; can improve thinking ability in some patients
Arimidex [anastrozole]	Z79.811	Aromatase inhibitor	Postmenopausal breast cancer
Aristospan [triamcinolone hexacetonide]	Z79.52	Corticosteroid	Severe inflammation
Arixtra [fondaparinux sodium]	Z79.01	Anticoagulant	Venous thrombosis and pulmonary embolism
Armonair Respiclick [fluticasone propionate]	Z79.51	Corticosteroid -- inhaled; anitasthmatic	Asthma
Arnuity Ellipta [fluticasone furoate]	Z79.51	Corticosteroid -inhaled; antiasthmatic	Prophylaxis and treatment of asthma
Aromasin [exemestane]	Z79.811	Aromatase inhibitor	Postmenopausal breast cancer
Arthrotec [diclofenac sodium/misoprostol]	Z79.1	Non-steroidal anti-inflammatory drug (NSAID)-prostaglandin combo	Treatment of patients with arthritis who may develop stomach ulcers from taking nonsteroidal anti-inflammatory drugs (NSAIDs) alone; used to help relieve some symptoms of arthritis, such as inflammation, swelling, stiffness, and joint pain
Asacol HD [mesalamine]		Antiinflammatory	Ulcerative colitis
Ashlyna [ethinyl estradiol/levonorgestrel]	Z79.3	Contraceptive	Prevention of pregnancy
Asmanex [mometasone furoate]	Z79.51	Corticosteroid -inhaled; antiasthmatic	Prophylaxis and treatment of asthma
Astagraf XL [tacrolimus]	Z79.899	Immunosuppressant	Prophylaxis of organ transplant rejection
Atelvia [risedronate sodium]	Z79.83	Bisphosphonate	Prevention of thinning of the bones (osteoporosis)
Atenolol [atenolol]		Beta blocker	Angina pectoris; hypertension; acute myocardial infarction

Drug	Z Code	Drug Action/Classification	Indications
Ativan [lorazepam]		Antianxiety; sedative/hypnotic	Anxiety disorder associated with depressive symptoms; controls tension, agitation, irritability, and insomnia
Atripla [efavirenz/emtricitabine/tenofovir disoproxil fumarate]	Z79.899	Antiviral	HIV
Atrovent HFA [ipratropium bromide]		Antiasthmatic/bronchodilator	Chronic bronchitis, emphysema; bronchial asthma
Augmentin [amoxicillin/clavulanate potassium]	Z79.2	Antibiotic	Middle ear, lower respiratory, sinus, skin and skin structures, and urinary tract infections
Avandia [rosiglitazone maleate]	Z79.84	Oral hypoglycemic	Diabetes mellitus
Avapro [irbesartan]		Antihypertensive	Hypertension
Avelox [moxifloxacin hydrochloride]	Z79.2	Antibiotic	Bacterial infections, specifically pneumonia; skin; intra-abdominal; plague; acute sinusitis; acute chronic bronchitis
Aviane-28 [ethinyl estradiol/levonorgestrel]	Z79.3	Contraceptive	Prevention of pregnancy
Avonex [interferon beta-1a]	Z79.899	Antiviral	Treatment of relapsing multiple sclerosis
Axid AR [nizatidine]		Histamine H2-receptor antagonist	Acid/peptic disorder; gastroesophageal reflux; duodenal, gastric, and peptic ulcers
Azactam [aztreonam]	Z79.2	Antibiotic	Severe bacterial infections
Azithromycin [azithromycin]	Z79.2	Antibiotic	Bacterial infections
Bactrim [sulfamethoxazole/trimethoprim]	Z79.2	Antibiotic	Treatment of urinary tract infections, acute otitis media, acute exacerbation of chronic bronchitis, shigellosis, and pneumocystis carinii
Balziva-28 [ethinyl estradiol/norethindrone]	Z79.3	Contraceptive	Prevention of pregnancy
Basaglar [insulin glargine]	Z79.4	Insulin	Diabetes mellitus
Bayer [acetylsalicylic acid]	Z79.82	Aspirin	Prophylaxis and treatment of heart attacks, angina or strokes; reduction of fever, pain and inflammation
Beconase AQ [beclomethasone dipropionate monohydrate]		Corticosteroid -inhaled/nasal	Perennial and seasonal allergies; vasomotor rhinitis
Bekyree [desogestrel/ethinyl estradiol]	Z79.3	Contraceptive	Prevention of pregnancy
Betaseron [interferon beta-1b]	Z79.899	Antiviral	Treatment of relapsing multiple sclerosis
Betoptic [betaxolol hydrochloride]		Beta blocker; ophthalmic glaucoma agent	Lowering of intraocular pressure; also used for treatment of ocular hypertension and chronic open-angle glaucoma
Bevyxxa	Z79.01	Anticoagulant	Prophylaxis of venous thromboembolism
Beyaz [drospirenone/ethinyl estradiol/levomefolate calcium]	Z79.3	Contraceptive	Prevention of pregnancy; acne
Biaxin XL [clarithromycin]	Z79.2	Antibiotic	Acid/peptic disorder or ulcer, acute exacerbation chronic bronchitis, human immunodeficiency virus, lower and upper respiratory tract infection, sinus infection, prophylaxis mycobacterium avium complex, pharyngitis, pneumonia, tonsillitis
Bijuva [estradiol/progesterone]	Z79.890	Estrogen/progesterone therapy	Menopausal symptoms
Biltricide [praziquantel]		Antiparasitic	Infections from Schistosoma species and liver flukes
Binosto [alendronate sodium]	Z79.83	Bisphosphonate	Prevention of thinning of the bones (osteoporosis)
Boniva [ibandronate sodium]	Z79.83	Bisphosphonate	Prevention of thinning of the bones (osteoporosis)
Breo Ellipta [fluticasone furoate/vilanterol trifenatate]	Z79.51	Corticosteroid -- inhaled; anitasthmatic	Maintenance treatment of asthma and COPD
Brevicon 28-day [ethinyl estradiol/norethindrone]	Z79.3	Contraceptive	Prevention of pregnancy; acne
Briellyn [ethinyl estradiol/norethindrone]	Z79.3	Contraceptive	Prevention of pregnancy
Brilinta [ticagrelor]	Z79.02	Antiplatelet	Unstable angina; heart attacks; prevention of blood clots
Brisdelle [paroxetine]		Selective serotonin reuptake inhibitor (SSRI)	Vasomotor symptoms related to menopause
Buprenex [buprenorphine hydrochloride]	Z79.891	Analgesic, narcotic	Moderate to severe pain
Buprenorphine HCl and Naloxone HCl [buprenorphine hydrochloride/naloxone hydrochloride]	Z79.891	Analgesic, narcotic	Moderate to severe pain
Buspirone HCl [buspirone hydrochloride]		Antianxiety	Generalized anxiety disorder
Butorphanol tartrate [butorphanol tartrate]	Z79.891	Analgesic, narcotic	Moderate to severe postsurgical pain

Drug	Z Code	Drug Action/Classification	Indications
Butrans [buprenorphine]	Z79.891	Analgesic, narcotic	Chronic pain
Byetta [exenatide]		Antidiabetic — injectable	Diabetes mellitus
Calan [verapamil hydrochloride]		Calcium channel blocker	Angina pectoris at rest and chronic stable, arrhythmia, atrial fibrillation, atrial flutter, paroxysmal supraventricular tachycardia, ventricular arrhythmia, hypertension
Caldolor [ibuprofen]	Z79.1	Nonsteroidal anti-inflammatory drug (NSAID)	Pain or fever relief
Cambia [diclofenac potassium]	Z79.1	Nonsteroidal anti-inflammatory drug (NSAID)	Migraine headaches
Camila [norethindrone]	Z79.3	Contraceptive	Prevention of pregnancy; menstrual disorders
Cardizem CD [diltiazem hydrochloride]		Calcium channel blocker	Chronic stable angina, atrial fibrillation, atrial flutter, hypertension, paroxysmal supraventricular tachycardia
Cardura [doxazosin mesylate]		Antihypertensive	Benign prostatic hyperplasia; hypertension
Catapres [clonidine hydrochloride]		Antihypertensive	Hypertension
Cefprozil [cefprozil]	Z79.2	Antibiotic	Acute exacerbation and chronic bronchitis, lower respiratory tract infection, upper respiratory tract infection, pharyngitis, tonsillitis
Ceftriaxone [ceftriaxone sodium]	Z79.2	Antibiotic	Bacterial infections
Celebrex [celecoxib]	Z79.1	Nonsteroidal anti-inflammatory drug (NSAID)	Relief of some symptoms caused by arthritis, such as inflammation, swelling, stiffness, and joint pain
Celestone Soluspan [betamethasone acetate/betamethasone sodium phosphate]	Z79.52	Corticosteroid; antiasthmatic	Asthma; severe inflammation
Celexa [citalopram hydrobromide]		Antidepressant	Depression
Cellcept [mycophenolate mofetil]	Z79.899	Immunosuppressant	Prophylaxis of organ transplant rejection
Centany [mupirocin]	Z79.2	Antibiotic	Skin infections
Cephalexin [cephalexin]	Z79.2	Antibiotic	Bacterial infections
Chantix [varenicline tartrate]		Smoking cessation aid	Nicotine addiction, smoking
Cimduo [lamivudine/tenofovir disoproxil fumarate]	Z79.899	Antiviral	HIV
Cipro [ciprofloxacin hydrochloride]	Z79.2	Antibiotic	Cystitis, infectious diarrhea, gonorrhea, bone and joint infection, gastrointestinal tract infection, lower and upper respiratory tract infection, sinus infection, urinary tract infection, nosocomial pneumonia, chronic prostatitis
Ciprofloxacin [ciprofloxacin]	Z79.2	Antibiotic	Bacterial infections
Clarithromycin [clarithromycin]	Z79.2	Antibiotic	Skin and respiratory bacterial infections
Claritin [loratadine]		Antihistamine	Seasonal allergic rhinitis; chronic idiopathic urticaria
Cleocin [clindamycin phosphate]	Z79.2	Antibiotic	Bacterial infections
Climara [estradiol]	Z79.890	Estrogen therapy	Osteoporosis prevention and to treat menopausal symptoms; vaginal and vulvar atrophy; hypoestrogenism; ovarian failure
Clindamycin [clindamycin phosphate]	Z79.2	Antibiotic	Bacterial infections
Clonazepam [clonazepam]		Anticonvulsant	Absence, akinetic and myoclonic epilepsy, Lennox-Gastaut syndrome
Clonidine HCl [clonidine hydrochloride]		Antihypertensive	Hypertension
Clopidogrel bisulfate [clopidogrel bisulfate]	Z79.02	Antiplatelet	Unstable angina; heart attacks; prevention of blood clots
Codeine [codeine sulfate]	Z79.891	Analgesic, narcotic	Mild to moderate pain
Cogentin [benztropine mesylate]		Antiparkinsonism	Parkinson's disease
Colace [docusate sodium]		Gastrointestinal agent; laxative, stool softener	Constipation
Colocort [hydrocortisone]	Z79.52	Corticosteroid	Inflammation of the colon
CombiPatch [ethinyl estradiol/norethindrone acetate]	Z79.890	Estrogen therapy	Menopause symptoms; vaginal and vulvar atrophy; osteoporosis prevention
Combivent respimat [ipratropium bromide/albuterol sulfate]		Antiasthmatic/bronchodilator	Chronic bronchitis, emphysema; bronchial asthma
Compro [prochlorperazine]		Antiemetic; antipsychotic	Nausea, vomiting, and manic phase of bipolar syndrome or schizophrenia
Copaxone [glatiramer acetate]		Immunostimulant	Treatment of relapsing multiple sclerosis
Coreg [carvedilol]		Beta blocker	Hypertension; chronic heart failure; left ventricular dysfunction following myocardial infarction

Drug	Z Code	Drug Action/Classification	Indications
Coreg CR [carvedilol phosphate]		Beta blocker	Hypertension; chronic heart failure; left ventricular dysfunction following myocardial infarction
Cortef [hydrocortisone]	Z79.52	Corticosteroid	Severe inflammation
Cortenema [hydrocortisone]	Z79.52	Corticosteroid	Inflammation of the colon
Cortifoam [hydrocortisone acetate]	Z79.52	Corticosteroid	Colon and rectum inflammation
Cortisone acetate [cortisone acetate]	Z79.52	Corticosteroid	Inflammation
Cortisporin [hydrocortisone acetate/neomycin sulfate/polymyxin B sulfate]		Topical anti-infective, topical steroid	Dermatosis
Cosentyx [secukinumab]	Z79.899	Immunosuppressant	Plaque psoriasis; psoriatic arthritis; ankylosing spondylitis
Coumadin [warfarin sodium]	Z79.01	Anticoagulant	Prophylaxis and treatment of venous thrombosis, treatment of atrial fibrillation with embolization (pulmonary embolism), arrhythmias, myocardial infarction, and stroke prevention
Cozaar [losartan potassium]		Antihypertensive	Hypertension
Crestor [rosuvastatin calcium]		HMG-CoA reductase inhibitor (statin)	Hypercholesterolemia; hyperlipidemia; hyperproteinemia
Crixivan [indinavir sulfate]	Z79.899	Antiviral	HIV, asymptomatic HIV
Cryselle [ethinyl estradiol/norgestrel]	Z79.3	Contraceptive	Prevention of pregnancy
Cubicin [daptomycin]	Z79.2	Antibiotic	Bacterial skin infections; *Staphylococcus aureus* bloodstream infections
Cyclafem [ethinyl estradiol/norethindrone]	Z79.3	Contraceptive	Prevention of pregnancy
Cyclessa [desogestrel/ethinyl estradiol]	Z79.3	Contraceptive	Prevention of pregnancy
Cyclosporine [cyclosporine]	Z79.899	Immunosuppressant	Prophylaxis of organ transplant rejection
Cyltezo [adalimumab-abdm]	Z79.899	Antirheumatic	Rheumatoid arthritis; juvenile idiopathic arthritis; psoriatic arthritis; Crohn's disease; ulcerative colitis; plaque psoriasis
Cymbalta [duloxetine hydrochloride]		Antidepressant, serotonin and norepinephrine reuptake inhibitor (SNRI)	Major depressive disorder; general anxiety disorder; fibromyalgia; diabetic peripheral neuropathy; chronic musculoskeletal pain
Cytomel [liothyronine sodium]		Thyroid hormone	Hypothyroidism or prevention of euthyroid goiters
Daptomycin [daptomycin]	Z79.2	Antibiotic	Skin and underlying tissue bacterial infections
Dasetta [ethinyl estradiol/norethindrone]	Z79.3	Contraceptive	Prevention of pregnancy
Daypro [oxaprozin]	Z79.1	Nonsteroidal anti-inflammatory drug (NSAID)	Osteoarthritis and rheumatoid arthritis
Daysee [ethinyl estradiol/levonorgestrel]	Z79.3	Contraceptive	Prevention of pregnancy
Delestrogen [estradiol valerate]	Z79.890	Estrogen therapy	Menopause symptoms
Demerol [meperidine hydrochloride]	Z79.891	Analgesic, narcotic	Moderate to severe pain
Depakote [divalproex sodium]		Anticonvulsant	Bipolar affective disorder; complex absence, complex partial and mixed pattern epilepsy; migraine headache
Depo-Medrol [methylprednisolone acetate]	Z79.52	Corticosteroid	Arthritis; joint disorders
Depo-Provera [medroxyprogesterone acetate]	Z79.3, Z79.890	Antineoplastic; contraceptive; progestin	Amenorrhea; carcinoma, endometrium, adjunct; carcinoma, renal; Prevention of pregnancy; hemorrhage
Depo-SubQ Provera [medroxyprogesterone acetate]	Z79.3	Contraceptive	Prevention of pregnancy; menstrual disorder pain
Descovy [emtricitabine/tenofovir alafenamide]	Z79.899	Antiretroviral	HIV
Desogen [desogestrel/ethinyl estradiol]	Z79.3	Contraceptive	Prevention of pregnancy
Detrol [tolterodine tartrate]		Muscarinic receptor antagonist	Overactive bladders in patients with urinary frequency, urgency, or urge incontinence
Dexamethasone Intensol [dexamethasone]	Z79.52	Corticosteroid	Arthritis; allergic disorders; breathing disorders; lupus
Dexilant [dexlansoprazole]		Proton pump inhibitor	Healing of erosive esophagitis; relieve of heartburn; treatment of non-erosive gastroesophageal reflux disease
Diabinese [chlorpropamide]	Z79.84	Oral hypoglycemic	Diabetes mellitus
Diaβeta [glyburide]	Z79.84	Oral hypoglycemic	Diabetes mellitus
Diclegis [doxylamine succinate/pyridoxine hydrochloride]		Antiemetic	Nausea/vomiting in pregnancy
Didronel [etidronate disodium]	Z79.83	Bisphosphonate	Paget's disease and irregular bone growth

Drug	Z Code	Drug Action/Classification	Indications
Dificid [fidaxomicin]	Z79.2	Antibiotic	Clostridium difficile
Diflucan [fluconazole]		Antifungal	Oropharyngeal and esophageal candidiasis and cryptococcal meningitis in AIDS patients
Digoxin [digoxin]		Cardiotonic glycoside	Heart failure, atrial flutter, atrial fibrillation, and supraventricular tachycardia
Dilantin [phenytoin sodium]		Anticonvulsant	Grand mal and psychomotor seizures
Dilaudid [hydromorphone hydrochloride]	Z79.891	Analgesic, narcotic	Moderate to severe pain
Diovan [valsartan]		Angiotensin II receptor blocker	Hypertension
Diskets [methadone hydrochloride]		Opioid agonist	Treatment of opioid addiction
Divigel [estradiol]	Z79.890	Estrogen therapy -topical	Menopause symptoms
Dolophine HCl [methadone hydrochloride]	Z79.891	Analgesic, narcotic; opioid agonist	Pain; treatment of opioid addiction
Doxycycline [doxycycline]	Z79.2	Antibiotic	Bacterial infections; acne
Duavee [bazedoxifene acetate/conjugated estrogens]	Z79.890	Estrogen therapy	Menopause symptoms; osteoporosis prevention
Duetact [glimepiride/pioglitazone hydrochloride]	Z79.84	Oral hypoglycemic	Diabetes mellitus
Duexis [famotidine/ibuprofen]	Z79.1	Nonsteroidal anti-inflammatory drug (NSAID)	Symptomatic treatment of osteoarthritis and rheumatoid arthritis; reduce risk of ulcers
Dulera [formoterol fumarate/mometasone furoate]	Z79.51	Corticosteroid -inhaled; antiasthmatic	Prophylaxis and treatment of asthma
Duragesic [fentanyl]	Z79.891	Analgesic, narcotic	Chronic pain
Duramorph PF [morphine sulfate]	Z79.891	Analgesic, narcotic	Moderate to severe pain
Durlaza [aspirin]	Z79.82	Aspirin	Prevention of heart attack, stroke, angina
Dynacin [minocycline hydrochloride]	Z79.2	Antibiotic	Severe acne treatment
E.E.S. [erythromycin ethylsuccinate]	Z79.2	Antibiotic	Bacterial infections
Effexor XR [venlafaxine hydrochloride]		Antidepressant, serotonin and norepinephrine reuptake inhibitors (SNRIs)	Major depressive disorder; social anxiety disorder; panic disorder
Effient [prasugrel hydrochloride]	Z79.02	Antiplatelet	Lessening of the chance of heart attack or stroke
Elestrin [estradiol]	Z79.890	Estrogen therapy	Menopause symptoms
Eligard [leuprolide acetate]	Z79.818	Agents affecting estrogen receptors and estrogen levels	Palliative treatment of prostate cancer symptoms
Elinest [norgestrel/ethinyl estradiol]	Z79.3	Contraceptive	Prevention of pregnancy
Eliquis [apixaban]	Z79.01	Anticoagulant	Venous thrombosis
Embeda [morphine sulfate/naltrexone hydrochloride]	Z79.891	Analgesic, narcotic	Moderate to severe pain
Emoquette [ethinyl estradiol/desogestrel]	Z79.3	Contraceptive	Prevention of pregnancy
Emtriva [emtricitabine]	Z79.899	Antiretroviral	HIV
Enbrel [etanercept]	Z79.899	Antirheumatic	Rheumatoid arthritis; polyarticular juvenile idiopathic arthritis; psoriatic arthritis; ankylosing spondylitis, plaque psoriasis
Enpresse-28 [ethinyl estradiol/levonorgestrel]	Z79.3	Contraceptive	Prevention of pregnancy
Enskyce [desogestrel/ethinyl estradiol]	Z79.3	Contraceptive	Prevention of pregnancy
Entocort EC [budesonide]	Z79.52	Corticosteroid	Crohn's disease; ulcerative colitis
Entresto [sacubitril/valsartan]		Angiotensin II receptor blocker; neprilysin inhibitor	Chronic heart failure
Entyvio [vedolizumab]	Z79.899	Immunosuppressant	Ulcerative colitis; Crohn's disease
Envarsus XR [tacrolimus]	Z79.899	Immunosuppressant	Prophylaxis of organ transplant rejection
Epinephrine [epinephrine]		Bronchodilator, cardiotonic	Most commonly, relief of distress due to bronchospasm and restoration of cardiac rhythm in cardiac arrest
Epivir, Epivir-HBV [lamivudine]	Z79.899	Antiretroviral	HIV, hepatitis B (HBV), asymptomatic HIV
Erelzi [etanercept-szzs]	Z79.899	Antirheumatic	Rheumatoid arthritis; polyarticular juvenile idiopathic arthritis; psoriatic arthritis; ankylosing spondylitis, plaque psoriasis
Errin [norethindrone]	Z79.3	Contraceptive	Prevention of pregnancy
Ertapenem [ertapenem sodium]	Z79.2	Antibiotic	Stomach, urinary tract, pelvis, skin and lung infections

Drug	Z Code	Drug Action/Classification	Indications
Ery-Tab [erythromycin]	Z79.2	Antibiotic	Bacterial infections
ERYC [erythromycin]	Z79.2	Antibiotic	Respiratory tract infections
Erygel [erythromycin]	Z79.2	Antibiotic, topical	Bacterial skin infections
EryPed [erythromycin ethylsuccinate]	Z79.2	Antibiotic	Bacterial infections; rheumatic fever attacks
Erythrocin [erythromycin lactobionate]	Z79.2	Antibiotic	Bacterial infections
Erythromycin [erythromycin]	Z79.2	Antibiotic	Respiratory tract infections
Estarylla [ethinyl estradiol/norgestimate]	Z79.3	Contraceptive	Prevention of pregnancy
Estrace [estradiol]	Z79.890	Estrogen therapy	Vaginal cream for treatment of vaginal and vulvar atrophy
EstroGel [estradiol]	Z79.890	Estrogen therapy -topical	Menopause symptoms
Estrostep Fe [ethinyl estradiol/norethindrone acetate]	Z79.3	Contraceptive	Prevention of pregnancy
Evista [raloxifene hydrochloride]	Z79.810	Selective estrogen receptor modulator (SERM)	Prevention of thinning of the bones (osteoporosis) only in postmenopausal women
Exalgo [hydromorphone hydrochloride]	Z79.891	Analgesic, narcotic	Moderate to severe pain
Exemestane [exemestane]	Z79.811	Aromatase inhibitor	Postmenopausal breast cancer
Factive [gemifloxacin mesylate]	Z79.2	Antibiotic	Bacterial lung infections
Falmina [ethinyl estradiol/levonorgestrel]	Z79.3	Contraceptive	Prevention of pregnancy
Fareston [toremifene citrate]	Z79.810	Selective estrogen receptor modulator (SERM)	Treatment of metastatic breast cancer in postmenopausal women
Farxiga [dapagliflozin propanediol]	Z79.84	Oral hypoglycemic	Diabetes mellitus
Faslodex [fulvestrant]	Z79.818	Agents affecting estrogen receptors and estrogen levels	Hormone-related breast cancer; metastatic breast cancer
Feldene [piroxicam]	Z79.1	Nonsteroidal anti-inflammatory drug (NSAID)	Treatment of pain and inflammation due to arthritis
Femara [letrozole]	Z79.811	Aromatase inhibitor	Postmenopausal breast cancer
Femcon Fe [ethinyl estradiol/norethindrone]	Z79.3	Contraceptive	Prevention of pregnancy; acne
Femhrt [ethinyl estradiol/norethindrone acetate]	Z79.3, Z79.890	Contraceptive; estrogen therapy	Prevention of pregnancy; menopause symptoms; osteoporosis prevention
Femring [estradiol acetate]	Z79.890	Estrogen therapy	Osteoporosis prevention and to treat menopausal symptoms; hypoestrogenism; ovarian failure
Fentanyl citrate [fentanyl citrate]	Z79.891	Analgesic, narcotic	Postprocedural or chronic pain
Fentora [fentanyl citrate]	Z79.891	Analgesic, narcotic	Breakthrough cancer pain
Fiasp [insulin aspart]	Z79.4	Insulin	Diabetes mellitus
Fioricet with codeine [acetaminophen/butalbital/caffeine/codeine phosphate]	Z79.891	Analgesic, narcotic	Tension headaches
Firmagon [degarelix]	Z79.890	Hormone therapy	Prostate cancer
Flagyl [metronidazole]	Z79.2	Antibiotic	Bacterial infections
Flavoxate HCl [flavoxate hydrochloride]		Urinary tract spasmolytic	Relief of dysuria, urgency, nocturia, suprapubic pain, frequency, and incontinence associated with cystitis, prostatitis, urethritis, and urethrocystitis/urethrotrigonitis
Flomax [tamsulosin hydrochloride]		Antiadrenergic	Benign prostatic hyperplasia
Flonase allergy relief [fluticasone propionate]		Corticosteroid -inhaled/nasal	Perennial and seasonal allergic rhinitis
Flovent HFA [fluticasone propionate]	Z79.51	Corticosteroid -inhaled; antiasthmatic	Asthma
Fortamet [metformin hydrochloride]	Z79.84	Oral hypoglycemic	Diabetes mellitus
Fortaz [ceftazidime]	Z79.2	Antibiotic	Pneumonia and lower respiratory infections
Fosamax [alendronate sodium]	Z79.83	Biophosphonate	Osteoporosis; Paget's disease
Fosinopril sodium [fosinopril sodium]		ACE inhibitor	Hypertension
Fosrenol [lanthanum carbonate]		Phosphate binder	End-stage renal disease (ESRD)
Fragmin [dalteparin sodium]	Z79.01	Anticoagulant	Prophylaxis and treatment of blood clots
Gengraf [cyclosporine]	Z79.899	Immunosuppressant	Prophylaxis of organ transplant rejection
Gentamicin sulfate [gentamicin sulfate]	Z79.2	Antibiotic	Severe bacterial infections
Gildagia [ethinyl estradiol/norethindrone]	Z79.3	Contraceptive	Prevention of pregnancy

Drug	Z Code	Drug Action/Classification	Indications
Gildess [ethinyl estradiol/norethindrone acetate]	Z79.3	Contraceptive	Prevention of pregnancy
Glimepiride [glimepiride]	Z79.84	Oral hypoglycemic	Diabetes mellitus
Glucophage [metformin hydrochloride]	Z79.84	Oral hypoglycemic	Diabetes mellitus
Glucotrol [glipizide]	Z79.84	Oral hypoglycemic	Diabetes mellitus
Glucovance [glyburide/metformin hydrochloride]	Z79.84	Oral hypoglycemic	Diabetes mellitus
Glumetza [metformin hydrochloride]	Z79.84	Oral hypoglycemic	Diabetes mellitus
Glyburide (micronized) [glyburide]	Z79.84	Oral hypoglycemic	Diabetes mellitus
Glynase [glyburide]	Z79.84	Oral hypoglycemic	Diabetes mellitus
Glyset [miglitol]	Z79.84	Oral hypoglycemic	Diabetes mellitus
Harvoni [ledipasvir/sofosbuvir]	Z79.899	Antiviral	Chronic hepatitis C
Heparin sodium [heparin sodium]	Z79.01	Anticoagulant	Prophylaxis and treatment of venous thrombosis, pulmonary embolism; prevention of cerebral thrombosis, and treatment of consumptive coagulopathies
Humalog [insulin lispro recombinant]	Z79.4	Insulin	Diabetes mellitus
Humira [adalimumab]	Z79.899	Antirheumatic	Rheumatoid arthritis; juvenile idiopathic arthritis; psoriatic arthritis; Crohn's disease; ulcerative colitis; plaque psoriasis; hidradenitis suppurativa; uveitis
Humulin R [insulin recombinant]	Z79.4	Insulin	Diabetes mellitus
Hydrochlorothiazide [hydrochlorothiazide]		Diuretic; antihypertensive	Management of hypertension and in adjunctive therapy for edema associated with congestive heart failure; hepatic cirrhosis; corticosteroid, and estrogen therapy
Hydrocodone [acetaminophen/hydrocodone bitartrate]	Z79.891	Analgesic, narcotic	Moderate to severe pain
Hydrocodone bitartrate and acetaminophen [acetaminophen/ hydrocodone bitartrate]	Z79.891	Analgesic, narcotic	Pain, moderate to severe
Hydrocortisone [hydrocortisone]	Z79.52	Corticosteroid	Addison's disease; arthritis; immune disorders; allergies; breathing problems
Hydromorphone HCl [hydromorphone hydrochloride]	Z79.891	Analgesic, narcotic	Moderate to severe pain
Hyrimoz [adalimumab-adaz]	Z79.899	Antirheumatic	Rheumatoid arthritis; juvenile idiopathic arthritis; psoriatic arthritis; Crohn's disease; ulcerative colitis; plaque psoriasis
Hyzaar [hydrochlorothiazide/ losartan potassium]		Antihypertensive	Hypertension
Ibuprofen [ibuprofen]	Z79.1	Nonsteroidal anti-inflammatory drug (NSAID)	Pain or fever relief
Imitrex [sumatriptan succinate]		Antimigraine	Migraine headache
Imuran [azathioprine]	Z79.899	Immunosuppressant	Rheumatoid arthritis
Inderal [propranolol hydrochloride]		Beta blocker	Angina pectoris; hypertension; cardiac arrhythmias
Indocin [indomethacin]	Z79.1	Nonsteroidal anti-inflammatory drug (NSAID)	Treatment of pain and inflammation
Integrilin [eptifibatide]	Z79.02	Antiplatelet	Unstable angina; heart attacks; prevention of blood clots
Intron A [interferon alfa 2-b]	Z79.899	Antineoplastic interferons; antiviral interferons	Cancer; hepatitis
Introvale [levonorgestrel/ethinyl estradiol]	Z79.3	Contraceptive	Prevention of pregnancy
Invanz [ertapeneum sodium]	Z79.2	Antibiotic	Stomach, urinary tract, pelvis, skin and lung infections
Invokamet [canagliflozin/metformin hydrochloride]	Z79.84	Oral hypoglycemic	Diabetes mellitus
Invokana [canagliflozin]	Z79.84	Oral hypoglycemic	Diabetes mellitus
Isoniazid [isoniazid]	Z79.2	Antibiotic	Tuberculosis
Isopto carpine [pilocarpine hydrochloride]		Cholinergic parasympathomimetic agent	Reduction of intraocular pressure in open-angle glaucoma or ocular hypertension; management of acute angle-closure glaucoma
Isordil [isosorbide dinitrate]		Smooth muscle relaxant	Acute anginal attacks
Isuprel [isoproterenol hydrochloride]		Adrenergic agent	Bronchodilator for asthma, chronic pulmonary emphysema, bronchitis, and other conditions accompanied by bronchospasm; can be used in cardiogenic shock cases

Drug	Z Code	Drug Action/Classification	Indications
Jantoven [warfarin sodium]	Z79.01	Anticoagulant	Prophylaxis and treatment of venous thrombosis, pulmonary embolism; prevention of cerebral thrombosis, and treatment of consumptive coagulopathies
Janumet [metformin hydrochloride/sitagliptin phosphate]	Z79.84	Oral hypoglycemic	Diabetes mellitus
Januvia [sitagliptin phosphate]	Z79.84	Oral hypoglycemic	Diabetes mellitus
Jencycla [norethindrone]	Z79.3	Contraceptive	Prevention of pregnancy
Jentadueto [linagliptin/metformin hydrochloride]]	Z79.84	Oral hypoglycemic	Diabetes mellitus
Junel [ethinyl estradiol/norethindrone acetate]	Z79.3	Contraceptive	Prevention of pregnancy
K-Tab [potassium chloride]		Replaces potassium and maintains potassium level	Hypokalemia
Kadian [morphine sulfate]	Z79.891	Analgesic, narcotic	Moderate to severe pain
Kariva [desogestrel/ethinyl estradiol]	Z79.3	Contraceptive	Prevention of pregnancy
Kazano [alogliptin benzoate/metformin hydrochloride]	Z79.84	Oral hypoglycemic	Diabetes mellitus
Keflex [cephalexin]	Z79.2	Antibiotic	Bone, middle ear, skin and skin structures, upper respiratory tract and urinary tract infections; acute prostatitis
Kelnor [ethynodiol diacetate/ethinyl estradiol]	Z79.3	Contraceptive	Prevention of pregnancy
Kenalog-10; Kenalog-40 [triamcinolone acetonide]	Z79.52	Corticosteroid	Gouty arthritis; bursitis; tenosynovitis; epicondylitis; rheumatoid arthritis; synovitis; osteoarthritis
Keytruda [pembrolizumab]	Z79.899	Antineoplastic	Cancer
Kimidess [ethinyl estradiol/desogestrel]	Z79.3	Contraceptive	Prevention of pregnancy
Klaron [sulfacetamide sodium]	Z79.2	Antibiotic, topical	Acne vulgaris
Klonopin [clonazepam]		Anticonvulsant; CNS depressant	Epilepsy; seizures; panic disorder
Klor-Con [potassium chloride]		Replaces potassium and maintains potassium level	Hypokalemia
Kombiglyze [metformin hydrochloride/saxagliptin hydrochloride]	Z79.84	Oral hypoglycemic	Diabetes mellitus
Kurvelo [ethinyl estradiol/levonorgestrel]	Z79.3	Contraceptive	Prevention of pregnancy; menstrual disorders
Kyleena [levonorgestrel]	Z79.3	Contraceptive	Prevention of pregnancy
Lamisil [terbinafine hydrochloride]		Antifungal	Tinea cruris (jock itch), T. pedis (athlete's foot), T. corporis (ringworm)
Lanoxin [digoxin]		Cardiotonic glycoside	Congestive heart failure
Lantus [insulin glargine recombinant]	Z79.4	Insulin	Diabetes mellitus
Larin [ethinyl estradiol/norethindrone acetate]	Z79.3	Contraceptive	Prevention of pregnancy
Lasix [furosemide]		Antihypertensive; diuretic	Management of edema associated with congestive heart failure, renal disease, including nephrotic syndrome and hypertension
Lazanda [fentanyl citrate]	Z79.891	Analgesics, narcotic	Breakthrough cancer pain
Lescol XL [fluvastatin sodium]		HMG-CoA reductase inhibitor (statin)	Hypercholesterolemia; hyperlipidemia; hyperlipoproteinemia
Lessina-28 [ethinyl estradiol/levonorgestrel]	Z79.3	Contraceptive	Prevention of pregnancy
Letrozole [letrozole]	Z79.811	Aromatase inhibitor	Postmenopausal breast cancer
Levemir [insulin detemir recombinant]	Z79.4	Insulin	Diabetes mellitus
Levonest [levonorgestrel/ethinyl estradiol]	Z79.3	Contraceptive	Prevention of pregnancy; menstrual disorders; acne
Levora [levonorgestrel/ethinyl estradiol]	Z79.3	Contraceptive	Prevention of pregnancy
Levothroid [levothyroxine sodium]		Thyroid hormone	Hypothyroidism
Levoxyl [levothyroxine sodium]		Thyroid hormone	Euthyroid goiter; hypothyroidism
Lexapro [escitalopram oxalate]		Antidepressant, selective serotonin reuptake inhibitor (SSRI)	Depression; anxiety
Lialda [mesalamine]		Antiinflammatory	Ulcerative colitis
Librium [chlordiazepoxide hydrochloride]		Antianxiety	Acute withdrawal symptoms, especially from alcohol, or for other anxiety-producing conditions

Drug	Z Code	Drug Action/Classification	Indications
Lidocaine HCl [lidocaine hydrochloride]		Antiarrhythmic	Management of ventricular arrhythmias or during cardiac manipulation, such as cardiac surgery
Liletta [levonorgestrel]	Z79.3	Contraceptive	Intrauterine device for prevention of pregnancy
Lincocin [lincocin hydrochloride]	Z79.2	Antibiotic	Severe bacterial infections
Lipitor [atorvastatin calcium]		HMG-CoA reductase inhibitor (statin)	Hypercholesterolemia; hyperlipidemia; hyperproteinemia
Lithium carbonate [lithium carbonate]		Antimanic	Control of manic episodes in bipolar disorders
Lo Loestrin Fe [ethinyl estradiol/norethindrone acetate]	Z79.3	Contraceptive	Prevention of pregnancy
Locoid [hydrocotisone butyrate]	Z79.52	Corticosteroid -topical	Atopic dermatitis; other dermatoses
Loestrin [ethinyl estradiol/norethindrone acetate]	Z79.3	Contraceptive	Prevention of pregnancy
Lomotil [diphenoxylate hydrochloride/atropine sulfate]		Antidiarrheal	Symptoms of chronic and functional diarrhea
Lopid [gemfibrozil]		Lipid regulating agent	Hypercholesterolemia, hyperlipidemia, hyperlipoproteinemia, hypertriglyceridemia
Lopressor [metoprolol tartrate]		Beta blocker	Angina pectoris; hypertension; acute myocardial infarction
Lorazepam [lorazepam]		Antianxiety; sedative/hypnotic	Anxiety disorder associated with depressive symptoms; controls tension, agitation, irritability, and insomnia
Loryna [drospirenone/ethinyl estradiol]	Z79.3	Contraceptive	Prevention of pregnancy
LoSeasonique [ethinyl estradiol/levonorgestrel]	Z79.3	Contraceptive	Prevention of pregnancy
Lotensin [benazepril hydrochloride]		ACE inhibitor	Hypertension
Lotrel [amlodipine besylate/benazepril hydrochloride]		Antihypertensive	Hypertension
Lotrisone [clotrimazole/ betamethasone dipropionate]		Antifungal-corticosteroid	Relief of redness, swelling, itching, and other discomfort of fungus infections
Lovastatin [lovastatin]		HMG-CoA reductase inhibitor (statin)	Hypercholesterolemia; hyperlipidemia; hyperlipoproteinemia
Lovenox [enoxaparin sodium]	Z79.01	Anticoagulant	Prophylaxis and treatment of venous thrombosis and pulmonary embolism
Low-Ogestrel-28 [norgestrel/ethinyl estradiol]	Z79.3	Contraceptive	Prevention of pregnancy
Lupron [leuprolide acetate]	Z79.818	Agents affecting estrogen receptors and estrogen levels	Endometriosis symptoms; uterine fibroids
Macrobid [nitrofuantoin]	Z79.2	Antibiotic	Urinary tract infections
Macrodantin [nitrofurantoin]	Z79.2	Antibiotic	Urinary tract infections
Marlissa [ethinyl estradiol/levonorgestrel]	Z79.3	Contraceptive	Prevention of pregnancy
Maxipime [cefepime hydrochloride]	Z79.2	Antibiotic	Bacterial infections
Meclizine hydrochloride [meclizine hydrochloride]		Antihistamine	Nausea and vomiting, and dizziness associated with motion sickness
Medrol [methylprednisolone]	Z79.52	Corticosteroid	Endocrine, rheumatic, hematologic disorders; collagen, dermatological, ophthalmic, respiratory, neoplastic, gastrointestinal, nervous system disorders; allergic and edematous states
Mefoxin [cefoxitin sodium]	Z79.2	Antibiotic	Bacterial infections
Megace ES [megestrol acetate]	Z79.818	Agents affecting estrogen receptors and estrogen levels	Endometrial or advanced breast cancers; weight loss due to AIDS
Menest [esteriefied estrogens]	Z79.890	Estrogen therapy	Menopause symptoms; ovarian failure
Menostar [estradiol]	Z79.890	Estrogen therapy	Menopause symptoms; osteoporosis prevention
Mepron [atovaquone]	Z79.2	Antibiotic	Pneumonia due to penumocystis jiroveci
Merrem [meropenem]	Z79.2	Antibiotic	Bacterial infections of skin or stomach; bacterial meningitis
Metformin [metformin hydrochloride]	Z79.84	Oral hypoglycemic	Diabetes mellitus
Methadone HCl [methadone hydrochloride]	Z79.891	Analgesic, narcotic; opioid agonist	Pain; treatment of opioid addiction
Methadose [methadone hydrochloride]	Z79.891	Analgesic, narcotic	Acute and chronic pain
Methergine [methylergonovine maleate]		Oxytocic agent	Routine management of postpartum hemorrhage after delivery of placenta
Methylprednisolone [methylprednisolone]	Z79.52	Corticosteroid	Inflammatory disorders

Drug	Z Code	Drug Action/Classification	Indications
Metronidazole [metronidazole]	Z79.2	Antibiotic	Bacterial infections
Miacalcin [calcitonin salmon]		Calcitonin; a peptide hormone	Hypercalcemia, osteoporosis, postmenopausal symptoms, Paget's disease
Microgestin [ethinyl estradiol/norethindrone acetate]	Z79.3	Contraceptive	Prevention of pregnancy
Micronor [norethindrone]	Z79.3	Contraceptive	Prevention of pregnancy
Minastrin [ethinyl estradiol/norethindrone acetate]	Z79.3	Contraceptive	Prevention of pregnancy
Minivelle [estradiol]	Z79.890	Estrogen therapy	Menopause symptoms; osteoporosis prevention
Minocin [minocycline hydrochloride]	Z79.2	Antibiotic	Bacterial infections; acne
Mirena [levonorgestrel]	Z79.3	Contraceptive	Intrauterine device for prevention of pregnancy; menstrual disorders
Mobic [meloxicam]	Z79.1	Nonsteroidal anti-inflammatory drug (NSAID)	Treatment of pain and inflammation due to osteoarthritis and rheumatoid arthritis
Modicon 28 [ethinyl estradiol/norethindrone]	Z79.3	Contraceptive	Prevention of pregnancy
Mono-Linyah [norgestimate/ethinyl estradiol]	Z79.3	Contraceptive	Prevention of pregnancy; menstrual disorders; acne
Monoclonal antibodies	Z79.899	Monoclonal antibodies	Cancer; prophylaxis of organ transplant rejection
Monodox [doxycycline]	Z79.2	Antibiotic	Bacterial infections; acne
Monoket [isosorbide mononitrate]		Antianginal; coronary vasodilator, nitrate	Angina pectoris
Monurol [fosfomycin tromethamine]	Z79.2	Antibiotic	Bacterial bladder infections
Morphabond ER [morphine sulfate]	Z79.891	Analgesics, narcotic	Pain
Morphine sulfate [morphine sulfate]	Z79.891	Analgesic, narcotic	Moderate to severe pain
Motrin IB [ibuprofen]	Z79.1	Nonsteroidal anti-inflammatory drug (NSAID)	Pain or fever relief
MS Contin [morphine sulfate]	Z79.891	Analgesic, narcotic	Moderate to severe pain
Multaq [dronedarone hydrochloride]		Cardiac rhythm regulator	Treatment of patients with recent episodes of atrial fibrillation or atrial flutter
Mycobutin [rifabutin]	Z79.2	Antibiotic	Mycobacterium avium complex (MAC) prophylactic in HIV patients
Mytesi [crofelemer]		Antidiarrheal	Diarrhea occurring in HIV/AIDs patient's on anti-retroviral therapy
Myzilra [ethinyl estradiol/levonorgestrel]	Z79.3	Contraceptive	Prevention of pregnancy
Nabumetone [nabumetone]	Z79.1	Non-steroidal anti-inflammatory drug (NSAID)	Osteoarthritis and rheumatoid arthritis
Nalfon [fenoprofen calcium]	Z79.1	Nonsteroidal anti-inflammatory drug (NSAID)	Pain or inflammation relief
Namzaric [memantine/donepezil hydrochlroides]		Acetylcholinesterase/cholinesterase inhibitors	Dementia due to Alzheimer's
Naprelan [naproxen sodium]	Z79.1	Nonsteroidal anti-inflammatory drug (NSAID)	Pain or inflammation relief
Naprosyn [naproxen]	Z79.1	Nonsteroidal anti-inflammatory drug (NSAID)	Rheumatoid, gouty arthritis and osteoarthritis; ankylosing spondylitis; bursitis; dysmenorrhea; pain, mild to moderate; tendonitis
Natazia [estradiol valerate/dienogest]	Z79.3	Contraceptive	Prevention of pregnancy; menstrual disorders
Nebupent [pentamidine isethionate]	Z79.2	Antibiotic	Severe bacterial lung infection in high risk patients with HIV
Nefazodone HCl [nefazodone hydrochloride]		Antidepressant	Depression
Nembutal sodium [pentobarbital sodium]		Sedative/hypnotic	Adjunct medication in diagnostic procedures or for emergency use with convulsive disorders
NeoProfen [ibuprofen lysine]	Z79.1	Nonsteroidal anti-inflammatory drug (NSAID)	Pain or fever relief
Neoral [cyclosporine]	Z79.899	Immunosuppressant	Prophylaxis of organ transplant rejection
Neurontin [gabapentin]		Anticonvulsant	Epilepsy, partial
Nexium [esomeprazole magnesium]		Proton pump inhibitor	Gastroesophageal reflux disease (GERD), erosive esophagitis
Nexplanon [etonogestrel]	Z79.3	Contraceptive	Implantable device used for prevention of pregnancy
Nitrofurantoin [nitrofurantoin]	Z79.2	Antibiotic	Bacterial urinary tract infections

Drug	Z Code	Drug Action/Classification	Indications
Nitropress [sodium nitroprusside]		Vasodilator	Potent, rapid action in reducing blood pressure in hypertensive crisis or for controlling bleeding during anesthesia by producing controlled hypotension
Nitrostat [nitroglycerin]		Muscle relaxant; antianginal; antihypertensive; coronary vasodilator	Prophylaxis and treatment of angina pectoris; heart failure associated with myocardial infarction; hypertension, perioperative; surgery, adjunct
Nor-QD [norethindrone]	Z79.3	Contraceptive	Prevention of pregnancy
Norco [acetaminophen/hydrocodone bitartrate]	Z79.891	Analgesic, narcotic	Moderate to severe pain
Norinyl [mestranol/norethisterone]	Z79.3	Contraceptive	Prevention of pregnancy
Norpace [disopyramide phosphate]		Antiarrhythmic	Coronary artery disease, for prevention, recurrence and control of unifocal, multifocal, and paired PVCs
Nortrel [ethinyl estradiol/norethindrone]	Z79.3	Contraceptive	Prevention of pregnancy
Norvasc [amlodipine besylate]		Calcium channel blocker	Hypertension, chronic stable angina, and vasospastic angina
Novolin [insulin recombinant]	Z79.4	Insulin	Diabetes mellitus
Novolog [insulin aspart recombinant]	Z79.4	Insulin	Diabetes mellitus
Nucynta [tapentadol hydrochloride]	Z79.891	Analgesic, narcotic	Moderate to severe pain
NuvaRing [etonogestrel/ethinyl estradiol]	Z79.3	Contraceptive	Vaginal ring for prevention of pregnancy
Ogestrel [norgestrel/ethinyl estradiol]	Z79.3	Contraceptive	Prevention of pregnancy
Onglyza [saxagliptin hydrochloride]	Z79.84	Oral hypoglycemic	Diabetes mellitus
Opana [oxymorphone hydrochloride]	Z79.891	Analgesic, narcotic	Moderate to severe pain
Oracea [doxycycline]	Z79.2	Antibiotic	Rosacea
Orapred ODT [prednisolone sodium phosphate]	Z79.52	Corticosteroid	Inflammatory disorders
Orbactiv [oritavancin diphosphate]	Z79.2	Antibiotic	Bacterial skin infections
Orencia [abatacept]	Z79.899	Antirheumatic	Rheumatoid arthritis; polyarticular juvenile idiopathic arthritis; psoriatic arthritis
Orilissa [elagolix]	Z79.890	Hormone therapy	Pain associated with endometriosis
Orphenadrine citrate [orphenadrine citrate]		Muscle relaxant	Acute spasms, tension, and post-trauma cases
Orsythia [ethinyl estradiol/levonorgestrel]	Z79.3	Contraceptive	Prevention of pregnancy
Ortho Cyclen-28 [ethinyl estradiol/norgestimate]	Z79.3	Contraceptive	Prevention of pregnancy
Ortho-Novum [norethindrone/ethinyl estradiol]	Z79.3	Contraceptive	Prevention of pregnancy
Ortho-Tri-Cyclen [ethinyl estradiol/norgestimate]	Z79.3	Contraceptive	Prevention of pregnancy
Oseni [alogliptin benzoate/pioglitazone hydrochloride]	Z79.84	Oral hypoglycemic	Diabetes mellitus
Osphena [ospemifene]	Z79.810, Z79.890	Selective estrogen receptor modulator (SERM)	Postmenopausal dyspareunia due to vaginal atrophy; osteoporosis prevention and treatment of menopausal symptoms
Otezla [apremilast]	Z79.899	Antirheumatic	Psoriatic arthritis; plaque psoriasis
Oxazepam [oxazepam]		Antianxiety	Anxiety, tension, and alcohol withdrawal
Oxycodone HCl [oxycodone hydrochloride]	Z79.891	Analgesic, narcotic	Moderate to severe pain
OxyContin [oxycodone hydrochloride]	Z79.891	Analgesic, narcotic	Moderate to severe pain
Ozempic [semaglutide]		Antidiabetic — injectable	Diabetes mellitus
Paxil [paroxetine hydrochloride]		Antidepressant	Anxiety with panic disorder and depression; obsessive-compulsive disorder
PediaPred [prednisolone sodium phosphate]	Z79.52	Corticosteroid	Inflammatory disorders
Pegintron [peginterferon alfa-2b]	Z79.899	Antiviral	Hepatitis C
Penicillin-VK [penicillin V potassium]	Z79.2	Antibiotic	Chorea, prevention; endocarditis, prevention, secondary to tooth extraction; erysipelas; infections of the skin and skin structures, upper respiratory tract; rheumatic fever, prophylaxis; scarlet fever; Vincent's gingivitis; Vincent's pharyngitis
Pentam [pentamidine isethionate]	Z79.2	Antibiotic	Severe bacterial lung infections

Drug	Z Code	Drug Action/Classification	Indications
Pepcid [famotidine]		Histamine H2-receptor inhibitor	Acid/peptic disorder; adenoma, secretory; gastroesophageal reflux; duodenal and gastric ulcer; Zollinger-Ellison syndrome
Percocet [oxycodone hydrochloride/acetaminophen]	Z79.891	Analgesic, narcotic	Pain, moderate to severe
Persantine [dipyridamole]	Z79.02	Antiplatelet	Therapy for chronic angina pectoris, preventing clots post heart valve surgery
Pfizerpen [penicillin g potassium]	Z79.2	Antibiotic	Severe bacterial infections
Phenobarbital [phenobarbital sodium]		Anticonvulsant	Grand mal epilepsy
Philith [ethinyl estradiol/norethindrone]	Z79.3	Contraceptive	Prevention of pregnancy
Pimtrea [desogestrel/ethinyl estradiol]	Z79.3	Contraceptive	Prevention of pregnancy
Pirmella [ethinyl estradiol/norethindrone]	Z79.3	Contraceptive	Prevention of pregnancy
Pitocin [oxytocin]		Uterotonic	Induction or stimulation of labor at term
Plan B One-Step [levonorgestrel]	Z79.3	Contraceptive	Prevention of pregnancy
Plavix [clopidogrel bisulfate]	Z79.02	Antiplatelet	Lessening of the chance of heart attack or stroke
Ponstel [mefenamic acid]	Z79.1	Nonsteroidal anti-inflammatory drug (NSAID)	Treatment of pain
Portia-28 [ethinyl estradiol/levonorgestrel]	Z79.3	Contraceptive	Prevention of pregnancy
Pradaxa [dabigatran etexilate mesylate]	Z79.01	Anticoagulant	Prophylaxis and treatment of blood clots in patients with atrial fibrillation
Prandimet [metformin hydrochloride/repaglinide]	Z79.84	Oral hypoglycemic	Diabetes mellitus
Prandin [repaglinide]	Z79.84	Oral hypoglycemic	Diabetes mellitus
Prasugrel [prasugrel hydrochloride]	Z79.02	Antiplatelet	Lessening the chance of heart attack or stroke
Pravachol [pravastatin sodium]		HMG-CoA reductase inhibitor (statin)	Hypercholesterolemia; hyperlipidemia; hyperlipoproteinemia
Precose [acarbose]	Z79.84	Oral hypoglycemic	Diabetes mellitus
Prednisolone [prednisolone]	Z79.52	Corticosteroid	Inflammatory disorders
Prednisone [prednisone]	Z79.52	Corticosteroid	Used for its immunosuppressant effects and for relief of inflammation; used in arthritis, polymyositis and other systemic diseases
Pregnyl [chorionic gonadotropin]		Gonadotropic hormone	Prepubertal cryptorchidism; hypogonadism; corpus luteum insufficiency and infertility
Prelone [prednisolone]	Z79.52	Corticosteroid	Inflammatory disorders
Prempro [conjugated estrogens/medroxyprogesterone acetate]	Z79.890	Estrogen/progesterone therapy	Menopause; osteoporosis; atrophic vaginitis
Prevacid [lansoprazole]		Proton pump inhibitor	Acid/peptic disorder, erosive esophagitis, duodenal ulcer, Zollinger-Ellison syndrome
Previfem [ethinyl estradiol/norgestimate]	Z79.3	Contraceptive	Prevention of pregnancy
Prezcobix [darunavir/cobicistat]	Z79.899	Antiviral	HIV
Prezista [darunavir ethanolate]	Z79.899	Antiviral	HIV
Priftin [rifapentine]	Z79.2	Antibiotic	Tuberculosis
Prilosec [omeprazole magnesium]		Proton pump inhibitor	Acid/peptic disorder; endocrine adenoma; erosive esophagitis; systemic mastocytosis; gastroesophageal reflux; duodenal, peptic and gastric ulcer; Zollinger-Ellison syndrome
Primaxin [cilastatin sodium/imipenem]	Z79.2	Antibiotic	Skin, stomach, female reproductive organs or lower respiratory tract infections
Prinivil [lisinopril]		ACE inhibitor	Congestive heart failure; hypertension
Pristiq [desvenlafaxine]		Antidepressant; serotonin and norepinephrine reuptake inhibitor (SNRI)	Major depressive disorder
Procardia [nifedipine]		Calcium channel blocker	Management of vasospastic angina and chronic stable angina, hypertension
Prograf [tacrolimus]	Z79.899	Immunosuppressant	Prophylaxis of organ transplant rejection
Prolia [denosumab]	Z79.899	Monoclonal antibody	Treatment and prevention of bone resorption and prevention of bone fracture

Drug	Z Code	Drug Action/Classification	Indications
Promethazine hydrochloride [promethazine hydrochloride]		Anesthesia, adjunct to; antiemetic; antihistamine; antitussive/expectorant; sedative/hypnotic; vertigo/motion sickness/vomiting	Anesthesia; adjunct; angioedema; conjunctivitis; dermographism; hypersensitivity, motion sickness; pain; perennial, seasonal, and allergic rhinitis; sedation, obstetrical; urticaria
Protonix [pantoprazole]		Proton pump inhibitor	Short-term treatment and maintenance therapy of erosive esophagitis associated with gastroesophageal reflux disease (GERD)
Protopic [tacrolimus]	Z79.899	Immunosuppressant	Atomic dermatitis (eczema)
Proventil-HFA [albuterol sulfate]		Antiasthmatic/bronchodilator	Asthma
Provera [medroxyprogesterone acetate]	Z79.3, Z79.890	Antineoplastic; contraceptive; progestin	Amenorrhea; carcinoma, endometrium, adjunct; carcinoma, renal; prevention of pregnancy; hemorrhage
Prozac [fluoxetine hydrochloride]		Selective serotonin reuptake inhibitor (SSRI)	Bulimia nervosa; depression; obsessive-compulsive disorder
Pulmicort [budesonide]	Z79.51	Corticosteroid -inhaled; antiasthmatic	Prophylaxis and treatment of asthma
Qnasl [beclomethasone dipropionate]		Corticosteroid -inhaled/nasal	Perennial and seasonal allergies; vasomotor rhinitis
Qtern [dapagliflozin propanediol/saxagliptin hydrochloride]	Z79.84	Oral hypoglycemic	Diabetes mellitus
Quartette [levonorgestrel/ethinyl estradiol]	Z79.3	Contraceptive	Prevention of pregnancy
Quasense [ethinyl estradiol/levonorgestrel]	Z79.3	Contraceptive	Prevention of pregnancy
Quinidine gluconate [quinidine gluconate]		Antiarrhythmic	Management of cardiac arrhythmias
Qvar [beclomethasone dipropionate]	Z79.51	Corticosteroid -inhaled; antiasthmatic	Prophylaxis and treatment of asthma
Raloxifene HCl [raloxifene hydrochloride]	Z79.810	Selective estrogen receptor modulator (SERM)	Prevention of thinning of the bones (osteoporosis) only in postmenopausal women
Rapaflo [silodosin]		Antiadrenergic	Benign prostatic hyperplasia
Rapamune [sirolimus]	Z79.899	Immunosuppressant	Prophylaxis of organ transplant rejection
Rayos [prednisone]	Z79.52	Corticosteroid; antiasthmatic	Arthritis; blood disorders; allergies; asthma
Rebetol [ribavirin]	Z79.899	Antiviral	Chronic hepatitis C
Rebif [interferon beta-1a]	Z79.899	Antiviral	Treatment of relapsing multiple sclerosis
Reclast [zoledronic acid]	Z79.83	Bisphosphonate	Prevention of thinning of the bones (osteoporosis); Paget's disease; bone cancer
Relenza [zanamivir]		Antiviral	Treat and prevent influenza A and B
Renvela [sevelamer carbonate]		Phosphate binder	Chronic kidney disease (CKD) on dialysis
Repaglinide [repaglinide]	Z79.84	Oral hypoglycemic	Diabetes mellitus
Reprexain [hydrocodone bitartrate/ibuprofen]	Z79.891	Analgesic, narcotic; nonsteroidal anti-inflammatory drug (NSAID)	Pain, inflammation or fever relief
Restasis [cyclosporine ophthalmic emulsion]		Antiinflammatory, ophthalmic	Ocular inflammation due to keratoconjunctivitis sicca
Restoril [temazepam]		Sedative/hypnotic	Insomnia
Retrovir [zidovudine]	Z79.899	Antiretroviral	Indicated in symptomatic HIV infection
Rifadin [rifampin]	Z79.2	Antibiotic	Tuberculosis
Rimactane [rifampin]	Z79.2	Antibiotic	Tuberculosis
Riomet [metformin hydrochloride]	Z79.84	Oral hypoglycemic	Diabetes mellitus
Risperdal [risperidone]		Antipsychotic/antimanic	Schizophrenia; bipolar I disorder
Ritalin [methylphenidate hydrochloride]		CNS stimulant	Depression; hyperkinetic activity in children
Roxicet [oxycodone hydrochloride/acetaminophen]	Z79.891	Analgesic, narcotic	Pain, moderate to severe
Roxicodone [oxycodone hydrochloride]	Z79.891	Analgesic, narcotic	Pain relief
Ryzodeg [insulin aspart/insulin degludec]	Z79.4	Insulin	Diabetes mellitus
Sabril [vigabatrin]		Anticonvulsant	Refractory complex partial seizures
Safyral [drospirenone/ethinyl estradiol/levomefolate calcium]	Z79.3	Contraceptive	Prevention of pregnancy
Sandimmune [cyclosporine]	Z79.899	Immunosuppressant	Prophylaxis of organ transplant rejection
Sarafem [fluoxetine hydrochloride]		Selective serotonin reuptake inhibitor (SSRI)	Premenstrual dysphoric disorder (PMDD)
Savaysa [edoxaban tosylate]	Z79.01	Anticoagulant	Prophylaxis and treatment of venous thrombosis, pulmonary embolism; prevention of blood clots due to atrial fibrillation

Drug	Z Code	Drug Action/Classification	Indications
Seasonale [levonorgestrel/ethinyl estradiol]	Z79.3	Contraceptive	Prevention of pregnancy
Seasonique [ethinyl estradiol/levonorgestrel]	Z79.3	Contraceptive	Prevention of pregnancy
Selfemra [fluoxetine hydrochloride]		Selective serotonin reuptake inhibitor (SSRI)	Premenstrual dysphoric disorder (PMDD)
Septra [sulfamethoxazole trimethoprim]	Z79.2	Antibiotic	Urinary tract infections, acute otitis media, acute exacerbations of chronic bronchitis, and shigellosis
Serevent [salmeterol xinafoate]		Bronchodilator	Asthma
Seromycin [cycloserine]	Z79.2	Antibiotic	Tuberculosis; urinary tract infections
Seroquel XR [quetiapine fumarate]		Antipsychotic	Schizophrenia; bipolar disorder; major depressive disorder
Setlakin [ethinyl estradiol/levonorgestrel]	Z79.3	Contraceptive	Prevention of pregnancy
Silvadene [silver sulfadiazine]	Z79.2	Antibiotic, topical	Wound sepsis due to second/third degree burns
Simulect [basiliximab]	Z79.899	Immunosuppressant	Prophylaxis of organ transplant rejection
Sinemet [carbidopa/levodopa]		Antiparkinsonism	Parkinson's disease
Singulair [montelukast sodium]		Antiasthmatic	Asthma; exercise-induced bronchoconstriction; perennial and seasonal allergic rhinitis
Sirolimus [sirolimus]	Z79.899	Immunosuppressant	Prophylaxis of organ transplant rejection
Sitagliptin [sitagliptin/metformin hydrochloride]	Z79.84	Oral hypoglycemic	Diabetes mellitus
Sivextro [tedizolid phosphate]	Z79.2	Antibiotic	Skin infections including MRSA
Skyla [levonorgestrel]	Z79.3	Contraceptive	Intrauterine device for prevention of pregnancy
Soliqua [insulin glargine/lixisenatide]	Z79.4	Insulin	Diabetes mellitus
Solodyn [minocycline hydrochloride]	Z79.2	Antibiotic	Bacterial infections
Soltamox [tamoxifen citrate]	Z79.810	Selective estrogen receptor modulator (SERM)	Breast cancer
Solu-Cortef [hydrocortisone sodium succinate]	Z79.52	Corticosteroid; antiasthmatic	Asthma; severe inflammation; allergic reactions
Solu-Medrol [methylprednisolone sodium succinate]	Z79.52	Corticosteroid	Anti-inflammatory and antiallergenic for shock and ulcerative colitis
Spiriva [tiotropium bromide]		Antiasthmatic/bronchodilator	Chronic obstructive pulmonary disease (COPD); asthma
Sprintec [norgestimate/ethinyl estradiol]	Z79.3	Contraceptive	Prevention of pregnancy
Starlix [nateglinide]	Z79.84	Oral hypoglycemic	Diabetes mellitus
Strattera [atomexetine hydrochloride]		CNS stimulant	Attention deficit hyperactivity disorder (ADHD)
Streptomycin sulfate [streptomycin sulfate]	Z79.2	Antibiotic	Severe bacterial infections
Sublimaze preservative free [fentanyl citrate]	Z79.891	Analgesic, narcotic	Pain relief
Supprelin LA [histrelin acetate]	Z79.818	Agents affecting estrogen receptors and estrogen levels	Precocious puberty
Suprax [cefixime]	Z79.2	Antibiotic	Bacterial infections
Sustiva [efavirenz]	Z79.899	Antiviral	HIV/AIDs
Syeda [drospirenone/ethinyl estradiol]	Z79.3	Contraceptive	Prevention of pregnancy
Sylatron [peginterferon alfa-2b]	Z79.899	Antineoplastic interferons; antiviral interferons	Prevention of recurrent malignant melanoma
Symbicort [budesonide/formoterol fumarate dihydrate]	Z79.51	Corticosteroid -inhaled; antiasthmatic	Prophylaxis and treatment of asthma and COPD
Symbyax [olanzapine/fluoxetine]		Antidepressant	Acute depressive episodes associated with bipolar I disorder; treatment resistant depression
Symtuza [darunavir/cobicistat/emtricitabine/tenofovir alafenamide]	Z79.899	Antiretroviral	HIV
Synarel [nafarelin acetate]	Z79.818	Agents affecting estrogen receptors and estrogen levels	Endometriosis symptoms; precocious puberty
Synercid [dalfopristin/quinupristin]	Z79.2	Antibiotic	Severe blood infections
Synjardy [empagliflozin/metformin hydrochloride]	Z79.84	Oral hypoglycemic	Diabetes mellitus
Synthroid [levothyroxine sodium]		Thyroid hormone	Hypothyroidism

Drug	Z Code	Drug Action/Classification	Indications
Tacrolimus [tacrolimus]	Z79.899	Immunosuppressant	Prophylaxis of organ transplant rejection
Tamiflu [oseltamivir phosphate]		Antiviral	Treatment and prevention of influenza A and B
Tamoxifen citrate [tamoxifen citrate]	Z79.810	Selective estrogen receptor modulator (SERM)	Metastatic breast cancer in postmenopausal women
Tazicef [ceftazidime]	Z79.2	Antibiotic	Confirmed or suspected bacterial infections
Teflaro [ceftaroline fosamil]	Z79.2	Antibiotic	Bacterial skin infections; pneumonia
Tegretol [carbamazepine]		Anticonvulsant; analgesic	Epilepsy, especially with complex symptomatology; specific analgesic for trigeminal neuralgia
Tenormin [atenolol]		Beta blocker	Angina pectoris; hypertension; acute myocardial infarction
Terazosin HCl [terazosin hydrochloride]		Antiadrenergic	Benign prostatic hypertrophy; hypertension
Testim [testosterone]	Z79.890	Testosterone therapy -topical	Primary hypogonadism; hypogonadotropic hypogonadism
Tetracycline HCl [tetracycline hydrochloride]	Z79.2	Antibiotic	Bacterial infections
Tiazac [diltiazem hydrochloride]		Calcium channel blocker	Chronic stable angina, atrial fibrillation, atrial flutter, hypertension, paroxysmal supraventricular tachycardia
Tivorbex [indomethacin]	Z79.1	Nonsteroidal anti-inflammatory drug (NSAID)	Treatment of pain, inflammation and joint stiffness
Tobradex [tobramycin/dexamethasone]		Aminoglycoside ocular anti-infective; anti-inflammatory	Infectious conjunctivitis; dermatosis, corticosteroid-responsive with secondary infection; foreign body in eye; corneal inflammation; uveitis
Tobramycin [dexamethasone/tobramycin]	Z79.2	Antibiotic	Bacterial eye infections
Topamax [topiramate]		Anticonvulsant	Epilepsy; primary generalized tonic-clonic seizures; seizures associated with Lennox-Gastaut syndrome; migraine headache
Toprol-XL [metoprolol succinate]		Beta blocker	Angina pectoris; hypertension
Toremifene citrate [toremifene citrate]	Z79.810	Selective estrogen receptor modulator (SERM)	Metastatic breast cancer in postmenopausal women
Torisel [temsirolimus]	Z79.899	Antineoplastic	Renal cell carcinoma
Toujeo Solostar [insulin glargine recombinant]	Z79.4	Insulin	Diabetes mellitus
Tradjenta [linagliptin]	Z79.84	Oral hypoglycemic	Diabetes mellitus
Trazodone HCl [trazodone hydrochloride]		Antidepressant	Depression
Trelegy Ellipta [fluticasone furoate/umeclidinium bromide/vilanterol trifenatate]	Z79.51	Corticosteroid -- inhaled; anitasthmatic	COPD
Trelstar [triptorelin pamoate]	Z79.818	Agents affecting estrogen receptors and estrogen levels	Palliative treatment of prostate cancer symptoms
Tresiba [insulin degludec]	Z79.4	Insulin	Diabetes mellitus
Tri-Estarylla [ethinyl estradiol/norgestimate]	Z79.3	Contraceptive	Prevention of pregnancy; acne
Tri-Legest [ethinyl estradiol/norethindrone acetate]	Z79.3	Contraceptive	Prevention of pregnancy
Tri-Linyah [ethinyl estradiol/norgestimate]	Z79.3	Contraceptive	Prevention of pregnancy
Tri-Lo-Estarylla [ethinyl estradiol/norgestimate]	Z79.3	Contraceptive	Prevention of pregnancy
Tri-Lo-Sprintec [ethinyl estradiol/norgestimate]	Z79.3	Contraceptive	Prevention of pregnancy
Tri-Norinyl 28-day [ethinyl estradiol/norethindrone]	Z79.3	Contraceptive	Prevention of pregnancy
Tri-Previfem [ethinyl estradiol/norgestimate]	Z79.3	Contraceptive	Prevention of pregnancy
Tri-Sprintec [ethinyl estradiol/norgestimate]	Z79.3	Contraceptive	Prevention of pregnancy; acne
Triamterene and hydrochlorothiazide [triamterene/ hydrochlorothiazide]		Antihypertensive; diuretic	Edema; hypertension
Trimethoprim [trimethoprim]	Z79.2	Antibiotic	Acute exacerbation chronic bronchitis; travelers' diarrhea; infections of the middle, lower respiratory tract, and urinary tract; pneumonia, pneumocystis; shigellosis

Drug	Z Code	Drug Action/Classification	Indications
Triptodur [triptorelin]	Z79.818	Agents affecting estrogen receptors and estrogen levels	Precocious puberty
Trivora-28 [ethinyl estradiol/ levonorgestrel]	Z79.3	Contraceptive	Prevention of pregnancy
Trokendi XR [topiramate]		Anticonvulsant	Epilepsy; primary generalized tonic-clonic seizures; seizures associated with Lennox-Gastaut syndrome; migraine headache
Trulicity [dulaglutide]		Antidiabetic -injectable	Diabetes mellitus
Truvada [emtricitabine/ tenofovir disoproxil fumarate]	Z79.899	Antiviral	Treatment and prevention of HIV
Tygacil [tigecycline]	Z79.2	Antibiotic	Bacterial skin or digestive system infections; pneumonia
Tylenol with codeine [acetaminophen/codeine phosphate]	Z79.891	Analgesic, narcotic	Pain and cough
Ultram [tramadol hydrochloride]	Z79.891	Analgesic, non-narcotic (opiate, narcotic-like)	Moderate to severe pain
Unasyn [ampicillin sodium/sulbactam sodium]	Z79.2	Antibiotic	Bacterial infections
Vabomere [meropenem; vaborbactam]	Z79.2	Antibiotic	Complicated urinary tract infections; pyelonephritis
Vagifem [estradiol]	Z79.890	Estrogen therapy	Menopause symptoms
Valium [diazepam]		Antianxiety; muscle relaxant; anticonvulsant	Anxiety, tension, withdrawal from alcohol, muscle spasms and anticonvulsant therapy; epilepsy, generalized tonic-clonic; status epilepticus; stiff-man syndrome; tetanus
Vancocin HCl [vancomycin hydrochloride]	Z79.2	Antibiotic	Severe bacterial infections
Vancomycin HCl [vancomycin hydrochloride]	Z79.2	Antibiotic	Severe bacterial infections
Vantas [histrelin acetate]	Z79.818	Agents affecting estrogen receptors and estrogen levels	Palliative treatment of prostate cancer symptoms
Vasotec [enalaprilat maleate]		ACE inhibitor	Congestive heart failure; hypertension
Velivet [desogestrel/ethinyl estradiol]	Z79.3	Contraceptive	Prevention of pregnancy
Venlafaxine HCl [venlafaxine hydrochloride]		Antidepressant, serotonin and norepinephrine reuptake inhibitor (SNRI)	Major depressive disorder; social anxiety disorder; panic disorder
Ventolin HFA [albuterol sulfate]		Antiasthmatic/bronchodilator	Asthma
Verapamil HCL [verapamil hydrochloride]		Calcium channel blocker	Angina pectoris, chronic stable angina, atrial fibrillation, atrial flutter, paroxysmal supraventricular tachycardia, ventricular arrhythmia, hypertension
Viagra [sildenafil citrate]		Phosphodiesterase-5 (PDE5) inhibitor	Erectile dysfunction
Vibativ [telavancin hydrochloride]	Z79.2	Antibiotic	Pneumonia; severe bacterial skin infections
Vibramycin [doxycycline calcium]	Z79.2	Antibiotic	Bacterial infections
Victoza [liraglutide]		Antidiabetic -injectable	Diabetes mellitus
Vienva [ethinyl estradiol/levonorgestrel]	Z79.3	Contraceptive	Prevention of pregnancy
Viorele [desogestrel/ethinyl estradiol]	Z79.3	Contraceptive	Prevention of pregnancy
Virazole [ribavirin]	Z79.899	Antiviral	Respiratory syncytial virus (RSV)
Viread [tenofovir disoproxil fumarate]	Z79.899	Antiviral	HIV; chronic hepatitis B
Vistaril [hydroxyzine pamoate]		Antianxiety; antiemetic	Treatment of nausea and vomiting, for reducing narcotic requirement in surgery and as tranquilizer for tension, anxiety, or agitation states
Vivelle [estradiol]	Z79.890	Estrogen therapy	Menopause symptoms; osteoporosis prevention
Voltaren [diclofenac sodium]	Z79.1	Nonsteroidal anti-inflammatory drug (NSAID)	Treatment of pain, inflammation and joint stiffness due to arthritis
Vytorin [ezetimibe/simvastatin]		HMG-CoA reductase inhibitor (statin); cholesterol absorption inhibitor	Hyperlipidemia; hypercholesterolemia
Warfarin [warfarin sodium]	Z79.01	Anticoagulant	Prophylaxis and treatment of venous thrombosis, treatment of atrial fibrillation with embolization (pulmonary embolism), arrhythmias, myocardial infarction, and stroke prevention
Wellbutrin SR, Wellbutrin XL [bupropion hydrochloride]		Antidepressant	Depression
Wera [ethinyl estradiol/norethindrone]	Z79.3	Contraceptive	Prevention of pregnancy
Xalatan [latanoprost]		Prostaglandin F2α analogue	Glaucoma, open-angle; ocular hypertension
Xanax, Xanax XR [alprazolam]		Antianxiety; sedative/hypnotic	Anxiety disorders with panic disorder and depression

Drug	Z Code	Drug Action/Classification	Indications
Xarelto [rivaraxaban]	Z79.01	Anticoagulant	Prophylaxis and treatment of venous thrombosis, pulmonary embolism; prevention of blood clots due to atrial fibrillation
Xeljanz [tofacitinib citrate]	Z79.899	Antirheumatic	Rheumatoid arthritis; psoriatic arthritis
Xgeva [denosumab]	Z79.899	Monoclonal antibody	Treatment and prevention of bone resorption and prevention of bone fracture
Xifaxan [rifaximin]	Z79.2	Antibiotic	E. coli diarrhea
Xigduo [dapagliflozin propanediol/metformin hydrochloride]	Z79.84	Oral hypoglycemic	Diabetes mellitus
Xultophy [insulin degludec/liraglutide]	Z79.4	Insulin	Diabetes mellitus
Xyrem [sodium oxybate]		CNS depressant; anoxiolytic/sedative/hypnotic	Cataplexy and/or excessive daytime sleepiness in narcolepsy
Xyzal [levocetirizine dihydrochloride]		Antihistamine	Perennial allergic rhinitis; chronic idiopathic urticaria
Yasmin [drospirenone/ethinyl estradiol]	Z79.3	Contraceptive	Prevention of pregnancy
Yaz [drospirenone/ethinyl estradiol]	Z79.3	Contraceptive	Prevention of pregnancy; menstrual disorders
Zantac [ranitidine hydrochloride]		Histamine H2-receptors inhibitor	Acid/peptic disorder, erosive esophagitis, gastrointestinal hypersecretion, mastocytosis, gastroesophageal reflux, peptic ulcer, Zollinger-Ellison syndrome
Zerbaxa [ceftolozane sulfate/tazobactam sodium]	Z79.2	Antibiotic	Complicated urinary tract and intra-abdominal infections
Zestoretic [lisinopril/hydrochlorothiazide]		ACE inhibitor	Congestive heart failure; hypertension
Zestril [lisinopril]		ACE inhibitor	Congestive heart failure; hypertension
Zetia [exetimibe]		Antihyperlipidemic	Hypercholesterolemia; sitosterolemia
Ziac [bisoprolol fumarate/hydrochlorothiazide]		Antihypertensive	Hypertension
Zinacef [cefuroxime sodium]	Z79.2	Antibiotic	Bacterial infections
Zipsor [diclofenac potassium]	Z79.1	Nonsteroidal anti-inflammatory drug (NSAID)	Pain and inflammation relief
Zithromax [azithromycin]	Z79.2	Antibiotic	Infections of the cervix, lower respiratory tract, skin and skin structures, urethra, nongonococcal; mycobacterium avium complex; pharyngitis, streptococcal pneumonia; tonsillitis
Zocor [simvastatin]		HMG-CoA reductase inhibitor (statin)	Hypercholesterolemia; hyperlipidemia; hyperlipoproteinemia; hypertriglyceridemia
Zoladex [goserelin acetate]	Z79.818	Agents affecting estrogen receptors and estrogen levels	Palliative treatment of prostate cancer and breast cancer symptoms; endometriosis
Zoloft [sertraline hydrochloride]		Antidepressant	Anxiety with panic disorder and depression; obsessive-compulsive disorder
Zometa [zoledronic acid]	Z79.83	Bisphosphonate	Multiple myeloma; Paget's disease
Zorvolex [diclofenac]	Z79.1	Nonsteroidal anti-inflammatory drug (NSAID)	Pain, inflammation or fever relief
Zosyn [piperacillin sodium/tazobactam sodium]	Z79.2	Antibiotic	Bacterial infections
Zovia [ethynodiol diacetate/ethinyl estradiol]	Z79.3	Contraceptive	Prevention of pregnancy
Zovirax [acyclovir]		Antiviral	Genital herpes and herpes zoster infections
Zubsolv [buprenorphine/naloxone]		Opioid agonist	Treatment of opioid addiction
Zyban [bupropion hydrochloride]		Smoking cessation aid	Nicotine addiction, smoking
Zyflo [zileuton]		Antiasthmatic	Asthma
Zyloprim [allopurinol]		Antigout	Gouty arthritis, renal calculus, hyperuricemia, hyperuricemia secondary to leukemia, hyperuricemia secondary to lymphoma
Zyprexa [olanzapine]		Antipsychotic/antimanic	Psychotic disorders; schizophrenia
Zyrtec allergy [cetirizine hydrochloride]		Antihistamine	Perennial and seasonal allergic rhinitis; chronic urticaria
Zyvox [linezolid]	Z79.2	Antibiotic	Severe bacterial infections

Appendix C: Z Codes for Long-Term Drug Use with Associated Drugs

This resource correlates the Z codes that are used to identify current long-term drug use with a list of drugs that are typically categorized to that class of drug. These lists are not all-inclusive, providing only the more commonly used drugs.

Z79.Ø1 Long term (current) use of anticoagulants
Angiomax
Argatroban
Arixtra
Bevyxxa
Coumadin
Eliquis
Fragmin
Heparin
Jantoven
Lovenox
Pradaxa
Savaysa
Warfarin
Xarelto

Z79.Ø2 Long term (current) use of antithrombotics/antiplatelets
Aggrastat
Aggrenox
Brilinta
Clopidogrel bisulfate
Effient
Integrilin
Persantine
Plavix
Prasugrel

Z79.1 Long term (current) use of non-steroidal anti-inflammatories (NSAID)
Advil
Aleve
Anaprox DS
Arthrotec
Caldolor
Cambia
Celebrex
Daypro
Duexis
Feldene
Ibuprofen
Indocin
Mobic
Motrin IB
Nabumetone
Nalfon
Naprelan
Naprosyn
NeoProfen
Ponstel
Tivorbex
Voltaren
Zipsor
Zorvolex

Z79.2 Long term (current) use of antibiotics
Altabax
Amikacin
Amoxicillin
Ampicillin
Ancef
Augmentin
Avelox
Azactam

Azithromycin
Bactrim
Biaxin XL
Cefprozil
Ceftriaxone
Centany
Cephalexin
Cipro
Ciprofloxacin
Clarithromycin
Cleocin
Clindamycin
Cubicin
Daptomycin
Dificid
Doxycycline
Dynacin
E.E.S.
Ertapenem
ERYC
Erygel
EryPed
Ery-Tab
Erythrocin
Erythromycin
Factive
Flagyl
Fortaz
Gentamicin sulfate
Invanz
Isoniazid
Keflex
Klaron
Lincocin
Macrobid
Macrodantin
Maxipime
Mefoxin
Mepron
Merrem
Metronidazole
Minocin
Monodox
Monurol
Mycobutin
Nebupent
Nitrofurantoin
Oracea
Orbactiv
Penicillin-VK
Pentam
Pfizerpen
Priftin
Primaxin
Rifadin
Rimactane
Septra
Seromycin
Silvadene
Sivextro
Solodyn
Streptomycin sulfate
Suprax

Synercid
Tazicef
Teflaro
Tetracycline HCl
Tobramycin
Trimethoprim
Tygacil
Unasyn
Vabomere
Vancocin HCl
Vancomycin HCl
Vibativ
Vibramycin
Xifaxan
Zerbaxa
Zinacef
Zithromax
Zosyn
Zyvox

Z79.3 Long term (current) use of hormonal contraceptives
Altavera
Alyacen
Aranelle
Ashlyna
Aviane-28
Balziva-28
Bekyree
Beyaz
Brevicon 28-day
Briellyn
Camila
Cryselle
Cyclafem
Cyclessa
Dasetta
Daysee
Depo-Provera
Depo-SubQ Provera
Desogen
Elinest
Emoquette
Enpresse-28
Enskyce
Errin
Estarylla
Estrostep Fe
Falmina
Femcon Fe
Femhrt
Gildagia
Gildess
Introvale
Jencycla
Junel
Kariva
Kelnor
Kimidess
Kurvelo
Kyleena
Larin
Lessina-28
Levonest

Appendix C: Z Codes for Long-Term Drug Use with Associated Drugs

Levora
Liletta
Lo Loestrin Fe
Loestrin
Loryna
LoSeasonique
Low-Ogestrel-28
Marlissa
Microgestin
Micronor
Minastrin
Mirena
Modicon 28
Mono-Linyah
Myzilra
Natazia
Nexplanon
Norinyl
Nor-QD
Nortrel
NuvaRing
Ogestrel
Orsythia
Ortho Cyclen-28
Ortho-Novum
Ortho-Tri-Cyclen
Philith
Pimtrea
Pirmella
Plan B One-Step
Portia-28
Previfem
Provera
Quartette
Quasense
Safyral
Seasonale
Seasonique
Setlakin
Skyla
Sprintec
Syeda
Tri-Estarylla
Tri-Legest
Tri-Linyah
Tri-Lo-Estarylla
Tri-Lo-Sprintec
Tri-Norinyl 28-day
Tri-Previfem
Tri-Sprintec
Trivora-28
Velivet
Vienva
Viorele
Wera
Yasmin
Yaz
Zovia

Z79.4 Long term (current) use of insulin
Admelog
Afrezza
Apidra
Basaglar
Fiasp
Humalog
Humulin R
Lantus

Levemir
Novolin
Novolog
Ryzodeg
Soliqua
Toujeo Solostar
Tresiba
Xultophy

Z79.51 Long term (current) use of inhaled steroids
Advair
Aerospan HFA
Alvesco
Airduo Respiclick
Armonair Respiclick
Arnuity Ellipta
Asmanex
Breo Ellipta
Dulera
Flovent
Pulmicort
Qvar
Symbicort
Trelegy Ellipta

Z79.52 Long term (current) use of systemic steroids
A-Methapred
Aristospan
Celestone Soluspan
Colocort
Cortef
Cortenema
Cortifoam
Cortisone acetate
Depo-Medrol
Dexamethasone Intensol
Entocort EC
Hydrocortisone
Kenalog-1Ø
Kenalog-4Ø
Locoid
Medrol
Methylprednisolone
Orapred ODT
PediaPred
Prednisolone
Prednisone
Prelone
Rayos
Solu-Cortef
Solu-Medrol

Z79.81Ø Long term (current) use of selective estrogen receptor modulators (SERMs)
Evista
Fareston
Osphena
Raloxifene HCl
Soltamox
Tamoxifen Citrate
Toremifene Citrate

Z79.811 Long term (current) use of aromatase inhibitors
Anastrozole
Arimidex
Aromasin
Exemestane

Femara
Letrozole

Z79.818 Long term (current) use of other agents affecting estrogen receptors and estrogen levels
Eligard
Faslodex
Lupron
Megace ES
Supprelin LA
Synarel
Trelstar
Triptodur
Vantas
Zoladex

Z79.82 Long term (current) use of aspirin
Bayer
Durlaza

Z79.83 Long term (current) use of bisphosphonates
Actonel
Atelvia
Binosto
Boniva
Didronel
Fosamax
Reclast
Zometa

Z79.84 Long term (current) use of oral hypoglycemic drugs
Acarbose
Actoplus Met
Actos
Amaryl
Avandia
Diabinese
DiaBeta
Duetact
Farxiga
Fortamet
Glimepiride
Glucophage
Glucotrol
Glucovance
Glumetza
Glyburide
Glynase
Glyset
Invokamet
Invokana
Janumet
Januvia
Jentadueto
Kazano
Kombiglyze
Metformin
Onglyza
Oseni
PrandiMet
Prandin
Precose
Qtern
Repaglinide
Riomet
Sitagliptin
Starlix
Synjardy

Tradjenta
Xigduo

Z79.890 Hormone replacement therapy
Activella
Alora
Androderm
AndroGel
Angeliq
Bijuva
Climara
CombiPatch
Delestrogen
Depo-Provera
Divigel
Duavee
Elestrin
Estrace
EstroGel
Femhrt
Femring
Firmagon
Menest
Menostar
Minivelle
Orlissa
Osphena
Prempro
Provera
Testim
Vagifem
Vivelle

Z79.891 Long term (current) use of opiate analgesic
Abstral
Acetaminophen with codeine
Buprenex
Buprenorphine HCl and Naloxone HCl
Butorphanol tartrate
Butrans
Codeine
Demerol
Dilaudid

Dolophine HCl
Duragesic
Duramorph PF
Embeda
Exalgo
Fentanyl Citrate
Fentora
Fioricet with codeine
Hydrocodone
Hydrocodone bitartrate and acetaminophen
Hydromorphone HCl
Kadian
Lazanda
Methadone HCl
Methadose
Morphabond ER
Morphine Sulfate
MS Contin
Norco
Nucynta
Opana
Oxycodone HCl
OxyContin
Percocet
Reprexain
Roxicet
Roxicodone
Sublimaze Preservative Free
Tylenol with codeine
Ultram

Z79.899 Other long term (current) drug therapy
Actimmune
Antineoplastic/chemotherapy
Astagraf XL
Atripla
Avonex
Betaseron
Cellcept
Cimduo
Cosentyx
Crixivan

Cyclosporine
Cyltezo
Descovy
Emtriva
Enbrel
Entyvio
Envarsus XR
Epivir
Erelzi
Gengraf
Harvoni
Humira
Hyrimoz
Imuran
Intron A
Keytruda
Monoclonal antibodies
Neoral
Orencia
Otezla
Pegintron
Prezcobix
Prezista
Prograf
Prolia
Protopic
Rapamune
Rebetol
Rebif
Retrovir
Sandimmune
Simulect
Sirolimus
Sustiva
Sylatron
Symtuza
Tacrolimus
Torisel
Truvada
Virazole
Viread
Xeljanz
Xgeva

Appendix D: Z Codes Only as Principal/First-Listed Diagnosis

Z00.00	Z01.20	Z02.5	Z04.2	Z34.81	Z38.66	Z52.000	Z52.811
Z00.01	Z01.21	Z02.6	Z04.3	Z34.82	Z38.68	Z52.001	Z52.812
Z00.110	Z01.30	Z02.71	Z04.41	Z34.83	Z38.69	Z52.008	Z52.813
Z00.111	Z01.31	Z02.79	Z04.42	Z34.90	Z38.7	Z52.010	Z52.819
Z00.121	Z01.411	Z02.81	Z04.6	Z34.91	Z38.8	Z52.011	Z52.89
Z00.129	Z01.419	Z02.82	Z04.71	Z34.92	Z39.0	Z52.018	Z76.1
Z00.2	Z01.42	Z02.83	Z04.72	Z34.93	Z39.1	Z52.090	Z76.2
Z00.3	Z01.810	Z02.89	Z04.81	Z38.00	Z39.2	Z52.091	Z99.12
Z00.5	Z01.811	Z02.9	Z04.82	Z38.01	Z40.00	Z52.098	
Z00.70	Z01.812	Z03.6	Z04.89	Z38.1	Z40.01	Z52.10	
Z00.71	Z01.818	Z03.71	Z04.9	Z38.2	Z40.02	Z52.11	
Z00.8	Z01.82	Z03.72	Z31.81	Z38.30	Z40.03	Z52.19	
Z01.00	Z01.83	Z03.73	Z31.83	Z38.31	Z40.09	Z52.20	
Z01.01	Z01.84	Z03.74	Z31.84	Z38.4	Z40.8	Z52.21	
Z01.020	Z01.89	Z03.75	Z33.2	Z38.5	Z40.9	Z52.29	
Z01.021	Z02.0	Z03.79	Z34.00	Z38.61	Z42.1	Z52.3	
Z01.10	Z02.1	Z03.810	Z34.01	Z38.62	Z42.8	Z52.4	
Z01.110	Z02.2	Z03.818	Z34.02	Z38.63	Z51.0	Z52.5	
Z01.118	Z02.3	Z03.89	Z34.03	Z38.64	Z51.11	Z52.6	
Z01.12	Z02.4	Z04.1	Z34.80	Z38.65	Z51.12	Z52.810	

Appendix E: Qualifications for Medicare Coverage of Home Health Services

The criteria that must be met by the patient to qualify for Medicare coverage of home health services are specified in the following sections of the Medicare Benefit Policy Manual (Pub. 100-02), Chapter 7 - Home Health Services.

Conditions to be Met for Coverage of Home Health Services

Medicare covers HHA services when the following criteria are met:

1. The person to whom the services are provided is an eligible Medicare beneficiary;
2. The HHA that is providing the services to the beneficiary has in effect a valid agreement to participate in the Medicare program;
3. The beneficiary qualifies for coverage of home health services as described in §30;
4. The services for which payment is claimed are covered as described in §§40 and 50;
5. Medicare is the appropriate payer; and
6. The services for which payment is claimed are not otherwise excluded from payment.

Reasonable and Necessary Services

Background: In enacting the Medicare program, Congress recognized that the physician would play an important role in determining utilization of services. The law requires that payment can be made only if a physician certifies the need for services and establishes a plan of care. The Secretary is responsible for ensuring that Medicare covers the claimed services, including determining whether they are "reasonable and necessary."

Determination of Coverage: The Medicare contractor's decision on whether care is reasonable and necessary is based on information reflected in the home health plan of care, the OASIS as required by 42 CFR 484.55 or a medical record of the individual patient. Medicare does not deny coverage solely on the basis of the reviewer's general inferences about patients with similar diagnoses or on data related to utilization generally, but bases it upon objective clinical evidence regarding the patient's individual need for care.

Coverage of skilled nursing care or therapy to perform a maintenance program does not turn on presence or absence of a patient's potential for improvement from nursing care or therapy, but rather on the patient's need for skilled care. Skilled care may be necessary to improve a patient's current condition, to maintain the patient's current condition, or to prevent or slow further deterioration of the patient's condition.

Impact of Other Available Caregivers and Other Available Coverage on Medicare Coverage of Home Health Services

Where the Medicare criteria for coverage of home health services are met, patients are entitled by law to coverage of reasonable and necessary home health services. Therefore, a patient is entitled to have the costs of reasonable and necessary services reimbursed by Medicare without regard to whether there is someone available to furnish the services. However, where a family member or other person is or will be providing services that adequately meet the patient's needs, it would not be reasonable and necessary for HHA personnel to furnish such services. Ordinarily it can be presumed that there is no able and willing person in the home to provide the services being rendered by the HHA unless the patient or family indicates otherwise and objects to the provision of the services by the HHA, or unless the HHA has first hand knowledge to the contrary.

Similarly, a patient is entitled to reasonable and necessary Medicare home health services even if the patient would qualify for institutional care (e.g., hospital care or skilled nursing facility care) and Medicare payment should be made for reasonable and necessary home health services where the patient is also receiving supplemental services that do not meet Medicare's definition of skilled nursing care or home health aide services.

Example 1: A patient who lives with an adult daughter and otherwise qualifies for Medicare coverage of home health services, requires the assistance of a home health aide for bathing and assistance with an exercise program to improve endurance. The daughter is unwilling to bathe her elderly father and assist him with the exercise program. Home health aide services would be reasonable and necessary.

Example 2: A patient who is being discharged from a hospital with a diagnosis of osteomyelitis and requires continuation of the I.V. antibiotic therapy that was begun in the hospital was found to meet the criteria for Medicare coverage of skilled nursing facility services. If the patient also meets the qualifying criteria for coverage of home health services, payment may be made for the reasonable and necessary home health services the patient needs, notwithstanding the availability of coverage in a skilled nursing facility.

Example 3: A patient who needs skilled nursing care on an intermittent basis also hires a licensed practical (vocational) nurse to provide nighttime assistance while family members sleep. The care provided by the nurse, as respite to the family members, does not require the skills of a licensed nurse (as defined in §40.1) and therefore has no impact on the beneficiary's eligibility for Medicare payment of home health services even though another third party insurer may pay for that nursing care.

Use of Utilization Screens and "Rules of Thumb"

Medicare recognizes that determinations of whether home health services are reasonable and necessary must be based on an assessment of each beneficiary's individual care needs. Therefore, denial of services based on numerical utilization screens, diagnostic screens, diagnosis or specific treatment norms is not appropriate.

Conditions Patient Must Meet to Qualify for Coverage of Home Health Services

To qualify for the Medicare home health benefit a Medicare beneficiary must meet the following requirements:

- Be confined to the home;
- Under the care of a physician;
- Receiving services under a plan of care established and periodically reviewed by a physician;
- Be in need of skilled nursing care on an intermittent basis or physical therapy or speech-language pathology; or
- Have a continuing need for occupational therapy.

For purposes of benefit eligibility, "intermittent" means skilled nursing care that is either provided or needed on fewer than seven days each week or less than eight hours of each day for periods of 21 days or less (with extensions in exceptional circumstances when the need for additional care is finite and predictable).

A patient must meet each of the criteria specified in this section. Patients who meet each of these criteria are eligible to have payment made on their behalf for services discussed in §§40 and 50.

Confined to the Home

For a patient to be eligible to receive covered home health services under both Part A and Part B, the law requires that a physician certify in all cases that the patient is confined to his/her home. For purposes of the statute, an individual shall be considered "confined to the home" (homebound) if the following two criteria are met:

1. Criterion-One:

   The patient must either:

   - Because of illness or injury, need the aid of supportive devices such as crutches, canes, wheelchairs, and walkers; the use of special transportation; or the assistance of another person in order to leave their place of residence

   OR

   - Have a condition such that leaving his or her home is medically contraindicated.

   If the patient meets one of the criterion-one conditions, then the patient must *also* meet two additional requirements defined in criterion two below.

2. Criterion-Two:

   - There must exist a normal inability to leave home;

   AND

   - Leaving home must require a considerable and taxing effort.

To clarify, in determining whether the patient meets criterion two of the homebound definition, the clinician needs to take into account the illness or injury for which the patient met criterion one and consider the illness or injury in the context of the patient's overall condition. The clinician is not required to include standardized phrases reflecting the patient's condition (e.g., repeating the words "taxing effort to leave the home") in the patient's chart, nor are such phrases sufficient, by themselves, to demonstrate that criterion two has been met. For example, longitudinal clinical information about the patient's health status is typically needed to sufficiently demonstrate a normal inability to leave the home and that leaving home requires a considerable and taxing effort. Such clinical information about the patient's overall health status may include, but is not limited to, such factors as the patient's diagnosis, duration of the patient's condition, clinical course (worsening or improvement), prognosis, nature and extent of functional limitations, other therapeutic interventions and results, etc.

If the patient does in fact leave the home, the patient may nevertheless be considered homebound if the absences from the home are infrequent or for periods of relatively short duration, or are attributable to the need to receive health care treatment. Absences attributable to the need to receive health care treatment include, but are not limited to:

- Attendance at adult day centers to receive medical care;
- Ongoing receipt of outpatient kidney dialysis; or
- The receipt of outpatient chemotherapy or radiation therapy.

Any absence of an individual from the home attributable to the need to receive health care treatment, including regular absences for the purpose of participating in therapeutic, psychosocial, or medical treatment in an adult day-care program that is licensed or certified by a State, or accredited to furnish adult day-care services in a State, shall not disqualify an individual from being considered to be confined to his home. Any other absence of an individual from the home shall not so disqualify an individual if the absence is of an infrequent or of relatively short duration. For purposes of the preceding sentence, any absence for the purpose of attending a religious service shall be deemed to be an absence of infrequent or short duration. It is expected that in most instances, absences from the home that occur will be for the purpose of receiving health care treatment. However, occasional absences from the home for nonmedical purposes, e.g., an occasional trip to the barber, a walk around the block or a drive, attendance at a family reunion, funeral, graduation, or other infrequent or unique event would not necessitate a finding that the patient is not homebound if the absences are undertaken on an infrequent basis or are of relatively short duration and do not indicate that the patient has the capacity to obtain the health care provided outside rather than in the home.

Some examples of homebound patients that illustrate the factors used to determine whether a homebound condition exists are listed below.

- A patient paralyzed from a stroke who is confined to a wheelchair or requires the aid of crutches in order to walk.
- A patient who is blind or senile and requires the assistance of another person in leaving their place of residence.
- A patient who has lost the use of their upper extremities and, therefore, is unable to open doors, use handrails on stairways, etc., and requires the assistance of another individual to leave their place of residence.
- A patient in the late stages of ALS or neurodegenerative disabilities. In determining whether the patient has the general inability to leave the home and leaves the home only infrequently or for periods of short duration, it is necessary (as is the case in determining whether skilled nursing services are intermittent) to look at the patient's condition over a period of time rather than for short periods within the home health stay. For example, a patient may leave the home (meeting both criteria listed above) more frequently during a short period when the patient has multiple appointments with health care professionals and medical tests in 1 week. So long as the patient's overall condition and experience is such that he or she meets these qualifications, he or she should be considered confined to the home.
- A patient who has just returned from a hospital stay involving surgery, who may be suffering from resultant weakness and pain because of the surgery and; therefore, their actions may be restricted by their physician to certain specified and limited activities (such as getting out of bed only for a specified period of time, walking stairs only once a day, etc.).
- A patient with arteriosclerotic heart disease of such severity that they must avoid all stress and physical activity.
- A patient with a psychiatric illness that is manifested in part by a refusal to leave home or is of such a nature that it would not be considered safe for the patient to leave home unattended, even if they have no physical limitations.

The aged person who does not often travel from home because of feebleness and insecurity brought on by advanced age would not be considered confined to the home for purposes of receiving home health services unless they meet one of the above conditions.

Although a patient must be confined to the home to be eligible for covered home health services, some services cannot be provided at the patient's residence because equipment is required that cannot be made available there. If the services required by an individual involve the use of such equipment, the HHA may make arrangements with a hospital, SNF, or a rehabilitation center to provide these services on an outpatient basis. (See §50.6.) However, even in these situations, for the services to be covered as home health services the patient must be considered confined to home and meet both criteria listed above.

If a question is raised as to whether a patient is confined to the home, the HHA will be requested to furnish the Medicare contractor with the information necessary to establish that the patient is homebound as defined above.

Place of Residence

A patient's residence is wherever he/she makes his/her home. This may be his/her own dwelling, an apartment, a relative's home, a home for the aged, or some other type of institution. However, an institution may not be considered a patient's residence if the institution meets the requirements of §§1861(e)(1) or 1819(a)(1) of the Act. Included in this group are hospitals and skilled nursing facilities. as well as most nursing facilities under Medicaid. (See the Medicare State Operations Manual, §2166.)

Thus, if a patient is in an institution or distinct part of an institution identified above, the patient is not entitled to have payment made for home health services under either Part A or Part B since these institutions may not be considered his/her residence. When a patient remains in a participating SNF following his/her discharge from active care, the facility may not be considered his/her residence for purposes of home health coverage.

A patient may have more than one home, and the Medicare rules do not prohibit a patient from having one or more places of residence. A patient, under a Medicare home health plan of care, who resides in more than one place of residence during an episode of Medicare covered home health services will not disqualify the patient's homebound status for purposes of eligibility. For example, a person may reside in a principal home and also a second vacation home, mobile home, or the home of a caretaker relative. The fact that the patient resides in more than one home and, as a result, must transit from one to the other, is not in itself, an indication that the patient is not homebound. The requirements of homebound must be met at each location (i.e., the patient must meet both criteria listed in section 30.1.1 above).

A – Assisted Living Facilities, Group Homes, and Personal Care Homes
An individual may be "confined to the home" for purposes of Medicare coverage of home health services if he or she resides in an institution that is not primarily engaged in providing to inpatients:

- Diagnostic and therapeutic services for medical diagnosis;
- Treatment;
- Care of injured, disabled or sick persons;
- Rehabilitation services or other skilled services needed to maintain a patient's current condition or to prevent or slow further deterioration; or
- Skilled nursing care or related services for patients who require medical or nursing care

If it is determined that the assisted living facility (also called personal care homes, group homes, etc.) in which the individuals reside are not primarily engaged in providing the above services, then Medicare will cover reasonable and necessary home health care furnished to these individuals.

If it is determined that the services furnished by the home health agency are duplicative of services furnished by an assisted living facility (also called personal care homes, group homes, etc.) when provision of such care is required of the facility under State licensure requirements, claims for such services should be denied under §1862(a)(1)(A) of the Act. Section 1862(a)(1)(A) excludes services that are not necessary for the diagnosis or treatment of illness or injury or to improve the functioning of a malformed body member from Medicare coverage. Services to people who already have access to appropriate care from a willing caregiver would not be considered reasonable and necessary to the treatment of the individual's illness or injury.

Medicare coverage would not be an optional substitute for the services that a facility that is required to provide by law to its patients or where the services are included in the base contract of the facility. An individual's choice to reside in such a facility is also a choice to accept the services it holds itself out as offering to its patients.

B – Day Care Centers and Patient's Place of Residence

The current statutory definition of homebound or confined does not imply that Medicare coverage has been expanded to include adult day care services.

The law does not permit an HHA to furnish a Medicare covered billable visit to a patient under a home health plan of care outside his or her home, except in those limited circumstances where the patient needs to use medical equipment that is too cumbersome to bring to the home. Section 1861(m) of the Act stipulates that home health services provided to a patient be provided to the patient on a visiting basis in a place of residence used as the individual's home. A licensed/certified day care center does not meet the definition of a place of residence.

C – State Licensure/Certification of Day Care Facilities

Per section 1861(m) of the Act, an adult day care center must be either licensed or certified by the State or accredited by a private accrediting body. State licensure or certification as an adult day care facility must be based on State interpretations of its process. For example, several States do not license adult day care facilities as a whole, but do certify some entities as Medicaid certified centers for purposes of providing adult day care under the Medicaid home and community based waiver program. It is the responsibility of the State to determine the necessary criteria for "State certification" in such a situation. A State could determine that Medicaid certification is an acceptable standard and consider its Medicaid certified adult day care facilities to be "State certified." On the other hand, a State could determine Medicaid certification to be insufficient and require other conditions to be met before the adult day care facility is considered "State certified."

D – Determination of the Therapeutic, Medical or Psychosocial Treatment of the Patient at the Day Care Facility

It is not the obligation of the HHA to determine whether the adult day care facility is providing psychosocial treatment, but only to assure that the adult day care center is licensed/certified by the State or accrediting body. The intent of the law, in extending the homebound exception status to attendance at such adult day care facilities, recognizes that they ordinarily furnish psychosocial services.

Services Are Provided Under a Plan of Care Established and Approved by a Physician

The HHA must be acting upon a physician plan of care that meets the requirements of this section for HHA services to be covered. For HHA services to be covered, the individualized plan of care must specify the services necessary to meet the patient-specific needs identified in the comprehensive assessment. In addition, the plan of care must include the identification of the responsible discipline(s) and the frequency and duration of all visits as well as those items listed in 42 CFR 484.60(a) that establish the need for such services. All care provided must be in accordance with the plan of care.

If the plan of care includes a course of treatment for therapy services: the course of therapy treatment must be established by the physician after any needed consultation with the qualified therapist; the plan must include measurable therapy treatment goals which pertain directly to the patient's illness or injury, and the patient's resultant impairments; the plan must include the expected duration of therapy services; and the plan must describe a course of treatment which is consistent with the qualified therapist's assessment of the patient's function.

The orders on the plan of care must specify the type of services to be provided to the patient, both with respect to the professional who will provide them and the nature of the individual services, as well as the frequency of the services.

Example 1: SN x 7/wk x 1 wk; 3/wk x 4 wk; 2/wk x 3 wk, (skilled nursing visits seven times per week for one week; three times per week for four weeks; and two times per week for three weeks) for skilled observation and evaluation of the surgical site, for teaching sterile dressing changes and to perform sterile dressing changes. The sterile change consists of (detail of procedure).

Orders for care may indicate a specific range in the frequency of visits to ensure that the most appropriate level of service is provided during the 60-day episode to home health patients. When a range of visits is ordered, the upper limit of the range is considered the specific frequency.

Example 2: SN x 2-4/wk x 4 wk; 1-2/wk x 4 wk for skilled observation and evaluation of the surgical site.

Orders for services to be furnished "as needed" or "PRN" must be accompanied by a description of the patient's medical signs and symptoms that would occasion a visit and a specific limit on the number of those visits to be made under the order before an additional physician order would have to be obtained.

The physician who signs the plan of care must be qualified to sign the physician certification as described in 42 CFR 424.22.

A – Initial Percentage Payment

If a physician signed plan of care is not available at the beginning of the episode, the HHA may submit a RAP for the initial percentage payment based on physician verbal orders OR a referral prescribing detailed orders for the services to be rendered that is signed and dated by the physician. If the RAP submission is based on physician verbal orders, the verbal order must be recorded in the plan of care, include a description of the patient's condition and the services to be provided by the home health agency, include an attestation (relating to the physician's orders and the date received per 42 CFR 409.43), and the plan of care is copied and immediately submitted to the physician. A billable visit must be rendered prior to the submission of a RAP.

B – Final Percentage Payment

The plan of care must be signed and dated by a physician as described who meets the certification and recertification requirements of 42 CFR 424.22 and before the claim for each episode for services is submitted for the final percentage payment. Any changes in the plan of care must be signed and dated by a physician.

Verbal Orders

When services are furnished based on a physician's oral order, the orders may be accepted and put in writing by personnel authorized to do so by applicable State and Federal laws and regulations, as well as by the HHA's internal policies. The orders must be signed and dated with the date of receipt by the registered nurse or qualified therapist (i.e., physical therapist, speech-language pathologist, occupational therapist, or medical social worker) responsible for furnishing or supervising the ordered services. The orders may be signed by the supervising registered nurse or qualified therapist after the services have been rendered, as long as HHA personnel who receive the oral orders notify that nurse or therapist before the service is rendered. Thus, the rendering of a service that is based on an oral order would not be delayed pending signature of the supervising nurse or therapist. Oral orders must be countersigned and dated by the physician before the HHA bills for the care in the same way as the plan of care.

Services that are provided from the beginning of the 60-day episode certification period based on a request for anticipated payment and before the physician signs the plan of care are considered to be provided under a plan of care established and approved by the physician where there is an oral order for the care prior to rendering the services which is documented in the medical record and where the services are included in a signed plan of care.

Services that are provided in the subsequent 60-day episode certification period are considered to be provided under the plan of care of the subsequent 60-day episode where there is an oral order before the services provided in the subsequent period are furnished and the order is reflected in the medical record. However, services that are provided after the expiration of a plan of care, but before the acquisition of an oral order or a signed plan of care, cannot be considered to be provided under a plan of care.

Example 1: The HHA acquires an oral order for I.V. medication administration for a patient to be performed on August 1. The HHA provides the I.V. medication administration August 1 and evaluates the patient's need for continued care. The physician signs the plan of care for the I.V. medication administration on August 15. The visit is covered since it is considered provided under a plan of care established and approved by the physician, and the HHA had acquired an oral order prior to the delivery of services.

Example 2: The patient is under a plan of care in which the physician orders I.V. medication administration every 2 weeks. The last day covered by the initial plan of care is July 31. The patient's next I.V. medication administration is scheduled for August 5 and the physician signs the plan of care for the new period on August 1. The I.V. medication administration on August 5 was provided under a plan of care established and approved by the physician. The episode begins on the 61 day regardless of the date of the first covered visit.

Example 3: The patient is under a plan of care in which the physician orders I.V. medication administration every two weeks. The last day covered by the plan of care is July 31. The patient's next I.V. medication administration is scheduled for August 5, and the physician does not sign the plan of care until August 6. The HHA acquires an oral order for the I.V. medication administration before the August 5 visit, and therefore the visit is considered to be provided under a plan of care established and approved by the physician. The episode begins on the 61st day regardless of the date of the first covered visit.

Any increase in the frequency of services or addition of new services during a certification period must be authorized by a physician by way of a written or oral order prior to the provision of the increased or additional services.

The plan of care must be reviewed and signed by the physician who established the plan of care, in consultation with HHA professional personnel, at least every 60 days. Each review of a patient's plan of care must contain the signature of the physician and the date of review.

The plan of care or oral order may be transmitted by facsimile machine. The HHA is not required to have the original signature on file. However, the HHA is responsible for obtaining original signatures if an issue surfaces that would require verification of an original signature.

HHAs that maintain patient records by computer rather than hard copy may use electronic signatures. However, all such entries must be appropriately authenticated and dated. Authentication must include signatures, written initials, or computer secure entry by a unique identifier of a primary author who has reviewed and approved the entry. The HHA must have safeguards to prevent unauthorized access to the records and a process for reconstruction of the records in the event of a system breakdown.

The plan of care is considered to be terminated if the patient does not receive at least one covered skilled nursing, physical therapy, speech-language pathology service, or occupational therapy visit in a 60-day period since these are qualifying services for the home health benefit. An exception is if the physician documents that the interval without such care is appropriate to the treatment of the patient's illness or injury.

Once patient eligibility has been confirmed and the plan of care contains physician orders for the qualifying service as well as other Medicare covered home health services, the qualifying service does not have to be rendered prior to the other Medicare covered home health services ordered in the plan of care. The sequence of visits performed by the disciplines must be dictated by the individual patient's plan of care. For example, for an eligible patient in an initial 60-day episode that has both physical therapy and occupational therapy orders in the plan of care, the sequence of the delivery of the type of therapy is irrelevant as long as the need for the qualifying service is established prior to the delivery of other Medicare covered services and the qualifying discipline provides a billable visit prior to transfer or discharge in accordance with 42 CFR 409.43(f).

Note: Dependent services provided after the final qualifying skilled service are not covered under the home health benefit, except when the dependent service was not followed by a qualifying skilled service due to unexpected inpatient admission, death of the patient, or some other unanticipated event.

Under the Care of a Physician

The patient must be under the care of a physician who is qualified to sign the physician certification and plan of care in accordance with 42 CFR 424.22.

A patient is expected to be under the care of the physician who signs the plan of care. It is expected, but not required for coverage, that in most instances, the physician who certifies the patient's eligibility for Medicare home health services, in accordance with §30.5 below, will be the same physician who establishes and signs the plan of care.

Needs Skilled Nursing Care on an Intermittent Basis (Other than Solely Venipuncture for the Purposes of Obtaining a Blood Sample) or Physical Therapy or Speech-Language Pathology Services or Has Continued Need for Occupational Therapy

The patient must need one of the following types of services:

1. Skilled nursing care that is
   - Reasonable and necessary as defined in §40.1;
   - Needed on an "intermittent" basis as defined in §40.1.3; and
   - Not solely needed for venipuncture for the purposes of obtaining blood sample as defined in §40.1.2.13; or
2. Physical therapy as defined in §40.2.2; or
3. Speech-language pathology services as defined in §40.2.3; or
4. Have a continuing need for occupational therapy as defined in §§40.2.4.

The patient has a continued need for occupational therapy when:

1. The services which the patient requires meet the definition of "occupational therapy" services of §40.2.4, and
2. The patient's eligibility for home health services has been established by virtue of a prior need for skilled nursing care (other than solely venipuncture for the purposes of obtaining a blood sample), speech-language pathology services, or physical therapy in the current or prior certification period.

Example: A patient who is recovering from a cerebrovascular accident (CVA) has an initial plan of care that called for physical therapy, speech-language pathology services, occupational therapy, and home health aide services. In the next certification period, the physician orders only occupational therapy and home health aide services because the patient no longer needs the skills of a physical therapist or a speech-language pathologist, but needs the services provided by the occupational therapist. The patient's need for occupational therapy qualifies him for home health services, including home health aide services (presuming that all other qualifying criteria are met), because in the prior certification period the beneficiary's eligibility for home health services was established by virtue of prior needs for physical therapy and speech-language pathology, and occupational therapy was initiated while the patient still required physical therapy and/or speech language-pathology.

Physician Certification

The HHA must be acting upon a plan of care as described in §30.2, and a physician certification or recertification that meets the requirements of this section for HHA services to be covered.

A certification (versus recertification) is considered to be any time that a Start of Care OASIS is completed to initiate care. In such instances, a physician must certify (attest) that:

1. The home health services are or were needed because the patient is or was confined to the home as defined in §30.1.1;
2. The patient needs or needed skilled nursing services on an intermittent basis (other than solely venipuncture for the purposes of obtaining a blood sample), or physical therapy, or speech-language pathology services. Where a patient's sole skilled service need is for skilled oversight of unskilled services (management and evaluation of the care plan as defined in §40.1.2.2), the physician must include a brief narrative describing the clinical justification of this need as part of the certification, or as a signed addendum to the certification;
3. A plan of care has been established and is periodically reviewed by a physician;
4. The services are or were furnished while the patient is or was under the care of a physician;
5. For episodes with starts of care beginning January 1, 2011 and later, in accordance with §30.5.1.1 below, a face-to-face encounter occurred no more than 90 days prior to or within 30 days after the start of the home health care, was related to the primary reason the patient requires home health services, and was performed by an allowed provider type. The certifying physician must also document the date of the encounter. Example Certification Statement:

> I certify that this patient is confined to his/her home and needs intermittent skilled nursing care, physical therapy and/or speech therapy or continues to need occupational therapy. The patient is under my care, and I have authorized services on this plan of care and will periodically review the plan. The patient had a face-to-face encounter with an allowed provider type on 11/01/2016 and the encounter was related to the primary reason for home health care.
>
> Physician's Signature and Date Signed: John Doe, MD 11/05/2016
>
> Physician's Name and Address
>
> John Doe, MD
> 2121 Washington Pkwy
> Suite 220
> Washington, DC 20000
>
> **Note:** *This represents one example of a valid certification statement. Certification statements can be included in varying forms or formats as long as the content requirements (#1-5 above) for the certification are met.*

If the patient is starting home health directly after discharge from an acute/post-acute care setting where the physician, with privileges, that cared for the patient in that setting is certifying the patient's eligibility for the home health benefit, but will not be following the patient after discharge, then the certifying physician must identify the community physician who will be following the patient after discharge. One of the criteria that must be met for a patient to be considered eligible for the home health benefit is that the patient must be under the care of a physician (number 4 listed above). Otherwise, the certification is not valid.

The certification must be complete prior to when an HHA bills Medicare for reimbursement; however, physicians should complete the certification when the plan of care is established, or as soon as possible thereafter. This is longstanding CMS policy as referenced in Pub 100-01, Medicare General Information, Eligibility, and Entitlement Manual, chapter 4, section 30.1. It is not acceptable for HHAs to wait until the end of a 60-day episode of care to obtain a completed certification/recertification.

Face-to-Face Encounter

1. Allowed provider types:

    As part of the certification of patient eligibility for the Medicare home health benefit, a face-to-face encounter with the patient must be performed by the certifying physician himself or herself, a physician that cared for the patient in the acute or post-acute care facility (with privileges who cared for the patient in an acute or post-acute care facility from which the patient was directly admitted to home health) or an allowed non-physician practitioner (NPP). NPPs who are allowed to perform the encounter are:

    – A nurse practitioner or a clinical nurse specialist working in accordance with State law and in collaboration with the certifying physician or in collaboration with an acute or post-acute care physician, with privileges, who cared for the patient in the acute or post-acute care facility from which the patient was directly admitted to home health;

    – A certified nurse midwife, as authorized by State law, under the supervision of the certifying physician or under the supervision of an acute or post-acute care physician with privileges who cared for the patient in the acute or post-acute care facility from which the patient was directly admitted to home health;

    – A physician assistant under the supervision of the certifying physician or under the supervision of an acute or post-acute care physician with privileges who cared for the patient in the acute or post-acute care facility from which the patient was directly admitted to home health.

    – NPPs performing the encounter are subject to the same financial restrictions with the HHA as the certifying physician, as described in 42 CFR 424.22(d).

2. Timeframe Requirements:

    The encounter must occur no more than 90 days prior to the home health start of care date or within 30 days after the start of care.

    In situations when a physician orders home health care for the patient based on a new condition that was not evident during a visit within the 90 days prior to start of care, the certifying physician or an allowed NPP must see the patient again within 30 days after admission. Specifically, if a patient saw the certifying physician or NPP within the 90 days prior to start of care, another encounter would be needed if the patient's condition had changed to the extent that standards of practice would indicate that the physician or a non-physician practitioner should examine the patient in order to establish an effective treatment plan.

3. Exceptional Circumstances:

    When a home health patient dies shortly after admission, before the face-to-face encounter occurs, if the contractor determines a good faith effort existed on the part of the HHA to facilitate/coordinate the encounter and if all other certification requirements are met, the certification is deemed to be complete.

4. Telehealth

    The face-to-face encounter can be performed via a telehealth service, in an approved originating site. An originating site is considered to be the location of an eligible Medicare beneficiary at the time the service is furnished via a telecommunications system occurs. Medicare beneficiaries are eligible for telehealth services only if they are presented from an originating site located in a rural health professional shortage area or in a county outside of a Metropolitan Statistical Area.

    Entities that participate in a Federal telemedicine demonstration project approved by (or receiving funding from) the Secretary of the Department of Health and Human Services as of December 31, 2000, qualify as originating sites regardless of geographic location.

    The originating sites authorized by law are: the office of a physician or practitioner; hospitals; Critical Access Hospitals (CAH); Rural Health Clinics (RHC); Federally Qualified Health Centers (FQHC); Hospital-based or CAH-based Renal Dialysis Centers (including satellites); Skilled Nursing Facilities (SNF); and Community Mental Health Centers (CMHC).

Supporting Documentation Requirements

As of January 1, 2015, documentation in the certifying physician's medical records and/or the acute/post-acute care facility's medical records (if the patient was directly admitted to home health) will be used as the basis upon which patient eligibility for the Medicare home health benefit will be determined. Documentation from the certifying physician's medical records and/or the acute/post-acute care facility's medical records (if the patient was directly admitted to home health) used to support the certification of home health eligibility must be provided, upon request, to the home health agency, review entities, and/or the

Centers for Medicare and Medicaid Services (CMS). In turn, an HHA must be able to provide, upon request, the supporting documentation that substantiates the eligibility for the Medicare home health benefit to review entities and/or CMS. If the documentation used as the basis for the certification of eligibility is not sufficient to demonstrate that the patient is or was eligible to receive services under the Medicare home health benefit, payment will not be rendered for home health services provided.

The certifying physician and/or the acute/post-acute care facility medical record for the patient must contain information that justifies the referral for Medicare home health services. This includes documentation that substantiates the patient's:

- Need for the skilled services; and

- Homebound status;

The certifying physician and/or the acute/post-acute care facility medical record (if the patient was directly admitted to home health) (if the patient was directly admitted to home health) for the patient must contain the actual clinical note for the face-to-face encounter visit that demonstrates that the encounter:

- Occurred within the required timeframe;

- Was related to the primary reason the patient requires home health services; and

- Was performed by an allowed provider type.

This information can be found most often in clinical and progress notes and discharge summaries. While the face-to-face encounter must be related to the primary reason for home health services, the patient's skilled need and homebound status can be substantiated through an examination of all submitted medical record documentation from the certifying physician, acute/post-acute care facility, and/or HHA (see below). The synthesis of progress notes, diagnostic findings, medications, nursing notes, etc., help to create a longitudinal clinical picture of the patient's health status.

- Information from the HHA, such as the plan of care required per 42 CFR §409.43 and the initial and/or comprehensive assessment of the patient required per 42 CFR §484.55, can be incorporated into the certifying physician's medical record for the patient and used to support the patient's homebound status and need for skilled care. However, this information must be corroborated by other medical record entries in the certifying physician's and/or the acute/post-acute care facility's medical record for the patient. This means that the appropriately incorporated HHA information, along with the certifying physician's and/or the acute/post-acute care facility's medical record, creates a clinically consistent picture that the patient is eligible for Medicare home health services.

- The certifying physician demonstrates the incorporation of the HHA information into his/her medical record for the patient by signing and dating the material. Once incorporated, the documentation from the HHA, in conjunction with the certifying physician and/or acute/post-acute care facility documentation must substantiate the patient's eligibility for home health services.

At the end of the 60-day episode, a decision must be made whether or not to recertify the patient for a subsequent 60-day episode. An eligible beneficiary who qualifies for a subsequent 60-day episode would start the subsequent 60-day episode on day 61. Under HH PPS, the plan of care must be reviewed and signed by the physician every 60 days unless one of the following occurs:

- A beneficiary transfers to another HHA;

- A discharge and return to home health during the 60-day episode.

For recertification of home health services, the physician must certify (attest) that:

- The home health services are or were needed because the patient is or was confined to the home as defined in §30.1;

- The patient needs or needed skilled nursing services on an intermittent basis (other than solely venipuncture for the purposes of obtaining a blood sample), or physical therapy, or speech-language pathology services; or continues to need occupational therapy after the need for skilled nursing care, physical therapy, or speech-language pathology services ceased. Where a patient's sole skilled service need is for skilled oversight of unskilled services (management and evaluation of the care plan as defined in §40.1.2.2), the physician must include a brief narrative describing the clinical justification of this need as part of the recertification, or as a signed addendum to the recertification;

- A plan of care has been established and is periodically reviewed by a physician; and

- The services are or were furnished while the patient is or was under the care of a physician.

Medicare does not limit the number of continuous episode recertifications for beneficiaries who continue to be eligible for the home health benefit. The physician certification may cover a period less than but not greater than 60 days. Because the updated home health plan of care must include the frequency and duration of visits to be made, the physician does not have to estimate how much longer skilled services will be needed for the recertification.

See §10.4 for counting initial and subsequent 60-day episodes and recertifications. See §10.5 for recertifications for split percentage payments.

The physician who signs the certification or recertification must be permitted to do so by 42 CFR 424.22.

Physician Billing for Certification and Recertification

Physician certification/recertification claims are Part B physician claims paid for under the Physician Fee Schedule. These claims are billed using HCPCS codes G0180 (certification) or G0179 (recertification). The descriptions of these two codes indicate that they are used to bill for certification or recertification of patient eligibility "for Medicare-covered home health services under a home health plan of care (patient not present), including contacts with the HHA and review of reports of patient status required by physicians to affirm the initial implementation of the plan of care that meets patient's needs, per certification period." As noted above, these codes are for physician certification or recertification for Medicare-covered home health services. If there are no Medicare-covered home health services, these codes should not be billed or paid. As such, physician claims for certification/recertification of eligibility for home health services (G0180 and G0179, respectively) will not be covered if the HHA claim itself was noncovered because the certification/recertification of eligibility was not complete or because there was insufficient documentation to support that the patient was eligible for the Medicare home health benefit.

Covered Services Under a Qualifying Home Health Plan of Care

Section 1861(m)of the Act governs the Medicare home health services that may be provided to eligible beneficiaries by or under arrangements made by a participating home health agency (HHA). Section 1861(m) describes home health services as

- Part-time or intermittent skilled nursing care (other than solely venipuncture for the purposes of obtaining a blood sample);
- Part-time or intermittent home health aide services;
- Physical therapy;
- Speech-language pathology;
- Occupational therapy;
- Medical social services;
- Medical supplies (including catheters, catheter supplies, ostomy bags, supplies related to ostomy care, and a covered osteoporosis drug (as defined in §1861(kk) of the Act), but excluding other drugs and biologicals);
- Durable medical equipment while under the plan of care established by physician;
- Medical services provided by an intern or resident-in-training under an approved teaching program of the hospital in the case of an HHA which is affiliated or under common control with a hospital; and
- Services at hospitals, skilled nursing facilities, or rehabilitation centers when they involve equipment too cumbersome to bring to the home.

Appendix F: Overview of the Patient-Driven Groupings Model (PDGM)

The Patient-Driven Groupings Model (PDGM) uses 30-day periods as a basis for payment. Figure 1 below provides an overview of how 30-day periods are categorized into 432 case-mix groups for the purposes of adjusting payment in the PDGM. In particular, 30-day periods are placed into different subgroups for each of the following broad categories:

- Admission source (two subgroups): community or institutional admission source
- Timing of the 30-day period (two subgroups): early or late
- Clinical grouping (twelve subgroups): musculoskeletal rehabilitation; neuro/stroke rehabilitation; wounds; medication management, teaching, and assessment (MMTA) — surgical aftercare; MMTA — cardiac and circulatory; MMTA — endocrine; MMTA — gastrointestinal tract and genitourinary system; MMTA — infectious disease, neoplasms, and blood-forming diseases; MMTA — respiratory; MMTA — other; behavioral health; or complex nursing interventions
- Functional impairment level (three subgroups): low, medium, or high
- Comorbidity adjustment (three subgroups): none, low, or high based on secondary diagnoses

In total, there are 2*2*12*3*3 = 432 possible case-mix adjusted payment groups. The remainder of this overview provides more detail on each PDGM grouping category and additional adjustments to payment that are made within the PDGM.

Figure 1. Structure of the PDGM

Admission Source and Timing (from claims)			
Community Early	Community Late	Institutional Early	Institutional Late

Clinical Grouping (from principal diagnosis reported on claim)		
Neuro Rehab	Wounds	Complex Nursing Interventions
MS Rehab	Behavioral Health	MMTA – Other
MMTA – Surgical Aftercare	MMTA – Cardiac and Circulatory	MMTA – Endocrine
MMTA – GI/GU	MMTA – Infectious Disease (includes neoplasms and blood forming diseases)	MMTA – Respiratory

Functional Impairment Level (from OASIS items)		
Low	Medium	High

Comorbidity Adjustment (from secondary diagnoses reported on claims)		
None	Low	High

HHRG (Home Health Resource Group)

Under the PDGM, a 30-day period is grouped into one (and only one) subcategory under each larger colored category. A 30-day period's combination of subcategories places the 30-day period into one of 432 different payment groups.

Timing

Under the PDGM, the first 30-day period is classified as early. All subsequent 30-day periods in the sequence (second or later) are classified as late. A sequence of 30-day periods continues until there is a gap of at least 60 days between the end of one 30-day period and the start of the next. When there is a gap of at least 60 days, the subsequent 30-day period is classified as being the first 30-day period of a new sequence (and therefore, is labeled as early). The comprehensive assessment must be completed within five days of the start of care date and updated no less frequently than during the last five days of every 60 days beginning with the start of care date (as currently required by the Medicare Conditions of Participation at 42 CFR 484.55). As a result, information obtained from the Outcome and Assessment Information Set (OASIS) used in the PDGM may not change over the two 30-day periods the OASIS covers. However, if a patient experiences a significant change in condition before the start of a subsequent, contiguous 30-day period, for example due to a fall, a follow-up assessment would be submitted at the start of a second 30-day period to reflect any changes in the patient's condition, including functional abilities, and the second 30-day claim would be grouped into its appropriate case-mix group accordingly.

Admission Source

Under the PDGM, each 30-day period is classified into one of two admission source categories — community or institutional — depending on what healthcare setting was utilized in the 14 days prior to home health admission. Late 30-day periods are always classified as a community admission unless there was an acute hospitalization in the 14 days prior to the late home health 30-day period. A post-acute stay in the 14 days prior to a late home health 30-day period would not be classified as an institutional admission unless the patient had been discharged from home health prior to post-acute stay.

Clinical Grouping

Under the PDGM, each 30-day period is grouped into one of twelve clinical groups based on the patient's principal diagnosis. The reported principal diagnosis provides information to describe the primary reason for which patients are receiving home health services under the Medicare home health benefit. Table 1 below describes the twelve clinical groups. These groups are designed to capture the most common types of care that home health agencies (HHAs) provide.

Table 1. PDGM Clinical Groups

Clinical Group	Primary Reason for Home Health Encounter is to Provide:
Musculoskeletal Rehabilitation	Therapy (PT/OT/SLP) for a musculoskeletal condition
Neuro/Stroke Rehabilitation	Therapy (PT/OT/SLP) for a neurological condition or stroke
Wounds — Post-Op Wound Aftercare and Skin/Non-Surgical Wound Care	Assessment, treatment and evaluation of a surgical wound(s); assessment, treatment and evaluation of non-surgical wounds, ulcers burns and other lesions
Complex Nursing Interventions	Assessment, treatment and evaluation of complex medical and surgical conditions
Behavioral Health Care	Assessment, treatment and evaluation of psychiatric and substance abuse conditions
Medication Management, Teach and Assessment (MMTA) • MMTA — Surgical Aftercare • MMTA — Cardiac/Circulatory • MMTA — Endocrine • MMTA — Gastrointestinal (GI)/Genitourinary (GU) • MMTA — Infectious Disease/Neoplasms/Blood-forming Diseases • MMTA — Respiratory • MMTA — Other	Assessment, evaluation, teaching, and medication management for a variety of medical and surgical conditions not classified in one of the above listed groups. The subgroups represent common clinical conditions that require home health services for medication management, teaching, and assessment.

Functional Impairment Level

The PDGM designates a functional impairment level for each 30-day period based on the following OASIS items:

- M1800   Grooming
- M1810   Current ability to dress upper body safely
- M1820   Current ability to dress lower body safely
- M1830   Bathing
- M1840   Toilet transferring
- M1850   Transferring
- M1860   Ambulation and locomotion
- M1033   Risk for hospitalization

CMS estimates a regression model that determines the relationship between the responses for the listed OASIS items and average 30-day period resource use. The coefficients from the regression are used to assign points to a 30-day period. Responses that indicate higher functional impairment and a higher risk of hospitalization are associated with having larger coefficients and are therefore assigned higher points. The points are then summed, and thresholds are applied to determine whether a 30-day period is assigned a low, medium, or high functional impairment level. Each clinical group is assigned a separate set of thresholds. On average, 30-day periods in the low level have responses for the listed OASIS items that are associated with the lowest resource use. On average, 30-day periods in the high level have responses on the above OASIS items that are associated with the highest resource use.

Comorbidity Adjustment

The PDGM includes a comorbidity adjustment category based on the presence of secondary diagnoses. Depending on a patient's secondary diagnoses, a 30-day period may receive no comorbidity adjustment, a low comorbidity adjustment, or a high comorbidity adjustment. Home health 30-day periods of care can receive a comorbidity adjustment under the following circumstances:

Low comorbidity adjustment: There is a reported secondary diagnosis that is associated with higher resource use, or;

High comorbidity adjustment: There are two or more secondary diagnoses that are associated with higher resource use when both are reported together compared to if they were reported separately. That is, the two diagnoses may interact with one another, resulting in higher resource use.

A 30-day period can have a low comorbidity adjustment or a high comorbidity adjustment, but not both. If a 30-day home health period of care does not have reported comorbidities that fall into one of the adjustments described above, there would be no comorbidity adjustment applied.

Determining Case-Mix Weights for the Patient-Driven Groupings Model

The case-mix weight for each of the 432 different payment groups under the PDGM are determined by estimating a regression where the dependent variable is the resource use of a 30-day period and the independent variables are categorical indicators representing the five dimensions of the model described above (timing of a 30-day period, admission source, clinical group, functional impairment level, and comorbidities). Case-mix weights are produced by dividing the predicted resource use for each PDGM payment group by the overall average resource use of all 30-day periods. The case-mix weights are then used to adjust the 30-day payment rate. Figure 2 describes how 30-day periods are paid and when payment adjustments are made.

Additional Payment Adjustments for the Patient-Driven Groupings Model

Payments for 30-day periods with a low number of visits are not case-mix adjusted, but instead paid on a per-visit basis using the national per-visit rates. Each of the 432 different PDGM payment groups has a threshold that determines if the 30-day period receives this Low-Utilization Payment Adjustment (LUPA). For each payment group, the 10th percentile value of visits is used to create a payment group specific LUPA threshold with a minimum threshold of at least two for each group. A 30-day

period with a total number of visits below the LUPA threshold are paid per-visit rather than being paid the case-mix adjusted 30-day payment rate. A 30-day period with a total number of visits at or above the LUPA threshold is paid the case-mix adjusted 30-day payment rate rather than being paid per-visit.

When a 30-day period of care involves an unusually large number or a costly mix of visits, the HHA may be eligible for an additional outlier payment (See Figure 3). Once the imputed cost of a 30-day period of care exceeds a threshold amount, the HHA receives a payment equal to 80 percent of the difference between the imputed costs and the threshold amount.

Payments would be adjusted if a beneficiary transfers from one home health agency to another or is discharged and readmitted to the same agency within 30 days of the original 30-day period start date. The case-mix adjusted payment for 30-day periods of that type is pro-rated based on the length of the 30-day period ending in transfer or discharge and readmission, resulting in a partial period payment.

Figure 2: How Payments and Adjustments are calculated for the PDGM

*   LUPA = Low Utilization Payment Adjustment

**   The wage-adjusted payment for a 30-day period is calculated by taking the case-mix adjusted 30-day payment amount and multiplying 76.1% of that payment by a wage-index value that controls for area wage differences. That value is then added to 23.9% of the case-mix adjusted base-payment to determine the wage-adjusted payment amount.

***   Outlier payment is in addition to the wage-adjusted and case-mix adjusted 30-day period payment.

Figure 3: Calculation of Outlier Payment

Calculate if Period Receives an Outlier Payment

Compute (1) Case-Mix and Wage-Adjusted Period Payment
Wage-adjusted national, standardized 30-day period
payment rate multiplied by the case-mix weight

Compute (2) Wage-Adjusted Fixed Dollar Loss Amount
Fixed dollar loss amount is equal to the fixed dollar loss ratio multiplied
by the national, standardized 30-day period payment rate

Compute (3) Outlier Threshold
Outlier threshold equals (2) wage-adjusted fixed dollar loss amount
plus (1) case-mix and wage-adjusted period payment

Compute (4) Wage-Adjusted Costs per 30-day Period
A wage-adjusted per-unit amount for each discipline is used to
calculate the cost of care (capped at 8 hours per day)
provided during a 30-day period)

**Are the (4) Wage-Adjusted Costs per 30-day
Period Greater than the (3) Outlier Threshold?**

YES
**Final Payment Equals (1) Case-Mix and Wage-Adjusted
Period Payment plus 80%* of the Difference Between the (4)
Wage-Adjusted Per Visit Rate and the (3) Outlier Threshold**

NO
**Final Payment Equals (1) Case-Mix and
Wage-Adjusted Period Payment**

*80% is referred to as the loss sharing ratio

Appendix G: OASIS Diagnosis Guidance

The Outcome and Assessment Information Set (OASIS-D) includes three OASIS M-items related to ICD-10-CM codes. These items are:

M1021 Primary Diagnosis

M1023 Other Diagnoses

M1028 Active Diagnoses-Comorbidities and Co-existing Conditions

The last item listed, M1028 Active Diagnoses-Comorbidities and Co-existing Conditions, while tied to specific ICD-10-CM related diagnostic conditions, does not require the assignment of ICD-10-CM codes.

CMS and all Medicare administrative contractors (MAC) require, for the purpose of payment and compliance, that all ICD-10-CM diagnoses assigned for a given episode be identically represented on the:

- OASIS-D comprehensive assessment
- Plan of care (POC), which is reviewed and signed by the certifying physician
- Home health claim submitted for the episode

The principal diagnosis reported on the claim must match the primary diagnosis code reported on the OASIS form item M1021 Primary Diagnosis. The home health agency enters the full ICD-10-CM codes for additional conditions if they coexisted at the time of the establishment of the plan of care. None of these other diagnoses may duplicate the principal diagnosis. Other diagnoses reported on the claim must match the additional diagnoses reported on the OASIS-D, form item M1023 Other Diagnoses. The diagnoses should be listed in the order that best reflects the seriousness of the patient's condition and justifies the disciplines and services provided and in accordance with the Official ICD-10-CM Guidelines for Coding and Reporting. The sequence of codes should follow ICD-10-CM guidelines for reporting manifestation codes. Therefore, if a manifestation code is part of the primary diagnosis, the first two diagnoses should match and appear in the same sequence on both forms.

The ICD-10-CM diagnoses entered onto the OASIS and claim form must be the full diagnosis code, all seven characters, where applicable. If the complete, valid code has fewer than the maximum number of characters, allowed on the form, it is not appropriate to fill it with zeros or other characters.

CMS has clarified "Active Diagnoses" for the purpose of assignment to M1021, M1023 and responses to M1028 with the following taken from Quarterly Q&As:

- Diagnoses that are the chief reason for home health services
- Comorbid condition that is addressed in the plan of care
- Conditions felt to have potential to affect the patient's responsiveness to treatment

Diagnoses felt to have the potential to affect the patient's responsiveness to treatment means that they have a direct relationship to the patient's current functional, cognitive mood, or behavior status; medical treatments; nurse monitoring; or risk of death at the time of assessment.

The following information can be found in the Outcome and Assessment Information Set OASIS-D Guidance Manual, effective January 1, 2019, chapter 3, section 3-C, "OASIS Item Guidance — Patient History and Diagnoses."

Chapter 3 contains item-by-item guidance for all OASIS items. Included here are *only* the items which pertain to assigning an ICD-10-CM diagnosis code, item M1021, M1023 and M1028.

Note: CY 2020 updates to the OASIS Guidance Manual were not available at the time this book was printed. Updated versions can be found at https://www.cms.gov/Medicare/Quality-Initiatives-Patient-Assessment-Instruments/HomeHealthQualityInits/HHQIOASISUserManual.html.

For each item, guidance is provided on the following topics:

ITEM INTENT: Describes the rationale for collecting the information, in the context of outcome and process quality measurement, care planning, outcome risk adjustment, or prospective payment rate adjustment.

TIME POINTS: Describes when the information is to be collected during the patient's home health episode of care.

RESPONSE-SPECIFIC INSTRUCTIONS: Describes how the clinician should decide which of the possible responses should apply. These instructions may not always provide definitive guidance for selecting responses in every case, because clinical judgement is often required to determine the most accurate response to a specific item.

DATA SOURCES/RESOURCES: Describes the potential sources of information that should be accessed during the assessment to determine the most accurate response to this specific item. May include other clinicians, administrative records, online guidance regarding coding or other assessment guidelines, or standards promulgated by professional or accrediting organizations.

In addition to the information provided in the tables, items M1021 and M1023 also have specific instructions related to reporting diagnoses in the various columns on the form which are as follows.

Diagnoses and Symptom Control:

List each diagnosis for which the patient is receiving home care in Column 1, and enter its ICD-10-CM code at the level of highest specificity in Column 2 (diagnosis codes only—no surgical or procedure codes allowed). Diagnoses are listed in the order that best reflects the seriousness of each condition and supports the disciplines and services provided. Rate the degree of symptom control for each condition in Column 2. ICD-10-C M sequencing requirements must be followed if multiple coding is indicated for any diagnoses.

Code each row according to the following directions for each column:

Column 1: Enter the description of the diagnosis. Sequencing of diagnoses should reflect the seriousness of each condition and support the disciplines and services provided.

Column 2: Enter the ICD-10-CM code for the condition described in Column 1 - no surgical or procedure codes allowed. Codes must be entered at the level of highest specificity and ICD-10-CM coding rules and sequencing requirements must be followed. Note that external cause codes (ICD-10-CM codes beginning with V, W, X, or Y) may not be reported in M1021 (Primary Diagnosis) but may be reported in M1023 (Secondary Diagnoses). Also note that when a Z-code is reported in Column 2, the code for the underlying condition can often be entered in Column 2, as long as it is an active on-going condition impacting home health care.

Rate the degree of symptom control for the condition listed in Column 1. Do not assign a symptom control rating if the diagnosis code is a V, W, X, Y or Z-code. Choose one value that represents the degree of symptom control appropriate for each diagnosis using the following scale:

0—Asymptomatic, no treatment needed at this time

1—Symptoms well controlled with current therapy

2—Symptoms controlled with difficulty, affecting daily functioning; patient needs ongoing monitoring

3—Symptoms poorly controlled; patient needs frequent adjustment in treatment and dose monitoring

4—Symptoms poorly controlled; history of re-hospitalizations

Note that the rating for symptom control in Column 2 should not be used to determine the sequencing of the diagnoses listed in Column 1. These are separate items and sequencing may not coincide.

M1028 draws information specifically related to diabetes mellitus (DM) and peripheral vascular disease (PVD)/ peripheral arterial disease (PAD). This item does not require the assignment of any ICD-10-CM codes but the assessing clinician must understand what ICD-10-CM codes are included for consideration when responding to the item for each of the comorbid conditions. The following information appears on the OASIS-D for item M1028, with instructions to check all that apply.

Peripheral vascular disease (PVD) or peripheral arterial disease (PAD)

Diabetes mellitus (DM)

None of the above

M1021

Item Intent	Time Points	Response-specific Instructions	Data Sources/resources

The intent of this item is to accurately report and code the patient's primary home health diagnosis and document the degree of symptom control for that diagnosis. The patient's primary home health diagnosis is defined as the chief reason the patient is receiving home care and the diagnosis most related to the current home health Plan of Care.	Start of care Resumption of care Follow-up	• HHA clinicians and coders must report the most current year's ICD-10-CM codes and comply with the ICD-10-CM Official Guidelines for Coding and Reporting when assigning primary diagnoses to the OASIS item M1021.
		
		  - The ICD-10-CM is a morbidity classification published by the United States for classifying diagnoses and reason for care in all health care settings. The ICD-10-CM is based on the ICD-10, the International Classification of Diseases published by the World Health Organization (WHO).
		  - The ICD-10-CM Official Guidelines for Coding and Reporting were developed by the Centers for Medicare & Medicaid Services (CMS) and the National Center for Health Statistics (NCHS). These guidelines are a set of rules that have been developed to accompany and complement the official conventions and instructions provided within the ICD-10-CM itself and should be used as a companion document to the official version of the ICD-10-CM Official Code Set.
		  - Adherence to the ICD-10-CM Official Guidelines for Coding and Reporting when assigning ICD-10-CM diagnosis codes is required under the Health Insurance Portability and Accountability Act (HIPAA). It is expected that each agency will ensure that diagnoses and ICD-10-CM codes reported in the OASIS data set meet these guidelines.
		• Identifying the patient's Primary Home Health Diagnoses
		
		  - The assessing clinician is expected to complete the patient's comprehensive assessment and understand the patient's overall medical condition and care needs before selecting and assigning diagnoses.
		  - The determination of the patient's primary home health diagnoses must be made by the assessing clinician based on the findings of the assessment, information in the medical record, and input from the physician.
		  - As noted in the Item Intent, the patient's primary diagnosis is defined as the chief reason the patient is receiving home care and the diagnosis most related to the current home health Plan of Care. The primary diagnosis may or may not relate to the patient's most recent hospital stay, but must relate to the skilled services (skilled nursing, physical therapy, occupational therapy, and speech language pathology) rendered by the HHA.
		  - When determining secondary diagnoses, the assessing clinician should consider diagnoses that are actively addressed in the Plan of Care as well as diagnoses that affect the patient's responsiveness to treatment and rehabilitative prognosis, even if the condition is not the focus of any home health treatment itself.
		  - Diagnoses may change during the course of the home health stay due to a change in the patient's health status or a change in the focus of home health care. At each required OASIS time point, the clinician must assess the patient's clinical status and determine the primary diagnosis based on patient status and treatment plan at the time of the assessment.
		  - Only current medical diagnoses should be reported as primary diagnosis in M1021. Diagnoses should be excluded if they are resolved or do not have the potential to impact the skilled services provided by the HHA. An example of a resolved condition is cholecystitis following a cholecystectomy.
		  - In addition to following the ICD-10-CM Official Guidelines for Coding and Reporting, selection of home health diagnoses must be performed in compliance with Medicare's rules and regulations for coverage and payment to ensure provider compliance with Section 1862(a)(1)(A) of the Social Security Act. Section 1862(a)(1)(A) excludes provider services from Medicare coverage and payment that "are not reasonable and necessary for diagnosis or treatment of illness or injury or to improve the functioning of a malformed body member."
			• Patient/caregiver interview
			• Physician
			• Physician orders
			• Referral information
			• Current medication list
			• Current ICD-10-CM Official Code Set and the ICD-10-CM Official Guidelines for Coding and Reporting should be the sources for coding.
			• For degree of symptom control, data sources may include patient/caregiver interview, physician, physical assessment, and review of past health history.

M1021 (Continued)

Item Intent	Time Points	Response-specific Instructions	Data Sources/resources
		• Reporting Primary Diagnosis in M1021 - At each required OASIS time point, the assessing clinician should enter the patient's current primary diagnosis in Column 1 of M1021. Complete Column 1 from top to bottom, leaving any blank entries at the bottom. • Reporting ICD-10-CM Codes in Column 2 of M1021 - The assessing clinician can enter the actual numeric ICD-10-CM codes for each diagnosis listed in Column 1 and 2 of M1021, once the assessment is completed and the diagnosis is entered in Column 1. Alternatively, a coding specialist in the agency may enter the actual numeric ICD-10-CM codes in Column 2, as long as the assessing clinician has determined the primary diagnosis in Column 1. - The correct process for selecting an ICD-10-CM code using the Alphabetic Index and the Tabular List is described in the ICD-10-CM Official Guidelines for Coding and Reporting. Follow the official conventions and instructions provided within the ICD-10-CM Official Code Set and the Official Guidelines to code each row in Column 2. - Each ICD-10-CM code must be entered at its highest level of specificity (diagnosis codes only - no surgical or procedure codes allowed). - ICD-10-CM does not allow external cause codes (ICD-10-CM codes beginning with V, W, X, or Y) to be reported in M1021 (Primary Diagnosis) but they may be reported in M1023 (Secondary Diagnoses). - Also note that when a Z-code is reported in Column 2, the code for the underlying condition may be entered in Column 2, as long as it is a current on-going condition that has a potential to impact the skilled services provided by the HHA. See the ICD-10-CM Official Guidelines for Coding and Reporting for complete instructions on code assignment and sequencing related to the use of Z-codes and use of multiple coding for a single condition (such as manifestation/etiology pairs). • Reporting the Symptom Control Rating in Column 2 of M1021 - At each required time point, the assessing clinician should record the symptom control rating for the primary diagnosis in column 2 of M1021. - Assessing degree of symptom control includes review of presenting signs and symptoms, type and number of medications, frequency of treatment readjustments, and frequency of contact with health care provider. Inquire about the degree to which each condition limits daily activities. Assess the patient to determine if symptoms are controlled by current treatments. Clarify which diagnoses/symptoms have been poorly controlled in the recent past. - Choose one value that represents the degree of symptom control appropriate for the diagnosis using the scale provided in the M1021 instructions.	

M1023

Item Intent	Time Points	Response-specific Instructions	Data Sources/resources

The intent of this item is to accurately report and code the patient's secondary home health diagnoses and document the degree of symptom control for each diagnosis. Secondary diagnoses are comorbid conditions that exist at the time of the assessment, that are actively addressed in the patient's Plan of Care, or that have the potential to affect the patient's responsiveness to treatment and rehabilitative prognosis.	Start of care
	Resumption of care
	Follow-up
		• HHA clinicians and coders must report the most current year's ICD-10-CM codes and comply with the ICD-10-CM Official Guidelines for Coding and Reporting when assigning secondary diagnoses to the OASIS items M1023. See Chapter 5 for link.
		
		  - The ICD-10-CM is a morbidity classification published by the United States for classifying diagnoses and reason for care in all health care settings. The ICD-10-CM is based on the ICD-10, the International Classification of Diseases published by the World Health Organization (WHO).
		  - The ICD-10-CM Official Guidelines for Coding and Reporting were developed by the Centers for Medicare & Medicaid Services (CMS) and the National Center for Health Statistics (NCHS). These guidelines are a set of rules that have been developed to accompany and complement the official conventions and instructions provided within the ICD-10-CM itself and should be used as a companion document to the official version of the ICD-10-CM Official Code Set.
		  - Adherence to the ICD-10-CM Official Guidelines for Coding and Reporting when assigning ICD-10-CM diagnosis codes is required under the Health Insurance Portability and Accountability Act (HIPAA). It is expected that each agency will ensure that diagnoses and ICD-10-CM codes reported in the OASIS data set meet these guidelines.
		• Identifying the patient's Secondary Home Health Diagnoses
		
		  - The assessing clinician is expected to complete the patient's comprehensive assessment and understand the patient's overall medical condition and care needs before selecting and assigning diagnoses.
		  - The determination of the patient's secondary home health diagnoses must be made by the assessing clinician based on the findings of the assessment, information in the medical record, and input from the physician.
		  - As noted in the Item Intent, the secondary diagnoses include coexisting conditions actively addressed in the patient's Plan of Care, and any comorbid conditions having the potential to affect the patient's responsiveness to treatment and rehabilitative prognosis. The secondary diagnoses may or may not be related to a patient's recent hospital stay, but must have the potential to impact the skilled services provided by the HHA.
		  - When determining secondary diagnoses, the assessing clinician should consider diagnoses that are actively addressed in the Plan of Care as well as diagnoses that affect the patient's responsiveness to treatment and rehabilitative prognosis, even if the condition is not the focus of any home health treatment itself.
		  - Diagnoses may change during the course of the home health stay due to a change in the patient's health status or a change in the focus of home health care. At each required OASIS time point, the clinician must assess the patient's clinical status and determine the secondary diagnoses based on patient status and treatment plan at the time of the assessment.
		  - Only current medical diagnoses should be reported as secondary diagnoses in M1023. Diagnoses should be excluded if they are resolved or do not have the potential to impact the skilled services provided by the HHA. An example of a resolved condition is cholecystitis following a cholecystectomy.
		  - In addition to following the ICD-10-CM Official Guidelines for Coding and Reporting, selection of home health diagnoses must be performed in compliance with Medicare's rules and regulations for coverage and payment to ensure provider compliance with Section 1862(a)(1)(A) of the Social Security Act. Section 1862(a)(1)(A) excludes provider services from Medicare coverage and payment that "are not reasonable and necessary for diagnosis or treatment of illness or injury or to improve the functioning of a malformed body member."
			• Patient/caregiver interview
			• Physician
			• Physician orders
			• Referral information
			• Current medication list
			• Current ICD-10-CM Official Code Set and the ICD-10-CM Official Guidelines for Coding and Reporting should be the source for coding.
			• For degree of symptom control, data sources may include patient/caregiver interview, physician, physical assessment, and review of past health history.

M1023 (Continued)

Item Intent	Time Points	Response-specific Instructions	Data Sources/resources

		• Reporting Secondary Diagnoses in M1023
		
		  - At each required OASIS time point, the assessing clinician should enter the patient's current secondary diagnoses in Column 1 of M1023. Complete Column 1 from top to bottom, leaving any blank entries at the bottom.
		  - Entry order of secondary diagnoses is determined by the degree that they impact the patient's health and need for home health care, rather than the degree of symptom control.
		• Reporting ICD-10-CM Codes in Column 2 of M1023
		
		  - The assessing clinician can enter the actual numeric ICD-10-CM codes for each diagnosis listed in Column 1 and 2 of M1023, once the assessment is completed and the diagnosis is entered in Column 1. Alternatively, a coding specialist in the agency may enter the actual numeric ICD-10-CM codes in Column 2, as long as the assessing clinician has determined the secondary diagnoses in Column 1.
		
		  - The correct process for selecting an ICD-10-CM code using the Alphabetic Index and the Tabular List is described in the ICD-10-CM Official Guidelines for Coding and Reporting. Follow the official conventions and instructions provided within the ICD-10-CM Official Code Set and the Official Guidelines to code each row in Column 2.
		  - Each ICD-10-CM code must be entered at its highest level of specificity (diagnosis codes only - no surgical or procedure codes allowed).
		  - ICD-10-CM does not allow external cause codes (ICD-10-CM codes beginning with V, W, X, or Y) to be reported in M1021 (Primary Diagnosis) but they may be reported in M1023 (Secondary Diagnoses).
		  - Also note that when a Z-code is reported in Column 2, the code for the underlying condition may be entered in Column 2, as long as it is a current on-going condition that has a potential to impact the skilled services provided by the HHA. See the ICD-10-CM Official Guidelines for Coding and Reporting for complete instructions on code assignment and sequencing related to the use of Z-codes and use of multiple coding for a single condition (such as manifestation/etiology pairs).
		• Reporting the Symptom Control Rating in Column 2 of M1023
		
		  - At each required time point, the assessing clinician should record the symptom control ratings for each secondary diagnosis in column 2 of M1023.
		  - Assessing degree of symptom control includes review of presenting signs and symptoms, type and number of medications, frequency of treatment readjustments, and frequency of contact with health care provider. Inquire about the degree to which each condition limits daily activities. Assess the patient to determine if symptoms are controlled by current treatments. Clarify which diagnoses/symptoms have been poorly controlled in the recent past.
		  - Choose one value that represents the degree of symptom control appropriate for each diagnosis using the scale provided in the M1023 instructions.	

M1028

Item Intent	Time Points	Response-specific Instructions	Data Sources/resources
This item identifies whether two specific diagnoses are present and active. These diagnoses influence a patient's functional outcomes or increase a patient's risk for development or worsening of pressure ulcer(s).	• Start of care • Resumption of care	• Complete only if M0100 = 01 Start of care or 03 Resumption of care • Select Response 1: if the patient has an active diagnosis of peripheral vascular disease or peripheral arterial disease, indicated by codes in the following category/subcategory: I70.2- I70.3- I70.4- I70.5- I70.6- I70.7- I70.91 I70.92 I73.- • Select Response 2: if the patient has an active diagnosis of diabetes mellitus indicated by codes in the following categories: E08 E09 E10 E11 E13	• Patient/caregiver interview • Physician • Physician orders • Current ICD-10-CM Official Code Set and the ICD-10-CM Official Guidelines for Coding and Reporting should be the source for coding

Appendix H: Patient-Driven Groupings Model (PDGM) Comorbid Conditions

This resource provides a comprehensive list of the ICD-10-CM codes that are considered comorbidities that interact with the primary diagnosis for the PDGM. If one of the reported secondary diagnosis codes is identified in the comorbidity low list, the period of care would receive a low comorbidity payment adjustment. If at least two of the reported secondary diagnosis codes are identified in the comorbidity high list, the period of care would receive a high comorbidity adjustment.

Note: An updated ICD-10-CM list was not available at the time this publication was printed and therefore does not reflect any FY 2020 code changes. An updated list of comorbidity high and low codes, including those codes effective October 1, 2019, can be found at: https://www.cms.gov/Medicare/Medicare-Fee-for-Service-Payment/HomeHealthPPS/HH-PDGM.html.

Comorbidity High

E08.40	E10.69	E11.69	E13.69	F34.9	I50.21	I69.098	I69.262
E08.42	E10.9	E11.9	E13.9	F39	I50.22	I69.110	I69.263
E09.40	E11.00	E13.00	F02.80	G04.1	I50.23	I69.111	I69.264
E09.42	E11.01	E13.01	F02.81	G20	I50.30	I69.112	I69.265
E10.10	E11.10	E13.10	F03.90	G21.11	I50.31	I69.113	I69.290
E10.11	E11.11	E13.11	F03.91	G21.19	I50.32	I69.114	I69.291
E10.21	E11.21	E13.21	F04	G21.2	I50.33	I69.115	I69.293
E10.22	E11.22	E13.22	F05	G21.3	I50.40	I69.118	I69.298
E10.29	E11.29	E13.29	F06.1	G21.4	I50.41	I69.120	I69.310
E10.319	E11.319	E13.319	F06.8	G21.8	I50.42	I69.121	I69.311
E10.3291	E11.3291	E13.3291	F30.10	G21.9	I50.43	I69.122	I69.312
E10.3292	E11.3292	E13.3292	F30.11	G35	I50.810	I69.123	I69.313
E10.3293	E11.3293	E13.3293	F30.12	G81.01	I50.811	I69.128	I69.314
E10.3391	E11.3391	E13.3391	F30.13	G81.02	I50.812	I69.131	I69.315
E10.3392	E11.3392	E13.3392	F30.2	G81.03	I50.813	I69.132	I69.318
E10.3393	E11.3393	E13.3393	F30.3	G81.04	I50.814	I69.133	I69.320
E10.3491	E11.3491	E13.3491	F30.4	G81.11	I50.82	I69.134	I69.321
E10.3492	E11.3492	E13.3492	F30.8	G81.12	I50.83	I69.141	I69.322
E10.3493	E11.3493	E13.3493	F30.9	G81.13	I50.84	I69.142	I69.323
E10.3521	E11.3521	E13.3521	F31.0	G81.14	I50.89	I69.143	I69.328
E10.3522	E11.3522	E13.3522	F31.10	G81.91	I50.9	I69.144	I69.331
E10.3523	E11.3523	E13.3523	F31.11	G81.92	I51.3	I69.151	I69.332
E10.3531	E11.3531	E13.3531	F31.12	G81.93	I51.89	I69.152	I69.333
E10.3532	E11.3532	E13.3532	F31.13	G81.94	I67.2	I69.153	I69.334
E10.3533	E11.3533	E13.3533	F31.2	G82.20	I67.81	I69.154	I69.341
E10.3541	E11.3541	E13.3541	F31.30	G82.21	I67.82	I69.161	I69.342
E10.3542	E11.3542	E13.3542	F31.31	G82.22	I67.89	I69.162	I69.343
E10.3543	E11.3543	E13.3543	F31.32	G82.50	I69.010	I69.163	I69.344
E10.3551	E11.3551	E13.3551	F31.4	G82.51	I69.011	I69.164	I69.351
E10.3552	E11.3552	E13.3552	F31.5	G82.52	I69.012	I69.165	I69.352
E10.3553	E11.3553	E13.3553	F31.60	G82.53	I69.013	I69.190	I69.353
E10.3591	E11.3591	E13.3591	F31.61	G82.54	I69.014	I69.191	I69.354
E10.3592	E11.3592	E13.3592	F31.62	I09.81	I69.015	I69.193	I69.361
E10.3593	E11.3593	E13.3593	F31.63	I11.0	I69.018	I69.198	I69.362
E10.36	E11.36	E13.36	F31.64	I12.0	I69.020	I69.210	I69.363
E10.37X1	E11.37X1	E13.37X1	F31.70	I12.9	I69.021	I69.211	I69.364
E10.37X2	E11.37X2	E13.37X2	F31.71	I13.0	I69.022	I69.212	I69.365
E10.37X3	E11.37X3	E13.37X3	F31.72	I13.10	I69.023	I69.213	I69.390
E10.39	E11.39	E13.39	F31.73	I13.11	I69.028	I69.214	I69.391
E10.40	E11.40	E13.40	F31.77	I13.2	I69.031	I69.215	I69.393
E10.41	E11.41	E13.41	F31.78	I20.0	I69.032	I69.218	I69.398
E10.42	E11.42	E13.42	F31.81	I20.1	I69.033	I69.220	I69.810
E10.43	E11.43	E13.43	F31.89	I20.8	I69.034	I69.221	I69.811
E10.44	E11.44	E13.44	F31.9	I20.9	I69.041	I69.222	I69.812
E10.49	E11.49	E13.49	F32.0	I24.0	I69.042	I69.223	I69.813
E10.51	E11.51	E13.51	F32.1	I24.1	I69.043	I69.228	I69.814
E10.52	E11.52	E13.52	F32.2	I24.8	I69.044	I69.231	I69.815
E10.59	E11.59	E13.59	F32.4	I24.9	I69.051	I69.232	I69.818
E10.610	E11.610	E13.610	F32.89	I25.10	I69.052	I69.233	I69.820
E10.618	E11.618	E13.618	F32.9	I48.0	I69.053	I69.234	I69.821
E10.620	E11.620	E13.620	F33.0	I48.3	I69.054	I69.241	I69.822
E10.621	E11.621	E13.621	F33.1	I48.4	I69.061	I69.242	I69.823
E10.622	E11.622	E13.622	F33.2	I48.91	I69.062	I69.243	I69.828
E10.628	E11.628	E13.628	F33.40	I48.92	I69.063	I69.244	I69.831
E10.630	E11.630	E13.630	F33.41	I49.5	I69.064	I69.251	I69.832
E10.638	E11.638	E13.638	F33.8	I49.8	I69.065	I69.252	I69.833
E10.641	E11.641	E13.641	F33.9	I49.9	I69.090	I69.253	I69.834
E10.649	E11.649	E13.649	F34.81	I50.1	I69.091	I69.254	I69.841
E10.65	E11.65	E13.65	F34.89	I50.20	I69.093	I69.261	I69.842

I69.843	I70.223	I70.631	I83.228	L03.123	L89.214	L97.214	L97.529
I69.844	I70.228	I70.632	I85.00	L03.124	L89.220	L97.215	L97.811
I69.851	I70.231	I70.633	I89.0	L03.125	L89.222	L97.216	L97.812
I69.852	I70.232	I70.634	I95.1	L03.126	L89.223	L97.218	L97.813
I69.853	I70.233	I70.635	I95.89	L03.221	L89.224	L97.219	L97.814
I69.854	I70.234	I70.638	I95.9	L03.222	L89.310	L97.221	L97.815
I69.861	I70.235	I70.639	I97.2	L03.311	L89.312	L97.222	L97.816
I69.862	I70.238	I70.641	J44.0	L03.312	L89.313	L97.223	L97.818
I69.863	I70.241	I70.642	J44.1	L03.313	L89.314	L97.224	L97.819
I69.864	I70.242	I70.643	J44.9	L03.314	L89.320	L97.225	L97.821
I69.865	I70.243	I70.644	J45.20	L03.315	L89.322	L97.226	L97.822
I69.890	I70.244	I70.645	J45.21	L03.316	L89.323	L97.228	L97.823
I69.891	I70.245	I70.648	J45.22	L03.317	L89.324	L97.229	L97.824
I69.893	I70.248	I70.649	J45.30	L03.319	L89.42	L97.311	L97.825
I69.898	I70.261	I70.731	J45.31	L03.321	L89.43	L97.312	L97.826
I69.910	I70.262	I70.732	J45.32	L03.322	L89.44	L97.313	L97.828
I69.911	I70.263	I70.733	J45.40	L03.323	L89.45	L97.314	L97.829
I69.912	I70.268	I70.734	J45.41	L03.324	L89.510	L97.315	L97.911
I69.913	I70.331	I70.735	J45.42	L03.325	L89.512	L97.316	L97.912
I69.914	I70.332	I70.738	J45.50	L03.326	L89.513	L97.318	L97.913
I69.915	I70.333	I70.739	J45.51	L03.327	L89.514	L97.319	L97.914
I69.918	I70.334	I70.741	J45.52	L03.329	L89.520	L97.321	L97.915
I69.920	I70.335	I70.742	J45.901	L03.811	L89.522	L97.322	L97.916
I69.921	I70.338	I70.743	J45.902	L03.818	L89.523	L97.323	L97.918
I69.922	I70.339	I70.744	J45.909	L03.891	L89.524	L97.324	L97.919
I69.923	I70.341	I70.745	J45.990	L03.898	L89.610	L97.325	L97.921
I69.928	I70.342	I70.748	J45.991	L89.010	L89.612	L97.326	L97.922
I69.931	I70.343	I70.749	J45.998	L89.012	L89.613	L97.328	L97.923
I69.932	I70.344	I70.90	J47.0	L89.013	L89.614	L97.329	L97.924
I69.933	I70.345	I70.91	J47.1	L89.014	L89.620	L97.411	L97.925
I69.934	I70.348	I71.2	J47.9	L89.020	L89.622	L97.412	L97.926
I69.941	I70.349	I71.4	L02.11	L89.022	L89.623	L97.413	L97.928
I69.942	I70.431	I71.6	L02.211	L89.023	L89.624	L97.414	L97.929
I69.943	I70.432	I73.9	L02.212	L89.024	L89.810	L97.415	L98.3
I69.944	I70.433	I79.0	L02.213	L89.102	L89.812	L97.416	N11.0
I69.951	I70.434	I83.011	L02.214	L89.103	L89.813	L97.418	N11.1
I69.952	I70.435	I83.012	L02.215	L89.104	L89.814	L97.419	N11.8
I69.953	I70.438	I83.013	L02.216	L89.110	L89.890	L97.421	N13.2
I69.954	I70.439	I83.014	L02.219	L89.112	L89.892	L97.422	N18.1
I69.961	I70.441	I83.015	L02.31	L89.113	L89.893	L97.423	N18.2
I69.962	I70.442	I83.018	L02.411	L89.114	L89.894	L97.424	N18.3
I69.963	I70.443	I83.021	L02.412	L89.120	L97.111	L97.425	N18.4
I69.964	I70.444	I83.022	L02.413	L89.122	L97.112	L97.426	N18.5
I69.965	I70.445	I83.023	L02.414	L89.123	L97.113	L97.428	N18.6
I69.990	I70.448	I83.024	L02.415	L89.124	L97.114	L97.429	N20.0
I69.991	I70.449	I83.025	L02.416	L89.130	L97.115	L97.511	N20.2
I69.993	I70.531	I83.028	L02.511	L89.132	L97.116	L97.512	N25.1
I69.998	I70.532	I83.11	L02.512	L89.133	L97.118	L97.513	N29
I70.0	I70.533	I83.12	L02.611	L89.134	L97.119	L97.514	N31.0
I70.1	I70.534	I83.211	L02.612	L89.140	L97.121	L97.515	N31.1
I70.201	I70.535	I83.212	L02.811	L89.142	L97.122	L97.516	N31.9
I70.202	I70.538	I83.213	L02.818	L89.143	L97.123	L97.518	N39.0
I70.203	I70.539	I83.214	L03.111	L89.144	L97.124	L97.519	N40.1
I70.208	I70.541	I83.215	L03.112	L89.150	L97.125	L97.521	R00.1
I70.211	I70.542	I83.218	L03.113	L89.152	L97.126	L97.522	
I70.212	I70.543	I83.221	L03.114	L89.153	L97.128	L97.523	
I70.213	I70.544	I83.222	L03.115	L89.154	L97.129	L97.524	
I70.218	I70.545	I83.223	L03.116	L89.210	L97.211	L97.525	
I70.221	I70.548	I83.224	L03.121	L89.212	L97.212	L97.526	
I70.222	I70.549	I83.225	L03.122	L89.213	L97.213	L97.528	

Comorbidity Low

C00.0	E08.3511	G21.19	H35.352	I26.99	I69.098	I69.311	I69.913
C00.1	E08.3512	G21.2	H35.353	I48.0	I69.110	I69.312	I69.914
C00.3	E08.3513	G21.3	H35.361	I48.3	I69.111	I69.313	I69.915
C00.4	E08.40	G21.4	H35.362	I48.4	I69.112	I69.314	I69.918
C00.8	E08.42	G21.8	H35.363	I48.91	I69.113	I69.315	I69.920
C01	E09.311	G21.9	H35.371	I48.92	I69.114	I69.318	I69.921
C02.0	E09.3211	G35	H35.372	I49.5	I69.115	I69.320	I69.922
C02.1	E09.3212	G62	H35.373	I49.8	I69.118	I69.321	I69.923
C02.2	E09.3213	G62.0	H35.381	I49.9	I69.120	I69.322	I69.928
C02.3	E09.3311	G62.1	H35.382	I50.1	I69.121	I69.323	I69.931
C02.4	E09.3312	G62.2	H35.383	I50.20	I69.122	I69.328	I69.932
C02.8	E09.3313	G62.8	H54.0	I50.21	I69.123	I69.331	I69.933
C02.9	E09.3411	G62.81	H54.0X	I50.22	I69.128	I69.332	I69.934
C03.1	E09.3412	G62.82	H54.0X3	I50.23	I69.131	I69.333	I69.941
C04.0	E09.3413	G62.89	H54.0X33	I50.30	I69.132	I69.334	I69.942
C04.1	E09.3511	G62.9	H54.0X34	I50.31	I69.133	I69.341	I69.943
C04.8	E09.3512	G81.01	H54.0X35	I50.32	I69.134	I69.342	I69.944
C04.9	E09.3513	G81.02	H54.0X4	I50.33	I69.141	I69.343	I69.951
C05.0	E09.40	G81.03	H54.0X43	I50.40	I69.142	I69.344	I69.952
C05.1	E09.42	G81.04	H54.0X44	I50.41	I69.143	I69.351	I69.953
C05.2	E10.311	G81.11	H54.0X45	I50.42	I69.144	I69.352	I69.954
C05.8	E10.3211	G81.12	H54.0X5	I50.43	I69.151	I69.353	I69.961
C05.9	E10.3212	G81.13	H54.0X53	I50.810	I69.152	I69.354	I69.962
C06.0	E10.3213	G81.14	H54.0X54	I50.811	I69.153	I69.361	I69.963
C06.1	E10.3311	G81.91	H54.0X55	I50.812	I69.154	I69.362	I69.964
C06.2	E10.3312	G81.92	H54.10	I50.813	I69.161	I69.363	I69.965
C06.80	E10.3313	G81.93	H54.11	I50.814	I69.162	I69.364	I69.990
C06.89	E10.3411	G81.94	H54.113	I50.82	I69.163	I69.365	I69.991
C06.9	E10.3412	G82.20	H54.1131	I50.83	I69.164	I69.390	I69.993
C07	E10.3413	G82.21	H54.1132	I50.84	I69.165	I69.391	I69.998
C08.0	E10.3511	G82.22	H54.114	I50.89	I69.190	I69.393	I70.231
C08.1	E10.3512	G82.50	H54.1141	I50.9	I69.191	I69.398	I70.232
C08.9	E10.3513	G82.51	H54.1142	I67.2	I69.193	I69.810	I70.233
C09.0	E10.40	G82.52	H54.115	I67.81	I69.198	I69.811	I70.234
C09.1	E10.42	G82.53	H54.1151	I67.82	I69.210	I69.812	I70.235
C09.8	E11.311	G82.54	H54.1152	I67.89	I69.211	I69.813	I70.238
C09.9	E11.3211	H35.30	H54.12	I69.010	I69.212	I69.814	I70.241
C10.0	E11.3212	H35.3110	H54.121	I69.011	I69.213	I69.815	I70.242
C10.1	E11.3213	H35.3111	H54.1213	I69.012	I69.214	I69.818	I70.243
C10.2	E11.3311	H35.3112	H54.1214	I69.013	I69.215	I69.820	I70.244
C10.3	E11.3312	H35.3113	H54.1215	I69.014	I69.218	I69.821	I70.245
C10.4	E11.3313	H35.3114	H54.122	I69.015	I69.220	I69.822	I70.248
C10.8	E11.3411	H35.3120	H54.1223	I69.018	I69.221	I69.823	I70.331
C10.9	E11.3412	H35.3121	H54.1224	I69.020	I69.222	I69.828	I70.332
C11.0	E11.3413	H35.3122	H54.1225	I69.021	I69.223	I69.831	I70.333
C11.1	E11.3511	H35.3123	H54.2	I69.022	I69.228	I69.832	I70.334
C11.2	E11.3512	H35.3124	H54.2X	I69.023	I69.231	I69.833	I70.335
C11.3	E11.3513	H35.3130	H54.2X1	I69.028	I69.232	I69.834	I70.338
C11.8	E11.40	H35.3131	H54.2X11	I69.031	I69.233	I69.841	I70.339
C12	E11.42	H35.3132	H54.2X12	I69.032	I69.234	I69.842	I70.341
C13.0	E13.311	H35.3133	H54.2X2	I69.033	I69.241	I69.843	I70.342
C13.1	E13.3211	H35.3134	H54.2X21	I69.034	I69.242	I69.844	I70.343
C13.2	E13.3212	H35.3210	H54.2X22	I69.041	I69.243	I69.851	I70.344
C13.8	E13.3213	H35.3211	H54.3	I69.042	I69.244	I69.852	I70.345
C13.9	E13.3311	H35.3212	H54.413A	I69.043	I69.251	I69.853	I70.348
C14.0	E13.3312	H35.3213	H54.414A	I69.044	I69.252	I69.854	I70.349
C14.2	E13.3313	H35.3220	H54.415A	I69.051	I69.253	I69.861	I70.431
C14.8	E13.3411	H35.3221	H54.42A3	I69.052	I69.254	I69.862	I70.432
E08.311	E13.3412	H35.3222	H54.42A4	I69.053	I69.261	I69.863	I70.433
E08.3211	E13.3413	H35.3223	H54.42A5	I69.054	I69.262	I69.864	I70.434
E08.3212	E13.3511	H35.3230	H54.511A	I69.061	I69.263	I69.865	I70.435
E08.3213	E13.3512	H35.3231	H54.512A	I69.062	I69.264	I69.890	I70.438
E08.3311	E13.3513	H35.3232	H54.52A1	I69.063	I69.265	I69.891	I70.439
E08.3312	E13.40	H35.3233	H54.52A2	I69.064	I69.290	I69.893	I70.441
E08.3313	E13.42	H35.341	H54.8	I69.065	I69.291	I69.898	I70.442
E08.3411	G04.1	H35.342	I09.81	I69.090	I69.293	I69.910	I70.443
E08.3412	G20	H35.343	I11.0	I69.091	I69.298	I69.911	I70.444
E08.3413	G21.11	H35.351	I26.09	I69.093	I69.310	I69.912	I70.445

Appendix H: Patient-Driven Groupings Model (PDGM) Comorbid Conditions

I70.448	I82.3	I82.611	I83.211	L03.313	L89.214	L97.124	L97.429
I70.449	I82.401	I82.612	I83.212	L03.314	L89.220	L97.125	L97.511
I70.531	I82.402	I82.613	I83.213	L03.315	L89.222	L97.126	L97.512
I70.532	I82.403	I82.621	I83.214	L03.316	L89.223	L97.128	L97.513
I70.533	I82.411	I82.622	I83.215	L03.317	L89.224	L97.129	L97.514
I70.534	I82.412	I82.623	I83.218	L03.319	L89.310	L97.211	L97.515
I70.535	I82.413	I82.701	I83.221	L03.321	L89.312	L97.212	L97.516
I70.538	I82.421	I82.702	I83.222	L03.322	L89.313	L97.213	L97.518
I70.539	I82.422	I82.703	I83.223	L03.323	L89.314	L97.214	L97.519
I70.541	I82.423	I82.711	I83.224	L03.324	L89.320	L97.215	L97.521
I70.542	I82.431	I82.712	I83.225	L03.325	L89.322	L97.216	L97.522
I70.543	I82.432	I82.713	I83.228	L03.326	L89.323	L97.218	L97.523
I70.544	I82.433	I82.721	I85.00	L03.327	L89.324	L97.219	L97.524
I70.545	I82.441	I82.722	I89.0	L03.329	L89.42	L97.221	L97.525
I70.548	I82.442	I82.723	I97.2	L03.811	L89.43	L97.222	L97.526
I70.549	I82.443	I82.811	L02.11	L03.818	L89.44	L97.223	L97.528
I70.631	I82.491	I82.812	L02.211	L03.891	L89.45	L97.224	L97.529
I70.632	I82.492	I82.813	L02.212	L03.898	L89.510	L97.225	L97.811
I70.633	I82.493	I82.890	L02.213	L89.010	L89.512	L97.226	L97.812
I70.634	I82.4Y1	I82.891	L02.214	L89.012	L89.513	L97.228	L97.813
I70.635	I82.4Y2	I82.A11	L02.215	L89.013	L89.514	L97.229	L97.814
I70.638	I82.4Y3	I82.A12	L02.216	L89.014	L89.520	L97.311	L97.815
I70.639	I82.4Z1	I82.A13	L02.219	L89.020	L89.522	L97.312	L97.816
I70.641	I82.4Z2	I82.A21	L02.31	L89.022	L89.523	L97.313	L97.818
I70.642	I82.4Z3	I82.A22	L02.411	L89.023	L89.524	L97.314	L97.819
I70.643	I82.501	I82.A23	L02.412	L89.024	L89.610	L97.315	L97.821
I70.644	I82.502	I82.B11	L02.413	L89.102	L89.612	L97.316	L97.822
I70.645	I82.503	I82.B12	L02.414	L89.103	L89.613	L97.318	L97.823
I70.648	I82.511	I82.B13	L02.415	L89.104	L89.614	L97.319	L97.824
I70.649	I82.512	I82.B21	L02.416	L89.110	L89.620	L97.321	L97.825
I70.731	I82.513	I82.B22	L02.511	L89.112	L89.622	L97.322	L97.826
I70.732	I82.521	I82.B23	L02.512	L89.113	L89.623	L97.323	L97.828
I70.733	I82.522	I82.C11	L02.611	L89.114	L89.624	L97.324	L97.829
I70.734	I82.523	I82.C12	L02.612	L89.120	L89.810	L97.325	L97.911
I70.735	I82.531	I82.C13	L02.811	L89.122	L89.812	L97.326	L97.912
I70.738	I82.532	I82.C21	L02.818	L89.123	L89.813	L97.328	L97.913
I70.739	I82.533	I82.C22	L03.111	L89.124	L89.814	L97.329	L97.914
I70.741	I82.541	I82.C23	L03.112	L89.130	L89.890	L97.411	L97.915
I70.742	I82.542	I83.011	L03.113	L89.132	L89.892	L97.412	L97.916
I70.743	I82.543	I83.012	L03.114	L89.133	L89.893	L97.413	L97.918
I70.744	I82.591	I83.013	L03.115	L89.134	L89.894	L97.414	L97.919
I70.745	I82.592	I83.014	L03.116	L89.140	L97.111	L97.415	L97.921
I70.748	I82.593	I83.015	L03.121	L89.142	L97.112	L97.416	L97.922
I70.749	I82.5Y1	I83.018	L03.122	L89.143	L97.113	L97.418	L97.923
I82.0	I82.5Y2	I83.021	L03.123	L89.144	L97.114	L97.419	L97.924
I82.1	I82.5Y3	I83.022	L03.124	L89.150	L97.115	L97.421	L97.925
I82.210	I82.5Z1	I83.023	L03.125	L89.152	L97.116	L97.422	L97.926
I82.211	I82.5Z2	I83.024	L03.126	L89.153	L97.118	L97.423	L97.928
I82.220	I82.5Z3	I83.025	L03.221	L89.154	L97.119	L97.424	L97.929
I82.221	I82.601	I83.028	L03.222	L89.210	L97.121	L97.425	L98.3
I82.290	I82.602	I83.11	L03.311	L89.212	L97.122	L97.426	R00.1
I82.291	I82.603	I83.12	L03.312	L89.213	L97.123	L97.428	

Appendix I: Patient-Driven Groupings Model (PDGM) Return-to-Provider Code List

This resource provides a comprehensive list of the ICD-10-CM codes that do not map to one of the 12 clinical grouping categories and therefore are not acceptable as the primary reason for home health care. These codes lack either the certainty or specificity required to properly categorize a resident under PDGM or describe underlying conditions that cannot be the main reason for home health care. When one of these codes is listed as the primary reason diagnosis code on the OASIS-D or as the principal diagnosis on the claim, the form should be returned to the provider to select an appropriate ICD-10-CM diagnosis code using the clinical grouping list provided by CMS.

Note: An updated ICD-10-CM list was not available at the time this publication was printed and therefore this list does not reflect any FY 2020 code changes. An updated list of the ICD-10-CM codes that map to each clinical grouping, including new codes effective October 1, 2019, can be found at: https://www.cms.gov/Medicare/Medicare-Fee-for-Service-Payment/HomeHealthPPS/HH-PDGM.html.

Note: All codes from chapter 20, "External Causes of Morbidity," have been removed from this list. Per official ICD-10-CM coding guidelines, external cause codes can never be sequenced as a first-listed code.

An asterisk [*] indicates that all codes within that category are return-to-provider codes. Refer to the ICD-10-CM Official Code Set for specific codes that fall in that category, including appropriate seventh-character (identifying the type of encounter) assignment when required.

A dash [-] after a code indicates that a seventh character (identifying the type of encounter) is required to complete the code. For the applicable seventh characters, refer to the ICD-10-CM Official Code Set. All applicable seventh characters for that subcategory are return-to-provider codes.

A18.10	C44.121	C50.619	C80.1	D22.9	D89.810	E21.5	F81*
A28.9	C44.131	C50.629	C80.2	D23.10	D89.811	E22.9	F84.9
A49*	C44.191	C50.819	D00.00	D23.20	D89.812	E23.2	F89
A64	C44.201	C50.829	D01.40	D23.30	D89.813	E23.7	F91.9
B03	C44.209	C50.919	D01.9	D23.60	E03.2	E25.9	F93.9
B34.8	C44.211	C50.929	D02.20	D23.70	E07.9	E26.9	F94.9
B34.9	C44.221	C56.9	D02.4	D23.9	E08*	E27.40	F95.9
B64	C44.291	C57.00	D03.10	D24.9	E09.8	E27.49	F98.9
B67.4	C44.300	C57.10	D03.20	D27.9	E10.3219	E27.9	F99
B67.7	C44.310	C57.20	D03.30	D28.9	E10.3299	E28.9	G01
B88.9	C44.320	C57.9	D03.60	D29.20	E10.3319	E29.9	G02
B89	C44.390	C60.0	D03.70	D29.30	E10.3399	E30.0	G03.8
B95.1	C44.601	C62.00	D03.9	D29.9	E10.3419	E30.1	G03.9
B95.2	C44.611	C62.10	D04.10	D30.00	E10.3499	E30.8	G05.3
B95.3	C44.621	C62.90	D04.20	D30.10	E10.3519	E30.9	G05.4
B95.4	C44.691	C63.00	D04.30	D30.20	E10.3529	E32.0	G07
B95.5	C44.701	C63.10	D04.60	D30.9	E10.3539	E32.9	G09
B95.61	C44.711	C63.9	D04.70	D31.00	E10.3549	E34.50 -	G13*
B95.62	C44.721	C64.9	D04.9	D31.10	E10.3559	E34.9	G24.9
B95.7	C44.791	C65.9	D05.00	D31.20	E10.3599	E35	G25.70
B95.8	C44.90	C66.9	D05.10	D31.30	E10.37X9	E56.9	G25.9
B96*	C44.91	C68.9	D05.80	D31.40	E10.8	E61.9	G31.9
B97*	C44.92	C69.00	D05.90	D31.50	E11.3219	E63.9	G32*
B99*	C44.99	C69.10	D07.30	D31.60	E11.3299	E64.9	G47.27
C00.2	C45.9	C69.20	D07.60	D31.90	E11.3319	E72.9	G47.36
C00.5	C46.50	C69.30	D09.10	D33.9	E11.3399	E74.9	G47.37
C00.9	C46.9	C69.40	D09.20	D35.00	E11.3419	E78.9	G47.421
C03.9	C47.10	C69.50	D09.9	D35.9	E11.3499	E79.8	G47.429
C06.9	C47.20	C69.60	D10.30	D36.9	E11.3519	E83.9	G47.54
C08.9	C49.10	C69.80	D11.9	D37.9	E11.3529	E88.9	G51.9
C09.1	C49.20	C69.90	D14.30	D38.6	E11.3539	F01*	G52.9
C34.10	C49.9	C72.20	D14.4	D39.10	E11.3549	F02*	G53
C34.30	C49.A0	C72.30	D15.9	D39.9	E11.3559	F04	G54.9
C34.80	C4A.10	C72.40	D16.00	D3A.00	E11.3599	F05	G55
C34.90	C4A.20	C72.50	D16.10	D40.10	E11.37X9	F06*	G56.00
C39.0	C4A.30	C74.10	D16.20	D40.9	E11.8	F07.0	G56.10
C39.9	C4A.60	C74.90	D16.30	D41.00	E13.3219	F09	G56.20
C40.00	C4A.70	C76.40	D16.9	D41.10	E13.3299	F10.11	G56.30
C40.10	C4A.9	C76.50	D17.20	D41.20	E13.3319	F11.11	G56.40
C40.20	C50.019	C77.9	D17.30	D41.9	E13.3399	F12.11	G56.80
C40.30	C50.029	C78.00	D17.9	D43.9	E13.3419	F13.11	G56.90
C40.80	C50.119	C78.30	D18.00	D44.10	E13.3499	F14.11	G57.00
C40.90	C50.129	C78.80	D19.9	D44.9	E13.3519	F15.11	G57.10
C43.10	C50.219	C79.00	D21.10	D48.60	E13.3529	F16.11	G57.20
C43.20	C50.229	C79.10	D21.20	D48.9	E13.3539	F18.11	G57.30
C43.30	C50.319	C79.40	D21.9	D49.519	E13.3549	F19.11	G57.40
C43.60	C50.329	C79.60	D22.10	D49.9	E13.3559	F40.10	G57.50
C43.70	C50.419	C79.70	D22.20	D57.3	E13.3599	F40.9	G57.60
C43.9	C50.429	C79.9	D22.30	D73.9	E13.37X9	F43.9	G57.70
C44.101	C50.519	C7A.00	D22.60	D75.9	E13.40	F69	G57.80
C44.111	C50.529	C7B.00	D22.70	D77	E13.8	F80.9	G57.90

G58.0	H02.019	H02.736	H05.319	H16.009	H20.029	H30.109	H35.3192
G58.9	H02.023	H02.739	H05.329	H16.019	H20.039	H30.119	H35.3193
G59	H02.026	H02.813	H05.339	H16.029	H20.049	H30.129	H35.3194
G61.9	H02.029	H02.816	H05.349	H16.039	H20.059	H30.139	H35.3210
G62.9	H02.033	H02.819	H05.359	H16.049	H20.10	H30.149	H35.3220
G63	H02.036	H02.823	H05.409	H16.059	H20.20	H30.20	H35.3290
G70.81	H02.039	H02.826	H05.419	H16.069	H20.819	H30.819	H35.3291
G70.9	H02.043	H02.829	H05.429	H16.079	H20.829	H30.899	H35.3292
G71.9	H02.046	H02.833	H05.50	H16.109	H21.00	H30.90	H35.3293
G73.1	H02.049	H02.836	H05.819	H16.119	H21.1X9	H31.009	H35.349
G73.3	H02.053	H02.839	H05.829	H16.129	H21.219	H31.019	H35.359
G73.7	H02.056	H02.843	H05.9	H16.139	H21.229	H31.029	H35.369
G81.00	H02.059	H02.846	H10.019	H16.149	H21.239	H31.099	H35.379
G81.10	H02.103	H02.849	H10.029	H16.209	H21.249	H31.109	H35.389
G81.90	H02.105	H02.853	H10.10	H16.219	H21.259	H31.119	H35.40
G83.10	H02.106	H02.856	H10.219	H16.229	H21.269	H31.129	H35.419
G83.20	H02.109	H02.859	H10.239	H16.239	H21.279	H31.309	H35.429
G83.30	H02.113	H02.863	H10.30	H16.249	H21.309	H31.319	H35.439
G83.9	H02.116	H02.866	H10.409	H16.259	H21.319	H31.329	H35.449
G90.519	H02.119	H02.869	H10.419	H16.269	H21.329	H31.409	H35.459
G90.529	H02.123	H02.873	H10.429	H16.299	H21.339	H31.419	H35.469
G90.9	H02.126	H02.876	H10.439	H16.309	H21.349	H31.429	H35.60
G91.4	H02.129	H02.879	H10.509	H16.319	H21.359	H31.9	H35.70
G91.9	H02.133	H02.883	H10.519	H16.329	H21.40	H32	H35.719
G93.82	H02.136	H02.886	H10.529	H16.339	H21.509	H33.009	H35.729
G93.9	H02.139	H02.889	H10.539	H16.399	H21.519	H33.019	H35.739
G94	H02.143	H02.9	H10.819	H16.409	H21.529	H33.029	H35.9
G95.20	H02.146	H04.009	H10.829	H16.419	H21.539	H33.039	H36
G95.9	H02.149	H04.019	H10.9	H16.429	H21.549	H33.049	H40.009
G96.9	H02.153	H04.029	H11.009	H16.439	H21.559	H33.059	H40.019
G99*	H02.156	H04.039	H11.019	H16.449	H21.569	H33.109	H40.029
H00.013	H02.159	H04.119	H11.029	H17.00	H21.9	H33.119	H40.039
H00.016	H02.203	H04.129	H11.039	H17.10	H22	H33.129	H40.049
H00.019	H02.206	H04.139	H11.049	H17.819	H25.019	H33.199	H40.059
H00.023	H02.209	H04.149	H11.059	H17.829	H25.039	H33.20	H40.069
H00.026	H02.213	H04.159	H11.069	H17.9	H25.049	H33.309	H40.1190
H00.029	H02.216	H04.169	H11.10	H18.009	H25.099	H33.319	H40.1191
H00.033	H02.219	H04.209	H11.119	H18.019	H25.10	H33.329	H40.1192
H00.036	H02.223	H04.219	H11.129	H18.029	H25.20	H33.339	H40.1193
H00.039	H02.226	H04.229	H11.139	H18.039	H25.819	H33.40	H40.1194
H00.13	H02.229	H04.309	H11.149	H18.049	H26.009	H34.00	H40.1290
H00.16	H02.233	H04.319	H11.159	H18.059	H26.019	H34.10	H40.1291
H00.19	H02.236	H04.329	H11.219	H18.069	H26.039	H34.219	H40.1292
H01.003	H02.239	H04.339	H11.229	H18.10	H26.049	H34.239	H40.1293
H01.006	H02.30	H04.419	H11.239	H18.219	H26.059	H34.8190	H40.1294
H01.009	H02.33	H04.429	H11.249	H18.229	H26.069	H34.8191	H40.1390
H01.013	H02.36	H04.439	H11.30	H18.239	H26.109	H34.8192	H40.1391
H01.016	H02.409	H04.519	H11.419	H18.319	H26.119	H34.829	H40.1392
H01.019	H02.419	H04.529	H11.429	H18.329	H26.129	H34.8390	H40.1393
H01.023	H02.429	H04.539	H11.439	H18.339	H26.139	H34.8391	H40.1394
H01.026	H02.439	H04.549	H11.449	H18.419	H26.219	H34.8392	H40.1490
H01.029	H02.513	H04.559	H11.819	H18.429	H26.229	H35.019	H40.1491
H01.113	H02.516	H04.569	H11.829	H18.449	H26.239	H35.029	H40.1492
H01.116	H02.519	H04.579	H11.9	H18.459	H26.40	H35.039	H40.1493
H01.119	H02.523	H04.619	H15.009	H18.469	H26.419	H35.049	H40.1494
H01.123	H02.526	H04.819	H15.019	H18.50	H26.499	H35.059	H40.159
H01.126	H02.529	H04.9	H15.029	H18.609	H26.9	H35.069	H40.219
H01.129	H02.533	H05.019	H15.039	H18.619	H27.00	H35.079	H40.2290
H01.133	H02.536	H05.029	H15.049	H18.629	H27.03	H35.109	H40.2291
H01.136	H02.539	H05.039	H15.059	H18.70	H27.10	H35.119	H40.2292
H01.139	H02.60	H05.049	H15.099	H18.719	H27.119	H35.129	H40.2293
H01.143	H02.63	H05.119	H15.109	H18.729	H27.129	H35.139	H40.2294
H01.146	H02.66	H05.129	H15.119	H18.739	H27.139	H35.149	H40.239
H01.149	H02.713	H05.219	H15.129	H18.799	H27.9	H35.159	H40.249
H01.9	H02.716	H05.229	H15.819	H18.819	H28	H35.169	H40.30X0
H02.003	H02.719	H05.239	H15.829	H18.829	H30.009	H35.179	H40.30X1
H02.006	H02.723	H05.249	H15.839	H18.839	H30.019	H35.20	H40.30X2
H02.009	H02.726	H05.259	H15.849	H18.899	H30.029	H35.30	H40.30X3
H02.013	H02.729	H05.269	H15.859	H18.9	H30.039	H35.3190	H40.30X4
H02.016	H02.733	H05.30	H15.9	H20.019	H30.049	H35.3191	H40.40X0

H40.40X1	H47.029	H59.099	H66.017	H81.399	I69.259	I77.70	I87.329
H40.40X2	H47.039	H59.119	H66.019	H81.8X9	I69.269	I77.9	I87.339
H40.40X3	H47.099	H59.129	H66.10	H81.90	I69.30	I78.9	I87.399
H40.40X4	H47.149	H59.219	H66.20	H81.91	I69.319	I79*	I87.9
H40.50X0	H47.219	H59.229	H66.3X9	H81.92	I69.339	I80.00	I88.9
H40.50X1	H47.239	H59.319	H66.40	H81.93	I69.349	I80.10	I89.9
H40.50X2	H47.299	H59.329	H66.90	H82*	I69.359	I80.209	I95.9
H40.50X3	H47.319	H59.339	H67*	H83.09	I69.369	I80.219	I99.9
H40.50X4	H47.329	H59.349	H68.009	H83.19	I69.80	I80.229	J17
H40.60X0	H47.339	H59.359	H68.019	H83.2X9	I69.819	I80.291	J34.9
H40.60X1	H47.399	H59.369	H68.029	H83.3X9	I69.839	I80.299	J35.9
H40.60X2	H47.519	H59.819	H68.109	H83.8X9	I69.849	I80.9	J38.00
H40.60X3	H47.529	H60.00	H68.119	H83.90	I69.859	I82.419	J94.9
H40.60X4	H47.539	H60.10	H68.129	H83.91	I69.869	I82.429	J95.00
H40.819	H47.619	H60.20	H68.139	H83.92	I69.90	I82.439	J98.9
H40.829	H47.629	H60.319	H69.00	H83.93	I69.919	I82.449	J99
H40.839	H47.639	H60.329	H69.80	H91.09	I69.939	I82.499	K00*
H42	H47.649	H60.339	H69.90	H91.10	I69.949	I82.4Y9	K01*
H43.00	H47.9	H60.399	H70.009	H91.20	I69.959	I82.4Z9	K02*
H43.10	H49.00	H60.40	H70.019	H91.8X9	I69.965	I82.509	K03*
H43.20	H49.10	H60.509	H70.099	H91.90	I69.969	I82.519	K04*
H43.319	H49.20	H60.519	H70.10	H92.09	I70.209	I82.529	K05*
H43.399	H49.30	H60.529	H70.209	H92.10	I70.219	I82.539	K06*
H43.819	H49.40	H60.539	H70.219	H92.20	I70.229	I82.549	K08*
H43.829	H49.819	H60.549	H70.229	H93.019	I70.239	I82.599	K09*
H43.9	H49.889	H60.559	H70.819	H93.099	I70.249	I82.5Y9	K11.9
H44.009	H51.20	H60.599	H70.899	H93.19	I70.269	I82.5Z9	K13.70
H44.019	H51.9	H60.60	H70.90	H93.219	I70.299	I82.609	K14.9
H44.029	H52.00	H60.8X9	H71.00	H93.229	I70.309	I82.619	K22.9
H44.119	H52.10	H60.90	H71.10	H93.239	I70.319	I82.629	K23
H44.129	H52.209	H61.009	H71.20	H93.249	I70.329	I82.709	K31.9
H44.139	H52.219	H61.019	H71.30	H93.299	I70.339	I82.719	K38.9
H44.20	H52.229	H61.029	H71.90	H93.3X9	I70.349	I82.729	K46.1
H44.2A9	H52.519	H61.039	H72.00	H93.8X9	I70.369	I82.819	K46.9
H44.2B9	H52.529	H61.109	H72.10	H93.90	I70.399	I82.90	K50.019
H44.2C9	H52.539	H61.119	H72.2X9	H93.91	I70.409	I82.91	K50.119
H44.2D9	H52.7	H61.129	H72.819	H93.92	I70.419	I82.A19	K50.819
H44.2E9	H53.009	H61.199	H72.829	H93.93	I70.429	I82.A29	K50.919
H44.30	H53.019	H61.20	H72.90	H93.A9	I70.439	I82.B19	K51.019
H44.319	H53.029	H61.309	H73.009	H94*	I70.449	I82.B29	K51.219
H44.329	H53.039	H61.319	H73.019	H95.00	I70.469	I82.C19	K51.319
H44.399	H53.049	H61.329	H73.099	H95.119	I70.499	I82.C29	K51.419
H44.419	H53.10	H61.399	H73.10	H95.129	I70.509	I83.001	K51.519
H44.429	H53.129	H61.819	H73.20	H95.139	I70.519	I83.002	K51.819
H44.439	H53.139	H61.899	H73.819	H95.199	I70.529	I83.003	K51.919
H44.449	H53.149	H61.90	H73.829	H95.819	I70.539	I83.004	K56.600
H44.50	H53.30	H61.91	H73.899	I21.A9	I70.549	I83.005	K56.601
H44.519	H53.419	H61.92	H73.90	I25.2	I70.569	I83.008	K56.609
H44.529	H53.429	H61.93	H74.09	I39	I70.599	I83.009	K62.9
H44.539	H53.439	H62.40	H74.19	I41	I70.609	I83.019	K63.9
H44.609	H53.459	H62.41	H74.20	I46.2	I70.619	I83.029	K66.9
H44.619	H53.469	H62.42	H74.319	I46.8	I70.629	I83.10	K67
H44.629	H53.489	H62.43	H74.329	I52	I70.639	I83.201	K71.9
H44.639	H53.50	H62.8X1	H74.399	I68.2	I70.649	I83.202	K76.9
H44.649	H53.60	H62.8X2	H74.40	I68.8	I70.669	I83.203	K77
H44.659	H53.9	H62.8X3	H74.8X9	I69.00	I70.699	I83.204	K82.9
H44.699	H54.40	H62.8X9	H74.90	I69.019	I70.709	I83.205	K83.9
H44.709	H54.50	H65.00	H74.91	I69.039	I70.719	I83.208	K86.9
H44.719	H54.60	H65.07	H74.92	I69.049	I70.729	I83.209	K87
H44.739	H54.7	H65.117	H74.93	I69.059	I70.739	I83.219	K92.9
H44.749	H57.059	H65.119	H75*	I69.069	I70.749	I83.229	K94.00
H44.759	H57.10	H65.197	H80.00	I69.119	I70.769	I83.819	K94.10
H44.799	H57.811	H65.199	H80.10	I69.139	I70.799	I83.90	K94.20
H44.819	H57.812	H65.20	H80.20	I69.149	I71.8	I87.009	K94.30
H44.829	H57.813	H65.30	H80.80	I69.159	I71.9	I87.019	L02.419
H44.9	H57.819	H65.419	H80.90	I69.169	I72.9	I87.029	L02.429
H46.00	H57.9	H65.499	H81.09	I69.20	I74.4	I87.039	L02.439
H46.10	H59.019	H65.90	H81.10	I69.219	I74.9	I87.099	L02.519
H46.9	H59.029	H66.007	H81.20	I69.239	I75.019	I87.309	L02.529
H47.019	H59.039	H66.009	H81.319	I69.249	I75.029	I87.319	L02.539

L02.619	L89.309	L97.801	M02.239	M05.579	M08.049	M10.429	M12.369
L02.629	L89.319	L97.802	M02.249	M05.619	M08.059	M10.439	M12.379
L02.639	L89.329	L97.803	M02.259	M05.629	M08.069	M10.449	M12.40
L02.91	L89.40	L97.804	M02.269	M05.639	M08.079	M10.459	M12.419
L02.92	L89.500	L97.805	M02.279	M05.649	M08.20	M10.469	M12.429
L02.93	L89.501	L97.806	M02.30	M05.659	M08.219	M10.479	M12.439
L03.019	L89.502	L97.808	M02.319	M05.669	M08.229	M11.00	M12.449
L03.029	L89.503	L97.809	M02.329	M05.679	M08.239	M11.019	M12.459
L03.039	L89.504	L97.901	M02.339	M05.711	M08.249	M11.029	M12.469
L03.049	L89.509	L97.902	M02.349	M05.719	M08.259	M11.039	M12.479
L03.119	L89.519	L97.903	M02.359	M05.729	M08.269	M11.049	M12.50
L03.129	L89.529	L97.904	M02.369	M05.739	M08.279	M11.059	M12.519
L03.90	L89.600	L97.905	M02.379	M05.749	M08.40	M11.069	M12.529
L03.91	L89.601	L97.906	M02.80	M05.759	M08.419	M11.079	M12.539
L04.9	L89.602	L97.908	M02.819	M05.769	M08.429	M11.10	M12.549
L14	L89.603	L97.909	M02.829	M05.779	M08.439	M11.119	M12.559
L29.9	L89.604	L98.9	M02.839	M05.80	M08.449	M11.121	M12.569
L45	L89.609	L99	M02.849	M05.819	M08.459	M11.129	M12.579
L49*	L89.619	M00.00	M02.859	M05.829	M08.469	M11.139	M12.80
L53.9	L89.629	M00.019	M02.869	M05.839	M08.479	M11.149	M12.819
L54	L89.819	M00.029	M02.879	M05.849	M08.80	M11.159	M12.829
L55.9	L89.899	M00.039	M02.9	M05.859	M08.819	M11.169	M12.839
L60.3	L89.90	M00.049	M04.9	M05.869	M08.829	M11.179	M12.849
L60.4	L89.91	M00.059	M05.00	M05.879	M08.839	M11.20	M12.859
L60.5	L89.92	M00.069	M05.019	M05.9	M08.849	M11.219	M12.869
L60.9	L89.93	M00.079	M05.029	M06.00	M08.859	M11.229	M12.879
L62	L89.94	M00.10	M05.039	M06.019	M08.869	M11.239	M13.10
L65.9	L89.95	M00.119	M05.049	M06.029	M08.879	M11.249	M13.119
L67.1	L90.9	M00.129	M05.059	M06.039	M08.90	M11.259	M13.129
L67.8	L91.9	M00.139	M05.069	M06.049	M08.919	M11.269	M13.139
L67.9	L94.9	M00.149	M05.079	M06.059	M08.929	M11.279	M13.149
L73.9	L97.101	M00.159	M05.10	M06.069	M08.939	M11.80	M13.159
L81.2	L97.102	M00.169	M05.119	M06.079	M08.949	M11.819	M13.169
L81.3	L97.103	M00.179	M05.129	M06.20	M08.959	M11.829	M13.179
L81.9	L97.104	M00.20	M05.139	M06.219	M08.969	M11.839	M13.829
L85.9	L97.105	M00.219	M05.149	M06.229	M08.979	M11.849	M13.839
L86	L97.106	M00.229	M05.159	M06.239	M10.00	M11.859	M13.849
L87.9	L97.108	M00.239	M05.169	M06.249	M10.019	M11.869	M13.859
L89.000	L97.109	M00.249	M05.179	M06.259	M10.029	M11.879	M13.869
L89.001	L97.201	M00.259	M05.20	M06.269	M10.039	M11.9	M13.879
L89.002	L97.202	M00.269	M05.219	M06.279	M10.049	M12.00	M14.60
L89.003	L97.203	M00.279	M05.229	M06.30	M10.059	M12.019	M14.619
L89.004	L97.204	M00.80	M05.239	M06.319	M10.069	M12.029	M14.629
L89.009	L97.205	M00.819	M05.249	M06.329	M10.079	M12.039	M14.639
L89.019	L97.206	M00.829	M05.259	M06.339	M10.10	M12.049	M14.649
L89.029	L97.208	M00.839	M05.269	M06.349	M10.119	M12.059	M14.659
L89.100	L97.209	M00.849	M05.279	M06.359	M10.129	M12.069	M14.669
L89.101	L97.302	M00.859	M05.30	M06.369	M10.139	M12.079	M14.679
L89.102	L97.303	M00.869	M05.319	M06.379	M10.149	M12.10	M14.80
L89.103	L97.304	M00.879	M05.329	M06.80	M10.159	M12.119	M14.811
L89.104	L97.305	M01*	M05.339	M06.819	M10.169	M12.129	M14.812
L89.109	L97.306	M02.00	M05.349	M06.829	M10.179	M12.139	M14.819
L89.119	L97.308	M02.019	M05.359	M06.839	M10.20	M12.149	M14.821
L89.129	L97.309	M02.029	M05.369	M06.849	M10.219	M12.159	M14.822
L89.139	L97.401	M02.039	M05.379	M06.859	M10.229	M12.169	M14.829
L89.149	L97.402	M02.049	M05.40	M06.869	M10.239	M12.179	M14.831
L89.159	L97.403	M02.059	M05.419	M06.879	M10.249	M12.20	M14.832
L89.200	L97.404	M02.069	M05.429	M06.9	M10.259	M12.219	M14.839
L89.201	L97.405	M02.079	M05.439	M07.60	M10.269	M12.229	M14.841
L89.202	L97.406	M02.10	M05.449	M07.619	M10.279	M12.239	M14.842
L89.203	L97.408	M02.119	M05.459	M07.629	M10.30	M12.249	M14.849
L89.204	L97.409	M02.129	M05.469	M07.639	M10.319	M12.259	M14.851
L89.209	L97.501	M02.139	M05.479	M07.649	M10.329	M12.269	M14.852
L89.219	L97.502	M02.149	M05.50	M07.659	M10.339	M12.279	M14.859
L89.229	L97.503	M02.159	M05.519	M07.669	M10.349	M12.30	M14.861
L89.300	L97.504	M02.169	M05.529	M07.679	M10.359	M12.319	M14.862
L89.301	L97.505	M02.179	M05.539	M08.00	M10.369	M12.329	M14.869
L89.302	L97.506	M02.20	M05.549	M08.019	M10.379	M12.339	M14.871
L89.303	L97.508	M02.219	M05.559	M08.029	M10.40	M12.349	M14.872
L89.304	L97.509	M02.229	M05.569	M08.039	M10.419	M12.359	M14.879

Appendix I: Patient-Driven Groupings Model (PDGM) Return-to-Provider Code List

M14.88	M1A.2390	M21.249	M23.649	M24.829	M25.571	M40.40	M60.005
M14.89	M1A.2391	M21.259	M23.679	M24.839	M25.572	M40.50	M60.009
M16.10	M1A.2490	M21.269	M23.8X9	M24.849	M25.579	M41.00	M60.019
M16.30	M1A.2491	M21.279	M23.90	M24.859	M25.60	M41.119	M60.029
M16.50	M1A.2590	M21.339	M23.91	M24.873	M25.611	M41.129	M60.039
M16.9	M1A.2591	M21.379	M23.92	M24.876	M25.612	M41.30	M60.043
M17.10	M1A.2690	M21.40	M24.00	M24.9	M25.619	M41.40	M60.044
M17.30	M1A.2691	M21.519	M24.019	M25.00	M25.621	M41.50	M60.045
M17.9	M1A.2790	M21.529	M24.029	M25.019	M25.622	M41.80	M60.046
M18.10	M1A.2791	M21.539	M24.039	M25.029	M25.629	M42.00	M60.059
M18.30	M1A.30X0	M21.549	M24.049	M25.039	M25.631	M42.10	M60.069
M18.50	M1A.30X1	M21.619	M24.059	M25.049	M25.632	M43.00	M60.072
M18.9	M1A.3190	M21.629	M24.073	M25.059	M25.639	M43.10	M60.075
M19.019	M1A.3191	M21.6X9	M24.076	M25.069	M25.641	M43.20	M60.078
M19.029	M1A.3290	M21.70	M24.10	M25.073	M25.642	M43.5X9	M60.10
M19.039	M1A.3291	M21.729	M24.119	M25.076	M25.649	M43.8X9	M60.119
M19.049	M1A.3390	M21.739	M24.129	M25.10	M25.651	M43.9	M60.129
M19.079	M1A.3391	M21.759	M24.139	M25.119	M25.652	M45.9	M60.132
M19.119	M1A.3490	M21.769	M24.149	M25.129	M25.659	M46.00	M60.139
M19.129	M1A.3491	M21.80	M24.159	M25.139	M25.661	M46.20	M60.149
M19.139	M1A.3590	M21.829	M24.173	M25.149	M25.662	M46.30	M60.159
M19.149	M1A.3591	M21.839	M24.176	M25.159	M25.669	M46.40	M60.169
M19.179	M1A.3690	M21.859	M24.20	M25.169	M25.671	M46.50	M60.179
M19.219	M1A.3691	M21.869	M24.219	M25.173	M25.672	M46.80	M60.20
M19.229	M1A.3790	M21.90	M24.229	M25.176	M25.673	M46.90	M60.219
M19.239	M1A.3791	M21.929	M24.239	M25.20	M25.674	M47.019	M60.229
M19.249	M1A.40X0	M21.939	M24.249	M25.219	M25.675	M47.029	M60.239
M19.279	M1A.40X1	M21.949	M24.259	M25.229	M25.676	M47.10	M60.249
M19.90	M1A.4190	M21.959	M24.273	M25.239	M25.70	M47.20	M60.259
M19.91	M1A.4191	M21.969	M24.276	M25.249	M25.719	M47.819	M60.269
M19.92	M1A.4290	M22.00	M24.30	M25.259	M25.729	M47.899	M60.279
M19.93	M1A.4291	M22.10	M24.319	M25.269	M25.739	M47.9	M60.80
M1A.00X0	M1A.4390	M22.2X9	M24.329	M25.279	M25.749	M48.00	M60.819
M1A.00X1	M1A.4391	M22.3X9	M24.339	M25.30	M25.759	M48.20	M60.829
M1A.0190	M1A.4490	M22.40	M24.349	M25.319	M25.769	M48.30	M60.839
M1A.0191	M1A.4491	M22.8X9	M24.359	M25.329	M25.773	M48.40X-	M60.849
M1A.0290	M1A.4591	M22.90	M24.369	M25.339	M25.776	M48.50X-	M60.859
M1A.0291	M1A.4690	M23.002	M24.373	M25.349	M25.80	M48.8X9	M60.869
M1A.0390	M1A.4691	M23.005	M24.376	M25.359	M25.819	M49.80	M60.879
M1A.0391	M1A.4790	M23.009	M24.40	M25.369	M25.829	M49.81	M60.9
M1A.0490	M1A.4791	M23.019	M24.419	M25.373	M25.839	M49.82	M61.00
M1A.0491	M20.001	M23.029	M24.429	M25.376	M25.849	M49.83	M61.019
M1A.0590	M20.002	M23.039	M24.439	M25.40	M25.859	M49.84	M61.029
M1A.0591	M20.009	M23.049	M24.443	M25.419	M25.869	M49.85	M61.039
M1A.0690	M20.019	M23.059	M24.446	M25.429	M25.879	M49.86	M61.049
M1A.0691	M20.029	M23.069	M24.459	M25.439	M25.9	M49.87	M61.059
M1A.0790	M20.039	M23.202	M24.469	M25.449	M26*	M49.88	M61.069
M1A.0791	M20.099	M23.205	M24.473	M25.459	M27.0	M49.89	M61.079
M1A.10X0	M20.10	M23.209	M24.476	M25.469	M27.1	M50.020	M61.10
M1A.10X1	M20.20	M23.219	M24.479	M25.473	M27.3	M50.10	M61.119
M1A.1190	M20.30	M23.229	M24.50	M25.476	M27.40	M50.120	M61.129
M1A.1191	M20.40	M23.239	M24.519	M25.50	M27.49	M50.20	M61.139
M1A.1290	M20.5X9	M23.249	M24.529	M25.511	M27.51	M50.220	M61.143
M1A.1291	M20.60	M23.259	M24.539	M25.512	M27.52	M50.30	M61.146
M1A.1390	M20.61	M23.269	M24.549	M25.519	M27.53	M50.320	M61.159
M1A.1391	M20.62	M23.302	M24.559	M25.521	M27.59	M50.80	M61.169
M1A.1490	M21.00	M23.305	M24.569	M25.522	M27.61	M50.820	M61.173
M1A.1491	M21.029	M23.309	M24.573	M25.529	M27.62	M50.90	M61.176
M1A.1590	M21.059	M23.319	M24.576	M25.531	M27.63	M50.920	M61.179
M1A.1591	M21.069	M23.329	M24.60	M25.532	M27.69	M53.2X9	M61.20
M1A.1690	M21.079	M23.339	M24.619	M25.539	M27.8	M53.80	M61.219
M1A.1691	M21.10	M23.349	M24.629	M25.541	M27.9	M53.9	M61.229
M1A.1790	M21.129	M23.359	M24.639	M25.542	M35.9	M54.00	M61.239
M1A.1791	M21.159	M23.369	M24.649	M25.549	M36.4	M54.10	M61.249
M1A.20X0	M21.169	M23.40	M24.659	M25.551	M36.8	M54.30	M61.259
M1A.20X1	M21.179	M23.50	M24.669	M25.552	M40.00	M54.40	M61.269
M1A.2190	M21.20	M23.609	M24.673	M25.559	M40.10	M54.5	M61.279
M1A.2191	M21.219	M23.619	M24.676	M25.561	M40.209	M54.6	M61.30
M1A.2290	M21.229	M23.629	M24.80	M25.562	M40.299	M54.9	M61.319
M1A.2291	M21.239	M23.639	M24.819	M25.569	M40.30	M60.002	M61.329

M61.339	M62.50	M66.319	M70.839	M75.90X	M84.319-	M85.169	M86.329
M61.349	M62.519	M66.329	M70.849	M76.00	M84.329-	M85.179	M86.339
M61.359	M62.529	M66.339	M70.859	M76.10	M84.339-	M85.2	M86.349
M61.369	M62.539	M66.349	M70.869	M76.20	M84.343-	M85.30	M86.359
M61.379	M62.549	M66.359	M70.879	M76.30	M84.346-	M85.319	M86.369
M61.40	M62.559	M66.369	M70.90	M76.40	M84.353-	M85.329	M86.379
M61.419	M62.569	M66.379	M70.919	M76.50	M84.359-	M85.339	M86.40
M61.429	M62.579	M66.80	M70.929	M76.60	M84.369-	M85.349	M86.419
M61.439	M62.81	M66.819	M70.939	M76.70	M84.373-	M85.359	M86.429
M61.449	M62.831	M66.829	M70.949	M76.819	M84.376-	M85.369	M86.439
M61.459	M62.838	M66.839	M70.959	M76.829	M84.379-	M85.379	M86.449
M61.469	M62.9	M66.849	M70.969	M76.899	M84.40X-	M85.40	M86.459
M61.479	M63*	M66.859	M70.979	M77.00	M84.419-	M85.419	M86.469
M61.50	M65.00	M66.869	M71.00	M77.10	M84.429-	M85.429	M86.479
M61.519	M65.019	M66.879	M71.019	M77.20	M84.439-	M85.439	M86.50
M61.529	M65.029	M66.9	M71.029	M77.30	M84.443-	M85.449	M86.519
M61.539	M65.039	M67.00	M71.039	M77.40	M84.446-	M85.459	M86.529
M61.549	M65.049	M67.20	M71.049	M77.50	M84.453-	M85.469	M86.539
M61.559	M65.059	M67.219	M71.059	M77.9	M84.459-	M85.479	M86.549
M61.569	M65.069	M67.229	M71.069	M79.601	M84.469-	M85.50	M86.559
M61.579	M65.079	M67.239	M71.079	M79.602	M84.473-	M85.519	M86.569
M61.9	M65.10	M67.249	M71.10	M79.603	M84.476-	M85.529	M86.579
M62.00	M65.119	M67.259	M71.119	M79.604	M84.479-	M85.539	M86.60
M62.019	M65.129	M67.269	M71.129	M79.605	M84.50X-	M85.549	M86.619
M62.029	M65.139	M67.279	M71.139	M79.606	M84.519-	M85.559	M86.629
M62.039	M65.149	M67.30	M71.149	M79.609	M84.529-	M85.569	M86.639
M62.049	M65.159	M67.319	M71.159	M79.621	M84.539-	M85.579	M86.649
M62.059	M65.169	M67.329	M71.169	M79.622	M84.549-	M85.619	M86.659
M62.069	M65.179	M67.339	M71.179	M79.629	M84.553-	M85.629	M86.669
M62.079	M65.20	M67.349	M71.20	M79.631	M84.559-	M85.639	M86.679
M62.10	M65.229	M67.359	M71.30	M79.632	M84.569-	M85.649	M86.9
M62.119	M65.239	M67.369	M71.319	M79.639	M84.573-	M85.659	M87.00
M62.129	M65.249	M67.379	M71.329	M79.641	M84.576-	M85.669	M87.011
M62.139	M65.259	M67.40	M71.339	M79.642	M84.60X-	M85.679	M87.019
M62.149	M65.269	M67.419	M71.349	M79.643	M84.619-	M85.80	M87.029
M62.159	M65.279	M67.429	M71.359	M79.644	M84.629-	M85.819	M87.033
M62.169	M65.30	M67.439	M71.379	M79.645	M84.639-	M85.829	M87.036
M62.179	M65.319	M67.449	M71.40	M79.646	M84.649-	M85.839	M87.039
M62.20	M65.329	M67.459	M71.429	M79.651	M84.653-	M85.849	M87.043
M62.219	M65.339	M67.469	M71.439	M79.652	M84.659-	M85.859	M87.046
M62.229	M65.349	M67.479	M71.449	M79.659	M84.669-	M85.869	M87.059
M62.239	M65.359	M67.50	M71.459	M79.661	M84.679-	M85.879	M87.063
M62.249	M65.80	M67.80	M71.469	M79.662	M84.676-	M85.9	M87.066
M62.259	M65.819	M67.819	M71.479	M79.669	M84.750-	M86.00	M87.073
M62.269	M65.829	M67.829	M71.50	M79.671	M84.753-	M86.019	M87.076
M62.279	M65.839	M67.839	M71.529	M79.672	M84.756-	M86.029	M87.079
M62.40	M65.849	M67.849	M71.539	M79.673	M84.759-	M86.039	M87.10
M62.411	M65.859	M67.859	M71.549	M79.674	M84.80	M86.049	M87.119
M62.412	M65.869	M67.869	M71.559	M79.675	M84.819	M86.059	M87.129
M62.419	M65.879	M67.879	M71.569	M79.676	M84.829	M86.069	M87.133
M62.421	M65.9	M67.90	M71.579	M79.9	M84.839	M86.079	M87.136
M62.422	M66.10	M67.919	M71.80	M79.A19	M84.849	M86.10	M87.139
M62.429	M66.119	M67.929	M71.819	M79.A29	M84.859	M86.119	M87.143
M62.431	M66.129	M67.939	M71.829	M80.00X-	M84.869	M86.129	M87.146
M62.432	M66.139	M67.949	M71.839	M80.019-	M84.879	M86.139	M87.159
M62.439	M66.143	M67.959	M71.849	M80.029-	M84.9	M86.149	M87.163
M62.441	M66.146	M67.969	M71.859	M80.039-	M85.00	M86.159	M87.166
M62.442	M66.159	M67.979	M71.869	M80.049-	M85.019	M86.169	M87.173
M62.449	M66.173	M70.039	M71.879	M80.059-	M85.029	M86.179	M87.176
M62.451	M66.176	M70.049	M71.9	M80.069-	M85.039	M86.20	M87.179
M62.452	M66.179	M70.10	M72.9	M80.079-	M85.049	M86.219	M87.20
M62.459	M66.20	M70.20	M75.00	M80.80X-	M85.059	M86.229	M87.219
M62.461	M66.219	M70.30	M75.100	M80.819-	M85.069	M86.239	M87.229
M62.462	M66.229	M70.40	M75.110	M80.829-	M85.079	M86.249	M87.233
M62.469	M66.239	M70.50	M75.120	M80.839-	M85.10	M86.259	M87.236
M62.471	M66.249	M70.60	M75.20	M80.849-	M85.119	M86.269	M87.239
M62.472	M66.259	M70.70	M75.30	M80.859-	M85.129	M86.279	M87.243
M62.479	M66.269	M70.80	M75.40	M80.869-	M85.139	M86.30	M87.246
M62.48	M66.279	M70.819	M75.50	M80.879-	M85.149	M86.319	M87.256
M62.49	M66.30	M70.829	M75.80	M04.30X	M85.159	M86.319	M87.263

M87.266	M89.419	M90.859	N00.9	N83.529	O23.90	O30.111	O40.9XX3
M87.273	M89.429	M90.869	N01.9	N83.9	O24.019	O30.112	O40.9XX4
M87.276	M89.439	M90.879	N02.9	N84.9	O24.119	O30.113	O40.9XX5
M87.279	M89.449	M91.10	N03.9	N85.9	O24.319	O30.119	O40.9XX9
M87.30	M89.459	M91.20	N04.9	N88.9	O24.819	O30.121	O41.00X0
M87.319	M89.469	M91.30	N05.9	N89.9	O24.919	O30.122	O41.00X1
M87.329	M89.479	M91.40	N06.9	N90.9	O25.10	O30.123	O41.00X2
M87.333	M89.50	M91.80	N07.9	N91.2	O26.00	O30.129	O41.00X3
M87.336	M89.519	M91.90	N08	N91.5	O26.10	O30.131	O41.00X4
M87.339	M89.529	M92.00	N13.729	N92.0	O26.20	O30.132	O41.00X5
M87.343	M89.539	M92.10	N13.739	N92.1	O26.30	O30.133	O41.00X9
M87.346	M89.549	M92.209	N16	N92.2	O26.40	O30.139	O41.1010
M87.353	M89.559	M92.219	N18.5	N92.3	O26.50	O30.191	O41.1011
M87.363	M89.569	M92.229	N18.6	N92.6	O26.612	O30.192	O41.1012
M87.366	M89.579	M92.299	N18.9	N93.9	O26.619	O30.193	O41.1013
M87.373	M89.60	M92.30	N19	N94.9	O26.719	O30.199	O41.1014
M87.376	M89.619	M92.40	N20.9	N95.9	O26.819	O30.201	O41.1015
M87.379	M89.629	M92.50	N21.9	N97.9	O26.829	O30.202	O41.1019
M87.80	M89.639	M92.60	N22	N98.9	O26.839	O30.203	O41.1020
M87.819	M89.649	M92.70	N25.9	O09.00	O26.849	O30.209	O41.1021
M87.829	M89.659	M92.9	N26.9	O09.10	O26.859	O30.211	O41.1022
M87.833	M89.669	M93.003	N27.9	O09.219	O26.879	O30.212	O41.1023
M87.836	M89.679	M93.013	N28.9	O09.299	O26.899	O30.213	O41.1024
M87.839	M89.70	M93.023	N29	O09.30	O26.90	O30.219	O41.1025
M87.843	M89.719	M93.033	N32.9	O09.40	O26.91	O30.221	O41.1029
M87.849	M89.729	M93.20	N33	O09.519	O26.92	O30.222	O41.1030
M87.859	M89.739	M93.219	N36.9	O09.529	O26.93	O30.223	O41.1031
M87.863	M89.749	M93.229	N37	O09.619	O28*	O30.229	O41.1032
M87.869	M89.759	M93.239	N39.43	O09.629	O29.019	O30.231	O41.1033
M87.873	M89.769	M93.249	N39.44	O09.70	O29.029	O30.232	O41.1034
M87.876	M89.779	M93.259	N39.45	O09.71	O29.099	O30.233	O41.1035
M87.879	M89.8X9	M93.269	N39.9	O09.72	O29.119	O30.239	O41.1039
M87.9	M89.9	M93.279	N41.9	O09.73	O29.129	O30.291	O41.1090
M88.819	M90.50	M93.80	N42.9	O09.819	O29.199	O30.292	O41.1091
M88.829	M90.511	M93.819	N43.3	O09.829	O29.219	O30.293	O41.1092
M88.839	M90.512	M93.829	N43.40	O09.899	O29.299	O30.299	O41.1093
M88.849	M90.519	M93.839	N46*	O09.90	O29.3X9	O30.801	O41.1094
M88.859	M90.521	M93.849	N48.32	O09.A0	O29.40	O30.802	O41.1095
M88.869	M90.522	M93.859	N48.9	O10.019	O29.5X9	O30.803	O41.1099
M88.879	M90.529	M93.869	N49.9	O10.119	O29.60	O30.809	O41.1290
M88.9	M90.531	M93.879	N50.819	O10.219	O29.8X9	O30.811	O41.1291
M89.00	M90.532	M93.90	N50.9	O10.319	O29.90	O30.812	O41.1292
M89.019	M90.539	M93.919	N51	O10.419	O29.91	O30.813	O41.1293
M89.029	M90.541	M93.929	N52.1	O10.919	O29.92	O30.819	O41.1294
M89.039	M90.542	M93.939	N53.9	O11.9	O29.93	O30.821	O41.1295
M89.049	M90.549	M93.949	N60.09	O12.00	O30.001	O30.822	O41.1299
M89.059	M90.551	M93.959	N60.19	O12.10	O30.002	O30.823	O41.1490
M89.069	M90.552	M93.969	N60.29	O12.20	O30.003	O30.829	O41.1491
M89.079	M90.559	M93.979	N60.39	O13.9	O30.009	O30.831	O41.1492
M89.129	M90.561	M93.98	N60.49	O14.00	O30.011	O30.832	O41.1493
M89.139	M90.562	M94.20	N60.89	O14.20	O30.012	O30.833	O41.1494
M89.159	M90.569	M94.219	N60.99	O14.90	O30.013	O30.839	O41.1495
M89.169	M90.571	M94.229	N63.0	O15.9	O30.019	O30.891	O41.1499
M89.20	M90.572	M94.239	N64.9	O16.9	O30.029	O30.892	O41.8X90
M89.219	M90.579	M94.249	N71.9	O22.00	O30.031	O30.893	O41.8X91
M89.229	M90.58	M94.259	N73.9	O22.10	O30.032	O30.899	O41.8X92
M89.239	M90.59	M94.269	N74	O22.20	O30.033	O30.90	O41.8X93
M89.249	M90.60	M94.279	N75.9	O22.30	O30.039	O30.91	O41.8X94
M89.259	M90.619	M94.359	N77.0	O22.40	O30.041	O30.92	O41.8X95
M89.269	M90.629	M94.8X9	N77.1	O22.50	O30.042	O30.93	O41.8X99
M89.279	M90.639	M94.9	N82.9	O22.8X9	O30.043	O31*	O41.90X0
M89.30	M90.649	M95.0	N83.00	O22.90	O30.049	O32*	O41.90X1
M89.319	M90.659	M95.10	N83.10	O23.00	O30.091	O33*	O41.90X2
M89.329	M90.669	M95.9	N83.209	O23.10	O30.092	O34*	O41.90X3
M89.339	M90.679	M96.629	N83.299	O23.20	O30.093	O35*	O41.90X4
M89.349	M90.80	M96.639	N83.319	O23.30	O30.099	O36*	O41.90X9
M89.359	M90.819	M96.669	N83.329	O23.40	O30.101	O40.1XX0	O41.91X0
M89.369	M90.829	M96.679	N83.339	O23.519	O30.102	O40.9XX0	O41.91X1
M89.379	M90.839	M97.9XX-	N83.40	O23.529	O30.103	O40.9XX1	O41.91X2
M89.40	M90.849	M99.9	N83.519	O23.599	O30.109	O40.9XX2	

O41.91X3	O60.10X9	O69.89X0	P11.2	Q51.9	Q93.9	R76*	S04.10X-
O41.91X4	O60.20X0	O69.89X1	P11.9	Q52.70	Q99.9	R77*	S04.20X-
O41.91X5	O60.20X1	O69.89X2	P12.9	Q52.9	R00*	R78*	S04.30X-
O41.91X9	O60.20X2	O69.89X3	P13.9	Q53.00	R01*	R79*	S04.40X-
O41.92X0	O60.20X3	O69.89X4	P14.9	Q53.10	R03*	R80*	S04.50X-
O41.92X1	O60.20X4	O69.89X5	P15.9	Q53.9	R04*	R81	S04.60X-
O41.92X2	O60.20X5	O69.89X9	P23.9	Q55.20	R05	R82*	S04.70X-
O41.92X3	O60.20X9	O69.9XX0	P27.9	Q55.9	R06*	R83*	S04.819-
O41.92X4	O61*	O69.9XX1	P28.9	Q60.2	R07*	R84*	S04.899-
O41.92X5	O62*	O69.9XX2	P29.30	Q60.5	R09*	R85*	S04.9XX-
O41.92X9	O63*	O69.9XX3	P29.38	Q61.9	R10*	R86*	S05.00X-
O41.93X0	O64*	O69.9XX4	P29.9	Q63.9	R11*	R87*	S05.01X-
O41.93X1	O65*	O69.9XX5	P35.9	Q64.70	R12	R88*	S05.02X-
O41.93X2	O66*	O71.00	P37.9	Q64.9	R13*	R89*	S05.10X-
O41.93X3	O69.0XX0	O71.9	P39.9	Q65.00	R14*	R90*	S05.11X-
O41.93X4	O69.0XX1	O74.9	P52.3	Q65.2	R15*	R91*	S05.12X-
O41.93X5	O69.0XX2	O75.82	P52.9	Q65.30	R16*	R92*	S05.20X-
O41.93X9	O69.0XX3	O75.9	P54.9	Q65.5	R17	R93*	S05.30X-
O42.00	O69.0XX4	O77.9	P55.9	Q65.9	R18*	R94*	S05.40X-
O42.019	O69.0XX5	O80	P56.90	Q66.50	R19*	R97*	S05.50X-
O42.10	O69.0XX9	O82	P61.9	Q66.80	R20*	R99	S05.60X-
O42.119	O69.1XX0	O91.219	P72.9	Q68.5	R21	S00*	S05.70X-
O42.90	O69.1XX1	O92.019	P74.9	Q69.9	R22*	S01.109-	S05.8X9-
O42.919	O69.1XX2	O92.119	P76.9	Q70.00	R23*	S01.119-	S05.90X-
O43.019	O69.1XX3	O92.20	P77.9	Q70.10	R25*	S01.129-	S05.91X-
O43.029	O69.1XX4	O92.70	P83.9	Q70.20	R26*	S01.139-	S05.92X-
O43.101	O69.1XX5	O98.019	P91.811	Q70.30	R27*	S01.149-	S06.1X7A
O43.102	O69.1XX9	O98.119	P91.9	Q70.31	R29*	S01.159-	S06.1X8A
O43.103	O69.2XX0	O98.219	P92.9	Q71.00	R30*	S01.309-	S06.2X7A
O43.109	O69.2XX1	O98.319	P94.9	Q71.10	R31*	S01.319-	S06.2X8A
O43.119	O69.2XX2	O98.419	P95	Q71.20	R32	S01.329-	S06.307A
O43.129	O69.2XX3	O98.519	P96.83	Q71.30	R33*	S01.339-	S06.308A
O43.199	O69.2XX4	O98.619	P96.9	Q71.40	R34	S01.349-	S06.317A
O43.219	O69.2XX5	O98.719	Q00*	Q71.50	R35*	S01.359-	S06.318A
O43.229	O69.2XX9	O98.819	Q01*	Q71.60	R36*	S01.409-	S06.327A
O43.239	O69.3XX0	O98.911	Q02	Q71.819	R37	S01.419-	S06.328A
O43.819	O69.3XX1	O98.912	Q03*	Q71.899	R39*	S01.429-	S06.337A
O43.899	O69.3XX2	O98.913	Q04*	Q72.10	R40*	S01.439-	S06.338A
O43.90	O69.3XX3	O98.919	Q06*	Q72.20	R41*	S01.449-	S06.346D
O43.91	O69.3XX4	O98.92	Q07.9	Q72.30	R42	S01.459-	S06.347A
O43.92	O69.3XX5	O98.93	Q10*	Q72.40	R43*	S01.90X-	S06.348A
O43.93	O69.3XX9	O99.019	Q11*	Q72.50	R44*	S01.91X-	S06.357A
O44.00	O69.4XX0	O99.119	Q12*	Q72.60	R45*	S01.92X-	S06.358A
O44.10	O69.4XX1	O99.210	Q13*	Q72.70	R46*	S01.93X-	S06.367A
O44.20	O69.4XX2	O99.280	Q14*	Q72.819	R47*	S01.94X-	S06.368A
O44.30	O69.4XX3	O99.310	Q15*	Q72.899	R48*	S01.95X-	S06.377A
O44.40	O69.4XX4	O99.320	Q16*	Q72.90	R49*	S02.109-	S06.378A
O44.50	O69.4XX5	O99.330	Q17*	Q73.0	R50*	S02.110-	S06.387A
O45.001	O69.4XX9	O99.340	Q18*	Q73.1	R51	S02.111-	S06.388A
O45.009	O69.5XX0	O99.350	Q20.9	Q73.8	R52	S02.112-	S06.4X7A
O45.019	O69.5XX1	O99.419	Q21.9	Q74.9	R53*	S02.118-	S06.4X8A
O45.029	O69.5XX2	O99.519	Q23.9	Q75.9	R54	S02.30X-	S06.5X7A
O45.099	O69.5XX3	O99.619	Q24.9	Q76.419	R55	S02.400-	S06.5X8A
O45.8X9	O69.5XX4	O99.719	Q25.40	Q76.429	R56*	S02.401-	S06.6X7A
O45.90	O69.5XX5	O99.840	Q25.9	Q76.9	R57*	S02.402-	S06.6X8A
O46.009	O69.5XX9	O9A.119	Q27.30	Q78.9	R58	S02.5XX-	S06.817A
O46.019	O69.81X0	O9A.219	Q27.9	Q79.9	R59*	S02.600-	S06.818A
O46.029	O69.81X1	O9A.319	Q28.9	Q80*	R60*	S02.610-	S06.827A
O46.099	O69.81X2	O9A.419	Q30.9	Q81.9	R61	S02.620-	S06.828A
O46.8X9	O69.81X3	O9A.519	Q31.9	Q82.9	R62*	S02.630-	S06.898A
O46.90	O69.81X4	P00.9	Q33.9	Q83.9	R63*	S02.640-	S06.9X0-
O47.00	O69.81X5	P03.9	Q34.9	Q84.1	R64	S02.650-	S06.9X1-
O47.9	O69.81X9	P04.9	Q35*	Q84.2	R65*	S02.670-	S06.9X2-
O60.00	O69.82X0	P05.00	Q36.9	Q84.3	R68*	S02.80X-	S06.9X3-
O60.10X0	O69.82X1	P05.10	Q37.9	Q84.4	R69	S03.00X-	S06.9X4-
O60.10X1	O69.82X2	P07.00	Q39.9	Q84.5	R70*	S03.2XX-	S06.9X5-
O60.10X2	O69.82X3	P07.10	Q40.3	Q84.6	R71*	S03.40X-	S06.9X6-
O60.10X3	O69.82X4	P07.20	Q40.9	Q84.9	R73*	S04.019-	S06.9X7A
O60.10X4	O69.82X5	P07.30	Q43.9	Q89.9	R74*	S04.039-	S06.9X8A
O60.10X5	O69.82X9	P10.9	Q45.9	Q92.9	R75	S04.049-	S06.9X9-

S08.119-	S20.109-	S20.97X-	S25.99X-	S30.867-	S33.100-	S36.508-	S42.023A
S08.129-	S20.111-	S21.009-	S26.00X-	S30.870-	S33.101-	S36.509-	S42.023B
S09.10X-	S20.112-	S21.019-	S26.10X-	S30.871-	S33.30X-	S36.519-	S42.023D
S09.11X-	S20.119-	S21.029-	S26.90X-	S30.872-	S34.101-	S36.529-	S42.023G
S09.19X-	S20.121-	S21.039-	S27.301-	S30.873-	S34.102-	S36.539-	S42.023K
S09.20X-	S20.122-	S21.049-	S27.302-	S30.874-	S34.103-	S36.599-	S42.023P
S09.301-	S20.129-	S21.059-	S27.309-	S30.875-	S34.104-	S36.60X-	S42.026-
S09.302-	S20.141-	S21.139-	S27.339-	S30.876-	S34.105-	S36.899-	S42.033-
S09.309-	S20.142-	S21.149-	S27.399-	S30.877-	S34.109-	S36.90X-	S42.036-
S09.319-	S20.149-	S21.159-	S27.401-	S30.91X-	S34.119-	S36.92X-	S42.109-
S09.399-	S20.151-	S21.239-	S27.402-	S30.92X-	S34.129-	S36.93X-	S42.113-
S09.90X-	S20.152-	S21.249-	S27.409-	S30.93X-	S34.139-	S36.99X-	S42.116-
S09.91X-	S20.159-	S21.259-	S27.419-	S30.94X-	S34.9XX-	S37.001-	S42.123-
S09.92X-	S20.161-	S21.339-	S27.429-	S30.95X-	S35.00X-	S37.002-	S42.126-
S09.93X-	S20.162-	S21.349-	S27.439-	S30.96X-	S35.10X-	S37.009-	S42.133-
S10*	S20.169-	S21.359-	S27.499-	S30.97X-	S35.219-	S37.029-	S42.136-
S11.93X-	S20.171-	S21.439-	S27.50X-	S30.98X-	S35.229-	S37.039-	S42.143-
S11.94X-	S20.172-	S21.449-	S27.60X-	S31.139-	S35.239-	S37.049-	S42.146-
S11.95X-	S20.179-	S21.459-	S27.809-	S31.149-	S35.299-	S37.059-	S42.153-
S14.101-	S20.20X-	S21.93X-	S27.819-	S31.159-	S35.319-	S37.099-	S42.156-
S14.102-	S20.219-	S21.94X-	S27.899-	S31.501-	S35.329-	S37.10X-	S42.199-
S14.103-	S20.229-	S21.95X-	S27.9XX-	S31.502-	S35.339-	S37.20X-	S42.209-
S14.104-	S20.301-	S22.39X-	S28.219-	S31.511-	S35.349-	S37.30X-	S42.213-
S14.105-	S20.302-	S22.49X-	S28.229-	S31.512-	S35.401-	S37.401-	S42.216-
S14.106-	S20.309-	S23.100-	S29.001-	S31.521-	S35.402-	S37.402-	S42.223-
S14.107-	S20.311-	S23.101-	S29.002-	S31.522-	S35.403-	S37.409-	S42.226-
S14.108-	S20.312-	S23.20X-	S29.009-	S31.531-	S35.404-	S37.429-	S42.239-
S14.109-	S20.319-	S23.29X-	S29.029-	S31.532-	S35.405-	S37.439-	S42.249-
S14.119-	S20.321-	S24.101-	S29.099-	S31.541-	S35.406-	S37.499-	S42.253-
S14.129-	S20.322-	S24.102-	S29.9XX-	S31.542-	S35.413-	S37.501-	S42.256-
S14.139-	S20.329-	S24.103-	S30.202D	S31.551-	S35.416-	S37.502-	S42.263-
S14.149-	S20.341-	S24.104-	S30.202S	S31.552-	S35.493-	S37.509-	S42.266-
S14.159-	S20.342-	S24.109-	S30.810-	S31.639-	S35.496-	S37.519-	S42.279-
S14.9XX-	S20.349-	S24.119-	S30.811-	S31.649-	S35.50X-	S37.529-	S42.293-
S15.001-	S20.351-	S24.139-	S30.812-	S31.659-	S35.513-	S37.539-	S42.296-
S15.002-	S20.352-	S24.149-	S30.813-	S31.801-	S35.516-	S37.599-	S42.309-
S15.009-	S20.359-	S24.159-	S30.814-	S31.802-	S35.533-	S37.60X-	S42.319-
S15.019A	S20.361-	S24.9XX-	S30.815-	S31.803-	S35.536-	S37.819-	S42.323-
S15.019S	S20.362-	S25.00X-	S30.816-	S31.804-	S35.8X9-	S37.829-	S42.326-
S15.029D	S20.369-	S25.101-	S30.817-	S31.805-	S35.90X-	S37.899-	S42.333-
S15.029S	S20.371-	S25.102-	S30.820-	S31.809-	S35.91X-	S37.90X-	S42.336-
S15.099-	S20.372-	S25.109-	S30.821-	S32.309-	S35.99X-	S37.92X-	S42.343-
S15.101-	S20.379-	S25.119-	S30.822-	S32.313-	S36.00X-	S37.93X-	S42.346-
S15.102-	S20.401-	S25.129-	S30.823-	S32.316-	S36.029-	S37.99X-	S42.353-
S15.109-	S20.402-	S25.199-	S30.824-	S32.399-	S36.039-	S38.001-	S42.356-
S15.119S	S20.409-	S25.20X-	S30.825-	S32.409-	S36.119-	S38.002-	S42.363-
S15.129A	S20.411-	S25.301-	S30.826-	S32.413-	S36.129-	S39.001-	S42.366-
S15.199-	S20.412-	S25.302-	S30.827-	S32.423-	S36.200-	S39.002-	S42.399-
S15.201-	S20.419-	S25.309-	S30.840-	S32.426-	S36.201-	S39.003-	S42.409-
S15.202-	S20.421-	S25.319-	S30.841-	S32.433-	S36.202-	S39.91X-	S42.413-
S15.209-	S20.422-	S25.329-	S30.842-	S32.436-	S36.209-	S39.92X-	S42.416-
S15.219-	S20.429-	S25.399-	S30.843-	S32.443-	S36.229-	S39.93X-	S42.423-
S15.229-	S20.441-	S25.401-	S30.844-	S32.446-	S36.239-	S39.94X-	S42.426-
S15.299-	S20.442-	S25.402-	S30.845-	S32.453-	S36.249-	S40*	S42.433-
S15.301-	S20.449-	S25.409-	S30.846-	S32.456-	S36.259-	S41.009-	S42.436-
S15.302-	S20.451-	S25.419-	S30.850-	S32.463-	S36.269-	S41.019-	S42.443-
S15.309-	S20.452-	S25.429-	S30.851-	S32.466-	S36.299D	S41.029-	S42.446-
S15.319-	S20.459-	S25.499-	S30.852-	S32.473-	S36.299S	S41.039-	S42.449-
S15.329-	S20.461-	S25.501-	S30.853-	S32.476-	S36.30X-	S41.049-	S42.453-
S15.399-	S20.462-	S25.502-	S30.854-	S32.483-	S36.400-	S41.059-	S42.456-
S15.9XX-	S20.469-	S25.509-	S30.855-	S32.486-	S36.408-	S41.109-	S42.463-
S16.8XX-	S20.471-	S25.519S	S30.856-	S32.499-	S36.409-	S41.119-	S42.466-
S16.9XX-	S20.472-	S25.599-	S30.857-	S32.509-	S36.419-	S41.129-	S42.473-
S17.9XX-	S20.479-	S25.801-	S30.860-	S32.519-	S36.429-	S41.139-	S42.476-
S19.9XX-	S20.90X-	S25.802-	S30.861-	S32.599-	S36.439-	S41.149-	S42.489-
S20.00X-	S20.91X-	S25.809-	S30.862-	S32.609-	S36.499-	S41.159-	S42.493-
S20.01X-	S20.92X-	S25.819-	S30.863-	S32.613-	S36.500-	S42.009-	S42.496-
S20.02X-	S20.94X-	S25.899-	S30.864-	S32.616-	S36.501-	S42.013-	S42.90X-
S20.101-	S20.95X-	S25.90X-	S30.865-	S32.699-	S36.502-	S42.016-	S43.003-
S20.102-	S20.96X-	S25.91X-	S30.866-	S32.9XX-	S36.503-	S42.019-	S43.006-

S43.013-	S45.901-	S49.149S	S52.389H	S53.133-	S56.301-	S59.911-	S62.209-
S43.016-	S45.902-	S49.199-	S52.389J	S53.136-	S56.302-	S59.912-	S62.213-
S43.023-	S45.909-	S49.80X-	S52.389K	S53.143-	S56.309-	S59.919-	S62.223-
S43.026-	S45.911-	S49.90X-	S52.389M	S53.146-	S56.319-	S60*	S62.226-
S43.033-	S45.912-	S49.91X-	S52.389N	S53.193-	S56.399-	S61.009-	S62.233-
S43.036-	S45.919-	S49.92X-	S52.389P	S53.196-	S56.401-	S61.019-	S62.236-
S43.083-	S45.991-	S50*	S52.389Q	S53.20X-	S56.402-	S61.029-	S62.243-
S43.086-	S45.992-	S51.009-	S52.389R	S53.30X-	S56.403-	S61.039-	S62.246-
S43.109-	S45.999-	S51.019-	S52.389S	S53.409-	S56.404-	S61.049-	S62.256-
S43.119-	S46.001-	S51.029-	S52.399-	S53.419-	S56.405-	S61.059-	S62.308-
S43.129-	S46.002-	S51.039-	S52.509-	S53.429-	S56.406-	S61.109-	S62.309-
S43.139-	S46.009-	S51.049-	S52.513-	S53.439-	S56.407-	S61.119-	S62.319B
S43.149-	S46.019-	S51.059-	S52.516-	S53.449-	S56.408-	S61.129-	S62.319D
S43.159-	S46.029-	S51.809-	S52.529-	S53.499-	S56.409-	S61.139-	S62.319G
S43.203-	S46.099-	S51.819-	S52.539-	S54.00X-	S56.419-	S61.149-	S62.319K
S43.206-	S46.101-	S51.829-	S52.549-	S54.10X-	S56.429-	S61.159-	S62.319P
S43.213-	S46.102-	S51.839-	S52.559-	S54.20X-	S56.499-	S61.209-	S62.319S
S43.216-	S46.109-	S51.849-	S52.569-	S54.30X-	S56.501-	S61.219-	S62.329-
S43.223-	S46.119-	S51.859-	S52.579-	S54.8X9-	S56.502-	S61.229-	S62.339-
S43.226-	S46.129-	S52.009-	S52.599-	S54.90X-	S56.509-	S61.239-	S62.349-
S43.303-	S46.199-	S52.019-	S52.609-	S54.91X-	S56.519-	S61.249-	S62.359-
S43.306-	S46.201-	S52.023-	S52.613-	S54.92X-	S56.529-	S61.259-	S62.369-
S43.313-	S46.202-	S52.026-	S52.616B	S55.001-	S56.599-	S61.309-	S62.399-
S43.316-	S46.209-	S52.033-	S52.616C	S55.002-	S56.801-	S61.319-	S62.509-
S43.393-	S46.219-	S52.036-	S52.616D	S55.009-	S56.802-	S61.329-	S62.513-
S43.396-	S46.229-	S52.043-	S52.616E	S55.019-	S56.809-	S61.339-	S62.516-
S43.409-	S46.299-	S52.046-	S52.616F	S55.099-	S56.819-	S61.349-	S62.523-
S43.419-	S46.301-	S52.099-	S52.616G	S55.101-	S56.829-	S61.359-	S62.526-
S43.429-	S46.302-	S52.109-	S52.616H	S55.102-	S56.899-	S61.409-	S62.609-
S43.439-	S46.309-	S52.119-	S52.616J	S55.109-	S56.901-	S61.419-	S62.619-
S43.499-	S46.319-	S52.123-	S52.616K	S55.119-	S56.902-	S61.429-	S62.629-
S43.50X-	S46.329-	S52.126-	S52.616M	S55.199-	S56.909-	S61.439-	S62.639-
S43.60X-	S46.399-	S52.133-	S52.616N	S55.201-	S56.991-	S61.449-	S62.649-
S43.80X-	S46.801-	S52.136-	S52.616P	S55.202-	S56.992-	S61.459-	S62.659-
S43.90X-	S46.802-	S52.189-	S52.616Q	S55.209-	S56.999-	S61.501A	S62.669-
S44.00X-	S46.809-	S52.209-	S52.616R	S55.219-	S57.00X-	S61.509-	S62.90X-
S44.10X-	S46.819-	S52.219-	S52.616S	S55.299-	S57.80X-	S61.519-	S63.003-
S44.20X-	S46.829-	S52.223-	S52.629-	S55.801-	S58.019-	S61.529-	S63.013-
S44.30X-	S46.899-	S52.226-	S52.699B	S55.802-	S58.029-	S61.539-	S63.023-
S44.40X-	S46.901-	S52.233-	S52.699C	S55.809-	S58.119-	S61.549-	S63.026-
S44.50X-	S46.902-	S52.236-	S52.699D	S55.819-	S58.129A	S61.559-	S63.033-
S44.8X9-	S46.909-	S52.241A	S52.699E	S55.899-	S58.129D	S62.009-	S63.036-
S44.90X-	S46.919-	S52.243-	S52.699F	S55.901-	S58.919-	S62.013-	S63.043-
S44.91X-	S46.929-	S52.246-	S52.699G	S55.902-	S58.929-	S62.016-	S63.046-
S44.92X-	S46.999-	S52.253-	S52.699H	S55.909-	S59.009-	S62.023-	S63.053-
S45.001-	S47.9XX-	S52.256-	S52.699J	S55.919-	S59.019-	S62.026-	S63.056-
S45.002-	S48.019-	S52.263-	S52.699K	S55.999-	S59.029-	S62.033-	S63.063-
S45.009-	S48.029-	S52.266-	S52.699M	S56.001-	S59.039-	S62.036-	S63.066-
S45.019-	S48.119-	S52.279-	S52.699N	S56.002-	S59.049-	S62.109-	S63.073-
S45.099-	S48.129-	S52.283-	S52.699P	S56.009-	S59.099-	S62.113-	S63.076-
S45.101-	S48.911-	S52.299-	S52.699Q	S56.029-	S59.109D	S62.116-	S63.093-
S45.102-	S48.912-	S52.309-	S52.699R	S56.099-	S59.109G	S62.123-	S63.096-
S45.109-	S48.919-	S52.319-	S52.699S	S56.101-	S59.109K	S62.126-	S63.103-
S45.119-	S48.921-	S52.323-	S52.90X-	S56.102-	S59.109P	S62.133-	S63.106-
S45.199-	S48.922-	S52.326-	S53.003-	S56.103-	S59.109S	S62.136-	S63.113-
S45.201-	S48.929-	S52.333-	S53.004-	S56.104-	S59.119-	S62.143-	S63.116-
S45.202-	S49.009-	S52.336-	S53.006-	S56.105-	S59.129-	S62.146-	S63.121-
S45.209-	S49.019-	S52.343-	S53.013-	S56.106-	S59.139-	S62.153-	S63.122-
S45.219-	S49.029-	S52.346-	S53.016-	S56.107-	S59.149-	S62.156-	S63.123-
S45.299-	S49.039-	S52.353-	S53.023-	S56.108-	S59.199-	S62.163A	S63.124-
S45.301-	S49.049-	S52.356-	S53.026-	S56.109-	S59.209-	S62.163B	S63.125-
S45.302-	S49.099-	S52.363-	S53.033-	S56.119-	S59.219-	S62.163D	S63.126-
S45.309-	S49.109-	S52.366-	S53.093-	S56.129-	S59.229-	S62.163G	S63.209-
S45.319-	S49.119-	S52.379-	S53.096-	S56.199-	S59.239-	S62.163K	S63.218S
S45.399-	S49.129-	S52.389B	S53.103-	S56.201-	S59.249-	S62.163P	S63.219-
S45.801-	S49.139-	S52.389C	S53.106-	S56.202-	S59.299-	S62.166-	S63.220-
S45.802-	S49.149D	S52.389D	S53.113-	S56.209-	S59.809-	S62.173-	S63.221-
S45.809-	S49.149G	S52.389E	S53.116-	S56.219-	S59.901-	S62.176-	S63.222-
S45.819-	S49.149K	S52.389F	S53.123-	S56.229-	S59.902-	S62.183-	S63.223-
S45.899-	S49.149P	S52.389G	S53.12G-	S56.299-	S59.909-	S62.186-	S63.224-

S63.225-	S65.319-	S66.402-	S72.023-	S72.356S	S75.902-	S81.009-	S82.446R
S63.226-	S65.399-	S66.409-	S72.026-	S72.363-	S75.909-	S81.019-	S82.446S
S63.227-	S65.401-	S66.419-	S72.033-	S72.366-	S75.919-	S81.029-	S82.453-
S63.228-	S65.402-	S66.429-	S72.036-	S72.399-	S75.991-	S81.039-	S82.456-
S63.229-	S65.409-	S66.499-	S72.043-	S72.409-	S75.992-	S81.049-	S82.463-
S63.239-	S65.419-	S66.500-	S72.046-	S72.413-	S75.999-	S81.059-	S82.466-
S63.249-	S65.499-	S66.501-	S72.059-	S72.416-	S76.001-	S81.809-	S82.499-
S63.259-	S65.500-	S66.502-	S72.063-	S72.423-	S76.002-	S81.819-	S82.53X-
S63.269-	S65.501-	S66.503-	S72.066B	S72.426-	S76.009-	S81.829-	S82.56X-
S63.270-	S65.502-	S66.504-	S72.066C	S72.433-	S76.019-	S81.839-	S82.63X-
S63.271-	S65.503-	S66.505-	S72.066D	S72.436-	S76.029-	S81.849-	S82.66X-
S63.272-	S65.504-	S66.506-	S72.066E	S72.443-	S76.099-	S81.859-	S82.819-
S63.273-	S65.505-	S66.507-	S72.066F	S72.446-	S76.101-	S82.009-	S82.829-
S63.274-	S65.506-	S66.508-	S72.066G	S72.453-	S76.102-	S82.013-	S82.839-
S63.275-	S65.507-	S66.509-	S72.066H	S72.456-	S76.109-	S82.016-	S82.843-
S63.276-	S65.508-	S66.519-	S72.066J	S72.463-	S76.119-	S82.023-	S82.846-
S63.277-	S65.509-	S66.529-	S72.066K	S72.466-	S76.129-	S82.026-	S82.853-
S63.278-	S65.519-	S66.599-	S72.066M	S72.479-	S76.199-	S82.033-	S82.856-
S63.279-	S65.599-	S66.801-	S72.066N	S72.499-	S76.201-	S82.036-	S82.863-
S63.289-	S65.801-	S66.802-	S72.066P	S72.8X9-	S76.202-	S82.043-	S82.866-
S63.299-	S65.802-	S66.809-	S72.066Q	S72.90X-	S76.209-	S82.046-	S82.873-
S63.309-	S65.809-	S66.819-	S72.066R	S73.001-	S76.219-	S82.099-	S82.876-
S63.319-	S65.819-	S66.829-	S72.066S	S73.002-	S76.229-	S82.109-	S82.899-
S63.329-	S65.899-	S66.899-	S72.099-	S73.003-	S76.299-	S82.113-	S82.90X-
S63.339-	S65.901-	S66.901-	S72.109-	S73.004-	S76.301-	S82.116-	S83.001-
S63.399-	S65.902-	S66.902-	S72.113-	S73.005-	S76.302-	S82.123-	S83.002-
S63.409-	S65.909-	S66.909-	S72.116D	S73.006-	S76.309-	S82.126-	S83.003-
S63.419-	S65.919-	S66.919-	S72.116E	S73.013-	S76.319-	S82.133-	S83.004-
S63.429-	S65.991-	S66.929-	S72.116F	S73.016-	S76.329-	S82.136-	S83.005-
S63.439-	S65.992-	S66.991-	S72.116G	S73.023-	S76.399-	S82.143-	S83.006-
S63.499-	S65.999-	S66.992-	S72.116H	S73.026-	S76.801-	S82.146-	S83.013-
S63.509-	S66.001-	S66.999-	S72.116J	S73.033-	S76.802-	S82.153-	S83.016-
S63.519-	S66.002-	S67.00X-	S72.116K	S73.036-	S76.809-	S82.156-	S83.093-
S63.529-	S66.009-	S67.10X-	S72.116M	S73.043-	S76.819-	S82.169-	S83.096-
S63.599-	S66.019-	S67.20X-	S72.116N	S73.046-	S76.829-	S82.199-	S83.101-
S63.609-	S66.029-	S67.30X-	S72.116P	S73.109-	S76.899-	S82.209-	S83.102-
S63.619-	S66.099-	S67.40X-	S72.116Q	S73.119-	S76.901-	S82.223-	S83.103-
S63.629-	S66.100-	S67.90X-	S72.116R	S73.129-	S76.902-	S82.226-	S83.104-
S63.639-	S66.101-	S68.019-	S72.116S	S73.199-	S76.909-	S82.233-	S83.105-
S63.649-	S66.102-	S68.029-	S72.123-	S74.00X-	S76.919-	S82.236-	S83.106-
S63.659-	S66.103-	S68.119-	S72.126-	S74.10X-	S76.929-	S82.243-	S83.113-
S63.689-	S66.104-	S68.129-	S72.133-	S74.20X-	S76.991-	S82.246-	S83.116-
S63.699-	S66.105-	S68.419-	S72.136-	S74.8X9-	S76.992-	S82.253-	S83.123-
S63.8X9-	S66.106-	S68.429-	S72.143-	S74.90X-	S76.999-	S82.256-	S83.126-
S63.90X-	S66.107-	S68.519-	S72.146-	S74.91X-	S77.00X-	S82.263-	S83.133-
S64.00X-	S66.108-	S68.529-	S72.23X-	S74.92X-	S77.10X-	S82.266-	S83.136-
S64.10X-	S66.109-	S68.619-	S72.24XA	S75.001-	S77.20X-	S82.299-	S83.143-
S64.20X-	S66.119-	S68.629-	S72.26X-	S75.002-	S78.019-	S82.309-	S83.146-
S64.30X-	S66.129-	S68.719-	S72.309-	S75.009-	S78.029-	S82.319-	S83.193-
S64.40X-	S66.199-	S68.729-	S72.323-	S75.019-	S78.119-	S82.399-	S83.196-
S64.8X9-	S66.201-	S69.80X-	S72.326-	S75.029-	S78.129-	S82.409-	S83.202-
S64.90X-	S66.202-	S69.82XS	S72.333-	S75.099-	S78.919-	S82.423-	S83.205-
S64.91X-	S66.209-	S69.90X-	S72.336-	S75.101-	S78.929-	S82.426-	S83.209-
S64.92X-	S66.219-	S69.91X-	S72.343-	S75.102-	S79.009-	S82.433-	S83.219-
S65.009-	S66.229-	S69.92X-	S72.346-	S75.109-	S79.019-	S82.436-	S83.229-
S65.019-	S66.299-	S70*	S72.353-	S75.119-	S79.099-	S82.442S	S83.239-
S65.099-	S66.300-	S71.009-	S72.356B	S75.129-	S79.109-	S82.443-	S83.249-
S65.101-	S66.301-	S71.019-	S72.356C	S75.199-	S79.119-	S82.446B	S83.259-
S65.102-	S66.302-	S71.029-	S72.356D	S75.201-	S79.129-	S82.446C	S83.269-
S65.109-	S66.303-	S71.039-	S72.356E	S75.202-	S79.139-	S82.446D	S83.279-
S65.119-	S66.304-	S71.049-	S72.356F	S75.209-	S79.149-	S82.446E	S83.289-
S65.199-	S66.305-	S71.059-	S72.356G	S75.219-	S79.199-	S82.446F	S83.30X-
S65.201-	S66.306-	S71.109-	S72.356H	S75.229-	S79.819-	S82.446G	S83.409-
S65.202-	S66.307-	S71.119-	S72.356J	S75.299-	S79.911-	S82.446H	S83.419-
S65.209-	S66.308-	S71.129-	S72.356K	S75.801-	S79.912-	S82.446J	S83.429-
S65.219-	S66.309-	S71.139-	S72.356M	S75.802-	S79.919-	S82.446K	S83.509-
S65.299-	S66.319-	S71.149-	S72.356N	S75.809-	S79.921-	S82.446M	S83.519-
S65.301-	S66.329-	S71.159-	S72.356P	S75.819-	S79.922-	S82.446N	S83.529-
S65.302-	S66.399-	S72.009-	S72.356Q	S75.899-	S79.929-	S82.446P	S83.60X-
S65.309-	S66.401-	S72.019-	S72.356R	S75.901-	S80*	S82.446Q	S83.8X9-

S83.90X-	S86.102-	S91.059-	S92.209-	S92.909-	S95.201-	S99.029-	T20.56X-
S84.00X-	S86.109-	S91.103-	S92.213-	S92.919-	S95.202-	S99.039-	T20.57X-
S84.10X-	S86.119-	S91.106-	S92.216-	S93.03X-	S95.209-	S99.049-	T20.59X-
S84.20X-	S86.129-	S91.109-	S92.223-	S93.06X-	S95.219-	S99.099-	T20.60X-
S84.809-	S86.199-	S91.113-	S92.226-	S93.101-	S95.299-	S99.109-	T20.611-
S84.90X-	S86.201-	S91.116-	S92.233-	S93.102-	S95.801-	S99.119-	T20.612-
S84.91X-	S86.202-	S91.119-	S92.236-	S93.103-	S95.802-	S99.129-	T20.619-
S84.92X-	S86.209-	S91.123-	S92.243-	S93.104-	S95.809-	S99.139-	T20.62X-
S85.001-	S86.219-	S91.126-	S92.246-	S93.105-	S95.819-	S99.149-	T20.63X-
S85.002-	S86.229-	S91.129-	S92.253-	S93.106-	S95.899-	S99.199-	T20.64X-
S85.009-	S86.299-	S91.133-	S92.256-	S93.113-	S95.901-	S99.209-	T20.65X-
S85.019-	S86.301-	S91.136-	S92.301A	S93.116-	S95.902-	S99.219-	T20.66X-
S85.099-	S86.302-	S91.139-	S92.301B	S93.119-	S95.909-	S99.229-	T20.67X-
S85.101-	S86.309-	S91.143-	S92.301G	S93.123-	S95.919-	S99.239-	T20.69X-
S85.102-	S86.319-	S91.146-	S92.301K	S93.126-	S95.991-	S99.249-	T20.70X-
S85.109-	S86.329-	S91.149-	S92.301P	S93.129-	S95.992-	S99.299-	T20.711-
S85.119-	S86.399-	S91.153-	S92.301S	S93.133-	S95.999-	S99.819-	T20.712-
S85.129-	S86.801-	S91.156-	S92.302A	S93.136-	S96.001-	S99.829-	T20.719-
S85.131-	S86.802-	S91.159-	S92.302B	S93.139-	S96.002-	S99.911-	T20.72X-
S85.132-	S86.809-	S91.203-	S92.302G	S93.143-	S96.009-	S99.912-	T20.73X-
S85.139A	S86.819-	S91.206-	S92.302K	S93.146-	S96.019-	S99.919-	T20.74X-
S85.139D	S86.829-	S91.209-	S92.302P	S93.149-	S96.029-	S99.921-	T20.75X-
S85.149-	S86.899-	S91.213-	S92.302S	S93.301-	S96.099-	S99.922-	T20.76X-
S85.159-	S86.901-	S91.216-	S92.309-	S93.302-	S96.101-	S99.929-	T20.77X-
S85.161-	S86.902-	S91.219-	S92.313-	S93.303-	S96.102-	T07*	T20.79X-
S85.162-	S86.909-	S91.223-	S92.316-	S93.304-	S96.109-	T14.8XX-	T21.00X-
S85.169-	S86.919-	S91.226-	S92.323-	S93.305-	S96.119-	T14.8XXD	T21.01X-
S85.179-	S86.929-	S91.229-	S92.326-	S93.306-	S96.129-	T14.8XXS	T21.02X-
S85.179S	S86.991-	S91.233-	S92.333-	S93.313-	S96.199-	T14.90X-	T21.03X-
S85.189-	S86.992-	S91.236-	S92.336-	S93.316-	S96.201-	T15.00X-	T21.04X-
S85.201-	S86.999-	S91.239-	S92.343-	S93.323-	S96.202-	T15.10X-	T21.05X-
S85.202-	S87.00X-	S91.243-	S92.346-	S93.326-	S96.209-	T15.80X-	T21.06X-
S85.209-	S87.80X-	S91.246-	S92.353-	S93.333-	S96.219-	T15.90X-	T21.07X-
S85.219-	S88.019-	S91.249-	S92.356-	S93.336-	S96.229-	T16.9XX-	T21.09X-
S85.299-	S88.029-	S91.253-	S92.403-	S93.409-	S96.299-	T20.00X-	T21.10X-
S85.301-	S88.119-	S91.256-	S92.406-	S93.419-	S96.801-	T20.011-	T21.20X-
S85.302-	S88.129-	S91.259-	S92.413-	S93.429-	S96.802-	T20.012-	T21.30X-
S85.309-	S88.919-	S91.309-	S92.416-	S93.439-	S96.809-	T20.019-	T21.40X-
S85.319-	S88.929-	S91.319-	S92.423-	S93.499-	S96.819-	T20.02XS	T21.41X-
S85.399-	S89.009-	S91.329-	S92.426-	S93.503-	S96.829-	T20.03X-	T21.42X-
S85.401-	S89.019-	S91.339-	S92.499-	S93.506-	S96.899-	T20.04X-	T21.43X-
S85.402-	S89.029-	S91.349-	S92.501A	S93.509-	S96.901-	T20.05X-	T21.44X-
S85.409-	S89.039-	S91.359-	S92.501B	S93.513-	S96.902-	T20.06X-	T21.45X-
S85.419-	S89.049-	S92.009-	S92.501G	S93.516-	S96.909-	T20.07X-	T21.46X-
S85.499-	S89.099-	S92.013-	S92.501K	S93.519-	S96.919-	T20.09X-	T21.47X-
S85.501-	S89.109-	S92.016-	S92.501P	S93.523-	S96.929-	T20.10X-	T21.49X-
S85.502-	S89.119-	S92.023-	S92.501S	S93.526-	S96.991-	T20.119-	T21.50X-
S85.509-	S89.129-	S92.026-	S92.502A	S93.529-	S96.992-	T20.20X-	T21.51X-
S85.519A	S89.139-	S92.033-	S92.502B	S93.609-	S96.999-	T20.219-	T21.52X-
S85.519D	S89.149-	S92.036-	S92.502G	S93.619-	S97.00X-	T20.30X-	T21.53X-
S85.599-	S89.199-	S92.043-	S92.502K	S93.629-	S97.101-	T20.319-	T21.54X-
S85.801-	S89.209-	S92.046-	S92.502P	S93.699-	S97.102-	T20.40X-	T21.55X-
S85.802-	S89.219-	S92.053-	S92.502S	S94.00X-	S97.109-	T20.411-	T21.56X-
S85.809-	S89.229-	S92.056-	S92.503-	S94.10X-	S97.119-	T20.412-	T21.57X-
S85.819-	S89.299-	S92.063-	S92.504-	S94.20X-	S97.129-	T20.419-	T21.59X-
S85.899-	S89.309-	S92.066-	S92.505A	S94.30X-	S97.80X-	T20.42X-	T21.60X-
S85.901-	S89.319-	S92.109-	S92.505B	S94.8X9-	S98.019-	T20.43X-	T21.61X-
S85.902-	S89.329-	S92.113-	S92.505G	S94.90X-	S98.029-	T20.44X-	T21.62X-
S85.909-	S89.399-	S92.116-	S92.505K	S94.91X-	S98.129-	T20.45X-	T21.63X-
S85.919-	S89.80X-	S92.123-	S92.505P	S94.92X-	S98.139-	T20.46X-	T21.64X-
S85.991-	S89.90X-	S92.126-	S92.505S	S95.001-	S98.149-	T20.47X-	T21.65X-
S85.992-	S89.91X-	S92.133-	S92.506-	S95.002-	S98.219-	T20.49X-	T21.66X-
S85.999-	S89.92X-	S92.136-	S92.513-	S95.009-	S98.229-	T20.50X-	T21.67X-
S86.001-	S90*	S92.143-	S92.516-	S95.019-	S98.319-	T20.511-	T21.69X-
S86.002-	S91.009A	S92.146-	S92.523-	S95.099-	S98.329-	T20.512-	T21.70X-
S86.009-	S91.009D	S92.153-	S92.526-	S95.101-	S98.919-	T20.519-	T21.71X-
S86.019-	S91.019-	S92.156-	S92.533-	S95.102-	S98.929-	T20.52X-	T21.72X-
S86.029-	S91.029-	S92.199-	S92.536-	S95.109-	S99.009-	T20.53X-	T21.73X-
S86.099-	S91.039-	S92.201-	S92.599-	S95.119-	S99.019-	T20.54X-	T21.74X-
S86.101-	S91.049-	S92.202-	S92.819-	S95.199-		T20.55X-	T21.75X-

T21.76X-	T22.511-	T23.019-	T23.419-	T23.671-	T24.402-	T25.099-	T26.52X-
T21.77X-	T22.512-	T23.021-	T23.421-	T23.672-	T24.409-	T25.119-	T26.60X-
T21.79X-	T22.519-	T23.022-	T23.422-	T23.679-	T24.411-	T25.129-	T26.61X-
T22.00X-	T22.521-	T23.029-	T23.429-	T23.691-	T24.412-	T25.139-	T26.62X-
T22.011-	T22.522-	T23.031-	T23.431-	T23.692-	T24.419-	T25.199-	T26.70X-
T22.012-	T22.529-	T23.032-	T23.432-	T23.699-	T24.421-	T25.219-	T26.71X-
T22.019-	T22.531-	T23.039-	T23.439-	T23.701-	T24.422-	T25.229-	T26.72X-
T22.021-	T22.532-	T23.041-	T23.441-	T23.702-	T24.429-	T25.239-	T26.80X-
T22.022-	T22.539-	T23.042-	T23.442-	T23.709-	T24.431-	T25.299-	T26.81X-
T22.029-	T22.541-	T23.049-	T23.449-	T23.711-	T24.432-	T25.319-	T26.82X-
T22.031-	T22.542-	T23.051-	T23.451-	T23.712-	T24.439-	T25.329-	T26.90X-
T22.032-	T22.549-	T23.052-	T23.452-	T23.719-	T24.491-	T25.339-	T26.91X-
T22.039-	T22.551-	T23.059-	T23.459-	T23.721-	T24.492-	T25.399-	T26.92X-
T22.041-	T22.552-	T23.061-	T23.461-	T23.722-	T24.499-	T25.411-	T27.3XX-
T22.042-	T22.559-	T23.062-	T23.462-	T23.729-	T24.501-	T25.412-	T27.7XXA
T22.049-	T22.561-	T23.069-	T23.469-	T23.731-	T24.502-	T25.419-	T27.7XXD
T22.051-	T22.562-	T23.071-	T23.471-	T23.732-	T24.509-	T25.421-	T28.40X-
T22.052-	T22.569-	T23.072-	T23.472-	T23.739-	T24.511-	T25.422-	T28.419-
T22.059-	T22.591-	T23.079-	T23.479-	T23.741-	T24.512-	T25.429-	T28.5XX-
T22.061-	T22.592-	T23.091-	T23.491-	T23.742-	T24.519-	T25.431-	T28.6XX-
T22.062-	T22.599-	T23.092-	T23.492-	T23.749-	T24.521-	T25.432-	T28.7XX-
T22.069-	T22.60X-	T23.099-	T23.499-	T23.751-	T24.522-	T25.439-	T28.8XX-
T22.091-	T22.611-	T23.101-	T23.501-	T23.752-	T24.529-	T25.491-	T28.90X-
T22.092-	T22.612-	T23.102-	T23.502-	T23.759-	T24.531-	T25.492-	T28.911-
T22.099-	T22.619-	T23.109-	T23.509-	T23.761-	T24.532-	T25.499-	T28.912-
T22.10X-	T22.621-	T23.119-	T23.511-	T23.762-	T24.539-	T25.511-	T28.919-
T22.119-	T22.622-	T23.129-	T23.512-	T23.769-	T24.591-	T25.512-	T28.99X-
T22.129-	T22.629-	T23.139-	T23.519-	T23.771-	T24.592-	T25.519-	T30*
T22.132S	T22.631-	T23.149-	T23.521-	T23.772-	T24.599-	T25.521-	T31*
T22.139-	T22.632-	T23.159-	T23.522-	T23.779-	T24.601-	T25.522-	T32*
T22.149-	T22.639-	T23.169-	T23.529-	T23.791-	T24.602-	T25.529-	T33.019-
T22.159-	T22.641-	T23.179-	T23.531-	T23.792-	T24.609-	T25.531-	T33.40X-
T22.169-	T22.642-	T23.199-	T23.532-	T23.799-	T24.611-	T25.532-	T33.519-
T22.20X-	T22.649-	T23.201-	T23.539-	T24.001-	T24.612-	T25.539-	T33.529-
T22.219-	T22.651-	T23.202-	T23.541-	T24.002-	T24.619-	T25.591-	T33.539-
T22.229-	T22.652-	T23.209-	T23.542-	T24.009-	T24.621-	T25.592-	T33.60X-
T22.239-	T22.659-	T23.219-	T23.549-	T24.011-	T24.622-	T25.599-	T33.70X-
T22.249-	T22.661-	T23.229-	T23.551-	T24.012-	T24.629-	T25.611-	T33.819-
T22.259-	T22.662-	T23.239-	T23.552-	T24.019-	T24.631-	T25.612-	T33.829-
T22.269-	T22.669-	T23.249-	T23.559-	T24.021-	T24.632-	T25.619-	T33.839-
T22.30X-	T22.691-	T23.259-	T23.561-	T24.022-	T24.639-	T25.621-	T33.90X-
T22.319-	T22.692-	T23.269-	T23.562-	T24.029-	T24.691-	T25.622-	T34.019-
T22.329-	T22.699-	T23.279-	T23.569-	T24.031-	T24.692-	T25.629-	T34.40X-
T22.339-	T22.70X-	T23.299-	T23.571-	T24.032-	T24.699-	T25.631-	T34.519-
T22.349-	T22.711-	T23.301-	T23.572-	T24.039-	T24.701-	T25.632-	T34.529-
T22.359-	T22.712-	T23.302-	T23.579-	T24.091-	T24.702-	T25.639-	T34.539-
T22.369-	T22.719-	T23.309-	T23.591-	T24.092-	T24.709-	T25.691-	T34.60X-
T22.40X-	T22.721-	T23.319-	T23.592-	T24.099-	T24.711-	T25.692-	T34.70X-
T22.411-	T22.722-	T23.329-	T23.599-	T24.101-	T24.712-	T25.699-	T34.819-
T22.412-	T22.729-	T23.339-	T23.601-	T24.102-	T24.719-	T25.711-	T34.829-
T22.419-	T22.731-	T23.349-	T23.602-	T24.109-	T24.721-	T25.712-	T34.839-
T22.421-	T22.732-	T23.359-	T23.609-	T24.119-	T24.722-	T25.719-	T34.90X-
T22.422-	T22.739-	T23.369-	T23.611-	T24.129-	T24.729-	T25.721-	T36.0X1A
T22.429-	T22.741-	T23.369D	T23.612-	T24.139-	T24.731-	T25.722-	T36.0X5-
T22.431-	T22.742-	T23.369S	T23.619-	T24.199-	T24.732-	T25.729-	T36.1X5-
T22.432-	T22.749-	T23.379-	T23.621-	T24.201-	T24.739-	T25.731-	T36.2X5-
T22.439-	T22.751-	T23.379D	T23.622-	T24.202-	T24.791-	T25.732-	T36.3X5-
T22.441-	T22.752-	T23.379S	T23.629-	T24.209-	T24.792-	T25.739-	T36.4X5-
T22.442-	T22.759-	T23.399-	T23.631-	T24.219-	T24.799-	T25.791-	T36.5X5-
T22.449-	T22.761-	T23.399D	T23.632-	T24.229-	T25.011-	T25.792-	T36.6X5-
T22.451-	T22.762-	T23.399S	T23.639-	T24.239-	T25.012-	T25.799-	T36.7X5-
T22.452-	T22.769-	T23.401-	T23.641-	T24.299-	T25.019-	T26.00X-	T36.8X5-
T22.459-	T22.791-	T23.401D	T23.642-	T24.301-	T25.021-	T26.10X-	T36.95X-
T22.461-	T22.792-	T23.401S	T23.649-	T24.302-	T25.022-	T26.20X-	T37.0X5-
T22.462-	T22.799-	T23.402-	T23.651-	T24.309-	T25.029-	T26.30X-	T37.1X5-
T22.469-	T23.001-	T23.402D	T23.652-	T24.319-	T25.031-	T26.40X-	T37.2X5-
T22.491-	T23.002-	T23.402S	T23.659-	T24.329-	T25.032-	T26.41X-	T37.3X5-
T22.492-	T23.009-	T23.409-	T23.661-	T24.339-	T25.039-	T26.42X-	T37.4X5-
T22.499-	T23.011-	T23.411-	T23.662-	T24.399-	T25.091-	T26.50X-	T37.5X5-
T22.50X-	T23.012-	T23.412-	T23.669-	T24.401-	T25.092-	T26.51X-	T37.8X5-

Appendix I: Patient-Driven Groupings Model (PDGM) Return-to-Provider Code List

T37.95X-	T42.75X-	T46.2X5-	T50.6X5-	T82.129-	T86.819	Z36*	Z51.89
T38.0X5-	T42.8X5-	T46.3X5-	T50.7X5-	T82.199-	T86.829	Z37*	Z52*
T38.1X5-	T43.015-	T46.4X5-	T50.8X5-	T82.319-	T86.839	Z38*	Z53*
T38.2X5-	T43.025-	T46.5X5-	T50.905-	T82.329-	T86.849	Z39*	Z55*
T38.3X5-	T43.1X5-	T46.6X5-	T50.995-	T82.339-	T86.859	Z3A*	Z56*
T38.4X5-	T43.205-	T46.7X5-	T50.-15-	T82.399-	T86.899	Z40*	Z57*
T38.5X5-	T43.215-	T46.8X5-	T50.-25-	T82.41X-	T86.90	Z41*	Z59*
T38.6X5-	T43.225-	T46.905-	T50.-95-	T82.42X-	T86.91	Z42*	Z60*
T38.7X5-	T43.295-	T46.995-	T50.B15-	T82.43X-	T86.92	Z43.9	Z62*
T38.805-	T43.3X5-	T47.0X5-	T50.B95-	T82.49X-	T86.93	Z44*	Z63*
T38.815-	T43.4X5-	T47.1X5-	T50.Z15-	T82.510-	T86.99	Z45.010	Z64*
T38.895-	T43.505-	T47.2X5-	T50.Z95-	T82.511-	T87.0X9	Z45.018	Z65*
T38.905-	T43.595-	T47.3X5-	T73.9XXD	T82.519-	T87.1X9	Z45.02	Z66
T38.995-	T43.605-	T47.4X5-	T73.9XXS	T82.520-	T87.30	Z45.09	Z67*
T39.015-	T43.615-	T47.5X5-	T74.61X-	T82.521-	T87.40	Z45.1	Z68*
T39.095-	T43.625-	T47.6X5-	T74.62X-	T82.529-	T87.50	Z45.31	Z69*
T39.1X5-	T43.635-	T47.7X5-	T74.91X-	T82.530-	T87.9	Z45.320	Z70*
T39.2X5-	T43.695-	T47.8X5-	T74.92X-	T82.531-	T88.7XX-	Z45.321	Z71*
T39.315-	T43.8X5-	T47.95X-	T75.00X-	T82.539-	T88.9XX-	Z45.328	Z72*
T39.395-	T43.95X-	T48.0X5-	T75.1XX-	T82.590-	Z00*	Z45.41	Z73*
T39.4X5-	T44.0X5-	T48.1X5-	T75.20X-	T82.591-	Z01*	Z45.42	Z74*
T39.8X5-	T44.1X5-	T48.205-	T76.61X-	T82.599-	Z02*	Z45.49	Z75*
T39.95X-	T44.2X5-	T48.295-	T76.62X-	T82.9XX-	Z03*	Z45.811	Z76*
T40.0X5-	T44.3X5-	T48.3X5-	T76.91X-	T83.9XX-	Z04*	Z45.812	Z77*
T40.2X5-	T44.4X5-	T48.4X5-	T76.92X-	T84.019-	Z05*	Z45.819	Z78*
T40.3X5-	T44.5X5-	T48.5X5-	T78.00X-	T84.029-	Z08	Z45.82	Z79*
T40.4X5-	T44.6X5-	T48.6X5-	T79.9XX-	T84.039-	Z09	Z45.89	Z80*
T40.5X5-	T44.7X5-	T48.905-	T79.-0X-	T84.059-	Z11*	Z45.9	Z81*
T40.605-	T44.8X5-	T48.995-	T79.-19-	T84.069-	Z12*	Z46.0	Z82*
T40.695-	T44.905-	T49.0X5-	T79.-29-	T84.099-	Z13*	Z46.1	Z83*
T40.7X5-	T44.995-	T49.1X5-	T80.219-	T84.119-	Z14*	Z46.2	Z84*
T40.905-	T45.0X5-	T49.2X5-	T81.12X-	T84.129-	Z15*	Z46.3	Z85*
T40.995-	T45.1X5-	T49.3X5-	T81.500-	T84.199-	Z16*	Z46.4	Z86*
T41.0X5-	T45.2X5-	T49.4X5-	T81.501-	T84.50X-	Z17*	Z46.51	Z87*
T41.1X5-	T45.3X5-	T49.5X5-	T81.502-	T84.60X-	Z18*	Z46.59	Z88*
T41.205-	T45.4X5-	T49.6X5D	T81.503-	T84.619-	Z19*	Z46.81	Z89*
T41.295-	T45.515-	T49.6X5S	T81.504-	T84.625S	Z20*	Z46.82	Z90*
T41.3X5-	T45.525-	T49.6X6A	T81.505-	T84.629-	Z21	Z46.89	Z91*
T41.45X-	T45.605-	T49.7X5-	T81.506-	T84.9XX-	Z22*	Z46.9	Z92*
T41.5X5-	T45.615-	T49.8X5-	T81.507-	T85.631D	Z23	Z47.2	Z93*
T42.0X5-	T45.625-	T49.95X-	T81.508-	T85.633D	Z28*	Z48.1	Z94*
T42.1X5-	T45.695-	T50.0X5-	T81.509-	T85.9XX-	Z29*	Z48.814	Z95*
T42.2X5-	T45.7X5-	T50.1X5-	T81.519-	T86.00	Z30*	Z48.89	Z96*
T42.3X5-	T45.8X5-	T50.2X5-	T81.599-	T86.10	Z31*	Z49*	
T42.4X5-	T45.95X-	T50.3X5-	T81.60X-	T86.20	Z32*	Z51.0	
T42.5X5-	T46.0X5-	T50.4X5-	T81.9XX-	T86.30	Z33*	Z51.6	
T42.6X5-	T46.1X5-	T50.5X5-	T82.119-	T86.40	Z34*	Z51.81	

Coverage of Hospice Services Under Hospital Insurance

CMS Manual Publication Number 100-04, *Medicare Claims Processing Manual*, Chapter 11

CMS Manual Publication 100-2, *Medicare Benefits Policy Manual*, Chapter 9

Requirements – General

Hospice care is a benefit under the hospital insurance program. To be eligible to elect hospice care under Medicare, an individual must be entitled to Part A of Medicare and be certified as being terminally ill. An individual is considered to be terminally ill if the medical prognosis is that the individual's life expectancy is six months or less if the illness runs its normal course. Only care provided by (or under arrangements made by) a Medicare certified hospice is covered under the Medicare hospice benefit.

The hospice admits a patient only on the recommendation of the medical director in consultation with, or with input from, the patient's attending physician (if any).

In reaching a decision to certify that the patient is terminally ill, the hospice medical director must consider at least the following information:

1. Diagnosis of the terminal condition of the patient.
2. Other health conditions, whether related or unrelated to the terminal condition.
3. Current clinically relevant information supporting all diagnoses.

Section §1814(a)(7) of the Social Security Act (the Act) specifies that certification of terminal illness for hospice benefits shall be based on the clinical judgment of the hospice medical director or physician member of the interdisciplinary group (IDG) and the individual's attending physician, if he/she has one, regarding the normal course of the individual's illness. No one other than a medical doctor or doctor of osteopathy can certify or re-certify a terminal illness. Predicting of life expectancy is not always exact. The fact that a beneficiary lives longer than expected in itself is not cause to terminate benefits. "Attending physician" is further defined in section 20.1 and 40.1.3.1.

An individual (or his authorized representative) must elect hospice care to receive it. An individual may elect to receive Medicare coverage for an unlimited number of election periods of hospice care. The periods consist of two 90-day periods, and an unlimited number of 60-day periods. If the individual (or authorized representative) elects to receive hospice care, he or she must file an election statement with a particular hospice. Hospices obtain election statements from the individual and file a Notice of Election with the A/B MAC (HHH), which transmits them to the Common Working File (CWF) in electronic format. Once the initial election is processed, CWF maintains the beneficiary in hospice status until a final claim indicates a discharge (alive or due to death) or until an election termination is received.

For the duration of the election of hospice care, an individual must waive all rights to Medicare payments for the following services:

- Hospice care provided by a hospice other than the hospice designated by the individual (unless provided under arrangements made by the designated hospice); and

- Any Medicare services that are related to the treatment of the terminal condition for which hospice care was elected or a related condition or services that are equivalent to hospice care, except for services provided by:

  1. The designated hospice (either directly or under arrangement);
  2. Another hospice under arrangements made by the designated hospice; or
  3. The individual's attending physician, who may be a nurse practitioner (NP), if that physician or nurse practitioner is not an employee of the designated hospice or receiving compensation from the hospice for those services.

Medicare services for a condition completely unrelated to the terminal condition for which hospice was elected remain available to the patient if he or she is eligible for such care.

Noncancer Hospice Care Eligibility Criteria

Medicare coverage of hospice care depends upon a physician's certification of an individual's prognosis of a life expectancy of six months or less if the terminal illness runs its normal course. Recognizing that determination of life expectancy during the course of a terminal illness is difficult, the following policies were originally developed by the Medicare home health and hospice administrative contractors (HHH MACs) and are included in the resource for guidance only. These medical criteria form a reasonable approach to the determination of prognosis for certain noncancer diagnoses and were found not to be in conflict with any existing CMS national coverage rules and/or regulations. However, some patients may not meet the criteria, yet still be appropriate for hospice care, because of other comorbidities or rapid decline. Coverage for these patients may be approved on an individual consideration basis.

The criteria in each of these policies are considered to be the most accurate parameters to determine Medicare coverage for these specific noncancer diagnoses. As of May 2016, there were four HHH areas handled by three HHH MACs.

Hospice Election

Each hospice designs and prints its election statement. The election statement must include the following items of information:

- Identification of the particular hospice that will provide care to the individual;
- The individual's or representative's (as applicable) acknowledgment that the individual has been given a full understanding of hospice care, particularly the palliative rather than curative nature of treatment;
- The individual's or representative's (as applicable) acknowledgment that the individual understands that certain Medicare services are waived by the election;
- The effective date of the election, which may be the first day of hospice care or a later date, but may be no earlier than the date of the election statement. An individual may not designate an effective date that is retroactive;
- The individual's designated attending physician (if any). Information identifying the attending physician recorded on the election statement should provide enough detail so that it is clear which physician or Nurse Practitioner (NP) was designated as the attending physician. This information should include, but is not limited to, the attending physician's full name, office address, NPI number, or any other detailed information to clearly identify the attending physician.
- The individual's acknowledgment that the designated attending physician was the individual's or representative's choice.
- The signature of the individual or representative.

An election to receive hospice care will be considered to continue through the initial election period and through the subsequent election periods without a break in care as long as the individual:

1. Remains in the care of a hospice;
2. Does not revoke the election; and
3. Is not discharged from the hospice.

For Medicare payment purposes, an election for Medicare hospice care must be made on or after the date that the hospice provider is Medicare-certified. As with any election, the hospice must fulfill all other admission requirements, such as certification or recertification, any required face-to-face encounters, or Conditions of Participation (CoP) assessments. See also Pub. 100-04, Medicare Claims Processing Manual, chapter 11, section 20.1.1.

An individual may change, once in each election period, the designation of the particular hospice from which he or she elects to receive hospice care. The change of the designated hospice is not considered a revocation of the election, but is a transfer. To change the designation of hospice programs, the individual must file, with the hospice from which he or she has received care and with the newly designated hospice, a signed statement that includes the following information:

- the name of the hospice from which the individual has received care,
- the name of the hospice from which they plan to receive care, and
- the date the change is to be effective.

As described in Pub. 100-04, Medicare Claims Processing Manual, chapter 11, section 20.1.1, when a hospice patient transfers to a new hospice, the receiving hospice must file a new Notice of Election; however, the benefit period dates are unaffected. The receiving hospice must complete all assessments required by the hospice conditions of participation as described in 42 CFR 418.54. Because the benefit period does not change in a transfer situation, if the patient is in the third or later benefit period and transfers hospices, a face-to-face encounter is not required if the receiving hospice can verify that the originating hospice had the encounter.

A change of ownership of a hospice is not considered a change in the patient's designation of a hospice and requires no action on the patient's part.

Medicare beneficiaries enrolled in managed care plans may elect hospice benefits. Federal regulations require that the Medicare contractor assigned the hospice specialty workload maintain payment responsibility for hospice services and may pay for other claims if that contractor is the geographically assigned Medicare contractor for the managed care enrollees who elect hospice; for specifics, see regulations at 42 CFR 417, Subpart P, 417.585, Special Rules: Hospice Care (b), and 42 CFR 417.531 Hospice Care Services (b). Institutional claims for services not related to the terminal illness would otherwise be the responsibility of another geographically assigned Medicare contractor.

Managed care enrollees who have elected hospice may revoke hospice election at any time, but claims will continue to be paid by fee-for-service contractors as if the beneficiary were a fee-for-service beneficiary until the first day of the month following the month in which hospice was revoked. As specified above, by regulation, the duration of payment responsibility by fee-for-service contractors extends through the remainder of the month in which hospice is revoked by hospice beneficiaries.

Part I. Decline in clinical status guidelines

Patients will be considered to have a life expectancy of six months or less if there is documented evidence of decline in clinical status based on the guidelines listed below. Since determination of decline presumes assessment of the patient's status over time, it is essential that both baseline and follow-up determinations be reported where appropriate. Baseline data may be established on admission to hospice or by using existing information from records. Other clinical variables not on this list may support a six-month or less life expectancy. These should be documented in the clinical record.

These changes in clinical variables apply to patients whose decline is not considered to be reversible. They are examples of findings that generally connote a poor prognosis. However, some are clearly more predictive of a poor prognosis than others; significant ongoing weight loss is a strong predictor, while decreased functional status is less so.

Progression of disease as documented by worsening clinical status, symptoms, signs and laboratory results.

1. Clinical Status

   a. Recurrent or intractable infections such as pneumonia, sepsis or upper urinary tract. National Government Services (NGS) adds: or pyelonephritis in place of upper urinary tract)

   b. Progressive inanition as documented by:

      1) Weight loss (NGS states weight loss of at least 10% body weight in the prior six months) not due to reversible causes such as depression or use of diuretics

      2) Decreasing anthropomorphic measurements (mid-arm circumference, abdominal girth), not due to reversible causes such as depression or use of diuretics

      3) Decreasing serum albumin or cholesterol

      4) Dysphagia leading to recurrent aspiration and/or inadequate oral intake documented by decreasing food portion consumption

2. Symptoms

   a. Dyspnea with increasing respiratory rate

   b. Cough, intractable

   c. Nausea/vomiting poorly responsive to treatment

   d. Diarrhea, intractable

   e. Pain requiring increasing doses of major analgesics more than briefly

3. Signs

   a. Decline in systolic blood pressure to below 90 or progressive postural hypotension

   b. Ascites

   c. Venous, arterial or lymphatic obstruction due to local progression or metastatic disease

   d. Edema

   e. Pleural/pericardial effusion

   f. Weakness

   g. Change in level of consciousness

4. Laboratory (When available. Lab testing is not required to establish hospice eligibility.)

   a. Increasing pCO2 or decreasing pO2 or decreasing SaO2

   b. Increasing calcium, creatinine or liver function studies

   c. Increasing tumor markers (e.g. CEA, PSA)

   d. Progressively decreasing or increasing serum sodium or increasing serum potassium

5. Decline in Karnofsky Performance Status (KPS) or Palliative Performance Score (PPS) (from <70% is stated by CGS)

6. Progressive decline in Functional Assessment Staging (FAST) for dementia (from ≥ 7A on the FAST)

7. Progression to dependence on assistance with additional activities of daily living. See Part II, Section B

8. Progressive stage 3-4 pressure ulcers in spite of optimal care

9. Increasing emergency room visits, hospitalizations, or physician's visits related to hospice primary diagnosis

Part II. Non-disease specific baseline guidelines (both of these should be met)

A. Physiologic impairment of functional status as demonstrated by: Karnofsky Performance Status (KPS) or Palliative Performance Score (PPS) < 70%. Note that two of the disease specific guidelines (HIV Disease, Stroke and Coma) establish a lower qualifying KPS or PPS.

B. Dependence on assistance for two or more activities of daily living (ADLs)

   1. Ambulation

   2. Continence

   3. Transfer

   4. Dressing

   5. Feeding

   6. Bathing

Part III. Co-morbidities

Although not the primary hospice diagnosis, the presence of disease such as the following, the severity of which is likely to contribute to a life expectancy of six months or less, should be considered in determining hospice eligibility.

   A. Chronic obstructive pulmonary disease

   B. Congestive heart failure

   C. Ischemic heart disease

   D. Diabetes mellitus

   E. Neurologic disease (CVA, ALS, MS, Parkinson's)

   F. Renal failure

   G. Liver Disease

   H. Neoplasia

   I. Acquired immune deficiency syndrome

   J. Dementia

(NGS adds: Refractory severe autoimmune disease [e.g., lupus or rheumatoid arthritis])

Hospice HIV Disease
L34566 Palmetto GBA (PGBA)

Indications and limitations of coverage and/or medical necessity:

Patients will be considered to be in the terminal stage of their illness (life expectancy of six months or less) if they meet the following criteria (1 and 2 must be present; factors from 3 will add supporting documentation):

1. CD4+ Count l00,000 copies/ml, plus one of the following:
   - CNS lymphoma
   - Untreated, or not responsive to treatment, wasting (loss of 33% lean body mass)
   - Mycobacterium avium complex (MAC) bacteremia, untreated, unresponsive to treatment, or treatment refused
   - Progressive multifocal leukoencephalopathy
   - Systemic lymphoma, with advanced HIV disease and partial response to chemotherapy
   - Visceral Kaposi's sarcoma unresponsive to therapy
   - Renal failure in the absence of dialysis
   - Cryptosporidium infection
   - Toxoplasmosis, unresponsive to therapy
2. Decreased performance status, as measured by the KarnofskyPerformance Status (KPS) scale, of less than or equal to 50%
3. Documentation of the following factors will support eligibility for hospice care:
   - Chronic persistent diarrhea for one year
   - Persistent serum albumin <2.5
   - Concomitant, active substance abuse
   - Age > 50 years
   - Absence of antiretroviral, chemotherapeutic and prophylactic drug therapy related specifically to HIV disease
   - Advanced AIDS dementia complex
   - Toxoplasmosis
   - Congestive heart failure, symptomatic at rest
   - Advanced liver disease

ICD-10-CM codes that support medical necessity

B20   Human immunodeficiency virus (HIV) disease

ICD-10 codes that do not support medical necessity

R75   Inconclusive laboratory evidence of human immunodeficiency virus (HIV)

Z20.5   Contact with and (suspected) exposure to viral hepatitis

Z20.6   Contact with and (suspected) exposure to human immunodeficiency virus (HIV)

Z20.828 Contact with and (suspected) exposure to other viral communicable diseases

Z21   Asymptomatic human immunodeficiency virus (HIV) infection status

Hospice Cardiopulmonary Conditions and Heart Disease
A53054, L34548-Palmetto GBA, L34538—CGS Administrators, LLC, L33393—National Government Services, Inc.

Indications and limitations of coverage and/or medical necessity:

Palmetto Criteria:

Cardiopulmonary conditions are associated with impairments, activity limitations, and disability. Their impact on any given individual depends on the individual's over-all health status. Health status includes measures of functioning, physical illness, mental wellbeing, as well as environmental factors, such as the availability of palliative care services. The objective of this policy is to present a framework for identifying, documenting, and communicating the unique health care needs of individuals with cardiopulmonary conditions and thus promote the over-all goal of the appropriate care for every person, every time.

Cardiopulmonary conditions may support a prognosis of six months or less under many clinical scenarios. Medicare rules and regulations addressing hospice services require the documentation of sufficient "clinical information and other documentation" to support the certification of individuals as having a terminal illness with a life expectancy of 6 or fewer months, if the illness runs its normal course. The identification of specific structural/functional impairments, together with any relevant activity limitations, should serve as the basis for palliative interventions and care-planning. Use of the International Classification of Functioning, Disability and Health (ICF) to help identify and document the unique service needs of individuals with cardiopulmonary conditions is suggested, but not required.

The health status changes associated with cardiopulmonary conditions can be characterized using categories contained in the ICF. The ICF contains domains (e.g., structures of cardiovascular and respiratory systems, functions of the cardiovascular and respiratory system, communication, mobility, and self-care) that allow for a comprehensive description of an individual's health status and service needs. Information addressing relevant ICF categories, defined within each of these domains, should form the core of the clinical record and be incorporated into the care plan, as appropriate.

Additionally the care plan may be impacted by relevant secondary and/or comorbid conditions. Secondary conditions are directly related to a primary condition. In the case of cardiopulmonary conditions, examples of secondary conditions could include delirium, pneumonia, stasis ulcers and pressure ulcers. Comorbid conditions affecting beneficiaries with cardiopulmonary conditions are, by definition, distinct from the primary condition itself. An example of a comorbid condition would be End Stage Renal Disease (ESRD).

The important roles of secondary and comorbid conditions are described below in order to facilitate their recognition and assist providers in documenting their impact. The identification and documentation of relevant secondary and comorbid conditions, together with the identification and description of associated structural/functional impairments, activity limitations, and environmental factors would help establish hospice eligibility and maintain a beneficiary-centered plan of care.

Secondary Conditions:

Cardiopulmonary conditions may be complicated by secondary conditions. The significance of a given secondary condition is best described by defining the structural/functional impairments—together with any limitation in activity and restriction in participation—related to the secondary condition. The occurrence of secondary conditions in beneficiaries with cardiopulmonary conditions results from the presence of impairments in such body functions as heart/respiratory rate and rhythm, contraction force of ventricular muscles, blood supply to the heart, sleep functions, and depth of respiration. These impairments contribute to the increased incidence of secondary conditions such as delirium, pneumonia, stasis ulcers and pressure ulcers observed in Medicare beneficiaries with cardiopulmonary conditions. Secondary conditions themselves may be associated with a new set of structural/functional impairments that may or may not respond/be amenable to treatment.

Ultimately, in order to support a hospice plan of care, the combined effects of the primary cardiopulmonary condition and any identified secondary condition(s) should be such that most beneficiaries with the identified impairments would have a prognosis of six months or less.

Comorbid Conditions:

The significance of a given comorbid condition is best described by defining the structural/functional impairments—together with any limitation in activity and restriction in participation—related to the comorbid condition. For example a beneficiary with a primary cardiopulmonary condition and ESRD could have specific ESRD-related impairments of water, mineral and electrolyte balance functions coexisting with the cardiopulmonary impairments associated with the primary cardiopulmonary condition (e.g., Aortic Stenosis, Chronic Obstructive Pulmonary Disease, or Heart Failure).

Ultimately, in order to support a hospice plan of care, the combined effects of the primary cardiopulmonary condition and any identified comorbid condition(s) should be such that most beneficiaries with the identified impairments would have a prognosis of six months or less.

The documentation of structural/functional impairments and activity limitations facilitate the selection of the most appropriate intervention strategies (palliative/hospice versus long-term disease management) and provide objective criteria for determining the effects of such interventions. The documentation of these variables is thus essential in the determination of reasonable and necessary Medicare Hospice Services.

CGS Criteria:

Patients will be considered to be in the terminal stage of heart disease (life expectancy of six months or less) if they meet the following criteria. (1 and 2 should be present. Factors from 3 will add supporting documentation.):

1. At the time of initial certification or recertification for hospice, the patient is or has been already optimally treated for heart disease or is not a candidate for a surgical procedure or has declined a procedure. (Optimally treated means that patients who are not on vasodilators have a medical reason for refusing these drugs, e.g., hypotension or renal disease.)
2. The patient is classified as New York Heart Association (NYHA) Class IV and may have significant symptoms of heart failure or angina at rest. (Class IV patients with heart disease have an inability to carry on any physical activity without discomfort. Symptoms of heart failure or of the anginal syndrome may be present even at rest. If any physical activity is undertaken, discomfort is increased.) Significant congestive heart failure may be documented by an ejection fraction of ≤20%, but is not required if not already available.
3. Documentation of the following factors will support but is not required to establish eligibility for hospice care:
   • Treatment resistant symptomatic supraventricular or ventricular arrhythmias;
   • History of cardiac arrest or resuscitation;
   • History of unexplained syncope;
   • Brain embolism of cardiac origin;
   • Concomitant HIV disease.

Stages of Heart Failure (HF)
[ACC/AHA Guidelines for the Evaluation and Management of Chronic Heart Failure in the Adult: Executive Summary A Report of the American College of Cardiology/American Heart Association Task Force on Practice Guidelines (Committee to Revise the 1995 Guidelines for the Evaluation and Management of Heart Failure)]

Stage A
Patients at high risk of developing HF because of the presence of conditions that are strongly associated with the development of HF. Such patients have no identified structural or functional abnormalities of the pericardium, myocardium, or cardiac valves and have never shown signs or symptoms of HF.

Example: Systemic hypertension; coronary artery disease; diabetes mellitus; history of cardiotoxic drug therapy or alcohol abuse; personal history of rheumatic fever; family history of cardiomyopathy.

Stage B
Patients who have developed structural heart disease that is strongly associated with the development of HF but who have never shown signs or symptoms of HF.

Example: Left ventricular hypertrophy or fibrosis; left ventricular dilatation or hypocontractility; asymptomatic valvular heart disease; previous myocardial infarction.

Stage C
Patients who have current or prior symptoms of HF associated with underlying structural heart disease.

Example: Dyspnea or fatigue due to left ventricular systolic dysfunction; asymptomatic patients who are undergoing treatment for prior symptoms of HF.

Stage D
Patients with advanced structural heart disease and marked symptoms of HF at rest despite maximal medical therapy and who require specialized interventions.

Example: Patients who are frequently hospitalized for HF or cannot be safely discharged from the hospital; patients in the hospital awaiting heart transplantation; patients at home receiving continuous intravenous support for symptom relief or being supported with a mechanical circulatory assist device; patients in a hospice setting for management of HF.

NYHA Functional Classification for Congestive Heart Failure
The New York Heart Association (NYHA) Functional Classification provides a simple way of classifying heart disease (originally cardiac failure). It places patients in one of four categories, based on how much they are limited during physical activity:

Class I: patients with no limitation of activities; they suffer no symptoms from ordinary activities.

Class II: patients with slight, mild limitation of activity; they are comfortable with rest or with mild exertion.

Class III: patients with marked limitation of activity; they are comfortable only at rest.

Class IV: patients who should be at complete rest, confined to bed or chair; any physical activity brings on discomfort and symptoms occur at rest.

Hospice Stroke and Coma
L33393, National Government Services (NGS), Inc.

Indications and limitations of coverage and/or medical necessity:

Patients will be considered to be in the terminal stage of stroke or coma (life expectancy of six months or less) if they meet the following criteria.

Stroke:

1. Poor functional status with Karnofsky score 40% or less;
2. Inability to maintain hydration and caloric intake with one of the following:
   • Weight loss > 10% in the last 6 months or > 7.5% in the last 3 months
   • Serum albumin < 2.5 gm/dl
   • Current history of pulmonary aspiration not responsive to speech language pathology intervention; Sequential calorie counts documenting inadequate caloric/fluid intake
   • Dysphagia severe enough to prevent patient from continuing fluids/foods necessary to sustain life and patient does not receive artificial nutrition and hydration

Coma (any etiology):

1. Comatose patients with any three of the following on day three of coma:
   • Abnormal brain stem response
   • Absent verbal response
   • Absent withdrawal response to pain
   • Serum creatinine >1.5 mg/dl

Documentation of the following factors will support eligibility for hospice care:

1. Documentation of medical complications, in the context of progressive clinical decline, within the previous 12 months, which support a terminal prognosis:
   • Aspiration pneumonia
   • Upper urinary tract infection (pyelonephritis)
   • Sepsis
   • Refractory stage 3-4 decubitus ulcers
   • Fever recurrent after antibiotics

Documentation of diagnostic imaging factors which support poor prognosis after stroke include:

A. For non-traumatic hemorrhagic stroke:
   • Large-volume hemorrhage on CT:
     – Infratentorial: ≥20 ml.
     – Supratentorial: ≥50 ml.
   • Ventricular extension of hemorrhage.
   • Surface area of involvement of hemorrhage ≥30% of cerebrum.
   • Midline shift ≥1.5 cm.
   • Obstructive hydrocephalus in patient who declines, or is not a candidate for, ventriculoperitoneal shunt.

B. For thrombotic/embolic stroke:
   • Large anterior infarcts with both cortical and subcortical involvement.
   • Large bihemispheric infarcts.
   • Basilar artery occlusion.
   • Bilateral vertebral artery occlusion.

Hospice Alzheimer's Disease and Related Disorders

L34538—CGS Administrators, LLC, L33393—National Government Services, Inc,
L34567—Palmetto GBA

The following criteria based on the FAST scale is from the PGBA local coverage determination.

The Reisberg Functional Assessment Staging (FAST) Scale has been used for many years to describe Medicare beneficiaries with Alzheimer's disease and a prognosis of six months or less. The FAST Scale is a 16-item scale designed to parallel the progressive activity limitations associated with Alzheimer's disease. Stage 7 identifies the threshold of activity limitation that would support a six-month prognosis. The FAST Scale does not address the impact of comorbid and secondary conditions. These two variables are thus considered separately by this policy.

FAST Scale Items:

Stage #1: (1) No difficulty, either subjectively or objectively

Stage #2: (2) Complains of forgetting location of objects; subjective work difficulties

Stage #3: (3) Decreased job functioning evident to coworkers; difficulty in traveling to new locations

Stage #4: (4) Decreased ability to perform complex tasks (e.g., planning dinner for guests; handling finances)

Stage #5: (5) Requires assistance in choosing proper clothing

Stage #6: (6) Decreased ability to dress, bathe, and toilet independently:

- Sub-stage 6a: Difficulty putting clothing on properly
- Sub-stage 6b: Unable to bathe properly; may develop fear of bathing
- Sub-stage 6c: Inability to handle mechanics of toileting (i.e., forgets to flush, does not wipe properly)
- Sub-stage 6d: Urinary incontinence
- Sub-stage 6e: Fecal incontinence

Stage #7: (7) Loss of speech, locomotion, and consciousness:

- Sub-stage 7a: Ability to speak limited (1 to 5 words a day)
- Sub-stage 7b: All intelligible vocabulary lost
- Sub-stage 7c: Non-ambulatory
- Sub-stage 7d: Unable to sit up independently
- Sub-stage 7e: Unable to smile
- Sub-stage 7f: Unable to hold head up

Comorbid Conditions:

The significance of a given comorbid condition is best described by defining the structural/functional impairments - together with any limitation in activity - related to the comorbid condition. For example, a beneficiary with Alzheimer's disease and clinically significant CHD or COPD would have specific impairments of cardiorespiratory function (e.g., dyspnea, orthopnea, wheezing, chest pain) which may or may not respond/be amenable to treatment. The identified impairments in cardiorespiratory function would be associated with both specific structural impairments of the coronary arteries or bronchial tree and may be associated with activity limitations (e.g., mobility, self-care). Ultimately, the combined effects of the Alzheimer's disease (stage 7 or beyond) and any comorbid condition should be such that most beneficiaries with Alzheimer's disease and similar impairments would have a prognosis of six months or less.

Secondary Conditions:

Alzheimer's disease may be complicated by secondary conditions. The significance of a given secondary condition is best described by defining the structural/functional impairments - together with any limitation in activity related to the secondary condition. The occurrence of secondary conditions in beneficiaries with Alzheimer's disease is facilitated by the presence of impairments in such body functions as mental functioning and movement functions. Such functional impairments contribute to the increased incidence of secondary conditions such as delirium and pressure ulcers observed in Medicare beneficiaries with Alzheimer's Disease. Secondary conditions themselves may be associated with a new set of structural/functional impairments that may or may not respond/be amenable to treatment. Ultimately, the combined effects of the Alzheimer's disease (stage 7 or beyond) and any secondary condition should be such that most beneficiaries with Alzheimer's disease and similar impairments would have a prognosis of six months or less.

The documentation of structural/functional impairments and activity limitations facilitate the selection of intervention strategies (palliative vs. curative) and provide objective criteria for determining the effects of such interventions. The documentation of these variables is thus essential in the determination of reasonable and necessary Medicare Hospice Services.

For beneficiaries with Alzheimer's disease to be eligible for hospice the individual should have a FAST level of greater than or equal to 7 and specific comorbid or secondary conditions meeting the above criteria.

ICD-10-CM codes that support medical necessity:

F03.90–F03.91	Unspecified dementia
G30.0–G30.9	Alzheimer's disease
G31.01	Pick's disease
G31.1	Senile degeneration of brain, not elsewhere classified
G31.85	Corticobasal degeneration

The following criteria are from the CGS and NGS local coverage determinations.

Patients will be considered to be in the terminal stage of dementia (life expectancy of six months or less) if they meet the following criteria. This section is specific for Alzheimer's disease and related disorders.

1. Patients with dementia should show all the following characteristics:

    a. Stage seven or beyond according to the Functional Assessment Staging Scale;

    b. Unable to ambulate without assistance;

    c. Unable to dress without assistance;

    d. Unable to bathe without assistance;

    e. Urinary and fecal incontinence, intermittent or constant;

    f. No consistently meaningful verbal communication: stereotypical phrases only or the ability to speak is limited to six or fewer intelligible words.

2. Patients should have had one of the following within the past 12 months:

    a. Aspiration pneumonia;

    b. Pyelonephritis or other upper urinary tract infection;

    c. Septicemia;

    d. Decubitus ulcers, multiple, stage 3-4;

    e. Fever, recurrent after antibiotics;

    f. Inability to maintain sufficient fluid and calorie intake with 10% weight loss during the previous six months or serum albumin < 2.5 gm/dl.

Hospice Amyotrophic Lateral Sclerosis (ALS) and Neurological Conditions

L34547—Palmetto GBA, L33393—National Government Services, L34538—CGS Administrators, LLC

Indications and limitations of coverage and/or medical necessity:

General Considerations:

1. ALS tends to progress in a linear fashion over time. Thus the overall rate of decline in each patient is fairly constant and predictable, unlike many other non-cancer diseases.

2. However, no single variable deteriorates at a uniform rate in all patients. Therefore, multiple clinical parameters are required to judge the progression of ALS.

3. Although ALS usually presents in a localized anatomical area, the location of initial presentation does not correlate with survival time. By the time patients become end-stage, muscle denervation has become widespread, affecting all areas of the body, and initial predominance patterns do not persist.

4. Progression of disease differs markedly from patient to patient. Some patients decline rapidly and die quickly; others progress more slowly. For this reason, the history of the rate of progression in individual patients is important to obtain to predict prognosis.

5. In end-stage ALS, two factors are critical in determining prognosis: ability to breathe, and to a lesser extent ability to swallow. The former can be managed by artificial ventilation, and the latter by gastrostomy or other artificial feeding, unless the patient has recurrent aspiration pneumonia. While not necessarily a

contraindication to hospice care, the decision to institute either artificial ventilation or artificial feeding will significantly alter six month prognosis.

6. Examination by a neurologist within three months of assessment for hospice is advised, both to confirm the diagnosis and to assist with prognosis.

CGS specifics:

Patients will be considered to be in the terminal stage of ALS (life expectancy of six months or less) if they meet the following criteria: (Must fulfill 1, 2, or 3.)

1. The patient must demonstrate critically impaired breathing capacity.

   a. Critically impaired breathing capacity as demonstrated by all the following characteristics occurring within the 12 months preceding initial hospice certification:

   – Vital capacity (VC) less than 30% of normal
   – Significant dyspnea at rest
   – Requiring supplemental oxygen at rest
   – Patient declines invasive artificial ventilation.

2. Patient must demonstrate both rapid progression of ALS and critical nutritional impairment.

   a. Rapid progression of ALS as demonstrated by all the following characteristics occurring within the 12 months preceding initial hospice certification:

   – Progression from independent ambulation to wheelchair or bed-bound status;
   – Progression from normal to barely intelligible or unintelligible speech;
   – Progression from normal to pureed diet;
   – Progression from independence in most or all activities of daily living (ADLs) to needing major assistance by caretaker in all ADLs.

   b. Critical nutritional impairment as demonstrated by all the following characteristics occurring within the 12 months preceding initial hospice certification:

   – Oral intake of nutrients and fluids insufficient to sustain life;
   – Continuing weight loss;
   – Dehydration or hypovolemia;
   – Absence of artificial feeding methods.

3. Patient must demonstrate both rapid progression of ALS and life-threatening complications

   a. Rapid progression of ALS, see 2.a. above.

   b. Life-threatening complications as demonstrated by one of the following characteristics occurring within the 12 months preceding initial hospice certification:

   – Recurrent aspiration pneumonia (with or without tube feedings);
   – Upper urinary tract infection, e.g., pyelonephritis;
   – Sepsis;
   – Recurrent fever after antibiotic therapy.;
   – Stage 3 or 4 decubitus ulcer(s).

NGS specifics:

Patients are considered eligible for Hospice care if they do not elect tracheostomy and invasive ventilation and display evidence of critically impaired respiratory function (with or without use of NIPPV) and/or severe nutritional insufficiency (with or without use of a gastrostomy tube).

Critically impaired respiratory function is as defined by:

1. FVC < 40% predicted (seated or supine) and 2 or more of the following symptoms and/or signs:

   • Dyspnea at rest
   • Orthopnea
   • Use of accessory respiratory musculature
   • Paradoxical abdominal motion
   • Respiratory rate > 20
   • Reduced speech/vocal volume
   • Weakened cough
   • Symptoms of sleep disordered breathing
   • Frequent awakening
   • Daytime somnolence / excessive daytime sleepiness

   • Unexplained headaches
   • Unexplained confusion
   • Unexplained anxiety
   • Unexplained nausea

2. If unable to perform the FVC test, patients meet this criterion if they manifest 3 or more of the above symptoms/signs.

Severe nutritional insufficiency is defined as:

1. Dysphagia with progressive weight loss of at least 5% of body weight with or without election for gastrostomy tube insertion.

   These revised criteria rely less on the measured FVC, and as such reflect the reality that not all patients with ALS can or will undertake regular pulmonary function tests.

Hospice Liver Disease

L34544—Palmetto GBA, L33393—National Government Services, L34538—CGS Administrators, LLC

Indications and limitations of coverage and/or medical necessity:

Patients will be considered to be in the terminal stage of liver disease (life expectancy of six months or less) if they meet the following criteria: (1 and 2 must be present, factors from 3 will lend supporting documentation.)

1. The patient should show both a and b:

   a. Prothrombin time prolonged more than 5 seconds over control, or International Normalized Ration (INR) >1.5;

   b. Serum albumin < 2.5 gm/dl.

2. End stage liver disease is present and the patient shows at least one of the following:

   a. Ascites, refractory to treatment or patient noncompliant;

   b. Spontaneous bacterial peritonitis;

   c. Hepatorenal syndrome (elevated creatinine and BUN with oliguria (< 400 ml/day) and urine sodium concentration <10 mEq/l);

   d. Hepatic encephalopathy, refractory to treatment, or patient noncompliant;

   e. Recurrent variceal bleeding, despite intensive therapy.

3. Documentation of the following factors will support eligibility for hospice care:

   a. Progressive malnutrition

   b. Muscle wasting with reduced strength and endurance

   c. Continued active alcoholism (>80 gm ethanol/day)

   d. Hepatocellular carcinoma

   e. HBsAg (Hepatitis B) positivity

   f. Hepatitis C refractory to interferon treatment.

Patients awaiting liver transplant who otherwise fit the above criteria may be certified for the Medicare hospice benefit, but if a donor organ is procured, the patient must be discharged from hospice.

ICD-10-CM codes that support medical necessity:

Code	Description
C22.0	Liver cell carcinoma
C22.2	Hepatoblastoma
C22.3–C22.7	Sarcoma of liver
C22.8	Malignant neoplasm of liver, primary, unspecified as to type
K70.2	Alcoholic fibrosis and sclerosis of liver
K70.30–K70.31	Alcoholic cirrhosis of liver
K70.41	Alcoholic hepatic failure with coma
K71.0–K71.9	Toxic liver disease
K72.01	Acute and subacute hepatic failure with coma
K72.11	Chronic hepatic failure with coma
K72.91	Hepatic failure, unspecified with coma
K73.0–K73.9	Chronic hepatitis not elsewhere classified
K74.0	Hepatic fibrosis
K74.3–K74.5	Biliary cirrhosis
K74.60–K74.69	Other and unspecified cirrhosis of liver
K75.2–K75.4	Hepatitis
K75.81	Nonalcoholic steatohepatitis (NASH)

K76.4 Peliosis hepatis
K76.7 Hepatorenal syndrome
K76.81 Hepatopulmonary syndrome
K83.Ø1 Primary sclerosing cholangitis

Hospice Renal Disease

L34559—Palmetto GBA, L33393—National Government Services, L34538—CGS Administrators, LLC

Indications and limitations of coverage and/or medical necessity:

Patients will be considered to be in the terminal stage of renal disease (life expectancy of six months or less) if they meet the following criteria:

CGS criteria:

Acute renal failure (1, 2, and 3 must be present; factors from 4 will lend supporting documentation):

1. The patient is not seeking dialysis or renal transplant;
2. Creatinine clearance <10 cc/min (<15 cc/min. for diabetes); based on measurement or calculation; or <15cc/min (<20cc/min for diabetics) with comorbidity of congestive heart failure;
3. Serum creatinine >8.0 mg/dl (>6.0 mg/dl for diabetes)
4. Comorbid conditions:
   - Mechanical ventilation;
   - Malignancy (other organ system);
   - Chronic lung disease;
   - Advanced cardiac disease;
   - Advanced liver disease;
   - Sepsis;
   - Immunosuppression/AIDS;
   - Albumin < 3.5 gm/dl;
   - Cachexia;
   - Platelet count < 25,000;
   - Disseminated intravascular coagulation;
   - Gastrointestinal bleeding.

Chronic renal failure (1, 2, and 3 must be present; factors from 4 will lend supporting documentation):

1. The patient is not seeking dialysis or renal transplant or is discontinuing dialysis;
2. Creatinine clearance <10 cc/min (<15 cc/min for diabetics) based on measurement or calculation; or < 15cc/min (< 20cc/min for diabetics) with co-morbidity of congestive heart failure
3. Serum creatinine > 8.0 mg/dl (> 6.0 mg/dl for diabetes);
4. Signs and symptoms of renal failure:
   - Uremia;
   - Oliguria (< 400 cc/24 hours);
   - Intractable hyperkalemia (> 7.0) not responsive to treatment;
   - Uremic pericarditis;
   - Hepatorenal syndrome;
   - Intractable fluid overload, not responsive to treatment.

NGS criteria:

Patients will be considered to be in the terminal stage of renal disease (life expectancy of six months or less) if they meet the following criteria.

Acute Renal Failure (1 and either 2, 3 or 4 should be present. Factors from 5 will lend supporting documentation.)

1. The patient is not seeking dialysis or renal transplant, or is discontinuing dialysis. As with any other condition, an individual with renal disease is eligible for the Hospice benefit if that individual has a prognosis of six months or less, if the illness runs its normal course. There is no regulation precluding patients on dialysis from electing Hospice care. However, the continuation of dialysis will significantly alter a patient's prognosis, and thus potentially impact that individual's eligibility.

   When an individual elects Hospice care for end stage renal disease (ESRD) or for a condition to which the need for dialysis is related, the Hospice agency is financially responsible for the dialysis. In such cases, there is no additional reimbursement beyond the per diem rate. The only situation in which a beneficiary may access both the Hospice benefit and the ESRD benefit is when the need for dialysis is not related to the patient's terminal illness.

2. Creatinine clearance <10 cc/min (<15 cc/min. for diabetics); or <15cc/min (<20cc/min for diabetics) with comorbidity of congestive heart failure.
3. Serum creatinine > 8.0 mg/dl (>6.0 mg/dl for diabetics).
4. Estimated glomerular filtration rate (GFR) <10 ml/min.
5. Comorbid conditions:
   a. Mechanical ventilation;
   b. Malignancy (other organ system);
   c. Chronic lung disease;
   d. Advanced cardiac disease;
   e. Advanced liver disease;
   f. Immunosuppression/AIDS;
   g. Albumin < 3.5 gm/dl;
   h. Platelet count < 25,000;
   i. Disseminated intravascular coagulation;
   j. Gastrointestinal bleeding.

Chronic Kidney Disease (1 and either 2, 3 or 4 should be present. Factors from 5 will lend supporting documentation.)

1. The patient is not seeking dialysis or renal transplant, or is discontinuing dialysis; As with any other condition, an individual with renal disease is eligible for the Hospice benefit if that individual has a prognosis of six months or less, if the illness runs its normal course. There is no regulation precluding patients on dialysis from electing Hospice care. However, the continuation of dialysis will significantly alter a patient's prognosis, and thus potentially impact that individual's eligibility.

   When an individual elects hospice care for end stage renal disease (ESRD) or for a condition to which the need for dialysis is related, the Hospice agency is financially responsible for the dialysis. In such cases, there is no additional reimbursement beyond the per diem rate. The only situation in which a beneficiary may access both the Hospice benefit and the ESRD benefit is when the need for dialysis is not related to the patient's terminal illness.

2. Creatinine clearance <10 cc/min (<15 cc/min for diabetics); or <15cc/min (<20cc/min for diabetics) with comorbidity of congestive heart failure.
3. Serum creatinine >8.0 mg/dl (>6.0 mg/dl for diabetics).
4. Signs and symptoms of renal failure:
   a. Uremia;
   b. Oliguria (<400 cc/24 hours);
   c. Intractable hyperkalemia (> 7.0) not responsive to treatment;
   d. Uremic pericarditis;
   e. Hepatorenal syndrome;
   f. Intractable fluid overload, not responsive to treatment.
5. Estimated glomerular filtration rate (GFR) <10 ml/min.

Indications and/or limitations of coverage:

Palmetto Criteria

End stage renal disease (ESRD) may support a prognosis of six months or less under many clinical scenarios. The identification of specific structural/functional impairments, together with any relevant activity limitations, should serve as the basis for palliative interventions and care planning. The structural and functional impairments associated with a primary diagnosis of ESRD are often complicated by comorbid and/or secondary conditions. Comorbid conditions affecting beneficiaries with ESRD are by definition distinct from the ESRD itself—examples include vascular disease manifested as coronary heart disease (CHD), peripheral vascular disease (PVD), and vascular dementia. Secondary conditions, on the other hand, are directly related to a primary condition. In the case of ESRD, examples include secondary hyperparathyroidism, calciphylaxis, nephrogenic systemic fibrosis, electrolyte abnormalities and anorexia. The important roles of comorbid and secondary conditions are described below in order to facilitate their recognition and assist providers in documenting their impact. Use of the *International Classification of Functioning, Disability and Health* (ICF) is suggested, but not required.

Medicare rules and regulations require the documentation of sufficient "clinical information and other documentation" to support the certification of individuals as having a terminal illness with a life expectancy of 6 or fewer months, if the illness runs its normal course. For beneficiaries with ESRD, the identification of relevant comorbid and secondary conditions, together with the identification and description of associated structural/functional impairments, activity limitations, and environmental factors would help establish hospice eligibility and maintain a beneficiary-centered plan of care.

Secondary Conditions:

ESRD may be complicated by secondary conditions. The significance of a given secondary condition is best described by defining the structural/functional impairments—together with any limitation in activity—related to the secondary condition. The occurrence of secondary conditions in beneficiaries with ESRD is facilitated by the presence of impairments in such body functions as urinary excretory function, water, mineral and electrolyte function, and endocrine gland functions. Such functional impairments contribute to the increased incidence of secondary conditions such as hyperkalemia, fluid overload, and secondary hyperparathyroidism observed in Medicare beneficiaries with ESRD. Secondary conditions themselves may be associated with a new set of structural/functional impairments that may or may not respond/be amenable to treatment. Ultimately, the combined effects of the ESRD and any secondary condition should be such that most beneficiaries with ESRD and similar impairments would have a prognosis of six months or less.

Comorbid Conditions:

The significance of a given comorbid condition is best described by defining the structural/functional impairments—together with any limitation in activity—related to the comorbid condition. For example, a beneficiary with ESRD and clinically significant CHD would have specific impairments of cardiovascular structure/function (e.g., narrowing of coronary arteries, dyspnea, orthopnea, chest pain) which may or may not respond/be amenable to treatment. The identified impairments in cardiovascular structure/function may be associated with activity limitations (e.g., mobility, self-care). Ultimately, the combined effects of the ESRD and any comorbid condition should be such that most beneficiaries with ESRD and similar impairments would have a prognosis of six months or less.

The documentation of structural/functional impairments and activity limitations facilitates the selection of intervention strategies (palliative vs. long-term disease management/curative) and provides objective criteria for determining the effects of such interventions. The documentation of these variables is thus essential in the determination of reasonable and necessary Medicare Hospice Services.

ICD-10-CM codes that support medical necessity:

I12.0	Hypertensive chronic kidney disease with stage 5 chronic kidney disease or end stage renal disease
I13.11	Hypertensive heart and chronic kidney disease without heart failure, with stage 5 chronic kidney disease, or end stage renal disease
I13.2	Hypertensive heart and chronic kidney disease with heart failure and with stage 5 chronic kidney disease, or end stage renal disease
N17.0	Acute kidney failure with tubular necrosis
N17.1	Acute kidney failure with acute cortical necrosis
N17.2	Acute kidney failure with medullary necrosis
N17.8	Other acute kidney failure
N17.9	Acute kidney failure, unspecified
N18.6	End stage renal disease
N19	Unspecified kidney failure

Hospice Pulmonary Disease
L33393—National Government Services, L34538—CGS Administrators, LLC

Indications and/or limitations of coverage:

Patients will be considered to be in the terminal stage of pulmonary disease (life expectancy of six months or less) if they meet the following criteria. The criteria refer to patients with various forms of advanced pulmonary disease who eventually follow a final common pathway for end stage pulmonary disease. (1 and 2 should be present. Documentation of 3, 4, and 5, will lend supporting documentation.):

1. Severe chronic lung disease as documented by both a and b:

   a. Disabling dyspnea at rest, poorly or unresponsive to bronchodilators, resulting in decreased functional capacity, e.g., bed to chair existence, fatigue, and cough: (Documentation of Forced Expiratory Volume in One Second (FEV1), after bronchodilator, less than 30% of predicted is objective evidence for disabling dyspnea, but is not necessary to obtain.)

   b. Progression of end stage pulmonary disease, as evidenced by increasing visits to the emergency department or hospitalizations for pulmonary infections and/or respiratory failure or increasing physician home visits prior to initial certification. (Documentation of serial decrease of FEV1>40 ml/year is objective evidence for disease progression, but is not necessary to obtain.)

2. Hypoxemia at rest on room air, as evidenced by pO2 =55 mmHg; or oxygen saturation =88%, determined either by arterial blood gases or oxygen saturation monitors; (These values may be obtained from recent hospital records.) OR Hypercapnia, as evidenced by pCO2 =50 mmHg. (This value may be obtained from recent [within 3 months] hospital records.)

3. Right heart failure (RHF) secondary to pulmonary disease (Cor pulmonale) (e.g., not secondary to left heart disease or valvulopathy).

4. Unintentional progressive weight loss of greater than 10% of body weight over the preceding six months.

5. Resting tachycardia >100/min.

Hospice the Adult Failure to Thrive Syndrome
L34558—Palmetto GBA.

Indications and/or limitations of coverage and medical necessity:

The adult failure to thrive syndrome is characterized by unexplained weight loss, malnutrition and disability. The syndrome has been associated with multiple primary conditions (e.g., infections and malignancies), but always includes two defining clinical elements, namely nutritional impairment and disability. The nutritional impairment and disability associated with the adult failure to thrive syndrome may be severe enough to have an impact on the patient's short-term survival.

The adult failure to thrive syndrome may manifest as an irreversible progression in the patient's nutritional impairment/disability despite a trial of therapy (i.e., treatment intended to affect the primary condition responsible for the patient's clinical presentation). The presence of comorbid conditions may hasten the patient's clinical progression and as such should be identified and addressed. This hospice policy addresses those cases where reversible causes of severe nutritional impairment and disability (i.e., the adult failure to thrive syndrome) have been excluded.

The Medicare Hospice Benefit is predicated upon physician-certification that an individual entitled to Part A of Medicare is terminally ill. An individual is considered to be terminally ill if the individual has a medical prognosis that his or her life expectancy is six months or less if the terminal illness runs its normal course. The medical criteria listed below would support a terminal prognosis for individuals with the adult failure to thrive syndrome. Medical criteria 1 and 2 are important indicators of nutritional and functional status respectively, and would thus support a terminal prognosis if met.

1. The nutritional impairment associated with the adult failure to thrive syndrome should be severe enough to impact a beneficiary's weight. It is expected that the Body Mass Index (BMI) of beneficiaries electing the Medicare Hospice Benefit for the adult failure to thrive syndrome will be below 22 kg/m 2 and that the patient is either declining enteral/parenteral nutritional support or has not responded to such nutritional support, despite an adequate caloric intake.

   BMI (kg/m 2) = 703 x (weight in pounds) divided by (height in inches) 2

2. The disability associated with the adult failure to thrive syndrome should be such that the individual is significantly disabled. Significant disability would be demonstrated by a Karnofsky or Palliative Performance Scale value less than or equal to 40%.

Both the beneficiary's BMI and level of disability should be determined using measurements/observations made within six months (180 days) of the most recent certification/recertification date. If enteral nutritional support has been instituted prior to the election of the Hospice Medicare Benefit and will be continued, the BMI and level of disability should be determined using measurements/observations made at the time of the initial certification and at each subsequent recertification.

At the time of recertification recumbent measurement(s) (anthropometry) such as mid-arm muscle area in cm 2 may be substituted for BMI with documentation as to why a BMI could not be measured. This information will be subject to review on a case by case basis.

In the event a beneficiary presenting with a nutritional impairment and disability does not meet the medical criteria listed above, but is still thought to be eligible for the Medicare Hospice Benefit, an alternate diagnosis that best describes the clinical circumstances of the individual beneficiary should be selected (e.g. R63.4 "abnormal loss of weight" and R64 "Cachexia").

ICD-10 Codes That Support Medical Necessity:

M62.84	Sarcopenia
R62.51	Failure to thrive (child)
R62.7	Adult failure to thrive
R63.4	Abnormal weight loss
R64	Cachexia

Source of Information

Social Security Act, Sections, 1102, 1812 (a)(4)and (d);1813 (a) (4); 1814 (a)(7) and (I); 1862 (a)(1),(6), and (9); 1861 (dd), 1871

42 CFR Part 418

CMS Manual Publication 100-2, Medicare Benefits Policy Chapter 9 Coverage of Hospice Services under Hospital Insurance, §10 Requirements

CMS Manual Publication 100-3, Medicare National Coverage Determinations

CMS Medicare Coverage Database:

http://www.cms.hhs.gov/mcd/search.asp? Search: Local Coverage, policies (LMRP/LCD); Final policies only Geographic area: all states Coverage topics: Hospice

Appendix K: Hospice Diagnosis and Quality Reporting Guidance

Highlights of the FY 2019 Hospice Final Rule

Hospice Wage Index

The hospice wage index is used to adjust payment rates for hospice agencies under the Medicare program to reflect local differences in area wage levels, based on the location where services are furnished. The hospice wage index utilizes the wage adjustment factors used by the Secretary for purposes of section 1886(d)(3)(E) of the Act for hospital wage adjustments. Our regulations at §418.306(c) require each labor market to be established using the most current hospital wage data available, including any changes made by Office of Management and Budget (OMB) to the Metropolitan Statistical Areas (MSAs) definitions.

CMS used the previous FY's hospital wage index data to calculate the hospice wage index values. For FY 2019, the hospice wage index will be based on the FY 2018 hospital pre-floor, pre-reclassified wage index. This means that the hospital wage data used for the hospice wage index is not adjusted to take into account any geographic reclassification of hospitals including those in accordance with section 1886(d)(8)(B) or 1886(d)(10) of the Act. The appropriate wage index value is applied to the labor portion of the payment rate based on the geographic area in which the beneficiary resides when receiving RHC or CHC. The appropriate wage index value is applied to the labor portion of the payment rate based on the geographic location of the facility for beneficiaries receiving GIP or IRC.

In the FY 2006 Hospice Wage Index final rule (70 FR45135), CMS adopted the policy that for urban labor markets without a hospital from which hospital wage index data could be derived, all of the CBSAs within the state would be used to calculate a statewide urban average pre-floor, pre-reclassified hospital wage index value to use as a reasonable proxy for these areas. For FY 2019, the only CBSA without a hospital from which hospital wage data can be derived is 25980, Hinesville-Fort Stewart, Georgia.

There exist some geographic areas where there were no hospitals, and thus, no hospital wage index data on which to base the calculation of the hospice wage index. In the FY 2008 Hospice Wage Index final rule (72 FR 50214), CMS implemented a methodology to update the hospice wage index for such areas. In cases where there was a rural area without rural hospital wage data, CMS used the average pre-floor, pre-reclassified hospital wage index data from all contiguous Core-Based Statistical Areas (CBSAs), to represent a reasonable proxy for the rural area. The term "contiguous" means sharing a border (72 FR 50217). Currently, the only rural area without a hospital from which hospital wage data could be derived is Puerto Rico. However, for rural Puerto Rico, CMS would not apply this methodology due to the distinct economic circumstances that exist there (for example, due to the close proximity to one another of almost all of Puerto Rico's various urban and non-urban areas, this methodology would produce a wage index for rural Puerto Rico that is higher than that in half of its urban areas); instead, CMS would continue to use the most recent wage index previously available for that area. For FY 2019, CMS will continue to use the most recent pre-floor, pre-reclassified hospital wage index value available for Puerto Rico, which is 0.4047.

As described in the August 8, 1997 Hospice Wage Index final rule (62 FR 42860), the pre-floor and pre-reclassified hospital wage index is used as the raw wage index for the hospice benefit. These raw wage index values are subject to application of the hospice floor to compute the hospice wage index used to determine payments to hospices. Pre-floor, pre-reclassified hospital wage index values below 0.8 are adjusted by a 15 percent increase subject to a maximum wage index value of 0.8. For example, if County A has a pre-floor, pre-reclassified hospital wage index value of 0.3994, CMS would multiply 0.3994 by 1.15, which equals 0.4593. Since 0.4593 is not greater than 0.8, then County A's hospice wage index would be 0.4593. In another example, if County B has a pre-floor, pre-reclassified hospital wage index value of 0.7440, CMS would multiply 0.7440 by 1.15 which equals 0.8556. Because 0.8556 is greater than 0.8, County B's hospice wage index would be 0.8.

On February 28, 2013, OMB issued OMB Bulletin No. 13-01, announcing revisions to the delineation of MSAs, Micropolitan Statistical Areas, and Combines Statistical Areas, and guidance on uses of the delineation in these areas. In the FY 2016 Hospice Wage Index and Payment Rate Update final rule (80 FR 47178), CMS adopted the OMB's new area delineations using a 1-year transition. Also in that final rule, CMS stated that beginning October 1, 2016, the wage index for all hospice payments would be fully based on the new OMB delineations.

On August 15, 2017, OMB issued bulletin No. 17–01, which announced that one Micropolitan Statistical Area, Twin Falls, Idaho, now qualifies as a Metropolitan Statistical Area. The new CBSA (46300) comprises the principal city of Twin Falls, Idaho, in Jerome County, Idaho, and Twin Falls County, Idaho. The FY 2019 hospice wage index value for CBSA 46300, Twin Falls, Idaho, will be 0.8000.

The hospice wage index applicable for FY 2019 (October 1, 2018, through September 30, 2019) is available on the CMS website at http://www.cms.gov/Medicare/Medicare-Fee-for-Service-Payment/Hospice/index.html.

The wage index applicable for FY 2018 is available on the CMS Web site at http://www.cms.gov/Medicare/Medicare-Fee-for-Service-Payment/Hospice/index.html. As of FY 2012, the wage index values applicable for the upcoming fiscal year and subsequent fiscal years are no longer published in the Federal Register (77 FR 44242). The hospice wage index for FY 2018 will be effective October 1, 2017 through September 30, 2018.

Hospice Payment Update Percentage

Section 4441(a) of the Balanced Budget Act of 1997 (BBA) (Pub. L. 105–33) amended section 1814(i)(1)(C)(ii)(VI) of the Act to establish updates to hospice rates for FYs 1998 through 2002. Hospice rates were to be updated by a factor equal to the inpatient hospital market basket percentage increase set out under section 1886(b)(3)(B)(iii) of the Act, minus 1 percentage point. Payment rates for FYs since 2002 have been updated according to section 1814(i)(1)(C)(ii)(VII) of the Act, which states that the update to the payment rates for subsequent FYs must be the inpatient market basket percentage increase for that FY. The Act historically required CMS to use the inpatient hospital market basket as the basis for the hospice payment rate update.

Section 3401(g) of the PPACA mandated that, starting with FY 2013 (and in subsequent FYs), the hospice payment update percentage would be annually reduced by changes in economy-wide productivity as specified in section 1886(b)(3)(B)(xi)(II) of the Act. The statute defines the productivity adjustment to be equal to the 10-year moving average of changes in annual economy-wide private nonfarm business multifactor productivity (MFP). In addition to the MFP adjustment, section 3401(g) of the ACA also mandated that in FY 2013 through FY 2019, the hospice payment update percentage would be reduced by an additional 0.3 percentage point (although for FY 2014 to FY 2019, the potential 0.3 percentage point reduction is subject to suspension under conditions specified in section 1814(i)(1)(C)(v) of the Act).

The hospice payment update percentage for FY 2019 is based on the inpatient hospital market basket update of 2.9 percent. Due to the requirements at sections 1886(b)(3)(B)(xi)(II) and 1814(i)(1)(C)(v) of the Act, the inpatient hospital market basket update for FY 2019 of 2.9 percent must be reduced by an MFP adjustment as mandated by the PPACA (0.8 percentage point for FY 2019). The inpatient hospital market basket update for FY 2019 is reduced further by 0.3 percentage point, as mandated by the PPACA. In effect, the hospice payment update percentage for FY 2019 is 1.8 percent.

Currently, the labor portion of the hospice payment rates is as follows: For RHC, 68.71 percent; for CHC, 68.71 percent; for General Inpatient Care, 64.01 percent; and for Respite Care, 54.13 percent. The non-labor portion is equal to 100 percent minus the labor portion for each level of care. Therefore, the non-labor portion of the payment rates is as follows: For RHC, 31.29 percent; for CHC, 31.29 percent; for General Inpatient Care, 35.99 percent; and for Respite Care, 45.87 percent. Beginning with cost reporting periods starting on or after October 1, 2014, freestanding hospice providers are required to submit cost data using CMS Form 1984-14 (https://www.cms.gov/Research-Statistics-Data-and-Systems/Downloadable-Public-Use-Files/Cost-Reports/Hospice-2014.html). CMS is currently analyzing this data for possible use in updating the labor portion of the hospice payment rates.

Hospice Payment Rates

There are four payment categories that are distinguished by the location and intensity of the services provided. The base payments are adjusted for geographic differences in wages by multiplying the labor share, which varies by category, of each base rate by the applicable hospice wage index. A hospice is paid the RHC rate for each day the beneficiary is enrolled in hospice, unless the hospice provides continuous home care (CHC), IRC, or general inpatient care (GIP). CHC is provided during a period of patient crisis to maintain the person at home; IRC is short-term care to allow the usual caregiver to rest and be relieved from caregiving; and GIP is to treat symptoms that cannot be managed in another setting.

As discussed in the FY 2016 Hospice Wage Index and Payment Rate Update final rule (80 FR 47172), CMS implemented two different RHC payment rates, one RHC rate for the first 60 days and a second RHC rate for days 61 and beyond. In addition, in the final rule, we adopted a Service Intensity Add-on (SIA) payment, when direct patient care is provided by a RN or social worker during the last 7 days of the beneficiary's life. The SIA payment is equal to the CHC hourly rate multiplied by the hours of nursing or social work provided (up to 4 hours total) that occurred on the day of service. In order to maintain budget neutrality, as required under section 1814(i)(6)(D)(ii) of the Act, the new RHC rates were adjusted by a SIA budget neutrality factor.

As discussed in the FY 2016 Hospice Wage Index and Rate Update final rule (80 FR 47177), CMS will continue to make the SIA payments budget neutral through an annual determination of the SIA budget neutrality factor (SBNF), which will then be applied to the RHC payment rates. The SBNF will be calculated for each FY using the most current and complete utilization data available at the time of rulemaking. For FY 2019, CMS calculated the SBNF using FY 2017 utilization data. For FY 2019, the SBNF that would apply to days 1 through 60 is calculated to be 0.9991. The SBNF that would apply to days 61 and beyond is calculated to be 0.9998.

In the FY 2017 Hospice Wage Index and Payment Rate Update final rule (81 FR 52156), CMS initiated a policy of applying a wage index standardization factor to hospice payments in order to eliminate the aggregate effect of annual variations in hospital wage data. In order to calculate the wage index standardization factor, CMS simulates total payments using the FY 2019 hospice wage index and compared it to its simulation of total payments using the FY 2018 hospice wage index. By dividing payments for each level of care using the FY 2019 wage index by payments for each level of care using the FY 2018 wage index, CMS obtained a wage index standardization factor for each level of care (RHC days 1-60, RHC days 61+, CHC, IRC, and GIP). The wage index standardization factors for each level of care are shown in the tables below.

Lastly, the hospice payment rates for hospices that submit the required quality data would be increased by the FY 2018 hospice payment update percentage of 1.0 percent as discussed in section III.B.2 of the FY2018 final rule.

FY 2019 Hospice RHC Payment Rates

CODE	DESCRIPTION	FY 2018 PAYMENT RATES	SIA BUDGET NEUTRALITY FACTOR	WAGE INDEX STANDARDIZATION FACTOR	FY 2019 HOSPICE PAYMENT UPDATE	FY 2019 PAYMENT RATES
651	Routine Home Care (days 1-60)	$192.78	x 0.9991	x 1.0009	x 1.018	$196.25
651	Routine Home Care (days 61+)	$151.41	x 0.9998	x 1.0007	x 1.018	$154.21

FY 2019 Hospice CHC, IRC, and GIP Payment Rates

CODE	DESCRIPTION	FY 2017 PAYMENT RATES	WAGE INDEX STANDARDIZATION FACTOR	FY 2018 HOSPICE PAYMENT UPDATE	FY 2018 PAYMENT RATES
652	Continuous Home Care Full Rate = 24 hours of care; $41.56 = FY 2019 hourly rate	$976.42	x 1.0034	x 1.018	$997.38
655	Inpatient Respite Care (IRC)	$172.78	x 1.0007	x 1.018	$176.01
656	General Inpatient Care (GIP)	$743.55	x 1.0015	x 1.018	$758.07

Sections 1814(i)(5)(A) through (C) of the Act require that hospices submit quality data, based on measures to be specified by the Secretary. In the FY 2012 Hospice Wage Index final rule (76 FR 47320 through 47324), CMS implemented a Hospice Quality Reporting Program (HQRP) as required by section 3004 of the Affordable Care Act. Hospices were required to begin collecting quality data in October 2012, and submit that quality data in 2013. Section 1814(i)(5)(A)(i) of the Act requires that beginning with FY 2014 and each subsequent FY, the Secretary shall reduce the market basket update by 2 percentage points for any hospice that does not comply with the quality data submission requirements with respect to that FY. The FY 2019 rates for hospices that do not submit the required quality data would be updated by the FY 2019 hospice payment update percentage of 1.8 percent minus 2 percentage points.

Hospice Cap Amount

As discussed in the FY 2016 Hospice Wage Index and Payment Rate Update final rule (80 FR 47183), CMS implemented changes mandated by the Improving Medicare Post-Acute Care Transformation Act of 2014 (IMPACT Act). Specifically, for accounting years that end after September 30, 2016 and before October 1, 2025, the hospice cap is updated by the hospice payment update percentage rather than using the consumer price index for urban consumers (CPI–U). The hospice cap amount for the 2019 cap year will be $29,205.44, which is equal to the 2018 cap amount ($28,689.04) updated by the FY 2019 hospice payment update percentage of 1.8 percent.

Previously Adopted Quality Measures for FY 2019 Payment Determination and Future Years

In the FY 2014 Hospice Wage Index final rule (78 FR 48257), and in compliance with section 1814(i)(5)(C) of the Act, CMS finalized the specific collection of data items that support the following 7 NQF-endorsed measures for hospice:

- NQF #1617 Patients Treated with an Opioid who are Given a Bowel Regimen,
- NQF #1634 Pain Screening,
- NQF #1637 Pain Assessment,
- NQF #1638 Dyspnea Treatment,
- NQF #1639 Dyspnea Screening,
- NQF #1641 Treatment Preferences,
- NQF #1647 Beliefs/Values Addressed (if desired by the patient).

CMS finalized the following two additional measures in the FY 2017 Hospice Wage Index final rule effective April 1, 2017. Data collected will, if not reported, affect payments for FY 2019 and subsequent years. (81 FR 52163 through 52173):

- Hospice Visits when Death is Imminent
- Hospice and Palliative Care Composite Process Measure—Comprehensive Assessment at Admission

The Hospice and Palliative Care Composite Process Measure — Comprehensive Assessment at Admission measure (hereafter referred to as "the Hospice Comprehensive Assessment Measure") underwent an off-cycle review by the NQF Palliative and End-of-Life Standing Committee and successfully received NQF endorsement in July 2017.

Data for the Hospice Visits When Death Is Imminent measure pair is being collected using new items added to the HIS V2.00.0, effective April 1, 2017. This one measure comprises a measure pair assessing hospice staff visits to patients at the end of life. Measure 1: Percentage of patients receiving at least one visit from registered nurses, physicians, nurse practitioners, or physician assistants in the last 3 days of life. Measure 2: Percentage of patients receiving at least two visits from medical social workers, chaplains or spiritual counselors, licensed practical nurses or hospice aides in the last 7 days of life. CMS will need at least 4 quarters of reliable data to conduct the necessary analyses to support submission to NQF. CMS will also need to assess the quality of data submitted in the first quarter of item implementation to determine whether they can be used in the analyses. CMS has begun analysis of the data, and, pending analysis, will submit the Hospice Visits When Death Is Imminent measure pair to NQF for endorsement review in accordance with NQF project timelines and call for measures. CMS will use a similar process to analyze and submit new quality measures to NQF for endorsement in future years. Providers will be notified of measure endorsement and public reporting through subregulatory channels.

In the FY 2015 Hospice Wage Index final rule (79 FR 50491 through 50496), CMS also finalized the Consumer Assessment of Healthcare Providers and Systems (CAHPS®) Hospice Survey to support quality measures based on patient and family experience of care. Please refer to section III.F.5 of the FY 2019 final rule for details regarding the CAHPS® Hospice Survey, including public reporting of selected survey measures.

Previously Finalized Quality Measures Affecting the FY 2019 Payment Determination and Subsequent Years

NQF No.	Hospice item set quality measure	Year the measure was first adopted for use in APU determination
1641	Treatment Preferences	FY 2016
1647	Beliefs/Values Addressed (if desired by the patient)	FY 2016
1634	Pain Screening	FY 2016
1637	Pain Assessment	FY 2016
1639	Dyspnea Screening	FY 2016
1638	Dyspnea Treatment	FY 2016
1617	Patients Treated with an Opioid Who Are Given a Bowel Regimen	FY 2016
3235	Hospice and Palliative Care Composite Process Measure—Comprehensive Assessment at Admission	FY 2019
TBD	Hospice Visits When Death is Imminent Measure Pair	FY 2019

CAHPS® Hospice Survey Participation Requirements for the FY 2023 APU and Subsequent Years

The CAHPS® Hospice Survey of CMS' HQRP is used to collect data on the experiences of hospice patients and the primary caregivers listed in their hospice records. Readers who want more information are referred to CMS's extensive discussion of the Hospice Experience of Care prior to the proposal for the public reporting of measures may refer to 79 FR 50452 and 78 FR 48261.

Background and Description of the CAHPS Hospice Survey

The CAHPS® Hospice Survey is the first standardized national survey available to collect information on patients' and informal caregivers' experience of hospice care. Patient centered experience measures are a key component of the CMS Quality Strategy, emphasizing patient-centered care by rating experience as a means to empower patients and their caregivers and improving the quality of their care. In addition, the survey introduces standard survey administration protocols that allow for fair comparisons across hospices.

Although the development of the CAHPS® Hospice Survey predates the Meaningful Measures initiative, it used many of the Meaningful Measure principles in its development. The overarching quality priority of "Strengthen Person and Family Engagement as Partners in Their Care" includes Meaningful Measure areas such as "Care Is Personalized and Aligned with Patient's Goals," "End of Life Care According to Preferences" and "Patient's Experience of Care." The survey questions were developed with input from caregivers of patients who died under hospice care. The survey focuses on topics that are meaningful to caregivers/patients and supports CMS's efforts to put the patient and their family members first.

Details regarding CAHPS Hospice Survey national implementation, survey administration, participation requirements, exemptions from the survey's requirements, hospice patient and caregiver eligibility criteria, fielding schedules, sampling requirements, survey instruments, and the languages that are available for the survey, are all available on the official CAHPS® Hospice Survey website: https://www.HospiceCAHPSsurvey.org, and in the CAHPS® Hospice Survey Quality Assurance Guidelines (QAG), which are posted on the website.

Overview of the CAHPS® Hospice Survey Measures

The CAHPS® Hospice Survey is administered after the patient is deceased and queries the decedent's primary, informal caregiver (usually a family member) regarding the patient and family experience of care, unlike the Hospital CAHPS® Survey deployed in 2006 (71 FR 48037 through 48039) and other subsequent CAHPS® surveys. National implementation of the CAHPS® Hospice Survey commenced January 1, 2015, as stated in the FY 2015 Hospice Wage Index and Payment Rate Update final rule (79 FR 50452).

The survey consists of 47 questions and is available (using the mailed version) in English, Spanish, Chinese, Russian, Portuguese, Vietnamese, Polish, and Korean. It covers topics such as access to care, communications, getting help for symptoms, and interactions with hospice staff. The survey also contains 2 global rating questions and asks for self-reported demographic information (race/ ethnicity, educational attainment level, languages spoken at home, among others). The CAHPS® Hospice Survey measures received NQF endorsement on October 26th, 2016 (NQF #2651). Measures derived from the CAHPS® Hospice Survey include 6 multi-item (composite) measures and 2 global ratings measures. They received NQF endorsement on October 26, 2016 (NQF #2651). CMS adopted these 8 survey based measures for the CY 2018 data collection period and for subsequent years. These 8 measures are reported on Hospice Compare.

Appendix L: Coding Issues for Long-Term Care (LTC)

The Uniform Hospital Discharge Data Set (UHDDS) definition of principal diagnosis, "that condition established after study to be chiefly responsible for occasioning the admission of the patient to the hospital for care," is applied across all nonoutpatient settings, including long-term care.

In a long-term care setting, the principal diagnosis is regarded as the "first-listed diagnosis" and is the diagnosis that is chiefly responsible for the admission to the facility, or the diagnosis that is chiefly responsible for continued residence in the facility and should be sequenced first. In addition, chronic conditions that affect a resident's care are also coded. The diagnoses present and the sequencing of these diagnoses depend on the point in time the coding is done as ICD-10-CM codes can be assigned upon admission; concurrently as diagnoses arise; or at the time of discharge, transfer, or death of the resident.

The following guidelines and examples have been developed and approved by the Cooperating Parties in conjunction with the Editorial Advisory Board of *Coding Clinic*, to standardize the process of data collection for LTC and to assist the coder in coding and reporting these cases using ICD-10-CM. This guidance appeared in *Coding Clinic for ICD-10-CM*, published by the American Hospital Association, 4Q, '12, 90-98; 4Q, '13, 129; 1Q, '14, 23; 3Q, '16, 16-17; 3Q, '17, 4.

Example 1:

The patient is discharged from the acute care hospital and admitted to the LTC facility with a diagnosis of acute cerebrovascular accident (CVA) with left-sided hemiparesis and dysphasia.

First listed diagnosis:
I69.354, Hemiplegia and hemiparesis following cerebral infarction affecting left non-dominant side

Additional diagnosis:
I69.321, Dysphasia following cerebral infarction

The hemiparesis and dysphasia are considered sequelae of the acute CVA for this LTC admission. Coding guidelines state that these "late effects" include neurologic deficits that persist after initial onset of conditions classifiable to categories I60-I67. Codes from I60-I67 are reserved for the initial (first) episode of care for the acute cerebrovascular disease. Coding guidelines also provide guidance as to the use of dominant/nondominant side for codes from category I69.

There is no time limit on when a late effect code may be used since the neurologic deficit caused by cerebrovascular disease may be present from the onset or may arise at any time after the onset of the condition classifiable to I60-I67. When the patient is admitted to LTC following treatment of an acute CVA, a code from subcategory I69.3, Sequelae of cerebral infarction, is assigned for the LTC admission.

Example 2:

A patient with progressive senile dementia, coronary artery disease, and congestive heart failure is admitted to a LTC facility after suffering a CVA and receiving treatment elsewhere. The patient has made a complete recovery from the CVA prior to admission to the LTC facility. She is admitted for long-term care because of her chronic illnesses and her deteriorating mental status.

First listed diagnosis:
F03.90, Unspecified dementia without behavioral disturbance

Additional diagnoses:
I50.9, Heart failure, unspecified

I25.10, Atherosclerotic heart disease of native coronary artery without angina pectoris

Z86.73, Personal history of transient ischemic attack (TIA), and cerebral infarction without residual deficits

Any of the patient's chronic diseases can be listed first, since each one could be considered chiefly responsible for LTC facility admission. Since this patient has no residuals from the CVA, a code from category I69, Sequelae of cerebrovascular disease, is inappropriate. Instead, code Z86.73, Personal history of transient ischemic attack (TIA), and cerebral infarction without residual deficits, may be assigned to identify the history of CVA without residual deficits.

Example 3:

A patient is admitted to the LTC facility for physical therapy from an acute care setting after treatment for acute pelvic and clavicular fractures.

First listed diagnosis:
S32.9XXD, Fracture of unspecified parts of lumbosacral spine and pelvis, subsequent encounter for fracture with routine healing

Additional diagnoses:
S42.009D, Fracture of unspecified part of unspecified clavicle, subsequent encounter for fracture with routine healing

The first-listed diagnosis for a patient admitted to LTC specifically for physical therapy following an injury should be the acute injury code with the appropriate 7th character for subsequent encounter. Assigning a Z code for any aftercare provided for traumatic fractures is inappropriate in ICD-10-CM. For further guidance on the application of the 7th characters for Chapter 19, refer to Section I.C.19.c., of the Official Guidelines for Coding and Reporting.

Either of these fractures could be the reason for the LTC admission and therefore either one could be assigned as the "first-listed" diagnosis. The appropriate procedure code(s) should also be assigned to show that physical therapy was provided.

Example 4:

A patient is admitted to LTC following hospital treatment of a traumatic fracture of the right femur in order to heal the fracture and regain strength.

First listed diagnosis:
S72.90XD, Unspecified fracture of right femur, subsequent encounter for closed fracture with routine healing

Additional diagnoses:
Code any other existing conditions that require treatment.

The patient is no longer receiving active treatment for the fracture and instead is receiving routine care while the fracture heals. The acute injury is still coded but with a 7th character of "D" signifying a subsequent encounter for fracture with routine healing. Do not assign an aftercare Z code.

Example 5:

A LTC patient develops a urinary tract infection during the LTC stay that was subsequently treated and resolved.

First listed diagnosis:
N39.0, Urinary tract infection, site not specified

Additional diagnoses:
Code any other existing conditions that require treatment.

The urinary tract infection would remain on the active problem list until resolution of the infection, after which it would no longer be correct to code or report it.

Example 6:

A patient returns to the LTC facility after hospitalization for pneumonia. The admission orders request "IV antibiotic continuation for three days, and then repeat x-ray to determine pneumonia status."

First listed diagnosis:
J18.9, Pneumonia, unspecified organism

Additional diagnoses:
Code any other existing conditions that require treatment.

Code the pneumonia until it is resolved, after which it should no longer be coded and reported.

Example 7:

After hospitalization for pneumonia, a nursing home resident is readmitted with orders for continued antibiotic regimen for pneumonia. Other specified residuals from a CVA several years ago are the chief reason for her original admission and continued residence in the LTC facility.

First listed diagnosis:
I69.3Ø, Unspecified sequelae of cerebral infarction

Additional diagnoses:
J18.9, Pneumonia, unspecified organism

Assign the appropriate code from subcategory I69.3, Sequelae of cerebral infarction, as the first-listed diagnosis to identify the residual neurologic deficits from the acute CVA. It is also appropriate to assign the code for the pneumonia as an additional diagnosis for as long as the patient receives treatment for the condition.

Example 8:

After surgical treatment in the acute care setting for a left wrist fracture sustained while a resident in a nursing home, the patient returns to the nursing home. The patient was admitted several years ago and has received continued care for Alzheimer's disease. Occupational therapy is ordered for the wrist, but the therapy is not the primary reason for the patient's admission.

First listed diagnosis:
G3Ø.9, Alzheimer's disease, unspecified

Additional diagnoses:
S62.1Ø2D, Fracture of unspecified carpal bone, left wrist, subsequent encounter for fracture with routine healing

W19.XXXD, Unspecified fall, subsequent encounter

Although the patient is receiving therapy for the wrist fracture, it is the Alzheimer's disease that is the reason the patient is continuing care in the nursing home and should be reported as the first-listed diagnosis, over the wrist fracture. However, the appropriate ICD-10-PCS procedure code should still be assigned to show that the patient received occupational therapy.

Example 9:

A patient is admitted to the LTC facility for convalescence following an acute illness or injury.

First listed diagnosis:
Z51.89, Encounter for other specified aftercare

Additional diagnoses:
Code any other existing conditions that require treatment.

Use only if the patient is admitted solely for convalescence and there is no information in the medical record identifying a more definitive diagnosis.

Selection of codes in all cases is based on documentation in the medical record of conditions treated. Codes for any late effects, signs, and symptoms present are assigned if documented.

Example 10:

A patient is transferred to a nursing home for convalescence and strengthening following coronary artery bypass surgery. The patient's degree of debility and inability to care for himself at home are the reasons for the nursing home admission.

First listed diagnosis:
Z48.812, Encounter for surgical aftercare following surgery on the circulatory system

Additional diagnoses:
Code any other existing conditions that require treatment.

Code any symptoms such as gait disturbance, weakness, or pain.

The condition that was treated surgically if still present would be coded.

Example 11:

A patient is transferred to a nursing home for convalescence following a hospitalization for an acute inferior wall myocardial infarction.

First listed diagnosis:
I21.19, ST elevation (STEMI) myocardial infarction involving other coronary artery of inferior wall

Additional diagnoses:
Code any other existing conditions that require treatment.

If the patient is in the recovery phase and requires continued care for the acute myocardial infarction, and is within the four-week time frame for the acute myocardial infarction (AMI), assign a code from category I21. This includes transfers to another acute setting or a postacute setting. If, however, the acute myocardial infarction occurred more than four weeks prior, assign instead code Z51.89, Encounter for other specified aftercare.

It would be inappropriate to assign code I22.1, Subsequent ST elevation (STEMI) myocardial infarction of inferior wall, for the long-term care admission. The codes in category (I22) are reserved for patients who have suffered an acute MI and experience a new acute MI within the four week time frame of the initial AMI. It is not for subsequent episodes of care.

Example 12:

The reason for admission to a nursing home is stated as "deconditioning".

First listed diagnosis:
Code whatever symptoms for deconditioning that the patient manifests, such as weakness, gait disturbance, etc.

Additional diagnoses:
Code any other existing conditions that require treatment.

Example 13:

The patient has a history of bowel perforation and obstruction, and is status post complex abdominal surgery due to intestinal anastomotic leak. She was transferred to the long-term care hospital (LTCH) for ongoing care of her abdominal wound. The patient presented with an enterocutaneous fistula with a large open abdominal wound and surgical wound dehiscence. Should the fistula be coded as a persistent postoperative fistula or according to the site of the fistula?

First listed diagnosis:
T81.83X-, Persistent postoperative fistula

Additional diagnoses:
K63.2, Fistula of intestine

T81.32X-, Disruption of internal operation (surgical) wound, not elsewhere classified

Assign codes T81.83X-, Persistent postoperative fistula, and K63.2, Fistula of intestine, for the enterocutaneous postsurgical fistula. Both codes are needed to show the postoperative complication and the specific site of the fistula. Assign also code T81.32X-, Disruption of internal operation (surgical) wound, not elsewhere classified, for the wound dehiscence. The assignment of the 7th character "A" depends on whether active treatment is still being provided.

Example 14:

A patient does not have a specific diagnosis, but is admitted to a LTC facility for symptoms such as weakness, debility, deterioration, or old age.

First listed diagnosis:
Code the symptoms related to the admission

Additional diagnoses:
Code any other existing conditions that require treatment.

Example 15:

The patient was transferred to a skilled nursing facility's rehabilitation unit for occupational therapy and physical therapy, following a prolonged stay at a long term care hospital (LTCH), where she was successfully weaned off mechanical ventilation. At the SNF, the patient received rehab due to deconditioning and debility. The provider documented that the patient presented with complex medical problems (i.e., chronic hypoxic respiratory failure, requiring supplemental oxygen, chronic obstructive pulmonary disease (COPD), tracheostomy status, type II diabetic neuropathy, and obesity). What are the appropriate code assignments for the rehabilitation stay at the SNF?

First Listed Diagnosis:
J96.11, Chronic respiratory failure with hypoxia

Additional diagnoses:
J44.9, Chronic obstructive pulmonary disease, unspecified

E11.40, Type 2 diabetes mellitus with diabetic neuropathy, unspecified

E66.9, Obesity, unspecified

Z99.81, Dependence on supplemental oxygen

Z93.0, Tracheostomy status

Assign code J96.11, Chronic respiratory failure with hypoxia, as the principal diagnosis. In this case, the underlying reason for the debility and deconditioning is coded as the principal diagnosis. Assign also codes J44.9, Chronic obstructive pulmonary disease, unspecified; E11.40, Type 2 diabetes mellitus with diabetic neuropathy, unspecified; E66.9, Obesity unspecified; Z99.81, Dependence on supplemental oxygen; and Z93.0, Tracheostomy status.

Example 16:

How should a nonhealing surgical wound be coded?

First listed diagnosis:
T81.89X-, Other complications of procedures, not elsewhere classified

Additional diagnoses:
Code also other conditions that require treatment.

ICD-10-CM does not provide a specific code to describe nonhealing surgical wound. Assign code T81.89X-, Other complications of procedures, not elsewhere classified, for an unspecified nonhealing surgical wound. If a postsurgical wound does not heal due to infection, assign code T81.4-, Infection following a procedure. If the wound was closed at one time and is no longer closed, it is coded as disruption. In that case, code T81.3-, Disruption of wound, not elsewhere classified, should be assigned.

Example 17:

A patient was admitted to an acute rehab facility for physical and occupational therapy following a total hip replacement (THR) due to a right intertrochanteric femur fracture. Since the hip joint was removed and replaced with a prosthetic, would the femoral fracture still be coded?

First listed diagnosis:
S72.141D, Displaced intertrochanteric fracture of right femur, subsequent encounter for closed fracture with routine healing

Additional diagnoses:
Z96.641, Presence of right artificial hip joint

Code any other existing conditions that require treatment

In this case, a total hip replacement was done to treat the traumatic fracture of the hip. The fracture is now in the healing and recovery phase after surgical treatment. Assign code S72.141D, Displaced intertrochanteric fracture of right femur, subsequent encounter for closed fracture with routine healing, as principal diagnosis. Assign also code Z96.641, Presence of right artificial hip joint.

The intent of ICD-10-CM's seventh character for fracture and other injuries is to track treatment through the various stages, as well as to track resource utilization and outcomes. There are clinical differences in joint replacement surgery performed because of a traumatic fracture versus elective joint replacement surgery. For example, an injury resulting in unexpected surgery might require more intensive rehabilitation than a hip replacement due to degenerative osteoarthritis of the hip.

Illustrations

Chapter 3. Diseases of the Blood and Blood-forming Organs and Certain Disorders Involving the Immune Mechanism (D5Ø–D89)

Red Blood Cells

White Blood Cell

Platelet

Coagulation

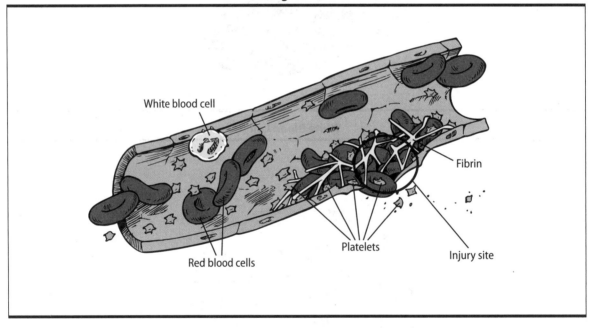

White blood cell

Fibrin

Red blood cells

Platelets

Injury site

Spleen Anatomical Location and External Structures

Spleen Interior Structures

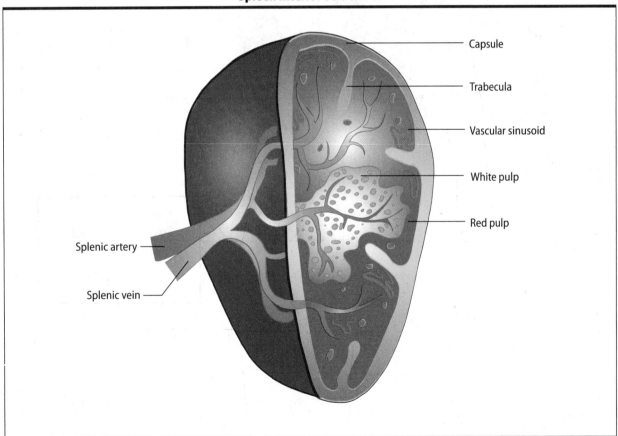

Chapter 4. Endocrine, Nutritional and Metabolic Diseases (E00–E89)

Endocrine System

Thyroid

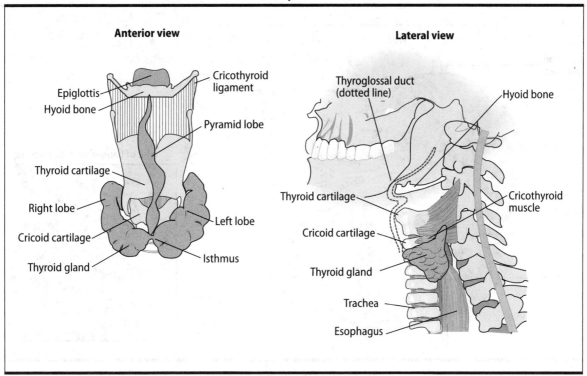

Anterior view

- Epiglottis
- Hyoid bone
- Cricothyroid ligament
- Pyramid lobe
- Thyroid cartilage
- Right lobe
- Left lobe
- Cricoid cartilage
- Isthmus
- Thyroid gland

Lateral view

- Thyroglossal duct (dotted line)
- Hyoid bone
- Thyroid cartilage
- Cricothyroid muscle
- Cricoid cartilage
- Thyroid gland
- Trachea
- Esophagus

Thyroid and Parathyroid Glands

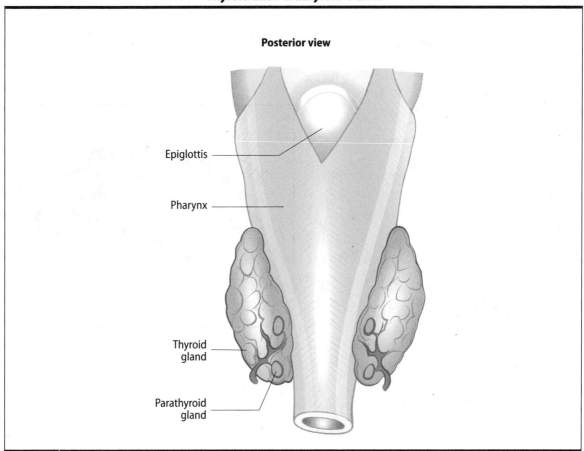

Posterior view

- Epiglottis
- Pharynx
- Thyroid gland
- Parathyroid gland

Pancreas

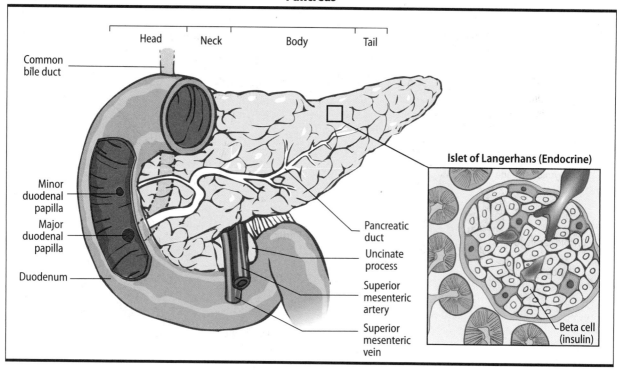

Anatomy of the Adrenal Gland

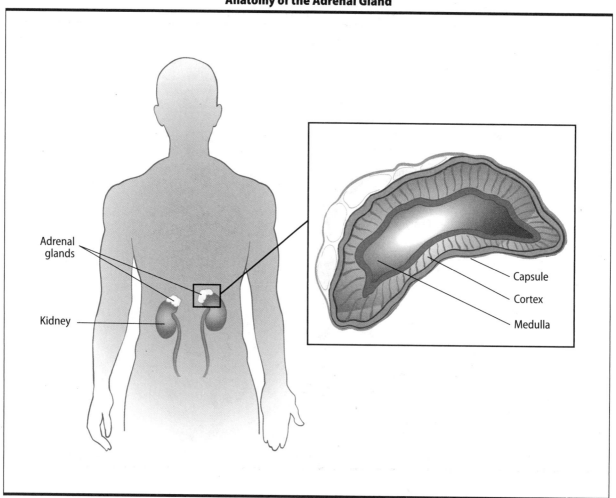

Structure of an Ovary

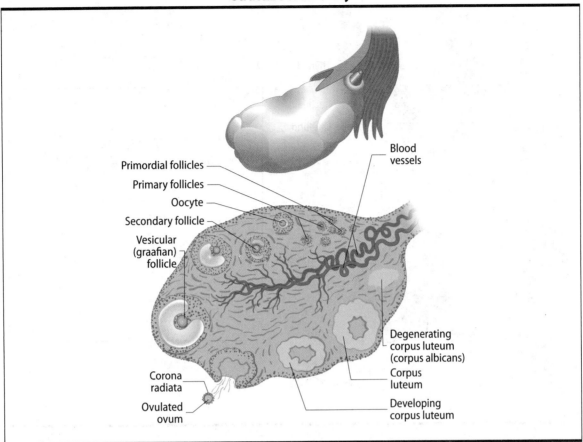

Testis and Associated Structures

Thymus

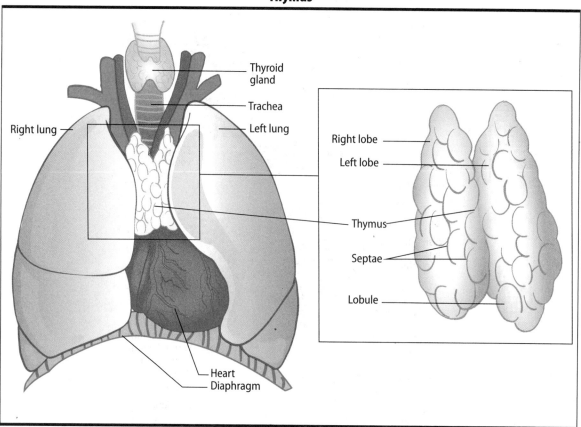

Chapter 6. Diseases of the Nervous System (GØØ–G99)

Brain

Cranial Nerves

Peripheral Nervous System

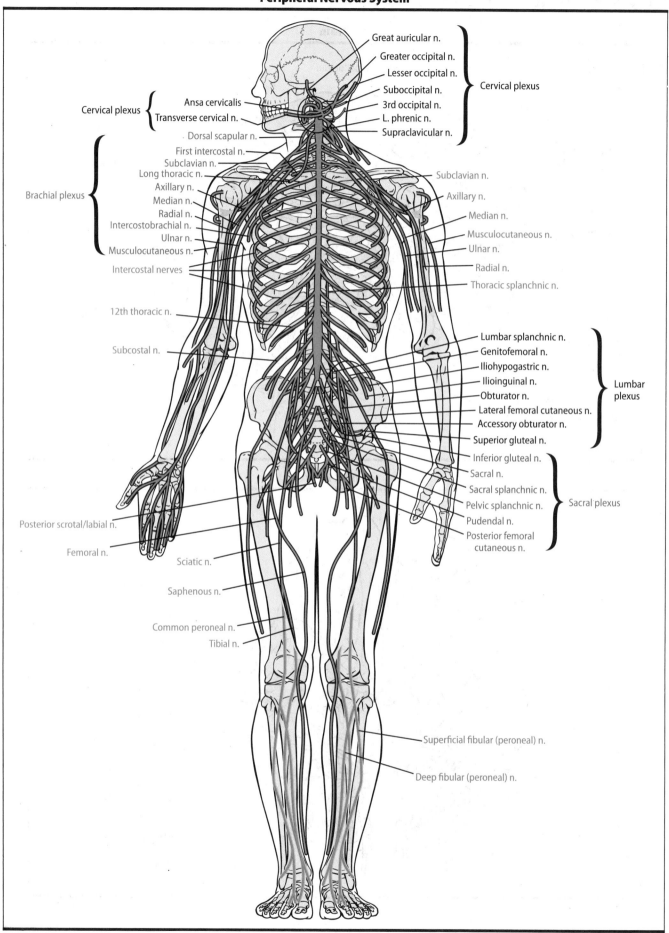

Great auricular n.
Greater occipital n.
Lesser occipital n.
Suboccipital n.
3rd occipital n.
L. phrenic n.
Supraclavicular n.

Cervical plexus

Cervical plexus
Ansa cervicalis
Transverse cervical n.
Dorsal scapular n.
First intercostal n.
Subclavian n.
Long thoracic n.
Axillary n.
Median n.
Radial n.
Intercostobrachial n.
Ulnar n.
Musculocutaneous n.
Intercostal nerves

Brachial plexus

Subclavian n.
Axillary n.
Median n.
Musculocutaneous n.
Ulnar n.
Radial n.
Thoracic splanchnic n.

12th thoracic n.

Subcostal n.

Lumbar splanchnic n.
Genitofemoral n.
Iliohypogastric n.
Ilioinguinal n.
Obturator n.
Lateral femoral cutaneous n.
Accessory obturator n.
Superior gluteal n.

Lumbar plexus

Inferior gluteal n.
Sacral n.
Sacral splanchnic n.
Pelvic splanchnic n.
Pudendal n.
Posterior femoral cutaneous n.

Sacral plexus

Posterior scrotal/labial n.
Femoral n.
Sciatic n.
Saphenous n.
Common peroneal n.
Tibial n.

Superficial fibular (peroneal) n.

Deep fibular (peroneal) n.

Spinal Cord and Spinal Nerves

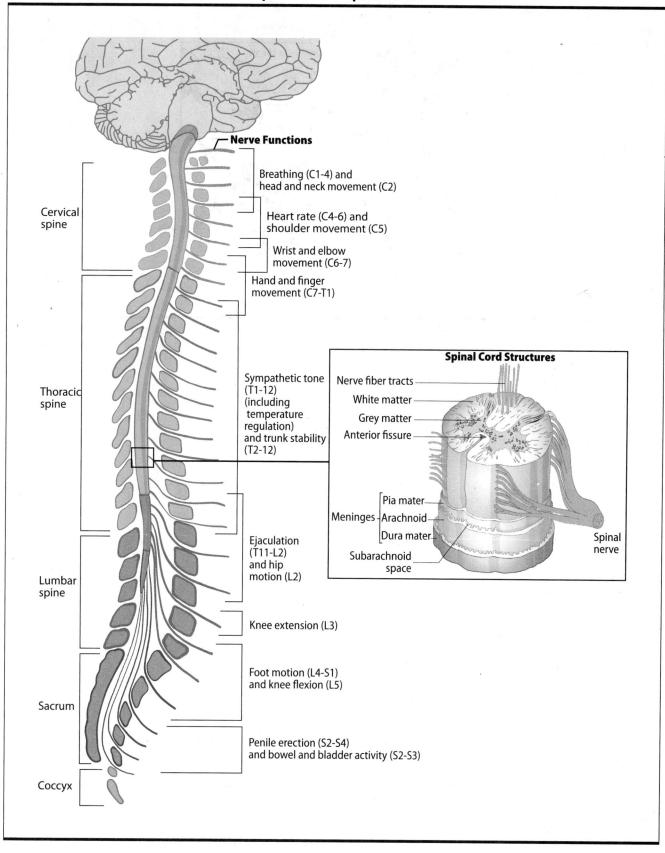

Nerve Functions

Breathing (C1-4) and head and neck movement (C2)

Heart rate (C4-6) and shoulder movement (C5)

Wrist and elbow movement (C6-7)

Hand and finger movement (C7-T1)

Cervical spine

Thoracic spine

Sympathetic tone (T1-12) (including temperature regulation) and trunk stability (T2-12)

Lumbar spine

Ejaculation (T11-L2) and hip motion (L2)

Knee extension (L3)

Foot motion (L4-S1) and knee flexion (L5)

Sacrum

Penile erection (S2-S4) and bowel and bladder activity (S2-S3)

Coccyx

Spinal Cord Structures

Nerve fiber tracts
White matter
Grey matter
Anterior fissure

Meninges — Pia mater, Arachnoid, Dura mater
Subarachnoid space
Spinal nerve

Nerve Cell

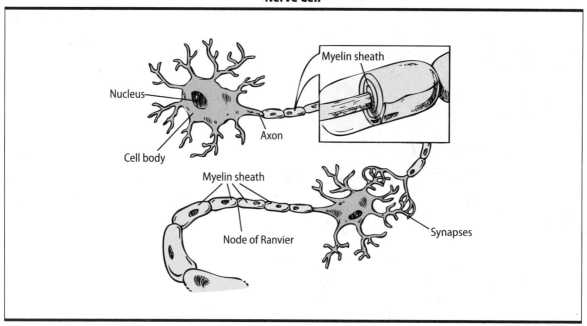

Chapter 7. Diseases of the Eye and Adnexa (H00–H59)

Eye

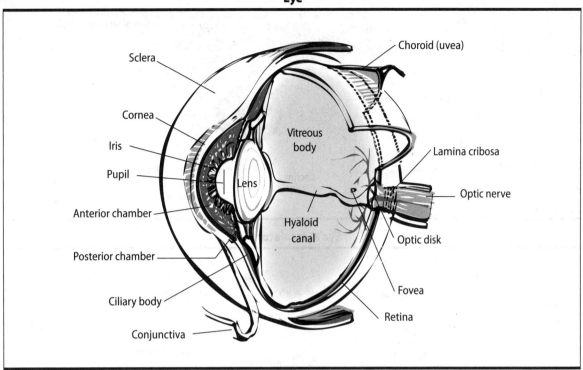

Posterior Pole of Globe/Flow of Aqueous Humor

Lacrimal System

Eye Musculature

Eyelid Structures

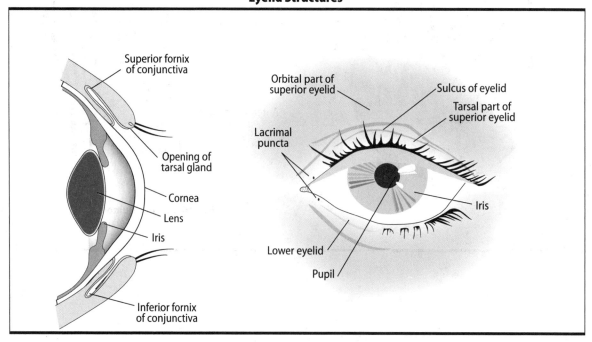

Chapter 8. Diseases of the Ear and Mastoid Process (H6Ø–H95)

Ear Anatomy

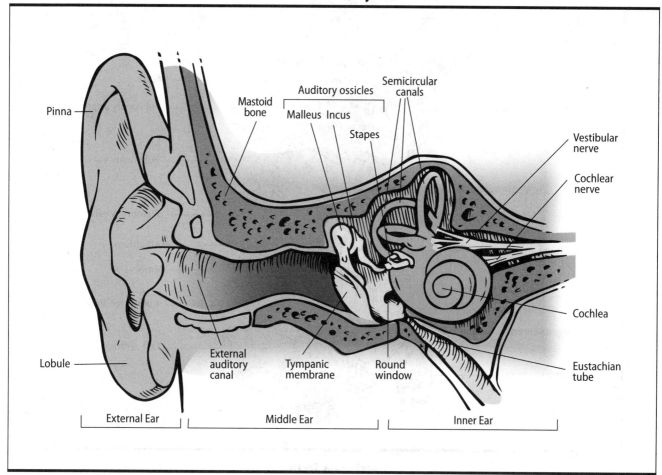

Chapter 9. Diseases of the Circulatory System (I00–I99)

Anatomy of the Heart

Heart Cross Section

Heart Valves

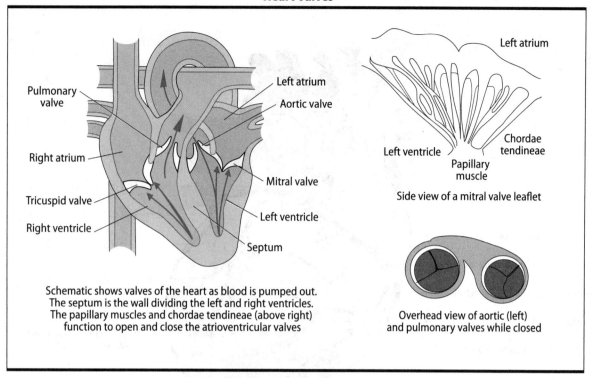

Schematic shows valves of the heart as blood is pumped out.
The septum is the wall dividing the left and right ventricles.
The papillary muscles and chordae tendineae (above right)
function to open and close the atrioventricular valves

Side view of a mitral valve leaflet

Overhead view of aortic (left)
and pulmonary valves while closed

Heart Conduction System

Coronary Arteries

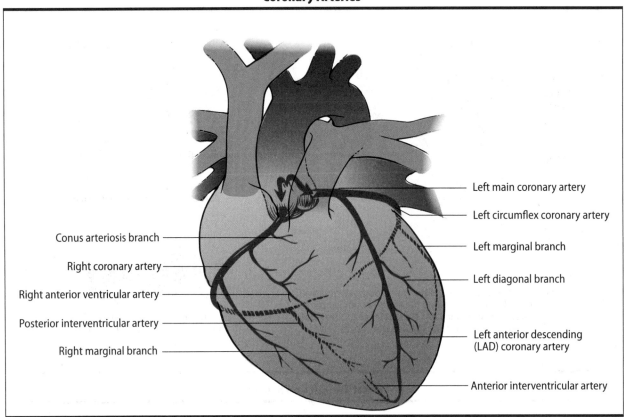

Left main coronary artery

Left circumflex coronary artery

Left marginal branch

Left diagonal branch

Left anterior descending (LAD) coronary artery

Anterior interventricular artery

Conus arteriosis branch

Right coronary artery

Right anterior ventricular artery

Posterior interventricular artery

Right marginal branch

Arteries

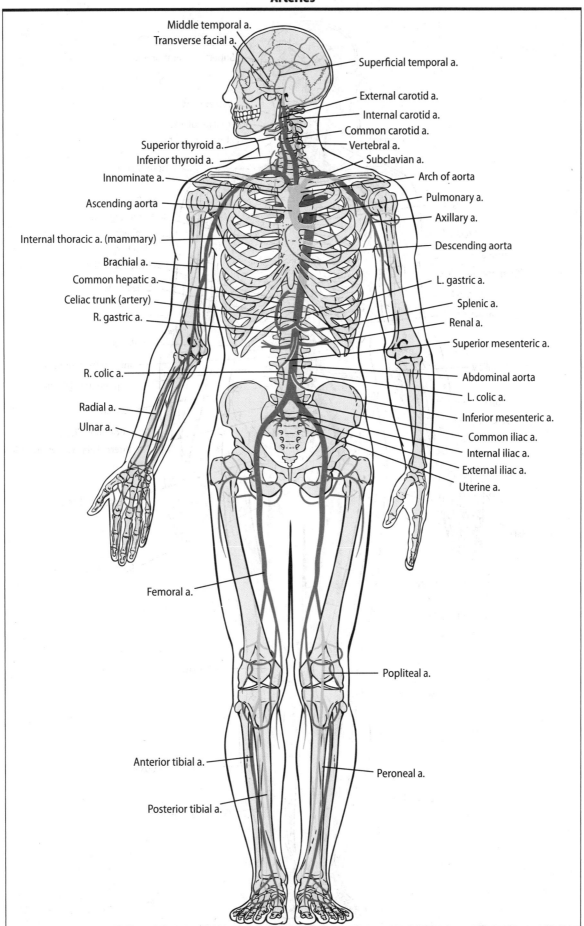

Middle temporal a.
Transverse facial a.
Superficial temporal a.
External carotid a.
Internal carotid a.
Common carotid a.
Vertebral a.
Superior thyroid a.
Inferior thyroid a.
Subclavian a.
Innominate a.
Arch of aorta
Ascending aorta
Pulmonary a.
Axillary a.
Internal thoracic a. (mammary)
Descending aorta
Brachial a.
Common hepatic a.
L. gastric a.
Celiac trunk (artery)
Splenic a.
R. gastric a.
Renal a.
Superior mesenteric a.
R. colic a.
Abdominal aorta
L. colic a.
Radial a.
Inferior mesenteric a.
Ulnar a.
Common iliac a.
Internal iliac a.
External iliac a.
Uterine a.
Femoral a.
Popliteal a.
Anterior tibial a.
Peroneal a.
Posterior tibial a.

Veins

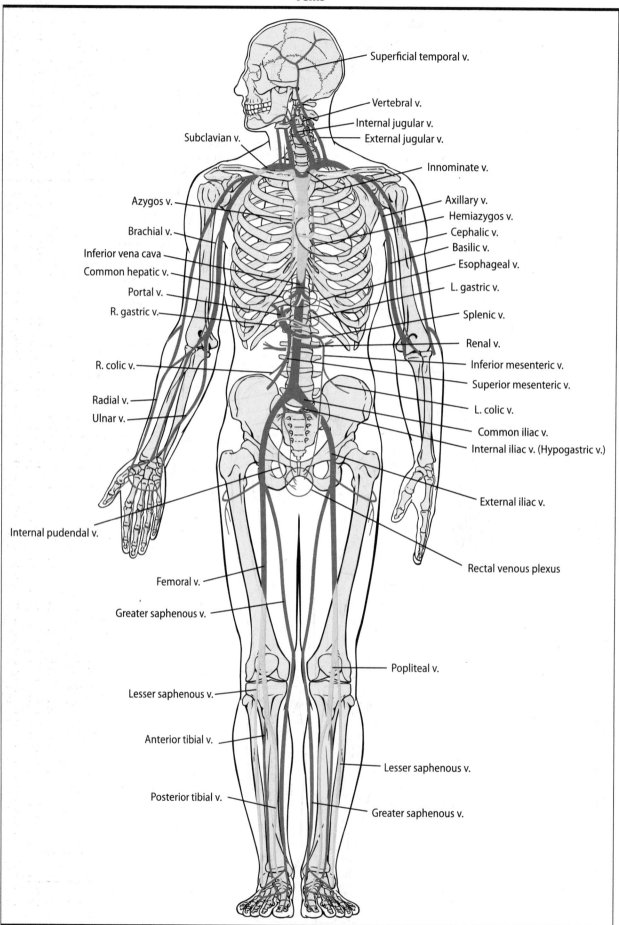

Internal Carotid and Vertebral Arteries and Branches

Side View

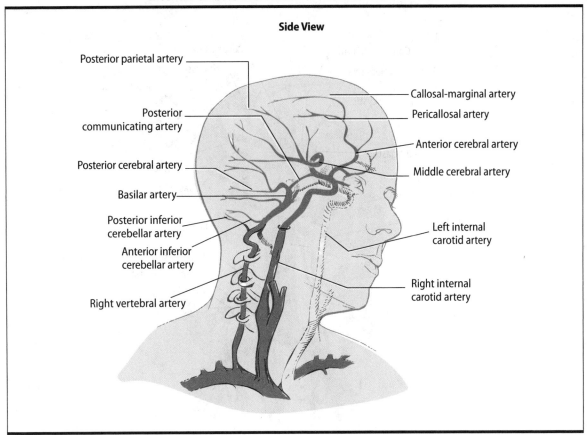

- Posterior parietal artery
- Posterior communicating artery
- Posterior cerebral artery
- Basilar artery
- Posterior inferior cerebellar artery
- Anterior inferior cerebellar artery
- Right vertebral artery
- Callosal-marginal artery
- Pericallosal artery
- Anterior cerebral artery
- Middle cerebral artery
- Left internal carotid artery
- Right internal carotid artery

External Carotid Artery and Branches

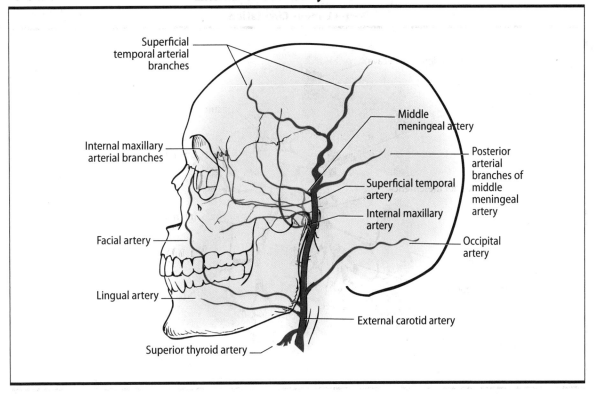

- Superficial temporal arterial branches
- Internal maxillary arterial branches
- Facial artery
- Lingual artery
- Superior thyroid artery
- Middle meningeal artery
- Superficial temporal artery
- Internal maxillary artery
- Posterior arterial branches of middle meningeal artery
- Occipital artery
- External carotid artery

Branches of Abdominal Aorta

Portal Venous Circulation

Lymphatic System

Axillary Lymph Nodes

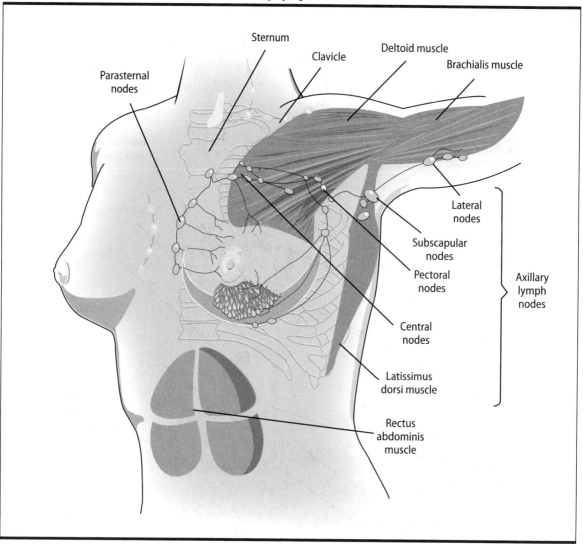

Lymphatic System of Head and Neck

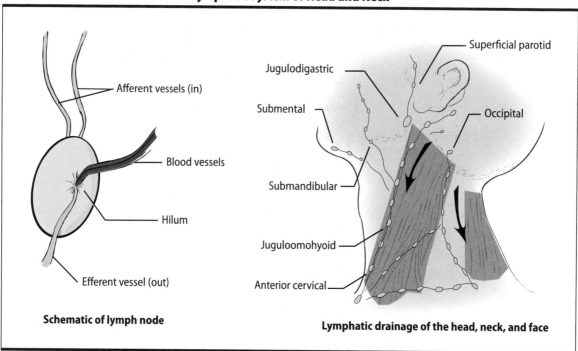

Schematic of lymph node

Lymphatic drainage of the head, neck, and face

Lymphatic Capillaries

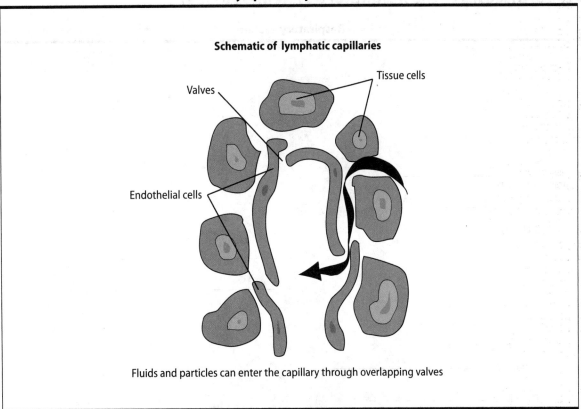

Schematic of lymphatic capillaries

Fluids and particles can enter the capillary through overlapping valves

Lymphatic Drainage

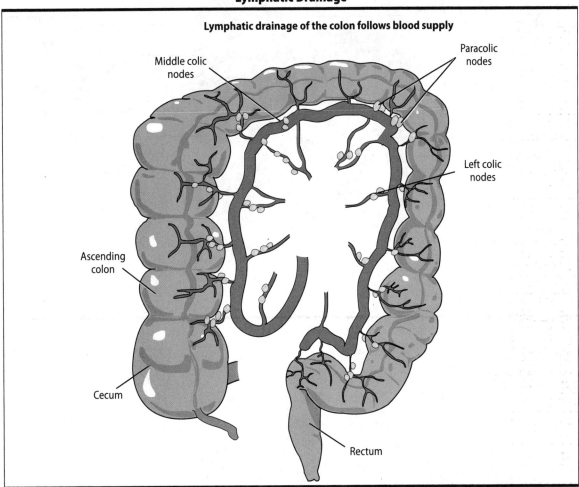

Lymphatic drainage of the colon follows blood supply

Chapter 10. Diseases of the Respiratory System (J00–J99)

Respiratory System

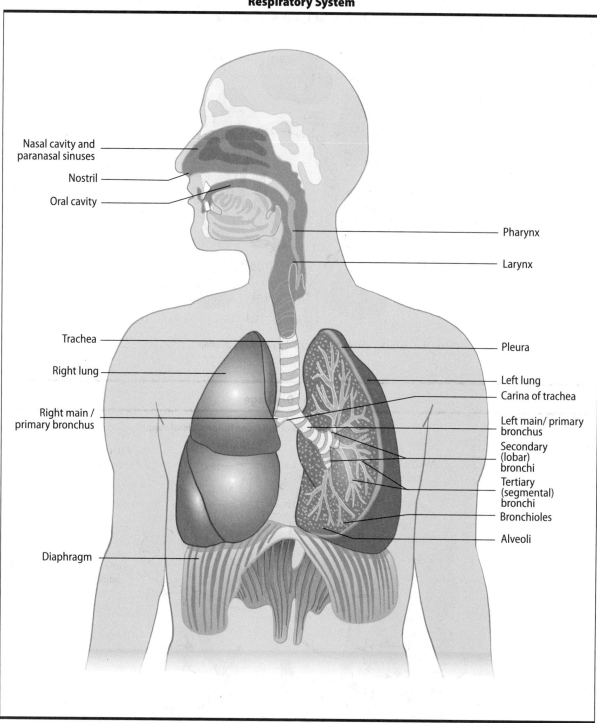

Nasal cavity and paranasal sinuses

Nostril

Oral cavity

Pharynx

Larynx

Trachea

Pleura

Right lung

Left lung

Carina of trachea

Right main / primary bronchus

Left main/ primary bronchus

Secondary (lobar) bronchi

Tertiary (segmental) bronchi

Bronchioles

Alveoli

Diaphragm

Upper Respiratory System

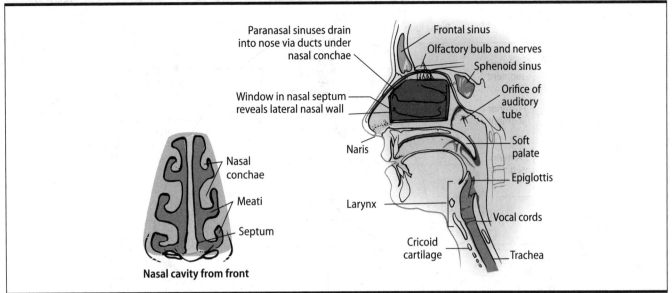

Paranasal sinuses drain into nose via ducts under nasal conchae

Window in nasal septum reveals lateral nasal wall

Frontal sinus

Olfactory bulb and nerves

Sphenoid sinus

Orifice of auditory tube

Naris

Soft palate

Nasal conchae

Meati

Septum

Larynx

Epiglottis

Vocal cords

Cricoid cartilage

Trachea

Nasal cavity from front

Lower Respiratory System

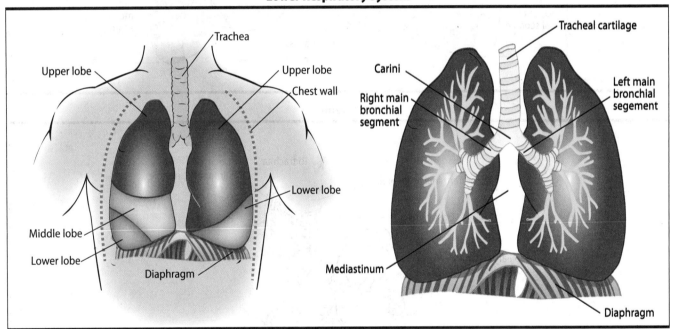

Trachea

Upper lobe

Upper lobe

Chest wall

Lower lobe

Middle lobe

Lower lobe

Diaphragm

Tracheal cartilage

Carini

Right main bronchial segment

Left main bronchial segement

Mediastinum

Diaphragm

Paranasal Sinuses

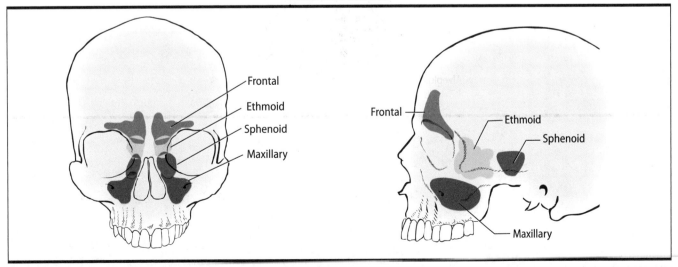

Frontal

Ethmoid

Sphenoid

Maxillary

Frontal

Ethmoid

Sphenoid

Maxillary

Lung Segments

Alveoli

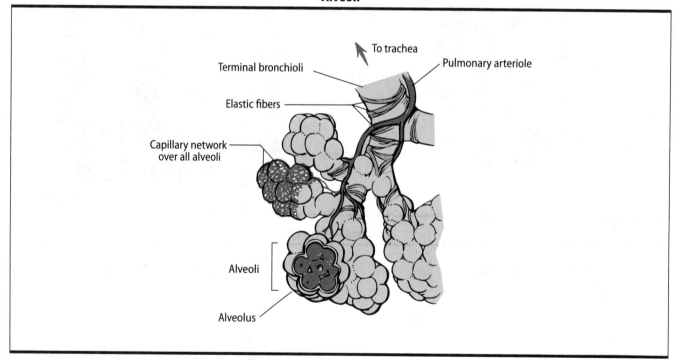

Chapter 11. Diseases of the Digestive System (K00–K95)

Digestive System

Omentum and Mesentery

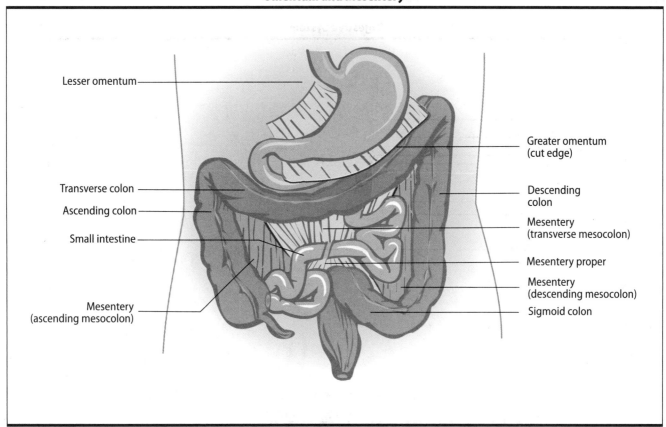

Lesser omentum

Transverse colon

Ascending colon

Small intestine

Mesentery
(ascending mesocolon)

Greater omentum
(cut edge)

Descending
colon

Mesentery
(transverse mesocolon)

Mesentery proper

Mesentery
(descending mesocolon)

Sigmoid colon

Peritoneum and Retroperitoneum

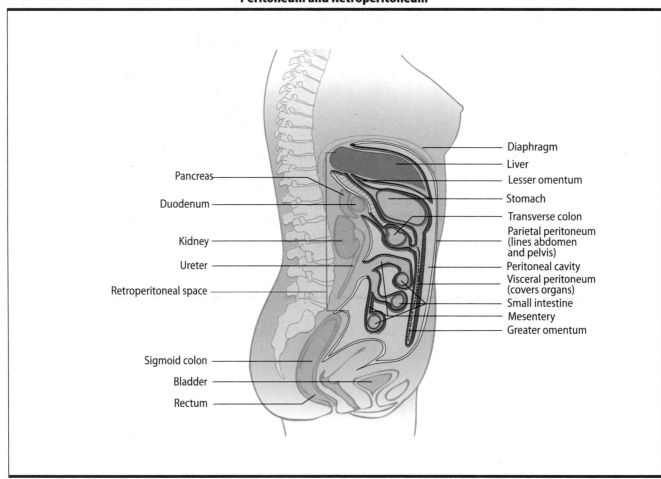

Pancreas

Duodenum

Kidney

Ureter

Retroperitoneal space

Sigmoid colon

Bladder

Rectum

Diaphragm

Liver

Lesser omentum

Stomach

Transverse colon

Parietal peritoneum
(lines abdomen
and pelvis)

Peritoneal cavity

Visceral peritoneum
(covers organs)

Small intestine

Mesentery

Greater omentum

Chapter 12. Diseases of the Skin and Subcutaneous Tissue (LØØ–L99)

Nail Anatomy

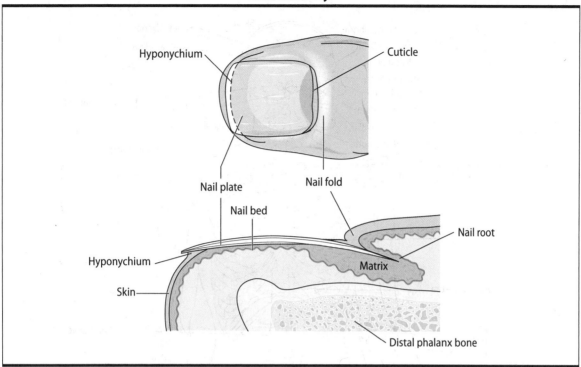

Skin and Subcutaneous Tissue

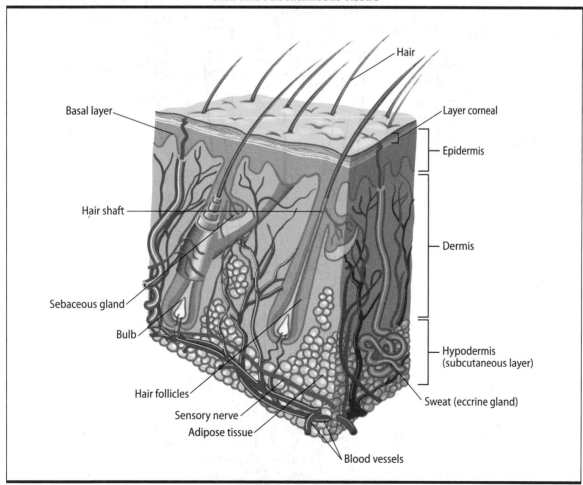

Chapter 13. Diseases of the Musculoskeletal System and Connective Tissue (MØØ–M99)

Bones and Joints

Shoulder Anterior View

Shoulder Posterior View

Elbow Anterior View

Elbow Posterior View

Hand

Hip Anterior View

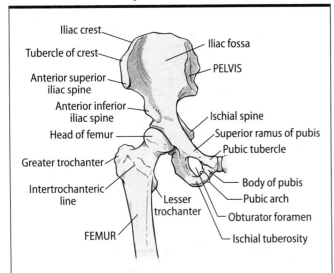

Iliac crest
Tubercle of crest
Anterior superior iliac spine
Anterior inferior iliac spine
Head of femur
Greater trochanter
Intertrochanteric line
FEMUR
Lesser trochanter
Iliac fossa
PELVIS
Ischial spine
Superior ramus of pubis
Pubic tubercle
Body of pubis
Pubic arch
Obturator foramen
Ischial tuberosity

Hip Posterior View

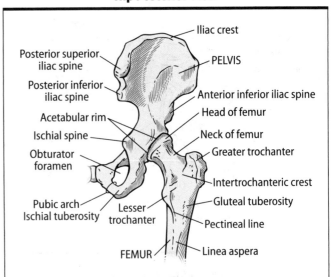

Posterior superior iliac spine
Posterior inferior iliac spine
Acetabular rim
Ischial spine
Obturator foramen
Pubic arch
Ischial tuberosity
Lesser trochanter
FEMUR
Iliac crest
PELVIS
Anterior inferior iliac spine
Head of femur
Neck of femur
Greater trochanter
Intertrochanteric crest
Gluteal tuberosity
Pectineal line
Linea aspera

Knee Anterior View

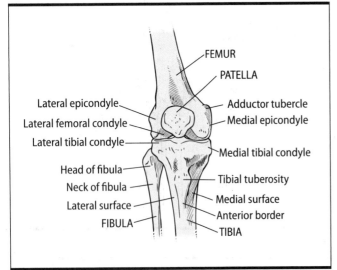

Lateral epicondyle
Lateral femoral condyle
Lateral tibial condyle
Head of fibula
Neck of fibula
Lateral surface
FIBULA
FEMUR
PATELLA
Adductor tubercle
Medial epicondyle
Medial tibial condyle
Tibial tuberosity
Medial surface
Anterior border
TIBIA

Knee Posterior View

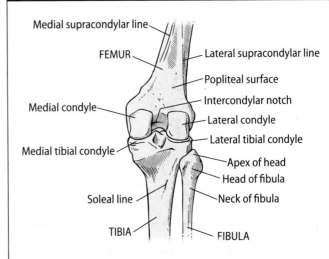

Medial supracondylar line
FEMUR
Medial condyle
Medial tibial condyle
Soleal line
TIBIA
Lateral supracondylar line
Popliteal surface
Intercondylar notch
Lateral condyle
Lateral tibial condyle
Apex of head
Head of fibula
Neck of fibula
FIBULA

Foot

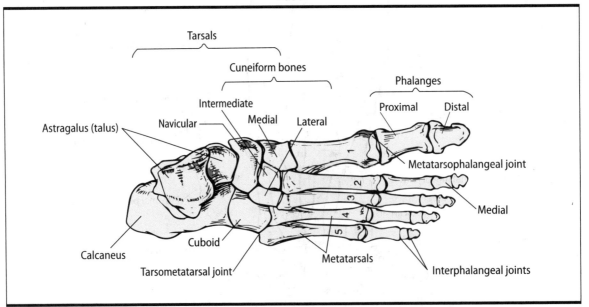

Tarsals
Cuneiform bones
Phalanges
Intermediate
Medial
Lateral
Proximal
Distal
Astragalus (talus)
Navicular
Metatarsophalangeal joint
Medial
Calcaneus
Cuboid
Tarsometatarsal joint
Metatarsals
Interphalangeal joints

Muscles

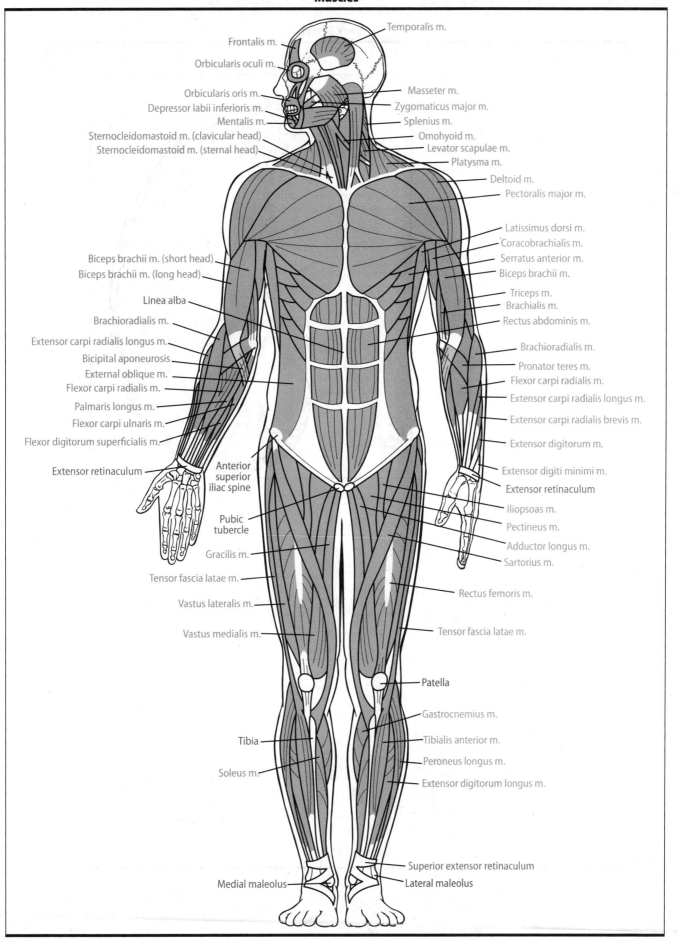

Chapter 14. Diseases of the Genitourinary System (NØØ–N99)

Urinary System

Male Genitourinary System

Female Internal Genitalia

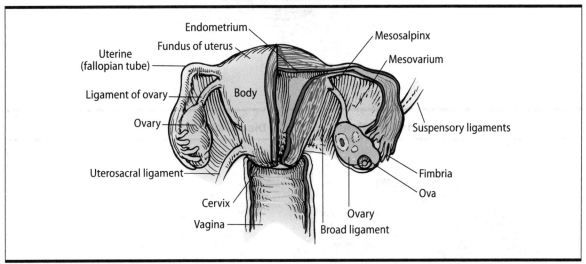

Female Genitourinary Tract Lateral View

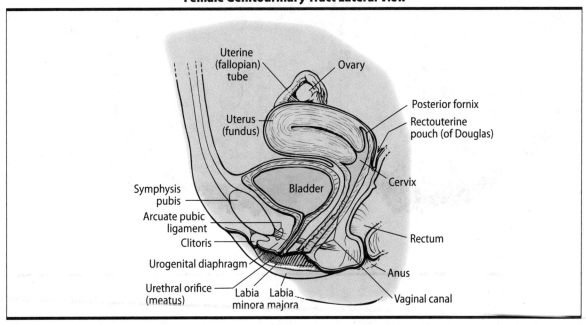

Chapter 15. Pregnancy, Childbirth and the Puerperium (O00–O9A)

Term Pregnancy – Single Gestation

Twin Gestation–Dichorionic–Diamniotic (DI-DI)

Twin Gestation–Monochorionic–Diamniotic (MO-DI)

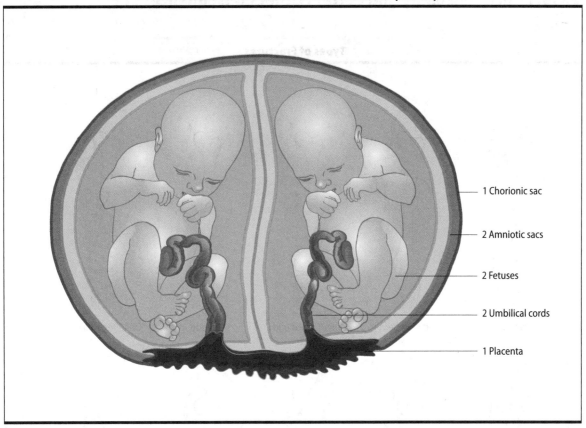

1 Chorionic sac

2 Amniotic sacs

2 Fetuses

2 Umbilical cords

1 Placenta

Twin Gestation–Monochorionic–Monoamniotic (MO-MO)

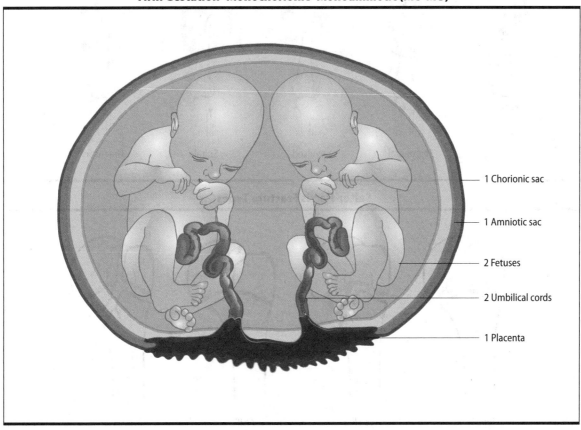

1 Chorionic sac

1 Amniotic sac

2 Fetuses

2 Umbilical cords

1 Placenta

Chapter 19. Injury, Poisoning and Certain Other Consequences of External Causes (S00–T88)

Types of Fractures

Normal   Transverse   Open/Compound   Oblique   Oblique displaced

Comminuted   Segmental   Avulsed   Spiral   Greenstick

Salter-Harris Fracture Types

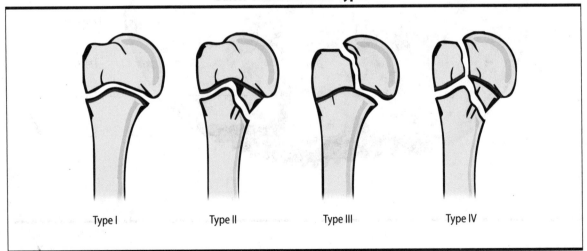

Type I   Type II   Type III   Type IV